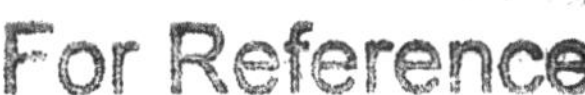

PETERSON'S GRADUATE PROGRAMS IN BIOLOGICAL/BIOMEDICAL SCIENCES & HEALTH-RELATED MEDICAL PROFESSIONS

2015

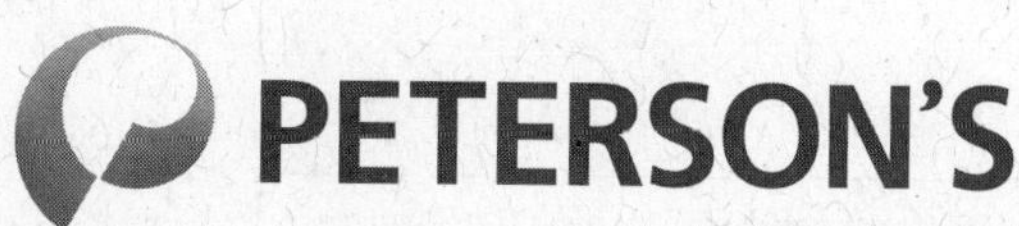

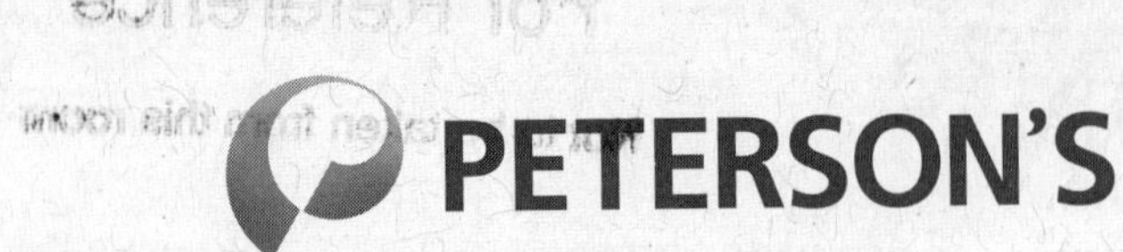

About Peterson's

Peterson's provides the accurate, dependable, high-quality education content and guidance you need to succeed. No matter where you are on your academic or professional path, you can rely on Peterson's print and digital publications for the most up-to-date education exploration data, expert test-prep tools, and top-notch career success resources—everything you need to achieve your goals.

For more information, contact Peterson's Publishing, 3 Columbia Circle, Suite 205, Albany, NY 12203-5158; 800-338-3282 Ext. 54229; or find us on the World Wide Web at www.petersonsbooks.com.

ISSN 1093-8443
ISBN: 978-0-7689-3880-7

Printed in the United States of America

10 9 8 7 6 5 4 3 2 1 17 16 15

Forty-ninth Edition

By producing this book on recycled paper (10% post-consumer waste) 80 trees were saved.

Sustainability—Its Importance to Peterson's

What does sustainability mean to Peterson's? As a leading publisher, we are aware that our business has a direct impact on vital resources—most importantly the raw material used to make our books. Peterson's is proud that its products are printed at SFI Chain-of-Custody certified facilities and that all of its books are printed on SFI certified paper with 10 percent post-consumer waste using vegetable-based ink.

Supporting the Sustainable Forestry Initiative® (SFI®) means that we only use vendors—from paper suppliers to printers—who have undergone rigorous certification audits by independent parties to demonstrate that they meet the standards.

Peterson's continuously strives to find new ways to incorporate responsible sourcing throughout all aspects of its business.

CONTENTS

A Note from the Peterson's Editors

The six volumes of Peterson's *Graduate and Professional Programs*, the only annually updated reference work of its kind, provide wideranging information on the graduate and professional programs offered by accredited colleges and universities in the United States, U.S. territories, and Canada and by those institutions outside the United States that are accredited by U.S. accrediting bodies. Nearly 36,000 individual academic and professional programs at more than 2,200 institutions are listed. Peterson's *Graduate and Professional Programs* have been used for more than forty years by prospective graduate and professional students, placement counselors, faculty advisers, and all others interested in postbaccalaureate education.

Graduate & Professional Programs: An Overview contains information on institutions as a whole, while the other books in the series are devoted to specific academic and professional fields:

Graduate Programs in the Humanities, Arts & Social Sciences
Graduate Programs in the Biological/Biomedical Sciences & Health-Related Medical Professions
Graduate Programs in the Physical Sciences, Mathematics, Agricultural Sciences, the Environment & Natural Resources
Graduate Programs in Engineering & Applied Sciences
Graduate Programs in Business, Education, Information Studies, Law & Social Work

The books may be used individually or as a set. For example, if you have chosen a field of study but do not know what institution you want to attend or if you have a college or university in mind but have not chosen an academic field of study, it is best to begin with the Overview guide.

Graduate & Professional Programs: An Overview presents several directories to help you identify programs of study that might interest you; you can then research those programs further in the other books in the series by using the Directory of Graduate and Professional Programs by Field, which lists 500 fields and gives the names of those institutions that offer graduate degree programs in each.

For geographical or financial reasons, you may be interested in attending a particular institution and will want to know what it has to offer. You should turn to the Directory of Institutions and Their Offerings, which lists the degree programs available at each institution. As in the Directory of Graduate and Professional Programs by Field, the level of degrees offered is also indicated.

All books in the series include advice on graduate education, including topics such as admissions tests, financial aid, and accreditation. **The Graduate Adviser** includes two essays and information about accreditation. The first essay, "The Admissions Process," discusses general admission requirements, admission tests, factors to consider when selecting a graduate school or program, when and how to apply, and how admission decisions are made. Special information for international students and tips for minority students are also included. The second essay, "Financial Support," is an overview of the broad range of support available at the graduate level. Fellowships, scholarships, and grants; assistantships and internships; federal and private loan programs, as well as Federal Work-Study; and the GI bill are detailed. This essay concludes with advice on applying for need-based financial aid. "Accreditation and Accrediting Agencies" gives information on accreditation and its purpose and lists institutional accrediting agencies first and then specialized accrediting agencies relevant to each volume's specific fields of study.

With information on more than 44,000 graduate programs in more than 500 disciplines, Peterson's *Graduate and Professional Programs* give you all the information you need about the programs that are of interest to you in three formats: **Profiles** (capsule summaries of basic information), **Displays** (information that an institution or program wants to emphasize), and **Close-Ups** (written by administrators, with more expansive information than the **Profiles**, emphasizing different aspects of the programs). By using these various formats of program information, coupled with **Appendixes** and **Indexes** covering directories and subject areas for all six books, you will find that these guides provide the most comprehensive, accurate, and up-to-date graduate study information available.

Peterson's publishes a full line of resources with information you need to guide you through the graduate admissions process. Peterson's publications can be found at college libraries and career centers and your local bookstore or library—or visit us on the Web at www.petersonsbooks.com. Peterson's books are now also available as ebooks.

Colleges and universities will be pleased to know that Peterson's helped you in your selection. Admissions staff members are more than happy to answer questions, address specific problems, and help in any way they can. The editors at Peterson's wish you great success in your graduate program search!

NOTICE: Certain portions of or information contained in this book have been submitted and paid for by the educational institution identified, and such institutions take full responsibility for the accuracy, timeliness, completeness and functionality of such contents. Such portions or information include (i) each display ad that comprises a half page of information covering a single educational institution or program and (ii) each two-page description or Close-Up of a graduate school or program that appear in the different sections of this guide. The "Close-Ups and Displays" are listed in various sections throughout the book.

THE GRADUATE ADVISER

The Admissions Process

Generalizations about graduate admissions practices are not always helpful because each institution has its own set of guidelines and procedures. Nevertheless, some broad statements can be made about the admissions process that may help you plan your strategy.

Factors Involved in Selecting a Graduate School or Program

Selecting a graduate school and a specific program of study is a complex matter. Quality of the faculty; program and course offerings; the nature, size, and location of the institution; admission requirements; cost; and the availability of financial assistance are among the many factors that affect one's choice of institution. Other considerations are job placement and achievements of the program's graduates and the institution's resources, such as libraries, laboratories, and computer facilities. If you are to make the best possible choice, you need to learn as much as you can about the schools and programs you are considering before you apply.

The following steps may help you narrow your choices.

- Talk to alumni of the programs or institutions you are considering to get their impressions of how well they were prepared for work in their fields of study.
- Remember that graduate school requirements change, so be sure to get the most up-to-date information possible.
- Talk to department faculty members and the graduate adviser at your undergraduate institution. They often have information about programs of study at other institutions.
- Visit the websites of the graduate schools in which you are interested to request a graduate catalog. Contact the department chair in your chosen field of study for additional information about the department and the field.
- Visit as many campuses as possible. Call ahead for an appointment with the graduate adviser in your field of interest and be sure to check out the facilities and talk to students.

General Requirements

Graduate schools and departments have requirements that applicants for admission must meet. Typically, these requirements include undergraduate transcripts (which provide information about undergraduate grade point average and course work applied toward a major), admission test scores, and letters of recommendation. Most graduate programs also ask for an essay or personal statement that describes your personal reasons for seeking graduate study. In some fields, such as art and music, portfolios or auditions may be required in addition to other evidence of talent. Some institutions require that the applicant have an undergraduate degree in the same subject as the intended graduate major.

Most institutions evaluate each applicant on the basis of the applicant's total record, and the weight accorded any given factor varies widely from institution to institution and from program to program.

The Application Process

You should begin the application process at least one year before you expect to begin your graduate study. Find out the application deadline for each institution (many are provided in the **Profile** section of this guide). Go to the institution's website and find out if you can apply online. If not, request a paper application form. Fill out this form thoroughly and neatly. Assume that the school needs all the information it is requesting and that the admissions officer will be sensitive to the neatness and overall quality of what you submit. Do not supply more information than the school requires.

The institution may ask at least one question that will require a three- or four-paragraph answer. Compose your response on the assumption that the admissions officer is interested in both what you think and how you express yourself. Keep your statement brief and to the point, but, at the same time, include all pertinent information about your past experiences and your educational goals. Individual statements vary greatly in style and content, which helps admissions officers differentiate among applicants. Many graduate departments give considerable weight to the statement in making their admissions decisions, so be sure to take the time to prepare a thoughtful and concise statement.

If recommendations are a part of the admissions requirements, carefully choose the individuals you ask to write them. It is generally best to ask current or former professors to write the recommendations, provided they are able to attest to your intellectual ability and motivation for doing the work required of a graduate student. It is advisable to provide stamped, preaddressed envelopes to people being asked to submit recommendations on your behalf.

Completed applications, including references, transcripts, and admission test scores, should be received at the institution by the specified date.

Be advised that institutions do not usually make admissions decisions until all materials have been received. Enclose a self-addressed postcard with your application, requesting confirmation of receipt. Allow at least ten days for the return of the postcard before making further inquiries.

If you plan to apply for financial support, it is imperative that you file your application early.

ADMISSION TESTS

The major testing program used in graduate admissions is the Graduate Record Examinations (GRE®) testing program, sponsored by the GRE Board and administered by Educational Testing Service, Princeton, New Jersey.

The Graduate Record Examinations testing program consists of a General Test and eight Subject Tests. The General Test measures critical thinking, verbal reasoning, quantitative reasoning, and analytical writing skills. It is offered as an Internet-based test (iBT) in the United States, Canada, and many other countries.

The GRE® revised General Test's questions were designed to reflect the kind of thinking that students need to do in graduate or business school and demonstrate that students are indeed ready for graduate-level work.

- **Verbal Reasoning**—Measures ability to analyze and evaluate written material and synthesize information obtained from it, analyze relationships among component parts of sentences, and recognize relationships among words and concepts.
- **Quantitative Reasoning**—Measures problem-solving ability, focusing on basic concepts of arithmetic, algebra, geometry, and data analysis.
- **Analytical Writing**—Measures critical thinking and analytical writing skills, specifically the ability to articulate and support complex ideas clearly and effectively.

The computer-delivered GRE® revised General Test is offered year-round at Prometric™ test centers and on specific dates at testing locations outside of the Prometric test center network. Appointments are scheduled on a first-come, first-served basis. The GRE® revised General Test is also offered as a paper-based test three times a year in areas where computer-based testing is not available.

You can take the computer-delivered GRE® revised General Test once every twenty-one days, up to five times within any continuous rolling twelve-month period (365 days)—even if you canceled your scores on a previously taken test. You may take the paper-delivered GRE® revised General Test as often as it is offered.

Three scores are reported on the revised General Test:

1. A **Verbal Reasoning score** is reported on a 130–170 score scale, in 1-point increments.
2. A **Quantitative Reasoning score** is reported on a 130–170 score scale, in 1-point increments.
3. An **Analytical Writing score** is reported on a 0–6 score level, in half-point increments.

The GRE® Subject Tests measure achievement and assume undergraduate majors or extensive background in the following eight disciplines:

- Biochemistry, Cell and Molecular Biology
- Biology
- Chemistry
- Computer Science
- Literature in English
- Mathematics
- Physics
- Psychology

The Subject Tests are available three times per year as paper-based administrations around the world. Testing time is approximately 2 hours and 50 minutes. You can obtain more information about the GRE® by visiting the ETS website at www.ets.org or consulting the *GRE® Information and Registration Bulletin*. The *Bulletin* can be obtained at many undergraduate colleges. You can also download it from the ETS website or obtain it by contacting Graduate Record Examinations, Educational Testing Service, P.O. Box 6000, Princeton, NJ 08541-6000; phone: 609-771-7670.

If you expect to apply for admission to a program that requires any of the GRE® tests, you should select a test date well in advance of the application deadline. Scores on the computer-based General Test are reported within ten to fifteen days; scores on the paper-based Subject Tests are reported within six weeks.

Another testing program, the Miller Analogies Test® (MAT®), is administered at more than 500 Controlled Testing Centers, licensed by Harcourt Assessment, Inc., in the United States, Canada, and other countries. The MAT® computer-based test is now available. Testing time is 60 minutes. The test consists of 120 partial analogies. You can obtain the *Candidate Information Booklet,* which contains a list of test centers and instructions for taking the test, from http://www.milleranalogies.com or by calling 800-328-5999 (toll-free).

Check the specific requirements of the programs to which you are applying.

How Admission Decisions Are Made

The program you apply to is directly involved in the admissions process. Although the final decision is usually made by the graduate dean (or an associate) or the faculty admissions committee, recommendations from faculty members in your intended field are important. At some institutions, an interview is incorporated into the decision process.

A Special Note for International Students

In addition to the steps already described, there are some special considerations for international students who intend to apply for graduate study in the United States. All graduate schools require an indication of competence in English. The purpose of the Test of English as a Foreign Language (TOEFL®) is to evaluate the English proficiency of people who are nonnative speakers of English and want to study at colleges and universities where English is the language of instruction. The TOEFL® is administered by Educational Testing Service (ETS) under the general direction of a policy board established by the College Board and the Graduate Record Examinations Board.

The TOEFL® iBT assesses the four basic language skills: listening, reading, writing, and speaking. It was administered for the first time in September 2005, and ETS continues to introduce the TOEFL® iBT in selected cities. The Internet-based test is administered at secure, official test centers. The testing time is approximately 4 hours. Because the TOEFL® iBT includes a speaking section, the Test of Spoken English (TSE) is no longer needed.

The TOEFL® is also offered in the paper-based format in areas of the world where Internet-based testing is not available. The paper-based TOEFL® consists of three sections—listening comprehension, structure and written expression, and reading comprehension. The testing time is approximately 3 hours. The Test of Written English (TWE®) is also given. The TWE® is a 30-minute essay that measures the examinee's ability to compose in English. Examinees receive a TWE® score separate from their TOEFL® score. The *Information Bulletin* contains information on local fees and registration procedures.

The TOEFL® paper-based test (TOEFL® PBT) began being phased out in mid-2012. For those who may have taken the TOEFL® PBT, scores remain valid for two years after the test date. The Test of Written English (TWE®) is also given. The TWE® is a 30-minute essay that measures the examinee's ability to compose in English. Examinees receive a TWE® score separate from their TOEFL® score. The Information Bulletin contains information on local fees and registration procedures.

Additional information and registration materials are available from TOEFL® Services, Educational Testing Service, P.O. Box 6151, Princeton, New Jersey 08541-6151. Phone: 609-771-7100. Website: www.toefl.org.

International students should apply especially early because of the number of steps required to complete the admissions process. Furthermore, many United States graduate schools have a limited number of spaces for international students, and many more students apply than the schools can accommodate.

International students may find financial assistance from institutions very limited. The U.S. government requires international applicants to submit a certification of support, which is a statement attesting to the applicant's financial resources. In addition, international students *must* have health insurance coverage.

Tips for Minority Students

Indicators of a university's values in terms of diversity are found both in its recruitment programs and its resources directed to student success. Important questions: Does the institution vigorously recruit minorities for its graduate programs? Is there funding available to help with the costs associated with visiting the school? Are minorities represented in the institution's brochures or website or on their faculty rolls? What campus-based resources or services (including assistance in locating housing or career counseling and placement) are available? Is funding available to members of underrepresented groups?

At the program level, it is particularly important for minority students to investigate the "climate" of a program under consideration. How many minority students are enrolled and how many have graduated? What opportunities are there to work with diverse faculty and mentors whose research interests match yours? How are conflicts resolved or concerns addressed? How interested are faculty in building strong and supportive relations with students? "Climate" concerns should be addressed by posing questions to various individuals, including faculty members, current students, and alumni.

Information is also available through various organizations, such as the Hispanic Association of Colleges & Universities (HACU), and publications such as *Diverse Issues in Higher Education* and *Hispanic Outlook* magazine. There are also books devoted to this topic, such as *The Multicultural Student's Guide to Colleges* by Robert Mitchell.

Financial Support

The range of financial support at the graduate level is very broad. The following descriptions will give you a general idea of what you might expect and what will be expected of you as a financial support recipient.

Fellowships, Scholarships, and Grants

These are usually outright awards of a few hundred to many thousands of dollars with no service to the institution required in return. Fellowships and scholarships are usually awarded on the basis of merit and are highly competitive. Grants are made on the basis of financial need or special talent in a field of study. Many fellowships, scholarships, and grants not only cover tuition, fees, and supplies but also include stipends for living expenses with allowances for dependents. However, the terms of each should be examined because some do not permit recipients to supplement their income with outside work. Fellowships, scholarships, and grants may vary in the number of years for which they are awarded.

In addition to the availability of these funds at the university or program level, many excellent fellowship programs are available at the national level and may be applied for before and during enrollment in a graduate program. A listing of many of these programs can be found at the Council of Graduate Schools' website: http://www. cgsnet.org. There is a wealth of information in the "Programs" and "Awards" sections.

Assistantships and Internships

Many graduate students receive financial support through assistantships, particularly involving teaching or research duties. It is important to recognize that such appointments should not be viewed simply as employment relationships but rather should constitute an integral and important part of a student's graduate education. As such, the appointments should be accompanied by strong faculty mentoring and increasingly responsible apprenticeship experiences. The specific nature of these appointments in a given program should be considered in selecting that graduate program.

TEACHING ASSISTANTSHIPS

These usually provide a salary and full or partial tuition remission and may also provide health benefits. Unlike fellowships, scholarships, and grants, which require no service to the institution, teaching assistantships require recipients to provide the institution with a specific amount of undergraduate teaching, ideally related to the student's field of study. Some teaching assistants are limited to grading papers, compiling bibliographies, taking notes, or monitoring laboratories. At some graduate schools, teaching assistants must carry lighter course loads than regular full-time students.

RESEARCH ASSISTANTSHIPS

These are very similar to teaching assistantships in the manner in which financial assistance is provided. The difference is that recipients are given basic research assignments in their disciplines rather than teaching responsibilities. The work required is normally related to the student's field of study; in most instances, the assistantship supports the student's thesis or dissertation research.

ADMINISTRATIVE INTERNSHIPS

These are similar to assistantships in application of financial assistance funds, but the student is given an assignment on a part-time basis, usually as a special assistant with one of the university's administrative offices. The assignment may not necessarily be directly related to the recipient's discipline.

RESIDENCE HALL AND COUNSELING ASSISTANTSHIPS

These assistantships are frequently assigned to graduate students in psychology, counseling, and social work, but they may be offered to students in other disciplines, especially if the student has worked in this capacity during his or her undergraduate years. Duties can vary from being available in a dean's office for a specific number of hours for consultation with undergraduates to living in campus residences and being responsible for both counseling and administrative tasks or advising student activity groups. Residence hall assistantships often include a room and board allowance and, in some cases, tuition assistance and stipends. Contact the Housing and Student Life Office for more information.

Health Insurance

The availability and affordability of health insurance is an important issue and one that should be considered in an applicant's choice of institution and program. While often included with assistantships and fellowships, this is not always the case and, even if provided, the benefits may be limited. It is important to note that the U.S. government requires international students to have health insurance.

The GI Bill

This provides financial assistance for students who are veterans of the United States armed forces. If you are a veteran, contact your local Veterans Administration office to determine your eligibility and to get full details about benefits. There are a number of programs that offer educational benefits to current military enlistees. Some states have tuition assistance programs for members of the National Guard. Contact the VA office at the college for more information.

Federal Work-Study Program (FWS)

Employment is another way some students finance their graduate studies. The federally funded Federal Work-Study Program provides eligible students with employment opportunities, usually in public and private nonprofit organizations. Federal funds pay up to 75 percent of the wages, with the remainder paid by the employing agency. FWS is available to graduate students who demonstrate financial need. Not all schools have these funds, and some only award them to undergraduates. Each school sets its application deadline and workstudy earnings limits. Wages vary and are related to the type of work done. You must file the Free Application for Federal Student Aid (FAFSA) to be eligible for this program.

Loans

Many graduate students borrow to finance their graduate programs when other sources of assistance (which do not have to be repaid) prove insufficient. You should always read and understand the terms of any loan program before submitting your application.

FEDERAL DIRECT LOANS

Federal Direct Stafford Loans. The Federal Direct Stafford Loan Program offers a variable-fixed interest rate loan to graduate students with the Department of Education acting as the lender. Students receive a new rate with each new loan, but that rate is fixed for the life of the loan. Beginning with loans made on or after July 1, 2013, the interest rate for loans made each July 1st to June 30th period are determined based on the last 10-year Treasury note auction prior to June 1st of that year, plus an added percentage. The interest rate can be no higher than 9.5%.

Beginning July 1, 2012, the Federal Direct Stafford Loan for graduate students is an unsubsidized loan. Under the *unsubsidized* program, the grad borrower pays the interest on the loan from the day proceeds are issued and is responsible for paying interest during all periods. If the borrower chooses not to pay the interest while in school, or during the grace periods, deferment, or forbearance, the interest accrues and will be capitalized.

Graduate students may borrow up to $20,500 per year through the Direct Stafford Loan Program, up to a cumulative maximum of $138,500, including undergraduate borrowing. No more than $65,000 of the $138,500 can be from subsidized loans that the grad borrower may have received for periods of enrollment that began before July 1, 2012, or for prior undergraduate borrowing. You may borrow up to the cost of attendance at the school in which you are enrolled or will attend, minus estimated financial assistance from other federal, state, and private sources, up to a maximum of $20,500. Grad borrowers who reach the aggregate loan limit over the course of their education cannot receive additional loans; however, if they repay some of their loans to bring the outstanding balance below the aggregate limit, they could be eligible to borrow again, up to that limit.

For Unsubsidized loans first disbursed on or after July 1, 2013, and before July 1, 2014, the interest rate is 5.41%. For those first disbursed on or after July 1, 2014, and before July 1, 2015, the interest rate is 6.21%.

A fee is deducted from the loan proceeds upon disbursement. Loans with a first disbursement on or after July 1, 2010 but before July 1, 2012, have a borrower origination fee of 1 percent. For loans disbursed after July 1, 2012, these fee deductions no longer apply. The Budget Control Act of 2011, signed into law on August 2, 2011, eliminated Direct Subsidized Loan eligibility for graduate and professional students for periods of enrollment beginning on or after July 1, 2012 and terminated the authority of the Department of Education to offer most repayment incentives to Direct Loan borrowers for loans disbursed on or after July 1, 2012.

Under the *subsidized* Federal Direct Stafford Loan Program, repayment begins six months after your last date of enrollment on at least a half-time basis. Under the *unsubsidized* program, repayment of interest begins within thirty days from disbursement of the loan proceeds, and repayment of the principal begins six months after your last enrollment on at least a half-time basis. Some borrowers may choose to defer interest payments while they are in school. The accrued interest is added to the loan balance when the borrower begins repayment. There are several repayment options.

Federal Perkins Loans. The Federal Perkins Loan is available to students demonstrating financial need and is administered directly by the school. Not all schools have these funds, and some may award them to undergraduates only. Eligibility is determined from the information you provide on the FAFSA. The school will notify you of your eligibility.

Eligible graduate students may borrow up to $8,000 per year, up to a maximum of $60,000, including undergraduate borrowing (even if your previous Perkins Loans have been repaid). The interest rate for Federal Perkins Loans is 5 percent, and no interest accrues while you remain in school at least half-time. Students who are attending less than half-time need to check with their school to determine the length of their grace period. There are no guarantee, loan, or disbursement fees. Repayment begins nine months after your last date of enrollment on at least a half-time basis and may extend over a maximum of ten years with no prepayment penalty.

Federal Direct Graduate PLUS Loans. Effective July 1, 2006, graduate and professional students are eligible for Graduate PLUS loans. This program allows students to borrow up to the cost of attendance, less any other aid received. These loans have a fixed interest rate, and interest begins to accrue at the time of disbursement. Beginning with loans made on or after July 1, 2013, the interest rate for loans made each July 1st to June 30th period are determined based on the last 10-year Treasury note auction prior to June 1st of that year. The interest rate can be no higher than 10.5%. The PLUS loans do involve a credit check; a PLUS borrower may obtain a loan with a cosigner if his or her credit is not good enough. Grad PLUS loans may be deferred while a student is in school and for the six months following a drop below half-time enrollment. For more information, you should contact a representative in your college's financial aid office.

Deferring Your Federal Loan Repayments. If you borrowed under the Federal Direct Stafford Loan Program, Federal Direct PLUS Loan Program, or the Federal Perkins Loan Program for previous undergraduate or graduate study, your payments may be deferred when you return to graduate school, depending on when you borrowed and under which program.

There are other deferment options available if you are temporarily unable to repay your loan. Information about these deferments is provided at your entrance and exit interviews. If you believe you are eligible for a deferment of your loan payments, you must contact your lender or loan servicer to request a deferment. The deferment must be filed prior to the time your payment is due, and it must be re-filed when it expires if you remain eligible for deferment at that time.

SUPPLEMENTAL (PRIVATE) LOANS

Many lending institutions offer supplemental loan programs and other financing plans, such as the ones described here, to students seeking additional assistance in meeting their education expenses. Some loan programs target all types of graduate students; others are designed specifically for business, law, or medical students. In addition, you can use private loans not specifically designed for education to help finance your graduate degree.

If you are considering borrowing through a supplemental or private loan program, you should carefully consider the terms and be sure to read the fine print. Check with the program sponsor for the most current terms that will be applicable to the amounts you intend to borrow for graduate study. Most supplemental loan programs for graduate study offer unsubsidized, credit-based loans. In general, a credit-ready borrower is one who has a satisfactory credit history or no credit history at all. A creditworthy borrower generally must pass a credit test to be eligible to borrow or act as a cosigner for the loan funds.

Many supplemental loan programs have minimum and maximum annual loan limits. Some offer amounts equal to the cost of attendance minus any other aid you will receive for graduate study. If you are planning to borrow for several years of graduate study, consider whether there is a cumulative or aggregate limit on the amount you may borrow. Often this cumulative or aggregate limit will include any amounts you borrowed and have not repaid for undergraduate or previous graduate study.

The combination of the annual interest rate, loan fees, and the repayment terms you choose will determine how much you will repay over time. Compare these features in combination before you decide which loan program to use. Some loans offer interest rates that are adjusted monthly, quarterly, or annually. Some offer interest rates that are lower during the in-school, grace, and deferment periods and then increase when you begin repayment. Some programs include a loan origination fee, which is usually deducted from the principal amount you receive when the loan is disbursed and must be repaid along with the interest and other principal when you graduate, withdraw from school, or drop below half-time study. Sometimes the loan fees are reduced if you borrow with a qualified cosigner. Some programs allow you to defer interest and/or principal payments while you are enrolled in graduate school. Many programs allow you to capitalize your interest payments; the interest due on your loan is added to the outstanding balance of your loan, so you don't have to repay immediately, but this increases the amount you owe. Other programs allow you to pay the interest as you go, which reduces the amount you later have to repay. The private loan market is very competitive, and your financial aid office can help you evaluate these programs.

Applying for Need-Based Financial Aid

Schools that award federal and institutional financial assistance based on need will require you to complete the FAFSA and, in some cases, an institutional financial aid application.

If you are applying for federal student assistance, you **must** complete the FAFSA. A service of the U.S. Department of Education, the FAFSA is free to all applicants. Most applicants apply online at www.fafsa.ed.gov. Paper applications are available at the financial aid office of your local college.

After your FAFSA information has been processed, you will receive a Student Aid Report (SAR). If you provided an e-mail address on the FAFSA, this will be sent to you electronically; otherwise, it will be mailed to your home address.

Follow the instructions on the SAR if you need to correct information reported on your original application. If your situation changes after you file your FAFSA, contact your financial aid officer to discuss amending your information. You can also appeal your financial aid award if you have extenuating circumstances.

If you would like more information on federal student financial aid, visit the FAFSA website or download the most recent version of *Funding Education Beyond High School: The Guide to Federal Student Aid* at http://studentaid.ed.gov/students/publications/student_guide/index.html. This guide is also available in Spanish.

The U.S. Department of Education also has a toll-free number for questions concerning federal student aid programs. The number is 1-800-4-FED AID (1-800-433-3243). If you are hearing impaired, call toll-free, 1-800-730-8913.

Summary

Remember that these are generalized statements about financial assistance at the graduate level. Because each institution allots its aid differently, you should communicate directly with the school and the specific department of interest to you. It is not unusual, for example, to find that an endowment vested within a specific department supports one or more fellowships. You may fit its requirements and specifications precisely.

Accreditation and Accrediting Agencies

Colleges and universities in the United States, and their individual academic and professional programs, are accredited by nongovernmental agencies concerned with monitoring the quality of education in this country. Agencies with both regional and national jurisdictions grant accreditation to institutions as a whole, while specialized bodies acting on a nationwide basis—often national professional associations—grant accreditation to departments and programs in specific fields.

Institutional and specialized accrediting agencies share the same basic concerns: the purpose an academic unit—whether university or program—has set for itself and how well it fulfills that purpose, the adequacy of its financial and other resources, the quality of its academic offerings, and the level of services it provides. Agencies that grant institutional accreditation take a broader view, of course, and examine university-wide or college-wide services with which a specialized agency may not concern itself.

Both types of agencies follow the same general procedures when considering an application for accreditation. The academic unit prepares a self-evaluation, focusing on the concerns mentioned above and usually including an assessment of both its strengths and weaknesses; a team of representatives of the accrediting body reviews this evaluation, visits the campus, and makes its own report; and finally, the accrediting body makes a decision on the application. Often, even when accreditation is granted, the agency makes a recommendation regarding how the institution or program can improve. All institutions and programs are also reviewed every few years to determine whether they continue to meet established standards; if they do not, they may lose their accreditation.

Accrediting agencies themselves are reviewed and evaluated periodically by the U.S. Department of Education and the Council for Higher Education Accreditation (CHEA). Recognized agencies adhere to certain standards and practices, and their authority in matters of accreditation is widely accepted in the educational community.

This does not mean, however, that accreditation is a simple matter, either for schools wishing to become accredited or for students deciding where to apply. Indeed, in certain fields the very meaning and methods of accreditation are the subject of a good deal of debate. For their part, those applying to graduate school should be aware of the safeguards provided by regional accreditation, especially in terms of degree acceptance and institutional longevity. Beyond this, applicants should understand the role that specialized accreditation plays in their field, as this varies considerably from one discipline to another. In certain professional fields, it is necessary to have graduated from a program that is accredited in order to be eligible for a license to practice, and in some fields the federal government also makes this a hiring requirement. In other disciplines, however, accreditation is not as essential, and there can be excellent programs that are not accredited. In fact, some programs choose not to seek accreditation, although most do.

Institutions and programs that present themselves for accreditation are sometimes granted the status of candidate for accreditation, or what is known as "preaccreditation." This may happen, for example, when an academic unit is too new to have met all the requirements for accreditation. Such status signifies initial recognition and indicates that the school or program in question is working to fulfill all requirements; it does not, however, guarantee that accreditation will be granted.

Institutional Accrediting Agencies—Regional

MIDDLE STATES ASSOCIATION OF COLLEGES AND SCHOOLS

Accredits institutions in Delaware, District of Columbia, Maryland, New Jersey, New York, Pennsylvania, Puerto Rico, and the Virgin Islands.

Dr. Elizabeth Sibolski, President
Middle States Commission on Higher Education
3624 Market Street, Second Floor West
Philadelphia, Pennsylvania 19104
Phone: 267-284-5000
Fax: 215-662-5501
E-mail: info@msche.org
Website: www.msche.org

NEW ENGLAND ASSOCIATION OF SCHOOLS AND COLLEGES

Accredits institutions in Connecticut, Maine, Massachusetts, New Hampshire, Rhode Island, and Vermont.

Dr. Barbara E. Brittingham, President/Director
Commission on Institutions of Higher Education
3 Burlington Woods Drive, Suite 100
Burlington, Massachusetts 01803-4531
Phone: 855-886-3272 or 781-425-7714
Fax: 781-425-1001
E-mail: cihe@neasc.org
Website: http://cihe.neasc.org

THE HIGHER LEARNING COMMISSION

Accredits institutions in Arizona, Arkansas, Colorado, Illinois, Indiana, Iowa, Kansas, Michigan, Minnesota, Missouri, Nebraska, New Mexico, North Dakota, Ohio, Oklahoma, South Dakota, West Virginia, Wisconsin, and Wyoming.

Dr. Barbara Gellman-Danley, President
The Higher Learning Commission
230 South LaSalle Street, Suite 7-500
Chicago, Illinois 60604-1413
Phone: 800-621-7440 or 312-263-0456
Fax: 312-263-7462
E-mail: info@hlcommission.org
Website: www.ncahlc.org

NORTHWEST COMMISSION ON COLLEGES AND UNIVERSITIES

Accredits institutions in Alaska, Idaho, Montana, Nevada, Oregon, Utah, and Washington.

Dr. Sandra E. Elman, President
8060 165th Avenue, NE, Suite 100
Redmond, Washington 98052
Phone: 425-558-4224
Fax: 425-376-0596
E-mail: selman@nwccu.org
Website: www.nwccu.org

SOUTHERN ASSOCIATION OF COLLEGES AND SCHOOLS

Accredits institutions in Alabama, Florida, Georgia, Kentucky, Louisiana, Mississippi, North Carolina, South Carolina, Tennessee, Texas, and Virginia.

Dr. Belle S. Wheelan, President
Commission on Colleges
1866 Southern Lane
Decatur, Georgia 30033-4097
Phone: 404-679-4500 Ext. 4504
Fax: 404-679-4558
E-mail: questions@sacscoc.org
Website: www.sacscoc.org

WESTERN ASSOCIATION OF SCHOOLS AND COLLEGES

Accredits institutions in California, Guam, and Hawaii.

Dr. Mary Ellen Petrisko, President
Accrediting Commission for Senior Colleges and Universities
985 Atlantic Avenue, Suite 100
Alameda, California 94501
Phone: 510-748-9001
Fax: 510-748-9797
E-mail: wasc@wascsenior.org
Website: http://www.wascsenior.org/

Institutional Accrediting Agencies—Other

ACCREDITING COUNCIL FOR INDEPENDENT COLLEGES AND SCHOOLS
Albert C. Gray, Ph.D., Executive Director and CEO
750 First Street, NE, Suite 980
Washington, DC 20002-4241
Phone: 202-336-6780
Fax: 202-842-2593
E-mail: info@acics.org
Website: www.acics.org

DISTANCE EDUCATION AND TRAINING COUNCIL (DETC)
Accrediting Commission
Leah Matthews, Executive Director
1601 18th Street, NW, Suite 2
Washington, DC 20009
Phone: 202-234-5100
Fax: 202-332-1386
E-mail: info@detc.org
Website: www.detc.org

Specialized Accrediting Agencies

ACUPUNCTURE AND ORIENTAL MEDICINE
Mark S. McKenzie, LAc MsOM DiplOM, Executive Director
Accreditation Commission for Acupuncture and Oriental Medicine
8941 Aztec Drive
Eden Prairie, Minnesota 55347
Phone: 952-212-2434
Fax: 301-313-0912
E-mail: coordinator@acaom.org
Website: www.acaom.org

ART AND DESIGN
Karen P. Moynahan, Executive Director
National Association of Schools of Art and Design (NASAD)
Commission on Accreditation
11250 Roger Bacon Drive, Suite 21
Reston, Virginia 20190-5248
Phone: 703-437-0700
Fax: 703-437-6312
E-mail: info@arts-accredit.org
Website: http://nasad.arts-accredit.org/

BUSINESS
Robert D. Reid, Executive Vice President and Chief Accreditation Officer
AACSB International—The Association to Advance Collegiate Schools of Business
777 South Harbour Island Boulevard, Suite 750
Tampa, Florida 33602
Phone: 813-769-6500
Fax: 813-769-6559
E-mail: bob@aacsb.edu
Website: www.aacsb.edu

CHIROPRACTIC
S. Ray Bennett, Director of Accreditation Services
Council on Chiropractic Education (CCE)
Commission on Accreditation
8049 North 85th Way
Scottsdale, Arizona 85258-4321
Phone: 480-443-8877 or 888-443-3506
Fax: 480-483-7333
E-mail: cce@cce-usa.org
Website: www.cce-usa.org

CLINICAL LABORATORY SCIENCES
Dianne M. Cearlock, Ph.D., Chief Executive Officer
National Accrediting Agency for Clinical Laboratory Sciences
5600 North River Road, Suite 720
Rosemont, Illinois 60018-5119
Phone: 773-714-8880 or 847-939-3597
Fax: 773-714-8886
E-mail: info@naacls.org
Website: www.naacls.org

CLINICAL PASTORAL EDUCATION
Trace Haythorn, Executive Director
Association for Clinical Pastoral Education, Inc.
1549 Clairmont Road, Suite 103
Decatur, Georgia 30033-4611
Phone: 404-320-1472
Fax: 404-320-0849
E-mail: acpe@acpe.edu
Website: www.acpe.edu

DANCE
Karen P. Moynahan, Executive Director
National Association of Schools of Dance (NASD)
Commission on Accreditation
11250 Roger Bacon Drive, Suite 21
Reston, Virginia 20190-5248
Phone: 703-437-0700
Fax: 703-437-6312
E-mail: info@arts-accredit.org
Website: http://nasd.arts-accredit.org

DENTISTRY
Dr. Sherin Tooks, Director
Commission on Dental Accreditation
American Dental Association
211 East Chicago Avenue, Suite 1900
Chicago, Illinois 60611
Phone: 312-440-4643 or 800-621-8099
E-mail: accreditation@ada.org
Website: www.ada.org

DIETETICS AND NUTRITION
Mary B. Gregoire, Ph.D., Executive Director; RD, FADA, FAND
Academy of Nutrition and Dietetics
Accreditation Council for Education in Nutrition and Dietetics (ACEND)
120 South Riverside Plaza, Suite 2000
Chicago, Illinois 60606-6995
Phone: 800-877-1600 Ext. 5400 or 312-899-0040
Fax: 312-899-4817
E-mail: acend@eatright.org
Website: www.eatright.org/ACEND

ENGINEERING
Michael Milligan, Ph.D., PE, Executive Director
Accreditation Board for Engineering and Technology, Inc. (ABET)
415 North Charles Street
Baltimore, Maryland 21201
Phone: 410-347-7700
E-mail: accreditation@abet.org
Website: www.abet.org

FORESTRY
Carol L. Redelsheimer
Director of Science and Education
Society of American Foresters
5400 Grosvenor Lane
Bethesda, Maryland 20814-2198
Phone: 301-897-8720 or 866-897-8720
Fax: 301-897-3690
E-mail: redelsheimerc@safnet.org
Website: www.safnet.org

HEALTH SERVICES ADMINISTRATION
Commission on Accreditation of Healthcare Management Education (CAHME)
Margaret Schulte, President and CEO
1700 Rockville Pike
Suite 400
Rockville, Maryland 20852
Phone: 301-998-6101
E-mail: info@cahme.org
Website: www.cahme.org

INTERIOR DESIGN
Holly Mattson, Executive Director
Council for Interior Design Accreditation
206 Grandview Avenue, Suite 350
Grand Rapids, Michigan 49503-4014
Phone: 616-458-0400
Fax: 616-458-0460
E-mail: info@accredit-id.org
Website: www.accredit-id.org

JOURNALISM AND MASS COMMUNICATIONS
Susanne Shaw, Executive Director
Accrediting Council on Education in Journalism and Mass Communications (ACEJMC)
School of Journalism
Stauffer-Flint Hall
University of Kansas
1435 Jayhawk Boulevard
Lawrence, Kansas 66045-7575
Phone: 785-864-3973
Fax: 785-864-5225
E-mail: sshaw@ku.edu
Website: http://www2.ku.edu/~acejmc/

LANDSCAPE ARCHITECTURE
Ronald C. Leighton, Executive Director
Landscape Architectural Accreditation Board (LAAB)
American Society of Landscape Architects (ASLA)
636 Eye Street, NW
Washington, DC 20001-3736
Phone: 202-898-2444 or 888-999-2752
Fax: 202-898-1185
E-mail: info@asla.org
Website: www.asla.org

LAW
Barry Currier, Managing Director of Accreditation & Legal Education
American Bar Association
321 North Clark Street, 21st Floor
Chicago, Illinois 60654
Phone: 312-988-6738
Fax: 312-988-5681
E-mail: legaled@americanbar.org
Website: http://www.americanbar.org/groups/legal_education/resources/accreditation.html

LIBRARY
Karen O'Brien, Director
Office for Accreditation
American Library Association
50 East Huron Street
Chicago, Illinois 60611-2795
Phone: 312-280-2432
Fax: 312-280-2433
E-mail: accred@ala.org
Website: www.ala.org/accreditation/

MARRIAGE AND FAMILY THERAPY
Tanya A. Tamarkin, Director of Educational Affairs
Commission on Accreditation for Marriage and Family Therapy Education
American Association for Marriage and Family Therapy
112 South Alfred Street
Alexandria, Virginia 22314-3061
Phone: 703-838-9808
Fax: 703-838-9805
E-mail: coamfte@aamft.org
Website: www.aamft.org

MEDICAL ILLUSTRATION
Commission on Accreditation of Allied Health Education Programs (CAAHEP)
Kathleen Megivern, Executive Director
1361 Park Street
Clearwater, Florida 33756
Phone: 727-210-2350
Fax: 727-210-2354
E-mail: mail@caahep.org
Website: www.caahep.org

MEDICINE
Liaison Committee on Medical Education (LCME)
Robert B. Hash, M.D., LCME Secretary
American Medical Association
Council on Medical Education
330 North Wabash Avenue, Suite 39300
Chicago, Illinois 60611-5885
Phone: 312-464-4933
E-mail: lcme@aamc.org
Website: www.ama-assn.org

Liaison Committee on Medical Education (LCME)
Heather Lent, M.A., Director
Accreditation Services
Association of American Medical Colleges
655 K Street, NW
Washington, DC 20001-2399
Phone: 202-828-0596
E-mail: lcme@aamc.org
Website: www.lcme.org

MUSIC
Karen P. Moynahan, Executive Director
National Association of Schools of Music (NASM)
Commission on Accreditation
11250 Roger Bacon Drive, Suite 21
Reston, Virginia 20190-5248
Phone: 703-437-0700
Fax: 703-437-6312
E-mail: info@arts-accredit.org
Website: http://nasm.arts-accredit.org/

NATUROPATHIC MEDICINE
Daniel Seitz, J.D., Ed.D., Executive Director
Council on Naturopathic Medical Education
P.O. Box 178
Great Barrington, Massachusetts 01230
Phone: 413-528-8877
E-mail: www.cnme.org/contact.html
Website: www.cnme.org

NURSE ANESTHESIA
Frank Gerbasi, Ph.D., CRNA, COA Executive Director
Council on Accreditation of Nurse Anesthesia Educational Programs (COA)
American Association of Nurse Anesthetists
222 South Prospect Avenue, Suite 304
Park Ridge, Illinois 60068-4001
Phone: 847-655-1160
Fax: 847-692-7137
E-mail: accreditation@coa.us.com
Website: http://home.coa.us.com

NURSE EDUCATION
Jennifer L. Butlin, Executive Director
Commission on Collegiate Nursing Education (CCNE)
One Dupont Circle, NW, Suite 530
Washington, DC 20036-1120
Phone: 202-887-6791
Fax: 202-887-8476
E-mail: jbutlin@aacn.nche.edu
Website: www.aacn.nche.edu/accreditation

NURSE MIDWIFERY
Heather L. Maurer, M.A., Executive Director
Accreditation Commission for Midwifery Education (ACME)
American College of Nurse-Midwives
8403 Colesville Road, Suite 1550
Silver Spring, Maryland 20910
Phone: 240-485-1800
Fax: 240-485-1818
E-mail: info@acnm.org
Website: www.midwife.org/Program-Accreditation

NURSE PRACTITIONER
Gay Johnson, CEO
National Association of Nurse Practitioners in Women's Health
Council on Accreditation
505 C Street, NE
Washington, DC 20002
Phone: 202-543-9693 Ext. 1
Fax: 202-543-9858
E-mail: info@npwh.org
Website: www.npwh.org

NURSING
Nell Ard, Ph.D., RN, CNE, Associate Director
Accreditation Commission for Education in Nursing (ACEN)
3343 Peachtree Road, NE, Suite 850
Atlanta, Georgia 30326
Phone: 404-975-5000
Fax: 404-975-5020
E-mail: info@acenursing.org
Website: www.acenursing.org

OCCUPATIONAL THERAPY
Heather Stagliano, DHSc, OTR/L, Director of Accreditation
The American Occupational Therapy Association, Inc.
4720 Montgomery Lane, Suite 200
Bethesda, Maryland 20814-3449
Phone: 301-652-6611 Ext. 2914
TDD: 800-377-8555
Fax: 301-652-7711
E-mail: accred@aota.org
Website: www.aota.org

OPTOMETRY
Joyce L. Urbeck, Administrative Director
Accreditation Council on Optometric Education (ACOE)
American Optometric Association
243 North Lindbergh Boulevard
St. Louis, Missouri 63141-7881
Phone: 800-365-7881
Fax: 314-991-4101
E-mail: accredit@aoa.org
Website: www.theacoe.org

OSTEOPATHIC MEDICINE
Konrad C. Miskowicz-Retz, Ph.D., CAE
Director, Department of Accreditation
Commission on Osteopathic College Accreditation (COCA)
American Osteopathic Association
142 East Ontario Street
Chicago, Illinois 60611
Phone: 312-202-8097
Fax: 312-202-8397
E-mail: predoc@osteopathic.org
Website: www.osteopathic.org

PHARMACY
Peter H. Vlasses, PharmD, Executive Director
Accreditation Council for Pharmacy Education
135 South LaSalle Street, Suite 4100
Chicago, Illinois 60603-4810
Phone: 312-664-3575
Fax: 312-664-4652
E-mail: csinfo@acpe-accredit.org
Website: www.acpe-accredit.org

PHYSICAL THERAPY
Mary Jane Harris, M.S., PT, Director
Commission on Accreditation in Physical Therapy Education (CAPTE)
American Physical Therapy Association (APTA)
1111 North Fairfax Street
Alexandria, Virginia 22314-1488
Phone: 703-684-2782 or 800-999-2782
TDD: 703-683-6748
Fax: 703-684-7343
E-mail: accreditation@apta.org
Website: www.capteonline.org

PHYSICIAN ASSISTANT STUDIES
John E. McCarty, Executive Director
Accreditation Review Commission on Education for the Physician Assistant, Inc. (ARC-PA)
12000 Findley Road, Suite 150
Johns Creek, Georgia 30097
Phone: 770-476-1224
Fax: 770-476-1738
E-mail: arc-pa@arc-pa.org
Website: www.arc-pa.org

PLANNING
Ms. Shonagh Merits, Executive Director
American Institute of Certified Planners/Association of Collegiate Schools of Planning/American Planning Association
Planning Accreditation Board (PAB)
2334 West Lawrence Avenue, Suite 209
Chicago, Illinois 60625
Phone: 773-334-7200
E-mail: smerits@planningaccreditationboard.org
Website: www.planningaccreditationboard.org

PODIATRIC MEDICINE
Alan R. Tinkleman, M.P.A., Executive Director
Council on Podiatric Medical Education (CPME)
American Podiatric Medical Association (APMA)
9312 Old Georgetown Road
Bethesda, Maryland 20814-1621
Phone: 301-571-9200
Fax: 301-571-4903
Website: www.cpme.org

PSYCHOLOGY AND COUNSELING
Susan Zlotlow, Ph.D., Associate Executive Director
Office of Program Consultation and Accreditation
American Psychological Association
750 First Street, NE
Washington, DC 20002-4242
Phone: 202-336-5979 or 800-374-2721
TDD/TTY: 202-336-6123
Fax: 202-336-5978
E-mail: apaaccred@apa.org
Website: www.apa.org/ed/accreditation

Carol L. Bobby, Ph.D., Executive Director
Council for Accreditation of Counseling and Related Educational Programs (CACREP)
1001 North Fairfax Street, Suite 510
Alexandria, Virginia 22314
Phone: 703-535-5990
Fax: 703-739-6209
E-mail: cacrep@cacrep.org
Website: www.cacrep.org

PUBLIC AFFAIRS AND ADMINISTRATION
Crystal Calarusse, Chief Accreditation Officer
Commission on Peer Review and Accreditation
National Association of Schools of Public Affairs and Administration
1029 Vermont Avenue, NW, Suite 1100
Washington, DC 20005
Phone: 202-628-8965
Fax: 202-626-4978
E-mail: copra@naspaa.org
Website: www.naspaa.org

PUBLIC HEALTH
Laura Rasar King, M.P.H., MCHES, Executive Director
Council on Education for Public Health
1010 Wayne Avenue, Suite 220
Silver Spring, Maryland 20910
Phone: 202-789-1050
Fax: 202-789-1895
E-mail: Lking@ceph.org
Website: www.ceph.org

REHABILITATION EDUCATION
Frank Lane, Ph.D., Executive Director
Council on Rehabilitation Education (CORE)
Commission on Standards and Accreditation
1699 Woodfield Road, Suite 300
Schaumburg, Illinois 60173
Phone: 847-944-1345
Fax: 847-944-1346
E-mail: lane@iit.edu
Website: www.core-rehab.org

SOCIAL WORK
Jo Ann Regan, Ph.D., Director
Office of Social Work Accreditation
Council on Social Work Education
1701 Duke Street, Suite 200
Alexandria, Virginia 22314
Phone: 703-683-8080
Fax: 703-683-8099
E-mail: info@cswe.org
Website: www.cswe.org

SPEECH-LANGUAGE PATHOLOGY AND AUDIOLOGY
Patrima L. Tice, Director of Accreditation
American Speech-Language-Hearing Association
Council on Academic Accreditation in Audiology and Speech-Language Pathology
2200 Research Boulevard
Rockville, Maryland 20850-3289
Phone: 301-296-5796
Fax: 301-296-8750
E-mail: ptice@asha.org
Website: www.asha.org/academic/accreditation/default.htm

TECHNOLOGY
Michale S. McComis, Ed.D., Executive Director
Accrediting Commission of Career Schools and Colleges
2101 Wilson Boulevard, Suite 302
Arlington, Virginia 22201
Phone: 703-247-4212
Fax: 703-247-4533
E-mail: mccomis@accsc.org
Website: www.accsc.org

TEACHER EDUCATION
James G. Cibulka, Ph.D., President
Council for the Accreditation of Educator Preparation
1140 19th Street, NW, Suite 400
Washington, DC 20036
Phone: 202-223-0077
E-mail: caep@caepnet.org
Website: www.caepnet.org

THEATER
Karen P. Moynahan, Executive Director
National Association of Schools of Theatre Commission on Accreditation
11250 Roger Bacon Drive, Suite 21
Reston, Virginia 20190
Phone: 703-437-0700
Fax: 703-437-6312
E-mail: info@arts-accredit.org
Website: http://nast.arts-accredit.org/

THEOLOGY
Keith Sharfman, Director
Association of Advanced Rabbinical and Talmudic Schools (AARTS)
Accreditation Commission
11 Broadway, Suite 405
New York, New York 10004
Phone: 212-363-1991
Fax: 212-533-5335
E-mail: k.sharfman.aarts@gmail.com

Daniel O. Aleshire, Executive Director
Association of Theological Schools in the United States and Canada (ATS)
Commission on Accrediting
10 Summit Park Drive
Pittsburgh, Pennsylvania 15275
Phone: 412-788-6505
Fax: 412-788-6510
E-mail: ats@ats.edu
Website: www.ats.edu

Paul Boatner, President
Transnational Association of Christian Colleges and Schools (TRACS)
Accreditation Commission
15935 Forest Road
Forest, Virginia 24551
Phone: 434-525-9539
Fax: 434-525-9538
E-mail: info@tracs.org
Website: www.tracs.org

VETERINARY MEDICINE
David Granstrom, Executive Director
Education and Research Division
American Veterinary Medical Association (AVMA)
Council on Education
1931 North Meacham Road, Suite 100
Schaumburg, Illinois 60173-4360
Phone: 847-925-8070 Ext. 6674
Fax: 847-925-9329
E-mail: info@avma.org
Website: www.avma.org

How to Use These Guides

As you identify the particular programs and institutions that interest you, you can use both the ***Graduate & Professional Programs: An Overview*** volume and the specialized volumes in the series to obtain detailed information.

- ***Graduate Programs in the Physical Sciences, Mathematics, Agricultural Sciences, the Environment & Natural Resources***
- ***Graduate Programs in Engineering & Applied Sciences***
- ***Graduate Programs the Humanities, Arts & Social Sciences***
- ***Graduate Programs in the Biological/Biomedical Sciences & Health-Related Professions***
- ***Graduate Programs in Business, Education, Information Studies, Law & Social Work***

Each of the specialized volumes in the series is divided into sections that contain one or more directories devoted to programs in a particular field. If you do not find a directory devoted to your field of interest in a specific volume, consult "Directories and Subject Areas" (located at the end of each volume). After you have identified the correct volume, consult the "Directories and Subject Areas in This Book" index, which shows (as does the more general directory) what directories cover subjects not specifically named in a directory or section title.

Each of the specialized volumes in the series has a number of general directories. These directories have entries for the largest unit at an institution granting graduate degrees in that field. For example, the general Engineering and Applied Sciences directory in the ***Graduate Programs in Engineering & Applied Sciences*** volume consists of **Profiles** for colleges, schools, and departments of engineering and applied sciences.

General directories are followed by other directories, or sections, that give more detailed information about programs in particular areas of the general field that has been covered. The general Engineering and Applied Sciences directory, in the previous example, is followed by nineteen sections with directories in specific areas of engineering, such as Chemical Engineering, Industrial/Management Engineering, and Mechanical Engineering.

Because of the broad nature of many fields, any system of organization is bound to involve a certain amount of overlap. Environmental studies, for example, is a field whose various aspects are studied in several types of departments and schools. Readers interested in such studies will find information on relevant programs in the ***Graduate Programs in the Biological/Biomedical Sciences & Health-Related Professions*** volume under Ecology and Environmental Biology and Environmental and Occupational Health; in the ***Graduate Programs in the Physical Sciences, Mathematics, Agricultural Sciences, the Environment & Natural Resources*** volume under Environmental Management and Policy and Natural Resources; and in the ***Graduate Programs in Engineering & Applied Sciences*** volume under Energy Management and Policy and Environmental Engineering. To help you find all of the programs of interest to you, the introduction to each section within the specialized volumes includes, if applicable, a paragraph suggesting other sections and directories with information on related areas of study.

Directory of Institutions with Programs in the Biological/ Biomedical Sciences & Health-Related Medical Professions

This directory lists institutions in alphabetical order and includes beneath each name the academic fields in which each institution offers graduate programs. The degree level in each field is also indicated, provided that the institution has supplied that information in response to Peterson's Annual Survey of Graduate and Professional Institutions.

An M indicates that a master's degree program is offered; a D indicates that a doctoral degree program is offered; an O signifies that other advanced degrees (e.g., certificates or specialist degrees) are offered; and an * (asterisk) indicates that a **Close-Up** and/or **Display** is located in this volume. See the index, "Close-Ups and Displays," for the specific page number.

Profiles of Academic and Professional Programs in the Specialized Volumes

Each section of **Profiles** has a table of contents that lists the Program Directories, **Displays**, and **Close-Ups.** Program Directories consist of the **Profiles** of programs in the relevant fields, with **Displays** following if programs have chosen to include them. **Close-Ups,** which are more individualized statements, are also listed for those graduate schools or programs that have chosen to submit them.

The **Profiles** found in the 500 directories in the specialized volumes provide basic data about the graduate units in capsule form for quick reference. To make these directories as useful as possible, **Profiles** are generally listed for an institution's smallest academic unit within a subject area. In other words, if an institution has a College of Liberal Arts that administers many related programs, the **Profile** for the individual program (e.g., Program in History), not the entire College, appears in the directory.

There are some programs that do not fit into any current directory and are not given individual **Profiles**. The directory structure is reviewed annually in order to keep this number to a minimum and to accommodate major trends in graduate education.

The following outline describes the **Profile** information found in the guides and explains how best to use that information. Any item that does not apply to or was not provided by a graduate unit is omitted from its listing. The format of the **Profiles** is constant, making it easy to compare one institution with another and one program with another.

Identifying Information. The institution's name, in boldface type, is followed by a complete listing of the administrative structure for that field of study. (For example, University of Akron, Buchtel College of Arts and Sciences, Department of Theoretical and Applied Mathematics, Program in Mathematics.) The last unit listed is the one to which all information in the **Profile** pertains. The institution's city, state, and zip code follow.

Offerings. Each field of study offered by the unit is listed with all postbaccalaureate degrees awarded. Degrees that are not preceded by a specific concentration are awarded in the general field listed in the unit name. Frequently, fields of study are broken down into subspecializations, and those appear following the degrees awarded; for example, "Offerings in secondary education (M.Ed.), including English education, mathematics education, science education." Students enrolled in the M.Ed. program would be able to specialize in any of the three fields mentioned.

Professional Accreditation. Some **Profiles** indicate whether a program is professionally accredited. Because it is possible for a program to receive or lose professional accreditation at any time, students entering fields in which accreditation is important to a career should verify the status of programs by contacting either the chairperson or the appropriate accrediting association.

Jointly Offered Degrees. Explanatory statements concerning programs that are offered in cooperation with other institutions are included in the list of degrees offered. This occurs most commonly on a regional basis (for example, two state universities offering a cooperative Ph.D. in special education) or where the specialized nature of the institutions encourages joint efforts (a J.D./M.B.A. offered by a law school at an institution with no formal business programs and an institution with a business school but lacking a law school). Only programs that are truly cooperative are listed; those involving only limited course work at another institution are not. Interested students should contact the heads of such units for further information.

Part-Time and Evening/Weekend Programs. When information regarding the availability of part-time or evening/weekend study appears in the **Profile**, it means that students are able to earn a degree exclusively through such study.

Postbaccalaureate Distance Learning Degrees. A postbaccalaureate distance learning degree program signifies that course requirements can be fulfilled with minimal or no on-campus study.

Faculty. Figures on the number of faculty members actively involved with graduate students through teaching or research are separated into full- and part-time as well as men and women whenever the information has been supplied.

Students. Figures for the number of students enrolled in graduate and professional programs pertain to the semester of highest enrollment from the 2013–14 academic year. These figures are broken down into full- and part-time and men and women whenever the data have been supplied. Information on the number of matriculated students enrolled in the unit who are members of a minority group or are international students appears here. The average age of the matriculated students is followed by the number of applicants, the percentage accepted, and the number enrolled for fall 2013.

Degrees Awarded. The number of degrees awarded in the calendar year is listed. Many doctoral programs offer a terminal master's degree if students leave the program after completing only part of the requirements for a doctoral degree; that is indicated here. All degrees are classified into one of four types: master's, doctoral, first professional, and other advanced degrees. A unit may award one or several degrees at a given level; however, the data are only collected by type and may therefore represent several different degree programs.

Degree Requirements. The information in this section is also broken down by type of degree, and all information for a degree level pertains to all degrees of that type unless otherwise specified. Degree requirements are collected in a simplified form to provide some very basic information on the nature of the program and on foreign language, thesis or dissertation, comprehensive exam, and registration requirements. Many units also provide a short list of additional requirements, such as fieldwork or an internship. For complete information on graduation requirements, contact the graduate school or program directly.

Entrance Requirements. Entrance requirements are broken down into the four degree levels of master's, doctoral, first professional, and other advanced degrees. Within each level, information may be provided in two basic categories: entrance exams and other requirements. The entrance exams are identified by the standard acronyms used by the testing agencies, unless they are not well known. Other entrance requirements are quite varied, but they often contain an undergraduate or graduate grade point average (GPA). Unless otherwise stated, the GPA is calculated on a 4.0 scale and is listed as a minimum required for admission. Additional exam requirements/recommendations for international students may be listed here. Application deadlines for domestic and international students, the application fee, and whether electronic applications are accepted may be listed here. Note that the deadline should be used for reference only; these dates are subject to change, and students interested in applying should always contact the graduate unit directly about application procedures and deadlines.

Expenses. The typical cost of study for the 2013–14 academic year is given in two basic categories: tuition and fees. Cost of study may be quite complex at a graduate institution. There are often sliding scales for part-time study, a different cost for first-year students, and other variables that make it impossible to completely cover the cost of study for each graduate program. To provide the most usable information, figures are given for full-time study for a full year where available and for part-time study in terms of a per-unit rate (per credit, per semester hour, etc.). Occasionally, variances may be noted in tuition and fees for reasons such as the type of program, whether courses are taken during the day or evening, whether courses are at the master's or doctoral level, or other institution-specific reasons. Expenses are usually subject to change; for exact costs at any given time, contact your chosen schools and programs directly. Keep in mind that the tuition of Canadian institutions is usually given in Canadian dollars.

Financial Support. This section contains data on the number of awards administered by the institution and given to graduate students during the 2013–14 academic year. The first figure given represents the total number of students receiving financial support enrolled in that unit. If the unit has provided information on graduate appointments, these are broken down into three major categories: fellowships give money to graduate students to cover the cost of study and living expenses and are not based on a work obligation or research commitment, research assistantships provide stipends to graduate students for assistance in a formal research project with a faculty member, and teaching assistantships provide stipends to graduate students for teaching or for assisting faculty members in teaching undergraduate classes. Within each category, figures are given for the total number of awards, the average yearly amount per award, and whether full or partial tuition reimbursements are awarded. In addition to graduate appointments, the availability of several other financial aid sources is covered in this section. Tuition waivers are routinely part of a graduate appointment, but units sometimes waive part or all of a student's tuition even if a graduate appointment is not available. Federal WorkStudy is made available to students who demonstrate need and meet the federal guidelines; this form of aid normally includes 10 or more hours of work per week in an office of the institution. Institutionally sponsored loans are low-interest loans available to graduate students to cover both educational and living expenses. Career-related internships or fieldwork offer money to students who are participating in a formal off-campus research project or practicum. Grants, scholarships, traineeships, unspecified assistantships, and other awards may also be noted. The availability of financial support to part-time students is also indicated here.

Some programs list the financial aid application deadline and the forms that need to be completed for students to be eligible for financial awards. There are two forms: FAFSA, the Free Application for Federal Student Aid, which is required for federal aid, and the CSS PROFILE®.

Faculty Research. Each unit has the opportunity to list several keyword phrases describing the current research involving faculty members and graduate students. Space limitations prevent the unit from listing complete information on all research programs. The total expenditure for funded research from the previous academic year may also be included.

Unit Head and Application Contact. The head of the graduate program for each unit may be listed with academic title, phone and fax numbers, and e-mail address. In addition to the unit head's contact information, many graduate programs also list a separate contact for application and admission information, followed by the graduate school, program, or department's website. If no unit head or application contact is given, you should contact the overall institution for information on graduate admissions.

Displays and Close-Ups

The **Displays** and **Close-Ups** are supplementary insertions submitted by deans, chairs, and other administrators who wish to offer an additional, more individualized statement to readers. A number of graduate school and program administrators have attached a **Display** ad near the **Profile** listing. Here you will find information that an institution or program wants to emphasize. The **Close-Ups** are by their very nature more expansive and flexible than the **Profiles**, and the administrators who have written them may emphasize different aspects of their programs. All of the **Close-Ups** are organized in the same way (with the exception of a few that describe research and training opportunities instead of degree programs), and in each one you will find information on the same basic topics, such as programs of study, research facilities, tuition and fees, financial aid, and application procedures. If an institution or program has submitted a **Close-Up**, a boldface cross-reference appears below its **Profile**. As with the **Displays**, all of the **Close-Ups** in the guides have been submitted by choice; the absence of a **Display** or **Close-Up** does not reflect any type of editorial judgment on the part of Peterson's, and their presence in the guides should not be taken as an indication of status, quality, or approval. Statements regarding a university's objectives and accomplishments are a reflection of its own beliefs and are not the opinions of the Peterson's editors.

Appendixes

This section contains two appendixes. The first, "Institutional Changes Since the 2014 Edition," lists institutions that have closed, merged, or changed their name or status since the last edition of the guides. The second, "Abbreviations Used in the Guides," gives abbreviations of degree names, along with what those abbreviations stand for. These appendixes are identical in all six volumes of ***Peterson's Graduate and Professional Programs***.

Indexes

There are three indexes presented here. The first index, "Close-Ups and Displays," gives page references for all programs that have chosen to place **Close-Ups** and **Displays** in this volume. It is arranged alphabetically by institution; within institutions, the arrangement is alphabetical by subject area. It is not an index to all programs in the book's directories of **Profiles**; readers must refer to the directories themselves for **Profile** information on programs that have not submitted the additional, more individualized statements. The second index, "Directories and Subject Areas in Other Books in This Series", gives book references for the directories in the specialized volumes and also includes cross-references for subject area names not used in the directory structure, for example, "Computing Technology (see Computer Science)." The third index, "Directories and Subject Areas in This Book," gives page references for the directories in this volume and cross-references for subject area names not used in this volume's directory structure.

Data Collection Procedures

The information published in the directories and **Profiles** of all the books is collected through Peterson's Annual Survey of Graduate and Professional Institutions. The survey is sent each spring to nearly 2,400 institutions offering postbaccalaureate degree programs, including accredited institutions in the United States, U.S. territories, and Canada and those institutions outside the United States that are accredited by U.S. accrediting bodies. Deans and other administrators complete these surveys, providing information on programs in the 500 academic and professional fields covered in the guides as well as overall institutional information. While every effort has been made to ensure the accuracy and completeness of the data, information is sometimes unavailable or changes occur after publication deadlines. All usable information received in time for publication has been included. The omission of any particular item from a directory or **Profile** signifies either that the item is not applicable to the institution or program or that information was not available. **Profiles** of programs scheduled to begin during the 2014–15 academic year cannot, obviously, include statistics on enrollment or, in many cases, the number of faculty members. If no usable data were submitted by an institution, its name, address, and program name appear in order to indicate the availability of graduate work.

Criteria for Inclusion in This Guide

To be included in this guide, an institution must have full accreditation or be a candidate for accreditation (preaccreditation) status by an institutional or specialized accrediting body recognized by the U.S. Department of Education or the Council for Higher Education Accreditation (CHEA). Institutional accrediting bodies, which review each institution as a whole, include the six regional associations of schools and colleges (Middle States, New England, North Central, Northwest, Southern, and Western), each of which is responsible for a specified portion of the United States and its territories. Other institutional accrediting bodies are national in scope and accredit specific kinds of institutions (e.g., Bible colleges, independent colleges, and rabbinical and Talmudic schools). Program registration by the New York State Board of Regents is considered to be the equivalent of institutional accreditation, since the board requires that all programs offered by an institution meet its standards before recognition is granted. A Canadian institution must be chartered and authorized to grant degrees by the provincial government, affiliated with a chartered institution, or accredited by a recognized U.S. accrediting body. This guide also includes institutions outside the United States that are accredited by these U.S. accrediting bodies. There are recognized specialized or professional accrediting bodies in more than fifty different fields, each of which is authorized to accredit institutions or specific programs in its particular field. For specialized institutions that offer programs in one field only, we designate this to be the equivalent of institutional accreditation. A full explanation of the accrediting process and complete information on recognized institutional (regional and national) and specialized accrediting bodies can be found online at www.chea.org or at www.ed.gov/admins/finaid/accred/index.html.

DIRECTORY OF INSTITUTIONS WITH PROGRAMS IN THE BIOLOGICAL/ BIOMEDICAL SCIENCES & HEALTH-RELATED MEDICAL PROFESSIONS

ABILENE CHRISTIAN UNIVERSITY
Communication Disorders M
Family Nurse Practitioner Studies M,O
Nursing and Healthcare Administration M,O
Nursing Education M,O
Nursing—General M,O

ACADEMY FOR FIVE ELEMENT ACUPUNCTURE
Acupuncture and Oriental Medicine M

ACADEMY OF CHINESE CULTURE AND HEALTH SCIENCES
Acupuncture and Oriental Medicine M

ACADIA UNIVERSITY
Biological and Biomedical Sciences—General M

ACUPUNCTURE & INTEGRATIVE MEDICINE COLLEGE, BERKELEY
Acupuncture and Oriental Medicine M

ACUPUNCTURE AND MASSAGE COLLEGE
Acupuncture and Oriental Medicine M

ADELPHI UNIVERSITY
Adult Nursing M
Biological and Biomedical Sciences—General M*
Communication Disorders M,D
Community Health M,O
Gerontological Nursing M
Nursing and Healthcare Administration M,O
Nursing Education M,O
Nursing—General D*
Nutrition M,D,O
Public Health—General M,O

ADLER SCHOOL OF PROFESSIONAL PSYCHOLOGY
Biopsychology M,D,O

ADVENTIST UNIVERSITY OF HEALTH SCIENCES
Nurse Anesthesia M

ALABAMA AGRICULTURAL AND MECHANICAL UNIVERSITY
Biological and Biomedical Sciences—General M
Communication Disorders M

ALABAMA STATE UNIVERSITY
Allied Health—General M,D
Biological and Biomedical Sciences—General M,D
Occupational Therapy M
Physical Therapy D
Rehabilitation Sciences M

ALASKA PACIFIC UNIVERSITY
Health Services Management and Hospital Administration M

ALBANY COLLEGE OF PHARMACY AND HEALTH SCIENCES
Cell Biology M
Clinical Laboratory Sciences/Medical Technology M
Health Services Research M,D
Molecular Biology M
Pharmaceutical Sciences M,D
Pharmacology M,D
Pharmacy M,D

ALBANY MEDICAL COLLEGE
Allopathic Medicine D
Bioethics M,D,O
Cardiovascular Sciences M,D
Cell Biology M,D
Immunology M,D
Microbiology M,D
Molecular Biology M,D
Neuroscience M,D
Nurse Anesthesia M
Pharmacology M,D
Physician Assistant Studies M

ALBANY STATE UNIVERSITY
Family Nurse Practitioner Studies M
Health Services Management and Hospital Administration M
Nursing Education M
Nursing—General M

ALBERT EINSTEIN COLLEGE OF MEDICINE
Allopathic Medicine D
Anatomy D
Biochemistry D
Biological and Biomedical Sciences—General D
Biophysics D
Cell Biology D
Clinical Research D
Computational Biology D
Developmental Biology D
Genetics D
Genomic Sciences D
Immunology D
Microbiology D
Molecular Biology D
Molecular Genetics D
Molecular Pharmacology D
Neurobiology D
Pathology D
Physiology D
Systems Biology D

ALCORN STATE UNIVERSITY
Biological and Biomedical Sciences—General M
Nursing—General M

ALDERSON BROADDUS UNIVERSITY
Physician Assistant Studies M

ALLEN COLLEGE
Acute Care/Critical Care Nursing M,D,O
Adult Nursing M,D,O
Community Health Nursing M,D,O
Family Nurse Practitioner Studies M,D,O
Gerontological Nursing M,D,O
Nursing and Healthcare Administration M,D,O
Nursing—General M,D,O
Psychiatric Nursing M,D,O
Public Health—General M,D,O

ALLIANT INTERNATIONAL UNIVERSITY–SAN DIEGO
Neuroscience M,D,O

ALLIANT INTERNATIONAL UNIVERSITY–SAN FRANCISCO
Pharmacology M

ALVERNIA UNIVERSITY
Occupational Therapy M

ALVERNO COLLEGE
Family Nurse Practitioner Studies M
Nursing Education M
Nursing—General M
Psychiatric Nursing M

AMERICAN COLLEGE OF ACUPUNCTURE AND ORIENTAL MEDICINE
Acupuncture and Oriental Medicine M

AMERICAN COLLEGE OF HEALTHCARE SCIENCES
Allied Health—General M,O
Nutrition M,O

AMERICAN COLLEGE OF TRADITIONAL CHINESE MEDICINE
Acupuncture and Oriental Medicine M,D,O

AMERICAN INTERCONTINENTAL UNIVERSITY ONLINE
Health Services Management and Hospital Administration M

AMERICAN INTERNATIONAL COLLEGE
Nursing and Healthcare Administration M
Nursing Education M
Nursing—General M
Occupational Therapy M
Physical Therapy D

AMERICAN MUSEUM OF NATURAL HISTORY–RICHARD GILDER GRADUATE SCHOOL
Biological and Biomedical Sciences—General D*

AMERICAN PUBLIC UNIVERSITY SYSTEM
Health Services Management and Hospital Administration M
Public Health—General M

AMERICAN SENTINEL UNIVERSITY
Health Services Management and Hospital Administration M
Nursing—General M

AMERICAN UNIVERSITY
Biological and Biomedical Sciences—General M,D,O
Biopsychology M,D,O
Health Promotion M,D,O
Neuroscience M,D,O
Nutrition M,D,O

AMERICAN UNIVERSITY OF ARMENIA
Public Health—General M

AMERICAN UNIVERSITY OF BEIRUT
Adult Nursing M
Allopathic Medicine M,D
Anatomy M,D
Biochemistry M,D
Biological and Biomedical Sciences—General M,D
Cell Biology M,D
Community Health Nursing M
Community Health M
Environmental and Occupational Health M
Epidemiology M
Genetics M,D
Health Promotion M
Health Services Management and Hospital Administration M
Immunology M,D
Microbiology M,D
Molecular Biology M,D
Neuroscience M,D
Nursing and Healthcare Administration M
Nursing—General M
Nutrition M
Pharmacology M,D
Psychiatric Nursing M
Public Health—General M
Toxicology M,D

AMERICAN UNIVERSITY OF HEALTH SCIENCES
Clinical Research M

ANDREWS UNIVERSITY
Allied Health—General M
Biological and Biomedical Sciences—General M
Nursing—General M
Nutrition M
Physical Therapy D

ANGELO STATE UNIVERSITY
Adult Nursing M
Biological and Biomedical Sciences—General M
Medical/Surgical Nursing M
Nursing Education M
Physical Therapy D

ANNA MARIA COLLEGE
Environmental and Occupational Health M

ANTIOCH UNIVERSITY NEW ENGLAND
Conservation Biology M

AOMA GRADUATE SCHOOL OF INTEGRATIVE MEDICINE
Acupuncture and Oriental Medicine M,D

APPALACHIAN COLLEGE OF PHARMACY
Pharmacy D

APPALACHIAN STATE UNIVERSITY
Biological and Biomedical Sciences—General M
Cell Biology M
Communication Disorders M
Molecular Biology M
Nutrition M
Rehabilitation Sciences M

AQUINAS COLLEGE
Health Services Management and Hospital Administration M

AQUINAS INSTITUTE OF THEOLOGY
Health Services Management and Hospital Administration M,D,O

ARCADIA UNIVERSITY
Community Health M
Physical Therapy D
Physician Assistant Studies M

ARGOSY UNIVERSITY, ATLANTA
Biopsychology M,D,O
Health Services Management and Hospital Administration M,D
Public Health—General M

ARGOSY UNIVERSITY, CHICAGO
Health Services Management and Hospital Administration M,D
Neuroscience D
Public Health—General M

ARGOSY UNIVERSITY, DALLAS
Health Services Management and Hospital Administration M,D,O
Public Health—General M

ARGOSY UNIVERSITY, DENVER
Health Services Management and Hospital Administration M,D
Public Health—General M

ARGOSY UNIVERSITY, HAWAI`I
Health Services Management and Hospital Administration M,D,O
Pharmacology M,O
Public Health—General M

ARGOSY UNIVERSITY, INLAND EMPIRE
Health Services Management and Hospital Administration M,D
Public Health—General M

ARGOSY UNIVERSITY, LOS ANGELES
Health Services Management and Hospital Administration M,D
Public Health—General M

ARGOSY UNIVERSITY, NASHVILLE
Health Services Management and Hospital Administration M,D
Public Health—General M

ARGOSY UNIVERSITY, ORANGE COUNTY
Health Services Management and Hospital Administration M,D,O
Public Health—General M

ARGOSY UNIVERSITY, PHOENIX
Health Services Management and Hospital Administration M,D
Neuroscience M,D
Public Health—General M

ARGOSY UNIVERSITY, SALT LAKE CITY
Health Services Management and Hospital Administration M,D
Public Health—General M

ARGOSY UNIVERSITY, SAN DIEGO
Public Health—General M

ARGOSY UNIVERSITY, SAN FRANCISCO BAY AREA
Health Services Management and Hospital Administration M,D
Public Health—General M

ARGOSY UNIVERSITY, SARASOTA
Health Services Management and Hospital Administration M,D,O
Public Health—General M

ARGOSY UNIVERSITY, SCHAUMBURG
Health Services Management and Hospital Administration M,D,O
Neuroscience M,D,O
Public Health—General M

ARGOSY UNIVERSITY, SEATTLE
Health Services Management and Hospital Administration M,D
Public Health—General M

ARGOSY UNIVERSITY, TAMPA
Health Services Management and Hospital Administration M,D
Neuroscience M,D
Public Health—General M

ARGOSY UNIVERSITY, TWIN CITIES
Biopsychology M,D,O
Health Services Management and Hospital Administration M,D
Public Health—General M

ARGOSY UNIVERSITY, WASHINGTON DC
Health Services Management and Hospital Administration M,D,O
Public Health—General M

ARIZONA SCHOOL OF ACUPUNCTURE AND ORIENTAL MEDICINE
Acupuncture and Oriental Medicine M

ARIZONA STATE UNIVERSITY AT THE TEMPE CAMPUS
Animal Behavior M,D
Biochemistry M,D
Biological and Biomedical Sciences—General M,D
Cell Biology M,D
Communication Disorders M,D
Community Health Nursing M,D,O
Community Health M,D,O
Computational Biology M,D
Evolutionary Biology M,D
Family Nurse Practitioner Studies M,D,O
International Health M,D,O
Microbiology M,D
Molecular Biology M,D
Neuroscience M,D
Nursing and Healthcare Administration M,D,O
Nursing—General M,D,O
Nutrition M,D,O
Psychiatric Nursing M,D,O
Public Health—General M,D,O

ARKANSAS STATE UNIVERSITY
Biological and Biomedical Sciences—General M,O
Communication Disorders M
Health Services Management and Hospital Administration M,D,O
Molecular Biology D
Nurse Anesthesia M,D,O
Nursing—General M,D,O
Physical Therapy D

ARKANSAS TECH UNIVERSITY
Nursing—General M

ARMSTRONG STATE UNIVERSITY
Acute Care/Critical Care Nursing M
Adult Nursing M
Communication Disorders M
Gerontological Nursing M
Health Services Management and Hospital Administration M,O
Nursing—General M
Physical Therapy D
Public Health—General M

ASHWORTH COLLEGE
Health Services Management and Hospital Administration M

ATHABASCA UNIVERSITY
Allied Health—General M,O
Nursing and Healthcare Administration M,O
Nursing—General M,O

ATLANTIC INSTITUTE OF ORIENTAL MEDICINE
Acupuncture and Oriental Medicine M

A.T. STILL UNIVERSITY
Allied Health—General M,D
Biological and Biomedical Sciences—General M,D
Communication Disorders M,D
Dentistry D
Health Services Management and Hospital Administration M,D
Occupational Therapy M,D
Oral and Dental Sciences M,D,O
Osteopathic Medicine M,D
Physical Therapy M,D
Physician Assistant Studies M,D
Public Health—General M,D

AUBURN UNIVERSITY
Anatomy M,D
Biochemistry M,D
Biological and Biomedical Sciences—General M,D
Botany M,D
Cell Biology M,D
Communication Disorders M,D
Entomology M,D
Health Promotion M,D,O
Microbiology M,D
Molecular Biology M,D
Nursing Education M
Nursing—General M
Nutrition M,D,O
Pathobiology M,D
Pharmaceutical Sciences M,D
Pharmacology M,D
Pharmacy D
Plant Pathology M,D
Radiation Biology M,D
Veterinary Medicine D
Veterinary Sciences M,D
Zoology M,D

AUBURN UNIVERSITY AT MONTGOMERY
Health Services Management and Hospital Administration M,D,O
Public Health—General M,D,O

AUGSBURG COLLEGE
- Community Health Nursing M
- Nursing—General M
- Physician Assistant Studies M
- Transcultural Nursing M

AURORA UNIVERSITY
- Nursing—General M,D

AUSTIN PEAY STATE UNIVERSITY
- Biological and Biomedical Sciences—General M
- Clinical Laboratory Sciences/Medical Technology M
- Community Health M
- Nursing and Healthcare Administration M
- Nursing Education M
- Nursing Informatics M
- Nursing—General M
- Public Health—General M
- Radiation Biology M

AVILA UNIVERSITY
- Health Services Management and Hospital Administration M

AZUSA PACIFIC UNIVERSITY
- Nursing Education M,D
- Nursing—General M,D
- Physical Therapy D

BAKER COLLEGE CENTER FOR GRADUATE STUDIES - ONLINE
- Health Services Management and Hospital Administration M,D

BALDWIN WALLACE UNIVERSITY
- Health Services Management and Hospital Administration M
- Physician Assistant Studies M

BALL STATE UNIVERSITY
- Biological and Biomedical Sciences—General M,D
- Communication Disorders M,D
- Health Promotion M
- Nursing—General M,D
- Physiology M

BANK STREET COLLEGE OF EDUCATION
- Maternal and Child Health M

BARRY UNIVERSITY
- Acute Care/Critical Care Nursing M,O
- Anatomy M
- Biological and Biomedical Sciences—General M
- Communication Disorders M
- Family Nurse Practitioner Studies M,O
- Health Services Management and Hospital Administration M,O
- Nurse Anesthesia M
- Nursing and Healthcare Administration M,D,O
- Nursing Education M,O
- Nursing—General M,D,O
- Occupational Therapy M
- Physician Assistant Studies M
- Podiatric Medicine D
- Public Health—General

BARUCH COLLEGE OF THE CITY UNIVERSITY OF NEW YORK
- Health Services Management and Hospital Administration M

BASTYR UNIVERSITY
- Acupuncture and Oriental Medicine M,D,O
- Naturopathic Medicine D
- Nurse Midwifery M,O
- Nutrition M,O

BAYLOR COLLEGE OF MEDICINE
- Allopathic Medicine D
- Biochemistry D
- Biological and Biomedical Sciences—General M,D
- Biophysics D
- Cancer Biology/Oncology D
- Cardiovascular Sciences D
- Cell Biology D
- Clinical Laboratory Sciences/Medical Technology M,D
- Computational Biology D
- Developmental Biology D
- Genetics D
- Human Genetics D
- Immunology D
- Microbiology D
- Molecular Biology D
- Molecular Biophysics D
- Molecular Medicine D
- Molecular Physiology D
- Neuroscience D
- Nurse Anesthesia D
- Pathology D
- Pharmacology D
- Physician Assistant Studies M
- Structural Biology D
- Translational Biology D
- Virology D

BAYLOR UNIVERSITY
- Allied Health—General M,D
- Biological and Biomedical Sciences—General M,D
- Communication Disorders M
- Community Health M,D
- Ecology D
- Emergency Medical Services D
- Environmental Biology M,D
- Family Nurse Practitioner Studies M,D
- Health Promotion M,D
- Health Services Management and Hospital Administration M
- Maternal and Child/Neonatal Nursing M,D
- Nurse Midwifery M,D
- Nursing—General M,D
- Nutrition M
- Physical Therapy D

BAY PATH COLLEGE
- Occupational Therapy M
- Physician Assistant Studies M

BELHAVEN UNIVERSITY (MS)
- Health Services Management and Hospital Administration M

BELLARMINE UNIVERSITY
- Family Nurse Practitioner Studies M,D
- Nursing and Healthcare Administration M,D
- Nursing Education M,D
- Nursing—General M,D
- Physical Therapy M,D

BELLEVUE UNIVERSITY
- Health Services Management and Hospital Administration M

BELLIN COLLEGE
- Family Nurse Practitioner Studies M
- Nursing Education M
- Nursing—General M

BELMONT UNIVERSITY
- Allied Health—General M,D
- Health Services Management and Hospital Administration M
- Nursing—General M,D
- Occupational Therapy M,D
- Pharmacy D
- Physical Therapy M,D

BEMIDJI STATE UNIVERSITY
- Biological and Biomedical Sciences—General M

BENEDICTINE UNIVERSITY
- Health Promotion M
- Health Services Management and Hospital Administration M
- Nursing—General M
- Nutrition M
- Public Health—General M

BENEDICTINE UNIVERSITY AT SPRINGFIELD
- Health Services Management and Hospital Administration M

BENNINGTON COLLEGE
- Allied Health—General O

BETHEL COLLEGE
- Nursing—General M

BETHEL UNIVERSITY (MN)
- Nurse Midwifery M,D,O
- Nursing and Healthcare Administration M,D,O
- Nursing Education M,D,O
- Nursing—General M,D,O
- Physician Assistant Studies M,D,O

BETHEL UNIVERSITY (TN)
- Physician Assistant Studies M

BINGHAMTON UNIVERSITY, STATE UNIVERSITY OF NEW YORK
- Biological and Biomedical Sciences—General M,D
- Biopsychology D
- Health Services Management and Hospital Administration M,D
- Nursing—General M,D,O

BLACK HILLS STATE UNIVERSITY
- Genomic Sciences M

BLESSING-RIEMAN COLLEGE OF NURSING
- Nursing—General M

BLOOMSBURG UNIVERSITY OF PENNSYLVANIA
- Adult Nursing M
- Biological and Biomedical Sciences—General M
- Communication Disorders M,D
- Community Health M
- Family Nurse Practitioner Studies M
- Nurse Anesthesia M
- Nursing and Healthcare Administration M
- Nursing—General M

BOISE STATE UNIVERSITY
- Biological and Biomedical Sciences—General M
- Environmental and Occupational Health M
- Health Promotion M
- Health Services Management and Hospital Administration M
- Health Services Research M
- Molecular Biology M,D
- Nursing—General M,O
- Public Health—General M,O

BOSTON COLLEGE
- Adult Nursing M,D
- Biochemistry M,D
- Biological and Biomedical Sciences—General D*
- Community Health Nursing M,D
- Forensic Nursing M,D
- Gerontological Nursing M,D
- Maternal and Child/Neonatal Nursing M,D
- Medical/Surgical Nursing M,D
- Nurse Anesthesia M,D
- Nursing—General M,D
- Pediatric Nursing M,D
- Psychiatric Nursing M,D

BOSTON UNIVERSITY
- Allied Health—General M,D
- Allopathic Medicine D
- Anatomy M,D
- Biochemistry M,D
- Bioethics M
- Biological and Biomedical Sciences—General M,D
- Biophysics M,D
- Biopsychology M
- Cell Biology M,D
- Clinical Research M
- Communication Disorders M,D
- Dental Hygiene M,D,O
- Dentistry M,D,O
- Environmental and Occupational Health M,D
- Epidemiology M,D
- Genetics D
- Genomic Sciences D
- Health Promotion D
- Health Services Management and Hospital Administration M,D
- Immunology D
- International Health M,D
- Maternal and Child Health M,D
- Medical Imaging M
- Molecular Biology M,D
- Molecular Medicine D
- Neurobiology M,D
- Neuroscience D
- Nutrition M,D
- Occupational Therapy M,D
- Oral and Dental Sciences M,D,O
- Pathology D
- Pharmaceutical Sciences M,D
- Pharmacology M,D
- Physical Therapy D
- Physician Assistant Studies M
- Physiology M,D
- Public Health—General M,D,O
- Rehabilitation Sciences M,D

BOWIE STATE UNIVERSITY
- Family Nurse Practitioner Studies M
- Nursing and Healthcare Administration M
- Nursing Education M
- Nursing—General M

BOWLING GREEN STATE UNIVERSITY
- Biological and Biomedical Sciences—General M,D
- Communication Disorders M,D
- Nutrition M
- Public Health—General M

BRADLEY UNIVERSITY
- Biological and Biomedical Sciences—General M
- Nurse Anesthesia M
- Nursing and Healthcare Administration M
- Nursing—General M
- Physical Therapy D

BRANDEIS UNIVERSITY
- Biochemistry D
- Biological and Biomedical Sciences—General M,D,O
- Biophysics D
- Cell Biology M,D
- Genetics M,D
- Health Services Management and Hospital Administration M
- International Health M,D
- Microbiology M,D
- Molecular Biology M,D
- Neurobiology M,D
- Neuroscience M,D

BRANDMAN UNIVERSITY
- Health Services Management and Hospital Administration M

BRENAU UNIVERSITY
- Family Nurse Practitioner Studies M
- Health Services Management and Hospital Administration M
- Nursing and Healthcare Administration M
- Nursing Education M
- Occupational Therapy M

BRIAR CLIFF UNIVERSITY
- Nursing—General M

BRIDGEWATER STATE UNIVERSITY
- Health Promotion M

BRIGHAM YOUNG UNIVERSITY
- Biochemistry M,D
- Biological and Biomedical Sciences—General M,D
- Communication Disorders M
- Developmental Biology M,D
- Family Nurse Practitioner Studies M
- Health Promotion M,D
- Microbiology M,D
- Molecular Biology M,D
- Neuroscience M,D
- Nursing—General M
- Nutrition M
- Physiology M,D

BROADVIEW UNIVERSITY–WEST JORDAN
- Health Services Management and Hospital Administration M

BROCK UNIVERSITY
- Allied Health—General M,D
- Biological and Biomedical Sciences—General M,D
- Neuroscience M,D

BROOKLYN COLLEGE OF THE CITY UNIVERSITY OF NEW YORK
- Biological and Biomedical Sciences—General M
- Communication Disorders M,D
- Community Health M
- Health Services Management and Hospital Administration M
- Nutrition M
- Public Health—General M

BROWN UNIVERSITY
- Allopathic Medicine D
- Biochemistry M,D
- Biological and Biomedical Sciences—General M,D
- Cell Biology M,D
- Community Health M,D
- Ecology D
- Epidemiology M,D
- Evolutionary Biology D
- Health Services Research D
- Molecular Biology M,D
- Molecular Pharmacology M,D
- Neuroscience D
- Pathobiology M,D
- Physiology M,D
- Public Health—General M

BRYAN COLLEGE OF HEALTH SCIENCES
- Nurse Anesthesia M

BUCKNELL UNIVERSITY
- Animal Behavior M
- Biological and Biomedical Sciences—General M

BUFFALO STATE COLLEGE, STATE UNIVERSITY OF NEW YORK
- Biological and Biomedical Sciences—General M
- Communication Disorders M

BUTLER UNIVERSITY
- Pharmaceutical Sciences M,D
- Pharmacy M,D
- Physician Assistant Studies M,D

CALIFORNIA BAPTIST UNIVERSITY
- Adult Nursing M
- Family Nurse Practitioner Studies M
- Health Promotion M
- Health Services Management and Hospital Administration M
- Nursing Education M
- Nursing—General M
- Nutrition M
- Public Health—General M

CALIFORNIA COAST UNIVERSITY
- Health Services Management and Hospital Administration M

CALIFORNIA INSTITUTE OF INTEGRAL STUDIES
- Ecology M,D

CALIFORNIA INSTITUTE OF TECHNOLOGY
- Biochemistry M,D
- Biological and Biomedical Sciences—General D
- Biophysics D
- Cell Biology D
- Developmental Biology D
- Genetics D
- Immunology D
- Molecular Biology D
- Molecular Biophysics M,D
- Neurobiology D
- Neuroscience M,D

CALIFORNIA INTERCONTINENTAL UNIVERSITY
- Health Services Management and Hospital Administration M,D

CALIFORNIA POLYTECHNIC STATE UNIVERSITY, SAN LUIS OBISPO
- Biochemistry M
- Biological and Biomedical Sciences—General M

CALIFORNIA SCHOOL OF PODIATRIC MEDICINE AT SAMUEL MERRITT UNIVERSITY
- Podiatric Medicine D

CALIFORNIA STATE POLYTECHNIC UNIVERSITY, POMONA
- Biological and Biomedical Sciences—General M

CALIFORNIA STATE UNIVERSITY, BAKERSFIELD
- Biological and Biomedical Sciences—General M
- Health Services Management and Hospital Administration M

CALIFORNIA STATE UNIVERSITY, CHICO
- Biological and Biomedical Sciences—General M

*M—masters degree; D—doctorate; O—other advanced degree; *—Close-Up and/or Display*

Program	Degrees
Botany	M
Communication Disorders	M
Health Services Management and Hospital Administration	M
Nursing—General	M
Nutrition	M

CALIFORNIA STATE UNIVERSITY, DOMINGUEZ HILLS

Program	Degrees
Biological and Biomedical Sciences—General	M
Nursing—General	M
Occupational Therapy	M

CALIFORNIA STATE UNIVERSITY, EAST BAY

Program	Degrees
Biochemistry	M
Biological and Biomedical Sciences—General	M
Communication Disorders	M
Health Services Management and Hospital Administration	M

CALIFORNIA STATE UNIVERSITY, FRESNO

Program	Degrees
Biological and Biomedical Sciences—General	M
Communication Disorders	M
Family Nurse Practitioner Studies	M
Health Promotion	M
Health Services Management and Hospital Administration	M
Nursing Education	M
Nursing—General	M
Physical Therapy	M,D
Public Health—General	M

CALIFORNIA STATE UNIVERSITY, FULLERTON

Program	Degrees
Biological and Biomedical Sciences—General	M
Communication Disorders	M
Nurse Anesthesia	M,D
Nursing and Healthcare Administration	M,D
Nursing Education	M,D
Nursing—General	M,D
Public Health—General	M
Women's Health Nursing	M,D

CALIFORNIA STATE UNIVERSITY, LONG BEACH

Program	Degrees
Biochemistry	M
Biological and Biomedical Sciences—General	M
Communication Disorders	M
Health Services Management and Hospital Administration	M
Microbiology	M
Nursing—General	M,D
Nutrition	M
Physical Therapy	D

CALIFORNIA STATE UNIVERSITY, LOS ANGELES

Program	Degrees
Biochemistry	M
Biological and Biomedical Sciences—General	M
Communication Disorders	M
Health Services Management and Hospital Administration	M
Nursing—General	M
Nutrition	M

CALIFORNIA STATE UNIVERSITY, NORTHRIDGE

Program	Degrees
Biochemistry	M
Biological and Biomedical Sciences—General	M
Communication Disorders	M
Environmental and Occupational Health	M
Health Services Management and Hospital Administration	M
Industrial Hygiene	M
Physical Therapy	M
Public Health—General	M

CALIFORNIA STATE UNIVERSITY, SACRAMENTO

Program	Degrees
Biological and Biomedical Sciences—General	M
Cell Biology	M
Communication Disorders	M
Conservation Biology	M
Developmental Biology	M
Molecular Biology	M
Nursing—General	M

CALIFORNIA STATE UNIVERSITY, SAN BERNARDINO

Program	Degrees
Biological and Biomedical Sciences—General	M
Health Services Management and Hospital Administration	M
Nursing—General	M
Public Health—General	M

CALIFORNIA STATE UNIVERSITY, SAN MARCOS

Program	Degrees
Biological and Biomedical Sciences—General	M

CALIFORNIA STATE UNIVERSITY, STANISLAUS

Program	Degrees
Conservation Biology	M
Ecology	M
Gerontological Nursing	M
Nursing Education	M
Nursing—General	M

CALIFORNIA UNIVERSITY OF PENNSYLVANIA

Program	Degrees
Communication Disorders	M
Rehabilitation Sciences	M

CAMBRIDGE COLLEGE

Program	Degrees
Health Services Management and Hospital Administration	M
School Nursing	M,D,O

CAMPBELL UNIVERSITY

Program	Degrees
Pharmaceutical Sciences	M,D
Pharmacy	M,D

CANADIAN COLLEGE OF NATUROPATHIC MEDICINE

Program	Degrees
Naturopathic Medicine	O*

CANADIAN MEMORIAL CHIROPRACTIC COLLEGE

Program	Degrees
Acupuncture and Oriental Medicine	O
Chiropractic	D,O

CANISIUS COLLEGE

Program	Degrees
Allied Health—General	M,O
Communication Disorders	M,O
Community Health	M,O
Nutrition	M,O
Zoology	M

CAPELLA UNIVERSITY

Program	Degrees
Environmental and Occupational Health	M,D
Epidemiology	D
Gerontological Nursing	M
Health Services Management and Hospital Administration	M,D
Nursing and Healthcare Administration	M
Nursing Education	M,D
Nursing—General	M,D

CAPITAL UNIVERSITY

Program	Degrees
Nursing and Healthcare Administration	M
Nursing—General	M

CARDINAL STRITCH UNIVERSITY

Program	Degrees
Nursing—General	M

CARIBBEAN UNIVERSITY

Program	Degrees
Gerontological Nursing	M,D
Pediatric Nursing	M,D

CARLETON UNIVERSITY

Program	Degrees
Biological and Biomedical Sciences—General	M,D
Neuroscience	M,D

CARLOS ALBIZU UNIVERSITY

Program	Degrees
Communication Disorders	M,D

CARLOW UNIVERSITY

Program	Degrees
Family Nurse Practitioner Studies	M,O
Health Services Management and Hospital Administration	M
Nursing and Healthcare Administration	M
Nursing Education	M
Nursing—General	D

CARNEGIE MELLON UNIVERSITY

Program	Degrees
Biochemistry	M,D
Biological and Biomedical Sciences—General	M,D
Biophysics	M,D
Biopsychology	D
Cell Biology	M,D
Computational Biology	M,D
Developmental Biology	M,D
Genetics	M,D
Health Services Management and Hospital Administration	M
Molecular Biology	M,D
Molecular Biophysics	D
Neurobiology	M,D
Neuroscience	D
Structural Biology	M,D

CARROLL UNIVERSITY

Program	Degrees
Physical Therapy	M,D
Physician Assistant Studies	M

CARSON-NEWMAN UNIVERSITY

Program	Degrees
Family Nurse Practitioner Studies	M
Nursing Education	M
Nursing—General	M

CASE WESTERN RESERVE UNIVERSITY

Program	Degrees
Acute Care/Critical Care Nursing	M,D
Allopathic Medicine	D
Anatomy	M
Anesthesiologist Assistant Studies	M
Biochemistry	M,D
Bioethics	M
Biological and Biomedical Sciences—General	M,D
Biophysics	M,D
Cancer Biology/Oncology	D
Cell Biology	M,D
Clinical Research	M
Communication Disorders	M,D
Dentistry	D
Epidemiology	M,D
Family Nurse Practitioner Studies	M,D
Genetics	D
Genomic Sciences	D
Gerontological Nursing	M,D
Health Services Research	M,D
Human Genetics	D
Immunology	M,D
Maternal and Child/Neonatal Nursing	M,D
Microbiology	D
Molecular Biology	D
Molecular Medicine	D
Molecular Physiology	M,D
Neurobiology	D
Neuroscience	D
Nurse Anesthesia	M
Nurse Midwifery	M,D
Nursing and Healthcare Administration	D
Nursing Education	M,D
Nursing—General	M,D
Nutrition	M,D
Oncology Nursing	M
Oral and Dental Sciences	M,O
Pathology	M,D
Pediatric Nursing	M,D
Pharmacology	D
Physiology	M,D
Psychiatric Nursing	M,D
Public Health—General	M
Virology	D
Women's Health Nursing	M,D

THE CATHOLIC UNIVERSITY OF AMERICA

Program	Degrees
Biological and Biomedical Sciences—General	M,D
Cell Biology	M,D
Clinical Laboratory Sciences/Medical Technology	M,D
Microbiology	M,D
Nursing—General	M,D,O

CEDAR CREST COLLEGE

Program	Degrees
Nursing and Healthcare Administration	M
Nursing Education	M
Nursing—General	M
Nutrition	O

CEDARS-SINAI MEDICAL CENTER

Program	Degrees
Biological and Biomedical Sciences—General	D
Translational Biology	D

CEDARVILLE UNIVERSITY

Program	Degrees
Family Nurse Practitioner Studies	M,D
International Health	M,D
Pharmacy	M,D

CENTRAL CONNECTICUT STATE UNIVERSITY

Program	Degrees
Biochemistry	O
Biological and Biomedical Sciences—General	M,O
Molecular Biology	M,O
Nurse Anesthesia	M,O

CENTRAL METHODIST UNIVERSITY

Program	Degrees
Nursing and Healthcare Administration	M
Nursing Education	M
Nursing—General	M

CENTRAL MICHIGAN UNIVERSITY

Program	Degrees
Biological and Biomedical Sciences—General	M
Communication Disorders	M,D
Conservation Biology	M
Health Services Management and Hospital Administration	M,D,O
International Health	M,D,O
Neuroscience	M,D
Nutrition	M,D,O
Physical Therapy	M,D
Physician Assistant Studies	M,D
Rehabilitation Sciences	M,D

CENTRAL WASHINGTON UNIVERSITY

Program	Degrees
Biological and Biomedical Sciences—General	M
Nutrition	M

CHAMPLAIN COLLEGE

Program	Degrees
Health Services Management and Hospital Administration	M

CHAPMAN UNIVERSITY

Program	Degrees
Communication Disorders	M,D,O
Nutrition	M
Physical Therapy	D
Physician Assistant Studies	M

CHARLES DREW UNIVERSITY OF MEDICINE AND SCIENCE

Program	Degrees
Allopathic Medicine	D
Public Health—General	M

CHATHAM UNIVERSITY

Program	Degrees
Biological and Biomedical Sciences—General	M
Environmental Biology	M
Nursing and Healthcare Administration	M,D
Nursing Education	M,D
Nursing—General	M,D
Occupational Therapy	M,D
Physical Therapy	D
Physician Assistant Studies	M

CHICAGO STATE UNIVERSITY

Program	Degrees
Biological and Biomedical Sciences—General	M
Nursing—General	M
Occupational Therapy	M
Pharmacy	D
Public Health—General	M

CHRISTIAN BROTHERS UNIVERSITY

Program	Degrees
Physician Assistant Studies	M

THE CITADEL, THE MILITARY COLLEGE OF SOUTH CAROLINA

Program	Degrees
Biological and Biomedical Sciences—General	M

CITY COLLEGE OF THE CITY UNIVERSITY OF NEW YORK

Program	Degrees
Biochemistry	M,D
Biological and Biomedical Sciences—General	M,D

CLAREMONT GRADUATE UNIVERSITY

Program	Degrees
Botany	M,D
Computational Biology	M,D
Health Promotion	M,D
Public Health—General	M,D

CLARION UNIVERSITY OF PENNSYLVANIA

Program	Degrees
Communication Disorders	M
Family Nurse Practitioner Studies	M,O
Nursing Education	M,O
Nursing—General	M
Rehabilitation Sciences	M

CLARK ATLANTA UNIVERSITY

Program	Degrees
Biological and Biomedical Sciences—General	M,D

CLARKE UNIVERSITY

Program	Degrees
Family Nurse Practitioner Studies	M,D,O
Nursing and Healthcare Administration	M,D,O
Nursing Education	M,D,O
Nursing—General	M,D,O
Physical Therapy	D

CLARKSON COLLEGE

Program	Degrees
Adult Nursing	M,O
Family Nurse Practitioner Studies	M,O
Nursing and Healthcare Administration	M,O
Nursing Education	M,O
Nursing—General	M,O

CLARKSON UNIVERSITY

Program	Degrees
Health Services Research	M
Physical Therapy	D
Physician Assistant Studies	M

CLARK UNIVERSITY

Program	Degrees
Biological and Biomedical Sciences—General	M,D

CLAYTON STATE UNIVERSITY

Program	Degrees
Health Services Management and Hospital Administration	M
Nursing—General	M

CLEARY UNIVERSITY

Program	Degrees
Health Services Management and Hospital Administration	M,O

CLEMSON UNIVERSITY

Program	Degrees
Biochemistry	D
Biological and Biomedical Sciences—General	M,D
Biophysics	M,D
Community Health	M
Ecology	M,D
Entomology	M,D
Environmental and Occupational Health	M
Evolutionary Biology	M,D
Genetics	M,D
Microbiology	M,D
Molecular Biology	D
Nursing—General	M,D
Nutrition	M
Plant Biology	M,D
Veterinary Sciences	M,D

CLEVELAND STATE UNIVERSITY

Program	Degrees
Allied Health—General	M
Bioethics	M,O
Biological and Biomedical Sciences—General	M,D
Communication Disorders	M
Community Health Nursing	M,D
Forensic Nursing	M,D
Health Services Management and Hospital Administration	M,O
Medical Imaging	M
Medical Physics	M
Medicinal and Pharmaceutical Chemistry	M,D
Molecular Medicine	M,D
Nursing Education	M,D
Nursing—General	M,D
Occupational Therapy	M
Physical Therapy	D
Physician Assistant Studies	M,D
Public Health—General	M

CLEVELAND UNIVERSITY–KANSAS CITY

Program	Degrees
Chiropractic	D
Health Promotion	M

COLD SPRING HARBOR LABORATORY, WATSON SCHOOL OF BIOLOGICAL SCIENCES

Program	Degrees
Biological and Biomedical Sciences—General	D*

THE COLLEGE AT BROCKPORT, STATE UNIVERSITY OF NEW YORK

Program	Degrees
Biological and Biomedical Sciences—General	M
Community Health	M
Health Services Management and Hospital Administration	M,O

COLLEGE OF CHARLESTON

Program	Degrees
Marine Biology	M

COLLEGE OF MOUNT SAINT VINCENT

Program	Degrees
Adult Nursing	M,O
Family Nurse Practitioner Studies	M,O
Gerontological Nursing	M,O
Nursing and Healthcare Administration	M,O
Nursing Education	M,O
Nursing—General	M,O

THE COLLEGE OF NEW JERSEY

Program	Degrees
Nursing—General	M,O

THE COLLEGE OF NEW ROCHELLE

Program	Degrees
Acute Care/Critical Care Nursing	M,O
Family Nurse Practitioner Studies	M,O
Nursing and Healthcare Administration	M,O
Nursing Education	M,O
Nursing—General	M,O

COLLEGE OF SAINT ELIZABETH
Health Services Management and Hospital Administration M
Nursing—General M
Nutrition M,O

COLLEGE OF SAINT MARY
Nursing—General M
Occupational Therapy M

THE COLLEGE OF SAINT ROSE
Communication Disorders M

THE COLLEGE OF ST. SCHOLASTICA
Nursing—General M,O
Occupational Therapy M
Physical Therapy D

COLLEGE OF STATEN ISLAND OF THE CITY UNIVERSITY OF NEW YORK
Adult Nursing M,O
Biological and Biomedical Sciences—General M
Gerontological Nursing M,O
Neuroscience M
Nursing Education O
Nursing—General M,O

THE COLLEGE OF WILLIAM AND MARY
Biological and Biomedical Sciences—General M
Computational Biology M,D
Medical Imaging M,D
Medical Physics M,D
Neuroscience M,D

COLORADO SCHOOL OF TRADITIONAL CHINESE MEDICINE
Acupuncture and Oriental Medicine M

COLORADO STATE UNIVERSITY
Biochemistry M,D
Biological and Biomedical Sciences—General M,D
Botany M,D
Cell Biology M,D
Conservation Biology M,D
Ecology M,D
Entomology M,D
Environmental and Occupational Health M,D
Immunology M,D
Microbiology M,D
Molecular Biology M,D
Neuroscience D
Nutrition M,D
Occupational Therapy M,D
Pathology M,D
Plant Pathology M,D
Radiation Biology M,D
Veterinary Medicine D
Veterinary Sciences M,D
Zoology M,D

COLORADO STATE UNIVERSITY–PUEBLO
Biochemistry M
Biological and Biomedical Sciences—General M
Nursing—General M

COLUMBIA SOUTHERN UNIVERSITY
Environmental and Occupational Health M
Health Services Management and Hospital Administration M

COLUMBIA UNIVERSITY
Acute Care/Critical Care Nursing M,O
Adult Nursing M,O
Allopathic Medicine M,D
Anatomy M,D
Biochemistry M,D
Bioethics M
Biological and Biomedical Sciences—General M,D,O*
Biophysics M,D
Cell Biology M,D
Community Health M,D
Conservation Biology M,D
Dentistry D
Developmental Biology M,D
Ecology M,D
Environmental and Occupational Health M,D
Epidemiology M,D
Evolutionary Biology M,D
Family Nurse Practitioner Studies M,O
Genetics M,D
Gerontological Nursing M,O
Health Services Management and Hospital Administration M
Maternal and Child Health M
Medical Physics M,D,O
Microbiology M,D
Molecular Biology D
Neurobiology D
Nurse Anesthesia M,O
Nurse Midwifery M
Nursing—General M,D,O
Nutrition M,D
Occupational Therapy M,D
Oral and Dental Sciences M,D,O
Pathobiology M,D
Pathology M,D
Pediatric Nursing M,O
Pharmaceutical Administration M
Pharmacology M,D
Physical Therapy D
Physiology M,D
Psychiatric Nursing M,O
Public Health—General M,D
Structural Biology D
Toxicology M,D

COLUMBUS STATE UNIVERSITY
Nursing—General M

THE COMMONWEALTH MEDICAL COLLEGE
Allied Health—General D
Biological and Biomedical Sciences—General M

CONCORDIA UNIVERSITY (CANADA)
Biological and Biomedical Sciences—General M,D,O
Genomic Sciences M,D,O

CONCORDIA UNIVERSITY, ST. PAUL
Health Services Management and Hospital Administration M

CONCORDIA UNIVERSITY WISCONSIN
Family Nurse Practitioner Studies M
Gerontological Nursing M
Health Services Management and Hospital Administration M
Nursing Education M
Nursing—General M
Occupational Therapy M
Physical Therapy M,D
Rehabilitation Sciences M

CONCORD UNIVERSITY
Health Promotion M

CONNECTICUT COLLEGE
Biopsychology M
Neuroscience M

COPENHAGEN BUSINESS SCHOOL
Health Services Management and Hospital Administration M,D

COPPIN STATE UNIVERSITY
Family Nurse Practitioner Studies M,O
Nursing—General M,O

CORNELL UNIVERSITY
Anatomy D
Animal Behavior D
Biochemistry M,D
Biological and Biomedical Sciences—General M,D
Biophysics D
Biopsychology D
Cell Biology D
Computational Biology D
Conservation Biology M,D
Developmental Biology M,D
Ecology M,D
Entomology M,D
Epidemiology M,D
Evolutionary Biology D
Genetics D
Genomic Sciences D
Health Services Management and Hospital Administration M,D
Immunology M,D
Infectious Diseases M,D
Microbiology D
Molecular Biology M,D
Molecular Medicine M,D
Neurobiology D
Nutrition M,D
Pharmacology M,D
Physiology M,D
Plant Biology M,D
Plant Molecular Biology M,D
Plant Pathology M,D
Plant Physiology M,D
Reproductive Biology M,D
Structural Biology M,D
Toxicology M,D
Veterinary Medicine D
Zoology D

COX COLLEGE
Family Nurse Practitioner Studies M
Nursing and Healthcare Administration M
Nursing Education M
Nursing—General M

CREIGHTON UNIVERSITY
Allied Health—General M,D
Allopathic Medicine D
Anatomy M
Biological and Biomedical Sciences—General M,D
Dentistry D
Immunology M,D
Medical Microbiology M,D
Nursing—General M,D
Occupational Therapy D
Pharmaceutical Sciences M,D
Pharmacology M,D
Pharmacy D
Physical Therapy D

CURRY COLLEGE
Nursing—General M

DAEMEN COLLEGE
Adult Nursing M,D,O
Health Services Management and Hospital Administration M
Medical/Surgical Nursing M,D,O
Nursing and Healthcare Administration M,D,O
Nursing Education M,D,O
Nursing—General M,D,O
Physical Therapy D,O
Physician Assistant Studies M

DALHOUSIE UNIVERSITY
Allopathic Medicine M,D
Anatomy M,D
Biochemistry M,D
Biological and Biomedical Sciences—General M,D
Biophysics M,D
Botany M
Communication Disorders M,D
Community Health M
Ecology M
Environmental Biology M
Epidemiology M
Health Services Management and Hospital Administration M,D
Immunology M,D
Microbiology M,D
Neurobiology M,D
Neuroscience M,D
Nursing—General M,D
Occupational Therapy M
Oral and Dental Sciences
Pathology M,D
Pharmacology M,D
Physical Therapy M
Physiology M,D
Plant Pathology M
Plant Physiology M

DALLAS BAPTIST UNIVERSITY
Health Services Management and Hospital Administration M

DARTMOUTH COLLEGE
Allopathic Medicine D
Biochemistry D
Biological and Biomedical Sciences—General D
Cancer Biology/Oncology D
Cardiovascular Sciences D
Cell Biology D
Ecology D
Evolutionary Biology D
Genetics D
Health Services Management and Hospital Administration M,D
Health Services Research M,D
Immunology
Microbiology D
Molecular Biology D
Molecular Medicine D
Molecular Pathogenesis D
Molecular Pharmacology D
Neuroscience D
Pharmaceutical Sciences D
Pharmacology D
Physiology D
Public Health—General M
Systems Biology D
Toxicology D

DAVENPORT UNIVERSITY
Health Services Management and Hospital Administration M
Public Health—General M

DEFIANCE COLLEGE
Health Services Management and Hospital Administration M

DELAWARE STATE UNIVERSITY
Biological and Biomedical Sciences—General M
Neuroscience M,D
Nursing—General M

DELTA STATE UNIVERSITY
Biological and Biomedical Sciences—General M
Family Nurse Practitioner Studies M
Health Services Management and Hospital Administration M
Nursing Education M
Nursing—General M

DEPAUL UNIVERSITY
Biological and Biomedical Sciences—General M,D
Family Nurse Practitioner Studies M,D
Health Services Management and Hospital Administration M
Nursing—General M,D
Public Health—General M

DESALES UNIVERSITY
Adult Nursing M,D,O
Family Nurse Practitioner Studies M,D,O
Health Services Management and Hospital Administration M
Nurse Midwifery M,D,O
Nursing and Healthcare Administration M,D,O
Nursing Education M,D,O
Nursing—General M,D,O
Physical Therapy M,D,O
Physician Assistant Studies M

DES MOINES UNIVERSITY
Anatomy M
Biological and Biomedical Sciences—General M
Health Services Management and Hospital Administration M
Osteopathic Medicine D
Physical Therapy D
Physician Assistant Studies M
Podiatric Medicine D
Public Health—General M

DOMINICAN COLLEGE
Allied Health—General M,D
Family Nurse Practitioner Studies M
Occupational Therapy M
Physical Therapy M,D

DOMINICAN UNIVERSITY OF CALIFORNIA
Biological and Biomedical Sciences—General M
Clinical Laboratory Sciences/Medical Technology M
Occupational Therapy M

DONGGUK UNIVERSITY LOS ANGELES
Acupuncture and Oriental Medicine M

DOWLING COLLEGE
Environmental Biology M
Health Services Management and Hospital Administration M,O
Microbiology M

DRAKE UNIVERSITY
Pharmacy D

DREW UNIVERSITY
Bioethics M,D,O
Biological and Biomedical Sciences—General M

DREXEL UNIVERSITY
Acute Care/Critical Care Nursing M
Allied Health—General M,D,O
Allopathic Medicine D
Biochemistry M,D
Biological and Biomedical Sciences—General M,D,O
Biopsychology M,D
Cell Biology M,D
Emergency Medical Services M
Epidemiology M,D,O
Family Nurse Practitioner Studies M
Genetics M,D
Immunology M,D
Microbiology M,D
Molecular Biology M,D
Molecular Medicine M
Neuroscience M,D
Nurse Anesthesia M
Nursing and Healthcare Administration M
Nursing Education M
Nursing—General M,D
Nutrition M
Pathobiology M,D
Pediatric Nursing M
Pharmaceutical Sciences M
Pharmacology M,D
Physical Therapy M,D,O
Physician Assistant Studies M
Psychiatric Nursing M
Public Health—General M,D,O
Veterinary Sciences M
Women's Health Nursing M

DUKE UNIVERSITY
Acute Care/Critical Care Nursing M,D,O
Adult Nursing M,D,O
Allopathic Medicine D
Anatomy D
Biochemistry D
Bioethics M
Biological and Biomedical Sciences—General D
Biopsychology D
Cancer Biology/Oncology D
Cell Biology D,O
Clinical Laboratory Sciences/Sciences/Medical Technology M
Clinical Research M
Computational Biology D,O
Developmental Biology O
Ecology D,O
Environmental and Occupational Health O
Family Nurse Practitioner Studies M,D,O
Genetics D
Genomic Sciences D
Gerontological Nursing M,D,O
Health Services Management and Hospital Administration M,O
Immunology D
International Health M
Maternal and Child/Neonatal Nursing M,D,O
Medical Physics M,D
Microbiology D
Molecular Biology D,O
Molecular Biophysics O
Molecular Genetics D
Neurobiology D
Neuroscience D,O
Nurse Anesthesia M,D,O
Nursing and Healthcare Administration M,D,O
Nursing Education M,D,O
Nursing Informatics M,D,O
Nursing—General D
Oncology Nursing M,D,O
Pathology M,D
Pediatric Nursing M,D,O
Pharmacology D
Physical Therapy D
Physician Assistant Studies M
Structural Biology O
Toxicology O

DUQUESNE UNIVERSITY
Allied Health—General M,D
Biochemistry M,D
Bioethics M,D,O
Biological and Biomedical Sciences—General M,D
Communication Disorders M,D
Community Health M
Family Nurse Practitioner Studies M,O
Forensic Nursing M,O
Health Services Management and Hospital Administration M,D
Medicinal and Pharmaceutical Chemistry M,D
Nursing Education M

*M—masters degree; D—doctorate; O—other advanced degree; *—Close-Up and/or Display*

Nursing—General M,D,O
Occupational Therapy M,D
Pharmaceutical Administration M
Pharmaceutical Sciences M,D
Pharmacology M,D
Pharmacy D
Physical Therapy M,D
Physician Assistant Studies M,D
Rehabilitation Sciences M,D

D'YOUVILLE COLLEGE
Chiropractic D
Community Health Nursing M,D,O
Family Nurse Practitioner Studies M,D,O
Health Services Management and Hospital Administration M,D,O
Nursing and Healthcare Administration M,D,O
Nursing Education M,D,O
Nursing—General M,D,O*
Nutrition M
Occupational Therapy M
Pharmacy D
Physical Therapy D,O
Physician Assistant Studies M

EAST CAROLINA UNIVERSITY
Allied Health—General M,D,O
Allopathic Medicine D
Anatomy D
Biochemistry M,D
Biological and Biomedical Sciences—General M,D
Biophysics M,D
Cell Biology D
Communication Disorders M,D
Community Health M,O
Environmental and Occupational Health M,D
Health Physics/Radiological Health M,D
Health Promotion M
Immunology M,D
Maternal and Child Health D
Medical Physics M,D
Microbiology M,D
Molecular Biology M,D
Nursing—General M,D,O
Nutrition M
Occupational Therapy M,D,O
Pathology D
Pharmacology D
Physical Therapy D
Physician Assistant Studies M
Physiology D
Public Health—General M
Rehabilitation Sciences M,D,O

EASTERN ILLINOIS UNIVERSITY
Biological and Biomedical Sciences—General M
Communication Disorders M
Nutrition M

EASTERN KENTUCKY UNIVERSITY
Allied Health—General M
Biological and Biomedical Sciences—General M
Communication Disorders M
Community Health M
Ecology M
Environmental and Occupational Health M
Family Nurse Practitioner Studies M
Health Promotion M
Health Services Management and Hospital Administration M
Nursing—General M
Nutrition M
Occupational Therapy M

EASTERN MENNONITE UNIVERSITY
Biological and Biomedical Sciences—General M
Health Services Management and Hospital Administration M
Nursing and Healthcare Administration M
Nursing—General M
School Nursing M

EASTERN MICHIGAN UNIVERSITY
Adult Nursing M,O
Biological and Biomedical Sciences—General M
Cell Biology M
Clinical Research M,O
Communication Disorders M
Ecology M
Health Promotion M,O
Health Services Management and Hospital Administration M,O
Molecular Biology M
Nursing and Healthcare Administration M,O
Nursing Education M,O
Nutrition M
Occupational Therapy M
Physiology M

EASTERN NEW MEXICO UNIVERSITY
Biochemistry M
Biological and Biomedical Sciences—General M
Botany M
Cell Biology M
Communication Disorders M
Ecology M
Microbiology M
Molecular Biology M
Nursing—General M
Zoology M

EASTERN UNIVERSITY
Health Services Management and Hospital Administration M
School Nursing M,O

EASTERN VIRGINIA MEDICAL SCHOOL
Allopathic Medicine D
Biological and Biomedical Sciences—General M,D
Medical/Surgical Nursing M
Physician Assistant Studies M
Public Health—General M
Reproductive Biology M
Vision Sciences O

EASTERN WASHINGTON UNIVERSITY
Biological and Biomedical Sciences—General M
Communication Disorders M
Dental Hygiene M
Occupational Therapy M
Physical Therapy D

EAST STROUDSBURG UNIVERSITY OF PENNSYLVANIA
Biological and Biomedical Sciences—General M
Communication Disorders M
Rehabilitation Sciences M

EAST TENNESSEE STATE UNIVERSITY
Allied Health—General M,D,O
Allopathic Medicine D
Anatomy D
Biochemistry D
Biological and Biomedical Sciences—General M,D
Communication Disorders M,D
Environmental and Occupational Health M,D
Health Services Management and Hospital Administration M,O
Microbiology M,D
Nutrition M
Pharmaceutical Sciences D
Pharmacology D
Pharmacy D
Physical Therapy D
Physiology D
Public Health—General M,D,O

EAST WEST COLLEGE OF NATURAL MEDICINE
Acupuncture and Oriental Medicine M

EDGEWOOD COLLEGE
Nursing—General M,D

EDINBORO UNIVERSITY OF PENNSYLVANIA
Biological and Biomedical Sciences—General M
Communication Disorders M
Family Nurse Practitioner Studies M,D
Nursing Education M,D
Nursing—General M,D

EDWARD VIA COLLEGE OF OSTEOPAHTIC MEDICINE–VIRGINIA CAMPUS
Osteopathic Medicine D

EDWARD VIA COLLEGE OF OSTEOPATHIC MEDICINE–CAROLINAS CAMPUS
Osteopathic Medicine D

ELIZABETH CITY STATE UNIVERSITY
Biological and Biomedical Sciences—General M

ELIZABETHTOWN COLLEGE
Occupational Therapy M

ELMEZZI GRADUATE SCHOOL OF MOLECULAR MEDICINE
Molecular Medicine D

ELMHURST COLLEGE
Communication Disorders M
Nursing—General M
Public Health—General M

ELMS COLLEGE
Communication Disorders M,O
Nursing and Healthcare Administration M
Nursing Education M
Nursing—General M

ELON UNIVERSITY
Physical Therapy D
Physician Assistant Studies M

EMBRY-RIDDLE AERONAUTICAL UNIVERSITY–WORLDWIDE
Environmental and Occupational Health M,O

EMERSON COLLEGE
Communication Disorders M

EMMANUEL COLLEGE (UNITED STATES)
Nursing and Healthcare Administration M
Nursing Education M
Nursing—General M
Pharmaceutical Administration M,O

EMORY UNIVERSITY
Adult Nursing M
Allied Health—General M,D
Allopathic Medicine D
Anesthesiologist Assistant Studies M
Animal Behavior D
Biochemistry D
Bioethics M
Biological and Biomedical Sciences—General D
Biophysics D
Cancer Biology/Oncology D
Cell Biology D
Clinical Research M

Developmental Biology D
Ecology D
Environmental and Occupational Health M,D
Epidemiology M,D
Evolutionary Biology D
Family Nurse Practitioner Studies M
Genetics D
Health Promotion M
Health Services Management and Hospital Administration M,D
Health Services Research M,D
Human Genetics M
Immunology D
International Health M
Microbiology D
Molecular Biology D
Molecular Genetics D
Molecular Pathogenesis D
Neuroscience D
Nurse Midwifery M
Nursing and Healthcare Administration M
Nursing—General M,D
Nutrition M,D
Pediatric Nursing M
Pharmacology D
Physical Therapy D
Physician Assistant Studies M
Public Health—General M,D
Women's Health Nursing M

EMPEROR'S COLLEGE OF TRADITIONAL ORIENTAL MEDICINE
Acupuncture and Oriental Medicine M,D

EMPORIA STATE UNIVERSITY
Biological and Biomedical Sciences—General M
Botany M
Cell Biology M
Environmental Biology M
Microbiology M
Zoology M

ENDICOTT COLLEGE
Nursing—General M

EXCELSIOR COLLEGE
Health Services Management and Hospital Administration M,O
Nursing Education M
Nursing Informatics M
Nursing—General M
Public Health—General M,O

FAIRFIELD UNIVERSITY
Family Nurse Practitioner Studies M,D
Nurse Anesthesia M,D
Nursing and Healthcare Administration M,D
Nursing—General M,D
Psychiatric Nursing M,D

FAIRLEIGH DICKINSON UNIVERSITY, COLLEGE AT FLORHAM
Biological and Biomedical Sciences—General M
Health Services Management and Hospital Administration M
Pharmacology M,O

FAIRLEIGH DICKINSON UNIVERSITY, METROPOLITAN CAMPUS
Biological and Biomedical Sciences—General M
Clinical Laboratory Sciences/Sciences/Medical Technology M
Health Services Management and Hospital Administration M
Nursing—General M,D,O
Pharmaceutical Administration M,O

FAIRMONT STATE UNIVERSITY
Health Promotion M

FAYETTEVILLE STATE UNIVERSITY
Biological and Biomedical Sciences—General M

FELICIAN COLLEGE
Adult Nursing M,O
Family Nurse Practitioner Studies M,O
Gerontological Nursing M,O
Health Services Management and Hospital Administration M
Nursing and Healthcare Administration M,D,O
Nursing Education M,O
Nursing—General M,D,O
School Nursing M,O

FERRIS STATE UNIVERSITY
Allied Health—General M
Nursing and Healthcare Administration M
Nursing Education M
Nursing Informatics M
Nursing—General M
Optometry D
Pharmacy D

FIELDING GRADUATE UNIVERSITY
Neuroscience M,D,O

FISK UNIVERSITY
Biological and Biomedical Sciences—General M

FITCHBURG STATE UNIVERSITY
Biological and Biomedical Sciences—General M,O
Forensic Nursing M,O

FIVE BRANCHES UNIVERSITY: GRADUATE SCHOOL OF TRADITIONAL CHINESE MEDICINE
Acupuncture and Oriental Medicine M

FLORIDA AGRICULTURAL AND MECHANICAL UNIVERSITY
Allied Health—General M
Biological and Biomedical Sciences—General M
Medicinal and Pharmaceutical Chemistry M,D
Nursing and Healthcare Administration M
Nursing—General M
Occupational Therapy M
Pharmaceutical Administration M,D
Pharmaceutical Sciences M,D
Pharmacology M,D
Pharmacy D
Physical Therapy M
Public Health—General M
Toxicology M,D

FLORIDA ATLANTIC UNIVERSITY
Adult Nursing M,D,O
Allopathic Medicine M,D
Biological and Biomedical Sciences—General M,D
Communication Disorders M
Family Nurse Practitioner Studies M,D,O
Gerontological Nursing M,D,O
Health Promotion M
Health Services Management and Hospital Administration M,D
Medical Physics M,D
Neuroscience D
Nursing and Healthcare Administration M,D,O
Nursing Education M,D,O
Nursing—General M,D,O

FLORIDA COLLEGE OF INTEGRATIVE MEDICINE
Acupuncture and Oriental Medicine M

FLORIDA GULF COAST UNIVERSITY
Allied Health—General M,D
Nurse Anesthesia M
Occupational Therapy M
Physical Therapy M,D

FLORIDA INSTITUTE OF TECHNOLOGY
Biochemistry M,D
Biological and Biomedical Sciences—General M,D
Cell Biology M
Conservation Biology M,D
Ecology M
Health Services Management and Hospital Administration M
Marine Biology M
Molecular Biology M

FLORIDA INTERNATIONAL UNIVERSITY
Allopathic Medicine M,D
Biological and Biomedical Sciences—General M,D
Communication Disorders M
Environmental and Occupational Health M,D
Epidemiology M,D
Health Promotion M,D
Health Services Management and Hospital Administration M,D
Nursing—General M,D
Nutrition M,D
Occupational Therapy M
Physical Therapy D
Public Health—General M,D

FLORIDA SOUTHERN COLLEGE
Adult Nursing M
Gerontological Nursing M
Nursing and Healthcare Administration M
Nursing Education M
Nursing—General M

FLORIDA STATE UNIVERSITY
Biochemistry M,D
Biological and Biomedical Sciences—General M,D
Cell Biology M,D
Communication Disorders M,D
Computational Biology D
Ecology M,D
Evolutionary Biology M,D
Family Nurse Practitioner Studies M,D,O
Health Services Management and Hospital Administration M,D,O
Molecular Biology M,D
Molecular Biophysics D
Neuroscience D
Nursing and Healthcare Administration M,D,O
Nursing Education M,D,O
Nursing—General M,D,O
Nutrition M,D
Plant Biology M,D
Public Health—General M
Structural Biology M,D

FONTBONNE UNIVERSITY
Communication Disorders M

FORDHAM UNIVERSITY
Biological and Biomedical Sciences—General M,D,O
Conservation Biology M,D,O

FORT HAYS STATE UNIVERSITY
Biological and Biomedical Sciences—General M
Communication Disorders M
Nursing—General M

FORT VALLEY STATE UNIVERSITY
Environmental and Occupational Health M
Public Health—General M

FRAMINGHAM STATE UNIVERSITY	
Health Services Management and Hospital Administration	M
Nursing and Healthcare Administration	M
Nursing Education	M
Nursing—General	M
Nutrition	M

FRANCISCAN UNIVERSITY OF STEUBENVILLE	
Nursing—General	M

FRANCIS MARION UNIVERSITY	
Family Nurse Practitioner Studies	M
Health Services Management and Hospital Administration	M
Nursing Education	M
Nursing—General	M

FRANKLIN PIERCE UNIVERSITY	
Health Services Management and Hospital Administration	M,D,O
Nursing—General	M,D,O
Physical Therapy	M,D,O
Physician Assistant Studies	M,D,O

FRIENDS UNIVERSITY	
Health Services Management and Hospital Administration	M

FRONTIER NURSING UNIVERSITY	
Family Nurse Practitioner Studies	M,D,O
Nurse Midwifery	M,D,O
Nursing—General	M,D,O
Women's Health Nursing	M,D,O

FROSTBURG STATE UNIVERSITY	
Biological and Biomedical Sciences—General	M
Conservation Biology	M
Ecology	M

FUTURE GENERATIONS GRADUATE SCHOOL	
Maternal and Child Health	M

GALLAUDET UNIVERSITY	
Communication Disorders	M,D,O
Neuroscience	M,D,O

GANNON UNIVERSITY	
Environmental and Occupational Health	M
Family Nurse Practitioner Studies	M,O
Nurse Anesthesia	M,O
Nursing and Healthcare Administration	M
Nursing—General	D
Occupational Therapy	M
Physical Therapy	D
Physician Assistant Studies	M

GARDNER-WEBB UNIVERSITY	
Nursing—General	M,D,O

GENEVA COLLEGE	
Cardiovascular Sciences	M

GEORGE FOX UNIVERSITY	
Physical Therapy	D

GEORGE MASON UNIVERSITY	
Biochemistry	M,D
Biological and Biomedical Sciences—General	M,D,O
Community Health	M,O
Computational Biology	M,D,O
Health Promotion	M
Health Services Management and Hospital Administration	M,O
International Health	M,O
Neuroscience	D
Nursing and Healthcare Administration	M,D,O
Nursing Education	M,D,O
Nursing—General	M,D,O
Nutrition	M,O
Public Health—General	M,O
Rehabilitation Sciences	D,O

GEORGETOWN UNIVERSITY	
Acute Care/Critical Care Nursing	M,D
Allopathic Medicine	D
Biochemistry	M,D
Biological and Biomedical Sciences—General	M,D
Epidemiology	M,O
Family Nurse Practitioner Studies	M,D
Health Promotion	M,D
Immunology	M,D
Infectious Diseases	M,D
International Health	M,D
Microbiology	M,D
Molecular Biology	M,D
Neuroscience	D
Nurse Anesthesia	M,D
Nurse Midwifery	M,D
Nursing Education	M,D
Nursing—General	M,D
Pharmacology	M,D
Public Health—General	M,D

THE GEORGE WASHINGTON UNIVERSITY	
Adult Nursing	M,D,O
Allopathic Medicine	D
Biochemistry	M,D
Biological and Biomedical Sciences—General	M,D
Communication Disorders	M
Environmental and Occupational Health	M
Epidemiology	M,D
Family Nurse Practitioner Studies	M,D,O
Health Services Management and Hospital Administration	M,D,O
Health Services Research	M,D
Immunology	D
Infectious Diseases	M
International Health	M
Microbiology	M,D
Molecular Biology	M,D
Molecular Genetics	M,D
Molecular Medicine	D
Nursing and Healthcare Administration	M,D,O
Nursing—General	M,D,O
Physical Therapy	D
Physician Assistant Studies	M
Public Health—General	M,O
Systems Biology	D
Toxicology	M

GEORGIA CAMPUS–PHILADELPHIA COLLEGE OF OSTEOPATHIC MEDICINE	
Osteopathic Medicine	D
Pharmacy	D*

GEORGIA COLLEGE & STATE UNIVERSITY	
Biological and Biomedical Sciences—General	M
Family Nurse Practitioner Studies	M,D
Health Promotion	M
Nursing—General	M,D

GEORGIA INSTITUTE OF TECHNOLOGY	
Biochemistry	M,D
Biological and Biomedical Sciences—General	M,D
Health Physics/Radiological Health	M,D
Health Services Management and Hospital Administration	M
Medical Physics	M,D
Physiology	M

GEORGIA REGENTS UNIVERSITY	
Allied Health—General	M
Allopathic Medicine	D
Anatomy	M,D
Biochemistry	M,D
Biological and Biomedical Sciences—General	M,D,O
Cardiovascular Sciences	M,D
Cell Biology	M,D
Clinical Research	M,O
Dental Hygiene	M
Dentistry	D
Family Nurse Practitioner Studies	M,O
Genomic Sciences	M,D
Molecular Biology	M,D
Molecular Medicine	M,D
Neuroscience	M,D
Nurse Anesthesia	M
Nursing and Healthcare Administration	M
Nursing—General	D
Oral and Dental Sciences	M,D
Pediatric Nursing	M,O
Pharmacology	M,D
Physiology	M,D
Public Health—General	M

GEORGIA SOUTHERN UNIVERSITY	
Allied Health—General	M,D
Biological and Biomedical Sciences—General	M
Community Health	M,D
Environmental and Occupational Health	M,D,O
Epidemiology	M,D
Family Nurse Practitioner Studies	M
Health Services Management and Hospital Administration	M,D
Nursing—General	D
Public Health—General	M,D

GEORGIA STATE UNIVERSITY	
Adult Nursing	M,D,O
Allied Health—General	M
Biochemistry	M,D
Biological and Biomedical Sciences—General	M,D
Cell Biology	M,D
Communication Disorders	M,D
Environmental Biology	M,D
Family Nurse Practitioner Studies	M,D,O
Health Services Management and Hospital Administration	M,D,O
Microbiology	M,D
Molecular Biology	M,D
Molecular Genetics	M,D
Neurobiology	M,D
Neuroscience	D
Nursing and Healthcare Administration	M,D,O
Nursing Informatics	M,D,O
Nursing—General	M,D,O
Nutrition	M
Pediatric Nursing	M,D,O
Physical Therapy	D
Physiology	M,D
Psychiatric Nursing	M,D,O
Public Health—General	M,D,O
Women's Health Nursing	M,D,O

GERSTNER SLOAN-KETTERING GRADUATE SCHOOL OF BIOMEDICAL SCIENCES	
Biological and Biomedical Sciences—General	D
Cancer Biology/Oncology	D*

GLOBE UNIVERSITY–WOODBURY	
Health Services Management and Hospital Administration	M

GODDARD COLLEGE	
Health Promotion	M

GOLDEY-BEACOM COLLEGE	
Health Services Management and Hospital Administration	M

GOLDFARB SCHOOL OF NURSING AT BARNES-JEWISH COLLEGE	
Adult Nursing	M
Health Services Management and Hospital Administration	M
Nurse Anesthesia	M
Nursing Education	M
Nursing—General	M
Oncology Nursing	M

GONZAGA UNIVERSITY	
Nurse Anesthesia	M
Nursing—General	M,D

GOODING INSTITUTE OF NURSE ANESTHESIA	
Nurse Anesthesia	M

GOSHEN COLLEGE	
Family Nurse Practitioner Studies	M
Nursing—General	M

GOUCHER COLLEGE	
Biological and Biomedical Sciences—General	O

GOVERNORS STATE UNIVERSITY	
Communication Disorders	M
Environmental Biology	M
Health Services Management and Hospital Administration	M
Nursing—General	M
Occupational Therapy	M
Physical Therapy	M,D

GRACELAND UNIVERSITY (IA)	
Family Nurse Practitioner Studies	M,D,O
Nursing Education	M,D,O
Nursing—General	M,D,O

THE GRADUATE CENTER, CITY UNIVERSITY OF NEW YORK	
Biochemistry	D
Biological and Biomedical Sciences—General	D
Biopsychology	D
Communication Disorders	D
Neuroscience	D
Nursing—General	D
Physical Therapy	D
Public Health—General	D

GRAMBLING STATE UNIVERSITY	
Family Nurse Practitioner Studies	M,O
Health Services Management and Hospital Administration	M
Nursing—General	M,O

GRAND CANYON UNIVERSITY	
Acute Care/Critical Care Nursing	M,O
Family Nurse Practitioner Studies	M,O
Health Services Management and Hospital Administration	M,O
Nursing Education	M,O
Nursing—General	M,O
Public Health—General	M

GRAND VALLEY STATE UNIVERSITY	
Allied Health—General	M,D
Biological and Biomedical Sciences—General	M
Cell Biology	M
Health Services Management and Hospital Administration	M,D
Molecular Biology	M
Nursing and Healthcare Administration	M,D
Nursing Education	M,D
Nursing—General	M,D
Occupational Therapy	M
Physical Therapy	D
Physician Assistant Studies	M

GRAND VIEW UNIVERSITY	
Nursing—General	M

GRANTHAM UNIVERSITY	
Health Services Management and Hospital Administration	M
Nursing and Healthcare Administration	M
Nursing Education	M
Nursing Informatics	M

GWYNEDD MERCY UNIVERSITY	
Adult Nursing	M
Family Nurse Practitioner Studies	M
Gerontological Nursing	M
Nursing—General	M
Oncology Nursing	M
Pediatric Nursing	M

HAMPTON UNIVERSITY	
Adult Nursing	M
Biological and Biomedical Sciences—General	M
Communication Disorders	M
Community Health Nursing	M
Environmental Biology	M
Gerontological Nursing	M
Health Services Management and Hospital Administration	M,D
Medical Physics	M,D
Nursing—General	M,D
Pediatric Nursing	M
Pharmacy	D
Physical Therapy	D
Psychiatric Nursing	M
Women's Health Nursing	M

HARDING UNIVERSITY	
Allied Health—General	M,D
Communication Disorders	M
Health Services Management and Hospital Administration	M
Pharmacy	D
Physical Therapy	D
Physician Assistant Studies	M

HARDIN-SIMMONS UNIVERSITY	
Family Nurse Practitioner Studies	M
Maternal and Child/Neonatal Nursing	M
Nursing—General	M
Physical Therapy	D

HARRISBURG UNIVERSITY OF SCIENCE AND TECHNOLOGY	
Health Services Management and Hospital Administration	M

HARVARD UNIVERSITY	
Allopathic Medicine	D
Biochemistry	D
Biological and Biomedical Sciences—General	M,D,O
Biophysics	D*
Biopsychology	D
Cell Biology	D
Dentistry	M,D,O
Environmental and Occupational Health	M,D
Epidemiology	M,D
Evolutionary Biology	D
Genetics	D
Genomic Sciences	D
Health Promotion	M,D
Health Services Management and Hospital Administration	M,D
International Health	M,D
Medical Physics	D
Microbiology	D
Molecular Biology	D
Molecular Genetics	D
Molecular Pharmacology	D
Neurobiology	D
Neuroscience	D
Nutrition	D
Oral and Dental Sciences	M,D,O
Pathology	D
Physiology	M,D
Public Health—General	M,D*
Structural Biology	D
Systems Biology	D

HAWAII COLLEGE OF ORIENTAL MEDICINE	
Acupuncture and Oriental Medicine	M

HAWAI`I PACIFIC UNIVERSITY	
Community Health Nursing	M
Family Nurse Practitioner Studies	M
Health Services Management and Hospital Administration	M
Nursing—General	M

HERZING UNIVERSITY ONLINE	
Health Services Management and Hospital Administration	M
Nursing and Healthcare Administration	M
Nursing Education	M
Nursing—General	M

HOFSTRA UNIVERSITY	
Allopathic Medicine	D
Biological and Biomedical Sciences—General	M,O
Communication Disorders	M,D
Community Health	M
Health Services Management and Hospital Administration	M,O
Medical Physics	M
Molecular Medicine	D
Physician Assistant Studies	M
Public Health—General	M

HOLY FAMILY UNIVERSITY	
Community Health Nursing	M
Health Services Management and Hospital Administration	M
Nursing and Healthcare Administration	M
Nursing Education	M
Nursing—General	M

HOLY NAMES UNIVERSITY	
Community Health Nursing	M,O
Family Nurse Practitioner Studies	M,O
Nursing and Healthcare Administration	M,O
Nursing Education	M,O
Nursing—General	M,O

HOOD COLLEGE	
Biological and Biomedical Sciences—General	M,O
Environmental Biology	M
Immunology	M,O
Microbiology	M,O
Molecular Biology	M,O

HOWARD UNIVERSITY	
Allopathic Medicine	D
Anatomy	M,D
Biochemistry	M,D
Biological and Biomedical Sciences—General	M,D
Biophysics	D
Biopsychology	M,D
Communication Disorders	M,D
Dentistry	D,O
Family Nurse Practitioner Studies	M,O
Microbiology	D

*M—masters degree; D—doctorate; O—other advanced degree; * Close-Up and/or Display*

- Molecular Biology M,D
- Nursing—General M,O
- Nutrition M,D
- Oral and Dental Sciences D,O
- Pharmacology M,D
- Pharmacy D
- Physiology D
- Public Health—General M

HUMBOLDT STATE UNIVERSITY
- Biological and Biomedical Sciences—General M
- Physical Therapy M

HUNTER COLLEGE OF THE CITY UNIVERSITY OF NEW YORK
- Adult Nursing M
- Biochemistry M,D
- Biological and Biomedical Sciences—General M,D
- Communication Disorders M
- Community Health Nursing M
- Community Health M
- Environmental and Occupational Health M
- Epidemiology M
- Gerontological Nursing M
- Health Services Management and Hospital Administration M
- Nursing—General M,O
- Nutrition M
- Psychiatric Nursing M,O
- Public Health—General M

HUNTINGTON COLLEGE OF HEALTH SCIENCES
- Nutrition M,D

HUSSON UNIVERSITY
- Community Health Nursing M,O
- Family Nurse Practitioner Studies M,O
- Health Services Management and Hospital Administration M
- Nursing Education M,O
- Nursing—General M,O
- Occupational Therapy M
- Pharmacy D
- Physical Therapy D
- Psychiatric Nursing M,O

ICAHN SCHOOL OF MEDICINE AT MOUNT SINAI
- Allopathic Medicine D
- Bioethics M
- Biological and Biomedical Sciences—General M,D
- Clinical Research M,D
- Community Health M,D
- Neuroscience M,D

IDAHO STATE UNIVERSITY
- Allied Health—General M,D,O
- Biological and Biomedical Sciences—General M,D
- Communication Disorders M,D,O
- Community Health O
- Dental Hygiene M
- Dentistry O
- Health Physics/Radiological Health M,D
- Medical Microbiology M,D
- Medicinal and Pharmaceutical Chemistry M,D
- Microbiology M,D
- Nursing—General M,O
- Nutrition M,O
- Occupational Therapy M
- Oral and Dental Sciences O
- Pharmaceutical Administration M,D
- Pharmaceutical Sciences M,D
- Pharmacology M,D
- Pharmacy M,D
- Physical Therapy D
- Physician Assistant Studies M
- Public Health—General M,O

ILLINOIS COLLEGE OF OPTOMETRY
- Optometry D

ILLINOIS INSTITUTE OF TECHNOLOGY
- Biochemistry M,D
- Biological and Biomedical Sciences—General M,D
- Cell Biology M,D
- Health Physics/Radiological Health M,D
- Medical Imaging M,D
- Microbiology M,D
- Molecular Biology M,D
- Molecular Biophysics M,D

ILLINOIS STATE UNIVERSITY
- Animal Behavior M,D
- Bacteriology M,D
- Biochemistry M,D
- Biological and Biomedical Sciences—General M,D
- Biophysics M,D
- Botany M,D
- Cell Biology M,D
- Communication Disorders M
- Conservation Biology M,D
- Developmental Biology M,D
- Ecology M,D
- Entomology M,D
- Evolutionary Biology M,D
- Family Nurse Practitioner Studies M,D,O
- Genetics M,D
- Immunology M,D
- Microbiology M,D
- Molecular Biology M,D
- Molecular Genetics M,D
- Neurobiology M,D
- Neuroscience M,D
- Nursing—General M,D,O
- Parasitology M,D
- Physiology M,D
- Plant Biology M,D
- Plant Molecular Biology M,D
- Structural Biology M,D
- Zoology M,D

IMMACULATA UNIVERSITY
- Health Promotion M
- Neuroscience M,D,O
- Nursing and Healthcare Administration M
- Nursing Education M
- Nursing—General M
- Nutrition M

INDEPENDENCE UNIVERSITY
- Community Health Nursing M
- Community Health M
- Gerontological Nursing M
- Health Promotion M
- Health Services Management and Hospital Administration M
- Nursing and Healthcare Administration M
- Nursing—General M
- Public Health—General M

INDIANA STATE UNIVERSITY
- Biological and Biomedical Sciences—General M,D
- Community Health M
- Ecology M,D
- Environmental and Occupational Health M
- Health Promotion M
- Microbiology M,D
- Nursing—General M
- Nutrition M
- Physiology M,D

INDIANA TECH
- Health Services Management and Hospital Administration M

INDIANA UNIVERSITY BLOOMINGTON
- Biochemistry M,D
- Biological and Biomedical Sciences—General M,D
- Cell Biology M,D
- Communication Disorders M,D
- Community Health M,D
- Ecology M,D,O
- Environmental and Occupational Health M,D
- Epidemiology M,D
- Evolutionary Biology M,D
- Genetics M,D
- Health Promotion M,D
- Health Services Management and Hospital Administration M,D
- Medical Physics M,D
- Microbiology M,D
- Molecular Biology M,D
- Neuroscience D
- Nutrition M,D
- Optometry M,D
- Plant Biology M,D
- Public Health—General M,D
- Toxicology M,D,O
- Zoology M,D

INDIANA UNIVERSITY EAST
- Nursing—General M

INDIANA UNIVERSITY KOKOMO
- Nursing and Healthcare Administration M
- Nursing Education M
- Nursing—General M
- Public Health—General M

INDIANA UNIVERSITY NORTHWEST
- Health Services Management and Hospital Administration M,O

INDIANA UNIVERSITY OF PENNSYLVANIA
- Biological and Biomedical Sciences—General M
- Communication Disorders M
- Environmental and Occupational Health M
- Health Services Management and Hospital Administration M,D
- Nursing and Healthcare Administration M
- Nursing Education M
- Nursing—General D
- Nutrition M

INDIANA UNIVERSITY–PURDUE UNIVERSITY FORT WAYNE
- Adult Nursing M,O
- Biological and Biomedical Sciences—General M
- Communication Disorders M
- Gerontological Nursing M,O
- Nursing and Healthcare Administration M,O
- Nursing Education M,O
- Nursing—General M,O
- Women's Health Nursing M,O

INDIANA UNIVERSITY–PURDUE UNIVERSITY INDIANAPOLIS
- Acute Care/Critical Care Nursing M,D
- Adult Nursing M,D
- Allopathic Medicine M,D
- Anatomy M,D
- Biochemistry M,D
- Bioethics M,O
- Biological and Biomedical Sciences—General M,D
- Biopsychology M,D
- Cell Biology M,D
- Community Health Nursing M,D
- Community Health M,D
- Dentistry M,D,O
- Environmental and Occupational Health M,D,O
- Epidemiology M,D
- Family Nurse Practitioner Studies M,D
- Health Services Management and Hospital Administration M,D
- Immunology M,D
- Maternal and Child/Neonatal Nursing M,D
- Microbiology M,D
- Molecular Biology D
- Molecular Genetics M,D
- Neurobiology D
- Nursing and Healthcare Administration M
- Nursing Education M
- Nursing—General M,D
- Nutrition M,D
- Occupational Therapy M,D
- Pathology M,D
- Pediatric Nursing M,D
- Pharmacology M,D
- Physical Therapy M,D
- Psychiatric Nursing M,D
- Public Health—General M,D
- Rehabilitation Sciences M,D
- Toxicology M,D
- Women's Health Nursing M,D

INDIANA UNIVERSITY SOUTH BEND
- Family Nurse Practitioner Studies M
- Nursing—General M

INDIANA WESLEYAN UNIVERSITY
- Health Services Management and Hospital Administration M,O
- Nursing and Healthcare Administration M,O
- Nursing Education M
- Nursing—General M

INSTITUTE OF CLINICAL ACUPUNCTURE AND ORIENTAL MEDICINE
- Acupuncture and Oriental Medicine M

INSTITUTE OF PUBLIC ADMINISTRATION
- Health Services Management and Hospital Administration M,O

INSTITUT FRANCO-EUROPÉEN DE CHIROPRATIQUE
- Chiropractic D

INSTITUTO TECNOLOGICO DE SANTO DOMINGO
- Allopathic Medicine M,D
- Bioethics M,O
- Health Promotion M,O
- Maternal and Child Health M,O
- Nutrition M,O

INTER AMERICAN UNIVERSITY OF PUERTO RICO, ARECIBO CAMPUS
- Acute Care/Critical Care Nursing M
- Medical/Surgical Nursing M
- Nurse Anesthesia M
- Nursing—General M

INTER AMERICAN UNIVERSITY OF PUERTO RICO, BAYAMÓN CAMPUS
- Ecology M

INTER AMERICAN UNIVERSITY OF PUERTO RICO, METROPOLITAN CAMPUS
- Clinical Laboratory Sciences/Medical Technology M
- Microbiology M
- Molecular Biology M

INTER AMERICAN UNIVERSITY OF PUERTO RICO SCHOOL OF OPTOMETRY
- Optometry D

IONA COLLEGE
- Health Services Management and Hospital Administration M,O

IOWA STATE UNIVERSITY OF SCIENCE AND TECHNOLOGY
- Biological and Biomedical Sciences—General M,D
- Biophysics M,D
- Cell Biology M,D
- Computational Biology M,D
- Developmental Biology M,D
- Ecology M,D
- Entomology M,D
- Evolutionary Biology M,D
- Genetics M,D
- Immunology M,D
- Microbiology M,D
- Molecular Biology M,D
- Molecular Genetics M,D
- Neuroscience M,D
- Nutrition M,D
- Pathology M,D
- Plant Biology M,D
- Plant Pathology M,D
- Structural Biology M,D
- Toxicology M,D
- Veterinary Medicine M
- Veterinary Sciences M,D

IRELL & MANELLA GRADUATE SCHOOL OF BIOLOGICAL SCIENCES
- Biological and Biomedical Sciences—General D*

ITHACA COLLEGE
- Allied Health—General M,D
- Communication Disorders M
- Occupational Therapy M
- Physical Therapy D

JACKSON STATE UNIVERSITY
- Biological and Biomedical Sciences—General M,D
- Communication Disorders M

JACKSONVILLE STATE UNIVERSITY
- Biological and Biomedical Sciences—General M
- Nursing—General M

JACKSONVILLE UNIVERSITY
- Nursing—General M,D
- Oral and Dental Sciences O

JAMES MADISON UNIVERSITY
- Biological and Biomedical Sciences—General M
- Communication Disorders M,D
- Nursing—General M
- Occupational Therapy M
- Physician Assistant Studies M

JEFFERSON COLLEGE OF HEALTH SCIENCES
- Nursing and Healthcare Administration M
- Nursing Education M
- Nursing—General M
- Occupational Therapy M
- Physician Assistant Studies M

JOHN CARROLL UNIVERSITY
- Biological and Biomedical Sciences—General M

JOHN HANCOCK UNIVERSITY
- Health Services Management and Hospital Administration M

JOHNS HOPKINS UNIVERSITY
- Allopathic Medicine D
- Anatomy D
- Biochemistry M,D
- Bioethics M,D
- Biological and Biomedical Sciences—General M,D
- Biophysics D
- Cardiovascular Sciences M,D
- Cell Biology D
- Clinical Research M,D
- Community Health M,D
- Developmental Biology D
- Environmental and Occupational Health M,D
- Epidemiology M,D
- Evolutionary Biology D
- Genetics M,D
- Health Services Management and Hospital Administration M,D,O
- Health Services Research M,D
- Human Genetics D
- Immunology M,D
- Infectious Diseases M,D
- International Health M,D
- Microbiology M,D
- Molecular Biology M,D
- Molecular Medicine D
- Neuroscience D
- Nursing—General M,D,O
- Nutrition M,D
- Pathobiology D
- Pathology D
- Pharmaceutical Sciences M
- Pharmacology D
- Physiology M,D
- Public Health—General M,D
- Toxicology M,D

JOHNSON & WALES UNIVERSITY
- Physician Assistant Studies M

JONES INTERNATIONAL UNIVERSITY
- Health Services Management and Hospital Administration M

KANSAS CITY UNIVERSITY OF MEDICINE AND BIOSCIENCES
- Bioethics M
- Biological and Biomedical Sciences—General M
- Osteopathic Medicine D

KANSAS STATE UNIVERSITY
- Biochemistry M,D
- Biological and Biomedical Sciences—General M,D
- Communication Disorders M,D,O
- Entomology M,D
- Genetics M,D
- Microbiology M,D
- Nutrition M,D
- Pathobiology M,D
- Physiology D
- Plant Pathology M,D
- Public Health—General M,D
- Veterinary Medicine D
- Veterinary Sciences M

KAPLAN UNIVERSITY, DAVENPORT CAMPUS
- Health Services Management and Hospital Administration M,O
- Nursing and Healthcare Administration M
- Nursing Education M
- Nursing—General M

KEAN UNIVERSITY
- Communication Disorders M
- Community Health Nursing M
- Health Services Management and Hospital Administration M
- Nursing and Healthcare Administration M
- Nursing—General M
- Occupational Therapy M
- School Nursing M

KECK GRADUATE INSTITUTE OF APPLIED LIFE SCIENCES
Biological and Biomedical Sciences—General M,D,O
Computational Biology M,D,O

KEENE STATE COLLEGE
Environmental and Occupational Health M,O

KEISER UNIVERSITY
Health Services Management and Hospital Administration M
Nursing—General M
Physician Assistant Studies M

KENNESAW STATE UNIVERSITY
Biochemistry M
Biological and Biomedical Sciences—General M
Health Services Management and Hospital Administration M
Nursing—General M,D

KENT STATE UNIVERSITY
Acute Care/Critical Care Nursing M,D
Adult Nursing M,D
Biochemistry M,D
Biological and Biomedical Sciences—General M,D
Cell Biology M,D
Communication Disorders M,D,O
Ecology M,D
Family Nurse Practitioner Studies M,D
Gerontological Nursing M,D
Health Promotion M,D
Molecular Biology M,D
Neuroscience M,D
Nursing and Healthcare Administration M,D
Nursing Education M,D
Nursing—General M,D
Nutrition M
Pediatric Nursing M,D
Pharmacology M,D
Physiology M,D
Podiatric Medicine D
Psychiatric Nursing M,D
Women's Health Nursing M,D

KETTERING COLLEGE
Physician Assistant Studies M

KEUKA COLLEGE
Nursing—General M
Occupational Therapy M

KING'S COLLEGE
Health Services Management and Hospital Administration M
Physician Assistant Studies M

LAKE ERIE COLLEGE
Health Services Management and Hospital Administration M

LAKE ERIE COLLEGE OF OSTEOPATHIC MEDICINE
Biological and Biomedical Sciences—General M,D,O
Osteopathic Medicine M,D,O
Pharmacy M,D,O

LAKE FOREST GRADUATE SCHOOL OF MANAGEMENT
Health Services Management and Hospital Administration M

LAKEHEAD UNIVERSITY
Biological and Biomedical Sciences—General M
Health Services Research M

LAKELAND COLLEGE
Health Services Management and Hospital Administration M

LAMAR UNIVERSITY
Biological and Biomedical Sciences—General M
Communication Disorders M,D
Health Services Management and Hospital Administration M
Nursing and Healthcare Administration M
Nursing Education M
Nursing—General M

LANGSTON UNIVERSITY
Physical Therapy D

LA ROCHE COLLEGE
Nurse Anesthesia M
Nursing and Healthcare Administration M
Nursing Education M
Nursing—General M

LA SALLE UNIVERSITY
Adult Nursing M,D,O
Communication Disorders M
Community Health Nursing M,D,O
Family Nurse Practitioner Studies M,D,O
Gerontological Nursing M,D,O
Nurse Anesthesia M,D,O
Nursing and Healthcare Administration M,D,O
Nursing Education M,D,O
Nursing—General M,D,O
Public Health—General M
School Nursing M,D,O

LASELL COLLEGE
Health Services Management and Hospital Administration M,O

LAURENTIAN UNIVERSITY
Biochemistry M
Biological and Biomedical Sciences—General M,D
Ecology M,D
Nursing—General M
Public Health—General D

LEBANESE AMERICAN UNIVERSITY
Pharmacy D

LEBANON VALLEY COLLEGE
Health Services Management and Hospital Administration M
Physical Therapy D

LEHIGH UNIVERSITY
Biochemistry M,D
Biological and Biomedical Sciences—General M,D
Cell Biology M,D
Health Services Management and Hospital Administration M
Molecular Biology M,D
Neuroscience M,D

LEHMAN COLLEGE OF THE CITY UNIVERSITY OF NEW YORK
Adult Nursing M
Biological and Biomedical Sciences—General M
Communication Disorders M
Gerontological Nursing M
Health Promotion M
Maternal and Child/Neonatal Nursing M
Nursing—General M
Nutrition M
Pediatric Nursing M

LE MOYNE COLLEGE
Gerontological Nursing M,O
Nursing and Healthcare Administration M,O
Nursing Education M,O
Nursing Informatics M,O
Nursing—General M,O
Physician Assistant Studies M

LENOIR-RHYNE UNIVERSITY
Occupational Therapy M

LESLEY UNIVERSITY
Ecology M,D,O

LETOURNEAU UNIVERSITY
Health Services Management and Hospital Administration M

LEWIS & CLARK COLLEGE
Communication Disorders M

LEWIS UNIVERSITY
Adult Nursing M,D
Environmental and Occupational Health M
Health Services Management and Hospital Administration M
Nursing and Healthcare Administration M,D
Nursing Education M,D
Nursing—General M,D

LIBERTY UNIVERSITY
Biological and Biomedical Sciences—General M,D
Health Promotion M,D
Health Services Management and Hospital Administration M,D
International Health M,D
Nursing and Healthcare Administration M,D
Nursing Education M,D
Nursing—General M,D
Nutrition M,D

LIFE CHIROPRACTIC COLLEGE WEST
Chiropractic D

LIFE UNIVERSITY
Chiropractic D
Nutrition M

LINCOLN MEMORIAL UNIVERSITY
Family Nurse Practitioner Studies M
Nurse Anesthesia M
Nursing—General M
Osteopathic Medicine D
Psychiatric Nursing M

LINDENWOOD UNIVERSITY
Health Services Management and Hospital Administration M,O

LINDENWOOD UNIVERSITY–BELLEVILLE
Health Services Management and Hospital Administration M

LIPSCOMB UNIVERSITY
Health Services Management and Hospital Administration M,O
Molecular Biology M
Nutrition M
Pharmacy D

LOCK HAVEN UNIVERSITY OF PENNSYLVANIA
Physician Assistant Studies M

LOGAN UNIVERSITY
Chiropractic M,D
Nutrition M
Rehabilitation Sciences M

LOMA LINDA UNIVERSITY
Adult Nursing M
Allied Health—General M,D
Allopathic Medicine M,D
Anatomy M,D
Biochemistry M,D
Bioethics M,O
Biological and Biomedical Sciences—General M,D
Communication Disorders M
Dentistry M,D,O
Environmental and Occupational Health M
Epidemiology M,D,O
Gerontological Nursing M
Health Promotion M,D
Health Services Management and Hospital Administration M
International Health M
Microbiology M,D
Nursing and Healthcare Administration M
Nursing—General M
Nutrition M,D
Occupational Therapy M,D
Oral and Dental Sciences M,O
Pathology M,D
Pediatric Nursing M
Pharmacology M,D
Pharmacy D
Physical Therapy M,D
Physician Assistant Studies M
Physiology M,D
Public Health—General M,D,O

LONG ISLAND UNIVERSITY–HUDSON AT ROCKLAND
Health Services Management and Hospital Administration M,O
Pharmaceutical Sciences M

LONG ISLAND UNIVERSITY–LIU BROOKLYN
Adult Nursing M,O
Biological and Biomedical Sciences—General M
Communication Disorders M
Community Health M
Health Services Management and Hospital Administration M
Nursing and Healthcare Administration M
Nursing—General M,O
Pharmaceutical Administration M
Pharmaceutical Sciences M,D
Pharmacology M,D
Physical Therapy D
Toxicology M,D

LONG ISLAND UNIVERSITY–LIU POST
Allied Health—General M,O
Biological and Biomedical Sciences—General M
Cardiovascular Sciences M
Clinical Laboratory Sciences/Medical Technology M
Communication Disorders M
Family Nurse Practitioner Studies M,O
Health Services Management and Hospital Administration M,O
Immunology M
Medicinal and Pharmaceutical Chemistry M
Microbiology M
Nursing—General M,O
Nutrition M,O
Perfusion M

LONGWOOD UNIVERSITY
Communication Disorders M

LOUISIANA STATE UNIVERSITY AND AGRICULTURAL & MECHANICAL COLLEGE
Biochemistry M,D
Biological and Biomedical Sciences—General M,D
Biopsychology M,D
Communication Disorders M,D
Entomology M,D
Medical Physics M,D
Plant Pathology M,D
Toxicology M,D
Veterinary Medicine D
Veterinary Sciences M,D

LOUISIANA STATE UNIVERSITY HEALTH SCIENCES CENTER
Adult Nursing M,D
Allopathic Medicine M,D
Anatomy M,D
Biological and Biomedical Sciences—General M,D
Cell Biology M,D
Communication Disorders M,D
Community Health Nursing M,D
Community Health M,D
Dentistry D
Developmental Biology M,D
Environmental and Occupational Health M,D
Epidemiology M,D
Health Services Management and Hospital Administration M,D
Human Genetics M,D
Immunology M,D
Microbiology M,D
Neurobiology M,D
Neuroscience M,D
Nurse Anesthesia M,D
Nursing—General M,D
Occupational Therapy M
Parasitology M,D
Pharmacology M,D
Physical Therapy D
Physiology M,D
Public Health—General M,D

LOUISIANA STATE UNIVERSITY HEALTH SCIENCES CENTER AT SHREVEPORT
Allopathic Medicine D
Anatomy M,D
Biochemistry M,D
Biological and Biomedical Sciences—General M
Cell Biology M,D
Immunology M,D
Microbiology M,D
Molecular Biology M,D
Pharmacology D
Physiology M,D

LOUISIANA STATE UNIVERSITY IN SHREVEPORT
Health Services Management and Hospital Administration M
Public Health—General M

LOUISIANA TECH UNIVERSITY
Biological and Biomedical Sciences—General M
Communication Disorders M,D
Molecular Biology M
Nutrition M

LOURDES UNIVERSITY
Nurse Anesthesia M
Nursing and Healthcare Administration M
Nursing Education M

LOYOLA MARYMOUNT UNIVERSITY
Bioethics M

LOYOLA UNIVERSITY CHICAGO
Acute Care/Critical Care Nursing M,O
Adult Nursing M,O
Allopathic Medicine D
Anatomy M,D
Biochemistry M,D
Bioethics D,O
Biological and Biomedical Sciences—General M,D
Cardiovascular Sciences M,O
Cell Biology M,D
Clinical Research M
Environmental and Occupational Health M,O
Family Nurse Practitioner Studies M
Health Services Management and Hospital Administration M,D,O
Immunology M
Infectious Diseases M,O
Microbiology M
Molecular Biology M,D
Molecular Physiology M,D
Neurobiology M,D
Neuroscience M,D
Nursing and Healthcare Administration M
Nursing Informatics D
Nursing—General M,D
Nutrition M,O
Oncology Nursing M,O
Pharmacology M
Physiology M,D
Public Health—General M
Women's Health Nursing M,O

LOYOLA UNIVERSITY MARYLAND
Communication Disorders M

LOYOLA UNIVERSITY NEW ORLEANS
Health Services Management and Hospital Administration M,D
Nursing—General M,D

LYNCHBURG COLLEGE
Nursing and Healthcare Administration M
Nursing Education M
Nursing—General M
Physical Therapy D

MADONNA UNIVERSITY
Adult Nursing M
Health Services Management and Hospital Administration M
Hospice Nursing M
Nursing and Healthcare Administration M
Nursing—General M

MALONE UNIVERSITY
Family Nurse Practitioner Studies M
Nursing—General M

MANCHESTER UNIVERSITY
Pharmacy D

MANSFIELD UNIVERSITY OF PENNSYLVANIA
Nursing—General M

MARIAN UNIVERSITY (IN)
Osteopathic Medicine D

MARIAN UNIVERSITY (WI)
Adult Nursing M
Nursing Education M
Nursing—General M

MARIETTA COLLEGE
Physician Assistant Studies M

MARLBORO COLLEGE
Health Services Management and Hospital Administration M

MARQUETTE UNIVERSITY
Acute Care/Critical Care Nursing M,D,O

*M—masters degree; D—doctorate; O—other advanced degree; *—Close-Up and/or Display*

Adult Nursing	M,D,O
Biological and Biomedical Sciences—General	M,D
Cardiovascular Sciences	M
Cell Biology	M,D
Communication Disorders	M,O
Dentistry	D
Developmental Biology	M,D
Ecology	M,D
Family Nurse Practitioner Studies	M,D,O
Genetics	M,D
Gerontological Nursing	M,D,O
Health Services Management and Hospital Administration	M,O
Microbiology	M,D
Molecular Biology	M,D
Neuroscience	M,D
Nurse Midwifery	M,D,O
Nursing and Healthcare Administration	M,D,O
Nursing—General	M,D,O
Oral and Dental Sciences	M,O
Pediatric Nursing	M,D,O
Physical Therapy	D
Physician Assistant Studies	M
Physiology	M,D
Rehabilitation Sciences	M,D

MARSHALL B. KETCHUM UNIVERSITY

Optometry	M,D
Vision Sciences	M,D

MARSHALL UNIVERSITY

Allopathic Medicine	D
Biological and Biomedical Sciences—General	M,D
Communication Disorders	M
Health Services Management and Hospital Administration	M
Nurse Anesthesia	D
Nursing—General	M
Nutrition	M
Pharmacy	D
Physical Therapy	D
Public Health—General	M

MARYLAND UNIVERSITY OF INTEGRATIVE HEALTH

Acupuncture and Oriental Medicine	M,O

MARYLHURST UNIVERSITY

Health Services Management and Hospital Administration	M

MARYMOUNT UNIVERSITY

Allied Health—General	M,D,O
Family Nurse Practitioner Studies	M,D,O
Health Promotion	M
Health Services Management and Hospital Administration	M
Nursing—General	M,D,O
Physical Therapy	D

MARYVILLE UNIVERSITY OF SAINT LOUIS

Adult Nursing	M,D
Allied Health—General	M,D,O
Family Nurse Practitioner Studies	M,D
Gerontological Nursing	M,D
Nursing Education	M,D
Nursing—General	M,D
Occupational Therapy	M
Physical Therapy	D

MARYWOOD UNIVERSITY

Communication Disorders	M
Health Promotion	M,D,O
Health Services Management and Hospital Administration	M
Nutrition	M,O
Physician Assistant Studies	M

MASSACHUSETTS INSTITUTE OF TECHNOLOGY

Biochemistry	D
Biological and Biomedical Sciences—General	M,D
Cell Biology	D
Communication Disorders	M,D
Computational Biology	D
Developmental Biology	D
Environmental Biology	M,D,O
Genetics	D
Genomic Sciences	M,D
Immunology	D
Medical Physics	M,D
Microbiology	D
Molecular Biology	D
Molecular Toxicology	D
Neurobiology	D
Neuroscience	D
Structural Biology	D
Systems Biology	D
Toxicology	M,D

MASSACHUSETTS SCHOOL OF PROFESSIONAL PSYCHOLOGY

Community Health	M,D,O
International Health	M,D,O

MAYO GRADUATE SCHOOL

Biochemistry	D
Biological and Biomedical Sciences—General	D
Cancer Biology/Oncology	D
Cell Biology	D
Genetics	D
Immunology	D
Molecular Biology	D
Molecular Pharmacology	D
Neuroscience	D
Structural Biology	D
Virology	D

MAYO MEDICAL SCHOOL

Allopathic Medicine	D

MAYO SCHOOL OF HEALTH SCIENCES

Nurse Anesthesia	D
Physical Therapy	D

MCGILL UNIVERSITY

Allopathic Medicine	M,D
Anatomy	M,D
Biochemistry	M,D
Bioethics	M,D,O
Biological and Biomedical Sciences—General	M,D
Cell Biology	M,D
Communication Disorders	M,D
Community Health	M,D,O
Dentistry	M,D,O
Entomology	M,D
Environmental and Occupational Health	M,D,O
Epidemiology	M,D,O
Family Nurse Practitioner Studies	M,D,O
Health Services Management and Hospital Administration	M,D,O
Human Genetics	M,D
Immunology	M,D
Medical Physics	M,D
Microbiology	M,D
Neuroscience	M,D
Nursing—General	M,D,O
Nutrition	M,D,O
Oral and Dental Sciences	M,D,O
Parasitology	M,D,O
Pathology	M,D
Pharmacology	M,D
Physiology	M,D
Rehabilitation Sciences	M,D,O

MCKENDREE UNIVERSITY

Nursing and Healthcare Administration	M
Nursing Education	M
Nursing—General	M

MCMASTER UNIVERSITY

Biochemistry	M,D
Biological and Biomedical Sciences—General	M,D
Cancer Biology/Oncology	M,D
Cardiovascular Sciences	M,D
Cell Biology	M,D
Genetics	M,D
Health Physics/Radiological Health	M,D
Health Services Research	M,D
Immunology	M,D
Medical Physics	M,D
Molecular Biology	M,D
Neuroscience	M,D
Nursing—General	M,D
Nutrition	M,D
Occupational Therapy	M
Pharmacology	M,D
Physical Therapy	M
Physiology	M,D
Rehabilitation Sciences	M,D
Virology	M,D

MCMURRY UNIVERSITY

Family Nurse Practitioner Studies	M
Nursing Education	M
Nursing—General	M

MCNEESE STATE UNIVERSITY

Family Nurse Practitioner Studies	M,O
Health Promotion	M
Nursing and Healthcare Administration	M,O
Nursing Education	M
Nursing—General	M,O
Nutrition	M
Psychiatric Nursing	M,O

MCPHS UNIVERSITY

Health Services Management and Hospital Administration	M
Nursing—General	M
Pharmaceutical Sciences	M,D
Pharmacology	M,D
Pharmacy	D
Physician Assistant Studies	M

MEDICAL COLLEGE OF WISCONSIN

Allopathic Medicine	D
Biochemistry	D
Bioethics	M,O
Biological and Biomedical Sciences—General	M,D,O
Biophysics	D
Clinical Laboratory Sciences/Medical Technology	M,D
Clinical Research	
Community Health	M,D,O
Epidemiology	M,D,O
Medical Imaging	D
Microbiology	M,D
Molecular Genetics	M,D
Neuroscience	D
Pharmacology	D
Physiology	D
Public Health—General	M,D,O
Toxicology	D

MEDICAL UNIVERSITY OF SOUTH CAROLINA

Adult Nursing	M,D
Allied Health—General	M,D
Allopathic Medicine	D
Biochemistry	M,D
Biological and Biomedical Sciences—General	M,D
Cancer Biology/Oncology	D
Cardiovascular Sciences	D
Cell Biology	D
Clinical Research	M
Dentistry	D
Developmental Biology	D
Epidemiology	M,D
Family Nurse Practitioner Studies	M,D
Genetics	D
Gerontological Nursing	M,D
Health Services Management and Hospital Administration	M,D
Immunology	M,D
International Health	M
Maternal and Child/Neonatal Nursing	M,D
Medical Imaging	D
Medicinal and Pharmaceutical Chemistry	D
Microbiology	M,D
Molecular Biology	M,D
Molecular Pharmacology	M,D
Neuroscience	M,D
Nurse Anesthesia	M
Nursing and Healthcare Administration	M
Nursing Education	M
Nursing—General	D
Occupational Therapy	M
Pathobiology	D
Pathology	M,D
Pharmacy	D
Physical Therapy	D
Physician Assistant Studies	M
Rehabilitation Sciences	D
Toxicology	D

MEHARRY MEDICAL COLLEGE

Allopathic Medicine	D
Biological and Biomedical Sciences—General	D
Cancer Biology/Oncology	D
Community Health	M
Dentistry	D
Environmental and Occupational Health	M
Health Services Management and Hospital Administration	M
Immunology	D
Microbiology	D
Neuroscience	D
Pharmacology	D

MEMORIAL UNIVERSITY OF NEWFOUNDLAND

Biochemistry	M,D
Biological and Biomedical Sciences—General	M,D,O
Biopsychology	M,D
Cancer Biology/Oncology	M,D
Cardiovascular Sciences	M,D
Clinical Research	M
Community Health	M,D,O
Epidemiology	M,D,O
Human Genetics	M,D
Immunology	M,D
Marine Biology	M,D
Neuroscience	M,D
Nursing—General	M,O
Pharmaceutical Sciences	M,D

MERCER UNIVERSITY

Allopathic Medicine	M,D
Environmental and Occupational Health	M,D
Nursing—General	M,D,O
Pharmaceutical Sciences	D
Pharmacy	D
Physical Therapy	M,D
Physician Assistant Studies	M,D
Public Health—General	M,D

MERCY COLLEGE

Allied Health—General	M,D
Communication Disorders	M
Health Services Management and Hospital Administration	M
Nursing and Healthcare Administration	M
Nursing Education	M
Nursing—General	M
Occupational Therapy	M
Physical Therapy	D
Physician Assistant Studies	M

MEREDITH COLLEGE

Nutrition	M,O

MESSIAH COLLEGE

Nursing Education	M

METHODIST UNIVERSITY

Physician Assistant Studies	M

METROPOLITAN STATE UNIVERSITY

Nursing and Healthcare Administration	M,D
Nursing Education	M,D
Nursing—General	M,D
Oral and Dental Sciences	M,D

MGH INSTITUTE OF HEALTH PROFESSIONS

Communication Disorders	M,O
Gerontological Nursing	M,D,O
Nursing Education	M,D,O
Nursing—General	M,D,O
Occupational Therapy	D
Pediatric Nursing	M,D,O
Physical Therapy	M,D,O
Psychiatric Nursing	M,D,O
Women's Health Nursing	M,D,O

MIAMI UNIVERSITY

Biochemistry	M,D
Biological and Biomedical Sciences—General	M,D
Botany	M,D
Cell Biology	M,D
Communication Disorders	M
Ecology	M,D
Environmental Biology	M,D
Microbiology	M,D
Molecular Biology	M,D
Structural Biology	M,D
Zoology	M,D

MICHIGAN STATE UNIVERSITY

Allopathic Medicine	D
Biochemistry	M,D
Biological and Biomedical Sciences—General	M,D
Cell Biology	M,D
Clinical Laboratory Sciences/Medical Technology	M
Communication Disorders	M,D
Ecology	D
Entomology	M,D
Epidemiology	M,D
Evolutionary Biology	D
Genetics	M,D
Microbiology	M,D
Molecular Biology	M,D
Molecular Genetics	M,D
Neuroscience	M,D
Nursing—General	M,D
Nutrition	M,D
Osteopathic Medicine	D
Pathobiology	M,D
Pathology	M,D
Pharmacology	M,D
Physiology	M,D
Plant Biology	M,D
Plant Pathology	M,D
Public Health—General	M
Structural Biology	D
Systems Biology	D
Toxicology	M,D
Veterinary Medicine	D
Veterinary Sciences	M,D
Zoology	M,D

MICHIGAN TECHNOLOGICAL UNIVERSITY

Biochemistry	D
Biological and Biomedical Sciences—General	M,D
Ecology	M,D
Molecular Biology	D
Plant Molecular Biology	M,D

MIDDLE TENNESSEE SCHOOL OF ANESTHESIA

Nurse Anesthesia	M,D

MIDDLE TENNESSEE STATE UNIVERSITY

Biological and Biomedical Sciences—General	M
Family Nurse Practitioner Studies	M,O
Health Services Management and Hospital Administration	O
Molecular Biology	D
Nursing and Healthcare Administration	M
Nursing Education	M
Nursing—General	M,O

MIDWEST COLLEGE OF ORIENTAL MEDICINE

Acupuncture and Oriental Medicine	M,O

MIDWESTERN STATE UNIVERSITY

Biological and Biomedical Sciences—General	M
Community Health	M
Family Nurse Practitioner Studies	M
Health Physics/Radiological Health	M
Health Services Management and Hospital Administration	M
Nursing Education	M
Nursing—General	M
Psychiatric Nursing	M

MIDWESTERN UNIVERSITY, DOWNERS GROVE CAMPUS

Allied Health—General	D
Biological and Biomedical Sciences—General	M
Dentistry	D
Occupational Therapy	M
Osteopathic Medicine	D
Pharmacy	D
Physical Therapy	D
Physician Assistant Studies	M

MIDWESTERN UNIVERSITY, GLENDALE CAMPUS

Allied Health—General	M,D
Biological and Biomedical Sciences—General	M
Cardiovascular Sciences	M
Dentistry	D
Nurse Anesthesia	M
Occupational Therapy	M
Optometry	D
Osteopathic Medicine	D
Pharmacy	D
Physical Therapy	D
Physician Assistant Studies	M
Podiatric Medicine	D

MIDWIVES COLLEGE OF UTAH

Nurse Midwifery	M

MILLERSVILLE UNIVERSITY OF PENNSYLVANIA

Family Nurse Practitioner Studies	M
Nursing Education	M
Nursing—General	M

MILLIGAN COLLEGE

Occupational Therapy	M

MILLIKIN UNIVERSITY

Nurse Anesthesia	M,D
Nursing and Healthcare Administration	M,D
Nursing Education	M,D
Nursing—General	M,D

MILLS COLLEGE

Biological and Biomedical Sciences—General	O

MILWAUKEE SCHOOL OF ENGINEERING
Cardiovascular Sciences M
Clinical Laboratory Sciences/Medical Technology M
Health Services Management and Hospital Administration M
Perfusion M

MINNESOTA STATE UNIVERSITY MANKATO
Allied Health—General M,D,O
Biological and Biomedical Sciences—General M
Communication Disorders M
Community Health M,O
Family Nurse Practitioner Studies M,D
Nursing—General M,D

MINNESOTA STATE UNIVERSITY MOORHEAD
Communication Disorders M
Nursing Education M
Nursing—General M,O

MINOT STATE UNIVERSITY
Communication Disorders M

MISERICORDIA UNIVERSITY
Allied Health—General M,D
Communication Disorders M
Nursing—General M
Occupational Therapy M,D
Physical Therapy D

MISSISSIPPI COLLEGE
Biochemistry M
Biological and Biomedical Sciences—General M
Health Services Management and Hospital Administration M

MISSISSIPPI STATE UNIVERSITY
Biochemistry M,D
Biological and Biomedical Sciences—General M,D
Entomology M,D
Genetics M,D
Health Promotion M,D
Molecular Biology M,D
Nutrition M,D
Plant Pathology M,D
Veterinary Medicine D
Veterinary Sciences M,D

MISSISSIPPI UNIVERSITY FOR WOMEN
Communication Disorders M,O
Nursing—General M,O

MISSISSIPPI VALLEY STATE UNIVERSITY
Environmental and Occupational Health M

MISSOURI SOUTHERN STATE UNIVERSITY
Dental Hygiene M
Nursing—General M

MISSOURI STATE UNIVERSITY
Biological and Biomedical Sciences—General M
Cell Biology M
Communication Disorders M,D
Family Nurse Practitioner Studies M
Health Services Management and Hospital Administration M
Molecular Biology M
Nurse Anesthesia M
Nursing Education M
Nursing—General M
Physical Therapy D
Physician Assistant Studies M
Public Health—General M

MISSOURI UNIVERSITY OF SCIENCE AND TECHNOLOGY
Biological and Biomedical Sciences—General M
Environmental Biology M

MISSOURI WESTERN STATE UNIVERSITY
Biological and Biomedical Sciences—General M
Nursing and Healthcare Administration M
Nursing—General M

MOLLOY COLLEGE
Adult Nursing M,D,O
Communication Disorders M
Family Nurse Practitioner Studies M,D,O
Health Services Management and Hospital Administration M
Nursing and Healthcare Administration M,D,O
Nursing Education M,D,O
Nursing Informatics M,D,O
Nursing—General M,D,O
Pediatric Nursing M,D,O
Psychiatric Nursing M,D,O

MONMOUTH UNIVERSITY
Adult Nursing M,D,O
Communication Disorders M,O
Family Nurse Practitioner Studies M,D,O
Forensic Nursing M,D,O
Gerontological Nursing M,D,O
Nursing and Healthcare Administration M,D,O
Nursing Education M,D,O
Nursing—General M,D,O
Physician Assistant Studies M,D,O
Psychiatric Nursing M,D,O
School Nursing M,D,O

MONROE COLLEGE
Public Health—General M

MONTANA STATE UNIVERSITY
Biochemistry M,D
Biological and Biomedical Sciences—General M,D
Ecology M,D
Family Nurse Practitioner Studies M,O
Immunology M,D
Infectious Diseases M,D
Microbiology M,D
Neuroscience M,D
Nursing and Healthcare Administration M,O
Nursing Education M,O
Plant Pathology M,D
Psychiatric Nursing M,O

MONTANA STATE UNIVERSITY BILLINGS
Health Services Management and Hospital Administration M

MONTANA TECH OF THE UNIVERSITY OF MONTANA
Industrial Hygiene M

MONTCLAIR STATE UNIVERSITY
Biochemistry M
Biological and Biomedical Sciences—General M,O
Communication Disorders M,D
Ecology M,O
Evolutionary Biology M,O
Molecular Biology M,O
Nutrition M,O
Pharmacology M
Physiology M,O
Public Health—General M

MORAVIAN COLLEGE
Allied Health—General M
Health Services Management and Hospital Administration M
Nursing and Healthcare Administration M
Nursing Education M
Nursing—General M

MOREHEAD STATE UNIVERSITY
Biological and Biomedical Sciences—General M

MOREHOUSE SCHOOL OF MEDICINE
Allopathic Medicine D
Biological and Biomedical Sciences—General M,D
Clinical Research M
Epidemiology M
Health Promotion M
Health Services Management and Hospital Administration M
International Health M
Public Health—General M

MORGAN STATE UNIVERSITY
Biological and Biomedical Sciences—General M,D
Environmental Biology D
Nursing—General M
Public Health—General M,D

MOUNT ALLISON UNIVERSITY
Biological and Biomedical Sciences—General M

MOUNT CARMEL COLLEGE OF NURSING
Acute Care/Critical Care Nursing M
Adult Nursing M
Family Nurse Practitioner Studies M
Gerontological Nursing M
Nursing and Healthcare Administration M
Nursing Education M
Nursing—General M

MOUNT MARTY COLLEGE
Nurse Anesthesia M
Nursing—General M

MOUNT MARY UNIVERSITY
Nursing and Healthcare Administration M
Nutrition M
Occupational Therapy M

MOUNT ST. JOSEPH UNIVERSITY
Health Promotion M,O
Nursing and Healthcare Administration M
Nursing Education M
Nursing—General M,D
Physical Therapy D

MOUNT SAINT MARY COLLEGE
Adult Nursing M,O
Family Nurse Practitioner Studies M,O
Nursing and Healthcare Administration M,O
Nursing Education M,O
Nursing—General M,O

MOUNT ST. MARY'S COLLEGE
Nursing—General M,D,O
Physical Therapy M,D,O

MOUNT ST. MARY'S UNIVERSITY
Health Services Management and Hospital Administration M

MOUNT SAINT VINCENT UNIVERSITY
Nutrition M

MURRAY STATE UNIVERSITY
Biological and Biomedical Sciences—General M,D
Communication Disorders M
Environmental and Occupational Health M
Family Nurse Practitioner Studies M
Industrial Hygiene M
Nurse Anesthesia M
Nursing—General M

NATIONAL COLLEGE OF MIDWIFERY
Nurse Midwifery M,D

NATIONAL COLLEGE OF NATURAL MEDICINE
Acupuncture and Oriental Medicine M
Naturopathic Medicine M,D

NATIONAL UNIVERSITY
Biological and Biomedical Sciences—General M,O
Communication Disorders M,O
Forensic Nursing M,D,O
Health Promotion M,D,O
Health Services Management and Hospital Administration M,D,O
Nurse Anesthesia M,D,O
Nursing and Healthcare Administration M,D,O
Nursing Informatics M,D,O
Nursing—General M,D,O
Public Health—General M,D,O

NATIONAL UNIVERSITY OF HEALTH SCIENCES
Acupuncture and Oriental Medicine M,D
Chiropractic M,D
Health Services Management and Hospital Administration M
Medical Imaging M
Naturopathic Medicine M,D

NAZARETH COLLEGE OF ROCHESTER
Communication Disorders M
Gerontological Nursing M
Nursing—General M
Physical Therapy M,D

NEBRASKA METHODIST COLLEGE
Health Promotion M
Health Services Management and Hospital Administration M
Nursing and Healthcare Administration M
Nursing Education M
Nursing—General M

NEBRASKA WESLEYAN UNIVERSITY
Nursing—General M

NEUMANN UNIVERSITY
Nursing—General M
Physical Therapy D

NEW CHARTER UNIVERSITY
Health Services Management and Hospital Administration M

NEW ENGLAND COLLEGE
Health Services Management and Hospital Administration M

THE NEW ENGLAND COLLEGE OF OPTOMETRY
Optometry M,D
Vision Sciences M,D

NEW ENGLAND INSTITUTE OF TECHNOLOGY
Occupational Therapy M

NEW ENGLAND SCHOOL OF ACUPUNCTURE
Acupuncture and Oriental Medicine M

NEW JERSEY CITY UNIVERSITY
Allied Health—General M
Community Health M
Health Services Management and Hospital Administration M

NEW JERSEY INSTITUTE OF TECHNOLOGY
Biological and Biomedical Sciences—General M,D
Computational Biology M,D
Health Services Management and Hospital Administration M,D
Medicinal and Pharmaceutical Chemistry M,D
Pharmaceutical Administration M,D
Pharmacology M,D

NEWMAN UNIVERSITY
Nurse Anesthesia M

NEW MEXICO INSTITUTE OF MINING AND TECHNOLOGY
Biological and Biomedical Sciences—General M

NEW MEXICO STATE UNIVERSITY
Adult Nursing M,D
Biological and Biomedical Sciences—General M,D
Communication Disorders M,D
Community Health Nursing M,D
Community Health M
Entomology M
Family Nurse Practitioner Studies M,D
Gerontological Nursing M,D
Health Services Management and Hospital Administration M
Molecular Biology M,D
Nursing—General M,D
Nutrition M
Plant Pathology M
Public Health—General M

NEW YORK ACADEMY OF ART
Anatomy M

NEW YORK CHIROPRACTIC COLLEGE
Acupuncture and Oriental Medicine M
Anatomy M
Chiropractic D
Health Physics/Radiological Health M
Nutrition M

NEW YORK COLLEGE OF HEALTH PROFESSIONS
Acupuncture and Oriental Medicine M

NEW YORK COLLEGE OF PODIATRIC MEDICINE
Podiatric Medicine D

NEW YORK COLLEGE OF TRADITIONAL CHINESE MEDICINE
Acupuncture and Oriental Medicine M

NEW YORK INSTITUTE OF TECHNOLOGY
Nutrition M,O
Occupational Therapy M
Osteopathic Medicine M,D
Physical Therapy D
Physician Assistant Studies M

NEW YORK MEDICAL COLLEGE
Allopathic Medicine D
Anatomy M,D
Biochemistry M,D
Biological and Biomedical Sciences—General M,D*
Cell Biology M,D
Communication Disorders M
Environmental and Occupational Health M,O
Epidemiology M
Health Promotion M,O
Health Services Management and Hospital Administration M,D,O
Immunology M,D
Industrial Hygiene O
International Health O
Microbiology M,D
Molecular Biology M,D
Pathology M,D
Pharmacology M,D
Physical Therapy D
Physiology M,D
Public Health—General M,D,O

NEW YORK UNIVERSITY
Acute Care/Critical Care Nursing M,D,O
Adult Nursing M,D,O
Allopathic Medicine M,D
Bioethics M
Biological and Biomedical Sciences—General M,D
Cancer Biology/Oncology M,D
Cell Biology D
Clinical Research M
Communication Disorders M,D
Community Health M
Computational Biology D
Dentistry D
Developmental Biology M,D
Environmental and Occupational Health M,D
Epidemiology M,D
Family Nurse Practitioner Studies M,D,O
Genetics M,D
Gerontological Nursing M,D,O
Health Promotion M,D,O
Health Services Management and Hospital Administration M,O
Immunology M,D
International Health M
Medical Imaging D
Microbiology M,D
Molecular Biology M,D
Molecular Biophysics D
Molecular Genetics M,D
Molecular Pharmacology D
Molecular Toxicology M,D
Neurobiology M,D
Neuroscience D
Nurse Midwifery M,D,O
Nursing Education M,O
Nursing Informatics M,O
Nursing—General M,D,O
Nutrition M,D
Occupational Therapy M,D
Oral and Dental Sciences M,D,O
Pathobiology D
Pediatric Nursing M,D,O
Physical Therapy M,D,O
Physiology D
Plant Biology M,D
Psychiatric Nursing M,D,O
Public Health—General M
Structural Biology D
Toxicology M,D

NICHOLLS STATE UNIVERSITY
Environmental Biology M
Family Nurse Practitioner Studies M
Marine Biology M
Nursing and Healthcare Administration M
Nursing—General M
Psychiatric Nursing M

NORTH CAROLINA AGRICULTURAL AND TECHNICAL STATE UNIVERSITY
Biological and Biomedical Sciences—General M

*M—masters degree; D—doctorate; O—other advanced degree; *—Close-Up and/or Display*

Program	Degrees
Environmental and Occupational Health	M
Nutrition	M

NORTH CAROLINA CENTRAL UNIVERSITY

Program	Degrees
Biological and Biomedical Sciences—General	M
Communication Disorders	M

NORTH CAROLINA STATE UNIVERSITY

Program	Degrees
Biochemistry	D
Biological and Biomedical Sciences—General	M,D,O
Botany	M,D
Cell Biology	M,D
Entomology	M,D
Epidemiology	M,D
Genetics	M,D
Genomic Sciences	M,D
Immunology	M,D
Infectious Diseases	M,D
Microbiology	M,D
Molecular Toxicology	M,D
Nutrition	M,D
Pathology	M,D
Pharmacology	M,D
Physiology	M,D
Plant Biology	M,D
Plant Pathology	M,D
Toxicology	M,D
Veterinary Medicine	M,D
Veterinary Sciences	M,D
Zoology	M,D

NORTH DAKOTA STATE UNIVERSITY

Program	Degrees
Biochemistry	M,D
Biological and Biomedical Sciences—General	M,D
Botany	M,D
Cell Biology	M,D
Ecology	M,D
Entomology	M,D
Epidemiology	M,D
Genomic Sciences	M,D
International Health	M,D
Microbiology	M,D
Molecular Biology	M,D
Molecular Pathogenesis	M,D
Nursing—General	M,D
Nutrition	M
Pathology	M,D
Pharmaceutical Sciences	M,D
Plant Pathology	M,D
Public Health—General	M,D
Veterinary Sciences	M,D
Zoology	M,D

NORTHEASTERN ILLINOIS UNIVERSITY

Program	Degrees
Biological and Biomedical Sciences—General	M

NORTHEASTERN STATE UNIVERSITY

Program	Degrees
Communication Disorders	M
Environmental and Occupational Health	M
Nursing Education	M
Occupational Therapy	M
Optometry	D

NORTHEASTERN UNIVERSITY

Program	Degrees
Acute Care/Critical Care Nursing	M,D,O
Allied Health—General	M,D,O
Biological and Biomedical Sciences—General	M,D
Communication Disorders	M,D,O
Marine Biology	M,D
Nursing and Healthcare Administration	M,D,O
Nursing—General	M,D,O
Nutrition	M
Pharmaceutical Sciences	M,D,O
Pharmacology	M,D,O
Physical Therapy	M,D,O
Physician Assistant Studies	M,D,O
Psychiatric Nursing	M,D,O
Public Health—General	M,D,O

NORTHEAST OHIO MEDICAL UNIVERSITY

Program	Degrees
Allopathic Medicine	D
Bioethics	M,D,O
Health Services Management and Hospital Administration	M,D,O
Pharmaceutical Administration	M,D,O
Pharmaceutical Sciences	M,D,O
Pharmacy	D
Public Health—General	M,D,O

NORTHERN ARIZONA UNIVERSITY

Program	Degrees
Allied Health—General	M,D,O
Biological and Biomedical Sciences—General	M,D
Communication Disorders	M
Family Nurse Practitioner Studies	M,D,O
Health Services Management and Hospital Administration	O
Nursing—General	M,D,O
Physical Therapy	D
Physician Assistant Studies	M
Public Health—General	O

NORTHERN ILLINOIS UNIVERSITY

Program	Degrees
Biological and Biomedical Sciences—General	M,D
Communication Disorders	M,D
Nursing—General	M
Nutrition	M
Physical Therapy	M,D
Public Health—General	M

NORTHERN KENTUCKY UNIVERSITY

Program	Degrees
Nursing—General	M,D,O

NORTHERN MICHIGAN UNIVERSITY

Program	Degrees
Biochemistry	M
Biological and Biomedical Sciences—General	M
Family Nurse Practitioner Studies	D
Health Services Management and Hospital Administration	M
Nursing—General	D

NORTH PARK UNIVERSITY

Program	Degrees
Adult Nursing	M
Nursing and Healthcare Administration	M
Nursing—General	M

NORTHWESTERN HEALTH SCIENCES UNIVERSITY

Program	Degrees
Acupuncture and Oriental Medicine	M
Chiropractic	D

NORTHWESTERN STATE UNIVERSITY OF LOUISIANA

Program	Degrees
Health Physics/Radiological Health	M
Nursing—General	M

NORTHWESTERN UNIVERSITY

Program	Degrees
Allopathic Medicine	
Biochemistry	D
Biological and Biomedical Sciences—General	D
Biophysics	D
Biopsychology	D
Cell Biology	D
Clinical Laboratory Sciences/Medical Technology	M
Clinical Research	M,O
Communication Disorders	M,D
Developmental Biology	D
Epidemiology	D
Health Services Management and Hospital Administration	M,D
Health Services Research	D
International Health	M
Molecular Biology	D
Neurobiology	M,D
Neuroscience	D
Physical Therapy	D
Physiology	M
Plant Biology	M,D
Public Health—General	M
Rehabilitation Sciences	D
Structural Biology	D
Systems Biology	D

NORTHWEST MISSOURI STATE UNIVERSITY

Program	Degrees
Biological and Biomedical Sciences—General	M

NORTHWEST NAZARENE UNIVERSITY

Program	Degrees
Health Services Management and Hospital Administration	M
Nursing and Healthcare Administration	M

NORWICH UNIVERSITY

Program	Degrees
Nursing and Healthcare Administration	M
Nursing Education	M
Nursing—General	M

NOTRE DAME DE NAMUR UNIVERSITY

Program	Degrees
Biological and Biomedical Sciences—General	O

NOVA SOUTHEASTERN UNIVERSITY

Program	Degrees
Allied Health—General	M,D
Biological and Biomedical Sciences—General	M,D,O
Communication Disorders	M,D,O
Dentistry	M,D,O
Marine Biology	M,D,O
Nursing Education	M,D
Nursing—General	M,D
Occupational Therapy	M,D
Optometry	M,D
Osteopathic Medicine	M,D,O
Pharmacology	M,D,O
Pharmacy	D*
Physical Therapy	M,D
Physician Assistant Studies	M,D
Public Health—General	M,D,O
Vision Sciences	M,D

OAKLAND UNIVERSITY

Program	Degrees
Adult Nursing	M
Allied Health—General	M,D,O
Biological and Biomedical Sciences—General	M,D
Environmental and Occupational Health	M
Family Nurse Practitioner Studies	M,O
Gerontological Nursing	M,O
Health Promotion	O
Maternal and Child Health	M,D,O
Medical Physics	M,D
Nurse Anesthesia	M,O
Nursing Education	M,O
Nursing—General	M,D,O
Physical Therapy	M,D,O

OCCIDENTAL COLLEGE

Program	Degrees
Biological and Biomedical Sciences—General	M

OHIO DOMINICAN UNIVERSITY

Program	Degrees
Physician Assistant Studies	M

OHIO NORTHERN UNIVERSITY

Program	Degrees
Pharmacy	D

THE OHIO STATE UNIVERSITY

Program	Degrees
Allied Health—General	M
Allopathic Medicine	D
Anatomy	M,D
Biochemistry	M,D
Biological and Biomedical Sciences—General	M,D
Biophysics	M,D
Cell Biology	M,D
Communication Disorders	M,D
Dental Hygiene	M,D
Dentistry	M,D
Developmental Biology	M,D
Ecology	M,D
Entomology	M,D
Evolutionary Biology	M,D
Genetics	M,D
Health Services Management and Hospital Administration	M,D
Immunology	D
Microbiology	M,D
Molecular Biology	M,D
Molecular Genetics	M,D
Neuroscience	D
Nursing—General	M,D
Nutrition	M,D
Occupational Therapy	M
Optometry	M,D
Oral and Dental Sciences	M,D
Pathobiology	M
Pathology	M
Pharmaceutical Administration	M,D
Pharmacology	M,D
Pharmacy	M,D
Physical Therapy	D
Plant Pathology	M,D
Public Health—General	M,D
Rehabilitation Sciences	M,D
Veterinary Sciences	M,D
Virology	D

OHIO UNIVERSITY

Program	Degrees
Acute Care/Critical Care Nursing	M
Biochemistry	M,D
Biological and Biomedical Sciences—General	M,D
Cell Biology	M,D
Communication Disorders	M,D
Ecology	M,D
Environmental Biology	M,D
Evolutionary Biology	M,D
Family Nurse Practitioner Studies	M
Health Services Management and Hospital Administration	M
Microbiology	M,D
Molecular Biology	M,D
Neuroscience	M,D
Nursing and Healthcare Administration	M
Nursing Education	M
Nursing—General	M
Nutrition	M
Osteopathic Medicine	D
Physical Therapy	D
Physiology	M,D
Plant Biology	M,D
Public Health—General	M

OKLAHOMA BAPTIST UNIVERSITY

Program	Degrees
Nursing Education	M
Nursing—General	M

OKLAHOMA CHRISTIAN UNIVERSITY

Program	Degrees
Health Services Management and Hospital Administration	M

OKLAHOMA CITY UNIVERSITY

Program	Degrees
Health Services Management and Hospital Administration	M,D
Nursing Education	M,D
Nursing—General	M,D

OKLAHOMA STATE UNIVERSITY

Program	Degrees
Biochemistry	M,D
Botany	M,D
Communication Disorders	M
Entomology	M,D
Microbiology	M,D
Molecular Biology	M,D
Molecular Genetics	M,D
Nutrition	M,D
Plant Pathology	M,D
Toxicology	M,D,O
Veterinary Medicine	D
Veterinary Sciences	M,D
Zoology	M,D

OKLAHOMA STATE UNIVERSITY CENTER FOR HEALTH SCIENCES

Program	Degrees
Biological and Biomedical Sciences—General	M,D
Health Services Management and Hospital Administration	M
Microbiology	M
Molecular Biology	M
Osteopathic Medicine	D
Pathology	M
Toxicology	M

OLD DOMINION UNIVERSITY

Program	Degrees
Allied Health—General	M,D
Biochemistry	M,D
Biological and Biomedical Sciences—General	M,D
Communication Disorders	M
Dental Hygiene	M
Ecology	D
Environmental and Occupational Health	M
Family Nurse Practitioner Studies	M,D
Health Promotion	M
Health Services Management and Hospital Administration	M
Health Services Research	D
Nurse Anesthesia	M
Nurse Midwifery	M,D
Nursing and Healthcare Administration	M,D
Nursing Education	M
Nursing—General	M,D
Physical Therapy	D
Public Health—General	M
Women's Health Nursing	M,D

OREGON COLLEGE OF ORIENTAL MEDICINE

Program	Degrees
Acupuncture and Oriental Medicine	M,D

OREGON HEALTH & SCIENCE UNIVERSITY

Program	Degrees
Allopathic Medicine	D
Biochemistry	M,D
Biological and Biomedical Sciences—General	M,D,O
Biopsychology	D
Cancer Biology/Oncology	D
Cell Biology	D
Clinical Research	M,O
Community Health Nursing	M,O
Computational Biology	M,D,O
Dentistry	D,O
Developmental Biology	D
Epidemiology	M,O
Family Nurse Practitioner Studies	M,O
Genetics	D
Gerontological Nursing	O
Health Services Management and Hospital Administration	M
Immunology	D
Microbiology	D
Molecular Biology	M,D
Neuroscience	D
Nurse Anesthesia	M
Nurse Midwifery	M,O
Nursing Education	M,O
Nursing—General	M,D,O
Nutrition	M,O
Oral and Dental Sciences	M,D,O
Pharmacology	D
Physician Assistant Studies	M
Physiology	D
Psychiatric Nursing	M,O

OREGON STATE UNIVERSITY

Program	Degrees
Allied Health—General	M,D
Biochemistry	M,D
Biophysics	M,D
Botany	M
Cell Biology	M,D
Environmental and Occupational Health	M,D
Epidemiology	M,D
Health Physics/Radiological Health	M,D
Health Promotion	M,D
Health Services Management and Hospital Administration	M,D
International Health	M,D
Medical Physics	M,D
Microbiology	M,D
Molecular Biology	M,D
Nutrition	M,D
Pharmaceutical Sciences	M,D
Pharmacy	D
Public Health—General	M,D
Toxicology	M,D
Veterinary Medicine	D
Veterinary Sciences	M,D
Zoology	M,D

OTTERBEIN UNIVERSITY

Program	Degrees
Family Nurse Practitioner Studies	M,D,O
Nurse Anesthesia	M,D,O
Nursing and Healthcare Administration	M,D,O
Nursing Education	M,D,O
Nursing—General	M,D,O

OUR LADY OF THE LAKE COLLEGE

Program	Degrees
Health Services Management and Hospital Administration	M
Nurse Anesthesia	M
Nursing and Healthcare Administration	M
Nursing Education	M
Nursing—General	M
Physician Assistant Studies	M

OUR LADY OF THE LAKE UNIVERSITY OF SAN ANTONIO

Program	Degrees
Communication Disorders	M
Health Services Management and Hospital Administration	M
Nursing and Healthcare Administration	M
Nursing Education	M
Nursing—General	M

PACE UNIVERSITY

Program	Degrees
Family Nurse Practitioner Studies	M,D,O
Health Services Management and Hospital Administration	M
Nursing and Healthcare Administration	M,D,O
Nursing Education	M,D,O
Nursing—General	M,D,O
Physician Assistant Studies	M

PACIFIC COLLEGE OF ORIENTAL MEDICINE

Program	Degrees
Acupuncture and Oriental Medicine	M,D

PACIFIC COLLEGE OF ORIENTAL MEDICINE–CHICAGO

Program	Degrees
Acupuncture and Oriental Medicine	M

PACIFIC COLLEGE OF ORIENTAL MEDICINE-NEW YORK

Program	Degrees
Acupuncture and Oriental Medicine	M

PACIFIC LUTHERAN UNIVERSITY

Program	Degrees
Family Nurse Practitioner Studies	M
Nursing and Healthcare Administration	M
Nursing—General	M

PACIFIC UNIVERSITY

Program	Degrees
Health Services Management and Hospital Administration	M
Occupational Therapy	M
Pharmacy	D
Physical Therapy	D
Physician Assistant Studies	M

PALM BEACH ATLANTIC UNIVERSITY

Program	Degrees
Pharmacy	D

PALMER COLLEGE OF CHIROPRACTIC
- Anatomy M
- Chiropractic D
- Clinical Research M

PALO ALTO UNIVERSITY
- Biopsychology D

PARKER UNIVERSITY
- Chiropractic D

PARK UNIVERSITY
- Health Services Management and Hospital Administration M,O
- International Health M,O

PENN STATE HARRISBURG
- Health Services Management and Hospital Administration M,D

PENN STATE HERSHEY MEDICAL CENTER
- Allopathic Medicine M,D
- Anatomy M,D
- Biochemistry M,D
- Biological and Biomedical Sciences—General M,D
- Health Services Research M
- Immunology M,D
- Molecular Genetics M,D
- Neuroscience M,D
- Public Health—General M
- Veterinary Sciences M
- Virology M,D

PENN STATE UNIVERSITY PARK
- Biochemistry M,D
- Biological and Biomedical Sciences—General M,D
- Biopsychology M,D
- Cell Biology M,D
- Communication Disorders M,D,O
- Developmental Biology M,D
- Ecology M,D
- Entomology M,D
- Genetics M,D
- Health Services Management and Hospital Administration M,D
- Immunology M,D
- Infectious Diseases M,D
- Microbiology M,D
- Molecular Biology M,D
- Molecular Medicine M,D
- Nursing—General M,D
- Nutrition M,D
- Pathobiology M,D
- Physiology M,D
- Plant Biology M,D
- Plant Pathology M,D
- Veterinary Sciences M,D

PFEIFFER UNIVERSITY
- Health Services Management and Hospital Administration M

PHILADELPHIA COLLEGE OF OSTEOPATHIC MEDICINE
- Biological and Biomedical Sciences—General M
- Biopsychology M,D,O
- Osteopathic Medicine D
- Pharmacy D
- Physician Assistant Studies M*

PHILADELPHIA UNIVERSITY
- Nurse Midwifery M,O
- Occupational Therapy M,D
- Physician Assistant Studies M

PIEDMONT COLLEGE
- Nursing and Healthcare Administration M
- Nursing Education M
- Nursing—General M

PITTSBURG STATE UNIVERSITY
- Biological and Biomedical Sciences—General M
- Nursing—General M

PLYMOUTH STATE UNIVERSITY
- Biological and Biomedical Sciences—General M
- Health Promotion M

POINT LOMA NAZARENE UNIVERSITY
- Biological and Biomedical Sciences—General M
- Family Nurse Practitioner Studies M,O
- Gerontological Nursing M,O
- Health Services Management and Hospital Administration M
- Maternal and Child/Neonatal Nursing M,O
- Nursing—General M,O
- Psychiatric Nursing M,O

PONCE SCHOOL OF MEDICINE & HEALTH SCIENCES
- Allopathic Medicine D
- Biological and Biomedical Sciences—General D
- Epidemiology M,D
- Public Health—General M,D

PONTIFICAL CATHOLIC UNIVERSITY OF PUERTO RICO
- Biological and Biomedical Sciences—General M
- Clinical Laboratory Sciences/Medical Technology O
- Medical/Surgical Nursing M
- Nursing—General M
- Psychiatric Nursing M

PONTIFICIA UNIVERSIDAD CATOLICA MADRE Y MAESTRA
- Allopathic Medicine D

PORTLAND STATE UNIVERSITY
- Biological and Biomedical Sciences—General M,D
- Communication Disorders M
- Health Promotion M,O
- Health Services Management and Hospital Administration M
- Public Health—General M,O

POST UNIVERSITY
- Health Services Management and Hospital Administration M

PRAIRIE VIEW A&M UNIVERSITY
- Biological and Biomedical Sciences—General M
- Family Nurse Practitioner Studies M
- Nursing and Healthcare Administration M
- Nursing Education M
- Nursing—General M
- Toxicology M

PRINCETON UNIVERSITY
- Computational Biology D
- Ecology D
- Evolutionary Biology D
- Marine Biology D
- Molecular Biology D
- Neuroscience D

PURDUE UNIVERSITY
- Allied Health—General M,D
- Anatomy M,D
- Biochemistry M,D
- Biological and Biomedical Sciences—General M,D
- Biophysics M,D
- Botany M,D
- Cancer Biology/Oncology D
- Cell Biology M,D
- Communication Disorders M,D
- Developmental Biology M,D
- Ecology M,D
- Entomology M,D
- Environmental and Occupational Health M,D
- Epidemiology M,D
- Evolutionary Biology M,D
- Genetics M,D
- Genomic Sciences D
- Health Physics/Radiological Health M,D
- Immunology M,D
- Medical Physics M,D
- Medicinal and Pharmaceutical Chemistry D
- Microbiology M,D
- Molecular Biology M,D
- Molecular Pharmacology D
- Neurobiology M,D
- Neuroscience D
- Nutrition M,D
- Pathobiology M,D
- Pathology M,D
- Pharmaceutical Administration M,D,O
- Pharmaceutical Sciences M,D
- Pharmacology M,D
- Pharmacy D
- Physiology M,D
- Plant Pathology M,D
- Plant Physiology M,D
- Public Health—General M,D
- Systems Biology D
- Toxicology M,D
- Veterinary Medicine D
- Veterinary Sciences M,D
- Virology M,D

PURDUE UNIVERSITY CALUMET
- Acute Care/Critical Care Nursing M
- Adult Nursing M
- Biological and Biomedical Sciences—General M
- Family Nurse Practitioner Studies M
- Nursing and Healthcare Administration M
- Nursing—General M

QUEENS COLLEGE OF THE CITY UNIVERSITY OF NEW YORK
- Biochemistry M
- Biological and Biomedical Sciences—General M
- Communication Disorders M

QUEEN'S UNIVERSITY AT KINGSTON
- Allopathic Medicine D
- Anatomy M,D
- Biochemistry M,D
- Biological and Biomedical Sciences—General M,D
- Cancer Biology/Oncology M,D
- Cardiovascular Sciences M,D
- Cell Biology M,D
- Epidemiology M,D
- Family Nurse Practitioner Studies M,D,O
- Health Services Management and Hospital Administration M,D
- Immunology M,D
- Microbiology M,D
- Molecular Biology M,D
- Molecular Medicine M,D
- Neurobiology M,D
- Neuroscience M,D
- Nursing—General M,D,O
- Occupational Therapy M,D
- Pathology M,D
- Pediatric Nursing M,D,O
- Pharmaceutical Sciences M,D
- Pharmacology M,D
- Physical Therapy M,D
- Physiology M,D
- Public Health—General M,D
- Rehabilitation Sciences M,D
- Reproductive Biology M,D
- Toxicology M,D
- Women's Health Nursing M,D,O

QUEENS UNIVERSITY OF CHARLOTTE
- Nursing and Healthcare Administration M
- Nursing—General M

QUINNIPIAC UNIVERSITY
- Adult Nursing M,D
- Allied Health—General M,D
- Anesthesiologist Assistant Studies M
- Biological and Biomedical Sciences—General M
- Cardiovascular Sciences M
- Cell Biology M
- Clinical Laboratory Sciences/Medical Technology M
- Community Health D
- Family Nurse Practitioner Studies M,D
- Health Physics/Radiological Health M
- Microbiology M
- Molecular Biology M
- Nursing—General M,D
- Occupational Therapy M
- Pathology M
- Perfusion M
- Physical Therapy D
- Physician Assistant Studies M

RADFORD UNIVERSITY
- Communication Disorders M
- Nursing—General M,D
- Occupational Therapy M
- Physical Therapy D

RAMAPO COLLEGE OF NEW JERSEY
- Nursing Education M
- Nursing—General M

REGIS COLLEGE (MA)
- Biological and Biomedical Sciences—General M,D,O
- Family Nurse Practitioner Studies M,D,O
- Health Services Management and Hospital Administration M,D,O
- Nursing Education M,D,O
- Nursing—General M,D,O

REGIS UNIVERSITY
- Allied Health—General M,D,O
- Biological and Biomedical Sciences—General M
- Health Services Management and Hospital Administration M,O
- Pharmacy D

RENSSELAER POLYTECHNIC INSTITUTE
- Biochemistry M,D
- Biological and Biomedical Sciences—General M,D
- Biophysics M,D

RESEARCH COLLEGE OF NURSING
- Adult Nursing M
- Family Nurse Practitioner Studies M
- Gerontological Nursing M
- Nursing and Healthcare Administration M
- Nursing Education M
- Nursing—General M

RESURRECTION UNIVERSITY
- Nursing—General M

RHODE ISLAND COLLEGE
- Biological and Biomedical Sciences—General M,O
- Nursing—General M

RICE UNIVERSITY
- Biochemistry M,D
- Cell Biology M,D
- Ecology M,D
- Evolutionary Biology M,D
- Health Services Management and Hospital Administration M

THE RICHARD STOCKTON COLLEGE OF NEW JERSEY
- Communication Disorders M
- Nursing—General M
- Occupational Therapy M
- Physical Therapy D

RIVIER UNIVERSITY
- Family Nurse Practitioner Studies M
- Nursing Education M
- Nursing—General M
- Psychiatric Nursing M

ROBERT MORRIS UNIVERSITY
- Nursing—General M,D

ROBERT MORRIS UNIVERSITY ILLINOIS
- Health Services Management and Hospital Administration M

ROBERTS WESLEYAN COLLEGE
- Health Services Management and Hospital Administration M
- Nursing and Healthcare Administration M
- Nursing Education M
- Nursing—General M

ROCHESTER INSTITUTE OF TECHNOLOGY
- Biological and Biomedical Sciences—General M
- Environmental and Occupational Health M
- Health Services Management and Hospital Administration M,O

THE ROCKEFELLER UNIVERSITY
- Biological and Biomedical Sciences—General M,D*

ROCKHURST UNIVERSITY
- Communication Disorders M
- Occupational Therapy M
- Physical Therapy D

ROCKY MOUNTAIN COLLEGE
- Physician Assistant Studies M

ROCKY MOUNTAIN UNIVERSITY OF HEALTH PROFESSIONS
- Family Nurse Practitioner Studies D
- Occupational Therapy D
- Physical Therapy D
- Physiology D

ROGER WILLIAMS UNIVERSITY
- Health Services Management and Hospital Administration M

ROOSEVELT UNIVERSITY
- Pharmacy D

ROSALIND FRANKLIN UNIVERSITY OF MEDICINE AND SCIENCE
- Allied Health—General M,D,O
- Allopathic Medicine D
- Anatomy M,D
- Biochemistry M,D
- Biological and Biomedical Sciences—General M,D
- Biophysics M,D
- Cell Biology M,D
- Health Services Management and Hospital Administration M,O
- Immunology M,D
- Medical Physics M
- Microbiology M,D
- Molecular Biology M,D
- Molecular Pharmacology M,D
- Neuroscience D
- Nurse Anesthesia M
- Nutrition M
- Pathology M
- Physical Therapy M,D
- Physician Assistant Studies M
- Physiology M,D
- Podiatric Medicine D
- Women's Health Nursing M,O

ROSEMAN UNIVERSITY OF HEALTH SCIENCES
- Dentistry M,D,O
- Pharmacy D

ROWAN UNIVERSITY
- Biological and Biomedical Sciences—General M
- Health Promotion M
- Osteopathic Medicine D
- School Nursing M,O

ROYAL ROADS UNIVERSITY
- Health Services Management and Hospital Administration O

RUSH UNIVERSITY
- Adult Nursing D
- Allopathic Medicine D
- Anatomy M,D
- Biochemistry M,D
- Bioethics M,O
- Cell Biology M,D
- Clinical Laboratory Sciences/Medical Technology M
- Communication Disorders M,D
- Community Health Nursing D,O
- Family Nurse Practitioner Studies D,O
- Gerontological Nursing D
- Health Services Management and Hospital Administration M,D
- Immunology M,D
- Maternal and Child/Neonatal Nursing D,O
- Medical Physics M,D
- Microbiology M,D
- Neuroscience M,D
- Nurse Anesthesia D
- Nursing and Healthcare Administration M
- Nursing—General M,D,O
- Nutrition M
- Occupational Therapy M
- Pediatric Nursing D,O
- Pharmaceutical Sciences M,D
- Pharmacology M,D
- Physician Assistant Studies M
- Physiology D
- Psychiatric Nursing D,O
- Virology M,D

RUTGERS, THE STATE UNIVERSITY OF NEW JERSEY, CAMDEN
- Biological and Biomedical Sciences—General M
- Computational Biology M,D
- Health Services Management and Hospital Administration M,O
- Physical Therapy D
- Public Health—General M,O

RUTGERS, THE STATE UNIVERSITY OF NEW JERSEY, NEWARK
- Adult Nursing M,D,O
- Allied Health—General M,D,O
- Allopathic Medicine D
- Biochemistry M,D

*M—masters degree; D—doctorate; O—other advanced degree; *—Close-Up and/or Display*

Biological and Biomedical Sciences—General M,D,O
Biopsychology D
Cancer Biology/Oncology D,O
Cell Biology D
Clinical Laboratory Sciences/Medical Technology M
Computational Biology M
Dentistry M,D,O
Developmental Biology D,O
Epidemiology M,O
Family Nurse Practitioner Studies M,D,O
Health Physics/Radiological Health M
Health Services Management and Hospital Administration M,D,O
Immunology D
Infectious Diseases D,O
Medical Imaging M
Microbiology D
Molecular Biology M,D
Molecular Genetics D
Molecular Medicine D
Molecular Pathology D
Neuroscience D
Nurse Anesthesia M,D,O
Nursing Informatics M
Nursing—General M,D,O
Nutrition M,D,O
Occupational Health Nursing M,D,O
Oral and Dental Sciences M,D,O
Pathology D
Pharmacology D
Physical Therapy D
Physician Assistant Studies M
Physiology D
Public Health—General M,O
Transcultural Nursing M,D,O
Women's Health Nursing M,D,O

RUTGERS, THE STATE UNIVERSITY OF NEW JERSEY, NEW BRUNSWICK

Allopathic Medicine D
Biochemistry M,D
Biological and Biomedical Sciences—General M,D
Biopsychology D
Cancer Biology/Oncology M,D
Cell Biology M,D
Clinical Laboratory Sciences/Medical Technology M
Computational Biology D
Developmental Biology M,D
Ecology M,D
Entomology M,D
Environmental and Occupational Health M,D,O
Environmental Biology M,D
Epidemiology M,D,O
Evolutionary Biology M,D
Genetics M,D
Health Services Management and Hospital Administration M,D,O
Immunology M,D
Marine Biology M,D
Medical Microbiology M,D
Medicinal and Pharmaceutical Chemistry M,D
Microbiology M,D
Molecular Biology M,D
Molecular Biophysics D
Molecular Genetics M,D
Molecular Pharmacology M,D
Molecular Physiology M,D
Neuroscience M,D
Nutrition M,D
Pharmaceutical Sciences M,D
Pharmacy M,D
Physiology M,D
Plant Biology M,D
Plant Molecular Biology M,D
Plant Pathology M,D
Public Health—General M,D,O
Reproductive Biology M,D
Systems Biology D
Toxicology M,D
Translational Biology M
Virology M,D

SACRED HEART UNIVERSITY

Family Nurse Practitioner Studies M,D
Health Services Management and Hospital Administration M,D
Nursing and Healthcare Administration M,D
Nursing Education M,D
Nursing—General M,D
Occupational Therapy M
Physical Therapy D

SAGE GRADUATE SCHOOL

Adult Nursing M,O
Community Health Nursing M,O
Community Health M,O
Family Nurse Practitioner Studies M,O
Gerontological Nursing M,D,O
Health Services Management and Hospital Administration M,D,O
Nursing and Healthcare Administration M,D,O
Nursing Education D
Nursing—General M,D,O
Nutrition M,O
Occupational Therapy M
Physical Therapy D
Psychiatric Nursing M,O

SAGINAW VALLEY STATE UNIVERSITY

Family Nurse Practitioner Studies M,D
Health Services Management and Hospital Administration M
Nursing and Healthcare Administration M
Nursing—General M
Occupational Therapy M

ST. AMBROSE UNIVERSITY

Communication Disorders M
Health Services Management and Hospital Administration M,D
Nursing—General M
Occupational Therapy M
Physical Therapy D

SAINT ANTHONY COLLEGE OF NURSING

Nursing—General M

ST. CATHARINE COLLEGE

Health Promotion M

ST. CATHERINE UNIVERSITY

Adult Nursing M,D
Gerontological Nursing M,D
Maternal and Child/Neonatal Nursing M,D
Nursing Education M,D
Nursing—General M,D
Occupational Therapy M,D
Pediatric Nursing M,D
Physical Therapy D
Physician Assistant Studies M
Public Health—General M

ST. CLOUD STATE UNIVERSITY

Biological and Biomedical Sciences—General M
Communication Disorders M

SAINT FRANCIS MEDICAL CENTER COLLEGE OF NURSING

Family Nurse Practitioner Studies M,D,O
Gerontological Nursing M,D,O
Maternal and Child/Neonatal Nursing M,D,O
Medical/Surgical Nursing M,D,O
Nursing and Healthcare Administration M,D,O
Nursing Education M,D,O
Nursing—General M,D,O
Psychiatric Nursing M,D,O

SAINT FRANCIS UNIVERSITY

Biological and Biomedical Sciences—General M
Occupational Therapy M
Physical Therapy D
Physician Assistant Studies M

ST. FRANCIS XAVIER UNIVERSITY

Biological and Biomedical Sciences—General M

ST. JOHN FISHER COLLEGE

Family Nurse Practitioner Studies M,O
Nursing Education M,O
Nursing—General M,D,O
Pharmacy D

ST. JOHN'S UNIVERSITY (NY)

Biological and Biomedical Sciences—General M,D
Communication Disorders M,D
Pharmaceutical Administration M
Pharmaceutical Sciences M,D
Public Health—General M
Toxicology M

ST. JOSEPH'S COLLEGE, LONG ISLAND CAMPUS

Health Services Management and Hospital Administration M,O
Nursing—General M

ST. JOSEPH'S COLLEGE, NEW YORK

Health Services Management and Hospital Administration M
Nursing—General M

SAINT JOSEPH'S COLLEGE OF MAINE

Family Nurse Practitioner Studies M,O
Health Services Management and Hospital Administration M
Nursing and Healthcare Administration M,O
Nursing Education M,O
Nursing—General M,O

SAINT JOSEPH'S UNIVERSITY

Biological and Biomedical Sciences—General M
Environmental and Occupational Health M,O
Health Services Management and Hospital Administration M,O
Nurse Anesthesia M,O
Nursing and Healthcare Administration M,O
School Nursing M,O

SAINT LEO UNIVERSITY

Health Services Management and Hospital Administration M

ST. LOUIS COLLEGE OF PHARMACY

Pharmacy D

SAINT LOUIS UNIVERSITY

Allied Health—General M,D,O
Allopathic Medicine D
Anatomy M,D
Biochemistry D
Bioethics D,O
Biological and Biomedical Sciences—General M,D
Communication Disorders M
Community Health M
Dentistry M
Health Services Management and Hospital Administration M,D
Immunology D
Microbiology D
Molecular Biology D
Nursing—General M,D,O
Nutrition M
Occupational Therapy M
Oral and Dental Sciences M
Pathology D
Pharmacology D
Physical Therapy M,D
Physician Assistant Studies M
Physiology D
Public Health—General M,D

SAINT MARY'S UNIVERSITY OF MINNESOTA

Environmental and Occupational Health M
Health Services Management and Hospital Administration M
Nurse Anesthesia M

SAINT PETER'S UNIVERSITY

Adult Nursing M,D,O
Health Services Management and Hospital Administration M
Nursing and Healthcare Administration M,D,O
Nursing—General M,D,O

ST. THOMAS UNIVERSITY

Health Services Management and Hospital Administration M,O

SAINT VINCENT COLLEGE

Nurse Anesthesia M
Nursing and Healthcare Administration M

SAINT XAVIER UNIVERSITY

Communication Disorders M
Health Services Management and Hospital Administration M,O
Nursing—General M,O

SALEM STATE UNIVERSITY

Gerontological Nursing M
Nursing and Healthcare Administration M
Nursing Education M
Nursing—General M
Occupational Therapy M

SALISBURY UNIVERSITY

Biological and Biomedical Sciences—General M
Nursing and Healthcare Administration M
Nursing Education M
Nursing—General M,D
Physiology M

SALUS UNIVERSITY

Communication Disorders D
Optometry D
Physician Assistant Studies M
Public Health—General M
Rehabilitation Sciences M,O
Vision Sciences M,O

SALVE REGINA UNIVERSITY

Health Services Management and Hospital Administration M,O

SAMFORD UNIVERSITY

Family Nurse Practitioner Studies M,D
Nurse Anesthesia M,D
Nursing and Healthcare Administration M,D
Nursing Education M,D
Nursing—General M,D
Pharmacy D

SAM HOUSTON STATE UNIVERSITY

Allied Health—General M
Biological and Biomedical Sciences—General M
Nutrition M

SAMRA UNIVERSITY OF ORIENTAL MEDICINE

Acupuncture and Oriental Medicine M,D

SAMUEL MERRITT UNIVERSITY

Family Nurse Practitioner Studies M,D,O
Nurse Anesthesia M,D,O
Nursing and Healthcare Administration M,D,O
Nursing—General M,D,O
Occupational Therapy M
Physical Therapy D
Physician Assistant Studies M

SAN DIEGO STATE UNIVERSITY

Biochemistry M,D
Biological and Biomedical Sciences—General M,D
Cell Biology M,D
Communication Disorders M,D
Ecology M,D
Emergency Medical Services M,D
Environmental and Occupational Health M,D
Epidemiology M,D
Health Physics/Radiological Health M
Health Promotion M,D
Health Services Management and Hospital Administration M,D
International Health M,D
Microbiology M
Molecular Biology M,D
Nursing—General M
Nutrition M
Pharmaceutical Administration M
Physical Therapy D
Public Health—General M,D
Toxicology M,D

SAN FRANCISCO STATE UNIVERSITY

Acute Care/Critical Care Nursing M,O
Biochemistry M
Biological and Biomedical Sciences—General M
Cell Biology M
Communication Disorders M
Community Health Nursing M,O
Developmental Biology M
Ecology M
Family Nurse Practitioner Studies M,O
Marine Biology M
Microbiology M
Molecular Biology M
Nursing and Healthcare Administration M,O
Nursing Education M,O
Nursing—General M,O
Pediatric Nursing M,O
Physical Therapy D
Physiology M
Public Health—General M
Women's Health Nursing M,O

SAN JOSE STATE UNIVERSITY

Biological and Biomedical Sciences—General M
Communication Disorders M
Ecology M
Gerontological Nursing M,O
Microbiology M
Molecular Biology M
Nursing and Healthcare Administration M,O
Nursing Education M,O
Nursing—General M,O
Nutrition M
Occupational Therapy M
Physiology M
Public Health—General M,O

SAN JUAN BAUTISTA SCHOOL OF MEDICINE

Allopathic Medicine M,D

SARAH LAWRENCE COLLEGE

Human Genetics M
Public Health—General M

SAYBROOK UNIVERSITY

Nutrition M,D,O

THE SCRIPPS RESEARCH INSTITUTE

Biological and Biomedical Sciences—General D

SEATTLE INSTITUTE OF ORIENTAL MEDICINE

Acupuncture and Oriental Medicine M

SEATTLE PACIFIC UNIVERSITY

Adult Nursing M,O
Family Nurse Practitioner Studies M,O
Gerontological Nursing M,O
Nursing and Healthcare Administration M,O
Nursing Education M,O
Nursing Informatics M,O
Nursing—General M,O

SEATTLE UNIVERSITY

Adult Nursing M
Community Health Nursing M
Family Nurse Practitioner Studies M
Gerontological Nursing M
Nurse Midwifery M
Nursing—General M,D
Psychiatric Nursing M
Public Health—General M,O

SETON HALL UNIVERSITY

Adult Nursing M,D
Allied Health—General D
Biochemistry M,D
Biological and Biomedical Sciences—General M,D
Communication Disorders M
Gerontological Nursing M,D
Health Services Management and Hospital Administration M,D,O
Microbiology M,D
Molecular Biology M,D
Neuroscience M,D
Nursing and Healthcare Administration M,D
Nursing Education M,D
Nursing—General M,D
Occupational Therapy M
Pediatric Nursing M,D
Physical Therapy D
Physician Assistant Studies M
School Nursing M,D

SETON HILL UNIVERSITY

Oral and Dental Sciences M
Physician Assistant Studies M

SHAWNEE STATE UNIVERSITY

Occupational Therapy M

SHENANDOAH UNIVERSITY

Allied Health—General M,D,O
Family Nurse Practitioner Studies M,D,O
Nursing Education M,D,O
Nursing—General M,D,O
Occupational Therapy M
Pharmacy D
Physical Therapy D
Physician Assistant Studies M
Psychiatric Nursing M,D,O

SHERMAN COLLEGE OF CHIROPRACTIC

Chiropractic D

SHIPPENSBURG UNIVERSITY OF PENNSYLVANIA

Biological and Biomedical Sciences—General M

SIENA HEIGHTS UNIVERSITY

Health Services Management and Hospital Administration M,O

SIMMONS COLLEGE
Health Promotion M,D,O
Health Services Management and Hospital Administration M
Nursing—General M,D,O
Nutrition M,D,O
Physical Therapy M,D,O

SIMON FRASER UNIVERSITY
Biochemistry M,D,O
Biological and Biomedical Sciences—General M,D,O
Entomology M,D,O
International Health M,D,O
Molecular Biology M,D,O
Public Health—General M,D,O
Toxicology M,D,O

SLIPPERY ROCK UNIVERSITY OF PENNSYLVANIA
Physical Therapy D

SMITH COLLEGE
Biological and Biomedical Sciences—General M

SONOMA STATE UNIVERSITY
Biochemistry M
Biological and Biomedical Sciences—General M
Cell Biology M
Ecology M
Environmental Biology M
Evolutionary Biology M
Family Nurse Practitioner Studies M
Health Promotion M
Molecular Biology M
Nursing—General M
Occupational Therapy M
Physical Therapy M

SOUTH BAYLO UNIVERSITY
Acupuncture and Oriental Medicine M

SOUTH CAROLINA STATE UNIVERSITY
Allied Health—General M
Communication Disorders M
Nutrition M

SOUTH COLLEGE
Physician Assistant Studies M

SOUTH DAKOTA STATE UNIVERSITY
Biological and Biomedical Sciences—General M,D
Microbiology M,D
Nursing—General M,D
Nutrition M,D
Pharmaceutical Sciences M,D
Pharmacy D
Veterinary Sciences M,D

SOUTHEASTERN LOUISIANA UNIVERSITY
Adult Nursing M,D
Biological and Biomedical Sciences—General M
Communication Disorders M
Family Nurse Practitioner Studies M,D
Nursing and Healthcare Administration M,D
Nursing Education M,D
Nursing—General M,D
Psychiatric Nursing M,D

SOUTHEASTERN OKLAHOMA STATE UNIVERSITY
Environmental and Occupational Health M

SOUTHEAST MISSOURI STATE UNIVERSITY
Biological and Biomedical Sciences—General M
Communication Disorders M
Health Services Management and Hospital Administration M
Nursing—General M
Nutrition M

SOUTHERN ADVENTIST UNIVERSITY
Acute Care/Critical Care Nursing M
Adult Nursing M
Family Nurse Practitioner Studies M
Health Services Management and Hospital Administration M
Nursing and Healthcare Administration M
Nursing—General M

SOUTHERN ARKANSAS UNIVERSITY–MAGNOLIA
Psychiatric Nursing M

SOUTHERN CALIFORNIA UNIVERSITY OF HEALTH SCIENCES
Acupuncture and Oriental Medicine M
Chiropractic D

SOUTHERN COLLEGE OF OPTOMETRY
Optometry D

SOUTHERN CONNECTICUT STATE UNIVERSITY
Biological and Biomedical Sciences—General M
Communication Disorders M
Nursing and Healthcare Administration M
Nursing Education M
Nursing—General M
Public Health—General M

SOUTHERN ILLINOIS UNIVERSITY CARBONDALE
Biochemistry M,D
Biological and Biomedical Sciences—General M,D
Communication Disorders M
Community Health M
Health Services Management and Hospital Administration M
Medical Physics M
Microbiology M,D
Molecular Biology M,D
Nutrition M
Pharmacology M,D
Physician Assistant Studies M
Physiology M,D
Plant Biology M,D
Zoology M,D

SOUTHERN ILLINOIS UNIVERSITY EDWARDSVILLE
Biological and Biomedical Sciences—General M
Communication Disorders M
Dentistry D
Family Nurse Practitioner Studies M,D,O
Nurse Anesthesia M,O
Nursing and Healthcare Administration M,O
Nursing Education M,O
Nursing—General M,D,O
Pharmacy D

SOUTHERN METHODIST UNIVERSITY
Biological and Biomedical Sciences—General M,D
Cell Biology M,D
Molecular Biology M,D
Physiology M

SOUTHERN NAZARENE UNIVERSITY
Health Services Management and Hospital Administration M
Nursing and Healthcare Administration M
Nursing Education M
Nursing—General M

SOUTHERN NEW HAMPSHIRE UNIVERSITY
Community Health M,O
Health Services Management and Hospital Administration M,O

SOUTHERN UNIVERSITY AND AGRICULTURAL AND MECHANICAL COLLEGE
Biochemistry M
Biological and Biomedical Sciences—General M
Family Nurse Practitioner Studies M,D,O
Gerontological Nursing M,D,O
Nursing and Healthcare Administration M,D,O
Nursing Education M,D,O
Nursing—General M,D,O

SOUTH UNIVERSITY (AL)
Health Services Management and Hospital Administration M
Nursing—General M

SOUTH UNIVERSITY
Family Nurse Practitioner Studies M
Health Services Management and Hospital Administration M
Nursing—General M

SOUTH UNIVERSITY
Adult Nursing M
Family Nurse Practitioner Studies M
Health Services Management and Hospital Administration M
Nursing Education M
Nursing—General M

SOUTH UNIVERSITY (GA)
Anesthesiologist Assistant Studies M
Health Services Management and Hospital Administration M
Nursing Education M
Nursing—General M
Pharmacy
Physician Assistant Studies M

SOUTH UNIVERSITY (MI)
Nursing—General M

SOUTH UNIVERSITY (SC)
Health Services Management and Hospital Administration M
Nursing—General M
Pharmacy D

SOUTH UNIVERSITY
Nursing—General M

SOUTHWEST ACUPUNCTURE COLLEGE
Acupuncture and Oriental Medicine M

SOUTHWEST BAPTIST UNIVERSITY
Health Services Management and Hospital Administration M
Physical Therapy D

SOUTHWEST COLLEGE OF NATUROPATHIC MEDICINE AND HEALTH SCIENCES
Naturopathic Medicine D

SOUTHWESTERN OKLAHOMA STATE UNIVERSITY
Allied Health—General M
Microbiology M
Pharmacy D

SPALDING UNIVERSITY
Adult Nursing M,O
Family Nurse Practitioner Studies M,O
Nursing and Healthcare Administration M,O
Nursing—General M,O
Occupational Therapy M
Pediatric Nursing M,O

SPRING ARBOR UNIVERSITY
Nursing—General M

SPRINGFIELD COLLEGE
Health Promotion M,D
Occupational Therapy M,O
Physical Therapy D
Physician Assistant Studies M

SPRING HILL COLLEGE
Nursing and Healthcare Administration M,O
Nursing—General M,O

STANFORD UNIVERSITY
Allopathic Medicine D
Biochemistry D
Biological and Biomedical Sciences—General M,D
Biophysics D
Cancer Biology/Oncology D
Developmental Biology D
Ecology M,D
Epidemiology M
Genetics M,D
Health Services Research M
Immunology D
International Health M
Microbiology D
Neuroscience D
Physiology D
Structural Biology D
Systems Biology D

STATE UNIVERSITY OF NEW YORK AT FREDONIA
Biological and Biomedical Sciences—General M
Communication Disorders M

STATE UNIVERSITY OF NEW YORK AT NEW PALTZ
Communication Disorders M

STATE UNIVERSITY OF NEW YORK AT PLATTSBURGH
Communication Disorders M

STATE UNIVERSITY OF NEW YORK COLLEGE AT ONEONTA
Biological and Biomedical Sciences—General M
Nutrition M

STATE UNIVERSITY OF NEW YORK COLLEGE OF ENVIRONMENTAL SCIENCE AND FORESTRY
Biochemistry M,D
Conservation Biology M,D
Ecology M,D
Entomology M,D
Environmental Biology M,D
Plant Pathology M,D

STATE UNIVERSITY OF NEW YORK COLLEGE OF OPTOMETRY
Optometry D
Vision Sciences D

STATE UNIVERSITY OF NEW YORK DOWNSTATE MEDICAL CENTER
Allopathic Medicine M,D
Biological and Biomedical Sciences—General M,D
Cell Biology D
Community Health M
Family Nurse Practitioner Studies M,O
Medical/Surgical Nursing M,O
Molecular Biology D
Neuroscience D
Nurse Anesthesia M
Nurse Midwifery M,O
Nursing—General M,O
Public Health—General M

STATE UNIVERSITY OF NEW YORK EMPIRE STATE COLLEGE
Nursing Education M

STATE UNIVERSITY OF NEW YORK INSTITUTE OF TECHNOLOGY
Family Nurse Practitioner Studies M,O
Nursing and Healthcare Administration M
Nursing Education M,O

STATE UNIVERSITY OF NEW YORK UPSTATE MEDICAL UNIVERSITY
Allopathic Medicine D
Anatomy M,D
Biochemistry M,D
Biological and Biomedical Sciences—General M,D
Cancer Biology/Oncology
Cardiovascular Sciences
Cell Biology M,D
Clinical Laboratory Sciences/Medical Technology M
Family Nurse Practitioner Studies M,O
Immunology M,D
Infectious Diseases
Microbiology M,D
Molecular Biology M,D
Neuroscience D
Nursing—General M,O
Pharmacology D
Physical Therapy D
Physiology M,D

STEPHEN F. AUSTIN STATE UNIVERSITY
Biological and Biomedical Sciences—General M
Communication Disorders M

STEVENS INSTITUTE OF TECHNOLOGY
Biochemistry M,D,O
Pharmaceutical Sciences M,O

STEVENSON UNIVERSITY
Nursing—General M

STONY BROOK UNIVERSITY, STATE UNIVERSITY OF NEW YORK
Adult Nursing M,D,O
Allopathic Medicine D
Anatomy D
Biochemistry M,D
Bioethics
Biological and Biomedical Sciences—General M,D,O
Biophysics D
Cell Biology M,D
Community Health M,D,O
Dentistry D,O
Developmental Biology M,D
Ecology M,D
Evolutionary Biology M,D
Family Nurse Practitioner Studies M,D,O
Genetics D
Health Services Management and Hospital Administration M,D,O
Immunology M,D
Maternal and Child/Neonatal Nursing M,D,O
Medical Physics M,D
Microbiology D
Molecular Biology M,D
Molecular Genetics D
Molecular Physiology D
Neuroscience M,D
Nurse Midwifery M,O
Nursing Education M,O
Nursing—General M,D,O
Nutrition M,O
Occupational Therapy M,D,O
Oral and Dental Sciences M,D,O
Pathology M,D
Pediatric Nursing M,D,O
Pharmacology D
Physical Therapy M,D,O
Physician Assistant Studies M,D,O
Physiology D
Psychiatric Nursing M,O
Public Health—General M,O
Structural Biology D
Women's Health Nursing M,D,O

STRAYER UNIVERSITY
Health Services Management and Hospital Administration M

SUFFOLK UNIVERSITY
Health Services Management and Hospital Administration M,O

SUL ROSS STATE UNIVERSITY
Biological and Biomedical Sciences—General M

SWEDISH INSTITUTE, COLLEGE OF HEALTH SCIENCES
Acupuncture and Oriental Medicine M

SYRACUSE UNIVERSITY
Biochemistry D
Biological and Biomedical Sciences—General M,D
Biophysics D
Communication Disorders M,D
Community Health M
Health Services Management and Hospital Administration O
International Health O
Maternal and Child Health M
Nutrition M
Public Health—General M,O
Structural Biology D

TARLETON STATE UNIVERSITY
Biological and Biomedical Sciences—General M
Clinical Laboratory Sciences/Medical Technology M
Nursing—General M

TEACHERS COLLEGE, COLUMBIA UNIVERSITY
Communication Disorders M,D
Neuroscience M
Nursing and Healthcare Administration M,D
Nutrition M,D
Physiology M,D

TEMPLE UNIVERSITY
Adult Nursing M,D
Allied Health—General M,D
Allopathic Medicine D
Biological and Biomedical Sciences—General M,D
Clinical Research M,D
Communication Disorders M,D
Community Health M,D
Dentistry D
Environmental and Occupational Health M,D
Epidemiology M,D
Family Nurse Practitioner Studies M,D
Health Services Management and Hospital Administration M,D
Medicinal and Pharmaceutical Chemistry M,D

*M—masters degree; D—doctorate; O—other advanced degree; *—Close-Up and/or Display*

Nursing and Healthcare Administration M,D
Nursing Education M,D
Nursing—General M,D
Occupational Therapy M,D
Oral and Dental Sciences M,O
Pharmaceutical Administration M
Pharmaceutical Sciences M
Pharmacy D
Physical Therapy D
Podiatric Medicine D
Public Health—General M,D

TENNESSEE STATE UNIVERSITY
Allied Health—General M,D
Biological and Biomedical Sciences—General M,D
Communication Disorders M
Family Nurse Practitioner Studies M
Nursing—General M
Occupational Therapy M
Physical Therapy D
Public Health—General M

TENNESSEE TECHNOLOGICAL UNIVERSITY
Biological and Biomedical Sciences—General M,D
Family Nurse Practitioner Studies M
Health Promotion M
Nursing and Healthcare Administration M
Nursing Education M
Nursing Informatics M
Nursing—General M

TEXAS A&M HEALTH SCIENCE CENTER
Biological and Biomedical Sciences—General M,D
Cell Biology D
Dental Hygiene M
Dentistry D
Environmental and Occupational Health M
Epidemiology M
Health Services Management and Hospital Administration M
Immunology D
Microbiology D
Molecular Biology D
Molecular Medicine D
Molecular Pathogenesis D
Neuroscience D
Oral and Dental Sciences M,D,O
Pharmacy D
Public Health—General M
Systems Biology D
Translational Biology D
Virology D

TEXAS A&M INTERNATIONAL UNIVERSITY
Biological and Biomedical Sciences—General M
Family Nurse Practitioner Studies M
Nursing—General M

TEXAS A&M UNIVERSITY
Biochemistry M,D
Biological and Biomedical Sciences—General M,D
Biopsychology M,D
Botany M,D
Entomology M,D
Epidemiology M
Health Physics/Radiological Health M,D
Microbiology M,D
Neuroscience M,D
Nutrition M,D
Pathobiology D
Pathology D
Physiology M,D
Plant Pathology M,D
Public Health—General M
Toxicology M,D
Veterinary Medicine M,D
Veterinary Sciences M
Zoology M,D

TEXAS A&M UNIVERSITY AT GALVESTON
Marine Biology M,D

TEXAS A&M UNIVERSITY–COMMERCE
Biological and Biomedical Sciences—General M,O
Health Promotion M,D

TEXAS A&M UNIVERSITY–CORPUS CHRISTI
Biological and Biomedical Sciences—General M
Family Nurse Practitioner Studies M
Health Services Management and Hospital Administration M
Nursing and Healthcare Administration M
Nursing—General M

TEXAS A&M UNIVERSITY–KINGSVILLE
Biological and Biomedical Sciences—General M
Communication Disorders M

TEXAS A&M UNIVERSITY–SAN ANTONIO
Health Services Management and Hospital Administration M

TEXAS CHIROPRACTIC COLLEGE
Chiropractic D

TEXAS CHRISTIAN UNIVERSITY
Adult Nursing M,D
Allied Health—General M,D
Biochemistry M,D
Biological and Biomedical Sciences—General M
Biophysics M,D
Communication Disorders M
Gerontological Nursing M,D
Neuroscience M,D
Nurse Anesthesia M,D
Nursing and Healthcare Administration M,D
Nursing Education M,D
Nursing—General M,D
Pediatric Nursing M,D

TEXAS HEALTH AND SCIENCE UNIVERSITY
Acupuncture and Oriental Medicine M

TEXAS SOUTHERN UNIVERSITY
Biological and Biomedical Sciences—General M
Health Services Management and Hospital Administration M
Pharmaceutical Sciences M,D
Pharmacy D
Toxicology M,D

TEXAS STATE UNIVERSITY
Allied Health—General M,D
Biochemistry M
Biological and Biomedical Sciences—General M
Communication Disorders M
Conservation Biology M
Health Services Management and Hospital Administration M
Health Services Research M
Marine Biology M,D
Nutrition M
Physical Therapy D

TEXAS TECH UNIVERSITY
Biological and Biomedical Sciences—General M,D
Health Services Management and Hospital Administration M,D
Microbiology M,D
Nutrition M,D
Toxicology M,D
Zoology M,D

TEXAS TECH UNIVERSITY HEALTH SCIENCES CENTER
Acute Care/Critical Care Nursing M,D,O
Allied Health—General M,D
Allopathic Medicine D
Biological and Biomedical Sciences—General M,D
Cell Biology M,D
Communication Disorders M,D
Family Nurse Practitioner Studies M,D,O
Gerontological Nursing M,D,O
Health Services Management and Hospital Administration M
Molecular Pathology M
Nursing and Healthcare Administration M,D,O
Nursing Education M,D,O
Nursing—General M,D,O
Occupational Therapy M
Pediatric Nursing M,D,O
Pharmaceutical Sciences M,D
Physical Therapy D
Physician Assistant Studies M
Rehabilitation Sciences D

TEXAS WESLEYAN UNIVERSITY
Health Services Management and Hospital Administration M
Nurse Anesthesia M,D

TEXAS WOMAN'S UNIVERSITY
Acute Care/Critical Care Nursing M,D
Adult Nursing M,D
Allied Health—General M,D
Biological and Biomedical Sciences—General M,D
Communication Disorders M
Family Nurse Practitioner Studies M,D
Health Services Management and Hospital Administration M,D
Molecular Biology M,D
Nursing and Healthcare Administration M,D
Nursing Education M,D
Nursing—General M,D
Nutrition M
Occupational Therapy M,D
Pediatric Nursing M,D
Physical Therapy D
Women's Health Nursing M,D

THOMAS EDISON STATE COLLEGE
Epidemiology O
Nursing Education O
Nursing—General M

THOMAS JEFFERSON UNIVERSITY
Allopathic Medicine D
Biochemistry D
Biological and Biomedical Sciences—General M,D,O
Biophysics D
Cancer Biology/Oncology D
Cell Biology M,D
Clinical Laboratory Sciences/Medical Technology M
Clinical Research O
Developmental Biology M,D
Genetics D
Genomic Sciences D
Health Physics/Radiological Health M
Health Services Management and Hospital Administration M,D,O
Health Services Research M,D,O
Immunology D
Infectious Diseases O
Microbiology M,D
Molecular Pharmacology D
Molecular Physiology D
Neuroscience D
Nursing—General M,D
Occupational Therapy M,D
Pharmacology M
Pharmacy D
Physical Therapy D
Public Health—General M,O
Structural Biology D

THOMAS UNIVERSITY
Nursing—General M

TIFFIN UNIVERSITY
Health Services Management and Hospital Administration M

TOURO COLLEGE
Communication Disorders M,D
Occupational Therapy M,D
Physical Therapy M,D
Physician Assistant Studies M,D

TOURO UNIVERSITY
Osteopathic Medicine M,D
Pharmacy M,D
Public Health—General M,D

TOWSON UNIVERSITY
Allied Health—General M
Biological and Biomedical Sciences—General M
Communication Disorders M,D
Environmental and Occupational Health D
Health Services Management and Hospital Administration O
Nursing Education M,O
Nursing—General M,O
Occupational Therapy M
Physician Assistant Studies M

TRENT UNIVERSITY
Biological and Biomedical Sciences—General M,D

TREVECCA NAZARENE UNIVERSITY
Health Services Management and Hospital Administration M,O
Physician Assistant Studies M

TRIDENT UNIVERSITY INTERNATIONAL
Clinical Research M,D,O
Environmental and Occupational Health M,D,O
Health Services Management and Hospital Administration M,D,O
International Health M,D,O
Nursing and Healthcare Administration M,D,O
Public Health—General M,D,O

TRINITY INTERNATIONAL UNIVERSITY
Bioethics M

TRINITY UNIVERSITY
Health Services Management and Hospital Administration M

TRINITY WASHINGTON UNIVERSITY
Public Health—General M

TRINITY WESTERN UNIVERSITY
Health Services Management and Hospital Administration M,O
Nursing—General M

TRI-STATE COLLEGE OF ACUPUNCTURE
Acupuncture and Oriental Medicine M,O

TROPICAL AGRICULTURE RESEARCH AND HIGHER EDUCATION CENTER
Conservation Biology M,D

TROY UNIVERSITY
Adult Nursing M,D,O
Biological and Biomedical Sciences—General M
Family Nurse Practitioner Studies M,D,O
Health Services Management and Hospital Administration M
Maternal and Child Health M,D,O
Nursing Informatics M,D,O
Nursing—General M,D,O

TRUMAN STATE UNIVERSITY
Biological and Biomedical Sciences—General M
Communication Disorders M

TUFTS UNIVERSITY
Allopathic Medicine D
Biochemistry D
Biological and Biomedical Sciences—General M,D
Cell Biology D
Clinical Research M,D
Dentistry D
Developmental Biology D
Environmental and Occupational Health M,D
Epidemiology M,D,O
Genetics D
Immunology D
Infectious Diseases M,D
International Health M,D
Microbiology D
Molecular Biology D
Molecular Physiology D
Neuroscience M,D
Nutrition M,D
Occupational Therapy M,D,O
Oral and Dental Sciences M,O
Pathology M,D
Pharmacology M,D
Physician Assistant Studies M,D
Public Health—General M,D
Reproductive Biology M,D
Veterinary Medicine M,D

TULANE UNIVERSITY
Allopathic Medicine D
Biochemistry M,D
Biological and Biomedical Sciences—General M,D
Cell Biology M,D
Ecology M,D
Environmental and Occupational Health M,D
Epidemiology M,D
Evolutionary Biology M,D
Health Services Management and Hospital Administration M,D
Human Genetics M,D
Immunology M,D
Infectious Diseases M,D,O
International Health M,D
Maternal and Child Health M,D
Microbiology M,D
Molecular Biology M,D
Neuroscience M,D
Nutrition M
Parasitology M,D,O
Pharmacology M,D
Physiology M,D
Public Health—General M,D,O
Structural Biology M,D

TUSKEGEE UNIVERSITY
Biological and Biomedical Sciences—General M,D
Nutrition M
Veterinary Medicine M,D
Veterinary Sciences M,D

UNIFORMED SERVICES UNIVERSITY OF THE HEALTH SCIENCES
Biological and Biomedical Sciences—General M,D
Cell Biology M,D
Environmental and Occupational Health M,D
Family Nurse Practitioner Studies M,D
Health Services Management and Hospital Administration M,D
Immunology D
Infectious Diseases D*
International Health M,D
Medical/Surgical Nursing M,D
Molecular Biology M,D*
Neuroscience D*
Nurse Anesthesia M,D
Nursing—General M,D
Psychiatric Nursing M,D
Public Health—General M,D
Zoology M,D

UNION COLLEGE (NE)
Physician Assistant Studies M

UNION GRADUATE COLLEGE
Bioethics M,O
Health Services Management and Hospital Administration M,O

UNION INSTITUTE & UNIVERSITY
Health Promotion M

UNION UNIVERSITY
Family Nurse Practitioner Studies M,D,O
Nurse Anesthesia M,D,O
Nursing and Healthcare Administration M,D,O
Nursing Education M,D,O
Nursing—General M,D,O

UNITED STATES UNIVERSITY
Family Nurse Practitioner Studies M

UNITED STATES UNIVERSITY
Nursing and Healthcare Administration M
Nursing Education M
Nursing—General M

UNIVERSIDAD ADVENTISTA DE LAS ANTILLAS
Medical/Surgical Nursing M

UNIVERSIDAD AUTONOMA DE GUADALAJARA
Allopathic Medicine D
Environmental and Occupational Health M,D

UNIVERSIDAD CENTRAL DEL CARIBE
Allopathic Medicine M,D
Anatomy M,D
Biochemistry M,D
Biological and Biomedical Sciences—General M,D
Cell Biology M,D
Immunology M,D
Microbiology M,D
Molecular Biology M,D
Pharmacology M,D
Physiology M,D

UNIVERSIDAD CENTRAL DEL ESTE
Allopathic Medicine D
Dentistry D

UNIVERSIDAD DE CIENCIAS MEDICAS
Allopathic Medicine M,D,O
Anatomy M,D,O
Biological and Biomedical Sciences—General M,D,O
Community Health M,D,O
Environmental and Occupational Health M,D,O
Health Services Management and Hospital Administration M,D,O
Pharmacy M,D,O

UNIVERSIDAD DE IBEROAMERICA
Acute Care/Critical Care Nursing M,D
Allopathic Medicine M,D

Health Services Management and Hospital Administration M,D
Neuroscience M,D

UNIVERSIDAD DE LAS AMÉRICAS PUEBLA
Clinical Laboratory Sciences/Medical Technology M

UNIVERSIDAD DEL TURABO
Adult Nursing M,O
Communication Disorders M
Environmental Biology M,D
Family Nurse Practitioner Studies M
Health Promotion M
Naturopathic Medicine D

UNIVERSIDAD IBEROAMERICANA
Allopathic Medicine D
Dentistry M,D

UNIVERSIDAD METROPOLITANA
Nursing and Healthcare Administration M,O
Nursing—General M,O
Oncology Nursing M,O

UNIVERSIDAD NACIONAL PEDRO HENRIQUEZ URENA
Allopathic Medicine D
Dentistry D
Ecology M

UNIVERSITÉ DE MONCTON
Biochemistry M
Biological and Biomedical Sciences—General M
Nutrition M

UNIVERSITÉ DE MONTRÉAL
Allopathic Medicine D
Biochemistry M,D,O
Bioethics M,D,O
Biological and Biomedical Sciences—General M,D
Cell Biology M,D
Communication Disorders M,O
Community Health M,D,O
Dental Hygiene O
Environmental and Occupational Health M
Genetics O
Health Services Management and Hospital Administration M,O
Immunology M,D
Microbiology M,D
Molecular Biology M,D
Neuroscience M,D
Nursing—General M,D,O
Nutrition M,D,O
Occupational Therapy O
Optometry D
Oral and Dental Sciences M,O
Pathology M,D
Pharmaceutical Sciences M,D,O
Pharmacology M,D
Physiology M,D
Public Health—General M,D,O
Rehabilitation Sciences O
Toxicology O
Veterinary Medicine D
Veterinary Sciences M,D
Virology D
Vision Sciences M,O

UNIVERSITÉ DE SHERBROOKE
Allopathic Medicine D
Biochemistry M,D
Biological and Biomedical Sciences—General M,D,O
Biophysics M,D
Cell Biology M,D
Clinical Laboratory Sciences/Medical Technology M,D
Immunology M,D
Microbiology M,D
Pharmacology M,D
Physiology M,D
Radiation Biology M,D

UNIVERSITÉ DU QUÉBEC À CHICOUTIMI
Genetics M

UNIVERSITÉ DU QUÉBEC À MONTRÉAL
Biological and Biomedical Sciences—General M,D
Environmental and Occupational Health O

UNIVERSITÉ DU QUÉBEC À RIMOUSKI
Nursing—General M,O

UNIVERSITÉ DU QUÉBEC À TROIS-RIVIÈRES
Biophysics M,D
Chiropractic D
Nursing—General M,O

UNIVERSITÉ DU QUÉBEC EN ABITIBI-TÉMISCAMINGUE
Biological and Biomedical Sciences—General M,D

UNIVERSITÉ DU QUÉBEC EN OUTAOUAIS
Nursing—General M,O

UNIVERSITÉ DU QUÉBEC, INSTITUT NATIONAL DE LA RECHERCHE SCIENTIFIQUE
Biological and Biomedical Sciences—General M,D
Immunology M,D
Medical Microbiology M,D
Microbiology M,D
Virology M,D

UNIVERSITÉ LAVAL
Allopathic Medicine D,O
Anatomy O
Anesthesiologist Assistant Studies O
Biochemistry M,D,O
Biological and Biomedical Sciences—General M,D,O
Cancer Biology/Oncology O
Cardiovascular Sciences O
Cell Biology M,D
Communication Disorders M
Community Health M,D,O
Dentistry D
Emergency Medical Services O
Environmental and Occupational Health O
Epidemiology M,D
Health Physics/Radiological Health O
Immunology M,D
Infectious Diseases O
Microbiology M,D
Molecular Biology M,D
Neurobiology M,D
Nursing—General M,D,O
Nutrition M,D
Oral and Dental Sciences M,O
Pathology O
Pharmaceutical Sciences M,D,O
Physiology M,D
Plant Biology M,D

UNIVERSITY AT ALBANY, STATE UNIVERSITY OF NEW YORK
Biochemistry M,D
Biological and Biomedical Sciences—General M,D
Biopsychology M,D,O
Cell Biology M,D
Conservation Biology M
Developmental Biology M,D
Ecology M,D
Environmental and Occupational Health M,D
Epidemiology M,D
Evolutionary Biology M,D
Genetics M,D
Health Services Management and Hospital Administration M
Immunology M,D
Molecular Biology M,D
Molecular Pathogenesis M,D
Neurobiology M,D
Neuroscience M,D
Public Health—General M,D
Structural Biology M,D
Toxicology M,D

UNIVERSITY AT BUFFALO, THE STATE UNIVERSITY OF NEW YORK
Adult Nursing M,D,O
Allied Health—General M,D,O
Allopathic Medicine D
Anatomy M,D
Biochemistry M,D
Biological and Biomedical Sciences—General M,D
Biophysics M,D
Cancer Biology/Oncology M
Cell Biology D
Clinical Laboratory Sciences/Medical Technology M
Communication Disorders M,D
Community Health M,D
Dentistry M,D,O
Ecology M,D,O
Epidemiology M,D
Evolutionary Biology M,D,O
Family Nurse Practitioner Studies M,D,O
Gerontological Nursing M,D,O
Health Services Management and Hospital Administration M,D,O
Immunology M,D
Medicinal and Pharmaceutical Chemistry M,D
Microbiology M,D
Molecular Biology D
Neuroscience M,D
Nurse Anesthesia M,D,O
Nursing and Healthcare Administration M,D,O
Nursing—General M,D,O
Nutrition M,D,O
Occupational Therapy M
Oral and Dental Sciences M,D,O
Pathology M,D
Pharmaceutical Sciences M,D
Pharmacology M,D
Pharmacy D
Physical Therapy D
Physiology M,D
Psychiatric Nursing M,D,O
Public Health—General M,D
Rehabilitation Sciences M,D,O
Structural Biology M,D
Toxicology M,D

THE UNIVERSITY OF AKRON
Biological and Biomedical Sciences—General M,D
Communication Disorders M,D
Health Services Management and Hospital Administration M
Nursing—General M,D
Nutrition M
Public Health—General M,D

THE UNIVERSITY OF ALABAMA
Biological and Biomedical Sciences—General M,D
Communication Disorders M
Community Health M
Health Promotion M,D
Nursing—General M,D
Nutrition M

THE UNIVERSITY OF ALABAMA AT BIRMINGHAM
Allied Health—General M,D
Allopathic Medicine D
Biochemistry D
Biological and Biomedical Sciences—General M,D
Cell Biology D
Clinical Laboratory Sciences/Medical Technology M,D
Dentistry D
Environmental and Occupational Health M,D
Epidemiology M,D
Genetics D
Health Promotion D
Health Services Management and Hospital Administration M,D
Health Services Research M,D
Industrial Hygiene M,D
Maternal and Child Health M,D
Microbiology D
Molecular Biology D
Molecular Genetics D
Molecular Physiology D
Neurobiology D
Neuroscience M,D
Nurse Anesthesia M,D
Nursing—General M,D
Nutrition M,D
Occupational Therapy M
Optometry D
Oral and Dental Sciences M
Pathology D
Pharmacology D
Physical Therapy D
Physician Assistant Studies M
Public Health—General M,D
Rehabilitation Sciences D
Toxicology M,D
Vision Sciences M,D

THE UNIVERSITY OF ALABAMA IN HUNTSVILLE
Acute Care/Critical Care Nursing M,D,O
Biological and Biomedical Sciences—General M,D
Family Nurse Practitioner Studies M,D,O
Health Services Management and Hospital Administration M,D,O
Nursing Education M,D,O
Nursing—General M,D,O

UNIVERSITY OF ALASKA ANCHORAGE
Biological and Biomedical Sciences—General M
Nursing—General M
Public Health—General M

UNIVERSITY OF ALASKA FAIRBANKS
Biochemistry M,D
Biological and Biomedical Sciences—General M,D
Botany M,D
Marine Biology M,D
Nutrition M,D
Zoology M,D

UNIVERSITY OF ALBERTA
Biochemistry M,D
Biological and Biomedical Sciences—General M,D
Cancer Biology/Oncology M,D
Cell Biology M,D
Clinical Laboratory Sciences/Medical Technology M,D
Communication Disorders M,D
Community Health M,D
Conservation Biology M,D
Dental Hygiene O
Dentistry D
Ecology M,D
Environmental and Occupational Health M,D
Environmental Biology M,D
Epidemiology M,D
Evolutionary Biology M,D
Genetics M,D
Health Physics/Radiological Health M,D
Health Promotion M,O
Health Services Management and Hospital Administration M,D
Health Services Research M,D
Immunology M,D
International Health M,D
Maternal and Child/Neonatal Nursing D
Medical Microbiology M,D
Medical Physics M,D
Microbiology M,D
Molecular Biology M,D
Neuroscience M,D
Nursing—General M,D
Occupational Therapy M,D
Oral and Dental Sciences M,D
Pathology M,D
Pharmaceutical Sciences M,D
Pharmacology M,D
Pharmacy M,D
Physical Therapy M,D
Physiology M,D
Plant Biology M,D
Public Health—General M,D
Rehabilitation Sciences D
Vision Sciences M,D

THE UNIVERSITY OF ARIZONA
Allopathic Medicine M,D
Biochemistry D
Biological and Biomedical Sciences—General M
Cancer Biology/Oncology D
Cell Biology M,D
Communication Disorders M,D
Ecology M,D
Entomology M,D
Epidemiology M,D
Evolutionary Biology M,D
Family Nurse Practitioner Studies M,D,O
Genetics M,D
Immunology M,D
Medical Physics M
Microbiology M,D
Molecular Biology M,D
Molecular Medicine M,D,O
Neuroscience D
Nursing—General M,D,O
Nutrition M,D
Perfusion M,D
Pharmaceutical Sciences M,D
Pharmacology M,D
Pharmacy D
Physiology M,D
Plant Pathology M,D
Public Health—General M,D

UNIVERSITY OF ARKANSAS
Biological and Biomedical Sciences—General M,D
Cell Biology M,D
Communication Disorders M
Community Health M,D
Entomology M,D
Health Promotion M,D
Molecular Biology M,D
Nursing—General M
Plant Pathology M

UNIVERSITY OF ARKANSAS AT LITTLE ROCK
Allied Health—General M
Biological and Biomedical Sciences—General M

UNIVERSITY OF ARKANSAS FOR MEDICAL SCIENCES
Allopathic Medicine D
Biochemistry M,D,O
Biological and Biomedical Sciences—General M,D,O
Communication Disorders M,D
Environmental and Occupational Health M,D,O
Epidemiology M,D,O
Health Physics/Radiological Health M,D
Health Promotion M,D,O
Health Services Management and Hospital Administration M,D,O
Health Services Research M,D,O
Immunology M,D,O
Microbiology M,D,O
Molecular Biology M,D,O
Molecular Biophysics M,D,O
Neurobiology M,D,O
Nursing—General D
Nutrition M,D,O
Pharmacology M,D,O
Pharmacy M,D
Physician Assistant Studies M,D
Physiology M,D,O
Public Health—General M,D,O
Toxicology M,D,O

UNIVERSITY OF BALTIMORE
Health Services Management and Hospital Administration M

UNIVERSITY OF BRIDGEPORT
Acupuncture and Oriental Medicine M
Chiropractic D
Dental Hygiene M
Naturopathic Medicine D
Nutrition M
Physician Assistant Studies M

THE UNIVERSITY OF BRITISH COLUMBIA
Allopathic Medicine M,D
Biochemistry M,D
Biopsychology M,D
Botany M,D
Cell Biology M,D
Communication Disorders M,D
Dentistry D
Developmental Biology M,D
Environmental and Occupational Health M,D
Epidemiology M,D
Genetics M,D
Health Services Management and Hospital Administration M,D
Immunology M,D
Microbiology M,D
Molecular Biology M,D
Neuroscience M,D
Nurse Anesthesia M,D
Nursing—General M,D
Nutrition M,D
Occupational Therapy M
Oral and Dental Sciences M,D,O
Pathology M,D
Pharmaceutical Sciences M,D
Pharmacology M,D
Pharmacy M,D
Public Health—General M,D
Rehabilitation Sciences M,D
Reproductive Biology M,D
Zoology M,D

*M—masters degree; D—doctorate; O—other advanced degree; *—Close-Up and/or Display*

UNIVERSITY OF CALGARY

Allopathic Medicine	D
Biochemistry	M,D
Biological and Biomedical Sciences—General	M,D
Cancer Biology/Oncology	M,D
Cardiovascular Sciences	M,D
Community Health	M,D
Genetics	M,D
Immunology	M,D
Infectious Diseases	M,D
Microbiology	M,D
Molecular Biology	M,D
Molecular Genetics	M,D
Neuroscience	M,D
Nursing—General	M,D,O
Pathology	M,D
Physiology	M,D

UNIVERSITY OF CALIFORNIA, BERKELEY

Allopathic Medicine	
Biochemistry	D
Biological and Biomedical Sciences—General	D
Biophysics	D
Cell Biology	D
Clinical Research	O
Environmental and Occupational Health	M,D
Epidemiology	M,D
Health Services Management and Hospital Administration	D
Immunology	D
Infectious Diseases	M,D
Microbiology	D
Molecular Biology	D
Molecular Toxicology	D
Neuroscience	D
Nutrition	D
Optometry	D,O
Physiology	D
Plant Biology	D
Public Health—General	M,D
Vision Sciences	M,D

UNIVERSITY OF CALIFORNIA, DAVIS

Allopathic Medicine	D
Animal Behavior	D
Biochemistry	M,D
Biophysics	M,D
Cell Biology	M,D
Clinical Research	M
Developmental Biology	M,D
Ecology	M,D
Entomology	M,D
Epidemiology	M,D
Evolutionary Biology	D
Genetics	M,D
Immunology	M,D
Maternal and Child Health	M
Microbiology	M,D
Molecular Biology	M,D
Neuroscience	D
Nutrition	M,D
Pathology	M,D
Pharmacology	M,D
Physiology	M,D
Plant Biology	M,D
Plant Pathology	M,D
Toxicology	M,D
Veterinary Medicine	D
Veterinary Sciences	M,O
Zoology	M

UNIVERSITY OF CALIFORNIA, IRVINE

Allopathic Medicine	D
Anatomy	M,D
Biochemistry	M,D
Biological and Biomedical Sciences—General	M,D
Biophysics	D
Cell Biology	M,D
Computational Biology	D
Developmental Biology	M,D
Ecology	M,D
Epidemiology	M,D
Evolutionary Biology	M,D
Genetics	D
Health Services Management and Hospital Administration	M
Medicinal and Pharmaceutical Chemistry	D
Microbiology	M,D
Molecular Biology	M,D
Molecular Genetics	M,D
Neurobiology	M,D
Neuroscience	D
Nursing—General	M
Pathology	D
Physiology	D
Public Health—General	M,D
Systems Biology	D
Toxicology	M,D

UNIVERSITY OF CALIFORNIA, LOS ANGELES

Allopathic Medicine	D
Anatomy	M,D
Biochemistry	M,D
Biological and Biomedical Sciences—General	M,D
Cell Biology	M,D
Clinical Research	M
Community Health	M,D
Dentistry	D,O
Developmental Biology	M,D
Ecology	M,D
Environmental and Occupational Health	M,D
Epidemiology	M,D
Evolutionary Biology	M,D
Health Services Management and Hospital Administration	M,D
Human Genetics	M,D
Immunology	M,D
Medical Physics	M,D
Microbiology	M,D
Molecular Biology	M,D
Molecular Genetics	M,D
Molecular Physiology	D
Molecular Toxicology	D
Neurobiology	M,D
Neuroscience	D
Nursing—General	M,D
Oral and Dental Sciences	M,D
Pathology	M,D
Pharmacology	M,D
Physiology	M,D
Public Health—General	M,D
Toxicology	D

UNIVERSITY OF CALIFORNIA, MERCED

Biochemistry	M,D
Biological and Biomedical Sciences—General	M,D
Systems Biology	M,D

UNIVERSITY OF CALIFORNIA, RIVERSIDE

Biochemistry	M,D
Biological and Biomedical Sciences—General	M,D
Botany	M,D
Cell Biology	M,D
Developmental Biology	M,D
Ecology	M,D
Entomology	M,D
Evolutionary Biology	M,D
Genetics	D
Genomic Sciences	D
Microbiology	M,D
Molecular Biology	M,D
Molecular Genetics	D
Neuroscience	D
Plant Biology	M,D
Plant Molecular Biology	M,D
Plant Pathology	M,D
Toxicology	M,D

UNIVERSITY OF CALIFORNIA, SAN DIEGO

Allopathic Medicine	D
Biochemistry	M,D
Biological and Biomedical Sciences—General	D
Biophysics	D
Clinical Laboratory Sciences/Medical Technology	M,D
Clinical Research	M
Communication Disorders	D
Ecology	D
Epidemiology	D
Evolutionary Biology	D
Health Physics/Radiological Health	M
Health Services Management and Hospital Administration	M
International Health	D
Marine Biology	M,D
Microbiology	D
Neuroscience	M,D
Pharmacy	D
Public Health—General	D
Systems Biology	D

UNIVERSITY OF CALIFORNIA, SAN FRANCISCO

Allopathic Medicine	D
Biochemistry	D
Biological and Biomedical Sciences—General	D
Biophysics	D
Cell Biology	D
Dentistry	D
Developmental Biology	D
Genetics	D
Genomic Sciences	D
Medicinal and Pharmaceutical Chemistry	D
Molecular Biology	D
Neuroscience	D
Nursing—General	M,D
Oral and Dental Sciences	M,D
Pharmaceutical Sciences	D
Pharmacology	D
Pharmacy	D
Physical Therapy	D

UNIVERSITY OF CALIFORNIA, SANTA BARBARA

Biochemistry	D
Biophysics	D
Cell Biology	M,D
Developmental Biology	M,D
Ecology	M,D
Evolutionary Biology	M,D
Marine Biology	M,D
Molecular Biology	M,D
Neuroscience	D
Pharmacology	M,D

UNIVERSITY OF CALIFORNIA, SANTA CRUZ

Biochemistry	M,D
Cell Biology	M,D
Developmental Biology	M,D
Ecology	M,D
Environmental Biology	M,D
Evolutionary Biology	M,D
Molecular Biology	M,D
Toxicology	M,D

UNIVERSITY OF CENTRAL ARKANSAS

Adult Nursing	M,O
Biological and Biomedical Sciences—General	M
Communication Disorders	M,D
Family Nurse Practitioner Studies	M,O
Nursing and Healthcare Administration	M,O
Nursing Education	M,O
Nursing—General	M,O
Occupational Therapy	M
Physical Therapy	D

UNIVERSITY OF CENTRAL FLORIDA

Adult Nursing	M,D,O
Allopathic Medicine	M,D
Biological and Biomedical Sciences—General	M,D,O
Communication Disorders	M,D,O
Conservation Biology	M,D,O
Family Nurse Practitioner Studies	M,D,O
Gerontological Nursing	M,D,O
Health Services Management and Hospital Administration	M,O
Nursing Education	M,D,O
Nursing—General	M,D,O
Physical Therapy	D

UNIVERSITY OF CENTRAL MISSOURI

Biological and Biomedical Sciences—General	M,D,O
Communication Disorders	M,D,O
Environmental and Occupational Health	M,D,O
Industrial Hygiene	M,D,O
Nursing—General	M,D,O

UNIVERSITY OF CENTRAL OKLAHOMA

Biological and Biomedical Sciences—General	M
Communication Disorders	M
Health Promotion	M
Nursing—General	M
Nutrition	M

UNIVERSITY OF CHARLESTON

Pharmacy	D
Physician Assistant Studies	M

UNIVERSITY OF CHICAGO

Allopathic Medicine	D
Anatomy	D
Biochemistry	D
Biological and Biomedical Sciences—General	D
Biophysics	D
Cancer Biology/Oncology	D
Cell Biology	D
Developmental Biology	D
Ecology	D
Evolutionary Biology	D
Genetics	D
Genomic Sciences	D
Health Promotion	M,D
Health Services Management and Hospital Administration	M,O
Human Genetics	D
Immunology	D
Medical Physics	D
Microbiology	D
Molecular Biology	D
Molecular Medicine	D
Molecular Pathogenesis	D
Molecular Physiology	D
Neurobiology	D
Neuroscience	D
Nutrition	D
Pathology	D
Pharmacology	D
Physiology	D
Systems Biology	D
Vision Sciences	D
Zoology	D

UNIVERSITY OF CINCINNATI

Acute Care/Critical Care Nursing	M,D
Adult Nursing	M,D
Allopathic Medicine	M,D
Biochemistry	M,D
Biological and Biomedical Sciences—General	M,D
Biophysics	D
Cancer Biology/Oncology	D
Cell Biology	D
Communication Disorders	M,D,O
Community Health Nursing	M,D
Developmental Biology	D
Environmental and Occupational Health	M,D
Epidemiology	M,D
Genomic Sciences	M,D
Health Physics/Radiological Health	M
Immunology	M,D
Industrial Hygiene	M,D
Maternal and Child/Neonatal Nursing	M,D
Medical Imaging	D
Medical Physics	M
Microbiology	M,D
Molecular Biology	M,D
Molecular Genetics	M,D
Molecular Medicine	D
Molecular Toxicology	M,D
Neuroscience	D
Nurse Anesthesia	M,D
Nurse Midwifery	M,D
Nursing and Healthcare Administration	M,D
Nursing—General	M,D
Nutrition	M
Occupational Health Nursing	M,D
Pathobiology	D
Pathology	D
Pediatric Nursing	M,D
Pharmaceutical Sciences	M,D
Pharmacology	D
Pharmacy	D
Physiology	D
Psychiatric Nursing	M,D
Rehabilitation Sciences	D
Women's Health Nursing	M,D

UNIVERSITY OF COLORADO BOULDER

Animal Behavior	M,D
Biochemistry	M,D
Cell Biology	M,D
Communication Disorders	M,D
Developmental Biology	M,D
Ecology	M,D
Evolutionary Biology	M,D
Genetics	M,D
Marine Biology	M,D
Medical Physics	M,D
Microbiology	M,D
Molecular Biology	M,D
Neurobiology	M,D
Physiology	M,D

UNIVERSITY OF COLORADO COLORADO SPRINGS

Adult Nursing	M,D
Biological and Biomedical Sciences—General	M
Gerontological Nursing	M,D
Health Promotion	M
Nursing Education	M,D
Nursing—General	M,D
Nutrition	M

UNIVERSITY OF COLORADO DENVER

Adult Nursing	M,D
Allopathic Medicine	D
Anatomy	M,D
Anesthesiologist Assistant Studies	M
Animal Behavior	M,D
Biochemistry	D
Biological and Biomedical Sciences—General	M,D
Biophysics	M,D
Cancer Biology/Oncology	D
Cell Biology	M,D
Clinical Laboratory Sciences/Medical Technology	M,D
Clinical Research	M,D
Community Health	M,D
Computational Biology	M,D
Dentistry	M,D
Developmental Biology	M,D
Ecology	M,D
Environmental and Occupational Health	M,D
Epidemiology	M,D
Evolutionary Biology	M,D
Family Nurse Practitioner Studies	M,D
Genetics	M,D
Health Services Management and Hospital Administration	M,D
Health Services Research	M,D
Immunology	D
International Health	M
Microbiology	M,D
Molecular Biology	M,D
Molecular Genetics	D
Neurobiology	M,D
Neuroscience	D
Nurse Midwifery	M,D
Nursing and Healthcare Administration	M,D
Nursing—General	M,D
Oral and Dental Sciences	M,D
Pediatric Nursing	M,D
Pharmaceutical Sciences	D
Pharmacology	D
Physical Therapy	D
Physician Assistant Studies	M
Physiology	D
Psychiatric Nursing	M,D
Public Health—General	M,D
Rehabilitation Sciences	D
Toxicology	D
Women's Health Nursing	M,D

UNIVERSITY OF CONNECTICUT

Allied Health—General	M
Biochemistry	M,D
Biological and Biomedical Sciences—General	D
Biophysics	M,D
Biopsychology	M,D,O
Botany	M,D
Cell Biology	M,D
Clinical Research	M
Communication Disorders	M,D
Developmental Biology	M,D
Ecology	M,D,O
Entomology	M,D
Environmental and Occupational Health	M
Genetics	M,D
Genomic Sciences	M
Health Services Management and Hospital Administration	M,D
Medicinal and Pharmaceutical Chemistry	M,D
Microbiology	M,D
Molecular Biology	M
Neurobiology	M,D
Neuroscience	M,D,O
Nursing—General	M,D,O
Nutrition	M,D
Oral and Dental Sciences	M
Pathobiology	M,D
Pharmaceutical Sciences	M,D
Pharmacology	M,D
Pharmacy	D
Physical Therapy	D
Physiology	M,D*
Plant Biology	M,D
Plant Molecular Biology	M,D
Public Health—General	M
Structural Biology	M,D
Toxicology	M,D
Zoology	M,D

UNIVERSITY OF CONNECTICUT HEALTH CENTER

Allopathic Medicine	D
Biochemistry	D
Biological and Biomedical Sciences—General	D*

Cell Biology D*
Clinical Research M
Dentistry D,O
Developmental Biology D
Genetics D*
Immunology D*
Molecular Biology D*
Neuroscience D*
Oral and Dental Sciences M,D*
Public Health—General M

UNIVERSITY OF DALLAS
Health Services Management and Hospital Administration M

UNIVERSITY OF DAYTON
Biological and Biomedical Sciences—General M,D
Physical Therapy M,D

UNIVERSITY OF DELAWARE
Adult Nursing M,O
Biochemistry M,D
Biological and Biomedical Sciences—General M,D
Cancer Biology/Oncology M,D
Cell Biology M,D
Developmental Biology M,D
Ecology M,D
Entomology M,D
Evolutionary Biology M,D
Family Nurse Practitioner Studies M,O
Genetics M,D
Gerontological Nursing M,O
Health Promotion M
HIV/AIDS Nursing M,O
Maternal and Child/Neonatal Nursing M,O
Microbiology M,D
Molecular Biology M,D
Neuroscience D
Nursing and Healthcare Administration M,O
Nursing—General M,O
Nutrition M
Oncology Nursing M,O
Pediatric Nursing M,O
Physical Therapy D
Physiology M,D
Psychiatric Nursing M,O
Women's Health Nursing M,O

UNIVERSITY OF DENVER
Biological and Biomedical Sciences—General M,D
Cell Biology M,D
Ecology M,D
Environmental and Occupational Health M,O
Evolutionary Biology M,D
Health Services Management and Hospital Administration M,O
International Health M,D,O
Molecular Biology M,D
Neuroscience D

UNIVERSITY OF DETROIT MERCY
Allied Health—General M,O
Biochemistry M
Dentistry D
Family Nurse Practitioner Studies M,O
Health Services Management and Hospital Administration M
Nurse Anesthesia M
Oral and Dental Sciences M,O
Physician Assistant Studies M

UNIVERSITY OF EVANSVILLE
Health Services Management and Hospital Administration M
Physical Therapy D

THE UNIVERSITY OF FINDLAY
Health Services Management and Hospital Administration M,D
Occupational Therapy M,D
Pharmacy M,D
Physical Therapy M,D
Physician Assistant Studies M,D

UNIVERSITY OF FLORIDA
Allied Health—General M,D,O
Allopathic Medicine D
Biochemistry D
Biological and Biomedical Sciences—General M,D
Botany M,D
Cell Biology M,D
Clinical Laboratory Sciences/Medical Technology M,D,O
Clinical Research M,D,O
Communication Disorders M,D
Dentistry D,O
Ecology M,D,O
Entomology M,D
Environmental and Occupational Health M,D,O
Epidemiology M,D,O
Genetics D
Health Services Management and Hospital Administration M,D
Health Services Research M,D
Immunology D
International Health M
Medical Physics M,D,O
Medicinal and Pharmaceutical Chemistry M,D
Microbiology M,D
Molecular Biology M,D
Molecular Genetics M
Neuroscience D
Nursing—General M,D
Nutrition M,D
Occupational Therapy M

Oral and Dental Sciences M,D,O
Pharmaceutical Administration M,D
Pharmaceutical Sciences M,D
Pharmacology M,D
Pharmacy M,D
Physical Therapy D
Physician Assistant Studies M
Physiology M,D
Plant Biology M,D
Plant Molecular Biology M,D
Plant Pathology M,D
Public Health—General M,D,O
Rehabilitation Sciences D
Toxicology M,D,O
Veterinary Medicine D
Veterinary Sciences M,D,O
Zoology M,D

UNIVERSITY OF GEORGIA
Anatomy M
Biochemistry M,D
Biological and Biomedical Sciences—General D
Cell Biology M,D
Communication Disorders M,D,O
Ecology M,D
Entomology M,D
Environmental and Occupational Health M
Genetics M,D
Genomic Sciences M,D
Health Promotion M,D
Health Services Management and Hospital Administration M
Infectious Diseases M,D
Microbiology M,D
Molecular Biology M,D
Neuroscience D
Nutrition M,D
Pathology M,D
Pharmaceutical Administration D
Pharmaceutical Sciences D
Pharmacology M,D
Pharmacy M,D,O
Physiology M,D
Plant Biology M,D
Plant Pathology M,D
Public Health—General D
Veterinary Medicine M,D
Veterinary Sciences M

UNIVERSITY OF GUAM
Biological and Biomedical Sciences—General M
Marine Biology M

UNIVERSITY OF GUELPH
Acute Care/Critical Care Nursing M,D,O
Anatomy M,D
Anesthesiologist Assistant Studies M,D,O
Biochemistry M,D
Biological and Biomedical Sciences—General M,D
Biophysics M,D
Botany M,D
Cardiovascular Sciences M,D,O
Cell Biology M,D
Ecology M,D
Emergency Medical Services M,D,O
Entomology M,D
Environmental Biology M,D
Epidemiology M,D
Evolutionary Biology M,D
Immunology M,D,O
Infectious Diseases M,D,O
Medical Imaging M,D,O
Microbiology M,D
Molecular Biology M,D
Molecular Genetics M,D
Neuroscience M,D,O
Nutrition M,D
Pathology M,D,O
Pharmacology M,D
Physiology M,D
Plant Pathology M,D
Toxicology M,D
Veterinary Medicine M,D,O
Veterinary Sciences M,D,O
Vision Sciences M,D,O
Zoology M,D

UNIVERSITY OF HARTFORD
Biological and Biomedical Sciences—General M
Community Health Nursing M
Neuroscience M
Nursing Education M
Nursing—General M
Physical Therapy M,D

UNIVERSITY OF HAWAII AT HILO
Conservation Biology M
Marine Biology M
Nursing—General D
Pharmaceutical Sciences D
Pharmacology M
Pharmacy D

UNIVERSITY OF HAWAII AT MANOA
Adult Nursing M,D,O
Allopathic Medicine D
Biological and Biomedical Sciences—General M,D
Botany M,D
Communication Disorders M
Community Health Nursing M,D,O
Conservation Biology M,D
Developmental Biology M,D
Ecology M,D
Entomology M,D
Epidemiology D
Evolutionary Biology M,D
Family Nurse Practitioner Studies M,D,O

Genetics M,D
Marine Biology M,D
Medical Microbiology M,D
Microbiology M,D
Molecular Biology M,D
Nursing and Healthcare Administration M,D,O
Nursing—General M,D,O
Nutrition M,D
Physiology M,D
Plant Pathology M,D
Public Health—General M,D,O
Reproductive Biology M,D
Zoology M,D

UNIVERSITY OF HOUSTON
Biochemistry M,D
Biological and Biomedical Sciences—General M,D
Communication Disorders M
Nutrition M,D
Optometry D
Pharmaceutical Administration M,D
Pharmaceutical Sciences M,D
Pharmacology M,D
Pharmacy M,D
Vision Sciences M,D

UNIVERSITY OF HOUSTON–CLEAR LAKE
Biological and Biomedical Sciences—General M
Health Services Management and Hospital Administration M

UNIVERSITY OF HOUSTON–VICTORIA
Biological and Biomedical Sciences—General M
Family Nurse Practitioner Studies M
Nursing and Healthcare Administration M
Nursing Education M
Nursing—General M

UNIVERSITY OF IDAHO
Biochemistry M,D
Biological and Biomedical Sciences—General M,D
Computational Biology M,D
Entomology M,D
Microbiology M,D
Molecular Biology M,D
Neuroscience M,D
Veterinary Sciences M,D

UNIVERSITY OF ILLINOIS AT CHICAGO
Acute Care/Critical Care Nursing M,O
Adult Nursing M,O
Allied Health—General M,D,O
Allopathic Medicine D
Anatomy
Biochemistry D
Biological and Biomedical Sciences—General M,D
Biophysics M,D
Cell Biology M,D
Community Health Nursing M,O
Community Health M,D
Dentistry D
Environmental and Occupational Health M,D
Epidemiology M,D
Family Nurse Practitioner Studies M,O
Genetics D
Gerontological Nursing M,O
Health Services Management and Hospital Administration M,D
Health Services Research M,D
Immunology D
Maternal and Child/Neonatal Nursing M,O
Microbiology D
Molecular Biology D
Molecular Genetics D
Neuroscience M,D
Nurse Midwifery M,O
Nursing and Healthcare Administration M,O
Nursing—General M,D,O
Nutrition M,D
Occupational Health Nursing M,O
Occupational Therapy M,D
Oral and Dental Sciences M,D
Pediatric Nursing M,O
Pharmaceutical Administration M,D
Pharmaceutical Sciences M,D
Pharmacology D
Pharmacy D
Physical Therapy M,D
Physiology M,D
Psychiatric Nursing M,O
Public Health—General M,D
Rehabilitation Sciences M,D
School Nursing M,O
Toxicology M
Women's Health Nursing M,O

UNIVERSITY OF ILLINOIS AT SPRINGFIELD
Biological and Biomedical Sciences—General M
Community Health M,O
Epidemiology M,O
Public Health—General M,O

UNIVERSITY OF ILLINOIS AT URBANA–CHAMPAIGN
Allopathic Medicine
Biochemistry M,D
Biological and Biomedical Sciences—General M,D
Biophysics M,D
Cell Biology D

Communication Disorders M,D
Community Health M,D
Computational Biology M,D
Conservation Biology M,D
Developmental Biology D
Ecology M,D
Entomology M,D
Evolutionary Biology M,D
Health Services Management and Hospital Administration M,D
Microbiology M,D
Molecular Physiology M,D
Neuroscience D
Nutrition M,D
Pathobiology M,D
Physiology M,D
Plant Biology M,D
Public Health—General M,D
Rehabilitation Sciences M,D
Veterinary Medicine D
Veterinary Sciences M,D
Zoology M,D

UNIVERSITY OF INDIANAPOLIS
Biological and Biomedical Sciences—General M
Family Nurse Practitioner Studies M,D
Maternal and Child/Neonatal Nursing M,D
Nurse Midwifery M,D
Nursing and Healthcare Administration M,D
Nursing Education M,D
Nursing—General M,D
Occupational Therapy M,D
Physical Therapy M,D
Public Health—General M,D
Women's Health Nursing M,D

THE UNIVERSITY OF IOWA
Allopathic Medicine D
Anatomy D
Bacteriology M,D
Biochemistry M,D
Biological and Biomedical Sciences—General M,D
Biophysics M,D
Cell Biology M,D
Clinical Research M,D
Communication Disorders M,D
Community Health M,D
Computational Biology M,D,O
Dentistry M,D,O
Environmental and Occupational Health M,D,O
Epidemiology M,D
Evolutionary Biology M,D
Genetics M,D
Health Services Management and Hospital Administration M,D
Immunology M,D
Industrial Hygiene M,D,O
Medicinal and Pharmaceutical Chemistry M,D
Microbiology M,D
Molecular Biology D
Neurobiology M,D
Neuroscience D
Nursing—General M,D
Oral and Dental Sciences M,D,O
Pathology M
Pharmaceutical Sciences M,D
Pharmacology M,D
Pharmacy M,D
Physical Therapy D
Physician Assistant Studies M
Physiology M,D
Public Health—General M,D,O
Radiation Biology M,D
Rehabilitation Sciences D
Toxicology M,D
Translational Biology M,D
Virology M,D

UNIVERSITY OF JAMESTOWN
Physical Therapy D

THE UNIVERSITY OF KANSAS
Adult Nursing M,D,O
Allied Health—General M,D,O
Allopathic Medicine D
Anatomy M,D
Biochemistry M,D
Biological and Biomedical Sciences—General M,D*
Biophysics M,D
Botany M,D
Cell Biology M,D
Clinical Research M
Communication Disorders M,D
Community Health Nursing M,D,O
Computational Biology D
Developmental Biology M,D
Ecology M,D
Entomology M,D
Environmental and Occupational Health M
Epidemiology M
Evolutionary Biology M,D
Gerontological Nursing M,D,O
Health Services Management and Hospital Administration M,D
Medicinal and Pharmaceutical Chemistry M,D
Microbiology M,D
Molecular Biology M,D
Neuroscience M,D
Nurse Anesthesia M,D
Nurse Midwifery M,D,O
Nursing and Healthcare Administration M,D,O
Nursing—General M,D,O

*M—masters degree; D—doctorate; O—other advanced degree; *—Close-Up and/or Display*

Nutrition M,D,O
Occupational Therapy M,D
Pathology M,D
Pharmaceutical Sciences M
Pharmacology M,D
Physical Therapy D
Physiology M,D
Psychiatric Nursing M,D,O
Public Health—General M
Rehabilitation Sciences M,D
Toxicology M,D

UNIVERSITY OF KENTUCKY
Allied Health—General M,D
Allopathic Medicine D
Anatomy D
Biochemistry D
Biological and Biomedical Sciences—General M,D
Clinical Research M
Communication Disorders M
Dentistry D
Entomology M,D
Epidemiology D
Health Physics/Radiological Health M
Health Promotion M,D
Health Services Management and Hospital Administration M
Immunology D
Medical Physics M
Microbiology D
Molecular Genetics D
Neurobiology D
Nursing—General D
Nutrition M,D
Oral and Dental Sciences M
Pharmaceutical Sciences M,D
Pharmacology D
Pharmacy D
Physical Therapy D
Physician Assistant Studies M
Physiology D
Plant Pathology M,D
Public Health—General M
Rehabilitation Sciences D
Toxicology M,D
Veterinary Sciences M,D

UNIVERSITY OF LA VERNE
Health Services Management and Hospital Administration M,D,O
Health Services Research M

UNIVERSITY OF LETHBRIDGE
Biochemistry M,D
Biological and Biomedical Sciences—General M,D
Molecular Biology M,D
Neuroscience M,D
Nursing—General M,D

UNIVERSITY OF LOUISIANA AT LAFAYETTE
Biological and Biomedical Sciences—General M,D
Communication Disorders M,D
Environmental Biology M,D
Evolutionary Biology M,D
Nursing—General M

UNIVERSITY OF LOUISIANA AT MONROE
Biological and Biomedical Sciences—General M
Communication Disorders M
Occupational Therapy M
Pharmacy D
Toxicology D

UNIVERSITY OF LOUISVILLE
Adult Nursing M,D
Allopathic Medicine D
Anatomy M,D
Biochemistry M,D
Biological and Biomedical Sciences—General M,D
Biophysics M,D
Clinical Research M,D,O
Communication Disorders M,D
Community Health M
Dentistry M,D
Environmental and Occupational Health M,D
Environmental Biology M,D
Epidemiology M,D
Family Nurse Practitioner Studies M,D
Health Promotion D
Health Services Management and Hospital Administration M,D
Immunology M,D
Maternal and Child/Neonatal Nursing M,D
Microbiology M,D
Molecular Biology M,D
Neurobiology M,D
Nursing—General M,D
Oral and Dental Sciences M,D
Pharmacology M,D
Physiology M,D
Psychiatric Nursing M,D
Public Health—General M,D
Toxicology M,D
Veterinary Sciences O

UNIVERSITY OF MAINE
Biochemistry M,D
Biological and Biomedical Sciences—General M,D
Botany M,D
Cell Biology M,D
Communication Disorders M
Ecology M,D
Entomology M,D
Family Nurse Practitioner Studies M,O
Genomic Sciences D
Marine Biology M,D

Microbiology M,D
Molecular Biology M,D
Neuroscience M,D
Nursing Education M,O
Nursing—General M,O
Nutrition M,D,O
Plant Pathology M,D
Toxicology M,D
Zoology M,D

UNIVERSITY OF MANAGEMENT AND TECHNOLOGY
Health Services Management and Hospital Administration M

THE UNIVERSITY OF MANCHESTER
Biochemistry M,D
Biological and Biomedical Sciences—General M,D
Biophysics M,D
Cancer Biology/Oncology M,D
Cell Biology M,D
Communication Disorders M,D
Dentistry M,D
Developmental Biology M,D
Ecology M,D
Environmental Biology M,D
Evolutionary Biology M,D
Genetics M,D
Immunology M,D
Microbiology M,D
Molecular Biology M,D
Molecular Genetics M,D
Neurobiology M,D
Neuroscience M,D
Nurse Midwifery M,D
Nursing—General M,D
Optometry M,D
Oral and Dental Sciences M,D
Pharmaceutical Sciences M,D
Pharmacology M,D
Pharmacy M,D
Physiology M,D
Public Health—General M,D
Structural Biology M,D
Toxicology M,D
Vision Sciences M,D

UNIVERSITY OF MANITOBA
Anatomy M,D
Biochemistry M,D
Biological and Biomedical Sciences—General M,D,O
Botany M,D
Cancer Biology/Oncology M
Community Health M,D,O
Dentistry D
Ecology M,D
Entomology M,D
Human Genetics M,D
Immunology M,D
Medical Microbiology M,D
Microbiology M,D
Nursing—General M
Nutrition M,D
Occupational Therapy M,D
Oral and Dental Sciences M,D
Pathology M
Pharmaceutical Sciences M,D
Pharmacology M,D
Physical Therapy M,D
Physiology M,D
Plant Physiology M,D
Rehabilitation Sciences M,D
Zoology M,D

UNIVERSITY OF MARY
Cardiovascular Sciences M
Family Nurse Practitioner Studies M
Health Services Management and Hospital Administration M
Nursing and Healthcare Administration M
Nursing Education M
Nursing—General M
Occupational Therapy M
Physical Therapy D

UNIVERSITY OF MARY HARDIN-BAYLOR
Family Nurse Practitioner Studies M,O
Nursing and Healthcare Administration M,O
Nursing Education M,D,O
Nursing—General M,O

UNIVERSITY OF MARYLAND, BALTIMORE
Allopathic Medicine D
Biochemistry M,D
Biological and Biomedical Sciences—General M,D
Cancer Biology/Oncology M,D
Cell Biology M,D
Clinical Laboratory Sciences/Medical Technology M
Clinical Research M,D,O
Community Health Nursing M
Dental Hygiene M
Dentistry D,O
Epidemiology M,D
Genomic Sciences M,D
Gerontological Nursing M
Health Services Research M,D
Human Genetics M,D
Immunology D
Maternal and Child/Neonatal Nursing M
Medical/Surgical Nursing M
Microbiology D
Molecular Biology M,D
Molecular Medicine M,D
Neurobiology D
Neuroscience D
Nurse Midwifery M
Nursing and Healthcare Administration M

Nursing Education M
Nursing—General M,D,O
Oral and Dental Sciences M,D,O
Pathology M
Pediatric Nursing M
Pharmaceutical Administration M,D
Pharmaceutical Sciences D
Pharmacology M,D
Pharmacy M,D
Physical Therapy D
Psychiatric Nursing M
Rehabilitation Sciences D
Toxicology M,D

UNIVERSITY OF MARYLAND, BALTIMORE COUNTY
Biochemistry M,D,O
Biological and Biomedical Sciences—General M,D,O
Cell Biology D
Epidemiology M,O
Health Services Management and Hospital Administration M,D,O
Molecular Biology M,D
Neuroscience D

UNIVERSITY OF MARYLAND, COLLEGE PARK
Biochemistry M,D
Biological and Biomedical Sciences—General M,D
Biophysics D
Cell Biology M,D
Communication Disorders M,D
Computational Biology D
Conservation Biology M
Ecology M,D
Entomology M,D
Environmental and Occupational Health M
Epidemiology M,D
Evolutionary Biology M,D
Genomic Sciences D
Health Services Management and Hospital Administration M,D
Maternal and Child Health M,D
Molecular Biology D
Molecular Genetics M,D
Neuroscience M,D
Nutrition M,D
Plant Biology M,D
Public Health—General M,D
Veterinary Medicine D
Veterinary Sciences M,D

UNIVERSITY OF MARYLAND EASTERN SHORE
Physical Therapy D
Rehabilitation Sciences M
Toxicology M,D

UNIVERSITY OF MARYLAND UNIVERSITY COLLEGE
Health Services Management and Hospital Administration M,O

UNIVERSITY OF MASSACHUSETTS AMHERST
Adult Nursing M,D
Animal Behavior M,D
Biochemistry M,D
Biological and Biomedical Sciences—General M,D
Cell Biology M,D
Communication Disorders M,D
Community Health Nursing M,D
Community Health M,D
Developmental Biology D
Environmental and Occupational Health M,D
Environmental Biology M,D
Epidemiology M,D
Evolutionary Biology M,D
Family Nurse Practitioner Studies M,D
Genetics M,D
Gerontological Nursing M,D
Health Services Management and Hospital Administration M,D
Microbiology M,D*
Molecular Biophysics D
Neuroscience M,D
Nursing and Healthcare Administration M,D
Nursing—General M,D
Nutrition M,D
Physiology M,D
Plant Biology M,D
Plant Molecular Biology M,D
Plant Physiology M,D
Public Health—General M,D

UNIVERSITY OF MASSACHUSETTS BOSTON
Biological and Biomedical Sciences—General M
Cell Biology D
Environmental Biology D
Health Services Management and Hospital Administration M,D,O
Molecular Biology D
Nursing—General M,D

UNIVERSITY OF MASSACHUSETTS DARTMOUTH
Adult Nursing M,D,O
Biochemistry M,D
Biological and Biomedical Sciences—General M
Clinical Laboratory Sciences/Medical Technology M,D
Community Health Nursing M,D,O
Gerontological Nursing M,D,O
Marine Biology M
Nursing and Healthcare Administration M,D,O

Nursing Education M,D,O
Nursing—General M,D,O

UNIVERSITY OF MASSACHUSETTS LOWELL
Allied Health—General M,D,O
Biochemistry M,D
Biological and Biomedical Sciences—General M,D
Clinical Laboratory Sciences/Medical Technology M,O
Epidemiology M,D,O
Family Nurse Practitioner Studies M
Gerontological Nursing M,O
Health Physics/Radiological Health M
Health Promotion D
Health Services Management and Hospital Administration M,O
Industrial Hygiene M,D,O
Nursing and Healthcare Administration D
Nursing—General M,D,O
Nutrition M,O
Pathology M,O
Physical Therapy D
Psychiatric Nursing M,O
Public Health—General M,O

UNIVERSITY OF MASSACHUSETTS WORCESTER
Adult Nursing M,D,O
Allopathic Medicine D
Biochemistry M,D
Biological and Biomedical Sciences—General M,D
Cancer Biology/Oncology M,D
Cell Biology M,D
Clinical Research M,D
Computational Biology M,D
Family Nurse Practitioner Studies M,D,O
Gerontological Nursing M,D,O
Health Services Research M,D
Immunology M,D
Microbiology M,D
Molecular Genetics M,D
Molecular Pharmacology M,D
Neuroscience M,D
Nursing and Healthcare Administration M,D,O
Nursing Education M,D,O
Nursing—General M,D,O
Translational Biology M,D
Virology M,D

UNIVERSITY OF MEMPHIS
Biological and Biomedical Sciences—General M,D
Communication Disorders M,D
Environmental and Occupational Health M
Epidemiology M
Family Nurse Practitioner Studies M,O
Health Promotion M
Health Services Management and Hospital Administration M
Nursing and Healthcare Administration M,O
Nursing Education M,O
Nursing Informatics M,O
Nursing—General M,O
Nutrition M
Public Health—General M

UNIVERSITY OF MIAMI
Acute Care/Critical Care Nursing M,D
Adult Nursing M,D
Allopathic Medicine D
Biochemistry D
Biological and Biomedical Sciences—General M,D
Biophysics D
Cancer Biology/Oncology D
Cell Biology D
Community Health D
Developmental Biology D
Environmental and Occupational Health M
Epidemiology M,D
Evolutionary Biology M,D
Family Nurse Practitioner Studies M,D
Genetics M,D
Immunology D
Marine Biology M,D
Microbiology D
Molecular Biology D
Neuroscience M,D
Nurse Anesthesia M,D
Nurse Midwifery M,D
Nursing—General M,D
Nutrition M
Pharmacology D
Physical Therapy D
Physiology D
Public Health—General M,D

UNIVERSITY OF MICHIGAN
Acute Care/Critical Care Nursing M,D,O
Adult Nursing M,D,O
Allopathic Medicine D
Biochemistry M,D
Biological and Biomedical Sciences—General D
Biophysics D
Biopsychology D
Cancer Biology/Oncology M,D
Cell Biology M,D
Clinical Research M
Conservation Biology M,D
Dental Hygiene M
Dentistry D
Developmental Biology M,D
Ecology M,D
Environmental and Occupational Health M,D
Epidemiology M,D
Evolutionary Biology M,D

Program	Degrees
Family Nurse Practitioner Studies	M,D,O
Gerontological Nursing	M,D,O
Health Physics/Radiological Health	M,D,O
Health Promotion	M,D
Health Services Management and Hospital Administration	M,D
Human Genetics	M,D
Immunology	M,D
Industrial Hygiene	M,D
International Health	M,D
Medicinal and Pharmaceutical Chemistry	D
Microbiology	M,D
Molecular Biology	M,D
Molecular Pathology	D
Neuroscience	D
Nurse Midwifery	M,D,O
Nursing and Healthcare Administration	M,D,O
Nursing—General	M,D,O
Nutrition	M,D
Oral and Dental Sciences	M,D
Pathology	D
Pediatric Nursing	M,D,O
Pharmaceutical Administration	D
Pharmaceutical Sciences	D
Pharmacology	M,D
Pharmacy	D
Physiology	M,D
Public Health—General	M,D
Toxicology	M,D

UNIVERSITY OF MICHIGAN–FLINT

Program	Degrees
Biochemistry	M
Biological and Biomedical Sciences—General	M
Family Nurse Practitioner Studies	M,D,O
Health Services Management and Hospital Administration	M,D,O
Nurse Anesthesia	M,D
Nursing—General	M,D,O
Physical Therapy	D
Public Health—General	M,D,O

UNIVERSITY OF MINNESOTA, DULUTH

Program	Degrees
Allopathic Medicine	D
Biochemistry	M,D
Biological and Biomedical Sciences—General	M,D
Biophysics	M,D
Communication Disorders	M
Immunology	M,D
Medical Microbiology	M,D
Molecular Biology	M,D
Pharmacology	M,D
Pharmacy	M,D
Physiology	M,D
Toxicology	M,D

UNIVERSITY OF MINNESOTA, TWIN CITIES CAMPUS

Program	Degrees
Adult Nursing	M
Allopathic Medicine	M,D
Animal Behavior	M,D
Biochemistry	D
Biological and Biomedical Sciences—General	M
Biophysics	M,D
Biopsychology	D
Cancer Biology/Oncology	D
Cell Biology	M,D
Clinical Laboratory Sciences/Medical Technology	M
Clinical Research	M
Communication Disorders	M,D
Community Health Nursing	M
Community Health	M
Conservation Biology	M,D
Dentistry	D
Developmental Biology	M,D
Ecology	M,D
Entomology	M,D
Environmental and Occupational Health	M,D,O
Epidemiology	M,D
Evolutionary Biology	M,D
Family Nurse Practitioner Studies	M
Genetics	M,D
Gerontological Nursing	M
Health Services Management and Hospital Administration	M,D
Health Services Research	M,D
Immunology	D
Industrial Hygiene	M,D
Infectious Diseases	M,D
International Health	M,D
Maternal and Child Health	M
Medical Physics	M,D
Medicinal and Pharmaceutical Chemistry	M,D
Microbiology	D
Molecular Biology	M,D
Neurobiology	M,D
Neuroscience	M,D
Nurse Anesthesia	M,D
Nurse Midwifery	M
Nursing and Healthcare Administration	M
Nursing—General	M,D
Nutrition	M,D
Occupational Health Nursing	M,D
Oral and Dental Sciences	M,D,O
Pediatric Nursing	M
Pharmaceutical Administration	M,D
Pharmaceutical Sciences	M,D
Pharmacology	M,D
Pharmacy	D
Physical Therapy	M,D
Physiology	D
Plant Biology	M,D
Plant Pathology	M,D
Psychiatric Nursing	M

Program	Degrees
Public Health—General	M,D,O
Structural Biology	D
Toxicology	M,D
Veterinary Medicine	D
Veterinary Sciences	M,D
Virology	D
Women's Health Nursing	M

UNIVERSITY OF MISSISSIPPI

Program	Degrees
Biological and Biomedical Sciences—General	M,D
Communication Disorders	M
Health Promotion	M,D
Medicinal and Pharmaceutical Chemistry	M,D
Nutrition	M
Pharmaceutical Administration	M,D
Pharmaceutical Sciences	M,D
Pharmacology	M,D
Pharmacy	D

UNIVERSITY OF MISSISSIPPI MEDICAL CENTER

Program	Degrees
Allied Health—General	M
Allopathic Medicine	D
Anatomy	M,D
Biochemistry	D
Biological and Biomedical Sciences—General	M,D
Biophysics	D
Dentistry	M,D
Microbiology	D
Neuroscience	D
Nursing—General	M,D
Occupational Therapy	M
Oral and Dental Sciences	M,D
Pathology	D
Pharmacology	D
Physical Therapy	M
Physiology	D
Toxicology	D

UNIVERSITY OF MISSOURI

Program	Degrees
Adult Nursing	M,D,O
Allopathic Medicine	D
Anatomy	M
Biochemistry	M,D
Biological and Biomedical Sciences—General	M,D
Cell Biology	M,D
Communication Disorders	M,D
Community Health	M,D
Conservation Biology	M,D,O
Ecology	M,D
Entomology	M,D
Evolutionary Biology	M,D
Family Nurse Practitioner Studies	M,D,O
Genetics	M,D
Gerontological Nursing	M,D,O
Health Physics/Radiological Health	M
Health Promotion	M,O
Health Services Management and Hospital Administration	M,D,O
Immunology	M,D
International Health	M,O
Medical Physics	M,D,O
Microbiology	M,D
Neurobiology	M,D
Neuroscience	M,D
Nursing and Healthcare Administration	M,D,O
Nursing—General	M,D,O
Nutrition	M,D
Occupational Therapy	M
Pathobiology	M,D
Pathology	M
Pediatric Nursing	M,D,O
Pharmacology	M,D
Physical Therapy	M,D
Physiology	M,D
Plant Biology	M,D
Psychiatric Nursing	M,D,O
Public Health—General	M,O
Veterinary Medicine	D
Veterinary Sciences	M,D

UNIVERSITY OF MISSOURI–KANSAS CITY

Program	Degrees
Adult Nursing	M,D
Allopathic Medicine	M,D
Anesthesiologist Assistant Studies	M,D
Biochemistry	D
Biological and Biomedical Sciences—General	M,D
Biophysics	D
Cell Biology	D
Dental Hygiene	M,D,O
Dentistry	M,D,O
Family Nurse Practitioner Studies	M,D
Gerontological Nursing	M,D
Maternal and Child/Neonatal Nursing	M,D
Molecular Biology	D
Nursing and Healthcare Administration	M,D
Nursing Education	M,D
Nursing—General	M,D
Oral and Dental Sciences	M,D,O
Pediatric Nursing	M,D
Pharmaceutical Sciences	D
Pharmacology	D
Pharmacy	D
Physician Assistant Studies	M,D
Toxicology	D
Women's Health Nursing	M,D

UNIVERSITY OF MISSOURI–ST. LOUIS

Program	Degrees
Adult Nursing	M,D,O
Biochemistry	M,D
Biological and Biomedical Sciences—General	M,D,O
Cell Biology	M,D,O

Program	Degrees
Conservation Biology	M,D,O
Ecology	M,D,O
Evolutionary Biology	M,D,O
Family Nurse Practitioner Studies	M,D,O
Health Services Management and Hospital Administration	M,O
Maternal and Child/Neonatal Nursing	M,D,O
Molecular Biology	M,D,O
Neuroscience	M,D,O
Nursing and Healthcare Administration	M,D,O
Nursing Education	M,D,O
Nursing—General	M,D,O
Optometry	D
Pediatric Nursing	M,D,O
Psychiatric Nursing	M,D,O
Women's Health Nursing	M,D,O

UNIVERSITY OF MOBILE

Program	Degrees
Nursing—General	M

THE UNIVERSITY OF MONTANA

Program	Degrees
Animal Behavior	M,D,O
Biochemistry	D
Biological and Biomedical Sciences—General	M,D
Cell Biology	D
Community Health	M
Developmental Biology	D
Ecology	M,D
Immunology	D
Medicinal and Pharmaceutical Chemistry	M,D
Microbiology	D
Molecular Biology	D
Neuroscience	M,D
Pharmaceutical Sciences	M,D
Pharmacy	M,D
Physical Therapy	D
Public Health—General	M,O
Toxicology	M,D
Zoology	M,D

UNIVERSITY OF MONTEVALLO

Program	Degrees
Communication Disorders	M

UNIVERSITY OF MOUNT UNION

Program	Degrees
Physician Assistant Studies	M

UNIVERSITY OF NEBRASKA AT KEARNEY

Program	Degrees
Biological and Biomedical Sciences—General	M
Communication Disorders	M

UNIVERSITY OF NEBRASKA AT OMAHA

Program	Degrees
Biological and Biomedical Sciences—General	M
Communication Disorders	M

UNIVERSITY OF NEBRASKA–LINCOLN

Program	Degrees
Biochemistry	M,D
Biological and Biomedical Sciences—General	M,D
Biopsychology	M,D
Communication Disorders	M,D
Entomology	M,D
Health Promotion	M,D
Nutrition	M,D
Toxicology	M,D
Veterinary Sciences	M,D

UNIVERSITY OF NEBRASKA MEDICAL CENTER

Program	Degrees
Allied Health—General	M,D,O
Allopathic Medicine	D,O
Anatomy	M,D
Biochemistry	M,D
Biological and Biomedical Sciences—General	M,D
Cancer Biology/Oncology	D
Cell Biology	M,D
Clinical Laboratory Sciences/Medical Technology	M,O
Dentistry	M,D,O
Environmental and Occupational Health	M,D
Genetics	M,D
Microbiology	M,D
Molecular Biology	M,D
Neuroscience	M,D
Nursing—General	D
Nutrition	O
Pathology	M,D
Perfusion	M
Pharmaceutical Sciences	M,D
Pharmacology	M,D
Pharmacy	D
Physical Therapy	D
Physician Assistant Studies	M
Physiology	M,D
Public Health—General	M

UNIVERSITY OF NEVADA, LAS VEGAS

Program	Degrees
Allied Health—General	M,D
Biochemistry	M,D
Biological and Biomedical Sciences—General	M,D
Community Health	M,D
Family Nurse Practitioner Studies	M,D,O
Health Physics/Radiological Health	M
Health Services Management and Hospital Administration	M
Nursing Education	M,D,O
Nursing—General	M,D,O
Pediatric Nursing	M,D,O
Physical Therapy	D
Public Health—General	M,D

UNIVERSITY OF NEVADA, RENO

Program	Degrees
Biochemistry	M,D
Biological and Biomedical Sciences—General	M

Program	Degrees
Cell Biology	M,D
Communication Disorders	M,D
Conservation Biology	D
Ecology	D
Environmental and Occupational Health	M,D
Evolutionary Biology	D
Molecular Biology	M,D
Molecular Pharmacology	D
Nursing—General	M,D
Nutrition	M
Physiology	D
Public Health—General	M,D

UNIVERSITY OF NEW BRUNSWICK FREDERICTON

Program	Degrees
Biological and Biomedical Sciences—General	M,D
Health Services Research	M
Nursing Education	M
Nursing—General	M

UNIVERSITY OF NEW BRUNSWICK SAINT JOHN

Program	Degrees
Biological and Biomedical Sciences—General	M,D

UNIVERSITY OF NEW ENGLAND

Program	Degrees
Biological and Biomedical Sciences—General	M
Dentistry	D
Nurse Anesthesia	M
Occupational Therapy	M
Osteopathic Medicine	D
Pharmacy	D
Physical Therapy	D
Physician Assistant Studies	M
Public Health—General	M,O

UNIVERSITY OF NEW HAMPSHIRE

Program	Degrees
Biochemistry	M,D
Biological and Biomedical Sciences—General	M,D
Communication Disorders	M
Family Nurse Practitioner Studies	M,D,O
Genetics	M,D
Microbiology	M,D
Nursing—General	M,D,O
Nutrition	M,D
Occupational Therapy	M,O
Plant Biology	M,D
Public Health—General	M,O
Zoology	M,D

UNIVERSITY OF NEW HAVEN

Program	Degrees
Cell Biology	M,O
Ecology	M,O
Environmental and Occupational Health	M,O
Health Services Management and Hospital Administration	M,O
Molecular Biology	M,O
Nutrition	M

UNIVERSITY OF NEW MEXICO

Program	Degrees
Allopathic Medicine	D
Biochemistry	M,D,O
Biological and Biomedical Sciences—General	M,D,O
Cell Biology	M,D,O
Clinical Laboratory Sciences/Medical Technology	M,O
Communication Disorders	M
Community Health	M
Dental Hygiene	M
Epidemiology	M
Genetics	M,D,O
Health Services Management and Hospital Administration	M
Microbiology	M,D,O
Molecular Biology	M,D,O
Neuroscience	M,D,O
Nursing—General	M,D
Nutrition	M
Occupational Therapy	M
Pathology	M,D,O
Pharmaceutical Sciences	M,D
Pharmacy	D
Physical Therapy	D
Physician Assistant Studies	M
Physiology	M,D,O
Public Health—General	M
Toxicology	M,D,O

UNIVERSITY OF NEW ORLEANS

Program	Degrees
Biological and Biomedical Sciences—General	M,D
Health Services Management and Hospital Administration	M

UNIVERSITY OF NORTH ALABAMA

Program	Degrees
Environmental and Occupational Health	M
Health Promotion	M
Health Services Management and Hospital Administration	M
Nursing—General	M

THE UNIVERSITY OF NORTH CAROLINA AT CHAPEL HILL

Program	Degrees
Adult Nursing	M,D,O
Allied Health—General	M,D
Allopathic Medicine	D
Biochemistry	M,D
Biological and Biomedical Sciences—General	M,D
Biophysics	M,D
Biopsychology	D
Botany	M,D
Cell Biology	M,D
Communication Disorders	M,D
Computational Biology	D
Dental Hygiene	M,D
Dentistry	D

*M—masters degree; D—doctorate; O—other advanced degree; *—Close-Up and/or Display*

Developmental Biology M,D
Ecology M,D
Environmental and Occupational Health M,D
Epidemiology M,D
Evolutionary Biology M,D
Family Nurse Practitioner Studies M,D,O
Genetics M,D
Health Promotion M
Health Services Management and Hospital Administration M,D
Immunology M,D
Industrial Hygiene M,D
Maternal and Child Health M,D
Microbiology M,D
Molecular Biology M,D
Molecular Physiology D
Neurobiology D
Neuroscience D
Nursing and Healthcare Administration M,D,O
Nursing—General M,D,O
Nutrition M,D
Occupational Health Nursing M
Occupational Therapy M,D
Oral and Dental Sciences M,D
Pathology D
Pediatric Nursing M,D,O
Pharmaceutical Sciences M,D
Pharmacology D
Physical Therapy M,D
Psychiatric Nursing M,D,O
Public Health—General M,D
Toxicology M,D

THE UNIVERSITY OF NORTH CAROLINA AT CHARLOTTE
Adult Nursing M,D,O
Biological and Biomedical Sciences—General M,D
Community Health M,D,O
Family Nurse Practitioner Studies M,D,O
Health Services Management and Hospital Administration M,D,O
Health Services Research D
Nurse Anesthesia M,D,O
Nursing Education M,D,O
Nursing—General M,D,O
Psychiatric Nursing M,D,O
Public Health—General M,D,O

THE UNIVERSITY OF NORTH CAROLINA AT GREENSBORO
Adult Nursing M,D,O
Biochemistry M
Biological and Biomedical Sciences—General M
Communication Disorders M,D
Community Health M,D
Gerontological Nursing M,D,O
Nurse Anesthesia M,D,O
Nursing and Healthcare Administration M,D,O
Nursing Education M,D,O
Nursing—General M,D,O
Nutrition M,D

THE UNIVERSITY OF NORTH CAROLINA AT PEMBROKE
Nursing and Healthcare Administration M
Nursing Education M
Nursing—General M

THE UNIVERSITY OF NORTH CAROLINA WILMINGTON
Biological and Biomedical Sciences—General M,D
Clinical Research M
Family Nurse Practitioner Studies M
Marine Biology M,D
Nursing—General M

UNIVERSITY OF NORTH DAKOTA
Allopathic Medicine D
Anatomy M,D
Biochemistry M,D
Biological and Biomedical Sciences—General M,D
Botany M,D
Cell Biology M,D
Clinical Laboratory Sciences/Medical Technology M
Communication Disorders M,D
Community Health Nursing M,D
Ecology M,D
Entomology M,D
Environmental Biology M,D
Family Nurse Practitioner Studies M,D
Genetics M,D
Gerontological Nursing M,D
Immunology M,D
Microbiology M,D
Molecular Biology M,D
Nurse Anesthesia M,D
Nursing Education M,D
Nursing—General M,D
Occupational Therapy M
Pharmacology M,D
Physical Therapy M,D
Physician Assistant Studies M
Physiology M,D
Psychiatric Nursing M,D
Public Health—General M,D
Zoology M,D

UNIVERSITY OF NORTHERN BRITISH COLUMBIA
Community Health M,D,O

UNIVERSITY OF NORTHERN COLORADO
Biological and Biomedical Sciences—General M
Communication Disorders M,D
Family Nurse Practitioner Studies M,D
Nursing Education M,D
Nursing—General M,D
Public Health—General M

UNIVERSITY OF NORTHERN IOWA
Biological and Biomedical Sciences—General M
Communication Disorders M
Health Promotion M

UNIVERSITY OF NORTH FLORIDA
Adult Nursing M,D,O
Allied Health—General M,D,O
Biological and Biomedical Sciences—General M
Communication Disorders M
Community Health M,O
Family Nurse Practitioner Studies M,D,O
Health Services Management and Hospital Administration M,O
Nurse Anesthesia M,D,O
Nursing and Healthcare Administration M,D,O
Nursing—General M,D,O
Nutrition M
Physical Therapy M,D
Public Health—General M,O

UNIVERSITY OF NORTH GEORGIA
Family Nurse Practitioner Studies M
Nursing Education M
Physical Therapy D

UNIVERSITY OF NORTH TEXAS
Biochemistry M,D,O
Biological and Biomedical Sciences—General M,D,O
Communication Disorders M,D,O
Health Services Management and Hospital Administration M,D,O
Molecular Biology M,D,O

UNIVERSITY OF NORTH TEXAS HEALTH SCIENCE CENTER AT FORT WORTH
Anatomy M,D
Biochemistry M,D
Biological and Biomedical Sciences—General M,D
Community Health M,D
Environmental and Occupational Health M,D
Epidemiology M,D
Genetics M,D
Health Services Management and Hospital Administration M,D
Immunology M,D
Microbiology M,D
Molecular Biology M,D
Osteopathic Medicine M,D
Pharmacology M,D
Physician Assistant Studies M
Physiology M,D
Public Health—General M,D

UNIVERSITY OF NOTRE DAME
Biochemistry M,D
Biological and Biomedical Sciences—General M,D
Cell Biology M,D
Ecology M,D
Evolutionary Biology M,D
Genetics M,D
Molecular Biology M,D
Parasitology M,D
Physiology M,D

UNIVERSITY OF OKLAHOMA
Biochemistry M,D
Biological and Biomedical Sciences—General M,D
Botany M,D
Ecology D
Evolutionary Biology D
Health Promotion M,D
Health Services Management and Hospital Administration M,O
Microbiology M,D
Neurobiology D

UNIVERSITY OF OKLAHOMA HEALTH SCIENCES CENTER
Allied Health—General M,D,O
Allopathic Medicine D
Biochemistry M,D
Biological and Biomedical Sciences—General M,D
Biopsychology M,D
Cell Biology M,D
Communication Disorders M,D,O
Dentistry D,O
Environmental and Occupational Health M,D
Epidemiology M,D
Health Physics/Radiological Health M,D
Health Promotion M,D
Health Services Management and Hospital Administration M,D
Immunology M,D
Medical Physics M,D
Microbiology M,D
Molecular Biology M,D
Neuroscience M,D
Nursing—General M
Nutrition M
Occupational Therapy M
Oral and Dental Sciences M
Pathology D
Pharmaceutical Sciences M,D
Pharmacy D
Physical Therapy M
Physiology M,D
Public Health—General M,D
Radiation Biology M,D
Rehabilitation Sciences M

UNIVERSITY OF OREGON
Biochemistry M,D
Biological and Biomedical Sciences—General M,D
Biopsychology M,D
Ecology M,D
Evolutionary Biology M,D
Genetics M,D
Marine Biology M,D
Molecular Biology M,D
Neuroscience M,D
Physiology M,D

UNIVERSITY OF OTTAWA
Allopathic Medicine M,D
Biochemistry M,D
Biological and Biomedical Sciences—General M,D
Cell Biology M,D
Communication Disorders M
Community Health M,D,O
Epidemiology M
Health Services Management and Hospital Administration M
Health Services Research D,O
Immunology M,D
Microbiology M,D
Molecular Biology M,D
Nursing—General M,D,O
Public Health—General D
Rehabilitation Sciences M

UNIVERSITY OF PENNSYLVANIA
Acute Care/Critical Care Nursing M
Adult Nursing M
Allopathic Medicine D
Biochemistry D
Bioethics M
Biological and Biomedical Sciences—General M,D
Cancer Biology/Oncology D
Cell Biology D
Clinical Laboratory Sciences/Medical Technology M
Computational Biology D
Dentistry D
Developmental Biology D
Epidemiology M
Family Nurse Practitioner Studies M,O
Genetics D
Genomic Sciences D
Health Services Management and Hospital Administration M,D
Health Services Research M
Immunology D
International Health M
Maternal and Child/Neonatal Nursing M,O
Medical Physics M,D
Microbiology D
Molecular Biology D
Molecular Biophysics D
Neuroscience D
Nurse Anesthesia M
Nurse Midwifery M
Nursing and Healthcare Administration M,D
Nursing—General M,D,O
Pediatric Nursing M
Pharmacology D
Physiology D
Psychiatric Nursing M
Public Health—General M
Veterinary Medicine D
Virology D
Women's Health Nursing M

UNIVERSITY OF PHOENIX–ATLANTA CAMPUS
Health Services Management and Hospital Administration M
Nursing Education M
Nursing—General M

UNIVERSITY OF PHOENIX–AUGUSTA CAMPUS
Health Services Management and Hospital Administration M
Nursing Education M
Nursing—General M

UNIVERSITY OF PHOENIX–AUSTIN CAMPUS
Health Services Management and Hospital Administration M
Nursing—General M

UNIVERSITY OF PHOENIX–BAY AREA CAMPUS
Gerontological Nursing M,D
Health Services Management and Hospital Administration M,D
Nursing and Healthcare Administration M,D
Nursing Education M,D
Nursing Informatics M,D
Nursing—General M,D

UNIVERSITY OF PHOENIX–BIRMINGHAM CAMPUS
Community Health M
Health Services Management and Hospital Administration M
Nursing Education M
Nursing—General M

UNIVERSITY OF PHOENIX–CENTRAL VALLEY CAMPUS
Community Health M
Health Services Management and Hospital Administration M
Nursing—General M

UNIVERSITY OF PHOENIX–CHARLOTTE CAMPUS
Health Services Management and Hospital Administration M
Nursing Education M
Nursing Informatics M
Nursing—General M

UNIVERSITY OF PHOENIX–CHATTANOOGA CAMPUS
Community Health M
Health Services Management and Hospital Administration M
Nursing—General M

UNIVERSITY OF PHOENIX–CHEYENNE CAMPUS
Health Services Management and Hospital Administration M
Nursing Education M
Nursing—General M

UNIVERSITY OF PHOENIX–CLEVELAND CAMPUS
Nursing—General M,D

UNIVERSITY OF PHOENIX–COLUMBUS GEORGIA CAMPUS
Nursing—General M

UNIVERSITY OF PHOENIX–COLUMBUS OHIO CAMPUS
Nursing—General M,D

UNIVERSITY OF PHOENIX–DENVER CAMPUS
Health Services Management and Hospital Administration M
Nursing—General M

UNIVERSITY OF PHOENIX–DES MOINES CAMPUS
Health Services Management and Hospital Administration M,D
Nursing Education M,D
Nursing Informatics M,D
Nursing—General M,D

UNIVERSITY OF PHOENIX–HAWAII CAMPUS
Community Health M
Family Nurse Practitioner Studies M
Health Services Management and Hospital Administration M
Nursing Education M
Nursing—General M

UNIVERSITY OF PHOENIX–HOUSTON CAMPUS
Health Services Management and Hospital Administration M
Nursing—General M

UNIVERSITY OF PHOENIX–IDAHO CAMPUS
Nursing Education M
Nursing—General M

UNIVERSITY OF PHOENIX–INDIANAPOLIS CAMPUS
Health Services Management and Hospital Administration M
Nursing Education M
Nursing—General M

UNIVERSITY OF PHOENIX–LAS VEGAS CAMPUS
Allied Health—General M

UNIVERSITY OF PHOENIX–LOUISIANA CAMPUS
Nursing—General M

UNIVERSITY OF PHOENIX–MEMPHIS CAMPUS
Health Services Management and Hospital Administration M,D
Nursing—General M,D

UNIVERSITY OF PHOENIX–MILWAUKEE CAMPUS
Health Services Management and Hospital Administration M

UNIVERSITY OF PHOENIX–NASHVILLE CAMPUS
Health Services Management and Hospital Administration M
Nursing—General M

UNIVERSITY OF PHOENIX–NEW MEXICO CAMPUS
Health Services Management and Hospital Administration M
Nursing Education M
Nursing—General M

UNIVERSITY OF PHOENIX–NORTH FLORIDA CAMPUS
Health Services Management and Hospital Administration M
Nursing Education M
Nursing—General M

UNIVERSITY OF PHOENIX–NORTHWEST ARKANSAS CAMPUS
Health Services Management and Hospital Administration M
Nursing Education M
Nursing—General M

UNIVERSITY OF PHOENIX–OKLAHOMA CITY CAMPUS
Nursing—General M

UNIVERSITY OF PHOENIX–OMAHA CAMPUS
Health Services Management and Hospital Administration M
Nursing—General M

UNIVERSITY OF PHOENIX–ONLINE CAMPUS
Family Nurse Practitioner Studies M,O

- Health Services Management and Hospital Administration M,D,O
- Nursing Education M,O
- Nursing—General M,D,O

UNIVERSITY OF PHOENIX–OREGON CAMPUS
- Health Services Management and Hospital Administration M
- Nursing—General M

UNIVERSITY OF PHOENIX–PHOENIX CAMPUS
- Family Nurse Practitioner Studies M,O
- Gerontological Nursing M,O
- Health Services Management and Hospital Administration M,O
- Nursing Education M,O
- Nursing Informatics M,O
- Nursing—General M,O

UNIVERSITY OF PHOENIX–PITTSBURGH CAMPUS
- Health Services Management and Hospital Administration M
- Nursing Education M
- Nursing—General M

UNIVERSITY OF PHOENIX–RICHMOND-VIRGINIA BEACH CAMPUS
- Health Services Management and Hospital Administration M
- Nursing Education M
- Nursing—General M

UNIVERSITY OF PHOENIX–SACRAMENTO VALLEY CAMPUS
- Family Nurse Practitioner Studies M
- Health Services Management and Hospital Administration M
- Nursing Education M
- Nursing—General M

UNIVERSITY OF PHOENIX–SAN ANTONIO CAMPUS
- Health Services Management and Hospital Administration M
- Nursing—General M

UNIVERSITY OF PHOENIX–SAN DIEGO CAMPUS
- Nursing Education M
- Nursing—General M

UNIVERSITY OF PHOENIX–SAVANNAH CAMPUS
- Health Services Management and Hospital Administration M
- Nursing Education M
- Nursing—General M

UNIVERSITY OF PHOENIX–SOUTHERN CALIFORNIA CAMPUS
- Family Nurse Practitioner Studies M,O
- Health Services Management and Hospital Administration M
- Nursing Education M,O
- Nursing Informatics M,O
- Nursing—General M,O

UNIVERSITY OF PHOENIX–SOUTHERN COLORADO CAMPUS
- Health Services Management and Hospital Administration M
- Nursing—General M

UNIVERSITY OF PHOENIX–SOUTH FLORIDA CAMPUS
- Health Services Management and Hospital Administration M
- Nursing Education M
- Nursing—General M

UNIVERSITY OF PHOENIX–SPRINGFIELD CAMPUS
- Health Services Management and Hospital Administration M
- Nursing—General M

UNIVERSITY OF PHOENIX–TULSA CAMPUS
- Nursing—General M

UNIVERSITY OF PHOENIX–UTAH CAMPUS
- Nursing Education M
- Nursing—General M

UNIVERSITY OF PHOENIX–WASHINGTON D.C. CAMPUS
- Health Services Management and Hospital Administration M,D
- Nursing and Healthcare Administration M,D
- Nursing Education M,D
- Nursing Informatics M,D
- Nursing—General M,D

UNIVERSITY OF PHOENIX–WEST FLORIDA CAMPUS
- Health Services Management and Hospital Administration M
- Nursing Education M
- Nursing—General M

UNIVERSITY OF PIKEVILLE
- Osteopathic Medicine D

UNIVERSITY OF PITTSBURGH
- Acute Care/Critical Care Nursing M,D
- Adult Nursing M,D
- Allopathic Medicine D
- Bioethics M
- Biological and Biomedical Sciences—General D
- Cell Biology D
- Clinical Laboratory Sciences/Medical Technology D
- Clinical Research M,O
- Communication Disorders M,D
- Community Health M,D,O
- Computational Biology D
- Dentistry M,D,O
- Developmental Biology D
- Ecology D
- Environmental and Occupational Health M,D,O
- Epidemiology M,D
- Evolutionary Biology D
- Family Nurse Practitioner Studies M,D
- Gerontological Nursing M,D
- Health Promotion M
- Health Services Management and Hospital Administration M,D,O
- Human Genetics M,D,O
- Immunology D
- Infectious Diseases M,D
- Maternal and Child/Neonatal Nursing M,D
- Microbiology M,D
- Molecular Biology D
- Molecular Biophysics D
- Molecular Genetics D
- Molecular Pathology D
- Molecular Pharmacology D
- Molecular Physiology D
- Neuroscience D
- Nurse Anesthesia M,D
- Nursing and Healthcare Administration M,D
- Nursing Informatics M,D
- Nursing—General M,D
- Nutrition M
- Occupational Therapy M
- Oral and Dental Sciences M,O
- Pathology D
- Pediatric Nursing M,D
- Pharmaceutical Sciences M,D
- Pharmacy D
- Physical Therapy M,D
- Physician Assistant Studies M
- Psychiatric Nursing M,D
- Public Health—General M,D,O
- Rehabilitation Sciences M,D
- Structural Biology D
- Systems Biology D
- Virology D

UNIVERSITY OF PORTLAND
- Health Services Management and Hospital Administration M
- Nursing Education M,D
- Nursing—General M,D

UNIVERSITY OF PRINCE EDWARD ISLAND
- Anatomy M,D
- Bacteriology M,D
- Biological and Biomedical Sciences—General M
- Epidemiology M,D
- Immunology M,D
- Parasitology M,D
- Pathology M,D
- Pharmacology M,D
- Physiology M,D
- Toxicology M,D
- Veterinary Medicine D
- Veterinary Sciences M,D
- Virology M,D

UNIVERSITY OF PUERTO RICO, MAYAGÜEZ CAMPUS
- Biological and Biomedical Sciences—General M

UNIVERSITY OF PUERTO RICO, MEDICAL SCIENCES CAMPUS
- Acute Care/Critical Care Nursing M
- Adult Nursing M
- Allied Health—General M,D,O
- Allopathic Medicine D
- Anatomy M,D
- Biochemistry M,D
- Biological and Biomedical Sciences—General M,D
- Clinical Laboratory Sciences/Medical Technology M,O
- Clinical Research M,O
- Communication Disorders M,D
- Community Health Nursing M
- Dentistry D
- Environmental and Occupational Health M,D
- Epidemiology M
- Family Nurse Practitioner Studies M
- Gerontological Nursing M
- Health Promotion O
- Health Services Management and Hospital Administration M
- Health Services Research M
- Industrial Hygiene M
- Maternal and Child Health M
- Maternal and Child/Neonatal Nursing M
- Microbiology M,D
- Nurse Midwifery M,O
- Nursing—General M
- Nutrition M,D,O
- Occupational Therapy M
- Oral and Dental Sciences O
- Pediatric Nursing M
- Pharmaceutical Sciences M,D
- Pharmacology M,D
- Pharmacy M,D
- Physical Therapy M
- Physiology M,D
- Psychiatric Nursing M
- Toxicology M,D

UNIVERSITY OF PUERTO RICO, RÍO PIEDRAS CAMPUS
- Biological and Biomedical Sciences—General M,D
- Cell Biology M,D
- Ecology M,D
- Evolutionary Biology M,D
- Genetics M,D
- Molecular Biology M,D
- Neuroscience M,D
- Nutrition M

UNIVERSITY OF PUGET SOUND
- Occupational Therapy M
- Physical Therapy D

UNIVERSITY OF REDLANDS
- Communication Disorders M

UNIVERSITY OF REGINA
- Biochemistry M,D
- Biological and Biomedical Sciences—General M,D
- Biophysics M,D
- Cancer Biology/Oncology M,D
- Health Services Management and Hospital Administration M,D,O
- Health Services Research M,D,O
- Nursing—General M

UNIVERSITY OF RHODE ISLAND
- Biochemistry M,D
- Biological and Biomedical Sciences—General M,D
- Cell Biology M,D
- Clinical Laboratory Sciences/Medical Technology M,D
- Communication Disorders M
- Family Nurse Practitioner Studies M,D
- Gerontological Nursing M,D
- Medicinal and Pharmaceutical Chemistry M,D
- Microbiology M,D
- Molecular Biology M,D
- Molecular Genetics M,D
- Nursing and Healthcare Administration M,D
- Nursing Education M,D
- Nursing—General M,D
- Nutrition M,D
- Pharmaceutical Sciences M,D
- Pharmacology M,D
- Pharmacy M,D
- Physical Therapy D
- Psychiatric Nursing M,D
- Toxicology M,D

UNIVERSITY OF ROCHESTER
- Acute Care/Critical Care Nursing M,D
- Adult Nursing M,D
- Allopathic Medicine D
- Anatomy D
- Biochemistry D
- Biological and Biomedical Sciences—General M,D
- Biophysics D
- Clinical Research M,D
- Computational Biology D
- Epidemiology D
- Family Nurse Practitioner Studies M,D
- Genetics D
- Genomic Sciences D
- Gerontological Nursing M,D
- Health Services Management and Hospital Administration M,D
- Health Services Research M,D
- Immunology M,D
- Maternal and Child/Neonatal Nursing M,D
- Microbiology M,D
- Molecular Biology D
- Neurobiology D
- Neuroscience D
- Nursing and Healthcare Administration M,D
- Nursing—General M,D
- Oral and Dental Sciences M
- Pathology D
- Pediatric Nursing M,D
- Pharmacology M,D
- Physiology M,D
- Psychiatric Nursing M,D
- Public Health—General M
- Structural Biology D
- Toxicology D

UNIVERSITY OF ST. AUGUSTINE FOR HEALTH SCIENCES
- Occupational Therapy M,D
- Physical Therapy D,O

UNIVERSITY OF ST. FRANCIS (IL)
- Family Nurse Practitioner Studies M,D,O
- Health Services Management and Hospital Administration M
- Nursing and Healthcare Administration M,D,O
- Nursing Education M,D,O
- Nursing—General M,D,O
- Physician Assistant Studies M,O
- Psychiatric Nursing M,D,O

UNIVERSITY OF SAINT FRANCIS (IN)
- Environmental and Occupational Health M
- Family Nurse Practitioner Studies M,O
- Health Services Management and Hospital Administration M
- Nursing—General M,O
- Physician Assistant Studies M

UNIVERSITY OF SAINT JOSEPH
- Biochemistry M
- Biological and Biomedical Sciences—General M
- Family Nurse Practitioner Studies M,D
- Nursing Education M,D
- Nursing—General M,D
- Nutrition M
- Pharmacy D
- Psychiatric Nursing M,D

UNIVERSITY OF SAINT MARY
- Health Services Management and Hospital Administration M
- Nursing and Healthcare Administration M
- Nursing Education M
- Nursing—General M
- Physical Therapy D

UNIVERSITY OF ST. THOMAS (MN)
- Health Services Management and Hospital Administration M

UNIVERSITY OF SAN DIEGO
- Adult Nursing M,D
- Communication Disorders M
- Family Nurse Practitioner Studies M,D
- Gerontological Nursing M,D
- Nursing and Healthcare Administration M,D
- Nursing—General M,D
- Pediatric Nursing M,D
- Psychiatric Nursing M,D

UNIVERSITY OF SAN FRANCISCO
- Biological and Biomedical Sciences—General M
- Family Nurse Practitioner Studies D
- Health Services Management and Hospital Administration M
- Nursing and Healthcare Administration M,D
- Nursing—General M,D
- Psychiatric Nursing D
- Public Health—General M

UNIVERSITY OF SASKATCHEWAN
- Allopathic Medicine D
- Anatomy M,D
- Biochemistry M,D
- Biological and Biomedical Sciences—General M,D
- Cell Biology M,D
- Community Health M,D
- Dentistry D
- Epidemiology M,D
- Health Services Management and Hospital Administration M
- Immunology M,D
- Microbiology M,D
- Nursing—General M
- Pathology M,D
- Pharmaceutical Sciences M,D
- Pharmacology M,D
- Physiology M,D
- Reproductive Biology M,D
- Toxicology M,D,O
- Veterinary Medicine M,D
- Veterinary Sciences M,D

THE UNIVERSITY OF SCRANTON
- Adult Nursing M,O
- Biochemistry M
- Family Nurse Practitioner Studies M,O
- Health Services Management and Hospital Administration M
- Nurse Anesthesia M,O
- Nursing—General M,O
- Occupational Therapy M
- Physical Therapy D

UNIVERSITY OF SIOUX FALLS
- Health Services Management and Hospital Administration M

UNIVERSITY OF SOUTH AFRICA
- Acute Care/Critical Care Nursing M,D
- Health Services Management and Hospital Administration M,D
- Maternal and Child/Neonatal Nursing M,D
- Medical/Surgical Nursing M,D
- Nurse Midwifery M,D
- Public Health—General M,D

UNIVERSITY OF SOUTH ALABAMA
- Adult Nursing M,D
- Allied Health—General M,D
- Allopathic Medicine D
- Biological and Biomedical Sciences—General M,D
- Communication Disorders M,D
- Community Health Nursing M,D
- Environmental and Occupational Health M
- Maternal and Child/Neonatal Nursing M,D
- Nursing—General M,D
- Occupational Therapy M
- Physical Therapy D
- Physician Assistant Studies M
- Toxicology M

UNIVERSITY OF SOUTH CAROLINA
- Acute Care/Critical Care Nursing M,O
- Adult Nursing M
- Allopathic Medicine D
- Biochemistry M,D
- Biological and Biomedical Sciences—General M,D,O
- Cell Biology M,D
- Communication Disorders M,D
- Community Health Nursing M

*M—masters degree; D—doctorate; O—other advanced degree; *—Close-Up and/or Display*

Developmental Biology M,D
Ecology M,D
Environmental and Occupational Health M,D
Epidemiology M,D
Evolutionary Biology M,D
Family Nurse Practitioner Studies M
Health Promotion M,D,O
Health Services Management and Hospital Administration M,D
Industrial Hygiene M,D
Medical/Surgical Nursing M
Molecular Biology M,D
Nurse Anesthesia M
Nursing and Healthcare Administration M
Nursing—General M,O
Pediatric Nursing M
Pharmaceutical Sciences M,D
Pharmacy D
Psychiatric Nursing M,O
Public Health—General M
Rehabilitation Sciences M,O
Women's Health Nursing M

THE UNIVERSITY OF SOUTH DAKOTA

Allied Health—General M,D,O
Allopathic Medicine D
Biological and Biomedical Sciences—General M,D
Cardiovascular Sciences M,D
Cell Biology M,D
Communication Disorders M,D
Health Services Management and Hospital Administration M
Immunology M,D
Microbiology M,D
Molecular Biology M,D
Neuroscience M,D
Occupational Therapy M
Pharmacology M,D
Physical Therapy D
Physician Assistant Studies M
Physiology M,D

UNIVERSITY OF SOUTHERN CALIFORNIA

Allopathic Medicine D
Biochemistry M
Biological and Biomedical Sciences—General M,D
Biophysics M
Clinical Research M,D,O
Computational Biology D
Dentistry D
Environmental and Occupational Health M
Environmental Biology M,D
Epidemiology M,D
Evolutionary Biology D
Genetics D
Health Promotion M
Health Services Management and Hospital Administration M,O
Health Services Research D
Immunology M
Infectious Diseases D
International Health M
Marine Biology M,D
Medical Imaging M,D
Microbiology M
Molecular Biology M,D
Molecular Pharmacology M,D
Neurobiology D
Neuroscience M,D
Occupational Therapy M,D
Oral and Dental Sciences M,D,O
Pathobiology M,D
Pathology M,D
Pharmaceutical Administration M
Pharmaceutical Sciences M,D,O
Pharmacy D
Physical Therapy M,D
Physician Assistant Studies M
Physiology M
Public Health—General M,D
Toxicology M,D

UNIVERSITY OF SOUTHERN INDIANA

Health Services Management and Hospital Administration M
Nursing—General M,D
Occupational Therapy M

UNIVERSITY OF SOUTHERN MAINE

Adult Nursing M,D,O
Biological and Biomedical Sciences—General M
Family Nurse Practitioner Studies M,D,O
Gerontological Nursing M,D,O
Health Services Management and Hospital Administration M
Immunology M
Molecular Biology M
Nursing and Healthcare Administration M,D,O
Nursing Education M,D,O
Nursing—General M,D,O
Occupational Therapy M,O
Psychiatric Nursing M,D,O
Public Health—General M,O

UNIVERSITY OF SOUTHERN MISSISSIPPI

Biochemistry M,D
Biological and Biomedical Sciences—General M,D
Clinical Laboratory Sciences/Medical Technology M
Communication Disorders M,D
Environmental and Occupational Health M
Environmental Biology M,D
Epidemiology M
Family Nurse Practitioner Studies M,D

Health Services Management and Hospital Administration M
Marine Biology M,D
Maternal and Child/Neonatal Nursing M,D
Microbiology M,D
Molecular Biology M,D
Nursing and Healthcare Administration M,D
Nursing—General M,D
Nutrition M,D
Psychiatric Nursing M,D
Public Health—General M

UNIVERSITY OF SOUTH FLORIDA

Acute Care/Critical Care Nursing M,D
Adult Nursing M,D
Allopathic Medicine M,D
Anatomy M,D
Bioethics O
Biological and Biomedical Sciences—General M,D
Biophysics M,D
Cancer Biology/Oncology M,D
Cardiovascular Sciences O
Cell Biology M,D
Clinical Research M,D,O
Communication Disorders M,D,O
Community Health M,D,O
Computational Biology M,D
Ecology M,D
Environmental and Occupational Health M,D,O
Environmental Biology M,D
Epidemiology M,D,O
Evolutionary Biology M,D
Family Nurse Practitioner Studies M,D
Gerontological Nursing M,D
Health Services Management and Hospital Administration M,D,O
Immunology M,D
International Health M,D,O
Maternal and Child Health O
Medical Microbiology M,D
Medical Physics M,D
Microbiology M,D
Molecular Biology M,D
Molecular Medicine M,D
Molecular Pharmacology M,D
Neuroscience M,D,O
Nurse Anesthesia M,D
Nursing and Healthcare Administration M,D
Nursing Education M,D
Nursing—General M,D
Nutrition M,D,O
Occupational Health Nursing M,D
Oncology Nursing M,D
Pathology M,D
Pediatric Nursing M,D
Pharmacology M,D
Pharmacy D,O
Physical Therapy D
Physiology M,D
Public Health—General M,D,O

THE UNIVERSITY OF TAMPA

Adult Nursing M
Family Nurse Practitioner Studies M
Nursing—General M

THE UNIVERSITY OF TENNESSEE

Anatomy M,D
Animal Behavior M,D
Biochemistry M,D
Bioethics M,D
Biological and Biomedical Sciences—General M,D
Communication Disorders M,D,O
Community Health M,D
Ecology M,D
Entomology M,D
Evolutionary Biology M,D
Genetics M,D
Genomic Sciences M,D
Health Promotion M
Health Services Management and Hospital Administration M
Microbiology M,D
Nursing—General M,D
Nutrition M
Physiology M,D
Plant Pathology M,D
Plant Physiology M,D
Public Health—General M
Veterinary Medicine D

THE UNIVERSITY OF TENNESSEE AT CHATTANOOGA

Family Nurse Practitioner Studies M,D,O
Nurse Anesthesia M,D,O
Nursing and Healthcare Administration M,D,O
Nursing Education M,D,O
Nursing—General M,D,O
Physical Therapy D

THE UNIVERSITY OF TENNESSEE AT MARTIN

Nutrition M

THE UNIVERSITY OF TENNESSEE HEALTH SCIENCE CENTER

Allied Health—General M,D
Allopathic Medicine D
Biological and Biomedical Sciences—General M,D
Clinical Laboratory Sciences/Medical Technology M,D
Communication Disorders M,D
Dentistry D
Epidemiology M,D
Health Services Research M,D
Nursing and Healthcare Administration M,D
Nursing—General M,D

Occupational Therapy M,D
Oral and Dental Sciences M,D
Pathology M,D
Pharmaceutical Sciences M,D
Pharmacology M,D
Pharmacy M,D
Physical Therapy M,D
Physician Assistant Studies M,D

THE UNIVERSITY OF TENNESSEE–OAK RIDGE NATIONAL LABORATORY

Biological and Biomedical Sciences—General M,D
Genomic Sciences M,D

THE UNIVERSITY OF TEXAS AT ARLINGTON

Biological and Biomedical Sciences—General M,D
Family Nurse Practitioner Studies M,D
Health Services Management and Hospital Administration M
Nursing and Healthcare Administration M,D
Nursing Education M,D
Nursing—General M,D

THE UNIVERSITY OF TEXAS AT AUSTIN

Adult Nursing M,D
Animal Behavior D
Biochemistry D
Biological and Biomedical Sciences—General M,D
Biopsychology D
Cell Biology D
Clinical Laboratory Sciences/Medical Technology M,D
Communication Disorders M,D
Community Health Nursing M,D
Ecology D
Evolutionary Biology D
Family Nurse Practitioner Studies M,D
Gerontological Nursing M,D
Maternal and Child/Neonatal Nursing M,D
Medicinal and Pharmaceutical Chemistry M,D
Microbiology D
Molecular Biology D
Neurobiology D
Neuroscience D
Nursing and Healthcare Administration M,D
Nursing Education M,D
Nursing—General M,D
Nutrition M,D
Pediatric Nursing M,D
Pharmaceutical Sciences M,D
Pharmacology M,D
Pharmacy D
Plant Biology M,D
Psychiatric Nursing M,D
Toxicology M,D

THE UNIVERSITY OF TEXAS AT BROWNSVILLE

Biological and Biomedical Sciences—General M
Community Health Nursing M
Nursing—General M

THE UNIVERSITY OF TEXAS AT DALLAS

Biological and Biomedical Sciences—General M,D
Cell Biology M,D
Communication Disorders M,D
Health Services Management and Hospital Administration M,D
Molecular Biology M,D
Neuroscience M,D

THE UNIVERSITY OF TEXAS AT EL PASO

Allied Health—General D
Biological and Biomedical Sciences—General M,D
Communication Disorders M
Family Nurse Practitioner Studies M,D,O
Health Services Management and Hospital Administration M,D,O
Nursing and Healthcare Administration M,D,O
Nursing Education M,D,O
Nursing—General M,D,O
Occupational Therapy M
Physical Therapy D

THE UNIVERSITY OF TEXAS AT SAN ANTONIO

Biological and Biomedical Sciences—General M,D
Cell Biology M,D
Molecular Biology M,D
Neurobiology M,D
Nutrition M

THE UNIVERSITY OF TEXAS AT TYLER

Biological and Biomedical Sciences—General M
Environmental and Occupational Health M
Family Nurse Practitioner Studies M,D
Health Services Management and Hospital Administration M
Nursing and Healthcare Administration M,D
Nursing Education M,D
Nursing—General M,D

THE UNIVERSITY OF TEXAS HEALTH SCIENCE CENTER AT HOUSTON

Allopathic Medicine D
Biochemistry M,D
Biological and Biomedical Sciences—General M,D
Cancer Biology/Oncology M,D
Cell Biology M,D

Dentistry M,D
Developmental Biology M,D
Genetics M,D
Human Genetics M,D
Immunology M,D
Medical Physics M,D
Microbiology M,D
Molecular Biology M,D
Molecular Genetics M,D
Molecular Pathology M,D
Neuroscience M,D
Nursing—General M,D
Public Health—General M,D,O
Virology M,D

THE UNIVERSITY OF TEXAS HEALTH SCIENCE CENTER AT SAN ANTONIO

Acute Care/Critical Care Nursing M,D,O
Allopathic Medicine M,D
Biochemistry M,D
Biological and Biomedical Sciences—General D
Cell Biology M,D
Clinical Laboratory Sciences/Medical Technology D
Clinical Research M
Communication Disorders M,D
Community Health Nursing M,D,O
Dentistry M,D,O
Family Nurse Practitioner Studies M,D,O
Gerontological Nursing M,D,O
Immunology D
Medical Physics M,D
Microbiology D
Molecular Medicine M,D
Neuroscience D
Nursing and Healthcare Administration M,D,O
Nursing Education M,D,O
Nursing—General M,D,O
Occupational Therapy M,D
Pediatric Nursing M,D,O
Pharmacology D
Physical Therapy M,D
Physician Assistant Studies M,D
Physiology M,D
Psychiatric Nursing M,D,O
Structural Biology M,D
Toxicology M,D

THE UNIVERSITY OF TEXAS MEDICAL BRANCH

Allied Health—General M,D
Allopathic Medicine D
Bacteriology D
Biochemistry D
Biological and Biomedical Sciences—General M,D
Biophysics D
Cell Biology D
Clinical Laboratory Sciences/Medical Technology M,D
Community Health M,D
Computational Biology D
Genetics D
Immunology M,D
Infectious Diseases D
Microbiology M,D
Molecular Biophysics M,D
Neuroscience D
Nursing—General M,D
Occupational Therapy M
Pathology D
Pharmacology M,D
Physical Therapy M,D
Physician Assistant Studies M
Physiology M,D
Public Health—General M
Rehabilitation Sciences M,D
Structural Biology D
Toxicology M,D
Virology D

THE UNIVERSITY OF TEXAS OF THE PERMIAN BASIN

Biological and Biomedical Sciences—General M

THE UNIVERSITY OF TEXAS–PAN AMERICAN

Adult Nursing M
Biological and Biomedical Sciences—General M
Communication Disorders M
Family Nurse Practitioner Studies M
Nursing—General M
Occupational Therapy M

THE UNIVERSITY OF TEXAS SOUTHWESTERN MEDICAL CENTER

Allopathic Medicine D
Biochemistry D
Biological and Biomedical Sciences—General M,D
Cancer Biology/Oncology D
Cell Biology D
Developmental Biology D
Genetics D
Immunology D
Microbiology D
Molecular Biophysics D
Neuroscience D
Nutrition M
Physical Therapy D
Physician Assistant Studies M

UNIVERSITY OF THE CUMBERLANDS

Physician Assistant Studies M

UNIVERSITY OF THE DISTRICT OF COLUMBIA

Cancer Biology/Oncology M
Communication Disorders M
Nutrition M

UNIVERSITY OF THE INCARNATE WORD

Biological and Biomedical Sciences—General	M
Health Promotion	M
Health Services Management and Hospital Administration	M
Nursing and Healthcare Administration	M,D
Nursing—General	M,D
Nutrition	M
Optometry	D
Pharmacy	D

UNIVERSITY OF THE PACIFIC

Biological and Biomedical Sciences—General	M
Communication Disorders	M
Dentistry	M,D,O
Pharmaceutical Sciences	M,D
Pharmacy	D
Physical Therapy	M,D

UNIVERSITY OF THE SACRED HEART

Environmental and Occupational Health	M
Occupational Health Nursing	M

UNIVERSITY OF THE SCIENCES

Biochemistry	M,D
Cell Biology	M,D
Health Services Management and Hospital Administration	M,D
Medicinal and Pharmaceutical Chemistry	M,D
Molecular Biology	D
Pharmaceutical Administration	M
Pharmaceutical Sciences	M,D
Pharmacology	M,D
Pharmacy	M,D
Public Health—General	M,D
Toxicology	M,D

THE UNIVERSITY OF TOLEDO

Biochemistry	M,D
Biological and Biomedical Sciences—General	M,D,O
Cancer Biology/Oncology	M,D
Cardiovascular Sciences	M,D
Communication Disorders	M,D
Community Health Nursing	M,O
Ecology	M,D
Environmental and Occupational Health	M,O
Epidemiology	M,O
Family Nurse Practitioner Studies	M,O
Genomic Sciences	M,O
Health Promotion	M,D,O
Health Services Management and Hospital Administration	M,O
Immunology	M,D
Industrial Hygiene	M,O
International Health	M,O
Medical Physics	M,D
Medicinal and Pharmaceutical Chemistry	M,D
Neuroscience	M,D
Nursing and Healthcare Administration	M,O
Nursing Education	M,O
Nursing—General	M,D,O
Nutrition	M,O
Occupational Therapy	M,D
Oral and Dental Sciences	M
Pathology	M,O
Pediatric Nursing	M,O
Pharmaceutical Administration	M
Pharmaceutical Sciences	M
Pharmacology	M,D
Physical Therapy	M,D
Physician Assistant Studies	M
Public Health—General	M,O

UNIVERSITY OF TORONTO

Allopathic Medicine	M,D
Biochemistry	M,D
Bioethics	M,D
Biophysics	M,D
Cell Biology	M,D
Communication Disorders	M,D
Dentistry	D
Ecology	M,D
Epidemiology	M,D
Evolutionary Biology	M,D
Health Physics/Radiological Health	M,D
Health Promotion	M,D
Health Services Management and Hospital Administration	M,D
Immunology	M,D
Molecular Genetics	M,D
Nursing—General	M,D
Nutrition	M,D
Occupational Therapy	M
Oral and Dental Sciences	M,D
Pathobiology	M,D
Pharmaceutical Sciences	M,D
Pharmacology	M,D
Physical Therapy	M
Physiology	M,D
Public Health—General	M,D
Rehabilitation Sciences	M,D
Systems Biology	M,D

THE UNIVERSITY OF TULSA

Biochemistry	M
Biological and Biomedical Sciences—General	M,D
Communication Disorders	M

UNIVERSITY OF UTAH

Allopathic Medicine	D
Anatomy	D
Biochemistry	M,D
Biological and Biomedical Sciences—General	M,D,O
Cancer Biology/Oncology	M,D
Clinical Laboratory Sciences/Medical Technology	M
Communication Disorders	M,D
Dentistry	D
Gerontological Nursing	M,O
Health Promotion	M,D
Health Services Management and Hospital Administration	M,D
Health Services Research	M,D
Human Genetics	M,D
Medical Physics	M,D
Medicinal and Pharmaceutical Chemistry	M,D
Molecular Biology	D
Neurobiology	D
Neuroscience	D
Nursing—General	M,D
Nutrition	M
Occupational Therapy	M,D
Pathology	M,D
Pharmaceutical Administration	M,D
Pharmaceutical Sciences	M,D
Pharmacology	D
Pharmacy	D
Physical Therapy	D
Physician Assistant Studies	M
Physiology	D
Public Health—General	M,D
Rehabilitation Sciences	D
Toxicology	D

UNIVERSITY OF VERMONT

Allied Health—General	M,D
Allopathic Medicine	D
Biological and Biomedical Sciences—General	M,D
Cell Biology	M,D
Clinical Laboratory Sciences/Medical Technology	M,D
Communication Disorders	M
Molecular Biology	M,D
Neuroscience	D
Nursing—General	M,D
Nutrition	M,D
Pathology	M
Pharmacology	M
Physical Therapy	D
Plant Biology	M,D

UNIVERSITY OF VICTORIA

Biochemistry	M,D
Biological and Biomedical Sciences—General	M,D
Family Nurse Practitioner Studies	M,D
Medical Physics	M,D
Microbiology	M,D
Nursing and Healthcare Administration	M,D
Nursing Education	M,D
Nursing—General	M,D

UNIVERSITY OF VIRGINIA

Acute Care/Critical Care Nursing	M,D
Allopathic Medicine	M,D
Biochemistry	D
Biological and Biomedical Sciences—General	M,D
Biophysics	M,D
Cell Biology	D
Clinical Research	M
Communication Disorders	M
Community Health	M,D
Health Services Management and Hospital Administration	M
Health Services Research	M
Microbiology	D
Molecular Genetics	D
Molecular Physiology	M,D
Neuroscience	D
Nursing and Healthcare Administration	M,D
Nursing—General	M,D
Pathology	D
Pharmacology	D
Physiology	D
Psychiatric Nursing	M,D
Public Health—General	M,D

UNIVERSITY OF WASHINGTON

Allopathic Medicine	D
Animal Behavior	D
Bacteriology	D
Biochemistry	D
Bioethics	M
Biological and Biomedical Sciences—General	M,D
Biophysics	D
Cell Biology	D*
Clinical Laboratory Sciences/Medical Technology	M
Clinical Research	M,D
Communication Disorders	M,D
Community Health	M,D
Dentistry	D
Ecology	M,D
Environmental and Occupational Health	M,D
Epidemiology	M,D
Genetics	M,D
Genomic Sciences	D
Health Services Management and Hospital Administration	M
Health Services Research	M,D
Immunology	D
International Health	M,D
Maternal and Child Health	M,D
Medicinal and Pharmaceutical Chemistry	D
Microbiology	D
Molecular Biology	D
Molecular Medicine	D
Neurobiology	D
Nursing—General	M,D,O
Nutrition	M,D
Occupational Therapy	M,D
Oral and Dental Sciences	M,D,O
Parasitology	D
Pathobiology	D
Pathology	D
Pharmaceutical Sciences	M,D
Pharmacology	D
Pharmacy	M,D
Physical Therapy	M,D
Physiology	D
Public Health—General	M
Rehabilitation Sciences	M,D
Structural Biology	D
Toxicology	M,D
Veterinary Sciences	M

UNIVERSITY OF WASHINGTON, BOTHELL

Nursing—General	M

UNIVERSITY OF WASHINGTON, TACOMA

Community Health Nursing	M
Nursing and Healthcare Administration	M
Nursing Education	M
Nursing—General	M

UNIVERSITY OF WATERLOO

Biochemistry	M,D
Biological and Biomedical Sciences—General	M,D
Optometry	M,D
Public Health—General	M
Vision Sciences	M,D

THE UNIVERSITY OF WESTERN ONTARIO

Allopathic Medicine	M,D
Anatomy	M,D
Biochemistry	M,D
Biological and Biomedical Sciences—General	M,D
Biophysics	M,D
Cell Biology	M,D
Communication Disorders	M
Dentistry	D
Epidemiology	M,D
Health Services Management and Hospital Administration	M,D
Immunology	M,D
Microbiology	M,D
Neuroscience	M,D
Nursing—General	M,D
Occupational Therapy	M
Oral and Dental Sciences	M
Pathology	M,D
Physical Therapy	M,O
Physiology	M,D

UNIVERSITY OF WESTERN STATES

Chiropractic	D

UNIVERSITY OF WEST FLORIDA

Biochemistry	M
Biological and Biomedical Sciences—General	M
Community Health	M
Environmental and Occupational Health	M
Environmental Biology	M
Nursing and Healthcare Administration	M,O
Nursing—General	M
Pharmaceutical Administration	M,O
Public Health—General	M

UNIVERSITY OF WEST GEORGIA

Biological and Biomedical Sciences—General	M
Communication Disorders	M,D,O
Health Services Management and Hospital Administration	M,D,O
Nursing Education	M,D,O
Nursing—General	M,D,O

UNIVERSITY OF WINDSOR

Biochemistry	M,D
Biological and Biomedical Sciences—General	M,D
Biopsychology	M,D
Nursing—General	M

UNIVERSITY OF WISCONSIN–EAU CLAIRE

Adult Nursing	M,D
Communication Disorders	M
Family Nurse Practitioner Studies	M,D
Gerontological Nursing	M,D
Nursing and Healthcare Administration	M,D
Nursing Education	M,D
Nursing—General	M,D

UNIVERSITY OF WISCONSIN–GREEN BAY

Nursing and Healthcare Administration	M

UNIVERSITY OF WISCONSIN–LA CROSSE

Biological and Biomedical Sciences—General	M
Cancer Biology/Oncology	M
Cell Biology	M
Community Health	M
Medical Microbiology	M
Microbiology	M
Molecular Biology	M
Nurse Anesthesia	M
Occupational Therapy	M
Physical Therapy	D
Physician Assistant Studies	M
Physiology	M
Rehabilitation Sciences	M

UNIVERSITY OF WISCONSIN–MADISON

Adult Nursing	D
Allopathic Medicine	D
Bacteriology	M
Biochemistry	M,D
Biological and Biomedical Sciences—General	M,D
Biophysics	D
Biopsychology	D
Botany	M,D
Cancer Biology/Oncology	D
Cell Biology	D
Communication Disorders	M,D
Community Health	M,D
Conservation Biology	M
Ecology	M
Entomology	M,D
Environmental Biology	M,D
Epidemiology	M,D
Genetics	M,D
Gerontological Nursing	D
Medical Microbiology	D
Medical Physics	M,D
Microbiology	D
Molecular Biology	D
Neurobiology	M,D
Neuroscience	M,D
Nursing—General	D
Nutrition	M,D
Occupational Therapy	M,D
Pathology	D*
Pediatric Nursing	D
Pharmaceutical Administration	M,D
Pharmaceutical Sciences	M,D
Pharmacology	D
Pharmacy	D
Physiology	M,D
Plant Pathology	M,D
Psychiatric Nursing	D
Toxicology	M,D
Veterinary Medicine	M,D
Veterinary Sciences	M,D
Zoology	M,D

UNIVERSITY OF WISCONSIN–MILWAUKEE

Allied Health—General	M,D,O
Biochemistry	M,D
Biological and Biomedical Sciences—General	M,D
Communication Disorders	M,O
Environmental and Occupational Health	D
Family Nurse Practitioner Studies	M,D,O
Health Promotion	M,D,O
Nursing—General	M,D,O
Occupational Therapy	M,O
Physical Therapy	D
Public Health—General	M,D,O

UNIVERSITY OF WISCONSIN–OSHKOSH

Adult Nursing	M
Biological and Biomedical Sciences—General	M
Botany	M
Family Nurse Practitioner Studies	M
Health Services Management and Hospital Administration	M
Microbiology	M
Nursing—General	M
Zoology	M

UNIVERSITY OF WISCONSIN–PARKSIDE

Molecular Biology	M

UNIVERSITY OF WISCONSIN–RIVER FALLS

Communication Disorders	M

UNIVERSITY OF WISCONSIN–STEVENS POINT

Communication Disorders	M,D
Health Promotion	M
Nutrition	M

UNIVERSITY OF WISCONSIN–STOUT

Industrial Hygiene	M
Nutrition	M

UNIVERSITY OF WISCONSIN–WHITEWATER

Communication Disorders	M
Environmental and Occupational Health	M

UNIVERSITY OF WYOMING

Botany	M,D
Cell Biology	D
Communication Disorders	M
Community Health	M,D
Computational Biology	D
Ecology	M,D
Entomology	M,D
Genetics	D
Health Promotion	M
Microbiology	D
Molecular Biology	M,D
Nursing—General	M
Nutrition	M
Pathobiology	M
Pharmacy	D
Physiology	M,D
Reproductive Biology	M,D
Zoology	M,D

URBANA UNIVERSITY

Nursing—General	M

*M—masters degree; D—doctorate; O—other advanced degree; *—Close-Up and/or Display*

URSULINE COLLEGE
Medical/Surgical Nursing M,D
Nursing and Healthcare Administration M,D
Nursing Education M,D
Nursing—General M,D

UTAH STATE UNIVERSITY
Biochemistry M,D
Biological and Biomedical Sciences—General M,D
Communication Disorders M,D,O
Ecology M,D
Nutrition M,D
Toxicology M,D
Veterinary Sciences M,D

UTAH VALLEY UNIVERSITY
Nursing—General M

UTICA COLLEGE
Health Services Management and Hospital Administration M
Occupational Therapy M
Physical Therapy D

VALDOSTA STATE UNIVERSITY
Health Services Management and Hospital Administration M

VALPARAISO UNIVERSITY
Health Services Management and Hospital Administration M
Nursing Education M,O
Nursing—General M,O

VANDERBILT UNIVERSITY
Acute Care/Critical Care Nursing M,D
Adult Nursing M,D
Allopathic Medicine M,D
Biochemistry M,D
Biological and Biomedical Sciences—General M,D
Biophysics M,D
Cancer Biology/Oncology M,D
Cell Biology M,D
Clinical Research M
Communication Disorders M,D
Developmental Biology M,D
Family Nurse Practitioner Studies M,D
Gerontological Nursing M,D
Health Physics/Radiological Health M,D
Human Genetics D
Immunology M,D
Maternal and Child/Neonatal Nursing M,D
Medical Physics M
Microbiology M,D
Molecular Biology M,D
Molecular Physiology M,D
Nurse Midwifery M,D
Nursing and Healthcare Administration M,D
Nursing Informatics M,D
Nursing—General M,D
Pathology D
Pediatric Nursing M,D
Pharmacology D
Psychiatric Nursing M,D
Public Health—General M
Women's Health Nursing M,D

VANGUARD UNIVERSITY OF SOUTHERN CALIFORNIA
Nursing—General M

VILLANOVA UNIVERSITY
Adult Nursing M,D,O
Biological and Biomedical Sciences—General M
Family Nurse Practitioner Studies M,D,O
Health Services Management and Hospital Administration M,D,O
Nurse Anesthesia M,D,O
Nursing and Healthcare Administration M,D,O
Nursing Education M,D,O
Nursing—General M,D,O
Pediatric Nursing M,D,O

VIRGINIA COLLEGE IN BIRMINGHAM
Health Services Management and Hospital Administration M

VIRGINIA COMMONWEALTH UNIVERSITY
Adult Nursing M,D,O
Allied Health—General D
Allopathic Medicine D
Anatomy D,O
Biochemistry M,D,O
Biological and Biomedical Sciences—General M,D,O
Biopsychology D
Clinical Laboratory Sciences/Medical Technology M,D
Community Health M,D
Dentistry M,D
Epidemiology M,D
Family Nurse Practitioner Studies M,O
Genetics M,D
Health Physics/Radiological Health D
Health Services Management and Hospital Administration M,D
Health Services Research D
Human Genetics M,D,O
Immunology M,D
Medical Physics M,D
Medicinal and Pharmaceutical Chemistry M,D
Microbiology M,D,O
Molecular Biology M,D
Neurobiology D
Neuroscience M,D,O
Nurse Anesthesia M,D
Nursing and Healthcare Administration M,D,O
Nursing Education M,D,O
Nursing—General M,D,O
Occupational Therapy M,D
Pathology D
Pediatric Nursing M,D,O
Pharmaceutical Administration M,D
Pharmaceutical Sciences M,D
Pharmacology M,D,O
Pharmacy D
Physical Therapy M,D
Physiology M,D,O
Psychiatric Nursing M,D,O
Public Health—General M,D
Rehabilitation Sciences D
Systems Biology D
Toxicology M,D,O
Women's Health Nursing M,D,O

VIRGINIA INTERNATIONAL UNIVERSITY
Health Services Management and Hospital Administration M,O

VIRGINIA POLYTECHNIC INSTITUTE AND STATE UNIVERSITY
Biological and Biomedical Sciences—General M,D
Entomology M,D
Genetics M,D
Nutrition M,D
Plant Pathology M,D
Plant Physiology M,D
Public Health—General M,D,O
Veterinary Medicine M,D,O
Veterinary Sciences M,D,O

VIRGINIA STATE UNIVERSITY
Biological and Biomedical Sciences—General M
Community Health M,D

VITERBO UNIVERSITY
Health Services Management and Hospital Administration M
Nursing—General M,D

WAGNER COLLEGE
Family Nurse Practitioner Studies O
Health Services Management and Hospital Administration M
Microbiology M
Nursing—General M
Physician Assistant Studies M

WAKE FOREST UNIVERSITY
Allopathic Medicine D
Anatomy D
Biochemistry D
Biological and Biomedical Sciences—General M,D
Cancer Biology/Oncology D
Genomic Sciences D
Health Services Research M
Human Genetics D
Immunology D
Microbiology D
Molecular Biology D
Molecular Genetics D
Molecular Medicine M,D
Neurobiology D
Neuroscience D
Pathobiology M,D
Pharmacology D
Physiology D

WALDEN UNIVERSITY
Adult Nursing M,D,O
Clinical Research M,D,O
Community Health M,D,O
Epidemiology M,D,O
Family Nurse Practitioner Studies M,D,O
Gerontological Nursing M,D,O
Health Promotion M,D,O
Health Services Management and Hospital Administration M,D,O
Nursing and Healthcare Administration M,D,O
Nursing Education M,D,O
Nursing Informatics M,D,O
Nursing—General M,D,O
Public Health—General M,D,O

WALLA WALLA UNIVERSITY
Biological and Biomedical Sciences—General M

WALSH UNIVERSITY
Health Services Management and Hospital Administration M,O
Nursing and Healthcare Administration M,D
Nursing Education M,D
Nursing—General M,D
Physical Therapy D

WASHBURN UNIVERSITY
Nursing and Healthcare Administration M,D
Nursing—General M,D

WASHINGTON ADVENTIST UNIVERSITY
Health Services Management and Hospital Administration M
Nursing and Healthcare Administration M
Nursing Education M
Nursing—General M

WASHINGTON STATE UNIVERSITY
Biochemistry M,D
Biological and Biomedical Sciences—General M
Biophysics M,D
Botany M,D
Entomology M,D
Health Promotion M,D
Immunology M,D
Neuroscience M,D
Nutrition M,D
Pharmacy M,D
Plant Molecular Biology M,D
Plant Pathology M,D
Veterinary Medicine M,D
Veterinary Sciences M
Zoology M,D

WASHINGTON STATE UNIVERSITY SPOKANE
Communication Disorders M
Community Health M,D
Family Nurse Practitioner Studies M,D
Health Services Management and Hospital Administration M
Nursing—General M,D
Nutrition M
Pharmaceutical Sciences D
Pharmacy D
Psychiatric Nursing M,D

WASHINGTON STATE UNIVERSITY TRI-CITIES
Nursing—General M,D

WASHINGTON STATE UNIVERSITY VANCOUVER
Nursing—General M

WASHINGTON UNIVERSITY IN ST. LOUIS
Allopathic Medicine D
Biochemistry D
Biological and Biomedical Sciences—General D
Cell Biology D
Clinical Research M
Communication Disorders M,D
Computational Biology D
Developmental Biology D
Ecology D
Environmental Biology D
Epidemiology M,D
Evolutionary Biology D
Genetics M,D
Genomic Sciences M
Health Services Research M,O
Human Genetics D
Immunology D
International Health M,D
Microbiology D
Molecular Biology D
Molecular Biophysics D
Molecular Genetics D
Molecular Pathogenesis D
Neuroscience D
Occupational Therapy M,D
Physical Therapy D
Plant Biology D
Public Health—General M,D
Rehabilitation Sciences D
Systems Biology D

WAYLAND BAPTIST UNIVERSITY
Health Services Management and Hospital Administration M
Nursing—General M

WAYNESBURG UNIVERSITY
Health Services Management and Hospital Administration M,D
Nursing and Healthcare Administration M,D
Nursing Education M,D
Nursing Informatics M,D
Nursing—General M,D

WAYNE STATE UNIVERSITY
Acute Care/Critical Care Nursing M
Adult Nursing M,O
Allopathic Medicine D
Anatomy M,D
Biochemistry M,D
Biological and Biomedical Sciences—General M,D
Biopsychology M,D
Cancer Biology/Oncology M,D
Cell Biology D
Communication Disorders M,D
Community Health Nursing M
Computational Biology M,D,O
Environmental and Occupational Health M,O
Evolutionary Biology M,D
Family Nurse Practitioner Studies M,D,O
Genetics D
Gerontological Nursing M
Health Physics/Radiological Health M,D
Health Services Management and Hospital Administration M
Immunology M,D
International Health O
Maternal and Child Health O
Maternal and Child/Neonatal Nursing M
Medical Physics M,D
Medicinal and Pharmaceutical Chemistry M,D
Microbiology M,D
Molecular Biology M,D
Neurobiology M,D
Neuroscience M,D
Nurse Anesthesia M,O
Nurse Midwifery M
Nursing Education O
Nursing—General D
Nutrition M,D
Occupational Therapy M
Pathology D
Pediatric Nursing M
Pharmaceutical Sciences M,D
Pharmacology M,D
Pharmacy M,D
Physical Therapy D
Physician Assistant Studies M
Physiology M,D
Psychiatric Nursing M
Public Health—General M,O
Reproductive Biology M,D
Toxicology M,D
Women's Health Nursing M

WEBER STATE UNIVERSITY
Health Physics/Radiological Health M
Health Services Management and Hospital Administration M
Nursing—General M

WEBSTER UNIVERSITY
Health Services Management and Hospital Administration M
Nurse Anesthesia M
Nursing—General M

WEILL CORNELL MEDICAL COLLEGE
Biochemistry M,D
Biological and Biomedical Sciences—General M,D
Biophysics M,D
Cell Biology M,D
Computational Biology D
Epidemiology M
Health Services Research M
Immunology M,D
Molecular Biology M,D
Neuroscience M,D
Pharmacology M,D
Physician Assistant Studies M
Physiology M,D
Structural Biology M,D
Systems Biology M,D

WESLEYAN UNIVERSITY
Biochemistry D
Biological and Biomedical Sciences—General D
Developmental Biology D
Ecology D
Evolutionary Biology D
Genetics D
Molecular Biology D
Molecular Biophysics D
Molecular Genetics D
Neurobiology D

WESLEY COLLEGE
Nursing—General M

WEST CHESTER UNIVERSITY OF PENNSYLVANIA
Biological and Biomedical Sciences—General M,O
Communication Disorders M,O
Community Health Nursing M,D
Community Health M,O
Environmental and Occupational Health M,O
Health Services Management and Hospital Administration M,O
Nursing and Healthcare Administration M,D
Nursing Education M,D
Nursing—General M,D
Nutrition M,O
Public Health—General M,O

WESTERN CAROLINA UNIVERSITY
Biological and Biomedical Sciences—General M
Communication Disorders M
Health Services Management and Hospital Administration M
Nursing Education M,O
Nursing—General M,O
Physical Therapy M,D

WESTERN CONNECTICUT STATE UNIVERSITY
Adult Nursing M
Biological and Biomedical Sciences—General M
Health Services Management and Hospital Administration M
Nursing Education D
Nursing—General M

WESTERN GOVERNORS UNIVERSITY
Health Services Management and Hospital Administration M
Nursing and Healthcare Administration M
Nursing Education M

WESTERN ILLINOIS UNIVERSITY
Biological and Biomedical Sciences—General M,O
Communication Disorders M
Health Services Management and Hospital Administration M,O
Marine Biology M,O
Zoology M,O

WESTERN KENTUCKY UNIVERSITY
Biological and Biomedical Sciences—General M
Communication Disorders M
Health Services Management and Hospital Administration M
Nursing—General M
Physical Therapy D
Public Health—General M

WESTERN MICHIGAN UNIVERSITY
Biological and Biomedical Sciences—General M,D
Communication Disorders M,D
Health Services Management and Hospital Administration M,D,O
Nursing—General M
Occupational Therapy M
Physician Assistant Studies M
Physiology M
Rehabilitation Sciences M

WESTERN NEW ENGLAND UNIVERSITY
Pharmacy D

WESTERN NEW MEXICO UNIVERSITY
Occupational Therapy M

WESTERN UNIVERSITY OF HEALTH SCIENCES
Allied Health—General M,D
Biological and Biomedical Sciences—General M
Dentistry D
Family Nurse Practitioner Studies M
Nursing and Healthcare Administration M
Nursing—General M,D
Optometry D
Osteopathic Medicine D
Pharmaceutical Sciences M
Pharmacy D
Physical Therapy D
Physician Assistant Studies M
Veterinary Medicine D

WESTERN WASHINGTON UNIVERSITY
Biological and Biomedical Sciences—General M
Communication Disorders M

WESTMINSTER COLLEGE (UT)
Family Nurse Practitioner Studies M
Nurse Anesthesia M
Nursing Education M
Nursing—General M
Public Health—General M

WEST TEXAS A&M UNIVERSITY
Biological and Biomedical Sciences—General M
Communication Disorders M
Family Nurse Practitioner Studies M
Nursing—General M

WEST VIRGINIA SCHOOL OF OSTEOPATHIC MEDICINE
Osteopathic Medicine D

WEST VIRGINIA UNIVERSITY
Allopathic Medicine D
Biochemistry M,D
Biological and Biomedical Sciences—General M,D
Cancer Biology/Oncology M,D
Cell Biology M,D
Communication Disorders M,D
Community Health M
Dentistry D
Developmental Biology M,D
Entomology M,D
Environmental and Occupational Health D
Environmental Biology M,D
Evolutionary Biology M,D
Genetics M,D
Genomic Sciences M,D
Health Promotion M,D
Human Genetics M,D
Immunology M,D
Industrial Hygiene M
Medicinal and Pharmaceutical Chemistry M,D
Microbiology M,D
Molecular Biology M,D
Neurobiology M,D
Neuroscience D
Nursing—General M,D,O
Nutrition M
Occupational Therapy M
Oral and Dental Sciences M
Pharmaceutical Administration M,D
Pharmaceutical Sciences M,D
Pharmacology M,D
Pharmacy M,D
Physical Therapy D
Physiology M,D
Plant Pathology M,D
Public Health—General M
Reproductive Biology M,D
Teratology M,D
Toxicology M,D

WEST VIRGINIA WESLEYAN COLLEGE
Family Nurse Practitioner Studies M,O
Nurse Midwifery M,O
Nursing and Healthcare Administration M,O
Nursing Education M,O
Nursing—General M,O
Psychiatric Nursing M,O

WHEELING JESUIT UNIVERSITY
Nursing—General M
Physical Therapy D

WICHITA STATE UNIVERSITY
Allied Health—General M,D
Biological and Biomedical Sciences—General M
Communication Disorders M,D
Nursing—General M,D
Physical Therapy D
Physician Assistant Studies M

WIDENER UNIVERSITY
Health Services Management and Hospital Administration M
Nursing—General M,D,O
Physical Therapy M,D

WILFRID LAURIER UNIVERSITY
Biological and Biomedical Sciences—General M
Health Promotion M
Neuroscience M,D

WILKES UNIVERSITY
Health Services Management and Hospital Administration M
Nursing—General M,D
Pharmacy D

WILLIAM CAREY UNIVERSITY
Nursing—General M

WILLIAM PATERSON UNIVERSITY OF NEW JERSEY
Biological and Biomedical Sciences—General M,D
Communication Disorders M,D
Nursing—General M,D

WILLIAM WOODS UNIVERSITY
Health Services Management and Hospital Administration M,D,O

WILMINGTON UNIVERSITY
Adult Nursing M,D
Family Nurse Practitioner Studies M,D
Gerontological Nursing M,D
Health Services Management and Hospital Administration M,D
Nursing and Healthcare Administration M,D
Nursing—General M,D

WINGATE UNIVERSITY
Pharmacy D

WINONA STATE UNIVERSITY
Adult Nursing M,D,O
Family Nurse Practitioner Studies M,D,O
Nursing and Healthcare Administration M,D,O
Nursing Education M,D,O
Nursing—General M,D,O

WINSTON-SALEM STATE UNIVERSITY
Nursing—General M
Occupational Therapy M
Physical Therapy M

WINTHROP UNIVERSITY
Biological and Biomedical Sciences—General M
Nutrition M

WON INSTITUTE OF GRADUATE STUDIES
Acupuncture and Oriental Medicine M

WOODS HOLE OCEANOGRAPHIC INSTITUTION
Marine Biology D

WORCESTER POLYTECHNIC INSTITUTE
Biochemistry M,D
Biological and Biomedical Sciences—General M,D
Computational Biology M,D

WORCESTER STATE UNIVERSITY
Communication Disorders M
Community Health Nursing M
Health Services Management and Hospital Administration M
Nursing Education M
Occupational Therapy M

WORLD MEDICINE INSTITUTE
Acupuncture and Oriental Medicine M

WRIGHT STATE UNIVERSITY
Acute Care/Critical Care Nursing M
Adult Nursing M
Allopathic Medicine D
Anatomy M
Biochemistry M
Biological and Biomedical Sciences—General M,D
Biophysics M
Community Health Nursing M
Family Nurse Practitioner Studies M
Health Promotion M
Health Services Management and Hospital Administration M
Immunology M
Medical Physics M
Microbiology M
Molecular Biology M
Nursing and Healthcare Administration M
Nursing—General M
Pediatric Nursing M
Pharmacology M
Physiology M
Public Health—General M
School Nursing M
Toxicology M

XAVIER UNIVERSITY
Family Nurse Practitioner Studies M
Forensic Nursing M
Health Services Management and Hospital Administration M
Nursing and Healthcare Administration M
Nursing Education M
Nursing—General M
Occupational Therapy M
School Nursing M

XAVIER UNIVERSITY OF LOUISIANA
Pharmacy D

YALE UNIVERSITY
Allopathic Medicine D
Biochemistry D
Biological and Biomedical Sciences—General D
Biophysics D
Cancer Biology/Oncology D
Cell Biology D
Computational Biology D
Developmental Biology D
Ecology D
Environmental and Occupational Health M,D
Epidemiology M,D
Evolutionary Biology D
Genetics D
Genomic Sciences D
Health Services Management and Hospital Administration M,D
Immunology D
Infectious Diseases D
International Health M,D
Microbiology D
Molecular Biology D
Molecular Biophysics D
Molecular Medicine D
Molecular Pathology D
Molecular Physiology D
Neurobiology D
Neuroscience D
Nursing—General M,D,O
Pathobiology D
Pathology M,D
Pharmacology D
Physician Assistant Studies M
Physiology D
Plant Biology D
Public Health—General M,D
Virology D

YORK COLLEGE OF PENNSYLVANIA
Adult Nursing M,D
Gerontological Nursing M,D
Health Services Management and Hospital Administration M
Nurse Anesthesia M,D
Nursing and Healthcare Administration M,D
Nursing Education M,D
Nursing—General M,D

YORK UNIVERSITY
Biological and Biomedical Sciences—General M,D
Nursing—General M

YO SAN UNIVERSITY OF TRADITIONAL CHINESE MEDICINE
Acupuncture and Oriental Medicine M

YOUNGSTOWN STATE UNIVERSITY
Anatomy M
Biochemistry M
Biological and Biomedical Sciences—General M
Environmental Biology M
Health Services Management and Hospital Administration M
Microbiology M
Molecular Biology M
Nursing—General M
Physical Therapy D
Physiology M

*M—masters degree; D—doctorate; O—other advanced degree; *—Close-Up and/or Display*

ACADEMIC AND PROFESSIONAL PROGRAMS IN THE BIOLOGICAL AND BIOMEDICAL SCIENCES

Section 1
Biological and Biomedical Sciences

This section contains a directory of institutions offering graduate work in biological and biomedical sciences, followed by in-depth entries submitted by institutions that chose to prepare detailed program descriptions. Additional information about programs listed in the directory but not augmented by an in-depth entry may be obtained by writing directly to the dean of a graduate school or chair of a department at the address given in the directory.

Programs in fields related to the biological and biomedical sciences may be found throughout this book. In the other guides in this series:

Graduate Programs in the Humanities, Arts & Social Sciences

See *Psychology and Counseling* and *Sociology, Anthropology, and Archaeology*

Graduate Programs in the Physical Sciences, Mathematics, Agricultural Sciences, the Environment & Natural Resources

See *Chemistry, Marine Sciences and Oceanography,* and *Mathematical Sciences*

Graduate Programs in Engineering & Applied Sciences

See *Agricultural Engineering and Bioengineering, Biomedical Engineering and Biotechnology, Civil and Environmental Engineering, Management of Engineering and Technology,* and *Ocean Engineering*

CONTENTS

Program Directory

Displays and Close-Ups

See also:

Biological and Biomedical Sciences—General

Acadia University, Faculty of Pure and Applied Science, Department of Biology, Wolfville, NS B4P 2R6, Canada. Offers M Sc. *Degree requirements:* For master's, comprehensive exam, thesis. *Entrance requirements:* For master's, minimum B-average in last 2 years of major. Additional exam requirements/recommendations for international students: Required—TOEFL (minimum score 580 paper-based; 93 iBT), IELTS (minimum score 6.5). *Faculty research:* Respiration physiology, estuaries and fisheries, limnology, plant biology, conservation biology.

Adelphi University, College of Arts and Sciences, Department of Biology, Garden City, NY 11530-0701. Offers MS. Part-time and evening/weekend programs available. *Students:* 24 full-time (18 women), 17 part-time (10 women); includes 14 minority (3 Black or African American, non-Hispanic/Latino; 7 Asian, non-Hispanic/Latino; 3 Hispanic/Latino; 1 Native Hawaiian or other Pacific Islander, non-Hispanic/Latino), 11 international. Average age 25. In 2013, 18 master's awarded. *Degree requirements:* For master's, thesis or alternative. *Entrance requirements:* For master's, bachelor's degree in biology or allied sciences, essay, 3 letters of recommendation, official transcripts. Additional exam requirements/recommendations for international students: Required—TOEFL (minimum score 550 paper-based; 80 iBT). *Application deadline:* For fall admission, 5/1 for international students; for spring admission, 12/1 for international students. Applications are processed on a rolling basis. Application fee: $50. Electronic applications accepted. *Expenses: Tuition:* Full-time $32,530; part-time $1010 per credit. *Required fees:* $1150. Tuition and fees vary according to degree level and program. *Financial support:* Research assistantships with full and partial tuition reimbursements, teaching assistantships, career-related internships or fieldwork, Federal Work-Study, institutionally sponsored loans, and unspecified assistantships available. Financial award application deadline: 2/15; financial award applicants required to submit FAFSA. *Faculty research:* Plant-animal interactions, physiology (plant, cornea), reproductive behavior, topics in evolution, fish biology. *Unit head:* Dr. Alan Schoenfeld, Chair, 516-877-4211, E-mail: schoenfeld@adelphi.edu. *Application contact:* Christine Murphy, Director of Admissions, 516-877-3050, Fax: 516-877-3039, E-mail: graduateadmissions@adelphi.edu.
Website: http://academics.adelphi.edu/artsci/bio/index.php

See Display below and Close-Up on page 109.

Alabama Agricultural and Mechanical University, School of Graduate Studies, School of Arts and Sciences, Department of Biology, Huntsville, AL 35811. Offers MS. Program offered jointly with The University of Alabama in Huntsville. Part-time and evening/weekend programs available. *Degree requirements:* For master's, comprehensive exam, thesis. *Entrance requirements:* For master's, GRE General Test. Additional exam requirements/recommendations for international students: Required—TOEFL (minimum score 500 paper-based; 61 iBT). Electronic applications accepted. *Faculty research:* Radiation and chemical mutagenesis, human cytogenetics, microbial biotechnology, microbial metabolism, environmental toxicology.

Alabama State University, College of Science, Mathematics and Technology, Department of Biological Sciences, Montgomery, AL 36101-0271. Offers MS, PhD. Part-time programs available. *Students:* 15 full-time (11 women), 15 part-time (8 women); includes 23 minority (all Black or African American, non-Hispanic/Latino), 4 international. Average age 33. 35 applicants, 34% accepted, 11 enrolled. In 2013, 2 master's, 3 doctorates awarded. *Degree requirements:* For master's, one foreign language, comprehensive exam, thesis. *Entrance requirements:* For master's, GRE General Test, GRE Subject Test, writing competency test. Additional exam requirements/recommendations for international students: Required—TOEFL (minimum score 500 paper-based). *Application deadline:* For fall admission, 7/15 for domestic students; for spring admission, 12/15 for domestic students. Applications are processed on a rolling basis. Application fee: $10. *Expenses:* Tuition, state resident: full-time $7958; part-time $343 per credit hour. Tuition, nonresident: full-time $14,132; part-time $686 per credit hour. *Required fees:* $446 per term. One-time fee: $1784 full-time; $892 part-time. Tuition and fees vary according to course load. *Financial support:* In 2013–14, 4 research assistantships with tuition reimbursements (averaging $12,000 per year) were awarded. *Faculty research:* Salmonella pseudomonas, cancer cells. *Total annual research expenditures:* $125,000. *Unit head:* Dr. Audrey Napier-Matthews, Chair, 334-229-4467, Fax: 334-229-1007, E-mail: anapier@alasu.edu. *Application contact:* Dr. Doris Screws, Dean of Graduate Studies, 334-229-4274, Fax: 334-229-4928, E-mail: dscrews@alasu.edu.
Website: http://www.alasu.edu/academics/colleges—departments/science-mathematics-technology/biological-sciences-department/index.aspx

Albert Einstein College of Medicine, Graduate Division of Biomedical Sciences, Bronx, NY 10461. Offers PhD, MD/PhD. *Degree requirements:* For doctorate, thesis/dissertation. *Entrance requirements:* For doctorate, GRE General Test. Additional exam requirements/recommendations for international students: Required—TOEFL.

Albert Einstein College of Medicine, Medical Scientist Training Program, Bronx, NY 10461. Offers MD/PhD.

Alcorn State University, School of Graduate Studies, School of Arts and Sciences, Department of Biology, Alcorn State, MS 39096-7500. Offers MS.

American Museum of Natural History–Richard Gilder Graduate School, Program in Comparative Biology, New York, NY 10024. Offers PhD. *Degree requirements:* For doctorate, thesis/dissertation, qualifying examination. *Entrance requirements:* For doctorate, GRE General Test (taken within the past five years); GRE Subject Test (recommended), BA, BS, or equivalent degree from accredited institution; official transcripts; essay;. Additional exam requirements/recommendations for international students: Required—TOEFL (minimum score 600 paper-based; 100 iBT), IELTS (minimum score 7).

See Display on next page and Close-Up on page 111.

American University, College of Arts and Sciences, Washington, DC 20016-8012. Offers addiction and addictive behavior (Certificate); anthropology (PhD); applied microeconomics (Certificate); applied statistics (Certificate); art history (MA); arts management (MA, Certificate); Asian studies (Certificate); audio production (Certificate); audio technology (MA); behavior, cognition, and neuroscience (PhD); bilingual education (MA, Certificate); biology (MA, MS); chemistry (MS); clinical psychology (PhD); computer science (MS, Certificate); creative writing (MFA); curriculum and instruction (M Ed, Certificate); economics (MA, PhD); environmental assessment (Certificate); environmental science (MS); ethics, peace, and global affairs (MA); gender analysis in economics (Certificate); health promotion management (MS); history (MA, PhD); international arts management (Certificate); international economic relations (Certificate); international economics (MA); international training and education (MA);

literature (MA); mathematics (MA); North American studies (Certificate); nutrition education (MS, Certificate); philosophy (MA); professional science: biotechnology (MS); professional science: environmental assessment (MS); professional science: quantitative analysis (MS); psychobiology of healing (Certificate); psychology (MA); psychology: general (PhD); public anthropology (MA, Certificate); public sociology (Certificate); social research (Certificate); sociology (MA); Spanish: Latin American studies (MA); special education: learning disabilities (MA); statistics (MS); studio art (MFA); teaching (MAT); teaching English as a foreign language (MA); teaching: early childhood (Certificate); teaching: elementary (Certificate); teaching: ESOL (Certificate); teaching: secondary (Certificate); technology in arts management (Certificate); TESOL (MA); translation: French (Certificate); translation: Russian (Certificate); translation: Spanish (Certificate); women's, gender, and sexuality studies (Certificate). Part-time and evening/weekend programs available. Postbaccalaureate distance learning degree programs offered (no on-campus study). *Faculty:* 358 full-time (187 women), 254 part-time/adjunct (127 women). *Students:* 627 full-time (411 women), 416 part-time (300 women); includes 206 minority (91 Black or African American, non-Hispanic/Latino; 5 American Indian or Alaska Native, non-Hispanic/Latino; 32 Asian, non-Hispanic/Latino; 64 Hispanic/Latino; 1 Native Hawaiian or other Pacific Islander, non-Hispanic/Latino; 13 Two or more races, non-Hispanic/Latino), 124 international. Average age 29. 1,672 applicants, 52% accepted, 361 enrolled. In 2013, 382 master's, 38 doctorates, 33 other advanced degrees awarded. Terminal master's awarded for partial completion of doctoral program. *Degree requirements:* For master's, comprehensive exam (for some programs), thesis (for some programs); for doctorate, comprehensive exam (for some programs), thesis/dissertation. *Entrance requirements:* For master's, GRE, minimum GPA of 3.0 in last 60 credit hours, letter of recommendation, statement of purpose, resume, unofficial transcript; for doctorate, GRE, minimum GPA of 3.0 for all graduate work, letter of recommendation, statement of purpose, resume, unofficial transcript. Additional exam requirements/recommendations for international students: Required—TOEFL (minimum score 600 paper-based; 100 iBT), IELTS (minimum score 7). *Application deadline:* For fall admission, 2/1 for domestic students; for spring admission, 10/1 for domestic students. Applications are processed on a rolling basis. Application fee: $55. Electronic applications accepted. *Expenses: Tuition:* Full-time $25,920; part-time $1482 per credit hour. *Required fees:* $430. Tuition and fees vary according to course load and program. *Financial support:* Fellowships, research assistantships with full and partial tuition reimbursements, teaching assistantships with full and partial tuition reimbursements, career-related internships or fieldwork, Federal Work-Study, institutionally sponsored loans, scholarships/grants, traineeships, tuition waivers (full and partial), and unspecified assistantships available. Support available to part-time students. Financial award applicants required to submit FAFSA. *Unit head:* Dr. Peter Starr, Dean, 202-885-2446, Fax: 202-885-2429, E-mail: pstarr@american.edu. *Application contact:* Kathleen Clowery, Associate Director, Graduate Enrollment Management, 202-885-3621, Fax: 202-885-1505, E-mail: clowery@american.edu.
Website: http://www.american.edu/cas/

American University of Beirut, Graduate Programs, Faculty of Arts and Sciences, Beirut, Lebanon. Offers anthropology (MA); Arab and Middle Eastern history (PhD); Arabic language and literature (MA, PhD); archaeology (MA); biology (MS); cell and molecular biology (PhD); chemistry (MS); clinical psychology (MA); computational sciences (MS); computer science (MS); economics (MA); education (MA); English language (MA); English literature (MA); environmental policy planning (MS); financial economics (MA); geology (MS); history (MA); mathematics (MA, MS); media studies (MA); Middle Eastern studies (MA); philosophy (MA); physics (MS); political studies (MA); psychology (MA); public administration (MA); sociology (MA); statistics (MA, MS); theoretical physics (PhD); transnational American studies (MA). Part-time programs available. *Faculty:* 88 full-time (22 women). *Students:* Average age 25. In 2013, 112 master's, 87 doctorates awarded. *Degree requirements:* For master's, one foreign language, comprehensive exam, thesis (for some programs); for doctorate, one foreign language, comprehensive exam, thesis/dissertation. *Entrance requirements:* For master's, GRE, letter of recommendation; for doctorate, GRE, letters of recommendation. Additional exam requirements/recommendations for international students: Required—TOEFL (minimum score 600 paper-based; 97 iBT), IELTS (minimum score 7). *Application deadline:* For fall admission, 4/30 for domestic students, 4/18 for international students; for spring admission, 11/1 for domestic and international students. Application fee: $50. *Expenses: Tuition:* Full-time $14,724; part-time $818 per credit. *Required fees:* $692. Tuition and fees vary according to course load and program. *Financial support:* Research assistantships, career-related internships or fieldwork, institutionally sponsored loans, scholarships/grants, health care benefits, and unspecified assistantships available. Financial award application deadline: 2/4; financial award applicants required to submit FAFSA. *Faculty research:* Modern Middle East history; Near Eastern archaeology; Islamic history; European history; software engineering; scientific computing; data mining; the applications of cooperative learning in language teaching and teacher education; world/comparative literature; rhetoric and composition; creative writing; public management; public policy and international affairs; hydrogeology; mineralogy, petrology, and geochemistry; tectonics and structural geology; cell and molecular biology; ecology. *Unit head:* Dr. Patrick McGreevy, Dean, 961-1374374 Ext. 3800, Fax: 961-1744461, E-mail: pm07@aub.edu.lb. *Application contact:* Dr. Salim Kanaan, Director, Admissions Office, 961-1-350000 Ext. 2590, Fax: 96-1-1750775, E-mail: sk00@aub.edu.lb.
Website: http://www.aub.edu.lb/fas/

American University of Beirut, Graduate Programs, Faculty of Medicine, Beirut, Lebanon. Offers anatomy, cell biology and human morphology (MS); biochemistry and medical genetics (MS); biomedical sciences (PhD); experimental pathology, immunology and microbiology (MS); medicine (MD); neuroscience (MS); pharmacology and toxicology (MS). Part-time programs available. *Faculty:* 259 full-time (78 women), 93 part-time/adjunct (16 women). *Students:* 364 full-time (165 women), 62 part-time (54 women). Average age 23. In 2013, 18 master's awarded. *Degree requirements:* For master's, one foreign language, comprehensive exam, thesis (for some programs); for doctorate, one foreign language, comprehensive exam, thesis/dissertation. *Entrance requirements:* For master's, letter of recommendation; for doctorate, MCAT, bachelor's degree. Additional exam requirements/recommendations for international students: Required—TOEFL (minimum score 600 paper-based; 100 iBT), IELTS (minimum score 7.5). *Application deadline:* For fall admission, 4/30 for domestic and international students; for spring admission, 11/1 for domestic and international students. Application fee: $50. *Expenses: Tuition:* Full-time $14,724; part-time $818 per credit. *Required fees:* $692. Tuition and fees vary according to course load and program. *Financial support:* In 2013–14, 242 students received support, including 60 teaching assistantships (averaging $4,000 per year); career-related internships or fieldwork, institutionally sponsored loans, scholarships/grants, health care benefits, and unspecified assistantships also available. Financial award application deadline: 2/2. *Faculty research:* Cancer research (targeted therapy, mechanisms of leukemogenesis, tumor cell extravasation and metastasis, cancer stem cells), stem cell research (regenerative medicine, drug discovery), genetic research (neurogenetics, hereditary cardiomyopathy, hemoglobinopathies, pharmacogenomics, proteomics), neuroscience research (pain, neurodegenerative disorder), metabolism (inflammation and metabolism, metabolic disorder, diabetes mellitus), vascular and renal biology, signal transduction. *Total annual*

research expenditures: $2.6 million. *Unit head:* Dr. Mohamed Sayegh, Dean, 961-1350000 Ext. 4700, Fax: 961-1744464, E-mail: msayegh@aub.edu.lb. *Application contact:* Dr. Salim Kanaan, Director, Admissions Office, 961-1-350000 Ext. 2594, Fax: 96-1-1750775, E-mail: sk00@aub.edu.lb.
Website: http://www.aub.edu.lb/fm/fm_home/Pages/index.aspx

Andrews University, School of Graduate Studies, College of Arts and Sciences, Department of Biology, Berrien Springs, MI 49104. Offers MAT, MS. *Faculty:* 9 full-time (3 women). *Students:* 3 full-time (2 women), 1 international. Average age 30. 7 applicants. In 2013, 2 master's awarded. *Degree requirements:* For master's, comprehensive exam, thesis. *Entrance requirements:* For master's, GRE Subject Test. Additional exam requirements/recommendations for international students: Required—TOEFL (minimum score 550 paper-based). *Application deadline:* Applications are processed on a rolling basis. Application fee: $40. *Financial support:* Fellowships, research assistantships, teaching assistantships, career-related internships or fieldwork, Federal Work-Study, and institutionally sponsored loans available. Financial award application deadline: 3/15. *Unit head:* Dr. Thomas Goodwin, Chairman, 269-471-3243. *Application contact:* Monica Wringer, Supervisor of Graduate Admission, 800-253-2874, Fax: 269-471-6321, E-mail: graduate@andrews.edu.

Angelo State University, College of Graduate Studies, College of Arts and Sciences, Department of Biology, San Angelo, TX 76909. Offers MS. Part-time and evening/weekend programs available. *Degree requirements:* For master's, comprehensive exam, thesis optional. *Entrance requirements:* For master's, GRE General Test, essay. Additional exam requirements/recommendations for international students: Required—TOEFL or IELTS. Electronic applications accepted. *Faculty research:* Texas poppy-mallow project, Chisos hedgehog cactus, skunks, reptiles, amphibians, rodents, seed germination, mammals.

Appalachian State University, Cratis D. Williams Graduate School, Department of Biology, Boone, NC 28608. Offers cell and molecular biology (MS); general biology (MS). Part-time programs available. *Degree requirements:* For master's, comprehensive exam, thesis. *Entrance requirements:* For master's, GRE General Test, 3 letters of recommendation. Additional exam requirements/recommendations for international students: Required—TOEFL (minimum score 570 paper-based; 79 iBT), IELTS (minimum score 6.5). Electronic applications accepted. *Faculty research:* Aquatic and terrestrial ecology, animal and plant physiology, behavior and systematics, immunology and cell biology, molecular biology and microbiology.

Arizona State University at the Tempe campus, College of Liberal Arts and Sciences, School of Life Sciences, Tempe, AZ 85287-4601. Offers animal behavior (PhD); applied ethics (biomedical and health ethics) (MA); biological design (PhD); biology (MS, PhD); biology (biology and society) (MS, PhD); environmental life sciences (PhD); evolutionary biology (PhD); human and social dimensions of science and technology (PhD); microbiology (PhD); molecular and cellular biology (PhD); neuroscience (PhD); philosophy (history and philosophy of science) (MA); sustainability (PhD). Terminal master's awarded for partial completion of doctoral program. *Degree requirements:* For master's, thesis (for some programs), interactive Program of Study (iPOS) submitted before completing 50 percent of required credit hours; for doctorate, variable foreign language requirement, comprehensive exam, thesis/dissertation, interactive Program of Study (iPOS) submitted before completing 50 percent of required credit hours. *Entrance requirements:* For master's and doctorate, GRE, minimum GPA of 3.0 or equivalent in last 2 years of work leading to bachelor's degree. Additional exam requirements/recommendations for international students: Required—TOEFL (minimum score 600 paper-based; 100 iBT). Electronic applications accepted.

Arizona State University at the Tempe campus, College of Technology and Innovation, Department of Applied Sciences and Mathematics, Mesa, AZ 85212. Offers applied biological sciences (MS). Part-time programs available. *Degree requirements:* For master's, thesis, oral defense, interactive Program of Study (iPOS) submitted before completing 50 percent of required credit hours. *Entrance requirements:* For master's, GRE (minimum combined score of 1080) or MAT (minimum score of 45), minimum GPA of 3.0 or equivalent in last 2 years of work leading to bachelor's degree, 3 letters of recommendation, resume, 18 hours of biological sciences or related courses, statement of intent. Additional exam requirements/recommendations for international students: Required—TOEFL (minimum score 83 iBT), TOEFL, IELTS, or PTE. Electronic applications accepted.

Arizona State University at the Tempe campus, Graduate College, Program in Biological Design, Tempe, AZ 85287-5001. Offers PhD. *Degree requirements:* For doctorate, comprehensive exam, thesis/dissertation, interactive Program of Study (iPOS) submitted before completing 50 percent of required credit hours. *Entrance requirements:* For doctorate, GRE, minimum GPA of 3.0 in the last 2 years of work leading to the bachelor's degree, 3 letters of recommendation, personal statement containing goals and prior/current research experience, resume. Additional exam requirements/recommendations for international students: Required—TOEFL (minimum score 550 paper-based; 80 iBT), IELTS (minimum score 6.5). Electronic applications accepted.

Arkansas State University, Graduate School, College of Sciences and Mathematics, Department of Biological Sciences, State University, AR 72467. Offers biological sciences (MA); biology (MS); biology education (MSE, SCCT); biotechnology (PSM). Part-time programs available. *Faculty:* 22 full-time (7 women). *Students:* 10 full-time (5 women), 17 part-time (9 women); includes 3 minority (1 Black or African American, non-Hispanic/Latino; 1 American Indian or Alaska Native, non-Hispanic/Latino; 1 Hispanic/Latino). Average age 29. 26 applicants, 23% accepted, 6 enrolled. In 2013, 12 master's awarded. *Degree requirements:* For master's, comprehensive exam, thesis (for some programs); for SCCT, comprehensive exam. *Entrance requirements:* For master's, GRE General Test, appropriate bachelor's degree, letters of reference, interview, official transcripts, immunization records, statement of educational objectives and career goals, teaching certificate (MSE); for SCCT, GRE General Test or MAT, interview, master's degree, letters of reference, official transcript, personal statement, immunization records. Additional exam requirements/recommendations for international students: Required—TOEFL (minimum score 550 paper-based; 79 iBT), IELTS (minimum score 6), PTE (minimum score 56). *Application deadline:* For fall admission, 7/1 for domestic and international students; for spring admission, 11/15 for domestic students, 11/14 for international students. Applications are processed on a rolling basis. Application fee: $30 ($40 for international students). Electronic applications accepted. *Expenses:* Tuition, state resident: full-time $4284; part-time $238 per credit hour. Tuition, nonresident: full-time $8568; part-time $476 per credit hour. *International tuition:* $9268 full-time. *Required fees:* $1098; $61 per credit hour. $25 per term. Tuition and fees vary according to course load and program. *Financial support:* In 2013–14, 12 students received support. Research assistantships, career-related internships or fieldwork, scholarships/grants, and unspecified assistantships available. Financial award application deadline: 7/1; financial award applicants required to submit FAFSA. *Unit head:* Dr. Thomas Risch, Chair, 870-972-3082, Fax: 870-972-2638, E-mail: trisch@astate.edu. *Application contact:* Vickey Ring, Graduate Admissions Coordinator, 870-972-3029, Fax: 870-972-3857, E-mail: vickeyring@astate.edu.
Website: http://www.astate.edu/college/sciences-and-mathematics/departments/biology/index.dot

A.T. Still University, Kirksville College of Osteopathic Medicine, Kirksville, MO 63501. Offers biomedical sciences (MS); osteopathic medicine (DO). *Accreditation:* AOsA. *Faculty:* 37 full-time (5 women), 36 part-time/adjunct (6 women). *Students:* 702 full-time (282 women), 10 part-time (3 women); includes 132 minority (13 Black or African American, non-Hispanic/Latino; 1 American Indian or Alaska Native, non-Hispanic/Latino; 69 Asian, non-Hispanic/Latino; 18 Hispanic/Latino; 31 Two or more races, non-Hispanic/Latino), 6 international. Average age 26. 4,110 applicants, 10% accepted, 172 enrolled. In 2013, 13 master's, 177 doctorates awarded. *Degree requirements:* For master's, thesis; for doctorate, Level 1 and 2 COMLEX-PE and CE exams. *Entrance requirements:* For master's, GRE, MCAT, or DAT, minimum undergraduate GPA of 2.65 (cumulative and science); for doctorate, MCAT, bachelor's degree with minimum GPA of 2.8 (cumulative and science) or 90 semester hours with minimum GPA of 3.5 (cumulative and science). Additional exam requirements/recommendations for international students: Recommended—TOEFL. *Application deadline:* For fall admission, 2/1 for domestic and international students; for summer admission, 2/1 for domestic students. Applications are processed on a rolling basis. Application fee: $70. Electronic applications accepted. *Expenses:* Contact institution. *Financial support:* In 2013–14, 230 students received support, including 23 fellowships with full tuition reimbursements available (averaging $49,817 per year); Federal Work-Study and scholarships/grants also available. Financial award application deadline: 5/1; financial award applicants required to submit FAFSA. *Faculty research:* Practice-based research network, antibiotic resistance, staphylococcus aureus, bacterial virulence and environmental survival, excitability of the exercise pressor reflex, clinical trials. *Total annual research expenditures:* $243,048. *Unit head:* Dr. Margaret WIlson, Dean, 660-626-2354, Fax: 660-626-2080, E-mail: mwilson@atsu.edu. *Application contact:* Donna Sparks, Associate Director, Admissions Processing, 660-626-2117, Fax: 660-626-2969, E-mail: admissions@atsu.edu.
Website: http://www.atsu.edu/kcom/

Auburn University, College of Veterinary Medicine and Graduate School, Graduate Programs in Veterinary Medicine, Auburn University, AL 36849. Offers biomedical sciences (MS, PhD), including anatomy, physiology and pharmacology (MS), biomedical sciences (PhD), clinical sciences (MS), large animal surgery and medicine (MS), pathobiology (MS), radiology (MS), small animal surgery and medicine (MS); DVM/MS. Part-time programs available. *Faculty:* 100 full-time (41 women), 4 part-time/adjunct (1 woman). *Students:* 24 full-time (16 women), 38 part-time (25 women); includes 5 minority (1 Black or African American, non-Hispanic/Latino; 1 American Indian or Alaska Native, non-Hispanic/Latino; 2 Asian, non-Hispanic/Latino; 1 Hispanic/Latino), 22 international. Average age 30. 36 applicants, 44% accepted, 13 enrolled. In 2013, 12 master's, 8 doctorates awarded. *Degree requirements:* For doctorate, thesis/dissertation. *Entrance requirements:* For master's, GRE General Test; for doctorate, GRE General Test, GRE Subject Test. *Application deadline:* For fall admission, 7/7 for domestic students; for spring admission, 11/24 for domestic students. Applications are processed on a rolling basis. Application fee: $50 ($60 for international students). Electronic applications accepted. *Expenses:* Tuition, state resident: full-time $8262; part-time $459 per credit hour. Tuition, nonresident: full-time $24,786; part-time $1377 per credit hour. Tuition and fees vary according to degree level and program. *Financial support:* Research assistantships, teaching assistantships, and Federal Work-Study available. Support available to part-time students. Financial award application deadline: 3/15; financial award applicants required to submit FAFSA. *Unit head:* Dr. Calvin Johnson, Acting Dean, 334-844-2650. *Application contact:* Dr. George Flowers, Dean of the Graduate School, 334-844-2125.

Auburn University, Graduate School, College of Sciences and Mathematics, Department of Biological Sciences, Auburn University, AL 36849. Offers botany (MS, PhD); microbiology (MS, PhD); zoology (MS, PhD). *Faculty:* 39 full-time (13 women), 1 (woman) part-time/adjunct. *Students:* 40 full-time (21 women), 66 part-time (26 women); includes 9 minority (2 Black or African American, non-Hispanic/Latino; 1 American Indian or Alaska Native, non-Hispanic/Latino; 4 Asian, non-Hispanic/Latino; 2 Hispanic/Latino), 17 international. Average age 28. 99 applicants, 31% accepted, 19 enrolled. In 2013, 10 master's, 11 doctorates awarded. *Entrance requirements:* For master's and doctorate, GRE General Test. Additional exam requirements/recommendations for international students: Required—TOEFL. *Application deadline:* For fall admission, 7/7 for domestic students; for spring admission, 11/24 for domestic students. Application fee: $50 ($60 for international students). Electronic applications accepted. *Expenses:* Tuition, state resident: full-time $8262; part-time $459 per credit hour. Tuition, nonresident: full-time $24,786; part-time $1377 per credit hour. Tuition and fees vary according to degree level and program. *Financial support:* Research assistantships and teaching assistantships available. Financial award applicants required to submit FAFSA. *Unit head:* Dr. Jack W. Feminella, Chair, 334-844-3906, Fax: 334-844-1645. *Application contact:* Dr. George Flowers, Dean of the Graduate School, 334-844-2125.

Austin Peay State University, College of Graduate Studies, College of Science and Mathematics, Department of Biology, Clarksville, TN 37044. Offers clinical laboratory science (MS); radiologic science (MS). Part-time programs available. *Faculty:* 12 full-time (5 women). *Students:* 5 full-time (4 women), 28 part-time (15 women); includes 3 minority (2 Black or African American, non-Hispanic/Latino; 1 Two or more races, non-Hispanic/Latino), 2 international. Average age 27. 15 applicants, 100% accepted, 12 enrolled. In 2013, 10 master's awarded. *Degree requirements:* For master's, comprehensive exam, thesis optional. *Entrance requirements:* For master's, GRE General Test, 3 letters of recommendation, minimum undergraduate GPA of 2.5. Additional exam requirements/recommendations for international students: Required—TOEFL (minimum score 500 paper-based). *Application deadline:* For fall admission, 8/5 priority date for domestic students. Applications are processed on a rolling basis. Application fee: $25. Electronic applications accepted. *Expenses:* Tuition, state resident: full-time $7500; part-time $375 per credit hour. Tuition, nonresident: full-time $20,800; part-time $1040 per credit hour. *Required fees:* $1284; $64.20 per credit hour. *Financial support:* In 2013–14, research assistantships with full tuition reimbursements (averaging $6,500 per year) were awarded; career-related internships or fieldwork, Federal Work-Study, institutionally sponsored loans, scholarships/grants, and unspecified assistantships also available. Support available to part-time students. Financial award application deadline: 3/1. *Faculty research:* Non-paint source pollution, amphibian biomonitoring, aquatic toxicology, biological indicators of water quality, taxonomy. *Unit head:* Dr. Don Dailey, Chair, 931-221-7781, Fax: 931-221-6323, E-mail: daileyd@apsu.edu. *Application contact:* June D. Lee, Graduate Coordinator, 800-859-4723, Fax: 931-221-7641, E-mail: gradadmissions@apsu.edu.
Website: http://www.apsu.edu/biology

Ball State University, Graduate School, College of Sciences and Humanities, Department of Biology, Muncie, IN 47306-1099. Offers biology (MA, MAE, MS); biology education (Ed D). *Faculty:* 19 full-time (5 women). *Students:* 20 full-time (8 women), 23 part-time (14 women); includes 2 minority (both Hispanic/Latino), 6 international. Average age 24. 49 applicants, 80% accepted, 13 enrolled. In 2013, 18 master's awarded. *Degree requirements:* For doctorate, thesis/dissertation. *Entrance requirements:* For master's, GRE General Test; for doctorate, GRE General Test, minimum graduate GPA of 3.2. Application fee: $50. *Financial support:* In 2013–14, 29 students received support, including 33 teaching assistantships with full and partial tuition reimbursements available (averaging $11,907 per year); research assistantships with full tuition reimbursements available and career-related internships or fieldwork also available. Financial award application deadline: 3/1. *Faculty research:* Aquatics and fisheries, tumors, water and air pollution, developmental biology and genetics. *Unit head:* Dr. Kemuel Badger, Chairman, 765-285-8820, Fax: 765-285-8804, E-mail: kbadger@bsu.edu. *Application contact:* Dr. Robert Morris, Associate Provost for Research and Dean of the Graduate School, 765-285-1300, E-mail: rmorris@bsu.edu. Website: http://cms.bsu.edu/Academics/CollegesandDepartments/Biology.aspx

Barry University, College of Health Sciences, Programs in Biology and Biomedical Sciences, Miami Shores, FL 33161-6695. Offers biology (MS); biomedical sciences (MS). Part-time and evening/weekend programs available. *Degree requirements:* For master's, comprehensive exam, thesis (for some programs). *Entrance requirements:* For master's, GRE General Test or Florida Teacher's Certification Exam (biology); GRE General Test, MCAT, or DAT (biomedical sciences). Electronic applications accepted. *Faculty research:* Genetics, immunology, anthropology.

Baylor College of Medicine, Graduate School of Biomedical Sciences, Houston, TX 77030-3498. Offers MS, PhD, MD/PhD. Terminal master's awarded for partial completion of doctoral program. *Degree requirements:* For master's, thesis; for doctorate, thesis/dissertation, public defense. *Entrance requirements:* For doctorate, GRE General Test, GRE Subject Test (strongly recommended), minimum GPA of 3.0. Additional exam requirements/recommendations for international students: Required—TOEFL. Electronic applications accepted. *Faculty research:* Cell and molecular biology of cardiac muscle, structural biophysics, gene expression and regulation, human genomes, viruses.

Baylor University, Graduate School, College of Arts and Sciences, Department of Biology, Waco, TX 76798. Offers biology (MA, MS, PhD); environmental biology (MS); limnology (MS). Part-time programs available. *Faculty:* 13 full-time (3 women). *Students:* 33 full-time (17 women), 4 part-time (all women); includes 9 minority (5 Asian, non-Hispanic/Latino; 4 Two or more races, non-Hispanic/Latino), 11 international. In 2013, 12 master's, 4 doctorates awarded. *Degree requirements:* For master's, thesis (for some programs); for doctorate, thesis/dissertation. *Entrance requirements:* For master's and doctorate, GRE General Test. Additional exam requirements/recommendations for international students: Required—TOEFL. *Application deadline:* For fall admission, 2/15 priority date for domestic and international students. Applications are processed on a rolling basis. Application fee: $25. *Expenses: Tuition:* Full-time $25,866; part-time $1437 per credit hour. *Required fees:* $2736; $152 per credit hour. Tuition and fees vary according to course load and program. *Financial support:* Research assistantships with full and partial tuition reimbursements, teaching assistantships with full and partial tuition reimbursements, career-related internships or fieldwork, Federal Work-Study, institutionally sponsored loans, and tuition waivers (full and partial) available. Support available to part-time students. Financial award application deadline: 2/28. *Faculty research:* Terrestrial ecology, aquatic ecology, genetics. *Unit head:* Dr. Ryan King, Graduate Program Director, 254-710-2150, Fax: 254-710-2969, E-mail: ryan_s_king@baylor.edu. *Application contact:* Tamara Lehmann, Academic Support Associate, 254-710-2578, Fax: 254-710-2969, E-mail: tamara_lehmann@baylor.edu.
Website: http://www.baylor.edu/biology/

Baylor University, Graduate School, Institute of Biomedical Studies, Waco, TX 76798. Offers MS, PhD. *Faculty:* 17 part-time/adjunct (3 women). *Students:* 23 full-time (5 women), 4 part-time (2 women); includes 6 minority (1 Black or African American, non-Hispanic/Latino; 3 Asian, non-Hispanic/Latino; 2 Hispanic/Latino), 14 international. Average age 24. 69 applicants, 10% accepted, 5 enrolled. In 2013, 3 master's, 1 doctorate awarded. *Degree requirements:* For master's, thesis (for some programs); for doctorate, thesis/dissertation. *Entrance requirements:* For master's and doctorate, GRE General Test. Additional exam requirements/recommendations for international students: Required—TOEFL (minimum score 550 paper-based). *Application deadline:* Applications are processed on a rolling basis. Application fee: $25. *Expenses: Tuition:* Full-time $25,866; part-time $1437 per credit hour. *Required fees:* $2736; $152 per credit hour. Tuition and fees vary according to course load and program. *Financial support:* In 2013–14, 22 students received support, including 11 research assistantships (averaging $20,000 per year), 11 teaching assistantships (averaging $20,000 per year); tuition waivers also available. *Unit head:* Dr. Chris Kearney, Graduate Program Director, 254-710-2131, Fax: 254-710-3878, E-mail: chris_kearney@baylor.edu. *Application contact:* Rhonda Bellert, Administrative Assistant, 254-710-2514, Fax: 254-710-2199, E-mail: rhonda_bellert@baylor.edu.
Website: http://www.baylor.edu/biomedical/

Bemidji State University, School of Graduate Studies, Bemidji, MN 56601. Offers biology (MS); education (MS); English (MA, MS); environmental studies (MS); mathematics (MS); mathematics (elementary and middle level education) (MS); special education (M Sp Ed, MS). Part-time programs available. Postbaccalaureate distance learning degree programs offered (no on-campus study). *Faculty:* 117 full-time (53 women), 20 part-time/adjunct (15 women). *Students:* 30 full-time (17 women), 157 part-time (108 women); includes 16 minority (2 Black or African American, non-Hispanic/Latino; 4 American Indian or Alaska Native, non-Hispanic/Latino; 2 Asian, non-Hispanic/Latino; 1 Hispanic/Latino; 7 Two or more races, non-Hispanic/Latino), 1 international. Average age 35. 73 applicants, 93% accepted, 38 enrolled. In 2013, 49 master's awarded. *Degree requirements:* For master's, comprehensive exam, thesis (for some programs). *Entrance requirements:* For master's, GRE; GMAT, letters of recommendation, letters of interest. Additional exam requirements/recommendations for international students: Required—TOEFL (minimum score 550 paper-based; 80 iBT). *Application deadline:* Applications are processed on a rolling basis. Application fee: $20. Electronic applications accepted. *Expenses:* Tuition, state resident: full-time $6941; part-time $365 per credit. Tuition, nonresident: full-time $6941; part-time $365 per credit. *Required fees:* $16 per credit. Tuition and fees vary according to program and reciprocity agreements. *Financial support:* In 2013–14, 131 students received support, including 18 research assistantships with partial tuition reimbursements available (averaging $12,889 per year), 23 teaching assistantships with partial tuition reimbursements available (averaging $12,889 per year); scholarships/grants and unspecified assistantships also available. Financial award application deadline: 3/31; financial award applicants required to submit FAFSA. *Faculty research:* Human performance, sport, and health: physical education teacher education, continuum models, spiritual health, intellectual health, resiliency, health priorities; psychology: health psychology, college student drinking behavior, micro-aggressions, infant cognition, false memories, leadership assessment; biology: structure and dynamics of forest communities, aquatic and riverine ecology, interaction between animal populations and aquatic environments, cellular motility. *Unit head:* Dr. James Barta, Interim Dean of Health Sciences and Human Ecology, 218-755-3874, Fax: 218-755-2258, E-mail: jbarta@bemidjistate.edu. *Application contact:* Joan Miller, Director, School of Graduate Studies, 218-755-2027, Fax: 218-755-2258, E-mail: jmiller@bemidjistate.edu.
Website: http://www.bemidjistate.edu/academics/graduate_studies/

Binghamton University, State University of New York, Graduate School, School of Arts and Sciences, Department of Biological Sciences, Vestal, NY 13850. Offers MA, MS, PhD. *Faculty:* 28 full-time (17 women), 6 part-time/adjunct (3 women). *Students:* 37 full-time (15 women), 37 part-time (21 women); includes 10 minority (2 Black or African American, non-Hispanic/Latino; 2 Asian, non-Hispanic/Latino; 4 Hispanic/Latino; 2 Native Hawaiian or other Pacific Islander, non-Hispanic/Latino), 17 international. Average age 27. 80 applicants, 34% accepted, 18 enrolled. In 2013, 8 master's, 10 doctorates awarded. Terminal master's awarded for partial completion of doctoral program. *Degree requirements:* For master's, thesis, oral exam, seminar presentation; for doctorate, comprehensive exam, thesis/dissertation. *Entrance requirements:* For master's and doctorate, GRE General Test, GRE Subject Test. Additional exam requirements/recommendations for international students: Required—TOEFL (minimum score 550 paper-based; 80 iBT). *Application deadline:* For fall admission, 1/15 priority date for domestic and international students; for spring admission, 10/15 priority date for domestic and international students. Applications are processed on a rolling basis. Application fee: $75. Electronic applications accepted. *Financial support:* In 2013–14, 40 students received support, including 6 research assistantships with full tuition reimbursements available (averaging $19,000 per year), 33 teaching assistantships with full tuition reimbursements available (averaging $17,500 per year); career-related internships or fieldwork, Federal Work-Study, institutionally sponsored loans, scholarships/grants, health care benefits, tuition waivers (full and partial), and unspecified assistantships also available. Financial award application deadline: 2/15; financial award applicants required to submit FAFSA. *Unit head:* Dr. Curt M. Pueschel, Chairperson, 607-777-2602, E-mail: curtp@binghamton.edu. *Application contact:* Kishan Zuber, Recruiting and Admissions Coordinator, 607-777-2151, Fax: 607-777-2501, E-mail: kzuber@binghamton.edu.

Bloomsburg University of Pennsylvania, School of Graduate Studies, College of Science and Technology, Department of Biological and Allied Health Sciences, Program in Biology, Bloomsburg, PA 17815-1301. Offers MS. *Faculty:* 8 full-time (3 women). *Students:* 4 full-time (0 women), 6 part-time (3 women); includes 1 minority (Asian, non-Hispanic/Latino), 1 international. Average age 29. 15 applicants, 40% accepted, 4 enrolled. In 2013, 2 master's awarded. *Degree requirements:* For master's, thesis optional. *Entrance requirements:* For master's, minimum QPA of 3.0, 2 letters of recommendation, personal statement, undergraduate degree in biology. Additional exam requirements/recommendations for international students: Required—TOEFL (minimum score 550 paper-based). *Application deadline:* Applications are processed on a rolling basis. Application fee: $35 ($60 for international students). Electronic applications accepted. *Expenses:* Tuition, state resident: full-time $7956; part-time $442 per credit. Tuition, nonresident: full-time $11,934; part-time $663 per credit. *Required fees:* $95.50 per credit. $55 per semester. Tuition and fees vary according to course load. *Financial support:* Unspecified assistantships available. *Unit head:* Dr. Thomas Klinger, MS Program Coordinator, 570-389-4118, Fax: 570-389-3028, E-mail: tklinger@bloomu.edu. *Application contact:* Jennifer Richard, Administrative Assistant, 570-389-4015, Fax: 570-389-3054, E-mail: jrichard@bloomu.edu.
Website: http://www.bloomu.edu/gradschool/biology

Boise State University, College of Arts and Sciences, Department of Biology, Boise, ID 83725-0399. Offers biology (MA, MS); raptor biology (MS). Part-time programs available. *Degree requirements:* For master's, thesis. *Entrance requirements:* For master's, GRE General Test, minimum GPA of 3.0. Electronic applications accepted. *Faculty research:* Soil and stream microbial ecology, avian ecology.

Boston College, Graduate School of Arts and Sciences, Department of Biology, Chestnut Hill, MA 02467-3800. Offers PhD, MBA/MS. *Faculty:* 19 full-time. *Students:* 54 full-time (30 women); includes 7 minority (1 Black or African American, non-Hispanic/Latino; 4 Asian, non-Hispanic/Latino; 1 Hispanic/Latino; 1 Two or more races, non-Hispanic/Latino), 14 international. 72 applicants, 35% accepted, 10 enrolled. In 2013, 4 doctorates awarded. *Degree requirements:* For doctorate, thesis/dissertation. *Entrance requirements:* For doctorate, GRE General Test, GRE Subject Test. Additional exam requirements/recommendations for international students: Required—TOEFL (minimum score 600 paper-based; 100 iBT). *Application deadline:* For fall admission, 1/2 priority date for domestic students, 1/2 for international students. Application fee: $75. Electronic applications accepted. *Financial support:* In 2013–14, fellowships with full tuition reimbursements (averaging $30,000 per year), research assistantships with full tuition reimbursements (averaging $30,000 per year), teaching assistantships with full tuition reimbursements (averaging $30,000 per year) were awarded; Federal Work-Study, scholarships/grants, health care benefits, and unspecified assistantships also available. Support available to part-time students. Financial award application deadline: 3/1; financial award applicants required to submit FAFSA. *Faculty research:* Molecular cell biology and genetics, cell cycle, neurobiology, developmental biology, structural and cellular biochemistry, vector biology, infectious disease, bioinformatics. *Unit head:* Dr. Thomas Chiles, Chairperson, 617-552-3540, E-mail: thomas.chiles@bc.edu. *Application contact:* Dr. Charlie Hoffman, Graduate Program Director, 617-552-2779, E-mail: charles.hoffman@bc.edu.
Website: http://www.bc.edu/biology

See Display on next page and Close-Up on page 113.

Boston University, Graduate School of Arts and Sciences, Department of Biology, Boston, MA 02215. Offers MA, PhD. *Students:* 82 full-time (49 women), 2 part-time (1 woman); includes 8 minority (1 Black or African American, non-Hispanic/Latino; 3 Asian, non-Hispanic/Latino; 3 Hispanic/Latino; 1 Two or more races, non-Hispanic/Latino), 2 international. Average age 28. 225 applicants, 13% accepted, 16 enrolled. In 2013, 16 master's, 5 doctorates awarded. Terminal master's awarded for partial completion of doctoral program. *Degree requirements:* For master's, one foreign language, thesis (for some programs); for doctorate, one foreign language, comprehensive exam, thesis/dissertation. *Entrance requirements:* For master's and doctorate, GRE General Test, GRE Subject Test, 3 letters of recommendation. Additional exam requirements/recommendations for international students: Required—TOEFL (minimum score 600 paper-based). *Application deadline:* For fall admission, 12/7 for domestic and international students. Application fee: $80. Electronic applications accepted. *Expenses: Tuition:* Full-time $43,970; part-time $1374 per credit hour. *Required fees:* $60 per semester. Tuition and fees vary according to class time, course level and program. *Financial support:* In 2013–14, 77 students received support, including 6 fellowships with full tuition reimbursements available (averaging $20,000 per year), 20 research assistantships with full tuition reimbursements available (averaging $20,000 per year), 51 teaching assistantships with full tuition reimbursements available (averaging $20,000 per year); Federal Work-Study, institutionally sponsored loans, scholarships/grants, traineeships, and health care benefits also available. Financial award application deadline: 12/7. *Unit head:* Michael Sorenson, Chairman, 617-353-3856, Fax: 617-353-6340, E-mail: msoren@bu.edu. *Application contact:* Meredith Canode, Academic Administrator, 617-353-2432, Fax: 617-353-6340, E-mail: mcanode@bu.edu.
Website: http://www.bu.edu/biology/

Boston University, School of Medicine, Division of Graduate Medical Sciences, Program in Biomedical Sciences (PiBS), Boston, MA 02118. Offers PhD. *Entrance requirements:* For doctorate, GRE. *Expenses: Tuition:* Full-time $43,970; part-time $1374 per credit hour. *Required fees:* $60 per semester. Tuition and fees vary according to class time, course level and program. *Financial support:* In 2013–14, fellowships (averaging $30,500 per year), research assistantships (averaging $30,500 per year), teaching assistantships (averaging $30,500 per year) were awarded. *Unit head:* Dr.

Biological and Biomedical Sciences—General

Linda Hyman, Associate Provost, 617-638-5255, Fax: 617-638-5740. *Application contact:* GMS Office of Admissions, 617-638-5255, Fax: 617-638-5740.
Website: http://www.bumc.bu.edu/gms/gateway/prospective/program-in-biomedical-sciences-track/

Bowling Green State University, Graduate College, College of Arts and Sciences, Department of Biological Sciences, Bowling Green, OH 43403. Offers MAT, MS, PhD. Part-time programs available. *Degree requirements:* For master's, thesis or alternative; for doctorate, comprehensive exam, thesis/dissertation. *Entrance requirements:* For master's and doctorate, GRE General Test. Additional exam requirements/recommendations for international students: Required—TOEFL. Electronic applications accepted. *Faculty research:* Aquatic ecology, endocrinology and neurophysiology, nitrogen fixation, photosynthesis.

Bradley University, Graduate School, College of Liberal Arts and Sciences, Department of Biology, Peoria, IL 61625-0002. Offers MS. Part-time programs available. *Degree requirements:* For master's, comprehensive exam, thesis. *Entrance requirements:* For master's, GRE General Test, 2 letters of recommendation. Additional exam requirements/recommendations for international students: Required—TOEFL (minimum score 550 paper-based). *Expenses: Tuition:* Full-time $14,580; part-time $810 per credit hour. Tuition and fees vary according to course load and program.

Brandeis University, Graduate School of Arts and Sciences, Department of Physics, Waltham, MA 02454-9110. Offers physics (MS, PhD); quantitative biology (PhD). Part-time programs available. Terminal master's awarded for partial completion of doctoral program. *Degree requirements:* For master's, thesis optional, qualifying exam, 1-year residency; for doctorate, comprehensive exam, thesis/dissertation, qualifying and advanced exams. *Entrance requirements:* For master's and doctorate, GRE General Test; GRE Subject Test (recommended), resume, 2 letters of recommendation, statement of purpose, transcript(s). Additional exam requirements/recommendations for international students: Required—TOEFL (minimum score 600 paper-based; 100 iBT), PTE (minimum score 68); Recommended—IELTS (minimum score 7). Electronic applications accepted. *Faculty research:* Astrophysics, condensed-matter and biophysics, high energy and gravitational theory, particle physics, microfluidics, radio astronomy, string theory.

Brandeis University, Graduate School of Arts and Sciences, Post-Baccalaureate Premedical Program, Waltham, MA 02454-9110. Offers Postbaccalaureate Certificate. *Entrance requirements:* For degree, GRE, ACT, or SAT, resume with paid and/or volunteer work relevant to field of medicine, letters of recommendation, transcript(s), statement of purpose. Electronic applications accepted. *Faculty research:* Health profession preparation, pre-medical, pre-veterinary, pre-dental, pre-optometry, pre-osteopathic.

Brandeis University, Graduate School of Arts and Sciences, Program in Biochemistry and Biophysics, Waltham, MA 02454. Offers biochemistry and biophysics (PhD); quantitative biology (PhD). Terminal master's awarded for partial completion of doctoral program. *Degree requirements:* For doctorate, thesis/dissertation, qualifying exams. *Entrance requirements:* For doctorate, GRE General Test, resume, 3 letters of recommendation, statement of purpose, transcript(s). Additional exam requirements/recommendations for international students: Required—TOEFL (minimum score 600 paper-based; 100 iBT), PTE (minimum score 68); Recommended—IELTS (minimum score 7). Electronic applications accepted. *Faculty research:* Macromolecular chemistry, structure and function, biochemistry, biophysics, biological macromolecules.

Brandeis University, Graduate School of Arts and Sciences, Program in Molecular and Cell Biology, Waltham, MA 02454-9110. Offers genetics (PhD); microbiology (PhD); molecular and cell biology (MS, PhD); molecular biology (PhD); neurobiology (PhD); quantitative biology (PhD). Terminal master's awarded for partial completion of doctoral program. *Degree requirements:* For master's, thesis or alternative, research project, research lab, or project lab; for doctorate, comprehensive exam, thesis/dissertation, journal clubs; research seminar; colloquia; qualifying exam. *Entrance requirements:* For master's, GRE General Test (or MCAT for applicants to the MS program), official transcript(s), resume, 3 letters of recommendation, statement of purpose; for doctorate, GRE General Test, official transcript(s), resume, 3 letters of recommendation, statement of purpose. Additional exam requirements/recommendations for international students: Required—TOEFL (minimum score 600 paper-based; 100 iBT), PTE (minimum score 68); Recommended—IELTS (minimum score 7). Electronic applications accepted. *Faculty research:* Structural biology; immunology; developmental biology; behavior and neurobiology; DNA replication, rearrangement, and repair; signal transduction, transcriptional regulation, and RNA processing; cancer and programmed cell death; cytoskeleton and molecular motors; nutrition.

Brandeis University, Graduate School of Arts and Sciences, Program in Neuroscience, Waltham, MA 02454-9110. Offers neuroscience (MS, PhD); quantitative biology (PhD). Terminal master's awarded for partial completion of doctoral program. *Degree requirements:* For master's, thesis optional, research project; for doctorate, comprehensive exam, thesis/dissertation, qualifying exams, teaching experience, journal club, research seminars. *Entrance requirements:* For master's and doctorate, GRE General Test, official transcript(s), statement of purpose, resume, 3 letters of recommendation. Additional exam requirements/recommendations for international students: Required—TOEFL (minimum score 600 paper-based; 100 iBT), PTE (minimum score 68); Recommended—IELTS (minimum score 7). Electronic applications accepted. *Faculty research:* Behavioral neuroscience, cellular and molecular neuroscience, cognitive neuroscience, computational and integrative neuroscience, systems neuroscience.

Brigham Young University, Graduate Studies, College of Life Sciences, Department of Biology, Provo, UT 84602. Offers biological science education (MS); biology (MS, PhD). *Faculty:* 22 full-time (2 women). *Students:* 44 full-time (14 women); includes 7 minority (1 American Indian or Alaska Native, non-Hispanic/Latino; 3 Asian, non-Hispanic/Latino; 3 Hispanic/Latino). Average age 29. 26 applicants, 54% accepted, 14 enrolled. In 2013, 3 master's, 2 doctorates awarded. *Degree requirements:* For master's, comprehensive exam, thesis, prospectus, defense of research, defense of thesis; for doctorate, comprehensive exam, thesis/dissertation, prospectus, defense of research, defense of dissertation. *Entrance requirements:* For master's and doctorate, GRE General Test, GRE Subject Test (biology), minimum GPA of 3.0 for last 60 credit hours of course work. Additional exam requirements/recommendations for international students: Required—TOEFL (minimum score 580 paper-based; 85 iBT). *Application deadline:* For fall admission, 1/15 for domestic and international students. Application fee: $50. Electronic applications accepted. *Expenses: Tuition:* Full-time $6130; part-time $340 per credit hour. Tuition and fees vary according to program and student's religious affiliation. *Financial support:* In 2013–14, 39 students received support, including 5 fellowships with full and partial tuition reimbursements available (averaging $14,000 per year), 35 research assistantships with full and partial tuition reimbursements available (averaging $6,214 per year), 44 teaching assistantships with full and partial tuition reimbursements available (averaging $6,244 per year); career-related internships or fieldwork, institutionally sponsored loans, scholarships/grants, health care benefits, tuition waivers (full and partial), and unspecified assistantships also available. Financial award application deadline: 3/1; financial award applicants required to submit FAFSA. *Faculty research:* Systematics, bioinformatics, ecology, evolution. *Total annual research expenditures:* $1.3 million. *Unit head:* Dr. Dennis K. Shiozawa, Chair, 801-422-4972, Fax: 801-422-0090, E-mail: dennis_shiozawa@byu.edu. *Application contact:* Gentri

Glaittli, Graduate Secretary, 801-422-7137, Fax: 801-422-0090, E-mail: biogradsec@byu.edu.
Website: http://biology.byu.edu/

Brock University, Faculty of Graduate Studies, Faculty of Mathematics and Science, Program in Biological Sciences, St. Catharines, ON L2S 3A1, Canada. Offers M Sc, PhD. Part-time programs available. *Degree requirements:* For master's, thesis; for doctorate, thesis/dissertation. *Entrance requirements:* For master's, honors B Sc in biology, minimum undergraduate GPA of 3.0; for doctorate, M Sc. Additional exam requirements/recommendations for international students: Required—TOEFL (minimum score 550 paper-based; 80 iBT), IELTS (minimum score 6.5), TWE (minimum score 4). Electronic applications accepted. *Faculty research:* Viticulture, neurobiology, ecology, molecular biology, molecular genetics.

Brooklyn College of the City University of New York, School of Education, Program in Middle Childhood Science Education, Brooklyn, NY 11210-2889. Offers biology (MA); chemistry (MA); earth science (MA); general science (MA); physics (MA). Part-time and evening/weekend programs available. *Entrance requirements:* For master's, LAST, interview, previous course work in education and mathematics, resume, 2 letters of recommendation, essay. Additional exam requirements/recommendations for international students: Required—TOEFL (minimum score 500 paper-based; 61 iBT). *Application deadline:* For fall admission, 7/15 priority date for domestic students, 6/1 priority date for international students; for spring admission, 11/15 priority date for domestic students, 10/1 priority date for international students. Applications are processed on a rolling basis. Application fee: $125. Electronic applications accepted. *Expenses: Tuition, area resident:* Full-time $4585; part-time $385 per credit. Tuition, state resident: full-time $4585; part-time $385 per credit. Tuition, nonresident: part-time $710 per credit. *Required fees:* $430; $153 per semester. Tuition and fees vary according to course load. *Financial support:* Federal Work-Study, institutionally sponsored loans, and scholarships/grants available. Support available to part-time students. Financial award application deadline: 5/1; financial award applicants required to submit FAFSA. *Faculty research:* Geometric thinking, mastery of basic facts, problem-solving strategies, history of mathematics. *Unit head:* Dr. Jennifer Adams, Program Head, 718-951-3637, E-mail: jadams@brooklyn.cuny.edu. *Application contact:* Dr. Jennifer Adams, Program Head, 718-951-3637, E-mail: jadams@brooklyn.cuny.edu.

Brooklyn College of the City University of New York, School of Natural and Behavioral Sciences, Department of Biology, Brooklyn, NY 11210-2889. Offers MA. In 2013, 5 master's awarded. *Degree requirements:* For master's, one foreign language, comprehensive exam, thesis. *Entrance requirements:* For master's, minimum GPA of 3.0, 2 letters of recommendation. Additional exam requirements/recommendations for international students: Required—TOEFL (minimum score 500 paper-based; 61 iBT). *Application deadline:* For fall admission, 7/31 for domestic students, 6/30 for international students; for spring admission, 12/15 for domestic students, 11/15 for international students. Applications are processed on a rolling basis. Application fee: $125. Electronic applications accepted. *Expenses: Tuition, area resident:* Full-time $4585; part-time $385 per credit. Tuition, state resident: full-time $4585; part-time $385 per credit. Tuition, nonresident: part-time $710 per credit. *Required fees:* $430; $153 per semester. Tuition and fees vary according to course load. *Financial support:* Federal Work-Study, institutionally sponsored loans, and scholarships/grants available. Support available to part-time students. Financial award application deadline: 5/1; financial award applicants required to submit FAFSA. *Faculty research:* Evolutionary biology, molecular biology of development, cell biology, comparative endocrinology, ecology. *Unit head:* Dan Eshel, Chairperson, 718-951-5396. *Application contact:* Hernan Sierra, Graduate Admissions Coordinator, 718-951-4536, Fax: 718-951-4506, E-mail: grads@brooklyn.cuny.edu.

Brown University, Graduate School, Division of Biology and Medicine, Providence, RI 02912. Offers AM, M Sc, MA, MPH, Sc M, MD, PhD, MD/PhD. Part-time programs available. Terminal master's awarded for partial completion of doctoral program. *Degree requirements:* For doctorate, thesis/dissertation. *Entrance requirements:* For master's and doctorate, GRE General Test. Additional exam requirements/recommendations for international students: Required—TOEFL. Electronic applications accepted.

Bucknell University, Graduate Studies, College of Arts and Sciences, Department of Biology, Lewisburg, PA 17837. Offers MS. *Degree requirements:* For master's, thesis. *Entrance requirements:* For master's, GRE General Test, GRE Subject Test, minimum GPA of 3.0. Additional exam requirements/recommendations for international students: Required—TOEFL (minimum score 600 paper-based).

Buffalo State College, State University of New York, The Graduate School, Faculty of Natural and Social Sciences, Department of Biology, Buffalo, NY 14222-1095. Offers biology (MA); secondary education (MS Ed), including biology. Evening/weekend programs available. *Degree requirements:* For master's, thesis (for some programs), project. *Entrance requirements:* For master's, minimum GPA of 2.75. Additional exam requirements/recommendations for international students: Required—TOEFL (minimum score 550 paper-based).

California Institute of Technology, Division of Biology, Pasadena, CA 91125-0001. Offers biochemistry and molecular biophysics (PhD); cell biology and biophysics (PhD); developmental biology (PhD); genetics (PhD); immunology (PhD); molecular biology (PhD); neurobiology (PhD). *Degree requirements:* For doctorate, thesis/dissertation, qualifying exam. *Entrance requirements:* For doctorate, GRE General Test. Additional exam requirements/recommendations for international students: Required—TOEFL. Electronic applications accepted. *Faculty research:* Molecular genetics of differentiation and development, structure of biological macromolecules, molecular and integrative neurobiology.

California Polytechnic State University, San Luis Obispo, College of Science and Mathematics, Department of Biological Sciences, San Luis Obispo, CA 93407. Offers MA, MS. Part-time programs available. *Faculty:* 5 full-time (2 women). *Students:* 14 full-time (5 women), 21 part-time (12 women); includes 3 minority (2 Hispanic/Latino; 1 Two or more races, non-Hispanic/Latino). Average age 24. 66 applicants, 27% accepted, 15 enrolled. In 2013, 9 master's awarded. *Degree requirements:* For master's, comprehensive exam (for some programs), thesis (for some programs). *Entrance requirements:* For master's, GRE General Test, minimum GPA of 3.0 in last 90 quarter units. Additional exam requirements/recommendations for international students: Required—TOEFL (minimum score 550 paper-based) or IELTS (minimum score 6). *Application deadline:* For fall admission, 2/1 for domestic students, 11/30 for international students. Applications are processed on a rolling basis. Application fee: $55. Electronic applications accepted. *Financial support:* Fellowships, research assistantships, teaching assistantships, career-related internships or fieldwork, and Federal Work-Study available. Support available to part-time students. Financial award application deadline: 3/2; financial award applicants required to submit FAFSA. *Faculty research:* Ancient fossil DNA, restoration ecology microbe biodiversity indices, biological inventories. *Unit head:* Dr. Emily Taylor, Graduate Coordinator, 805-756-2616, Fax: 805-756-1419, E-mail: etaylor@calpoly.edu. *Application contact:* Dr. James Maraviglia, Associate Vice Provost for Marketing and Enrollment Development, 805-756-2311, Fax: 805-756-5400, E-mail: admissions@calpoly.edu.
Website: http://bio.calpoly.edu/

California State Polytechnic University, Pomona, Academic Affairs, College of Science, Program in Biological Sciences, Pomona, CA 91768-2557. Offers MS. Part-time programs available. *Students:* 32 full-time (19 women), 45 part-time (25 women); includes 36 minority (2 Black or African American, non-Hispanic/Latino; 1 American Indian or Alaska Native, non-Hispanic/Latino; 14 Asian, non-Hispanic/Latino; 18 Hispanic/Latino; 1 Two or more races, non-Hispanic/Latino), 8 international. Average age 27. 45 applicants, 47% accepted, 19 enrolled. In 2013, 24 master's awarded. *Degree requirements:* For master's, thesis. *Entrance requirements:* For master's, GRE General Test. *Application deadline:* For fall admission, 5/1 priority date for domestic students; for winter admission, 10/15 priority date for domestic students; for spring admission, 1/20 priority date for domestic students. Applications are processed on a rolling basis. Application fee: $55. Electronic applications accepted. *Expenses:* Tuition, state resident: full-time $6738. Tuition, nonresident: full-time $12,690. *Required fees:* $878; $248 per credit hour. *Financial support:* Career-related internships or fieldwork, Federal Work-Study, and institutionally sponsored loans available. Support available to part-time students. Financial award application deadline: 3/2; financial award applicants required to submit FAFSA. *Unit head:* Dr. Steve Alas, Graduate Coordinator, 909-869-4546, Fax: 909-869-4078, E-mail: alas@csupomona.edu. *Application contact:* Deborah L. Brandon, Executive Director, Admissions and Outreach, 909-869-3427, Fax: 909-869-5315, E-mail: dlbrandon@csupomona.edu.
Website: http://www.csupomona.edu/~biology/gradprog/

California State University, Bakersfield, Division of Graduate Studies, School of Natural Sciences, Mathematics, and Engineering, Program in Biology, Bakersfield, CA 93311. Offers MS. *Entrance requirements:* For master's, GRE, minimum undergraduate GPA of 3.0 in last 90 quarter units, 3 letters of recommendation. Additional exam requirements/recommendations for international students: Required—TOEFL. *Application deadline:* Applications are processed on a rolling basis. *Financial support:* Teaching assistantships available. *Unit head:* Dr. Anna L. Jacobsen, Graduate Coordinator, 661-654-2572, E-mail: ajacobsen@csub.edu. *Application contact:* Debbie Blowers, Assistant Director of Admissions, 661-664-3381, E-mail: dblowers@csub.edu.
Website: http://www.csub.edu/biology/index.html

California State University, Chico, Office of Graduate Studies, College of Natural Sciences, Department of Biological Sciences, Program in Biological Sciences, Chico, CA 95929-0722. Offers MS. *Degree requirements:* For master's, thesis, thesis and presentation. *Entrance requirements:* For master's, GRE General Test, GRE Subject Test (biology), 2 letters of recommendation, statement of purpose. Additional exam requirements/recommendations for international students: Required—TOEFL (minimum score 550 paper-based; 80 iBT), IELTS (minimum score 6.5), PTE. Electronic applications accepted.

California State University, Dominguez Hills, College of Natural and Behavioral Sciences, Department of Biology, Carson, CA 90747-0001. Offers MS. Part-time and evening/weekend programs available. *Faculty:* 2 full-time (1 woman). *Students:* 8 full-time (5 women), 17 part-time (9 women); includes 14 minority (2 Black or African American, non-Hispanic/Latino; 10 Hispanic/Latino; 2 Two or more races, non-Hispanic/Latino), 6 international. Average age 30. 7 applicants. In 2013, 12 master's awarded. *Degree requirements:* For master's, thesis. *Entrance requirements:* For master's, minimum GPA of 2.75. Additional exam requirements/recommendations for international students: Required—TOEFL (minimum score 550 paper-based). *Application deadline:* For fall admission, 6/1 for domestic students, 5/1 for international students; for spring admission, 12/15 for domestic students, 10/1 for international students. Application fee: $55. Electronic applications accepted. *Expenses:* Tuition, state resident: full-time $6738. Tuition, nonresident: full-time $13,434. *Required fees:* $622. *Faculty research:* Cancer biology, infectious diseases, ecology of native plants, remediation, community ecology. *Unit head:* Dr. John Thomlinson, Chair, 310-243-3381, Fax: 310-243-2350, E-mail: jthomlinson@csudh.edu. *Application contact:* Dr. Getachew Kidane, Graduate Program Coordinator, 310-243-3564, Fax: 310-243-2350, E-mail: gkidane@csudh.edu.
Website: http://www4.csudh.edu/biology/

California State University, East Bay, Office of Academic Programs and Graduate Studies, College of Science, Department of Biological Sciences, Hayward, CA 94542-3000. Offers biological sciences (MS); marine science (MS). Part-time programs available. *Degree requirements:* For master's, thesis. *Entrance requirements:* For master's, GRE General and Subject Tests, minimum GPA of 3.0 in field, 2.75 overall; 3 letters of reference; statement of purpose. Additional exam requirements/recommendations for international students: Required—TOEFL (minimum score 550 paper-based). Electronic applications accepted.

California State University, Fresno, Division of Graduate Studies, College of Science and Mathematics, Department of Biology, Fresno, CA 93740-8027. Offers biology (MA); biotechnology (MBT). Part-time and evening/weekend programs available. *Degree requirements:* For master's, thesis. *Entrance requirements:* For master's, GRE General Test, GRE Subject Test, minimum GPA of 2.5 in last 60 units. Additional exam requirements/recommendations for international students: Required—TOEFL. Electronic applications accepted. *Faculty research:* Genome neuroscience, ecology conflict resolution, biomechanics, cell death, vibrio cholerae.

California State University, Fullerton, Graduate Studies, College of Natural Science and Mathematics, Department of Biological Science, Fullerton, CA 92834-9480. Offers biology (MS); biotechnology (MBT). Part-time programs available. *Students:* 5 full-time (2 women), 50 part-time (31 women); includes 27 minority (2 Black or African American, non-Hispanic/Latino; 16 Asian, non-Hispanic/Latino; 8 Hispanic/Latino; 1 Two or more races, non-Hispanic/Latino), 3 international. Average age 28. 78 applicants, 27% accepted, 13 enrolled. In 2013, 22 master's awarded. *Degree requirements:* For master's, thesis. *Entrance requirements:* For master's, GRE General and Subject Tests, MCAT, or DAT, minimum GPA of 3.0 in biology. Application fee: $55. *Financial support:* Research assistantships, teaching assistantships, career-related internships or fieldwork, Federal Work-Study, institutionally sponsored loans, and scholarships/grants available. Support available to part-time students. Financial award application deadline: 3/1; financial award applicants required to submit FAFSA. *Faculty research:* Glycosidase release and the block to polyspermy in ascidian eggs. *Unit head:* Dr. Katherine Dickson, Acting Chair, 657-278-3614. *Application contact:* Admissions/Applications, 657-278-2371.

California State University, Long Beach, Graduate Studies, College of Natural Sciences and Mathematics, Department of Biological Sciences, Long Beach, CA 90840. Offers biology (MS); microbiology (MS). Part-time programs available. *Entrance requirements:* For master's, GRE Subject Test, minimum GPA of 3.0. Electronic applications accepted.

California State University, Los Angeles, Graduate Studies, College of Natural and Social Sciences, Department of Biological Sciences, Los Angeles, CA 90032-8530. Offers biology (MS). Part-time and evening/weekend programs available. *Faculty:* 4 full-time (2 women), 8 part-time/adjunct (4 women). *Students:* 34 full-time (23 women), 52 part-time (32 women); includes 60 minority (5 Black or African American, non-Hispanic/Latino; 16 Asian, non-Hispanic/Latino; 37 Hispanic/Latino; 2 Two or more races, non-Hispanic/Latino), 7 international. Average age 28. 102 applicants, 39% accepted, 30 enrolled. In 2013, 25 master's awarded. *Degree requirements:* For master's,

comprehensive exam or thesis. *Entrance requirements:* Additional exam requirements/recommendations for international students: Required—TOEFL (minimum score 500 paper-based). *Application deadline:* For fall admission, 5/1 for domestic and international students. Applications are processed on a rolling basis. Application fee: $55. *Financial support:* Federal Work-Study available. Support available to part-time students. Financial award application deadline: 3/1. *Faculty research:* Ecology, environmental biology, cell and molecular biology, physiology, medical microbiology. *Unit head:* Dr. Nancy McQueen, Chair, 323-343-2050, Fax: 323-343-6451, E-mail: nmcquee@exchange.calstatela.edu. *Application contact:* Dr. Larry Fritz, Dean of Graduate Studies, 323-343-3820, Fax: 323-343-5653, E-mail: lfritz@calstatela.edu.
Website: http://www.calstatela.edu/academic/biol/

California State University, Northridge, Graduate Studies, College of Science and Mathematics, Department of Biology, Northridge, CA 91330. Offers MS. *Degree requirements:* For master's, thesis, seminar. *Entrance requirements:* For master's, GRE Subject Test, GRE General Test. Additional exam requirements/recommendations for international students: Required—TOEFL. *Faculty research:* Cell adhesion, cancer research, fishery research.

California State University, Sacramento, Office of Graduate Studies, College of Natural Sciences and Mathematics, Department of Biological Sciences, Sacramento, CA 95819. Offers biological conservation (MS); marine science (MS); molecular and cellular biology (MS); stem cell (MA). Part-time programs available. *Degree requirements:* For master's, thesis, writing proficiency exam. *Entrance requirements:* For master's, GRE, bachelor's degree in biology or equivalent; minimum GPA of 3.0 in biology, 2.75 overall during last 2 years of course work. Additional exam requirements/recommendations for international students: Required—TOEFL. *Application deadline:* For fall admission, 2/1 for domestic students, 3/1 for international students; for spring admission, 9/30 for international students. Applications are processed on a rolling basis. Application fee: $55. Electronic applications accepted. *Financial support:* Research assistantships, teaching assistantships, career-related internships or fieldwork, and Federal Work-Study available. Support available to part-time students. Financial award application deadline: 3/1; financial award applicants required to submit FAFSA. *Unit head:* Jennifer Lundmark, Chair, 916-278-6535, E-mail: lundmark@csus.edu. *Application contact:* Jose Martinez, Graduate Admissions Supervisor, 916-278-7871, E-mail: martinj@skymail.csus.edu.
Website: http://www.csus.edu/bios

California State University, San Bernardino, Graduate Studies, College of Natural Sciences, Department of Biology, San Bernardino, CA 92407-2397. Offers MS. Part-time programs available. *Students:* 13 full-time (6 women), 16 part-time (12 women); includes 8 minority (3 Asian, non-Hispanic/Latino; 4 Hispanic/Latino; 1 Two or more races, non-Hispanic/Latino), 3 international. Average age 26. 28 applicants, 39% accepted, 8 enrolled. In 2013, 5 master's awarded. *Degree requirements:* For master's, thesis or alternative, advancement to candidacy. *Entrance requirements:* For master's, minimum GPA of 3.0. *Application deadline:* For fall admission, 8/31 priority date for domestic students. Application fee: $55. *Financial support:* Fellowships, research assistantships, teaching assistantships, and career-related internships or fieldwork available. *Faculty research:* Ecology, molecular biology, physiology, cell biology, neurobiology. *Unit head:* Dr. David M. Polcyn, Chair, 909-537-5313, Fax: 909-537-7038, E-mail: dpolcyn@csusb.edu. *Application contact:* Dr. Jeffrey Thompson, Dean of Graduate Studies, 909-537-5058, E-mail: jthompso@csusb.edu.

California State University, San Marcos, College of Science and Mathematics, Program in Biological Sciences, San Marcos, CA 92096-0001. Offers MS. Part-time programs available. *Degree requirements:* For master's, thesis. *Entrance requirements:* For master's, GRE Subject Test, minimum GPA of 2.7 in mathematics and science or 3.0 in last 35 units of mathematics and science. Tuition and fees vary according to program. *Faculty research:* Gene regulation of life states, carbon cycling, genetic markers of viral infection, neurobiology.

Carleton University, Faculty of Graduate Studies, Faculty of Science, Department of Biology, Ottawa, ON K1S 5B6, Canada. Offers M Sc, PhD. Programs offered jointly with University of Ottawa. *Degree requirements:* For master's, thesis, seminar; for doctorate, comprehensive exam, thesis/dissertation, seminar. *Entrance requirements:* For master's, honors degree in science; for doctorate, M Sc. Additional exam requirements/recommendations for international students: Required—TOEFL. *Faculty research:* Biochemical, structural, and genetic regulation in cells; behavioral ecology; insect taxonomy; physiology of cells.

Carnegie Mellon University, Mellon College of Science, Department of Biological Sciences, Pittsburgh, PA 15213-3891. Offers biochemistry (PhD); biophysics (PhD); cell and developmental biology (PhD); computational biology (MS, PhD); genetics (PhD); molecular biology (PhD); neuroscience (PhD); structural biology (PhD). *Degree requirements:* For doctorate, comprehensive exam, thesis/dissertation. *Entrance requirements:* For doctorate, GRE General Test, GRE Subject Test, interview. *Application deadline:* Applications are processed on a rolling basis. Application fee: $0. Electronic applications accepted. *Financial support:* Fellowships, research assistantships, teaching assistantships, and traineeships available. *Faculty research:* Genetic structure, function, and regulation; protein structure and function; biological membranes; biological spectroscopy. *Unit head:* John L. Woolford, Acting Department Head, 412-268-3193, E-mail: jw17@andrew.cmu.edu. *Application contact:* Ena Miceli, Graduate Programs Manager, 412-268-33012, E-mail: emiceli@andrew.cmu.edu.
Website: http://www.bio.cmu.edu/

Case Western Reserve University, School of Graduate Studies, Department of Biology, Cleveland, OH 44106. Offers MS, PhD. Part-time programs available. *Faculty:* 23 full-time (11 women), 5 part-time/adjunct (3 women). *Students:* 65 full-time (29 women), 11 part-time (8 women); includes 8 minority (4 Black or African American, non-Hispanic/Latino; 2 Asian, non-Hispanic/Latino; 2 Hispanic/Latino), 27 international. Average age 27. 98 applicants, 35% accepted, 23 enrolled. In 2013, 20 master's, 2 doctorates awarded. Terminal master's awarded for partial completion of doctoral program. *Degree requirements:* For master's, thesis or alternative; for doctorate, thesis/dissertation. *Entrance requirements:* For master's and doctorate, GRE General Test, GRE Subject Test, statement of objectives; three letters of recommendation. Additional exam requirements/recommendations for international students: Required—TOEFL (minimum score 577 paper-based; 90 iBT); Recommended—IELTS (minimum score 7). *Application deadline:* For fall admission, 1/7 priority date for domestic students. Applications are processed on a rolling basis. Application fee: $50. Electronic applications accepted. *Financial support:* Fellowships, research assistantships, teaching assistantships, career-related internships or fieldwork, Federal Work-Study, scholarships/grants, tuition waivers, unspecified assistantships, and stipends available. Financial award application deadline: 1/7; financial award applicants required to submit FAFSA. *Faculty research:* Cellular, developmental, and molecular biology; genetics; genetic engineering; biotechnology; ecology. *Unit head:* Christopher Cullis, Chairman, 216-368-3557, Fax: 216-368-4762, E-mail: christopher.cullis@case.edu. *Application contact:* Julia Brown, Program Coordinator, 216-368-3556, Fax: 216-368-4672, E-mail: jab12@case.edu.
Website: http://www.case.edu/artsci/biol/

Case Western Reserve University, School of Medicine and School of Graduate Studies, Graduate Programs in Medicine, Biomedical Sciences Training Program, Cleveland, OH 44106. Offers PhD. *Degree requirements:* For doctorate, thesis/dissertation. *Entrance requirements:* For doctorate, GRE General Test. Additional exam requirements/recommendations for international students: Required—TOEFL. Electronic applications accepted. *Faculty research:* Biochemistry, molecular biology, immunology, genetics, neurosciences.

Case Western Reserve University, School of Medicine and School of Graduate Studies, Graduate Programs in Medicine, Department of Biochemistry, Program in RNA Biology, Cleveland, OH 44106. Offers PhD. *Degree requirements:* For doctorate, comprehensive exam, thesis/dissertation. *Entrance requirements:* For doctorate, GRE. Additional exam requirements/recommendations for international students: Required—TOEFL (minimum score 550 paper-based).

Case Western Reserve University, School of Medicine, Medical Scientist Training Program, Cleveland, OH 44106. Offers MD/PhD. Electronic applications accepted. *Faculty research:* Biomedical research.

The Catholic University of America, School of Arts and Sciences, Department of Biology, Washington, DC 20064. Offers cell and microbial biology (MS, PhD), including cell biology, microbiology; clinical laboratory science (MS, PhD); MSLS/MS. Part-time programs available. *Faculty:* 9 full-time (4 women), 5 part-time/adjunct (4 women). *Students:* 27 full-time (19 women), 36 part-time (22 women); includes 12 minority (7 Black or African American, non-Hispanic/Latino; 2 Asian, non-Hispanic/Latino; 2 Hispanic/Latino; 1 Two or more races, non-Hispanic/Latino), 36 international. Average age 30. 66 applicants, 56% accepted, 19 enrolled. In 2013, 10 master's, 3 doctorates awarded. *Degree requirements:* For master's, comprehensive exam, thesis or alternative; for doctorate, comprehensive exam, thesis/dissertation. *Entrance requirements:* For master's and doctorate, GRE General Test, GRE Subject Test, statement of purpose, official copies of academic transcripts, three letters of recommendation. Additional exam requirements/recommendations for international students: Required—TOEFL (minimum score 580 paper-based). *Application deadline:* For fall admission, 8/1 priority date for domestic students, 7/15 for international students; for spring admission, 12/1 priority date for domestic students, 10/15 for international students. Applications are processed on a rolling basis. Application fee: $55. Electronic applications accepted. *Expenses: Tuition:* Full-time $38,500; part-time $1490 per credit hour. *Required fees:* $400; $1525 per credit hour. One-time fee: $425. Tuition and fees vary according to program. *Financial support:* Fellowships, research assistantships, teaching assistantships, Federal Work-Study, scholarships/grants, tuition waivers (full and partial), and unspecified assistantships available. Financial award application deadline: 2/1; financial award applicants required to submit FAFSA. *Faculty research:* Cell and microbiology, molecular biology of cell proliferation, cellular effects of electromagnetic radiation, biotechnology. *Total annual research expenditures:* $1.5 million. *Unit head:* Dr. Venigalla Rao, Chair, 202-319-5271, Fax: 202-319-5721, E-mail: rao@cua.edu. *Application contact:* Andrew Woodall, Director of Graduate Admissions, 202-319-5057, Fax: 202-319-6533, E-mail: cua-admissions@cua.edu.
Website: http://biology.cua.edu/

Cedars-Sinai Medical Center, Graduate Program in Biomedical Sciences and Translational Medicine, Los Angeles, CA 90048. Offers PhD. *Degree requirements:* For doctorate, comprehensive exam, thesis/dissertation. *Entrance requirements:* For doctorate, GRE, 3 letters of recommendation. Additional exam requirements/recommendations for international students: Required—TOEFL (minimum score 550 paper-based; 80 iBT), IELTS (minimum score 6.5). Electronic applications accepted. *Faculty research:* Immunology and infection, neuroscience, cardiovascular science, cancer, human genetics.

Central Connecticut State University, School of Graduate Studies, School of Arts and Sciences, Department of Biology, New Britain, CT 06050-4010. Offers biological sciences (MA, MS), including anesthesia (MS), ecology and environmental sciences (MA), general biology (MA), health sciences (MS), professional education (MS); biology (Certificate). Part-time and evening/weekend programs available. *Faculty:* 4 full-time (0 women), 2 part-time/adjunct (both women). *Students:* 130 full-time (85 women), 34 part-time (23 women); includes 25 minority (9 Black or African American, non-Hispanic/Latino; 11 Asian, non-Hispanic/Latino; 3 Hispanic/Latino; 2 Two or more races, non-Hispanic/Latino), 1 international. Average age 30. 30 applicants, 67% accepted, 11 enrolled. In 2013, 46 master's, 10 other advanced degrees awarded. *Degree requirements:* For master's, comprehensive exam, thesis or alternative; for Certificate, qualifying exam. *Entrance requirements:* For master's and Certificate, minimum undergraduate GPA of 2.7, essay, letters of recommendation. Additional exam requirements/recommendations for international students: Required—TOEFL (minimum score 550 paper-based; 79 iBT). *Application deadline:* For fall admission, 6/1 for domestic students, 5/1 for international students; for spring admission, 11/1 for domestic and international students. Applications are processed on a rolling basis. Application fee: $50. Electronic applications accepted. Part-time tuition and fees vary according to degree level. *Financial support:* In 2013–14, 2 students received support, including 2 research assistantships; career-related internships or fieldwork, Federal Work-Study, scholarships/grants, and unspecified assistantships also available. Support available to part-time students. Financial award application deadline: 3/1; financial award applicants required to submit FAFSA. *Faculty research:* Environmental science, anesthesia, health sciences, zoology, animal behavior. *Unit head:* Dr. Douglas Carter, Chair, 860-832-2645, E-mail: carterd@ccsu.edu. *Application contact:* Patricia Gardner, Associate Director of Graduate Studies, 860-832-2350, Fax: 860-832-2362, E-mail: graduateadmissions@ccsu.edu.
Website: http://www.ccsu.edu/page.cfm?p=14516

Central Michigan University, College of Graduate Studies, College of Science and Technology, Department of Biology, Mount Pleasant, MI 48859. Offers biology (MS); conservation biology (MS). Part-time programs available. *Degree requirements:* For master's, thesis or alternative. *Entrance requirements:* For master's, GRE, bachelor's degree with a major in biological science, minimum GPA of 3.0. Electronic applications accepted. *Faculty research:* Conservation biology, morphology and taxonomy of aquatic plants, molecular biology and genetics, microbials and invertebrate ecology, vertebrates.

Central Washington University, Graduate Studies and Research, College of the Sciences, Department of Biological Sciences, Ellensburg, WA 98926. Offers MS. Part-time programs available. *Degree requirements:* For master's, thesis. *Entrance requirements:* For master's, GRE General Test, minimum GPA of 3.0. Additional exam requirements/recommendations for international students: Required—TOEFL (minimum score 550 paper-based; 79 iBT). Electronic applications accepted.

Chatham University, Program in Biology, Pittsburgh, PA 15232-2826. Offers environmental biology (MS); human biology (MS). Part-time programs available. *Faculty:* 1 (woman) part-time/adjunct. *Students:* 45 full-time (33 women), 5 part-time (all women); includes 14 minority (6 Black or African American, non-Hispanic/Latino; 3 Asian, non-Hispanic/Latino; 4 Hispanic/Latino; 1 Two or more races, non-Hispanic/Latino), 6 international. Average age 25. 83 applicants, 66% accepted, 35 enrolled. In 2013, 20 master's awarded. *Degree requirements:* For master's, thesis optional. *Entrance requirements:* For master's, 3 letters of recommendation. Additional exam requirements/

recommendations for international students: Required—TOEFL (minimum score 600 paper-based; 100 iBT), IELTS (minimum score 7), TWE. *Application deadline:* For fall admission, 4/1 priority date for domestic and international students; for spring admission, 11/1 priority date for domestic students, 10/1 priority date for international students. Applications are processed on a rolling basis. Application fee: $45. Electronic applications accepted. Application fee is waived when completed online. *Expenses: Tuition:* Full-time $14,886; part-time $827 per credit hour. One-time fee: $396 full-time. *Financial support:* Applicants required to submit FAFSA. *Faculty research:* Molecular evolution of iron homeostasis, characteristics of soil bacterial communities, gene flow through seed movement, role of gonadotropins in spermatogonial proliferation, phosphatid/linositol metabolism in epithelial cells. *Unit head:* Dr. Lisa Lambert, Director, 412-365-1217, E-mail: lambert@chatham.edu. *Application contact:* Ashlee Bartko, Senior Assistant Director of Graduate Admission, 412-365-1115, Fax: 412-365-1609, E-mail: gradadmissions@chatham.edu.
Website: http://www.chatham.edu/departments/sciences/graduate/biology

Chicago State University, School of Graduate and Professional Studies, College of Arts and Sciences, Department of Biological Sciences, Chicago, IL 60628. Offers MS. Part-time and evening/weekend programs available. *Degree requirements:* For master's, thesis. *Entrance requirements:* For master's, minimum GPA of 3.0, 15 credit hours in biological sciences. *Faculty research:* Molecular genetics of gene complexes, mammalian immune cell function, genetics of agriculturally important microbes, environmental toxicology, neuromuscular physiology.

The Citadel, The Military College of South Carolina, Citadel Graduate College, Department of Biology, Charleston, SC 29409. Offers MA. *Accreditation:* NCATE. Part-time and evening/weekend programs available. *Faculty:* 4 full-time (1 woman). *Students:* 8 full-time (3 women), 11 part-time (6 women); includes 2 minority (both Black or African American, non-Hispanic/Latino). Average age 28. In 2013, 12 master's awarded. *Entrance requirements:* For master's, GRE (minimum score 900) or MAT (raw score 40), minimum undergraduate GPA of 2.5. Additional exam requirements/recommendations for international students: Required—TOEFL (minimum score 550 paper-based). *Application deadline:* Applications are processed on a rolling basis. Application fee: $30. Electronic applications accepted. *Expenses: Tuition, area resident:* Part-time $525 per credit hour. Tuition, state resident: part-time $525 per credit hour. Tuition, nonresident: part-time $865 per credit hour. *Financial support:* Health care benefits and unspecified assistantships available. Support available to part-time students. Financial award application deadline: 7/1; financial award applicants required to submit FAFSA. *Faculty research:* Genetic control of parasite-host interactions, mechanisms of development of antibiotic resistance in pseudomonas aeruginosa, interaction of visual and vocal signals in avian mate choice and competition, effects of pollutants on salt marsh animals, structure and function of mitochondrial histone H3 protein, development of cardiac conduction tissue in tadpoles with left-right axis perturbation, evolution and ecology of barnacles and marine hosts. *Unit head:* Dr. John E. Weinstein, Department Head, 843-953-5203, Fax: 843-953-7264, E-mail: john.weinstein@citadel.edu. *Application contact:* Dr. Robert H. McNamara, Associate Provost, The Citadel Graduate College, 843-953-5089, Fax: 843-953-7630, E-mail: cgc@citadel.edu.
Website: http://www.citadel.edu/root/biology

City College of the City University of New York, Graduate School, College of Liberal Arts and Science, Division of Science, Department of Biology, New York, NY 10031-9198. Offers MA, PhD. PhD program offered jointly with Graduate School and University Center of the City University of New York. Part-time programs available. Terminal master's awarded for partial completion of doctoral program. *Degree requirements:* For master's, thesis or alternative; for doctorate, one foreign language, thesis/dissertation, teaching experience. *Entrance requirements:* For doctorate, GRE General Test. Additional exam requirements/recommendations for international students: Required—TOEFL (minimum score 500 paper-based; 61 iBT). Electronic applications accepted. *Faculty research:* Animal behavior, ecology, genetics, neurobiology, molecular biology.

Clark Atlanta University, School of Arts and Sciences, Department of Biology, Atlanta, GA 30314. Offers MS, PhD. Part-time programs available. *Faculty:* 8 full-time (4 women). *Students:* 20 full-time (15 women), 13 part-time (11 women); includes 24 minority (23 Black or African American, non-Hispanic/Latino; 1 Asian, non-Hispanic/Latino), 9 international. Average age 28. 18 applicants, 44% accepted, 8 enrolled. In 2013, 4 doctorates awarded. Terminal master's awarded for partial completion of doctoral program. *Degree requirements:* For master's, one foreign language, thesis; for doctorate, 2 foreign languages, thesis/dissertation. *Entrance requirements:* For master's, GRE General Test, minimum GPA of 2.5; for doctorate, GRE General Test, minimum graduate GPA of 3.0. Additional exam requirements/recommendations for international students: Required—TOEFL (minimum score 500 paper-based; 61 iBT). *Application deadline:* For fall admission, 4/1 for domestic and international students; for spring admission, 11/1 for domestic and international students. Applications are processed on a rolling basis. Application fee: $40 ($55 for international students). Electronic applications accepted. *Expenses: Tuition:* Full-time $14,616; part-time $812 per credit hour. *Required fees:* $706; $353 per semester. *Financial support:* In 2013–14, 6 research assistantships were awarded; career-related internships or fieldwork, Federal Work-Study, scholarships/grants, traineeships, and unspecified assistantships also available. Support available to part-time students. Financial award application deadline: 4/30; financial award applicants required to submit FAFSA. *Faculty research:* Regulation of amino-DNA, cellular regulations. *Unit head:* Dr. Marjorie Campbell, Chairperson, 404-880-6190, E-mail: mcampbell@cau.edu. *Application contact:* Michelle Clark-Davis, Graduate Program Admissions, 404-880-6605, E-mail: cauadmissions@cau.edu.

Clark University, Graduate School, Department of Biology, Worcester, MA 01610-1477. Offers MS, PhD. *Faculty:* 14 full-time (4 women). *Students:* 26 full-time (15 women), 4 part-time (1 woman); includes 2 minority (1 Asian, non-Hispanic/Latino; 1 Hispanic/Latino), 7 international. Average age 28. 23 applicants, 35% accepted, 8 enrolled. In 2013, 7 master's awarded. *Degree requirements:* For master's, thesis; for doctorate, thesis/dissertation. *Entrance requirements:* For master's and doctorate, GRE General Test. Additional exam requirements/recommendations for international students: Required—TOEFL. *Application deadline:* For fall admission, 2/15 priority date for domestic students. Applications are processed on a rolling basis. Application fee: $50. Electronic applications accepted. *Expenses: Tuition:* Full-time $39,200; part-time $1225 per credit hour. *Financial support:* In 2013–14, 6 research assistantships with full tuition reimbursements (averaging $19,825 per year), 13 teaching assistantships with full tuition reimbursements (averaging $19,825 per year) were awarded; fellowships, scholarships/grants, and tuition waivers (full and partial) also available. *Faculty research:* Nitrogen assimilation in marine algae, polyporale taxonomies, fungal evolutionary history, drug discovery, taste sensitivities, biodiversity inventories. *Total annual research expenditures:* $900,000. *Unit head:* Dr. Susan Foster, Chair, 508-793-7204. *Application contact:* Paula Kupstas, Department Secretary, 508-793-7173, Fax: 528-793-7174, E-mail: pkupstas@clarku.edu.
Website: http://www.clarku.edu/departments/biology/phd/index.cfm

Clemson University, Graduate School, College of Agriculture, Forestry and Life Sciences, Department of Biological Sciences, Online Master of Biological Sciences Program, Clemson, SC 29634. Offers MBS. Postbaccalaureate distance learning degree programs offered (no on-campus study). *Students:* 63 part-time (42 women); includes 11 minority (7 Black or African American, non-Hispanic/Latino; 1 Asian, non-Hispanic/Latino; 2 Hispanic/Latino; 1 Two or more races, non-Hispanic/Latino). Average age 36. 41 applicants, 98% accepted, 30 enrolled. In 2013, 17 degrees awarded. *Entrance requirements:* For master's, GRE, two letters of recommendation, resume. Additional exam requirements/recommendations for international students: Required—TOEFL (minimum score 550 paper-based; 80 iBT). Application fee: $70 ($80 for international students). *Unit head:* Dr. Alfred Wheeler, Chair, 864-656-1415, Fax: 864-656-0435, E-mail: wheeler@clemson.edu. *Application contact:* Jay Lyn Martin, Coordinator for Graduate Program, 864-656-3587, Fax: 864-656-0435, E-mail: gradbio@clemson.edu.
Website: http://www.clemson.edu/cafls/departments/biosci/graduates/biol_online/index.html

Clemson University, Graduate School, College of Agriculture, Forestry and Life Sciences, Department of Biological Sciences, Program in Biological Sciences, Clemson, SC 29634. Offers MS, PhD. *Students:* 31 full-time (19 women), 147 part-time (101 women); includes 15 minority (4 Black or African American, non-Hispanic/Latino; 1 Asian, non-Hispanic/Latino; 5 Hispanic/Latino; 5 Two or more races, non-Hispanic/Latino), 9 international. Average age 33. 137 applicants, 70% accepted, 84 enrolled. In 2013, 6 master's, 3 doctorates awarded. *Degree requirements:* For master's, thesis optional; for doctorate, comprehensive exam, thesis/dissertation. *Entrance requirements:* For master's and doctorate, GRE General Test. Additional exam requirements/recommendations for international students: Required—TOEFL, IELTS. *Application deadline:* For fall admission, 1/15 for domestic students, 4/15 for international students. Applications are processed on a rolling basis. Application fee: $70 ($80 for international students). Electronic applications accepted. *Financial support:* In 2013–14, 27 students received support, including 3 fellowships with full and partial tuition reimbursements available (averaging $16,167 per year), 3 research assistantships with partial tuition reimbursements available (averaging $18,167 per year), 23 teaching assistantships with partial tuition reimbursements available (averaging $18,452 per year); career-related internships or fieldwork, institutionally sponsored loans, scholarships/grants, health care benefits, and unspecified assistantships also available. Support available to part-time students. Financial award application deadline: 3/15; financial award applicants required to submit FAFSA. *Unit head:* Dr. Alfred Wheeler, Department Chair, 864-656-1415, Fax: 864-656-0435, E-mail: wheeler@clemson.edu. *Application contact:* Jay Lyn Martin, Coordinator for Graduate Program, 864-656-3587, Fax: 864-656-0435, E-mail: gradbio@clemson.edu.
Website: http://www.clemson.edu/cafls/departments/biosci/

Cleveland State University, College of Graduate Studies, College of Sciences and Health Professions, Department of Biological, Geological, and Environmental Sciences, Cleveland, OH 44115. Offers biology (MS); environmental science (MS); regulatory biology (PhD); JD/MS. Part-time programs available. *Faculty:* 17 full-time (4 women), 40 part-time/adjunct (14 women). *Students:* 4 full-time (1 woman), 87 part-time (48 women); includes 9 minority (2 Black or African American, non-Hispanic/Latino; 5 Asian, non-Hispanic/Latino; 1 Hispanic/Latino; 1 Two or more races, non-Hispanic/Latino), 42 international. Average age 30. 76 applicants, 37% accepted, 11 enrolled. In 2013, 12 master's, 4 doctorates awarded. Terminal master's awarded for partial completion of doctoral program. *Degree requirements:* For master's, comprehensive exam (for some programs), thesis, thesis defense; for doctorate, comprehensive exam, thesis/dissertation, dissertation defense. *Entrance requirements:* For master's, GRE General Test, 3 letters of recommendation; for doctorate, GRE General Test, 3 letters of recommendation; 1-2 page essay; statement of career goals and research interests. Additional exam requirements/recommendations for international students: Required—TOEFL (minimum score 525 paper-based), IELTS (minimum score 6.5). *Application deadline:* For fall admission, 4/1 priority date for domestic and international students; for spring admission, 12/1 priority date for domestic students. Applications are processed on a rolling basis. Application fee: $30. Electronic applications accepted. *Expenses:* Tuition, state resident: full-time $8335; part-time $521 per credit hour. Tuition, nonresident: full-time $15,670; part-time $979 per credit hour. *Required fees:* $50; $25 per semester. *Financial support:* In 2013–14, 33 students received support, including 30 research assistantships with full and partial tuition reimbursements available (averaging $21,000 per year), 33 teaching assistantships with full and partial tuition reimbursements available (averaging $21,000 per year); institutionally sponsored loans and unspecified assistantships also available. *Faculty research:* Molecular and cell biology, immunology, urban ecology, cancer biology, reproductive health, and environmental science. *Unit head:* Dr. Crystal Weyman, Chair, 216-687-2120, Fax: 216-687-6972, E-mail: c.weyman@csuohio.edu. *Application contact:* Dr. Girish Shukla, Associate Professor and Graduate Program Director, 216-687-2395, Fax: 216-687-6972, E-mail: g.shukla@csuohio.edu.
Website: http://www.csuohio.edu/sciences/dept/biology/index.html

Cold Spring Harbor Laboratory, Watson School of Biological Sciences, Graduate Program, Cold Spring Harbor, NY 11724. Offers PhD. *Faculty:* 56 full-time (10 women). *Students:* 51 full-time (23 women); includes 4 minority (1 Black or African American, non-Hispanic/Latino; 1 Asian, non-Hispanic/Latino; 2 Hispanic/Latino), 31 international. Average age 27. 274 applicants, 11% accepted, 12 enrolled. In 2013, 10 doctorates awarded. *Median time to degree:* Of those who began their doctoral program in fall 2005, 100% received their degree in 8 years or less. *Degree requirements:* For doctorate, comprehensive exam, thesis/dissertation, lab rotations, teaching experience, qualifying exam, postdoctoral proposals. *Entrance requirements:* For doctorate, GRE (recommended). Additional exam requirements/recommendations for international students: Required—TOEFL or IELTS. *Application deadline:* For fall admission, 12/1 for domestic and international students. Application fee: $60. Electronic applications accepted. *Financial support:* In 2013–14, 51 students received support, including 54 fellowships with full tuition reimbursements available (averaging $31,500 per year); health care benefits and tuition waivers (full) also available. Financial award application deadline: 12/1. *Faculty research:* Genetics and genomics, neurobiology, cancer, plant biology, molecular biology, quantitative biology, bioinformatics. *Application contact:* E-mail: gradschool@cshl.edu.
Website: http://www.cshl.edu/gradschool/

See Display on next page and Close-Up on page 117.

The College at Brockport, State University of New York, School of Science and Mathematics, Department of Biology, Brockport, NY 14420-2997. Offers MS, PSM. Part-time programs available. *Faculty:* 6 full-time (1 woman). *Students:* 6 full-time (2 women), 5 part-time (3 women); includes 2 minority (1 Black or African American, non-Hispanic/Latino; 1 Hispanic/Latino). 11 applicants, 64% accepted, 5 enrolled. In 2013, 9 master's awarded. *Degree requirements:* For master's, comprehensive exam, thesis or alternative. *Entrance requirements:* For master's, GRE General or Subject Test (biology, biochemistry, cell and molecular biology), letters of recommendation, minimum GPA of 3.0, scientific writing sample, statement of objectives. Additional exam requirements/recommendations for international students: Required—TOEFL (minimum score 550 paper-based; 79 iBT), IELTS (minimum score 6.5). *Application deadline:* For fall admission, 7/15 priority date for domestic and international students; for spring admission, 11/15 priority date for domestic and international students; for summer admission, 7/15 priority date for domestic students, 6/15 priority date for international

students. Application fee: $50. Electronic applications accepted. *Expenses:* Tuition, state resident: full-time $9870. Tuition, nonresident: full-time $18,350. *Required fees:* $1848. *Financial support:* In 2013–14, 7 teaching assistantships with full tuition reimbursements (averaging $6,000 per year) were awarded; Federal Work-Study, scholarships/grants, and unspecified assistantships also available. Support available to part-time students. Financial award application deadline: 3/15; financial award applicants required to submit FAFSA. *Faculty research:* Microbiology, molecular genetics, cellular biology developmental biology, animal physiology. *Unit head:* Dr. Rey Sia, Chairperson, 585-395-2783, Fax: 585-395-2741, E-mail: rsia@brockport.edu. *Application contact:* Dr. Adam Rich, Graduate Program Director, 585-395-5740, Fax: 585-395-2741, E-mail: arich@brockport.edu.
Website: http://www.brockport.edu/biology/graduate/

College of Staten Island of the City University of New York, Graduate Programs, Program in Biology, Staten Island, NY 10314-6600. Offers MS. Part-time programs available. *Faculty:* 6 full-time (1 woman), 2 part-time/adjunct (1 woman). *Students:* 10. Average age 32. 12 applicants, 42% accepted, 5 enrolled. In 2013, 2 master's awarded. *Entrance requirements:* For master's, GRE General Test, GRE Subject Test (biology), bachelor's degrees with minimum GPA of 3.0 in science and math courses, 2.75 overall; 2 letters of recommendation. Additional exam requirements/recommendations for international students: Required—TOEFL (minimum score 550 paper-based; 79 iBT), IELTS (minimum score 6.5). *Application deadline:* For fall admission, 4/15 for domestic and international students; for spring admission, 11/25 for domestic and international students. Applications are processed on a rolling basis. Application fee: $125. Electronic applications accepted. *Expenses:* Tuition, state resident: full-time $9240; part-time $385 per credit hour. Tuition, nonresident: full-time $17,040; part-time $710 per credit hour. *Required fees:* $428; $128 per term. *Financial support:* Federal Work-Study and scholarships/grants available. Support available to part-time students. Financial award applicants required to submit FAFSA. *Faculty research:* Field surveys for offshore wind. *Total annual research expenditures:* $368,463. *Unit head:* Dr. Lisa Manne, Graduate Program Coordinator, 718-982-3855, Fax: 718-982-3852, E-mail: lisa.manne@csi.cuny.edu. *Application contact:* Sasha Spence, Assistant Director for Graduate Admissions, 718-982-2019, Fax: 718-982-2500, E-mail: sasha.spence@csi.cuny.edu.
Website: http://www.csi.cuny.edu/departments/biology/graduate.html

The College of William and Mary, Faculty of Arts and Sciences, Department of Biology, Williamsburg, VA 23187-8795. Offers MS. Part-time programs available. *Faculty:* 26 full-time (9 women), 3 part-time/adjunct (2 women). *Students:* 19 full-time (14 women); includes 4 minority (1 American Indian or Alaska Native, non-Hispanic/Latino; 1 Asian, non-Hispanic/Latino; 2 Two or more races, non-Hispanic/Latino), 1 international. Average age 24. 30 applicants, 47% accepted, 8 enrolled. In 2013, 11 master's awarded. *Degree requirements:* For master's, comprehensive exam, thesis (for some programs). *Entrance requirements:* For master's, GRE Subject Test, GRE General Test, minimum GPA of 3.0. Additional exam requirements/recommendations for international students: Required—TOEFL. *Application deadline:* For fall admission, 2/1 priority date for domestic and international students. Application fee: $45. Electronic applications accepted. *Expenses:* Tuition, state resident: full-time $7120; part-time $405 per credit hour. Tuition, nonresident: full-time $21,639; part-time $1050 per credit hour. *Required fees:* $4764. *Financial support:* In 2013–14, 7 teaching assistantships with full tuition reimbursements (averaging $13,500 per year) were awarded; Federal Work-Study, institutionally sponsored loans, and unspecified assistantships also available. Financial award application deadline: 2/1; financial award applicants required to submit FAFSA. *Faculty research:* Cellular and molecular biology, genetics, ecology, organismal biology, physiology. *Total annual research expenditures:* $2.2 million. *Unit head:* Dr. Lizabeth A. Allison, Chair, 757-221-2207, Fax: 757-221-6483, E-mail: laalli@wm.edu. *Application contact:* Dr. Matthew Wawersik, Graduate Director, 757-221-2237, Fax: 757-221-6483, E-mail: mjwawe@wm.edu.
Website: http://www.wm.edu/biology/

Colorado State University, College of Veterinary Medicine and Biomedical Sciences, Department of Biomedical Sciences, Fort Collins, CO 80523-1680. Offers MS, PhD. *Faculty:* 24 full-time (6 women), 3 part-time/adjunct (1 woman). *Students:* 67 full-time (37 women), 27 part-time (10 women); includes 15 minority (1 American Indian or Alaska Native, non-Hispanic/Latino; 4 Asian, non-Hispanic/Latino; 7 Hispanic/Latino; 3 Two or more races, non-Hispanic/Latino), 6 international. Average age 29. 164 applicants, 47% accepted, 63 enrolled. In 2013, 55 master's, 5 doctorates awarded. Terminal master's awarded for partial completion of doctoral program. *Degree requirements:* For master's, comprehensive exam (for some programs), thesis (for some programs); for doctorate, thesis/dissertation. *Entrance requirements:* For master's, GRE General Test, GRE Subject Test, MCAT, DAT, or other standardized test or professional school entrance exam, bachelor's degree, minimum GPA of 3.0; for doctorate, GRE General Test, GRE Subject Test, bachelor's or professional degree, minimum GPA of 3.0. Additional exam requirements/recommendations for international students: Required—TOEFL (minimum score 550 paper-based; 80 iBT). *Application deadline:* For fall admission, 4/1 for domestic and international students; for winter admission, 9/1 for domestic students. Application fee: $50. Electronic applications accepted. *Expenses:* Tuition, state resident: full-time $9075.40; part-time $504 per credit. Tuition, nonresident: full-time $22,248; part-time $1236 per credit. *Required fees:* $1819; $60 per credit. *Financial support:* In 2013–14, 37 students received support, including 7 fellowships with full tuition reimbursements available (averaging $32,563 per year), 25 research assistantships with full and partial tuition reimbursements available (averaging $15,221 per year), 5 teaching assistantships with full tuition reimbursements available (averaging $6,636 per year); Federal Work-Study, scholarships/grants, traineeships, and unspecified assistantships also available. Financial award application deadline: 4/1. *Faculty research:* Developmental neurobiology, reproductive physiology, equine reproduction, molecular endocrinology, neurophysiology. *Total annual research expenditures:* $6.8 million. *Unit head:* Dr. Colin M. Clay, Chair, 970-491-7571, Fax: 970-491-3557, E-mail: colin.clay@colostate.edu. *Application contact:* Erin Bisenius, Graduate Education Coordinator, 970-491-6188, Fax: 970-491-7569, E-mail: erin.bisenius@colostate.edu.
Website: http://csu-cvmbs.colostate.edu/academics/bms/Pages/default.aspx

Colorado State University, Graduate School, College of Natural Sciences, Department of Biology, Fort Collins, CO 80523-1878. Offers botany (MS, PhD); zoology (MS, PhD). *Faculty:* 25 full-time (10 women), 1 part-time/adjunct (0 women). *Students:* 18 full-time (11 women), 25 part-time (15 women); includes 6 minority (4 Asian, non-Hispanic/Latino; 2 Hispanic/Latino), 6 international. Average age 30. 45 applicants, 27% accepted, 10 enrolled. In 2013, 5 master's, 7 doctorates awarded. Terminal master's awarded for partial completion of doctoral program. *Degree requirements:* For master's, comprehensive exam, thesis; for doctorate, comprehensive exam, thesis/dissertation. *Entrance requirements:* For master's and doctorate, GRE General Test (minimum scores above 70th percentile), 2 transcripts, 3 letters of recommendation, statement of educational goals/research interests, minimum GPA of 3.0. Additional exam requirements/recommendations for international students: Required—TOEFL (minimum score 550 paper-based; 80 iBT), IELTS (minimum score 6.5). *Application deadline:* For fall admission, 1/15 priority date for domestic and international students; for spring admission, 11/1 priority date for domestic and international students. Applications are processed on a rolling basis. Application fee: $50. Electronic applications accepted. *Expenses:* Tuition, state resident: full-time $9075.40; part-time $504 per credit. Tuition, nonresident: full-time $22,248; part-time $1236 per credit. *Required fees:* $1819; $60 per credit. *Financial support:* In 2013–14, 106 students received support, including 19

fellowships (averaging $31,747 per year), 22 research assistantships with full tuition reimbursements available (averaging $10,909 per year), 65 teaching assistantships with full tuition reimbursements available (averaging $13,683 per year); career-related internships or fieldwork, Federal Work-Study, institutionally sponsored loans, scholarships/grants, traineeships, health care benefits, and unspecified assistantships also available. Financial award application deadline: 3/1; financial award applicants required to submit FAFSA. *Faculty research:* Organismal interactions in infectious disease, stream ecology, muscle protein structure, molecular evolution, plant biotechnology. *Total annual research expenditures:* $9.7 million. *Unit head:* Dr. Michael Antolin, Professor and Interim Chair, 970-491-1911, Fax: 970-491-0649, E-mail: michael.antolin@colostate.edu. *Application contact:* Dorothy Ramirez, Graduate Coordinator, 970-491-1923, Fax: 970-491-0649, E-mail: dorothy.ramirez@colostate.edu.
Website: http://www.biology.colostate.edu/

Colorado State University–Pueblo, College of Science and Mathematics, Pueblo, CO 81001-4901. Offers applied natural science (MS), including biochemistry, biology, chemistry. Part-time and evening/weekend programs available. *Degree requirements:* For master's, comprehensive exam (for some programs), thesis (for some programs), internship report (if non-thesis). *Entrance requirements:* For master's, GRE General Test (minimum score 1000), 2 letters of reference, minimum GPA of 3.0. Additional exam requirements/recommendations for international students: Required—TOEFL (minimum score 500 paper-based), IELTS (minimum score 5). *Faculty research:* Fungal cell walls, molecular biology, bioactive materials synthesis, atomic force microscopy-surface chemistry, nanoscience.

Columbia University, College of Physicians and Surgeons, New York, NY 10032. Offers M Phil, MA, MS, DN Sc, DPT, Ed D, MD, PhD, Adv C, MBA/MS, MD/DDS, MD/MPH, MD/MS, MD/PhD, MPH/MS. Part-time programs available. *Entrance requirements:* For master's, GRE General Test. Additional exam requirements/recommendations for international students: Required—TOEFL. *Expenses:* Contact institution.

Columbia University, Graduate School of Arts and Sciences, Department of Biological Sciences, New York, NY 10027. Offers PhD, MD/PhD. *Degree requirements:* For doctorate, comprehensive exam, thesis/dissertation, teaching experience. *Entrance requirements:* For doctorate, GRE General Test, GRE Subject Test (recommended), letters of recommendation. Additional exam requirements/recommendations for international students: Required—TOEFL (minimum score 600 paper-based; 100 iBT). *Application deadline:* For fall admission, 1/4 for domestic students. Application fee: $100. *Financial support:* Fellowships, teaching assistantships, Federal Work-Study, institutionally sponsored loans, and health care benefits available. Support available to part-time students. Financial award application deadline: 12/1; financial award applicants required to submit FAFSA. *Unit head:* Sarah Kim Fein, Program Coordinator, 212-854-2313, Fax: 212-865-8246, E-mail: sarah@biology.columbia.edu. *Application contact:* Robert Furno, Assistant Dean for Admissions, 212-854-4738, Fax: 212-854-2863, E-mail: ref8@columbia.edu.
Website: http://www.columbia.edu/cu/biology/

See Display below and Close-Up on page 119.

The Commonwealth Medical College, Graduate Programs in Medicine, Scranton, PA 18509. Offers biomedical sciences (MBS). *Students:* 55 full-time (26 women). *Entrance requirements:* For master's, bachelor's degree; coursework in biology with lab, organic chemistry with lab, inorganic chemistry with lab, physics with lab, and English; official transcripts; three letters of recommendation. *Application deadline:* Applications are processed on a rolling basis. Application fee: $55. Electronic applications accepted. *Expenses: Tuition:* Full-time $50,000. *Required fees:* $6112. Tuition and fees vary according to degree level, program and student level. *Application contact:* Jillian Golaszewski, Enrollment Management Recruiter, 570-504-7000, Fax: 570-504-2794, E-mail: jgolaszewski@tcmedc.org.
Website: http://www.tcmc.edu/mbs

Concordia University, School of Graduate Studies, Faculty of Arts and Science, Department of Biology, Montréal, QC H3G 1M8, Canada. Offers biology (M Sc, PhD); biotechnology and genomics (Diploma). *Degree requirements:* For master's, thesis; for doctorate, thesis/dissertation, pedagogical training. *Entrance requirements:* For master's, honors degree in biology; for doctorate, M Sc in life science. *Faculty research:* Cell biology, animal physiology, ecology, microbiology/molecular biology, plant physiology/biochemistry and biotechnology.

Cornell University, Graduate School, Graduate Fields of Comparative Biomedical Sciences, Field of Comparative Biomedical Sciences, Ithaca, NY 14853-0001. Offers cellular and molecular medicine (MS, PhD); developmental and reproductive biology (MS, PhD); infectious diseases (MS, PhD); population medicine and epidemiology (MS, PhD); structural and functional biology (MS, PhD). *Faculty:* 104 full-time (32 women). *Students:* 32 full-time (22 women); includes 3 minority (1 Asian, non-Hispanic/Latino; 2 Hispanic/Latino), 12 international. Average age 29. 47 applicants, 23% accepted, 6 enrolled. In 2013, 2 master's, 12 doctorates awarded. *Degree requirements:* For master's, thesis; for doctorate, comprehensive exam, thesis/dissertation. *Entrance requirements:* For master's and doctorate, GRE General Test, 2 letters of recommendation. Additional exam requirements/recommendations for international students: Required—TOEFL (minimum score 550 paper-based; 77 iBT). *Application deadline:* For fall admission, 12/15 for domestic students. Application fee: $95. Electronic applications accepted. *Financial support:* In 2013–14, 18 students received support, including 3 fellowships with full tuition reimbursements available, 14 research assistantships with full tuition reimbursements available, 1 teaching assistantship with full tuition reimbursement available; institutionally sponsored loans, scholarships/grants, health care benefits, tuition waivers (full and partial), and unspecified assistantships also available. Financial award applicants required to submit FAFSA. *Faculty research:* Receptors and signal transduction, viral and bacterial infectious diseases, tumor metastasis, clinical sciences/nutritional disease, developmental/neurological disorders. *Unit head:* Director of Graduate Studies, 607-253-3276, Fax: 607-253-3756. *Application contact:* Graduate Field Assistant, 607-253-3276, Fax: 607-253-3756, E-mail: graduate_edcvm@cornell.edu.
Website: http://www.gradschool.cornell.edu/fields.php?id-64&a-2

Creighton University, School of Medicine and Graduate School, Graduate Programs in Medicine, Department of Biomedical Sciences, Omaha, NE 68178-0001. Offers MS, PhD, MD/PhD. *Faculty:* 24 full-time (4 women), 2 part-time/adjunct (1 woman). *Students:* 16 full-time (7 women), 9 international. Average age 25. 26 applicants, 19% accepted, 3 enrolled. In 2013, 1 master's, 2 doctorates awarded. Terminal master's awarded for partial completion of doctoral program. *Degree requirements:* For master's, thesis; for doctorate, thesis/dissertation. *Entrance requirements:* For master's, GRE General Test (minimum 50th percentile), three recommendations; for doctorate, GRE General Test (minimum score: 50th percentile), three recommendations. Additional exam requirements/recommendations for international students: Required—TOEFL. *Application deadline:* For fall admission, 6/1 priority date for domestic students, 5/1 priority date for international students; for spring admission, 11/1 priority date for domestic students, 10/1 priority date for international students. Applications are processed on a rolling basis. Application fee: $50. Electronic applications accepted. *Expenses: Tuition:* Full-time $13,608; part-time $756 per credit hour. *Required fees:* $149 per semester. Tuition and fees vary according to course load, campus/location, program, reciprocity agreements and student's religious affiliation. *Financial support:* In 2013–14, 16 students received support, including 16 fellowships with tuition reimbursements available (averaging $23,868 per year); research assistantships with tuition reimbursements available, teaching assistantships with tuition reimbursements available, institutionally sponsored loans, and tuition waivers (full) also available. *Faculty research:* Molecular biology and gene transfection. *Total annual research expenditures:* $4.4 million. *Unit head:* Dr. John Yee, Chairman, 402-280-2916, Fax: 402-280-2690, E-mail: johnyee@creighton.edu. *Application contact:* Dr. Philip Brauer, Program Director, 402-280-2839, Fax: 402-280-2690, E-mail: prbrauer@creighton.edu. Website: http://medschool.creighton.edu/medicine/departments/biomedicalsciences/

Dalhousie University, Faculty of Graduate Studies and Faculty of Medicine, Graduate Programs in Medicine, Halifax, NS B3H 4R2, Canada. Offers M Sc, PhD. *Degree requirements:* For master's, thesis; for doctorate, thesis/dissertation. *Entrance requirements:* Additional exam requirements/recommendations for international students: Required—1 of 5 approved tests: TOEFL, IELTS, CANTEST, CAEL, Michigan English Language Assessment Battery. Electronic applications accepted. *Expenses:* Contact institution.

Dalhousie University, Faculty of Science, Department of Biology, Halifax, NS B3H 4R2, Canada. Offers M Sc, PhD. Terminal master's awarded for partial completion of doctoral program. *Degree requirements:* For master's, thesis; for doctorate, thesis/dissertation. *Entrance requirements:* Additional exam requirements/recommendations for international students: Required—TOEFL, IELTS, CANTEST, CAEL, or Michigan English Language Assessment Battery. Electronic applications accepted. *Faculty research:* Marine biology, ecology, animal physiology, plant physiology, microbiology (cell, molecular, genetics, development).

Dartmouth College, Graduate Program in Molecular and Cellular Biology, Department of Biological Sciences, Hanover, NH 03755. Offers PhD, MD/PhD. *Entrance requirements:* For doctorate, GRE General Test, letters of recommendation. Additional exam requirements/recommendations for international students: Required—TOEFL (minimum score 450 paper-based; 90 iBT) or IELTS (minimum score 7). Electronic applications accepted.

Delaware State University, Graduate Programs, Department of Biological Sciences, Program in Biological Sciences, Dover, DE 19901-2277. Offers MS. *Entrance requirements:* For master's, GRE, prerequisite undergraduate courses. Additional exam requirements/recommendations for international students: Required—TOEFL.

Delta State University, Graduate Programs, College of Arts and Sciences, Division of Biological and Physical Sciences, Cleveland, MS 38733-0001. Offers natural sciences (MSNS). Part-time programs available. *Faculty:* 12 full-time (5 women). *Students:* 11 full-time (10 women), 3 part-time (1 woman); includes 9 minority (7 Black or African American, non-Hispanic/Latino; 1 Hispanic/Latino; 1 Two or more races, non-Hispanic/Latino). Average age 27. 36 applicants, 92% accepted, 22 enrolled. In 2013, 2 master's awarded. *Degree requirements:* For master's, research project or thesis. *Entrance requirements:* For master's, GRE General Test. *Application deadline:* For fall admission, 8/1 priority date for domestic students; for spring admission, 12/1 priority date for domestic students. Applications are processed on a rolling basis. Application fee: $0. *Expenses:* Tuition, state resident: full-time $3006; part-time $334 per credit hour. Tuition, nonresident: full-time $3006; part-time $334 per credit hour. *Financial support:* Research assistantships, career-related internships or fieldwork, Federal Work-Study, and institutionally sponsored loans available. Support available to part-time students. Financial award application deadline: 6/1. *Unit head:* Dr. Barry E. Campbell, Chair, 662-846-4240, Fax: 662-846-4798. *Application contact:* Dr. Beverly Moon, Dean of Graduate Studies, 662-846-4873, Fax: 662-846-4313, E-mail: grad-info@deltastate.edu. Website: http://www.deltastate.edu/pages/296.asp

DePaul University, College of Science and Health, Chicago, IL 60614. Offers applied mathematics (MS); applied statistics (MS); biological sciences (MA, MS); chemistry (MS); mathematics education (MA); mathematics for teaching (MS); nursing (MS); nursing practice (DNP); physics (MS); psychology (MS); pure mathematics (MS); science education (MS); MA/PhD. *Faculty:* 66 full-time (40 women), 23 part-time/adjunct (21 women). *Students:* 485 full-time (338 women), 207 part-time (132 women); includes 198 minority (55 Black or African American, non-Hispanic/Latino; 1 American Indian or Alaska Native, non-Hispanic/Latino; 64 Asian, non-Hispanic/Latino; 53 Hispanic/Latino; 2 Native Hawaiian or other Pacific Islander, non-Hispanic/Latino; 23 Two or more races, non-Hispanic/Latino), 48 international. Average age 29. In 2013, 244 master's, 20 doctorates awarded. *Application deadline:* Applications are processed on a rolling basis. Application fee: $40. Electronic applications accepted. Tuition and fees vary according to course level, course load and degree level. *Financial support:* Applicants required to submit FAFSA. *Application contact:* Ann Spittle, Director of Graduate Admission, 773-325-7315, Fax: 312-476-3244, E-mail: graddepaul@depaul.edu. Website: http://csh.depaul.edu/

Des Moines University, College of Osteopathic Medicine, Program in Biomedical Sciences, Des Moines, IA 50312-4104. Offers MS.

Dominican University of California, School of Health and Natural Sciences, Program in Biological Sciences, San Rafael, CA 94901-2298. Offers MS. *Faculty:* 3 full-time (0 women), 6 part-time/adjunct (2 women). *Students:* 18 full-time (11 women), 1 part-time (0 women); includes 8 minority (4 Asian, non-Hispanic/Latino; 4 Hispanic/Latino), 3 international. Average age 25. 26 applicants, 46% accepted, 8 enrolled. *Degree requirements:* For master's, thesis. *Entrance requirements:* For master's, GRE, BS in biology, biological sciences or biomedical sciences; minimum GPA of 3.0 in last 60 units. Additional exam requirements/recommendations for international students: Required—TOEFL (minimum score 550 paper-based; 80 iBT), IELTS (minimum score 6.5). *Application deadline:* For fall admission, 3/15 priority date for domestic and international students. Applications are processed on a rolling basis. Electronic applications accepted. Application fee is waived when completed online. *Financial support:* Research assistantships, teaching assistantships, and career-related internships or fieldwork available. Financial award application deadline: 3/2; financial award applicants required to submit FAFSA. *Unit head:* Dr. Randall Hall, Chair, Natural Science and Mathematics, 415-482-1911, Fax: 415-482-1972, E-mail: randall.hall@dominican.edu. *Application contact:* Shannon Lovelace-White, Assistant Vice President, Graduate and Adult Admissions, 415-485-3204, Fax: 415-485-3214, E-mail: shannon.lovelace-white@dominican.edu.
Website: http://www.dominican.edu/academics/hns/sciencemath/graduate/copy_of_msbio

Drew University, Caspersen School of Graduate Studies, Program in Education, Madison, NJ 07940-1493. Offers biology (MAT); chemistry (MAT); English (MAT); French (MAT); Italian (MAT); math (MAT); physics (MAT); social studies (MAT); Spanish (MAT); theatre arts (MAT). Part-time programs available. *Degree requirements:* For master's, student teaching internship and seminar. *Entrance requirements:* For master's, transcripts, statement of purpose, three letters of recommendation. Additional exam requirements/recommendations for international students: Required—TOEFL. *Expenses:* Contact institution.

Drexel University, College of Arts and Sciences, Department of Biology, Philadelphia, PA 19104-2875. Offers biological sciences (MS, PhD); human nutrition (MS). Part-time programs available. *Degree requirements:* For doctorate, thesis/dissertation. *Entrance requirements:* For master's and doctorate, GRE General Test. Additional exam requirements/recommendations for international students: Required—TOEFL. Electronic applications accepted. *Faculty research:* Genetic engineering, physiological ecology.

Drexel University, College of Medicine, Biomedical Graduate Programs, Philadelphia, PA 19129. Offers MLAS, MMS, MS, PhD, Certificate, MD/PhD. Part-time programs available. Terminal master's awarded for partial completion of doctoral program. *Degree requirements:* For master's, comprehensive exam; for doctorate, thesis/dissertation, qualifying exam. *Entrance requirements:* For master's and doctorate, GRE General Test. Additional exam requirements/recommendations for international students: Required—TOEFL. Electronic applications accepted. *Expenses:* Contact institution.

Drexel University, College of Medicine, MD/PhD Program, Philadelphia, PA 19104-2875. Offers MD/PhD. Electronic applications accepted.

Drexel University, School of Biomedical Engineering, Science and Health Systems, Program in Biomedical Science, Philadelphia, PA 19104-2875. Offers MS, PhD. *Degree requirements:* For master's, thesis (for some programs); for doctorate, thesis/dissertation. Electronic applications accepted.

Duke University, Graduate School, Department of Biology, Durham, NC 27708. Offers PhD. *Faculty:* 50. *Students:* 72 full-time (41 women); includes 8 minority (1 American Indian or Alaska Native, non-Hispanic/Latino; 3 Asian, non-Hispanic/Latino; 4 Hispanic/Latino), 28 international. 107 applicants, 17% accepted, 7 enrolled. In 2013, 12 doctorates awarded. *Degree requirements:* For doctorate, one foreign language, thesis/dissertation. *Entrance requirements:* For doctorate, GRE General Test, GRE Subject Test (recommended). Additional exam requirements/recommendations for international students: Required—TOEFL (minimum score 577 paper-based; 90 iBT) or IELTS (minimum score 7). *Application deadline:* For fall admission, 12/8 priority date for domestic and international students. Application fee: $80. Electronic applications accepted. *Financial support:* Fellowships, research assistantships, teaching assistantships, and Federal Work-Study available. Financial award application deadline: 12/8. *Unit head:* Sonke Johnsen, Director of Graduate Studies, 919-684-3649, Fax: 919-660-7293, E-mail: aslzoo@duke.edu. *Application contact:* Elizabeth Hutton, Director of Admissions, 919-684-3913, Fax: 919-684-2277, E-mail: grad-admissions@duke.edu. Website: http://www.biology.duke.edu/

Duquesne University, Bayer School of Natural and Environmental Sciences, Department of Biological Sciences, Pittsburgh, PA 15282-0001. Offers MS, PhD, MS/MS. Part-time programs available. *Faculty:* 16 full-time (5 women). *Students:* 32 full-time (18 women), 1 part-time (0 women); includes 2 minority (1 Asian, non-Hispanic/Latino; 1 Two or more races, non-Hispanic/Latino), 9 international. Average age 28. 47 applicants, 23% accepted, 9 enrolled. In 2013, 2 master's, 3 doctorates awarded. Terminal master's awarded for partial completion of doctoral program. *Degree requirements:* For master's, thesis (for some programs), 32 credit hours (for non-thesis option); for doctorate, thesis/dissertation. *Entrance requirements:* For master's, GRE General Test; GRE Subject Test in biology, biochemistry, or cell and molecular biology (recommended), BS in biological sciences or related field, 3 letters of recommendation, official transcripts, statement of purpose; for doctorate, GRE General Test; GRE Subject Test in biology, biochemistry, or cell and molecular biology (recommended), BS or MS in biological sciences or related field, 3 letters of recommendation, statement of purpose, official transcripts. Additional exam requirements/recommendations for international students: Required—TOEFL (minimum score 90 iBT). *Application deadline:* For fall admission, 1/15 for domestic students, 2/15 for international students. Applications are processed on a rolling basis. Application fee: $0 ($40 for international students). Electronic applications accepted. *Expenses:* Contact institution. *Financial support:* In 2013–14, 34 students received support, including 1 fellowship with full tuition reimbursement available (averaging $23,675 per year), 2 research assistantships with full tuition reimbursements available (averaging $23,175 per year), 31 teaching assistantships with full tuition reimbursements available (averaging $23,175 per year); scholarships/grants, tuition waivers (partial), and unspecified assistantships also available. Financial award application deadline: 5/31. *Faculty research:* Cell and developmental biology, molecular biology and genetics, evolution, ecology, physiology and microbiology. *Total annual research expenditures:* $856,750. *Unit head:* Dr. Joseph McCormick, Chair, 412-396-5657, Fax: 412-396-5907, E-mail: mccormick@duq.edu. *Application contact:* Heather Costello, Graduate Academic Advisor, 412-396-6339, Fax: 412-396-4881, E-mail: costelloh@duq.edu.
Website: http://www.duq.edu/academics/schools/natural-and-environmental-sciences/academic-programs/biological-sciences

East Carolina University, Brody School of Medicine, Department of Biochemistry and Molecular Biology, Greenville, NC 27858-4353. Offers biochemistry and molecular biology (PhD); biomedical science (MS). *Degree requirements:* For doctorate, comprehensive exam, thesis/dissertation. *Entrance requirements:* For doctorate, GRE General Test. Additional exam requirements/recommendations for international students: Required—TOEFL. *Application deadline:* For fall admission, 6/1 priority date for domestic students. Applications are processed on a rolling basis. Application fee: $50. *Expenses:* Tuition, state resident: full-time $4223. Tuition, nonresident: full-time $16,540. *Required fees:* $2184. *Financial support:* Fellowships with full and partial tuition reimbursements available. Financial award application deadline: 6/1. *Faculty research:* Gene regulation, development and differentiation, contractility and motility, macromolecular interactions, cancer. *Unit head:* Dr. Phillip H. Pekala, Chairman, 252-744-2684, Fax: 252-744-3383, E-mail: pekalap@ecu.edu. *Application contact:* Dr. Phillip H. Pekala, Chairman, 252-744-2684, Fax: 252-744-3383, E-mail: pekalap@ecu.edu. Website: http://www.ecu.edu/cs-dhs/biochemistry/Graduate-Program-Information.cfm

East Carolina University, Graduate School, Thomas Harriot College of Arts and Sciences, Department of Biology, Greenville, NC 27858-4353. Offers biology (MS); molecular biology and biotechnology (MS). Part-time programs available. *Degree requirements:* For master's, one foreign language, comprehensive exam, thesis. *Entrance requirements:* For master's, GRE General Test, GRE Subject Test. Additional exam requirements/recommendations for international students: Required—TOEFL. *Application deadline:* For fall admission, 6/1 priority date for domestic students; for spring admission, 10/15 for domestic students. Applications are processed on a rolling basis. Application fee: $50. *Expenses:* Tuition, state resident: full-time $4223. Tuition, nonresident: full-time $16,540. *Required fees:* $2184. *Financial support:* Fellowships with partial tuition reimbursements, research assistantships with partial tuition reimbursements, teaching assistantships with partial tuition reimbursements, career-related internships or fieldwork, Federal Work-Study, scholarships/grants, and unspecified assistantships available. Support available to part-time students. Financial award application deadline: 6/1. *Faculty research:* Biochemistry, microbiology, cell biology. *Unit head:* Dr. Jeff McKinnon, Chair, 252-328-6718, E-mail: mckinnonj@ecu.edu. *Application contact:* Dean of Graduate School, 252-328-6012, Fax: 252-328-6071, E-mail: gradschool@ecu.edu.
Website: http://www.ecu.edu/cs-cas/biology/graduate.cfm

Eastern Illinois University, Graduate School, College of Sciences, Department of Biological Sciences, Charleston, IL 61920-3099. Offers MS. *Degree requirements:* For master's, exam. *Expenses: Tuition, area resident:* Part-time $283 per credit hour.

Tuition, state resident: part-time $283 per credit hour. Tuition, nonresident: part-time $679 per credit hour.

Eastern Kentucky University, The Graduate School, College of Arts and Sciences, Department of Biological Sciences, Richmond, KY 40475-3102. Offers biological sciences (MS); ecology (MS). Part-time programs available. *Degree requirements:* For master's, thesis. *Entrance requirements:* For master's, GRE General Test, minimum GPA of 2.5. *Faculty research:* Systematics, ecology, and biodiversity; animal behavior; protein structure and molecular genetics; biomonitoring and aquatic toxicology; pathogenesis of microbes and parasites.

Eastern Mennonite University, Program in Biomedicine, Harrisonburg, VA 22802-2462. Offers MA. Electronic applications accepted.

Eastern Michigan University, Graduate School, College of Arts and Sciences, Department of Biology, Ypsilanti, MI 48197. Offers cell and molecular biology (MS); community college biology teaching (MS); ecology and organismal biology (MS); general biology (MS); water resources (MS). Part-time and evening/weekend programs available. Postbaccalaureate distance learning degree programs offered (minimal on-campus study). *Faculty:* 19 full-time (4 women). *Students:* 11 full-time (6 women), 31 part-time (18 women); includes 3 minority (1 Black or African American, non-Hispanic/Latino; 1 Asian, non-Hispanic/Latino; 1 Hispanic/Latino), 6 international. Average age 26. 56 applicants, 59% accepted, 20 enrolled. In 2013, 13 master's awarded. *Entrance requirements:* For master's, GRE General Test, GRE Subject Test. Additional exam requirements/recommendations for international students: Required—TOEFL. *Application deadline:* Applications are processed on a rolling basis. Application fee: $35. *Expenses:* Tuition, state resident: full-time $12,300; part-time $466 per credit hour. Tuition, nonresident: full-time $23,159; part-time $918 per credit hour. *Required fees:* $71 per credit hour. $46 per semester. One-time fee: $100. Tuition and fees vary according to course level and degree level. *Financial support:* Fellowships, research assistantships with full tuition reimbursements, teaching assistantships with full tuition reimbursements, career-related internships or fieldwork, Federal Work-Study, institutionally sponsored loans, scholarships/grants, tuition waivers (partial), and unspecified assistantships available. Support available to part-time students. Financial award applicants required to submit FAFSA. *Unit head:* Dr. Daniel Clemans, Department Head, 734-487-4242, Fax: 734-487-9235, E-mail: dclemans@emich.edu. *Application contact:* Dr. David Kass, Graduate Coordinator, 734-487-4242, Fax: 734-487-9235, E-mail: dkass@emich.edu.
Website: http://www.emich.edu/biology

Eastern New Mexico University, Graduate School, College of Liberal Arts and Sciences, Department of Biology, Portales, NM 88130. Offers applied ecology (MS); botany (MS); cell, molecular biology and biotechnology (MS); microbiology (MS); zoology (MS). Part-time programs available. *Degree requirements:* For master's, comprehensive exam, thesis optional. *Entrance requirements:* For master's, GRE, minimum GPA of 3.0, 2 letters of recommendation, statement of research interest, bachelor's degree related to field of study or proof of common knowledge. Additional exam requirements/recommendations for international students: Required—TOEFL (minimum score 550 paper-based; 79 iBT), IELTS (minimum score 6). Electronic applications accepted.

Eastern Virginia Medical School, Doctoral Program in Biomedical Sciences, Norfolk, VA 23501-1980. Offers PhD. *Students:* 14 full-time (10 women); includes 5 minority (2 Black or African American, non-Hispanic/Latino; 2 Asian, non-Hispanic/Latino; 1 Hispanic/Latino). 20 applicants, 3 enrolled. In 2013, 1 doctorate awarded. *Degree requirements:* For doctorate, thesis/dissertation. *Entrance requirements:* For doctorate, GRE General Test. Additional exam requirements/recommendations for international students: Required—TOEFL. *Application deadline:* For fall admission, 2/1 for domestic students. Applications are processed on a rolling basis. Application fee: $60. Electronic applications accepted. *Expenses:* Contact institution. *Financial support:* Research assistantships with full tuition reimbursements available. *Unit head:* Dr. Earl Godfrey, Director, 757-446-5609, Fax: 757-446-6179, E-mail: godfreew@evms.edu. *Application contact:* Kathleen Wilkinson, Administrative Support Coordinator, 757-446-5076, Fax: 757-446-6179, E-mail: wilkinkd@evms.edu.
Website: http://www.evms.edu/education/doctoral_programs/biomedical_sciences/

Eastern Virginia Medical School, Master's Program in Biomedical Sciences Research, Norfolk, VA 23501-1980. Offers MS. *Faculty:* 57. *Students:* 9 full-time (4 women), 2 part-time (both women); includes 3 minority (1 Black or African American, non-Hispanic/Latino; 2 Two or more races, non-Hispanic/Latino). 35 applicants, 5 enrolled. In 2013, 9 master's awarded. *Degree requirements:* For master's, comprehensive exam (for some programs), thesis optional. *Entrance requirements:* For master's, GRE. Additional exam requirements/recommendations for international students: Required—TOEFL. *Application deadline:* For fall admission, 3/1 for domestic students. Applications are processed on a rolling basis. Application fee: $60. Electronic applications accepted. *Expenses:* Contact institution. *Unit head:* Dr. Earl Godfrey, Director, 757-446-5609, Fax: 757-624-2255, E-mail: godfreew@evms.edu. *Application contact:* Kathleen Wilkinson, Administrative Support Coordinator, 757-446-5076, Fax: 757-446-6179, E-mail: wilkinkd@evms.edu.
Website: http://evms.edu/education/masters_programs/biomedical_sciences_research_masters_program/

Eastern Virginia Medical School, Master's Program in Clinical Embryology and Andrology, Norfolk, VA 23501-1980. Offers MS. Postbaccalaureate distance learning degree programs offered (minimal on-campus study). *Faculty:* 12 full-time, 8 part-time/adjunct. *Students:* 44 full-time (35 women), 15 part-time (10 women); includes 28 minority (4 Black or African American, non-Hispanic/Latino; 21 Asian, non-Hispanic/Latino; 2 Hispanic/Latino; 1 Two or more races, non-Hispanic/Latino). 44 applicants, 27 enrolled. In 2013, 20 master's awarded. *Entrance requirements:* Additional exam requirements/recommendations for international students: Required—TOEFL (minimum score 550 paper-based; 80 iBT). *Application deadline:* For fall admission, 1/14 for domestic and international students. Applications are processed on a rolling basis. Application fee: $60. Electronic applications accepted. *Expenses:* Contact institution. *Unit head:* Dr. Jacob Mayer, Director, 757-446-5049, Fax: 757-446-5905. *Application contact:* Prof. Helena Russell, Administrator, 757-446-8482, Fax: 757-446-6179, E-mail: russelhi@evms.edu.
Website: http://evms.edu/education/masters_programs/clinical_embryology_andrology_program/

Eastern Virginia Medical School, Medical Master's Program in Biomedical Sciences, Norfolk, VA 23501-1980. Offers MS. *Faculty:* 25. *Students:* 66 full-time (24 women); includes 36 minority (1 Black or African American, non-Hispanic/Latino; 28 Asian, non-Hispanic/Latino; 7 Two or more races, non-Hispanic/Latino). 311 applicants, 66 enrolled. In 2013, 38 master's awarded. *Entrance requirements:* For master's, MCAT. *Application deadline:* For fall admission, 4/1 for domestic students. Applications are processed on a rolling basis. Application fee: $60. Electronic applications accepted. *Expenses:* Contact institution. *Financial support:* Institutionally sponsored loans available. Financial award applicants required to submit FAFSA. *Unit head:* Dr. Donald Meyer, Director, 757-446-5615, Fax: 757-446-6179, E-mail: meyerdc@evms.edu. *Application contact:* Amber Donlan, Administrative Support Coordinator, 757-446-5944, Fax: 757-446-6179, E-mail: donlanae@evms.edu.
Website: http://www.evms.edu/education/masters_programs/medical_masters_program/

Eastern Washington University, Graduate Studies, College of Science, Health and Engineering, Department of Biology, Cheney, WA 99004-2431. Offers MS. *Faculty:* 15 full-time (6 women). *Students:* 17 full-time (10 women), 3 part-time (2 women); includes 1 minority (Asian, non-Hispanic/Latino). Average age 36. 30 applicants, 30% accepted, 9 enrolled. In 2013, 13 master's awarded. *Degree requirements:* For master's, comprehensive exam, thesis. *Entrance requirements:* For master's, GRE General Test, minimum GPA of 3.0. *Application deadline:* For fall admission, 4/1 priority date for domestic students; for spring admission, 1/15 for domestic students. Applications are processed on a rolling basis. Application fee: $50. *Financial support:* In 2013–14, 12 teaching assistantships with partial tuition reimbursements (averaging $7,000 per year) were awarded; career-related internships or fieldwork, Federal Work-Study, institutionally sponsored loans, scholarships/grants, health care benefits, tuition waivers (partial), and unspecified assistantships also available. Support available to part-time students. Financial award application deadline: 2/1; financial award applicants required to submit FAFSA. *Faculty research:* Ecology of Eastern Washington Channeled Scablands, Columbia River fisheries, biotechnology applied to vaccines, role of mycorrhiza in plant nutrition, exercise and estrous cycles. *Unit head:* Dr. Flash Gibson, Chair, 509-359-2348, Fax: 509-359-6867. *Application contact:* Dr. Ross Black, Graduate Adviser, 509-359-2339.
Website: http://www.ewu.edu/cshe/programs/biology.xml

East Stroudsburg University of Pennsylvania, Graduate College, College of Arts and Sciences, Department of Biology, East Stroudsburg, PA 18301-2999. Offers M Ed, MS. Part-time and evening/weekend programs available. *Faculty:* 8 full-time (2 women). *Students:* 15 full-time (7 women), 4 part-time (1 woman); includes 1 minority (Two or more races, non-Hispanic/Latino), 1 international. Average age 28. 28 applicants, 68% accepted, 7 enrolled. In 2013, 9 master's awarded. *Degree requirements:* For master's, comprehensive exam, thesis or alternative. *Entrance requirements:* For master's, GRE, resume, undergraduate major in life science (or equivalent), completion of organic chemistry (minimum two semesters), 3 letters of recommendation, letter of intent. Additional exam requirements/recommendations for international students: Required—TOEFL (minimum score 560 paper-based; 83 iBT) or IELTS. *Application deadline:* For fall admission, 7/31 for domestic students, 6/30 priority date for international students; for spring admission, 11/30 for domestic students, 10/31 for international students. Applications are processed on a rolling basis. Application fee: $50. Electronic applications accepted. *Expenses:* Tuition, state resident: full-time $7956; part-time $442 per credit. Tuition, nonresident: full-time $11,934; part-time $663 per credit. *Required fees:* $2129; $118 per credit. *Financial support:* Research assistantships with full and partial tuition reimbursements, Federal Work-Study, and institutionally sponsored loans available. Financial award application deadline: 3/1; financial award applicants required to submit FAFSA. *Unit head:* Dr. Jane Huffman, Graduate Coordinator, 570-422-3725, Fax: 570-422-3724, E-mail: jhuffman@po-box.esu.edu. *Application contact:* Kevin Quintero, Graduate Admission Coordinator, 570-422-3536, Fax: 570-422-3711, E-mail: kquintero@esu.edu.
Website: http://www4.esu.edu/academics/departments/biology/graduate_programs/index.cfm

East Tennessee State University, James H. Quillen College of Medicine, Department of Biomedical Sciences, Johnson City, TN 37614. Offers anatomy (PhD); biochemistry (PhD); microbiology (PhD); pharmaceutical sciences (PhD); pharmacology (PhD); physiology (PhD); quantitative biosciences (PhD). *Faculty:* 43 full-time (11 women), 1 (woman) part-time/adjunct. *Students:* 31 full-time (17 women), 4 part-time (1 woman); includes 6 minority (2 Black or African American, non-Hispanic/Latino; 3 Asian, non-Hispanic/Latino; 1 Hispanic/Latino), 9 international. Average age 29. 53 applicants, 17% accepted, 8 enrolled. In 2013, 6 doctorates awarded. *Degree requirements:* For doctorate, thesis/dissertation, comprehensive qualifying exam. *Entrance requirements:* For doctorate, GRE General Test, GRE Subject Test. Additional exam requirements/recommendations for international students: Required—TOEFL (minimum score 550 paper-based; 79 iBT). *Application deadline:* For fall admission, 3/15 priority date for domestic students, 3/1 priority date for international students. Application fee: $35 ($45 for international students). Electronic applications accepted. *Expenses:* Contact institution. *Financial support:* In 2013–14, 30 students received support, including 30 research assistantships with full tuition reimbursements available (averaging $19,000 per year); career-related internships or fieldwork, institutionally sponsored loans, scholarships/grants, and unspecified assistantships also available. Financial award application deadline: 7/1; financial award applicants required to submit FAFSA. *Faculty research:* Cardiovascular, infectious disease, neurosciences, cancer, immunology. *Unit head:* Dr. Mitchell E. Robinson, Associate Dean/Program Director, 423-439-2031, Fax: 423-439-2140, E-mail: robinson@etsu.edu. *Application contact:* Shella Bennett, Graduate Specialist, 423-439-4708, Fax: 423-439-5624, E-mail: bennetsg@etsu.edu.
Website: http://www.etsu.edu/com/dbms/

East Tennessee State University, School of Graduate Studies, College of Arts and Sciences, Department of Biological Sciences, Johnson City, TN 37614. Offers biology (MS); biomedical sciences (MS); microbiology (MS); paleontology (MS). *Faculty:* 21 full-time (5 women), 6 part-time/adjunct (1 woman). *Students:* 36 full-time (15 women), 6 part-time (3 women); includes 2 minority (1 Black or African American, non-Hispanic/Latino; 1 Asian, non-Hispanic/Latino), 18 international. Average age 27. 64 applicants, 42% accepted, 24 enrolled. In 2013, 8 master's awarded. *Degree requirements:* For master's, comprehensive exam, thesis. *Entrance requirements:* For master's, GRE General Test or GRE Subject Test, minimum GPA of 3.0, undergraduate degree in life or physical sciences, two letters of recommendation. Additional exam requirements/recommendations for international students: Required—TOEFL (minimum score 550 paper-based; 79 iBT). *Application deadline:* For fall admission, 4/1 for domestic students, 2/1 for international students; for spring admission, 9/1 for domestic students, 7/1 for international students. Application fee: $35 ($45 for international students). Electronic applications accepted. *Expenses:* Tuition, state resident: full-time $7900; part-time $395 per credit hour. Tuition, nonresident: full-time $21,960; part-time $1098 per credit hour. *Required fees:* $1345; $84 per credit hour. *Financial support:* In 2013–14, 36 students received support, including 2 research assistantships with full tuition reimbursements available (averaging $9,000 per year), 30 teaching assistantships with full tuition reimbursements available (averaging $8,500 per year); institutionally sponsored loans, scholarships/grants, and unspecified assistantships also available. Financial award application deadline: 7/1; financial award applicants required to submit FAFSA. *Faculty research:* Neuroethology, chronobiology, molecular biology, behavioral ecology, systematics, paleobotany. *Unit head:* Dr. Darrell Moore, Interim Chair, 423-439-4329, Fax: 423-439-5958, E-mail: moored@etsu.edu. *Application contact:* Gail Powers, Graduate Specialist, 423-439-4703, Fax: 423-439-5624, E-mail: powersg@etsu.edu.

Edinboro University of Pennsylvania, Department of Biology and Health Services, Edinboro, PA 16444. Offers biology (MS). Part-time and evening/weekend programs available. *Degree requirements:* For master's, thesis or alternative, competency exam.

Biological and Biomedical Sciences—General

Entrance requirements: For master's, GRE or MAT, minimum QPA of 2.5. *Application deadline:* Applications are processed on a rolling basis. Application fee: $30. Electronic applications accepted. *Expenses:* Tuition, state resident: part-time $454 per credit hour. Tuition, nonresident: part-time $681 per credit hour. *Required fees:* $143.55 per credit hour. Part-time tuition and fees vary according to campus/location and program. *Financial support:* Research assistantships with full and partial tuition reimbursements, Federal Work-Study, scholarships/grants, and unspecified assistantships available. Support available to part-time students. Financial award application deadline: 2/15; financial award applicants required to submit FAFSA. *Faculty research:* Microbiology, molecular biology, zoology, botany, ecology. *Unit head:* Dr. John Ashley, Chairperson, 814-732-2500, E-mail: jashley@edinboro.edu. *Application contact:* Dr. John Ashley, Chairperson, 814-732-2500, E-mail: jashley@edinboro.edu.
Website: http://www.edinboro.edu/departments/biology/

Elizabeth City State University, School of Mathematics, Science and Technology, Master of Science in Biology/Biological Science Program, Elizabeth City, NC 27909-7806. Offers biological sciences (MS); biology education (MS). Part-time and evening/weekend programs available. *Faculty:* 8 full-time (1 woman), 1 (woman) part-time/adjunct. *Students:* 3 full-time (1 woman), 17 part-time (11 women); includes 14 minority (12 Black or African American, non-Hispanic/Latino; 1 Asian, non-Hispanic/Latino; 1 Two or more races, non-Hispanic/Latino). Average age 30. 10 applicants, 70% accepted, 5 enrolled. In 2013, 10 master's awarded. *Degree requirements:* For master's, thesis. *Entrance requirements:* For master's, GRE, minimum GPA of 3.0, 3 letters of recommendation, 2 official transcripts from all undergraduate/graduate schools attended, typewritten one-page expository description of student educational preparation, research interests and career aspirations. Additional exam requirements/recommendations for international students: Required—TOEFL (minimum score 550 paper-based, 80 iBT) or IELTS (minimum score 6.5). *Application deadline:* For fall admission, 7/15 priority date for domestic and international students; for spring admission, 11/15 priority date for domestic and international students; for summer admission, 3/15 priority date for domestic and international students. Applications are processed on a rolling basis. Application fee: $30. Electronic applications accepted. *Expenses:* Tuition, state resident: full-time $2916; part-time $364.48 per credit. Tuition, nonresident: full-time $14,199; part-time $1774.83 per credit. *Required fees:* $2972.23; $206.58 per credit. $571.06 per semester. *Financial support:* In 2013–14, 18 students received support. Scholarships/grants available. Financial award application deadline: 6/30; financial award applicants required to submit FAFSA. *Faculty research:* Apoptosis and cancer, plant bioengineering, development of biofuels, microbial degradation, developmental toxicology. *Unit head:* Dr. Gloria Payne, Chair, 252-335-3595, Fax: 252-335-3697, E-mail: gepayne@mail.ecsu.edu. *Application contact:* Dr. Paula S. Viltz, Interim Dean, School of Education & Psychology and Graduate Education, 252-335-3455, Fax: 252-335-3146, E-mail: psviltz@mail.ecsu.edu.

Emory University, Laney Graduate School, Division of Biological and Biomedical Sciences, Atlanta, GA 30322-1100. Offers PhD. *Degree requirements:* For doctorate, comprehensive exam, thesis/dissertation. *Entrance requirements:* For doctorate, GRE General Test, minimum GPA of 3.0 in science course work (recommended). Additional exam requirements/recommendations for international students: Required—TOEFL. Electronic applications accepted. *Expenses:* Contact institution. *Faculty research:* Biochemistry, cancer; genetics; immunology and microbiology; neuroscience and pharmacology; nutrition; population biology and ecology.

Emporia State University, Department of Biological Sciences, Emporia, KS 66801-5415. Offers botany (MS); environmental biology (MS); general biology (MS); microbial and cellular biology (MS); zoology (MS). Part-time programs available. *Faculty:* 13 full-time (3 women). *Students:* 32 full-time (16 women), 7 part-time (1 woman); includes 2 minority (1 Black or African American, non-Hispanic/Latino; 1 Asian, non-Hispanic/Latino), 18 international. 25 applicants, 88% accepted, 3 enrolled. In 2013, 8 master's awarded. *Degree requirements:* For master's, comprehensive exam or thesis. *Entrance requirements:* For master's, GRE, appropriate undergraduate degree, interview, letters of reference. Additional exam requirements/recommendations for international students: Required—TOEFL (minimum score 520 paper-based; 68 iBT). *Application deadline:* For fall admission, 8/15 priority date for domestic students. Applications are processed on a rolling basis. Application fee: $30 ($75 for international students). Electronic applications accepted. *Expenses: Tuition, area resident:* Part-time $220 per credit hour. Tuition, state resident: part-time $220 per credit hour. Tuition, nonresident: part-time $685 per credit hour. *Required fees:* $73 per credit hour. *Financial support:* In 2013–14, 5 research assistantships with full tuition reimbursements (averaging $7,371 per year), 9 teaching assistantships with full tuition reimbursements (averaging $7,950 per year) were awarded; career-related internships or fieldwork, Federal Work-Study, institutionally sponsored loans, health care benefits, and unspecified assistantships also available. Financial award application deadline: 3/15; financial award applicants required to submit FAFSA. *Faculty research:* Fisheries, range, and wildlife management; aquatic, plant, grassland, vertebrate, and invertebrate ecology; mammalian and plant systematics, taxonomy, and evolution; immunology, virology, and molecular biology. *Unit head:* Dr. R. Brent Thomas, Chair, 620-341-5311, Fax: 620-341-5608, E-mail: rthomas2@emporia.edu. *Application contact:* Dr. Scott Crupper, Graduate Coordinator, 620-341-5621, Fax: 620-341-5607, E-mail: scrupper@emporia.edu.
Website: http://www.emporia.edu/info/degrees-courses/grad/biology

Fairleigh Dickinson University, College at Florham, Maxwell Becton College of Arts and Sciences, Department of Biological and Allied Health Sciences, Program in Biology, Madison, NJ 07940-1099. Offers MS.

Fairleigh Dickinson University, Metropolitan Campus, University College: Arts, Sciences, and Professional Studies, School of Natural Sciences, Program in Biology, Teaneck, NJ 07666-1914. Offers MS.

Fayetteville State University, Graduate School, Department of Biological Sciences, Fayetteville, NC 28301-4298. Offers biology (MS). Part-time and evening/weekend programs available. *Faculty:* 11 full-time (4 women), 2 part-time/adjunct (1 woman). *Students:* 6 full-time (4 women), 9 part-time (7 women); includes 10 minority (6 Black or African American, non-Hispanic/Latino; 3 Hispanic/Latino; 1 Two or more races, non-Hispanic/Latino). Average age 27. 1 applicant, 100% accepted, 1 enrolled. In 2013, 3 master's awarded. *Degree requirements:* For master's, comprehensive exam, thesis, internship. *Entrance requirements:* For master's, GRE General Test. *Application deadline:* For fall admission, 4/15 for domestic students; for spring admission, 10/15 for domestic students. Applications are processed on a rolling basis. Application fee: $40. Electronic applications accepted. *Faculty research:* Genetic and quantitative trait loci (QTL) mapping of important agronomic traits in soybean and other plant species such as disease resistance, yield, and phyto-pharmaceuticals; dinosaur paleobiology, dinosaur systematic, and the evolution/creation controversy; coral reef toxins in education; animal behavior and physiology; forensic science, DNA fingerprinting, and latent evidence. *Total annual research expenditures:* $170,000. *Unit head:* Dr. Abdelmajid Kassem, Chairperson, 910-672-1691, E-mail: mkassem@uncfsu.edu. *Application contact:* Katrina Hoffman, Graduate Admissions Officer, 910-672-1374, Fax: 910-672-1470, E-mail: khoffma1@uncfsu.edu.

Fisk University, Division of Graduate Studies, Department of Biology, Nashville, TN 37208-3051. Offers MA. Part-time programs available. *Degree requirements:* For master's, comprehensive exam, thesis. *Entrance requirements:* For master's, GRE. Electronic applications accepted. *Faculty research:* Cell biology, topographical imaging, serotonin receptors in rats, enzyme assays, developmental biology.

Fitchburg State University, Division of Graduate and Continuing Education, Programs in Biology and Teaching Biology (Secondary Level), Fitchburg, MA 01420-2697. Offers MA, MAT, Certificate. *Accreditation:* NCATE. Part-time and evening/weekend programs available. *Entrance requirements:* Additional exam requirements/recommendations for international students: Required—TOEFL (minimum score 550 paper-based; 79 iBT). Electronic applications accepted.

Florida Agricultural and Mechanical University, Division of Graduate Studies, Research, and Continuing Education, College of Arts and Sciences, Department of Biology, Tallahassee, FL 32307-3200. Offers MS. Part-time programs available. *Degree requirements:* For master's, comprehensive exam, thesis. *Entrance requirements:* For master's, GRE General Test, minimum GPA of 3.0. Additional exam requirements/recommendations for international students: Required—TOEFL (minimum score 550 paper-based).

Florida Atlantic University, Charles E. Schmidt College of Medicine, Boca Raton, FL 33431-0991. Offers biomedical science (MS); medicine (MD). Part-time programs available. *Faculty:* 13 full-time (5 women), 4 part-time/adjunct (0 women). *Students:* 220 full-time (120 women), 16 part-time (10 women); includes 79 minority (16 Black or African American, non-Hispanic/Latino; 26 Asian, non-Hispanic/Latino; 33 Hispanic/Latino; 4 Two or more races, non-Hispanic/Latino), 1 international. Average age 25. 3,109 applicants, 3% accepted, 78 enrolled. In 2013, 24 master's awarded. *Degree requirements:* For master's, thesis (for some programs); for doctorate, comprehensive exam. *Entrance requirements:* For master's, GRE, minimum GPA of 3.0; for doctorate, MCAT, AMCAS application, letters of recommendation, interview. *Application deadline:* For fall admission, 5/1 for domestic students, 3/15 for international students; for spring admission, 10/1 for domestic and international students. Application fee: $30. Electronic applications accepted. *Expenses:* Tuition, state resident: full-time $6660; part-time $370 per credit hour. Tuition, nonresident: full-time $18,450; part-time $1025 per credit hour. Tuition and fees vary according to course load. *Financial support:* In 2013–14, 1 student received support. Fellowships and research assistantships available. Financial award applicants required to submit FAFSA. *Faculty research:* Osteoarthritis, aging, breast cancer, HIV/AIDS, cardiometabolic risk in psychiatry. *Unit head:* Dr. David J. Bjorkman, Dean, 561-297-4341. *Application contact:* Julie Sivigny, Academic Program Specialist for Graduate Studies, 561-297-2216, E-mail: jsivigny@fau.edu.
Website: http://med.fau.edu/

Florida Atlantic University, Charles E. Schmidt College of Science, Department of Biological Sciences, Boca Raton, FL 33431-0991. Offers biology (MS, MST); business biotechnology (MS); environmental science (MS); integrative biology (PhD). Part-time programs available. *Faculty:* 36 full-time (7 women), 3 part-time/adjunct (1 woman). *Students:* 82 full-time (53 women), 63 part-time (37 women); includes 31 minority (3 Black or African American, non-Hispanic/Latino; 7 Asian, non-Hispanic/Latino; 18 Hispanic/Latino; 3 Two or more races, non-Hispanic/Latino), 15 international. Average age 30. 126 applicants, 20% accepted, 20 enrolled. In 2013, 32 master's, 15 doctorates awarded. *Degree requirements:* For master's, thesis (for some programs). *Entrance requirements:* For master's, GRE General Test, minimum GPA of 3.0. Additional exam requirements/recommendations for international students: Required—TOEFL (minimum score 500 paper-based; 61 iBT), IELTS (minimum score 6). *Application deadline:* For fall admission, 3/15 for domestic and international students; for spring admission, 10/1 for domestic and international students. Application fee: $30. *Expenses:* Tuition, state resident: full-time $6660; part-time $370 per credit hour. Tuition, nonresident: full-time $18,450; part-time $1025 per credit hour. Tuition and fees vary according to course load. *Financial support:* Fellowships, research assistantships, teaching assistantships with tuition reimbursements, career-related internships or fieldwork, and Federal Work-Study available. *Faculty research:* Ecology of the Everglades, molecular biology and biotechnology, marine biology. *Unit head:* Dr. Rodney K. Murphey, Chair, 561-297-3320, Fax: 561-297-2749. *Application contact:* Becky Dixon, Graduate Program Assistant, 561-297-3230.
Website: http://www.science.fau.edu/biology/

Florida Institute of Technology, Graduate Programs, College of Science, Department of Biological Sciences, Melbourne, FL 32901-6975. Offers biological science (PhD); biotechnology (MS); cell and molecular biology (MS); conservation technology (MS); ecology (MS); marine biology (MS). Part-time programs available. *Faculty:* 16 full-time (1 woman), 1 (woman) part-time/adjunct. *Students:* 73 full-time (39 women), 14 part-time (11 women); includes 4 minority (1 Asian, non-Hispanic/Latino; 2 Hispanic/Latino; 1 Two or more races, non-Hispanic/Latino), 34 international. Average age 27. 204 applicants, 34% accepted, 38 enrolled. In 2013, 29 master's, 1 doctorate awarded. *Degree requirements:* For master's, thesis (for some programs), research, seminar, internship, or summer lab; for doctorate, comprehensive exam, thesis/dissertation, dissertations seminar, publications. *Entrance requirements:* For master's, GRE General Test, 3 letters of recommendation, minimum GPA of 3.0, resume, statement of objectives; for doctorate, GRE General Test, resume, 3 letters of recommendation, minimum GPA of 3.2, statement of objectives. Additional exam requirements/recommendations for international students: Required—TOEFL (minimum score 550 paper-based; 79 iBT). *Application deadline:* For fall admission, 3/1 for domestic students, 4/1 for international students; for spring admission, 9/1 for domestic and international students. Applications are processed on a rolling basis. Electronic applications accepted. *Expenses: Tuition:* Full-time $20,214; part-time $1123 per credit. Tuition and fees vary according to campus/location. *Financial support:* In 2013–14, 12 research assistantships with full and partial tuition reimbursements (averaging $11,687 per year), 22 teaching assistantships with full and partial tuition reimbursements (averaging $13,947 per year) were awarded; fellowships, career-related internships or fieldwork, institutionally sponsored loans, tuition waivers (partial), unspecified assistantships, and tuition remissions also available. Support available to part-time students. Financial award application deadline: 3/1; financial award applicants required to submit FAFSA. *Faculty research:* Initiation of protein synthesis in eukaryotic cells, fixation of radioactive carbon, changes in DNA molecule, endangered or threatened avian and mammalian species, hydroacoustics and feeding preference of the West Indian manatee. *Total annual research expenditures:* $1.4 million. *Unit head:* Dr. Richard B. Aronson, Department Head, 321-674-8034, Fax: 321-674-7238, E-mail: raronson@fit.edu. *Application contact:* Cheryl A. Brown, Associate Director of Graduate Admissions, 321-674-7581, Fax: 321-723-9468, E-mail: cbrown@fit.edu.
Website: http://cos.fit.edu/biology/

Florida International University, College of Arts and Sciences, Department of Biological Sciences, Miami, FL 33199. Offers MS, PhD. Part-time programs available. *Degree requirements:* For master's, thesis; for doctorate, comprehensive exam, thesis/dissertation. *Entrance requirements:* For master's, GRE General Test, 2 letters of recommendation, minimum GPA of 3.0, faculty sponsor; for doctorate, GRE General Test, 3 letters of recommendation, faculty sponsor with dissertation advisor status, minimum GPA of 3.0. Additional exam requirements/recommendations for international students: Required—TOEFL (minimum score 550 paper-based; 80 iBT). Electronic applications accepted.

Florida State University, The Graduate School, College of Arts and Sciences, Department of Biological Science, Tallahassee, FL 32306-4295. Offers cell and molecular biology (MS, PhD); ecology and evolutionary biology (MS, PhD); plant biology (MS, PhD); science teaching (MST), including community college science teaching, secondary science teaching; structural biology (MS, PhD). *Faculty:* 45 full-time (14 women). *Students:* 110 full-time (53 women); includes 11 minority (2 Black or African American, non-Hispanic/Latino; 1 Asian, non-Hispanic/Latino; 8 Hispanic/Latino), 26 international. 245 applicants, 18% accepted, 21 enrolled. In 2013, 7 master's, 9 doctorates awarded. Terminal master's awarded for partial completion of doctoral program. *Degree requirements:* For master's, comprehensive exam, thesis, teaching experience, seminar presentations; for doctorate, comprehensive exam, thesis/dissertation, teaching experience; seminar presentations. *Entrance requirements:* For master's and doctorate, GRE General Test, minimum upper-division GPA of 3.0. Additional exam requirements/recommendations for international students: Required—TOEFL (minimum score 600 paper-based; 92 iBT). *Application deadline:* For fall admission, 12/1 for domestic and international students. Application fee: $30. Electronic applications accepted. *Expenses:* Tuition, state resident: part-time $403.51 per credit hour. Tuition, nonresident: part-time $1004.85 per credit hour. *Required fees:* $75.81 per credit hour. One-time fee: $20 part-time. Tuition and fees vary according to course load, campus/location and student level. *Financial support:* In 2013–14, 109 students received support, including 9 fellowships with full tuition reimbursements available (averaging $30,000 per year), 27 research assistantships with full tuition reimbursements available (averaging $21,500 per year), 73 teaching assistantships with full tuition reimbursements available (averaging $21,500 per year); scholarships/grants, traineeships, and unspecified assistantships also available. Financial award application deadline: 12/1; financial award applicants required to submit FAFSA. *Faculty research:* Cell and molecular biology and genetics, ecology and evolutionary biology, plant science, structural biology. *Unit head:* Dr. Debra A. Fadool, Professor and Associate Chair, 850-644-4775, Fax: 850-644-9829, E-mail: dfadool@bio.fsu.edu. *Application contact:* Judy Bowers, Coordinator, Graduate Affairs, 850-644-3023, Fax: 850-644-9829, E-mail: gradinfo@bio.fsu.edu.
Website: http://www.bio.fsu.edu/

Florida State University, The Graduate School, College of Arts and Sciences, Department of Mathematics, Tallahassee, FL 32304. Offers applied computational mathematics (MS, PhD); biomathematics (MS, PhD); financial mathematics (MS, PhD); pure mathematics (MS, PhD). Part-time programs available. *Faculty:* 33 full-time (4 women). *Students:* 117 full-time (35 women), 9 part-time (3 women); includes 63 minority (6 Black or African American, non-Hispanic/Latino; 46 Asian, non-Hispanic/Latino; 5 Hispanic/Latino; 6 Two or more races, non-Hispanic/Latino), 48 international. 275 applicants, 28% accepted, 32 enrolled. In 2013, 37 master's, 16 doctorates awarded. Terminal master's awarded for partial completion of doctoral program. *Degree requirements:* For master's, comprehensive exam (for some programs), thesis optional; for doctorate, comprehensive exam (for some programs), thesis/dissertation, candidacy exam (including written qualifying examinations which differ by degree concentration). *Entrance requirements:* For master's and doctorate, GRE General Test, minimum upper-division GPA of 3.0, 4-year bachelor's degree. Additional exam requirements/recommendations for international students: Required—TOEFL (minimum score 550 paper-based; 80 iBT), IELTS (minimum score 6.5). *Application deadline:* For fall admission, 1/31 priority date for domestic and international students; for spring admission, 10/1 for domestic students, 11/1 for international students. Applications are processed on a rolling basis. Application fee: $30. Electronic applications accepted. *Expenses:* Tuition, state resident: part-time $403.51 per credit hour. Tuition, nonresident: part-time $1004.85 per credit hour. *Required fees:* $75.81 per credit hour. One-time fee: $20 part-time. Tuition and fees vary according to course load, campus/location and student level. *Financial support:* In 2013–14, 105 students received support, including 8 fellowships with full tuition reimbursements available (averaging $22,600 per year), 13 research assistantships with full tuition reimbursements available (averaging $22,000 per year), 83 teaching assistantships with full tuition reimbursements available (averaging $19,300 per year); career-related internships or fieldwork, institutionally sponsored loans, scholarships/grants, health care benefits, tuition waivers (full and partial), and unspecified assistantships also available. *Faculty research:* Low-dimensional and geometric topology, mathematical modeling in neuroscience, computational stochastics and Monte Carlo methods, mathematical physics, applied analysis. *Total annual research expenditures:* $185,302. *Unit head:* Dr. Xiaoming Wang, Chairperson, 850-645-3338, Fax: 850-644-4053, E-mail: wxm@math.fsu.edu. *Application contact:* Dr. Giray Okten, Associate Chair for Graduate Studies, 850-644-8713, Fax: 850-644-4053, E-mail: okten@math.fsu.edu.
Website: http://www.math.fsu.edu/

Florida State University, The Graduate School, College of Arts and Sciences, Department of Scientific Computing, Tallahassee, FL 32306-4120. Offers computational science (MS, PSM, PhD), including atmospheric science (PhD), biochemistry (PhD), biological science (PhD), computational molecular biology/bioinformatics (PSM), computational science (PhD), geological science (PhD), materials science (PhD), physics (PhD). Part-time programs available. *Faculty:* 14 full-time (2 women). *Students:* 28 full-time (5 women), 4 part-time (0 women); includes 12 minority (10 Asian, non-Hispanic/Latino; 2 Hispanic/Latino). Average age 28. 28 applicants, 43% accepted, 7 enrolled. In 2013, 11 master's, 5 doctorates awarded. Terminal master's awarded for partial completion of doctoral program. *Degree requirements:* For master's, thesis (for some programs); for doctorate, comprehensive exam, thesis/dissertation. *Entrance requirements:* For master's and doctorate, GRE General Test, knowledge of at least one object-oriented computing language, 3 letters of recommendation. Additional exam requirements/recommendations for international students: Required—TOEFL (minimum score 550 paper-based; 80 iBT). *Application deadline:* For fall admission, 1/15 for domestic and international students. Application fee: $30. Electronic applications accepted. *Expenses:* Tuition, state resident: part-time $403.51 per credit hour. Tuition, nonresident: part-time $1004.85 per credit hour. *Required fees:* $75.81 per credit hour. One-time fee: $20 part-time. Tuition and fees vary according to course load, campus/location and student level. *Financial support:* In 2013–14, 32 students received support, including 12 research assistantships with full tuition reimbursements available (averaging $20,000 per year), 17 teaching assistantships with full tuition reimbursements available (averaging $20,000 per year); scholarships/grants and unspecified assistantships also available. Financial award application deadline: 4/15. *Faculty research:* Morphometrics, mathematical and systems biology, mining proteomic and metabolic data, computational materials research, advanced 4-D Var data-assimilation methods in dynamic meteorology and oceanography, computational fluid dynamics, astrophysics. *Unit head:* Dr. Max Gunzburger, Chair, 850-644-1010, E-mail: mgunzburger@fsu.edu. *Application contact:* Maribel Amwake, Academic Coordinator, 850-644-0143, Fax: 850-644-0098, E-mail: mamwake@fsu.edu.
Website: http://www.sc.fsu.edu

Fordham University, Graduate School of Arts and Sciences, Department of Biological Sciences, New York, NY 10458. Offers biological sciences (MS, PhD); conservation biology (Graduate Certificate). Part-time and evening/weekend programs available. *Faculty:* 18 full-time (2 women). *Students:* 56 full-time (35 women), 3 part-time (2 women); includes 2 minority (1 Asian, non-Hispanic/Latino; 1 Hispanic/Latino), 17 international. Average age 29. 99 applicants, 39% accepted, 16 enrolled. In 2013, 11 master's, 2 doctorates awarded. Terminal master's awarded for partial completion of doctoral program. *Degree requirements:* For master's, one foreign language, comprehensive exam, thesis optional; for doctorate, one foreign language, comprehensive exam, thesis/dissertation. *Entrance requirements:* For master's and doctorate, GRE General Test, GRE Subject Test (recommended). Additional exam requirements/recommendations for international students: Required—TOEFL (minimum score 550 paper-based). *Application deadline:* For fall admission, 1/4 priority date for domestic students; for spring admission, 11/1 for domestic students. Application fee: $70. Electronic applications accepted. *Financial support:* In 2013–14, 28 students received support, including 3 fellowships with full and partial tuition reimbursements available (averaging $29,000 per year), 39 teaching assistantships with full and partial tuition reimbursements available (averaging $28,319 per year); Federal Work-Study, institutionally sponsored loans, scholarships/grants, tuition waivers (full and partial), and unspecified assistantships also available. Support available to part-time students. Financial award application deadline: 1/4; financial award applicants required to submit FAFSA. *Faculty research:* Avian ecology, behavioral ecology, and conservation biology; plant, community and ecosystem responses to invasive organisms; neurobiology and ion channel disorders; biochemical, physiological and morphological basis of pattern formation; behavioral, physiological and biochemical adaptations of mammals to extreme environments; evolutionary ecology, functional morphology and ichthyology; genotypic response to biogeographic and anthropogenic factors; community-based sustainable resource use. *Total annual research expenditures:* $1.5 million. *Unit head:* Dr. James Lewis, Chair, 718-817-3642, Fax: 718-817-3645, E-mail: jdlewis@fordham.edu. *Application contact:* Bernadette Valentino-Morrison, Director of Graduate Admissions, 718-817-4419, Fax: 718-817-3566, E-mail: valentinomor@fordham.edu.

Fort Hays State University, Graduate School, College of Health and Life Sciences, Department of Biological Sciences, Program in Biology, Hays, KS 67601-4099. Offers MS. Part-time programs available. *Degree requirements:* For master's, comprehensive exam, thesis optional. *Entrance requirements:* Additional exam requirements/recommendations for international students: Required—TOEFL (minimum score 550 paper-based). Electronic applications accepted.

Frostburg State University, Graduate School, College of Liberal Arts and Sciences, Department of Biology, Frostburg, MD 21532-1099. Offers applied ecology and conservation biology (MS); fisheries and wildlife management (MS). Part-time and evening/weekend programs available. *Degree requirements:* For master's, thesis. *Entrance requirements:* For master's, GRE General Test, resume. Additional exam requirements/recommendations for international students: Required—TOEFL. Electronic applications accepted. *Expenses: Tuition, area resident:* Part-time $340 per credit hour. Tuition, state resident: part-time $340 per credit hour. Tuition, nonresident: part-time $437 per credit hour. *Faculty research:* Molecular and morphological evolution, ecology and behavior of birds, conservation genetics of amphibians and fishes, biology of endangered species.

George Mason University, College of Science, Programs in Biomedical Sciences, Fairfax, VA 22030. Offers MS, Advanced Certificate. Programs offered jointly with Georgetown University. *Faculty:* 5 full-time (1 woman). *Students:* 85 full-time (50 women), 1 part-time (0 women); includes 57 minority (26 Black or African American, non-Hispanic/Latino; 22 Asian, non-Hispanic/Latino; 6 Hispanic/Latino; 3 Two or more races, non-Hispanic/Latino), 1 international. Average age 23. 406 applicants, 50% accepted, 85 enrolled. In 2013, 16 master's, 63 other advanced degrees awarded. *Entrance requirements:* For master's, MCAT or GRE, BA/BS in related field with minimum GPA of 3.0; 3 letters of recommendation; expanded goals statement; resume; 2 official copies of transcripts; for Advanced Certificate, bachelor's degree in related field with minimum GPA of 3.0; 3 letters of recommendation; resume; expanded goals statement; 2 official copies of transcripts. Additional exam requirements/recommendations for international students: Required—TOEFL (minimum score 570 paper-based; 88 iBT), IELTS (minimum score 6.5), PTE. *Application deadline:* For fall admission, 4/15 priority date for domestic students. Application fee: $65 ($80 for international students). Electronic applications accepted. *Expenses:* Contact institution. *Financial support:* Application deadline: 3/1; applicants required to submit FAFSA. *Faculty research:* Systems medicine. *Unit head:* Donna M. Fox, Director, 703-993-8797, Fax: 703-993-1993, E-mail: dfox1@gmu.edu. *Application contact:* Tanneh Kamara, Program Coordinator, 703-993-7136, Fax: 703-993-7139, E-mail: tkamara@gmu.edu.
Website: http://georgesquared.gmu.edu/ms-biomedical-sciences-curriculum/

George Mason University, College of Science, School of Systems Biology, Fairfax, VA 22030. Offers bioinformatics and computational biology (MS, PhD, Graduate Certificate); biology (MS); biosciences (PhD). *Faculty:* 11 full-time (2 women), 1 part-time/adjunct (0 women). *Students:* 75 full-time (34 women), 71 part-time (35 women); includes 33 minority (5 Black or African American, non-Hispanic/Latino; 1 American Indian or Alaska Native, non-Hispanic/Latino; 22 Asian, non-Hispanic/Latino; 4 Hispanic/Latino; 1 Native Hawaiian or other Pacific Islander, non-Hispanic/Latino), 38 international. Average age 31. 153 applicants, 45% accepted, 32 enrolled. In 2013, 20 master's, 15 doctorates, 2 other advanced degrees awarded. *Degree requirements:* For master's, research project or thesis; for doctorate, comprehensive exam, thesis/dissertation. *Entrance requirements:* For master's, GRE, resume; 3 letters of recommendation; expanded goals statement; 2 copies of official transcripts; bachelor's degree in related field with minimum GPA of 3.0 in last 60 hours; for doctorate, GRE, self-assessment form; resume; 3 letters of recommendation; expanded goals statement; 2 copies of official transcripts; bachelor's degree in related field with minimum GPA of 3.0 in last 60 hours; for Graduate Certificate, resume; 2 copies of official transcripts. Additional exam requirements/recommendations for international students: Required—TOEFL (minimum score 570 paper-based; 88 iBT), IELTS (minimum score 6.5), PTE. Application fee: $65 ($80 for international students). Electronic applications accepted. *Expenses:* Tuition, state resident: full-time $9350; part-time $390 per credit. Tuition, nonresident: full-time $25,754; part-time $1073 per credit. *Required fees:* $2688; $112 per credit. *Financial support:* In 2013–14, 50 students received support, including 15 fellowships (averaging $3,801 per year), 23 research assistantships with full and partial tuition reimbursements available (averaging $14,040 per year), 33 teaching assistantships with full and partial tuition reimbursements available (averaging $14,053 per year); career-related internships or fieldwork, Federal Work-Study, scholarships/grants, unspecified assistantships, and health care benefits (for full-time research or teaching assistantship recipients) also available. Support available to part-time students. Financial award application deadline: 3/1; financial award applicants required to submit FAFSA. *Faculty research:* Functional genomics of chronic human diseases, ecology of vector-borne infectious diseases, neurogenetics, molecular biology, computational modeling, proteomics, chronic metabolic diseases, nanotechnology. *Total annual research expenditures:* $886,819. *Unit head:* Dr. James D. Willett, Director, 703-993-8311, Fax: 703-993-8976, E-mail: jwillett@gmu.edu. *Application contact:* Diane St. Germain, Graduate Student Services Coordinator, 703-993-4263, Fax: 703-993-8976, E-mail: dstgerma@gmu.edu.
Website: http://ssb.gmu.edu/

George Mason University, School of Policy, Government, and International Affairs, Department of Public and International Affairs, Fairfax, VA 22030. Offers administration

of justice (Certificate); association management (Certificate); biodefense (MS, PhD); critical analysis and strategic response to terrorism (Certificate); emergency management and homeland security (Certificate); nonprofit management (Certificate); political science (MA, PhD); public administration (MPA); public management (Certificate). *Accreditation:* NASPAA (one or more programs are accredited). *Faculty:* 39 full-time (10 women), 35 part-time/adjunct (10 women). *Students:* 174 full-time (89 women), 281 part-time (162 women); includes 105 minority (34 Black or African American, non-Hispanic/Latino; 22 Asian, non-Hispanic/Latino; 35 Hispanic/Latino; 2 Native Hawaiian or other Pacific Islander, non-Hispanic/Latino; 12 Two or more races, non-Hispanic/Latino), 19 international. Average age 30. 415 applicants, 68% accepted, 144 enrolled. In 2013, 136 master's, 3 doctorates, 8 other advanced degrees awarded. *Entrance requirements:* For master's, GRE, GMAT or LSAT (for MPA); GRE (for MS in biodefense and MA in political science), expanded goals statement; 3 letters of recommendation; official transcripts; resume (for MPA); writing sample (for MS, MA); for doctorate, GRE (taken within the last 5 years), 3 letters of recommendation; expanded goals statement; resume; official transcript; writing sample; for Certificate, GRE, GMAT or LSAT, expanded goals statement; 3 letters of recommendation; official transcripts; resume. Additional exam requirements/recommendations for international students: Required—TOEFL (minimum score 570 paper-based; 88 iBT), IELTS (minimum score 6.5), PTE. Application fee: $65 ($80 for international students). Electronic applications accepted. *Expenses:* Contact institution. *Financial support:* In 2013–14, 32 students received support, including 1 fellowship (averaging $2,500 per year), 14 research assistantships with full and partial tuition reimbursements available (averaging $15,364 per year), 18 teaching assistantships with full and partial tuition reimbursements available (averaging $12,562 per year); career-related internships or fieldwork, Federal Work-Study, scholarships/grants, unspecified assistantships, and health care benefits (for full-time research or teaching assistantship recipients) also available. Support available to part-time students. Financial award application deadline: 3/1; financial award applicants required to submit FAFSA. *Faculty research:* The Rehnquist Court and economic liberties; intersection of economic development with high-tech industry, telecommunications, and entrepreneurism; political economy of development; violence, terrorism and U.S. foreign policy; international security issues. *Total annual research expenditures:* $503,888. *Unit head:* Dr. Priscilla Regan, Chair, 703-993-1419, Fax: 703-993-1399, E-mail: pregan@gmu.edu. *Application contact:* Peg Koback, Education Support Specialist, 703-993-3707, Fax: 703-993-1399, E-mail: mkoback@gmu.edu.
Website: http://pia.gmu.edu/

Georgetown University, GeorgeSquared Special Master's Program, Washington, DC 20057. Offers MS. Program offered jointly with George Mason University. *Application deadline:* For fall admission, 6/15 for domestic students. Applications are processed on a rolling basis. *Application contact:* Graduate School Admissions Office, 202-687-5568, E-mail: gsquared@gmu.edu.
Website: http://georgesquared.georgetown.edu/

Georgetown University, Graduate School of Arts and Sciences, Department of Biology, Washington, DC 20057. Offers PhD. Terminal master's awarded for partial completion of doctoral program. *Degree requirements:* For doctorate, comprehensive exam, thesis/dissertation. *Entrance requirements:* For doctorate, GRE General Test, GRE Subject Test (biology). Additional exam requirements/recommendations for international students: Required—TOEFL (minimum score 550 paper-based). *Application deadline:* For fall admission, 1/3 priority date for domestic students. Application fee: $50. Electronic applications accepted. *Financial support:* Fellowships, research assistantships with full tuition reimbursements, teaching assistantships with full tuition reimbursements, scholarships/grants, health care benefits, and unspecified assistantships available. Financial award application deadline: 2/1; financial award applicants required to submit FAFSA. *Faculty research:* Parasitology, ecology, evaluation and behavior, neuroscience and development, cell and molecular biology, immunology. *Unit head:* Dr. Steven Singer, Chair, 202-687-9884, E-mail: steven.singer@georgetown.edu. *Application contact:* Graduate School Admissions Office, 202-687-5568.

Georgetown University, National Institutes of Health Sponsored Programs, GU-NIH Graduate Partnership Programs in Biomedical Sciences, Washington, DC 20057. Offers MS, PhD, MD/PhD, MS/PhD. *Entrance requirements:* For doctorate, GRE General Test. Additional exam requirements/recommendations for international students: Required—TOEFL. Application fee: $50 ($55 for international students). *Financial support:* Career-related internships or fieldwork available. *Application contact:* Graduate School Admissions Office, 202-687-5568.

The George Washington University, Columbian College of Arts and Sciences, Department of Anthropology, Program in Hominid Paleobiology, Washington, DC 20052. Offers MS, PhD. Part-time and evening/weekend programs available. Terminal master's awarded for partial completion of doctoral program. *Degree requirements:* For master's, comprehensive exam, thesis; for doctorate, thesis/dissertation, general exam. *Entrance requirements:* For master's, GRE General Test, bachelor's degree in field, minimum GPA of 3.0; for doctorate, GRE General Test, minimum GPA of 3.0. Additional exam requirements/recommendations for international students: Required—TOEFL (minimum score 550 paper-based). Electronic applications accepted.

The George Washington University, Columbian College of Arts and Sciences, Department of Biological Sciences, Washington, DC 20052. Offers MS, PhD. Part-time and evening/weekend programs available. *Faculty:* 25 full-time (8 women). *Students:* 15 full-time (9 women), 21 part-time (11 women); includes 5 minority (2 Asian, non-Hispanic/Latino; 1 Hispanic/Latino; 2 Two or more races, non-Hispanic/Latino), 17 international. Average age 29. 118 applicants, 10% accepted, 8 enrolled. In 2013, 4 master's, 5 doctorates awarded. Terminal master's awarded for partial completion of doctoral program. *Degree requirements:* For master's, comprehensive exam; for doctorate, thesis/dissertation, general exam. *Entrance requirements:* For master's and doctorate, GRE General Test, minimum GPA of 3.0. Additional exam requirements/recommendations for international students: Required—TOEFL (minimum score 550 paper-based; 80 iBT). *Application deadline:* For fall admission, 1/2 priority date for domestic and international students; for spring admission, 10/1 priority date for domestic and international students. Applications are processed on a rolling basis. Application fee: $75. Electronic applications accepted. *Financial support:* In 2013–14, 25 students received support. Fellowships with full tuition reimbursements available, teaching assistantships with full tuition reimbursements available, Federal Work-Study, and tuition waivers available. Financial award application deadline: 1/2. *Faculty research:* Systematics, evolution, ecology, developmental biology, cell/molecular biology. *Total annual research expenditures:* $900,000. *Unit head:* Dr. Diana Lipscomb, Chair, 202-994-5828, Fax: 202-994-6100, E-mail: biodl@gwu.edu.

The George Washington University, Columbian College of Arts and Sciences, Institute for Biomedical Sciences, Washington, DC 20037. Offers biochemistry and systems biology (PhD); microbiology and immunology (PhD); molecular medicine (PhD), including molecular and cellular oncology, neurosciences, pharmacology and physiology. Part-time and evening/weekend programs available. *Degree requirements:* For doctorate, thesis/dissertation. *Entrance requirements:* For doctorate, GRE General Test, minimum GPA of 3.0. Additional exam requirements/recommendations for international students: Required—TOEFL (minimum score 600 paper-based; 80 iBT). Electronic applications accepted.

Georgia College & State University, Graduate School, College of Arts and Sciences, Department of Biology, Milledgeville, GA 31061. Offers MS. Part-time programs available. *Students:* 23 full-time (7 women), 6 part-time (2 women); includes 4 minority (2 Black or African American, non-Hispanic/Latino; 2 Hispanic/Latino), 4 international. Average age 26. In 2013, 29 master's awarded. *Degree requirements:* For master's, thesis optional, minimum GPA of 3.0. *Entrance requirements:* For master's, GRE (minimum score of 800), 30 hours of undergraduate course work in biological science. Additional exam requirements/recommendations for international students: Recommended—TOEFL (minimum score 550 paper-based; 79 iBT). *Application deadline:* For fall admission, 7/1 priority date for domestic students, 4/1 for international students; for spring admission, 11/15 priority date for domestic students, 9/1 for international students. Applications are processed on a rolling basis. Application fee: $40. Electronic applications accepted. *Financial support:* In 2013–14, 19 research assistantships with tuition reimbursements were awarded; career-related internships or fieldwork and unspecified assistantships also available. Support available to part-time students. Financial award application deadline: 3/1; financial award applicants required to submit FAFSA. *Faculty research:* Molecular genetics, cell biology, environmental microbiology, microbial ecology. *Unit head:* Dr. Indiren Pillay, Chair, 478-445-0809, E-mail: indiren.pillayll@gcsu.edu. *Application contact:* Dr. Chris Skelton, Graduate Coordinator, 478-445-2440, E-mail: chris.skelton@gcsu.edu.

Georgia Institute of Technology, Graduate Studies and Research, College of Sciences, School of Biology, Atlanta, GA 30332-0001. Offers applied biology (MS, PhD); bioinformatics (MS, PhD); biology (MS). Part-time programs available. Terminal master's awarded for partial completion of doctoral program. *Degree requirements:* For master's, thesis; for doctorate, thesis/dissertation, qualifying exam. *Entrance requirements:* For master's, GRE General Test, minimum GPA of 2.9; for doctorate, GRE General Test, minimum GPA of 3.0. Additional exam requirements/recommendations for international students: Required—TOEFL. Electronic applications accepted. *Faculty research:* Microbiology, molecular and cell biology, ecology.

Georgia Regents University, The Graduate School, Augusta, GA 30912. Offers M Ed, MAT, MBA, MCTS, MPH, MS, MSN, DNP, PhD, CCTS, Ed S, Post-Master's Certificate. Part-time programs available. Postbaccalaureate distance learning degree programs offered (no on-campus study). *Faculty:* 225 full-time (74 women), 7 part-time/adjunct (4 women). *Students:* 642 full-time (477 women), 384 part-time (295 women); includes 306 minority (170 Black or African American, non-Hispanic/Latino; 86 Asian, non-Hispanic/Latino; 35 Hispanic/Latino; 15 Two or more races, non-Hispanic/Latino), 85 international. Average age 32. 451 applicants, 44% accepted, 125 enrolled. In 2013, 104 master's, 33 doctorates awarded. *Degree requirements:* For doctorate, thesis/dissertation. *Entrance requirements:* For master's and doctorate, GRE General Test. Additional exam requirements/recommendations for international students: Required—TOEFL. Application fee: $50. Electronic applications accepted. *Financial support:* In 2013–14, 10 fellowships with partial tuition reimbursements (averaging $26,000 per year), 111 research assistantships with partial tuition reimbursements (averaging $23,000 per year) were awarded; teaching assistantships, career-related internships or fieldwork, Federal Work-Study, institutionally sponsored loans, scholarships/grants, traineeships, and unspecified assistantships also available. Support available to part-time students. Financial award application deadline: 5/31; financial award applicants required to submit FAFSA. *Faculty research:* Cancer, cardiovascular biology, neurosciences, inflammation/infection, diabetes. *Total annual research expenditures:* $331,986. *Unit head:* Dr. Gretchen B. Caughman, Dean, 706-721-3278, Fax: 706-721-6829, E-mail: gcaughma@mail.mcg.edu. *Application contact:* Heather Metress, Interim Director of Admissions, 706-721-2725, Fax: 706-721-7279, E-mail: hmetress@georgiahealth.edu.
Website: http://www.gru.edu/gradstudies/index.php

Georgia Southern University, Jack N. Averitt College of Graduate Studies, College of Science and Mathematics, Department of Biology, Statesboro, GA 30460. Offers MS. Part-time programs available. *Faculty:* 30 full-time (8 women). *Students:* 50 full-time (32 women), 12 part-time (6 women); includes 9 minority (2 Black or African American, non-Hispanic/Latino; 1 American Indian or Alaska Native, non-Hispanic/Latino; 1 Asian, non-Hispanic/Latino; 4 Hispanic/Latino; 1 Two or more races, non-Hispanic/Latino). Average age 26. 35 applicants, 51% accepted, 15 enrolled. In 2013, 13 master's awarded. *Degree requirements:* For master's, comprehensive exam, thesis optional, terminal exam. *Entrance requirements:* For master's, GRE General Test, GRE Subject Test (preferred), minimum GPA of 2.8, BS in biology, 2 letters of reference. Additional exam requirements/recommendations for international students: Required—TOEFL (minimum score 550 paper-based; 80 iBT). *Application deadline:* For fall admission, 3/1 priority date for domestic and international students; for spring admission, 10/1 priority date for domestic students, 10/1 for international students. Applications are processed on a rolling basis. Application fee: $50. Electronic applications accepted. *Expenses:* Tuition, state resident: full-time $7068; part-time $270 per semester hour. Tuition, nonresident: full-time $26,446; part-time $1077 per semester hour. *Required fees:* $2092. *Financial support:* In 2013–14, 36 students received support, including research assistantships with partial tuition reimbursements available (averaging $10,000 per year), teaching assistantships with partial tuition reimbursements available (averaging $10,000 per year); career-related internships or fieldwork, Federal Work-Study, scholarships/grants, tuition waivers (partial), and unspecified assistantships also available. Support available to part-time students. Financial award application deadline: 4/15; financial award applicants required to submit FAFSA. *Faculty research:* Behavior, evolution and ecology, molecular biology, physiology, parasitology, vector-borne diseases, natural resources, coastal plain science. *Total annual research expenditures:* $420,563. *Unit head:* Dr. Stephen Vives, Department Chair, 912-478-5487, Fax: 912-478-0845, E-mail: svives@georgiasouthern.edu. *Application contact:* Amanda Gilliland, Coordinator for Graduate Student Recruitment, 912-478-5384, Fax: 912-478-0740, E-mail: gradadmissions@georgiasouthern.edu.
Website: http://www.bio.georgiasouthern.edu

Georgia State University, College of Arts and Sciences, Department of Biology, Atlanta, GA 30302-3083. Offers applied and environmental microbiology (MS, PhD), including applied and environmental microbiology, bioinformatics (MS); cellular and molecular biology and physiology (MS, PhD), including bioinformatics (MS), cellular and molecular biology and physiology; molecular genetics and biochemistry (MS, PhD), including bioinformatics (MS), molecular genetics and biochemistry; neurobiology and behavior (MS, PhD), including bioinformatics (MS), neurobiology and behavior. Part-time programs available. *Faculty:* 39 full-time (15 women). *Students:* 242 full-time (154 women), 31 part-time (21 women); includes 113 minority (60 Black or African American, non-Hispanic/Latino; 34 Asian, non-Hispanic/Latino; 10 Hispanic/Latino; 9 Two or more races, non-Hispanic/Latino), 76 international. Average age 28. 242 applicants, 58% accepted, 103 enrolled. In 2013, 87 master's, 15 doctorates awarded. Terminal master's awarded for partial completion of doctoral program. *Degree requirements:* For master's, comprehensive exam (for some programs), thesis optional; for doctorate, comprehensive exam, thesis/dissertation. *Entrance requirements:* For master's, GRE. Additional exam requirements/recommendations for international students: Required—

TOEFL (minimum score 550 paper-based; 82 iBT) or IELTS (minimum score 7). *Application deadline:* For fall admission, 6/1 priority date for domestic and international students; for spring admission, 10/1 priority date for domestic and international students. Applications are processed on a rolling basis. Application fee: $50. Electronic applications accepted. *Expenses: Tuition, area resident:* Full-time $4176; part-time $348 per credit hour. Tuition, state resident: full-time $14,544; part-time $1212 per credit hour. Tuition, nonresident: full-time $14,544; part-time $1212 per credit hour. Tuition and fees vary according to course load and program. *Financial support:* In 2013–14, fellowships with full tuition reimbursements (averaging $2,200 per year), research assistantships with full tuition reimbursements (averaging $20,000 per year), teaching assistantships with full tuition reimbursements (averaging $5,400 per year) were awarded; unspecified assistantships also available. Financial award application deadline: 3/1. *Faculty research:* Applied and environmental microbiology, cell biology and immunology, molecular pathogenesis, protein modeling, neurobiology and behavior. *Unit head:* Dr. Sidney Crow, Professor and Chair, 404-413-5300, E-mail: scrow@gsu.edu. *Application contact:* Ritu Aneja, Director of Graduate Studies, 404-413-5300, Fax: 404-413-5301, E-mail: raneja@gsu.edu.
Website: http://biology.gsu.edu/

Georgia State University, College of Arts and Sciences, MD/PhD Program, Atlanta, GA 30302-3083. Offers MD/PhD. *Expenses: Tuition, area resident:* Full-time $4176; part-time $348 per credit hour. Tuition, state resident: full-time $14,544; part-time $1212 per credit hour. Tuition, nonresident: full-time $14,544; part-time $1212 per credit hour. Tuition and fees vary according to course load and program. *Unit head:* Dr. William J. Long, Dean, 404-413-5114, Fax: 404-413-5117, E-mail: long@gsu.edu. *Application contact:* Amber Amari, Director, Graduate and Scheduling Services, 404-413-5037, E-mail: aamari@gsu.edu.

Georgia State University, College of Education, Department of Middle and Secondary Education, Atlanta, GA 30302-3083. Offers curriculum and instruction (Ed D); English education (MAT); mathematics education (M Ed, MAT); middle level education (MAT); reading, language and literacy education (M Ed, MAT), including reading instruction (M Ed); science education (M Ed, MAT), including biology (MAT), broad field science (MAT), chemistry (MAT), earth science (MAT), physics (MAT); social studies education (M Ed, MAT), including economics (MAT), geography (MAT), history (MAT), political science (MAT); teaching and learning (PhD), including language and literacy, mathematics education, music education, science education, social studies education, teaching and teacher education. *Accreditation:* NCATE. Part-time and evening/weekend programs available. Postbaccalaureate distance learning degree programs offered (minimal on-campus study). *Faculty:* 27 full-time (19 women). *Students:* 181 full-time (113 women), 203 part-time (145 women); includes 161 minority (127 Black or African American, non-Hispanic/Latino; 1 American Indian or Alaska Native, non-Hispanic/Latino; 10 Asian, non-Hispanic/Latino; 11 Hispanic/Latino; 1 Native Hawaiian or other Pacific Islander, non-Hispanic/Latino; 11 Two or more races, non-Hispanic/Latino), 9 international. Average age 36. 2 applicants, 50% accepted, 1 enrolled. In 2013, 213 master's, 17 doctorates awarded. *Degree requirements:* For master's, comprehensive exam (for some programs), thesis or alternative, exit portfolio; for doctorate, comprehensive exam, thesis/dissertation. *Entrance requirements:* For master's, GRE; GACE I (for initial teacher preparation programs), baccalaureate degree or equivalent, resume, goals statement, two letters of recommendation, minimum undergraduate GPA of 2.5; proof of initial teacher certification in the content area (for M Ed); for doctorate, GRE, resume, goals statement, writing sample, two letters of recommendation, minimum graduate GPA of 3.3, interview. Additional exam requirements/recommendations for international students: Required—TOEFL (minimum score 550 paper-based; 79 iBT) or IELTS (minimum score 6.5). *Application deadline:* For fall admission, 1/15 priority date for domestic and international students; for spring admission, 10/1 for domestic and international students. Application fee: $50. Electronic applications accepted. *Expenses: Tuition, area resident:* Full-time $4176; part-time $348 per credit hour. Tuition, state resident: full-time $14,544; part-time $1212 per credit hour. Tuition, nonresident: full-time $14,544; part-time $1212 per credit hour. Tuition and fees vary according to course load and program. *Financial support:* In 2013–14, fellowships with full tuition reimbursements (averaging $19,667 per year), research assistantships with full tuition reimbursements (averaging $5,436 per year), teaching assistantships with full tuition reimbursements (averaging $2,779 per year) were awarded; career-related internships or fieldwork, Federal Work-Study, scholarships/grants, health care benefits, tuition waivers (full and partial), and unspecified assistantships also available. Financial award application deadline: 3/15. *Faculty research:* Teacher education in language and literacy, mathematics, science, and social studies in urban middle and secondary school settings; learning technologies in school, community, and corporate settings; multicultural education and education for social justice; urban education; international education. *Unit head:* Dr. Dana L. Fox, Chair, 404-413-8060, Fax: 404-413-8063, E-mail: dfox@gsu.edu. *Application contact:* Bobbie Turner, Administrative Coordinator I, 404-413-8405, Fax: 404-413-8063, E-mail: bnturner@gsu.edu.
Website: http://mse.education.gsu.edu/

Gerstner Sloan-Kettering Graduate School of Biomedical Sciences, Program in Cancer Biology, New York, NY 10021. Offers PhD. *Faculty:* 134 full-time (23 women). *Students:* 64 full-time (32 women); includes 6 minority (1 Black or African American, non-Hispanic/Latino; 4 Asian, non-Hispanic/Latino; 1 Hispanic/Latino), 4 international. *Degree requirements:* For doctorate, thesis/dissertation. *Entrance requirements:* For doctorate, GRE, transcripts, three letters of recommendation. Additional exam requirements/recommendations for international students: Required—TOEFL. *Application deadline:* For fall admission, 12/1 for domestic students. Electronic applications accepted. *Financial support:* Fellowship package including stipend ($33,773), full-tuition scholarship, first-year allowance, and comprehensive medical and dental insurance available. *Faculty research:* Biochemistry and molecular biology, biophysics/structural biology, computational biology, genetics, immunology. *Unit head:* Linda Burnley, Associate Dean, 646-888-6639, E-mail: burnleyl@sloankettering.edu. *Application contact:* Main Office, 646-888-6639, Fax: 646-422-2351, E-mail: gradstudies@sloankettering.edu.

See Display on page 188 and Close-Up on page 237.

Goucher College, Post-Baccalaureate Premedical Program, Baltimore, MD 21204-2794. Offers Certificate. *Faculty:* 10 full-time (4 women). *Students:* 34 full-time (20 women). Average age 25. 381 applicants, 12% accepted, 32 enrolled. *Entrance requirements:* For degree, GRE, SAT or ACT. *Application deadline:* Applications are processed on a rolling basis. Application fee: $60. *Expenses:* Contact institution. *Financial support:* In 2013–14, 6 students received support, including 8 fellowships (averaging $4,000 per year); institutionally sponsored loans and scholarships/grants also available. Financial award application deadline: 3/1; financial award applicants required to submit FAFSA. *Unit head:* Betsy Merideth, Director, 800-414-3437, Fax: 410-337-6461, E-mail: bmerideth@goucher.edu. *Application contact:* Theresa Reifsnider, Program Assistant, 800-414-3437, Fax: 410-337-6461, E-mail: pbpm@goucher.edu.
Website: http://www.goucher.edu/postbac/

The Graduate Center, City University of New York, Graduate Studies, Program in Biology, New York, NY 10016-4039. Offers PhD. *Degree requirements:* For doctorate, thesis/dissertation, teaching experience. *Entrance requirements:* For doctorate, GRE General Test. Additional exam requirements/recommendations for international students: Required—TOEFL. Electronic applications accepted.

Grand Valley State University, College of Liberal Arts and Sciences, Biology Department, Allendale, MI 49401-9403. Offers MS. Part-time programs available. *Degree requirements:* For master's, comprehensive exam, thesis or alternative. *Entrance requirements:* For master's, GRE General Test, 3 letters of reference. Additional exam requirements/recommendations for international students: Required—TOEFL. Electronic applications accepted. *Faculty research:* Natural resources conservation biology, aquatic sciences, terrestrial ecology, behavioral biology.

Grand Valley State University, College of Liberal Arts and Sciences, Department of Biomedical Sciences, Allendale, MI 49401-9403. Offers MHS. Part-time programs available. *Degree requirements:* For master's, thesis, qualifying exam. *Entrance requirements:* For master's, GRE General Test, minimum GPA of 3.0. Additional exam requirements/recommendations for international students: Required—TOEFL. Electronic applications accepted. *Faculty research:* Cell regulation, neurobiology, parasitology, virology, microbial pathogenicity.

Hampton University, Graduate College, Department of Biological Sciences, Hampton, VA 23668. Offers biology (MS); environmental science (MS); medical science (MS). Part-time and evening/weekend programs available. *Degree requirements:* For master's, thesis optional. *Entrance requirements:* For master's, GRE General Test. *Faculty research:* Marine ecology, microbial and chemical pollution, pesticide problems.

Harvard University, Extension School, Cambridge, MA 02138-3722. Offers applied sciences (CAS); biotechnology (ALM); educational technologies (ALM); educational technology (CET); English for graduate and professional studies (DGP); environmental management (ALM, CEM); information technology (ALM); journalism (ALM); liberal arts (ALM); management (ALM, CM); mathematics for teaching (ALM); museum studies (ALM); premedical studies (Diploma); publication and communication (CPC). Part-time and evening/weekend programs available. *Degree requirements:* For master's, thesis. *Entrance requirements:* For master's, 3 completed graduate courses with grade of B or higher. Additional exam requirements/recommendations for international students: Required—TOEFL (minimum score 600 paper-based), TWE (minimum score 5). *Expenses:* Contact institution.

Harvard University, Graduate School of Arts and Sciences, Department of Organismic and Evolutionary Biology, Cambridge, MA 02138. Offers biology (PhD). *Degree requirements:* For doctorate, 2 foreign languages, public presentation of thesis research, exam. *Entrance requirements:* For doctorate, GRE General Test, GRE Subject Test (recommended), 7 courses in biology, chemistry, physics, mathematics, computer science, or geology. Additional exam requirements/recommendations for international students: Required—TOEFL. *Expenses: Tuition:* Full-time $38,888. *Required fees:* $958. Tuition and fees vary according to campus/location, program and student level.

Harvard University, Graduate School of Arts and Sciences, Division of Medical Sciences, Boston, MA 02115. Offers biological chemistry and molecular pharmacology (PhD); cell biology (PhD); genetics (PhD); microbiology and molecular genetics (PhD); pathology (PhD), including experimental pathology. *Degree requirements:* For doctorate, thesis/dissertation. *Entrance requirements:* For doctorate, GRE General Test, GRE Subject Test. Additional exam requirements/recommendations for international students: Required—TOEFL. *Expenses: Tuition:* Full-time $38,888. *Required fees:* $958. Tuition and fees vary according to campus/location, program and student level.

Harvard University, Harvard School of Public Health, PhD Program in Biological Sciences in Public Health, Boston, MA 02115. Offers PhD. *Faculty:* 22 full-time (9 women), 28 part-time/adjunct (6 women). *Students:* 55 full-time (39 women); includes 13 minority (4 Black or African American, non-Hispanic/Latino; 3 Asian, non-Hispanic/Latino; 3 Hispanic/Latino; 3 Two or more races, non-Hispanic/Latino), 15 international. Average age 27. 438 applicants, 12% accepted, 40 enrolled. In 2013, 32 doctorates awarded. *Degree requirements:* For doctorate, qualifying examination, dissertation/defense. *Entrance requirements:* For doctorate, GRE General Test. Additional exam requirements/recommendations for international students: Required—TOEFL. *Application deadline:* For fall admission, 12/8 for domestic students. *Expenses: Tuition:* Full-time $38,888. *Required fees:* $958. Tuition and fees vary according to campus/location, program and student level. *Financial support:* Fellowships, research assistantships, teaching assistantships, institutionally sponsored loans, and tuition waivers (full) available. Financial award application deadline: 1/1. *Faculty research:* Nutrition biochemistry, molecular and cellular toxicology, cardiovascular disease, cancer biology, immunology and infectious diseases, environmental health physiology. *Unit head:* Carole Knapp, Administrator, 617-432-2932.

Hofstra University, College of Liberal Arts and Sciences, Department of Biology, Hempstead, NY 11549. Offers biology (MA, MS); urban ecology (MA, MS).

Hofstra University, School of Education, Programs in Teaching - Secondary Education, Hempstead, NY 11549. Offers business education (MS Ed); education technology (Advanced Certificate); English education (MA, MS Ed); foreign language and TESOL (MS Ed); foreign language education (MA, MS Ed), including French, German, Russian, Spanish; mathematics education (MA, MS Ed); science education (MA, MS Ed), including biology, chemistry, earth science, geology, physics; secondary education (Advanced Certificate); social studies education (MA, MS Ed); technology for learning (MA).

Hood College, Graduate School, Program in Biomedical Science, Frederick, MD 21701-8575. Offers biomedical science (MS), including biotechnology/molecular biology, microbiology/immunology/virology, regulatory compliance; regulatory compliance (Certificate). Part-time and evening/weekend programs available. *Faculty:* 3 full-time (1 woman), 14 part-time/adjunct (6 women). *Students:* 5 full-time (2 women), 91 part-time (57 women); includes 17 minority (10 Black or African American, non-Hispanic/Latino; 4 Asian, non-Hispanic/Latino; 2 Hispanic/Latino; 1 Two or more races, non-Hispanic/Latino), 6 international. Average age 31. 60 applicants, 52% accepted, 21 enrolled. In 2013, 12 master's, 4 other advanced degrees awarded. *Degree requirements:* For master's, comprehensive exam, thesis or alternative. *Entrance requirements:* For master's, bachelor's degree in biology; minimum GPA of 2.75; undergraduate course work in cell biology, chemistry, organic chemistry, and genetics. Additional exam requirements/recommendations for international students: Required—TOEFL (minimum score 575 paper-based; 89 iBT), IELTS (minimum score 6.5). *Application deadline:* For fall admission, 7/15 priority date for domestic students, 7/15 for international students; for spring admission, 12/1 priority date for domestic students, 12/1 for international students. Applications are processed on a rolling basis. Application fee: $35. Electronic applications accepted. Application fee is waived when completed online. *Expenses: Tuition:* Part-time $405 per credit. *Required fees:* $100 per semester. *Financial support:* In 2013–14, 3 students received support, including 3 research assistantships with full tuition reimbursements available (averaging $10,609 per year); tuition waivers (partial) and unspecified assistantships also available. Financial award applicants required to submit FAFSA. *Unit head:* Dr. Rachel Bagni, Director, 301-696-3650, Fax: 301-696-3597, E-mail: bagni@hood.edu. *Application contact:* Dr. Maria

Biological and Biomedical Sciences—General

Green Cowles, Dean of Graduate School, 301-696-3811, Fax: 301-696-3597, E-mail: gofurther@hood.edu.
Website: http://www.hood.edu/graduate

Howard University, Graduate School, Department of Biology, Washington, DC 20059-0002. Offers MS, PhD. Part-time programs available. *Degree requirements:* For master's, thesis, qualifying exams; for doctorate, thesis/dissertation, qualifying exams. *Entrance requirements:* For master's and doctorate, GRE General Test, minimum GPA of 3.0. Additional exam requirements/recommendations for international students: Required—TOEFL. Electronic applications accepted. *Faculty research:* Physiology, molecular biology, cell biology, microbiology, environmental biology.

Humboldt State University, Academic Programs, College of Natural Resources and Sciences, Department of Biological Sciences, Arcata, CA 95521-8299. Offers MA. *Degree requirements:* For master's, project or thesis. *Entrance requirements:* For master's, GRE General Test, appropriate bachelor's degree, minimum GPA of 2.5, 3 letters of recommendation. Additional exam requirements/recommendations for international students: Required—TOEFL (minimum score 500 paper-based). *Faculty research:* Plant ecology, DNA sequencing, invertebrates.

Hunter College of the City University of New York, Graduate School, School of Arts and Sciences, Department of Biological Sciences, New York, NY 10065-5085. Offers MA, PhD. PhD offered jointly with Graduate School and University Center of the City University of New York. Part-time programs available. *Faculty:* 15 full-time (8 women). *Students:* 8 full-time (5 women), 20 part-time (14 women); includes 13 minority (2 Black or African American, non-Hispanic/Latino; 8 Asian, non-Hispanic/Latino; 3 Hispanic/Latino), 3 international. Average age 26. 29 applicants, 62% accepted, 8 enrolled. In 2013, 29 master's awarded. Terminal master's awarded for partial completion of doctoral program. *Degree requirements:* For master's, one foreign language, comprehensive exam or thesis. *Entrance requirements:* For master's, GRE, 1 year of course work in organic chemistry (including laboratory), college physics, calculus; undergraduate major in biology, botany, physiology, zoology, chemistry or physics. Additional exam requirements/recommendations for international students: Required—TOEFL. *Application deadline:* For fall admission, 4/1 for domestic students, 2/1 for international students; for spring admission, 11/1 for domestic students, 9/1 for international students. Application fee: $125. *Financial support:* Fellowships, research assistantships, teaching assistantships, scholarships/grants, and tuition waivers (partial) available. Support available to part-time students. *Faculty research:* Analysis of prokaryotic and eukaryotic DNA, protein structure, mammalian DNA replication, oncogene expression, neuroscience. *Unit head:* Dr. Shirley Raps, Chairperson, 212-772-5293, E-mail: raps@genectr.hunter.cuny.edu. *Application contact:* William Zlata, Director for Graduate Admissions, 212-772-4482, Fax: 212-650-3336, E-mail: admissions@hunter.cuny.edu.

Icahn School of Medicine at Mount Sinai, Graduate School of Biological Sciences, New York, NY 10029-6504. Offers biomedical sciences (MS, PhD); clinical research education (MS, PhD); community medicine (MPH); genetic counseling (MS); neurosciences (PhD); MD/PhD. Terminal master's awarded for partial completion of doctoral program. *Degree requirements:* For master's, thesis; for doctorate, comprehensive exam, thesis/dissertation. *Entrance requirements:* For master's, GRE General Test; for doctorate, GRE General Test, GRE Subject Test, 3 years of college pre-med course work. Additional exam requirements/recommendations for international students: Required—TOEFL. Electronic applications accepted. *Faculty research:* Cancer, genetics and genomics, immunology, neuroscience, developmental and stem cell biology, translational research.

Idaho State University, Office of Graduate Studies, College of Science and Engineering, Department of Biological Sciences, Pocatello, ID 83209-8007. Offers biology (MNS, MS, DA, PhD); clinical laboratory science (MS); microbiology (MS). *Accreditation:* NAACLS. Part-time programs available. *Degree requirements:* For master's, comprehensive exam, thesis; for doctorate, comprehensive exam, thesis/dissertation, 9 credits of internship (for DA). *Entrance requirements:* For master's, GRE General Test, minimum GPA of 3.0 in all upper division classes; for doctorate, GRE General Test, GRE Subject Test (biology), diagnostic exam (DA), minimum GPA of 3.0 in all upper division classes. Additional exam requirements/recommendations for international students: Required—TOEFL (minimum score 550 paper-based; 80 iBT). Electronic applications accepted. *Faculty research:* Ecology, plant and animal physiology, plant and animal developmental biology, immunology, molecular biology, bioinfomatics.

Illinois Institute of Technology, Graduate College, College of Science and Letters, Department of Biological and Chemical Sciences, Biology Division, Chicago, IL 60616. Offers biochemistry (MBS, MS); biology (PhD); biotechnology (MBS, MS); cell and molecular biology (MBS, MS); microbiology (MB, MS); molecular biochemistry and biophysics (PhD); molecular biology and biophysics (MS). Part-time and evening/weekend programs available. Postbaccalaureate distance learning degree programs offered (minimal on-campus study). Terminal master's awarded for partial completion of doctoral program. *Degree requirements:* For master's, comprehensive exam, thesis (for some programs); for doctorate, comprehensive exam, thesis/dissertation. *Entrance requirements:* For master's, GRE General Test (minimum score 1000 Quantitative and Verbal, 2.5 Analytical Writing), minimum undergraduate GPA of 3.0; for doctorate, GRE General Test (minimum score 1200 Quantitative and Verbal, 3.0 Analytical Writing), minimum undergraduate GPA of 3.0. Additional exam requirements/recommendations for international students: Required—TOEFL (minimum score 523 paper-based; 70 iBT); Recommended—IELTS (minimum score 5.5). Electronic applications accepted. *Faculty research:* Structure and biophysics of macromolecular systems; efficacy and mechanism of action of chemopreventive agents in experimental carcinogenesis of breast, colon, lung and prostate; study of fundamental structural biochemistry problems that have direct links to the understanding and treatment of disease; spectroscopic techniques for the study of multi-domain proteins; molecular mechanisms of cancer and cancer gene therapy.

Illinois State University, Graduate School, College of Arts and Sciences, Department of Biological Sciences, Normal, IL 61790-2200. Offers animal behavior (MS); bacteriology (MS); biochemistry (MS); biological sciences (MS); biology (PhD); biophysics (MS); biotechnology (MS); botany (MS, PhD); cell biology (MS); conservation biology (MS); developmental biology (MS); ecology (MS, PhD); entomology (MS); evolutionary biology (MS); genetics (MS, PhD); immunology (MS); microbiology (MS, PhD); molecular biology (MS); molecular genetics (MS); neurobiology (MS); neuroscience (MS); parasitology (MS); physiology (MS, PhD); plant biology (MS); plant molecular biology (MS); plant sciences (MS); structural biology (MS); zoology (MS, PhD). Part-time programs available. *Degree requirements:* For master's, thesis or alternative; for doctorate, variable foreign language requirement, thesis/dissertation, 2 terms of residency. *Entrance requirements:* For master's, GRE General Test, minimum GPA of 2.6 in last 60 hours of course work; for doctorate, GRE General Test. *Faculty research:* Redoc balance and drug development in schistosoma mansoni, control of the growth of listeria monocytogenes at low temperature, regulation of cell expansion and microtubule function by SPRI, CRUI: physiology and fitness consequences of different life history phenotypes.

Indiana State University, College of Graduate and Professional Studies, College of Arts and Sciences, Department of Biology, Terre Haute, IN 47809. Offers ecology (PhD); life sciences (MS); microbiology (PhD); physiology (PhD); science education (MS). *Faculty:* 23 full-time (6 women), 1 (woman) part-time/adjunct. *Students:* 73 full-time (31 women), 15 part-time (6 women); includes 7 minority (6 Asian, non-Hispanic/Latino; 1 Hispanic/Latino), 17 international. Average age 26. 63 applicants, 65% accepted, 40 enrolled. In 2013, 9 master's, 5 doctorates awarded. *Degree requirements:* For master's, thesis (for some programs); for doctorate, comprehensive exam, thesis/dissertation. *Entrance requirements:* For master's and doctorate, GRE General Test. *Application deadline:* For fall admission, 7/1 priority date for domestic students; for spring admission, 11/1 priority date for domestic students. Applications are processed on a rolling basis. Application fee: $35. Electronic applications accepted. *Financial support:* In 2013–14, 9 research assistantships with partial tuition reimbursements (averaging $7,500 per year), 19 teaching assistantships with partial tuition reimbursements (averaging $8,000 per year) were awarded; Federal Work-Study, institutionally sponsored loans, and tuition waivers (partial) also available. Financial award application deadline: 3/1; financial award applicants required to submit FAFSA. *Unit head:* Dr. Arthur M. Halpern, Interim Chairperson, 812-237-2400. *Application contact:* Dr. Jay Gatrell, Dean, 800-444-GRAD, Fax: 812-237-8060, E-mail: jay.gatrell@indstate.edu.

Indiana University Bloomington, University Graduate School, College of Arts and Sciences, Department of Biology, Bloomington, IN 47405. Offers biology teaching (MAT); biotechnology (MA); evolution, ecology, and behavior (MA, PhD); genetics (PhD); microbiology (MA, PhD); molecular, cellular, and developmental biology (PhD); plant sciences (MA, PhD); zoology (MA, PhD). *Faculty:* 58 full-time (15 women), 21 part-time/adjunct (6 women). *Students:* 166 full-time (94 women), 2 part-time (both women); includes 22 minority (8 Black or African American, non-Hispanic/Latino; 3 Asian, non-Hispanic/Latino; 10 Hispanic/Latino; 1 Two or more races, non-Hispanic/Latino), 47 international. Average age 27. 261 applicants, 23% accepted, 32 enrolled. In 2013, 17 master's, 20 doctorates awarded. Terminal master's awarded for partial completion of doctoral program. *Degree requirements:* For master's, thesis, oral defense; for doctorate, thesis/dissertation, oral defense. *Entrance requirements:* For master's and doctorate, GRE General Test. Additional exam requirements/recommendations for international students: Required—TOEFL (minimum score 100 iBT). *Application deadline:* For fall admission, 1/5 priority date for domestic students, 12/1 priority date for international students. Application fee: $55 ($65 for international students). Electronic applications accepted. *Financial support:* In 2013–14, fellowships with tuition reimbursements (averaging $24,000 per year), research assistantships with tuition reimbursements (averaging $21,000 per year), teaching assistantships with tuition reimbursements (averaging $22,000 per year) were awarded; scholarships/grants, traineeships, health care benefits, and unspecified assistantships also available. Financial award application deadline: 1/5. *Faculty research:* Evolution, ecology and behavior; microbiology; molecular biology and genetics; plant biology. *Unit head:* Dr. Clay Fuqua, Chair, 812-856-6005, Fax: 812-855-6082, E-mail: cfuqua@indiana.edu. *Application contact:* Tracey D. Stohr, Graduate Student Recruitment Coordinator, 812-856-6303, Fax: 812-855-6082, E-mail: gradbio@indiana.edu.
Website: http://www.bio.indiana.edu/

Indiana University of Pennsylvania, School of Graduate Studies and Research, College of Natural Sciences and Mathematics, Department of Biology, Program in Biology, Indiana, PA 15705-1087. Offers MS. Part-time programs available. *Faculty:* 12 full-time (3 women). *Students:* 25 full-time (12 women), 4 part-time (2 women); includes 2 minority (both Black or African American, non-Hispanic/Latino), 9 international. Average age 28. 43 applicants, 28% accepted, 8 enrolled. In 2013, 8 master's awarded. *Degree requirements:* For master's, comprehensive exam, thesis optional. *Entrance requirements:* For master's, 2 letters of recommendation. Additional exam requirements/recommendations for international students: Required—TOEFL (minimum score 550 paper-based). *Application deadline:* Applications are processed on a rolling basis. Application fee: $50. Electronic applications accepted. *Expenses:* Tuition, state resident: full-time $3978; part-time $442 per credit. Tuition, nonresident: full-time $5967; part-time $663 per credit. *Required fees:* $2080; $115.55 per credit. $93 per semester. Tuition and fees vary according to degree level and program. *Financial support:* In 2013–14, 1 fellowship with full tuition reimbursement (averaging $1,000 per year), 7 research assistantships with full and partial tuition reimbursements (averaging $4,978 per year) were awarded; career-related internships or fieldwork, Federal Work-Study, scholarships/grants, and unspecified assistantships also available. Financial award application deadline: 4/15; financial award applicants required to submit FAFSA. *Unit head:* Dr. Joe Duchamp, Graduate Coordinator, 724-357-1299, E-mail: jduchamp@iup.edu.
Website: http://www.iup.edu/grad/biology/default.aspx

Indiana University–Purdue University Fort Wayne, College of Arts and Sciences, Department of Biology, Fort Wayne, IN 46805-1499. Offers MS. Part-time and evening/weekend programs available. *Faculty:* 16 full-time (2 women), 1 (woman) part-time/adjunct. *Students:* 13 full-time (9 women), 16 part-time (9 women); includes 2 minority (both Hispanic/Latino), 4 international. Average age 26. 16 applicants, 88% accepted, 8 enrolled. In 2013, 18 master's awarded. *Degree requirements:* For master's, thesis optional. *Entrance requirements:* For master's, GRE General Test, minimum GPA of 3.0, major or minor in biology, three letters of recommendation. Additional exam requirements/recommendations for international students: Required—TOEFL (minimum score 550 paper-based; 79 iBT), TWE. *Application deadline:* For fall admission, 4/15 priority date for domestic students, 2/15 priority date for international students; for spring admission, 8/15 priority date for domestic and international students. Applications are processed on a rolling basis. Application fee: $55 ($60 for international students). Electronic applications accepted. *Financial support:* In 2013–14, 2 research assistantships with partial tuition reimbursements (averaging $13,322 per year), 17 teaching assistantships with partial tuition reimbursements (averaging $13,322 per year) were awarded; scholarships/grants and unspecified assistantships also available. Support available to part-time students. Financial award application deadline: 3/1; financial award applicants required to submit FAFSA. *Faculty research:* Agaronia propatula, biological hypothesis testing, Pacific leatherback turtles. *Total annual research expenditures:* $107,985. *Unit head:* Dr. Frank Paladino, Chair/Professor, 260-481-6304, Fax: 260-481-6087, E-mail: paladino@ipfw.edu.
Website: http://www.ipfw.edu/biology

Indiana University–Purdue University Indianapolis, School of Science, Department of Biology, Indianapolis, IN 46202-2896. Offers MS, PhD. PhD offered jointly with Purdue University. Part-time and evening/weekend programs available. *Faculty:* 7 full-time (2 women). *Students:* 94 full-time (44 women), 22 part-time (14 women); includes 21 minority (3 Black or African American, non-Hispanic/Latino; 12 Asian, non-Hispanic/Latino; 5 Hispanic/Latino; 1 Two or more races, non-Hispanic/Latino), 26 international. Average age 25. 155 applicants, 49% accepted, 67 enrolled. In 2013, 87 master's awarded. Terminal master's awarded for partial completion of doctoral program. *Degree requirements:* For master's, thesis (for some programs); for doctorate, thesis/dissertation. *Entrance requirements:* For master's and doctorate, GRE General Test. *Application deadline:* For fall admission, 6/1 for domestic students. Application fee: $55 ($65 for international students). *Financial support:* Fellowships with partial tuition reimbursements, research assistantships with partial tuition reimbursements, teaching assistantships with partial tuition reimbursements, and career-related internships or fieldwork available. Financial award application deadline: 4/1. *Faculty research:* Cell and model membranes, cell and molecular biology, immunology, oncology, developmental biology. *Unit head:* Dr. Simon Atkinson, Chair, 317-274-0582. *Application contact:* Xianxhong Wang, Graduate Director, 317-278-5174, E-mail: xzwang@iupui.edu. Website: http://biology.iupui.edu/graduate/degrees

Iowa State University of Science and Technology, Department of Biomedical Sciences, Ames, IA 50011. Offers MS, PhD. *Entrance requirements:* For master's and doctorate, GRE General Test. Additional exam requirements/recommendations for international students: Required—TOEFL (minimum score 590 paper-based; 79 iBT), IELTS (minimum score 6.5). Electronic applications accepted. *Faculty research:* Cerebella research; endocrine physiology; memory, learning and associated diseases; ion-channels and dry resistance; glia-neuron signaling; neurobiology of pain.

Irell & Manella Graduate School of Biological Sciences, Graduate Program, Duarte, CA 91010. Offers PhD. *Degree requirements:* For doctorate, comprehensive exam, thesis/dissertation. *Entrance requirements:* For doctorate, GRE General Test; GRE Subject Test (recommended), 2 years of course work in chemistry (general and organic); 1 year course work each in biochemistry, general biology, and general physics; 2 semesters of course work in mathematics; significant research laboratory experience. Additional exam requirements/recommendations for international students: Required—TOEFL. Electronic applications accepted. *Faculty research:* DNA damage and repair, protein structure, cancer biology, T cells and immunology, RNA splicing and binding.

See Display on this page and Close-Up on page 115.

Jackson State University, Graduate School, College of Science, Engineering and Technology, Department of Biology, Jackson, MS 39217. Offers environmental science (MS, PhD). Part-time and evening/weekend programs available. *Degree requirements:* For master's, comprehensive exam, thesis (alternative accepted for MST); for doctorate, comprehensive exam, thesis/dissertation. *Entrance requirements:* For master's, GRE General Test; for doctorate, MAT. Additional exam requirements/recommendations for international students: Required—TOEFL (minimum score 520 paper-based; 67 iBT). *Faculty research:* Comparative studies on the carbohydrate composition of marine macroalgae, host-parasite relationship between the spruce budworm and entomepathogen fungus.

Jacksonville State University, College of Graduate Studies and Continuing Education, College of Arts and Sciences, Department of Biology, Jacksonville, AL 36265-1602. Offers MS. Part-time and evening/weekend programs available. *Degree requirements:* For master's, comprehensive exam, thesis (for some programs). *Entrance requirements:* For master's, GRE General Test or MAT. Additional exam requirements/recommendations for international students: Required—TOEFL (minimum score 61 iBT). Electronic applications accepted.

James Madison University, The Graduate School, College of Science and Mathematics, Department of Biology, Harrisonburg, VA 22807. Offers MS. Part-time programs available. *Faculty:* 20 full-time (10 women), 1 (woman) part-time/adjunct. *Students:* 17 full-time (8 women), 1 part-time (0 women); includes 3 minority (2 Hispanic/Latino; 1 Two or more races, non-Hispanic/Latino). Average age 27. In 2013, 5 master's awarded. *Degree requirements:* For master's, thesis (for some programs). *Entrance requirements:* For master's, GRE General Test, GRE Subject Test, 3 letters of recommendation. Additional exam requirements/recommendations for international students: Required—TOEFL. *Application deadline:* For fall admission, 2/15 for domestic students. Applications are processed on a rolling basis. Application fee: $55. Electronic applications accepted. *Financial support:* In 2013–14, 15 students received support. Federal Work-Study and 15 graduate assistantships (averaging $7530) available. Financial award application deadline: 3/1; financial award applicants required to submit FAFSA. *Faculty research:* Evolutionary ecology, gene regulation, microbial ecology, plant development, biomechanics. *Unit head:* Dr. Judith A. Dilts, Interim Academic Unit Head, 540-568-3508, E-mail: diltsja@jmu.edu. *Application contact:* Dr. Jon Kastendiek, Interim Graduate Director, 540-568-6225.

John Carroll University, Graduate School, Department of Biology, University Heights, OH 44118-4581. Offers MA, MS. Part-time programs available. *Degree requirements:* For master's, essay or thesis, seminar. *Entrance requirements:* For master's, undergraduate major in biology, 1 semester of biochemistry, minimum 2.5 GPA. Electronic applications accepted. *Faculty research:* Algal ecology, systematics, molecular genetics, neurophysiology, behavioral ecology.

Johns Hopkins University, National Institutes of Health Sponsored Programs, Baltimore, MD 21218-2699. Offers biology (PhD), including biochemistry, biophysics, cell biology, developmental biology, genetic biology, molecular biology; cell, molecular, and developmental biology and biophysics (PhD). *Faculty:* 25 full-time (4 women). *Students:* 126 full-time (72 women); includes 36 minority (3 Black or African American, non-Hispanic/Latino; 1 American Indian or Alaska Native, non-Hispanic/Latino; 21 Asian, non-Hispanic/Latino; 11 Hispanic/Latino), 19 international. 282 applicants, 26% accepted, 36 enrolled. In 2013, 15 doctorates awarded. *Degree requirements:* For doctorate, comprehensive exam, thesis/dissertation. *Entrance requirements:* For doctorate, GRE General Test. Additional exam requirements/recommendations for international students: Required—TOEFL (minimum score 600 paper-based), TWE. *Application deadline:* For fall admission, 12/15 priority date for domestic students. Application fee: $60. Electronic applications accepted. *Financial support:* In 2013–14, 24 fellowships (averaging $23,000 per year), 93 research assistantships (averaging $23,000 per year), 22 teaching assistantships (averaging $23,000 per year) were awarded; Federal Work-Study, institutionally sponsored loans, scholarships/grants, traineeships, health care benefits, tuition waivers (partial), and unspecified assistantships also available. Financial award application deadline: 4/15; financial award applicants required to submit FAFSA. *Faculty research:* Protein and nucleic acid biochemistry and biophysical chemistry, molecular biology and development. *Total annual research expenditures:* $11.2 million. *Unit head:* Dr. Allen Shearn, Chair, 410-516-4693, Fax: 410-516-5213, E-mail: bio_cals@jhu.edu. *Application contact:* Joan Miller, Academic Affairs Manager, 410-516-5502, Fax: 410-516-5213, E-mail: joan@jhu.edu.

Johns Hopkins University, School of Medicine, Graduate Programs in Medicine, Baltimore, MD 21218-2699. Offers MA, PhD, MD/PhD. *Faculty:* 258 full-time (77 women), 31 part-time/adjunct (12 women). *Students:* 831 full-time (412 women); includes 227 minority (32 Black or African American, non-Hispanic/Latino; 2 American Indian or Alaska Native, non-Hispanic/Latino; 127 Asian, non-Hispanic/Latino; 44 Hispanic/Latino; 22 Two or more races, non-Hispanic/Latino), 235 international. Average age 27. 1,850 applicants, 15% accepted, 132 enrolled. In 2013, 27 master's, 137 doctorates awarded. *Degree requirements:* For doctorate, thesis/dissertation. *Entrance requirements:* Additional exam requirements/recommendations for international students: Required—TOEFL. *Application deadline:* For fall admission, 1/10 for domestic students, 1/10 priority date for international students. Application fee: $85. Electronic applications accepted. *Expenses:* Contact institution. *Financial support:* Fellowships, research assistantships, teaching assistantships, career-related internships or fieldwork,

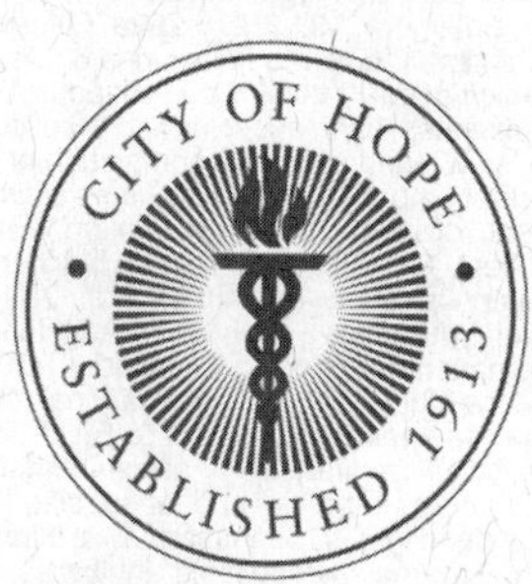

IRELL & MANELLA GRADUATE SCHOOL OF BIOLOGICAL SCIENCES

Earn your doctorate where you and your research will have the greatest impact.

The Irell and Manella Graduate School of Biological Sciences at City of Hope offers a Doctor of Philosophy (Ph.D.) degree in Biological Sciences.

City of Hope ranks in the top 5 percent of U.S. institutions in NIH research funding

TRAIN IN TWO BROADLY DEFINED TRACKS:

Molecular and Cellular Biology
- Stem cell research
- Endocrinology and metabolism
- Chromatin structure and repair
- Tumor biology
- Immunology
- Virology
- Neurosciences

Chemical Biology
- Protein structure
  - X-ray crystallography
  - NMR
  - Computational modeling
- Small molecule synthesis
- Bioconjugate chemistry
- Analytical biological instrumentation

Enjoy a $32,000 stipend per year, plus paid insurance

Publish in top-level journals

Attend national and international meetings

FOR MORE INFORMATION AND TO APPLY, VISIT www.cityofhope.org/gradschool

Biological and Biomedical Sciences—General

Federal Work-Study, institutionally sponsored loans, and tuition waivers (full) available. Financial award applicants required to submit FAFSA.

Johns Hopkins University, Zanvyl Krieger School of Arts and Sciences, Chemistry-Biology Interface Program, Baltimore, MD 21218-2699. Offers PhD. *Faculty:* 32 full-time (7 women). *Students:* 28 full-time (10 women); includes 6 minority (1 American Indian or Alaska Native, non-Hispanic/Latino; 3 Asian, non-Hispanic/Latino; 2 Hispanic/Latino). Average age 26. 83 applicants, 10% accepted, 4 enrolled. In 2013, 4 doctorates awarded. Terminal master's awarded for partial completion of doctoral program. *Degree requirements:* For doctorate, comprehensive exam, thesis/dissertation, 8 one-semester courses, research proposal, graduate board oral exam. *Entrance requirements:* For doctorate, GRE General Test, GRE Subject Test in biochemistry, cell and molecular biology, biology or chemistry (strongly recommended), 3 letters of recommendation, transcripts, statement of purpose, interview. Additional exam requirements/recommendations for international students: Required—TOEFL. *Application deadline:* For fall admission, 1/15 for domestic and international students. Applications are processed on a rolling basis. Application fee: $75. Electronic applications accepted. *Financial support:* Fellowships, teaching assistantships, Federal Work-Study, scholarships/grants, health care benefits, and unspecified assistantships available. Financial award application deadline: 4/15; financial award applicants required to submit FAFSA. *Faculty research:* Enzyme mechanisms, inhibitors, and metabolic pathways; DNA replication, damaged, and repair; using small molecules to probe signal transduction, gene regulation, angiogenesis, and other biological processes; synthetic methods and medicinal chemistry; synthetic modeling of metalloenzymes. *Unit head:* Dr. Steve Rokita, Director, 410-516-5793, Fax: 410-516-8420, E-mail: rokita@jhu.edu. *Application contact:* Lauren McGhee, Academic Coordinator, 410-516-7427, Fax: 410-516-8420, E-mail: lauren.mcghee@jhu.edu.
Website: http://www.cbi.jhu.edu

Johns Hopkins University, Zanvyl Krieger School of Arts and Sciences, Department of Biology, Baltimore, MD 21218. Offers PhD. *Faculty:* 35 full-time (12 women), 8 part-time/adjunct (2 women). *Students:* 105 full-time (57 women); includes 28 minority (2 Black or African American, non-Hispanic/Latino; 17 Asian, non-Hispanic/Latino; 6 Hispanic/Latino; 3 Two or more races, non-Hispanic/Latino), 16 international. Average age 26. 158 applicants, 30% accepted, 19 enrolled. In 2013, 23 doctorates awarded. Terminal master's awarded for partial completion of doctoral program. *Degree requirements:* For doctorate, comprehensive exam, thesis/dissertation. *Entrance requirements:* For doctorate, GRE General Test. Additional exam requirements/recommendations for international students: Required—TOEFL (minimum score 600 paper-based), IELTS, TWE. *Application deadline:* For fall admission, 12/7 for domestic and international students. Application fee: $75. Electronic applications accepted. *Financial support:* In 2013–14, 98 students received support, including 3 fellowships with tuition reimbursements available (averaging $29,218 per year), 81 research assistantships with tuition reimbursements available (averaging $29,218 per year), 38 teaching assistantships with tuition reimbursements available (averaging $29,218 per year); Federal Work-Study, institutionally sponsored loans, scholarships/grants, traineeships, health care benefits, tuition waivers (full), and unspecified assistantships also available. Financial award application deadline: 4/15; financial award applicants required to submit FAFSA. *Faculty research:* Cell biology, molecular biology and development, biochemistry, developmental biology, biophysics, genetics. *Total annual research expenditures:* $7.2 million. *Unit head:* Dr. Beverly R. Wendland, Chair, 410-516-4693, Fax: 410-516-5213, E-mail: bwendland@jhu.edu. *Application contact:* Joan Miller, Academic Affairs Administrator, 410-516-5502, Fax: 410-516-5213, E-mail: joan@jhu.edu.
Website: http://cmdb.jhu.edu

Kansas City University of Medicine and Biosciences, College of Biosciences, Kansas City, MO 64106-1453. Offers bioethics (MA); biomedical sciences (MS). Part-time programs available. *Degree requirements:* For master's, comprehensive exam, thesis (for some programs). *Entrance requirements:* For master's, MCAT, GRE.

Kansas State University, College of Veterinary Medicine, Department of Diagnostic Medicine/Pathobiology, Manhattan, KS 66506. Offers biomedical science (MS); diagnostic medicine/pathobiology (PhD). *Faculty:* 23 full-time (6 women), 5 part-time/adjunct (3 women). *Students:* 30 full-time (11 women), 7 part-time (4 women); includes 3 minority (1 Black or African American, non-Hispanic/Latino; 1 Hispanic/Latino; 1 Native Hawaiian or other Pacific Islander, non-Hispanic/Latino), 15 international. Average age 32. 14 applicants, 29% accepted, 3 enrolled. In 2013, 1 doctorate awarded. Terminal master's awarded for partial completion of doctoral program. *Degree requirements:* For doctorate, thesis/dissertation. *Entrance requirements:* For master's and doctorate, interviews. Additional exam requirements/recommendations for international students: Required—TOEFL (minimum score 550 paper-based). *Application deadline:* For fall admission, 2/1 priority date for domestic and international students; for spring admission, 8/1 priority date for domestic and international students. Applications are processed on a rolling basis. Application fee: $50 ($75 for international students). Electronic applications accepted. *Financial support:* In 2013–14, 22 research assistantships (averaging $21,849 per year) were awarded; Federal Work-Study, institutionally sponsored loans, and scholarships/grants also available. Financial award application deadline: 3/1; financial award applicants required to submit FAFSA. *Faculty research:* Infectious disease of animals, food safety and security, epidemiology and public health, toxicology, pathology. *Total annual research expenditures:* $9.2 million. *Unit head:* M. M. Chengappa, Head, 785-532-4403, E-mail: chengap@ksu.edu. *Application contact:* T. G. Nagaraja, Director, 785-532-1214, E-mail: tnagaraj@ksu.edu.
Website: http://www.vet.k-state.edu/education/dmp/

Kansas State University, Graduate School, College of Arts and Sciences, Division of Biology, Manhattan, KS 66506. Offers biology (MS, PhD); microbiology (PhD). *Faculty:* 73 full-time (18 women), 26 part-time/adjunct (6 women). *Students:* 57 full-time (32 women), 4 part-time (2 women); includes 5 minority (1 Black or African American, non-Hispanic/Latino; 4 Hispanic/Latino), 13 international. Average age 27. 109 applicants, 7% accepted, 5 enrolled. In 2013, 4 master's, 7 doctorates awarded. Terminal master's awarded for partial completion of doctoral program. *Degree requirements:* For master's, thesis; for doctorate, thesis/dissertation. *Entrance requirements:* For master's, GRE General Test, minimum undergraduate GPA of 3.0; for doctorate, GRE General Test, minimum GPA of 3.0. Additional exam requirements/recommendations for international students: Required—TOEFL (minimum score 550 paper-based). *Application deadline:* For fall admission, 12/15 priority date for domestic and international students; for spring admission, 8/1 priority date for domestic and international students. Applications are processed on a rolling basis. Application fee: $50 ($75 for international students). Electronic applications accepted. *Financial support:* In 2013–14, 11 fellowships with full tuition reimbursements (averaging $30,000 per year), 28 research assistantships with full tuition reimbursements (averaging $20,020 per year), 27 teaching assistantships with full tuition reimbursements (averaging $20,020 per year) were awarded; institutionally sponsored loans, scholarships/grants, and health care benefits also available. Support available to part-time students. Financial award application deadline: 3/1; financial award applicants required to submit FAFSA. *Faculty research:* Ecology, genetics, developmental biology, microbiology, cell biology. *Total annual research expenditures:* $9.3 million. *Unit head:* Brian Spooner, Director/Professor, Division of Biology, 785-532-6615, Fax: 785-532-6653, E-mail: biology@ksu.edu. *Application contact:* Dave Rintoul, Graduate Program Director, 785-532-6615, Fax: 785-532-6653, E-mail: drintoul@ksu.edu.
Website: http://www.k-state.edu/biology/

Keck Graduate Institute of Applied Life Sciences, Bioscience Program, Claremont, CA 91711. Offers applied life science (PhD); bioscience (MBS); bioscience management (Certificate); computational systems biology (PhD). *Degree requirements:* For master's, comprehensive exam, project. *Entrance requirements:* For master's, GRE General Test or MCAT. Additional exam requirements/recommendations for international students: Required—TOEFL. Electronic applications accepted. *Faculty research:* Computational biology, drug discovery and development, molecular and cellular biology, biomedical engineering, biomaterials and tissue engineering.

Kennesaw State University, College of Science and Mathematics, Program in Integrative Biology, Kennesaw, GA 30144-5591. Offers MS. *Students:* 12 full-time (6 women), 1 (woman) part-time; includes 1 minority (Hispanic/Latino). Average age 28. 12 applicants, 75% accepted, 7 enrolled. *Degree requirements:* For master's, thesis. *Entrance requirements:* For master's, GRE, two letters of recommendation, official transcript, statement of interest. Additional exam requirements/recommendations for international students: Required—TOEFL (minimum score 550 paper-based; 80 iBT), IELTS (minimum score 6.5). *Application deadline:* For fall admission, 2/1 for domestic and international students. Application fee: $60. Electronic applications accepted. *Expenses:* Tuition, state resident: full-time $4806; part-time $267 per semester hour. Tuition, nonresident: full-time $17,298; part-time $961 per semester hour. *Required fees:* $1834; $784.50 per semester. *Financial support:* In 2013–14, 11 students received support, including 5 research assistantships with full tuition reimbursements available (averaging $12,000 per year); unspecified assistantships also available. Financial award application deadline: 4/1; financial award applicants required to submit FAFSA. *Unit head:* Dr. Joe Dirnberger, Coordinator, 770-423-6546, E-mail: jdirnber@kennesaw.edu. *Application contact:* Admissions Counselor, 770-420-4377, Fax: 770-423-6885, E-mail: ksugrad@kennesaw.edu.
Website: http://biology.kennesaw.edu/MSIB/

Kennesaw State University, Leland and Clarice C. Bagwell College of Education, Program in Teaching, Kennesaw, GA 30144-5591. Offers art education (MAT); biology (MAT); chemistry (MAT); foreign language education (Chinese and Spanish) (MAT); physics (MAT); secondary English (MAT); secondary mathematics (MAT); special education (MAT); teaching English to speakers of other languages (MAT). Part-time and evening/weekend programs available. *Students:* 82 full-time (59 women), 16 part-time (12 women); includes 28 minority (14 Black or African American, non-Hispanic/Latino; 4 Asian, non-Hispanic/Latino; 7 Hispanic/Latino; 1 Native Hawaiian or other Pacific Islander, non-Hispanic/Latino; 2 Two or more races, non-Hispanic/Latino), 3 international. Average age 35. 28 applicants, 68% accepted, 15 enrolled. In 2013, 54 master's awarded. *Entrance requirements:* For master's, GRE, GACE I (state certificate exam), minimum GPA of 2.75, 2 recommendations, resume. Additional exam requirements/recommendations for international students: Required—TOEFL (minimum score 550 paper-based; 80 iBT), IELTS (minimum score 6). *Application deadline:* For fall admission, 6/1 for domestic and international students; for spring admission, 3/1 for domestic and international students; for summer admission, 4/15 for domestic and international students. Applications are processed on a rolling basis. Application fee: $60. Electronic applications accepted. *Expenses:* Tuition, state resident: full-time $4806; part-time $267 per semester hour. Tuition, nonresident: full-time $17,298; part-time $961 per semester hour. *Required fees:* $1834; $784.50 per semester. *Financial support:* In 2013–14, 2 research assistantships with tuition reimbursements (averaging $8,000 per year) were awarded; unspecified assistantships also available. Financial award application deadline: 4/1; financial award applicants required to submit FAFSA. *Unit head:* Dr. Jillian Ford, Director, 770-499-3093, E-mail: graded@kennesaw.edu. *Application contact:* Melinda Ross, Admissions Counselor, 770-423-6122, Fax: 770-423-6885, E-mail: ksugrad@kennesaw.edu.
Website: http://www.kennesaw.edu

Kent State University, College of Arts and Sciences, Department of Biological Sciences, Kent, OH 44242-0001. Offers ecology (MS, PhD); physiology (MS, PhD). *Degree requirements:* For master's, thesis; for doctorate, thesis/dissertation. *Entrance requirements:* For master's, GRE General Test, minimum GPA of 3.0; for doctorate, GRE General Test, minimum GPA of 3.25. Additional exam requirements/recommendations for international students: Required—TOEFL (minimum score 600 paper-based). Electronic applications accepted.

Kent State University, School of Biomedical Sciences, Kent, OH 44242-0001. Offers MS, PhD. Terminal master's awarded for partial completion of doctoral program. *Degree requirements:* For master's, thesis; for doctorate, thesis/dissertation. *Entrance requirements:* For master's and doctorate, GRE General Test. Electronic applications accepted.

Lake Erie College of Osteopathic Medicine, Professional Programs, Erie, PA 16509-1025. Offers biomedical sciences (Postbaccalaureate Certificate); medical education (MS); osteopathic medicine (DO); pharmacy (Pharm D). *Accreditation:* ACPE; AOsA. *Degree requirements:* For doctorate, comprehensive exam, National Osteopathic Medical Licensing Exam, Levels 1 and 2; for Postbaccalaureate Certificate, comprehensive exam, North American Pharmacist Licensure Examination (NAPLEX). *Entrance requirements:* For doctorate, MCAT, minimum GPA of 3.2, letters of recommendation; for Postbaccalaureate Certificate, PCAT, letters of recommendation, minimum GPA of 3.5. Electronic applications accepted. *Faculty research:* Cardiac smooth and skeletal muscle mechanics, chemotherapeutics and vitamins, osteopathic manipulation.

Lakehead University, Graduate Studies, Faculty of Social Sciences and Humanities, Department of Biology, Thunder Bay, ON P7B 5E1, Canada. Offers M Sc. Part-time and evening/weekend programs available. *Degree requirements:* For master's, thesis, department seminary, oral examination. *Entrance requirements:* For master's, minimum B average. Additional exam requirements/recommendations for international students: Required—TOEFL. *Faculty research:* Systematics and biogeography, wildlife parasitology, plant physiology and biochemistry, plant ecology, fishery biology.

Lamar University, College of Graduate Studies, College of Arts and Sciences, Department of Biology, Beaumont, TX 77710. Offers MS. Part-time and evening/weekend programs available. *Degree requirements:* For master's, thesis. *Entrance requirements:* For master's, GRE General Test, minimum GPA of 2.5 in last 60 hours of undergraduate course work. Additional exam requirements/recommendations for international students: Required—TOEFL. *Faculty research:* Microbiology, limnology, vertebrate ecology, invertebrate hemoglobin, ornithology.

Laurentian University, School of Graduate Studies and Research, Programme in Biology, Sudbury, ON P3E 2C6, Canada. Offers biology (M Sc); boreal ecology (PhD). Part-time programs available. *Degree requirements:* For master's, thesis. *Entrance requirements:* For master's, honors degree with second class or better. *Faculty research:* Recovery of acid-stressed lakes, effects of climate change, origin and maintenance of biocomplexity, radionuclide dynamics, cytogenetic studies of plants.

Lehigh University, College of Arts and Sciences, Department of Biological Sciences, Bethlehem, PA 18015. Offers biochemistry (PhD); cell and molecular biology (PhD); integrative biology and neuroscience (PhD); molecular biology (MS). Part-time programs available. Postbaccalaureate distance learning degree programs offered (no on-campus study). *Faculty:* 18 full-time (9 women). *Students:* 38 full-time (20 women), 30 part-time (23 women); includes 8 minority (4 Black or African American, non-Hispanic/Latino; 2 Asian, non-Hispanic/Latino; 2 Hispanic/Latino), 5 international. Average age 29. 54 applicants, 41% accepted, 11 enrolled. In 2013, 8 master's, 5 doctorates awarded. Terminal master's awarded for partial completion of doctoral program. *Degree requirements:* For master's, research report; for doctorate, comprehensive exam, thesis/dissertation. *Entrance requirements:* For doctorate, GRE General Test. Additional exam requirements/recommendations for international students: Required—TOEFL. *Application deadline:* For fall admission, 12/15 for domestic and international students. Applications are processed on a rolling basis. Application fee: $75. Electronic applications accepted. *Financial support:* In 2013–14, 2 fellowships with full tuition reimbursements (averaging $24,500 per year), 8 research assistantships with full tuition reimbursements (averaging $23,750 per year), 20 teaching assistantships with full tuition reimbursements (averaging $23,750 per year) were awarded; scholarships/grants and unspecified assistantships also available. Financial award application deadline: 12/15. *Faculty research:* Gene expression, cytoskeleton and cell structure, cell cycle and growth regulation, neuroscience, animal behavior, microbiology. *Total annual research expenditures:* $1.7 million. *Unit head:* Dr. Murray Itzkowitz, Chairperson, 610-758-3680, Fax: 610-758-4004, E-mail: mi00@lehigh.edu. *Application contact:* Dr. Mary Kathryn Iovine, Graduate Coordinator, 610-758-6981, Fax: 610-758-4004, E-mail: mki3@lehigh.edu.
Website: http://www.lehigh.edu/~inbios/

Lehman College of the City University of New York, School of Natural and Social Sciences, Department of Biological Sciences, Program in Biology, Bronx, NY 10468-1589. Offers MA.

Liberty University, School of Health Sciences, Lynchburg, VA 24515. Offers biomedical sciences (MS); clinical mental health counseling (MA); global health (MPH); health promotion (MPH); human services (MA), including addictions and recovery, business, Christian ministry, criminal justice, crisis response and trauma, executive leadership, health and wellness, life coaching, marriage and family, military resilience; marriage and family therapy (MA); nurse educator (MS); nursing (MSN); nursing administration (MSN); nutrition (MPH); pastoral care and counseling (PhD); professional counseling (MA, PhD). *Students:* 2,830 full-time (2,293 women), 6,275 part-time (5,051 women); includes 1,677 minority (1,178 Black or African American, non-Hispanic/Latino; 19 American Indian or Alaska Native, non-Hispanic/Latino; 36 Asian, non-Hispanic/Latino; 278 Hispanic/Latino; 7 Native Hawaiian or other Pacific Islander, non-Hispanic/Latino; 159 Two or more races, non-Hispanic/Latino), 177 international. Average age 37. 9,147 applicants, 50% accepted, 2939 enrolled. In 2013, 2,618 master's, 11 doctorates awarded. *Degree requirements:* For master's, thesis (for some programs); for doctorate, thesis/dissertation. *Entrance requirements:* For doctorate, MAT or GRE, minimum GPA of 3.25 in master's program, 2-3 recommendations, writing samples (for some programs), letter of intent, professional vitae. Additional exam requirements/recommendations for international students: Required—TOEFL (minimum score 600 paper-based; 100 iBT). Application fee: $50. *Expenses: Tuition:* Full-time $9630; part-time $535 per credit hour. *Required fees:* $175 per term. One-time fee: $50. Tuition and fees vary according to course load, degree level, campus/location and program. *Application contact:* Jay Bridge, Director of Admissions, 800-424-9595, Fax: 800-628-7977, E-mail: gradadmissions@liberty.edu.

Loma Linda University, School of Science and Technology, Department of Biological and Earth Sciences, Loma Linda, CA 92350. Offers MS, PhD. *Degree requirements:* For master's, comprehensive exam, thesis; for doctorate, comprehensive exam, thesis/dissertation. *Entrance requirements:* For master's, minimum GPA of 3.0. Additional exam requirements/recommendations for international students: Required—TOEFL (minimum score 550 paper-based).

Long Island University–LIU Brooklyn, Richard L. Conolly College of Liberal Arts and Sciences, Department of Biology, Brooklyn, NY 11201-8423. Offers MS. Part-time and evening/weekend programs available. *Degree requirements:* For master's, thesis or alternative. *Entrance requirements:* For master's, 2 letters of recommendation. Additional exam requirements/recommendations for international students: Required—TOEFL (minimum score 500 paper-based). Electronic applications accepted.

Long Island University–LIU Post, College of Liberal Arts and Sciences, Department of Biology, Brookville, NY 11548-1300. Offers biology (MS); biology education (MS); genetic counseling (MS). Part-time and evening/weekend programs available. *Degree requirements:* For master's, thesis optional. *Entrance requirements:* For master's, GRE General Test, minimum GPA of 2.75 in major. Electronic applications accepted. *Faculty research:* Immunology, molecular biology, systematics, behavioral ecology, microbiology.

Long Island University–LIU Post, School of Health Professions and Nursing, Department of Biomedical Sciences, Brookville, NY 11548-1300. Offers cardiovascular perfusion (MS); clinical laboratory management (MS); medical biology (MS), including hematology, immunology, medical biology, medical chemistry, medical microbiology. Part-time and evening/weekend programs available. Postbaccalaureate distance learning degree programs offered. *Degree requirements:* For master's, thesis. *Entrance requirements:* For master's, minimum GPA of 2.75 in major. Electronic applications accepted.

Louisiana State University and Agricultural & Mechanical College, Graduate School, College of Science, Department of Biological Sciences, Baton Rouge, LA 70803. Offers biochemistry (MS, PhD); biological science (MS, PhD); science (MNS). Part-time programs available. *Faculty:* 61 full-time (10 women), 1 (woman) part-time/adjunct. *Students:* 126 full-time (51 women), 10 part-time (7 women); includes 14 minority (4 Black or African American, non-Hispanic/Latino; 3 Asian, non-Hispanic/Latino; 4 Hispanic/Latino; 3 Two or more races, non-Hispanic/Latino), 54 international. Average age 29. 98 applicants, 30% accepted, 19 enrolled. In 2013, 1 master's, 25 doctorates awarded. Terminal master's awarded for partial completion of doctoral program. *Degree requirements:* For doctorate, thesis/dissertation. *Entrance requirements:* For master's and doctorate, GRE General Test, minimum GPA of 3.0. Additional exam requirements/recommendations for international students: Required—TOEFL (minimum score 550 paper-based; 79 IBT), IELTS (minimum score 6.5), or PTE (minimum score 59). *Application deadline:* For fall admission, 5/15 for domestic and international students; for spring admission, 10/15 for domestic and international students. Applications are processed on a rolling basis. Application fee: $25. Electronic applications accepted. *Financial support:* In 2013–14, 134 students received support, including 12 fellowships with full and partial tuition reimbursements available (averaging $38,765 per year), 30 research assistantships with full and partial tuition reimbursements available (averaging $22,757 per year), 84 teaching assistantships with full and partial tuition reimbursements available (averaging $19,694 per year); Federal Work-Study, institutionally sponsored loans, health care benefits, and unspecified assistantships also available. Support available to part-time students. Financial award applicants required to submit FAFSA. *Faculty research:* Biochemistry and molecular biology, cell developmental and integrative biology, systematics, ecology and evolutionary biology. *Total annual research expenditures:* $9.9 million. *Unit head:* Dr. Joe Sibenaller, Chair, 225-578-1765, Fax: 225-578-7299, E-mail: zojose@lsu.edu. *Application contact:* Dr. Michael E. Hellberg, Associate Chairman, 225-578-1240, Fax: 225-578-7299, E-mail: mhellbe@lsu.edu.
Website: http://www.biology.lsu.edu/

Louisiana State University Health Sciences Center, School of Graduate Studies in New Orleans, New Orleans, LA 70112-2223. Offers MPH, MS, PhD, MD/PhD. Part-time and evening/weekend programs available. Terminal master's awarded for partial completion of doctoral program. *Degree requirements:* For master's, comprehensive exam, thesis; for doctorate, comprehensive exam, thesis/dissertation. *Entrance requirements:* For master's and doctorate, GRE General Test. Additional exam requirements/recommendations for international students: Required—TOEFL.

Louisiana State University Health Sciences Center at Shreveport, Master of Science in Biomedical Sciences Program, Shreveport, LA 71130-3932. Offers MS. *Faculty:* 59 full-time (5 women), 12 part-time/adjunct (0 women). *Students:* 5 full-time (4 women); includes 2 minority (both Black or African American, non-Hispanic/Latino). 3 applicants, 33% accepted. In 2013, 1 master's awarded. Terminal master's awarded for partial completion of doctoral program. *Degree requirements:* For master's, thesis. *Entrance requirements:* For master's, GRE. Additional exam requirements/recommendations for international students: Required—TOEFL, IELTS. *Application deadline:* For fall admission, 1/15 for domestic students. Application fee: $0. *Financial support:* Tuition waivers available. *Faculty research:* Cardiovascular, cancer, neuroscience, genetics, virology, immunology. *Unit head:* Dr. Sandra C. Roerig, Dean, School of Graduate Studies, 318-675-7676, E-mail: shvgraduatestudies@lsuhsc.edu. *Application contact:* Laura Mackowiak, Coordinator of Graduate Studies, 318-675-7674, Fax: 318-675-4343, E-mail: shvgraduatestudies@lsuhsc.edu.
Website: http://www.lsuhscshreveport.edu/gradschool

Louisiana Tech University, Graduate School, College of Applied and Natural Sciences, School of Biological Sciences, Ruston, LA 71272. Offers biology (MS); molecular sciences and nanotechnology (MS). Part-time programs available. *Degree requirements:* For master's, thesis or alternative. *Entrance requirements:* For master's, GRE General Test, GRE Subject Test. *Application deadline:* For fall admission, 7/29 priority date for domestic students; for spring admission, 2/3 for domestic students. Applications are processed on a rolling basis. Application fee: $20 ($30 for international students). *Financial support:* Fellowships, research assistantships, and teaching assistantships available. Financial award application deadline: 2/1. *Faculty research:* Genetics, animal biology, plant biology, physiology biocontrol. *Unit head:* Dr. William Campbell, Director, 318-257-4573, Fax: 318-257-5060, E-mail: campbell@latech.edu.
Website: http://ans.latech.edu/bls.html

Loyola University Chicago, Graduate School, Department of Biology, Chicago, IL 60660. Offers biology (MA, MS); medical sciences (MA). *Faculty:* 18 full-time (6 women). *Students:* 79 full-time (40 women), 1 (woman) part-time; includes 26 minority (1 Black or African American, non-Hispanic/Latino; 19 Asian, non-Hispanic/Latino; 4 Hispanic/Latino; 2 Two or more races, non-Hispanic/Latino). Average age 25. 335 applicants, 47% accepted, 66 enrolled. In 2013, 57 master's awarded. *Degree requirements:* For master's, thesis (for some programs). *Entrance requirements:* For master's, GRE General Test, 3 letters of recommendation. Additional exam requirements/recommendations for international students: Required—TOEFL. *Application deadline:* For fall admission, 6/1 for domestic and international students. Applications are processed on a rolling basis. Application fee: $50. Electronic applications accepted. *Expenses: Tuition:* Full-time $16,740; part-time $930 per credit. *Required fees:* $135 per semester. *Financial support:* In 2013–14, 7 students received support, including 7 fellowships with full tuition reimbursements available (averaging $16,000 per year); Federal Work-Study and institutionally sponsored loans also available. Financial award application deadline: 2/1; financial award applicants required to submit FAFSA. *Faculty research:* Evolution, development, aquatic biology, molecular biology and genetics, cell biology, neurobiology. *Total annual research expenditures:* $2.5 million. *Unit head:* Dr. Terry Grande, Graduate Program Director, 773-583-5649, Fax: 773-508-3646, E-mail: tgrande@luc.edu. *Application contact:* Ron Martin, Assistant Director of Enrollment Management, 312-915-8950, Fax: 312-915-8905, E-mail: gradapp@luc.edu.
Website: http://www.luc.edu/biology/

Loyola University Chicago, Graduate School, Integrated Programs in Biomedical Science, Chicago, IL 60660. Offers MS, PhD. *Students:* 62 full-time (36 women); includes 11 minority (4 Black or African American, non-Hispanic/Latino; 4 Asian, non-Hispanic/Latino; 1 Hispanic/Latino; 2 Two or more races, non-Hispanic/Latino), 6 international. Average age 25. 214 applicants, 21% accepted, 18 enrolled. In 2013, 9 master's, 13 doctorates awarded. *Expenses: Tuition:* Full-time $16,740; part-time $930 per credit. *Required fees:* $135 per semester. *Unit head:* Dr. Samuel Attoh, Dean, 773-508-3459, Fax: 773-508-2460, E-mail: sattoh@luc.edu. *Application contact:* Ron Martin, Associate Director of Enrollment Management, 312-915-8950, Fax: 312-915-8905, E-mail: gradapp@luc.edu.

Marquette University, Graduate School, College of Arts and Sciences, Department of Biology, Milwaukee, WI 53201-1881. Offers cell biology (MS, PhD); developmental biology (MS, PhD); ecology (MS, PhD); epithelial physiology (MS, PhD); genetics (MS, PhD); microbiology (MS, PhD); molecular biology (MS, PhD); muscle and exercise physiology (MS, PhD); neuroscience (PhD). *Faculty:* 21 full-time (9 women), 3 part-time/adjunct (0 women). *Students:* 34 full-time (16 women), 4 part-time (1 woman), 15 international. Average age 27. 70 applicants, 23% accepted, 5 enrolled. In 2013, 1 master's, 6 doctorates awarded. Terminal master's awarded for partial completion of doctoral program. *Degree requirements:* For master's, comprehensive exam, thesis, 1 year of teaching experience or equivalent; for doctorate, thesis/dissertation, 1 year of teaching experience or equivalent, qualifying exam. *Entrance requirements:* For master's and doctorate, GRE General Test, GRE Subject Test, official transcripts from all current and previous colleges/universities except Marquette, statement of professional goals and aspirations, three letters of recommendation. Additional exam requirements/recommendations for international students: Required—TOEFL (minimum score 530 paper-based). *Application deadline:* For fall admission, 12/15 for domestic and international students. Application fee: $50. Electronic applications accepted. *Financial support:* In 2013–14, 39 students received support, including 6 fellowships (averaging $1,208 per year), 4 research assistantships with full tuition reimbursements available (averaging $21,750 per year), 29 teaching assistantships with full tuition reimbursements available (averaging $21,750 per year); scholarships/grants, health care benefits, tuition waivers (full and partial), and unspecified assistantships also available. Support available to part-time students. Financial award application deadline: 2/15. *Faculty research:* Neurobiology, neuroendocrinology, epithelial physiology, neuropeptide interactions, synaptic transmission. *Total annual research expenditures:* $1.5 million. *Unit head:* Dr. Dale Noel, Chair and Professor, 414-288-1748. *Application contact:* Dr. Michelle Mynlieff, Professor, 414-288-1467.
Website: http://www.marquette.edu/biology/

Marshall University, Academic Affairs Division, College of Science, Department of Biological Science, Huntington, WV 25755. Offers MA, MS. *Students:* 28 full-time (19 women), 2 part-time (1 woman); includes 3 minority (2 Black or African American, non-

Biological and Biomedical Sciences—General

Hispanic/Latino; 1 Hispanic/Latino), 1 international. Average age 25. In 2013, 9 master's awarded. *Degree requirements:* For master's, thesis (for some programs). *Entrance requirements:* For master's, GRE General Test. Application fee: $40. *Financial support:* Career-related internships or fieldwork available. *Unit head:* Dr. David Mallory, Chairperson, 304-696-2353, E-mail: mallory@marshall.edu. *Application contact:* Information Contact, 304-746-1900, Fax: 304-746-1902, E-mail: services@marshall.edu.

Marshall University, Joan C. Edwards School of Medicine and Academic Affairs Division, Program in Biomedical Sciences, Huntington, WV 25755. Offers MS, PhD. Terminal master's awarded for partial completion of doctoral program. *Degree requirements:* For master's, comprehensive exam, thesis optional; for doctorate, thesis/dissertation, written and oral qualifying exams. *Entrance requirements:* For master's, GRE General Test or MCAT (medical science), 1 year of course work in biology, physics, chemistry, and organic chemistry and associated labs; for doctorate, GRE General Test, 1 year of course work in biology, physics, chemistry, and organic chemistry and associated labs. Additional exam requirements/recommendations for international students: Required—TOEFL (minimum score 525 paper-based). *Expenses:* Contact institution. *Faculty research:* Neurosciences, cardiopulmonary science, molecular biology, toxicology, endocrinology.

Massachusetts Institute of Technology, School of Engineering, Harvard-MIT Health Sciences and Technology Program, Cambridge, MA 02139-4307. Offers health sciences and technology (SM, PhD, Sc D), including bioastronautics (PhD, Sc D), bioinformatics and integrative genomics (PhD, Sc D), medical engineering and medical physics (PhD, Sc D), speech and hearing bioscience and technology (PhD, Sc D). *Students:* 281 full-time (115 women), 10 part-time (0 women); includes 84 minority (1 Black or African American, non-Hispanic/Latino; 1 American Indian or Alaska Native, non-Hispanic/Latino; 68 Asian, non-Hispanic/Latino; 11 Hispanic/Latino; 3 Two or more races, non-Hispanic/Latino), 48 international. Average age 26. 180 applicants, 17% accepted, 18 enrolled. In 2013, 7 master's, 20 doctorates awarded. Terminal master's awarded for partial completion of doctoral program. *Degree requirements:* For master's, thesis; for doctorate, comprehensive exam, thesis/dissertation. *Entrance requirements:* For doctorate, GRE General Test (for medical engineering and medical physics). Additional exam requirements/recommendations for international students: Required—TOEFL (minimum score 600 paper-based; 100 iBT), IELTS (minimum score 7). *Application deadline:* For fall admission, 12/15 for domestic and international students. Application fee: $75. Electronic applications accepted. *Expenses: Tuition:* Full-time $43,210; part-time $670 per credit hour. *Required fees:* $288. *Financial support:* In 2013–14, 144 students received support, including 66 fellowships (averaging $35,700 per year), 49 research assistantships (averaging $31,300 per year), 1 teaching assistantship (averaging $33,300 per year); Federal Work-Study, institutionally sponsored loans, scholarships/grants, traineeships, health care benefits, and unspecified assistantships also available. Financial award application deadline: 12/15. *Faculty research:* Signal processing, biomedical imaging, drug delivery, medical devices, medical diagnostics, regenerative biomedical technologies. *Unit head:* Emery N. Brown, Director, 617-452-4091. *Application contact:* Emery N. Brown, Director, 617-452-4091.
Website: http://hst.mit.edu/

Massachusetts Institute of Technology, School of Science, Department of Biology, Cambridge, MA 02139-4307. Offers biochemistry (PhD); biological oceanography (PhD); biology (PhD); biophysical chemistry and molecular structure (PhD); cell biology (PhD); computational and systems biology (PhD); developmental biology (PhD); genetics (PhD); immunology (PhD); microbiology (PhD); molecular biology (PhD); neurobiology (PhD). *Faculty:* 58 full-time (15 women). *Students:* 261 full-time (133 women); includes 77 minority (3 Black or African American, non-Hispanic/Latino; 1 American Indian or Alaska Native, non-Hispanic/Latino; 32 Asian, non-Hispanic/Latino; 32 Hispanic/Latino; 9 Two or more races, non-Hispanic/Latino), 46 international. Average age 26. 651 applicants, 15% accepted, 39 enrolled. In 2013, 25 doctorates awarded. *Degree requirements:* For doctorate, comprehensive exam, thesis/dissertation, two semesters as a teaching assistant. *Entrance requirements:* For doctorate, GRE General Test. Additional exam requirements/recommendations for international students: Required—TOEFL (minimum score 577 paper-based), IELTS (minimum score 6.5). *Application deadline:* For fall admission, 12/1 for domestic and international students. Application fee: $75. Electronic applications accepted. *Expenses: Tuition:* Full-time $43,210; part-time $670 per credit hour. *Required fees:* $288. *Financial support:* In 2013–14, 252 students received support, including 135 fellowships (averaging $36,800 per year), 122 research assistantships (averaging $35,500 per year), 1 teaching assistantship; Federal Work-Study, institutionally sponsored loans, scholarships/grants, traineeships, health care benefits, and unspecified assistantships also available. *Faculty research:* Cellular, developmental and molecular (plant and animal) biology; biochemistry, bioengineering, biophysics and structural biology; classical and molecular genetics, stem cell and epigenetics; immunology and microbiology; cancer biology, molecular medicine, neurobiology and human disease; computational and systems biology. *Total annual research expenditures:* $44.5 million. *Unit head:* Alan Grossman, Interim Head, 617-253-4701. *Application contact:* Biology Education Office, 617-253-3717, Fax: 617-258-9329, E-mail: gradbio@mit.edu.
Website: https://biology.mit.edu/

Mayo Graduate School, Graduate Programs in Biomedical Sciences, Rochester, MN 55905. Offers PhD, MD/PhD. *Degree requirements:* For doctorate, oral defense of dissertation, qualifying oral and written exam. *Entrance requirements:* For doctorate, GRE, 1 year of chemistry, biology, calculus, and physics. Additional exam requirements/recommendations for international students: Required—TOEFL. Electronic applications accepted.

McGill University, Faculty of Graduate and Postdoctoral Studies, Faculty of Medicine, Department of Medicine, Montréal, QC H3A 2T5, Canada. Offers experimental medicine (M Sc, PhD), including bioethics (M Sc), experimental medicine.

McGill University, Faculty of Graduate and Postdoctoral Studies, Faculty of Science, Department of Biology, Montréal, QC H3A 2T5, Canada. Offers bioinformatics (M Sc, PhD); environment (M Sc, PhD); neo-tropical environment (M Sc, PhD).

McMaster University, Faculty of Health Sciences, Department of Biochemistry and Biomedical Sciences, Hamilton, ON L8S 4M2, Canada. Offers M Sc, PhD. Terminal master's awarded for partial completion of doctoral program. *Degree requirements:* For master's, thesis; for doctorate, comprehensive exam, thesis/dissertation. *Entrance requirements:* For master's and doctorate, minimum B+ average. Additional exam requirements/recommendations for international students: Required—TOEFL (minimum score 550 paper-based). *Faculty research:* Molecular and cell biology, biomolecular structure and function, molecular pharmacology and toxicology.

McMaster University, Faculty of Health Sciences and School of Graduate Studies, Program in Medical Sciences, Hamilton, ON L8S 4M2, Canada. Offers blood and vascular (M Sc, PhD); genetics and cancer (M Sc, PhD); immunity and infection (M Sc, PhD); metabolism and nutrition (M Sc, PhD); neurosciences and behavioral sciences (M Sc, PhD); physiology/pharmacology (M Sc, PhD); MD/PhD. *Degree requirements:* For master's, thesis; for doctorate, comprehensive exam, thesis/dissertation. *Entrance requirements:* For master's, honors B Sc, B+ average in related field; for doctorate, M Sc, minimum B+ average. Additional exam requirements/recommendations for international students: Required—TOEFL (minimum score 580 paper-based; 92 iBT).

McMaster University, School of Graduate Studies, Faculty of Science, Department of Biology, Hamilton, ON L8S 4M2, Canada. Offers M Sc, PhD. Part-time programs available. *Degree requirements:* For master's, thesis; for doctorate, comprehensive exam, thesis/dissertation. *Entrance requirements:* Additional exam requirements/recommendations for international students: Required—TOEFL (minimum score 550 paper-based).

Medical College of Wisconsin, Graduate School of Biomedical Sciences, Milwaukee, WI 53226-0509. Offers MA, MPH, MS, PhD, Graduate Certificate, MD/PhD. Part-time and evening/weekend programs available. Postbaccalaureate distance learning degree programs offered (minimal on-campus study). *Degree requirements:* For master's, comprehensive exam (for some programs), thesis (for some programs); for doctorate, comprehensive exam, thesis/dissertation. *Entrance requirements:* For master's and doctorate, GRE General Test. Additional exam requirements/recommendations for international students: Required—TOEFL. Electronic applications accepted. *Faculty research:* Clinical and translational science, genomics and proteomics, cancer.

Medical College of Wisconsin, Interdisciplinary Program in Biomedical Sciences, Milwaukee, WI 53226-0509. Offers PhD.

Medical University of South Carolina, College of Graduate Studies, Charleston, SC 29425. Offers MS, PhD, DMD/PhD, MD/PhD, Pharm D/PhD. Terminal master's awarded for partial completion of doctoral program. *Degree requirements:* For master's, thesis; for doctorate, thesis/dissertation, oral and written exams. *Entrance requirements:* For doctorate, GRE General Test, interview. Additional exam requirements/recommendations for international students: Required—TOEFL (minimum score 600 paper-based; 100 iBT). Electronic applications accepted. *Expenses:* Contact institution. *Faculty research:* Cell signaling and cancer biology, drug discovery and toxicology, biochemistry and genetics, macromolecular structure, neurosciences, microbiology and immunology.

Meharry Medical College, School of Graduate Studies, Program in Biomedical Sciences, Nashville, TN 37208-9989. Offers cancer biology (PhD); microbiology and immunology (PhD); neuroscience (PhD); pharmacology (PhD); MD/PhD. *Degree requirements:* For doctorate, comprehensive exam, thesis/dissertation. *Entrance requirements:* For doctorate, GRE General Test, GRE Subject Test. *Faculty research:* Molecular mechanisms of biological systems and their relationship to human diseases, regulatory biological and cellular structure and function, genetic regulation of growth and cellular metabolism.

Memorial University of Newfoundland, Faculty of Medicine and School of Graduate Studies, Graduate Programs in Medicine, St. John's, NL A1C 5S7, Canada. Offers M Sc, PhD, Diploma, MD/PhD. Part-time programs available. *Degree requirements:* For master's, thesis; for doctorate, comprehensive exam, thesis/dissertation, oral defense of thesis. *Entrance requirements:* For master's, MD or B Sc; for doctorate, MD or M Sc; for Diploma, bachelor's degree in health-related field. Additional exam requirements/recommendations for international students: Required—TOEFL (minimum score 550 paper-based). Electronic applications accepted. *Faculty research:* Human genetics, community health, clinical epidemial, cancer, immunology, cardiovascular and immol sciences, applied health services research, neuroscience.

Memorial University of Newfoundland, School of Graduate Studies, Department of Biology, St. John's, NL A1C 5S7, Canada. Offers biology (M Sc, PhD); marine biology (M Sc, PhD). Part-time programs available. *Degree requirements:* For master's, thesis; for doctorate, comprehensive exam, thesis/dissertation, oral defense of thesis. *Entrance requirements:* For master's, honors degree (minimum 2nd class standing) in related field. Electronic applications accepted. *Faculty research:* Northern flora and fauna, especially cold ocean and boreal environments.

Miami University, College of Arts and Science, Department of Biology, Oxford, OH 45056. Offers biological sciences (MAT); biology (MS, PhD); botany (MAT, MS, PhD); cell, molecular and structural biology (MS, PhD); ecology, evolution and environmental biology (PhD); zoology (MA, MS, PhD). Part-time programs available. Postbaccalaureate distance learning degree programs offered. *Students:* 89 full-time (49 women), 612 part-time (502 women); includes 63 minority (9 Black or African American, non-Hispanic/Latino; 2 American Indian or Alaska Native, non-Hispanic/Latino; 6 Asian, non-Hispanic/Latino; 27 Hispanic/Latino; 1 Native Hawaiian or other Pacific Islander, non-Hispanic/Latino; 18 Two or more races, non-Hispanic/Latino), 35 international. Average age 34. In 2013, 133 master's, 4 doctorates awarded. *Entrance requirements:* For master's and doctorate, GRE General Test. Additional exam requirements/recommendations for international students: Recommended—TOEFL (minimum score 80 iBT), IELTS (minimum score 6.5), TSE (minimum score 54). *Application deadline:* For fall admission, 1/15 for domestic and international students. Application fee: $50. Electronic applications accepted. *Expenses:* Tuition, state resident: full-time $12,634; part-time $526 per credit hour. Tuition, nonresident: full-time $27,892; part-time $1162 per credit hour. Part-time tuition and fees vary according to course load, campus/location and program. *Financial support:* Fellowships with full tuition reimbursements, research assistantships with full tuition reimbursements, teaching assistantships with full tuition reimbursements, Federal Work-Study, health care benefits, tuition waivers (full), and unspecified assistantships available. Financial award application deadline: 1/15; financial award applicants required to submit FAFSA. *Unit head:* Dr. Douglas Meikle, Chair, 513-529-3103, E-mail: meikled@miamioh.edu.
Website: http://miamioh.edu/cas/about/biology

Michigan State University, College of Human Medicine and The Graduate School, Graduate Programs in Human Medicine, East Lansing, MI 48824. Offers biochemistry and molecular biology (MS, PhD); epidemiology (MS, PhD); microbiology (MS); microbiology and molecular genetics (PhD); pharmacology and toxicology (MS, PhD); physiology (MS, PhD); public health (MPH). *Entrance requirements:* Additional exam requirements/recommendations for international students: Required—TOEFL.

Michigan State University, College of Osteopathic Medicine and The Graduate School, Graduate Studies in Osteopathic Medicine, East Lansing, MI 48824. Offers biochemistry and molecular biology (MS, PhD); microbiology (MS); microbiology and molecular genetics (PhD); pharmacology and toxicology (MS, PhD), including integrative pharmacology (MS), pharmacology and toxicology, pharmacology and toxicology-environmental toxicology (PhD); physiology (MS, PhD).

Michigan State University, College of Veterinary Medicine and The Graduate School, Graduate Programs in Veterinary Medicine, Program in Comparative Medicine and Integrative Biology, East Lansing, MI 48824. Offers comparative medicine and integrative biology (MS, PhD); comparative medicine and integrative biology–environmental toxicology (PhD). *Entrance requirements:* Additional exam requirements/recommendations for international students: Required—TOEFL. Electronic applications accepted.

Michigan Technological University, Graduate School, College of Sciences and Arts, Department of Biological Sciences, Houghton, MI 49931. Offers MS, PhD. Part-time programs available. Terminal master's awarded for partial completion of doctoral program. *Degree requirements:* For master's, comprehensive exam (for some programs), thesis (for some programs); for doctorate, comprehensive exam, thesis/dissertation. *Entrance requirements:* For master's and doctorate, GRE, statement of purpose, official transcripts, 2 letters of recommendation. Additional exam requirements/recommendations for international students: Required—TOEFL (minimum score 79 iBT) or IELTS. Electronic applications accepted. *Faculty research:* Aquatic ecology, biological control, predator-prey interactions, environmental microbiology, microbial and plant biochemistry, genomics and bioinformatics.

Middle Tennessee State University, College of Graduate Studies, College of Basic and Applied Sciences, Department of Biology, Murfreesboro, TN 37132. Offers MS. Part-time and evening/weekend programs available. Postbaccalaureate distance learning degree programs offered. *Faculty:* 32 full-time (6 women), 3 part-time/adjunct (0 women). *Students:* 9 full-time (5 women), 34 part-time (18 women); includes 5 minority (3 Asian, non-Hispanic/Latino; 2 Two or more races, non-Hispanic/Latino). 44 applicants, 45% accepted. In 2013, 8 master's awarded. *Degree requirements:* For master's, comprehensive exam, thesis. *Entrance requirements:* For master's, GRE. Additional exam requirements/recommendations for international students: Required—TOEFL (minimum score 525 paper-based; 71 iBT) or IELTS (minimum score 6). *Application deadline:* For fall admission, 6/1 for domestic and international students. Applications are processed on a rolling basis. Application fee: $25 ($30 for international students). Electronic applications accepted. *Financial support:* In 2013–14, 30 students received support. Tuition waivers available. Support available to part-time students. Financial award application deadline: 5/1; financial award applicants required to submit FAFSA. *Faculty research:* Molecular biosciences. *Unit head:* Dr. Lynn Boyd, Chair, 615-898-2847, Fax: 615-898-5093, E-mail: lynn.boyd@mtsu.edu. *Application contact:* Dr. Michael D. Allen, Vice Provost for Research/Dean, 615-898-2840, Fax: 615-904-8020, E-mail: michael.allen@mtsu.edu.

Midwestern State University, Graduate School, College of Science and Mathematics, Department of Biology, Wichita Falls, TX 76308. Offers MS. Part-time and evening/weekend programs available. *Degree requirements:* For master's, comprehensive exam, thesis. *Entrance requirements:* For master's, GRE General Test, MAT or GMAT. Additional exam requirements/recommendations for international students: Required—TOEFL (minimum score 550 paper-based). *Application deadline:* For fall admission, 7/1 priority date for domestic students, 4/1 for international students; for spring admission, 11/1 priority date for domestic students, 8/1 for international students. Applications are processed on a rolling basis. Application fee: $35 ($50 for international students). Electronic applications accepted. *Expenses:* Tuition, state resident: full-time $3627; part-time $201.50 per credit hour. Tuition, nonresident: full-time $10,899; part-time $605.50 per credit hour. *Required fees:* $1357. *Financial support:* Teaching assistantships with partial tuition reimbursements, career-related internships or fieldwork, Federal Work-Study, institutionally sponsored loans, scholarships/grants, tuition waivers (partial), and unspecified assistantships available. Support available to part-time students. Financial award application deadline: 3/1; financial award applicants required to submit FAFSA. *Faculty research:* Molecular analysis of flora and fauna, mineral toxicity in plants, embryonic patterning and cell signaling, animal physiology, mammalogy. *Unit head:* William Cook, Chair, 940-397-4192, E-mail: william.cook@mwsu.edu.
Website: http://www.mwsu.edu/academics/scienceandmath/biology/index

Midwestern University, Downers Grove Campus, College of Health Sciences, Illinois Campus, Master of Arts Program in Biomedical Sciences, Downers Grove, IL 60515-1235. Offers MA. *Entrance requirements:* For master's, GRE General Test, MCAT, PCAT, DAT, OAT or other professional exam, bachelor's degree, minimum cumulative GPA of 2.75.

Midwestern University, Downers Grove Campus, College of Health Sciences, Illinois Campus, Program in Biomedical Sciences, Downers Grove, IL 60515-1235. Offers MBS. Part-time programs available. *Entrance requirements:* For master's, GRE General Test, MCAT or PCAT, 2 letters of recommendation.

Midwestern University, Glendale Campus, College of Health Sciences, Arizona Campus, MA Program in Biomedical Sciences, Glendale, AZ 85308. Offers MA. *Entrance requirements:* For master's, GRE General Test, MCAT, or other professional exam, bachelor's degree, minimum cumulative GPA of 2.75.

Midwestern University, Glendale Campus, College of Health Sciences, Arizona Campus, MBS Program in Biomedical Sciences, Glendale, AZ 85308. Offers MBS. *Expenses:* Contact institution.

Mills College, Graduate Studies, Pre-Medical Studies Program, Oakland, CA 94613-1000. Offers Certificate. Part-time programs available. *Faculty:* 10 full-time (7 women), 12 part-time/adjunct (9 women). *Students:* 62 full-time (39 women), 5 part-time (3 women); includes 18 minority (8 Asian, non-Hispanic/Latino; 7 Hispanic/Latino; 3 Two or more races, non-Hispanic/Latino). Average age 26. 152 applicants, 76% accepted, 38 enrolled. In 2013, 36 Certificates awarded. *Entrance requirements:* For degree, SAT/ACT or GRE General Test, bachelor's degree in a non-science area. Additional exam requirements/recommendations for international students: Required—TOEFL (minimum score 550 paper-based; 80 iBT) or IELTS (minimum score 6). *Application deadline:* For fall admission, 2/1 priority date for domestic students, 12/15 for international students. Applications are processed on a rolling basis. Application fee: $50. Electronic applications accepted. *Expenses: Tuition:* Full-time $29,860. *Required fees:* $1134. Part-time tuition and fees vary according to course load, degree level and program. *Financial support:* In 2013–14, 42 students received support, including 29 fellowships with full and partial tuition reimbursements available (averaging $4,616 per year), 10 teaching assistantships with full and partial tuition reimbursements available (averaging $3,522 per year); institutionally sponsored loans and scholarships/grants also available. Support available to part-time students. Financial award application deadline: 2/1; financial award applicants required to submit FAFSA. *Faculty research:* Antifungal compounds and their modes of action, organic chemistry-spectroscopy and organic chemistry reaction mechanisms, oceanography, physics and chemistry education, cell-cell and cell-extracellular matrix interactions. *Total annual research expenditures:* $277,899. *Unit head:* Dr. John Brabson, Chair of Pre-Medical Program, 510-430-2203, Fax: 510-430-2159, E-mail: johnb@mills.edu. *Application contact:* Shrim Bathey, Director of Graduate Admission, 510-430-3309, Fax: 510-430-2159, E-mail: grad-admission@mills.edu.
Website: http://www.mills.edu/premed

Minnesota State University Mankato, College of Graduate Studies and Research, College of Science, Engineering and Technology, Department of Biological Sciences, Mankato, MN 56001. Offers biology (MS); biology education (MS); environmental sciences (MS). Part-time programs available. *Students:* 9 full-time (4 women), 24 part-time (11 women). *Degree requirements:* For master's, one foreign language, comprehensive exam, thesis or alternative. *Entrance requirements:* For master's, minimum GPA of 3.0 during previous 2 years of course work. Additional exam requirements/recommendations for international students: Required—TOEFL. *Application deadline:* For fall admission, 7/1 priority date for domestic students; for spring admission, 11/1 for domestic students. Applications are processed on a rolling basis. Application fee: $40. Electronic applications accepted. *Financial support:* Fellowships, research assistantships with full tuition reimbursements, teaching assistantships with full tuition reimbursements, career-related internships or fieldwork, Federal Work-Study, institutionally sponsored loans, and unspecified assistantships available. Support available to part-time students. Financial award application deadline: 3/15; financial award applicants required to submit FAFSA. *Faculty research:* Limnology, enzyme analysis, membrane engineering, converters. *Unit head:* Dr. Penny Knoblich, Graduate Coordinator, 507-389-5736. *Application contact:* 507-389-2321, E-mail: grad@mnsu.edu.

Mississippi College, Graduate School, College of Arts and Sciences, School of Science and Mathematics, Department of Biological Sciences, Clinton, MS 39058. Offers biological science (M Ed); biology (MCS); biology-biological sciences (MS); biology-medical sciences (MS). Part-time programs available. *Degree requirements:* For master's, comprehensive exam, thesis optional. *Entrance requirements:* For master's, GRE General Test, minimum GPA of 2.5. Additional exam requirements/recommendations for international students: Recommended—TOEFL, IELTS. Electronic applications accepted.

Mississippi State University, College of Arts and Sciences, Department of Biological Sciences, Mississippi State, MS 39762. Offers MS, PhD. MS offered online only. Postbaccalaureate distance learning degree programs offered (minimal on-campus study). *Faculty:* 10 full-time (5 women), 1 part-time/adjunct (0 women). *Students:* 40 full-time (19 women), 93 part-time (59 women); includes 19 minority (10 Black or African American, non-Hispanic/Latino; 3 Asian, non-Hispanic/Latino; 2 Hispanic/Latino; 4 Two or more races, non-Hispanic/Latino), 12 international. Average age 33. 188 applicants, 37% accepted, 60 enrolled. In 2013, 33 master's, 3 doctorates awarded. Terminal master's awarded for partial completion of doctoral program. *Degree requirements:* For master's, one foreign language, thesis, comprehensive oral or written exam; for doctorate, one foreign language, thesis/dissertation, comprehensive oral or written exam. *Entrance requirements:* For master's, GRE General Test, minimum GPA of 2.75 on last 60 hours of undergraduate courses; for doctorate, GRE General Test. Additional exam requirements/recommendations for international students: Required—TOEFL (minimum score 550 paper-based; 79 iBT); Recommended—IELTS (minimum score 6.5). *Application deadline:* For fall admission, 7/1 for domestic students, 5/1 for international students; for spring admission, 11/1 for domestic students, 9/1 for international students. Applications are processed on a rolling basis. Application fee: $60. Electronic applications accepted. *Financial support:* In 2013–14, 3 research assistantships with full and partial tuition reimbursements (averaging $16,767 per year), 37 teaching assistantships with full and partial tuition reimbursements (averaging $15,285 per year) were awarded; Federal Work-Study, institutionally sponsored loans, scholarships/grants, and unspecified assistantships also available. Financial award applicants required to submit FAFSA. *Faculty research:* Botany, zoology, microbiology, ecology. *Total annual research expenditures:* $3.2 million. *Unit head:* Dr. Nancy Reichert, Professor/Head/General Biology Coordinator, 662-325-3483, Fax: 662-325-7939, E-mail: nar1@biology.msstate.edu. *Application contact:* Dr. Gary Ervin, Professor/Graduate Coordinator, 662-325-1203, Fax: 662-325-7939, E-mail: grad_studies@biology.msstate.edu.
Website: http://www.biology.msstate.edu

Missouri State University, Graduate College, College of Natural and Applied Sciences, Department of Biology, Springfield, MO 65897. Offers biology (MS); natural and applied science (MNAS), including biology (MNAS, MS Ed); secondary education (MS Ed), including biology (MNAS, MS Ed). *Faculty:* 16 full-time (4 women), 8 part-time/adjunct (2 women). *Students:* 17 full-time (10 women), 28 part-time (15 women), 3 international. Average age 28. 27 applicants, 48% accepted, 12 enrolled. In 2013, 18 master's awarded. *Degree requirements:* For master's, comprehensive exam, thesis or alternative. *Entrance requirements:* For master's, GRE (MS, MNAS), 24 hours of course work in biology (MS); minimum GPA of 3.0 (MS, MNAS), 9-12 teacher certification (MS Ed). Additional exam requirements/recommendations for international students: Required—TOEFL (minimum score 550 paper-based; 79 iBT). *Application deadline:* For fall admission, 7/20 priority date for domestic students, 5/1 for international students; for spring admission, 12/20 priority date for domestic students, 9/1 for international students. Applications are processed on a rolling basis. Application fee: $35 ($50 for international students). Electronic applications accepted. *Expenses:* Tuition, state resident: full-time $4500; part-time $250 per credit hour. Tuition, nonresident: full-time $9018; part-time $501 per credit hour. *Required fees:* $361 per semester. Tuition and fees vary according to course level, course load and program. *Financial support:* In 2013–14, 18 research assistantships with full tuition reimbursements (averaging $10,128 per year), 18 teaching assistantships with full tuition reimbursements (averaging $9,226 per year) were awarded; Federal Work-Study, institutionally sponsored loans, scholarships/grants, and unspecified assistantships also available. Financial award application deadline: 3/31; financial award applicants required to submit FAFSA. *Faculty research:* Hibernation physiology of bats, behavioral ecology of salamanders, mussel conservation, plant evolution and systematics, cellular/molecular mechanisms involved in migraine pathology. *Unit head:* Dr. S. Alicia Mathis, Head, 417-836-5126, Fax: 417-836-6934, E-mail: biology@missouristate.edu. *Application contact:* Misty Stewart, Coordinator of Graduate Recruitment, 417-836-6079, Fax: 417-836-6200, E-mail: mistystewart@missouristate.edu.
Website: http://biology.missouristate.edu/

Missouri University of Science and Technology, Graduate School, Department of Biological Sciences, Rolla, MO 65409. Offers applied and environmental biology (MS). *Entrance requirements:* For master's, GRE (minimum score 600 quantitative, 4 writing). Additional exam requirements/recommendations for international students: Required—TOEFL (minimum score 570 paper-based).

Missouri Western State University, Program in Applied Science, St. Joseph, MO 64507-2294. Offers chemistry (MAS); engineering technology management (MAS); human factors and usability testing (MAS); industrial life science (MAS); information technology management (MAS); sport and fitness management (MAS). Part-time programs available. *Students:* 38 full-time (11 women), 24 part-time (10 women); includes 7 minority (4 Black or African American, non-Hispanic/Latino; 1 Asian, non-Hispanic/Latino; 1 Hispanic/Latino; 1 Two or more races, non-Hispanic/Latino), 21 international. Average age 28. 60 applicants, 90% accepted, 37 enrolled. In 2013, 15 master's awarded. *Entrance requirements:* Additional exam requirements/recommendations for international students: Recommended—TOEFL (minimum score 500 paper-based; 61 iBT), IELTS (minimum score 5.5). *Application deadline:* For fall admission, 7/15 for domestic students, 6/15 for international students; for spring admission, 10/1 for domestic students, 10/15 for international students. Applications are processed on a rolling basis. Application fee: $45 ($50 for international students). Electronic applications accepted. *Expenses:* Tuition, state resident: full-time $6019; part-time $300.96 per credit hour. Tuition, nonresident: full-time $11,194; part-time $559.71 per credit hour. *Required fees:* $542; $99 per credit hour. $176 per semester. Tuition and fees vary according to course load and program. *Financial support:* Scholarships/grants and unspecified assistantships available. Support available to part-time students. *Unit head:* Dr. Benjamin D. Caldwell, Dean of the Graduate School, 816-271-4394, Fax: 816-271-4525, E-mail: graduate@missouriwestern.edu. *Application* *contact:* Dr. Benjamin D. Caldwell, Dean of the Graduate School, 816-271-4394, Fax: 816-271-4525, E-mail: graduate@missouriwestern.edu.

Montana State University, College of Graduate Studies, College of Letters and Science, Department of Cell Biology and Neuroscience, Bozeman, MT 59717. Offers biological sciences (PhD); neuroscience (MS, PhD). Part-time programs available. *Degree requirements:* For master's, comprehensive exam; for doctorate, comprehensive exam, thesis/dissertation. *Entrance requirements:* For master's and doctorate, GRE General Test. Additional exam requirements/recommendations for international students: Required—TOEFL (minimum score 550 paper-based). Electronic applications accepted. *Faculty research:* Development of the nervous system, neuronal mechanisms of visual perception, ion channel biophysics, mechanisms of sensory coding, neuroinformatics.

Montclair State University, The Graduate School, College of Science and Mathematics, Department of Biology and Molecular Biology, Montclair, NJ 07043-1624. Offers biology (MS), including biological science education, biology, ecology and evolution, physiology; molecular biology (MS, Certificate). Part-time and evening/weekend programs available. *Degree requirements:* For master's, comprehensive exam, thesis or alternative. *Entrance requirements:* For master's, GRE General Test, 24 credits of course work in undergraduate biology, 2 letters of recommendation, teaching certificate (biology sciences education concentration); for Certificate, 2 letters of recommendation, essay. Additional exam requirements/recommendations for international students: Required—TOEFL (minimum score 83 iBT) or IELTS. Electronic applications accepted. *Faculty research:* Ecosystem biology, molecular biology, signal transduction, neuroscience, aquatic and coastal biology.

Morehead State University, Graduate Programs, College of Science and Technology, Department of Biology and Chemistry, Morehead, KY 40351. Offers biology (MS); biology regional analysis (MS). Part-time programs available. *Degree requirements:* For master's, comprehensive exam, thesis optional, oral and written final exams. *Entrance requirements:* For master's, GRE General Test, minimum GPA of 3.0 in biology, 2.5 overall; undergraduate major/minor in biology, environmental science, or equivalent. Additional exam requirements/recommendations for international students: Required—TOEFL (minimum score 525 paper-based). Electronic applications accepted. *Faculty research:* Atherosclerosis, RNA evolution, cancer biology, water quality/ecology, immunoparasitology.

Morehouse School of Medicine, Graduate Programs in Biomedical Sciences, Atlanta, GA 30310-1495. Offers biomedical research (MS); biomedical sciences (PhD); biomedical technology (MS). *Faculty:* 52 full-time (17 women), 7 part-time/adjunct (2 women). *Students:* 33 full-time (25 women); includes 30 minority (16 Black or African American, non-Hispanic/Latino; 1 Asian, non-Hispanic/Latino; 12 Hispanic/Latino; 1 Two or more races, non-Hispanic/Latino). Average age 28. 37 applicants, 27% accepted, 5 enrolled. In 2013, 2 doctorates awarded. *Degree requirements:* For master's, thesis (for some programs); for doctorate, thesis/dissertation. *Entrance requirements:* For doctorate, GRE General Test. Additional exam requirements/recommendations for international students: Required—TOEFL (minimum score 550 paper-based). *Application deadline:* For fall admission, 10/1 for domestic and international students; for spring admission, 2/1 for domestic and international students. Application fee: $50. Electronic applications accepted. *Expenses:* Contact institution. *Financial support:* Fellowships with full and partial tuition reimbursements, career-related internships or fieldwork, institutionally sponsored loans, scholarships/grants, traineeships, health care benefits, and tuition waivers (full) available. Financial award application deadline: 5/1; financial award applicants required to submit FAFSA. *Unit head:* Dr. Douglas Paulsen, Director, 404-752-1559. *Application contact:* Brandon Hunter, Director of Admissions, 404-752-1650, Fax: 404-752-1512, E-mail: phdadmissions@msm.edu.
Website: http://www.msm.edu/Education/GEBS/GEBSOverview.php

Morgan State University, School of Graduate Studies, School of Computer, Mathematical, and Natural Sciences, Department of Biology, Baltimore, MD 21251. Offers bioenvironmental science (PhD); biology (MS); science education (MS). *Degree requirements:* For master's, comprehensive exam, thesis. *Entrance requirements:* For master's, minimum GPA of 3.0.

Mount Allison University, Department of Biology, Sackville, NB E4L 1E4, Canada. Offers M Sc. *Degree requirements:* For master's, thesis. *Entrance requirements:* For master's, honors degree. *Faculty research:* Ecology, evolution, physiology, behavior, biochemistry.

Murray State University, College of Science, Engineering and Technology, Program in Biological Sciences, Murray, KY 42071. Offers MAT, MS, PhD. PhD offered jointly with University of Louisville. Part-time programs available. *Degree requirements:* For master's, comprehensive exam, thesis optional. *Entrance requirements:* For master's, GRE General Test. Additional exam requirements/recommendations for international students: Required—TOEFL. *Faculty research:* Aquatic and terrestrial ecology, molecular systematics, micro ecology, cell biology and metabolism, palentology.

National University, Academic Affairs, College of Letters and Sciences, La Jolla, CA 92037-1011. Offers applied linguistics (MA); biology (MS); counseling psychology (MA), including licensed professional clinical counseling, marriage and family therapy; creative writing (MFA); English (MA), including Gothic studies, rhetoric; film studies (MA); forensic and crime science (Certificate); forensic studies (MFS), including criminalistics, investigation; gerontology (MA); history (MA); human behavior (MA); mathematics for educators (MS); performance psychology (MA); strategic communications (MA). Part-time and evening/weekend programs available. Postbaccalaureate distance learning degree programs offered (no on-campus study). *Faculty:* 62 full-time (29 women), 95 part-time/adjunct (54 women). *Students:* 708 full-time (525 women), 409 part-time (269 women); includes 503 minority (151 Black or African American, non-Hispanic/Latino; 8 American Indian or Alaska Native, non-Hispanic/Latino; 64 Asian, non-Hispanic/Latino; 221 Hispanic/Latino; 4 Native Hawaiian or other Pacific Islander, non-Hispanic/Latino; 55 Two or more races, non-Hispanic/Latino), 6 international. Average age 35. 265 applicants, 100% accepted, 204 enrolled. In 2013, 594 master's awarded. *Degree requirements:* For master's, thesis (for some programs). *Entrance requirements:* For master's, interview, minimum GPA of 2.5. Additional exam requirements/recommendations for international students: Required—TOEFL (minimum score 550 paper-based; 79 iBT), IELTS (minimum score 6). *Application deadline:* Applications are processed on a rolling basis. Application fee: $60 ($65 for international students). Electronic applications accepted. *Expenses: Tuition:* Full-time $13,824; part-time $1728 per course. One-time fee: $160. *Financial support:* Career-related internships or fieldwork, institutionally sponsored loans, scholarships/grants, and tuition waivers (partial) available. Support available to part-time students. Financial award application deadline: 6/30; financial award applicants required to submit FAFSA. *Unit head:* College of Letters and Sciences, 800-628-8648, E-mail: cols@nu.edu. *Application contact:* Louis Cruz, Interim Vice President for Enrollment Services, 800-628-8648, E-mail: advisor@nu.edu.
Website: http://www.nu.edu/OurPrograms/CollegeOfLettersAndSciences.html

New Jersey Institute of Technology, College of Science and Liberal Arts, Newark, NJ 07102. Offers applied mathematics (MS); applied physics (M Sc, PhD); applied statistics (MS); biology (MS, PhD); biostatistics (MS); chemistry (MS, PhD); computational biology (MS); environmental science (MS, PhD); history (MA, MAT); materials science and engineering (MS, PhD); mathematical and computational finance (MS); mathematics science (PhD); pharmaceutical chemistry (MS); professional and technical communications (MS). Part-time and evening/weekend programs available. *Faculty:* 150 full-time (33 women), 76 part-time/adjunct (27 women). *Students:* 245 full-time (97 women), 115 part-time (49 women); includes 75 minority (26 Black or African American, non-Hispanic/Latino; 1 American Indian or Alaska Native, non-Hispanic/Latino; 35 Asian, non-Hispanic/Latino; 12 Hispanic/Latino; 1 Native Hawaiian or other Pacific Islander, non-Hispanic/Latino), 189 international. Average age 30. 754 applicants, 59% accepted, 109 enrolled. In 2013, 104 master's, 29 doctorates awarded. Terminal master's awarded for partial completion of doctoral program. *Degree requirements:* For master's, thesis optional; for doctorate, thesis/dissertation. *Entrance requirements:* For master's, GRE General Test; for doctorate, GRE General Test, minimum graduate GPA of 3.5. Additional exam requirements/recommendations for international students: Required—TOEFL (minimum score 550 paper-based; 79 iBT). *Application deadline:* For fall admission, 6/1 priority date for domestic students, 5/1 priority date for international students; for spring admission, 11/15 priority date for domestic and international students. Applications are processed on a rolling basis. Application fee: $65. Electronic applications accepted. *Expenses:* Tuition, state resident: full-time $17,384; part-time $945 per credit. Tuition, nonresident: full-time $25,404; part-time $1341 per credit. *Required fees:* $2396; $118 per credit. *Financial support:* Fellowships with full tuition reimbursements, research assistantships with full tuition reimbursements, and teaching assistantships with full tuition reimbursements available. Financial award application deadline: 1/15. *Total annual research expenditures:* $6.9 million. *Unit head:* Dr. Fadi P. Deek, Dean, 973-596-3676, Fax: 973-565-0586, E-mail: fadi.deek@njit.edu. *Application contact:* Kathryn Kelly, Director of Admissions, 973-596-3300, Fax: 973-596-3461, E-mail: admissions@njit.edu.
Website: http://csla.njit.edu/

New Mexico Institute of Mining and Technology, Graduate Studies, Department of Biology, Socorro, NM 87801. Offers MS. Part-time programs available. *Degree requirements:* For master's, thesis. *Entrance requirements:* For master's, GRE General Test. Additional exam requirements/recommendations for international students: Required—TOEFL (minimum score 540 paper-based). Electronic applications accepted. *Expenses:* Tuition, state resident: full-time $5270; part-time $292.80 per credit hour. Tuition, nonresident: full-time $16,833; part-time $968.51 per credit hour. *Required fees:* $648. Part-time tuition and fees vary according to course load. *Faculty research:* Molecular biology, evolution and evolutionary ecology, immunology, endocrinology.

New Mexico State University, Graduate School, College of Agricultural, Consumer and Environmental Sciences, Department of Animal and Range Sciences, Las Cruces, NM 88003. Offers animal science (MS, PhD); domestic animal biology (M Ag); range science (M Ag, MS, PhD). Part-time programs available. *Faculty:* 17 full-time (5 women). *Students:* 28 full-time (17 women), 5 part-time (1 woman); includes 8 minority (all Hispanic/Latino), 9 international. Average age 28. 20 applicants, 70% accepted, 12 enrolled. In 2013, 8 master's, 3 doctorates awarded. *Degree requirements:* For master's, thesis, seminar, experimental statistics; for doctorate, thesis/dissertation, research tool. *Entrance requirements:* For master's, minimum GPA of 3.0 in last 60 hours of undergraduate course work (MS); for doctorate, minimum graduate GPA of 3.2, MS with thesis. Additional exam requirements/recommendations for international students: Required—TOEFL (minimum score 550 paper-based; 79 iBT), IELTS (minimum score 6.5). *Application deadline:* For fall admission, 2/15 priority date for domestic and international students; for winter admission, 10/1 priority date for domestic and international students; for spring admission, 11/1 for domestic and international students. Applications are processed on a rolling basis. Application fee: $40 ($50 for international students). Electronic applications accepted. *Expenses:* Tuition, state resident: full-time $5398; part-time $224.90 per credit. Tuition, nonresident: full-time $18,821; part-time $784.20 per credit. *Required fees:* $1310; $54.60 per credit. *Financial support:* In 2013–14, 26 students received support, including 1 fellowship (averaging $4,050 per year), 5 research assistantships (averaging $18,679 per year), 18 teaching assistantships (averaging $16,019 per year); career-related internships or fieldwork, Federal Work-Study, scholarships/grants, traineeships, health care benefits, and unspecified assistantships also available. Support available to part-time students. Financial award application deadline: 3/15. *Faculty research:* Reproductive physiology, ruminant nutrition, nutrition toxicology, range ecology, wildland hydrology. *Total annual research expenditures:* $3.7 million. *Unit head:* Dr. Tim Ross, Head, 575-646-2515, Fax: 575-646-5441, E-mail: tross@nmsu.edu. *Application contact:* Coordinator, 575-646-2736, Fax: 575-646-7721, E-mail: gradinfo@nmsu.edu.
Website: http://aces.nmsu.edu/academics/anrs

New Mexico State University, Graduate School, College of Arts and Sciences, Department of Biology, Las Cruces, NM 88003-8001. Offers biology (MS, PhD); biotechnology and business (MS). Part-time programs available. *Faculty:* 23 full-time (11 women). *Students:* 60 full-time (35 women), 11 part-time (7 women); includes 18 minority (1 Black or African American, non-Hispanic/Latino; 3 American Indian or Alaska Native, non-Hispanic/Latino; 13 Hispanic/Latino; 1 Two or more races, non-Hispanic/Latino), 19 international. Average age 30. 34 applicants, 50% accepted, 14 enrolled. In 2013, 9 master's, 11 doctorates awarded. *Degree requirements:* For master's, thesis (for some programs), defense or oral exam; for doctorate, comprehensive exam, thesis/dissertation, qualifying exam. *Entrance requirements:* Additional exam requirements/recommendations for international students: Required—TOEFL (minimum score 550 paper-based; 79 iBT), IELTS (minimum score 6.5). *Application deadline:* For fall admission, 1/15 priority date for domestic students, 1/15 for international students; for spring admission, 10/4 priority date for domestic students, 10/4 for international students. Applications are processed on a rolling basis. Application fee: $40 ($50 for international students). Electronic applications accepted. *Expenses:* Tuition, state resident: full-time $5398; part-time $224.90 per credit. Tuition, nonresident: full-time $18,821; part-time $784.20 per credit. *Required fees:* $1310; $54.60 per credit. *Financial support:* In 2013–14, 54 students received support, including 6 fellowships (averaging $4,050 per year), 10 research assistantships (averaging $15,919 per year), 36 teaching assistantships (averaging $16,098 per year); Federal Work-Study, scholarships/grants, health care benefits, and unspecified assistantships also available. Support available to part-time students. Financial award application deadline: 1/15. *Faculty research:* Microbiology, cell and organismal physiology, ecology and ethology, evolution, genetics, developmental biology. *Total annual research expenditures:* $3 million. *Unit head:* Dr. Ralph Preszler, Head, 575-646-3611, Fax: 575-646-5665, E-mail: rpreszle@nmsu.edu. *Application contact:* Gloria Valencia, Administrative Assistant, 575-646-3611, Fax: 575-646-5665, E-mail: gvalenci@nmsu.edu.
Website: http://biology-web.nmsu.edu/

New York Medical College, Graduate School of Basic Medical Sciences, Valhalla, NY 10595-1691. Offers MS, PhD, MD/PhD. Part-time and evening/weekend programs available. *Faculty:* 91 full-time (16 women), 5 part-time/adjunct (2 women). *Students:* 142 full-time (80 women); includes 69 minority (14 Black or African American, non-Hispanic/Latino; 1 American Indian or Alaska Native, non-Hispanic/Latino; 41 Asian, non-Hispanic/Latino; 13 Hispanic/Latino). Average age 26. 379 applicants, 44% accepted, 52 enrolled. In 2013, 52 master's, 17 doctorates awarded. Terminal master's awarded for partial completion of doctoral program. *Degree requirements:* For master's, thesis; for doctorate, comprehensive exam, thesis/dissertation. *Entrance requirements:* For master's, GRE General Test, MCAT, or DAT; for doctorate, GRE General Test. Additional exam requirements/recommendations for international students: Required—TOEFL. *Application deadline:* For fall admission, 7/1 priority date for domestic students, 5/1 priority date for international students; for spring admission, 12/1 priority date for domestic students, 9/15 priority date for international students. Applications are processed on a rolling basis. Application fee: $75 ($100 for international students). Electronic applications accepted. *Expenses: Tuition:* Full-time $49,170; part-time $910 per credit. Tuition and fees vary according to program. *Financial support:* In 2013–14, fellowships with full tuition reimbursements (averaging $25,500 per year), research assistantships with full tuition reimbursements (averaging $25,500 per year) were awarded; Federal Work-Study, scholarships/grants, tuition waivers (full), and health benefits (for PhD candidates only) also available. Support available to part-time students. Financial award applicants required to submit FAFSA. *Faculty research:* Cardiovascular science, infectious diseases, neuroscience, cancer, cell signaling. *Unit head:* Dr. Francis L. Belloni, Dean, 914-594-4110, Fax: 914-594-4944, E-mail: francis_belloni@nymc.edu. *Application contact:* Valerie Romeo-Messana, Director of Admissions, 914-594-4110, Fax: 914-594-4944, E-mail: v_romeomessana@nymc.edu.

See Display below and Close-Up on page 121.

New York University, Graduate School of Arts and Science, Department of Biology, New York, NY 10012-1019. Offers biology (PhD); biomedical journalism (MS); cancer and molecular biology (PhD); computational biology (PhD); computers in biological research (MS); developmental genetics (PhD); general biology (MS); immunology and microbiology (PhD); molecular genetics (PhD); neurobiology (PhD); oral biology (MS); plant biology (PhD); recombinant DNA technology (MS); MS/MBA. Part-time programs available. *Faculty:* 24 full-time (5 women). *Students:* 161 full-time (88 women), 28 part-time (15 women); includes 41 minority (5 Black or African American, non-Hispanic/Latino; 23 Asian, non-Hispanic/Latino; 9 Hispanic/Latino; 4 Two or more races, non-Hispanic/Latino), 80 international. Average age 27. 412 applicants, 54% accepted, 65 enrolled. In 2013, 77 master's, 9 doctorates awarded. Terminal master's awarded for partial completion of doctoral program. *Degree requirements:* For master's, thesis or alternative, qualifying paper; for doctorate, comprehensive exam, thesis/dissertation. *Entrance requirements:* For master's and doctorate, GRE General Test. Additional exam requirements/recommendations for international students: Required—TOEFL. *Application deadline:* For fall admission, 12/1 priority date for domestic students, 12/1 for international students. Application fee: $95. *Expenses: Tuition:* Full-time $35,856; part-time $1494 per unit. *Required fees:* $1408; $64 per unit. $473 per term. Tuition and fees vary according to course load and program. *Financial support:* Fellowships with tuition reimbursements, research assistantships with tuition reimbursements, teaching assistantships with tuition reimbursements, career-related internships or fieldwork, Federal Work-Study, institutionally sponsored loans, scholarships/grants, health care benefits, and unspecified assistantships available. Financial award application deadline: 12/1; financial award applicants required to submit FAFSA. *Faculty research:* Genomics, molecular and cell biology, development and molecular genetics, molecular evolution of plants and animals. *Unit head:* Stephen Small, Chair, 212-998-8200, Fax: 212-995-4015, E-mail: biology.admissions@nyu.edu. *Application contact:* Justin Blau, Director of Graduate Studies, PhD Programs, 212-998-8200, Fax: 212-995-4015, E-mail: biology.admissions@nyu.edu.
Website: http://biology.as.nyu.edu/

New York University, Graduate School of Arts and Science, Department of Environmental Medicine, New York, NY 10012-1019. Offers environmental health sciences (MS, PhD), including biostatistics (PhD), environmental hygiene (MS), epidemiology (PhD), ergonomics and biomechanics (PhD), exposure assessment and health effects (PhD), molecular toxicology/carcinogenesis (PhD), toxicology. Part-time programs available. *Faculty:* 26 full-time (7 women). *Students:* 55 full-time (34 women), 13 part-time (3 women); includes 16 minority (1 Black or African American, non-Hispanic/Latino; 8 Asian, non-Hispanic/Latino; 6 Hispanic/Latino; 1 Two or more races, non-Hispanic/Latino), 23 international. Average age 31. 69 applicants, 55% accepted, 18 enrolled. In 2013, 14 master's, 7 doctorates awarded. Terminal master's awarded for partial completion of doctoral program. *Degree requirements:* For master's, thesis or alternative; for doctorate, one foreign language, thesis/dissertation, oral and written exams. *Entrance requirements:* For master's and doctorate, GRE General Test, minimum GPA of 3.0; bachelor's degree in biological, physical, or engineering science. Additional exam requirements/recommendations for international students: Required—TOEFL. *Application deadline:* For fall admission, 12/18 for domestic and international students. Application fee: $95. *Expenses: Tuition:* Full-time $35,856; part-time $1494 per unit. *Required fees:* $1408; $64 per unit. $473 per term. Tuition and fees vary according to course load and program. *Financial support:* Fellowships with tuition reimbursements, teaching assistantships with tuition reimbursements, career-related internships or fieldwork, Federal Work-Study, institutionally sponsored loans, and health care benefits available. Financial award application deadline: 12/18; financial award applicants required to submit FAFSA. *Unit head:* Dr. Max Costa, Chair, 845-731-3661, Fax: 845-351-2058, E-mail: ehs@env.med.nyu.edu. *Application contact:* Dr. Jerome J. Solomon, Director of Graduate Studies, 845-731-3661, Fax: 845-351-2058, E-mail: ehs@env.med.nyu.edu.
Website: http://environmental-medicine.med.nyu.edu/

New York University, School of Medicine and Graduate School of Arts and Science, Medical Scientist Training Program, New York, NY 10012-1019. Offers MD/MS, MD/PhD. Students must be accepted by both the School of Medicine and the Graduate School of Arts and Science. *Faculty:* 170 full-time (36 women). *Students:* 340 applicants, 7% accepted, 9 enrolled. *Application deadline:* For fall admission, 10/15 for domestic students. Application fee: $100. Electronic applications accepted. *Expenses:* Contact institution. *Financial support:* In 2013–14, 29 fellowships with full tuition reimbursements (averaging $27,000 per year), 47 research assistantships with full tuition reimbursements (averaging $25,000 per year) were awarded; teaching assistantships, health care benefits, and unspecified assistantships also available. *Faculty research:* Neurosciences, cell biology and molecular genetics, structural biology, microbial pathogenesis and host defense. *Total annual research expenditures:* $13 million. *Unit head:* Dr. Rodney E. Ulane, Director, 212-263-2149, Fax: 212-263-3766, E-mail: rodney.ulane@med.nyu.edu. *Application contact:* Cindy D. Meador, Academic Coordinator, 212-263-3767, E-mail: cindy.meador@med.nyu.edu.
Website: http://med.nyu.edu/mdphd

New York University, Steinhardt School of Culture, Education, and Human Development, Department of Teaching and Learning, Clinically Rich Integrated Science Program (CRISP), New York, NY 10003. Offers biology (MA), including teaching biology grades 7-12; chemistry (MA), including teaching chemistry grades 7-12; physics (MA), including teaching physics grades 7-12. Part-time and evening/weekend programs available. *Faculty:* 4 full-time (3 women). *Students:* 22 full-time (14 women), 1 part-time (0 women); includes 8 minority (3 Black or African American, non-Hispanic/Latino; 3 Asian, non-Hispanic/Latino; 2 Hispanic/Latino), 2 international. Average age 27. 42 applicants, 64% accepted, 19 enrolled. In 2013, 9 master's awarded. *Degree requirements:* For master's, thesis (for some programs). *Entrance requirements:* Additional exam requirements/recommendations for international students: Required—TOEFL (minimum score 100 iBT). *Application deadline:* For fall admission, 2/1 priority date for domestic and international students; for spring admission, 10/1 for domestic and international students. Applications are processed on a rolling basis. Application fee: $75. Electronic applications accepted. *Expenses: Tuition:* Full-time $35,856; part-time

$1494 per unit. *Required fees:* $1408; $64 per unit. $473 per term. Tuition and fees vary according to course load and program. *Financial support:* Career-related internships or fieldwork, Federal Work-Study, institutionally sponsored loans, scholarships/grants, and tuition waivers (partial) available. Support available to part-time students. Financial award application deadline: 2/1; financial award applicants required to submit FAFSA. *Faculty research:* Science curriculum development, gender and ethnicity, technology use, history and philosophy of school science, science in urban schools. *Unit head:* Dr. Pamela Fraser-Abder, Director, 212-998-5870, Fax: 212-995-4049. *Application contact:* 212-998-5030, Fax: 212-995-4328, E-mail: steinhardt.gradadmissions@nyu.edu.
Website: http://steinhardt.nyu.edu/teachlearn/crisp

North Carolina Agricultural and Technical State University, School of Graduate Studies, College of Arts and Sciences, Department of Biology, Greensboro, NC 27411. Offers biology (MS); biology education (MAT). Part-time and evening/weekend programs available. *Degree requirements:* For master's, comprehensive exam, thesis (for some programs), qualifying exam. *Entrance requirements:* For master's, GRE General Test, personal statement. *Faculty research:* Physical ecology, cytochemistry, botany, parasitology, microbiology.

North Carolina Central University, College of Science and Technology, Department of Biology, Durham, NC 27707-3129. Offers MS. *Degree requirements:* For master's, one foreign language, comprehensive exam, thesis. *Entrance requirements:* For master's, GRE, minimum GPA of 3.0 in major, 2.5 overall. Additional exam requirements/recommendations for international students: Required—TOEFL.

North Carolina State University, College of Veterinary Medicine, Program in Comparative Biomedical Sciences, Raleigh, NC 27695. Offers cell biology (MS, PhD); infectious disease (MS, PhD); pathology (MS, PhD); pharmacology (MS, PhD); population medicine (MS, PhD). Part-time programs available. *Degree requirements:* For master's, thesis; for doctorate, thesis/dissertation. *Entrance requirements:* For master's and doctorate, GRE General Test. Additional exam requirements/recommendations for international students: Required—TOEFL (minimum score 550 paper-based). Electronic applications accepted. *Expenses:* Contact institution. *Faculty research:* Infectious diseases, cell biology, pharmacology and toxicology, genomics, pathology and population medicine.

North Carolina State University, Graduate School, College of Agriculture and Life Sciences, Raleigh, NC 27695. Offers M Tox, MAE, MB, MBAE, MFG, MFM, MFS, MG, MMB, MN, MP, MS, MZS, Ed D, PhD, Certificate. Part-time programs available. Electronic applications accepted.

North Dakota State University, College of Graduate and Interdisciplinary Studies, College of Science and Mathematics, Department of Biological Sciences, Fargo, ND 58108. Offers biology (MS); botany (MS, PhD); cellular and molecular biology (PhD); genomics (PhD); zoology (MS, PhD). *Faculty:* 17 full-time (9 women), 1 part-time/adjunct (0 women). *Students:* 20 full-time (10 women), 3 part-time (all women); includes 2 minority (1 American Indian or Alaska Native, non-Hispanic/Latino; 1 Two or more races, non-Hispanic/Latino), 1 international. Average age 32. 9 applicants, 11% accepted, 1 enrolled. In 2013, 4 master's awarded. *Degree requirements:* For master's, thesis; for doctorate, thesis/dissertation. *Entrance requirements:* For master's and doctorate, GRE General Test. Additional exam requirements/recommendations for international students: Required—TOEFL. *Application deadline:* For fall admission, 1/15 for domestic students. Applications are processed on a rolling basis. Application fee: $35. Electronic applications accepted. *Financial support:* Fellowships with full tuition reimbursements, research assistantships with full tuition reimbursements, teaching assistantships with full tuition reimbursements, career-related internships or fieldwork, Federal Work-Study, institutionally sponsored loans, scholarships/grants, tuition waivers (full), and unspecified assistantships available. Support available to part-time students. Financial award application deadline: 4/15; financial award applicants required to submit FAFSA. *Faculty research:* Comparative endocrinology, physiology, behavioral ecology, plant cell biology, aquatic biology. *Unit head:* Dr. Wendy Reed, Head, 701-231-7087, E-mail: wendy.reed@ndsu.edu. *Application contact:* Sonya Goergen, Marketing, Recruitment, and Public Relations Coordinator, 701-231-7033, Fax: 701-231-6524.
Website: http://biology.ndsu.nodak.edu/

Northeastern Illinois University, College of Graduate Studies and Research, College of Arts and Sciences, Program in Biology, Chicago, IL 60625-4699. Offers MS. Part-time and evening/weekend programs available. *Degree requirements:* For master's, comprehensive exam, thesis optional. *Entrance requirements:* For master's, minimum GPA of 2.75. Additional exam requirements/recommendations for international students: Required—TOEFL (minimum score 550 paper-based; 79 iBT). Electronic applications accepted. *Faculty research:* Paleoecology and freshwater biology, protein biosynthesis and targeting, microbial growth and physiology, molecular biology of antibody production, reptilian neurobiology.

Northeastern University, College of Science, Department of Biology, Boston, MA 02115-5096. Offers bioinformatics (MS, PSM); biology (MS, PhD); biotechnology (MS, PSM); marine biology (MS). Terminal master's awarded for partial completion of doctoral program. *Degree requirements:* For master's, thesis (for some programs); for doctorate, thesis/dissertation, qualifying exam. *Entrance requirements:* For master's and doctorate, GRE General Test. Additional exam requirements/recommendations for international students: Required—TOEFL (minimum score 100 iBT). Electronic applications accepted. *Faculty research:* Biochemistry, marine sciences, molecular biology, microbiology and immunology neurobiology, cellular and molecular biology, biochemistry, marine biochemistry and ecology, microbiology, neurobiology, biotechnology.

Northern Arizona University, Graduate College, College of Engineering, Forestry and Natural Sciences, Department of Biological Sciences, Flagstaff, AZ 86011. Offers MS, PhD. *Faculty:* 45 full-time (15 women), 6 part-time/adjunct (5 women). *Students:* 88 full-time (43 women), 19 part-time (10 women); includes 14 minority (1 American Indian or Alaska Native, non-Hispanic/Latino; 3 Asian, non-Hispanic/Latino; 6 Hispanic/Latino; 4 Two or more races, non-Hispanic/Latino), 5 international. Average age 31. 67 applicants, 48% accepted, 23 enrolled. In 2013, 13 master's, 4 doctorates awarded. *Degree requirements:* For master's, thesis, oral exam; for doctorate, thesis/dissertation. *Entrance requirements:* For master's and doctorate, GRE General Test. Additional exam requirements/recommendations for international students: Required—TOEFL (minimum score 550 paper-based; 80 iBT), IELTS (minimum score 7). *Application deadline:* For fall admission, 2/15 priority date for domestic and international students. Application fee: $65. Electronic applications accepted. *Financial support:* In 2013–14, 2 fellowships, 22 research assistantships with full tuition reimbursements (averaging $13,164 per year), 73 teaching assistantships with full tuition reimbursements (averaging $13,164 per year) were awarded; Federal Work-Study, scholarships/grants, traineeships, health care benefits, tuition waivers (full and partial), and unspecified assistantships also available. Financial award applicants required to submit FAFSA. *Faculty research:* Genetic levels of trophic levels, plant hybrid zones, insect biodiversity, natural history and cognition of wild jays. *Total annual research expenditures:* $2.2 million. *Unit head:* Dr. Maribeth Watwood, Chair, 928-523-9322, Fax: 928-523-7500, E-mail: maribeth.watwood@nau.edu. *Application contact:* Singne Slayton, Administrative Assistant, 928-523-0896, Fax: 928-523-7500, E-mail: singne.slayton@nau.edu.
Website: http://nau.edu/cefns/natsci/biology/

Northern Illinois University, Graduate School, College of Liberal Arts and Sciences, Department of Biological Sciences, De Kalb, IL 60115-2854. Offers MS, PhD. Part-time programs available. *Faculty:* 30 full-time (6 women), 7 part-time/adjunct (1 woman). *Students:* 48 full-time (24 women), 24 part-time (13 women); includes 11 minority (1 Black or African American, non-Hispanic/Latino; 3 Asian, non-Hispanic/Latino; 5 Hispanic/Latino; 2 Two or more races, non-Hispanic/Latino), 9 international. Average age 29. 78 applicants, 38% accepted, 16 enrolled. In 2013, 16 master's, 3 doctorates awarded. Terminal master's awarded for partial completion of doctoral program. *Degree requirements:* For master's, comprehensive exam, thesis optional; for doctorate, thesis/dissertation, candidacy exam, dissertation defense. *Entrance requirements:* For master's, GRE General Test, bachelor's degree in related field, minimum GPA of 2.75; for doctorate, GRE General Test, bachelor's or master's degree in related field; minimum undergraduate GPA of 2.75, graduate 3.2. Additional exam requirements/recommendations for international students: Required—TOEFL (minimum score 550 paper-based). *Application deadline:* For fall admission, 6/1 for domestic students, 5/1 for international students; for spring admission, 11/1 for domestic students, 10/1 for international students. Applications are processed on a rolling basis. Application fee: $40. Electronic applications accepted. *Financial support:* In 2013–14, 6 research assistantships with full tuition reimbursements, 37 teaching assistantships with full tuition reimbursements were awarded; fellowships with full tuition reimbursements, career-related internships or fieldwork, Federal Work-Study, scholarships/grants, tuition waivers (full), and unspecified assistantships also available. Support available to part-time students. Financial award applicants required to submit FAFSA. *Faculty research:* Plant molecular biology, neurosecretory control, ethnobotany, organellar genomes, carbon metabolism. *Unit head:* Dr. Barrie P. Bode, Chair, 815-753-1753, Fax: 815-753-0461, E-mail: bodebp@niu.edu. *Application contact:* Dr. Thomas Sims, Director of Graduate Studies, 815-753-7873.
Website: http://www.bios.niu.edu/

Northern Michigan University, College of Graduate Studies, College of Arts and Sciences, Department of Biology, Marquette, MI 49855-5301. Offers biochemistry (MS); biology (MS). Part-time programs available. *Faculty:* 15 full-time (3 women). *Students:* 34. Average age 27. 20 applicants, 90% accepted, 14 enrolled. In 2013, 5 master's awarded. *Degree requirements:* For master's, thesis. *Entrance requirements:* For master's, GRE, minimum GPA of 3.0; references; coursework in biology and other sciences, faculty member as mentor. Additional exam requirements/recommendations for international students: Required—TOEFL (minimum score 550 paper-based; 79 iBT), IELTS (minimum score 6.5). *Application deadline:* For fall admission, 5/1 for domestic students; for winter admission, 11/1 for domestic students; for spring admission, 3/17 for domestic students. Applications are processed on a rolling basis. Application fee: $50. Electronic applications accepted. *Expenses:* Tuition, state resident: part-time $427 per credit. Tuition, nonresident: part-time $614.50 per credit. *Required fees:* $325 per semester. Tuition and fees vary according to course load and program. *Financial support:* In 2013–14, 19 students received support, including 1 research assistantship, 19 teaching assistantships; career-related internships or fieldwork, Federal Work-Study, institutionally sponsored loans, tuition waivers, and unspecified assistantships also available. Support available to part-time students. Financial award application deadline: 3/1. *Faculty research:* Evolutionary genetics, neurobiology, conservation biology, fisheries and wildlife, microbiology. *Unit head:* Dr. Jill B.K. Leonard, Graduate Program Director, 906-227-1619, E-mail: jileonar@nmu.edu. *Application contact:* Dr. Brian Cherry, Assistant Provost of Graduate Education and Research, 906-227-2300, Fax: 906-227-2315, E-mail: graduate@nmu.edu.
Website: http://www.nmu.edu/biology/

Northwestern University, Fienberg School of Medicine, Combined MD/PhD Medical Scientist Training Program, Evanston, IL 60208. Offers MD/PhD. Application must be made to both The Graduate School and the Medical School. *Accreditation:* LCME/AMA. Electronic applications accepted. *Faculty research:* Cardiovascular epidemiology, cancer epidemiology, nutritional interventions for the prevention of cardiovascular disease and cancer, women's health, outcomes research.

Northwestern University, Fienberg School of Medicine and Interdepartmental Programs, Integrated Graduate Programs in the Life Sciences, Chicago, IL 60611. Offers biostatistics (PhD); epidemiology (PhD); health and biomedical informatics (PhD); health services and outcomes research (PhD); healthcare quality and patient safety (PhD); translational outcomes in science (PhD). *Degree requirements:* For doctorate, comprehensive exam, thesis/dissertation, written and oral qualifying exams. *Entrance requirements:* For doctorate, GRE General Test. Additional exam requirements/recommendations for international students: Required—TOEFL (minimum score 600 paper-based). Electronic applications accepted.

Northwestern University, The Graduate School, Interdisciplinary Biological Sciences Program (IBiS), Evanston, IL 60208. Offers biochemistry (PhD); bioengineering and biotechnology (PhD); biotechnology (PhD); cell and molecular biology (PhD); developmental and systems biology (PhD); nanotechnology (PhD); neurobiology (PhD); structural biology and biophysics (PhD). *Degree requirements:* For doctorate, thesis/dissertation, qualifying exam. *Entrance requirements:* For doctorate, GRE General Test. Additional exam requirements/recommendations for international students: Required—TOEFL (minimum score 600 paper-based). *Application deadline:* For fall admission, 12/15 for domestic and international students. Applications are processed on a rolling basis. Application fee: $95. Electronic applications accepted. *Financial support:* Fellowships, research assistantships, teaching assistantships, career-related internships or fieldwork, institutionally sponsored loans, scholarships/grants, traineeships, health care benefits, and unspecified assistantships available. Financial award application deadline: 12/31; financial award applicants required to submit FAFSA. *Faculty research:* Biophysics/structural biology, cell/molecular biology, synthetic biology, developmental systems biology, chemical biology/nanotechnology. *Unit head:* Dr. Deborah Klos Dehring, Associate Director, 847-467-0451, E-mail: d-klos@northwestern.edu. *Application contact:* Cathy Prullage, Program Manager, 847-491-4301, E-mail: ibis@northwestern.edu.
Website: http://www.biochem.northwestern.edu/ibis/

Northwest Missouri State University, Graduate School, College of Arts and Sciences, Department of Natural Sciences, Maryville, MO 64468-6001. Offers biology (MS); teaching: science (MS Ed). Part-time programs available. *Degree requirements:* For master's, comprehensive exam, thesis. *Entrance requirements:* For master's, GRE General Test, minimum GPA of 3.0 in last 60 hours or 2.75 overall, writing sample. Additional exam requirements/recommendations for international students: Required—TOEFL (minimum score 550 paper-based).

Notre Dame de Namur University, Division of Academic Affairs, College of Arts and Sciences, Department of Natural Sciences, Belmont, CA 94002-1908. Offers premedical studies (Certificate). *Entrance requirements:* Additional exam requirements/recommendations for international students: Required—TOEFL (minimum score 550 paper-based; 79 iBT). Electronic applications accepted.

Nova Southeastern University, College of Medical Sciences, Fort Lauderdale, FL 33314-7796. Offers biomedical sciences (MBS). *Students:* 27 full-time (11 women); includes 13 minority (1 Black or African American, non-Hispanic/Latino; 5 Asian, non-Hispanic/Latino; 7 Hispanic/Latino). Average age 25. In 2013, 5 master's awarded. *Degree requirements:* For master's, thesis. *Entrance requirements:* For master's, MCAT, DAT, minimum GPA of 2.5. *Application deadline:* For fall admission, 4/15 for domestic students. Applications are processed on a rolling basis. Application fee: $50. *Expenses:* Contact institution. *Financial support:* Application deadline: 8/7; applicants required to submit FAFSA. *Faculty research:* Neurophysiology, mucosal immunology, allergies involving the lungs, cardiovascular physiology parasitology. *Unit head:* Dr. Harold E. Laubach, Dean, 954-262-1303, Fax: 954-262-1802, E-mail: harold@nova.edu. *Application contact:* Lori B. Dribin, PhD, Assistant Dean for Student Affairs, 954-262-1341, Fax: 954-262-1802, E-mail: lorib@nova.edu.

Nova Southeastern University, Oceanographic Center, Fort Lauderdale, FL 33314-7796. Offers biological sciences (MS); coastal studies (Certificate); coastal zone management (MS); marine and coastal climate change (Certificate); marine and coastal studies (MA); marine biology (MS); marine biology and oceanography (PhD), including marine biology, oceanography; marine environmental sciences (MS). Part-time and evening/weekend programs available. Postbaccalaureate distance learning degree programs offered (no on-campus study). *Faculty:* 16 full-time (2 women), 22 part-time/adjunct (11 women). *Students:* 121 full-time (74 women), 128 part-time (83 women); includes 33 minority (6 Black or African American, non-Hispanic/Latino; 1 American Indian or Alaska Native, non-Hispanic/Latino; 7 Asian, non-Hispanic/Latino; 11 Hispanic/Latino; 8 Two or more races, non-Hispanic/Latino), 5 international. Average age 29. 79 applicants, 57% accepted, 26 enrolled. In 2013, 38 master's, 8 other advanced degrees awarded. *Degree requirements:* For master's, thesis; for doctorate, comprehensive exam, thesis/dissertation, departmental qualifying exam. *Entrance requirements:* For master's, GRE General Test, 3 letters of recommendation, BS/BA in natural science (for marine biology program), BS/BA in biology (for biological sciences program), minor in the natural sciences or equivalent (for coastal zone management and marine environmental sciences); for doctorate, GRE General Test, master's degree. Additional exam requirements/recommendations for international students: Required—TOEFL (minimum score 550 paper-based). *Application deadline:* Applications are processed on a rolling basis. Application fee: $50. *Expenses:* Contact institution. *Financial support:* In 2013–14, 2 fellowships with full and partial tuition reimbursements (averaging $16,300 per year), 50 research assistantships with full and partial tuition reimbursements (averaging $19,000 per year) were awarded; teaching assistantships, career-related internships or fieldwork, Federal Work-Study, scholarships/grants, health care benefits, tuition waivers (full and partial), and unspecified assistantships also available. Support available to part-time students. Financial award applicants required to submit FAFSA. *Faculty research:* Physical, geological, chemical, and biological oceanography. *Unit head:* Dr. Richard Dodge, Dean, 954-262-3600, Fax: 954-262-4020, E-mail: dodge@nsu.nova.edu. *Application contact:* Dr. Richard Spieler, Associate Dean of Academic Programs, 954-262-3600, Fax: 954-262-4020, E-mail: spieler@nova.edu.
Website: http://www.nova.edu/ocean/

Oakland University, Graduate Study and Lifelong Learning, College of Arts and Sciences, Department of Biological Sciences, Rochester, MI 48309-4401. Offers biological sciences (MA, MS); biomedical sciences: biological communications (PhD). *Faculty:* 19 full-time (6 women), 2 part-time/adjunct (both women). *Students:* 46 full-time (27 women), 14 part-time (8 women); includes 7 minority (1 Black or African American, non-Hispanic/Latino; 1 American Indian or Alaska Native, non-Hispanic/Latino; 5 Asian, non-Hispanic/Latino), 11 international. Average age 26. 102 applicants, 33% accepted, 25 enrolled. In 2013, 4 master's awarded. *Degree requirements:* For master's, thesis. *Entrance requirements:* For master's, GRE Subject Test, GRE General Test, minimum GPA of 3.0. Additional exam requirements/recommendations for international students: Required—TOEFL (minimum score 550 paper-based). *Application deadline:* Applications are processed on a rolling basis. Application fee: $0. Electronic applications accepted. *Expenses:* Contact institution. *Financial support:* Federal Work-Study, institutionally sponsored loans, and tuition waivers (full) available. Financial award application deadline: 3/1; financial award applicants required to submit FAFSA. *Faculty research:* Mechanisms of RSC recruitment and its role in transcription. *Total annual research expenditures:* $889,811. *Unit head:* Dr. Arik Dvir, Chair, 248-370-3580, Fax: 248-370-4225, E-mail: dvir@oakland.edu. *Application contact:* Dr. Doug Wendell, Associate Professor, 248-370-4457, E-mail: wendell@oakland.edu.
Website: http://www2.oakland.edu/biology

Occidental College, Graduate Studies, Department of Biology, Los Angeles, CA 90041-3314. Offers MA. Part-time programs available. *Degree requirements:* For master's, thesis, final exam. *Entrance requirements:* For master's, GRE General Test, GRE Subject Test, minimum GPA of 3.0. Additional exam requirements/recommendations for international students: Required—TOEFL (minimum score 625 paper-based). *Expenses:* Contact institution.

The Ohio State University, College of Medicine, School of Biomedical Science, Biomedical Sciences Graduate Program, Columbus, OH 43210. Offers immunology (PhD); medical genetics (PhD); molecular virology (PhD); pharmacology (PhD). *Students:* 109 full-time (55 women), 9 part-time (6 women); includes 24 minority (5 Black or African American, non-Hispanic/Latino; 1 American Indian or Alaska Native, non-Hispanic/Latino; 10 Asian, non-Hispanic/Latino; 6 Hispanic/Latino; 1 Native Hawaiian or other Pacific Islander, non-Hispanic/Latino; 1 Two or more races, non-Hispanic/Latino), 4 international. Average age 27. In 2013, 20 doctorates awarded. *Degree requirements:* For doctorate, thesis/dissertation. *Entrance requirements:* For doctorate, GRE General Test; GRE Subject Test in biochemistry, cell and molecular biology (recommended for some programs). Additional exam requirements/recommendations for international students: Required—TOEFL (minimum score 600 paper-based; 100 iBT), Michigan English Language Assessment Battery (minimum score 86); Recommended—IELTS (minimum score 8). *Application deadline:* For fall admission, 12/13 priority date for domestic students, 11/1 priority date for international students. Applications are processed on a rolling basis. Application fee: $60 ($70 for international students). Electronic applications accepted. *Financial support:* In 2013–14, 53 students received support, including 4 fellowships with full tuition reimbursements available (averaging $19,000 per year), 49 research assistantships with full tuition reimbursements available (averaging $19,000 per year); scholarships/grants and unspecified assistantships also available. Financial award application deadline: 1/15. *Unit head:* Joanna Groden, Co-Director, 614-688-4301, Fax: 614-292-6226, E-mail: ibgp@osumc.edu. *Application contact:* Graduate Admissions, 614-292-9444, Fax: 614-292-3895, E-mail: domestic.grad@osu.edu.
Website: http://www.ibgp.org

The Ohio State University, Graduate School, College of Arts and Sciences, Division of Natural and Mathematical Sciences, Department of Mathematics, Columbus, OH 43210. Offers computational sciences (MMS); mathematical biosciences (MMS); mathematics (PhD); mathematics for educators (MMS). *Faculty:* 61. *Students:* 126 full-time (32 women), 8 part-time (1 woman); includes 8 minority (3 Asian, non-Hispanic/Latino; 3 Hispanic/Latino; 2 Two or more races, non-Hispanic/Latino), 64 international. Average age 26. In 2013, 15 master's, 9 doctorates awarded. *Degree requirements:* For master's, thesis optional; for doctorate, one foreign language, thesis/dissertation. *Entrance requirements:* For master's, GRE General Test; for doctorate, GRE General Test (recommended), GRE Subject Test (mathematics). Additional exam requirements/recommendations for international students: Required—TOEFL (minimum score 550 paper-based; 79 iBT), Michigan English Language Assessment Battery (minimum score 82); Recommended—IELTS (minimum score 7). *Application deadline:* For fall admission, 12/15 priority date for domestic and international students. Applications are processed on a rolling basis. Application fee: $60 ($70 for international students). Electronic applications accepted. *Financial support:* Fellowships with tuition reimbursements, research assistantships with tuition reimbursements, teaching assistantships with tuition reimbursements, Federal Work-Study, institutionally sponsored loans, and unspecified assistantships available. Support available to part-time students. *Unit head:* Luis Casian, Chair, 614-292-7173, E-mail: casian@math.ohio-state.edu. *Application contact:* Roman Nitze, Graduate Studies Coordinator, 614-292-6274, Fax: 614-292-1479, E-mail: nitze.1@osu.edu.
Website: http://www.math.osu.edu/

Ohio University, Graduate College, College of Arts and Sciences, Department of Biological Sciences, Athens, OH 45701-2979. Offers biological sciences (MS, PhD); cell biology and physiology (MS, PhD); ecology and evolutionary biology (MS, PhD); exercise physiology and muscle biology (MS, PhD); microbiology (MS, PhD); neuroscience (MS, PhD). Terminal master's awarded for partial completion of doctoral program. *Degree requirements:* For master's, comprehensive exam, thesis, 1 quarter of teaching experience; for doctorate, comprehensive exam, thesis/dissertation, 2 quarters of teaching experience. *Entrance requirements:* For master's, GRE General Test, names of three faculty members whose research interests most closely match the applicant's interest; for doctorate, GRE General Test, essay concerning prior training, research interest and career goals, plus names of three faculty members whose research interests most closely match the applicant's interest. Additional exam requirements/recommendations for international students: Required—TOEFL (minimum score 620 paper-based; 105 iBT) or IELTS (minimum score 7.5). Electronic applications accepted. *Faculty research:* Ecology and evolutionary biology, exercise physiology and muscle biology, neurobiology, cell biology, physiology.

Oklahoma State University Center for Health Sciences, Program in Biomedical Sciences, Tulsa, OK 74107. Offers MS, PhD, DO/PhD. Part-time programs available. *Faculty:* 39 full-time (9 women), 1 part-time/adjunct (0 women). *Students:* 21 full-time (13 women), 8 part-time (4 women); includes 5 minority (3 Black or African American, non-Hispanic/Latino; 1 American Indian or Alaska Native, non-Hispanic/Latino; 1 Hispanic/Latino), 2 international. Average age 31. 20 applicants, 45% accepted, 8 enrolled. In 2013, 6 master's, 1 doctorate awarded. *Degree requirements:* For master's, thesis; for doctorate, thesis/dissertation, comprehensive, oral and written exam. *Entrance requirements:* For master's, GRE General Test, minimum GPA of 3.0; for doctorate, GRE General Test, MCAT, minimum GPA of 3.0. Additional exam requirements/recommendations for international students: Required—TOEFL (minimum score 79 iBT). *Application deadline:* For fall admission, 2/15 for domestic students, 2/1 for international students; for winter admission, 9/15 for domestic and international students; for spring admission, 11/1 for domestic and international students. Application fee: $40 ($75 for international students). *Expenses:* Tuition, state resident: full-time $22,127; part-time $178 per credit hour. Tuition, nonresident: full-time $43,572; part-time $728 per credit hour. *Required fees:* $910.79; $200 per semester. *Financial support:* In 2013–14, 18 students received support, including 12 research assistantships with full tuition reimbursements available (averaging $21,180 per year), 2 teaching assistantships with full tuition reimbursements available (averaging $21,180 per year); Federal Work-Study and tuition waivers (full) also available. Financial award application deadline: 4/1; financial award applicants required to submit FAFSA. *Faculty research:* Neuroscience, cell biology, cell signaling, infectious disease, virology, neurotoxicology. *Total annual research expenditures:* $1.7 million. *Unit head:* Dr. Randall L. Davis, Director, 918-561-8408, Fax: 918-561-8276. *Application contact:* Patrick Anderson, Coordinator of Graduate Admissions, 800-677-1972, Fax: 918-561-8243, E-mail: patrick.anderson@okstate.edu.

Old Dominion University, College of Sciences, Master of Science in Biology Program, Norfolk, VA 23529. Offers MS. Part-time programs available. *Faculty:* 22 full-time (4 women), 23 part-time/adjunct (2 women). *Students:* 30 full-time (18 women), 11 part-time (4 women); includes 5 minority (1 Black or African American, non-Hispanic/Latino; 1 Asian, non-Hispanic/Latino; 3 Hispanic/Latino), 2 international. Average age 27. 25 applicants, 48% accepted, 10 enrolled. In 2013, 14 master's awarded. *Degree requirements:* For master's, comprehensive exam, thesis optional. *Entrance requirements:* For master's, GRE General Test, MCAT, minimum GPA of 3.0. Additional exam requirements/recommendations for international students: Required—TOEFL (minimum score 550 paper-based; 79 iBT). *Application deadline:* For fall admission, 2/1 priority date for domestic and international students; for winter admission, 6/1 priority date for domestic and international students; for spring admission, 10/1 priority date for domestic and international students. Application fee: $50. Electronic applications accepted. *Expenses:* Tuition, state resident: full-time $9888; part-time $412 per credit. Tuition, nonresident: full-time $25,152; part-time $1048 per credit. *Required fees:* $59 per semester. One-time fee: $50. *Financial support:* In 2013–14, 2 fellowships (averaging $6,575 per year), 10 research assistantships with partial tuition reimbursements (averaging $15,000 per year), 8 teaching assistantships with partial tuition reimbursements (averaging $15,000 per year) were awarded; career-related internships or fieldwork and scholarships/grants also available. Support available to part-time students. Financial award application deadline: 2/1; financial award applicants required to submit FAFSA. *Faculty research:* Wetland ecology, systematics and ecology of vertebrates, marine biology, molecular and cellular microbiology, cell biology, immunology, physiological and reproductive biology. *Total annual research expenditures:* $2 million. *Unit head:* Dr. Robert Ratzlaff, Graduate Program Director, 757-683-4361, Fax: 757-683-5283, E-mail: biolgpd@odu.edu. *Application contact:* William Heffelfinger, Director of Graduate Admissions, 757-683-5554, Fax: 757-683-3255, E-mail: gradadmit@odu.edu.
Website: http://sci.odu.edu/biology/academics/bio-ms.shtml

Old Dominion University, College of Sciences, Program in Biomedical Sciences, Norfolk, VA 23529. Offers PhD. Program offered jointly with Eastern Virginia Medical School. *Faculty:* 29 full-time (8 women). *Students:* 32 full-time (16 women), 2 part-time (0 women); includes 7 minority (3 Black or African American, non-Hispanic/Latino; 1 Asian, non-Hispanic/Latino; 2 Hispanic/Latino; 1 Two or more races, non-Hispanic/Latino), 17 international. Average age 34. 18 applicants, 22% accepted, 4 enrolled. In 2013, 4 doctorates awarded. *Degree requirements:* For doctorate, comprehensive exam, thesis/dissertation. *Entrance requirements:* For doctorate, GRE General Test, minimum GPA of 3.0. Additional exam requirements/recommendations for international students: Required—TOEFL (minimum score 79 iBT). *Application deadline:* For fall admission, 2/1 priority date for domestic and international students. Application fee: $50. Electronic applications accepted. *Expenses:* Tuition, state resident: full-time $9888; part-time $412 per credit. Tuition, nonresident: full-time $25,152; part-time $1048 per credit. *Required fees:* $59 per semester. One-time fee: $50. *Financial support:* In 2013–14, 2 fellowships with full tuition reimbursements (averaging $18,000 per year), 2 research assistantships with full tuition reimbursements (averaging $18,000 per year), 4

teaching assistantships with full tuition reimbursements (averaging $15,000 per year) were awarded; career-related internships or fieldwork, scholarships/grants, tuition waivers (partial), and unspecified assistantships also available. Support available to part-time students. Financial award application deadline: 2/15; financial award applicants required to submit FAFSA. *Faculty research:* Systems biology and biophysics, pure and applied biomedical sciences, biological chemistry, clinical chemistry, cell biology and molecular pathogenesis. *Total annual research expenditures:* $3.7 million. *Unit head:* Dr. Robert Ratzlaff, Graduate Program Director, 757-683-4361, Fax: 757-683-5283, E-mail: bimdgpd@odu.edu. *Application contact:* William Heffelfinger, Director of Graduate Admissions, 757-683-5554, Fax: 757-683-3255, E-mail: gradadmit@odu.edu.
Website: http://sci.odu.edu/biology/academics/phdmed.shtml

Oregon Health & Science University, School of Medicine, Graduate Programs in Medicine, Portland, OR 97239-3098. Offers MBA, MBST, MCR, MPAS, MPH, MS, MSCNU, PhD, Certificate, Graduate Certificate. Part-time programs available. *Faculty:* 567 full-time (219 women), 331 part-time/adjunct (110 women). *Students:* 379 full-time (232 women), 424 part-time (243 women); includes 175 minority (19 Black or African American, non-Hispanic/Latino; 2 American Indian or Alaska Native, non-Hispanic/Latino; 85 Asian, non-Hispanic/Latino; 40 Hispanic/Latino; 3 Native Hawaiian or other Pacific Islander, non-Hispanic/Latino; 26 Two or more races, non-Hispanic/Latino), 61 international. Average age 34. 1,874 applicants, 15% accepted, 263 enrolled. In 2013, 159 master's, 37 doctorates, 130 other advanced degrees awarded. Terminal master's awarded for partial completion of doctoral program. *Degree requirements:* For master's, thesis or capstone experience; for doctorate, comprehensive exam, thesis/dissertation, qualifying exam. *Entrance requirements:* For master's, GRE General Test (minimum scores: 153 [500 old version] Verbal/148 [600 old version] Quantitative/4.5 Analytical), MCAT or GMAT (for some programs); for doctorate, GRE General Test (minimum scores: 153 [500 old version] Verbal/148 [600 old version] Quantitative/4.5 Analytical). Additional exam requirements/recommendations for international students: Required—TOEFL. *Application deadline:* Applications are processed on a rolling basis. Application fee: $70. Electronic applications accepted. *Expenses:* Contact institution. *Financial support:* Fellowships, research assistantships, teaching assistantships, scholarships/grants, health care benefits, and full tuition and stipends (for PhD students) available. *Unit head:* Dr. Allison Fryer, Associate Dean for Graduate Studies, 503-494-6222, Fax: 503-494-3400, E-mail: somgrad@ohsu.edu. *Application contact:* Lorie Gookin, Admissions Coordinator, 503-494-6222, Fax: 503-494-3400, E-mail: somgrad@ohsu.edu.

Penn State Hershey Medical Center, College of Medicine, Graduate School Programs in the Biomedical Sciences, Hershey, PA 17033. Offers MPH, MS, PhD, MD/PhD, PhD/MBA. Terminal master's awarded for partial completion of doctoral program. *Degree requirements:* For master's, thesis or alternative; for doctorate, comprehensive exam, thesis/dissertation, oral exam. *Entrance requirements:* For master's, GRE; for doctorate, GRE, minimum GPA of 3.0. Additional exam requirements/recommendations for international students: Required—TOEFL (minimum score 550 paper-based; 80 iBT). *Application deadline:* For fall admission, 1/31 priority date for domestic students, 2/1 priority date for international students. Applications are processed on a rolling basis. Application fee: $65. Electronic applications accepted. *Expenses:* Contact institution. *Financial support:* In 2013–14, 3 fellowships with full tuition reimbursements (averaging $26,500 per year), 37 research assistantships with full tuition reimbursements (averaging $23,028 per year) were awarded; career-related internships or fieldwork, scholarships/grants, health care benefits, tuition waivers (full), and unspecified assistantships also available. Financial award applicants required to submit FAFSA. *Unit head:* Dr. Michael Verderame, Associate Dean of Graduate Studies, 717-531-8892, Fax: 717-531-0786, E-mail: grad-hmc@psu.edu. *Application contact:* Kathleen M. Simon, Administrative Assistant, 717-531-8892, Fax: 717-531-0786, E-mail: grad-hmc@psu.edu.
Website: http://www.pennstatehershey.org/web/gsa/home

Penn State University Park, Graduate School, Eberly College of Science, Department of Biology, University Park, PA 16802. Offers MS, PhD. *Unit head:* Dr. Daniel J. Larson, Dean, 814-865-9591, Fax: 814-865-3634, E-mail: djlarson@psu.edu. *Application contact:* Cynthia E. Nicosia, Director, Graduate Enrollment Services, 814-865-1834, Fax: 814-863-4627, E-mail: cey1@psu.edu.
Website: http://bio.psu.edu/

Penn State University Park, Graduate School, Intercollege Graduate Programs, Intercollege Graduate Program in Integrative Biosciences, University Park, PA 16802. Offers MS, PhD. *Unit head:* Dr. Regina Vasilatos-Younken, Interim Dean, 814-865-2516, Fax: 814-863-4627, E-mail: rxv@psu.edu. *Application contact:* Cynthia E. Nicosia, Director, Graduate Enrollment Services, 814-865-1834, Fax: 814-863-4627, E-mail: cey1@psu.edu.

Philadelphia College of Osteopathic Medicine, Graduate and Professional Programs, Graduate Programs in Biomedical Sciences, Philadephia, PA 19131. Offers MS. Evening/weekend programs available. *Faculty:* 25 full-time (14 women). *Students:* 92 full-time (43 women); includes 34 minority (8 Black or African American, non-Hispanic/Latino; 11 Asian, non-Hispanic/Latino; 3 Hispanic/Latino; 12 Two or more races, non-Hispanic/Latino). Average age 26. 346 applicants, 53% accepted, 75 enrolled. In 2013, 13 master's awarded. *Degree requirements:* For master's, thesis optional. *Entrance requirements:* For master's, GRE, MCAT, DAT, OAT, PCAT, pre-medical prerequisite coursework; biochemistry (recommended). Additional exam requirements/recommendations for international students: Required—TOEFL (minimum score 79 iBT). *Application deadline:* For fall admission, 7/15 for domestic students. Applications are processed on a rolling basis. Application fee: $50. Electronic applications accepted. *Financial support:* In 2013–14, 59 students received support. Federal Work-Study, institutionally sponsored loans, and scholarships/grants available. Financial award application deadline: 3/15; financial award applicants required to submit FAFSA. *Faculty research:* Neuroscience and neurodegenerative disorders, inflammation and allergic response to food allergens, cardiovascular function and disease, bone and joint disorders, cancer biology. *Total annual research expenditures:* $533,489. *Unit head:* Dr. Marcus Bell, Chair, 215-871-6834, Fax: 215-871-6865, E-mail: marcusbe@pcom.edu. *Application contact:* Kari A. Shotwell, Director of Admissions, 215-871-6700, Fax: 215-871-6719, E-mail: karis@pcom.edu.
Website: http://www.pcom.edu

Pittsburg State University, Graduate School, College of Arts and Sciences, Department of Biology, Pittsburg, KS 66762. Offers MS. *Degree requirements:* For master's, thesis or alternative.

Plymouth State University, College of Graduate Studies, Graduate Studies in Education, Program in Science, Plymouth, NH 03264-1595. Offers applied meteorology (MS); biology (MS); clinical mental health counseling (MS); environmental science and policy (MS); science education (MS).

Point Loma Nazarene University, Department of Biology, San Diego, CA 92106-2899. Offers MA, MS. Part-time programs available. *Students:* 1 (woman) full-time, 16 part-time (10 women); includes 5 minority (1 American Indian or Alaska Native, non-Hispanic/Latino; 4 Hispanic/Latino). Average age 34. 6 applicants, 67% accepted, 3 enrolled. In 2013, 5 master's awarded. *Entrance requirements:* For master's, BA/BS in science field, letters of recommendation, essay, interview. Additional exam requirements/recommendations for international students: Required—TOEFL. *Application deadline:* For fall admission, 7/4 priority date for domestic students; for spring admission, 12/8 priority date for domestic students; for summer admission, 5/23 priority date for domestic students. Applications are processed on a rolling basis. Application fee: $50. Electronic applications accepted. *Expenses: Tuition:* Full-time $6900; part-time $567 per credit hour. *Financial support:* Applicants required to submit FAFSA. *Unit head:* Dr. Dianne Anderson, Director of Master's Program in Biology, 619-849-2705, E-mail: dianneanderson@pointloma.edu. *Application contact:* Laura Leinweber, Graduate Enrollment Counselor, 866-692-4723, E-mail: lauraleinweber@pointloma.edu.
Website: http://www.pointloma.edu/discover/graduate-school-san-diego/san-diego-graduate-programs-masters-degree-san-diego/biology

Ponce School of Medicine & Health Sciences, Program in Biomedical Sciences, Ponce, PR 00732-7004. Offers PhD. *Faculty:* 6 full-time (1 woman). *Students:* 27 full-time (16 women); includes 26 minority (all Hispanic/Latino), 1 international. Average age 30. 7 applicants, 57% accepted, 3 enrolled. In 2013, 6 doctorates awarded. *Degree requirements:* For doctorate, one foreign language, comprehensive exam, thesis/dissertation. *Entrance requirements:* For doctorate, GRE General Test, proficiency in Spanish and English, minimum overall GPA of 3.0, 3 letters of recommendation, minimum of 35 credits in science. *Application deadline:* For fall admission, 1/15 for domestic and international students. Application fee: $150. *Financial support:* In 2013–14, 8 students received support, including 1 fellowship with full tuition reimbursement available (averaging $7,399 per year); research assistantships, tuition waivers (partial), and unspecified assistantships also available. Financial award application deadline: 4/30; financial award applicants required to submit FAFSA. *Unit head:* Dr. Jose Torres, Director, PhD Program in Biomedical Sciences, 787-840-2158, E-mail: jtorres@psm.edu. *Application contact:* Maria Colon, Admissions Officer, 787-840-2575 Ext. 2143, E-mail: mcolon@psm.edu.

Pontifical Catholic University of Puerto Rico, College of Sciences, Department of Biology, Ponce, PR 00717-0777. Offers environmental sciences (MS). *Degree requirements:* For master's, thesis. *Entrance requirements:* For master's, GRE, 2 letters of recommendation, interview, minimum GPA of 2.75.

Portland State University, Graduate Studies, College of Liberal Arts and Sciences, Department of Biology, Portland, OR 97207-0751. Offers MA, MS, PhD. *Faculty:* 21 full-time (6 women), 7 part-time/adjunct (3 women). *Students:* 46 full-time (25 women), 13 part-time (4 women); includes 6 minority (1 American Indian or Alaska Native, non-Hispanic/Latino; 1 Asian, non-Hispanic/Latino; 3 Hispanic/Latino; 1 Two or more races, non-Hispanic/Latino), 3 international. Average age 31. 63 applicants, 19% accepted, 10 enrolled. In 2013, 13 master's, 4 doctorates awarded. *Degree requirements:* For master's, one foreign language, thesis; for doctorate, thesis/dissertation. *Entrance requirements:* For master's, GRE General Test, GRE Subject Test, minimum GPA of 3.0 in upper-division course work or 2.75 overall, 2 letters of reference; for doctorate, GRE General Test, GRE Subject Test, minimum GPA of 3.5 in science. Additional exam requirements/recommendations for international students: Required—TOEFL (minimum score 550 paper-based). *Application deadline:* For fall admission, 2/15 for domestic and international students; for winter admission, 9/1 for domestic students, 7/1 for international students; for spring admission, 11/1 for domestic and international students. Applications are processed on a rolling basis. Application fee: $50. *Expenses:* Tuition, state resident: full-time $9207; part-time $341 per credit. Tuition, nonresident: full-time $14,391; part-time $533 per credit. *Required fees:* $1263; $22 per credit. $98 per quarter. One-time fee: $150. Tuition and fees vary according to program. *Financial support:* In 2013–14, 4 teaching assistantships with full tuition reimbursements (averaging $7,500 per year) were awarded; Federal Work-Study, scholarships/grants, tuition waivers (partial), and unspecified assistantships also available. Support available to part-time students. Financial award application deadline: 3/1; financial award applicants required to submit FAFSA. *Faculty research:* Genetic diversity and natural population, vertebrate temperature regulation, water balance and sensory physiology, trace elements and aquatic ecology, molecular genetics. *Total annual research expenditures:* $2.1 million. *Unit head:* Dr. Jason Podrabsky, Chair, 503-725-5772, E-mail: jpod@pdx.edu. *Application contact:* Amy Jolstead, Office Specialist, 503-725-8757, Fax: 503-725-3888, E-mail: amyj@pdx.edu.
Website: http://www.bio.pdx.edu/

Prairie View A&M University, College of Arts and Sciences, Department of Biology, Prairie View, TX 77446-0519. Offers bio-environmental toxicology (MS); biology (MS). Part-time and evening/weekend programs available. *Faculty:* 5 full-time (2 women). *Students:* 1 (woman) part-time; minority (Black or African American, non-Hispanic/Latino). Average age 25. In 2013, 8 master's awarded. *Degree requirements:* For master's, comprehensive exam, thesis optional. *Entrance requirements:* For master's, GRE General Test. Additional exam requirements/recommendations for international students: Required—TOEFL. *Application deadline:* For fall admission, 7/1 for domestic and international students; for spring admission, 11/1 for domestic and international students. Applications are processed on a rolling basis. Application fee: $50. Electronic applications accepted. *Expenses:* Tuition, state resident: full-time $3776; part-time $209.77 per credit hour. Tuition, nonresident: full-time $10,183; part-time $565.77 per credit hour. *Required fees:* $2037; $446.50 per credit hour. *Financial support:* In 2013–14, 3 students received support, including 3 teaching assistantships (averaging $13,440 per year); Federal Work-Study and unspecified assistantships also available. Financial award application deadline: 4/1; financial award applicants required to submit FAFSA. *Faculty research:* Genomics, hypertension, control of gene express, proteins, ligands that interact with hormone receptors, prostate cancer, renin-angiotensin yeast metabolism. *Unit head:* Dr. Harriette Howard-Lee-Block, Head, 936-261-3160, Fax: 936-261-3179, E-mail: hlblock@pvamu.edu. *Application contact:* Dr. Seab A. Smith, Associate Professor, 936-261-3169, Fax: 936-261-3179, E-mail: sasmith@pvamu.edu.

Purdue University, Graduate School, Biomedical Sciences Interdisciplinary Graduate Program, West Lafayette, IN 47907. Offers PhD. Program offered jointly by School of Veterinary Medicine and Weldon School of Biomedical Engineering. *Students:* 11 full-time (6 women), 1 part-time (0 women); includes 1 minority (Hispanic/Latino), 4 international. Average age 27. 25 applicants, 20% accepted, 4 enrolled. *Degree requirements:* For doctorate, thesis/dissertation, seminars, teaching experience. *Entrance requirements:* For doctorate, GRE General Test (minimum scores: verbal 550, quantitative 700), minimum undergraduate GPA of 3.0. Additional exam requirements/recommendations for international students: Required—TOEFL (minimum score 550 paper-based; 77 iBT); Recommended—TWE. *Application deadline:* For fall admission, 12/15 priority date for domestic and international students. Applications are processed on a rolling basis. Application fee: $60 ($75 for international students). Electronic applications accepted. *Financial support:* Fellowships, research assistantships, and teaching assistantships available. Support available to part-time students. *Unit head:* Harm HogenEsch, Head, 765-496-3487, Fax: 765-496-1261, E-mail: hogenesch@purdue.edu. *Application contact:* Sandra M. May, Graduate Contact for Admissions, 765-494-7054, E-mail: smmay@purdue.edu.
Website: http://www.gradschool.purdue.edu/BSDT/

Purdue University, Graduate School, College of Science, Department of Biological Sciences, West Lafayette, IN 47907. Offers biochemistry (PhD); biophysics (PhD); cell and developmental biology (PhD); ecology, evolutionary and population biology (MS, PhD), including ecology, evolutionary biology, population biology; genetics (MS, PhD); microbiology (MS, PhD); molecular biology (PhD); neurobiology (MS, PhD); plant physiology (PhD). *Faculty:* 50 full-time (13 women), 5 part-time/adjunct (1 woman). *Students:* 111 full-time (61 women), 5 part-time (0 women); includes 9 minority (1 Black or African American, non-Hispanic/Latino; 5 Asian, non-Hispanic/Latino; 3 Hispanic/Latino), 62 international. Average age 27. 170 applicants, 19% accepted, 17 enrolled. In 2013, 9 master's, 18 doctorates awarded. Terminal master's awarded for partial completion of doctoral program. *Degree requirements:* For master's, thesis (for some programs); for doctorate, thesis/dissertation, seminars, teaching experience. *Entrance requirements:* For master's, GRE General Test (minimum analytical writing score of 3.5), minimum undergraduate GPA of 3.0; for doctorate, GRE General Test (minimum analytical writing score of 3.5), minimum undergraduate GPA of 3.5. Additional exam requirements/recommendations for international students: Required—TOEFL (minimum score 600 paper-based; 107 iBT for MS, 80 iBT for PhD). *Application deadline:* For fall admission, 12/7 for domestic and international students. Applications are processed on a rolling basis. Application fee: $60 ($75 for international students). Electronic applications accepted. *Financial support:* Fellowships, research assistantships, and teaching assistantships available. Support available to part-time students. Financial award application deadline: 2/15; financial award applicants required to submit FAFSA. *Unit head:* Dr. Richard J. Kuhn, Head, 765-494-4407, E-mail: kuhnr@purdue.edu. *Application contact:* Georgina E. Rupp, Graduate Coordinator, 765-494-8142, Fax: 765-494-0876, E-mail: ruppg@purdue.edu.
Website: http://www.bio.purdue.edu/

Purdue University, Graduate School, PULSe - Purdue University Life Sciences Program, West Lafayette, IN 47907. Offers biomolecular structure and biophysics (PhD); biotechnology (PhD); chemical biology (PhD); chromatin and regulation of gene expression (PhD); integrative neuroscience (PhD); integrative plant sciences (PhD); membrane biology (PhD); microbiology (PhD); molecular evolutionary and cancer biology (PhD); molecular evolutionary genetics (PhD); molecular virology (PhD). *Students:* 154 full-time (78 women), 1 part-time (0 women); includes 23 minority (5 Black or African American, non-Hispanic/Latino; 5 Asian, non-Hispanic/Latino; 10 Hispanic/Latino; 3 Two or more races, non-Hispanic/Latino), 73 international. Average age 26. 239 applicants, 33% accepted, 40 enrolled. *Entrance requirements:* For doctorate, GRE, minimum undergraduate GPA of 3.0. Additional exam requirements/recommendations for international students: Required—TOEFL (minimum score 550 paper-based; 77 iBT). *Application deadline:* For fall admission, 1/15 priority date for domestic and international students. Applications are processed on a rolling basis. Application fee: $60 ($75 for international students). Electronic applications accepted. *Financial support:* In 2013–14, research assistantships with tuition reimbursements (averaging $22,500 per year), teaching assistantships with tuition reimbursements (averaging $22,500 per year) were awarded. *Unit head:* Dr. Christine A. Hrycyna, Head, 765-494-7322, E-mail: hrycyna@purdue.edu. *Application contact:* Colleen Gabauer, Graduate Contact, 765-494-9256, E-mail: cgabauer@purdue.edu.
Website: http://www.gradschool.purdue.edu/pulse

Purdue University Calumet, Graduate Studies Office, School of Engineering, Mathematics, and Science, Department of Biological Sciences, Hammond, IN 46323-2094. Offers biology (MS); biology teaching (MS); biotechnology (MS). *Entrance requirements:* For master's, GRE. Additional exam requirements/recommendations for international students: Required—TOEFL. Electronic applications accepted. *Faculty research:* Cell biology, molecular biology, genetics, microbiology, neurophysiology.

Queens College of the City University of New York, Division of Graduate Studies, Mathematics and Natural Sciences Division, Department of Biology, Flushing, NY 11367-1597. Offers MA. Part-time and evening/weekend programs available. *Degree requirements:* For master's, comprehensive exam, thesis or alternative, qualifying exam. *Entrance requirements:* For master's, minimum GPA of 3.0. Additional exam requirements/recommendations for international students: Required—TOEFL.

Queen's University at Kingston, School of Graduate Studies, Faculty of Arts and Sciences, Department of Biology, Kingston, ON K7L 3N6, Canada. Offers M Sc, PhD. Part-time programs available. *Degree requirements:* For master's, thesis; for doctorate, comprehensive exam, thesis/dissertation. *Entrance requirements:* Additional exam requirements/recommendations for international students: Required—TOEFL. *Faculty research:* Limnology, plant morphogenesis, nitrogen fixation, cell cycle, genetics.

Quinnipiac University, School of Health Sciences, Program in Medical Laboratory Sciences, Hamden, CT 06518-1940. Offers biomedical sciences (MHS); laboratory management (MHS); microbiology (MHS). Part-time and evening/weekend programs available. *Faculty:* 14 full-time (6 women), 20 part-time/adjunct (8 women). *Students:* 66 full-time (36 women), 30 part-time (13 women); includes 20 minority (7 Black or African American, non-Hispanic/Latino; 8 Asian, non-Hispanic/Latino; 4 Hispanic/Latino; 1 Two or more races, non-Hispanic/Latino), 41 international. 79 applicants, 73% accepted, 38 enrolled. In 2013, 47 master's awarded. *Degree requirements:* For master's, comprehensive exam, thesis optional. *Entrance requirements:* For master's, minimum GPA of 2.75; bachelor's degree in biological, medical, or health sciences. Additional exam requirements/recommendations for international students: Required—TOEFL (minimum score 575 paper-based; 90 iBT), IELTS (minimum score 6.5). *Application deadline:* For fall admission, 7/30 priority date for domestic students, 4/30 priority date for international students; for spring admission, 12/15 priority date for domestic students, 9/15 priority date for international students. Applications are processed on a rolling basis. Application fee: $45. Electronic applications accepted. *Expenses: Tuition:* Part-time $920 per credit. *Required fees:* $37 per credit. *Financial support:* In 2013–14, 7 students received support. Career-related internships or fieldwork, Federal Work-Study, scholarships/grants, and unspecified assistantships available. Support available to part-time students. Financial award application deadline: 6/1; financial award applicants required to submit FAFSA. *Faculty research:* ACL injury mechanism and running injuries and performance; transcriptional activators upstream stimulatory factor (USF); identification of novel antimicrobials; vaccines, formites and opportunistic pathogens; molecular biology of the Lyme Disease agent, Borrelia burgdorferi; molecular and microscopic techniques in host-pathogen interactions; non-invasive vascular biology, external pneumatic compression, sports performance. *Application contact:* Office of Graduate Admissions, 800-462-1944, Fax: 203-582-3443, E-mail: graduate@quinnipiac.edu.
Website: http://www.quinnipiac.edu/gradmedlab

Regis College, School of Nursing, Science and Health Professions, Weston, MA 02493. Offers applied behavior analysis (MS); biomedical sciences (MS); health administration (MS); nurse practitioner (Certificate); nursing (MS, DNP); nursing education (Certificate). Part-time and evening/weekend programs available. *Degree requirements:* For master's, thesis. *Entrance requirements:* For master's, GRE General Test or MAT, minimum GPA of 3.0; for doctorate, MAT or GRE if GPA from master's lower than 3.5. Additional exam requirements/recommendations for international students: Required—TOEFL (minimum score 550 paper-based). Electronic applications accepted. *Faculty research:* Health policy, education, aging, job satisfaction, psychiatric nursing, critical thinking.

Regis University, Regis College, Denver, CO 80221-1099. Offers biomedical sciences (MS); education (MA). *Accreditation:* Teacher Education Accreditation Council. Part-time programs available. *Faculty:* 11 full-time (8 women), 24 part-time/adjunct (23 women). *Students:* 41 full-time (24 women), 52 part-time (47 women); includes 14 minority (2 Black or African American, non-Hispanic/Latino; 3 Asian, non-Hispanic/Latino; 9 Hispanic/Latino). Average age 38. 195 applicants, 100% accepted, 165 enrolled. In 2013, 36 master's awarded. *Degree requirements:* For master's, thesis (for some programs), capstone presentation. *Entrance requirements:* For master's, official transcript reflecting baccalaureate degree awarded from U.S.-based regionally-accredited college or university. Additional exam requirements/recommendations for international students: Required—TOEFL (minimum score 550 paper-based; 82 iBT). *Application deadline:* For fall admission, 4/15 priority date for domestic students, 7/1 priority date for international students; for spring admission, 12/15 priority date for domestic students. Applications are processed on a rolling basis. Application fee: $75. Electronic applications accepted. *Expenses:* Contact institution. *Financial support:* In 2013–14, 2 students received support. Federal Work-Study and scholarships/grants available. Financial award application deadline: 4/15; financial award applicants required to submit FAFSA. *Unit head:* Dr. Stephen Doty, Interim Academic Dean, 303-458-4040. *Application contact:* Sarah Engel, Director of Admissions, 303-458-4900, Fax: 303-964-5534, E-mail: regisadm@regis.edu.
Website: http://www.regis.edu/RC.aspx

Rensselaer Polytechnic Institute, Graduate School, School of Science, Program in Biology, Troy, NY 12180-3590. Offers MS, PhD. *Faculty:* 17 full-time (6 women), 1 part-time/adjunct (0 women). *Students:* 30 full-time (13 women), 3 part-time (0 women), 6 international. Average age 29. 94 applicants, 32% accepted, 12 enrolled. In 2013, 12 master's, 4 doctorates awarded. Terminal master's awarded for partial completion of doctoral program. *Degree requirements:* For master's, comprehensive exam, thesis optional; for doctorate, comprehensive exam, thesis/dissertation. *Entrance requirements:* For master's and doctorate, GRE. Additional exam requirements/recommendations for international students: Required—TOEFL (minimum score 570 paper-based; 88 iBT), IELTS (minimum score 6.5), PTE (minimum score 60). *Application deadline:* For fall admission, 1/1 priority date for domestic and international students. Applications are processed on a rolling basis. Application fee: $75. Electronic applications accepted. *Expenses: Tuition:* Full-time $45,100; part-time $1879 per credit hour. *Required fees:* $1983. *Financial support:* In 2013–14, 16 students received support, including research assistantships (averaging $18,500 per year), teaching assistantships (averaging $18,500 per year); fellowships also available. Financial award application deadline: 1/1. *Faculty research:* Biochemistry; bioinformatics; biophysics; cancer biology; computational biology; ecology and environmental sciences; microbiology; molecular, cell, and developmental biology; neuroscience; stem cells; structural biology. *Total annual research expenditures:* $825,366. *Unit head:* Dr. Lee Ligon, Graduate Program Director, 518-276-3458, E-mail: ligonl@rpi.edu. *Application contact:* Office of Graduate Admissions, 518-276-6216, E-mail: gradadmissions@rpi.edu.
Website: http://www.rpi.edu/dept/bio/

Rhode Island College, School of Graduate Studies, Faculty of Arts and Sciences, Department of Biology, Providence, RI 02908-1991. Offers biology (MA); modern biological sciences (CGS). Part-time programs available. *Faculty:* 7 full-time (6 women). *Students:* 6 part-time (4 women); includes 1 minority (Hispanic/Latino). Average age 27. In 2013, 4 master's awarded. *Degree requirements:* For master's, thesis. *Entrance requirements:* For master's, GRE General and Subject Tests. Additional exam requirements/recommendations for international students: Recommended—TOEFL (minimum score 550 paper-based; 79 iBT). *Application deadline:* For fall admission, 3/1 for domestic students. Applications are processed on a rolling basis. Application fee: $50. *Expenses:* Tuition, state resident: full-time $8928; part-time $372 per credit hour. Tuition, nonresident: full-time $17,376; part-time $724 per credit hour. *Required fees:* $602; $22 per credit. $72 per term. *Financial support:* In 2013–14, 3 teaching assistantships with full tuition reimbursements (averaging $3,500 per year) were awarded; career-related internships or fieldwork, Federal Work-Study, scholarships/grants, health care benefits, and unspecified assistantships also available. Support available to part-time students. Financial award application deadline: 5/15; financial award applicants required to submit FAFSA. *Unit head:* Dr. Lloyd Matsumoto, Chair, 401-456-8010, E-mail: biology@ric.edu. *Application contact:* Graduate Studies, 401-456-8700.
Website: http://www.ric.edu/biology/index.php

Rochester Institute of Technology, Graduate Enrollment Services, College of Science, Thomas H. Gosnell School of Life Sciences, Rochester, NY 14623-5603. Offers bioinformatics (MS); environmental science (MS). Part-time programs available. *Students:* 22 full-time (12 women), 15 part-time (9 women); includes 5 minority (3 American Indian or Alaska Native, non-Hispanic/Latino; 2 Hispanic/Latino), 12 international. Average age 27. 61 applicants, 48% accepted, 15 enrolled. In 2013, 12 master's awarded. *Degree requirements:* For master's, thesis or alternative. *Entrance requirements:* Additional exam requirements/recommendations for international students: Required—TOEFL (minimum score 570 paper-based; 88 iBT) or IELTS (minimum score 6.5). *Application deadline:* For fall admission, 2/15 priority date for domestic and international students. Applications are processed on a rolling basis. Application fee: $60. Electronic applications accepted. *Expenses: Tuition:* Full-time $37,236; part-time $1552 per credit hour. *Required fees:* $250. *Financial support:* Fellowships with partial tuition reimbursements, research assistantships with partial tuition reimbursements, teaching assistantships with partial tuition reimbursements, career-related internships or fieldwork, scholarships/grants, and unspecified assistantships available. Support available to part-time students. Financial award applicants required to submit FAFSA. *Faculty research:* Bioinformatics software development, bioscience, biomedical research, environmental research examining the human relationship to nature and developing solutions that prevent or reverse environmental deterioration. *Unit head:* Gary Skuse, Associate Head, School of Life Sciences, 585-475-6725, Fax: 585-475-2533, E-mail: biology@rit.edu. *Application contact:* Diane Ellison, Assistant Vice President, Graduate Enrollment Services, 585-475-2229, Fax: 585-475-7164, E-mail: gradinfo@rit.edu.
Website: http://www.rit.edu/cos/lifesciences/

The Rockefeller University, Graduate Program in Biomedical Sciences, New York, NY 10021-6399. Offers MS, PhD, MD/PhD. *Faculty:* 96 full-time (21 women), 168 part-time/adjunct (47 women). *Students:* 201 full-time (84 women); includes 35 minority (5 Black or African American, non-Hispanic/Latino; 14 Asian, non-Hispanic/Latino; 13 Hispanic/Latino; 3 Two or more races, non-Hispanic/Latino), 77 international. Average age 29. 719 applicants, 10% accepted, 26 enrolled. In 2013, 5 master's, 17 doctorates awarded. Terminal master's awarded for partial completion of doctoral program. *Degree requirements:* For master's, thesis; for doctorate, thesis/dissertation. *Entrance requirements:* For doctorate, GRE General Test; GRE Subject Test (strongly recommended), three letters of recommendation, official college or university transcripts, personal essay. Additional exam requirements/recommendations for international

students: Required—TOEFL. *Application deadline:* For fall and winter admission, 12/1 for domestic and international students. Application fee: $50. Electronic applications accepted. *Financial support:* Fellowships with full tuition reimbursements, institutionally sponsored loans, scholarships/grants, traineeships, and health care benefits available. *Unit head:* Dr. Sidney Strickland, Dean of Graduate Studies, 212-327-8086, Fax: 212-327-8505, E-mail: phd@rockefeller.edu. *Application contact:* Kristen Cullen, Graduate Admissions Administrator/Registrar, 212-327-8088, Fax: 212-327-8505, E-mail: kristen.cullen@rockefeller.edu.
Website: http://www.rockefeller.edu/graduate/

See Display on this page and Close-Up on page 123.

Rosalind Franklin University of Medicine and Science, College of Health Professions, Department of Interprofessional Healthcare Studies, Biomedical Sciences Program, North Chicago, IL 60064-3095. Offers MS. *Entrance requirements:* For master's, MCAT, DAT, OAT, PCAT or GRE, BS in chemistry, physics, biology. Additional exam requirements/recommendations for international students: Required—TOEFL.

Rosalind Franklin University of Medicine and Science, School of Graduate and Postdoctoral Studies - Interdisciplinary Graduate Program in Biomedical Sciences, North Chicago, IL 60064-3095. Offers MS, PhD, DPM/PhD, MD/PhD. *Students:* 39 full-time (20 women); includes 18 minority (15 American Indian or Alaska Native, non-Hispanic/Latino; 2 Asian, non-Hispanic/Latino; 1 Hispanic/Latino), 21 international. Average age 29. 66 applicants, 15% accepted, 5 enrolled. In 2013, 4 doctorates awarded. Terminal master's awarded for partial completion of doctoral program. *Degree requirements:* For master's, comprehensive exam, thesis, publication; for doctorate, comprehensive exam, thesis/dissertation. *Entrance requirements:* For master's and doctorate, GRE General Test. Additional exam requirements/recommendations for international students: Required—TOEFL, TWE. *Application deadline:* For fall admission, 12/31 priority date for domestic and international students. Application fee: $0. Electronic applications accepted. *Expenses:* Contact institution. *Financial support:* In 2013–14, 38 fellowships (averaging $28,000 per year) were awarded; career-related internships or fieldwork, Federal Work-Study, traineeships, health care benefits, tuition waivers (full and partial), and unspecified assistantships also available. Financial award applicants required to submit FAFSA. *Faculty research:* Extracellular matrix, nutrition and mood, neuropsychopharmacology, membrane transport, brain metabolism. *Unit head:* Dr. Joseph X. DiMario, Dean, 847-578-8493, E-mail: joseph.dimario@rosalindfranklin.edu. *Application contact:* Caryn F. Wickersheim, Senior Administrative Assistant, School of Graduate and Professional Studies Dean's Office, 847-578-8493, E-mail: igpbs@rosalindfranklin.edu.
Website: http://www.rosalindfranklin.edu/SGPS

Rowan University, Graduate School, College of Liberal Arts and Sciences, Department of Biological Science, Glassboro, NJ 08028-1701. Offers MS. *Faculty:* 3 full-time (1 woman), 4 part-time/adjunct (1 woman). *Students:* 36 part-time (35 women); includes 13 minority (9 Black or African American, non-Hispanic/Latino; 1 American Indian or Alaska Native, non-Hispanic/Latino; 1 Asian, non-Hispanic/Latino; 2 Hispanic/Latino). Average age 39. 55 applicants, 78% accepted, 39 enrolled. Application fee: $65. *Expenses: Tuition, area resident:* Part-time $638 per credit. Tuition, state resident: full-time $5742. *Required fees:* $142 per credit. Tuition and fees vary according to course level and program. *Unit head:* Dr. Horacio Sosa, Dean, College of Graduate and Continuing Education, 856-256-4747, Fax: 856-256-5638, E-mail: sosa@rowan.edu. *Application contact:* Admissions and Enrollment Services, 856-256-5435, Fax: 856-256-5637, E-mail: cgceadmissions@rowan.edu.

Rutgers, The State University of New Jersey, Camden, Graduate School of Arts and Sciences, Program in Biology, Camden, NJ 08102. Offers MS. Part-time and evening/weekend programs available. *Degree requirements:* For master's, comprehensive exam, thesis (for some programs), 30 credits. *Entrance requirements:* For master's, GRE General Test, GRE Subject Test (recommended), 3 letters of recommendation; statement of personal, professional and academic goals; biology or related undergraduate degree (preferred). Additional exam requirements/recommendations for international students: Required—TOEFL, IELTS. Electronic applications accepted. *Faculty research:* Neurobiology, biochemistry, ecology, developmental biology, biological signaling mechanisms.

Rutgers, The State University of New Jersey, Newark, Graduate School of Biomedical Sciences, Newark, NJ 07107. Offers biodefense (Certificate); biomedical engineering (PhD); biomedical sciences (multidisciplinary) (PhD); cellular biology, neuroscience and physiology (PhD), including neuroscience, physiology, biophysics, cardiovascular biology, molecular pharmacology, stem cell biology; infection, immunity and inflammation (PhD), including immunology, infectious disease, microbiology, oral biology; molecular biology, genetics and cancer (PhD), including biochemistry, molecular genetics, cancer biology, radiation biology, bioinformatics; neuroscience (Certificate); pharmacological sciences (Certificate); stem cell (Certificate); DMD/PhD; MD/PhD. PhD in biomedical engineering offered jointly with New Jersey Institute of Technology. Part-time and evening/weekend programs available. Terminal master's awarded for partial completion of doctoral program. *Degree requirements:* For doctorate, thesis/dissertation, qualifying exam. *Entrance requirements:* For doctorate, GRE General Test. Additional exam requirements/recommendations for international students: Required—TOEFL. Electronic applications accepted.

Rutgers, The State University of New Jersey, Newark, Graduate School, Program in Biology, Newark, NJ 07102. Offers MS, PhD. Part-time and evening/weekend programs available. Terminal master's awarded for partial completion of doctoral program. *Degree requirements:* For master's, comprehensive exam, thesis optional; for doctorate, thesis/dissertation, qualifying exam. *Entrance requirements:* For master's, GRE General Test, minimum undergraduate B average; for doctorate, GRE General Test, GRE Subject Test, minimum B average. Electronic applications accepted. *Faculty research:* Cell-cytoskeletal elements, development and regeneration in the nervous system, cellular trafficking, environmental stressors and their impact on development, opportunistic parasitic infections in AIDS.

Rutgers, The State University of New Jersey, Newark, Graduate School, Program in Computational Biology, Newark, NJ 07102. Offers MS. Program offered jointly with New Jersey Institute of Technology. *Entrance requirements:* For master's, GRE, minimum undergraduate B average. Additional exam requirements/recommendations for international students: Required—TOEFL.

Rutgers, The State University of New Jersey, New Brunswick, Graduate School-New Brunswick, BioMaPS Institute for Quantitative Biology, Piscataway, NJ 08854-8097. Offers computational biology and molecular biophysics (PhD). *Degree requirements:* For doctorate, comprehensive exam, thesis/dissertation. *Entrance requirements:* For doctorate, GRE. Additional exam requirements/recommendations for international students: Required—TOEFL. Electronic applications accepted. *Faculty research:* Structural biology, systems biology, bioinformatics, translational medicine, genomics.

Rutgers, The State University of New Jersey, New Brunswick, Graduate School of Biomedical Sciences, Piscataway, NJ 08854-5635. Offers biochemistry and molecular biology (MS, PhD); biomedical engineering (MS, PhD); biomedical science (MS); cellular and molecular pharmacology (MS, PhD); clinical and translational science (MS); environmental sciences/exposure assessment (PhD); molecular genetics, microbiology and immunology (MS, PhD); neuroscience (MS, PhD); physiology and integrative biology (MS, PhD); toxicology (PhD); MD/PhD. Terminal master's awarded for partial completion of doctoral program. *Degree requirements:* For master's, thesis (for some programs), ethics training; for doctorate, comprehensive exam, thesis/dissertation, ethics training. *Entrance requirements:* For master's, GRE General Test, MCAT, DAT; for doctorate, GRE General Test. Additional exam requirements/recommendations for international students: Required—TOEFL. Electronic applications accepted.

St. Cloud State University, School of Graduate Studies, College of Science and Engineering, Department of Biology, St. Cloud, MN 56301-4498. Offers MA, MS. *Degree requirements:* For master's, comprehensive exam (for some programs), thesis or alternative. *Entrance requirements:* For master's, GRE General Test, minimum GPA of 2.75. Additional exam requirements/recommendations for international students: Recommended—TOEFL (minimum score 550 paper-based), IELTS (minimum score 6.5). Electronic applications accepted.

Saint Francis University, Department of Physician Assistant Sciences, Medical Science Program, Loretto, PA 15940-0600. Offers MMS. Part-time and evening/weekend programs available. Postbaccalaureate distance learning degree programs offered (no on-campus study). *Faculty:* 2 full-time (both women), 6 part-time/adjunct (5 women). *Students:* 126 part-time (90 women); includes 42 minority (11 Black or African American, non-Hispanic/Latino; 1 American Indian or Alaska Native, non-Hispanic/Latino; 13 Asian, non-Hispanic/Latino; 14 Hispanic/Latino; 3 Two or more races, non-Hispanic/Latino). Average age 31. 45 applicants, 80% accepted, 36 enrolled. In 2013, 111 master's awarded. *Degree requirements:* For master's, thesis or alternative, successful completion of affiliate PA program, minimum GPA of 2.8 in program. *Entrance requirements:* For master's, enrollment in affiliate PA program, bachelor's degree with minimum GPA of 2.5, resume, transcript. Additional exam requirements/recommendations for international students: Recommended—TOEFL (minimum score 80 iBT). *Application deadline:* For fall admission, 6/15 for domestic students; for spring admission, 11/15 for domestic students; for summer admission, 3/15 for domestic students. Applications are processed on a rolling basis. Application fee: $0. Electronic applications accepted. *Expenses:* Contact institution. *Financial support:* Available to part-time students. Applicants required to submit FAFSA. *Faculty research:* Health care policy, physician assistant practice roles, health promotion/disease prevention, public health epidemiology. *Unit head:* Deborah E. Budash, Director, 814-472-3919, Fax: 814-472-3066, E-mail: dbudash@francis.edu. *Application contact:* Jean A. Kline, Administrative Assistant, 814-472-3357, Fax: 814-472-3066, E-mail: jkline@francis.edu.
Website: http://francis.edu/master-of-medical-science/

St. Francis Xavier University, Graduate Studies, Department of Biology, Antigonish, NS B2G 2W5, Canada. Offers M Sc. *Degree requirements:* For master's, thesis. *Entrance requirements:* For master's, 2 letters of recommendation. Additional exam requirements/recommendations for international students: Required—TOEFL (minimum score 580 paper-based). *Faculty research:* Cellular, whole organism, and population levels; marine photosynthesis; biophysical mechanisms; aquatic biology.

St. John's University, St. John's College of Liberal Arts and Sciences, Department of Biological Sciences, Queens, NY 11439. Offers MS, PhD. Part-time and evening/weekend programs available. *Students:* 34 full-time (22 women), 4 part-time (1 woman); includes 7 minority (1 Black or African American, non-Hispanic/Latino; 4 Asian, non-Hispanic/Latino; 2 Hispanic/Latino), 21 international. Average age 27. 69 applicants, 23% accepted, 9 enrolled. In 2013, 12 master's, 3 doctorates awarded. *Degree requirements:* For master's, comprehensive exam, thesis optional, residency; for doctorate, comprehensive exam, thesis/dissertation, residency. *Entrance requirements:* For master's, GRE, minimum GPA of 3.0, 2 letters of recommendation, transcript, bachelor's degree; for doctorate, GRE General Test, GRE Subject Test, minimum GPA of 3.0 (undergraduate), 3.5 (graduate); 3 letters of recommendation, writing sample, MS in biology, transcript. Additional exam requirements/recommendations for international students: Required—TOEFL (minimum score 600 paper-based; 100 iBT), IELTS (minimum score 5.5). *Application deadline:* For fall admission, 5/1 priority date for domestic and international students; for spring admission, 11/1 priority date for domestic and international students. Applications are processed on a rolling basis. Application fee: $70. Electronic applications accepted. *Expenses: Tuition:* Full-time $19,800; part-time $1100 per credit. *Required fees:* $170 per semester. *Financial support:* Fellowships, research assistantships, and scholarships/grants available. Support available to part-time students. Financial award application deadline: 3/1; financial award applicants required to submit FAFSA. *Faculty research:* Regulation of gene transcription, immunology and inflammation, cancer research, infectious diseases, molecular control of developmental processes, signal transduction, neurobiology and neurodegenerative diseases. *Total annual research expenditures:* $300,000. *Unit head:* Dr. Ales Vancura, Chair, 718-990-1679, E-mail: vancuraa@stjohns.edu. *Application contact:* Robert Medrano, Director of Graduate Admission, 718-990-1601, Fax: 718-990-5686, E-mail: gradhelp@stjohns.edu.

Saint Joseph's University, College of Arts and Sciences, Department of Biology, Philadelphia, PA 19131-1395. Offers MA, MS. Part-time programs available. *Faculty:* 11 full-time (3 women), 2 part-time/adjunct (both women). *Students:* 9 full-time (5 women), 10 part-time (5 women); includes 6 minority (1 Black or African American, non-Hispanic/Latino; 3 Hispanic/Latino; 2 Two or more races, non-Hispanic/Latino). Average age 25. 37 applicants, 70% accepted, 10 enrolled. In 2013, 12 master's awarded. *Degree requirements:* For master's, comprehensive exam (for some programs), thesis (for some programs), minimum GPA of 3.0, completion of degree within 5 years. *Entrance requirements:* For master's, GRE, 2 letters of recommendation, transcript, personal statement, resume. Additional exam requirements/recommendations for international students: Required—TOEFL (minimum score 550 paper-based; 80 iBT), IELTS (minimum score 6.5). *Application deadline:* For fall admission, 7/15 priority date for domestic students, 7/15 for international students; for spring admission, 11/15 priority date for domestic students, 11/15 for international students. Applications are processed on a rolling basis. Application fee: $35. Electronic applications accepted. *Expenses: Tuition:* Part-time $786 per credit hour. Tuition and fees vary according to degree level and program. *Financial support:* Research assistantships with tuition reimbursements and unspecified assistantships available. Financial award applicants required to submit FAFSA. *Faculty research:* Life science, undergraduate science education, confocal microscope for research and training, telomere biology, bridging the gap in racial disparities in colorectal cancer. *Total annual research expenditures:* $248,885. *Unit head:* Dr. James Watrous, Director, 610-660-1829, E-mail: jwatrous@sju.edu. *Application contact:* Elisabeth Woodward, Director of Marketing and Admissions, Graduate Arts and Sciences, 610-660-3131, Fax: 610-660-3230, E-mail: gradstudies@sju.edu.
Website: http://sju.edu/majors-programs/graduate-arts-sciences/masters/biology-ma-and-ms

Saint Louis University, Graduate Education, College of Arts and Sciences and Graduate Education, Department of Biology, St. Louis, MO 63103-2097. Offers MS, MS-R, PhD. *Degree requirements:* For master's, comprehensive exam, thesis (for some programs); for doctorate, thesis/dissertation, preliminary exams. *Entrance requirements:* For master's, GRE General Test, letters of recommendation, resume; for doctorate, GRE General Test, letters of recommendation, resumé, statement, transcripts. Additional exam requirements/recommendations for international students: Required—TOEFL (minimum score 550 paper-based). Electronic applications accepted. *Faculty research:* Systematics, speciation, evolution, community ecology, conservation biology, molecular signaling.

Saint Louis University, Graduate Education and School of Medicine, Graduate Program in Biomedical Sciences, St. Louis, MO 63103-2097. Offers MS-R, PhD. *Degree requirements:* For doctorate, comprehensive exam, thesis/dissertation. *Entrance requirements:* For doctorate, GRE. Additional exam requirements/recommendations for international students: Required—TOEFL. Electronic applications accepted. *Faculty research:* Biochemistry and molecular biology, physiology and pharmacology, virology, pathology, immunology.

Salisbury University, Program in Applied Biology, Salisbury, MD 21801-6837. Offers MS. Part-time programs available. *Faculty:* 12 full-time (5 women). *Students:* 8 full-time (5 women), 4 part-time (2 women). Average age 26. 9 applicants, 22% accepted, 2 enrolled. In 2013, 2 master's awarded. *Degree requirements:* For master's, thesis optional. *Entrance requirements:* For master's, GRE (with scores at or above 50th percentile), undergraduate degree with minimum cumulative GPA of 3.0 in biology or related field, 3 letters of recommendation, personal statement, writing sample, letter from graduate advisor. Additional exam requirements/recommendations for international students: Required—TOEFL (minimum score 550 paper-based; 79 iBT), IELTS (minimum score 6.5). *Application deadline:* For fall admission, 3/1 priority date for domestic and international students; for spring admission, 10/1 priority date for domestic and international students. Application fee: $50. Electronic applications accepted. *Expenses:* Tuition, state resident: part-time $342 per credit hour. Tuition, nonresident: part-time $631 per credit hour. *Required fees:* $76 per credit hour. Tuition and fees vary according to program. *Financial support:* In 2013–14, 6 teaching assistantships with full tuition reimbursements (averaging $9,750 per year) were awarded; career-related internships or fieldwork, institutionally sponsored loans, scholarships/grants, and unspecified assistantships also available. Support available to part-time students. Financial award application deadline: 3/1; financial award applicants required to submit FAFSA. *Faculty research:* Molecular genetics, cell biology, organismal biology, animal behavior, microbiology. *Unit head:* Dr. Stephen Genrich, Chair of Biological Sciences, 410-543-6423, E-mail: scgenrich@salisbury.edu. *Application contact:* Sandra Ramses, Program Management Specialist, 410-543-6054, E-mail: shramses@salisbury.edu.
Website: http://www.salisbury.edu/biology/MS_Applied_Biology.html

Sam Houston State University, College of Sciences, Department of Biology, Huntsville, TX 77341. Offers MA, MS. Part-time programs available. *Faculty:* 18 full-time (6 women). *Students:* 1 (woman) full-time, 28 part-time (19 women); includes 2 minority (both Two or more races, non-Hispanic/Latino), 2 international. Average age 27. 21 applicants, 57% accepted, 4 enrolled. In 2013, 8 master's awarded. *Degree requirements:* For master's, comprehensive exam, thesis (for some programs). *Entrance requirements:* For master's, GRE General Test. Additional exam requirements/recommendations for international students: Required—TOEFL (minimum score 550 paper-based; 79 iBT), IELTS (minimum score 6.5). *Application deadline:* For fall admission, 8/1 for domestic students, 6/25 for international students; for spring admission, 12/1 for domestic students, 11/12 for international students. Applications are processed on a rolling basis. Application fee: $45 ($75 for international students). Electronic applications accepted. *Financial support:* In 2013–14, 18 research assistantships (averaging $8,609 per year), 13 teaching assistantships (averaging $7,317 per year) were awarded; career-related internships or fieldwork, Federal Work-Study, institutionally sponsored loans, scholarships/grants, and unspecified assistantships also available. Support available to part-time students. Financial award application deadline: 5/31; financial award applicants required to submit FAFSA. *Unit head:* Dr. Chad Hargrave, Chair, 936-294-1538, Fax: 936-294-1598, E-mail: cwh005@shsu.edu. *Application contact:* Dr. Sibyl Bucheli, Advisor, 936-294-1554, E-mail: bucheli@shsu.edu.
Website: http://www.shsu.edu/~bio_www/

San Diego State University, Graduate and Research Affairs, College of Sciences, Department of Biology, San Diego, CA 92182. Offers biology (MA, MS), including ecology (MS), molecular biology (MS), physiology (MS), systematics/evolution (MS); cell and molecular biology (PhD); ecology (MS, PhD); microbiology (MS). Terminal master's awarded for partial completion of doctoral program. *Degree requirements:* For master's, thesis; for doctorate, thesis/dissertation. *Entrance requirements:* For master's, GRE General Test, GRE Subject Test, resume or curriculum vitae, 2 letters of recommendation. Additional exam requirements/recommendations for international students: Required—TOEFL. Electronic applications accepted.

San Francisco State University, Division of Graduate Studies, College of Science and Engineering, Department of Biology, San Francisco, CA 94132-1722. Offers biomedical science (MS); cell and molecular biology (MS); ecology, evolution, and conservation biology (MS); marine biology (MS); marine science (MS); microbiology (MS); physiology and behavioral biology (MS); science (PSM), including biotechnology, stem cell science. *Application deadline:* Applications are processed on a rolling basis. *Unit head:* Dr. Michael A. Goldman, Chair, 415-338-1549, E-mail: goldman@sfsu.edu. *Application contact:* Dr. Robert Patterson, Graduate Coordinator, 415-338-1237, E-mail: patters@sfsu.edu.
Website: http://biology.sfsu.edu/

San Jose State University, Graduate Studies and Research, College of Science, Department of Biological Sciences, San Jose, CA 95192-0001. Offers biological sciences (MA, MS); molecular biology and microbiology (MS); organismal biology, conservation and ecology (MS); physiology (MS). Part-time programs available. *Entrance requirements:* For master's, GRE. Electronic applications accepted. *Faculty research:* Systemic physiology, molecular genetics, SEM studies, toxicology, large mammal ecology.

The Scripps Research Institute, Kellogg School of Science and Technology, La Jolla, CA 92037. Offers chemical and biological sciences (PhD). *Degree requirements:* For doctorate, thesis/dissertation. *Entrance requirements:* For doctorate, GRE General Test, GRE Subject Test, 3 letters of recommendation, official transcripts. Additional exam requirements/recommendations for international students: Required—TOEFL. Electronic applications accepted. *Faculty research:* Molecular structure and function, plant biology, immunology, bioorganic chemistry and molecular design, synthetic organic chemistry and natural product synthesis.

Seton Hall University, College of Arts and Sciences, Department of Biological Sciences, South Orange, NJ 07079-2697. Offers biology (MS); biology/business administration (MS); microbiology (MS); molecular bioscience (PhD); molecular bioscience/neuroscience (PhD). Part-time and evening/weekend programs available. *Degree requirements:* For master's, thesis optional; for doctorate, comprehensive exam, thesis/dissertation. *Entrance requirements:* For master's and doctorate, GRE or MS from accredited university in the U.S. Additional exam requirements/recommendations for international students: Required—TOEFL. Electronic applications accepted. *Faculty* *research:* Neurobiology, genetics, immunology, molecular biology, cellular physiology, toxicology, microbiology, bioinformatics.

Shippensburg University of Pennsylvania, School of Graduate Studies, College of Arts and Sciences, Department of Biology, Shippensburg, PA 17257-2299. Offers MS. Part-time and evening/weekend programs available. *Faculty:* 12 full-time (5 women). *Students:* 29 full-time (17 women), 3 part-time (2 women); includes 3 minority (2 Black or African American, non-Hispanic/Latino; 1 Asian, non-Hispanic/Latino), 5 international. Average age 27. 42 applicants, 33% accepted, 10 enrolled. In 2013, 14 master's awarded. *Degree requirements:* For master's, thesis, oral thesis defense, seminar, minimum QPA of 3.0. *Entrance requirements:* For master's, minimum GPA of 2.75; essay; 400-500 word statement of purpose; 33 credits of course work in biology; minimum 4 courses/labs in chemistry including both inorganic and organic chemistry or biochemistry; calculus I and two lab courses in physics (recommended). Additional exam requirements/recommendations for international students: Required—TOEFL (minimum score 580 paper-based); Recommended—IELTS (minimum score 6). *Application deadline:* For fall admission, 4/30 for international students; for spring admission, 9/30 for international students. Applications are processed on a rolling basis. Application fee: $45. Electronic applications accepted. *Expenses: Tuition, area resident:* Part-time $442 per credit. Tuition, state resident: part-time $442 per credit. Tuition, nonresident: part-time $663 per credit. *Required fees:* $127 per credit. *Financial support:* In 2013–14, 14 research assistantships with full tuition reimbursements (averaging $5,000 per year) were awarded; career-related internships or fieldwork, scholarships/grants, unspecified assistantships, and resident hall director and student payroll positions also available. Support available to part-time students. Financial award application deadline: 3/1; financial award applicants required to submit FAFSA. *Unit head:* Dr. Theo S. Light, Graduate Coordinator, 717-477-1401, Fax: 717-477-4064, E-mail: tsligh@ship.edu. *Application contact:* Jeremy R. Goshorn, Assistant Dean of Graduate Admissions, 717-477-1231, Fax: 717-477-4016, E-mail: jrgoshorn@ship.edu.
Website: http://www.ship.edu/biology/

Simon Fraser University, Office of Graduate Studies, Faculty of Science, Department of Biological Sciences, Burnaby, BC V5A 1S6, Canada. Offers bioinformatics (Graduate Diploma); biological sciences (M Sc, PhD); environmental toxicology (MET); pest management (MPM). *Faculty:* 47 full-time (15 women). *Students:* 138 full-time (70 women). 29 applicants, 59% accepted, 15 enrolled. In 2013, 27 master's, 13 doctorates awarded. *Degree requirements:* For master's, thesis; for doctorate, thesis/dissertation, candidacy exam; for Graduate Diploma, practicum. *Entrance requirements:* For master's, minimum GPA of 3.0 (on scale of 4.33), or 3.33 based on last 60 credits of undergraduate courses; for doctorate, minimum GPA of 3.5 (on scale of 4.33); for Graduate Diploma, minimum GPA of 2.5 (on scale of 4.33), or 2.67 based on the last 60 credits of undergraduate courses. Additional exam requirements/recommendations for international students: Recommended—TOEFL (minimum score 580 paper-based; 93 iBT), IELTS (minimum score 7), TWE (minimum score 5). *Application deadline:* For fall admission, 6/1 for domestic and international students; for winter admission, 10/1 for domestic and international students; for spring admission, 2/1 for domestic and international students. Applications are processed on a rolling basis. Application fee: $90 ($125 for international students). Electronic applications accepted. *Expenses: Tuition, area resident:* Full-time $5084 Canadian dollars. *Required fees:* $840 Canadian dollars. *Financial support:* In 2013–14, 68 students received support, including 77 fellowships (averaging $6,250 per year), teaching assistantships (averaging $5,608 per year); research assistantships and scholarships/grants also available. *Faculty research:* Cell biology, wildlife ecology, environmental and evolutionary physiology, environmental toxicology, pest management. *Unit head:* Dr. Julian Guttman, Graduate Chair, 778-782-4459, Fax: 778-782-3496, E-mail: bisc-grad-chair@sfu.ca. *Application contact:* Marlene Nguyen, Graduate Secretary, 778-782-3120, Fax: 778-782-3496, E-mail: biscgrad@sfu.ca.
Website: http://www.sfu.ca/biology

Smith College, Graduate and Special Programs, Department of Biological Sciences, Northampton, MA 01063. Offers MAT, MS. Part-time programs available. *Faculty:* 14 full-time (5 women), 3 part-time/adjunct (1 woman). *Students:* 2 full-time (both women), 6 part-time (all women); includes 2 minority (1 Black or African American, non-Hispanic/Latino; 1 Hispanic/Latino), 1 international. Average age 29. 5 applicants, 80% accepted, 3 enrolled. In 2013, 3 master's awarded. *Degree requirements:* For master's, one foreign language, thesis (for some programs). *Entrance requirements:* For master's, GRE General Test, GRE Subject Test. Additional exam requirements/recommendations for international students: Required—TOEFL (minimum score 595 paper-based; 97 iBT). *Application deadline:* For fall admission, 1/15 for domestic and international students; for spring admission, 12/1 for domestic students. Application fee: $60. *Expenses: Tuition:* Full-time $32,160; part-time $1340 per credit. *Financial support:* In 2013–14, 7 students received support, including 7 research assistantships with full tuition reimbursements available (averaging $13,370 per year); fellowships with full tuition reimbursements available, career-related internships or fieldwork, institutionally sponsored loans, and scholarships/grants also available. Support available to part-time students. Financial award application deadline: 1/15; financial award applicants required to submit CSS PROFILE or FAFSA. *Unit head:* Steven Williams, Graduate Student Advisor, 413-585-3826, E-mail: swilliam@smith.edu. *Application contact:* Ruth Morgan, Administrative Assistant, 413-585-3050, Fax: 413-585-3054, E-mail: rmorgan@smith.edu.
Website: http://www.smith.edu/biology/

Sonoma State University, School of Science and Technology, Department of Biology, Rohnert Park, CA 94928. Offers biochemistry (MA); ecology (MS); environmental biology (MS); evolutionary biology (MS); functional morphology (MS); molecular and cell biology (MS); organismal biology (MS). Part-time programs available. *Faculty:* 9 full-time (1 woman). *Students:* 4 full-time (2 women), 21 part-time (14 women); includes 5 minority (1 American Indian or Alaska Native, non-Hispanic/Latino; 1 Asian, non-Hispanic/Latino; 2 Hispanic/Latino; 1 Two or more races, non-Hispanic/Latino), 2 international. Average age 29. 23 applicants, 65% accepted, 6 enrolled. In 2013, 6 master's awarded. *Degree requirements:* For master's, thesis or alternative, oral exam. *Entrance requirements:* For master's, GRE General Test, GRE Subject Test, minimum GPA of 3.0. Additional exam requirements/recommendations for international students: Required—TOEFL (minimum score 500 paper-based). *Application deadline:* For fall admission, 11/30 for domestic students. Applications are processed on a rolling basis. Application fee: $55. *Expenses:* Tuition, state resident: full-time $8500. Tuition, nonresident: full-time $12,964. *Required fees:* $1762. *Financial support:* In 2013–14, 1 fellowship (averaging $1,520 per year), 6 research assistantships (averaging $3,562 per year), 22 teaching assistantships (averaging $6,738 per year) were awarded; career-related internships or fieldwork, Federal Work-Study, and tuition waivers (full) also available. Financial award application deadline: 3/2; financial award applicants required to submit FAFSA. *Faculty research:* Plant physiology, comparative physiology, community ecology, restoration ecology, marine ecology, conservation genetics, primate behavior, behavioral ecology, developmental biology, plant and animal systematics. *Total annual research expenditures:* $4,400. *Unit head:* Dr. Nathan Rank, Chair, 707-664-3053, E-mail: nathan.rank@sonoma.edu. *Application contact:* Dr. Derek Girman, Graduate Adviser, 707-664-3055, E-mail: derek.girman@sonoma.edu.
Website: http://www.sonoma.edu/biology/graduate

South Dakota State University, Graduate School, College of Agriculture and Biological Sciences, Department of Animal and Range Sciences, Brookings, SD 57007. Offers animal science (MS, PhD); biological sciences (PhD). Part-time programs available. *Degree requirements:* For master's, thesis, oral exam; for doctorate, comprehensive exam, thesis/dissertation, preliminary oral and written exams. *Entrance requirements:* Additional exam requirements/recommendations for international students: Required—TOEFL (minimum score 550 paper-based; 79 iBT). *Faculty research:* Ruminant and nonruminant nutrition, meat science, reproductive physiology, range utilization, ecology genetics, muscle biology, animal production.

South Dakota State University, Graduate School, College of Agriculture and Biological Sciences, Department of Biology and Microbiology, Brookings, SD 57007. Offers biological sciences (MS, PhD). Part-time programs available. *Degree requirements:* For master's, thesis (for some programs), oral exam; for doctorate, comprehensive exam, thesis/dissertation, oral exam. *Entrance requirements:* For master's and doctorate, GRE General Test. Additional exam requirements/recommendations for international students: Required—TOEFL (minimum score 600 paper-based; 100 iBT). *Faculty research:* Ecosystem ecology; plant, animal and microbial genomics; animal infectious disease, microbial bioproducts.

South Dakota State University, Graduate School, College of Agriculture and Biological Sciences, Department of Dairy Science, Brookings, SD 57007. Offers animal sciences (MS, PhD); biological sciences (MS, PhD). Part-time programs available. *Degree requirements:* For master's, thesis, oral exam; for doctorate, comprehensive exam, thesis/dissertation, preliminary oral and written exams. *Entrance requirements:* Additional exam requirements/recommendations for international students: Required—TOEFL (minimum score 550 paper-based). *Faculty research:* Dairy cattle nutrition, energy metabolism, food safety, dairy processing technology.

South Dakota State University, Graduate School, College of Agriculture and Biological Sciences, Department of Veterinary and Biomedical Sciences, Brookings, SD 57007. Offers biological sciences (MS, PhD). Part-time and evening/weekend programs available. *Degree requirements:* For master's, thesis (for some programs), oral exam; for doctorate, comprehensive exam, thesis/dissertation, preliminary oral and written exams. *Entrance requirements:* Additional exam requirements/recommendations for international students: Required—TOEFL (minimum score 525 paper-based; 71 iBT). *Faculty research:* Infectious disease, food animal, virology, immunology.

South Dakota State University, Graduate School, College of Engineering, Department of Agricultural and Biosystems Engineering, Brookings, SD 57007. Offers biological sciences (MS, PhD); engineering (MS). PhD offered jointly with Iowa State University of Science and Technology. Part-time programs available. *Degree requirements:* For master's, thesis (for some programs), oral exam; for doctorate, thesis/dissertation, preliminary oral and written exams. *Entrance requirements:* For master's and doctorate, engineering degree. Additional exam requirements/recommendations for international students: Required—TOEFL (minimum score 550 paper-based; 79 iBT). *Faculty research:* Water resources, food engineering, natural resources engineering, machine design, bioprocess engineering.

South Dakota State University, Graduate School, College of Pharmacy, Department of Pharmaceutical Sciences, Brookings, SD 57007. Offers biological science (MS); pharmaceutical sciences (PhD). *Degree requirements:* For master's, thesis, oral exam; for doctorate, comprehensive exam, thesis/dissertation, oral exam. *Entrance requirements:* For master's and doctorate, GRE General Test. Additional exam requirements/recommendations for international students: Required—TOEFL (minimum score 550 paper-based). *Faculty research:* Drugs of abuse, anti-cancer drugs, sustained drug delivery, drug metabolism.

Southeastern Louisiana University, College of Science and Technology, Department of Biological Sciences, Hammond, LA 70402. Offers biology (MS). Part-time programs available. *Faculty:* 15 full-time (4 women), 1 part-time/adjunct (0 women). *Students:* 11 full-time (9 women), 8 part-time (5 women); includes 2 minority (1 Black or African American, non-Hispanic/Latino; 1 Hispanic/Latino). Average age 25. 26 applicants, 46% accepted, 7 enrolled. In 2013, 7 master's awarded. *Degree requirements:* For master's, comprehensive exam, thesis (for some programs). *Entrance requirements:* For master's, GRE General Test (minimum score 1000), minimum GPA of 3.0; 30 hours of undergraduate biology courses; two letters of recommendation; curriculum vitae; letter of intent. Additional exam requirements/recommendations for international students: Required—TOEFL (minimum score 500 paper-based; 61 iBT). *Application deadline:* For fall admission, 7/15 priority date for domestic students, 6/1 priority date for international students; for spring admission, 12/1 priority date for domestic students, 10/1 priority date for international students. Applications are processed on a rolling basis. Application fee: $20 ($30 for international students). Electronic applications accepted. *Expenses:* Tuition, state resident: full-time $5047. Tuition, nonresident: full-time $17,066. *Required fees:* $1213. Tuition and fees vary according to degree level. *Financial support:* In 2013–14, 4 research assistantships (averaging $8,425 per year), 14 teaching assistantships (averaging $7,741 per year) were awarded; career-related internships or fieldwork, Federal Work-Study, institutionally sponsored loans, scholarships/grants, traineeships, and unspecified assistantships also available. Support available to part-time students. Financial award application deadline: 5/1; financial award applicants required to submit FAFSA. *Faculty research:* Evolutionary biology, ecology, molecular biology, morphology and physiology, microbiology and immunology. *Total annual research expenditures:* $563,541. *Unit head:* Dr. Christopher Beachy, Department Head, 985-549-3740, Fax: 985-549-3851, E-mail: christopher.beachy@selu.edu. *Application contact:* Sandra Meyers, Graduate Admissions Analyst, 985-549-5620, Fax: 985-549-5632, E-mail: admissions@selu.edu.
Website: http://www.selu.edu/acad_research/depts/biol

Southeast Missouri State University, School of Graduate Studies, Department of Biology, Cape Girardeau, MO 63701-4799. Offers MNS. Part-time programs available. *Faculty:* 14 full-time (5 women), 1 part-time/adjunct (0 women). *Students:* 23 full-time (13 women), 12 part-time (4 women); includes 1 minority (Black or African American, non-Hispanic/Latino), 8 international. Average age 27. 27 applicants, 59% accepted, 13 enrolled. In 2013, 9 master's awarded. *Degree requirements:* For master's, comprehensive exam (for some programs), thesis (for some programs), either thesis and oral defense, or research paper and comprehensive exam. *Entrance requirements:* For master's, GRE General Test, minimum undergraduate GPA of 2.5, 2.75 in last 30 hours of undergraduate course work in science and mathematics; 2 letters of recommendation; faculty sponsor agreement. Additional exam requirements/recommendations for international students: Required—TOEFL (minimum score 550 paper-based; 79 iBT), IELTS (minimum score 6), PTE (minimum score 53). *Application deadline:* For fall admission, 4/1 for domestic and international students; for spring admission, 10/1 for domestic and international students; for summer admission, 4/1 for domestic students. Applications are processed on a rolling basis. Application fee: $30 ($40 for international students). Electronic applications accepted. *Expenses:* Tuition, state resident: full-time $5139; part-time $285.50 per credit hour. Tuition, nonresident: full-time $9099; part-time $505.50 per credit hour. *Financial support:* In 2013–14, 25 students received support, including 19 teaching assistantships with full tuition reimbursements available (averaging $8,144 per year); career-related internships or fieldwork, Federal Work-Study, scholarships/grants, traineeships, tuition waivers (full),

and unspecified assistantships also available. Financial award application deadline: 6/30; financial award applicants required to submit FAFSA. *Faculty research:* Evolutionary ecology, animal behavior and ecology, case-based learning, plant systematics and physiology, genetics. *Total annual research expenditures:* $609,925. *Unit head:* Dr. James E. Champine, Department of Biology Chair and Professor, 573-651-2171, Fax: 573-651-2382, E-mail: jchampine@semo.edu. *Application contact:* Dr. Dustin Siegel, Department of Biology Graduate Coordinator, 573-651-2262, Fax: 573-651-2382, E-mail: dsiegel@semo.edu.
Website: http://www.semo.edu/biology/

Southern Connecticut State University, School of Graduate Studies, School of Arts and Sciences, Department of Biology, New Haven, CT 06515-1355. Offers MS. Part-time and evening/weekend programs available. *Degree requirements:* For master's, thesis optional. *Entrance requirements:* For master's, previous course work in biology, chemistry, and mathematics; interview. Electronic applications accepted.

Southern Illinois University Carbondale, Graduate School, College of Science, Biological Sciences Program, Carbondale, IL 62901-4701. Offers MS. *Students:* 5 full-time (1 woman); includes 4 minority (all Black or African American, non-Hispanic/Latino). Average age 25. 1 applicant, 100% accepted, 1 enrolled. In 2013, 1 master's awarded. *Degree requirements:* For master's, thesis or alternative. *Entrance requirements:* For master's, GRE General Test, minimum GPA of 2.7. Additional exam requirements/recommendations for international students: Required—TOEFL. *Application deadline:* Applications are processed on a rolling basis. Application fee: $50. *Financial support:* Fellowships with full tuition reimbursements, research assistantships with full tuition reimbursements, teaching assistantships with full tuition reimbursements, Federal Work-Study, institutionally sponsored loans, and tuition waivers (full) available. Support available to part-time students. *Faculty research:* Molecular mechanisms of mutagenesis, reproductive endocrinology, avian energetics and nutrition, developmental plant physiology. *Unit head:* Dr. Harold Bardo, Graduate Director, 618-453-1650, E-mail: hbardo@siumed.edu.

Southern Illinois University Carbondale, Graduate School, Graduate Program in Medicine, Carbondale, IL 62901-4701. Offers molecular, cellular and systemic physiology (MS); pharmacology (MS, PhD); physician assistant studies (MSPA); physiology (MS, PhD). *Faculty:* 31 full-time (5 women). *Students:* 86 full-time (60 women), 18 part-time (14 women); includes 4 minority (1 Black or African American, non-Hispanic/Latino; 2 Asian, non-Hispanic/Latino; 1 Hispanic/Latino), 22 international. 72 applicants, 8% accepted, 6 enrolled. In 2013, 30 master's, 4 doctorates awarded. Terminal master's awarded for partial completion of doctoral program. *Degree requirements:* For master's, thesis; for doctorate, thesis/dissertation. *Entrance requirements:* For master's, minimum GPA of 3.0; for doctorate, minimum GPA of 3.25. Additional exam requirements/recommendations for international students: Required—TOEFL. Application fee: $50. *Financial support:* In 2013–14, 27 students received support, including 12 fellowships with full tuition reimbursements available, 1 research assistantship with full tuition reimbursement available, 10 teaching assistantships with full tuition reimbursements available; institutionally sponsored loans and tuition waivers (full) also available. *Faculty research:* Cardiovascular physiology, neurophysiology of hearing. *Unit head:* Dr. Prema Narayan, Director of Graduate Studies, 618-453-4567, E-mail: pnarayan@siumed.edu. *Application contact:* Pamela Jacobini, Office Manager, 618-453-1512, E-mail: pjacobini@siumed.edu.

Southern Illinois University Edwardsville, Graduate School, College of Arts and Sciences, Department of Biological Sciences, Program in Biology, Edwardsville, IL 62026-0001. Offers MA, MS. Part-time programs available. *Faculty:* 25 full-time (6 women). *Students:* 19 full-time (8 women), 52 part-time (37 women); includes 9 minority (4 Asian, non-Hispanic/Latino; 2 Hispanic/Latino; 3 Two or more races, non-Hispanic/Latino), 2 international. 21 applicants, 86% accepted. In 2013, 20 master's awarded. *Degree requirements:* For master's, thesis (for some programs). *Entrance requirements:* For master's, GRE. Additional exam requirements/recommendations for international students: Required—TOEFL (minimum score 550 paper-based, 79 iBT), IELTS (minimum score 6.5), Michigan Test of English Language Proficiency or PTE. *Application deadline:* For fall admission, 7/18 for domestic students, 6/1 for international students; for spring admission, 12/12 for domestic students, 10/1 for international students; for summer admission, 4/24 for domestic students, 3/1 for international students. Applications are processed on a rolling basis. Application fee: $30. Electronic applications accepted. *Expenses:* Tuition, state resident: full-time $3551. Tuition, nonresident: full-time $8378. *Financial support:* In 2013–14, 39 students received support, including 5 research assistantships with full tuition reimbursements available (averaging $9,585 per year), 34 teaching assistantships with full tuition reimbursements available (averaging $9,585 per year); fellowships with full tuition reimbursements available, career-related internships or fieldwork, institutionally sponsored loans, scholarships/grants, and unspecified assistantships also available. Financial award application deadline: 3/1; financial award applicants required to submit FAFSA. *Unit head:* Dr. Rick Essner, Director, 618-650-3468, E-mail: ressner@siue.edu. *Application contact:* Melissa K. Mace, Assistant Director of Graduate and International Recruitment, 618-650-2756, Fax: 618-650-3618, E-mail: mmace@siue.edu.
Website: http://www.siue.edu/BIOLOGY/graduate.htm

Southern Methodist University, Dedman College of Humanities and Sciences, Department of Biological Sciences, Dallas, TX 75275. Offers molecular and cellular biology (MA, MS, PhD). Terminal master's awarded for partial completion of doctoral program. *Degree requirements:* For master's, thesis (for MS), oral exam; for doctorate, thesis/dissertation, qualifying exam. *Entrance requirements:* For master's, GRE General Test (minimum score 1200), minimum GPA of 3.0; for doctorate, GRE General Test (minimum score: 1200), minimum GPA of 3.0. Additional exam requirements/recommendations for international students: Required—TOEFL (minimum score 550 paper-based). Electronic applications accepted. *Faculty research:* Free radicals and aging, protein structure, chromatin structure, signal processes, retroviral pathogenesis.

Southern University and Agricultural and Mechanical College, Graduate School, College of Sciences, Department of Biology, Baton Rouge, LA 70813. Offers MS. *Degree requirements:* For master's, comprehensive exam, thesis. *Entrance requirements:* For master's, GRE General Test. Additional exam requirements/recommendations for international students: Required—TOEFL (minimum score 525 paper-based). *Faculty research:* Toxicology, neuroendocrinology, mycotoxin, virology.

Stanford University, School of Humanities and Sciences, Department of Biology, Stanford, CA 94305-9991. Offers MS, PhD. Terminal master's awarded for partial completion of doctoral program. *Degree requirements:* For doctorate, thesis/dissertation, oral exam. *Entrance requirements:* For master's, GRE General Test; for doctorate, GRE General Test, GRE Subject Test. Additional exam requirements/recommendations for international students: Required—TOEFL. Electronic applications accepted. *Expenses: Tuition:* Full-time $42,690; part-time $949 per credit. *Required fees:* $185.

Stanford University, School of Medicine, Graduate Programs in Medicine, Stanford, CA 94305-9991. Offers MS, PhD. Terminal master's awarded for partial completion of doctoral program. *Degree requirements:* For master's, thesis; for doctorate, thesis/dissertation. *Entrance requirements:* For master's, GRE General Test or MCAT. Additional exam requirements/recommendations for international students: Required—TOEFL. Electronic applications accepted. *Expenses: Tuition:* Full-time $42,690; part-time $949 per credit. *Required fees:* $185.

State University of New York at Fredonia, Graduate Studies, Department of Biology, Fredonia, NY 14063-1136. Offers MS, MS Ed. Part-time and evening/weekend programs available. *Degree requirements:* For master's, thesis optional. *Expenses:* Tuition, state resident: full-time $7398; part-time $411 per credit hour. Tuition, nonresident: full-time $13,770; part-time $765 per credit hour. *Required fees:* $1143.90; $63.55 per credit hour. Tuition and fees vary according to course load.

State University of New York College at Oneonta, Graduate Education, Department of Biology, Oneonta, NY 13820-4015. Offers MA. Part-time and evening/weekend programs available. *Degree requirements:* For master's, comprehensive exam. *Entrance requirements:* For master's, GRE General Test, GRE Subject Test.

State University of New York Downstate Medical Center, School of Graduate Studies, Brooklyn, NY 11203-2098. Offers MS, PhD, MD/PhD. *Degree requirements:* For doctorate, thesis/dissertation. *Entrance requirements:* For doctorate, GRE. Additional exam requirements/recommendations for international students: Required—TOEFL. *Faculty research:* Cellular and molecular neurobiology, role of oncogenes in early cardiogenesis, mechanism of gene regulation, cardiovascular physiology, yeast molecular genetics.

State University of New York Upstate Medical University, College of Graduate Studies, Syracuse, NY 13210-2334. Offers MS, PhD, MD/PhD. Terminal master's awarded for partial completion of doctoral program. *Degree requirements:* For master's, thesis; for doctorate, comprehensive exam, thesis/dissertation. *Entrance requirements:* For master's, GRE General Test, interview; for doctorate, GRE General Test, telephone interview. Additional exam requirements/recommendations for international students: Required—TOEFL. Electronic applications accepted. *Faculty research:* Cancer, disorders of the nervous system, infectious diseases, diabetes/metabolic disorders/cardiovascular diseases.

Stephen F. Austin State University, Graduate School, College of Sciences and Mathematics, Department of Biology, Nacogdoches, TX 75962. Offers MS. *Degree requirements:* For master's, comprehensive exam, thesis optional. *Entrance requirements:* For master's, GRE General Test, minimum GPA of 2.8 in last 60 hours, 2.5 overall. Additional exam requirements/recommendations for international students: Required—TOEFL.

Stony Brook University, State University of New York, Stony Brook University Medical Center, Health Sciences Center, School of Medicine and Graduate School, Graduate Programs in Medicine, Stony Brook, NY 11794. Offers MS, PhD, Advanced Certificate. *Students:* 100 full-time (48 women), 4 part-time (all women); includes 37 minority (14 Black or African American, non-Hispanic/Latino; 12 Asian, non-Hispanic/Latino; 11 Hispanic/Latino), 15 international. 173 applicants, 29% accepted, 32 enrolled. In 2013, 28 master's, 17 doctorates awarded. *Degree requirements:* For doctorate, thesis/dissertation, exam. *Entrance requirements:* For doctorate, GRE General Test. Additional exam requirements/recommendations for international students: Required—TOEFL. *Application deadline:* For fall admission, 1/15 for domestic students; for spring admission, 10/1 for domestic students. Application fee: $100. Electronic applications accepted. *Expenses:* Contact institution. *Financial support:* Fellowships, research assistantships, teaching assistantships, career-related internships or fieldwork, and Federal Work-Study available. Financial award application deadline: 3/15. *Unit head:* Dr. Kenneth Kaushansky, Dean and Senior Vice President of Health Sciences, 631-444-2113, Fax: 631-444-6032. *Application contact:* Melissa Jordan, Assistant Dean, 631-632-9712, Fax: 631-632-7243, E-mail: melissa.jordan@stonybrook.edu.

Stony Brook University, State University of New York, Stony Brook University Medical Center, Health Sciences Center, School of Medicine, Medical Scientist Training Program, Stony Brook, NY 11794. Offers MD/PhD. *Application deadline:* For fall admission, 1/15 for domestic students. *Expenses:* Tuition, state resident: full-time $9870; part-time $411 per credit. Tuition, nonresident: full-time $18,350; part-time $765 per credit. *Financial support:* Tuition waivers (full) available. *Unit head:* Dr. Michael A. Frohman, Director, Medical Scientist Training Program, 631-444-3219, Fax: 631-444-6229, E-mail: michael.frohman@stonybrook.edu. *Application contact:* Carron Allen, Program Administrator, 631-444-3219, Fax: 631-444-3492, E-mail: carron.kaufman@stonybrook.edu.
Website: http://www.pharm.stonybrook.edu/mstp/

Sul Ross State University, School of Arts and Sciences, Department of Biology, Alpine, TX 79832. Offers MS. Part-time programs available. *Degree requirements:* For master's, thesis optional. *Entrance requirements:* For master's, GRE General Test, minimum GPA of 2.5 in last 60 hours of undergraduate work. *Faculty research:* Plant-animal interaction, Chihuahuan desert biology, insect biological control, plant and animal systematics, wildlife biology.

Syracuse University, College of Arts and Sciences, Program in Biology, Syracuse, NY 13244. Offers MS, PhD. Part-time programs available. *Students:* 41 full-time (27 women), 2 part-time (1 woman); includes 2 minority (1 Asian, non-Hispanic/Latino; 1 Two or more races, non-Hispanic/Latino), 19 international. Average age 26. 97 applicants, 24% accepted, 10 enrolled. In 2013, 1 master's, 5 doctorates awarded. Terminal master's awarded for partial completion of doctoral program. *Degree requirements:* For master's, thesis; for doctorate, thesis/dissertation. *Entrance requirements:* For master's and doctorate, GRE General Test, GRE Subject Test (recommended), interview. Additional exam requirements/recommendations for international students: Required—TOEFL (minimum score 100 iBT). *Application deadline:* For fall admission, 12/15 priority date for domestic students, 12/14 priority date for international students. Application fee: $75. Electronic applications accepted. *Financial support:* Fellowships with full and partial tuition reimbursements, research assistantships with full and partial tuition reimbursements, and teaching assistantships with full and partial tuition reimbursements available. Financial award application deadline: 1/10; financial award applicants required to submit FAFSA. *Faculty research:* Cell signaling, plant ecosystem ecology, aquatic ecology, genetics and molecular biology of color vision, ion transport by cell membranes. *Unit head:* Dr. Steve Dorus, Graduate Program Director, 315-443-7091, E-mail: biology@syr.edu. *Application contact:* Information Contact, 315-443-9154.
Website: http://biology.syr.edu/

Tarleton State University, College of Graduate Studies, College of Science and Technology, Department of Biological Sciences, Stephenville, TX 76402. Offers biology (MS). Part-time and evening/weekend programs available. *Faculty:* 6 full-time (2 women), 1 part-time/adjunct (0 women). *Students:* 9 full-time (5 women), 13 part-time (9 women); includes 2 minority (1 Black or African American, non-Hispanic/Latino; 1 Hispanic/Latino), 1 international. Average age 28. 14 applicants, 93% accepted, 10 enrolled. In 2013, 1 master's awarded. *Degree requirements:* For master's, comprehensive exam, thesis (for some programs). *Entrance requirements:* For master's, GRE General Test, minimum GPA of 3.0. Additional exam requirements/recommendations for international students: Required—TOEFL (minimum score 550 paper-based; 80 iBT). *Application deadline:* For fall admission, 8/15 priority date for domestic students; for spring admission, 1/7 for domestic students. Applications are

processed on a rolling basis. Application fee: $30 ($130 for international students). Electronic applications accepted. *Expenses:* Tuition, state resident: full-time $3312; part-time $184 per credit hour. Tuition, nonresident: full-time $9144; part-time $508 per credit hour. *Required fees:* $1916. Tuition and fees vary according to course load and campus/location. *Financial support:* Research assistantships, teaching assistantships, career-related internships or fieldwork, and Federal Work-Study available. Support available to part-time students. Financial award application deadline: 5/1; financial award applicants required to submit FAFSA. *Unit head:* Dr. Phil Sudman, Head, 254-968-9154, Fax: 254-968-9157, E-mail: sudman@tarleton.edu. *Application contact:* Information Contact, 254-968-9104, Fax: 254-968-9670, E-mail: gradoffice@tarleton.edu.
Website: http://www.tarleton.edu/COSTWEB/biology/

Temple University, College of Science and Technology, Department of Biology, Philadelphia, PA 19122. Offers biology (MS, PhD); biotechnology (MS). *Faculty:* 44 full-time (17 women), 24 part-time/adjunct (12 women). *Students:* 38 full-time (19 women), 5 part-time (3 women); includes 7 minority (2 Black or African American, non-Hispanic/Latino; 4 Asian, non-Hispanic/Latino; 1 Hispanic/Latino), 13 international. 81 applicants, 22% accepted, 12 enrolled. In 2013, 2 doctorates awarded. Terminal master's awarded for partial completion of doctoral program. *Degree requirements:* For master's, comprehensive exam (for some programs), thesis (for some programs); for doctorate, comprehensive exam (for some programs), thesis/dissertation. *Entrance requirements:* For master's and doctorate, GRE General Test, minimum GPA of 3.0. Additional exam requirements/recommendations for international students: Required—TOEFL (minimum score 550 paper-based; 79 iBT). *Application deadline:* For fall admission, 1/15 for domestic students, 12/15 for international students; for spring admission, 10/15 for domestic students, 8/1 for international students. Applications are processed on a rolling basis. Application fee: $60. *Financial support:* Fellowships, research assistantships, teaching assistantships, Federal Work-Study, and tuition waivers (full) available. Financial award application deadline: 1/15; financial award applicants required to submit FAFSA. *Faculty research:* Membrane proteins, genetics, molecular biology, neuroscience, aquatic biology. *Unit head:* Dr. Allen Nicholson, Chair, 215-204-8854, Fax: 215-204-6646, E-mail: biology@temple.edu. *Application contact:* Regee Neely, Administrative Assistant, 215-204-8854, E-mail: rneely@temple.edu.
Website: https://bio.cst.temple.edu/

Temple University, School of Medicine, Biomedical Sciences Programs, Philadephia, PA 19122. Offers MS, PhD, MD/PhD. *Faculty:* 102 full-time (30 women). *Students:* 59 full-time (36 women), 2 part-time (0 women); includes 16 minority (6 Black or African American, non-Hispanic/Latino; 7 Asian, non-Hispanic/Latino; 2 Hispanic/Latino; 1 Two or more races, non-Hispanic/Latino), 18 international. 197 applicants, 22% accepted, 25 enrolled. In 2013, 1 master's awarded. Terminal master's awarded for partial completion of doctoral program. *Degree requirements:* For master's, thesis optional; for doctorate, thesis/dissertation, research seminars. *Entrance requirements:* For master's and doctorate, GRE General Test, minimum undergraduate GPA of 3.0. Additional exam requirements/recommendations for international students: Required—TOEFL. *Application deadline:* For fall admission, 2/15 for domestic and international students. Application fee: $60. Electronic applications accepted. *Expenses:* Contact institution. *Financial support:* In 2013–14, 70 fellowships with full tuition reimbursements (averaging $26,500 per year), 41 research assistantships with full tuition reimbursements (averaging $26,500 per year) were awarded; scholarships/grants and health care benefits also available. Financial award application deadline: 2/15; financial award applicants required to submit FAFSA. *Faculty research:* Translational medicine, molecular biology and immunology of autoimmune disease and cancer, cardiovascular and pulmonary disease pathophysiology, biology of substance abuse, causes and consequences of obesity, molecular mechanisms of neurological dysfunction. *Unit head:* Dr. Scott K. Shore, Associate Dean for Graduate Studies, 215-707-2423, Fax: 215-707-5072, E-mail: sks@temple.edu. *Application contact:* Tracy Burton, Office of Admissions, 215-707-2423, E-mail: tusmgrad@temple.edu.
Website: http://www.temple.edu/medicine/biomedical_sciences/index.htm

Tennessee State University, The School of Graduate Studies and Research, College of Agriculture, Human and Natural Sciences, Department of Biological Sciences, Nashville, TN 37209-1561. Offers MS, PhD. *Degree requirements:* For master's, thesis optional; for doctorate, thesis/dissertation. *Entrance requirements:* For master's, GRE General Test, GRE Subject Test, minimum GPA of 3.0; for doctorate, GRE General Test, GRE Subject Test. *Faculty research:* Cellular and molecular biology and agribiology.

Tennessee Technological University, College of Graduate Studies, College of Arts and Sciences, Department of Biology, Cookeville, TN 38505. Offers fish, game, and wildlife management (MS). Part-time programs available. *Faculty:* 22 full-time (2 women). *Students:* 5 full-time (2 women), 11 part-time (4 women). Average age 25. 18 applicants, 28% accepted, 5 enrolled. In 2013, 2 degrees awarded. *Degree requirements:* For master's, thesis. *Entrance requirements:* For master's, GRE. Additional exam requirements/recommendations for international students: Required—TOEFL (minimum score 527 paper-based; 71 iBT), IELTS (minimum score 5.5), PTE (minimum score 48), or TOEIC (Test of English as an International Communication). *Application deadline:* For fall admission, 8/1 for domestic students, 5/1 for international students; for spring admission, 12/1 for domestic students, 10/1 for international students. Applications are processed on a rolling basis. Application fee: $35 ($40 for international students). Electronic applications accepted. *Expenses:* Tuition, state resident: full-time $9347; part-time $465 per credit hour. Tuition, nonresident: full-time $23,635; part-time $1152 per credit hour. *Financial support:* In 2013–14, 17 research assistantships (averaging $9,000 per year), 8 teaching assistantships (averaging $7,500 per year) were awarded. Financial award application deadline: 4/1. *Faculty research:* Aquatics, environmental studies. *Unit head:* Dr. Steven Bradford Cook, Interim Chairperson, 931-372-3134, Fax: 931-372-6257, E-mail: sbcook@tntech.edu. *Application contact:* Shelia K. Kendrick, Coordinator of Graduate Studies, 931-372-3808, Fax: 931-372-3497, E-mail: skendrick@tntech.edu.

Tennessee Technological University, College of Graduate Studies, School of Environmental Studies, Department of Environmental Sciences, Cookeville, TN 38505. Offers biology (PhD); chemistry (PhD). Part-time programs available. *Students:* 4 full-time (0 women), 10 part-time (5 women); includes 2 minority (1 Black or African American, non-Hispanic/Latino; 1 Hispanic/Latino), 5 international. 714 applicants, 1% accepted, 1 enrolled. In 2013, 5 doctorates awarded. *Degree requirements:* For doctorate, comprehensive exam, thesis/dissertation. *Entrance requirements:* For doctorate, GRE. Additional exam requirements/recommendations for international students: Required—TOEFL (minimum score 527 paper-based; 71 iBT), IELTS (minimum score 5.5), PTE (minimum score 48), or TOEIC (Test of English as an International Communication). *Application deadline:* For fall admission, 8/1 for domestic students, 5/1 for international students; for spring admission, 12/1 for domestic students, 10/2 for international students. Applications are processed on a rolling basis. Application fee: $35 ($40 for international students). Electronic applications accepted. *Expenses:* Tuition, state resident: full-time $9347; part-time $465 per credit hour. Tuition, nonresident: full-time $23,635; part-time $1152 per credit hour. *Financial support:* In 2013–14, 5 research assistantships (averaging $10,000 per year), 3 teaching assistantships (averaging $10,000 per year) were awarded; fellowships also available. Financial award application deadline: 4/1. *Unit head:* Dr. Dennis B. George, Director, 931-372-3609, E-mail: dgeorge@tntech.edu. *Application contact:* Shelia K. Kendrick, Coordinator of Graduate Studies, 931-372-3808, Fax: 931-372-3497, E-mail: skendrick@tntech.edu.

Texas A&M Health Science Center, Baylor College of Dentistry, Department of Biomedical Sciences, College Station, TX 77840. Offers MS, PhD. Part-time programs available. Terminal master's awarded for partial completion of doctoral program. *Degree requirements:* For master's, thesis; for doctorate, thesis/dissertation. *Entrance requirements:* For master's, GRE General Test; for doctorate, GRE General Test, DDS or DMD. Additional exam requirements/recommendations for international students: Required—TOEFL. *Faculty research:* Craniofacial biology, aging, neuroscience, physiology, molecular/cellular biology.

Texas A&M Health Science Center, Institute of Biosciences and Technology, Houston, TX 77030-3303. Offers medical sciences (PhD). Degree awarded by the Graduate School for Biomedical Sciences. *Degree requirements:* For doctorate, thesis/dissertation. *Entrance requirements:* For doctorate, GRE General Test. Additional exam requirements/recommendations for international students: Required—TOEFL, TWE. *Expenses:* Contact institution. *Faculty research:* Cancer biology, DNA structure, extracellular matrix biology, development, birth defects.

Texas A&M International University, Office of Graduate Studies and Research, College of Arts and Sciences, Department of Biology and Chemistry, Laredo, TX 78041-1900. Offers biology (MS). *Faculty:* 6 full-time (1 woman). *Students:* 21 full-time (14 women), 13 part-time (7 women); includes 30 minority (2 Black or African American, non-Hispanic/Latino; 28 Hispanic/Latino), 2 international. Average age 28. 25 applicants, 52% accepted, 10 enrolled. In 2013, 1 master's awarded. *Degree requirements:* For master's, comprehensive exam, thesis (for some programs). *Entrance requirements:* Additional exam requirements/recommendations for international students: Required—TOEFL (minimum score 79 iBT). *Application deadline:* For fall admission, 4/30 for domestic and international students; for spring admission, 11/30 for domestic students, 10/1 for international students. Applications are processed on a rolling basis. Application fee: $35 ($50 for international students). *Expenses:* Tuition, state resident: full-time $5184. *International tuition:* $11,556 full-time. *Financial support:* In 2013–14, 11 students received support, including 3 research assistantships, 8 teaching assistantships. *Unit head:* Dr. Daniel Mott, Chair, 956-326-2583. *Application contact:* Suzanne Hansen-Alford, Director of Graduate Recruiting, 956-326-3023, E-mail: salford@tamiu.edu.
Website: http://www.tamiu.edu/coas/depts/biochem/

Texas A&M University, College of Science, Department of Biology, College Station, TX 77843. Offers biology (MS, PhD); botany (MS, PhD); microbiology (MS, PhD); zoology (MS, PhD). *Faculty:* 40. *Students:* 94 full-time (54 women), 7 part-time (4 women); includes 10 minority (1 Black or African American, non-Hispanic/Latino; 3 Asian, non-Hispanic/Latino; 6 Hispanic/Latino), 49 international. Average age 29. 120 applicants, 25% accepted, 19 enrolled. In 2013, 5 master's, 16 doctorates awarded. *Degree requirements:* For master's, thesis or alternative; for doctorate, comprehensive exam, thesis/dissertation. *Entrance requirements:* For master's and doctorate, GRE General Test. Additional exam requirements/recommendations for international students: Required—TOEFL. *Application deadline:* For fall admission, 1/15 for domestic students. Applications are processed on a rolling basis. Application fee: $50 ($75 for international students). Electronic applications accepted. *Expenses:* Tuition, state resident: full-time $4078; part-time $226.55 per credit hour. Tuition, nonresident: full-time $10,450; part-time $580.55 per credit hour. *Required fees:* $2328; $278.50 per credit hour. $642.45 per semester. *Financial support:* Fellowships, research assistantships, and teaching assistantships available. Financial award application deadline: 4/1; financial award applicants required to submit FAFSA. *Unit head:* Dr. Tom McKnight, Department Head, 979-845-3896, Fax: 979-845-2891, E-mail: mcknight@bio.tamu.edu. *Application contact:* Dr. Arne Lekven, Graduate Advisor, 979-458-3461, Fax: 979-845-2891, E-mail: alekven@bio.tamu.edu.
Website: http://www.bio.tamu.edu/index.html

Texas A&M University, College of Veterinary Medicine and Biomedical Sciences, Department of Veterinary Physiology and Pharmacology, College Station, TX 77843. Offers biomedical science (MS, PhD); toxicology (PhD). *Faculty:* 16. *Students:* 25 full-time (13 women), 3 part-time (2 women); includes 6 minority (1 Black or African American, non-Hispanic/Latino; 2 Asian, non-Hispanic/Latino; 2 Hispanic/Latino; 1 Two or more races, non-Hispanic/Latino), 9 international. Average age 28. 6 applicants, 100% accepted, 6 enrolled. In 2013, 6 master's, 3 doctorates awarded. *Entrance requirements:* For master's and doctorate, GRE General Test. Additional exam requirements/recommendations for international students: Required—TOEFL. Application fee: $50 ($75 for international students). *Expenses:* Tuition, state resident: full-time $4078; part-time $226.55 per credit hour. Tuition, nonresident: full-time $10,450; part-time $580.55 per credit hour. *Required fees:* $2328; $278.50 per credit hour. $642.45 per semester. *Financial support:* Fellowships, research assistantships, and teaching assistantships available. Financial award application deadline: 4/1; financial award applicants required to submit FAFSA. *Faculty research:* Gamete and embryo physiology, endocrinology, equine laminitis. *Unit head:* Dr. John Stallone, Head, 979-862-3065, E-mail: john-n-stallone@exchange.tamu.edu. *Application contact:* Graduate Admissions, 979-845-1044, E-mail: admissions@tamu.edu.
Website: http://vetmed.tamu.edu/vtpp

Texas A&M University–Commerce, Graduate School, College of Science, Engineering and Agriculture, Department of Biological and Environmental Sciences, Commerce, TX 75429-3011. Offers biological sciences (M Ed, MS); environmental sciences (Certificate). *Degree requirements:* For master's, comprehensive exam, thesis (for some programs). *Entrance requirements:* For master's, GRE General Test. Electronic applications accepted. *Expenses:* Tuition, state resident: full-time $3630; part-time $2420 per year. Tuition, nonresident: full-time $9948; part-time $6632.16 per year. *Required fees:* $1006 per year. Tuition and fees vary according to course load. *Faculty research:* Microbiology, botany, environmental science, birds.

Texas A&M University–Corpus Christi, Graduate Studies and Research, College of Science and Technology, Program in Biology, Corpus Christi, TX 78412-5503. Offers MS.

Texas A&M University–Kingsville, College of Graduate Studies, College of Arts and Sciences, Department of Biology, Program in Biology, Kingsville, TX 78363. Offers MS. *Faculty:* 5 full-time (0 women), 1 part-time/adjunct (0 women). *Students:* 12 full-time (5 women), 5 part-time (1 woman); includes 8 minority (all Hispanic/Latino), 3 international. Average age 24. 18 applicants, 83% accepted, 6 enrolled. In 2013, 7 master's awarded. *Degree requirements:* For master's, comprehensive exam, thesis or alternative. *Entrance requirements:* For master's, GRE General Test, minimum GPA of 3.0. Additional exam requirements/recommendations for international students: Required—TOEFL. *Application deadline:* Applications are processed on a rolling basis. Application fee: $35 ($50 for international students). Electronic applications accepted. *Financial support:* Career-related internships or fieldwork and Federal Work-Study available. Support available to part-time students. Financial award applicants required to submit

FAFSA. *Unit head:* Dr. James Pierce, Chair, 361-593-3803, E-mail: kfjrp00@tamuk.edu. *Application contact:* Director of Admissions, 361-593-2315.

Texas Christian University, College of Science and Engineering, Department of Biology, Fort Worth, TX 76129. Offers MA, MS. Part-time programs available. *Faculty:* 12 full-time (3 women), 1 part-time/adjunct (0 women). *Students:* 5 full-time (3 women), 10 part-time (6 women); includes 1 minority (Hispanic/Latino), 4 international. Average age 27. 15 applicants, 73% accepted, 7 enrolled. In 2013, 7 master's awarded. *Degree requirements:* For master's, comprehensive exam, thesis (for some programs). *Entrance requirements:* For master's, GRE General Test. Additional exam requirements/recommendations for international students: Required—TOEFL (minimum score 560 paper-based). *Application deadline:* For fall admission, 1/15 priority date for domestic and international students; for spring admission, 7/15 priority date for domestic and international students. Applications are processed on a rolling basis. Application fee: $60. Electronic applications accepted. *Expenses: Tuition:* Part-time $1270 per credit hour. Tuition and fees vary according to course load and program. *Financial support:* In 2013–14, 12 students received support, including 11 teaching assistantships with full tuition reimbursements available (averaging $15,500 per year). Financial award application deadline: 1/15. *Faculty research:* Invasive species, anthrax, mercury in biota, ecological impact of wind turbines, aging. *Total annual research expenditures:* $460,351. *Unit head:* Dr. Ray Drenner, Chairperson, 817-257-7165, E-mail: r.drenner@tcu.edu. *Application contact:* Dr. Magnus Rittby, Associate Dean, College of Science and Engineering, 817-257-7729, E-mail: m.rittby@tcu.edu.
Website: http://www.bio.tcu.edu/

Texas Southern University, School of Science and Technology, Department of Biology, Houston, TX 77004-4584. Offers MS. Part-time and evening/weekend programs available. *Faculty:* 5 full-time (2 women), 4 part-time/adjunct (2 women). *Students:* 18 full-time (12 women), 15 part-time (10 women); includes 31 minority (30 Black or African American, non-Hispanic/Latino; 1 Asian, non-Hispanic/Latino), 1 international. Average age 28. 35 applicants, 40% accepted, 9 enrolled. In 2013, 9 master's awarded. *Degree requirements:* For master's, one foreign language, comprehensive exam, thesis. *Entrance requirements:* For master's, GRE General Test, minimum GPA of 2.5. Additional exam requirements/recommendations for international students: Required—TOEFL. *Application deadline:* For fall admission, 7/1 for domestic and international students; for spring admission, 11/1 for domestic and international students. Applications are processed on a rolling basis. Application fee: $50 ($75 for international students). Electronic applications accepted. *Financial support:* In 2013–14, 3 research assistantships (averaging $13,500 per year), 5 teaching assistantships (averaging $4,160 per year) were awarded; fellowships, career-related internships or fieldwork, scholarships/grants, and unspecified assistantships also available. Financial award application deadline: 5/1. *Faculty research:* Microbiology, cell and molecular biology, biochemistry, biochemical virology, biophysics. *Unit head:* Dr. Warren Williams, Interim Chair, 713-313-4322, E-mail: williams_we@tsu.edu. *Application contact:* Helen Pittman-Cockrell, Administrative Assistant, 713-313-7005, E-mail: pittman_hj@tsu.edu.
Website: http://www.cost.tsu.edu/WebPages/Department_Site.php?Department=Biology

Texas State University, Graduate School, College of Science and Engineering, Department of Biology, Program in Biology, San Marcos, TX 78666. Offers M Ed, MA, MS. *Faculty:* 10 full-time (2 women), 1 part-time/adjunct (0 women). *Students:* 34 full-time (16 women), 6 part-time (3 women); includes 8 minority (2 Asian, non-Hispanic/Latino; 6 Hispanic/Latino), 8 international. Average age 29. 22 applicants, 68% accepted, 12 enrolled. In 2013, 12 master's awarded. *Degree requirements:* For master's, comprehensive exam, thesis (for some programs). *Entrance requirements:* For master's, GRE General Test (minimum score 1000 preferred), minimum GPA of 3.0 in last 60 hours of undergraduate work. Additional exam requirements/recommendations for international students: Required—TOEFL (minimum score 550 paper-based; 78 iBT). *Application deadline:* For fall admission, 6/15 for domestic students, 6/1 for international students; for spring admission, 10/15 for domestic students, 10/1 for international students. Applications are processed on a rolling basis. Application fee: $40 ($90 for international students). Electronic applications accepted. *Expenses:* Tuition, state resident: full-time $6663; part-time $278 per credit hour. Tuition, nonresident: full-time $15,159; part-time $632 per credit hour. *Required fees:* $1872; $54 per credit hour. $306 per term. Tuition and fees vary according to course load. *Financial support:* In 2013–14, 26 students received support, including 3 research assistantships (averaging $17,880 per year), 26 teaching assistantships (averaging $12,749 per year); Federal Work-Study, institutionally sponsored loans, scholarships/grants, health care benefits, and unspecified assistantships also available. Support available to part-time students. Financial award application deadline: 4/1. *Unit head:* Dr. David Lemke, Graduate Advisor, 512-245-2178, E-mail: dl10@txstate.edu. *Application contact:* Dr. Andrea Golato, Dean of the Graduate School, 512-245-2581, Fax: 512-245-8365, E-mail: jw02@swt.edu.
Website: http://www.bio.txstate.edu/

Texas State University, Graduate School, Emmett and Miriam McCoy College of Business Administration, Program in Human Resource Management, San Marcos, TX 78666. Offers MS. *Students:* 2 full-time (1 woman), 6 part-time (all women); includes 2 minority (1 Asian, non-Hispanic/Latino; 1 Hispanic/Latino), 1 international. Average age 31. 14 applicants, 29% accepted, 3 enrolled. *Degree requirements:* For master's, comprehensive exam, thesis optional. *Entrance requirements:* For master's, GRE (minimum score 1000 verbal and quantitative preferred), bachelor's degree in biology or related field, minimum GPA of 3.0 in last 60 hours of undergraduate work. Additional exam requirements/recommendations for international students: Required—TOEFL (minimum score 550 paper-based; 78 iBT). *Application deadline:* For fall admission, 6/15 priority date for domestic students, 6/1 for international students; for spring admission, 10/15 priority date for domestic students, 10/1 for international students. Applications are processed on a rolling basis. Application fee: $40 ($90 for international students). *Expenses:* Tuition, state resident: full-time $6663; part-time $278 per credit hour. Tuition, nonresident: full-time $15,159; part-time $632 per credit hour. *Required fees:* $1872; $54 per credit hour. $306 per term. Tuition and fees vary according to course load. *Financial support:* In 2013–14, 2 students received support. Research assistantships, teaching assistantships, Federal Work-Study, institutionally sponsored loans, scholarships/grants, health care benefits, and unspecified assistantships available. Support available to part-time students. Financial award application deadline: 4/1; financial award applicants required to submit FAFSA. *Unit head:* Dr. William Chittenden, Graduate Advisor, 512-245-3591, E-mail: wc10@txstate.edu. *Application contact:* Dr. Andrea Golato, Dean of Graduate School, 512-245-2581, Fax: 512-245-8365, E-mail: gradcollege@txstate.edu.
Website: http://www.gradcollege.txstate.edu/bhrm.html

Texas Tech University, Graduate School, College of Arts and Sciences, Department of Biological Sciences, Lubbock, TX 79409-3131. Offers biology (MS, PhD); environmental sustainability and natural resources management (PSM); microbiology (MS); zoology (MS, PhD). Part-time programs available. *Faculty:* 37 full-time (6 women), 1 (woman) part-time/adjunct. *Students:* 93 full-time (50 women), 10 part-time (7 women); includes 7 minority (1 Black or African American, non-Hispanic/Latino; 3 Asian, non-Hispanic/Latino; 3 Hispanic/Latino), 45 international. Average age 30. 59 applicants, 32% accepted, 7 enrolled. In 2013, 13 master's, 12 doctorates awarded. *Degree requirements:* For master's, thesis or alternative; for doctorate, thesis/dissertation. *Entrance requirements:* For master's and doctorate, GRE General Test. Additional exam requirements/recommendations for international students: Required—TOEFL (minimum score 550 paper-based; 79 iBT). *Application deadline:* For fall admission, 6/1 priority date for domestic students, 1/15 priority date for international students; for spring admission, 9/1 priority date for domestic students, 6/15 priority date for international students. Applications are processed on a rolling basis. Application fee: $60. Electronic applications accepted. *Expenses:* Tuition, state resident: full-time $6062; part-time $252.57 per credit hour. Tuition, nonresident: full-time $14,558; part-time $606.57 per credit hour. *Required fees:* $2655; $35 per credit hour. $907.50 per semester. Tuition and fees vary according to course load. *Financial support:* In 2013–14, 100 students received support, including 69 fellowships (averaging $1,404 per year), 16 research assistantships (averaging $4,232 per year), 78 teaching assistantships (averaging $4,702 per year). Financial award application deadline: 4/15; financial award applicants required to submit FAFSA. *Faculty research:* Biodiversity and evolution, climate change in arid ecosystems, plant biology and biotechnology, animal communication and behavior, zoonotic and emerging diseases. *Total annual research expenditures:* $2.1 million. *Unit head:* Dr. Llewellyn D. Densmore, Chair, 806-742-2715, Fax: 806-742-2963, E-mail: lou.densmore@ttu.edu. *Application contact:* Dr. Randall M. Jeter, Graduate Adviser, 806-742-2710 Ext. 270, Fax: 806-742-2963, E-mail: randall.jeter@ttu.edu.
Website: http://www.biol.ttu.edu/default.aspx

Texas Tech University Health Sciences Center, Graduate School of Biomedical Sciences, Lubbock, TX 79430-0002. Offers MS, PhD, MD/PhD, MS/PhD. Terminal master's awarded for partial completion of doctoral program. *Degree requirements:* For master's, thesis; for doctorate, thesis/dissertation. *Entrance requirements:* For master's and doctorate, GRE General Test, minimum GPA of 3.0. Additional exam requirements/recommendations for international students: Required—TOEFL (minimum score 550 paper-based). Electronic applications accepted. *Faculty research:* Genetics of neurological disorders, hemodynamics to prevent DVT, toxin A synthesis, DA neurons, peroxidases.

Texas Woman's University, Graduate School, College of Arts and Sciences, Department of Biology, Denton, TX 76201. Offers biology (MS); molecular biology (PhD). Part-time programs available. *Faculty:* 11 full-time (9 women), 3 part-time/adjunct (1 woman). *Students:* 9 full-time (8 women), 40 part-time (29 women); includes 9 minority (3 Black or African American, non-Hispanic/Latino; 1 American Indian or Alaska Native, non-Hispanic/Latino; 3 Asian, non-Hispanic/Latino; 2 Hispanic/Latino), 18 international. Average age 31. 17 applicants, 59% accepted, 5 enrolled. In 2013, 6 master's, 1 doctorate awarded. Terminal master's awarded for partial completion of doctoral program. *Degree requirements:* For master's, comprehensive exam, thesis; for doctorate, comprehensive exam, thesis/dissertation, residency. *Entrance requirements:* For master's, GRE General Test (preferred minimum score 149 [425 old version] verbal, 141 [425 old version] quantitative), 3 letters of reference; letter of interest; for doctorate, GRE General Test (preferred minimum score 153 [500 old version] verbal, 144 [500 old version] quantitative), 3 letters of reference, letter of interest. Additional exam requirements/recommendations for international students: Required—TOEFL (minimum score 550 paper-based; 79 iBT). *Application deadline:* For fall admission, 2/1 priority date for domestic students, 2/1 for international students. Applications are processed on a rolling basis. Application fee: $50 ($75 for international students). Electronic applications accepted. *Expenses:* Tuition, state resident: full-time $4182; part-time $233.32 per credit hour. Tuition, nonresident: full-time $10,716; part-time $595.32 per credit hour. *Financial support:* In 2013–14, 7 students received support, including 51 research assistantships (averaging $15,652 per year); career-related internships or fieldwork, Federal Work-Study, institutionally sponsored loans, scholarships/grants, traineeships, health care benefits, and unspecified assistantships also available. Support available to part-time students. Financial award application deadline: 3/1; financial award applicants required to submit FAFSA. *Faculty research:* Computational biology, protein-protein Interactions, chromatin structure and regulation, regulation of RNA synthesis, virus-host interactions, regulation of axon growth and guidance in neurons, estrogen compounds in plants, regulation of gene expression in male reproductive tissues, female gonadal hormones in the development of anxiety and depression, electron microscopy. *Total annual research expenditures:* $447,324. *Unit head:* Dr. Sarah McIntire, Chair, 940-898-2352, Fax: 940-898-2382, E-mail: smcintire@twu.edu. *Application contact:* Dr. Samuel Wheeler, Assistant Director of Admissions, 940-898-3188, Fax: 940-898-3081, E-mail: wheelersr@twu.edu.
Website: http://www.twu.edu/biology

Thomas Jefferson University, Jefferson Graduate School of Biomedical Sciences, Philadelphia, PA 19107. Offers MS, PhD, Certificate, MD/PhD. Part-time and evening/weekend programs available. *Faculty:* 190 full-time (53 women), 37 part-time/adjunct (15 women). *Students:* 180 full-time (92 women), 109 part-time (66 women); includes 52 minority (11 Black or African American, non-Hispanic/Latino; 32 Asian, non-Hispanic/Latino; 8 Hispanic/Latino; 1 Native Hawaiian or other Pacific Islander, non-Hispanic/Latino), 34 international. Average age 29. 627 applicants, 26% accepted, 94 enrolled. In 2013, 38 master's, 19 doctorates, 3 other advanced degrees awarded. Terminal master's awarded for partial completion of doctoral program. *Degree requirements:* For master's, thesis; for doctorate, comprehensive exam, thesis/dissertation. *Entrance requirements:* For master's, GRE or MCAT; for doctorate, GRE or MCAT, minimum GPA of 3.2; for Certificate, SAT/ACT. Additional exam requirements/recommendations for international students: Required—TOEFL (minimum score 100 iBT). *Application deadline:* For fall admission, 1/15 priority date for domestic and international students; for winter admission, 6/1 priority date for international students; for spring admission, 9/1 priority date for international students. Applications are processed on a rolling basis. Application fee: $75. Electronic applications accepted. *Financial support:* In 2013–14, 122 fellowships with full tuition reimbursements (averaging $56,052 per year) were awarded; Federal Work-Study, institutionally sponsored loans, scholarships/grants, and traineeships also available. Support available to part-time students. Financial award application deadline: 5/1; financial award applicants required to submit FAFSA. *Unit head:* Dr. Gerald B. Grunwald, Dean, 215-503-4191, Fax: 215-503-6690, E-mail: gerald.grunwald@jefferson.edu. *Application contact:* Marc E. Stearns, Director of Admissions, 215-503-0155, Fax: 215-503-3433, E-mail: jgsbs-info@jefferson.edu.
Website: http://www.jefferson.edu/Biomedical_Sciences/

Towson University, Program in Biology, Towson, MD 21252-0001. Offers MS. Part-time and evening/weekend programs available. *Students:* 23 full-time (17 women), 27 part-time (14 women); includes 13 minority (10 Black or African American, non-Hispanic/Latino; 2 Asian, non-Hispanic/Latino; 1 Two or more races, non-Hispanic/Latino), 6 international. *Degree requirements:* For master's, thesis optional. *Entrance requirements:* For master's, GRE General Test (for thesis students), minimum GPA of 3.0, 24 credits in related course work, 3 letters of recommendation, minimum 24 units in biology, coursework in chemistry, organic chemistry, and physics, personal statement, official transcripts. Application fee: $45. Electronic applications accepted. *Financial support:* Application deadline: 4/1. *Unit head:* Dr. John Lapolla, Graduate Program Co-

Director, 410-704-3121, E-mail: jlapolla@towson.edu. *Application contact:* Alicia Arkell-Kleis, Information Contact, 410-704-6004, E-mail: grads@towson.edu.
Website: http://grad.towson.edu/program/master/biol-ms/

Trent University, Graduate Studies, Program in Applications of Modeling in the Natural and Social Sciences, Peterborough, ON K9J 7B8, Canada. Offers applications of modeling in the natural and social sciences (MA); biology (M Sc, PhD); chemistry (M Sc); computer studies (M Sc); geography (M Sc, PhD); physics (M Sc). Part-time programs available. *Degree requirements:* For master's, thesis. *Entrance requirements:* For master's, honours degree. *Faculty research:* Computation of heat transfer, atmospheric physics, statistical mechanics, stress and coping, evolutionary ecology.

Trent University, Graduate Studies, Program in Environmental and Life Sciences and Program in Applications of Modeling in the Natural and Social Sciences, Department of Biology, Peterborough, ON K9J 7B8, Canada. Offers M Sc, PhD. Part-time programs available. *Degree requirements:* For master's, thesis; for doctorate, thesis/dissertation. *Entrance requirements:* For master's, honours degree; for doctorate, master's degree. *Faculty research:* Aquatic and behavioral ecology, hydrology and limnology, human impact on ecosystems, behavioral ecology of birds, ecology of fish.

Troy University, Graduate School, College of Arts and Sciences, Program in Environmental and Biological Sciences, Troy, AL 36082. Offers biological science (MS); environmental analysis and management (MS); environmental policy (MS); environmental science (MS). Part-time and evening/weekend programs available. *Faculty:* 8 full-time (1 woman), 2 part-time/adjunct (1 woman). *Students:* 8 full-time (all women), 37 part-time (21 women); includes 18 minority (13 Black or African American, non-Hispanic/Latino; 2 Asian, non-Hispanic/Latino; 2 Hispanic/Latino; 1 Two or more races, non-Hispanic/Latino). Average age 26. 37 applicants, 51% accepted, 19 enrolled. In 2013, 7 master's awarded. *Degree requirements:* For master's, comprehensive exam (for some programs), thesis (for some programs), comprehensive exam or thesis, minimum GPA of 3.0, admission to candidacy. *Entrance requirements:* For master's, GRE (minimum score of 850 on old exam or 290 on new exam), MAT (minimum score of 385) or GMAT (minimum score of 380), bachelor's degree; minimum undergraduate GPA of 2.5 or 3.0 on last 30 semester hours. Additional exam requirements/recommendations for international students: Required—TOEFL (minimum score 523 paper-based; 70 iBT), IELTS (minimum score 6). *Application deadline:* Applications are processed on a rolling basis. Application fee: $50. Electronic applications accepted. *Expenses:* Tuition, state resident: full-time $6084; part-time $338 per credit hour. Tuition, nonresident: full-time $12,168; part-time $676 per credit hour. *Required fees:* $630; $35 per credit hour. $50 per semester. *Unit head:* Dr. Glenn Cohen, Chairman, 334-670-3660, Fax: 334-670-3401, E-mail: gcohen@troy.edu. *Application contact:* Brenda K. Campbell, Director of Graduate Admissions, 334-670-3178, Fax: 334-670-3733, E-mail: bcamp@troy.edu.

Truman State University, Graduate School, School of Arts and Letters, Program in Biology, Kirksville, MO 63501-4221. Offers MS. *Degree requirements:* For master's, comprehensive exam, thesis. *Entrance requirements:* For master's, GRE General Test, minimum GPA of 3.0. Additional exam requirements/recommendations for international students: Required—TOEFL (minimum score 550 paper-based). Electronic applications accepted.

Tufts University, Cummings School of Veterinary Medicine, North Grafton, MA 01536. Offers animals and public policy (MS); biomedical sciences (PhD), including digestive diseases, infectious diseases, neuroscience and reproductive biology, pathology; conservation medicine (MS); veterinary medicine (DVM); DVM/MPH; DVM/MS. *Accreditation:* AVMA (one or more programs are accredited). *Faculty:* 98 full-time (45 women), 13 part-time/adjunct (7 women). *Students:* 426 full-time (364 women); includes 60 minority (5 Black or African American, non-Hispanic/Latino; 1 American Indian or Alaska Native, non-Hispanic/Latino; 32 Asian, non-Hispanic/Latino; 20 Hispanic/Latino; 2 Two or more races, non-Hispanic/Latino), 4 international. Average age 25. 899 applicants, 29% accepted, 119 enrolled. In 2013, 85 master's, 2 doctorates awarded. *Degree requirements:* For master's, thesis (for some programs); for doctorate, comprehensive exam, thesis/dissertation (for some programs). *Entrance requirements:* For master's and doctorate, GRE General Test. Additional exam requirements/recommendations for international students: Required—TOEFL or IELTS. *Application deadline:* For fall admission, 11/1 for domestic and international students. Application fee: $70. Electronic applications accepted. *Expenses:* Contact institution. *Financial support:* In 2013–14, 230 students received support, including 7 research assistantships with full tuition reimbursements available (averaging $25,000 per year), 6 teaching assistantships (averaging $5,000 per year); career-related internships or fieldwork, Federal Work-Study, institutionally sponsored loans, scholarships/grants, and institutional aid awards, health care benefits for PhD students also available. Financial award application deadline: 4/15; financial award applicants required to submit FAFSA. *Faculty research:* Oncology, veterinary ethics, international veterinary medicine, veterinary genomics, pathogenesis of Clostridium difficile, wildlife fertility control. *Unit head:* Dr. Deborah T. Kochevar, Dean, 508-839-5302, Fax: 508-839-2953, E-mail: deborah.kochevar@tufts.edu. *Application contact:* Rebecca Russo, Director of Admissions, 508-839-7920, Fax: 508-887-4820, E-mail: vetadmissions@tufts.edu.
Website: http://www.tufts.edu/

Tufts University, Graduate School of Arts and Sciences, Department of Biology, Medford, MA 02155. Offers biology (MS, PhD); soft materials robotics (PhD). Part-time programs available. *Faculty:* 23 full-time. *Students:* 48 full-time (31 women); includes 6 minority (2 Asian, non-Hispanic/Latino; 4 Hispanic/Latino), 6 international. Average age 27. 140 applicants, 8% accepted, 9 enrolled. In 2013, 2 master's, 4 doctorates awarded. Terminal master's awarded for partial completion of doctoral program. *Degree requirements:* For master's, thesis (for some programs); for doctorate, thesis/dissertation. *Entrance requirements:* For master's and doctorate, GRE General Test. Additional exam requirements/recommendations for international students: Required—TOEFL (minimum score 550 paper-based; 80 iBT), IELTS (minimum score 6.5). *Application deadline:* For fall admission, 12/15 for domestic and international students; for spring admission, 10/15 for domestic students, 9/15 for international students. Applications are processed on a rolling basis. Application fee: $75. Electronic applications accepted. *Financial support:* Fellowships, research assistantships with full and partial tuition reimbursements, teaching assistantships with full and partial tuition reimbursements, Federal Work-Study, scholarships/grants, tuition waivers (partial), and unspecified assistantships available. Financial award application deadline: 1/15; financial award applicants required to submit FAFSA. *Unit head:* Dr. Sergei Mirkin, Chair, 617-627-3195. *Application contact:* Kelly McLaughlin, Graduate Advisor, 617-627-3195.
Website: http://www.ase.tufts.edu/biology

Tufts University, Sackler School of Graduate Biomedical Sciences, Boston, MA 02111. Offers MS, PhD, DVM/PhD, MD/PhD. *Faculty:* 200 full-time (60 women). *Students:* 217 full-time (124 women), 3 part-time (2 women); includes 47 minority (4 Black or African American, non-Hispanic/Latino; 28 Asian, non-Hispanic/Latino; 7 Hispanic/Latino; 8 Two or more races, non-Hispanic/Latino), 44 international. Average age 33. 690 applicants, 15% accepted, 45 enrolled. In 2013, 16 master's, 20 doctorates awarded. Terminal master's awarded for partial completion of doctoral program. *Degree requirements:* For master's, comprehensive exam (for some programs), thesis; for doctorate, thesis/dissertation. *Entrance requirements:* For doctorate, GRE General Test, 3 letters of reference. Additional exam requirements/recommendations for international students: Required—TOEFL (minimum score 600 paper-based; 100 iBT). *Application deadline:* For fall admission, 12/15 for domestic and international students. Application fee: $70. Electronic applications accepted. *Expenses:* Contact institution. *Financial support:* In 2013–14, 183 students received support, including 183 research assistantships with full tuition reimbursements available (averaging $31,000 per year); health care benefits also available. Financial award application deadline: 12/15. *Unit head:* Dr. Naomi Rosenberg, Dean, 617-636-6767, Fax: 617-636-0375, E-mail: naomi.rosenberg@tufts.edu. *Application contact:* Kellie Melchin, Associate Director of Admissions, 617-636-6767, Fax: 617-636-0375, E-mail: sackler-school@tufts.edu.
Website: http://sackler.tufts.edu/

Tulane University, School of Medicine and School of Liberal Arts, Graduate Programs in Biomedical Sciences, New Orleans, LA 70118-5669. Offers MBS, MS, PhD, MD/MS, MD/PhD. *Degree requirements:* For doctorate, thesis/dissertation. *Entrance requirements:* For master's, GRE General Test, minimum B average in undergraduate course work; for doctorate, GRE General Test. Additional exam requirements/recommendations for international students: Required—TOEFL. *Expenses:* Contact institution.

Tuskegee University, Graduate Programs, College of Arts and Sciences, Department of Biology, Tuskegee, AL 36088. Offers MS. *Degree requirements:* For master's, thesis. *Entrance requirements:* For master's, GRE General Test, GRE Subject Test. Additional exam requirements/recommendations for international students: Required—TOEFL (minimum score 500 paper-based). *Application deadline:* For fall admission, 7/15 for domestic students. Applications are processed on a rolling basis. Application fee: $25 ($35 for international students). *Financial support:* Fellowships, teaching assistantships, Federal Work-Study, and institutionally sponsored loans available. Support available to part-time students. Financial award application deadline: 4/15. *Unit head:* Dr. John P. Davidson, Head, 334-727-8822. *Application contact:* Dr. Cynthia Sellers-Simon, Vice President for Student Affairs and Enrollment Management, 334-724-4746, Fax: 334-727-5750, E-mail: sellersc@mytu.tuskegee.edu.

Tuskegee University, Graduate Programs, Program in Integrative Biosciences, Tuskegee, AL 36088. Offers PhD. *Degree requirements:* For doctorate, thesis/dissertation. *Entrance requirements:* For doctorate, GRE General Test, GRE Subject Test, minimum cumulative GPA of 3.0, 3.4 in upper-division courses; 3 letters of recommendation; resume or curriculum vitae. Additional exam requirements/recommendations for international students: Required—TOEFL (minimum score 500 paper-based). *Application deadline:* For fall admission, 12/15 for domestic students, 3/1 for international students. Application fee: $35. Electronic applications accepted. *Unit head:* Dr. Deloris Alexander, Director, 334-552-0690, E-mail: dalexander@mytu.tuskegee.edu. *Application contact:* Dr. Cynthia Sellers-Simon, Vice President for Student Affairs and Enrollment Management, 334-724-4746, Fax: 334-727-5750, E-mail: sellersc@mytu.tuskegee.edu.
Website: http://www.tuskegee.edu/phd_program_in_integrative_biosciences.aspx

Uniformed Services University of the Health Sciences, School of Medicine, Graduate Programs in the Biomedical Sciences and Public Health, Bethesda, MD 20814. Offers emerging infectious diseases (PhD); medical and clinical psychology (PhD), including clinical psychology, medical psychology; molecular and cell biology (MS, PhD); neuroscience (PhD); preventive medicine and biometrics (MPH, MS, MSPH, MTMH, Dr PH, PhD), including environmental health sciences (PhD), healthcare administration and policy (MS), medical zoology (PhD), public health (MPH, MSPH, Dr PH), tropical medicine and hygiene (MTMH). *Faculty:* 372 full-time (119 women), 4,044 part-time/adjunct (908 women). *Students:* 240 full-time (133 women); includes 40 minority (15 Black or African American, non-Hispanic/Latino; 13 Asian, non-Hispanic/Latino; 12 Hispanic/Latino), 30 international. Average age 25. 598 applicants, 17% accepted, 77 enrolled. In 2013, 19 master's, 50 doctorates awarded. Terminal master's awarded for partial completion of doctoral program. *Degree requirements:* For master's, comprehensive exam, thesis or alternative; for doctorate, comprehensive exam, thesis/dissertation, qualifying exam. *Entrance requirements:* For master's, GRE General Test; for doctorate, GRE General Test, minimum GPA of 3.0. Additional exam requirements/recommendations for international students: Required—TOEFL. *Application deadline:* For fall admission, 1/1 priority date for domestic and international students. Applications are processed on a rolling basis. Application fee: $0. Electronic applications accepted. *Financial support:* In 2013–14, fellowships with full tuition reimbursements (averaging $27,000 per year), research assistantships with full tuition reimbursements (averaging $27,000 per year) were awarded; career-related internships or fieldwork, scholarships/grants, health care benefits, and tuition waivers (full) also available. *Unit head:* Dr. Eleanor S. Metcalf, Associate Dean, 301-295-1104, E-mail: emetcalf@usuhs.edu. *Application contact:* Tina Finley, Administrative Officer, 301-295-3642, Fax: 301-295-6772, E-mail: netina.finley@usuhs.edu.
Website: http://www.usuhs.mil/graded

Universidad Central del Caribe, School of Medicine, Program in Biomedical Sciences, Bayamón, PR 00960-6032. Offers anatomy and cell biology (MA, MS); biochemistry (MS); biomedical sciences (MA); cellular and molecular biology (PhD); microbiology and immunology (MA, MS); pharmacology (MS); physiology (MS).

Universidad de Ciencias Medicas, Graduate Programs, San Jose, Costa Rica. Offers dermatology (SP); family health (MS); health service center administration (MHA); human anatomy (MS); medical and surgery (MD); occupational medicine (MS); pharmacy (Pharm D). Part-time programs available. *Degree requirements:* For master's, thesis; for doctorate and SP, comprehensive exam. *Entrance requirements:* For master's, MD or bachelor's degree; for doctorate, admissions test; for SP, admissions test, MD.

Université de Moncton, Faculty of Sciences, Department of Biology, Moncton, NB E1A 3E9, Canada. Offers M Sc. *Degree requirements:* For master's, one foreign language, thesis. *Entrance requirements:* For master's, minimum GPA of 3.0. Electronic applications accepted. *Faculty research:* Terrestrial ecology, aquatic ecology, marine biology, aquaculture, ethology, biotechnology.

Université de Montréal, Faculty of Arts and Sciences, Department of Biological Sciences, Montréal, QC H3C 3J7, Canada. Offers M Sc, PhD. Part-time programs available. *Degree requirements:* For master's, thesis; for doctorate, thesis/dissertation, general exam. *Entrance requirements:* For doctorate, MS in biology or related field. Electronic applications accepted. *Faculty research:* Fresh water ecology, plant biotechnology, neurobiology, genetics, cell physiology.

Université de Montréal, Faculty of Medicine, Programs in Biomedical Sciences, Montréal, QC H3C 3J7, Canada. Offers M Sc, PhD. *Degree requirements:* For master's, thesis; for doctorate, thesis/dissertation, general exam. *Entrance requirements:* For master's and doctorate, proficiency in French, knowledge of English. Electronic applications accepted.

Université de Sherbrooke, Faculty of Medicine and Health Sciences, Graduate Programs in Medicine, Sherbrooke, QC J1H 5N4, Canada. Offers M Sc, PhD. Part-time programs available. Terminal master's awarded for partial completion of doctoral program. *Degree requirements:* For master's, thesis; for doctorate, thesis/dissertation. Electronic applications accepted. *Expenses:* Contact institution.

Université de Sherbrooke, Faculty of Sciences, Department of Biology, Sherbrooke, QC J1K 2R1, Canada. Offers M Sc, PhD, Diploma. *Degree requirements:* For master's, thesis; for doctorate, comprehensive exam, thesis/dissertation. *Entrance requirements:* For doctorate, master's degree. Electronic applications accepted. *Faculty research:* Microbiology, ecology, molecular biology, cell biology, biotechnology.

Université du Québec à Montréal, Graduate Programs, Program in Biology, Montréal, QC H3C 3P8, Canada. Offers M Sc, PhD. Part-time programs available. *Degree requirements:* For master's, thesis; for doctorate, thesis/dissertation. *Entrance requirements:* For master's, appropriate bachelor's degree or equivalent, proficiency in French; for doctorate, appropriate master's degree or equivalent, proficiency in French.

Université du Québec en Abitibi-Témiscamingue, Graduate Programs, Program in Environmental Sciences, Rouyn-Noranda, QC J9X 5E4, Canada. Offers biology (MS); environmental sciences (PhD); sustainable forest ecosystem management (MS).

Université du Québec, Institut National de la Recherche Scientifique, Graduate Programs, Research Center–INRS–Institut Armand-Frappier, Laval, QC H7V 1B7, Canada. Offers applied microbiology (M Sc); biology (PhD); experimental health sciences (M Sc); virology and immunology (M Sc, PhD). Programs given in French. Part-time programs available. *Faculty:* 45 full-time. *Students:* 126 full-time (78 women), 11 part-time (7 women), 52 international. Average age 30. In 2013, 19 master's, 12 doctorates awarded. *Degree requirements:* For master's, thesis; for doctorate, thesis/dissertation. *Entrance requirements:* For master's, appropriate bachelor's degree, proficiency in French; for doctorate, appropriate master's degree, proficiency in French. *Application deadline:* For fall admission, 3/30 for domestic and international students; for winter admission, 11/1 for domestic and international students; for spring admission, 3/1 for domestic and international students. Application fee: $45 Canadian dollars. Electronic applications accepted. *Financial support:* In 2013–14, fellowships (averaging $16,500 per year) were awarded; research assistantships also available. *Faculty research:* Immunity, infection and cancer; toxicology and environmental biotechnology; molecular pharmacochemistry. *Unit head:* Charles Dozois, Director, 450-687-5010, Fax: 450-686-5566, E-mail: charles.dozois@iaf.inrs.ca. *Application contact:* Sylvie Richard, Registrar, 418-654-2518, Fax: 418-654-3858, E-mail: sylvie.richard@adm.inrs.ca. Website: http://www.iaf.inrs.ca

Université Laval, Faculty of Medicine, Graduate Programs in Medicine, Québec, QC G1K 7P4, Canada. Offers M Sc, PhD, Diploma. *Degree requirements:* For doctorate, comprehensive exam, thesis/dissertation. *Entrance requirements:* For doctorate, knowledge of French, comprehension of written English; for Diploma, knowledge of French. Electronic applications accepted.

Université Laval, Faculty of Sciences and Engineering, Department of Biology, Programs in Biology, Québec, QC G1K 7P4, Canada. Offers M Sc, PhD. Terminal master's awarded for partial completion of doctoral program. *Degree requirements:* For master's, thesis; for doctorate, comprehensive exam, thesis/dissertation. *Entrance requirements:* For master's and doctorate, knowledge of French and English. Electronic applications accepted.

University at Albany, State University of New York, College of Arts and Sciences, Department of Biological Sciences, Albany, NY 12222-0001. Offers biodiversity, conservation, and policy (MS); ecology, evolution, and behavior (MS, PhD); forensic molecular biology (MS); molecular, cellular, developmental, and neural biology (MS, PhD). *Degree requirements:* For master's, one foreign language; for doctorate, one foreign language, thesis/dissertation. *Entrance requirements:* For master's and doctorate, GRE General Test. Additional exam requirements/recommendations for international students: Required—TOEFL (minimum score 550 paper-based). Electronic applications accepted. *Faculty research:* Interferon, neural development, RNA self-splicing, behavioral ecology, DNA repair enzymes.

University at Albany, State University of New York, School of Public Health, Department of Biomedical Sciences, Albany, NY 12222-0001. Offers biochemistry, molecular biology, and genetics (MS, PhD); cell and molecular structure (MS, PhD); immunobiology and immunochemistry (MS, PhD); molecular pathogenesis (MS, PhD); neuroscience (MS, PhD). *Degree requirements:* For master's, thesis; for doctorate, comprehensive exam, thesis/dissertation. *Entrance requirements:* For master's and doctorate, GRE General Test, 3 letters of reference. Additional exam requirements/recommendations for international students: Required—TOEFL (minimum score 600 paper-based). Electronic applications accepted. *Faculty research:* Geno expression; RNA processing; membrane transport; immune response regulation; etiology of AIDS, Lyme disease, epilepsy.

University at Buffalo, the State University of New York, Graduate School, College of Arts and Sciences, Department of Biological Sciences, Buffalo, NY 14260. Offers MA, MS, PhD. *Faculty:* 27 full-time (8 women), 5 part-time/adjunct (3 women). *Students:* 83 full-time (38 women); includes 39 minority (6 Black or African American, non-Hispanic/Latino; 1 American Indian or Alaska Native, non-Hispanic/Latino; 32 Asian, non-Hispanic/Latino), 1 international. Average age 26. 167 applicants, 19% accepted, 24 enrolled. In 2013, 20 master's, 4 doctorates awarded. Terminal master's awarded for partial completion of doctoral program. *Degree requirements:* For master's, thesis, research rotation, seminar; for doctorate, comprehensive exam, thesis/dissertation, oral candidacy exam, research, seminar. *Entrance requirements:* For master's and doctorate, GRE General Test, 2 semesters of course work in calculus, course work in chemistry through organic chemistry, strong biology background. Additional exam requirements/recommendations for international students: Required—TOEFL (minimum score 600 paper-based; 100 iBT). *Application deadline:* For fall admission, 1/1 priority date for domestic and international students; for spring admission, 11/1 for domestic and international students. Applications are processed on a rolling basis. Application fee: $75. Electronic applications accepted. *Financial support:* In 2013–14, 59 students received support, including 5 fellowships (averaging $6,000 per year), 17 research assistantships with full tuition reimbursements available (averaging $23,500 per year), 39 teaching assistantships with full tuition reimbursements available (averaging $22,800 per year); scholarships/grants, health care benefits, and unspecified assistantships also available. *Faculty research:* Biochemistry, bioinformatics, biophysics, biotechnology, botany, cell biology, developmental biology, evolutionary biology, genetics, genomics, molecular biology, microbiology, neuroscience, physiology, plant physiology, plant sciences, structural biology, virology, zoology. *Total annual research expenditures:* $2.7 million. *Unit head:* Dr. Gerald Koudelka, Chairman, 716-645-4940, Fax: 716-645-2975, E-mail: koudelka@buffalo.edu. *Application contact:* Dr. Michael Yu, Director of Graduate Studies, 716-645-4931, Fax: 716-645-2975, E-mail: mcyu@buffalo.edu. Website: http://www.biologicalsciences.buffalo.edu/

University at Buffalo, the State University of New York, Graduate School, Graduate Programs in Cancer Research and Biomedical Sciences at Roswell Park Cancer Institute, Interdisciplinary Master of Science Program in Natural and Biomedical Sciences at Roswell Park Cancer Institute, Buffalo, NY 14260. Offers biomedical sciences and cancer research (MS). Part-time programs available. *Faculty:* 124 full-time (36 women), 24 part-time/adjunct (8 women). *Students:* 50 full-time (27 women); includes 6 minority (4 Black or African American, non-Hispanic/Latino; 1 Asian, non-Hispanic/Latino; 1 Two or more races, non-Hispanic/Latino), 20 international. 82 applicants, 50% accepted, 28 enrolled. In 2013, 29 master's awarded. *Degree requirements:* For master's, thesis, oral defense of thesis based on research project. *Entrance requirements:* For master's, GRE General Test. Additional exam requirements/recommendations for international students: Required—TOEFL (minimum score 79 iBT). *Application deadline:* For fall admission, 3/1 priority date for domestic and international students. Application fee: $75. Electronic applications accepted. *Financial support:* Application deadline: 2/28. *Faculty research:* Biochemistry, oncology, pathology, biophysics, pharmacology, molecular biology, cellular biology, genetics, bioinformatics, immunology, therapeutic development, epidemiology. *Unit head:* Dr. Norman J. Karin, Associate Dean, 716-845-2339, Fax: 716-845-8178, E-mail: norman.karin@roswellpark.org. *Application contact:* Dr. Norman J. Karin, Associate Dean, 716-845-2339, Fax: 716-845-8178, E-mail: norman.karin@roswellpark.org. Website: http://www.roswellpark.edu/education/interdisciplinary-masters

University at Buffalo, the State University of New York, Graduate School, School of Medicine and Biomedical Sciences, Graduate Programs in Medicine and Biomedical Sciences, Buffalo, NY 14260. Offers MA, MS, PhD, MD/PhD. *Faculty:* 132 full-time (37 women), 12 part-time/adjunct (2 women). *Students:* 183 full-time (84 women), 4 part-time (2 women); includes 52 minority (8 Black or African American, non-Hispanic/Latino; 2 American Indian or Alaska Native, non-Hispanic/Latino; 39 Asian, non-Hispanic/Latino; 3 Hispanic/Latino), 40 international. Average age 28. 621 applicants, 20% accepted, 52 enrolled. In 2013, 30 master's, 16 doctorates awarded. Terminal master's awarded for partial completion of doctoral program. *Degree requirements:* For master's, comprehensive exam (for some programs), thesis (for some programs); for doctorate, comprehensive exam, thesis/dissertation. *Entrance requirements:* For master's, GRE General Test; for doctorate, GRE General Test, 3 letters of recommendation. Additional exam requirements/recommendations for international students: Required—TOEFL (minimum score 600 paper-based; 100 iBT). *Application deadline:* For fall admission, 2/1 priority date for domestic and international students. Applications are processed on a rolling basis. Application fee: $75. Electronic applications accepted. *Expenses:* Contact institution. *Financial support:* In 2013–14, 44 students received support, including 12 fellowships with full tuition reimbursements available (averaging $9,325 per year), 88 research assistantships with full tuition reimbursements available (averaging $25,000 per year), 7 teaching assistantships with full tuition reimbursements available (averaging $12,128 per year); career-related internships or fieldwork, Federal Work-Study, institutionally sponsored loans, scholarships/grants, traineeships, health care benefits, and unspecified assistantships also available. Financial award application deadline: 2/1; financial award applicants required to submit FAFSA. *Faculty research:* Neuroscience; molecular, cell, and structural biology; microbial pathogenesis; cardiopulmonary physiology; biochemistry, biotechnology and clinical laboratory science. *Total annual research expenditures:* $23.1 million. *Unit head:* Dr. Anthony Campagnari, Senior Associate Dean for Research and Graduate Education, 716-829-3398, Fax: 716-829-2437, E-mail: aac@buffalo.edu. *Application contact:* Elizabeth A. White, Administrative Director, 716-829-3399, Fax: 716-829-2437, E-mail: bethw@buffalo.edu.

University at Buffalo, the State University of New York, Graduate School, School of Medicine and Biomedical Sciences, PhD Program in Biomedical Sciences, Buffalo, NY 14260. Offers PhD. *Students:* 13 full-time (3 women); includes 5 minority (1 Black or African American, non-Hispanic/Latino; 1 American Indian or Alaska Native, non-Hispanic/Latino; 2 Asian, non-Hispanic/Latino; 1 Hispanic/Latino), 2 international. 304 applicants, 13% accepted, 13 enrolled. *Degree requirements:* For doctorate, comprehensive exam, thesis/dissertation. *Entrance requirements:* For doctorate, GRE General Test, 3 letters of recommendation. Additional exam requirements/recommendations for international students: Required—TOEFL (minimum score 600 paper-based; 100 iBT). *Application deadline:* For fall admission, 1/10 priority date for domestic and international students. Applications are processed on a rolling basis. Application fee: $75. Electronic applications accepted. *Financial support:* In 2013–14, 13 students received support. Scholarships/grants, traineeships, health care benefits, and unspecified assistantships available. Financial award application deadline: 1/10. *Faculty research:* Molecular, cell and structural biology; pharmacology and toxicology; neurosciences; microbiology; pathogenesis and disease. *Unit head:* Dr. Mark Sutton, Director, 716-829-3398, Fax: 716-829-2437, E-mail: smbs-gradprog@buffalo.edu. *Application contact:* Elizabeth A. White, Administrative Director, 716-829-3399, Fax: 716-829-2437, E-mail: bethw@buffalo.edu. Website: http://medicine.buffalo.edu/phdprogram

The University of Akron, Graduate School, Buchtel College of Arts and Sciences, Department of Biology, Akron, OH 44325. Offers biology (MS); integrated bioscience (PhD). Part-time programs available. *Faculty:* 17 full-time (3 women), 4 part-time/adjunct (1 woman). *Students:* 56 full-time (22 women), 2 part-time (1 woman); includes 6 minority (2 Black or African American, non-Hispanic/Latino; 1 Asian, non-Hispanic/Latino; 1 Hispanic/Latino; 2 Two or more races, non-Hispanic/Latino), 15 international. Average age 28. 47 applicants, 32% accepted, 13 enrolled. In 2013, 6 master's, 5 doctorates awarded. *Degree requirements:* For master's, thesis optional, oral defense of thesis, oral exam, seminars; for doctorate, thesis/dissertation, oral defense of dissertation, seminars. *Entrance requirements:* For master's, GRE, baccalaureate degree in biology or the equivalent; minimum GPA of 3.0 overall and in biology; letter of interest; letter from potential biology adviser; for doctorate, GRE, minimum overall GPA of 3.0, letters of recommendation, personal statement of career goals and research interest. Additional exam requirements/recommendations for international students: Required—TOEFL (minimum score 550 paper-based; 79 iBT). *Application deadline:* Applications are processed on a rolling basis. Application fee: $40 ($60 for international students). Electronic applications accepted. *Expenses:* Tuition, state resident: full-time $7430; part-time $412.80 per credit hour. Tuition, nonresident: full-time $12,722; part-time $706.80 per credit hour. *Required fees:* $53 per credit hour. $12 per semester. Tuition and fees vary according to course load and program. *Financial support:* In 2013–14, 3 research assistantships, 12 teaching assistantships with full tuition reimbursements were awarded. *Faculty research:* Behavior/neuroscience, ecology-evolution, genetics, molecular biology, physiology. *Total annual research expenditures:* $1.4 million. *Unit head:* Dr. Monte Turner, Interim Chair, 330-972-7155, E-mail: meturner@uakron.edu. *Application contact:* Dr. Todd Blackledge, Graduate Director, 330-972-4264, E-mail: blackledge@uakron.edu. Website: http://www.uakron.edu/biology/

The University of Alabama, Graduate School, College of Arts and Sciences, Department of Biological Sciences, Tuscaloosa, AL 35487. Offers MS, PhD. *Faculty:* 33 full-time (15 women), 4 part-time/adjunct (2 women). *Students:* 67 full-time (34 women), 15 part-time (8 women); includes 9 minority (6 Black or African American, non-Hispanic/Latino; 1 Asian, non-Hispanic/Latino; 1 Hispanic/Latino; 1 Two or more races, non-Hispanic/Latino), 18 international. Average age 28. 71 applicants, 31% accepted, 13 enrolled. In 2013, 14 master's, 3 doctorates awarded. Terminal master's awarded for partial completion of doctoral program. *Degree requirements:* For master's, comprehensive exam, thesis optional; for doctorate, comprehensive exam, thesis/dissertation, written and oral candidacy exams. *Entrance requirements:* For master's and doctorate, GRE General Test, minimum GPA of 3.0. Additional exam requirements/recommendations for international students: Required—TOEFL (minimum score 550 paper-based; 80 iBT). *Application deadline:* For fall admission, 12/5 priority date for

domestic and international students; for spring admission, 12/5 priority date for domestic students, 9/5 priority date for international students. Applications are processed on a rolling basis. Application fee: $50 ($60 for international students). Electronic applications accepted. *Expenses:* Tuition, state resident: full-time $9450. Tuition, nonresident: full-time $23,950. *Financial support:* In 2013–14, 23 fellowships with full tuition reimbursements (averaging $18,000 per year), 21 research assistantships with full tuition reimbursements (averaging $21,000 per year), 44 teaching assistantships with full tuition reimbursements (averaging $17,000 per year) were awarded; scholarships/grants, health care benefits, and unspecified assistantships also available. Financial award application deadline: 7/1; financial award applicants required to submit FAFSA. *Faculty research:* Molecular and cellular biology, developmental genetics, ecology, evolutionary biology, systematics. *Total annual research expenditures:* $2.9 million. *Unit head:* Dr. Patrica A. Sobecky, Chair, 205-348-1807, Fax: 205-348-1786, E-mail: psobecky@as.ua.edu. *Application contact:* Dr. Stevan Marcus, Graduate Program Director, 205-348-8094, Fax: 205-348-1786, E-mail: smarcus@as.ua.edu.
Website: http://bsc.ua.edu

The University of Alabama at Birmingham, College of Arts and Sciences, Program in Biology, Birmingham, AL 35294-1170. Offers MS, PhD. Terminal master's awarded for partial completion of doctoral program. *Degree requirements:* For master's, comprehensive exam (for some programs), thesis (for some programs); for doctorate, thesis/dissertation. *Entrance requirements:* For master's and doctorate, GRE General Test, previous course work in biology, calculus, organic chemistry, and physics; letters of recommendation. Additional exam requirements/recommendations for international students: Required—TOEFL, TWE. Electronic applications accepted.

The University of Alabama at Birmingham, Graduate Programs in Joint Health Sciences, Program in Basic Medical Sciences, Birmingham, AL 35294. Offers MSBMS. *Entrance requirements:* For master's, GRE. Electronic applications accepted.

The University of Alabama in Huntsville, School of Graduate Studies, College of Science, Department of Biological Sciences, Huntsville, AL 35899. Offers biology (MS); biotechnology science and engineering (PhD); education (MS). Part-time and evening/weekend programs available. *Faculty:* 11 full-time (1 woman). *Students:* 23 full-time (16 women), 14 part-time (10 women); includes 4 minority (1 Black or African American, non-Hispanic/Latino; 1 American Indian or Alaska Native, non-Hispanic/Latino; 1 Asian, non-Hispanic/Latino; 1 Two or more races, non-Hispanic/Latino), 6 international. Average age 30. 39 applicants, 44% accepted, 11 enrolled. In 2013, 9 master's awarded. *Degree requirements:* For master's, comprehensive exam, thesis or alternative, oral and written exams. *Entrance requirements:* For master's, GRE General Test, previous course work in biochemistry and organic chemistry, minimum GPA of 3.0. Additional exam requirements/recommendations for international students: Required—TOEFL (minimum score 550 paper-based; 80 iBT), IELTS (minimum score 6.5). *Application deadline:* For fall admission, 7/15 priority date for domestic students, 4/1 priority date for international students; for spring admission, 11/30 for domestic students, 9/1 priority date for international students. Applications are processed on a rolling basis. Application fee: $50. Electronic applications accepted. *Expenses:* Tuition, state resident: full-time $8912; part-time $540 per credit hour. Tuition, nonresident: full-time $20,774; part-time $1252 per credit hour. *Required fees:* $148 per semester. One-time fee: $150. *Financial support:* In 2013–14, 20 students received support, including 2 fellowships with full tuition reimbursements available (averaging $11,000 per year), 3 research assistantships (averaging $10,976 per year), 16 teaching assistantships with full and partial tuition reimbursements available (averaging $8,743 per year); career-related internships or fieldwork, Federal Work-Study, institutionally sponsored loans, scholarships/grants, health care benefits, tuition waivers (full and partial), and unspecified assistantships also available. Support available to part-time students. Financial award application deadline: 4/1; financial award applicants required to submit FAFSA. *Faculty research:* Physiology, microbiology, genomics and protemics, ecology and evolution, drug discovery. *Total annual research expenditures:* $1.1 million. *Unit head:* Dr. Debra M. Moriarity, Interim Chair, 256-824-6045, Fax: 256-824-6305, E-mail: moriard@uah.edu. *Application contact:* Kim Gray, Graduate Studies Admissions Manager, 256-824-6002, Fax: 256-824-6405, E-mail: deangrad@uah.edu.
Website: http://www.uah.edu/colleges/science/biology/

University of Alaska Anchorage, College of Arts and Sciences, Department of Biological Sciences, Anchorage, AK 99508. Offers MS. Part-time programs available. *Students:* 6 full-time (5 women), 20 part-time (17 women); includes 1 minority (American Indian or Alaska Native, non-Hispanic/Latino). *Degree requirements:* For master's, comprehensive exam, thesis. *Entrance requirements:* For master's, GRE General Test, GRE Subject Test, bachelor's degree in biology, chemistry or equivalent science. Additional exam requirements/recommendations for international students: Required—TOEFL (minimum score 550 paper-based). *Application deadline:* For fall admission, 7/1 priority date for domestic and international students; for spring admission, 11/1 priority date for domestic and international students. Applications are processed on a rolling basis. Application fee: $45. *Financial support:* Research assistantships, teaching assistantships, Federal Work-Study, scholarships/grants, traineeships, health care benefits, and unspecified assistantships available. Support available to part-time students. Financial award application deadline: 4/1; financial award applicants required to submit FAFSA. *Faculty research:* Taxonomy and vegetative analysis in Alaskan ecosystems, fish environment and seafood, biochemistry, arctic ecology, vertebrate ecology. *Unit head:* Fred Rainey, Director, 907-786-4987, E-mail: farainey@uaa.alaska.edu. *Application contact:* Dr. Jocelyn Krebs, Graduate Program Director, 907-786-1556, Fax: 907-786-1314, E-mail: jecrebs@uaa.alaska.edu.
Website: http://www.uaa.alaska.edu/biological-sciences/

University of Alaska Fairbanks, College of Natural Sciences and Mathematics, Department of Biology and Wildlife, Fairbanks, AK 99775-6100. Offers biological sciences (MS, PhD), including biology, botany, wildlife biology (PhD), zoology; biology (MAT, MS); wildlife biology (MS). Part-time programs available. *Faculty:* 21 full-time (9 women). *Students:* 73 full-time (39 women), 29 part-time (17 women); includes 7 minority (1 Asian, non-Hispanic/Latino; 4 Hispanic/Latino; 2 Two or more races, non-Hispanic/Latino), 5 international. Average age 31. 47 applicants, 21% accepted, 10 enrolled. In 2013, 12 master's, 8 doctorates awarded. *Degree requirements:* For master's, comprehensive exam, thesis, oral exam, oral defense; for doctorate, comprehensive exam, thesis/dissertation, oral exam, oral defense. *Entrance requirements:* For master's and doctorate, GRE General Test, GRE Subject Test (biology). Additional exam requirements/recommendations for international students: Required—TOEFL (minimum score 550 paper-based; 80 iBT), TWE. *Application deadline:* For fall admission, 6/1 for domestic students, 3/1 for international students; for spring admission, 10/15 for domestic students, 9/1 for international students. Applications are processed on a rolling basis. Application fee: $60. Electronic applications accepted. *Expenses:* Tuition, state resident: full-time $7254; part-time $403 per credit. Tuition, nonresident: full-time $14,814; part-time $823 per credit. Tuition and fees vary according to course level, course load and reciprocity agreements. *Financial support:* In 2013–14, 33 research assistantships with tuition reimbursements (averaging $15,138 per year), 21 teaching assistantships with tuition reimbursements (averaging $8,654 per year) were awarded; fellowships with tuition reimbursements, career-related internships or fieldwork, Federal Work-Study, scholarships/grants, health care benefits, and unspecified assistantships also available. Support available to part-time students. Financial award application deadline: 7/1; financial award applicants required to submit FAFSA. *Faculty research:* Plant-herbivore interactions, plant metabolic defenses, insect manufacture of glycerol, ice nucleators, structure and functions of arctic and subarctic freshwater ecosystems. *Unit head:* Diane Wagner, Department Chair, 907-474-7671, Fax: 907-474-6716, E-mail: uaf-bw-dept@alaska.edu. *Application contact:* Libby Eddy, Registrar and Director of Admissions, 907-474-7500, Fax: 907-474-7097, E-mail: admissions@uaf.edu.
Website: http://www.bw.uaf.edu

University of Alberta, Faculty of Graduate Studies and Research, Department of Biological Sciences, Edmonton, AB T6G 2E1, Canada. Offers environmental biology and ecology (M Sc, PhD); microbiology and biotechnology (M Sc, PhD); molecular biology and genetics (M Sc, PhD); physiology and cell biology (M Sc, PhD); plant biology (M Sc, PhD); systematics and evolution (M Sc, PhD). Terminal master's awarded for partial completion of doctoral program. *Degree requirements:* For master's, thesis; for doctorate, thesis/dissertation. *Entrance requirements:* Additional exam requirements/recommendations for international students: Required—TOEFL.

University of Alberta, Faculty of Medicine and Dentistry and Faculty of Graduate Studies and Research, Graduate Programs in Medicine, Edmonton, AB T6G 2E1, Canada. Offers M Sc, MD, PhD. Part-time programs available. *Degree requirements:* For doctorate, thesis/dissertation (for some programs). *Faculty research:* Basic, clinical, and applied biomedicine.

The University of Arizona, College of Science, Department of Molecular and Cellular Biology and Eller College of Management, Program in Applied Biosciences, Tucson, AZ 85721. Offers PSM. Part-time programs available. *Students:* 26 full-time (14 women), 10 part-time (5 women); includes 10 minority (2 Asian, non-Hispanic/Latino; 6 Hispanic/Latino; 2 Two or more races, non-Hispanic/Latino), 5 international. Average age 27. 34 applicants, 59% accepted, 14 enrolled. In 2013, 4 master's awarded. *Degree requirements:* For master's, thesis or alternative, internship, colloquium, business courses. *Entrance requirements:* For master's, 3 letters of recommendation. Additional exam requirements/recommendations for international students: Required—TOEFL (minimum score 600 paper-based; 90 iBT). *Application deadline:* For fall admission, 2/1 for domestic students, 12/1 for international students. Application fee: $75. Electronic applications accepted. *Expenses:* Tuition, state resident: full-time $11,526. Tuition, nonresident: full-time $27,398. *Financial support:* Career-related internships or fieldwork, Federal Work-Study, scholarships/grants, health care benefits, and unspecified assistantships available. *Faculty research:* Biotechnology, bioinformatics, pharmaceuticals, agriculture, oncology. *Unit head:* Dr. Kathleen Dixon, Department Head, 520-621-7563, Fax: 520-621-3709, E-mail: dixonk@email.arizona.edu. *Application contact:* Maryloo Myers, Graduate Coordinator, 520-621-4521, E-mail: myersm@email.arizona.edu.
Website: http://appliedbiosci.arizona.edu/

University of Arkansas, Graduate School, J. William Fulbright College of Arts and Sciences, Department of Biological Sciences, Fayetteville, AR 72701-1201. Offers MA, MS, PhD. *Degree requirements:* For doctorate, one foreign language, thesis/dissertation. *Entrance requirements:* For master's and doctorate, GRE Subject Test. Electronic applications accepted.

University of Arkansas at Little Rock, Graduate School, College of Science and Mathematics, Program in Biology, Little Rock, AR 72204-1099. Offers MS. *Expenses:* Tuition, state resident: full-time $5690; part-time $284.50 per credit hour. Tuition, nonresident: full-time $13,030; part-time $651.50 per credit hour. *Required fees:* $1121; $672 per term. One-time fee: $40 full-time.

University of Arkansas for Medical Sciences, Graduate School, Little Rock, AR 72205. Offers biochemistry and molecular biology (MS, PhD); bioinformatics (MS, PhD); cellular physiology and molecular biophysics (MS, PhD); clinical nutrition (MS); interdisciplinary biomedical sciences (MS, PhD, Certificate); interdisciplinary toxicology (MS); microbiology and immunology (PhD); neurobiology and developmental sciences (PhD); pharmacology (PhD); MD/PhD. Bioinformatics programs hosted jointly with the University of Arkansas at Little Rock. Part-time programs available. *Faculty:* 397 full-time (205 women). *Students:* 196 full-time (126 women), 117 part-time (87 women); includes 65 minority (38 Black or African American, non-Hispanic/Latino; 1 American Indian or Alaska Native, non-Hispanic/Latino; 21 Asian, non-Hispanic/Latino; 4 Hispanic/Latino; 1 Two or more races, non-Hispanic/Latino), 57 international. 455 applicants, 27% accepted, 89 enrolled. In 2013, 41 master's, 18 doctorates, 28 other advanced degrees awarded. Terminal master's awarded for partial completion of doctoral program. *Degree requirements:* For master's, comprehensive exam (for some programs), thesis (for some programs); for doctorate, thesis/dissertation. *Entrance requirements:* For master's and doctorate, GRE. Additional exam requirements/recommendations for international students: Required—TOEFL. *Application deadline:* Applications are processed on a rolling basis. Application fee: $0. Electronic applications accepted. *Expenses:* Contact institution. *Financial support:* In 2013–14, 120 research assistantships (averaging $24,000 per year) were awarded; career-related internships or fieldwork, Federal Work-Study, and traineeships also available. Support available to part-time students. Financial award applicants required to submit FAFSA. *Unit head:* Dr. Robert E. McGehee, Jr., Dean, 501-686-5454. *Application contact:* Dr. Kristen Sterba, Assistant Dean, Office of Graduate Student Recruiting and Retention, 501-526-7396, E-mail: kmsterba@uams.edu.
Website: http://www.uams.edu/gradschool/

University of Calgary, Cumming School of Medicine and Faculty of Graduate Studies, Medical Science Graduate Program, Calgary, AB T2N 1N4, Canada. Offers cancer biology (M Sc, PhD); critical care medicine (M Sc, PhD); joint injury and arthritis (M Sc, PhD); molecular and medical genetics (M Sc, PhD); mountain medicine and high altitude physiology (M Sc, PhD); pathologists' assistant (M Sc, PhD). *Degree requirements:* For master's, thesis; for doctorate, thesis/dissertation, candidacy exam. *Entrance requirements:* For master's, minimum undergraduate GPA of 3.2; for doctorate, minimum graduate GPA of 3.2. Additional exam requirements/recommendations for international students: Required—TOEFL (minimum score 600 paper-based). Electronic applications accepted. *Faculty research:* Cancer biology, immunology, joint injury and arthritis, medical education, population genomics.

University of Calgary, Faculty of Graduate Studies, Faculty of Science, Department of Biological Sciences, Calgary, AB T2N 1N4, Canada. Offers M Sc, PhD. Part-time programs available. *Degree requirements:* For master's, thesis; for doctorate, thesis/dissertation, candidacy exam. *Entrance requirements:* Additional exam requirements/recommendations for international students: Required—TOEFL. Electronic applications accepted. *Faculty research:* Biochemistry; cellular, molecular, and microbial biology; botany; ecology; zoology.

University of California, Berkeley, Graduate Division, College of Letters and Science, Department of Integrative Biology, Berkeley, CA 94720-1500. Offers PhD. *Degree requirements:* For doctorate, thesis/dissertation, oral qualifying exam. *Entrance requirements:* For doctorate, GRE General Test, GRE Subject Test, 3 letters of recommendation. Additional exam requirements/recommendations for international students: Required—TOEFL. *Faculty research:* Morphology, physiology, development of plants and animals, behavior, ecology.

University of California, Irvine, School of Biological Sciences, Irvine, CA 92697. Offers MS, PhD, MD/PhD. *Students:* 229 full-time (117 women), 3 part-time (1 woman); includes 92 minority (2 Black or African American, non-Hispanic/Latino; 45 Asian, non-Hispanic/Latino; 35 Hispanic/Latino; 2 Native Hawaiian or other Pacific Islander, non-Hispanic/Latino; 8 Two or more races, non-Hispanic/Latino), 20 international. Average age 27. 479 applicants, 24% accepted, 51 enrolled. In 2013, 26 master's, 40 doctorates awarded. *Degree requirements:* For doctorate, thesis/dissertation. *Entrance requirements:* For master's and doctorate, GRE General Test, GRE Subject Test, minimum GPA of 3.0. Additional exam requirements/recommendations for international students: Required—TOEFL (minimum score 550 paper-based). *Application deadline:* For fall admission, 12/15 for domestic and international students. Applications are processed on a rolling basis. Application fee: $80 ($100 for international students). Electronic applications accepted. *Financial support:* Fellowships with full tuition reimbursements, research assistantships with full tuition reimbursements, teaching assistantships with full tuition reimbursements, career-related internships or fieldwork, institutionally sponsored loans, scholarships/grants, traineeships, health care benefits, and unspecified assistantships available. Financial award application deadline: 3/1; financial award applicants required to submit FAFSA. *Faculty research:* Molecular biology and biochemistry, developmental and cell biology, physiology and biophysics, neurosciences, ecology and evolutionary biology. *Unit head:* Prof. Albert F. Bennett, Dean, 949-824-5315, Fax: 949-824-3035, E-mail: abennett@uci.edu. *Application contact:* Prof. Michael R. Mulligan, Associate Dean, 949-824-8433, Fax: 949-824-4709, E-mail: rmmullig@uci.edu.
Website: http://www.bio.uci.edu/

University of California, Los Angeles, David Geffen School of Medicine and Graduate Division, Graduate Programs in Medicine, Los Angeles, CA 90095. Offers MS, PhD, MD/PhD. Terminal master's awarded for partial completion of doctoral program. *Degree requirements:* For doctorate, thesis/dissertation, written and oral qualifying exams. Electronic applications accepted. *Expenses:* Contact institution.

University of California, Los Angeles, Graduate Division, College of Letters and Science, Department of Ecology and Evolutionary Biology, Los Angeles, CA 90095. Offers MA, PhD. Terminal master's awarded for partial completion of doctoral program. *Degree requirements:* For master's, comprehensive exam or thesis; for doctorate, thesis/dissertation, oral and written qualifying exams; 3 quarters of teaching experience. *Entrance requirements:* For master's and doctorate, GRE General Test, GRE Subject Test (biology), bachelor's degree; minimum undergraduate GPA of 3.0 (or its equivalent if letter grade system not used). Additional exam requirements/recommendations for international students: Required—TOEFL. Electronic applications accepted.

University of California, Merced, Graduate Division, School of Natural Sciences, Merced, CA 95343. Offers applied mathematics (MS, PhD); chemistry and chemical biology (MS, PhD); physics (MS, PhD); quantitative and systems biology (MS, PhD). *Students:* 133 full-time (52 women); includes 48 minority (3 Black or African American, non-Hispanic/Latino; 16 Asian, non-Hispanic/Latino; 22 Hispanic/Latino; 1 Native Hawaiian or other Pacific Islander, non-Hispanic/Latino; 6 Two or more races, non-Hispanic/Latino), 29 international. Average age 28. 143 applicants, 45% accepted, 33 enrolled. In 2013, 1 master's, 8 doctorates awarded. *Degree requirements:* For master's, variable foreign language requirement, comprehensive exam, thesis (for some programs); for doctorate, variable foreign language requirement, comprehensive exam, thesis/dissertation. *Entrance requirements:* For master's and doctorate, GRE. Additional exam requirements/recommendations for international students: Required—TOEFL (minimum score 550 paper-based; 68 iBT); Recommended—IELTS. *Expenses:* Tuition, state resident: full-time $6405. Tuition, nonresident: full-time $13,956. *Financial support:* In 2013–14, 30 fellowships with full and partial tuition reimbursements (averaging $8,646 per year) were awarded; scholarships/grants also available. *Unit head:* Dr. Juan Meza, Dean, 209-228-4487, Fax: 209-228-4060, E-mail: jcmeza@ucmerced.edu. *Application contact:* Carrie King, Graduate Admissions and Academic Services Manager, 209-228-4613, Fax: 209-228-6906, E-mail: cking7@ucmerced.edu.

University of California, Riverside, Graduate Division, Department of Biology, Riverside, CA 92521-0102. Offers evolution, ecology and organismal biology (MS, PhD). Terminal master's awarded for partial completion of doctoral program. *Degree requirements:* For master's, thesis, oral defense of thesis; for doctorate, thesis/dissertation, 3 quarters of teaching experience, qualifying exams. *Entrance requirements:* For master's and doctorate, GRE General Test, minimum GPA of 3.2. Additional exam requirements/recommendations for international students: Required—TOEFL (minimum score 550 paper-based, 80 iBT) or IELTS. Electronic applications accepted. *Faculty research:* Ecology, evolutionary biology, physiology, quantitative genetics, conservation biology.

University of California, Riverside, Graduate Division, Program in Biomedical Sciences, Riverside, CA 92521-0102. Offers PhD. *Faculty:* 41 full-time (14 women). *Students:* 15 full-time (6 women); includes 11 minority (1 Black or African American, non-Hispanic/Latino; 8 Asian, non-Hispanic/Latino; 2 Hispanic/Latino). Average age 31. 48 applicants, 25% accepted, 4 enrolled. In 2013, 3 doctorates awarded. *Degree requirements:* For doctorate, thesis/dissertation, qualifying exams. *Entrance requirements:* For doctorate, GRE General Test, minimum GPA of 3.2. Additional exam requirements/recommendations for international students: Required—TOEFL (minimum score 550 paper-based; 80 iBT). *Application deadline:* For fall admission, 12/15 priority date for domestic students, 5/1 for international students. Application fee: $80 ($100 for international students). Electronic applications accepted. *Financial support:* In 2013–14, fellowships with tuition reimbursements (averaging $12,000 per year), research assistantships with tuition reimbursements (averaging $18,000 per year), teaching assistantships with tuition reimbursements (averaging $16,500 per year) were awarded; scholarships/grants also available. Financial award application deadline: 2/1; financial award applicants required to submit FAFSA. *Faculty research:* Cancer cell biology; chronic inflammatory and autoimmune disease; cytokine, chemokine and endocrine biology in health and disease; microbiology, parasitology and vector borne diseases; neurodegeneration. *Unit head:* Dr. David Lo, Graduate Advisor and Program Director, 951-827-4553, E-mail: david.lo@ucr.edu. *Application contact:* John Herring, Student Affairs Officer, 951-827-2441, E-mail: john.herring@ucr.edu.
Website: http://medschool.ucr.edu/graduate/

University of California, San Diego, Office of Graduate Studies, Department of Physics, La Jolla, CA 92093. Offers biophysics (PhD); multi-scale biology (PhD); physics (PhD). *Students:* 180 full-time (20 women), 2 part-time (1 woman); includes 30 minority (4 Black or African American, non-Hispanic/Latino; 18 Asian, non-Hispanic/Latino; 8 Hispanic/Latino), 45 international. 526 applicants, 24% accepted, 32 enrolled. In 2013, 22 doctorates awarded. *Degree requirements:* For doctorate, comprehensive exam, thesis/dissertation, teaching assistantship. *Entrance requirements:* For doctorate, GRE General Test, GRE Subject Test. Additional exam requirements/recommendations for international students: Required—TOEFL, IELTS. *Application deadline:* For fall admission, 12/16 for domestic students. Application fee: $80 ($100 for international students). Electronic applications accepted. *Expenses:* Tuition, state resident: full-time $11,220; part-time $1870 per quarter. Tuition, nonresident: full-time $26,322; part-time $4387 per quarter. *Required fees:* $519.50 per quarter. Part-time tuition and fees vary according to course load and program. *Financial support:* Research assistantships, teaching assistantships, scholarships/grants, and unspecified assistantships available. Financial award applicants required to submit FAFSA. *Faculty research:* Astrophysics/astronomy, biophysics, condensed matter, elementary particles, plasma physics. *Unit head:* Dimitri Basov, Chair, 858-534-6832, E-mail: chair@physics.ucsd.edu. *Application contact:* Hilari Ford, Graduate Coordinator, 858-534-3293, E-mail: hford@ucsd.edu.
Website: http://physics.ucsd.edu/

University of California, San Diego, Office of Graduate Studies, Division of Biological Sciences, La Jolla, CA 92093. Offers anthropogeny (PhD); bioinformatics (PhD); biology (PhD); ecology, behavior and evolution (PhD); microbiology (PhD). *Students:* 285 full-time (154 women), 8 part-time (4 women); includes 70 minority (2 Black or African American, non-Hispanic/Latino; 3 American Indian or Alaska Native, non-Hispanic/Latino; 51 Asian, non-Hispanic/Latino; 13 Hispanic/Latino; 1 Native Hawaiian or other Pacific Islander, non-Hispanic/Latino), 30 international. 626 applicants, 24% accepted, 85 enrolled. In 2013, 32 doctorates awarded. *Degree requirements:* For doctorate, thesis/dissertation, 3 quarters of teaching assistantship. *Entrance requirements:* For doctorate, GRE General Test; GRE Subject Test (recommended). Additional exam requirements/recommendations for international students: Required—TOEFL, IELTS. *Application deadline:* For fall admission, 12/4 for domestic students. Application fee: $80 ($100 for international students). Electronic applications accepted. *Expenses:* Tuition, state resident: full-time $11,220; part-time $1870 per quarter. Tuition, nonresident: full-time $26,322; part-time $4387 per quarter. *Required fees:* $519.50 per quarter. Part-time tuition and fees vary according to course load and program. *Financial support:* Fellowships, research assistantships, teaching assistantships, and scholarships/grants available. Financial award applicants required to submit FAFSA. *Faculty research:* Ecology, behavior and evolution; microbiology; bioinformatics; multi-scale biology; anthropogeny. *Unit head:* William McGinnis, Dean, 858-822-0458, E-mail: wmcginnis@ucsd.edu. *Application contact:* Cathy Pugh, Graduate Coordinator, 858-534-0181, E-mail: gradprog@biology.ucsd.edu.
Website: http://biology.ucsd.edu/

University of California, San Diego, School of Medicine and Office of Graduate Studies, Graduate Studies in Biomedical Sciences, La Jolla, CA 92093. Offers anthropogeny (PhD); bioinformatics (PhD); multi-scale biology (PhD). *Students:* 178 full-time (95 women), 4 part-time (2 women); includes 76 minority (11 Black or African American, non-Hispanic/Latino; 45 Asian, non-Hispanic/Latino; 20 Hispanic/Latino), 4 international. 379 applicants, 21% accepted, 32 enrolled. In 2013, 30 doctorates awarded. *Degree requirements:* For doctorate, thesis/dissertation, 1-quarter teaching assistantship. *Entrance requirements:* For doctorate, GRE General Test; GRE Subject Test in either biology, biochemistry, cell and molecular biology or chemistry (recommended). Additional exam requirements/recommendations for international students: Required—TOEFL, IELTS. *Application deadline:* For fall admission, 12/2 for domestic students. Application fee: $80 ($100 for international students). Electronic applications accepted. *Expenses:* Tuition, state resident: full-time $11,220; part-time $1870 per quarter. Tuition, nonresident: full-time $26,322; part-time $4387 per quarter. *Required fees:* $519.50 per quarter. Part-time tuition and fees vary according to course load and program. *Financial support:* Fellowships, research assistantships, teaching assistantships, scholarships/grants, health care benefits, unspecified assistantships, and stipends available. Financial award applicants required to submit FAFSA. *Faculty research:* Genetics, microbiology and immunology, molecular cell biology, molecular pharmacology, molecular pathology. *Unit head:* Deborah Spector, Chair, 858-822-4003, E-mail: dspector@ucsd.edu. *Application contact:* Leanne Nordeman, Student Affairs Coordinator, 858-534-3982, E-mail: biomedsci@ucsd.edu.
Website: http://biomedsci.ucsd.edu

University of California, San Diego, School of Medicine, Medical Scientist Training Program, La Jolla, CA 92093. Offers MD/PhD. *Expenses:* Tuition, state resident: full-time $11,220; part-time $1870 per quarter. Tuition, nonresident: full-time $26,322; part-time $4387 per quarter. *Required fees:* $519.50 per quarter. Part-time tuition and fees vary according to course load and program.

University of California, San Francisco, Graduate Division, Biomedical Sciences Graduate Program, San Francisco, CA 94143. Offers PhD. *Degree requirements:* For doctorate, thesis/dissertation. *Entrance requirements:* For doctorate, GRE General Test, three letters of recommendation, official transcripts. Additional exam requirements/recommendations for international students: Required—TOEFL, IELTS. *Application deadline:* For fall admission, 12/1 for domestic students. Application fee: $80 ($100 for international students). *Expenses:* Tuition, state resident: full-time $11,220. Tuition, nonresident: full-time $26,322. *Required fees:* $5204. Full-time tuition and fees vary according to degree level and program. *Financial support:* Fellowships, research assistantships, and teaching assistantships available. Financial award application deadline: 1/10. *Faculty research:* Cancer biology and cell signaling, developmental and stem cell biology, human genetics, immunology, neurobiology, tissue/organ biology and endocrinology, vascular and cardiac biology, virology and microbial pathogenesis. *Unit head:* Jason Cyster, Co-Director, 415-502-6427, E-mail: jason.cyster@ucsf.edu. *Application contact:* Jason Cyster, Co-Director, 415-502-6427, E-mail: jason.cyster@ucsf.edu.
Website: http://bms.ucsf.edu/

University of California, San Francisco, School of Medicine, San Francisco, CA 94143-0410. Offers MD, PhD, MD/MPH, MD/MS, MD/PhD. *Accreditation:* LCME/AMA (one or more programs are accredited). *Faculty:* 2,031 full-time (678 women), 128 part-time/adjunct (41 women). *Students:* 632 full-time (341 women); includes 331 minority (44 Black or African American, non-Hispanic/Latino; 124 Asian, non-Hispanic/Latino; 100 Hispanic/Latino; 24 Native Hawaiian or other Pacific Islander, non-Hispanic/Latino; 39 Two or more races, non-Hispanic/Latino). Average age 24. 6,926 applicants, 4% accepted, 149 enrolled. In 2013, 163 doctorates awarded. *Entrance requirements:* For doctorate, MCAT (for MD), interview (for MD). *Application deadline:* For fall admission, 10/15 for domestic students. Applications are processed on a rolling basis. Application fee: $60 ($80 for international students). Electronic applications accepted. *Expenses:* Contact institution. *Financial support:* In 2013–14, 543 students received support. Federal Work-Study, institutionally sponsored loans, scholarships/grants, and tuition waivers (partial) available. Financial award application deadline: 2/1; financial award applicants required to submit FAFSA. *Faculty research:* Neurosciences, human genetics, developmental biology, social/behavioral/policy sciences, immunology. *Total annual research expenditures:* $414.4 million. *Unit head:* Dr. Sam Hawgood, Dean, 415-476-2342, Fax: 415-476-0689, E-mail: sam.hawgood@ucsf.edu. *Application contact:* Hallen Chung, Director of Admissions, 415-476-8090, Fax: 415-476-5490, E-mail: chungh@medsch.ucsf.edu.
Website: http://www.medschool.ucsf.edu/

University of Central Arkansas, Graduate School, College of Natural Sciences and Math, Department of Biological Science, Conway, AR 72035-0001. Offers MS. Part-time programs available. *Degree requirements:* For master's, comprehensive exam, thesis optional. *Entrance requirements:* For master's, GRE General Test, minimum GPA of 2.7. Additional exam requirements/recommendations for international students: Required—TOEFL (minimum score 550 paper-based; 80 iBT). Electronic applications accepted.

Biological and Biomedical Sciences—General

University of Central Florida, College of Medicine, Burnett School of Biomedical Sciences, Orlando, FL 32816. Offers biomedical sciences (MS, PhD); biotechnology (MS). *Students:* 86 full-time (44 women), 9 part-time (5 women); includes 22 minority (4 Black or African American, non-Hispanic/Latino; 1 American Indian or Alaska Native, non-Hispanic/Latino; 10 Asian, non-Hispanic/Latino; 7 Hispanic/Latino), 28 international. Average age 28. 132 applicants, 33% accepted, 27 enrolled. In 2013, 21 master's, 10 doctorates awarded. *Financial support:* In 2013–14, 73 students received support, including 20 fellowships (averaging $5,600 per year), 52 research assistantships (averaging $11,100 per year), 38 teaching assistantships (averaging $9,900 per year). *Unit head:* Dr. Richard Peppler, Interim Director, 407-226-1000, E-mail: pep@ucf.edu. *Application contact:* Barbara Rodriguez Lamas, Director, Admissions and Student Services, 407-823-2766, Fax: 407-823-6442, E-mail: gradadmissions@ucf.edu.
Website: http://www.biomed.ucf.edu/

University of Central Florida, College of Sciences, Department of Biology, Orlando, FL 32816. Offers biology (MS); conservation biology (MS, PhD, Certificate). Part-time and evening/weekend programs available. *Faculty:* 22 full-time (8 women), 11 part-time/adjunct (5 women). *Students:* 58 full-time (35 women), 14 part-time (10 women); includes 8 minority (2 Asian, non-Hispanic/Latino; 5 Hispanic/Latino; 1 Two or more races, non-Hispanic/Latino), 6 international. Average age 29. 81 applicants, 38% accepted, 16 enrolled. In 2013, 9 master's, 4 doctorates, 1 other advanced degree awarded. *Degree requirements:* For master's, comprehensive exam, thesis or alternative, field exam. *Entrance requirements:* For master's, GRE General Test, minimum GPA of 3.0 in last 60 hours. Additional exam requirements/recommendations for international students: Required—TOEFL. *Application deadline:* For fall admission, 3/1 priority date for domestic students; for spring admission, 10/15 for domestic students. Application fee: $30. Electronic applications accepted. *Financial support:* In 2013–14, 53 students received support, including 16 fellowships with partial tuition reimbursements available (averaging $3,500 per year), 15 research assistantships with partial tuition reimbursements available (averaging $7,400 per year), 43 teaching assistantships with partial tuition reimbursements available (averaging $11,800 per year); career-related internships or fieldwork, Federal Work-Study, institutionally sponsored loans, tuition waivers (partial), and unspecified assistantships also available. Financial award application deadline: 3/1; financial award applicants required to submit FAFSA. *Unit head:* Dr. Laurence von Kalm, Interim Chair, 407-823-6684, Fax: 407-823-5769, E-mail: lvonkalm@ucf.edu. *Application contact:* Barbara Rodriguez Lamas, Associate Director, Admissions and Student Services, 407-823-2766, Fax: 407-823-6442, E-mail: gradadmissions@ucf.edu.
Website: http://biology.cos.ucf.edu/

University of Central Missouri, The Graduate School, Warrensburg, MO 6409. Offers accountancy (MA); accounting (MBA); applied mathematics (MS); aviation safety (MA); biology (MS); business administration (MBA); career and technical education leadership (MS); college student personnel administration (MS); communication (MA); computer science (MS); counseling (MS); criminal justice (MS); educational leadership (Ed D); educational technology (MS); elementary and early childhood education (MSE); English (MA); environmental studies (MA); finance (MBA); history (MA); human services/educational technology (Ed S); human services/learning resources (Ed S); human services/professional counseling (Ed S); industrial hygiene (MS); industrial management (MS); information systems (MBA); information technology (MS); kinesiology (MS); library science and information services (MS); literacy education (MSE); marketing (MBA); mathematics (MS); music (MA); occupational safety management (MS); psychology (MS); rural family nursing (MS); school administration (MSE); social gerontology (MS); sociology (MA); special education (MSE); speech language pathology (MS); superintendency (Ed S); teaching (MAT); teaching English as a second language (MA); technology (MS); technology management (PhD); theatre (MA). Part-time programs available. *Faculty:* 233. *Students:* 890 full-time (396 women), 1,486 part-time (1,001 women); includes 192 minority (97 Black or African American, non-Hispanic/Latino; 9 American Indian or Alaska Native, non-Hispanic/Latino; 32 Asian, non-Hispanic/Latino; 40 Hispanic/Latino; 3 Native Hawaiian or other Pacific Islander, non-Hispanic/Latino; 11 Two or more races, non-Hispanic/Latino), 539 international. Average age 31. 1,953 applicants, 75% accepted. In 2013, 719 master's, 58 other advanced degrees awarded. *Degree requirements:* For master's and Ed S, comprehensive exam (for some programs), thesis (for some programs). *Entrance requirements:* Additional exam requirements/recommendations for international students: Required—TOEFL (minimum score 550 paper-based; 79 iBT). *Application deadline:* For fall admission, 6/1 for domestic students; for spring admission, 10/1 for domestic and international students. Applications are processed on a rolling basis. Application fee: $30 ($75 for international students). Electronic applications accepted. *Expenses:* Tuition, state resident: full-time $7326; part-time $276.25 per credit hour. Tuition, nonresident: full-time $13,956; part-time $552.50 per credit hour. *Required fees:* $29 per credit hour. *Financial support:* In 2013–14, 118 students received support, including 271 research assistantships with full and partial tuition reimbursements available (averaging $7,500 per year), 109 teaching assistantships with full and partial tuition reimbursements available (averaging $7,500 per year); career-related internships or fieldwork, Federal Work-Study, scholarships/grants, and administrative and laboratory assistantships also available. Support available to part-time students. Financial award application deadline: 3/1; financial award applicants required to submit FAFSA. *Unit head:* Dr. Joseph Vaughn, Assistant Provost for Research/Dean, 660-543-4092, Fax: 660-543-4778, E-mail: vaughn@ucmo.edu. *Application contact:* Brittany Lawrence, Graduate Student Services Coordinator, 660-543-4621, Fax: 660-543-4778, E-mail: gradinfo@ucmo.edu.
Website: http://www.ucmo.edu/graduate/

University of Central Oklahoma, The Jackson College of Graduate Studies, College of Mathematics and Science, Department of Biology, Edmond, OK 73034-5209. Offers MS. Part-time programs available. *Faculty:* 10 full-time (2 women), 3 part-time/adjunct (1 woman). *Students:* 5 full-time (2 women), 12 part-time (9 women); includes 2 minority (1 Black or African American, non-Hispanic/Latino; 1 Hispanic/Latino), 1 international. Average age 30. 8 applicants, 75% accepted, 1 enrolled. In 2013, 1 master's awarded. *Degree requirements:* For master's, thesis. *Entrance requirements:* For master's, GRE General Test, GRE Subject Test (biology), faculty commitment to mentor. Additional exam requirements/recommendations for international students: Required—TOEFL (minimum score 550 paper-based; 79 iBT), IELTS (minimum score 6.5). *Application deadline:* For fall admission, 7/1 for international students; for spring admission, 11/1 for international students. Applications are processed on a rolling basis. Application fee: $50. Electronic applications accepted. *Expenses:* Tuition, state resident: full-time $4137; part-time $206.85 per credit hour. Tuition, nonresident: full-time $10,359; part-time $517.95 per credit hour. *Required fees:* $481. Tuition and fees vary according to course load and program. *Financial support:* In 2013–14, 12 students received support, including 2 research assistantships with partial tuition reimbursements available (averaging $7,394 per year), 10 teaching assistantships with partial tuition reimbursements available (averaging $4,141 per year); Federal Work-Study, scholarships/grants, tuition waivers (partial), and unspecified assistantships also available. Financial award application deadline: 3/31; financial award applicants required to submit FAFSA. *Unit head:* Dr. Gloria Caddell, Chair, 405-974-5827, Fax: 405-974-3824, E-mail: gcaddell@uco.edu. *Application contact:* Dr. Richard Bernard, Dean, Graduate College, 405-974-3493, Fax: 405-974-3852, E-mail: gradcoll@uco.edu.
Website: http://www.biology.uco.edu/

University of Chicago, Division of Biological Sciences, The Interdisciplinary Scientist Training Program, Chicago, IL 60637-1513. Offers PhD. *Degree requirements:* For doctorate, thesis/dissertation, ethics class, 2 teaching assistantships. *Entrance requirements:* Additional exam requirements/recommendations for international students: Required—TOEFL (minimum score 600 paper-based; 104 iBT), IELTS (minimum score 7). Electronic applications accepted.

University of Cincinnati, Graduate School, College of Medicine, Biomedical Sciences Flex Option Program, Cincinnati, OH 45221. Offers PhD. *Degree requirements:* For doctorate, thesis/dissertation, qualifying exam. *Entrance requirements:* For doctorate, GRE, 2 letters of recommendation. Additional exam requirements/recommendations for international students: Required—TOEFL. Electronic applications accepted. *Faculty research:* Environmental health, developmental biology, cell and molecular biology, immunobiology, molecular genetics.

University of Cincinnati, Graduate School, College of Medicine, Graduate Programs in Biomedical Sciences, Cincinnati, OH 45221. Offers MS, PhD. Terminal master's awarded for partial completion of doctoral program. *Degree requirements:* For master's, thesis; for doctorate, thesis/dissertation, qualifying exam. *Entrance requirements:* For master's and doctorate, GRE General Test. Additional exam requirements/recommendations for international students: Required—TOEFL (minimum score 600 paper-based; 100 iBT). Electronic applications accepted. *Expenses:* Contact institution. *Faculty research:* Cancer, cardiovascular, metabolic disorders, neuroscience, computational medicine.

University of Cincinnati, Graduate School, College of Medicine, Physician Scientist Training Program, Cincinnati, OH 45221. Offers MD/PhD. *Entrance requirements:* Additional exam requirements/recommendations for international students: Required—TOEFL. Electronic applications accepted.

University of Cincinnati, Graduate School, McMicken College of Arts and Sciences, Department of Biological Sciences, Cincinnati, OH 45221-0006. Offers MS, PhD. Part-time programs available. Terminal master's awarded for partial completion of doctoral program. *Degree requirements:* For master's, thesis; for doctorate, comprehensive exam, thesis/dissertation. *Entrance requirements:* For master's and doctorate, GRE General Test, BS in biology, chemistry, or equivalent. Additional exam requirements/recommendations for international students: Required—TOEFL (minimum score 600 paper-based; 100 iBT). Electronic applications accepted. *Faculty research:* Physiology and development, cell and molecular, ecology and evolutionary.

University of Colorado Colorado Springs, College of Letters, Arts and Sciences, Master of Sciences Program, Colorado Springs, CO 80933-7150. Offers biology (M Sc); chemistry (M Sc); health promotion (M Sc); mathematics (M Sc); physics (M Sc); sports medicine (M Sc), including strength and conditioning; sports nutrition (M Sc). Part-time programs available. *Students:* 50 full-time (36 women), 35 part-time (23 women); includes 12 minority (1 Black or African American, non-Hispanic/Latino; 1 American Indian or Alaska Native, non-Hispanic/Latino; 3 Asian, non-Hispanic/Latino; 5 Hispanic/Latino; 2 Two or more races, non-Hispanic/Latino), 11 international. Average age 29. 122 applicants, 47% accepted, 36 enrolled. In 2013, 37 master's awarded. *Degree requirements:* For master's, thesis or alternative. *Entrance requirements:* For master's, minimum GPA of 2.75. Additional exam requirements/recommendations for international students: Required—TOEFL (minimum score 525 paper-based). *Application deadline:* For fall admission, 3/1 priority date for domestic students; for spring admission, 12/1 for domestic students. Applications are processed on a rolling basis. Application fee: $60 ($75 for international students). Electronic applications accepted. *Expenses:* Contact institution. *Financial support:* In 2013–14, 21 students received support, including 21 fellowships (averaging $2,600 per year); research assistantships, teaching assistantships, career-related internships or fieldwork, Federal Work-Study, and scholarships/grants also available. Support available to part-time students. Financial award application deadline: 3/1; financial award applicants required to submit FAFSA. *Faculty research:* Biomechanics and physiology of elite athletic training, genetic engineering in yeast and bacteria including phage display and DNA repair, immunology and cell biology, synthetic organic chemistry. *Total annual research expenditures:* $38,075. *Unit head:* Dr. Peter A. Braza, Dean, 719-255-4550, Fax: 719-255-4200, E-mail: pbraza@uccs.edu. *Application contact:* Taryn Bailey, Graduate Recruitment Specialist, 719-255-3702, Fax: 719-255-3037, E-mail: gradinfo@uccs.edu.

University of Colorado Denver, College of Liberal Arts and Sciences, Department of Integrative Biology, Denver, CO 80217. Offers animal behavior (MS); biology (MS); cell and developmental biology (MS); ecology (MS); evolutionary biology (MS); genetics (MS); integrative and systems biology (PhD); microbiology (MS); molecular biology (MS); neurobiology (MS); plant systematics (MS). Part-time programs available. *Faculty:* 21 full-time (7 women), 3 part-time/adjunct (2 women). *Students:* 18 full-time (11 women), 5 part-time (all women); includes 5 minority (1 Black or African American, non-Hispanic/Latino; 2 Hispanic/Latino; 2 Two or more races, non-Hispanic/Latino), 1 international. Average age 29. 25 applicants, 44% accepted, 11 enrolled. In 2013, 13 master's awarded. *Degree requirements:* For master's, comprehensive exam, thesis, 30-32 credit hours. *Entrance requirements:* For master's, GRE General Test (minimum score in 50th percentile in each section), BA/BS from accredited institution awarded within the last 10 years; minimum undergraduate GPA of 3.0; prerequisite courses: 1 year each of general biology and general chemistry; 1 semester each of general genetics, general ecology, and cell biology; and a structure/function course. Additional exam requirements/recommendations for international students: Required—TOEFL (minimum score 537 paper-based; 75 iBT); Recommended—IELTS (minimum score 6.5). *Application deadline:* For fall admission, 2/1 for domestic and international students. Application fee: $50 ($75 for international students). Electronic applications accepted. *Financial support:* In 2013–14, 8 students received support. Fellowships, research assistantships, teaching assistantships, Federal Work-Study, institutionally sponsored loans, scholarships/grants, and traineeships available. Financial award application deadline: 4/1; financial award applicants required to submit FAFSA. *Faculty research:* Molecular developmental biology; quantitative ecology, biogeography, and population dynamics; environmental signaling and endocrine disruption; speciation, the evolution of reproductive isolation, and hybrid zones; evolutionary, behavioral, and conservation ecology. *Unit head:* Dr. John Swallow, Biology Department Chair, 303-556-6154, E-mail: john.swallow@ucdenver.edu. *Application contact:* Timberley Roane, Associate Professor/Director of MS in Biology Program, 303-556-6592, E-mail: timberley.roane@ucdenver.edu.
Website: http://www.ucdenver.edu/academics/colleges/CLAS/Departments/biology/Programs/MasterofScience/Pages/BiologyMasterOfScience.aspx

University of Colorado Denver, School of Medicine, Biomedical Sciences Program, Aurora, CO 80045. Offers MS, PhD. *Students:* 27 full-time (17 women), 3 part-time (2 women); includes 7 minority (2 Black or African American, non-Hispanic/Latino; 2 Asian, non-Hispanic/Latino; 3 Hispanic/Latino), 2 international. Average age 27. 165 applicants, 10% accepted, 9 enrolled. In 2013, 9 master's awarded. Terminal master's awarded for partial completion of doctoral program. *Degree requirements:* For master's

and doctorate, comprehensive exam. *Entrance requirements:* For master's, GRE, three letters of recommendation; for doctorate, GRE, minimum undergraduate GPA of 3.0; prerequisite coursework in organic chemistry, biology, biochemistry, physics, and calculus; letters of recommendation; interview. Additional exam requirements/recommendations for international students: Required—TOEFL (minimum score 550 paper-based; 80 iBT). *Application deadline:* For fall admission, 12/1 for domestic students, 11/1 for international students. Application fee: $50 ($75 for international students). Electronic applications accepted. *Expenses:* Contact institution. *Financial support:* In 2013–14, 7 students received support. Fellowships, research assistantships, teaching assistantships, Federal Work-Study, institutionally sponsored loans, scholarships/grants, traineeships, health care benefits, tuition waivers (full), and unspecified assistantships available. Financial award applicants required to submit FAFSA. *Unit head:* Heide Ford, Director, 303-724-3509, E-mail: heide.ford@ucdenver.edu. *Application contact:* Elizabeth Bowen, Program Administrator, 303-724-3565, E-mail: elizabeth.bowen@ucdenver.edu.
Website: http://www.ucdenver.edu/academics/colleges/Graduate-School/academic-programs/Biomedical/Pages/Welcome.aspx

University of Connecticut, Graduate School, University of Connecticut Health Center, Field of Biomedical Science, Storrs, CT 06269. Offers PhD. *Degree requirements:* For doctorate, thesis/dissertation. *Entrance requirements:* For doctorate, GRE General Test, GRE Subject Test. Additional exam requirements/recommendations for international students: Required—TOEFL (minimum score 550 paper-based). Electronic applications accepted.

University of Connecticut Health Center, Graduate School and School of Medicine, Combined Degree Program in Biomedical Sciences, Farmington, CT 06030. Offers MD/PhD. *Entrance requirements:* Additional exam requirements/recommendations for international students: Required—TOEFL (minimum score 600 paper-based). *Expenses:* Contact institution.

University of Connecticut Health Center, Graduate School, Programs in Biomedical Sciences, Farmington, CT 06030. Offers PhD, DMD/PhD, MD/PhD. *Degree requirements:* For doctorate, comprehensive exam, thesis/dissertation. *Entrance requirements:* For doctorate, GRE General Test. Additional exam requirements/recommendations for international students: Required—TOEFL (minimum score 600 paper-based). Electronic applications accepted.

See Display below and Close-Up on page 125.

University of Connecticut Health Center, Graduate School, Programs in Biomedical Sciences - Integrated, Farmington, CT 06030. Offers PhD, DMD/PhD, MD/PhD. *Degree requirements:* For doctorate, comprehensive exam, thesis/dissertation. *Entrance requirements:* For doctorate, GRE General Test. Additional exam requirements/recommendations for international students: Required—TOEFL (minimum score 600 paper-based). Electronic applications accepted.

University of Dayton, Department of Biology, Dayton, OH 45469-1300. Offers MS, PhD. *Faculty:* 16 full-time (5 women). *Students:* 21 full-time (13 women), 8 international. Average age 26. 63 applicants, 8% accepted, 5 enrolled. In 2013, 4 master's, 4 doctorates awarded. Terminal master's awarded for partial completion of doctoral program. *Degree requirements:* For master's, comprehensive exam, thesis; for doctorate, comprehensive exam, thesis/dissertation. *Entrance requirements:* For master's and doctorate, GRE General Test, minimum undergraduate GPA of 3.0. Additional exam requirements/recommendations for international students: Required—TOEFL (minimum score 550 paper-based; 80 iBT). *Application deadline:* For fall admission, 3/1 priority date for domestic students, 5/1 priority date for international students; for winter admission, 10/15 priority date for domestic and international students; for spring admission, 11/1 priority date for international students. Applications are processed on a rolling basis. Application fee: $50 for international students. Electronic applications accepted. *Expenses: Tuition:* Full-time $10,296; part-time $858 per credit hour. *Required fees:* $50; $25. *Financial support:* In 2013–14, 5 research assistantships with full tuition reimbursements (averaging $18,760 per year), 12 teaching assistantships with full tuition reimbursements (averaging $18,760 per year) were awarded; institutionally sponsored loans, health care benefits, and unspecified assistantships also available. Financial award application deadline: 3/1; financial award applicants required to submit FAFSA. *Faculty research:* Tissue regeneration and developmental biology; cancer and stem cell biology; microbiology and immunology; molecular genetics, evolution and bioinformatics; environmental and restoration ecology. *Unit head:* Dr. Jayne B. Robinson, Chair, 937-229-2521, Fax: 937-229-2021. *Application contact:* Dr. Amit Singh, Director, Biology Graduate Programs, 937-229-2894, Fax: 937-229-2021, E-mail: asingh1@udayton.edu.
Website: http://www.udayton.edu/artssciences/biology/

University of Delaware, College of Arts and Sciences, Department of Biological Sciences, Newark, DE 19716. Offers biotechnology (MS); cancer biology (MS, PhD); cell and extracellular matrix biology (MS, PhD); cell and systems physiology (MS, PhD); developmental biology (MS, PhD); ecology and evolution (MS, PhD); microbiology (MS, PhD); molecular biology and genetics (MS, PhD). Terminal master's awarded for partial completion of doctoral program. *Degree requirements:* For master's, thesis, preliminary exam; for doctorate, comprehensive exam, thesis/dissertation, preliminary exam. *Entrance requirements:* For master's and doctorate, GRE General Test. Additional exam requirements/recommendations for international students: Required—TOEFL (minimum score 600 paper-based); Recommended—TWE. Electronic applications accepted. *Faculty research:* Microorganisms, bone, cancer metastasis, developmental biology, cell biology, DNA.

University of Denver, Division of Natural Sciences and Mathematics, Department of Biological Sciences, Denver, CO 80208-9010. Offers biomedical sciences (PSM); cell and molecular biology (MS, PhD); ecology and evolution (MS, PhD). Part-time programs available. *Faculty:* 23 full-time (8 women). *Students:* 1 (woman) full-time, 21 part-time (13 women); includes 3 minority (all Hispanic/Latino), 7 international. Average age 27. 50 applicants, 22% accepted, 10 enrolled. In 2013, 5 master's, 2 doctorates awarded. Terminal master's awarded for partial completion of doctoral program. *Degree requirements:* For master's, comprehensive exam (for some programs), thesis; for doctorate, one foreign language, comprehensive exam (for some programs), thesis/dissertation. *Entrance requirements:* For master's and doctorate, GRE General Test, bachelor's degree in biology or related field, transcripts, personal statement, three letters of recommendation. Additional exam requirements/recommendations for international students: Required—TOEFL (minimum score 570 paper-based; 88 iBT). *Application deadline:* For fall admission, 1/1 priority date for domestic and international students. Applications are processed on a rolling basis. Application fee: $60. Electronic applications accepted. *Financial support:* In 2013–14, 19 students received support, including 3 research assistantships with full and partial tuition reimbursements available (averaging $22,448 per year), 15 teaching assistantships with full and partial tuition reimbursements available (averaging $25,161 per year); Federal Work-Study, institutionally sponsored loans, scholarships/grants, and unspecified assistantships also available. Support available to part-time students. Financial award application deadline: 2/15; financial award applicants required to submit FAFSA. *Faculty research:* Molecular biology, cell biology, neurobiology, ecology, molecular evolution. *Unit head:* Dr. Joseph Angleson, Chair, 303-871-3463, Fax: 303-871-3471, E-mail: jangleso@du.edu. *Application contact:* Randi Flageolle, Assistant to the Chair, 303-871-3457, Fax: 303-871-3471, E-mail: rflageol@du.edu.
Website: http://www.du.edu/nsm/departments/biologicalsciences/index.html

Biological and Biomedical Sciences—General

University of Florida, College of Medicine and Graduate School, Interdisciplinary Program in Biomedical Sciences, Gainesville, FL 32610-0229. Offers MS, PhD, MD/PhD. *Degree requirements:* For doctorate, comprehensive exam, thesis/dissertation. *Entrance requirements:* For doctorate, GRE General Test, minimum GPA of 3.0, biochemistry before enrollment. Additional exam requirements/recommendations for international students: Required—TOEFL, IELTS. Electronic applications accepted. *Expenses:* Contact institution.

University of Georgia, Biomedical and Health Sciences Institute, Athens, GA 30602. Offers neuroscience (PhD). *Entrance requirements:* For doctorate, GRE, official transcripts, 3 letters of recommendation, statement of interest. Additional exam requirements/recommendations for international students: Required—TOEFL.

University of Guam, Office of Graduate Studies, College of Natural and Applied Sciences, Program in Biology, Mangilao, GU 96923. Offers tropical marine biology (MS). *Degree requirements:* For master's, comprehensive exam, thesis. *Entrance requirements:* For master's, GRE General Test, GRE Subject Test. Additional exam requirements/recommendations for international students: Required—TOEFL. *Faculty research:* Maintenance and ecology of coral reefs.

University of Guelph, Graduate Studies, College of Biological Science, Guelph, ON N1G 2W1, Canada. Offers M Sc, PhD. Part-time programs available. *Degree requirements:* For master's, thesis (for some programs); for doctorate, comprehensive exam (for some programs), thesis/dissertation. *Entrance requirements:* Additional exam requirements/recommendations for international students: Required—TOEFL (minimum score 550 paper-based). Electronic applications accepted.

University of Hartford, College of Arts and Sciences, Department of Biology, West Hartford, CT 06117-1599. Offers biology (MS); neuroscience (MS). Part-time and evening/weekend programs available. *Degree requirements:* For master's, comprehensive exam, thesis optional, oral exams. *Entrance requirements:* For master's, GRE or MCAT. Additional exam requirements/recommendations for international students: Required—TOEFL (minimum score 550 paper-based). Electronic applications accepted. *Faculty research:* Neurobiology of aging, central actions of neural steroids, neuroendocrine control of reproduction, retinopathies in sharks, plasticity in the central nervous system.

University of Hawaii at Manoa, John A. Burns School of Medicine and Graduate Division, Graduate Programs in Biomedical Sciences, Honolulu, HI 96822. Offers MS, PhD. Part-time programs available. Terminal master's awarded for partial completion of doctoral program. *Degree requirements:* For master's, thesis optional; for doctorate, comprehensive exam, thesis/dissertation. *Entrance requirements:* For master's and doctorate, GRE General Test. Additional exam requirements/recommendations for international students: Required—TOEFL (minimum score 500 paper-based; 61 iBT), IELTS (minimum score 5). *Expenses:* Contact institution.

University of Houston, College of Natural Sciences and Mathematics, Department of Biology and Biochemistry, Houston, TX 77204. Offers biochemistry (MA, PhD); biology (MA). Terminal master's awarded for partial completion of doctoral program. *Degree requirements:* For master's, comprehensive exam (for some programs), thesis optional; for doctorate, comprehensive exam (for some programs), thesis/dissertation. *Entrance requirements:* For master's and doctorate, GRE. Additional exam requirements/recommendations for international students: Required—TOEFL (minimum score 550 paper-based; 79 iBT), IELTS (minimum score 6.5). Electronic applications accepted. *Faculty research:* Cell and molecular biology, ecology and evolution, biochemical and biophysical sciences, chemical biology.

University of Houston–Clear Lake, School of Science and Computer Engineering, Program in Biological Sciences, Houston, TX 77058-1002. Offers MS. Part-time and evening/weekend programs available. *Entrance requirements:* For master's, GRE General Test. Additional exam requirements/recommendations for international students: Required—TOEFL (minimum score 550 paper-based).

University of Houston–Victoria, School of Arts and Sciences, Program in Biomedical Sciences, Victoria, TX 77901-4450. Offers biological sciences (MS); biomedical sciences (MS); forensic science (MS). *Expenses:* Tuition, state resident: full-time $4534; part-time $251 per credit hour. Tuition, nonresident: full-time $10,906; part-time $606 per contact hour. *Required fees:* $68 per semester hour. Tuition and fees vary according to course load. *Unit head:* Dr. Richard Gunasekera, Director, 361-570-4201, E-mail: gunasekerar@uhv.edu. *Application contact:* Tracey Fox, Director of Services, 361-570-4233, Fax: 361-580-5507, E-mail: foxt@uhv.edu.
Website: http://www.uhv.edu/asa/graduate/MSBiomedicalScience.aspx

University of Idaho, College of Graduate Studies, College of Science, Department of Biological Sciences, Moscow, ID 83844-3051. Offers biology (MS, PhD); microbiology, molecular biology and biochemistry (MS, PhD). *Faculty:* 12 full-time. *Students:* 20 full-time, 3 part-time. Average age 31. In 2013, 2 master's, 5 doctorates awarded. *Degree requirements:* For doctorate, one foreign language, thesis/dissertation. *Entrance requirements:* For master's, GRE, minimum GPA of 2.8; for doctorate, GRE, minimum undergraduate GPA of 2.8, 3.0 graduate. Additional exam requirements/recommendations for international students: Required—TOEFL. *Application deadline:* For fall admission, 8/1 for domestic students; for spring admission, 12/15 for domestic students. Applications are processed on a rolling basis. Application fee: $60. Electronic applications accepted. *Expenses:* Tuition, state resident: full-time $5596; part-time $363 per credit hour. Tuition, nonresident: full-time $18,672; part-time $1089 per credit hour. *Financial support:* Research assistantships and teaching assistantships available. Financial award applicants required to submit FAFSA. *Faculty research:* Animal behavior development, germ cell development, evolutionary biology, fish reproductive biology, molecular mechanisms. *Unit head:* Dr. James J. Nagler, Interim Department Chair, 208-885-6280, E-mail: biosci@uidaho.edu. *Application contact:* Stephanie Thomas, Graduate Recruitment Coordinator, 208-885-4001, Fax: 208-885-4406, E-mail: gadms@uidaho.edu.
Website: http://www.uidaho.edu/sci/biology

University of Illinois at Chicago, College of Medicine and Graduate College, Graduate Programs in Medicine, Chicago, IL 60607-7128. Offers MHPE, MS, PhD, MD/MS, MD/PhD. Part-time programs available. *Students:* 133 full-time (72 women), 109 part-time (71 women); includes 41 minority (10 Black or African American, non-Hispanic/Latino; 16 Asian, non-Hispanic/Latino; 11 Hispanic/Latino; 4 Two or more races, non-Hispanic/Latino), 69 international. Average age 34. 523 applicants, 21% accepted, 64 enrolled. In 2013, 40 master's, 41 doctorates awarded. Terminal master's awarded for partial completion of doctoral program. *Degree requirements:* For master's, thesis; for doctorate, thesis/dissertation. *Entrance requirements:* For master's and doctorate, GRE General Test. *Application deadline:* For fall admission, 3/1 priority date for domestic students, 2/15 for international students. *Expenses:* Contact institution. *Financial support:* In 2013–14, 14 fellowships with full tuition reimbursements were awarded; research assistantships with full tuition reimbursements, teaching assistantships with full tuition reimbursements, career-related internships or fieldwork, Federal Work-Study, institutionally sponsored loans, scholarships/grants, traineeships, tuition waivers (full), and unspecified assistantships also available. Financial award application deadline: 3/1; financial award applicants required to submit FAFSA. *Unit head:* Dr. Dimitri T. Azar, Head, 312-996-3500, Fax: 312-996-9006, E-mail: dtazar@uic.edu. *Application contact:* Jackie Perry, Graduate College Receptionist, 312-413-2550, Fax: 312-413-0185, E-mail: gradcoll@uic.edu.
Website: http://www.medicine.uic.edu/

University of Illinois at Chicago, Graduate College, College of Liberal Arts and Sciences, Department of Biological Sciences, Chicago, IL 60607-7128. Offers MS, PhD. *Faculty:* 39 full-time (17 women), 3 part-time/adjunct (1 woman). *Students:* 100 full-time (67 women), 5 part-time (4 women); includes 20 minority (4 Black or African American, non-Hispanic/Latino; 5 Asian, non-Hispanic/Latino; 10 Hispanic/Latino; 1 Two or more races, non-Hispanic/Latino), 23 international. Average age 29. 152 applicants, 21% accepted, 15 enrolled. In 2013, 7 master's, 18 doctorates awarded. *Degree requirements:* For master's, thesis; for doctorate, thesis/dissertation, preliminary exam. *Entrance requirements:* For master's and doctorate, GRE General Test, GRE Subject Test, previous course work in physics, calculus, and organic chemistry; minimum GPA of 2.75. Additional exam requirements/recommendations for international students: Required—TOEFL. *Application deadline:* For fall admission, 1/1 for domestic and international students. Applications are processed on a rolling basis. Application fee: $40 ($50 for international students). Electronic applications accepted. *Expenses:* Tuition, state resident: full-time $11,066; part-time $3689 per term. Tuition, nonresident: full-time $23,064; part-time $7688 per term. *Required fees:* $3004; $1190 per term. Tuition and fees vary according to course level and program. *Financial support:* In 2013–14, 1 fellowship with full tuition reimbursement was awarded; research assistantships with full tuition reimbursements, teaching assistantships with full tuition reimbursements, career-related internships or fieldwork, Federal Work-Study, scholarships/grants, traineeships, tuition waivers (full), and unspecified assistantships also available. Financial award application deadline: 3/1; financial award applicants required to submit FAFSA. *Faculty research:* Classical and molecular genetic analysis, modulation of synaptic transmission, molecular ecology, landscape genetics, conservation biology, ecophysiology, plant nutrition and global climate change, predator-prey interactions and urban wildlife, genetic studies of Drosophila, glutamate signaling in Drosophila, molecular mechanisms of exocytosis and endocytosis, global change biology, plant and ecosystem physiology, isotope ecology, respiration, community. *Total annual research expenditures:* $4.4 million. *Unit head:* Prof. Brian K. Kay, Head, 312-996-4249, E-mail: bkay@uic.edu. *Application contact:* Prof. Aixa Alfonso, Director of Graduate Studies, 312-355-0318, E-mail: aalfonso@uic.edu.
Website: http://www.uic.edu/depts/bios/

University of Illinois at Springfield, Graduate Programs, College of Liberal Arts and Sciences, Program in Biology, Springfield, IL 62703-5407. Offers MS. Part-time and evening/weekend programs available. *Faculty:* 2 full-time (0 women). *Students:* 9 full-time (7 women), 12 part-time (5 women); includes 1 minority (Black or African American, non-Hispanic/Latino), 1 international. Average age 26. 34 applicants, 26% accepted, 7 enrolled. In 2013, 11 master's awarded. *Degree requirements:* For master's, project or thesis. *Entrance requirements:* For master's, GRE General Test, GRE Subject Test (biology), minimum undergraduate GPA of 3.0, 3 letters of reference. Additional exam requirements/recommendations for international students: Required—TOEFL (minimum score 500 paper-based; 61 iBT). *Application deadline:* Applications are processed on a rolling basis. Application fee: $60 ($75 for international students). Electronic applications accepted. *Expenses:* Tuition, state resident: full-time $7440. Tuition, nonresident: full-time $15,744. *Required fees:* $2985.60. *Financial support:* In 2013–14, fellowships with full tuition reimbursements (averaging $9,900 per year), research assistantships with full tuition reimbursements (averaging $9,550 per year), teaching assistantships with full tuition reimbursements (averaging $9,700 per year) were awarded; career-related internships or fieldwork, Federal Work-Study, scholarships/grants, health care benefits, and unspecified assistantships also available. Support available to part-time students. Financial award application deadline: 11/15; financial award applicants required to submit FAFSA. *Unit head:* Dr. Amy B. McEuen, Acting Program Administrator, 217-206-7341, Fax: 217-206-6217, E-mail: mceuen.amy@uis.edu. *Application contact:* Dr. Lynn Pardie, Office of Graduate Studies, 800-252-8533, Fax: 217-206-7623, E-mail: lpard1@uis.edu.
Website: http://www.uis.edu/biology

University of Illinois at Urbana–Champaign, Graduate College, College of Liberal Arts and Sciences, School of Chemical Sciences, Champaign, IL 61820. Offers MA, MS, PhD, MS/JD, MS/MBA. *Students:* 403 (147 women). Application fee: $75 ($90 for international students). *Expenses:* Contact institution. *Unit head:* Jonathan Sweedler, Director, 217-333-5070, Fax: 217-333-2685, E-mail: jsweedle@illinois.edu. *Application contact:* Cheryl Kappes, Office Manager, 217-333-5070, Fax: 217-333-3120, E-mail: dambache@illinois.edu.
Website: http://www.scs.illinois.edu/

University of Illinois at Urbana–Champaign, Graduate College, College of Liberal Arts and Sciences, School of Integrative Biology, Champaign, IL 61820. Offers MS, MST, PSM, PhD. Part-time programs available. Postbaccalaureate distance learning degree programs offered (no on-campus study). *Students:* 156 (75 women). Application fee: $75 ($90 for international students). *Unit head:* Evan De Lucia, Director, 217-333-6177, Fax: 217-244-1224, E-mail: delucia@illinois.edu. *Application contact:* Kimberly Leigh, Office Manager, 217-333-2910, Fax: 217-244-1224, E-mail: kaleigh@illinois.edu.
Website: http://sib.illinois.edu/

University of Indianapolis, Graduate Programs, College of Arts and Sciences, Department of Biology, Indianapolis, IN 46227-3697. Offers human biology (MS). Part-time and evening/weekend programs available. *Faculty:* 3 full-time (0 women), 1 (woman) part-time/adjunct. *Students:* 10 full-time (8 women), 7 part-time (all women); includes 1 minority (Asian, non-Hispanic/Latino). Average age 27. In 2013, 3 master's awarded. *Degree requirements:* For master's, thesis. *Entrance requirements:* For master's, GRE General Test, 3 letters of recommendation; minimum GPA of 3.0; BA/BS in anthropology, biology, human biology or closely-related field, resume. Additional exam requirements/recommendations for international students: Required—TOEFL (minimum score 550 paper-based). *Application deadline:* For fall admission, 1/15 for domestic and international students. Applications are processed on a rolling basis. Application fee: $30. *Expenses: Tuition:* Full-time $5436; part-time $810 per credit hour. *Financial support:* Federal Work-Study, scholarships/grants, and tuition waivers (full and partial) available. Support available to part-time students. Financial award application deadline: 5/1; financial award applicants required to submit FAFSA. *Unit head:* Dr. L. Mark Harrison, Chairperson, 317-788-3264, E-mail: harrison@uindy.edu. *Application contact:* Dr. Stephen P. Nawrocki, Director, Graduate Program in Human Biology, 317-788-3486, Fax: 317-788-3480, E-mail: snawrocki@uindy.edu.
Website: http://biology.uindy.edu/mshumanbio/

The University of Iowa, Graduate College, College of Liberal Arts and Sciences, Department of Biology, Iowa City, IA 52242-1324. Offers biology (MS, PhD); cell and developmental biology (MS, PhD); evolution (MS, PhD); genetics (MS, PhD); neurobiology (MS, PhD). Terminal master's awarded for partial completion of doctoral program. *Degree requirements:* For master's, thesis optional, exam; for doctorate, comprehensive exam, thesis/dissertation. *Entrance requirements:* For master's and doctorate, GRE General Test, minimum GPA of 3.0. Additional exam requirements/recommendations for international students: Required—TOEFL (minimum score 600 paper-based; 100 iBT). Electronic applications accepted. *Faculty research:* Neurobiology, evolutionary biology, genetics, cell and developmental biology.

The University of Iowa, Roy J. and Lucille A. Carver College of Medicine and Graduate College, Biosciences Program, Iowa City, IA 52242-1316. Offers anatomy and cell biology (PhD); biochemistry (PhD); biology (PhD); biomedical engineering (PhD); chemistry (PhD); free radical and radiation biology (PhD); genetics (PhD); human toxicology (PhD); immunology (PhD); microbiology (PhD); molecular and cellular biology (PhD); molecular physiology and biophysics (PhD); neuroscience (PhD); pharmacology (PhD); physical therapy and rehabilitation science (PhD); rehabilitation science (PhD); speech and hearing (PhD). *Faculty:* 332 full-time. *Students:* 8 full-time (3 women); includes 2 minority (1 Black or African American, non-Hispanic/Latino; 1 Asian, non-Hispanic/Latino), 1 international. 200 applicants. *Degree requirements:* For doctorate, thesis/dissertation. *Entrance requirements:* For doctorate, GRE General Test, minimum GPA of 3.0. Additional exam requirements/recommendations for international students: Required—TOEFL (minimum score 600 paper-based; 100 iBT). *Application deadline:* For fall admission, 1/1 priority date for domestic and international students. Applications are processed on a rolling basis. Application fee: $60 ($100 for international students). Electronic applications accepted. *Expenses:* Contact institution. *Financial support:* In 2013–14, 8 students received support, including 8 research assistantships with full tuition reimbursements available (averaging $26,000 per year); fellowships, teaching assistantships, health care benefits, and unspecified assistantships also available. *Unit head:* Dr. Douglas Spitz, Director, 319-335-8001, E-mail: douglas-spitz@uiowa.edu. *Application contact:* Jodi Graff, Director, Admissions and First-Year Experience, 319-335-8306, E-mail: biosciences-admissions@uiowa.edu.
Website: http://www.medicine.uiowa.edu/biosciences/

The University of Iowa, Roy J. and Lucille A. Carver College of Medicine and Graduate College, Graduate Programs in Medicine, Iowa City, IA 52242-1316. Offers MA, MPAS, MS, DPT, PhD, JD/MHA, MBA/MHA, MD/JD, MD/PhD, MHA/MA, MHA/MS, MPH/MHA, MS/MA, MS/MS. Part-time programs available. *Faculty:* 137 full-time (31 women), 115 part-time/adjunct (51 women). *Students:* 297 full-time (160 women), 4 part-time (1 woman); includes 40 minority (7 Black or African American, non-Hispanic/Latino; 1 American Indian or Alaska Native, non-Hispanic/Latino; 25 Asian, non-Hispanic/Latino; 5 Hispanic/Latino; 1 Native Hawaiian or other Pacific Islander, non-Hispanic/Latino; 1 Two or more races, non-Hispanic/Latino), 19 international. 1,366 applicants, 7% accepted, 80 enrolled. In 2013, 32 master's, 29 doctorates awarded. *Degree requirements:* For doctorate, thesis/dissertation. Electronic applications accepted. *Expenses:* Contact institution. *Financial support:* In 2013–14, 156 students received support, including fellowships (averaging $26,000 per year), research assistantships (averaging $26,000 per year), teaching assistantships (averaging $26,000 per year); career-related internships or fieldwork, Federal Work-Study, institutionally sponsored loans, health care benefits, and tuition waivers (full and partial) also available. Support available to part-time students. Financial award applicants required to submit FAFSA. *Unit head:* Dr. Debra A. Schwinn, Dean, 319-384-4590, Fax: 319-335-8318, E-mail: debra-schwinn@uiowa.edu. *Application contact:* Betty Wood, Associate Director of Admissions, 319-335-1525, Fax: 319-335-1535, E-mail: admissions@uiowa.edu.

The University of Iowa, Roy J. and Lucille A. Carver College of Medicine and Graduate College, Medical Scientist Training Program, Iowa City, IA 52242-1316. Offers MD/PhD. *Faculty:* 155 full-time (36 women), 2 part-time/adjunct (0 women). *Students:* 72 full-time (26 women); includes 25 minority (1 Black or African American, non-Hispanic/Latino; 2 American Indian or Alaska Native, non-Hispanic/Latino; 15 Asian, non-Hispanic/Latino; 6 Hispanic/Latino; 1 Native Hawaiian or other Pacific Islander, non-Hispanic/Latino). Average age 24. 200 applicants, 16% accepted, 13 enrolled. *Application deadline:* For fall admission, 12/15 priority date for domestic students. Applications are processed on a rolling basis. Electronic applications accepted. Application fee is waived when completed online. *Financial support:* In 2013–14, 43 students received support, including 12 fellowships with full tuition reimbursements available (averaging $22,032 per year), 43 research assistantships with full tuition reimbursements available (averaging $3,468 per year); scholarships/grants, traineeships, health care benefits, unspecified assistantships, and travel awards also available. *Faculty research:* Structure and function of ion channels, molecular genetics of human disease, neurobiology of pain, viral immunology and immunopathology, epidemiology of aging and cancer, human learning and memory, structural enzymology. *Total annual research expenditures:* $2 million. *Unit head:* Dr. Steven R. Lentz, Director, 319-356-4048, Fax: 319-335-6634, E-mail: steven-lentz@uiowa.edu. *Application contact:* Leslie Harrington, Administrative Director, 319-335-8304, Fax: 319-335-6634, E-mail: mstp@uiowa.edu.
Website: http://www.medicine.uiowa.edu/mstp

The University of Kansas, University of Kansas Medical Center, School of Medicine, Interdisciplinary Graduate Program in Biomedical Sciences (IGPBS), Kansas City, KS 66160. Offers MA, MPH, MS, PhD, MD/MPH, MD/MS, MD/PhD. *Students:* 19 full-time (9 women); includes 1 minority (Hispanic/Latino), 10 international. Average age 26. 135 applicants, 24% accepted, 16 enrolled. Terminal master's awarded for partial completion of doctoral program. *Degree requirements:* For master's, thesis; for doctorate, comprehensive exam, thesis/dissertation. *Entrance requirements:* For master's and doctorate, GRE. Additional exam requirements/recommendations for international students: Required—TOEFL. *Application deadline:* For fall admission, 1/5 priority date for domestic and international students. Applications are processed on a rolling basis. Application fee: $60. Electronic applications accepted. *Financial support:* In 2013–14, 3 research assistantships with full tuition reimbursements, 18 teaching assistantships with full tuition reimbursements were awarded; scholarships/grants and unspecified assistantships also available. Financial award application deadline: 3/1; financial award applicants required to submit FAFSA. *Faculty research:* Cardiovascular biology, neurosciences, signal transduction and cancer biology, molecular biology and genetics, developmental biology. *Unit head:* Dr. Michael J. Werle, Director, 913-588-7491, Fax: 913-588-2710, E-mail: mwerle@kumc.edu. *Application contact:* Miranda Olenhouse, Coordinator, 913-588-2719, Fax: 913-588-2711, E-mail: molenhouse@kumc.edu.
Website: http://www.kumc.edu/igpbs.html

See Display below and Close-Up on page 127.

University of Kentucky, Graduate School, College of Arts and Sciences, Program in Biology, Lexington, KY 40506-0032. Offers MS, PhD. *Degree requirements:* For master's, comprehensive exam, thesis optional; for doctorate, comprehensive exam, thesis/dissertation. *Entrance requirements:* For master's, GRE General Test, minimum undergraduate GPA of 2.75; for doctorate, GRE General Test, minimum graduate GPA of 3.0. Additional exam requirements/recommendations for international students: Required—TOEFL (minimum score 550 paper-based). Electronic applications accepted. *Faculty research:* General biology, microbiology, &ITDrosophila&RO molecular genetics, molecular virology, multiple loci inheritance.

University of Kentucky, Graduate School, Graduate School Programs from the College of Medicine, Lexington, KY 40506-0032. Offers MS, PhD, MD/PhD. *Degree requirements:* For master's, comprehensive exam, thesis (for some programs); for doctorate, comprehensive exam, thesis/dissertation. *Entrance requirements:* For master's, GRE General Test, minimum undergraduate GPA of 2.75; for doctorate, GRE General Test, minimum undergraduate GPA of 3.0. Additional exam requirements/recommendations for international students: Required—TOEFL (minimum score 550 paper-based). Electronic applications accepted.

University of Lethbridge, School of Graduate Studies, Lethbridge, AB T1K 3M4, Canada. Offers accounting (MScM); addictions counseling (M Sc); agricultural biotechnology (M Sc); agricultural studies (M Sc, MA); anthropology (MA); archaeology

(M Sc, MA); art (MA, MFA); biochemistry (M Sc); biological sciences (M Sc); biomolecular science (PhD); biosystems and biodiversity (PhD); Canadian studies (MA); chemistry (M Sc); computer science (M Sc); computer science and geographical information science (M Sc); counseling (MC); counseling psychology (M Ed); dramatic arts (MA); earth, space, and physical science (PhD); economics (MA); education (MA); educational leadership (M Ed); English (MA); environmental science (M Sc); evolution and behavior (PhD); exercise science (M Sc); finance (MScM); French (MA); French/German (MA); French/Spanish (MA); general education (M Ed); general management (MScM); geography (M Sc, MA); German (MA); health sciences (M Sc); human resource management and labour relations (MScM); individualized multidisciplinary (M Sc, MA); information systems (MScM); international management (MScM); kinesiology (M Sc, MA); marketing (MScM); mathematics (M Sc); modern languages (MA); music (M Mus, MA); Native American studies (MA); neuroscience (M Sc, PhD); new media (MA, MFA); nursing (M Sc); philosophy (MA); physics (M Sc); policy and strategy (MScM); political science (MA); psychology (M Sc, MA); religious studies (MA); sociology (MA); theatre and dramatic arts (MFA); theoretical and computational science (PhD); urban and regional studies (MA); women and gender studies (MA). Part-time and evening/weekend programs available. *Degree requirements:* For doctorate, comprehensive exam, thesis/dissertation. *Entrance requirements:* For master's, GMAT (for M Sc in management), bachelor's degree in related field, minimum GPA of 3.0 during previous 20 graded semester courses, 2 years teaching or related experience (M Ed); for doctorate, master's degree, minimum graduate GPA of 3.5. Additional exam requirements/recommendations for international students: Required—TOEFL. Application fee: $60 Canadian dollars. *Financial support:* Fellowships, research assistantships, teaching assistantships, scholarships/grants, health care benefits, and unspecified assistantships available. *Faculty research:* Movement and brain plasticity, gibberellin physiology, photosynthesis, carbon cycling, molecular properties of main-group ring components. *Application contact:* School of Graduate Studies, 403-329-2793, Fax: 403-332-5239, E-mail: sgsinquiries@uleth.ca.
Website: http://www.uleth.ca/graduatestudies/

University of Louisiana at Lafayette, College of Sciences, Department of Biology, Lafayette, LA 70504. Offers biology (MS); environmental and evolutionary biology (PhD). Terminal master's awarded for partial completion of doctoral program. *Degree requirements:* For master's, thesis; for doctorate, 2 foreign languages, comprehensive exam, thesis/dissertation. *Entrance requirements:* For master's, GRE General Test, minimum GPA of 2.75; for doctorate, GRE General Test, GRE Subject Test, minimum GPA of 3.0. Additional exam requirements/recommendations for international students: Required—TOEFL (minimum score 550 paper-based). Electronic applications accepted. *Faculty research:* Structure and ultrastructure, system biology, ecology, processes, environmental physiology.

University of Louisiana at Monroe, Graduate School, College of Arts, Education, and Sciences, Department of Biology, Monroe, LA 71209-0001. Offers MS. *Entrance requirements:* For master's, GRE General Test, minimum GPA of 2.5. Additional exam requirements/recommendations for international students: Required—TOEFL (minimum score 500 paper-based; 61 iBT); Recommended—IELTS (minimum score 5.5). *Application deadline:* For fall admission, 8/24 priority date for domestic students, 3/1 for international students; for winter admission, 12/14 priority date for domestic students, 4/1 for international students; for spring admission, 1/19 for domestic students, 8/1 for international students. Applications are processed on a rolling basis. Application fee: $20 ($30 for international students). Electronic applications accepted. *Expenses:* Tuition, state resident: full-time $6607. Tuition, nonresident: full-time $17,179. Full-time tuition and fees vary according to program. *Financial support:* Teaching assistantships, career-related internships or fieldwork, Federal Work-Study, and unspecified assistantships available. Financial award application deadline: 4/1; financial award applicants required to submit FAFSA. *Faculty research:* Fish systematics and zoogeography, taxonomy and distribution of Louisiana plants, aquatic biology, secondary succession, microbial ecology. *Unit head:* Dr. Sushma Krishnamurthy, Head, 318-342-1813, Fax: 318-342-1790, E-mail: krishnamurthy@ulm.edu. *Application contact:* Dr. Kim Marie Tolson, Graduate Coordinator, 318-342-1805, Fax: 318-342-1790, E-mail: tolson@ulm.edu.
Website: http://www.ulm.edu/biology/

University of Louisville, Graduate School, College of Arts and Sciences, Department of Biology, Louisville, KY 40292-0001. Offers biology (MS); environmental biology (PhD). *Students:* 48 full-time (24 women), 5 part-time (2 women); includes 4 minority (2 Black or African American, non-Hispanic/Latino; 1 Asian, non-Hispanic/Latino; 1 Two or more races, non-Hispanic/Latino), 9 international. Average age 30. 43 applicants, 60% accepted, 15 enrolled. In 2013, 2 master's awarded. *Degree requirements:* For master's, thesis (for some programs); for doctorate, thesis/dissertation. *Entrance requirements:* For master's and doctorate, GRE General Test. Additional exam requirements/recommendations for international students: Required—TOEFL (minimum score 550 paper-based; 79 iBT). *Application deadline:* For fall admission, 5/1 priority date for international students; for spring admission, 11/1 priority date for international students; for summer admission, 4/1 priority date for international students. Applications are processed on a rolling basis. Application fee: $60. Electronic applications accepted. *Expenses:* Tuition, state resident: full-time $10,788; part-time $599 per credit hour. Tuition, nonresident: full-time $22,446; part-time $1247 per credit hour. *Required fees:* $196. Tuition and fees vary according to program and reciprocity agreements. *Financial support:* Fellowships, research assistantships, and teaching assistantships available. *Unit head:* Dr. Ronald Fell, Chair, 502-852-6771, Fax: 502-852-0725, E-mail: rdfell@louisville.edu. *Application contact:* Libby Leggett, Director, Graduate Admissions, 502-852-3101, Fax: 502-852-6536, E-mail: gradadm@louisville.edu.

University of Maine, Graduate School, College of Natural Sciences, Forestry, and Agriculture, Department of Molecular and Biomedical Sciences, Orono, ME 04469. Offers biochemistry (MPS, MS); biochemistry and molecular biology (PhD); microbiology (MPS, MS, PhD). *Faculty:* 30 full-time (6 women), 20 part-time/adjunct (4 women). *Students:* 26 full-time (17 women), 4 part-time (3 women); includes 3 minority (2 Asian, non-Hispanic/Latino; 1 Native Hawaiian or other Pacific Islander, non-Hispanic/Latino), 5 international. Average age 31. 7 applicants, 100% accepted, 5 enrolled. In 2013, 5 master's, 4 doctorates awarded. *Degree requirements:* For master's, thesis (for some programs); for doctorate, comprehensive exam, thesis/dissertation. *Entrance requirements:* For master's and doctorate, GRE General Test. Additional exam requirements/recommendations for international students: Required—TOEFL. *Application deadline:* For fall admission, 2/1 priority date for domestic students. Applications are processed on a rolling basis. Application fee: $65. Electronic applications accepted. *Expenses:* Tuition, state resident: full-time $7524. Tuition, nonresident: full-time $23,112. *Required fees:* $1970. *Financial support:* In 2013–14, 16 students received support, including 5 research assistantships with full tuition reimbursements available (averaging $22,000 per year), 10 teaching assistantships with full tuition reimbursements available (averaging $19,000 per year); tuition waivers (full and partial) also available. Financial award application deadline: 3/1. *Total annual research expenditures:* $242,844. *Unit head:* Dr. Robert Gundersen, Chair, 207-581-2802, Fax: 207-581-2801. *Application contact:* Scott G. Delcourt, Associate Dean of the Graduate School, 207-581-3291, Fax: 207-581-3232, E-mail: graduate@maine.edu.
Website: http://umaine.edu/biomed/

University of Maine, Graduate School, College of Natural Sciences, Forestry, and Agriculture, School of Biology and Ecology, Orono, ME 04469. Offers biological sciences (PhD); botany and plant pathology (MS); ecology and environmental science (MS, PhD); entomology (MS); plant science (PhD); zoology (MS, PhD). Part-time programs available. *Faculty:* 33 full-time (13 women), 26 part-time/adjunct (5 women). *Students:* 66 full-time (40 women), 4 part-time (2 women); includes 4 minority (1 American Indian or Alaska Native, non-Hispanic/Latino; 2 Asian, non-Hispanic/Latino; 1 Hispanic/Latino), 7 international. Average age 30. 97 applicants, 25% accepted, 17 enrolled. In 2013, 8 master's, 3 doctorates awarded. Terminal master's awarded for partial completion of doctoral program. *Degree requirements:* For master's, thesis (for some programs); for doctorate, comprehensive exam, thesis/dissertation. *Entrance requirements:* For master's and doctorate, GRE General Test. Additional exam requirements/recommendations for international students: Required—TOEFL. *Application deadline:* For fall admission, 2/1 priority date for domestic students. Applications are processed on a rolling basis. Application fee: $65. Electronic applications accepted. *Expenses:* Tuition, state resident: full-time $7524. Tuition, nonresident: full-time $23,112. *Required fees:* $1970. *Financial support:* In 2013–14, 66 students received support, including 3 fellowships with full tuition reimbursements available (averaging $25,000 per year), 28 research assistantships with full tuition reimbursements available (averaging $14,600 per year), 21 teaching assistantships with full tuition reimbursements available (averaging $14,600 per year); career-related internships or fieldwork, Federal Work-Study, institutionally sponsored loans, and tuition waivers (full and partial) also available. Financial award application deadline: 3/1. *Total annual research expenditures:* $569,533. *Unit head:* Dr. Ellie Groden, Director, 207-581-2551, Fax: 207-581-2537. *Application contact:* Scott G. Delcourt, Associate Dean of the Graduate School, 207-581-3291, Fax: 207-581-3232, E-mail: graduate@maine.edu.
Website: http://sbe.umaine.edu/

University of Maine, Graduate School, Graduate School of Biomedical Science and Engineering, Orono, ME 04469. Offers bioinformatics (PSM); biomedical engineering (PhD); cell and molecular biology (PhD); neuroscience (PhD); toxicology (PhD). *Faculty:* 39 full-time (10 women), 31 part-time/adjunct (8 women). *Students:* 31 full-time (18 women), 5 part-time (4 women), 11 international. Average age 30. 57 applicants, 16% accepted, 7 enrolled. In 2013, 5 doctorates awarded. *Degree requirements:* For doctorate, comprehensive exam, thesis/dissertation. *Entrance requirements:* For doctorate, GRE General Test, master's degree. Additional exam requirements/recommendations for international students: Required—TOEFL. *Application deadline:* For fall admission, 1/1 for domestic students. Application fee: $65. *Expenses:* Tuition, state resident: full-time $7524. Tuition, nonresident: full-time $23,112. *Required fees:* $1970. *Financial support:* In 2013–14, 16 students received support, including 1 fellowship with full tuition reimbursement available (averaging $18,000 per year), 13 research assistantships with full tuition reimbursements available (averaging $21,000 per year), 2 teaching assistantships (averaging $20,000 per year). *Faculty research:* Biomedical engineering, toxicology, neuroscience, cell and molecular biology, bioinformatics. *Total annual research expenditures:* $650,000. *Unit head:* Dr. David Neivandt, Director, 207-581-2803. *Application contact:* Scott G. Delcourt, Associate Dean of the Graduate School, 207-581-3291, Fax: 207-581-3232, E-mail: graduate@maine.edu.
Website: http://gsbse.umaine.edu/

The University of Manchester, Faculty of Life Sciences, Manchester, United Kingdom. Offers adaptive organismal biology (M Phil, PhD); animal biology (M Phil, PhD); biochemistry (M Phil, PhD); bioinformatics (M Phil, PhD); biomolecular sciences (M Phil, PhD); biotechnology (M Phil, PhD); cell biology (M Phil, PhD); cell matrix research (M Phil, PhD); channels and transporters (M Phil, PhD); developmental biology (M Phil, PhD); Egyptology (M Phil, PhD); environmental biology (M Phil, PhD); evolutionary biology (M Phil, PhD); gene expression (M Phil, PhD); genetics (M Phil, PhD); history of science, technology and medicine (M Phil, PhD); immunology (M Phil, PhD); integrative neurobiology and behavior (M Phil, PhD); membrane trafficking (M Phil, PhD); microbiology (M Phil, PhD); molecular and cellular neuroscience (M Phil, PhD); molecular biology (M Phil, PhD); molecular cancer studies (M Phil, PhD); neuroscience (M Phil, PhD); ophthalmology (M Phil, PhD); optometry (M Phil, PhD); organelle function (M Phil, PhD); pharmacology (M Phil, PhD); physiology (M Phil, PhD); plant sciences (M Phil, PhD); stem cell research (M Phil, PhD); structural biology (M Phil, PhD); systems neuroscience (M Phil, PhD); toxicology (M Phil, PhD).

The University of Manchester, School of Chemical Engineering and Analytical Science, Manchester, United Kingdom. Offers biocatalysis (M Phil, PhD); chemical engineering (M Phil, PhD); chemical engineering and analytical science (M Phil, D Eng, PhD); colloids, crystals, interfaces and materials (M Phil, PhD); environment and sustainable technology (M Phil, PhD); instrumentation (M Phil, PhD); multi-scale modeling (M Phil, PhD); process integration (M Phil, PhD); systems biology (M Phil, PhD).

The University of Manchester, School of Materials, Manchester, United Kingdom. Offers advanced aerospace materials engineering (M Sc); advanced metallic systems (PhD); biomedical materials (M Phil, M Sc, PhD); ceramics and glass (M Phil, M Sc, PhD); composite materials (M Sc, PhD); corrosion and protection (M Phil, M Sc, PhD); materials (M Phil, PhD); metallic materials (M Phil, M Sc, PhD); nanostructural materials (M Phil, M Sc, PhD); paper science (M Phil, M Sc, PhD); polymer science and engineering (M Phil, M Sc, PhD); technical textiles (M Sc); textile design, fashion and management (M Phil, M Sc, PhD); textile science and technology (M Phil, M Sc, PhD); textiles (M Phil, PhD); textiles and fashion (M Ent).

The University of Manchester, School of Medicine, Manchester, United Kingdom. Offers M Phil, PhD.

University of Manitoba, Faculty of Graduate Studies, Faculty of Science, Department of Biological Sciences, Winnipeg, MB R3T 2N2, Canada. Offers botany (M Sc, PhD); ecology (M Sc, PhD); zoology (M Sc, PhD).

University of Manitoba, Faculty of Medicine and Faculty of Graduate Studies, Graduate Programs in Medicine, Winnipeg, MB R3T 2N2, Canada. Offers M Sc, MPH, PhD, G Dip, MD/PhD. *Accreditation:* LCME/AMA. Part-time programs available. *Expenses:* Contact institution.

University of Maryland, Baltimore, Graduate School, Graduate Program in Life Sciences, Baltimore, MD 21201. Offers biochemistry and molecular biology (MS, PhD), including biochemistry; epidemiology (PhD); gerontology (PhD); molecular medicine (MS, PhD), including cancer biology (PhD), cell and molecular physiology (PhD), human genetics and genomic medicine (PhD), molecular medicine (MS), molecular toxicology and pharmacology (PhD); molecular microbiology and immunology (PhD); neuroscience (PhD); physical rehabilitation science (PhD); toxicology (MS, PhD); MD/MS; MD/PhD. *Students:* 287 full-time (156 women), 71 part-time (42 women); includes 91 minority (27 Black or African American, non-Hispanic/Latino; 39 Asian, non-Hispanic/Latino; 15 Hispanic/Latino; 10 Two or more races, non-Hispanic/Latino), 45 international. Average age 29. 633 applicants, 23% accepted, 71 enrolled. In 2013, 31 master's, 42 doctorates awarded. *Degree requirements:* For master's, comprehensive exam (for some programs), thesis (for some programs); for doctorate, comprehensive exam, thesis/dissertation. *Entrance requirements:* For master's and doctorate, GRE. Additional exam

requirements/recommendations for international students: Required—TOEFL (minimum score 550 paper-based; 80 iBT); Recommended—IELTS (minimum score 7). *Application deadline:* For fall admission, 12/14 for domestic students, 1/15 for international students. Application fee: $75. Electronic applications accepted. *Financial support:* In 2013–14, research assistantships with partial tuition reimbursements (averaging $25,000 per year) were awarded; fellowships, scholarships/grants, health care benefits, and unspecified assistantships also available. Financial award application deadline: 3/1; financial award applicants required to submit FAFSA. *Faculty research:* Cancer, reproduction, cardiovascular, immunology. *Unit head:* Dr. Dudley Strickland, Assistant Dean for Graduate Studies, 410-706-8010. *Application contact:* Keith T. Brooks, Assistant Dean, 410-706-7131, Fax: 410-706-3473, E-mail: kbrooks@umaryland.edu.
Website: http://lifesciences.umaryland.edu

University of Maryland, Baltimore County, Graduate School, College of Arts, Humanities and Social Sciences, Department of Education, Program in Teaching, Baltimore, MD 21250. Offers early childhood education (MAT); elementary education (MAT); secondary education (MAT), including art, biology, chemistry, choral music, classical foreign language, dance, earth/space science, English, instrumental music, mathematics, modern foreign language, physical science, physics, social studies, theatre. Part-time and evening/weekend programs available. *Faculty:* 24 full-time (18 women), 25 part-time/adjunct (19 women). *Students:* 49 full-time (34 women), 35 part-time (23 women); includes 19 minority (9 Black or African American, non-Hispanic/Latino; 3 Asian, non-Hispanic/Latino; 6 Hispanic/Latino; 1 Two or more races, non-Hispanic/Latino). Average age 30. 40 applicants, 95% accepted, 35 enrolled. In 2013, 106 master's awarded. *Degree requirements:* For master's, comprehensive exam (for some programs), thesis (for some programs). *Entrance requirements:* For master's, PRAXIS I or SAT (minimum score of 1000), minimum GPA of 3.0. Additional exam requirements/recommendations for international students: Required—TOEFL. *Application deadline:* For fall admission, 6/1 for domestic students; for spring admission, 11/1 for domestic students. Applications are processed on a rolling basis. Application fee: $50. Electronic applications accepted. One-time fee: $200 full-time. *Financial support:* In 2013–14, 6 students received support, including teaching assistantships with full and partial tuition reimbursements available (averaging $12,000 per year); career-related internships or fieldwork, Federal Work-Study, scholarships/grants, tuition waivers, and unspecified assistantships also available. Financial award application deadline: 3/1. *Faculty research:* STEM teacher education, culturally sensitive pedagogy, ESOL/bilingual education, early childhood education, language, literacy and culture. *Unit head:* Dr. Susan M. Blunck, Graduate Program Director, 410-455-2869, Fax: 410-455-3986, E-mail: blunck@umbc.edu. *Application contact:* Dr. Susan M. Blunck, Graduate Program Director, 410-455-2869, Fax: 410-455-3986, E-mail: blunck@umbc.edu.
Website: http://www.umbc.edu/education/

University of Maryland, Baltimore County, Graduate School, College of Natural and Mathematical Sciences, Department of Biological Sciences, Baltimore, MD 21250. Offers applied molecular biology (MS); biological sciences (MS, PhD); biotechnology (MPS), including biotechnology; biotechnology (Graduate Certificate), including biotechnology management; marine-estuarine-environmental sciences (MS); molecular and cell biology (PhD); neuroscience and cognitive sciences (PhD). *Faculty:* 26 full-time (11 women). *Students:* 81 full-time (48 women), 9 part-time (5 women); includes 25 minority (12 Black or African American, non-Hispanic/Latino; 6 Asian, non-Hispanic/Latino; 3 Hispanic/Latino; 1 Native Hawaiian or other Pacific Islander, non-Hispanic/Latino; 3 Two or more races, non-Hispanic/Latino), 19 international. Average age 27. 201 applicants, 36% accepted, 43 enrolled. In 2013, 8 master's, 9 doctorates awarded. Terminal master's awarded for partial completion of doctoral program. *Degree requirements:* For master's, thesis; for doctorate, thesis/dissertation. *Entrance requirements:* For master's and doctorate, GRE General Test, minimum GPA of 3.0. Additional exam requirements/recommendations for international students: Required—TOEFL (minimum score 80 iBT). *Application deadline:* For fall admission, 1/1 priority date for domestic and international students. Application fee: $50. Electronic applications accepted. One-time fee: $200 full-time. *Financial support:* In 2013–14, 59 students received support, including 6 fellowships with full tuition reimbursements available (averaging $23,000 per year), 10 research assistantships with full tuition reimbursements available (averaging $22,746 per year), 43 teaching assistantships with full tuition reimbursements available (averaging $21,726 per year); career-related internships or fieldwork and tuition waivers also available. *Unit head:* Dr. Philip Farabaugh, Chairman, 410-455-3081, Fax: 410-455-3875, E-mail: farabaug@umbc.edu. *Application contact:* Dr. Stephen Miller, Director, 410-455-3381, Fax: 410-455-3875, E-mail: biograd@umbc.edu.

University of Maryland, College Park, Academic Affairs, College of Computer, Mathematical and Natural Sciences, Department of Biology, PhD Program in Biological Sciences, College Park, MD 20742. Offers behavior, ecology, evolution, and systematics (PhD); computational biology, bioinformatics, and genomics (PhD); molecular and cellular biology (PhD); physiological systems (PhD). *Students:* 104 full-time (59 women), 4 part-time (1 woman); includes 21 minority (2 Black or African American, non-Hispanic/Latino; 1 American Indian or Alaska Native, non-Hispanic/Latino; 9 Asian, non-Hispanic/Latino; 7 Hispanic/Latino; 2 Two or more races, non-Hispanic/Latino), 34 international. 365 applicants, 13% accepted, 20 enrolled. In 2013, 5 doctorates awarded. *Degree requirements:* For doctorate, comprehensive exam, thesis/dissertation, thesis work presentation in seminar. *Entrance requirements:* For doctorate, GRE General Test; GRE Subject Test in biology (recommended), academic transcripts, statement of purpose/research interests, 3 letters of recommendation. Additional exam requirements/recommendations for international students: Required—TOEFL. *Application deadline:* For fall admission, 12/15 for domestic and international students. Applications are processed on a rolling basis. Application fee: $75. Electronic applications accepted. *Expenses:* Tuition, state resident: full-time $10,314; part-time $573 per credit hour. Tuition, nonresident: full-time $22,248; part-time $1236 per credit. *Required fees:* $1446; $403.15 per semester. Tuition and fees vary according to program. *Financial support:* In 2013–14, 21 fellowships with full and partial tuition reimbursements (averaging $27,603 per year), 25 research assistantships (averaging $19,557 per year), 55 teaching assistantships (averaging $18,959 per year) were awarded. *Unit head:* Dr. Charles F. Delwiche, Director, 301-405-6884, E-mail: bisidirector@umd.edu. *Application contact:* Dr. Charles A. Caramello, Dean of Graduate School, 301-405-0358, Fax: 301-314-9305, E-mail: ccaramel@umd.edu.
Website: http://www.bisi.umd.edu/

University of Maryland, College Park, Academic Affairs, College of Computer, Mathematical and Natural Sciences, Department of Biology, Program in Biology, College Park, MD 20742. Offers MS, PhD. Part-time and evening/weekend programs available. *Students:* 20 full-time (12 women); includes 2 minority (both Two or more races, non-Hispanic/Latino), 5 international. In 2013, 2 master's, 8 doctorates awarded. Terminal master's awarded for partial completion of doctoral program. *Degree requirements:* For master's, comprehensive exam, thesis optional; for doctorate, thesis/dissertation, oral exam. *Expenses:* Tuition, state resident: full-time $10,314; part-time $573 per credit hour. Tuition, nonresident: full-time $22,248; part-time $1236 per credit. *Required fees:* $1446; $403.15 per semester. Tuition and fees vary according to program. *Financial support:* In 2013–14, 4 fellowships with full tuition reimbursements (averaging $24,276 per year), 4 research assistantships with tuition reimbursements (averaging $19,810 per year), 6 teaching assistantships with tuition reimbursements (averaging $19,618 per year) were awarded. Financial award application deadline: 2/1; financial award applicants required to submit FAFSA. *Unit head:* Dr. Gerald S. Wilkinson, Chair, 301-405-6884, E-mail: wilkinso@umd.edu. *Application contact:* Dr. Charles A. Caramello, Dean of Graduate School, 301-405-0358, Fax: 301-314-9305, E-mail: ccaramel@umd.edu.

University of Maryland, College Park, Academic Affairs, College of Computer, Mathematical and Natural Sciences, Program in Life Sciences, College Park, MD 20742. Offers MLS. *Students:* 10 full-time (5 women), 58 part-time (41 women); includes 15 minority (7 Black or African American, non-Hispanic/Latino; 2 Asian, non-Hispanic/Latino; 3 Hispanic/Latino; 3 Two or more races, non-Hispanic/Latino), 5 international. 26 applicants, 77% accepted, 13 enrolled. In 2013, 23 master's awarded. *Degree requirements:* For master's, scholarly paper. *Entrance requirements:* For master's, 1 year of teaching experience, letters of recommendation. *Application deadline:* Applications are processed on a rolling basis. Application fee: $75. Electronic applications accepted. *Expenses:* Tuition, state resident: full-time $10,314; part-time $573 per credit hour. Tuition, nonresident: full-time $22,248; part-time $1236 per credit. *Required fees:* $1446; $403.15 per semester. Tuition and fees vary according to program. *Financial support:* Fellowships, research assistantships, teaching assistantships, Federal Work-Study, and scholarships/grants available. Support available to part-time students. Financial award applicants required to submit FAFSA. *Faculty research:* Genetic engineering, gene therapy, ecology, biocomplexity. *Unit head:* Dr. Paul J. Smith, Associate Dean, 301-405-2327, Fax: 301-314-9949, E-mail: pjs@umd.edu. *Application contact:* Dr. Charles A. Caramello, Dean of Graduate School, 301-405-0358, Fax: 301-314-9305, E-mail: ccaramel@umd.edu.

University of Massachusetts Amherst, Graduate School, College of Natural Sciences, Department of Animal Biotechnology and Biomedical Sciences, Amherst, MA 01003. Offers MS, PhD. Part-time programs available. *Faculty:* 22 full-time (10 women). *Students:* 16 full-time (8 women), 7 international. Average age 30. 38 applicants, 11% accepted, 4 enrolled. In 2013, 3 master's, 5 doctorates awarded. Terminal master's awarded for partial completion of doctoral program. *Degree requirements:* For master's, thesis or alternative; for doctorate, comprehensive exam, thesis/dissertation. *Entrance requirements:* For doctorate, GRE General Test. Additional exam requirements/recommendations for international students: Required—TOEFL (minimum score 550 paper-based; 80 iBT), IELTS (minimum score 6.5). *Application deadline:* For fall admission, 1/15 for domestic and international students; for spring admission, 10/1 for domestic and international students. Applications are processed on a rolling basis. Application fee: $75. Electronic applications accepted. *Financial support:* Fellowships with full and partial tuition reimbursements, research assistantships with full and partial tuition reimbursements, teaching assistantships with full and partial tuition reimbursements, career-related internships or fieldwork, Federal Work-Study, scholarships/grants, traineeships, health care benefits, tuition waivers (full and partial), and unspecified assistantships available. Support available to part-time students. Financial award application deadline: 1/15. *Unit head:* Dr. Lisa Minter, Graduate Program Director, 413-577-1193, Fax: 413-577-1150. *Application contact:* Lindsay DeSantis, Supervisor of Admissions, 413-545-0722, Fax: 413-577-0010, E-mail: gradadm@grad.umass.edu.
Website: http://www.vasci.umass.edu/graduate-program-overview

University of Massachusetts Boston, Office of Graduate Studies, College of Science and Mathematics, Program in Biology, Boston, MA 02125-3393. Offers MS. Part-time and evening/weekend programs available. *Degree requirements:* For master's, thesis, oral exams. *Entrance requirements:* For master's, GRE General Test, GRE Subject Test, minimum GPA of 2.75. *Faculty research:* Microbial ecology, population and conservation genetics energetics of insect locomotion, science education, evolution and ecology of marine invertebrates.

University of Massachusetts Boston, Office of Graduate Studies, College of Science and Mathematics, Program in Biotechnology and Biomedical Science, Boston, MA 02125-3393. Offers MS. Part-time and evening/weekend programs available. *Degree requirements:* For master's, comprehensive exam, thesis optional, oral exams. *Entrance requirements:* For master's, GRE General Test, GRE Subject Test, minimum GPA of 2.75, 3.0 in science and math. *Faculty research:* Evolutionary and molecular immunology, molecular genetics, tissue culture, computerized laboratory technology.

University of Massachusetts Dartmouth, Graduate School, College of Arts and Sciences, Department of Biology, North Dartmouth, MA 02747-2300. Offers biology (MS); marine biology (MS). Part-time programs available. *Faculty:* 18 full-time (6 women), 1 (woman) part-time/adjunct. *Students:* 7 full-time (all women), 13 part-time (10 women); includes 3 minority (2 Hispanic/Latino; 1 Two or more races, non-Hispanic/Latino). Average age 27. 24 applicants, 42% accepted, 4 enrolled. In 2013, 9 master's awarded. *Degree requirements:* For master's, thesis. *Entrance requirements:* For master's, GRE, statement of purpose (minimum of 300 words), resume, 3 letters of recommendation, official transcripts. Additional exam requirements/recommendations for international students: Required—TOEFL (minimum score 533 paper-based; 72 iBT). *Application deadline:* For fall admission, 2/15 priority date for domestic students, 1/15 priority date for international students. Applications are processed on a rolling basis. Application fee: $60. Electronic applications accepted. *Expenses:* Tuition, state resident: full-time $2071; part-time $86.29 per credit. Tuition, nonresident: full-time $8099; part-time $337.46 per credit. Tuition and fees vary according to course load and reciprocity agreements. *Financial support:* In 2013–14, 2 research assistantships with full tuition reimbursements (averaging $10,200 per year), 10 teaching assistantships with full tuition reimbursements (averaging $14,400 per year) were awarded; Federal Work-Study and unspecified assistantships also available. Support available to part-time students. Financial award application deadline: 3/1; financial award applicants required to submit FAFSA. *Faculty research:* Shark biology, marine mammal biology, domestication of fish, cell body, fish biology. *Total annual research expenditures:* $1.5 million. *Unit head:* Dr. Diego Bernal, Graduate Program Director, 508-999-8307, Fax: 508-999-8196, E-mail: dbernal@umassd.edu. *Application contact:* Steven Briggs, Director of Marketing and Recruitment for Graduate Studies, 508-999-8604, Fax: 508-999-8183, E-mail: graduate@umassd.edu.
Website: http://www.umassd.edu/cas/biology/

University of Massachusetts Lowell, College of Sciences, Department of Biological Sciences, Lowell, MA 01854-2881. Offers biochemistry (PhD); biological sciences (MS); biotechnology (MS). Part-time programs available. *Degree requirements:* For master's, thesis; for doctorate, thesis/dissertation. *Entrance requirements:* For master's and doctorate, GRE General Test. Electronic applications accepted.

University of Massachusetts Worcester, Graduate School of Biomedical Sciences, Worcester, MA 01655-0115. Offers biochemistry and molecular pharmacology (PhD); bioinformatics and computational biology (PhD); cancer biology (PhD); cell biology (PhD); clinical and population health research (PhD); clinical investigation (MS); immunology and virology (PhD); interdisciplinary biomedical research (PhD); millennium (PhD); molecular genetics and microbiology (PhD); neuroscience (PhD); translational science (PhD); MD/PhD. *Faculty:* 1,388 full-time (521 women), 309 part-time/adjunct (198 women). *Students:* 385 full-time (210 women); includes 53 minority (13 Black or

African American, non-Hispanic/Latino; 30 Asian, non-Hispanic/Latino; 10 Hispanic/Latino), 138 international. Average age 28. 491 applicants, 19% accepted, 39 enrolled. In 2013, 5 master's, 50 doctorates awarded. Terminal master's awarded for partial completion of doctoral program. *Median time to degree:* Of those who began their doctoral program in fall 2005, 67% received their degree in 8 years or less. *Degree requirements:* For master's, comprehensive exam, thesis; for doctorate, comprehensive exam, thesis/dissertation. *Entrance requirements:* For master's, MD, PhD, DVM, or PharmD; for doctorate, GRE General Test, bachelor's degree. Additional exam requirements/recommendations for international students: Required—TOEFL (minimum score 100 iBT) or IELTS (minimum score 7.5). *Application deadline:* For fall admission, 12/15 for domestic and international students; for spring admission, 5/15 for domestic students. Application fee: $80. Electronic applications accepted. *Expenses:* Contact institution. *Financial support:* In 2013–14, 431 students received support, including research assistantships with full tuition reimbursements available (averaging $29,500 per year); scholarships/grants, health care benefits, tuition waivers (full), and unspecified assistantships also available. Financial award application deadline: 5/16. *Faculty research:* RNA interference, cell/molecular/developmental biology, bioinformatics, clinical/translational research, infectious disease. *Total annual research expenditures:* $245.9 million. *Unit head:* Dr. Anthony Carruthers, Dean, 508-856-4135, E-mail: anthony.carruthers@umassmed.edu. *Application contact:* Dr. Kendall Knight, Associate Dean and Interim Director of Admissions and Recruitment, 508-856-5628, Fax: 508-856-3659, E-mail: kendall.knight@umassmed.edu.
Website: http://www.umassmed.edu/gsbs/

University of Memphis, Graduate School, College of Arts and Sciences, Department of Biology, Memphis, TN 38152. Offers MS, PhD. *Faculty:* 17 full-time (1 woman), 1 (woman) part-time/adjunct. *Students:* 38 full-time (25 women), 10 part-time (5 women); includes 3 minority (1 Black or African American, non-Hispanic/Latino; 2 Asian, non-Hispanic/Latino), 12 international. Average age 29. 28 applicants, 64% accepted, 10 enrolled. In 2013, 8 master's, 4 doctorates awarded. Terminal master's awarded for partial completion of doctoral program. *Degree requirements:* For master's, comprehensive exam, thesis (for some programs); for doctorate, one foreign language, comprehensive exam, thesis/dissertation. *Entrance requirements:* For master's, GRE General Test; for doctorate, GRE General Test, master's degree. Additional exam requirements/recommendations for international students: Required—TOEFL (minimum score 550 paper-based; 79 iBT). *Application deadline:* For fall admission, 2/1 for domestic and international students; for spring admission, 10/15 for domestic and international students. Applications are processed on a rolling basis. Application fee: $35 ($60 for international students). Electronic applications accepted. *Financial support:* In 2013–14, 16 students received support. Research assistantships with full tuition reimbursements available, teaching assistantships with full tuition reimbursements available, Federal Work-Study, scholarships/grants, and unspecified assistantships available. Financial award application deadline: 2/15; financial award applicants required to submit FAFSA. *Faculty research:* Protein trafficking and signal transduction; animal behavior and communication, neurobiology, and circadian clock function; phylogenetics, evolution, and ecology; causation and prevention of cancer; reproductive biology. *Unit head:* Dr. Randall Bayer, Chairman, 901-678-2596, Fax: 901-678-4746, E-mail: rbayer@memphis.edu. *Application contact:* Dr. Melvin Beck, Professor and Graduate Studies Coordinator, 901-678-2970, Fax: 901-678-4457, E-mail: mbeck@memphis.edu.
Website: http://www.memphis.edu/biology/

University of Miami, Graduate School, College of Arts and Sciences, Department of Biology, Coral Gables, FL 33124. Offers biology (MS, PhD); genetics and evolution (MS, PhD). Terminal master's awarded for partial completion of doctoral program. *Degree requirements:* For master's, comprehensive exam (for some programs), thesis (for some programs); for doctorate, thesis/dissertation, oral and written qualifying exam. *Entrance requirements:* For master's, GRE General Test, 3 letters of recommendation, research papers; for doctorate, GRE General Test, 3 letters of recommendation, research papers, sponsor letter. Additional exam requirements/recommendations for international students: Required—TOEFL (minimum score 550 paper-based; 59 iBT). Electronic applications accepted. *Faculty research:* Neuroscience to ethology; plants, vertebrates and mycorrhizae; phylogenies, life histories and species interactions; molecular biology, gene expression and populations; cells, auditory neurons and vertebrate locomotion.

University of Michigan, Medical School and Rackham Graduate School, Medical Scientist Training Program, Ann Arbor, MI 48109. Offers MD/PhD. *Accreditation:* LCME/AMA. *Students:* 91 full-time (30 women); includes 39 minority (4 Black or African American, non-Hispanic/Latino; 35 Asian, non-Hispanic/Latino). 360 applicants, 11% accepted, 15 enrolled. *Application deadline:* For fall admission, 10/15 for domestic students. Applications are processed on a rolling basis. Application fee: $160. Electronic applications accepted. Tuition and fees vary according to course level, course load, degree level, program and student level. *Financial support:* In 2013–14, 91 students received support, including 72 fellowships with full tuition reimbursements available (averaging $28,500 per year), 16 research assistantships with full tuition reimbursements available (averaging $28,500 per year), 3 teaching assistantships with full tuition reimbursements available (averaging $28,500 per year); scholarships/grants, traineeships, and health care benefits also available. *Unit head:* Dr. Ronald J. Koenig, Director, 734-764-6176, Fax: 734-764-8180, E-mail: rkoenig@umich.edu. *Application contact:* Laurie Koivupalo, Administrative Associate, 734-764-6176, Fax: 734-764-8180, E-mail: lkoivupl@umich.edu.
Website: http://www.med.umich.edu/medschool/mstp/

University of Michigan, Rackham Graduate School, Program in Biomedical Sciences (PIBS), Ann Arbor, MI 48109-5619. Offers MS, PhD. *Faculty:* 508 full-time. *Students:* 60 full-time (37 women); includes 15 minority (3 Black or African American, non-Hispanic/Latino; 5 Asian, non-Hispanic/Latino; 4 Hispanic/Latino; 1 Native Hawaiian or other Pacific Islander, non-Hispanic/Latino; 2 Two or more races, non-Hispanic/Latino), 13 international. Average age 24. 819 applicants, 21% accepted, 60 enrolled. *Degree requirements:* For doctorate, thesis/dissertation, oral defense of dissertation, preliminary exam. *Entrance requirements:* For doctorate, GRE General Test, 3 letters of recommendation, research experience. Additional exam requirements/recommendations for international students: Required—TOEFL (minimum score 84 iBT). *Application deadline:* For fall admission, 12/1 for domestic and international students. Application fee: $75 ($90 for international students). Electronic applications accepted. Tuition and fees vary according to course level, course load, degree level, program and student level. *Financial support:* In 2013–14, 60 students received support, including 60 fellowships with full tuition reimbursements available (averaging $28,500 per year); scholarships/grants, health care benefits, tuition waivers (full), and unspecified assistantships also available. Financial award application deadline: 12/1. *Faculty research:* Genetics, cellular and molecular biology, microbial pathogenesis, cancer biology, neuroscience. *Unit head:* Dr. Lori L. Isom, Assistant Dean/Director/Professor of Molecular and Integrative Physiology and Pharmacology, 734-615-7005, Fax: 734-647-7022, E-mail: lisom@umich.edu. *Application contact:* Michelle S. Melis, Director of Student Life, 734-615-6538, Fax: 734-647-7022, E-mail: msmtegan@umich.edu.
Website: http://www.med.umich.edu/pibs/

University of Michigan–Flint, College of Arts and Sciences, Program in Biology, Flint, MI 48502-1950. Offers MS. Part-time programs available. *Faculty:* 9 full-time (3 women), 1 part-time/adjunct (0 women). *Students:* 16 full-time (10 women), 13 part-time (9 women); includes 4 minority (1 Black or African American, non-Hispanic/Latino; 2 Asian, non-Hispanic/Latino; 1 Two or more races, non-Hispanic/Latino), 5 international. Average age 30. 22 applicants, 45% accepted, 9 enrolled. In 2013, 5 master's awarded. *Degree requirements:* For master's, thesis or alternative. *Entrance requirements:* For master's, GRE, minimum undergraduate GPA of 3.0 in prerequisites. Additional exam requirements/recommendations for international students: Required—TOEFL (minimum score 560 paper-based; 84 iBT), IELTS (minimum score 6.5). *Application deadline:* For fall admission, 8/1 for domestic students, 5/1 for international students; for winter admission, 11/15 for domestic students, 9/1 for international students; for spring admission, 3/15 for domestic students, 1/1 for international students; for summer admission, 5/15 for domestic students. Applications are processed on a rolling basis. Application fee: $55. Electronic applications accepted. *Expenses:* Contact institution. *Financial support:* Federal Work-Study, scholarships/grants, and unspecified assistantships available. Support available to part-time students. Financial award application deadline: 3/1; financial award applicants required to submit FAFSA. *Unit head:* Dr. Joseph Sucic, Director, 810-762-3360, Fax: 810-762-3310, E-mail: jsucic@umflint.edu. *Application contact:* Bradley T. Maki, Director of Graduate Admissions, 810-762-3171, Fax: 810-766-6789, E-mail: bmaki@umflint.edu.
Website: http://www.umflint.edu/graduateprograms/biology.htm

University of Minnesota, Duluth, Graduate School, Swenson College of Science and Engineering, Department of Biology, Integrated Biosciences Program, Duluth, MN 55812-2496. Offers MS, PhD. Terminal master's awarded for partial completion of doctoral program. *Degree requirements:* For master's, thesis, seminar; for doctorate, comprehensive exam, thesis/dissertation, written and oral exam, seminar, written thesis. *Entrance requirements:* For master's, GRE, 1 year of biology, physics, and chemistry; 1 semester of calculus; for doctorate, GRE, 1 year each of chemistry, biology, physics, calculus, and advanced chemistry. Additional exam requirements/recommendations for international students: Required—TOEFL (minimum score 550 paper-based; 79 iBT). Electronic applications accepted. *Faculty research:* Ecology, organizational and population biology; cell, molecular and physiological biology.

University of Minnesota, Twin Cities Campus, Graduate School, College of Biological Sciences, Biological Science Program, Minneapolis, MN 55455-0213. Offers MBS. Part-time and evening/weekend programs available. *Entrance requirements:* For master's, 2 years of work experience. Electronic applications accepted. *Expenses:* Contact institution.

University of Minnesota, Twin Cities Campus, Graduate School, Stem Cell Biology Graduate Program, Minneapolis, MN 55455-3007. Offers MS. *Degree requirements:* For master's, thesis. *Entrance requirements:* For master's, GRE, BS, BA, or foreign equivalent in biological sciences or related field; minimum undergraduate GPA of 3.2. Additional exam requirements/recommendations for international students: Required—TOEFL (minimum score 580 paper-based, with a minimum score of 4 in the TWE, or 94 Internet-based, with a minimum score of 22 on each of the reading and listening, 26 on the speaking, and 26 on the writing section. *Faculty research:* Stem cell and developmental biology; embryonic stem cells; iPS cells; muscle satellite cells; hematopoietic stem cells; neuronal stem cells; cardiovascular, kidney and limb development; regenerating systems.

University of Mississippi, Graduate School, College of Liberal Arts, Department of Biology, University, MS 38677. Offers MS, PhD. *Faculty:* 29 full-time (10 women), 1 (woman) part-time/adjunct. *Students:* 39 full-time (16 women), 2 part-time (1 woman); includes 1 minority (Two or more races, non-Hispanic/Latino), 5 international. In 2013, 1 master's, 1 doctorate awarded. *Degree requirements:* For master's, thesis; for doctorate, thesis/dissertation. *Entrance requirements:* For master's and doctorate, GRE General Test, GRE Subject Test, minimum GPA of 3.0. Additional exam requirements/recommendations for international students: Required—TOEFL. *Application deadline:* For fall admission, 4/1 for domestic students; for spring admission, 10/1 for domestic students. Applications are processed on a rolling basis. Application fee: $40. Electronic applications accepted. *Financial support:* Research assistantships, teaching assistantships, and scholarships/grants available. Financial award application deadline: 3/1; financial award applicants required to submit FAFSA. *Faculty research:* Freshwater biology, including ecology and evolutionary biology; environmental and applied biology. *Unit head:* Dr. Paul Lago, Interim Chair, 662-915-7203, Fax: 662-915-5144, E-mail: biology@olemiss.edu. *Application contact:* Dr. Christy M. Wyandt, Associate Dean, 662-915-7474, Fax: 662-915-7577, E-mail: cwyandt@olemiss.edu.

University of Mississippi Medical Center, School of Graduate Studies in the Health Sciences, Jackson, MS 39216-4505. Offers MS, PhD, MD/PhD. Part-time programs available. *Faculty:* 101 full-time (28 women), 6 part-time/adjunct (3 women). *Students:* 242 full-time (144 women), 5 part-time (3 women); includes 93 minority (39 Black or African American, non-Hispanic/Latino; 50 Asian, non-Hispanic/Latino; 2 Hispanic/Latino; 2 Two or more races, non-Hispanic/Latino), 39 international. Average age 28. 186 applicants, 38% accepted, 62 enrolled. In 2013, 56 master's, 79 doctorates awarded. Terminal master's awarded for partial completion of doctoral program. *Degree requirements:* For master's, thesis (for some programs); for doctorate, comprehensive exam, thesis/dissertation, first authored publication. *Entrance requirements:* For master's and doctorate, GRE. Additional exam requirements/recommendations for international students: Required—TOEFL (minimum score 550 paper-based; 79 iBT), IELTS (minimum score 6.5), PTE (minimum score 53). *Application deadline:* For fall admission, 6/1 for domestic and international students; for spring admission, 10/1 for domestic and international students; for summer admission, 4/1 for domestic and international students. Applications are processed on a rolling basis. Application fee: $25. *Financial support:* In 2013–14, 52 students received support, including research assistantships with full and partial tuition reimbursements available (averaging $24,150 per year). Financial award application deadline: 4/15; financial award applicants required to submit FAFSA. *Faculty research:* Immunology; protein chemistry and biosynthesis; cardiovascular, renal, and endocrine physiology; rehabilitation therapy on immune system/hypothalamic/adrenal axis interaction. *Total annual research expenditures:* $11.3 million. *Unit head:* Libby Spence, PhD, Dean, 601-984-1204, Fax: 601-815-9440, E-mail: lspence@umc.edu. *Application contact:* Barbara Westerfield, Director, Student Records/Registrar, 601-984-1080, Fax: 601-984-1079, E-mail: bwesterfield@umc.edu.
Website: http://www.umc.edu/graduateschool/

University of Missouri, Graduate School, College of Arts and Science, Division of Biological Sciences, Columbia, MO 65211. Offers evolutionary biology and ecology (MA, PhD); genetic, cellular and developmental biology (MA, PhD); neurobiology and behavior (MA, PhD). *Faculty:* 40 full-time (11 women), 1 part-time/adjunct (0 women). *Students:* 70 full-time (32 women), 3 part-time (2 women); includes 12 minority (4 Black or African American, non-Hispanic/Latino; 1 American Indian or Alaska Native, non-Hispanic/Latino; 2 Asian, non-Hispanic/Latino; 3 Hispanic/Latino; 2 Two or more races, non-Hispanic/Latino), 5 international. Average age 28. 46 applicants, 28% accepted, 13 enrolled. In 2013, 7 master's, 13 doctorates awarded. Terminal master's awarded for partial completion of doctoral program. *Degree requirements:* For master's, thesis; for

doctorate, comprehensive exam, thesis/dissertation. *Entrance requirements:* For master's and doctorate, GRE General Test (minimum score 1200 verbal and quantitative), minimum GPA of 3.0. Additional exam requirements/recommendations for international students: Required—TOEFL (minimum score 600 paper-based; 100 iBT). *Application deadline:* For fall admission, 12/15 priority date for domestic and international students. Applications are processed on a rolling basis. Application fee: $55 ($75 for international students). Electronic applications accepted. *Financial support:* Fellowships with full tuition reimbursements, research assistantships with full tuition reimbursements, teaching assistantships with full tuition reimbursements, institutionally sponsored loans, traineeships, health care benefits, and unspecified assistantships available. *Faculty research:* Evolutionary biology, ecology and behavior; genetic, cellular, molecular and developmental biology; neurobiology and behavior; plant sciences. *Unit head:* Dr. John C. Walker, Division Director, 573-882-3583, E-mail: walkerj@missouri.edu. *Application contact:* Nila Emerich, Application Contact, 800-553-5698, E-mail: emerichn@missouri.edu.
Website: http://biology.missouri.edu/graduate-studies/

University of Missouri, School of Medicine and Graduate School, Graduate Programs in Medicine, Columbia, MO 65211. Offers family and community medicine (MS); health administration (MS); medical pharmacology and physiology (MS, PhD); molecular microbiology and immunology (MS, PhD); pathology and anatomical sciences (MS). Part-time programs available. *Faculty:* 71 full-time (16 women), 12 part-time/adjunct (4 women). *Students:* 55 full-time (30 women), 3 part-time (all women); includes 6 minority (4 Black or African American, non-Hispanic/Latino; 1 American Indian or Alaska Native, non-Hispanic/Latino; 1 Hispanic/Latino), 25 international. Average age 28. 73 applicants, 16% accepted, 11 enrolled. In 2013, 1 master's, 13 doctorates awarded. *Degree requirements:* For doctorate, thesis/dissertation. *Entrance requirements:* For master's and doctorate, GRE General Test, minimum GPA of 3.0. Additional exam requirements/recommendations for international students: Required—TOEFL. *Application deadline:* Applications are processed on a rolling basis. Application fee: $55 ($75 for international students). *Expenses:* Contact institution. *Financial support:* Fellowships, research assistantships, teaching assistantships, career-related internships or fieldwork, and institutionally sponsored loans available. *Faculty research:* HIV enzymes, calcium and heart function, gene study and Muscular Dystrophy, military medical training using simulation technology, clinical and translational science. *Unit head:* William M. Crist, Dean Emeritus, 573-884-8733, E-mail: cristwm@missouri.edu. *Application contact:* Charles Rudkin, Graduate Programs Assistant, 573-882-4637, E-mail: rudkinc@health.missouri.edu.
Website: http://som.missouri.edu/departments.shtml

University of Missouri–Kansas City, School of Biological Sciences, Kansas City, MO 64110-2499. Offers biology (MA); cell biology and biophysics (PhD); cellular and molecular biology (MS); molecular biology and biochemistry (PhD). PhD (interdisciplinary) offered through the School of Graduate Studies. Part-time and evening/weekend programs available. *Faculty:* 34 full-time (9 women), 3 part-time/adjunct (all women). *Students:* 11 full-time (6 women), 36 part-time (23 women); includes 7 minority (4 Asian, non-Hispanic/Latino; 2 Hispanic/Latino; 1 Two or more races, non-Hispanic/Latino), 3 international. Average age 29. 41 applicants, 56% accepted, 10 enrolled. In 2013, 26 master's awarded. *Degree requirements:* For doctorate, comprehensive exam, thesis/dissertation. *Entrance requirements:* For master's, GRE, minimum GPA of 3.0; for doctorate, GRE General Test. Additional exam requirements/recommendations for international students: Required—TOEFL (minimum score 550 paper-based; 80 iBT). *Application deadline:* For fall admission, 2/15 priority date for domestic and international students. Applications are processed on a rolling basis. Application fee: $45 ($50 for international students). *Expenses:* Tuition, state resident: full-time $6073; part-time $337.40 per credit hour. Tuition, nonresident: full-time $15,680; part-time $871.10 per credit hour. *Required fees:* $97.59 per credit hour. Full-time tuition and fees vary according to program. *Financial support:* In 2013–14, 19 research assistantships with full tuition reimbursements (averaging $23,424 per year), 14 teaching assistantships with full tuition reimbursements (averaging $17,639 per year) were awarded; Federal Work-Study, institutionally sponsored loans, scholarships/grants, tuition waivers (full and partial), and unspecified assistantships also available. Support available to part-time students. Financial award application deadline: 3/1; financial award applicants required to submit FAFSA. *Faculty research:* Structural biology, molecular genetics. *Unit head:* Dr. Theodore White, Dean, 816-235-2538, Fax: 816-235-5158, E-mail: whitetc@umkc.edu. *Application contact:* Information Contact, 816-235-1330, Fax: 816-235-5158, E-mail: sbsgradrecruit@umkc.edu.
Website: http://sbs.umkc.edu/

University of Missouri–St. Louis, College of Arts and Sciences, Department of Biology, St. Louis, MO 63121. Offers biotechnology (Certificate); cell and molecular biology (MS, PhD); ecology, evolution and systematics (MS, PhD); tropical biology and conservation (Certificate). Part-time programs available. *Faculty:* 33 full-time (13 women), 9 part-time/adjunct (1 woman). *Students:* 52 full-time (23 women), 58 part-time (29 women); includes 13 minority (9 Black or African American, non-Hispanic/Latino; 3 Asian, non-Hispanic/Latino; 1 Hispanic/Latino), 30 international. Average age 28. 113 applicants, 42% accepted, 22 enrolled. In 2013, 31 master's, 5 doctorates, 4 other advanced degrees awarded. *Degree requirements:* For master's, thesis or alternative; for doctorate, thesis/dissertation, 1 semester of teaching experience. *Entrance requirements:* For master's, 3 letters of recommendation; for doctorate, GRE General Test, 3 letters of recommendation. Additional exam requirements/recommendations for international students: Required—TOEFL (minimum score 79 iBT), IELTS (minimum score 6.5). *Application deadline:* For fall admission, 12/15 priority date for domestic and international students; for spring admission, 12/1 priority date for domestic and international students. Applications are processed on a rolling basis. Application fee: $50 ($40 for international students). Electronic applications accepted. *Expenses:* Tuition, state resident: full-time $7364; part-time $409.10 per credit hour. Tuition, nonresident: full-time $19,162; part-time $1008.50 per credit hour. *Financial support:* In 2013–14, 13 research assistantships with full and partial tuition reimbursements (averaging $17,000 per year), 23 teaching assistantships with full and partial tuition reimbursements (averaging $17,000 per year) were awarded; fellowships with full tuition reimbursements, career-related internships or fieldwork, and Federal Work-Study also available. Support available to part-time students. Financial award application deadline: 2/1. *Faculty research:* Molecular biology, microbial genetics, animal behavior, tropical ecology, plant systematics. *Unit head:* Dr. Teresa Thiel, Director of Graduate Studies, 314-516-6200, Fax: 314-516-6233, E-mail: thiel@umsl.edu. *Application contact:* 314-516-5458, Fax: 314-516-6996, E-mail: gradadm@umsl.edu.
Website: http://www.umsl.edu/divisions/artscience/biology/

The University of Montana, Graduate School, College of Health Professions and Biomedical Sciences, Skaggs School of Pharmacy, Department of Biomedical and Pharmaceutical Sciences, Missoula, MT 59812-0002. Offers biomedical sciences (PhD); medicinal chemistry (MS, PhD); molecular and cellular toxicology (MS, PhD); neuroscience (PhD); pharmaceutical sciences (MS). *Accreditation:* ACPE. *Degree requirements:* For master's, oral defense of thesis; for doctorate, research dissertation defense. *Entrance requirements:* For master's and doctorate, GRE General Test. Additional exam requirements/recommendations for international students: Required—TOEFL (minimum score 540 paper-based). *Application deadline:* For fall admission, 3/1 priority date for domestic and international students. Applications are processed on a rolling basis. Application fee: $45. Electronic applications accepted. *Financial support:* Teaching assistantships with full and partial tuition reimbursements, Federal Work-Study, scholarships/grants, and tuition waivers (full and partial) available. Financial award application deadline: 3/1. *Faculty research:* Cardiovascular pharmacology, medicinal chemistry, neurosciences, environmental toxicology, pharmacogenetics, cancer. *Unit head:* Dr. Richard Bridges, Chair, 406-243-4972, E-mail: richard.bridges@umontana.edu. *Application contact:* Information Contact, E-mail: gradschl@mso.umt.edu.
Website: http://www.umt.edu/pharmsci/

The University of Montana, Graduate School, College of Humanities and Sciences, Division of Biological Sciences, Missoula, MT 59812-0002. Offers cellular, molecular and microbial biology (PhD), including cellular and developmental biology, microbial evolution and ecology, microbiology and immunology, molecular biology and biochemistry; organismal biology and ecology (MS, PhD); systems ecology (MS, PhD). Terminal master's awarded for partial completion of doctoral program. *Degree requirements:* For master's, thesis; for doctorate, thesis/dissertation. *Entrance requirements:* For master's and doctorate, GRE General Test. Additional exam requirements/recommendations for international students: Required—TOEFL. *Application deadline:* For fall admission, 2/1 priority date for domestic students. Applications are processed on a rolling basis. Application fee: $45. *Financial support:* Research assistantships with full tuition reimbursements, teaching assistantships with full tuition reimbursements, Federal Work-Study, and unspecified assistantships available. Financial award application deadline: 3/1; financial award applicants required to submit FAFSA. *Faculty research:* Biochemistry/microbiology, organismal biology, ecology. *Unit head:* Charles Janson, Chair, 406-243-5122, E-mail: charles.janson@mso.umt.edu. *Application contact:* Information Contact, E-mail: gradschl@mso.umt.edu.

University of Nebraska at Kearney, Graduate Programs, College of Natural and Social Sciences, Department of Biology, Kearney, NE 68849. Offers biology (MS); science/math education (MA Ed). Part-time and evening/weekend programs available. Postbaccalaureate distance learning degree programs offered (no on-campus study). *Degree requirements:* For master's, thesis optional. *Entrance requirements:* For master's, GRE (for thesis option and for online program applicants if undergraduate GPA is below 2.75), letter of interest. Additional exam requirements/recommendations for international students: Required—TOEFL (minimum score 550 paper-based; 79 iBT). Electronic applications accepted. *Faculty research:* Pollution injury, molecular biology-viral gene expression, prairie range condition modeling, evolution of symbiotic nitrogen fixation.

University of Nebraska at Omaha, Graduate Studies, College of Arts and Sciences, Department of Biology, Omaha, NE 68182. Offers MS. Part-time programs available. *Faculty:* 23 full-time (6 women). *Students:* 8 full-time (6 women), 17 part-time (10 women); includes 3 minority (1 Black or African American, non-Hispanic/Latino; 2 Hispanic/Latino), 1 international. Average age 27. 17 applicants, 53% accepted, 4 enrolled. In 2013, 6 master's awarded. *Degree requirements:* For master's, comprehensive exam (for some programs), thesis (for some programs). *Entrance requirements:* For master's, GRE General Test, minimum GPA of 3.0, transcripts, 24 undergraduate biology hours, 3 letters of recommendation, statement of purpose. Additional exam requirements/recommendations for international students: Required—TOEFL, IELTS, PTE. *Application deadline:* For fall admission, 2/15 priority date for domestic students; for spring admission, 10/15 priority date for domestic students; for summer admission, 2/15 for domestic students. Applications are processed on a rolling basis. Application fee: $45. Electronic applications accepted. *Financial support:* In 2013–14, 17 students received support, including 17 teaching assistantships with tuition reimbursements available; fellowships, research assistantships with tuition reimbursements available, Federal Work-Study, institutionally sponsored loans, scholarships/grants, tuition waivers (partial), and unspecified assistantships also available. Support available to part-time students. Financial award application deadline: 3/1; financial award applicants required to submit FAFSA. *Unit head:* Dr. William Tapprich, Chairperson, 402-554-2641. *Application contact:* Dr. Ann Antlfinger, Graduate Program Chair, 402-554-2256, E-mail: graduate@unomaha.edu.

University of Nebraska–Lincoln, Graduate College, College of Agricultural Sciences and Natural Resources, School of Veterinary Medicine and Biomedical Sciences, Lincoln, NE 68588. Offers veterinary science (MS). MS, PhD offered jointly with University of Nebraska Medical Center. Postbaccalaureate distance learning degree programs offered (minimal on-campus study). *Degree requirements:* For master's, thesis optional; for doctorate, comprehensive exam, thesis/dissertation. *Entrance requirements:* For master's, GRE General Test; for doctorate, GRE General Test, MCAT, or VCAT. Additional exam requirements/recommendations for international students: Required—TOEFL (minimum score 550 paper-based). Electronic applications accepted. *Faculty research:* Virology, immunobiology, molecular biology, mycotoxins, ocular degeneration.

University of Nebraska–Lincoln, Graduate College, College of Arts and Sciences, School of Biological Sciences, Lincoln, NE 68588. Offers MA, MS, PhD. *Degree requirements:* For master's, thesis optional; for doctorate, comprehensive exam, thesis/dissertation. *Entrance requirements:* For master's and doctorate, GRE General Test. Additional exam requirements/recommendations for international students: Required—TOEFL (minimum score 550 paper-based). Electronic applications accepted. *Faculty research:* Behavior, botany, and zoology; ecology and evolutionary biology; genetics; cellular and molecular biology; microbiology.

University of Nebraska Medical Center, Biomedical Research Training Program, Omaha, NE 68198. Offers MD/PhD. *Entrance requirements:* Additional exam requirements/recommendations for international students: Required—TOEFL (minimum score 600 paper-based). Electronic applications accepted. *Expenses: Required fees:* $300 per semester. Tuition and fees vary according to program. *Faculty research:* Neuroscience, cancer, cardiovascular immunology, genetics.

University of Nebraska Medical Center, Medical Sciences Interdepartmental Area, Omaha, NE 68198-7810. Offers MS, PhD. Part-time programs available. Terminal master's awarded for partial completion of doctoral program. *Degree requirements:* For master's, comprehensive exam, thesis; for doctorate, comprehensive exam, thesis/dissertation. *Entrance requirements:* For master's and doctorate, GRE General Test. Additional exam requirements/recommendations for international students: Required—TOEFL (minimum score 550 paper-based). *Expenses: Required fees:* $300 per semester. Tuition and fees vary according to program. *Faculty research:* Molecular genetics, oral biology, veterinary pathology, newborn medicine, immunology.

University of Nevada, Las Vegas, Graduate College, College of Science, School of Life Sciences, Las Vegas, NV 89154-4004. Offers biological sciences (MS, PhD). Part-time programs available. *Faculty:* 11 full-time (3 women), 2 part-time/adjunct (0 women). *Students:* 32 full-time (18 women), 6 part-time (1 woman); includes 12 minority (1 Black or African American, non-Hispanic/Latino; 1 Asian, non-Hispanic/Latino; 6 Hispanic/Latino; 1 Native Hawaiian or other Pacific Islander, non-Hispanic/Latino; 3 Two or more races, non-Hispanic/Latino), 3 international. Average age 31. 34 applicants, 50% accepted, 11 enrolled. In 2013, 4 master's, 6 doctorates awarded. *Degree requirements:*

Biological and Biomedical Sciences—General

For master's, thesis, oral exam; for doctorate, one foreign language, comprehensive exam, thesis/dissertation. *Entrance requirements:* For master's and doctorate, GRE General Test. Additional exam requirements/recommendations for international students: Required—TOEFL (minimum score 550 paper-based; 80 iBT), IELTS (minimum score 7). *Application deadline:* For fall admission, 1/15 for domestic students, 5/1 for international students; for spring admission, 10/1 for international students. Application fee: $60 ($95 for international students). Electronic applications accepted. *Expenses:* Tuition, state resident: full-time $4752; part-time $264 per credit. Tuition, nonresident: full-time $18,662; part-time $554.50 per credit. *International tuition:* $18,952 full-time. *Required fees:* $532; $12 per credit. $266 per semester. One-time fee: $35. Tuition and fees vary according to course load and program. *Financial support:* In 2013–14, 33 students received support, including 2 fellowships with full tuition reimbursements available (averaging $15,000 per year), 6 research assistantships with partial tuition reimbursements available (averaging $11,639 per year), 25 teaching assistantships with partial tuition reimbursements available (averaging $16,230 per year); institutionally sponsored loans, scholarships/grants, health care benefits, and unspecified assistantships also available. Financial award application deadline: 3/1. *Faculty research:* Environmental and medical microbiology; biodiversity, evolution, and ecological sustainability; cell and molecular biology; integrative physiology. *Total annual research expenditures:* $3.7 million. *Unit head:* Dr. Dennis Bazylinski, Chair, 702-895-3399, Fax: 702-895-3956, E-mail: dennis.bazylinski@unlv.edu. *Application contact:* Graduate College Admissions Evaluator, 702-895-3320, Fax: 702-895-4180, E-mail: gradcollege@unlv.edu.
Website: http://sols.unlv.edu/

University of Nevada, Reno, Graduate School, College of Science, Department of Biology, Reno, NV 89557. Offers MS. *Degree requirements:* For master's, thesis optional. *Entrance requirements:* For master's, GRE General Test, minimum GPA of 2.75. Additional exam requirements/recommendations for international students: Required—TOEFL (minimum score 500 paper-based; 61 iBT), IELTS (minimum score 6). Electronic applications accepted. *Faculty research:* Gene expression, stress protein genes, secretory proteins, conservation biology, behavioral ecology.

University of New Brunswick Fredericton, School of Graduate Studies, Faculty of Science, Department of Biology, Fredericton, NB E3B 5A3, Canada. Offers M Sc, PhD. Part-time programs available. *Faculty:* 25 full-time (6 women), 56 part-time/adjunct (17 women). *Students:* 47 full-time (28 women), 5 part-time (3 women). In 2013, 10 master's, 1 doctorate awarded. *Degree requirements:* For master's, thesis; for doctorate, thesis/dissertation. *Entrance requirements:* For master's, minimum GPA of 3.0; undergraduate degree (B Sc or equivalent preferred); for doctorate, minimum GPA of 3.0; undergraduate and/or master's degree in related discipline. Additional exam requirements/recommendations for international students: Required—TWE (minimum score 4), TOEFL (minimum score 600 paper-based) or IELTS (minimum score 7). *Application deadline:* For fall admission, 3/1 for domestic students. Applications are processed on a rolling basis. Application fee: $50 Canadian dollars. Electronic applications accepted. *Financial support:* In 2013–14, 112 research assistantships with tuition reimbursements, 51 teaching assistantships were awarded; fellowships also available. *Faculty research:* Evolutionary biology, aquatic ecology, wildlife and conservation biology, marine biology, algae and plant biology. *Unit head:* Dr. Les C. Cwynar, Director of Graduate Studies, 506-452-6197, Fax: 506-453-3583, E-mail: biodogs@unb.ca. *Application contact:* Heidi Stewart, Graduate Secretary, 506-458-7488, E-mail: scigrad@unb.ca.
Website: http://go.unb.ca/gradprograms

University of New Brunswick Saint John, Department of Biology, Saint John, NB E2L 4L5, Canada. Offers biology (M Sc, PhD). Part-time programs available. *Faculty:* 14 full-time (1 woman). *Students:* 41 full-time (23 women), 4 part-time (2 women). In 2013, 8 master's, 1 doctorate awarded. *Degree requirements:* For master's, thesis; for doctorate, comprehensive exam, thesis/dissertation. *Entrance requirements:* For master's, B Sc, minimum GPA of 3.0; for doctorate, M Sc, minimum GPA of 3.0. Additional exam requirements/recommendations for international students: Required—TOEFL (minimum score 600 paper-based), TWE (minimum score 4). *Application deadline:* For fall admission, 2/15 for domestic and international students. Applications are processed on a rolling basis. Application fee: $50 Canadian dollars. Electronic applications accepted. *Financial support:* In 2013–14, 32 fellowships, 41 research assistantships, 83 teaching assistantships were awarded; scholarships/grants and unspecified assistantships also available. *Faculty research:* Marine and environmental biology (including assessing impacts of anthropogenic stressors on aquatic and terrestrial systems using molecular through ecological endpoints), evolution, natural products chemistry. *Unit head:* Dr. Kate Frego, Director of Graduate Studies, 506-648-5566, Fax: 506-648-5811, E-mail: frego@unb.ca. *Application contact:* Kim Banks, Secretary, 506-648-5605, Fax: 506-648-5811, E-mail: kbanks@unb.ca.
Website: http://go.unb.ca/gradprograms

University of New England, College of Arts and Sciences, Programs in Professional Science, Biddeford, ME 04005-9526. Offers MS. *Faculty:* 7 full-time (2 women). *Students:* 6 full-time (1 woman), 1 part-time (0 women); includes 2 minority (both Two or more races, non-Hispanic/Latino). Average age 23. 9 applicants, 56% accepted, 5 enrolled. *Degree requirements:* For master's, thesis. *Entrance requirements:* For master's, GRE. *Application deadline:* For fall admission, 2/1 for domestic students. Application fee: $40. *Financial support:* Application deadline: 5/1; applicants required to submit FAFSA. *Unit head:* Dr. A. Christine Brown, Chair/Professor, 207-602-2617, E-mail: sbrown@une.edu. *Application contact:* Dr. Cynthia Forrest, Vice President for Student Affairs, 207-221-4225, Fax: 207-523-1925, E-mail: gradadmissions@une.edu.
Website: http://www.une.edu/cas/biology/graduate/index.cfm

University of New Hampshire, Graduate School, College of Life Sciences and Agriculture, Department of Biological Sciences, Durham, NH 03824. Offers animal science (MS); plant biology (MS, PhD); zoology (MS, PhD). Part-time programs available. *Faculty:* 27 full-time (4 women). *Students:* 24 full-time (19 women), 37 part-time (20 women); includes 5 minority (1 Asian, non-Hispanic/Latino; 2 Hispanic/Latino; 2 Two or more races, non-Hispanic/Latino), 4 international. Average age 31. 64 applicants, 22% accepted, 12 enrolled. In 2013, 17 master's, 12 doctorates awarded. *Degree requirements:* For doctorate, thesis/dissertation. *Entrance requirements:* For master's and doctorate, GRE General Test. Additional exam requirements/recommendations for international students: Required—TOEFL (minimum score 550 paper-based; 80 iBT). *Application deadline:* For fall admission, 6/1 for domestic students, 4/1 for international students; for spring admission, 12/1 for domestic students. Applications are processed on a rolling basis. Application fee: $65. Electronic applications accepted. *Expenses:* Tuition, state resident: full-time $13,500; part-time $750 per credit hour. Tuition, nonresident: full-time $26,200; part-time $1100 per credit hour. *Required fees:* $1741; $435.25 per term. Tuition and fees vary according to course level, course load, campus/location and program. *Financial support:* In 2013–14, 40 students received support, including 3 fellowships, 11 research assistantships, 25 teaching assistantships. *Unit head:* Chris Neefus, Dean, 603-862-1990. *Application contact:* Diane Lavalliere, Administrative Assistant, 603-862-2100, Fax: 603-862-0275, E-mail: grad.school@unh.edu.
Website: http://www.biolsci.unh.edu/

University of New Mexico, Graduate School, College of Arts and Sciences, Department of Biology, Albuquerque, NM 87131. Offers MS, PhD. *Faculty:* 55 full-time (16 women), 8 part-time/adjunct (5 women). *Students:* 90 full-time (58 women), 28 part-time (13 women); includes 28 minority (1 American Indian or Alaska Native, non-Hispanic/Latino; 6 Asian, non-Hispanic/Latino; 21 Hispanic/Latino), 9 international. Average age 32. 88 applicants, 23% accepted, 19 enrolled. In 2013, 6 master's, 9 doctorates awarded. *Degree requirements:* For master's, comprehensive exam, thesis optional; for doctorate, comprehensive exam, thesis/dissertation. *Entrance requirements:* For master's and doctorate, GRE General Test, minimum GPA of 3.2, letters of recommendation. Additional exam requirements/recommendations for international students: Required—TOEFL (minimum score 550 paper-based; 79 iBT). *Application deadline:* For fall admission, 1/3 priority date for domestic and international students. Applications are processed on a rolling basis. Application fee: $50. Electronic applications accepted. *Financial support:* In 2013–14, 94 students received support, including 5 fellowships with full tuition reimbursements available (averaging $13,267 per year), 50 research assistantships with full tuition reimbursements available (averaging $12,045 per year), 56 teaching assistantships with full tuition reimbursements available (averaging $11,214 per year); Federal Work-Study, scholarships/grants, health care benefits, and unspecified assistantships also available. Financial award application deadline: 1/3; financial award applicants required to submit FAFSA. *Faculty research:* Aquatic ecology, behavioral ecology, botany, cell biology, comparative biology, conservation biology, developmental biology, ecology, evolutionary biology, genetics, genomics, global change biology, immunology, invertebrate biology, mathematical biology, microbiology, molecular evolution, paleobiology, parasitology, physiological ecology, plant biology, systematics, vertebrate biology. *Total annual research expenditures:* $10.8 million. *Unit head:* Dr. Robert D. Miller, Chair, 505-277-2496, Fax: 505-277-0304, E-mail: rdmiller@unm.edu. *Application contact:* Cheryl Martin, Graduate Program Coordinator, 505-277-1712, Fax: 505-277-0304, E-mail: cherylm@unm.edu.
Website: http://biology.unm.edu/

University of New Mexico, School of Medicine, Program in Biomedical Sciences, Albuquerque, NM 87131-5196. Offers biochemistry and molecular biology (MS, PhD); cell biology and physiology (MS, PhD); clinical and translational science (Certificate); molecular genetics and microbiology (MS, PhD); neuroscience (MS, PhD); pathology (MS, PhD); toxicology (MS, PhD); university science teaching (Certificate). Part-time programs available. *Students:* 73 full-time (39 women), 14 part-time (9 women); includes 24 minority (1 Black or African American, non-Hispanic/Latino; 1 American Indian or Alaska Native, non-Hispanic/Latino; 2 Asian, non-Hispanic/Latino; 17 Hispanic/Latino; 1 Native Hawaiian or other Pacific Islander, non-Hispanic/Latino; 2 Two or more races, non-Hispanic/Latino), 16 international. Average age 29. 89 applicants, 20% accepted, 17 enrolled. In 2013, 7 master's, 17 doctorates awarded. Terminal master's awarded for partial completion of doctoral program. *Degree requirements:* For master's, thesis; for doctorate, comprehensive exam, thesis/dissertation, qualifying exam at the end of year 1/core curriculum. *Entrance requirements:* For master's and doctorate, GRE General Test, minimum undergraduate GPA of 3.0. Additional exam requirements/recommendations for international students: Required—TOEFL. *Application deadline:* For fall admission, 3/1 priority date for domestic and international students. Applications are processed on a rolling basis. Application fee: $50. Electronic applications accepted. *Financial support:* In 2013–14, 94 students received support, including 28 fellowships with full and partial tuition reimbursements available (averaging $22,000 per year), 73 research assistantships with full tuition reimbursements available (averaging $23,000 per year), 8 teaching assistantships (averaging $2,800 per year); career-related internships or fieldwork, Federal Work-Study, institutionally sponsored loans, scholarships/grants, traineeships, health care benefits, and unspecified assistantships also available. Financial award application deadline: 1/1; financial award applicants required to submit FAFSA. *Faculty research:* Infectious disease/immunity, cancer biology, cardiovascular and metabolic diseases, brain and behavioral illness, environmental health. *Unit head:* Dr. Helen J. Hathaway, Program Director, 505-272-1887, Fax: 505-272-2412, E-mail: hhathaway@salud.unm.edu. *Application contact:* Mary Fenton, Admissions Coordinator, 505-272-1887, Fax: 505-272-2412, E-mail: mfenton@salud.unm.edu.
Website: http://hsc.unm.edu/research/brep/bsgpabout.shtm

University of New Orleans, Graduate School, College of Sciences, Department of Biological Sciences, New Orleans, LA 70148. Offers MS, PhD. *Degree requirements:* For master's, one foreign language, thesis. *Entrance requirements:* For master's, GRE General Test. Additional exam requirements/recommendations for international students: Required—TOEFL (minimum score 550 paper-based; 79 iBT), IELTS (minimum score 6.5). Electronic applications accepted. *Faculty research:* Biochemistry, genetics, vertebrate and invertebrate systematics and ecology, cell and mammalian physiology, morphology.

The University of North Carolina at Chapel Hill, Graduate School, College of Arts and Sciences, Department of Biology, Chapel Hill, NC 27599. Offers botany (MA, MS, PhD); cell biology, development, and physiology (MA, MS, PhD); cell motility and cytoskeleton (PhD); ecology and behavior (MA, MS, PhD); genetics and molecular biology (MA, MS, PhD); morphology, systematics, and evolution (MA, MS, PhD). Terminal master's awarded for partial completion of doctoral program. *Degree requirements:* For master's, comprehensive exam, thesis (for some programs); for doctorate, comprehensive exam, thesis/dissertation. *Entrance requirements:* For master's, GRE General Test, GRE Subject Test, 2 semesters of calculus or statistics; 2 semesters of physics, organic chemistry; 3 semesters of biology; for doctorate, GRE General Test, GRE Subject Test, 2 semesters calculus or statistics, 2 semesters physics, organic chemistry, 3 semesters of biology. Additional exam requirements/recommendations for international students: Required—TOEFL (minimum score 550 paper-based). Electronic applications accepted. *Faculty research:* Gene expression, biomechanics, yeast genetics, plant ecology, plant molecular biology.

The University of North Carolina at Chapel Hill, School of Medicine and Graduate School, Graduate Programs in Medicine, Chapel Hill, NC 27599. Offers allied health sciences (MPT, MS, Au D, DPT, PhD), including human movement science (MS, PhD), occupational science (MS, PhD), physical therapy (MPT, MS, DPT), rehabilitation counseling and psychology (MS), speech and hearing sciences (MS, Au D, PhD); biochemistry and biophysics (MS, PhD); bioinformatics and computational biology (PhD); biomedical engineering (MS, PhD); cell and developmental biology (PhD); cell and molecular physiology (PhD); genetics and molecular biology (PhD); microbiology and immunology (MS, PhD), including immunology, microbiology; neurobiology (PhD); pathology and laboratory medicine (PhD), including experimental pathology; pharmacology (PhD); MD/PhD. Postbaccalaureate distance learning degree programs offered. Terminal master's awarded for partial completion of doctoral program. *Degree requirements:* For master's, comprehensive exam; for doctorate, thesis/dissertation. Electronic applications accepted. *Expenses:* Contact institution.

The University of North Carolina at Charlotte, The Graduate School, College of Liberal Arts and Sciences, Department of Biological Sciences, Charlotte, NC 28223-0001. Offers MA, MS, PhD. Part-time and evening/weekend programs available. *Faculty:* 23 full-time (9 women). *Students:* 20 full-time (10 women), 20 part-time (13 women); includes 4 minority (1 Black or African American, non-Hispanic/Latino; 1

Hispanic/Latino; 2 Two or more races, non-Hispanic/Latino), 6 international. Average age 29. 40 applicants, 45% accepted, 10 enrolled. In 2013, 8 master's, 8 doctorates awarded. Terminal master's awarded for partial completion of doctoral program. *Degree requirements:* For master's, thesis, 30-32 semester hours with minimum GPA of 3.0; for doctorate, thesis/dissertation. *Entrance requirements:* For master's, GRE General Test, minimum GPA of 3.0 in undergraduate major, 2.75 overall; for doctorate, GRE General Test, minimum GPA of 3.5 in biology; 3.0 in chemistry, math, and overall. Additional exam requirements/recommendations for international students: Required—TOEFL (minimum score 557 paper-based; 83 iBT). *Application deadline:* For fall admission, 1/15 for domestic and international students; for spring admission, 7/1 for domestic and international students. Application fee: $75. Electronic applications accepted. *Expenses:* Tuition, state resident: full-time $3522. Tuition, nonresident: full-time $16,051. *Required fees:* $2585. Tuition and fees vary according to course load and program. *Financial support:* In 2013–14, 28 students received support, including 4 fellowships (averaging $24,667 per year), 4 research assistantships (averaging $5,986 per year), 20 teaching assistantships (averaging $8,675 per year); career-related internships or fieldwork, institutionally sponsored loans, and scholarships/grants also available. Support available to part-time students. Financial award application deadline: 4/1; financial award applicants required to submit FAFSA. *Faculty research:* The role of the neuropeptide substance P in microbially induced central nervous system (CNS) inflammation, the mechanism of enhanced metastasis induced by arthritis, the use of plant-derived vaccines. *Total annual research expenditures:* $2 million. *Unit head:* Dr. Martin G. Klotz, Chair, 704-687-8686, Fax: 704-687-3128, E-mail: chknobla@uncc.edu. *Application contact:* Kathy B. Giddings, Director of Graduate Admissions, 704-687-5503, Fax: 704-687-1668, E-mail: gradadm@uncc.edu.
Website: http://biology.uncc.edu/graduate-programs

The University of North Carolina at Greensboro, Graduate School, College of Arts and Sciences, Department of Biology, Greensboro, NC 27412-5001. Offers MS. *Degree requirements:* For master's, thesis. *Entrance requirements:* For master's, GRE General Test, GRE Subject Test. Additional exam requirements/recommendations for international students: Required—TOEFL. Electronic applications accepted. *Faculty research:* Environmental biology, biochemistry, animal ecology, vertebrate reproduction.

The University of North Carolina Wilmington, College of Arts and Sciences, Department of Biology and Marine Biology, Wilmington, NC 28403-3297. Offers biology (MS); marine biology (MS, PhD). Part-time programs available. *Faculty:* 29 full-time (9 women). *Students:* 5 full-time (4 women), 67 part-time (34 women); includes 5 minority (1 Asian, non-Hispanic/Latino; 4 Hispanic/Latino), 2 international. Average age 28. 76 applicants, 25% accepted, 18 enrolled. In 2013, 13 master's, 5 doctorates awarded. *Degree requirements:* For master's, comprehensive exam, thesis; for doctorate, comprehensive exam, thesis/dissertation. *Entrance requirements:* For master's, GRE General Test, GRE Subject Test, minimum B average in undergraduate major; for doctorate, GRE General Test, minimum B average in undergraduate major and graduate courses. Additional exam requirements/recommendations for international students: Required—TOEFL (minimum score 550 paper-based; 79 iBT), IELTS (minimum score 6.5). *Application deadline:* For fall admission, 3/15 for domestic students. Applications are processed on a rolling basis. Application fee: $60. Electronic applications accepted. *Expenses:* Tuition, state resident: full-time $4163. Tuition, nonresident: full-time $16,098. *Financial support:* In 2013–14, 24 research assistantships with full and partial tuition reimbursements (averaging $14,000 per year), 36 teaching assistantships with full and partial tuition reimbursements (averaging $14,000 per year) were awarded; career-related internships or fieldwork and Federal Work-Study also available. Support available to part-time students. Financial award application deadline: 3/15. *Faculty research:* Ecology, physiology, cell and molecular biology, systematics, biomechanics. *Total annual research expenditures:* $3.1 million. *Unit head:* Dr. Chris Finelli, Chair, 910-962-3487, E-mail: finellic@uncw.edu. *Application contact:* Dr. Stephen Kinsey, Graduate Coordinator, 910-962-7398, Fax: 910-962-4066, E-mail: kinseys@uncw.edu.
Website: http://www.uncw.edu/bio/graduate.html

University of North Dakota, Graduate School, College of Arts and Sciences, Department of Biology, Grand Forks, ND 58202. Offers botany (MS, PhD); ecology (MS, PhD); entomology (MS, PhD); environmental biology (MS, PhD); fisheries/wildlife (MS, PhD); genetics (MS, PhD); zoology (MS, PhD). Terminal master's awarded for partial completion of doctoral program. *Degree requirements:* For master's, thesis, final exam; for doctorate, comprehensive exam, thesis/dissertation, final exam. *Entrance requirements:* For master's, GRE General Test, GRE Subject Test, minimum GPA of 3.0; for doctorate, GRE General Test, GRE Subject Test, minimum GPA of 3.5. Additional exam requirements/recommendations for international students: Required—TOEFL (minimum score 550 paper-based; 79 iBT), IELTS (minimum score 6.5). Electronic applications accepted. *Faculty research:* Population biology, wildlife ecology, RNA processing, hormonal control of behavior.

University of Northern Colorado, Graduate School, College of Natural and Health Sciences, School of Biological Sciences, Program in Biology, Greeley, CO 80639. Offers MS. Part-time programs available. *Degree requirements:* For master's, comprehensive exam. *Entrance requirements:* For master's, GRE General Test, 3 letters of recommendation. Electronic applications accepted.

University of Northern Iowa, Graduate College, College of Humanities, Arts and Sciences, Department of Biology, Program in Biology, Cedar Falls, IA 50614. Offers MA, MS. *Students:* 17 full-time (6 women), 5 part-time (0 women). 29 applicants, 34% accepted, 7 enrolled. In 2013, 5 master's awarded. *Degree requirements:* For master's, comprehensive exam, thesis. Application fee: $50 ($70 for international students). *Unit head:* Dr. David Saunders, Coordinator, 319-273-2456, E-mail: david.saunders@uni.edu. *Application contact:* Laurie S. Russell, Record Analyst, 319-273-2623, Fax: 319-273-2885, E-mail: laurie.russell@uni.edu.
Website: http://www.grad.uni.edu/degrees-programs/programs/biology-ms

University of North Florida, College of Arts and Sciences, Department of Biology, Jacksonville, FL 32224. Offers MA, MS. Part-time programs available. *Faculty:* 21 full-time (7 women), 1 (woman) part-time/adjunct. *Students:* 18 full-time (14 women), 21 part-time (12 women); includes 9 minority (1 Black or African American, non-Hispanic/Latino; 1 Asian, non-Hispanic/Latino; 4 Hispanic/Latino; 3 Two or more races, non-Hispanic/Latino). Average age 28. 37 applicants, 46% accepted, 11 enrolled. In 2013, 19 master's awarded. *Degree requirements:* For master's, thesis (for some programs). *Entrance requirements:* For master's, GRE General Test, minimum GPA of 3.0 in last 60 hours, letters of recommendation. Additional exam requirements/recommendations for international students: Required—TOEFL (minimum score 570 paper-based). Application fee: $30. Electronic applications accepted. *Expenses:* Tuition, state resident: full-time $9794; part-time $408.10 per credit hour. Tuition, nonresident: full-time $22,383; part-time $932.61 per credit hour. *Required fees:* $2020; $84.20 per credit hour. Tuition and fees vary according to course load and program. *Financial support:* In 2013–14, 8 students received support, including 2 research assistantships (averaging $1,388 per year), 8 teaching assistantships (averaging $6,002 per year); Federal Work-Study, scholarships/grants, and unspecified assistantships also available. Support available to part-time students. Financial award application deadline: 4/1; financial award applicants required to submit FAFSA. *Total annual research expenditures:* $629,633. *Unit head:* Dr. Daniel Moon, Chair, 904-620-2239, Fax: 904-620-3885, E-mail: dmoon@unf.edu. *Application contact:* Dr. Amanda Pascale, Director, The Graduate School, 904-620-1360, Fax: 904-620-1362, E-mail: graduateschool@unf.edu.
Website: http://www.unf.edu/coas/biology/

University of North Texas, Robert B. Toulouse School of Graduate Studies, Denton, TN 76203-5017. Offers accounting (MS, PhD); applied anthropology (MA, MS); applied behavior analysis (Certificate); applied technology and performance improvement (M Ed, MS, PhD); art education (MA, PhD); art history (MA); art museum education (Certificate); arts leadership (Certificate); audiology (Au D); behavior analysis (MS); biochemistry and molecular biology (MS, PhD); biology (MA, MS, PhD); business (PhD); business computer information systems (PhD); chemistry (MS, PhD); clinical psychology (PhD); communication studies (MA, MS); computer engineering (MS); computer science (MS); computer science and engineering (PhD); counseling (M Ed, MS, PhD), including clinical mental health counseling (MS), college and university counseling (M Ed, MS), elementary school counseling (M Ed, MS), secondary school counseling (M Ed, MS); counseling psychology (PhD); creative writing (MA); criminal justice (MS); curriculum and instruction (M Ed, PhD), including curriculum studies (PhD), early childhood studies (PhD), language and literacy studies (PhD); decision sciences (MBA); design (MA, MFA), including fashion design (MFA), innovation studies, interior design (MFA); early childhood studies (MS); economics (MS); educational leadership (M Ed, Ed D, PhD); educational psychology (MS), including family studies, gifted and talented (MS, PhD), human development, learning and cognition, research, measurement and evaluation; educational research (PhD), including gifted and talented (MS, PhD), human development and family studies, psychological aspects of sports and exercise, research, measurement and statistics; electrical engineering (MS); emergency management (MPA); engineering systems (MS); English (MA, PhD); environmental science (MS, PhD); experimental psychology (PhD); finance (MBA, MS, PhD); financial management (MPA); French (MA); health psychology and behavioral medicine (PhD); health services management (MBA); higher education (M Ed, Ed D, PhD); history (MA, MS, PhD), including European history (PhD), military history (PhD), United States history (PhD); hospitality management (MS); human resources management (MPA); information science (MS, PhD); information technologies (MBA); information technology and decision sciences (MS); interdisciplinary studies (MA, MS); international sustainable tourism (MS); jazz studies (MM); journalism (MA, MJ, Graduate Certificate), including interactive and virtual digital communication (Graduate Certificate), narrative journalism (Graduate Certificate), public relations (Graduate Certificate); kinesiology (MS); learning technologies (MS, PhD); library science (MS); local government management (MPA); logistics and supply chain management (MBA, PhD); long-term care, senior housing, and aging services (MA, MS); management science (PhD); marketing (MBA, PhD); materials science and engineering (MS, PhD); mathematics (MA, PhD); merchandising (MS); music (MA, MM Ed, PhD), including ethnomusicology (MA), music education (MM Ed, PhD), music theory (MA, PhD), musicology (MA, PhD), performance (MA); nonprofit management (MPA); operations and supply chain management (MBA); performance (MM, DMA); philosophy (MA, PhD); physics (MS, PhD); political science (MA, MS, PhD); public administration and management (PhD), including emergency management, nonprofit management, public financial management, urban management; radio, television and film (MA, MFA); recreation, event and sport management (MS); rehabilitation counseling (MS, Certificate); sociology (MA, MS, PhD); Spanish (MA); special education (M Ed, PhD), including autism intervention (PhD), emotional/behavioral disorders (PhD), mild/moderate disabilities (PhD); speech-language pathology (MA, MS); strategic management (MBA); studio art (MFA); taxation (MS); teaching (M Ed); MBA/MS; MS/MPH; MSES/MBA. Part-time and evening/weekend programs available. Postbaccalaureate distance learning degree programs offered. *Faculty:* 661 full-time (213 women), 240 part-time/adjunct (144 women). *Students:* 3,106 full-time (1,620 women), 3,543 part-time (2,221 women); includes 1,740 minority (533 Black or African American, non-Hispanic/Latino; 15 American Indian or Alaska Native, non-Hispanic/Latino; 286 Asian, non-Hispanic/Latino; 746 Hispanic/Latino; 3 Native Hawaiian or other Pacific Islander, non-Hispanic/Latino; 157 Two or more races, non-Hispanic/Latino), 1,145 international. Average age 32. 6,289 applicants, 43% accepted, 1751 enrolled. In 2013, 1,778 master's, 239 doctorates, 10 other advanced degrees awarded. Terminal master's awarded for partial completion of doctoral program. *Degree requirements:* For master's, variable foreign language requirement, comprehensive exam (for some programs), thesis (for some programs); for doctorate, variable foreign language requirement, comprehensive exam (for some programs), thesis/dissertation; for other advanced degree, variable foreign language requirement, comprehensive exam (for some programs). *Entrance requirements:* For master's and doctorate, GRE, GMAT. Additional exam requirements/recommendations for international students: Required—TOEFL (minimum score 550 paper-based; 79 iBT). *Application deadline:* For fall admission, 7/15 for domestic students, 3/15 for international students; for spring admission, 11/15 for domestic students, 9/15 for international students; for summer admission, 5/1 for domestic students. Applications are processed on a rolling basis. Application fee: $60. Electronic applications accepted. *Financial support:* Fellowships with partial tuition reimbursements, research assistantships with partial tuition reimbursements, teaching assistantships, career-related internships or fieldwork, Federal Work-Study, institutionally sponsored loans, scholarships/grants, health care benefits, and library assistantships available. Support available to part-time students. Financial award applicants required to submit FAFSA. *Unit head:* Mark Wardell, Dean, 940-565-2383, E-mail: mark.wardell@unt.edu. *Application contact:* Toulouse School of Graduate Studies, 940-565-2383, Fax: 940-565-2141, E-mail: gradsch@unt.edu.
Website: http://tsgs.unt.edu/

University of North Texas Health Science Center at Fort Worth, Graduate School of Biomedical Sciences, Fort Worth, TX 76107-2699. Offers anatomy and cell biology (MS, PhD); biochemistry and molecular biology (MS, PhD); biomedical sciences (MS, PhD); biotechnology (MS); forensic genetics (MS); integrative physiology (MS, PhD); medical science (MS); microbiology and immunology (MS, PhD); pharmacology (MS, PhD); science education (MS); DO/MS; DO/PhD. Terminal master's awarded for partial completion of doctoral program. *Degree requirements:* For master's, thesis; for doctorate, thesis/dissertation. *Entrance requirements:* For master's and doctorate, GRE General Test. Additional exam requirements/recommendations for international students: Required—TOEFL. *Expenses:* Contact institution. *Faculty research:* Alzheimer's disease, aging, eye diseases, cancer, cardiovascular disease.

University of Notre Dame, Graduate School, College of Science, Department of Biological Sciences, Notre Dame, IN 46556. Offers aquatic ecology, evolution and environmental biology (MS, PhD); cellular and molecular biology (MS, PhD); genetics (MS, PhD); physiology (MS, PhD); vector biology and parasitology (MS, PhD). Terminal master's awarded for partial completion of doctoral program. *Degree requirements:* For master's, comprehensive exam, thesis; for doctorate, comprehensive exam, thesis/dissertation, candidacy exam. *Entrance requirements:* For master's and doctorate, GRE General Test. Additional exam requirements/recommendations for international students: Required—TOEFL (minimum score 600 paper-based; 80 iBT). Electronic applications accepted. *Faculty research:* Tropical disease, molecular genetics, neurobiology, evolutionary biology, aquatic biology.

Biological and Biomedical Sciences—General

University of Oklahoma, College of Arts and Sciences, Department of Biology, Program in Biology, Norman, OK 73019. Offers bioinformatics (MS, PhD); biology (MS, PhD); natural science (M Nat Sci). *Students:* 14 full-time (5 women), 17 part-time (9 women); includes 1 minority (Asian, non-Hispanic/Latino), 7 international. Average age 26. 23 applicants, 43% accepted, 10 enrolled. In 2013, 7 master's, 3 doctorates awarded. *Degree requirements:* For master's, thesis, course in biostatistics; for doctorate, comprehensive exam, thesis/dissertation, course in biostatistics; 2 semesters as teaching assistant. *Entrance requirements:* For master's and doctorate, GRE, transcripts, 3 letters of recommendation, personal statement. Additional exam requirements/recommendations for international students: Required—TOEFL (minimum score 79 iBT). *Application deadline:* For fall admission, 12/15 for domestic and international students. Application fee: $50 ($100 for international students). Electronic applications accepted. *Expenses:* Tuition, state resident: full-time $4205; part-time $175.20 per credit hour. Tuition, nonresident: full-time $16,205; part-time $675.20 per credit hour. *Required fees:* $2745; $103.85 per credit hour. $126.50 per semester. *Financial support:* In 2013–14, 24 students received support. Scholarships/grants, health care benefits, and unspecified assistantships available. Financial award application deadline: 6/1; financial award applicants required to submit FAFSA. *Faculty research:* Geographical ecology; evolution, cellular and behavioral neurobiology; evolutionary and molecular genetics; evolution of development. *Unit head:* Dr. Randall Hewes, Chair, 405-325-6200, Fax: 405-325-6202, E-mail: biology@ou.edu. *Application contact:* Dr. Rosemary Knapp, Director of Graduate Studies, 405-325-4389, Fax: 405-325-6202, E-mail: biologygrad@ou.edu.
Website: http://biology.ou.edu

University of Oklahoma Health Sciences Center, College of Medicine and Graduate College, Graduate Programs in Medicine, Oklahoma City, OK 73190. Offers biochemistry and molecular biology (MS, PhD), including biochemistry, molecular biology; cell biology (MS, PhD); medical sciences (MS); microbiology and immunology (MS, PhD), including immunology, microbiology; neuroscience (MS, PhD); pathology (PhD); physiology (MS, PhD); psychiatry and behavioral sciences (MS, PhD), including biological psychology; radiological sciences (MS, PhD), including medical radiation physics; MD/PhD. Part-time programs available. *Faculty:* 63 full-time (21 women), 1 part-time/adjunct (0 women). *Students:* 262 full-time (205 women), 92 part-time (44 women); includes 65 minority (5 Black or African American, non-Hispanic/Latino; 5 American Indian or Alaska Native, non-Hispanic/Latino; 23 Asian, non-Hispanic/Latino; 13 Hispanic/Latino; 1 Native Hawaiian or other Pacific Islander, non-Hispanic/Latino; 18 Two or more races, non-Hispanic/Latino), 41 international. Average age 27. 679 applicants, 16% accepted, 5 enrolled. In 2013, 88 master's, 25 doctorates awarded. Terminal master's awarded for partial completion of doctoral program. *Degree requirements:* For doctorate, thesis/dissertation. *Entrance requirements:* For doctorate, GRE General Test, 3 letters of recommendation. Additional exam requirements/recommendations for international students: Required—TOEFL. *Application deadline:* For fall admission, 12/15 for domestic students. Application fee: $25 ($50 for international students). *Expenses:* Contact institution. *Financial support:* In 2013–14, 74 research assistantships (averaging $18,000 per year) were awarded; fellowships, teaching assistantships, career-related internships or fieldwork, Federal Work-Study, institutionally sponsored loans, and tuition waivers (full and partial) also available. Support available to part-time students. *Faculty research:* Behavior and drugs, structure and function of endothelium, genetics and behavior, gene structure and function, action of antibiotics. *Unit head:* Dr. Dewayne Andrews, Executive Dean, 405-271-2265. *Application contact:* Dr. James J. Tomasek, Dean of the Graduate College, 405-271-2085, Fax: 405-271-1155, E-mail: james-tomasek@ouhsc.edu.

University of Oregon, Graduate School, College of Arts and Sciences, Department of Biology, Eugene, OR 97403. Offers ecology and evolution (MA, MS, PhD); marine biology (MA, MS, PhD); molecular, cellular and genetic biology (PhD); neuroscience and development (PhD). Terminal master's awarded for partial completion of doctoral program. *Degree requirements:* For master's, thesis (for some programs); for doctorate, thesis/dissertation. *Entrance requirements:* For master's and doctorate, GRE General Test, minimum GPA of 3.2. Additional exam requirements/recommendations for international students: Required—TOEFL. *Faculty research:* Developmental neurobiology; evolution, population biology, and quantitative genetics; regulation of gene expression; biochemistry of marine organisms.

University of Ottawa, Faculty of Graduate and Postdoctoral Studies, Faculty of Science, Ottawa-Carleton Institute of Biology, Ottawa, ON K1N 6N5, Canada. Offers M Sc, PhD. M Sc, PhD offered jointly with Carleton University. Part-time programs available. *Degree requirements:* For master's, thesis, seminar; for doctorate, comprehensive exam, thesis/dissertation, seminar. *Entrance requirements:* For master's, honors B Sc degree or equivalent, minimum B average; for doctorate, honors B Sc with minimum B+ average or M Sc with minimum B+ average. Electronic applications accepted. *Faculty research:* Physiology/biochemistry, cellular and molecular biology, ecology, behavior and systematics.

University of Pennsylvania, Perelman School of Medicine, Biomedical Graduate Studies, Philadelphia, PA 19104. Offers MS, PhD, MD/PhD, VMD/PhD. *Faculty:* 904. *Students:* 833 full-time (450 women), 35 part-time (20 women); includes 250 minority (37 Black or African American, non-Hispanic/Latino; 2 American Indian or Alaska Native, non-Hispanic/Latino; 163 Asian, non-Hispanic/Latino; 43 Hispanic/Latino; 5 Two or more races, non-Hispanic/Latino), 86 international. Average age 31. 1,215 applicants, 23% accepted, 157 enrolled. In 2013, 104 master's, 92 doctorates awarded. Terminal master's awarded for partial completion of doctoral program. *Degree requirements:* For doctorate, thesis/dissertation. *Entrance requirements:* For doctorate, GRE General Test. Additional exam requirements/recommendations for international students: Required—TOEFL. *Application deadline:* For fall admission, 12/1 priority date for domestic and international students. Applications are processed on a rolling basis. Application fee: $80. Electronic applications accepted. *Expenses:* Contact institution. *Financial support:* In 2013–14, 730 students received support. Fellowships, research assistantships, scholarships/grants, traineeships, and unspecified assistantships available. *Unit head:* Dr. Michael P. Nusbaum, Director, 215-898-1585, E-mail: nusbaum@mail.med.upenn.edu. *Application contact:* Kai Evenson, Admissions Coordinator, 215-746-6349, E-mail: kevenson@mail.med.upenn.edu.
Website: http://www.med.upenn.edu/bgs/

University of Pennsylvania, School of Arts and Sciences, Graduate Group in Biology, Philadelphia, PA 19104. Offers PhD. *Faculty:* 41 full-time (9 women), 6 part-time/adjunct (0 women). *Students:* 49 full-time (25 women); includes 9 minority (5 Asian, non-Hispanic/Latino; 2 Hispanic/Latino; 2 Two or more races, non-Hispanic/Latino), 26 international. 220 applicants, 11% accepted, 8 enrolled. In 2013, 7 doctorates awarded. *Degree requirements:* For doctorate, thesis/dissertation. *Entrance requirements:* For doctorate, GRE General Test, GRE Subject Test. Additional exam requirements/recommendations for international students: Required—TOEFL. *Application deadline:* For fall admission, 12/1 priority date for domestic students. Application fee: $70. Electronic applications accepted. *Financial support:* Fellowships, research assistantships, teaching assistantships, institutionally sponsored loans, scholarships/grants, traineeships, health care benefits, and unspecified assistantships available. Financial award application deadline: 12/15. *Unit head:* Dr. Ralph M. Rosen, Associate Dean for Graduate Studies, 215-898-7156, Fax: 215-573-8068, E-mail: grad-dean@sas.upenn.edu. *Application contact:* Arts and Sciences Graduate Admissions, 215-573-5816, Fax: 215-573-8068, E-mail: gdasadmis@sas.upenn.edu.
Website: http://www.bio.upenn.edu

University of Pittsburgh, Dietrich School of Arts and Sciences, Department of Biological Sciences, Pittsburgh, PA 15260. Offers ecology and evolution (PhD); molecular, cellular, and developmental biology (PhD). *Faculty:* 25 full-time (6 women). *Students:* 68 full-time (32 women); includes 9 minority (2 Black or African American, non-Hispanic/Latino; 1 American Indian or Alaska Native, non-Hispanic/Latino; 4 Asian, non-Hispanic/Latino; 2 Hispanic/Latino), 15 international. Average age 23. 214 applicants, 11% accepted, 14 enrolled. In 2013, 10 doctorates awarded. *Degree requirements:* For doctorate, comprehensive exam, thesis/dissertation, completion of research integrity module. *Entrance requirements:* For doctorate, GRE General Test, GRE Subject Test. Additional exam requirements/recommendations for international students: Required—TOEFL (minimum score 90 iBT). *Application deadline:* For fall admission, 1/3 priority date for domestic students, 12/9 priority date for international students. Applications are processed on a rolling basis. Application fee: $0 ($50 for international students). Electronic applications accepted. *Expenses:* Tuition, state resident: full-time $19,964; part-time $807 per credit. Tuition, nonresident: full-time $32,686; part-time $1337 per credit. *Required fees:* $740; $200. Tuition and fees vary according to program. *Financial support:* In 2013–14, 54 fellowships with full tuition reimbursements (averaging $30,682 per year), 93 research assistantships with full tuition reimbursements (averaging $26,580 per year), 38 teaching assistantships with full tuition reimbursements (averaging $25,659 per year) were awarded; Federal Work-Study, scholarships/grants, traineeships, and health care benefits also available. *Faculty research:* Molecular biology, cell biology, molecular biophysics, developmental biology, ecology and evolution. *Total annual research expenditures:* $1.2 million. *Unit head:* Dr. Paula J. Grabowski, Professor and Chair, 412-624-4350, Fax: 412-624-4759, E-mail: pag4@pitt.edu. *Application contact:* Cathleen M. Barr, Graduate Administrator, 412-624-4268, Fax: 412-624-4759, E-mail: cbarr@pitt.edu.
Website: http://www.biology.pitt.edu/

University of Pittsburgh, Dietrich School of Arts and Sciences, Program in Computational Modeling and Simulation, Pittsburgh, PA 15260. Offers bioengineering (PhD); biological science (PhD); chemical and petroleum engineering (PhD); civil and environmental engineering (PhD); computer science (PhD); economics (PhD); industrial engineering (PhD); mathematics (PhD); mechanical engineering and materials science (PhD); physics and astronomy (PhD); psychology (PhD); statistics (PhD). Part-time programs available. *Faculty:* 4 full-time (0 women). *Students:* 5 full-time (2 women), 1 part-time (0 women), 5 international. Average age 22. 14 applicants, 14% accepted, 2 enrolled. *Degree requirements:* For doctorate, comprehensive exam, thesis/dissertation, preliminary exam. *Entrance requirements:* For doctorate, GRE, statement of purpose, transcripts for all college-level institutions attended, three letters of reference. Additional exam requirements/recommendations for international students: Required—TOEFL (minimum score 90 iBT), IELTS (minimum score 7). *Application deadline:* For fall admission, 2/21 for domestic and international students. Applications are processed on a rolling basis. Application fee: $0 ($50 for international students). Electronic applications accepted. *Expenses:* Tuition, state resident: full-time $19,964; part-time $807 per credit. Tuition, nonresident: full-time $32,686; part-time $1337 per credit. *Required fees:* $740; $200. Tuition and fees vary according to program. *Financial support:* In 2013–14, 5 students received support, including 3 fellowships with tuition reimbursements available (averaging $25,500 per year), 2 research assistantships with tuition reimbursements available (averaging $26,000 per year). *Unit head:* Kathleen Blee, Associate Dean, Graduate Studies and Research, 412-624-3939, Fax: 412-624-6855. *Application contact:* Dave R. Carmen, Administrative Secretary, 412-624-6094, Fax: 412-624-6855, E-mail: drc41@pitt.edu.
Website: http://cmsp.pitt.edu/

University of Pittsburgh, School of Medicine, Graduate Programs in Medicine, Interdisciplinary Biomedical Graduate Program, Pittsburgh, PA 15260. Offers PhD. *Faculty:* 273 full-time (74 women). *Students:* 23 full-time (15 women); includes 5 minority (2 Black or African American, non-Hispanic/Latino; 1 Asian, non-Hispanic/Latino; 2 Hispanic/Latino), 6 international. Average age 25. 517 applicants, 13% accepted, 22 enrolled. *Degree requirements:* For doctorate, comprehensive exam, thesis/dissertation. *Entrance requirements:* For doctorate, GRE General Test, GRE Subject Test, minimum QPA of 3.0. Additional exam requirements/recommendations for international students: Required—TOEFL (minimum score 600 paper-based; 100 iBT), IELTS (minimum score 7). *Application deadline:* For fall admission, 1/1 priority date for domestic and international students. Application fee: $50. Electronic applications accepted. *Expenses:* Tuition, state resident: full-time $19,964; part-time $807 per credit. Tuition, nonresident: full-time $32,686; part-time $1337 per credit. *Required fees:* $740; $200. Tuition and fees vary according to program. *Financial support:* In 2013–14, 23 research assistantships with full tuition reimbursements (averaging $26,010 per year) were awarded; institutionally sponsored loans, scholarships/grants, traineeships, health care benefits, and unspecified assistantships also available. *Faculty research:* Cell biology and molecular physiology, cellular and molecular pathology, immunology, molecular genetics and developmental biology, molecular pharmacology and molecular virology and microbiology. *Unit head:* Dr. John P. Horn, Associate Dean for Graduate Studies, 412-648-8957, Fax: 412-648-1077, E-mail: gradstudies@medschool.pitt.edu. *Application contact:* Graduate Studies Administrator, 412-648-8957, Fax: 412-648-1077, E-mail: gradstudies@medschool.pitt.edu.
Website: http://www.gradbiomed.pitt.edu/

University of Prince Edward Island, Faculty of Science, Charlottetown, PE C1A 4P3, Canada. Offers biology (M Sc); chemistry (M Sc). *Degree requirements:* For master's, thesis. *Entrance requirements:* Additional exam requirements/recommendations for international students: Required—TOEFL (minimum score 550 paper-based; 80 iBT), Canadian Academic English Language Assessment, Michigan English Language Assessment Battery, Canadian Test of English for Scholars and Trainees. *Faculty research:* Ecology and wildlife biology, molecular, genetics and biotechnology, organametallic, bio-organic, supramolecular and synthetic organic chemistry, neurobiology and stoke materials science.

University of Puerto Rico, Mayagüez Campus, Graduate Studies, College of Arts and Sciences, Department of Biology, Mayagüez, PR 00681-9000. Offers MS. Part-time programs available. *Faculty:* 35 full-time (13 women), 2 part-time/adjunct (1 woman). *Students:* 51 full-time (32 women), 13 part-time (5 women). 18 applicants, 83% accepted, 14 enrolled. In 2013, 16 master's awarded. *Degree requirements:* For master's, one foreign language, comprehensive exam, thesis. *Entrance requirements:* For master's, GRE General Test, BS in biology or its equivalent; minimum GPA of 3.0 in biology courses. Additional exam requirements/recommendations for international students: Required—TOEFL. *Application deadline:* For fall admission, 2/15 for domestic and international students; for spring admission, 9/15 for domestic and international students. Applications are processed on a rolling basis. Application fee: $25. *Expenses: Tuition, area resident:* Full-time $2466; part-time $822 per year. *International tuition:* $6371 full-time. *Required fees:* $1095; $1095. Tuition and fees vary according to course level, course load and reciprocity agreements. *Financial support:* In 2013–14, 43

students received support, including 4 research assistantships with tuition reimbursements available (averaging $8,048 per year), 39 teaching assistantships with tuition reimbursements available (averaging $8,968 per year); fellowships with full tuition reimbursements available, Federal Work-Study, institutionally sponsored loans, and unspecified assistantships also available. *Faculty research:* Herpetology, entomology, microbiology, immunology, botany. *Total annual research expenditures:* $2.1 million. *Unit head:* Dr. Nannette Difoot, Director, 787-265-3837, Fax: 787-834-3673, E-mail: nanette.difoot@upr.edu. *Application contact:* Alicia Collazo, Secretary, 787-832-4040 Ext. 3900, Fax: 787-265-1225.
Website: http://biology.uprm.edu

University of Puerto Rico, Medical Sciences Campus, School of Medicine, Division of Graduate Studies, San Juan, PR 00936-5067. Offers MS, PhD. Terminal master's awarded for partial completion of doctoral program. *Degree requirements:* For master's, one foreign language, thesis; for doctorate, one foreign language, comprehensive exam, thesis/dissertation. *Entrance requirements:* For master's and doctorate, GRE General Test, GRE Subject Test, interview, 3 letters of recommendation, minimum GPA of 3.0. Electronic applications accepted. *Expenses:* Contact institution.

University of Puerto Rico, Río Piedras Campus, College of Natural Sciences, Department of Biology, San Juan, PR 00931-3300. Offers ecology/systematics (MS, PhD); evolution/genetics (MS, PhD); molecular/cellular biology (MS, PhD); neuroscience (MS, PhD). Part-time programs available. *Degree requirements:* For master's, one foreign language, comprehensive exam, thesis; for doctorate, one foreign language, comprehensive exam, thesis/dissertation. *Entrance requirements:* For master's, GRE Subject Test, interview, minimum GPA of 3.0, letter of recommendation; for doctorate, GRE Subject Test, interview, master's degree, minimum GPA of 3.0, letter of recommendation. *Faculty research:* Environmental, poblational and systematic biology.

University of Regina, Faculty of Graduate Studies and Research, Faculty of Science, Department of Biology, Regina, SK S4S 0A2, Canada. Offers M Sc, PhD. Part-time programs available. *Faculty:* 15 full-time (3 women), 16 part-time/adjunct (2 women). *Students:* 29 full-time (18 women), 5 part-time (3 women). 28 applicants, 43% accepted. In 2013, 10 master's, 1 doctorate awarded. *Degree requirements:* For master's, thesis; for doctorate, comprehensive exam, thesis/dissertation. *Entrance requirements:* Additional exam requirements/recommendations for international students: Required—TOEFL (minimum score 580 paper-based; 80 iBT), IELTS (minimum score 6.5). *Application deadline:* Applications are processed on a rolling basis. Application fee: $100. Electronic applications accepted. *Expenses: Tuition, area resident:* Full-time $4338 Canadian dollars. *International tuition:* $7338 Canadian dollars full-time. *Required fees:* $449.25 Canadian dollars. *Financial support:* In 2013–14, 13 fellowships (averaging $6,462 per year), 1 research assistantship (averaging $6,000 per year), 10 teaching assistantships (averaging $2,402 per year) were awarded; scholarships/grants also available. Financial award application deadline: 6/15. *Faculty research:* Aquatic and terrestrial ecology, molecular and population genetics, developmental biology, microbiology, plant physiology and morphology. *Unit head:* Dr. Mark Brigham, Department Head, 306-585-4255, Fax: 306-337-2410, E-mail: mark.brigham@uregina.ca. *Application contact:* Dr. Chris Somers, Graduate Program Coordinator, 306-585-4580, Fax: 306-337-2410, E-mail: chris.somers@uregina.ca.
Website: http://www.uregina.ca/science/biology/

University of Rhode Island, Graduate School, College of the Environment and Life Sciences, Department of Biological Sciences, Kingston, RI 02881. Offers MS, PhD. Part-time programs available. *Faculty:* 19 full-time (9 women). *Students:* 82 full-time (50 women), 12 part-time (4 women); includes 6 minority (2 Black or African American, non-Hispanic/Latino; 1 American Indian or Alaska Native, non-Hispanic/Latino; 2 Asian, non-Hispanic/Latino; 1 Two or more races, non-Hispanic/Latino), 13 international. In 2013, 3 master's, 5 doctorates awarded. *Degree requirements:* For master's, comprehensive exam (for some programs), thesis optional; for doctorate, comprehensive exam, thesis/dissertation. *Entrance requirements:* For master's and doctorate, GRE, 2 letters of recommendation. Additional exam requirements/recommendations for international students: Required—TOEFL (minimum score 550 paper-based). *Application deadline:* For fall admission, 4/15 for domestic students, 1/15 for international students. Application fee: $65. Electronic applications accepted. *Expenses:* Tuition, state resident: full-time $11,532; part-time $641 per credit. Tuition, nonresident: full-time $23,606; part-time $1311 per credit. *Required fees:* $1388; $36 per credit. $35 per semester. One-time fee: $130. *Financial support:* In 2013–14, 7 research assistantships with full and partial tuition reimbursements (averaging $15,112 per year), 8 teaching assistantships with full and partial tuition reimbursements (averaging $13,279 per year) were awarded. Financial award application deadline: 1/15; financial award applicants required to submit FAFSA. *Faculty research:* Physiological constraints on predators in the Antarctics, effects of CO2 absorption in salt water particularly as it impacts pteropods. *Total annual research expenditures:* $1.2 million. *Unit head:* Dr. Alison Roberts, Chairperson, 401-874-4098, Fax: 401-874-2065, E-mail: aroberts@uri.edu. *Application contact:* Dr. Scott McWilliams, Graduate Program Director, 401-874-7531, Fax: 401-874-5787, E-mail: srmcwilliams@uri.edu.
Website: http://www.uri.edu/cels/bio/

University of Rochester, School of Arts and Sciences, Department of Biology, Rochester, NY 14627. Offers MS, PhD. *Faculty:* 20 full-time (5 women). *Students:* 52 full-time (22 women), 1 part-time (0 women); includes 4 minority (1 Asian, non-Hispanic/Latino; 1 Hispanic/Latino; 2 Two or more races, non-Hispanic/Latino), 35 international. 89 applicants, 29% accepted, 9 enrolled. In 2013, 7 master's, 4 doctorates awarded. Terminal master's awarded for partial completion of doctoral program. *Degree requirements:* For doctorate, thesis/dissertation, qualifying exam. *Entrance requirements:* For master's and doctorate, GRE General Test, GRE Subject Test (highly recommended). Additional exam requirements/recommendations for international students: Required—TOEFL. *Application deadline:* For fall admission, 1/1 priority date for domestic and international students. Application fee: $60. Electronic applications accepted. *Expenses: Tuition:* Full-time $44,580; part-time $1394 per credit hour. *Required fees:* $492. *Financial support:* Fellowships, research assistantships, teaching assistantships, and tuition scholarships (for PhD students) available. Financial award application deadline: 1/1. *Faculty research:* Molecular, cellular, and developmental biology; genetics, ecology and evolutionary biology. *Unit head:* Gloria Culver, Chair, 585-276-3602. *Application contact:* Cindy Landry, Graduate Program Administrative Assistant, 585-275-7991.
Website: http://www.rochester.edu/College/BIO/graduate.html

University of Rochester, School of Medicine and Dentistry, Graduate Programs in Medicine and Dentistry, Interdepartmental Program in Translational Biomedical Science, Rochester, NY 14627. Offers PhD. *Expenses: Tuition:* Full-time $44,580; part-time $1394 per credit hour. *Required fees:* $492.

University of Saint Joseph, Department of Biology, West Hartford, CT 06117-2700. Offers MS. Part-time programs available. Postbaccalaureate distance learning degree programs offered (no on-campus study). *Degree requirements:* For master's, comprehensive exam, thesis or alternative. *Entrance requirements:* For master's, 2 letters of recommendation. *Application deadline:* Applications are processed on a rolling basis. Application fee: $50. Electronic applications accepted. Application fee is waived when completed online. *Financial support:* Unspecified assistantships available. Support available to part-time students. Financial award applicants required to submit FAFSA. *Unit head:* Dr. Melissa Marcucci, Chair, 860-231-5248, E-mail: mmarcucci@usj.edu. *Application contact:* Graduate Admissions Office, 860-231-5261, E-mail: graduate@usj.edu.
Website: http://www.usj.edu/index.php/academics/schools/school-of-health-natural-sciences/biology

University of San Francisco, College of Arts and Sciences, Biology Program, San Francisco, CA 94117-1080. Offers MS. *Faculty:* 6 full-time (4 women). *Students:* 6 full-time (5 women), 1 (woman) part-time; includes 4 minority (3 Asian, non-Hispanic/Latino; 1 Hispanic/Latino). Average age 25. 23 applicants, 4% accepted, 1 enrolled. In 2013, 3 master's awarded. *Degree requirements:* For master's, thesis. *Entrance requirements:* For master's, GRE General Test, GRE Subject Test, BS in biology or the equivalent. *Application deadline:* For fall admission, 3/15 for domestic students; for spring admission, 10/15 for domestic students. Application fee: $55 ($65 for international students). *Expenses: Tuition:* Full-time $21,150; part-time $1175 per unit. Tuition and fees vary according to course load, campus/location and program. *Financial support:* In 2013–14, 7 students received support. Teaching assistantships, career-related internships or fieldwork, Federal Work-Study, institutionally sponsored loans, and tuition waivers available. Financial award application deadline: 3/2; financial award applicants required to submit FAFSA. *Unit head:* Dr. James Sikes, Chair, 415-422-6755, Fax: 415-422-6363. *Application contact:* Mark Landerghini, Information Contact, 415-422-5101, Fax: 415-422-2217, E-mail: asgraduate@usfca.edu.
Website: http://www.usfca.edu/artsci/biog/

University of Saskatchewan, College of Graduate Studies and Research, College of Arts and Science, Department of Biology, Saskatoon, SK S7N 5A2, Canada. Offers M Sc, PhD. *Degree requirements:* For master's, thesis (for some programs); for doctorate, comprehensive exam (for some programs), thesis/dissertation. *Entrance requirements:* Additional exam requirements/recommendations for international students: Required—TOEFL (minimum score 80 iBT); Recommended—IELTS (minimum score 6.5). Electronic applications accepted. *Expenses: Tuition, area resident:* Full-time $3585 Canadian dollars; part-time $585 Canadian dollars per course. Tuition, nonresident: part-time $877 Canadian dollars per course. *International tuition:* $5377 Canadian dollars full-time. *Required fees:* $889.51 Canadian dollars.

University of Saskatchewan, Western College of Veterinary Medicine and College of Graduate Studies and Research, Graduate Programs in Veterinary Medicine, Department of Veterinary Biomedical Sciences, Saskatoon, SK S7N 5A2, Canada. Offers veterinary anatomy (M Sc); veterinary biomedical sciences (M Vet Sc); veterinary physiological sciences (M Sc, PhD). *Degree requirements:* For master's, thesis; for doctorate, comprehensive exam (for some programs), thesis/dissertation. *Entrance requirements:* Additional exam requirements/recommendations for international students: Required—TOEFL (minimum score 80 iBT); Recommended—IELTS (minimum score 6.5). Electronic applications accepted. *Expenses: Tuition, area resident:* Full-time $3585 Canadian dollars; part-time $585 Canadian dollars per course. Tuition, nonresident: part-time $877 Canadian dollars per course. *International tuition:* $5377 Canadian dollars full-time. *Required fees:* $889.51 Canadian dollars. *Faculty research:* Toxicology, animal reproduction, pharmacology, chloride channels, pulmonary pathobiology.

University of South Alabama, College of Medicine and Graduate School, Interdisciplinary Graduate Program in Basic Medical Sciences, Mobile, AL 36688-0002. Offers PhD. *Faculty:* 33 full-time (7 women). *Students:* 52 full-time (28 women), 2 part-time (both women); includes 8 minority (4 Black or African American, non-Hispanic/Latino; 1 American Indian or Alaska Native, non-Hispanic/Latino; 1 Asian, non-Hispanic/Latino; 2 Hispanic/Latino), 6 international. 42 applicants, 24% accepted, 10 enrolled. In 2013, 7 doctorates awarded. *Degree requirements:* For doctorate, comprehensive exam, thesis/dissertation. *Entrance requirements:* For doctorate, GRE, three semesters or quarters of undergraduate work in physics, general chemistry, organic chemistry, biology, English composition, and mathematics (including statistics and calculus) with minimum GPA of 3.0. Additional exam requirements/recommendations for international students: Required—TOEFL. *Application deadline:* For fall admission, 4/1 for domestic students, 3/31 for international students. Applications are processed on a rolling basis. Application fee: $0. *Expenses:* Contact institution. *Financial support:* Fellowships, research assistantships, and institutionally sponsored loans available. Financial award application deadline: 4/1; financial award applicants required to submit FAFSA. *Faculty research:* Microcirculation, molecular biology, cell biology, growth control. *Unit head:* Dr. Ronald Balczon, Director of College of Medicine Graduate Studies, 251-460-6153, Fax: 251-460-6071, E-mail: rbalzon@usouthal.edu. *Application contact:* Dr. B. Keith Harrison, Dean of the Graduate School, 251-460-6310, Fax: 251-461-1513, E-mail: kharriso@usouthal.edu.
Website: http://www.southalabama.edu/com/

University of South Alabama, Graduate School, College of Arts and Sciences, Department of Biological Sciences, Mobile, AL 36688-0002. Offers MS. Part-time programs available. *Faculty:* 4 full-time (2 women). *Students:* 6 full-time (0 women), 4 part-time (2 women); includes 1 minority (Asian, non-Hispanic/Latino). 12 applicants, 17% accepted, 2 enrolled. In 2013, 7 master's awarded. *Degree requirements:* For master's, one foreign language, comprehensive exam, thesis optional. *Entrance requirements:* For master's, GRE Subject Test, minimum GPA of 3.0. Additional exam requirements/recommendations for international students: Required—TOEFL (minimum score 600 paper-based). *Application deadline:* For fall admission, 7/15 priority date for domestic students, 6/15 for international students; for spring admission, 12/1 for domestic students, 11/1 for international students. Applications are processed on a rolling basis. Application fee: $35. *Expenses:* Tuition, state resident: full-time $8976; part-time $374 per credit hour. Tuition, nonresident: full-time $17,952; part-time $748 per credit hour. *Financial support:* Fellowships, research assistantships, and teaching assistantships available. Support available to part-time students. Financial award application deadline: 4/1. *Faculty research:* Aquatic and marine biology, molecular biochemistry, plant and animal taxonomy. *Unit head:* Dr. John Freeman, Chair, 251-460-6331. *Application contact:* Dr. Brian Axsmith, Graduate Coordinator, 251-460-6331, E-mail: baxsmith@jaguar1.usouthal.edu.
Website: http://www.southalabama.edu/biology

University of South Carolina, The Graduate School, College of Arts and Sciences, Department of Biological Sciences, Columbia, SC 29208. Offers biology (MS, PhD); biology education (IMA, MAT); ecology, evolution and organismal biology (MS, PhD); molecular, cellular, and developmental biology (MS, PhD). IMA and MAT offered in cooperation with the College of Education. Terminal master's awarded for partial completion of doctoral program. *Degree requirements:* For master's, one foreign language, thesis (for some programs); for doctorate, one foreign language, thesis/dissertation. *Entrance requirements:* For master's and doctorate, GRE General Test, minimum GPA of 3.0 in science. Electronic applications accepted. *Faculty research:* Marine ecology, population and evolutionary biology, molecular biology and genetics, development.

University of South Carolina, School of Medicine and The Graduate School, Graduate Programs in Medicine, Columbia, SC 29208. Offers biomedical science (MBS, PhD); genetic counseling (MS); nurse anesthesia (MNA); rehabilitation counseling (MRC,

Biological and Biomedical Sciences—General

Certificate), including psychiatric rehabilitation (Certificate), rehabilitation counseling (MRC). Terminal master's awarded for partial completion of doctoral program. *Degree requirements:* For master's, comprehensive exam, thesis (for some programs), practicum; for doctorate, comprehensive exam, thesis/dissertation. *Entrance requirements:* For master's, doctorate, and Certificate, GRE General Test. Electronic applications accepted. *Expenses:* Contact institution. *Faculty research:* Cardiovascular diseases, oncology, neuroscience, psychiatric rehabilitation, genetics.

University of South Carolina, School of Medicine and The Graduate School, Graduate Programs in Medicine, Graduate Program in Biomedical Science, Doctoral Program in Biomedical Science, Columbia, SC 29208. Offers PhD. *Degree requirements:* For doctorate, comprehensive exam, thesis/dissertation. *Entrance requirements:* For doctorate, GRE General Test. Electronic applications accepted. *Faculty research:* Cancer, neuroscience, cardiovascular, reproductive, immunology.

University of South Carolina, School of Medicine and The Graduate School, Graduate Programs in Medicine, Graduate Program in Biomedical Science, Master's Program in Biomedical Science, Columbia, SC 29208. Offers MBS. *Degree requirements:* For master's, comprehensive exam, thesis. *Entrance requirements:* For master's, GRE General Test. Electronic applications accepted. *Faculty research:* Cardiovascular diseases, oncology, reproductive biology, neuroscience, microbiology.

The University of South Dakota, Graduate School, College of Arts and Sciences, Department of Biology, Vermillion, SD 57069-2390. Offers MA, MS, PhD. *Degree requirements:* For master's, comprehensive exam (for some programs), thesis (for some programs); for doctorate, comprehensive exam, thesis/dissertation. *Entrance requirements:* For master's, GRE Subject Test, GRE General Test, minimum GPA of 2.7; for doctorate, GRE General Test, GRE Subject Test, minimum GPA of 2.7. Additional exam requirements/recommendations for international students: Required—TOEFL (minimum score 550 paper-based; 70 iBT). Electronic applications accepted. *Faculty research:* Evolutionary and ecological informatics, neuroscience, stress physiology.

The University of South Dakota, Graduate School, School of Medicine and Graduate School, Biomedical Sciences Graduate Program, Vermillion, SD 57069-2390. Offers cardiovascular research (MS, PhD); cellular and molecular biology (MS, PhD); molecular microbiology and immunology (MS, PhD); neuroscience (MS, PhD); physiology and pharmacology (MS, PhD). Terminal master's awarded for partial completion of doctoral program. *Degree requirements:* For master's, thesis; for doctorate, comprehensive exam, thesis/dissertation. *Entrance requirements:* For master's and doctorate, GRE General Test, minimum GPA of 3.0. Additional exam requirements/recommendations for international students: Required—TOEFL (minimum score 550 paper-based; 80 iBT), IELTS (minimum score 6). Electronic applications accepted. *Expenses:* Contact institution. *Faculty research:* Molecular biology, microbiology, neuroscience, cellular biology, physiology.

University of Southern California, Graduate School, Dana and David Dornsife College of Letters, Arts and Sciences, Department of Biological Sciences, Los Angeles, CA 90089. Offers biology (MS); computational molecular biology (MS); integrative and evolutionary biology (PhD); marine biology and biological oceanography (MS, PhD), including marine and environmental biology (MS), marine biology and biological oceanography (PhD); molecular and computational biology (PhD), including biology, computational biology and bioinformatics, molecular biology; neurobiology (PhD). Terminal master's awarded for partial completion of doctoral program. *Degree requirements:* For master's, comprehensive exam (for some programs), research paper; for doctorate, thesis/dissertation, qualifying examination, dissertation defense. *Entrance requirements:* For master's, GRE, 3 letters of recommendation, personal statement, resume, minimum GPA of 3.0; for doctorate, GRE, 3 letters of recommendation, resume, minimum GPA of 3.0. Additional exam requirements/recommendations for international students: Required—TOEFL (minimum score 600 paper-based; 100 iBT). Electronic applications accepted. *Faculty research:* Microarray data analysis, microbial ecology and genetics, integrative organismal and behavioral biology and ecology, stem cell pluipotency, cancer cell biology.

University of Southern California, Keck School of Medicine and Graduate School, Graduate Programs in Medicine, Los Angeles, CA 90089. Offers MPAP, MPH, MS, PhD. *Faculty:* 236 full-time (68 women), 7 part-time/adjunct (2 women). *Students:* 701 full-time (454 women), 32 part-time (24 women); includes 289 minority (36 Black or African American, non-Hispanic/Latino; 3 American Indian or Alaska Native, non-Hispanic/Latino; 157 Asian, non-Hispanic/Latino; 75 Hispanic/Latino; 4 Native Hawaiian or other Pacific Islander, non-Hispanic/Latino; 14 Two or more races, non-Hispanic/Latino), 224 international. Average age 27. 1,747 applicants, 23% accepted, 235 enrolled. In 2013, 188 master's, 49 doctorates awarded. Terminal master's awarded for partial completion of doctoral program. *Entrance requirements:* For master's, GRE General Test, minimum GPA of 3.0; for doctorate, GRE General Test (minimum combined Verbal and Quantitative score of 1000), minimum GPA of 3.0. Additional exam requirements/recommendations for international students: Required—TOEFL (minimum score 600 paper-based; 100 iBT). *Application deadline:* Applications are processed on a rolling basis. Application fee: $85. Electronic applications accepted. *Financial support:* In 2013–14, 25 fellowships with tuition reimbursements (averaging $31,000 per year), 183 research assistantships with full and partial tuition reimbursements (averaging $31,000 per year), 33 teaching assistantships with full and partial tuition reimbursements (averaging $31,000 per year) were awarded; career-related internships or fieldwork, Federal Work-Study, institutionally sponsored loans, scholarships/grants, traineeships, health care benefits, and unspecified assistantships also available. Support available to part-time students. Financial award application deadline: 5/4; financial award applicants required to submit CSS PROFILE or FAFSA. *Unit head:* Dr. Peggy Farnham, Associate Dean for Graduate Affairs, 323-442-8015, Fax: 323-442-7739, E-mail: pfarnham@usc.edu. *Application contact:* Marisela Zuniga, Administrative Coordinator, 323-442-1607, Fax: 323-442-1199, E-mail: mzuniga@usc.edu.
Website: http://keck.usc.edu/

University of Southern Maine, College of Science, Technology, and Health, Program in Biology, Portland, ME 04104-9300. Offers MS. *Faculty:* 4 full-time (2 women). *Students:* 3 full-time (2 women), 4 part-time (3 women); includes 2 minority (1 Asian, non-Hispanic/Latino; 1 Two or more races, non-Hispanic/Latino), 1 international. Average age 28. 7 applicants, 43% accepted, 1 enrolled. In 2013, 5 master's awarded. Application fee: $65. *Expenses:* Tuition, state resident: part-time $380 per credit. Tuition, nonresident: part-time $1026 per credit. Part-time tuition and fees vary according to program. *Faculty research:* Salt marsh plant ecology, marine microbial ecology, brain development, ecophysiology of marine cyanobacteria, evolution of mammalian social behavior. *Unit head:* Dr. Douglas Currie, Associate Professor and Graduate Program Coordinator, 207-228-8192, E-mail: dcurrie@usm.maine.edu. *Application contact:* Mary Sloan, Assistant Dean of Graduate Studies and Director of Graduate Admissions, 207-780-4386, E-mail: gradstudies@usm.maine.edu.
Website: http://www.usm.maine.edu/bio

University of Southern Mississippi, Graduate School, College of Science and Technology, Department of Biological Sciences, Hattiesburg, MS 39406-0001. Offers environmental biology (MS, PhD); marine biology (MS, PhD); microbiology (MS, PhD); molecular biology (MS, PhD). *Faculty:* 27 full-time (6 women). *Students:* 63 full-time (26 women), 4 part-time (all women); includes 4 minority (1 Black or African American, non-Hispanic/Latino; 1 Hispanic/Latino; 2 Two or more races, non-Hispanic/Latino), 17 international. Average age 32. 43 applicants, 30% accepted, 12 enrolled. In 2013, 12 master's, 9 doctorates awarded. Terminal master's awarded for partial completion of doctoral program. *Degree requirements:* For master's, comprehensive exam, thesis; for doctorate, comprehensive exam, thesis/dissertation. *Entrance requirements:* For master's, GRE General Test, minimum GPA of 3.0 on last 60 hours; for doctorate, GRE General Test, minimum GPA of 3.5. Additional exam requirements/recommendations for international students: Required—TOEFL, IELTS. *Application deadline:* For fall admission, 3/1 priority date for domestic students, 3/1 for international students; for spring admission, 1/10 priority date for domestic and international students. Applications are processed on a rolling basis. Application fee: $50. *Financial support:* In 2013–14, 25 research assistantships with full tuition reimbursements (averaging $9,700 per year), 33 teaching assistantships with full tuition reimbursements (averaging $10,600 per year) were awarded; Federal Work-Study, scholarships/grants, health care benefits, and unspecified assistantships also available. Financial award application deadline: 3/15; financial award applicants required to submit FAFSA. *Unit head:* Dr. Glenmore Shearer, Chair, 601-266-4748, Fax: 601-266-5797. *Application contact:* Dr. Jake Schaefer, Director of Graduate Studies, 601-266-4748, Fax: 601-266-5797.
Website: http://www.usm.edu/graduateschool/table.php

University of South Florida, College of Arts and Sciences, Department of Cell Biology, Microbiology, and Molecular Biology, Tampa, FL 33620-9951. Offers biology (MS), including cell and molecular biology; cancer biology (PhD); cell and molecular biology (PhD); microbiology (MS). *Faculty:* 19 full-time (5 women), 1 part-time/adjunct (0 women). *Students:* 77 full-time (46 women), 3 part-time (1 woman); includes 8 minority (5 Asian, non-Hispanic/Latino; 3 Hispanic/Latino), 19 international. Average age 27. 155 applicants, 17% accepted, 17 enrolled. In 2013, 19 master's, 12 doctorates awarded. *Degree requirements:* For master's, thesis or alternative; for doctorate, comprehensive exam, thesis/dissertation. *Entrance requirements:* For master's and doctorate, GRE General Test, minimum GPA of 3.0, extensive background in biology or chemistry. Additional exam requirements/recommendations for international students: Required—TOEFL (minimum score 550 paper-based; 79 iBT) or IELTS (minimum score 6.5). *Application deadline:* For fall admission, 2/1 for domestic students, 1/1 for international students. Application fee: $30. *Financial support:* Career-related internships or fieldwork, health care benefits, and unspecified assistantships available. Financial award application deadline: 4/1. *Faculty research:* Cell biology, microbiology and molecular biology: basic and applied science in bacterial pathogenesis, genome integrity and mechanisms of aging, structural and computational biology; cancer biology: immunology, cancer control, signal transduction, drug discovery, genomics. *Total annual research expenditures:* $1.9 million. *Unit head:* Dr. James Garey, Professor/Chair, 813-974-7103, Fax: 813-974-1614, E-mail: garey@usf.edu. *Application contact:* Dr. Kenneth Wright, Associate Professor of Cancer Biology, H. Lee Moffitt Cancer Center and Research Institute, 813-745-3918, Fax: 813-974-1614, E-mail: ken.wright@moffitt.org.
Website: http://biology.usf.edu/cmmb/

University of South Florida, College of Arts and Sciences, Department of Integrative Biology, Tampa, FL 33620-9951. Offers biology (MS), including ecology and evolution (MS, PhD), environmental and ecological microbiology (MS, PhD), physiology and morphology (MS, PhD); integrative biology (PhD), including ecology and evolution (MS, PhD), environmental and ecological microbiology (MS, PhD), physiology and morphology (MS, PhD). Part-time programs available. *Faculty:* 16 full-time (4 women), 1 part-time/adjunct (0 women). *Students:* 40 full-time (24 women), 7 part-time (4 women); includes 6 minority (5 Hispanic/Latino; 1 Two or more races, non-Hispanic/Latino), 3 international. Average age 29. 59 applicants, 29% accepted, 11 enrolled. In 2013, 4 master's, 5 doctorates awarded. *Degree requirements:* For master's, comprehensive exam, thesis (for some programs); for doctorate, comprehensive exam, thesis/dissertation. *Entrance requirements:* For master's and doctorate, GRE General Test (minimum preferred scores of 153 verbal, 148 quantitative, 4.5 analytical/500 verbal and 600 quantitative with 4.5 in analytical writing on old scoring), minimum GPA of 3.0 in last 60 hours of BS. Additional exam requirements/recommendations for international students: Required—TOEFL (minimum score 570 paper-based; 88 iBT). *Application deadline:* For fall admission, 2/15 priority date for domestic students, 1/2 for international students; for spring admission, 8/1 for domestic students, 6/1 for international students. Application fee: $30. Electronic applications accepted. *Financial support:* Research assistantships, teaching assistantships, and unspecified assistantships available. Financial award application deadline: 6/30; financial award applicants required to submit FAFSA. *Faculty research:* Marine ecology, ecosystem responses to urbanization, biomechanical and physiological mechanisms of animal movement, population biology and conservation, microbial ecology and public health microbiology, natural diversity of parasites and herbivores; ecosystems, vertebrates, disturbance ecology, functional and ecological morphology of feeding in fishes, rare amphibians and reptiles, genomics in ecological experiments, ecotoxicology, global carbon cycle, plant-animal interactions. *Total annual research expenditures:* $968,227. *Unit head:* Dr. Peter Stiling, Chair, Department of Integrative Biology, 813-974-6229, Fax: 813-974-3263, E-mail: pstiling@usf.edu. *Application contact:* Christine Brubaker, Graduate Program Specialist, Department of Integrative Biology, 813-974-4747, Fax: 813-974-3263, E-mail: brubaker@usf.edu.
Website: http://biology.usf.edu/ib/grad/

University of South Florida, Morsani College of Medicine and Graduate School, Graduate Programs in Medical Sciences, Tampa, FL 33620-9951. Offers aging and neuroscience (MSMS); allergy, immunology and infectious disease (PhD); anatomy (MSMS, PhD); athletic training (MSMS); bioinformatics and computational biology (MSBCB); biotechnology (MSB); clinical and translational research (MSMS, PhD); health informatics (MSHI, MSMS); health science (MSMS); interdisciplinary medical sciences (MSMS); medical microbiology and immunology (MSMS); metabolic and nutritional medicine (MSMS); molecular medicine (MSMS, PhD); molecular pharmacology and physiology (PhD); neurology (PhD); pathology and laboratory medicine (PhD); pharmacology and therapeutics (PhD); physiology and biophysics (PhD); women's health (MSMS). *Students:* 336 full-time (182 women), 39 part-time (21 women); includes 170 minority (45 Black or African American, non-Hispanic/Latino; 54 Asian, non-Hispanic/Latino; 59 Hispanic/Latino; 2 Native Hawaiian or other Pacific Islander, non-Hispanic/Latino; 10 Two or more races, non-Hispanic/Latino), 17 international. Average age 26. 1,066 applicants, 44% accepted, 250 enrolled. In 2013, 191 master's, 12 doctorates awarded. Terminal master's awarded for partial completion of doctoral program. *Degree requirements:* For master's, comprehensive exam, thesis; for doctorate, comprehensive exam, thesis/dissertation. *Entrance requirements:* For master's, GRE General Test or GMAT, bachelor's degree or equivalent from regionally-accredited university with minimum GPA of 3.0 in upper-division sciences coursework; prerequisites in general biology, general chemistry, general physics, organic chemistry, quantitative analysis, and integral and differential calculus; for doctorate, GRE General Test (minimum score of 600 quantitative), bachelor's degree from regionally-accredited university with minimum GPA of 3.0 in upper-division sciences coursework; 3 letters of recommendation; personal interview; 1-2 page personal statement; prerequisites in

biology, chemistry, physics, organic chemistry, quantitative analysis, and integral/differential calculus. Additional exam requirements/recommendations for international students: Required—TOEFL (minimum score 550 paper-based; 79 iBT) or IELTS (minimum score 6.5). *Application deadline:* For fall admission, 2/15 for domestic students, 1/2 for international students. Application fee: $30. *Expenses:* Contact institution. *Faculty research:* Anatomy, biochemistry, cancer biology, cardiovascular disease, cell biology, immunology, microbiology, molecular biology, neuroscience, pharmacology, physiology. *Unit head:* Dr. Michael Barber, Professor and Associate Dean for Graduate and Postdoctoral Affairs, 813-974-9908, Fax: 813-974-4317, E-mail: mbarber@health.usf.edu. *Application contact:* Dr. Eric Bennett, Graduate Director, PhD Program in Medical Sciences, 813-974-1545, Fax: 813-974-4317, E-mail: esbennet@health.usf.edu.
Website: http://health.usf.edu/nocms/medicine/graduatestudies/

The University of Tennessee, Graduate School, College of Arts and Sciences, Program in Life Sciences, Knoxville, TN 37996. Offers genome science and technology (MS, PhD); plant physiology and genetics (MS, PhD). *Degree requirements:* For doctorate, one foreign language, thesis/dissertation. *Entrance requirements:* For master's and doctorate, GRE General Test, minimum GPA of 2.7. Additional exam requirements/recommendations for international students: Required—TOEFL. Electronic applications accepted. *Expenses:* Tuition, state resident: full-time $9540; part-time $531 per credit hour. Tuition, nonresident: full-time $27,728; part-time $1542 per credit hour. *Required fees:* $1404; $67 per credit hour.

The University of Tennessee, Graduate School, Intercollegiate Programs, Program in Comparative and Experimental Medicine, Knoxville, TN 37996. Offers MS, PhD. *Degree requirements:* For master's, thesis; for doctorate, thesis/dissertation. *Entrance requirements:* For master's and doctorate, GRE General Test, minimum GPA of 2.7. Additional exam requirements/recommendations for international students: Required—TOEFL. Electronic applications accepted. *Expenses:* Tuition, state resident: full-time $9540; part-time $531 per credit hour. Tuition, nonresident: full-time $27,728; part-time $1542 per credit hour. *Required fees:* $1404; $67 per credit hour.

The University of Tennessee Health Science Center, College of Graduate Health Sciences, Memphis, TN 38163-0002. Offers biomedical engineering (MS, PhD); biomedical sciences (PhD); dental sciences (MDS); epidemiology (MS); health outcomes and policy research (PhD); laboratory research and management (MS); nursing science (PhD); pharmaceutical sciences (PhD); pharmacology (MS); speech and hearing science (PhD); DDS/PhD; DNP/PhD; MD/PhD; Pharm D/PhD. *Faculty:* 318 full-time (92 women), 59 part-time/adjunct (16 women). *Students:* 220 full-time (102 women), 22 part-time (13 women); includes 194 minority (22 Black or African American, non-Hispanic/Latino; 161 Asian, non-Hispanic/Latino; 7 Hispanic/Latino; 3 Native Hawaiian or other Pacific Islander, non-Hispanic/Latino; 1 Two or more races, non-Hispanic/Latino), 106 international. Average age 25. 404 applicants, 17% accepted, 64 enrolled. In 2013, 13 master's, 25 doctorates awarded. Terminal master's awarded for partial completion of doctoral program. *Degree requirements:* For master's, comprehensive exam, thesis; for doctorate, comprehensive exam, thesis/dissertation, oral and written preliminary and comprehensive exams. *Entrance requirements:* For master's and doctorate, GRE General Test, minimum GPA of 3.0. Additional exam requirements/recommendations for international students: Required—TOEFL (minimum score 79 iBT); Recommended—IELTS (minimum score 6.5). *Application deadline:* For fall admission, 5/15 priority date for domestic students. Applications are processed on a rolling basis. Application fee: $0. Electronic applications accepted. *Financial support:* In 2013–14, 125 students received support, including 125 research assistantships (averaging $23,000 per year); career-related internships or fieldwork, Federal Work-Study, institutionally sponsored loans, and tuition waivers (full and partial) also available. Support available to part-time students. Financial award application deadline: 2/25; financial award applicants required to submit FAFSA. *Unit head:* Dr. Donald B. Thomason, Dean, 901-448-5538, E-mail: dthomaso@uthsc.edu. *Application contact:* William Carter, Director for Admissions, 901-448-1687, E-mail: wcarte17@uthsc.edu.
Website: http://www.uthsc.edu/grad/

The University of Tennessee–Oak Ridge National Laboratory, Graduate Program in Genome Science and Technology, Knoxville, TN 37966. Offers life sciences (MS, PhD). *Students:* Average age 30. *Degree requirements:* For master's, thesis; for doctorate, comprehensive exam, thesis/dissertation. *Entrance requirements:* For master's and doctorate, GRE General Test. Additional exam requirements/recommendations for international students: Required—TOEFL. *Application deadline:* For fall admission, 1/15 priority date for domestic students, 2/1 for international students. Electronic applications accepted. *Financial support:* Fellowships, research assistantships with full tuition reimbursements, institutionally sponsored loans, health care benefits, tuition waivers (full), and unspecified assistantships available. Financial award application deadline: 3/31. *Faculty research:* Genetics/genomics, structural biology/proteomics, computational biology/bioinformatics, bioanalytical technologies. *Unit head:* Roger Gray, Director, 865-974-9561, E-mail: rgray17@utk.edu. *Application contact:* Roger Gray, Program Resource Specialist, 865-974-9561, Fax: 865-974-5037, E-mail: rgray17@utk.edu.
Website: http://gst.tennessee.edu

The University of Texas at Arlington, Graduate School, College of Science, Department of Biology, Arlington, TX 76019. Offers biology (MS); quantitative biology (PhD). Part-time and evening/weekend programs available. *Degree requirements:* For master's, thesis, oral defense of thesis; for doctorate, comprehensive exam, thesis/dissertation, oral defense of dissertation. *Entrance requirements:* For master's and doctorate, GRE General Test. Additional exam requirements/recommendations for international students: Required—TOEFL (minimum score 550 paper-based; 79 iBT). Electronic applications accepted. *Faculty research:* Cellular and microbiology, comparative genomics, evolution and ecology.

The University of Texas at Austin, Graduate School, College of Natural Sciences, School of Biological Sciences, Austin, TX 78712-1111. Offers ecology, evolution and behavior (PhD); microbiology (PhD); plant biology (MA, PhD). *Entrance requirements:* For master's and doctorate, GRE General Test. Electronic applications accepted.

The University of Texas at Brownsville, Graduate Studies, College of Science, Mathematics and Technology, Brownsville, TX 78520-4991. Offers biological sciences (MS); biology (MSIS); computer science (MSIS); computer sciences (MS); mathematics (MS); physics (MS). Part-time and evening/weekend programs available. Postbaccalaureate distance learning degree programs offered (no on-campus study). *Faculty:* 54 full-time (8 women). *Students:* 43 full-time (17 women), 82 part-time (39 women); includes 90 minority (1 Black or African American, non-Hispanic/Latino; 2 American Indian or Alaska Native, non-Hispanic/Latino; 7 Asian, non-Hispanic/Latino; 80 Hispanic/Latino), 13 international. 87 applicants, 54% accepted, 44 enrolled. In 2013, 37 master's awarded. *Degree requirements:* For master's, comprehensive exam (for some programs), thesis optional, project (for some programs). *Entrance requirements:* For master's, GRE General Test, letters of recommendation. Additional exam requirements/recommendations for international students: Required—TOEFL (minimum score 550 paper-based; 77 iBT). *Application deadline:* For fall admission, 7/1 priority date for domestic students, 7/1 for international students; for spring admission, 12/1 priority date for domestic students, 12/1 for international students. Applications are processed on a rolling basis. Application fee: $30. Electronic applications accepted. *Expenses:* Tuition, state resident: full-time $3444; part-time $1148 per semester. Tuition, nonresident: full-time $9816. *Required fees:* $1018; $221 per credit hour. $401 per semester. *Financial support:* In 2013–14, 40 students received support, including 3 research assistantships with partial tuition reimbursements available (averaging $10,000 per year); Federal Work-Study, scholarships/grants, tuition waivers (partial), and unspecified assistantships also available. Support available to part-time students. Financial award application deadline: 3/1; financial award applicants required to submit FAFSA. *Faculty research:* Fish, insects, barrier islands, algae. *Unit head:* Dr. Mikhail M. Bouniaev, Dean, 956-882-6701, Fax: 956-882-6657, E-mail: mikhail.bouniaev@utb.edu. *Application contact:* Mari Montelongo, Graduate Studies Specialist, 956-882-7787, Fax: 956-882-7279, E-mail: mari.montelongo@utb.edu.
Website: http://www.utb.edu/vpaa/csmt/Pages/UTB-College-of-Science-Mathematics-and-Technology.aspx

The University of Texas at Dallas, School of Natural Sciences and Mathematics, Department of Biology, Richardson, TX 75080. Offers bioinformatics and computational biology (MS); biotechnology (MS); molecular and cell biology (MS, PhD). Part-time and evening/weekend programs available. *Faculty:* 20 full-time (3 women), 1 (woman) part-time/adjunct. *Students:* 99 full-time (63 women), 15 part-time (7 women); includes 10 minority (1 Black or African American, non-Hispanic/Latino; 6 Asian, non-Hispanic/Latino; 3 Hispanic/Latino), 77 international. Average age 27. 381 applicants, 23% accepted, 48 enrolled. In 2013, 49 master's, 3 doctorates awarded. *Degree requirements:* For master's, thesis optional; for doctorate, thesis/dissertation, publishable paper. *Entrance requirements:* For master's and doctorate, GRE (minimum combined score of 1000 on verbal and quantitative). Additional exam requirements/recommendations for international students: Required—TOEFL (minimum score 550 paper-based; 80 iBT). *Application deadline:* For fall admission, 7/15 for domestic students, 5/1 priority date for international students; for spring admission, 11/15 for domestic students, 9/1 priority date for international students. Applications are processed on a rolling basis. Application fee: $50 ($100 for international students). Electronic applications accepted. *Expenses:* Tuition, state resident: full-time $11,940; part-time $663.33 per credit hour. Tuition, nonresident: full-time $21,606; part-time $1200.33 per credit hour. *Financial support:* In 2013–14, 57 students received support, including 12 research assistantships with partial tuition reimbursements available (averaging $20,867 per year), 44 teaching assistantships with partial tuition reimbursements available (averaging $15,300 per year); career-related internships or fieldwork, Federal Work-Study, institutionally sponsored loans, scholarships/grants, and unspecified assistantships also available. Support available to part-time students. Financial award application deadline: 4/30; financial award applicants required to submit FAFSA. *Faculty research:* Role of mitochondria in neurodegenerative diseases, protein-DNA interactions in site-specific recombination, eukaryotic gene expression, bio-nanotechnology, sickle cell research. *Unit head:* Dr. Stephen Spiro, Department Head, 972-883-6032, Fax: 972-883-2502, E-mail: stephen.spiro@utdallas.edu. *Application contact:* Dr. Lawrence Reitzer, Graduate Advisor, 972-883-2502, Fax: 972-883-2402, E-mail: reitzer@utdallas.edu.
Website: http://www.utdallas.edu/biology/

The University of Texas at El Paso, Graduate School, College of Science, Department of Biological Sciences, El Paso, TX 79968-0001. Offers bioinformatics (MS); biological sciences (MS, PhD). Part-time and evening/weekend programs available. *Degree requirements:* For master's, thesis; for doctorate, thesis/dissertation. *Entrance requirements:* For master's, GRE, minimum GPA of 3.0, letters of recommendation; for doctorate, GRE, statement of purpose, letters of recommendation. Additional exam requirements/recommendations for international students: Required—TOEFL; Recommended—IELTS. Electronic applications accepted.

The University of Texas at San Antonio, College of Sciences, Department of Biology, San Antonio, TX 78249-0617. Offers biology (MS); biotechnology (MS); cell and molecular biology (PhD); neurobiology (PhD). *Faculty:* 46 full-time (9 women), 15 part-time/adjunct (10 women). *Students:* 116 full-time (56 women), 62 part-time (34 women); includes 70 minority (7 Black or African American, non-Hispanic/Latino; 1 American Indian or Alaska Native, non-Hispanic/Latino; 10 Asian, non-Hispanic/Latino; 49 Hispanic/Latino; 2 Native Hawaiian or other Pacific Islander, non-Hispanic/Latino; 1 Two or more races, non-Hispanic/Latino), 34 international. Average age 29. 176 applicants, 53% accepted, 43 enrolled. In 2013, 47 master's, 6 doctorates awarded. Terminal master's awarded for partial completion of doctoral program. *Degree requirements:* For master's, comprehensive exam, thesis or alternative; for doctorate, comprehensive exam, thesis/dissertation. *Entrance requirements:* For master's, GRE General Test, bachelor's degree with 18 credit hours in field of study or in another appropriate field of study; for doctorate, GRE General Test, 3 letters of recommendation, statement of purpose, resume. Additional exam requirements/recommendations for international students: Required—TOEFL (minimum score 500 paper-based; 100 iBT), IELTS (minimum score 5). *Application deadline:* For fall admission, 7/1 for domestic students, 4/1 for international students; for spring admission, 11/1 for domestic students, 9/1 for international students. Application fee: $45 ($80 for international students). Electronic applications accepted. *Expenses:* Tuition, state resident: full-time $4671. Tuition, nonresident: full-time $8708. *International tuition:* $17,415 full-time. *Required fees:* $1924.60. Tuition and fees vary according to course load and degree level. *Financial support:* In 2013–14, 42 students received support, including 14 fellowships (averaging $26,142 per year), 19 research assistantships (averaging $24,350 per year), 9 teaching assistantships (averaging $24,350 per year). *Faculty research:* Development of human and veterinary vaccines against a fungal disease, mammalian germ cells and stem cells, dopamine neuron physiology and addiction, plant biochemistry, dendritic computation and synaptic plasticity. *Total annual research expenditures:* $2.1 million. *Unit head:* Dr. Edwin J. Barea-Rodriguez, Chair, 210-458-4511, Fax: 210-458-5658, E-mail: edwin.barea@utsa.edu. *Application contact:* Rene Munguia, Jr., Senior Program Coordinator, 210-458-4642, Fax: 210-458-5658, E-mail: rene.munguia@utsa.edu.
Website: http://bio.utsa.edu/

The University of Texas at Tyler, College of Arts and Sciences, Department of Biology, Tyler, TX 75799-0001. Offers biology (MS); interdisciplinary studies (MSIS). *Degree requirements:* For master's, comprehensive exam, thesis, oral qualifying exam, thesis defense. *Entrance requirements:* For master's, GRE General Test, GRE Subject Test, bachelor's degree in biology or equivalent. Additional exam requirements/recommendations for international students: Required—TOEFL. Electronic applications accepted. *Faculty research:* Phenotypic plasticity and heritability of life history traits, invertebrate ecology and genetics, systematics and phylogenetics of reptiles, hibernation physiology in turtles, landscape ecology, host-microbe interaction, outer membrane proteins in bacteria.

The University of Texas Health Science Center at Houston, Graduate School of Biomedical Sciences, Houston, TX 77225-0036. Offers MS, PhD, MD/PhD. Terminal master's awarded for partial completion of doctoral program. *Degree requirements:* For master's, thesis; for doctorate, thesis/dissertation. *Entrance requirements:* For master's and doctorate, GRE General Test. Additional exam requirements/recommendations for international students: Required—TOEFL. Electronic applications accepted. *Expenses:* Tuition, state resident: full-time $3474; part-time $193 per credit hour. Tuition, nonresident: full-time $13,644; part-time $758 per credit hour. *Required fees:* $226.30; $87 per credit hour. *Faculty research:* Biomedical sciences.

The University of Texas Health Science Center at San Antonio, Graduate School of Biomedical Sciences, Integrated Multidisciplinary Graduate Program, San Antonio, TX 78229-3900. Offers PhD. *Faculty:* 143 full-time (38 women), 42 part-time/adjunct (8 women). *Students:* 29 full-time (17 women); includes 11 minority (3 Black or African American, non-Hispanic/Latino; 5 Asian, non-Hispanic/Latino; 3 Hispanic/Latino), 5 international. Average age 26. 379 applicants, 15% accepted, 21 enrolled. *Degree requirements:* For doctorate, comprehensive exam, thesis/dissertation. *Entrance requirements:* For doctorate, GRE, bachelor's degree. Additional exam requirements/recommendations for international students: Required—TOEFL (minimum score 560 paper-based; 68 iBT). *Application deadline:* For fall admission, 1/15 priority date for domestic students, 1/15 for international students. Applications are processed on a rolling basis. Application fee: $0. Electronic applications accepted. *Financial support:* In 2013–14, 3 students received support. Federal Work-Study and scholarships/grants available. Financial award application deadline: 6/30; financial award applicants required to submit FAFSA. *Faculty research:* Neurophysiology, neurodegenerative disorders, bioinformatics and computational biochemistry, enzymology and metabolic regulation, caloric restriction and dietary intervention in aging. *Unit head:* Dr. Reto Asmis, Associate Dean, 210-567-3714, Fax: 210-567-3719, E-mail: asmis@uthscsa.edu. *Application contact:* Dr. Nicquet Blake, Assistant Dean for Graduate Student Recruitment, 210-567-3722, Fax: 210-567-3719, E-mail: blaken@uthscsa.edu.
Website: http://gsbs.uthscsa.edu/main/graduate/phd/imgp/overview

The University of Texas Medical Branch, Graduate School of Biomedical Sciences, Galveston, TX 77555. Offers MA, MMS, MPH, MS, PhD, MD/PhD. Terminal master's awarded for partial completion of doctoral program. *Degree requirements:* For master's, comprehensive exam (for some programs), thesis or alternative; for doctorate, comprehensive exam, thesis/dissertation. *Entrance requirements:* For master's and doctorate, GRE General Test, 3 letters of recommendation. Additional exam requirements/recommendations for international students: Required—TOEFL (minimum score 550 paper-based; 80 iBT), IELTS (minimum score 6.5). Electronic applications accepted. *Expenses:* Contact institution.

The University of Texas of the Permian Basin, Office of Graduate Studies, College of Arts and Sciences, Department of Biology, Odessa, TX 79762-0001. Offers MS. Part-time and evening/weekend programs available. *Degree requirements:* For master's, comprehensive exam, thesis or alternative. *Entrance requirements:* For master's, GRE General Test. Additional exam requirements/recommendations for international students: Required—TOEFL (minimum score 550 paper-based).

The University of Texas–Pan American, College of Science and Mathematics, Department of Biology, Edinburg, TX 78539. Offers MS. Part-time and evening/weekend programs available. *Faculty:* 7 full-time (1 woman). *Students:* 15 full-time (8 women), 31 part-time (14 women); includes 43 minority (2 Asian, non-Hispanic/Latino; 40 Hispanic/Latino; 1 Two or more races, non-Hispanic/Latino). Average age 30. 25 applicants, 76% accepted, 14 enrolled. In 2013, 6 master's awarded. *Degree requirements:* For master's, comprehensive exam, thesis optional, minimum GPA of 3.0 overall and in all higher biology courses. *Entrance requirements:* For master's, GRE General Test, 24 hours of undergraduate courses in biological sciences or closely-related disciplines with minimum GPA of 3.0. Additional exam requirements/recommendations for international students: Required—TOEFL (minimum score 500 paper-based; 61 iBT); Recommended—IELTS (minimum score 5.5). *Application deadline:* For fall admission, 6/1 for domestic and international students; for spring admission, 11/1 for domestic students, 10/1 for international students; for summer admission, 5/1 for domestic students, 3/1 for international students. Applications are processed on a rolling basis. Application fee: $50. Electronic applications accepted. *Expenses:* Tuition, state resident: full-time $5986; part-time $333 per credit hour. Tuition, nonresident: full-time $12,358; part-time $687 per credit hour. *Required fees:* $782. Tuition and fees vary according to program. *Financial support:* Teaching assistantships, institutionally sponsored loans, and unspecified assistantships available. Financial award application deadline: 6/1. *Faculty research:* Flora and fauna of South Padre Island, plant taxonomy of Rio Grande Valley. *Unit head:* Dr. Fred Zaidan, Chair, 956-665-3537, Fax: 956-665-3657, E-mail: fzaidan@utpa.edu. *Application contact:* Dr. Zen Faulkes, Program Director, 956-665-2614, Fax: 956-665-3657, E-mail: zfaulkes@utpa.edu.
Website: http://portal.utpa.edu/utpa_main/daa_home/cose_home/biology_home/biology_graduate

The University of Texas Southwestern Medical Center, Southwestern Graduate School of Biomedical Sciences, Clinical Science Program, Dallas, TX 75390. Offers MCS, MSCS. Part-time programs available. *Students:* 3 full-time (1 woman), 37 part-time (17 women); includes 13 minority (3 Black or African American, non-Hispanic/Latino; 1 American Indian or Alaska Native, non-Hispanic/Latino; 6 Asian, non-Hispanic/Latino; 3 Hispanic/Latino), 5 international. Average age 29. 16 applicants, 88% accepted, 14 enrolled. In 2013, 9 master's awarded. *Degree requirements:* For master's, 1-year clinical research project. *Entrance requirements:* For master's, graduate degree in biomedical science. *Application deadline:* For fall admission, 7/15 for domestic students; for spring admission, 12/15 for domestic students. Applications are processed on a rolling basis. Electronic applications accepted. *Unit head:* Dr. Milton Packer, Chair, 214-648-0491, Fax: 214-648-6417, E-mail: milton.packer@utsouthwestern.edu.

The University of Texas Southwestern Medical Center, Southwestern Graduate School of Biomedical Sciences, Division of Basic Science, Dallas, TX 75390. Offers biological chemistry (PhD); biomedical engineering (MS, PhD); cancer biology (PhD); cell regulation (PhD); genetics and development (PhD); immunology (PhD); integrative biology (PhD); molecular biophysics (PhD); molecular microbiology (PhD); neuroscience (PhD); MD/PhD. *Faculty:* 278 full-time (70 women), 10 part-time/adjunct (0 women). *Students:* 59 full-time (32 women); includes 12 minority (2 Black or African American, non-Hispanic/Latino; 2 Asian, non-Hispanic/Latino; 6 Hispanic/Latino; 2 Two or more races, non-Hispanic/Latino), 28 international. Average age 26. 1,229 applicants, 9% accepted. *Degree requirements:* For doctorate, thesis/dissertation, qualifying exam. *Entrance requirements:* For doctorate, GRE General Test, research experience. Additional exam requirements/recommendations for international students: Required—TOEFL. *Application deadline:* For fall admission, 12/15 priority date for domestic and international students. Application fee: $0. Electronic applications accepted. *Financial support:* Fellowships, research assistantships, institutionally sponsored loans, and traineeships available. *Unit head:* Associate Dean, 214-648-6708, Fax: 214-648-2102. *Application contact:* -, Fax: -.
Website: http://www.utsouthwestern.edu/education/graduate-school/application-and-admissions/basic-sciences.html

The University of Texas Southwestern Medical Center, Southwestern Graduate School of Biomedical Sciences, Medical Scientist Training Program, Dallas, TX 75390. Offers PhD, MD/PhD. *Students:* 12 full-time (4 women), 14 part-time (5 women); includes 13 minority (2 Black or African American, non-Hispanic/Latino; 8 Asian, non-Hispanic/Latino; 2 Hispanic/Latino; 1 Two or more races, non-Hispanic/Latino). Average age 25. *Application deadline:* For fall admission, 11/1 for domestic students. Application fee: $0. Electronic applications accepted. *Financial support:* Application deadline: 3/1. *Unit head:* Dr. Andrew Zinn, Associate Dean, 214-648-2057, Fax: 214-648-2814, E-mail: dennis.mckearin@utsouthwestern.edu. *Application contact:* Robin Downing, Education Coordinator, 214-648-6764, Fax: 214-648-2814, E-mail: robin.downing@utsouthwestern.edu.
Website: http://www.utsouthwestern.edu/utsw/cda/dept21839/files/21914.html

University of the Incarnate Word, School of Graduate Studies and Research, School of Mathematics, Science, and Engineering, Program in Biology, San Antonio, TX 78209-6397. Offers MA, MS. Part-time and evening/weekend programs available. *Faculty:* 5 full-time (3 women). *Students:* 2 full-time (both women), 4 part-time (all women); includes 5 minority (all Hispanic/Latino), 1 international. Average age 27. 14 applicants, 21% accepted, 2 enrolled. In 2013, 3 master's awarded. *Degree requirements:* For master's, comprehensive exam (for MA); thesis defense (for MS). *Entrance requirements:* For master's, GRE Subject Test (biology), minimum GPA of 3.0 in biology or GRE (minimum combined score 1000 Verbal and Quantitative), 8 hours of principles of chemistry, 6 hours of organic chemistry, 12 upper-division hours in biology. Additional exam requirements/recommendations for international students: Required—TOEFL (minimum score 560 paper-based; 83 iBT). *Application deadline:* Applications are processed on a rolling basis. Application fee: $20. Electronic applications accepted. *Expenses: Tuition:* Part-time $815 per credit hour. *Required fees:* $86 per credit hour. One-time fee: $40 part-time. Tuition and fees vary according to degree level and program. *Financial support:* Federal Work-Study and scholarships/grants available. Financial award applicants required to submit FAFSA. *Faculty research:* Regeneration of nervous system elements, social behaviors of electric fish, gene expression in human cells, transmission of pathogenic protozoa, human DNA response to cancer fighting molecules. *Total annual research expenditures:* $1.2 million. *Unit head:* Dr. David Foglesong, Graduate Program Director, 210-283-5033, Fax: 210-829-3153, E-mail: davidf@uiwtx.edu. *Application contact:* Andrea Cyterski-Acosta, Dean of Enrollment, 210-829-6005, Fax: 210-829-3921, E-mail: admis@uiwtx.edu.
Website: http://www.uiw.edu/biology/graduate_program.htm

University of the Pacific, College of the Pacific, Department of Biological Sciences, Stockton, CA 95211-0197. Offers MS. *Faculty:* 17 full-time (5 women). *Students:* 26 part-time (12 women); includes 18 minority (1 Black or African American, non-Hispanic/Latino; 1 American Indian or Alaska Native, non-Hispanic/Latino; 13 Asian, non-Hispanic/Latino; 3 Hispanic/Latino), 1 international. Average age 24. 21 applicants, 52% accepted, 9 enrolled. In 2013, 10 master's awarded. *Degree requirements:* For master's, thesis. *Entrance requirements:* For master's, GRE General Test, GRE Subject Test. Additional exam requirements/recommendations for international students: Required—TOEFL. *Application deadline:* For fall admission, 3/1 priority date for domestic students; for spring admission, 10/1 priority date for domestic students. Applications are processed on a rolling basis. Application fee: $75. *Financial support:* In 2013–14, 25 teaching assistantships were awarded; institutionally sponsored loans also available. Support available to part-time students. Financial award application deadline: 3/1; financial award applicants required to submit FAFSA. *Unit head:* Dr. Gregg Jongeward, Co-Chairman, 209-946-3022. *Application contact:* Information Contact, 209-946-2261.

The University of Toledo, College of Graduate Studies, College of Medicine and Life Sciences, Interdepartmental Programs, Toledo, OH 43606-3390. Offers bioinformatics and proteomics/genomics (MSBS); biomarkers and bioinformatics (Certificate); biomarkers and diagnostics (PSM); human donation sciences (MSBS); medical sciences (MSBS); MD/MSBS. *Faculty:* 44. *Students:* 60 full-time (27 women), 3 part-time (2 women); includes 19 minority (4 Black or African American, non-Hispanic/Latino; 13 Asian, non-Hispanic/Latino; 2 Hispanic/Latino). Average age 24. 200 applicants, 41% accepted, 57 enrolled. In 2013, 55 master's awarded. *Degree requirements:* For master's, thesis or alternative. *Entrance requirements:* For master's, GRE, minimum undergraduate GPA of 3.0, three letters of recommendation, statement of purpose, transcripts from all prior institutions attended, resume; for Certificate, minimum undergraduate GPA of 3.0, three letters of recommendation, statement of purpose, transcripts from all prior institutions attended, resume. Additional exam requirements/recommendations for international students: Required—TOEFL (minimum score 550 paper-based; 80 iBT). *Application deadline:* For fall admission, 1/15 priority date for domestic and international students. Application fee: $45 ($75 for international students). Electronic applications accepted. *Financial support:* In 2013–14, 2 research assistantships with full tuition reimbursements (averaging $10,000 per year) were awarded; scholarships/grants also available. *Unit head:* Dr. Ronald McGinnis, Interim Dean, 419-383-4243, E-mail: ronald.mcginnis@utoledo.edu. *Application contact:* Admissions Analyst, 419-383-4112, Fax: 419-383-6140.
Website: http://www.utoledo.edu/med/grad/

The University of Toledo, College of Graduate Studies, College of Natural Sciences and Mathematics, Department of Biological Sciences, Toledo, OH 43606-3390. Offers biology (MS, PhD). Part-time programs available. *Faculty:* 27. *Students:* 68 full-time (30 women), 25 part-time (15 women); includes 3 minority (1 Asian, non-Hispanic/Latino; 2 Two or more races, non-Hispanic/Latino), 41 international. Average age 28. 78 applicants, 38% accepted, 24 enrolled. In 2013, 13 master's, 10 doctorates awarded. *Degree requirements:* For master's, thesis or alternative; for doctorate, thesis/dissertation. *Entrance requirements:* For master's and doctorate, GRE General Test, GRE Subject Test, minimum cumulative point-hour ratio of 2.7 for all previous academic work, three letters of recommendation, statement of purpose, transcripts from all prior institutions attended. Additional exam requirements/recommendations for international students: Required—TOEFL (minimum score 550 paper-based; 80 iBT). *Application deadline:* For fall admission, 1/15 priority date for domestic and international students. Applications are processed on a rolling basis. Application fee: $45 ($75 for international students). Electronic applications accepted. *Financial support:* In 2013–14, 8 research assistantships with full and partial tuition reimbursements (averaging $10,713 per year), 42 teaching assistantships with full and partial tuition reimbursements (averaging $14,888 per year) were awarded; fellowships, Federal Work-Study, institutionally sponsored loans, scholarships/grants, tuition waivers (full), and unspecified assistantships also available. Support available to part-time students. *Faculty research:* Biochemical parasitology, physiological ecology, animal physiology. *Unit head:* Dr. Doug Leaman, Chair, 419-530-2066, E-mail: douglas.leaman@utoledo.edu. *Application contact:* Graduate School Office, 419-530-4723, Fax: 419-530-4724, E-mail: grdsch@utnet.utoledo.edu.
Website: http://www.utoledo.edu/nsm/bio/

The University of Toledo, College of Graduate Studies, College of Natural Sciences and Mathematics, Department of Environmental Sciences, Toledo, OH 43606-3390. Offers biology (MS, PhD), including ecology; geology (MS), including earth surface processes. Part-time programs available. *Faculty:* 51. *Students:* 5 full-time (2 women), 1 (woman) part-time, 2 international. Average age 28. 2 applicants, 100% accepted, 2 enrolled. In 2013, 5 master's awarded. *Degree requirements:* For master's, thesis or alternative. *Entrance requirements:* For master's, GRE General Test, minimum cumulative point-hour ratio of 2.7 for all previous academic work, three letters of recommendation, statement of purpose, transcripts from all prior institutions attended. Additional exam requirements/recommendations for international students: Required—TOEFL (minimum score 550 paper-based; 80 iBT). *Application deadline:* For fall admission, 1/15 priority date for domestic and international students. Applications are processed on a rolling basis. Application fee: $45 ($75 for international students).

Electronic applications accepted. *Financial support:* In 2013–14, 4 teaching assistantships with full and partial tuition reimbursements (averaging $10,850 per year) were awarded; Federal Work-Study, institutionally sponsored loans, scholarships/grants, tuition waivers (full), and unspecified assistantships also available. Support available to part-time students. *Faculty research:* Environmental geochemistry, geophysics, petrology and mineralogy, paleontology, geohydrology. *Unit head:* Dr. Timothy G. Fisher, Chair, 419-530-2883, E-mail: timothy.fisher@utoledo.edu. *Application contact:* Graduate School Office, 419-530-4723, Fax: 419-530-4724, E-mail: grdsch@utnet.utoledo.edu.
Website: http://www.utoledo.edu/nsm/envsciences/

The University of Tulsa, Graduate School, College of Arts and Sciences, School of Urban Education, Program in Teaching Arts, Tulsa, OK 74104-3189. Offers art (MTA); biology (MTA); English (MTA); history (MTA); mathematics (MTA). Part-time programs available. *Students:* 1 full-time (0 women), 1 part-time (0 women); includes 1 minority (Black or African American, non-Hispanic/Latino). Average age 30. 2 applicants, 100% accepted, 2 enrolled. *Entrance requirements:* For master's, GRE General Test. Additional exam requirements/recommendations for international students: Required—TOEFL (minimum score 577 paper-based), IELTS (minimum score 6.5). *Application deadline:* Applications are processed on a rolling basis. Application fee: $40. Electronic applications accepted. *Expenses: Tuition:* Full-time $19,566; part-time $1087 per credit hour. *Required fees:* $1690; $5 per credit hour. $160 per semester. Tuition and fees vary according to course load. *Financial support:* In 2013–14, 1 student received support, including 1 research assistantship with full and partial tuition reimbursement available (averaging $12,766 per year); fellowships with full and partial tuition reimbursements available, teaching assistantships with full and partial tuition reimbursements available, career-related internships or fieldwork, Federal Work-Study, scholarships/grants, health care benefits, tuition waivers (full and partial), and unspecified assistantships also available. Support available to part-time students. Financial award application deadline: 2/1; financial award applicants required to submit FAFSA. *Unit head:* Dr. Kara Gae Neal, Chair, 918-631-2238, Fax: 918-631-3721, E-mail: karagae-neal@utulsa.edu. *Application contact:* Dr. David Brown, Advisor, 918-631-2719, Fax: 918-631-2133, E-mail: david-brown@utulsa.edu.

The University of Tulsa, Graduate School, College of Engineering and Natural Sciences, Department of Biological Science, Tulsa, OK 74104-3189. Offers MS, MTA, PhD, JD/MS. Part-time programs available. *Faculty:* 13 full-time (2 women). *Students:* 18 full-time (9 women), 1 (woman) part-time; includes 2 minority (both American Indian or Alaska Native, non-Hispanic/Latino), 7 international. Average age 31. 18 applicants, 22% accepted, 3 enrolled. In 2013, 1 master's, 4 doctorates awarded. Terminal master's awarded for partial completion of doctoral program. *Degree requirements:* For master's, thesis, oral exams; for doctorate, comprehensive exam, thesis/dissertation. *Entrance requirements:* For master's and doctorate, GRE General Test. Additional exam requirements/recommendations for international students: Required—TOEFL (minimum score 550 paper-based; 80 iBT), IELTS (minimum score 6). *Application deadline:* Applications are processed on a rolling basis. Application fee: $40. Electronic applications accepted. *Expenses: Tuition:* Full-time $19,566; part-time $1087 per credit hour. *Required fees:* $1690; $5 per credit hour. $160 per semester. Tuition and fees vary according to course load. *Financial support:* In 2013–14, 16 students received support, including 10 fellowships with full and partial tuition reimbursements available (averaging $1,922 per year), 4 research assistantships with full and partial tuition reimbursements available (averaging $13,529 per year), 12 teaching assistantships with full and partial tuition reimbursements available (averaging $12,958 per year); career-related internships or fieldwork, Federal Work-Study, scholarships/grants, health care benefits, tuition waivers (full and partial), and unspecified assistantships also available. Support available to part-time students. Financial award application deadline: 2/1; financial award applicants required to submit FAFSA. *Faculty research:* Aerobiology, animal behavior and behavioral ecology, cell and molecular biology, ecology, developmental biology, genetics, herpetology, glycobiology, immunology, microbiology, morphology, mycology, ornithology, molecular systematic and virology. *Total annual research expenditures:* $438,686. *Unit head:* Dr. Estelle Levetin, Chairperson, 918-631-2764, Fax: 918-631-2762, E-mail: estelle-levetin@utulsa.edu. *Application contact:* Dr. Harrington Wells, Advisor, 918-631-3071, Fax: 918-631-2762, E-mail: harrington-wells@utulsa.edu.
Website: http://www.utulsa.edu/academics/colleges/college-of-engineering-and-natural-sciences/departments-and-schools/Department-of-Biological-Science.aspx

University of Utah, Graduate School, College of Science, Department of Biology, Salt Lake City, UT 84112. Offers MS, PhD. Part-time programs available. *Faculty:* 42 full-time (8 women), 31 part-time/adjunct (13 women). *Students:* 60 full-time (29 women), 21 part-time (6 women); includes 9 minority (2 Black or African American, non-Hispanic/Latino; 1 American Indian or Alaska Native, non-Hispanic/Latino; 2 Asian, non-Hispanic/Latino; 1 Hispanic/Latino; 3 Two or more races, non-Hispanic/Latino), 23 international. Average age 29. 145 applicants, 14% accepted, 10 enrolled. In 2013, 15 master's, 8 doctorates awarded. Terminal master's awarded for partial completion of doctoral program. *Degree requirements:* For master's, comprehensive exam, thesis; for doctorate, comprehensive exam, thesis/dissertation. *Entrance requirements:* For master's and doctorate, GRE General Test, minimum GPA of 3.0. Additional exam requirements/recommendations for international students: Required—TOEFL (minimum score 500 paper-based; 80 iBT). *Application deadline:* For fall admission, 1/5 for domestic and international students. Application fee: $55 ($65 for international students). Electronic applications accepted. Application fee is waived when completed online. *Expenses:* Tuition, state resident: full-time $5259. Tuition, nonresident: full-time $18,569. *Required fees:* $841. Tuition and fees vary according to course load. *Financial support:* In 2013–14, 90 students received support, including 24 fellowships with full tuition reimbursements available (averaging $26,000 per year), 30 research assistantships with full tuition reimbursements available (averaging $26,000 per year), 32 teaching assistantships with full tuition reimbursements available (averaging $18,000 per year); career-related internships or fieldwork, scholarships/grants, traineeships, and health care benefits also available. Financial award application deadline: 3/15; financial award applicants required to submit FAFSA. *Faculty research:* Ecology, evolutionary biology, cell and developmental biology, physiology and organismal biology, molecular biology, biochemistry, microbiology, plant biology, neurobiology, genetics. *Total annual research expenditures:* $10 million. *Unit head:* Dr. Niel Vickers, Department Chair, 801-585-1930, E-mail: vickers@biology.utah.edu. *Application contact:* Shannon Nielsen, Administrative Program Coordinator, 801-581-5636, Fax: 801-581-4668, E-mail: shannon.nielsen@bioscience.utah.edu.
Website: http://www.biology.utah.edu

University of Utah, School of Medicine and Graduate School, Graduate Programs in Medicine, Salt Lake City, UT 84112-1107. Offers M Phil, M Stat, MPAS, MPH, MS, MSPH, PhD, Certificate. Part-time programs available. *Degree requirements:* For doctorate, thesis/dissertation. *Entrance requirements:* For doctorate, MCAT. Electronic applications accepted. *Expenses:* Tuition, state resident: full-time $5259. Tuition, nonresident: full-time $18,569. *Required fees:* $841. Tuition and fees vary according to course load. *Faculty research:* Molecular biology, biochemistry, cell biology, immunology, bioengineering.

University of Vermont, College of Medicine and Graduate College, Graduate Programs in Medicine, Burlington, VT 05405. Offers clinical and translational science (MS, PhD); neuroscience (PhD); pathology (MS); pharmacology (MS). *Students:* 46 (21 women); includes 7 minority (1 Black or African American, non-Hispanic/Latino; 6 Hispanic/Latino), 7 international. 64 applicants, 22% accepted, 6 enrolled. In 2013, 1 master's, 9 doctorates awarded. *Degree requirements:* For master's, thesis; for doctorate, thesis/dissertation. *Entrance requirements:* For master's and doctorate, GRE General Test. Additional exam requirements/recommendations for international students: Required—TOEFL (minimum score 550 paper-based; 80 iBT). *Application deadline:* For fall admission, 4/1 priority date for domestic students, 4/1 for international students. Applications are processed on a rolling basis. Application fee: $65. Electronic applications accepted. *Financial support:* Fellowships, research assistantships, teaching assistantships, traineeships, and analytical assistantships available. Financial award application deadline: 3/1. *Unit head:* Dr. Frederick C. Morin, Dean, 802-656-2156. *Application contact:* Ralph Swenson, Director of Graduate Admissions, 802-656-2699, Fax: 802-656-0519, E-mail: graduate.admissions@uvm.edu.

University of Vermont, Graduate College, Cellular, Molecular and Biomedical Sciences Program, Burlington, VT 05405. Offers MS, PhD. *Students:* 39 (13 women); includes 6 minority (1 Black or African American, non-Hispanic/Latino; 4 Asian, non-Hispanic/Latino; 1 Hispanic/Latino), 11 international. 106 applicants, 22% accepted, 5 enrolled. In 2013, 3 master's, 10 doctorates awarded. *Degree requirements:* For master's, thesis; for doctorate, thesis/dissertation. *Entrance requirements:* For master's and doctorate, GRE General Test. Additional exam requirements/recommendations for international students: Required—TOEFL (minimum score 550 paper-based; 80 iBT). *Application deadline:* For fall admission, 12/1 priority date for domestic students, 12/1 for international students. Application fee: $65. Electronic applications accepted. *Financial support:* Fellowships, research assistantships, teaching assistantships, and career-related internships or fieldwork available. Financial award application deadline: 3/1. *Unit head:* Prof. Nick Heintz, Coordinator, 802-656-9673.

University of Vermont, Graduate College, College of Arts and Sciences, Department of Biology, Burlington, VT 05405. Offers biology (MS, PhD); biology education (MST). *Faculty:* 17. *Students:* 38 (18 women); includes 4 minority (1 Asian, non-Hispanic/Latino; 3 Hispanic/Latino), 11 international. 55 applicants, 24% accepted, 8 enrolled. In 2013, 3 master's, 3 doctorates awarded. *Degree requirements:* For master's, thesis; for doctorate, thesis/dissertation. *Entrance requirements:* For master's and doctorate, GRE General Test. Additional exam requirements/recommendations for international students: Required—TOEFL (minimum score 550 paper-based; 80 iBT). *Application deadline:* For fall admission, 12/15 priority date for domestic students, 12/15 for international students. Applications are processed on a rolling basis. Application fee: $65. Electronic applications accepted. *Financial support:* Fellowships, research assistantships, and teaching assistantships available. Financial award application deadline: 3/1. *Unit head:* Dr. Jim Vigoreaux, Chairperson, 802-656-2922. *Application contact:* Dr. Judith Van Houten, Coordinator, 802-656-2922.

University of Victoria, Faculty of Graduate Studies, Faculty of Science, Department of Biology, Victoria, BC V8W 2Y2, Canada. Offers M Sc, PhD. *Degree requirements:* For master's, thesis, seminar; for doctorate, thesis/dissertation, seminar, candidacy exam. *Entrance requirements:* For master's and doctorate, GRE General Test, minimum B+ average in previous 2 years of biology course work. Additional exam requirements/recommendations for international students: Required—TOEFL (minimum score 575 paper-based), IELTS (minimum score 7). Electronic applications accepted. *Faculty research:* Neurobiology of vertebrates and invertebrates, physiology, reproduction and tissue culture of forest trees, evolution and ecology, cell and molecular biology, molecular biology of environmental health.

University of Virginia, College and Graduate School of Arts and Sciences, Department of Biology, Charlottesville, VA 22903. Offers MA, MS, PhD. *Faculty:* 34 full-time (8 women), 1 part-time/adjunct (0 women). *Students:* 46 full-time (29 women); includes 3 minority (1 Black or African American, non-Hispanic/Latino; 1 Asian, non-Hispanic/Latino; 1 Hispanic/Latino), 14 international. Average age 26. 115 applicants, 17% accepted, 10 enrolled. In 2013, 1 master's, 8 doctorates awarded. *Degree requirements:* For master's, thesis; for doctorate, thesis/dissertation. *Entrance requirements:* For master's and doctorate, GRE General Test, GRE Subject Test (recommended), 2 letters of recommendation. Additional exam requirements/recommendations for international students: Required—TOEFL (minimum score 600 paper-based; 90 iBT), IELTS (minimum score 7). *Application deadline:* For fall admission, 12/21 for domestic and international students. Applications are processed on a rolling basis. Application fee: $60. Electronic applications accepted. *Expenses:* Tuition, state resident: part-time $334 per credit hour. Tuition, nonresident: part-time $1224 per credit hour. *Financial support:* Fellowships, research assistantships, and teaching assistantships available. Financial award applicants required to submit FAFSA. *Faculty research:* Ecology and evolution, neurobiology and behavior, molecular genetics, cell development. *Unit head:* Laura Galloway, Chair, 434-982-5010, Fax: 434-982-5626, E-mail: lgalloway@virginia.edu. *Application contact:* Dorothy Schafer, Director of Graduate Studies, 434-982-5297, Fax: 434-982-5626, E-mail: das9w@virginia.edu.
Website: http://bio.virginia.edu/

University of Virginia, School of Medicine, Department of Molecular Physiology and Biological Physics, Program in Biological and Physical Sciences, Charlottesville, VA 22903. Offers MS. In 2013, 23 master's awarded. *Entrance requirements:* For master's, GRE General Test. Additional exam requirements/recommendations for international students: Required—TOEFL. *Application deadline:* Applications are processed on a rolling basis. Application fee: $60. Electronic applications accepted. *Expenses:* Tuition, state resident: part-time $334 per credit hour. Tuition, nonresident: part-time $1224 per credit hour. *Financial support:* Applicants required to submit FAFSA. *Unit head:* Dr. Mark Yeager, Chair, 434-924-5108, Fax: 434-982-1616, E-mail: my3r@virginia.edu. *Application contact:* Director of Graduate Studies, E-mail: physiograd@virginia.edu.
Website: http://www.healthsystem.virginia.edu/internet/physio/

University of Washington, Graduate School, College of Arts and Sciences, Department of Biology, Seattle, WA 98195. Offers PhD.

University of Washington, Graduate School, School of Medicine, Graduate Programs in Medicine, Seattle, WA 98195. Offers MA, MOT, MPO, MS, DPT, PhD. Part-time programs available. *Degree requirements:* For doctorate, thesis/dissertation. *Entrance requirements:* For doctorate, GRE. Electronic applications accepted. *Expenses:* Contact institution.

University of Waterloo, Graduate Studies, Faculty of Science, Department of Biology, Waterloo, ON N2L 3G1, Canada. Offers M Sc, PhD. Part-time programs available. *Degree requirements:* For master's, thesis, seminar, proposal; for doctorate, comprehensive exam, thesis/dissertation, seminar, proposal. *Entrance requirements:* For master's, honor's degree; for doctorate, master's degree. Additional exam requirements/recommendations for international students: Required—TOEFL (minimum score 580 paper-based; 90 iBT), TWE (minimum score 4). Electronic applications accepted. *Faculty research:* Biosystematics, ecology and limnology, molecular and cellular biology, biochemistry, physiology.

Biological and Biomedical Sciences—General

The University of Western Ontario, Faculty of Graduate Studies, Biosciences Division, Department of Biology, London, ON N6A 5B8, Canada. Offers M Sc, PhD. *Degree requirements:* For master's, thesis; for doctorate, thesis/dissertation. *Entrance requirements:* For doctorate, M Sc or equivalent. Additional exam requirements/recommendations for international students: Required—TOEFL. *Faculty research:* Ecology systematics, plant biochemistry and physiology, yeast genetics, molecular biology.

University of West Florida, College of Arts and Sciences: Sciences, School of Allied Health and Life Sciences, Department of Biology, Pensacola, FL 32514-5750. Offers biological chemistry (MS); biology (MS); biology education (MST); biotechnology (MS); coastal zone studies (MS); environmental biology (MS). *Degree requirements:* For master's, thesis. *Entrance requirements:* For master's, GRE (minimum score: verbal 450, quantitative 550), official transcripts; BS in biology or related field; letter of interest; relevant past experience; three letters of recommendation from individuals who can evaluate applicant's academic ability. Additional exam requirements/recommendations for international students: Required—TOEFL (minimum score 550 paper-based).

University of West Georgia, College of Science and Mathematics, Department of Biology, Carrollton, GA 30118. Offers MS. Part-time programs available. *Faculty:* 9 full-time (2 women). *Students:* 13 full-time (6 women), 6 part-time (5 women); includes 6 minority (4 Black or African American, non-Hispanic/Latino; 1 Asian, non-Hispanic/Latino; 1 Hispanic/Latino). Average age 27. 15 applicants, 73% accepted, 5 enrolled. In 2013, 11 master's awarded. *Degree requirements:* For master's, comprehensive exam (for some programs), thesis (for some programs). *Entrance requirements:* For master's, GRE General Test, minimum GPA of 2.8, undergraduate degree in biology. Additional exam requirements/recommendations for international students: Required—TOEFL (minimum score 523 paper-based; 69 iBT); Recommended—IELTS (minimum score 6). *Application deadline:* For fall admission, 6/1 for domestic and international students; for spring admission, 11/15 for domestic students, 10/15 for international students. Applications are processed on a rolling basis. Application fee: $40. Electronic applications accepted. *Expenses:* Tuition, state resident: full-time $4600; part-time $192 per semester hour. Tuition, nonresident: full-time $17,880; part-time $745 per semester hour. *Required fees:* $1858; $46.34 per semester hour. $512 per semester. Tuition and fees vary according to course load, degree level, campus/location and program. *Financial support:* In 2013–14, 8 teaching assistantships with full tuition reimbursements (averaging $8,000 per year) were awarded; scholarships/grants and unspecified assistantships also available. Financial award application deadline: 4/1; financial award applicants required to submit FAFSA. *Faculty research:* Molecular systematics, animal physiology, marine ecology, plant ecology, animal behavior. *Unit head:* Dr. Christopher Tabit, Chair, 678-839-4022, Fax: 678-839-6548, E-mail: ctabit@westga.edu. *Application contact:* Alice Wesley, Departmental Assistant, 678-839-5192, E-mail: awesley@westga.edu.
Website: http://www.westga.edu/biology/

University of Windsor, Faculty of Graduate Studies, Faculty of Science, Department of Biological Sciences, Windsor, ON N9B 3P4, Canada. Offers M Sc, PhD. Part-time programs available. *Degree requirements:* For master's, thesis; for doctorate, comprehensive exam, thesis/dissertation. *Entrance requirements:* For master's and doctorate, minimum B average. Additional exam requirements/recommendations for international students: Required—TOEFL (minimum score 560 paper-based). Electronic applications accepted. *Faculty research:* Great Lakes Institute: aquatic ecotoxicology, regulation and development of the olfactory system, mating system evolution, signal transduction, aquatic ecology.

University of Wisconsin–La Crosse, Graduate Studies, College of Science and Health, Department of Biology, La Crosse, WI 54601-3742. Offers aquatic sciences (MS); biology (MS); cellular and molecular biology (MS); clinical microbiology (MS); microbiology (MS); nurse anesthesia (MS); physiology (MS). Part-time programs available. *Faculty:* 22 full-time (8 women), 3 part-time/adjunct (1 woman). *Students:* 21 full-time (13 women), 37 part-time (24 women); includes 7 minority (2 Asian, non-Hispanic/Latino; 4 Hispanic/Latino; 1 Two or more races, non-Hispanic/Latino), 5 international. Average age 28. 107 applicants, 26% accepted, 25 enrolled. In 2013, 16 master's awarded. *Degree requirements:* For master's, comprehensive exam, thesis. *Entrance requirements:* For master's, GRE General Test, minimum GPA of 2.85. Additional exam requirements/recommendations for international students: Required—TOEFL (minimum score 550 paper-based; 79 iBT). *Application deadline:* For fall admission, 2/1 priority date for domestic and international students; for spring admission, 1/4 priority date for domestic and international students. Applications are processed on a rolling basis. Electronic applications accepted. *Financial support:* Research assistantships with partial tuition reimbursements, Federal Work-Study, scholarships/grants, health care benefits, and tuition waivers (partial) available. Support available to part-time students. Financial award application deadline: 3/15; financial award applicants required to submit FAFSA. *Unit head:* Dr. Thomas Volk, Coordinator of Graduate Studies, 608-785-6972, Fax: 608-785-6959, E-mail: volk.thom@uwlax.edu. *Application contact:* Corey Sjoquist, Director of Admissions, 608-785-8939, E-mail: admissions@uwlax.edu.
Website: http://uwlax.edu/biology/

University of Wisconsin–Madison, School of Medicine and Public Health and Graduate School, Graduate Programs in Medicine, Madison, WI 53705. Offers biomolecular chemistry (MS, PhD); cancer biology (PhD); epidemiology (MS, PhD); genetics and medical genetics (MS, PhD), including genetics (PhD), medical genetics (MS); medical physics (MS, PhD), including health physics (MS), medical physics; microbiology (PhD); molecular and cellular pharmacology (PhD); neuroscience (PhD); pathology and laboratory medicine (PhD); physiology (PhD); population health (MS, PhD), including population health; DPT/MPH; DVM/MPH; MD/MPH; MD/PhD; MPA/MPH; MS/MPH; Pharm D/MPH. Part-time programs available. Postbaccalaureate distance learning degree programs offered (minimal on-campus study). Terminal master's awarded for partial completion of doctoral program. Application fee: $45. Electronic applications accepted. *Expenses:* Contact institution. *Financial support:* Fellowships with full tuition reimbursements, research assistantships with full tuition reimbursements, teaching assistantships with full tuition reimbursements, scholarships/grants, traineeships, and tuition waivers (full) available. *Unit head:* Dr. Richard L. Moss, Senior Associate Dean for Basic Research, Biotechnology and Graduate Studies, 608-265-0523, Fax: 608-265-0522, E-mail: rlmoss@wisc.edu. *Application contact:* Information Contact, 608-262-2433, Fax: 608-262-5134, E-mail: gradadmiss@mail.bascom.wisc.edu.
Website: http://www.med.wisc.edu

University of Wisconsin–Madison, School of Medicine and Public Health, Medical Scientist Training Program, Madison, WI 53705-2221. Offers MD/PhD. *Accreditation:* LCME/AMA. *Faculty:* 380 full-time (80 women). *Students:* 79 full-time (29 women); includes 26 minority (7 Black or African American, non-Hispanic/Latino; 16 Asian, non-Hispanic/Latino; 3 Hispanic/Latino). 269 applicants, 12% accepted, 6 enrolled. *Application deadline:* For fall admission, 12/1 for domestic students. Applications are processed on a rolling basis. Application fee: $54. Electronic applications accepted. *Expenses:* Tuition, state resident: full-time $10,728; part-time $790 per credit. Tuition, nonresident: full-time $24,054; part-time $1623 per credit. *Required fees:* $1130; $119 per credit. *Financial support:* In 2013–14, 79 students received support, including fellowships with full tuition reimbursements available (averaging $24,500 per year), research assistantships with full tuition reimbursements available (averaging $24,500 per year); traineeships and health care benefits also available. *Unit head:* Dr. Anna Huttenlocher, Director, 608-265-4642, Fax: 608-262-8418, E-mail: huttenlocher@wisc.edu. *Application contact:* Paul Cook, Program Administrator, 608-262-6321, Fax: 608-262-4226, E-mail: pscook@wisc.edu.
Website: http://mstp.med.wisc.edu/

University of Wisconsin–Milwaukee, Graduate School, College of Health Sciences, PhD Program in Health Sciences, Milwaukee, WI 53201-0413. Offers PhD. *Faculty:* 8 full-time (4 women), 1 part-time/adjunct (0 women). *Students:* 22 full-time (12 women), 4 part-time (3 women); includes 4 minority (1 Asian, non-Hispanic/Latino; 3 Two or more races, non-Hispanic/Latino), 8 international. Average age 31. 26 applicants, 65% accepted, 11 enrolled. In 2013, 7 doctorates awarded. *Degree requirements:* For doctorate, comprehensive exam, thesis/dissertation. *Entrance requirements:* For doctorate, GRE. Additional exam requirements/recommendations for international students: Required—TOEFL (minimum score 600 paper-based), IELTS (minimum score 6.5). Application fee: $56 ($96 for international students). *Financial support:* In 2013–14, 4 fellowships, 5 research assistantships, 3 teaching assistantships were awarded; project assistantships also available. *Unit head:* Paula M. Rhyner, Program Representative, 414-229-4878, E-mail: prhyner@uwm.edu. *Application contact:* Roger O. Smith, General Information Contact, 414-229-6697, Fax: 414-229-6697, E-mail: smithro@uwm.edu.
Website: http://www4.uwm.edu/chs/academics/phd_health_sciences/

University of Wisconsin–Milwaukee, Graduate School, College of Health Sciences, Program in Biomedical Sciences, Milwaukee, WI 53211. Offers MS. *Accreditation:* NAACLS. Part-time programs available. *Faculty:* 8 full-time (4 women). *Students:* 9 full-time (6 women), 6 part-time (all women); includes 2 minority (1 Asian, non-Hispanic/Latino; 1 Two or more races, non-Hispanic/Latino), 4 international. Average age 29. 42 applicants, 14% accepted, 4 enrolled. *Degree requirements:* For master's, thesis. *Entrance requirements:* For master's, GRE General Test. Additional exam requirements/recommendations for international students: Required—TOEFL (minimum score 550 paper-based; 79 iBT), IELTS (minimum score 6.5). *Application deadline:* For fall admission, 1/1 priority date for domestic students; for spring admission, 9/1 for domestic students. Applications are processed on a rolling basis. Application fee: $56 ($96 for international students). *Financial support:* In 2013–14, 6 teaching assistantships were awarded; fellowships, research assistantships, career-related internships or fieldwork, and unspecified assistantships also available. Support available to part-time students. Financial award application deadline: 4/15. *Unit head:* Jeri-Anne Lyons, Representative, 414-229-3812, E-mail: jlyons@uwm.edu. *Application contact:* Roger O. Smith, General Information Contact, 414-229-6697, Fax: 414-229-6697, E-mail: smithro@uwm.edu.
Website: http://www4.uwm.edu/chs/academics/biomedical_sciences/bms_masters/

University of Wisconsin–Milwaukee, Graduate School, College of Letters and Sciences, Department of Biological Sciences, Milwaukee, WI 53201-0413. Offers MS, PhD. *Faculty:* 31 full-time (10 women). *Students:* 38 full-time (21 women), 27 part-time (16 women); includes 6 minority (2 Asian, non-Hispanic/Latino; 4 Two or more races, non-Hispanic/Latino), 23 international. Average age 29. 80 applicants, 24% accepted, 12 enrolled. In 2013, 9 master's, 7 doctorates awarded. *Degree requirements:* For master's, thesis; for doctorate, thesis/dissertation, 1 foreign language or data analysis proficiency. *Entrance requirements:* For master's and doctorate, GRE General Test. Additional exam requirements/recommendations for international students: Required—TOEFL (minimum score 550 paper-based; 79 iBT), IELTS (minimum score 6.5). *Application deadline:* For fall admission, 3/1 priority date for domestic students. Applications are processed on a rolling basis. Application fee: $56 ($96 for international students). *Financial support:* In 2013–14, 3 fellowships, 9 research assistantships, 67 teaching assistantships were awarded; career-related internships or fieldwork, unspecified assistantships, and project assistantships also available. Support available to part-time students. Financial award application deadline: 4/15; financial award applicants required to submit FAFSA. *Unit head:* Daad Saffarini, Department Chair, 414-229-4279, E-mail: daads@uwm.edu. *Application contact:* General Information Contact, 414-229-4982, Fax: 414-229-6967, E-mail: gradschool@uwm.edu.
Website: http://www.uwm.edu/dept/biology/

University of Wisconsin–Oshkosh, Graduate Studies, College of Letters and Science, Department of Biology and Microbiology, Oshkosh, WI 54901. Offers biology (MS), including botany, microbiology, zoology. *Degree requirements:* For master's, comprehensive exam, thesis. *Entrance requirements:* For master's, GRE General Test, minimum GPA of 3.0, BS in biology. Additional exam requirements/recommendations for international students: Required—TOEFL (minimum score 550 paper-based; 79 iBT). Electronic applications accepted.

Utah State University, School of Graduate Studies, College of Science, Department of Biology, Logan, UT 84322. Offers biology (MS, PhD); ecology (MS, PhD). Part-time programs available. *Degree requirements:* For master's, thesis; for doctorate, thesis/dissertation. *Entrance requirements:* For master's and doctorate, GRE General Test, minimum GPA of 3.0. Additional exam requirements/recommendations for international students: Required—TOEFL (minimum score 575 paper-based). *Faculty research:* Plant, insect, microbial, and animal biology.

Vanderbilt University, Graduate School, Department of Biological Sciences, Nashville, TN 37240-1001. Offers MS, PhD, MD/PhD. *Faculty:* 20 full-time (2 women). *Students:* 51 full-time (30 women); includes 12 minority (3 Black or African American, non-Hispanic/Latino; 6 Asian, non-Hispanic/Latino; 3 Hispanic/Latino), 17 international. Average age 26. 161 applicants, 7% accepted, 7 enrolled. In 2013, 4 master's, 10 doctorates awarded. Terminal master's awarded for partial completion of doctoral program. *Degree requirements:* For master's, thesis; for doctorate, thesis/dissertation, final and qualifying exams. *Entrance requirements:* For master's and doctorate, GRE General Test. Additional exam requirements/recommendations for international students: Required—TOEFL (minimum score 570 paper-based; 88 iBT). *Application deadline:* For fall admission, 1/15 for domestic and international students. Electronic applications accepted. *Financial support:* Fellowships with full and partial tuition reimbursements, research assistantships with full tuition reimbursements, teaching assistantships with full tuition reimbursements, Federal Work-Study, institutionally sponsored loans, scholarships/grants, traineeships, and health care benefits available. Financial award application deadline: 1/15; financial award applicants required to submit CSS PROFILE or FAFSA. *Faculty research:* Protein structure and function, protein transport, membrane ion channels and receptors, signal transduction, posttranscriptional control of gene expression, DNA replication and recombination, biological clocks, development, neurobiology, vector biology, insect physiology, ecology and evolution, bioinformatics. *Unit head:* Dr. Katherine Friedman, Director of Graduate Studies, 615-322-5143, Fax: 615-343-6707, E-mail: katherine.friedman@vanderbilt.edu. *Application contact:* Leslie L. Maxwell, Program Coordinator, 615-343-3076, Fax: 615-343-6707, E-mail: leslie.l.maxwell@vanderbilt.edu.
Website: http://sitemason.vanderbilt.edu/biosci/grad/

Vanderbilt University, School of Medicine and Graduate School, Medical Scientist Training Program, Nashville, TN 37240-1001. Offers MD/PhD. *Entrance requirements:*

Additional exam requirements/recommendations for international students: Recommended—TOEFL. Electronic applications accepted. *Expenses:* Contact institution. *Faculty research:* Cancer biology, neurosciences, microbiology, biochemistry, metabolism/diabetics.

Villanova University, Graduate School of Liberal Arts and Sciences, Department of Biology, Villanova, PA 19085-1699. Offers MA, MS. Part-time and evening/weekend programs available. *Students:* 52 full-time (32 women), 12 part-time (6 women); includes 8 minority (3 Asian, non-Hispanic/Latino; 5 Hispanic/Latino), 2 international. Average age 26. 38 applicants, 76% accepted, 20 enrolled. In 2013, 12 master's awarded. *Degree requirements:* For master's, comprehensive exam (for some programs), thesis (for some programs). *Entrance requirements:* For master's, GRE General Test, minimum GPA of 3.0, 3 recommendation letters. *Application deadline:* For fall admission, 3/1 priority date for domestic students, 5/1 for international students; for spring admission, 11/15 priority date for domestic students, 10/15 for international students; for summer admission, 5/1 for domestic students, 4/1 for international students. Applications are processed on a rolling basis. Application fee: $50. Electronic applications accepted. *Financial support:* Research assistantships with tuition reimbursements, teaching assistantships with tuition reimbursements, scholarships/grants, health care benefits, and unspecified assistantships available. Financial award applicants required to submit FAFSA. *Unit head:* Dr. Aaron Bauer, Chair, 610-519-4857. *Application contact:* Dr. Adele Lindenmeyr, Dean, Graduate School of Liberal Arts and Sciences, 610-519-7093, Fax: 610-519-7096.
Website: http://www.villanova.edu/artsci/biology/graduate/

Virginia Commonwealth University, Graduate School, College of Humanities and Sciences, Department of Biology, Richmond, VA 23284-9005. Offers MS. Part-time programs available. *Degree requirements:* For master's, thesis. *Entrance requirements:* For master's, GRE General Test, BS in biology or related field. Additional exam requirements/recommendations for international students: Required—TOEFL (minimum score 600 paper-based; 100 iBT) or IELTS (minimum score 6.5). *Faculty research:* Molecular and cellular biology, terrestrial and aquatic ecology, systematics, physiology and developmental biology.

Virginia Commonwealth University, Graduate School, School of Life Sciences, Richmond, VA 23284-9005. Offers M Env Sc, MB, MS, PhD. *Entrance requirements:* For master's and doctorate, GRE. Additional exam requirements/recommendations for international students: Required—TOEFL (minimum score 600 paper-based; 100 iBT). Electronic applications accepted.

Virginia Commonwealth University, Medical College of Virginia-Professional Programs, School of Medicine, School of Medicine Graduate Programs, Richmond, VA 23284-9005. Offers MPH, MS, PhD, Certificate, MD/MPH, MD/PhD. Part-time programs available. Terminal master's awarded for partial completion of doctoral program. *Degree requirements:* For doctorate, thesis/dissertation, comprehensive oral and written exams. *Entrance requirements:* For doctorate, GRE General Test, MCAT.

Virginia Commonwealth University, Program in Pre-Medical Basic Health Sciences, Richmond, VA 23284-9005. Offers anatomy (CBHS); biochemistry (CBHS); human genetics (CBHS); microbiology (CBHS); pharmacology (CBHS); physiology (CBHS). *Entrance requirements:* For degree, GRE, MCAT or DAT, course work in organic chemistry, minimum undergraduate GPA of 2.8. Additional exam requirements/recommendations for international students: Required—TOEFL (minimum score 600 paper-based). Electronic applications accepted.

Virginia Polytechnic Institute and State University, Graduate School, College of Science, Blacksburg, VA 24061. Offers biological sciences (MS, PhD); biomedical technology development and management (MS); chemistry (MS, PhD); economics (MA, PhD); geosciences (MS, PhD); mathematics (MS, PhD); physics (MS, PhD); psychology (MS, PhD); statistics (MS, PhD). *Faculty:* 272 full-time (74 women), 1 (woman) part-time/adjunct. *Students:* 558 full-time (223 women), 39 part-time (20 women); includes 54 minority (14 Black or African American, non-Hispanic/Latino; 10 Asian, non-Hispanic/Latino; 17 Hispanic/Latino; 13 Two or more races, non-Hispanic/Latino), 253 international. Average age 27. 1,123 applicants, 18% accepted, 112 enrolled. In 2013, 82 master's, 80 doctorates awarded. *Degree requirements:* For master's, comprehensive exam (for some programs), thesis (for some programs); for doctorate, comprehensive exam (for some programs), thesis/dissertation (for some programs). *Entrance requirements:* For master's and doctorate, GRE/GMAT (may vary by department). Additional exam requirements/recommendations for international students: Required—TOEFL (minimum score 550 paper-based). *Application deadline:* For fall admission, 8/1 for domestic students, 4/1 for international students; for spring admission, 1/1 for domestic students, 9/1 for international students. Applications are processed on a rolling basis. Application fee: $75. Electronic applications accepted. *Expenses:* Tuition, state resident: full-time $11,185; part-time $621.50 per credit hour. Tuition, nonresident: full-time $22,146; part-time $1230.25 per credit hour. *Required fees:* $2442; $449.25 per semester. Tuition and fees vary according to course load, campus/location and program. *Financial support:* In 2013–14, 1 fellowship with full tuition reimbursement (averaging $5,313 per year), 163 research assistantships with full tuition reimbursements (averaging $20,937 per year), 345 teaching assistantships with full tuition reimbursements (averaging $17,975 per year) were awarded. Financial award application deadline: 3/1; financial award applicants required to submit FAFSA. *Total annual research expenditures:* $25 million. *Unit head:* Dr. Lay Nam Chang, Dean, 540-231-5422, Fax: 540-231-3380, E-mail: laynam@vt.edu. *Application contact:* Diane Stearns, Assistant to the Dean, 540-231-7515, Fax: 540-231-3380, E-mail: dstearns@vt.edu.
Website: http://www.science.vt.edu/

Virginia State University, School of Graduate Studies, Research, and Outreach, School of Engineering, Science and Technology, Department of Biology, Petersburg, VA 23806-0001. Offers MS. *Degree requirements:* For master's, one foreign language, thesis. *Entrance requirements:* For master's, GRE General Test. *Faculty research:* Schwann cell cultures, selection of apios as an alternative crop, systematic botany, flowers of three species of wild ginger.

Wake Forest University, Graduate School of Arts and Sciences, Department of Biology, Winston-Salem, NC 27109. Offers MS, PhD. Part-time programs available. *Degree requirements:* For master's, one foreign language, thesis; for doctorate, 2 foreign languages, comprehensive exam, thesis/dissertation. *Entrance requirements:* For master's and doctorate, GRE General Test. Additional exam requirements/recommendations for international students: Required—TOEFL (minimum score 79 iBT). Electronic applications accepted. *Faculty research:* Cell biology, ecology, parasitology, immunology.

Wake Forest University, School of Medicine and Graduate School of Arts and Sciences, Graduate Programs in Medicine, Winston-Salem, NC 27109. Offers MS, PhD, MD/PhD. *Degree requirements:* For master's, thesis; for doctorate, thesis/dissertation. *Entrance requirements:* For master's and doctorate, GRE General Test. Additional exam requirements/recommendations for international students: Required—TOEFL. Electronic applications accepted. *Expenses:* Contact institution. *Faculty research:* Atherosclerosis, cardiovascular physiology, pharmacology, neuroanatomy, endocrinology.

Walla Walla University, Graduate School, Department of Biological Sciences, College Place, WA 99324-1198. Offers biology (MS). *Degree requirements:* For master's, thesis. *Entrance requirements:* For master's, GRE General Test, GRE Subject Test, minimum GPA of 2.75. Additional exam requirements/recommendations for international students: Required—TOEFL (minimum score 550 paper-based; 79 iBT). Electronic applications accepted. *Faculty research:* Marine biology, plant development, neurobiology, animal physiology, behavior.

Washington State University, Graduate School, College of Arts and Sciences, Program in Biology, Pullman, WA 99164-4236. Offers MS. *Degree requirements:* For master's, comprehensive exam (for some programs), thesis (for some programs), oral examination. *Entrance requirements:* For master's, GRE, three letters of recommendation, official transcripts from each university-level school attended, minimum GPA of 3.0. Additional exam requirements/recommendations for international students: Required—TOEFL, IELTS. *Faculty research:* Student learning styles.

Washington University in St. Louis, Graduate School of Arts and Sciences, Division of Biology and Biomedical Sciences, St. Louis, MO 63130-4899. Offers biochemistry (PhD); computational and molecular biophysics (PhD); computational and systems biology (PhD); developmental, regenerative, and stem cell biology (PhD); evolution, ecology and population biology (PhD), including ecology, environmental biology, evolutionary biology, genetics; human and statistical genetics (PhD); immunology (PhD); molecular cell biology (PhD); molecular genetics and genomics (PhD); molecular microbiology and microbial pathogenesis (PhD); neurosciences (PhD); plant biology (PhD); MD/PhD. *Degree requirements:* For doctorate, thesis/dissertation. *Entrance requirements:* For doctorate, GRE General Test, GRE Subject Test. Electronic applications accepted.

Wayne State University, College of Liberal Arts and Sciences, Department of Biological Sciences, Detroit, MI 48202. Offers biological sciences (MA, MS); cell development and neurobiology (PhD); evolution and organismal biology (PhD); molecular biology and biotechnology (PhD); molecular biotechnology (MS). Fall application deadline for PhD is December 1. *Faculty:* 26 full-time (9 women). *Students:* 66 full-time (37 women), 8 part-time (3 women); includes 8 minority (1 Black or African American, non-Hispanic/Latino; 5 Asian, non-Hispanic/Latino; 1 Hispanic/Latino; 1 Two or more races, non-Hispanic/Latino), 41 international. Average age 29. 270 applicants, 14% accepted, 14 enrolled. In 2013, 14 master's, 8 doctorates awarded. Terminal master's awarded for partial completion of doctoral program. *Degree requirements:* For master's, thesis (for some programs); for doctorate, thesis/dissertation. *Entrance requirements:* For master's, GRE (for MS applicants), minimum GPA of 3.0; adequate preparation in biological sciences and supporting courses in chemistry, physics and mathematics; curriculum vitae; for doctorate, GRE, three letters of reference, statement of goals and career objectives, bachelor's or master's degree in biological or other science. Additional exam requirements/recommendations for international students: Required—TOEFL (minimum score 550 paper-based; 79 iBT), TWE (minimum score 5.5), Michigan English Language Assessment Battery (minimum score 85); Recommended—IELTS (minimum score 6.5). *Application deadline:* For fall admission, 4/1 for domestic students, 3/1 for international students. Applications are processed on a rolling basis. Application fee: $0. Electronic applications accepted. *Expenses:* Tuition, state resident: part-time $554.15 per credit. Tuition, nonresident: part-time $1200.35 per credit. *Required fees:* $42.15 per credit. $268.30 per semester. Tuition and fees vary according to course load and program. *Financial support:* In 2013–14, 55 students received support, including 3 fellowships with tuition reimbursements available (averaging $16,842 per year), 9 research assistantships with tuition reimbursements available (averaging $18,582 per year), 49 teaching assistantships with tuition reimbursements available (averaging $18,488 per year); institutionally sponsored loans, scholarships/grants, health care benefits, and unspecified assistantships also available. Financial award application deadline: 3/31; financial award applicants required to submit FAFSA. *Faculty research:* Transcription and chromatin remodeling, genomic and developmental evolution, community and landscape ecology and environmental degradation, microbiology and virology, cell and neurobiology. *Total annual research expenditures:* $1.7 million. *Unit head:* Dr. David Njus, Professor and Chair, 313-577-2783, Fax: 313-577-6891, E-mail: dnjus@wayne.edu. *Application contact:* Rose Mary Priest, Office Services Clerk, 313-577-6818, Fax: 313-577-6891, E-mail: rpriest@wayne.edu.
Website: http://clasweb.clas.wayne.edu/biology

Weill Cornell Medical College, Weill Cornell Graduate School of Medical Sciences, New York, NY 10065. Offers MS, PhD. Terminal master's awarded for partial completion of doctoral program. *Degree requirements:* For master's, comprehensive exam, thesis (for some programs); for doctorate, thesis/dissertation, final exam. *Entrance requirements:* For doctorate, GRE General Test. Additional exam requirements/recommendations for international students: Required—TOEFL. Electronic applications accepted. *Expenses:* Contact institution.

Weill Cornell Medical College, Weill Cornell/Rockefeller/Sloan-Kettering Tri-Institutional MD-PhD Program, New York, NY 10065. Offers MD/PhD. Offered jointly with The Rockefeller University and Sloan-Kettering Institute. Electronic applications accepted. *Expenses:* Contact institution. *Faculty research:* Neuroscience, pharmacology, immunology, structural biology, genetics.

Wesleyan University, Graduate Studies, Department of Biology, Middletown, CT 06459. Offers cell and developmental genetics (PhD); evolution and ecology (PhD); neurobiology and behavior (PhD). *Degree requirements:* For doctorate, variable foreign language requirement, thesis/dissertation. *Entrance requirements:* For doctorate, GRE. Additional exam requirements/recommendations for international students: Required—TOEFL. *Faculty research:* Microbial population genetics, genetic basis of evolutionary adaptation, genetic regulation of differentiation and pattern formation in &ITdrosophila&RO.

West Chester University of Pennsylvania, College of Arts and Sciences, Department of Biology, West Chester, PA 19383. Offers MS, Teaching Certificate. Part-time and evening/weekend programs available. *Faculty:* 9 full-time (2 women). *Students:* 10 full-time (7 women), 22 part-time (11 women); includes 6 minority (1 Black or African American, non-Hispanic/Latino; 1 Asian, non-Hispanic/Latino; 3 Hispanic/Latino; 1 Two or more races, non-Hispanic/Latino), 2 international. Average age 29. 32 applicants, 81% accepted, 14 enrolled. In 2013, 15 master's awarded. *Degree requirements:* For master's, comprehensive exam, thesis (for some programs). *Entrance requirements:* For master's, two letters of reference. Additional exam requirements/recommendations for international students: Required—TOEFL (minimum score 550 paper-based; 80 iBT). *Application deadline:* For fall admission, 4/15 priority date for domestic students, 3/15 for international students; for spring admission, 10/15 priority date for domestic students, 9/1 for international students. Applications are processed on a rolling basis. Application fee: $45. Electronic applications accepted. *Expenses:* Tuition, state resident: full-time $7956; part-time $442 per credit. Tuition, nonresident: full-time $11,934; part-time $663 per credit. *Required fees:* $2134.20; $106.24 per credit. Tuition and fees vary according to campus/location and program. *Financial support:* Unspecified assistantships available. Support available to part-time students. Financial award application deadline: 2/15; financial award applicants required to submit FAFSA. *Faculty research:* Medical microbiology, molecular genetics and physiology of living systems, mammalian

biomechanics, invertebrate and vertebrate animal systems, aquatic and terrestrial ecology. *Unit head:* Dr. Jack Waber, Chair, 610-436-2319, E-mail: jwaber@wcupa.edu. *Application contact:* Dr. Xin Fan, Graduate Coordinator, 610-436-2281, E-mail: xfan@wcupa.edu.
Website: http://bio.wcupa.edu/biology/index.php

Western Carolina University, Graduate School, College of Arts and Sciences, Department of Biology, Cullowhee, NC 28723. Offers MS. Part-time and evening/weekend programs available. *Degree requirements:* For master's, thesis. *Entrance requirements:* For master's, GRE General Test, appropriate undergraduate degree, 3 letters of recommendation. Additional exam requirements/recommendations for international students: Required—TOEFL (minimum score 550 paper-based; 79 iBT). *Faculty research:* Pathogen interactions, gene expression, plant community ecology, restoration ecology, ornithology, herpetology.

Western Connecticut State University, Division of Graduate Studies, School of Arts and Sciences, Department of Biological and Environmental Sciences, Danbury, CT 06810-6885. Offers MA. Part-time programs available. *Degree requirements:* For master's, comprehensive exam or thesis, completion of program in 6 years. *Entrance requirements:* For master's, minimum GPA of 2.5. Additional exam requirements/recommendations for international students: Recommended—TOEFL (minimum score 550 paper-based; 79 iBT), IELTS (minimum score 6). *Expenses:* Contact institution. *Faculty research:* Biology, taxonomy and evolution of aquatic flowering plants; aquatic plant reproductive systems, the spread of invasive aquatic plants, aquatic plant structure, and the taxonomy of water starworts (Callitrichaceae) and riverweeds (Podostemaceae).

Western Illinois University, School of Graduate Studies, College of Arts and Sciences, Department of Biological Sciences, Macomb, IL 61455-1390. Offers biological sciences (MS); environmental geographic information systems (Certificate); zoo and aquarium studies (Certificate). Part-time programs available. *Students:* 52 full-time (40 women), 27 part-time (19 women); includes 3 minority (1 Black or African American, non-Hispanic/Latino; 2 Hispanic/Latino), 4 international. Average age 26. In 2013, 14 master's, 17 other advanced degrees awarded. *Degree requirements:* For master's, thesis or alternative. *Entrance requirements:* Additional exam requirements/recommendations for international students: Required—TOEFL (minimum score 550 paper-based; 80 iBT); Recommended—IELTS. *Application deadline:* Applications are processed on a rolling basis. Application fee: $30. Electronic applications accepted. *Financial support:* In 2013–14, 29 students received support, including 9 research assistantships with full tuition reimbursements available (averaging $7,544 per year), 20 teaching assistantships with full tuition reimbursements available (averaging $8,688 per year). Financial award applicants required to submit FAFSA. *Unit head:* Dr. Charles Lydeard, Chairperson, 309-298-1546. *Application contact:* Dr. Nancy Parsons, Associate Provost and Director of Graduate Studies, 309-298-1806, Fax: 309-298-2345, E-mail: grad-office@wiu.edu.
Website: http://wiu.edu/biology

Western Kentucky University, Graduate Studies, Ogden College of Science and Engineering, Department of Biology, Bowling Green, KY 42101. Offers MS. Postbaccalaureate distance learning degree programs offered. *Degree requirements:* For master's, comprehensive exam, thesis optional, research tool. *Entrance requirements:* For master's, GRE General Test, minimum GPA of 2.75. Additional exam requirements/recommendations for international students: Required—TOEFL (minimum score 555 paper-based; 79 iBT). *Faculty research:* Phytoremediation, culturing of salt water organisms, PCR-based standards, biological monitoring (water) bioremediation, genetic diversity.

Western Michigan University, Graduate College, College of Arts and Sciences, Department of Biological Sciences, Kalamazoo, MI 49008. Offers MS, PhD. *Degree requirements:* For master's, thesis, oral exam; for doctorate, thesis/dissertation, oral exam. *Entrance requirements:* For master's and doctorate, GRE General Test.

Western Michigan University, Graduate College, College of Arts and Sciences, Mallinson Institute for Science Education, Kalamazoo, MI 49008. Offers science education (MA, PhD); science education: biological sciences (PhD); science education: chemistry (PhD); science education: geosciences (PhD); science education: physical geography (PhD); science education: physics (PhD). *Degree requirements:* For doctorate, thesis/dissertation, oral and written exams. *Entrance requirements:* For master's, undergraduate degree in a science or science education, teacher certification (or appropriate education courses); for doctorate, GRE General Test, master's degree in a science or science education. Additional exam requirements/recommendations for international students: Recommended—TOEFL. Electronic applications accepted. *Faculty research:* History and philosophy of science, curriculum and instruction, science content learning, college science teaching and learning, social and cultural factors in science education.

Western University of Health Sciences, Graduate College of Biomedical Sciences, Master of Science in Biomedical Sciences Program, Pomona, CA 91766-1854. Offers MS. *Faculty:* 4 full-time (1 woman). *Students:* 12 full-time (all women); includes 7 minority (1 Black or African American, non-Hispanic/Latino; 3 Asian, non-Hispanic/Latino; 2 Hispanic/Latino; 1 Two or more races, non-Hispanic/Latino). Average age 24. 31 applicants, 29% accepted, 8 enrolled. In 2013, 1 master's awarded. *Degree requirements:* For master's, comprehensive exam (for some programs), thesis. *Entrance requirements:* For master's, GRE, minimum overall GPA of 3.0; letters of recommendation; personal statement; resume; BS in pharmacy, chemistry, biology or related scientific area. Additional exam requirements/recommendations for international students: Required—TOEFL. *Application deadline:* For fall admission, 4/1 for domestic students. Application fee: $50. Electronic applications accepted. *Unit head:* Dr. Guru Betageri, Assistant Dean, Graduate College of Biomedical Sciences, 909-469-5682, E-mail: gbetageri@westernu.edu. *Application contact:* Kathryn Ford, Director of Admission, 909-469-5335, Fax: 909-469-5570, E-mail: admissions@westernu.edu.
Website: https://www.westernu.edu/biomedical-sciences/biomedical-sciences-academics/biomedical-sciences-msbs/

Western University of Health Sciences, Graduate College of Biomedical Sciences, Master of Science in Medical Sciences Program, Pomona, CA 91766-1854. Offers MS. *Faculty:* 1 (woman) full-time. *Students:* 33 full-time (14 women); includes 27 minority (7 Black or African American, non-Hispanic/Latino; 8 Asian, non-Hispanic/Latino; 9 Hispanic/Latino; 1 Native Hawaiian or other Pacific Islander, non-Hispanic/Latino; 2 Two or more races, non-Hispanic/Latino), 1 international. Average age 27. 283 applicants, 14% accepted, 32 enrolled. In 2013, 34 master's awarded. *Degree requirements:* For master's, comprehensive exam (for some programs). *Entrance requirements:* For master's, GRE, MCAT, OAT, or DAT, minimum overall GPA of 2.5; letters of recommendation; personal statement; resume; transcripts; bachelor's degree. Additional exam requirements/recommendations for international students: Required—TOEFL (minimum score 89 iBT). *Application deadline:* For fall admission, 3/1 for domestic students. Application fee: $50. Electronic applications accepted. *Unit head:* Jodi Olson, Director, Master's Program in Clinical Sciences, 909-706-3842, Fax: 909-469-5577, E-mail: olsonj@westernu.edu. *Application contact:* Kathryn Ford, Director of Admission, 909-469-5335, Fax: 909-469-5570, E-mail: admissions@westernu.edu.
Website: http://prospective.westernu.edu/medical-sciences/welcome-4/

Western Washington University, Graduate School, College of Sciences and Technology, Department of Biology, Bellingham, WA 98225-5996. Offers MS. Part-time programs available. *Degree requirements:* For master's, thesis. *Entrance requirements:* For master's, GRE General Test, GRE Subject Test (biology), minimum GPA of 3.0 in last 60 semester hours or last 90 quarter hours. Additional exam requirements/recommendations for international students: Required—TOEFL (minimum score 567 paper-based). Electronic applications accepted. *Faculty research:* Organismal biology, ecology and evolutionary biology, marine biology, cell and molecular biology, developmental biology, larval ecology, microzoo planton, symbiosis.

West Texas A&M University, College of Agriculture, Science and Engineering, Department of Life, Earth, and Environmental Sciences, Program in Biology, Canyon, TX 79016-0001. Offers MS. Part-time programs available. *Degree requirements:* For master's, comprehensive exam, thesis optional. *Entrance requirements:* For master's, GRE General Test. Additional exam requirements/recommendations for international students: Required—TOEFL (minimum score 550 paper-based). Electronic applications accepted. *Faculty research:* Aeroallergen concentration, scorpions, kangaroo mice, seed anatomy with light and scanning electron microscope.

West Virginia University, Eberly College of Arts and Sciences, Department of Biology, Morgantown, WV 26506. Offers cell and molecular biology (MS, PhD); environmental and evolutionary biology (MS, PhD); forensic biology (MS, PhD); genomic biology (MS, PhD); neurobiology (MS, PhD). Terminal master's awarded for partial completion of doctoral program. *Degree requirements:* For master's, thesis, final exam; for doctorate, thesis/dissertation, preliminary and final exams. *Entrance requirements:* For master's, GRE General Test, GRE Subject Test, minimum GPA of 3.0; for doctorate, GRE General Test, minimum GPA of 3.0. Additional exam requirements/recommendations for international students: Required—TOEFL. *Faculty research:* Environmental biology, genetic engineering, developmental biology, global change, biodiversity.

West Virginia University, School of Medicine, Graduate Programs at the Health Sciences Center, Morgantown, WV 26506. Offers MS, PhD, MD/PhD. Part-time and evening/weekend programs available. Postbaccalaureate distance learning degree programs offered (minimal on-campus study). *Expenses:* Contact institution.

Wichita State University, Graduate School, Fairmount College of Liberal Arts and Sciences, Department of Biological Sciences, Wichita, KS 67260. Offers MS. Part-time programs available. *Application deadline:* For fall admission, 3/1 for domestic and international students; for spring admission, 10/1 for domestic students, 8/1 for international students. *Unit head:* Dr. William J. Hendry, III, Chair, 316-978-3111, Fax: 316-978-3772, E-mail: william.hendry@wichita.edu. *Application contact:* Jordan Oleson, Admissions Coordinator, 316-978-3095, E-mail: jordan.oleson@wichita.edu.
Website: http://www.wichita.edu/

Wilfrid Laurier University, Faculty of Graduate and Postdoctoral Studies, Faculty of Science, Department of Biology, Waterloo, ON N2L 3C5, Canada. Offers integrative biology (M Sc). *Degree requirements:* For master's, thesis. *Entrance requirements:* For master's, honours BA in last two years of undergraduate studies with a minimum B average. Additional exam requirements/recommendations for international students: Required—TOEFL (minimum score 89 iBT). Electronic applications accepted. *Faculty research:* Genetic/development, anatomy/physiology, ecology/environment, evolution.

William Paterson University of New Jersey, College of Science and Health, Wayne, NJ 07470-8420. Offers biotechnology (MS); communication disorders (MS); exercise and sports studies (MS); general biology (MS); nursing (MSN); nursing practice (DNP). Part-time and evening/weekend programs available. *Faculty:* 29 full-time (10 women), 10 part-time/adjunct (1 woman). *Students:* 67 full-time (56 women), 160 part-time (138 women); includes 76 minority (19 Black or African American, non-Hispanic/Latino; 26 Asian, non-Hispanic/Latino; 29 Hispanic/Latino; 2 Two or more races, non-Hispanic/Latino). Average age 35. 490 applicants, 33% accepted, 83 enrolled. In 2013, 51 master's awarded. *Degree requirements:* For master's, comprehensive exam (for some programs), thesis (for some programs), non-thesis internship/practicum (for some programs). *Entrance requirements:* For master's, GRE/MAT, minimum GPA of 2.75; for doctorate, GRE/MAT, minimum GPA of 3.3. Additional exam requirements/recommendations for international students: Required—TOEFL (minimum score 550 paper-based; 79 iBT), IELTS (minimum score 6). *Application deadline:* For fall admission, 6/1 for domestic students, 5/1 for international students; for spring admission, 11/1 for domestic students, 10/1 for international students. Applications are processed on a rolling basis. Application fee: $50. Electronic applications accepted. *Financial support:* Research assistantships with full tuition reimbursements, career-related internships or fieldwork, and unspecified assistantships available. Support available to part-time students. Financial award application deadline: 4/1; financial award applicants required to submit FAFSA. *Faculty research:* Human biomechanics, autism, nanomaterials, health and environment, red-tide causing algae. *Unit head:* Dr. Kenneth Wolf, Dean, 973-720-2194, E-mail: wolfk@wpunj.edu. *Application contact:* Christina Aiello, Assistant Director, Graduate Admissions, 973-720-2506, Fax: 973-720-2035, E-mail: aielloc@wpunj.edu.
Website: http://www.wpunj.edu/cosh

Winthrop University, College of Arts and Sciences, Department of Biology, Rock Hill, SC 29733. Offers MS. Part-time programs available. *Degree requirements:* For master's, thesis optional. *Entrance requirements:* For master's, GRE General Test. Electronic applications accepted. *Faculty research:* Anatomy of marsupials; oxygen consumption, respiratory quotient and mechanical efficiency; bioremediation with microbial mats; floristic survey.

Worcester Polytechnic Institute, Graduate Studies and Research, Department of Biology and Biotechnology, Worcester, MA 01609-2280. Offers biology and biotechnology (MS); biotechnology (PhD). *Faculty:* 10 full-time (5 women). *Students:* 16 full-time (8 women), 4 part-time (3 women); includes 1 minority (Asian, non-Hispanic/Latino), 8 international. 88 applicants, 13% accepted, 7 enrolled. In 2013, 2 master's, 1 doctorate awarded. Terminal master's awarded for partial completion of doctoral program. *Degree requirements:* For master's, thesis; for doctorate, comprehensive exam, thesis/dissertation, qualifying exam. *Entrance requirements:* For master's and doctorate, GRE General Test, 3 letters of recommendation, statement of purpose. Additional exam requirements/recommendations for international students: Required—TOEFL (minimum score 563 paper-based; 84 iBT), IELTS (minimum score 7). *Application deadline:* For fall admission, 1/1 priority date for domestic and international students. Application fee: $70. Electronic applications accepted. *Financial support:* Research assistantships, teaching assistantships, career-related internships or fieldwork, institutionally sponsored loans, scholarships/grants, and unspecified assistantships available. Financial award application deadline: 1/1; financial award applicants required to submit FAFSA. *Unit head:* Dr. Joseph Duffy, Head, 508-831-4111, Fax: 508-831-5936, E-mail: jduffy@wpi.edu. *Application contact:* Dr. Luis Vidali, Graduate Coordinator, 508-831-4111, Fax: 508-831-5936, E-mail: lvidali@wpi.edu.
Website: http://www.wpi.edu/Academics/Depts/BBT/

Wright State University, School of Graduate Studies, College of Science and Mathematics, Department of Biological Sciences, Dayton, OH 45435. Offers biological sciences (MS); environmental sciences (MS). *Degree requirements:* For master's, thesis optional. *Entrance requirements:* Additional exam requirements/recommendations for international students: Required—TOEFL.

Wright State University, School of Graduate Studies, College of Science and Mathematics and School of Medicine, Program in Biomedical Sciences, Dayton, OH 45435. Offers PhD. *Degree requirements:* For doctorate, thesis/dissertation. *Entrance requirements:* For doctorate, GRE General Test. Additional exam requirements/recommendations for international students: Required—TOEFL.

Yale University, School of Medicine and Graduate School of Arts and Sciences, Combined Program in Biological and Biomedical Sciences (BBS), New Haven, CT 06520. Offers PhD, MD/PhD. *Degree requirements:* For doctorate, thesis/dissertation. *Entrance requirements:* For doctorate, GRE General Test. Additional exam requirements/recommendations for international students: Required—TOEFL. Electronic applications accepted. *Expenses:* Contact institution.

York University, Faculty of Graduate Studies, Faculty of Science, Program in Biology, Toronto, ON M3J 1P3, Canada. Offers M Sc, PhD. Part-time and evening/weekend programs available. *Degree requirements:* For master's, thesis or alternative; for doctorate, comprehensive exam, thesis/dissertation, preliminary exam. *Application deadline:* Applications are processed on a rolling basis. Application fee: $80. Electronic applications accepted. *Financial support:* Fellowships, research assistantships, teaching assistantships, career-related internships or fieldwork, and fee bursaries available. *Unit head:* Samuel Benchimol, Chair, 416-736-2100 Ext. 20726, E-mail: biochair@yorku.ca. *Application contact:* Cristalina Del Biondo, Graduate Program Assistant, 416-736-2100 Ext. 22342, E-mail: delbiond@yorku.ca.
Website: http://www.biol.yorku.ca/grad/

Youngstown State University, Graduate School, College of Science, Technology, Engineering and Mathematics, Department of Biological Sciences, Youngstown, OH 44555-0001. Offers environmental biology (MS); molecular biology, microbiology, and genetic (MS); physiology and anatomy (MS). Part-time programs available. *Degree requirements:* For master's, comprehensive exam, thesis, oral review. *Entrance requirements:* For master's, GRE General Test, minimum GPA of 2.7. Additional exam requirements/recommendations for international students: Required—TOEFL. *Faculty research:* Cell biology, neurophysiology, molecular biology, neurobiology, gene regulation.

ADELPHI UNIVERSITY

College of the Arts and Sciences
Program in Biology

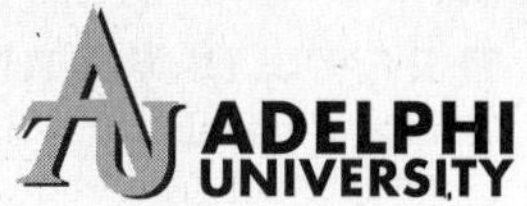

Program of Study

Adelphi's Master of Science in Biology prepares students for doctoral study and entrance into professional schools of medicine, dentistry, and veterinary medicine. The program also qualifies future educators for certification and expands the knowledge base of experienced teachers. Other graduates acquire the tools and skills necessary for successful careers in research, public health, and environmental law. At Adelphi, students gain a broad foundation in biology, practical experience, and the fundamental skills of scientific research. Laboratory courses emphasize contemporary scientific techniques and integrate technology into the learning experience. Faculty members work closely with students as mentors, ensuring a personal academic experience and career guidance. It is possible to fulfill degree requirements on the basis of either full- or part-time study, with completion in one to two years of full-time study.

There are two paths to the M.S. in Biology—the research thesis (33 credits) and the nonthesis option (36 credits). Requirements are subject to change. Most courses are offered in the evening, for the convenience of the working student. Adelphi students have opportunities to gain professional experience through internships at many hospitals, laboratories, private medical and dental practices, and research institutions in the area.

Students seeking a graduate degree and New York State teaching certification for secondary-level teaching (grades 7 through 12) can complete required course work for a Master of Arts degree through Adelphi's graduate program in biology in conjunction with the Ruth S. Ammon School of Education. Students who successfully complete the program are awarded a Master of Arts from the Ammon School of Education.

Adelphi also offers an M.S. in Biology with a concentration in biotechnology. This innovative program prepares students for careers in this rapidly expanding and dynamic discipline of biotechnology and in the related fields of pharmaceuticals, biomedical research, cancer research, and laboratory medicine. Students may pursue a research thesis track or a scholarly paper track; a limited number of teaching assistantships are available.

Research Facilities

Departmental laboratory facilities include modern equipment for the study of molecular biology, cell and tissue culture, and scanning and transmission electron microscopy. Students use these facilities for graduate research in cellular and molecular biology, immunology, genetics, evolution, and ecology.

The University's primary research holdings are at Swirbul Library and include 603,000 volumes (including bound periodicals and government publications); 806,000 items in microformats; 35,000 audiovisual items; and online access to more than 80,000 e-book titles, 76,000 electronic journal titles, and 265 research databases.

Value

Earning an Adelphi degree means joining a growing network of more than 90,000 alumni. For the eighth straight year, Adelphi was designated a Best Buy by the *Fiske Guide to Colleges*, one of only twenty private universities nationwide to earn that distinction. *The Princeton Review* also named Adelphi a Best College in the Northeast, and *Forbes* magazine named Adelphi a Top College. According to payscale.com's 2013 College Education ROI rankings, Adelphi ranks in the top 15 percent of colleges and universities nationwide for return on investment. The numbers speak for themselves—91 percent of Adelphi's undergraduates receive financial aid or scholarships.

Financial Aid

Adelphi University offers a wide variety of federal aid programs, state grants, scholarship and fellowship programs, on- and off-campus employment, and teaching and research assistantships. More information is available online at ecampus.adelphi.edu/sfs.

Cost of Study

For the 2014–15 academic year, the tuition rate is $1,055 per credit. University fees range from $330 to $575 per semester.

Living and Housing Costs

The University assists single and married students in finding suitable accommodations whenever possible. The cost of living is dependent on location and the number of rooms rented.

Location

Located in Garden City, New York, just 23 miles from Manhattan, where students can take advantage of numerous cultural and internship opportunities, Adelphi's 75-acre suburban campus is known for the beauty of its landscape and architecture. The campus is a short walk from the Long Island Rail Road and is convenient to New York's major airports and several major highways. Off-campus centers are located in Manhattan, the Hudson Valley, and Suffolk County.

The University and The College

Founded in 1896, Adelphi is a fully accredited, private university with nearly 8,000 undergraduate, graduate, and returning-adult students in the arts and sciences, business, clinical psychology, education, nursing, and social work. Students come from forty states and forty-five countries.

Mindful of the cultural inheritance of the past, the College of Arts and Sciences encompasses those realms of inquiry that have characterized the modern pursuit of knowledge. The faculty members of the College place a high priority on students' intellectual development in and out of the classroom and structure programs to foster that growth. Students analyze original research and other creative work, develop firsthand facility with creative and research methodologies, undertake collaborative work with peers and mentors, engage in serious internships, and hone communicative skills.

Applying

Applicants must hold a bachelor's degree in biology or an allied field (or its equivalent) and show promise of successful achievement in the field. A student must submit a completed application, a $50 application fee, official college transcripts and two letters of recommendation.

Correspondence and Information

800-ADELPHI (toll-free)
academics.adelphi.edu/artsci/bio/graduate-biology.php

THE FACULTY AND THEIR RESEARCH

Tandra Chakraborty, Ph.D., Calcutta, India. Interplay between endocrinology and neurobiology; estrogen metabolism; obesity, hypoglycemia.

Jonna Coombs, Ph.D., Penn State University. Bioremediation; microbial ecology.

Deborah Cooperstein, Ph.D., CUNY. Cellular physiology; biochemistry.

Matthias Foellmer, Ph.D., Concordia University. Behavioral ecology: mating systems in spiders; salt marsh community ecology; biostatistics.

Aaren Freeman, Ph.D., University of New Hampshire. Marine biology and ecology; evolutionary processes.

Heather Liwanag, Ph.D., University of California, Santa Cruz. Comparative physiology in ecological and evolutionary context.

George Russell, Ph.D., Harvard University. Genetics; biochemistry; molecular genetics.

Alan Schoenfeld, Ph.D., Yeshiva University (Einstein). Cancer biology; cell biology; molecular genetics.

Aram Stump, Ph.D., University of Notre Dame. Genomics; molecular genetics; genetics and evolution.

Eugenia Villa-Cuesta, Ph.D., Universidad Autonoma de Madrid. Genetics; molecular biology.

Andrea Ward, Ph.D., University of Massachusetts Amherst. Functional morphology in fishes; comparative vertebrate anatomy; evolution and development.

Benjamin Weeks, Ph.D., University of Connecticut. Developmental biology; environmental toxicology; developmental neurotoxicology.

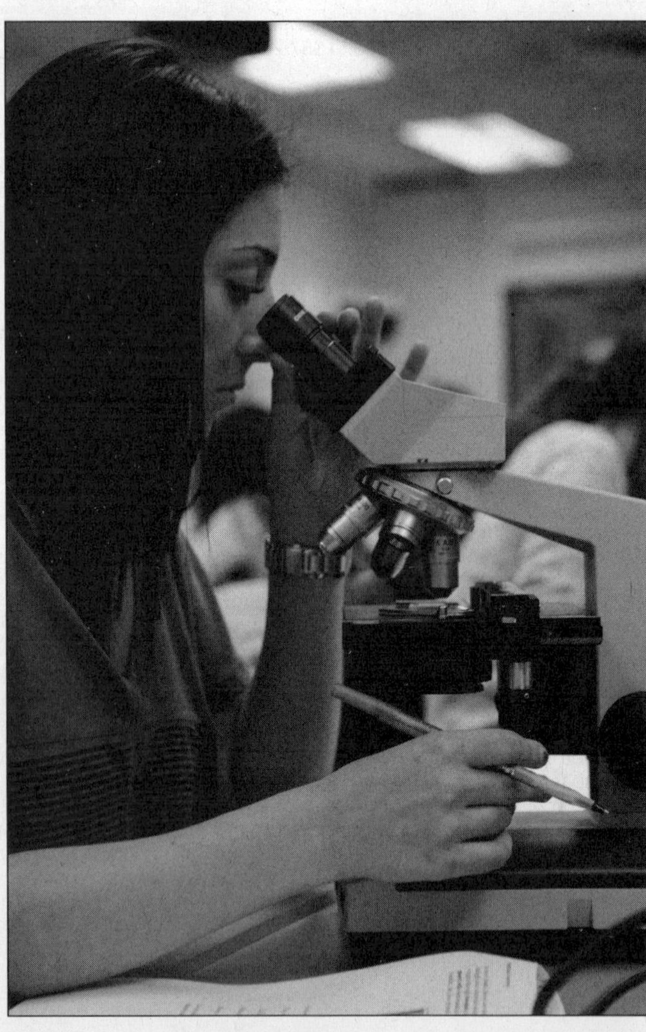

Laboratory courses emphasize contemporary scientific techniques and integrate technology into the learning experience.

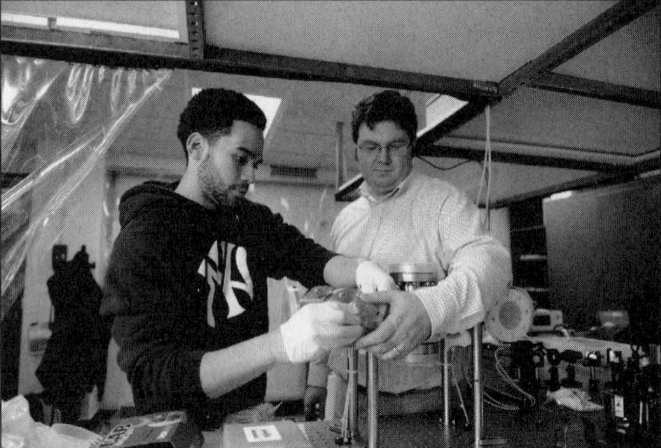

Faculty members work closely with students as mentors, ensuring a personal academic experience and career guidance.

AMERICAN MUSEUM OF NATURAL HISTORY

Richard Gilder Graduate School
Ph.D. Program in Comparative Biology

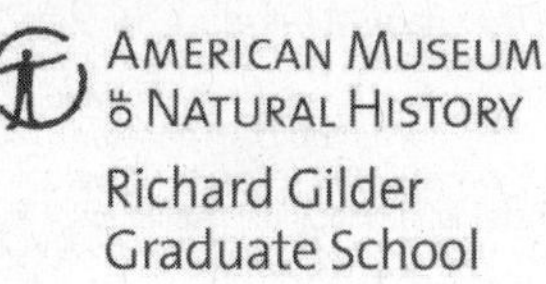

Program of Study

The Ph.D. Program in Comparative Biology is designed to educate the next generation of biologists through an integrated approach that focuses on the history, evolutionary relationships, and interactions among organisms. The Richard Gilder Graduate School is housed in a refurbished complex in the American Museum of Natural History. Training and research opportunities exist across a wide array of disciplines in comparative biology, incorporating research in systematic and evolutionary biology, paleontology, conservation biology, comparative genomics, computational biology, Earth history, anthropology, and biological and cultural diversity. Global fieldwork with AMNH faculty provides exceptional research opportunities for students.

The normal course of study is four years. Students earn a minimum of 62 credits through a combination of coursework, teaching assistantships, and individual dissertation research. As a distinctive strength of the program, students can begin working on their own research as early as their first semester. To ensure this, students are matched to faculty members' research programs and/or laboratories upon admission. The curriculum provides students with the environment, tools, and experiences to prepare them for a career in research and teaching, as well as for an array of other fields. It is novel, highly flexible, collections-centered, and, where appropriate, field-based. The program provides students with broad exposure to the conceptual bases, language, tools, and methods for studying life, as well as the ability to undertake and complete intensive individual investigations.

This is the first doctoral program offered at a museum in the Western hemisphere, allowing students to take advantage of the Museum's internationally recognized collections and scientists.

Research Facilities

The American Museum of Natural History provides exceptional support facilities for research for students, with collections of more than 32 million specimens and artifacts. The Museum houses one of the largest natural history libraries in the world, providing access to over 500,000 printed items and over 4,000 serial titles, more than 1,200 of which are available on-line. AMNH is exceptionally well equipped for research in comparative biology, with three state-of-the-art molecular laboratories in the Sackler Institute for Comparative Genomics, powerful parallel computing facilities, the Ambrose Monell Frozen Tissue Collection, paleontological labs, an imaging and microscopy laboratory, and the Southwestern Research Station, a field station that attracts top field biologists and their students from many universities annually. The Museum also is an Associate Member of the New York Genome Center. The Richard Gilder Graduate School also is served by significant instructional space and resources, which include numerous classrooms and laboratories, and many informal spaces located throughout the institution.

Financial Aid

Students typically are fully funded, with tuition, a competitive stipend for a full twelve months per year, some research support, and health insurance (presuming satisfactory progress in the program). The Museum provides this commitment through a combination of generous philanthropic support and foundation and governmental training grants to the institution or individual students. Students are expected to be highly competitive for foundation-based fellowships, U.S. federal or New York State grants, or international governmental support. This exceptional level of support allows students to focus on research, while receiving training in teaching in both formal academic and informal public settings.

Cost of Study

AMNH generally provides full financial support to the students matriculating in the Comparative Biology Ph.D. Program. Each AMNH-supported student is awarded a tuition fellowship and receives an annual stipend and research funding, as well as health insurance, through the Richard Gilder Graduate School and/or extramural funds.

Living and Housing Costs

The AMNH does not provide graduate student housing; however, there are numerous housing options available in the nearby area. The Museum also has entered into a special partnership with International House to ensure that at least two years of housing is available for all students entering the Museum's Comparative Biology Ph.D. Program. The graduate school can provide housing referral services, listing searches, and placement assistance.

Student Group

The graduate student body includes doctoral students matriculated in the AMNH Comparative Biology Ph.D. program, doctoral students matriculated at partner universities, and other students taking courses at, or receiving fellowships from, the Richard Gilder Graduate School. The program is limited to around 4 or 5 new students each year. This novel accelerated four-year program is designed to attract exceptionally motivated and qualified U.S. and international students who have demonstrated proficiency in academics and original research.

Student Outcomes

There is a diverse array of U.S. and international career opportunities for graduates from Comparative Biology Ph.D. Program, from conventional academic careers to employment by government agencies and the private sector, including postdoctoral research, high school or college faculty appointments, and museum curation. Recent program graduates are employed at the Royal Ontario Museum, Harvard, Columbia, Nagoya University (Japan), U.S. Geological Survey, Cold Spring Harbor Laboratories, and California Academy of Sciences.

Location

The AMNH is located in Manhattan at 79th Street overlooking beautiful Central Park. One of the world's great cities, New York provides a nearly limitless array of cultural and entertainment activities. An unmatched variety of restaurants, museums, bars, theaters, parks, and galleries provides a rich cultural backdrop for a city of 8 million people representing more than 200 different nationalities.

The Museum and The Graduate School

Since its founding in 1869, the American Museum of Natural History has been dedicated to a joint mission of science and public education, and it provides a unique platform for communicating the results of current research to the public. The Richard Gilder Graduate School and its new and novel Ph.D. Program in Comparative Biology, the first Ph.D. degree-granting program for any museum in the western hemisphere, offers unique opportunities for students to participate in AMNH's research and educational missions as part of their course of study.

Applying

The annual application deadline for the Comparative Biology Ph.D. Program is December 15. Application requires submission of the following items: online application, application cover page, statement of academic purpose, official transcripts from each undergraduate and graduate institution attended, GRE scores, three letters of recommendation, TOEFL or IELTS scores (required of non-native English speakers only), and a nonrefundable application fee. Onsite applicant interviews may be scheduled in early to mid-February, with notification of admission typically occurring in late February or early March.

Correspondence and Information

The Richard Gilder Graduate School
American Museum of Natural History
Central Park West at 79th Street
New York, New York 10024
Phone: 212-769-5055
Fax: 212-769-5257
E-mail: Info-rggs@amnh.org
Website: http://www.amnh.org/our-research/richard-gilder-graduate-school/amnh-ph.d.-program

THE FACULTY AND THEIR RESEARCH

Professorial/Curatorial Faculty

George F. Barrowclough, Associate Professor and Associate Curator, Vertebrate Zoology (Ornithology); Ph.D., Minnesota, 1980. Evolution and systematics of birds.

James M. Carpenter, Professor, Division Chair and Peter J. Solomon Family Curator, Invertebrate Zoology; Ph.D., Cornell, 1983. Phylogenetic relationships, taxonomy and behavior of Hymenoptera.

Joel L. Cracraft, Professor, Chair, and Lamont Curator, Vertebrate Zoology (Ornithology); Ph.D., Columbia, 1969. Evolution and systematics of birds; biogeography.

Alex de Voogt, Assistant Professor and Assistant Curator, Anthropology; Ph.D., Leiden (Netherlands), 2005. Dispersal of board games; development and history of scripts.

Robert DeSalle, Professor and Curator, Invertebrate Zoology; Ph.D., Washington (St. Louis), 1984. Molecular systematics; microbial evolution; genomics.

Denton S. Ebel, Professor, Chair (Physical Sciences), and Curator (Earth and Planetary Sciences); Ph.D., Purdue, 1993. Meteoritics; thermodynamic modeling; solar system origin.

John J. Flynn, Dean of the RGGS, Professor, and Frick Curator, Paleontology; Ph.D., Columbia, 1983. Phylogeny and evolution of mammals; Mesozoic vertebrates; geochronology; paleobiology.

Darrel R. Frost, Professor and Curator-in-Charge, Vertebrate Zoology (Herpetology); Ph.D., Kansas, 1998. Evolutionary origins and diversification of amphibians and reptiles; epistemological issues of knowledge claims in evolutionary biology.

David A. Grimaldi, Professor and Curator, Invertebrate Zoology; Ph.D., Cornell, 1986. Insect evolutionary history; amber fossils; evolutionary radiations; paleoclimate, origins and evolution of tropical forest ecosystems.

American Museum of Natural History

George E. Harlow, Professor and Curator, Physical Sciences, Earth and Planetary Sciences; Ph.D., Princeton, 1977. Chemistry and structure of minerals, their origins, and records of geological processes; gems.
Melanie J. Hopkins, Assistant Professor and Assistant Curator, Paleontology; Ph.D., Chicago, 2010. Morphological evolution, phylogeny, and diversity of marine arthropods; quantitative paleobiology methods; global change biology; paleoecology.
Laurel Kendall, Professor, Division Chair, and Curator, Anthropology; Ph.D., Columbia, 1979. Popular religion and its material manifestations in East and Southeast Asia; production and consumption of sacred objects in contemporary market economies.
Eunsoo Kim, Assistant Professor and Assistant Curator, Invertebrate Zoology; Ph.D., Wisconsin–Madison, 2006. Diversity, genomics, evolution, and ecology of single-celled eukaryotic flagellates; symbiosis; origin of photosynthetic eukaryotes.
Neil H. Landman, Professor and Curator-in-Charge (Fossil Invertebrates), Paleontology; Ph.D., Yale, 1982. Evolution, life history, and systematics of externally shelled cephalopods; Cretaceous/Paleogene boundary.
Mordecai-Mark Mac Low, Professor and Curator, Physical Sciences (Astrophysics); Ph.D., Colorado at Boulder, 1989. Formation of planets, stars, and galaxies; numerical and computational modeling and simulations.
Ross D.E. MacPhee, Professor and Curator, Vertebrate Zoology (Mammalogy); Ph.D., Alberta, 1977. Paleobiogeography; extinction and cranial developmental biology of mammals and other vertebrates.
John G. Maisey, Professor, Axelrod Research Curator, and Curator-in-Charge (Fossil Fish), Paleontology; Ph.D., London (University College), 1974. Anatomy, phylogeny, origins, and evolution of sharks.
Edmond A. Mathez, Professor and Curator, Physical Sciences (Earth and Planetary Sciences); Ph.D., Washington (Seattle), 1981. Petrology of layered mafic intrusions; volatile and platinum group element geochemistry; mantle petrology; evolution of early earth.
Jin Meng, Professor and Curator-in-Charge (Fossil Mammals), Paleontology; Ph.D., Columbia, 1991. Morphology, systematics, and evolution of mammals (Mesozoic and Paleogene); Asian Tertiary stratigraphy and biochronology.
Jennifer E. Newell, Assistant Professor and Assistant Curator, Anthropology; Ph.D., Australian National University, 2005. Pacific ethnography; material culture and relationship between Pacific Islanders and their environments.
Mark A. Norell, Professor, Chair (Paleontology), and Curator-in-Charge, (Fossil Amphibians, Reptiles, and Birds); Ph.D., Yale, 1988. Evolution of non-avian dinosaurs; lizard phylogeny; Asian Mesozoic faunas; phylogenetic theory and methods.
Michael J. Novacek, Professor, Senior Vice President, Provost of Science, and Curator, Paleontology; Ph.D., Berkeley, 1978. Patterns of evolution and relationships among mammals; paleontological, anatomical, and molecular methods.
Rebecca Oppenheimer, Professor and Curator, Physical Sciences (Astrophysics); Ph.D., Caltech, 1999. Comparative exoplanetary science; faint white dwarfs; astronomical instrumentation development.
Susan L. Perkins, Associate Professor and Associate Curator, Invertebrate Zoology; Ph.D., Vermont, 2000. Microbiology; systematics, evolution, biogeography, and genomics of parasites; symbiosis.
Lorenzo Prendini, Professor and Curator, Invertebrate Zoology; Ph.D., Cape Town, 2001. Systematics, biogeography, and evolution of scorpions and other arachnids; evolution of insect-plant associations; phylogenetic theory and methods.
Christopher J. Raxworthy, Associate Professor, Associate Dean of Science for Education and Exhibition, and Associate Curator, Vertebrate Zoology (Herpetology); Ph.D., Open University, 1989. Systematics, biogeography, ecology, ethology, and conservation biology of reptiles and amphibians; GIS methods.
Brian G. Richmond, Professor and Curator, Anthropology; Ph.D., SUNY at Stony Brook, 1998. Biological anthropology; human and ape evolution; evolution of human bipedalism; functional anatomy and biomechanics.
Estefanía Rodriguez, Assistant Professor and Assistant Curator, Invertebrate Zoology; Ph.D., Seville, 2007. Morphological diversity, systematics, evolutionary history, biogeography, reproduction, and ecology of sea anemones.
Jerome G. Rozen, Professor and Curator, Invertebrate Zoology; Ph.D., Berkeley, 1955. Biology, immature stages and evolutionary relationships of bees; comparative biology of solitary and cleptoparasitic bees.
Scott A. Schaefer, Professor, Associate Dean of Science for Collections, and Curator, Vertebrate Zoology (Ichthyology); Ph.D., Chicago, 1986. Systematics, biogeography and evolutionary morphology of tropical freshwater fishes (Africa, South America).
Michael M. Shara, Professor and Curator, Physical Sciences (Astrophysics); Ph.D., Tel Aviv, 1977. Structure and evolution of novae and supernovae; star collisions; star populations inhabiting star clusters and galaxies.
Mark E. Siddall, Professor and Curator, Invertebrate Zoology; Ph.D., Toronto, 1994. Evolution of leeches and their blood-feeding behavior; protozoan parasitology.
Nancy B. Simmons, Professor and Curator-in-Charge, Vertebrate Zoology (Mammalogy); Ph.D., Berkeley, 1989. Morphology and evolutionary biology of living and fossil bats; database tools and crowd sourcing for large-scale phenomic tree-of-life projects.
Brian T. Smith, Assistant Professor and Assistant Curator, Vertebrate Zoology (Ornithology); Ph.D., Nevada, 2011. Evolutionary history of birds; phylogenomics, biogeography, and statistical modeling.
John S. Sparks, Professor and Curator-in-Charge, Vertebrate Zoology (Ichthyology); Ph.D., Michigan, 2001. Systematics, evolution, and biogeography of freshwater and nearshore and deep-sea marine fishes; bioluminescence and biofluorescence.
Charles S. Spencer, Professor and Curator, Anthropology; Ph.D., Michigan, 1981. Development of pre-Columbian complex societies in Mexico and Venezuela; ecological anthropology and cultural evolution.
Melanie L.J. Stiassny, Professor and Herbert R. and Evelyn Axelrod Research Curator, Vertebrate Zoology (Ichthyology); Ph.D., London, 1980. Systematics, diversity, and evolutionary morphology of tropical freshwater fish faunas; teleostean tree of life.
David Hurst Thomas, Professor and Curator, Anthropology; Ph.D., California, Davis, 1971. Archaeology; St. Catherine's Island; Mission San Marcos; Great Basin; Gatecliff Shelter; relationship between Native American and anthropological communities.
Robert S. Voss, Professor and Curator, Vertebrate Zoology, Mammalogy; Ph.D., Michigan, 1983. Marsupial evolution; systematics and biogeography of Neotropical mammals of moist-forest habitats, Amazonia, and the Andes.
James D. Webster, Professor and Curator, Physical Sciences (Earth and Planetary Sciences); Ph.D., Arizona State, 1987. Volcanoes, magma volatile chemistry, hydrothermal fluids, and mineral deposits; experimental petrology and geochemistry.
Ward C. Wheeler, Professor and Curator, Invertebrate Zoology; Ph.D., Harvard, 1988. Systematic theory and its application to the historical relationships of metazoans; genomics; theoretical, algorithmic, and computational phylogenetics.
Peter M. Whiteley, Professor and Curator, Anthropology; Ph.D., New Mexico, 1982. Ethnography and history of Native North American cultures; kinship systems; application of phylogenetic methods to language evolution study.

Affiliated and Adjunct Faculty

George Amato, Affiliated Professor and Director, Sackler Institute for Comparative Genomics; Ph.D., Yale, 1994. Conservation genetics; molecular ecology; taxonomy, phylogeny, and molecular analyses to determine units of conservation.
Mary E. Blair, Affiliated Professor and Assistant Director, Center for Biodiversity and Conservation; Ph.D., Columbia, 2011. Conservation biology of primates and other mammals; molecular and GIS methods; evolutionary processes and biodiversity.
Robert F. Rockwell, Adjunct Professor; Ph.D., Queen's at Kingston, 1975. Population biology and ecology.
Eleanor J. Sterling, Affiliated Professor and Chief Conservation Scientist, Center for Biodiversity and Conservation; Ph.D., Yale, 1993. Behavioral ecology of endangered mammals, turtles, and tortoises; biogeography and its application to conservation.

Emeriti Faculty

Robert L. Carneiro, Professor Emeritus and Curator Emeritus, Anthropology; Ph.D., Michigan, 1957. South American ethnology, cultural evolution, and political evolution.
Niles Eldredge, Professor Emeritus and Curator Emeritus, Paleontology; Ph.D., Columbia, 1969. Trilobites; evolutionary theory; extinction, evolution, and biodiversity.
Lee H. Herman, Professor Emeritus and Curator Emeritus, Invertebrate Zoology; Ph.D., Catholic University, 1967. Systematics of rove beetles.
Norman I. Platnick, Professor Emeritus and Peter J. Solomon Family Curator Emeritus, Invertebrate Zoology; Ph.D., Harvard, 1973. Arachnid phylogeny, historical biogeography and conservation; spider family Oonopidae (goblin spiders).
Randall T. Schuh, Professor Emeritus and George T. Willett Curator Emeritus, Invertebrate Zoology; Ph.D., Connecticut, 1971. Phylogeny, classification and systematic study of Heteroptera (true bugs); plant-herbivore-parasitoid interactions; systematic methods.
Ian Tattersall, Professor Emeritus and Curator Emeritus, Anthropology; Ph.D., Yale, 1971. Species variety and higher-taxa relationships within hominid and lemuriform primate groups.

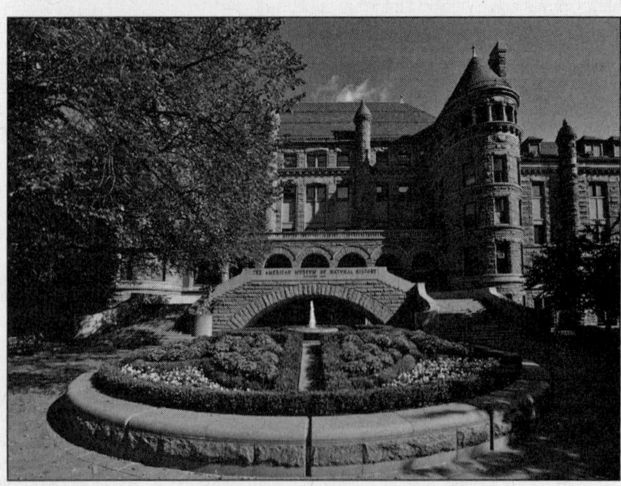

BOSTON COLLEGE

Biology Department

BOSTON COLLEGE

Programs of Study

The Department offers a program of study leading to a Ph.D. degree in biology. Basic areas of study include biochemistry, cellular and developmental biology, genetics, cell cycle, vector biology, and neurobiology.

The Ph.D. program provides an in-depth training experience. Core course work is provided in cell biology, biochemistry, molecular biology, genetics, and bioinformatics. Advanced electives are available in all areas of faculty expertise. Seminar courses provide students with ongoing training in critical thinking and oral presentation of scientific data. Research experience is provided by working in close cooperation with faculty members, postdoctoral fellows, and senior students in a collaborative, supportive environment.

Research Facilities

The Department, in Higgins Hall, is well-equipped for modern molecular, genomic, and proteomic research; biochemistry; imaging; and bioinformatics.

Departmental genomics and proteomics infrastructure includes capacities for Beckman and LiCor DNA sequencing and DNA fragment polymorphism analysis and Alpha-Innotech two-dimensional gel proteomic analysis. The College possesses state-of-the-art cell culture and protein purification systems, including the BioCad SPRINT perfusion chromatography system, HPLC, FPLC, and preparative isoelectric focusing.

Imaging facilities include a Leica confocal microscope, a Phillips transmission electron microscope, departmental and individual laboratory Zeiss and Nikon fluorescence and Nomarski compound microscopes, Molecular Dynamics phosphoimager and densitometer workstations, and X-ray diffraction capability. The digital graphics and image processing facility includes numerous Macintosh workstations with multiprocessor CPU configurations, coupled with high-resolution scanners. A large-format poster printer and dye sublimation printers support preparation of high-quality posters and print communications.

The departmental bioinformatics computing platform consists of a 132 CPU-core cluster and 7 terabytes of local data storage. It is available free of charge to faculty, graduate students, and other researchers. In addition, faculty, students, and staff have access to the College's central computing cluster, and individual laboratories may have their own dedicated computing systems.

Financial Aid

Graduate assistantships (teaching and research based) are available with full tuition remission. Stipends are $30,000 per calendar year.

Cost of Study

For the 2014–15 academic year, tuition and fees for a full-time student are $1,398 per credit, 100 percent of which is covered by tuition remission for students receiving financial aid.

Living and Housing Costs

The Housing Office provides an extensive list of off-campus housing options, including off-campus graduate housing. Most graduate students rent rooms or apartments near Chestnut Hill; many biology students share apartments with other students in the program. Average monthly expenses (rent, food, utilities) for the academic year (nine months) are $2,105 for students.

Student Group

The enrollment at Boston College is 14,500, including 4,200 students enrolled in the various graduate schools. There are 50 graduate students in the Ph.D. program. The graduate students are geographically and ethnically diverse.

Location

Boston College is located in the Chestnut Hill section of Newton, an attractive residential area about 5 miles from the heart of Boston, with easy access to the city by public transportation. The Boston area, with its numerous educational and biomedical research institutions, offers countless outstanding seminars, lectures, colloquia, and concerts throughout the year. A wide variety of cultural and recreational opportunities can be found close to the campus.

The College

Founded in Massachusetts in 1863, Boston College currently includes the Graduate School of Arts and Sciences and graduate schools of law, social work, management, nursing, and education. Its expanding campus is graced with many attractive Gothic buildings. Boston College has a strong tradition of academic excellence and service to the community.

Applying

Preference is given to completed applications received prior to January 1. Admission is granted on the basis of academic background and demonstrated aptitude in biology and related disciplines. A year of organic chemistry, physics, and mathematics and a solid background in biology are highly recommended for admission. Scores on the Graduate Record Examinations General Test and the Subject Test in biology are required.

Correspondence and Information

Professor Charles Hoffman
Director, Graduate Program
Biology Department
Higgins Hall
Boston College
Chestnut Hill, Massachusetts 02467-3961
Phone: 617-552-3540
E-mail: gradbio@bc.edu
Website: http://www.bc.edu/biology

Boston College

THE GRADUATE RESEARCH FACULTY

Anthony T. Annunziato, Professor; Ph.D., Massachusetts Amherst, 1979. Biochemistry/molecular biology; DNA replication and nucleosome assembly in mammalian cells.

David R. Burgess, Professor; Ph.D., California, Davis, 1974. Spatial and temporal regulation of cytokinesis; role of the actin- and microtubule-based cytoskeletons in early development.

Hugh P. Cam, Assistant Professor; Ph.D., Harvard 2003. Epigenetic control of higher-order genome organization and chromatin structures.

Thomas C. Chiles, Professor and Chairman of Biology, The DeLuca Chair in Biology, Vice Provost for Research; Ph.D., Florida, 1988. Cell biology, signal transduction; cell-cycle control, gene regulation in mature B lymphocytes.

Peter G. Clote, Professor; Ph.D., Duke, 1979. Algorithms and mathematical modeling in computational biology: genomic motif detection, protein folding on lattice models, RNA secondary structure, functional genomics via gene expression profile.

Eric S. Folker, Assistant Professor; Ph.D Notre Dame. Cellular organization; mechanisms of nuclear movement and the role of nuclear movement in muscle development and disease pathogenesis.

Marc-Jan Gubbels, Assistant Professor; Ph.D., Utrecht (Netherlands), 2000. Genetics and cell biology of the apicomplexan parasite *Toxoplasma gondii.*

Charles Hoffman, Professor; Ph.D., Tufts, 1986. Signal transduction and transcriptional regulation in fission yeast; analysis of PKA and MAPK signal pathways in nutrient monitoring.

Welkin Johnson, Professor; Ph.D., Tufts, 1998. Retroviruses; primate lentiviruses (HIV and SIV); co-evolution of viruses and their hosts.

Daniel Kirschner, Professor; Ph.D., Harvard, 1972. Structural biochemistry of amyloids and myelin sheath; neurodegenerative diseases; peripheral demyelinating neuropathies.

Laura Anne Lowery, Assistant Professor; Ph.D., MIT. Cytoskeletal dynamics during cell migration; axon outgrowth; development of the nervous system.

Michelle Meyer, Assistant Professor; Ph.D., Caltech, 2006. Bioinformatic discovery and experimental characterization of RNA-based gene regulatory mechanisms.

Junona Moroianu, Associate Professor; Ph.D., Rockefeller, 1996. Cell biology; molecular mechanisms of nucleocytoplasmic transport of cellular and viral macromolecules in mammalian cells.

Marc A. T. Muskavitch, Professor; Ph.D., Stanford, 1981. Developmental biology: intercellular signaling and cell-fate specification in *Drosophila;* host-parasite interactions in *Anopheles.*

Thomas N. Seyfried, Professor; Ph.D., Illinois, 1976. Neurogenetics: use of genetics and neurochemistry in neural membrane function and developmental neurobiology.

Timothy van Opijnen, Assistant Professor; Ph.D., Amsterdam (the Netherlands). Microbial systems biology; drug/gene interaction networks and the development of new antimicrobials; the development of genome-wide next generation sequencing strategies to link genotypes to phenotypes;and engineering of bacteria with new traits and novel applicability.

Kenneth C. Williams, Associate Professor; Ph.D., McGill, 1993. Central nervous system macrophages; neuroAIDS; AIDS pathogenesis; monocyte/macrophage biology.

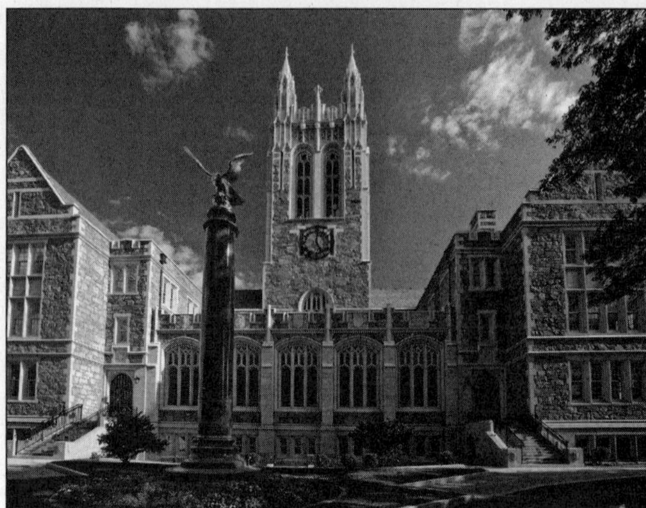

Higgins Hall, home of the Biology Department.

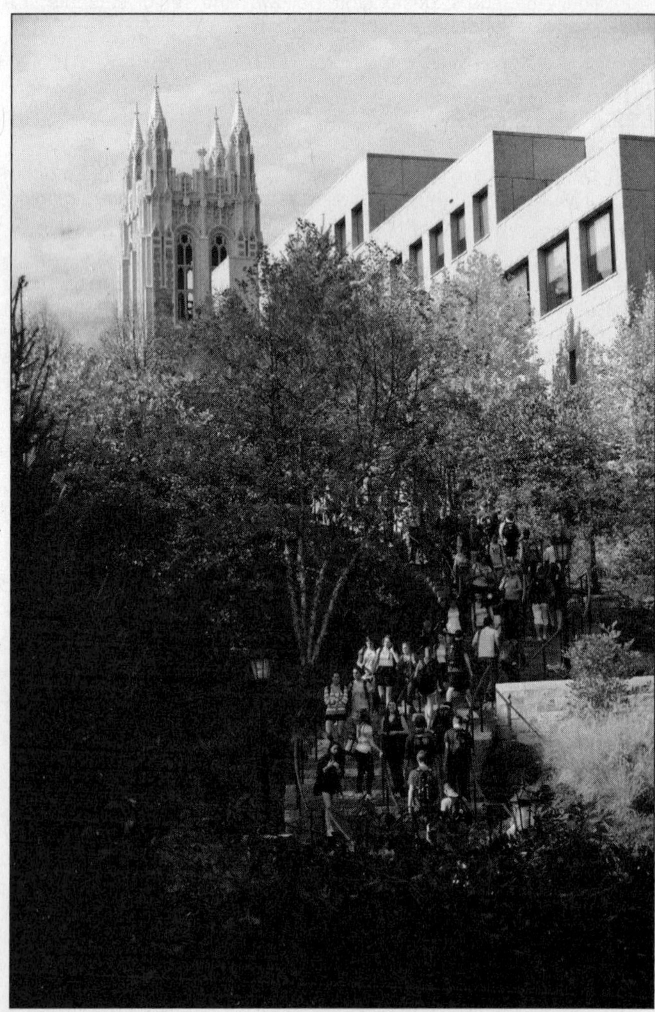

Students find a blend of the old and the new at Boston College.

CITY OF HOPE NATIONAL MEDICAL CENTER BECKMAN RESEARCH INSTITUTE

Irell & Manella Graduate School of Biological Sciences

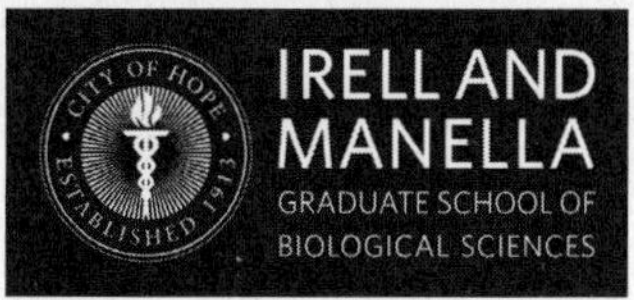

Programs of Study

The mission of the City of Hope Graduate School of Biological Sciences is to train students to be outstanding research scientists in chemical, molecular, and cellular biology. Graduates of this program are awarded the degree of Doctor of Philosophy in biological sciences and are equipped to address fundamental questions in the life sciences and biomedicine for careers in academia, industry, and government. The time spent in the program is devoted to full-time study and research. During the first year, the student completes the core curriculum and three laboratory rotations (eight to ten weeks each). The core curriculum contains biochemistry, molecular biology, cell biology, and biostatistics/bioinformatics. One Advanced Topics course is taken during spring of the first year. After the first year, the student prepares and orally defends a research proposal based on an original topic not related to previous work conducted by the student, and in the second year students prepare and defend a research proposal based on their actual thesis topic. Two additional Advanced Topics courses are required after the first year and students are required to take a literature-based journal club every year after the first year. Students also participate in courses on scientific communication and on the responsible conduct of research. After successfully completing the core curriculum and research proposal, students concentrate the majority of their time on their individual dissertation laboratory research project. The written thesis/dissertation must be presented by the student for examination by 4 members of the City of Hope staff and 1 qualified member from an outside institution.

Research Facilities

City of Hope is a premier medical center, one of forty-one National Cancer Institute–designated Comprehensive Cancer Centers. Its Beckman Research Institute launched the biotech industry by creating the first human recombinant gene products, insulin and growth hormone, which are now used by millions of people worldwide. State-of-the-art facilities include mass spectrometry, NMR, molecular modeling, cell sorting, DNA sequencing, molecular pathology, scanning and transmission electron microscopy, confocal microscopy, and molecular imaging. The Lee Graff Medical and Scientific Library allows access to the latest biomedical information via its journal and book collection, document delivery, interlibrary loans, and searches of online databases.

Financial Aid

All students in the Graduate School receive a fellowship of $32,000 per year as well as paid health and dental insurance.

Cost of Study

There are no tuition charges. A student services fee of $50 per semester ($150 per year) is the student's only financial obligation to City of Hope.

Living and Housing Costs

The School has limited, low-cost housing available. Living in student housing provides easy access to campus resources and a connection to the vibrant campus community. Additional housing is available within the immediate area at an average cost of $700 to $1,000 per month.

Student Group

The Graduate School faculty consists of 76 of City of Hope's investigators. Seventy-five graduate students were working toward the Ph.D. degree in biological sciences in 2013–14.

Student Outcomes

Graduates have gone on to work as postdoctoral fellows at California Institute of Technology; Harvard University; Scripps Research Institute; Stanford University; University of California, Los Angeles; University of California, San Diego; University of California, Irvine; Genentech; University of Southern California; and Washington University in St. Louis. Graduates have also found positions with Wyeth-Ayerst Research; Allergan, Inc.; and the U.S. Biodefense and its subsidiary, Stem Cell Research Institute of California, Inc.

Location

City of Hope is located 25 miles northeast of downtown Los Angeles, minutes away from Pasadena and close to beaches, mountains, and many recreational and cultural activities.

The Medical Center and The Institute

City of Hope was founded in 1913, initially as a tuberculosis sanatorium. Research programs were initiated in 1951, and, in 1983, the Beckman Research Institute of City of Hope was established with support from the Arnold and Mabel Beckman Foundation. The Institute comprises basic science research groups within the Divisions of Biology, Immunology, Molecular Medicine, and Neurosciences, among others.

Applying

The deadline for application is January 1 for classes starting in August. Applying early is advisable. Candidates must submit transcripts, three letters of recommendation, and take the Graduate Record Examination (General Test required, Subject Test recommended). For further information and an application, students should contact the School at the address listed in this description.

Correspondence and Information

City of Hope
Irell & Manella Graduate School of Biological Sciences
1500 East Duarte Road
Duarte, California 91010
United States
Phone: 877-715-GRAD or 626-256-4673 Ext. 63899
Fax: 626-301-8105
E-mail: gradschool@coh.org
Website: http://www.cityofhope.org/gradschool

THE FACULTY AND THEIR RESEARCH

Professors

David K. Ann, Ph.D. Molecular mechanisms of maintaining genomic integrity.

Michael E. Barish, Ph.D. Physiological and imaging studies of brain tumors and their interactions with neural stem cells.

Ravi Bhatia, M.D. Regulation of normal and malignant hematopoietic stem cell growth.

Edouard M. Cantin, Ph.D. Herpes simplex virus infections in the nervous system.

Saswati Chatterjee, Ph.D. Adeno-associated virus vectors for stem-cell gene therapy.

Shiuan Chen, Ph.D. Hormones and cancer.

Yuan Chen, Ph.D. Ubiquitin-like modifications.

Don J. Diamond, Ph.D. Translational research in cancer vaccines.

Richard W. Ermel, D.V.M., Ph.D. Comparative medicine.

Stephen J. Forman, M.D. T-Cell immunotherapy for treatment of cancer.

David Horne, Ph.D. Developing natural products as novel anticancer agents.

Keiichi Itakura, Ph.D. Functions of Mrf-1 and Mrf-2.

Richard Jove, Ph.D. Development of molecular targeted therapeutics.

Susan E. Kane, Ph.D. Drug resistance and cancer.

Peter P. Lee, Ph.D. The impact of cancer on immune system.

Ren-Jang Lin, Ph.D. RNA splicing and post-transcriptional gene regulation.

Chih-Pin Liu, Ph.D. Immune regulation of autoimmune disease and tumor.

Linda Malkas, Ph.D. The selective targeting of cancer cells.

Marcia M. Miller, Ph.D. Molecular immunogenetics.

Rama Natarajan, Ph.D. Diabetic vascular complications.

Susan Neuhausen, Ph.D. Genetic epidemiology of complex diseases.

Timothy R. O'Connor, Ph.D. DNA repair.

Gerd P. Pfeifer, Ph.D. Molecular mechanisms of cancer.

Arthur D. Riggs, Ph.D. Epigenetics, chromatin structure, and X chromosome inactivation.

John J. Rossi, Ph.D. The biology and applications of small RNAs.

Paul M. Salvaterra, Ph.D. Modeling Alzheimer-type neurogeneration.

Binghui Shen, Ph.D. The study of DNA replication and repair nucleases in genome stability and cancers.

John E. Shively, Ph.D. Structure, function, and regulation of carcinoembryonic antigen genes.

Judith Singer-Sam, Ph.D. Epigenetics and disorders of the CNS.

Steven S. Smith, Ph.D. Cancer epigenetics.

Cy A. Stein, M.D, Ph.D. Cellular delivery of therapeutic oligonucleotides.

John Termini, Ph.D. Mutagenesis and carcinogenesis.

Nagarajan Vaidehi, Ph.D. Predicting protein structure and dynamics for drug discovery.

Jeffrey N. Weitzel, M.D. Genetic predisposition to cancer.

Jiing-Kuan Yee, Ph.D. Vectors for gene therapy.

Yun Yen, M.D., Ph.D. Novel molecular-targeted cancer therapies.

Hua Yu, Ph.D. Stat 3 and the tumor microenvironment.

John A. Zaia, M.D. Genetic and other anti-HIV therapy.

Associate and Assistant Professors

Karen S. Aboody, M.D. Neural stem cells—therapeutic applications.

Adam M. Bailis, Ph.D. Homologous recombination governs genome dynamics and tumor suppression.

Jacob Berlin, Ph.D. Nanoparticles for the diagnosis and treatment of cancer.

Mark Boldin, Ph.D. Noncoding RNA control of inflammation and cancer.

Ching-Cheng Chen, Ph.D. Cellular and molecular characterization of the hematopoietic niche.

Wen Yong Chen, Ph.D. Epigenetics, cancer, and aging.

Warren Chow, M.D., FACP. Cell signaling and cancer.

Carlotta A. Glackin, Ph.D. Understanding gene regulation from stem cells.

Robert Hickey, Ph.D. Identification and clinical translation of molecular signatures of disease.

Wendong Huang, Ph.D. Metabolic regulation, cancer, and aging.

Janice Huss, Ph.D. The role of orphan nuclear receptors in cardiac and skeletal muscle biology.

Rahul Jandial, M.D, Ph.D. Breast-to-brain cancer metastasis.

Jeremy Jones, Ph.D. The androgen receptor in human disease.

Markus Kalkum, Dr. Rer. Nat. (Ph.D.) Biodefense and emerging infectious diseases.

Joseph Kim, M.D. Uncovering the roots of pancreatic cancer.

Mei Kong, Ph.D. Signal transduction and cancer metabolism.

Marcin Kortylewski, Ph.D. Immune cells as targets for cancer therapy.

Hsun Teresa Ku, Ph.D. Pancreatic endocrine stem cells.

Ya-Huei Kuo, Ph.D. Molecular genetics of hematopoietic stem cells and leukemia stem cells.

Yilun Liu, Ph.D. Human RECQ helicases in aging and cancer prevention.

Qiang Lu, Ph.D. Understanding the mechanisms that control self-renewal and differentiation of neural progenitor/stem cells.

Edward M. Newman, Ph.D. Biochemical pharmacology of antimetabolites.

Vu Ngo, Ph.D. Molecular pathogenesis of lymphoid malignancies.

Andrei Rodin, Ph.D. Engineering biological networks using systems biology data.

Dustin E. Schones, Ph.D. Epigenomics of development and disease.

Yanhong Shi, Ph.D. Nuclear receptors in neural stem cells and adult neurogenesis.

Jeremy M. Stark, Ph.D. Factors and pathways that influence mammalian chromosomal stability.

Zuoming Sun, Ph.D. Mechanisms regulating T cell-mediated immunity.

Timothy W. Synold, Pharm.D. Pharmacokinetics and pharmacodynamics of anti-cancer drugs.

Piroska E. Szabó, Ph.D. Mechanisms of genomic imprinting and environmental reproductive biology.

Tijana Talisman, Ph.D. Super-resolution microscopy in drug discovery.

Shizhen Emily Wang, Ph.D. Outsmarting breast cancer.

John C. Williams, Ph.D. Structural biology and biophysics.

Defu Zeng, M.D. Transplantation immune tolerance.

COLD SPRING HARBOR LABORATORY

Watson School of Biological Sciences

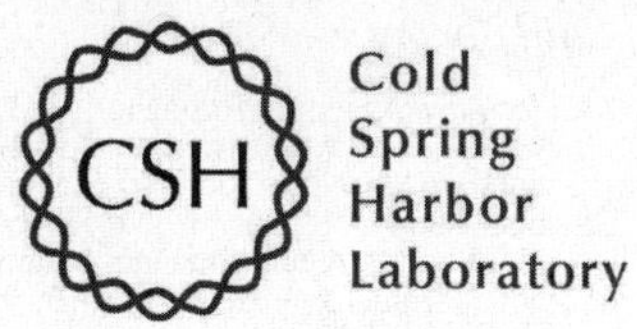

Program of Study

The Watson School of Biological Sciences at Cold Spring Harbor Laboratory (CSHL) offers an accredited Ph.D. program for motivated students of outstanding ability and intellect. The School aims to produce graduates in the biological sciences who are likely to become world leaders in science and society. The curriculum takes advantage of the unique and flexible environment of CSHL and includes the following innovative features: approximately four to five years from matriculation to Ph.D. degree; a broad representation of the biological sciences; core courses completed in the first semester; course work and laboratory rotations in separate phases; emphasis on the principles of scientific reasoning and logic; continued advanced course instruction throughout the graduate curriculum; and two-tier mentoring.

The program provides an exciting and intensive educational experience. The curriculum trains students to be self-reliant; students learn to identify and acquire the knowledge they need for their research and career. The course work is varied, allowing students to progress from gaining competence in a range of research areas to becoming experts in their chosen fields.

Research at CSHL focuses on molecular biology and cancer, neuroscience, quantitative biology, plant biology, and genetics and genomics. Students may choose any CSHL faculty member's laboratory for their thesis research.

Requirements for the award of the Ph.D. degree are successful completion of all coursework, laboratory rotations, teaching at CSHL's Dolan DNA Learning Center, the qualifying exam, thesis research, and defense of a written thesis that describes original research.

Research Facilities

CSHL has state-of-the-art research facilities, including an extensive network of shared resources through CSHL's status as a National Cancer Institute Cancer Center. There are several libraries on campus, providing a large collection of print and digital resources, as well as library services such as database searching and reference and interlibrary loan services. The information technology department supports computer resources campus-wide and maintains a high-performance cluster.

Financial Aid

The Watson School of Biological Sciences supports each student with an annual stipend, computer, books, health benefits, affordable housing, subsidized food, and funds for research costs. Students are encouraged to apply for independent funding through fellowships from federal and private sources.

Cost of Study

The Watson School provides full remission of all tuition fees for accepted students. Each student receives a stipend and research costs.

Living and Housing Costs

Students have access to CSHL's network of affordable on- and off-campus housing. Single graduate students live in single rooms in shared houses with housekeeping services; married students live in apartments. First-year Watson School students are offered rooms in the Townsend Knight House or the Cutting House, restored homes located on the shore of Cold Spring Harbor opposite the Laboratory campus. CSHL has on-campus child daycare. Recreational activities on campus include a fitness room, tennis and volleyball courts, a private beach, boats, and quiet roads for running or walking. The Laboratory sponsors classical music performances for its scientists and the neighboring community.

Student Group

The class size is approximately 10 students per year. Over the years, students have come to the School from across the United States and all over the world. Approximately half of Watson School students are international. There are no restrictions on citizenship.

Location

The Laboratory is located on the wooded north shore of Long Island, 35 miles east of New York City. CSHL's main campus is about 5 miles from the town of Huntington, which has a diverse selection of restaurants, shops, bars, and movie theaters.

The Laboratory

Since its inception in 1890, CSHL has been a leader in biology education. The CSHL Press publishes internationally recognized books and journals. The Dolan DNA Learning Center educates K–12 students and teachers about molecular biology and genetics. The Undergraduate Research Program hosts exceptional undergraduates from around the world for a summer research experience. CSHL's Meetings and Courses offers more than twenty-five advanced courses in biology and numerous international conferences, bringing more than 10,000 scientists to CSHL each year. In addition to the Watson School Ph.D. students, CSHL hosts visiting graduate students from institutions around the world and particularly from nearby Stony Brook University.

Applying

Applicants must have received a baccalaureate degree or equivalent from an accredited university or college prior to matriculation. Admission is based on the perceived ability of the applicant to excel in this doctoral program, without regard to gender, race, color, ethnic origin, sexual orientation, disability, or marital status. Suitable applicants are assessed on the basis of their academic record, recommendations from their mentors, and an on-site interview. Students must ensure that the School receives all application materials (transcripts, examination scores, letters of recommendation, etc.) no later than December 1 for the following Fall term. All applicants must apply online. Further information about the School and the application procedure may be found at http://www.cshl.edu/gradschool.

Correspondence and Information

Kimberly Creteur
Admissions Coordinator
Cold Spring Harbor Laboratory
Watson School of Biological Sciences
One Bungtown Road
Cold Spring Harbor, New York 11724
Phone: 516-367-6890
Fax: 516-367-6919
E-mail: gradschool@cshl.edu
Website: http://www.cshl.edu/gradschool

THE FACULTY AND THEIR RESEARCH

Research Faculty

Dinu Florin Albeanu, Assistant Professor; Ph.D., Harvard, 2008. Neuronal circuits; sensory coding and synaptic plasticity; neuronal correlates of behavior; olfactory processing.

Gurinder Singh "Mickey" Atwal, Assistant Professor; Ph.D., Cornell, 2002. Population genetics; bioinformatics; cancer; stochastic processes; statistical mechanics and information theory.

Anne Churchland, Assistant Professor; Ph.D., California, San Francisco, 2003. Decision-making; electrophysiology; sensory processing; vision; audition; neural computation; modeling; behavior.

Josh Dubnau, Associate Professor; Ph.D., Columbia, 1995. Learning; memory; genetics; behavior.

Mikala Egeblad, Associate Professor; Ph.D., Copenhagen, 2000. Tumor microenvironment; intravital imaging; tumor-associated myeloid cells; breast cancer.

Grigori Enikolopov, Associate Professor; Ph.D., Russian Academy of Sciences (Moscow), 1978. Stem cells; neurogenesis; development; signal transduction.

Doug Fearon, Professor; M.D.; Johns Hopkins, 1968. Cancer and immunology.

Hiro Furukawa, Associate Professor; Ph.D., Tokyo, 2001. Membrane proteins, X-ray crystallography, electrophysiology, neurodegenerative disease.

Jesse Gillis, Assistant Professor; Ph.D., Toronto, 2007. Gene networks; gene function prediction; guilt by association; neuropsychiatric; hub genes; multifunctionality; computational genomics.

Thomas Gingeras, Professor; Ph.D., NYU, 1976. Genome-wide organization of transcription and the functional roles of nonprotein coding RNAs.

Chris Hammell, Assistant Professor; Ph.D., Dartmouth, 2002. Post-transcriptional gene regulation; control of animal developmental timing; RNA biology.

Molly Hammell, Assistant Professor; Ph.D., Dartmouth, 2003. Gene regulatory networks; integrated genomic analysis; bioinformatics; RNA biology; small RNAs.

Gregory Hannon, Professor; Ph.D., Case Western Reserve, 1992. Growth control in mammalian cells; post-transcriptional gene silencing.

Z. Josh Huang, Professor; Ph.D., Brandeis, 1994. Development and function of the GABAergic inhibitory circuitry in neocortex; cortical circuits; mouse genetics; developmental plasticity; neurogenomics; autism.

Cold Spring Harbor Laboratory

Ivan Iossifov, Assistant Professor; Ph.D., Columbia, 2008. Computational biology; molecular networks; human genetics; human disease; applied statistical and machine learning; biomedical text-mining; molecular evolution.
David Jackson, Professor; Ph.D., East Anglia (England), 1991. Plant development; genetics; stem cell signaling; genomics and imaging.
Leemor Joshua-Tor, Professor; Ph.D., Weizmann (Israel), 1991. Structural biology; nucleic acid regulation; RNAi; molecular recognition; X-ray crystallography.
Adam Kepecs, Associate Professor; Ph.D., Brandeis, 2002. Decision-making; neural circuits; behavioral electrophysiology; theoretical neuroscience; neuroeconomics.
Alexei Koulakov, Professor; Ph.D., Minnesota, 1998. Theoretical neurobiology; quantitative principles of cortical design; computer science; applied mathematics.
Adrian R. Krainer, Professor; Ph.D., Harvard, 1986. Posttranscriptional control of gene expression; pre-mRNA splicing mechanisms, fidelity and genetic diseases; alternative splicing; RNA-protein interactions; cancer.
Alexander Krasnitz, Assistant Professor; Ph.D., Tel Aviv University, 1990. Genomics of cancer; machine learning for biology; inference from noisy biological data; large-scale numerical computing.
Dan Levy, Assistant Professor; Ph.D., Berkeley, 2005. Human genetics; mathematical modeling; algorithm development.
Bo Li, Associate Professor; Ph.D., British Columbia, 2003. Neuroscience; glutamatergic synapse; synaptic plasticity; schizophrenia; depression; rodent models of psychiatric disorders.
Zachary Lippman, Associate Professor; Ph.D., Watson School of Biological Sciences at Cold Spring Harbor Laboratory, 2004. Plant development; genetics; molecular mechanisms of phase transitions for flowering time and inflorescence branching; heterosis.
Gholson Lyon, Assistant Professor; M.D., Cornell, Weill, 2004; Ph.D., Rockefeller, 2003. Human genetics; neuropsychiatric diseases; whole genome sequencing; biochemistry; amino-terminal acetylation of proteins.
Robert Martienssen, Professor; Ph.D., Cambridge, 1986. Epigenetics; DNA methylation; chromatin and chromosome biology; transposable elements; RNA interference; stem cells; germline specification; plant genomics; plant evolution; aquatic plants.
W. Richard McCombie, Professor; Ph.D., Michigan, 1982. Genomics of psychiatric disorders; genomics of cancer; computational genomics; plant genomics.
Alea A. Mills, Professor; Ph.D., California, Irvine, 1997. Cancer; development; aging; senescence; epigenetics.
Partha P. Mitra, Professor; Ph.D., Harvard, 1993. Neuroinformatics; theoretical engineering; animal communications; neural prostheses; brain imaging; developmental linguistics.
Pavel Osten, Associate Professor; M.D., Charles University (Prague), 1991; Ph.D., SUNY Downstate Medical Center, 1995. Neurobiology of autism and schizophrenia; gene expression-based mapping of brain activity; anatomical mapping of brain connectivity; high throughput microscopy.
Darryl J. Pappin, Associate Professor; Ph.D., Leeds (United Kingdom), 1984. Proteomics; mass spectrometry; protein chemistry.
Michael C. Schatz, Assistant Professor; Ph.D., Maryland, College Park. Genomics; genome assembly and validation; sequence alignment; high performance and multicore computing; parallel algorithms; cloud computing.
Stephen Shea, Assistant Professor; Ph.D., Chicago, 2004. Olfaction; audition; communication behaviors; *in vivo* electrophysiology; individual recognition.
Adam Siepel, Professor; Ph.D., California, Santa Cruz, 2005. Quantitative biology.
Raffaella Sordella, Associate Professor; Ph.D., Turin, 1998. Molecular therapeutics; signal transduction.
David L. Spector, Professor; Ph.D., Rutgers, 1980. Cell biology; gene expression; nuclear structure; microscopy; noncoding RNAs.
Arne Stenlund, Associate Professor; Ph.D., Uppsala (Sweden), 1984. Papillomavirus; cancer; DNA replication.
Bruce Stillman, President and Professor; Ph.D., Australian National, 1979. DNA replication; chromatin assembly; biochemistry; yeast genetics; cancer; cell cycle.
Marja Timmermans, Professor; Ph.D., Rutgers, 1996. Plant development; epigenetic regulation of stem cell fate; pattern formation via small RNAs.
Nicholas Tonks, Professor; Ph.D., Dundee (Scotland), 1985. Posttranslational modification; phosphorylation; phosphatases; signal transduction; protein structure and function.
Jessica Tollkuhn, Assistant Professor; Ph.D., California, San Diego, 2006. Neuroscience.
Lloyd Trotman, Associate Professor; Ph.D., Zurich, 2001. Senescence and tumor progression; cancer modeling and treatment; cancer visualization; PTEN regulation.
Glenn Turner, Associate Professor; Ph.D., Caltech, 2000. Neural coding; learning and memory; sensory processing; *Drosophila;* electrophysiology.
David Tuveson, Professor; M.D., Ph.D., Johns Hopkins, 1994. Pancreatic cancer; experimental therapeutics; diagnostics; mouse models; cancer genetics.
Chris Vakoc, Assistant Professor; M.D., Ph.D., Pennsylvania, 2007. Chromatin; transcriptional regulation; acute myeloid leukemia; BET bromodomains; lysine methyltransferases.
Linda Van Aelst, Professor; Ph.D., Leuven (Belgium), 1991. Signal transduction; Ras and Rho proteins; tumorigenesis; neural development.
Doreen Ware, Associate Professor; Ph.D., Ohio State, 2000. Computational biology; comparative genomics; genome evolution; diversity; gene regulation; plant biology.
Michael Wigler, Professor; Ph.D., Columbia, 1978. Human genetic disorders; population genetics; cancer genomics.
Anthony Zador, Professor; M.D./Ph.D., Yale, 1994. Neural circuits; sensory processing, attention and decision making; attention; molecular tool development; connectomics.
Hongwu Zheng, Assistant Professor; Ph.D., Boston University, 2003. Malignant gliomagenesis; animal modeling; stem cell renewal/differentiation; genetic and epigenetic regulation.
Yi Zhong, Professor; Ph.D., Iowa, 1991. Neurophysiology; *Drosophila;* learning and memory; neurofibromatosis; signal transduction.

Non-Research Faculty
Alexander A. F. Gann, Dean WSBS; Ph.D., Edinburgh, 1989.
Terri Grodzicker, Dean of Academic Affairs; Ph.D., Columbia, 1969.
John R. Inglis, Executive Director, CSHL Press; Ph.D., Edinburgh, 1976.
David A. Micklos, Executive Director, DNA Learning Center; M.A., Maryland, 1982.
David J. Stewart, Director, Meetings and Courses; Ph.D., Cambridge, 1988.
Jan A. Witkowski, Executive Director, Banbury Center; Ph.D., London, 1972.

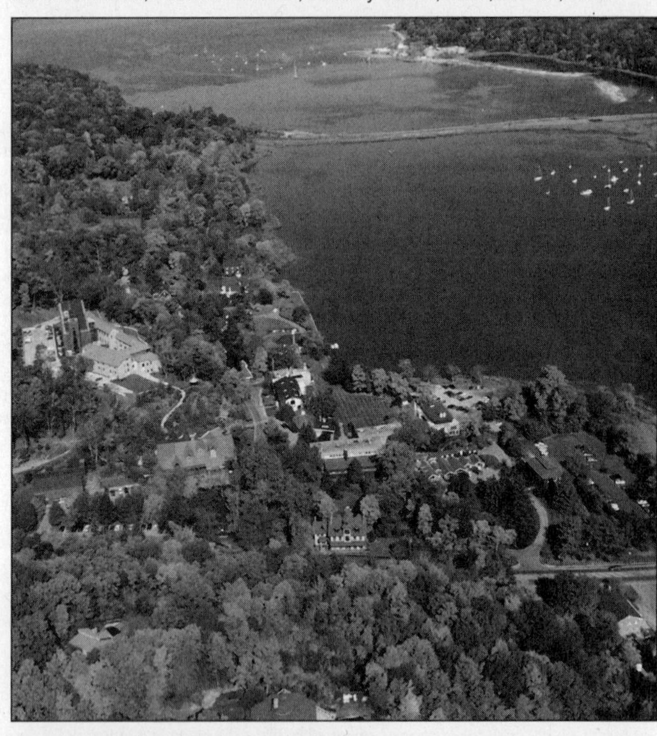

The campus of Cold Spring Harbor Laboratory.

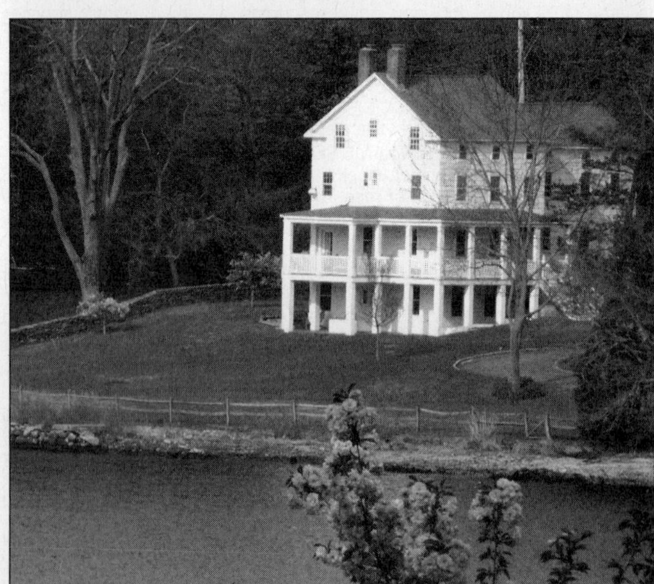

Townsend Knight House: first-year student housing.

COLUMBIA UNIVERSITY

Graduate School of Arts and Sciences
Department of Biological Sciences

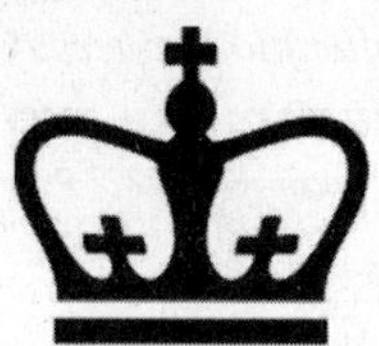

Program of Study

The Department offers training leading to a Ph.D. in cellular, molecular, developmental, computational, and structural biology as well as genetics, molecular biophysics, and neurobiology. The graduate program provides each student with a solid background in contemporary biology and an in-depth knowledge of one or more of the above areas. The specific nature and scheduling of courses taken during the first two graduate years are determined by the student's consultation with the graduate student adviser, taking into account the background and specific research interests of the student. During the first year, all students take an intensive core course that provides a solid background in structural biology, cell biology, genetics, molecular biology, and bioinformatics.

Beginning in the first year, graduate students attend advanced seminar courses, including the preresearch seminar, which is a forum for faculty-student research discussion. Important components of graduate education include the ability to analyze critically the contemporary research literature and to present such analyses effectively through oral and written presentations. Students acquire training in these skills through participation in advanced-level seminars and journal clubs, as well as through presentation and defense of original research proposals during the spring semester of the second year of graduate study or the fall semester of the third year.

Beginning in the first year of graduate work, students also engage in research training. Students may choose laboratories in the Department of Biological Sciences on Columbia's main Morningside Heights Campus or in about twenty-five other laboratories, including many at Columbia's Health Sciences Campus. To inform incoming students of research opportunities, faculty members discuss ongoing research projects with them in the preresearch seminar held in the autumn term of the first year. All students are required to participate in ongoing research in up to three different laboratories during the first year. The choice of a dissertation sponsor is made after consultation between the student and potential faculty advisers, and intensive research begins following the spring term of the student's first year. Each student is assigned a Ph.D. Advisory Committee made up of the student's sponsor and 2 other faculty members.

Research Facilities

The Department of Biological Sciences is located in the Sherman Fairchild Center for the Life Sciences. The building provides nearly 78,000 square feet of laboratory space for the Department's laboratories, as well as extensive shared instrument facilities, including extensive sophisticated microscopy, X-ray diffraction, fluorescence-activated cell sorting (FACS), real-time PCR analysis, mass spectrometry, infrared scanning, phosphorimaging, and microinjection, as well as housing and care of research animals, including transgenic mice. In addition, several laboratories are located in the nearby new state-of-the-art Northwest Corner interdisciplinary science building.

Financial Aid

All accepted students receive generous stipends, complete tuition exemption, and medical insurance. Special fellowships with larger stipends are also available (e.g., to members of minority groups).

Cost of Study

Tuition and fees are paid for all graduate students accepted into the Department.

Living and Housing Costs

Most students live in University-owned, subsidized apartments within easy walking distance of the laboratories. In addition, both the Morningside and Health Sciences Campuses are easily reached by public transportation from all areas of the city.

Student Group

There are about 100 graduate students and 60 postdoctoral fellows in the Department.

Location

New York is the cultural center of the country and offers unrivaled opportunities for attending concerts, operas, plays, and sporting events, for visiting outstanding museums, and for varied, affordable dining. Many excellent beaches, ski slopes, and state and national parks are within reasonable driving distance.

The University and The Department

Columbia was established as King's College in 1754 and has grown into one of the major universities of the world. The Department is located on the beautiful main campus in Morningside Heights, which combines the advantages of an urban setting and a peaceful college-town atmosphere.

Applying

Undergraduate training in one of the natural or physical sciences is recommended, although successful students have come from computer science or engineering backgrounds, as well. It is desirable for students to have had at least one year of calculus, as well as courses in organic and physical chemistry, physics, genetics, biochemistry, and cell biology. Any deficiencies may be made up while in graduate school. The Graduate Record Examinations (GRE) is required, as is the Test of English as a Foreign Language (TOEFL) for international applicants whose native language is not English and who do not hold an undergraduate degree from a U.S. college. The GRE Subject Test in biology, biochemistry, chemistry, computer science, or physics is highly recommended. Completed applications should be returned by January 5 for admission to the fall semester. Applications will be reviewed in the order received, so those submitting complete applications earlier have a better chance of being invited for an interview. Application forms and additional information can be obtained from the Department's website.

Columbia University is an Equal Opportunity/Affirmative Action institution.

Correspondence and Information

Graduate Student Adviser
Department of Biological Sciences
Columbia University
1212 Amsterdam Avenue, Mail Code 2402
Sherman Fairchild Center, Room 600
New York, New York 10027
United States
Phone: 212-854-2313
Fax: 212-865-8246
E-mail: biology@columbia.edu
Website: http://www.columbia.edu/cu/biology/

Columbia University

THE FACULTY AND THEIR RESEARCH

J. Chloë Bulinski, Professor; Ph.D., Wisconsin, 1980. Dynamics and functions of microtubules during myogenic differentiation and cell-cycle progression.

Harmen Bussemaker, Associate Professor; Ph.D., Utrecht (Netherlands), 1995. Data-driven modeling of transcriptional and posttranscriptional networks based on biophysical principles.

Martin Chalfie, Professor; Ph.D., Harvard, 1977; Member, National Academy of Sciences and Nobel Laureate in Chemistry 2008. Developmental genetics of identified nerve cells in *Caenorhabditis elegans;* genetic analysis of cell differentiation, mechanosensory transduction, synapse specification, and aging.

Lawrence A. Chasin, Professor; Ph.D., MIT, 1967. Pre-mRNA splicing in cultured mammalian cells.

Lars Dietrich, Assistant Professor, Ph.D., Heidelberg (Germany), 2004. Bacterial models for biological shape and pattern formation.

Julio Fernandez, Professor; Ph.D., Berkeley, 1982. Study of the cellular events that lead to the release of histamine or catecholamine-containing secretory granules from single, isolated mast cells or chromaffin cells; analysis of single-protein elasticity by atomic force microscopy (AFM).

Stuart Firestein, Professor; Ph.D., Berkeley, 1988. Cellular and molecular physiology of transduction; coding and neuronal regeneration in the vertebrate olfactory system.

Joachim Frank, Professor and Howard Hughes Medical Institute Investigator; Ph.D., Munich Technical, 1970; Member, National Academy of Sciences. Cryoelectron microscopy and three-dimensional reconstruction for the study of the mechanism of protein biosynthesis.

Tulle Hazelrigg, Professor; Ph.D., Indiana, 1982. mRNA localization in *Drosophila* oocytes.

John F. Hunt, Professor; Ph.D., Yale, 1993. Structural genomics and biophysical studies of the molecular mechanism of transmembrane transport.

Songtao Jia, Associate Professor; Ph.D., UCLA, 2003. Epigenetic regulation of the genome.

Daniel D. Kalderon, Professor; Ph.D., London, 1984. Molecular mechanisms of cellular interactions mediated by cAMP-dependent protein kinase (PKA) in *Drosophila;* roles of PKA in hedgehog signaling and in generating anterior/posterior polarity in oocytes.

Darcy B. Kelley, Professor and Howard Hughes Medical Institute Professor; Ph.D., Rockefeller, 1975. Sexual differentiation of the nervous system; molecular analyses of androgen-regulated development in neurons and muscle; neuroethology of vocal communication; evolution of the nuclear receptor family.

James L. Manley, Professor; Ph.D., SUNY at Stony Brook, 1976. Regulation of mRNA synthesis in animal cells; biochemical and genetic analysis of mechanisms and control of mRNA transcription, splicing, and polyadenylation; developmental control of gene expression.

Elizabeth Miller, Associate Professor; Ph.D., La Trobe (Australia), 1999. Protein folding, assembly, and the regulation of intracellular protein transport.

Dana Pe'er, Associate Professor; Ph.D., Hebrew (Israel), 2003. Function and organization of molecular networks.

Carol L. Prives, Professor; Ph.D., McGill, 1968; Member, National Academy of Sciences and National Institute of Medicine. Structure and function of the p53 tumor suppressor protein and p53 family members; studies on cell cycle and apoptosis; stress-activated signaling and control of proteolysis.

Ron Prywes, Professor; Ph.D., MIT, 1984. Normal and cancerous mechanisms of regulation of cellular proliferation and gene expression; signal transduction and activation of transcription factors; activation of transcription by the ER stress/unfolded protein response.

Molly Przeworski, Professor; Ph.D., Chicago, 2000. Population genetics, evolutionary genetics, meiotic recombination.

Ozgur Sahin, Associate Professor of Biological Sciences and Physics; Ph.D., Stanford, 2005. Mechanical investigations of biological systems for energy, environment, and biological research.

Guy Sella, Associate Professor; Ph.D., Tel Aviv (Israel), 2001. Evolutionary genetics of adaptation, disease risk and other quantitative traits.

Michael P. Sheetz, Professor; Ph.D., Caltech, 1972. Lasker Award for Basic Medical Research 2012. Motility studies of cells and microtubule motor proteins, with an emphasis on the force-dependent interactions relevant to transformed cells and neuron pathfinding, using laser tweezers.

Brent Stockwell, Associate Professor and Howard Hughes Medical Institute Investigator; Ph.D., Harvard, 1997. Diagramming disease networks with chemical and biological tools.

Liang Tong, Professor; Ph.D., Berkeley, 1989. Structural biology of proteins involved in human diseases (obesity, diabetes, cancer); structural biology of proteins involved in pre-mRNA 3'-end processing.

Alexander A. Tzagoloff, Professor of Biological Sciences; Ph.D., Columbia, 1962. Energy-coupling mechanisms; structure of membrane enzymes; biogenesis of mitochondria; genetics of mitochondria in yeast.

Jian Yang, Professor; Ph.D., Washington (Seattle), 1991. Structure and function of ion channels; molecular mechanisms of ion channel regulation and localization.

Rafael Yuste, Professor and Howard Hughes Medical Institute Investigator; M.D., Madrid, 1987; Ph.D., Rockefeller, 1992. Development and function of the cortical microcircuitry.

Additional Faculty Sponsors for Ph.D. Research

Richard Axel, Biochemistry and Molecular Biophysics/Pathology and Cell Biology; Howard Hughes Medical Institute Investigator and Nobel Laureate in Physiology or Medicine 2004; Member, National Academy of Sciences. Central and peripheral organization of the olfactory system.

Richard J. Baer, Pathology and Cell Biology. The pathogenesis of hereditary breast cancer.

Andrea Califano, Biomedical Informatics. Study of gene regulatory and signaling networks in mammalian cellular contexts using computational methods.

Virginia Cornish, Chemistry. Development of in vivo selection strategies for evolving proteins with novel catalytic properties.

Riccardo Dalla-Favera, Genetics and Development, and Microbiology and Immunology. Molecular genetics of cancer; molecular pathogenesis of lymphoma and leukemia.

Jonathan E. Dworkin, Microbiology and Immunology. Bacterial signaling and interactions with the host.

Jean Gautier, Genetics and Development/Institute for Cancer Genetics. Cell cycle and cell death during early development.

Ruben L. Gonzalez Jr., Chemistry. Single molecule biophysics.

Eric C. Greene, Biochemistry and Molecular Biophysics; Howard Hughes Medical Institute Investigator. Molecular mechanisms of DNA recombination and repair; single-molecule fluorescence microscopy and other biochemical approaches.

Lloyd Greene, Pathology and Cell Biology. Mechanisms of neuronal differentiation and degeneration and their regulation by external growth factors.

Iva Greenwald, Biochemistry and Molecular Biophysics; Howard Hughes Medical Institute Investigator; Member, National Academy of Sciences, Development and cell-cell interactions.

Wesley Grueber, Physiology and Cellular Biophysics/Neuroscience. Molecular basis of nervous system development and function in *Drosophila.*

Wei Gu, Pathology and Cell Biology. P53 in tumor suppression and aging.

René Hen, Pharmacology. Serotonin receptors and behavior.

Christopher Henderson, Rehabilitation and Regenerative Medicine. Motor neuron biology and disease: developmental mechanisms and therapeutic targets for ALS and SMA.

Wayne Hendrickson, Biochemistry and Molecular Biophysics; Howard Hughes Medical Institute Investigator; Member, National Academy of Sciences. Macromolecular structure; X-ray crystallography.

Oliver Hobert, Biochemistry and Molecular Biophysics; Howard Hughes Medical Institute Investigator. Nervous system development and function.

Thomas Jessell, Biochemistry and Molecular Biophysics; Howard Hughes Medical Institute Investigator; Member, National Academy of Sciences. Molecular mechanisms of neural differentiation.

Laura Johnston, Genetics and Development. Control of growth and cell division during development.

Eric Kandel, Physiology and Cellular Biophysics/Psychiatry/Biochemistry and Molecular Biophysics; Howard Hughes Medical Institute Investigator and Nobel Laureate in Physiology or Medicine 2000; Member, National Academy of Sciences. Cell and molecular mechanisms of associative and nonassociative learning.

Richard Mann, Biochemistry and Molecular Biophysics. Transcriptional control.

Ann McDermott, Chemistry/Biological Sciences/Chemical Engineering; Member, National Academy of Sciences. Solid-state NMR of enzyme active sites and model systems.

Arthur G. Palmer, Biochemistry and Molecular Biophysics. Biomolecular dynamics, structure, and function; NMR spectroscopy.

Liam Paninski, Statistics. Statistical analysis of neural and imaging data.

Virginia Papaioannou, Genetics and Development. Genetic control of mammalian development in the peri-implantation period.

Itsik Pe'er, Computer Science. Novel computational methods in human genetics.

Rodney Rothstein, Genetics and Development. Yeast genetics; mechanisms of genetic recombination; control of genome stability; functional genomics.

Christian Schindler, Microbiology/Medicine. JAK-STAT signaling and immune response.

Steve Siegelbaum, Pharmacology; Howard Hughes Medical Institute Investigator. Molecular studies of ion channel structure and function; synaptic transmission and plasticity in the mammalian brain.

Gary Struhl, Genetics and Development; Howard Hughes Medical Institute Investigator; Member, National Academy of Sciences. Developmental genetics in *Drosophila.*

Lorraine Symington, Microbiology. Homologous recombination in the yeast *Saccharomyces cerevisiae.*

Richard Vallee, Pathology and Cell Biology. Motor proteins in axonal transport, brain developmental disease, and synaptic function.

Charles Zuker, Biochemistry and Molecular Biophysics/Neuroscience. Signal processing, information transfer, and coding mechanisms in sensory systems.

NEW YORK MEDICAL COLLEGE

Graduate School of Basic Medical Sciences

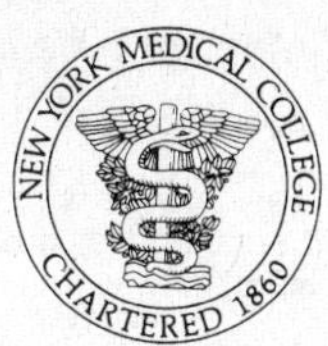

Programs of Study

The Graduate School of Basic Medical Sciences (GSBMS) of New York Medical College offers programs leading to the M.S. and Ph.D. degrees in biochemistry and molecular biology, cell biology, microbiology and immunology, pathology, pharmacology, and physiology plus an interdisciplinary M.S. degree in basic medical sciences. The full-time faculty of 80 basic medical scientists, with their individual and collaborative research programs, great depth of knowledge, and classroom experience, provide an intellectually challenging yet supportive environment to those students with the requisite talent and motivation. These internal assets are supplemented by the Graduate School's plentiful access to other experts—in clinical research, the pharmaceutical and biotechnology industry, and public health—who are available to participate in its research and educational activities.

Ph.D. degrees are awarded in six basic medical sciences. During the first year, students undertake an interdisciplinary core curriculum of courses and rotate through laboratories throughout the Graduate School. After this first year, students choose their major discipline of study and dissertation sponsor, complete the remaining didactic requirements in the chosen discipline, and begin intensive research training. Formal course work is usually substantially completed within two years, after which the student completes the qualifying exam, forms a dissertation advisory committee, presents a formal thesis proposal, and devotes his or her primary effort to the dissertation research project.

The M.S. degree requires completion of 30 to 32 credits, depending upon the discipline and specific track chosen. Two M.S. degree sequences are available: (1) a research program consisting of 25 didactic (i.e., classroom-based) credits, up to 5 research credits, and a research thesis or (2) a program consisting of 29 to 32 didactic credits and a scholarly literature review. The M.S. degree is earned on a full- or part-time basis with classes offered in the evening. The interdisciplinary M.S. program, with two separate tracks, is particularly suitable for students who want to prepare for a career in medicine, dentistry, or other health professions. The traditional track is a two-year program consisting entirely of evening classes. The accelerated track allows highly qualified candidates to take preclinical medical school courses during the day; they complete the didactic portion of the program within one year.

The **Department of Cell Biology** offers training in cell biology and neuroscience leading to careers in academia and industry. Ongoing research includes studies of oncogene expression and cytokines; intracellular mechanisms of pulmonary arterial hypertension; modulation of neuronal and astrocytic signaling; hemorrhage and neuroprotection in the developing brain; aging and preservation of oocytes and ovarian tissue; growth control in skeletal muscle; signal transduction in a variety of tissues, including platelets, the retina, muscle cells, and the *Drosophila* nervous system; intracellular protein trafficking and degradation; cytoskeletal and receptor function; the development and regeneration of the visual system; apoptosis in glaucoma; extracellular matrices and limb development; spinal cord injury; molecular mechanisms of neuroplasticity; learning and memory; Alzheimer's disease; and modulation of seizures.

The **Department of Biochemistry and Molecular Biology** provides students with a solid foundation in the concepts and applications of modern biochemistry and molecular biology. Areas of research include protein structure and function, enzyme reaction mechanisms, regulation of gene expression, mechanisms of hormone action and cell signaling, enzymology, mechanisms of DNA replication and repair, cell-cycle regulation, control of cell growth, molecular biology of cancer cells and the cancer process, mechanisms of nutrition and cancer prevention, molecular neurobiology and studies of neurodegenerative disorders, and the aging process.

The **Department of Pathology** offers a vigorous multidisciplinary milieu for training in experimental pathology. The programs focus on the comprehensive study of pathogenic mechanisms of human disease. Areas of interest in the department include examination of the underlying mechanisms involved in biochemical toxicology, cancer cell biology, cell-cycle regulation and apoptosis, chemical carcinogenesis, and tissue engineering.

In the **Department of Microbiology and Immunology**, students acquire a broad expanse of knowledge in microbiology, molecular biology, and immunology as well as depth in a particular elective field. Areas available for thesis research include molecular biology of tumor cells, cancer vaccines, the role of stem cells in cancer, bacterial genetics, pathogenesis of infectious disease, structure and function of influenza virus antigens, molecular virology, and the biochemistry and genetics of emerging bacterial pathogens.

The **Department of Pharmacology** emphasizes training in research methods for examining the mechanism of action of drugs at the systemic, cellular, and subcellular levels. Areas of research include investigation into the therapeutic and pathophysiologic role of bioactive lipids (eicosanoids) in cancer, ophthalmology, and cardiovascular diseases including hypertension, kidney disease, stroke, diabetes, atherosclerosis and inflammatory conditions, cytochrome P-450 function and control, patch-clamp analysis of ion transport, and the roles of vasoactive hormones and inflammatory cytokines in hypertension end-organ damage and cardiovascular function.

The **Department of Physiology** provides students with an understanding of the function of the body's cells and organ systems and the mechanisms for regulation of these functions. Research opportunities include cellular neurophysiology, regulation of sleep and awake states, neural and endocrine control of the heart and circulation, microcirculation, the physiology of gene expression, heart failure, and the physiological effects of oxygen metabolites.

Research Facilities

The College has an extensive laboratory complex in the basic medical and clinical sciences. The Basic Sciences Building houses research laboratories with core facilities for protein sequencing, mass spectrometry, gas or liquid (HPLC) chromatography, confocal and intravital microscopy, cell cytometry, and other advanced research techniques, as well as a biosafety level-3 laboratory and stem cell laboratory. The Health Sciences Library, which maintains 200,000 volumes, has an extensive collection of print and electronic journals, and a variety of online databases and search engines. The campus also offers a fully accredited comparative medicine facility, a well-equipped and staffed instrumentation shop, a variety of classrooms and conference rooms, a bookstore, a cafeteria, and student lounges.

Financial Aid

Federal and state loan programs are available for M.S. students. Ph.D. students receive a stipend, full tuition remission, medical insurance, and combinations of College fellowships and research assistantships. The Office of Student Financial Planning should be consulted for information on federal and state loan programs.

Cost of Study

In 2014–15, tuition is $975 per credit, or $15,600 annually, for a full-time master's student taking 8 credits per semester. The Accelerated Master's Program has an annual tuition rate of $36,330. Annual Ph.D. tuition is $26,600 before candidacy (first two years) and $4,000 after candidacy. Comprehensive medical insurance is available on an annual basis (July–June) for individuals ($4,818), student plus spouse ($9,222), or family ($13,492) coverage. Insurance premiums are prorated for master's students beginning studies in August.

Living and Housing Costs

The student residences on the Valhalla campus are comprised of a garden-style apartment complex and a five-building suite-style complex. The costs range from $810 to $865 per month for furnished suite-style apartments and $630 to $1,125 for unfurnished single-student apartments. Married student apartment costs range from $1,330 for a one-bedroom apartment, $1,490 for a two-bedroom apartment, and $1,890 for a three-bedroom apartment (families with children). All apartments include kitchens with a full-size refrigerator, microwave, and an oven/stove. A student center, in the center of the complex, offers a coin-operated laundry room and an exercise center with a weight room and cardio-fitness room equipped with Stairmasters, treadmills, and stationary bicycles. Students interested in applying for housing should contact the Associate Director of Student and Residential Life, Administration Building (phone: 914-594-4832 or e-mail: housing@nymc.edu), well in advance in order to make housing arrangements. Housing is not guaranteed. There is a limited number of rooms and apartments available for graduate students on campus.

Student Group

The total College enrollment in fall 2013 was more than 1,400. There were 31 Ph.D. and 110 M.S. students in the Graduate School of Basic Medical Sciences.

New York Medical College

Location

The College is located on a large suburban campus in Valhalla, New York, near the Westchester Medical Center. It is 5 miles from White Plains, 25 miles north of New York City, and is easily accessible by car or public transportation.

The College

New York Medical College, a member of the Touro College and University System, was established in 1860 and is one of the largest medical schools in the country. Graduate education at the College began informally in 1910. Graduate degrees were offered as early as 1938, and a graduate division was established in 1963.

Applying

Applications for admission may be submitted from September 1 through July 1. For optimal review of credentials and consideration for financial aid and housing, however, applications for fall enrollment into Ph.D. programs should be received by January 1. International applicants to the Master's program should complete their application no later than May 1. Specific admissions requirements are available on the College website at: http://www.nymc.edu/Academics/SchoolOfBasicMedicalSciences/Admissions/Requirements.html. Students must apply online at the College website. Ph.D. applicants must submit GRE General Test scores. Applicants for the Accelerated Master's Program must submit scores for the Medical College Admission Test (MCAT). Applicants for other M.S. programs may submit GRE, MCAT, or DAT (Dental Admission Test) scores. International students are required to submit results of the TOEFL. Transcripts from all post-secondary institutions attended (undergraduate and graduate) and two letters of recommendation from teachers or scientists personally familiar with the applicant must be submitted directly by the school or recommenders separately.

Correspondence and Information

Francis L. Belloni, Ph.D., Dean
Graduate School of Basic Medical Sciences
Basic Sciences Building, Room A41
New York Medical College
Valhalla, New York 10595
United States
E-mail: gsbms_apply@nymc.edu
Website: http://www.nymc.edu/gsbms/

THE GRADUATE FACULTY AND THEIR RESEARCH

Biochemistry and Molecular Biology. E. Y. C. Lee, Ph.D., Professor and Chairman: enzymology, structure-function relationships, and regulation of ser/thr protein phosphatases. A. J. L. Cooper, Ph.D., Professor: amino acid chemistry and biochemistry; biochemical mechanisms underlying neurological diseases. M. Y. W. Lee, Ph.D., Professor: DNA replication, polymerases, and repair; cell-cycle regulation. S. C. Olson, Ph.D., Associate Professor: signal transduction; regulation of phospholipase D pathway by protein kinase C and G proteins. J. T. Pinto, Ph.D., Professor: effects of chemopreventive agents, dietary factors, and xenobiotic substances on oxidation/reduction capacity in human cells. E. L. Sabban, Ph.D., Professor: molecular neurobiology; molecular mechanisms of stress; cloning and regulation of gene expression for catecholamine-synthesizing enzymes and neuropeptides. J. M. Wu, Ph.D., Professor and Master's Program Director: regulation of gene expression in leukemic and prostate cancer cells; cell-cycle control; chemoprevention by fenretinide and resveratrol. Z. Zhang, Ph.D., Assistant Professor and Ph.D. Program Director: X-ray crystallography; stem cell factor; quinone reductase 2.

Cell Biology and Anatomy. J. D. Etlinger, Ph.D., Professor and Chairman: skeletal muscle growth and atrophy; intracellular proteolysis in erythroid and muscle cells; role of proteasomes and ubiquitin; spinal cord injury. P. Ballabh, M.D., Professor: germinal matrix hemorrhage, pericytes. V. A. Fried, Ph.D., Professor and Graduate Program Director: ubiquitin and cellular regulation; cytoskeletal structure and functions. F. L. Hannan, Ph.D., Assistant Professor: *Drosophila melanogaster;* learning and memory; Ras-MAPK and mTOR pathways in neurological disorders, including neurofibromatosis; J. Kang, M.D., Ph.D., Associate Professor: astrocyte-mediated modulation of inhibitory synaptic transmission; interplay between excitatory and inhibitory synapses; properties of gap junction, K^+, and $GABA_A$ channels. M. Kumarasiri, Ph.D., Assistant Professor: protein turnover, ubiquitin-conjugated enzymes. K. M. Lerea, Ph.D., Associate Professor and Interdisciplinary Program Director: mechanisms of signal transduction; role of protein ser/thr kinases and phosphatases in integrin functions and platelet activation. S. A. Newman, Ph.D., Professor: physical and molecular mechanisms of development and evolution; pattern formation in the vertebrate limb; collagen assembly. K. Oktay, M.D., Professor: preservation by freezing and transplantation of oocytes and ovarian tissues to protect these cells from damage due to radiation and chemotherapy. P. B. Sehgal, M.D., Ph.D., Professor: interleukin-6; p53; gene expression; signal transduction (STAT3); cellular mechanisms of pulmonary arterial hypertension. S. C. Sharma, Ph.D., Professor: genetic approaches to regeneration of adult CNS neurons. A. D. Springer, Ph.D., Professor: engineering models of retinal development; optic nerve regeneration. P. K. Stanton, Ph.D., Professor: neuronal plasticity; long-term depression and potentiation of synaptic strength; synaptic functional changes in epilepsy; mechanisms of ischemia-induced delayed neuronal death. L. Velíšek, M.D., Ph.D., Professor, Accelerated Master's Program Director, and M.D./Ph.D. Program Director: epilepsy and epileptogenesis; epileptic syndromes of childhood; role of prenatal corticosteroids and stress in brain development and function; hypothalamic peptides and neuronal excitability. J. Velíšková, M.D., Ph.D., Professor: mechanisms of estrogen effects on neuronal excitability; seizures and epilepsy; neuroprotection; and synaptic plasticity; estrogen regulation of neuropeptideY and metabotropic glutamate receptor-NR2B subunit-containing NMDA receptor interactions. R. J. Zeman, Ph.D., Associate Professor: β_2-adrenoceptors in musculoskeletal growth; mechanisms of spinal cord injury; regulation of intracellular calcium.

Pathology. J. T. Fallon, M.D., Ph.D., Professor and Chairman: cardiovascular pathology; ischemic heart disease; experimental vascular injury; immunopathology of human myocarditis and allograft rejection. A. N. Arnold, Ph.D., Assistant Professor: transplantation immunology and histocompatibility. A. Bokhari, M.B.B.S., Assistant Clinical Professor: neonatal and pediatric pathology. P. M. Chander, M.B.B.S., Professor: pathogenesis of renal and vascular damage in stroke-prone spontaneously hypertensive rats; pathogenesis of HIV-associated nephropathy. Z. Darzynkiewicz, M.D., Ph.D., Professor: development of new methods of cell analysis using flow cytometry; analysis of cell-cycle specificity of antitumor drugs. M. Iatropoulos, M.D., Ph.D., Research Professor: comparative mechanisms of toxicity and carcinogenesis. P. A. Lucas, Ph.D., Research Associate Professor: wound healing and tissue engineering. F. H. Moy, Ph.D., Associate Professor of Clinical Pathology and Graduate Program Director: biostatistics and epidemiology, methodology, and applications in clinical trials and risk assessment. G. Wang, M.D., Clinical Assistant Professor: cytokines in Lyme carditis; antibacterial properties of treated fabrics; daptomycin-nonsusceptible enterococci. G. M. Williams, M.D., Professor: mechanisms of carcinogenesis; metabolic and genetic effects of chemical carcinogens.

Microbiology and Immunology. I. S. Schwartz, Ph.D., Professor and Chairman: molecular pathogenesis of Lyme disease and other emerging bacterial pathogens; functional genomics. C. S. Bakshi, D.V.M., Ph.D., Assistant Professor: immuno-pathogenesis of *Francisella tularensis*, respiratory infection. R. Banerjee, Ph.D., Assistant Professor: molecular virology and molecular oncology. D. Bessen, Ph.D., Professor: molecular pathogenesis, epidemiology, and evolutionary biology of group A *Streptococcus* (GAS); role of GAS infection in pediatric neuropsychiatric disorders. D. J. Bucher, Ph.D., Associate Professor: structure, function, and immunochemistry of viral antigens. F. C. Cabello, M.D., Professor: microbial genetics; infectious disease; recombinant DNA. R. J. Dattwyler, M.D., Professor: oral wildlife bait vaccine, Lyme disease, Yersinia pestis. J. Geliebter, Ph.D., Professor: immunology and molecular biology of thyroid and prostate cancer. C. V. Hamby, Ph.D., Associate Professor: molecular biology and immunology of human tumors. D. Mordue, Ph.D., Assistant Professor: cellular and molecular strategies used by intracellular pathogens to establish and maintain infection. M. M. Petzke, Ph.D., Assistant Professor: Lyme disease; bacterial pathogenesis; innate immunity; dendritic cells; interferons; pattern recognition receptors; functional genomics. R. K. Tiwari, Ph.D., Professor and Graduate Program Director: tumor immunology and chemoprevention and therapy using stem cells and tumor microenvironment in thyroid cancer, breast cancer, prostate cancer and melanoma. X. Zhou, M.D., Ph.D., Associate Professor: tumor immunology; immunotherapy; adoptive cell therapy; Sleeping Beauty transposon; micro RNAs; lymphozyte development; hematopoietic stem cells; stem cell transplantation.

Pharmacology. M. L. Schwartzman, Ph.D., Professor and Chairwoman: cytochrome P-450 metabolism of arachidonic acid in inflammation and hypertension. M. A. Carroll, Ph.D., Professor: renal cytochrome P-450 metabolites of arachidonic acid. N. R. Ferreri, Ph.D., Professor: cytokine production and function in the kidney and vascular smooth muscle. M. S. Goligorsky, M.D., Ph.D., Professor: basic mechanisms of endothelial dysfunction, its prevention and reversal; translation of bench findings to clinical physiology and pharmacology. A. M. Guo, Ph.D., Assistant Professor: cytochrome P-450-derived eicosanoids (20-HETE) in angiogenesis and cancer growth; regulation of endothelial precursor cell function. M. A. Inchiosa Jr., Ph.D., Professor: biochemical pharmacology of muscle. D. Lin, M.D., Ph.D., Research Assistant Professor: microRNA, renal K^+ secretion and Na^+ reabsorption. A. Nasjletti, M.D., Professor and Ph.D. Program Director: hormonal mediators of blood pressure regulation. C. A. Powers, Ph.D., Professor: neuroendocrinology. C. T. Stier, Ph.D., Associate Professor and M.S. Program Director: pharmacological protection against vascular damage and stroke. W. Wang, M.D., Professor: regulation of renal electrolytes transport.

Physiology. T. H. Hintze, Ph.D., Professor and Chairman: cardiovascular functions in chronically instrumented animals. F. L. Belloni, Ph.D., Professor: vascular and cardiac actions of adenosine; biomedical and research ethics. John G. Edwards, Ph.D., Associate Professor: physiological control of gene transcription; regulation of transcription factors; cardiac hypertrophy; exercise biochemistry and overload alterations of the myocardial phenotype. C. A. Eisenberg, Ph.D., Associate Professor: phenotypic potential of "adult" stem cells. L. M. Eisenberg, Ph.D., Professor: molecular mechanisms controlling the phenotypic direction of differentiating stem cells. A. Huang, M.D., Ph.D., Associate Professor of Physiology: role of estrogens in vascular function. A. Koller, M.D., Professor: regulation of blood flow in the microcirculation. C. S. Leonard, Ph.D., Professor: neuronal integration; synaptic and nonsynaptic neuromodulation; nitric oxide in the CNS; brain cholinergic systems; neural basis of sleep and wakefulness. E. J. Messina, Ph.D., Professor: microvascular control and regulation of smooth-muscle reactivity. M. Mozzor, B.A., Instructor: radiation physics. S. S. Passo, Ph.D., Professor: neuroendocrine control of blood pressure. S. J. Popilskis, D.V.M., DACLAM, Assistant Professor: comparative medicine. W. N. Ross, Ph.D., Professor: regional properties of neurons. J. M. Stewart, M.D., Ph.D., Professor: orthostatic hypotension. D. Sun, M.D., Ph.D., Associate Professor: role of endothelial stress on coronary arteriolar function. C. I. Thompson, Ph.D., Professor and Graduate Program Director: renal hemodynamics and GFR control. M. S. Wolin, Ph.D., Professor: vascular regulation via cyclic GMP, metabolites, and oxygen tension.

THE ROCKEFELLER UNIVERSITY

Graduate Programs

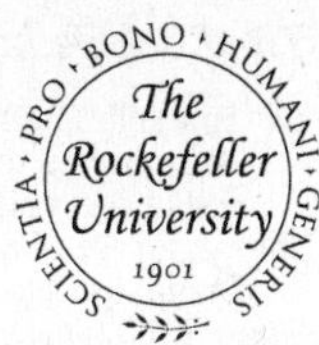

Programs of Study

Graduate education leading to the Ph.D. is offered to outstanding students regarded as potential leaders in their scientific fields. The University's research covers a wide range of biomedical and related sciences, including chemical and structural biology; genetics and genomics; immunology, virology, and microbiology; medical sciences, systems physiology and human genetics; molecular and cell biology; neurosciences and behavior; organismal biology, evolution, ethology, and ecology; physical, mathematical, and computational biology; and stem cells, development, regeneration, and aging, as summarized by the faculty list in this description. Students work closely with a faculty of active scientists and are encouraged to learn through a combination of course work, tutorial guidance, and apprenticeship in research laboratories. Graduate Fellows spend the first two years engaged in a flexible combination of courses geared toward academic qualification while conducting research in laboratories pertaining to their area of scientific interest. They choose a laboratory for thesis research by the end of the first year and devote their remaining time to pursuit of significant experimental or theoretical research, culminating in a dissertation and thesis defense. Students can spend full time in research; there are no teaching or other service obligations.

The faculties of the Rockefeller University, Weill Medical College of Cornell University, the Weill Graduate School of Medical Sciences of Cornell University, and Sloan-Kettering Institute collaborate in offering a combined M.D./Ph.D. program in the biomedical sciences to about 90 students. This program, conducted on the adjacent campuses of these three institutions in New York City, normally requires six or seven years of study and leads to an M.D. degree conferred by Cornell University and a Ph.D. degree conferred by either the Rockefeller University or the Weill Graduate School of Cornell University, depending upon the organizational affiliation of the student's adviser.

Research Facilities

The University and its affiliate Howard Hughes Medical Institute maintain a full range of laboratories and services for the research activities of the professional staff and students. Facilities include clinical and animal research centers on campus, a library, computing services, a field research center in Dutchess County, the Aaron Diamond AIDS Research Center (ADARC), as well as new centers for human genetics, studies in physics and biology, biochemistry and structural biology, immunology and immune diseases, sensory neuroscience, and Alzheimer's disease research.

Financial Aid

Each student accepted into the Ph.D. program receives a stipend ($36,000 in 2014–15) that is adequate to meet all living expenses. Students also receive an annual budget of $1,500 that can be used for travel, books and journals, computer purchases, and lab supplies.

Cost of Study

The University provides full remission of all tuition and fees for all accepted students.

Living and Housing Costs

On-campus housing is available for all students at subsidized rates. The stipend is designed to cover the cost of food, housing, and other basic living expenses. Students may elect to live off campus, but rents in the vicinity are very high.

Student Group

There are 184 graduate students, of whom 156 are enrolled in the Ph.D. program and 28 in the Ph.D. phase of the combined M.D./Ph.D. program. It is the policy of the Rockefeller University to support equality of educational opportunity. No individual is denied admission to the University or otherwise discriminated against with respect to any program of the University because of creed, color, national or ethnic origin, race, sex, or disability.

Student Outcomes

Graduates of the Rockefeller University have excelled in their professions. Two graduates have been awarded the Nobel Prize, and 29 graduates are members of the National Academy of Sciences. Most Ph.D. graduates move to postdoctoral positions at academic and research centers and subsequently have careers in academics, biotechnology, and the pharmaceutical industry. A few have pursued careers in medicine, law, and business. Almost all M.D./Ph.D. graduates first complete residencies in medical specialties, and most become medical scientists at major academic and medical research centers.

Location

The University is situated between 62nd and 68th streets in Manhattan, overlooking the East River. Despite its central metropolitan location, the 15-acre campus has a distinctive nonurban character, featuring gardens, picnic areas, fountains, and a tennis court. In addition to administrative and residential buildings, there are seven large laboratory buildings and a forty-bed hospital that serves as a clinical research center. Immediate neighbors are the New York Hospital, the Weill Medical College of Cornell University, Memorial Hospital, and the Sloan-Kettering Institute for Cancer Research. The wide range of institutions in New York City affords unlimited opportunities in research specialties, library facilities, and cultural resources.

The University

The Rockefeller University is dedicated to benefiting humankind through scientific research and its application. Founded in 1901 by John D. Rockefeller as the Rockefeller Institute for Medical Research, it rapidly became a source of major scientific innovation in treating and preventing human disease. Since 1954, the institute has extended its function by offering graduate work at the doctoral level to a select group of qualified students.

Laboratories, rather than departments, are the fundamental units of the University. The absence of departmental barriers between laboratories encourages interdisciplinary, problem-oriented approaches to research and facilitates intellectual interaction and collaboration. The collegial atmosphere fosters independence and initiative in students. In addition to the 184 doctoral students, there are 350 postdoctoral associates and fellows and a faculty of 73 full, associate, and assistant professors on campus who head laboratories.

Applying

Applications for the M.D./Ph.D. program must be completed by September 30; those for the Ph.D. program must be completed by December 1. Applicants are required to submit a personal statement describing research experience and goals as well as reasons for pursuing graduate study at The Rockefeller University. Also required are official transcripts and at least three letters of recommendation. Official GRE General Test scores are required and Subject Test scores are highly recommended for admission to the Ph.D. program. MCAT scores are required for the M.D./Ph.D. program. Further information about each program and details on application procedures may be obtained from the programs' respective websites. This information is also available on the University website, from which application forms and instructions can be downloaded (https://graduateapplication.rockefeller.edu).

Correspondence and Information

The Rockefeller University
The David Rockefeller Graduate Program
Kristen E. Cullen
Graduate Admissions Administrator and Registrar
1230 York Avenue
New York, New York 10065
Phone: 212-327-8086
E-mail: phd@rockefeller.edu
Website: http://www.rockefeller.edu/graduate
https://www.facebook.com/rockefelleruniversity
https://twitter.com/rockefelleruniv

LABORATORY HEADS AND THEIR RESEARCH

C. David Allis, Ph.D. (Chromatin Biology and Epigenetics). Studies the role of DNA packaging proteins in gene expression and DNA replication and repair.

Cori Bargmann, Ph.D. (Neural Circuits and Behavior). Studies the relationship between genes, neural circuits and behavior in *C. elegans*.

Paul Bieniasz, Ph.D. (Retrovirology) Studies the biology and evolution of retroviruses, including HIV, and genetics of host-virus interactions.

Günter Blobel, M.D., Ph.D. (Cell Biology). Uses genetic, biochemical, and ultrastructural methods to elucidate mechanisms of protein production and regulation.

Sean Brady, Ph.D. (Genetically Encoded Small Molecules). Discovers and characterizes new small molecules from microbial sources.

Jan L. Breslow, M.D. (Biochemical Genetics and Metabolism). Investigates the genetic basis of atherosclerotic disease.

The Rockefeller University

Ali Brivanlou, Ph.D. (Stem Cell Biology and Molecular Embryology). Researches the molecular events and cellular interactions that establish cell fate in vertebrate embryogenesis.
Jean-Laurent Casanova, M.D., Ph.D. (Human Genetics of Infectious Diseases). Researches the genetic basis of pediatric infectious diseases.
Brian T. Chait, D.Phil. (Mass Spectrometry and Gaseous Ion Chemistry). Uses mass spectrometry as a tool for studying biomolecules and protein interactions.
Jue Chen, Ph.D. (Membrane Biology and Biophysics). Combines structural and function techniques to study ABC membrane transporter proteins in health and disease.
Nam-Hai Chua, Ph.D. (Plant Molecular Biology). Studies molecular signaling pathways involved in plants' response to stress, light and infection.
Joel Cohen, Ph.D., Dr.P.H. (Populations). Studies interactions among groups of living beings in order to develop concepts helpful for understanding populations.
Barry Coller, M.D. (Blood and Vascular Biology). Investigates the role of blood platelets and the mechanisms of blood cell adhesion in vascular disease.
Frederick P. Cross, Ph.D. (Cell Cycle Genetics). Investigates the molecular basis of cell cycle control.
Robert B. Darnell, M.D., Ph.D. (Molecular Neuro-Oncology). Works to understand human autoimmune responses to cancer and neurologic disease.
Seth Darst, Ph.D. (Molecular Biophysics). Investigates the structure, function and regulation of the bacterial transcription machinery.
Titia de Lange, Ph.D. (Cell Biology and Genetics). Studies how telomeres protect chromosome ends from the DNA damage response.
Mitchell J. Feigenbaum, Ph.D. (Mathematical Physics). Develops mathematical descriptions and predictions of natural events that exhibit erratic behavior.
Vincent A. Fischetti, Ph.D. (Bacterial Pathogenesis and Immunology). Investigates bacterial infectious disease and the use of phage enzymes to block infection.
Winrich Freiwald, Ph.D. (Neural Systems). Researches the neural processes of object recognition and attention.
Jeffrey M. Friedman, M.D., Ph.D. (Molecular Genetics). Studies the molecular mechanisms that regulate food intake and body weight.
Elaine Fuchs, Ph.D. (Mammalian Cell Biology and Development). Investigates molecular mechanisms of skin stem cells, how they make and repair tissues, and how cancers develop.
Hinonori Funabiki, Ph.D. (Chromosome and Cell Biology). Studies signaling events in chromosome segregation in mitosis.
David C. Gadsby, Ph.D. (Cardiac and Membrane Physiology). Works to understand how ion transport proteins function in cells.
Charles D. Gilbert, M.D., Ph.D. (Neurobiology). Studies neural mechanisms of visual perception, learning and memory.
Joseph G. Gleeson, M.D. (Pediatric Brain Disease). Studies the causes of recessive brain disorders in children using high-throughput sequencing.
Konstantin A. Goulianos, Ph.D. (Experimental High-Energy Physics). Studies interactions among basic constituents of matter in order to explore the evolution and fate of the universe.
Paul Greengard, Ph.D. (Molecular and Cellular Neuroscience). Researches the molecular basis of communication between neurons in the mammalian brain.
Howard C. Hang, Ph.D. (Chemical Biology and Microbial Pathogenesis). Develops chemical tools for the study of microbe-host interaction.
Mary E. Hatten, Ph.D. (Developmental Neurobiology). Investigates mechanisms of neuronal differentiation and migration during embryonic development.
Nathaniel Heintz, Ph.D. (Molecular Biology). Investigates histological and functional aspects of the mammalian brain in health and disease.
David D. Ho, M.D. (Dynamics of HIV/SIV Replication). Pursues the development of drugs and vaccines to prevent HIV transmission.
A. James Hudspeth, M.D., Ph.D. (Sensory Neuroscience). Studies neural mechanisms of hearing and pursues treatments for hearing loss.
Tarun Kapoor, Ph.D. (Chemistry and Cell Biology). Investigates molecular and physical mechanisms of cell division.
Sebastian Klinge, Ph.D. (Protein and Nucleic Acid Chemistry). Studies the structure and function of macromolecular complexes involved in eukaryotic ribosome assembly.
Bruce W. Knight Jr. (Biophysics). Develops mathematical descriptions of the nerve networks involved in visual perception.
M. Magda Konarska, Ph.D. (Molecular Biology and Biochemistry). Investigates mechanisms of RNA splicing and the role of splicing in RNA transcription.
Mary Jeanne Kreek, M.D. (Biology of Addictive Diseases). Investigates the genetic basis of, and novel treatments for, addictive diseases.
Daniel Kronauer, Ph.D. (Insect Social Evolution). Studies evolution in insect societies at the level of the gene, individual, and colony.
James G. Krueger, M.D., Ph.D. (Investigative Dermatology). Uses psoriasis as a model to investigate the pathogenesis of inflammatory disease and autoimmunity.
Stanislas Leibler, Ph.D. (Living Matter). Conducts quantitative analyses of microbial systems on cellular and population levels.
Albert J. Libchaber, Ph.D. (Experimental Condensed-Matter Physics). Applies mathematical models to biological systems at organismal, cellular, and molecular levels.
Roderick MacKinnon, M.D. (Molecular Neurobiology and Biophysics). Studies principles underlying electricity in biology, particularly the passage of ions across cell membranes.
Marcelo Magnasco, Ph.D. (Mathematical Physics). Creates computational and mathematical models to describe neurophysiological systems and living organisms.
Gaby Maimon, Ph.D. (Integrative Brain Function). Studies electrical activity and computation underlying behavior in *Drosophila*.
Luciano Marraffini, Ph.D. (Bacteriology). Investigates the exchange of genetic material among bacteria.
Bruce S. McEwen, Ph.D. (Neuroendocrinology). Studies molecular mechanisms underlying effects of stress and sex hormones on the brain.
Daniel Mucida, Ph.D. (Mucosal Immunology). Investigates mechanisms of immune activity and tolerance in intestinal mucosa.
Fernando Nottebohm, Ph.D. (Animal Behavior). Investigates the biology of vocal learning and neuronal replacement in songbirds.
Michel C. Nussenzweig, M.D., Ph.D. (Molecular Immunology). Studies molecular aspects of adaptive and innate immune responses.
Michael O'Donnell, Ph.D. (DNA Replication). Studies molecular mechanisms of DNA replication, recombination, and repair.
F. Nina Papavasiliou, Ph.D. (Lymphocyte Biology). Studies RNA editing and DNA mutation as creators of information diversity in biological systems.
Donald W. Pfaff, Ph.D. (Neurobiology and Behavior). Studies steroid hormone effects on nerve cells regulating specific natural behaviors and overall CNS arousal.
Jeffrey V. Ravetch, M.D., Ph.D. (Molecular Genetics and Immunology). Investigates mechanisms of the functional diversity of antibodies in host defense and immunotherapy.
George N. Reeke Jr., Ph.D. (Biological Modeling). Uses computational modeling to understand complex biological or neurological functions.
Charles Rice, Ph.D. (Virology). Investigates mechanisms of hepatitis C virus infection and replication.
Robert G. Roeder, Ph.D. (Biochemistry and Molecular Biology). Studies the proteins and enzymes that execute and regulate gene transcription.
Michael P. Rout, Ph.D. (Cellular and Structural Cell Biology). Researches the structure of nuclear pore complexes and their role in oncogenic and developmental defects.
Vanessa Ruta, Ph.D. (Neurophysiology and Behavior).Investigates neural circuits that underlie innate and learned behaviors.
Thomas P. Sakmar, M.D. (Chemical Biology and Signal Transduction). Conducts biological and chemical investigations of G protein coupled receptors.
Shai Shaham, Ph.D. (Developmental Genetics). Investigates the role of glial cells in nervous system development and function.
Eric Siggia, Ph.D. (Theoretical Condensed-Matter Physics). Uses bioinformatics to study regulatory patterns in gene expression.
Sanford M. Simon, Ph.D. (Cellular Biophysics). Uses imaging techniques and other biophysical tools to study single events in biological systems.
Agata Smogorzewska, M.D., Ph.D. (Genome Maintenance). Uses Fanconia anemia as a backdrop to investigate DNA repair mechanisms in aging and cancer.
C. Erec Stebbins, Ph.D. (Structural Microbiology). Examines the targeting of host machineries by bacterial virulence factors.
Hermann Steller, Ph.D. (Apoptosis and Cancer Biology). Investigates signaling pathways underlying apoptosis.
Sidney Strickland, Ph.D. (Neurobiology and Genetics). Investigates neurovascular dysfunction in Alzheimer's disease and hemorrhagic stroke.
Alexander Tarakhovsky, M.D., Ph.D. (Immune Cell Epigenetics and Signaling). Investigates the epigenetic control of immune gene expression.
Sohail Tavazoie, M.D., Ph.D. (Systems Cancer Biology). Uses a variety of laboratory and clinical approaches to study the processes of cancer metastasis.
Marc Tessier-Lavigne, Ph.D. (Brain Development and Repair). Investigates nerve circuit formation and regeneration and the mechanisms underlying nerve cell death.
Alexander Tomasz, Ph.D. (Microbiology and Infectious Diseases). Tracks and studies mechanisms of bacterial antibiotic resistance.
Thomas Tuschl, Ph.D. (RNA Molecular Biology). Investigates gene regulatory mechanisms triggered by double-stranded RNA and RNA-binding proteins.
Leslie Vosshall, Ph.D. (Neurogenetics and Behavior). Investigates how odor stimuli are processed and perceived.
Michael W. Young, Ph.D. (Genetics). Investigates the genetic regulation of biological clocks that underlie many activities of living organisms.

UCONN HEALTH

Graduate Programs in Biomedical Sciences

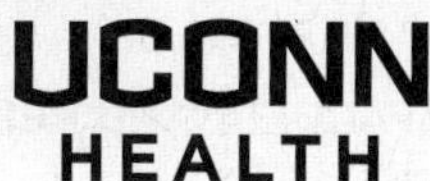

Programs of Study

Work leading to the Ph.D. degree in biomedical sciences and master's degrees in dental sciences, public health, and clinical and translational research is offered through Graduate School faculty members associated with the Schools of Medicine and Dental Medicine at the UConn Health in Farmington. A combined-degree program with the School of Medicine offers an M.D./Ph.D. degree to qualified students interested in academic medicine and research. The School of Dental Medicine offers a D.M.D./Ph.D. and a Combined Certificate Training Ph.D. program for students with advanced dental degrees. In addition, the Schools of Medicine and Dental Medicine, in conjunction with the Public Health Program, offer a combined program leading to the M.D./M.P.H. or D.M.D./M.P.H. Ph.D. students apply to the Integrated Admissions Mode, which offers a first year of study in the basic science curriculum prior to the selection of an area of concentration in which to pursue the Ph.D. thesis work.

Research Facilities

Programs are located at UConn Health in Farmington. A wide range of general and specialized equipment and expertise in the biological, biochemical, and biophysical sciences is available. Students have access to all facilities and equipment necessary for the pursuit of their research programs. In addition, major institutional resources include central small-animal facilities and the Lyman Maynard Stowe Library that contains approximately 200,000 volumes and 450 CAI programs and subscribes to more than 1,700 current periodicals.

Financial Aid

Support for doctoral students engaged in full-time degree programs at UConn Health is provided on a competitive basis. Graduate research assistantships for 2014–15 provide a stipend of $29,000 per year, which includes a waiver of tuition/most University fees for the fall and spring semesters and the option of participating in a student health insurance plan. While financial aid is offered competitively, UConn Health makes every possible effort to address the financial needs of all doctoral students during their period of training.

Cost of Study

For 2014–15, tuition is $12,202 per year for full-time students who are Connecticut residents and $32,258 per year for full-time students who are out-of-state residents. General University fees are added to the cost of tuition for students who do not receive a tuition waiver. These costs are usually met by traineeships or research assistantships for doctoral students.

Living and Housing Costs

There is a wide range of affordable housing options in the greater Hartford area within easy commuting distance of the campus, including an extensive complex that is adjacent to UConn Health. Costs range from $700 to $1,000 per month for a one-bedroom unit; 2 or more students sharing an apartment usually pay less. University housing is not available on campus.

Student Group

Approximately 550 students in the Schools of Medicine and Dental Medicine, 400 graduate students in the Ph.D. and master's programs, and numerous postdoctoral fellows use the facilities in Farmington.

Location

UConn Health is located in the historic town of Farmington, Connecticut. Set in the beautiful New England countryside on a hill overlooking the Farmington Valley, it is close to ski areas, hiking trails, and facilities for boating, fishing, and swimming. Connecticut's capital city of Hartford, 7 miles east of Farmington, is the center of an urban region of approximately 800,000 people. The beaches of the Long Island Sound are about 50 minutes away to the south, and the beautiful Berkshires are a short drive to the northwest. New York City and Boston can be reached within 2½ hours by car. Hartford is the home of the acclaimed Hartford Stage Company, TheatreWorks, the Hartford Symphony and Chamber orchestras, two ballet companies, an opera company, the Wadsworth Athenaeum (the oldest public art museum in the nation), the Mark Twain house, the Hartford Civic Center, and many other interesting cultural and recreational facilities. The area is also home to several branches of the University of Connecticut, Trinity College, and the University of Hartford, which includes the Hartt School of Music. Bradley International Airport (about 30 minutes from campus) serves the Hartford/Springfield area with frequent airline connections to major cities in this country and abroad. Frequent bus and rail service is also available from Hartford.

The Health Center

The 200-acre UConn Health campus at Farmington houses a division of the University of Connecticut Graduate School, as well as the School of Medicine and Dental Medicine. The campus also includes the John Dempsey Hospital, associated clinics, and extensive medical research facilities, all in a centralized facility with more than 1 million square feet of floor space. The Academic Research Building, built in 1999, is an impressive eleven-story structure providing 170,000 square feet of laboratory space. In addition, renovations are underway in the main Laboratory building, converting existing lab space into state-of-the-art open lab areas. There are more than 260 full-time members at UConn Health. The institution has a strong commitment to graduate study within an environment that promotes social and intellectual interaction among the various educational programs. Graduate students are represented on various administrative committees concerned with curricular affairs, and the Graduate Student Organization (GSO) represents graduate students' needs and concerns to the faculty and administration, in addition to fostering social contact among graduate students at UConn Health.

Applying

Prospective students should check with their degree program of interest for specific admission requirements. For the biomedical science Ph.D. program, applications for admission should be submitted via the online application system and should be filed together with transcripts, three letters of recommendation, a personal statement, and recent results from the General Test of the Graduate Record Examinations. International students must take the Test of English as a Foreign Language (TOEFL) to satisfy Graduate School requirements. The deadline for completed applications and receipt of all supplemental materials is **December 1** for the Ph.D. in Biomedical Science program. Note that GRE and TOEFL exams taken after the due date will not be accepted for consideration for admission. In accordance with the laws of the state of Connecticut and of the United States, UConn Health does not discriminate against any person in its educational and employment activities on the grounds of race, color, creed, national origin, sex, age, or physical disability. Details and contact information for additional degree programs is available online at grad.uchc.edu.

Correspondence and Information

Graduate Admissions Office
Ph.D. in Biomedical Science Program
UConn Health
263 Farmington Ave., MC 3906
Farmington, Connecticut 06030-3906
United States
Phone: 860-679-4509
E-mail: BiomedSciAdmissions@uchc.edu
Website: http://grad.uchc.edu/prospective/programs/phd_biosci/index.html

FACULTY AND RESEARCH AREAS

Biomedical Science Ph.D. Research Areas:

UConn Health's graduate faculty of more than 150 members is drawn from both the basic and clinical departments of the Schools of Medicine and Dental Medicine.

Cell Analysis and Modeling (CAM). This program is designed to train students from diverse disciplinary backgrounds in the cutting-edge research techniques that comprise the interdisciplinary research of modern cell biology. Faculty members associated with this area explore complex biological systems using computational cell biology, optical imaging, and other quantitative approaches to analyze processes in living cells. The CAM program is particularly strong in the following areas of research: cellular modeling (analysis and simulation, data integration, modeling movies boundaries, modularity and multistate complexes, molecular flux in crowded spaces, stochastic modeling and discrete particles); biophysics (biological signaling platforms, in vivo nanofabrication); optical imaging (fluorescent correlation spectroscopy, optical probe development, second harmonic generation, single-molecule imaging); cell biology (cellular tissues and development, cytoskeletal dynamics, RNA trafficking, signal transduction, molecular medicine). John H. Carson, Professor of Molecular, Microbial, and Structural Biology and Program Director.

Cell Biology. This interdisciplinary program offers the student the opportunity to bring modern molecular and physical techniques to bear on problems in cell biology. Faculty members' research spans a broad range of interests in the areas of eukaryotic cell biology and related clinical aspects. The program is particularly strong in the following areas of research: angiogenesis, cancer biology, gene expression, molecular medicine, reproductive biology, signal transduction, vascular biology, optical methods, proteomics, and computer modeling of complex biological systems. Guo-Hua Fong, Associate Professor of Cell Biology and Center for Vascular Biology and Program Director.

Genetics and Developmental Biology. This program emphasizes cellular and molecular bases of differentiation and development and includes opportunities in molecular human genetics. Research opportunities are available in the biology of human embryonic stem cells, mapping and cloning of genes responsible for human disease, RNA processing (including RNA editing, alternative splicing, antisense regulation, and RNA interference), the molecular mechanisms of aging, signal transduction pathways, microbial pathogenesis, developmental neurobiology, cell differentiation, musculoskeletal development, morphogenesis and pattern formation, reproductive biology, and endocrinology. Blanka Rogina, Associate Professor of Genetics and Developmental Biology and Program Director.

Immunology. The central focus of this program is to train the student to become an independent investigator and educator who will provide research and educational contributions to basic, applied, or clinical immunology through lectures, seminars, laboratory rotations, research presentations, and a concentration on laboratory research. Research in the program is focused on the cellular and molecular aspects of immune system structure and function in animal models and in humans. Areas of emphasis include molecular immunology (mechanisms of antigen presentation, major histocompatibility complex genetics and function, cytokines and cytokine receptors, and tumor antigens), cellular immunology (biochemical mechanisms and biological aspects of signal transduction of lymphocytes and granulocytes; cellular and molecular requirements for thymic T-lymphocyte development, selection, and activation; cytokines in B- and T-cell development; regulation of antitumor immunity; immunoparasitology, including parasite genetics and immune recognition of parasite antigens; and mechanisms of inflammation), organ-based immunology (immune effector mechanisms of the intestine, lymphocyte interactions in the lung, and immune regulation of the eye), immunity to infectious agents (viruses, bacteria, and parasites, including vector-borne organisms), and autoimmunity (animal models of autoimmune disease and effector mechanisms in human autoimmunity). H. Leonardo Aguila, Associate Professor of Immunology and Program Director.

Molecular Biology and Biochemistry. This program uniquely bridges modern molecular biology, microbiology, biochemistry, cell biology, and structural biology. Research in this program is directed toward explaining biological phenomena at the molecular level. The program includes four major areas of concentration and research: relation of the structure of macromolecules to their function, biosynthesis of macromolecules, biochemical genetics, and assembly of macromolecules into complex cellular structures. Chris Heinen, Associate Professor of Medicine and Program Director.

Neuroscience. This interdepartmental program offers comprehensive conceptual and experimental training in molecular, systems, and behavioral neuroscience. The faculty members of the neuroscience program engage in research that involves cellular, molecular, and developmental neurobiology; neuroanatomy; neuroimaging; neurophysiology; neurochemistry; neuroendocrinology; neuropharmacology; and neuropathology. Zhao-Wen Wang, Associate Professor of Genetics and Developmental Biology and Program Director.

Skeletal, Craniofacial, and Oral Biology. This program offers interdisciplinary research training in the areas of skeletal, craniofacial, and oral biology, emphasizing contemporary research technologies in cell, molecular, and developmental biology; genetics; and biochemistry. Areas of research include regulation of the formation, outgrowth, and patterning of the developing limb; control of cartilage differentiation, endochondral ossification, osteogenesis, and joint formation; molecular regulation of gene expression in bone; homeobox gene regulation of osteoblast differentiation; gene therapy of bone diseases; hormonal and cytokine regulation of bone growth, formation, and remodeling; control of craniofacial skeletogenesis and tooth development; signal transduction and intracellular signaling pathways; cellular and molecular aspects of the pathogenesis of inflammatory disease; microbiology, pathogenesis, and immunology of caries and periodontal disease; neural structure and function in the gustatory system; biomaterial development for tissue engineering; bone cell–implant interactions; differentiation of human embryonic stem cells into skeletal tissues; and analysis of oral and mucosal function and disease. Caroline Dealy, Associate Professor, Center for Regenerative Medicine and Skeletal Development and Program Director.

Combined Degree Programs:

Combined M.D./Ph.D. Program. This program is designed for students interested in careers in medical research and academic medicine. It enables students to acquire competence in both the basic science and clinical aspects of their chosen fields. The program allows a student to combine the curricula of two schools in a way that meets the specific degree requirements of each, and yet it allows the completion of both in a period less than that needed if the two curricula were taken in sequence. Entry into the program is limited to a small number of unusually well qualified students who are either currently enrolled in the medical school or who have been accepted into the first-year class. Carol Pilbeam, Professor of Medicine and Program Director.

Combined D.M.D./Ph.D. Program. This program is designed for students interested in careers in dental research and academic dental medicine. It enables students to acquire competence in both the basic science and clinical aspects of their chosen fields. The program allows a student to combine the curricula of two schools in a way that meets the specific degree requirements of each, and yet it allows the completion of both in a period less than that needed if the two curricula were taken in sequence. Entry into the program is limited to a small number of unusually well qualified students who are either currently enrolled in the dental school or who have been accepted into the first-year class. Mina Mina, Professor of Orthodontics, Oral and Maxillofacial Surgery, Pediatric Dentistry, and Advanced Education and Program Director.

Combined M.D./M.P.H. or D.M.D./M.P.H. Program. A joint-degree program leading to the Master of Public Health in addition to the Doctor of Medicine or the Doctor of Dental Medicine is sponsored by the Graduate Program in Public Health and the Schools of Medicine and Dental Medicine. The joint-degree program has been developed to prepare future physicians and dentists to deal creatively with the rapidly changing environment of medicine and health care. It is possible to complete the degree requirements for both programs during the four years of medical or dental school. David Gregorio, Professor of Community Medicine and Health Care and Program Director.

Other Degree Programs:

Clinical and Translational Research. The Master of Science degree program in clinical and translational research is administered in the Department of Medicine and stresses clinical research methods and research practicum in order to provide practical research training in preparation for independent research. The program is offered to individuals who have a health-related terminal degree (M.D., D.M.D., or Ph.D.) or who are involved in an M.D., D.M.D., or Ph.D. program in a health-related field and are in good standing. The master's program is based on both course work and research experience, but no research thesis is required. Students are required to sit for a final examination, which may entail the oral defense of a grant application and a manuscript. Lisa Godin (godin@nso.uchc.edu).

Dental Science. The Master of Dental Science degree program is an interdepartmental program whose primary objective is to provide instruction in dental science that will enhance the student's ability to instruct and undertake research in dental schools. This program provides an opportunity for cooperative study and research between dentistry, the basic sciences, and allied health fields. Both M.Dent.Sc. and oral biology Ph.D. students may combine their work in these programs with advanced clinical training in endodontics, orthodontics, oral pathology, pedodontics, periodontics, oral medicine, oral radiology, and oral and maxillofacial surgery. Arthur Hand, Assistant Dean for Medical and Graduate Education.

Public Health. This multidisciplinary master's program, accredited by the Council for Education in Public Health, is based in the Department of Community Medicine and Health Care. It offers a core curriculum in epidemiology, biostatistics, health administration, environmental health, the sociomedical sciences, health law, and electives in these and related areas. A Ph.D. program in public health is also offered. David Gregorio, Professor of Community Medicine and Health Care and Program Director.

THE UNIVERSITY OF KANSAS MEDICAL CENTER

Interdisciplinary Graduate Program in Biomedical Sciences

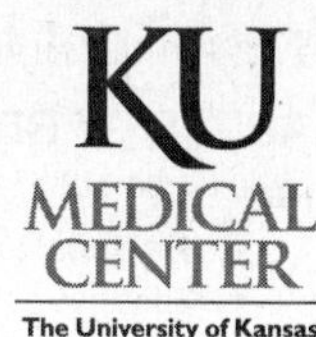

Programs of Study

At the University of Kansas Medical Center (KUMC), students pursue graduate studies on the cutting edge of biomedical research. Students have the opportunity to develop research skills and earn a Ph.D. degree in a broad range of biomedical research areas, including neuroscience; protein structure and function; pharmacology and toxicology; and viral, microbial, molecular, cellular, developmental, reproductive, immunological, renal, and physiological biology. Research also includes many clinically related studies that focus on a wide range of human diseases. The graduate program is a partnership between KUMC (http://www.kumc.edu/igpbs) and the nearby Stowers Institute for Medical Research (http://www.stowers-institute.org); students may conduct their research at either institution.

Graduate students pursuing a Ph.D. degree in biomedical sciences are admitted through the Interdisciplinary Graduate Program in Biomedical Sciences (IGPBS). This program is responsible for the first-year, highly integrated curriculum that allows each student to experience current areas of biomedical science before selecting a laboratory in which to carry out his or her doctoral research. In addition to the fundamental principles essential to the biomedical sciences, students receive an introduction to practical aspects of research, including biographics, bioethics, appropriate use of animals in research, laboratory safety, and procedures for human studies research. Faculty members also present their research programs to students through a research seminar series, giving students the opportunity to evaluate each research program. Following this introduction, each student selects three laboratory rotations that are completed during the first year. Laboratory rotations expose students to potential research advisers and to the principles and procedures of cutting-edge laboratory techniques, and they allow students to decide which laboratory best fits their needs. At the beginning of the second year, each student selects a research adviser for their doctoral research. At this time, the student also enters one of eight graduate programs.

Research Facilities

State-of-the-art technology and equipment is available through a variety of core research facilities, including DNA microarray technology, laser capture microdissection, rodent behavioral testing facilities, bioinformatics, transgenic mouse laboratories, fluorescence-activated cell sorting, molecular neurobiology, mass spectrometry, a highly automated histological and immunohistochemistry core, FT-IR microspectroscopy, electron microscopy, confocal microscopes for live cell imaging and spectral separation, noninvasive magnetic resonance spectroscopy, functional magnetic resonance imaging, and magnetoencephalography.

Financial Aid

Teaching and research assistantships are available. Students admitted into the IGPBS are awarded $24,000 in financial support and given a tuition waiver. Student travel awards are also available as pupils progress through the program.

Cost of Study

Students accepted into the IGPBS receive a tuition waiver upon meeting enrollment requirements. Students are responsible for campus and library fees, estimated at $473 per academic year.

Living and Housing Costs

Multiple options are available near the KUMC campus. Current housing costs are between $450 and $800 per month.

Student Group

Twenty-five percent of the students enrolled in the IGPBS are from international locales. The age range of students generally falls between 22 and 32 years.

Student Outcomes

Upon graduation from KUMC, students can expect to obtain a position in the biotechnology, academic, or governmental career fields.

Location

The University of Kansas Medical Center is located at 39th Avenue and Rainbow Boulevard in Kansas City, Kansas. It is on the border of Kansas and Missouri, with quick access to Westport, the Country Club Plaza, the Nelson-Atkins Museum of Art, and the Kansas City Art Institute.

The Graduate Program

The Interdisciplinary Graduate Program in Biomedical Sciences is an educational program within the School of Medicine at the University of Kansas Medical Center. It consists of eight degree-granting departments or programs. The IGPBS is made up of the Departments of Anatomy and Cell Biology; Biochemistry and Molecular Biology; Microbiology, Molecular Genetics, and Immunology; Pathology and Laboratory Medicine; Molecular and Integrative Physiology; Pharmacology, Toxicology, and Therapeutics; the Neuroscience Graduate Program; and the Training Program in Environmental Toxicology.

Applying

Students who are interested in the IGPBS may apply online at http://www.kumc.edu/igpbs. Applications must be received by January 4, although applications received after that date will be considered until the class is filled.

Correspondence and Information

Director
Interdisciplinary Graduate Program in Biomedical Sciences
5015 Wescoe, MS3025
The University of Kansas Medical Center
3901 Rainbow Boulevard
Kansas City, Kansas 66160-7836
Phone: 913-588-2719
800-408-2039 (toll-free)
Fax: 913-588-2711
E-mail: igpbs@kumc.edu
Website: http://www.kumc.edu/igpbs

The University of Kansas Medical Center

AREAS OF RESEARCH

Faculty members at KUMC have the following areas of research emphasis:

- Bacterial and viral pathogenesis
- Biophysics
- Imaging
- Immunology
- Metabolism in health and disease
- Molecular biology and genetics
- Pharmacological sciences
- Structural biology
- Toxicology and environmental health
- Translational medicine
- Transcription, chromatin, and epigenetics
- Cancer biology
- Cardiovascular biology
- Cell and developmental biology
- Liver biology
- Musculoskeletal biology
- Neurosciences
- Personalized medicine
- Renal biology
- Reproductive biology
- Signal transduction
- Stem cell biology

Section 2
Anatomy

This section contains a directory of institutions offering graduate work in anatomy. Additional information about programs listed in the directory may be obtained by writing directly to the dean of a graduate school or chair of a department at the address given in the directory.

For programs offering related work, see also in this book *Allied Health; Biomedical Sciences; Cell, Molecular, and Structural Biology; Dentistry and Dental Sciences; Genetics, Developmental Biology, and Reproductive Biology; Neuroscience and Neurobiology; Pathology and Pathobiology; Physiology; Veterinary Medicine and Sciences;* and *Zoology.* In another guide in this series:

Graduate Programs in the Humanities, Arts & Social Sciences
See *Sociology, Anthropology, and Archaeology*

CONTENTS

Program Directory

Anatomy

Albert Einstein College of Medicine, Graduate Division of Biomedical Sciences, Department of Anatomy and Structural Biology, Bronx, NY 10461. Offers anatomy (PhD); cell and developmental biology (PhD); MD/PhD. *Degree requirements:* For doctorate, thesis/dissertation. *Entrance requirements:* For doctorate, GRE General Test. Additional exam requirements/recommendations for international students: Required—TOEFL. Electronic applications accepted. *Faculty research:* Cell motility, cell membranes and membrane-cytoskeletal interactions as applied to processing of pancreatic hormones, mechanisms of secretion.

American University of Beirut, Graduate Programs, Faculty of Medicine, Beirut, Lebanon. Offers anatomy, cell biology and human morphology (MS); biochemistry and medical genetics (MS); biomedical sciences (PhD); experimental pathology, immunology and microbiology (MS); medicine (MD); neuroscience (MS); pharmacology and toxicology (MS). Part-time programs available. *Faculty:* 259 full-time (78 women), 93 part-time/adjunct (16 women). *Students:* 364 full-time (165 women), 62 part-time (54 women). Average age 23. In 2013, 18 master's awarded. *Degree requirements:* For master's, one foreign language, comprehensive exam, thesis (for some programs); for doctorate, one foreign language, comprehensive exam, thesis/dissertation. *Entrance requirements:* For master's, letter of recommendation; for doctorate, MCAT, bachelor's degree. Additional exam requirements/recommendations for international students: Required—TOEFL (minimum score 600 paper-based; 100 iBT), IELTS (minimum score 7.5). *Application deadline:* For fall admission, 4/30 for domestic and international students; for spring admission, 11/1 for domestic and international students. Application fee: $50. *Expenses: Tuition:* Full-time $14,724; part-time $818 per credit. *Required fees:* $692. Tuition and fees vary according to course load and program. *Financial support:* In 2013–14, 242 students received support, including 60 teaching assistantships (averaging $4,000 per year); career-related internships or fieldwork, institutionally sponsored loans, scholarships/grants, health care benefits, and unspecified assistantships also available. Financial award application deadline: 2/2. *Faculty research:* Cancer research (targeted therapy, mechanisms of leukemogenesis, tumor cell extravasation and metastasis, cancer stem cells), stem cell research (regenerative medicine, drug discovery), genetic research (neurogenetics, hereditary cardiomyopathy, hemoglobinopathies, pharmacogenomics, proteomics), neuroscience research (pain, neurodegenerative disorder), metabolism (inflammation and metabolism, metabolic disorder, diabetes mellitus), vascular and renal biology, signal transduction. *Total annual research expenditures:* $2.6 million. *Unit head:* Dr. Mohamed Sayegh, Dean, 961-1350000 Ext. 4700, Fax: 961-1744464, E-mail: msayegh@aub.edu.lb. *Application contact:* Dr. Salim Kanaan, Director, Admissions Office, 961-1-350000 Ext. 2594, Fax: 96-1-1750775, E-mail: sk00@aub.edu.lb.
Website: http://www.aub.edu.lb/fm/fm_home/Pages/index.aspx

Auburn University, College of Veterinary Medicine and Graduate School, Graduate Programs in Veterinary Medicine, Auburn University, AL 36849. Offers biomedical sciences (MS, PhD), including anatomy, physiology and pharmacology (MS), biomedical sciences (PhD), clinical sciences (MS), large animal surgery and medicine (MS), pathobiology (MS), radiology (MS), small animal surgery and medicine (MS); DVM/MS. Part-time programs available. *Faculty:* 100 full-time (41 women), 4 part-time/adjunct (1 woman). *Students:* 24 full-time (16 women), 38 part-time (25 women); includes 5 minority (1 Black or African American, non-Hispanic/Latino; 1 American Indian or Alaska Native, non-Hispanic/Latino; 2 Asian, non-Hispanic/Latino; 1 Hispanic/Latino), 22 international. Average age 30. 36 applicants, 44% accepted, 13 enrolled. In 2013, 12 master's, 8 doctorates awarded. *Degree requirements:* For doctorate, thesis/dissertation. *Entrance requirements:* For master's, GRE General Test; for doctorate, GRE General Test, GRE Subject Test. *Application deadline:* For fall admission, 7/7 for domestic students; for spring admission, 11/24 for domestic students. Applications are processed on a rolling basis. Application fee: $50 ($60 for international students). Electronic applications accepted. *Expenses:* Tuition, state resident: full-time $8262; part-time $459 per credit hour. Tuition, nonresident: full-time $24,786; part-time $1377 per credit hour. Tuition and fees vary according to degree level and program. *Financial support:* Research assistantships, teaching assistantships, and Federal Work-Study available. Support available to part-time students. Financial award application deadline: 3/15; financial award applicants required to submit FAFSA. *Unit head:* Dr. Calvin Johnson, Acting Dean, 334-844-2650. *Application contact:* Dr. George Flowers, Dean of the Graduate School, 334-844-2125.

Barry University, School of Podiatric Medicine, Program in Anatomy, Miami Shores, FL 33161-6695. Offers MS. *Entrance requirements:* For master's, GRE.

Boston University, College of Health and Rehabilitation Sciences: Sargent College, Department of Health Sciences, Programs in Human Physiology, Boston, MA 02215. Offers MS, PhD. *Faculty:* 10 full-time (9 women), 5 part-time/adjunct (2 women). *Students:* 7 full-time (6 women), 4 part-time (2 women); includes 5 minority (2 Black or African American, non-Hispanic/Latino; 2 Asian, non-Hispanic/Latino; 1 Hispanic/Latino). Average age 25. 40 applicants, 48% accepted, 6 enrolled. In 2013, 5 master's, 5 doctorates awarded. Terminal master's awarded for partial completion of doctoral program. *Degree requirements:* For master's, thesis or alternative; for doctorate, comprehensive exam, thesis/dissertation. *Entrance requirements:* For master's, GRE General Test, minimum GPA of 3.0; for doctorate, GRE General Test. Additional exam requirements/recommendations for international students: Required—TOEFL (minimum score 550 paper-based; 84 iBT). *Application deadline:* For fall admission, 1/15 priority date for domestic and international students; for spring admission, 10/1 for domestic and international students. Applications are processed on a rolling basis. Application fee: $80. Electronic applications accepted. *Expenses: Tuition:* Full-time $43,970; part-time $1374 per credit hour. *Required fees:* $60 per semester. Tuition and fees vary according to class time, course level and program. *Financial support:* In 2013–14, 1 fellowship with full tuition reimbursement (averaging $20,000 per year), 1 research assistantship with full tuition reimbursement (averaging $18,000 per year) were awarded; teaching assistantships, career-related internships or fieldwork, Federal Work-Study, institutionally sponsored loans, scholarships/grants, and tuition waivers (partial) also available. Support available to part-time students. Financial award application deadline: 4/15; financial award applicants required to submit FAFSA. *Faculty research:* Skeletal muscle, neural systems, smooth muscle, muscular dystrophy. *Total annual research expenditures:* $1.3 million. *Unit head:* Dr. Kathleen Morgan, Chair, 617-353-2717, E-mail: kmorgan@bu.edu. *Application contact:* Sharon Sankey, Director, Student Services, 617-353-2713, Fax: 617-353-7500, E-mail: ssankey@bu.edu.

Boston University, School of Medicine, Division of Graduate Medical Sciences, Department of Anatomy and Neurobiology, Boston, MA 02118. Offers MA, PhD, MD/PhD. Part-time programs available. Terminal master's awarded for partial completion of doctoral program. *Degree requirements:* For master's, thesis; for doctorate, thesis/dissertation. *Application deadline:* For fall admission, 1/15 for domestic students; for spring admission, 10/15 for domestic students. *Expenses: Tuition:* Full-time $43,970; part-time $1374 per credit hour. *Required fees:* $60 per semester. Tuition and fees vary according to class time, course level and program. *Unit head:* Dr. Mark Moss, Chairman, 617-638-4200, Fax: 617-638-4216. *Application contact:* Patricia Jones, Financial Coordinator, 617-414-2315, E-mail: psterlin@bu.edu.
Website: http://www.bumc.bu.edu/anatneuro/

Case Western Reserve University, School of Medicine and School of Graduate Studies, Graduate Programs in Medicine, Department of Anatomy, Cleveland, OH 44106. Offers applied anatomy (MS); biological anthropology (MS); cellular biology (MS); MD/MS. Part-time programs available. *Degree requirements:* For master's, comprehensive exam, thesis (for some programs). *Entrance requirements:* For master's, GRE General Test. Additional exam requirements/recommendations for international students: Required—TOEFL. *Faculty research:* Hypoxia, cell injury, biochemical aberration occurrences in ischemic tissue, human functional morphology, evolutionary morphology.

Columbia University, College of Physicians and Surgeons, Department of Anatomy and Cell Biology, New York, NY 10032. Offers anatomy (M Phil, MA, PhD); anatomy and cell biology (PhD); MD/PhD. Only candidates for the PhD are admitted. Terminal master's awarded for partial completion of doctoral program. *Degree requirements:* For doctorate, thesis/dissertation, oral exam. *Entrance requirements:* For master's and doctorate, GRE General Test. Additional exam requirements/recommendations for international students: Required—TOEFL. *Faculty research:* Protein sorting, membrane biophysics, muscle energetics, neuroendocrinology, developmental biology, cytoskeleton, transcription factors.

Cornell University, Graduate School, Graduate Fields of Agriculture and Life Sciences, Field of Zoology and Wildlife Conservation, Ithaca, NY 14853-0001. Offers animal cytology (PhD); comparative and functional anatomy (PhD); developmental biology (PhD); ecology (PhD); histology (PhD); wildlife conservation (PhD). *Faculty:* 21 full-time (6 women). *Students:* 4 full-time (3 women), 1 part-time (0 women); includes 2 minority (1 Hispanic/Latino; 1 Two or more races, non-Hispanic/Latino), 1 international. Average age 26. 18 applicants, 6% accepted, 1 enrolled. In 2013, 1 doctorate awarded. *Degree requirements:* For doctorate, comprehensive exam, thesis/dissertation, 2 semesters of teaching experience. *Entrance requirements:* For doctorate, GRE General Test, GRE Subject Test (biology), 2 letters of recommendation. Additional exam requirements/recommendations for international students: Required—TOEFL (minimum score 550 paper-based; 77 iBT). *Application deadline:* For fall admission, 2/1 priority date for domestic students. Application fee: $95. Electronic applications accepted. *Financial support:* In 2013–14, 4 students received support, including 3 research assistantships with full tuition reimbursements available, 1 teaching assistantship with full tuition reimbursement available; fellowships with full tuition reimbursements available, institutionally sponsored loans, scholarships/grants, health care benefits, tuition waivers (full and partial), and unspecified assistantships also available. Financial award applicants required to submit FAFSA. *Faculty research:* Organismal biology, functional morphology, biomechanics, comparative vertebrate anatomy, comparative invertebrate anatomy, paleontology. *Unit head:* Director of Graduate Studies, 607-253-3276, Fax: 607-253-3756. *Application contact:* Graduate Field Assistant, 607-253-3276, Fax: 607-253-3756, E-mail: graduate_edcvm@cornell.edu.
Website: http://www.gradschool.cornell.edu/fields.php?id-65&a-2

Creighton University, School of Medicine and Graduate School, Graduate Programs in Medicine, Program in Clinical Anatomy, Omaha, NE 68178-0001. Offers MS. *Faculty:* 8 full-time (3 women). *Students:* 25 full-time (5 women); includes 1 minority (Asian, non-Hispanic/Latino). Average age 25. 45 applicants, 36% accepted, 14 enrolled. In 2013, 12 master's awarded. *Degree requirements:* For master's, comprehensive exam, thesis or alternative. *Entrance requirements:* For master's, GRE, MCAT or DAT. Additional exam requirements/recommendations for international students: Required—TOEFL. *Application deadline:* For spring admission, 4/15 for domestic and international students. Application fee: $50. Electronic applications accepted. *Expenses: Tuition:* Full-time $13,608; part-time $756 per credit hour. *Required fees:* $149 per semester. Tuition and fees vary according to course load, campus/location, program, reciprocity agreements and student's religious affiliation. *Financial support:* Fellowships, research assistantships, teaching assistantships, and tuition waivers (partial) available. *Faculty research:* Neural crest cell migration; ontogenetic and phylogenetic nervous system development; skeletal biology. *Unit head:* Dr. Deniz Yilmazer-Hanke, Director, 402-280-2965, Fax: 402-280-2690, E-mail: denizyilmazer-hanke@creighton.edu. *Application contact:* Katy Traver, Program Coordinator, 402-280-2542, Fax: 402-280-2670, E-mail: katy@creighton.edu.

Dalhousie University, Faculty of Graduate Studies and Faculty of Medicine, Graduate Programs in Medicine, Department of Anatomy and Neurobiology, Halifax, NS B3H 4R2, Canada. Offers M Sc, PhD. *Degree requirements:* For master's, thesis; for doctorate, thesis/dissertation. *Entrance requirements:* For master's and doctorate, GRE (recommended), minimum A- average. Additional exam requirements/recommendations for international students: Required—1 of 5 approved tests: TOEFL, IELTS, CANTEST, CAEL, Michigan English Language Assessment Battery. Electronic applications accepted. *Faculty research:* Neuroscience histology, cell biology, neuroendocrinology, evolutionary biology.

Des Moines University, College of Osteopathic Medicine, Program in Anatomy, Des Moines, IA 50312-4104. Offers MS.

Duke University, Graduate School, Department of Evolutionary Anthropology, Durham, NC 27708. Offers cellular and molecular biology (PhD); gross anatomy and physical anthropology (PhD), including comparative morphology of human and non-human primates, primate social behavior, vertebrate paleontology; neuroanatomy (PhD). *Faculty:* 12. *Students:* 16 full-time (9 women); includes 5 minority (2 Black or African American, non-Hispanic/Latino; 1 Asian, non-Hispanic/Latino; 2 Hispanic/Latino). 69 applicants, 6% accepted, 3 enrolled. In 2013, 1 degree awarded. *Median time to degree:* Of those who began their doctoral program in fall 2005, 87% received their degree in 8 years or less. *Degree requirements:* For doctorate, one foreign language, thesis/dissertation. *Entrance requirements:* For doctorate, GRE General Test. Additional exam requirements/recommendations for international students: Required—TOEFL (minimum score 577 paper-based; 90 iBT) or IELTS (minimum score 7). *Application deadline:* For fall admission, 12/8 priority date for domestic and international students. Application fee: $80. Electronic applications accepted. *Financial support:* Fellowships, teaching assistantships, and Federal Work-Study available. Financial award application deadline: 12/31. *Unit head:* Richard Kay, Director of Graduate Studies, 919-684-4124, Fax: 919-684-8542, E-mail: mlsquire@duke.edu. *Application contact:* Elizabeth Hutton, Director of Admissions, 919-684-3913, Fax: 919-684-2277, E-mail: grad-admissions@duke.edu.
Website: http://evolutionaryanthropology.duke.edu/

East Carolina University, Brody School of Medicine, Department of Anatomy and Cell Biology, Greenville, NC 27858-4353. Offers PhD. *Degree requirements:* For doctorate, comprehensive exam, thesis/dissertation. *Entrance requirements:* For doctorate, GRE General Test. Additional exam requirements/recommendations for international students: Required—TOEFL. *Application deadline:* For fall admission, 6/1 priority date for domestic students. Applications are processed on a rolling basis. Application fee: $50. *Expenses:* Tuition, state resident: full-time $4223. Tuition, nonresident: full-time $16,540. *Required fees:* $2184. *Financial support:* Fellowships with full tuition reimbursements and health care benefits available. Financial award application deadline: 6/1. *Faculty research:* Kinesin motors during slow matogensis, mitochondria and peroxisomes in obesity, ovarian innervation, tight junction function and regulation. *Unit head:* Dr. Cheryl Knudson, Chairman, 252-744-2852, Fax: 252-744-2850, E-mail: knudsonc@ecu.edu. *Application contact:* Dr. Ron Dudek, Senior Director of Graduate Studies, 252-744-2863, Fax: 252-744-2850, E-mail: dudekr@ecu.edu.
Website: http://www.ecu.edu/cs-dhs/anatomy/gradProg.cfm

East Tennessee State University, James H. Quillen College of Medicine, Department of Biomedical Sciences, Johnson City, TN 37614. Offers anatomy (PhD); biochemistry (PhD); microbiology (PhD); pharmaceutical sciences (PhD); pharmacology (PhD); physiology (PhD); quantitative biosciences (PhD). *Faculty:* 43 full-time (11 women), 1 (woman) part-time/adjunct. *Students:* 31 full-time (17 women), 4 part-time (1 woman); includes 6 minority (2 Black or African American, non-Hispanic/Latino; 3 Asian, non-Hispanic/Latino; 1 Hispanic/Latino), 9 international. Average age 29. 53 applicants, 17% accepted, 8 enrolled. In 2013, 6 doctorates awarded. *Degree requirements:* For doctorate, thesis/dissertation, comprehensive qualifying exam. *Entrance requirements:* For doctorate, GRE General Test, GRE Subject Test. Additional exam requirements/recommendations for international students: Required—TOEFL (minimum score 550 paper-based; 79 iBT). *Application deadline:* For fall admission, 3/15 priority date for domestic students, 3/1 priority date for international students. Application fee: $35 ($45 for international students). Electronic applications accepted. *Expenses:* Contact institution. *Financial support:* In 2013–14, 30 students received support, including 30 research assistantships with full tuition reimbursements available (averaging $19,000 per year); career-related internships or fieldwork, institutionally sponsored loans, scholarships/grants, and unspecified assistantships also available. Financial award application deadline: 7/1; financial award applicants required to submit FAFSA. *Faculty research:* Cardiovascular, infectious disease, neurosciences, cancer, immunology. *Unit head:* Dr. Mitchell E. Robinson, Associate Dean/Program Director, 423-439-2031, Fax: 423-439-2140, E-mail: robinson@etsu.edu. *Application contact:* Shella Bennett, Graduate Specialist, 423-439-4708, Fax: 423-439-5624, E-mail: bennetsg@etsu.edu.
Website: http://www.etsu.edu/com/dbms/

Georgia Regents University, The Graduate School, Program in Cellular Biology and Anatomy, Augusta, GA 30912. Offers MS, PhD. *Faculty:* 15 full-time (6 women), 3 part-time/adjunct (1 woman). *Students:* 12 full-time (9 women); includes 7 minority (1 Black or African American, non-Hispanic/Latino; 5 Asian, non-Hispanic/Latino; 1 Hispanic/Latino), 4 international. Average age 29. In 2013, 2 doctorates awarded. *Degree requirements:* For doctorate, comprehensive exam, thesis/dissertation. *Entrance requirements:* For doctorate, GRE General Test. Additional exam requirements/recommendations for international students: Required—TOEFL (minimum score 550 paper-based; 79 iBT). *Application deadline:* For fall admission, 1/15 for domestic and international students. Applications are processed on a rolling basis. Application fee: $50. *Financial support:* In 2013–14, 2 students received support, including 1 fellowship with partial tuition reimbursement available (averaging $26,000 per year), 9 research assistantships with partial tuition reimbursements available (averaging $23,000 per year); teaching assistantships with partial tuition reimbursements available, Federal Work-Study, institutionally sponsored loans, and scholarships/grants also available. Support available to part-time students. Financial award application deadline: 5/31; financial award applicants required to submit FAFSA. *Faculty research:* Eye disease, developmental biology, cell injury and death, stroke and neurotoxicity, diabetic complications. *Total annual research expenditures:* $2.8 million. *Unit head:* Dr. Sally S. Atherton, Chair and Professor, 706-721-3731, Fax: 706-721-6120, E-mail: satherton@georgiahealth.edu. *Application contact:* Dr. Patricia L. Cameron, Acting Vice Dean, 706-721-3279, E-mail: pcameron@georgiahealth.edu.
Website: http://www.gru.edu/mcg/cba/gradstudents/

Howard University, Graduate School, Department of Anatomy, Washington, DC 20059-0002. Offers MS, PhD. *Degree requirements:* For master's, comprehensive exam, thesis, teaching experience; for doctorate, comprehensive exam, thesis/dissertation, teaching experience. *Entrance requirements:* For master's and doctorate, GRE General Test, minimum GPA of 3.0. Additional exam requirements/recommendations for international students: Required—TOEFL (minimum score 550 paper-based). Electronic applications accepted. *Faculty research:* Neural control of function, mammalian evolution and paleontology, cellular differentiation, cellular and neuronal communication, development, cell biology, molecular biology, anatomy.

Indiana University–Purdue University Indianapolis, Indiana University School of Medicine, Department of Anatomy and Cell Biology, Indianapolis, IN 46202-2896. Offers MS, PhD, MD/PhD. *Faculty:* 14 full-time (1 woman). *Students:* 14 full-time (9 women); includes 2 minority (both Two or more races, non-Hispanic/Latino), 3 international. Average age 29. 16 applicants, 38% accepted, 4 enrolled. In 2013, 3 doctorates awarded. *Degree requirements:* For master's, thesis or alternative; for doctorate, thesis/dissertation. *Entrance requirements:* For master's and doctorate, GRE General Test. *Application deadline:* For fall admission, 1/15 priority date for domestic students. Application fee: $55 ($65 for international students). *Financial support:* Fellowships, research assistantships, teaching assistantships, Federal Work-Study, institutionally sponsored loans, tuition waivers (partial), and stipends available. Financial award application deadline: 2/15. *Faculty research:* Acoustic reflex control, osteoarthritis and bone disease, diabetes, kidney diseases, cellular and molecular neurobiology. *Unit head:* Dr. Kathryn Jones, Chair, 317-274-7495, E-mail: kjjones1@iupui.edu. *Application contact:* Dr. James Williams, Graduate Adviser, 317-274-3423, Fax: 317-278-2040, E-mail: williams@anatomy.iupui.edu.
Website: http://anatomy.iupui.edu/

Johns Hopkins University, School of Medicine, Graduate Programs in Medicine, Center for Functional Anatomy and Evolution, Baltimore, MD 21218-2699. Offers PhD. *Faculty:* 5 full-time (1 woman), 2 part-time/adjunct (1 woman). *Students:* 10 full-time (9 women), 3 international. Average age 26. 25 applicants, 16% accepted, 2 enrolled. In 2013, 3 doctorates awarded. *Degree requirements:* For doctorate, comprehensive exam, thesis/dissertation, oral exams. *Entrance requirements:* For doctorate, GRE. Additional exam requirements/recommendations for international students: Required—TOEFL. *Application deadline:* For fall admission, 1/10 for domestic and international students. Application fee: $85. *Financial support:* Fellowships, teaching assistantships, career-related internships or fieldwork, institutionally sponsored loans, health care benefits, and tuition waivers (full) available. *Faculty research:* Vertebrate evolution, functional anatomy, primate evolution, vertebrate paleobiology, vertebrate morphology. *Unit head:* Dr. Kenneth D. Rose, Director, 410-955-7172, Fax: 410-614-9030, E-mail: kdrose@jhmi.edu. *Application contact:* Catherine L. Will, Coordinator, Graduate Student Affairs, 410-614-3385, E-mail: grad_study@som.adm.jhu.edu.

Loma Linda University, School of Medicine, Department of Pathology and Human Anatomy, Loma Linda, CA 92350. Offers MS, PhD. Part-time programs available. Terminal master's awarded for partial completion of doctoral program. *Degree requirements:* For master's, thesis; for doctorate, 2 foreign languages, thesis/dissertation. *Entrance requirements:* For master's and doctorate, GRE General Test. Additional exam requirements/recommendations for international students: Required—TOEFL (minimum score 550 paper-based). *Faculty research:* Neuroendocrine system, histochemistry and image analysis, effect of age and diabetes on PNS, electron microscopy, histology.

Louisiana State University Health Sciences Center, School of Graduate Studies in New Orleans, Department of Cell Biology and Anatomy, New Orleans, LA 70112-2223. Offers cell biology and anatomy (MS, PhD), including cell biology, developmental biology, neurobiology and anatomy; MD/PhD. *Degree requirements:* For master's, comprehensive exam, thesis; for doctorate, comprehensive exam, thesis/dissertation. *Entrance requirements:* For master's and doctorate, GRE General Test, GRE Subject Test, minimum undergraduate GPA of 3.0. Additional exam requirements/recommendations for international students: Required—TOEFL. *Faculty research:* Visual system organization, neural development, plasticity of sensory systems, information processing through the nervous system, visuomotor integration.

Louisiana State University Health Sciences Center at Shreveport, Department of Cellular Biology and Anatomy, Shreveport, LA 71130-3932. Offers MS, PhD, MD/PhD. *Faculty:* 14 full-time (2 women). *Students:* 10 full-time (6 women); includes 4 minority (3 Black or African American, non-Hispanic/Latino; 1 Asian, non-Hispanic/Latino), 2 international. Average age 28. 6 applicants, 17% accepted, 1 enrolled. In 2013, 2 doctorates awarded. Terminal master's awarded for partial completion of doctoral program. *Degree requirements:* For master's, thesis; for doctorate, thesis/dissertation. *Entrance requirements:* For master's and doctorate, GRE General Test. Additional exam requirements/recommendations for international students: Required—TOEFL. *Application deadline:* For fall admission, 5/1 priority date for domestic students. Applications are processed on a rolling basis. *Financial support:* In 2013–14, 9 students received support, including 10 research assistantships (averaging $24,000 per year); institutionally sponsored loans also available. Financial award application deadline: 5/1. *Faculty research:* Cancer biology, redox biology, neurosciences, immunobiology, cardiovascular sciences. *Unit head:* Dr. William Mayhan, Chairman, 318-675-5313. *Application contact:* Dr. Sumitra Miriyala, Graduate Recruiter, 318-675-6940, Fax: 318-675-5889, E-mail: smiriy@lsuhsc.edu.
Website: http://www.lsuhscshreveport.edu/CellularBiologyandAnatomy/AnatomyHome.aspx

Loyola University Chicago, Graduate School, Department of Cell Biology, Neurobiology and Anatomy, Chicago, IL 60660. Offers MS, PhD. Part-time programs available. *Faculty:* 16 full-time (6 women), 9 part-time/adjunct (4 women). *Students:* 16 full-time (6 women); includes 3 minority (2 Black or African American, non-Hispanic/Latino; 1 Hispanic/Latino), 1 international. Average age 27. 17 applicants, 24% accepted. In 2013, 1 master's, 6 doctorates awarded. Terminal master's awarded for partial completion of doctoral program. *Degree requirements:* For master's, thesis; for doctorate, comprehensive exam, thesis/dissertation. *Entrance requirements:* For master's, GRE General Test, minimum GPA of 3.0; for doctorate, GRE General Test, GRE Subject Test (biology), minimum GPA of 3.0. Additional exam requirements/recommendations for international students: Required—TOEFL (minimum score 600 paper-based). *Application deadline:* For fall admission, 5/1 priority date for domestic and international students. Applications are processed on a rolling basis. Application fee: $50. Electronic applications accepted. *Expenses: Tuition:* Full-time $16,740; part-time $930 per credit. *Required fees:* $135 per semester. *Financial support:* In 2013–14, 5 fellowships with full tuition reimbursements (averaging $23,000 per year), 5 research assistantships with full tuition reimbursements (averaging $23,000 per year) were awarded; Federal Work-Study and unspecified assistantships also available. Financial award application deadline: 5/1; financial award applicants required to submit FAFSA. *Faculty research:* Brain steroids, immunology, neuroregeneration, cytokines. *Total annual research expenditures:* $1 million. *Unit head:* Dr. Phong Le, Head, 708-216-3603, Fax: 708-216-3913, E-mail: ple@lumc.edu. *Application contact:* Ginny Hayes, Graduate Program Secretary, 708-216-3353, Fax: 708-216-3913, E-mail: vhayes@lumc.edu.

McGill University, Faculty of Graduate and Postdoctoral Studies, Faculty of Medicine, Department of Anatomy and Cell Biology, Montréal, QC H3A 2T5, Canada. Offers M Sc, PhD.

New York Academy of Art, Master of Fine Arts Program, New York, NY 10013-2911. Offers drawing (MFA), including anatomy, printmaking; painting (MFA), including anatomy, printmaking; sculpture (MFA), including anatomy, printmaking. *Accreditation:* NASAD. *Degree requirements:* For master's, thesis. *Entrance requirements:* For master's, slide portfolio, two letters of recommendation, essay, official undergraduate transcripts. Additional exam requirements/recommendations for international students: Required—TOEFL, IELTS. Application fee is waived when completed online.

New York Chiropractic College, Program in Clinical Anatomy, Seneca Falls, NY 13148-0800. Offers MS. *Degree requirements:* For master's, thesis. *Entrance requirements:* For master's, minimum GPA of 3.0, DC, bachelor's degree or equivalent. *Application deadline:* Applications are processed on a rolling basis. Application fee: $0. Electronic applications accepted. *Financial support:* Fellowships with full tuition reimbursements available. Financial award applicants required to submit FAFSA. *Faculty research:* Bone histology, biomechanics, craniofacial growth and anatomy, skeletal morphology. *Unit head:* Dr. Jennette J. Ball, Director, 315-568-3292, E-mail: jball@nycc.edu. *Application contact:* Dr. Jennette J. Ball, Director, 315-568-3292, E-mail: jball@nycc.edu.
Website: http://www.nycc.edu/AcademicPrograms_MSCAprogram.htm

New York Chiropractic College, Program in Human Anatomy and Physiology Instruction, Seneca Falls, NY 13148-0800. Offers MS. Postbaccalaureate distance learning degree programs offered. *Financial support:* Applicants required to submit FAFSA. *Unit head:* Dr. Robert A. Crocker, Director, 516-796-4800, E-mail: rcrocker@nycc.edu. *Application contact:* Kimberly McCrea, Assistant Director of Admissions for Online Programs, 717-387-3146, E-mail: kmccrea@nycc.edu.
Website: http://www.nycc.edu/AcademicPrograms_MSHAPIprogram.htm

New York Medical College, Graduate School of Basic Medical Sciences, Cell Biology and Anatomy Master's Program, Valhalla, NY 10595-1691. Offers MS, PhD, MD/PhD. Part-time and evening/weekend programs available. *Faculty:* 16 full-time (2 women), 2 part-time/adjunct (1 woman). *Students:* 2 full-time (both women); includes 1 minority (Asian, non-Hispanic/Latino). Average age 25. 5 applicants, 100% accepted, 1 enrolled. Terminal master's awarded for partial completion of doctoral program. *Degree requirements:* For master's, thesis; for doctorate, comprehensive exam, thesis/dissertation. *Entrance requirements:* For master's, GRE General Test, MCAT, or DAT. Additional exam requirements/recommendations for international students: Required—TOEFL. *Application deadline:* For fall admission, 7/1 priority date for domestic students, 5/1 priority date for international students; for spring admission, 12/1 for domestic students, 10/1 for international students. Applications are processed on a rolling basis.

Application fee: $75 ($100 for international students). Electronic applications accepted. *Expenses: Tuition:* Full-time $49,170; part-time $910 per credit. Tuition and fees vary according to program. *Financial support:* Federal Work-Study and scholarships/grants available. Support available to part-time students. Financial award applicants required to submit FAFSA. *Faculty research:* Mechanisms of growth control in skeletal muscle, cartilage differentiation, cytoskeletal functions, signal transduction pathways, neuronal development and plasticity. *Unit head:* Dr. Victor Fried, Program Director, 914-594-4005, Fax: 914-594-4944, E-mail: victor_fried@nymc.edu. *Application contact:* Valerie Romeo-Messana, Director of Admissions, 914-594-4110, Fax: 914-594-4944, E-mail: v_romeomessana@nymc.edu.

New York Medical College, Graduate School of Basic Medical Sciences, Integrated PhD Program, Valhalla, NY 10595-1691. Offers biochemistry and molecular biology (PhD); cell biology and anatomy (PhD); microbiology and immunology (PhD); pathology (PhD); pharmacology (PhD); physiology (PhD). *Faculty:* 91 full-time (16 women), 5 part-time/adjunct (2 women). *Students:* 31 full-time (21 women); includes 17 minority (4 Black or African American, non-Hispanic/Latino; 11 Asian, non-Hispanic/Latino; 2 Hispanic/Latino). Average age 27. 56 applicants, 36% accepted, 9 enrolled. In 2013, 17 doctorates awarded. *Degree requirements:* For doctorate, comprehensive exam, thesis/dissertation. *Entrance requirements:* For doctorate, GRE General Test. Additional exam requirements/recommendations for international students: Required—TOEFL. *Application deadline:* For fall admission, 1/1 priority date for domestic and international students. Applications are processed on a rolling basis. Application fee: $75 ($100 for international students). Electronic applications accepted. *Expenses: Tuition:* Full-time $49,170; part-time $910 per credit. Tuition and fees vary according to program. *Financial support:* In 2013–14, fellowships with full tuition reimbursements (averaging $25,500 per year), research assistantships with full tuition reimbursements (averaging $25,500 per year) were awarded; Federal Work-Study, scholarships/grants, traineeships, health care benefits, and tuition waivers (full) also available. Financial award applicants required to submit FAFSA. *Faculty research:* Cardiovascular sciences, infectious diseases, neuroscience, cancer and cell signaling. *Unit head:* Dr. Francis L. Belloni, Dean, 914-594-4110, Fax: 914-594-4944, E-mail: francis_belloni@nymc.edu. *Application contact:* Valerie Romeo-Messana, Director of Admissions, 914-594-4110, Fax: 914-594-4944, E-mail: v_romeomessana@nymc.edu.

The Ohio State University, College of Medicine, School of Health and Rehabilitation Sciences, Program in Anatomy, Columbus, OH 43210. Offers MS, PhD. *Faculty:* 6. *Students:* 25 full-time (16 women), 4 part-time (2 women); includes 4 minority (1 Asian, non-Hispanic/Latino; 3 Two or more races, non-Hispanic/Latino), 3 international. Average age 28. In 2013, 6 master's awarded. Terminal master's awarded for partial completion of doctoral program. *Degree requirements:* For doctorate, thesis/dissertation. *Entrance requirements:* For master's and doctorate, GRE General Test. Additional exam requirements/recommendations for international students: Required—TOEFL (minimum score 600 paper-based; 100 iBT), Michigan English Language Assessment Battery (minimum score 86); Recommended—IELTS (minimum score 8). *Application deadline:* For fall admission, 12/13 priority date for domestic students, 11/30 priority date for international students; for spring admission, 10/1 for domestic and international students. Applications are processed on a rolling basis. Application fee: $60 ($70 for international students). Electronic applications accepted. *Financial support:* In 2013–14, 2 students received support. Fellowships with tuition reimbursements available, research assistantships with tuition reimbursements available, teaching assistantships with tuition reimbursements available, and Federal Work-Study available. Financial award application deadline: 1/10. *Faculty research:* Cell biology, biomechanical trauma, computer-assisted instruction. *Total annual research expenditures:* $407,610. *Unit head:* Dr. Amanda Agnew, Graduate Studies Committee Chair, 614-366-2005, Fax: 614-292-7659, E-mail: agnew.17@osu.edu. *Application contact:* Graduate Admissions, 614-292-9444, Fax: 614-292-3895, E-mail: gradadmissions@osu.edu.
Website: http://medicine.osu.edu/hrs/anatomy

Palmer College of Chiropractic, Division of Graduate Studies, Davenport, IA 52803-5287. Offers clinical research (MS). *Degree requirements:* For master's, 2 mentored practicum projects. *Entrance requirements:* For master's, GRE General Test, minimum GPA of 2.5, bachelor's and doctoral-level health professions degrees. Additional exam requirements/recommendations for international students: Required—TOEFL. Electronic applications accepted. *Expenses:* Contact institution. *Faculty research:* Chiropractic clinical research.

Penn State Hershey Medical Center, College of Medicine, Graduate School Programs in the Biomedical Sciences, Program in Anatomy, Hershey, PA 17033. Offers MS, PhD. *Students:* 14 full-time (11 women); includes 1 minority (Hispanic/Latino), 1 international. 21 applicants, 24% accepted, 5 enrolled. In 2013, 2 master's, 1 doctorate awarded. Terminal master's awarded for partial completion of doctoral program. *Degree requirements:* For master's, thesis or alternative; for doctorate, comprehensive exam, thesis/dissertation. *Entrance requirements:* For master's and doctorate, GRE General Test or MCAT, minimum GPA of 3.0. Additional exam requirements/recommendations for international students: Required—TOEFL (minimum score 500 paper-based). *Application deadline:* For fall admission, 1/31 priority date for domestic students, 2/1 priority date for international students. Applications are processed on a rolling basis. Application fee: $65. Electronic applications accepted. *Financial support:* In 2013–14, research assistantships with full tuition reimbursements (averaging $24,544 per year) were awarded; fellowships with full tuition reimbursements, scholarships/grants, health care benefits, and unspecified assistantships also available. Financial award applicants required to submit FAFSA. *Faculty research:* Developmental biology, stem cell, cancer-basic science and clinical application, wound healing, angiogenesis. *Unit head:* Dr. Patricia J. McLaughlin, Program Director, 717-531-0003, Fax: 717-531-0306, E-mail: anat-grad-hmc@psu.edu. *Application contact:* Dee Clarke, Program Assistant, 717-531-0003, Fax: 717-531-0306, E-mail: anat-grad-hmc@psu.edu.
Website: http://www.pennstatehershey.org/web/anatomy/home

Purdue University, School of Veterinary Medicine and Graduate School, Graduate Programs in Veterinary Medicine, Department of Basic Medical Sciences, West Lafayette, IN 47907. Offers anatomy (MS, PhD); pharmacology (MS, PhD); physiology (MS, PhD). Part-time programs available. Terminal master's awarded for partial completion of doctoral program. *Degree requirements:* For master's, thesis; for doctorate, thesis/dissertation. *Entrance requirements:* For master's and doctorate, GRE General Test. Additional exam requirements/recommendations for international students: Required—TOEFL. Electronic applications accepted. *Faculty research:* Development and regeneration, tissue injury and shock, biomedical engineering, ovarian function, bone and cartilage biology, cell and molecular biology.

Queen's University at Kingston, School of Graduate Studies, Faculty of Health Sciences, Department of Anatomy and Cell Biology, Kingston, ON K7L 3N6, Canada. Offers biology of reproduction (M Sc, PhD); cancer (M Sc, PhD); cardiovascular pathophysiology (M Sc, PhD); cell and molecular biology (M Sc, PhD); drug metabolism (M Sc, PhD); endocrinology (M Sc, PhD); motor control (M Sc, PhD); neural regeneration (M Sc, PhD); neurophysiology (M Sc, PhD). Part-time programs available. *Degree requirements:* For master's, thesis; for doctorate, one foreign language, comprehensive exam, thesis/dissertation. *Entrance requirements:* Additional exam requirements/recommendations for international students: Required—TOEFL. Electronic applications accepted. *Faculty research:* Human kinetics, neuroscience, reproductive biology, cardiovascular.

Rosalind Franklin University of Medicine and Science, School of Graduate and Postdoctoral Studies - Interdisciplinary Graduate Program in Biomedical Sciences, Department of Cell Biology and Anatomy, North Chicago, IL 60064-3095. Offers MS, PhD, MD/PhD. Terminal master's awarded for partial completion of doctoral program. *Degree requirements:* For master's, comprehensive exam, thesis, qualifying exam; for doctorate, comprehensive exam, thesis/dissertation, original research project. *Entrance requirements:* For master's and doctorate, GRE General Test, minimum GPA of 3.0. Additional exam requirements/recommendations for international students: Required—TOEFL, TWE. *Faculty research:* Neuroscience, molecular biology.

Rush University, Graduate College, Division of Anatomy and Cell Biology, Chicago, IL 60612-3832. Offers MS, PhD, MD/MS, MD/PhD. Terminal master's awarded for partial completion of doctoral program. *Degree requirements:* For master's, thesis; for doctorate, comprehensive exam, thesis/dissertation, preliminary exam, dissertation proposal. *Entrance requirements:* For master's, GRE General Test, minimum GPA of 3.0, bachelor's degree in biology or chemistry (preferred), interview; for doctorate, GRE General Test, minimum GPA of 3.0, interview. Additional exam requirements/recommendations for international students: Required—TOEFL. Electronic applications accepted. *Faculty research:* Incontinence following vaginal distension, knee replacement, biomimetric materials, injured spinal motoneurons, implant fixation.

Saint Louis University, Graduate Education and School of Medicine, Graduate Program in Biomedical Sciences and Graduate Education, Center for Anatomical Science and Education, St. Louis, MO 63103-2097. Offers anatomy (MS-R, PhD). *Degree requirements:* For master's, comprehensive exam, thesis; for doctorate, comprehensive exam, thesis/dissertation, departmental qualifying exams. *Entrance requirements:* For master's, GRE General Test, letters of recommendation, resume; for doctorate, GRE General Test, letters of recommendation, resumé, goal statement, transcripts. Additional exam requirements/recommendations for international students: Required—TOEFL (minimum score 525 paper-based). *Faculty research:* Neurodegenerative diseases, cerebellar cortical circuitry, neurogenesis, evolutionary anatomy.

State University of New York Upstate Medical University, College of Graduate Studies, Program in Cell and Developmental Biology, Syracuse, NY 13210-2334. Offers anatomy (MS, PhD); MD/PhD. Terminal master's awarded for partial completion of doctoral program. *Degree requirements:* For master's, thesis; for doctorate, comprehensive exam, thesis/dissertation. *Entrance requirements:* For master's, GRE General Test, interview; for doctorate, GRE General Test, telephone interview. Additional exam requirements/recommendations for international students: Required—TOEFL. Electronic applications accepted. *Faculty research:* Cancer, disorders of the nervous system, infectious diseases, diabetes/metabolic disorders/cardiovascular diseases.

Stony Brook University, State University of New York, Stony Brook University Medical Center, Health Sciences Center, School of Medicine and Graduate School, Graduate Programs in Medicine, Department of Anatomical Sciences, Stony Brook, NY 11794. Offers PhD. *Faculty:* 15 full-time (5 women). *Students:* 8 full-time (4 women), 1 (woman) part-time, 1 international. Average age 30. 15 applicants, 13% accepted, 2 enrolled. *Degree requirements:* For doctorate, comprehensive exam, thesis/dissertation. *Entrance requirements:* For doctorate, GRE General Test, GRE Subject Test, BA in life sciences, minimum GPA of 3.0. Additional exam requirements/recommendations for international students: Required—TOEFL. *Application deadline:* For fall admission, 1/15 for domestic students; for spring admission, 10/1 for domestic students. Application fee: $100. *Expenses:* Tuition, state resident: full-time $9870; part-time $411 per credit. Tuition, nonresident: full-time $18,350; part-time $765 per credit. *Financial support:* In 2013–14, 3 fellowships, 9 research assistantships were awarded; teaching assistantships and Federal Work-Study also available. Financial award application deadline: 3/15. *Faculty research:* Biological membranes, biomechanics of locomotion, systematics and evolutionary history of primates. *Total annual research expenditures:* $618,725. *Unit head:* Dr. William Jungers, Chair, 631-444-3114, Fax: 631-444-3947, E-mail: william.jungers@stonybrook.edu. *Application contact:* Christine Johnson, Coordinator, 631-444-3114, Fax: 631-444-3947, E-mail: christine.johnson@stonybrook.edu.
Website: http://www.anat.stonybrook.edu/

Universidad Central del Caribe, School of Medicine, Program in Biomedical Sciences, Bayamón, PR 00960-6032. Offers anatomy and cell biology (MA, MS); biochemistry (MS); biomedical sciences (MA); cellular and molecular biology (PhD); microbiology and immunology (MA, MS); pharmacology (MS); physiology (MS).

Universidad de Ciencias Medicas, Graduate Programs, San Jose, Costa Rica. Offers dermatology (SP); family health (MS); health service center administration (MHA); human anatomy (MS); medical and surgery (MD); occupational medicine (MS); pharmacy (Pharm D). Part-time programs available. *Degree requirements:* For master's, thesis; for doctorate and SP, comprehensive exam. *Entrance requirements:* For master's, MD or bachelor's degree; for doctorate, admissions test; for SP, admissions test, MD.

Université Laval, Faculty of Medicine, Post-Professional Programs in Medical Studies, Québec, QC G1K 7P4, Canada. Offers anatomy–pathology (DESS); anesthesiology (DESS); cardiology (DESS); care of older people (Diploma); clinical research (DESS); community health (DESS); dermatology (DESS); diagnostic radiology (DESS); emergency medicine (Diploma); family medicine (DESS); general surgery (DESS); geriatrics (DESS); hematology (DESS); internal medicine (DESS); maternal and fetal medicine (Diploma); medical biochemistry (DESS); medical microbiology and infectious diseases (DESS); medical oncology (DESS); nephrology (DESS); neurology (DESS); neurosurgery (DESS); obstetrics and gynecology (DESS); ophthalmology (DESS); orthopedic surgery (DESS); oto-rhino-laryngology (DESS); palliative medicine (Diploma); pediatrics (DESS); plastic surgery (DESS); psychiatry (DESS); pulmonary medicine (DESS); radiology–oncology (DESS); thoracic surgery (DESS); urology (DESS). *Degree requirements:* For other advanced degree, comprehensive exam. *Entrance requirements:* For degree, knowledge of French. Electronic applications accepted.

University at Buffalo, the State University of New York, Graduate School, School of Medicine and Biomedical Sciences, Graduate Programs in Medicine and Biomedical Sciences, Department of Pathology and Anatomical Sciences, Buffalo, NY 14214. Offers anatomical sciences (MA, PhD); pathology (MA, PhD). Part-time programs available. *Faculty:* 16 full-time (5 women). *Students:* 6 full-time (1 woman). Average age 29. 18 applicants, 17% accepted, 3 enrolled. In 2013, 2 master's, 2 doctorates awarded. *Degree requirements:* For master's, thesis; for doctorate, comprehensive exam, thesis/dissertation. *Entrance requirements:* For master's and doctorate, GRE, MCAT, or DAT, 3 letters of recommendation. Additional exam requirements/recommendations for international students: Required—TOEFL (minimum score 600 paper-based; 100 iBT). *Application deadline:* For fall admission, 3/1 priority date for domestic and international students. Application fee: $75. *Financial support:* In 2013–14, 2 students received

support, including 1 research assistantship with full tuition reimbursement available (averaging $24,900 per year), 1 teaching assistantship with full tuition reimbursement available (averaging $24,900 per year); health care benefits also available. Financial award application deadline: 2/1; financial award applicants required to submit FAFSA. *Faculty research:* Immunopathology-immunobiology, experimental hypertension, neuromuscular disease, molecular pathology, cell motility and cytoskeleton. *Unit head:* Dr. John E. Tomaszewski, Department Chair, 716-829-2846, Fax: 716-829-2911, E-mail: johntoma@buffalo.edu. *Application contact:* Graduate Program Coordinator, 716-829-2846, Fax: 716-829-2911, E-mail: ubpathad@buffalo.edu.
Website: http://wings.buffalo.edu/smbs/path/

University of California, Irvine, School of Medicine and School of Biological Sciences, Department of Anatomy and Neurobiology, Irvine, CA 92697. Offers biological sciences (MS, PhD); MD/PhD. *Faculty:* 26 full-time (13 women), 2 part-time/adjunct (1 woman). *Students:* 26 full-time (13 women), 2 part-time (1 woman); includes 10 minority (9 Asian, non-Hispanic/Latino; 1 Hispanic/Latino), 4 international. Average age 27. In 2013, 1 master's, 7 doctorates awarded. *Degree requirements:* For doctorate, thesis/dissertation. *Entrance requirements:* For master's and doctorate, GRE General Test, GRE Subject Test. Additional exam requirements/recommendations for international students: Required—TOEFL (minimum score 550 paper-based). *Application deadline:* For fall admission, 1/15 priority date for domestic students, 1/15 for international students. Applications are processed on a rolling basis. Application fee: $80 ($100 for international students). Electronic applications accepted. *Financial support:* Fellowships, research assistantships with full tuition reimbursements, teaching assistantships, institutionally sponsored loans, traineeships, health care benefits, and unspecified assistantships available. Financial award application deadline: 3/1; financial award applicants required to submit FAFSA. *Faculty research:* Neurotransmitter immunocytochemistry, intracellular physiology, molecular neurobiology, forebrain organization and development, structure and function of sensory and motor systems. *Unit head:* Prof. Ivan Soltesz, Professor and Chair, 949-824-3957, Fax: 949-824-9860, E-mail: isoltesz@uci.edu. *Application contact:* Sara Johnson, Chief Administrative Officer, 949-824-6340, Fax: 949-824-8549, E-mail: sara.johnson@uci.edu.

University of California, Los Angeles, David Geffen School of Medicine and Graduate Division, Graduate Programs in Medicine, Department of Neurobiology, Los Angeles, CA 90095. Offers MS, PhD. Terminal master's awarded for partial completion of doctoral program. *Degree requirements:* For master's, comprehensive exam; for doctorate, thesis/dissertation, oral and written qualifying exams; 2 quarters of teaching experience. *Entrance requirements:* For doctorate, GRE General Test; GRE Subject Test, bachelor's degree; minimum undergraduate GPA of 3.0 (or its equivalent if letter grade system not used). Additional exam requirements/recommendations for international students: Required—TOEFL. Electronic applications accepted.

University of Chicago, Division of Biological Sciences, Darwinian Sciences Cluster: Ecological, Integrative and Evolutionary Biology, Department of Organismal Biology and Anatomy, Chicago, IL 60637-1513. Offers integrative biology (PhD). *Degree requirements:* For doctorate, thesis/dissertation, ethics class, 2 teaching assistantships. *Entrance requirements:* For doctorate, GRE General Test. Additional exam requirements/recommendations for international students: Required—TOEFL (minimum score 600 paper-based; 104 iBT), IELTS (minimum score 7). Electronic applications accepted. *Faculty research:* Ecological physiology, evolution of fossil reptiles, vertebrate paleontology.

University of Colorado Denver, School of Medicine, Program in Cell Biology, Stem Cells, and Developmental Biology, Aurora, CO 80045. Offers cell biology, stem cells, and developmental biology (PhD); modern human anatomy (MS). *Students:* 30 full-time (16 women), 1 part-time (0 women); includes 3 minority (all Hispanic/Latino), 5 international. Average age 28. 33 applicants, 15% accepted, 5 enrolled. In 2013, 2 doctorates awarded. *Degree requirements:* For doctorate, comprehensive exam, thesis/dissertation, at least 30 credit hours of coursework and 30 credit hours of thesis research; laboratory rotations. *Entrance requirements:* For doctorate, GRE, minimum GPA of 3.0; 3 letters of reference; prerequisite coursework in organic chemistry, biology, biochemistry, physics and calculus; research experience (highly recommended). Additional exam requirements/recommendations for international students: Required—TOEFL (minimum score 550 paper-based; 80 iBT). *Application deadline:* For fall admission, 12/1 for domestic students, 11/1 priority date for international students. Application fee: $50 ($75 for international students). Electronic applications accepted. *Expenses:* Contact institution. *Financial support:* In 2013–14, 31 students received support. Fellowships, research assistantships, teaching assistantships, Federal Work-Study, institutionally sponsored loans, scholarships/grants, traineeships, health care benefits, and tuition waivers (full) available. Financial award application deadline: 3/15; financial award applicants required to submit FAFSA. *Faculty research:* Development and repair of the vertebrate nervous system; molecular, genetic and developmental mechanisms involved in the patterning of the early spinal cord (neural plate) during vertebrate embryogenesis; structural analysis of protein glycosylation using NMR and mass spectrometry; small RNAs and post-transcriptional gene regulation during nematode gametogenesis and early development; diabetes-mediated changes in cardiovascular gene expression and functional exercise capacity. *Total annual research expenditures:* $5.7 million. *Unit head:* Dr. Wendy Macklin, Department Chair, 303-724-3426, E-mail: wendy.macklin@ucdenver.edu. *Application contact:* Kenton Owsley, Program Administrator, 303-724-3468, Fax: 303-724-3420, E-mail: kenton.owsley@ucdenver.edu.
Website: http://www.ucdenver.edu/academics/colleges/medicalschool/programs/CSD/Pages/CSD.aspx

University of Georgia, College of Veterinary Medicine, Department of Veterinary Anatomy and Radiology, Athens, GA 30602. Offers veterinary anatomy (MS). *Degree requirements:* For master's, thesis. *Entrance requirements:* For master's, GRE General Test. Electronic applications accepted.

University of Guelph, Ontario Veterinary College and Graduate Studies, Graduate Programs in Veterinary Sciences, Department of Biomedical Sciences, Guelph, ON N1G 2W1, Canada. Offers morphology (M Sc, DV Sc, PhD); neuroscience (M Sc, DV Sc, PhD); pharmacology (M Sc, DV Sc, PhD); physiology (M Sc, DV Sc, PhD); toxicology (M Sc, DV Sc, PhD). Part-time programs available. *Degree requirements:* For master's, thesis; for doctorate, comprehensive exam, thesis/dissertation. *Entrance requirements:* For master's, honors B Sc, minimum 75% average in last 20 courses; for doctorate, M Sc with thesis from accredited institution. Additional exam requirements/recommendations for international students: Required—TOEFL (minimum score 550 paper-based; 89 iBT). Electronic applications accepted. *Faculty research:* Cellular morphology; endocrine, vascular and reproductive physiology; clinical pharmacology; veterinary toxicology; developmental biology, neuroscience.

University of Illinois at Chicago, College of Medicine and Graduate College, Graduate Programs in Medicine, Department of Anatomy and Cell Biology, Chicago, IL 60612. Offers MD/PhD. *Faculty:* 14 full-time (6 women), 11 part-time/adjunct (5 women). *Students:* 11 full-time (8 women); includes 2 minority (both Hispanic/Latino), 3 international. Average age 29. 17 applicants, 6% accepted. *Entrance requirements:* Additional exam requirements/recommendations for international students: Required—TOEFL (minimum score 550 paper-based). *Application deadline:* For fall admission, 5/15 for domestic students, 2/15 for international students. Applications are processed on a rolling basis. Application fee: $50 ($60 for international students). Electronic applications accepted. *Expenses:* Tuition, state resident: full-time $11,066; part-time $3689 per term. Tuition, nonresident: full-time $23,064; part-time $7688 per term. *Required fees:* $3004; $1190 per term. Tuition and fees vary according to course level and program. *Financial support:* Research or teaching assistantships with stipend of $24,000 per year, plus a tuition waiver available. *Faculty research:* Synapses, axonal transport, neurodegenerative diseases. *Total annual research expenditures:* $5.1 million. *Unit head:* Scott T. Brady, Head, 312-996-3313. *Application contact:* Dr. Ernesto R. Bongarzone, Associate Professor/Director of Graduate Studies, 312-996-6791, Fax: 312-413-0354, E-mail: ebongarz@uic.edu.
Website: http://www.anatomy.uic.edu/

The University of Iowa, Roy J. and Lucille A. Carver College of Medicine and Graduate College, Biosciences Program, Iowa City, IA 52242-1316. Offers anatomy and cell biology (PhD); biochemistry (PhD); biology (PhD); biomedical engineering (PhD); chemistry (PhD); free radical and radiation biology (PhD); genetics (PhD); human toxicology (PhD); immunology (PhD); microbiology (PhD); molecular and cellular biology (PhD); molecular physiology and biophysics (PhD); neuroscience (PhD); pharmacology (PhD); physical therapy and rehabilitation science (PhD); rehabilitation science (PhD); speech and hearing (PhD). *Faculty:* 332 full-time. *Students:* 8 full-time (3 women); includes 2 minority (1 Black or African American, non-Hispanic/Latino; 1 Asian, non-Hispanic/Latino), 1 international. 200 applicants. *Degree requirements:* For doctorate, thesis/dissertation. *Entrance requirements:* For doctorate, GRE General Test, minimum GPA of 3.0. Additional exam requirements/recommendations for international students: Required—TOEFL (minimum score 600 paper-based; 100 iBT). *Application deadline:* For fall admission, 1/1 priority date for domestic and international students. Applications are processed on a rolling basis. Application fee: $60 ($100 for international students). Electronic applications accepted. *Expenses:* Contact institution. *Financial support:* In 2013–14, 8 students received support, including 8 research assistantships with full tuition reimbursements available (averaging $26,000 per year); fellowships, teaching assistantships, health care benefits, and unspecified assistantships also available. *Unit head:* Dr. Douglas Spitz, Director, 319-335-8001, E-mail: douglas-spitz@uiowa.edu. *Application contact:* Jodi Graff, Director, Admissions and First-Year Experience, 319-335-8306, E-mail: biosciences-admissions@uiowa.edu.
Website: http://www.medicine.uiowa.edu/biosciences/

The University of Iowa, Roy J. and Lucille A. Carver College of Medicine and Graduate College, Graduate Programs in Medicine, Department of Anatomy and Cell Biology, Iowa City, IA 52242-1316. Offers PhD. *Faculty:* 20 full-time (3 women). *Students:* 17 full-time (6 women); includes 7 minority (2 Black or African American, non-Hispanic/Latino; 1 American Indian or Alaska Native, non-Hispanic/Latino; 4 Asian, non-Hispanic/Latino), 1 international. Average age 28. 116 applicants. In 2013, 4 doctorates awarded. *Degree requirements:* For doctorate, comprehensive exam, thesis/dissertation. *Entrance requirements:* For doctorate, GRE General Test, minimum GPA of 3.0. Additional exam requirements/recommendations for international students: Required—TOEFL (minimum score 600 paper-based; 100 iBT). *Application deadline:* For fall admission, 1/15 priority date for domestic and international students. Applications are processed on a rolling basis. Application fee: $60 ($100 for international students). Electronic applications accepted. *Financial support:* In 2013–14, 17 students received support, including fellowships with full tuition reimbursements available (averaging $26,000 per year), 17 research assistantships with full tuition reimbursements available (averaging $26,000 per year), teaching assistantships with full tuition reimbursements available (averaging $26,000 per year); institutionally sponsored loans, scholarships/grants, and health care benefits also available. Financial award application deadline: 3/1. *Faculty research:* Biology of differentiation and transformation, developmental and vascular cell biology, neurobiology. *Total annual research expenditures:* $6.6 million. *Unit head:* Dr. John F. Engelhardt, Professor/Chair/Department Executive Officer, 319-335-7744, Fax: 319-335-7770, E-mail: john-engelhardt@uiowa.edu. *Application contact:* Julie A. Stark, Administrative Services Coordinator, 319-335-7744, Fax: 319-335-7770, E-mail: julie-stark@uiowa.edu.
Website: http://www.medicine.uiowa.edu/acb/

The University of Kansas, University of Kansas Medical Center, School of Medicine, Department of Anatomy and Cell Biology, Kansas City, KS 66160. Offers MA, PhD, MD/PhD. *Faculty:* 31. *Students:* 14 full-time (9 women); includes 1 minority (Hispanic/Latino), 5 international. Average age 27. In 2013, 4 doctorates awarded. Terminal master's awarded for partial completion of doctoral program. *Degree requirements:* For doctorate, comprehensive exam, thesis/dissertation. *Entrance requirements:* For doctorate, GRE. Additional exam requirements/recommendations for international students: Required—TOEFL. *Application deadline:* For fall admission, 1/15 priority date for domestic students. Applications are processed on a rolling basis. Application fee: $0. Electronic applications accepted. *Financial support:* Fellowships, research assistantships with full tuition reimbursements, teaching assistantships with full tuition reimbursements, institutionally sponsored loans, health care benefits, and unspecified assistantships available. Financial award application deadline: 3/1; financial award applicants required to submit FAFSA. *Faculty research:* Development of the synapse and neuromuscular junction, pain perception and diabetic neuropathies, cardiovascular and kidney development, reproductive immunology, post-fertilization signaling events. *Total annual research expenditures:* $8.7 million. *Unit head:* Dr. Dale R. Abrahamson, Chairman, 913-588-7000, Fax: 913-588-2710, E-mail: dabrahamson@kumc.edu. *Application contact:* Dr. Margaret Petroff, Associate Professor, 913-588-2781, Fax: 913-588-2710, E-mail: mpetroff@kumc.edu.
Website: http://www.kumc.edu/school-of-medicine/anatomy-and-cell-biology.html

University of Kentucky, Graduate School, Graduate School Programs from the College of Medicine, Department of Anatomy and Neurobiology, Lexington, KY 40506-0032. Offers PhD. *Degree requirements:* For doctorate, comprehensive exam, thesis/dissertation. *Entrance requirements:* For doctorate, GRE General Test, minimum undergraduate GPA of 2.75. Additional exam requirements/recommendations for international students: Required—TOEFL (minimum score 550 paper-based). Electronic applications accepted. *Faculty research:* Neuroendocrinology, developmental neurobiology, neurotrophic substances, neural plasticity and trauma, neurobiology of aging.

University of Louisville, School of Medicine, Department of Anatomical Sciences and Neurobiology, Louisville, KY 40292-0001. Offers MS, PhD, MD/PhD. *Students:* 25 full-time (16 women), 9 part-time (4 women); includes 9 minority (1 Black or African American, non-Hispanic/Latino; 3 Asian, non-Hispanic/Latino; 1 Hispanic/Latino; 4 Two or more races, non-Hispanic/Latino), 8 international. Average age 29. 39 applicants, 31% accepted, 9 enrolled. In 2013, 3 master's, 2 doctorates awarded. Terminal master's awarded for partial completion of doctoral program. *Degree requirements:* For master's, thesis; for doctorate, comprehensive exam, thesis/dissertation. *Entrance requirements:* For master's and doctorate, GRE General Test (minimum score of 1000 verbal and quantitative), minimum GPA of 3.0. Additional exam requirements/recommendations for international students: Required—TOEFL. *Application deadline:* For fall admission, 1/15 priority date for domestic students; for spring admission, 4/15 priority date for domestic and international students. Applications are processed on a rolling basis. Application fee: $60. Electronic applications accepted. *Expenses:* Tuition, state resident: full-time $10,788; part-time $599 per credit hour. Tuition, nonresident: full-time $22,446; part-time $1247 per credit hour. *Required fees:* $196. Tuition and fees vary according to program and reciprocity agreements. *Financial support:* Fellowships with full tuition reimbursements, research assistantships with full tuition reimbursements, health care benefits, and unspecified assistantships available. Financial award application deadline: 4/15. *Faculty research:* Human adult neural stem cells, development and plasticity of the nervous system, organization of the dorsal thalamus, electrophysiology/neuroanatomy of central neurons mediating control of reproductive and pelvic organs, normal neural mechanisms and plasticity following injury and/or chronic pain, differentiation and regeneration of motor neurons and oligodendrocytes. *Total annual research expenditures:* $4 million. *Unit head:* Dr. Fred J. Roisen, Chair, 502-852-5165, Fax: 502-852-6228, E-mail: fjrois01@gwise.louisville.edu. *Application contact:* Dr. Charles Hubscher, Director of Graduate Studies, 502-852-3058, Fax: 502-852-6228, E-mail: chhub01@louisville.edu.

University of Manitoba, Faculty of Medicine and Faculty of Graduate Studies, Graduate Programs in Medicine, Department of Human Anatomy and Cell Science, Winnipeg, MB R3T 2N2, Canada. Offers M Sc, PhD. *Degree requirements:* For master's, thesis; for doctorate, one foreign language, thesis/dissertation.

University of Mississippi Medical Center, School of Graduate Studies in the Health Sciences, Department of Anatomy, Jackson, MS 39216-4505. Offers clinical anatomy (MS, PhD); MD/PhD. *Students:* Average age 29. *Degree requirements:* For doctorate, comprehensive exam, thesis/dissertation, first authored publication. *Entrance requirements:* For doctorate, GRE General Test, minimum GPA of 3.0, personal statement. Additional exam requirements/recommendations for international students: Required—TOEFL. *Application deadline:* For fall admission, 1/31 priority date for domestic and international students. Application fee: $10. *Financial support:* In 2013–14, research assistantships (averaging $16,559 per year) were awarded. Financial award application deadline: 3/15. *Faculty research:* Systems neuroscience with emphasis on motor and sensory, cell biology with emphasis on cell-matrix interactions, development of cardiovascular system, biology of glial cells. *Unit head:* Michael Lehman, Chair, 601-984-1607, Fax: 601-984-1655, E-mail: mlehman@umc.edu.
Website: http://www.umc.edu/ClinAnatProgram/

University of Missouri, School of Medicine and Graduate School, Graduate Programs in Medicine, Department of Pathology and Anatomical Sciences, Columbia, MO 65211. Offers MS. *Faculty:* 22 full-time (8 women), 7 part-time/adjunct (3 women). *Students:* 2 applicants. *Entrance requirements:* For master's, GRE (minimum Verbal and Analytical score of 1250), letters of recommendation, minimum GPA of 3.5. Additional exam requirements/recommendations for international students: Required—TOEFL. Application fee: $55 ($75 for international students). Electronic applications accepted. *Faculty research:* Anatomic pathology, cancer biology, diabetes, integrative anatomy, laboratory medicine, neurobiology, tissue procurement core. *Unit head:* Dr. Lester Layfield, Chair, 573-882-8915, E-mail: layfieldl@missouri.edu. *Application contact:* Dr. Carol V. Ward, Director of Graduate Studies, 573-884-7303, E-mail: wardcv@missouri.edu.
Website: http://pathology-anatomy.missouri.edu/

University of Nebraska Medical Center, Department of Genetics, Cell Biology and Anatomy, Omaha, NE 68198-5805. Offers MS, PhD. Part-time programs available. Terminal master's awarded for partial completion of doctoral program. *Degree requirements:* For master's, comprehensive exam, thesis; for doctorate, comprehensive exam, thesis/dissertation. *Entrance requirements:* For master's and doctorate, GRE General Test. Additional exam requirements/recommendations for international students: Required—TOEFL (minimum score 550 paper-based). Electronic applications accepted. *Expenses: Required fees:* $300 per semester. Tuition and fees vary according to program. *Faculty research:* Hematology, immunology, developmental biology, genetics cancer biology, neuroscience.

University of North Dakota, Graduate School and Graduate School, Graduate Programs in Medicine, Department of Anatomy and Cell Biology, Grand Forks, ND 58202. Offers MS, PhD. *Degree requirements:* For master's, thesis, final exam; for doctorate, comprehensive exam, thesis/dissertation, final exam. *Entrance requirements:* For master's and doctorate, GRE General Test, minimum GPA of 3.0. Additional exam requirements/recommendations for international students: Required—TOEFL (minimum score 550 paper-based; 79 iBT), IELTS (minimum score 6.5). Electronic applications accepted. *Faculty research:* Coronary vessel, vasculogenesis, acellular glomerular and retinal microvessel membranes, ependymal cells, cardiac muscle.

University of North Texas Health Science Center at Fort Worth, Graduate School of Biomedical Sciences, Fort Worth, TX 76107-2699. Offers anatomy and cell biology (MS, PhD); biochemistry and molecular biology (MS, PhD); biomedical sciences (MS, PhD); biotechnology (MS); forensic genetics (MS); integrative physiology (MS, PhD); medical science (MS); microbiology and immunology (MS, PhD); pharmacology (MS, PhD); science education (MS); DO/MS; DO/PhD. Terminal master's awarded for partial completion of doctoral program. *Degree requirements:* For master's, thesis; for doctorate, thesis/dissertation. *Entrance requirements:* For master's and doctorate, GRE General Test. Additional exam requirements/recommendations for international students: Required—TOEFL. *Expenses:* Contact institution. *Faculty research:* Alzheimer's disease, aging, eye diseases, cancer, cardiovascular disease.

University of Prince Edward Island, Atlantic Veterinary College, Graduate Program in Veterinary Medicine, Charlottetown, PE C1A 4P3, Canada. Offers anatomy (M Sc, PhD); bacteriology (M Sc, PhD); clinical pharmacology (M Sc, PhD); clinical sciences (M Sc, PhD); epidemiology (M Sc, PhD), including reproduction; fish health (M Sc, PhD); food animal nutrition (M Sc, PhD); immunology (M Sc, PhD); microanatomy (M Sc, PhD); parasitology (M Sc, PhD); pathology (M Sc, PhD); pharmacology (M Sc, PhD); physiology (M Sc, PhD); toxicology (M Sc, PhD); veterinary science (M Vet Sc); virology (M Sc, PhD). Part-time programs available. *Degree requirements:* For master's, thesis; for doctorate, thesis/dissertation. *Entrance requirements:* For master's, DVM, B Sc honors degree, or equivalent; for doctorate, M Sc. Additional exam requirements/recommendations for international students: Required—TOEFL (minimum score 550 paper-based; 80 iBT). *Expenses:* Contact institution. *Faculty research:* Animal health management, infectious diseases, fin fish and shellfish health, basic biomedical sciences, ecosystem health.

University of Puerto Rico, Medical Sciences Campus, School of Medicine, Division of Graduate Studies, Department of Anatomy and Neurobiology, San Juan, PR 00936-5067. Offers anatomy (MS, PhD). *Degree requirements:* For master's, one foreign language, comprehensive exam, thesis; for doctorate, one foreign language, comprehensive exam, thesis/dissertation. *Entrance requirements:* For master's and doctorate, GRE General Test, GRE Subject Test, interview, minimum GPA of 3.0, 3 letters of recommendation. Electronic applications accepted. *Faculty research:* Neurobiology, primatology, visual system, muscle structure.

University of Rochester, School of Medicine and Dentistry, Graduate Programs in Medicine and Dentistry, Department of Neurobiology and Anatomy, Programs in Neurobiology and Anatomy, Rochester, NY 14627. Offers PhD, MD/MS. *Degree requirements:* For doctorate, thesis/dissertation, qualifying exam. *Entrance requirements:* For doctorate, GRE General Test. *Expenses: Tuition:* Full-time $44,580; part-time $1394 per credit hour. *Required fees:* $492.

University of Saskatchewan, College of Medicine, Department of Anatomy and Cell Biology, Saskatoon, SK S7N 5A2, Canada. Offers M Sc, PhD. *Degree requirements:* For master's, thesis; for doctorate, thesis/dissertation. *Entrance requirements:* Additional exam requirements/recommendations for international students: Required—TOEFL. *Expenses: Tuition, area resident:* Full-time $3585 Canadian dollars; part-time $585 Canadian dollars per course. Tuition, nonresident: part-time $877 Canadian dollars per course. *International tuition:* $5377 Canadian dollars full-time. *Required fees:* $889.51 Canadian dollars.

University of Saskatchewan, Western College of Veterinary Medicine and College of Graduate Studies and Research, Graduate Programs in Veterinary Medicine, Department of Veterinary Biomedical Sciences, Saskatoon, SK S7N 5A2, Canada. Offers veterinary anatomy (M Sc); veterinary biomedical sciences (M Vet Sc); veterinary physiological sciences (M Sc, PhD). *Degree requirements:* For master's, thesis; for doctorate, comprehensive exam (for some programs), thesis/dissertation. *Entrance requirements:* Additional exam requirements/recommendations for international students: Required—TOEFL (minimum score 80 iBT); Recommended—IELTS (minimum score 6.5). Electronic applications accepted. *Expenses: Tuition, area resident:* Full-time $3585 Canadian dollars; part-time $585 Canadian dollars per course. Tuition, nonresident: part-time $877 Canadian dollars per course. *International tuition:* $5377 Canadian dollars full-time. *Required fees:* $889.51 Canadian dollars. *Faculty research:* Toxicology, animal reproduction, pharmacology, chloride channels, pulmonary pathobiology.

University of South Florida, Morsani College of Medicine and Graduate School, Graduate Programs in Medical Sciences, Tampa, FL 33620-9951. Offers aging and neuroscience (MSMS); allergy, immunology and infectious disease (PhD); anatomy (MSMS, PhD); athletic training (MSMS); bioinformatics and computational biology (MSBCB); biotechnology (MSB); clinical and translational research (MSMS, PhD); health informatics (MSHI, MSMS); health science (MSMS); interdisciplinary medical sciences (MSMS); medical microbiology and immunology (MSMS); metabolic and nutritional medicine (MSMS); molecular medicine (MSMS, PhD); molecular pharmacology and physiology (PhD); neurology (PhD); pathology and laboratory medicine (PhD); pharmacology and therapeutics (PhD); physiology and biophysics (PhD); women's health (MSMS). *Students:* 336 full-time (182 women), 39 part-time (21 women); includes 170 minority (45 Black or African American, non-Hispanic/Latino; 54 Asian, non-Hispanic/Latino; 59 Hispanic/Latino; 2 Native Hawaiian or other Pacific Islander, non-Hispanic/Latino; 10 Two or more races, non-Hispanic/Latino), 17 international. Average age 26. 1,066 applicants, 44% accepted, 250 enrolled. In 2013, 191 master's, 12 doctorates awarded. Terminal master's awarded for partial completion of doctoral program. *Degree requirements:* For master's, comprehensive exam, thesis; for doctorate, comprehensive exam, thesis/dissertation. *Entrance requirements:* For master's, GRE General Test or GMAT, bachelor's degree or equivalent from regionally-accredited university with minimum GPA of 3.0 in upper-division sciences coursework; prerequisites in general biology, general chemistry, general physics, organic chemistry, quantitative analysis, and integral and differential calculus; for doctorate, GRE General Test (minimum score of 600 quantitative), bachelor's degree from regionally-accredited university with minimum GPA of 3.0 in upper-division sciences coursework; 3 letters of recommendation; personal interview; 1-2 page personal statement; prerequisites in biology, chemistry, physics, organic chemistry, quantitative analysis, and integral/differential calculus. Additional exam requirements/recommendations for international students: Required—TOEFL (minimum score 550 paper-based; 79 iBT) or IELTS (minimum score 6.5). *Application deadline:* For fall admission, 2/15 for domestic students, 1/2 for international students. Application fee: $30. *Expenses:* Contact institution. *Faculty research:* Anatomy, biochemistry, cancer biology, cardiovascular disease, cell biology, immunology, microbiology, molecular biology, neuroscience, pharmacology, physiology. *Unit head:* Dr. Michael Barber, Professor and Associate Dean for Graduate and Postdoctoral Affairs, 813-974-9908, Fax: 813-974-4317, E-mail: mbarber@health.usf.edu. *Application contact:* Dr. Eric Bennett, Graduate Director, PhD Program in Medical Sciences, 813-974-1545, Fax: 813-974-4317, E-mail: esbennet@health.usf.edu.
Website: http://health.usf.edu/nocms/medicine/graduatestudies/

The University of Tennessee, Graduate School, College of Agricultural Sciences and Natural Resources, Department of Animal Science, Knoxville, TN 37996. Offers animal anatomy (PhD); breeding (MS, PhD); management (MS, PhD); nutrition (MS, PhD); physiology (MS, PhD). Part-time programs available. *Degree requirements:* For master's, thesis; for doctorate, thesis/dissertation. *Entrance requirements:* For master's and doctorate, GRE General Test, minimum GPA of 2.7. Additional exam requirements/recommendations for international students: Required—TOEFL. Electronic applications accepted. *Expenses:* Tuition, state resident: full-time $9540; part-time $531 per credit hour. Tuition, nonresident: full-time $27,728; part-time $1542 per credit hour. *Required fees:* $1404; $67 per credit hour.

University of Utah, School of Medicine and Graduate School, Graduate Programs in Medicine, Department of Neurobiology and Anatomy, Salt Lake City, UT 84112-1107. Offers PhD. Part-time programs available. Terminal master's awarded for partial completion of doctoral program. *Degree requirements:* For doctorate, comprehensive exam, thesis/dissertation. *Entrance requirements:* For doctorate, GRE General Test. Additional exam requirements/recommendations for international students: Required—TOEFL. *Expenses:* Tuition, state resident: full-time $5259. Tuition, nonresident: full-time $18,569. *Required fees:* $841. Tuition and fees vary according to course load. *Faculty research:* Neuroscience, neuroanatomy, developmental neurobiology, neurogenetics.

The University of Western Ontario, Faculty of Graduate Studies, Biosciences Division, Department of Anatomy and Cell Biology, London, ON N6A 5B8, Canada. Offers anatomy and cell biology (M Sc, PhD); clinical anatomy (M Sc). *Degree requirements:* For master's, thesis; for doctorate, comprehensive exam, thesis/dissertation. *Entrance requirements:* For master's, honors degree or equivalent in biological sciences; for doctorate, master's degree. Additional exam requirements/recommendations for international students: Required—TOEFL. *Faculty research:* Cell and molecular biology, developmental biology, neuroscience, immunobiology and cancer.

Virginia Commonwealth University, Medical College of Virginia-Professional Programs, School of Medicine, School of Medicine Graduate Programs, Department of Anatomy and Neurobiology, Program in Anatomy and Neurobiology, Richmond, VA 23284-9005. Offers PhD. *Accreditation:* APTA. *Degree requirements:* For doctorate, thesis/dissertation. *Entrance requirements:* For doctorate, GRE, MCAT or DAT. Electronic applications accepted.

Virginia Commonwealth University, Program in Pre-Medical Basic Health Sciences, Richmond, VA 23284-9005. Offers anatomy (CBHS); biochemistry (CBHS); human genetics (CBHS); microbiology (CBHS); pharmacology (CBHS); physiology (CBHS). *Entrance requirements:* For degree, GRE, MCAT or DAT, course work in organic chemistry, minimum undergraduate GPA of 2.8. Additional exam requirements/

recommendations for international students: Required—TOEFL (minimum score 600 paper-based). Electronic applications accepted.

Wake Forest University, School of Medicine and Graduate School of Arts and Sciences, Graduate Programs in Medicine, Department of Neurobiology and Anatomy, Winston-Salem, NC 27109. Offers PhD, MD/PhD. *Degree requirements:* For doctorate, thesis/dissertation. *Entrance requirements:* For doctorate, GRE General Test. Additional exam requirements/recommendations for international students: Required—TOEFL. Electronic applications accepted. *Faculty research:* Sensory neurobiology, reproductive endocrinology, regulatory processes in cell biology.

Wayne State University, School of Medicine, Graduate Programs in Medicine, Department of Anatomy and Cell Biology, Detroit, MI 48202. Offers anatomy (MS, PhD); MD/PhD. *Students:* 9 full-time (7 women); includes 2 minority (1 Black or African American, non-Hispanic/Latino; 1 Hispanic/Latino), 5 international. Average age 29. 28 applicants, 14% accepted, 1 enrolled. In 2013, 1 master's, 4 doctorates awarded. *Degree requirements:* For doctorate, thesis/dissertation. *Entrance requirements:* For master's, GRE General Test, minimum GPA of 3.0 undergraduate and in life science coursework, research experience, three letters of faculty recommendation, personal statement, resume; for doctorate, GRE General Test, minimum GPA of 3.0 undergraduate and in life science coursework, research experience, three letters of faculty recommendation, personal statement, resume, interview. Additional exam requirements/recommendations for international students: Required—TOEFL (minimum score 100 iBT), IELTS (minimum score 6.5), TWE (minimum score 5.5). *Application deadline:* For fall admission, 3/1 for domestic and international students; for winter admission, 10/1 for domestic students, 9/1 for international students; for spring admission, 2/1 for domestic students, 1/1 for international students. Applications are processed on a rolling basis. Application fee: $0. Electronic applications accepted. *Expenses:* Contact institution. *Financial support:* In 2013–14, 7 students received support, including 3 fellowships with tuition reimbursements available (averaging $22,003 per year), 5 research assistantships with tuition reimbursements available (averaging $22,116 per year); Federal Work-Study, scholarships/grants, health care benefits, and unspecified assistantships also available. Financial award application deadline: 3/31; financial award applicants required to submit FAFSA. *Faculty research:* Molecular mechanisms of corneal wound healing, cell biology of ocular tumors, genetic regulation of ocular development, retinal synaptic organization and function, molecular mechanisms controlling development and regenerative capacity of retina, brain and spinal cord plasticity and function following injury and disease. *Unit head:* Dr. Linda D. Hazlett, Professor/Chair, 313-577-1061, E-mail: lhazlett@med.wayne.edu. *Application contact:* Dr. Paul D. Walker, Professor and Graduate Director of Anatomy and Cell Biology, 313-577-5678, E-mail: pdwalker@med.wayne.edu.
Website: http://gradprograms.med.wayne.edu/program-spotlight.php?id=27

Wright State University, School of Graduate Studies, College of Science and Mathematics, Department of Neuroscience, Cell Biology, and Physiology, Dayton, OH 45435. Offers anatomy (MS); physiology and biophysics (MS). *Degree requirements:* For master's, thesis optional. *Entrance requirements:* Additional exam requirements/recommendations for international students: Required—TOEFL. *Faculty research:* Reproductive cell biology, neurobiology of pain, neurohistochemistry.

Youngstown State University, Graduate School, College of Science, Technology, Engineering and Mathematics, Department of Biological Sciences, Youngstown, OH 44555-0001. Offers environmental biology (MS); molecular biology, microbiology, and genetic (MS); physiology and anatomy (MS). Part-time programs available. *Degree requirements:* For master's, comprehensive exam, thesis, oral review. *Entrance requirements:* For master's, GRE General Test, minimum GPA of 2.7. Additional exam requirements/recommendations for international students: Required—TOEFL. *Faculty research:* Cell biology, neurophysiology, molecular biology, neurobiology, gene regulation.

Section 3
Biochemistry

This section contains a directory of institutions offering graduate work in biochemistry. Additional information about programs listed in the directory but not augmented by an in-depth entry may be obtained by writing directly to the dean of a graduate school or chair of a department at the address given in the directory.

For programs offering related work, see also in this book *Allied Health; Biological and Biomedical Sciences; Biophysics; Botany and Plant Biology; Cell, Molecular, and Structural Biology; Genetics, Developmental Biology, and Reproductive Biology; Microbiological Sciences; Neuroscience and Neurobiology; Nutrition; Pathology and Pathobiology; Pharmacology and Toxicology; Pharmacy and Pharmaceutical Sciences;* and *Physiology.* In the other guides in this series:

Graduate Programs in the Physical Sciences, Mathematics, Agricultural Sciences, the Environment & Natural Resources

See *Agricultural and Food Sciences, Chemistry,* and *Physics*

Graduate Programs in Engineering & Applied Sciences

See *Agricultural Engineering and Bioengineering, Biomedical Engineering and Biotechnology, Chemical Engineering,* and *Materials Sciences and Engineering*

CONTENTS

Program Directory

Display and Close-Up

See:

Biochemistry

Albert Einstein College of Medicine, Graduate Division of Biomedical Sciences, Department of Biochemistry, Bronx, NY 10461-1602. Offers PhD, MD/PhD. *Degree requirements:* For doctorate, thesis/dissertation. *Entrance requirements:* For doctorate, GRE General Test. Additional exam requirements/recommendations for international students: Required—TOEFL. *Faculty research:* Biochemical mechanisms, enzymology, protein chemistry, bio-organic chemistry, molecular genetics.

American University of Beirut, Graduate Programs, Faculty of Medicine, Beirut, Lebanon. Offers anatomy, cell biology and human morphology (MS); biochemistry and medical genetics (MS); biomedical sciences (PhD); experimental pathology, immunology and microbiology (MS); medicine (MD); neuroscience (MS); pharmacology and toxicology (MS). Part-time programs available. *Faculty:* 259 full-time (78 women), 93 part-time/adjunct (16 women). *Students:* 364 full-time (165 women), 62 part-time (54 women). Average age 23. In 2013, 18 master's awarded. *Degree requirements:* For master's, one foreign language, comprehensive exam, thesis (for some programs); for doctorate, one foreign language, comprehensive exam, thesis/dissertation. *Entrance requirements:* For master's, letter of recommendation; for doctorate, MCAT, bachelor's degree. Additional exam requirements/recommendations for international students: Required—TOEFL (minimum score 600 paper-based; 100 iBT), IELTS (minimum score 7.5). *Application deadline:* For fall admission, 4/30 for domestic and international students; for spring admission, 11/1 for domestic and international students. Application fee: $50. *Expenses: Tuition:* Full-time $14,724; part-time $818 per credit. *Required fees:* $692. Tuition and fees vary according to course load and program. *Financial support:* In 2013–14, 242 students received support, including 60 teaching assistantships (averaging $4,000 per year); career-related internships or fieldwork, institutionally sponsored loans, scholarships/grants, health care benefits, and unspecified assistantships also available. Financial award application deadline: 2/2. *Faculty research:* Cancer research (targeted therapy, mechanisms of leukemogenesis, tumor cell extravasation and metastasis, cancer stem cells), stem cell research (regenerative medicine, drug discovery), genetic research (neurogenetics, hereditary cardiomyopathy, hemoglobinopathies, pharmacogenomics, proteomics), neuroscience research (pain, neurodegenerative disorder), metabolism (inflammation and metabolism, metabolic disorder, diabetes mellitus), vascular and renal biology, signal transduction. *Total annual research expenditures:* $2.6 million. *Unit head:* Dr. Mohamed Sayegh, Dean, 961-1350000 Ext. 4700, Fax: 961-1744464, E-mail: msayegh@aub.edu.lb. *Application contact:* Dr. Salim Kanaan, Director, Admissions Office, 961-1-350000 Ext. 2594, Fax: 96-1-1750775, E-mail: sk00@aub.edu.lb.
Website: http://www.aub.edu.lb/fm/fm_home/Pages/index.aspx

Arizona State University at the Tempe campus, College of Liberal Arts and Sciences, Department of Chemistry and Biochemistry, Tempe, AZ 85287-1604. Offers biochemistry (MS, PhD); chemistry (MS, PhD); nanoscience (PSM). Terminal master's awarded for partial completion of doctoral program. *Degree requirements:* For master's, thesis, interactive Program of Study (iPOS) submitted before completing 50 percent of required credit hours; for doctorate, comprehensive exam, thesis/dissertation, interactive Program of Study (iPOS) submitted before completing 50 percent of required credit hours. *Entrance requirements:* For master's and doctorate, GRE, minimum GPA of 3.0 or equivalent in last 2 years of work leading to bachelor's degree. Additional exam requirements/recommendations for international students: Required—TOEFL, IELTS, or PTE. Electronic applications accepted.

Auburn University, Graduate School, College of Sciences and Mathematics, Department of Chemistry and Biochemistry, Auburn University, AL 36849. Offers analytical chemistry (MS, PhD); biochemistry (MS, PhD); inorganic chemistry (MS, PhD); organic chemistry (MS, PhD); physical chemistry (MS, PhD). Part-time programs available. *Faculty:* 28 full-time (5 women), 1 part-time/adjunct (0 women). *Students:* 43 full-time (18 women), 19 part-time (9 women); includes 10 minority (7 Black or African American, non-Hispanic/Latino; 1 American Indian or Alaska Native, non-Hispanic/Latino; 1 Asian, non-Hispanic/Latino; 1 Hispanic/Latino), 36 international. Average age 27. 34 applicants, 71% accepted, 20 enrolled. In 2013, 17 doctorates awarded. *Degree requirements:* For master's, thesis (for some programs); for doctorate, thesis/dissertation, oral and written exams. *Entrance requirements:* For master's and doctorate, GRE General Test. *Application deadline:* For fall admission, 7/7 for domestic students; for spring admission, 11/24 for domestic students. Applications are processed on a rolling basis. Application fee: $50 ($60 for international students). Electronic applications accepted. *Expenses:* Tuition, state resident: full-time $8262; part-time $459 per credit hour. Tuition, nonresident: full-time $24,786; part-time $1377 per credit hour. Tuition and fees vary according to degree level and program. *Financial support:* Fellowships, research assistantships, and teaching assistantships available. Financial award application deadline: 3/15; financial award applicants required to submit FAFSA. *Unit head:* Dr. J. V. Ortiz, Chair, 334-844-4043, Fax: 334-844-4043. *Application contact:* Dr. George Flowers, Dean of the Graduate School, 334-844-2125.
Website: http://www.auburn.edu/cosam/departments/chemistry/

Baylor College of Medicine, Graduate School of Biomedical Sciences, Department of Biochemistry and Molecular Biology, Houston, TX 77030-3498. Offers PhD, MD/PhD. *Degree requirements:* For doctorate, thesis/dissertation, public defense. *Entrance requirements:* For doctorate, GRE General Test, GRE Subject Test (strongly recommended), minimum GPA of 3.0. Additional exam requirements/recommendations for international students: Required—TOEFL. Electronic applications accepted. *Faculty research:* DNA repair, homologous recombination, gene therapy, trinucleotide repeat diseases, retinitis pigmentosa.

Baylor College of Medicine, Graduate School of Biomedical Sciences, Interdepartmental Program in Cell and Molecular Biology, Houston, TX 77030-3498. Offers biochemistry (PhD); cell and molecular biology (PhD); genetics (PhD); human genetics (PhD); immunology (PhD); microbiology (PhD); virology (PhD); MD/PhD. *Degree requirements:* For doctorate, thesis/dissertation, public defense. *Entrance requirements:* For doctorate, GRE General Test, GRE Subject Test (strongly recommended), minimum GPA of 3.0. Additional exam requirements/recommendations for international students: Required—TOEFL. Electronic applications accepted. *Faculty research:* Molecular and cellular biology; cancer, aging and stem cells; genomics and proteomics; microbiome, molecular microbiology; infectious disease, immunology and translational research.

Boston College, Graduate School of Arts and Sciences, Department of Chemistry, Chestnut Hill, MA 02467-3800. Offers biochemistry (PhD); inorganic chemistry (PhD); organic chemistry (PhD); physical chemistry (PhD); science education (MST). *Students:* 97 full-time (44 women); includes 7 minority (6 Asian, non-Hispanic/Latino; 1 Hispanic/Latino), 36 international. 216 applicants, 34% accepted, 22 enrolled. In 2013, 3 master's, 20 doctorates awarded. *Degree requirements:* For doctorate, thesis/dissertation, qualifying exam. *Entrance requirements:* For doctorate, GRE General Test, GRE Subject Test. Additional exam requirements/recommendations for international students: Required—TOEFL (minimum score 600 paper-based; 100 iBT), IELTS (minimum score 7). *Application deadline:* For fall admission, 1/2 for domestic and international students. Application fee: $70. Electronic applications accepted. *Financial support:* In 2013–14, fellowships with full tuition reimbursements (averaging $27,500 per year), research assistantships with full tuition reimbursements (averaging $27,500 per year), teaching assistantships with full tuition reimbursements (averaging $27,500 per year) were awarded; Federal Work-Study, health care benefits, and unspecified assistantships also available. Support available to part-time students. Financial award application deadline: 3/1; financial award applicants required to submit FAFSA. *Unit head:* Dr. Amir Hoveyda, Chairperson, 617-552-1735, E-mail: amir.hoveyda@bc.edu. *Application contact:* Dr. Marc Snapper, Graduate Program Director, 617-552-8096, Fax: 617-552-0833, E-mail: marc.snapper@bc.edu.
Website: http://www.bc.edu/schools/cas/chemistry/

Boston University, Graduate School of Arts and Sciences, Molecular Biology, Cell Biology, and Biochemistry Program (MCBB), Boston, MA 02215. Offers MA, PhD. *Students:* 34 full-time (16 women), 2 part-time (1 woman); includes 10 minority (2 Black or African American, non-Hispanic/Latino; 2 Asian, non-Hispanic/Latino; 5 Hispanic/Latino; 1 Two or more races, non-Hispanic/Latino), 9 international. Average age 27. 96 applicants, 16% accepted, 8 enrolled. In 2013, 2 master's, 5 doctorates awarded. Terminal master's awarded for partial completion of doctoral program. *Degree requirements:* For master's, one foreign language, thesis (for some programs); for doctorate, one foreign language, comprehensive exam, thesis/dissertation. *Entrance requirements:* For master's and doctorate, GRE General Test, GRE Subject Test, 3 letters of recommendation. Additional exam requirements/recommendations for international students: Required—TOEFL (minimum score 600 paper-based). *Application deadline:* For fall admission, 12/7 for domestic and international students. Application fee: $80. Electronic applications accepted. *Expenses: Tuition:* Full-time $43,970; part-time $1374 per credit hour. *Required fees:* $60 per semester. Tuition and fees vary according to class time, course level and program. *Financial support:* In 2013–14, 32 students received support, including 4 fellowships with full tuition reimbursements available (averaging $20,000 per year), 12 research assistantships with full tuition reimbursements available (averaging $20,000 per year), 4 teaching assistantships with full tuition reimbursements available (averaging $20,000 per year); Federal Work-Study, scholarships/grants, traineeships, and health care benefits also available. Financial award application deadline: 12/7; financial award applicants required to submit FAFSA. *Unit head:* Dr. Ulla Hansen, Director, 617-353-2432, Fax: 617-353-6340, E-mail: uhansen@bu.edu. *Application contact:* Meredith Canode, Academic Administrator, 617-353-2432, Fax: 617-353-6340, E-mail: mcanode@bu.edu.
Website: http://www.bu.edu/mcbb/

Brandeis University, Graduate School of Arts and Sciences, Program in Biochemistry and Biophysics, Waltham, MA 02454. Offers biochemistry and biophysics (PhD); quantitative biology (PhD). Terminal master's awarded for partial completion of doctoral program. *Degree requirements:* For doctorate, thesis/dissertation, qualifying exams. *Entrance requirements:* For doctorate, GRE General Test, resume, 3 letters of recommendation, statement of purpose, transcript(s). Additional exam requirements/recommendations for international students: Required—TOEFL (minimum score 600 paper-based; 100 iBT), PTE (minimum score 68); Recommended—IELTS (minimum score 7). Electronic applications accepted. *Faculty research:* Macromolecular chemistry, structure and function, biochemistry, biophysics, biological macromolecules.

Brigham Young University, Graduate Studies, College of Physical and Mathematical Sciences, Department of Chemistry and Biochemistry, Provo, UT 84602. Offers biochemistry (MS, PhD); chemistry (MS, PhD). *Faculty:* 29 full-time (2 women). *Students:* 101 full-time (41 women); includes 1 minority (Asian, non-Hispanic/Latino), 56 international. Average age 29. 75 applicants, 41% accepted, 16 enrolled. In 2013, 2 master's, 14 doctorates awarded. *Degree requirements:* For master's, thesis; for doctorate, comprehensive exam, thesis/dissertation, qualifying exam. *Entrance requirements:* For master's and doctorate, GRE General Test, minimum GPA of 3.0 in last 60 hours. Additional exam requirements/recommendations for international students: Required—TOEFL (minimum score 580 paper-based; 85 iBT), IELTS (minimum score 7); Recommended—TWE. *Application deadline:* For fall admission, 2/1 priority date for domestic and international students. Applications are processed on a rolling basis. Application fee: $50. Electronic applications accepted. *Expenses: Tuition:* Full-time $6130; part-time $340 per credit hour. Tuition and fees vary according to program and student's religious affiliation. *Financial support:* In 2013–14, 101 students received support, including 12 fellowships with full tuition reimbursements available (averaging $21,250 per year), 55 research assistantships with full tuition reimbursements available (averaging $21,250 per year), 34 teaching assistantships with full tuition reimbursements available (averaging $21,250 per year); institutionally sponsored loans, scholarships/grants, health care benefits, tuition waivers (full), unspecified assistantships, and supplementary awards also available. Financial award application deadline: 2/1. *Faculty research:* Separation science, molecular recognition, organic synthesis and biomedical application, biochemistry and molecular biology, molecular spectroscopy. *Total annual research expenditures:* $5.6 million. *Unit head:* Dr. Gregory F. Burton, Chair, 801-422-4917, Fax: 801-422-0153, E-mail: gburton@byu.edu. *Application contact:* Dr. Paul B. Farnsworth, Graduate Coordinator, 801-422-6502, Fax: 801-422-0153, E-mail: pbfarnsw@byu.edu.
Website: http://www.chem.byu.edu/

Brown University, Graduate School, Division of Biology and Medicine, Department of Molecular Biology, Cell Biology, and Biochemistry, Providence, RI 02912. Offers MA, PhD. Part-time programs available. Terminal master's awarded for partial completion of doctoral program. *Degree requirements:* For master's, thesis (for some programs); for doctorate, one foreign language, thesis/dissertation, preliminary exam. *Entrance requirements:* For master's and doctorate, GRE General Test, GRE Subject Test. Additional exam requirements/recommendations for international students: Required—TOEFL. Electronic applications accepted. *Faculty research:* Molecular genetics, gene regulation.

California Institute of Technology, Division of Biology and Division of Chemistry and Chemical Engineering, Biochemistry and Molecular Biophysics Graduate Option, Pasadena, CA 91125-0001. Offers PhD. *Degree requirements:* For doctorate, thesis/dissertation, qualifying exam. *Entrance requirements:* For doctorate, GRE General Test. Additional exam requirements/recommendations for international students: Required—TOEFL. Electronic applications accepted.

California Institute of Technology, Division of Chemistry and Chemical Engineering, Pasadena, CA 91125-0001. Offers biochemistry and molecular biophysics (MS, PhD); chemical engineering (MS, PhD); chemistry (MS, PhD). *Faculty:* 44 full-time (8 women).

Students: 314 full-time (107 women). Average age 26. 823 applicants, 19% accepted, 56 enrolled. In 2013, 8 master's, 49 doctorates awarded. Terminal master's awarded for partial completion of doctoral program. *Degree requirements:* For master's, thesis; for doctorate, thesis/dissertation. *Entrance requirements:* For doctorate, GRE, BS. Additional exam requirements/recommendations for international students: Required—TOEFL; Recommended—IELTS, TWE. *Application deadline:* For fall admission, 1/1 for domestic and international students. Application fee: $100. Electronic applications accepted. *Financial support:* In 2013–14, 298 students received support. Fellowships, research assistantships, teaching assistantships, Federal Work-Study, institutionally sponsored loans, scholarships/grants, traineeships, health care benefits, and unspecified assistantships available. Financial award application deadline: 1/15. *Unit head:* Prof. Jacqueline K. Barton, Chair, Division of Chemistry and Chemical Engineering, 626-395-3646, Fax: 626-395-6948, E-mail: jkbarton@caltech.edu. *Application contact:* Natalie Gilmore, Graduate Office, 626-395-3812, Fax: 626-577-9246, E-mail: ngilmore@its.caltech.edu.
Website: http://cce.caltech.edu/

California Polytechnic State University, San Luis Obispo, College of Science and Mathematics, Department of Chemistry and Biochemistry, San Luis Obispo, CA 93407. Offers polymers and coating science (MS). Part-time programs available. *Faculty:* 2 full-time (1 woman). *Students:* 4 full-time (1 woman), 6 part-time (1 woman); includes 3 minority (1 Asian, non-Hispanic/Latino; 1 Hispanic/Latino; 1 Two or more races, non-Hispanic/Latino), 1 international. Average age 22. 8 applicants, 75% accepted, 5 enrolled. In 2013, 7 master's awarded. *Degree requirements:* For master's, comprehensive exam (for some programs), thesis (for some programs), comprehensive oral exam. *Entrance requirements:* For master's, minimum GPA of 2.5 in last 90 quarter units of course work. Additional exam requirements/recommendations for international students: Required—TOEFL (minimum score 550 paper-based) or IELTS (minimum score 6). *Application deadline:* For fall admission, 7/1 for domestic students, 11/30 for international students; for winter admission, 11/1 for domestic students, 6/30 for international students; for spring admission, 2/1 for domestic students. Applications are processed on a rolling basis. Application fee: $55. Electronic applications accepted. *Financial support:* Fellowships, research assistantships, career-related internships or fieldwork, Federal Work-Study, and scholarships/grants available. Support available to part-time students. Financial award application deadline: 3/2; financial award applicants required to submit FAFSA. *Faculty research:* Polymer physical chemistry and analysis, polymer synthesis, coatings formulation. *Unit head:* Dr. Ray Fernando, Graduate Coordinator, 805-756-2395, Fax: 805-756-5500, E-mail: rhfernan@calpoly.edu. *Application contact:* Dr. James Maraviglia, Associate Vice Provost for Marketing and Enrollment Development, 805-756-2311, Fax: 805-756-5400, E-mail: admissions@calpoly.edu.
Website: http://www.chemistry.calpoly.edu/

California State University, East Bay, Office of Academic Programs and Graduate Studies, College of Science, Department of Chemistry and Biochemistry, Hayward, CA 94542-3000. Offers chemistry (MS), including biochemistry, chemistry. *Degree requirements:* For master's, comprehensive exam or thesis. *Entrance requirements:* For master's, minimum GPA of 2.6 in field during previous 2 years of course work. Additional exam requirements/recommendations for international students: Required—TOEFL (minimum score 550 paper-based). Electronic applications accepted.

California State University, Long Beach, Graduate Studies, College of Natural Sciences and Mathematics, Department of Chemistry and Biochemistry, Long Beach, CA 90840. Offers biochemistry (MS); chemistry (MS). Part-time programs available. *Degree requirements:* For master's, thesis, departmental qualifying exam. Electronic applications accepted. *Faculty research:* Enzymology, organic synthesis, molecular modeling, environmental chemistry, reaction kinetics.

California State University, Los Angeles, Graduate Studies, College of Natural and Social Sciences, Department of Chemistry and Biochemistry, Los Angeles, CA 90032-8530. Offers analytical chemistry (MS); biochemistry (MS); chemistry (MS); inorganic chemistry (MS); organic chemistry (MS); physical chemistry (MS). Part-time and evening/weekend programs available. *Faculty:* 4 part-time/adjunct (1 woman). *Students:* 20 full-time (8 women), 31 part-time (13 women); includes 32 minority (3 Black or African American, non-Hispanic/Latino; 9 Asian, non-Hispanic/Latino; 20 Hispanic/Latino), 7 international. Average age 29. 46 applicants, 61% accepted, 19 enrolled. In 2013, 16 master's awarded. *Degree requirements:* For master's, one foreign language, comprehensive exam or thesis. *Entrance requirements:* Additional exam requirements/recommendations for international students: Required—TOEFL. *Application deadline:* For fall admission, 5/1 for domestic and international students. Applications are processed on a rolling basis. Application fee: $55. *Financial support:* Federal Work-Study available. Support available to part-time students. Financial award application deadline: 3/1. *Faculty research:* Intercalation of heavy metal, carborane chemistry, conductive polymers and fabrics, titanium reagents, computer modeling and synthesis. *Unit head:* Dr. Robert L. Vellanoweth, Chair, 323-343-2300, Fax: 323-343-6490, E-mail: rvellan@calstatela.edu. *Application contact:* Dr. Larry Fritz, Dean of Graduate Studies, 323-343-3827, Fax: 323-343-5653, E-mail: lfritz@calstatela.edu.
Website: http://www.calstatela.edu/dept/chem/index.htm

California State University, Northridge, Graduate Studies, College of Science and Mathematics, Department of Chemistry and Biochemistry, Northridge, CA 91330. Offers biochemistry (MS); chemistry (MS), including chemistry, environmental chemistry. *Degree requirements:* For master's, thesis. *Entrance requirements:* For master's, GRE General Test or minimum GPA of 3.0. Additional exam requirements/recommendations for international students: Required—TOEFL. Electronic applications accepted.

Carnegie Mellon University, Mellon College of Science, Department of Biological Sciences, Pittsburgh, PA 15213-3891. Offers biochemistry (PhD); biophysics (PhD); cell and developmental biology (PhD); computational biology (MS, PhD); genetics (PhD); molecular biology (PhD); neuroscience (PhD); structural biology (PhD). *Degree requirements:* For doctorate, comprehensive exam, thesis/dissertation. *Entrance requirements:* For doctorate, GRE General Test, GRE Subject Test, interview. *Application deadline:* Applications are processed on a rolling basis. Application fee: $0. Electronic applications accepted. *Financial support:* Fellowships, research assistantships, teaching assistantships, and traineeships available. *Faculty research:* Genetic structure, function, and regulation; protein structure and function; biological membranes; biological spectroscopy. *Unit head:* John L. Woolford, Acting Department Head, 412-268-3193, E-mail: jw17@andrew.cmu.edu. *Application contact:* Ena Miceli, Graduate Programs Manager, 412-268-33012, E-mail: emiceli@andrew.cmu.edu.
Website: http://www.bio.cmu.edu/

Carnegie Mellon University, Mellon College of Science, Department of Chemistry, Pittsburgh, PA 15213-3891. Offers atmospheric chemistry (PhD); bioinorganic chemistry (PhD); bioorganic chemistry and chemical biology (PhD); biophysical chemistry (PhD); catalysis (PhD); green and environmental chemistry (PhD); materials and nanoscience (PhD); renewable energy (PhD); sensors, probes, and imaging (PhD); spectroscopy and single molecule analysis (PhD); theoretical and computational chemistry (PhD). Part-time programs available. Terminal master's awarded for partial completion of doctoral program. *Degree requirements:* For doctorate, thesis/dissertation, departmental qualifying and oral exams, teaching experience. *Entrance requirements:* For doctorate, GRE General Test, GRE Subject Test. Additional exam requirements/recommendations for international students: Required—TOEFL. *Application deadline:* For fall admission, 1/15 priority date for domestic students. Applications are processed on a rolling basis. Application fee: $0. Electronic applications accepted. *Financial support:* Fellowships, research assistantships, and teaching assistantships available. *Faculty research:* Physical and theoretical chemistry, chemical synthesis, biophysical/bioinorganic chemistry. *Unit head:* Dr. Richard D. McCullough, Dean, 412-268-6400, E-mail: rm5g@andrew.cmu.edu. *Application contact:* Valerie Bridge, Graduate Program Specialist, 412-268-3150, Fax: 412-268-1061, E-mail: vbog@andrew.cmu.edu.
Website: http://www.chem.cmu.edu/grad/

Case Western Reserve University, School of Medicine and School of Graduate Studies, Graduate Programs in Medicine, Department of Biochemistry, Cleveland, OH 44106. Offers biochemical research (MS); biochemistry (MS, PhD); RNA biology (PhD); MD/PhD. Part-time programs available. Terminal master's awarded for partial completion of doctoral program. *Degree requirements:* For master's, thesis (for some programs); for doctorate, thesis/dissertation. *Entrance requirements:* For master's and doctorate, GRE General Test. Additional exam requirements/recommendations for international students: Required—TOEFL. Electronic applications accepted. *Faculty research:* Regulation of metabolism, regulation of gene expression and protein synthesis, cell biology, molecular biology, structural biology.

Case Western Reserve University, School of Medicine and School of Graduate Studies, Graduate Programs in Medicine, Department of Nutrition, Cleveland, OH 44106. Offers dietetics (MS); nutrition (MS, PhD), including molecular nutrition (PhD), nutrition and biochemistry (PhD); public health nutrition (MS). Part-time programs available. Terminal master's awarded for partial completion of doctoral program. *Degree requirements:* For master's, thesis (for some programs); for doctorate, thesis/dissertation. *Entrance requirements:* For master's, GRE General Test; for doctorate, GRE General Test, GRE Subject Test. Additional exam requirements/recommendations for international students: Required—TOEFL. *Faculty research:* Fatty acid metabolism, application of gene therapy to nutritional problems, dietary intake methodology, nutrition and physical fitness, metabolism during infancy and pregnancy.

Central Connecticut State University, School of Graduate Studies, School of Arts and Sciences, Department of Chemistry and Biochemistry, New Britain, CT 06050-4010. Offers Certificate. Part-time and evening/weekend programs available. *Faculty:* 1 full-time (0 women). *Students:* 1 (woman) part-time; minority (Two or more races, non-Hispanic/Latino). Average age 26. 1 applicant, 100% accepted, 1 enrolled. *Degree requirements:* For Certificate, qualifying exam. *Entrance requirements:* Additional exam requirements/recommendations for international students: Required—TOEFL (minimum score 550 paper-based; 79 iBT). *Application deadline:* For fall admission, 6/1 for domestic students, 5/1 for international students; for spring admission, 11/1 for domestic and international students. Applications are processed on a rolling basis. Application fee: $50. Electronic applications accepted. Part-time tuition and fees vary according to degree level. *Unit head:* Dr. Barry Westcott, Chair, 860-832-2675, E-mail: westcottb@ccsu.edu. *Application contact:* Patricia Gardner, Associate Director of Graduate Studies, 860-832-2350, Fax: 860-832-2362, E-mail: graduateadmissions@ccsu.edu.
Website: http://www.ccsu.edu/page.cfm?p=1972

City College of the City University of New York, Graduate School, College of Liberal Arts and Science, Division of Science, Department of Chemistry, Program in Biochemistry, New York, NY 10031-9198. Offers MA, PhD. PhD program offered jointly with Graduate School and University Center of the City University of New York. Terminal master's awarded for partial completion of doctoral program. *Degree requirements:* For doctorate, one foreign language, thesis/dissertation. *Entrance requirements:* For doctorate, GRE. Additional exam requirements/recommendations for international students: Required—TOEFL (minimum score 550 paper-based; 79 iBT). Electronic applications accepted. *Faculty research:* Fatty acid metabolism, lectins, gene structure.

Clemson University, Graduate School, College of Agriculture, Forestry and Life Sciences, Department of Genetics and Biochemistry, Program in Biochemistry and Molecular Biology, Clemson, SC 29634. Offers PhD. *Students:* 17 full-time (10 women); includes 1 minority (Asian, non-Hispanic/Latino), 8 international. Average age 27. 38 applicants, 18% accepted, 4 enrolled. In 2013, 3 doctorates awarded. *Degree requirements:* For doctorate, comprehensive exam, thesis/dissertation. *Entrance requirements:* For doctorate, GRE General Test. Additional exam requirements/recommendations for international students: Required—TOEFL. *Application deadline:* For fall admission, 1/1 for domestic students; for spring admission, 9/1 for domestic students. Applications are processed on a rolling basis. Application fee: $70 ($80 for international students). Electronic applications accepted. *Expenses:* Contact institution. *Financial support:* In 2013–14, 17 students received support, including 3 fellowships with full and partial tuition reimbursements available (averaging $13,778 per year), 10 research assistantships with partial tuition reimbursements available (averaging $15,495 per year), 6 teaching assistantships with partial tuition reimbursements available (averaging $15,625 per year); career-related internships or fieldwork, institutionally sponsored loans, scholarships/grants, health care benefits, and unspecified assistantships also available. Support available to part-time students. Financial award application deadline: 3/15; financial award applicants required to submit FAFSA. *Faculty research:* Biomembranes, protein structure, molecular biology of plants, APYA and stress response. *Unit head:* Dr. Keith Murphy, Chair, 864-656-6237, Fax: 864-656-0435, E-mail: kmurph2@clemson.edu. *Application contact:* Sheryl Banks, Administrative Coordinator, 864-656-6878, E-mail: sherylb@clemson.edu.
Website: http://www.clemson.edu/genbiochem

Colorado State University, Graduate School, College of Natural Sciences, Department of Biochemistry and Molecular Biology, Fort Collins, CO 80523-1870. Offers biochemistry (MS, PhD). *Faculty:* 12 full-time (5 women), 1 part-time/adjunct (0 women). *Students:* 18 full-time (13 women), 22 part-time (10 women); includes 5 minority (2 Asian, non-Hispanic/Latino; 1 Hispanic/Latino; 2 Two or more races, non-Hispanic/Latino), 9 international. Average age 28. 70 applicants, 13% accepted, 8 enrolled. In 2013, 6 master's, 4 doctorates awarded. Terminal master's awarded for partial completion of doctoral program. *Degree requirements:* For master's, comprehensive exam, thesis (for some programs); for doctorate, comprehensive exam, thesis/dissertation, comprehensive oral exam at the end of second year. *Entrance requirements:* For master's, GRE General Test, minimum GPA of 3.25; 3 letters of recommendation; resume, mentor letter of support, statement of purpose, transcripts; for doctorate, GRE (minimum combined score of 600 on verbal and quantitative sections), minimum GPA of 3.0; one year of biology, organic chemistry, physics, calculus, and biochemistry; 3 letters of recommendation; bachelor's degree, transcripts, statement of purpose, resume. Additional exam requirements/recommendations for international students: Required—TOEFL (minimum score 550 paper-based; 80 iBT). *Application deadline:* For fall and spring admission, 1/1 priority date for domestic and international students. Application fee: $50. Electronic applications accepted. *Expenses:* Tuition, state resident: full-time $9075.40; part-time $504 per credit. Tuition, nonresident: full-time $22,248; part-time $1236 per credit. *Required fees:* $1819; $60 per credit. *Financial support:* In 2013–14, 46 students received support, including 4 fellowships (averaging $36,360 per year), 31 research assistantships with tuition reimbursements available (averaging $11,005 per year), 11 teaching assistantships with tuition reimbursements

available (averaging $15,718 per year); health care benefits and unspecified assistantships also available. Financial award application deadline: 1/1; financial award applicants required to submit FAFSA. *Faculty research:* Neurodegenerative diseases, gene regulation and cancer, antivirals, retrovirus assembly, yeast prions (models for human amyloid diseases). *Total annual research expenditures:* $5.7 million. *Unit head:* Dr. P. Shing Ho, Chair, 970-491-0569, Fax: 970-491-0494, E-mail: shing.ho@colostate.edu. *Application contact:* Neda Amidon, Graduate Contact, 970-491-6841, Fax: 970-491-0494, E-mail: neda.amidon@colostate.edu.
Website: http://www.bmb.colostate.edu/

Colorado State University–Pueblo, College of Science and Mathematics, Pueblo, CO 81001-4901. Offers applied natural science (MS), including biochemistry, biology, chemistry. Part-time and evening/weekend programs available. *Degree requirements:* For master's, comprehensive exam (for some programs), thesis (for some programs), internship report (if non-thesis). *Entrance requirements:* For master's, GRE General Test (minimum score 1000), 2 letters of reference, minimum GPA of 3.0. Additional exam requirements/recommendations for international students: Required—TOEFL (minimum score 500 paper-based), IELTS (minimum score 5). *Faculty research:* Fungal cell walls, molecular biology, bioactive materials synthesis, atomic force microscopy-surface chemistry, nanoscience.

Columbia University, College of Physicians and Surgeons, Department of Biochemistry and Molecular Biophysics, New York, NY 10032. Offers biochemistry and molecular biophysics (M Phil, PhD); biophysics (PhD); MD/PhD. Only candidates for the PhD are admitted. *Degree requirements:* For doctorate, one foreign language, thesis/dissertation. *Entrance requirements:* For master's and doctorate, GRE General Test. Additional exam requirements/recommendations for international students: Required—TOEFL.

Cornell University, Graduate School, Graduate Fields of Agriculture and Life Sciences, Field of Biochemistry, Molecular and Cell Biology, Ithaca, NY 14853-0001. Offers biochemistry (PhD); biophysics (PhD); cell biology (PhD); molecular biology (PhD). *Faculty:* 20 full-time (19 women). *Students:* 87 full-time (43 women); includes 17 minority (7 Asian, non-Hispanic/Latino; 6 Hispanic/Latino; 4 Two or more races, non-Hispanic/Latino), 28 international. Average age 26. 238 applicants, 20% accepted, 20 enrolled. In 2013, 17 doctorates awarded. *Degree requirements:* For doctorate, comprehensive exam, thesis/dissertation, 2 semesters of teaching experience. *Entrance requirements:* For doctorate, GRE General Test, GRE Subject Test (biology, chemistry, physics, biochemistry, cell and molecular biology), 3 letters of recommendation. Additional exam requirements/recommendations for international students: Required—TOEFL (minimum score 600 paper-based; 77 iBT). *Application deadline:* For fall admission, 1/5 for domestic students. Application fee: $95. Electronic applications accepted. *Financial support:* In 2013–14, 62 students received support, including 8 fellowships with full tuition reimbursements available, 38 research assistantships with full tuition reimbursements available, 16 teaching assistantships with full tuition reimbursements available; institutionally sponsored loans, scholarships/grants, health care benefits, tuition waivers (full and partial), and unspecified assistantships also available. Financial award applicants required to submit FAFSA. *Faculty research:* Biophysics, structural biology. *Unit head:* Director of Graduate Studies, 607-255-2100, Fax: 607-255-2100. *Application contact:* Graduate Field Assistant, 607-255-2100, Fax: 607-255-2100, E-mail: bmcb@cornell.edu.
Website: http://www.gradschool.cornell.edu/fields.php?id-43&a-2

Cornell University, Graduate School, Graduate Fields of Agriculture and Life Sciences, Field of Plant Biology, Ithaca, NY 14853-0001. Offers cytology (MS, PhD); paleobotany (MS, PhD); plant biochemistry (MS, PhD); plant cell biology (MS, PhD); plant ecology (MS, PhD); plant molecular biology (MS, PhD); plant morphology, anatomy and biomechanics (MS, PhD); plant physiology (MS, PhD); systematic botany (MS, PhD). *Faculty:* 49 full-time (14 women). *Students:* 33 full-time (20 women); includes 5 minority (1 Black or African American, non-Hispanic/Latino; 3 Hispanic/Latino; 1 Two or more races, non-Hispanic/Latino), 16 international. Average age 27. 71 applicants, 23% accepted, 10 enrolled. In 2013, 2 doctorates awarded. *Degree requirements:* For doctorate, comprehensive exam, thesis/dissertation. *Entrance requirements:* For doctorate, GRE General Test, GRE Subject Test in biology (recommended), 3 letters of recommendation. Additional exam requirements/recommendations for international students: Required—TOEFL (minimum score 610 paper-based; 77 iBT). *Application deadline:* For fall admission, 1/15 priority date for domestic students. Application fee: $95. Electronic applications accepted. *Financial support:* In 2013–14, 25 students received support, including 7 fellowships with full tuition reimbursements available, 9 research assistantships with full tuition reimbursements available, 9 teaching assistantships with full tuition reimbursements available; institutionally sponsored loans, scholarships/grants, health care benefits, tuition waivers (full and partial), and unspecified assistantships also available. Financial award applicants required to submit FAFSA. *Faculty research:* Plant cell biology/cytology; plant molecular biology; plant morphology/anatomy/biomechanics; plant physiology, systematic botany, paleobotany; plant ecology, ethnobotany, plant biochemistry, photosynthesis. *Unit head:* Director of Graduate Studies, 607-255-2131. *Application contact:* Graduate Field Assistant, 607-255-2131, E-mail: plbio@cornell.edu.
Website: http://www.gradschool.cornell.edu/fields.php?id-45&a-2

Cornell University, Graduate School, Graduate Fields of Arts and Sciences, Field of Chemistry and Chemical Biology, Ithaca, NY 14853-0001. Offers analytical chemistry (PhD); bio-organic chemistry (PhD); biophysical chemistry (PhD); chemical biology (PhD); chemical physics (PhD); inorganic chemistry (PhD); materials chemistry (PhD); organic chemistry (PhD); organometallic chemistry (PhD); physical chemistry (PhD); polymer chemistry (PhD); theoretical chemistry (PhD). *Faculty:* 49 full-time (7 women). *Students:* 155 full-time (61 women); includes 27 minority (2 Black or African American, non-Hispanic/Latino; 1 American Indian or Alaska Native, non-Hispanic/Latino; 11 Asian, non-Hispanic/Latino; 6 Hispanic/Latino; 7 Two or more races, non-Hispanic/Latino), 40 international. Average age 25. 273 applicants, 32% accepted, 34 enrolled. In 2013, 24 doctorates awarded. *Degree requirements:* For doctorate, comprehensive exam, thesis/dissertation. *Entrance requirements:* For doctorate, GRE General Test, GRE Subject Test (chemistry), 3 letters of recommendation. Additional exam requirements/recommendations for international students: Required—TOEFL (minimum score 600 paper-based; 77 iBT). *Application deadline:* For fall admission, 1/10 for domestic students. Application fee: $95. Electronic applications accepted. *Financial support:* In 2013–14, 129 students received support, including 1 fellowship with full tuition reimbursement available, 62 research assistantships with full tuition reimbursements available, 66 teaching assistantships with full tuition reimbursements available; institutionally sponsored loans, scholarships/grants, health care benefits, tuition waivers (full and partial), and unspecified assistantships also available. Financial award applicants required to submit FAFSA. *Faculty research:* Analytical, organic, inorganic, physical, materials, chemical biology. *Unit head:* Director of Graduate Studies, 607-255-4139, Fax: 607-255-4137. *Application contact:* Graduate Field Assistant, 607-255-4139, Fax: 607-255-4137, E-mail: chemgrad@cornell.edu.
Website: http://www.gradschool.cornell.edu/fields.php?id-26&a-2

Dalhousie University, Faculty of Medicine, Department of Biochemistry and Molecular Biology, Halifax, NS B3H 4R2, Canada. Offers M Sc, PhD. *Degree requirements:* For master's, thesis, demonstrating/teaching experience, oral defense, seminar; for doctorate, comprehensive exam, thesis/dissertation, demonstrating/teaching experience, oral defense, seminar, 2 short grant proposals in year 3. *Entrance requirements:* For master's and doctorate, GRE. Additional exam requirements/recommendations for international students: Required—1 of 5 approved tests: TOEFL, IELTS, CANTEST, CAEL, Michigan English Language Assessment Battery. Electronic applications accepted. *Expenses:* Contact institution. *Faculty research:* Gene expression and cell regulation; lipids, lipoproteins, and membranes; molecular evolution; proteins, molecular cell biology and molecular genetics; structure, function, and metabolism of biomolecules.

Dartmouth College, Graduate Program in Molecular and Cellular Biology, Department of Biochemistry, Hanover, NH 03755. Offers PhD, MD/PhD. *Entrance requirements:* For doctorate, GRE General Test, letters of recommendation. Additional exam requirements/recommendations for international students: Required—TOEFL (minimum score 450 paper-based; 90 iBT) or IELTS (minimum score 7). Electronic applications accepted.

Drexel University, College of Medicine, Biomedical Graduate Programs, Program in Biochemistry, Philadelphia, PA 19104-2875. Offers MS, PhD, MD/PhD. Part-time programs available. Terminal master's awarded for partial completion of doctoral program. *Degree requirements:* For master's, comprehensive exam, thesis; for doctorate, thesis/dissertation, qualifying exam. *Entrance requirements:* For master's, GRE General Test, minimum GPA of 2.75; for doctorate, GRE General Test, minimum GPA of 3.0. Additional exam requirements/recommendations for international students: Required—TOEFL. Electronic applications accepted.

Duke University, Graduate School, Department of Biochemistry, Durham, NC 27710. Offers crystallography of macromolecules (PhD); enzyme mechanisms (PhD); lipid biochemistry (PhD); membrane structure and function (PhD); molecular genetics (PhD); neurochemistry (PhD); nucleic acid structure and function (PhD); protein structure and function (PhD). *Faculty:* 30. *Students:* 63 full-time (26 women); includes 35 minority (4 Black or African American, non-Hispanic/Latino; 30 American Indian or Alaska Native, non-Hispanic/Latino; 1 Asian, non-Hispanic/Latino), 27 international. 90 applicants, 17% accepted, 5 enrolled. In 2013, 15 doctorates awarded. *Degree requirements:* For doctorate, thesis/dissertation. *Entrance requirements:* For doctorate, GRE General Test, GRE Subject Test (recommended). Additional exam requirements/recommendations for international students: Required—TOEFL (minimum score 577 paper-based; 90 iBT) or IELTS (minimum score 7). *Application deadline:* For fall admission, 12/8 priority date for domestic and international students. Application fee: $80. Electronic applications accepted. *Financial support:* Fellowships, research assistantships, teaching assistantships, and Federal Work-Study available. Financial award application deadline: 12/8. *Unit head:* Leonard Spicer, Director of Graduate Studies, 919-681-8770, Fax: 919-684-8885, E-mail: norfleet@duke.edu. *Application contact:* Elizabeth Hutton, Director of Admissions, 919-684-3913, Fax: 919-684-2277, E-mail: grad-admissions@duke.edu.
Website: http://www.biochem.duke.edu/

Duquesne University, Bayer School of Natural and Environmental Sciences, Department of Chemistry and Biochemistry, Pittsburgh, PA 15282-0001. Offers chemistry (MS, PhD). Part-time programs available. *Faculty:* 15 full-time (4 women). *Students:* 43 full-time (19 women), 2 part-time (1 woman); includes 6 minority (2 Black or African American, non-Hispanic/Latino; 2 Asian, non-Hispanic/Latino; 2 Hispanic/Latino), 6 international. Average age 27. 56 applicants, 41% accepted, 12 enrolled. In 2013, 3 master's, 6 doctorates awarded. Terminal master's awarded for partial completion of doctoral program. *Degree requirements:* For master's, thesis (for some programs); for doctorate, thesis/dissertation. *Entrance requirements:* For master's, GRE General Test, BS in chemistry or related field, 3 letters of recommendation, official transcripts, statement of purpose; for doctorate, GRE General Test, BS in chemistry or related field, statement of purpose, official transcripts, 3 letters of recommendation with recommendation forms. Additional exam requirements/recommendations for international students: Required—TOEFL (minimum score 100 iBT). *Application deadline:* For fall admission, 2/15 priority date for domestic students, 2/15 for international students; for spring admission, 10/1 priority date for domestic students, 10/1 for international students. Applications are processed on a rolling basis. Application fee: $0 ($40 for international students). Electronic applications accepted. *Expenses:* Contact institution. *Financial support:* In 2013–14, 38 students received support, including 1 fellowship with tuition reimbursement available (averaging $23,675 per year), 11 research assistantships with full tuition reimbursements available (averaging $23,175 per year), 26 teaching assistantships with full tuition reimbursements available (averaging $23,175 per year); scholarships/grants and unspecified assistantships also available. Financial award application deadline: 5/31. *Faculty research:* Computational physical chemistry, bioinorganic chemistry, analytical chemistry, biophysics, synthetic organic chemistry. *Total annual research expenditures:* $2.2 million. *Unit head:* Dr. Ralph Wheeler, Chair, 412-396-6341, Fax: 412-396-5683, E-mail: wheeler7@duq.edu. *Application contact:* Heather Costello, Graduate Academic Advisor, 412-396-6339, Fax: 412-396-4881, E-mail: costelloh@duq.edu.
Website: http://www.duq.edu/academics/schools/natural-and-environmental-sciences/academic-programs/chemistry-and-biochemistry

East Carolina University, Brody School of Medicine, Department of Biochemistry and Molecular Biology, Greenville, NC 27858-4353. Offers biochemistry and molecular biology (PhD); biomedical science (MS). *Degree requirements:* For doctorate, comprehensive exam, thesis/dissertation. *Entrance requirements:* For doctorate, GRE General Test. Additional exam requirements/recommendations for international students: Required—TOEFL. *Application deadline:* For fall admission, 6/1 priority date for domestic students. Applications are processed on a rolling basis. Application fee: $50. *Expenses:* Tuition, state resident: full-time $4223. Tuition, nonresident: full-time $16,540. *Required fees:* $2184. *Financial support:* Fellowships with full and partial tuition reimbursements available. Financial award application deadline: 6/1. *Faculty research:* Gene regulation, development and differentiation, contractility and motility, macromolecular interactions, cancer. *Unit head:* Dr. Phillip H. Pekala, Chairman, 252-744-2684, Fax: 252-744-3383, E-mail: pekalap@ecu.edu. *Application contact:* Dr. Phillip H. Pekala, Chairman, 252-744-2684, Fax: 252-744-3383, E-mail: pekalap@ecu.edu.
Website: http://www.ecu.edu/cs-dhs/biochemistry/Graduate-Program-Information.cfm

Eastern New Mexico University, Graduate School, College of Liberal Arts and Sciences, Department of Physical Sciences, Portales, NM 88130. Offers chemistry (MS), including analytical, biochemistry, inorganic, organic, physical. Part-time programs available. *Degree requirements:* For master's, thesis optional, seminar, oral and written comprehensive exams. *Entrance requirements:* For master's, ACS placement examination, minimum GPA of 3.0; 2 letters of recommendation; personal statement of career goals; bachelor's degree with one year minimum each of general, organic, and analytical chemistry. Additional exam requirements/recommendations for international students: Required—TOEFL (minimum score 550 paper-based; 79 iBT), IELTS (minimum score 6). Electronic applications accepted. *Faculty research:* Synfuel, electrochemistry, protein chemistry.

East Tennessee State University, James H. Quillen College of Medicine, Department of Biomedical Sciences, Johnson City, TN 37614. Offers anatomy (PhD); biochemistry (PhD); microbiology (PhD); pharmaceutical sciences (PhD); pharmacology (PhD);

physiology (PhD); quantitative biosciences (PhD). *Faculty:* 43 full-time (11 women), 1 (woman) part-time/adjunct. *Students:* 31 full-time (17 women), 4 part-time (1 woman); includes 6 minority (2 Black or African American, non-Hispanic/Latino; 3 Asian, non-Hispanic/Latino; 1 Hispanic/Latino), 9 international. Average age 29. 53 applicants, 17% accepted, 8 enrolled. In 2013, 6 doctorates awarded. *Degree requirements:* For doctorate, thesis/dissertation, comprehensive qualifying exam. *Entrance requirements:* For doctorate, GRE General Test, GRE Subject Test. Additional exam requirements/recommendations for international students: Required—TOEFL (minimum score 550 paper-based; 79 iBT). *Application deadline:* For fall admission, 3/15 priority date for domestic students, 3/1 priority date for international students. Application fee: $35 ($45 for international students). Electronic applications accepted. *Expenses:* Contact institution. *Financial support:* In 2013–14, 30 students received support, including 30 research assistantships with full tuition reimbursements available (averaging $19,000 per year); career-related internships or fieldwork, institutionally sponsored loans, scholarships/grants, and unspecified assistantships also available. Financial award application deadline: 7/1; financial award applicants required to submit FAFSA. *Faculty research:* Cardiovascular, infectious disease, neurosciences, cancer, immunology. *Unit head:* Dr. Mitchell E. Robinson, Associate Dean/Program Director, 423-439-2031, Fax: 423-439-2140, E-mail: robinson@etsu.edu. *Application contact:* Shella Bennett, Graduate Specialist, 423-439-4708, Fax: 423-439-5624, E-mail: bennetsg@etsu.edu. Website: http://www.etsu.edu/com/dbms/

Emory University, Laney Graduate School, Division of Biological and Biomedical Sciences, Program in Biochemistry, Cell and Developmental Biology, Atlanta, GA 30322. Offers PhD. *Degree requirements:* For doctorate, comprehensive exam, thesis/dissertation. *Entrance requirements:* For doctorate, GRE General Test, minimum GPA of 3.0 in science course work (recommended). Additional exam requirements/recommendations for international students: Required—TOEFL. Electronic applications accepted. *Faculty research:* Signal transduction, molecular biology, enzymes and cofactors, receptor and ion channel function, membrane biology.

Florida Institute of Technology, Graduate Programs, College of Science, Department of Chemistry, Melbourne, FL 32901-6975. Offers biochemistry (MS); chemistry (MS, PhD). Part-time programs available. *Faculty:* 7 full-time (1 woman), 1 part-time/adjunct (0 women). *Students:* 44 full-time (22 women), 14 part-time (8 women); includes 1 minority (Black or African American, non-Hispanic/Latino), 47 international. Average age 28. 84 applicants, 60% accepted, 17 enrolled. In 2013, 8 master's, 4 doctorates awarded. Terminal master's awarded for partial completion of doctoral program. *Degree requirements:* For master's, comprehensive exam, thesis, research proposal, oral examination in defense of the thesis, proficiency examination; for doctorate, comprehensive exam, thesis/dissertation, oral defense of dissertation, dissertation research publishable to standards, complete original research study. *Entrance requirements:* For master's, proficiency exams, minimum GPA of 3.0, 3 letters of recommendation, resume, statement of objectives; for doctorate, minimum GPA of 3.3, resume, 3 letters of recommendation, statement of objectives. Additional exam requirements/recommendations for international students: Required—TOEFL (minimum score 550 paper-based; 79 iBT). *Application deadline:* For fall admission, 4/1 for international students; for spring admission, 9/30 for international students. Applications are processed on a rolling basis. Electronic applications accepted. *Expenses: Tuition:* Full-time $20,214; part-time $1123 per credit. Tuition and fees vary according to campus/location. *Financial support:* In 2013–14, 7 research assistantships with full and partial tuition reimbursements (averaging $7,630 per year), 15 teaching assistantships with full and partial tuition reimbursements (averaging $9,561 per year) were awarded; career-related internships or fieldwork, institutionally sponsored loans, tuition waivers (partial), unspecified assistantships, and tuition remissions also available. Support available to part-time students. Financial award application deadline: 3/1; financial award applicants required to submit FAFSA. *Faculty research:* Energy storage applications, marine and organic chemistry, stereochemistry, medicinal chemistry, environmental chemistry. *Total annual research expenditures:* $668,972. *Unit head:* Dr. Michael W. Babich, Department Head, 321-674-8046, Fax: 321-674-8951, E-mail: babich@fit.edu. *Application contact:* Cheryl A. Brown, Associate Director of Graduate Admissions, 321-674-7581, Fax: 321-723-9468, E-mail: cbrown@fit.edu. Website: http://cos.fit.edu/chemistry/

Florida State University, The Graduate School, College of Arts and Sciences, Department of Chemistry and Biochemistry, Tallahassee, FL 32306-4390. Offers analytical chemistry (MS, PhD); biochemistry (MS, PhD); inorganic chemistry (MS, PhD); materials chemistry (PhD); organic chemistry (MS, PhD); physical chemistry (MS, PhD). *Faculty:* 37 full-time (4 women), 2 part-time/adjunct (1 woman). *Students:* 136 full-time (44 women), 4 part-time (0 women); includes 19 minority (4 Black or African American, non-Hispanic/Latino; 5 Asian, non-Hispanic/Latino; 6 Hispanic/Latino; 4 Two or more races, non-Hispanic/Latino), 49 international. Average age 25. 150 applicants, 53% accepted, 35 enrolled. In 2013, 7 master's, 24 doctorates awarded. Terminal master's awarded for partial completion of doctoral program. *Median time to degree:* Of those who began their doctoral program in fall 2005, 68% received their degree in 8 years or less. *Degree requirements:* For master's, comprehensive exam, thesis (for some programs); for doctorate, comprehensive exam, thesis/dissertation. *Entrance requirements:* For master's and doctorate, GRE General Test (minimum scores: 150 verbal, 151 quantitative; 1100 total on the old scale), minimum GPA of 3.1 in undergraduate course work. Additional exam requirements/recommendations for international students: Required—TOEFL (minimum score 90 iBT). *Application deadline:* For fall admission, 12/15 priority date for domestic and international students; for spring admission, 9/15 for domestic and international students. Applications are processed on a rolling basis. Application fee: $30. Electronic applications accepted. *Expenses:* Contact institution. *Financial support:* In 2013–14, 139 students received support, including 7 fellowships with full and partial tuition reimbursements available (averaging $10,000 per year), 28 research assistantships with full tuition reimbursements available (averaging $20,000 per year), 107 teaching assistantships with full tuition reimbursements available (averaging $20,000 per year); health care benefits also available. Financial award application deadline: 12/15; financial award applicants required to submit FAFSA. *Faculty research:* Bioanalytical chemistry, including separations, microfluidics, petroleomics; materials chemistry, including magnets, polymers, catalysts, nanomaterials; spectroscopy, including NMR and EPR, ultrafast, Raman, and mass spectrometry; organic synthesis, natural products, photochemistry, and supramolecular chemistry; biochemistry, with focus on structural biology, metabolomics, and anticancer drugs. *Total annual research expenditures:* $8.2 million. *Unit head:* Dr. Timothy Logan, Chairman, 850-644-3810, Fax: 850-644-8281, E-mail: gradinfo@chem.fsu.edu. *Application contact:* Dr. Michael Shatruk, Associate Chair for Graduate Studies, 850-417-8417, Fax: 850-644-8281, E-mail: gradinfo@chem.fsu.edu. Website: http://www.chem.fsu.edu/

Florida State University, The Graduate School, College of Arts and Sciences, Department of Scientific Computing, Tallahassee, FL 32306-4120. Offers computational science (MS, PSM, PhD), including atmospheric science (PhD), biochemistry (PhD), biological science (PhD), computational molecular biology/bioinformatics (PSM), computational science (PhD), geological science (PhD), materials science (PhD), physics (PhD). Part-time programs available. *Faculty:* 14 full-time (2 women). *Students:* 28 full-time (5 women), 4 part-time (0 women); includes 12 minority (10 Asian, non-Hispanic/Latino; 2 Hispanic/Latino). Average age 28. 28 applicants, 43% accepted, 7 enrolled. In 2013, 11 master's, 5 doctorates awarded. Terminal master's awarded for partial completion of doctoral program. *Degree requirements:* For master's, thesis (for some programs); for doctorate, comprehensive exam, thesis/dissertation. *Entrance requirements:* For master's and doctorate, GRE General Test, knowledge of at least one object-oriented computing language, 3 letters of recommendation. Additional exam requirements/recommendations for international students: Required—TOEFL (minimum score 550 paper-based; 80 iBT). *Application deadline:* For fall admission, 1/15 for domestic and international students. Application fee: $30. Electronic applications accepted. *Expenses:* Tuition, state resident: part-time $403.51 per credit hour. Tuition, nonresident: part-time $1004.85 per credit hour. *Required fees:* $75.81 per credit hour. One-time fee: $20 part-time. Tuition and fees vary according to course load, campus/location and student level. *Financial support:* In 2013–14, 32 students received support, including 12 research assistantships with full tuition reimbursements available (averaging $20,000 per year), 17 teaching assistantships with full tuition reimbursements available (averaging $20,000 per year); scholarships/grants and unspecified assistantships also available. Financial award application deadline: 4/15. *Faculty research:* Morphometrics, mathematical and systems biology, mining proteomic and metabolic data, computational materials research, advanced 4-D Var data-assimilation methods in dynamic meteorology and oceanography, computational fluid dynamics, astrophysics. *Unit head:* Dr. Max Gunzburger, Chair, 850-644-1010, E-mail: mgunzburger@fsu.edu. *Application contact:* Maribel Amwake, Academic Coordinator, 850-644-0143, Fax: 850-644-0098, E-mail: mamwake@fsu.edu. Website: http://www.sc.fsu.edu

George Mason University, College of Science, Department of Chemistry and Biochemistry, Fairfax, VA 22030. Offers chemistry (MS); chemistry and biochemistry (PhD). *Faculty:* 17 full-time (4 women), 2 part-time/adjunct (1 woman). *Students:* 25 full-time (13 women), 26 part-time (9 women); includes 16 minority (5 Black or African American, non-Hispanic/Latino; 1 American Indian or Alaska Native, non-Hispanic/Latino; 5 Asian, non-Hispanic/Latino; 4 Hispanic/Latino; 1 Two or more races, non-Hispanic/Latino), 6 international. Average age 29. 68 applicants, 50% accepted, 15 enrolled. In 2013, 18 master's, 1 doctorate awarded. *Degree requirements:* For master's, thesis or alternative; for doctorate, comprehensive exam, thesis/dissertation, exit seminar. *Entrance requirements:* For master's, GRE, bachelor's degree in related field; 2 official copies of transcripts; expanded goals statement; 3 letters of recommendation; resume for those whose bachelor's degree is 5 years or older; for doctorate, GRE, undergraduate degree in related field; BS with minimum GPA of 3.0; 3 letters of recommendation; 2 copies of official transcripts; expanded goals statement; resume. Additional exam requirements/recommendations for international students: Required—TOEFL (minimum score 570 paper-based; 88 iBT), IELTS (minimum score 6.5), PTE. *Application deadline:* For fall admission, 4/15 priority date for domestic students; for spring admission, 11/1 priority date for domestic students. Application fee: $65 ($80 for international students). Electronic applications accepted. *Expenses:* Tuition, state resident: full-time $9350; part-time $390 per credit. Tuition, nonresident: full-time $25,754; part-time $1073 per credit. *Required fees:* $2688; $112 per credit. *Financial support:* In 2013–14, 23 students received support, including 2 fellowships (averaging $11,250 per year), 5 research assistantships with full and partial tuition reimbursements available (averaging $16,401 per year), 18 teaching assistantships with full and partial tuition reimbursements available (averaging $13,411 per year); career-related internships or fieldwork, Federal Work-Study, scholarships/grants, unspecified assistantships, and health care benefits (for full-time research or teaching assistantship recipients) also available. Support available to part-time students. Financial award application deadline: 3/1; financial award applicants required to submit FAFSA. *Faculty research:* Electroanalytical techniques for the study of toxic species in the environment, problems associated with the solid-gas interface, applying peptide/protein engineering principles to investigate biomolecules, enzymes, isoprene biosynthesis, contaminants in the aquatic environment, radioactivity, middle distillate fuels. *Total annual research expenditures:* $185,203. *Unit head:* John A. Schreifels, Chair, 703-993-1082, Fax: 703-993-1055, E-mail: jschreif@gmu.edu. *Application contact:* Robert Honeychuck, Graduate Coordinator, 703-993-1076, Fax: 703-993-1055, E-mail: rhoneych@gmu.edu. Website: http://chemistry.gmu.edu/

Georgetown University, Graduate School of Arts and Sciences, Department of Chemistry, Washington, DC 20057. Offers analytical chemistry (PhD); biochemistry (PhD); computational chemistry (PhD); inorganic chemistry (PhD); materials chemistry (PhD); organic chemistry (PhD); theoretical chemistry (PhD). Terminal master's awarded for partial completion of doctoral program. *Degree requirements:* For doctorate, comprehensive exam, thesis/dissertation. *Entrance requirements:* For doctorate, GRE General Test. Additional exam requirements/recommendations for international students: Required—TOEFL. *Application deadline:* For fall admission, 8/1 priority date for domestic students. Applications are processed on a rolling basis. Application fee: $0. *Financial support:* Fellowships, research assistantships, teaching assistantships, Federal Work-Study, institutionally sponsored loans, scholarships/grants, tuition waivers (full and partial), and lectureships available. Support available to part-time students. Financial award application deadline: 7/1. *Unit head:* Dr. Yuye Tong, Chair, 202-687-5872, Fax: 202-687-6209, E-mail: yyt@georgetown.edu. *Application contact:* Graduate School Admissions Office, 202-687-5568.

Georgetown University, Graduate School of Arts and Sciences, Programs in Biomedical Sciences, Department of Biochemistry and Molecular Biology, Washington, DC 20057. Offers MS, PhD. *Degree requirements:* For doctorate, comprehensive exam, thesis/dissertation. *Entrance requirements:* For doctorate, GRE General Test. Additional exam requirements/recommendations for international students: Required—TOEFL. *Application deadline:* Applications are processed on a rolling basis. Application fee: $50 ($55 for international students). *Unit head:* Dr. Elliot Crooke, Chair, 202-687-1644. *Application contact:* Graduate School Admissions Office, 202-687-5568.

The George Washington University, Columbian College of Arts and Sciences, Institute for Biomedical Sciences, Program in Biochemistry and Systems Biology, Washington, DC 20037. Offers PhD. *Students:* 4 full-time (2 women), 3 part-time (1 woman); includes 3 minority (2 Asian, non-Hispanic/Latino; 1 Hispanic/Latino), 1 international. Average age 30. In 2013, 1 doctorate awarded. Terminal master's awarded for partial completion of doctoral program. *Degree requirements:* For doctorate, thesis/dissertation, general exam. *Entrance requirements:* For doctorate, GRE General Test, interview, minimum GPA of 3.0. Additional exam requirements/recommendations for international students: Required—TOEFL (minimum score 600 paper-based). *Application deadline:* For fall admission, 12/15 priority date for domestic and international students; for spring admission, 10/1 priority date for domestic and international students. Applications are processed on a rolling basis. Application fee: $75. Electronic applications accepted. *Financial support:* In 2013–14, 3 students received support. Fellowships, Federal Work-Study, institutionally sponsored loans, and tuition waivers available. Financial award application deadline: 2/1. *Unit head:* Dr. Eric Hoffman, Director, 202-476-6029, E-mail: ehoffman@cnmcresearch.org. *Application contact:* Information Contact, 202-994-7120, Fax: 202-994-6100, E-mail: genetics@gwu.edu. Website: http://www.gwumc.edu/ibs/fields/biochemgenetics.html

Biochemistry

The George Washington University, School of Medicine and Health Sciences, Department of Biochemistry and Molecular Biology, Washington, DC 20037. Offers biochemistry and molecular biology (MS); biochemistry and molecular genetics (PhD); molecular biochemistry and bioinformatics (MS). *Degree requirements:* For master's, comprehensive exam; for doctorate, thesis/dissertation, general exam. *Entrance requirements:* For master's, GRE General Test, interview, minimum GPA of 3.0; for doctorate, GRE General Test, minimum GPA of 3.0. Additional exam requirements/recommendations for international students: Required—TOEFL (minimum score 550 paper-based).

Georgia Institute of Technology, Graduate Studies and Research, College of Sciences, School of Chemistry and Biochemistry, Atlanta, GA 30332-0001. Offers MS, MS Chem, PhD. Terminal master's awarded for partial completion of doctoral program. *Degree requirements:* For master's, thesis (for some programs); for doctorate, thesis/dissertation. *Entrance requirements:* For master's and doctorate, GRE General Test, GRE Subject Test, minimum GPA of 2.7. Additional exam requirements/recommendations for international students: Required—TOEFL. Electronic applications accepted. *Faculty research:* Inorganic, organic, physical, and analytical chemistry.

Georgia Regents University, The Graduate School, Program in Biochemistry and Molecular Biology, Augusta, GA 30912. Offers MS, PhD. *Faculty:* 13 full-time (2 women). *Students:* 14 full-time (8 women); includes 9 minority (8 Asian, non-Hispanic/Latino; 1 Hispanic/Latino), 7 international. Average age 30. In 2013, 4 doctorates awarded. *Degree requirements:* For doctorate, comprehensive exam, thesis/dissertation. *Entrance requirements:* For doctorate, GRE General Test. Additional exam requirements/recommendations for international students: Required—TOEFL (minimum score 550 paper-based; 79 iBT). *Application deadline:* For fall admission, 1/15 for domestic and international students. Application fee: $50. Electronic applications accepted. *Financial support:* In 2013–14, 8 research assistantships with partial tuition reimbursements (averaging $23,000 per year) were awarded; Federal Work-Study, institutionally sponsored loans, and scholarships/grants also available. Support available to part-time students. Financial award application deadline: 5/31; financial award applicants required to submit FAFSA. *Faculty research:* Bacterial pathogenesis, eye diseases, vitamins and amino acid transporters, transcriptional control and molecular oncology, tumor biology. *Total annual research expenditures:* $3.8 million. *Unit head:* Dr. Vadivel Ganapathy, Chair/Professor, 706-721-7652, Fax: 706-721-9947, E-mail: vganapat@georgiahealth.edu. *Application contact:* Dr. Patricia L. Cameron, Acting Vice Dean, 706-721-3279, E-mail: pcameron@georgiahealth.edu.
Website: http://www.gru.edu/mcg/bmb/students/

Georgia State University, College of Arts and Sciences, Department of Biology, Program in Molecular Genetics and Biochemistry, Atlanta, GA 30302-3083. Offers bioinformatics (MS); molecular genetics and biochemistry (MS, PhD). Part-time programs available. Terminal master's awarded for partial completion of doctoral program. *Degree requirements:* For master's, comprehensive exam (for some programs), thesis optional; for doctorate, comprehensive exam, thesis/dissertation. *Entrance requirements:* For master's and doctorate, GRE. Additional exam requirements/recommendations for international students: Required—TOEFL (minimum score 550 paper-based; 82 iBT) or IELTS (minimum score 7). *Application deadline:* For fall admission, 7/1 priority date for domestic students, 6/1 priority date for international students; for spring admission, 11/15 priority date for domestic students, 10/15 priority date for international students. Applications are processed on a rolling basis. Application fee: $50. Electronic applications accepted. *Expenses: Tuition, area resident:* Full-time $4176; part-time $348 per credit hour. Tuition, state resident: full-time $14,544; part-time $1212 per credit hour. Tuition, nonresident: full-time $14,544; part-time $1212 per credit hour. Tuition and fees vary according to course load and program. *Financial support:* In 2013–14, fellowships with full tuition reimbursements (averaging $22,000 per year), research assistantships with full tuition reimbursements (averaging $20,000 per year) were awarded. Financial award application deadline: 12/3. *Faculty research:* Gene regulation, microbial pathogenesis, molecular transport, protein modeling, viral pathogenesis. *Unit head:* Dr. Parjit Kaur, Professor, 404-413-5432, Fax: 404-413-5301. *Application contact:* LaTesha Warren, Graduate Coordinator, 404-413-5314, Fax: 404-413-5301, E-mail: lwarren@gsu.edu.
Website: http://biology.gsu.edu/

Georgia State University, College of Arts and Sciences, Department of Chemistry, Atlanta, GA 30302-3083. Offers analytical chemistry (MS, PhD); biochemistry (MS, PhD); bioinformatics (MS, PhD); biophysical chemistry (PhD); computational chemistry (MS, PhD); geochemistry (PhD); organic/medicinal chemistry (MS, PhD); physical chemistry (MS). PhD in geochemistry offered jointly with Department of Geology. Part-time programs available. *Faculty:* 23 full-time (4 women). *Students:* 145 full-time (71 women), 9 part-time (5 women); includes 42 minority (23 Black or African American, non-Hispanic/Latino; 1 American Indian or Alaska Native, non-Hispanic/Latino; 10 Asian, non-Hispanic/Latino; 5 Hispanic/Latino; 3 Two or more races, non-Hispanic/Latino), 77 international. Average age 27. 120 applicants, 67% accepted, 54 enrolled. In 2013, 23 master's, 12 doctorates awarded. Terminal master's awarded for partial completion of doctoral program. *Degree requirements:* For master's, one foreign language, comprehensive exam (for some programs), thesis (for some programs); for doctorate, one foreign language, comprehensive exam, thesis/dissertation. *Entrance requirements:* For master's and doctorate, GRE. Additional exam requirements/recommendations for international students: Required—TOEFL (minimum score 550 paper-based; 80 iBT) or IELTS (minimum score 6.5). *Application deadline:* For fall admission, 7/1 priority date for domestic and international students; for winter admission, 11/15 priority date for domestic and international students; for spring admission, 4/15 priority date for domestic and international students. Applications are processed on a rolling basis. Application fee: $50. Electronic applications accepted. *Expenses: Tuition, area resident:* Full-time $4176; part-time $348 per credit hour. Tuition, state resident: full-time $14,544; part-time $1212 per credit hour. Tuition, nonresident: full-time $14,544; part-time $1212 per credit hour. Tuition and fees vary according to course load and program. *Financial support:* Fellowships with full tuition reimbursements, research assistantships with full tuition reimbursements, and teaching assistantships with full tuition reimbursements available. *Faculty research:* Analytical chemistry, biological/biochemistry, biophysical/computational chemistry, chemical education, organic/medicinal chemistry. *Unit head:* Dr. Binghe Wang, Department Chair, 404-413-5500, Fax: 404-413-5506, E-mail: chemchair@gsu.edu. *Application contact:* Rita S. Bennett, Academic Specialist, 404-413-5497, Fax: 404-413-5505, E-mail: rsb423@gsu.edu.
Website: http://chemistry.gsu.edu/

The Graduate Center, City University of New York, Graduate Studies, Program in Biochemistry, New York, NY 10016-4039. Offers PhD. *Degree requirements:* For doctorate, thesis/dissertation, field experience. *Entrance requirements:* For doctorate, GRE General Test. Additional exam requirements/recommendations for international students: Required—TOEFL. Electronic applications accepted.

Harvard University, Graduate School of Arts and Sciences, Department of Chemistry and Chemical Biology, Cambridge, MA 02138. Offers biochemical chemistry (PhD); inorganic chemistry (PhD); organic chemistry (PhD); physical chemistry (PhD). *Degree requirements:* For doctorate, thesis/dissertation, cumulative exams. *Entrance requirements:* For doctorate, GRE General Test, GRE Subject Test. Additional exam requirements/recommendations for international students: Required—TOEFL. *Expenses: Tuition:* Full-time $38,888. *Required fees:* $958. Tuition and fees vary according to campus/location, program and student level.

Harvard University, Graduate School of Arts and Sciences, Division of Medical Sciences, Boston, MA 02115. Offers biological chemistry and molecular pharmacology (PhD); cell biology (PhD); genetics (PhD); microbiology and molecular genetics (PhD); pathology (PhD), including experimental pathology. *Degree requirements:* For doctorate, thesis/dissertation. *Entrance requirements:* For doctorate, GRE General Test, GRE Subject Test. Additional exam requirements/recommendations for international students: Required—TOEFL. *Expenses: Tuition:* Full-time $38,888. *Required fees:* $958. Tuition and fees vary according to campus/location, program and student level.

Howard University, College of Medicine, Department of Biochemistry and Molecular Biology, Washington, DC 20059-0002. Offers biochemistry and molecular biology (PhD); biotechnology (MS); MD/PhD. Part-time programs available. *Degree requirements:* For master's, externship; for doctorate, comprehensive exam, thesis/dissertation. *Entrance requirements:* For master's and doctorate, GRE General Test, minimum GPA of 3.0. *Faculty research:* Cellular and molecular biology of olfaction, gene regulation and expression, enzymology, NMR spectroscopy of molecular structure, hormone regulation/metabolism.

Howard University, Graduate School, Department of Chemistry, Washington, DC 20059-0002. Offers analytical chemistry (MS, PhD); atmospheric (MS, PhD); biochemistry (MS, PhD); environmental (MS, PhD); inorganic chemistry (MS, PhD); organic chemistry (MS, PhD); physical chemistry (MS, PhD). Terminal master's awarded for partial completion of doctoral program. *Degree requirements:* For master's, comprehensive exam, thesis, teaching experience; for doctorate, comprehensive exam, thesis/dissertation, teaching experience. *Entrance requirements:* For master's, GRE General Test, minimum GPA of 2.7; for doctorate, GRE General Test, minimum GPA of 3.0. Additional exam requirements/recommendations for international students: Required—TOEFL. Electronic applications accepted. *Faculty research:* Synthetic organics, materials, natural products, mass spectrometry.

Hunter College of the City University of New York, Graduate School, School of Arts and Sciences, Department of Chemistry, Program in Biochemistry, New York, NY 10065-5085. Offers MA, PhD. Part-time programs available. *Faculty:* 8 full-time (5 women). *Students:* 9 part-time (8 women); includes 2 minority (both Hispanic/Latino), 4 international. Average age 27. 7 applicants, 57% accepted, 3 enrolled. In 2013, 2 master's awarded. *Degree requirements:* For master's, comprehensive exam or thesis. *Entrance requirements:* For master's, GRE General Test, 1 year of course work in chemistry, quantitative analysis, organic chemistry, physical chemistry, biology, biochemistry lecture and laboratory. Additional exam requirements/recommendations for international students: Required—TOEFL. *Application deadline:* For fall admission, 4/1 for domestic students; for spring admission, 11/1 for domestic students. Application fee: $125. *Financial support:* Teaching assistantships, Federal Work-Study, scholarships/grants, and tuition waivers (partial) available. Support available to part-time students. *Faculty research:* Protein/nucleic acid interactions, physical properties of iron-sulfur proteins, neurotransmitter receptors and ion channels, Drosophila melanogaster, requirements of DNA synthesis, oncogenes. *Unit head:* Yuiia Xu, Adviser, 212-772-4310. *Application contact:* William Zlata, Director for Graduate Admissions, 212-772-4482, Fax: 212-650-3336, E-mail: admissions@hunter.cuny.edu.

Illinois Institute of Technology, Graduate College, College of Science and Letters, Department of Biological and Chemical Sciences, Biology Division, Chicago, IL 60616. Offers biochemistry (MBS, MS); biology (PhD); biotechnology (MBS, MS); cell and molecular biology (MBS, MS); microbiology (MB, MS); molecular biochemistry and biophysics (PhD); molecular biology and biophysics (MS). Part-time and evening/weekend programs available. Postbaccalaureate distance learning degree programs offered (minimal on-campus study). Terminal master's awarded for partial completion of doctoral program. *Degree requirements:* For master's, comprehensive exam, thesis (for some programs); for doctorate, comprehensive exam, thesis/dissertation. *Entrance requirements:* For master's, GRE General Test (minimum score 1000 Quantitative and Verbal, 2.5 Analytical Writing), minimum undergraduate GPA of 3.0; for doctorate, GRE General Test (minimum score 1200 Quantitative and Verbal, 3.0 Analytical Writing), minimum undergraduate GPA of 3.0. Additional exam requirements/recommendations for international students: Required—TOEFL (minimum score 523 paper-based; 70 iBT); Recommended—IELTS (minimum score 5.5). Electronic applications accepted. *Faculty research:* Structure and biophysics of macromolecular systems; efficacy and mechanism of action of chemopreventive agents in experimental carcinogenesis of breast, colon, lung and prostate; study of fundamental structural biochemistry problems that have direct links to the understanding and treatment of disease; spectroscopic techniques for the study of multi-domain proteins; molecular mechanisms of cancer and cancer gene therapy.

Illinois State University, Graduate School, College of Arts and Sciences, Department of Biological Sciences, Normal, IL 61790-2200. Offers animal behavior (MS); bacteriology (MS); biochemistry (MS); biological sciences (MS); biology (PhD); biophysics (MS); biotechnology (MS); botany (MS, PhD); cell biology (MS); conservation biology (MS); developmental biology (MS); ecology (MS, PhD); entomology (MS); evolutionary biology (MS); genetics (MS, PhD); immunology (MS); microbiology (MS, PhD); molecular biology (MS); molecular genetics (MS); neurobiology (MS); neuroscience (MS); parasitology (MS); physiology (MS, PhD); plant biology (MS); plant molecular biology (MS); plant sciences (MS); structural biology (MS); zoology (MS, PhD). Part-time programs available. *Degree requirements:* For master's, thesis or alternative; for doctorate, variable foreign language requirement, thesis/dissertation, 2 terms of residency. *Entrance requirements:* For master's, GRE General Test, minimum GPA of 2.6 in last 60 hours of course work; for doctorate, GRE General Test. *Faculty research:* Redoc balance and drug development in schistosoma mansoni, control of the growth of listeria monocytogenes at low temperature, regulation of cell expansion and microtubule function by SPRI, CRUI: physiology and fitness consequences of different life history phenotypes.

Indiana University Bloomington, University Graduate School, College of Arts and Sciences, Department of Chemistry, Bloomington, IN 47405. Offers analytical chemistry (PhD); chemical biology (PhD); chemistry (MAT); inorganic chemistry (PhD); materials chemistry (PhD); organic chemistry (PhD); physical chemistry (PhD). *Faculty:* 42 full-time (4 women). *Students:* 189 full-time (80 women), 6 part-time (5 women); includes 17 minority (6 Black or African American, non-Hispanic/Latino; 7 Asian, non-Hispanic/Latino; 2 Hispanic/Latino; 2 Two or more races, non-Hispanic/Latino), 60 international. Average age 27. 220 applicants, 40% accepted, 19 enrolled. In 2013, 12 master's, 20 doctorates awarded. Terminal master's awarded for partial completion of doctoral program. *Degree requirements:* For master's, thesis; for doctorate, thesis/dissertation. *Entrance requirements:* For master's and doctorate, GRE General Test, GRE Subject Test. Additional exam requirements/recommendations for international students: Required—TOEFL. *Application deadline:* For fall admission, 1/15 priority date for domestic students, 12/1 for international students. Applications are processed on a rolling basis. Application fee: $55 ($65 for international students). Electronic applications accepted. *Financial support:* In 2013–14, 10 fellowships with full tuition reimbursements, 66 research assistantships with full tuition reimbursements, 108

teaching assistantships with full tuition reimbursements were awarded; Federal Work-Study and institutionally sponsored loans also available. *Faculty research:* Synthesis of complex natural products, organic reaction mechanisms, organic electrochemistry, transitive-metal chemistry, solid-state and surface chemistry. *Total annual research expenditures:* $7.7 million. *Unit head:* Dr. David Giedroc, Chairperson, 812-855-6239, E-mail: chemchair@indiana.edu. *Application contact:* Dalane Anderson, Admissions Coordinator, 812-855-2069, Fax: 812-855-8385, E-mail: chemgrad@indiana.edu.
Website: http://www.chem.indiana.edu/

Indiana University Bloomington, University Graduate School, College of Arts and Sciences, Interdisciplinary Biochemistry Graduate Program, Bloomington, IN 47405. Offers PhD. *Faculty:* 59 full-time (16 women). *Students:* 70 full-time (31 women), 3 part-time (2 women); includes 9 minority (3 Black or African American, non-Hispanic/Latino; 1 American Indian or Alaska Native, non-Hispanic/Latino; 3 Asian, non-Hispanic/Latino; 2 Two or more races, non-Hispanic/Latino), 34 international. Average age 26. 93 applicants, 30% accepted, 13 enrolled. In 2013, 7 doctorates awarded. Terminal master's awarded for partial completion of doctoral program. *Degree requirements:* For doctorate, comprehensive exam, thesis/dissertation, Test of English Proficiency for International Associate Instructor Candidates (TEPAIC)(for international students). *Entrance requirements:* For doctorate, GRE. Additional exam requirements/recommendations for international students: Required—TOEFL (minimum score 550 paper-based; 79 iBT). *Application deadline:* For fall admission, 1/15 priority date for domestic students, 12/1 priority date for international students. Application fee: $55 ($65 for international students). Electronic applications accepted. *Financial support:* In 2013–14, 10 students received support, including 19 fellowships with full tuition reimbursements available (averaging $23,000 per year), 5 research assistantships with full tuition reimbursements available (averaging $10,883 per year), 1 teaching assistantship with full tuition reimbursement available (averaging $10,883 per year); scholarships/grants, health care benefits, tuition waivers (full), and unspecified assistantships also available. *Faculty research:* Biochemistry of genes and genomes, microbial biochemistry and virology, structural biology, chemical biology, cellular and medicinal biochemistry, plant biochemistry. *Unit head:* Dr. Carl E. Bauer, Chair, Molecular and Cellular Biochemistry Department, 812-856-0192, Fax: 812-856-5710, E-mail: bchem@indiana.edu. *Application contact:* Susanne Kindred, Administrative Assistant, 812-856-1301, Fax: 812-856-5710, E-mail: bchem@indiana.edu.
Website: http://www.indiana.edu/~mcbdept/graduate/#3

Indiana University–Purdue University Indianapolis, Indiana University School of Medicine, Department of Biochemistry and Molecular Biology, Indianapolis, IN 46202-2896. Offers PhD, MD/MS, MD/PhD. *Faculty:* 53 full-time (36 women). *Students:* 44 full-time (20 women), 9 part-time (6 women); includes 6 minority (1 Black or African American, non-Hispanic/Latino; 3 Asian, non-Hispanic/Latino; 2 Hispanic/Latino), 25 international. Average age 32. 3 applicants, 33% accepted. In 2013, 9 doctorates awarded. Terminal master's awarded for partial completion of doctoral program. *Degree requirements:* For doctorate, thesis/dissertation. *Entrance requirements:* For doctorate, GRE General Test, GRE Subject Test (recommended), previous course work in organic chemistry. *Application deadline:* For fall admission, 1/15 priority date for domestic students. Applications are processed on a rolling basis. Application fee: $55 ($65 for international students). *Financial support:* Fellowships with tuition reimbursements, research assistantships with tuition reimbursements, teaching assistantships, Federal Work-Study, institutionally sponsored loans, scholarships/grants, and tuition waivers (partial) available. Support available to part-time students. Financial award application deadline: 2/1. *Faculty research:* Metabolic regulation, enzymology, peptide and protein chemistry, cell biology, signal transduction. *Unit head:* Dr. Zhong-Yin Zhang, Chairman, 317-274-7151. *Application contact:* Director of Admissions, 317-274-3772, E-mail: inmedadm@iupui.edu.
Website: http://www.biochemistry.iu.edu/

Indiana University–Purdue University Indianapolis, School of Science, Department of Chemistry and Chemical Biology, Indianapolis, IN 46202-2896. Offers MS, PhD, MD/PhD. MD/PhD offered jointly with Indiana University School of Medicine and Purdue University. Part-time and evening/weekend programs available. *Faculty:* 10 full-time (2 women). *Students:* 19 full-time (11 women), 14 part-time (5 women); includes 2 minority (1 Asian, non-Hispanic/Latino; 1 Two or more races, non-Hispanic/Latino), 10 international. Average age 31. 20 applicants, 10% accepted, 2 enrolled. In 2013, 7 master's awarded. Terminal master's awarded for partial completion of doctoral program. *Degree requirements:* For master's, thesis (for some programs); for doctorate, thesis/dissertation. *Entrance requirements:* For master's and doctorate, minimum GPA of 3.0. Additional exam requirements/recommendations for international students: Required—TOEFL. *Application deadline:* Applications are processed on a rolling basis. Application fee: $55 ($65 for international students). *Financial support:* Fellowships with partial tuition reimbursements, research assistantships with partial tuition reimbursements, teaching assistantships with partial tuition reimbursements, career-related internships or fieldwork, institutionally sponsored loans, tuition waivers (partial), and cooperative positions available. Financial award application deadline: 3/1. *Faculty research:* Analytical, biological, inorganic, organic, and physical chemistry. *Total annual research expenditures:* $1.6 million. *Unit head:* Nigel Richards, Chair, 317-274-6624, E-mail: ngrichar@iupui.edu. *Application contact:* Kitty O'Doherty, Graduate Administrator, 317-274-8969, E-mail: czinski@iupui.edu.
Website: http://www.chem.iupui.edu/

Johns Hopkins University, Bloomberg School of Public Health, Department of Biochemistry and Molecular Biology, Baltimore, MD 21205. Offers MHS, Sc M, PhD. Part-time programs available. *Faculty:* 16 full-time (3 women), 5 part-time/adjunct (3 women). *Students:* 76 full-time (51 women), 4 part-time (2 women); includes 40 minority (8 Black or African American, non-Hispanic/Latino; 18 Asian, non-Hispanic/Latino; 10 Hispanic/Latino; 4 Two or more races, non-Hispanic/Latino), 12 international. Average age 25. 96 applicants, 67% accepted, 38 enrolled. In 2013, 42 master's, 5 doctorates awarded. *Degree requirements:* For master's, thesis; for doctorate, comprehensive exam, thesis/dissertation, oral and written exams. *Entrance requirements:* For master's, MCAT or GRE, 3 letters of recommendation, curriculum vitae; for doctorate, GRE General Test, 3 letters of recommendation, curriculum vitae. Additional exam requirements/recommendations for international students: Required—TOEFL (minimum score 600 paper-based). *Application deadline:* For fall admission, 12/15 priority date for domestic students, 12/15 for international students; for spring admission, 6/1 for domestic and international students. Applications are processed on a rolling basis. Application fee: $45. Electronic applications accepted. *Financial support:* Fellowships with tuition reimbursements, research assistantships with tuition reimbursements, teaching assistantships, Federal Work-Study, institutionally sponsored loans, scholarships/grants, health care benefits, and stipends available. Financial award application deadline: 3/15; financial award applicants required to submit FAFSA. *Faculty research:* DNA replication, repair, structure, carcinogenesis, protein structure, enzyme catalysts, reproductive biology. *Total annual research expenditures:* $6 million. *Unit head:* Dr. Pierre Coulombe, Chairman, 410-955-3671, Fax: 410-955-2926, E-mail: pcoulomb@jhsph.edu. *Application contact:* Sharon Gaston, Senior Academic Program Administrator, 410-955-3672, Fax: 410-955-2926, E-mail: sgaston@jhsph.edu.
Website: http://www.jhsph.edu/dept/bmb/

Johns Hopkins University, National Institutes of Health Sponsored Programs, Baltimore, MD 21218-2699. Offers biology (PhD), including biochemistry, biophysics, cell biology, developmental biology, genetic biology, molecular biology; cell, molecular, and developmental biology and biophysics (PhD). *Faculty:* 25 full-time (4 women). *Students:* 126 full-time (72 women); includes 36 minority (3 Black or African American, non-Hispanic/Latino; 1 American Indian or Alaska Native, non-Hispanic/Latino; 21 Asian, non-Hispanic/Latino; 11 Hispanic/Latino), 19 international. 282 applicants, 26% accepted, 36 enrolled. In 2013, 15 doctorates awarded. *Degree requirements:* For doctorate, comprehensive exam, thesis/dissertation. *Entrance requirements:* For doctorate, GRE General Test. Additional exam requirements/recommendations for international students: Required—TOEFL (minimum score 600 paper-based), TWE. *Application deadline:* For fall admission, 12/15 priority date for domestic students. Application fee: $60. Electronic applications accepted. *Financial support:* In 2013–14, 24 fellowships (averaging $23,000 per year), 93 research assistantships (averaging $23,000 per year), 22 teaching assistantships (averaging $23,000 per year) were awarded; Federal Work-Study, institutionally sponsored loans, scholarships/grants, traineeships, health care benefits, tuition waivers (partial), and unspecified assistantships also available. Financial award application deadline: 4/15; financial award applicants required to submit FAFSA. *Faculty research:* Protein and nucleic acid biochemistry and biophysical chemistry, molecular biology and development. *Total annual research expenditures:* $11.2 million. *Unit head:* Dr. Allen Shearn, Chair, 410-516-4693, Fax: 410-516-5213, E-mail: bio_cals@jhu.edu. *Application contact:* Joan Miller, Academic Affairs Manager, 410-516-5502, Fax: 410-516-5213, E-mail: joan@jhu.edu.

Johns Hopkins University, School of Medicine, Graduate Programs in Medicine, Department of Biological Chemistry, Baltimore, MD 21205. Offers PhD. *Faculty:* 16 full-time (5 women). *Students:* 19 full-time (7 women), 15 international. Average age 27. 14 applicants, 21% accepted, 2 enrolled. In 2013, 5 doctorates awarded. *Degree requirements:* For doctorate, thesis/dissertation. *Entrance requirements:* For doctorate, GRE General Test. Additional exam requirements/recommendations for international students: Required—TOEFL. *Application deadline:* For winter admission, 1/15 priority date for domestic and international students. Application fee: $75. Electronic applications accepted. *Financial support:* Research assistantships, health care benefits, and tuition waivers (full) available. Financial award application deadline: 1/1. *Faculty research:* Cell adhesion, genetics, signal transduction and RNA metabolism, enzyme structure and function, gene expression. *Unit head:* Dr. Denise Montell, Co-Director, 410-614-2016, Fax: 410-614-8375, E-mail: dmontell@jhmi.edu. *Application contact:* Wendy Seno, Program Coordinator, 410-614-2976, Fax: 410-614-8375, E-mail: wendy@jnmi.edu.
Website: http://www.hopkinsmedicine.org/biochem/

Johns Hopkins University, School of Medicine, Graduate Programs in Medicine, Program in Biochemistry, Cellular and Molecular Biology, Baltimore, MD 21205. Offers PhD. *Faculty:* 101 full-time (35 women). *Students:* 128 full-time (67 women); includes 30 minority (9 Black or African American, non-Hispanic/Latino; 1 American Indian or Alaska Native, non-Hispanic/Latino; 11 Asian, non-Hispanic/Latino; 8 Hispanic/Latino; 1 Two or more races, non-Hispanic/Latino), 36 international. Average age 26. 118 applicants, 31% accepted, 19 enrolled. In 2013, 23 doctorates awarded. *Degree requirements:* For doctorate, comprehensive exam, thesis/dissertation. *Entrance requirements:* For doctorate, GRE General Test. Additional exam requirements/recommendations for international students: Required—TOEFL. *Application deadline:* For winter admission, 1/10 for domestic and international students. Applications are processed on a rolling basis. Application fee: $80. Electronic applications accepted. *Financial support:* Fellowships, research assistantships, traineeships, and tuition waivers (full) available. Financial award application deadline: 12/31. *Faculty research:* Developmental biology, genomics/proteomics, protein targeting, signal transduction, structural biology. *Unit head:* Dr. Carolyn Machamer, Director, 410-955-3466, Fax: 410-614-8842, E-mail: machamer@jhmi.edu. *Application contact:* Dr. Jeff Corden, Admissions Director, 410-955-3506, Fax: 410-614-8842, E-mail: jcorden@jhmi.edu.
Website: http://bcmb.bs.jhmi.edu/Pages/default.aspx

Kansas State University, Graduate School, College of Arts and Sciences, Department of Biochemistry and Molecular Biophysics, Manhattan, KS 66506. Offers MS, PhD. Part-time programs available. *Faculty:* 13 full-time (2 women), 1 part-time/adjunct (0 women). *Students:* 30 full-time (14 women), 6 part-time (2 women); includes 3 minority (2 Black or African American, non-Hispanic/Latino; 1 Hispanic/Latino), 20 international. Average age 28. 26 applicants, 27% accepted, 6 enrolled. In 2013, 1 master's, 3 doctorates awarded. *Degree requirements:* For master's, thesis; for doctorate, thesis/dissertation. *Entrance requirements:* For master's, GRE General Test, minimum GPA of 3.0 for junior and senior year; for doctorate, GRE General Test, minimum undergraduate GPA of 3.0 or an excellent postgraduate record. Additional exam requirements/recommendations for international students: Required—TOEFL (minimum score 550 paper-based; 79 iBT). *Application deadline:* For fall admission, 2/1 priority date for domestic students, 12/15 priority date for international students; for spring admission, 8/1 for domestic and international students. Applications are processed on a rolling basis. Application fee: $50 ($75 for international students). Electronic applications accepted. *Financial support:* In 2013–14, 27 research assistantships (averaging $18,080 per year), 12 teaching assistantships (averaging $19,243 per year) were awarded; Federal Work-Study, institutionally sponsored loans, and scholarships/grants also available. Support available to part-time students. Financial award application deadline: 3/1; financial award applicants required to submit FAFSA. *Faculty research:* Protein structure/function, insect biochemistry, computational biochemistry, molecular mechanisms in cancer, membrane and lipids biochemistry. *Total annual research expenditures:* $1.8 million. *Unit head:* Dr. Phillip Klebba, Head, 785-532-6121, Fax: 785-532-7278, E-mail: peklebba@ksu.edu. *Application contact:* Dr. Michal Zolkiewski, Director, 785-532-3083, Fax: 785-532-7278, E-mail: michalz@ksu.edu.
Website: http://www.k-state.edu/bmb/

Kansas State University, Graduate School, College of Arts and Sciences, Department of Chemistry, Manhattan, KS 66506. Offers analytical chemistry (MS); biological chemistry (MS); chemistry (PhD); inorganic chemistry (MS); materials chemistry (MS); organic chemistry (MS); physical chemistry (MS). *Faculty:* 38 full-time (5 women), 1 part-time/adjunct (0 women). *Students:* 62 full-time (33 women), 3 part-time (2 women); includes 2 minority (1 Black or African American, non-Hispanic/Latino; 1 Asian, non-Hispanic/Latino), 54 international. Average age 28. 78 applicants, 38% accepted, 16 enrolled. In 2013, 3 master's, 9 doctorates awarded. Terminal master's awarded for partial completion of doctoral program. *Degree requirements:* For master's, thesis; for doctorate, thesis/dissertation. *Entrance requirements:* For master's and doctorate, GRE, minimum GPA of 3.0. Additional exam requirements/recommendations for international students: Required—TOEFL (minimum score 550 paper-based). *Application deadline:* For fall admission, 2/1 priority date for domestic and international students; for spring admission, 8/1 priority date for domestic and international students. Applications are processed on a rolling basis. Application fee: $50 ($75 for international students). Electronic applications accepted. *Financial support:* In 2013–14, 39 research assistantships (averaging $18,182 per year), 24 teaching assistantships with full tuition reimbursements (averaging $18,106 per year) were awarded; institutionally sponsored loans and scholarships/grants also available. Support available to part-time students.

Biochemistry

Financial award application deadline: 3/1; financial award applicants required to submit FAFSA. *Faculty research:* Inorganic chemistry, organic and biological chemistry, analytical chemistry, physical chemistry, materials chemistry and nanotechnology. *Total annual research expenditures:* $2.5 million. *Unit head:* Eric Maatta, Head, 785-532-6665, Fax: 785-532-6666, E-mail: eam@ksu.edu. *Application contact:* Christer Aakeroy, Director, 785-532-6096, Fax: 785-532-6666, E-mail: aakeroy@ksu.edu.
Website: http://www.k-state.edu/chem/

Kennesaw State University, College of Science and Mathematics, Program in Chemical Sciences, Kennesaw, GA 30144-5591. Offers biochemistry (MS); chemistry (MS). *Students:* 6 full-time (2 women); includes 1 minority (Hispanic/Latino). Average age 23. 14 applicants, 64% accepted, 6 enrolled. *Degree requirements:* For master's, thesis. *Entrance requirements:* For master's, GRE. Additional exam requirements/recommendations for international students: Required—TOEFL (minimum score 550 paper-based; 80 iBT), IELTS (minimum score 6.5). *Application deadline:* For fall admission, 3/1 for domestic and international students. Application fee: $60. Electronic applications accepted. *Expenses:* Tuition, state resident: full-time $4806; part-time $267 per semester hour. Tuition, nonresident: full-time $17,298; part-time $961 per semester hour. *Required fees:* $1834; $784.50 per semester. *Financial support:* In 2013–14, 6 students received support, including 6 teaching assistantships with full tuition reimbursements available (averaging $12,000 per year); unspecified assistantships also available. Financial award application deadline: 4/1; financial award applicants required to submit FAFSA. *Unit head:* Dr. Chris Dockery, Director, 470-578-6159, E-mail: mscb@kennesaw.edu. *Application contact:* Admissions Counselor, 770-420-4377, Fax: 770-423-6885, E-mail: ksugrad@kennesaw.edu.
Website: http://chemistry.kennesaw.edu/mscb/

Kent State University, College of Arts and Sciences, Department of Chemistry and Biochemistry, Kent, OH 44242-0001. Offers analytical chemistry (MS, PhD); biochemistry (MS, PhD); chemistry (MA); inorganic chemistry (MS, PhD); organic chemistry (MS, PhD); physical chemistry (MS, PhD). Terminal master's awarded for partial completion of doctoral program. *Degree requirements:* For master's, comprehensive exam, thesis; for doctorate, comprehensive exam, thesis/dissertation. *Entrance requirements:* For master's and doctorate, placement exam, GRE General Test, GRE Subject Test (recommended), minimum GPA of 2.75. Additional exam requirements/recommendations for international students: Required—TOEFL (minimum score 525 paper-based; 71 iBT). Electronic applications accepted. *Faculty research:* Biological chemistry, materials chemistry, molecular spectroscopy.

Laurentian University, School of Graduate Studies and Research, Programme in Chemistry and Biochemistry, Sudbury, ON P3E 2C6, Canada. Offers analytical chemistry (M Sc); biochemistry (M Sc); environmental chemistry (M Sc); organic chemistry (M Sc); physical/theoretical chemistry (M Sc). Part-time programs available. *Degree requirements:* For master's, thesis or alternative. *Entrance requirements:* For master's, honors degree with minimum second class. *Faculty research:* Cell cycle checkpoints, kinetic modeling, toxicology to metal stress, quantum chemistry, biogeochemistry metal speciation.

Lehigh University, College of Arts and Sciences, Department of Biological Sciences, Bethlehem, PA 18015. Offers biochemistry (PhD); cell and molecular biology (PhD); integrative biology and neuroscience (PhD); molecular biology (MS). Part-time programs available. Postbaccalaureate distance learning degree programs offered (no on-campus study). *Faculty:* 18 full-time (9 women). *Students:* 38 full-time (20 women), 30 part-time (23 women); includes 8 minority (4 Black or African American, non-Hispanic/Latino; 2 Asian, non-Hispanic/Latino; 2 Hispanic/Latino), 5 international. Average age 29. 54 applicants, 41% accepted, 11 enrolled. In 2013, 8 master's, 5 doctorates awarded. Terminal master's awarded for partial completion of doctoral program. *Degree requirements:* For master's, research report; for doctorate, comprehensive exam, thesis/dissertation. *Entrance requirements:* For doctorate, GRE General Test. Additional exam requirements/recommendations for international students: Required—TOEFL. *Application deadline:* For fall admission, 12/15 for domestic and international students. Applications are processed on a rolling basis. Application fee: $75. Electronic applications accepted. *Financial support:* In 2013–14, 2 fellowships with full tuition reimbursements (averaging $24,500 per year), 8 research assistantships with full tuition reimbursements (averaging $23,750 per year), 20 teaching assistantships with full tuition reimbursements (averaging $23,750 per year) were awarded; scholarships/grants and unspecified assistantships also available. Financial award application deadline: 12/15. *Faculty research:* Gene expression, cytoskeleton and cell structure, cell cycle and growth regulation, neuroscience, animal behavior, microbiology. *Total annual research expenditures:* $1.7 million. *Unit head:* Dr. Murray Itzkowitz, Chairperson, 610-758-3680, Fax: 610-758-4004, E-mail: mi00@lehigh.edu. *Application contact:* Dr. Mary Kathryn Iovine, Graduate Coordinator, 610-758-6981, Fax: 610-758-4004, E-mail: mki3@lehigh.edu.
Website: http://www.lehigh.edu/~inbios/

Loma Linda University, School of Medicine, Department of Biochemistry/Microbiology, Loma Linda, CA 92350. Offers MS, PhD. Part-time programs available. *Degree requirements:* For master's, thesis or alternative; for doctorate, thesis/dissertation. *Entrance requirements:* For master's and doctorate, GRE General Test. Additional exam requirements/recommendations for international students: Required—TOEFL (minimum score 550 paper-based). *Faculty research:* Physical chemistry of macromolecules, biochemistry of endocrine system, biochemical mechanism of bone volume regulation.

Louisiana State University and Agricultural & Mechanical College, Graduate School, College of Science, Department of Biological Sciences, Baton Rouge, LA 70803. Offers biochemistry (MS, PhD); biological science (MS, PhD); science (MNS). Part-time programs available. *Faculty:* 61 full-time (10 women), 1 (woman) part-time/adjunct. *Students:* 126 full-time (51 women), 10 part-time (7 women); includes 14 minority (4 Black or African American, non-Hispanic/Latino; 3 Asian, non-Hispanic/Latino; 4 Hispanic/Latino; 3 Two or more races, non-Hispanic/Latino), 54 international. Average age 29. 98 applicants, 30% accepted, 19 enrolled. In 2013, 1 master's, 25 doctorates awarded. Terminal master's awarded for partial completion of doctoral program. *Degree requirements:* For doctorate, thesis/dissertation. *Entrance requirements:* For master's and doctorate, GRE General Test, minimum GPA of 3.0. Additional exam requirements/recommendations for international students: Required—TOEFL (minimum score 550 paper-based; 79 IBT), IELTS (minimum score 6.5), or PTE (minimum score 59). *Application deadline:* For fall admission, 5/15 for domestic and international students; for spring admission, 10/15 for domestic and international students. Applications are processed on a rolling basis. Application fee: $25. Electronic applications accepted. *Financial support:* In 2013–14, 134 students received support, including 12 fellowships with full and partial tuition reimbursements available (averaging $38,765 per year), 30 research assistantships with full and partial tuition reimbursements available (averaging $22,757 per year), 84 teaching assistantships with full and partial tuition reimbursements available (averaging $19,694 per year); Federal Work-Study, institutionally sponsored loans, health care benefits, and unspecified assistantships also available. Support available to part-time students. Financial award applicants required to submit FAFSA. *Faculty research:* Biochemistry and molecular biology, cell developmental and integrative biology, systematics, ecology and evolutionary biology. *Total annual research expenditures:* $9.9 million. *Unit head:* Dr. Joe Sibenaller, Chair, 225-578-1765, Fax: 225-578-7299, E-mail: zojose@lsu.edu. *Application contact:* Dr. Michael E. Hellberg, Associate Chairman, 225-578-1240, Fax: 225-578-7299, E-mail: mhellbe@lsu.edu.
Website: http://www.biology.lsu.edu/

Louisiana State University Health Sciences Center at Shreveport, Department of Biochemistry and Molecular Biology, Shreveport, LA 71130-3932. Offers MS, PhD, MD/PhD. *Faculty:* 13 full-time (2 women), 3 part-time/adjunct (1 woman). *Students:* 17 full-time (9 women); includes 10 minority (all Asian, non-Hispanic/Latino), 12 international. Average age 26. 16 applicants, 13% accepted, 2 enrolled. In 2013, 1 master's, 2 doctorates awarded. *Degree requirements:* For master's, thesis; for doctorate, thesis/dissertation. *Entrance requirements:* For master's and doctorate, GRE General Test. Additional exam requirements/recommendations for international students: Required—TOEFL. *Application deadline:* For fall admission, 1/15 priority date for domestic students, 1/15 for international students. Applications are processed on a rolling basis. *Financial support:* In 2013–14, 4 fellowships (averaging $28,000 per year), 13 research assistantships (averaging $26,000 per year) were awarded. *Faculty research:* Metabolite transport, regulation of translation and transcription, prokaryotic molecular genetics, cell matrix biochemistry, yeast molecular genetics, oncogenes, prostate cancer, oxalate nephrotoxicity. *Unit head:* Dr. Hari K. Koul, Head, 318-675-5160, Fax: 318-675-5180. *Application contact:* Sandra Darby, Coordinator, 318-675-5160, Fax: 318-675-5180, E-mail: sdarb4@lsuhsc.edu.
Website: http://www.shrevebiochem.com

Loyola University Chicago, Graduate School, Program in Molecular and Cellular Biochemistry, Chicago, IL 60660. Offers MS, PhD. *Faculty:* 23 full-time (11 women). *Students:* 3 full-time (1 woman); includes 1 minority (Asian, non-Hispanic/Latino), 1 international. Average age 29. In 2013, 2 master's, 3 doctorates awarded. *Degree requirements:* For master's, oral and written reports; for doctorate, comprehensive exam, thesis/dissertation. *Entrance requirements:* For master's and doctorate, GRE General Test. Additional exam requirements/recommendations for international students: Required—TOEFL (minimum score 600 paper-based). *Application deadline:* For fall admission, 3/30 priority date for domestic students, 3/30 for international students. Applications are processed on a rolling basis. Application fee: $50. Electronic applications accepted. *Expenses: Tuition:* Full-time $16,740; part-time $930 per credit. *Required fees:* $135 per semester. *Financial support:* In 2013–14, 5 students received support, including 5 fellowships with full tuition reimbursements available, 11 research assistantships with full tuition reimbursements available; Federal Work-Study, institutionally sponsored loans, and scholarships/grants also available. Financial award application deadline: 3/30. *Faculty research:* Molecular oncology, molecular neurochemical mechanisms of brain development and alcohol addiction, biochemistry of RNA and protein synthesis and intracellular protein degradation, developmentally regulated genes, neurotransmitters and cell-cell interactions. *Unit head:* Dr. William H. Simmons, Chief, 708-216-3362, Fax: 708-216-8523, E-mail: hsimmon@lumc.edu. *Application contact:* Ashyia D. Paul, Administrative Secretary, 708-216-3360, Fax: 708-216-8523, E-mail: apaul@lumc.edu.

Massachusetts Institute of Technology, School of Science, Department of Biology, Cambridge, MA 02139-4307. Offers biochemistry (PhD); biological oceanography (PhD); biology (PhD); biophysical chemistry and molecular structure (PhD); cell biology (PhD); computational and systems biology (PhD); developmental biology (PhD); genetics (PhD); immunology (PhD); microbiology (PhD); molecular biology (PhD); neurobiology (PhD). *Faculty:* 58 full-time (15 women). *Students:* 261 full-time (133 women); includes 77 minority (3 Black or African American, non-Hispanic/Latino; 1 American Indian or Alaska Native, non-Hispanic/Latino; 32 Asian, non-Hispanic/Latino; 32 Hispanic/Latino; 9 Two or more races, non-Hispanic/Latino), 46 international. Average age 26. 651 applicants, 15% accepted, 39 enrolled. In 2013, 25 doctorates awarded. *Degree requirements:* For doctorate, comprehensive exam, thesis/dissertation, two semesters as a teaching assistant. *Entrance requirements:* For doctorate, GRE General Test. Additional exam requirements/recommendations for international students: Required—TOEFL (minimum score 577 paper-based), IELTS (minimum score 6.5). *Application deadline:* For fall admission, 12/1 for domestic and international students. Application fee: $75. Electronic applications accepted. *Expenses: Tuition:* Full-time $43,210; part-time $670 per credit hour. *Required fees:* $288. *Financial support:* In 2013–14, 252 students received support, including 135 fellowships (averaging $36,800 per year), 122 research assistantships (averaging $35,500 per year), 1 teaching assistantship; Federal Work-Study, institutionally sponsored loans, scholarships/grants, traineeships, health care benefits, and unspecified assistantships also available. *Faculty research:* Cellular, developmental and molecular (plant and animal) biology; biochemistry, bioengineering, biophysics and structural biology; classical and molecular genetics, stem cell and epigenetics; immunology and microbiology; cancer biology, molecular medicine, neurobiology and human disease; computational and systems biology. *Total annual research expenditures:* $44.5 million. *Unit head:* Alan Grossman, Interim Head, 617-253-4701. *Application contact:* Biology Education Office, 617-253-3717, Fax: 617-258-9329, E-mail: gradbio@mit.edu.
Website: https://biology.mit.edu/

Massachusetts Institute of Technology, School of Science, Department of Chemistry, Cambridge, MA 02139-4307. Offers biological chemistry (PhD, Sc D); inorganic chemistry (PhD, Sc D); organic chemistry (PhD, Sc D); physical chemistry (PhD, Sc D). *Faculty:* 26 full-time (5 women). *Students:* 218 full-time (73 women), 1 part-time (0 women); includes 47 minority (4 Black or African American, non-Hispanic/Latino; 2 American Indian or Alaska Native, non-Hispanic/Latino; 27 Asian, non-Hispanic/Latino; 10 Hispanic/Latino; 4 Two or more races, non-Hispanic/Latino), 72 international. Average age 26. 617 applicants, 18% accepted, 36 enrolled. In 2013, 28 doctorates awarded. *Degree requirements:* For doctorate, comprehensive exam, thesis/dissertation. *Entrance requirements:* For doctorate, GRE General Test. Additional exam requirements/recommendations for international students: Required—IELTS (minimum score 7); Recommended—TOEFL (minimum score 600 paper-based). *Application deadline:* For fall admission, 12/15 for domestic and international students. Application fee: $75. Electronic applications accepted. *Expenses: Tuition:* Full-time $43,210; part-time $670 per credit hour. *Required fees:* $288. *Financial support:* In 2013–14, 205 students received support, including 76 fellowships (averaging $34,900 per year), 100 research assistantships (averaging $32,800 per year), 40 teaching assistantships (averaging $34,900 per year); Federal Work-Study, institutionally sponsored loans, scholarships/grants, traineeships, health care benefits, and unspecified assistantships also available. *Faculty research:* Synthetic organic and organometallic chemistry including catalysis; biological chemistry including bioorganic chemistry; physical chemistry including chemical dynamics, theoretical chemistry and biophysical chemistry; inorganic chemistry including synthesis, catalysis, bioinorganic and physical inorganic chemistry; materials chemistry including surface science, nanoscience and polymers. *Total annual research expenditures:* $24.8 million. *Unit head:* Prof. Sylvia T. Ceyer, Head, 617-253-1803, Fax: 617-258-7500. *Application contact:* Graduate Administrator, 617-253-1845, Fax: 617-258-0241, E-mail: chemgradeducation@mit.edu.
Website: http://web.mit.edu/chemistry/www/

Mayo Graduate School, Graduate Programs in Biomedical Sciences, Programs in Biochemistry, Structural Biology, Cell Biology, and Genetics, Rochester, MN 55905.

Offers biochemistry and structural biology (PhD); cell biology and genetics (PhD); molecular biology (PhD). *Degree requirements:* For doctorate, oral defense of dissertation, qualifying oral and written exam. *Entrance requirements:* For doctorate, GRE, 1 year of chemistry, biology, calculus, and physics. Additional exam requirements/recommendations for international students: Required—TOEFL. Electronic applications accepted. *Faculty research:* Gene structure and function, membranes and receptors/cytoskeleton, oncogenes and growth factors, protein structure and function, steroid hormonal action.

McGill University, Faculty of Graduate and Postdoctoral Studies, Faculty of Medicine, Department of Biochemistry, Montréal, QC H3A 2T5, Canada. Offers M Sc, PhD.

McGill University, Faculty of Graduate and Postdoctoral Studies, Faculty of Science, Department of Chemistry, Montréal, QC H3A 2T5, Canada. Offers chemical biology (M Sc, PhD); chemistry (M Sc, PhD).

McMaster University, Faculty of Health Sciences, Department of Biochemistry and Biomedical Sciences, Hamilton, ON L8S 4M2, Canada. Offers M Sc, PhD. Terminal master's awarded for partial completion of doctoral program. *Degree requirements:* For master's, thesis; for doctorate, comprehensive exam, thesis/dissertation. *Entrance requirements:* For master's and doctorate, minimum B+ average. Additional exam requirements/recommendations for international students: Required—TOEFL (minimum score 550 paper-based). *Faculty research:* Molecular and cell biology, biomolecular structure and function, molecular pharmacology and toxicology.

Medical College of Wisconsin, Graduate School of Biomedical Sciences, Department of Biochemistry, Milwaukee, WI 53226-0509. Offers PhD, MD/PhD. *Degree requirements:* For doctorate, comprehensive exam, thesis/dissertation. *Entrance requirements:* For doctorate, GRE, official transcripts, three letters of recommendation. Additional exam requirements/recommendations for international students: Required—TOEFL. *Faculty research:* Enzymology, macromolecular structure and synthesis, nucleic acids, molecular and cell biology.

Medical University of South Carolina, College of Graduate Studies, Department of Biochemistry and Molecular Biology, Charleston, SC 29425. Offers MS, PhD, MD/PhD. Terminal master's awarded for partial completion of doctoral program. *Degree requirements:* For master's, thesis, oral exam/thesis defense; for doctorate, thesis/dissertation, oral and written exams/dissertation defense. *Entrance requirements:* For master's, GRE General Test; for doctorate, GRE General Test, interview, minimum GPA of 3.0. Additional exam requirements/recommendations for international students: Required—TOEFL (minimum score 600 paper-based; 100 iBT). Electronic applications accepted. *Faculty research:* Lipid biochemistry, DNA replication, nucleic acids, protein structure.

Memorial University of Newfoundland, School of Graduate Studies, Department of Biochemistry, St. John's, NL A1C 5S7, Canada. Offers biochemistry (M Sc, PhD); food science (M Sc, PhD). Part-time programs available. *Degree requirements:* For master's, thesis; for doctorate, comprehensive exam, thesis/dissertation, oral defense of thesis. *Entrance requirements:* For master's, 2nd class degree in related field; for doctorate, M Sc. Electronic applications accepted. *Faculty research:* Toxicology, cell and molecular biology, food engineering, marine biotechnology, lipid biology.

Miami University, College of Arts and Science, Department of Chemistry and Biochemistry, Oxford, OH 45056. Offers MS, PhD. *Students:* 61 full-time (27 women), 1 part-time (0 women); includes 3 minority (2 Black or African American, non-Hispanic/Latino; 1 Asian, non-Hispanic/Latino), 27 international. Average age 27. In 2013, 3 master's, 15 doctorates awarded. *Entrance requirements:* For master's and doctorate, GRE General Test; GRE Subject Test (recommended). Additional exam requirements/recommendations for international students: Recommended—TOEFL (minimum score 80 iBT), IELTS (minimum score 6.5), TSE (minimum score 54). *Application deadline:* Applications are processed on a rolling basis. Application fee: $50. Electronic applications accepted. *Expenses:* Tuition, state resident: full-time $12,634; part-time $526 per credit hour. Tuition, nonresident: full-time $27,892; part-time $1162 per credit hour. Part-time tuition and fees vary according to course load, campus/location and program. *Financial support:* Fellowships with full tuition reimbursements, research assistantships with full tuition reimbursements, teaching assistantships with full tuition reimbursements, Federal Work-Study, institutionally sponsored loans, tuition waivers (full), and unspecified assistantships available. Financial award application deadline: 2/15; financial award applicants required to submit FAFSA. *Unit head:* Dr. Michael Crowder, Professor and Chair, 513-529-7274, E-mail: crowdemw@miamioh.edu. *Application contact:* Dr. Stacey Lowery Bretz, Professor, 513-529-3731, E-mail: bretzsl@miamioh.edu.
Website: http://www.chemistry.MiamiOH.edu

Michigan State University, College of Human Medicine and The Graduate School, Graduate Programs in Human Medicine, East Lansing, MI 48824. Offers biochemistry and molecular biology (MS, PhD); epidemiology (MS, PhD); microbiology (MS); microbiology and molecular genetics (PhD); pharmacology and toxicology (MS, PhD); physiology (MS, PhD); public health (MPH). *Entrance requirements:* Additional exam requirements/recommendations for international students: Required—TOEFL.

Michigan State University, College of Osteopathic Medicine and The Graduate School, Graduate Studies in Osteopathic Medicine, East Lansing, MI 48824. Offers biochemistry and molecular biology (MS, PhD); microbiology (MS); microbiology and molecular genetics (PhD); pharmacology and toxicology (MS, PhD), including integrative pharmacology (MS), pharmacology and toxicology, pharmacology and toxicology-environmental toxicology (PhD); physiology (MS, PhD).

Michigan State University, The Graduate School, College of Agriculture and Natural Resources, MSU-DOE Plant Research Laboratory, East Lansing, MI 48824. Offers biochemistry and molecular biology (PhD); cellular and molecular biology (PhD); crop and soil sciences (PhD); genetics (PhD); microbiology and molecular genetics (PhD); plant biology (PhD); plant physiology (PhD). Offered jointly with the Department of Energy. *Degree requirements:* For doctorate, comprehensive exam, thesis/dissertation, laboratory rotation, defense of dissertation. *Entrance requirements:* For doctorate, GRE General Test, acceptance into one of the affiliated department programs; 3 letters of recommendation; bachelor's degree or equivalent in life sciences, chemistry, biochemistry, or biophysics; research experience. Electronic applications accepted. *Faculty research:* Role of hormones in the regulation of plant development and physiology, molecular mechanisms associated with signal recognition, development and application of genetic methods and materials, protein routing and function.

Michigan State University, The Graduate School, College of Natural Science and Graduate Programs in Human Medicine and Graduate Studies in Osteopathic Medicine, Department of Biochemistry and Molecular Biology, East Lansing, MI 48824. Offers biochemistry and molecular biology (MS, PhD); biochemistry and molecular biology/environmental toxicology (PhD). *Entrance requirements:* Additional exam requirements/recommendations for international students: Required—TOEFL. Electronic applications accepted.

Michigan Technological University, Graduate School, Interdisciplinary Programs, Houghton, MI 49931. Offers atmospheric sciences (PhD); biochemistry and molecular biology (PhD); computational science and engineering (PhD); environmental engineering (PhD). *Degree requirements:* For doctorate, comprehensive exam, thesis/dissertation. *Entrance requirements:* For doctorate, GRE, statement of purpose, official transcripts, 3 letters of recommendation. Additional exam requirements/recommendations for international students: Required—TOEFL or IELTS.

Mississippi College, Graduate School, College of Arts and Sciences, School of Science and Mathematics, Department of Chemistry and Biochemistry, Clinton, MS 39058. Offers MCS, MS. Part-time programs available. *Degree requirements:* For master's, comprehensive exam, thesis (for some programs). *Entrance requirements:* For master's, GRE. Additional exam requirements/recommendations for international students: Recommended—TOEFL, IELTS. Electronic applications accepted.

Mississippi State University, College of Agriculture and Life Sciences, Department of Biochemistry, Molecular Biology, Entomology and Plant Pathology, Mississippi State, MS 39762. Offers agriculture life sciences (MS), including biochemistry (MS, PhD), entomology (MS, PhD), plant pathology (MS, PhD); life science (PhD), including biochemistry (MS, PhD), entomology (MS, PhD), plant pathology (MS, PhD); molecular biology (PhD). *Faculty:* 23 full-time (1 woman). *Students:* 43 full-time (16 women), 17 part-time (10 women); includes 5 minority (4 Black or African American, non-Hispanic/Latino; 1 Hispanic/Latino), 14 international. Average age 29. 62 applicants, 18% accepted, 10 enrolled. In 2013, 11 master's, 4 doctorates awarded. Terminal master's awarded for partial completion of doctoral program. *Degree requirements:* For master's, thesis (for some programs), final oral exam; for doctorate, thesis/dissertation, preliminary oral and written exam. *Entrance requirements:* For master's, GRE General Test, minimum GPA of 2.75; for doctorate, GRE. Additional exam requirements/recommendations for international students: Required—TOEFL (minimum score 500 paper-based; 61 iBT); Recommended—IELTS (minimum score 5.5). *Application deadline:* For fall admission, 7/1 for domestic students, 5/1 for international students; for spring admission, 11/1 for domestic students, 9/1 for international students. Applications are processed on a rolling basis. Application fee: $60. Electronic applications accepted. *Financial support:* In 2013–14, 35 research assistantships with full tuition reimbursements (averaging $16,388 per year) were awarded; Federal Work-Study, institutionally sponsored loans, and unspecified assistantships also available. Financial award application deadline: 4/1; financial award applicants required to submit FAFSA. *Faculty research:* Fish nutrition, plant and animal molecular biology, plant biochemistry, enzymology, lipid metabolism, chromatin, cell wall synthesis in rice, a model grass bioenergy species and the source of rice stover residues using reverse genetic and functional genomic and proteomic approaches. *Unit head:* Dr. Scott T. Willard, Professor and Department Head, 662-325-2640, Fax: 662-325-8664, E-mail: swilliard@ads.msstate.edu. *Application contact:* Dr. Din-Pow Ma, Professor/Graduate Coordinator, 662-325-7739, Fax: 662-325-8664, E-mail: dm1@ra.msstate.edu.
Website: http://www.biochemistry.msstate.edu

Montana State University, College of Graduate Studies, College of Letters and Science, Department of Chemistry and Biochemistry, Bozeman, MT 59717. Offers biochemistry (MS, PhD); chemistry (MS, PhD). Part-time programs available. *Degree requirements:* For master's, comprehensive exam, thesis (for some programs); for doctorate, comprehensive exam, thesis/dissertation. *Entrance requirements:* For master's and doctorate, GRE General Test, transcripts, letter of recommendation. Additional exam requirements/recommendations for international students: Required—TOEFL (minimum score 550 paper-based). Electronic applications accepted. *Faculty research:* Proteomics, nano-materials chemistry, computational chemistry, optical spectroscopy, photochemistry.

Montclair State University, The Graduate School, College of Science and Mathematics, Department of Chemistry and Biochemistry, Program in Pharmaceutical Biochemistry, Montclair, NJ 07043-1624. Offers MS. Part-time and evening/weekend programs available. *Entrance requirements:* For master's, GRE General Test, 24 undergraduate credits in chemistry, 2 letters of recommendation, essay. Electronic applications accepted. *Faculty research:* Enzyme kinetics, enzyme expression, pharmaceutical biochemistry, medicinal chemistry, biophysical chemistry.

New York Medical College, Graduate School of Basic Medical Sciences, Biochemistry and Molecular Biology Master's Program, Valhalla, NY 10595-1691. Offers MS, PhD, MD/PhD. Part-time and evening/weekend programs available. *Faculty:* 10 full-time (4 women), 2 part-time/adjunct (0 women). *Students:* 5 full-time (1 woman); includes 3 minority (2 Asian, non-Hispanic/Latino; 1 Hispanic/Latino). Average age 25. 8 applicants, 100% accepted, 4 enrolled. In 2013, 4 master's awarded. Terminal master's awarded for partial completion of doctoral program. *Degree requirements:* For master's, thesis; for doctorate, comprehensive exam, thesis/dissertation. *Entrance requirements:* For master's, GRE General Test, MCAT, or DAT. Additional exam requirements/recommendations for international students: Required—TOEFL. *Application deadline:* For fall admission, 7/1 priority date for domestic students, 5/1 priority date for international students; for spring admission, 12/1 for domestic students, 10/1 for international students. Applications are processed on a rolling basis. Application fee: $75 ($100 for international students). Electronic applications accepted. *Expenses: Tuition:* Full-time $49,170; part-time $910 per credit. Tuition and fees vary according to program. *Financial support:* Federal Work-Study and scholarships/grants available. Support available to part-time students. Financial award applicants required to submit FAFSA. *Faculty research:* Expression, mechanisms of hormone action and cell signaling, enzymology, mechanisms of DNA replication and repair, cell cycle regulation, control of cell growth, molecular biology of cancer cells and the cancer process, mechanisms of nutrition and cancer prevention, molecular neurobiology and studies of neurodegenerative disorders, the aging process. *Unit head:* Dr. Joseph Wu, Program Director, 914-594-4891, Fax: 914-594-4944, E-mail: joseph_wu@nymc.edu. *Application contact:* Valerie Romeo-Messana, Director of Admissions, 914-594-4110, Fax: 914-594-4944, E-mail: v_romeomessana@nymc.edu.

New York Medical College, Graduate School of Basic Medical Sciences, Integrated PhD Program, Valhalla, NY 10595-1691. Offers biochemistry and molecular biology (PhD); cell biology and anatomy (PhD); microbiology and immunology (PhD); pathology (PhD); pharmacology (PhD); physiology (PhD). *Faculty:* 91 full-time (16 women), 5 part-time/adjunct (2 women). *Students:* 31 full-time (21 women); includes 17 minority (4 Black or African American, non-Hispanic/Latino; 11 Asian, non-Hispanic/Latino; 2 Hispanic/Latino). Average age 27. 56 applicants, 36% accepted, 9 enrolled. In 2013, 17 doctorates awarded. *Degree requirements:* For doctorate, comprehensive exam, thesis/dissertation. *Entrance requirements:* For doctorate, GRE General Test. Additional exam requirements/recommendations for international students: Required—TOEFL. *Application deadline:* For fall admission, 1/1 priority date for domestic and international students. Applications are processed on a rolling basis. Application fee: $75 ($100 for international students). Electronic applications accepted. *Expenses: Tuition:* Full-time $49,170; part-time $910 per credit. Tuition and fees vary according to program. *Financial support:* In 2013–14, fellowships with full tuition reimbursements (averaging $25,500 per year), research assistantships with full tuition reimbursements (averaging $25,500 per year) were awarded; Federal Work-Study, scholarships/grants, traineeships, health care benefits, and tuition waivers (full) also available. Financial award applicants required to submit FAFSA. *Faculty research:* Cardiovascular sciences, infectious diseases, neuroscience, cancer and cell signaling. *Unit head:* Dr. Francis L. Belloni, Dean, 914-594-4110, Fax: 914-594-4944, E-mail: francis_belloni@nymc.edu.

Biochemistry

Application contact: Valerie Romeo-Messana, Director of Admissions, 914-594-4110, Fax: 914-594-4944, E-mail: v_romeomessana@nymc.edu.

North Carolina State University, Graduate School, College of Agriculture and Life Sciences, Department of Biochemistry, Raleigh, NC 27695. Offers PhD. *Degree requirements:* For doctorate, thesis/dissertation. *Entrance requirements:* For doctorate, GRE General Test. Additional exam requirements/recommendations for international students: Required—TOEFL. Electronic applications accepted. *Faculty research:* Regulation of gene expression, structure and function of proteins and nucleic acids, molecular biology, high-field NMR, bioinorganic chemistry.

North Dakota State University, College of Graduate and Interdisciplinary Studies, College of Science and Mathematics, Department of Biochemistry and Molecular Biology, Program in Biochemistry, Fargo, ND 58108. Offers MS, PhD. Part-time programs available. *Students:* 15 full-time (10 women), 6 part-time (2 women); includes 1 minority (Asian, non-Hispanic/Latino), 8 international. Average age 28. 23 applicants, 35% accepted, 5 enrolled. *Degree requirements:* For master's, thesis; for doctorate, thesis/dissertation. *Entrance requirements:* Additional exam requirements/recommendations for international students: Required—TOEFL (minimum score 550 paper-based). *Application deadline:* For fall admission, 3/1 priority date for domestic and international students; for spring admission, 9/1 priority date for domestic and international students. Applications are processed on a rolling basis. Application fee: $35. Electronic applications accepted. *Financial support:* In 2013–14, 4 research assistantships with full tuition reimbursements (averaging $19,000 per year), 5 teaching assistantships with full tuition reimbursements (averaging $19,000 per year) were awarded; career-related internships or fieldwork, Federal Work-Study, and institutionally sponsored loans also available. Financial award application deadline: 4/15. *Unit head:* Dr. Gregory Cook, Chair, 701-231-8694, Fax: 701-231-8831, E-mail: gregory.cook@ndsu.edu. *Application contact:* Sonya Goergen, Marketing, Recruitment, and Public Relations Coordinator, 701-231-7033, Fax: 701-231-6524.

Northern Michigan University, College of Graduate Studies, College of Arts and Sciences, Department of Biology, Marquette, MI 49855-5301. Offers biochemistry (MS); biology (MS). Part-time programs available. *Faculty:* 15 full-time (3 women). *Students:* 34. Average age 27. 20 applicants, 90% accepted, 14 enrolled. In 2013, 5 master's awarded. *Degree requirements:* For master's, thesis. *Entrance requirements:* For master's, GRE, minimum GPA of 3.0; references; coursework in biology and other sciences, faculty member as mentor. Additional exam requirements/recommendations for international students: Required—TOEFL (minimum score 550 paper-based; 79 iBT), IELTS (minimum score 6.5). *Application deadline:* For fall admission, 5/1 for domestic students; for winter admission, 11/1 for domestic students; for spring admission, 3/17 for domestic students. Applications are processed on a rolling basis. Application fee: $50. Electronic applications accepted. *Expenses:* Tuition, state resident: part-time $427 per credit. Tuition, nonresident: part-time $614.50 per credit. *Required fees:* $325 per semester. Tuition and fees vary according to course load and program. *Financial support:* In 2013–14, 19 students received support, including 1 research assistantship, 19 teaching assistantships; career-related internships or fieldwork, Federal Work-Study, institutionally sponsored loans, tuition waivers, and unspecified assistantships also available. Support available to part-time students. Financial award application deadline: 3/1. *Faculty research:* Evolutionary genetics, neurobiology, conservation biology, fisheries and wildlife, microbiology. *Unit head:* Dr. Jill B.K. Leonard, Graduate Program Director, 906-227-1619, E-mail: jileonar@nmu.edu. *Application contact:* Dr. Brian Cherry, Assistant Provost of Graduate Education and Research, 906-227-2300, Fax: 906-227-2315, E-mail: graduate@nmu.edu.
Website: http://www.nmu.edu/biology/

Northwestern University, The Graduate School, Interdisciplinary Biological Sciences Program (IBiS), Evanston, IL 60208. Offers biochemistry (PhD); bioengineering and biotechnology (PhD); biotechnology (PhD); cell and molecular biology (PhD); developmental and systems biology (PhD); nanotechnology (PhD); neurobiology (PhD); structural biology and biophysics (PhD). *Degree requirements:* For doctorate, thesis/dissertation, qualifying exam. *Entrance requirements:* For doctorate, GRE General Test. Additional exam requirements/recommendations for international students: Required—TOEFL (minimum score 600 paper-based). *Application deadline:* For fall admission, 12/15 for domestic and international students. Applications are processed on a rolling basis. Application fee: $95. Electronic applications accepted. *Financial support:* Fellowships, research assistantships, teaching assistantships, career-related internships or fieldwork, institutionally sponsored loans, scholarships/grants, traineeships, health care benefits, and unspecified assistantships available. Financial award application deadline: 12/31; financial award applicants required to submit FAFSA. *Faculty research:* Biophysics/structural biology, cell/molecular biology, synthetic biology, developmental systems biology, chemical biology/nanotechnology. *Unit head:* Dr. Deborah Klos Dehring, Associate Director, 847-467-0451, E-mail: d-klos@northwestern.edu. *Application contact:* Cathy Prullage, Program Manager, 847-491-4301, E-mail: ibis@northwestern.edu.
Website: http://www.biochem.northwestern.edu/ibis/

The Ohio State University, Graduate School, College of Arts and Sciences, Division of Natural and Mathematical Sciences, Biochemistry Program, Columbus, OH 43210. Offers PhD. *Students:* 85 full-time (37 women), 2 part-time (0 women); includes 3 minority (1 Black or African American, non-Hispanic/Latino; 2 Asian, non-Hispanic/Latino), 33 international. Average age 26. In 2013, 9 doctorates awarded. Terminal master's awarded for partial completion of doctoral program. *Degree requirements:* For doctorate, thesis/dissertation. *Entrance requirements:* For doctorate, GRE General Test. Additional exam requirements/recommendations for international students: Required—TOEFL (minimum score 620 paper-based; 105 iBT); Recommended—IELTS (minimum score 8). *Application deadline:* For fall admission, 12/13 priority date for domestic students, 11/30 priority date for international students. Applications are processed on a rolling basis. Application fee: $60 ($70 for international students). Electronic applications accepted. *Financial support:* Fellowships with tuition reimbursements, research assistantships with tuition reimbursements, and teaching assistantships with tuition reimbursements available. *Unit head:* Thomas Magliery, PhD, Program Director, 614-292-2120, Fax: 614-292-6511, E-mail: ibba.1@osu.edu. *Application contact:* Graduate Admissions, 614-292-9444, Fax: 614-292-3895, E-mail: gradadmissions@osu.edu.
Website: http://osbp.osu.edu/

The Ohio State University, Graduate School, College of Arts and Sciences, Division of Natural and Mathematical Sciences, Departments of Chemistry and Biochemistry, Columbus, OH 43210. Offers biochemistry (MS); chemistry (MS, PhD). *Faculty:* 47. *Students:* 242 full-time (81 women), 7 part-time (2 women); includes 24 minority (8 Black or African American, non-Hispanic/Latino; 1 American Indian or Alaska Native, non-Hispanic/Latino; 6 Asian, non-Hispanic/Latino; 6 Hispanic/Latino; 3 Two or more races, non-Hispanic/Latino), 119 international. Average age 25. In 2013, 6 master's, 28 doctorates awarded. *Degree requirements:* For master's, thesis optional; for doctorate, thesis/dissertation. *Entrance requirements:* For master's and doctorate, GRE General Test. Additional exam requirements/recommendations for international students: Required—TOEFL (minimum score 550 paper-based; 79 iBT), Michigan English Language Assessment Battery (minimum score 82); Recommended—IELTS (minimum score 7). *Application deadline:* For fall admission, 12/16 for domestic and international students; for winter admission, 12/1 for domestic students, 11/1 for international students; for spring admission, 3/1 for domestic students, 2/1 for international students. Applications are processed on a rolling basis. Application fee: $60 ($70 for international students). Electronic applications accepted. *Financial support:* Fellowships, research assistantships, teaching assistantships, Federal Work-Study, and institutionally sponsored loans available. Support available to part-time students. *Unit head:* Dr. Susan V. Olesik, Chair, 614-292-0733, E-mail: olesik.1@osu.edu. *Application contact:* Dr. Claudia Turro, Vice Chair, 614-292-6708, Fax: 614-292-1685, E-mail: turro.1@osu.edu.
Website: https://chemistry.osu.edu/

Ohio University, Graduate College, College of Arts and Sciences, Department of Chemistry and Biochemistry, Athens, OH 45701-2979. Offers MS, PhD. *Degree requirements:* For master's, comprehensive exam, thesis, exam; for doctorate, comprehensive exam, thesis/dissertation, exam. *Entrance requirements:* For master's and doctorate, GRE. Additional exam requirements/recommendations for international students: Required—TOEFL (minimum score 550 paper-based; 80 iBT) or IELTS (minimum score 6.5). Electronic applications accepted. *Faculty research:* Materials, RNA, synthesis, carbohydrate, mass spectrometry.

Oklahoma State University, College of Agricultural Science and Natural Resources, Department of Biochemistry and Molecular Biology, Stillwater, OK 74078. Offers MS, PhD. *Faculty:* 24 full-time (8 women), 3 part-time/adjunct (1 woman). *Students:* 4 full-time (2 women), 24 part-time (9 women); includes 5 minority (2 Asian, non-Hispanic/Latino; 2 Hispanic/Latino; 1 Two or more races, non-Hispanic/Latino), 15 international. Average age 28. 61 applicants, 7% accepted, 3 enrolled. In 2013, 7 master's, 4 doctorates awarded. *Degree requirements:* For master's, thesis, oral exam; for doctorate, comprehensive exam, thesis/dissertation. *Entrance requirements:* For master's and doctorate, GRE or GMAT. Additional exam requirements/recommendations for international students: Required—TOEFL (minimum score 550 paper-based; 79 iBT). *Application deadline:* For fall admission, 3/1 priority date for international students; for spring admission, 8/1 priority date for international students. Applications are processed on a rolling basis. Application fee: $40 ($75 for international students). Electronic applications accepted. *Expenses:* Tuition, state resident: full-time $4272; part-time $178 per credit hour. Tuition, nonresident: full-time $17,472; part-time $709 per credit hour. *Required fees:* $2413.20; $100.55 per credit hour. One-time fee: $50 full-time. Part-time tuition and fees vary according to course load and campus/location. *Financial support:* In 2013–14, 26 research assistantships (averaging $18,865 per year), 2 teaching assistantships (averaging $18,801 per year) were awarded; career-related internships or fieldwork, Federal Work-Study, scholarships/grants, health care benefits, tuition waivers (partial), and unspecified assistantships also available. Support available to part-time students. Financial award application deadline: 3/1; financial award applicants required to submit FAFSA. *Unit head:* Dr. John Gustafson, Department Head, 405-744-6189, Fax: 405-744-7799, E-mail: john.gustafson@okstate.edu.
Website: http://biochemistry.okstate.edu/

Old Dominion University, College of Sciences, Program in Chemistry, Norfolk, VA 23529. Offers analytical chemistry (MS); biochemistry (MS); chemistry (PhD); environmental chemistry (MS); organic chemistry (MS); physical chemistry (MS). Part-time and evening/weekend programs available. *Faculty:* 19 full-time (5 women). *Students:* 38 full-time (20 women), 3 part-time (all women); includes 3 minority (2 Black or African American, non-Hispanic/Latino; 1 Two or more races, non-Hispanic/Latino), 14 international. Average age 27. 35 applicants, 60% accepted, 8 enrolled. In 2013, 4 master's, 1 doctorate awarded. *Degree requirements:* For master's, comprehensive exam, thesis. *Entrance requirements:* For master's, GRE General Test, minimum GPA of 3.0 in major, 2.5 overall; for doctorate, GRE General Test. Additional exam requirements/recommendations for international students: Required—TOEFL. *Application deadline:* For fall admission, 7/1 for domestic students, 1/15 for international students; for spring admission, 11/1 for domestic students, 8/15 for international students. Applications are processed on a rolling basis. Application fee: $30. Electronic applications accepted. *Expenses:* Tuition, state resident: full-time $9888; part-time $412 per credit. Tuition, nonresident: full-time $25,152; part-time $1048 per credit. *Required fees:* $59 per semester. One-time fee: $50. *Financial support:* In 2013–14, 6 students received support, including fellowships (averaging $18,000 per year), research assistantships with tuition reimbursements available (averaging $21,000 per year), teaching assistantships with tuition reimbursements available (averaging $18,000 per year); career-related internships or fieldwork, scholarships/grants, and unspecified assistantships also available. Financial award application deadline: 2/15; financial award applicants required to submit FAFSA. *Faculty research:* Biogeochemistry, materials chemistry, computational chemistry, organic chemistry, biofuels. *Total annual research expenditures:* $2.6 million. *Unit head:* Dr. John Donat, Graduate Program Director, 757-683-4098, Fax: 757-683-4628, E-mail: chemgpd@odu.edu.

Oregon Health & Science University, School of Medicine, Graduate Programs in Medicine, Department of Environmental and Biomolecular Systems, Portland, OR 97239-3098. Offers biochemistry and molecular biology (MS, PhD); environmental science and engineering (MS, PhD). Part-time programs available. *Faculty:* 12 full-time (4 women), 2 part-time/adjunct (1 woman). *Students:* 27 full-time (18 women), 2 part-time (both women); includes 9 minority (1 Black or African American, non-Hispanic/Latino; 1 American Indian or Alaska Native, non-Hispanic/Latino; 1 Asian, non-Hispanic/Latino; 5 Hispanic/Latino; 1 Two or more races, non-Hispanic/Latino), 4 international. Average age 31. 24 applicants, 17% accepted, 4 enrolled. In 2013, 2 master's, 1 doctorate awarded. Terminal master's awarded for partial completion of doctoral program. *Degree requirements:* For master's, thesis (for some programs); for doctorate, comprehensive exam, thesis/dissertation, qualifying exam. *Entrance requirements:* For master's and doctorate, GRE General Test (minimum scores: 500 Verbal/600 Quantitative/4.5 Analytical) or MCAT (for some programs). Additional exam requirements/recommendations for international students: Required—TOEFL. *Application deadline:* For fall admission, 7/15 for domestic students, 5/15 for international students; for winter admission, 10/15 for domestic students, 9/15 for international students; for spring admission, 1/15 for domestic students, 12/15 for international students. Applications are processed on a rolling basis. Application fee: $70. Electronic applications accepted. *Financial support:* Health care benefits and full tuition and stipends (for PhD students) available. *Unit head:* Dr. Paul Tratnyek, Program Director, 503-748-1070, E-mail: info@ebs.ogi.edu. *Application contact:* Nancy Christie, Program Coordinator, 503-748-1070, E-mail: info@ebs.ogi.edu.

Oregon Health & Science University, School of Medicine, Graduate Programs in Medicine, Program in Molecular and Cellular Biosciences, Department of Biochemistry and Molecular Biology, Portland, OR 97239-3098. Offers PhD. *Faculty:* 10 full-time (2 women). *Students:* 10 full-time (4 women), 1 (woman) part-time, 2 international. Average age 28. In 2013, 1 doctorate awarded. *Degree requirements:* For doctorate, comprehensive exam, thesis/dissertation, qualifying exam. *Entrance requirements:* For doctorate, GRE General Test (minimum scores: 153 Verbal/148 Quantitative/4.5 Analytical). Additional exam requirements/recommendations for international students: Required—TOEFL. Electronic applications accepted. *Financial support:* Health care benefits, tuition waivers (full), and full tuition and stipends (for PhD students) available.

Faculty research: Protein structure, membrane proteins, metabolic regulation, molecular basis of disease, signal transduction mechanisms. *Unit head:* Dr. David Farrens, Program Director, 503-494-7781, E-mail: farrensd@ohsu.edu. *Application contact:* Valerie Scott, Administrative Coordinator, 503-494-8632, E-mail: wroblews@ohsu.edu.
Website: http://www.ohsu.edu/som-biochem/

Oregon State University, College of Science, Program in Biochemistry and Biophysics, Corvallis, OR 97331. Offers MA, MAIS, MS, PhD. *Faculty:* 17 full-time (6 women). *Students:* 27 full-time (12 women); includes 3 minority (1 Black or African American, non-Hispanic/Latino; 1 American Indian or Alaska Native, non-Hispanic/Latino; 1 Asian, non-Hispanic/Latino), 7 international. Average age 27. 23 applicants, 43% accepted, 7 enrolled. In 2013, 2 degrees awarded. *Degree requirements:* For master's, thesis optional; for doctorate, thesis/dissertation, exams. *Entrance requirements:* For master's and doctorate, GRE, minimum GPA of 3.0. Additional exam requirements/recommendations for international students: Required—TOEFL (minimum score 600 paper-based). *Application deadline:* For fall admission, 1/15 for domestic students. Application fee: $60. *Expenses:* Tuition, state resident: full-time $11,664; part-time $432 per credit hour. Tuition, nonresident: full-time $19,197; part-time $711 per credit hour. *Required fees:* $1446; $443 per quarter. One-time fee: $300. Tuition and fees vary according to course load and program. *Financial support:* Research assistantships, teaching assistantships, and institutionally sponsored loans available. Support available to part-time students. Financial award application deadline: 2/1. *Faculty research:* DNA and deoxyribonucleotide metabolism, cell growth control, receptors and membranes, protein structure and function. *Unit head:* Dr. Gary Merrill, Chair, 541-737-4511, Fax: 541-737-0481, E-mail: merrillg@science.oregonstate.edu. *Application contact:* Dr. Michael Freitag, Chair of Graduate Admissions, 541-737-4511, Fax: 541-737-0481, E-mail: freitagm@cgrb.oregonstate.edu.
Website: http://biochem.science.oregonstate.edu/about-graduate-program

Penn State Hershey Medical Center, College of Medicine, Graduate School Programs in the Biomedical Sciences, Graduate Program in Biomedical Sciences, Hershey, PA 17033. Offers biochemistry and molecular genetics (MS, PhD); biomedical sciences (MS, PhD); translational therapeutics (MS, PhD); virology and immunology (MS, PhD); MD/PhD; PhD/MBA. *Students:* 40 full-time (22 women); includes 7 minority (2 Black or African American, non-Hispanic/Latino; 2 Asian, non-Hispanic/Latino; 1 Hispanic/Latino; 2 Two or more races, non-Hispanic/Latino), 10 international. 215 applicants, 20% accepted, 14 enrolled. Terminal master's awarded for partial completion of doctoral program. *Degree requirements:* For master's, thesis (for some programs); for doctorate, comprehensive exam, thesis/dissertation, candidacy exam. *Entrance requirements:* For doctorate, GRE General Test. Additional exam requirements/recommendations for international students: Required—TOEFL (minimum score 550 paper-based; 80 iBT). *Application deadline:* For fall admission, 2/1 for domestic and international students. Applications are processed on a rolling basis. Application fee: $65. Electronic applications accepted. *Financial support:* In 2013–14, research assistantships (averaging $24,544 per year) were awarded; fellowships, scholarships/grants, health care benefits, and unspecified assistantships also available. Financial award applicants required to submit FAFSA. *Unit head:* Dr. Ralph L. Keil, Chair, 717-531-8595, Fax: 717-531-0388, E-mail: rlk9@psu.edu. *Application contact:* Kristin E. Smith, Enrollment Support Manager, 717-531-0003, Fax: 717-531-0388, E-mail: kec17@psu.edu.
Website: http://med.psu.edu/web/biomedical-sciences/home

Penn State University Park, Graduate School, Eberly College of Science, Department of Biochemistry and Molecular Biology, University Park, PA 16802. Offers biochemistry, microbiology, and molecular biology (MS, PhD); biotechnology (MBIOT). *Unit head:* Dr. Daniel J. Larson, Dean, 814-865-9591, Fax: 814-865-3634, E-mail: djlarson@psu.edu. *Application contact:* Cynthia E. Nicosia, Director, Graduate Enrollment Services, 814-865-1834, Fax: 814-863-4627, E-mail: cey1@psu.edu.
Website: http://bmb.psu.edu/

Purdue University, College of Pharmacy and Pharmacal Sciences and Graduate School, Graduate Programs in Pharmacy and Pharmacal Sciences, Department of Medicinal Chemistry and Molecular Pharmacology, West Lafayette, IN 47907. Offers biophysical and computational chemistry (PhD); cancer research (PhD); immunology and infectious disease (PhD); medicinal biochemistry and molecular biology (PhD); medicinal chemistry and chemical biology (PhD); molecular pharmacology (PhD); neuropharmacology, neurodegeneration, and neurotoxicity (PhD); systems biology and functional genomics (PhD). *Faculty:* 23 full-time (3 women), 6 part-time/adjunct (1 woman). *Students:* 50 full-time (21 women), 3 part-time (2 women); includes 1 minority (Asian, non-Hispanic/Latino), 30 international. Average age 26. 147 applicants, 20% accepted, 13 enrolled. In 2013, 12 doctorates awarded. *Degree requirements:* For doctorate, thesis/dissertation. *Entrance requirements:* For doctorate, GRE General Test; GRE Subject Test in biology, biochemistry, and chemistry (recommended), minimum undergraduate GPA of 3.0. Additional exam requirements/recommendations for international students: Required—TOEFL (minimum score 550 paper-based; 77 iBT); Recommended—TWE. *Application deadline:* For fall admission, 2/1 for domestic and international students. Applications are processed on a rolling basis. Application fee: $60 ($75 for international students). Electronic applications accepted. *Financial support:* Fellowships, research assistantships, teaching assistantships, and traineeships available. Support available to part-time students. Financial award applicants required to submit FAFSA. *Faculty research:* Drug design and development, cancer research, drug synthesis and analysis, chemical pharmacology, environmental toxicology. *Unit head:* Dr. Richard F. Borch, Head, 765-494-1403, E-mail: borch@purdue.edu. *Application contact:* Dr. Janine C. Mott, Graduate Contact, 765-494-1269, E-mail: jmott@purdue.edu.

Purdue University, Graduate School, College of Agriculture, Department of Biochemistry, West Lafayette, IN 47907. Offers MS, PhD. *Faculty:* 20 full-time (7 women). *Students:* 42 full-time (22 women); includes 4 minority (3 Asian, non-Hispanic/Latino; 1 Hispanic/Latino), 20 international. Average age 26. 80 applicants, 16% accepted, 6 enrolled. In 2013, 4 doctorates awarded. Terminal master's awarded for partial completion of doctoral program. *Degree requirements:* For doctorate, thesis/dissertation, preliminary and qualifying exams. *Entrance requirements:* For doctorate, GRE General Test, minimum undergraduate GPA of 3.0 or equivalent. Additional exam requirements/recommendations for international students: Required—TOEFL (minimum score 600 paper-based; 77 iBT). *Application deadline:* For fall admission, 1/15 priority date for domestic and international students; for spring admission, 9/30 for domestic and international students. Applications are processed on a rolling basis. Application fee: $60 ($75 for international students). Electronic applications accepted. *Financial support:* Fellowships, research assistantships, and teaching assistantships available. Support available to part-time students. Financial award application deadline: 4/15; financial award applicants required to submit FAFSA. *Faculty research:* Molecular biology and post-translational modifications of neuropeptides, membrane transport proteins. *Unit head:* Dr. Clint C. Chapple, Head, 765-494-0494, E-mail: chapple@purdue.edu. *Application contact:* Kristi L. Trimble, Graduate Contact for Admissions, 765-494-1636, E-mail: trimblek@purdue.edu.
Website: https://ag.purdue.edu/biochem

Purdue University, Graduate School, PULSe - Purdue University Life Sciences Program, West Lafayette, IN 47907. Offers biomolecular structure and biophysics (PhD); biotechnology (PhD); chemical biology (PhD); chromatin and regulation of gene expression (PhD); integrative neuroscience (PhD); integrative plant sciences (PhD); membrane biology (PhD); microbiology (PhD); molecular evolutionary and cancer biology (PhD); molecular evolutionary genetics (PhD); molecular virology (PhD). *Students:* 154 full-time (78 women), 1 part-time (0 women); includes 23 minority (5 Black or African American, non-Hispanic/Latino; 5 Asian, non-Hispanic/Latino; 10 Hispanic/Latino; 3 Two or more races, non-Hispanic/Latino), 73 international. Average age 26. 239 applicants, 33% accepted, 40 enrolled. *Entrance requirements:* For doctorate, GRE, minimum undergraduate GPA of 3.0. Additional exam requirements/recommendations for international students: Required—TOEFL (minimum score 550 paper-based; 77 iBT). *Application deadline:* For fall admission, 1/15 priority date for domestic and international students. Applications are processed on a rolling basis. Application fee: $60 ($75 for international students). Electronic applications accepted. *Financial support:* In 2013–14, research assistantships with tuition reimbursements (averaging $22,500 per year), teaching assistantships with tuition reimbursements (averaging $22,500 per year) were awarded. *Unit head:* Dr. Christine A. Hrycyna, Head, 765-494-7322, E-mail: hrycyna@purdue.edu. *Application contact:* Colleen Gabauer, Graduate Contact, 765-494-9256, E-mail: cgabauer@purdue.edu.
Website: http://www.gradschool.purdue.edu/pulse

Queens College of the City University of New York, Division of Graduate Studies, Mathematics and Natural Sciences Division, Department of Chemistry and Biochemistry, Flushing, NY 11367-1597. Offers biochemistry (MA); chemistry (MA). Part-time and evening/weekend programs available. *Degree requirements:* For master's, comprehensive exam. *Entrance requirements:* For master's, GRE, previous course work in calculus and physics, minimum GPA of 3.0. Additional exam requirements/recommendations for international students: Required—TOEFL.

Queen's University at Kingston, School of Graduate Studies, Faculty of Health Sciences, Department of Biochemistry, Kingston, ON K7L 3N6, Canada. Offers M Sc, PhD. Part-time programs available. *Degree requirements:* For master's, thesis, research proposal; for doctorate, comprehensive exam, thesis/dissertation, research proposal. *Entrance requirements:* For master's, GRE (if undergraduate degree is not from a Canadian University); for doctorate, GRE required if undergraduate degree is not from a Canadian University. Additional exam requirements/recommendations for international students: Required—TOEFL (minimum score 580 paper-based). Electronic applications accepted. *Faculty research:* Gene expression, protein structure, enzyme activity, signal transduction.

Rensselaer Polytechnic Institute, Graduate School, School of Science, Program in Biochemistry and Biophysics, Troy, NY 12180-3590. Offers MS, PhD. *Faculty:* 8 full-time (7 women). *Students:* 8 full-time (3 women), 1 international. Average age 28. 40 applicants, 15% accepted, 1 enrolled. In 2013, 1 doctorate awarded. Terminal master's awarded for partial completion of doctoral program. *Degree requirements:* For master's, thesis optional; for doctorate, comprehensive exam, thesis/dissertation. *Entrance requirements:* For master's and doctorate, GRE. Additional exam requirements/recommendations for international students: Required—TOEFL (minimum score 600 paper-based; 100 iBT), IELTS (minimum score 7), PTE (minimum score 68). *Application deadline:* For fall admission, 1/1 priority date for domestic and international students; for spring admission, 8/15 priority date for domestic and international students. Applications are processed on a rolling basis. Application fee: $75. Electronic applications accepted. *Expenses: Tuition:* Full-time $45,100; part-time $1879 per credit hour. *Required fees:* $1983. *Financial support:* In 2013–14, 6 students received support, including research assistantships (averaging $18,500 per year), teaching assistantships (averaging $18,500 per year); fellowships also available. Financial award application deadline: 1/1. *Faculty research:* Biochemistry; bioinformatics; biophysics; cancer biology; computational biology; molecular, cell, and developmental biology; neuroscience; protein folding; stem cells; structural biology. *Total annual research expenditures:* $1.2 million. *Unit head:* Dr. Chunyu Wang, Graduate Program Director, 518-276-3497, E-mail: wangc5@rpi.edu. *Application contact:* Office of Graduate Admissions, 518-276-6216, E-mail: gradadmissions@rpi.edu.
Website: http://www.rpi.edu/dept/bcbp/

Rice University, Graduate Programs, Wiess School of Natural Sciences, Department of Biochemistry and Cell Biology, Houston, TX 77251-1892. Offers MA, PhD. Terminal master's awarded for partial completion of doctoral program. *Degree requirements:* For master's, thesis; for doctorate, thesis/dissertation. *Entrance requirements:* For master's and doctorate, GRE. Additional exam requirements/recommendations for international students: Required—TOEFL (minimum score 600 paper-based; 90 iBT). Electronic applications accepted. *Expenses:* Contact institution. *Faculty research:* Steroid metabolism, protein structure NMR, biophysics, cell growth and movement.

Rosalind Franklin University of Medicine and Science, School of Graduate and Postdoctoral Studies - Interdisciplinary Graduate Program in Biomedical Sciences, Department of Biochemistry and Molecular Biology, North Chicago, IL 60064-3095. Offers MS, PhD, MD/PhD. Terminal master's awarded for partial completion of doctoral program. *Degree requirements:* For master's, comprehensive exam, thesis; for doctorate, comprehensive exam, thesis/dissertation. *Entrance requirements:* For master's and doctorate, GRE General Test, minimum GPA of 3.0. Additional exam requirements/recommendations for international students: Required—TOEFL, TWE. Electronic applications accepted. *Faculty research:* Structure of control enzymes, extracellular matrix, glucose metabolism, gene expression, ATP synthesis.

Rush University, Graduate College, Division of Biochemistry, Chicago, IL 60612-3832. Offers MS, PhD, MD/PhD. *Degree requirements:* For doctorate, thesis/dissertation, preliminary exam. *Entrance requirements:* For doctorate, GRE General Test. Additional exam requirements/recommendations for international students: Required—TOEFL. Electronic applications accepted. *Faculty research:* Biochemistry of extracellular matrix, connective tissue biosynthesis and degradation, molecular biology of connective tissue components, cartilage, arthritis.

Rutgers, The State University of New Jersey, Newark, Graduate School of Biomedical Sciences, Department of Biochemistry and Molecular Biology, Newark, NJ 07107. Offers MS, PhD. *Degree requirements:* For master's, thesis; for doctorate, thesis/dissertation, qualifying exam. *Entrance requirements:* For master's and doctorate, GRE General Test. Additional exam requirements/recommendations for international students: Required—TOEFL. Electronic applications accepted.

Rutgers, The State University of New Jersey, Newark, Graduate School, Program in Chemistry, Newark, NJ 07102. Offers analytical chemistry (MS, PhD); biochemistry (MS, PhD); inorganic chemistry (MS, PhD); organic chemistry (MS, PhD); physical chemistry (MS, PhD). Part-time and evening/weekend programs available. Terminal master's awarded for partial completion of doctoral program. *Degree requirements:* For master's, thesis optional, cumulative exams; for doctorate, thesis/dissertation, exams, research proposal. *Entrance requirements:* For master's and doctorate, GRE General Test, minimum undergraduate B average. Additional exam requirements/recommendations for international students: Required—TOEFL. Electronic applications accepted. *Faculty research:* Medicinal chemistry, natural products, isotope effects, biophysics and biorganic approaches to enzyme mechanisms, organic and organometallic synthesis.

Biochemistry

Rutgers, The State University of New Jersey, New Brunswick, Graduate School-New Brunswick, Department of Chemistry and Chemical Biology, Piscataway, NJ 08854-8097. Offers biological chemistry (MS, PhD); inorganic chemistry (MS, PhD); organic chemistry (MS, PhD); physical chemistry (MS, PhD). Part-time and evening/weekend programs available. Terminal master's awarded for partial completion of doctoral program. *Degree requirements:* For master's, thesis or alternative, exam; for doctorate, thesis/dissertation, 1 year residency. *Entrance requirements:* For master's and doctorate, GRE General Test, GRE Subject Test. Additional exam requirements/recommendations for international students: Required—TOEFL. Electronic applications accepted. *Faculty research:* Biophysical organic/bioorganic, inorganic/bioinorganic, theoretical, and solid-state/surface chemistry.

Rutgers, The State University of New Jersey, New Brunswick, Graduate School-New Brunswick, Programs in the Molecular Biosciences, Piscataway, NJ 08854-8097. Offers biochemistry (PhD); cell and developmental biology (MS, PhD); microbiology and molecular genetics (MS, PhD), including applied microbiology, clinical microbiology (MS), clinical mircobiology (PhD), computational molecular biology (PhD), immunology, microbial biochemistry, molecular genetics, virology. MS, PhD offered jointly with University of Medicine and Dentistry of New Jersey.

Rutgers, The State University of New Jersey, New Brunswick, Graduate School of Biomedical Sciences, Program in Biochemistry, Piscataway, NJ 08854-5635. Offers MS, PhD, MD/PhD. PhD, MS offered jointly with Rutgers, The State University of New Jersey, New Brunswick. Terminal master's awarded for partial completion of doctoral program. *Degree requirements:* For master's, thesis, qualifying exam; for doctorate, thesis/dissertation, qualifying exam. *Entrance requirements:* For master's and doctorate, GRE General Test. Additional exam requirements/recommendations for international students: Required—TOEFL. Electronic applications accepted. *Faculty research:* Signal transduction, regulation of RNA, polymerase II transcribed genes, developmental gene expression.

Saint Louis University, Graduate Education and School of Medicine, Graduate Program in Biomedical Sciences and Graduate Education, Department of Biochemistry and Molecular Biology, St. Louis, MO 63103-2097. Offers PhD. *Degree requirements:* For doctorate, comprehensive exam, thesis/dissertation, departmental qualifying exams. *Entrance requirements:* For doctorate, GRE General Test, GRE Subject Test (optional), letters of recommendation, resume, interview. Additional exam requirements/recommendations for international students: Required—TOEFL (minimum score 525 paper-based). Electronic applications accepted. *Faculty research:* Transcription, chromatin modification and regulation of gene expression; structure/function of proteins and enzymes, including x-ray crystallography; inflammatory mediators in pathenogenesis of diabetes and arteriosclerosis; cellular signaling in response to growth factors, opiates and angiogenic mediators; genomics and proteomics of Cryptococcus neoformans.

San Diego State University, Graduate and Research Affairs, College of Sciences, Department of Chemistry and Biochemistry, San Diego, CA 92182. Offers MA, MS, PhD. PhD offered jointly with University of California, San Diego. Terminal master's awarded for partial completion of doctoral program. *Degree requirements:* For doctorate, thesis/dissertation. *Entrance requirements:* For master's, GRE General Test, bachelor's degree in related field, 3 letters of reference; for doctorate, GRE General Test, GRE Subject Test. Additional exam requirements/recommendations for international students: Required—TOEFL. Electronic applications accepted. *Faculty research:* Nonlinear, laser, and electrochemistry; surface reaction dynamics; catalysis, synthesis, and organometallics; proteins, enzymology, and gene expression regulation.

San Francisco State University, Division of Graduate Studies, College of Science and Engineering, Department of Chemistry and Biochemistry, San Francisco, CA 94132-1722. Offers chemistry (MS), including biochemistry. Part-time programs available. *Application deadline:* Applications are processed on a rolling basis. Electronic applications accepted. *Unit head:* Dr. Jane DeWitt, Chair, 415-338-1288, Fax: 415-338-2384, E-mail: gradchem@sfsu.edu. *Application contact:* Dr. Andrew Ichimura, Graduate Coordinator, 415-405-0721, Fax: 415-338-2384, E-mail: ichimura@sfsu.edu.
Website: http://www.chembiochem.sfsu.edu/0home/0layout.php

Seton Hall University, College of Arts and Sciences, Department of Chemistry and Biochemistry, South Orange, NJ 07079-2697. Offers analytical chemistry (MS, PhD); biochemistry (MS, PhD); chemistry (MS); inorganic chemistry (MS, PhD); organic chemistry (MS, PhD); physical chemistry (MS, PhD). Part-time and evening/weekend programs available. Terminal master's awarded for partial completion of doctoral program. *Degree requirements:* For master's, thesis optional; for doctorate, comprehensive exam, thesis/dissertation. *Entrance requirements:* Additional exam requirements/recommendations for international students: Required—TOEFL. Electronic applications accepted. *Faculty research:* DNA metal reactions; chromatography; bioinorganic, biophysical, organometallic, polymer chemistry; heterogeneous catalyst; synthetic organic and carbohydrate chemistry.

Simon Fraser University, Office of Graduate Studies, Faculty of Science, Department of Molecular Biology and Biochemistry, Burnaby, BC V5A 1S6, Canada. Offers bioinformatics (Graduate Diploma); molecular biology and biochemistry (M Sc, PhD). *Faculty:* 29 full-time (10 women). *Students:* 75 full-time (40 women). 12 applicants, 75% accepted, 8 enrolled. In 2013, 13 master's, 12 doctorates awarded. *Degree requirements:* For master's, thesis; for doctorate, thesis/dissertation; for Graduate Diploma, practicum. *Entrance requirements:* For master's, minimum GPA of 3.0 (on scale of 4.33), or 3.33 based on last 60 credits of undergraduate courses; for doctorate, minimum GPA of 3.5; for Graduate Diploma, minimum GPA of 2.5 (on scale of 4.33), or 2.67 based on the last 60 credits of undergraduate courses. Additional exam requirements/recommendations for international students: Recommended—TOEFL (minimum score 580 paper-based; 100 iBT), IELTS (minimum score 7.5), TWE (minimum score 5). *Application deadline:* Applications are processed on a rolling basis. Application fee: $90 ($125 for international students). Electronic applications accepted. *Expenses: Tuition, area resident:* Full-time $5084 Canadian dollars. *Required fees:* $840 Canadian dollars. *Financial support:* In 2013–14, 45 students received support, including 48 fellowships (averaging $6,250 per year), teaching assistantships (averaging $5,608 per year); research assistantships and scholarships/grants also available. *Faculty research:* Genomics and bioinformatics, cell and developmental biology, structural biology/biochemistry, immunology, nucleic acid function. *Unit head:* Dr. Michel Leroux, Graduate Chair, 778-782-6683, Fax: 778-782-5583, E-mail: mbb-grad-chair@sfu.ca. *Application contact:* Mimi Fourie, Graduate Secretary, 778-782-5631, Fax: 778-782-5583, E-mail: mbb@sfu.ca.
Website: http://www.sfu.ca/mbb

Sonoma State University, School of Science and Technology, Department of Biology, Rohnert Park, CA 94928. Offers biochemistry (MA); ecology (MS); environmental biology (MS); evolutionary biology (MS); functional morphology (MS); molecular and cell biology (MS); organismal biology (MS). Part-time programs available. *Faculty:* 9 full-time (1 woman). *Students:* 4 full-time (2 women), 21 part-time (14 women); includes 5 minority (1 American Indian or Alaska Native, non-Hispanic/Latino; 1 Asian, non-Hispanic/Latino; 2 Hispanic/Latino; 1 Two or more races, non-Hispanic/Latino), 2 international. Average age 29. 23 applicants, 65% accepted, 6 enrolled. In 2013, 6 master's awarded. *Degree requirements:* For master's, thesis or alternative, oral exam. *Entrance requirements:* For master's, GRE General Test, GRE Subject Test, minimum GPA of 3.0. Additional exam requirements/recommendations for international students: Required—TOEFL (minimum score 500 paper-based). *Application deadline:* For fall admission, 11/30 for domestic students. Applications are processed on a rolling basis. Application fee: $55. *Expenses:* Tuition, state resident: full-time $8500. Tuition, nonresident: full-time $12,964. *Required fees:* $1762. *Financial support:* In 2013–14, 1 fellowship (averaging $1,520 per year), 6 research assistantships (averaging $3,562 per year), 22 teaching assistantships (averaging $6,738 per year) were awarded; career-related internships or fieldwork, Federal Work-Study, and tuition waivers (full) also available. Financial award application deadline: 3/2; financial award applicants required to submit FAFSA. *Faculty research:* Plant physiology, comparative physiology, community ecology, restoration ecology, marine ecology, conservation genetics, primate behavior, behavioral ecology, developmental biology, plant and animal systematics. *Total annual research expenditures:* $4,400. *Unit head:* Dr. Nathan Rank, Chair, 707-664-3053, E-mail: nathan.rank@sonoma.edu. *Application contact:* Dr. Derek Girman, Graduate Adviser, 707-664-3055, E-mail: derek.girman@sonoma.edu.
Website: http://www.sonoma.edu/biology/graduate

Southern Illinois University Carbondale, Graduate School, College of Science, Department of Chemistry and Biochemistry, Carbondale, IL 62901-4701. Offers MS, PhD. Part-time programs available. *Faculty:* 18 full-time (1 woman), 2 part-time/adjunct (0 women). *Students:* 42 full-time (17 women), 16 part-time (8 women); includes 2 minority (both Asian, non-Hispanic/Latino), 37 international. Average age 25. 29 applicants, 17% accepted, 4 enrolled. In 2013, 3 master's, 3 doctorates awarded. Terminal master's awarded for partial completion of doctoral program. *Degree requirements:* For master's, one foreign language, thesis; for doctorate, variable foreign language requirement, thesis/dissertation. *Entrance requirements:* For master's, minimum GPA of 2.7; for doctorate, GRE General Test, minimum GPA of 3.25. Additional exam requirements/recommendations for international students: Required—TOEFL. *Application deadline:* Applications are processed on a rolling basis. Application fee: $50. *Financial support:* In 2013–14, 17 research assistantships with full tuition reimbursements, 23 teaching assistantships with full tuition reimbursements were awarded; fellowships with full tuition reimbursements, Federal Work-Study, institutionally sponsored loans, and tuition waivers (full) also available. Support available to part-time students. *Faculty research:* Materials, separations, computational chemistry, synthetics. *Total annual research expenditures:* $1 million. *Unit head:* Gary Kinsel, Chair, 618-453-6482, Fax: 618-453-6408. *Application contact:* Doug Coons, Office Specialist, 618-453-6496, Fax: 618-453-6408, E-mail: dcoons@chem.siu.edu.

Southern Illinois University Carbondale, Graduate School, College of Science, Program in Molecular Biology, Microbiology, and Biochemistry, Carbondale, IL 62901-4701. Offers MS, PhD. *Faculty:* 16 full-time (2 women). *Students:* 40 full-time (27 women), 39 part-time (21 women); includes 6 minority (2 Black or African American, non-Hispanic/Latino; 4 Asian, non-Hispanic/Latino), 50 international. Average age 25. 143 applicants, 6% accepted, 5 enrolled. In 2013, 5 master's, 4 doctorates awarded. *Degree requirements:* For master's, thesis; for doctorate, thesis/dissertation. *Entrance requirements:* For master's, GRE, minimum GPA of 2.7; for doctorate, GRE, minimum GPA of 3.25. Additional exam requirements/recommendations for international students: Required—TOEFL. *Application deadline:* Applications are processed on a rolling basis. Application fee: $50. *Financial support:* In 2013–14, 40 students received support, including 3 fellowships with full tuition reimbursements available, 24 research assistantships with full tuition reimbursements available, 12 teaching assistantships with full tuition reimbursements available; Federal Work-Study and institutionally sponsored loans also available. Support available to part-time students. Financial award application deadline: 3/1. *Faculty research:* Prokaryotic gene regulation and expression; eukaryotic gene regulation; microbial, phylogenetic, and metabolic diversity; immune responses to tumors, pathogens, and autoantigens; protein folding and structure. *Unit head:* Dr. Judy Davie, Director, 618-453-5002, E-mail: jdavie@siumed.edu. *Application contact:* Cindy Filla, Office Systems Specialist, 618-453-8911, E-mail: cfilla@siumed.edu.
Website: http://mbmb.siu.edu/

Southern University and Agricultural and Mechanical College, Graduate School, College of Sciences, Department of Chemistry, Baton Rouge, LA 70813. Offers analytical chemistry (MS); biochemistry (MS); environmental sciences (MS); inorganic chemistry (MS); organic chemistry (MS); physical chemistry (MS). *Degree requirements:* For master's, thesis. *Entrance requirements:* For master's, GMAT or GRE General Test. Additional exam requirements/recommendations for international students: Required—TOEFL (minimum score 525 paper-based). *Faculty research:* Synthesis of macrocyclic ligands, latex accelerators, anticancer drugs, biosensors, absorption isotheums, isolation of specific enzymes from plants.

Stanford University, School of Medicine, Graduate Programs in Medicine, Department of Biochemistry, Stanford, CA 94305-9991. Offers PhD. *Degree requirements:* For doctorate, thesis/dissertation. *Entrance requirements:* For doctorate, GRE General Test, GRE Subject Test (biology or chemistry). Additional exam requirements/recommendations for international students: Required—TOEFL. Electronic applications accepted. *Expenses: Tuition:* Full-time $42,690; part-time $949 per credit. *Required fees:* $185. *Faculty research:* DNA replication, recombination, and gene regulation; methods of isolating, analyzing, and altering genes and genomes; protein structure, protein folding, and protein processing; protein targeting and transport in the cell; intercellular signaling.

Stanford University, School of Medicine, Graduate Programs in Medicine, Department of Chemical and Systems Biology, Stanford, CA 94305-9991. Offers PhD. *Degree requirements:* For doctorate, thesis/dissertation, qualifying examination. *Entrance requirements:* For doctorate, GRE General Test, GRE Subject Test. Additional exam requirements/recommendations for international students: Required—TOEFL. Electronic applications accepted. *Expenses: Tuition:* Full-time $42,690; part-time $949 per credit. *Required fees:* $185. *Faculty research:* Action of drugs such as epinephrine, cell differentiation and development, microsomal enzymes, neuropeptide gene expression.

State University of New York College of Environmental Science and Forestry, Department of Chemistry, Syracuse, NY 13210-2779. Offers biochemistry (MPS, MS, PhD); environmental chemistry (MPS, MS, PhD); organic chemistry of natural products (MPS, MS, PhD); polymer chemistry (MPS, MS, PhD). *Faculty:* 17 full-time (2 women). *Students:* 42 full-time (23 women), 2 part-time (1 woman); includes 14 minority (2 Black or African American, non-Hispanic/Latino; 12 Asian, non-Hispanic/Latino). 43 applicants, 65% accepted, 5 enrolled. In 2013, 7 master's, 4 doctorates awarded. *Degree requirements:* For master's, thesis; for doctorate, comprehensive exam, thesis/dissertation. *Entrance requirements:* For master's and doctorate, GRE General Test, GRE Subject Test, minimum GPA of 3.0. Additional exam requirements/recommendations for international students: Required—TOEFL (minimum score 550 paper-based; 80 iBT), IELTS (minimum score 6). *Application deadline:* For fall admission, 2/1 priority date for domestic and international students; for spring admission, 11/1 priority date for domestic and international students. Applications are processed on a rolling basis. Application fee: $60. Electronic applications accepted. *Expenses:* Tuition, state resident: full-time $10,370; part-time $432 per credit hour.

Tuition, nonresident: full-time $20,190; part-time $841 per credit hour. *Required fees:* $44 per credit hour. *Financial support:* In 2013–14, 40 students received support, including 5 fellowships with full tuition reimbursements available (averaging $4,000 per year), 19 research assistantships with full tuition reimbursements available (averaging $20,000 per year), 44 teaching assistantships with full tuition reimbursements available (averaging $21,300 per year); Federal Work-Study, institutionally sponsored loans, scholarships/grants, health care benefits, unspecified assistantships, and departmental tuition assistance also available. Financial award application deadline: 6/30; financial award applicants required to submit FAFSA. *Faculty research:* Polymer chemistry, biochemistry, environmental chemistry, natural products chemistry. *Total annual research expenditures:* $1.8 million. *Unit head:* Prof. Gregory Boyer, Chair, 315-470-6825, Fax: 315-470-6856, E-mail: glboyer@esf.edu. *Application contact:* Scott Shannon, Associate Provost for Instruction/Dean of the Graduate School, 315-470-6599, Fax: 315-470-6978, E-mail: sshannon@esf.edu.
Website: http://www.esf.edu/chemistry

State University of New York Upstate Medical University, College of Graduate Studies, Program in Biochemistry and Molecular Biology, Syracuse, NY 13210-2334. Offers biochemistry (MS); biochemistry and molecular biology (PhD); MD/PhD. Terminal master's awarded for partial completion of doctoral program. *Degree requirements:* For master's, thesis; for doctorate, comprehensive exam, thesis/dissertation. *Entrance requirements:* For master's, GRE General Test, interview; for doctorate, GRE General Test, telephone interview. Additional exam requirements/recommendations for international students: Required—TOEFL. Electronic applications accepted. *Faculty research:* Enzymology, membrane structure and functions, developmental biochemistry.

Stevens Institute of Technology, Graduate School, Charles V. Schaefer Jr. School of Engineering, Department of Chemistry, Chemical Biology and Biomedical Engineering, Hoboken, NJ 07030. Offers analytical chemistry (PhD, Certificate); bioinformatics (PhD, Certificate); biomedical chemistry (Certificate); biomedical engineering (M Eng, Certificate); chemical biology (MS, PhD, Certificate); chemical physiology (Certificate); chemistry (MS, PhD); organic chemistry (PhD); physical chemistry (PhD); polymer chemistry (PhD, Certificate). Part-time and evening/weekend programs available. Postbaccalaureate distance learning degree programs offered (no on-campus study). Terminal master's awarded for partial completion of doctoral program. *Degree requirements:* For master's, thesis or alternative; for doctorate, one foreign language, thesis/dissertation; for Certificate, project or thesis. *Entrance requirements:* Additional exam requirements/recommendations for international students: Required—TOEFL. Electronic applications accepted. *Faculty research:* Biochemical reaction engineering, polymerization engineering, reactor design, biochemical process control and synthesis.

Stony Brook University, State University of New York, Graduate School, College of Arts and Sciences, Department of Biochemistry and Cell Biology, Biochemistry and Cell Biology Program, Stony Brook, NY 11794. Offers MS. Part-time programs available. *Students:* 25 full-time (14 women), 2 part-time (1 woman); includes 7 minority (4 Asian, non-Hispanic/Latino; 2 Hispanic/Latino; 1 Two or more races, non-Hispanic/Latino), 6 international. 125 applicants, 14% accepted, 13 enrolled. In 2013, 7 master's awarded. *Degree requirements:* For master's, thesis. *Entrance requirements:* For master's, three letters of recommendation, BS or BA in a life science related field with minimum B average, personal statement. Additional exam requirements/recommendations for international students: Required—TOEFL (minimum score 550 paper-based; 90 iBT). *Application deadline:* For fall admission, 4/1 for domestic and international students. Applications are processed on a rolling basis. Electronic applications accepted. *Expenses:* Tuition, state resident: full-time $9870; part-time $411 per credit. Tuition, nonresident: full-time $18,350; part-time $765 per credit. *Unit head:* Prof. Robert Haltiwanger, Director, 631-632-7336, Fax: 631-632-9730, E-mail: robert.haltiwanger@stonybrook.edu. *Application contact:* Diana Berger, Coordinator, 631-632-8585, Fax: 631-632-9730, E-mail: diana.berger@stonybrook.edu.
Website: http://www.stonybrook.edu/commcms/biochem/education/graduate/overview.html

Stony Brook University, State University of New York, Graduate School, College of Arts and Sciences, Department of Biochemistry and Cell Biology, Molecular and Cellular Biology Program, Stony Brook, NY 11794. Offers biochemistry and molecular biology (PhD); biological sciences (MA); immunology and pathology (PhD); molecular and cellular biology (PhD). *Faculty:* 23 full-time (7 women), 1 part-time/adjunct (0 women). *Students:* 75 full-time (42 women); includes 7 minority (5 Asian, non-Hispanic/Latino; 2 Hispanic/Latino), 46 international. Average age 30. 211 applicants, 15% accepted, 8 enrolled. In 2013, 13 master's, 15 doctorates awarded. *Degree requirements:* For doctorate, comprehensive exam, thesis/dissertation, teaching experience. *Entrance requirements:* For doctorate, GRE General Test, GRE Subject Test. Additional exam requirements/recommendations for international students: Required—TOEFL. *Application deadline:* For fall admission, 1/15 for domestic students; for spring admission, 10/1 for domestic students. Application fee: $100. *Expenses:* Tuition, state resident: full-time $9870; part-time $411 per credit. Tuition, nonresident: full-time $18,350; part-time $765 per credit. *Financial support:* In 2013–14, 22 fellowships, 18 research assistantships, 12 teaching assistantships were awarded; Federal Work-Study also available. *Unit head:* Prof. Robert Haltiwanger, Chair, 631-632-8560, E-mail: robert.haltiwanger@stonybrook.edu. *Application contact:* Joann DeLucia-Conlon, Coordinator, 631-632-8613, Fax: 631-632-9730, E-mail: joann.delucia-conlon@stonybrook.edu.

Stony Brook University, State University of New York, Graduate School, College of Arts and Sciences, Department of Biochemistry and Cell Biology, Program in Biochemistry and Structural Biology, Stony Brook, NY 11794. Offers PhD. *Students:* 32 full-time (11 women); includes 4 minority (1 Asian, non-Hispanic/Latino; 2 Hispanic/Latino; 1 Native Hawaiian or other Pacific Islander, non-Hispanic/Latino), 14 international. Average age 27. 57 applicants, 30% accepted, 13 enrolled. In 2013, 7 doctorates awarded. *Entrance requirements:* For doctorate, GRE. Additional exam requirements/recommendations for international students: Required—TOEFL. *Application deadline:* For fall admission, 1/15 for domestic students; for spring admission, 10/1 for domestic students. Application fee: $100. *Expenses:* Tuition, state resident: full-time $9870; part-time $411 per credit. Tuition, nonresident: full-time $18,350; part-time $765 per credit. *Financial support:* In 2013–14, 4 fellowships, 25 research assistantships, 5 teaching assistantships were awarded. *Unit head:* Prof. Robert Haltiwanger, Chair, 631-632-7336, Fax: 631-632-9730, E-mail: robert.haltiwanger@stonybrook.edu. *Application contact:* Joann DeLucia-Conlon, 631-632-8613, Fax: 631-632-8575, E-mail: joann.delucia-conlon@stonybrook.edu.
Website: http://www.stonybrook.edu/commcms/biochem/education/graduate/overview.html

Syracuse University, College of Arts and Sciences, Program in Structural Biology, Biochemistry and Biophysics, Syracuse, NY 13244. Offers PhD. *Students:* 3 full-time (1 woman), 1 part-time (0 women), 1 international. Average age 33. 4 applicants, 25% accepted. In 2013, 2 doctorates awarded. *Degree requirements:* For doctorate, comprehensive exam, thesis/dissertation. *Entrance requirements:* For doctorate, GRE General Test, GRE Subject Test. Additional exam requirements/recommendations for international students: Required—TOEFL (minimum score 100 iBT). *Application deadline:* For fall admission, 12/15 priority date for domestic and international students. Application fee: $75. Electronic applications accepted. *Financial support:* Fellowships with full tuition reimbursements, research assistantships with full and partial tuition reimbursements, teaching assistantships with full and partial tuition reimbursements, and tuition waivers available. Financial award application deadline: 1/1; financial award applicants required to submit FAFSA. *Unit head:* Prof. Liviu Movileanu, Director of Graduate Studies, 315-443-8078, Fax: 315-443-2012, E-mail: lmovilea@syr.edu.
Website: http://sb3.syr.edu/

Texas A&M University, College of Agriculture and Life Sciences, Department of Biochemistry and Biophysics, College Station, TX 77843. Offers biochemistry (MS, PhD). *Faculty:* 32. *Students:* 140 full-time (61 women), 8 part-time (4 women); includes 17 minority (5 Black or African American, non-Hispanic/Latino; 3 Asian, non-Hispanic/Latino; 8 Hispanic/Latino; 1 Two or more races, non-Hispanic/Latino), 43 international. Average age 28. 129 applicants, 41% accepted, 37 enrolled. In 2013, 12 master's, 11 doctorates awarded. *Entrance requirements:* For master's and doctorate, GRE General Test. Additional exam requirements/recommendations for international students: Required—TOEFL. *Application deadline:* For fall admission, 2/1 priority date for domestic students, 12/1 priority date for international students. Applications are processed on a rolling basis. Application fee: $50 ($75 for international students). Electronic applications accepted. *Expenses:* Tuition, state resident: full-time $4078; part-time $226.55 per credit hour. Tuition, nonresident: full-time $10,450; part-time $580.55 per credit hour. *Required fees:* $2328; $278.50 per credit hour. $642.45 per semester. *Financial support:* In 2013–14, 6 fellowships with tuition reimbursements (averaging $20,000 per year), 70 research assistantships with partial tuition reimbursements (averaging $20,000 per year) were awarded; teaching assistantships with partial tuition reimbursements, institutionally sponsored loans, scholarships/grants, traineeships, and unspecified assistantships also available. Financial award application deadline: 2/1; financial award applicants required to submit FAFSA. *Faculty research:* Enzymology, gene expression, protein structure, plant biochemistry. *Unit head:* Dr. Gregory D. Reinhart, Department Head, 979-862-2263, Fax: 979-845-9274, E-mail: gdr@tamu.edu. *Application contact:* Rafael Almanzar, Graduate Advisor, 979-845-1779, Fax: 979-845-9274.
Website: http://biochemistry.tamu.edu/

Texas Christian University, College of Science and Engineering, Department of Chemistry, Fort Worth, TX 76129. Offers biochemistry (MS, PhD); chemistry (MA); inorganic chemistry (MS, PhD); organic chemistry (MS, PhD); physical chemistry (MS, PhD). Part-time programs available. *Faculty:* 11 full-time (2 women). *Students:* 25 part-time (12 women); includes 2 minority (1 Asian, non-Hispanic/Latino; 1 Hispanic/Latino), 13 international. Average age 28. 19 applicants, 21% accepted, 2 enrolled. In 2013, 3 doctorates awarded. *Degree requirements:* For master's, thesis; for doctorate, thesis/dissertation, literature seminar, cumulative exams, research progress report, original proposal. *Entrance requirements:* For master's and doctorate, GRE General Test. Additional exam requirements/recommendations for international students: Required—TOEFL (minimum score 80 iBT). *Application deadline:* For fall admission, 2/1 priority date for domestic and international students; for spring admission, 9/1 priority date for domestic and international students. Application fee: $60. Electronic applications accepted. *Expenses: Tuition:* Part-time $1270 per credit hour. Tuition and fees vary according to course load and program. *Financial support:* In 2013–14, 16 students received support, including 16 teaching assistantships with full tuition reimbursements available; tuition waivers (full and partial) and unspecified assistantships also available. Financial award application deadline: 2/1. *Faculty research:* Phase transitions and transport properties of bio/macromolecular solutions, nanoscale biomaterials, electronic structure theory, synthetic methodology and total synthesis of natural products, chemistry and biology of (bio)polymers. *Unit head:* Dr. Robert Neilson, Chairperson/Professor, 817-257-7345, Fax: 817-257-5851, E-mail: r.neilson@tcu.edu. *Application contact:* Dr. Sergei V. Dzyuba, Director of Graduate Studies/Assistant Professor, 817-257-6218, Fax: 817-257-5851, E-mail: s.dzyuba@tcu.edu.
Website: http://www.chm.tcu.edu/

Texas State University, Graduate School, College of Science and Engineering, Department of Chemistry and Biochemistry, Program in Biochemistry, San Marcos, TX 78666. Offers MS. *Faculty:* 7 full-time (4 women). *Students:* 17 full-time (8 women), 6 part-time (2 women); includes 9 minority (1 Black or African American, non-Hispanic/Latino; 2 Asian, non-Hispanic/Latino; 5 Hispanic/Latino; 1 Two or more races, non-Hispanic/Latino), 3 international. Average age 27. 22 applicants, 64% accepted, 9 enrolled. In 2013, 6 master's awarded. *Degree requirements:* For master's, thesis. *Entrance requirements:* For master's, minimum GPA of 2.75 in last 60 hours of course work. Additional exam requirements/recommendations for international students: Required—TOEFL (minimum score 550 paper-based; 78 iBT). *Application deadline:* For fall admission, 6/15 priority date for domestic students, 6/1 priority date for international students; for spring admission, 10/15 priority date for domestic students, 10/1 priority date for international students. Applications are processed on a rolling basis. Application fee: $40 ($90 for international students). Electronic applications accepted. *Expenses:* Tuition, state resident: full-time $6663; part-time $278 per credit hour. Tuition, nonresident: full-time $15,159; part-time $632 per credit hour. *Required fees:* $1872; $54 per credit hour. $306 per term. Tuition and fees vary according to course load. *Financial support:* In 2013–14, 15 students received support, including 4 research assistantships (averaging $12,710 per year), 13 teaching assistantships (averaging $12,164 per year); Federal Work-Study, institutionally sponsored loans, scholarships/grants, health care benefits, and unspecified assistantships also available. Support available to part-time students. Financial award application deadline: 4/1; financial award applicants required to submit FAFSA. *Unit head:* Dr. Chad Booth, Graduate Advisor, 512-245-8789, Fax: 512-245-2374, E-mail: chadbooth@txstate.edu. *Application contact:* Dr. Andrea Golato, Dean of Graduate School, 512-245-2581, Fax: 512-245-8365, E-mail: gradcollege@txstate.edu.
Website: http://www.txstate.edu/chemistry/

Thomas Jefferson University, Jefferson Graduate School of Biomedical Sciences, PhD Program in Biochemistry and Molecular Pharmacology, Philadelphia, PA 19107. Offers PhD. *Faculty:* 68 full-time (19 women), 1 (woman) part-time/adjunct. *Students:* 36 full-time (21 women); includes 9 minority (all Asian, non-Hispanic/Latino), 9 international. Average age 24. 64 applicants, 34% accepted, 6 enrolled. In 2013, 4 doctorates awarded. *Degree requirements:* For doctorate, comprehensive exam, thesis/dissertation. *Entrance requirements:* For doctorate, GRE General Test or MCAT, minimum GPA of 3.2. Additional exam requirements/recommendations for international students: Required—TOEFL (minimum score 100 iBT) or IELTS. *Application deadline:* For fall admission, 1/2 priority date for domestic and international students. Applications are processed on a rolling basis. Application fee: $75. Electronic applications accepted. *Financial support:* In 2013–14, 36 students received support, including 36 fellowships with full tuition reimbursements available (averaging $56,052 per year); Federal Work-Study, institutionally sponsored loans, scholarships/grants, traineeships, and stipends also available. Financial award application deadline: 5/1; financial award applicants required to submit FAFSA. *Faculty research:* Signal transduction and molecular genetics, translational biochemistry, human mitochondrial genetics, molecular biology of protein-RNA interaction, mammalian mitochondrial biogenesis and function. *Unit head:* Dr. Michael J. Root, Program Director, 215-503-4564, Fax: 215-923-2117, E-mail:

michael.root@jefferson.edu. *Application contact:* Marc E. Stearns, Director of Admissions, 215-503-0155, Fax: 215-503-3433, E-mail: jgsbs-info@jefferson.edu. Website: http://www.jefferson.edu/university/biomedical_sciences/programs/phd/biochemistry_pharmacology.html

Tufts University, Sackler School of Graduate Biomedical Sciences, Biochemistry Program, Medford, MA 02155. Offers PhD. *Faculty:* 25 full-time (6 women). *Students:* 12 full-time (7 women); includes 3 minority (all Asian, non-Hispanic/Latino), 1 international. Average age 29. In 2013, 2 doctorates awarded. Terminal master's awarded for partial completion of doctoral program. *Degree requirements:* For doctorate, comprehensive exam, thesis/dissertation. *Entrance requirements:* For doctorate, GRE, 3 letters of recommendation. Additional exam requirements/recommendations for international students: Required—TOEFL (minimum score 600 paper-based; 100 iBT). *Application deadline:* For fall admission, 12/15 for domestic and international students. Application fee: $70. Electronic applications accepted. *Financial support:* In 2013–14, 12 students received support, including 12 research assistantships with full tuition reimbursements available (averaging $31,000 per year); health care benefits also available. Financial award application deadline: 12/15. *Faculty research:* Structure-based drug design based on nuclear magnetic resonance (NMR) analysis; mechanism of protein action using x-ray crystallography; biochemical basis of cell death; molecular basis of gene function including DNA replication, molecular bases of cancer. *Unit head:* Dr. Larry Feig, Program Director, 617-636-6956, Fax: 617-636-2409, E-mail: larry.feig@tufts.edu. *Application contact:* Kellie Melchin, Associate Director of Admissions, 617-636-6767, Fax: 617-636-0375, E-mail: sackler-school@tufts.edu.
Website: http://sackler.tufts.edu/Academics/Degree-Programs/PhD-Programs/Biochemistry

Tulane University, School of Medicine and School of Liberal Arts, Graduate Programs in Biomedical Sciences, Department of Biochemistry, New Orleans, LA 70118-5669. Offers MS, PhD, MD/PhD. MS and PhD offered through the Graduate School. *Degree requirements:* For master's, thesis; for doctorate, 2 foreign languages, thesis/dissertation. *Entrance requirements:* For master's, GRE General Test, GRE Subject Test, minimum B average in undergraduate course work; for doctorate, GRE General Test, GRE Subject Test. Additional exam requirements/recommendations for international students: Required—TOEFL. Electronic applications accepted. *Faculty research:* Nucleic acid chemistry, complex carbohydrates biochemistry.

Universidad Central del Caribe, School of Medicine, Program in Biomedical Sciences, Bayamón, PR 00960-6032. Offers anatomy and cell biology (MA, MS); biochemistry (MS); biomedical sciences (MA); cellular and molecular biology (PhD); microbiology and immunology (MA, MS); pharmacology (MS); physiology (MS).

Université de Moncton, Faculty of Sciences, Department of Chemistry and Biochemistry, Moncton, NB E1A 3E9, Canada. Offers biochemistry (M Sc); chemistry (M Sc). Part-time programs available. *Degree requirements:* For master's, one foreign language, thesis. *Entrance requirements:* For master's, minimum GPA of 3.0. Electronic applications accepted. *Faculty research:* Environmental contaminants, natural products synthesis, nutraceutical, organic catalysis, molecular biology of cancer.

Université de Montréal, Faculty of Medicine, Department of Biochemistry, Montréal, QC H3C 3J7, Canada. Offers biochemistry (M Sc, PhD); clinical biochemistry (DEPD). Terminal master's awarded for partial completion of doctoral program. *Degree requirements:* For master's, thesis; for doctorate, thesis/dissertation, general exam. *Entrance requirements:* For master's and doctorate, proficiency in French, knowledge of English; for DEPD, proficiency in French. Electronic applications accepted.

Université de Sherbrooke, Faculty of Medicine and Health Sciences, Graduate Programs in Medicine, Department of Biochemistry, Sherbrooke, QC J1H 5N4, Canada. Offers M Sc, PhD. Terminal master's awarded for partial completion of doctoral program. *Degree requirements:* For master's, thesis; for doctorate, thesis/dissertation. Electronic applications accepted. *Faculty research:* RNA structure-function, chromatin and gene expression, genetic diseases.

Université Laval, Faculty of Medicine, Post-Professional Programs in Medical Studies, Québec, QC G1K 7P4, Canada. Offers anatomy–pathology (DESS); anesthesiology (DESS); cardiology (DESS); care of older people (Diploma); clinical research (DESS); community health (DESS); dermatology (DESS); diagnostic radiology (DESS); emergency medicine (Diploma); family medicine (DESS); general surgery (DESS); geriatrics (DESS); hematology (DESS); internal medicine (DESS); maternal and fetal medicine (Diploma); medical biochemistry (DESS); medical microbiology and infectious diseases (DESS); medical oncology (DESS); nephrology (DESS); neurology (DESS); neurosurgery (DESS); obstetrics and gynecology (DESS); ophthalmology (DESS); orthopedic surgery (DESS); oto-rhino-laryngology (DESS); palliative medicine (Diploma); pediatrics (DESS); plastic surgery (DESS); psychiatry (DESS); pulmonary medicine (DESS); radiology–oncology (DESS); thoracic surgery (DESS); urology (DESS). *Degree requirements:* For other advanced degree, comprehensive exam. *Entrance requirements:* For degree, knowledge of French. Electronic applications accepted.

Université Laval, Faculty of Sciences and Engineering, Department of Biochemistry and Microbiology, Programs in Biochemistry, Québec, QC G1K 7P4, Canada. Offers M Sc, PhD. Terminal master's awarded for partial completion of doctoral program. *Degree requirements:* For master's, thesis; for doctorate, comprehensive exam, thesis/dissertation. *Entrance requirements:* For master's and doctorate, knowledge of French, comprehension of written English. Electronic applications accepted.

University at Albany, State University of New York, School of Public Health, Department of Biomedical Sciences, Program in Biochemistry, Molecular Biology, and Genetics, Albany, NY 12222-0001. Offers MS, PhD. *Degree requirements:* For master's, thesis; for doctorate, thesis/dissertation. *Entrance requirements:* For master's and doctorate, GRE General Test, GRE Subject Test.

University at Buffalo, the State University of New York, Graduate School, School of Medicine and Biomedical Sciences, Graduate Programs in Medicine and Biomedical Sciences, Department of Biochemistry, Buffalo, NY 14260. Offers MA, PhD. *Faculty:* 21 full-time (7 women), 1 (woman) part-time/adjunct. *Students:* 31 full-time (15 women), 19 international. Average age 26. 22 applicants, 32% accepted, 3 enrolled. In 2013, 2 doctorates awarded. Terminal master's awarded for partial completion of doctoral program. *Degree requirements:* For master's, thesis optional; for doctorate, comprehensive exam, thesis/dissertation. *Entrance requirements:* For master's, GRE General Test; for doctorate, GRE General Test, 3 letters of recommendation. Additional exam requirements/recommendations for international students: Required—TOEFL (minimum score 600 paper-based; 100 iBT). *Application deadline:* For fall admission, 2/1 priority date for domestic and international students. Applications are processed on a rolling basis. Application fee: $50. Electronic applications accepted. *Financial support:* In 2013–14, 3 fellowships with full tuition reimbursements (averaging $5,000 per year), 24 research assistantships with full tuition reimbursements (averaging $25,000 per year), teaching assistantships with full tuition reimbursements (averaging $25,000 per year) were awarded; Federal Work-Study, institutionally sponsored loans, scholarships/grants, health care benefits, and unspecified assistantships also available. Financial award application deadline: 2/1; financial award applicants required to submit FAFSA. *Faculty research:* Gene expression, proteins and metalloenzymes, biochemical endocrinology. *Total annual research expenditures:* $4.4 million. *Unit head:* Dr. Mark R. O'Brian, Interim Chair, 716-829-3200, Fax: 716-829-2725, E-mail: mrobrian@buffalo.edu. *Application contact:* Dr. Gabriela K. Popescu, Director of Graduate Studies, 716-829-3807, Fax: 716-829-2725, E-mail: popescu@buffalo.edu.
Website: http://www.smbs.buffalo.edu/bch/

The University of Alabama at Birmingham, Graduate Programs in Joint Health Sciences, Program in Biochemistry and Molecular Genetics, Birmingham, AL 35294. Offers PhD. *Degree requirements:* For doctorate, thesis/dissertation. *Entrance requirements:* For doctorate, GRE General Test, interview, letters of recommendation, minimum GPA of 3.0. Additional exam requirements/recommendations for international students: Required—TOEFL (minimum score 600 paper-based; 100 iBT). Electronic applications accepted.

University of Alaska Fairbanks, College of Natural Sciences and Mathematics, Department of Chemistry and Biochemistry, Fairbanks, AK 99775-6160. Offers biochemistry and molecular biology (MS, PhD); chemistry (MA, MS); environmental chemistry (MS, PhD). Part-time programs available. *Faculty:* 8 full-time (1 woman). *Students:* 27 full-time (17 women), 3 part-time (all women); includes 4 minority (1 Asian, non-Hispanic/Latino; 2 Hispanic/Latino; 1 Two or more races, non-Hispanic/Latino), 8 international. Average age 29. 32 applicants, 25% accepted, 8 enrolled. In 2013, 2 master's, 3 doctorates awarded. *Degree requirements:* For master's, comprehensive exam, thesis or alternative; for doctorate, comprehensive exam, thesis/dissertation, oral defense. *Entrance requirements:* Additional exam requirements/recommendations for international students: Required—TOEFL (minimum score 550 paper-based). *Application deadline:* For fall admission, 6/1 for domestic students, 3/1 for international students; for spring admission, 10/15 for domestic students, 9/1 for international students. Applications are processed on a rolling basis. Application fee: $60. Electronic applications accepted. *Expenses:* Tuition, state resident: full-time $7254; part-time $403 per credit. Tuition, nonresident: full-time $14,814; part-time $823 per credit. Tuition and fees vary according to course level, course load and reciprocity agreements. *Financial support:* In 2013–14, 9 research assistantships with tuition reimbursements (averaging $12,111 per year), 15 teaching assistantships with tuition reimbursements (averaging $17,372 per year) were awarded; fellowships with tuition reimbursements, Federal Work-Study, scholarships/grants, health care benefits, and unspecified assistantships also available. Support available to part-time students. Financial award application deadline: 7/1; financial award applicants required to submit FAFSA. *Faculty research:* Atmospheric aerosols, cold adaptation, hibernation and neuroprotection, liganogated ion channels, arctic contaminants. *Unit head:* Bill Simpson, Department Chair, 907-474-5510, Fax: 907-474-5640, E-mail: uaf-chem-biochem@alaska.edu. *Application contact:* Libby Eddy, Registrar and Director of Admissions, 907-474-7500, Fax: 907-474-7097, E-mail: admissions@uaf.edu.
Website: http://www.uaf.edu/chem

University of Alberta, Faculty of Medicine and Dentistry and Faculty of Graduate Studies and Research, Graduate Programs in Medicine, Department of Biochemistry, Edmonton, AB T6G 2E1, Canada. Offers M Sc, PhD. Terminal master's awarded for partial completion of doctoral program. *Degree requirements:* For master's, thesis; for doctorate, thesis/dissertation. *Entrance requirements:* For master's and doctorate, minimum GPA of 3.3. Additional exam requirements/recommendations for international students: Required—TOEFL (minimum score 550 paper-based). *Faculty research:* Proteins, nucleic acids, membranes, regulation of gene expression, receptors.

The University of Arizona, College of Science, Department of Chemistry and Biochemistry, Tucson, AZ 85721. Offers biochemistry (PhD); chemistry (PhD). Part-time programs available. *Faculty:* 32 full-time (6 women), 4 part-time/adjunct (2 women). *Students:* 178 full-time (72 women), 5 part-time (3 women); includes 25 minority (3 Black or African American, non-Hispanic/Latino; 1 American Indian or Alaska Native, non-Hispanic/Latino; 2 Asian, non-Hispanic/Latino; 9 Hispanic/Latino; 1 Native Hawaiian or other Pacific Islander, non-Hispanic/Latino; 9 Two or more races, non-Hispanic/Latino), 69 international. Average age 28. 240 applicants, 35% accepted, 36 enrolled. In 2013, 18 doctorates awarded. *Degree requirements:* For doctorate, comprehensive exam, thesis/dissertation. *Entrance requirements:* For doctorate, GRE General Test, 3 letters of recommendation, statement of purpose. Additional exam requirements/recommendations for international students: Required—TOEFL (minimum score 550 paper-based; 79 iBT). *Application deadline:* For fall admission, 2/1 for domestic students, 1/1 for international students; for spring admission, 10/15 for domestic and international students. Applications are processed on a rolling basis. Application fee: $75. Electronic applications accepted. *Expenses:* Tuition, state resident: full-time $11,526. Tuition, nonresident: full-time $27,398. *Financial support:* In 2013–14, 43 research assistantships with full tuition reimbursements (averaging $24,349 per year), 103 teaching assistantships with full tuition reimbursements (averaging $24,878 per year) were awarded; institutionally sponsored loans, scholarships/grants, health care benefits, tuition waivers (partial), and unspecified assistantships also available. Financial award applicants required to submit FAFSA. *Faculty research:* Analytical, inorganic, organic, physical chemistry, biological chemistry. *Total annual research expenditures:* $8.5 million. *Unit head:* Dr. Vicki Wysocki, Head, 520-621-2628, Fax: 520-621-8407, E-mail: vwysocki@u.arizona.edu. *Application contact:* Lori Boyd, Senior Program Coordinator, 800-545-5814, Fax: 520-621-8407, E-mail: chemistry@arizona.edu.
Website: http://www.chem.arizona.edu/

University of Arkansas for Medical Sciences, Graduate School, Little Rock, AR 72205. Offers biochemistry and molecular biology (MS, PhD); bioinformatics (MS, PhD); cellular physiology and molecular biophysics (MS, PhD); clinical nutrition (MS); interdisciplinary biomedical sciences (MS, PhD, Certificate); interdisciplinary toxicology (MS); microbiology and immunology (PhD); neurobiology and developmental sciences (PhD); pharmacology (PhD); MD/PhD. Bioinformatics programs hosted jointly with the University of Arkansas at Little Rock. Part-time programs available. *Faculty:* 397 full-time (205 women). *Students:* 196 full-time (126 women), 117 part-time (87 women); includes 65 minority (38 Black or African American, non-Hispanic/Latino; 1 American Indian or Alaska Native, non-Hispanic/Latino; 21 Asian, non-Hispanic/Latino; 4 Hispanic/Latino; 1 Two or more races, non-Hispanic/Latino), 57 international. 455 applicants, 27% accepted, 89 enrolled. In 2013, 41 master's, 18 doctorates, 28 other advanced degrees awarded. Terminal master's awarded for partial completion of doctoral program. *Degree requirements:* For master's, comprehensive exam (for some programs), thesis (for some programs); for doctorate, thesis/dissertation. *Entrance requirements:* For master's and doctorate, GRE. Additional exam requirements/recommendations for international students: Required—TOEFL. *Application deadline:* Applications are processed on a rolling basis. Application fee: $0. Electronic applications accepted. *Expenses:* Contact institution. *Financial support:* In 2013–14, 120 research assistantships (averaging $24,000 per year) were awarded; career-related internships or fieldwork, Federal Work-Study, and traineeships also available. Support available to part-time students. Financial award applicants required to submit FAFSA. *Unit head:* Dr. Robert E. McGehee, Jr., Dean, 501-686-5454. *Application contact:* Dr. Kristen Sterba, Assistant Dean, Office of Graduate Student Recruiting and Retention, 501-526-7396, E-mail: kmsterba@uams.edu.
Website: http://www.uams.edu/gradschool/

The University of British Columbia, Faculty of Medicine, Department of Biochemistry and Molecular Biology, Vancouver, BC V6T 1Z1, Canada. Offers M Sc, PhD. *Degree requirements:* For master's, thesis; for doctorate, comprehensive exam, thesis/dissertation. *Entrance requirements:* For master's, first class B Sc; for doctorate, master's or first class honors bachelor's degree in biochemistry. Additional exam requirements/recommendations for international students: Required—TOEFL (minimum score 625 paper-based). Electronic applications accepted. *Expenses: Tuition, area resident:* Full-time $8000 Canadian dollars. *Faculty research:* Membrane biochemistry, protein structure/function, signal transduction, biochemistry.

University of Calgary, Cumming School of Medicine and Faculty of Graduate Studies, Department of Biochemistry and Molecular Biology, Calgary, AB T2N 1N4, Canada. Offers M Sc, PhD. *Degree requirements:* For master's, thesis; for doctorate, thesis/dissertation, candidacy exam. *Entrance requirements:* For master's and doctorate, GRE General Test, minimum GPA of 3.2. Additional exam requirements/recommendations for international students: Required—TOEFL. Electronic applications accepted. *Faculty research:* Molecular and developmental genetics; molecular biology of disease; genomics, proteomics and bioinformatics; cell signaling and structure.

University of California, Berkeley, Graduate Division, Group in Comparative Biochemistry, Berkeley, CA 94720-1500. Offers PhD. *Degree requirements:* For doctorate, thesis/dissertation, qualifying exam. *Entrance requirements:* For doctorate, GRE General Test, GRE Subject Test, minimum GPA of 3.0, 3 letters of recommendation. Additional exam requirements/recommendations for international students: Required—TOEFL.

University of California, Davis, Graduate Studies, Graduate Group in Biochemistry and Molecular Biology, Davis, CA 95616. Offers MS, PhD. Terminal master's awarded for partial completion of doctoral program. *Degree requirements:* For master's, comprehensive exam (for some programs), thesis (for some programs); for doctorate, thesis/dissertation. *Entrance requirements:* For master's and doctorate, GRE General Test, GRE Subject Test. Additional exam requirements/recommendations for international students: Required—TOEFL (minimum score 550 paper-based). Electronic applications accepted. *Faculty research:* Gene expression, protein structure, molecular virology, protein synthesis, enzymology, membrane transport and structural biology.

University of California, Irvine, School of Biological Sciences, Department of Molecular Biology and Biochemistry, Irvine, CA 92697. Offers biological science (MS); biological sciences (PhD); biotechnology (MS); MD/PhD. *Students:* 59 full-time (28 women), 1 part-time (0 women); includes 28 minority (1 Black or African American, non-Hispanic/Latino; 14 Asian, non-Hispanic/Latino; 12 Hispanic/Latino; 1 Native Hawaiian or other Pacific Islander, non-Hispanic/Latino), 4 international. Average age 28. In 2013, 6 master's, 10 doctorates awarded. *Degree requirements:* For doctorate, thesis/dissertation. *Entrance requirements:* For master's, GRE, minimum GPA of 3.0; for doctorate, GRE General Test, GRE Subject Test, minimum GPA of 3.0. Additional exam requirements/recommendations for international students: Required—TOEFL (minimum score 550 paper-based). *Application deadline:* For fall admission, 12/15 priority date for domestic students, 12/15 for international students. Applications are processed on a rolling basis. Application fee: $80 ($100 for international students). Electronic applications accepted. *Financial support:* Fellowships, research assistantships with full tuition reimbursements, teaching assistantships, institutionally sponsored loans, traineeships, health care benefits, and unspecified assistantships available. Financial award application deadline: 3/1; financial award applicants required to submit FAFSA. *Faculty research:* Structure and synthesis of nucleic acids and proteins, regulation, virology, biochemical genetics, gene organization. *Unit head:* Prof. Christopher Hughes, Chair, 949-824-8771, Fax: 949-824-8551, E-mail: cchughes@uci.edu. *Application contact:* Morgan Oldham, Student Affairs Assistant, 949-826-6034, Fax: 949-824-8551, E-mail: morgano@uci.edu.
Website: http://www.bio.uci.edu/

University of California, Irvine, School of Biological Sciences and School of Medicine, Interdisciplinary Graduate Program in Cellular and Molecular Biosciences, Irvine, CA 92697. Offers PhD. *Degree requirements:* For doctorate, thesis/dissertation, teaching assignment, preliminary exam. *Entrance requirements:* For doctorate, GRE General Test, three letters of recommendation, interview. Additional exam requirements/recommendations for international students: Required—TOEFL or IELTS. *Application deadline:* For fall admission, 12/8 for domestic and international students. Application fee: $60 ($80 for international students). Electronic applications accepted. *Expenses:* Contact institution. *Financial support:* Fellowships with full tuition reimbursements, institutionally sponsored loans, scholarships/grants, tuition waivers (full), unspecified assistantships, and stipends available. Financial award application deadline: 1/1; financial award applicants required to submit FAFSA. *Faculty research:* Cellular biochemistry; gene structure and expression; protein structure, function, and design; molecular genetics; pathogenesis and inherited disease. *Unit head:* Dr. David Fruman, Director, 949-824-1947, Fax: 949-824-1965, E-mail: dfruman@uci.edu. *Application contact:* Renee Frigo, Administrator, 949-824-8145, Fax: 949-824-1965, E-mail: rfrigo@uci.edu.
Website: http://cmb.uci.edu/

University of California, Irvine, School of Medicine and School of Biological Sciences, Department of Biological Chemistry, Irvine, CA 92697. Offers biological sciences (MS, PhD). *Students:* 22 full-time (8 women); includes 11 minority (3 Black or African American, non-Hispanic/Latino; 5 Asian, non-Hispanic/Latino; 3 Hispanic/Latino), 4 international. Average age 28. 1 applicant. In 2013, 1 master's, 13 doctorates awarded. *Degree requirements:* For doctorate, thesis/dissertation. *Entrance requirements:* For master's, minimum GPA of 3.0; for doctorate, GRE General Test, GRE Subject Test, minimum GPA of 3.0. Additional exam requirements/recommendations for international students: Required—TOEFL (minimum score 550 paper-based). *Application deadline:* For fall admission, 1/15 priority date for domestic students, 1/15 for international students. Application fee: $80 ($100 for international students). Electronic applications accepted. *Financial support:* Fellowships, research assistantships with full tuition reimbursements, teaching assistantships, institutionally sponsored loans, traineeships, health care benefits, and unspecified assistantships available. Financial award application deadline: 3/1; financial award applicants required to submit FAFSA. *Faculty research:* RNA splicing, mammalian chromosomal organization, membrane-hormone interactions, regulation of protein synthesis, molecular genetics of metabolic processes. *Unit head:* Dr. Eva Yhp Lee, Chair/Professor, 949-824-9766, Fax: 949-824-9767, E-mail: elee@uci.edu. *Application contact:* Kyoko Yokomori, Graduate Faculty Advisor, 949-824-8215, Fax: 949-824-2688, E-mail: kyokomor@uci.edu.
Website: http://www.bio.uci.edu/

University of California, Los Angeles, David Geffen School of Medicine and Graduate Division, Graduate Programs in Medicine, Department of Biological Chemistry, Los Angeles, CA 90095. Offers MS, PhD. Terminal master's awarded for partial completion of doctoral program. *Degree requirements:* For master's, comprehensive exam or thesis; for doctorate, thesis/dissertation, oral and written qualifying exams; 2 quarters of teaching experience. *Entrance requirements:* For master's and doctorate, GRE General Test, bachelor's degree; minimum undergraduate GPA of 3.0 (or its equivalent if letter grade system not used). Additional exam requirements/recommendations for international students: Required—TOEFL. Electronic applications accepted.

University of California, Los Angeles, Graduate Division, College of Letters and Science, Department of Chemistry and Biochemistry, Program in Biochemistry and Molecular Biology, Los Angeles, CA 90095. Offers MS, PhD. Terminal master's awarded for partial completion of doctoral program. *Degree requirements:* For master's, comprehensive exam or thesis; for doctorate, thesis/dissertation, oral and written qualifying exams; 3 quarters of teaching experience. *Entrance requirements:* For doctorate, GRE General Test, GRE Subject Test (recommended), bachelor's degree; minimum undergraduate GPA of 3.0 (or its equivalent if letter grade system not used). Additional exam requirements/recommendations for international students: Required—TOEFL. Electronic applications accepted.

University of California, Los Angeles, Graduate Division, College of Letters and Science and David Geffen School of Medicine, UCLA ACCESS to Programs in the Molecular, Cellular and Integrative Life Sciences, Los Angeles, CA 90095. Offers biochemistry and molecular biology (PhD); biological chemistry (PhD); cellular and molecular pathology (PhD); human genetics (PhD); microbiology, immunology, and molecular genetics (PhD); molecular biology (PhD); molecular toxicology (PhD); molecular, cellular and integrative physiology (PhD); neurobiology (PhD); oral biology (PhD); physiology (PhD). *Degree requirements:* For doctorate, thesis/dissertation, oral and written qualifying exams. *Entrance requirements:* For doctorate, GRE General Test, bachelor's degree; minimum undergraduate GPA of 3.0 (or its equivalent if letter grade system not used). Additional exam requirements/recommendations for international students: Required—TOEFL. Electronic applications accepted.

University of California, Merced, Graduate Division, School of Natural Sciences, Merced, CA 95343. Offers applied mathematics (MS, PhD); chemistry and chemical biology (MS, PhD); physics (MS, PhD); quantitative and systems biology (MS, PhD). *Students:* 133 full-time (52 women); includes 48 minority (3 Black or African American, non-Hispanic/Latino; 16 Asian, non-Hispanic/Latino; 22 Hispanic/Latino; 1 Native Hawaiian or other Pacific Islander, non-Hispanic/Latino; 6 Two or more races, non-Hispanic/Latino), 29 international. Average age 28. 143 applicants, 45% accepted, 33 enrolled. In 2013, 1 master's, 8 doctorates awarded. *Degree requirements:* For master's, variable foreign language requirement, comprehensive exam, thesis (for some programs); for doctorate, variable foreign language requirement, comprehensive exam, thesis/dissertation. *Entrance requirements:* For master's and doctorate, GRE. Additional exam requirements/recommendations for international students: Required—TOEFL (minimum score 550 paper-based; 68 iBT); Recommended—IELTS. *Expenses:* Tuition, state resident: full-time $6405. Tuition, nonresident: full-time $13,956. *Financial support:* In 2013–14, 30 fellowships with full and partial tuition reimbursements (averaging $8,646 per year) were awarded; scholarships/grants also available. *Unit head:* Dr. Juan Meza, Dean, 209-228-4487, Fax: 209-228-4060, E-mail: jcmeza@ucmerced.edu. *Application contact:* Carrie King, Graduate Admissions and Academic Services Manager, 209-228-4613, Fax: 209-228-6906, E-mail: cking7@ucmerced.edu.

University of California, Riverside, Graduate Division, Department of Biochemistry, Riverside, CA 92521-0102. Offers biochemistry and molecular biology (MS, PhD). Part-time programs available. Terminal master's awarded for partial completion of doctoral program. *Degree requirements:* For master's, comprehensive exams or thesis; for doctorate, comprehensive exam, thesis/dissertation, 2 quarters of teaching experience, qualifying exams. *Entrance requirements:* For master's and doctorate, GRE General Test, minimum GPA of 3.25. Additional exam requirements/recommendations for international students: Required—TOEFL (minimum score 550 paper-based; 80 iBT). Electronic applications accepted. *Faculty research:* Structural biology and molecular biophysics, signal transduction, plant biochemistry and molecular biology, gene expression and metabolic regulation, molecular toxicology and pathogenesis.

University of California, San Diego, Office of Graduate Studies, Department of Chemistry and Biochemistry, La Jolla, CA 92093. Offers chemistry (MS, PhD). PhD offered jointly with San Diego State University. *Students:* 268 full-time (99 women), 2 part-time (1 woman); includes 88 minority (10 Black or African American, non-Hispanic/Latino; 1 American Indian or Alaska Native, non-Hispanic/Latino; 55 Asian, non-Hispanic/Latino; 21 Hispanic/Latino; 1 Native Hawaiian or other Pacific Islander, non-Hispanic/Latino), 29 international. 567 applicants, 30% accepted, 55 enrolled. In 2013, 61 master's, 26 doctorates awarded. *Degree requirements:* For doctorate, thesis/dissertation. *Entrance requirements:* For doctorate, GRE General Test, GRE Subject Test. Additional exam requirements/recommendations for international students: Required—TOEFL, IELTS. *Application deadline:* For fall admission, 12/15 priority date for domestic students. Application fee: $80 ($100 for international students). Electronic applications accepted. *Expenses:* Tuition, state resident: full-time $11,220; part-time $1870 per quarter. Tuition, nonresident: full-time $26,322; part-time $4387 per quarter. *Required fees:* $519.50 per quarter. Part-time tuition and fees vary according to course load and program. *Financial support:* Research assistantships, teaching assistantships, and scholarships/grants available. Financial award applicants required to submit FAFSA. *Faculty research:* Analytical and atmospheric chemistry, cellular and systems biochemistry, chemical biology, structural biology and biophysics, theoretical and computational chemistry. *Unit head:* Seth M. Cohen, Chair, 858-822-5596, E-mail: chaircohen@ucsd.edu. *Application contact:* Jeanine Sun, Graduate Coordinator, 858-822-6014, E-mail: jesun@ucsd.edu.
Website: https://www-chem.ucsd.edu/

University of California, San Francisco, Graduate Division and School of Medicine, Tetrad Graduate Program, Biochemistry and Molecular Biology Track, San Francisco, CA 94143. Offers PhD, MD/PhD. *Degree requirements:* For doctorate, thesis/dissertation. *Entrance requirements:* For doctorate, GRE General Test, GRE Subject Test. Additional exam requirements/recommendations for international students: Required—TOEFL. *Application deadline:* For fall admission, 12/1 for domestic students. Application fee: $40. *Expenses:* Contact institution. *Financial support:* Fellowships available. Financial award application deadline: 2/1. *Faculty research:* Structural biology, genetics, cell biology, cell physiology, metabolism. *Unit head:* Dr. Peter Walter, Chair, 415-476-5017. *Application contact:* Dr. Peter Walter, Chair, 415-476-5017.
Website: http://tetrad.ucsf.edu/

University of California, San Francisco, School of Pharmacy and Graduate Division, Chemistry and Chemical Biology Graduate Program, San Francisco, CA 94143. Offers PhD. *Degree requirements:* For doctorate, thesis/dissertation. *Entrance requirements:* For doctorate, GRE General Test, minimum GPA of 3.0, bachelor's degree. Additional exam requirements/recommendations for international students: Required—TOEFL (minimum score 550 paper-based; 80 iBT). *Application deadline:* For fall admission, 12/1 for domestic and international students. Applications are processed on a rolling basis. Application fee: $80 ($100 for international students). Electronic applications accepted. *Expenses:* Tuition, state resident: full-time $11,220. Tuition, nonresident: full-time $26,322. *Required fees:* $5204. Full-time tuition and fees vary according to degree level and program. *Financial support:* In 2013–14, fellowships with full tuition reimbursements (averaging $32,500 per year), research assistantships with full tuition reimbursements (averaging $32,500 per year) were awarded; teaching assistantships with partial tuition reimbursements, institutionally sponsored loans, scholarships/grants, traineeships, and tuition waivers (full) also available. Financial award application deadline: 5/15. *Faculty research:* Macromolecular structure function and dynamics, computational chemistry and biology, biological chemistry and synthetic biology, chemical biology and molecular

design, nanomolecular design. *Unit head:* Dr. Charles S. Craik, Director, 415-476-8146, E-mail: craik@cgl.ucsf.edu. *Application contact:* Julia Molla, Administrator, 415-476-1914, Fax: 415-514-1546, E-mail: julia.molla@ucsf.edu.
Website: http://ccb.ucsf.edu/

University of California, Santa Barbara, Graduate Division, College of Letters and Sciences, Division of Mathematics, Life, and Physical Sciences, Interdepartmental Graduate Program in Biomolecular Science and Engineering, Santa Barbara, CA 93106-2014. Offers biochemistry and molecular biology (PhD), including biochemistry and molecular biology, biophysics and bioengineering. *Faculty:* 35 full-time (3 women), 3 part-time/adjunct (all women). *Students:* 26 full-time (13 women); includes 5 minority (4 Asian, non-Hispanic/Latino; 1 Hispanic/Latino), 2 international. Average age 29. 98 applicants, 17% accepted, 6 enrolled. In 2013, 6 doctorates awarded. Terminal master's awarded for partial completion of doctoral program. *Degree requirements:* For doctorate, thesis/dissertation. *Entrance requirements:* For doctorate, GRE General Test. Additional exam requirements/recommendations for international students: Required—TOEFL (minimum score 630 paper-based; 109 iBT), IELTS (minimum score 7). *Application deadline:* For fall admission, 12/15 for domestic and international students. Application fee: $80 ($100 for international students). Electronic applications accepted. *Expenses:* Tuition, state resident: part-time $5148.26 per quarter. Tuition, nonresident: part-time $10,182.26 per quarter. *Financial support:* In 2013–14, 28 students received support, including 16 fellowships with full and partial tuition reimbursements available (averaging $11,321 per year), 31 research assistantships with full and partial tuition reimbursements available (averaging $14,777 per year), 16 teaching assistantships with full and partial tuition reimbursements available (averaging $6,307 per year); Federal Work-Study, traineeships, health care benefits, tuition waivers (full and partial), and unspecified assistantships also available. Financial award application deadline: 12/15; financial award applicants required to submit FAFSA. *Faculty research:* Biochemistry and molecular biology, biophysics, biomaterials, bioengineering, systems biology. *Unit head:* Prof. Omar A. Saleh, Director/Professor, 805-893-8814, E-mail: saleh@engineering.ucsb.edu. *Application contact:* Nicole McCoy, 805-893-8499, E-mail: nicole.mccoy@lifesci.ucsb.edu.
Website: http://www.bmse.ucsb.edu/

University of California, Santa Cruz, Division of Graduate Studies, Division of Physical and Biological Sciences, Department of Chemistry and Biochemistry, Santa Cruz, CA 95064. Offers MS, PhD. *Degree requirements:* For master's, thesis optional; for doctorate, one foreign language, thesis/dissertation, qualifying exam. *Entrance requirements:* For master's and doctorate, GRE General Test, GRE Subject Test. Additional exam requirements/recommendations for international students: Required—TOEFL (minimum score 570 paper-based; 89 iBT); Recommended—IELTS (minimum score 8). Electronic applications accepted. *Faculty research:* Marine chemistry; biochemistry; inorganic, organic, and physical chemistry.

University of Chicago, Division of Biological Sciences, Molecular Biosciences Cluster, Department of Biochemistry and Molecular Biology, Chicago, IL 60637-1513. Offers PhD, MD/PhD. *Degree requirements:* For doctorate, thesis/dissertation, ethics class, 2 teaching assistantships. *Entrance requirements:* For doctorate, GRE General Test, GRE Subject Test. Additional exam requirements/recommendations for international students: Required—TOEFL (minimum score 600 paper-based; 104 iBT), IELTS (minimum score 7). Electronic applications accepted. *Faculty research:* Molecular biology, gene expression, and DNA-protein interactions; membrane biochemistry, molecular endocrinology, and transmembrane signaling; enzyme mechanisms, physical biochemistry, and structural biology.

University of Cincinnati, Graduate School, College of Medicine, Graduate Programs in Biomedical Sciences, Department of Molecular Genetics, Biochemistry and Microbiology, Cincinnati, OH 45221. Offers MS, PhD. Terminal master's awarded for partial completion of doctoral program. *Degree requirements:* For master's, thesis or alternative; for doctorate, thesis/dissertation, qualifying exam. *Entrance requirements:* For master's and doctorate, GRE General Test. Additional exam requirements/recommendations for international students: Required—TOEFL (minimum score 600 paper-based; 100 iBT), TWE. Electronic applications accepted. *Faculty research:* Cancer biology and developmental genetics, gene regulation and chromosome structure, microbiology and pathogenic mechanisms, structural biology, membrane biochemistry and signal transduction.

University of Cincinnati, Graduate School, McMicken College of Arts and Sciences, Department of Chemistry, Cincinnati, OH 45221. Offers analytical chemistry (MS, PhD); biochemistry (MS, PhD); inorganic chemistry (MS, PhD); organic chemistry (MS, PhD); physical chemistry (MS, PhD); polymer chemistry (MS, PhD); sensors (PhD). Part-time and evening/weekend programs available. Terminal master's awarded for partial completion of doctoral program. *Degree requirements:* For master's, thesis optional; for doctorate, comprehensive exam, thesis/dissertation. *Entrance requirements:* For master's and doctorate, GRE General Test. Additional exam requirements/recommendations for international students: Required—TOEFL (minimum score 580 paper-based). Electronic applications accepted. *Faculty research:* Biomedical chemistry, laser chemistry, surface science, chemical sensors, synthesis.

University of Colorado Boulder, Graduate School, College of Arts and Sciences, Department of Chemistry and Biochemistry, Boulder, CO 80309. Offers biochemistry (PhD); chemistry (MS). *Faculty:* 40 full-time (6 women). *Students:* 240 full-time (98 women), 1 part-time (0 women); includes 34 minority (2 Black or African American, non-Hispanic/Latino; 8 Asian, non-Hispanic/Latino; 17 Hispanic/Latino; 7 Two or more races, non-Hispanic/Latino), 47 international. Average age 27. 556 applicants, 10% accepted, 49 enrolled. In 2013, 4 master's, 27 doctorates awarded. Terminal master's awarded for partial completion of doctoral program. *Degree requirements:* For master's, comprehensive exam or thesis; for doctorate, comprehensive exam, thesis/dissertation, cumulative exam. *Entrance requirements:* For master's, GRE General Test, GRE Subject Test, minimum undergraduate GPA of 2.75; for doctorate, GRE General Test, GRE Subject Test, minimum GPA of 3.0. *Application deadline:* For fall admission, 12/15 for domestic and international students. Applications are processed on a rolling basis. Application fee: $50 ($60 for international students). Electronic applications accepted. *Financial support:* In 2013–14, 533 students received support, including 68 fellowships (averaging $9,011 per year), 149 research assistantships with full and partial tuition reimbursements available (averaging $29,263 per year), 83 teaching assistantships with full and partial tuition reimbursements available (averaging $29,025 per year); institutionally sponsored loans, scholarships/grants, health care benefits, and unspecified assistantships also available. Financial award applicants required to submit FAFSA. *Faculty research:* Physical chemistry, biochemistry: proteins, organic chemistry, nucleic acid. *Total annual research expenditures:* $21.8 million.
Website: http://chem.colorado.edu

University of Colorado Denver, School of Medicine, Biochemistry Program, Aurora, CO 80045. Offers biochemistry (PhD); biochemistry and molecular genetics (PhD). *Students:* 14 full-time (5 women); includes 1 minority (Hispanic/Latino), 1 international. Average age 31. 2 applicants, 100% accepted, 2 enrolled. In 2013, 3 doctorates awarded. *Degree requirements:* For doctorate, comprehensive exam, thesis/dissertation, 30 credit hours each of coursework and thesis research. *Entrance requirements:* For doctorate, GRE, minimum of three letters of recommendation from qualified referees. Additional exam requirements/recommendations for international students: Required—TOEFL (minimum score 550 paper-based; 80 iBT). *Application deadline:* For fall admission, 12/1 for domestic students. Applications are processed on a rolling basis. Application fee: $50 ($75 for international students). Electronic applications accepted. *Expenses:* Contact institution. *Financial support:* In 2013–14, 14 students received support. Fellowships, research assistantships, teaching assistantships, Federal Work-Study, institutionally sponsored loans, scholarships/grants, traineeships, health care benefits, tuition waivers (full), and unspecified assistantships available. Financial award application deadline: 3/15; financial award applicants required to submit FAFSA. *Faculty research:* DNA damage, cancer and neurodegeneration, molecular mechanisms of pro-MRNA splicing, yeast RNA polymerases, DNA replication. *Total annual research expenditures:* $8.6 million. *Unit head:* Dr. Mark Johnston, Professor and Chair, 303-724-3203, Fax: 303-724-3215, E-mail: mark.johnston@ucdenver.edu. *Application contact:* Jennifer Spaulding, Administrative Assistant, 303-724-3201, Fax: 303-724-3215, E-mail: jennifer.spaulding@ucdenver.edu.
Website: http://www.ucdenver.edu/academics/colleges/medicalschool/departments/biochemistry/Pages/Home.aspx

University of Connecticut, Graduate School, College of Liberal Arts and Sciences, Department of Molecular and Cell Biology, Field of Biochemistry, Storrs, CT 06269. Offers MS, PhD. Terminal master's awarded for partial completion of doctoral program. *Degree requirements:* For master's, comprehensive exam; for doctorate, thesis/dissertation. *Entrance requirements:* For master's and doctorate, GRE General Test, GRE Subject Test. Additional exam requirements/recommendations for international students: Required—TOEFL (minimum score 550 paper-based). Electronic applications accepted.

University of Connecticut Health Center, Graduate School, Programs in Biomedical Sciences, Graduate Program in Molecular Biology and Biochemistry, Farmington, CT 06030. Offers PhD, DMD/PhD, MD/PhD. *Degree requirements:* For doctorate, comprehensive exam, thesis/dissertation. *Entrance requirements:* For doctorate, GRE General Test. Additional exam requirements/recommendations for international students: Required—TOEFL (minimum score 600 paper-based). Electronic applications accepted. *Faculty research:* Molecular biology, structural biology, protein biochemistry, microbial physiology and pathogenesis.

See Display on page 224 and Close-Up on page 245.

University of Delaware, College of Arts and Sciences, Department of Chemistry and Biochemistry, Newark, DE 19716. Offers biochemistry (MA, MS, PhD); chemistry (MA, MS, PhD). Part-time programs available. Terminal master's awarded for partial completion of doctoral program. *Degree requirements:* For master's, one foreign language, thesis (for some programs); for doctorate, one foreign language, thesis/dissertation, cumulative exam. *Entrance requirements:* For master's and doctorate, GRE General Test. Additional exam requirements/recommendations for international students: Required—TOEFL (minimum score 600 paper-based). Electronic applications accepted. *Faculty research:* Micro-organisms, bone, cancer metastosis, developmental biology, cell biology, molecular biology.

University of Detroit Mercy, College of Engineering and Science, Department of Chemistry and Biochemistry, Detroit, MI 48221. Offers chemistry (MS). Evening/weekend programs available. *Degree requirements:* For master's, thesis. *Entrance requirements:* For master's, GRE General Test, minimum GPA of 3.0. *Faculty research:* Polymer and physical chemistry, industrial aspects of chemistry.

University of Florida, College of Medicine and Graduate School, Interdisciplinary Program in Biomedical Sciences, Concentration in Biochemistry and Molecular Biology, Gainesville, FL 32611. Offers PhD. *Degree requirements:* For doctorate, thesis/dissertation. *Entrance requirements:* For doctorate, GRE General Test, minimum GPA of 3.0, biochemistry before enrollment. Additional exam requirements/recommendations for international students: Required—TOEFL. Electronic applications accepted. *Expenses:* Tuition, state resident: full-time $12,640. Tuition, nonresident: full-time $30,000. *Faculty research:* Gene expression, metabolic regulation, structural biology, enzyme mechanism, membrane transporters.

University of Georgia, Franklin College of Arts and Sciences, Department of Biochemistry and Molecular Biology, Athens, GA 30602. Offers MS, PhD. *Degree requirements:* For master's, one foreign language, thesis; for doctorate, one foreign language, thesis/dissertation. *Entrance requirements:* For master's and doctorate, GRE General Test. Additional exam requirements/recommendations for international students: Required—TOEFL. Electronic applications accepted.

University of Guelph, Graduate Studies, College of Biological Science, Department of Molecular and Cellular Biology, Guelph, ON N1G 2W1, Canada. Offers biochemistry (M Sc, PhD); biophysics (M Sc, PhD); botany (M Sc, PhD); microbiology (M Sc, PhD); molecular biology and genetics (M Sc, PhD). *Degree requirements:* For master's, thesis, research proposal; for doctorate, comprehensive exam, thesis/dissertation, research proposal. *Entrance requirements:* For master's, minimum B-average during previous 2 years of coursework; for doctorate, minimum A-average. Additional exam requirements/recommendations for international students: Required—TOEFL (minimum score 550 paper-based), IELTS (minimum score 6.5). Electronic applications accepted. *Faculty research:* Physiology, structure, genetics, and ecology of microbes; virology and microbial technology.

University of Guelph, Graduate Studies, College of Physical and Engineering Science, Guelph-Waterloo Centre for Graduate Work in Chemistry and Biochemistry, Guelph, ON N1G 2W1, Canada. Offers M Sc, PhD. M Sc, PhD offered jointly with University of Waterloo. Part-time programs available. *Degree requirements:* For master's, thesis; for doctorate, thesis/dissertation. *Faculty research:* Inorganic, analytical, biological, physical/theoretical, polymer, and organic chemistry.

University of Houston, College of Natural Sciences and Mathematics, Department of Biology and Biochemistry, Houston, TX 77204. Offers biochemistry (MA, PhD); biology (MA). Terminal master's awarded for partial completion of doctoral program. *Degree requirements:* For master's, comprehensive exam (for some programs), thesis optional; for doctorate, comprehensive exam (for some programs), thesis/dissertation. *Entrance requirements:* For master's and doctorate, GRE. Additional exam requirements/recommendations for international students: Required—TOEFL (minimum score 550 paper-based; 79 iBT), IELTS (minimum score 6.5). Electronic applications accepted. *Faculty research:* Cell and molecular biology, ecology and evolution, biochemical and biophysical sciences, chemical biology.

University of Idaho, College of Graduate Studies, College of Science, Department of Biological Sciences, Moscow, ID 83844-3051. Offers biology (MS, PhD); microbiology, molecular biology and biochemistry (MS, PhD). *Faculty:* 12 full-time. *Students:* 20 full-time, 3 part-time. Average age 31. In 2013, 2 master's, 5 doctorates awarded. *Degree requirements:* For doctorate, one foreign language, thesis/dissertation. *Entrance requirements:* For master's, GRE, minimum GPA of 2.8; for doctorate, GRE, minimum undergraduate GPA of 2.8, 3.0 graduate. Additional exam requirements/recommendations for international students: Required—TOEFL. *Application deadline:* For fall admission, 8/1 for domestic students; for spring admission, 12/15 for domestic

students. Applications are processed on a rolling basis. Application fee: $60. Electronic applications accepted. *Expenses:* Tuition, state resident: full-time $5596; part-time $363 per credit hour. Tuition, nonresident: full-time $18,672; part-time $1089 per credit hour. *Financial support:* Research assistantships and teaching assistantships available. Financial award applicants required to submit FAFSA. *Faculty research:* Animal behavior development, germ cell development, evolutionary biology, fish reproductive biology, molecular mechanisms. *Unit head:* Dr. James J. Nagler, Interim Department Chair, 208-885-6280, E-mail: biosci@uidaho.edu. *Application contact:* Stephanie Thomas, Graduate Recruitment Coordinator, 208-885-4001, Fax: 208-885-4406, E-mail: gadms@uidaho.edu.
Website: http://www.uidaho.edu/sci/biology

University of Illinois at Chicago, College of Medicine and Graduate College, Graduate Programs in Medicine, Department of Biochemistry and Molecular Genetics, Chicago, IL 60607-7128. Offers PhD, MD/PhD. *Faculty:* 32 full-time (11 women), 6 part-time/adjunct (1 woman). *Students:* 31 full-time (17 women), 1 (woman) part-time; includes 5 minority (4 Asian, non-Hispanic/Latino; 1 Hispanic/Latino), 16 international. Average age 29. 7 applicants, 86% accepted, 3 enrolled. In 2013, 10 doctorates awarded. Terminal master's awarded for partial completion of doctoral program. *Degree requirements:* For doctorate, thesis/dissertation. *Entrance requirements:* For doctorate, GRE General Test. Additional exam requirements/recommendations for international students: Required—TOEFL. *Application deadline:* For fall admission, 3/1 priority date for domestic students, 2/15 for international students. Applications are processed on a rolling basis. Application fee: $40 ($50 for international students). Electronic applications accepted. *Expenses:* Tuition, state resident: full-time $11,066; part-time $3689 per term. Tuition, nonresident: full-time $23,064; part-time $7688 per term. *Required fees:* $3004; $1190 per term. Tuition and fees vary according to course level and program. *Financial support:* In 2013–14, 22 students received support. Fellowships with full tuition reimbursements available, research assistantships with full tuition reimbursements available, teaching assistantships with full tuition reimbursements available, career-related internships or fieldwork, Federal Work-Study, institutionally sponsored loans, traineeships, tuition waivers (full), and unspecified assistantships available. Financial award application deadline: 3/1; financial award applicants required to submit FAFSA. *Faculty research:* Nature of cellular components, control of metabolic processes, regulation of gene expression. *Total annual research expenditures:* $6.9 million. *Unit head:* Dr. Jack Kaplan, Head, 312-355-2732, E-mail: kaplanj@uic.edu. *Application contact:* Dr. Karen Colley, Co-Director of Graduate Studies, 312-996-7756.
Website: http://www.uic.edu/com/bcmg/

University of Illinois at Urbana–Champaign, Graduate College, College of Liberal Arts and Sciences, School of Chemical Sciences, Champaign, IL 61820. Offers MA, MS, PhD, MS/JD, MS/MBA. *Students:* 403 (147 women). Application fee: $75 ($90 for international students). *Expenses:* Contact institution. *Unit head:* Jonathan Sweedler, Director, 217-333-5070, Fax: 217-333-2685, E-mail: jsweedle@illinois.edu. *Application contact:* Cheryl Kappes, Office Manager, 217-333-5070, Fax: 217-333-3120, E-mail: dambache@illinois.edu.
Website: http://www.scs.illinois.edu/

University of Illinois at Urbana–Champaign, Graduate College, College of Liberal Arts and Sciences, School of Molecular and Cellular Biology, Department of Biochemistry, Champaign, IL 61820. Offers MS, PhD. *Students:* 69 (32 women). Application fee: $75 ($90 for international students). *Unit head:* James Morrissey, Head, 217-333-2013, Fax: 217-333-8920, E-mail: jhmorris@illinois.edu. *Application contact:* Satish K. Nair, Associate Professor, 217-333-6041, Fax: 217-244-5858, E-mail: snair@illinois.edu.
Website: http://mcb.illinois.edu/departments/biochemistry/index.html

The University of Iowa, Roy J. and Lucille A. Carver College of Medicine and Graduate College, Biosciences Program, Iowa City, IA 52242-1316. Offers anatomy and cell biology (PhD); biochemistry (PhD); biology (PhD); biomedical engineering (PhD); chemistry (PhD); free radical and radiation biology (PhD); genetics (PhD); human toxicology (PhD); immunology (PhD); microbiology (PhD); molecular and cellular biology (PhD); molecular physiology and biophysics (PhD); neuroscience (PhD); pharmacology (PhD); physical therapy and rehabilitation science (PhD); rehabilitation science (PhD); speech and hearing (PhD). *Faculty:* 332 full-time. *Students:* 8 full-time (3 women); includes 2 minority (1 Black or African American, non-Hispanic/Latino; 1 Asian, non-Hispanic/Latino), 1 international. 200 applicants. *Degree requirements:* For doctorate, thesis/dissertation. *Entrance requirements:* For doctorate, GRE General Test, minimum GPA of 3.0. Additional exam requirements/recommendations for international students: Required—TOEFL (minimum score 600 paper-based; 100 iBT). *Application deadline:* For fall admission, 1/1 priority date for domestic and international students. Applications are processed on a rolling basis. Application fee: $60 ($100 for international students). Electronic applications accepted. *Expenses:* Contact institution. *Financial support:* In 2013–14, 8 students received support, including 8 research assistantships with full tuition reimbursements available (averaging $26,000 per year); fellowships, teaching assistantships, health care benefits, and unspecified assistantships also available. *Unit head:* Dr. Douglas Spitz, Director, 319-335-8001, E-mail: douglas-spitz@uiowa.edu. *Application contact:* Jodi Graff, Director, Admissions and First-Year Experience, 319-335-8306, E-mail: biosciences-admissions@uiowa.edu.
Website: http://www.medicine.uiowa.edu/biosciences/

The University of Iowa, Roy J. and Lucille A. Carver College of Medicine and Graduate College, Graduate Programs in Medicine, Department of Biochemistry, Iowa City, IA 52240. Offers MS, MD/PhD. *Faculty:* 20 full-time (7 women), 8 part-time/adjunct (1 woman). *Students:* 27 full-time (11 women); includes 2 minority (both Asian, non-Hispanic/Latino), 10 international. Average age 27. 61 applicants, 13% accepted, 5 enrolled. In 2013, 1 master's awarded. *Degree requirements:* For master's, thesis. *Entrance requirements:* For master's, GRE General Test. Additional exam requirements/recommendations for international students: Required—TOEFL (minimum score 600 paper-based; 100 iBT). *Application deadline:* For winter admission, 1/1 priority date for domestic and international students. Applications are processed on a rolling basis. Application fee: $60 ($100 for international students). Electronic applications accepted. Application fee is waived when completed online. *Financial support:* In 2013–14, research assistantships with full tuition reimbursements (averaging $26,000 per year) were awarded; institutionally sponsored loans, scholarships/grants, traineeships, tuition waivers, and unspecified assistantships also available. *Faculty research:* Regulation of gene expression, protein structure, membrane structure/function, DNA structure and replication. *Total annual research expenditures:* $5.1 million. *Unit head:* Dr. Charles M. Brenner, Chair and Department Executive Officer, 319-335-7934, Fax: 319-335-9570, E-mail: charles-brenner@uiowa.edu. *Application contact:* Admissions Committee, 319-335-7932, Fax: 319-335-9570, E-mail: biochem@uiowa.edu.
Website: http://www.biochem.uiowa.edu/

The University of Kansas, Graduate Studies, College of Liberal Arts and Sciences, Department of Molecular Biosciences, Lawrence, KS 66045. Offers biochemistry and biophysics (MA, PhD); microbiology (MA, PhD); molecular, cellular, and developmental biology (MA, PhD). *Faculty:* 34. *Students:* 52 full-time (28 women); includes 5 minority (2 Asian, non-Hispanic/Latino; 3 Hispanic/Latino), 23 international. Average age 27. 96 applicants, 25% accepted, 13 enrolled. In 2013, 3 master's, 9 doctorates awarded. Terminal master's awarded for partial completion of doctoral program. *Degree requirements:* For master's, comprehensive exam, thesis; for doctorate, comprehensive exam, thesis/dissertation. *Entrance requirements:* For master's and doctorate, GRE General Test. Additional exam requirements/recommendations for international students: Required—TOEFL or IELTS. *Application deadline:* For fall admission, 12/15 for domestic and international students. Application fee: $55 ($65 for international students). Electronic applications accepted. *Financial support:* Fellowships with tuition reimbursements, research assistantships with tuition reimbursements, teaching assistantships with tuition reimbursements, health care benefits, and unspecified assistantships available. Financial award application deadline: 3/1. *Faculty research:* Structure and function of proteins, genetics of organism development, molecular genetics, neurophysiology, molecular virology and pathogenics, developmental biology, cell biology. *Unit head:* Dr. Mark Richter, Chair, 785-864-3334, E-mail: richter@ku.edu. *Application contact:* John Connolly, Graduate Admissions Contact, 785-864-4311, E-mail: jconnolly@ku.edu.
Website: http://www.molecularbiosciences.ku.edu/

The University of Kansas, University of Kansas Medical Center, School of Medicine, Department of Biochemistry and Molecular Biology, Kansas City, KS 66160. Offers MS, PhD, MD/PhD. *Faculty:* 18. *Students:* 9 full-time (4 women), 6 international. Average age 27. In 2013, 1 doctorate awarded. Terminal master's awarded for partial completion of doctoral program. *Degree requirements:* For master's, thesis, oral defense of thesis; for doctorate, thesis/dissertation, comprehensive oral and written exam. *Entrance requirements:* Additional exam requirements/recommendations for international students: Required—TOEFL. Application fee: $0. Electronic applications accepted. *Financial support:* Fellowships, research assistantships with partial tuition reimbursements, teaching assistantships with full and partial tuition reimbursements, traineeships, health care benefits, and unspecified assistantships available. Financial award application deadline: 3/1; financial award applicants required to submit FAFSA. *Faculty research:* Determination of portion structure, underlying bases for interaction of proteins with their target, mapping allosteric circuiting within proteins, mechanism of action of transcription factors, renal signal transduction. *Total annual research expenditures:* $2.1 million. *Unit head:* Dr. Gerald M. Carlson, Chairman, 913-588-7005, Fax: 913-588-9896, E-mail: gcarlson@kumc.edu. *Application contact:* Dr. Liskin Swint-Kruse, Associate Professor, 913-588-0399, Fax: 913-588-9896, E-mail: lswint-kruse@kumc.edu.
Website: http://www.kumc.edu/school-of-medicine/biochemistry-and-molecular-biology.html

University of Kentucky, Graduate School, Graduate School Programs from the College of Medicine, Program in Molecular and Cellular Biochemistry, Lexington, KY 40506-0032. Offers PhD, MD/PhD. *Degree requirements:* For doctorate, comprehensive exam, thesis/dissertation. *Entrance requirements:* For doctorate, GRE General Test, minimum undergraduate GPA of 2.75. Additional exam requirements/recommendations for international students: Required—TOEFL (minimum score 550 paper-based). Electronic applications accepted.

University of Lethbridge, School of Graduate Studies, Lethbridge, AB T1K 3M4, Canada. Offers accounting (MScM); addictions counseling (M Sc); agricultural biotechnology (M Sc); agricultural studies (M Sc, MA); anthropology (MA); archaeology (M Sc, MA); art (MA, MFA); biochemistry (M Sc); biological sciences (M Sc); biomolecular science (PhD); biosystems and biodiversity (PhD); Canadian studies (MA); chemistry (M Sc); computer science (M Sc); computer science and geographical information science (M Sc); counseling (MC); counseling psychology (M Ed); dramatic arts (MA); earth, space, and physical science (PhD); economics (MA); education (MA); educational leadership (M Ed); English (MA); environmental science (M Sc); evolution and behavior (PhD); exercise science (M Sc); finance (MScM); French (MA); French/German (MA); French/Spanish (MA); general education (M Ed); general management (MScM); geography (M Sc, MA); German (MA); health sciences (M Sc); human resource management and labour relations (MScM); individualized multidisciplinary (M Sc, MA); information systems (MScM); international management (MScM); kinesiology (M Sc, MA); marketing (MScM); mathematics (M Sc); modern languages (MA); music (M Mus, MA); Native American studies (MA); neuroscience (M Sc, PhD); new media (MA, MFA); nursing (M Sc); philosophy (MA); physics (M Sc); policy and strategy (MScM); political science (MA); psychology (M Sc, MA); religious studies (MA); sociology (MA); theatre and dramatic arts (MFA); theoretical and computational science (PhD); urban and regional studies (MA); women and gender studies (MA). Part-time and evening/weekend programs available. *Degree requirements:* For doctorate, comprehensive exam, thesis/dissertation. *Entrance requirements:* For master's, GMAT (for M Sc in management), bachelor's degree in related field, minimum GPA of 3.0 during previous 20 graded semester courses, 2 years teaching or related experience (M Ed); for doctorate, master's degree, minimum graduate GPA of 3.5. Additional exam requirements/recommendations for international students: Required—TOEFL. Application fee: $60 Canadian dollars. *Financial support:* Fellowships, research assistantships, teaching assistantships, scholarships/grants, health care benefits, and unspecified assistantships available. *Faculty research:* Movement and brain plasticity, gibberellin physiology, photosynthesis, carbon cycling, molecular properties of main-group ring components. *Application contact:* School of Graduate Studies, 403-329-2793, Fax: 403-332-5239, E-mail: sgsinquiries@uleth.ca.
Website: http://www.uleth.ca/graduatestudies/

University of Louisville, Graduate School, College of Arts and Sciences, Department of Chemistry, Louisville, KY 40292-0001. Offers analytical chemistry (MS, PhD); biochemistry (MS, PhD); chemical physics (PhD); inorganic chemistry (MS, PhD); organic chemistry (MS, PhD); physical chemistry (MS, PhD). *Students:* 44 full-time (14 women), 6 part-time (1 woman); includes 2 minority (1 Hispanic/Latino; 1 Two or more races, non-Hispanic/Latino), 35 international. Average age 30. 49 applicants, 45% accepted, 12 enrolled. In 2013, 5 master's, 5 doctorates awarded. Terminal master's awarded for partial completion of doctoral program. *Degree requirements:* For master's, variable foreign language requirement, comprehensive exam, thesis optional; for doctorate, variable foreign language requirement, comprehensive exam, thesis/dissertation. *Entrance requirements:* For master's and doctorate, GRE General Test, BA or BS coursework. Additional exam requirements/recommendations for international students: Required—TOEFL (minimum score 550 paper-based; 79 iBT). *Application deadline:* For fall admission, 3/15 for domestic students, 5/1 priority date for international students; for winter admission, 9/15 for domestic and international students; for spring admission, 11/1 priority date for international students; for summer admission, 4/1 priority date for international students. Applications are processed on a rolling basis. Application fee: $60. Electronic applications accepted. *Expenses:* Tuition, state resident: full-time $10,788; part-time $599 per credit hour. Tuition, nonresident: full-time $22,446; part-time $1247 per credit hour. *Required fees:* $196. Tuition and fees vary according to program and reciprocity agreements. *Financial support:* Fellowships with full tuition reimbursements, research assistantships with full tuition reimbursements, teaching assistantships with full tuition reimbursements, career-related internships or fieldwork, scholarships/grants, traineeships, health care benefits, and unspecified assistantships available. Support available to part-time students. Financial award application deadline: 3/15. *Faculty research:* Computational chemistry, biophysics nuclear magnetic resonance, synthetic organic chemistry, synthetic inorganic chemistry, medicinal chemistry, protein chemistry, enzymology, nanochemistry, electrochemistry, analytical chemistry, synthetic biology, bioinformatics. *Unit head:* Dr. Richard J. Wittebort, Professor/Chair, 502-852-6613. *Application contact:* Libby Leggett, Director, Graduate Admissions, 502-852-3101, Fax: 502-852-6536, E-mail: gradadm@louisville.edu.

University of Louisville, School of Medicine, Department of Biochemistry and Molecular Biology, Louisville, KY 40292-0001. Offers MS, PhD, MD/PhD. *Students:* 28 full-time (13 women), 8 part-time (4 women); includes 4 minority (2 Black or African American, non-Hispanic/Latino; 1 Asian, non-Hispanic/Latino; 1 Hispanic/Latino), 9 international. Average age 30. 34 applicants, 21% accepted, 9 enrolled. In 2013, 5 master's, 4 doctorates awarded. Terminal master's awarded for partial completion of doctoral program. *Degree requirements:* For master's, thesis; for doctorate, comprehensive exam, thesis/dissertation, one first author publication. *Entrance requirements:* For master's and doctorate, GRE General Test (minimum score of 1000 verbal and quantitative), minimum GPA of 3.0. Additional exam requirements/recommendations for international students: Required—TOEFL. *Application deadline:* For fall admission, 4/15 for domestic and international students. Applications are processed on a rolling basis. Application fee: $60. Electronic applications accepted. *Expenses:* Tuition, state resident: full-time $10,788; part-time $599 per credit hour. Tuition, nonresident: full-time $22,446; part-time $1247 per credit hour. *Required fees:* $196. Tuition and fees vary according to program and reciprocity agreements. *Financial support:* In 2013–14, 12 fellowships with full tuition reimbursements (averaging $22,000 per year), 23 research assistantships with full tuition reimbursements (averaging $22,000 per year) were awarded; teaching assistantships with tuition reimbursements, scholarships/grants, traineeships, tuition waivers (full and partial), and unspecified assistantships also available. Financial award application deadline: 4/15. *Faculty research:* Genetic regulatory mechanisms, microRNAs, vesicular trafficking in cancer metastasis and angiogenesis, ribosome biogenesis and disease, regulation of foreign compound metabolism/lipid and steroid metabolism. *Unit head:* Dr. Ronald G. Gregg, Chair, 502-852-5217, Fax: 502-852-6222, E-mail: rggreg02@gwise.louisville.edu. *Application contact:* Dr. William L. Dean, Information Contact, 502-852-5227, Fax: 502-852-6222, E-mail: wldean01@gwise.louisville.edu.

University of Maine, Graduate School, College of Natural Sciences, Forestry, and Agriculture, Department of Molecular and Biomedical Sciences, Orono, ME 04469. Offers biochemistry (MPS, MS); biochemistry and molecular biology (PhD); microbiology (MPS, MS, PhD). *Faculty:* 30 full-time (6 women), 20 part-time/adjunct (4 women). *Students:* 26 full-time (17 women), 4 part-time (3 women); includes 3 minority (2 Asian, non-Hispanic/Latino; 1 Native Hawaiian or other Pacific Islander, non-Hispanic/Latino), 5 international. Average age 31. 7 applicants, 100% accepted, 5 enrolled. In 2013, 5 master's, 4 doctorates awarded. *Degree requirements:* For master's, thesis (for some programs); for doctorate, comprehensive exam, thesis/dissertation. *Entrance requirements:* For master's and doctorate, GRE General Test. Additional exam requirements/recommendations for international students: Required—TOEFL. *Application deadline:* For fall admission, 2/1 priority date for domestic students. Applications are processed on a rolling basis. Application fee: $65. Electronic applications accepted. *Expenses:* Tuition, state resident: full-time $7524. Tuition, nonresident: full-time $23,112. *Required fees:* $1970. *Financial support:* In 2013–14, 16 students received support, including 5 research assistantships with full tuition reimbursements available (averaging $22,000 per year), 10 teaching assistantships with full tuition reimbursements available (averaging $19,000 per year); tuition waivers (full and partial) also available. Financial award application deadline: 3/1. *Total annual research expenditures:* $242,844. *Unit head:* Dr. Robert Gundersen, Chair, 207-581-2802, Fax: 207-581-2801. *Application contact:* Scott G. Delcourt, Associate Dean of the Graduate School, 207-581-3291, Fax: 207-581-3232, E-mail: graduate@maine.edu. Website: http://umaine.edu/biomed/

The University of Manchester, Faculty of Life Sciences, Manchester, United Kingdom. Offers adaptive organismal biology (M Phil, PhD); animal biology (M Phil, PhD); biochemistry (M Phil, PhD); bioinformatics (M Phil, PhD); biomolecular sciences (M Phil, PhD); biotechnology (M Phil, PhD); cell biology (M Phil, PhD); cell matrix research (M Phil, PhD); channels and transporters (M Phil, PhD); developmental biology (M Phil, PhD); Egyptology (M Phil, PhD); environmental biology (M Phil, PhD); evolutionary biology (M Phil, PhD); gene expression (M Phil, PhD); genetics (M Phil, PhD); history of science, technology and medicine (M Phil, PhD); immunology (M Phil, PhD); integrative neurobiology and behavior (M Phil, PhD); membrane trafficking (M Phil, PhD); microbiology (M Phil, PhD); molecular and cellular neuroscience (M Phil, PhD); molecular biology (M Phil, PhD); molecular cancer studies (M Phil, PhD); neuroscience (M Phil, PhD); ophthalmology (M Phil, PhD); optometry (M Phil, PhD); organelle function (M Phil, PhD); pharmacology (M Phil, PhD); physiology (M Phil, PhD); plant sciences (M Phil, PhD); stem cell research (M Phil, PhD); structural biology (M Phil, PhD); systems neuroscience (M Phil, PhD); toxicology (M Phil, PhD).

The University of Manchester, School of Chemistry, Manchester, United Kingdom. Offers biological chemistry (PhD); chemistry (M Ent, M Phil, M Sc, D Ent, PhD); inorganic chemistry (PhD); materials chemistry (PhD); nanoscience (PhD); nuclear fission (PhD); organic chemistry (PhD); physical chemistry (PhD); theoretical chemistry (PhD).

University of Manitoba, Faculty of Medicine and Faculty of Graduate Studies, Graduate Programs in Medicine, Department of Biochemistry and Medical Genetics, Winnipeg, MB R3T 2N2, Canada. Offers M Sc, PhD. Terminal master's awarded for partial completion of doctoral program. *Degree requirements:* For master's, thesis; for doctorate, thesis/dissertation. *Faculty research:* Cancer, gene expression, membrane lipids, metabolic control, genetic diseases.

University of Maryland, Baltimore, Graduate School, Graduate Program in Life Sciences, Program in Biochemistry and Molecular Biology, Baltimore, MD 21201. Offers biochemistry (MS, PhD); MD/PhD. *Students:* 26 full-time (11 women), 3 part-time (1 woman); includes 8 minority (3 Black or African American, non-Hispanic/Latino; 1 Asian, non-Hispanic/Latino; 3 Hispanic/Latino; 1 Two or more races, non-Hispanic/Latino), 4 international. Average age 27. 47 applicants, 17% accepted, 3 enrolled. In 2013, 1 master's, 7 doctorates awarded. *Degree requirements:* For doctorate, comprehensive exam, thesis/dissertation. *Entrance requirements:* For doctorate, GRE General Test. Additional exam requirements/recommendations for international students: Required—TOEFL (minimum score 550 paper-based; 80 iBT); Recommended—IELTS (minimum score 7). *Application deadline:* For fall admission, 1/15 for domestic and international students. Application fee: $75. Electronic applications accepted. *Financial support:* In 2013–14, research assistantships with full tuition reimbursements (averaging $25,000 per year) were awarded; fellowships, health care benefits, and unspecified assistantships also available. Financial award application deadline: 3/1; financial award applicants required to submit FAFSA. *Faculty research:* Membrane transport, hormonal regulation, protein structure, molecular virology. *Unit head:* Dr. Gerald Wilson, Professor/Director, 410-706-8904. *Application contact:* Kiriaki Cozmo, Program Coordinator, 410-706-7340, Fax: 410-706-8297, E-mail: kicozmo@som.umaryland.edu. Website: http://biochemistry.umaryland.edu

University of Maryland, Baltimore County, Graduate School, College of Natural and Mathematical Sciences, Department of Chemistry and Biochemistry, Baltimore, MD 21250. Offers biochemistry (PhD); chemistry (MS, PhD); chemistry and biochemistry (Postbaccalaureate Certificate). Part-time programs available. *Faculty:* 19 full-time (4 women), 3 part-time/adjunct (0 women). *Students:* 51 full-time (23 women), 3 part-time (1 woman); includes 11 minority (5 Black or African American, non-Hispanic/Latino; 3 Asian, non-Hispanic/Latino; 3 Hispanic/Latino), 12 international. Average age 26. 79 applicants, 32% accepted, 12 enrolled. In 2013, 3 master's, 7 doctorates awarded. Terminal master's awarded for partial completion of doctoral program. *Degree requirements:* For master's, comprehensive exam (for some programs), thesis (for some programs); for doctorate, comprehensive exam, thesis/dissertation. *Entrance requirements:* For master's, GRE General Test, minimum GPA of 3.0; for doctorate, GRE General Test, GRE Subject Test (recommended), minimum GPA of 3.0. Additional exam requirements/recommendations for international students: Required—TOEFL (minimum score 550 paper-based; 80 iBT). *Application deadline:* For fall admission, 6/1 priority date for domestic students, 1/1 priority date for international students; for spring admission, 11/1 priority date for domestic students, 5/1 for international students. Applications are processed on a rolling basis. Application fee: $50. Electronic applications accepted. One-time fee: $200 full-time. *Financial support:* In 2013–14, 3 fellowships with full tuition reimbursements (averaging $24,000 per year), 19 research assistantships with full tuition reimbursements (averaging $21,420 per year), 29 teaching assistantships with full tuition reimbursements (averaging $21,420 per year) were awarded; health care benefits also available. *Faculty research:* Protein structures, bio-organic chemistry, enzyme catalysis, molecular biology, metabolism, nanotechnology. *Total annual research expenditures:* $4.1 million. *Unit head:* Dr. Zeev Rosenzweig, Director, Graduate Program, 410-455-2491, Fax: 410-455-2608, E-mail: chemgrad@umbc.edu. *Application contact:* Patricia Gagne, Graduate Coordinator, 866-PhD-UMBC, Fax: 410-455-2608, E-mail: pgagne1@umbc.edu.
Website: http://www.umbc.edu/chem

University of Maryland, College Park, Academic Affairs, College of Computer, Mathematical and Natural Sciences, Department of Chemistry and Biochemistry, Biochemistry Program, College Park, MD 20742. Offers MS, PhD. Part-time and evening/weekend programs available. *Students:* 49 full-time (22 women), 1 (woman) part-time; includes 10 minority (3 Black or African American, non-Hispanic/Latino; 6 Asian, non-Hispanic/Latino; 1 Two or more races, non-Hispanic/Latino), 21 international. 96 applicants, 30% accepted, 14 enrolled. In 2013, 2 master's, 11 doctorates awarded. Terminal master's awarded for partial completion of doctoral program. *Degree requirements:* For master's, thesis or alternative; for doctorate, thesis/dissertation, 2 seminar presentations, oral exam. *Entrance requirements:* For master's and doctorate, GRE General Test, GRE Subject Test (recommended), minimum GPA of 3.0, 3 letters of recommendation. Additional exam requirements/recommendations for international students: Required—TOEFL. *Application deadline:* For fall admission, 1/15 for domestic and international students; for spring admission, 6/1 for domestic and international students. Applications are processed on a rolling basis. Application fee: $75. Electronic applications accepted. *Expenses:* Tuition, state resident: full-time $10,314; part-time $573 per credit hour. Tuition, nonresident: full-time $22,248; part-time $1236 per credit. *Required fees:* $1446; $403.15 per semester. Tuition and fees vary according to program. *Financial support:* In 2013–14, 5 fellowships with full and partial tuition reimbursements (averaging $13,226 per year), 11 research assistantships (averaging $20,164 per year), 33 teaching assistantships (averaging $19,370 per year) were awarded; Federal Work-Study also available. Support available to part-time students. Financial award applicants required to submit FAFSA. *Faculty research:* Analytical biochemistry, immunochemistry, drug metabolism, biosynthesis of proteins, mass spectrometry. *Unit head:* Dr. Michael Doyle, Chairperson, 301-405-1795, Fax: 301-314-2779, E-mail: mdoyle3@umd.edu. *Application contact:* Dr. Charles A. Caramello, Dean of Graduate School, 301-405-0358, Fax: 301-314-9305, E-mail: ccaramel@umd.edu.

University of Massachusetts Amherst, Graduate School, College of Natural Sciences, Department of Biochemistry and Molecular Biology, Amherst, MA 01003. Offers MS, PhD. Part-time programs available. *Faculty:* 21 full-time (10 women). *Students:* 2 part-time (1 woman); includes 1 minority (Hispanic/Latino). Average age 29. In 2013, 1 master's awarded. Terminal master's awarded for partial completion of doctoral program. *Degree requirements:* For master's, thesis or alternative; for doctorate, comprehensive exam, thesis/dissertation. *Entrance requirements:* Additional exam requirements/recommendations for international students: Required—TOEFL (minimum score 550 paper-based; 80 iBT), IELTS (minimum score 6.5). *Application deadline:* For fall admission, 2/1 for domestic and international students; for spring admission, 10/1 for domestic and international students. Applications are processed on a rolling basis. Application fee: $75. Electronic applications accepted. *Financial support:* Fellowships with full and partial tuition reimbursements, research assistantships with full and partial tuition reimbursements, teaching assistantships with full and partial tuition reimbursements, career-related internships or fieldwork, Federal Work-Study, scholarships/grants, traineeships, health care benefits, tuition waivers (full and partial), and unspecified assistantships available. Support available to part-time students. Financial award application deadline: 2/1. *Unit head:* Dr. Danny Schnell, Graduate Program Director, 413-545-0352, Fax: 413-545-3291. *Application contact:* Lindsay DeSantis, Supervisor of Admissions, 413-545-0722, Fax: 413-577-0010, E-mail: gradadm@grad.umass.edu.
Website: http://www.biochem.umass.edu/graduate

University of Massachusetts Amherst, Graduate School, Interdisciplinary Programs, Program in Molecular and Cellular Biology, Amherst, MA 01003. Offers biological chemistry and molecular biophysics (PhD); biomedicine (PhD); cellular and developmental biology (PhD). Part-time programs available. *Students:* 72 full-time (41 women); includes 15 minority (4 Black or African American, non-Hispanic/Latino; 5 Asian, non-Hispanic/Latino; 4 Hispanic/Latino; 2 Two or more races, non-Hispanic/Latino), 28 international. Average age 27. 160 applicants, 23% accepted, 20 enrolled. In 2013, 13 doctorates awarded. Terminal master's awarded for partial completion of doctoral program. *Degree requirements:* For doctorate, comprehensive exam, thesis/dissertation. *Entrance requirements:* For doctorate, GRE General Test. Additional exam requirements/recommendations for international students: Required—TOEFL (minimum score 550 paper-based; 80 iBT), IELTS (minimum score 6.5). *Application deadline:* For fall admission, 12/1 for domestic and international students. Applications are processed on a rolling basis. Application fee: $75. Electronic applications accepted. *Financial support:* Fellowships with full and partial tuition reimbursements, research assistantships with full and partial tuition reimbursements, teaching assistantships with full and partial tuition reimbursements, career-related internships or fieldwork, Federal Work-Study, scholarships/grants, traineeships, health care benefits, tuition waivers (full and partial), and unspecified assistantships available. Support available to part-time students. Financial award application deadline: 12/1; financial award applicants required to submit FAFSA. *Unit head:* Dr. Barbara Osborne, Graduate Program Director, 413-545-3246, Fax: 413-545-1812, E-mail: mcb@mcb.umass.edu. *Application contact:* Lindsay DeSantis, Supervisor of Admissions, 413-545-0722, Fax: 413-577-0010, E-mail: gradadm@grad.umass.edu.
Website: http://www.bio.umass.edu/mcb/

University of Massachusetts Amherst, Graduate School, Interdisciplinary Programs, Program in Plant Biology, Amherst, MA 01003. Offers biochemistry and metabolism (MS, PhD); cell biology and physiology (MS, PhD); environmental, ecological and

integrative biology (MS, PhD); genetics and evolution (MS, PhD). *Students:* 20 full-time (11 women), 9 international. Average age 28. 72 applicants, 17% accepted, 2 enrolled. In 2013, 1 master's, 2 doctorates awarded. *Degree requirements:* For master's, thesis; for doctorate, 2 foreign languages, comprehensive exam, thesis/dissertation. *Entrance requirements:* For master's and doctorate, GRE General Test. Additional exam requirements/recommendations for international students: Required—TOEFL (minimum score 550 paper-based; 80 iBT), IELTS (minimum score 6.5). *Application deadline:* For fall admission, 12/15 for domestic and international students; for spring admission, 10/1 for domestic and international students. Applications are processed on a rolling basis. Application fee: $75. Electronic applications accepted. *Financial support:* Fellowships with full and partial tuition reimbursements, research assistantships with full and partial tuition reimbursements, teaching assistantships with full and partial tuition reimbursements, career-related internships or fieldwork, Federal Work-Study, scholarships/grants, traineeships, health care benefits, tuition waivers (full and partial), and unspecified assistantships available. Support available to part-time students. Financial award application deadline: 12/15; financial award applicants required to submit FAFSA. *Unit head:* Dr. Elsbeth L. Walker, Graduate Program Director, 413-577-3217, Fax: 413-545-3243, E-mail: pb@bio.umass.edu. *Application contact:* Lindsay DeSantis, Supervisor of Admissions, 413-545-0722, Fax: 413-577-0010, E-mail: gradadm@grad.umass.edu.
Website: http://www.bio.umass.edu/plantbio/

University of Massachusetts Dartmouth, Graduate School, College of Arts and Sciences, Department of Chemistry and Biochemistry, North Dartmouth, MA 02747-2300. Offers MS, PhD. Part-time programs available. *Faculty:* 15 full-time (3 women), 3 part-time/adjunct (2 women). *Students:* 17 full-time (9 women), 14 part-time (7 women); includes 4 minority (1 Black or African American, non-Hispanic/Latino; 3 Asian, non-Hispanic/Latino), 17 international. Average age 27. 29 applicants, 79% accepted, 10 enrolled. In 2013, 4 master's awarded. *Degree requirements:* For master's, comprehensive exam (for some programs), thesis or project; for doctorate, thesis/dissertation (for some programs). *Entrance requirements:* For master's and doctorate, GRE (recommended), statement of purpose (minimum of 300 words), resume, 2 letters of recommendation, official transcripts. Additional exam requirements/recommendations for international students: Required—TOEFL (minimum score 550 paper-based). *Application deadline:* For fall admission, 3/15 priority date for domestic students, 2/15 priority date for international students; for spring admission, 11/1 priority date for domestic students, 10/1 priority date for international students. Applications are processed on a rolling basis. Application fee: $60. Electronic applications accepted. *Expenses:* Tuition, state resident: full-time $2071; part-time $86.29 per credit. Tuition, nonresident: full-time $8099; part-time $337.46 per credit. Tuition and fees vary according to course load and reciprocity agreements. *Financial support:* In 2013–14, 7 research assistantships with full tuition reimbursements (averaging $10,038 per year), 24 teaching assistantships with full and partial tuition reimbursements (averaging $10,542 per year) were awarded; Federal Work-Study and unspecified assistantships also available. Support available to part-time students. Financial award application deadline: 3/1; financial award applicants required to submit FAFSA. *Faculty research:* Bioanalytical chemistry, biochemistry and molecular biology, inorganic chemistry, organic analytical chemistry, physical chemistry. *Total annual research expenditures:* $1.8 million. *Unit head:* Dr. Yuegang Zuo, Graduate Program Director, 508-999-8959, Fax: 508-999-9167, E-mail: yzuo@umassd.edu. *Application contact:* Steven Briggs, Director of Marketing and Recruitment for Graduate Studies, 508-999-8604, Fax: 508-999-8183, E-mail: graduate@umassd.edu.
Website: http://www.umassd.edu/cas/chemistry/

University of Massachusetts Lowell, College of Sciences, Department of Biological Sciences, Lowell, MA 01854-2881. Offers biochemistry (PhD); biological sciences (MS); biotechnology (MS). Part-time programs available. *Degree requirements:* For master's, thesis; for doctorate, thesis/dissertation. *Entrance requirements:* For master's and doctorate, GRE General Test. Electronic applications accepted.

University of Massachusetts Lowell, College of Sciences, Department of Chemistry, Lowell, MA 01854-2881. Offers analytical chemistry (PhD); biochemistry (PhD); chemistry (MS, PhD); environmental studies (PhD); green chemistry (PhD); inorganic chemistry (PhD); organic chemistry (PhD); polymer science (MS). Terminal master's awarded for partial completion of doctoral program. *Degree requirements:* For master's, thesis; for doctorate, 2 foreign languages, thesis/dissertation. *Entrance requirements:* For master's and doctorate, GRE General Test. Electronic applications accepted.

University of Massachusetts Worcester, Graduate School of Biomedical Sciences, Worcester, MA 01655-0115. Offers biochemistry and molecular pharmacology (PhD); bioinformatics and computational biology (PhD); cancer biology (PhD); cell biology (PhD); clinical and population health research (PhD); clinical investigation (MS); immunology and virology (PhD); interdisciplinary biomedical research (PhD); millennium (PhD); molecular genetics and microbiology (PhD); neuroscience (PhD); translational science (PhD); MD/PhD. *Faculty:* 1,388 full-time (521 women), 309 part-time/adjunct (198 women). *Students:* 385 full-time (210 women); includes 53 minority (13 Black or African American, non-Hispanic/Latino; 30 Asian, non-Hispanic/Latino; 10 Hispanic/Latino), 138 international. Average age 28. 491 applicants, 19% accepted, 39 enrolled. In 2013, 5 master's, 50 doctorates awarded. Terminal master's awarded for partial completion of doctoral program. *Median time to degree:* Of those who began their doctoral program in fall 2005, 67% received their degree in 8 years or less. *Degree requirements:* For master's, comprehensive exam, thesis; for doctorate, comprehensive exam, thesis/dissertation. *Entrance requirements:* For master's, MD, PhD, DVM, or PharmD; for doctorate, GRE General Test, bachelor's degree. Additional exam requirements/recommendations for international students: Required—TOEFL (minimum score 100 iBT) or IELTS (minimum score 7.5). *Application deadline:* For fall admission, 12/15 for domestic and international students; for spring admission, 5/15 for domestic students. Application fee: $80. Electronic applications accepted. *Expenses:* Contact institution. *Financial support:* In 2013–14, 431 students received support, including research assistantships with full tuition reimbursements available (averaging $29,500 per year); scholarships/grants, health care benefits, tuition waivers (full), and unspecified assistantships also available. Financial award application deadline: 5/16. *Faculty research:* RNA interference, cell/molecular/developmental biology, bioinformatics, clinical/translational research, infectious disease. *Total annual research expenditures:* $245.9 million. *Unit head:* Dr. Anthony Carruthers, Dean, 508-856-4135, E-mail: anthony.carruthers@umassmed.edu. *Application contact:* Dr. Kendall Knight, Associate Dean and Interim Director of Admissions and Recruitment, 508-856-5628, Fax: 508-856-3659, E-mail: kendall.knight@umassmed.edu.
Website: http://www.umassmed.edu/gsbs/

University of Miami, Graduate School, Miller School of Medicine, Graduate Programs in Medicine, Department of Biochemistry and Molecular Biology, Coral Gables, FL 33124. Offers PhD, MD/PhD. *Degree requirements:* For doctorate, comprehensive exam, thesis/dissertation, proposition exams. *Faculty research:* Macromolecule metabolism, molecular genetics, protein folding and 3-D structure, regulation of gene expression and enzyme function, signal transduction and developmental biology.

University of Michigan, Rackham Graduate School, College of Literature, Science, and the Arts, Department of Chemistry, Ann Arbor, MI 48109-1055. Offers analytical chemistry (PhD); chemical biology (PhD); inorganic chemistry (PhD); material chemistry (PhD); organic chemistry (PhD); physical chemistry (PhD). *Faculty:* 37 full-time (10 women), 15 part-time/adjunct (1 woman). *Students:* 232 full-time (102 women); includes 31 minority (19 Asian, non-Hispanic/Latino; 5 Hispanic/Latino; 7 Two or more races, non-Hispanic/Latino), 59 international. 596 applicants, 30% accepted, 57 enrolled. In 2013, 35 doctorates awarded. *Degree requirements:* For doctorate, comprehensive exam, thesis/dissertation, oral defense of dissertation, organic cumulative proficiency exams. *Entrance requirements:* For doctorate, GRE General Test, GRE Subject Test (recommended), 3 letters of recommendation. Additional exam requirements/recommendations for international students: Required—TOEFL (minimum score 560 paper-based; 84 iBT). *Application deadline:* For fall admission, 12/15 for domestic and international students. Applications are processed on a rolling basis. Application fee: $0 ($90 for international students). Electronic applications accepted. Tuition and fees vary according to course level, course load, degree level, program and student level. *Financial support:* In 2013–14, 232 students received support, including 14 fellowships with full tuition reimbursements available (averaging $27,900 per year), 82 research assistantships with full tuition reimbursements available (averaging $27,900 per year), 136 teaching assistantships with full tuition reimbursements available (averaging $27,900 per year); career-related internships or fieldwork, scholarships/grants, traineeships, health care benefits, and unspecified assistantships also available. *Faculty research:* Biological catalysis, protein engineering, chemical sensors, de novo metalloprotein design, supramolecular architecture. *Unit head:* Dr. Carol A. Fierke, Chair, 734-763-9681, Fax: 734-647-4847. *Application contact:* Cornelius Wright, Manager of Student Services, 734-764-7278, Fax: 734-647-4865, E-mail: chemadmissions@umich.edu.
Website: http://www.lsa.umich.edu/chem/

University of Michigan, Rackham Graduate School, Program in Biomedical Sciences (PIBS), Department of Biological Chemistry, Ann Arbor, MI 48109-0600. Offers MS, PhD. *Faculty:* 44 full-time (9 women), 2 part-time/adjunct (0 women). *Students:* 35 full-time (14 women); includes 8 minority (2 Black or African American, non-Hispanic/Latino; 1 Asian, non-Hispanic/Latino; 3 Hispanic/Latino; 2 Two or more races, non-Hispanic/Latino), 4 international. Average age 27. 95 applicants, 32% accepted, 10 enrolled. In 2013, 1 master's, 9 doctorates awarded. Terminal master's awarded for partial completion of doctoral program. *Degree requirements:* For master's, thesis; for doctorate, comprehensive exam, thesis/dissertation. *Entrance requirements:* For master's, bachelor's degree; for doctorate, GRE, bachelor's degree. Additional exam requirements/recommendations for international students: Required—TOEFL (minimum score 84 iBT). *Application deadline:* For fall admission, 12/1 for domestic and international students. Application fee: $75 ($90 for international students). Electronic applications accepted. *Expenses:* Contact institution. *Financial support:* In 2013–14, 1 student received support, including 1 fellowship with full tuition reimbursement available (averaging $28,800 per year), 33 research assistantships with full tuition reimbursements available (averaging $28,500 per year), 11 teaching assistantships with partial tuition reimbursements available; traineeships, health care benefits, tuition waivers, and unspecified assistantships also available. *Faculty research:* Biochemical signaling, structural enzymology, protein processing and folding, regulation of gene expression. *Total annual research expenditures:* $5.3 million. *Unit head:* Melinda K. Warden, Administrative Director, Healthcare, 734-763-0185, Fax: 734-763-4581, E-mail: mkwarden@umich.edu. *Application contact:* Elizabeth L. Goodwin, Graduate Program Manager, 734-764-8594, Fax: 734-763-4581, E-mail: egoodwin@umich.edu.
Website: http://www.biochem.med.umich.edu/

University of Michigan, Rackham Graduate School, Program in Chemical Biology, Ann Arbor, MI 48109-2216. Offers cancer chemical biology (MS); chemical biology (PhD). *Faculty:* 46 full-time (10 women), 1 (woman) part-time/adjunct. *Students:* 54 full-time (22 women); includes 13 minority (3 Black or African American, non-Hispanic/Latino; 4 Asian, non-Hispanic/Latino; 3 Hispanic/Latino; 3 Two or more races, non-Hispanic/Latino), 8 international. Average age 26. 79 applicants, 57% accepted, 18 enrolled. In 2013, 2 master's, 8 doctorates awarded. *Degree requirements:* For doctorate, thesis/dissertation. *Entrance requirements:* Additional exam requirements/recommendations for international students: Required—TOEFL (minimum score 600 paper-based; 102 iBT). *Application deadline:* For fall admission, 12/15 priority date for domestic and international students. Applications are processed on a rolling basis. Application fee: $75 ($90 for international students). Electronic applications accepted. Tuition and fees vary according to course level, course load, degree level, program and student level. *Financial support:* In 2013–14, 46 students received support, including fellowships with full tuition reimbursements available (averaging $28,500 per year), research assistantships with full tuition reimbursements available (averaging $28,500 per year); career-related internships or fieldwork, scholarships/grants, traineeships, health care benefits, and unspecified assistantships also available. *Faculty research:* Chemical genetics, structural enzymology, signal transduction, biological catalysis, biomolecular structure, function and recognition. *Unit head:* Prof. Anna Mapp, Program Director, 734-763-7175, Fax: 734-615-1252, E-mail: chemicalbiology@umich.edu. *Application contact:* Admissions Office, 734-764-8129, E-mail: rackadmis@umich.edu.
Website: http://www.chembio.umich.edu/

University of Michigan–Flint, College of Arts and Sciences, Flint, MI 48502-1950. Offers arts administration (MA), including museum and visual arts, performance; biochemistry (MS); biology (MS); chemistry (MS); computer science and information systems (MS), including computer science, information systems; English language and literature (MA), including literature, writing and rhetoric; liberal studies (MA), including American culture, American theatre; mathematics (MA); social sciences (MA), including gender studies, global studies, U.S. history and politics. Part-time programs available. *Faculty:* 47 full-time (20 women), 20 part-time/adjunct (8 women). *Students:* 65 full-time (33 women), 315 part-time (174 women); includes 72 minority (43 Black or African American, non-Hispanic/Latino; 1 American Indian or Alaska Native, non-Hispanic/Latino; 6 Asian, non-Hispanic/Latino; 8 Hispanic/Latino; 1 Native Hawaiian or other Pacific Islander, non-Hispanic/Latino; 13 Two or more races, non-Hispanic/Latino), 53 international. Average age 33. 219 applicants, 54% accepted, 64 enrolled. In 2013, 131 master's awarded. *Degree requirements:* For master's, thesis optional. *Entrance requirements:* Additional exam requirements/recommendations for international students: Required—TOEFL (minimum score 560 paper-based; 84 iBT), IELTS (minimum score 6.5). *Application deadline:* For fall admission, 8/1 for domestic students, 5/1 for international students; for winter admission, 11/15 for domestic students, 9/1 for international students; for spring admission, 3/15 for domestic students, 1/1 for international students. Applications are processed on a rolling basis. Application fee: $55. Electronic applications accepted. *Expenses:* Contact institution. *Financial support:* Federal Work-Study, scholarships/grants, and unspecified assistantships available. Support available to part-time students. Financial award application deadline: 3/1; financial award applicants required to submit FAFSA. *Faculty research:* Household hazardous waste, e. coli, invasive aquatic species, small heterafullerene molecules, cantor-derived elevation and terrain slope. *Unit head:* Dr. Albert C. Price, Interim Dean, 810-762-6514, Fax: 810-762-3006, E-mail: acprice@umflint.edu. *Application contact:* Bradley T. Maki, Director of Graduate Admissions, 810-762-3171, Fax: 810-766-6789, E-mail: bmaki@umflint.edu.
Website: http://www.umflint.edu/graduateprograms/

Biochemistry

University of Minnesota, Duluth, Graduate School, Swenson College of Science and Engineering, Department of Chemistry and Biochemistry, Duluth, MN 55812-2496. Offers MS. Part-time programs available. *Degree requirements:* For master's, thesis. *Entrance requirements:* For master's, bachelor's degree in chemistry, minimum GPA of 3.0. Additional exam requirements/recommendations for international students: Required—TOEFL (minimum score 550 paper-based; 79 iBT), IELTS (minimum score 6.5). *Faculty research:* Physical, inorganic, organic, and analytical chemistry; biochemistry and molecular biology.

University of Minnesota, Duluth, Medical School, Department of Biochemistry, Molecular Biology and Biophysics, Duluth, MN 55812-2496. Offers biochemistry, molecular biology and biophysics (MS); biology and biophysics (PhD); social, administrative, and clinical pharmacy (MS, PhD); toxicology (MS, PhD). Terminal master's awarded for partial completion of doctoral program. *Degree requirements:* For master's, comprehensive exam, thesis; for doctorate, comprehensive exam, thesis/dissertation. *Entrance requirements:* For master's and doctorate, GRE General Test. Additional exam requirements/recommendations for international students: Required—TOEFL. Electronic applications accepted. *Faculty research:* Intestinal cancer biology; hepatotoxins and mitochondriopathies; toxicology; cell cycle regulation in stem cells; neurobiology of brain development, trace metal function and blood-brain barrier; hibernation biology.

University of Minnesota, Twin Cities Campus, Graduate School, College of Biological Sciences, Biochemistry, Molecular Biology and Biophysics Graduate Program, Minneapolis, MN 55455-0213. Offers PhD. *Degree requirements:* For doctorate, thesis/dissertation. *Entrance requirements:* For doctorate, GRE, 3 letters of recommendation, more than 1 semester of laboratory experience. Additional exam requirements/recommendations for international students: Required—TOEFL (minimum score 625 paper-based; 108 iBT with writing subsection 25 and reading subsection 25) or IELTS (minimum score 7). Electronic applications accepted. *Faculty research:* Microbial biochemistry, biotechnology, molecular biology, regulatory biochemistry, structural biology and biophysics, physical biochemistry, enzymology, physiological chemistry.

University of Mississippi Medical Center, School of Graduate Studies in the Health Sciences, Department of Biochemistry, Jackson, MS 39216-4505. Offers PhD, MD/PhD. *Faculty:* 9 full-time (0 women). *Students:* 17 full-time (7 women); includes 1 minority (Black or African American, non-Hispanic/Latino), 9 international. Average age 27. 7 applicants, 43% accepted. *Degree requirements:* For doctorate, thesis/dissertation, first authored publication. *Entrance requirements:* For doctorate, GRE General Test, minimum GPA of 3.0. Additional exam requirements/recommendations for international students: Required—TOEFL. *Application deadline:* For fall admission, 3/1 priority date for domestic students. Application fee: $10. *Financial support:* In 2013–14, research assistantships (averaging $24,150 per year) were awarded. Financial award application deadline: 3/31. *Faculty research:* Structural biology, regulation of gene expression, enzymology of redox reactions, mechanism of anti cancer drugs, function of nuclear substructure. *Total annual research expenditures:* $1.4 million. *Unit head:* Dr. John Correia, Chairman, 601-984-1500, Fax: 601-984-1501, E-mail: jcorreia@umc.edu. *Application contact:* Dr. Drazen Raucher, Director, 601-984-1510, Fax: 601-984-1501, E-mail: draucher@umc.edu.
Website: http://www.umc.edu/biochemistry/

University of Missouri, Graduate School, College of Agriculture, Food and Natural Resources, Department of Biochemistry, Columbia, MO 65211. Offers MS, PhD. *Faculty:* 32 full-time (11 women), 5 part-time/adjunct (2 women). *Students:* 44 full-time (18 women), 2 part-time (0 women); includes 1 minority (Asian, non-Hispanic/Latino), 24 international. Average age 27. 37 applicants, 19% accepted, 7 enrolled. In 2013, 2 master's, 3 doctorates awarded. Terminal master's awarded for partial completion of doctoral program. *Degree requirements:* For master's, thesis; for doctorate, comprehensive exam, thesis/dissertation. *Entrance requirements:* For master's and doctorate, GRE, minimum GPA of 3.0; undergraduate research; 3 letters of reference; 500-word personal statement. Additional exam requirements/recommendations for international students: Required—TOEFL (minimum score 620 paper-based; 95 iBT). *Application deadline:* For fall admission, 1/15 priority date for domestic students, 1/15 for international students. Application fee: $55 ($75 for international students). Electronic applications accepted. *Financial support:* Fellowships with tuition reimbursements, research assistantships with tuition reimbursements, teaching assistantships with tuition reimbursements, institutionally sponsored loans, scholarships/grants, health care benefits, and unspecified assistantships available. Support available to part-time students. *Faculty research:* Gene expression; molecular medicine; plant sciences; receptors and signaling; macromolecular synthesis, assembly and localization; structural and chemical biology; proteomics, genomics and combinatorial chemistry; enzymology, nutrition and metabolism. *Unit head:* Dr. Gerald Hazelbauer, Department Chair, 573-882-4845, E-mail: hazelbauerg@missouri.edu. *Application contact:* Angela Nation, Executive Assistant, 573-882-4845, E-mail: nationa@missouri.edu.
Website: http://biochem.missouri.edu/grad-program/index.php

University of Missouri–Kansas City, School of Biological Sciences, Program in Molecular Biology and Biochemistry, Kansas City, MO 64110-2499. Offers PhD. Offered through the School of Graduate Studies. *Faculty:* 34 full-time (9 women), 3 part-time/adjunct (all women). *Students:* 11 full-time (6 women), 7 part-time (5 women); includes 7 minority (4 Asian, non-Hispanic/Latino; 2 Hispanic/Latino; 1 Two or more races, non-Hispanic/Latino), 3 international. Average age 26. 43 applicants, 33% accepted, 10 enrolled. *Degree requirements:* For doctorate, comprehensive exam, thesis/dissertation. *Entrance requirements:* For doctorate, GRE General Test, bachelor's degree in chemistry, biology, or a related discipline; minimum GPA of 3.0. Additional exam requirements/recommendations for international students: Required—TOEFL (minimum score 550 paper-based; 80 iBT). *Application deadline:* For fall admission, 2/15 priority date for domestic and international students. Application fee: $45 ($50 for international students). *Expenses:* Tuition, state resident: full-time $6073; part-time $337.40 per credit hour. Tuition, nonresident: full-time $15,680; part-time $871.10 per credit hour. *Required fees:* $97.59 per credit hour. Full-time tuition and fees vary according to program. *Financial support:* In 2013–14, 18 research assistantships with full tuition reimbursements (averaging $23,281 per year), 14 teaching assistantships with full and partial tuition reimbursements (averaging $17,639 per year) were awarded; scholarships/grants, tuition waivers (full and partial), and unspecified assistantships also available. Financial award application deadline: 3/1; financial award applicants required to submit FAFSA. *Unit head:* Dr. Xiao-Qiang Yu, Interim Head, 816-235-6379, E-mail: yux@umkc.edu. *Application contact:* Karen Bame, Graduate Programs Officer, 816-235-2243, Fax: 816-235-5595, E-mail: bamek@umkc.edu.
Website: http://sbs.umkc.edu/

University of Missouri–St. Louis, College of Arts and Sciences, Department of Chemistry and Biochemistry, St. Louis, MO 63121. Offers chemistry (MS, PhD), including biochemistry, inorganic chemistry, organic chemistry, physical chemistry. Part-time and evening/weekend programs available. *Faculty:* 20 full-time (3 women), 6 part-time/adjunct (1 woman). *Students:* 39 full-time (17 women), 24 part-time (14 women); includes 8 minority (2 Black or African American, non-Hispanic/Latino; 1 Asian, non-Hispanic/Latino; 3 Hispanic/Latino; 1 Native Hawaiian or other Pacific Islander, non-Hispanic/Latino; 1 Two or more races, non-Hispanic/Latino), 13 international. Average age 29. 51 applicants, 49% accepted, 12 enrolled. In 2013, 12 master's, 8 doctorates awarded. Terminal master's awarded for partial completion of doctoral program. *Degree requirements:* For master's, thesis optional; for doctorate, thesis/dissertation. *Entrance requirements:* For master's, 2 letters of recommendation; for doctorate, GRE General Test, 3 letters of recommendation. Additional exam requirements/recommendations for international students: Required—TOEFL (minimum score 550 paper-based; 79 iBT), IELTS (minimum score 6.5). *Application deadline:* For fall admission, 7/1 priority date for domestic and international students; for spring admission, 12/1 priority date for domestic and international students. Applications are processed on a rolling basis. Application fee: $35 ($40 for international students). Electronic applications accepted. *Expenses:* Tuition, state resident: full-time $7364; part-time $409.10 per credit hour. Tuition, nonresident: full-time $19,162; part-time $1008.50 per credit hour. *Financial support:* In 2013–14, 14 research assistantships with full and partial tuition reimbursements (averaging $13,500 per year), 22 teaching assistantships with full and partial tuition reimbursements (averaging $13,500 per year) were awarded; fellowships with full and partial tuition reimbursements also available. *Faculty research:* Metallaborane chemistry, serum transferrin chemistry, natural products chemistry, organic synthesis. *Unit head:* Dr. Janet Wilking, Director of Graduate Studies, 314-516-5311, Fax: 314-516-5342, E-mail: gradchem@umsl.edu. *Application contact:* Graduate Admissions, 314-516-5458, Fax: 314-516-6996, E-mail: gradadm@umsl.edu.
Website: http://www.umsl.edu/chemistry/

The University of Montana, Graduate School, College of Humanities and Sciences, Division of Biological Sciences, Program in Cellular, Molecular and Microbial Biology, Missoula, MT 59812-0002. Offers cellular and developmental biology (PhD); microbial evolution and ecology (PhD); microbiology and immunology (PhD); molecular biology and biochemistry (PhD). Terminal master's awarded for partial completion of doctoral program. *Degree requirements:* For doctorate, variable foreign language requirement, thesis/dissertation. *Entrance requirements:* For doctorate, GRE General Test. *Application deadline:* For fall admission, 2/1 for domestic students. Application fee: $45. *Financial support:* In 2013–14, research assistantships with tuition reimbursements (averaging $9,400 per year), teaching assistantships with full tuition reimbursements (averaging $9,400 per year) were awarded; Federal Work-Study and tuition waivers (full and partial) also available. Financial award application deadline: 3/1; financial award applicants required to submit FAFSA. *Faculty research:* Ribosome structure, medical microbiology/pathogenesis, microbial ecology/environmental microbiology. *Unit head:* Charles Janson, Chair, 406-243-5122, E-mail: charles.janson@mso.umt.edu. *Application contact:* Information Contact, E-mail: gradschl@mso.umt.edu.
Website: http://www.biology.umt.edu/

University of Nebraska–Lincoln, Graduate College, College of Agricultural Sciences and Natural Resources and College of Arts and Sciences, Department of Biochemistry, Lincoln, NE 68588. Offers MS, PhD. Terminal master's awarded for partial completion of doctoral program. *Degree requirements:* For master's, thesis optional; for doctorate, comprehensive exam, thesis/dissertation. *Entrance requirements:* For master's and doctorate, GRE General Test, GRE Subject Test. Additional exam requirements/recommendations for international students: Required—TOEFL (minimum score 550 paper-based). Electronic applications accepted. *Faculty research:* Molecular genetics, enzymology, photosynthesis, molecular virology, structural biology.

University of Nebraska–Lincoln, Graduate College, College of Arts and Sciences, Department of Chemistry, Lincoln, NE 68588. Offers analytical chemistry (PhD); biochemistry (PhD); chemistry (MS); inorganic chemistry (PhD); materials chemistry (PhD); organic chemistry (PhD); physical chemistry (PhD). *Degree requirements:* For master's, one foreign language, thesis optional, departmental qualifying exam; for doctorate, one foreign language, comprehensive exam, thesis/dissertation, departmental qualifying exams. *Entrance requirements:* For master's and doctorate, GRE. Additional exam requirements/recommendations for international students: Required—TOEFL (minimum score 550 paper-based). Electronic applications accepted. *Faculty research:* Bioorganic and bioinorganic chemistry, biophysical and bioanalytical chemistry, structure-function of DNA and proteins, organometallics, mass spectrometry.

University of Nebraska Medical Center, Department of Biochemistry and Molecular Biology, Omaha, NE 68198. Offers MS, PhD. Terminal master's awarded for partial completion of doctoral program. *Degree requirements:* For master's, comprehensive exam, thesis; for doctorate, comprehensive exam, thesis/dissertation. *Entrance requirements:* For master's and doctorate, GRE General Test. Additional exam requirements/recommendations for international students: Required—TOEFL (minimum score 550 paper-based). Electronic applications accepted. *Expenses: Required fees:* $300 per semester. Tuition and fees vary according to program. *Faculty research:* Recombinant DNA, cancer biology, diabetes and drug metabolism, biochemical endocrinology.

University of Nevada, Las Vegas, Graduate College, College of Science, Department of Chemistry, Las Vegas, NV 89154-4003. Offers biochemistry (MS); chemistry (MS, PhD); radiochemistry (PhD). Part-time programs available. *Faculty:* 14 full-time (4 women). *Students:* 40 full-time (22 women), 10 part-time (4 women); includes 7 minority (4 Black or African American, non-Hispanic/Latino; 2 Asian, non-Hispanic/Latino; 1 Hispanic/Latino), 8 international. Average age 29. 35 applicants, 26% accepted, 9 enrolled. In 2013, 2 master's, 8 doctorates awarded. *Degree requirements:* For master's, thesis. *Entrance requirements:* For master's and doctorate, GRE General Test. Additional exam requirements/recommendations for international students: Required—TOEFL (minimum score 550 paper-based; 80 iBT), IELTS (minimum score 7). *Application deadline:* For fall admission, 2/1 for domestic students, 5/1 for international students; for spring admission, 10/1 for domestic and international students. Application fee: $60 ($95 for international students). Electronic applications accepted. *Expenses:* Tuition, state resident: full-time $4752; part-time $264 per credit. Tuition, nonresident: full-time $18,662; part-time $554.50 per credit. *International tuition:* $18,952 full-time. *Required fees:* $532; $12 per credit. $266 per semester. One-time fee: $35. Tuition and fees vary according to course load and program. *Financial support:* In 2013–14, 49 students received support, including 31 research assistantships with partial tuition reimbursements available (averaging $16,286 per year), 18 teaching assistantships with partial tuition reimbursements available (averaging $18,668 per year); institutionally sponsored loans, scholarships/grants, health care benefits, and unspecified assistantships also available. Financial award application deadline: 3/1. *Faculty research:* Material science, biochemistry, chemical education, physical chemistry and theoretical computation, analytical and organic chemistry. *Total annual research expenditures:* $1.9 million. *Unit head:* Dr. David Hatchett, Chair/Professor, 702-895-4226, Fax: 702-895-4072, E-mail: david.hatchett@unlv.edu. *Application contact:* Graduate Coordinator, 702-895-3320, Fax: 702-895-4180, E-mail: gradcollege@unlv.edu.
Website: http://www.unlv.edu/chemistry

University of Nevada, Reno, Graduate School, College of Agriculture, Biotechnology and Natural Resources, Program in Biochemistry, Reno, NV 89557. Offers MS, PhD. Terminal master's awarded for partial completion of doctoral program. *Degree requirements:* For master's, thesis; for doctorate, thesis/dissertation. *Entrance requirements:* For master's, GRE General Test, minimum GPA of 2.75; for doctorate, GRE General Test, minimum GPA of 3.0. Additional exam requirements/

recommendations for international students: Required—TOEFL (minimum score 500 paper-based; 61 iBT), IELTS (minimum score 6). Electronic applications accepted. *Faculty research:* Cancer research, insect biochemistry, plant biochemistry, enzymology.

University of New Hampshire, Graduate School, College of Life Sciences and Agriculture, Department of Molecular, Cellular and Biomedical Sciences, Program in Biochemistry, Durham, NH 03824. Offers MS, PhD. Part-time programs available. *Faculty:* 21 full-time. *Students:* 19 full-time (9 women), 1 (woman) part-time; includes 3 minority (1 Black or African American, non-Hispanic/Latino; 2 Asian, non-Hispanic/Latino), 4 international. Average age 29. 40 applicants, 10% accepted, 2 enrolled. In 2013, 1 master's, 1 doctorate awarded. Terminal master's awarded for partial completion of doctoral program. *Degree requirements:* For master's, thesis; for doctorate, one foreign language, thesis/dissertation. *Entrance requirements:* For master's and doctorate, GRE General Test. Additional exam requirements/recommendations for international students: Required—TOEFL (minimum score 550 paper-based; 80 iBT). *Application deadline:* For fall admission, 1/15 priority date for domestic students. Applications are processed on a rolling basis. Application fee: $65. Electronic applications accepted. *Expenses:* Tuition, state resident: full-time $13,500; part-time $750 per credit hour. Tuition, nonresident: full-time $26,200; part-time $1100 per credit hour. *Required fees:* $1741; $435.25 per term. Tuition and fees vary according to course level, course load, campus/location and program. *Financial support:* In 2013–14, 17 students received support, including 1 fellowship, 5 research assistantships, 11 teaching assistantships; career-related internships or fieldwork, Federal Work-Study, scholarships/grants, and tuition waivers (full and partial) also available. Support available to part-time students. Financial award application deadline: 2/15. *Faculty research:* General areas of molecular biology, cellular biology, and biochemistry, with specific research programs in eukaryotic gene regulation; reproductive physiology; molecular population genetics; macromolecular interactions; cell signaling pathways in cancer and leukemia; evolution of eukaryotic genomes; glycobiology; protein kinases and phosphatases in plant signaling; mass spectrometry-based proteomics; chromatin biology; DNA repair mechanisms; etiology of vascular disease; sensory transduction. *Unit head:* Dr. Rick Cote, Chairperson, 603-862-2470. *Application contact:* Flora Joyal, Administrative Assistant, 603-862-2103, E-mail: flora.joyal@unh.edu.
Website: http://biochemistry.unh.edu/

University of New Mexico, School of Medicine, Program in Biomedical Sciences, Albuquerque, NM 87131-5196. Offers biochemistry and molecular biology (MS, PhD); cell biology and physiology (MS, PhD); clinical and translational science (Certificate); molecular genetics and microbiology (MS, PhD); neuroscience (MS, PhD); pathology (MS, PhD); toxicology (MS, PhD); university science teaching (Certificate). Part-time programs available. *Students:* 73 full-time (39 women), 14 part-time (9 women); includes 24 minority (1 Black or African American, non-Hispanic/Latino; 1 American Indian or Alaska Native, non-Hispanic/Latino; 2 Asian, non-Hispanic/Latino; 17 Hispanic/Latino; 1 Native Hawaiian or other Pacific Islander, non-Hispanic/Latino; 2 Two or more races, non-Hispanic/Latino), 16 international. Average age 29. 89 applicants, 20% accepted, 17 enrolled. In 2013, 7 master's, 17 doctorates awarded. Terminal master's awarded for partial completion of doctoral program. *Degree requirements:* For master's, thesis; for doctorate, comprehensive exam, thesis/dissertation, qualifying exam at the end of year 1/core curriculum. *Entrance requirements:* For master's and doctorate, GRE General Test, minimum undergraduate GPA of 3.0. Additional exam requirements/recommendations for international students: Required—TOEFL. *Application deadline:* For fall admission, 3/1 priority date for domestic and international students. Applications are processed on a rolling basis. Application fee: $50. Electronic applications accepted. *Financial support:* In 2013–14, 94 students received support, including 28 fellowships with full and partial tuition reimbursements available (averaging $22,000 per year), 73 research assistantships with full tuition reimbursements available (averaging $23,000 per year), 8 teaching assistantships (averaging $2,800 per year); career-related internships or fieldwork, Federal Work-Study, institutionally sponsored loans, scholarships/grants, traineeships, health care benefits, and unspecified assistantships also available. Financial award application deadline: 1/1; financial award applicants required to submit FAFSA. *Faculty research:* Infectious disease/immunity, cancer biology, cardiovascular and metabolic diseases, brain and behavioral illness, environmental health. *Unit head:* Dr. Helen J. Hathaway, Program Director, 505-272-1887, Fax: 505-272-2412, E-mail: hhathaway@salud.unm.edu. *Application contact:* Mary Fenton, Admissions Coordinator, 505-272-1887, Fax: 505-272-2412, E-mail: mfenton@salud.unm.edu.
Website: http://hsc.unm.edu/research/brep/bsgpabout.shtm

The University of North Carolina at Chapel Hill, School of Medicine and Graduate School, Graduate Programs in Medicine, Department of Biochemistry and Biophysics, Chapel Hill, NC 27599. Offers MS, PhD. Terminal master's awarded for partial completion of doctoral program. *Degree requirements:* For master's, comprehensive exam, thesis; for doctorate, comprehensive exam, thesis/dissertation. *Entrance requirements:* For master's and doctorate, GRE General Test, GRE Subject Test (recommended), minimum GPA of 3.0. Additional exam requirements/recommendations for international students: Required—TOEFL. Electronic applications accepted.

The University of North Carolina at Greensboro, Graduate School, College of Arts and Sciences, Department of Chemistry and Biochemistry, Greensboro, NC 27412-5001. Offers biochemistry (MS); chemistry (MS). *Degree requirements:* For master's, one foreign language, thesis. *Entrance requirements:* For master's, GRE General Test. Additional exam requirements/recommendations for international students: Required—TOEFL. Electronic applications accepted. *Faculty research:* Synthesis of novel cyclopentadienes, molybdenum hydroxylase-cata ladder polymers, vinyl silicones.

University of North Dakota, Graduate School and Graduate School, Graduate Programs in Medicine, Department of Biochemistry and Molecular Biology, Grand Forks, ND 58202. Offers MS, PhD. *Degree requirements:* For master's, thesis, final exam; for doctorate, comprehensive exam, thesis/dissertation, final exam. *Entrance requirements:* For master's and doctorate, GRE General Test, minimum GPA of 3.0. Additional exam requirements/recommendations for international students: Required—TOEFL (minimum score 550 paper-based; 79 iBT), IELTS (minimum score 6.5). Electronic applications accepted. *Faculty research:* Glucose-6-phosphatase, guanine nucleotides, carbohydrate and lipid metabolism, cytoskeletal proteins, chromatin structure.

University of North Texas, Robert B. Toulouse School of Graduate Studies, Denton, TN 76203-5017. Offers accounting (MS, PhD); applied anthropology (MA, MS); applied behavior analysis (Certificate); applied technology and performance improvement (M Ed, MS, PhD); art education (MA, PhD); art history (MA); art museum education (Certificate); arts leadership (Certificate); audiology (Au D); behavior analysis (MS); biochemistry and molecular biology (MS, PhD); biology (MA, MS, PhD); business (PhD); business computer information systems (PhD); chemistry (MS, PhD); clinical psychology (PhD); communication studies (MA, MS); computer engineering (MS); computer science (MS); computer science and engineering (PhD); counseling (M Ed, MS, PhD), including clinical mental health counseling (MS), college and university counseling (M Ed, MS), elementary school counseling (M Ed, MS), secondary school counseling (M Ed, MS); counseling psychology (PhD); creative writing (MA); criminal justice (MS); curriculum and instruction (M Ed, PhD), including curriculum studies (PhD), early childhood studies (PhD), language and literacy studies (PhD); decision sciences (MBA); design (MA, MFA), including fashion design (MFA), innovation studies, interior design (MFA); early childhood studies (MS); economics (MS); educational leadership (M Ed, Ed D, PhD); educational psychology (MS), including family studies, gifted and talented (MS, PhD), human development, learning and cognition, research, measurement and evaluation; educational research (PhD), including gifted and talented (MS, PhD), human development and family studies, psychological aspects of sports and exercise, research, measurement and statistics; electrical engineering (MS); emergency management (MPA); engineering systems (MS); English (MA, PhD); environmental science (MS, PhD); experimental psychology (PhD); finance (MBA, MS, PhD); financial management (MPA); French (MA); health psychology and behavioral medicine (PhD); health services management (MBA); higher education (M Ed, Ed D, PhD); history (MA, MS, PhD), including European history (PhD), military history (PhD), United States history (PhD); hospitality management (MS); human resources management (MPA); information science (MS, PhD); information technologies (MBA); information technology and decision sciences (MS); interdisciplinary studies (MA, MS); international sustainable tourism (MS); jazz studies (MM); journalism (MA, MJ, Graduate Certificate), including interactive and virtual digital communication (Graduate Certificate), narrative journalism (Graduate Certificate), public relations (Graduate Certificate); kinesiology (MS); learning technologies (MS, PhD); library science (MS); local government management (MPA); logistics and supply chain management (MBA, PhD); long-term care, senior housing, and aging services (MA, MS); management science (PhD); marketing (MBA, PhD); materials science and engineering (MS, PhD); mathematics (MA, PhD); merchandising (MS); music (MA, MM Ed, PhD), including ethnomusicology (MA), music education (MM Ed, PhD), music theory (MA, PhD), musicology (MA, PhD), performance (MA); nonprofit management (MPA); operations and supply chain management (MBA); performance (MM, DMA); philosophy (MA, PhD); physics (MS, PhD); political science (MA, MS, PhD); public administration and management (PhD), including emergency management, nonprofit management, public financial management, urban management; radio, television and film (MA, MFA); recreation, event and sport management (MS); rehabilitation counseling (MS, Certificate); sociology (MA, MS, PhD); Spanish (MA); special education (M Ed, PhD), including autism intervention (PhD), emotional/behavioral disorders (PhD), mild/moderate disabilities (PhD); speech-language pathology (MA, MS); strategic management (MBA); studio art (MFA); taxation (MS); teaching (M Ed); MBA/MS; MS/MPH; MSES/MBA. Part-time and evening/weekend programs available. Postbaccalaureate distance learning degree programs offered. *Faculty:* 661 full-time (213 women), 240 part-time/adjunct (144 women). *Students:* 3,106 full-time (1,620 women), 3,543 part-time (2,221 women); includes 1,740 minority (533 Black or African American, non-Hispanic/Latino; 15 American Indian or Alaska Native, non-Hispanic/Latino; 286 Asian, non-Hispanic/Latino; 746 Hispanic/Latino; 3 Native Hawaiian or other Pacific Islander, non-Hispanic/Latino; 157 Two or more races, non-Hispanic/Latino), 1,145 international. Average age 32. 6,289 applicants, 43% accepted, 1751 enrolled. In 2013, 1,778 master's, 239 doctorates, 10 other advanced degrees awarded. Terminal master's awarded for partial completion of doctoral program. *Degree requirements:* For master's, variable foreign language requirement, comprehensive exam (for some programs), thesis (for some programs); for doctorate, variable foreign language requirement, comprehensive exam (for some programs), thesis/dissertation; for other advanced degree, variable foreign language requirement, comprehensive exam (for some programs). *Entrance requirements:* For master's and doctorate, GRE, GMAT. Additional exam requirements/recommendations for international students: Required—TOEFL (minimum score 550 paper-based; 79 iBT). *Application deadline:* For fall admission, 7/15 for domestic students, 3/15 for international students; for spring admission, 11/15 for domestic students, 9/15 for international students; for summer admission, 5/1 for domestic students. Applications are processed on a rolling basis. Application fee: $60. Electronic applications accepted. *Financial support:* Fellowships with partial tuition reimbursements, research assistantships with partial tuition reimbursements, teaching assistantships, career-related internships or fieldwork, Federal Work-Study, institutionally sponsored loans, scholarships/grants, health care benefits, and library assistantships available. Support available to part-time students. Financial award applicants required to submit FAFSA. *Unit head:* Mark Wardell, Dean, 940-565-2383, E-mail: mark.wardell@unt.edu. *Application contact:* Toulouse School of Graduate Studies, 940-565-2383, Fax: 940-565-2141, E-mail: gradsch@unt.edu.
Website: http://tsgs.unt.edu/

University of North Texas Health Science Center at Fort Worth, Graduate School of Biomedical Sciences, Fort Worth, TX 76107-2699. Offers anatomy and cell biology (MS, PhD); biochemistry and molecular biology (MS, PhD); biomedical sciences (MS, PhD); biotechnology (MS); forensic genetics (MS); integrative physiology (MS, PhD); medical science (MS); microbiology and immunology (MS, PhD); pharmacology (MS, PhD); science education (MS); DO/MS; DO/PhD. Terminal master's awarded for partial completion of doctoral program. *Degree requirements:* For master's, thesis; for doctorate, thesis/dissertation. *Entrance requirements:* For master's and doctorate, GRE General Test. Additional exam requirements/recommendations for international students: Required—TOEFL. *Expenses:* Contact institution. *Faculty research:* Alzheimer's disease, aging, eye diseases, cancer, cardiovascular disease.

University of Notre Dame, Graduate School, College of Science, Department of Chemistry and Biochemistry, Notre Dame, IN 46556. Offers biochemistry (MS, PhD); inorganic chemistry (MS, PhD); organic chemistry (MS, PhD); physical chemistry (MS, PhD). Terminal master's awarded for partial completion of doctoral program. *Degree requirements:* For master's, comprehensive exam, thesis; for doctorate, thesis/dissertation, qualifying exam. *Entrance requirements:* For master's and doctorate, GRE General Test, GRE Subject Test (strongly recommended). Additional exam requirements/recommendations for international students: Required—TOEFL (minimum score 600 paper-based; 80 iBT). Electronic applications accepted. *Faculty research:* Reaction design and mechanistic studies; reactive intermediates; synthesis, structure and reactivity of organometallic cluster complexes and biologically active natural products; bioorganic chemistry; enzymology.

University of Oklahoma, College of Arts and Sciences, Department of Chemistry and Biochemistry, Norman, OK 73019. Offers bioinformatics (MS); chemistry (PhD). Part-time programs available. *Faculty:* 25 full-time (5 women). *Students:* 66 full-time (22 women), 23 part-time (9 women); includes 12 minority (4 Black or African American, non-Hispanic/Latino; 1 American Indian or Alaska Native, non-Hispanic/Latino; 1 Asian, non-Hispanic/Latino; 5 Hispanic/Latino; 1 Two or more races, non-Hispanic/Latino), 29 international. Average age 26. 107 applicants, 23% accepted, 21 enrolled. In 2013, 14 master's, 13 doctorates awarded. Terminal master's awarded for partial completion of doctoral program. *Degree requirements:* For master's, comprehensive exam (for some programs), thesis (for some programs); for doctorate, comprehensive exam, thesis/dissertation. *Entrance requirements:* For master's and doctorate, GRE, minimum GPA of 3.0. Additional exam requirements/recommendations for international students: Required—TOEFL (minimum score 79 iBT). *Application deadline:* For fall admission, 1/15 for domestic and international students; for spring admission, 9/1 for domestic students, 9/15 for international students. Application fee: $50 ($100 for international students). Electronic applications accepted. *Expenses:* Tuition, state resident: full-time $4205; part-time $175.20 per credit hour. Tuition, nonresident: full-time $16,205; part-

time $675.20 per credit hour. *Required fees:* $2745; $103.85 per credit hour. $126.50 per semester. *Financial support:* In 2013–14, 84 students received support, including 4 fellowships with full tuition reimbursements available (averaging $5,000 per year), 15 research assistantships with partial tuition reimbursements available (averaging $15,432 per year), 65 teaching assistantships with partial tuition reimbursements available (averaging $16,853 per year); institutionally sponsored loans, scholarships/grants, health care benefits, tuition waivers (full), and unspecified assistantships also available. Support available to part-time students. Financial award application deadline: 6/1; financial award applicants required to submit FAFSA. *Faculty research:* Structural biology, synthesis and catalysis, natural products, membrane biochemistry, genomics. *Total annual research expenditures:* $8.2 million. *Unit head:* Dr. George Richter-Addo, Professor and Chair, 405-325-4811, Fax: 405-325-6111, E-mail: grichteraddo@ou.edu. *Application contact:* Angelika Tietz, Graduate Program Assistant, 405-325-4811 Ext. 62946, Fax: 405-325-6111, E-mail: atietz@ou.edu.
Website: http://chem.ou.edu

University of Oklahoma Health Sciences Center, College of Medicine and Graduate College, Graduate Programs in Medicine, Department of Biochemistry and Molecular Biology, Oklahoma City, OK 73190. Offers biochemistry (MS, PhD); molecular biology (MS, PhD). Part-time programs available. *Faculty:* 8 full-time (2 women). *Students:* 1 (woman) full-time, 22 part-time (12 women); includes 2 minority (1 Asian, non-Hispanic/Latino; 1 Two or more races, non-Hispanic/Latino), 9 international. Average age 28. 7 applicants, 14% accepted, 1 enrolled. In 2013, 1 master's, 5 doctorates awarded. Terminal master's awarded for partial completion of doctoral program. *Degree requirements:* For master's, thesis; for doctorate, thesis/dissertation. *Entrance requirements:* For master's, GRE General Test, 2 letters of recommendation; for doctorate, GRE General Test, 3 letters of recommendation. Additional exam requirements/recommendations for international students: Required—TOEFL. *Application deadline:* For fall admission, 1/31 for domestic students. Application fee: $50. *Expenses:* Tuition, state resident: full-time $3504; part-time $175.20 per credit hour. Tuition, nonresident: full-time $13,504; part-time $675.20 per credit hour. *Required fees:* $1545; $52.70 per credit hour. $245.25 per semester. Tuition and fees vary according to course load. *Financial support:* In 2013–14, 20 research assistantships (averaging $18,000 per year) were awarded; institutionally sponsored loans also available. Support available to part-time students. Financial award application deadline: 3/31; financial award applicants required to submit FAFSA. *Faculty research:* Gene expression, regulation of transcription, enzyme evolution, melanogenesis, signal transduction. *Unit head:* Dr. Paul H. Weigel, Chair, 405-271-2227, E-mail: paul-weigel@ouhsc.edu. *Application contact:* Dr. Gillian Air, Graduate Liaison, 405-271-2227, Fax: 405-271-3092, E-mail: gillian-air@ouhsc.edu.

University of Oregon, Graduate School, College of Arts and Sciences, Department of Chemistry, Eugene, OR 97403. Offers biochemistry (MA, MS, PhD); chemistry (MA, MS, PhD). Terminal master's awarded for partial completion of doctoral program. *Degree requirements:* For doctorate, thesis/dissertation. *Entrance requirements:* For master's and doctorate, GRE General Test, minimum GPA of 3.0. Additional exam requirements/recommendations for international students: Required—TOEFL. *Faculty research:* Organic chemistry, organometallic chemistry, inorganic chemistry, physical chemistry, materials science, biochemistry, chemical physics, molecular or cell biology.

University of Ottawa, Faculty of Graduate and Postdoctoral Studies, Faculty of Medicine, Department of Biochemistry, Microbiology and Immunology, Ottawa, ON K1N 6N5, Canada. Offers biochemistry (M Sc, PhD); microbiology and immunology (M Sc, PhD). *Degree requirements:* For master's, thesis; for doctorate, comprehensive exam, thesis/dissertation, seminar. *Entrance requirements:* For master's, honors degree or equivalent, minimum B average; for doctorate, master's degree, minimum B+ average. Electronic applications accepted. *Faculty research:* General biochemistry, molecular biology, microbiology, host biology, nutrition and metabolism.

University of Pennsylvania, Perelman School of Medicine, Biomedical Graduate Studies, Graduate Group in Biochemistry and Molecular Biophysics, Philadelphia, PA 19104. Offers PhD, MD/PhD, VMD/PhD. *Faculty:* 76. *Students:* 86 full-time (34 women); includes 19 minority (11 Asian, non-Hispanic/Latino; 8 Hispanic/Latino), 12 international. 93 applicants, 35% accepted, 9 enrolled. In 2013, 7 doctorates awarded. *Degree requirements:* For doctorate, thesis/dissertation. *Entrance requirements:* For doctorate, GRE General Test. Additional exam requirements/recommendations for international students: Required—TOEFL. *Application deadline:* For fall admission, 12/1 priority date for domestic and international students. Applications are processed on a rolling basis. Application fee: $80. Electronic applications accepted. *Financial support:* In 2013–14, 76 students received support. Fellowships, research assistantships, scholarships/grants, traineeships, and unspecified assistantships available. *Faculty research:* Biochemistry of cell differentiation, tissue culture, intermediary metabolism, structure of proteins and nucleic acids, biochemical genetics. *Unit head:* Dr. Kathryn Ferguson, Chairperson, 215-573-1207. *Application contact:* Ruth Keris, Administrator, 215-898-4829.
Website: http://www.med.upenn.edu/bmbgrad/

University of Puerto Rico, Medical Sciences Campus, School of Medicine, Division of Graduate Studies, Department of Biochemistry, San Juan, PR 00936-5067. Offers MS, PhD. *Degree requirements:* For master's, thesis; for doctorate, comprehensive exam, thesis/dissertation. *Entrance requirements:* For master's and doctorate, GRE General Test, GRE Subject Test, interview, minimum GPA of 3.0. Electronic applications accepted. *Faculty research:* Genetics, cell and molecular biology, cancer biology, protein structure/function, glycosilation of proteins.

University of Regina, Faculty of Graduate Studies and Research, Faculty of Science, Department of Chemistry and Biochemistry, Regina, SK S4S 0A2, Canada. Offers analytical/environmental chemistry (M Sc, PhD); biophysics of biological interfaces (M Sc, PhD); enzymology/chemical biology (M Sc, PhD); inorganic/organometallic chemistry (M Sc, PhD); signal transduction and mechanisms of cancer cell regulation (M Sc, PhD); supramolecular organic photochemistry and photophysics (M Sc, PhD); synthetic organic chemistry (M Sc, PhD); theoretical/computational chemistry (M Sc, PhD). *Faculty:* 11 full-time (2 women), 4 part-time/adjunct (0 women). *Students:* 12 full-time (9 women), 1 part-time (0 women). 25 applicants, 36% accepted. In 2013, 3 master's awarded. *Degree requirements:* For master's, thesis; for doctorate, thesis/dissertation. *Entrance requirements:* Additional exam requirements/recommendations for international students: Required—TOEFL (minimum score 580 paper-based; 80 iBT), IELTS (minimum score 6.5). *Application deadline:* Applications are processed on a rolling basis. Application fee: $100. Electronic applications accepted. *Expenses: Tuition, area resident:* Full-time $4338 Canadian dollars. *International tuition:* $7338 Canadian dollars full-time. *Required fees:* $449.25 Canadian dollars. *Financial support:* In 2013–14, 5 fellowships (averaging $7,000 per year), 8 teaching assistantships (averaging $2,456 per year) were awarded; research assistantships and scholarships/grants also available. Financial award application deadline: 6/15. *Faculty research:* Asymmetric synthesis and methodology, theoretical and computational chemistry, biophysical biochemistry, analytical and environmental chemistry, chemical biology. *Unit head:* Dr. Renata Raina-Fulton, Department Head, 306-585-4012, Fax: 306-337-2409, E-mail: renata.raina@uregina.ca. *Application contact:* Dr. Brian Sterenberg, Graduate Program Coordinator, 306-585-4106, Fax: 306-337-2409, E-mail: brian.sterenberg@uregina.ca.
Website: http://www.uregina.ca/science/chem-biochem/

University of Rhode Island, Graduate School, College of the Environment and Life Sciences, Department of Cell and Molecular Biology, Kingston, RI 02881. Offers biochemistry (MS, PhD); clinical laboratory sciences (MS), including biotechnology, clinical laboratory science, cytopathology; microbiology (MS, PhD); molecular genetics (MS, PhD). Part-time programs available. *Faculty:* 17 full-time (8 women), 2 part-time/adjunct (1 woman). *Students:* 19 full-time (11 women), 40 part-time (23 women); includes 14 minority (4 Black or African American, non-Hispanic/Latino; 1 American Indian or Alaska Native, non-Hispanic/Latino; 7 Asian, non-Hispanic/Latino; 2 Hispanic/Latino), 5 international. In 2013, 20 master's, 2 doctorates awarded. *Degree requirements:* For master's, comprehensive exam (for some programs), thesis optional; for doctorate, comprehensive exam, thesis/dissertation. *Entrance requirements:* For master's and doctorate, GRE, 2 letters of recommendation. Additional exam requirements/recommendations for international students: Required—TOEFL (minimum score 550 paper-based). *Application deadline:* For fall admission, 7/15 for domestic students, 2/1 for international students; for spring admission, 11/15 for domestic students, 7/15 for international students. Application fee: $65. Electronic applications accepted. *Expenses:* Tuition, state resident: full-time $11,532; part-time $641 per credit. Tuition, nonresident: full-time $23,606; part-time $1311 per credit. *Required fees:* $1388; $36 per credit. $35 per semester. One-time fee: $130. *Financial support:* In 2013–14, 5 research assistantships with full and partial tuition reimbursements (averaging $12,078 per year), 2 teaching assistantships with full and partial tuition reimbursements (averaging $11,883 per year) were awarded. Financial award application deadline: 2/1; financial award applicants required to submit FAFSA. *Faculty research:* Genomics. *Total annual research expenditures:* $6.7 million. *Unit head:* Dr. Gongqing Sun, Chairperson, 401-874-5937, Fax: 401-874-2202, E-mail: gsun@mail.uri.edu. *Application contact:* Graduate Admissions, 401-874-2872, E-mail: gradadm@etal.uri.edu.
Website: http://cels.uri.edu/cmb/

University of Rochester, School of Medicine and Dentistry, Graduate Programs in Medicine and Dentistry, Department of Biochemistry and Biophysics, Programs in Biochemistry, Rochester, NY 14627. Offers biochemistry and molecular biology (PhD). Terminal master's awarded for partial completion of doctoral program. *Degree requirements:* For doctorate, thesis/dissertation, qualifying exam. *Entrance requirements:* For doctorate, GRE General Test. *Expenses: Tuition:* Full-time $44,580; part-time $1394 per credit hour. *Required fees:* $492.

University of Saint Joseph, Department of Chemistry, West Hartford, CT 06117-2700. Offers biochemistry (MS); chemistry (MS). Part-time and evening/weekend programs available. Postbaccalaureate distance learning degree programs offered (no on-campus study). *Degree requirements:* For master's, comprehensive exam, thesis optional. *Entrance requirements:* For master's, 2 letters of recommendation, official undergraduate transcript. *Application deadline:* Applications are processed on a rolling basis. Application fee: $50. Electronic applications accepted. Application fee is waived when completed online. *Financial support:* Career-related internships or fieldwork and unspecified assistantships available. Support available to part-time students. Financial award applicants required to submit FAFSA. *Unit head:* Dr. Leonidas Jones, Chair, 860-231-5212, E-mail: ljones@usj.edu. *Application contact:* Graduate Admissions Office, 860-231-5261, E-mail: graduate@usj.edu.
Website: http://www.usj.edu/academics/schools/school-of-health-natural-sciences/chemistry/

University of Saskatchewan, College of Medicine, Department of Biochemistry, Saskatoon, SK S7N 5A2, Canada. Offers M Sc, PhD. *Degree requirements:* For master's, thesis; for doctorate, thesis/dissertation. *Entrance requirements:* Additional exam requirements/recommendations for international students: Required—TOEFL. *Expenses: Tuition, area resident:* Full-time $3585 Canadian dollars; part-time $585 Canadian dollars per course. Tuition, nonresident: part-time $877 Canadian dollars per course. *International tuition:* $5377 Canadian dollars full-time. *Required fees:* $889.51 Canadian dollars.

The University of Scranton, College of Graduate and Continuing Education, Department of Chemistry, Program in Biochemistry, Scranton, PA 18510. Offers MA, MS. Part-time and evening/weekend programs available. *Faculty:* 10 full-time (3 women), 1 part-time/adjunct (0 women). *Students:* 24 full-time (13 women), 6 part-time (3 women); includes 4 minority (2 Black or African American, non-Hispanic/Latino; 1 Hispanic/Latino; 1 Two or more races, non-Hispanic/Latino), 3 international. Average age 25. 27 applicants, 44% accepted. In 2013, 9 master's awarded. *Degree requirements:* For master's, comprehensive exam (for some programs), thesis (for some programs), capstone experience. *Entrance requirements:* For master's, minimum GPA of 3.0. Additional exam requirements/recommendations for international students: Required—TOEFL (minimum score 500 paper-based), IELTS (minimum score 6). *Application deadline:* Applications are processed on a rolling basis. Application fee: $0. *Financial support:* Fellowships, teaching assistantships with full and partial tuition reimbursements, career-related internships or fieldwork, Federal Work-Study, and unspecified assistantships available. Support available to part-time students. Financial award application deadline: 3/1. *Unit head:* Dr. Joan Wasilewski, Director, 570-941-7705, Fax: 570-941-7510, E-mail: joan.wasilewski@scranton.edu. *Application contact:* Dr. Christopher A. Baumann, Director, 570-941-6389, Fax: 570-941-7510, E-mail: cab@scranton.edu.

University of South Carolina, The Graduate School, College of Arts and Sciences, Department of Chemistry and Biochemistry, Columbia, SC 29208. Offers IMA, MAT, MS, PhD. IMA and MAT offered in cooperation with the College of Education. Part-time programs available. Terminal master's awarded for partial completion of doctoral program. *Degree requirements:* For master's, comprehensive exam, thesis; for doctorate, comprehensive exam, thesis/dissertation. *Entrance requirements:* For master's and doctorate, GRE General Test. Additional exam requirements/recommendations for international students: Required—TOEFL. Electronic applications accepted. *Faculty research:* Spectroscopy, crystallography, organic and organometallic synthesis, analytical chemistry, materials.

University of Southern California, Keck School of Medicine and Graduate School, Graduate Programs in Medicine, Department of Biochemistry and Molecular Biology, Los Angeles, CA 90089. Offers MS. *Faculty:* 22 full-time (4 women). *Students:* 30 full-time (23 women); includes 4 minority (all Asian, non-Hispanic/Latino), 26 international. Average age 24. 51 applicants, 55% accepted, 17 enrolled. In 2013, 16 master's awarded. Terminal master's awarded for partial completion of doctoral program. *Degree requirements:* For master's, thesis. *Entrance requirements:* For master's, GRE General Test, minimum GPA of 3.0. Additional exam requirements/recommendations for international students: Required—TOEFL (minimum score 600 paper-based; 100 iBT). *Application deadline:* For fall admission, 4/15 priority date for domestic and international students. Applications are processed on a rolling basis. Application fee: $85. Electronic applications accepted. *Financial support:* Application deadline: 5/4; applicants required to submit CSS PROFILE or FAFSA. *Faculty research:* Molecular genetics, gene expression, membrane biochemistry, metabolic regulation, cancer biology. *Total annual*

research expenditures: $9.3 million. *Unit head:* Dr. Michael R. Stallcup, Chair, 323-442-1145, Fax: 323-442-1224, E-mail: stallcup@usc.edu. *Application contact:* Janet Stoeckert, Administrative Director, Basic Science Departments, 323-442-3568, Fax: 323-442-1610, E-mail: janet.stoeckert@usc.edu.
Website: http://www.usc.edu/medicine/biochemistry/

University of Southern Mississippi, Graduate School, College of Science and Technology, Department of Chemistry and Biochemistry, Hattiesburg, MS 39406-0001. Offers analytical chemistry (MS, PhD); biochemistry (MS, PhD); inorganic chemistry (MS, PhD); organic chemistry (MS, PhD); physical chemistry (MS, PhD). *Faculty:* 16 full-time (4 women). *Students:* 27 full-time (9 women), 1 part-time (0 women); includes 2 minority (1 Black or African American, non-Hispanic/Latino; 1 Two or more races, non-Hispanic/Latino), 10 international. Average age 28. 23 applicants, 22% accepted, 5 enrolled. In 2013, 1 master's, 1 doctorate awarded. *Degree requirements:* For master's, comprehensive exam, thesis; for doctorate, comprehensive exam, thesis/dissertation. *Entrance requirements:* For master's, GRE General Test, minimum GPA of 2.75 in last 60 hours; for doctorate, GRE General Test, minimum GPA of 3.5. Additional exam requirements/recommendations for international students: Required—TOEFL, IELTS. *Application deadline:* For fall admission, 3/1 priority date for domestic students, 3/1 for international students. Applications are processed on a rolling basis. Application fee: $50. *Financial support:* In 2013–14, 3 research assistantships with full tuition reimbursements (averaging $17,000 per year), 19 teaching assistantships with full tuition reimbursements (averaging $20,700 per year) were awarded; fellowships, Federal Work-Study, institutionally sponsored loans, scholarships/grants, health care benefits, and unspecified assistantships also available. Support available to part-time students. Financial award application deadline: 3/15; financial award applicants required to submit FAFSA. *Faculty research:* Plant biochemistry, photo chemistry, polymer chemistry, x-ray analysis, enzyme chemistry. *Unit head:* Dr. Sabine Heinhorst, Chair, 601-266-4701, Fax: 601-266-6075. *Application contact:* Shonna Breland, Manager of Graduate School Admissions, 601-266-6567, Fax: 601-266-5138.
Website: http://www.usm.edu/graduateschool/table.php

The University of Tennessee, Graduate School, College of Arts and Sciences, Department of Biochemistry, Cellular and Molecular Biology, Knoxville, TN 37996. Offers MS, PhD. Terminal master's awarded for partial completion of doctoral program. *Degree requirements:* For master's, thesis; for doctorate, thesis/dissertation. *Entrance requirements:* For master's and doctorate, GRE General Test, minimum GPA of 2.7. Additional exam requirements/recommendations for international students: Required—TOEFL. Electronic applications accepted. *Expenses:* Tuition, state resident: full-time $9540; part-time $531 per credit hour. Tuition, nonresident: full-time $27,728; part-time $1542 per credit hour. *Required fees:* $1404; $67 per credit hour.

The University of Texas at Austin, Graduate School, College of Natural Sciences, Department of Chemistry and Biochemistry, Program in Biochemistry, Austin, TX 78712-1111. Offers PhD. *Entrance requirements:* For doctorate, GRE General Test.

The University of Texas Health Science Center at Houston, Graduate School of Biomedical Sciences, Program in Biochemistry and Molecular Biology, Houston, TX 77225-0036. Offers MS, PhD, MD/PhD. Terminal master's awarded for partial completion of doctoral program. *Degree requirements:* For master's, thesis; for doctorate, thesis/dissertation. *Entrance requirements:* For master's and doctorate, GRE General Test. Additional exam requirements/recommendations for international students: Required—TOEFL. Electronic applications accepted. *Expenses:* Tuition, state resident: full-time $3474; part-time $193 per credit hour. Tuition, nonresident: full-time $13,644; part-time $758 per credit hour. *Required fees:* $226.30; $87 per credit hour. *Faculty research:* Biochemistry, membrane biology, macromolecular structure, structural biophysics, molecular models of human disease, molecular biology of the cell.

The University of Texas Health Science Center at San Antonio, Graduate School of Biomedical Sciences, Department of Biochemistry, San Antonio, TX 78229. Offers MS, PhD. *Faculty:* 31 full-time (6 women), 6 part-time/adjunct (1 woman). *Students:* 1 full-time (0 women), all international. Average age 28. In 2013, 1 master's awarded. *Degree requirements:* For master's, thesis; for doctorate, comprehensive exam, thesis/dissertation. *Entrance requirements:* For master's and doctorate, GRE General Test. Additional exam requirements/recommendations for international students: Required—TOEFL (minimum score 560 paper-based; 68 iBT). *Application deadline:* For fall admission, 1/15 priority date for domestic and international students. Applications are processed on a rolling basis. Application fee: $0. Electronic applications accepted. *Financial support:* Application deadline: 6/30; applicants required to submit FAFSA. *Faculty research:* Protein structure and function, lipid biochemistry, metabolic regulation, immunology, membrane assembly. *Total annual research expenditures:* $5.7 million. *Unit head:* Dr. Bruce J. Nicholson, Department Chair, 210-567-3770, Fax: 210-567-6595, E-mail: nicholsonb@uthscsa.edu. *Application contact:* Dr. Rui Sousa, Chairman, Committee on Graduate Studies, 210-567-2506, Fax: 210-567-6595, E-mail: sousa@uthscsa.edu.
Website: http://www.biochem.uthscsa.edu/

The University of Texas Medical Branch, Graduate School of Biomedical Sciences, Program in Biochemistry and Molecular Biology, Galveston, TX 77555. Offers biochemistry (PhD); bioinformatics (PhD); biophysics (PhD); cell biology (PhD); computational biology (PhD); structural biology (PhD). *Degree requirements:* For doctorate, thesis/dissertation. *Entrance requirements:* Additional exam requirements/recommendations for international students: Required—TOEFL (minimum score 550 paper-based). Electronic applications accepted.

The University of Texas Southwestern Medical Center, Southwestern Graduate School of Biomedical Sciences, Division of Basic Science, Program in Biological Chemistry, Dallas, TX 75390. Offers PhD. *Faculty:* 44 full-time (9 women), 1 part-time/adjunct (0 women). *Students:* 43 full-time (13 women); includes 11 minority (4 Asian, non-Hispanic/Latino; 7 Hispanic/Latino), 15 international. Average age 27. In 2013, 11 doctorates awarded. *Degree requirements:* For doctorate, thesis/dissertation, qualifying exam. *Entrance requirements:* For doctorate, GRE General Test, minimum GPA of 3.0. Additional exam requirements/recommendations for international students: Required—TOEFL. *Application deadline:* For fall admission, 12/15 priority date for domestic students. Application fee: $0. Electronic applications accepted. *Financial support:* Fellowships, research assistantships, and institutionally sponsored loans available. *Faculty research:* Regulation of gene expression, protein trafficking, molecular neurobiology, protein structure and function, metabolic regulation.
Website: http://www.utsouthwestern.edu/education/graduate-school/programs/phd-degrees/biological-chemistry/training-track/index.html

University of the Sciences, College of Graduate Studies, Program in Chemistry, Biochemistry and Pharmacognosy, Philadelphia, PA 19104-4495. Offers biochemistry (MS, PhD); chemistry (MS, PhD); pharmacognosy (MS, PhD). Part-time programs available. *Faculty:* 10 full-time (1 woman), 1 part-time/adjunct (0 women). *Students:* 30 full-time (15 women), 15 part-time (10 women); includes 7 minority (4 Black or African American, non-Hispanic/Latino; 3 Asian, non-Hispanic/Latino), 6 international. Average age 28. 52 applicants, 83% accepted, 9 enrolled. In 2013, 4 master's, 2 doctorates awarded. *Degree requirements:* For master's, thesis, qualifying exams; for doctorate, comprehensive exam, thesis/dissertation, qualifying exams. *Entrance requirements:* For master's and doctorate, GRE General Test, GRE Subject Test. Additional exam requirements/recommendations for international students: Required—TOEFL, TWE. *Application deadline:* For fall admission, 5/1 for international students; for winter admission, 10/1 for international students; for spring admission, 3/1 for international students. Applications are processed on a rolling basis. Application fee: $50. *Expenses:* Contact institution. *Financial support:* In 2013–14, 17 students received support, including 1 fellowship with full tuition reimbursement available, 2 research assistantships with full tuition reimbursements available (averaging $13,884 per year), 11 teaching assistantships with full tuition reimbursements available (averaging $18,836 per year); institutionally sponsored loans, scholarships/grants, and tuition waivers (full) also available. Financial award application deadline: 5/1. *Faculty research:* Organic and medicinal synthesis, mass spectroscopy use in protein analysis, study of analogues of taxol, cholesteryl esters. *Unit head:* Dr. Shenaz Tejani-Butt, Associate Dean, Graduate Studies, E-mail: graduate@usciences.edu. *Application contact:* Christopher Miciek, Associate Director, Graduate Admissions, 215-596-8597, E-mail: c.miciek@usciences.edu.

The University of Toledo, College of Graduate Studies, College of Natural Sciences and Mathematics, Department of Chemistry, Toledo, OH 43606-3390. Offers analytical chemistry (MS, PhD); biological chemistry (MS, PhD); inorganic chemistry (MS, PhD); organic chemistry (MS, PhD); physical chemistry (MS, PhD). Part-time programs available. *Faculty:* 22. *Students:* 69 full-time (21 women), 7 part-time (2 women); includes 3 minority (1 Asian, non-Hispanic/Latino; 2 Hispanic/Latino), 50 international. Average age 27. 98 applicants, 29% accepted, 20 enrolled. In 2013, 9 master's, 8 doctorates awarded. *Degree requirements:* For master's, thesis or alternative; for doctorate, thesis/dissertation. *Entrance requirements:* For master's and doctorate, GRE General Test, GRE Subject Test, minimum cumulative point-hour ratio of 2.7 for all previous academic work, three letters of recommendation, statement of purpose, transcripts from all prior institutions attended. Additional exam requirements/recommendations for international students: Required—TOEFL (minimum score 550 paper-based; 80 iBT). *Application deadline:* For fall admission, 1/15 priority date for domestic and international students. Applications are processed on a rolling basis. Application fee: $45 ($75 for international students). Electronic applications accepted. *Financial support:* In 2013–14, 15 research assistantships with full and partial tuition reimbursements (averaging $11,633 per year), 39 teaching assistantships with full and partial tuition reimbursements (averaging $15,336 per year) were awarded; Federal Work-Study, institutionally sponsored loans, scholarships/grants, tuition waivers (full), and unspecified assistantships also available. Support available to part-time students. *Faculty research:* Enzymology, materials chemistry, crystallography, theoretical chemistry. *Unit head:* Dr. Ronald Viola, Chair, 419-530-1582, Fax: 419-530-4033, E-mail: ronald.viola@utoledo.edu. *Application contact:* Graduate School Office, 419-530-4723, Fax: 419-530-4724, E-mail: grdsch@utnet.utoledo.edu.
Website: http://www.utoledo.edu/nsm/

The University of Toledo, College of Graduate Studies, College of Pharmacy and Pharmaceutical Sciences, Program in Medicinal and Biological Chemistry, Toledo, OH 43606-3390. Offers MS, PhD. Terminal master's awarded for partial completion of doctoral program. *Degree requirements:* For master's, thesis; for doctorate, thesis/dissertation. *Entrance requirements:* For master's and doctorate, GRE General Test. Additional exam requirements/recommendations for international students: Required—TOEFL (minimum score 550 paper-based; 80 iBT). Electronic applications accepted. *Faculty research:* Neuroscience, molecular modeling, immunotoxicology, organic synthesis, peptide biochemistry.

University of Toronto, Faculty of Medicine, Department of Biochemistry, Toronto, ON M5S 1A1, Canada. Offers M Sc, PhD. *Degree requirements:* For master's, thesis, oral examination of thesis; for doctorate, thesis/dissertation, oral defense of thesis. *Entrance requirements:* For master's, B Sc in biochemistry or molecular biology, minimum B+ average, letters of reference. Additional exam requirements/recommendations for international students: Required—TOEFL (minimum score 580 paper-based; 93 iBT), TWE (minimum score 5). Electronic applications accepted.

The University of Tulsa, Graduate School, College of Engineering and Natural Sciences, Department of Chemistry and Biochemistry, Program in Biochemistry, Tulsa, OK 74104-3189. Offers MS. Part-time programs available. *Faculty:* 2 full-time (0 women). *Students:* 5 full-time (3 women), 3 international. Average age 25. 5 applicants, 40% accepted, 1 enrolled. In 2013, 2 master's awarded. *Degree requirements:* For master's, thesis (for some programs). *Entrance requirements:* For master's, GRE General Test. Additional exam requirements/recommendations for international students: Required—TOEFL (minimum score 550 paper-based; 80 iBT), IELTS (minimum score 6). *Application deadline:* Applications are processed on a rolling basis. Application fee: $40. Electronic applications accepted. *Expenses:* Tuition: Full-time $19,566; part-time $1087 per credit hour. *Required fees:* $1690; $5 per credit hour. $160 per semester. Tuition and fees vary according to course load. *Financial support:* In 2013–14, 3 students received support, including 1 fellowship (averaging $6,500 per year), 3 teaching assistantships (averaging $10,638 per year); career-related internships or fieldwork, Federal Work-Study, scholarships/grants, health care benefits, and unspecified assistantships also available. Support available to part-time students. Financial award application deadline: 2/1; financial award applicants required to submit FAFSA. *Unit head:* Dr. Dale C. Teeters, Chairperson and Advisor, 918-631-2515, Fax: 918-631-3404, E-mail: dale-teeters@utulsa.edu. *Application contact:* Dr. Robert Sheaff, Advisor, 918-631-2319, Fax: 918-631-3404, E-mail: robert-sheaff@utulsa.edu.

University of Utah, School of Medicine and Graduate School, Graduate Programs in Medicine, Department of Biochemistry, Salt Lake City, UT 84112-1107. Offers MS, PhD. Terminal master's awarded for partial completion of doctoral program. *Degree requirements:* For master's, thesis; for doctorate, thesis/dissertation. *Entrance requirements:* For doctorate, GRE Subject Test, minimum GPA of 3.0. Additional exam requirements/recommendations for international students: Required—TOEFL. Electronic applications accepted. *Expenses:* Tuition, state resident: full-time $5259. Tuition, nonresident: full-time $18,569. *Required fees:* $841. Tuition and fees vary according to course load. *Faculty research:* Protein structure and function, nucleic acid structure and function, nucleic acid enzymology, RNA modification, protein turnover.

University of Victoria, Faculty of Graduate Studies, Faculty of Science, Department of Biochemistry and Microbiology, Victoria, BC V8W 2Y2, Canada. Offers biochemistry (M Sc, PhD); microbiology (M Sc, PhD). *Degree requirements:* For master's, thesis, seminar; for doctorate, thesis/dissertation, seminar, candidacy exam. *Entrance requirements:* For master's, GRE General Test, minimum B+ average; for doctorate, GRE General Test, minimum B+ average, M Sc. Additional exam requirements/recommendations for international students: Required—TOEFL (minimum score 600 paper-based). Electronic applications accepted. *Faculty research:* Molecular pathogenesis, prokaryotic, eukaryotic, macromolecular interactions, microbial surfaces, virology, molecular genetics.

University of Virginia, School of Medicine, Department of Biochemistry and Molecular Genetics, Charlottesville, VA 22903. Offers biochemistry (PhD); MD/PhD. *Faculty:* 24 full-time (3 women), 2 part-time/adjunct (both women). *Students:* 28 full-time (15 women); includes 4 minority (2 Hispanic/Latino; 2 Two or more races, non-Hispanic/Latino), 7 international. Average age 26. In 2013, 6 doctorates awarded. *Degree*

requirements: For doctorate, thesis/dissertation, written research proposal and defense. *Entrance requirements:* For doctorate, GRE General Test, 3 letters of recommendation. Additional exam requirements/recommendations for international students: Recommended—TOEFL (minimum score 630 paper-based; 90 iBT). Application fee: $60. Electronic applications accepted. *Expenses:* Tuition, state resident: part-time $334 per credit hour. Tuition, nonresident: part-time $1224 per credit hour. *Financial support:* Fellowships, health care benefits, and tuition waivers (full) available. Financial award applicants required to submit FAFSA. *Unit head:* Anindya Dutta, Chair, 434-924-1940, Fax: 434-924-5069, E-mail: ad8q@virginia.edu. *Application contact:* Biomedical Sciences Graduate Studies, E-mail: bims@virginia.edu.
Website: http://www.virginia.edu/bmg/

University of Washington, Graduate School, School of Medicine, Graduate Programs in Medicine, Department of Biochemistry, Seattle, WA 98195. Offers PhD. *Degree requirements:* For doctorate, thesis/dissertation. *Entrance requirements:* For doctorate, GRE General Test, GRE Subject Test (biology, chemistry, biochemistry, or cell and molecular biology), minimum GPA of 3.0. Additional exam requirements/recommendations for international students: Required—TOEFL. Electronic applications accepted. *Faculty research:* Blood coagulation, structure and function of enzymes, fertilization events, interaction of plants with bacteria, protein structure.

University of Waterloo, Graduate Studies, Faculty of Science, Guelph-Waterloo Centre for Graduate Work in Chemistry and Biochemistry, Waterloo, ON N2L 3G1, Canada. Offers M Sc, PhD. M Sc, PhD offered jointly with University of Guelph. Part-time programs available. *Degree requirements:* For master's and doctorate, project or thesis. *Entrance requirements:* For master's, GRE, honors degree, minimum B average; for doctorate, GRE, master's degree, minimum B average. Additional exam requirements/recommendations for international students: Required—TOEFL, TWE. Electronic applications accepted. *Faculty research:* Polymer, physical, inorganic, organic, and theoretical chemistry.

The University of Western Ontario, Faculty of Graduate Studies, Biosciences Division, Department of Biochemistry, London, ON N6A 5B8, Canada. Offers M Sc, PhD. *Degree requirements:* For master's, thesis; for doctorate, thesis/dissertation. *Entrance requirements:* For master's, minimum B+ average in last 2 years of undergraduate study; for doctorate, M Sc or an external scholarship winner.

University of West Florida, College of Arts and Sciences: Sciences, School of Allied Health and Life Sciences, Department of Biology, Pensacola, FL 32514-5750. Offers biological chemistry (MS); biology (MS); biology education (MST); biotechnology (MS); coastal zone studies (MS); environmental biology (MS). *Degree requirements:* For master's, thesis. *Entrance requirements:* For master's, GRE (minimum score: verbal 450, quantitative 550), official transcripts; BS in biology or related field; letter of interest; relevant past experience; three letters of recommendation from individuals who can evaluate applicant's academic ability. Additional exam requirements/recommendations for international students: Required—TOEFL (minimum score 550 paper-based).

University of Windsor, Faculty of Graduate Studies, Faculty of Science, Department of Chemistry and Biochemistry, Windsor, ON N9B 3P4, Canada. Offers M Sc, PhD. Part-time programs available. *Degree requirements:* For master's, thesis; for doctorate, comprehensive exam, thesis/dissertation. *Entrance requirements:* For master's and doctorate, minimum B average. Additional exam requirements/recommendations for international students: Required—TOEFL (minimum score 560 paper-based). Electronic applications accepted. *Faculty research:* Molecular biology/recombinant DNA techniques (PCR, cloning mutagenesis), No/02 detectors, western immunoblotting and detection, CD/NMR protein/peptide structure determination, confocal/electron microscopes.

University of Wisconsin–Madison, Graduate School, College of Agricultural and Life Sciences, Department of Biochemistry, Madison, WI 53706. Offers PhD. Terminal master's awarded for partial completion of doctoral program. *Degree requirements:* For doctorate, thesis/dissertation. *Entrance requirements:* For doctorate, GRE General Test, GRE Subject Test (recommended). Additional exam requirements/recommendations for international students: Required—TOEFL. Electronic applications accepted. *Expenses:* Tuition, state resident: full-time $10,728; part-time $790 per credit. Tuition, nonresident: full-time $24,054; part-time $1623 per credit. *Required fees:* $1130; $119 per credit. *Faculty research:* Molecular structure of vitamins and hormones, enzymology, NMR spectroscopy, protein structure, molecular genetics.

University of Wisconsin–Madison, School of Medicine and Public Health and Graduate School, Graduate Programs in Medicine, Department of Biomolecular Chemistry, Madison, WI 53706-1380. Offers MS, PhD. *Faculty:* 16 full-time (4 women). *Students:* 24 full-time (15 women); includes 2 minority (both Hispanic/Latino), 6 international. Average age 25. 275 applicants, 16% accepted, 12 enrolled. In 2013, 5 doctorates awarded. Terminal master's awarded for partial completion of doctoral program. *Degree requirements:* For master's, thesis; for doctorate, thesis/dissertation. *Entrance requirements:* For doctorate, GRE. *Application deadline:* For fall admission, 12/1 priority date for domestic students. Application fee: $56. Electronic applications accepted. *Expenses:* Tuition, state resident: full-time $10,728; part-time $790 per credit. Tuition, nonresident: full-time $24,054; part-time $1623 per credit. *Required fees:* $1130; $119 per credit. *Financial support:* In 2013–14, fellowships with full tuition reimbursements (averaging $20,000 per year), research assistantships with full tuition reimbursements (averaging $26,000 per year), teaching assistantships with full tuition reimbursements (averaging $27,640 per year) were awarded; traineeships, health care benefits, and tuition waivers (full) also available. *Faculty research:* Membrane biochemistry, protein folding and translocation, gene expression, signal transduction, cell growth and differentiation. *Total annual research expenditures:* $3.4 million. *Unit head:* Dr. Patricia Kiley, Chair, 608-262-1347, Fax: 608-262-5253, E-mail: pjkiley@wisc.edu. *Application contact:* Elyse Meuer, Student Services Coordinator, 608-262-1347, Fax: 608-262-5253, E-mail: eemeuer@wisc.edu.
Website: http://www.bmolchem.wisc.edu

University of Wisconsin–Milwaukee, Graduate School, College of Letters and Sciences, Department of Chemistry, Milwaukee, WI 53201-0413. Offers biogeochemistry (PhD); chemistry (MS, PhD). *Faculty:* 20 full-time (4 women). *Students:* 53 full-time (24 women), 16 part-time (8 women); includes 8 minority (5 Asian, non-Hispanic/Latino; 3 Two or more races, non-Hispanic/Latino), 33 international. Average age 31. 74 applicants, 28% accepted, 7 enrolled. In 2013, 7 master's, 11 doctorates awarded. *Degree requirements:* For master's, thesis or alternative; for doctorate, thesis/dissertation. *Entrance requirements:* For doctorate, GRE General Test. Additional exam requirements/recommendations for international students: Required—TOEFL (minimum score 600 paper-based; 79 iBT), IELTS (minimum score 6.5). *Application deadline:* For fall admission, 1/1 priority date for domestic students; for spring admission, 9/1 for domestic students. Applications are processed on a rolling basis. Application fee: $56 ($96 for international students). *Financial support:* In 2013–14, 3 fellowships, 30 research assistantships, 46 teaching assistantships were awarded; career-related internships or fieldwork, unspecified assistantships, and project assistantships also available. Support available to part-time students. Financial award application deadline: 4/15; financial award applicants required to submit FAFSA. *Faculty research:* Analytical chemistry, biochemistry, inorganic chemistry, organic chemistry, physical chemistry. *Unit head:* Peter Geissinger, Department Chair, 414-229-5230, Fax: 414-229-5530, E-mail: geissing@uwm.edu. *Application contact:* General Information Contact, 414-229-4982, Fax: 414-229-6967, E-mail: gradschool@uwm.edu.
Website: http://www.uwm.edu/dept/chemistry/

Utah State University, School of Graduate Studies, College of Science, Department of Chemistry and Biochemistry, Logan, UT 84322. Offers biochemistry (MS, PhD); chemistry (MS, PhD). Part-time programs available. Terminal master's awarded for partial completion of doctoral program. *Degree requirements:* For master's, thesis, oral and written exams; for doctorate, thesis/dissertation, oral and written exams. *Entrance requirements:* For master's and doctorate, GRE General Test, minimum GPA of 3.0. Additional exam requirements/recommendations for international students: Required—TOEFL. *Faculty research:* Analytical, inorganic, organic, and physical chemistry; iron in asbestos chemistry and carcinogenicity; dicopper complexes; photothermal spectrometry; metal molecule clusters.

Vanderbilt University, Graduate School and School of Medicine, Department of Biochemistry, Nashville, TN 37240-1001. Offers MS, PhD, MD/PhD. *Faculty:* 19 full-time (1 woman). *Students:* 39 full-time (19 women); includes 9 minority (2 Black or African American, non-Hispanic/Latino; 2 Asian, non-Hispanic/Latino; 3 Hispanic/Latino; 2 Two or more races, non-Hispanic/Latino), 4 international. Average age 27. In 2013, 1 master's, 4 doctorates awarded. Terminal master's awarded for partial completion of doctoral program. *Degree requirements:* For master's, thesis; for doctorate, thesis/dissertation, preliminary, qualifying, and final exams. *Entrance requirements:* For master's, GRE General Test; for doctorate, GRE General Test, GRE Subject Test (recommended). Additional exam requirements/recommendations for international students: Required—TOEFL (minimum score 570 paper-based; 88 iBT). *Application deadline:* For fall admission, 1/15 for domestic and international students. Application fee: $0. Electronic applications accepted. *Financial support:* Fellowships with full tuition reimbursements, research assistantships with full tuition reimbursements, Federal Work-Study, institutionally sponsored loans, scholarships/grants, traineeships, and tuition waivers (partial) available. Financial award application deadline: 1/15; financial award applicants required to submit CSS PROFILE or FAFSA. *Faculty research:* Protein chemistry, carcinogenesis, metabolism, toxicology, receptors and signaling, DNA recognition and transcription. *Unit head:* Prof. John David York, Director of Department of Biochemistry, 615-322-3318, Fax: 615-322-4349, E-mail: john.york@vanderbilt.edu. *Application contact:* Walter B. Bieschke, Program Coordinator for Graduate Admissions, 615-342-0236, E-mail: vandygrad@vanderbilt.edu.
Website: https://medschool.vanderbilt.edu/biochemistry/

Vanderbilt University, School of Medicine, Program in Chemical and Physical Biology, Nashville, TN 37240-1001. Offers PhD. *Degree requirements:* For doctorate, comprehensive exam, thesis/dissertation, dissertation defense. *Entrance requirements:* For doctorate, GRE, 3 letters of recommendation, official transcripts. Additional exam requirements/recommendations for international students: Required—TOEFL. Electronic applications accepted. *Faculty research:* Mathematical modeling, enzyme kinetics, structural biology, genomics, proteomics and mass spectrometry.

Virginia Commonwealth University, Medical College of Virginia-Professional Programs, School of Medicine, School of Medicine Graduate Programs, Department of Biochemistry, Richmond, VA 23284-9005. Offers biochemistry (MS, PhD); molecular biology (MS, PhD); MD/PhD. *Degree requirements:* For master's, thesis; for doctorate, thesis/dissertation, comprehensive oral and written exams. *Entrance requirements:* For master's and doctorate, GRE, MCAT or DAT. Electronic applications accepted. *Faculty research:* Molecular biology, peptide/protein chemistry, neurochemistry, enzyme mechanisms, macromolecular structure determination.

Virginia Commonwealth University, Program in Pre-Medical Basic Health Sciences, Richmond, VA 23284-9005. Offers anatomy (CBHS); biochemistry (CBHS); human genetics (CBHS); microbiology (CBHS); pharmacology (CBHS); physiology (CBHS). *Entrance requirements:* For degree, GRE, MCAT or DAT, course work in organic chemistry, minimum undergraduate GPA of 2.8. Additional exam requirements/recommendations for international students: Required—TOEFL (minimum score 600 paper-based). Electronic applications accepted.

Wake Forest University, School of Medicine and Graduate School of Arts and Sciences, Graduate Programs in Medicine, Department of Biochemistry, Winston-Salem, NC 27109. Offers PhD, MD/PhD. *Degree requirements:* For doctorate, thesis/dissertation. *Entrance requirements:* For doctorate, GRE General Test. Additional exam requirements/recommendations for international students: Required—TOEFL. Electronic applications accepted. *Faculty research:* Biomembranes, cancer, biophysics.

Washington State University, College of Veterinary Medicine, Program in Molecular Biosciences, Pullman, WA 99164. Offers PSM, PhD. Postbaccalaureate distance learning degree programs offered. *Faculty:* 30 full-time (11 women), 28 part-time/adjunct (6 women). *Students:* 53 full-time (24 women), 16 part-time (9 women); includes 10 minority (3 Black or African American, non-Hispanic/Latino; 3 Asian, non-Hispanic/Latino; 3 Hispanic/Latino; 1 Two or more races, non-Hispanic/Latino), 3 international. Average age 28. 94 applicants, 19% accepted, 10 enrolled. In 2013, 4 master's, 4 doctorates awarded. Terminal master's awarded for partial completion of doctoral program. *Degree requirements:* For master's, thesis or alternative, oral exam; for doctorate, comprehensive exam, thesis/dissertation, oral exam, written exam. *Entrance requirements:* For master's and doctorate, GRE General Test, minimum GPA of 3.0. Additional exam requirements/recommendations for international students: Required—TOEFL (minimum score 100 iBT). *Application deadline:* For fall admission, 12/15 for domestic and international students. Application fee: $75. Electronic applications accepted. *Financial support:* In 2013–14, 9 fellowships with full tuition reimbursements (averaging $22,032 per year), 23 research assistantships with full tuition reimbursements (averaging $22,194 per year), 20 teaching assistantships with full tuition reimbursements (averaging $22,194 per year) were awarded; career-related internships or fieldwork, Federal Work-Study, institutionally sponsored loans, traineeships, and health care benefits also available. Financial award application deadline: 4/1; financial award applicants required to submit FAFSA. *Faculty research:* Gene regulation, signal transduction, protein export, reproductive biology, DNA repair. *Total annual research expenditures:* $5.8 million. *Unit head:* Dr. Jonathan Jones, Director, 509-335-8724, Fax: 509-335-9688, E-mail: jcr.jones@vetmed.wsu.edu. *Application contact:* Kelly G. McGovern, Coordinator, 509-335-4566, E-mail: mcgoverk@wsu.edu.

Washington University in St. Louis, Graduate School of Arts and Sciences, Division of Biology and Biomedical Sciences, Program in Biochemistry, St. Louis, MO 63130-4899. Offers PhD. *Degree requirements:* For doctorate, thesis/dissertation. *Entrance requirements:* For doctorate, GRE General Test, GRE Subject Test. Electronic applications accepted.

Wayne State University, College of Liberal Arts and Sciences, Department of Chemistry, Detroit, MI 48202. Offers analytical chemistry (PhD); biochemistry (PhD); chemistry (MA, MS); inorganic chemistry (PhD); organic chemistry (PhD); physical chemistry (PhD). *Students:* 160 full-time (76 women), 1 part-time (0 women); includes 10 minority (3 Black or African American, non-Hispanic/Latino; 1 American Indian or Alaska Native, non-Hispanic/Latino; 2 Asian, non-Hispanic/Latino; 2 Hispanic/Latino; 2

Two or more races, non-Hispanic/Latino), 112 international. Average age 27. 405 applicants, 13% accepted, 32 enrolled. In 2013, 8 master's, 21 doctorates awarded. *Degree requirements:* For master's, thesis (for some programs), oral exam; for doctorate, thesis/dissertation, oral exam. *Entrance requirements:* For master's, GRE (strongly recommended), admission to Graduate School, 1 year of physics, math through calculus, general chemistry (8 credits), organic chemistry (8 credits), physical chemistry (6 credits), quantitative analysis (4 credits), advanced chemistry (3 credits); advanced biology (for biochemistry applicants); minimum undergraduate GPA of 2.75 in chemistry and cognate sciences; for doctorate, GRE (strongly recommended), admission to Graduate School, minimum undergraduate GPA of 3.0 in chemistry and cognate science. Additional exam requirements/recommendations for international students: Required—TOEFL (minimum score 90 iBT), TWE (minimum score 5.5), Michigan English Language Assessment Battery (minimum score 85); Recommended—IELTS (minimum score 6.5). *Application deadline:* For fall admission, 2/10 priority date for domestic students, 1/10 priority date for international students; for winter admission, 10/1 for domestic students, 9/1 for international students; for spring admission, 2/1 for domestic students, 1/1 for international students. Applications are processed on a rolling basis. Application fee: $0. Electronic applications accepted. *Expenses:* Tuition, state resident: part-time $554.15 per credit. Tuition, nonresident: part-time $1200.35 per credit. *Required fees:* $42.15 per credit. $268.30 per semester. Tuition and fees vary according to course load and program. *Financial support:* In 2013–14, 125 students received support, including 10 fellowships with tuition reimbursements available (averaging $24,211 per year), 55 research assistantships with tuition reimbursements available (averaging $20,153 per year), 82 teaching assistantships with tuition reimbursements available (averaging $21,487 per year); scholarships/grants, health care benefits, and unspecified assistantships also available. Financial award application deadline: 3/31; financial award applicants required to submit FAFSA. *Faculty research:* Natural products synthesis, molecular biology, molecular mechanics calculations, organometallic chemistry, experimental physical chemistry. *Total annual research expenditures:* $6.4 million. *Unit head:* Dr. James Rigby, Chair, 313-577-3472, Fax: 313-577-8822, E-mail: aa392@wayne.edu. *Application contact:* Melissa Barton, Graduate Academic Services Officer, 313-577-2844, E-mail: melissa@wayne.edu.
Website: http://chem.wayne.edu/

Wayne State University, School of Medicine, Graduate Programs in Medicine, Department of Biochemistry and Molecular Biology, Detroit, MI 48202. Offers MS, PhD, MD/PhD. *Students:* 25 full-time (13 women); includes 5 minority (2 Black or African American, non-Hispanic/Latino; 2 Asian, non-Hispanic/Latino; 1 Two or more races, non-Hispanic/Latino), 10 international. Average age 26. 113 applicants, 18% accepted, 9 enrolled. In 2013, 7 master's, 1 doctorate awarded. Terminal master's awarded for partial completion of doctoral program. *Degree requirements:* For master's, thesis; for doctorate, thesis/dissertation. *Entrance requirements:* For master's, GRE, BA or BS in biology, chemistry, or (if approved) physics or mathematics with minimum GPA of 2.6 from accredited university; three letters of recommendation; personal statement, admission to the Graduate School; for doctorate, GRE, BA or BS in biology, chemistry or physics (preferred), undergraduate degree with minimum GPA of 3.0, admission to the Graduate School. Additional exam requirements/recommendations for international students: Required—TOEFL (minimum score 600 paper-based; 100 iBT). *Application deadline:* For fall admission, 2/1 for domestic and international students. Application fee: $0. Electronic applications accepted. *Expenses:* Contact institution. *Financial support:* In 2013–14, 11 students received support, including 3 fellowships with tuition reimbursements available (averaging $22,811 per year), 10 research assistantships with tuition reimbursements available (averaging $22,594 per year); scholarships/grants, health care benefits, and unspecified assistantships also available. Financial award application deadline: 3/31; financial award applicants required to submit FAFSA. *Faculty research:* Cancer biology, structural biology and drug design, molecular evolution, viral and fungal metabolism/resistance, cardiovascular disease, computational biology. *Unit head:* Dr. Bharati Mitra, Professor and Chair, Department of Biochemistry and Molecular Biology, 313-577-1512, Fax: 313-577-2765, E-mail: bmitra@med.wayne.edu. *Application contact:* Dr. David Evans, Graduate Program Director, 313-577-5712, E-mail: drevans@med.wayne.edu.
Website: http://gradprograms.med.wayne.edu/program-spotlight.php?id=28

Weill Cornell Medical College, Weill Cornell Graduate School of Medical Sciences, Biochemistry, Cell and Molecular Biology Allied Program, New York, NY 10065. Offers MS, PhD. Terminal master's awarded for partial completion of doctoral program. *Degree requirements:* For master's, comprehensive exam; for doctorate, thesis/dissertation, final exam. *Entrance requirements:* For doctorate, GRE General Test, background in genetics, molecular biology, chemistry, or biochemistry. Additional exam requirements/recommendations for international students: Required—TOEFL. Electronic applications accepted. *Faculty research:* Molecular structure determination, protein structure, gene structure, stem cell biology, control of gene expression, DNA replication, chromosome maintenance, RNA biosynthesis.

Weill Cornell Medical College, Weill Cornell Graduate School of Medical Sciences, Tri-Institutional Training Program in Chemical Biology, New York, NY 10065. Offers PhD. Program offered jointly with The Rockefeller University and Sloan-Kettering Institute. *Degree requirements:* For doctorate, comprehensive exam, thesis/dissertation. *Entrance requirements:* For doctorate, GRE General Test, 3 letters of recommendation. Additional exam requirements/recommendations for international students: Required—TOEFL (minimum score 600 paper-based; 90 iBT). Electronic applications accepted. *Faculty research:* Bio-organic chemistry, biological chemistry/biochemistry, biophysical chemistry, bio-analytical chemistry, computational chemistry and biology.

Wesleyan University, Graduate Studies, Department of Chemistry, Middletown, CT 06459-0180. Offers biochemistry (PhD); chemical physics (PhD); inorganic chemistry (PhD); organic chemistry (PhD); physical chemistry (PhD); theoretical chemistry (PhD). Terminal master's awarded for partial completion of doctoral program. *Degree requirements:* For doctorate, thesis/dissertation, proposal. *Entrance requirements:* For doctorate, GRE General Test, 3 recommendations. Additional exam requirements/recommendations for international students: Required—TOEFL. Electronic applications accepted.

Wesleyan University, Graduate Studies, Department of Molecular Biology and Biochemistry, Middletown, CT 06459. Offers biochemistry (PhD); molecular biology (PhD); molecular biophysics (PhD); molecular genetics (PhD). *Degree requirements:* For doctorate, comprehensive exam, thesis/dissertation. *Entrance requirements:* For doctorate, GRE General Test, GRE Subject Test. Additional exam requirements/recommendations for international students: Required—TOEFL. Electronic applications accepted. *Faculty research:* The olfactory system and new frontiers in genome research, chromosome structure and gene expression.

West Virginia University, School of Medicine, Graduate Programs at the Health Sciences Center, Interdisciplinary Graduate Programs in Biomedical Sciences, Program in Biochemistry and Molecular Biology, Morgantown, WV 26506. Offers MS, PhD, MD/PhD. *Degree requirements:* For doctorate, comprehensive exam, thesis/dissertation. *Entrance requirements:* For doctorate, GRE General Test, minimum GPA of 3.0. Additional exam requirements/recommendations for international students: Required—TOEFL. Electronic applications accepted. *Faculty research:* Regulation of gene expression, cell survival mechanisms, signal transduction, regulation of metabolism, sensory neuroscience.

Worcester Polytechnic Institute, Graduate Studies and Research, Department of Chemistry and Biochemistry, Worcester, MA 01609-2280. Offers biochemistry (MS, PhD); chemistry (MS, PhD). Evening/weekend programs available. *Faculty:* 9 full-time (1 woman), 1 part-time/adjunct (0 women). *Students:* 17 full-time (9 women); includes 1 minority (Two or more races, non-Hispanic/Latino), 8 international. 40 applicants, 3% accepted, 1 enrolled. In 2013, 1 master's, 2 doctorates awarded. *Degree requirements:* For master's, thesis; for doctorate, comprehensive exam, thesis/dissertation. *Entrance requirements:* For master's and doctorate, GRE General Test, 3 letters of recommendation, statement of purpose. Additional exam requirements/recommendations for international students: Required—TOEFL (minimum score 563 paper-based; 84 iBT), IELTS (minimum score 7). *Application deadline:* For fall admission, 1/1 priority date for domestic and international students; for spring admission, 10/1 priority date for domestic and international students. Applications are processed on a rolling basis. Application fee: $70. Electronic applications accepted. *Financial support:* Research assistantships, teaching assistantships, career-related internships or fieldwork, institutionally sponsored loans, scholarships/grants, and unspecified assistantships available. Financial award application deadline: 1/1; financial award applicants required to submit FAFSA. *Unit head:* Dr. Arne Gericke, Department Head, 508-831-5371, Fax: 508-831-5933, E-mail: agericke@wpi.edu. *Application contact:* Dr. George Kaminski, Graduate Coordinator, 508-831-5371, Fax: 508-831-5933, E-mail: gkaminski@wpi.edu.
Website: http://www.wpi.edu/Academics/Depts/Chemistry/

Wright State University, School of Graduate Studies, College of Science and Mathematics, Department of Biochemistry and Molecular Biology, Dayton, OH 45435. Offers MS. *Degree requirements:* For master's, thesis. *Entrance requirements:* Additional exam requirements/recommendations for international students: Required—TOEFL. *Faculty research:* Regulation of gene expression, macromolecular structural function, NMR imaging, visual biochemistry.

Yale University, Graduate School of Arts and Sciences, Department of Geology and Geophysics, New Haven, CT 06520. Offers biogeochemistry (PhD); climate dynamics (PhD); geochemistry (PhD); geophysics (PhD); meteorology (PhD); oceanography (PhD); paleontology (PhD); paleooceanography (PhD); petrology (PhD); tectonics (PhD). *Degree requirements:* For doctorate, thesis/dissertation. *Entrance requirements:* For doctorate, GRE General Test. Additional exam requirements/recommendations for international students: Required—TOEFL.

Yale University, Graduate School of Arts and Sciences, Department of Molecular Biophysics and Biochemistry, New Haven, CT 06520. Offers PhD. *Degree requirements:* For doctorate, thesis/dissertation. *Entrance requirements:* For doctorate, GRE General Test, GRE Subject Test.

Yale University, Graduate School of Arts and Sciences, Department of Molecular, Cellular, and Developmental Biology, Program in Biochemistry, Molecular Biology and Chemical Biology, New Haven, CT 06520. Offers PhD. *Degree requirements:* For doctorate, thesis/dissertation. *Entrance requirements:* For doctorate, GRE General Test, GRE Subject Test.

Yale University, School of Medicine and Graduate School of Arts and Sciences, Combined Program in Biological and Biomedical Sciences (BBS), Molecular Biophysics and Biochemistry Track, New Haven, CT 06520. Offers PhD, MD/PhD. *Degree requirements:* For doctorate, thesis/dissertation. *Entrance requirements:* For doctorate, GRE General Test. Additional exam requirements/recommendations for international students: Required—TOEFL. Electronic applications accepted.

Youngstown State University, Graduate School, College of Science, Technology, Engineering and Mathematics, Department of Chemistry, Youngstown, OH 44555-0001. Offers analytical chemistry (MS); biochemistry (MS); chemistry education (MS); inorganic chemistry (MS); organic chemistry (MS); physical chemistry (MS). Part-time programs available. *Degree requirements:* For master's, thesis. *Entrance requirements:* For master's, bachelor's degree in chemistry, minimum GPA of 2.7. Additional exam requirements/recommendations for international students: Required—TOEFL. *Faculty research:* Analysis of antioxidants, chromatography, defects and disorder in crystalline oxides, hydrogen bonding, novel organic and organometallic materials.

Section 4
Biophysics

This section contains a directory of institutions offering graduate work in biophysics, followed by an in-depth entry submitted by an institution that chose to prepare a detailed program description. Additional information about programs listed in the directory but not augmented by an in-depth entry may be obtained by writing directly to the dean of a graduate school or chair of a department at the address given in the directory.

For programs offering related work, see also in this book *Allied Health; Biochemistry; Biological and Biomedical Sciences; Cell, Molecular, and Structural Biology; Optometry and Vision Sciences; Neuroscience and Neurobiology; Physiology;* and *Public Health.* In the other guides in this series:

Graduate Programs in the Physical Sciences, Mathematics, Agricultural Sciences, the Environment & Natural Resources

See *Chemistry* and *Physics*

Graduate Programs in Engineering & Applied Sciences

See *Agricultural Engineering and Bioengineering* and *Biomedical Engineering and Biotechnology*

CONTENTS

Program Directories

Display and Close-Up

Biophysics

Albert Einstein College of Medicine, Graduate Division of Biomedical Sciences, Department of Physiology and Biophysics, Bronx, NY 10461. Offers PhD, MD/PhD. *Degree requirements:* For doctorate, thesis/dissertation. *Entrance requirements:* For doctorate, GRE General Test. Additional exam requirements/recommendations for international students: Required—TOEFL. *Faculty research:* Biophysical and biochemical basis of body function at the subcellular, cellular, organ, and whole-body level.

Baylor College of Medicine, Graduate School of Biomedical Sciences, Department of Molecular Physiology and Biophysics, Houston, TX 77030-3498. Offers cardiovascular sciences (PhD); molecular physiology and biophysics (PhD); MD/PhD. *Degree requirements:* For doctorate, thesis/dissertation, public defense. *Entrance requirements:* For doctorate, GRE General Test, GRE Subject Test (strongly recommended), minimum GPA of 3.0. Additional exam requirements/recommendations for international students: Required—TOEFL. Electronic applications accepted. *Faculty research:* Cardiovascular disease; skeletal muscle disease (myasthenia gravis, muscular dystrophy, malignant hyperthermia, central core disease); cancer; Alzheimer's disease; developmental diseases of the nervous system, eye and heart; diabetes; motor neuron disease (amyotrophic lateral sclerosis and spinal muscular atrophy); asthma; autoimmune diseases.

Boston University, School of Medicine, Division of Graduate Medical Sciences, Department of Physiology and Biophysics, Boston, MA 02118. Offers MA, PhD, MD/PhD. Part-time programs available. Terminal master's awarded for partial completion of doctoral program. *Degree requirements:* For master's, thesis; for doctorate, thesis/dissertation. *Application deadline:* For fall admission, 1/15 for domestic students; for spring admission, 10/15 for domestic students. *Expenses: Tuition:* Full-time $43,970; part-time $1374 per credit hour. *Required fees:* $60 per semester. Tuition and fees vary according to class time, course level and program. *Faculty research:* X-ray scattering, NMR spectroscopy, protein crystallography, structural electron. *Unit head:* Dr. David Atkinson, Chairman, 617-638-4015, Fax: 617-638-4041, E-mail: atkinson@bu.edu. *Application contact:* Dr. Esther Bullitt, Associate Professor, 617-638-5037, E-mail: bullitt@bu.edu.
Website: http://www.bumc.bu.edu/phys-biophys/

Brandeis University, Graduate School of Arts and Sciences, Program in Biochemistry and Biophysics, Waltham, MA 02454. Offers biochemistry and biophysics (PhD); quantitative biology (PhD). Terminal master's awarded for partial completion of doctoral program. *Degree requirements:* For doctorate, thesis/dissertation, qualifying exams. *Entrance requirements:* For doctorate, GRE General Test, resume, 3 letters of recommendation, statement of purpose, transcript(s). Additional exam requirements/recommendations for international students: Required—TOEFL (minimum score 600 paper-based; 100 iBT), PTE (minimum score 68); Recommended—IELTS (minimum score 7). Electronic applications accepted. *Faculty research:* Macromolecular chemistry, structure and function, biochemistry, biophysics, biological macromolecules.

California Institute of Technology, Division of Biology, Program in Cell Biology and Biophysics, Pasadena, CA 91125-0001. Offers PhD. *Degree requirements:* For doctorate, thesis/dissertation, qualifying exam. *Entrance requirements:* For doctorate, GRE General Test.

Carnegie Mellon University, Mellon College of Science, Department of Biological Sciences, Pittsburgh, PA 15213-3891. Offers biochemistry (PhD); biophysics (PhD); cell and developmental biology (PhD); computational biology (MS, PhD); genetics (PhD); molecular biology (PhD); neuroscience (PhD); structural biology (PhD). *Degree requirements:* For doctorate, comprehensive exam, thesis/dissertation. *Entrance requirements:* For doctorate, GRE General Test, GRE Subject Test, interview. *Application deadline:* Applications are processed on a rolling basis. Application fee: $0. Electronic applications accepted. *Financial support:* Fellowships, research assistantships, teaching assistantships, and traineeships available. *Faculty research:* Genetic structure, function, and regulation; protein structure and function; biological membranes; biological spectroscopy. *Unit head:* John L. Woolford, Acting Department Head, 412-268-3193, E-mail: jw17@andrew.cmu.edu. *Application contact:* Ena Miceli, Graduate Programs Manager, 412-268-33012, E-mail: emiceli@andrew.cmu.edu.
Website: http://www.bio.cmu.edu/

Case Western Reserve University, School of Medicine and School of Graduate Studies, Graduate Programs in Medicine, Department of Physiology and Biophysics, Cleveland, OH 44106. Offers cell and molecular physiology (MS); cell physiology (PhD); molecular/cellular biophysics (PhD); physiology and biophysics (PhD); systems physiology (PhD); MD/PhD. Terminal master's awarded for partial completion of doctoral program. *Degree requirements:* For master's, thesis; for doctorate, thesis/dissertation. *Entrance requirements:* For master's, GRE General Test, minimum GPA of 3.28; for doctorate, GRE General Test, minimum GPA of 3.6. Additional exam requirements/recommendations for international students: Required—TOEFL. Electronic applications accepted. *Faculty research:* Cardiovascular physiology, calcium metabolism, epithelial cell biology.

Clemson University, Graduate School, College of Engineering and Science, Department of Physics and Astronomy, Clemson, SC 29634. Offers physics (MS, PhD), including astronomy and astrophysics, atmospheric physics, biophysics. Part-time programs available. *Faculty:* 23 full-time (3 women). *Students:* 63 full-time (17 women), 1 part-time (0 women); includes 2 minority (both Hispanic/Latino), 31 international. Average age 25. 85 applicants, 35% accepted, 16 enrolled. In 2013, 14 master's, 6 doctorates awarded. Terminal master's awarded for partial completion of doctoral program. *Median time to degree:* Of those who began their doctoral program in fall 2005, 71% received their degree in 8 years or less. *Degree requirements:* For master's, thesis or alternative; for doctorate, thesis/dissertation. *Entrance requirements:* For master's and doctorate, GRE General Test. Additional exam requirements/recommendations for international students: Required—TOEFL. *Application deadline:* For fall admission, 1/15 priority date for domestic students; for spring admission, 9/15 priority date for domestic students. Applications are processed on a rolling basis. Application fee: $70 ($80 for international students). Electronic applications accepted. *Financial support:* In 2013–14, 60 students received support, including 3 fellowships with full and partial tuition reimbursements available (averaging $2,133 per year), 18 research assistantships with partial tuition reimbursements available (averaging $27,824 per year), 44 teaching assistantships with partial tuition reimbursements available (averaging $14,298 per year); career-related internships or fieldwork, institutionally sponsored loans, scholarships/grants, health care benefits, and unspecified assistantships also available. Support available to part-time students. Financial award application deadline: 6/1; financial award applicants required to submit FAFSA. *Faculty research:* Radiation physics, solid-state physics, nuclear physics, radar and lidar studies of atmosphere. *Total annual research expenditures:* $4.3 million. *Unit head:* Dr. Peter Barnes, Chair, 864-656-3419, Fax: 864-656-0805, E-mail: peterb@clemson.edu. *Application contact:* Graduate Coordinator, 864-656-6702, Fax: 864-656-0805, E-mail: physgradinfo-l@clemson.edu.
Website: http://physicsnt.clemson.edu/

Columbia University, College of Physicians and Surgeons, Department of Biochemistry and Molecular Biophysics, New York, NY 10032. Offers biochemistry and molecular biophysics (M Phil, PhD); biophysics (PhD); MD/PhD. Only candidates for the PhD are admitted. *Degree requirements:* For doctorate, one foreign language, thesis/dissertation. *Entrance requirements:* For master's and doctorate, GRE General Test. Additional exam requirements/recommendations for international students: Required—TOEFL.

Columbia University, College of Physicians and Surgeons, Department of Physiology and Cellular Biophysics, New York, NY 10032. Offers M Phil, MA, PhD, MD/PhD. Only candidates for the PhD are admitted. Terminal master's awarded for partial completion of doctoral program. *Degree requirements:* For doctorate, thesis/dissertation. *Entrance requirements:* For master's and doctorate, GRE General Test. Additional exam requirements/recommendations for international students: Required—TOEFL. *Faculty research:* Membrane physiology, cellular biology, cardiovascular physiology, neurophysiology.

Columbia University, College of Physicians and Surgeons, Integrated Program in Cellular, Molecular, Structural and Genetic Studies, New York, NY 10032. Offers PhD. Terminal master's awarded for partial completion of doctoral program. *Degree requirements:* For doctorate, thesis/dissertation. *Entrance requirements:* For doctorate, GRE General Test, GRE Subject Test. Additional exam requirements/recommendations for international students: Required—TOEFL. *Expenses:* Contact institution. *Faculty research:* Transcription, macromolecular sorting, gene expression during development, cellular interaction.

Cornell University, Graduate School, Graduate Fields of Agriculture and Life Sciences, Field of Biochemistry, Molecular and Cell Biology, Ithaca, NY 14853-0001. Offers biochemistry (PhD); biophysics (PhD); cell biology (PhD); molecular biology (PhD). *Faculty:* 20 full-time (19 women). *Students:* 87 full-time (43 women); includes 17 minority (7 Asian, non-Hispanic/Latino; 6 Hispanic/Latino; 4 Two or more races, non-Hispanic/Latino), 28 international. Average age 26. 238 applicants, 20% accepted, 20 enrolled. In 2013, 17 doctorates awarded. *Degree requirements:* For doctorate, comprehensive exam, thesis/dissertation, 2 semesters of teaching experience. *Entrance requirements:* For doctorate, GRE General Test, GRE Subject Test (biology, chemistry, physics, biochemistry, cell and molecular biology), 3 letters of recommendation. Additional exam requirements/recommendations for international students: Required—TOEFL (minimum score 600 paper-based; 77 iBT). *Application deadline:* For fall admission, 1/5 for domestic students. Application fee: $95. Electronic applications accepted. *Financial support:* In 2013–14, 62 students received support, including 8 fellowships with full tuition reimbursements available, 38 research assistantships with full tuition reimbursements available, 16 teaching assistantships with full tuition reimbursements available; institutionally sponsored loans, scholarships/grants, health care benefits, tuition waivers (full and partial), and unspecified assistantships also available. Financial award applicants required to submit FAFSA. *Faculty research:* Biophysics, structural biology. *Unit head:* Director of Graduate Studies, 607-255-2100, Fax: 607-255-2100. *Application contact:* Graduate Field Assistant, 607-255-2100, Fax: 607-255-2100, E-mail: bmcb@cornell.edu.
Website: http://www.gradschool.cornell.edu/fields.php?id-43&a-2

Cornell University, Graduate School, Graduate Fields of Agriculture and Life Sciences, Field of Biophysics, Ithaca, NY 14853-0001. Offers PhD. *Faculty:* 34 full-time (5 women). *Students:* 17 full-time (7 women); includes 2 minority (1 Asian, non-Hispanic/Latino; 1 Hispanic/Latino), 4 international. Average age 27. 24 applicants, 46% accepted, 2 enrolled. In 2013, 2 doctorates awarded. *Degree requirements:* For doctorate, comprehensive exam, thesis/dissertation. *Entrance requirements:* For doctorate, GRE General Test, GRE Subject Test (physics or chemistry preferred), 3 letters of recommendation. Additional exam requirements/recommendations for international students: Required—TOEFL (minimum score 550 paper-based; 77 iBT). *Application deadline:* For fall admission, 1/15 for domestic students. Application fee: $95. Electronic applications accepted. *Financial support:* In 2013–14, 10 students received support, including 2 fellowships with full tuition reimbursements available, 6 research assistantships with full tuition reimbursements available, 2 teaching assistantships with full tuition reimbursements available; institutionally sponsored loans, scholarships/grants, health care benefits, tuition waivers (full and partial), and unspecified assistantships also available. Financial award applicants required to submit FAFSA. *Faculty research:* Protein structure and function, biomolecular and cellular function, membrane biophysics, signal transduction, computational biology. *Unit head:* Director of Graduate Studies, 607-255-2100, E-mail: biophysics@cornell.edu. *Application contact:* Graduate Field Assistant, 610-255-2100, E-mail: biophysics@cornell.edu.
Website: http://www.gradschool.cornell.edu/fields.php?id-68&a-2

Dalhousie University, Faculty of Medicine, Department of Physiology and Biophysics, Halifax, NS B3H 1X5, Canada. Offers M Sc, PhD, M Sc/PhD. *Degree requirements:* For master's, thesis; for doctorate, thesis/dissertation. *Entrance requirements:* For master's and doctorate, GRE Subject Test (for international students). Additional exam requirements/recommendations for international students: Required—1 of 5 approved tests: TOEFL, IELTS, CANTEST, CAEL, Michigan English Language Assessment Battery. Electronic applications accepted. *Faculty research:* Computer modeling, reproductive and endocrine physiology, cardiovascular physiology, neurophysiology, membrane biophysics.

East Carolina University, Graduate School, Thomas Harriot College of Arts and Sciences, Department of Physics, Greenville, NC 27858-4353. Offers applied physics (MS); biomedical physics (PhD); health physics (MS); medical physics (MS). Part-time programs available. *Degree requirements:* For master's, one foreign language, comprehensive exam. *Entrance requirements:* For master's, GRE General Test. Additional exam requirements/recommendations for international students: Required—TOEFL. *Application deadline:* Applications are processed on a rolling basis. Application fee: $50. *Expenses:* Tuition, state resident: full-time $4223. Tuition, nonresident: full-time $16,540. *Required fees:* $2184. *Financial support:* Research assistantships with partial tuition reimbursements, teaching assistantships with partial tuition reimbursements, and Federal Work-Study available. Support available to part-time students. Financial award application deadline: 6/1. *Unit head:* Dr. John Sutherland, Chair, 252-328-6739, E-mail: sutherlandj@ecu.edu. *Application contact:* Dean of Graduate School, 252-328-6012, Fax: 252-328-6071, E-mail: gradschool@ecu.edu.
Website: http://www.ecu.edu/cs-cas/physics/Graduate-Program.cfm#

Emory University, Laney Graduate School, Department of Physics, Atlanta, GA 30322-1100. Offers biophysics (PhD); experimental condensed matter physics (PhD); theoretical and computational statistical physics (PhD); MS/PhD. *Degree requirements:* For doctorate, thesis/dissertation, qualifier proposal. *Entrance requirements:* For doctorate, GRE General Test, minimum GPA of 3.0. Additional exam requirements/recommendations for international students: Required—TOEFL (minimum score 600 paper-based). Electronic applications accepted. *Faculty research:* Experimental studies of the structure and function of metalloproteins, soft condensed matter, granular materials, biophotonics and fluorescence correlation spectroscopy, single molecule studies of DNA-protein systems.

Harvard University, Graduate School of Arts and Sciences, Committee on Biophysics, Cambridge, MA 02138. Offers PhD. *Degree requirements:* For doctorate, thesis/dissertation, exam, qualifying paper. *Entrance requirements:* For doctorate, GRE General Test, GRE Subject Test (recommended). Additional exam requirements/recommendations for international students: Required—TOEFL. *Expenses: Tuition:* Full-time $38,888. *Required fees:* $958. Tuition and fees vary according to campus/location, program and student level. *Faculty research:* Structural molecular biology, cell and membrane biophysics, molecular genetics, physical biochemistry, mathematical biophysics.

See Display on this page and Close-Up on page 173.

Howard University, Graduate School, Department of Physiology and Biophysics, Washington, DC 20059-0002. Offers biophysics (PhD); physiology (PhD). *Degree requirements:* For doctorate, comprehensive exam, thesis/dissertation. *Entrance requirements:* For doctorate, GRE General Test, minimum B average in field. *Faculty research:* Cardiovascular physiology, pulmonary physiology, renal physiology, neurophysiology, endocrinology.

Illinois State University, Graduate School, College of Arts and Sciences, Department of Biological Sciences, Normal, IL 61790-2200. Offers animal behavior (MS); bacteriology (MS); biochemistry (MS); biological sciences (MS); biology (PhD); biophysics (MS); biotechnology (MS); botany (MS, PhD); cell biology (MS); conservation biology (MS); developmental biology (MS); ecology (MS, PhD); entomology (MS); evolutionary biology (MS); genetics (MS, PhD); immunology (MS); microbiology (MS, PhD); molecular biology (MS); molecular genetics (MS); neurobiology (MS); neuroscience (MS); parasitology (MS); physiology (MS, PhD); plant biology (MS); plant molecular biology (MS); plant sciences (MS); structural biology (MS); zoology (MS, PhD). Part-time programs available. *Degree requirements:* For master's, thesis or alternative; for doctorate, variable foreign language requirement, thesis/dissertation, 2 terms of residency. *Entrance requirements:* For master's, GRE General Test, minimum GPA of 2.6 in last 60 hours of course work; for doctorate, GRE General Test. *Faculty research:* Redoc balance and drug development in schistosoma mansoni, control of the growth of listeria monocytogenes at low temperature, regulation of cell expansion and microtubule function by SPRI, CRUI: physiology and fitness consequences of different life history phenotypes.

Iowa State University of Science and Technology, Program in Biophysics, Ames, IA 50011. Offers MS, PhD. *Entrance requirements:* For master's, GRE. Additional exam requirements/recommendations for international students: Required—TOEFL (minimum score 550 paper-based; 79 iBT), IELTS (minimum score 6.5). Electronic applications accepted.

Johns Hopkins University, National Institutes of Health Sponsored Programs, Baltimore, MD 21218-2699. Offers biology (PhD), including biochemistry, biophysics, cell biology, developmental biology, genetic biology, molecular biology; cell, molecular, and developmental biology and biophysics (PhD). *Faculty:* 25 full-time (4 women). *Students:* 126 full-time (72 women); includes 36 minority (3 Black or African American, non-Hispanic/Latino; 1 American Indian or Alaska Native, non-Hispanic/Latino; 21 Asian, non-Hispanic/Latino; 11 Hispanic/Latino), 19 international. 282 applicants, 26% accepted, 36 enrolled. In 2013, 15 doctorates awarded. *Degree requirements:* For doctorate, comprehensive exam, thesis/dissertation. *Entrance requirements:* For doctorate, GRE General Test. Additional exam requirements/recommendations for international students: Required—TOEFL (minimum score 600 paper-based), TWE. *Application deadline:* For fall admission, 12/15 priority date for domestic students. Application fee: $60. Electronic applications accepted. *Financial support:* In 2013–14, 24 fellowships (averaging $23,000 per year), 93 research assistantships (averaging $23,000 per year), 22 teaching assistantships (averaging $23,000 per year) were awarded; Federal Work-Study, institutionally sponsored loans, scholarships/grants, traineeships, health care benefits, tuition waivers (partial), and unspecified assistantships also available. Financial award application deadline: 4/15; financial award applicants required to submit FAFSA. *Faculty research:* Protein and nucleic acid biochemistry and biophysical chemistry, molecular biology and development. *Total annual research expenditures:* $11.2 million. *Unit head:* Dr. Allen Shearn, Chair, 410-516-4693, Fax: 410-516-5213, E-mail: bio_cals@jhu.edu. *Application contact:* Joan Miller, Academic Affairs Manager, 410-516-5502, Fax: 410-516-5213, E-mail: joan@jhu.edu.

Johns Hopkins University, Zanvyl Krieger School of Arts and Sciences, Thomas C. Jenkins Department of Biophysics, Baltimore, MD 21218-2699. Offers PhD. *Faculty:* 10 full-time (4 women). *Students:* 61 full-time (18 women); includes 14 minority (7 Asian, non-Hispanic/Latino; 6 Hispanic/Latino; 1 Two or more races, non-Hispanic/Latino), 4 international. Average age 26. 89 applicants, 17% accepted, 10 enrolled. In 2013, 9 doctorates awarded. *Degree requirements:* For doctorate, comprehensive exam, thesis/dissertation. *Entrance requirements:* For doctorate, GRE General Test. Additional exam requirements/recommendations for international students: Required—TOEFL (minimum score 600 paper-based), IELTS; Recommended—TWE. *Application deadline:* For fall admission, 1/2 for domestic and international students. Application fee: $75. Electronic applications accepted. *Financial support:* In 2013–14, fellowships with full tuition reimbursements (averaging $29,218 per year), research assistantships (averaging $29,218 per year) were awarded; scholarships/grants, traineeships, and health care benefits also available. Financial award application deadline: 4/15. *Faculty research:* Application of thermodynamics and kinetics, NMR spectroscopy, X-ray crystallography and computational methods to examine the function and structural and physical properties of proteins and nucleic acids. *Unit head:* Dr. Bertrand Garcia-Moreno, Professor and Department Chair, 410-516-7245, Fax: 410-516-4118, E-mail: bertrand@jhu.edu. *Application contact:* Ranice H. Crosby, Coordinator, Graduate Admissions, 410-516-5197, Fax: 410-516-4118, E-mail: crosbyr@jhu.edu.
Website: http://biophysics.jhu.edu/

Medical College of Wisconsin, Graduate School of Biomedical Sciences, Department of Biophysics, Milwaukee, WI 53226-0509. Offers PhD.

Medical College of Wisconsin, Graduate School of Biomedical Sciences, Program in Biophysics, Milwaukee, WI 53226-0509. Offers PhD, MD/PhD. Part-time programs available. *Degree requirements:* For doctorate, thesis/dissertation, oral exam. *Entrance requirements:* For doctorate, GRE General Test. Additional exam requirements/recommendations for international students: Required—TOEFL. Electronic applications accepted. *Faculty research:* X-ray crystallography, electron spin resonance and membrane structure, protein and membrane dynamics, magnetic resonance imaging, free radical biology.

Northwestern University, The Graduate School, Interdisciplinary Biological Sciences Program (IBiS), Evanston, IL 60208. Offers biochemistry (PhD); bioengineering and biotechnology (PhD); biotechnology (PhD); cell and molecular biology (PhD); developmental and systems biology (PhD); nanotechnology (PhD); neurobiology (PhD); structural biology and biophysics (PhD). *Degree requirements:* For doctorate, thesis/dissertation, qualifying exam. *Entrance requirements:* For doctorate, GRE General Test. Additional exam requirements/recommendations for international students: Required—TOEFL (minimum score 600 paper-based). *Application deadline:* For fall admission, 12/15 for domestic and international students. Applications are processed on a rolling basis. Application fee: $95. Electronic applications accepted. *Financial support:* Fellowships, research assistantships, teaching assistantships, career-related internships or fieldwork, institutionally sponsored loans, scholarships/grants, traineeships, health care benefits, and unspecified assistantships available. Financial award application deadline: 12/31; financial award applicants required to submit FAFSA. *Faculty research:* Biophysics/structural biology, cell/molecular biology, synthetic biology, developmental systems biology, chemical biology/nanotechnology. *Unit head:* Dr. Deborah Klos Dehring, Associate Director, 847-467-0451, E-mail: d-klos@northwestern.edu. *Application contact:* Cathy Prullage, Program Manager, 847-491-4301, E-mail: ibis@northwestern.edu.
Website: http://www.biochem.northwestern.edu/ibis/

The Ohio State University, Graduate School, College of Arts and Sciences, Division of Natural and Mathematical Sciences, Program in Biophysics, Columbus, OH 43210. Offers MS, PhD. *Students:* 33 full-time (11 women), 2 part-time (1 woman); includes 3 minority (all Asian, non-Hispanic/Latino), 17 international. Average age 28. In 2013, 1 master's, 7 doctorates awarded. *Degree requirements:* For master's, thesis optional; for doctorate, thesis/dissertation. *Entrance requirements:* For master's and doctorate, GRE General Test. Additional exam requirements/recommendations for international students: Required—TOEFL (minimum score 600 paper-based; 100 iBT), Michigan English Language Assessment Battery (minimum score 86); Recommended—IELTS (minimum score 8). *Application deadline:* For fall admission, 11/30 priority date for domestic and international students; for winter admission, 12/1 for domestic students, 11/1 for international students; for spring admission, 12/6 for domestic students, 11/11 for international students; for summer admission, 4/4 for domestic students, 3/7 for international students. Applications are processed on a rolling basis. Application fee: $60 ($70 for international students). Electronic applications accepted. *Financial support:* Fellowships with tuition reimbursements, research assistantships with tuition reimbursements, teaching assistantships with tuition reimbursements, Federal Work-Study, and institutionally sponsored loans available. Support available to part-time students. *Unit head:* Jeffrey Kuret, 614-688-5899, E-mail: kuret.3@osu.edu. *Application contact:* Lakisha Mays, Program Administrator, 614-292-5626, Fax: 614-688-3555, E-mail: mays.63@osu.edu.
Website: http://biophysics.osu.edu/

Oregon State University, College of Science, Program in Biochemistry and Biophysics, Corvallis, OR 97331. Offers MA, MAIS, MS, PhD. *Faculty:* 17 full-time (6 women). *Students:* 27 full-time (12 women); includes 3 minority (1 Black or African American, non-Hispanic/Latino; 1 American Indian or Alaska Native, non-Hispanic/Latino; 1 Asian, non-Hispanic/Latino), 7 international. Average age 27. 23 applicants, 43% accepted, 7 enrolled. In 2013, 2 degrees awarded. *Degree requirements:* For master's, thesis optional; for doctorate, thesis/dissertation, exams. *Entrance requirements:* For master's and doctorate, GRE, minimum GPA of 3.0. Additional exam requirements/recommendations for international students: Required—TOEFL (minimum score 600 paper-based). *Application deadline:* For fall admission, 1/15 for domestic students. Application fee: $60. *Expenses:* Tuition, state resident: full-time $11,664; part-time $432 per credit hour. Tuition, nonresident: full-time $19,197; part-time $711 per credit hour. *Required fees:* $1446; $443 per quarter. One-time fee: $300. Tuition and fees vary according to course load and program. *Financial support:* Research assistantships, teaching assistantships, and institutionally sponsored loans available. Support available to part-time students. Financial award application deadline: 2/1. *Faculty research:* DNA and deoxyribonucleotide metabolism, cell growth control, receptors and membranes, protein structure and function. *Unit head:* Dr. Gary Merrill, Chair, 541-737-4511, Fax: 541-737-0481, E-mail: merrillg@science.oregonstate.edu. *Application contact:* Dr. Michael Freitag, Chair of Graduate Admissions, 541-737-4511, Fax: 541-737-0481, E-mail: freitagm@cgrb.oregonstate.edu.
Website: http://biochem.science.oregonstate.edu/about-graduate-program

Purdue University, Graduate School, College of Science, Department of Biological Sciences, West Lafayette, IN 47907. Offers biochemistry (PhD); biophysics (PhD); cell and developmental biology (PhD); ecology, evolutionary and population biology (MS, PhD), including ecology, evolutionary biology, population biology; genetics (MS, PhD); microbiology (MS, PhD); molecular biology (PhD); neurobiology (MS, PhD); plant physiology (PhD). *Faculty:* 50 full-time (13 women), 5 part-time/adjunct (1 woman). *Students:* 111 full-time (61 women), 5 part-time (0 women); includes 9 minority (1 Black or African American, non-Hispanic/Latino; 5 Asian, non-Hispanic/Latino; 3 Hispanic/Latino), 62 international. Average age 27. 170 applicants, 19% accepted, 17 enrolled. In 2013, 9 master's, 18 doctorates awarded. Terminal master's awarded for partial completion of doctoral program. *Degree requirements:* For master's, thesis (for some programs); for doctorate, thesis/dissertation, seminars, teaching experience. *Entrance requirements:* For master's, GRE General Test (minimum analytical writing score of 3.5), minimum undergraduate GPA of 3.0; for doctorate, GRE General Test (minimum analytical writing score of 3.5), minimum undergraduate GPA of 3.5. Additional exam requirements/recommendations for international students: Required—TOEFL (minimum score 600 paper-based; 107 iBT for MS, 80 iBT for PhD). *Application deadline:* For fall admission, 12/7 for domestic and international students. Applications are processed on a rolling basis. Application fee: $60 ($75 for international students). Electronic applications accepted. *Financial support:* Fellowships, research assistantships, and teaching assistantships available. Support available to part-time students. Financial award application deadline: 2/15; financial award applicants required to submit FAFSA. *Unit head:* Dr. Richard J. Kuhn, Head, 765-494-4407, E-mail: kuhnr@purdue.edu. *Application contact:* Georgina E. Rupp, Graduate Coordinator, 765-494-8142, Fax: 765-494-0876, E-mail: ruppg@purdue.edu.
Website: http://www.bio.purdue.edu/

Purdue University, Graduate School, PULSe - Purdue University Life Sciences Program, West Lafayette, IN 47907. Offers biomolecular structure and biophysics (PhD); biotechnology (PhD); chemical biology (PhD); chromatin and regulation of gene expression (PhD); integrative neuroscience (PhD); integrative plant sciences (PhD); membrane biology (PhD); microbiology (PhD); molecular evolutionary and cancer biology (PhD); molecular evolutionary genetics (PhD); molecular virology (PhD). *Students:* 154 full-time (78 women), 1 part-time (0 women); includes 23 minority (5 Black or African American, non-Hispanic/Latino; 5 Asian, non-Hispanic/Latino; 10 Hispanic/Latino; 3 Two or more races, non-Hispanic/Latino), 73 international. Average age 26. 239 applicants, 33% accepted, 40 enrolled. *Entrance requirements:* For doctorate, GRE, minimum undergraduate GPA of 3.0. Additional exam requirements/recommendations for international students: Required—TOEFL (minimum score 550 paper-based; 77 iBT). *Application deadline:* For fall admission, 1/15 priority date for domestic and international students. Applications are processed on a rolling basis. Application fee: $60 ($75 for international students). Electronic applications accepted. *Financial support:* In 2013–14, research assistantships with tuition reimbursements (averaging $22,500 per year), teaching assistantships with tuition reimbursements (averaging $22,500 per year) were awarded. *Unit head:* Dr. Christine A. Hrycyna, Head, 765-494-7322, E-mail: hrycyna@purdue.edu. *Application contact:* Colleen Gabauer, Graduate Contact, 765-494-9256, E-mail: cgabauer@purdue.edu.
Website: http://www.gradschool.purdue.edu/pulse

Rensselaer Polytechnic Institute, Graduate School, School of Science, Program in Biochemistry and Biophysics, Troy, NY 12180-3590. Offers MS, PhD. *Faculty:* 8 full-time (7 women). *Students:* 8 full-time (3 women), 1 international. Average age 28. 40 applicants, 15% accepted, 1 enrolled. In 2013, 1 doctorate awarded. Terminal master's awarded for partial completion of doctoral program. *Degree requirements:* For master's, thesis optional; for doctorate, comprehensive exam, thesis/dissertation. *Entrance requirements:* For master's and doctorate, GRE. Additional exam requirements/recommendations for international students: Required—TOEFL (minimum score 600 paper-based; 100 iBT), IELTS (minimum score 7), PTE (minimum score 68). *Application deadline:* For fall admission, 1/1 priority date for domestic and international students; for spring admission, 8/15 priority date for domestic and international students. Applications are processed on a rolling basis. Application fee: $75. Electronic applications accepted. *Expenses: Tuition:* Full-time $45,100; part-time $1879 per credit hour. *Required fees:* $1983. *Financial support:* In 2013–14, 6 students received support, including research assistantships (averaging $18,500 per year), teaching assistantships (averaging $18,500 per year); fellowships also available. Financial award application deadline: 1/1. *Faculty research:* Biochemistry; bioinformatics; biophysics; cancer biology; computational biology; molecular, cell, and developmental biology; neuroscience; protein folding; stem cells; structural biology. *Total annual research expenditures:* $1.2 million. *Unit head:* Dr. Chunyu Wang, Graduate Program Director, 518-276-3497, E-mail: wangc5@rpi.edu. *Application contact:* Office of Graduate Admissions, 518-276-6216, E-mail: gradadmissions@rpi.edu.
Website: http://www.rpi.edu/dept/bcbp/

Rosalind Franklin University of Medicine and Science, School of Graduate and Postdoctoral Studies - Interdisciplinary Graduate Program in Biomedical Sciences, Department of Physiology and Biophysics, North Chicago, IL 60064-3095. Offers MS, PhD, MD/PhD. Terminal master's awarded for partial completion of doctoral program. *Degree requirements:* For master's, comprehensive exam, thesis; for doctorate, comprehensive exam, thesis/dissertation. *Entrance requirements:* For master's and doctorate, GRE General Test. Additional exam requirements/recommendations for international students: Required—TOEFL, TWE. *Faculty research:* Membrane transport, mechanisms of cellular regulation, brain metabolism, peptide metabolism.

Stanford University, School of Humanities and Sciences, Program in Biophysics, Stanford, CA 94305-9991. Offers PhD. *Degree requirements:* For doctorate, thesis/dissertation, oral exam. *Entrance requirements:* For doctorate, GRE General Test, GRE Subject Test. Additional exam requirements/recommendations for international students: Required—TOEFL. Electronic applications accepted. *Expenses: Tuition:* Full-time $42,690; part-time $949 per credit. *Required fees:* $185.

Stony Brook University, State University of New York, Stony Brook University Medical Center, Health Sciences Center, School of Medicine and Graduate School, Graduate Programs in Medicine, Department of Physiology and Biophysics, Stony Brook, NY 11794. Offers PhD. *Faculty:* 17 full-time (6 women). *Students:* 27 full-time (16 women), 2 part-time (both women); includes 16 minority (11 Black or African American, non-Hispanic/Latino; 2 Asian, non-Hispanic/Latino; 3 Hispanic/Latino), 3 international. Average age 29. 4 applicants, 25% accepted, 1 enrolled. In 2013, 1 doctorate awarded. *Degree requirements:* For doctorate, comprehensive exam, thesis/dissertation. *Entrance requirements:* For doctorate, GRE General Test, GRE Subject Test, BS in related field, minimum GPA of 3.0, recommendation. Additional exam requirements/recommendations for international students: Required—TOEFL (minimum score 550 paper-based). *Application deadline:* For fall admission, 1/15 for domestic students; for spring admission, 10/1 for domestic students. Application fee: $100. *Expenses:* Tuition, state resident: full-time $9870; part-time $411 per credit. Tuition, nonresident: full-time $18,350; part-time $765 per credit. *Financial support:* In 2013–14, 4 fellowships, 10 research assistantships were awarded; teaching assistantships and Federal Work-Study also available. Financial award application deadline: 3/15. *Faculty research:* Cellular electrophysiology, membrane permeation and transport, metabolic endocrinology. *Total annual research expenditures:* $7.3 million. *Unit head:* Dr. Peter Brink, Chair, 631-444-3124, Fax: 631-444-3432, E-mail: peter.brink@stonybrook.edu. *Application contact:* Odalis Hernandez, Coordinator, 631-444-3057, Fax: 631-444-3432, E-mail: odalis.hernandez@stonybrook.edu.
Website: http://pnb.informatics.stonybrook.edu/

Syracuse University, College of Arts and Sciences, Program in Structural Biology, Biochemistry and Biophysics, Syracuse, NY 13244. Offers PhD. *Students:* 3 full-time (1 woman), 1 part-time (0 women), 1 international. Average age 33. 4 applicants, 25% accepted. In 2013, 2 doctorates awarded. *Degree requirements:* For doctorate, comprehensive exam, thesis/dissertation. *Entrance requirements:* For doctorate, GRE General Test, GRE Subject Test. Additional exam requirements/recommendations for international students: Required—TOEFL (minimum score 100 iBT). *Application deadline:* For fall admission, 12/15 priority date for domestic and international students. Application fee: $75. Electronic applications accepted. *Financial support:* Fellowships with full tuition reimbursements, research assistantships with full and partial tuition reimbursements, teaching assistantships with full and partial tuition reimbursements, and tuition waivers available. Financial award application deadline: 1/1; financial award applicants required to submit FAFSA. *Unit head:* Prof. Liviu Movileanu, Director of Graduate Studies, 315-443-8078, Fax: 315-443-2012, E-mail: lmovilea@syr.edu.
Website: http://sb3.syr.edu/

Texas Christian University, College of Science and Engineering, Department of Physics and Astronomy, Fort Worth, TX 76129. Offers physics (MA, MS, PhD), including astrophysics (PhD), biophysics (PhD), business (PhD), physics (PhD); PhD/MBA. *Faculty:* 7 full-time (0 women). *Students:* 20 part-time (8 women); includes 2 minority (1 Asian, non-Hispanic/Latino; 1 Hispanic/Latino), 11 international. Average age 32. 27 applicants, 26% accepted, 6 enrolled. In 2013, 2 doctorates awarded. Terminal master's awarded for partial completion of doctoral program. *Degree requirements:* For master's, comprehensive exam, thesis; for doctorate, comprehensive exam, thesis/dissertation, paper submitted to scientific journal. *Entrance requirements:* For master's and doctorate, GRE General Test, minimum GPA of 3.0. Additional exam requirements/recommendations for international students: Required—TOEFL (minimum score 600 paper-based). *Application deadline:* For fall admission, 2/1 for domestic and international students; for spring admission, 10/1 for domestic and international students. Applications are processed on a rolling basis. Application fee: $60. Electronic applications accepted. *Expenses: Tuition:* Part-time $1270 per credit hour. Tuition and fees vary according to course load and program. *Financial support:* In 2013–14, 16 students received support, including 1 research assistantship with full tuition

reimbursement available (averaging $20,500 per year), 11 teaching assistantships with full tuition reimbursements available (averaging $19,500 per year); scholarships/grants, tuition waivers, and unspecified assistantships also available. Financial award application deadline: 2/1. *Faculty research:* Biophysics, astrophysics, molecular physics, solid state physics, spectroscopy. *Total annual research expenditures:* $225,000. *Unit head:* Dr. William R. Graham, Professor and Chair, 817-257-7375 Ext. 6383, Fax: 817-257-7742, E-mail: w.graham@tcu.edu. *Application contact:* Dr. Yuri Strzhemechny, Associate Professor/Director, Graduate Program, 817-257-7375 Ext. 5793, Fax: 817-257-7742, E-mail: y.strzhemechny@tcu.edu.
Website: http://www.phys.tcu.edu/grad_program.asp

Thomas Jefferson University, Jefferson Graduate School of Biomedical Sciences, Program in Molecular Physiology and Biophysics, Philadelphia, PA 19107. Offers PhD. *Faculty:* 10 full-time (5 women). *Students:* 1 full-time (0 women). *Degree requirements:* For doctorate, comprehensive exam, thesis/dissertation. *Entrance requirements:* For doctorate, GRE General Test, minimum GPA of 3.2. Additional exam requirements/recommendations for international students: Required—TOEFL (minimum score 100 iBT). *Application deadline:* For fall admission, 1/15 for domestic and international students. *Financial support:* In 2013–14, 1 fellowship with full tuition reimbursement (averaging $56,052 per year) was awarded; Federal Work-Study, institutionally sponsored loans, scholarships/grants, traineeships, and stipends also available. Support available to part-time students. Financial award application deadline: 5/1; financial award applicants required to submit FAFSA. *Faculty research:* Cardiovascular physiology, smooth muscle physiology, pathophysiology of myocardial ischemia, endothelial cell physiology, molecular biology of ion channel physiology. *Total annual research expenditures:* $893,526. *Unit head:* Dr. Thomas M. Butler, Program Director, 215-503-6583, E-mail: thomas.butler@jefferson.edu. *Application contact:* Marc E. Stearns, Director of Admissions, 215-503-0155, Fax: 215-503-3433, E-mail: jgsbs-info@jefferson.edu.
Website: http://www.jefferson.edu/jmc/departments/physiology.html

Université de Sherbrooke, Faculty of Medicine and Health Sciences, Graduate Programs in Medicine, Department of Physiology and Biophysics, Sherbrooke, QC J1H 5N4, Canada. Offers M Sc, PhD. Terminal master's awarded for partial completion of doctoral program. *Degree requirements:* For master's, thesis; for doctorate, thesis/dissertation. Electronic applications accepted. *Faculty research:* Ion channels, neurological basis of pain, insulin resistance, obesity.

Université du Québec à Trois-Rivières, Graduate Programs, Program in Biophysics and Cellular Biology, Trois-Rivières, QC G9A 5H7, Canada. Offers M Sc, PhD. Part-time programs available. *Degree requirements:* For master's, thesis; for doctorate, thesis/dissertation. *Entrance requirements:* For master's, appropriate bachelor's degree, proficiency in French; for doctorate, appropriate master's degree, proficiency in French.

University at Buffalo, the State University of New York, Graduate School, Graduate Programs in Cancer Research and Biomedical Sciences at Roswell Park Cancer Institute, Department of Molecular and Cellular Biophysics and Biochemistry at Roswell Park Cancer Institute, Buffalo, NY 14260. Offers PhD. *Faculty:* 23 full-time (3 women), 3 part-time/adjunct (1 woman). *Students:* 19 full-time (9 women), 1 part-time (0 women); includes 3 minority (all Asian, non-Hispanic/Latino), 4 international. 11 applicants, 45% accepted, 3 enrolled. In 2013, 3 doctorates awarded. *Degree requirements:* For doctorate, comprehensive exam, thesis/dissertation, oral defense of disseration. *Entrance requirements:* For doctorate, GRE General Test. Additional exam requirements/recommendations for international students: Required—TOEFL (minimum score 79 iBT). *Application deadline:* For fall admission, 1/5 priority date for domestic and international students. Application fee: $75. Electronic applications accepted. *Financial support:* In 2013–14, 19 research assistantships with full tuition reimbursements (averaging $25,000 per year) were awarded; scholarships/grants, health care benefits, and unspecified assistantships also available. Financial award application deadline: 1/5. *Faculty research:* MRI research, structural and function of biomolecules, photodynamic therapy, DNA damage and repair, heat-shock proteins and vaccine research. *Unit head:* Dr. Eugene Kandel, Director of Graduate Studies, 716-845-3530, E-mail: eugene.kandel@roswellpark.org. *Application contact:* Dr. Norman J. Karin, Associate Dean, 716-845-2339, Fax: 716-845-8178, E-mail: norman.karin@roswellpark.org.
Website: http://www.roswellpark.edu/education/phd-programs/molecular-cellular-biophysics-and-biochemistry

University at Buffalo, the State University of New York, Graduate School, School of Medicine and Biomedical Sciences, Graduate Programs in Medicine and Biomedical Sciences, Department of Physiology and Biophysics, Buffalo, NY 14214. Offers biophysics (MS, PhD); physiology (MA, PhD). *Faculty:* 19 full-time (4 women). *Students:* 25 full-time (5 women); includes 9 minority (all Asian, non-Hispanic/Latino). Average age 29. 59 applicants, 46% accepted, 10 enrolled. In 2013, 2 master's, 2 doctorates awarded. Terminal master's awarded for partial completion of doctoral program. *Degree requirements:* For master's, thesis, oral exam, project; for doctorate, thesis/dissertation, oral and written qualifying exam or 2 research proposals. *Entrance requirements:* For master's and doctorate, GRE General Test, unofficial transcripts, 3 letters of recommendation, personal statement, curriculum vitae. Additional exam requirements/recommendations for international students: Required—TOEFL (minimum score 600 paper-based; 100 iBT). *Application deadline:* For fall admission, 2/1 priority date for domestic and international students. Applications are processed on a rolling basis. Application fee: $75. Electronic applications accepted. *Financial support:* In 2013–14, 1 student received support, including 12 research assistantships with full and partial tuition reimbursements available (averaging $25,000 per year); Federal Work-Study, institutionally sponsored loans, health care benefits, and unspecified assistantships also available. Financial award application deadline: 2/1; financial award applicants required to submit FAFSA. *Faculty research:* Neurosciences, ion channels, cardiac physiology, renal/epithelial transport, cardiopulmonary exercise. *Total annual research expenditures:* $2.4 million. *Unit head:* Dr. Perry M. Hogan, Chair, 716-829-2738, Fax: 716-829-2344, E-mail: phogan@buffalo.edu. *Application contact:* Samantha A. Greenwood, Faculty Support Coordinator, 716-829-2738, Fax: 716-829-2344, E-mail: sagreenw@buffalo.edu.
Website: http://www.smbs.buffalo.edu/phb/

University of California, Berkeley, Graduate Division, College of Letters and Science, Group in Biophysics, Berkeley, CA 94720-1500. Offers PhD. *Degree requirements:* For doctorate, thesis/dissertation, qualifying exam. *Entrance requirements:* For doctorate, GRE General Test, minimum GPA of 3.0, 3 letters of recommendation.

University of California, Davis, Graduate Studies, Graduate Group in Biophysics, Davis, CA 95616. Offers MS, PhD. *Degree requirements:* For doctorate, thesis/dissertation. *Entrance requirements:* For master's and doctorate, GRE General Test, GRE Subject Test. Additional exam requirements/recommendations for international students: Required—TOEFL (minimum score 550 paper-based). Electronic applications accepted. *Faculty research:* Molecular structure, protein structure/function relationships, spectroscopy.

University of California, Irvine, School of Medicine and School of Biological Sciences, Department of Physiology and Biophysics, Irvine, CA 92697. Offers biological sciences (PhD); MD/PhD. *Students:* 11 full-time (5 women); includes 5 minority (3 Asian, non-Hispanic/Latino; 1 Hispanic/Latino; 1 Native Hawaiian or other Pacific Islander, non-Hispanic/Latino), 1 international. Average age 28. In 2013, 4 doctorates awarded. *Degree requirements:* For doctorate, thesis/dissertation. *Entrance requirements:* For doctorate, GRE General Test, GRE Subject Test, minimum GPA of 3.0. Additional exam requirements/recommendations for international students: Required—TOEFL (minimum score 550 paper-based). *Application deadline:* For fall admission, 1/15 priority date for domestic students, 1/15 for international students. Application fee: $80 ($100 for international students). Electronic applications accepted. *Financial support:* Fellowships, research assistantships with full tuition reimbursements, teaching assistantships, institutionally sponsored loans, traineeships, health care benefits, and unspecified assistantships available. Financial award application deadline: 3/1; financial award applicants required to submit FAFSA. *Faculty research:* Membrane physiology, exercise physiology, regulation of hormone biosynthesis and action, endocrinology, ion channels and signal transduction. *Unit head:* Prof. Michael Cahalan, Chairman, 949-824-7776, Fax: 949-824-3143, E-mail: mcahalan@uci.edu. *Application contact:* Jamie K. Matsuno-Rich, Assistant Director, 949-824-3484, Fax: 949-824-2636, E-mail: jmrich@uci.edu.
Website: http://www.physiology.uci.edu/

University of California, San Diego, Office of Graduate Studies, Department of Physics, La Jolla, CA 92093. Offers biophysics (PhD); multi-scale biology (PhD); physics (PhD). *Students:* 180 full-time (20 women), 2 part-time (1 woman); includes 30 minority (4 Black or African American, non-Hispanic/Latino; 18 Asian, non-Hispanic/Latino; 8 Hispanic/Latino), 45 international. 526 applicants, 24% accepted, 32 enrolled. In 2013, 22 doctorates awarded. *Degree requirements:* For doctorate, comprehensive exam, thesis/dissertation, teaching assistantship. *Entrance requirements:* For doctorate, GRE General Test, GRE Subject Test. Additional exam requirements/recommendations for international students: Required—TOEFL, IELTS. *Application deadline:* For fall admission, 12/16 for domestic students. Application fee: $80 ($100 for international students). Electronic applications accepted. *Expenses:* Tuition, state resident: full-time $11,220; part-time $1870 per quarter. Tuition, nonresident: full-time $26,322; part-time $4387 per quarter. *Required fees:* $519.50 per quarter. Part-time tuition and fees vary according to course load and program. *Financial support:* Research assistantships, teaching assistantships, scholarships/grants, and unspecified assistantships available. Financial award applicants required to submit FAFSA. *Faculty research:* Astrophysics/astronomy, biophysics, condensed matter, elementary particles, plasma physics. *Unit head:* Dimitri Basov, Chair, 858-534-6832, E-mail: chair@physics.ucsd.edu. *Application contact:* Hilari Ford, Graduate Coordinator, 858-534-3293, E-mail: hford@ucsd.edu.
Website: http://physics.ucsd.edu/

University of California, San Francisco, School of Pharmacy and School of Medicine, Program in Biophysics, San Francisco, CA 94143. Offers PhD. *Degree requirements:* For doctorate, thesis/dissertation. *Entrance requirements:* For doctorate, GRE General Test; GRE Subject Test (recommended), bachelor's degree with minimum GPA of 3.0. Additional exam requirements/recommendations for international students: Required—TOEFL. *Application deadline:* For fall admission, 12/1 for domestic students. Application fee: $80 ($100 for international students). Electronic applications accepted. *Expenses:* Tuition, state resident: full-time $11,220. Tuition, nonresident: full-time $26,322. *Required fees:* $5204. Full-time tuition and fees vary according to degree level and program. *Financial support:* In 2013–14, fellowships with full tuition reimbursements (averaging $32,500 per year), research assistantships with full tuition reimbursements (averaging $32,500 per year) were awarded; traineeships, health care benefits, tuition waivers (full), unspecified assistantships, and stipends also available. *Faculty research:* Structural biology, proteomics and genomics, biophysical approaches to cell biology, complex biological systems, computational and theoretical biophysics, membrane biophysics, protein engineering and synthetic biology. *Unit head:* Dr. Matthew Jacobson, Director, 415-514-9811, E-mail: matt.jacobson@ucsf.edu. *Application contact:* Rebecca Brown, Administrator, 415-476-6671, Fax: 415-476-1902, E-mail: rebecca.brown3@ucsf.edu.
Website: http://biophysics.ucsf.edu/

University of California, Santa Barbara, Graduate Division, College of Letters and Sciences, Division of Mathematics, Life, and Physical Sciences, Interdepartmental Graduate Program in Biomolecular Science and Engineering, Santa Barbara, CA 93106-2014. Offers biochemistry and molecular biology (PhD), including biochemistry and molecular biology, biophysics and bioengineering. *Faculty:* 35 full-time (3 women), 3 part-time/adjunct (all women). *Students:* 26 full-time (13 women); includes 5 minority (4 Asian, non-Hispanic/Latino; 1 Hispanic/Latino), 2 international. Average age 29. 98 applicants, 17% accepted, 6 enrolled. In 2013, 6 doctorates awarded. Terminal master's awarded for partial completion of doctoral program. *Degree requirements:* For doctorate, thesis/dissertation. *Entrance requirements:* For doctorate, GRE General Test. Additional exam requirements/recommendations for international students: Required—TOEFL (minimum score 630 paper-based; 109 iBT), IELTS (minimum score 7). *Application deadline:* For fall admission, 12/15 for domestic and international students. Application fee: $80 ($100 for international students). Electronic applications accepted. *Expenses:* Tuition, state resident: part-time $5148.26 per quarter. Tuition, nonresident: part-time $10,182.26 per quarter. *Financial support:* In 2013–14, 28 students received support, including 16 fellowships with full and partial tuition reimbursements available (averaging $11,321 per year), 31 research assistantships with full and partial tuition reimbursements available (averaging $14,777 per year), 16 teaching assistantships with full and partial tuition reimbursements available (averaging $6,307 per year); Federal Work-Study, traineeships, health care benefits, tuition waivers (full and partial), and unspecified assistantships also available. Financial award application deadline: 12/15; financial award applicants required to submit FAFSA. *Faculty research:* Biochemistry and molecular biology, biophysics, biomaterials, bioengineering, systems biology. *Unit head:* Prof. Omar A. Saleh, Director/Professor, 805-893-8814, E-mail: saleh@engineering.ucsb.edu. *Application contact:* Nicole McCoy, 805-893-8499, E-mail: nicole.mccoy@lifesci.ucsb.edu.
Website: http://www.bmse.ucsb.edu/

University of Chicago, Division of the Physical Sciences, Graduate Program in Biophysical Science, Chicago, IL 60637-1513. Offers PhD. *Degree requirements:* For doctorate, comprehensive exam, thesis/dissertation, ethics class, 2 teaching assistantships. *Entrance requirements:* Additional exam requirements/recommendations for international students: Required—IELTS (minimum score 7); Recommended—TOEFL (minimum score 600 paper-based; 104 iBT). Electronic applications accepted.

University of Cincinnati, Graduate School, College of Medicine, Graduate Programs in Biomedical Sciences, Department of Pharmacology and Cell Biophysics, Cincinnati, OH 45221. Offers cell biophysics (PhD); pharmacology (PhD). *Degree requirements:* For doctorate, thesis/dissertation, qualifying exam. *Entrance requirements:* For doctorate, GRE General Test. Additional exam requirements/recommendations for international students: Required—TOEFL. Electronic applications accepted. *Faculty research:* Lipoprotein research, enzyme regulation, electrophysiology, gene actuation.

University of Colorado Denver, School of Medicine, Graduate Program in Genetic Counseling, Aurora, CO 80045. Offers biophysics and genetics (MS, PhD). *Students:* 12 full-time (all women); includes 2 minority (1 Asian, non-Hispanic/Latino; 1 Hispanic/

Latino). Average age 26. 72 applicants, 8% accepted, 6 enrolled. In 2013, 5 master's awarded. *Degree requirements:* For master's, 44 core semester hours, project or thesis; for doctorate, comprehensive exam, thesis/dissertation, 30 hours each of didactic course work and research credits. *Entrance requirements:* For master's, GRE, minimum undergraduate GPA of 3.0; 4 letters of recommendation; prerequisite coursework in biology, general chemistry, general biochemistry, general genetics, general psychology; experience in counseling and laboratory settings and strong understanding of genetic counseling field (highly recommended); for doctorate, GRE, three letters of recommendation, laboratory research experience and solid undergraduate foundation in mathematics and biological sciences. Additional exam requirements/recommendations for international students: Required—TOEFL (minimum score 570 paper-based; 89 iBT). *Application deadline:* For fall admission, 1/1 for domestic students, 12/1 for international students. Application fee: $50 ($75 for international students). Electronic applications accepted. *Expenses:* Contact institution. *Financial support:* In 2013–14, 7 students received support. Fellowships, research assistantships, teaching assistantships, career-related internships or fieldwork, Federal Work-Study, institutionally sponsored loans, scholarships/grants, traineeships, and unspecified assistantships available. Financial award application deadline: 4/1; financial award applicants required to submit FAFSA. *Faculty research:* Psychosocial aspects of genetic counseling, clinical cytogenetics and molecular genetics, human inborn errors of metabolism, congenital malformations and disorders of the newborn, cancer genetics and genetic counseling. *Unit head:* Carol Walton, Director, 303-724-2370, E-mail: carol.walton@ucdenver.edu. *Application contact:* Associate Dean for Admissions, 303-724-8025, E-mail: somadmin@ucdenver.edu.
Website: http://www.ucdenver.edu/academics/colleges/Graduate-School/academic-programs/genetic-counseling/Pages/default.aspx

University of Connecticut, Graduate School, College of Liberal Arts and Sciences, Department of Molecular and Cell Biology, Field of Biophysics and Structural Biology, Storrs, CT 06269. Offers MS, PhD. Terminal master's awarded for partial completion of doctoral program. *Degree requirements:* For master's, comprehensive exam; for doctorate, thesis/dissertation. *Entrance requirements:* For master's and doctorate, GRE General Test, GRE Subject Test. Additional exam requirements/recommendations for international students: Required—TOEFL (minimum score 550 paper-based). Electronic applications accepted.

University of Guelph, Graduate Studies, Biophysics Interdepartmental Group, Guelph, ON N1G 2W1, Canada. Offers M Sc, PhD. *Degree requirements:* For master's, thesis; for doctorate, comprehensive exam, thesis/dissertation. *Entrance requirements:* For master's, minimum B average during previous 2 years of course work; for doctorate, minimum B+ average. Additional exam requirements/recommendations for international students: Required—TOEFL (minimum score 550 paper-based). Electronic applications accepted. *Faculty research:* Molecular, cellular, structural, and computational biophysics.

University of Guelph, Graduate Studies, College of Biological Science, Department of Molecular and Cellular Biology, Guelph, ON N1G 2W1, Canada. Offers biochemistry (M Sc, PhD); biophysics (M Sc, PhD); botany (M Sc, PhD); microbiology (M Sc, PhD); molecular biology and genetics (M Sc, PhD). *Degree requirements:* For master's, thesis, research proposal; for doctorate, comprehensive exam, thesis/dissertation, research proposal. *Entrance requirements:* For master's, minimum B-average during previous 2 years of coursework; for doctorate, minimum A-average. Additional exam requirements/recommendations for international students: Required—TOEFL (minimum score 550 paper-based), IELTS (minimum score 6.5). Electronic applications accepted. *Faculty research:* Physiology, structure, genetics, and ecology of microbes; virology and microbial technology.

University of Illinois at Chicago, College of Medicine and Graduate College, Graduate Programs in Medicine, Department of Physiology and Biophysics, Chicago, IL 60607-7128. Offers MS, PhD. *Faculty:* 19 full-time (5 women), 3 part-time/adjunct (1 woman). *Students:* 14 full-time (6 women); includes 4 minority (1 Asian, non-Hispanic/Latino; 3 Hispanic/Latino), 3 international. Average age 28. 12 applicants, 42% accepted, 3 enrolled. In 2013, 3 master's, 4 doctorates awarded. Terminal master's awarded for partial completion of doctoral program. *Degree requirements:* For master's, thesis; for doctorate, thesis/dissertation. *Entrance requirements:* For master's and doctorate, GRE General Test. Additional exam requirements/recommendations for international students: Required—TOEFL. *Application deadline:* For fall admission, 1/15 priority date for domestic students, 2/15 for international students. Applications are processed on a rolling basis. Application fee: $40 ($50 for international students). Electronic applications accepted. *Expenses:* Tuition, state resident: full-time $11,066; part-time $3689 per term. Tuition, nonresident: full-time $23,064; part-time $7688 per term. *Required fees:* $3004; $1190 per term. Tuition and fees vary according to course level and program. *Financial support:* In 2013–14, 5 fellowships with full tuition reimbursements were awarded; research assistantships with full tuition reimbursements, teaching assistantships with full tuition reimbursements, Federal Work-Study, traineeships, and tuition waivers (full) also available. Financial award application deadline: 3/1; financial award applicants required to submit FAFSA. *Faculty research:* Neuroscience, endocrinology and reproduction, cell physiology, exercise physiology, NMR, cardiovascular physiology and metabolism, cytoskeleton and vascular biology, gastrointestinal and epithelial cell biology, reproductive and endocrine sciences. *Total annual research expenditures:* $7.5 million. *Unit head:* Prof. R. John Solaro, Department Head, 312-996-7620, Fax: 312-996-1414, E-mail: solarorj@uic.edu. *Application contact:* Jackie Perry, Graduate College Receptionist, 312-413-2550, Fax: 312-413-0185, E-mail: gradcoll@uic.edu.
Website: http://www.physiology.uic.edu/

University of Illinois at Urbana–Champaign, Graduate College, College of Liberal Arts and Sciences, School of Molecular and Cellular Biology, Center for Biophysics and Computational Biology, Champaign, IL 61820. Offers MS, PhD. *Students:* 52 (13 women). Application fee: $75 ($90 for international students). *Unit head:* Taekjip Ha, Director, 217-265-0717, Fax: 217-244-3186, E-mail: tjha@illinois.edu. *Application contact:* Cynthia Dodds, Office Administrator, 217-333-1630, Fax: 217-244-6615, E-mail: dodds@illinois.edu.
Website: http://biophysics.illinois.edu/

The University of Iowa, Roy J. and Lucille A. Carver College of Medicine and Graduate College, Graduate Programs in Medicine, Department of Molecular Physiology and Biophysics, Iowa City, IA 52240. Offers MS, PhD. *Faculty:* 17 full-time (3 women), 17 part-time/adjunct (2 women). *Students:* 19 full-time (4 women); includes 4 minority (all Asian, non-Hispanic/Latino), 3 international. Average age 25. In 2013, 1 master's, 1 doctorate awarded. *Degree requirements:* For master's, comprehensive exam; for doctorate, comprehensive exam, thesis/dissertation. *Entrance requirements:* For master's, GRE General Test; for doctorate, GRE. Additional exam requirements/recommendations for international students: Required—TOEFL. *Application deadline:* For fall admission, 4/1 for domestic students, 3/1 for international students; for spring admission, 10/1 for domestic students, 9/1 for international students. Applications are processed on a rolling basis. Application fee: $60 ($80 for international students). Electronic applications accepted. *Financial support:* In 2013–14, 1 fellowship with full tuition reimbursement (averaging $25,500 per year), 17 research assistantships with full tuition reimbursements (averaging $25,500 per year) were awarded; traineeships also available. Financial award application deadline: 4/1. *Faculty research:* Cellular and molecular endocrinology, membrane structure and function, cardiac cell electrophysiology, regulation of gene expression, neurophysiology. *Unit head:* Dr. Kevin P. Campbell, Chair and Department Executive Officer, 319-335-7800, Fax: 319-335-7330, E-mail: kevin-campbell@uiowa.edu. *Application contact:* Dr. Mark Stamnes, Director of Graduate Studies, 319-335-7858, Fax: 319-335-7330, E-mail: mark-stamnes@uiowa.edu.
Website: http://www.physiology.uiowa.edu/

The University of Kansas, Graduate Studies, College of Liberal Arts and Sciences, Department of Molecular Biosciences, Lawrence, KS 66045. Offers biochemistry and biophysics (MA, PhD); microbiology (MA, PhD); molecular, cellular, and developmental biology (MA, PhD). *Faculty:* 34. *Students:* 52 full-time (28 women); includes 5 minority (2 Asian, non-Hispanic/Latino; 3 Hispanic/Latino), 23 international. Average age 27. 96 applicants, 25% accepted, 13 enrolled. In 2013, 3 master's, 9 doctorates awarded. Terminal master's awarded for partial completion of doctoral program. *Degree requirements:* For master's, comprehensive exam, thesis; for doctorate, comprehensive exam, thesis/dissertation. *Entrance requirements:* For master's and doctorate, GRE General Test. Additional exam requirements/recommendations for international students: Required—TOEFL or IELTS. *Application deadline:* For fall admission, 12/15 for domestic and international students. Application fee: $55 ($65 for international students). Electronic applications accepted. *Financial support:* Fellowships with tuition reimbursements, research assistantships with tuition reimbursements, teaching assistantships with tuition reimbursements, health care benefits, and unspecified assistantships available. Financial award application deadline: 3/1. *Faculty research:* Structure and function of proteins, genetics of organism development, molecular genetics, neurophysiology, molecular virology and pathogenics, developmental biology, cell biology. *Unit head:* Dr. Mark Richter, Chair, 785-864-3334, E-mail: richter@ku.edu. *Application contact:* John Connolly, Graduate Admissions Contact, 785-864-4311, E-mail: jconnolly@ku.edu.
Website: http://www.molecularbiosciences.ku.edu/

University of Louisville, School of Medicine, Department of Physiology and Biophysics, Louisville, KY 40292-0001. Offers MS, PhD, MD/PhD. *Students:* 31 full-time (9 women), 7 part-time (5 women); includes 8 minority (3 Black or African American, non-Hispanic/Latino; 4 Asian, non-Hispanic/Latino; 1 Two or more races, non-Hispanic/Latino), 7 international. Average age 28. 25 applicants, 52% accepted, 10 enrolled. In 2013, 13 master's, 6 doctorates awarded. Terminal master's awarded for partial completion of doctoral program. *Degree requirements:* For master's, thesis; for doctorate, comprehensive exam, thesis/dissertation. *Entrance requirements:* For master's and doctorate, GRE General Test (minimum score of 1000 verbal and quantitative), minimum GPA of 3.0. Additional exam requirements/recommendations for international students: Required—TOEFL. *Application deadline:* For fall admission, 1/15 priority date for domestic students. Applications are processed on a rolling basis. Application fee: $60. Electronic applications accepted. *Expenses:* Tuition, state resident: full-time $10,788; part-time $599 per credit hour. Tuition, nonresident: full-time $22,446; part-time $1247 per credit hour. *Required fees:* $196. Tuition and fees vary according to program and reciprocity agreements. *Financial support:* Fellowships with full tuition reimbursements and research assistantships with full tuition reimbursements available. Financial award application deadline: 4/15. *Faculty research:* Control of microvascular function during normal and disease states; mechanisms of cellular adhesive interactions on endothelial cells lining blood vessels; changes in blood rheological properties and mechanisms associated with increased blood fibrinogen content; role of nutrition in microvascular control mechanisms; mechanism of cardiovascular-renal remodeling in hypertension, diabetes, and heart failure. *Unit head:* Dr. Irving G. Joshua, Chair, 502-852-5371, Fax: 502-852-6239, E-mail: igjosh01@gwise.louisville.edu. *Application contact:* Dr. William Wead, Director of Admissions, 502-852-7571, Fax: 502-852-6849, E-mail: wbwead01@gwise.louisville.edu.
Website: http://louisville.edu/medschool/physiology/

The University of Manchester, School of Physics and Astronomy, Manchester, United Kingdom. Offers astronomy and astrophysics (M Sc, PhD); biological physics (M Sc, PhD); condensed matter physics (M Sc, PhD); nonlinear and liquid crystals physics (M Sc, PhD); nuclear physics (M Sc, PhD); particle physics (M Sc, PhD); photon physics (M Sc, PhD); physics (M Sc, PhD); theoretical physics (M Sc, PhD).

University of Maryland, College Park, Academic Affairs, College of Computer, Mathematical and Natural Sciences, Department of Biology, PhD Program in Biological Sciences, College Park, MD 20742. Offers behavior, ecology, evolution, and systematics (PhD); computational biology, bioinformatics, and genomics (PhD); molecular and cellular biology (PhD); physiological systems (PhD). *Students:* 104 full-time (59 women), 4 part-time (1 woman); includes 21 minority (2 Black or African American, non-Hispanic/Latino; 1 American Indian or Alaska Native, non-Hispanic/Latino; 9 Asian, non-Hispanic/Latino; 7 Hispanic/Latino; 2 Two or more races, non-Hispanic/Latino), 34 international. 365 applicants, 13% accepted, 20 enrolled. In 2013, 5 doctorates awarded. *Degree requirements:* For doctorate, comprehensive exam, thesis/dissertation, thesis work presentation in seminar. *Entrance requirements:* For doctorate, GRE General Test; GRE Subject Test in biology (recommended), academic transcripts, statement of purpose/research interests, 3 letters of recommendation. Additional exam requirements/recommendations for international students: Required—TOEFL. *Application deadline:* For fall admission, 12/15 for domestic and international students. Applications are processed on a rolling basis. Application fee: $75. Electronic applications accepted. *Expenses:* Tuition, state resident: full-time $10,314; part-time $573 per credit hour. Tuition, nonresident: full-time $22,248; part-time $1236 per credit. *Required fees:* $1446; $403.15 per semester. Tuition and fees vary according to program. *Financial support:* In 2013–14, 21 fellowships with full and partial tuition reimbursements (averaging $27,603 per year), 25 research assistantships (averaging $19,557 per year), 55 teaching assistantships (averaging $18,959 per year) were awarded. *Unit head:* Dr. Charles F. Delwiche, Director, 301-405-6884, E-mail: bisidirector@umd.edu. *Application contact:* Dr. Charles A. Caramello, Dean of Graduate School, 301-405-0358, Fax: 301-314-9305, E-mail: ccaramel@umd.edu.
Website: http://www.bisi.umd.edu/

University of Maryland, College Park, Academic Affairs, College of Computer, Mathematical and Natural Sciences, Institute for Physical Science and Technology, Program in Biophysics, College Park, MD 20742. Offers PhD. *Students:* 21 full-time (6 women), 1 (woman) part-time; includes 2 minority (1 Asian, non-Hispanic/Latino; 1 Two or more races, non-Hispanic/Latino), 14 international. 26 applicants, 50% accepted, 6 enrolled. In 2013, 1 doctorate awarded. *Application deadline:* For fall admission, 1/15 for domestic and international students. Application fee: $75. *Expenses:* Tuition, state resident: full-time $10,314; part-time $573 per credit hour. Tuition, nonresident: full-time $22,248; part-time $1236 per credit. *Required fees:* $1446; $403.15 per semester. Tuition and fees vary according to program. *Financial support:* In 2013–14, 3 fellowships with full and partial tuition reimbursements (averaging $56,533 per year), 7 research assistantships (averaging $20,653 per year), 9 teaching assistantships (averaging $18,244 per year) were awarded; Federal Work-Study and scholarships/grants also available. Support available to part-time students. Financial award applicants required to submit FAFSA. *Unit head:* Wolfgang Losert, Director, 301-405-0629, Fax: 301-314-9363, E-mail: wlosert@umd.edu. *Application contact:* Dr. Charles A. Caramello, Dean of the Graduate School, 301-405-0376, Fax: 301-314-9305, E-mail: ccaramel@umd.edu.

University of Miami, Graduate School, Miller School of Medicine, Graduate Programs in Medicine, Department of Physiology and Biophysics, Coral Gables, FL 33124. Offers PhD, MD/PhD. *Degree requirements:* For doctorate, thesis/dissertation, qualifying exam. *Entrance requirements:* For doctorate, GRE General Test, minimum GPA of 3.0 in sciences. Additional exam requirements/recommendations for international students: Required—TOEFL. *Faculty research:* Cell and membrane physiology, cell-to-cell communication, molecular neurobiology, neuroimmunology, neural development.

University of Michigan, Rackham Graduate School, College of Literature, Science, and the Arts, Department of Biophysics, Ann Arbor, MI 48109. Offers PhD. *Degree requirements:* For doctorate, thesis/dissertation, oral defense of dissertation, preliminary exam. *Entrance requirements:* For doctorate, GRE General Test, GRE Subject Test. Additional exam requirements/recommendations for international students: Required—TOEFL. Electronic applications accepted. Tuition and fees vary according to course level, course load, degree level, program and student level. *Faculty research:* Structural biology, computational biophysics, physical chemistry, cellular biophysics.

University of Minnesota, Duluth, Medical School, Department of Biochemistry, Molecular Biology and Biophysics, Duluth, MN 55812-2496. Offers biochemistry, molecular biology and biophysics (MS); biology and biophysics (PhD); social, administrative, and clinical pharmacy (MS, PhD); toxicology (MS, PhD). Terminal master's awarded for partial completion of doctoral program. *Degree requirements:* For master's, comprehensive exam, thesis; for doctorate, comprehensive exam, thesis/dissertation. *Entrance requirements:* For master's and doctorate, GRE General Test. Additional exam requirements/recommendations for international students: Required—TOEFL. Electronic applications accepted. *Faculty research:* Intestinal cancer biology; hepatotoxins and mitochondriopathies; toxicology; cell cycle regulation in stem cells; neurobiology of brain development, trace metal function and blood-brain barrier; hibernation biology.

University of Minnesota, Twin Cities Campus, Graduate School, College of Biological Sciences, Biochemistry, Molecular Biology and Biophysics Graduate Program, Minneapolis, MN 55455-0213. Offers PhD. *Degree requirements:* For doctorate, thesis/dissertation. *Entrance requirements:* For doctorate, GRE, 3 letters of recommendation, more than 1 semester of laboratory experience. Additional exam requirements/recommendations for international students: Required—TOEFL (minimum score 625 paper-based; 108 iBT with writing subsection 25 and reading subsection 25) or IELTS (minimum score 7). Electronic applications accepted. *Faculty research:* Microbial biochemistry, biotechnology, molecular biology, regulatory biochemistry, structural biology and biophysics, physical biochemistry, enzymology, physiological chemistry.

University of Minnesota, Twin Cities Campus, Graduate School, Program in Biophysical Sciences and Medical Physics, Minneapolis, MN 55455-0213. Offers MS, PhD. Part-time programs available. *Degree requirements:* For master's, thesis optional, research paper, oral exam; for doctorate, thesis/dissertation, oral/written preliminary exam, oral final exam. *Faculty research:* Theoretical biophysics, radiological physics, cellular and molecular biophysics.

University of Mississippi Medical Center, School of Graduate Studies in the Health Sciences, Department of Physiology and Biophysics, Jackson, MS 39216-4505. Offers PhD, MD/PhD. *Faculty:* 20 full-time (5 women). *Students:* 7 full-time (2 women); includes 2 minority (1 Black or African American, non-Hispanic/Latino; 1 Asian, non-Hispanic/Latino). Average age 25. 10 applicants, 30% accepted, 3 enrolled. *Degree requirements:* For doctorate, thesis/dissertation, first authored publication. *Entrance requirements:* For doctorate, GRE General Test, minimum GPA of 3.0. *Application deadline:* For fall admission, 8/1 for domestic students. Applications are processed on a rolling basis. Application fee: $10. *Financial support:* In 2013–14, 7 students received support, including 7 research assistantships with full tuition reimbursements available (averaging $24,150 per year); health care benefits also available. Financial award application deadline: 4/1. *Faculty research:* Cardiovascular, renal, endocrine, and cellular neurophysiology; molecular physiology. *Unit head:* Dr. John E. Hall, Chairman, 601-984-1801, Fax: 601-984-1817. *Application contact:* Dr. Michael J. Ryan, Director, 601-984-1801, Fax: 601-984-1817, E-mail: mjryan@umc.edu.
Website: http://www.umc.edu/Education/Schools/Medicine/Basic_Science/Physiology_and_Biophysics/Graduate_Program%28Physiology%29/Academics.aspx

University of Missouri–Kansas City, School of Biological Sciences, Program in Cell Biology and Biophysics, Kansas City, MO 64110-2499. Offers PhD. Offered through the School of Graduate Studies. *Faculty:* 34 full-time (9 women), 3 part-time/adjunct (all women). *Students:* 4 full-time (2 women), 9 part-time (4 women), 9 international. Average age 29. 3 applicants, 100% accepted, 3 enrolled. *Degree requirements:* For doctorate, comprehensive exam, thesis/dissertation. *Entrance requirements:* For doctorate, GRE General Test, bachelor's degree in chemistry, biology or related field; minimum GPA of 3.0. Additional exam requirements/recommendations for international students: Required—TOEFL (minimum score 550 paper-based; 80 iBT). *Application deadline:* For fall admission, 2/15 priority date for domestic and international students. Applications are processed on a rolling basis. Application fee: $45 ($50 for international students). Electronic applications accepted. *Expenses:* Tuition, state resident: full-time $6073; part-time $337.40 per credit hour. Tuition, nonresident: full-time $15,680; part-time $871.10 per credit hour. *Required fees:* $97.59 per credit hour. Full-time tuition and fees vary according to program. *Financial support:* Fellowships with full tuition reimbursements, research assistantships with full tuition reimbursements, teaching assistantships with full and partial tuition reimbursements, scholarships/grants, tuition waivers (full and partial), and unspecified assistantships available. Financial award application deadline: 3/1; financial award applicants required to submit FAFSA. *Unit head:* Dr. Marilyn Yoder, Interim Head, 816-235-5247, E-mail: sbsgradrecruit@umkc.edu. *Application contact:* Mary Flores, Information Contact, 816-235-5247, Fax: 816-235-5158, E-mail: lasterlo@umkc.edu.
Website: http://sbs.umkc.edu/

The University of North Carolina at Chapel Hill, School of Medicine and Graduate School, Graduate Programs in Medicine, Department of Biochemistry and Biophysics, Chapel Hill, NC 27599. Offers MS, PhD. Terminal master's awarded for partial completion of doctoral program. *Degree requirements:* For master's, comprehensive exam, thesis; for doctorate, comprehensive exam, thesis/dissertation. *Entrance requirements:* For master's and doctorate, GRE General Test, GRE Subject Test (recommended), minimum GPA of 3.0. Additional exam requirements/recommendations for international students: Required—TOEFL. Electronic applications accepted.

University of Regina, Faculty of Graduate Studies and Research, Faculty of Science, Department of Chemistry and Biochemistry, Regina, SK S4S 0A2, Canada. Offers analytical/environmental chemistry (M Sc, PhD); biophysics of biological interfaces (M Sc, PhD); enzymology/chemical biology (M Sc, PhD); inorganic/organometallic chemistry (M Sc, PhD); signal transduction and mechanisms of cancer cell regulation (M Sc, PhD); supramolecular organic photochemistry and photophysics (M Sc, PhD); synthetic organic chemistry (M Sc, PhD); theoretical/computational chemistry (M Sc, PhD). *Faculty:* 11 full-time (2 women), 4 part-time/adjunct (0 women). *Students:* 12 full-time (9 women), 1 part-time (0 women). 25 applicants, 36% accepted. In 2013, 3 master's awarded. *Degree requirements:* For master's, thesis; for doctorate, thesis/dissertation. *Entrance requirements:* Additional exam requirements/recommendations for international students: Required—TOEFL (minimum score 580 paper-based; 80 iBT), IELTS (minimum score 6.5). *Application deadline:* Applications are processed on a rolling basis. Application fee: $100. Electronic applications accepted. *Expenses: Tuition, area resident:* Full-time $4338 Canadian dollars. *International tuition:* $7338 Canadian dollars full-time. *Required fees:* $449.25 Canadian dollars. *Financial support:* In 2013–14, 5 fellowships (averaging $7,000 per year), 8 teaching assistantships (averaging $2,456 per year) were awarded; research assistantships and scholarships/grants also available. Financial award application deadline: 6/15. *Faculty research:* Asymmetric synthesis and methodology, theoretical and computational chemistry, biophysical biochemistry, analytical and environmental chemistry, chemical biology. *Unit head:* Dr. Renata Raina-Fulton, Department Head, 306-585-4012, Fax: 306-337-2409, E-mail: renata.raina@uregina.ca. *Application contact:* Dr. Brian Sterenberg, Graduate Program Coordinator, 306-585-4106, Fax: 306-337-2409, E-mail: brian.sterenberg@uregina.ca.
Website: http://www.uregina.ca/science/chem-biochem/

University of Rochester, School of Medicine and Dentistry, Graduate Programs in Medicine and Dentistry, Department of Biochemistry and Biophysics, Programs in Biophysics, Rochester, NY 14627. Offers biophysics, structural and computational biology (PhD). Terminal master's awarded for partial completion of doctoral program. *Degree requirements:* For doctorate, thesis/dissertation, qualifying exam. *Entrance requirements:* For doctorate, GRE General Test. *Expenses: Tuition:* Full-time $44,580; part-time $1394 per credit hour. *Required fees:* $492.

University of Southern California, Keck School of Medicine and Graduate School, Graduate Programs in Medicine, Department of Physiology and Biophysics, Los Angeles, CA 90089. Offers MS. *Faculty:* 13 full-time (2 women). *Students:* 6 full-time (2 women), 4 international. Average age 27. 6 applicants, 17% accepted, 1 enrolled. In 2013, 2 master's awarded. *Degree requirements:* For master's, thesis optional. *Entrance requirements:* For master's, GRE General Test, minimum GPA of 3.0. Additional exam requirements/recommendations for international students: Required—TOEFL (minimum score 600 paper-based; 100 iBT). *Application deadline:* For fall admission, 12/1 priority date for domestic and international students. Application fee: $85. Electronic applications accepted. *Financial support:* Federal Work-Study, institutionally sponsored loans, scholarships/grants, traineeships, health care benefits, and unspecified assistantships available. Financial award application deadline: 5/4. *Faculty research:* Endocrinology and metabolism, neurophysiology, mathematical modeling, cell transport, autoimmunity and cancer immunotherapy. *Total annual research expenditures:* $4.5 million. *Unit head:* Dr. Berislav Zlokavic, Chair, 323-442-2566, Fax: 323-442-2230, E-mail: zlokovic@usc.edu. *Application contact:* Janet Stoeckert, Administrative Director, Basic Sciences Departments, 323-442-3568, Fax: 323-442-1610, E-mail: janet.stoeckert@usc.edu.

University of South Florida, Morsani College of Medicine and Graduate School, Graduate Programs in Medical Sciences, Tampa, FL 33620-9951. Offers aging and neuroscience (MSMS); allergy, immunology and infectious disease (PhD); anatomy (MSMS, PhD); athletic training (MSMS); bioinformatics and computational biology (MSBCB); biotechnology (MSB); clinical and translational research (MSMS, PhD); health informatics (MSHI, MSMS); health science (MSMS); interdisciplinary medical sciences (MSMS); medical microbiology and immunology (MSMS); metabolic and nutritional medicine (MSMS); molecular medicine (MSMS, PhD); molecular pharmacology and physiology (PhD); neurology (PhD); pathology and laboratory medicine (PhD); pharmacology and therapeutics (PhD); physiology and biophysics (PhD); women's health (MSMS). *Students:* 336 full-time (182 women), 39 part-time (21 women); includes 170 minority (45 Black or African American, non-Hispanic/Latino; 54 Asian, non-Hispanic/Latino; 59 Hispanic/Latino; 2 Native Hawaiian or other Pacific Islander, non-Hispanic/Latino; 10 Two or more races, non-Hispanic/Latino), 17 international. Average age 26. 1,066 applicants, 44% accepted, 250 enrolled. In 2013, 191 master's, 12 doctorates awarded. Terminal master's awarded for partial completion of doctoral program. *Degree requirements:* For master's, comprehensive exam, thesis; for doctorate, comprehensive exam, thesis/dissertation. *Entrance requirements:* For master's, GRE General Test or GMAT, bachelor's degree or equivalent from regionally-accredited university with minimum GPA of 3.0 in upper-division sciences coursework; prerequisites in general biology, general chemistry, general physics, organic chemistry, quantitative analysis, and integral and differential calculus; for doctorate, GRE General Test (minimum score of 600 quantitative), bachelor's degree from regionally-accredited university with minimum GPA of 3.0 in upper-division sciences coursework; 3 letters of recommendation; personal interview; 1-2 page personal statement; prerequisites in biology, chemistry, physics, organic chemistry, quantitative analysis, and integral/differential calculus. Additional exam requirements/recommendations for international students: Required—TOEFL (minimum score 550 paper-based; 79 iBT) or IELTS (minimum score 6.5). *Application deadline:* For fall admission, 2/15 for domestic students, 1/2 for international students. Application fee: $30. *Expenses:* Contact institution. *Faculty research:* Anatomy, biochemistry, cancer biology, cardiovascular disease, cell biology, immunology, microbiology, molecular biology, neuroscience, pharmacology, physiology. *Unit head:* Dr. Michael Barber, Professor and Associate Dean for Graduate and Postdoctoral Affairs, 813-974-9908, Fax: 813-974-4317, E-mail: mbarber@health.usf.edu. *Application contact:* Dr. Eric Bennett, Graduate Director, PhD Program in Medical Sciences, 813-974-1545, Fax: 813-974-4317, E-mail: esbennet@health.usf.edu.
Website: http://health.usf.edu/nocms/medicine/graduatestudies/

The University of Texas Medical Branch, Graduate School of Biomedical Sciences, Program in Biochemistry and Molecular Biology, Galveston, TX 77555. Offers biochemistry (PhD); bioinformatics (PhD); biophysics (PhD); cell biology (PhD); computational biology (PhD); structural biology (PhD). *Degree requirements:* For doctorate, thesis/dissertation. *Entrance requirements:* Additional exam requirements/recommendations for international students: Required—TOEFL (minimum score 550 paper-based). Electronic applications accepted.

University of Toronto, Faculty of Medicine, Department of Medical Biophysics, Toronto, ON M5S 1A1, Canada. Offers M Sc, PhD. *Degree requirements:* For master's, thesis; for doctorate, thesis/dissertation. *Entrance requirements:* For master's and doctorate, resume, 2 letters of reference. Additional exam requirements/recommendations for international students: Required—TOEFL (minimum score 620 paper-based), TWE (minimum score 5). Electronic applications accepted.

University of Virginia, School of Medicine, Department of Molecular Physiology and Biological Physics, Charlottesville, VA 22903. Offers biological and physical sciences (MS); physiology (PhD); MD/PhD. *Faculty:* 27 full-time (6 women), 1 part-time/adjunct (0 women). *Students:* 5 full-time (3 women). Average age 27. In 2013, 23 master's, 6 doctorates awarded. *Entrance requirements:* For doctorate, GRE General Test, GRE Subject Test. Additional exam requirements/recommendations for international students: Required—TOEFL. *Application deadline:* For fall admission, 2/15 for domestic and international students. Applications are processed on a rolling basis. Application fee: $60. Electronic applications accepted. *Expenses:* Tuition, state resident: part-time

$334 per credit hour. Tuition, nonresident: part-time $1224 per credit hour. *Financial support:* Fellowships, research assistantships, and teaching assistantships available. Financial award applicants required to submit FAFSA. *Unit head:* Dr. Mark Yeager, Chair, 434-924-5108, Fax: 434-982-1616, E-mail: my3r@virginia.edu. *Application contact:* Director of Graduate Studies, E-mail: physiograd@virginia.edu.
Website: http://www.healthsystem.virginia.edu/internet/physio/

University of Virginia, School of Medicine, Interdisciplinary Program in Biophysics, Charlottesville, VA 22908. Offers PhD. *Students:* 14 full-time (6 women); includes 2 minority (1 Asian, non-Hispanic/Latino; 1 Hispanic/Latino), 6 international. Average age 27. In 2013, 2 doctorates awarded. *Degree requirements:* For doctorate, thesis/dissertation, research proposal, oral defense. *Entrance requirements:* For doctorate, GRE General Test, GRE Subject Test (recommended), 2 or more letters of recommendation. Additional exam requirements/recommendations for international students: Required—TOEFL. *Application deadline:* For fall admission, 4/15 for domestic and international students. Applications are processed on a rolling basis. Application fee: $60. Electronic applications accepted. *Expenses:* Tuition, state resident: part-time $334 per credit hour. Tuition, nonresident: part-time $1224 per credit hour. *Financial support:* Fellowships with full tuition reimbursements, research assistantships with full tuition reimbursements, teaching assistantships with full tuition reimbursements, and tuition waivers (full) available. Financial award application deadline: 1/15; financial award applicants required to submit FAFSA. *Faculty research:* Structural biology and structural genomics, structural biology of membrane proteins and membrane biophysics, spectroscopy and thermodynamics of macromolecular interactions, high resolution imaging and cell biophysics. *Unit head:* Dr. Robert K. Nakamoto, Director of the Biophysics Program, 434-982-0279, E-mail: rkn3c@virginia.edu. *Application contact:* Biomedical Sciences Graduate Program, E-mail: biophysicsuva@virginia.edu.
Website: http://www.medicine.virginia.edu/education/phd/scbb-new-biophysics/welcome-to-biophysics-at-uva.html

University of Washington, Graduate School, School of Medicine, Graduate Programs in Medicine, Department of Physiology and Biophysics, Seattle, WA 98195. Offers PhD. *Degree requirements:* For doctorate, thesis/dissertation. *Entrance requirements:* For doctorate, GRE General Test. Additional exam requirements/recommendations for international students: Required—TOEFL (minimum score 580 paper-based; 70 iBT). *Faculty research:* Membrane and cell biophysics, neuroendocrinology, cardiovascular and respiratory physiology, systems neurophysiology and behavior, molecular physiology.

The University of Western Ontario, Faculty of Graduate Studies, Biosciences Division, Department of Medical Biophysics, London, ON N6A 5B8, Canada. Offers M Sc, PhD. *Degree requirements:* For master's, thesis; for doctorate, thesis/dissertation. *Entrance requirements:* Additional exam requirements/recommendations for international students: Required—TOEFL. *Faculty research:* Haemodynamics and cardiovascular biomechanics, microcirculation, orthopedic biomechanics, radiobiology, medical imaging.

University of Wisconsin–Madison, Graduate School, Program in Biophysics, Madison, WI 53706-1380. Offers PhD. *Degree requirements:* For doctorate, comprehensive exam, thesis/dissertation. *Entrance requirements:* For doctorate, GRE General Test, minimum GPA of 3.0. Additional exam requirements/recommendations for international students: Required—TOEFL (minimum score 600 paper-based). Electronic applications accepted. *Expenses:* Tuition, state resident: full-time $10,728; part-time $790 per credit. Tuition, nonresident: full-time $24,054; part-time $1623 per credit. *Required fees:* $1130; $119 per credit. *Faculty research:* NMR spectroscopy, high-speed automated DNA sequencing, x-ray crystallography, neuronal signaling and exocytosis, protein structure.

Vanderbilt University, Graduate School and School of Medicine, Department of Molecular Physiology and Biophysics, Nashville, TN 37240-1001. Offers MS, PhD, MD/PhD. *Faculty:* 35 full-time (8 women). *Students:* 42 full-time (27 women); includes 9 minority (3 Black or African American, non-Hispanic/Latino; 4 Hispanic/Latino; 2 Two or more races, non-Hispanic/Latino), 1 international. Average age 26. In 2013, 7 doctorates awarded. *Degree requirements:* For doctorate, comprehensive exam, thesis/dissertation, preliminary, qualifying, and final exams. *Entrance requirements:* For doctorate, GRE General Test, GRE Subject Test (recommended). Additional exam requirements/recommendations for international students: Required—TOEFL (minimum score 570 paper-based; 88 iBT). *Application deadline:* For fall admission, 1/15 for domestic and international students. Application fee: $0. Electronic applications accepted. *Financial support:* Fellowships with full tuition reimbursements, research assistantships with full tuition reimbursements, Federal Work-Study, institutionally sponsored loans, scholarships/grants, traineeships, health care benefits, and tuition waivers (partial) available. Financial award application deadline: 1/15; financial award applicants required to submit CSS PROFILE or FAFSA. *Faculty research:* Biophysics, cell signaling and gene regulation, human genetics, diabetes and obesity, neuroscience. *Unit head:* Prof. Roger D. Cone, Chair of the Department of Molecular Physiology and Biophysics, 615-936-7085, Fax: 615-343-0490, E-mail: roger.cone@vanderbilt.edu. *Application contact:* Walter B. Bieschke, Program Coordinator for Graduate Admissions, 615-342-0236, E-mail: walter.bieschke@vanderbilt.edu.
Website: http://www.mc.vanderbilt.edu/root/vumc.php?site-MPB

Vanderbilt University, School of Medicine, Program in Chemical and Physical Biology, Nashville, TN 37240-1001. Offers PhD. *Degree requirements:* For doctorate, comprehensive exam, thesis/dissertation, dissertation defense. *Entrance requirements:* For doctorate, GRE, 3 letters of recommendation, official transcripts. Additional exam requirements/recommendations for international students: Required—TOEFL. Electronic applications accepted. *Faculty research:* Mathematical modeling, enzyme kinetics, structural biology, genomics, proteomics and mass spectrometry.

Washington State University, College of Veterinary Medicine, Program in Molecular Biosciences, Pullman, WA 99164. Offers PSM, PhD. Postbaccalaureate distance learning degree programs offered. *Faculty:* 30 full-time (11 women), 28 part-time/adjunct (6 women). *Students:* 53 full-time (24 women), 16 part-time (9 women); includes 10 minority (3 Black or African American, non-Hispanic/Latino; 3 Asian, non-Hispanic/Latino; 3 Hispanic/Latino; 1 Two or more races, non-Hispanic/Latino), 3 international. Average age 28. 94 applicants, 19% accepted, 10 enrolled. In 2013, 4 master's, 4 doctorates awarded. Terminal master's awarded for partial completion of doctoral program. *Degree requirements:* For master's, thesis or alternative, oral exam; for doctorate, comprehensive exam, thesis/dissertation, oral exam, written exam. *Entrance requirements:* For master's and doctorate, GRE General Test, minimum GPA of 3.0. Additional exam requirements/recommendations for international students: Required—TOEFL (minimum score 100 iBT). *Application deadline:* For fall admission, 12/15 for domestic and international students. Application fee: $75. Electronic applications accepted. *Financial support:* In 2013–14, 9 fellowships with full tuition reimbursements (averaging $22,032 per year), 23 research assistantships with full tuition reimbursements (averaging $22,194 per year), 20 teaching assistantships with full tuition reimbursements (averaging $22,194 per year) were awarded; career-related internships or fieldwork, Federal Work-Study, institutionally sponsored loans, traineeships, and health care benefits also available. Financial award application deadline: 4/1; financial award applicants required to submit FAFSA. *Faculty research:* Gene regulation, signal transduction, protein export, reproductive biology, DNA repair. *Total annual research expenditures:* $5.8 million. *Unit head:* Dr. Jonathan Jones, Director, 509-335-8724, Fax: 509-335-9688, E-mail: jcr.jones@vetmed.wsu.edu. *Application contact:* Kelly G. McGovern, Coordinator, 509-335-4566, E-mail: mcgoverk@wsu.edu.

Weill Cornell Medical College, Weill Cornell Graduate School of Medical Sciences, Physiology, Biophysics and Systems Biology Program, New York, NY 10065. Offers MS, PhD. Terminal master's awarded for partial completion of doctoral program. *Degree requirements:* For master's, comprehensive exam; for doctorate, thesis/dissertation, final exam. *Entrance requirements:* For doctorate, GRE General Test, introductory courses in biology, inorganic and organic chemistry, physics, and mathematics. Additional exam requirements/recommendations for international students: Required—TOEFL. *Faculty research:* Receptor-mediated regulation of cell function, molecular properties of channels or receptors, bioinformatics, mathematical modeling.

Wright State University, School of Graduate Studies, College of Science and Mathematics, Department of Neuroscience, Cell Biology, and Physiology, Dayton, OH 45435. Offers anatomy (MS); physiology and biophysics (MS). *Degree requirements:* For master's, thesis optional. *Entrance requirements:* Additional exam requirements/recommendations for international students: Required—TOEFL. *Faculty research:* Reproductive cell biology, neurobiology of pain, neurohistochemistry.

Yale University, Graduate School of Arts and Sciences, Department of Molecular Biophysics and Biochemistry, New Haven, CT 06520. Offers PhD. *Degree requirements:* For doctorate, thesis/dissertation. *Entrance requirements:* For doctorate, GRE General Test, GRE Subject Test.

Molecular Biophysics

Baylor College of Medicine, Graduate School of Biomedical Sciences, Program in Structural and Computational Biology and Molecular Biophysics, Houston, TX 77030-3498. Offers PhD, MD/PhD. MD/PhD offered jointly with Rice University and University of Houston. *Degree requirements:* For doctorate, thesis/dissertation, public defense. *Entrance requirements:* For doctorate, GRE General Test, GRE Subject Test (strongly recommended), minimum GPA of 3.0. Additional exam requirements/recommendations for international students: Required—TOEFL. Electronic applications accepted. *Faculty research:* Computational biology, structural biology, biophysics.

California Institute of Technology, Division of Biology and Division of Chemistry and Chemical Engineering, Biochemistry and Molecular Biophysics Graduate Option, Pasadena, CA 91125-0001. Offers PhD. *Degree requirements:* For doctorate, thesis/dissertation, qualifying exam. *Entrance requirements:* For doctorate, GRE General Test. Additional exam requirements/recommendations for international students: Required—TOEFL. Electronic applications accepted.

California Institute of Technology, Division of Chemistry and Chemical Engineering, Pasadena, CA 91125-0001. Offers biochemistry and molecular biophysics (MS, PhD); chemical engineering (MS, PhD); chemistry (MS, PhD). *Faculty:* 44 full-time (8 women). *Students:* 314 full-time (107 women). Average age 26. 823 applicants, 19% accepted, 56 enrolled. In 2013, 8 master's, 49 doctorates awarded. Terminal master's awarded for partial completion of doctoral program. *Degree requirements:* For master's, thesis; for doctorate, thesis/dissertation. *Entrance requirements:* For doctorate, GRE, BS. Additional exam requirements/recommendations for international students: Required—TOEFL; Recommended—IELTS, TWE. *Application deadline:* For fall admission, 1/1 for domestic and international students. Application fee: $100. Electronic applications accepted. *Financial support:* In 2013–14, 298 students received support. Fellowships, research assistantships, teaching assistantships, Federal Work-Study, institutionally sponsored loans, scholarships/grants, traineeships, health care benefits, and unspecified assistantships available. Financial award application deadline: 1/15. *Unit head:* Prof. Jacqueline K. Barton, Chair, Division of Chemistry and Chemical Engineering, 626-395-3646, Fax: 626-395-6948, E-mail: jkbarton@caltech.edu. *Application contact:* Natalie Gilmore, Graduate Office, 626-395-3812, Fax: 626-577-9246, E-mail: ngilmore@its.caltech.edu.
Website: http://cce.caltech.edu/

Carnegie Mellon University, Mellon College of Science, Joint Pitt + CMU Molecular Biophysics and Structural Biology Graduate Program, Pittsburgh, PA 15213-3891. Offers PhD. Program offered jointly with University of Pittsburgh. *Degree requirements:* For doctorate, comprehensive exam, thesis/dissertation. *Entrance requirements:* For doctorate, GRE General Test. Additional exam requirements/recommendations for international students: Required—TOEFL (minimum score 600 paper-based; 100 iBT), IELTS (minimum score 7). *Application deadline:* For fall admission, 12/15 priority date for domestic and international students. Application fee: $0. Electronic applications accepted. *Financial support:* Fellowships with full tuition reimbursements, research assistantships with full tuition reimbursements, institutionally sponsored loans, scholarships/grants, traineeships, and unspecified assistantships available. *Faculty research:* Structural biology, protein dynamics and folding, computational biophysics, molecular informatics, membrane biophysics and ion channels, NMR, x-ray crystallography cryaelectron microscopy. *Unit head:* Dr. Gordon Rule, Director, 412-268-1839, Fax: 412-268-7129, E-mail: rule@andrew.cmu.edu. *Application contact:* Dr. Gordon Rule, Director, 412-268-1839, Fax: 412-268-7129, E-mail: rule@andrew.cmu.edu.
Website: http://www.mbsb.pitt.edu/

Duke University, Graduate School, University Program in Structural Biology and Biophysics, Durham, NC 27710. Offers Certificate. Students must be enrolled in a participating PhD program (biochemistry, cell biology, chemistry, molecular genetics, neurobiology, pharmacology). *Faculty:* 28. *Students:* 2 full-time (0 women). 32 applicants, 16% accepted, 2 enrolled. *Entrance requirements:* For degree, GRE General

Test. Additional exam requirements/recommendations for international students: Required—TOEFL (minimum score 577 paper-based; 90 iBT) or IELTS (minimum score 7). *Application deadline:* For fall admission, 12/8 priority date for domestic and international students. Application fee: $80. *Financial support:* Application deadline: 12/8. *Unit head:* Harold P. Erickson, Director of Graduate Studies, 919-684-6559, Fax: 919-684-8346, E-mail: carol.richardson@duke.edu. *Application contact:* Elizabeth Hutton, Director of Admissions, 919-684-3913, Fax: 919-684-2277, E-mail: grad-admissions@duke.edu.
Website: http://sbb.duke.edu

Florida State University, The Graduate School, College of Arts and Sciences, Program in Molecular Biophysics, Tallahassee, FL 32306. Offers computational structural biology (PhD); molecular biophysics (PhD). *Faculty:* 34 full-time (7 women). *Students:* 25 full-time (8 women); includes 2 minority (both Hispanic/Latino), 12 international. Average age 29. 24 applicants, 33% accepted, 5 enrolled. In 2013, 4 doctorates awarded. *Degree requirements:* For doctorate, comprehensive exam, thesis/dissertation, teaching 1 term in professor's major department. *Entrance requirements:* For doctorate, GRE General Test. Additional exam requirements/recommendations for international students: Required—TOEFL (minimum score 600 paper-based; 90 iBT). *Application deadline:* For fall admission, 12/15 for domestic and international students. Applications are processed on a rolling basis. Application fee: $30. Electronic applications accepted. *Expenses:* Tuition, state resident: part-time $403.51 per credit hour. Tuition, nonresident: part-time $1004.85 per credit hour. *Required fees:* $75.81 per credit hour. One-time fee: $20 part-time. Tuition and fees vary according to course load, campus/location and student level. *Financial support:* In 2013–14, 24 students received support, including 1 fellowship with full and partial tuition reimbursement available (averaging $23,000 per year), 18 research assistantships with full and partial tuition reimbursements available (averaging $23,500 per year), 6 teaching assistantships with full and partial tuition reimbursements available (averaging $23,500 per year); scholarships/grants, health care benefits, and unspecified assistantships also available. Financial award applicants required to submit FAFSA. *Faculty research:* Protein and nucleic acid structure and function, membrane protein structure, computational biophysics, 3-D image reconstruction. *Total annual research expenditures:* $2.3 million. *Unit head:* Dr. Hong Li, Director, 850-644-6785, Fax: 850-644-7244, E-mail: hli4@fsu.edu. *Application contact:* Lyn Kittle, Academic Coordinator, Graduate Programs, 850-644-1012, Fax: 850-644-7244, E-mail: lkittle@fsu.edu.
Website: http://www.sb.fsu.edu/graduate-program

Illinois Institute of Technology, Graduate College, College of Science and Letters, Department of Biological and Chemical Sciences, Biology Division, Chicago, IL 60616. Offers biochemistry (MBS, MS); biology (PhD); biotechnology (MBS, MS); cell and molecular biology (MBS, MS); microbiology (MB, MS); molecular biochemistry and biophysics (PhD); molecular biology and biophysics (MS). Part-time and evening/weekend programs available. Postbaccalaureate distance learning degree programs offered (minimal on-campus study). Terminal master's awarded for partial completion of doctoral program. *Degree requirements:* For master's, comprehensive exam, thesis (for some programs); for doctorate, comprehensive exam, thesis/dissertation. *Entrance requirements:* For master's, GRE General Test (minimum score 1000 Quantitative and Verbal, 2.5 Analytical Writing), minimum undergraduate GPA of 3.0; for doctorate, GRE General Test (minimum score 1200 Quantitative and Verbal, 3.0 Analytical Writing), minimum undergraduate GPA of 3.0. Additional exam requirements/recommendations for international students: Required—TOEFL (minimum score 523 paper-based; 70 iBT); Recommended—IELTS (minimum score 5.5). Electronic applications accepted. *Faculty research:* Structure and biophysics of macromolecular systems; efficacy and mechanism of action of chemopreventive agents in experimental carcinogenesis of breast, colon, lung and prostate; study of fundamental structural biochemistry problems that have direct links to the understanding and treatment of disease; spectroscopic techniques for the study of multi-domain proteins; molecular mechanisms of cancer and cancer gene therapy.

New York University, School of Medicine and Graduate School of Arts and Science, Sackler Institute of Graduate Biomedical Sciences, Program in Molecular Biophysics, New York, NY 10012-1019. Offers PhD. *Faculty:* 21 full-time (2 women). *Students:* 13 full-time (6 women); includes 1 minority (Black or African American, non-Hispanic/Latino), 4 international. Average age 30. In 2013, 4 doctorates awarded. *Degree requirements:* For doctorate, thesis/dissertation, qualifying examination. *Entrance requirements:* For doctorate, GRE General Test, GRE Subject Test in biology or chemistry (recommended). Additional exam requirements/recommendations for international students: Required—TOEFL. *Application deadline:* For fall admission, 2/1 for domestic students. Application fee: $85. *Expenses: Tuition:* Full-time $35,856; part-time $1494 per unit. *Required fees:* $1408; $64 per unit. $473 per term. Tuition and fees vary according to course load and program. *Financial support:* Research assistantships with full tuition reimbursements, institutionally sponsored loans, and health care benefits available. *Faculty research:* Receptor tyrosine kinases, biophysics of t-cell activation, ion transport and cell-cell interactions. *Unit head:* Dr. Joel D. Oppenheim, Senior Associate Dean for Graduate Studies, 212-263-8001, Fax: 212-263-7600. *Application contact:* Michael Escosia, Admissions Associate, 212-263-5648, E-mail: sackler-info@med.nyu.edu.
Website: http://www.med.nyu.edu/Sackler/

Rutgers, The State University of New Jersey, New Brunswick, Graduate School-New Brunswick, BioMaPS Institute for Quantitative Biology, Piscataway, NJ 08854-8097. Offers computational biology and molecular biophysics (PhD). *Degree requirements:* For doctorate, comprehensive exam, thesis/dissertation. *Entrance requirements:* For doctorate, GRE. Additional exam requirements/recommendations for international students: Required—TOEFL. Electronic applications accepted. *Faculty research:* Structural biology, systems biology, bioinformatics, translational medicine, genomics.

University of Arkansas for Medical Sciences, Graduate School, Little Rock, AR 72205. Offers biochemistry and molecular biology (MS, PhD); bioinformatics (MS, PhD); cellular physiology and molecular biophysics (MS, PhD); clinical nutrition (MS); interdisciplinary biomedical sciences (MS, PhD, Certificate); interdisciplinary toxicology (MS); microbiology and immunology (PhD); neurobiology and developmental sciences (PhD); pharmacology (PhD); MD/PhD. Bioinformatics programs hosted jointly with the University of Arkansas at Little Rock. Part-time programs available. *Faculty:* 397 full-time (205 women). *Students:* 196 full-time (126 women), 117 part-time (87 women); includes 65 minority (38 Black or African American, non-Hispanic/Latino; 1 American Indian or Alaska Native, non-Hispanic/Latino; 21 Asian, non-Hispanic/Latino; 4 Hispanic/Latino; 1 Two or more races, non-Hispanic/Latino), 57 international. 455 applicants, 27% accepted, 89 enrolled. In 2013, 41 master's, 18 doctorates, 28 other advanced degrees awarded. Terminal master's awarded for partial completion of doctoral program. *Degree requirements:* For master's, comprehensive exam (for some programs), thesis (for some programs); for doctorate, thesis/dissertation. *Entrance requirements:* For master's and doctorate, GRE. Additional exam requirements/recommendations for international students: Required—TOEFL. *Application deadline:* Applications are processed on a rolling basis. Application fee: $0. Electronic applications accepted. *Expenses:* Contact institution. *Financial support:* In 2013–14, 120 research assistantships (averaging $24,000 per year) were awarded; career-related internships or fieldwork, Federal Work-Study, and traineeships also available. Support available to part-time students. Financial award applicants required to submit FAFSA. *Unit head:* Dr. Robert E. McGehee, Jr., Dean, 501-686-5454. *Application contact:* Dr. Kristen Sterba, Assistant Dean, Office of Graduate Student Recruiting and Retention, 501-526-7396, E-mail: kmsterba@uams.edu.
Website: http://www.uams.edu/gradschool/

University of Massachusetts Amherst, Graduate School, Interdisciplinary Programs, Program in Molecular and Cellular Biology, Amherst, MA 01003. Offers biological chemistry and molecular biophysics (PhD); biomedicine (PhD); cellular and developmental biology (PhD). Part-time programs available. *Students:* 72 full-time (41 women); includes 15 minority (4 Black or African American, non-Hispanic/Latino; 5 Asian, non-Hispanic/Latino; 4 Hispanic/Latino; 2 Two or more races, non-Hispanic/Latino), 28 international. Average age 27. 160 applicants, 23% accepted, 20 enrolled. In 2013, 13 doctorates awarded. Terminal master's awarded for partial completion of doctoral program. *Degree requirements:* For doctorate, comprehensive exam, thesis/dissertation. *Entrance requirements:* For doctorate, GRE General Test. Additional exam requirements/recommendations for international students: Required—TOEFL (minimum score 550 paper-based; 80 iBT), IELTS (minimum score 6.5). *Application deadline:* For fall admission, 12/1 for domestic and international students. Applications are processed on a rolling basis. Application fee: $75. Electronic applications accepted. *Financial support:* Fellowships with full and partial tuition reimbursements, research assistantships with full and partial tuition reimbursements, teaching assistantships with full and partial tuition reimbursements, career-related internships or fieldwork, Federal Work-Study, scholarships/grants, traineeships, health care benefits, tuition waivers (full and partial), and unspecified assistantships available. Support available to part-time students. Financial award application deadline: 12/1; financial award applicants required to submit FAFSA. *Unit head:* Dr. Barbara Osborne, Graduate Program Director, 413-545-3246, Fax: 413-545-1812, E-mail: mcb@mcb.umass.edu. *Application contact:* Lindsay DeSantis, Supervisor of Admissions, 413-545-0722, Fax: 413-577-0010, E-mail: gradadm@grad.umass.edu.
Website: http://www.bio.umass.edu/mcb/

University of Pennsylvania, Perelman School of Medicine, Biomedical Graduate Studies, Graduate Group in Biochemistry and Molecular Biophysics, Philadelphia, PA 19104. Offers PhD, MD/PhD, VMD/PhD. *Faculty:* 76. *Students:* 86 full-time (34 women); includes 19 minority (11 Asian, non-Hispanic/Latino; 8 Hispanic/Latino), 12 international. 93 applicants, 35% accepted, 9 enrolled. In 2013, 7 doctorates awarded. *Degree requirements:* For doctorate, thesis/dissertation. *Entrance requirements:* For doctorate, GRE General Test. Additional exam requirements/recommendations for international students: Required—TOEFL. *Application deadline:* For fall admission, 12/1 priority date for domestic and international students. Applications are processed on a rolling basis. Application fee: $80. Electronic applications accepted. *Financial support:* In 2013–14, 76 students received support. Fellowships, research assistantships, scholarships/grants, traineeships, and unspecified assistantships available. *Faculty research:* Biochemistry of cell differentiation, tissue culture, intermediary metabolism, structure of proteins and nucleic acids, biochemical genetics. *Unit head:* Dr. Kathryn Ferguson, Chairperson, 215-573-1207. *Application contact:* Ruth Keris, Administrator, 215-898-4829.
Website: http://www.med.upenn.edu/bmbgrad/

University of Pittsburgh, School of Medicine and Dietrich School of Arts and Sciences, Molecular Biophysics and Structural Biology Graduate Program, Pittsburgh, PA 15260. Offers PhD. PhD jointly offered by the University of Pittsburgh and Carnegie Mellon University. *Faculty:* 52 full-time (15 women). *Students:* 22 full-time (10 women); includes 3 minority (1 Asian, non-Hispanic/Latino; 1 Hispanic/Latino; 1 Native Hawaiian or other Pacific Islander, non-Hispanic/Latino), 5 international. Average age 25. 85 applicants, 8% accepted, 5 enrolled. In 2013, 2 doctorates awarded. *Degree requirements:* For doctorate, comprehensive exam, thesis/dissertation. *Entrance requirements:* For doctorate, GRE General Test. Additional exam requirements/recommendations for international students: Required—TOEFL (minimum score 600 paper-based; 100 iBT), IELTS (minimum score 7). *Application deadline:* For fall admission, 1/15 priority date for domestic and international students. Application fee: $0. Electronic applications accepted. *Expenses:* Tuition, state resident: full-time $19,964; part-time $807 per credit. Tuition, nonresident: full-time $32,686; part-time $1337 per credit. *Required fees:* $740; $200. Tuition and fees vary according to program. *Financial support:* In 2013–14, 2 fellowships with full tuition reimbursements (averaging $25,575 per year), 20 research assistantships with full tuition reimbursements (averaging $26,010 per year) were awarded; institutionally sponsored loans, scholarships/grants, traineeships, and unspecified assistantships also available. *Faculty research:* Structural biology, protein dynamics and folding, computational biophysics, molecular informatics, membrane biophysics and ion channels, x-ray crystallography cryaelectron microscopy. *Unit head:* Dr. James Conway, Director, 412-648-8957, Fax: 412-648-1077, E-mail: mbsbinfo@medschool.pitt.edu. *Application contact:* Susanna T. Godwin, Program Coordinator, 412-648-8957, Fax: 412-648-1077, E-mail: mbsbinfo@medschool.pitt.edu.
Website: http://www.mbsb.pitt.edu

The University of Texas Medical Branch, Graduate School of Biomedical Sciences, Program in Cellular Physiology and Molecular Biophysics, Galveston, TX 77555. Offers MS, PhD. *Degree requirements:* For master's, thesis or alternative; for doctorate, thesis/dissertation. *Entrance requirements:* For master's and doctorate, GRE General Test. Additional exam requirements/recommendations for international students: Required—TOEFL (minimum score 550 paper-based). Electronic applications accepted.

The University of Texas Southwestern Medical Center, Southwestern Graduate School of Biomedical Sciences, Division of Basic Science, Program in Molecular Biophysics, Dallas, TX 75390. Offers PhD. *Faculty:* 34 full-time (6 women). *Students:* 38 full-time (12 women), 1 part-time (0 women); includes 3 minority (2 Asian, non-Hispanic/Latino; 1 Hispanic/Latino), 19 international. Average age 26. In 2013, 4 doctorates awarded. *Degree requirements:* For doctorate, thesis/dissertation, qualifying exam. *Entrance requirements:* For doctorate, GRE General Test, minimum GPA of 3.0. Additional exam requirements/recommendations for international students: Required—TOEFL. *Application deadline:* For fall admission, 12/15 priority date for domestic students. Applications are processed on a rolling basis. Application fee: $0. Electronic applications accepted. *Financial support:* Fellowships, research assistantships, institutionally sponsored loans, and traineeships available. *Faculty research:* Optical spectroscopy, x-ray crystallography, protein chemistry, ion channels, contractile and cytoskeletal proteins. *Unit head:* Dr. Kevin Gardner, Chair, 214-645-6365, Fax: 214-645-6353, E-mail: kevin.gardner@utsouthwestern.edu.
Website: http://www.utsouthwestern.edu/education/graduate-school/programs/phd-degrees/molecular-biophysics/index.html

Washington University in St. Louis, Graduate School of Arts and Sciences, Division of Biology and Biomedical Sciences, Program in Computational and Molecular Biophysics, St. Louis, MO 63130-4899. Offers PhD. *Degree requirements:* For doctorate, thesis/dissertation. *Entrance requirements:* For doctorate, GRE General Test, GRE Subject Test. Electronic applications accepted.

Molecular Biophysics

Wesleyan University, Graduate Studies, Department of Molecular Biology and Biochemistry, Middletown, CT 06459. Offers biochemistry (PhD); molecular biology (PhD); molecular biophysics (PhD); molecular genetics (PhD). *Degree requirements:* For doctorate, comprehensive exam, thesis/dissertation. *Entrance requirements:* For doctorate, GRE General Test, GRE Subject Test. Additional exam requirements/recommendations for international students: Required—TOEFL. Electronic applications accepted. *Faculty research:* The olfactory system and new frontiers in genome research, chromosome structure and gene expression.

Yale University, School of Medicine and Graduate School of Arts and Sciences, Combined Program in Biological and Biomedical Sciences (BBS), Molecular Biophysics and Biochemistry Track, New Haven, CT 06520. Offers PhD, MD/PhD. *Degree requirements:* For doctorate, thesis/dissertation. *Entrance requirements:* For doctorate, GRE General Test. Additional exam requirements/recommendations for international students: Required—TOEFL. Electronic applications accepted.

Radiation Biology

Auburn University, College of Veterinary Medicine and Graduate School, Graduate Programs in Veterinary Medicine, Auburn University, AL 36849. Offers biomedical sciences (MS, PhD), including anatomy, physiology and pharmacology (MS), biomedical sciences (PhD), clinical sciences (MS), large animal surgery and medicine (MS), pathobiology (MS), radiology (MS), small animal surgery and medicine (MS); DVM/MS. Part-time programs available. *Faculty:* 100 full-time (41 women), 4 part-time/adjunct (1 woman). *Students:* 24 full-time (16 women), 38 part-time (25 women); includes 5 minority (1 Black or African American, non-Hispanic/Latino; 1 American Indian or Alaska Native, non-Hispanic/Latino; 2 Asian, non-Hispanic/Latino; 1 Hispanic/Latino), 22 international. Average age 30. 36 applicants, 44% accepted, 13 enrolled. In 2013, 12 master's, 8 doctorates awarded. *Degree requirements:* For doctorate, thesis/dissertation. *Entrance requirements:* For master's, GRE General Test; for doctorate, GRE General Test, GRE Subject Test. *Application deadline:* For fall admission, 7/7 for domestic students; for spring admission, 11/24 for domestic students. Applications are processed on a rolling basis. Application fee: $50 ($60 for international students). Electronic applications accepted. *Expenses:* Tuition, state resident: full-time $8262; part-time $459 per credit hour. Tuition, nonresident: full-time $24,786; part-time $1377 per credit hour. Tuition and fees vary according to degree level and program. *Financial support:* Research assistantships, teaching assistantships, and Federal Work-Study available. Support available to part-time students. Financial award application deadline: 3/15; financial award applicants required to submit FAFSA. *Unit head:* Dr. Calvin Johnson, Acting Dean, 334-844-2650. *Application contact:* Dr. George Flowers, Dean of the Graduate School, 334-844-2125.

Austin Peay State University, College of Graduate Studies, College of Science and Mathematics, Department of Biology, Clarksville, TN 37044. Offers clinical laboratory science (MS); radiologic science (MS). Part-time programs available. *Faculty:* 12 full-time (5 women). *Students:* 5 full-time (4 women), 28 part-time (15 women); includes 3 minority (2 Black or African American, non-Hispanic/Latino; 1 Two or more races, non-Hispanic/Latino), 2 international. Average age 27. 15 applicants, 100% accepted, 12 enrolled. In 2013, 10 master's awarded. *Degree requirements:* For master's, comprehensive exam, thesis optional. *Entrance requirements:* For master's, GRE General Test, 3 letters of recommendation, minimum undergraduate GPA of 2.5. Additional exam requirements/recommendations for international students: Required—TOEFL (minimum score 500 paper-based). *Application deadline:* For fall admission, 8/5 priority date for domestic students. Applications are processed on a rolling basis. Application fee: $25. Electronic applications accepted. *Expenses:* Tuition, state resident: full-time $7500; part-time $375 per credit hour. Tuition, nonresident: full-time $20,800; part-time $1040 per credit hour. *Required fees:* $1284; $64.20 per credit hour. *Financial support:* In 2013–14, research assistantships with full tuition reimbursements (averaging $6,500 per year) were awarded; career-related internships or fieldwork, Federal Work-Study, institutionally sponsored loans, scholarships/grants, and unspecified assistantships also available. Support available to part-time students. Financial award application deadline: 3/1. *Faculty research:* Non-paint source pollution, amphibian biomonitoring, aquatic toxicology, biological indicators of water quality, taxonomy. *Unit head:* Dr. Don Dailey, Chair, 931-221-7781, Fax: 931-221-6323, E-mail: daileyd@apsu.edu. *Application contact:* June D. Lee, Graduate Coordinator, 800-859-4723, Fax: 931-221-7641, E-mail: gradadmissions@apsu.edu.
Website: http://www.apsu.edu/biology

Colorado State University, College of Veterinary Medicine and Biomedical Sciences, Department of Environmental and Radiological Health Sciences, Fort Collins, CO 80523-1681. Offers environmental health (MS, PhD); radiological health sciences (MS, PhD). Part-time programs available. *Faculty:* 26 full-time (8 women), 1 part-time/adjunct (0 women). *Students:* 74 full-time (51 women), 38 part-time (22 women); includes 9 minority (2 American Indian or Alaska Native, non-Hispanic/Latino; 2 Asian, non-Hispanic/Latino; 4 Hispanic/Latino; 1 Two or more races, non-Hispanic/Latino), 7 international. Average age 31. 75 applicants, 72% accepted, 36 enrolled. In 2013, 56 master's, 2 doctorates awarded. Terminal master's awarded for partial completion of doctoral program. *Degree requirements:* For master's, comprehensive exam (for some programs), thesis (for some programs), publishable paper; for doctorate, comprehensive exam, thesis/dissertation, publishable paper. *Entrance requirements:* For master's, GRE General Test, 1 year of course work in biology lab and chemistry lab, 1 semester of course work in organic chemistry, course work in calculus, resume, 3 letters of recommendation, bachelor's degree, minimum GPA 3.0, transcripts, written statement; for doctorate, GRE General Test, 1 year of course work in biology lab and chemistry lab, 1 semester of course work in organic chemistry, course work in calculus, resume, 3 letters of recommendation, evidence of research capability, bachelor's degree, minimum GPA 3.0, transcripts, written statement. Additional exam requirements/recommendations for international students: Required—TOEFL (minimum score 550 paper-based; 80 iBT), IELTS. *Application deadline:* For fall admission, 6/30 for domestic and international students; for spring admission, 11/1 for domestic and international students. Applications are processed on a rolling basis. Application fee: $50. Electronic applications accepted. *Expenses:* Tuition, state resident: full-time $9075.40; part-time $504 per credit. Tuition, nonresident: full-time $22,248; part-time $1236 per credit. *Required fees:* $1819; $60 per credit. *Financial support:* In 2013–14, 32 students received support, including 19 fellowships with tuition reimbursements available (averaging $35,529 per year), 12 research assistantships with tuition reimbursements available (averaging $21,110 per year), 1 teaching assistantship with tuition reimbursement available (averaging $14,875 per year); scholarships/grants, traineeships, and unspecified assistantships also available. Financial award application deadline: 4/30. *Faculty research:* Air pollution commuter study, dietary interventions for improved gut health and immunity, agricultural health and safety, impacts of space travel on the human body, radiation protection and Fukushima accident. *Total annual research expenditures:* $7.9 million. *Unit head:* Dr. Jac A. Nickoloff, Professor/Department Head, 970-491-6674, Fax: 970-491-0623, E-mail: j.nickoloff@colostate.edu. *Application contact:* Jeanne A. Brockway, Graduate Program Coordinator, 970-491-5003, Fax: 970-491-2940, E-mail: jeanne.brockway@colostate.edu.
Website: http://csu-cvmbs.colostate.edu/academics/erhs/Pages/graduate-studies.aspx

Université de Sherbrooke, Faculty of Medicine and Health Sciences, Graduate Programs in Medicine, Program in Radiobiology, Sherbrooke, QC J1H 5N4, Canada. Offers M Sc, PhD. Terminal master's awarded for partial completion of doctoral program. *Degree requirements:* For master's, thesis; for doctorate, thesis/dissertation. Electronic applications accepted. *Faculty research:* DNA repair, physiochemical actions of radiation, radiopharmacy, phototherapy, imaging.

The University of Iowa, Roy J. and Lucille A. Carver College of Medicine and Graduate College, Biosciences Program, Iowa City, IA 52242-1316. Offers anatomy and cell biology (PhD); biochemistry (PhD); biology (PhD); biomedical engineering (PhD); chemistry (PhD); free radical and radiation biology (PhD); genetics (PhD); human toxicology (PhD); immunology (PhD); microbiology (PhD); molecular and cellular biology (PhD); molecular physiology and biophysics (PhD); neuroscience (PhD); pharmacology (PhD); physical therapy and rehabilitation science (PhD); rehabilitation science (PhD); speech and hearing (PhD). *Faculty:* 332 full-time. *Students:* 8 full-time (3 women); includes 2 minority (1 Black or African American, non-Hispanic/Latino; 1 Asian, non-Hispanic/Latino), 1 international. 200 applicants. *Degree requirements:* For doctorate, thesis/dissertation. *Entrance requirements:* For doctorate, GRE General Test, minimum GPA of 3.0. Additional exam requirements/recommendations for international students: Required—TOEFL (minimum score 600 paper-based; 100 iBT). *Application deadline:* For fall admission, 1/1 priority date for domestic and international students. Applications are processed on a rolling basis. Application fee: $60 ($100 for international students). Electronic applications accepted. *Expenses:* Contact institution. *Financial support:* In 2013–14, 8 students received support, including 8 research assistantships with full tuition reimbursements available (averaging $26,000 per year); fellowships, teaching assistantships, health care benefits, and unspecified assistantships also available. *Unit head:* Dr. Douglas Spitz, Director, 319-335-8001, E-mail: douglas-spitz@uiowa.edu. *Application contact:* Jodi Graff, Director, Admissions and First-Year Experience, 319-335-8306, E-mail: biosciences-admissions@uiowa.edu.
Website: http://www.medicine.uiowa.edu/biosciences/

The University of Iowa, Roy J. and Lucille A. Carver College of Medicine and Graduate College, Graduate Programs in Medicine, Program in Free Radical and Radiation Biology, Iowa City, IA 52242-1316. Offers MS. Part-time programs available. *Faculty:* 6 full-time (1 woman). *Students:* 11 full-time (6 women); includes 5 minority (4 Asian, non-Hispanic/Latino; 1 Hispanic/Latino). Average age 27. 11 applicants, 18% accepted, 1 enrolled. In 2013, 1 master's awarded. *Degree requirements:* For master's, thesis. *Entrance requirements:* For master's, GRE. Additional exam requirements/recommendations for international students: Required—TOEFL. *Application deadline:* For fall admission, 5/31 priority date for domestic and international students; for spring admission, 10/31 for domestic and international students. Applications are processed on a rolling basis. Application fee: $60 ($100 for international students). *Financial support:* In 2013–14, fellowships with partial tuition reimbursements (averaging $26,000 per year), research assistantships with tuition reimbursements (averaging $26,000 per year) were awarded; traineeships, health care benefits, tuition waivers (partial), and unspecified assistantships also available. *Faculty research:* Radiation injury and cellular repair, cell proliferation kinetics, free radical biology, tumor control, positron emission tomography (PET) imaging, electron paramagnetic resonance (EPR). *Total annual research expenditures:* $1 million. *Unit head:* Dr. Douglas Spitz, Director, 319-335-8019, Fax: 319-335-8039. *Application contact:* Jennifer K. DeWitte, Grant and Program Administrator, 319-335-8164, Fax: 319-335-8039, E-mail: jennifer-dewitte@uiowa.edu.
Website: http://www.uiowa.edu/~frrbp/

University of Oklahoma Health Sciences Center, College of Medicine and Graduate College, Graduate Programs in Medicine, Department of Radiological Sciences, Oklahoma City, OK 73190. Offers medical radiation physics (MS, PhD), including diagnostic radiology, nuclear medicine, radiation therapy, ultrasound. Part-time programs available. *Faculty:* 11 full-time (2 women). *Students:* 1 full-time (0 women), 10 part-time (1 woman); includes 2 minority (1 Asian, non-Hispanic/Latino; 1 Two or more races, non-Hispanic/Latino). Average age 27. 28 applicants, 18% accepted, 5 enrolled. In 2013, 2 master's, 1 doctorate awarded. Terminal master's awarded for partial completion of doctoral program. *Degree requirements:* For master's, thesis; for doctorate, thesis/dissertation. *Entrance requirements:* For master's, GRE General Test; for doctorate, GRE General Test, 3 letters of recommendation. Additional exam requirements/recommendations for international students: Required—TOEFL. *Application deadline:* For fall admission, 4/1 priority date for domestic students; for spring admission, 10/1 for domestic students. Applications are processed on a rolling basis. Application fee: $50. *Expenses:* Tuition, state resident: full-time $3504; part-time $175.20 per credit hour. Tuition, nonresident: full-time $13,504; part-time $675.20 per credit hour. *Required fees:* $1545; $52.70 per credit hour. $245.25 per semester. Tuition and fees vary according to course load. *Financial support:* In 2013–14, 2 research assistantships (averaging $17,000 per year) were awarded; fellowships, career-related internships or fieldwork, and institutionally sponsored loans also available. Support available to part-time students. Financial award application deadline: 7/1. *Faculty research:* Monte Carlo applications in radiation therapy, observer-performed studies in diagnostic radiology, error analysis in gated cardiac nuclear medicine studies, nuclear medicine absorbed fraction determinations. *Unit head:* Dr. Susan Edwards, Chair, 405-271-5132, E-mail: susan-edwards@ouhsc.edu. *Application contact:* Dr. Jagadeesh Sonnad, Graduate Liaison, 405-270-8001, E-mail: jagadeesh-sonnad@ouhsc.edu.

HARVARD UNIVERSITY

Biophysics Program

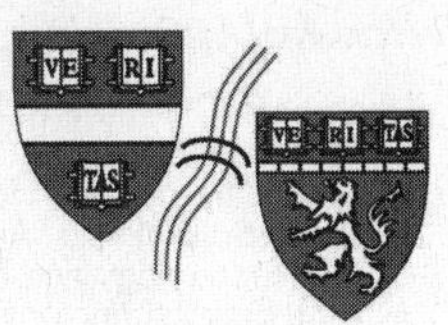

Program of Study

The Committee on Higher Degrees in Biophysics offers a program of study leading to the Ph.D. degree. The committee comprises senior representatives of the Departments of Chemistry and Chemical Biology, Physics, and Molecular and Cellular Biology; the School of Engineering and Applied Sciences; and the Division of Medical Sciences. Students receive sufficient training in physics, biology, and chemistry to enable them to apply the concepts and methods of the physical sciences to the solution of biological problems.

An initial goal of the Biophysics Program is to provide an introduction through courses and seminars to several of the diverse areas of biophysics, such as structural molecular biology, cell and membrane biophysics, neurobiology, molecular genetics, physical biochemistry, and theoretical biophysics. The program is flexible, and special effort has been devoted to minimizing course work and other formal requirements. Students engage in several research rotations during their first two years. The qualifying examination is taken at the end of the second year to determine admission to candidacy. Students undertake dissertation research as early as possible in the field and subject of their choice. Opportunities for dissertation research are available in a number of special fields. The Ph.D. requires not less than three years devoted to advanced studies, including dissertation research and the dissertation. The Committee on Higher Degrees in Biophysics anticipates that it takes an average of five years, with the maximum being six years, to complete this program.

Research Facilities

Many more of the University's modern research facilities are available to the biophysics student because of the interdepartmental nature of the program. Research programs may be pursued in the Departments of Chemistry and Chemical Biology, Molecular and Cellular Biology, Applied Physics, and Engineering Sciences in Cambridge as well as in the Departments of Biological Chemistry and Molecular Pharmacology, Genetics, Microbiology, Neurobiology, and Cell Biology in the Harvard Medical School Division of Medical Sciences. Research may also be pursued in the Harvard School of Public Health, the Dana Farber Cancer Institute, Children's Hospital, Massachusetts General Hospital, Beth Israel Hospital, and more than ten other Harvard-affiliated institutions located throughout the cities.

Financial Aid

In 2014–15, all graduate students receive a stipend ($34,608 for twelve months) and full tuition and health fees ($43,774). A semester of teaching is required in the second year. Students are strongly encouraged to apply for fellowships from such sources as the National Science Foundation, the NDSEG, the Hertz Foundation, and the Ford Foundation. Full-time Ph.D. candidates in good academic standing are guaranteed full financial support through their sixth year of study or throughout their academic program if less than six years.

Cost of Study

Tuition and health fees for the 2014–15 academic year are $43,774. After two years in residence, students are eligible for a reduced rate (currently $13,866).

Living and Housing Costs

Accommodations in graduate residence halls are available at rents ranging from $6,478 to $10,174 per academic year. In addition, there are approximately 1,500 apartments available for graduate students in Harvard-owned buildings. Applications may be obtained from the Harvard University Housing Office, which also maintains a list of available private rooms, houses, and apartments in the vicinity.

Student Group

On average, the program enrolls 58 students annually. Currently, 12 women and 11 international students are enrolled in the program. Biophysics students intermingle in both their research and their social life with graduate students from the many other departments where research in the biophysical sciences is carried out.

Location

The Biophysics Program maintains a dual-campus orientation in the neighboring cities of Cambridge and Boston. Their proximity provides for a wide range of academic, cultural, extracurricular, and recreational opportunities, and the large numbers of theaters, museums, libraries, and universities contribute to enrich the scientific and cultural life of students. Because New England is compact in area, it is easy to reach countryside, mountains, and seacoast for winter and summer sports or just for a change of scenery.

The University

Established in 1636 in the Massachusetts Bay Colony, Harvard has grown to become a complex of many facilities whose educational vitality, social commitment, and level of cultural achievement contribute to make the University a leader in the academic world. Comprising more than 15,000 students and 3,000 faculty members, Harvard appeals to self-directed, resourceful students of diverse beliefs and backgrounds.

Applying

Students must apply by December 1, 2014, to be considered for admission in September 2015. Scores on the General Test of the Graduate Record Examinations are required except in rare circumstances. GRE Subject Tests are recommended. Due to the early application deadline, applicants should plan to take the GRE test no later than October to ensure that original scores are received by December 1. Information about Graduate School fellowships and scholarships, admission procedures, and graduate study at Harvard may be obtained by writing to the Admissions Office.

Correspondence and Information

For information on the program:
Harvard Biophysics Program
Building C2, Room 122
Harvard Medical School Campus
240 Longwood Avenue
Boston, Massachusetts 02115
United States
E-mail: biophys@fas.harvard.edu
Website: http://fas.harvard.edu/~biophys

For application forms for admission and financial aid (applications accepted online only):
Admissions Office
Graduate School of Arts and Sciences
Holyoke Center
Harvard University
1350 Massachusetts Avenue
Cambridge, Massachusetts 02138
United States
E-mail: admiss@fas.harvard.edu
Website: http://www.gsas.harvard.edu

THE FACULTY AND THEIR RESEARCH

The following faculty members accept students for degree work in biophysics. Thesis research with other faculty members is possible by arrangement.

John Assad, Ph.D., Professor of Neurobiology. Mechanisms of visual processing in the visual cortex of awake behaving monkeys.

Frederick M. Ausubel, Ph.D., Professor of Genetics. Molecular biology of microbial pathogenesis in plants and animals.

Harvard University

Stephen C. Blacklow, M.D., Ph.D., Gustavus Adolphus Pfeiffer Professor of Biological Chemistry and Molecular Pharmacology. Molecular basis for specificity in protein folding and protein-protein interactions.
Martha L. Bulyk, Ph.D., Associate Professor of Medicine and Health Sciences and Technology and of Pathology. Computational methods; genomic and proteomic technologies in the study of DNA-protein interactions.
James J. Chou, Ph.D., Associate Professor of Biological Chemistry and Molecular Pharmacology. NMR spectroscopy on membrane-associated proteins and peptides.
George McDonald Church, Ph.D., Professor of Genetics. Human and microbial functional genomics; genotyping; gene expression regulatory network models.
David E. Clapham, M.D., Ph.D., Professor of Pediatrics and of Neurobiology. Intracellular signal transduction.
Adam E. Cohen, Ph.D., Assistant Professor of Chemistry and Chemical Biology and of Physics. Analysis of structure and function of nicotinic acetylcholine receptors.
Jonathan B. Cohen, Ph.D., Professor of Neurobiology. Structure and function of ligand-gated ion channels.
David P. Corey, Ph.D., Professor of Neurobiology. Ion channels in neural cell membranes.
Vladimir Denic, Ph.D., Assistant Professor of Molecular and Cellular Biology. Structural diversification of very long-chain fatty acids.
Michael M. Desai, Ph.D., Assistant Professor of Organismic and Evolutionary Biology and of Physics. Theoretical and experimental approaches to study genetic variation within populations.
Michael J. Eck, M.D., Ph.D., Professor of Biological Chemistry and Molecular Pharmacology. Structural studies of proteins involved in signal transduction pathways.
Florian Engert, Ph.D., Associate Professor of Molecular and Cellular Biology. Synaptic plasticity and neuronal networks.
Conor L. Evans, Ph.D., Assistant Professor of Dermatology. Development and application of optical detection, treatment, and monitoring approaches targeting major human diseases.
Rachelle Gaudet, Ph.D., Associate Professor of Molecular and Cellular Biology. Structural studies of the stereochemistry of signaling and transport through biological membranes.
David E. Golan, M.D., Ph.D., Professor of Biological Chemistry and Molecular Pharmacology and of Medicine. Membrane dynamics; membrane structure; cellular adhesion.
Stephen C. Harrison, Ph.D., Professor of Biological Chemistry and Molecular Pharmacology. Structure of viruses and viral membranes; protein-DNA interactions; structural aspects of signal transduction and membrane traffic; X-ray diffraction.
James M. Hogle, Ph.D., Professor of Biological Chemistry and Molecular Pharmacology. Structure and function of viruses and virus-related proteins; X-ray crystallography.
Sun Hur, Ph.D., Assistant Professor of Biological Chemistry and Molecular Pharmacology. Principles of self versus nonself RNA discrimination by the immune system.
Donald E. Ingber, M.D., Ph.D., Professor of Bioengineering and Judah Folkman Professor of Vascular Biology. Research in integrin signaling, cytoskeleton, and control of angiogenesis.
Tomas Kirchhausen, Ph.D., Professor of Cell Biology. Molecular mechanisms of membrane traffic; X-ray crystallography; chemical genetics.
Andrew J. M. Kiruluta, Ph.D., Associate Professor of Radiology. Novel theory and experiments in NMR spectroscopy.
Roy Kishony, Ph.D., Associate Professor of Systems Biology. System-level genetic networks.
Nancy Kleckner, Ph.D., Herchel Smith Professor of Molecular Biology. Chromosome metabolism in bacteria and yeast.
Roberto G. Kolter, Ph.D., Professor of Microbiology and Molecular Genetics. DNA protection from oxidative damage; cell-cell communication in biofilms; microbial evolution.
Gabriel Kreiman, Ph.D., Assistant Professor of Neurology. Transcriptional regulatory circuits and neuronal circuits in visual recognition.
Galit Lahav, Ph.D., Associate Professor of Systems Biology. Dynamics of network motifs in single living human cells.
Andres Leschziner, Ph.D., Assistant Professor of Molecular and Cellular Biology. Structural biology of ATP-dependent chromatin remodeling.
Erel Levine, Ph.D., Assistant Professor of Physics. Communication in and between cells and organisms.
David R. Liu, Ph.D., Professor of Chemistry and Chemical Biology. Organic chemistry and chemical biology.
Jun S. Liu, Ph.D., Professor of Statistics. Stochastic processes, probability theory, and statistical inference.
Joseph J. Loparo, Ph.D., Assistant Professor of Biological Chemistry and Molecular Pharmacology. Developing novel single-molecule methods to study multiprotein complexes.
Jarrod Marto, Ph.D., Assistant Professor of Biological Chemistry and Molecular Pharmacology. Quantitative proteomics of cancer progression.
Keith W. Miller, Ph.D., Mallinckrodt Professor of Pharmacology, Department of Anesthesia. Molecular mechanisms of regulatory conformation changes and drug action on membrane receptors and channels, using rapid kinetics, time-resolved photolabeling, and spectroscopy (EPR, fluorescence, NMR); characterization of lipid-protein interactions in membrane proteins.
Timothy Mitchison, Ph.D., Hasib Sabbagh Professor of Systems Biology. Cytoskeleton dynamics; mechanism of mitosis and cell locomotion; small-molecule inhibitors.
Andrew W. Murray, Ph.D., Herchel Smith Professor of Molecular Genetics. Regulation of mitosis.
Venkatesh N. Murthy, Ph.D., Professor of Molecular and Cellular Biology. Mechanisms of synaptic transmission and plasticity.
Daniel J. Needleman, Ph.D., Assistant Professor of Applied Physics. Physics of macromolecular assemblies and subcellular organization.
Bence P. Olveczky, Ph.D., Assistant Professor of Organismic and Evolutionary Biology. Neurobiology of vocal learning.
Erin K. O'Shea, Ph.D., Professor of Molecular and Cellular Biology and of Chemistry and Chemical Biology. Quantitative analysis of regulatory networks.
David Pellman, M.D., Professor of Cell Biology. The mechanics and regulation of mitosis.
Mara Prentiss, Ph.D., Professor of Physics. Exploitation of optical manipulation to measure adhesion properties, including virus cell binding.
Sharad Ramanathan, Ph.D., Associate Professor of Molecular and Cellular Biology. Decision-making in cells and organisms.
Tom A. Rapoport, Ph.D., Professor of Cell Biology. Mechanism of how proteins are transported across the endoplasmic reticulum membrane.
Samara L. Reck-Peterson, Ph.D., Assistant Professor of Cell Biology. Single molecule studies of cellular motors.
Gary Ruvkun, Ph.D., Professor of Genetics. Genetic control of developmental timing, neurogenesis, and neural function.
Bernardo L. Sabatini, Ph.D., Associate Professor of Neurobiology. Regulation of synaptic transmission and dendritic function in the mammalian brain.
Aravinthan D. T. Samuel, Ph.D., Associate Professor of Physics. Topics in biophysics, neurobiology, and animal behavior.
Stuart L. Schreiber, Ph.D., Morris Loeb Professor of Chemistry and Chemical Biology. Forward and reverse chemical genetics: using small molecules to explore biology.
Brian Seed, Ph.D., Professor of Genetics. Genetic analysis of signal transduction in the immune system.
Jagesh V. Shah, Ph.D., Assistant Professor of Systems Biology, Assistant Professor of Health Sciences and Technology, and Assistant Professor of Medicine. Quantitative models of cellular behavior to investigate protein function.
Eugene Shakhnovich, Ph.D., Professor of Chemistry and Chemical Biology. Theory and experiments in protein folding and design; theory of molecular evolution; rational drug design and physical chemistry of protein-ligand interactions; theory of complex systems.
William Shih, Ph.D., Associate Professor of Biological Chemistry and Molecular Pharmacology. Biomolecular nanotechnology.
Steven E. Shoelson, M.D., Ph.D., Professor of Medicine. Structural and cellular biology of insulin signal transduction, insulin, resistance, diabetes, and obesity.
Pamela Silver, Ph.D., Professor of Systems Biology. Nucleocytoplasmic transport; RNA-protein interactions; protein methylation; cell-based small-molecule screens.
Timothy A. Springer, Ph.D., Latham Family Professor of Pathology. Molecular biology of immune cell interactions.
Hanno Steen, Ph.D., Assistant Professor of Pathology. Cell cycle studies using mass spectrometric and proteomic technology.
Shamil R. Sunyaev, Ph.D., Associate Professor of Genetics. Population genetic variation and genomic divergence, with a focus on protein coding regions.
Jack W. Szostak, Ph.D., Professor of Genetics. Directed evolution; information content and molecular function; self-replicating systems.
Naoshige Uchida, Ph.D., Associate Professor of Molecular and Cellular Biology. Sensory information in neuronal processes.
Gregory L. Verdine, Ph.D., Erving Professor of Chemistry. Protein–nucleic acid interactions; transcriptional regulation; X-ray crystallography.
Gerhard Wagner, Ph.D., Elkan Blout Professor of Biological Chemistry and Molecular Pharmacology. Protein and nucleic acid structure, interaction, and mobility; NMR spectroscopy.
John R. Wakeley, Ph.D., Professor of Organismic and Evolutionary Biology. Theoretical population genetics.
Johannes C. Walter, Ph.D., Professor of Biological Chemistry and Molecular Pharmacology. Maintenance of genome stability in S phase.
Thomas Walz, Ph.D., Professor of Cell Biology. High-resolution electron microscopy.
George M. Whitesides, Ph.D., Mallinckrodt Professor of Chemistry. Molecular pharmacology; biosurface chemistry; virology.
Wesley P. Wong, Ph.D., Assistant Professor of Biological Chemistry and Molecular Pharmacology. Understanding physical basis of how biological systems work at the nanoscale, focused on the role of mechanical force.
Kai Wucherpfennig, M.D., Ph.D., Professor of Neurology. Basic mechanisms of T cell mediated autoimmune diseases.
Xiaoliang Sunney Xie, Ph.D., Mallinckrodt Professor of Chemistry and Chemical Biology. Single-molecule spectroscopy and dynamics; molecular interaction and chemical dynamics in biological systems.
Gary Yellen, Ph.D., Professor of Neurobiology. Molecular physiology of ion channels: functional motions, drug interactions, and electrophysiological mechanisms.
Xaiowei Zhuang, Ph.D., Professor of Chemistry and Chemical Biology and of Physics. Single-molecule biophysics.

Section 5
Botany and Plant Biology

This section contains a directory of institutions offering graduate work in botany and plant biology. Additional information about programs listed in the directory may be obtained by writing directly to the dean of a graduate school or chair of a department at the address given in the directory.

For programs offering related work, see also in this book *Biochemistry; Biological and Biomedical Sciences; Cell, Molecular, and Structural Biology; Ecology, Environmental Biology, and Evolutionary Biology; Entomology; Genetics, Developmental Biology, and Reproductive Biology;* and *Microbiological Sciences.* In the other guides in this series:

Graduate Programs in the Humanities, Arts & Social Sciences
See *Architecture (Landscape Architecture)* and *Economics (Agricultural Economics and Agribusiness)*

Graduate Programs in the Physical Sciences, Mathematics, Agricultural Sciences, the Environment & Natural Resources
See *Agricultural and Food Sciences*

Graduate Programs in Engineering & Applied Sciences
See *Agricultural Engineering* and *Bioengineering*

CONTENTS

Program Directories

Botany

Auburn University, Graduate School, College of Sciences and Mathematics, Department of Biological Sciences, Auburn University, AL 36849. Offers botany (MS, PhD); microbiology (MS, PhD); zoology (MS, PhD). *Faculty:* 39 full-time (13 women), 1 (woman) part-time/adjunct. *Students:* 40 full-time (21 women), 66 part-time (26 women); includes 9 minority (2 Black or African American, non-Hispanic/Latino; 1 American Indian or Alaska Native, non-Hispanic/Latino; 4 Asian, non-Hispanic/Latino; 2 Hispanic/Latino), 17 international. Average age 28. 99 applicants, 31% accepted, 19 enrolled. In 2013, 10 master's, 11 doctorates awarded. *Entrance requirements:* For master's and doctorate, GRE General Test. Additional exam requirements/recommendations for international students: Required—TOEFL. *Application deadline:* For fall admission, 7/7 for domestic students; for spring admission, 11/24 for domestic students. Application fee: $50 ($60 for international students). Electronic applications accepted. *Expenses:* Tuition, state resident: full-time $8262; part-time $459 per credit hour. Tuition, nonresident: full-time $24,786; part-time $1377 per credit hour. Tuition and fees vary according to degree level and program. *Financial support:* Research assistantships and teaching assistantships available. Financial award applicants required to submit FAFSA. *Unit head:* Dr. Jack W. Feminella, Chair, 334-844-3906, Fax: 334-844-1645. *Application contact:* Dr. George Flowers, Dean of the Graduate School, 334-844-2125.

California State University, Chico, Office of Graduate Studies, College of Natural Sciences, Department of Biological Sciences, Program in Botany, Chico, CA 95929-0722. Offers MS. *Degree requirements:* For master's, thesis, thesis and presentation. *Entrance requirements:* For master's, GRE General Test, GRE Subject Test (biology), two letters of recommendation, statement of purpose. Additional exam requirements/recommendations for international students: Required—TOEFL (minimum score 550 paper-based; 80 iBT), IELTS (minimum score 6.5), PTE. Electronic applications accepted.

Claremont Graduate University, Graduate Programs, Program in Botany, Claremont, CA 91711-6160. Offers MS, PhD. Part-time programs available. *Faculty:* 5 full-time (3 women). *Students:* 17 full-time (10 women), 1 (woman) part-time; includes 3 minority (1 American Indian or Alaska Native, non-Hispanic/Latino; 2 Hispanic/Latino), 3 international. Average age 31. In 2013, 1 doctorate awarded. Terminal master's awarded for partial completion of doctoral program. *Entrance requirements:* For master's and doctorate, GRE General Test. Additional exam requirements/recommendations for international students: Required—TOEFL (minimum score 550 paper-based; 80 iBT). *Application deadline:* For fall admission, 2/1 priority date for domestic and international students. Applications are processed on a rolling basis. Application fee: $80. Electronic applications accepted. *Expenses: Tuition:* Full-time $40,560; part-time $1690 per credit. *Required fees:* $275 per semester. Tuition and fees vary according to program. *Financial support:* Fellowships, research assistantships, Federal Work-Study, institutionally sponsored loans, scholarships/grants, and tuition waivers (full) available. Support available to part-time students. Financial award application deadline: 2/15; financial award applicants required to submit FAFSA. *Unit head:* Lucinda McDade, Director of Research/Chair, 909-625-8767 Ext. 234, Fax: 909-626-3489, E-mail: lucinda.mcdade@cgu.edu. *Application contact:* Linda Worlow, Program Coordinator, 909-625-8767 Ext. 241, Fax: 909-626-3489, E-mail: botany@cgu.edu.
Website: http://www.cgu.edu/pages/1311.asp

Colorado State University, Graduate School, College of Natural Sciences, Department of Biology, Fort Collins, CO 80523-1878. Offers botany (MS, PhD); zoology (MS, PhD). *Faculty:* 25 full-time (10 women), 1 part-time/adjunct (0 women). *Students:* 18 full-time (11 women), 25 part-time (15 women); includes 6 minority (4 Asian, non-Hispanic/Latino; 2 Hispanic/Latino), 6 international. Average age 30. 45 applicants, 27% accepted, 10 enrolled. In 2013, 5 master's, 7 doctorates awarded. Terminal master's awarded for partial completion of doctoral program. *Degree requirements:* For master's, comprehensive exam, thesis; for doctorate, comprehensive exam, thesis/dissertation. *Entrance requirements:* For master's and doctorate, GRE General Test (minimum scores above 70th percentile), 2 transcripts, 3 letters of recommendation, statement of educational goals/research interests, minimum GPA of 3.0. Additional exam requirements/recommendations for international students: Required—TOEFL (minimum score 550 paper-based; 80 iBT), IELTS (minimum score 6.5). *Application deadline:* For fall admission, 1/15 priority date for domestic and international students; for spring admission, 11/1 priority date for domestic and international students. Applications are processed on a rolling basis. Application fee: $50. Electronic applications accepted. *Expenses:* Tuition, state resident: full-time $9075.40; part-time $504 per credit. Tuition, nonresident: full-time $22,248; part-time $1236 per credit. *Required fees:* $1819; $60 per credit. *Financial support:* In 2013–14, 106 students received support, including 19 fellowships (averaging $31,747 per year), 22 research assistantships with full tuition reimbursements available (averaging $10,909 per year), 65 teaching assistantships with full tuition reimbursements available (averaging $13,683 per year); career-related internships or fieldwork, Federal Work-Study, institutionally sponsored loans, scholarships/grants, traineeships, health care benefits, and unspecified assistantships also available. Financial award application deadline: 3/1; financial award applicants required to submit FAFSA. *Faculty research:* Organismal interactions in infectious disease, stream ecology, muscle protein structure, molecular evolution, plant biotechnology. *Total annual research expenditures:* $9.7 million. *Unit head:* Dr. Michael Antolin, Professor and Interim Chair, 970-491-1911, Fax: 970-491-0649, E-mail: michael.antolin@colostate.edu. *Application contact:* Dorothy Ramirez, Graduate Coordinator, 970-491-1923, Fax: 970-491-0649, E-mail: dorothy.ramirez@colostate.edu.
Website: http://www.biology.colostate.edu/

Dalhousie University, Faculty of Agriculture, Halifax, NS B3H 4R2, Canada. Offers agriculture (M Sc), including air quality, animal behavior, animal molecular genetics, animal nutrition, animal technology, aquaculture, botany, crop management, crop physiology, ecology, environmental microbiology, food science, horticulture, nutrient management, pest management, physiology, plant biotechnology, plant pathology, soil chemistry, soil fertility, waste management and composting, water quality. Part-time programs available. *Degree requirements:* For master's, thesis, ATC Exam Teaching Assistantship. *Entrance requirements:* For master's, honors B Sc, minimum GPA of 3.0. Additional exam requirements/recommendations for international students: Required—TOEFL (minimum score 580 paper-based; 92 iBT), IELTS, Michigan English Language Assessment Battery, CanTEST, CAEL. *Faculty research:* Bio-product development, organic agriculture, nutrient management, air and water quality, agricultural biotechnology.

Eastern New Mexico University, Graduate School, College of Liberal Arts and Sciences, Department of Biology, Portales, NM 88130. Offers applied ecology (MS); botany (MS); cell, molecular biology and biotechnology (MS); microbiology (MS); zoology (MS). Part-time programs available. *Degree requirements:* For master's, comprehensive exam, thesis optional. *Entrance requirements:* For master's, GRE, minimum GPA of 3.0, 2 letters of recommendation, statement of research interest, bachelor's degree related to field of study or proof of common knowledge. Additional exam requirements/recommendations for international students: Required—TOEFL (minimum score 550 paper-based; 79 iBT), IELTS (minimum score 6). Electronic applications accepted.

Emporia State University, Department of Biological Sciences, Emporia, KS 66801-5415. Offers botany (MS); environmental biology (MS); general biology (MS); microbial and cellular biology (MS); zoology (MS). Part-time programs available. *Faculty:* 13 full-time (3 women). *Students:* 32 full-time (16 women), 7 part-time (1 woman); includes 2 minority (1 Black or African American, non-Hispanic/Latino; 1 Asian, non-Hispanic/Latino), 18 international. 25 applicants, 88% accepted, 3 enrolled. In 2013, 8 master's awarded. *Degree requirements:* For master's, comprehensive exam or thesis. *Entrance requirements:* For master's, GRE, appropriate undergraduate degree, interview, letters of reference. Additional exam requirements/recommendations for international students: Required—TOEFL (minimum score 520 paper-based; 68 iBT). *Application deadline:* For fall admission, 8/15 priority date for domestic students. Applications are processed on a rolling basis. Application fee: $30 ($75 for international students). Electronic applications accepted. *Expenses: Tuition, area resident:* Part-time $220 per credit hour. Tuition, state resident: part-time $220 per credit hour. Tuition, nonresident: part-time $685 per credit hour. *Required fees:* $73 per credit hour. *Financial support:* In 2013–14, 5 research assistantships with full tuition reimbursements (averaging $7,371 per year), 9 teaching assistantships with full tuition reimbursements (averaging $7,950 per year) were awarded; career-related internships or fieldwork, Federal Work-Study, institutionally sponsored loans, health care benefits, and unspecified assistantships also available. Financial award application deadline: 3/15; financial award applicants required to submit FAFSA. *Faculty research:* Fisheries, range, and wildlife management; aquatic, plant, grassland, vertebrate, and invertebrate ecology; mammalian and plant systematics, taxonomy, and evolution; immunology, virology, and molecular biology. *Unit head:* Dr. R. Brent Thomas, Chair, 620-341-5311, Fax: 620-341-5608, E-mail: rthomas2@emporia.edu. *Application contact:* Dr. Scott Crupper, Graduate Coordinator, 620-341-5621, Fax: 620-341-5607, E-mail: scrupper@emporia.edu.
Website: http://www.emporia.edu/info/degrees-courses/grad/biology

Illinois State University, Graduate School, College of Arts and Sciences, Department of Biological Sciences, Normal, IL 61790-2200. Offers animal behavior (MS); bacteriology (MS); biochemistry (MS); biological sciences (MS); biology (PhD); biophysics (MS); biotechnology (MS); botany (MS, PhD); cell biology (MS); conservation biology (MS); developmental biology (MS); ecology (MS, PhD); entomology (MS); evolutionary biology (MS); genetics (MS, PhD); immunology (MS); microbiology (MS, PhD); molecular biology (MS); molecular genetics (MS); neurobiology (MS); neuroscience (MS); parasitology (MS); physiology (MS, PhD); plant biology (MS); plant molecular biology (MS); plant sciences (MS); structural biology (MS); zoology (MS, PhD). Part-time programs available. *Degree requirements:* For master's, thesis or alternative; for doctorate, variable foreign language requirement, thesis/dissertation, 2 terms of residency. *Entrance requirements:* For master's, GRE General Test, minimum GPA of 2.6 in last 60 hours of course work; for doctorate, GRE General Test. *Faculty research:* Redoc balance and drug development in schistosoma mansoni, control of the growth of listeria monocytogenes at low temperature, regulation of cell expansion and microtubule function by SPRI, CRUI: physiology and fitness consequences of different life history phenotypes.

Miami University, College of Arts and Science, Department of Biology, Oxford, OH 45056. Offers biological sciences (MAT); biology (MS, PhD); botany (MAT, MS, PhD); cell, molecular and structural biology (MS, PhD); ecology, evolution and environmental biology (PhD); zoology (MA, MS, PhD). Part-time programs available. Postbaccalaureate distance learning degree programs offered. *Students:* 89 full-time (49 women), 612 part-time (502 women); includes 63 minority (9 Black or African American, non-Hispanic/Latino; 2 American Indian or Alaska Native, non-Hispanic/Latino; 6 Asian, non-Hispanic/Latino; 27 Hispanic/Latino; 1 Native Hawaiian or other Pacific Islander, non-Hispanic/Latino; 18 Two or more races, non-Hispanic/Latino), 35 international. Average age 34. In 2013, 133 master's, 4 doctorates awarded. *Entrance requirements:* For master's and doctorate, GRE General Test. Additional exam requirements/recommendations for international students: Recommended—TOEFL (minimum score 80 iBT), IELTS (minimum score 6.5), TSE (minimum score 54). *Application deadline:* For fall admission, 1/15 for domestic and international students. Application fee: $50. Electronic applications accepted. *Expenses:* Tuition, state resident: full-time $12,634; part-time $526 per credit hour. Tuition, nonresident: full-time $27,892; part-time $1162 per credit hour. Part-time tuition and fees vary according to course load, campus/location and program. *Financial support:* Fellowships with full tuition reimbursements, research assistantships with full tuition reimbursements, teaching assistantships with full tuition reimbursements, Federal Work-Study, health care benefits, tuition waivers (full), and unspecified assistantships available. Financial award application deadline: 1/15; financial award applicants required to submit FAFSA. *Unit head:* Dr. Douglas Meikle, Chair, 513-529-3103, E-mail: meikled@miamioh.edu.
Website: http://miamioh.edu/cas/about/biology

North Carolina State University, Graduate School, College of Agriculture and Life Sciences, Department of Plant Biology, Raleigh, NC 27695. Offers MS, PhD. Part-time programs available. Terminal master's awarded for partial completion of doctoral program. *Degree requirements:* For master's, thesis (for some programs); for doctorate, thesis/dissertation. *Entrance requirements:* For master's and doctorate, GRE. Additional exam requirements/recommendations for international students: Required—TOEFL. Electronic applications accepted. *Faculty research:* Plant molecular and cell biology, aquatic ecology, community ecology, restoration, systematics plant pathogen and environmental interactions.

North Dakota State University, College of Graduate and Interdisciplinary Studies, College of Science and Mathematics, Department of Biological Sciences, Fargo, ND 58108. Offers biology (MS); botany (MS, PhD); cellular and molecular biology (PhD); genomics (PhD); zoology (MS, PhD). *Faculty:* 17 full-time (9 women), 1 part-time/adjunct (0 women). *Students:* 20 full-time (10 women), 3 part-time (all women); includes 2 minority (1 American Indian or Alaska Native, non-Hispanic/Latino; 1 Two or more races, non-Hispanic/Latino), 1 international. Average age 32. 9 applicants, 11% accepted, 1 enrolled. In 2013, 4 master's awarded. *Degree requirements:* For master's, thesis; for doctorate, thesis/dissertation. *Entrance requirements:* For master's and doctorate, GRE General Test. Additional exam requirements/recommendations for international students: Required—TOEFL. *Application deadline:* For fall admission, 1/15 for domestic students. Applications are processed on a rolling basis. Application fee: $35. Electronic applications accepted. *Financial support:* Fellowships with full tuition reimbursements, research assistantships with full tuition reimbursements, teaching assistantships with full tuition reimbursements, career-related internships or fieldwork, Federal Work-Study, institutionally sponsored loans, scholarships/grants, tuition waivers (full), and unspecified assistantships available. Support available to part-time students. Financial award application deadline: 4/15; financial award applicants required to submit FAFSA. *Faculty research:* Comparative endocrinology, physiology, behavioral ecology, plant cell biology, aquatic biology. *Unit head:* Dr. Wendy Reed, Head, 701-231-7087, E-mail: wendy.reed@ndsu.edu. *Application contact:* Sonya Goergen, Marketing, Recruitment, and Public Relations Coordinator, 701-231-7033, Fax: 701-231-6524. Website: http://biology.ndsu.nodak.edu/

Oklahoma State University, College of Arts and Sciences, Department of Botany, Stillwater, OK 74078. Offers botany (MS); environmental science (MS, PhD); plant science (PhD). *Faculty:* 13 full-time (3 women), 2 part-time/adjunct (1 woman). *Students:* 2 full-time (0 women), 14 part-time (7 women); includes 4 minority (1 American Indian or Alaska Native, non-Hispanic/Latino; 3 Two or more races, non-Hispanic/Latino). Average age 31. 4 applicants, 25% accepted, 1 enrolled. In 2013, 2 master's awarded. *Degree requirements:* For master's, thesis; for doctorate, comprehensive exam, thesis/dissertation. *Entrance requirements:* For master's and doctorate, GRE or GMAT. Additional exam requirements/recommendations for international students: Required—TOEFL (minimum score 550 paper-based; 79 iBT). *Application deadline:* For fall admission, 3/1 priority date for international students; for spring admission, 8/1 priority date for international students. Applications are processed on a rolling basis. Application fee: $40 ($75 for international students). Electronic applications accepted. *Expenses:* Tuition, state resident: full-time $4272; part-time $178 per credit hour. Tuition, nonresident: full-time $17,472; part-time $709 per credit hour. *Required fees:* $2413.20; $100.55 per credit hour. One-time fee: $50 full-time. Part-time tuition and fees vary according to course load and campus/location. *Financial support:* In 2013–14, 2 research assistantships (averaging $20,004 per year), 10 teaching assistantships (averaging $19,932 per year) were awarded; career-related internships or fieldwork, Federal Work-Study, scholarships/grants, health care benefits, tuition waivers (partial), and unspecified assistantships also available. Support available to part-time students. Financial award application deadline: 3/1; financial award applicants required to submit FAFSA. *Faculty research:* Ethnobotany, developmental genetics of Arabidopsis, biological roles of Plasmodesmata, community ecology and biodiversity, nutrient cycling in grassland ecosystems. *Unit head:* Dr. Linda Watson, Department Head, 405-744-5559, Fax: 405-744-7074, E-mail: linda.watson10@okstate.edu. *Application contact:* Ming Yang, Coordinator for the Botany MS Program, 405-744-9508, E-mail: ming.yang@okstate.edu.
Website: http://botany.okstate.edu

Oregon State University, College of Agricultural Sciences, Program in Applied Systematics in Botany, Corvallis, OR 97331. Offers PSM. Part-time programs available. *Faculty:* 28 full-time (8 women), 4 part-time/adjunct (1 woman). *Students:* 1 (woman) full-time, 1 (woman) part-time. 1 applicant, 100% accepted, 1 enrolled. In 2013, 1 master's awarded. *Entrance requirements:* For master's, GRE. Additional exam requirements/recommendations for international students: Required—TOEFL (minimum score 80 iBT), IELTS (minimum score 6.5). *Application deadline:* For fall admission, 2/15 for domestic students. Application fee: $60. *Expenses:* Contact institution. *Unit head:* Dr. Aaron Liston, Director, 541-737-5301, E-mail: listona@science.oregonstate.edu.

Purdue University, Graduate School, College of Agriculture, Department of Botany and Plant Pathology, West Lafayette, IN 47907. Offers MS, PhD. Part-time programs available. *Faculty:* 20 full-time (7 women), 2 part-time/adjunct (1 woman). *Students:* 43 full-time (21 women), 3 part-time (1 woman); includes 1 minority (Asian, non-Hispanic/Latino), 21 international. Average age 27. 61 applicants, 21% accepted, 6 enrolled. In 2013, 9 master's, 4 doctorates awarded. Terminal master's awarded for partial completion of doctoral program. *Degree requirements:* For master's, thesis; for doctorate, thesis/dissertation. *Entrance requirements:* For master's, GRE General Test, minimum undergraduate GPA of 3.0 or equivalent; for doctorate, GRE, minimum undergraduate GPA of 3.0 or equivalent. Additional exam requirements/recommendations for international students: Required—TOEFL (minimum score 550 paper-based; 77 iBT); Recommended—TWE. *Application deadline:* For fall admission, 4/15 priority date for domestic and international students; for spring admission, 12/15 for domestic students, 9/15 for international students; for summer admission, 4/15 for domestic students, 2/15 for international students. Applications are processed on a rolling basis. Application fee: $60 ($75 for international students). Electronic applications accepted. *Financial support:* In 2013–14, 30 students received support. Fellowships with full tuition reimbursements available, research assistantships with full tuition reimbursements available, teaching assistantships with full tuition reimbursements available, and career-related internships or fieldwork available. Support available to part-time students. Financial award application deadline: 3/1; financial award applicants required to submit FAFSA. *Faculty research:* Biotechnology, plant growth, weed control, crop improvement, plant physiology. *Unit head:* Dr. Peter B. Goldsbrough, Head, 765-494-4615, Fax: 765-494-0363, E-mail: goldsbrough@purdue.edu. *Application contact:* Tyson J. McFall, Graduate Contact, 765-494-0352, E-mail: tjmcfall@purdue.edu.
Website: https://ag.purdue.edu/btny

Texas A&M University, College of Science, Department of Biology, College Station, TX 77843. Offers biology (MS, PhD); botany (MS, PhD); microbiology (MS, PhD); zoology (MS, PhD). *Faculty:* 40. *Students:* 94 full-time (54 women), 7 part-time (4 women); includes 10 minority (1 Black or African American, non-Hispanic/Latino; 3 Asian, non-Hispanic/Latino; 6 Hispanic/Latino), 49 international. Average age 29. 120 applicants, 25% accepted, 19 enrolled. In 2013, 5 master's, 16 doctorates awarded. *Degree requirements:* For master's, thesis or alternative; for doctorate, comprehensive exam, thesis/dissertation. *Entrance requirements:* For master's and doctorate, GRE General Test. Additional exam requirements/recommendations for international students: Required—TOEFL. *Application deadline:* For fall admission, 1/15 for domestic students. Applications are processed on a rolling basis. Application fee: $50 ($75 for international students). Electronic applications accepted. *Expenses:* Tuition, state resident: full-time $4078; part-time $226.55 per credit hour. Tuition, nonresident: full-time $10,450; part-time $580.55 per credit hour. *Required fees:* $2328; $278.50 per credit hour. $642.45 per semester. *Financial support:* Fellowships, research assistantships, and teaching assistantships available. Financial award application deadline: 4/1; financial award applicants required to submit FAFSA. *Unit head:* Dr. Tom McKnight, Department Head, 979-845-3896, Fax: 979-845-2891, E-mail: mcknight@bio.tamu.edu. *Application contact:* Dr. Arne Lekven, Graduate Advisor, 979-458-3461, Fax: 979-845-2891, E-mail: alekven@bio.tamu.edu.
Website: http://www.bio.tamu.edu/index.html

University of Alaska Fairbanks, College of Natural Sciences and Mathematics, Department of Biology and Wildlife, Fairbanks, AK 99775-6100. Offers biological sciences (MS, PhD), including biology, botany, wildlife biology (PhD), zoology; biology (MAT, MS); wildlife biology (MS). Part-time programs available. *Faculty:* 21 full-time (9 women). *Students:* 73 full-time (39 women), 29 part-time (17 women); includes 7 minority (1 Asian, non-Hispanic/Latino; 4 Hispanic/Latino; 2 Two or more races, non-Hispanic/Latino), 5 international. Average age 31. 47 applicants, 21% accepted, 10 enrolled. In 2013, 12 master's, 8 doctorates awarded. *Degree requirements:* For master's, comprehensive exam, thesis, oral exam, oral defense; for doctorate, comprehensive exam, thesis/dissertation, oral exam, oral defense. *Entrance requirements:* For master's and doctorate, GRE General Test, GRE Subject Test (biology). Additional exam requirements/recommendations for international students: Required—TOEFL (minimum score 550 paper-based; 80 iBT), TWE. *Application deadline:* For fall admission, 6/1 for domestic students, 3/1 for international students; for spring admission, 10/15 for domestic students, 9/1 for international students. Applications are processed on a rolling basis. Application fee: $60. Electronic applications accepted. *Expenses:* Tuition, state resident: full-time $7254; part-time $403 per credit. Tuition, nonresident: full-time $14,814; part-time $823 per credit. Tuition and fees vary according to course level, course load and reciprocity agreements. *Financial support:* In 2013–14, 33 research assistantships with tuition reimbursements (averaging $15,138 per year), 21 teaching assistantships with tuition reimbursements (averaging $8,654 per year) were awarded; fellowships with tuition reimbursements, career-related internships or fieldwork, Federal Work-Study, scholarships/grants, health care benefits, and unspecified assistantships also available. Support available to part-time students. Financial award application deadline: 7/1; financial award applicants required to submit FAFSA. *Faculty research:* Plant-herbivore interactions, plant metabolic defenses, insect manufacture of glycerol, ice nucleators, structure and functions of arctic and subarctic freshwater ecosystems. *Unit head:* Diane Wagner, Department Chair, 907-474-7671, Fax: 907-474-6716, E-mail: uaf-bw-dept@alaska.edu. *Application contact:* Libby Eddy, Registrar and Director of Admissions, 907-474-7500, Fax: 907-474-7097, E-mail: admissions@uaf.edu.
Website: http://www.bw.uaf.edu

The University of British Columbia, Faculty of Science, Department of Botany, Vancouver, BC V6T 1Z1, Canada. Offers M Sc, PhD. *Degree requirements:* For master's, thesis; for doctorate, comprehensive exam, thesis/dissertation. *Entrance requirements:* Additional exam requirements/recommendations for international students: Required—TOEFL. Electronic applications accepted. *Expenses: Tuition, area resident:* Full-time $8000 Canadian dollars. *Faculty research:* Plant ecology, evolution and systematics, cell and developmental biology, plant physiology/biochemistry, genetics.

University of California, Riverside, Graduate Division, Department of Botany and Plant Sciences, Riverside, CA 92521-0102. Offers plant biology (MS, PhD), including plant cell, molecular, and developmental biology (PhD), plant ecology (PhD), plant genetics (PhD). Part-time programs available. *Faculty:* 40 full-time (13 women). *Students:* 66 full-time (40 women); includes 12 minority (5 Asian, non-Hispanic/Latino; 7 Hispanic/Latino), 24 international. Average age 29. In 2013, 3 master's, 3 doctorates awarded. Terminal master's awarded for partial completion of doctoral program. *Degree requirements:* For master's, comprehensive exams or thesis; for doctorate, thesis/dissertation, qualifying exams. *Entrance requirements:* For master's and doctorate, GRE General Test, minimum GPA of 3.2. Additional exam requirements/recommendations for international students: Required—TOEFL (minimum score 550 paper-based; 80 iBT). *Application deadline:* For fall admission, 5/1 for domestic students, 2/1 for international students; for winter admission, 2/1 for domestic students, 7/1 for international students; for spring admission, 12/1 for domestic students, 10/1 for international students. Applications are processed on a rolling basis. Application fee: $80 ($100 for international students). Electronic applications accepted. *Financial support:* In 2013–14, fellowships with tuition reimbursements (averaging $12,000 per year), research assistantships with tuition reimbursements (averaging $23,000 per year), teaching assistantships with tuition reimbursements (averaging $16,500 per year) were awarded; career-related internships or fieldwork, Federal Work-Study, institutionally sponsored loans, scholarships/grants, and tuition waivers (full and partial) also available. *Faculty research:* Agricultural plant biology; biochemistry and physiology; cellular, molecular and developmental biology; ecology, evolution, systematics and ethnobotany; genetics, genomics and bioinformatics. *Unit head:* Dr. Mikeal Roose, Chair, 951-827-4413. *Application contact:* Jammy Yang, Graduate Program Assistant, 800-735-0717, Fax: 951-827-5517, E-mail: deidra.kornfeld@ucr.edu.
Website: http://www.plantbiology.ucr.edu/

University of Connecticut, Graduate School, College of Liberal Arts and Sciences, Department of Ecology and Evolutionary Biology, Storrs, CT 06269. Offers botany (MS, PhD); ecology (MS, PhD); entomology (MS, PhD); zoology (MS, PhD). Terminal master's awarded for partial completion of doctoral program. *Degree requirements:* For master's, comprehensive exam; for doctorate, thesis/dissertation. *Entrance requirements:* For master's and doctorate, GRE General Test, GRE Subject Test. Additional exam requirements/recommendations for international students: Required—TOEFL (minimum score 550 paper-based). Electronic applications accepted.

University of Florida, Graduate School, College of Liberal Arts and Sciences, Department of Biology, Gainesville, FL 32611. Offers botany (MS, MST, PhD), including botany; zoology (MS, MST, PhD), including animal molecular and cellular biology (PhD), tropical conservation and development (MS), wetland sciences (MS), zoology. *Faculty:* 31 full-time (9 women), 26 part-time/adjunct (9 women). *Students:* 99 full-time (44 women), 6 part-time (4 women); includes 14 minority (2 Black or African American, non-Hispanic/Latino; 1 American Indian or Alaska Native, non-Hispanic/Latino; 5 Asian, non-Hispanic/Latino; 6 Hispanic/Latino), 35 international. Average age 31. 74 applicants, 32% accepted, 18 enrolled. In 2013, 4 master's, 13 doctorates awarded. *Degree requirements:* For master's, comprehensive exam (for some programs), thesis; for doctorate, comprehensive exam, thesis/dissertation. *Entrance requirements:* For master's and doctorate, GRE General Test, minimum GPA of 3.0. Additional exam requirements/recommendations for international students: Required—TOEFL (minimum score 550 paper-based; 80 iBT), IELTS (minimum score 6). *Application deadline:* For fall admission, 12/1 for domestic and international students. Applications are processed on a rolling basis. Application fee: $30. Electronic applications accepted. *Expenses:* Tuition, state resident: full-time $12,640. Tuition, nonresident: full-time $30,000. *Financial support:* In 2013–14, 98 students received support, including 7 fellowships (averaging $22,150 per year), 34 research assistantships (averaging $19,000 per year), 66 teaching assistantships (averaging $16,250 per year); unspecified assistantships also available. Financial award application deadline: 12/15; financial award applicants required to submit FAFSA. *Faculty research:* Ecology, evolution, genetics, molecular and cellular biology, physiology. *Unit head:* Craig Osenberg, PhD, Professor and Chair, 352-392-9201, Fax: 352-392-3704, E-mail: osenberg@ufl.edu. *Application contact:* William T. Barbazuk, PhD, Associate Professor/Graduate Coordinator, 352-273-8624, Fax: 352-392-3704, E-mail: bbarbazuk@ufl.edu.
Website: http://www.biology.ufl.edu/

University of Guelph, Graduate Studies, College of Biological Science, Department of Integrative Biology, Botany and Zoology, Guelph, ON N1G 2W1, Canada. Offers botany (M Sc, PhD); zoology (M Sc, PhD). Part-time programs available. *Degree requirements:* For master's, thesis, research proposal; for doctorate, thesis/dissertation, research proposal, qualifying exam. *Entrance requirements:* For master's, minimum B average during previous 2 years of course work. Additional exam requirements/recommendations for international students: Required—TOEFL (minimum score 550 paper-based), IELTS (minimum score 6.5). Electronic applications accepted. *Faculty research:* Aquatic science, environmental physiology, parasitology, wildlife biology, management.

Botany

University of Guelph, Graduate Studies, College of Biological Science, Department of Molecular and Cellular Biology, Guelph, ON N1G 2W1, Canada. Offers biochemistry (M Sc, PhD); biophysics (M Sc, PhD); botany (M Sc, PhD); microbiology (M Sc, PhD); molecular biology and genetics (M Sc, PhD). *Degree requirements:* For master's, thesis, research proposal; for doctorate, comprehensive exam, thesis/dissertation, research proposal. *Entrance requirements:* For master's, minimum B-average during previous 2 years of coursework; for doctorate, minimum A-average. Additional exam requirements/recommendations for international students: Required—TOEFL (minimum score 550 paper-based), IELTS (minimum score 6.5). Electronic applications accepted. *Faculty research:* Physiology, structure, genetics, and ecology of microbes; virology and microbial technology.

University of Hawaii at Manoa, Graduate Division, College of Natural Sciences, Department of Botany, Honolulu, HI 96822. Offers MS, PhD. Part-time programs available. Terminal master's awarded for partial completion of doctoral program. *Degree requirements:* For master's, one foreign language, thesis optional, presentation; for doctorate, one foreign language, comprehensive exam, thesis/dissertation, presentation. *Entrance requirements:* For master's and doctorate, GRE General Test, GRE Subject Test (biology). Additional exam requirements/recommendations for international students: Required—TOEFL (minimum score 540 paper-based; 76 iBT), IELTS (minimum score 5). *Faculty research:* Plant ecology, evolution, systematics, conservation biology, ethnobotany.

The University of Kansas, Graduate Studies, College of Liberal Arts and Sciences, Department of Ecology and Evolutionary Biology, Lawrence, KS 66045. Offers botany (MA, PhD); ecology and evolutionary biology (MA, PhD); entomology (MA, PhD). *Faculty:* 35. *Students:* 57 full-time (25 women); includes 3 minority (all Two or more races, non-Hispanic/Latino), 19 international. Average age 29. 48 applicants, 29% accepted, 10 enrolled. In 2013, 9 doctorates awarded. Terminal master's awarded for partial completion of doctoral program. *Degree requirements:* For master's, comprehensive exam, thesis (for some programs), 30-36 credits, thesis presentation; for doctorate, comprehensive exam, thesis/dissertation, residency, responsible scholarship and research skills, final exam, dissertation defense. *Entrance requirements:* For master's, GRE General Test, bachelor's degree with minimum undergraduate GPA of 3.0; for doctorate, GRE General Test, bachelor's degree; minimum undergraduate/graduate GPA of 3.0. Additional exam requirements/recommendations for international students: Required—TOEFL or IELTS. *Application deadline:* For fall admission, 12/1 for domestic and international students; for spring admission, 9/15 for domestic and international students. Application fee: $55 ($65 for international students). Electronic applications accepted. *Financial support:* In 2013–14, 8 fellowships with full and partial tuition reimbursements, 22 research assistantships with full and partial tuition reimbursements, 32 teaching assistantships with full and partial tuition reimbursements were awarded; scholarships/grants, traineeships, health care benefits, and unspecified assistantships also available. Financial award application deadline: 12/1. *Faculty research:* Ecology and global change, diversity and macroevolution, evolutionary mechanisms, systematics/phylogenetics, biogeography. *Unit head:* Dr. Christopher H. Haufler, Chair, 785-864-3255, Fax: 785-864-5860, E-mail: vulgare@ku.edu. *Application contact:* Aagje Ashe, Graduate Coordinator, 785-864-2362, Fax: 785-864-5860, E-mail: a4ashe@ku.edu.
Website: http://eeb.ku.edu/

University of Maine, Graduate School, College of Natural Sciences, Forestry, and Agriculture, School of Biology and Ecology, Orono, ME 04469. Offers biological sciences (PhD); botany and plant pathology (MS); ecology and environmental science (MS, PhD); entomology (MS); plant science (PhD); zoology (MS, PhD). Part-time programs available. *Faculty:* 33 full-time (13 women), 26 part-time/adjunct (5 women). *Students:* 66 full-time (40 women), 4 part-time (2 women); includes 4 minority (1 American Indian or Alaska Native, non-Hispanic/Latino; 2 Asian, non-Hispanic/Latino; 1 Hispanic/Latino), 7 international. Average age 30. 97 applicants, 25% accepted, 17 enrolled. In 2013, 8 master's, 3 doctorates awarded. Terminal master's awarded for partial completion of doctoral program. *Degree requirements:* For master's, thesis (for some programs); for doctorate, comprehensive exam, thesis/dissertation. *Entrance requirements:* For master's and doctorate, GRE General Test. Additional exam requirements/recommendations for international students: Required—TOEFL. *Application deadline:* For fall admission, 2/1 priority date for domestic students. Applications are processed on a rolling basis. Application fee: $65. Electronic applications accepted. *Expenses:* Tuition, state resident: full-time $7524. Tuition, nonresident: full-time $23,112. *Required fees:* $1970. *Financial support:* In 2013–14, 66 students received support, including 3 fellowships with full tuition reimbursements available (averaging $25,000 per year), 28 research assistantships with full tuition reimbursements available (averaging $14,600 per year), 21 teaching assistantships with full tuition reimbursements available (averaging $14,600 per year); career-related internships or fieldwork, Federal Work-Study, institutionally sponsored loans, and tuition waivers (full and partial) also available. Financial award application deadline: 3/1. *Total annual research expenditures:* $569,533. *Unit head:* Dr. Ellie Groden, Director, 207-581-2551, Fax: 207-581-2537. *Application contact:* Scott G. Delcourt, Associate Dean of the Graduate School, 207-581-3291, Fax: 207-581-3232, E-mail: graduate@maine.edu.
Website: http://sbe.umaine.edu/

University of Manitoba, Faculty of Graduate Studies, Faculty of Science, Department of Biological Sciences, Winnipeg, MB R3T 2N2, Canada. Offers botany (M Sc, PhD); ecology (M Sc, PhD); zoology (M Sc, PhD).

The University of North Carolina at Chapel Hill, Graduate School, College of Arts and Sciences, Department of Biology, Chapel Hill, NC 27599. Offers botany (MA, MS, PhD); cell biology, development, and physiology (MA, MS, PhD); cell motility and cytoskeleton (PhD); ecology and behavior (MA, MS, PhD); genetics and molecular biology (MA, MS, PhD); morphology, systematics, and evolution (MA, MS, PhD). Terminal master's awarded for partial completion of doctoral program. *Degree requirements:* For master's, comprehensive exam, thesis (for some programs); for doctorate, comprehensive exam, thesis/dissertation. *Entrance requirements:* For master's, GRE General Test, GRE Subject Test, 2 semesters of calculus or statistics; 2 semesters of physics, organic chemistry; 3 semesters of biology; for doctorate, GRE General Test, GRE Subject Test, 2 semesters calculus or statistics, 2 semesters physics, organic chemistry, 3 semesters of biology. Additional exam requirements/recommendations for international students: Required—TOEFL (minimum score 550 paper-based). Electronic applications accepted. *Faculty research:* Gene expression, biomechanics, yeast genetics, plant ecology, plant molecular biology.

University of North Dakota, Graduate School, College of Arts and Sciences, Department of Biology, Grand Forks, ND 58202. Offers botany (MS, PhD); ecology (MS, PhD); entomology (MS, PhD); environmental biology (MS, PhD); fisheries/wildlife (MS, PhD); genetics (MS, PhD); zoology (MS, PhD). Terminal master's awarded for partial completion of doctoral program. *Degree requirements:* For master's, thesis, final exam; for doctorate, comprehensive exam, thesis/dissertation, final exam. *Entrance requirements:* For master's, GRE General Test, GRE Subject Test, minimum GPA of 3.0; for doctorate, GRE General Test, GRE Subject Test, minimum GPA of 3.5. Additional exam requirements/recommendations for international students: Required—TOEFL (minimum score 550 paper-based; 79 iBT), IELTS (minimum score 6.5). Electronic applications accepted. *Faculty research:* Population biology, wildlife ecology, RNA processing, hormonal control of behavior.

University of Oklahoma, College of Arts and Sciences, Department of Microbiology and Plant Biology, Program in Botany, Norman, OK 73019. Offers bioinformatics (MS, PhD); botany (MS, PhD). *Students:* 12 full-time (9 women), 9 part-time (3 women); includes 3 minority (2 American Indian or Alaska Native, non-Hispanic/Latino; 1 Hispanic/Latino), 10 international. Average age 27. 13 applicants, 31% accepted, 3 enrolled. In 2013, 5 master's, 1 doctorate awarded. Terminal master's awarded for partial completion of doctoral program. *Degree requirements:* For master's, thesis; for doctorate, one foreign language, comprehensive exam, thesis/dissertation. *Entrance requirements:* For master's and doctorate, GRE, 3 recommendation letters, letter of intent, bachelor's degree. Additional exam requirements/recommendations for international students: Required—TOEFL (minimum score 80 iBT). *Application deadline:* For fall admission, 4/1 for domestic and international students; for spring admission, 9/1 for domestic and international students. Application fee: $50 ($100 for international students). Electronic applications accepted. *Expenses:* Tuition, state resident: full-time $4205; part-time $175.20 per credit hour. Tuition, nonresident: full-time $16,205; part-time $675.20 per credit hour. *Required fees:* $2745; $103.85 per credit hour. $126.50 per semester. *Financial support:* In 2013–14, 20 students received support. Federal Work-Study, institutionally sponsored loans, scholarships/grants, health care benefits, and unspecified assistantships available. Support available to part-time students. Financial award application deadline: 6/1; financial award applicants required to submit FAFSA. *Faculty research:* Ecology, evolution, and systematics of plants, molecular biology of plant stress and reproduction, global change, biology and ecosystem modeling, plant structure and development, science education. *Unit head:* Dr. Gordon Uno, Professor/Department Chair, 405-325-4321, Fax: 405-325-7619, E-mail: guno@ou.edu. *Application contact:* Adell Hopper, Staff Assistant, 405-325-4322, Fax: 405-325-7619, E-mail: ahopper@ou.edu.
Website: http://mpbio.ou.edu/

University of Wisconsin–Madison, Graduate School, College of Letters and Science, Department of Botany, Madison, WI 53706-1380. Offers MS, PhD. Part-time programs available. Terminal master's awarded for partial completion of doctoral program. *Degree requirements:* For master's, thesis; for doctorate, one foreign language, thesis/dissertation. *Entrance requirements:* For master's and doctorate, GRE General Test. Electronic applications accepted. *Expenses:* Tuition, state resident: full-time $10,728; part-time $790 per credit. Tuition, nonresident: full-time $24,054; part-time $1623 per credit. *Required fees:* $1130; $119 per credit. *Faculty research:* Taxonomy and systematics; ecology; structural botany; physiological, cellular, and molecular biology.

University of Wisconsin–Oshkosh, Graduate Studies, College of Letters and Science, Department of Biology and Microbiology, Oshkosh, WI 54901. Offers biology (MS), including botany, microbiology, zoology. *Degree requirements:* For master's, comprehensive exam, thesis. *Entrance requirements:* For master's, GRE General Test, minimum GPA of 3.0, BS in biology. Additional exam requirements/recommendations for international students: Required—TOEFL (minimum score 550 paper-based; 79 iBT). Electronic applications accepted.

University of Wyoming, College of Arts and Sciences, Department of Botany, Laramie, WY 82071. Offers botany (MS, PhD); botany/water resources (MS). Part-time programs available. Terminal master's awarded for partial completion of doctoral program. *Degree requirements:* For master's, thesis; for doctorate, thesis/dissertation. *Entrance requirements:* For master's and doctorate, GRE General Test, minimum GPA of 3.0. Additional exam requirements/recommendations for international students: Required—TOEFL. Electronic applications accepted. *Faculty research:* Ecology, systematics, physiology, mycology, genetics.

Washington State University, Graduate School, College of Arts and Sciences, Program in Botany, Pullman, WA 99164-4236. Offers MS, PhD. *Degree requirements:* For master's, comprehensive exam (for some programs), thesis, oral exam; for doctorate, comprehensive exam, thesis/dissertation, oral exam. *Entrance requirements:* For master's and doctorate, GRE General Test, GRE Subject Test (recommended), three letters of recommendation, official transcripts from each university-level school attended, minimum GPA of 3.0. Additional exam requirements/recommendations for international students: Required—TOEFL, IELTS. *Faculty research:* Photosynthesis, plant physiology, plant ion transport, plant phylogenetics, population genetics, community and ecosystem ecology.

Plant Biology

Clemson University, Graduate School, College of Agriculture, Forestry and Life Sciences, School of Agricultural, Forest, and Environmental Sciences, Program in Plant and Environmental Sciences, Clemson, SC 29634. Offers MS, PhD. *Students:* 54 full-time (23 women), 6 part-time (2 women); includes 2 minority (1 Hispanic/Latino; 1 Two or more races, non-Hispanic/Latino), 24 international. Average age 27. 36 applicants, 67% accepted, 15 enrolled. In 2013, 9 master's, 5 doctorates awarded. *Degree requirements:* For master's, thesis; for doctorate, comprehensive exam, thesis/dissertation. *Entrance requirements:* For master's, GRE General Test, bachelor's degree in biological science or related disciplines; for doctorate, GRE General Test. Additional exam requirements/recommendations for international students: Required—TOEFL, IELTS. *Application deadline:* Applications are processed on a rolling basis. Electronic applications accepted. *Expenses:* Contact institution. *Financial support:* In 2013–14, 42 students received support, including 3 fellowships with full and partial tuition reimbursements available (averaging $7,333 per year), 25 research assistantships with partial tuition reimbursements available (averaging $15,335 per year), 12 teaching assistantships with partial tuition reimbursements available (averaging $13,163 per year); career-related internships or fieldwork, institutionally sponsored loans, scholarships/grants, health care benefits, and unspecified

assistantships also available. Support available to part-time students. Financial award application deadline: 3/15; financial award applicants required to submit FAFSA. *Faculty research:* Sustainable agroecology, horticulture and turfgrass, physiology and pathology of plants. *Unit head:* Dr. Patricia Layton, School Director, 864-656-3302, Fax: 864-656-3304, E-mail: playton@clemson.edu. *Application contact:* Dr. Halina Knap, Coordinator, 864-656-3523, Fax: 864-656-3443, E-mail: hskrpsk@clemson.edu.
Website: http://www.clemson.edu/cafls/departments/pes/

Cornell University, Graduate School, Graduate Fields of Agriculture and Life Sciences, Field of Plant Biology, Ithaca, NY 14853-0001. Offers cytology (MS, PhD); paleobotany (MS, PhD); plant biochemistry (MS, PhD); plant cell biology (MS, PhD); plant ecology (MS, PhD); plant molecular biology (MS, PhD); plant morphology, anatomy and biomechanics (MS, PhD); plant physiology (MS, PhD); systematic botany (MS, PhD). *Faculty:* 49 full-time (14 women). *Students:* 33 full-time (20 women); includes 5 minority (1 Black or African American, non-Hispanic/Latino; 3 Hispanic/Latino; 1 Two or more races, non-Hispanic/Latino), 16 international. Average age 27. 71 applicants, 23% accepted, 10 enrolled. In 2013, 2 doctorates awarded. *Degree requirements:* For doctorate, comprehensive exam, thesis/dissertation. *Entrance requirements:* For doctorate, GRE General Test, GRE Subject Test in biology (recommended), 3 letters of recommendation. Additional exam requirements/recommendations for international students: Required—TOEFL (minimum score 610 paper-based; 77 iBT). *Application deadline:* For fall admission, 1/15 priority date for domestic students. Application fee: $95. Electronic applications accepted. *Financial support:* In 2013–14, 25 students received support, including 7 fellowships with full tuition reimbursements available, 9 research assistantships with full tuition reimbursements available, 9 teaching assistantships with full tuition reimbursements available; institutionally sponsored loans, scholarships/grants, health care benefits, tuition waivers (full and partial), and unspecified assistantships also available. Financial award applicants required to submit FAFSA. *Faculty research:* Plant cell biology/cytology; plant molecular biology; plant morphology/anatomy/biomechanics; plant physiology, systematic botany, paleobotany; plant ecology, ethnobotany, plant biochemistry, photosynthesis. *Unit head:* Director of Graduate Studies, 607-255-2131. *Application contact:* Graduate Field Assistant, 607-255-2131, E-mail: plbio@cornell.edu.
Website: http://www.gradschool.cornell.edu/fields.php?id-45&a-2

Florida State University, The Graduate School, College of Arts and Sciences, Department of Biological Science, Specialization in Plant Biology, Tallahassee, FL 32306-4295. Offers MS, PhD. *Faculty:* 10 full-time (5 women). *Students:* 13 full-time (6 women); includes 2 minority (both Hispanic/Latino), 5 international. In 2013, 1 master's, 2 doctorates awarded. Terminal master's awarded for partial completion of doctoral program. *Degree requirements:* For master's, comprehensive exam, thesis, teaching experience, seminar presentation; for doctorate, comprehensive exam, thesis/dissertation, teaching experience, seminar presentation. *Entrance requirements:* For master's and doctorate, GRE General Test, minimum upper-division GPA of 3.0. Additional exam requirements/recommendations for international students: Required—TOEFL (minimum score 600 paper-based; 92 iBT). *Application deadline:* For fall admission, 12/1 for domestic and international students. Application fee: $30. Electronic applications accepted. *Expenses:* Tuition, state resident: part-time $403.51 per credit hour. Tuition, nonresident: part-time $1004.85 per credit hour. *Required fees:* $75.81 per credit hour. One-time fee: $20 part-time. Tuition and fees vary according to course load, campus/location and student level. *Financial support:* In 2013–14, 13 students received support, including 5 research assistantships with full tuition reimbursements available (averaging $21,500 per year), 8 teaching assistantships with full tuition reimbursements available (averaging $21,500 per year). Financial award application deadline: 12/1; financial award applicants required to submit FAFSA. *Faculty research:* Plant cell and molecular biology; plant population ecology and evolution; meiosis in higher plants; plant systematics, evolution, ecology, and biogeography; plant-environment interaction; community ecology; plant-insect interactions; rhizobial/plant symbiotic interactions; cell fate specification and reprogramming in plants; evolutionary and developmental biology; plant-environment interaction. *Unit head:* Dr. Debra A. Fadool, Professor and Associate Chairman for Graduate Studies, 850-644-4775, Fax: 850-644-9829, E-mail: dfadool@bio.fsu.edu. *Application contact:* Judy Bowers, Coordinator, Graduate Affairs, 850-644-3023, Fax: 850-644-9829, E-mail: gradinfo@bio.fsu.edu.
Website: http://bio.fsu.edu

Illinois State University, Graduate School, College of Arts and Sciences, Department of Biological Sciences, Normal, IL 61790-2200. Offers animal behavior (MS); bacteriology (MS); biochemistry (MS); biological sciences (MS); biology (PhD); biophysics (MS); biotechnology (MS); botany (MS, PhD); cell biology (MS); conservation biology (MS); developmental biology (MS); ecology (MS, PhD); entomology (MS); evolutionary biology (MS); genetics (MS, PhD); immunology (MS); microbiology (MS, PhD); molecular biology (MS); molecular genetics (MS); neurobiology (MS); neuroscience (MS); parasitology (MS); physiology (MS, PhD); plant biology (MS); plant molecular biology (MS); plant sciences (MS); structural biology (MS); zoology (MS, PhD). Part-time programs available. *Degree requirements:* For master's, thesis or alternative; for doctorate, variable foreign language requirement, thesis/dissertation, 2 terms of residency. *Entrance requirements:* For master's, GRE General Test, minimum GPA of 2.6 in last 60 hours of course work; for doctorate, GRE General Test. *Faculty research:* Redoc balance and drug development in schistosoma mansoni, control of the growth of listeria monocytogenes at low temperature, regulation of cell expansion and microtubule function by SPRI, CRUI: physiology and fitness consequences of different life history phenotypes.

Indiana University Bloomington, University Graduate School, College of Arts and Sciences, Department of Biology, Bloomington, IN 47405. Offers biology teaching (MAT); biotechnology (MA); evolution, ecology, and behavior (MA, PhD); genetics (PhD); microbiology (MA, PhD); molecular, cellular, and developmental biology (PhD); plant sciences (MA, PhD); zoology (MA, PhD). *Faculty:* 58 full-time (15 women), 21 part-time/adjunct (6 women). *Students:* 166 full-time (94 women), 2 part-time (both women); includes 22 minority (8 Black or African American, non-Hispanic/Latino; 3 Asian, non-Hispanic/Latino; 10 Hispanic/Latino; 1 Two or more races, non-Hispanic/Latino), 47 international. Average age 27. 261 applicants, 23% accepted, 32 enrolled. In 2013, 17 master's, 20 doctorates awarded. Terminal master's awarded for partial completion of doctoral program. *Degree requirements:* For master's, thesis, oral defense; for doctorate, thesis/dissertation, oral defense. *Entrance requirements:* For master's and doctorate, GRE General Test. Additional exam requirements/recommendations for international students: Required—TOEFL (minimum score 100 iBT). *Application deadline:* For fall admission, 1/5 priority date for domestic students, 12/1 priority date for international students. Application fee: $55 ($65 for international students). Electronic applications accepted. *Financial support:* In 2013–14, fellowships with tuition reimbursements (averaging $24,000 per year), research assistantships with tuition reimbursements (averaging $21,000 per year), teaching assistantships with tuition reimbursements (averaging $22,000 per year) were awarded; scholarships/grants, traineeships, health care benefits, and unspecified assistantships also available. Financial award application deadline: 1/5. *Faculty research:* Evolution, ecology and behavior; microbiology; molecular biology and genetics; plant biology. *Unit head:* Dr. Clay Fuqua, Chair, 812-856-6005, Fax: 812-855-6082, E-mail: cfuqua@indiana.edu. *Application contact:* Tracey D. Stohr, Graduate Student Recruitment Coordinator, 812-856-6303, Fax: 812-855-6082, E-mail: gradbio@indiana.edu.
Website: http://www.bio.indiana.edu/

Iowa State University of Science and Technology, Program in Plant Biology, Ames, IA 50011. Offers MS, PhD. *Degree requirements:* For master's, thesis; for doctorate, thesis/dissertation. *Entrance requirements:* For master's and doctorate, GRE General Test. Additional exam requirements/recommendations for international students: Required—TOEFL (minimum score 550 paper-based; 79 iBT), IELTS (minimum score 6.5). Electronic applications accepted.

Michigan State University, The Graduate School, College of Agriculture and Natural Resources, MSU-DOE Plant Research Laboratory, East Lansing, MI 48824. Offers biochemistry and molecular biology (PhD); cellular and molecular biology (PhD); crop and soil sciences (PhD); genetics (PhD); microbiology and molecular genetics (PhD); plant biology (PhD); plant physiology (PhD). Offered jointly with the Department of Energy. *Degree requirements:* For doctorate, comprehensive exam, thesis/dissertation, laboratory rotation, defense of dissertation. *Entrance requirements:* For doctorate, GRE General Test, acceptance into one of the affiliated department programs; 3 letters of recommendation; bachelor's degree or equivalent in life sciences, chemistry, biochemistry, or biophysics; research experience. Electronic applications accepted. *Faculty research:* Role of hormones in the regulation of plant development and physiology, molecular mechanisms associated with signal recognition, development and application of genetic methods and materials, protein routing and function.

Michigan State University, The Graduate School, College of Natural Science and College of Agriculture and Natural Resources, Department of Plant Biology, East Lansing, MI 48824. Offers plant biology (MS, PhD); plant breeding, genetics and biotechnology - plant biology (MS, PhD). *Entrance requirements:* Additional exam requirements/recommendations for international students: Required—TOEFL. Electronic applications accepted. *Faculty research:* Physiological, molecular, and biochemical mechanisms; systematics; inheritance; ecology and geohistory.

New York University, Graduate School of Arts and Science, Department of Biology, New York, NY 10012-1019. Offers biology (PhD); biomedical journalism (MS); cancer and molecular biology (PhD); computational biology (PhD); computers in biological research (MS); developmental genetics (PhD); general biology (MS); immunology and microbiology (PhD); molecular genetics (PhD); neurobiology (PhD); oral biology (MS); plant biology (PhD); recombinant DNA technology (MS); MS/MBA. Part-time programs available. *Faculty:* 24 full-time (5 women). *Students:* 161 full-time (88 women), 28 part-time (15 women); includes 41 minority (5 Black or African American, non-Hispanic/Latino; 23 Asian, non-Hispanic/Latino; 9 Hispanic/Latino; 4 Two or more races, non-Hispanic/Latino), 80 international. Average age 27. 412 applicants, 54% accepted, 65 enrolled. In 2013, 77 master's, 9 doctorates awarded. Terminal master's awarded for partial completion of doctoral program. *Degree requirements:* For master's, thesis or alternative, qualifying paper; for doctorate, comprehensive exam, thesis/dissertation. *Entrance requirements:* For master's and doctorate, GRE General Test. Additional exam requirements/recommendations for international students: Required—TOEFL. *Application deadline:* For fall admission, 12/1 priority date for domestic students, 12/1 for international students. Application fee: $95. *Expenses: Tuition:* Full-time $35,856; part-time $1494 per unit. *Required fees:* $1408; $64 per unit. $473 per term. Tuition and fees vary according to course load and program. *Financial support:* Fellowships with tuition reimbursements, research assistantships with tuition reimbursements, teaching assistantships with tuition reimbursements, career-related internships or fieldwork, Federal Work-Study, institutionally sponsored loans, scholarships/grants, health care benefits, and unspecified assistantships available. Financial award application deadline: 12/1; financial award applicants required to submit FAFSA. *Faculty research:* Genomics, molecular and cell biology, development and molecular genetics, molecular evolution of plants and animals. *Unit head:* Stephen Small, Chair, 212-998-8200, Fax: 212-995-4015, E-mail: biology.admissions@nyu.edu. *Application contact:* Justin Blau, Director of Graduate Studies, PhD Programs, 212-998-8200, Fax: 212-995-4015, E-mail: biology.admissions@nyu.edu.
Website: http://biology.as.nyu.edu/

North Carolina State University, Graduate School, College of Agriculture and Life Sciences, Department of Plant Biology, Raleigh, NC 27695. Offers MS, PhD. Part-time programs available. Terminal master's awarded for partial completion of doctoral program. *Degree requirements:* For master's, thesis (for some programs); for doctorate, thesis/dissertation. *Entrance requirements:* For master's and doctorate, GRE. Additional exam requirements/recommendations for international students: Required—TOEFL. Electronic applications accepted. *Faculty research:* Plant molecular and cell biology, aquatic ecology, community ecology, restoration, systematics plant pathogen and environmental interactions.

Northwestern University, The Graduate School, Judd A. and Marjorie Weinberg College of Arts and Sciences, Program in Plant Biology and Conservation, Evanston, IL 60208. Offers MA, PhD. Program held jointly with Chicago Botanic Garden.

Ohio University, Graduate College, College of Arts and Sciences, Department of Environmental and Plant Biology, Athens, OH 45701-2979. Offers MS, PhD. Part-time programs available. *Degree requirements:* For master's, thesis, 2 terms of teaching experience; for doctorate, comprehensive exam, thesis/dissertation, 2 terms of teaching experience. *Entrance requirements:* For master's, GRE General Test, minimum GPA of 3.0; for doctorate, GRE General Test, minimum GPA of 3.2. Additional exam requirements/recommendations for international students: Required—TOEFL (minimum score 620 paper-based; 105 iBT) or IELTS (minimum score 7.5). Electronic applications accepted. *Faculty research:* Eastern deciduous forest ecology, evolutionary developmental plant biology, phylogenetic systematics, plant cell wall biotechnology.

Penn State University Park, Graduate School, Intercollege Graduate Programs, Intercollege Graduate Program in Plant Biology, University Park, PA 16802. Offers MS, PhD. *Unit head:* Dr. Regina Vasilatos-Younken, Interim Dean, 814-865-2516, Fax: 814-863-4627, E-mail: rxv@psu.edu. *Application contact:* Cynthia E. Nicosia, Director, Graduate Enrollment Services, 814-865-1834, Fax: 814-863-4627, E-mail: cey1@psu.edu.

Rutgers, The State University of New Jersey, New Brunswick, Graduate School-New Brunswick, Program in Plant Biology, Piscataway, NJ 08854-8097. Offers horticulture and plant technology (MS, PhD); molecular and cellular biology (MS, PhD); organismal and population biology (MS, PhD); plant pathology (MS, PhD). Part-time programs available. Terminal master's awarded for partial completion of doctoral program. *Degree requirements:* For master's, comprehensive exam, thesis or alternative; for doctorate, comprehensive exam, thesis/dissertation. *Entrance requirements:* For master's and doctorate, GRE General Test, GRE Subject Test (recommended). Additional exam requirements/recommendations for international students: Required—TOEFL (minimum score 600 paper-based). Electronic applications accepted. *Faculty research:* Molecular biology and biochemistry of plants, plant development and genomics, plant protection, plant improvement, plant management of horticultural and field crops.

Southern Illinois University Carbondale, Graduate School, College of Science, Department of Plant Biology, Carbondale, IL 62901-4701. Offers MS, PhD. *Faculty:* 13

full-time (2 women). *Students:* 11 full-time (3 women), 30 part-time (17 women); includes 8 minority (2 Black or African American, non-Hispanic/Latino; 4 Asian, non-Hispanic/Latino; 2 Hispanic/Latino), 4 international. Average age 25. 11 applicants, 55% accepted, 6 enrolled. In 2013, 4 master's, 7 doctorates awarded. *Degree requirements:* For master's, thesis; for doctorate, one foreign language, thesis/dissertation. *Entrance requirements:* For master's, GRE General Test, minimum GPA of 2.7; for doctorate, GRE General Test, minimum GPA of 3.25. Additional exam requirements/recommendations for international students: Required—TOEFL. *Application deadline:* Applications are processed on a rolling basis. Application fee: $50. *Financial support:* In 2013–14, 24 students received support, including 4 fellowships with full tuition reimbursements available, 6 research assistantships with full tuition reimbursements available, 13 teaching assistantships with full tuition reimbursements available; Federal Work-Study, institutionally sponsored loans, and tuition waivers (full) also available. Support available to part-time students. *Faculty research:* Algal toxins, ethnobotany, community and wetland ecology, morphogenesis, systematics and evolution. *Total annual research expenditures:* $524,140. *Unit head:* Dr. Stephen Ebbs, Interim Chair, 618-453-3226, E-mail: sebbs@plant.siu.edu. *Application contact:* David Gibson, Director of Graduate Studies, 618-453-3231, E-mail: dgibson@plant.siu.edu.

Université Laval, Faculty of Agricultural and Food Sciences, Program in Plant Biology, Québec, QC G1K 7P4, Canada. Offers M Sc, PhD. Terminal master's awarded for partial completion of doctoral program. *Degree requirements:* For master's, thesis (for some programs); for doctorate, comprehensive exam, thesis/dissertation. *Entrance requirements:* For master's and doctorate, knowledge of French and English. Electronic applications accepted.

University of Alberta, Faculty of Graduate Studies and Research, Department of Biological Sciences, Edmonton, AB T6G 2E1, Canada. Offers environmental biology and ecology (M Sc, PhD); microbiology and biotechnology (M Sc, PhD); molecular biology and genetics (M Sc, PhD); physiology and cell biology (M Sc, PhD); plant biology (M Sc, PhD); systematics and evolution (M Sc, PhD). Terminal master's awarded for partial completion of doctoral program. *Degree requirements:* For master's, thesis; for doctorate, thesis/dissertation. *Entrance requirements:* Additional exam requirements/recommendations for international students: Required—TOEFL.

University of California, Berkeley, Graduate Division, College of Natural Resources, Department of Plant and Microbial Biology, Berkeley, CA 94720-1500. Offers plant biology (PhD). *Degree requirements:* For doctorate, thesis/dissertation, qualifying exam, seminar presentation. *Entrance requirements:* For doctorate, GRE General Test, minimum GPA of 3.0, 3 letters of recommendation. *Faculty research:* Development, molecular biology, genetics, microbial biology, mycology.

University of California, Davis, Graduate Studies, Graduate Group in Plant Biology, Davis, CA 95616. Offers MS, PhD. *Degree requirements:* For master's, comprehensive exam (for some programs), thesis (for some programs); for doctorate, thesis/dissertation. *Entrance requirements:* For master's, GRE General Test, GRE Subject Test (biology), minimum GPA of 3.0; for doctorate, GRE General Test, GRE Subject Test (biology). Additional exam requirements/recommendations for international students: Required—TOEFL (minimum score 550 paper-based). Electronic applications accepted. *Faculty research:* Cell and molecular biology, ecology, systematics and evolution, integrative plant and crop physiology, plant development and structure.

University of California, Riverside, Graduate Division, Department of Botany and Plant Sciences, Riverside, CA 92521-0102. Offers plant biology (MS, PhD), including plant cell, molecular, and developmental biology (PhD), plant ecology (PhD), plant genetics (PhD). Part-time programs available. *Faculty:* 40 full-time (13 women). *Students:* 66 full-time (40 women); includes 12 minority (5 Asian, non-Hispanic/Latino; 7 Hispanic/Latino), 24 international. Average age 29. In 2013, 3 master's, 3 doctorates awarded. Terminal master's awarded for partial completion of doctoral program. *Degree requirements:* For master's, comprehensive exams or thesis; for doctorate, thesis/dissertation, qualifying exams. *Entrance requirements:* For master's and doctorate, GRE General Test, minimum GPA of 3.2. Additional exam requirements/recommendations for international students: Required—TOEFL (minimum score 550 paper-based; 80 iBT). *Application deadline:* For fall admission, 5/1 for domestic students, 2/1 for international students; for winter admission, 2/1 for domestic students, 7/1 for international students; for spring admission, 12/1 for domestic students, 10/1 for international students. Applications are processed on a rolling basis. Application fee: $80 ($100 for international students). Electronic applications accepted. *Financial support:* In 2013–14, fellowships with tuition reimbursements (averaging $12,000 per year), research assistantships with tuition reimbursements (averaging $23,000 per year), teaching assistantships with tuition reimbursements (averaging $16,500 per year) were awarded; career-related internships or fieldwork, Federal Work-Study, institutionally sponsored loans, scholarships/grants, and tuition waivers (full and partial) also available. *Faculty research:* Agricultural plant biology; biochemistry and physiology; cellular, molecular and developmental biology; ecology, evolution, systematics and ethnobotany; genetics, genomics and bioinformatics. *Unit head:* Dr. Mikeal Roose, Chair, 951-827-4413. *Application contact:* Jammy Yang, Graduate Program Assistant, 800-735-0717, Fax: 951-827-5517, E-mail: deidra.kornfeld@ucr.edu.
Website: http://www.plantbiology.ucr.edu/

University of Connecticut, Graduate School, College of Liberal Arts and Sciences, Department of Molecular and Cell Biology, Field of Plant Cell and Molecular Biology, Storrs, CT 06269. Offers MS, PhD. *Degree requirements:* For doctorate, thesis/dissertation. *Entrance requirements:* For master's and doctorate, GRE General Test, GRE Subject Test. Additional exam requirements/recommendations for international students: Required—TOEFL.

University of Florida, Graduate School, College of Agricultural and Life Sciences and College of Liberal Arts and Sciences, Program in Plant Molecular and Cellular Biology, Gainesville, FL 32611. Offers MS, PhD. *Students:* 28 full-time (16 women); includes 4 minority (1 Black or African American, non-Hispanic/Latino; 2 Asian, non-Hispanic/Latino; 1 Hispanic/Latino), 16 international. Average age 28. 52 applicants, 17% accepted, 5 enrolled. In 2013, 2 master's, 2 doctorates awarded. *Degree requirements:* For master's, thesis; for doctorate, comprehensive exam, thesis/dissertation, first author peer-reviewed publication. *Entrance requirements:* For master's and doctorate, GRE General Test, minimum GPA of 3.0. Additional exam requirements/recommendations for international students: Required—TOEFL (minimum score 550 paper-based; 80 iBT), IELTS (minimum score 6). *Application deadline:* For fall admission, 1/3 priority date for domestic students, 1/3 for international students; for spring admission, 8/1 for domestic and international students. Applications are processed on a rolling basis. Application fee: $30. Electronic applications accepted. *Expenses:* Tuition, state resident: full-time $12,640. Tuition, nonresident: full-time $30,000. *Financial support:* In 2013–14, 27 students received support, including 2 fellowships (averaging $18,550 per year), 35 research assistantships (averaging $14,590 per year); unspecified assistantships also available. Financial award applicants required to submit FAFSA. *Faculty research:* The understanding of molecular and cellular mechanisms that mediate plant development, adaptation, and evolution including bioinformatics, genomics, proteomics, genetics, biochemistry, breeding, physiology and molecular and cellular biology. *Unit head:* A. Mark Settles, PhD, Director, 352-392-7571, Fax: 352-392-4726, E-mail: settles@ufl.edu. *Application contact:* Anna-Lisa Paul, PhD, Graduate Coordinator, 352-273-4855, E-mail: alp@ufl.edu.
Website: http://pmcb.ifas.ufl.edu/

University of Georgia, Franklin College of Arts and Sciences, Department of Plant Biology, Athens, GA 30602. Offers MS, PhD. *Degree requirements:* For master's, thesis; for doctorate, one foreign language, thesis/dissertation. *Entrance requirements:* For master's and doctorate, GRE General Test. Electronic applications accepted.

University of Illinois at Urbana–Champaign, Graduate College, College of Liberal Arts and Sciences, School of Integrative Biology, Department of Plant Biology, Champaign, IL 61820. Offers plant biology (MS, PhD); plant biotechnology (PSM). *Students:* 45 (20 women). Application fee: $75 ($90 for international students). *Unit head:* Feng Sheng Hu, Head, 217-244-2982, Fax: 217-244-7246, E-mail: fhu@illinois.edu. *Application contact:* Rayme T. Dorsey, Office Specialist, 217-333-3261, Fax: 217-244-7246, E-mail: rdorsey@illinois.edu.
Website: http://www.life.illinois.edu/plantbio/

University of Illinois at Urbana–Champaign, Graduate College, College of Liberal Arts and Sciences, School of Integrative Biology, Program in Physiological and Molecular Plant Biology, Champaign, IL 61820. Offers PhD. *Students:* 3 full-time (1 woman), 2 international. Application fee: $75 ($90 for international students). *Unit head:* Stephen Moose, Director, 217-244-6308, Fax: 217-244-1224, E-mail: smoose@illinois.edu. *Application contact:* Kimberly Leigh, Office Manager, 217-333-8208, Fax: 217-244-1224, E-mail: kaleigh@illinois.edu.
Website: http://www.life.illinois.edu/plantbio/pmpb/

University of Maryland, College Park, Academic Affairs, College of Computer, Mathematical and Natural Sciences, Department of Cell Biology and Molecular Genetics, College Park, MD 20742. Offers cell biology and molecular genetics (MS, PhD); molecular and cellular biology (PhD); plant biology (MS, PhD). Part-time and evening/weekend programs available. *Faculty:* 79 full-time (28 women), 3 part-time/adjunct (2 women). *Students:* 42 full-time (24 women), 1 (woman) part-time; includes 7 minority (1 Black or African American, non-Hispanic/Latino; 5 Asian, non-Hispanic/Latino; 1 Hispanic/Latino), 17 international. In 2013, 2 master's, 14 doctorates awarded. Terminal master's awarded for partial completion of doctoral program. *Degree requirements:* For master's, thesis; for doctorate, thesis/dissertation. *Entrance requirements:* For master's, GRE General Test, minimum GPA of 3.0, 3 letters of recommendation; for doctorate, GRE General Test. Additional exam requirements/recommendations for international students: Required—TOEFL. *Application deadline:* For fall admission, 12/15 for domestic and international students. Applications are processed on a rolling basis. Application fee: $75. Electronic applications accepted. *Expenses:* Tuition, state resident: full-time $10,314; part-time $573 per credit hour. Tuition, nonresident: full-time $22,248; part-time $1236 per credit. *Required fees:* $1446; $403.15 per semester. Tuition and fees vary according to program. *Financial support:* In 2013–14, 3 fellowships with full tuition reimbursements (averaging $31,090 per year), 20 research assistantships (averaging $19,508 per year), 25 teaching assistantships (averaging $19,474 per year) were awarded; Federal Work-Study and scholarships/grants also available. Support available to part-time students. Financial award applicants required to submit FAFSA. *Faculty research:* Cytoskeletal activity, membrane biology, cell division, genetics and genomics, virology. *Total annual research expenditures:* $7.7 million. *Unit head:* Norma Andrews, Chair, 301-405-8418, E-mail: andrewsn@umd.edu. *Application contact:* Dr. Charles A. Caramello, Dean of Graduate School, 301-405-0358, Fax: 301-314-9305, E-mail: ccaramel@umd.edu.

University of Massachusetts Amherst, Graduate School, Interdisciplinary Programs, Program in Plant Biology, Amherst, MA 01003. Offers biochemistry and metabolism (MS, PhD); cell biology and physiology (MS, PhD); environmental, ecological and integrative biology (MS, PhD); genetics and evolution (MS, PhD). *Students:* 20 full-time (11 women), 9 international. Average age 28. 72 applicants, 17% accepted, 2 enrolled. In 2013, 1 master's, 2 doctorates awarded. *Degree requirements:* For master's, thesis; for doctorate, 2 foreign languages, comprehensive exam, thesis/dissertation. *Entrance requirements:* For master's and doctorate, GRE General Test. Additional exam requirements/recommendations for international students: Required—TOEFL (minimum score 550 paper-based; 80 iBT), IELTS (minimum score 6.5). *Application deadline:* For fall admission, 12/15 for domestic and international students; for spring admission, 10/1 for domestic and international students. Applications are processed on a rolling basis. Application fee: $75. Electronic applications accepted. *Financial support:* Fellowships with full and partial tuition reimbursements, research assistantships with full and partial tuition reimbursements, teaching assistantships with full and partial tuition reimbursements, career-related internships or fieldwork, Federal Work-Study, scholarships/grants, traineeships, health care benefits, tuition waivers (full and partial), and unspecified assistantships available. Support available to part-time students. Financial award application deadline: 12/15; financial award applicants required to submit FAFSA. *Unit head:* Dr. Elsbeth L. Walker, Graduate Program Director, 413-577-3217, Fax: 413-545-3243, E-mail: pb@bio.umass.edu. *Application contact:* Lindsay DeSantis, Supervisor of Admissions, 413-545-0722, Fax: 413-577-0010, E-mail: gradadm@grad.umass.edu.
Website: http://www.bio.umass.edu/plantbio/

University of Minnesota, Twin Cities Campus, Graduate School, College of Biological Sciences, Program in Plant Biological Sciences, Minneapolis, MN 55455-0213. Offers MS, PhD. Part-time programs available. Terminal master's awarded for partial completion of doctoral program. *Degree requirements:* For master's, thesis or alternative; for doctorate, thesis/dissertation, written and oral preliminary exams. *Entrance requirements:* For master's and doctorate, GRE General Test. Additional exam requirements/recommendations for international students: Required—TOEFL. Electronic applications accepted. *Faculty research:* Cell and molecular biology; plant physiology; plant structure, diversity, and development; ecology, systematics, evolution and genomics.

University of Missouri, Graduate School, College of Agriculture, Food and Natural Resources, Division of Plant Sciences, Columbia, MO 65211. Offers crop, soil and pest management (MS, PhD); entomology (MS, PhD); horticulture (MS, PhD); plant biology and genetics (MS, PhD); plant stress biology (MS, PhD). *Faculty:* 40 full-time (11 women). *Students:* 71 full-time (32 women), 12 part-time (3 women); includes 5 minority (2 Black or African American, non-Hispanic/Latino; 1 American Indian or Alaska Native, non-Hispanic/Latino; 1 Hispanic/Latino; 1 Two or more races, non-Hispanic/Latino), 35 international. Average age 28. 78 applicants, 27% accepted, 17 enrolled. In 2013, 10 master's, 10 doctorates awarded. Terminal master's awarded for partial completion of doctoral program. *Degree requirements:* For master's, thesis; for doctorate, comprehensive exam, thesis/dissertation. *Entrance requirements:* For master's and doctorate, GRE General Test, minimum GPA of 3.0; bachelor's degree from accredited college. Additional exam requirements/recommendations for international students: Required—TOEFL (minimum score 500 paper-based; 61 iBT), IELTS (minimum score 5.5). *Application deadline:* For fall admission, 1/15 priority date for domestic students, 1/15 for international students. Applications are processed on a rolling basis. Application fee: $55 ($75 for international students). Electronic applications accepted. *Financial support:* In 2013–14, 2 fellowships with tuition reimbursements, 59 research assistantships with tuition reimbursements, 1 teaching assistantship with tuition

reimbursement were awarded; institutionally sponsored loans, scholarships/grants, health care benefits, and unspecified assistantships also available. Support available to part-time students. *Faculty research:* Crop, soil and pest management; entomology; horticulture; plant biology and genetics; plant microbiology and pathology. *Unit head:* Dr. Michael Collins, Director, 573-882-1957, E-mail: collinsm@missouri.edu. *Application contact:* Dr. James Schoelz, Director of Graduate Studies, 573-882-1185, E-mail: schoelzj@missouri.edu.
Website: http://plantsci.missouri.edu/graduate/

University of New Hampshire, Graduate School, College of Life Sciences and Agriculture, Department of Biological Sciences, Program in Plant Biology, Durham, NH 03824. Offers MS, PhD. Part-time programs available. *Faculty:* 27 full-time. *Students:* 9 full-time (8 women), 8 part-time (2 women); includes 1 minority (Two or more races, non-Hispanic/Latino), 2 international. Average age 31. 16 applicants, 25% accepted, 3 enrolled. In 2013, 3 master's, 1 doctorate awarded. Terminal master's awarded for partial completion of doctoral program. *Degree requirements:* For master's, thesis; for doctorate, thesis/dissertation. *Entrance requirements:* For master's and doctorate, GRE General Test, GRE Subject Test. Additional exam requirements/recommendations for international students: Required—TOEFL (minimum score 550 paper-based; 80 iBT). *Application deadline:* For fall admission, 6/1 priority date for domestic students, 4/1 for international students; for spring admission, 12/1 for domestic students. Applications are processed on a rolling basis. Application fee: $65. Electronic applications accepted. *Expenses:* Tuition, state resident: full-time $13,500; part-time $750 per credit hour. Tuition, nonresident: full-time $26,200; part-time $1100 per credit hour. *Required fees:* $1741; $435.25 per term. Tuition and fees vary according to course level, course load, campus/location and program. *Financial support:* In 2013–14, 12 students received support, including 1 fellowship, 3 research assistantships, 8 teaching assistantships; career-related internships or fieldwork, Federal Work-Study, scholarships/grants, and tuition waivers (full and partial) also available. Support available to part-time students. Financial award application deadline: 2/15. *Unit head:* Dr. Larry Harris, Chairperson, 603-862-3897. *Application contact:* Diane Lavalliere, Administrative Assistant, 603-862-4095, E-mail: diane.lavallier@unh.edu.
Website: http://www.plant.unh.edu/

The University of Texas at Austin, Graduate School, College of Natural Sciences, School of Biological Sciences, Program in Plant Biology, Austin, TX 78712-1111. Offers MA, PhD. *Entrance requirements:* For master's and doctorate, GRE General Test, minimum GPA of 3.0. Additional exam requirements/recommendations for international students: Required—TOEFL. Electronic applications accepted. *Faculty research:* Systematics, plant molecular biology, psychology, ecology, evolution.

University of Vermont, Graduate College, College of Agriculture and Life Sciences, Department of Plant Biology, Burlington, VT 05405. Offers field naturalist (MS); plant biology (MS, PhD). *Students:* 18 (10 women); includes 1 minority (Asian, non-Hispanic/Latino), 6 international. 34 applicants, 21% accepted, 4 enrolled. In 2013, 10 master's, 2 doctorates awarded. *Entrance requirements:* For master's and doctorate, GRE. Additional exam requirements/recommendations for international students: Required—TOEFL (minimum score 550 paper-based; 80 iBT). *Application deadline:* For fall admission, 12/1 priority date for domestic students, 12/1 for international students. Application fee: $65. Electronic applications accepted. *Unit head:* Dr. David Barrington, Interim Chairperson, 802-656-2930. *Application contact:* Mary Tierney, Director/Coordinator, 802-656-2930.

Washington University in St. Louis, Graduate School of Arts and Sciences, Division of Biology and Biomedical Sciences, Program in Plant Biology, St. Louis, MO 63130-4899. Offers PhD. *Degree requirements:* For doctorate, thesis/dissertation. *Entrance requirements:* For doctorate, GRE General Test, GRE Subject Test. Electronic applications accepted.

Yale University, Graduate School of Arts and Sciences, Department of Molecular, Cellular, and Developmental Biology, Program in Plant Sciences, New Haven, CT 06520. Offers PhD. *Degree requirements:* For doctorate, thesis/dissertation. *Entrance requirements:* For doctorate, GRE General Test, GRE Subject Test.

Plant Molecular Biology

Cornell University, Graduate School, Graduate Fields of Agriculture and Life Sciences, Field of Plant Biology, Ithaca, NY 14853-0001. Offers cytology (MS, PhD); paleobotany (MS, PhD); plant biochemistry (MS, PhD); plant cell biology (MS, PhD); plant ecology (MS, PhD); plant molecular biology (MS, PhD); plant morphology, anatomy and biomechanics (MS, PhD); plant physiology (MS, PhD); systematic botany (MS, PhD). *Faculty:* 49 full-time (14 women). *Students:* 33 full-time (20 women); includes 5 minority (1 Black or African American, non-Hispanic/Latino; 3 Hispanic/Latino; 1 Two or more races, non-Hispanic/Latino), 16 international. Average age 27. 71 applicants, 23% accepted, 10 enrolled. In 2013, 2 doctorates awarded. *Degree requirements:* For doctorate, comprehensive exam, thesis/dissertation. *Entrance requirements:* For doctorate, GRE General Test, GRE Subject Test in biology (recommended), 3 letters of recommendation. Additional exam requirements/recommendations for international students: Required—TOEFL (minimum score 610 paper-based; 77 iBT). *Application deadline:* For fall admission, 1/15 priority date for domestic students. Application fee: $95. Electronic applications accepted. *Financial support:* In 2013–14, 25 students received support, including 7 fellowships with full tuition reimbursements available, 9 research assistantships with full tuition reimbursements available, 9 teaching assistantships with full tuition reimbursements available; institutionally sponsored loans, scholarships/grants, health care benefits, tuition waivers (full and partial), and unspecified assistantships also available. Financial award applicants required to submit FAFSA. *Faculty research:* Plant cell biology/cytology; plant molecular biology; plant morphology/anatomy/biomechanics; plant physiology, systematic botany, paleobotany; plant ecology, ethnobotany, plant biochemistry, photosynthesis. *Unit head:* Director of Graduate Studies, 607-255-2131. *Application contact:* Graduate Field Assistant, 607-255-2131, E-mail: plbio@cornell.edu.
Website: http://www.gradschool.cornell.edu/fields.php?id-45&a-2

Illinois State University, Graduate School, College of Arts and Sciences, Department of Biological Sciences, Normal, IL 61790-2200. Offers animal behavior (MS); bacteriology (MS); biochemistry (MS); biological sciences (MS); biology (PhD); biophysics (MS); biotechnology (MS); botany (MS, PhD); cell biology (MS); conservation biology (MS); developmental biology (MS); ecology (MS, PhD); entomology (MS); evolutionary biology (MS); genetics (MS, PhD); immunology (MS); microbiology (MS, PhD); molecular biology (MS); molecular genetics (MS); neurobiology (MS); neuroscience (MS); parasitology (MS); physiology (MS, PhD); plant biology (MS); plant molecular biology (MS); plant sciences (MS); structural biology (MS); zoology (MS, PhD). Part-time programs available. *Degree requirements:* For master's, thesis or alternative; for doctorate, variable foreign language requirement, thesis/dissertation, 2 terms of residency. *Entrance requirements:* For master's, GRE General Test, minimum GPA of 2.6 in last 60 hours of course work; for doctorate, GRE General Test. *Faculty research:* Redoc balance and drug development in schistosoma mansoni, control of the growth of listeria monocytogenes at low temperature, regulation of cell expansion and microtubule function by SPRI, CRUI: physiology and fitness consequences of different life history phenotypes.

Michigan Technological University, Graduate School, School of Forest Resources and Environmental Science, Houghton, MI 49931. Offers applied ecology (MS); forest ecology and management (MS); forest science (PhD); forestry (MF, MS); molecular genetics and biotechnology (MS, PhD). *Accreditation:* SAF. Part-time programs available. Terminal master's awarded for partial completion of doctoral program. *Degree requirements:* For master's, comprehensive exam (for some programs), thesis (for some programs); for doctorate, comprehensive exam, thesis/dissertation. *Entrance requirements:* For master's and doctorate, GRE (minimum scores: 500 in verbal, 500 quantitative, 3.5 in analytical), statement of purpose, official transcripts, 3 letters of recommendation, resume/curriculum vitae. Additional exam requirements/recommendations for international students: Required—TOEFL (minimum score 79 iBT) or IELTS. Electronic applications accepted. *Faculty research:* Forest molecular genetics and biotechnology, forestry, forest ecology and management, applied ecology, wood science.

Rutgers, The State University of New Jersey, New Brunswick, Graduate School-New Brunswick, Program in Plant Biology, Piscataway, NJ 08854-8097. Offers horticulture and plant technology (MS, PhD); molecular and cellular biology (MS, PhD); organismal and population biology (MS, PhD); plant pathology (MS, PhD). Part-time programs available. Terminal master's awarded for partial completion of doctoral program. *Degree requirements:* For master's, comprehensive exam, thesis or alternative; for doctorate, comprehensive exam, thesis/dissertation. *Entrance requirements:* For master's and doctorate, GRE General Test, GRE Subject Test (recommended). Additional exam requirements/recommendations for international students: Required—TOEFL (minimum score 600 paper-based). Electronic applications accepted. *Faculty research:* Molecular biology and biochemistry of plants, plant development and genomics, plant protection, plant improvement, plant management of horticultural and field crops.

University of California, Riverside, Graduate Division, Department of Botany and Plant Sciences, Riverside, CA 92521-0102. Offers plant biology (MS, PhD), including plant cell, molecular, and developmental biology (PhD), plant ecology (PhD), plant genetics (PhD). Part-time programs available. *Faculty:* 40 full-time (13 women). *Students:* 66 full-time (40 women); includes 12 minority (5 Asian, non-Hispanic/Latino; 7 Hispanic/Latino), 24 international. Average age 29. In 2013, 3 master's, 3 doctorates awarded. Terminal master's awarded for partial completion of doctoral program. *Degree requirements:* For master's, comprehensive exams or thesis; for doctorate, thesis/dissertation, qualifying exams. *Entrance requirements:* For master's and doctorate, GRE General Test, minimum GPA of 3.2. Additional exam requirements/recommendations for international students: Required—TOEFL (minimum score 550 paper-based; 80 iBT). *Application deadline:* For fall admission, 5/1 for domestic students, 2/1 for international students; for winter admission, 2/1 for domestic students, 7/1 for international students; for spring admission, 12/1 for domestic students, 10/1 for international students. Applications are processed on a rolling basis. Application fee: $80 ($100 for international students). Electronic applications accepted. *Financial support:* In 2013–14, fellowships with tuition reimbursements (averaging $12,000 per year), research assistantships with tuition reimbursements (averaging $23,000 per year), teaching assistantships with tuition reimbursements (averaging $16,500 per year) were awarded; career-related internships or fieldwork, Federal Work-Study, institutionally sponsored loans, scholarships/grants, and tuition waivers (full and partial) also available. *Faculty research:* Agricultural plant biology; biochemistry and physiology; cellular, molecular and developmental biology; ecology, evolution, systematics and ethnobotany; genetics, genomics and bioinformatics. *Unit head:* Dr. Mikeal Roose, Chair, 951-827-4413. *Application contact:* Jammy Yang, Graduate Program Assistant, 800-735-0717, Fax: 951-827-5517, E-mail: deidra.kornfeld@ucr.edu.
Website: http://www.plantbiology.ucr.edu/

University of Connecticut, Graduate School, College of Liberal Arts and Sciences, Department of Molecular and Cell Biology, Field of Plant Cell and Molecular Biology, Storrs, CT 06269. Offers MS, PhD. *Degree requirements:* For doctorate, thesis/dissertation. *Entrance requirements:* For master's and doctorate, GRE General Test, GRE Subject Test. Additional exam requirements/recommendations for international students: Required—TOEFL.

University of Florida, Graduate School, College of Agricultural and Life Sciences and College of Liberal Arts and Sciences, Program in Plant Molecular and Cellular Biology, Gainesville, FL 32611. Offers MS, PhD. *Students:* 28 full-time (16 women); includes 4 minority (1 Black or African American, non-Hispanic/Latino; 2 Asian, non-Hispanic/Latino; 1 Hispanic/Latino), 16 international. Average age 28. 52 applicants, 17% accepted, 5 enrolled. In 2013, 2 master's, 2 doctorates awarded. *Degree requirements:* For master's, thesis; for doctorate, comprehensive exam, thesis/dissertation, first author peer-reviewed publication. *Entrance requirements:* For master's and doctorate, GRE General Test, minimum GPA of 3.0. Additional exam requirements/recommendations for international students: Required—TOEFL (minimum score 550 paper-based; 80 iBT), IELTS (minimum score 6). *Application deadline:* For fall admission, 1/3 priority date for domestic students, 1/3 for international students; for spring admission, 8/1 for domestic and international students. Applications are processed on a rolling basis. Application fee: $30. Electronic applications accepted. *Expenses:* Tuition, state resident: full-time $12,640. Tuition, nonresident: full-time $30,000. *Financial support:* In 2013–14, 27 students received support, including 2 fellowships (averaging $18,550 per year), 35 research assistantships (averaging $14,590 per year); unspecified assistantships also available. Financial award applicants required to submit FAFSA. *Faculty research:* The understanding of molecular and cellular mechanisms that mediate plant development, adaptation, and evolution including bioinformatics, genomics, proteomics, genetics, biochemistry, breeding, physiology and molecular and cellular biology. *Unit head:* A. Mark Settles, PhD, Director, 352-392-7571, Fax: 352-392-4726, E-mail: settles@ufl.edu.

Application contact: Anna-Lisa Paul, PhD, Graduate Coordinator, 352-273-4855, E-mail: alp@ufl.edu.
Website: http://pmcb.ifas.ufl.edu/

University of Massachusetts Amherst, Graduate School, Interdisciplinary Programs, Program in Plant Biology, Amherst, MA 01003. Offers biochemistry and metabolism (MS, PhD); cell biology and physiology (MS, PhD); environmental, ecological and integrative biology (MS, PhD); genetics and evolution (MS, PhD). *Students:* 20 full-time (11 women), 9 international. Average age 28. 72 applicants, 17% accepted, 2 enrolled. In 2013, 1 master's, 2 doctorates awarded. *Degree requirements:* For master's, thesis; for doctorate, 2 foreign languages, comprehensive exam, thesis/dissertation. *Entrance requirements:* For master's and doctorate, GRE General Test. Additional exam requirements/recommendations for international students: Required—TOEFL (minimum score 550 paper-based; 80 iBT), IELTS (minimum score 6.5). *Application deadline:* For fall admission, 12/15 for domestic and international students; for spring admission, 10/1 for domestic and international students. Applications are processed on a rolling basis. Application fee: $75. Electronic applications accepted. *Financial support:* Fellowships with full and partial tuition reimbursements, research assistantships with full and partial tuition reimbursements, teaching assistantships with full and partial tuition reimbursements, career-related internships or fieldwork, Federal Work-Study, scholarships/grants, traineeships, health care benefits, tuition waivers (full and partial), and unspecified assistantships available. Support available to part-time students. Financial award application deadline: 12/15; financial award applicants required to submit FAFSA. *Unit head:* Dr. Elsbeth L. Walker, Graduate Program Director, 413-577-3217, Fax: 413-545-3243, E-mail: pb@bio.umass.edu. *Application contact:* Lindsay DeSantis, Supervisor of Admissions, 413-545-0722, Fax: 413-577-0010, E-mail: gradadm@grad.umass.edu.
Website: http://www.bio.umass.edu/plantbio/

Washington State University, Graduate School, College of Agricultural, Human, and Natural Resource Sciences, Molecular Plant Sciences Graduate Program, Pullman, WA 99164. Offers MS, PhD. Terminal master's awarded for partial completion of doctoral program. *Degree requirements:* For master's, comprehensive exam (for some programs), thesis (for some programs), oral exam, written exam; for doctorate, comprehensive exam, thesis/dissertation, oral exam, written exam. *Entrance requirements:* For master's and doctorate, GRE General Test. Additional exam requirements/recommendations for international students: Required—TOEFL, IELTS. *Faculty research:* Cell response to environmental signals, transport of amino acids, regulation of synthesis of defense proteins.

Plant Pathology

Auburn University, Graduate School, College of Agriculture, Department of Entomology and Plant Pathology, Auburn University, AL 36849. Offers entomology (M Ag, MS, PhD); plant pathology (M Ag, MS, PhD). Part-time programs available. *Faculty:* 15 full-time (5 women). *Students:* 25 full-time (10 women), 8 part-time (3 women), 18 international. Average age 29. 23 applicants, 30% accepted, 7 enrolled. In 2013, 5 master's, 4 doctorates awarded. *Degree requirements:* For master's, thesis (for some programs); for doctorate, one foreign language, thesis/dissertation. *Entrance requirements:* For master's, GRE General Test; for doctorate, GRE General Test, GRE Subject Test, master's degree with thesis. *Application deadline:* For fall admission, 7/7 for domestic students; for spring admission, 11/24 for domestic students. Applications are processed on a rolling basis. Application fee: $50 ($60 for international students). Electronic applications accepted. *Expenses:* Tuition, state resident: full-time $8262; part-time $459 per credit hour. Tuition, nonresident: full-time $24,786; part-time $1377 per credit hour. Tuition and fees vary according to degree level and program. *Financial support:* Research assistantships, teaching assistantships, and Federal Work-Study available. Support available to part-time students. Financial award application deadline: 3/15; financial award applicants required to submit FAFSA. *Faculty research:* Pest management, biological control, systematics, medical entomology. *Unit head:* Dr. Arthur Appel, Chair, 334-844-5006. *Application contact:* Dr. George Flowers, Dean of the Graduate School, 334-844-2125.

Colorado State University, Graduate School, College of Agricultural Sciences, Department of Bioagricultural Sciences and Pest Management, Fort Collins, CO 80523-1177. Offers entomology (MS, PhD); plant pathology and weed science (MS, PhD). Part-time programs available. Postbaccalaureate distance learning degree programs offered (minimal on-campus study). *Faculty:* 19 full-time (5 women). *Students:* 12 full-time (9 women), 17 part-time (6 women); includes 3 minority (1 Black or African American, non-Hispanic/Latino; 2 Hispanic/Latino), 5 international. Average age 33. 8 applicants, 63% accepted, 5 enrolled. In 2013, 5 master's, 5 doctorates awarded. *Degree requirements:* For master's, comprehensive exam, thesis; for doctorate, comprehensive exam, thesis/dissertation. *Entrance requirements:* For master's and doctorate, GRE General Test, minimum GPA of 3.0, letters of recommendation, essay, transcripts. Additional exam requirements/recommendations for international students: Required—TOEFL (minimum score 550 paper-based; 79 iBT). *Application deadline:* For fall admission, 1/15 priority date for domestic students, 1/1 priority date for international students; for spring admission, 9/1 priority date for domestic and international students. Applications are processed on a rolling basis. Application fee: $50. Electronic applications accepted. *Expenses:* Tuition, state resident: full-time $9075.40; part-time $504 per credit. Tuition, nonresident: full-time $22,248; part-time $1236 per credit. *Required fees:* $1819; $60 per credit. *Financial support:* In 2013–14, 35 students received support, including 4 fellowships with full tuition reimbursements available (averaging $47,570 per year), 20 research assistantships with full tuition reimbursements available (averaging $14,408 per year), 11 teaching assistantships with full tuition reimbursements available (averaging $13,798 per year). Financial award application deadline: 1/15; financial award applicants required to submit FAFSA. *Faculty research:* Genomics and molecular biology, ecology and biodiversity, biology and management of invasive species, integrated pest management. *Total annual research expenditures:* $3.1 million. *Unit head:* Dr. Thomas O. Holtzer, Department Head and Professor, 970-491-5261, Fax: 970-491-3862, E-mail: thomas.holtzer@colostate.edu. *Application contact:* Janet Dill, Administrative Assistant III, 970-491-0402, Fax: 970-491-3862, E-mail: janet.dill@colostate.edu.
Website: http://bspm.agsci.colostate.edu/

Cornell University, Graduate School, Graduate Fields of Agriculture and Life Sciences, Field of Plant Pathology and Plant-Microbe Biology, Ithaca, NY 14853-0001. Offers fungal and oomycete biology (MPS, MS, PhD); plant microbe pathology (MPS, MS, PhD); plant pathology (MPS, MS, PhD). *Faculty:* 48 full-time (18 women). *Students:* 35 full-time (22 women); includes 5 minority (1 Asian, non-Hispanic/Latino; 3 Hispanic/Latino; 1 Two or more races, non-Hispanic/Latino), 10 international. Average age 28. 44 applicants, 23% accepted, 8 enrolled. In 2013, 3 master's, 3 doctorates awarded. *Degree requirements:* For master's, thesis (MS), project paper (MPS); for doctorate, comprehensive exam, thesis/dissertation. *Entrance requirements:* For master's and doctorate, GRE General Test, GRE Subject Test (biology recommended), 3 letters of recommendation. Additional exam requirements/recommendations for international students: Required—TOEFL (minimum score 550 paper-based; 77 iBT). *Application deadline:* For fall admission, 1/15 priority date for domestic students. Applications are processed on a rolling basis. Application fee: $95. Electronic applications accepted. *Financial support:* In 2013–14, 32 students received support, including 5 fellowships with full tuition reimbursements available, 22 research assistantships with full tuition reimbursements available, 5 teaching assistantships with full tuition reimbursements available; institutionally sponsored loans, scholarships/grants, health care benefits, tuition waivers (full and partial), and unspecified assistantships also available. Financial award applicants required to submit FAFSA. *Faculty research:* Plant pathology; mycology; molecular plant pathology; plant disease epidemiology, ecological and environmental plant pathology; plant disease epidemiology and simulation modeling. *Unit head:* Director of Graduate Studies, 607-255-3259, Fax: 607-255-4471. *Application contact:* Graduate Field Assistant, 607-255-3259, Fax: 607-255-4471, E-mail: plpathology@cornell.edu.
Website: http://www.gradschool.cornell.edu/fields.php?id-59&a-2

Dalhousie University, Faculty of Agriculture, Halifax, NS B3H 4R2, Canada. Offers agriculture (M Sc), including air quality, animal behavior, animal molecular genetics, animal nutrition, animal technology, aquaculture, botany, crop management, crop physiology, ecology, environmental microbiology, food science, horticulture, nutrient management, pest management, physiology, plant biotechnology, plant pathology, soil chemistry, soil fertility, waste management and composting, water quality. Part-time programs available. *Degree requirements:* For master's, thesis, ATC Exam Teaching Assistantship. *Entrance requirements:* For master's, honors B Sc, minimum GPA of 3.0. Additional exam requirements/recommendations for international students: Required—TOEFL (minimum score 580 paper-based; 92 iBT), IELTS, Michigan English Language Assessment Battery, CanTEST, CAEL. *Faculty research:* Bio-product development, organic agriculture, nutrient management, air and water quality, agricultural biotechnology.

Iowa State University of Science and Technology, Department of Plant Pathology, Ames, IA 50011. Offers MS, PhD. *Entrance requirements:* For master's and doctorate, GRE General Test, resume. Additional exam requirements/recommendations for international students: Required—TOEFL (minimum score 550 paper-based; 79 iBT), IELTS (minimum score 6.5). Electronic applications accepted.

Kansas State University, Graduate School, College of Agriculture, Department of Plant Pathology, Manhattan, KS 66506. Offers genetics (MS, PhD); plant pathology (MS, PhD). *Faculty:* 21 full-time (5 women), 5 part-time/adjunct (0 women). *Students:* 30 full-time (10 women); includes 1 minority (Asian, non-Hispanic/Latino), 20 international. Average age 28. 27 applicants, 22% accepted, 3 enrolled. In 2013, 2 doctorates awarded. Terminal master's awarded for partial completion of doctoral program. *Degree requirements:* For master's, thesis, oral exam; for doctorate, thesis/dissertation, preliminary exams. *Entrance requirements:* For master's and doctorate, minimum undergraduate GPA of 3.0. Additional exam requirements/recommendations for international students: Required—TOEFL (minimum score 550 paper-based; 79 iBT). *Application deadline:* For fall admission, 5/15 priority date for domestic students, 11/1 priority date for international students; for spring admission, 10/15 priority date for domestic students, 6/1 priority date for international students; for summer admission, 3/1 for domestic students, 10/18 for international students. Applications are processed on a rolling basis. Application fee: $50 ($75 for international students). Electronic applications accepted. *Financial support:* In 2013–14, 30 research assistantships with full tuition reimbursements (averaging $24,600 per year) were awarded; Federal Work-Study, institutionally sponsored loans, and scholarships/grants also available. Support available to part-time students. Financial award application deadline: 3/1; financial award applicants required to submit FAFSA. *Faculty research:* Applied microbiology, microbial genetics, microbial ecology/epidemiology, integrated pest management, plant genetics/genomics/molecular biology. *Total annual research expenditures:* $6.3 million. *Unit head:* Dr. John Leslie, Head, 785-532-6176, Fax: 785-532-5692, E-mail: jfl@ksu.edu. *Application contact:* Dr. Bill Bockus, Chair of Graduate Selection Committee, 785-532-1378, Fax: 785-532-5692, E-mail: bockus@ksu.edu.
Website: http://www.plantpath.ksu.edu/p.aspx

Louisiana State University and Agricultural & Mechanical College, Graduate School, College of Agriculture, Department of Plant Pathology and Crop Physiology, Baton Rouge, LA 70803. Offers plant health (MS, PhD). *Faculty:* 18 full-time (1 woman). *Students:* 25 full-time (12 women), 2 part-time (1 woman), 19 international. Average age 31. 14 applicants, 29% accepted, 4 enrolled. In 2013, 6 master's, 4 doctorates awarded. Terminal master's awarded for partial completion of doctoral program. *Degree requirements:* For master's, thesis; for doctorate, thesis/dissertation. *Entrance requirements:* For master's and doctorate, GRE General Test, minimum GPA of 3.0. Additional exam requirements/recommendations for international students: Required—TOEFL (minimum score 550 paper-based; 79 IBT), IELTS (minimum score 6.5), or PTE (minimum score 59). *Application deadline:* For fall admission, 1/25 priority date for domestic students, 5/15 for international students; for spring admission, 10/15 for international students. Applications are processed on a rolling basis. Application fee: $50 ($70 for international students). Electronic applications accepted. *Financial support:* In 2013–14, 27 students received support, including 24 research assistantships with partial tuition reimbursements available (averaging $18,160 per year); fellowships, teaching assistantships with partial tuition reimbursements available, career-related internships or fieldwork, Federal Work-Study, health care benefits, and tuition waivers (full) also available. Support available to part-time students. Financial award applicants required to submit FAFSA. *Faculty research:* Plant health and protection, weed biology and management, crop physiology and biotechnology. *Total annual research expenditures:* $5,233. *Unit head:* Dr. Lawrence Datnoff, Chair, 225-578-1464, Fax: 225-763-5573, E-mail: ldatno1@lsu.edu. *Application contact:* Dr. Raymond Schneider, Graduate Adviser, 225-578-4880, Fax: 225-578-1415, E-mail: rschneider@agcenter.lsu.edu.
Website: http://www.lsu.edu/ppcp/

Michigan State University, The Graduate School, College of Agriculture and Natural Resources and College of Natural Science, Department of Plant Pathology, East Lansing, MI 48824. Offers MS, PhD. *Entrance requirements:* Additional exam requirements/recommendations for international students: Required—TOEFL.

Mississippi State University, College of Agriculture and Life Sciences, Department of Biochemistry, Molecular Biology, Entomology and Plant Pathology, Mississippi State, MS 39762. Offers agriculture life sciences (MS), including biochemistry (MS, PhD), entomology (MS, PhD), plant pathology (MS, PhD); life science (PhD), including biochemistry (MS, PhD), entomology (MS, PhD), plant pathology (MS, PhD); molecular biology (PhD). *Faculty:* 23 full-time (1 woman). *Students:* 43 full-time (16 women), 17 part-time (10 women); includes 5 minority (4 Black or African American, non-Hispanic/Latino; 1 Hispanic/Latino), 14 international. Average age 29. 62 applicants, 18% accepted, 10 enrolled. In 2013, 11 master's, 4 doctorates awarded. Terminal master's awarded for partial completion of doctoral program. *Degree requirements:* For master's, thesis (for some programs), final oral exam; for doctorate, thesis/dissertation, preliminary oral and written exam. *Entrance requirements:* For master's, GRE General Test, minimum GPA of 2.75; for doctorate, GRE. Additional exam requirements/recommendations for international students: Required—TOEFL (minimum score 500 paper-based; 61 iBT); Recommended—IELTS (minimum score 5.5). *Application deadline:* For fall admission, 7/1 for domestic students, 5/1 for international students; for spring admission, 11/1 for domestic students, 9/1 for international students. Applications are processed on a rolling basis. Application fee: $60. Electronic applications accepted. *Financial support:* In 2013–14, 35 research assistantships with full tuition reimbursements (averaging $16,388 per year) were awarded; Federal Work-Study, institutionally sponsored loans, and unspecified assistantships also available. Financial award application deadline: 4/1; financial award applicants required to submit FAFSA. *Faculty research:* Fish nutrition, plant and animal molecular biology, plant biochemistry, enzymology, lipid metabolism, chromatin, cell wall synthesis in rice, a model grass bioenergy species and the source of rice stover residues using reverse genetic and functional genomic and proteomic approaches. *Unit head:* Dr. Scott T. Willard, Professor and Department Head, 662-325-2640, Fax: 662-325-8664, E-mail: swilliard@ads.msstate.edu. *Application contact:* Dr. Din-Pow Ma, Professor/Graduate Coordinator, 662-325-7739, Fax: 662-325-8664, E-mail: dm1@ra.msstate.edu.
Website: http://www.biochemistry.msstate.edu

Montana State University, College of Graduate Studies, College of Agriculture, Department of Plant Sciences and Plant Pathology, Bozeman, MT 59717. Offers plant pathology (MS); plant sciences (MS, PhD), including plant genetics (PhD), plant pathology (PhD). Part-time programs available. *Degree requirements:* For master's, comprehensive exam; for doctorate, comprehensive exam, thesis/dissertation. *Entrance requirements:* For master's, GRE General Test, minimum GPA of 3.0; for doctorate, GRE General Test. Additional exam requirements/recommendations for international students: Required—TOEFL (minimum score 550 paper-based). Electronic applications accepted. *Faculty research:* Plant genetics, plant metabolism, plant microbe interactions, plant pathology, entomology research.

New Mexico State University, Graduate School, College of Agricultural, Consumer and Environmental Sciences, Department of Entomology, Plant Pathology and Weed Science, Las Cruces, NM 88003-8001. Offers agricultural biology (MS). Part-time programs available. *Faculty:* 10 full-time (2 women). *Students:* 7 full-time (3 women), 2 part-time (1 woman); includes 2 minority (both Hispanic/Latino), 1 international. Average age 26. 2 applicants, 100% accepted, 2 enrolled. In 2013, 4 master's awarded. *Degree requirements:* For master's, comprehensive exam, thesis. *Entrance requirements:* For master's, GRE General Test. Additional exam requirements/recommendations for international students: Required—TOEFL (minimum score 550 paper-based; 79 iBT), IELTS (minimum score 6.5). *Application deadline:* For fall admission, 7/1 priority date for domestic students; for spring admission, 11/1 priority date for domestic students. Applications are processed on a rolling basis. Application fee: $40 ($50 for international students). Electronic applications accepted. *Expenses:* Tuition, state resident: full-time $5398; part-time $224.90 per credit. Tuition, nonresident: full-time $18,821; part-time $784.20 per credit. *Required fees:* $1310; $54.60 per credit. *Financial support:* In 2013–14, 7 students received support, including 7 research assistantships (averaging $20,908 per year); career-related internships or fieldwork, Federal Work-Study, health care benefits, and unspecified assistantships also available. Financial award application deadline: 3/1. *Faculty research:* Integrated pest management; biology/ecology of plants, insects, nematodes, microorganisms; pesticide metabolism and environmental fate; urban pest management; management of pest resistance to pesticides. *Total annual research expenditures:* $2.7 million. *Unit head:* Dr. Gerald K. Sims, Interim Head, 575-646-3225, Fax: 575-646-8087, E-mail: gksims@nmsu.edu. *Application contact:* Cindy Bullard, Intermediate Administrative Assistant/Recruiting Contact, 575-646-1145, Fax: 575-646-8087, E-mail: cbullard@nmsu.edu.
Website: http://eppws.nmsu.edu/

North Carolina State University, Graduate School, College of Agriculture and Life Sciences, Department of Plant Pathology, Raleigh, NC 27695. Offers MS, PhD. Terminal master's awarded for partial completion of doctoral program. *Degree requirements:* For master's, thesis (for some programs); for doctorate, thesis/dissertation. *Entrance requirements:* For master's and doctorate, GRE. Additional exam requirements/recommendations for international students: Required—TOEFL. Electronic applications accepted. *Faculty research:* Microbe-plant interactions, biology of plant pathogens, pathogen evaluation, host-plant resistance, genomics.

North Dakota State University, College of Graduate and Interdisciplinary Studies, College of Agriculture, Food Systems, and Natural Resources, Department of Plant Pathology, Fargo, ND 58108. Offers MS, PhD. Part-time programs available. *Faculty:* 15 full-time (3 women). *Students:* 40 full-time (19 women), 7 part-time (5 women); includes 3 minority (1 Black or African American, non-Hispanic/Latino; 1 Hispanic/Latino; 1 Two or more races, non-Hispanic/Latino), 28 international. Average age 30. 18 applicants, 61% accepted, 6 enrolled. In 2013, 2 master's, 3 doctorates awarded. *Degree requirements:* For master's, thesis; for doctorate, thesis/dissertation. *Entrance requirements:* Additional exam requirements/recommendations for international students: Required—TOEFL (minimum score 550 paper-based; 79 iBT). *Application deadline:* For fall admission, 5/1 for international students; for winter admission, 8/1 for international students. Applications are processed on a rolling basis. Application fee: $35. Electronic applications accepted. *Financial support:* In 2013–14, 19 research assistantships with full tuition reimbursements were awarded; Federal Work-Study and institutionally sponsored loans also available. Financial award application deadline: 4/15. *Faculty research:* Electron microscopy, disease physiology, molecular biology, genetic resistance, tissue culture. *Unit head:* Dr. Jack Rasmussen, Chair, 701-231-8362, Fax: 701-231-7851, E-mail: jack.rasmussen@ndsu.edu. *Application contact:* Sonya Goergen, Marketing, Recruitment, and Public Relations Coordinator, 701-231-7033, Fax: 701-231-6524.

The Ohio State University, Graduate School, College of Food, Agricultural, and Environmental Sciences, Department of Plant Pathology, Columbus, OH 43210. Offers MPHM, MS, PhD. MPHM offered jointly with Department of Entomology. *Faculty:* 16. *Students:* 29 full-time (15 women), 2 part-time (0 women); includes 4 minority (1 Black or African American, non-Hispanic/Latino; 1 Asian, non-Hispanic/Latino; 1 Hispanic/Latino; 1 Two or more races, non-Hispanic/Latino), 12 international. Average age 28. In 2013, 9 master's, 3 doctorates awarded. *Degree requirements:* For master's, thesis optional; for doctorate, thesis/dissertation. *Entrance requirements:* For master's and doctorate, GRE General Test. Additional exam requirements/recommendations for international students: Required—TOEFL (minimum score 550 paper-based; 79 iBT), Michigan English Language Assessment Battery (minimum score 82); Recommended—IELTS (minimum score 7). *Application deadline:* For fall admission, 12/13 priority date for domestic students, 11/30 priority date for international students; for spring admission, 12/6 for domestic students, 11/11 for international students; for summer admission, 4/4 for domestic students, 3/7 for international students. Applications are processed on a rolling basis. Application fee: $60 ($70 for international students). Electronic applications accepted. *Financial support:* Fellowships with tuition reimbursements, research assistantships with tuition reimbursements, teaching assistantships with tuition reimbursements, Federal Work-Study, and institutionally sponsored loans available. Support available to part-time students. *Unit head:* Laurence Madden, Associate Chair, 330-263-3839, E-mail: madden.1@osu.edu. *Application contact:* Graduate Admissions, 614-292-6031, Fax: 614-292-3656, E-mail: gradadmissions@osu.edu.
Website: http://plantpath.osu.edu/

Oklahoma State University, College of Agricultural Science and Natural Resources, Department of Entomology and Plant Pathology, Stillwater, OK 74078. Offers entomology (PhD); entomology and plant pathology (MS); plant pathology (PhD). *Faculty:* 30 full-time (11 women). *Students:* 5 full-time (3 women), 35 part-time (15 women); includes 5 minority (1 Black or African American, non-Hispanic/Latino; 1 American Indian or Alaska Native, non-Hispanic/Latino; 1 Asian, non-Hispanic/Latino; 1 Hispanic/Latino; 1 Two or more races, non-Hispanic/Latino), 15 international. Average age 30. 22 applicants, 32% accepted, 6 enrolled. In 2013, 5 master's, 4 doctorates awarded. *Degree requirements:* For master's, thesis or alternative; for doctorate, comprehensive exam, thesis/dissertation. *Entrance requirements:* For master's and doctorate, GRE or GMAT. Additional exam requirements/recommendations for international students: Required—TOEFL (minimum score 550 paper-based; 79 iBT). *Application deadline:* For fall admission, 3/1 priority date for international students; for spring admission, 8/1 priority date for international students. Applications are processed on a rolling basis. Application fee: $40 ($75 for international students). Electronic applications accepted. *Expenses:* Tuition, state resident: full-time $4272; part-time $178 per credit hour. Tuition, nonresident: full-time $17,472; part-time $709 per credit hour. *Required fees:* $2413.20; $100.55 per credit hour. One-time fee: $50 full-time. Part-time tuition and fees vary according to course load and campus/location. *Financial support:* In 2013–14, 36 research assistantships (averaging $17,554 per year), 1 teaching assistantship (averaging $18,504 per year) were awarded; career-related internships or fieldwork, Federal Work-Study, scholarships/grants, health care benefits, tuition waivers (partial), and unspecified assistantships also available. Support available to part-time students. Financial award application deadline: 3/1; financial award applicants required to submit FAFSA. *Unit head:* Dr. Phillip Mulder, Jr., Department Head, 405-744-5527, Fax: 405-744-6039, E-mail: phil.mulder@okstate.edu. *Application contact:* Dr. Brad Kard, Graduate Coordinator, 405-744-2142, Fax: 405-744-6039, E-mail: brad.kard@okstate.edu.
Website: http://entoplp.okstate.edu/

Penn State University Park, Graduate School, College of Agricultural Sciences, Department of Plant Pathology and Environmental Microbiology, University Park, PA 16802. Offers plant pathology (MS, PhD). *Unit head:* Dr. Barbara J. Christ, Interim Dean, 814-865-2541, Fax: 814-865-3103, E-mail: ebf@psu.edu. *Application contact:* Cynthia E. Nicosia, Director of Graduate Enrollment Services, 814-865-1834, Fax: 814-863-4627, E-mail: cey1@psu.edu.
Website: http://plantpath.psu.edu/

Purdue University, Graduate School, College of Agriculture, Department of Botany and Plant Pathology, West Lafayette, IN 47907. Offers MS, PhD. Part-time programs available. *Faculty:* 20 full-time (7 women), 2 part-time/adjunct (1 woman). *Students:* 43 full-time (21 women), 3 part-time (1 woman); includes 1 minority (Asian, non-Hispanic/Latino), 21 international. Average age 27. 61 applicants, 21% accepted, 6 enrolled. In 2013, 9 master's, 4 doctorates awarded. Terminal master's awarded for partial completion of doctoral program. *Degree requirements:* For master's, thesis; for doctorate, thesis/dissertation. *Entrance requirements:* For master's, GRE General Test, minimum undergraduate GPA of 3.0 or equivalent; for doctorate, GRE, minimum undergraduate GPA of 3.0 or equivalent. Additional exam requirements/recommendations for international students: Required—TOEFL (minimum score 550 paper-based; 77 iBT); Recommended—TWE. *Application deadline:* For fall admission, 4/15 priority date for domestic and international students; for spring admission, 12/15 for domestic students, 9/15 for international students; for summer admission, 4/15 for domestic students, 2/15 for international students. Applications are processed on a rolling basis. Application fee: $60 ($75 for international students). Electronic applications accepted. *Financial support:* In 2013–14, 30 students received support. Fellowships with full tuition reimbursements available, research assistantships with full tuition reimbursements available, teaching assistantships with full tuition reimbursements available, and career-related internships or fieldwork available. Support available to part-time students. Financial award application deadline: 3/1; financial award applicants required to submit FAFSA. *Faculty research:* Biotechnology, plant growth, weed control, crop improvement, plant physiology. *Unit head:* Dr. Peter B. Goldsbrough, Head, 765-494-4615, Fax: 765-494-0363, E-mail: goldsbrough@purdue.edu. *Application contact:* Tyson J. McFall, Graduate Contact, 765-494-0352, E-mail: tjmcfall@purdue.edu.
Website: https://ag.purdue.edu/btny

Rutgers, The State University of New Jersey, New Brunswick, Graduate School-New Brunswick, Program in Plant Biology, Piscataway, NJ 08854-8097. Offers horticulture and plant technology (MS, PhD); molecular and cellular biology (MS, PhD); organismal and population biology (MS, PhD); plant pathology (MS, PhD). Part-time programs available. Terminal master's awarded for partial completion of doctoral program. *Degree requirements:* For master's, comprehensive exam, thesis or alternative; for doctorate, comprehensive exam, thesis/dissertation. *Entrance requirements:* For master's and doctorate, GRE General Test, GRE Subject Test (recommended). Additional exam requirements/recommendations for international students: Required—TOEFL (minimum score 600 paper-based). Electronic applications accepted. *Faculty research:* Molecular biology and biochemistry of plants, plant development and genomics, plant protection, plant improvement, plant management of horticultural and field crops.

State University of New York College of Environmental Science and Forestry, Department of Environmental and Forest Biology, Syracuse, NY 13210-2779. Offers applied ecology (MPS); chemical ecology (MPS, MS, PhD); conservation biology (MPS, MS, PhD); ecology (MPS, MS, PhD); entomology (MPS, MS, PhD); environmental interpretation (MPS, MS, PhD); environmental physiology (MPS, MS, PhD); fish and wildlife biology and management (MPS, MS, PhD); forest pathology and mycology (MPS, MS, PhD); plant biotechnology (MPS); plant science and biotechnology (MPS, MS, PhD). *Faculty:* 32 full-time (10 women). *Students:* 105 full-time (54 women), 31 part-time (16 women); includes 9 minority (2 Black or African American, non-Hispanic/Latino; 3 American Indian or Alaska Native, non-Hispanic/Latino; 2 Hispanic/Latino; 1 Native

Hawaiian or other Pacific Islander, non-Hispanic/Latino; 1 Two or more races, non-Hispanic/Latino), 17 international. Average age 28. In 2013, 15 master's, 7 doctorates awarded. *Degree requirements:* For master's, thesis (for some programs), capstone seminar; for doctorate, comprehensive exam, thesis/dissertation, capstone seminar. *Entrance requirements:* For master's and doctorate, GRE General Test, minimum GPA of 3.0. Additional exam requirements/recommendations for international students: Required—TOEFL (minimum score 550 paper-based; 80 iBT), IELTS (minimum score 6). *Application deadline:* For fall admission, 2/1 priority date for domestic and international students; for spring admission, 11/1 priority date for domestic and international students. Applications are processed on a rolling basis. Application fee: $60. *Expenses:* Tuition, state resident: full-time $10,370; part-time $432 per credit hour. Tuition, nonresident: full-time $20,190; part-time $841 per credit hour. *Required fees:* $44 per credit hour. *Financial support:* In 2013–14, 4 fellowships with full and partial tuition reimbursements, 36 research assistantships with full and partial tuition reimbursements, 39 teaching assistantships with full and partial tuition reimbursements (averaging $11,490 per year) were awarded; Federal Work-Study, institutionally sponsored loans, scholarships/grants, health care benefits, and unspecified assistantships also available. Financial award application deadline: 6/30. *Faculty research:* Ecology, conservation biology, fish and wildlife biology and management, plant science, entomology. *Total annual research expenditures:* $4.1 million. *Unit head:* Dr. Donald J. Leopold, Chair, 315-470-6760, Fax: 315-470-6934, E-mail: djleopold@esf.edu. *Application contact:* Dr. Danilo D. Fernando, Director, Graduate Program/Associate Professor, 315-470-6746, Fax: 315-470-6934, E-mail: dfernando@esf.edu.
Website: http://www.esf.edu/efb/grad/default.asp

Texas A&M University, College of Agriculture and Life Sciences, Department of Plant Pathology and Microbiology, College Station, TX 77843. Offers MS, PhD. Part-time programs available. Postbaccalaureate distance learning degree programs offered. *Faculty:* 14. *Students:* 22 full-time (8 women), 12 part-time (9 women); includes 6 minority (2 Black or African American, non-Hispanic/Latino; 2 Asian, non-Hispanic/Latino; 2 Hispanic/Latino), 11 international. Average age 29. 39 applicants, 26% accepted, 8 enrolled. In 2013, 9 master's, 6 doctorates awarded. *Degree requirements:* For master's, comprehensive exam (for some programs), thesis; for doctorate, comprehensive exam, thesis/dissertation. *Entrance requirements:* For master's and doctorate, GRE General Test, letters of recommendation, BS/BA in biological sciences. *Application deadline:* Applications are processed on a rolling basis. Application fee: $50 ($75 for international students). *Expenses:* Tuition, state resident: full-time $4078; part-time $226.55 per credit hour. Tuition, nonresident: full-time $10,450; part-time $580.55 per credit hour. *Required fees:* $2328; $278.50 per credit hour. $642.45 per semester. *Financial support:* In 2013–14, research assistantships with partial tuition reimbursements (averaging $16,800 per year), teaching assistantships with partial tuition reimbursements (averaging $16,800 per year) were awarded; fellowships, career-related internships or fieldwork, Federal Work-Study, institutionally sponsored loans, and unspecified assistantships also available. Support available to part-time students. Financial award application deadline: 4/1; financial award applicants required to submit FAFSA. *Faculty research:* Plant disease control, population biology of plant pathogens, disease epidemiology, molecular genetics of host/parasite interactions. *Unit head:* Leland S. Pierson, III, Professor and Department Head, 979-845-8288, Fax: 979-845-6483, E-mail: lspierson@tamu.edu. *Application contact:* Dr. Wo-Bo Shim, Associate Professor, 979-458-2190, E-mail: wbshim@tamu.edu.
Website: http://plantpathology.tamu.edu/

The University of Arizona, College of Agriculture and Life Sciences, School of Plant Sciences, Program in Plant Pathology, Tucson, AZ 85721. Offers MS, PhD. Part-time programs available. *Faculty:* 19 full-time (5 women), 1 part-time/adjunct (0 women). *Students:* 10 full-time (6 women); includes 4 minority (2 Asian, non-Hispanic/Latino; 2 Two or more races, non-Hispanic/Latino), 2 international. Average age 29. 16 applicants, 19% accepted, 2 enrolled. In 2013, 1 master's, 3 doctorates awarded. *Degree requirements:* For master's, thesis optional; for doctorate, thesis/dissertation. *Entrance requirements:* For master's, GRE (recommended), minimum GPA of 3.0, academic resume, 3 letters of recommendation; for doctorate, GRE (recommended), minimum GPA of 3.0, academic resume, statement of purpose, 3 letters of recommendation. Additional exam requirements/recommendations for international students: Required—TOEFL (minimum score 550 paper-based; 79 iBT). *Application deadline:* For fall admission, 12/1 for domestic and international students; for spring admission, 6/1 for domestic and international students. Applications are processed on a rolling basis. Application fee: $75. Electronic applications accepted. *Expenses:* Tuition, state resident: full-time $11,526. Tuition, nonresident: full-time $27,398. *Financial support:* In 2013–14, 8 research assistantships with full tuition reimbursements (averaging $19,951 per year), 10 teaching assistantships with full tuition reimbursements (averaging $20,520 per year) were awarded; fellowships, Federal Work-Study, and institutionally sponsored loans also available. *Faculty research:* Fungal molecular biology, ecology of soil-borne plant pathogens, plant virology, plant bacteriology, plant/pathogen interactions. *Total annual research expenditures:* $8 million. *Unit head:* Dr. Karen Schumaker, Director, 520-621-9635, Fax: 520-621-7186, E-mail: schumake@email.arizona.edu. *Application contact:* Georgina Lambert, Graduate Coordinator, 520-621-1219, Fax: 520-621-7186, E-mail: georgina@cals.arizona.edu.
Website: http://cals.arizona.edu/spls/graduate

University of Arkansas, Graduate School, Dale Bumpers College of Agricultural, Food and Life Sciences, Department of Plant Pathology, Fayetteville, AR 72701-1201. Offers MS. *Degree requirements:* For master's, thesis. Electronic applications accepted.

University of California, Davis, Graduate Studies, Program in Plant Pathology, Davis, CA 95616. Offers MS, PhD. Terminal master's awarded for partial completion of doctoral program. *Degree requirements:* For master's, comprehensive exam (for some programs), thesis (for some programs); for doctorate, thesis/dissertation. *Entrance requirements:* For master's and doctorate, GRE General Test. Additional exam requirements/recommendations for international students: Required—TOEFL (minimum score 550 paper-based). Electronic applications accepted. *Faculty research:* Soil microbiology; diagnosis etiology and control of plant diseases; genomics and molecular biology of plant microbe interactions; biotechnology, ecology of plant pathogens and epidemiology of diseases in agricultural and native ecosystems.

University of California, Riverside, Graduate Division, Department of Plant Pathology, Riverside, CA 92521-0102. Offers MS, PhD. *Faculty:* 15 full-time (3 women). *Students:* 15 full-time (6 women); includes 3 minority (1 Asian, non-Hispanic/Latino; 2 Hispanic/Latino), 10 international. Average age 30. 21 applicants, 19% accepted, 2 enrolled. In 2013, 1 master's, 3 doctorates awarded. Terminal master's awarded for partial completion of doctoral program. *Degree requirements:* For master's, comprehensive exams or thesis; for doctorate, thesis/dissertation, qualifying exams. *Entrance requirements:* For master's and doctorate, GRE General Test (minimum score 1100 or approximately 300 on new scoring scale), minimum GPA of 3.2. Additional exam requirements/recommendations for international students: Required—TOEFL (minimum score 550 paper-based; 80 iBT). *Application deadline:* For fall admission, 5/1 for domestic students, 2/1 for international students; for winter admission, 9/1 for domestic students, 7/1 for international students; for spring admission, 12/1 for domestic students, 10/1 for international students. Applications are processed on a rolling basis. Application fee: $85 ($100 for international students). Electronic applications accepted. *Financial support:* In 2013–14, 7 students received support, including fellowships with full and partial tuition reimbursements available (averaging $12,000 per year), research assistantships with full and partial tuition reimbursements available (averaging $18,081 per year), teaching assistantships with full and partial tuition reimbursements available (averaging $16,500 per year); career-related internships or fieldwork, institutionally sponsored loans, scholarships/grants, health care benefits, tuition waivers (full and partial), and unspecified assistantships also available. *Faculty research:* Host-pathogen interactions, biological control and integrated approaches to disease management, fungicide behavior, molecular genetics. *Unit head:* Dr. Katherine Borkovich, Chair, 951-827-2753. *Application contact:* Jammy Yang, Student Affairs Officer, 800-735-0717, Fax: 951-827-5688, E-mail: plantpa@urc.edu.
Website: http://www.plantpathology.ucr.edu/

University of Florida, Graduate School, College of Agricultural and Life Sciences, Department of Plant Pathology, Gainesville, FL 32611. Offers MS, PhD. Part-time programs available. *Faculty:* 34 full-time (8 women), 6 part-time/adjunct (2 women). *Students:* 38 full-time (20 women), 4 part-time (2 women); includes 5 minority (1 Asian, non-Hispanic/Latino; 4 Hispanic/Latino), 27 international. Average age 30. 46 applicants, 20% accepted, 9 enrolled. In 2013, 6 master's, 3 doctorates awarded. Terminal master's awarded for partial completion of doctoral program. *Degree requirements:* For master's, comprehensive exam (for some programs), thesis optional; for doctorate, comprehensive exam, thesis/dissertation. *Entrance requirements:* For master's and doctorate, GRE General Test, minimum GPA of 3.0. Additional exam requirements/recommendations for international students: Required—TOEFL (minimum score 550 paper-based; 80 iBT), IELTS (minimum score 6). *Application deadline:* For fall admission, 2/1 priority date for domestic students, 2/1 for international students; for winter admission, 2/1 for domestic and international students; for spring admission, 10/1 for domestic students, 9/1 for international students. Applications are processed on a rolling basis. Application fee: $30. Electronic applications accepted. *Expenses:* Tuition, state resident: full-time $12,640. Tuition, nonresident: full-time $30,000. *Financial support:* In 2013–14, 30 students received support, including 1 fellowship (averaging $21,525 per year), 34 research assistantships (averaging $17,000 per year); career-related internships or fieldwork also available. Financial award application deadline: 2/1; financial award applicants required to submit FAFSA. *Faculty research:* Epidemiology, molecular biology of host-parasite interactions, bacteriology, virology, post-harvest diseases. *Unit head:* Rosemary Loria, PhD, Chair, 352-273-4634, Fax: 352-392-6532, E-mail: loria@ufl.edu. *Application contact:* Jeffrey B. Jones, PhD, Graduate Coordinator, 352-273-4673 Ext. 213, Fax: 352-392-6532, E-mail: jbjones@ufl.edu.
Website: http://plantpath.ifas.ufl.edu/

University of Georgia, College of Agricultural and Environmental Sciences, Department of Plant Pathology, Athens, GA 30602. Offers MS, PhD. *Degree requirements:* For master's, thesis (MS); for doctorate, one foreign language, thesis/dissertation. *Entrance requirements:* For master's and doctorate, GRE General Test. Electronic applications accepted.

University of Guelph, Graduate Studies, Ontario Agricultural College, Department of Environmental Biology, Guelph, ON N1G 2W1, Canada. Offers entomology (M Sc, PhD); environmental microbiology and biotechnology (M Sc, PhD); environmental toxicology (M Sc, PhD); plant and forest systems (M Sc, PhD); plant pathology (M Sc, PhD). Part-time programs available. *Degree requirements:* For master's, thesis; for doctorate, comprehensive exam, thesis/dissertation. *Entrance requirements:* For master's, minimum 75% average during previous 2 years of course work; for doctorate, minimum 75% average. Additional exam requirements/recommendations for international students: Required—TOEFL or IELTS. Electronic applications accepted. *Faculty research:* Entomology, environmental microbiology and biotechnology, environmental toxicology, forest ecology, plant pathology.

University of Hawaii at Manoa, Graduate Division, College of Tropical Agriculture and Human Resources, Department of Plant and Environmental Protection Sciences, Program in Tropical Plant Pathology, Honolulu, HI 96822. Offers MS, PhD. Part-time programs available. *Degree requirements:* For master's, thesis optional; for doctorate, comprehensive exam, thesis/dissertation. *Entrance requirements:* For master's and doctorate, GRE General Test. Additional exam requirements/recommendations for international students: Required—TOEFL (minimum score 540 paper-based; 76 iBT), IELTS (minimum score 5).

University of Kentucky, Graduate School, College of Agriculture, Food and Environment, Program in Plant Pathology, Lexington, KY 40506-0032. Offers MS, PhD. *Degree requirements:* For master's, comprehensive exam, thesis; for doctorate, comprehensive exam, thesis/dissertation. *Entrance requirements:* For master's, GRE General Test, minimum undergraduate GPA of 2.75; for doctorate, GRE General Test, minimum graduate GPA of 3.0. Additional exam requirements/recommendations for international students: Required—TOEFL (minimum score 550 paper-based). Electronic applications accepted. *Faculty research:* Molecular biology of viruses and fungi, biochemistry and physiology of disease resistance, plant transformation, disease ecology, forest pathology.

University of Maine, Graduate School, College of Natural Sciences, Forestry, and Agriculture, School of Biology and Ecology, Orono, ME 04469. Offers biological sciences (PhD); botany and plant pathology (MS); ecology and environmental science (MS, PhD); entomology (MS); plant science (PhD); zoology (MS, PhD). Part-time programs available. *Faculty:* 33 full-time (13 women), 26 part-time/adjunct (5 women). *Students:* 66 full-time (40 women), 4 part-time (2 women); includes 4 minority (1 American Indian or Alaska Native, non-Hispanic/Latino; 2 Asian, non-Hispanic/Latino; 1 Hispanic/Latino), 7 international. Average age 30. 97 applicants, 25% accepted, 17 enrolled. In 2013, 8 master's, 3 doctorates awarded. Terminal master's awarded for partial completion of doctoral program. *Degree requirements:* For master's, thesis (for some programs); for doctorate, comprehensive exam, thesis/dissertation. *Entrance requirements:* For master's and doctorate, GRE General Test. Additional exam requirements/recommendations for international students: Required—TOEFL. *Application deadline:* For fall admission, 2/1 priority date for domestic students. Applications are processed on a rolling basis. Application fee: $65. Electronic applications accepted. *Expenses:* Tuition, state resident: full-time $7524. Tuition, nonresident: full-time $23,112. *Required fees:* $1970. *Financial support:* In 2013–14, 66 students received support, including 3 fellowships with full tuition reimbursements available (averaging $25,000 per year), 28 research assistantships with full tuition reimbursements available (averaging $14,600 per year), 21 teaching assistantships with full tuition reimbursements available (averaging $14,600 per year); career-related internships or fieldwork, Federal Work-Study, institutionally sponsored loans, and tuition waivers (full and partial) also available. Financial award application deadline: 3/1. *Total annual research expenditures:* $569,533. *Unit head:* Dr. Ellie Groden, Director, 207-581-2551, Fax: 207-581-2537. *Application contact:* Scott G. Delcourt, Associate Dean of the Graduate School, 207-581-3291, Fax: 207-581-3232, E-mail: graduate@maine.edu.
Website: http://sbe.umaine.edu/

University of Minnesota, Twin Cities Campus, Graduate School, College of Food, Agricultural and Natural Resource Sciences, Department of Plant Pathology, Saint Paul,

MN 55108. Offers MS, PhD. Part-time programs available. *Faculty:* 17 full-time (7 women), 10 part-time/adjunct (3 women). *Students:* 19 full-time (6 women), 2 part-time (both women); includes 5 minority (all Asian, non-Hispanic/Latino), 4 international. 18 applicants, 33% accepted, 6 enrolled. In 2013, 1 master's, 5 doctorates awarded. Terminal master's awarded for partial completion of doctoral program. *Degree requirements:* For master's, comprehensive exam, thesis; for doctorate, comprehensive exam, thesis/dissertation. *Entrance requirements:* For master's and doctorate, GRE General Test. Additional exam requirements/recommendations for international students: Required—TOEFL (minimum score 550 paper-based; 79 iBT), IELTS (minimum score 6.5). *Application deadline:* For fall admission, 1/10 priority date for domestic and international students; for spring admission, 5/1 priority date for domestic students, 5/10 priority date for international students. Applications are processed on a rolling basis. Application fee: $75 ($95 for international students). Electronic applications accepted. *Financial support:* In 2013–14, 2 students received support, including fellowships with full tuition reimbursements available (averaging $40,000 per year), research assistantships with full and partial tuition reimbursements available (averaging $40,000 per year), teaching assistantships with full and partial tuition reimbursements available (averaging $40,000 per year); career-related internships or fieldwork, scholarships/grants, traineeships, health care benefits, and unspecified assistantships also available. Support available to part-time students. Financial award application deadline: 1/10. *Faculty research:* Plant disease management, disease resistance, product deterioration, international agriculture, molecular biology. *Total annual research expenditures:* $2,915. *Unit head:* Dr. Robert Blanchette, Director of Graduate Studies, 612-625-4735, Fax: 612-625-0202, E-mail: robertb@umn.edu. *Application contact:* Anne Lageson, Program Coordinator, 612-625-8200, Fax: 612-625-9728, E-mail: lages001@umn.edu.
Website: http://plpa.cfans.umn.edu/

The University of Tennessee, Graduate School, College of Agricultural Sciences and Natural Resources, Department of Entomology and Plant Pathology, Knoxville, TN 37996. Offers entomology (MS, PhD); integrated pest management and bioactive natural products (PhD); plant pathology (MS, PhD). Part-time programs available. *Degree requirements:* For master's, thesis, seminar. *Entrance requirements:* For master's, GRE General Test, minimum GPA of 2.7, 3 reference letters, letter of intent; for doctorate, GRE General Test, minimum GPA of 2.7, 3 reference letters, letter of intent, proposed dissertation research. Additional exam requirements/recommendations for international students: Required—TOEFL. Electronic applications accepted. *Expenses:* Tuition, state resident: full-time $9540; part-time $531 per credit hour. Tuition, nonresident: full-time $27,728; part-time $1542 per credit hour. *Required fees:* $1404; $67 per credit hour.

University of Wisconsin–Madison, Graduate School, College of Agricultural and Life Sciences, Department of Plant Pathology, Madison, WI 53706-1380. Offers MS, PhD. Part-time programs available. Terminal master's awarded for partial completion of doctoral program. *Degree requirements:* For master's, thesis; for doctorate, thesis/dissertation. *Entrance requirements:* For master's and doctorate, GRE. Additional exam requirements/recommendations for international students: Required—TOEFL. Electronic applications accepted. *Expenses:* Tuition, state resident: full-time $10,728; part-time $790 per credit. Tuition, nonresident: full-time $24,054; part-time $1623 per credit. *Required fees:* $1130; $119 per credit. *Faculty research:* Plant disease, plant health, plant-microbe interactions, plant disease management, biological control.

Virginia Polytechnic Institute and State University, Graduate School, College of Agriculture and Life Sciences, Blacksburg, VA 24061. Offers agricultural and applied economics (MS); agricultural and life sciences (MS); animal and poultry science (MS, PhD); crop and soil environmental sciences (MS, PhD); dairy science (MS); entomology (PhD); horticulture (MS, PhD); human nutrition, foods and exercise (MS, PhD); life sciences (MS, PhD); plant pathology, physiology and weed science (PhD). *Faculty:* 234 full-time (66 women), 1 (woman) part-time/adjunct. *Students:* 347 full-time (188 women), 80 part-time (53 women); includes 53 minority (19 Black or African American, non-Hispanic/Latino; 1 American Indian or Alaska Native, non-Hispanic/Latino; 19 Asian, non-Hispanic/Latino; 7 Hispanic/Latino; 7 Two or more races, non-Hispanic/Latino), 106 international. Average age 29. 410 applicants, 35% accepted, 111 enrolled. In 2013, 80 master's, 44 doctorates awarded. *Degree requirements:* For master's, comprehensive exam (for some programs), thesis (for some programs); for doctorate, comprehensive exam (for some programs), thesis/dissertation (for some programs). *Entrance requirements:* For master's and doctorate, GRE/GMAT (may vary by department). Additional exam requirements/recommendations for international students: Required—TOEFL (minimum score 550 paper-based). *Application deadline:* For fall admission, 8/1 for domestic students, 4/1 for international students; for spring admission, 1/1 for domestic students, 9/1 for international students. Applications are processed on a rolling basis. Application fee: $75. Electronic applications accepted. *Expenses:* Tuition, state resident: full-time $11,185; part-time $621.50 per credit hour. Tuition, nonresident: full-time $22,146; part-time $1230.25 per credit hour. *Required fees:* $2442; $449.25 per semester. Tuition and fees vary according to course load, campus/location and program. *Financial support:* In 2013–14, 1 fellowship with full tuition reimbursement (averaging $19,278 per year), 232 research assistantships with full tuition reimbursements (averaging $19,370 per year), 83 teaching assistantships with full tuition reimbursements (averaging $18,677 per year) were awarded. Financial award application deadline: 3/1; financial award applicants required to submit FAFSA. *Total annual research expenditures:* $44.3 million. *Unit head:* Dr. Alan L. Grant, Dean, 540-231-4152, Fax: 540-231-4163, E-mail: algrant@vt.edu. *Application contact:* Sheila Norman, Administrative Assistant, 540-231-4152, Fax: 540-231-4163, E-mail: snorman@vt.edu.
Website: http://www.cals.vt.edu/

Washington State University, Graduate School, College of Agricultural, Human, and Natural Resource Sciences, Department of Plant Pathology, Pullman, WA 99164. Offers MS, PhD. Terminal master's awarded for partial completion of doctoral program. *Degree requirements:* For master's, comprehensive exam (for some programs), thesis (for some programs), oral exam; for doctorate, comprehensive exam, thesis/dissertation, oral exam. *Entrance requirements:* For master's and doctorate, GRE, statement of purpose. Additional exam requirements/recommendations for international students: Required—TOEFL (minimum score 550 paper-based), IELTS. Electronic applications accepted. *Faculty research:* Biology of fungi, bacteria, and viruses; diseases of plants; genetics of fungi, bacteria, and viruses.

West Virginia University, Davis College of Agriculture, Forestry and Consumer Sciences, Division of Plant and Soil Sciences, Morgantown, WV 26506. Offers agricultural sciences (PhD), including animal and food sciences, plant and soil sciences; agronomy (MS); entomology (MS); environmental microbiology (MS); horticulture (MS); plant pathology (MS). *Degree requirements:* For master's, thesis. *Entrance requirements:* For master's, GRE, minimum GPA of 2.5. Additional exam requirements/recommendations for international students: Required—TOEFL. *Faculty research:* Water quality, reclamation of disturbed land, crop production, pest control, environmental protection.

Plant Physiology

Cornell University, Graduate School, Graduate Fields of Agriculture and Life Sciences, Field of Plant Biology, Ithaca, NY 14853-0001. Offers cytology (MS, PhD); paleobotany (MS, PhD); plant biochemistry (MS, PhD); plant cell biology (MS, PhD); plant ecology (MS, PhD); plant molecular biology (MS, PhD); plant morphology, anatomy and biomechanics (MS, PhD); plant physiology (MS, PhD); systematic botany (MS, PhD). *Faculty:* 49 full-time (14 women). *Students:* 33 full-time (20 women); includes 5 minority (1 Black or African American, non-Hispanic/Latino; 3 Hispanic/Latino; 1 Two or more races, non-Hispanic/Latino), 16 international. Average age 27. 71 applicants, 23% accepted, 10 enrolled. In 2013, 2 doctorates awarded. *Degree requirements:* For doctorate, comprehensive exam, thesis/dissertation. *Entrance requirements:* For doctorate, GRE General Test, GRE Subject Test in biology (recommended), 3 letters of recommendation. Additional exam requirements/recommendations for international students: Required—TOEFL (minimum score 610 paper-based; 77 iBT). *Application deadline:* For fall admission, 1/15 priority date for domestic students. Application fee: $95. Electronic applications accepted. *Financial support:* In 2013–14, 25 students received support, including 7 fellowships with full tuition reimbursements available, 9 research assistantships with full tuition reimbursements available, 9 teaching assistantships with full tuition reimbursements available; institutionally sponsored loans, scholarships/grants, health care benefits, tuition waivers (full and partial), and unspecified assistantships also available. Financial award applicants required to submit FAFSA. *Faculty research:* Plant cell biology/cytology; plant molecular biology; plant morphology/anatomy/biomechanics; plant physiology, systematic botany, paleobotany; plant ecology, ethnobotany, plant biochemistry, photosynthesis. *Unit head:* Director of Graduate Studies, 607-255-2131. *Application contact:* Graduate Field Assistant, 607-255-2131, E-mail: plbio@cornell.edu.
Website: http://www.gradschool.cornell.edu/fields.php?id-45&a-2

Dalhousie University, Faculty of Agriculture, Halifax, NS B3H 4R2, Canada. Offers agriculture (M Sc), including air quality, animal behavior, animal molecular genetics, animal nutrition, animal technology, aquaculture, botany, crop management, crop physiology, ecology, environmental microbiology, food science, horticulture, nutrient management, pest management, physiology, plant biotechnology, plant pathology, soil chemistry, soil fertility, waste management and composting, water quality. Part-time programs available. *Degree requirements:* For master's, thesis, ATC Exam Teaching Assistantship. *Entrance requirements:* For master's, honors B Sc, minimum GPA of 3.0. Additional exam requirements/recommendations for international students: Required—TOEFL (minimum score 580 paper-based; 92 iBT), IELTS, Michigan English Language Assessment Battery, CanTEST, CAEL. *Faculty research:* Bio-product development, organic agriculture, nutrient management, air and water quality, agricultural biotechnology.

Purdue University, Graduate School, College of Science, Department of Biological Sciences, West Lafayette, IN 47907. Offers biochemistry (PhD); biophysics (PhD); cell and developmental biology (PhD); ecology, evolutionary and population biology (MS, PhD), including ecology, evolutionary biology, population biology; genetics (MS, PhD); microbiology (MS, PhD); molecular biology (PhD); neurobiology (MS, PhD); plant physiology (PhD). *Faculty:* 50 full-time (13 women), 5 part-time/adjunct (1 woman). *Students:* 111 full-time (61 women), 5 part-time (0 women); includes 9 minority (1 Black or African American, non-Hispanic/Latino; 5 Asian, non-Hispanic/Latino; 3 Hispanic/Latino), 62 international. Average age 27. 170 applicants, 19% accepted, 17 enrolled. In 2013, 9 master's, 18 doctorates awarded. Terminal master's awarded for partial completion of doctoral program. *Degree requirements:* For master's, thesis (for some programs); for doctorate, thesis/dissertation, seminars, teaching experience. *Entrance requirements:* For master's, GRE General Test (minimum analytical writing score of 3.5), minimum undergraduate GPA of 3.0; for doctorate, GRE General Test (minimum analytical writing score of 3.5), minimum undergraduate GPA of 3.5. Additional exam requirements/recommendations for international students: Required—TOEFL (minimum score 600 paper-based; 107 iBT for MS, 80 iBT for PhD). *Application deadline:* For fall admission, 12/7 for domestic and international students. Applications are processed on a rolling basis. Application fee: $60 ($75 for international students). Electronic applications accepted. *Financial support:* Fellowships, research assistantships, and teaching assistantships available. Support available to part-time students. Financial award application deadline: 2/15; financial award applicants required to submit FAFSA. *Unit head:* Dr. Richard J. Kuhn, Head, 765-494-4407, E-mail: kuhnr@purdue.edu. *Application contact:* Georgina E. Rupp, Graduate Coordinator, 765-494-8142, Fax: 765-494-0876, E-mail: ruppg@purdue.edu.
Website: http://www.bio.purdue.edu/

University of Manitoba, Faculty of Graduate Studies, Faculty of Agricultural and Food Sciences, Department of Plant Science, Winnipeg, MB R3T 2N2, Canada. Offers agronomy and plant protection (M Sc, PhD); horticulture (M Sc, PhD); plant breeding and genetics (M Sc, PhD); plant physiology-biochemistry (M Sc, PhD). *Degree requirements:* For master's, thesis; for doctorate, one foreign language, thesis/dissertation.

University of Massachusetts Amherst, Graduate School, Interdisciplinary Programs, Program in Plant Biology, Amherst, MA 01003. Offers biochemistry and metabolism (MS, PhD); cell biology and physiology (MS, PhD); environmental, ecological and integrative biology (MS, PhD); genetics and evolution (MS, PhD). *Students:* 20 full-time (11 women), 9 international. Average age 28. 72 applicants, 17% accepted, 2 enrolled. In 2013, 1 master's, 2 doctorates awarded. *Degree requirements:* For master's, thesis; for doctorate, 2 foreign languages, comprehensive exam, thesis/dissertation. *Entrance requirements:* For master's and doctorate, GRE General Test. Additional exam requirements/recommendations for international students: Required—TOEFL (minimum score 550 paper-based; 80 iBT), IELTS (minimum score 6.5). *Application deadline:* For fall admission, 12/15 for domestic and international students; for spring admission, 10/1 for domestic and international students. Applications are processed on a rolling basis. Application fee: $75. Electronic applications accepted. *Financial support:* Fellowships

with full and partial tuition reimbursements, research assistantships with full and partial tuition reimbursements, teaching assistantships with full and partial tuition reimbursements, career-related internships or fieldwork, Federal Work-Study, scholarships/grants, traineeships, health care benefits, tuition waivers (full and partial), and unspecified assistantships available. Support available to part-time students. Financial award application deadline: 12/15; financial award applicants required to submit FAFSA. *Unit head:* Dr. Elsbeth L. Walker, Graduate Program Director, 413-577-3217, Fax: 413-545-3243, E-mail: pb@bio.umass.edu. *Application contact:* Lindsay DeSantis, Supervisor of Admissions, 413-545-0722, Fax: 413-577-0010, E-mail: gradadm@grad.umass.edu.
Website: http://www.bio.umass.edu/plantbio/

The University of Tennessee, Graduate School, College of Arts and Sciences, Program in Life Sciences, Knoxville, TN 37996. Offers genome science and technology (MS, PhD); plant physiology and genetics (MS, PhD). *Degree requirements:* For doctorate, one foreign language, thesis/dissertation. *Entrance requirements:* For master's and doctorate, GRE General Test, minimum GPA of 2.7. Additional exam requirements/recommendations for international students: Required—TOEFL. Electronic applications accepted. *Expenses:* Tuition, state resident: full-time $9540; part-time $531 per credit hour. Tuition, nonresident: full-time $27,728; part-time $1542 per credit hour. *Required fees:* $1404; $67 per credit hour.

Virginia Polytechnic Institute and State University, Graduate School, College of Agriculture and Life Sciences, Blacksburg, VA 24061. Offers agricultural and applied economics (MS); agricultural and life sciences (MS); animal and poultry science (MS, PhD); crop and soil environmental sciences (MS, PhD); dairy science (MS); entomology (PhD); horticulture (MS, PhD); human nutrition, foods and exercise (MS, PhD); life sciences (MS, PhD); plant pathology, physiology and weed science (PhD). *Faculty:* 234 full-time (66 women), 1 (woman) part-time/adjunct. *Students:* 347 full-time (188 women), 80 part-time (53 women); includes 53 minority (19 Black or African American, non-Hispanic/Latino; 1 American Indian or Alaska Native, non-Hispanic/Latino; 19 Asian, non-Hispanic/Latino; 7 Hispanic/Latino; 7 Two or more races, non-Hispanic/Latino), 106 international. Average age 29. 410 applicants, 35% accepted, 111 enrolled. In 2013, 80 master's, 44 doctorates awarded. *Degree requirements:* For master's, comprehensive exam (for some programs), thesis (for some programs); for doctorate, comprehensive exam (for some programs), thesis/dissertation (for some programs). *Entrance requirements:* For master's and doctorate, GRE/GMAT (may vary by department). Additional exam requirements/recommendations for international students: Required—TOEFL (minimum score 550 paper-based). *Application deadline:* For fall admission, 8/1 for domestic students, 4/1 for international students; for spring admission, 1/1 for domestic students, 9/1 for international students. Applications are processed on a rolling basis. Application fee: $75. Electronic applications accepted. *Expenses:* Tuition, state resident: full-time $11,185; part-time $621.50 per credit hour. Tuition, nonresident: full-time $22,146; part-time $1230.25 per credit hour. *Required fees:* $2442; $449.25 per semester. Tuition and fees vary according to course load, campus/location and program. *Financial support:* In 2013–14, 1 fellowship with full tuition reimbursement (averaging $19,278 per year), 232 research assistantships with full tuition reimbursements (averaging $19,370 per year), 83 teaching assistantships with full tuition reimbursements (averaging $18,677 per year) were awarded. Financial award application deadline: 3/1; financial award applicants required to submit FAFSA. *Total annual research expenditures:* $44.3 million. *Unit head:* Dr. Alan L. Grant, Dean, 540-231-4152, Fax: 540-231-4163, E-mail: algrant@vt.edu. *Application contact:* Sheila Norman, Administrative Assistant, 540-231-4152, Fax: 540-231-4163, E-mail: snorman@vt.edu.
Website: http://www.cals.vt.edu/

Section 6
Cell, Molecular, and Structural Biology

This section contains a directory of institutions offering graduate work in cell, molecular, and structural biology, followed by in-depth entries submitted by institutions that chose to prepare detailed program descriptions. Additional information about programs listed in the directory but not augmented by an in-depth entry may be obtained by writing directly to the dean of a graduate school or chair of a department at the address given in the directory.

For programs offering related work, see also in this book *Anatomy; Biochemistry; Biological and Biomedical Sciences; Biophysics; Botany and Plant Biology; Genetics, Developmental Biology, and Reproductive Biology; Microbiological Sciences; Pathology and Pathobiology; Pharmacology and Toxicology; Pharmacy and Pharmaceutical Sciences; Physiology;* and *Veterinary Medicine and Sciences.* In the other guides in this series:

Graduate Programs in the Physical Sciences, Mathematics, Agricultural Sciences, the Environment & Natural Resources

See *Chemistry*

Graduate Programs in Engineering & Applied Sciences

See *Agricultural Engineering and Bioengineering* and *Biomedical Engineering and Biotechnology*

CONTENTS

Program Directories

Displays and Close-Ups

Cancer Biology/Oncology

Baylor College of Medicine, Graduate School of Biomedical Sciences, Program in Translational Biology and Molecular Medicine, Houston, TX 77030-3498. Offers PhD. *Degree requirements:* For doctorate, thesis/dissertation, public defense. *Entrance requirements:* For doctorate, GRE, minimum GPA of 3.0. Additional exam requirements/recommendations for international students: Required—TOEFL. Electronic applications accepted. *Faculty research:* Molecular medicine, translational biology, human disease biology and therapy.

Case Western Reserve University, School of Medicine and School of Graduate Studies, Graduate Programs in Medicine, Programs in Molecular and Cellular Basis of Disease/Pathology, Cancer Biology Training Program, Cleveland, OH 44106. Offers PhD, MD/PhD. *Degree requirements:* For doctorate, comprehensive exam, thesis/dissertation. *Entrance requirements:* For doctorate, GRE. Additional exam requirements/recommendations for international students: Required—TOEFL (minimum score 550 paper-based).

Dartmouth College, Program in Experimental and Molecular Medicine, Cancer Biology and Molecular Therapeutics Track, Hanover, NH 03755. Offers PhD.

Duke University, Graduate School, University Program in Molecular Cancer Biology, Durham, NC 27710. Offers PhD. *Faculty:* 50. *Students:* 44 full-time (27 women); includes 8 minority (2 Black or African American, non-Hispanic/Latino; 3 Asian, non-Hispanic/Latino; 3 Hispanic/Latino), 13 international. 77 applicants, 14% accepted, 2 enrolled. In 2013, 9 doctorates awarded. *Degree requirements:* For doctorate, thesis/dissertation. *Entrance requirements:* For doctorate, GRE General Test, GRE Subject Test in biology or biochemistry, cell and molecular biology (recommended). Additional exam requirements/recommendations for international students: Required—TOEFL (minimum score 577 paper-based; 90 iBT) or IELTS (minimum score 7). *Application deadline:* For fall admission, 12/8 priority date for domestic and international students. Application fee: $80. Electronic applications accepted. *Financial support:* Fellowships and research assistantships available. Financial award application deadline: 12/31. *Unit head:* Ann Marie Pendergast, Director of Graduate Studies, 919-613-8600, Fax: 919-681-7767, E-mail: baize@duke.edu. *Application contact:* Elizabeth Hutton, Director of Admissions, 919-684-3913, Fax: 919-684-2277, E-mail: grad-admissions@duke.edu. Website: http://pharmacology.mc.duke.edu/grad/mcb.html

Emory University, Laney Graduate School, Division of Biological and Biomedical Sciences, Program in Cancer Biology, Atlanta, GA 30322. Offers PhD. *Degree requirements:* For doctorate, comprehensive exam, thesis/dissertation. *Entrance requirements:* For doctorate, GRE General Test, minimum GPA of 3.0 in science course work (recommended). Additional exam requirements/recommendations for international students: Required—TOEFL. Electronic applications accepted. *Expenses:* Contact institution. *Faculty research:* Basic and translational cancer research, molecular and cellular biology, genetics and epigenetics, signal transduction, genetic engineering and nanotechnologies.

Gerstner Sloan-Kettering Graduate School of Biomedical Sciences, Program in Cancer Biology, New York, NY 10021. Offers PhD. *Faculty:* 134 full-time (23 women). *Students:* 64 full-time (32 women); includes 6 minority (1 Black or African American, non-Hispanic/Latino; 4 Asian, non-Hispanic/Latino; 1 Hispanic/Latino), 4 international. *Degree requirements:* For doctorate, thesis/dissertation. *Entrance requirements:* For doctorate, GRE, transcripts, three letters of recommendation. Additional exam requirements/recommendations for international students: Required—TOEFL. *Application deadline:* For fall admission, 12/1 for domestic students. Electronic applications accepted. *Financial support:* Fellowship package including stipend ($33,773), full-tuition scholarship, first-year allowance, and comprehensive medical and dental insurance available. *Faculty research:* Biochemistry and molecular biology, biophysics/structural biology, computational biology, genetics, immunology. *Unit head:* Linda Burnley, Associate Dean, 646-888-6639, E-mail: burnleyl@sloankettering.edu. *Application contact:* Main Office, 646-888-6639, Fax: 646-422-2351, E-mail: gradstudies@sloankettering.edu.

See Display below and Close-Up on page 237.

Mayo Graduate School, Graduate Programs in Biomedical Sciences, Program in Tumor Biology, Rochester, MN 55905. Offers PhD. *Degree requirements:* For doctorate, oral defense of dissertation, qualifying oral and written exam. *Entrance requirements:* For doctorate, GRE, 1 year of chemistry, biology, calculus, and physics. Additional exam requirements/recommendations for international students: Required—TOEFL. Electronic applications accepted.

McMaster University, Faculty of Health Sciences and School of Graduate Studies, Program in Medical Sciences, Genetics and Cancer Area, Hamilton, ON L8S 4M2, Canada. Offers M Sc, PhD, MD/PhD. *Degree requirements:* For master's, thesis; for doctorate, comprehensive exam, thesis/dissertation. *Entrance requirements:* For master's, honors B Sc, B+ average in related field; for doctorate, M Sc, minimum B+ average, students with proven research experience and an A average may be admitted with a B Sc degree. Additional exam requirements/recommendations for international students: Required—TOEFL (minimum score 580 paper-based; 92 iBT).

Medical University of South Carolina, College of Graduate Studies, Program in Molecular and Cellular Biology and Pathobiology, Charleston, SC 29425. Offers cancer biology (PhD); cardiovascular biology (PhD); cardiovascular imaging (PhD); cell regulation (PhD); craniofacial biology (PhD); genetics and development (PhD); marine biomedicine (PhD); DMD/PhD; MD/PhD. *Degree requirements:* For doctorate, thesis/dissertation, oral and written exams. *Entrance requirements:* For doctorate, GRE General Test, interview, minimum GPA of 3.0. Additional exam requirements/recommendations for international students: Required—TOEFL (minimum score 600 paper-based; 100 iBT). Electronic applications accepted.

Meharry Medical College, School of Graduate Studies, Program in Biomedical Sciences, Cancer Biology Emphasis, Nashville, TN 37208-9989. Offers PhD, MD/PhD. *Degree requirements:* For doctorate, comprehensive exam, thesis/dissertation. *Entrance requirements:* For doctorate, GRE. *Faculty research:* Regulation of metabolism, enzymology, signal transduction, physical biochemistry.

Memorial University of Newfoundland, Faculty of Medicine and School of Graduate Studies, Graduate Programs in Medicine, Division of Biomedical Sciences, St. John's, NL A1C 5S7, Canada. Offers cancer (M Sc, PhD); cardiovascular (M Sc, PhD); immunology (M Sc, PhD); neuroscience (M Sc, PhD). Part-time programs available. *Degree requirements:* For master's, thesis; for doctorate, comprehensive exam, thesis/dissertation, oral defense of thesis. *Entrance requirements:* For master's, MD or B Sc; for doctorate, MD or M Sc. Additional exam requirements/recommendations for international students: Required—TOEFL. *Faculty research:* Neuroscience, immunology, cardiovascular, and cancer.

New York University, Graduate School of Arts and Science, Department of Biology, New York, NY 10012-1019. Offers biology (PhD); biomedical journalism (MS); cancer and molecular biology (PhD); computational biology (PhD); computers in biological research (MS); developmental genetics (PhD); general biology (MS); immunology and microbiology (PhD); molecular genetics (PhD); neurobiology (PhD); oral biology (MS); plant biology (PhD); recombinant DNA technology (MS); MS/MBA. Part-time programs available. *Faculty:* 24 full-time (5 women). *Students:* 161 full-time (88 women), 28 part-time (15 women); includes 41 minority (5 Black or African American, non-Hispanic/Latino; 23 Asian, non-Hispanic/Latino; 9 Hispanic/Latino; 4 Two or more races, non-Hispanic/Latino), 80 international. Average age 27. 412 applicants, 54% accepted, 65 enrolled. In 2013, 77 master's, 9 doctorates awarded. Terminal master's awarded for partial completion of doctoral program. *Degree requirements:* For master's, thesis or alternative, qualifying paper; for doctorate, comprehensive exam, thesis/dissertation. *Entrance requirements:* For master's and doctorate, GRE General Test. Additional exam requirements/recommendations for international students: Required—TOEFL. *Application deadline:* For fall admission, 12/1 priority date for domestic students, 12/1 for international students. Application fee: $95. *Expenses: Tuition:* Full-time $35,856; part-time $1494 per unit. *Required fees:* $1408; $64 per unit. $473 per term. Tuition and fees vary according to course load and program. *Financial support:* Fellowships with tuition reimbursements, research assistantships with tuition reimbursements, teaching assistantships with tuition reimbursements, career-related internships or fieldwork, Federal Work-Study, institutionally sponsored loans, scholarships/grants, health care benefits, and unspecified assistantships available. Financial award application deadline: 12/1; financial award applicants required to submit FAFSA. *Faculty research:* Genomics, molecular and cell biology, development and molecular genetics, molecular evolution of plants and animals. *Unit head:* Stephen Small, Chair, 212-998-8200, Fax: 212-995-4015, E-mail: biology.admissions@nyu.edu. *Application contact:* Justin Blau, Director of Graduate Studies, PhD Programs, 212-998-8200, Fax: 212-995-4015, E-mail: biology.admissions@nyu.edu.
Website: http://biology.as.nyu.edu/

New York University, School of Medicine and Graduate School of Arts and Science, Sackler Institute of Graduate Biomedical Sciences, Program in Molecular Oncology and Tumor Immunology, New York, NY 10012-1019. Offers immunology (PhD); molecular oncology (PhD); MD/PhD. *Faculty:* 51 full-time (16 women). *Students:* 23 full-time (10 women); includes 5 minority (2 Black or African American, non-Hispanic/Latino; 1 Asian, non-Hispanic/Latino; 2 Hispanic/Latino), 7 international. Average age 28. In 2013, 9 doctorates awarded. *Degree requirements:* For doctorate, one foreign language, thesis/dissertation, qualifying exam. *Entrance requirements:* For doctorate, GRE General Test, GRE Subject Test. Additional exam requirements/recommendations for international students: Required—TOEFL. *Application deadline:* For fall admission, 2/1 for domestic students. Applications are processed on a rolling basis. Application fee: $85. Electronic applications accepted. *Expenses: Tuition:* Full-time $35,856; part-time $1494 per unit. *Required fees:* $1408; $64 per unit. $473 per term. Tuition and fees vary according to course load and program. *Financial support:* Tuition waivers (full) available. *Faculty research:* Stem cells, immunology, genome instability, DNA damage checkpoints. *Unit head:* Dr. Joel D. Oppenheim, Senior Associate Dean for Graduate Studies, 212-263-8001, Fax: 212-263-7600. *Application contact:* Dr. David Levy, Graduate Adviser, 212-263-8192, Fax: 212-263-8211, E-mail: david.levy@med.nyu.edu.

Oregon Health & Science University, School of Medicine, Graduate Programs in Medicine, Program in Molecular and Cellular Biosciences, Cancer Biology Program, Portland, OR 97239-3098. Offers PhD. *Faculty:* 39 full-time (8 women), 1 (woman) part-time/adjunct. *Students:* 16 full-time (10 women); includes 4 minority (1 Black or African American, non-Hispanic/Latino; 2 Asian, non-Hispanic/Latino; 1 Two or more races, non-Hispanic/Latino), 3 international. Average age 28. *Degree requirements:* For doctorate, comprehensive exam, thesis/dissertation, qualifying exam. *Entrance requirements:* For doctorate, GRE General Test (minimum scores: 158 Verbal/148 Quantitative/4.5 Analytical). Additional exam requirements/recommendations for international students: Required—TOEFL. Electronic applications accepted. *Financial support:* Health care benefits and full tuition and stipends (for PhD students) available. *Faculty research:* Signal transduction, apoptosis, carcinogenesis, genome integrity, tumor micro-environment. *Unit head:* Dr. Matthew Thayer, Program Leader, 503-494-2447, E-mail: thayerm@ohsu.edu. *Application contact:* Lola Bichler, Program Coordinator, 503-494-5824, E-mail: bichler@ohsu.edu.
Website: http://www.ohsu.edu/cancerbio

Purdue University, Graduate School, PULSe - Purdue University Life Sciences Program, West Lafayette, IN 47907. Offers biomolecular structure and biophysics (PhD); biotechnology (PhD); chemical biology (PhD); chromatin and regulation of gene expression (PhD); integrative neuroscience (PhD); integrative plant sciences (PhD); membrane biology (PhD); microbiology (PhD); molecular evolutionary and cancer biology (PhD); molecular evolutionary genetics (PhD); molecular virology (PhD). *Students:* 154 full-time (78 women), 1 part-time (0 women); includes 23 minority (5 Black or African American, non-Hispanic/Latino; 5 Asian, non-Hispanic/Latino; 10 Hispanic/Latino; 3 Two or more races, non-Hispanic/Latino), 73 international. Average age 26. 239 applicants, 33% accepted, 40 enrolled. *Entrance requirements:* For doctorate, GRE, minimum undergraduate GPA of 3.0. Additional exam requirements/recommendations for international students: Required—TOEFL (minimum score 550 paper-based; 77 iBT). *Application deadline:* For fall admission, 1/15 priority date for domestic and international students. Applications are processed on a rolling basis. Application fee: $60 ($75 for international students). Electronic applications accepted. *Financial support:* In 2013–14, research assistantships with tuition reimbursements (averaging $22,500 per year), teaching assistantships with tuition reimbursements (averaging $22,500 per year) were awarded. *Unit head:* Dr. Christine A. Hrycyna, Head, 765-494-7322, E-mail: hrycyna@purdue.edu. *Application contact:* Colleen Gabauer, Graduate Contact, 765-494-9256, E-mail: cgabauer@purdue.edu.
Website: http://www.gradschool.purdue.edu/pulse

Queen's University at Kingston, School of Graduate Studies, Faculty of Health Sciences, Department of Anatomy and Cell Biology, Kingston, ON K7L 3N6, Canada. Offers biology of reproduction (M Sc, PhD); cancer (M Sc, PhD); cardiovascular pathophysiology (M Sc, PhD); cell and molecular biology (M Sc, PhD); drug metabolism (M Sc, PhD); endocrinology (M Sc, PhD); motor control (M Sc, PhD); neural regeneration (M Sc, PhD); neurophysiology (M Sc, PhD). Part-time programs available. *Degree requirements:* For master's, thesis; for doctorate, one foreign language, comprehensive exam, thesis/dissertation. *Entrance requirements:* Additional exam requirements/recommendations for international students: Required—TOEFL. Electronic applications accepted. *Faculty research:* Human kinetics, neuroscience, reproductive biology, cardiovascular.

Rutgers, The State University of New Jersey, Newark, Graduate School of Biomedical Sciences, Newark, NJ 07107. Offers biodefense (Certificate); biomedical engineering (PhD); biomedical sciences (multidisciplinary) (PhD); cellular biology, neuroscience and physiology (PhD), including neuroscience, physiology, biophysics, cardiovascular biology, molecular pharmacology, stem cell biology; infection, immunity and inflammation (PhD), including immunology, infectious disease, microbiology, oral biology; molecular biology, genetics and cancer (PhD), including biochemistry, molecular genetics, cancer biology, radiation biology, bioinformatics; neuroscience (Certificate); pharmacological sciences (Certificate); stem cell (Certificate); DMD/PhD; MD/PhD. PhD in biomedical engineering offered jointly with New Jersey Institute of Technology. Part-time and evening/weekend programs available. Terminal master's awarded for partial completion of doctoral program. *Degree requirements:* For doctorate, thesis/dissertation, qualifying exam. *Entrance requirements:* For doctorate, GRE General Test. Additional exam requirements/recommendations for international students: Required—TOEFL. Electronic applications accepted.

Rutgers, The State University of New Jersey, New Brunswick, Graduate School-New Brunswick, Program in Endocrinology and Animal Biosciences, Piscataway, NJ 08854-8097. Offers MS, PhD. Terminal master's awarded for partial completion of doctoral program. *Degree requirements:* For master's, thesis; for doctorate, comprehensive exam, thesis/dissertation. *Entrance requirements:* For master's and doctorate, GRE General Test. Additional exam requirements/recommendations for international students: Required—TOEFL. Electronic applications accepted. *Faculty research:* Comparative and behavioral endocrinology, epigenetic regulation of the endocrine system, exercise physiology and immunology, fetal and neonatal developmental programming, mammary gland biology and breast cancer, neuroendocrinology and alcohol studies, reproductive and developmental toxicology.

Stanford University, School of Medicine, Graduate Programs in Medicine, Program in Cancer Biology, Stanford, CA 94305-9991. Offers PhD. *Degree requirements:* For doctorate, thesis/dissertation, qualifying examination. *Entrance requirements:* For doctorate, GRE General Test, GRE Subject Test. Additional exam requirements/recommendations for international students: Required—TOEFL. Electronic applications accepted. *Expenses: Tuition:* Full-time $42,690; part-time $949 per credit. *Required fees:* $185.

State University of New York Upstate Medical University, College of Graduate Studies, Major Research Areas of the College of Graduate Studies, Syracuse, NY 13210-2334.

Thomas Jefferson University, Jefferson Graduate School of Biomedical Sciences, PhD Program in Genetics, Genomics and Cancer Biology, Philadelphia, PA 19107. Offers PhD. *Faculty:* 48 full-time (16 women), 4 part-time/adjunct (3 women). *Students:* 16 full-time (8 women); includes 4 minority (2 Asian, non-Hispanic/Latino; 2 Hispanic/Latino), 1 international. 41 applicants, 24% accepted, 4 enrolled. In 2013, 5 doctorates awarded. *Degree requirements:* For doctorate, comprehensive exam, thesis/dissertation. *Entrance requirements:* For doctorate, GRE General Test, minimum GPA of 3.2. Additional exam requirements/recommendations for international students: Required—TOEFL (minimum score 100 iBT) or IELTS. *Application deadline:* For fall admission, 1/5 priority date for domestic and international students. Applications are processed on a rolling basis. Application fee: $75. Electronic applications accepted. *Financial support:* In 2013–14, 16 students received support, including 16 fellowships with full tuition reimbursements available (averaging $56,052 per year); Federal Work-Study, institutionally sponsored loans, scholarships/grants, traineeships, and stipends also available. Support available to part-time students. Financial award application deadline: 5/1; financial award applicants required to submit FAFSA. *Faculty research:* Functional genomics, cancer susceptibility, cell cycle, regulation oncogenes and tumor suppressor genes, genetics of neoplastic disease. *Unit head:* Dr. Linda D. Siracusa, Program Director, 215-503-4536, E-mail: linda.siracusa@jefferson.edu. *Application contact:* Marc E. Stearns, Director of Admissions, 215-503-0155, Fax: 215-503-3433, E-mail: jgsbs-info@jefferson.edu.
Website: http://www.jefferson.edu/university/biomedical_sciences/programs/phd/genetics.html

Université Laval, Faculty of Medicine, Post-Professional Programs in Medical Studies, Québec, QC G1K 7P4, Canada. Offers anatomy–pathology (DESS); anesthesiology (DESS); cardiology (DESS); care of older people (Diploma); clinical research (DESS); community health (DESS); dermatology (DESS); diagnostic radiology (DESS); emergency medicine (Diploma); family medicine (DESS); general surgery (DESS); geriatrics (DESS); hematology (DESS); internal medicine (DESS); maternal and fetal medicine (Diploma); medical biochemistry (DESS); medical microbiology and infectious diseases (DESS); medical oncology (DESS); nephrology (DESS); neurology (DESS); neurosurgery (DESS); obstetrics and gynecology (DESS); ophthalmology (DESS); orthopedic surgery (DESS); oto-rhino-laryngology (DESS); palliative medicine (Diploma); pediatrics (DESS); plastic surgery (DESS); psychiatry (DESS); pulmonary medicine (DESS); radiology–oncology (DESS); thoracic surgery (DESS); urology (DESS). *Degree requirements:* For other advanced degree, comprehensive exam. *Entrance requirements:* For degree, knowledge of French. Electronic applications accepted.

University at Buffalo, the State University of New York, Graduate School, Graduate Programs in Cancer Research and Biomedical Sciences at Roswell Park Cancer Institute, Interdisciplinary Master of Science Program in Natural and Biomedical Sciences at Roswell Park Cancer Institute, Buffalo, NY 14260. Offers biomedical sciences and cancer research (MS). Part-time programs available. *Faculty:* 124 full-time (36 women), 24 part-time/adjunct (8 women). *Students:* 50 full-time (27 women); includes 6 minority (4 Black or African American, non-Hispanic/Latino; 1 Asian, non-Hispanic/Latino; 1 Two or more races, non-Hispanic/Latino), 20 international. 82 applicants, 50% accepted, 28 enrolled. In 2013, 29 master's awarded. *Degree requirements:* For master's, thesis, oral defense of thesis based on research project. *Entrance requirements:* For master's, GRE General Test. Additional exam requirements/recommendations for international students: Required—TOEFL (minimum score 79 iBT). *Application deadline:* For fall admission, 3/1 priority date for domestic and international students. Application fee: $75. Electronic applications accepted. *Financial support:* Application deadline: 2/28. *Faculty research:* Biochemistry, oncology, pathology, biophysics, pharmacology, molecular biology, cellular biology, genetics, bioinformatics, immunology, therapeutic development, epidemiology. *Unit head:* Dr. Norman J. Karin, Associate Dean, 716-845-2339, Fax: 716-845-8178, E-mail: norman.karin@roswellpark.org. *Application contact:* Dr. Norman J. Karin, Associate Dean, 716-845-2339, Fax: 716-845-8178, E-mail: norman.karin@roswellpark.org.
Website: http://www.roswellpark.edu/education/interdisciplinary-masters

University of Alberta, Faculty of Medicine and Dentistry and Faculty of Graduate Studies and Research, Graduate Programs in Medicine, Department of Oncology, Edmonton, AB T6G 2E1, Canada. Offers M Sc, PhD. Terminal master's awarded for partial completion of doctoral program. *Degree requirements:* For master's, thesis; for doctorate, thesis/dissertation. *Entrance requirements:* For master's and doctorate, minimum GPA of 7.0 on a 9.0 scale, B SC. Additional exam requirements/recommendations for international students: Required—TOEFL (minimum score 600 paper-based). Electronic applications accepted. *Faculty research:* Experimental oncology, radiation oncology, medical physics, medical oncology.

The University of Arizona, Graduate Interdisciplinary Programs, Graduate Interdisciplinary Program in Cancer Biology, Tucson, AZ 85721. Offers PhD. *Students:* 10 full-time (5 women), 7 part-time (5 women); includes 4 minority (2 Hispanic/Latino; 2

Two or more races, non-Hispanic/Latino), 4 international. Average age 28. 13 applicants, 23% accepted, 3 enrolled. In 2013, 6 doctorates awarded. *Degree requirements:* For doctorate, comprehensive exam, thesis/dissertation. *Entrance requirements:* For doctorate, GRE General Test, 3 letters of recommendation. Additional exam requirements/recommendations for international students: Required—TOEFL (minimum score 550 paper-based; 79 iBT). *Application deadline:* For fall admission, 12/1 for domestic and international students. Applications are processed on a rolling basis. Application fee: $75. Electronic applications accepted. *Expenses:* Tuition, state resident: full-time $11,526. Tuition, nonresident: full-time $27,398. *Financial support:* In 2013–14, 7 research assistantships with full tuition reimbursements (averaging $23,675 per year) were awarded; institutionally sponsored loans, scholarships/grants, traineeships, health care benefits, tuition waivers (full), and unspecified assistantships also available. *Faculty research:* Differential gene expression, DNA-protein cross linking, cell growth regulation steroid, receptor proteins. *Unit head:* Dr. Jesse Tim Martinez, Chairman, 520-626-7479, E-mail: jmartinez@uacc.arizona.edu. *Application contact:* Anne Cione, Senior Program Coordinator, 520-626-7479, Fax: 520-626-4979, E-mail: acione@azcc.arizona.edu.
Website: http://www.azcc.arizona.edu/academics/cbio

University of Calgary, Cumming School of Medicine and Faculty of Graduate Studies, Medical Science Graduate Program, Calgary, AB T2N 1N4, Canada. Offers cancer biology (M Sc, PhD); critical care medicine (M Sc, PhD); joint injury and arthritis (M Sc, PhD); molecular and medical genetics (M Sc, PhD); mountain medicine and high altitude physiology (M Sc, PhD); pathologists' assistant (M Sc, PhD). *Degree requirements:* For master's, thesis; for doctorate, thesis/dissertation, candidacy exam. *Entrance requirements:* For master's, minimum undergraduate GPA of 3.2; for doctorate, minimum graduate GPA of 3.2. Additional exam requirements/recommendations for international students: Required—TOEFL (minimum score 600 paper-based). Electronic applications accepted. *Faculty research:* Cancer biology, immunology, joint injury and arthritis, medical education, population genomics.

University of Chicago, Division of Biological Sciences, Biomedical Sciences Cluster: Cancer Biology, Immunology, Molecular Metabolism and Nutrition, Pathology, and Microbiology, Committee on Cancer Biology, Chicago, IL 60637-1513. Offers PhD. *Degree requirements:* For doctorate, thesis/dissertation, ethics class, 2 teaching assistantships. *Entrance requirements:* For doctorate, GRE General Test. Additional exam requirements/recommendations for international students: Required—TOEFL (minimum score 600 paper-based; 104 iBT), IELTS (minimum score 7). Electronic applications accepted. *Faculty research:* Cancer genetics, apoptosis, signal transduction, tumor biology, cell cycle regulation.

University of Cincinnati, Graduate School, College of Medicine, Graduate Programs in Biomedical Sciences, Graduate Program in Cell and Cancer Biology, Cincinnati, OH 45221. Offers PhD. *Degree requirements:* For doctorate, thesis/dissertation, qualifying exam. *Entrance requirements:* For doctorate, GRE General Test. Additional exam requirements/recommendations for international students: Required—TOEFL. Electronic applications accepted. *Faculty research:* Cancer biology, cell and molecular biology, breast cancer, pancreatic cancer, drug discovery.

University of Colorado Denver, School of Medicine, Program in Cancer Biology, Aurora, CO 80045. Offers PhD. *Students:* 25 full-time (18 women), 1 (woman) part-time; includes 5 minority (3 Asian, non-Hispanic/Latino; 2 Two or more races, non-Hispanic/Latino), 6 international. Average age 27. 30 applicants, 13% accepted, 4 enrolled. In 2013, 5 doctorates awarded. *Degree requirements:* For doctorate, comprehensive exam, thesis/dissertation, 3 laboratory rotations. *Entrance requirements:* For doctorate, GRE General Test, interview, minimum undergraduate GPA of 3.0. Additional exam requirements/recommendations for international students: Required—TOEFL (minimum score 550 paper-based; 80 iBT). *Application deadline:* For fall admission, 12/1 for domestic students, 11/1 priority date for international students. Application fee: $50 ($75 for international students). Electronic applications accepted. *Expenses:* Contact institution. *Financial support:* In 2013–14, 25 students received support. Fellowships with full tuition reimbursements available, research assistantships, teaching assistantships, Federal Work-Study, institutionally sponsored loans, scholarships/grants, traineeships, health care benefits, tuition waivers (full), and unspecified assistantships available. Financial award application deadline: 3/15; financial award applicants required to submit FAFSA. *Faculty research:* Signal transduction by tyrosine kinases, estrogen and progesterone receptors in breast cancer, mechanism of mitochondrial DNA replication in the mammalian cell. *Total annual research expenditures:* $9 million. *Unit head:* Dr. Mary Reyland, Director, Cancer Biology Program, 303-724-4572, E-mail: mary.reyland@ucdenver.edu. *Application contact:* Deanne Sylvester, Program Administrator, 303-724-3244, E-mail: deanne.sylvester@ucdenver.edu.
Website: http://www.ucdenver.edu/academics/colleges/Graduate-School/academic-programs/cancerbiology/Pages/cancerbiologyprogram.aspx

University of Delaware, College of Arts and Sciences, Department of Biological Sciences, Newark, DE 19716. Offers biotechnology (MS); cancer biology (MS, PhD); cell and extracellular matrix biology (MS, PhD); cell and systems physiology (MS, PhD); developmental biology (MS, PhD); ecology and evolution (MS, PhD); microbiology (MS, PhD); molecular biology and genetics (MS, PhD). Terminal master's awarded for partial completion of doctoral program. *Degree requirements:* For master's, thesis, preliminary exam; for doctorate, comprehensive exam, thesis/dissertation, preliminary exam. *Entrance requirements:* For master's and doctorate, GRE General Test. Additional exam requirements/recommendations for international students: Required—TOEFL (minimum score 600 paper-based); Recommended—TWE. Electronic applications accepted. *Faculty research:* Microorganisms, bone, cancer metastasis, developmental biology, cell biology, DNA.

The University of Manchester, Faculty of Life Sciences, Manchester, United Kingdom. Offers adaptive organismal biology (M Phil, PhD); animal biology (M Phil, PhD); biochemistry (M Phil, PhD); bioinformatics (M Phil, PhD); biomolecular sciences (M Phil, PhD); biotechnology (M Phil, PhD); cell biology (M Phil, PhD); cell matrix research (M Phil, PhD); channels and transporters (M Phil, PhD); developmental biology (M Phil, PhD); Egyptology (M Phil, PhD); environmental biology (M Phil, PhD); evolutionary biology (M Phil, PhD); gene expression (M Phil, PhD); genetics (M Phil, PhD); history of science, technology and medicine (M Phil, PhD); immunology (M Phil, PhD); integrative neurobiology and behavior (M Phil, PhD); membrane trafficking (M Phil, PhD); microbiology (M Phil, PhD); molecular and cellular neuroscience (M Phil, PhD); molecular biology (M Phil, PhD); molecular cancer studies (M Phil, PhD); neuroscience (M Phil, PhD); ophthalmology (M Phil, PhD); optometry (M Phil, PhD); organelle function (M Phil, PhD); pharmacology (M Phil, PhD); physiology (M Phil, PhD); plant sciences (M Phil, PhD); stem cell research (M Phil, PhD); structural biology (M Phil, PhD); systems neuroscience (M Phil, PhD); toxicology (M Phil, PhD).

The University of Manchester, School of Dentistry, Manchester, United Kingdom. Offers basic dental sciences (cancer studies) (M Phil, PhD); basic dental sciences (molecular genetics) (M Phil, PhD); basic dental sciences (stem cell biology) (M Phil, PhD); biomaterials sciences and dental technology (M Phil, PhD); dental public health/community dentistry (M Phil, PhD); dental science (clinical) (PhD); endodontology (M Phil, PhD); fixed and removable prosthodontics (M Phil, PhD); operative dentistry (M Phil, PhD); oral and maxillofacial surgery (M Phil, PhD); oral radiology (M Phil, PhD); orthodontics (M Phil, PhD); restorative dentistry (M Phil, PhD).

University of Manitoba, Faculty of Graduate Studies, Faculty of Nursing, Winnipeg, MB R3T 2N2, Canada. Offers cancer nursing (MN); nursing (MN). *Degree requirements:* For master's, thesis.

University of Maryland, Baltimore, Graduate School, Graduate Program in Life Sciences, Program in Molecular Medicine, Baltimore, MD 21201. Offers cancer biology (PhD); cell and molecular physiology (PhD); human genetics and genomic medicine (PhD); molecular medicine (MS); molecular toxicology and pharmacology (PhD); MD/PhD. *Students:* 91 full-time (49 women), 14 part-time (8 women); includes 32 minority (10 Black or African American, non-Hispanic/Latino; 12 Asian, non-Hispanic/Latino; 5 Hispanic/Latino; 5 Two or more races, non-Hispanic/Latino), 9 international. Average age 27. 180 applicants, 33% accepted, 24 enrolled. In 2013, 10 master's, 15 doctorates awarded. *Degree requirements:* For doctorate, comprehensive exam, thesis/dissertation. *Entrance requirements:* For master's and doctorate, GRE. Additional exam requirements/recommendations for international students: Required—TOEFL (minimum score 600 paper-based; 100 iBT); Recommended—IELTS (minimum score 7). *Application deadline:* For fall admission, 12/1 priority date for domestic students, 1/15 for international students. Application fee: $75. Electronic applications accepted. *Financial support:* In 2013–14, research assistantships with partial tuition reimbursements (averaging $25,000 per year) were awarded; fellowships also available. Financial award application deadline: 3/1; financial award applicants required to submit FAFSA. *Unit head:* Dr. Toni Antalis, Director, 410-706-8222, E-mail: tantalis@som.umaryland.edu. *Application contact:* Sharron Graves, Program Coordinator, 410-706-6044, Fax: 410-706-6040, E-mail: sgraves@som.umaryland.edu.
Website: http://molecularmedicine.umaryland.edu

University of Massachusetts Worcester, Graduate School of Biomedical Sciences, Worcester, MA 01655-0115. Offers biochemistry and molecular pharmacology (PhD); bioinformatics and computational biology (PhD); cancer biology (PhD); cell biology (PhD); clinical and population health research (PhD); clinical investigation (MS); immunology and virology (PhD); interdisciplinary biomedical research (PhD); millennium (PhD); molecular genetics and microbiology (PhD); neuroscience (PhD); translational science (PhD); MD/PhD. *Faculty:* 1,388 full-time (521 women), 309 part-time/adjunct (198 women). *Students:* 385 full-time (210 women); includes 53 minority (13 Black or African American, non-Hispanic/Latino; 30 Asian, non-Hispanic/Latino; 10 Hispanic/Latino), 138 international. Average age 28. 491 applicants, 19% accepted, 39 enrolled. In 2013, 5 master's, 50 doctorates awarded. Terminal master's awarded for partial completion of doctoral program. *Median time to degree:* Of those who began their doctoral program in fall 2005, 67% received their degree in 8 years or less. *Degree requirements:* For master's, comprehensive exam, thesis; for doctorate, comprehensive exam, thesis/dissertation. *Entrance requirements:* For master's, MD, PhD, DVM, or PharmD; for doctorate, GRE General Test, bachelor's degree. Additional exam requirements/recommendations for international students: Required—TOEFL (minimum score 100 iBT) or IELTS (minimum score 7.5). *Application deadline:* For fall admission, 12/15 for domestic and international students; for spring admission, 5/15 for domestic students. Application fee: $80. Electronic applications accepted. *Expenses:* Contact institution. *Financial support:* In 2013–14, 431 students received support, including research assistantships with full tuition reimbursements available (averaging $29,500 per year); scholarships/grants, health care benefits, tuition waivers (full), and unspecified assistantships also available. Financial award application deadline: 5/16. *Faculty research:* RNA interference, cell/molecular/developmental biology, bioinformatics, clinical/translational research, infectious disease. *Total annual research expenditures:* $245.9 million. *Unit head:* Dr. Anthony Carruthers, Dean, 508-856-4135, E-mail: anthony.carruthers@umassmed.edu. *Application contact:* Dr. Kendall Knight, Associate Dean and Interim Director of Admissions and Recruitment, 508-856-5628, Fax: 508-856-3659, E-mail: kendall.knight@umassmed.edu.
Website: http://www.umassmed.edu/gsbs/

University of Miami, Graduate School, Miller School of Medicine, Program in Cancer Biology, Coral Gables, FL 33124. Offers PhD, MD/PhD.

University of Michigan, Rackham Graduate School, Program in Biomedical Sciences (PIBS), Program in Cancer Biology, Ann Arbor, MI 48109. Offers PhD. *Faculty:* 41 full-time (12 women). *Students:* 14 full-time (11 women); includes 5 minority (1 Black or African American, non-Hispanic/Latino; 2 Asian, non-Hispanic/Latino; 2 Hispanic/Latino), 1 international. Average age 28. 60 applicants, 13% accepted, 4 enrolled. In 2013, 1 doctorate awarded. *Degree requirements:* For doctorate, thesis/dissertation, preliminary examination, oral defense of dissertation. *Entrance requirements:* For doctorate, GRE General Test, three letters of recommendation, research experience, personal and research statements. Additional exam requirements/recommendations for international students: Required—TOEFL (minimum score 84 iBT). *Application deadline:* For fall admission, 12/1 for domestic and international students. Application fee: $75 ($90 for international students). Electronic applications accepted. Tuition and fees vary according to course level, course load, degree level, program and student level. *Financial support:* In 2013–14, 14 students received support, including 4 fellowships with full tuition reimbursements available (averaging $28,500 per year), 10 research assistantships with full tuition reimbursements available (averaging $28,500 per year); scholarships/grants, health care benefits, tuition waivers (full), and unspecified assistantships also available. Financial award application deadline: 12/1. *Faculty research:* Tumor immunology, viral oncogenesis, cell biology, genetics, epidemiology, pathology, bioinformatics. *Unit head:* Dr. Michael Imperiale, Director, 734-763-9162, Fax: 734-615-6560, E-mail: imperial@umich.edu. *Application contact:* Michelle S. Melis, Director of Student Life, Programs in Biomedical Sciences (PIBS), 734-615-6538, Fax: 734-647-7022, E-mail: msmtegan@umich.edu.
Website: http://www.med.umich.edu/cancerbio/

University of Michigan, Rackham Graduate School, Program in Chemical Biology, Ann Arbor, MI 48109-2216. Offers cancer chemical biology (MS); chemical biology (PhD). *Faculty:* 46 full-time (10 women), 1 (woman) part-time/adjunct. *Students:* 54 full-time (22 women); includes 13 minority (3 Black or African American, non-Hispanic/Latino; 4 Asian, non-Hispanic/Latino; 3 Hispanic/Latino; 3 Two or more races, non-Hispanic/Latino), 8 international. Average age 26. 79 applicants, 57% accepted, 18 enrolled. In 2013, 2 master's, 8 doctorates awarded. *Degree requirements:* For doctorate, thesis/dissertation. *Entrance requirements:* Additional exam requirements/recommendations for international students: Required—TOEFL (minimum score 600 paper-based; 102 iBT). *Application deadline:* For fall admission, 12/15 priority date for domestic and international students. Applications are processed on a rolling basis. Application fee: $75 ($90 for international students). Electronic applications accepted. Tuition and fees vary according to course level, course load, degree level, program and student level. *Financial support:* In 2013–14, 46 students received support, including fellowships with full tuition reimbursements available (averaging $28,500 per year), research assistantships with full tuition reimbursements available (averaging $28,500 per year); career-related internships or fieldwork, scholarships/grants, traineeships, health care benefits, and unspecified assistantships also available. *Faculty research:* Chemical genetics, structural enzymology, signal transduction, biological catalysis, biomolecular structure, function and recognition. *Unit head:* Prof. Anna Mapp, Program Director, 734-

763-7175, Fax: 734-615-1252, E-mail: chemicalbiology@umich.edu. *Application contact:* Admissions Office, 734-764-8129, E-mail: rackadmis@umich.edu.
Website: http://www.chembio.umich.edu/

University of Minnesota, Twin Cities Campus, Graduate School, PhD Program in Microbiology, Immunology and Cancer Biology, Minneapolis, MN 55455-0213. Offers PhD. *Degree requirements:* For doctorate, thesis/dissertation. *Entrance requirements:* For doctorate, GRE General Test. Additional exam requirements/recommendations for international students: Required—TOEFL (minimum score 600 paper-based). Electronic applications accepted. *Faculty research:* Virology, microbiology, cancer biology, immunology.

University of Nebraska Medical Center, Program in Cancer Research, Omaha, NE 68198-7810. Offers PhD. Terminal master's awarded for partial completion of doctoral program. *Degree requirements:* For doctorate, comprehensive exam, thesis/dissertation. *Entrance requirements:* For doctorate, GRE, 3 letters of reference; course work in chemistry, biology, physics and mathematics. Additional exam requirements/recommendations for international students: Required—TOEFL (minimum score 550 paper-based). Electronic applications accepted. *Expenses: Required fees:* $300 per semester. Tuition and fees vary according to program. *Faculty research:* DNA repair, tumor immunology, signal transduction, structural biology, gene expression.

University of Pennsylvania, Perelman School of Medicine, Biomedical Graduate Studies, Graduate Group in Cell and Molecular Biology, Philadelphia, PA 19104. Offers cancer biology (PhD); cell biology and physiology (PhD); developmental stem cell regenerative biology (PhD); gene therapy and vaccines (PhD); genetics and gene regulation (PhD); microbiology, virology, and parasitology (PhD); MD/PhD; VMD/PhD. *Faculty:* 321. *Students:* 352 full-time (205 women); includes 99 minority (11 Black or African American, non-Hispanic/Latino; 65 Asian, non-Hispanic/Latino; 21 Hispanic/Latino; 2 Two or more races, non-Hispanic/Latino), 45 international. 488 applicants, 20% accepted, 40 enrolled. In 2013, 41 doctorates awarded. *Degree requirements:* For doctorate, thesis/dissertation. *Entrance requirements:* For doctorate, GRE General Test. Additional exam requirements/recommendations for international students: Required—TOEFL. *Application deadline:* For fall admission, 12/1 priority date for domestic and international students. Applications are processed on a rolling basis. Application fee: $80. Electronic applications accepted. *Financial support:* In 2013–14, 352 students received support. Fellowships, research assistantships, scholarships/grants, traineeships, and unspecified assistantships available. *Unit head:* Dr. Daniel Kessler, Graduate Group Chair, 215-898-1478. *Application contact:* Meagan Schofer, Coordinator, 215-898-4360.
Website: http://www.med.upenn.edu/camb/

University of Regina, Faculty of Graduate Studies and Research, Faculty of Science, Department of Chemistry and Biochemistry, Regina, SK S4S 0A2, Canada. Offers analytical/environmental chemistry (M Sc, PhD); biophysics of biological interfaces (M Sc, PhD); enzymology/chemical biology (M Sc, PhD); inorganic/organometallic chemistry (M Sc, PhD); signal transduction and mechanisms of cancer cell regulation (M Sc, PhD); supramolecular organic photochemistry and photophysics (M Sc, PhD); synthetic organic chemistry (M Sc, PhD); theoretical/computational chemistry (M Sc, PhD). *Faculty:* 11 full-time (2 women), 4 part-time/adjunct (0 women). *Students:* 12 full-time (9 women), 1 part-time (0 women). 25 applicants, 36% accepted. In 2013, 3 master's awarded. *Degree requirements:* For master's, thesis; for doctorate, thesis/dissertation. *Entrance requirements:* Additional exam requirements/recommendations for international students: Required—TOEFL (minimum score 580 paper-based; 80 iBT), IELTS (minimum score 6.5). *Application deadline:* Applications are processed on a rolling basis. Application fee: $100. Electronic applications accepted. *Expenses: Tuition, area resident:* Full-time $4338 Canadian dollars. *International tuition:* $7338 Canadian dollars full-time. *Required fees:* $449.25 Canadian dollars. *Financial support:* In 2013–14, 5 fellowships (averaging $7,000 per year), 8 teaching assistantships (averaging $2,456 per year) were awarded; research assistantships and scholarships/grants also available. Financial award application deadline: 6/15. *Faculty research:* Asymmetric synthesis and methodology, theoretical and computational chemistry, biophysical biochemistry, analytical and environmental chemistry, chemical biology. *Unit head:* Dr. Renata Raina-Fulton, Department Head, 306-585-4012, Fax: 306-337-2409, E-mail: renata.raina@uregina.ca. *Application contact:* Dr. Brian Sterenberg, Graduate Program Coordinator, 306-585-4106, Fax: 306-337-2409, E-mail: brian.sterenberg@uregina.ca.
Website: http://www.uregina.ca/science/chem-biochem/

University of South Florida, College of Arts and Sciences, Department of Cell Biology, Microbiology, and Molecular Biology, Tampa, FL 33620-9951. Offers biology (MS), including cell and molecular biology; cancer biology (PhD); cell and molecular biology (PhD); microbiology (MS). *Faculty:* 19 full-time (5 women), 1 part-time/adjunct (0 women). *Students:* 77 full-time (46 women), 3 part-time (1 woman); includes 8 minority (5 Asian, non-Hispanic/Latino; 3 Hispanic/Latino), 19 international. Average age 27. 155 applicants, 17% accepted, 17 enrolled. In 2013, 19 master's, 12 doctorates awarded. *Degree requirements:* For master's, thesis or alternative; for doctorate, comprehensive exam, thesis/dissertation. *Entrance requirements:* For master's and doctorate, GRE General Test, minimum GPA of 3.0, extensive background in biology or chemistry. Additional exam requirements/recommendations for international students: Required—TOEFL (minimum score 550 paper-based; 79 iBT) or IELTS (minimum score 6.5). *Application deadline:* For fall admission, 2/1 for domestic students, 1/1 for international students. Application fee: $30. *Financial support:* Career-related internships or fieldwork, health care benefits, and unspecified assistantships available. Financial award application deadline: 4/1. *Faculty research:* Cell biology, microbiology and molecular biology: basic and applied science in bacterial pathogenesis, genome integrity and mechanisms of aging, structural and computational biology; cancer biology: immunology, cancer control, signal transduction, drug discovery, genomics. *Total annual research expenditures:* $1.9 million. *Unit head:* Dr. James Garey, Professor/Chair, 813-974-7103, Fax: 813-974-1614, E-mail: garey@usf.edu. *Application contact:* Dr. Kenneth Wright, Associate Professor of Cancer Biology, H. Lee Moffitt Cancer Center and Research Institute, 813-745-3918, Fax: 813-974-1614, E-mail: ken.wright@moffitt.org.
Website: http://biology.usf.edu/cmmb/

The University of Texas Health Science Center at Houston, Graduate School of Biomedical Sciences, Program in Cancer Biology, Houston, TX 77225-0036. Offers MS, PhD, MD/PhD. Terminal master's awarded for partial completion of doctoral program. *Degree requirements:* For master's, thesis; for doctorate, thesis/dissertation. *Entrance requirements:* For master's and doctorate, GRE General Test. Additional exam requirements/recommendations for international students: Required—TOEFL. Electronic applications accepted. *Expenses:* Tuition, state resident: full-time $3474; part-time $193 per credit hour. Tuition, nonresident: full-time $13,644; part-time $758 per credit hour. *Required fees:* $226.30; $87 per credit hour. *Faculty research:* Cancer metastasis, signal transduction, therapeutic resistance, cell cycle deregulation, cancer markers and target.

The University of Texas Health Science Center at Houston, Graduate School of Biomedical Sciences, Program in Molecular Carcinogenesis, Houston, TX 77225-0036. Offers MS, PhD, MD/PhD. Terminal master's awarded for partial completion of doctoral program. *Degree requirements:* For master's, thesis; for doctorate, thesis/dissertation. *Entrance requirements:* For master's and doctorate, GRE General Test. Additional exam requirements/recommendations for international students: Required—TOEFL. Electronic applications accepted. *Expenses:* Tuition, state resident: full-time $3474; part-time $193 per credit hour. Tuition, nonresident: full-time $13,644; part-time $758 per credit hour. *Required fees:* $226.30; $87 per credit hour. *Faculty research:* Carcinogenesis, mutagenesis, epigenetics, mouse models, cancer prevention.

The University of Texas Southwestern Medical Center, Southwestern Graduate School of Biomedical Sciences, Division of Basic Science, Program in Cancer Biology, Dallas, TX 75390. Offers PhD. *Faculty:* 85 full-time (16 women), 2 part-time/adjunct (0 women). *Students:* 62 full-time (29 women), 2 part-time (1 woman); includes 18 minority (1 Black or African American, non-Hispanic/Latino; 9 Asian, non-Hispanic/Latino; 8 Hispanic/Latino), 24 international. Average age 27. In 2013, 12 doctorates awarded. *Degree requirements:* For doctorate, thesis/dissertation, qualifying examination. *Unit head:* Dr. Jerry Shay, Chair, 214-648-3282, E-mail: jerry.shay@utsouthwestern.edu. *Application contact:* 214-648-5617, Fax: 214-648-3289, E-mail: admissions@utsouthwestern.edu.
Website: http://www.utsouthwestern.edu/graduateschool/cancerbiology.html

University of the District of Columbia, College of Arts and Sciences, Department of Biological and Environmental Sciences, Program in Cancer Biology, Prevention and Control, Washington, DC 20008-1175. Offers MS. Program offered in partnership with Lombardi Comprehensive Cancer Center at Georgetown University. *Expenses: Tuition, area resident:* Full-time $7883.28; part-time $437.96 per credit hour. Tuition, state resident: full-time $8923.14. Tuition, nonresident: full-time $15,163; part-time $842.40 per credit hour. *Required fees:* $620; $30 per credit hour.

The University of Toledo, College of Graduate Studies, College of Medicine and Life Sciences, Department of Biochemistry and Cancer Biology, Toledo, OH 43606-3390. Offers cancer biology (MSBS, PhD); MD/MSBS; MD/PhD. *Faculty:* 16. *Students:* 19 full-time (14 women), 2 part-time (1 woman); includes 2 minority (1 Asian, non-Hispanic/Latino; 1 Hispanic/Latino), 13 international. Average age 26. 27 applicants, 30% accepted, 5 enrolled. In 2013, 4 doctorates awarded. Terminal master's awarded for partial completion of doctoral program. *Degree requirements:* For master's, thesis, qualifying exam; for doctorate, thesis/dissertation, qualifying exam. *Entrance requirements:* For master's and doctorate, GRE, minimum undergraduate GPA of 3.0, three letters of recommendation, statement of purpose, transcripts from all prior institutions attended; resume. Additional exam requirements/recommendations for international students: Required—TOEFL (minimum score 550 paper-based; 80 iBT). *Application deadline:* For fall admission, 1/15 priority date for domestic and international students. Application fee: $45 ($75 for international students). Electronic applications accepted. *Financial support:* In 2013–14, 21 research assistantships with full tuition reimbursements (averaging $22,032 per year) were awarded; Federal Work-Study, institutionally sponsored loans, scholarships/grants, tuition waivers (full), and unspecified assistantships also available. *Unit head:* Dr. William Maltese, Track Director, 419-383-4161, E-mail: william.maltese@utoledo.edu. *Application contact:* Admissions Analyst, 419-383-4112, Fax: 419-383-6140.
Website: http://www.utoledo.edu/med/grad/

University of Utah, School of Medicine and Graduate School, Graduate Programs in Medicine, Department of Oncological Sciences, Salt Lake City, UT 84112-1107. Offers M Phil, MS, PhD. Terminal master's awarded for partial completion of doctoral program. *Degree requirements:* For master's, thesis (for some programs); for doctorate, thesis/dissertation. *Entrance requirements:* For master's and doctorate, GRE General Test, GRE Subject Test, minimum GPA of 3.0. Additional exam requirements/recommendations for international students: Required—TOEFL. *Expenses:* Tuition, state resident: full-time $5259. Tuition, nonresident: full-time $18,569. *Required fees:* $841. Tuition and fees vary according to course load. *Faculty research:* Molecular basis of cell growth and differences, regulation of gene expression, biochemical mechanics of DNA replication, molecular biology and biochemistry of signal transduction, somatic cell genetics.

University of Wisconsin–La Crosse, Graduate Studies, College of Science and Health, Department of Health Professions, Program in Medical Dosimetry, La Crosse, WI 54601-3742. Offers MS. Postbaccalaureate distance learning degree programs offered (no on-campus study). *Faculty:* 1 (woman) full-time. *Students:* 21 full-time (9 women); includes 6 minority (2 Black or African American, non-Hispanic/Latino; 2 Asian, non-Hispanic/Latino; 2 Hispanic/Latino). Average age 30. 29 applicants, 45% accepted, 13 enrolled. In 2013, 13 master's awarded. *Entrance requirements:* For master's, American Registry of Radiologic Technologists test, Medical Dosimetrist Certification Board Exam. Additional exam requirements/recommendations for international students: Required—TOEFL (minimum score 600 paper-based; 100 iBT). *Application deadline:* For fall admission, 12/1 priority date for domestic students, 11/1 priority date for international students. Electronic applications accepted. *Expenses:* Contact institution. *Financial support:* Federal Work-Study and scholarships/grants available. Support available to part-time students. Financial award applicants required to submit FAFSA. *Unit head:* Nishele Lenards, Program Director, 608-785-8470, E-mail: nlenards@uwlax.edu. *Application contact:* Corey Sjoquist, Director of Admissions, 608-785-8939, E-mail: admissions@uwlax.edu.
Website: http://www.uwlax.edu/md/

University of Wisconsin–Madison, School of Medicine and Public Health and Graduate School, Graduate Programs in Medicine, Program in Cancer Biology, Madison, WI 53706. Offers PhD. *Faculty:* 51 full-time (15 women). *Students:* 31 full-time (18 women); includes 8 minority (1 Asian, non-Hispanic/Latino; 4 Hispanic/Latino; 3 Native Hawaiian or other Pacific Islander, non-Hispanic/Latino), 8 international. 200 applicants, 8% accepted, 5 enrolled. In 2013, 1 doctorate awarded. *Degree requirements:* For doctorate, comprehensive exam, thesis/dissertation. *Entrance requirements:* For doctorate, GRE General Test. Additional exam requirements/recommendations for international students: Required—TOEFL (minimum score 580 paper-based; 92 iBT). *Application deadline:* For fall admission, 12/1 priority date for domestic and international students. Application fee: $56. Electronic applications accepted. *Expenses:* Tuition, state resident: full-time $10,728; part-time $790 per credit. Tuition, nonresident: full-time $24,054; part-time $1623 per credit. *Required fees:* $1130; $119 per credit. *Financial support:* In 2013–14, 31 students received support, including fellowships with full tuition reimbursements available (averaging $25,500 per year), research assistantships with full tuition reimbursements available (averaging $25,500 per year); traineeships, health care benefits, and unspecified assistantships also available. Financial award application deadline: 12/1. *Faculty research:* Cancer genetics, tumor virology, chemical carcinogenesis, signal transduction, cell cycle. *Total annual research expenditures:* $18 million. *Unit head:* Dr. James Shull, Director, 608-262-2177, Fax: 608-262-2824, E-mail: shull@oncology.wisc.edu. *Application contact:* Katie Roemer, Administrative Program Manager, 608-262-4682, Fax: 608-262-2824, E-mail: kjroemer@oncology.wisc.edu.
Website: http://www.cancerbiology.wisc.edu/

Vanderbilt University, Graduate School, Department of Cancer Biology, Nashville, TN 37240-1001. Offers MS, PhD, MD/PhD. *Faculty:* 11 full-time (6 women). *Students:* 45 full-time (31 women); includes 15 minority (9 Black or African American, non-Hispanic/Latino; 2 Asian, non-Hispanic/Latino; 3 Hispanic/Latino; 1 Two or more races, non-Hispanic/Latino), 6 international. Average age 27. In 2013, 1 master's, 7 doctorates

awarded. *Degree requirements:* For doctorate, thesis/dissertation, final and qualifying exams. *Entrance requirements:* For master's and doctorate, GRE General Test. Additional exam requirements/recommendations for international students: Required—TOEFL (minimum score 570 paper-based; 88 iBT). *Application deadline:* For fall admission, 1/15 for domestic and international students. Application fee: $0. Electronic applications accepted. *Financial support:* Fellowships with full and partial tuition reimbursements, research assistantships with full and partial tuition reimbursements, Federal Work-Study, institutionally sponsored loans, scholarships/grants, traineeships, and health care benefits available. Financial award application deadline: 1/15; financial award applicants required to submit CSS PROFILE or FAFSA. *Faculty research:* Microenvironmental influences on cellular phenotype, in particular as it relates to host/tumor interactions, tumor-stroma interactions, angiogenesis, growth factor and cytokine signaling, oncogenes, tumor suppressors, matrix and matrix degradation, cell adhesion, metastasis. *Unit head:* Dr. Jin Chen, Director of Graduate Studies, 615-343-3819, Fax: 615-936-2911, E-mail: jin.chen@vanderbilt.edu. *Application contact:* Tracy Tveit, Graduate Program Coordinator, 615-936-2910, Fax: 615-936-2911, E-mail: tracy.s.tveit@vanderbilt.edu.
Website: https://medschool.vanderbilt.edu/cancer-biology/

Wake Forest University, School of Medicine and Graduate School of Arts and Sciences, Graduate Programs in Medicine, Department of Cancer Biology, Winston-Salem, NC 27109. Offers PhD, MD/PhD. *Degree requirements:* For doctorate, thesis/dissertation. *Entrance requirements:* For doctorate, GRE General Test. Additional exam requirements/recommendations for international students: Required—TOEFL. Electronic applications accepted. *Faculty research:* Cancer research, mechanisms of carcinogenesis, signal transduction and regulation of cell growth.

Wayne State University, School of Medicine, Graduate Programs in Medicine, Cancer Biology Graduate Program, Detroit, MI 48202. Offers MS, PhD. *Students:* 31 full-time (16 women); includes 6 minority (4 Black or African American, non-Hispanic/Latino; 1 Asian, non-Hispanic/Latino; 1 Two or more races, non-Hispanic/Latino), 1 international. Average age 27. 70 applicants, 7% accepted, 3 enrolled. In 2013, 1 master's, 5 doctorates awarded. *Degree requirements:* For doctorate, thesis/dissertation. *Entrance requirements:* For master's and doctorate, GRE General Test, statement of purpose, detailed description of research experience, resume, three letters of recommendation, background in one of the chemical or biological sciences, bachelor's or master's degree with minimum GPA of 3.0, admission to Graduate School. Additional exam requirements/recommendations for international students: Required—TOEFL (minimum score 550 paper-based; 100 iBT), TWE (minimum score 5.5), Michigan English Language Assessment Battery (minimum score 85); Recommended—IELTS (minimum score 6.5). *Application deadline:* For fall admission, 3/1 for domestic and international students. Application fee: $0. Electronic applications accepted. *Expenses:* Contact institution. *Financial support:* In 2013–14, 26 students received support, including 13 fellowships with tuition reimbursements available (averaging $22,562 per year), 17 research assistantships with tuition reimbursements available (averaging $22,762 per year); scholarships/grants, health care benefits, and unspecified assistantships also available. Financial award application deadline: 3/31; financial award applicants required to submit FAFSA. *Faculty research:* Molecular therapeutics, molecular imaging and diagnostics, tumor microenvironment, population studies. *Unit head:* Dr. George Brush, Director, 313-578-4300, E-mail: brushg@karmanos.org. *Application contact:* E-mail: cancerbio@karmanos.org.
Website: http://cancerbiologyprogram.med.wayne.edu/

Wayne State University, School of Medicine, Graduate Programs in Medicine, Department of Radiation Oncology, Detroit, MI 48202. Offers medical physics (PhD); radiological physics (MS). Part-time and evening/weekend programs available. *Students:* 25 full-time (3 women), 12 part-time (3 women); includes 10 minority (6 Asian, non-Hispanic/Latino; 2 Hispanic/Latino; 2 Two or more races, non-Hispanic/Latino), 10 international. Average age 30. 85 applicants, 27% accepted, 14 enrolled. In 2013, 12 master's, 1 doctorate awarded. Terminal master's awarded for partial completion of doctoral program. *Degree requirements:* For master's, thesis, essay, exit exam; for doctorate, thesis/dissertation, qualifying exam. *Entrance requirements:* For master's and doctorate, GRE General Test, BS in physics or related area, admission to the Graduate School. Additional exam requirements/recommendations for international students: Required—TOEFL (minimum score 550 paper-based); Recommended—TWE (minimum score 6). *Application deadline:* For fall admission, 1/15 for domestic students, 6/1 for international students; for winter admission, 10/1 for international students; for spring admission, 2/1 for international students. Application fee: $0. Electronic applications accepted. *Expenses:* Contact institution. *Financial support:* In 2013–14, 5 students received support, including 5 research assistantships (averaging $17,373 per year); fellowships, teaching assistantships, scholarships/grants, health care benefits, and unspecified assistantships also available. Financial award application deadline: 3/31; financial award applicants required to submit FAFSA. *Unit head:* Harold E. Kim, MD, Associate Professor and Interim Chair, 313-745-1538, E-mail: kimh@wayne.edu. *Application contact:* Dr. Jay Burmeister, Director, 313-745-2483, E-mail: burmeist@wayne.edu.
Website: http://radiationoncology.med.wayne.edu/

West Virginia University, Davis College of Agriculture, Forestry and Consumer Sciences, Interdisciplinary Program in Genetics and Developmental Biology, Morgantown, WV 26506. Offers animal breeding (MS, PhD); biochemical and molecular genetics (MS, PhD); cytogenetics (MS, PhD); descriptive embryology (MS, PhD); developmental genetics (MS); experimental morphogenesis/teratology (MS); human genetics (MS, PhD); immunogenetics (MS, PhD); life cycles of animals and plants (MS, PhD); molecular aspects of development (MS, PhD); mutagenesis (MS, PhD); oncology (MS, PhD); plant genetics (MS, PhD); population and quantitative genetics (MS, PhD); regeneration (MS, PhD); teratology (PhD); toxicology (MS, PhD). *Degree requirements:* For master's, thesis; for doctorate, comprehensive exam, thesis/dissertation. *Entrance requirements:* For master's, GRE or MCAT, minimum GPA of 2.75. Additional exam requirements/recommendations for international students: Required—TOEFL.

West Virginia University, School of Medicine, Graduate Programs at the Health Sciences Center, Interdisciplinary Graduate Programs in Biomedical Sciences, Program in Cancer Cell Biology, Morgantown, WV 26506. Offers PhD, MD/PhD. *Degree requirements:* For doctorate, comprehensive exam, thesis/dissertation. *Entrance requirements:* For doctorate, GRE General Test, minimum GPA of 3.0. Additional exam requirements/recommendations for international students: Required—TOEFL. Electronic applications accepted. *Faculty research:* Cellular signaling, tumor microenvironment, cancer therapeutics.

Yale University, School of Medicine and Graduate School of Arts and Sciences, Combined Program in Biological and Biomedical Sciences (BBS), Pharmacological Sciences and Molecular Medicine Track, New Haven, CT 06520. Offers PhD, MD/PhD. *Degree requirements:* For doctorate, thesis/dissertation. *Entrance requirements:* For doctorate, GRE General Test. Additional exam requirements/recommendations for international students: Required—TOEFL. Electronic applications accepted.

Cell Biology

Albany College of Pharmacy and Health Sciences, School of Health Sciences, Albany, NY 12208. Offers clinical laboratory sciences (MS); cytotechnology and molecular cytology (MS); molecular biosciences (MS). *Students:* 14 full-time (10 women), 5 part-time (2 women), 7 international. Average age 25. 53 applicants, 64% accepted, 13 enrolled. In 2013, 20 master's awarded. *Degree requirements:* For master's, thesis. *Entrance requirements:* For master's, GRE, minimum GPA of 3.0. Additional exam requirements/recommendations for international students: Required—TOEFL (minimum score 84 iBT). *Application deadline:* For fall admission, 4/15 for domestic and international students. Applications are processed on a rolling basis. Application fee: $75. Electronic applications accepted. *Financial support:* Federal Work-Study and scholarships/grants available. Support available to part-time students. Financial award application deadline: 3/1; financial award applicants required to submit FAFSA. *Unit head:* Dr. Martha Hass, Dean of Graduate Studies, 518-694-7238. *Application contact:* Ann Bruno, Coordinator, Graduate Programs, 518-694-7130, E-mail: graduate@acphs.edu.
Website: http://acphs.edu/academics/schools-departments/school-arts-and-sciences

Albany Medical College, Center for Cell Biology and Cancer Research, Albany, NY 12208-3479. Offers MS, PhD. Part-time programs available. Terminal master's awarded for partial completion of doctoral program. *Degree requirements:* For master's, thesis; for doctorate, comprehensive exam, thesis/dissertation. *Entrance requirements:* For master's and doctorate, GRE General Test, all transcripts, letters of recommendation. Additional exam requirements/recommendations for international students: Required—TOEFL. *Faculty research:* Cancer cell biology, tissue remodeling, signal transduction, gene regulation, cell adhesion, angiogenesis.

Albert Einstein College of Medicine, Graduate Division of Biomedical Sciences, Department of Anatomy and Structural Biology, Bronx, NY 10461. Offers anatomy (PhD); cell and developmental biology (PhD); MD/PhD. *Degree requirements:* For doctorate, thesis/dissertation. *Entrance requirements:* For doctorate, GRE General Test. Additional exam requirements/recommendations for international students: Required—TOEFL. Electronic applications accepted. *Faculty research:* Cell motility, cell membranes and membrane-cytoskeletal interactions as applied to processing of pancreatic hormones, mechanisms of secretion.

Albert Einstein College of Medicine, Graduate Division of Biomedical Sciences, Department of Cell Biology, Bronx, NY 10461. Offers PhD, MD/PhD. *Degree requirements:* For doctorate, thesis/dissertation. *Entrance requirements:* For doctorate, GRE General Test. Additional exam requirements/recommendations for international students: Required—TOEFL. *Faculty research:* Molecular and genetic basis of gene expression in animal cells; expression of differentiated traits of albumin, hemoglobin, myosin, and immunoglobin.

American University of Beirut, Graduate Programs, Faculty of Arts and Sciences, Beirut, Lebanon. Offers anthropology (MA); Arab and Middle Eastern history (PhD); Arabic language and literature (MA, PhD); archaeology (MA); biology (MS); cell and molecular biology (PhD); chemistry (MS); clinical psychology (MA); computational sciences (MS); computer science (MS); economics (MA); education (MA); English language (MA); English literature (MA); environmental policy planning (MS); financial economics (MA); geology (MS); history (MA); mathematics (MA, MS); media studies (MA); Middle Eastern studies (MA); philosophy (MA); physics (MS); political studies (MA); psychology (MA); public administration (MA); sociology (MA); statistics (MA, MS); theoretical physics (PhD); transnational American studies (MA). Part-time programs available. *Faculty:* 88 full-time (22 women). *Students:* Average age 25. In 2013, 112 master's, 87 doctorates awarded. *Degree requirements:* For master's, one foreign language, comprehensive exam, thesis (for some programs); for doctorate, one foreign language, comprehensive exam, thesis/dissertation. *Entrance requirements:* For master's, GRE, letter of recommendation; for doctorate, GRE, letters of recommendation. Additional exam requirements/recommendations for international students: Required—TOEFL (minimum score 600 paper-based; 97 iBT), IELTS (minimum score 7). *Application deadline:* For fall admission, 4/30 for domestic students, 4/18 for international students; for spring admission, 11/1 for domestic and international students. Application fee: $50. *Expenses: Tuition:* Full-time $14,724; part-time $818 per credit. *Required fees:* $692. Tuition and fees vary according to course load and program. *Financial support:* Research assistantships, career-related internships or fieldwork, institutionally sponsored loans, scholarships/grants, health care benefits, and unspecified assistantships available. Financial award application deadline: 2/4; financial award applicants required to submit FAFSA. *Faculty research:* Modern Middle East history; Near Eastern archaeology; Islamic history; European history; software engineering; scientific computing; data mining; the applications of cooperative learning in language teaching and teacher education; world/comparative literature; rhetoric and composition; creative writing; public management; public policy and international affairs; hydrogeology; mineralogy, petrology, and geochemistry; tectonics and structural geology; cell and molecular biology; ecology. *Unit head:* Dr. Patrick McGreevy, Dean, 961-1374374 Ext. 3800, Fax: 961-1744461, E-mail: pm07@aub.edu.lb. *Application contact:* Dr. Salim Kanaan, Director, Admissions Office, 961-1-350000 Ext. 2590, Fax: 96-1-1750775, E-mail: sk00@aub.edu.lb.
Website: http://www.aub.edu.lb/fas/

American University of Beirut, Graduate Programs, Faculty of Medicine, Beirut, Lebanon. Offers anatomy, cell biology and human morphology (MS); biochemistry and medical genetics (MS); biomedical sciences (PhD); experimental pathology, immunology and microbiology (MS); medicine (MD); neuroscience (MS); pharmacology and toxicology (MS). Part-time programs available. *Faculty:* 259 full-time (78 women), 93 part-time/adjunct (16 women). *Students:* 364 full-time (165 women), 62 part-time (54 women). Average age 23. In 2013, 18 master's awarded. *Degree requirements:* For master's, one foreign language, comprehensive exam, thesis (for some programs); for doctorate, one foreign language, comprehensive exam, thesis/dissertation. *Entrance requirements:* For master's, letter of recommendation; for doctorate, MCAT, bachelor's degree. Additional exam requirements/recommendations for international students:

Required—TOEFL (minimum score 600 paper-based; 100 iBT), IELTS (minimum score 7.5). *Application deadline:* For fall admission, 4/30 for domestic and international students; for spring admission, 11/1 for domestic and international students. Application fee: $50. *Expenses: Tuition:* Full-time $14,724; part-time $818 per credit. *Required fees:* $692. Tuition and fees vary according to course load and program. *Financial support:* In 2013–14, 242 students received support, including 60 teaching assistantships (averaging $4,000 per year); career-related internships or fieldwork, institutionally sponsored loans, scholarships/grants, health care benefits, and unspecified assistantships also available. Financial award application deadline: 2/2. *Faculty research:* Cancer research (targeted therapy, mechanisms of leukemogenesis, tumor cell extravasation and metastasis, cancer stem cells), stem cell research (regenerative medicine, drug discovery), genetic research (neurogenetics, hereditary cardiomyopathy, hemoglobinopathies, pharmacogenomics, proteomics), neuroscience research (pain, neurodegenerative disorder), metabolism (inflammation and metabolism, metabolic disorder, diabetes mellitus), vascular and renal biology, signal transduction. *Total annual research expenditures:* $2.6 million. *Unit head:* Dr. Mohamed Sayegh, Dean, 961-1350000 Ext. 4700, Fax: 961-1744464, E-mail: msayegh@aub.edu.lb. *Application contact:* Dr. Salim Kanaan, Director, Admissions Office, 961-1-350000 Ext. 2594, Fax: 96-1-1750775, E-mail: sk00@aub.edu.lb.
Website: http://www.aub.edu.lb/fm/fm_home/Pages/index.aspx

Appalachian State University, Cratis D. Williams Graduate School, Department of Biology, Boone, NC 28608. Offers cell and molecular biology (MS); general biology (MS). Part-time programs available. *Degree requirements:* For master's, comprehensive exam, thesis. *Entrance requirements:* For master's, GRE General Test, 3 letters of recommendation. Additional exam requirements/recommendations for international students: Required—TOEFL (minimum score 570 paper-based; 79 iBT), IELTS (minimum score 6.5). Electronic applications accepted. *Faculty research:* Aquatic and terrestrial ecology, animal and plant physiology, behavior and systematics, immunology and cell biology, molecular biology and microbiology.

Arizona State University at the Tempe campus, College of Liberal Arts and Sciences, School of Life Sciences, Tempe, AZ 85287-4601. Offers animal behavior (PhD); applied ethics (biomedical and health ethics) (MA); biological design (PhD); biology (MS, PhD); biology (biology and society) (MS, PhD); environmental life sciences (PhD); evolutionary biology (PhD); human and social dimensions of science and technology (PhD); microbiology (PhD); molecular and cellular biology (PhD); neuroscience (PhD); philosophy (history and philosophy of science) (MA); sustainability (PhD). Terminal master's awarded for partial completion of doctoral program. *Degree requirements:* For master's, thesis (for some programs), interactive Program of Study (iPOS) submitted before completing 50 percent of required credit hours; for doctorate, variable foreign language requirement, comprehensive exam, thesis/dissertation, interactive Program of Study (iPOS) submitted before completing 50 percent of required credit hours. *Entrance requirements:* For master's and doctorate, GRE, minimum GPA of 3.0 or equivalent in last 2 years of work leading to bachelor's degree. Additional exam requirements/recommendations for international students: Required—TOEFL (minimum score 600 paper-based; 100 iBT). Electronic applications accepted.

Auburn University, Graduate School, Interdepartmental Programs, Auburn University, AL 36849. Offers applied economics (PhD); cell and molecular biology (PhD); real estate development (MRED); sociology and rural sociology (MA, MS), including rural sociology (MS), sociology. Part-time programs available. *Students:* 42 full-time (21 women), 35 part-time (8 women); includes 15 minority (12 Black or African American, non-Hispanic/Latino; 1 American Indian or Alaska Native, non-Hispanic/Latino; 2 Asian, non-Hispanic/Latino), 30 international. Average age 32. 80 applicants, 68% accepted, 33 enrolled. In 2013, 21 master's, 6 doctorates awarded. *Entrance requirements:* For master's, GRE General Test. *Application deadline:* For fall admission, 7/7 for domestic students; for spring admission, 11/24 for domestic students. Applications are processed on a rolling basis. Application fee: $50 ($60 for international students). Electronic applications accepted. *Expenses:* Tuition, state resident: full-time $8262; part-time $459 per credit hour. Tuition, nonresident: full-time $24,786; part-time $1377 per credit hour. Tuition and fees vary according to degree level and program. *Financial support:* Fellowships, research assistantships, teaching assistantships, and Federal Work-Study available. Support available to part-time students. Financial award application deadline: 3/15; financial award applicants required to submit FAFSA. *Unit head:* Dr. George Flowers, Dean, 334-844-4700, E-mail: gradadm@auburn.edu. *Application contact:* Dr. George Flowers, Dean of the Graduate School, 334-844-2125.

Baylor College of Medicine, Graduate School of Biomedical Sciences, Department of Molecular and Cellular Biology, Houston, TX 77030-3498. Offers PhD, MD/PhD. *Degree requirements:* For doctorate, thesis/dissertation, public defense, qualifying exam. *Entrance requirements:* For doctorate, GRE General Test, GRE Subject Test (strongly recommended), minimum GPA of 3.0. Additional exam requirements/recommendations for international students: Required—TOEFL. Electronic applications accepted. *Faculty research:* Hormone action, development, cancer, gene therapy, neurobiology.

Baylor College of Medicine, Graduate School of Biomedical Sciences, Interdepartmental Program in Cell and Molecular Biology, Houston, TX 77030-3498. Offers biochemistry (PhD); cell and molecular biology (PhD); genetics (PhD); human genetics (PhD); immunology (PhD); microbiology (PhD); virology (PhD); MD/PhD. *Degree requirements:* For doctorate, thesis/dissertation, public defense. *Entrance requirements:* For doctorate, GRE General Test, GRE Subject Test (strongly recommended), minimum GPA of 3.0. Additional exam requirements/recommendations for international students: Required—TOEFL. Electronic applications accepted. *Faculty research:* Molecular and cellular biology; cancer, aging and stem cells; genomics and proteomics; microbiome, molecular microbiology; infectious disease, immunology and translational research.

Baylor College of Medicine, Graduate School of Biomedical Sciences, Program in Developmental Biology, Houston, TX 77030-3498. Offers PhD, MD/PhD. *Degree requirements:* For doctorate, thesis/dissertation, public defense. *Entrance requirements:* For doctorate, GRE General Test, GRE Subject Test (strongly recommended), minimum GPA of 3.0. Additional exam requirements/recommendations for international students: Required—TOEFL. Electronic applications accepted. *Faculty research:* Stem cells, cancer, neurobiology, organogenesis, genetics of model organisms.

Boston University, Graduate School of Arts and Sciences, Molecular Biology, Cell Biology, and Biochemistry Program (MCBB), Boston, MA 02215. Offers MA, PhD. *Students:* 34 full-time (16 women), 2 part-time (1 woman); includes 10 minority (2 Black or African American, non-Hispanic/Latino; 2 Asian, non-Hispanic/Latino; 5 Hispanic/Latino; 1 Two or more races, non-Hispanic/Latino), 9 international. Average age 27. 96 applicants, 16% accepted, 8 enrolled. In 2013, 2 master's, 5 doctorates awarded. Terminal master's awarded for partial completion of doctoral program. *Degree requirements:* For master's, one foreign language, thesis (for some programs); for doctorate, one foreign language, comprehensive exam, thesis/dissertation. *Entrance requirements:* For master's and doctorate, GRE General Test, GRE Subject Test, 3 letters of recommendation. Additional exam requirements/recommendations for international students: Required—TOEFL (minimum score 600 paper-based). *Application deadline:* For fall admission, 12/7 for domestic and international students. Application fee: $80. Electronic applications accepted. *Expenses: Tuition:* Full-time $43,970; part-time $1374 per credit hour. *Required fees:* $60 per semester. Tuition and fees vary according to class time, course level and program. *Financial support:* In 2013–14, 32 students received support, including 4 fellowships with full tuition reimbursements available (averaging $20,000 per year), 12 research assistantships with full tuition reimbursements available (averaging $20,000 per year), 4 teaching assistantships with full tuition reimbursements available (averaging $20,000 per year); Federal Work-Study, scholarships/grants, traineeships, and health care benefits also available. Financial award application deadline: 12/7; financial award applicants required to submit FAFSA. *Unit head:* Dr. Ulla Hansen, Director, 617-353-2432, Fax: 617-353-6340, E-mail: uhansen@bu.edu. *Application contact:* Meredith Canode, Academic Administrator, 617-353-2432, Fax: 617-353-6340, E-mail: mcanode@bu.edu.
Website: http://www.bu.edu/mcbb/

Boston University, School of Medicine, Division of Graduate Medical Sciences, Department of Biochemistry, Boston, MA 02118. Offers MA, PhD, MD/PhD. Part-time programs available. Terminal master's awarded for partial completion of doctoral program. *Degree requirements:* For master's, thesis or alternative; for doctorate, thesis/dissertation. *Application deadline:* For fall admission, 1/15 for domestic students; for spring admission, 10/15 for domestic students. *Expenses: Tuition:* Full-time $43,970; part-time $1374 per credit hour. *Required fees:* $60 per semester. Tuition and fees vary according to class time, course level and program. *Unit head:* Dr. David A. Harris, Chair, 617-638-5090. *Application contact:* Dr. Barbara Schreiber, Director of the Graduate Program, 617-638-5094, E-mail: schreibe@bu.edu.
Website: http://www.bumc.bu.edu/biochemistry/

Boston University, School of Medicine, Division of Graduate Medical Sciences, Program in Cell and Molecular Biology, Boston, MA 02118. Offers PhD. *Degree requirements:* For doctorate, thesis/dissertation. *Application deadline:* For fall admission, 1/15 for domestic students; for spring admission, 10/15 for domestic students. *Expenses: Tuition:* Full-time $43,970; part-time $1374 per credit hour. *Required fees:* $60 per semester. Tuition and fees vary according to class time, course level and program. *Financial support:* Scholarships/grants and traineeships available. Financial award applicants required to submit FAFSA. *Unit head:* Dr. Vickery Trinkaus-Randall, Director, 617-638-6099, Fax: 617-638-5337, E-mail: vickery@bu.edu. *Application contact:* GMS Admissions Office, 617-638-5255, Fax: 617-638-5740, E-mail: natashah@bu.edu.
Website: http://www.bumc.bu.edu/cmbio/

Brandeis University, Graduate School of Arts and Sciences, Program in Molecular and Cell Biology, Waltham, MA 02454-9110. Offers genetics (PhD); microbiology (PhD); molecular and cell biology (MS, PhD); molecular biology (PhD); neurobiology (PhD); quantitative biology (PhD). Terminal master's awarded for partial completion of doctoral program. *Degree requirements:* For master's, thesis or alternative, research project, research lab, or project lab; for doctorate, comprehensive exam, thesis/dissertation, journal clubs; research seminar; colloquia; qualifying exam. *Entrance requirements:* For master's, GRE General Test (or MCAT for applicants to the MS program), official transcript(s), resume, 3 letters of recommendation, statement of purpose; for doctorate, GRE General Test, official transcript(s), resume, 3 letters of recommendation, statement of purpose. Additional exam requirements/recommendations for international students: Required—TOEFL (minimum score 600 paper-based; 100 iBT), PTE (minimum score 68); Recommended—IELTS (minimum score 7). Electronic applications accepted. *Faculty research:* Structural biology; immunology; developmental biology; behavior and neurobiology; DNA replication, rearrangement, and repair; signal transduction, transcriptional regulation, and RNA processing; cancer and programmed cell death; cytoskeleton and molecular motors; nutrition.

Brown University, Graduate School, Division of Biology and Medicine, Department of Molecular Biology, Cell Biology, and Biochemistry, Providence, RI 02912. Offers MA, PhD. Part-time programs available. Terminal master's awarded for partial completion of doctoral program. *Degree requirements:* For master's, thesis (for some programs); for doctorate, one foreign language, thesis/dissertation, preliminary exam. *Entrance requirements:* For master's and doctorate, GRE General Test, GRE Subject Test. Additional exam requirements/recommendations for international students: Required—TOEFL. Electronic applications accepted. *Faculty research:* Molecular genetics, gene regulation.

California Institute of Technology, Division of Biology, Program in Cell Biology and Biophysics, Pasadena, CA 91125-0001. Offers PhD. *Degree requirements:* For doctorate, thesis/dissertation, qualifying exam. *Entrance requirements:* For doctorate, GRE General Test.

California State University, Sacramento, Office of Graduate Studies, College of Natural Sciences and Mathematics, Department of Biological Sciences, Sacramento, CA 95819. Offers biological conservation (MS); marine science (MS); molecular and cellular biology (MS); stem cell (MA). Part-time programs available. *Degree requirements:* For master's, thesis, writing proficiency exam. *Entrance requirements:* For master's, GRE, bachelor's degree in biology or equivalent; minimum GPA of 3.0 in biology, 2.75 overall during last 2 years of course work. Additional exam requirements/recommendations for international students: Required—TOEFL. *Application deadline:* For fall admission, 2/1 for domestic students, 3/1 for international students; for spring admission, 9/30 for international students. Applications are processed on a rolling basis. Application fee: $55. Electronic applications accepted. *Financial support:* Research assistantships, teaching assistantships, career-related internships or fieldwork, and Federal Work-Study available. Support available to part-time students. Financial award application deadline: 3/1; financial award applicants required to submit FAFSA. *Unit head:* Jennifer Lundmark, Chair, 916-278-6535, E-mail: lundmark@csus.edu. *Application contact:* Jose Martinez, Graduate Admissions Supervisor, 916-278-7871, E-mail: martinj@skymail.csus.edu.
Website: http://www.csus.edu/bios

Carnegie Mellon University, Mellon College of Science, Department of Biological Sciences, Pittsburgh, PA 15213-3891. Offers biochemistry (PhD); biophysics (PhD); cell and developmental biology (PhD); computational biology (MS, PhD); genetics (PhD); molecular biology (PhD); neuroscience (PhD); structural biology (PhD). *Degree requirements:* For doctorate, comprehensive exam, thesis/dissertation. *Entrance requirements:* For doctorate, GRE General Test, GRE Subject Test, interview. *Application deadline:* Applications are processed on a rolling basis. Application fee: $0. Electronic applications accepted. *Financial support:* Fellowships, research assistantships, teaching assistantships, and traineeships available. *Faculty research:* Genetic structure, function, and regulation; protein structure and function; biological membranes; biological spectroscopy. *Unit head:* John L. Woolford, Acting Department Head, 412-268-3193, E-mail: jw17@andrew.cmu.edu. *Application contact:* Ena Miceli, Graduate Programs Manager, 412-268-33012, E-mail: emiceli@andrew.cmu.edu.
Website: http://www.bio.cmu.edu/

Case Western Reserve University, School of Medicine and School of Graduate Studies, Graduate Programs in Medicine, Department of Anatomy, Cleveland, OH 44106. Offers applied anatomy (MS); biological anthropology (MS); cellular biology (MS); MD/MS. Part-time programs available. *Degree requirements:* For master's, comprehensive exam, thesis (for some programs). *Entrance requirements:* For master's,

GRE General Test. Additional exam requirements/recommendations for international students: Required—TOEFL. *Faculty research:* Hypoxia, cell injury, biochemical aberration occurrences in ischemic tissue, human functional morphology, evolutionary morphology.

Case Western Reserve University, School of Medicine and School of Graduate Studies, Graduate Programs in Medicine, Department of Molecular Biology and Microbiology, Cleveland, OH 44106-4960. Offers cellular biology (PhD); microbiology (PhD); molecular biology (PhD); molecular virology (PhD); MD/PhD. Students are admitted to an integrated Biomedical Sciences Training Program involving 11 basic science programs at Case Western Reserve University. *Degree requirements:* For doctorate, thesis/dissertation. *Entrance requirements:* For doctorate, GRE General Test, GRE Subject Test. Additional exam requirements/recommendations for international students: Required—TOEFL. Electronic applications accepted. *Faculty research:* Gene expression in eukaryotic and prokaryotic systems; microbial physiology; intracellular transport and signaling; mechanisms of oncogenesis; molecular mechanisms of RNA processing, editing, and catalysis.

Case Western Reserve University, School of Medicine and School of Graduate Studies, Graduate Programs in Medicine, Program in Cell Biology, Cleveland, OH 44106. Offers PhD. *Degree requirements:* For doctorate, thesis/dissertation. *Entrance requirements:* For doctorate, GRE General Test, GRE Subject Test, previous course work in biochemistry. Additional exam requirements/recommendations for international students: Required—TOEFL. Electronic applications accepted. *Faculty research:* Macromolecular transport, membrane traffic, signal transduction, nuclear organization, lipid metabolism.

Case Western Reserve University, School of Medicine and School of Graduate Studies, Graduate Programs in Medicine, Programs in Molecular and Cellular Basis of Disease/Pathology, Cleveland, OH 44106. Offers cancer biology (PhD); cell biology (MS, PhD); immunology (MS, PhD); pathology (MS, PhD); MD/PhD. Terminal master's awarded for partial completion of doctoral program. *Degree requirements:* For master's, thesis; for doctorate, thesis/dissertation. *Entrance requirements:* For master's and doctorate, GRE General Test, GRE Subject Test. Additional exam requirements/recommendations for international students: Required—TOEFL (minimum score 550 paper-based). Electronic applications accepted. *Faculty research:* Neurobiology, molecular biology, cancer biology, biomaterials, biocompatibility.

The Catholic University of America, School of Arts and Sciences, Department of Biology, Washington, DC 20064. Offers cell and microbial biology (MS, PhD), including cell biology, microbiology; clinical laboratory science (MS, PhD); MSLS/MS. Part-time programs available. *Faculty:* 9 full-time (4 women), 5 part-time/adjunct (4 women). *Students:* 27 full-time (19 women), 36 part-time (22 women); includes 12 minority (7 Black or African American, non-Hispanic/Latino; 2 Asian, non-Hispanic/Latino; 2 Hispanic/Latino; 1 Two or more races, non-Hispanic/Latino), 36 international. Average age 30. 66 applicants, 56% accepted, 19 enrolled. In 2013, 10 master's, 3 doctorates awarded. *Degree requirements:* For master's, comprehensive exam, thesis or alternative; for doctorate, comprehensive exam, thesis/dissertation. *Entrance requirements:* For master's and doctorate, GRE General Test, GRE Subject Test, statement of purpose, official copies of academic transcripts, three letters of recommendation. Additional exam requirements/recommendations for international students: Required—TOEFL (minimum score 580 paper-based). *Application deadline:* For fall admission, 8/1 priority date for domestic students, 7/15 for international students; for spring admission, 12/1 priority date for domestic students, 10/15 for international students. Applications are processed on a rolling basis. Application fee: $55. Electronic applications accepted. *Expenses: Tuition:* Full-time $38,500; part-time $1490 per credit hour. *Required fees:* $400; $1525 per credit hour. One-time fee: $425. Tuition and fees vary according to program. *Financial support:* Fellowships, research assistantships, teaching assistantships, Federal Work-Study, scholarships/grants, tuition waivers (full and partial), and unspecified assistantships available. Financial award application deadline: 2/1; financial award applicants required to submit FAFSA. *Faculty research:* Cell and microbiology, molecular biology of cell proliferation, cellular effects of electromagnetic radiation, biotechnology. *Total annual research expenditures:* $1.5 million. *Unit head:* Dr. Venigalla Rao, Chair, 202-319-5271, Fax: 202-319-5721, E-mail: rao@cua.edu. *Application contact:* Andrew Woodall, Director of Graduate Admissions, 202-319-5057, Fax: 202-319-6533, E-mail: cua-admissions@cua.edu.
Website: http://biology.cua.edu/

Colorado State University, Graduate School, Program in Cell and Molecular Biology, Fort Collins, CO 80523-1618. Offers MS, PhD. *Students:* 28 full-time (18 women), 50 part-time (27 women); includes 11 minority (2 Black or African American, non-Hispanic/Latino; 8 Hispanic/Latino; 1 Two or more races, non-Hispanic/Latino), 28 international. Average age 30. 54 applicants, 17% accepted, 9 enrolled. In 2013, 2 master's, 3 doctorates awarded. Terminal master's awarded for partial completion of doctoral program. *Degree requirements:* For master's, comprehensive exam (for some programs), thesis; for doctorate, comprehensive exam, thesis/dissertation. *Entrance requirements:* For master's and doctorate, GRE General Test, GRE Subject Test in biology (strongly recommended), minimum GPA of 3.0; BA/BS in biology, biochemistry, physics; calculus sequence, letters of recommendation. Additional exam requirements/recommendations for international students: Required—TOEFL (minimum score 625 paper-based; 107 iBT). *Application deadline:* For fall admission, 1/1 priority date for domestic and international students. Applications are processed on a rolling basis. Application fee: $50. Electronic applications accepted. *Expenses:* Tuition, state resident: full-time $9075.40; part-time $504 per credit. Tuition, nonresident: full-time $22,248; part-time $1236 per credit. *Required fees:* $1819; $60 per credit. *Financial support:* In 2013–14, 7 students received support, including 4 research assistantships with full tuition reimbursements available (averaging $22,765 per year), 3 teaching assistantships with full tuition reimbursements available (averaging $16,380 per year); tuition waivers (full) also available. Financial award application deadline: 1/1. *Faculty research:* Cancer biology, genomics and computational biology, infectious diseases, metabolic regulation, neuroscience and molecular physiology, plant biology, regulation of gene expression, reproductive and developmental biology. *Total annual research expenditures:* $2,294. *Unit head:* Dr. Howard Liber, Director, 970-491-0580, Fax: 970-491-2194, E-mail: howard.liber@colostate.edu. *Application contact:* Lori Williams, Graduate Coordinator, 970-491-0241, Fax: 970-491-2194, E-mail: lori.williams@colostate.edu.
Website: http://cmb.colostate.edu/

Columbia University, College of Physicians and Surgeons, Department of Anatomy and Cell Biology, New York, NY 10032. Offers anatomy (M Phil, MA, PhD); anatomy and cell biology (PhD); MD/PhD. Only candidates for the PhD are admitted. Terminal master's awarded for partial completion of doctoral program. *Degree requirements:* For doctorate, thesis/dissertation, oral exam. *Entrance requirements:* For master's and doctorate, GRE General Test. Additional exam requirements/recommendations for international students: Required—TOEFL. *Faculty research:* Protein sorting, membrane biophysics, muscle energetics, neuroendocrinology, developmental biology, cytoskeleton, transcription factors.

Columbia University, College of Physicians and Surgeons, Integrated Program in Cellular, Molecular, Structural and Genetic Studies, New York, NY 10032. Offers PhD. Terminal master's awarded for partial completion of doctoral program. *Degree requirements:* For doctorate, thesis/dissertation. *Entrance requirements:* For doctorate, GRE General Test, GRE Subject Test. Additional exam requirements/recommendations for international students: Required—TOEFL. *Expenses:* Contact institution. *Faculty research:* Transcription, macromolecular sorting, gene expression during development, cellular interaction.

Cornell University, Graduate School, Graduate Fields of Agriculture and Life Sciences, Field of Biochemistry, Molecular and Cell Biology, Ithaca, NY 14853-0001. Offers biochemistry (PhD); biophysics (PhD); cell biology (PhD); molecular biology (PhD). *Faculty:* 20 full-time (19 women). *Students:* 87 full-time (43 women); includes 17 minority (7 Asian, non-Hispanic/Latino; 6 Hispanic/Latino; 4 Two or more races, non-Hispanic/Latino), 28 international. Average age 26. 238 applicants, 20% accepted, 20 enrolled. In 2013, 17 doctorates awarded. *Degree requirements:* For doctorate, comprehensive exam, thesis/dissertation, 2 semesters of teaching experience. *Entrance requirements:* For doctorate, GRE General Test, GRE Subject Test (biology, chemistry, physics, biochemistry, cell and molecular biology), 3 letters of recommendation. Additional exam requirements/recommendations for international students: Required—TOEFL (minimum score 600 paper-based; 77 iBT). *Application deadline:* For fall admission, 1/5 for domestic students. Application fee: $95. Electronic applications accepted. *Financial support:* In 2013–14, 62 students received support, including 8 fellowships with full tuition reimbursements available, 38 research assistantships with full tuition reimbursements available, 16 teaching assistantships with full tuition reimbursements available; institutionally sponsored loans, scholarships/grants, health care benefits, tuition waivers (full and partial), and unspecified assistantships also available. Financial award applicants required to submit FAFSA. *Faculty research:* Biophysics, structural biology. *Unit head:* Director of Graduate Studies, 607-255-2100, Fax: 607-255-2100. *Application contact:* Graduate Field Assistant, 607-255-2100, Fax: 607-255-2100, E-mail: bmcb@cornell.edu.
Website: http://www.gradschool.cornell.edu/fields.php?id-43&a-2

Cornell University, Graduate School, Graduate Fields of Agriculture and Life Sciences, Field of Computational Biology, Ithaca, NY 14853-0001. Offers computational behavioral biology (PhD); computational biology (PhD); computational cell biology (PhD); computational ecology (PhD); computational genetics (PhD); computational macromolecular biology (PhD); computational organismal biology (PhD). *Faculty:* 37 full-time (5 women). *Students:* 26 full-time (8 women); includes 8 minority (5 Asian, non-Hispanic/Latino; 1 Hispanic/Latino; 1 Native Hawaiian or other Pacific Islander, non-Hispanic/Latino; 1 Two or more races, non-Hispanic/Latino), 8 international. Average age 25. 171 applicants, 13% accepted, 10 enrolled. *Degree requirements:* For doctorate, comprehensive exam, thesis/dissertation, 2 semesters of teaching experience. *Entrance requirements:* For doctorate, GRE General Test, GRE Subject Test (biology), 2 letters of recommendation. Additional exam requirements/recommendations for international students: Required—TOEFL (minimum score 550 paper-based; 77 iBT). *Application deadline:* For fall admission, 2/1 priority date for domestic students. Application fee: $95. Electronic applications accepted. *Financial support:* In 2013–14, 22 students received support, including 20 research assistantships with full tuition reimbursements available, 2 teaching assistantships with full tuition reimbursements available; fellowships with full tuition reimbursements available, institutionally sponsored loans, scholarships/grants, health care benefits, tuition waivers (full and partial), and unspecified assistantships also available. Financial award applicants required to submit FAFSA. *Faculty research:* Computational behavioral biology, computational biology, computational cell biology, computational ecology, computational genetics, computational macromolecular biology, computational organismal biology. *Unit head:* Dr. Andrew Clark, Director of Graduate Studies, 607-255-5488, E-mail: ac347@cornell.edu. *Application contact:* Graduate School Application Requests, 607-255-5816, E-mail: gradadmissions@cornell.edu.
Website: http://www.gradschool.cornell.edu/fields.php?id-4A

Cornell University, Graduate School, Graduate Fields of Agriculture and Life Sciences, Field of Zoology and Wildlife Conservation, Ithaca, NY 14853-0001. Offers animal cytology (PhD); comparative and functional anatomy (PhD); developmental biology (PhD); ecology (PhD); histology (PhD); wildlife conservation (PhD). *Faculty:* 21 full-time (6 women). *Students:* 4 full-time (3 women), 1 part-time (0 women); includes 2 minority (1 Hispanic/Latino; 1 Two or more races, non-Hispanic/Latino), 1 international. Average age 26. 18 applicants, 6% accepted, 1 enrolled. In 2013, 1 doctorate awarded. *Degree requirements:* For doctorate, comprehensive exam, thesis/dissertation, 2 semesters of teaching experience. *Entrance requirements:* For doctorate, GRE General Test, GRE Subject Test (biology), 2 letters of recommendation. Additional exam requirements/recommendations for international students: Required—TOEFL (minimum score 550 paper-based; 77 iBT). *Application deadline:* For fall admission, 2/1 priority date for domestic students. Application fee: $95. Electronic applications accepted. *Financial support:* In 2013–14, 4 students received support, including 3 research assistantships with full tuition reimbursements available, 1 teaching assistantship with full tuition reimbursement available; fellowships with full tuition reimbursements available, institutionally sponsored loans, scholarships/grants, health care benefits, tuition waivers (full and partial), and unspecified assistantships also available. Financial award applicants required to submit FAFSA. *Faculty research:* Organismal biology, functional morphology, biomechanics, comparative vertebrate anatomy, comparative invertebrate anatomy, paleontology. *Unit head:* Director of Graduate Studies, 607-253-3276, Fax: 607-253-3756. *Application contact:* Graduate Field Assistant, 607-253-3276, Fax: 607-253-3756, E-mail: graduate_edcvm@cornell.edu.
Website: http://www.gradschool.cornell.edu/fields.php?id-65&a-2

Dartmouth College, Graduate Program in Molecular and Cellular Biology, Hanover, NH 03755. Offers PhD, MD/PhD. *Entrance requirements:* For doctorate, GRE General Test, letters of recommendation. Additional exam requirements/recommendations for international students: Required—TOEFL (minimum score 450 paper-based; 90 iBT) or IELTS (minimum score 7). Electronic applications accepted.

Drexel University, College of Medicine, Biomedical Graduate Programs, Interdisciplinary Program in Molecular and Cell Biology and Genetics, Philadelphia, PA 19104-2875. Offers MS, PhD, MD/PhD. Terminal master's awarded for partial completion of doctoral program. *Degree requirements:* For master's, comprehensive exam, thesis; for doctorate, thesis/dissertation, qualifying exam. *Entrance requirements:* For master's, GRE General Test, minimum GPA of 2.75; for doctorate, GRE General Test, minimum GPA of 3.0. Additional exam requirements/recommendations for international students: Required—TOEFL. Electronic applications accepted. *Faculty research:* Molecular anatomy, biochemistry, medical biotechnology, molecular pathology, microbiology and immunology.

Duke University, Graduate School, Department of Cell Biology, Durham, NC 27710. Offers PhD. *Faculty:* 15. *Students:* 32 full-time (17 women); includes 8 minority (1 American Indian or Alaska Native, non-Hispanic/Latino; 4 Asian, non-Hispanic/Latino; 3 Hispanic/Latino), 4 international. In 2013, 3 doctorates awarded. *Degree requirements:* For doctorate, thesis/dissertation. *Entrance requirements:* For doctorate, GRE General Test, GRE Subject Test in biology, chemistry, cell and molecular biology (recommended). Additional exam requirements/recommendations for international students: Required—TOEFL (minimum score 577 paper-based; 90 iBT) or IELTS

(minimum score 7). *Application deadline:* For fall admission, 12/8 priority date for domestic and international students. Applications are processed on a rolling basis. Application fee: $80. Electronic applications accepted. *Financial support:* Fellowships, research assistantships, teaching assistantships, and Federal Work-Study available. Financial award application deadline: 12/8. *Unit head:* Terry Lechler, Director of Graduate Studies, 919-684-8085, Fax: 919-684-8592, E-mail: jacquelyn.soderling@duke.edu. *Application contact:* Elizabeth Hutton, Director of Admissions, 919-684-3913, Fax: 919-684-2277, E-mail: grad-admissions@duke.edu.
Website: http://www.cellbio.duke.edu/

Duke University, Graduate School, Department of Evolutionary Anthropology, Durham, NC 27708. Offers cellular and molecular biology (PhD); gross anatomy and physical anthropology (PhD), including comparative morphology of human and non-human primates, primate social behavior, vertebrate paleontology; neuroanatomy (PhD). *Faculty:* 12. *Students:* 16 full-time (9 women); includes 5 minority (2 Black or African American, non-Hispanic/Latino; 1 Asian, non-Hispanic/Latino; 2 Hispanic/Latino). 69 applicants, 6% accepted, 3 enrolled. In 2013, 1 degree awarded. *Median time to degree:* Of those who began their doctoral program in fall 2005, 87% received their degree in 8 years or less. *Degree requirements:* For doctorate, one foreign language, thesis/dissertation. *Entrance requirements:* For doctorate, GRE General Test. Additional exam requirements/recommendations for international students: Required—TOEFL (minimum score 577 paper-based; 90 iBT) or IELTS (minimum score 7). *Application deadline:* For fall admission, 12/8 priority date for domestic and international students. Application fee: $80. Electronic applications accepted. *Financial support:* Fellowships, teaching assistantships, and Federal Work-Study available. Financial award application deadline: 12/31. *Unit head:* Richard Kay, Director of Graduate Studies, 919-684-4124, Fax: 919-684-8542, E-mail: mlsquire@duke.edu. *Application contact:* Elizabeth Hutton, Director of Admissions, 919-684-3913, Fax: 919-684-2277, E-mail: grad-admissions@duke.edu.
Website: http://evolutionaryanthropology.duke.edu/

Duke University, Graduate School, Program in Cell and Molecular Biology, Durham, NC 27710. Offers Certificate. Students must be enrolled in a participating PhD program (biology, cell biology, immunology, molecular genetics, neurobiology, pathology, pharmacology). *Faculty:* 146. *Students:* 17 full-time (10 women); includes 2 minority (both Black or African American, non-Hispanic/Latino), 4 international. 190 applicants, 19% accepted, 14 enrolled. *Entrance requirements:* Additional exam requirements/recommendations for international students: Required—TOEFL (minimum score 577 paper-based; 90 iBT) or IELTS (minimum score 7). *Application deadline:* For fall admission, 12/8 priority date for domestic and international students. Application fee: $80. Electronic applications accepted. *Financial support:* Fellowships available. Financial award application deadline: 12/8. *Unit head:* Dr. Meta Kuehn, Director of Graduate Studies, 919-684-6559, Fax: 919-684-8346, E-mail: carol.richardson@duke.edu. *Application contact:* Elizabeth Hutton, Director of Admissions, 919-684-3913, Fax: 919-684-3913, E-mail: grad-admissions@duke.edu.
Website: http://cmb.duke.edu/

East Carolina University, Brody School of Medicine, Department of Anatomy and Cell Biology, Greenville, NC 27858-4353. Offers PhD. *Degree requirements:* For doctorate, comprehensive exam, thesis/dissertation. *Entrance requirements:* For doctorate, GRE General Test. Additional exam requirements/recommendations for international students: Required—TOEFL. *Application deadline:* For fall admission, 6/1 priority date for domestic students. Applications are processed on a rolling basis. Application fee: $50. *Expenses:* Tuition, state resident: full-time $4223. Tuition, nonresident: full-time $16,540. *Required fees:* $2184. *Financial support:* Fellowships with full tuition reimbursements and health care benefits available. Financial award application deadline: 6/1. *Faculty research:* Kinesin motors during slow matogensis, mitochondria and peroxisomes in obesity, ovarian innervation, tight junction function and regulation. *Unit head:* Dr. Cheryl Knudson, Chairman, 252-744-2852, Fax: 252-744-2850, E-mail: knudsonc@ecu.edu. *Application contact:* Dr. Ron Dudek, Senior Director of Graduate Studies, 252-744-2863, Fax: 252-744-2850, E-mail: dudekr@ecu.edu.
Website: http://www.ecu.edu/cs-dhs/anatomy/gradProg.cfm

Eastern Michigan University, Graduate School, College of Arts and Sciences, Department of Biology, Ypsilanti, MI 48197. Offers cell and molecular biology (MS); community college biology teaching (MS); ecology and organismal biology (MS); general biology (MS); water resources (MS). Part-time and evening/weekend programs available. Postbaccalaureate distance learning degree programs offered (minimal on-campus study). *Faculty:* 19 full-time (4 women). *Students:* 11 full-time (6 women), 31 part-time (18 women); includes 3 minority (1 Black or African American, non-Hispanic/Latino; 1 Asian, non-Hispanic/Latino; 1 Hispanic/Latino), 6 international. Average age 26. 56 applicants, 59% accepted, 20 enrolled. In 2013, 13 master's awarded. *Entrance requirements:* For master's, GRE General Test, GRE Subject Test. Additional exam requirements/recommendations for international students: Required—TOEFL. *Application deadline:* Applications are processed on a rolling basis. Application fee: $35. *Expenses:* Tuition, state resident: full-time $12,300; part-time $466 per credit hour. Tuition, nonresident: full-time $23,159; part-time $918 per credit hour. *Required fees:* $71 per credit hour. $46 per semester. One-time fee: $100. Tuition and fees vary according to course level and degree level. *Financial support:* Fellowships, research assistantships with full tuition reimbursements, teaching assistantships with full tuition reimbursements, career-related internships or fieldwork, Federal Work-Study, institutionally sponsored loans, scholarships/grants, tuition waivers (partial), and unspecified assistantships available. Support available to part-time students. Financial award applicants required to submit FAFSA. *Unit head:* Dr. Daniel Clemans, Department Head, 734-487-4242, Fax: 734-487-9235, E-mail: dclemans@emich.edu. *Application contact:* Dr. David Kass, Graduate Coordinator, 734-487-4242, Fax: 734-487-9235, E-mail: dkass@emich.edu.
Website: http://www.emich.edu/biology

Eastern New Mexico University, Graduate School, College of Liberal Arts and Sciences, Department of Biology, Portales, NM 88130. Offers applied ecology (MS); botany (MS); cell, molecular biology and biotechnology (MS); microbiology (MS); zoology (MS). Part-time programs available. *Degree requirements:* For master's, comprehensive exam, thesis optional. *Entrance requirements:* For master's, GRE, minimum GPA of 3.0, 2 letters of recommendation, statement of research interest, bachelor's degree related to field of study or proof of common knowledge. Additional exam requirements/recommendations for international students: Required—TOEFL (minimum score 550 paper-based; 79 iBT), IELTS (minimum score 6). Electronic applications accepted.

Emory University, Laney Graduate School, Division of Biological and Biomedical Sciences, Program in Biochemistry, Cell and Developmental Biology, Atlanta, GA 30322. Offers PhD. *Degree requirements:* For doctorate, comprehensive exam, thesis/dissertation. *Entrance requirements:* For doctorate, GRE General Test, minimum GPA of 3.0 in science course work (recommended). Additional exam requirements/recommendations for international students: Required—TOEFL. Electronic applications accepted. *Faculty research:* Signal transduction, molecular biology, enzymes and cofactors, receptor and ion channel function, membrane biology.

Emporia State University, Department of Biological Sciences, Emporia, KS 66801-5415. Offers botany (MS); environmental biology (MS); general biology (MS); microbial and cellular biology (MS); zoology (MS). Part-time programs available. *Faculty:* 13 full-time (3 women). *Students:* 32 full-time (16 women), 7 part-time (1 woman); includes 2 minority (1 Black or African American, non-Hispanic/Latino; 1 Asian, non-Hispanic/Latino), 18 international. 25 applicants, 88% accepted, 3 enrolled. In 2013, 8 master's awarded. *Degree requirements:* For master's, comprehensive exam or thesis. *Entrance requirements:* For master's, GRE, appropriate undergraduate degree, interview, letters of reference. Additional exam requirements/recommendations for international students: Required—TOEFL (minimum score 520 paper-based; 68 iBT). *Application deadline:* For fall admission, 8/15 priority date for domestic students. Applications are processed on a rolling basis. Application fee: $30 ($75 for international students). Electronic applications accepted. *Expenses: Tuition, area resident:* Part-time $220 per credit hour. Tuition, state resident: part-time $220 per credit hour. Tuition, nonresident: part-time $685 per credit hour. *Required fees:* $73 per credit hour. *Financial support:* In 2013–14, 5 research assistantships with full tuition reimbursements (averaging $7,371 per year), 9 teaching assistantships with full tuition reimbursements (averaging $7,950 per year) were awarded; career-related internships or fieldwork, Federal Work-Study, institutionally sponsored loans, health care benefits, and unspecified assistantships also available. Financial award application deadline: 3/15; financial award applicants required to submit FAFSA. *Faculty research:* Fisheries, range, and wildlife management; aquatic, plant, grassland, vertebrate, and invertebrate ecology; mammalian and plant systematics, taxonomy, and evolution; immunology, virology, and molecular biology. *Unit head:* Dr. R. Brent Thomas, Chair, 620-341-5311, Fax: 620-341-5608, E-mail: rthomas2@emporia.edu. *Application contact:* Dr. Scott Crupper, Graduate Coordinator, 620-341-5621, Fax: 620-341-5607, E-mail: scrupper@emporia.edu.
Website: http://www.emporia.edu/info/degrees-courses/grad/biology

Florida Institute of Technology, Graduate Programs, College of Science, Department of Biological Sciences, Program in Cell and Molecular Biology, Melbourne, FL 32901-6975. Offers MS. Part-time programs available. *Faculty:* 16 full-time (1 woman), 1 (woman) part-time/adjunct. *Students:* 1 (woman) full-time, 3 part-time (2 women), 1 international. Average age 24. 47 applicants. In 2013, 1 master's awarded. *Degree requirements:* For master's, thesis. *Entrance requirements:* For master's, GRE General Test, 3 letters of recommendation, minimum GPA of 3.0, resume, statement of objectives. Additional exam requirements/recommendations for international students: Required—TOEFL (minimum score 550 paper-based; 79 iBT). *Application deadline:* For fall admission, 4/1 for international students; for spring admission, 9/1 for international students. Applications are processed on a rolling basis. Electronic applications accepted. *Expenses: Tuition:* Full-time $20,214; part-time $1123 per credit. Tuition and fees vary according to campus/location. *Financial support:* Career-related internships or fieldwork, institutionally sponsored loans, tuition waivers (partial), unspecified assistantships, and tuition remissions available. Support available to part-time students. Financial award application deadline: 3/1; financial award applicants required to submit FAFSA. *Faculty research:* Changes in DNA molecule and differential expression of genetic information during aging. *Total annual research expenditures:* $1.4 million. *Unit head:* Dr. Richard B. Aronson, Department Head, 321-674-8034, Fax: 321-674-7238, E-mail: raronson@fit.edu. *Application contact:* Cheryl A. Brown, Associate Director of Graduate Admission, 321-674-7581, Fax: 321-723-9468, E-mail: cbrown@fit.edu.
Website: http://cos.fit.edu/biology/grad/catalog.php

Florida State University, The Graduate School, College of Arts and Sciences, Department of Biological Science, Specialization in Cell and Molecular Biology, Tallahassee, FL 32306-4295. Offers MS, PhD. *Faculty:* 25 full-time (7 women). *Students:* 62 full-time (28 women); includes 7 minority (1 Black or African American, non-Hispanic/Latino; 1 Asian, non-Hispanic/Latino; 5 Hispanic/Latino), 23 international. 113 applicants, 20% accepted, 9 enrolled. In 2013, 1 master's, 3 doctorates awarded. Terminal master's awarded for partial completion of doctoral program. *Degree requirements:* For master's, comprehensive exam, thesis, teaching experience, seminar presentation; for doctorate, comprehensive exam, thesis/dissertation, teaching experience; seminar presentation. *Entrance requirements:* For master's and doctorate, GRE General Test, minimum upper-division GPA of 3.0. Additional exam requirements/recommendations for international students: Required—TOEFL (minimum score 600 paper-based; 92 iBT). *Application deadline:* For fall admission, 12/1 for domestic and international students. Application fee: $30. Electronic applications accepted. *Expenses:* Tuition, state resident: part-time $403.51 per credit hour. Tuition, nonresident: part-time $1004.85 per credit hour. *Required fees:* $75.81 per credit hour. One-time fee: $20 part-time. Tuition and fees vary according to course load, campus/location and student level. *Financial support:* In 2013–14, 62 students received support, including 2 fellowships with full tuition reimbursements available (averaging $30,000 per year), 17 research assistantships with full tuition reimbursements available (averaging $21,500 per year), 43 teaching assistantships with full tuition reimbursements available (averaging $21,500 per year); scholarships/grants and unspecified assistantships also available. Financial award application deadline: 12/1; financial award applicants required to submit FAFSA. *Faculty research:* Molecular biology; genetics and genomics; developmental biology and gene expression; cell structure, function, and motility; cellular and organismal physiology; biophysical and structural biology. *Unit head:* Dr. Debra A. Fadool, Professor and Associate Chair, 850-644-4775, Fax: 850-644-9829, E-mail: dfadool@bio.fsu.edu. *Application contact:* Judy Bowers, Coordinator, Graduate Affairs, 850-644-3023, Fax: 850-644-9829, E-mail: gradinfo@bio.fsu.edu.
Website: http://www.bio.fsu.edu/cmb/

Georgia Regents University, The Graduate School, Program in Cellular Biology and Anatomy, Augusta, GA 30912. Offers MS, PhD. *Faculty:* 15 full-time (6 women), 3 part-time/adjunct (1 woman). *Students:* 12 full-time (9 women); includes 7 minority (1 Black or African American, non-Hispanic/Latino; 5 Asian, non-Hispanic/Latino; 1 Hispanic/Latino), 4 international. Average age 29. In 2013, 2 doctorates awarded. *Degree requirements:* For doctorate, comprehensive exam, thesis/dissertation. *Entrance requirements:* For doctorate, GRE General Test. Additional exam requirements/recommendations for international students: Required—TOEFL (minimum score 550 paper-based; 79 iBT). *Application deadline:* For fall admission, 1/15 for domestic and international students. Applications are processed on a rolling basis. Application fee: $50. *Financial support:* In 2013–14, 2 students received support, including 1 fellowship with partial tuition reimbursement available (averaging $26,000 per year), 9 research assistantships with partial tuition reimbursements available (averaging $23,000 per year); teaching assistantships with partial tuition reimbursements available, Federal Work-Study, institutionally sponsored loans, and scholarships/grants also available. Support available to part-time students. Financial award application deadline: 5/31; financial award applicants required to submit FAFSA. *Faculty research:* Eye disease, developmental biology, cell injury and death, stroke and neurotoxicity, diabetic complications. *Total annual research expenditures:* $2.8 million. *Unit head:* Dr. Sally S. Atherton, Chair and Professor, 706-721-3731, Fax: 706-721-6120, E-mail: satherton@georgiahealth.edu. *Application contact:* Dr. Patricia L. Cameron, Acting Vice Dean, 706-721-3279, E-mail: pcameron@georgiahealth.edu.
Website: http://www.gru.edu/mcg/cba/gradstudents/

Georgia State University, College of Arts and Sciences, Department of Biology, Program in Cellular and Molecular Biology and Physiology, Atlanta, GA 30302-3083. Offers bioinformatics (MS); cellular and molecular biology and physiology (MS, PhD). Part-time programs available. Terminal master's awarded for partial completion of

doctoral program. *Degree requirements:* For master's, comprehensive exam (for some programs), thesis optional; for doctorate, comprehensive exam, thesis/dissertation. *Entrance requirements:* For master's and doctorate, GRE. Additional exam requirements/recommendations for international students: Required—TOEFL (minimum score 550 paper-based; 82 iBT) or IELTS (minimum score 7). *Application deadline:* For fall admission, 7/1 priority date for domestic students, 6/1 priority date for international students; for spring admission, 11/15 priority date for domestic students, 10/15 priority date for international students. Applications are processed on a rolling basis. Application fee: $50. Electronic applications accepted. *Expenses: Tuition, area resident:* Full-time $4176; part-time $348 per credit hour. Tuition, state resident: full-time $14,544; part-time $1212 per credit hour. Tuition, nonresident: full-time $14,544; part-time $1212 per credit hour. Tuition and fees vary according to course load and program. *Financial support:* In 2013–14, fellowships with full tuition reimbursements (averaging $22,000 per year), research assistantships with full tuition reimbursements (averaging $20,000 per year) were awarded. Financial award application deadline: 12/3. *Faculty research:* Membrane transport, viral infection, molecular immunology, protein modeling, gene regulation. *Unit head:* Dr. Julia Hilliard, Professor, 404-413-6560, Fax: 404-413-5301, E-mail: jhilliard@gsu.edu. *Application contact:* LaTesha Warren, Graduate Coordinator, 404-413-5314, Fax: 404-413-5301, E-mail: lwarren@gsu.edu.
Website: http://biology.gsu.edu/

Grand Valley State University, College of Liberal Arts and Sciences, Program in Cell and Molecular Biology, Allendale, MI 49401-9403. Offers MS. *Entrance requirements:* For master's, minimum GPA of 3.0. *Faculty research:* Plant cell biology, plant development, cell/signal integration.

Harvard University, Graduate School of Arts and Sciences, Department of Molecular and Cellular Biology, Cambridge, MA 02138. Offers PhD. *Degree requirements:* For doctorate, thesis/dissertation, oral exam. *Entrance requirements:* For doctorate, GRE General Test, GRE Subject Test (recommended). Additional exam requirements/recommendations for international students: Required—TOEFL. *Expenses: Tuition:* Full-time $38,888. *Required fees:* $958. Tuition and fees vary according to campus/location, program and student level.

Harvard University, Graduate School of Arts and Sciences, Division of Medical Sciences, Boston, MA 02115. Offers biological chemistry and molecular pharmacology (PhD); cell biology (PhD); genetics (PhD); microbiology and molecular genetics (PhD); pathology (PhD), including experimental pathology. *Degree requirements:* For doctorate, thesis/dissertation. *Entrance requirements:* For doctorate, GRE General Test, GRE Subject Test. Additional exam requirements/recommendations for international students: Required—TOEFL. *Expenses: Tuition:* Full-time $38,888. *Required fees:* $958. Tuition and fees vary according to campus/location, program and student level.

Illinois Institute of Technology, Graduate College, College of Science and Letters, Department of Biological and Chemical Sciences, Biology Division, Chicago, IL 60616. Offers biochemistry (MBS, MS); biology (PhD); biotechnology (MBS, MS); cell and molecular biology (MBS, MS); microbiology (MB, MS); molecular biochemistry and biophysics (PhD); molecular biology and biophysics (MS). Part-time and evening/weekend programs available. Postbaccalaureate distance learning degree programs offered (minimal on-campus study). Terminal master's awarded for partial completion of doctoral program. *Degree requirements:* For master's, comprehensive exam, thesis (for some programs); for doctorate, comprehensive exam, thesis/dissertation. *Entrance requirements:* For master's, GRE General Test (minimum score 1000 Quantitative and Verbal, 2.5 Analytical Writing), minimum undergraduate GPA of 3.0; for doctorate, GRE General Test (minimum score 1200 Quantitative and Verbal, 3.0 Analytical Writing), minimum undergraduate GPA of 3.0. Additional exam requirements/recommendations for international students: Required—TOEFL (minimum score 523 paper-based; 70 iBT); Recommended—IELTS (minimum score 5.5). Electronic applications accepted. *Faculty research:* Structure and biophysics of macromolecular systems; efficacy and mechanism of action of chemopreventive agents in experimental carcinogenesis of breast, colon, lung and prostate; study of fundamental structural biochemistry problems that have direct links to the understanding and treatment of disease; spectroscopic techniques for the study of multi-domain proteins; molecular mechanisms of cancer and cancer gene therapy.

Illinois State University, Graduate School, College of Arts and Sciences, Department of Biological Sciences, Normal, IL 61790-2200. Offers animal behavior (MS); bacteriology (MS); biochemistry (MS); biological sciences (MS); biology (PhD); biophysics (MS); biotechnology (MS); botany (MS, PhD); cell biology (MS); conservation biology (MS); developmental biology (MS); ecology (MS, PhD); entomology (MS); evolutionary biology (MS); genetics (MS, PhD); immunology (MS); microbiology (MS, PhD); molecular biology (MS); molecular genetics (MS); neurobiology (MS); neuroscience (MS); parasitology (MS); physiology (MS, PhD); plant biology (MS); plant molecular biology (MS); plant sciences (MS); structural biology (MS); zoology (MS, PhD). Part-time programs available. *Degree requirements:* For master's, thesis or alternative; for doctorate, variable foreign language requirement, thesis/dissertation, 2 terms of residency. *Entrance requirements:* For master's, GRE General Test, minimum GPA of 2.6 in last 60 hours of course work; for doctorate, GRE General Test. *Faculty research:* Redoc balance and drug development in schistosoma mansoni, control of the growth of listeria monocytogenes at low temperature, regulation of cell expansion and microtubule function by SPRI, CRUI: physiology and fitness consequences of different life history phenotypes.

Indiana University Bloomington, University Graduate School, College of Arts and Sciences, Department of Biology, Bloomington, IN 47405. Offers biology teaching (MAT); biotechnology (MA); evolution, ecology, and behavior (MA, PhD); genetics (PhD); microbiology (MA, PhD); molecular, cellular, and developmental biology (PhD); plant sciences (MA, PhD); zoology (MA, PhD). *Faculty:* 58 full-time (15 women), 21 part-time/adjunct (6 women). *Students:* 166 full-time (94 women), 2 part-time (both women); includes 22 minority (8 Black or African American, non-Hispanic/Latino; 3 Asian, non-Hispanic/Latino; 10 Hispanic/Latino; 1 Two or more races, non-Hispanic/Latino), 47 international. Average age 27. 261 applicants, 23% accepted, 32 enrolled. In 2013, 17 master's, 20 doctorates awarded. Terminal master's awarded for partial completion of doctoral program. *Degree requirements:* For master's, thesis, oral defense; for doctorate, thesis/dissertation, oral defense. *Entrance requirements:* For master's and doctorate, GRE General Test. Additional exam requirements/recommendations for international students: Required—TOEFL (minimum score 100 iBT). *Application deadline:* For fall admission, 1/5 priority date for domestic students, 12/1 priority date for international students. Application fee: $55 ($65 for international students). Electronic applications accepted. *Financial support:* In 2013–14, fellowships with tuition reimbursements (averaging $24,000 per year), research assistantships with tuition reimbursements (averaging $21,000 per year), teaching assistantships with tuition reimbursements (averaging $22,000 per year) were awarded; scholarships/grants, traineeships, health care benefits, and unspecified assistantships also available. Financial award application deadline: 1/5. *Faculty research:* Evolution, ecology and behavior; microbiology; molecular biology and genetics; plant biology. *Unit head:* Dr. Clay Fuqua, Chair, 812-856-6005, Fax: 812-855-6082, E-mail: cfuqua@indiana.edu. *Application contact:* Tracey D. Stohr, Graduate Student Recruitment Coordinator, 812-856-6303, Fax: 812-855-6082, E-mail: gradbio@indiana.edu.
Website: http://www.bio.indiana.edu/

Indiana University–Purdue University Indianapolis, Indiana University School of Medicine, Department of Anatomy and Cell Biology, Indianapolis, IN 46202-2896. Offers MS, PhD, MD/PhD. *Faculty:* 14 full-time (1 woman). *Students:* 14 full-time (9 women); includes 2 minority (both Two or more races, non-Hispanic/Latino), 3 international. Average age 29. 16 applicants, 38% accepted, 4 enrolled. In 2013, 3 doctorates awarded. *Degree requirements:* For master's, thesis or alternative; for doctorate, thesis/dissertation. *Entrance requirements:* For master's and doctorate, GRE General Test. *Application deadline:* For fall admission, 1/15 priority date for domestic students. Application fee: $55 ($65 for international students). *Financial support:* Fellowships, research assistantships, teaching assistantships, Federal Work-Study, institutionally sponsored loans, tuition waivers (partial), and stipends available. Financial award application deadline: 2/15. *Faculty research:* Acoustic reflex control, osteoarthritis and bone disease, diabetes, kidney diseases, cellular and molecular neurobiology. *Unit head:* Dr. Kathryn Jones, Chair, 317-274-7495, E-mail: kjjones1@iupui.edu. *Application contact:* Dr. James Williams, Graduate Adviser, 317-274-3423, Fax: 317-278-2040, E-mail: williams@anatomy.iupui.edu.
Website: http://anatomy.iupui.edu/

Iowa State University of Science and Technology, Program in Molecular, Cellular, and Developmental Biology, Ames, IA 50011. Offers MS, PhD. *Entrance requirements:* For master's and doctorate, GRE General Test. Additional exam requirements/recommendations for international students: Required—TOEFL (minimum score 580 paper-based; 85 iBT), IELTS (minimum score 7). Electronic applications accepted.

Johns Hopkins University, National Institutes of Health Sponsored Programs, Baltimore, MD 21218-2699. Offers biology (PhD), including biochemistry, biophysics, cell biology, developmental biology, genetic biology, molecular biology; cell, molecular, and developmental biology and biophysics (PhD). *Faculty:* 25 full-time (4 women). *Students:* 126 full-time (72 women); includes 36 minority (3 Black or African American, non-Hispanic/Latino; 1 American Indian or Alaska Native, non-Hispanic/Latino; 21 Asian, non-Hispanic/Latino; 11 Hispanic/Latino), 19 international. 282 applicants, 26% accepted, 36 enrolled. In 2013, 15 doctorates awarded. *Degree requirements:* For doctorate, comprehensive exam, thesis/dissertation. *Entrance requirements:* For doctorate, GRE General Test. Additional exam requirements/recommendations for international students: Required—TOEFL (minimum score 600 paper-based), TWE. *Application deadline:* For fall admission, 12/15 priority date for domestic students. Application fee: $60. Electronic applications accepted. *Financial support:* In 2013–14, 24 fellowships (averaging $23,000 per year), 93 research assistantships (averaging $23,000 per year), 22 teaching assistantships (averaging $23,000 per year) were awarded; Federal Work-Study, institutionally sponsored loans, scholarships/grants, traineeships, health care benefits, tuition waivers (partial), and unspecified assistantships also available. Financial award application deadline: 4/15; financial award applicants required to submit FAFSA. *Faculty research:* Protein and nucleic acid biochemistry and biophysical chemistry, molecular biology and development. *Total annual research expenditures:* $11.2 million. *Unit head:* Dr. Allen Shearn, Chair, 410-516-4693, Fax: 410-516-5213, E-mail: bio_cals@jhu.edu. *Application contact:* Joan Miller, Academic Affairs Manager, 410-516-5502, Fax: 410-516-5213, E-mail: joan@jhu.edu.

Johns Hopkins University, School of Medicine, Graduate Programs in Medicine, Graduate Program in Cellular and Molecular Medicine, Baltimore, MD 21218-2699. Offers PhD. *Faculty:* 125 full-time (29 women). *Students:* 125 full-time (76 women); includes 49 minority (4 Black or African American, non-Hispanic/Latino; 1 American Indian or Alaska Native, non-Hispanic/Latino; 30 Asian, non-Hispanic/Latino; 8 Hispanic/Latino; 6 Two or more races, non-Hispanic/Latino), 19 international. Average age 27. 143 applicants, 39% accepted, 21 enrolled. In 2013, 25 doctorates awarded. *Degree requirements:* For doctorate, comprehensive exam, thesis/dissertation, oral exam. *Entrance requirements:* For doctorate, GRE. Additional exam requirements/recommendations for international students: Required—TOEFL. *Application deadline:* For winter admission, 1/1 for domestic students. Application fee: $85. Electronic applications accepted. *Financial support:* Fellowships, scholarships/grants, health care benefits, and tuition waivers (full) available. *Faculty research:* Cellular and molecular basis of disease. *Total annual research expenditures:* $100 million. *Unit head:* Dr. Rajini Rao, Director, 410-955-4732, Fax: 410-614-7294, E-mail: rrao@jhmi.edu. *Application contact:* Leslie Lichter-Mason, Admissions Administrator, 410-614-0391, Fax: 410-614-7294, E-mail: llichte2@jhmi.edu.
Website: http://cmm.jhmi.edu

Johns Hopkins University, School of Medicine, Graduate Programs in Medicine, Program in Biochemistry, Cellular and Molecular Biology, Baltimore, MD 21205. Offers PhD. *Faculty:* 101 full-time (35 women). *Students:* 128 full-time (67 women); includes 30 minority (9 Black or African American, non-Hispanic/Latino; 1 American Indian or Alaska Native, non-Hispanic/Latino; 11 Asian, non-Hispanic/Latino; 8 Hispanic/Latino; 1 Two or more races, non-Hispanic/Latino), 36 international. Average age 26. 118 applicants, 31% accepted, 19 enrolled. In 2013, 23 doctorates awarded. *Degree requirements:* For doctorate, comprehensive exam, thesis/dissertation. *Entrance requirements:* For doctorate, GRE General Test. Additional exam requirements/recommendations for international students: Required—TOEFL. *Application deadline:* For winter admission, 1/10 for domestic and international students. Applications are processed on a rolling basis. Application fee: $80. Electronic applications accepted. *Financial support:* Fellowships, research assistantships, traineeships, and tuition waivers (full) available. Financial award application deadline: 12/31. *Faculty research:* Developmental biology, genomics/proteomics, protein targeting, signal transduction, structural biology. *Unit head:* Dr. Carolyn Machamer, Director, 410-955-3466, Fax: 410-614-8842, E-mail: machamer@jhmi.edu. *Application contact:* Dr. Jeff Corden, Admissions Director, 410-955-3506, Fax: 410-614-8842, E-mail: jcorden@jhmi.edu.
Website: http://bcmb.bs.jhmi.edu/Pages/default.aspx

Kent State University, School of Biomedical Sciences, Program in Cellular and Molecular Biology, Kent, OH 44242-0001. Offers MS, PhD. Offered in cooperation with Northeastern Ohio Universities College of Medicine. Terminal master's awarded for partial completion of doctoral program. *Degree requirements:* For master's, thesis; for doctorate, thesis/dissertation. *Entrance requirements:* For master's, GRE General Test, letter of recommendation, minimum GPA of 3.0; for doctorate, GRE General Test, letter of recommendation, minimum GPA of 3.0, MS. Additional exam requirements/recommendations for international students: Required—TOEFL. Electronic applications accepted. *Faculty research:* Molecular genetics, molecular endocrinology, virology and tumor biology, P450 enzymology and catalysis, membrane structure and function.

Lehigh University, College of Arts and Sciences, Department of Biological Sciences, Bethlehem, PA 18015. Offers biochemistry (PhD); cell and molecular biology (PhD); integrative biology and neuroscience (PhD); molecular biology (MS). Part-time programs available. Postbaccalaureate distance learning degree programs offered (no on-campus study). *Faculty:* 18 full-time (9 women). *Students:* 38 full-time (20 women), 30 part-time (23 women); includes 8 minority (4 Black or African American, non-Hispanic/Latino; 2 Asian, non-Hispanic/Latino; 2 Hispanic/Latino), 5 international. Average age 29. 54

applicants, 41% accepted, 11 enrolled. In 2013, 8 master's, 5 doctorates awarded. Terminal master's awarded for partial completion of doctoral program. *Degree requirements:* For master's, research report; for doctorate, comprehensive exam, thesis/dissertation. *Entrance requirements:* For doctorate, GRE General Test. Additional exam requirements/recommendations for international students: Required—TOEFL. *Application deadline:* For fall admission, 12/15 for domestic and international students. Applications are processed on a rolling basis. Application fee: $75. Electronic applications accepted. *Financial support:* In 2013–14, 2 fellowships with full tuition reimbursements (averaging $24,500 per year), 8 research assistantships with full tuition reimbursements (averaging $23,750 per year), 20 teaching assistantships with full tuition reimbursements (averaging $23,750 per year) were awarded; scholarships/grants and unspecified assistantships also available. Financial award application deadline: 12/15. *Faculty research:* Gene expression, cytoskeleton and cell structure, cell cycle and growth regulation, neuroscience, animal behavior, microbiology. *Total annual research expenditures:* $1.7 million. *Unit head:* Dr. Murray Itzkowitz, Chairperson, 610-758-3680, Fax: 610-758-4004, E-mail: mi00@lehigh.edu. *Application contact:* Dr. Mary Kathryn Iovine, Graduate Coordinator, 610-758-6981, Fax: 610-758-4004, E-mail: mki3@lehigh.edu.
Website: http://www.lehigh.edu/~inbios/

Louisiana State University Health Sciences Center, School of Graduate Studies in New Orleans, Department of Cell Biology and Anatomy, New Orleans, LA 70112-2223. Offers cell biology and anatomy (MS, PhD), including cell biology, developmental biology, neurobiology and anatomy; MD/PhD. *Degree requirements:* For master's, comprehensive exam, thesis; for doctorate, comprehensive exam, thesis/dissertation. *Entrance requirements:* For master's and doctorate, GRE General Test, GRE Subject Test, minimum undergraduate GPA of 3.0. Additional exam requirements/recommendations for international students: Required—TOEFL. *Faculty research:* Visual system organization, neural development, plasticity of sensory systems, information processing through the nervous system, visuomotor integration.

Louisiana State University Health Sciences Center at Shreveport, Department of Cellular Biology and Anatomy, Shreveport, LA 71130-3932. Offers MS, PhD, MD/PhD. *Faculty:* 14 full-time (2 women). *Students:* 10 full-time (6 women); includes 4 minority (3 Black or African American, non-Hispanic/Latino; 1 Asian, non-Hispanic/Latino), 2 international. Average age 28. 6 applicants, 17% accepted, 1 enrolled. In 2013, 2 doctorates awarded. Terminal master's awarded for partial completion of doctoral program. *Degree requirements:* For master's, thesis; for doctorate, thesis/dissertation. *Entrance requirements:* For master's and doctorate, GRE General Test. Additional exam requirements/recommendations for international students: Required—TOEFL. *Application deadline:* For fall admission, 5/1 priority date for domestic students. Applications are processed on a rolling basis. *Financial support:* In 2013–14, 9 students received support, including 10 research assistantships (averaging $24,000 per year); institutionally sponsored loans also available. Financial award application deadline: 5/1. *Faculty research:* Cancer biology, redox biology, neurosciences, immunobiology, cardiovascular sciences. *Unit head:* Dr. William Mayhan, Chairman, 318-675-5313. *Application contact:* Dr. Sumitra Miriyala, Graduate Recruiter, 318-675-6940, Fax: 318-675-5889, E-mail: smiriy@lsuhsc.edu.
Website: http://www.lsuhscshreveport.edu/CellularBiologyandAnatomy/AnatomyHome.aspx

Loyola University Chicago, Graduate School, Department of Cell Biology, Neurobiology and Anatomy, Chicago, IL 60660. Offers MS, PhD. Part-time programs available. *Faculty:* 16 full-time (6 women), 9 part-time/adjunct (4 women). *Students:* 16 full-time (6 women); includes 3 minority (2 Black or African American, non-Hispanic/Latino; 1 Hispanic/Latino), 1 international. Average age 27. 17 applicants, 24% accepted. In 2013, 1 master's, 6 doctorates awarded. Terminal master's awarded for partial completion of doctoral program. *Degree requirements:* For master's, thesis; for doctorate, comprehensive exam, thesis/dissertation. *Entrance requirements:* For master's, GRE General Test, minimum GPA of 3.0; for doctorate, GRE General Test, GRE Subject Test (biology), minimum GPA of 3.0. Additional exam requirements/recommendations for international students: Required—TOEFL (minimum score 600 paper-based). *Application deadline:* For fall admission, 5/1 priority date for domestic and international students. Applications are processed on a rolling basis. Application fee: $50. Electronic applications accepted. *Expenses: Tuition:* Full-time $16,740; part-time $930 per credit. *Required fees:* $135 per semester. *Financial support:* In 2013–14, 5 fellowships with full tuition reimbursements (averaging $23,000 per year), 5 research assistantships with full tuition reimbursements (averaging $23,000 per year) were awarded; Federal Work-Study and unspecified assistantships also available. Financial award application deadline: 5/1; financial award applicants required to submit FAFSA. *Faculty research:* Brain steroids, immunology, neuroregeneration, cytokines. *Total annual research expenditures:* $1 million. *Unit head:* Dr. Phong Le, Head, 708-216-3603, Fax: 708-216-3913, E-mail: ple@lumc.edu. *Application contact:* Ginny Hayes, Graduate Program Secretary, 708-216-3353, Fax: 708-216-3913, E-mail: vhayes@lumc.edu.

Marquette University, Graduate School, College of Arts and Sciences, Department of Biology, Milwaukee, WI 53201-1881. Offers cell biology (MS, PhD); developmental biology (MS, PhD); ecology (MS, PhD); epithelial physiology (MS, PhD); genetics (MS, PhD); microbiology (MS, PhD); molecular biology (MS, PhD); muscle and exercise physiology (MS, PhD); neuroscience (PhD). *Faculty:* 21 full-time (9 women), 3 part-time/adjunct (0 women). *Students:* 34 full-time (16 women), 4 part-time (1 woman), 15 international. Average age 27. 70 applicants, 23% accepted, 5 enrolled. In 2013, 1 master's, 6 doctorates awarded. Terminal master's awarded for partial completion of doctoral program. *Degree requirements:* For master's, comprehensive exam, thesis, 1 year of teaching experience or equivalent; for doctorate, thesis/dissertation, 1 year of teaching experience or equivalent, qualifying exam. *Entrance requirements:* For master's and doctorate, GRE General Test, GRE Subject Test, official transcripts from all current and previous colleges/universities except Marquette, statement of professional goals and aspirations, three letters of recommendation. Additional exam requirements/recommendations for international students: Required—TOEFL (minimum score 530 paper-based). *Application deadline:* For fall admission, 12/15 for domestic and international students. Application fee: $50. Electronic applications accepted. *Financial support:* In 2013–14, 39 students received support, including 6 fellowships (averaging $1,208 per year), 4 research assistantships with full tuition reimbursements available (averaging $21,750 per year), 29 teaching assistantships with full tuition reimbursements available (averaging $21,750 per year); scholarships/grants, health care benefits, tuition waivers (full and partial), and unspecified assistantships also available. Support available to part-time students. Financial award application deadline: 2/15. *Faculty research:* Neurobiology, neuroendocrinology, epithelial physiology, neuropeptide interactions, synaptic transmission. *Total annual research expenditures:* $1.5 million. *Unit head:* Dr. Dale Noel, Chair and Professor, 414-288-1748. *Application contact:* Dr. Michelle Mynlieff, Professor, 414-288-1467.
Website: http://www.marquette.edu/biology/

Massachusetts Institute of Technology, School of Science, Department of Biology, Cambridge, MA 02139-4307. Offers biochemistry (PhD); biological oceanography (PhD); biology (PhD); biophysical chemistry and molecular structure (PhD); cell biology (PhD); computational and systems biology (PhD); developmental biology (PhD); genetics (PhD); immunology (PhD); microbiology (PhD); molecular biology (PhD); neurobiology (PhD). *Faculty:* 58 full-time (15 women). *Students:* 261 full-time (133 women); includes 77 minority (3 Black or African American, non-Hispanic/Latino; 1 American Indian or Alaska Native, non-Hispanic/Latino; 32 Asian, non-Hispanic/Latino; 32 Hispanic/Latino; 9 Two or more races, non-Hispanic/Latino), 46 international. Average age 26. 651 applicants, 15% accepted, 39 enrolled. In 2013, 25 doctorates awarded. *Degree requirements:* For doctorate, comprehensive exam, thesis/dissertation, two semesters as a teaching assistant. *Entrance requirements:* For doctorate, GRE General Test. Additional exam requirements/recommendations for international students: Required—TOEFL (minimum score 577 paper-based), IELTS (minimum score 6.5). *Application deadline:* For fall admission, 12/1 for domestic and international students. Application fee: $75. Electronic applications accepted. *Expenses: Tuition:* Full-time $43,210; part-time $670 per credit hour. *Required fees:* $288. *Financial support:* In 2013–14, 252 students received support, including 135 fellowships (averaging $36,800 per year), 122 research assistantships (averaging $35,500 per year), 1 teaching assistantship; Federal Work-Study, institutionally sponsored loans, scholarships/grants, traineeships, health care benefits, and unspecified assistantships also available. *Faculty research:* Cellular, developmental and molecular (plant and animal) biology; biochemistry, bioengineering, biophysics and structural biology; classical and molecular genetics, stem cell and epigenetics; immunology and microbiology; cancer biology, molecular medicine, neurobiology and human disease; computational and systems biology. *Total annual research expenditures:* $44.5 million. *Unit head:* Alan Grossman, Interim Head, 617-253-4701. *Application contact:* Biology Education Office, 617-253-3717, Fax: 617-258-9329, E-mail: gradbio@mit.edu.
Website: https://biology.mit.edu/

Mayo Graduate School, Graduate Programs in Biomedical Sciences, Programs in Biochemistry, Structural Biology, Cell Biology, and Genetics, Rochester, MN 55905. Offers biochemistry and structural biology (PhD); cell biology and genetics (PhD); molecular biology (PhD). *Degree requirements:* For doctorate, oral defense of dissertation, qualifying oral and written exam. *Entrance requirements:* For doctorate, GRE, 1 year of chemistry, biology, calculus, and physics. Additional exam requirements/recommendations for international students: Required—TOEFL. Electronic applications accepted. *Faculty research:* Gene structure and function, membranes and receptors/cytoskeleton, oncogenes and growth factors, protein structure and function, steroid hormonal action.

McGill University, Faculty of Graduate and Postdoctoral Studies, Faculty of Medicine, Department of Anatomy and Cell Biology, Montréal, QC H3A 2T5, Canada. Offers M Sc, PhD.

McMaster University, Faculty of Health Sciences and School of Graduate Studies, Program in Medical Sciences, Metabolism and Nutrition Area, Hamilton, ON L8S 4M2, Canada. Offers M Sc, PhD, MD/PhD. *Degree requirements:* For master's, thesis; for doctorate, comprehensive exam, thesis/dissertation. *Entrance requirements:* For master's, honors B Sc, B+ average in related field; for doctorate, M Sc, minimum B+ average, students with proven research experience and an A average may be admitted with a B Sc degree. Additional exam requirements/recommendations for international students: Required—TOEFL (minimum score 580 paper-based; 92 iBT).

Medical University of South Carolina, College of Graduate Studies, Program in Molecular and Cellular Biology and Pathobiology, Charleston, SC 29425. Offers cancer biology (PhD); cardiovascular biology (PhD); cardiovascular imaging (PhD); cell regulation (PhD); craniofacial biology (PhD); genetics and development (PhD); marine biomedicine (PhD); DMD/PhD; MD/PhD. *Degree requirements:* For doctorate, thesis/dissertation, oral and written exams. *Entrance requirements:* For doctorate, GRE General Test, interview, minimum GPA of 3.0. Additional exam requirements/recommendations for international students: Required—TOEFL (minimum score 600 paper-based; 100 iBT). Electronic applications accepted.

Miami University, College of Arts and Science, Department of Biology, Oxford, OH 45056. Offers biological sciences (MAT); biology (MS, PhD); botany (MAT, MS, PhD); cell, molecular and structural biology (MS, PhD); ecology, evolution and environmental biology (PhD); zoology (MA, MS, PhD). Part-time programs available. Postbaccalaureate distance learning degree programs offered. *Students:* 89 full-time (49 women), 612 part-time (502 women); includes 63 minority (9 Black or African American, non-Hispanic/Latino; 2 American Indian or Alaska Native, non-Hispanic/Latino; 6 Asian, non-Hispanic/Latino; 27 Hispanic/Latino; 1 Native Hawaiian or other Pacific Islander, non-Hispanic/Latino; 18 Two or more races, non-Hispanic/Latino), 35 international. Average age 34. In 2013, 133 master's, 4 doctorates awarded. *Entrance requirements:* For master's and doctorate, GRE General Test. Additional exam requirements/recommendations for international students: Recommended—TOEFL (minimum score 80 iBT), IELTS (minimum score 6.5), TSE (minimum score 54). *Application deadline:* For fall admission, 1/15 for domestic and international students. Application fee: $50. Electronic applications accepted. *Expenses:* Tuition, state resident: full-time $12,634; part-time $526 per credit hour. Tuition, nonresident: full-time $27,892; part-time $1162 per credit hour. Part-time tuition and fees vary according to course load, campus/location and program. *Financial support:* Fellowships with full tuition reimbursements, research assistantships with full tuition reimbursements, teaching assistantships with full tuition reimbursements, Federal Work-Study, health care benefits, tuition waivers (full), and unspecified assistantships available. Financial award application deadline: 1/15; financial award applicants required to submit FAFSA. *Unit head:* Dr. Douglas Meikle, Chair, 513-529-3103, E-mail: meikled@miamioh.edu.
Website: http://miamioh.edu/cas/about/biology

Michigan State University, The Graduate School, College of Agriculture and Natural Resources, MSU-DOE Plant Research Laboratory, East Lansing, MI 48824. Offers biochemistry and molecular biology (PhD); cellular and molecular biology (PhD); crop and soil sciences (PhD); genetics (PhD); microbiology and molecular genetics (PhD); plant biology (PhD); plant physiology (PhD). Offered jointly with the Department of Energy. *Degree requirements:* For doctorate, comprehensive exam, thesis/dissertation, laboratory rotation, defense of dissertation. *Entrance requirements:* For doctorate, GRE General Test, acceptance into one of the affiliated department programs; 3 letters of recommendation; bachelor's degree or equivalent in life sciences, chemistry, biochemistry, or biophysics; research experience. Electronic applications accepted. *Faculty research:* Role of hormones in the regulation of plant development and physiology, molecular mechanisms associated with signal recognition, development and application of genetic methods and materials, protein routing and function.

Michigan State University, The Graduate School, College of Natural Science, Program in Cell and Molecular Biology, East Lansing, MI 48824. Offers cell and molecular biology (MS, PhD); cell and molecular biology/environmental toxicology (PhD). *Entrance requirements:* Additional exam requirements/recommendations for international students: Required—TOEFL. Electronic applications accepted.

Missouri State University, Graduate College, College of Health and Human Services, Department of Biomedical Sciences, Program in Cell and Molecular Biology, Springfield, MO 65897. Offers MS. Part-time programs available. *Students:* 10 full-time (7 women), 11 part-time (6 women); includes 1 minority (Two or more races, non-Hispanic/Latino), 3

international. Average age 24. 13 applicants, 85% accepted, 8 enrolled. In 2013, 6 master's awarded. *Degree requirements:* For master's, thesis or alternative, oral and written exams. *Entrance requirements:* For master's, GRE General Test, 2 semesters of course work in organic chemistry and physics, 1 semester of course work in calculus, minimum GPA of 3.0 in last 60 hours of course work. Additional exam requirements/recommendations for international students: Required—TOEFL (minimum score 550 paper-based; 79 iBT). *Application deadline:* For fall admission, 7/20 priority date for domestic students, 5/1 for international students; for spring admission, 12/20 priority date for domestic students, 9/1 for international students. Applications are processed on a rolling basis. Application fee: $35 ($50 for international students). Electronic applications accepted. *Expenses:* Tuition, state resident: full-time $4500; part-time $250 per credit hour. Tuition, nonresident: full-time $9018; part-time $501 per credit hour. *Required fees:* $361 per semester. Tuition and fees vary according to course level, course load and program. *Financial support:* In 2013–14, 15 teaching assistantships with full tuition reimbursements (averaging $8,324 per year) were awarded; career-related internships or fieldwork, Federal Work-Study, institutionally sponsored loans, scholarships/grants, and unspecified assistantships also available. Support available to part-time students. Financial award application deadline: 3/31; financial award applicants required to submit FAFSA. *Faculty research:* Extracellular matrix membrane protein, P2 nucleotide receptors, double stranded RNA viruses. *Unit head:* Dr. Scott Zimmernan, Program Director, 417-836-5478, Fax: 417-836-5588, E-mail: scottzimmerman@missouristate.edu. *Application contact:* Misty Stewart, Coordinator of Graduate Admissions and Recruitment, 417-836-6079, Fax: 417-836-6200, E-mail: mistystewart@missouristate.edu.
Website: http://www.missouristate.edu/bms/CMB/

New York Medical College, Graduate School of Basic Medical Sciences, Cell Biology and Anatomy Master's Program, Valhalla, NY 10595-1691. Offers MS, PhD, MD/PhD. Part-time and evening/weekend programs available. *Faculty:* 16 full-time (2 women), 2 part-time/adjunct (1 woman). *Students:* 2 full-time (both women); includes 1 minority (Asian, non-Hispanic/Latino). Average age 25. 5 applicants, 100% accepted, 1 enrolled. Terminal master's awarded for partial completion of doctoral program. *Degree requirements:* For master's, thesis; for doctorate, comprehensive exam, thesis/dissertation. *Entrance requirements:* For master's, GRE General Test, MCAT, or DAT. Additional exam requirements/recommendations for international students: Required—TOEFL. *Application deadline:* For fall admission, 7/1 priority date for domestic students, 5/1 priority date for international students; for spring admission, 12/1 for domestic students, 10/1 for international students. Applications are processed on a rolling basis. Application fee: $75 ($100 for international students). Electronic applications accepted. *Expenses: Tuition:* Full-time $49,170; part-time $910 per credit. Tuition and fees vary according to program. *Financial support:* Federal Work-Study and scholarships/grants available. Support available to part-time students. Financial award applicants required to submit FAFSA. *Faculty research:* Mechanisms of growth control in skeletal muscle, cartilage differentiation, cytoskeletal functions, signal transduction pathways, neuronal development and plasticity. *Unit head:* Dr. Victor Fried, Program Director, 914-594-4005, Fax: 914-594-4944, E-mail: victor_fried@nymc.edu. *Application contact:* Valerie Romeo-Messana, Director of Admissions, 914-594-4110, Fax: 914-594-4944, E-mail: v_romeomessana@nymc.edu.

New York Medical College, Graduate School of Basic Medical Sciences, Integrated PhD Program, Valhalla, NY 10595-1691. Offers biochemistry and molecular biology (PhD); cell biology and anatomy (PhD); microbiology and immunology (PhD); pathology (PhD); pharmacology (PhD); physiology (PhD). *Faculty:* 91 full-time (16 women), 5 part-time/adjunct (2 women). *Students:* 31 full-time (21 women); includes 17 minority (4 Black or African American, non-Hispanic/Latino; 11 Asian, non-Hispanic/Latino; 2 Hispanic/Latino). Average age 27. 56 applicants, 36% accepted, 9 enrolled. In 2013, 17 doctorates awarded. *Degree requirements:* For doctorate, comprehensive exam, thesis/dissertation. *Entrance requirements:* For doctorate, GRE General Test. Additional exam requirements/recommendations for international students: Required—TOEFL. *Application deadline:* For fall admission, 1/1 priority date for domestic and international students. Applications are processed on a rolling basis. Application fee: $75 ($100 for international students). Electronic applications accepted. *Expenses: Tuition:* Full-time $49,170; part-time $910 per credit. Tuition and fees vary according to program. *Financial support:* In 2013–14, fellowships with full tuition reimbursements (averaging $25,500 per year), research assistantships with full tuition reimbursements (averaging $25,500 per year) were awarded; Federal Work-Study, scholarships/grants, traineeships, health care benefits, and tuition waivers (full) also available. Financial award applicants required to submit FAFSA. *Faculty research:* Cardiovascular sciences, infectious diseases, neuroscience, cancer and cell signaling. *Unit head:* Dr. Francis L. Belloni, Dean, 914-594-4110, Fax: 914-594-4944, E-mail: francis_belloni@nymc.edu. *Application contact:* Valerie Romeo-Messana, Director of Admissions, 914-594-4110, Fax: 914-594-4944, E-mail: v_romeomessana@nymc.edu.

New York University, School of Medicine and Graduate School of Arts and Science, Sackler Institute of Graduate Biomedical Sciences, Program in Cellular and Molecular Biology, New York, NY 10012-1019. Offers PhD, MD/PhD. *Faculty:* 55 full-time (18 women). *Students:* 30 full-time (14 women); includes 12 minority (2 Black or African American, non-Hispanic/Latino; 1 American Indian or Alaska Native, non-Hispanic/Latino; 5 Asian, non-Hispanic/Latino; 4 Hispanic/Latino), 11 international. Average age 27. In 2013, 4 doctorates awarded. *Degree requirements:* For doctorate, comprehensive exam, thesis/dissertation, qualifying exams. *Entrance requirements:* For doctorate, GRE General Test. Additional exam requirements/recommendations for international students: Required—TOEFL. *Application deadline:* For fall admission, 1/4 priority date for domestic students. Applications are processed on a rolling basis. Application fee: $85. *Expenses: Tuition:* Full-time $35,856; part-time $1494 per unit. *Required fees:* $1408; $64 per unit. $473 per term. Tuition and fees vary according to course load and program. *Financial support:* Fellowships with tuition reimbursements, research assistantships with tuition reimbursements, and teaching assistantships with tuition reimbursements available. *Faculty research:* Membrane and organelle structure and biogenesis, intracellular transport and processing of proteins, cellular recognition and cell adhesion, oncogene structure and function, action of growth factors. *Total annual research expenditures:* $1.9 million. *Unit head:* Dr. Daniel Rifkin, Director, 212-263-5109, E-mail: rifkind01@popmail.med.nyu.edu. *Application contact:* Lynette Wilson, Information Contact, 212-263-7684, Fax: 212-263-8139, E-mail: wilsoe01@popmail.med.nyu.edu.

North Carolina State University, College of Veterinary Medicine, Program in Comparative Biomedical Sciences, Raleigh, NC 27695. Offers cell biology (MS, PhD); infectious disease (MS, PhD); pathology (MS, PhD); pharmacology (MS, PhD); population medicine (MS, PhD). Part-time programs available. *Degree requirements:* For master's, thesis; for doctorate, thesis/dissertation. *Entrance requirements:* For master's and doctorate, GRE General Test. Additional exam requirements/recommendations for international students: Required—TOEFL (minimum score 550 paper-based). Electronic applications accepted. *Expenses:* Contact institution. *Faculty research:* Infectious diseases, cell biology, pharmacology and toxicology, genomics, pathology and population medicine.

North Dakota State University, College of Graduate and Interdisciplinary Studies, College of Science and Mathematics, Department of Biological Sciences, Fargo, ND 58108. Offers biology (MS); botany (MS, PhD); cellular and molecular biology (PhD); genomics (PhD); zoology (MS, PhD). *Faculty:* 17 full-time (9 women), 1 part-time/adjunct (0 women). *Students:* 20 full-time (10 women), 3 part-time (all women); includes 2 minority (1 American Indian or Alaska Native, non-Hispanic/Latino; 1 Two or more races, non-Hispanic/Latino), 1 international. Average age 32. 9 applicants, 11% accepted, 1 enrolled. In 2013, 4 master's awarded. *Degree requirements:* For master's, thesis; for doctorate, thesis/dissertation. *Entrance requirements:* For master's and doctorate, GRE General Test. Additional exam requirements/recommendations for international students: Required—TOEFL. *Application deadline:* For fall admission, 1/15 for domestic students. Applications are processed on a rolling basis. Application fee: $35. Electronic applications accepted. *Financial support:* Fellowships with full tuition reimbursements, research assistantships with full tuition reimbursements, teaching assistantships with full tuition reimbursements, career-related internships or fieldwork, Federal Work-Study, institutionally sponsored loans, scholarships/grants, tuition waivers (full), and unspecified assistantships available. Support available to part-time students. Financial award application deadline: 4/15; financial award applicants required to submit FAFSA. *Faculty research:* Comparative endocrinology, physiology, behavioral ecology, plant cell biology, aquatic biology. *Unit head:* Dr. Wendy Reed, Head, 701-231-7087, E-mail: wendy.reed@ndsu.edu. *Application contact:* Sonya Goergen, Marketing, Recruitment, and Public Relations Coordinator, 701-231-7033, Fax: 701-231-6524.
Website: http://biology.ndsu.nodak.edu/

North Dakota State University, College of Graduate and Interdisciplinary Studies, Interdisciplinary Program in Cellular and Molecular Biology, Fargo, ND 58108. Offers PhD. Program offered in cooperation with 11 departments in the university. *Students:* 8 full-time (6 women), 2 part-time (both women); includes 1 minority (Asian, non-Hispanic/Latino), 5 international. Average age 28. 34 applicants, 6% accepted, 2 enrolled. In 2013, 2 doctorates awarded. *Degree requirements:* For doctorate, thesis/dissertation. *Entrance requirements:* For doctorate, GRE. Additional exam requirements/recommendations for international students: Required—TOEFL (minimum score 525 paper-based; 71 iBT). *Application deadline:* Applications are processed on a rolling basis. Application fee: $35. Electronic applications accepted. *Financial support:* Fellowships with full tuition reimbursements, research assistantships with full tuition reimbursements, teaching assistantships with full tuition reimbursements, and unspecified assistantships available. Financial award application deadline: 3/15. *Faculty research:* Plant and animal cell biology, gene regulation, molecular genetics, plant and animal virology. *Unit head:* Dr. Mark Sheridan, Director, 701-231-7087, E-mail: ndsu.cmb@ndsu.edu. *Application contact:* Sonya Goergen, Marketing, Recruitment, and Public Relations Coordinator, 701-231-7033, Fax: 701-231-6524.
Website: http://www.ndsu.edu/cellularmolecularbiology/

Northwestern University, The Graduate School, Interdisciplinary Biological Sciences Program (IBiS), Evanston, IL 60208. Offers biochemistry (PhD); bioengineering and biotechnology (PhD); biotechnology (PhD); cell and molecular biology (PhD); developmental and systems biology (PhD); nanotechnology (PhD); neurobiology (PhD); structural biology and biophysics (PhD). *Degree requirements:* For doctorate, thesis/dissertation, qualifying exam. *Entrance requirements:* For doctorate, GRE General Test. Additional exam requirements/recommendations for international students: Required—TOEFL (minimum score 600 paper-based). *Application deadline:* For fall admission, 12/15 for domestic and international students. Applications are processed on a rolling basis. Application fee: $95. Electronic applications accepted. *Financial support:* Fellowships, research assistantships, teaching assistantships, career-related internships or fieldwork, institutionally sponsored loans, scholarships/grants, traineeships, health care benefits, and unspecified assistantships available. Financial award application deadline: 12/31; financial award applicants required to submit FAFSA. *Faculty research:* Biophysics/structural biology, cell/molecular biology, synthetic biology, developmental systems biology, chemical biology/nanotechnology. *Unit head:* Dr. Deborah Klos Dehring, Associate Director, 847-467-0451, E-mail: d-klos@northwestern.edu. *Application contact:* Cathy Prullage, Program Manager, 847-491-4301, E-mail: ibis@northwestern.edu.
Website: http://www.biochem.northwestern.edu/ibis/

The Ohio State University, Graduate School, College of Arts and Sciences, Division of Natural and Mathematical Sciences, Department of Molecular Genetics, Columbus, OH 43210. Offers cell and developmental biology (MS, PhD); genetics (MS, PhD); molecular biology (MS, PhD). *Faculty:* 29. *Students:* 35 full-time (15 women); includes 3 minority (1 Black or African American, non-Hispanic/Latino; 2 Asian, non-Hispanic/Latino), 16 international. Average age 26. In 2013, 1 master's, 2 doctorates awarded. *Degree requirements:* For master's, thesis; for doctorate, thesis/dissertation. *Entrance requirements:* For doctorate, GRE General Test, GRE Subject Test in biology or chemistry (recommended). Additional exam requirements/recommendations for international students: Required—TOEFL (minimum score 550 paper-based; 79 iBT), Michigan English Language Assessment Battery (minimum score 82); Recommended—IELTS (minimum score 7). *Application deadline:* For fall admission, 12/13 priority date for domestic students, 11/30 priority date for international students; for winter admission, 12/1 for domestic students, 11/1 for international students; for spring admission, 3/1 for domestic students, 2/1 for international students. Applications are processed on a rolling basis. Application fee: $60 ($70 for international students). Electronic applications accepted. *Financial support:* Fellowships with tuition reimbursements, research assistantships with tuition reimbursements, teaching assistantships with tuition reimbursements, Federal Work-Study, and institutionally sponsored loans available. Support available to part-time students. *Unit head:* Dr. Anita Hopper, Chair, 614-688-3306, Fax: 614-292-4466, E-mail: hopper.64@osu.edu. *Application contact:* Graduate Admissions, 614-292-9444, Fax: 614-292-3895, E-mail: gradadmissions@osu.edu.
Website: https://molgen.osu.edu/

The Ohio State University, Graduate School, College of Arts and Sciences, Division of Natural and Mathematical Sciences, Program in Molecular, Cellular and Developmental Biology, Columbus, OH 43210. Offers MS, PhD. *Faculty:* 172. *Students:* 117 full-time (67 women), 5 part-time (1 woman); includes 13 minority (1 Black or African American, non-Hispanic/Latino; 6 Asian, non-Hispanic/Latino; 4 Hispanic/Latino; 2 Two or more races, non-Hispanic/Latino), 60 international. Average age 27. In 2013, 2 master's, 15 doctorates awarded. Terminal master's awarded for partial completion of doctoral program. *Degree requirements:* For master's, thesis; for doctorate, thesis/dissertation. *Entrance requirements:* For doctorate, GRE General Test, GRE Subject Test in any science (desired, preferably biology or chemistry, biochemistry or cell and molecular biology). Additional exam requirements/recommendations for international students: Required—TOEFL (minimum score 600 paper-based; 85 iBT); Recommended—IELTS (minimum score 8). *Application deadline:* For fall admission, 12/13 priority date for domestic students, 11/30 priority date for international students; for winter admission, 12/1 for domestic students, 11/1 for international students; for spring admission, 3/1 for domestic students, 2/1 for international students. Applications are processed on a rolling basis. Application fee: $60 ($70 for international students). Electronic applications accepted. *Financial support:* Fellowships with tuition reimbursements, research assistantships with tuition reimbursements, and teaching assistantships with tuition reimbursements available. *Unit head:* David Bisaro, Director, 614-292-2804, Fax: 614-

292-7817, E-mail: bisaro.1@osu.edu. *Application contact:* Graduate Admissions, 614-292-9444, Fax: 614-292-3895, E-mail: gradadmissions@osu.edu.
Website: http://mcdb.osu.edu/

Ohio University, Graduate College, College of Arts and Sciences, Department of Biological Sciences, Athens, OH 45701-2979. Offers biological sciences (MS, PhD); cell biology and physiology (MS, PhD); ecology and evolutionary biology (MS, PhD); exercise physiology and muscle biology (MS, PhD); microbiology (MS, PhD); neuroscience (MS, PhD). Terminal master's awarded for partial completion of doctoral program. *Degree requirements:* For master's, comprehensive exam, thesis, 1 quarter of teaching experience; for doctorate, comprehensive exam, thesis/dissertation, 2 quarters of teaching experience. *Entrance requirements:* For master's, GRE General Test, names of three faculty members whose research interests most closely match the applicant's interest; for doctorate, GRE General Test, essay concerning prior training, research interest and career goals, plus names of three faculty members whose research interests most closely match the applicant's interest. Additional exam requirements/recommendations for international students: Required—TOEFL (minimum score 620 paper-based; 105 iBT) or IELTS (minimum score 7.5). Electronic applications accepted. *Faculty research:* Ecology and evolutionary biology, exercise physiology and muscle biology, neurobiology, cell biology, physiology.

Ohio University, Graduate College, College of Arts and Sciences, Interdisciplinary Graduate Program in Molecular and Cellular Biology, Athens, OH 45701-2979. Offers MS, PhD. *Degree requirements:* For master's, comprehensive exam, thesis, research proposal, teaching experience; for doctorate, comprehensive exam, thesis/dissertation, research proposal, teaching experience. *Entrance requirements:* For master's and doctorate, GRE General Test. Additional exam requirements/recommendations for international students: Required—TOEFL (minimum score 620 paper-based; 105 iBT); Recommended—TWE. Electronic applications accepted. *Faculty research:* Animal biotechnology, plant molecular biology RNA, immunology, cellular genetics, biochemistry of signal transduction, cancer research, membrane transport, bioinformatics, bioengineering, chemical biology and drug discovery, diabetes, microbiology, neuroscience.

Oregon Health & Science University, School of Medicine, Graduate Programs in Medicine, Program in Molecular and Cellular Biosciences, Department of Cell and Developmental Biology, Portland, OR 97239-3098. Offers PhD. *Faculty:* 8 full-time (3 women), 36 part-time/adjunct (7 women). *Students:* 16 full-time (10 women), 1 (woman) part-time; includes 2 minority (both Two or more races, non-Hispanic/Latino), 5 international. Average age 29. In 2013, 5 doctorates awarded. *Degree requirements:* For doctorate, comprehensive exam, thesis/dissertation, qualifying exam. *Entrance requirements:* For doctorate, GRE General Test (minimum scores: 153 Verbal/148 Quantitative/4.5 Analytical) or MCAT. Additional exam requirements/recommendations for international students: Required—TOEFL. *Financial support:* Health care benefits, tuition waivers (full), and full tuition and stipends available. *Faculty research:* Developmental mechanisms, molecular biology of cancer, molecular neurobiology, intracellular signaling, growth factors and development. *Unit head:* Dr. Richard Maurer, Program Director, 503-494-7811, E-mail: maurerr@ohsu.edu. *Application contact:* Lola Bichler, Program Coordinator, 503-494-5824, E-mail: bichler@ohsu.edu.
Website: http://www.ohsu.edu/cellbio

Oregon State University, Interdisciplinary/Institutional Programs, Program in Molecular and Cellular Biology, Corvallis, OR 97331. Offers MS, PhD. *Students:* 31 full-time (17 women), 1 part-time (0 women); includes 5 minority (2 Asian, non-Hispanic/Latino; 2 Hispanic/Latino; 1 Two or more races, non-Hispanic/Latino), 11 international. Average age 29. 125 applicants, 9% accepted, 6 enrolled. In 2013, 1 master's, 8 doctorates awarded. *Degree requirements:* For doctorate, thesis/dissertation, oral and written qualifying exams. *Entrance requirements:* For master's and doctorate, GRE. Additional exam requirements/recommendations for international students: Required—TOEFL (minimum score 80 iBT), IELTS (minimum score 6.5). *Application deadline:* For fall admission, 6/1 for domestic students. Application fee: $60. *Expenses:* Tuition, state resident: full-time $11,664; part-time $432 per credit hour. Tuition, nonresident: full-time $19,197; part-time $711 per credit hour. *Required fees:* $1446; $443 per quarter. One-time fee: $300. Tuition and fees vary according to course load and program. *Financial support:* Fellowships, career-related internships or fieldwork, Federal Work-Study, and institutionally sponsored loans available. Support available to part-time students. *Unit head:* Dr. Barbara Taylor, Director, Molecular and Cellular Biology Graduate Program, 541-737-5344, E-mail: taylorb@science.oregonstate.edu. *Application contact:* Gail Millimaki, Molecular and Cellular Biology Advisor, 541-737-3799, E-mail: mcb@science.oregonstate.edu.
Website: http://www.mcb.oregonstate.edu/

Penn State University Park, Graduate School, Intercollege Graduate Programs, Intercollege Graduate Program in Cell and Developmental Biology, University Park, PA 16802. Offers MS, PhD. *Degree requirements:* For doctorate, thesis/dissertation, laboratory rotations, research project. *Unit head:* Dr. Regina Vasilatos-Younken, Interim Dean, 814-865-2516, Fax: 814-863-4627, E-mail: rxv@psu.edu. *Application contact:* Cynthia E. Nicosia, Director, Graduate Enrollment Services, 814-865-1834, Fax: 814-863-4627, E-mail: cey1@psu.edu.

Purdue University, Graduate School, College of Science, Department of Biological Sciences, West Lafayette, IN 47907. Offers biochemistry (PhD); biophysics (PhD); cell and developmental biology (PhD); ecology, evolutionary and population biology (MS, PhD), including ecology, evolutionary biology, population biology; genetics (MS, PhD); microbiology (MS, PhD); molecular biology (PhD); neurobiology (MS, PhD); plant physiology (PhD). *Faculty:* 50 full-time (13 women), 5 part-time/adjunct (1 woman). *Students:* 111 full-time (61 women), 5 part-time (0 women); includes 9 minority (1 Black or African American, non-Hispanic/Latino; 5 Asian, non-Hispanic/Latino; 3 Hispanic/Latino), 62 international. Average age 27. 170 applicants, 19% accepted, 17 enrolled. In 2013, 9 master's, 18 doctorates awarded. Terminal master's awarded for partial completion of doctoral program. *Degree requirements:* For master's, thesis (for some programs); for doctorate, thesis/dissertation, seminars, teaching experience. *Entrance requirements:* For master's, GRE General Test (minimum analytical writing score of 3.5), minimum undergraduate GPA of 3.0; for doctorate, GRE General Test (minimum analytical writing score of 3.5), minimum undergraduate GPA of 3.5. Additional exam requirements/recommendations for international students: Required—TOEFL (minimum score 600 paper-based; 107 iBT for MS, 80 iBT for PhD). *Application deadline:* For fall admission, 12/7 for domestic and international students. Applications are processed on a rolling basis. Application fee: $60 ($75 for international students). Electronic applications accepted. *Financial support:* Fellowships, research assistantships, and teaching assistantships available. Support available to part-time students. Financial award application deadline: 2/15; financial award applicants required to submit FAFSA. *Unit head:* Dr. Richard J. Kuhn, Head, 765-494-4407, E-mail: kuhnr@purdue.edu. *Application contact:* Georgina E. Rupp, Graduate Coordinator, 765-494-8142, Fax: 765-494-0876, E-mail: ruppg@purdue.edu.
Website: http://www.bio.purdue.edu/

Queen's University at Kingston, School of Graduate Studies, Faculty of Health Sciences, Department of Anatomy and Cell Biology, Kingston, ON K7L 3N6, Canada. Offers biology of reproduction (M Sc, PhD); cancer (M Sc, PhD); cardiovascular pathophysiology (M Sc, PhD); cell and molecular biology (M Sc, PhD); drug metabolism (M Sc, PhD); endocrinology (M Sc, PhD); motor control (M Sc, PhD); neural regeneration (M Sc, PhD); neurophysiology (M Sc, PhD). Part-time programs available. *Degree requirements:* For master's, thesis; for doctorate, one foreign language, comprehensive exam, thesis/dissertation. *Entrance requirements:* Additional exam requirements/recommendations for international students: Required—TOEFL. Electronic applications accepted. *Faculty research:* Human kinetics, neuroscience, reproductive biology, cardiovascular.

Quinnipiac University, College of Arts and Sciences, Program in Molecular and Cell Biology, Hamden, CT 06518-1940. Offers MS. Part-time and evening/weekend programs available. *Faculty:* 12 full-time (6 women), 19 part-time/adjunct (8 women). *Students:* 24 full-time (11 women), 21 part-time (13 women); includes 8 minority (1 American Indian or Alaska Native, non-Hispanic/Latino; 3 Asian, non-Hispanic/Latino; 4 Hispanic/Latino), 15 international. 43 applicants, 42% accepted, 7 enrolled. In 2013, 19 master's awarded. *Degree requirements:* For master's, thesis optional. *Entrance requirements:* For master's, bachelor's degree in biological, medical, or health sciences; minimum GPA of 2.75. Additional exam requirements/recommendations for international students: Required—TOEFL (minimum score 575 paper-based; 90 iBT), IELTS (minimum score 6.5). *Application deadline:* For fall admission, 7/30 priority date for domestic students, 4/15 priority date for international students; for spring admission, 12/15 priority date for domestic students, 9/15 priority date for international students. Applications are processed on a rolling basis. Application fee: $45. Electronic applications accepted. *Expenses: Tuition:* Part-time $920 per credit. *Required fees:* $37 per credit. *Financial support:* In 2013–14, 2 students received support. Career-related internships or fieldwork, Federal Work-Study, scholarships/grants, and unspecified assistantships available. Support available to part-time students. Financial award application deadline: 6/1; financial award applicants required to submit FAFSA. *Unit head:* Dr. Michelle Geremia, Director, E-mail: michelle.geremia@quinnipiac.edu. *Application contact:* Office of Graduate Admissions, 800-462-1944, Fax: 203-582-3443, E-mail: graduate@quinnipiac.edu.
Website: http://www.quinnipiac.edu/gradmolecular

Rice University, Graduate Programs, Wiess School of Natural Sciences, Department of Biochemistry and Cell Biology, Houston, TX 77251-1892. Offers MA, PhD. Terminal master's awarded for partial completion of doctoral program. *Degree requirements:* For master's, thesis; for doctorate, thesis/dissertation. *Entrance requirements:* For master's and doctorate, GRE. Additional exam requirements/recommendations for international students: Required—TOEFL (minimum score 600 paper-based; 90 iBT). Electronic applications accepted. *Expenses:* Contact institution. *Faculty research:* Steroid metabolism, protein structure NMR, biophysics, cell growth and movement.

Rosalind Franklin University of Medicine and Science, School of Graduate and Postdoctoral Studies - Interdisciplinary Graduate Program in Biomedical Sciences, Department of Cell Biology and Anatomy, North Chicago, IL 60064-3095. Offers MS, PhD, MD/PhD. Terminal master's awarded for partial completion of doctoral program. *Degree requirements:* For master's, comprehensive exam, thesis, qualifying exam; for doctorate, comprehensive exam, thesis/dissertation, original research project. *Entrance requirements:* For master's and doctorate, GRE General Test, minimum GPA of 3.0. Additional exam requirements/recommendations for international students: Required—TOEFL, TWE. *Faculty research:* Neuroscience, molecular biology.

Rush University, Graduate College, Division of Anatomy and Cell Biology, Chicago, IL 60612-3832. Offers MS, PhD, MD/MS, MD/PhD. Terminal master's awarded for partial completion of doctoral program. *Degree requirements:* For master's, thesis; for doctorate, comprehensive exam, thesis/dissertation, preliminary exam, dissertation proposal. *Entrance requirements:* For master's, GRE General Test, minimum GPA of 3.0, bachelor's degree in biology or chemistry (preferred), interview; for doctorate, GRE General Test, minimum GPA of 3.0, interview. Additional exam requirements/recommendations for international students: Required—TOEFL. Electronic applications accepted. *Faculty research:* Incontinence following vaginal distension, knee replacement, biomimetric materials, injured spinal motoneurons, implant fixation.

Rutgers, The State University of New Jersey, Newark, Graduate School of Biomedical Sciences, Department of Cell Biology and Molecular Medicine, Newark, NJ 07107. Offers PhD. *Degree requirements:* For doctorate, thesis/dissertation, qualifying exam. *Entrance requirements:* For doctorate, GRE General Test. Additional exam requirements/recommendations for international students: Required—TOEFL. Electronic applications accepted.

Rutgers, The State University of New Jersey, New Brunswick, Graduate School-New Brunswick, Programs in the Molecular Biosciences, Program in Cell and Developmental Biology, Piscataway, NJ 08854-8097. Offers MS, PhD. MS, PhD offered jointly with University of Medicine and Dentistry of New Jersey. Part-time programs available. Terminal master's awarded for partial completion of doctoral program. *Degree requirements:* For master's, thesis; for doctorate, thesis/dissertation, written qualifying exam. *Entrance requirements:* For master's, GRE General Test; for doctorate, GRE General Test, GRE Subject Test (recommended), minimum GPA of 3.0. Additional exam requirements/recommendations for international students: Required—TOEFL. Electronic applications accepted. *Faculty research:* Signal transduction and regulation of gene expression, developmental biology, cellular biology, developmental genetics, neurobiology.

San Diego State University, Graduate and Research Affairs, College of Sciences, Department of Biology, San Diego, CA 92182. Offers biology (MA, MS), including ecology (MS), molecular biology (MS), physiology (MS), systematics/evolution (MS); cell and molecular biology (PhD); ecology (MS, PhD); microbiology (MS). Terminal master's awarded for partial completion of doctoral program. *Degree requirements:* For master's, thesis; for doctorate, thesis/dissertation. *Entrance requirements:* For master's, GRE General Test, GRE Subject Test, resume or curriculum vitae, 2 letters of recommendation. Additional exam requirements/recommendations for international students: Required—TOEFL. Electronic applications accepted.

San Diego State University, Graduate and Research Affairs, College of Sciences, Molecular Biology Institute, Program in Cell and Molecular Biology, San Diego, CA 92182. Offers PhD. Program offered jointly with University of California, San Diego. *Degree requirements:* For doctorate, thesis/dissertation, oral comprehensive qualifying exam. *Entrance requirements:* For doctorate, GRE General Test, GRE Subject Test, resumé or curriculum vitae, 3 letters of recommendation. Electronic applications accepted. *Faculty research:* Structure/dynamics of protein kinesis, chromatin structure and DNA methylation membrane biochemistry, secretory protein targeting, molecular biology of cardiac myocytes.

San Francisco State University, Division of Graduate Studies, College of Science and Engineering, Department of Biology, Program in Cell and Molecular Biology, San Francisco, CA 94132-1722. Offers MS. *Application deadline:* Applications are processed on a rolling basis. *Unit head:* Dr. Diana Chu, Program Coordinator, 415-405-3487, E-mail: chud@sfsu.edu. *Application contact:* Dr. Robert Patterson, Graduate Coordinator, 415-338-1237, E-mail: patters@sfsu.edu.
Website: http://biology.sfsu.edu/programs/graduate

Cell Biology

Sonoma State University, School of Science and Technology, Department of Biology, Rohnert Park, CA 94928. Offers biochemistry (MA); ecology (MS); environmental biology (MS); evolutionary biology (MS); functional morphology (MS); molecular and cell biology (MS); organismal biology (MS). Part-time programs available. *Faculty:* 9 full-time (1 woman). *Students:* 4 full-time (2 women), 21 part-time (14 women); includes 5 minority (1 American Indian or Alaska Native, non-Hispanic/Latino; 1 Asian, non-Hispanic/Latino; 2 Hispanic/Latino; 1 Two or more races, non-Hispanic/Latino), 2 international. Average age 29. 23 applicants, 65% accepted, 6 enrolled. In 2013, 6 master's awarded. *Degree requirements:* For master's, thesis or alternative, oral exam. *Entrance requirements:* For master's, GRE General Test, GRE Subject Test, minimum GPA of 3.0. Additional exam requirements/recommendations for international students: Required—TOEFL (minimum score 500 paper-based). *Application deadline:* For fall admission, 11/30 for domestic students. Applications are processed on a rolling basis. Application fee: $55. *Expenses:* Tuition, state resident: full-time $8500. Tuition, nonresident: full-time $12,964. *Required fees:* $1762. *Financial support:* In 2013–14, 1 fellowship (averaging $1,520 per year), 6 research assistantships (averaging $3,562 per year), 22 teaching assistantships (averaging $6,738 per year) were awarded; career-related internships or fieldwork, Federal Work-Study, and tuition waivers (full) also available. Financial award application deadline: 3/2; financial award applicants required to submit FAFSA. *Faculty research:* Plant physiology, comparative physiology, community ecology, restoration ecology, marine ecology, conservation genetics, primate behavior, behavioral ecology, developmental biology, plant and animal systematics. *Total annual research expenditures:* $4,400. *Unit head:* Dr. Nathan Rank, Chair, 707-664-3053, E-mail: nathan.rank@sonoma.edu. *Application contact:* Dr. Derek Girman, Graduate Adviser, 707-664-3055, E-mail: derek.girman@sonoma.edu.
Website: http://www.sonoma.edu/biology/graduate

Southern Methodist University, Dedman College of Humanities and Sciences, Department of Biological Sciences, Dallas, TX 75275. Offers molecular and cellular biology (MA, MS, PhD). Terminal master's awarded for partial completion of doctoral program. *Degree requirements:* For master's, thesis (for MS), oral exam; for doctorate, thesis/dissertation, qualifying exam. *Entrance requirements:* For master's, GRE General Test (minimum score 1200), minimum GPA of 3.0; for doctorate, GRE General Test (minimum score: 1200), minimum GPA of 3.0. Additional exam requirements/recommendations for international students: Required—TOEFL (minimum score 550 paper-based). Electronic applications accepted. *Faculty research:* Free radicals and aging, protein structure, chromatin structure, signal processes, retroviral pathogenesis.

State University of New York Downstate Medical Center, School of Graduate Studies, Program in Molecular and Cellular Biology, Brooklyn, NY 11203-2098. Offers PhD, MD/PhD. Affiliation with a particular PhD degree-granting program is deferred to the second year. *Degree requirements:* For doctorate, comprehensive exam, thesis/dissertation. *Entrance requirements:* For doctorate, GRE General Test. Additional exam requirements/recommendations for international students: Recommended—TOEFL. *Faculty research:* Mechanism of gene regulation, molecular virology.

State University of New York Upstate Medical University, College of Graduate Studies, Program in Cell and Developmental Biology, Syracuse, NY 13210-2334. Offers anatomy (MS, PhD); MD/PhD. Terminal master's awarded for partial completion of doctoral program. *Degree requirements:* For master's, thesis; for doctorate, comprehensive exam, thesis/dissertation. *Entrance requirements:* For master's, GRE General Test, interview; for doctorate, GRE General Test, telephone interview. Additional exam requirements/recommendations for international students: Required—TOEFL. Electronic applications accepted. *Faculty research:* Cancer, disorders of the nervous system, infectious diseases, diabetes/metabolic disorders/cardiovascular diseases.

Stony Brook University, State University of New York, Graduate School, College of Arts and Sciences, Department of Biochemistry and Cell Biology, Biochemistry and Cell Biology Program, Stony Brook, NY 11794. Offers MS. Part-time programs available. *Students:* 25 full-time (14 women), 2 part-time (1 woman); includes 7 minority (4 Asian, non-Hispanic/Latino; 2 Hispanic/Latino; 1 Two or more races, non-Hispanic/Latino), 6 international. 125 applicants, 14% accepted, 13 enrolled. In 2013, 7 master's awarded. *Degree requirements:* For master's, thesis. *Entrance requirements:* For master's, three letters of recommendation, BS or BA in a life science related field with minimum B average, personal statement. Additional exam requirements/recommendations for international students: Required—TOEFL (minimum score 550 paper-based; 90 iBT). *Application deadline:* For fall admission, 4/1 for domestic and international students. Applications are processed on a rolling basis. Electronic applications accepted. *Expenses:* Tuition, state resident: full-time $9870; part-time $411 per credit. Tuition, nonresident: full-time $18,350; part-time $765 per credit. *Unit head:* Prof. Robert Haltiwanger, Director, 631-632-7336, Fax: 631-632-9730, E-mail: robert.haltiwanger@stonybrook.edu. *Application contact:* Diana Berger, Coordinator, 631-632-8585, Fax: 631-632-9730, E-mail: diana.berger@stonybrook.edu.
Website: http://www.stonybrook.edu/commcms/biochem/education/graduate/overview.html

Stony Brook University, State University of New York, Graduate School, College of Arts and Sciences, Department of Biochemistry and Cell Biology, Molecular and Cellular Biology Program, Stony Brook, NY 11794. Offers biochemistry and molecular biology (PhD); biological sciences (MA); immunology and pathology (PhD); molecular and cellular biology (PhD). *Faculty:* 23 full-time (7 women), 1 part-time/adjunct (0 women). *Students:* 75 full-time (42 women); includes 7 minority (5 Asian, non-Hispanic/Latino; 2 Hispanic/Latino), 46 international. Average age 30. 211 applicants, 15% accepted, 8 enrolled. In 2013, 13 master's, 15 doctorates awarded. *Degree requirements:* For doctorate, comprehensive exam, thesis/dissertation, teaching experience. *Entrance requirements:* For doctorate, GRE General Test, GRE Subject Test. Additional exam requirements/recommendations for international students: Required—TOEFL. *Application deadline:* For fall admission, 1/15 for domestic students; for spring admission, 10/1 for domestic students. Application fee: $100. *Expenses:* Tuition, state resident: full-time $9870; part-time $411 per credit. Tuition, nonresident: full-time $18,350; part-time $765 per credit. *Financial support:* In 2013–14, 22 fellowships, 18 research assistantships, 12 teaching assistantships were awarded; Federal Work-Study also available. *Unit head:* Prof. Robert Haltiwanger, Chair, 631-632-8560, E-mail: robert.haltiwanger@stonybrook.edu. *Application contact:* Joann DeLucia-Conlon, Coordinator, 631-632-8613, Fax: 631-632-9730, E-mail: joann.delucia-conlon@stonybrook.edu.

Texas A&M Health Science Center, College of Medicine, Department of Molecular and Cellular Medicine, College Station, TX 77840. Offers PhD. *Degree requirements:* For doctorate, thesis/dissertation. *Entrance requirements:* For doctorate, GRE General Test. *Faculty research:* Immunology, cell and membrane biology, protein biochemistry, molecular genetics, parasitology, vertebrate embryogenesis and microbiology.

Texas A&M Health Science Center, College of Medicine, Program in Cell and Molecular Biology, College Station, TX 77840. Offers PhD.

Texas Tech University Health Sciences Center, Graduate School of Biomedical Sciences, Program in Biomedical Sciences, Lubbock, TX 79430. Offers MS, PhD, MD/PhD, MS/PhD. Terminal master's awarded for partial completion of doctoral program. *Degree requirements:* For master's, comprehensive exam, thesis; for doctorate, comprehensive exam, thesis/dissertation. *Entrance requirements:* For master's and doctorate, GRE General Test, minimum GPA of 3.0. Additional exam requirements/recommendations for international students: Required—TOEFL (minimum score 550 paper-based). Electronic applications accepted. *Faculty research:* Biochemical endocrinology, neurobiology, molecular biology, reproductive biology, biology of developing systems.

Thomas Jefferson University, Jefferson Graduate School of Biomedical Sciences, MS Program in Cell and Developmental Biology, Philadelphia, PA 19107. Offers MS. Part-time and evening/weekend programs available. *Faculty:* 44 full-time (14 women), 27 part-time/adjunct (11 women). *Students:* 15 part-time (12 women); includes 2 minority (both Black or African American, non-Hispanic/Latino), 2 international. 12 applicants, 58% accepted, 4 enrolled. In 2013, 2 master's awarded. *Degree requirements:* For master's, thesis, clerkship. *Entrance requirements:* For master's, GRE General Test or MCAT, minimum GPA of 3.0. Additional exam requirements/recommendations for international students: Required—TOEFL (minimum score 100 iBT) or IELTS (minimum score 7). *Application deadline:* For fall admission, 8/1 priority date for domestic students, 3/1 priority date for international students; for winter admission, 12/1 priority date for domestic students, 6/1 priority date for international students; for spring admission, 4/1 priority date for domestic students. Applications are processed on a rolling basis. Application fee: $75. Electronic applications accepted. *Financial support:* Federal Work-Study and institutionally sponsored loans available. Support available to part-time students. Financial award application deadline: 5/1; financial award applicants required to submit FAFSA. *Faculty research:* Developmental biology, cell biology, planning and management, drug development. *Unit head:* Dr. Gerald B. Grunwald, Dean and Program Director, 215-503-4191, Fax: 215-503-6690, E-mail: gerald.grunwald@jefferson.edu. *Application contact:* Marc E. Stearns, Director of Admissions, 215-503-0155, Fax: 215-503-3433, E-mail: jgsbs-info@jefferson.edu.
Website: http://www.jefferson.edu/university/biomedical_sciences/programs/masters/cell-developmental-bio.html

Thomas Jefferson University, Jefferson Graduate School of Biomedical Sciences, PhD Program in Cell and Developmental Biology, Philadelphia, PA 19107. Offers PhD. *Faculty:* 75 full-time (17 women). *Students:* 29 full-time (14 women); includes 5 minority (1 Black or African American, non-Hispanic/Latino; 3 Asian, non-Hispanic/Latino; 1 Hispanic/Latino), 4 international. 40 applicants, 15% accepted, 3 enrolled. In 2013, 5 doctorates awarded. *Degree requirements:* For doctorate, comprehensive exam, thesis/dissertation. *Entrance requirements:* For doctorate, GRE General Test, minimum GPA of 3.2. Additional exam requirements/recommendations for international students: Required—TOEFL (minimum score 100 iBT). *Application deadline:* For fall admission, 1/5 priority date for domestic and international students. Applications are processed on a rolling basis. Application fee: $75. Electronic applications accepted. *Financial support:* In 2013–14, 29 students received support, including 29 fellowships with full tuition reimbursements available (averaging $56,052 per year); Federal Work-Study, institutionally sponsored loans, scholarships/grants, traineeships, and stipends also available. Support available to part-time students. Financial award application deadline: 5/1; financial award applicants required to submit FAFSA. *Unit head:* Dr. Jan B. Hoek, Program Director, 215-503-5016, Fax: 215-923-2218, E-mail: joannes.hoek@jefferson.edu. *Application contact:* Marc E. Stearns, Director of Admissions, 215-503-0155, Fax: 215-503-3433, E-mail: jgsbs-info@jefferson.edu.
Website: http://www.jefferson.edu/university/biomedical_sciences/programs/phd/cell_biology.html

Tufts University, Sackler School of Graduate Biomedical Sciences, Cell, Molecular, and Developmental Biology Program, Medford, MA 02155. Offers PhD. *Faculty:* 45 full-time (15 women). *Students:* 25 full-time (10 women); includes 8 minority (1 Black or African American, non-Hispanic/Latino; 5 Asian, non-Hispanic/Latino; 1 Hispanic/Latino; 1 Two or more races, non-Hispanic/Latino), 5 international. Average age 29. In 2013, 3 doctorates awarded. Terminal master's awarded for partial completion of doctoral program. *Degree requirements:* For doctorate, comprehensive exam, thesis/dissertation. *Entrance requirements:* For doctorate, GRE General Test, 3 letters of reference. Additional exam requirements/recommendations for international students: Required—TOEFL (minimum score 600 paper-based; 100 iBT). *Application deadline:* For fall admission, 12/15 for domestic and international students. Application fee: $70. Electronic applications accepted. *Financial support:* In 2013–14, 25 students received support, including 25 research assistantships with full tuition reimbursements available (averaging $31,000 per year); fellowships and health care benefits also available. *Faculty research:* Reproduction and hormone action, control of gene expression, cell-matrix and cell-cell interactions, growth control and tumorigenesis, cytoskeleton and contractile proteins. *Unit head:* Dr. John Castellot, Program Director, 617-636-0303, Fax: 617-636-0375. *Application contact:* Kellie Johnston, Associate Director of Admissions, 617-636-6767, Fax: 617-636-0375, E-mail: sackler-school@tufts.edu.
Website: http://sackler.tufts.edu/Academics/Degree-Programs/PhD-Programs/Cell-Molecular-and-Developmental-Biology

Tulane University, School of Medicine and School of Liberal Arts, Graduate Programs in Biomedical Sciences, Department of Structural and Cellular Biology, New Orleans, LA 70118-5669. Offers MS, PhD, MD/PhD. MS and PhD offered through the Graduate School. *Degree requirements:* For master's, one foreign language, thesis; for doctorate, 2 foreign languages, thesis/dissertation. *Entrance requirements:* For master's, GRE General Test, minimum B average in undergraduate course work; for doctorate, GRE General Test. Additional exam requirements/recommendations for international students: Required—TOEFL. Electronic applications accepted. *Faculty research:* Reproductive endocrinology, visual neuroscience, neural response to altered hormones.

Tulane University, School of Medicine and School of Liberal Arts, Graduate Programs in Biomedical Sciences, Interdisciplinary Graduate Program in Molecular and Cellular Biology, New Orleans, LA 70118-5669. Offers PhD, MD/PhD. PhD offered through the Graduate School. *Degree requirements:* For doctorate, thesis/dissertation. *Entrance requirements:* For doctorate, GRE General Test, GRE Subject Test. Additional exam requirements/recommendations for international students: Required—TOEFL. Electronic applications accepted. *Faculty research:* Developmental biology, neuroscience, virology.

Tulane University, School of Science and Engineering, Department of Cell and Molecular Biology, New Orleans, LA 70118-5669. Offers MS, PhD. Terminal master's awarded for partial completion of doctoral program. *Degree requirements:* For doctorate, thesis/dissertation. *Entrance requirements:* For master's, GRE General Test, minimum B average in undergraduate course work; for doctorate, GRE General Test. Additional exam requirements/recommendations for international students: Required—TOEFL. Electronic applications accepted.

Uniformed Services University of the Health Sciences, School of Medicine, Graduate Programs in the Biomedical Sciences and Public Health, Graduate Program in Molecular and Cell Biology, Bethesda, MD 20814-4799. Offers MS, PhD. *Faculty:* 43 full-time (11 women), 3 part-time/adjunct (0 women). *Students:* 26 full-time (13 women); includes 6 minority (2 Asian, non-Hispanic/Latino; 4 Hispanic/Latino), 11 international. Average age 26. 34 applicants, 35% accepted, 4 enrolled. In 2013, 4 doctorates awarded. *Degree requirements:* For doctorate, comprehensive exam, thesis/

dissertation, qualifying exam. *Entrance requirements:* For doctorate, GRE General Test, minimum GPA of 3.0. Additional exam requirements/recommendations for international students: Required—TOEFL. *Application deadline:* For fall admission, 1/1 priority date for domestic and international students. Applications are processed on a rolling basis. Application fee: $0. Electronic applications accepted. *Financial support:* In 2013–14, fellowships with full tuition reimbursements (averaging $27,000 per year) were awarded; scholarships/grants, health care benefits, and tuition waivers (full) also available. *Faculty research:* Immunology, biochemistry, cancer biology, stem cell biology. *Unit head:* Dr. Mary Lou Cutler, Director, 301-295-3453, Fax: 301-295-1996, E-mail: mary.cutler@usuhs.edu. *Application contact:* Tina Finley, Administrative Assistant, 301-295-3642, Fax: 301-295-1996, E-mail: netina.finley@usuhs.edu.
Website: http://www.usuhs.mil/mcb/index.html

See Display on page 221 and Close-Up on page 239.

Universidad Central del Caribe, School of Medicine, Program in Biomedical Sciences, Bayamón, PR 00960-6032. Offers anatomy and cell biology (MA, MS); biochemistry (MS); biomedical sciences (MA); cellular and molecular biology (PhD); microbiology and immunology (MA, MS); pharmacology (MS); physiology (MS).

Université de Montréal, Faculty of Medicine, Department of Pathology and Cellular Biology, Montréal, QC H3C 3J7, Canada. Offers M Sc, PhD. Terminal master's awarded for partial completion of doctoral program. *Degree requirements:* For master's, thesis; for doctorate, thesis/dissertation, general exam. *Entrance requirements:* For master's and doctorate, proficiency in French, knowledge of English. Electronic applications accepted. *Faculty research:* Immunopathology, cardiovascular pathology, oncogenetics, cellular neurocytology, muscular dystrophy.

Université de Sherbrooke, Faculty of Medicine and Health Sciences, Graduate Programs in Medicine, Department of Anatomy and Cell Biology, Sherbrooke, QC J1H 5N4, Canada. Offers cell biology (M Sc, PhD). Terminal master's awarded for partial completion of doctoral program. *Degree requirements:* For master's, thesis; for doctorate, thesis/dissertation. Electronic applications accepted. *Faculty research:* Biology of the gut epithelium, signal transduction, gene expression and differentiation, intestinal inflammation, vascular and skeletal muscle cell biology.

Université Laval, Faculty of Medicine, Graduate Programs in Medicine, Programs in Cellular and Molecular Biology, Québec, QC G1K 7P4, Canada. Offers M Sc, PhD. Terminal master's awarded for partial completion of doctoral program. *Degree requirements:* For master's, thesis; for doctorate, comprehensive exam, thesis/dissertation. *Entrance requirements:* For master's and doctorate, knowledge of French, comprehension of written English. Electronic applications accepted. *Faculty research:* Oral bacterial metabolism, sugar transport.

University at Albany, State University of New York, College of Arts and Sciences, Department of Biological Sciences, Specialization in Molecular, Cellular, Developmental, and Neural Biology, Albany, NY 12222-0001. Offers MS, PhD. *Degree requirements:* For master's, one foreign language; for doctorate, one foreign language, thesis/dissertation. *Entrance requirements:* For master's and doctorate, GRE General Test.

University at Albany, State University of New York, School of Public Health, Department of Biomedical Sciences, Program in Cell and Molecular Structure, Albany, NY 12222-0001. Offers MS, PhD. *Degree requirements:* For master's, thesis; for doctorate, thesis/dissertation. *Entrance requirements:* For master's and doctorate, GRE General Test, GRE Subject Test.

University at Buffalo, the State University of New York, Graduate School, Graduate Programs in Cancer Research and Biomedical Sciences at Roswell Park Cancer Institute, Department of Cellular and Molecular Biology at Roswell Park Cancer Institute, Buffalo, NY 14260. Offers PhD. *Faculty:* 20 full-time (2 women), 5 part-time/adjunct (1 woman). *Students:* 18 full-time (9 women); includes 3 minority (1 Black or African American, non-Hispanic/Latino; 1 Asian, non-Hispanic/Latino; 1 Hispanic/Latino), 3 international. 74 applicants, 8% accepted, 2 enrolled. In 2013, 3 doctorates awarded. *Degree requirements:* For doctorate, comprehensive exam, thesis/dissertation, oral defense of disseration. *Entrance requirements:* For doctorate, GRE General Test. Additional exam requirements/recommendations for international students: Required—TOEFL (minimum score 79 iBT). *Application deadline:* For fall admission, 1/5 priority date for domestic and international students; for winter admission, 12/30 for domestic and international students. Application fee: $75. Electronic applications accepted. *Financial support:* In 2013–14, 18 students received support, including 18 research assistantships with full tuition reimbursements available (averaging $25,000 per year); scholarships/grants, health care benefits, and unspecified assistantships also available. Financial award application deadline: 1/5. *Faculty research:* Cancer genetics, chromatin structure and replication, regulation of transcription, human gene mapping, genetic and structural approaches to regulation of gene expression. *Unit head:* Dr. Dominic J. Smiraglia, Director of Graduate Studies, 716-845-1347, Fax: 716-845-1698, E-mail: dominic.smiraglia@roswellpark.org. *Application contact:* Dr. Norman J. Karin, Associate Dean, 716-845-2339, Fax: 716-845-8178, E-mail: norman.karin@roswellpark.org.
Website: http://www.roswellpark.edu/education/phd-programs/cellular-molecular-biology

The University of Alabama at Birmingham, Graduate Programs in Joint Health Sciences, Program in Cell Biology, Birmingham, AL 35294. Offers PhD. *Degree requirements:* For doctorate, variable foreign language requirement, comprehensive exam, thesis/dissertation. *Entrance requirements:* For doctorate, GRE General Test, interview, evaluation forms. Electronic applications accepted.

The University of Alabama at Birmingham, Graduate Programs in Joint Health Sciences, Program in Cellular and Molecular Physiology, Birmingham, AL 35294. Offers PhD. *Degree requirements:* For doctorate, comprehensive exam, thesis/dissertation.

University of Alberta, Faculty of Graduate Studies and Research, Department of Biological Sciences, Edmonton, AB T6G 2E1, Canada. Offers environmental biology and ecology (M Sc, PhD); microbiology and biotechnology (M Sc, PhD); molecular biology and genetics (M Sc, PhD); physiology and cell biology (M Sc, PhD); plant biology (M Sc, PhD); systematics and evolution (M Sc, PhD). Terminal master's awarded for partial completion of doctoral program. *Degree requirements:* For master's, thesis; for doctorate, thesis/dissertation. *Entrance requirements:* Additional exam requirements/recommendations for international students: Required—TOEFL.

University of Alberta, Faculty of Medicine and Dentistry and Faculty of Graduate Studies and Research, Graduate Programs in Medicine, Department of Cell Biology, Edmonton, AB T6G 2E1, Canada. Offers cell and molecular biology (M Sc, PhD). Terminal master's awarded for partial completion of doctoral program. *Degree requirements:* For master's, thesis; for doctorate, thesis/dissertation. *Entrance requirements:* For master's and doctorate, 3 letters of reference, curriculum vitae. Additional exam requirements/recommendations for international students: Required—TOEFL (minimum score 600 paper-based). *Faculty research:* Protein targeting, membrane trafficking, signal transduction, cell growth and division, cell-cell interaction and development.

The University of Arizona, College of Science, Department of Molecular and Cellular Biology, Tucson, AZ 85721. Offers applied biosciences (PSM); molecular and cellular biology (MS, PhD). Evening/weekend programs available. *Faculty:* 14 full-time (5 women). *Students:* 36 full-time (16 women); includes 13 minority (2 Black or African American, non-Hispanic/Latino; 2 Asian, non-Hispanic/Latino; 3 Hispanic/Latino; 6 Two or more races, non-Hispanic/Latino), 5 international. Average age 28. 34 applicants, 74% accepted, 13 enrolled. In 2013, 8 master's, 3 doctorates awarded. Terminal master's awarded for partial completion of doctoral program. *Degree requirements:* For master's, thesis; for doctorate, thesis/dissertation. *Entrance requirements:* For master's, 3 letters of recommendation; for doctorate, 3 letters of recommendation, statement of purpose. Additional exam requirements/recommendations for international students: Required—TOEFL (minimum score 600 paper-based; 90 iBT), IELTS (minimum score 7). *Application deadline:* For fall admission, 1/1 for domestic and international students. Applications are processed on a rolling basis. Application fee: $75. Electronic applications accepted. *Expenses:* Tuition, state resident: full-time $11,526. Tuition, nonresident: full-time $27,398. *Financial support:* In 2013–14, 15 research assistantships with full tuition reimbursements (averaging $24,838 per year), 5 teaching assistantships with full tuition reimbursements (averaging $22,587 per year) were awarded; career-related internships or fieldwork, scholarships/grants, health care benefits, and unspecified assistantships also available. *Faculty research:* Plant molecular biology, cellular and molecular aspects of development, genetics of bacteria and lower eukaryotes. *Total annual research expenditures:* $5.5 million. *Unit head:* Tricia Serio, Department Head, 520-621-1519, E-mail: bmcb@email.arizona.edu. *Application contact:* 520-621-1519, E-mail: bmcb@email.arizona.edu.
Website: http://bmcb.biology.arizona.edu/

University of Arkansas, Graduate School, Interdisciplinary Program in Cell and Molecular Biology, Fayetteville, AR 72701-1201. Offers MS, PhD. *Degree requirements:* For doctorate, thesis/dissertation. Electronic applications accepted.

The University of British Columbia, Faculty of Medicine, Department of Cellular and Physiological Sciences, Vancouver, BC V6T 1Z3, Canada. Offers M Sc, PhD. *Faculty:* 29 full-time (5 women), 2 part-time/adjunct (0 women). *Students:* 69 full-time (38 women); includes 26 minority (all Asian, non-Hispanic/Latino), 17 international. 26 applicants, 35% accepted, 8 enrolled. In 2013, 4 master's, 1 doctorate awarded. *Degree requirements:* For master's, thesis, oral defense; for doctorate, comprehensive exam, thesis/dissertation, oral defense. *Entrance requirements:* For master's, minimum overall B+ average in third- and fourth-year courses; for doctorate, minimum overall B+ average in a master's degree (or equivalent) from an approved institution with clear evidence of research ability or potential. Additional exam requirements/recommendations for international students: Required—TOEFL (minimum score 550 paper-based), IELTS (minimum score 6.5). *Application deadline:* For fall admission, 4/1 priority date for domestic students, 3/9 priority date for international students. Application fee: $90 ($150 for international students). *Expenses: Tuition, area resident:* Full-time $8000 Canadian dollars. *Financial support:* In 2013–14, 9 fellowships with full tuition reimbursements (averaging $16,000 per year), 8 research assistantships with partial tuition reimbursements (averaging $17,000 per year), 18 teaching assistantships with full tuition reimbursements (averaging $7,500 per year) were awarded; Federal Work-Study, institutionally sponsored loans, scholarships/grants, traineeships, tuition waivers (full), and unspecified assistantships also available. Financial award application deadline: 9/30. *Total annual research expenditures:* $3.8 million. *Unit head:* Dr. Christian Naus, Head, 604-822-2498. *Application contact:* Vincy Yung, Student Academic Services Application Clerk, 604-822-3907, Fax: 604-822-5802, E-mail: grad.admissions@ubc.ca.
Website: http://www.cell.ubc.ca/

University of California, Berkeley, Graduate Division, College of Letters and Science, Department of Molecular and Cell Biology, Berkeley, CA 94720-1500. Offers PhD. *Faculty:* 94 full-time (28 women), 1 part-time/adjunct (0 women). *Students:* 243 full-time (126 women); includes 75 minority (5 Black or African American, non-Hispanic/Latino; 4 American Indian or Alaska Native, non-Hispanic/Latino; 29 Asian, non-Hispanic/Latino; 24 Hispanic/Latino; 4 Native Hawaiian or other Pacific Islander, non-Hispanic/Latino; 9 Two or more races, non-Hispanic/Latino), 29 international. Average age 26. 687 applicants, 16% accepted, 37 enrolled. In 2013, 37 doctorates awarded. *Degree requirements:* For doctorate, comprehensive exam, thesis/dissertation, qualifying exam, 2 semesters of teaching. *Entrance requirements:* For doctorate, GRE General Test, GRE Subject Test (recommended), minimum GPA of 3.0. Additional exam requirements/recommendations for international students: Required—TOEFL (minimum score 570 paper-based; 68 iBT), IELTS (minimum score 7). *Application deadline:* For fall admission, 12/1 for domestic and international students. Applications are processed on a rolling basis. Application fee: $80 ($100 for international students). Electronic applications accepted. *Financial support:* In 2013–14, fellowships with full tuition reimbursements (averaging $31,000 per year), research assistantships with full tuition reimbursements (averaging $31,000 per year), teaching assistantships with full tuition reimbursements (averaging $31,000 per year) were awarded; scholarships/grants, traineeships, health care benefits, tuition waivers (full), and unspecified assistantships also available. Financial award application deadline: 12/1; financial award applicants required to submit FAFSA. *Faculty research:* Biochemistry, biophysics and structural biology; cell and developmental biology; genetics, genomics and development; immunology and pathogenesis; neurobiology. *Unit head:* Tanya Sullivan, Student Services Manager, 510-642-5252. *Application contact:* Berta Parra, Graduate Student Adviser, 510-642-5252, E-mail: mcbgao@berkeley.edu.
Website: http://mcb.berkeley.edu/

University of California, Davis, Graduate Studies, Graduate Group in Cell and Developmental Biology, Davis, CA 95616. Offers MS, PhD. *Degree requirements:* For master's, comprehensive exam (for some programs), thesis (for some programs); for doctorate, thesis/dissertation. *Entrance requirements:* For doctorate, GRE General Test, GRE Subject Test. Additional exam requirements/recommendations for international students: Required—TOEFL (minimum score 550 paper-based). Electronic applications accepted. *Faculty research:* Molecular basis of cell function and development.

University of California, Irvine, School of Biological Sciences, Department of Developmental and Cell Biology, Irvine, CA 92697. Offers biological sciences (MS, PhD). *Students:* 37 full-time (19 women); includes 23 minority (13 Asian, non-Hispanic/Latino; 9 Hispanic/Latino; 1 Native Hawaiian or other Pacific Islander, non-Hispanic/Latino), 1 international. Average age 29. In 2013, 4 master's, 12 doctorates awarded. *Degree requirements:* For doctorate, thesis/dissertation. *Entrance requirements:* For master's and doctorate, GRE General Test, GRE Subject Test, minimum GPA of 3.0. Additional exam requirements/recommendations for international students: Required—TOEFL (minimum score 550 paper-based). *Application deadline:* For fall admission, 12/15 priority date for domestic and international students. Application fee: $80 ($100 for international students). Electronic applications accepted. *Financial support:* Fellowships, research assistantships with full tuition reimbursements, teaching assistantships, institutionally sponsored loans, traineeships, health care benefits, and unspecified assistantships available. Financial award application deadline: 3/1; financial award applicants required to submit FAFSA. *Faculty research:* Genetics and development, oncogene signaling pathways, gene regulation, tissue regeneration and molecular genetics. *Unit head:* Prof. Diane K. O'Dowd, Department Chair, 949-824-4562, Fax: 949-824-1105, E-mail: dkodowd@uci.edu. *Application contact:* Grace Kuei, Personnel Manager, 949-824-6677, Fax: 949-824-4709, E-mail: jlmarsh@uci.edu.
Website: http://devcell.bio.uci.edu/

Cell Biology

University of California, Irvine, School of Biological Sciences and School of Medicine, Interdisciplinary Graduate Program in Cellular and Molecular Biosciences, Irvine, CA 92697. Offers PhD. *Degree requirements:* For doctorate, thesis/dissertation, teaching assignment, preliminary exam. *Entrance requirements:* For doctorate, GRE General Test, three letters of recommendation, interview. Additional exam requirements/recommendations for international students: Required—TOEFL or IELTS. *Application deadline:* For fall admission, 12/8 for domestic and international students. Application fee: $60 ($80 for international students). Electronic applications accepted. *Expenses:* Contact institution. *Financial support:* Fellowships with full tuition reimbursements, institutionally sponsored loans, scholarships/grants, tuition waivers (full), unspecified assistantships, and stipends available. Financial award application deadline: 1/1; financial award applicants required to submit FAFSA. *Faculty research:* Cellular biochemistry; gene structure and expression; protein structure, function, and design; molecular genetics; pathogenesis and inherited disease. *Unit head:* Dr. David Fruman, Director, 949-824-1947, Fax: 949-824-1965, E-mail: dfruman@uci.edu. *Application contact:* Renee Frigo, Administrator, 949-824-8145, Fax: 949-824-1965, E-mail: rfrigo@uci.edu.
Website: http://cmb.uci.edu/

University of California, Los Angeles, David Geffen School of Medicine and Graduate Division, Graduate Programs in Medicine, Department of Neurobiology, Los Angeles, CA 90095. Offers MS, PhD. Terminal master's awarded for partial completion of doctoral program. *Degree requirements:* For master's, comprehensive exam; for doctorate, thesis/dissertation, oral and written qualifying exams; 2 quarters of teaching experience. *Entrance requirements:* For doctorate, GRE General Test; GRE Subject Test, bachelor's degree; minimum undergraduate GPA of 3.0 (or its equivalent if letter grade system not used). Additional exam requirements/recommendations for international students: Required—TOEFL. Electronic applications accepted.

University of California, Los Angeles, Graduate Division, College of Letters and Science, Department of Molecular, Cell and Developmental Biology, Los Angeles, CA 90095. Offers MA, PhD. Terminal master's awarded for partial completion of doctoral program. *Degree requirements:* For master's, comprehensive exam, thesis; for doctorate, thesis/dissertation, oral and written qualifying exams; 2 quarters of teaching experience. *Entrance requirements:* For doctorate, GRE General Test. Additional exam requirements/recommendations for international students: Required—TOEFL. Electronic applications accepted.

University of California, Los Angeles, Graduate Division, College of Letters and Science and David Geffen School of Medicine, UCLA ACCESS to Programs in the Molecular, Cellular and Integrative Life Sciences, Los Angeles, CA 90095. Offers biochemistry and molecular biology (PhD); biological chemistry (PhD); cellular and molecular pathology (PhD); human genetics (PhD); microbiology, immunology, and molecular genetics (PhD); molecular biology (PhD); molecular toxicology (PhD); molecular, cellular and integrative physiology (PhD); neurobiology (PhD); oral biology (PhD); physiology (PhD). *Degree requirements:* For doctorate, thesis/dissertation, oral and written qualifying exams. *Entrance requirements:* For doctorate, GRE General Test, bachelor's degree; minimum undergraduate GPA of 3.0 (or its equivalent if letter grade system not used). Additional exam requirements/recommendations for international students: Required—TOEFL. Electronic applications accepted.

University of California, Riverside, Graduate Division, Program in Cell, Molecular, and Developmental Biology, Riverside, CA 92521-0102. Offers MS, PhD. Terminal master's awarded for partial completion of doctoral program. *Degree requirements:* For master's, thesis, oral defense of thesis; for doctorate, thesis/dissertation, oral defense of thesis, qualifying exams, 2 quarters of teaching experience. *Entrance requirements:* For master's and doctorate, GRE General Test, minimum GPA of 3.2. Additional exam requirements/recommendations for international students: Required—TOEFL (minimum score 550 paper-based; 80 iBT). Electronic applications accepted.

University of California, San Francisco, Graduate Division and School of Medicine, Tetrad Graduate Program, Cell Biology Track, San Francisco, CA 94143. Offers PhD, MD/PhD. *Degree requirements:* For doctorate, thesis/dissertation. *Entrance requirements:* For doctorate, GRE General Test, GRE Subject Test. Additional exam requirements/recommendations for international students: Required—TOEFL. *Application deadline:* For fall admission, 12/1 for domestic students. Application fee: $40. *Expenses:* Contact institution. *Financial support:* Application deadline: 2/1. *Unit head:* Robert Edwards, Co-Director, 415-502-5687. *Application contact:* Robert Edwards, Co-Director, 415-502-5687.

University of California, Santa Barbara, Graduate Division, College of Letters and Sciences, Division of Mathematics, Life, and Physical Sciences, Department of Molecular, Cellular, and Developmental Biology, Santa Barbara, CA 93106-9625. Offers molecular, cellular, and developmental biology (MA, PhD); pharmacology/biotechnology (MA); MA/PhD. *Faculty:* 29 full-time (3 women), 4 part-time/adjunct (0 women). *Students:* 48 full-time (23 women); includes 8 minority (2 Black or African American, non-Hispanic/Latino; 3 Asian, non-Hispanic/Latino; 3 Hispanic/Latino), 1 international. Average age 29. 182 applicants, 18% accepted, 11 enrolled. In 2013, 7 master's, 7 doctorates awarded. Terminal master's awarded for partial completion of doctoral program. *Degree requirements:* For master's, comprehensive exam (for some programs), thesis (for some programs); for doctorate, comprehensive exam, thesis/dissertation. *Entrance requirements:* For master's and doctorate, GRE General Test, 3 letters of recommendation, statement of purpose, personal achievements/contributions statement, resume/curriculum vitae, transcripts for post-secondary institutions attended. Additional exam requirements/recommendations for international students: Required—TOEFL (minimum score 550 paper-based; 80 iBT), IELTS (minimum score 7). *Application deadline:* For fall admission, 12/15 priority date for domestic and international students. Application fee: $80 ($100 for international students). Electronic applications accepted. *Expenses:* Tuition, state resident: part-time $5148.26 per quarter. Tuition, nonresident: part-time $10,182.26 per quarter. *Financial support:* In 2013–14, 3 students received support, including 3 fellowships with full and partial tuition reimbursements available (averaging $22,000 per year), 40 research assistantships with full and partial tuition reimbursements available (averaging $26,250 per year), 46 teaching assistantships with partial tuition reimbursements available (averaging $17,655 per year); career-related internships or fieldwork, Federal Work-Study, institutionally sponsored loans, scholarships/grants, traineeships, health care benefits, and unspecified assistantships also available. Financial award application deadline: 3/13; financial award applicants required to submit FAFSA. *Faculty research:* Microbiology, neurobiology (including stem cell research), developmental, virology, cell biology. *Unit head:* Dr. William Smith, Chair, 805-893-7698, E-mail: wililam.smith@lifesci.ucsb.edu. *Application contact:* Nicole McCoy, Graduate Program Advisor, 805-893-8499, E-mail: nicole.mccoy@lifesci.ucsb.edu.
Website: https://www.mcdb.ucsb.edu/grad

University of California, Santa Cruz, Division of Graduate Studies, Division of Physical and Biological Sciences, Program in Molecular, Cellular, and Developmental Biology, Santa Cruz, CA 95064. Offers MA, PhD. Terminal master's awarded for partial completion of doctoral program. *Degree requirements:* For master's, thesis; for doctorate, thesis/dissertation, qualifying exam. *Entrance requirements:* For master's and doctorate, GRE General Test, 3 letters of recommendation, interview. Additional exam requirements/recommendations for international students: Required—TOEFL (minimum score 550 paper-based; 83 iBT); Recommended—IELTS (minimum score 8). Electronic applications accepted. *Faculty research:* RNA biology, chromatin and chromosome biology, neurobiology, stem cell biology and differentiation, cell structure and function.

University of Chicago, Division of Biological Sciences, Molecular Biosciences Cluster, Graduate Program in Cell and Molecular Biology, Chicago, IL 60637-1513. Offers PhD. *Degree requirements:* For doctorate, thesis/dissertation, ethics class, 2 teaching assistantships. *Entrance requirements:* For doctorate, GRE General Test. Additional exam requirements/recommendations for international students: Required—TOEFL (minimum score 600 paper-based; 104 iBT), IELTS (minimum score 7). Electronic applications accepted. *Faculty research:* Gene expression, chromosome structure, animal viruses, plant molecular genetics.

University of Cincinnati, Graduate School, College of Medicine, Graduate Programs in Biomedical Sciences, Graduate Program in Cell and Cancer Biology, Cincinnati, OH 45221. Offers PhD. *Degree requirements:* For doctorate, thesis/dissertation, qualifying exam. *Entrance requirements:* For doctorate, GRE General Test. Additional exam requirements/recommendations for international students: Required—TOEFL. Electronic applications accepted. *Faculty research:* Cancer biology, cell and molecular biology, breast cancer, pancreatic cancer, drug discovery.

University of Colorado Boulder, Graduate School, College of Arts and Sciences, Department of Molecular, Cellular, and Developmental Biology, Boulder, CO 80309. Offers cellular structure and function (MA, PhD); developmental biology (MA, PhD); molecular biology (MA, PhD). *Faculty:* 25 full-time (7 women). *Students:* 64 full-time (36 women), 1 part-time (0 women); includes 5 minority (2 Asian, non-Hispanic/Latino; 2 Hispanic/Latino; 1 Native Hawaiian or other Pacific Islander, non-Hispanic/Latino), 9 international. Average age 27. 311 applicants, 12% accepted, 11 enrolled. In 2013, 2 master's, 11 doctorates awarded. Terminal master's awarded for partial completion of doctoral program. *Degree requirements:* For master's, comprehensive exam, thesis or alternative; for doctorate, comprehensive exam, thesis/dissertation. *Entrance requirements:* For master's, GRE General Test, GRE Subject Test, minimum undergraduate GPA of 3.0; for doctorate, GRE General Test, GRE Subject Test. *Application deadline:* For fall admission, 12/1 for domestic students, 12/15 for international students. Application fee: $50 ($60 for international students). Electronic applications accepted. *Financial support:* In 2013–14, 154 students received support, including 32 fellowships (averaging $6,403 per year), 62 research assistantships with full and partial tuition reimbursements available (averaging $30,807 per year), 11 teaching assistantships with full and partial tuition reimbursements available (averaging $27,393 per year); institutionally sponsored loans, scholarships/grants, health care benefits, and unspecified assistantships also available. Financial award application deadline: 2/1; financial award applicants required to submit FAFSA. *Faculty research:* Molecular biology, cellular biology, genetics, biological sciences, gene cloning. *Total annual research expenditures:* $14.8 million.
Website: http://mcdb.colorado.edu/

University of Colorado Denver, College of Liberal Arts and Sciences, Department of Integrative Biology, Denver, CO 80217. Offers animal behavior (MS); biology (MS); cell and developmental biology (MS); ecology (MS); evolutionary biology (MS); genetics (MS); integrative and systems biology (PhD); microbiology (MS); molecular biology (MS); neurobiology (MS); plant systematics (MS). Part-time programs available. *Faculty:* 21 full-time (7 women), 3 part-time/adjunct (2 women). *Students:* 18 full-time (11 women), 5 part-time (all women); includes 5 minority (1 Black or African American, non-Hispanic/Latino; 2 Hispanic/Latino; 2 Two or more races, non-Hispanic/Latino), 1 international. Average age 29. 25 applicants, 44% accepted, 11 enrolled. In 2013, 13 master's awarded. *Degree requirements:* For master's, comprehensive exam, thesis, 30-32 credit hours. *Entrance requirements:* For master's, GRE General Test (minimum score in 50th percentile in each section), BA/BS from accredited institution awarded within the last 10 years; minimum undergraduate GPA of 3.0; prerequisite courses: 1 year each of general biology and general chemistry; 1 semester each of general genetics, general ecology, and cell biology; and a structure/function course. Additional exam requirements/recommendations for international students: Required—TOEFL (minimum score 537 paper-based; 75 iBT); Recommended—IELTS (minimum score 6.5). *Application deadline:* For fall admission, 2/1 for domestic and international students. Application fee: $50 ($75 for international students). Electronic applications accepted. *Financial support:* In 2013–14, 8 students received support. Fellowships, research assistantships, teaching assistantships, Federal Work-Study, institutionally sponsored loans, scholarships/grants, and traineeships available. Financial award application deadline: 4/1; financial award applicants required to submit FAFSA. *Faculty research:* Molecular developmental biology; quantitative ecology, biogeography, and population dynamics; environmental signaling and endocrine disruption; speciation, the evolution of reproductive isolation, and hybrid zones; evolutionary, behavioral, and conservation ecology. *Unit head:* Dr. John Swallow, Biology Department Chair, 303-556-6154, E-mail: john.swallow@ucdenver.edu. *Application contact:* Timberley Roane, Associate Professor/Director of MS in Biology Program, 303-556-6592, E-mail: timberley.roane@ucdenver.edu.
Website: http://www.ucdenver.edu/academics/colleges/CLAS/Departments/biology/Programs/MasterofScience/Pages/BiologyMasterOfScience.aspx

University of Colorado Denver, School of Medicine, Program in Cell Biology, Stem Cells, and Developmental Biology, Aurora, CO 80045. Offers cell biology, stem cells, and developmental biology (PhD); modern human anatomy (MS). *Students:* 30 full-time (16 women), 1 part-time (0 women); includes 3 minority (all Hispanic/Latino), 5 international. Average age 28. 33 applicants, 15% accepted, 5 enrolled. In 2013, 2 doctorates awarded. *Degree requirements:* For doctorate, comprehensive exam, thesis/dissertation, at least 30 credit hours of coursework and 30 credit hours of thesis research; laboratory rotations. *Entrance requirements:* For doctorate, GRE, minimum GPA of 3.0; 3 letters of reference; prerequisite coursework in organic chemistry, biology, biochemistry, physics and calculus; research experience (highly recommended). Additional exam requirements/recommendations for international students: Required—TOEFL (minimum score 550 paper-based; 80 iBT). *Application deadline:* For fall admission, 12/1 for domestic students, 11/1 priority date for international students. Application fee: $50 ($75 for international students). Electronic applications accepted. *Expenses:* Contact institution. *Financial support:* In 2013–14, 31 students received support. Fellowships, research assistantships, teaching assistantships, Federal Work-Study, institutionally sponsored loans, scholarships/grants, traineeships, health care benefits, and tuition waivers (full) available. Financial award application deadline: 3/15; financial award applicants required to submit FAFSA. *Faculty research:* Development and repair of the vertebrate nervous system; molecular, genetic and developmental mechanisms involved in the patterning of the early spinal cord (neural plate) during vertebrate embryogenesis; structural analysis of protein glycosylation using NMR and mass spectrometry; small RNAs and post-transcriptional gene regulation during nematode gametogenesis and early development; diabetes-mediated changes in cardiovascular gene expression and functional exercise capacity. *Total annual research expenditures:* $5.7 million. *Unit head:* Dr. Wendy Macklin, Department Chair, 303-724-3426, E-mail: wendy.macklin@ucdenver.edu. *Application contact:* Kenton Owsley,

Program Administrator, 303-724-3468, Fax: 303-724-3420, E-mail: kenton.owsley@ucdenver.edu.
Website: http://www.ucdenver.edu/academics/colleges/medicalschool/programs/CSD/Pages/CSD.aspx

University of Connecticut, Graduate School, College of Liberal Arts and Sciences, Department of Molecular and Cell Biology, Field of Cell and Developmental Biology, Storrs, CT 06269. Offers MS, PhD. *Degree requirements:* For doctorate, thesis/dissertation. *Entrance requirements:* For master's and doctorate, GRE General Test, GRE Subject Test. Additional exam requirements/recommendations for international students: Required—TOEFL (minimum score 550 paper-based). Electronic applications accepted.

University of Connecticut Health Center, Graduate School, Graduate Program in Cell Analysis and Modeling, Farmington, CT 06030. Offers PhD. *Degree requirements:* For doctorate, comprehensive exam, thesis/dissertation. *Entrance requirements:* For doctorate, GRE General Test. Additional exam requirements/recommendations for international students: Required—TOEFL (minimum score 600 paper-based). Electronic applications accepted.

See Display below and Close-Up on page 241.

University of Connecticut Health Center, Graduate School, Programs in Biomedical Sciences, Graduate Program in Cell Biology, Farmington, CT 06030. Offers PhD, DMD/PhD, MD/PhD. *Degree requirements:* For doctorate, comprehensive exam, thesis/dissertation. *Entrance requirements:* For doctorate, GRE General Test. Additional exam requirements/recommendations for international students: Required—TOEFL (minimum score 600 paper-based). Electronic applications accepted. *Faculty research:* Vascular biology, computational biology, cytoskeleton and molecular motors, reproductive biology, signal transduction.

See Display below and Close-Up on page 243.

University of Delaware, College of Arts and Sciences, Department of Biological Sciences, Newark, DE 19716. Offers biotechnology (MS); cancer biology (MS, PhD); cell and extracellular matrix biology (MS, PhD); cell and systems physiology (MS, PhD); developmental biology (MS, PhD); ecology and evolution (MS, PhD); microbiology (MS, PhD); molecular biology and genetics (MS, PhD). Terminal master's awarded for partial completion of doctoral program. *Degree requirements:* For master's, thesis, preliminary exam; for doctorate, comprehensive exam, thesis/dissertation, preliminary exam. *Entrance requirements:* For master's and doctorate, GRE General Test. Additional exam requirements/recommendations for international students: Required—TOEFL (minimum score 600 paper-based); Recommended—TWE. Electronic applications accepted. *Faculty research:* Microorganisms, bone, cancer metastasis, developmental biology, cell biology, DNA.

University of Denver, Division of Natural Sciences and Mathematics, Department of Biological Sciences, Denver, CO 80208-9010. Offers biomedical sciences (PSM); cell and molecular biology (MS, PhD); ecology and evolution (MS, PhD). Part-time programs available. *Faculty:* 23 full-time (8 women). *Students:* 1 (woman) full-time, 21 part-time (13 women); includes 3 minority (all Hispanic/Latino), 7 international. Average age 27. 50 applicants, 22% accepted, 10 enrolled. In 2013, 5 master's, 2 doctorates awarded. Terminal master's awarded for partial completion of doctoral program. *Degree requirements:* For master's, comprehensive exam (for some programs), thesis; for doctorate, one foreign language, comprehensive exam (for some programs), thesis/dissertation. *Entrance requirements:* For master's and doctorate, GRE General Test, bachelor's degree in biology or related field, transcripts, personal statement, three letters of recommendation. Additional exam requirements/recommendations for international students: Required—TOEFL (minimum score 570 paper-based; 88 iBT). *Application deadline:* For fall admission, 1/1 priority date for domestic and international students. Applications are processed on a rolling basis. Application fee: $60. Electronic applications accepted. *Financial support:* In 2013–14, 19 students received support, including 3 research assistantships with full and partial tuition reimbursements available (averaging $22,448 per year), 15 teaching assistantships with full and partial tuition reimbursements available (averaging $25,161 per year); Federal Work-Study, institutionally sponsored loans, scholarships/grants, and unspecified assistantships also available. Support available to part-time students. Financial award application deadline: 2/15; financial award applicants required to submit FAFSA. *Faculty research:* Molecular biology, cell biology, neurobiology, ecology, molecular evolution. *Unit head:* Dr. Joseph Angleson, Chair, 303-871-3463, Fax: 303-871-3471, E-mail: jangleso@du.edu. *Application contact:* Randi Flageolle, Assistant to the Chair, 303-871-3457, Fax: 303-871-3471, E-mail: rflageol@du.edu.
Website: http://www.du.edu/nsm/departments/biologicalsciences/index.html

University of Florida, College of Medicine and Graduate School, Interdisciplinary Program in Biomedical Sciences, Concentration in Molecular Cell Biology, Gainesville, FL 32611. Offers PhD. *Degree requirements:* For doctorate, thesis/dissertation. *Entrance requirements:* For doctorate, GRE General Test, minimum GPA of 3.0, biochemistry before enrollment. Additional exam requirements/recommendations for international students: Required—TOEFL, IELTS. Electronic applications accepted. *Expenses:* Tuition, state resident: full-time $12,640. Tuition, nonresident: full-time $30,000.

University of Florida, Graduate School, College of Agricultural and Life Sciences, Department of Animal Sciences, Interdisciplinary Concentration in Animal Molecular and Cellular Biology, Gainesville, FL 32611. Offers MS, PhD. *Students:* 13 full-time (9 women), 3 part-time (2 women); includes 2 minority (both Hispanic/Latino), 10 international. Average age 29. 7 applicants, 71% accepted, 4 enrolled. In 2013, 1 master's, 4 doctorates awarded. *Entrance requirements:* For master's and doctorate, GRE General Test, minimum GPA of 3.0. Additional exam requirements/recommendations for international students: Required—TOEFL (minimum score 550 paper-based; 80 iBT), IELTS (minimum score 6). Application fee: $30. Electronic applications accepted. *Expenses:* Tuition, state resident: full-time $12,640. Tuition, nonresident: full-time $30,000. *Financial support:* In 2013–14, 11 students received support, including 1 fellowship (averaging $12,000 per year), 11 research assistantships (averaging $18,775 per year). Financial award applicants required to submit FAFSA. *Unit head:* Geoffrey E. Dahl, PhD, Professor and Department Chair, 352-392-1981, Fax: 352-392-5595, E-mail: gdahl@ufl.edu. *Application contact:* Office of Admissions, 352-392-1365, E-mail: webrequests@admissions.ufl.edu.
Website: http://www.animal.ufl.edu/amcb/

University of Florida, Graduate School, College of Agricultural and Life Sciences, Department of Microbiology and Cell Science, Gainesville, FL 32611. Offers MS, PhD. *Faculty:* 26 full-time (7 women), 4 part-time/adjunct (0 women). *Students:* 55 full-time (32 women), 4 part-time (2 women); includes 13 minority (5 Black or African American, non-Hispanic/Latino; 1 American Indian or Alaska Native, non-Hispanic/Latino; 2 Asian, non-Hispanic/Latino; 5 Hispanic/Latino), 26 international. Average age 28. 82 applicants, 20% accepted, 14 enrolled. In 2013, 3 master's, 4 doctorates awarded. *Degree requirements:* For master's, comprehensive exam, thesis (for some programs); for doctorate, comprehensive exam, thesis/dissertation. *Entrance requirements:* For master's, GRE General Test, minimum GPA of 3.0; for doctorate, GRE General Test, minimum GPA of 3.0. Additional exam requirements/recommendations for international students: Required—TOEFL (minimum score 550 paper-based; 80 iBT), IELTS (minimum score 6). *Application deadline:* For fall admission, 6/1 priority date for domestic students. Applications are processed on a rolling basis. Application fee: $30. Electronic applications accepted. *Expenses:* Tuition, state resident: full-time $12,640.

Tuition, nonresident: full-time $30,000. *Financial support:* In 2013–14, 46 students received support, including 5 fellowships (averaging $25,325 per year), 33 research assistantships (averaging $23,830 per year), 10 teaching assistantships (averaging $22,350 per year). Financial award applicants required to submit FAFSA. *Faculty research:* Biomass conversion, membrane and cell wall chemistry, plant biochemistry and genetics. *Unit head:* Eric Triplett, PhD, Professor and Chair, 352-392-1906, Fax: 352-392-5922, E-mail: ewt@ufl.edu. *Application contact:* Tony Romeo, PhD, Graduate Coordinator, 352-392-2400, Fax: 352-392-5922, E-mail: tromeo@ufl.edu.
Website: http://microcell.ufl.edu/

University of Florida, Graduate School, College of Liberal Arts and Sciences, Department of Biology, Gainesville, FL 32611. Offers botany (MS, MST, PhD), including botany; zoology (MS, MST, PhD), including animal molecular and cellular biology (PhD), tropical conservation and development (MS), wetland sciences (MS), zoology. *Faculty:* 31 full-time (9 women), 26 part-time/adjunct (9 women). *Students:* 99 full-time (44 women), 6 part-time (4 women); includes 14 minority (2 Black or African American, non-Hispanic/Latino; 1 American Indian or Alaska Native, non-Hispanic/Latino; 5 Asian, non-Hispanic/Latino; 6 Hispanic/Latino), 35 international. Average age 31. 74 applicants, 32% accepted, 18 enrolled. In 2013, 4 master's, 13 doctorates awarded. *Degree requirements:* For master's, comprehensive exam (for some programs), thesis; for doctorate, comprehensive exam, thesis/dissertation. *Entrance requirements:* For master's and doctorate, GRE General Test, minimum GPA of 3.0. Additional exam requirements/recommendations for international students: Required—TOEFL (minimum score 550 paper-based; 80 iBT), IELTS (minimum score 6). *Application deadline:* For fall admission, 12/1 for domestic and international students. Applications are processed on a rolling basis. Application fee: $30. Electronic applications accepted. *Expenses:* Tuition, state resident: full-time $12,640. Tuition, nonresident: full-time $30,000. *Financial support:* In 2013–14, 98 students received support, including 7 fellowships (averaging $22,150 per year), 34 research assistantships (averaging $19,000 per year), 66 teaching assistantships (averaging $16,250 per year); unspecified assistantships also available. Financial award application deadline: 12/15; financial award applicants required to submit FAFSA. *Faculty research:* Ecology, evolution, genetics, molecular and cellular biology, physiology. *Unit head:* Craig Osenberg, PhD, Professor and Chair, 352-392-9201, Fax: 352-392-3704, E-mail: osenberg@ufl.edu. *Application contact:* William T. Barbazuk, PhD, Associate Professor/Graduate Coordinator, 352-273-8624, Fax: 352-392-3704, E-mail: bbarbazuk@ufl.edu.
Website: http://www.biology.ufl.edu/

University of Georgia, Franklin College of Arts and Sciences, Department of Cellular Biology, Athens, GA 30602. Offers MS, PhD. *Degree requirements:* For master's, thesis; for doctorate, one foreign language, thesis/dissertation. *Entrance requirements:* For master's and doctorate, GRE General Test. Electronic applications accepted.

University of Guelph, Graduate Studies, College of Biological Science, Department of Molecular and Cellular Biology, Guelph, ON N1G 2W1, Canada. Offers biochemistry (M Sc, PhD); biophysics (M Sc, PhD); botany (M Sc, PhD); microbiology (M Sc, PhD); molecular biology and genetics (M Sc, PhD). *Degree requirements:* For master's, thesis, research proposal; for doctorate, comprehensive exam, thesis/dissertation, research proposal. *Entrance requirements:* For master's, minimum B-average during previous 2 years of coursework; for doctorate, minimum A-average. Additional exam requirements/recommendations for international students: Required—TOEFL (minimum score 550 paper-based), IELTS (minimum score 6.5). Electronic applications accepted. *Faculty research:* Physiology, structure, genetics, and ecology of microbes; virology and microbial technology.

University of Illinois at Chicago, College of Medicine and Graduate College, Graduate Programs in Medicine, Department of Anatomy and Cell Biology, Chicago, IL 60612. Offers MD/PhD. *Faculty:* 14 full-time (6 women), 11 part-time/adjunct (5 women). *Students:* 11 full-time (8 women); includes 2 minority (both Hispanic/Latino), 3 international. Average age 29. 17 applicants, 6% accepted. *Entrance requirements:* Additional exam requirements/recommendations for international students: Required—TOEFL (minimum score 550 paper-based). *Application deadline:* For fall admission, 5/15 for domestic students, 2/15 for international students. Applications are processed on a rolling basis. Application fee: $50 ($60 for international students). Electronic applications accepted. *Expenses:* Tuition, state resident: full-time $11,066; part-time $3689 per term. Tuition, nonresident: full-time $23,064; part-time $7688 per term. *Required fees:* $3004; $1190 per term. Tuition and fees vary according to course level and program. *Financial support:* Research or teaching assistantships with stipend of $24,000 per year, plus a tuition waiver available. *Faculty research:* Synapses, axonal transport, neurodegenerative diseases. *Total annual research expenditures:* $5.1 million. *Unit head:* Scott T. Brady, Head, 312-996-3313. *Application contact:* Dr. Ernesto R. Bongarzone, Associate Professor/Director of Graduate Studies, 312-996-6791, Fax: 312-413-0354, E-mail: ebongarz@uic.edu.
Website: http://www.anatomy.uic.edu/

University of Illinois at Chicago, Graduate College, Program in Neuroscience, Chicago, IL 60612. Offers cellular and systems neuroscience and cell biology (PhD); neuroscience (MS). *Students:* 17 full-time (9 women); includes 3 minority (1 Asian, non-Hispanic/Latino; 1 Hispanic/Latino; 1 Two or more races, non-Hispanic/Latino), 3 international. Average age 28. 63 applicants, 13% accepted, 6 enrolled. In 2013, 5 doctorates awarded. *Expenses:* Tuition, state resident: full-time $11,066; part-time $3689 per term. Tuition, nonresident: full-time $23,064; part-time $7688 per term. *Required fees:* $3004; $1190 per term. Tuition and fees vary according to course level and program. *Unit head:* Dr. Daniel Corcos, Program Chair, 312-355-1708, Fax: 312-423-3699, E-mail: dcorcos@uic.edu. *Application contact:* Perry Clark, Program Coordinator, 312-413-0185, Fax: 312-413-0354, E-mail: pclark5@uic.edu.
Website: http://www.uic.edu/depts/neurosci/

University of Illinois at Urbana–Champaign, Graduate College, College of Liberal Arts and Sciences, School of Molecular and Cellular Biology, Department of Cell and Developmental Biology, Champaign, IL 61820. Offers PhD. *Students:* 56 (31 women). Application fee: $75 ($90 for international students). *Unit head:* Jie Chen, Head, 217-265-0674, Fax: 217-244-1648, E-mail: jchen@illinois.edu. *Application contact:* Shannon J. Croft, 217-244-8116, Fax: 217-244-1648, E-mail: shannon9@illinois.edu.
Website: http://mcb.illinois.edu/departments/cdb/

The University of Iowa, Graduate College, College of Liberal Arts and Sciences, Department of Biology, Iowa City, IA 52242-1324. Offers biology (MS, PhD); cell and developmental biology (MS, PhD); evolution (MS, PhD); genetics (MS, PhD); neurobiology (MS, PhD). Terminal master's awarded for partial completion of doctoral program. *Degree requirements:* For master's, thesis optional, exam; for doctorate, comprehensive exam, thesis/dissertation. *Entrance requirements:* For master's and doctorate, GRE General Test, minimum GPA of 3.0. Additional exam requirements/recommendations for international students: Required—TOEFL (minimum score 600 paper-based; 100 iBT). Electronic applications accepted. *Faculty research:* Neurobiology, evolutionary biology, genetics, cell and developmental biology.

The University of Iowa, Graduate College, Program in Molecular and Cellular Biology, Iowa City, IA 52242-1316. Offers PhD. *Degree requirements:* For doctorate, comprehensive exam, thesis/dissertation. *Entrance requirements:* For doctorate, GRE General Test, minimum GPA of 3.0. Additional exam requirements/recommendations for international students: Required—TOEFL (minimum score 600 paper-based; 100 iBT). Electronic applications accepted. *Faculty research:* Regulation of gene expression, inherited human genetic diseases, signal transduction mechanisms, structural biology and function.

The University of Iowa, Roy J. and Lucille A. Carver College of Medicine and Graduate College, Biosciences Program, Iowa City, IA 52242-1316. Offers anatomy and cell biology (PhD); biochemistry (PhD); biology (PhD); biomedical engineering (PhD); chemistry (PhD); free radical and radiation biology (PhD); genetics (PhD); human toxicology (PhD); immunology (PhD); microbiology (PhD); molecular and cellular biology (PhD); molecular physiology and biophysics (PhD); neuroscience (PhD); pharmacology (PhD); physical therapy and rehabilitation science (PhD); rehabilitation science (PhD); speech and hearing (PhD). *Faculty:* 332 full-time. *Students:* 8 full-time (3 women); includes 2 minority (1 Black or African American, non-Hispanic/Latino; 1 Asian, non-Hispanic/Latino), 1 international. 200 applicants. *Degree requirements:* For doctorate, thesis/dissertation. *Entrance requirements:* For doctorate, GRE General Test, minimum GPA of 3.0. Additional exam requirements/recommendations for international students: Required—TOEFL (minimum score 600 paper-based; 100 iBT). *Application deadline:* For fall admission, 1/1 priority date for domestic and international students. Applications are processed on a rolling basis. Application fee: $60 ($100 for international students). Electronic applications accepted. *Expenses:* Contact institution. *Financial support:* In 2013–14, 8 students received support, including 8 research assistantships with full tuition reimbursements available (averaging $26,000 per year); fellowships, teaching assistantships, health care benefits, and unspecified assistantships also available. *Unit head:* Dr. Douglas Spitz, Director, 319-335-8001, E-mail: douglas-spitz@uiowa.edu. *Application contact:* Jodi Graff, Director, Admissions and First-Year Experience, 319-335-8306, E-mail: biosciences-admissions@uiowa.edu.
Website: http://www.medicine.uiowa.edu/biosciences/

The University of Iowa, Roy J. and Lucille A. Carver College of Medicine and Graduate College, Graduate Programs in Medicine, Department of Anatomy and Cell Biology, Iowa City, IA 52242-1316. Offers PhD. *Faculty:* 20 full-time (3 women). *Students:* 17 full-time (6 women); includes 7 minority (2 Black or African American, non-Hispanic/Latino; 1 American Indian or Alaska Native, non-Hispanic/Latino; 4 Asian, non-Hispanic/Latino), 1 international. Average age 28. 116 applicants. In 2013, 4 doctorates awarded. *Degree requirements:* For doctorate, comprehensive exam, thesis/dissertation. *Entrance requirements:* For doctorate, GRE General Test, minimum GPA of 3.0. Additional exam requirements/recommendations for international students: Required—TOEFL (minimum score 600 paper-based; 100 iBT). *Application deadline:* For fall admission, 1/15 priority date for domestic and international students. Applications are processed on a rolling basis. Application fee: $60 ($100 for international students). Electronic applications accepted. *Financial support:* In 2013–14, 17 students received support, including fellowships with full tuition reimbursements available (averaging $26,000 per year), 17 research assistantships with full tuition reimbursements available (averaging $26,000 per year), teaching assistantships with full tuition reimbursements available (averaging $26,000 per year); institutionally sponsored loans, scholarships/grants, and health care benefits also available. Financial award application deadline: 3/1. *Faculty research:* Biology of differentiation and transformation, developmental and vascular cell biology, neurobiology. *Total annual research expenditures:* $6.6 million. *Unit head:* Dr. John F. Engelhardt, Professor/Chair/Department Executive Officer, 319-335-7744, Fax: 319-335-7770, E-mail: john-engelhardt@uiowa.edu. *Application contact:* Julie A. Stark, Administrative Services Coordinator, 319-335-7744, Fax: 319-335-7770, E-mail: julie-stark@uiowa.edu.
Website: http://www.medicine.uiowa.edu/acb/

The University of Kansas, Graduate Studies, College of Liberal Arts and Sciences, Department of Molecular Biosciences, Lawrence, KS 66045. Offers biochemistry and biophysics (MA, PhD); microbiology (MA, PhD); molecular, cellular, and developmental biology (MA, PhD). *Faculty:* 34. *Students:* 52 full-time (28 women); includes 5 minority (2 Asian, non-Hispanic/Latino; 3 Hispanic/Latino), 23 international. Average age 27. 96 applicants, 25% accepted, 13 enrolled. In 2013, 3 master's, 9 doctorates awarded. Terminal master's awarded for partial completion of doctoral program. *Degree requirements:* For master's, comprehensive exam, thesis; for doctorate, comprehensive exam, thesis/dissertation. *Entrance requirements:* For master's and doctorate, GRE General Test. Additional exam requirements/recommendations for international students: Required—TOEFL or IELTS. *Application deadline:* For fall admission, 12/15 for domestic and international students. Application fee: $55 ($65 for international students). Electronic applications accepted. *Financial support:* Fellowships with tuition reimbursements, research assistantships with tuition reimbursements, teaching assistantships with tuition reimbursements, health care benefits, and unspecified assistantships available. Financial award application deadline: 3/1. *Faculty research:* Structure and function of proteins, genetics of organism development, molecular genetics, neurophysiology, molecular virology and pathogenics, developmental biology, cell biology. *Unit head:* Dr. Mark Richter, Chair, 785-864-3334, E-mail: richter@ku.edu. *Application contact:* John Connolly, Graduate Admissions Contact, 785-864-4311, E-mail: jconnolly@ku.edu.
Website: http://www.molecularbiosciences.ku.edu/

The University of Kansas, University of Kansas Medical Center, School of Medicine, Department of Anatomy and Cell Biology, Kansas City, KS 66160. Offers MA, PhD, MD/PhD. *Faculty:* 31. *Students:* 14 full-time (9 women); includes 1 minority (Hispanic/Latino), 5 international. Average age 27. In 2013, 4 doctorates awarded. Terminal master's awarded for partial completion of doctoral program. *Degree requirements:* For doctorate, comprehensive exam, thesis/dissertation. *Entrance requirements:* For doctorate, GRE. Additional exam requirements/recommendations for international students: Required—TOEFL. *Application deadline:* For fall admission, 1/15 priority date for domestic students. Applications are processed on a rolling basis. Application fee: $0. Electronic applications accepted. *Financial support:* Fellowships, research assistantships with full tuition reimbursements, teaching assistantships with full tuition reimbursements, institutionally sponsored loans, health care benefits, and unspecified assistantships available. Financial award application deadline: 3/1; financial award applicants required to submit FAFSA. *Faculty research:* Development of the synapse and neuromuscular junction, pain perception and diabetic neuropathies, cardiovascular and kidney development, reproductive immunology, post-fertilization signaling events. *Total annual research expenditures:* $8.7 million. *Unit head:* Dr. Dale R. Abrahamson, Chairman, 913-588-7000, Fax: 913-588-2710, E-mail: dabrahamson@kumc.edu. *Application contact:* Dr. Margaret Petroff, Associate Professor, 913-588-2781, Fax: 913-588-2710, E-mail: mpetroff@kumc.edu.
Website: http://www.kumc.edu/school-of-medicine/anatomy-and-cell-biology.html

University of Maine, Graduate School, Graduate School of Biomedical Science and Engineering, Orono, ME 04469. Offers bioinformatics (PSM); biomedical engineering (PhD); cell and molecular biology (PhD); neuroscience (PhD); toxicology (PhD). *Faculty:* 39 full-time (10 women), 31 part-time/adjunct (8 women). *Students:* 31 full-time (18 women), 5 part-time (4 women), 11 international. Average age 30. 57 applicants, 16% accepted, 7 enrolled. In 2013, 5 doctorates awarded. *Degree requirements:* For doctorate, comprehensive exam, thesis/dissertation. *Entrance requirements:* For

doctorate, GRE General Test, master's degree. Additional exam requirements/recommendations for international students: Required—TOEFL. *Application deadline:* For fall admission, 1/1 for domestic students. Application fee: $65. *Expenses:* Tuition, state resident: full-time $7524. Tuition, nonresident: full-time $23,112. *Required fees:* $1970. *Financial support:* In 2013–14, 16 students received support, including 1 fellowship with full tuition reimbursement available (averaging $18,000 per year), 13 research assistantships with full tuition reimbursements available (averaging $21,000 per year), 2 teaching assistantships (averaging $20,000 per year). *Faculty research:* Biomedical engineering, toxicology, neuroscience, cell and molecular biology, bioinformatics. *Total annual research expenditures:* $650,000. *Unit head:* Dr. David Neivandt, Director, 207-581-2803. *Application contact:* Scott G. Delcourt, Associate Dean of the Graduate School, 207-581-3291, Fax: 207-581-3232, E-mail: graduate@maine.edu.
Website: http://gsbse.umaine.edu/

The University of Manchester, Faculty of Life Sciences, Manchester, United Kingdom. Offers adaptive organismal biology (M Phil, PhD); animal biology (M Phil, PhD); biochemistry (M Phil, PhD); bioinformatics (M Phil, PhD); biomolecular sciences (M Phil, PhD); biotechnology (M Phil, PhD); cell biology (M Phil, PhD); cell matrix research (M Phil, PhD); channels and transporters (M Phil, PhD); developmental biology (M Phil, PhD); Egyptology (M Phil, PhD); environmental biology (M Phil, PhD); evolutionary biology (M Phil, PhD); gene expression (M Phil, PhD); genetics (M Phil, PhD); history of science, technology and medicine (M Phil, PhD); immunology (M Phil, PhD); integrative neurobiology and behavior (M Phil, PhD); membrane trafficking (M Phil, PhD); microbiology (M Phil, PhD); molecular and cellular neuroscience (M Phil, PhD); molecular biology (M Phil, PhD); molecular cancer studies (M Phil, PhD); neuroscience (M Phil, PhD); ophthalmology (M Phil, PhD); optometry (M Phil, PhD); organelle function (M Phil, PhD); pharmacology (M Phil, PhD); physiology (M Phil, PhD); plant sciences (M Phil, PhD); stem cell research (M Phil, PhD); structural biology (M Phil, PhD); systems neuroscience (M Phil, PhD); toxicology (M Phil, PhD).

University of Maryland, Baltimore, Graduate School, Graduate Program in Life Sciences, Program in Molecular Medicine, Baltimore, MD 21201. Offers cancer biology (PhD); cell and molecular physiology (PhD); human genetics and genomic medicine (PhD); molecular medicine (MS); molecular toxicology and pharmacology (PhD); MD/PhD. *Students:* 91 full-time (49 women), 14 part-time (8 women); includes 32 minority (10 Black or African American, non-Hispanic/Latino; 12 Asian, non-Hispanic/Latino; 5 Hispanic/Latino; 5 Two or more races, non-Hispanic/Latino), 9 international. Average age 27. 180 applicants, 33% accepted, 24 enrolled. In 2013, 10 master's, 15 doctorates awarded. *Degree requirements:* For doctorate, comprehensive exam, thesis/dissertation. *Entrance requirements:* For master's and doctorate, GRE. Additional exam requirements/recommendations for international students: Required—TOEFL (minimum score 600 paper-based; 100 iBT); Recommended—IELTS (minimum score 7). *Application deadline:* For fall admission, 12/1 priority date for domestic students, 1/15 for international students. Application fee: $75. Electronic applications accepted. *Financial support:* In 2013–14, research assistantships with partial tuition reimbursements (averaging $25,000 per year) were awarded; fellowships also available. Financial award application deadline: 3/1; financial award applicants required to submit FAFSA. *Unit head:* Dr. Toni Antalis, Director, 410-706-8222, E-mail: tantalis@som.umaryland.edu. *Application contact:* Sharron Graves, Program Coordinator, 410-706-6044, Fax: 410-706-6040, E-mail: sgraves@som.umaryland.edu.
Website: http://molecularmedicine.umaryland.edu

University of Maryland, Baltimore County, Graduate School, College of Natural and Mathematical Sciences, Department of Biological Sciences, Program in Molecular and Cell Biology, Baltimore, MD 21250. Offers PhD. *Faculty:* 26 full-time (11 women). *Students:* 7 full-time (4 women), 1 international. Average age 29. 25 applicants, 12% accepted. In 2013, 3 doctorates awarded. *Degree requirements:* For doctorate, thesis/dissertation. *Entrance requirements:* For doctorate, GRE General Test, GRE Subject Test, minimum GPA of 3.0. Additional exam requirements/recommendations for international students: Required—TOEFL (minimum score 80 iBT). *Application deadline:* For fall admission, 1/1 priority date for domestic and international students. Application fee: $50. Electronic applications accepted. One-time fee: $200 full-time. *Financial support:* In 2013–14, 7 students received support, including 3 fellowships with full tuition reimbursements available (averaging $25,000 per year), 4 teaching assistantships with full tuition reimbursements available (averaging $22,726 per year). *Unit head:* Dr. Stephen Miller, Graduate Program Director, 410-455-3381, Fax: 410-455-3875, E-mail: biograd@umbc.edu. *Application contact:* Dr. Stephen Miller, Director, 410-455-3381, Fax: 410-455-3875, E-mail: biograd@umbc.edu.
Website: http://biology.umbc.edu

University of Maryland, College Park, Academic Affairs, College of Computer, Mathematical and Natural Sciences, Department of Biology, PhD Program in Biological Sciences, College Park, MD 20742. Offers behavior, ecology, evolution, and systematics (PhD); computational biology, bioinformatics, and genomics (PhD); molecular and cellular biology (PhD); physiological systems (PhD). *Students:* 104 full-time (59 women), 4 part-time (1 woman); includes 21 minority (2 Black or African American, non-Hispanic/Latino; 1 American Indian or Alaska Native, non-Hispanic/Latino; 9 Asian, non-Hispanic/Latino; 7 Hispanic/Latino; 2 Two or more races, non-Hispanic/Latino), 34 international. 365 applicants, 13% accepted, 20 enrolled. In 2013, 5 doctorates awarded. *Degree requirements:* For doctorate, comprehensive exam, thesis/dissertation, thesis work presentation in seminar. *Entrance requirements:* For doctorate, GRE General Test; GRE Subject Test in biology (recommended), academic transcripts, statement of purpose/research interests, 3 letters of recommendation. Additional exam requirements/recommendations for international students: Required—TOEFL. *Application deadline:* For fall admission, 12/15 for domestic and international students. Applications are processed on a rolling basis. Application fee: $75. Electronic applications accepted. *Expenses:* Tuition, state resident: full-time $10,314; part-time $573 per credit hour. Tuition, nonresident: full-time $22,248; part-time $1236 per credit. *Required fees:* $1446; $403.15 per semester. Tuition and fees vary according to program. *Financial support:* In 2013–14, 21 fellowships with full and partial tuition reimbursements (averaging $27,603 per year), 25 research assistantships (averaging $19,557 per year), 55 teaching assistantships (averaging $18,959 per year) were awarded. *Unit head:* Dr. Charles F. Delwiche, Director, 301-405-6884, E-mail: bisidirector@umd.edu. *Application contact:* Dr. Charles A. Caramello, Dean of Graduate School, 301-405-0358, Fax: 301-314-9305, E-mail: ccaramel@umd.edu.
Website: http://www.bisi.umd.edu/

University of Maryland, College Park, Academic Affairs, College of Computer, Mathematical and Natural Sciences, Department of Cell Biology and Molecular Genetics, Program in Cell Biology and Molecular Genetics, College Park, MD 20742. Offers MS, PhD. *Students:* 24 full-time (12 women); includes 2 minority (both Asian, non-Hispanic/Latino), 8 international. In 2013, 2 master's, 11 doctorates awarded. *Degree requirements:* For master's, thesis; for doctorate, thesis/dissertation, exams. *Expenses:* Tuition, state resident: full-time $10,314; part-time $573 per credit hour. Tuition, nonresident: full-time $22,248; part-time $1236 per credit. *Required fees:* $1446; $403.15 per semester. Tuition and fees vary according to program. *Financial support:* In 2013–14, 1 fellowship with full tuition reimbursement (averaging $40,429 per year), 11 research assistantships (averaging $19,284 per year), 15 teaching assistantships (averaging $19,550 per year) were awarded. Financial award applicants required to submit FAFSA. *Faculty research:* Cytoskeletal activity, membrane biology, cell division, genetics and genomics, virology. *Unit head:* Norma Andrews, Chair, 301-405-8418, E-mail: andrewsn@umd.edu. *Application contact:* Dr. Charles A. Caramello, Dean of Graduate School, 301-405-0358, Fax: 301-314-9305, E-mail: ccaramel@umd.edu.

University of Maryland, College Park, Academic Affairs, College of Computer, Mathematical and Natural Sciences, Department of Cell Biology and Molecular Genetics, Program in Molecular and Cellular Biology, College Park, MD 20742. Offers PhD. Part-time and evening/weekend programs available. *Students:* 18 full-time (12 women), 1 (woman) part-time; includes 5 minority (1 Black or African American, non-Hispanic/Latino; 3 Asian, non-Hispanic/Latino; 1 Hispanic/Latino), 9 international. In 2013, 3 doctorates awarded. *Degree requirements:* For doctorate, thesis/dissertation, exam, public service. *Expenses:* Tuition, state resident: full-time $10,314; part-time $573 per credit hour. Tuition, nonresident: full-time $22,248; part-time $1236 per credit. *Required fees:* $1446; $403.15 per semester. Tuition and fees vary according to program. *Financial support:* In 2013–14, 2 fellowships with full tuition reimbursements (averaging $26,421 per year), 9 research assistantships (averaging $19,782 per year), 10 teaching assistantships (averaging $19,360 per year) were awarded. Financial award applicants required to submit FAFSA. *Faculty research:* Monoclonal antibody production, oligonucleotide synthesis, macronolular processing, signal transduction, developmental biology. *Unit head:* Norma Andrews, Chair, 301-405-8418, E-mail: andrewsn@umd.edu. *Application contact:* Dr. Charles A. Caramello, Dean of Graduate School, 301-405-0358, Fax: 301-314-9305, E-mail: ccaramel@umd.edu.

University of Massachusetts Amherst, Graduate School, Interdisciplinary Programs, Program in Molecular and Cellular Biology, Amherst, MA 01003. Offers biological chemistry and molecular biophysics (PhD); biomedicine (PhD); cellular and developmental biology (PhD). Part-time programs available. *Students:* 72 full-time (41 women); includes 15 minority (4 Black or African American, non-Hispanic/Latino; 5 Asian, non-Hispanic/Latino; 4 Hispanic/Latino; 2 Two or more races, non-Hispanic/Latino), 28 international. Average age 27. 160 applicants, 23% accepted, 20 enrolled. In 2013, 13 doctorates awarded. Terminal master's awarded for partial completion of doctoral program. *Degree requirements:* For doctorate, comprehensive exam, thesis/dissertation. *Entrance requirements:* For doctorate, GRE General Test. Additional exam requirements/recommendations for international students: Required—TOEFL (minimum score 550 paper-based; 80 iBT), IELTS (minimum score 6.5). *Application deadline:* For fall admission, 12/1 for domestic and international students. Applications are processed on a rolling basis. Application fee: $75. Electronic applications accepted. *Financial support:* Fellowships with full and partial tuition reimbursements, research assistantships with full and partial tuition reimbursements, teaching assistantships with full and partial tuition reimbursements, career-related internships or fieldwork, Federal Work-Study, scholarships/grants, traineeships, health care benefits, tuition waivers (full and partial), and unspecified assistantships available. Support available to part-time students. Financial award application deadline: 12/1; financial award applicants required to submit FAFSA. *Unit head:* Dr. Barbara Osborne, Graduate Program Director, 413-545-3246, Fax: 413-545-1812, E-mail: mcb@mcb.umass.edu. *Application contact:* Lindsay DeSantis, Supervisor of Admissions, 413-545-0722, Fax: 413-577-0010, E-mail: gradadm@grad.umass.edu.
Website: http://www.bio.umass.edu/mcb/

University of Massachusetts Amherst, Graduate School, Interdisciplinary Programs, Program in Plant Biology, Amherst, MA 01003. Offers biochemistry and metabolism (MS, PhD); cell biology and physiology (MS, PhD); environmental, ecological and integrative biology (MS, PhD); genetics and evolution (MS, PhD). *Students:* 20 full-time (11 women), 9 international. Average age 28. 72 applicants, 17% accepted, 2 enrolled. In 2013, 1 master's, 2 doctorates awarded. *Degree requirements:* For master's, thesis; for doctorate, 2 foreign languages, comprehensive exam, thesis/dissertation. *Entrance requirements:* For master's and doctorate, GRE General Test. Additional exam requirements/recommendations for international students: Required—TOEFL (minimum score 550 paper-based; 80 iBT), IELTS (minimum score 6.5). *Application deadline:* For fall admission, 12/15 for domestic and international students; for spring admission, 10/1 for domestic and international students. Applications are processed on a rolling basis. Application fee: $75. Electronic applications accepted. *Financial support:* Fellowships with full and partial tuition reimbursements, research assistantships with full and partial tuition reimbursements, teaching assistantships with full and partial tuition reimbursements, career-related internships or fieldwork, Federal Work-Study, scholarships/grants, traineeships, health care benefits, tuition waivers (full and partial), and unspecified assistantships available. Support available to part-time students. Financial award application deadline: 12/15; financial award applicants required to submit FAFSA. *Unit head:* Dr. Elsbeth L. Walker, Graduate Program Director, 413-577-3217, Fax: 413-545-3243, E-mail: pb@bio.umass.edu. *Application contact:* Lindsay DeSantis, Supervisor of Admissions, 413-545-0722, Fax: 413-577-0010, E-mail: gradadm@grad.umass.edu.
Website: http://www.bio.umass.edu/plantbio/

University of Massachusetts Boston, Office of Graduate Studies, College of Science and Mathematics, Track in Molecular, Cellular and Organismal Biology, Boston, MA 02125-3393. Offers PhD.

University of Massachusetts Worcester, Graduate School of Biomedical Sciences, Worcester, MA 01655-0115. Offers biochemistry and molecular pharmacology (PhD); bioinformatics and computational biology (PhD); cancer biology (PhD); cell biology (PhD); clinical and population health research (PhD); clinical investigation (MS); immunology and virology (PhD); interdisciplinary biomedical research (PhD); millennium (PhD); molecular genetics and microbiology (PhD); neuroscience (PhD); translational science (PhD); MD/PhD. *Faculty:* 1,388 full-time (521 women), 309 part-time/adjunct (198 women). *Students:* 385 full-time (210 women); includes 53 minority (13 Black or African American, non-Hispanic/Latino; 30 Asian, non-Hispanic/Latino; 10 Hispanic/Latino), 138 international. Average age 28. 491 applicants, 19% accepted, 39 enrolled. In 2013, 5 master's, 50 doctorates awarded. Terminal master's awarded for partial completion of doctoral program. *Median time to degree:* Of those who began their doctoral program in fall 2005, 67% received their degree in 8 years or less. *Degree requirements:* For master's, comprehensive exam, thesis; for doctorate, comprehensive exam, thesis/dissertation. *Entrance requirements:* For master's, MD, PhD, DVM, or PharmD; for doctorate, GRE General Test, bachelor's degree. Additional exam requirements/recommendations for international students: Required—TOEFL (minimum score 100 iBT) or IELTS (minimum score 7.5). *Application deadline:* For fall admission, 12/15 for domestic and international students; for spring admission, 5/15 for domestic students. Application fee: $80. Electronic applications accepted. *Expenses:* Contact institution. *Financial support:* In 2013–14, 431 students received support, including research assistantships with full tuition reimbursements available (averaging $29,500 per year); scholarships/grants, health care benefits, tuition waivers (full), and unspecified assistantships also available. Financial award application deadline: 5/16. *Faculty research:* RNA interference, cell/molecular/developmental biology, bioinformatics, clinical/translational research, infectious disease. *Total annual research*

expenditures: $245.9 million. *Unit head:* Dr. Anthony Carruthers, Dean, 508-856-4135, E-mail: anthony.carruthers@umassmed.edu. *Application contact:* Dr. Kendall Knight, Associate Dean and Interim Director of Admissions and Recruitment, 508-856-5628, Fax: 508-856-3659, E-mail: kendall.knight@umassmed.edu.
Website: http://www.umassmed.edu/gsbs/

University of Miami, Graduate School, Miller School of Medicine, Graduate Programs in Medicine, Department of Cell Biology and Anatomy, Coral Gables, FL 33124. Offers molecular cell and developmental biology (PhD); MD/PhD. *Degree requirements:* For doctorate, thesis/dissertation. *Entrance requirements:* For doctorate, GRE General Test, GRE Subject Test. Additional exam requirements/recommendations for international students: Required—TOEFL. Electronic applications accepted.

University of Michigan, Rackham Graduate School, College of Literature, Science, and the Arts, Department of Molecular, Cellular, and Developmental Biology, Ann Arbor, MI 48109. Offers MS, PhD. Part-time programs available. *Faculty:* 35 full-time (11 women). *Students:* 77 full-time (40 women), 2 part-time (1 woman); includes 10 minority (4 Asian, non-Hispanic/Latino; 5 Hispanic/Latino; 1 Native Hawaiian or other Pacific Islander, non-Hispanic/Latino), 42 international. Average age 27. 100 applicants, 25% accepted, 12 enrolled. In 2013, 5 master's, 7 doctorates awarded. Terminal master's awarded for partial completion of doctoral program. *Degree requirements:* For master's, 24 credits with at least 16 in molecular, cellular, and developmental biology and 4 in a cognate field; for doctorate, thesis/dissertation, preliminary exam, oral defense. *Entrance requirements:* For master's and doctorate, GRE General Test. Additional exam requirements/recommendations for international students: Required—TOEFL (minimum score 560 paper-based; 83 iBT). *Application deadline:* For fall admission, 1/5 for domestic and international students; for winter admission, 11/1 for domestic and international students; for spring admission, 4/1 for domestic and international students. Applications are processed on a rolling basis. Application fee: $75 ($90 for international students). Electronic applications accepted. Tuition and fees vary according to course level, course load, degree level, program and student level. *Financial support:* In 2013–14, 13 fellowships with full tuition reimbursements (averaging $28,500 per year), 31 research assistantships with full tuition reimbursements (averaging $28,500 per year), 17 teaching assistantships with full tuition reimbursements (averaging $28,500 per year) were awarded; health care benefits also available. *Faculty research:* Cell biology, microbiology, neurobiology and physiology, developmental biology and plant molecular biology. *Total annual research expenditures:* $7.8 million. *Unit head:* Dr. Robert J. Denver, Department Chair, 734-764-7476, Fax: 734-615-6337, E-mail: rdenver@umich.edu. *Application contact:* Mary Carr, Graduate Coordinator, 734-615-1635, Fax: 734-764-0884, E-mail: carrmm@umich.edu.
Website: http://www.mcdb.lsa.umich.edu

University of Michigan, Rackham Graduate School, Program in Biomedical Sciences (PIBS), Department of Cell and Developmental Biology, Ann Arbor, MI 48109-2200. Offers PhD. *Faculty:* 39 full-time (11 women). *Students:* 16 full-time (9 women); includes 8 minority (7 Asian, non-Hispanic/Latino; 1 Hispanic/Latino). Average age 29. 57 applicants, 18% accepted, 6 enrolled. In 2013, 10 doctorates awarded. *Degree requirements:* For doctorate, thesis/dissertation, oral defense of dissertation, preliminary exam. *Entrance requirements:* For doctorate, GRE General Test, 3 letters of recommendation, research experience. Additional exam requirements/recommendations for international students: Required—TOEFL (minimum score 84 iBT). *Application deadline:* For fall admission, 12/1 for domestic and international students. Application fee: $75 ($90 for international students). Electronic applications accepted. Tuition and fees vary according to course level, course load, degree level, program and student level. *Financial support:* In 2013–14, fellowships (averaging $28,500 per year) were awarded; scholarships/grants, health care benefits, tuition waivers (full), and unspecified assistantships also available. Financial award application deadline: 12/1. *Faculty research:* Cell signaling, stem cells, organogenesis, cell biology, developmental genetics. *Total annual research expenditures:* $4 million. *Unit head:* Dr. Deborah L. Gumucio, Professor/Interim Chair, 734-647-0172, Fax: 734-763-1166, E-mail: dgumucio@umich.edu. *Application contact:* Michelle S. Melis, Director of Student Life, 734-615-6538, Fax: 734-647-7022, E-mail: msmtegan@umich.edu.
Website: http://cdb.med.umich.edu/

University of Michigan, Rackham Graduate School, Program in Biomedical Sciences (PIBS), Interdisciplinary Program in Cellular and Molecular Biology, Ann Arbor, MI 48109. Offers PhD. *Faculty:* 169 part-time/adjunct (47 women). *Students:* 64 full-time (36 women); includes 17 minority (2 Black or African American, non-Hispanic/Latino; 1 American Indian or Alaska Native, non-Hispanic/Latino; 8 Asian, non-Hispanic/Latino; 6 Hispanic/Latino). Average age 26. In 2013, 19 doctorates awarded. *Degree requirements:* For doctorate, comprehensive exam, thesis/dissertation, preliminary exam; oral defense of dissertation. *Entrance requirements:* For doctorate, GRE General Test. *Application deadline:* For fall admission, 12/1 for domestic students. Application fee: $75 ($90 for international students). Tuition and fees vary according to course level, course load, degree level, program and student level. *Financial support:* In 2013–14, 64 students received support, including 15 fellowships with full tuition reimbursements available (averaging $28,500 per year), 41 research assistantships with full tuition reimbursements available (averaging $28,500 per year), 8 teaching assistantships with full tuition reimbursements available (averaging $28,500 per year); scholarships/grants also available. *Faculty research:* Genetics, genomics, gene regulation, models of disease, microbes. *Total annual research expenditures:* $20 million. *Unit head:* Dr. Robert S. Fuller, Director, 734-764-5428, Fax: 734-647-6232, E-mail: bfuller@umich.edu. *Application contact:* Catherine A. Mitchell, Senior Student Services Associate I, 734-764-5428, Fax: 734-647-6232, E-mail: cmbgrad@umich.edu.
Website: http://www.med.umich.edu/cmb/

University of Minnesota, Twin Cities Campus, Graduate School, Program in Molecular, Cellular, Developmental Biology and Genetics, Minneapolis, MN 55455-0213. Offers genetic counseling (MS); molecular, cellular, developmental biology and genetics (PhD). Terminal master's awarded for partial completion of doctoral program. *Degree requirements:* For master's, thesis optional; for doctorate, thesis/dissertation. *Entrance requirements:* For master's and doctorate, GRE General Test. Additional exam requirements/recommendations for international students: Required—TOEFL (minimum score 625 paper-based; 80 iBT). Electronic applications accepted. *Faculty research:* Membrane receptors and membrane transport, cell interactions, cytoskeleton and cell mobility, regulation of gene expression, plant cell and molecular biology.

University of Minnesota, Twin Cities Campus, Graduate School, Stem Cell Biology Graduate Program, Minneapolis, MN 55455-3007. Offers MS. *Degree requirements:* For master's, thesis. *Entrance requirements:* For master's, GRE, BS, BA, or foreign equivalent in biological sciences or related field; minimum undergraduate GPA of 3.2. Additional exam requirements/recommendations for international students: Required—TOEFL (minimum score 580 paper-based, with a minimum score of 4 in the TWE, or 94 Internet-based, with a minimum score of 22 on each of the reading and listening, 26 on the speaking, and 26 on the writing section. *Faculty research:* Stem cell and developmental biology; embryonic stem cells; iPS cells; muscle satellite cells; hematopoietic stem cells; neuronal stem cells; cardiovascular, kidney and limb development; regenerating systems.

University of Missouri, Graduate School, College of Arts and Science, Division of Biological Sciences, Columbia, MO 65211. Offers evolutionary biology and ecology (MA, PhD); genetic, cellular and developmental biology (MA, PhD); neurobiology and behavior (MA, PhD). *Faculty:* 40 full-time (11 women), 1 part-time/adjunct (0 women). *Students:* 70 full-time (32 women), 3 part-time (2 women); includes 12 minority (4 Black or African American, non-Hispanic/Latino; 1 American Indian or Alaska Native, non-Hispanic/Latino; 2 Asian, non-Hispanic/Latino; 3 Hispanic/Latino; 2 Two or more races, non-Hispanic/Latino), 5 international. Average age 28. 46 applicants, 28% accepted, 13 enrolled. In 2013, 7 master's, 13 doctorates awarded. Terminal master's awarded for partial completion of doctoral program. *Degree requirements:* For master's, thesis; for doctorate, comprehensive exam, thesis/dissertation. *Entrance requirements:* For master's and doctorate, GRE General Test (minimum score 1200 verbal and quantitative), minimum GPA of 3.0. Additional exam requirements/recommendations for international students: Required—TOEFL (minimum score 600 paper-based; 100 iBT). *Application deadline:* For fall admission, 12/15 priority date for domestic and international students. Applications are processed on a rolling basis. Application fee: $55 ($75 for international students). Electronic applications accepted. *Financial support:* Fellowships with full tuition reimbursements, research assistantships with full tuition reimbursements, teaching assistantships with full tuition reimbursements, institutionally sponsored loans, traineeships, health care benefits, and unspecified assistantships available. *Faculty research:* Evolutionary biology, ecology and behavior; genetic, cellular, molecular and developmental biology; neurobiology and behavior; plant sciences. *Unit head:* Dr. John C. Walker, Division Director, 573-882-3583, E-mail: walkerj@missouri.edu. *Application contact:* Nila Emerich, Application Contact, 800-553-5698, E-mail: emerichn@missouri.edu.
Website: http://biology.missouri.edu/graduate-studies/

University of Missouri–Kansas City, School of Biological Sciences, Program in Cell Biology and Biophysics, Kansas City, MO 64110-2499. Offers PhD. Offered through the School of Graduate Studies. *Faculty:* 34 full-time (9 women), 3 part-time/adjunct (all women). *Students:* 4 full-time (2 women), 9 part-time (4 women), 9 international. Average age 29. 3 applicants, 100% accepted, 3 enrolled. *Degree requirements:* For doctorate, comprehensive exam, thesis/dissertation. *Entrance requirements:* For doctorate, GRE General Test, bachelor's degree in chemistry, biology or related field; minimum GPA of 3.0. Additional exam requirements/recommendations for international students: Required—TOEFL (minimum score 550 paper-based; 80 iBT). *Application deadline:* For fall admission, 2/15 priority date for domestic and international students. Applications are processed on a rolling basis. Application fee: $45 ($50 for international students). Electronic applications accepted. *Expenses:* Tuition, state resident: full-time $6073; part-time $337.40 per credit hour. Tuition, nonresident: full-time $15,680; part-time $871.10 per credit hour. *Required fees:* $97.59 per credit hour. Full-time tuition and fees vary according to program. *Financial support:* Fellowships with full tuition reimbursements, research assistantships with full tuition reimbursements, teaching assistantships with full and partial tuition reimbursements, scholarships/grants, tuition waivers (full and partial), and unspecified assistantships available. Financial award application deadline: 3/1; financial award applicants required to submit FAFSA. *Unit head:* Dr. Marilyn Yoder, Interim Head, 816-235-5247, E-mail: sbsgradrecruit@umkc.edu. *Application contact:* Mary Flores, Information Contact, 816-235-5247, Fax: 816-235-5158, E-mail: lasterlo@umkc.edu.
Website: http://sbs.umkc.edu/

University of Missouri–St. Louis, College of Arts and Sciences, Department of Biology, St. Louis, MO 63121. Offers biotechnology (Certificate); cell and molecular biology (MS, PhD); ecology, evolution and systematics (MS, PhD); tropical biology and conservation (Certificate). Part-time programs available. *Faculty:* 33 full-time (13 women), 9 part-time/adjunct (1 woman). *Students:* 52 full-time (23 women), 58 part-time (29 women); includes 13 minority (9 Black or African American, non-Hispanic/Latino; 3 Asian, non-Hispanic/Latino; 1 Hispanic/Latino), 30 international. Average age 28. 113 applicants, 42% accepted, 22 enrolled. In 2013, 31 master's, 5 doctorates, 4 other advanced degrees awarded. *Degree requirements:* For master's, thesis or alternative; for doctorate, thesis/dissertation, 1 semester of teaching experience. *Entrance requirements:* For master's, 3 letters of recommendation; for doctorate, GRE General Test, 3 letters of recommendation. Additional exam requirements/recommendations for international students: Required—TOEFL (minimum score 79 iBT), IELTS (minimum score 6.5). *Application deadline:* For fall admission, 12/15 priority date for domestic and international students; for spring admission, 12/1 priority date for domestic and international students. Applications are processed on a rolling basis. Application fee: $50 ($40 for international students). Electronic applications accepted. *Expenses:* Tuition, state resident: full-time $7364; part-time $409.10 per credit hour. Tuition, nonresident: full-time $19,162; part-time $1008.50 per credit hour. *Financial support:* In 2013–14, 13 research assistantships with full and partial tuition reimbursements (averaging $17,000 per year), 23 teaching assistantships with full and partial tuition reimbursements (averaging $17,000 per year) were awarded; fellowships with full tuition reimbursements, career-related internships or fieldwork, and Federal Work-Study also available. Support available to part-time students. Financial award application deadline: 2/1. *Faculty research:* Molecular biology, microbial genetics, animal behavior, tropical ecology, plant systematics. *Unit head:* Dr. Teresa Thiel, Director of Graduate Studies, 314-516-6200, Fax: 314-516-6233, E-mail: thiel@umsl.edu. *Application contact:* 314-516-5458, Fax: 314-516-6996, E-mail: gradadm@umsl.edu.
Website: http://www.umsl.edu/divisions/artscience/biology/

The University of Montana, Graduate School, College of Humanities and Sciences, Division of Biological Sciences, Program in Cellular, Molecular and Microbial Biology, Missoula, MT 59812-0002. Offers cellular and developmental biology (PhD); microbial evolution and ecology (PhD); microbiology and immunology (PhD); molecular biology and biochemistry (PhD). Terminal master's awarded for partial completion of doctoral program. *Degree requirements:* For doctorate, variable foreign language requirement, thesis/dissertation. *Entrance requirements:* For doctorate, GRE General Test. *Application deadline:* For fall admission, 2/1 for domestic students. Application fee: $45. *Financial support:* In 2013–14, research assistantships with tuition reimbursements (averaging $9,400 per year), teaching assistantships with full tuition reimbursements (averaging $9,400 per year) were awarded; Federal Work-Study and tuition waivers (full and partial) also available. Financial award application deadline: 3/1; financial award applicants required to submit FAFSA. *Faculty research:* Ribosome structure, medical microbiology/pathogenesis, microbial ecology/environmental microbiology. *Unit head:* Charles Janson, Chair, 406-243-5122, E-mail: charles.janson@mso.umt.edu. *Application contact:* Information Contact, E-mail: gradschl@mso.umt.edu.
Website: http://www.biology.umt.edu/

University of Nebraska Medical Center, Department of Genetics, Cell Biology and Anatomy, Omaha, NE 68198-5805. Offers MS, PhD. Part-time programs available. Terminal master's awarded for partial completion of doctoral program. *Degree requirements:* For master's, comprehensive exam, thesis; for doctorate, comprehensive exam, thesis/dissertation. *Entrance requirements:* For master's and doctorate, GRE General Test. Additional exam requirements/recommendations for international students: Required—TOEFL (minimum score 550 paper-based). Electronic applications accepted. *Expenses: Required fees:* $300 per semester. Tuition and fees vary according to program. *Faculty research:* Hematology, immunology, developmental biology, genetics cancer biology, neuroscience.

University of Nevada, Reno, Graduate School, Interdisciplinary Program in Cell and Molecular Biology, Reno, NV 89557. Offers MS, PhD. Terminal master's awarded for partial completion of doctoral program. *Degree requirements:* For master's, thesis; for doctorate, thesis/dissertation. *Entrance requirements:* For master's, GRE Subject Test (recommended), minimum GPA of 2.75; for doctorate, GRE Subject Test (recommended), minimum GPA of 3.0. Additional exam requirements/recommendations for international students: Required—TOEFL (minimum score 500 paper-based; 61 iBT), IELTS (minimum score 6). Electronic applications accepted. *Faculty research:* Cellular biology, biophysics, cancer, microbiology, insect biochemistry.

University of New Haven, Graduate School, College of Arts and Sciences, Program in Cellular and Molecular Biology, West Haven, CT 06516-1916. Offers MS, Graduate Certificate. Part-time and evening/weekend programs available. *Students:* 30 full-time (23 women), 9 part-time (6 women); includes 8 minority (5 Black or African American, non-Hispanic/Latino; 1 Asian, non-Hispanic/Latino; 1 Hispanic/Latino; 1 Two or more races, non-Hispanic/Latino), 16 international. 72 applicants, 68% accepted, 24 enrolled. In 2013, 19 master's, 1 other advanced degree awarded. *Degree requirements:* For master's, thesis or alternative. *Entrance requirements:* Additional exam requirements/recommendations for international students: Required—TOEFL (minimum score 80 iBT), IELTS, PTE (minimum score 53). *Application deadline:* For fall admission, 5/31 for international students; for winter admission, 10/15 for international students; for spring admission, 1/15 for international students. Applications are processed on a rolling basis. Application fee: $75. Electronic applications accepted. Application fee is waived when completed online. *Expenses: Tuition:* Full-time $21,600; part-time $800 per credit hour. *Required fees:* $45 per trimester. *Financial support:* Research assistantships with partial tuition reimbursements, teaching assistantships with partial tuition reimbursements, career-related internships or fieldwork, Federal Work-Study, scholarships/grants, and unspecified assistantships available. Support available to part-time students. Financial award application deadline: 5/1; financial award applicants required to submit FAFSA. *Unit head:* Dr. Roman Zajac, Chair, 203-932-7114, E-mail: rzajac@newhaven.edu. *Application contact:* Eloise Gormley, Director of Graduate Admissions, 203-932-7440, E-mail: gradinfo@newhaven.edu.
Website: http://www.newhaven.edu/4724/

University of New Mexico, School of Medicine, Program in Biomedical Sciences, Albuquerque, NM 87131-5196. Offers biochemistry and molecular biology (MS, PhD); cell biology and physiology (MS, PhD); clinical and translational science (Certificate); molecular genetics and microbiology (MS, PhD); neuroscience (MS, PhD); pathology (MS, PhD); toxicology (MS, PhD); university science teaching (Certificate). Part-time programs available. *Students:* 73 full-time (39 women), 14 part-time (9 women); includes 24 minority (1 Black or African American, non-Hispanic/Latino; 1 American Indian or Alaska Native, non-Hispanic/Latino; 2 Asian, non-Hispanic/Latino; 17 Hispanic/Latino; 1 Native Hawaiian or other Pacific Islander, non-Hispanic/Latino; 2 Two or more races, non-Hispanic/Latino), 16 international. Average age 29. 89 applicants, 20% accepted, 17 enrolled. In 2013, 7 master's, 17 doctorates awarded. Terminal master's awarded for partial completion of doctoral program. *Degree requirements:* For master's, thesis; for doctorate, comprehensive exam, thesis/dissertation, qualifying exam at the end of year 1/core curriculum. *Entrance requirements:* For master's and doctorate, GRE General Test, minimum undergraduate GPA of 3.0. Additional exam requirements/recommendations for international students: Required—TOEFL. *Application deadline:* For fall admission, 3/1 priority date for domestic and international students. Applications are processed on a rolling basis. Application fee: $50. Electronic applications accepted. *Financial support:* In 2013–14, 94 students received support, including 28 fellowships with full and partial tuition reimbursements available (averaging $22,000 per year), 73 research assistantships with full tuition reimbursements available (averaging $23,000 per year), 8 teaching assistantships (averaging $2,800 per year); career-related internships or fieldwork, Federal Work-Study, institutionally sponsored loans, scholarships/grants, traineeships, health care benefits, and unspecified assistantships also available. Financial award application deadline: 1/1; financial award applicants required to submit FAFSA. *Faculty research:* Infectious disease/immunity, cancer biology, cardiovascular and metabolic diseases, brain and behavioral illness, environmental health. *Unit head:* Dr. Helen J. Hathaway, Program Director, 505-272-1887, Fax: 505-272-2412, E-mail: hhathaway@salud.unm.edu. *Application contact:* Mary Fenton, Admissions Coordinator, 505-272-1887, Fax: 505-272-2412, E-mail: mfenton@salud.unm.edu.
Website: http://hsc.unm.edu/research/brep/bsgpabout.shtm

The University of North Carolina at Chapel Hill, Graduate School, College of Arts and Sciences, Department of Biology, Chapel Hill, NC 27599. Offers botany (MA, MS, PhD); cell biology, development, and physiology (MA, MS, PhD); cell motility and cytoskeleton (PhD); ecology and behavior (MA, MS, PhD); genetics and molecular biology (MA, MS, PhD); morphology, systematics, and evolution (MA, MS, PhD). Terminal master's awarded for partial completion of doctoral program. *Degree requirements:* For master's, comprehensive exam, thesis (for some programs); for doctorate, comprehensive exam, thesis/dissertation. *Entrance requirements:* For master's, GRE General Test, GRE Subject Test, 2 semesters of calculus or statistics; 2 semesters of physics, organic chemistry; 3 semesters of biology; for doctorate, GRE General Test, GRE Subject Test, 2 semesters calculus or statistics, 2 semesters physics, organic chemistry, 3 semesters of biology. Additional exam requirements/recommendations for international students: Required—TOEFL (minimum score 550 paper-based). Electronic applications accepted. *Faculty research:* Gene expression, biomechanics, yeast genetics, plant ecology, plant molecular biology.

The University of North Carolina at Chapel Hill, School of Medicine and Graduate School, Graduate Programs in Medicine, Department of Cell and Developmental Biology, Chapel Hill, NC 27599. Offers PhD. *Degree requirements:* For doctorate, comprehensive exam, thesis/dissertation. *Entrance requirements:* For doctorate, GRE General Test, GRE Subject Test. Electronic applications accepted. *Faculty research:* Cell adhesion, motility and cytoskeleton; molecular analysis of signal transduction; development biology and toxicology; reproductive biology; cell and molecular imaging.

University of North Dakota, Graduate School and Graduate School, Graduate Programs in Medicine, Department of Anatomy and Cell Biology, Grand Forks, ND 58202. Offers MS, PhD. *Degree requirements:* For master's, thesis, final exam; for doctorate, comprehensive exam, thesis/dissertation, final exam. *Entrance requirements:* For master's and doctorate, GRE General Test, minimum GPA of 3.0. Additional exam requirements/recommendations for international students: Required—TOEFL (minimum score 550 paper-based; 79 iBT), IELTS (minimum score 6.5). Electronic applications accepted. *Faculty research:* Coronary vessel, vasculogenesis, acellular glomerular and retinal microvessel membranes, ependymal cells, cardiac muscle.

University of Notre Dame, Graduate School, College of Science, Department of Biological Sciences, Notre Dame, IN 46556. Offers aquatic ecology, evolution and environmental biology (MS, PhD); cellular and molecular biology (MS, PhD); genetics (MS, PhD); physiology (MS, PhD); vector biology and parasitology (MS, PhD). Terminal master's awarded for partial completion of doctoral program. *Degree requirements:* For master's, comprehensive exam, thesis; for doctorate, comprehensive exam, thesis/dissertation, candidacy exam. *Entrance requirements:* For master's and doctorate, GRE General Test. Additional exam requirements/recommendations for international students: Required—TOEFL (minimum score 600 paper-based; 80 iBT). Electronic applications accepted. *Faculty research:* Tropical disease, molecular genetics, neurobiology, evolutionary biology, aquatic biology.

University of Oklahoma Health Sciences Center, College of Medicine and Graduate College, Graduate Programs in Medicine, Department of Cell Biology, Oklahoma City, OK 73190. Offers MS, PhD. *Faculty:* 8 full-time (4 women). *Students:* 24 part-time (14 women); includes 4 minority (2 Asian, non-Hispanic/Latino; 1 Hispanic/Latino; 1 Native Hawaiian or other Pacific Islander, non-Hispanic/Latino), 6 international. Average age 29. 5 applicants. In 2013, 1 master's, 8 doctorates awarded. *Degree requirements:* For master's, thesis; for doctorate, thesis/dissertation. *Entrance requirements:* For doctorate, GRE General Test, GRE Subject Test, 3 letters of recommendation. Additional exam requirements/recommendations for international students: Required—TOEFL. *Application deadline:* For fall admission, 1/31 for domestic students. Application fee: $50. *Expenses:* Tuition, state resident: full-time $3504; part-time $175.20 per credit hour. Tuition, nonresident: full-time $13,504; part-time $675.20 per credit hour. *Required fees:* $1545; $52.70 per credit hour. $245.25 per semester. Tuition and fees vary according to course load. *Financial support:* In 2013–14, 5 research assistantships (averaging $18,000 per year) were awarded; teaching assistantships, career-related internships or fieldwork, and institutionally sponsored loans also available. Support available to part-time students. Financial award application deadline: 7/1. *Faculty research:* Neurobiology, reproductive, neuronal plasticity, extracellular matrix, neuroendocrinology. *Unit head:* Dr. Lawrence Rothblum, Chair, 405-271-2377, E-mail: larence-rothblum@ouhsc.edu. *Application contact:* Dr. Leo Tsiokias, Graduate Liaison, 405-271-8001, E-mail: leo-tsiokas@ouhsc.edu.

University of Ottawa, Faculty of Graduate and Postdoctoral Studies, Faculty of Medicine, Department of Cellular and Molecular Medicine, Ottawa, ON K1H 8M5, Canada. Offers M Sc, PhD. *Degree requirements:* For master's, thesis, seminar; for doctorate, comprehensive exam, thesis/dissertation, seminar. *Entrance requirements:* For master's, honors degree or equivalent, minimum B average; for doctorate, master's degree, minimum B+ average. Electronic applications accepted. *Faculty research:* Physiology, pharmacology, growth and development.

University of Pennsylvania, Perelman School of Medicine, Biomedical Graduate Studies, Graduate Group in Cell and Molecular Biology, Philadelphia, PA 19104. Offers cancer biology (PhD); cell biology and physiology (PhD); developmental stem cell regenerative biology (PhD); gene therapy and vaccines (PhD); genetics and gene regulation (PhD); microbiology, virology, and parasitology (PhD); MD/PhD; VMD/PhD. *Faculty:* 321. *Students:* 352 full-time (205 women); includes 99 minority (11 Black or African American, non-Hispanic/Latino; 65 Asian, non-Hispanic/Latino; 21 Hispanic/Latino; 2 Two or more races, non-Hispanic/Latino), 45 international. 488 applicants, 20% accepted, 40 enrolled. In 2013, 41 doctorates awarded. *Degree requirements:* For doctorate, thesis/dissertation. *Entrance requirements:* For doctorate, GRE General Test. Additional exam requirements/recommendations for international students: Required—TOEFL. *Application deadline:* For fall admission, 12/1 priority date for domestic and international students. Applications are processed on a rolling basis. Application fee: $80. Electronic applications accepted. *Financial support:* In 2013–14, 352 students received support. Fellowships, research assistantships, scholarships/grants, traineeships, and unspecified assistantships available. *Unit head:* Dr. Daniel Kessler, Graduate Group Chair, 215-898-1478. *Application contact:* Meagan Schofer, Coordinator, 215-898-4360.
Website: http://www.med.upenn.edu/camb/

University of Pittsburgh, Dietrich School of Arts and Sciences, Department of Biological Sciences, Program in Molecular, Cellular, and Developmental Biology, Pittsburgh, PA 15260. Offers PhD. *Faculty:* 19 full-time (4 women). *Students:* 45 full-time (24 women); includes 5 minority (1 Black or African American, non-Hispanic/Latino; 3 Asian, non-Hispanic/Latino; 1 Hispanic/Latino), 14 international. Average age 23. 180 applicants, 9% accepted, 8 enrolled. In 2013, 6 doctorates awarded. *Degree requirements:* For doctorate, comprehensive exam, thesis/dissertation, completion of research integrity module. *Entrance requirements:* For doctorate, GRE General Test, GRE Subject Test. Additional exam requirements/recommendations for international students: Required—TOEFL (minimum score 90 iBT). *Application deadline:* For fall admission, 1/3 priority date for domestic students, 12/9 priority date for international students. Applications are processed on a rolling basis. Application fee: $0 ($50 for international students). Electronic applications accepted. *Expenses:* Tuition, state resident: full-time $19,964; part-time $807 per credit. Tuition, nonresident: full-time $32,686; part-time $1337 per credit. *Required fees:* $740; $200. Tuition and fees vary according to program. *Financial support:* In 2013–14, 26 fellowships with full tuition reimbursements (averaging $30,682 per year), 79 research assistantships with full tuition reimbursements (averaging $26,544 per year), 18 teaching assistantships with full tuition reimbursements (averaging $25,716 per year) were awarded; Federal Work-Study, scholarships/grants, traineeships, health care benefits, and tuition waivers (full) also available. *Unit head:* Dr. Jeffrey G. Lawrence, Professor, 412-624-4204, Fax: 412-624-4759, E-mail: jlawrenc@pitt.edu. *Application contact:* Cathleen M. Barr, Graduate Administrator, 412-624-4268, Fax: 412-624-4759, E-mail: cbarr@pitt.edu.
Website: http://www.biology.pitt.edu/graduate/mcdb-program

University of Pittsburgh, School of Medicine, Graduate Programs in Medicine, Cell Biology and Molecular Physiology Graduate Program, Pittsburgh, PA 15260. Offers PhD. *Faculty:* 45 full-time (10 women). *Students:* 3 full-time (2 women). Average age 30. 517 applicants, 13% accepted, 22 enrolled. In 2013, 3 doctorates awarded. *Degree requirements:* For doctorate, comprehensive exam, thesis/dissertation. *Entrance requirements:* For doctorate, GRE General Test, GRE Subject Test, minimum QPA of 3.0. Additional exam requirements/recommendations for international students: Required—TOEFL (minimum score 600 paper-based; 100 iBT), IELTS (minimum score 7). *Application deadline:* For fall admission, 1/1 priority date for domestic and international students. Application fee: $50. Electronic applications accepted. *Expenses:* Tuition, state resident: full-time $19,964; part-time $807 per credit. Tuition, nonresident: full-time $32,686; part-time $1337 per credit. *Required fees:* $740; $200. Tuition and fees vary according to program. *Financial support:* In 2013–14, 1 research assistantship with full tuition reimbursement (averaging $26,010 per year), 2 teaching assistantships with full tuition reimbursements (averaging $26,010 per year) were awarded; institutionally sponsored loans, scholarships/grants, traineeships, health care benefits, and unspecified assistantships also available. *Faculty research:* Genetic disorders of ion channels, regulation of gene expression/development, membrane traffic of proteins and lipids, reproductive biology, signal transduction in diabetes and metabolism. *Unit head:* Dr. Donna B. Stolz, Graduate Program Director, 412-383-7283, Fax: 412-648-2927, E-mail: dstolz@pitt.edu. *Application contact:* Graduate Studies Administrator, 412-648-8957, Fax: 412-648-1077, E-mail: gradstudies@medschool.pitt.edu.
Website: http://www.gradbiomed.pitt.edu

University of Puerto Rico, Río Piedras Campus, College of Natural Sciences, Department of Biology, San Juan, PR 00931-3300. Offers ecology/systematics (MS, PhD); evolution/genetics (MS, PhD); molecular/cellular biology (MS, PhD); neuroscience (MS, PhD). Part-time programs available. *Degree requirements:* For master's, one foreign language, comprehensive exam, thesis; for doctorate, one foreign language, comprehensive exam, thesis/dissertation. *Entrance requirements:* For master's, GRE Subject Test, interview, minimum GPA of 3.0, letter of recommendation; for doctorate, GRE Subject Test, interview, master's degree, minimum GPA of 3.0, letter of recommendation. *Faculty research:* Environmental, poblational and systematic biology.

University of Rhode Island, Graduate School, College of the Environment and Life Sciences, Department of Cell and Molecular Biology, Kingston, RI 02881. Offers biochemistry (MS, PhD); clinical laboratory sciences (MS), including biotechnology, clinical laboratory science, cytopathology; microbiology (MS, PhD); molecular genetics (MS, PhD). Part-time programs available. *Faculty:* 17 full-time (8 women), 2 part-time/adjunct (1 woman). *Students:* 19 full-time (11 women), 40 part-time (23 women); includes 14 minority (4 Black or African American, non-Hispanic/Latino; 1 American Indian or Alaska Native, non-Hispanic/Latino; 7 Asian, non-Hispanic/Latino; 2 Hispanic/Latino), 5 international. In 2013, 20 master's, 2 doctorates awarded. *Degree requirements:* For master's, comprehensive exam (for some programs), thesis optional; for doctorate, comprehensive exam, thesis/dissertation. *Entrance requirements:* For master's and doctorate, GRE, 2 letters of recommendation. Additional exam requirements/recommendations for international students: Required—TOEFL (minimum score 550 paper-based). *Application deadline:* For fall admission, 7/15 for domestic students, 2/1 for international students; for spring admission, 11/15 for domestic students, 7/15 for international students. Application fee: $65. Electronic applications accepted. *Expenses:* Tuition, state resident: full-time $11,532; part-time $641 per credit. Tuition, nonresident: full-time $23,606; part-time $1311 per credit. *Required fees:* $1388; $36 per credit. $35 per semester. One-time fee: $130. *Financial support:* In 2013–14, 5 research assistantships with full and partial tuition reimbursements (averaging $12,078 per year), 2 teaching assistantships with full and partial tuition reimbursements (averaging $11,883 per year) were awarded. Financial award application deadline: 2/1; financial award applicants required to submit FAFSA. *Faculty research:* Genomics. *Total annual research expenditures:* $6.7 million. *Unit head:* Dr. Gongqing Sun, Chairperson, 401-874-5937, Fax: 401-874-2202, E-mail: gsun@mail.uri.edu. *Application contact:* Graduate Admissions, 401-874-2872, E-mail: gradadm@etal.uri.edu.
Website: http://cels.uri.edu/cmb/

University of Saskatchewan, College of Medicine, Department of Anatomy and Cell Biology, Saskatoon, SK S7N 5A2, Canada. Offers M Sc, PhD. *Degree requirements:* For master's, thesis; for doctorate, thesis/dissertation. *Entrance requirements:* Additional exam requirements/recommendations for international students: Required—TOEFL. *Expenses: Tuition, area resident:* Full-time $3585 Canadian dollars; part-time $585 Canadian dollars per course. Tuition, nonresident: part-time $877 Canadian dollars per course. *International tuition:* $5377 Canadian dollars full-time. *Required fees:* $889.51 Canadian dollars.

University of South Carolina, The Graduate School, College of Arts and Sciences, Department of Biological Sciences, Graduate Training Program in Molecular, Cellular, and Developmental Biology, Columbia, SC 29208. Offers MS, PhD. *Degree requirements:* For master's, one foreign language, thesis; for doctorate, one foreign language, thesis/dissertation. *Entrance requirements:* For master's and doctorate, GRE General Test, minimum GPA of 3.0 in science. Electronic applications accepted. *Faculty research:* Marine ecology, population and evolutionary biology, molecular biology and genetics, development.

The University of South Dakota, Graduate School, School of Medicine and Graduate School, Biomedical Sciences Graduate Program, Cellular and Molecular Biology Group, Vermillion, SD 57069-2390. Offers MS, PhD. Terminal master's awarded for partial completion of doctoral program. *Degree requirements:* For master's, thesis; for doctorate, comprehensive exam, thesis/dissertation. *Entrance requirements:* For master's and doctorate, GRE General Test, GRE Subject Test, minimum GPA of 3.0. Additional exam requirements/recommendations for international students: Required—TOEFL (minimum score 550 paper-based; 80 iBT), IELTS (minimum score 6). Electronic applications accepted. *Expenses:* Contact institution. *Faculty research:* Molecular aspects of protein and DNA, neurochemistry and energy transduction, gene regulation, cellular development.

University of South Florida, College of Arts and Sciences, Department of Cell Biology, Microbiology, and Molecular Biology, Tampa, FL 33620-9951. Offers biology (MS), including cell and molecular biology; cancer biology (PhD); cell and molecular biology (PhD); microbiology (MS). *Faculty:* 19 full-time (5 women), 1 part-time/adjunct (0 women). *Students:* 77 full-time (46 women), 3 part-time (1 woman); includes 8 minority (5 Asian, non-Hispanic/Latino; 3 Hispanic/Latino), 19 international. Average age 27. 155 applicants, 17% accepted, 17 enrolled. In 2013, 19 master's, 12 doctorates awarded. *Degree requirements:* For master's, thesis or alternative; for doctorate, comprehensive exam, thesis/dissertation. *Entrance requirements:* For master's and doctorate, GRE General Test, minimum GPA of 3.0, extensive background in biology or chemistry. Additional exam requirements/recommendations for international students: Required—TOEFL (minimum score 550 paper-based; 79 iBT) or IELTS (minimum score 6.5). *Application deadline:* For fall admission, 2/1 for domestic students, 1/1 for international students. Application fee: $30. *Financial support:* Career-related internships or fieldwork, health care benefits, and unspecified assistantships available. Financial award application deadline: 4/1. *Faculty research:* Cell biology, microbiology and molecular biology: basic and applied science in bacterial pathogenesis, genome integrity and mechanisms of aging, structural and computational biology; cancer biology: immunology, cancer control, signal transduction, drug discovery, genomics. *Total annual research expenditures:* $1.9 million. *Unit head:* Dr. James Garey, Professor/Chair, 813-974-7103, Fax: 813-974-1614, E-mail: garey@usf.edu. *Application contact:* Dr. Kenneth Wright, Associate Professor of Cancer Biology, H. Lee Moffitt Cancer Center and Research Institute, 813-745-3918, Fax: 813-974-1614, E-mail: ken.wright@moffitt.org.
Website: http://biology.usf.edu/cmmb/

The University of Texas at Austin, Graduate School, Institute for Cellular and Molecular Biology, Austin, TX 78712-1111. Offers PhD.

The University of Texas at Dallas, School of Natural Sciences and Mathematics, Department of Biology, Richardson, TX 75080. Offers bioinformatics and computational biology (MS); biotechnology (MS); molecular and cell biology (MS, PhD). Part-time and evening/weekend programs available. *Faculty:* 20 full-time (3 women), 1 (woman) part-time/adjunct. *Students:* 99 full-time (63 women), 15 part-time (7 women); includes 10 minority (1 Black or African American, non-Hispanic/Latino; 6 Asian, non-Hispanic/Latino; 3 Hispanic/Latino), 77 international. Average age 27. 381 applicants, 23% accepted, 48 enrolled. In 2013, 49 master's, 3 doctorates awarded. *Degree requirements:* For master's, thesis optional; for doctorate, thesis/dissertation, publishable paper. *Entrance requirements:* For master's and doctorate, GRE (minimum combined score of 1000 on verbal and quantitative). Additional exam requirements/recommendations for international students: Required—TOEFL (minimum score 550 paper-based; 80 iBT). *Application deadline:* For fall admission, 7/15 for domestic students, 5/1 priority date for international students; for spring admission, 11/15 for domestic students, 9/1 priority date for international students. Applications are processed on a rolling basis. Application fee: $50 ($100 for international students). Electronic applications accepted. *Expenses:* Tuition, state resident: full-time $11,940; part-time $663.33 per credit hour. Tuition, nonresident: full-time $21,606; part-time $1200.33 per credit hour. *Financial support:* In 2013–14, 57 students received support, including 12 research assistantships with partial tuition reimbursements available (averaging $20,867 per year), 44 teaching assistantships with partial tuition reimbursements available (averaging $15,300 per year); career-related internships or fieldwork, Federal Work-Study, institutionally sponsored loans, scholarships/grants, and unspecified assistantships also available. Support available to part-time students. Financial award application deadline: 4/30; financial award applicants required to submit FAFSA. *Faculty research:* Role of mitochondria in neurodegenerative diseases, protein-DNA interactions in site-specific recombination, eukaryotic gene expression, bio-nanotechnology, sickle cell research. *Unit head:* Dr. Stephen Spiro, Department Head, 972-883-6032, Fax: 972-883-2502, E-mail: stephen.spiro@utdallas.edu. *Application contact:* Dr. Lawrence Reitzer, Graduate Advisor, 972-883-2502, Fax: 972-883-2402, E-mail: reitzer@utdallas.edu.
Website: http://www.utdallas.edu/biology/

The University of Texas at San Antonio, College of Sciences, Department of Biology, San Antonio, TX 78249-0617. Offers biology (MS); biotechnology (MS); cell and molecular biology (PhD); neurobiology (PhD). *Faculty:* 46 full-time (9 women), 15 part-time/adjunct (10 women). *Students:* 116 full-time (56 women), 62 part-time (34 women); includes 70 minority (7 Black or African American, non-Hispanic/Latino; 1 American Indian or Alaska Native, non-Hispanic/Latino; 10 Asian, non-Hispanic/Latino; 49 Hispanic/Latino; 2 Native Hawaiian or other Pacific Islander, non-Hispanic/Latino; 1 Two or more races, non-Hispanic/Latino), 34 international. Average age 29. 176 applicants, 53% accepted, 43 enrolled. In 2013, 47 master's, 6 doctorates awarded. Terminal master's awarded for partial completion of doctoral program. *Degree requirements:* For master's, comprehensive exam, thesis or alternative; for doctorate, comprehensive exam, thesis/dissertation. *Entrance requirements:* For master's, GRE General Test, bachelor's degree with 18 credit hours in field of study or in another appropriate field of study; for doctorate, GRE General Test, 3 letters of recommendation, statement of purpose, resume. Additional exam requirements/recommendations for international students: Required—TOEFL (minimum score 500 paper-based; 100 iBT), IELTS (minimum score 5). *Application deadline:* For fall admission, 7/1 for domestic students, 4/1 for international students; for spring admission, 11/1 for domestic students, 9/1 for international students. Application fee: $45 ($80 for international students). Electronic applications accepted. *Expenses:* Tuition, state resident: full-time $4671. Tuition, nonresident: full-time $8708. *International tuition:* $17,415 full-time. *Required fees:* $1924.60. Tuition and fees vary according to course load and degree level. *Financial support:* In 2013–14, 42 students received support, including 14 fellowships (averaging $26,142 per year), 19 research assistantships (averaging $24,350 per year), 9 teaching assistantships (averaging $24,350 per year). *Faculty research:* Development of human and veterinary vaccines against a fungal disease, mammalian germ cells and stem cells, dopamine neuron physiology and addiction, plant biochemistry, dendritic computation and synaptic plasticity. *Total annual research expenditures:* $2.1 million. *Unit head:* Dr. Edwin J. Barea-Rodriguez, Chair, 210-458-4511, Fax: 210-458-5658, E-mail: edwin.barea@utsa.edu. *Application contact:* Rene Munguia, Jr., Senior Program Coordinator, 210-458-4642, Fax: 210-458-5658, E-mail: rene.munguia@utsa.edu.
Website: http://bio.utsa.edu/

The University of Texas Health Science Center at Houston, Graduate School of Biomedical Sciences, Program in Cell and Regulatory Biology, Houston, TX 77225-0036. Offers MS, PhD, MD/PhD. Terminal master's awarded for partial completion of doctoral program. *Degree requirements:* For master's, thesis; for doctorate, thesis/dissertation. *Entrance requirements:* For master's and doctorate, GRE General Test. Additional exam requirements/recommendations for international students: Required—TOEFL. Electronic applications accepted. *Expenses:* Tuition, state resident: full-time $3474; part-time $193 per credit hour. Tuition, nonresident: full-time $13,644; part-time $758 per credit hour. *Required fees:* $226.30; $87 per credit hour. *Faculty research:* Pharmacology, cell biology, physiology, signal transduction, systems biology.

The University of Texas Health Science Center at San Antonio, Graduate School of Biomedical Sciences, Department of Cellular and Structural Biology, San Antonio, TX 78229-3900. Offers MS, PhD. *Faculty:* 51 full-time (24 women), 11 part-time/adjunct (5 women). *Students:* 56 full-time (39 women), 10 part-time (7 women); includes 24 minority (3 Black or African American, non-Hispanic/Latino; 12 Asian, non-Hispanic/Latino; 9 Hispanic/Latino), 20 international. Average age 28. In 2013, 4 master's, 10 doctorates awarded. *Degree requirements:* For master's, thesis; for doctorate, comprehensive exam, thesis/dissertation. *Entrance requirements:* For master's, GRE (minimum cumulative Verbal plus Quantitative score of 1000), minimum undergraduate GPA of 3.0; for doctorate, GRE General Test, previous course work in biology, chemistry, physics, and calculus. Additional exam requirements/recommendations for international students: Required—TOEFL (minimum score 550 paper-based; 68 iBT). *Application deadline:* For fall admission, 3/1 priority date for domestic and international students. Applications are processed on a rolling basis. Application fee: $0. Electronic applications accepted. *Financial support:* In 2013–14, 7 students received support. Federal Work-Study and scholarships/grants available. Financial award application deadline: 6/30; financial award applicants required to submit FAFSA. *Faculty research:* Human/molecular genetics, endocrinology and neurobiology, cell biology, stem cell biology, cancer biology, biology of aging. *Total annual research expenditures:* $7.5 million. *Unit head:* Dr. Christi A. Walter, Department Chair, 210-567-3800, Fax: 210-567-0073, E-mail: walter@uthscsa.edu. *Application contact:* Dr. Babatunde Oyajobi, Committee on Graduate Studies Chair, 210-567-0909, Fax: 210-567-0073, E-mail: oyajobi@uthscsa.edu.
Website: http://www.uthscsa.edu/csb/

The University of Texas Medical Branch, Graduate School of Biomedical Sciences, Program in Biochemistry and Molecular Biology, Galveston, TX 77555. Offers biochemistry (PhD); bioinformatics (PhD); biophysics (PhD); cell biology (PhD); computational biology (PhD); structural biology (PhD). *Degree requirements:* For doctorate, thesis/dissertation. *Entrance requirements:* Additional exam requirements/recommendations for international students: Required—TOEFL (minimum score 550 paper-based). Electronic applications accepted.

The University of Texas Southwestern Medical Center, Southwestern Graduate School of Biomedical Sciences, Division of Basic Science, Program in Cell Regulation, Dallas, TX 75390. Offers PhD. *Faculty:* 47 full-time (12 women), 2 part-time/adjunct (0 women). *Students:* 29 full-time (17 women), 2 part-time (0 women); includes 5 minority (2 Black or African American, non-Hispanic/Latino; 1 Asian, non-Hispanic/Latino; 1 Hispanic/Latino; 1 Two or more races, non-Hispanic/Latino), 11 international. Average age 26. In 2013, 14 doctorates awarded. *Degree requirements:* For doctorate, thesis/dissertation, qualifying exam. *Entrance requirements:* For doctorate, GRE General Test, minimum GPA of 3.0. Additional exam requirements/recommendations for international students: Required—TOEFL. *Application deadline:* For fall admission, 12/15 priority date for domestic students. Applications are processed on a rolling basis. Application fee: $0. Electronic applications accepted. *Financial support:* Fellowships, research assistantships, institutionally sponsored loans, and traineeships available. *Faculty research:* Molecular and cellular approaches to regulatory biology, receptor-effector coupling, membrane structure, function, and assembly. *Unit head:* Dr. Paul Sternweis,

Chair, 214-645-6149, Fax: 214-645-6131, E-mail: paul.sternweis@utsouthwestern.edu. *Application contact:* 214-648-5617, Fax: 214-648-3289, E-mail: admissions@utsouthwestern.edu.
Website: http://www.utsouthwestern.edu/education/graduate-school/programs/phd-degrees/cell-regulation/index.html

University of the Sciences, College of Graduate Studies, Misher College of Arts and Sciences, Program in Cell and Molecular Biology, Philadelphia, PA 19104-4495. Offers PhD. *Students:* 18. In 2013, 1 doctorate awarded. *Entrance requirements:* Additional exam requirements/recommendations for international students: Required—TOEFL, TWE. *Expenses: Tuition:* Part-time $1447 per credit. Tuition and fees vary according to campus/location and program. *Unit head:* Dr. Shenaz Tejani-Butt, Associate Dean, Professional Studies, 215-596-8886, Fax: 215-895-1185, E-mail: graduate@usciences.edu. *Application contact:* Christopher Miciek, Associate Director, Graduate Admissions, 215-596-8597, E-mail: c.miciek@usciences.edu.

University of the Sciences, College of Graduate Studies, Program in Cell Biology and Biotechnology, Philadelphia, PA 19104-4495. Offers cell and molecular biology (PhD); cell biology (MS). Part-time and evening/weekend programs available. *Faculty:* 8 full-time (1 woman), 3 part-time/adjunct (all women). *Students:* 4 full-time (3 women), 10 part-time (8 women); includes 2 minority (both Asian, non-Hispanic/Latino), 2 international. Average age 28. In 2013, 5 master's awarded. *Degree requirements:* For master's, thesis (for some programs). *Entrance requirements:* For master's, GRE General Test. Additional exam requirements/recommendations for international students: Required—TOEFL, TWE. *Application deadline:* For fall admission, 5/1 for international students; for winter admission, 10/1 for international students; for spring admission, 3/1 for international students. Applications are processed on a rolling basis. Application fee: $50. *Expenses:* Contact institution. *Financial support:* In 2013–14, 7 students received support, including 5 teaching assistantships with full tuition reimbursements available (averaging $17,638 per year); scholarships/grants and tuition waivers (partial) also available. Financial award application deadline: 5/1. *Faculty research:* Invertebrate cell adhesion, plant-microbe interactions, natural product mechanisms, cell signal transduction, gene regulation and organization. *Unit head:* Dr. Shenaz Tejani-Butt, Associate Dean, Graduate Studies, E-mail: graduate@usciences.edu. *Application contact:* Christopher Miciek, Associate Director, Graduate Admissions, 215-596-8597, E-mail: c.miciek@usciences.edu.

University of Toronto, School of Graduate Studies, Faculty of Arts and Science, Department of Cell and Systems Biology, Toronto, ON M5S 1A1, Canada. Offers M Sc, PhD. *Degree requirements:* For master's, thesis, thesis defense; for doctorate, thesis/dissertation, thesis defense, oral thesis examination. *Entrance requirements:* For master's, minimum B+ average in final year, B overall, 3 letters of reference. Additional exam requirements/recommendations for international students: Required—TOEFL (minimum score 580 paper-based; 93 iBT), TWE (minimum score 5). Electronic applications accepted.

University of Vermont, Graduate College, Cellular, Molecular and Biomedical Sciences Program, Burlington, VT 05405. Offers MS, PhD. *Students:* 39 (13 women); includes 6 minority (1 Black or African American, non-Hispanic/Latino; 4 Asian, non-Hispanic/Latino; 1 Hispanic/Latino), 11 international. 106 applicants, 22% accepted, 5 enrolled. In 2013, 3 master's, 10 doctorates awarded. *Degree requirements:* For master's, thesis; for doctorate, thesis/dissertation. *Entrance requirements:* For master's and doctorate, GRE General Test. Additional exam requirements/recommendations for international students: Required—TOEFL (minimum score 550 paper-based; 80 iBT). *Application deadline:* For fall admission, 12/1 priority date for domestic students, 12/1 for international students. Application fee: $65. Electronic applications accepted. *Financial support:* Fellowships, research assistantships, teaching assistantships, and career-related internships or fieldwork available. Financial award application deadline: 3/1. *Unit head:* Prof. Nick Heintz, Coordinator, 802-656-9673.

University of Virginia, School of Medicine, Department of Cell Biology, Charlottesville, VA 22903. Offers PhD, MD/PhD. *Faculty:* 22 full-time (8 women), 3 part-time/adjunct (1 woman). *Students:* 13 full-time (9 women); includes 2 minority (both Black or African American, non-Hispanic/Latino), 6 international. Average age 27. In 2013, 9 doctorates awarded. *Degree requirements:* For doctorate, one foreign language, thesis/dissertation. *Entrance requirements:* For doctorate, GRE General Test, GRE Subject Test (recommended), 2 letters of recommendation. Additional exam requirements/recommendations for international students: Required—TOEFL. *Application deadline:* For fall admission, 4/15 for domestic and international students. Applications are processed on a rolling basis. Application fee: $60. Electronic applications accepted. *Expenses:* Tuition, state resident: part-time $334 per credit hour. Tuition, nonresident: part-time $1224 per credit hour. *Financial support:* Application deadline: 1/15; applicants required to submit FAFSA. *Unit head:* Dr. Barry M. Gumbiner, Chairman, 434-924-2731, Fax: 434-982-3912, E-mail: bmg4n@virginia.edu. *Application contact:* Biomedical Sciences Graduate Study, E-mail: bims@virginia.edu.
Website: http://www.medicine.virginia.edu/basic-science/departments/cell-biology

University of Washington, Graduate School, School of Medicine, Graduate Programs in Medicine, Program in Molecular and Cellular Biology, Seattle, WA 98195. Offers PhD. Offered jointly with Fred Hutchinson Cancer Research Center. *Degree requirements:* For doctorate, thesis/dissertation. *Entrance requirements:* For doctorate, GRE General Test. Additional exam requirements/recommendations for international students: Required—TOEFL. Electronic applications accepted.

See Display on this page and Close-Up on page 247.

The University of Western Ontario, Faculty of Graduate Studies, Biosciences Division, Department of Anatomy and Cell Biology, London, ON N6A 5B8, Canada. Offers anatomy and cell biology (M Sc, PhD); clinical anatomy (M Sc). *Degree requirements:* For master's, thesis; for doctorate, comprehensive exam, thesis/dissertation. *Entrance requirements:* For master's, honors degree or equivalent in biological sciences; for doctorate, master's degree. Additional exam requirements/recommendations for international students: Required—TOEFL. *Faculty research:* Cell and molecular biology, developmental biology, neuroscience, immunobiology and cancer.

University of Wisconsin–La Crosse, Graduate Studies, College of Science and Health, Department of Biology, La Crosse, WI 54601-3742. Offers aquatic sciences (MS); biology (MS); cellular and molecular biology (MS); clinical microbiology (MS); microbiology (MS); nurse anesthesia (MS); physiology (MS). Part-time programs available. *Faculty:* 22 full-time (8 women), 3 part-time/adjunct (1 woman). *Students:* 21 full-time (13 women), 37 part-time (24 women); includes 7 minority (2 Asian, non-Hispanic/Latino; 4 Hispanic/Latino; 1 Two or more races, non-Hispanic/Latino), 5 international. Average age 28. 107 applicants, 26% accepted, 25 enrolled. In 2013, 16 master's awarded. *Degree requirements:* For master's, comprehensive exam, thesis. *Entrance requirements:* For master's, GRE General Test, minimum GPA of 2.85. Additional exam requirements/recommendations for international students: Required—TOEFL (minimum score 550 paper-based; 79 iBT). *Application deadline:* For fall admission, 2/1 priority date for domestic and international students; for spring admission, 1/4 priority date for domestic and international students. Applications are processed on a rolling basis. Electronic applications accepted. *Financial support:* Research assistantships with partial tuition reimbursements, Federal Work-Study,

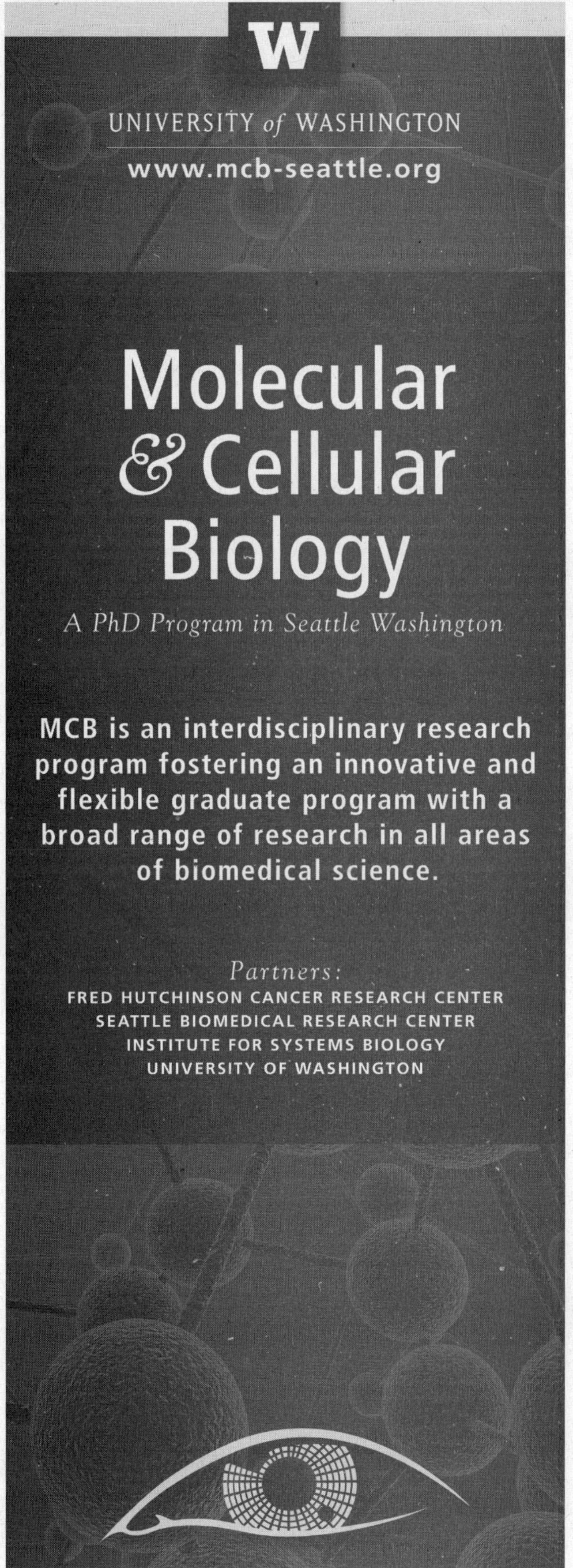

scholarships/grants, health care benefits, and tuition waivers (partial) available. Support available to part-time students. Financial award application deadline: 3/15; financial award applicants required to submit FAFSA. *Unit head:* Dr. Thomas Volk, Coordinator of Graduate Studies, 608-785-6972, Fax: 608-785-6959, E-mail: volk.thom@uwlax.edu. *Application contact:* Corey Sjoquist, Director of Admissions, 608-785-8939, E-mail: admissions@uwlax.edu.
Website: http://uwlax.edu/biology/

University of Wisconsin–Madison, Graduate School, Program in Cellular and Molecular Biology, Madison, WI 53706-1596. Offers PhD. *Degree requirements:* For doctorate, comprehensive exam, thesis/dissertation. *Entrance requirements:* For doctorate, GRE General Test, GRE Subject Test (recommended), minimum GPA of 3.0, lab experience. Additional exam requirements/recommendations for international students: Required—TOEFL (minimum score 580 paper-based; 92 iBT). Electronic applications accepted. *Expenses:* Tuition, state resident: full-time $10,728; part-time $790 per credit. Tuition, nonresident: full-time $24,054; part-time $1623 per credit. *Required fees:* $1130; $119 per credit. *Faculty research:* Virology, cancer biology, transcriptional mechanisms, plant biology, immunology.

University of Wyoming, Graduate Program in Molecular and Cellular Life Sciences, Laramie, WY 82071. Offers PhD. *Degree requirements:* For doctorate, thesis/dissertation, four eight-week laboratory rotations, comprehensive basic practical exam, two-part qualifying exam, seminars, symposium.

Vanderbilt University, Graduate School and School of Medicine, Department of Cell and Developmental Biology, Nashville, TN 37240-1001. Offers MS, PhD, MD/PhD. *Faculty:* 19 full-time (7 women). *Students:* 74 full-time (43 women); includes 9 minority (3 Black or African American, non-Hispanic/Latino; 3 Asian, non-Hispanic/Latino; 1 Hispanic/Latino; 1 Native Hawaiian or other Pacific Islander, non-Hispanic/Latino; 1 Two or more races, non-Hispanic/Latino), 9 international. Average age 27. In 2013, 2 master's, 9 doctorates awarded. Terminal master's awarded for partial completion of doctoral program. *Degree requirements:* For master's, thesis or alternative; for doctorate, thesis/dissertation, preliminary, qualifying, and final exams. *Entrance requirements:* For master's, GRE General Test; for doctorate, GRE General Test, GRE Subject Test (recommended). Additional exam requirements/recommendations for international students: Required—TOEFL (minimum score 570 paper-based; 88 iBT). *Application deadline:* For fall admission, 1/15 for domestic and international students. Application fee: $0. Electronic applications accepted. *Financial support:* Fellowships with full and partial tuition reimbursements, research assistantships with full and partial tuition reimbursements, career-related internships or fieldwork, Federal Work-Study, institutionally sponsored loans, scholarships/grants, traineeships, health care benefits, and tuition waivers (partial) available. Financial award application deadline: 1/15; financial award applicants required to submit CSS PROFILE or FAFSA. *Faculty research:* Cancer biology, cell cycle regulation, cell signaling, cytoskeletal biology, developmental biology, neurobiology, proteomics, stem cell biology, structural biology, reproductive biology, trafficking and transport, medical education and gross anatomy. *Unit head:* Dr. Kathleen Gould, Director of Graduate Studies, 615-343-9502, Fax: 615-343-4539, E-mail: kathy.gould@vanderbilt.edu. *Application contact:* Elaine Caine, Administrative Assistant, 615-322-2294, Fax: 615-343-4539, E-mail: elaine.caine@vanderbilt.edu.
Website: http://www.mc.vanderbilt.edu/cdb/

Washington University in St. Louis, Graduate School of Arts and Sciences, Division of Biology and Biomedical Sciences, Program in Molecular Cell Biology, St. Louis, MO 63130-4899. Offers PhD. *Degree requirements:* For doctorate, thesis/dissertation. *Entrance requirements:* For doctorate, GRE General Test, GRE Subject Test. Electronic applications accepted.

Wayne State University, School of Medicine, Graduate Programs in Medicine, Program in Molecular Biology and Genetics, Detroit, MI 48201. Offers bioinformatics and computational biology (PhD); cellular neuroscience (PhD); MD/PhD. *Students:* 21 full-time (11 women), 1 part-time (0 women); includes 1 minority (Hispanic/Latino), 3 international. Average age 27. 45 applicants, 13% accepted, 4 enrolled. In 2013, 5 doctorates awarded. Terminal master's awarded for partial completion of doctoral program. *Degree requirements:* For doctorate, thesis/dissertation. *Entrance requirements:* For doctorate, GRE General Test, GRE Subject Test (chemistry or biology), minimum GPA of 3.0, strong background in one of the chemical or biological sciences, three letters of recommendation, personal statement, interview. Additional exam requirements/recommendations for international students: Required—TOEFL (minimum score 550 paper-based; 79 iBT), Michigan English Language Assessment Battery (minimum score 85); Recommended—IELTS (minimum score 6.5), TWE (minimum score 5.5). *Application deadline:* For fall admission, 3/1 for domestic students, 5/1 for international students; for winter admission, 10/1 for domestic students, 9/1 for international students; for spring admission, 2/1 for domestic students, 1/1 for international students. Applications are processed on a rolling basis. Application fee: $0. Electronic applications accepted. *Expenses:* Tuition, state resident: part-time $554.15 per credit. Tuition, nonresident: part-time $1200.35 per credit. *Required fees:* $42.15 per credit. $268.30 per semester. Tuition and fees vary according to course load and program. *Financial support:* In 2013–14, 18 students received support. Fellowships with tuition reimbursements available, research assistantships with tuition reimbursements available, teaching assistantships with tuition reimbursements available, scholarships/grants, and unspecified assistantships available. Financial award application deadline: 3/31; financial award applicants required to submit FAFSA. *Faculty research:* Human gene mapping, genome organization and sequencing, gene regulation, molecular evolution. *Total annual research expenditures:* $2.6 million. *Unit head:* Dr. Lawrence Grossman, Director, 313-577-5323, E-mail: l.grossman@wayne.edu. *Application contact:* Dr. Gregory Kapatos, Professor, Director for Education, and Graduate Officer, 313-577-5965, Fax: 313-993-4269, E-mail: gkapato@med.wayne.edu.
Website: http://genetics.wayne.edu/students/mdphd.php

Weill Cornell Medical College, Weill Cornell Graduate School of Medical Sciences, Biochemistry, Cell and Molecular Biology Allied Program, New York, NY 10065. Offers MS, PhD. Terminal master's awarded for partial completion of doctoral program. *Degree requirements:* For master's, comprehensive exam; for doctorate, thesis/dissertation, final exam. *Entrance requirements:* For doctorate, GRE General Test, background in genetics, molecular biology, chemistry, or biochemistry. Additional exam requirements/recommendations for international students: Required—TOEFL. Electronic applications accepted. *Faculty research:* Molecular structure determination, protein structure, gene structure, stem cell biology, control of gene expression, DNA replication, chromosome maintenance, RNA biosynthesis.

West Virginia University, Eberly College of Arts and Sciences, Department of Biology, Morgantown, WV 26506. Offers cell and molecular biology (MS, PhD); environmental and evolutionary biology (MS, PhD); forensic biology (MS, PhD); genomic biology (MS, PhD); neurobiology (MS, PhD). Terminal master's awarded for partial completion of doctoral program. *Degree requirements:* For master's, thesis, final exam; for doctorate, thesis/dissertation, preliminary and final exams. *Entrance requirements:* For master's, GRE General Test, GRE Subject Test, minimum GPA of 3.0; for doctorate, GRE General Test, minimum GPA of 3.0. Additional exam requirements/recommendations for international students: Required—TOEFL. *Faculty research:* Environmental biology, genetic engineering, developmental biology, global change, biodiversity.

Yale University, Graduate School of Arts and Sciences, Department of Cell Biology, New Haven, CT 06520. Offers PhD. *Degree requirements:* For doctorate, thesis/dissertation. *Entrance requirements:* For doctorate, GRE General Test. *Expenses:* Contact institution.

Yale University, Graduate School of Arts and Sciences, Department of Molecular, Cellular, and Developmental Biology, Program in Cellular and Developmental Biology, New Haven, CT 06520. Offers PhD. *Degree requirements:* For doctorate, thesis/dissertation. *Entrance requirements:* For doctorate, GRE General Test, GRE Subject Test.

Yale University, School of Medicine and Graduate School of Arts and Sciences, Combined Program in Biological and Biomedical Sciences (BBS), Molecular Cell Biology, Genetics, and Development Track, New Haven, CT 06520. Offers PhD, MD/PhD. *Entrance requirements:* Additional exam requirements/recommendations for international students: Required—TOEFL.

Molecular Biology

Albany College of Pharmacy and Health Sciences, School of Health Sciences, Albany, NY 12208. Offers clinical laboratory sciences (MS); cytotechnology and molecular cytology (MS); molecular biosciences (MS). *Students:* 14 full-time (10 women), 5 part-time (2 women), 7 international. Average age 25. 53 applicants, 64% accepted, 13 enrolled. In 2013, 20 master's awarded. *Degree requirements:* For master's, thesis. *Entrance requirements:* For master's, GRE, minimum GPA of 3.0. Additional exam requirements/recommendations for international students: Required—TOEFL (minimum score 84 iBT). *Application deadline:* For fall admission, 4/15 for domestic and international students. Applications are processed on a rolling basis. Application fee: $75. Electronic applications accepted. *Financial support:* Federal Work-Study and scholarships/grants available. Support available to part-time students. Financial award application deadline: 3/1; financial award applicants required to submit FAFSA. *Unit head:* Dr. Martha Hass, Dean of Graduate Studies, 518-694-7238. *Application contact:* Ann Bruno, Coordinator, Graduate Programs, 518-694-7130, E-mail: graduate@acphs.edu.
Website: http://acphs.edu/academics/schools-departments/school-arts-and-sciences

Albany Medical College, Center for Cell Biology and Cancer Research, Albany, NY 12208-3479. Offers MS, PhD. Part-time programs available. Terminal master's awarded for partial completion of doctoral program. *Degree requirements:* For master's, thesis; for doctorate, comprehensive exam, thesis/dissertation. *Entrance requirements:* For master's and doctorate, GRE General Test, all transcripts, letters of recommendation. Additional exam requirements/recommendations for international students: Required—TOEFL. *Faculty research:* Cancer cell biology, tissue remodeling, signal transduction, gene regulation, cell adhesion, angiogenesis.

Albert Einstein College of Medicine, Graduate Division of Biomedical Sciences, Department of Developmental and Molecular Biology, Bronx, NY 10461. Offers PhD, MD/PhD. *Degree requirements:* For doctorate, thesis/dissertation. *Entrance requirements:* For doctorate, GRE General Test. Additional exam requirements/recommendations for international students: Required—TOEFL. *Faculty research:* DNA, RNA, and protein synthesis in prokaryotes and eukaryotes; chemical and enzymatic alteration of RNA; glycoproteins.

American University of Beirut, Graduate Programs, Faculty of Arts and Sciences, Beirut, Lebanon. Offers anthropology (MA); Arab and Middle Eastern history (PhD); Arabic language and literature (MA, PhD); archaeology (MA); biology (MS); cell and molecular biology (PhD); chemistry (MS); clinical psychology (MA); computational sciences (MS); computer science (MS); economics (MA); education (MA); English language (MA); English literature (MA); environmental policy planning (MS); financial economics (MA); geology (MS); history (MA); mathematics (MA, MS); media studies (MA); Middle Eastern studies (MA); philosophy (MA); physics (MS); political studies (MA); psychology (MA); public administration (MA); sociology (MA); statistics (MA, MS); theoretical physics (PhD); transnational American studies (MA). Part-time programs available. *Faculty:* 88 full-time (22 women). *Students:* Average age 25. In 2013, 112 master's, 87 doctorates awarded. *Degree requirements:* For master's, one foreign language, comprehensive exam, thesis (for some programs); for doctorate, one foreign language, comprehensive exam, thesis/dissertation. *Entrance requirements:* For master's, GRE, letter of recommendation; for doctorate, GRE, letters of recommendation. Additional exam requirements/recommendations for international students: Required—TOEFL (minimum score 600 paper-based; 97 iBT), IELTS (minimum score 7). *Application deadline:* For fall admission, 4/30 for domestic students, 4/18 for international students; for spring admission, 11/1 for domestic and international students. Application fee: $50. *Expenses: Tuition:* Full-time $14,724; part-time $818 per credit. *Required fees:* $692. Tuition and fees vary according to course load and program. *Financial support:* Research assistantships, career-related internships or fieldwork, institutionally sponsored loans, scholarships/grants, health care benefits, and unspecified assistantships available. Financial award application deadline: 2/4; financial award applicants required to submit FAFSA. *Faculty research:* Modern Middle East history; Near Eastern archaeology; Islamic history; European history; software engineering; scientific computing; data mining; the applications of cooperative learning in language teaching and teacher education; world/comparative literature; rhetoric and composition; creative writing; public management; public policy and international affairs; hydrogeology; mineralogy, petrology, and geochemistry; tectonics and structural geology; cell and molecular biology; ecology. *Unit head:* Dr. Patrick McGreevy, Dean, 961-1374374 Ext. 3800, Fax: 961-1744461, E-mail: pm07@aub.edu.lb. *Application contact:* Dr. Salim Kanaan, Director, Admissions Office, 961-1-350000 Ext. 2590, Fax: 96-1-1750775, E-mail: sk00@aub.edu.lb.
Website: http://www.aub.edu.lb/fas/

Appalachian State University, Cratis D. Williams Graduate School, Department of Biology, Boone, NC 28608. Offers cell and molecular biology (MS); general biology (MS). Part-time programs available. *Degree requirements:* For master's, comprehensive exam, thesis. *Entrance requirements:* For master's, GRE General Test, 3 letters of recommendation. Additional exam requirements/recommendations for international students: Required—TOEFL (minimum score 570 paper-based; 79 iBT), IELTS (minimum score 6.5). Electronic applications accepted. *Faculty research:* Aquatic and terrestrial ecology, animal and plant physiology, behavior and systematics, immunology and cell biology, molecular biology and microbiology.

Arizona State University at the Tempe campus, College of Liberal Arts and Sciences, School of Life Sciences, Tempe, AZ 85287-4601. Offers animal behavior (PhD); applied ethics (biomedical and health ethics) (MA); biological design (PhD); biology (MS, PhD); biology (biology and society) (MS, PhD); environmental life sciences (PhD); evolutionary biology (PhD); human and social dimensions of science and technology (PhD); microbiology (PhD); molecular and cellular biology (PhD); neuroscience (PhD); philosophy (history and philosophy of science) (MA); sustainability (PhD). Terminal master's awarded for partial completion of doctoral program. *Degree requirements:* For master's, thesis (for some programs), interactive Program of Study (iPOS) submitted before completing 50 percent of required credit hours; for doctorate, variable foreign language requirement, comprehensive exam, thesis/dissertation, interactive Program of Study (iPOS) submitted before completing 50 percent of required credit hours. *Entrance requirements:* For master's and doctorate, GRE, minimum GPA of 3.0 or equivalent in last 2 years of work leading to bachelor's degree. Additional exam requirements/recommendations for international students: Required—TOEFL (minimum score 600 paper-based; 100 iBT). Electronic applications accepted.

Arkansas State University, Graduate School, College of Sciences and Mathematics, Program in Molecular Biosciences, State University, AR 72467. Offers PhD. Part-time programs available. *Faculty:* 1 full-time (0 women). *Students:* 18 full-time (9 women); includes 1 minority (American Indian or Alaska Native, non-Hispanic/Latino), 11 international. Average age 29. 15 applicants, 13% accepted, 2 enrolled. In 2013, 4 doctorates awarded. *Degree requirements:* For doctorate, comprehensive exam, thesis/dissertation. *Entrance requirements:* For doctorate, GRE, appropriate bachelor's or master's degree, interview, letters of reference, official transcripts, personal statement, immunization records. Additional exam requirements/recommendations for international students: Required—TOEFL (minimum score 550 paper-based; 79 iBT), IELTS (minimum score 6), PTE (minimum score 56). *Application deadline:* For fall admission, 2/15 for domestic and international students; for spring admission, 11/15 for domestic students, 11/14 for international students. Applications are processed on a rolling basis. Application fee: $50. Electronic applications accepted. *Expenses:* Tuition, state resident: full-time $4284; part-time $238 per credit hour. Tuition, nonresident: full-time $8568; part-time $476 per credit hour. *International tuition:* $9268 full-time. *Required fees:* $1098; $61 per credit hour. $25 per term. Tuition and fees vary according to course load and program. *Financial support:* In 2013–14, 2 students received support. Fellowships, research assistantships, teaching assistantships, career-related internships or fieldwork, scholarships/grants, and unspecified assistantships available. Financial award application deadline: 7/1; financial award applicants required to submit FAFSA. *Unit head:* Dr. Malathia Srivatsan, Assistant Director of Arkansas Biosciences Institute, 870-972-2007, Fax: 870-972-3827, E-mail: msrivatsan@astate.edu. *Application contact:* Vickey Ring, Graduate Admissions Coordinator, 870-972-3029, Fax: 870-972-3857, E-mail: vickeyring@astate.edu.
Website: http://www.astate.edu/college/sciences-and-mathematics/doctoral-programs/molecular-biosciences/

Auburn University, Graduate School, Interdepartmental Programs, Auburn University, AL 36849. Offers applied economics (PhD); cell and molecular biology (PhD); real estate development (MRED); sociology and rural sociology (MA, MS), including rural sociology (MS), sociology. Part-time programs available. *Students:* 42 full-time (21 women), 35 part-time (8 women); includes 15 minority (12 Black or African American, non-Hispanic/Latino; 1 American Indian or Alaska Native, non-Hispanic/Latino; 2 Asian, non-Hispanic/Latino), 30 international. Average age 32. 80 applicants, 68% accepted, 33 enrolled. In 2013, 21 master's, 6 doctorates awarded. *Entrance requirements:* For master's, GRE General Test. *Application deadline:* For fall admission, 7/7 for domestic students; for spring admission, 11/24 for domestic students. Applications are processed on a rolling basis. Application fee: $50 ($60 for international students). Electronic applications accepted. *Expenses:* Tuition, state resident: full-time $8262; part-time $459 per credit hour. Tuition, nonresident: full-time $24,786; part-time $1377 per credit hour. Tuition and fees vary according to degree level and program. *Financial support:* Fellowships, research assistantships, teaching assistantships, and Federal Work-Study available. Support available to part-time students. Financial award application deadline: 3/15; financial award applicants required to submit FAFSA. *Unit head:* Dr. George Flowers, Dean, 334-844-4700, E-mail: gradadm@auburn.edu. *Application contact:* Dr. George Flowers, Dean of the Graduate School, 334-844-2125.

Baylor College of Medicine, Graduate School of Biomedical Sciences, Department of Biochemistry and Molecular Biology, Houston, TX 77030-3498. Offers PhD, MD/PhD. *Degree requirements:* For doctorate, thesis/dissertation, public defense. *Entrance requirements:* For doctorate, GRE General Test, GRE Subject Test (strongly recommended), minimum GPA of 3.0. Additional exam requirements/recommendations for international students: Required—TOEFL. Electronic applications accepted. *Faculty research:* DNA repair, homologous recombination, gene therapy, trinucleotide repeat diseases, retinitis pigmentosa.

Baylor College of Medicine, Graduate School of Biomedical Sciences, Department of Molecular and Cellular Biology, Houston, TX 77030-3498. Offers PhD, MD/PhD. *Degree requirements:* For doctorate, thesis/dissertation, public defense, qualifying exam. *Entrance requirements:* For doctorate, GRE General Test, GRE Subject Test (strongly recommended), minimum GPA of 3.0. Additional exam requirements/recommendations for international students: Required—TOEFL. Electronic applications accepted. *Faculty research:* Hormone action, development, cancer, gene therapy, neurobiology.

Baylor College of Medicine, Graduate School of Biomedical Sciences, Interdepartmental Program in Cell and Molecular Biology, Houston, TX 77030-3498. Offers biochemistry (PhD); cell and molecular biology (PhD); genetics (PhD); human genetics (PhD); immunology (PhD); microbiology (PhD); virology (PhD); MD/PhD. *Degree requirements:* For doctorate, thesis/dissertation, public defense. *Entrance requirements:* For doctorate, GRE General Test, GRE Subject Test (strongly recommended), minimum GPA of 3.0. Additional exam requirements/recommendations for international students: Required—TOEFL. Electronic applications accepted. *Faculty research:* Molecular and cellular biology; cancer, aging and stem cells; genomics and proteomics; microbiome, molecular microbiology; infectious disease, immunology and translational research.

Baylor College of Medicine, Graduate School of Biomedical Sciences, Program in Developmental Biology, Houston, TX 77030-3498. Offers PhD, MD/PhD. *Degree requirements:* For doctorate, thesis/dissertation, public defense. *Entrance requirements:* For doctorate, GRE General Test, GRE Subject Test (strongly recommended), minimum GPA of 3.0. Additional exam requirements/recommendations for international students: Required—TOEFL. Electronic applications accepted. *Faculty research:* Stem cells, cancer, neurobiology, organogenesis, genetics of model organisms.

Boise State University, College of Arts and Sciences, Department of Chemistry and Biochemistry, Boise, ID 83725-0399. Offers biomolecular sciences (PhD); chemistry (MS).

Boston University, Graduate School of Arts and Sciences, Molecular Biology, Cell Biology, and Biochemistry Program (MCBB), Boston, MA 02215. Offers MA, PhD. *Students:* 34 full-time (16 women), 2 part-time (1 woman); includes 10 minority (2 Black or African American, non-Hispanic/Latino; 2 Asian, non-Hispanic/Latino; 5 Hispanic/Latino; 1 Two or more races, non-Hispanic/Latino), 9 international. Average age 27. 96 applicants, 16% accepted, 8 enrolled. In 2013, 2 master's, 5 doctorates awarded. Terminal master's awarded for partial completion of doctoral program. *Degree requirements:* For master's, one foreign language, thesis (for some programs); for doctorate, one foreign language, comprehensive exam, thesis/dissertation. *Entrance requirements:* For master's and doctorate, GRE General Test, GRE Subject Test, 3 letters of recommendation. Additional exam requirements/recommendations for international students: Required—TOEFL (minimum score 600 paper-based). *Application deadline:* For fall admission, 12/7 for domestic and international students. Application fee: $80. Electronic applications accepted. *Expenses: Tuition:* Full-time $43,970; part-time $1374 per credit hour. *Required fees:* $60 per semester. Tuition and fees vary according to class time, course level and program. *Financial support:* In 2013–14, 32 students received support, including 4 fellowships with full tuition reimbursements available (averaging $20,000 per year), 12 research assistantships with full tuition reimbursements available (averaging $20,000 per year), 4 teaching assistantships with full tuition reimbursements available (averaging $20,000 per year); Federal Work-Study, scholarships/grants, traineeships, and health care benefits also available. Financial award application deadline: 12/7; financial award applicants required to submit FAFSA. *Unit head:* Dr. Ulla Hansen, Director, 617-353-2432, Fax: 617-353-6340, E-mail: uhansen@bu.edu. *Application contact:* Meredith Canode, Academic Administrator, 617-353-2432, Fax: 617-353-6340, E-mail: mcanode@bu.edu.
Website: http://www.bu.edu/mcbb/

Boston University, School of Medicine, Division of Graduate Medical Sciences, Department of Biochemistry, Boston, MA 02118. Offers MA, PhD, MD/PhD. Part-time programs available. Terminal master's awarded for partial completion of doctoral program. *Degree requirements:* For master's, thesis or alternative; for doctorate, thesis/dissertation. *Application deadline:* For fall admission, 1/15 for domestic students; for spring admission, 10/15 for domestic students. *Expenses: Tuition:* Full-time $43,970; part-time $1374 per credit hour. *Required fees:* $60 per semester. Tuition and fees vary according to class time, course level and program. *Unit head:* Dr. David A. Harris, Chair, 617-638-5090. *Application contact:* Dr. Barbara Schreiber, Director of the Graduate Program, 617-638-5094, E-mail: schreibe@bu.edu.
Website: http://www.bumc.bu.edu/biochemistry/

Boston University, School of Medicine, Division of Graduate Medical Sciences, Program in Cell and Molecular Biology, Boston, MA 02118. Offers PhD. *Degree requirements:* For doctorate, thesis/dissertation. *Application deadline:* For fall admission, 1/15 for domestic students; for spring admission, 10/15 for domestic students. *Expenses: Tuition:* Full-time $43,970; part-time $1374 per credit hour. *Required fees:* $60 per semester. Tuition and fees vary according to class time, course level and program. *Financial support:* Scholarships/grants and traineeships available. Financial award applicants required to submit FAFSA. *Unit head:* Dr. Vickery Trinkaus-Randall, Director, 617-638-6099, Fax: 617-638-5337, E-mail: vickery@bu.edu. *Application contact:* GMS Admissions Office, 617-638-5255, Fax: 617-638-5740, E-mail: natashah@bu.edu.
Website: http://www.bumc.bu.edu/cmbio/

Brandeis University, Graduate School of Arts and Sciences, Program in Molecular and Cell Biology, Waltham, MA 02454-9110. Offers genetics (PhD); microbiology (PhD); molecular and cell biology (MS, PhD); molecular biology (PhD); neurobiology (PhD); quantitative biology (PhD). Terminal master's awarded for partial completion of doctoral program. *Degree requirements:* For master's, thesis or alternative, research project, research lab, or project lab; for doctorate, comprehensive exam, thesis/dissertation, journal clubs; research seminar; colloquia; qualifying exam. *Entrance requirements:* For master's, GRE General Test (or MCAT for applicants to the MS program), official transcript(s), resume, 3 letters of recommendation, statement of purpose; for doctorate, GRE General Test, official transcript(s), resume, 3 letters of recommendation, statement of purpose. Additional exam requirements/recommendations for international students: Required—TOEFL (minimum score 600 paper-based; 100 iBT), PTE (minimum score 68); Recommended—IELTS (minimum score 7). Electronic applications accepted. *Faculty research:* Structural biology; immunology; developmental biology; behavior and neurobiology; DNA replication, rearrangement, and repair; signal transduction, transcriptional regulation, and RNA processing; cancer and programmed cell death; cytoskeleton and molecular motors; nutrition.

Brigham Young University, Graduate Studies, College of Life Sciences, Department of Microbiology and Molecular Biology, Provo, UT 84602. Offers MS, PhD. *Faculty:* 15 full-time (3 women). *Students:* 28 full-time (11 women); includes 4 minority (3 Hispanic/Latino; 1 Native Hawaiian or other Pacific Islander, non-Hispanic/Latino), 2 international. Average age 28. 35 applicants, 34% accepted, 12 enrolled. In 2013, 4 master's awarded. Terminal master's awarded for partial completion of doctoral program. *Degree requirements:* For master's, comprehensive exam, thesis; for doctorate, comprehensive exam, thesis/dissertation. *Entrance requirements:* For master's, GRE General Test, minimum GPA of 3.0 during previous 2 years; for doctorate, GRE General Test, minimum GPA of 3.0. Additional exam requirements/recommendations for international students: Required—TOEFL (minimum score 580 paper-based; 85 iBT), IELTS (minimum score 7). *Application deadline:* For fall admission, 12/15 priority date for domestic and international students. Application fee: $50. Electronic applications accepted. *Expenses: Tuition:* Full-time $6130; part-time $340 per credit hour. Tuition and fees vary according to program and student's religious affiliation. *Financial support:* In 2013–14, 19 students received support, including 16 research assistantships with full tuition reimbursements available (averaging $21,000 per year), 2 teaching assistantships with full and partial tuition reimbursements available (averaging $18,000 per year); institutionally sponsored loans, scholarships/grants, health care benefits, and unspecified assistantships also available. Financial award application deadline: 2/1. *Faculty research:* Immunobiology, molecular genetics, molecular virology, cancer biology, pathogenic and environmental microbiology. *Total annual research expenditures:* $778,143. *Unit head:* Dr. Laura Bridgewater, Chair, 801-422-2434, Fax: 801-422-0519, E-mail: laura_bridgewater@byu.edu. *Application contact:* Dr. Joel Griffitts, Graduate Coordinator, 801-422-7997, Fax: 801-422-0519, E-mail: joel_griffitts@byu.edu.
Website: http://mmbio.byu.edu/

Brown University, Graduate School, Division of Biology and Medicine, Department of Molecular Biology, Cell Biology, and Biochemistry, Providence, RI 02912. Offers MA, PhD. Part-time programs available. Terminal master's awarded for partial completion of doctoral program. *Degree requirements:* For master's, thesis (for some programs); for doctorate, one foreign language, thesis/dissertation, preliminary exam. *Entrance* *requirements:* For master's and doctorate, GRE General Test, GRE Subject Test. Additional exam requirements/recommendations for international students: Required—TOEFL. Electronic applications accepted. *Faculty research:* Molecular genetics, gene regulation.

California Institute of Technology, Division of Biology, Program in Molecular Biology, Pasadena, CA 91125-0001. Offers PhD. *Degree requirements:* For doctorate, thesis/dissertation, qualifying exam. *Entrance requirements:* For doctorate, GRE General Test.

California State University, Sacramento, Office of Graduate Studies, College of Natural Sciences and Mathematics, Department of Biological Sciences, Sacramento, CA 95819. Offers biological conservation (MS); marine science (MS); molecular and cellular biology (MS); stem cell (MA). Part-time programs available. *Degree requirements:* For master's, thesis, writing proficiency exam. *Entrance requirements:* For master's, GRE, bachelor's degree in biology or equivalent; minimum GPA of 3.0 in biology, 2.75 overall during last 2 years of course work. Additional exam requirements/recommendations for international students: Required—TOEFL. *Application deadline:* For fall admission, 2/1 for domestic students, 3/1 for international students; for spring admission, 9/30 for international students. Applications are processed on a rolling basis. Application fee: $55. Electronic applications accepted. *Financial support:* Research assistantships, teaching assistantships, career-related internships or fieldwork, and Federal Work-Study available. Support available to part-time students. Financial award application deadline: 3/1; financial award applicants required to submit FAFSA. *Unit head:* Jennifer Lundmark, Chair, 916-278-6535, E-mail: lundmark@csus.edu. *Application contact:* Jose Martinez, Graduate Admissions Supervisor, 916-278-7871, E-mail: martinj@skymail.csus.edu.
Website: http://www.csus.edu/bios

Carnegie Mellon University, Mellon College of Science, Department of Biological Sciences, Pittsburgh, PA 15213-3891. Offers biochemistry (PhD); biophysics (PhD); cell and developmental biology (PhD); computational biology (MS, PhD); genetics (PhD); molecular biology (PhD); neuroscience (PhD); structural biology (PhD). *Degree requirements:* For doctorate, comprehensive exam, thesis/dissertation. *Entrance requirements:* For doctorate, GRE General Test, GRE Subject Test, interview. *Application deadline:* Applications are processed on a rolling basis. Application fee: $0. Electronic applications accepted. *Financial support:* Fellowships, research assistantships, teaching assistantships, and traineeships available. *Faculty research:* Genetic structure, function, and regulation; protein structure and function; biological membranes; biological spectroscopy. *Unit head:* John L. Woolford, Acting Department Head, 412-268-3193, E-mail: jw17@andrew.cmu.edu. *Application contact:* Ena Miceli, Graduate Programs Manager, 412-268-33012, E-mail: emiceli@andrew.cmu.edu.
Website: http://www.bio.cmu.edu/

Case Western Reserve University, School of Medicine and School of Graduate Studies, Graduate Programs in Medicine, Department of Molecular Biology and Microbiology, Cleveland, OH 44106-4960. Offers cellular biology (PhD); microbiology (PhD); molecular biology (PhD); molecular virology (PhD); MD/PhD. Students are admitted to an integrated Biomedical Sciences Training Program involving 11 basic science programs at Case Western Reserve University. *Degree requirements:* For doctorate, thesis/dissertation. *Entrance requirements:* For doctorate, GRE General Test, GRE Subject Test. Additional exam requirements/recommendations for international students: Required—TOEFL. Electronic applications accepted. *Faculty research:* Gene expression in eukaryotic and prokaryotic systems; microbial physiology; intracellular transport and signaling; mechanisms of oncogenesis; molecular mechanisms of RNA processing, editing, and catalysis.

Central Connecticut State University, School of Graduate Studies, School of Technology, Department of Biomolecular Sciences, New Britain, CT 06050-4010. Offers MS, Certificate. Part-time and evening/weekend programs available. *Faculty:* 8 full-time (3 women), 1 (woman) part-time/adjunct. *Students:* 14 full-time (8 women), 13 part-time (6 women); includes 12 minority (4 Black or African American, non-Hispanic/Latino; 4 Asian, non-Hispanic/Latino; 3 Hispanic/Latino; 1 Two or more races, non-Hispanic/Latino), 1 international. Average age 29. 41 applicants, 71% accepted, 18 enrolled. In 2013, 15 master's awarded. *Degree requirements:* For master's, comprehensive exam, thesis or alternative; for Certificate, qualifying exam. *Entrance requirements:* For master's, minimum undergraduate GPA of 2.7, essay, letters of recommendation; for Certificate, essay. Additional exam requirements/recommendations for international students: Required—TOEFL (minimum score 550 paper-based; 79 iBT). *Application deadline:* For fall admission, 6/1 for domestic students, 5/1 for international students; for spring admission, 11/1 for domestic and international students. Applications are processed on a rolling basis. Application fee: $50. Electronic applications accepted. Part-time tuition and fees vary according to degree level. *Financial support:* In 2013–14, 6 students received support, including 3 research assistantships; career-related internships or fieldwork, Federal Work-Study, scholarships/grants, and unspecified assistantships also available. Support available to part-time students. Financial award application deadline: 3/1; financial award applicants required to submit FAFSA. *Unit head:* Dr. James Mulrooney, Chair, 860-832-3560, E-mail: mulrooneyj@ccsu.edu. *Application contact:* Patricia Gardner, Associate Director of Graduate Studies, 860-832-2350, Fax: 860-832-2362, E-mail: graduateadmissions@ccsu.edu.
Website: http://www.ccsu.edu/page.cfm?p=6494

Clemson University, Graduate School, College of Agriculture, Forestry and Life Sciences, Department of Genetics and Biochemistry, Program in Biochemistry and Molecular Biology, Clemson, SC 29634. Offers PhD. *Students:* 17 full-time (10 women); includes 1 minority (Asian, non-Hispanic/Latino), 8 international. Average age 27. 38 applicants, 18% accepted, 4 enrolled. In 2013, 3 doctorates awarded. *Degree requirements:* For doctorate, comprehensive exam, thesis/dissertation. *Entrance requirements:* For doctorate, GRE General Test. Additional exam requirements/recommendations for international students: Required—TOEFL. *Application deadline:* For fall admission, 1/1 for domestic students; for spring admission, 9/1 for domestic students. Applications are processed on a rolling basis. Application fee: $70 ($80 for international students). Electronic applications accepted. *Expenses:* Contact institution. *Financial support:* In 2013–14, 17 students received support, including 3 fellowships with full and partial tuition reimbursements available (averaging $13,778 per year), 10 research assistantships with partial tuition reimbursements available (averaging $15,495 per year), 6 teaching assistantships with partial tuition reimbursements available (averaging $15,625 per year); career-related internships or fieldwork, institutionally sponsored loans, scholarships/grants, health care benefits, and unspecified assistantships also available. Support available to part-time students. Financial award application deadline: 3/15; financial award applicants required to submit FAFSA. *Faculty research:* Biomembranes, protein structure, molecular biology of plants, APYA and stress response. *Unit head:* Dr. Keith Murphy, Chair, 864-656-6237, Fax: 864-656-0435, E-mail: kmurph2@clemson.edu. *Application contact:* Sheryl Banks, Administrative Coordinator, 864-656-6878, E-mail: sherylb@clemson.edu.
Website: http://www.clemson.edu/genbiochem

Colorado State University, Graduate School, Program in Cell and Molecular Biology, Fort Collins, CO 80523-1618. Offers MS, PhD. *Students:* 28 full-time (18 women), 50 part-time (27 women); includes 11 minority (2 Black or African American, non-Hispanic/Latino; 8 Hispanic/Latino; 1 Two or more races, non-Hispanic/Latino), 28 international. Average age 30. 54 applicants, 17% accepted, 9 enrolled. In 2013, 2 master's, 3 doctorates awarded. Terminal master's awarded for partial completion of doctoral program. *Degree requirements:* For master's, comprehensive exam (for some programs), thesis; for doctorate, comprehensive exam, thesis/dissertation. *Entrance requirements:* For master's and doctorate, GRE General Test, GRE Subject Test in biology (strongly recommended), minimum GPA of 3.0; BA/BS in biology, biochemistry, physics; calculus sequence, letters of recommendation. Additional exam requirements/recommendations for international students: Required—TOEFL (minimum score 625 paper-based; 107 iBT). *Application deadline:* For fall admission, 1/1 priority date for domestic and international students. Applications are processed on a rolling basis. Application fee: $50. Electronic applications accepted. *Expenses:* Tuition, state resident: full-time $9075.40; part-time $504 per credit. Tuition, nonresident: full-time $22,248; part-time $1236 per credit. *Required fees:* $1819; $60 per credit. *Financial support:* In 2013–14, 7 students received support, including 4 research assistantships with full tuition reimbursements available (averaging $22,765 per year), 3 teaching assistantships with full tuition reimbursements available (averaging $16,380 per year); tuition waivers (full) also available. Financial award application deadline: 1/1. *Faculty research:* Cancer biology, genomics and computational biology, infectious diseases, metabolic regulation, neuroscience and molecular physiology, plant biology, regulation of gene expression, reproductive and developmental biology. *Total annual research expenditures:* $2,294. *Unit head:* Dr. Howard Liber, Director, 970-491-0580, Fax: 970-491-2194, E-mail: howard.liber@colostate.edu. *Application contact:* Lori Williams, Graduate Coordinator, 970-491-0241, Fax: 970-491-2194, E-mail: lori.williams@colostate.edu.
Website: http://cmb.colostate.edu/

Columbia University, College of Physicians and Surgeons, Integrated Program in Cellular, Molecular, Structural and Genetic Studies, New York, NY 10032. Offers PhD. Terminal master's awarded for partial completion of doctoral program. *Degree requirements:* For doctorate, thesis/dissertation. *Entrance requirements:* For doctorate, GRE General Test, GRE Subject Test. Additional exam requirements/recommendations for international students: Required—TOEFL. *Expenses:* Contact institution. *Faculty research:* Transcription, macromolecular sorting, gene expression during development, cellular interaction.

Cornell University, Graduate School, Graduate Fields of Agriculture and Life Sciences, Field of Biochemistry, Molecular and Cell Biology, Ithaca, NY 14853-0001. Offers biochemistry (PhD); biophysics (PhD); cell biology (PhD); molecular biology (PhD). *Faculty:* 20 full-time (19 women). *Students:* 87 full-time (43 women); includes 17 minority (7 Asian, non-Hispanic/Latino; 6 Hispanic/Latino; 4 Two or more races, non-Hispanic/Latino), 28 international. Average age 26. 238 applicants, 20% accepted, 20 enrolled. In 2013, 17 doctorates awarded. *Degree requirements:* For doctorate, comprehensive exam, thesis/dissertation, 2 semesters of teaching experience. *Entrance requirements:* For doctorate, GRE General Test, GRE Subject Test (biology, chemistry, physics, biochemistry, cell and molecular biology), 3 letters of recommendation. Additional exam requirements/recommendations for international students: Required—TOEFL (minimum score 600 paper-based; 77 iBT). *Application deadline:* For fall admission, 1/5 for domestic students. Application fee: $95. Electronic applications accepted. *Financial support:* In 2013–14, 62 students received support, including 8 fellowships with full tuition reimbursements available, 38 research assistantships with full tuition reimbursements available, 16 teaching assistantships with full tuition reimbursements available; institutionally sponsored loans, scholarships/grants, health care benefits, tuition waivers (full and partial), and unspecified assistantships also available. Financial award applicants required to submit FAFSA. *Faculty research:* Biophysics, structural biology. *Unit head:* Director of Graduate Studies, 607-255-2100, Fax: 607-255-2100. *Application contact:* Graduate Field Assistant, 607-255-2100, Fax: 607-255-2100, E-mail: bmcb@cornell.edu.
Website: http://www.gradschool.cornell.edu/fields.php?id-43&a-2

Cornell University, Graduate School, Graduate Fields of Agriculture and Life Sciences and Graduate Fields of Human Ecology, Field of Nutrition, Ithaca, NY 14853-0001. Offers animal nutrition (MPS, PhD); community nutrition (MPS, PhD); human nutrition (MPS, PhD); international nutrition (MPS, PhD); molecular biochemistry (MPS, PhD). *Faculty:* 55 full-time (29 women). *Students:* 64 full-time (57 women); includes 16 minority (6 Black or African American, non-Hispanic/Latino; 4 Asian, non-Hispanic/Latino; 3 Hispanic/Latino; 3 Two or more races, non-Hispanic/Latino), 19 international. Average age 28. 112 applicants, 12% accepted, 10 enrolled. In 2013, 1 master's, 9 doctorates awarded. *Degree requirements:* For master's, thesis (MS), project papers (MPS); for doctorate, comprehensive exam, thesis/dissertation. *Entrance requirements:* For master's and doctorate, GRE General Test, previous course work in organic chemistry (with laboratory) and biochemistry; 2 letters of recommendation. Additional exam requirements/recommendations for international students: Required—TOEFL (minimum score 550 paper-based; 77 iBT). *Application deadline:* For fall admission, 1/10 priority date for domestic students; for spring admission, 10/1 for domestic students. Application fee: $95. Electronic applications accepted. *Financial support:* In 2013–14, 41 students received support, including 9 fellowships with full tuition reimbursements available, 6 research assistantships with full tuition reimbursements available, 26 teaching assistantships with full tuition reimbursements available; institutionally sponsored loans, scholarships/grants, health care benefits, tuition waivers (full and partial), and unspecified assistantships also available. Financial award applicants required to submit FAFSA. *Faculty research:* Nutritional biochemistry, experimental human and animal nutrition, international nutrition, community nutrition. *Unit head:* Director of Graduate Studies, 607-255-2528, Fax: 607-255-0178. *Application contact:* Graduate Field Assistant, 607-255-2628, Fax: 607-225-0178, E-mail: nutrition_gfr@cornell.edu.
Website: http://www.gradschool.cornell.edu/fields.php?id-56&a-2

Dartmouth College, Graduate Program in Molecular and Cellular Biology, Hanover, NH 03755. Offers PhD, MD/PhD. *Entrance requirements:* For doctorate, GRE General Test, letters of recommendation. Additional exam requirements/recommendations for international students: Required—TOEFL (minimum score 450 paper-based; 90 iBT) or IELTS (minimum score 7). Electronic applications accepted.

Drexel University, College of Medicine, Biomedical Graduate Programs, Interdisciplinary Program in Molecular and Cell Biology and Genetics, Philadelphia, PA 19104-2875. Offers MS, PhD, MD/PhD. Terminal master's awarded for partial completion of doctoral program. *Degree requirements:* For master's, comprehensive exam, thesis; for doctorate, thesis/dissertation, qualifying exam. *Entrance requirements:* For master's, GRE General Test, minimum GPA of 2.75; for doctorate, GRE General Test, minimum GPA of 3.0. Additional exam requirements/recommendations for international students: Required—TOEFL. Electronic applications accepted. *Faculty research:* Molecular anatomy, biochemistry, medical biotechnology, molecular pathology, microbiology and immunology.

Duke University, Graduate School, Department of Evolutionary Anthropology, Durham, NC 27708. Offers cellular and molecular biology (PhD); gross anatomy and physical anthropology (PhD), including comparative morphology of human and non-human primates, primate social behavior, vertebrate paleontology; neuroanatomy (PhD). *Faculty:* 12. *Students:* 16 full-time (9 women); includes 5 minority (2 Black or African American, non-Hispanic/Latino; 1 Asian, non-Hispanic/Latino; 2 Hispanic/Latino). 69

applicants, 6% accepted, 3 enrolled. In 2013, 1 degree awarded. *Median time to degree:* Of those who began their doctoral program in fall 2005, 87% received their degree in 8 years or less. *Degree requirements:* For doctorate, one foreign language, thesis/dissertation. *Entrance requirements:* For doctorate, GRE General Test. Additional exam requirements/recommendations for international students: Required—TOEFL (minimum score 577 paper-based; 90 iBT) or IELTS (minimum score 7). *Application deadline:* For fall admission, 12/8 priority date for domestic and international students. Application fee: $80. Electronic applications accepted. *Financial support:* Fellowships, teaching assistantships, and Federal Work-Study available. Financial award application deadline: 12/31. *Unit head:* Richard Kay, Director of Graduate Studies, 919-684-4124, Fax: 919-684-8542, E-mail: mlsquire@duke.edu. *Application contact:* Elizabeth Hutton, Director of Admissions, 919-684-3913, Fax: 919-684-2277, E-mail: grad-admissions@duke.edu. Website: http://evolutionaryanthropology.duke.edu/

Duke University, Graduate School, Program in Cell and Molecular Biology, Durham, NC 27710. Offers Certificate. Students must be enrolled in a participating PhD program (biology, cell biology, immunology, molecular genetics, neurobiology, pathology, pharmacology). *Faculty:* 146. *Students:* 17 full-time (10 women); includes 2 minority (both Black or African American, non-Hispanic/Latino), 4 international. 190 applicants, 19% accepted, 14 enrolled. *Entrance requirements:* Additional exam requirements/recommendations for international students: Required—TOEFL (minimum score 577 paper-based; 90 iBT) or IELTS (minimum score 7). *Application deadline:* For fall admission, 12/8 priority date for domestic and international students. Application fee: $80. Electronic applications accepted. *Financial support:* Fellowships available. Financial award application deadline: 12/8. *Unit head:* Dr. Meta Kuehn, Director of Graduate Studies, 919-684-6559, Fax: 919-684-8346, E-mail: carol.richardson@duke.edu. *Application contact:* Elizabeth Hutton, Director of Admissions, 919-684-3913, Fax: 919-684-3913, E-mail: grad-admissions@duke.edu. Website: http://cmb.duke.edu/

East Carolina University, Brody School of Medicine, Department of Biochemistry and Molecular Biology, Greenville, NC 27858-4353. Offers biochemistry and molecular biology (PhD); biomedical science (MS). *Degree requirements:* For doctorate, comprehensive exam, thesis/dissertation. *Entrance requirements:* For doctorate, GRE General Test. Additional exam requirements/recommendations for international students: Required—TOEFL. *Application deadline:* For fall admission, 6/1 priority date for domestic students. Applications are processed on a rolling basis. Application fee: $50. *Expenses:* Tuition, state resident: full-time $4223. Tuition, nonresident: full-time $16,540. *Required fees:* $2184. *Financial support:* Fellowships with full and partial tuition reimbursements available. Financial award application deadline: 6/1. *Faculty research:* Gene regulation, development and differentiation, contractility and motility, macromolecular interactions, cancer. *Unit head:* Dr. Phillip H. Pekala, Chairman, 252-744-2684, Fax: 252-744-3383, E-mail: pekalap@ecu.edu. *Application contact:* Dr. Phillip H. Pekala, Chairman, 252-744-2684, Fax: 252-744-3383, E-mail: pekalap@ecu.edu. Website: http://www.ecu.edu/cs-dhs/biochemistry/Graduate-Program-Information.cfm

East Carolina University, Graduate School, Thomas Harriot College of Arts and Sciences, Department of Biology, Greenville, NC 27858-4353. Offers biology (MS); molecular biology and biotechnology (MS). Part-time programs available. *Degree requirements:* For master's, one foreign language, comprehensive exam, thesis. *Entrance requirements:* For master's, GRE General Test, GRE Subject Test. Additional exam requirements/recommendations for international students: Required—TOEFL. *Application deadline:* For fall admission, 6/1 priority date for domestic students; for spring admission, 10/15 for domestic students. Applications are processed on a rolling basis. Application fee: $50. *Expenses:* Tuition, state resident: full-time $4223. Tuition, nonresident: full-time $16,540. *Required fees:* $2184. *Financial support:* Fellowships with partial tuition reimbursements, research assistantships with partial tuition reimbursements, teaching assistantships with partial tuition reimbursements, career-related internships or fieldwork, Federal Work-Study, scholarships/grants, and unspecified assistantships available. Support available to part-time students. Financial award application deadline: 6/1. *Faculty research:* Biochemistry, microbiology, cell biology. *Unit head:* Dr. Jeff McKinnon, Chair, 252-328-6718, E-mail: mckinnonj@ecu.edu. *Application contact:* Dean of Graduate School, 252-328-6012, Fax: 252-328-6071, E-mail: gradschool@ecu.edu. Website: http://www.ecu.edu/cs-cas/biology/graduate.cfm

Eastern Michigan University, Graduate School, College of Arts and Sciences, Department of Biology, Ypsilanti, MI 48197. Offers cell and molecular biology (MS); community college biology teaching (MS); ecology and organismal biology (MS); general biology (MS); water resources (MS). Part-time and evening/weekend programs available. Postbaccalaureate distance learning degree programs offered (minimal on-campus study). *Faculty:* 19 full-time (4 women). *Students:* 11 full-time (6 women), 31 part-time (18 women); includes 3 minority (1 Black or African American, non-Hispanic/Latino; 1 Asian, non-Hispanic/Latino; 1 Hispanic/Latino), 6 international. Average age 26. 56 applicants, 59% accepted, 20 enrolled. In 2013, 13 master's awarded. *Entrance requirements:* For master's, GRE General Test, GRE Subject Test. Additional exam requirements/recommendations for international students: Required—TOEFL. *Application deadline:* Applications are processed on a rolling basis. Application fee: $35. *Expenses:* Tuition, state resident: full-time $12,300; part-time $466 per credit hour. Tuition, nonresident: full-time $23,159; part-time $918 per credit hour. *Required fees:* $71 per credit hour. $46 per semester. One-time fee: $100. Tuition and fees vary according to course level and degree level. *Financial support:* Fellowships, research assistantships with full tuition reimbursements, teaching assistantships with full tuition reimbursements, career-related internships or fieldwork, Federal Work-Study, institutionally sponsored loans, scholarships/grants, tuition waivers (partial), and unspecified assistantships available. Support available to part-time students. Financial award applicants required to submit FAFSA. *Unit head:* Dr. Daniel Clemans, Department Head, 734-487-4242, Fax: 734-487-9235, E-mail: dclemans@emich.edu. *Application contact:* Dr. David Kass, Graduate Coordinator, 734-487-4242, Fax: 734-487-9235, E-mail: dkass@emich.edu. Website: http://www.emich.edu/biology

Eastern New Mexico University, Graduate School, College of Liberal Arts and Sciences, Department of Biology, Portales, NM 88130. Offers applied ecology (MS); botany (MS); cell, molecular biology and biotechnology (MS); microbiology (MS); zoology (MS). Part-time programs available. *Degree requirements:* For master's, comprehensive exam, thesis optional. *Entrance requirements:* For master's, GRE, minimum GPA of 3.0, 2 letters of recommendation, statement of research interest, bachelor's degree related to field of study or proof of common knowledge. Additional exam requirements/recommendations for international students: Required—TOEFL (minimum score 550 paper-based; 79 iBT), IELTS (minimum score 6). Electronic applications accepted.

Emory University, Laney Graduate School, Division of Biological and Biomedical Sciences, Program in Genetics and Molecular Biology, Atlanta, GA 30322-1100. Offers PhD. *Degree requirements:* For doctorate, comprehensive exam, thesis/dissertation. *Entrance requirements:* For doctorate, GRE General Test, minimum GPA of 3.0 in science course work (recommended). Additional exam requirements/recommendations for international students: Required—TOEFL. Electronic applications accepted. *Faculty research:* Gene regulation, genetic combination, developmental regulation.

Florida Institute of Technology, Graduate Programs, College of Science, Department of Biological Sciences, Program in Cell and Molecular Biology, Melbourne, FL 32901-6975. Offers MS. Part-time programs available. *Faculty:* 16 full-time (1 woman), 1 (woman) part-time/adjunct. *Students:* 1 (woman) full-time, 3 part-time (2 women), 1 international. Average age 24. 47 applicants. In 2013, 1 master's awarded. *Degree requirements:* For master's, thesis. *Entrance requirements:* For master's, GRE General Test, 3 letters of recommendation, minimum GPA of 3.0, resume, statement of objectives. Additional exam requirements/recommendations for international students: Required—TOEFL (minimum score 550 paper-based; 79 iBT). *Application deadline:* For fall admission, 4/1 for international students; for spring admission, 9/1 for international students. Applications are processed on a rolling basis. Electronic applications accepted. *Expenses: Tuition:* Full-time $20,214; part-time $1123 per credit. Tuition and fees vary according to campus/location. *Financial support:* Career-related internships or fieldwork, institutionally sponsored loans, tuition waivers (partial), unspecified assistantships, and tuition remissions available. Support available to part-time students. Financial award application deadline: 3/1; financial award applicants required to submit FAFSA. *Faculty research:* Changes in DNA molecule and differential expression of genetic information during aging. *Total annual research expenditures:* $1.4 million. *Unit head:* Dr. Richard B. Aronson, Department Head, 321-674-8034, Fax: 321-674-7238, E-mail: raronson@fit.edu. *Application contact:* Cheryl A. Brown, Associate Director of Graduate Admission, 321-674-7581, Fax: 321-723-9468, E-mail: cbrown@fit.edu. Website: http://cos.fit.edu/biology/grad/catalog.php

Florida State University, The Graduate School, College of Arts and Sciences, Department of Biological Science, Specialization in Cell and Molecular Biology, Tallahassee, FL 32306-4295. Offers MS, PhD. *Faculty:* 25 full-time (7 women). *Students:* 62 full-time (28 women); includes 7 minority (1 Black or African American, non-Hispanic/Latino; 1 Asian, non-Hispanic/Latino; 5 Hispanic/Latino), 23 international. 113 applicants, 20% accepted, 9 enrolled. In 2013, 1 master's, 3 doctorates awarded. Terminal master's awarded for partial completion of doctoral program. *Degree requirements:* For master's, comprehensive exam, thesis, teaching experience, seminar presentation; for doctorate, comprehensive exam, thesis/dissertation, teaching experience; seminar presentation. *Entrance requirements:* For master's and doctorate, GRE General Test, minimum upper-division GPA of 3.0. Additional exam requirements/recommendations for international students: Required—TOEFL (minimum score 600 paper-based; 92 iBT). *Application deadline:* For fall admission, 12/1 for domestic and international students. Application fee: $30. Electronic applications accepted. *Expenses:* Tuition, state resident: part-time $403.51 per credit hour. Tuition, nonresident: part-time $1004.85 per credit hour. *Required fees:* $75.81 per credit hour. One-time fee: $20 part-time. Tuition and fees vary according to course load, campus/location and student level. *Financial support:* In 2013–14, 62 students received support, including 2 fellowships with full tuition reimbursements available (averaging $30,000 per year), 17 research assistantships with full tuition reimbursements available (averaging $21,500 per year), 43 teaching assistantships with full tuition reimbursements available (averaging $21,500 per year); scholarships/grants and unspecified assistantships also available. Financial award application deadline: 12/1; financial award applicants required to submit FAFSA. *Faculty research:* Molecular biology; genetics and genomics; developmental biology and gene expression; cell structure, function, and motility; cellular and organismal physiology; biophysical and structural biology. *Unit head:* Dr. Debra A. Fadool, Professor and Associate Chair, 850-644-4775, Fax: 850-644-9829, E-mail: dfadool@bio.fsu.edu. *Application contact:* Judy Bowers, Coordinator, Graduate Affairs, 850-644-3023, Fax: 850-644-9829, E-mail: gradinfo@bio.fsu.edu. Website: http://www.bio.fsu.edu/cmb/

Florida State University, The Graduate School, College of Arts and Sciences, Department of Scientific Computing, Tallahassee, FL 32306-4120. Offers computational science (MS, PSM, PhD), including atmospheric science (PhD), biochemistry (PhD), biological science (PhD), computational molecular biology/bioinformatics (PSM), computational science (PhD), geological science (PhD), materials science (PhD), physics (PhD). Part-time programs available. *Faculty:* 14 full-time (2 women). *Students:* 28 full-time (5 women), 4 part-time (0 women); includes 12 minority (10 Asian, non-Hispanic/Latino; 2 Hispanic/Latino). Average age 28. 28 applicants, 43% accepted, 7 enrolled. In 2013, 11 master's, 5 doctorates awarded. Terminal master's awarded for partial completion of doctoral program. *Degree requirements:* For master's, thesis (for some programs); for doctorate, comprehensive exam, thesis/dissertation. *Entrance requirements:* For master's and doctorate, GRE General Test, knowledge of at least one object-oriented computing language, 3 letters of recommendation. Additional exam requirements/recommendations for international students: Required—TOEFL (minimum score 550 paper-based; 80 iBT). *Application deadline:* For fall admission, 1/15 for domestic and international students. Application fee: $30. Electronic applications accepted. *Expenses:* Tuition, state resident: part-time $403.51 per credit hour. Tuition, nonresident: part-time $1004.85 per credit hour. *Required fees:* $75.81 per credit hour. One-time fee: $20 part-time. Tuition and fees vary according to course load, campus/location and student level. *Financial support:* In 2013–14, 32 students received support, including 12 research assistantships with full tuition reimbursements available (averaging $20,000 per year), 17 teaching assistantships with full tuition reimbursements available (averaging $20,000 per year); scholarships/grants and unspecified assistantships also available. Financial award application deadline: 4/15. *Faculty research:* Morphometrics, mathematical and systems biology, mining proteomic and metabolic data, computational materials research, advanced 4-D Var data-assimilation methods in dynamic meteorology and oceanography, computational fluid dynamics, astrophysics. *Unit head:* Dr. Max Gunzburger, Chair, 850-644-1010, E-mail: mgunzburger@fsu.edu. *Application contact:* Maribel Amwake, Academic Coordinator, 850-644-0143, Fax: 850-644-0098, E-mail: mamwake@fsu.edu. Website: http://www.sc.fsu.edu

Georgetown University, Graduate School of Arts and Sciences, Programs in Biomedical Sciences, Department of Biochemistry and Molecular Biology, Washington, DC 20057. Offers MS, PhD. *Degree requirements:* For doctorate, comprehensive exam, thesis/dissertation. *Entrance requirements:* For doctorate, GRE General Test. Additional exam requirements/recommendations for international students: Required—TOEFL. *Application deadline:* Applications are processed on a rolling basis. Application fee: $50 ($55 for international students). *Unit head:* Dr. Elliot Crooke, Chair, 202-687-1644. *Application contact:* Graduate School Admissions Office, 202-687-5568.

The George Washington University, School of Medicine and Health Sciences, Department of Biochemistry and Molecular Biology, Washington, DC 20037. Offers biochemistry and molecular biology (MS); biochemistry and molecular genetics (PhD); molecular biochemistry and bioinformatics (MS). *Degree requirements:* For master's, comprehensive exam; for doctorate, thesis/dissertation, general exam. *Entrance requirements:* For master's, GRE General Test, interview, minimum GPA of 3.0; for doctorate, GRE General Test, minimum GPA of 3.0. Additional exam requirements/recommendations for international students: Required—TOEFL (minimum score 550 paper-based).

Molecular Biology

Georgia Regents University, The Graduate School, Program in Biochemistry and Molecular Biology, Augusta, GA 30912. Offers MS, PhD. *Faculty:* 13 full-time (2 women). *Students:* 14 full-time (8 women); includes 9 minority (8 Asian, non-Hispanic/Latino; 1 Hispanic/Latino), 7 international. Average age 30. In 2013, 4 doctorates awarded. *Degree requirements:* For doctorate, comprehensive exam, thesis/dissertation. *Entrance requirements:* For doctorate, GRE General Test. Additional exam requirements/recommendations for international students: Required—TOEFL (minimum score 550 paper-based; 79 iBT). *Application deadline:* For fall admission, 1/15 for domestic and international students. Application fee: $50. Electronic applications accepted. *Financial support:* In 2013–14, 8 research assistantships with partial tuition reimbursements (averaging $23,000 per year) were awarded; Federal Work-Study, institutionally sponsored loans, and scholarships/grants also available. Support available to part-time students. Financial award application deadline: 5/31; financial award applicants required to submit FAFSA. *Faculty research:* Bacterial pathogenesis, eye diseases, vitamins and amino acid transporters, transcriptional control and molecular oncology, tumor biology. *Total annual research expenditures:* $3.8 million. *Unit head:* Dr. Vadivel Ganapathy, Chair/Professor, 706-721-7652, Fax: 706-721-9947, E-mail: vganapat@georgiahealth.edu. *Application contact:* Dr. Patricia L. Cameron, Acting Vice Dean, 706-721-3279, E-mail: pcameron@georgiahealth.edu.
Website: http://www.gru.edu/mcg/bmb/students/

Georgia State University, College of Arts and Sciences, Department of Biology, Program in Cellular and Molecular Biology and Physiology, Atlanta, GA 30302-3083. Offers bioinformatics (MS); cellular and molecular biology and physiology (MS, PhD). Part-time programs available. Terminal master's awarded for partial completion of doctoral program. *Degree requirements:* For master's, comprehensive exam (for some programs), thesis optional; for doctorate, comprehensive exam, thesis/dissertation. *Entrance requirements:* For master's and doctorate, GRE. Additional exam requirements/recommendations for international students: Required—TOEFL (minimum score 550 paper-based; 82 iBT) or IELTS (minimum score 7). *Application deadline:* For fall admission, 7/1 priority date for domestic students, 6/1 priority date for international students; for spring admission, 11/15 priority date for domestic students, 10/15 priority date for international students. Applications are processed on a rolling basis. Application fee: $50. Electronic applications accepted. *Expenses: Tuition, area resident:* Full-time $4176; part-time $348 per credit hour. Tuition, state resident: full-time $14,544; part-time $1212 per credit hour. Tuition, nonresident: full-time $14,544; part-time $1212 per credit hour. Tuition and fees vary according to course load and program. *Financial support:* In 2013–14, fellowships with full tuition reimbursements (averaging $22,000 per year), research assistantships with full tuition reimbursements (averaging $20,000 per year) were awarded. Financial award application deadline: 12/3. *Faculty research:* Membrane transport, viral infection, molecular immunology, protein modeling, gene regulation. *Unit head:* Dr. Julia Hilliard, Professor, 404-413-6560, Fax: 404-413-5301, E-mail: jhilliard@gsu.edu. *Application contact:* LaTesha Warren, Graduate Coordinator, 404-413-5314, Fax: 404-413-5301, E-mail: lwarren@gsu.edu.
Website: http://biology.gsu.edu/

Grand Valley State University, College of Liberal Arts and Sciences, Program in Cell and Molecular Biology, Allendale, MI 49401-9403. Offers MS. *Entrance requirements:* For master's, minimum GPA of 3.0. *Faculty research:* Plant cell biology, plant development, cell/signal integration.

Harvard University, Graduate School of Arts and Sciences, Department of Molecular and Cellular Biology, Cambridge, MA 02138. Offers PhD. *Degree requirements:* For doctorate, thesis/dissertation, oral exam. *Entrance requirements:* For doctorate, GRE General Test, GRE Subject Test (recommended). Additional exam requirements/recommendations for international students: Required—TOEFL. *Expenses: Tuition:* Full-time $38,888. *Required fees:* $958. Tuition and fees vary according to campus/location, program and student level.

Harvard University, Graduate School of Arts and Sciences, Program in Chemical Biology, Cambridge, MA 02138. Offers PhD. *Expenses: Tuition:* Full-time $38,888. *Required fees:* $958. Tuition and fees vary according to campus/location, program and student level.

Hood College, Graduate School, Program in Biomedical Science, Frederick, MD 21701-8575. Offers biomedical science (MS), including biotechnology/molecular biology, microbiology/immunology/virology, regulatory compliance; regulatory compliance (Certificate). Part-time and evening/weekend programs available. *Faculty:* 3 full-time (1 woman), 14 part-time/adjunct (6 women). *Students:* 5 full-time (2 women), 91 part-time (57 women); includes 17 minority (10 Black or African American, non-Hispanic/Latino; 4 Asian, non-Hispanic/Latino; 2 Hispanic/Latino; 1 Two or more races, non-Hispanic/Latino), 6 international. Average age 31. 60 applicants, 52% accepted, 21 enrolled. In 2013, 12 master's, 4 other advanced degrees awarded. *Degree requirements:* For master's, comprehensive exam, thesis or alternative. *Entrance requirements:* For master's, bachelor's degree in biology; minimum GPA of 2.75; undergraduate course work in cell biology, chemistry, organic chemistry, and genetics. Additional exam requirements/recommendations for international students: Required—TOEFL (minimum score 575 paper-based; 89 iBT), IELTS (minimum score 6.5). *Application deadline:* For fall admission, 7/15 priority date for domestic students, 7/15 for international students; for spring admission, 12/1 priority date for domestic students, 12/1 for international students. Applications are processed on a rolling basis. Application fee: $35. Electronic applications accepted. Application fee is waived when completed online. *Expenses: Tuition:* Part-time $405 per credit. *Required fees:* $100 per semester. *Financial support:* In 2013–14, 3 students received support, including 3 research assistantships with full tuition reimbursements available (averaging $10,609 per year); tuition waivers (partial) and unspecified assistantships also available. Financial award applicants required to submit FAFSA. *Unit head:* Dr. Rachel Bagni, Director, 301-696-3650, Fax: 301-696-3597, E-mail: bagni@hood.edu. *Application contact:* Dr. Maria Green Cowles, Dean of Graduate School, 301-696-3811, Fax: 301-696-3597, E-mail: gofurther@hood.edu.
Website: http://www.hood.edu/graduate

Howard University, College of Medicine, Department of Biochemistry and Molecular Biology, Washington, DC 20059-0002. Offers biochemistry and molecular biology (PhD); biotechnology (MS); MD/PhD. Part-time programs available. *Degree requirements:* For master's, externship; for doctorate, comprehensive exam, thesis/dissertation. *Entrance requirements:* For master's and doctorate, GRE General Test, minimum GPA of 3.0. *Faculty research:* Cellular and molecular biology of olfaction, gene regulation and expression, enzymology, NMR spectroscopy of molecular structure, hormone regulation/metabolism.

Illinois Institute of Technology, Graduate College, College of Science and Letters, Department of Biological and Chemical Sciences, Biology Division, Chicago, IL 60616. Offers biochemistry (MBS, MS); biology (PhD); biotechnology (MBS, MS); cell and molecular biology (MBS, MS); microbiology (MB, MS); molecular biochemistry and biophysics (PhD); molecular biology and biophysics (MS). Part-time and evening/weekend programs available. Postbaccalaureate distance learning degree programs offered (minimal on-campus study). Terminal master's awarded for partial completion of doctoral program. *Degree requirements:* For master's, comprehensive exam, thesis (for some programs); for doctorate, comprehensive exam, thesis/dissertation. *Entrance requirements:* For master's, GRE General Test (minimum score 1000 Quantitative and Verbal, 2.5 Analytical Writing), minimum undergraduate GPA of 3.0; for doctorate, GRE General Test (minimum score 1200 Quantitative and Verbal, 3.0 Analytical Writing), minimum undergraduate GPA of 3.0. Additional exam requirements/recommendations for international students: Required—TOEFL (minimum score 523 paper-based; 70 iBT); Recommended—IELTS (minimum score 5.5). Electronic applications accepted. *Faculty research:* Structure and biophysics of macromolecular systems; efficacy and mechanism of action of chemopreventive agents in experimental carcinogenesis of breast, colon, lung and prostate; study of fundamental structural biochemistry problems that have direct links to the understanding and treatment of disease; spectroscopic techniques for the study of multi-domain proteins; molecular mechanisms of cancer and cancer gene therapy.

Illinois State University, Graduate School, College of Arts and Sciences, Department of Biological Sciences, Normal, IL 61790-2200. Offers animal behavior (MS); bacteriology (MS); biochemistry (MS); biological sciences (MS); biology (PhD); biophysics (MS); biotechnology (MS); botany (MS, PhD); cell biology (MS); conservation biology (MS); developmental biology (MS); ecology (MS, PhD); entomology (MS); evolutionary biology (MS); genetics (MS, PhD); immunology (MS); microbiology (MS, PhD); molecular biology (MS); molecular genetics (MS); neurobiology (MS); neuroscience (MS); parasitology (MS); physiology (MS, PhD); plant biology (MS); plant molecular biology (MS); plant sciences (MS); structural biology (MS); zoology (MS, PhD). Part-time programs available. *Degree requirements:* For master's, thesis or alternative; for doctorate, variable foreign language requirement, thesis/dissertation, 2 terms of residency. *Entrance requirements:* For master's, GRE General Test, minimum GPA of 2.6 in last 60 hours of course work; for doctorate, GRE General Test. *Faculty research:* Redoc balance and drug development in schistosoma mansoni, control of the growth of listeria monocytogenes at low temperature, regulation of cell expansion and microtubule function by SPRI, CRUI: physiology and fitness consequences of different life history phenotypes.

Indiana University Bloomington, University Graduate School, College of Arts and Sciences, Department of Biology, Bloomington, IN 47405. Offers biology teaching (MAT); biotechnology (MA); evolution, ecology, and behavior (MA, PhD); genetics (PhD); microbiology (MA, PhD); molecular, cellular, and developmental biology (PhD); plant sciences (MA, PhD); zoology (MA, PhD). *Faculty:* 58 full-time (15 women), 21 part-time/adjunct (6 women). *Students:* 166 full-time (94 women), 2 part-time (both women); includes 22 minority (8 Black or African American, non-Hispanic/Latino; 3 Asian, non-Hispanic/Latino; 10 Hispanic/Latino; 1 Two or more races, non-Hispanic/Latino), 47 international. Average age 27. 261 applicants, 23% accepted, 32 enrolled. In 2013, 17 master's, 20 doctorates awarded. Terminal master's awarded for partial completion of doctoral program. *Degree requirements:* For master's, thesis, oral defense; for doctorate, thesis/dissertation, oral defense. *Entrance requirements:* For master's and doctorate, GRE General Test. Additional exam requirements/recommendations for international students: Required—TOEFL (minimum score 100 iBT). *Application deadline:* For fall admission, 1/5 priority date for domestic students, 12/1 priority date for international students. Application fee: $55 ($65 for international students). Electronic applications accepted. *Financial support:* In 2013–14, fellowships with tuition reimbursements (averaging $24,000 per year), research assistantships with tuition reimbursements (averaging $21,000 per year), teaching assistantships with tuition reimbursements (averaging $22,000 per year) were awarded; scholarships/grants, traineeships, health care benefits, and unspecified assistantships also available. Financial award application deadline: 1/5. *Faculty research:* Evolution, ecology and behavior; microbiology; molecular biology and genetics; plant biology. *Unit head:* Dr. Clay Fuqua, Chair, 812-856-6005, Fax: 812-855-6082, E-mail: cfuqua@indiana.edu. *Application contact:* Tracey D. Stohr, Graduate Student Recruitment Coordinator, 812-856-6303, Fax: 812-855-6082, E-mail: gradbio@indiana.edu.
Website: http://www.bio.indiana.edu/

Indiana University–Purdue University Indianapolis, Indiana University School of Medicine, Department of Biochemistry and Molecular Biology, Indianapolis, IN 46202-2896. Offers PhD, MD/MS, MD/PhD. *Faculty:* 53 full-time (36 women). *Students:* 44 full-time (20 women), 9 part-time (6 women); includes 6 minority (1 Black or African American, non-Hispanic/Latino; 3 Asian, non-Hispanic/Latino; 2 Hispanic/Latino), 25 international. Average age 32. 3 applicants, 33% accepted. In 2013, 9 doctorates awarded. Terminal master's awarded for partial completion of doctoral program. *Degree requirements:* For doctorate, thesis/dissertation. *Entrance requirements:* For doctorate, GRE General Test, GRE Subject Test (recommended), previous course work in organic chemistry. *Application deadline:* For fall admission, 1/15 priority date for domestic students. Applications are processed on a rolling basis. Application fee: $55 ($65 for international students). *Financial support:* Fellowships with tuition reimbursements, research assistantships with tuition reimbursements, teaching assistantships, Federal Work-Study, institutionally sponsored loans, scholarships/grants, and tuition waivers (partial) available. Support available to part-time students. Financial award application deadline: 2/1. *Faculty research:* Metabolic regulation, enzymology, peptide and protein chemistry, cell biology, signal transduction. *Unit head:* Dr. Zhong-Yin Zhang, Chairman, 317-274-7151. *Application contact:* Director of Admissions, 317-274-3772, E-mail: inmedadm@iupui.edu.
Website: http://www.biochemistry.iu.edu/

Inter American University of Puerto Rico, Metropolitan Campus, Graduate Programs, Program in Medical Technology, San Juan, PR 00919-1293. Offers administration of clinical laboratories (MS); molecular microbiology (MS). *Accreditation:* NAACLS. Part-time programs available. *Degree requirements:* For master's, comprehensive exam. *Entrance requirements:* For master's, BS in medical technology, minimum GPA of 2.5. Electronic applications accepted.

Iowa State University of Science and Technology, Bioinformatics and Computational Biology Program, Ames, IA 50011. Offers MS, PhD. *Degree requirements:* For doctorate, thesis/dissertation. *Entrance requirements:* For master's and doctorate, GRE General Test. Additional exam requirements/recommendations for international students: Recommended—TOEFL, IELTS. Electronic applications accepted. *Faculty research:* Functional and structural genomics, genome evolution, macromolecular structure and function, mathematical biology and biological statistics, metabolic and developmental networks.

Iowa State University of Science and Technology, Program in Molecular, Cellular, and Developmental Biology, Ames, IA 50011. Offers MS, PhD. *Entrance requirements:* For master's and doctorate, GRE General Test. Additional exam requirements/recommendations for international students: Required—TOEFL (minimum score 580 paper-based; 85 iBT), IELTS (minimum score 7). Electronic applications accepted.

Johns Hopkins University, Bloomberg School of Public Health, Department of Biochemistry and Molecular Biology, Baltimore, MD 21205. Offers MHS, Sc M, PhD. Part-time programs available. *Faculty:* 16 full-time (3 women), 5 part-time/adjunct (3 women). *Students:* 76 full-time (51 women), 4 part-time (2 women); includes 40 minority (8 Black or African American, non-Hispanic/Latino; 18 Asian, non-Hispanic/Latino; 10 Hispanic/Latino; 4 Two or more races, non-Hispanic/Latino), 12 international. Average age 25. 96 applicants, 67% accepted, 38 enrolled. In 2013, 42 master's, 5 doctorates awarded. *Degree requirements:* For master's, thesis; for doctorate, comprehensive

exam, thesis/dissertation, oral and written exams. *Entrance requirements:* For master's, MCAT or GRE, 3 letters of recommendation, curriculum vitae; for doctorate, GRE General Test, 3 letters of recommendation, curriculum vitae. Additional exam requirements/recommendations for international students: Required—TOEFL (minimum score 600 paper-based). *Application deadline:* For fall admission, 12/15 priority date for domestic students, 12/15 for international students; for spring admission, 6/1 for domestic and international students. Applications are processed on a rolling basis. Application fee: $45. Electronic applications accepted. *Financial support:* Fellowships with tuition reimbursements, research assistantships with tuition reimbursements, teaching assistantships, Federal Work-Study, institutionally sponsored loans, scholarships/grants, health care benefits, and stipends available. Financial award application deadline: 3/15; financial award applicants required to submit FAFSA. *Faculty research:* DNA replication, repair, structure, carcinogenesis, protein structure, enzyme catalysts, reproductive biology. *Total annual research expenditures:* $6 million. *Unit head:* Dr. Pierre Coulombe, Chairman, 410-955-3671, Fax: 410-955-2926, E-mail: pcoulomb@jhsph.edu. *Application contact:* Sharon Gaston, Senior Academic Program Administrator, 410-955-3672, Fax: 410-955-2926, E-mail: sgaston@jhsph.edu.
Website: http://www.jhsph.edu/dept/bmb/

Johns Hopkins University, National Institutes of Health Sponsored Programs, Baltimore, MD 21218-2699. Offers biology (PhD), including biochemistry, biophysics, cell biology, developmental biology, genetic biology, molecular biology; cell, molecular, and developmental biology and biophysics (PhD). *Faculty:* 25 full-time (4 women). *Students:* 126 full-time (72 women); includes 36 minority (3 Black or African American, non-Hispanic/Latino; 1 American Indian or Alaska Native, non-Hispanic/Latino; 21 Asian, non-Hispanic/Latino; 11 Hispanic/Latino), 19 international. 282 applicants, 26% accepted, 36 enrolled. In 2013, 15 doctorates awarded. *Degree requirements:* For doctorate, comprehensive exam, thesis/dissertation. *Entrance requirements:* For doctorate, GRE General Test. Additional exam requirements/recommendations for international students: Required—TOEFL (minimum score 600 paper-based), TWE. *Application deadline:* For fall admission, 12/15 priority date for domestic students. Application fee: $60. Electronic applications accepted. *Financial support:* In 2013–14, 24 fellowships (averaging $23,000 per year), 93 research assistantships (averaging $23,000 per year), 22 teaching assistantships (averaging $23,000 per year) were awarded; Federal Work-Study, institutionally sponsored loans, scholarships/grants, traineeships, health care benefits, tuition waivers (partial), and unspecified assistantships also available. Financial award application deadline: 4/15; financial award applicants required to submit FAFSA. *Faculty research:* Protein and nucleic acid biochemistry and biophysical chemistry, molecular biology and development. *Total annual research expenditures:* $11.2 million. *Unit head:* Dr. Allen Shearn, Chair, 410-516-4693, Fax: 410-516-5213, E-mail: bio_cals@jhu.edu. *Application contact:* Joan Miller, Academic Affairs Manager, 410-516-5502, Fax: 410-516-5213, E-mail: joan@jhu.edu.

Johns Hopkins University, School of Medicine, Graduate Programs in Medicine, Department of Pharmacology and Molecular Sciences, Baltimore, MD 21205. Offers PhD. *Faculty:* 42 full-time (8 women). *Students:* 52 full-time (27 women); includes 15 minority (3 Black or African American, non-Hispanic/Latino; 9 Asian, non-Hispanic/Latino; 2 Hispanic/Latino; 1 Two or more races, non-Hispanic/Latino), 10 international. Average age 26. 76 applicants, 17% accepted, 9 enrolled. In 2013, 6 doctorates awarded. *Degree requirements:* For doctorate, comprehensive exam, thesis/dissertation, departmental seminar. *Entrance requirements:* For doctorate, GRE General Test. Additional exam requirements/recommendations for international students: Required—TOEFL. *Application deadline:* For fall admission, 1/10 for domestic and international students. Application fee: $85. Electronic applications accepted. *Unit head:* Dr. Philip A. Cole, Chairman, 410-614-0540, Fax: 410-614-7717, E-mail: pcole@jhmi.edu. *Application contact:* Dr. James T. Stivers, Director of Admissions, 410-955-7117, Fax: 410-955-3023, E-mail: jstivers@jhmi.edu.
Website: http://www.hopkinsmedicine.org/pharmacology/

Johns Hopkins University, School of Medicine, Graduate Programs in Medicine, Predoctoral Training Program in Human Genetics, Baltimore, MD 21218-2699. Offers PhD, MD/PhD. *Faculty:* 59 full-time (14 women). *Students:* 71 full-time (47 women); includes 15 minority (2 Black or African American, non-Hispanic/Latino; 6 Asian, non-Hispanic/Latino; 4 Hispanic/Latino; 3 Two or more races, non-Hispanic/Latino), 14 international. Average age 27. 64 applicants, 28% accepted, 11 enrolled. In 2013, 21 doctorates awarded. Terminal master's awarded for partial completion of doctoral program. *Degree requirements:* For doctorate, comprehensive exam, thesis/dissertation. *Entrance requirements:* For doctorate, GRE General Test, GRE Subject Test. Additional exam requirements/recommendations for international students: Recommended—TOEFL. *Application deadline:* For fall admission, 1/1 priority date for domestic and international students. Application fee: $85. Electronic applications accepted. *Financial support:* Fellowships, teaching assistantships, and health care benefits available. *Faculty research:* Human, mammalian, and molecular genetics, bioinformatics, genomics. *Unit head:* Dr. David Valle, Director, 410-955-4260, Fax: 410-955-7397, E-mail: muscelli@jhmi.edu. *Application contact:* Sandy Muscelli, Administrator, 410-955-4260, Fax: 410-955-7397, E-mail: muscelli@jhmi.edu.
Website: http://humangenetics.jhmi.edu/

Johns Hopkins University, School of Medicine, Graduate Programs in Medicine, Program in Biochemistry, Cellular and Molecular Biology, Baltimore, MD 21205. Offers PhD. *Faculty:* 101 full-time (35 women). *Students:* 128 full-time (67 women); includes 30 minority (9 Black or African American, non-Hispanic/Latino; 1 American Indian or Alaska Native, non-Hispanic/Latino; 11 Asian, non-Hispanic/Latino; 8 Hispanic/Latino; 1 Two or more races, non-Hispanic/Latino), 36 international. Average age 26. 118 applicants, 31% accepted, 19 enrolled. In 2013, 23 doctorates awarded. *Degree requirements:* For doctorate, comprehensive exam, thesis/dissertation. *Entrance requirements:* For doctorate, GRE General Test. Additional exam requirements/recommendations for international students: Required—TOEFL. *Application deadline:* For winter admission, 1/10 for domestic and international students. Applications are processed on a rolling basis. Application fee: $80. Electronic applications accepted. *Financial support:* Fellowships, research assistantships, traineeships, and tuition waivers (full) available. Financial award application deadline: 12/31. *Faculty research:* Developmental biology, genomics/proteomics, protein targeting, signal transduction, structural biology. *Unit head:* Dr. Carolyn Machamer, Director, 410-955-3466, Fax: 410-614-8842, E-mail: machamer@jhmi.edu. *Application contact:* Dr. Jeff Corden, Admissions Director, 410-955-3506, Fax: 410-614-8842, E-mail: jcorden@jhmi.edu.
Website: http://bcmb.bs.jhmi.edu/Pages/default.aspx

Kent State University, School of Biomedical Sciences, Program in Cellular and Molecular Biology, Kent, OH 44242-0001. Offers MS, PhD. Offered in cooperation with Northeastern Ohio Universities College of Medicine. Terminal master's awarded for partial completion of doctoral program. *Degree requirements:* For master's, thesis; for doctorate, thesis/dissertation. *Entrance requirements:* For master's, GRE General Test, letter of recommendation, minimum GPA of 3.0; for doctorate, GRE General Test, letter of recommendation, minimum GPA of 3.0, MS. Additional exam requirements/recommendations for international students: Required—TOEFL. Electronic applications accepted. *Faculty research:* Molecular genetics, molecular endocrinology, virology and tumor biology, P450 enzymology and catalysis, membrane structure and function.

Lehigh University, College of Arts and Sciences, Department of Biological Sciences, Bethlehem, PA 18015. Offers biochemistry (PhD); cell and molecular biology (PhD); integrative biology and neuroscience (PhD); molecular biology (MS). Part-time programs available. Postbaccalaureate distance learning degree programs offered (no on-campus study). *Faculty:* 18 full-time (9 women). *Students:* 38 full-time (20 women), 30 part-time (23 women); includes 8 minority (4 Black or African American, non-Hispanic/Latino; 2 Asian, non-Hispanic/Latino; 2 Hispanic/Latino), 5 international. Average age 29. 54 applicants, 41% accepted, 11 enrolled. In 2013, 8 master's, 5 doctorates awarded. Terminal master's awarded for partial completion of doctoral program. *Degree requirements:* For master's, research report; for doctorate, comprehensive exam, thesis/dissertation. *Entrance requirements:* For doctorate, GRE General Test. Additional exam requirements/recommendations for international students: Required—TOEFL. *Application deadline:* For fall admission, 12/15 for domestic and international students. Applications are processed on a rolling basis. Application fee: $75. Electronic applications accepted. *Financial support:* In 2013–14, 2 fellowships with full tuition reimbursements (averaging $24,500 per year), 8 research assistantships with full tuition reimbursements (averaging $23,750 per year), 20 teaching assistantships with full tuition reimbursements (averaging $23,750 per year) were awarded; scholarships/grants and unspecified assistantships also available. Financial award application deadline: 12/15. *Faculty research:* Gene expression, cytoskeleton and cell structure, cell cycle and growth regulation, neuroscience, animal behavior, microbiology. *Total annual research expenditures:* $1.7 million. *Unit head:* Dr. Murray Itzkowitz, Chairperson, 610-758-3680, Fax: 610-758-4004, E-mail: mi00@lehigh.edu. *Application contact:* Dr. Mary Kathryn Iovine, Graduate Coordinator, 610-758-6981, Fax: 610-758-4004, E-mail: mki3@lehigh.edu.
Website: http://www.lehigh.edu/~inbios/

Lipscomb University, Program in Biomolecular Science, Nashville, TN 37204-3951. Offers MS. Part-time and evening/weekend programs available. *Faculty:* 4 full-time (3 women). *Students:* 21 full-time (14 women), 1 (woman) part-time; includes 9 minority (4 Black or African American, non-Hispanic/Latino; 4 Asian, non-Hispanic/Latino; 1 Two or more races, non-Hispanic/Latino). Average age 24. 9 applicants, 89% accepted, 8 enrolled. In 2013, 7 master's awarded. *Degree requirements:* For master's, capstone project. *Entrance requirements:* For master's, GRE (minimum of 300/1000 on prior scoring system), MCAT (minimum of 24), DAT (minimum of 17), BS in related field, transcripts, minimum undergraduate GPA of 3.0, 2 letters of recommendation, resume. Additional exam requirements/recommendations for international students: Required—TOEFL (minimum score 570 paper-based). *Application deadline:* For fall admission, 8/1 for domestic students; for winter admission, 12/14 for domestic students; for spring admission, 5/14 for domestic students. Applications are processed on a rolling basis. Application fee: $50 ($75 for international students). Electronic applications accepted. *Expenses: Tuition:* Full-time $15,570; part-time $865 per credit hour. Tuition and fees vary according to degree level and program. *Financial support:* Teaching assistantships and unspecified assistantships available. Financial award applicants required to submit FAFSA. *Unit head:* Dr. Kent Gallaher, Director, 615-966-5721, E-mail: kent.gallaher@lipscomb.edu. *Application contact:* Waleska Rehbein, Administrative Assistant, 615-966-5330, E-mail: waleska.rehbein@lipscomb.edu.
Website: http://www.lipscomb.edu/biology/Graduate-Program

Louisiana State University Health Sciences Center at Shreveport, Department of Biochemistry and Molecular Biology, Shreveport, LA 71130-3932. Offers MS, PhD, MD/PhD. *Faculty:* 13 full-time (2 women), 3 part-time/adjunct (1 woman). *Students:* 17 full-time (9 women); includes 10 minority (all Asian, non-Hispanic/Latino), 12 international. Average age 26. 16 applicants, 13% accepted, 2 enrolled. In 2013, 1 master's, 2 doctorates awarded. *Degree requirements:* For master's, thesis; for doctorate, thesis/dissertation. *Entrance requirements:* For master's and doctorate, GRE General Test. Additional exam requirements/recommendations for international students: Required—TOEFL. *Application deadline:* For fall admission, 1/15 priority date for domestic students, 1/15 for international students. Applications are processed on a rolling basis. *Financial support:* In 2013–14, 4 fellowships (averaging $28,000 per year), 13 research assistantships (averaging $26,000 per year) were awarded. *Faculty research:* Metabolite transport, regulation of translation and transcription, prokaryotic molecular genetics, cell matrix biochemistry, yeast molecular genetics, oncogenes, prostate cancer, oxalate nephrotoxicity. *Unit head:* Dr. Hari K. Koul, Head, 318-675-5160, Fax: 318-675-5180. *Application contact:* Sandra Darby, Coordinator, 318-675-5160, Fax: 318-675-5180, E-mail: sdarb4@lsuhsc.edu.
Website: http://www.shrevebiochem.com

Louisiana Tech University, Graduate School, College of Applied and Natural Sciences, School of Biological Sciences, Ruston, LA 71272. Offers biology (MS); molecular sciences and nanotechnology (MS). Part-time programs available. *Degree requirements:* For master's, thesis or alternative. *Entrance requirements:* For master's, GRE General Test, GRE Subject Test. *Application deadline:* For fall admission, 7/29 priority date for domestic students; for spring admission, 2/3 for domestic students. Applications are processed on a rolling basis. Application fee: $20 ($30 for international students). *Financial support:* Fellowships, research assistantships, and teaching assistantships available. Financial award application deadline: 2/1. *Faculty research:* Genetics, animal biology, plant biology, physiology biocontrol. *Unit head:* Dr. William Campbell, Director, 318-257-4573, Fax: 318-257-5060, E-mail: campbell@latech.edu.
Website: http://ans.latech.edu/bls.html

Loyola University Chicago, Graduate School, Program in Molecular Biology, Maywood, IL 60153. Offers MS, PhD. *Faculty:* 28 full-time (5 women). *Students:* 13 full-time (9 women); includes 2 minority (both Two or more races, non-Hispanic/Latino), 3 international. Average age 27. 21 applicants, 19% accepted, 3 enrolled. In 2013, 1 master's, 2 doctorates awarded. Terminal master's awarded for partial completion of doctoral program. *Degree requirements:* For master's, comprehensive exam (for some programs), thesis; for doctorate, comprehensive exam, thesis/dissertation, 48 credit hours. *Entrance requirements:* For master's, GRE General Test, statement of purpose, transcripts, 3 letters of recommendation; for doctorate, GRE General Test, 3 letters of recommendation. Additional exam requirements/recommendations for international students: Required—TOEFL (minimum score 600 paper-based). *Application deadline:* For fall admission, 3/1 for domestic and international students. Applications are processed on a rolling basis. Application fee: $40. Electronic applications accepted. *Expenses: Tuition:* Full-time $16,740; part-time $930 per credit. *Required fees:* $135 per semester. *Financial support:* In 2013–14, 7 students received support, including fellowships (averaging $23,000 per year); research assistantships, Federal Work-Study, institutionally sponsored loans, scholarships/grants, and health care benefits also available. Financial award application deadline: 2/15; financial award applicants required to submit FAFSA. *Faculty research:* Cell cycle regulation, molecular immunology, molecular genetics, molecular oncology, molecular virology. *Total annual research expenditures:* $3,500. *Unit head:* Dr. Manuel O. Diaz, Director, 708-327-3172, Fax: 708-216-6505, E-mail: mdiaz@luc.edu. *Application contact:* Dr. Mitchell Denning, Graduate Program Director, 708-327-3358, E-mail: mdennin@lumc.edu.
Website: http://www.luc.edu/biomed

Molecular Biology

Marquette University, Graduate School, College of Arts and Sciences, Department of Biology, Milwaukee, WI 53201-1881. Offers cell biology (MS, PhD); developmental biology (MS, PhD); ecology (MS, PhD); epithelial physiology (MS, PhD); genetics (MS, PhD); microbiology (MS, PhD); molecular biology (MS, PhD); muscle and exercise physiology (MS, PhD); neuroscience (PhD). *Faculty:* 21 full-time (9 women), 3 part-time/adjunct (0 women). *Students:* 34 full-time (16 women), 4 part-time (1 woman), 15 international. Average age 27. 70 applicants, 23% accepted, 5 enrolled. In 2013, 1 master's, 6 doctorates awarded. Terminal master's awarded for partial completion of doctoral program. *Degree requirements:* For master's, comprehensive exam, thesis, 1 year of teaching experience or equivalent; for doctorate, thesis/dissertation, 1 year of teaching experience or equivalent, qualifying exam. *Entrance requirements:* For master's and doctorate, GRE General Test, GRE Subject Test, official transcripts from all current and previous colleges/universities except Marquette, statement of professional goals and aspirations, three letters of recommendation. Additional exam requirements/recommendations for international students: Required—TOEFL (minimum score 530 paper-based). *Application deadline:* For fall admission, 12/15 for domestic and international students. Application fee: $50. Electronic applications accepted. *Financial support:* In 2013–14, 39 students received support, including 6 fellowships (averaging $1,208 per year), 4 research assistantships with full tuition reimbursements available (averaging $21,750 per year), 29 teaching assistantships with full tuition reimbursements available (averaging $21,750 per year); scholarships/grants, health care benefits, tuition waivers (full and partial), and unspecified assistantships also available. Support available to part-time students. Financial award application deadline: 2/15. *Faculty research:* Neurobiology, neuroendocrinology, epithelial physiology, neuropeptide interactions, synaptic transmission. *Total annual research expenditures:* $1.5 million. *Unit head:* Dr. Dale Noel, Chair and Professor, 414-288-1748. *Application contact:* Dr. Michelle Mynlieff, Professor, 414-288-1467.
Website: http://www.marquette.edu/biology/

Massachusetts Institute of Technology, School of Science, Department of Biology, Cambridge, MA 02139-4307. Offers biochemistry (PhD); biological oceanography (PhD); biology (PhD); biophysical chemistry and molecular structure (PhD); cell biology (PhD); computational and systems biology (PhD); developmental biology (PhD); genetics (PhD); immunology (PhD); microbiology (PhD); molecular biology (PhD); neurobiology (PhD). *Faculty:* 58 full-time (15 women). *Students:* 261 full-time (133 women); includes 77 minority (3 Black or African American, non-Hispanic/Latino; 1 American Indian or Alaska Native, non-Hispanic/Latino; 32 Asian, non-Hispanic/Latino; 32 Hispanic/Latino; 9 Two or more races, non-Hispanic/Latino), 46 international. Average age 26. 651 applicants, 15% accepted, 39 enrolled. In 2013, 25 doctorates awarded. *Degree requirements:* For doctorate, comprehensive exam, thesis/dissertation, two semesters as a teaching assistant. *Entrance requirements:* For doctorate, GRE General Test. Additional exam requirements/recommendations for international students: Required—TOEFL (minimum score 577 paper-based), IELTS (minimum score 6.5). *Application deadline:* For fall admission, 12/1 for domestic and international students. Application fee: $75. Electronic applications accepted. *Expenses: Tuition:* Full-time $43,210; part-time $670 per credit hour. *Required fees:* $288. *Financial support:* In 2013–14, 252 students received support, including 135 fellowships (averaging $36,800 per year), 122 research assistantships (averaging $35,500 per year), 1 teaching assistantship; Federal Work-Study, institutionally sponsored loans, scholarships/grants, traineeships, health care benefits, and unspecified assistantships also available. *Faculty research:* Cellular, developmental and molecular (plant and animal) biology; biochemistry, bioengineering, biophysics and structural biology; classical and molecular genetics, stem cell and epigenetics; immunology and microbiology; cancer biology, molecular medicine, neurobiology and human disease; computational and systems biology. *Total annual research expenditures:* $44.5 million. *Unit head:* Alan Grossman, Interim Head, 617-253-4701. *Application contact:* Biology Education Office, 617-253-3717, Fax: 617-258-9329, E-mail: gradbio@mit.edu.
Website: https://biology.mit.edu/

Mayo Graduate School, Graduate Programs in Biomedical Sciences, Programs in Biochemistry, Structural Biology, Cell Biology, and Genetics, Rochester, MN 55905. Offers biochemistry and structural biology (PhD); cell biology and genetics (PhD); molecular biology (PhD). *Degree requirements:* For doctorate, oral defense of dissertation, qualifying oral and written exam. *Entrance requirements:* For doctorate, GRE, 1 year of chemistry, biology, calculus, and physics. Additional exam requirements/recommendations for international students: Required—TOEFL. Electronic applications accepted. *Faculty research:* Gene structure and function, membranes and receptors/cytoskeleton, oncogenes and growth factors, protein structure and function, steroid hormonal action.

McMaster University, Faculty of Health Sciences and School of Graduate Studies, Program in Medical Sciences, Hamilton, ON L8S 4M2, Canada. Offers blood and vascular (M Sc, PhD); genetics and cancer (M Sc, PhD); immunity and infection (M Sc, PhD); metabolism and nutrition (M Sc, PhD); neurosciences and behavioral sciences (M Sc, PhD); physiology/pharmacology (M Sc, PhD); MD/PhD. *Degree requirements:* For master's, thesis; for doctorate, comprehensive exam, thesis/dissertation. *Entrance requirements:* For master's, honors B Sc, B+ average in related field; for doctorate, M Sc, minimum B+ average. Additional exam requirements/recommendations for international students: Required—TOEFL (minimum score 580 paper-based; 92 iBT).

Medical University of South Carolina, College of Graduate Studies, Department of Biochemistry and Molecular Biology, Charleston, SC 29425. Offers MS, PhD, MD/PhD. Terminal master's awarded for partial completion of doctoral program. *Degree requirements:* For master's, thesis, oral exam/thesis defense; for doctorate, thesis/dissertation, oral and written exams/dissertation defense. *Entrance requirements:* For master's, GRE General Test; for doctorate, GRE General Test, interview, minimum GPA of 3.0. Additional exam requirements/recommendations for international students: Required—TOEFL (minimum score 600 paper-based; 100 iBT). Electronic applications accepted. *Faculty research:* Lipid biochemistry, DNA replication, nucleic acids, protein structure.

Medical University of South Carolina, College of Graduate Studies, Program in Molecular and Cellular Biology and Pathobiology, Charleston, SC 29425. Offers cancer biology (PhD); cardiovascular biology (PhD); cardiovascular imaging (PhD); cell regulation (PhD); craniofacial biology (PhD); genetics and development (PhD); marine biomedicine (PhD); DMD/PhD; MD/PhD. *Degree requirements:* For doctorate, thesis/dissertation, oral and written exams. *Entrance requirements:* For doctorate, GRE General Test, interview, minimum GPA of 3.0. Additional exam requirements/recommendations for international students: Required—TOEFL (minimum score 600 paper-based; 100 iBT). Electronic applications accepted.

Miami University, College of Arts and Science, Department of Biology, Oxford, OH 45056. Offers biological sciences (MAT); biology (MS, PhD); botany (MAT, MS, PhD); cell, molecular and structural biology (MS, PhD); ecology, evolution and environmental biology (PhD); zoology (MA, MS, PhD). Part-time programs available. Postbaccalaureate distance learning degree programs offered. *Students:* 89 full-time (49 women), 612 part-time (502 women); includes 63 minority (9 Black or African American, non-Hispanic/Latino; 2 American Indian or Alaska Native, non-Hispanic/Latino; 6 Asian, non-Hispanic/Latino; 27 Hispanic/Latino; 1 Native Hawaiian or other Pacific Islander, non-Hispanic/Latino; 18 Two or more races, non-Hispanic/Latino), 35 international. Average age 34. In 2013, 133 master's, 4 doctorates awarded. *Entrance requirements:* For master's and doctorate, GRE General Test. Additional exam requirements/recommendations for international students: Recommended—TOEFL (minimum score 80 iBT), IELTS (minimum score 6.5), TSE (minimum score 54). *Application deadline:* For fall admission, 1/15 for domestic and international students. Application fee: $50. Electronic applications accepted. *Expenses:* Tuition, state resident: full-time $12,634; part-time $526 per credit hour. Tuition, nonresident: full-time $27,892; part-time $1162 per credit hour. Part-time tuition and fees vary according to course load, campus/location and program. *Financial support:* Fellowships with full tuition reimbursements, research assistantships with full tuition reimbursements, teaching assistantships with full tuition reimbursements, Federal Work-Study, health care benefits, tuition waivers (full), and unspecified assistantships available. Financial award application deadline: 1/15; financial award applicants required to submit FAFSA. *Unit head:* Dr. Douglas Meikle, Chair, 513-529-3103, E-mail: meikled@miamioh.edu.
Website: http://miamioh.edu/cas/about/biology

Michigan State University, The Graduate School, College of Agriculture and Natural Resources, MSU-DOE Plant Research Laboratory, East Lansing, MI 48824. Offers biochemistry and molecular biology (PhD); cellular and molecular biology (PhD); crop and soil sciences (PhD); genetics (PhD); microbiology and molecular genetics (PhD); plant biology (PhD); plant physiology (PhD). Offered jointly with the Department of Energy. *Degree requirements:* For doctorate, comprehensive exam, thesis/dissertation, laboratory rotation, defense of dissertation. *Entrance requirements:* For doctorate, GRE General Test, acceptance into one of the affiliated department programs; 3 letters of recommendation; bachelor's degree or equivalent in life sciences, chemistry, biochemistry, or biophysics; research experience. Electronic applications accepted. *Faculty research:* Role of hormones in the regulation of plant development and physiology, molecular mechanisms associated with signal recognition, development and application of genetic methods and materials, protein routing and function.

Michigan State University, The Graduate School, College of Natural Science and Graduate Programs in Human Medicine and Graduate Studies in Osteopathic Medicine, Department of Biochemistry and Molecular Biology, East Lansing, MI 48824. Offers biochemistry and molecular biology (MS, PhD); biochemistry and molecular biology/environmental toxicology (PhD). *Entrance requirements:* Additional exam requirements/recommendations for international students: Required—TOEFL. Electronic applications accepted.

Michigan State University, The Graduate School, College of Natural Science, Program in Cell and Molecular Biology, East Lansing, MI 48824. Offers cell and molecular biology (MS, PhD); cell and molecular biology/environmental toxicology (PhD). *Entrance requirements:* Additional exam requirements/recommendations for international students: Required—TOEFL. Electronic applications accepted.

Michigan Technological University, Graduate School, Interdisciplinary Programs, Houghton, MI 49931. Offers atmospheric sciences (PhD); biochemistry and molecular biology (PhD); computational science and engineering (PhD); environmental engineering (PhD). *Degree requirements:* For doctorate, comprehensive exam, thesis/dissertation. *Entrance requirements:* For doctorate, GRE, statement of purpose, official transcripts, 3 letters of recommendation. Additional exam requirements/recommendations for international students: Required—TOEFL or IELTS.

Middle Tennessee State University, College of Graduate Studies, College of Basic and Applied Sciences, Interdisciplinary Program in Molecular Biosciences, Murfreesboro, TN 37132. Offers PhD. *Students:* 8 full-time (4 women), 18 part-time (10 women); includes 12 minority (2 Black or African American, non-Hispanic/Latino; 1 American Indian or Alaska Native, non-Hispanic/Latino; 6 Asian, non-Hispanic/Latino; 1 Hispanic/Latino; 2 Two or more races, non-Hispanic/Latino). 20 applicants, 85% accepted. *Unit head:* Dr. Robert W. Fischer, Jr., Dean, 615-898-2613, Fax: 615-898-2615, E-mail: bud.fischer@mtsu.edu. *Application contact:* Dr. Michael D. Allen, Vice Provost for Research/Dean, 615-898-2840, Fax: 615-904-8020, E-mail: michael.allen@mtsu.edu.

Mississippi State University, College of Agriculture and Life Sciences, Department of Biochemistry, Molecular Biology, Entomology and Plant Pathology, Mississippi State, MS 39762. Offers agriculture life sciences (MS), including biochemistry (MS, PhD), entomology (MS, PhD), plant pathology (MS, PhD); life science (PhD), including biochemistry (MS, PhD), entomology (MS, PhD), plant pathology (MS, PhD); molecular biology (PhD). *Faculty:* 23 full-time (1 woman). *Students:* 43 full-time (16 women), 17 part-time (10 women); includes 5 minority (4 Black or African American, non-Hispanic/Latino; 1 Hispanic/Latino), 14 international. Average age 29. 62 applicants, 18% accepted, 10 enrolled. In 2013, 11 master's, 4 doctorates awarded. Terminal master's awarded for partial completion of doctoral program. *Degree requirements:* For master's, thesis (for some programs), final oral exam; for doctorate, thesis/dissertation, preliminary oral and written exam. *Entrance requirements:* For master's, GRE General Test, minimum GPA of 2.75; for doctorate, GRE. Additional exam requirements/recommendations for international students: Required—TOEFL (minimum score 500 paper-based; 61 iBT); Recommended—IELTS (minimum score 5.5). *Application deadline:* For fall admission, 7/1 for domestic students, 5/1 for international students; for spring admission, 11/1 for domestic students, 9/1 for international students. Applications are processed on a rolling basis. Application fee: $60. Electronic applications accepted. *Financial support:* In 2013–14, 35 research assistantships with full tuition reimbursements (averaging $16,388 per year) were awarded; Federal Work-Study, institutionally sponsored loans, and unspecified assistantships also available. Financial award application deadline: 4/1; financial award applicants required to submit FAFSA. *Faculty research:* Fish nutrition, plant and animal molecular biology, plant biochemistry, enzymology, lipid metabolism, chromatin, cell wall synthesis in rice, a model grass bioenergy species and the source of rice stover residues using reverse genetic and functional genomic and proteomic approaches. *Unit head:* Dr. Scott T. Willard, Professor and Department Head, 662-325-2640, Fax: 662-325-8664, E-mail: swilliard@ads.msstate.edu. *Application contact:* Dr. Din-Pow Ma, Professor/Graduate Coordinator, 662-325-7739, Fax: 662-325-8664, E-mail: dm1@ra.msstate.edu.
Website: http://www.biochemistry.msstate.edu

Missouri State University, Graduate College, College of Health and Human Services, Department of Biomedical Sciences, Program in Cell and Molecular Biology, Springfield, MO 65897. Offers MS. Part-time programs available. *Students:* 10 full-time (7 women), 11 part-time (6 women); includes 1 minority (Two or more races, non-Hispanic/Latino), 3 international. Average age 24. 13 applicants, 85% accepted, 8 enrolled. In 2013, 6 master's awarded. *Degree requirements:* For master's, thesis or alternative, oral and written exams. *Entrance requirements:* For master's, GRE General Test, 2 semesters of course work in organic chemistry and physics, 1 semester of course work in calculus, minimum GPA of 3.0 in last 60 hours of course work. Additional exam requirements/recommendations for international students: Required—TOEFL (minimum score 550 paper-based; 79 iBT). *Application deadline:* For fall admission, 7/20 priority date for domestic students, 5/1 for international students; for spring admission, 12/20 priority date for domestic students, 9/1 for international students. Applications are processed on a rolling basis. Application fee: $35 ($50 for international students). Electronic applications accepted. *Expenses:* Tuition, state resident: full-time $4500; part-time $250

per credit hour. Tuition, nonresident: full-time $9018; part-time $501 per credit hour. *Required fees:* $361 per semester. Tuition and fees vary according to course level, course load and program. *Financial support:* In 2013–14, 15 teaching assistantships with full tuition reimbursements (averaging $8,324 per year) were awarded; career-related internships or fieldwork, Federal Work-Study, institutionally sponsored loans, scholarships/grants, and unspecified assistantships also available. Support available to part-time students. Financial award application deadline: 3/31; financial award applicants required to submit FAFSA. *Faculty research:* Extracellular matrix membrane protein, P2 nucleotide receptors, double stranded RNA viruses. *Unit head:* Dr. Scott Zimmernan, Program Director, 417-836-5478, Fax: 417-836-5588, E-mail: scottzimmerman@missouristate.edu. *Application contact:* Misty Stewart, Coordinator of Graduate Admissions and Recruitment, 417-836-6079, Fax: 417-836-6200, E-mail: mistystewart@missouristate.edu.
Website: http://www.missouristate.edu/bms/CMB/

Montclair State University, The Graduate School, College of Science and Mathematics, Department of Biology and Molecular Biology, Montclair, NJ 07043-1624. Offers biology (MS), including biological science education, biology, ecology and evolution, physiology; molecular biology (MS, Certificate). Part-time and evening/weekend programs available. *Degree requirements:* For master's, comprehensive exam, thesis or alternative. *Entrance requirements:* For master's, GRE General Test, 24 credits of course work in undergraduate biology, 2 letters of recommendation, teaching certificate (biology sciences education concentration); for Certificate, 2 letters of recommendation, essay. Additional exam requirements/recommendations for international students: Required—TOEFL (minimum score 83 iBT) or IELTS. Electronic applications accepted. *Faculty research:* Ecosystem biology, molecular biology, signal transduction, neuroscience, aquatic and coastal biology.

New Mexico State University, Graduate School, Program in Molecular Biology, Las Cruces, NM 88003-8001. Offers MS, PhD. *Students:* 14 full-time (8 women), 4 part-time (3 women); includes 2 minority (both Hispanic/Latino), 7 international. Average age 30. 3 applicants. In 2013, 2 master's, 2 doctorates awarded. *Degree requirements:* For master's, thesis, oral seminars; for doctorate, comprehensive exam, thesis/dissertation, oral seminars. *Entrance requirements:* For master's and doctorate, GRE General Test, minimum GPA of 3.3. Additional exam requirements/recommendations for international students: Required—TOEFL (minimum score 550 paper-based; 79 iBT), IELTS (minimum score 6.5). *Application deadline:* For fall admission, 12/15 for domestic and international students; for spring admission, 1/15 for domestic and international students. Applications are processed on a rolling basis. Application fee: $40 ($50 for international students). Electronic applications accepted. *Expenses:* Tuition, state resident: full-time $5398; part-time $224.90 per credit. Tuition, nonresident: full-time $18,821; part-time $784.20 per credit. *Required fees:* $1310; $54.60 per credit. *Financial support:* In 2013–14, 12 students received support, including 1 fellowship (averaging $4,050 per year), 2 research assistantships (averaging $17,069 per year), 9 teaching assistantships (averaging $15,334 per year); career-related internships or fieldwork, Federal Work-Study, scholarships/grants, health care benefits, and unspecified assistantships also available. Financial award application deadline: 2/1. *Faculty research:* Emerging pathogens, plant-molecular biology and virology, molecular symbiotic interactions, cell and organismal biology, applied and environmental microbiology. *Unit head:* Dr. Charles Brad Shuster, Director, 575-646-1325, Fax: 575-646-8087, E-mail: cshuster@nmsu.edu. *Application contact:* Nancy McDow, Program Secretary, 575-646-3437, Fax: 575-646-5170, E-mail: nancyt@nmsu.edu.
Website: http://molb.research.nmsu.edu

New York Medical College, Graduate School of Basic Medical Sciences, Biochemistry and Molecular Biology Master's Program, Valhalla, NY 10595-1691. Offers MS, PhD, MD/PhD. Part-time and evening/weekend programs available. *Faculty:* 10 full-time (4 women), 2 part-time/adjunct (0 women). *Students:* 5 full-time (1 woman); includes 3 minority (2 Asian, non-Hispanic/Latino; 1 Hispanic/Latino). Average age 25. 8 applicants, 100% accepted, 4 enrolled. In 2013, 4 master's awarded. Terminal master's awarded for partial completion of doctoral program. *Degree requirements:* For master's, thesis; for doctorate, comprehensive exam, thesis/dissertation. *Entrance requirements:* For master's, GRE General Test, MCAT, or DAT. Additional exam requirements/recommendations for international students: Required—TOEFL. *Application deadline:* For fall admission, 7/1 priority date for domestic students, 5/1 priority date for international students; for spring admission, 12/1 for domestic students, 10/1 for international students. Applications are processed on a rolling basis. Application fee: $75 ($100 for international students). Electronic applications accepted. *Expenses: Tuition:* Full-time $49,170; part-time $910 per credit. Tuition and fees vary according to program. *Financial support:* Federal Work-Study and scholarships/grants available. Support available to part-time students. Financial award applicants required to submit FAFSA. *Faculty research:* Expression, mechanisms of hormone action and cell signaling, enzymology, mechanisms of DNA replication and repair, cell cycle regulation, control of cell growth, molecular biology of cancer cells and the cancer process, mechanisms of nutrition and cancer prevention, molecular neurobiology and studies of neurodegenerative disorders, the aging process. *Unit head:* Dr. Joseph Wu, Program Director, 914-594-4891, Fax: 914-594-4944, E-mail: joseph_wu@nymc.edu. *Application contact:* Valerie Romeo-Messana, Director of Admissions, 914-594-4110, Fax: 914-594-4944, E-mail: v_romeomessana@nymc.edu.

New York Medical College, Graduate School of Basic Medical Sciences, Integrated PhD Program, Valhalla, NY 10595-1691. Offers biochemistry and molecular biology (PhD); cell biology and anatomy (PhD); microbiology and immunology (PhD); pathology (PhD); pharmacology (PhD); physiology (PhD). *Faculty:* 91 full-time (16 women), 5 part-time/adjunct (2 women). *Students:* 31 full-time (21 women); includes 17 minority (4 Black or African American, non-Hispanic/Latino; 11 Asian, non-Hispanic/Latino; 2 Hispanic/Latino). Average age 27. 56 applicants, 36% accepted, 9 enrolled. In 2013, 17 doctorates awarded. *Degree requirements:* For doctorate, comprehensive exam, thesis/dissertation. *Entrance requirements:* For doctorate, GRE General Test. Additional exam requirements/recommendations for international students: Required—TOEFL. *Application deadline:* For fall admission, 1/1 priority date for domestic and international students. Applications are processed on a rolling basis. Application fee: $75 ($100 for international students). Electronic applications accepted. *Expenses: Tuition:* Full-time $49,170; part-time $910 per credit. Tuition and fees vary according to program. *Financial support:* In 2013–14, fellowships with full tuition reimbursements (averaging $25,500 per year), research assistantships with full tuition reimbursements (averaging $25,500 per year) were awarded; Federal Work-Study, scholarships/grants, traineeships, health care benefits, and tuition waivers (full) also available. Financial award applicants required to submit FAFSA. *Faculty research:* Cardiovascular sciences, infectious diseases, neuroscience, cancer and cell signaling. *Unit head:* Dr. Francis L. Belloni, Dean, 914-594-4110, Fax: 914-594-4944, E-mail: francis_belloni@nymc.edu. *Application contact:* Valerie Romeo-Messana, Director of Admissions, 914-594-4110, Fax: 914-594-4944, E-mail: v_romeomessana@nymc.edu.

New York University, Graduate School of Arts and Science, Department of Biology, New York, NY 10012-1019. Offers biology (PhD); biomedical journalism (MS); cancer and molecular biology (PhD); computational biology (PhD); computers in biological research (MS); developmental genetics (PhD); general biology (MS); immunology and microbiology (PhD); molecular genetics (PhD); neurobiology (PhD); oral biology (MS); plant biology (PhD); recombinant DNA technology (MS); MS/MBA. Part-time programs available. *Faculty:* 24 full-time (5 women). *Students:* 161 full-time (88 women), 28 part-time (15 women); includes 41 minority (5 Black or African American, non-Hispanic/Latino; 23 Asian, non-Hispanic/Latino; 9 Hispanic/Latino; 4 Two or more races, non-Hispanic/Latino), 80 international. Average age 27. 412 applicants, 54% accepted, 65 enrolled. In 2013, 77 master's, 9 doctorates awarded. Terminal master's awarded for partial completion of doctoral program. *Degree requirements:* For master's, thesis or alternative, qualifying paper; for doctorate, comprehensive exam, thesis/dissertation. *Entrance requirements:* For master's and doctorate, GRE General Test. Additional exam requirements/recommendations for international students: Required—TOEFL. *Application deadline:* For fall admission, 12/1 priority date for domestic students, 12/1 for international students. Application fee: $95. *Expenses: Tuition:* Full-time $35,856; part-time $1494 per unit. *Required fees:* $1408; $64 per unit. $473 per term. Tuition and fees vary according to course load and program. *Financial support:* Fellowships with tuition reimbursements, research assistantships with tuition reimbursements, teaching assistantships with tuition reimbursements, career-related internships or fieldwork, Federal Work-Study, institutionally sponsored loans, scholarships/grants, health care benefits, and unspecified assistantships available. Financial award application deadline: 12/1; financial award applicants required to submit FAFSA. *Faculty research:* Genomics, molecular and cell biology, development and molecular genetics, molecular evolution of plants and animals. *Unit head:* Stephen Small, Chair, 212-998-8200, Fax: 212-995-4015, E-mail: biology.admissions@nyu.edu. *Application contact:* Justin Blau, Director of Graduate Studies, PhD Programs, 212-998-8200, Fax: 212-995-4015, E-mail: biology.admissions@nyu.edu.
Website: http://biology.as.nyu.edu/

New York University, School of Medicine and Graduate School of Arts and Science, Sackler Institute of Graduate Biomedical Sciences, Program in Cellular and Molecular Biology, New York, NY 10012-1019. Offers PhD, MD/PhD. *Faculty:* 55 full-time (18 women). *Students:* 30 full-time (14 women); includes 12 minority (2 Black or African American, non-Hispanic/Latino; 1 American Indian or Alaska Native, non-Hispanic/Latino; 5 Asian, non-Hispanic/Latino; 4 Hispanic/Latino), 11 international. Average age 27. In 2013, 4 doctorates awarded. *Degree requirements:* For doctorate, comprehensive exam, thesis/dissertation, qualifying exams. *Entrance requirements:* For doctorate, GRE General Test. Additional exam requirements/recommendations for international students: Required—TOEFL. *Application deadline:* For fall admission, 1/4 priority date for domestic students. Applications are processed on a rolling basis. Application fee: $85. *Expenses: Tuition:* Full-time $35,856; part-time $1494 per unit. *Required fees:* $1408; $64 per unit. $473 per term. Tuition and fees vary according to course load and program. *Financial support:* Fellowships with tuition reimbursements, research assistantships with tuition reimbursements, and teaching assistantships with tuition reimbursements available. *Faculty research:* Membrane and organelle structure and biogenesis, intracellular transport and processing of proteins, cellular recognition and cell adhesion, oncogene structure and function, action of growth factors. *Total annual research expenditures:* $1.9 million. *Unit head:* Dr. Daniel Rifkin, Director, 212-263-5109, E-mail: rifkind01@popmail.med.nyu.edu. *Application contact:* Lynette Wilson, Information Contact, 212-263-7684, Fax: 212-263-8139, E-mail: wilsoe01@popmail.med.nyu.edu.

North Dakota State University, College of Graduate and Interdisciplinary Studies, College of Science and Mathematics, Department of Biological Sciences, Fargo, ND 58108. Offers biology (MS); botany (MS, PhD); cellular and molecular biology (PhD); genomics (PhD); zoology (MS, PhD). *Faculty:* 17 full-time (9 women), 1 part-time/adjunct (0 women). *Students:* 20 full-time (10 women), 3 part-time (all women); includes 2 minority (1 American Indian or Alaska Native, non-Hispanic/Latino; 1 Two or more races, non-Hispanic/Latino), 1 international. Average age 32. 9 applicants, 11% accepted, 1 enrolled. In 2013, 4 master's awarded. *Degree requirements:* For master's, thesis; for doctorate, thesis/dissertation. *Entrance requirements:* For master's and doctorate, GRE General Test. Additional exam requirements/recommendations for international students: Required—TOEFL. *Application deadline:* For fall admission, 1/15 for domestic students. Applications are processed on a rolling basis. Application fee: $35. Electronic applications accepted. *Financial support:* Fellowships with full tuition reimbursements, research assistantships with full tuition reimbursements, teaching assistantships with full tuition reimbursements, career-related internships or fieldwork, Federal Work-Study, institutionally sponsored loans, scholarships/grants, tuition waivers (full), and unspecified assistantships available. Support available to part-time students. Financial award application deadline: 4/15; financial award applicants required to submit FAFSA. *Faculty research:* Comparative endocrinology, physiology, behavioral ecology, plant cell biology, aquatic biology. *Unit head:* Dr. Wendy Reed, Head, 701-231-7087, E-mail: wendy.reed@ndsu.edu. *Application contact:* Sonya Goergen, Marketing, Recruitment, and Public Relations Coordinator, 701-231-7033, Fax: 701-231-6524.
Website: http://biology.ndsu.nodak.edu/

North Dakota State University, College of Graduate and Interdisciplinary Studies, Interdisciplinary Program in Cellular and Molecular Biology, Fargo, ND 58108. Offers PhD. Program offered in cooperation with 11 departments in the university. *Students:* 8 full-time (6 women), 2 part-time (both women); includes 1 minority (Asian, non-Hispanic/Latino), 5 international. Average age 28. 34 applicants, 6% accepted, 2 enrolled. In 2013, 2 doctorates awarded. *Degree requirements:* For doctorate, thesis/dissertation. *Entrance requirements:* For doctorate, GRE. Additional exam requirements/recommendations for international students: Required—TOEFL (minimum score 525 paper-based; 71 iBT). *Application deadline:* Applications are processed on a rolling basis. Application fee: $35. Electronic applications accepted. *Financial support:* Fellowships with full tuition reimbursements, research assistantships with full tuition reimbursements, teaching assistantships with full tuition reimbursements, and unspecified assistantships available. Financial award application deadline: 3/15. *Faculty research:* Plant and animal cell biology, gene regulation, molecular genetics, plant and animal virology. *Unit head:* Dr. Mark Sheridan, Director, 701-231-7087, E-mail: ndsu.cmb@ndsu.edu. *Application contact:* Sonya Goergen, Marketing, Recruitment, and Public Relations Coordinator, 701-231-7033, Fax: 701-231-6524.
Website: http://www.ndsu.edu/cellularmolecularbiology/

Northwestern University, The Graduate School, Interdisciplinary Biological Sciences Program (IBiS), Evanston, IL 60208. Offers biochemistry (PhD); bioengineering and biotechnology (PhD); biotechnology (PhD); cell and molecular biology (PhD); developmental and systems biology (PhD); nanotechnology (PhD); neurobiology (PhD); structural biology and biophysics (PhD). *Degree requirements:* For doctorate, thesis/dissertation, qualifying exam. *Entrance requirements:* For doctorate, GRE General Test. Additional exam requirements/recommendations for international students: Required—TOEFL (minimum score 600 paper-based). *Application deadline:* For fall admission, 12/15 for domestic and international students. Applications are processed on a rolling basis. Application fee: $95. Electronic applications accepted. *Financial support:* Fellowships, research assistantships, teaching assistantships, career-related internships or fieldwork, institutionally sponsored loans, scholarships/grants, traineeships, health care benefits, and unspecified assistantships available. Financial award application deadline: 12/31; financial award applicants required to submit FAFSA. *Faculty research:* Biophysics/structural biology, cell/molecular biology, synthetic biology,

developmental systems biology, chemical biology/nanotechnology. *Unit head:* Dr. Deborah Klos Dehring, Associate Director, 847-467-0451, E-mail: d-klos@northwestern.edu. *Application contact:* Cathy Prullage, Program Manager, 847-491-4301, E-mail: ibis@northwestern.edu.
Website: http://www.biochem.northwestern.edu/ibis/

The Ohio State University, Graduate School, College of Arts and Sciences, Division of Natural and Mathematical Sciences, Department of Molecular Genetics, Columbus, OH 43210. Offers cell and developmental biology (MS, PhD); genetics (MS, PhD); molecular biology (MS, PhD). *Faculty:* 29. *Students:* 35 full-time (15 women); includes 3 minority (1 Black or African American, non-Hispanic/Latino; 2 Asian, non-Hispanic/Latino), 16 international. Average age 26. In 2013, 1 master's, 2 doctorates awarded. *Degree requirements:* For master's, thesis; for doctorate, thesis/dissertation. *Entrance requirements:* For doctorate, GRE General Test, GRE Subject Test in biology or chemistry (recommended). Additional exam requirements/recommendations for international students: Required—TOEFL (minimum score 550 paper-based; 79 iBT), Michigan English Language Assessment Battery (minimum score 82); Recommended—IELTS (minimum score 7). *Application deadline:* For fall admission, 12/13 priority date for domestic students, 11/30 priority date for international students; for winter admission, 12/1 for domestic students, 11/1 for international students; for spring admission, 3/1 for domestic students, 2/1 for international students. Applications are processed on a rolling basis. Application fee: $60 ($70 for international students). Electronic applications accepted. *Financial support:* Fellowships with tuition reimbursements, research assistantships with tuition reimbursements, teaching assistantships with tuition reimbursements, Federal Work-Study, and institutionally sponsored loans available. Support available to part-time students. *Unit head:* Dr. Anita Hopper, Chair, 614-688-3306, Fax: 614-292-4466, E-mail: hopper.64@osu.edu. *Application contact:* Graduate Admissions, 614-292-9444, Fax: 614-292-3895, E-mail: gradadmissions@osu.edu.
Website: https://molgen.osu.edu/

The Ohio State University, Graduate School, College of Arts and Sciences, Division of Natural and Mathematical Sciences, Program in Molecular, Cellular and Developmental Biology, Columbus, OH 43210. Offers MS, PhD. *Faculty:* 172. *Students:* 117 full-time (67 women), 5 part-time (1 woman); includes 13 minority (1 Black or African American, non-Hispanic/Latino; 6 Asian, non-Hispanic/Latino; 4 Hispanic/Latino; 2 Two or more races, non-Hispanic/Latino), 60 international. Average age 27. In 2013, 2 master's, 15 doctorates awarded. Terminal master's awarded for partial completion of doctoral program. *Degree requirements:* For master's, thesis; for doctorate, thesis/dissertation. *Entrance requirements:* For doctorate, GRE General Test, GRE Subject Test in any science (desired, preferably biology or chemistry, biochemistry or cell and molecular biology). Additional exam requirements/recommendations for international students: Required—TOEFL (minimum score 600 paper-based; 85 iBT); Recommended—IELTS (minimum score 8). *Application deadline:* For fall admission, 12/13 priority date for domestic students, 11/30 priority date for international students; for winter admission, 12/1 for domestic students, 11/1 for international students; for spring admission, 3/1 for domestic students, 2/1 for international students. Applications are processed on a rolling basis. Application fee: $60 ($70 for international students). Electronic applications accepted. *Financial support:* Fellowships with tuition reimbursements, research assistantships with tuition reimbursements, and teaching assistantships with tuition reimbursements available. *Unit head:* David Bisaro, Director, 614-292-2804, Fax: 614-292-7817, E-mail: bisaro.1@osu.edu. *Application contact:* Graduate Admissions, 614-292-9444, Fax: 614-292-3895, E-mail: gradadmissions@osu.edu.
Website: http://mcdb.osu.edu/

Ohio University, Graduate College, College of Arts and Sciences, Interdisciplinary Graduate Program in Molecular and Cellular Biology, Athens, OH 45701-2979. Offers MS, PhD. *Degree requirements:* For master's, comprehensive exam, thesis, research proposal, teaching experience; for doctorate, comprehensive exam, thesis/dissertation, research proposal, teaching experience. *Entrance requirements:* For master's and doctorate, GRE General Test. Additional exam requirements/recommendations for international students: Required—TOEFL (minimum score 620 paper-based; 105 iBT); Recommended—TWE. Electronic applications accepted. *Faculty research:* Animal biotechnology, plant molecular biology RNA, immunology, cellular genetics, biochemistry of signal transduction, cancer research, membrane transport, bioinformatics, bioengineering, chemical biology and drug discovery, diabetes, microbiology, neuroscience.

Oklahoma State University, College of Agricultural Science and Natural Resources, Department of Biochemistry and Molecular Biology, Stillwater, OK 74078. Offers MS, PhD. *Faculty:* 24 full-time (8 women), 3 part-time/adjunct (1 woman). *Students:* 4 full-time (2 women), 24 part-time (9 women); includes 5 minority (2 Asian, non-Hispanic/Latino; 2 Hispanic/Latino; 1 Two or more races, non-Hispanic/Latino), 15 international. Average age 28. 61 applicants, 7% accepted, 3 enrolled. In 2013, 7 master's, 4 doctorates awarded. *Degree requirements:* For master's, thesis, oral exam; for doctorate, comprehensive exam, thesis/dissertation. *Entrance requirements:* For master's and doctorate, GRE or GMAT. Additional exam requirements/recommendations for international students: Required—TOEFL (minimum score 550 paper-based; 79 iBT). *Application deadline:* For fall admission, 3/1 priority date for international students; for spring admission, 8/1 priority date for international students. Applications are processed on a rolling basis. Application fee: $40 ($75 for international students). Electronic applications accepted. *Expenses:* Tuition, state resident: full-time $4272; part-time $178 per credit hour. Tuition, nonresident: full-time $17,472; part-time $709 per credit hour. *Required fees:* $2413.20; $100.55 per credit hour. One-time fee: $50 full-time. Part-time tuition and fees vary according to course load and campus/location. *Financial support:* In 2013–14, 26 research assistantships (averaging $18,865 per year), 2 teaching assistantships (averaging $18,801 per year) were awarded; career-related internships or fieldwork, Federal Work-Study, scholarships/grants, health care benefits, tuition waivers (partial), and unspecified assistantships also available. Support available to part-time students. Financial award application deadline: 3/1; financial award applicants required to submit FAFSA. *Unit head:* Dr. John Gustafson, Department Head, 405-744-6189, Fax: 405-744-7799, E-mail: john.gustafson@okstate.edu.
Website: http://biochemistry.okstate.edu/

Oklahoma State University Center for Health Sciences, Graduate Program in Forensic Sciences, Tulsa, OK 74107. Offers forensic biology/DNA (MS); forensic document examination/forensic pathology (MS); forensic psychology (MS); forensic science administration (MS); microbiology (MS); trace evidence/forensic toxicology (MS). Part-time and evening/weekend programs available. Postbaccalaureate distance learning degree programs offered (no on-campus study). *Faculty:* 4 full-time (0 women), 14 part-time/adjunct (6 women). *Students:* 4 full-time (0 women), 14 part-time (6 women); includes 7 minority (4 American Indian or Alaska Native, non-Hispanic/Latino; 3 Hispanic/Latino), 3 international. Average age 31. 28 applicants, 50% accepted, 5 enrolled. In 2013, 5 master's awarded. *Degree requirements:* For master's, comprehensive exam, thesis (for some programs), creative component (for non-thesis options). *Entrance requirements:* For master's, MAT (for options in forensic science administration and forensic document examination) or GRE General Test, professional experience (for options in forensic science administration and forensic document examination). Additional exam requirements/recommendations for international students: Required—TOEFL (minimum score 100 iBT) or IELTS (minimum score 7.0). *Application deadline:* For fall admission, 3/1 for domestic and international students; for spring admission, 10/1 for domestic and international students; for summer admission, 7/1 for domestic and international students. Applications are processed on a rolling basis. Application fee: $40 ($75 for international students). Electronic applications accepted. *Expenses:* Tuition, state resident: full-time $22,127; part-time $178 per credit hour. Tuition, nonresident: full-time $43,572; part-time $728 per credit hour. *Required fees:* $910.79; $200 per semester. *Financial support:* In 2013–14, 14 students received support, including 8 research assistantships (averaging $12,000 per year); career-related internships or fieldwork, Federal Work-Study, and tuition waivers (partial) also available. Support available to part-time students. Financial award application deadline: 4/1; financial award applicants required to submit FAFSA. *Faculty research:* Studies on the variability in chromosomal DNA; development/enhancement of accessory methods useful for forensic DNA typing; development of universal methods useful for discriminating pathogenic bacteria; forensic dentistry; transmission of microbial diseases by dentures, protective athletic mouth-guards, band wind instruments, and infant pacifiers; changes in ecologies and antibiotic sensitivities of aerobic microorganisms; forensic toxicology and trace chemical method development. *Total annual research expenditures:* $58,000. *Unit head:* Dr. Robert W. Allen, Director, 918-561-1108, Fax: 918-561-8414. *Application contact:* Cathy Newsome, Coordinator, 918-561-1108, Fax: 918-561-8414, E-mail: cathy.newsome@okstate.edu.
Website: http://www.healthsciences.okstate.edu/forensic/index.cfm

Oregon Health & Science University, School of Medicine, Graduate Programs in Medicine, Department of Environmental and Biomolecular Systems, Portland, OR 97239-3098. Offers biochemistry and molecular biology (MS, PhD); environmental science and engineering (MS, PhD). Part-time programs available. *Faculty:* 12 full-time (4 women), 2 part-time/adjunct (1 woman). *Students:* 27 full-time (18 women), 2 part-time (both women); includes 9 minority (1 Black or African American, non-Hispanic/Latino; 1 American Indian or Alaska Native, non-Hispanic/Latino; 1 Asian, non-Hispanic/Latino; 5 Hispanic/Latino; 1 Two or more races, non-Hispanic/Latino), 4 international. Average age 31. 24 applicants, 17% accepted, 4 enrolled. In 2013, 2 master's, 1 doctorate awarded. Terminal master's awarded for partial completion of doctoral program. *Degree requirements:* For master's, thesis (for some programs); for doctorate, comprehensive exam, thesis/dissertation, qualifying exam. *Entrance requirements:* For master's and doctorate, GRE General Test (minimum scores: 500 Verbal/600 Quantitative/4.5 Analytical) or MCAT (for some programs). Additional exam requirements/recommendations for international students: Required—TOEFL. *Application deadline:* For fall admission, 7/15 for domestic students, 5/15 for international students; for winter admission, 10/15 for domestic students, 9/15 for international students; for spring admission, 1/15 for domestic students, 12/15 for international students. Applications are processed on a rolling basis. Application fee: $70. Electronic applications accepted. *Financial support:* Health care benefits and full tuition and stipends (for PhD students) available. *Unit head:* Dr. Paul Tratnyek, Program Director, 503-748-1070, E-mail: info@ebs.ogi.edu. *Application contact:* Nancy Christie, Program Coordinator, 503-748-1070, E-mail: info@ebs.ogi.edu.

Oregon Health & Science University, School of Medicine, Graduate Programs in Medicine, Program in Molecular and Cellular Biosciences, Department of Biochemistry and Molecular Biology, Portland, OR 97239-3098. Offers PhD. *Faculty:* 10 full-time (2 women). *Students:* 10 full-time (4 women), 1 (woman) part-time, 2 international. Average age 28. In 2013, 1 doctorate awarded. *Degree requirements:* For doctorate, comprehensive exam, thesis/dissertation, qualifying exam. *Entrance requirements:* For doctorate, GRE General Test (minimum scores: 153 Verbal/148 Quantitative/4.5 Analytical). Additional exam requirements/recommendations for international students: Required—TOEFL. Electronic applications accepted. *Financial support:* Health care benefits, tuition waivers (full), and full tuition and stipends (for PhD students) available. *Faculty research:* Protein structure, membrane proteins, metabolic regulation, molecular basis of disease, signal transduction mechanisms. *Unit head:* Dr. David Farrens, Program Director, 503-494-7781, E-mail: farrensd@ohsu.edu. *Application contact:* Valerie Scott, Administrative Coordinator, 503-494-8632, E-mail: wroblews@ohsu.edu.
Website: http://www.ohsu.edu/som-biochem/

Oregon State University, Interdisciplinary/Institutional Programs, Program in Molecular and Cellular Biology, Corvallis, OR 97331. Offers MS, PhD. *Students:* 31 full-time (17 women), 1 part-time (0 women); includes 5 minority (2 Asian, non-Hispanic/Latino; 2 Hispanic/Latino; 1 Two or more races, non-Hispanic/Latino), 11 international. Average age 29. 125 applicants, 9% accepted, 6 enrolled. In 2013, 1 master's, 8 doctorates awarded. *Degree requirements:* For doctorate, thesis/dissertation, oral and written qualifying exams. *Entrance requirements:* For master's and doctorate, GRE. Additional exam requirements/recommendations for international students: Required—TOEFL (minimum score 80 iBT), IELTS (minimum score 6.5). *Application deadline:* For fall admission, 6/1 for domestic students. Application fee: $60. *Expenses:* Tuition, state resident: full-time $11,664; part-time $432 per credit hour. Tuition, nonresident: full-time $19,197; part-time $711 per credit hour. *Required fees:* $1446; $443 per quarter. One-time fee: $300. Tuition and fees vary according to course load and program. *Financial support:* Fellowships, career-related internships or fieldwork, Federal Work-Study, and institutionally sponsored loans available. Support available to part-time students. *Unit head:* Dr. Barbara Taylor, Director, Molecular and Cellular Biology Graduate Program, 541-737-5344, E-mail: taylorb@science.oregonstate.edu. *Application contact:* Gail Millimaki, Molecular and Cellular Biology Advisor, 541-737-3799, E-mail: mcb@science.oregonstate.edu.
Website: http://www.mcb.oregonstate.edu/

Penn State University Park, Graduate School, Eberly College of Science, Department of Biochemistry and Molecular Biology, University Park, PA 16802. Offers biochemistry, microbiology, and molecular biology (MS, PhD); biotechnology (MBIOT). *Unit head:* Dr. Daniel J. Larson, Dean, 814-865-9591, Fax: 814-865-3634, E-mail: djlarson@psu.edu. *Application contact:* Cynthia E. Nicosia, Director, Graduate Enrollment Services, 814-865-1834, Fax: 814-863-4627, E-mail: cey1@psu.edu.
Website: http://bmb.psu.edu/

Princeton University, Graduate School, Department of Molecular Biology, Princeton, NJ 08544-1019. Offers PhD. *Degree requirements:* For doctorate, thesis/dissertation. *Entrance requirements:* For doctorate, GRE General Test. Additional exam requirements/recommendations for international students: Required—TOEFL (minimum score 600 paper-based). Electronic applications accepted. *Faculty research:* Genetics, virology, biochemistry.

Purdue University, College of Pharmacy and Pharmacal Sciences and Graduate School, Graduate Programs in Pharmacy and Pharmacal Sciences, Department of Medicinal Chemistry and Molecular Pharmacology, West Lafayette, IN 47907. Offers biophysical and computational chemistry (PhD); cancer research (PhD); immunology and infectious disease (PhD); medicinal biochemistry and molecular biology (PhD); medicinal chemistry and chemical biology (PhD); molecular pharmacology (PhD); neuropharmacology, neurodegeneration, and neurotoxicity (PhD); systems biology and functional genomics (PhD). *Faculty:* 23 full-time (3 women), 6 part-time/adjunct (1 woman). *Students:* 50 full-time (21 women), 3 part-time (2 women); includes 1 minority

(Asian, non-Hispanic/Latino), 30 international. Average age 26. 147 applicants, 20% accepted, 13 enrolled. In 2013, 12 doctorates awarded. *Degree requirements:* For doctorate, thesis/dissertation. *Entrance requirements:* For doctorate, GRE General Test; GRE Subject Test in biology, biochemistry, and chemistry (recommended), minimum undergraduate GPA of 3.0. Additional exam requirements/recommendations for international students: Required—TOEFL (minimum score 550 paper-based; 77 iBT); Recommended—TWE. *Application deadline:* For fall admission, 2/1 for domestic and international students. Applications are processed on a rolling basis. Application fee: $60 ($75 for international students). Electronic applications accepted. *Financial support:* Fellowships, research assistantships, teaching assistantships, and traineeships available. Support available to part-time students. Financial award applicants required to submit FAFSA. *Faculty research:* Drug design and development, cancer research, drug synthesis and analysis, chemical pharmacology, environmental toxicology. *Unit head:* Dr. Richard F. Borch, Head, 765-494-1403, E-mail: borch@purdue.edu. *Application contact:* Dr. Janine C. Mott, Graduate Contact, 765-494-1269, E-mail: jmott@purdue.edu.

Purdue University, Graduate School, College of Science, Department of Biological Sciences, West Lafayette, IN 47907. Offers biochemistry (PhD); biophysics (PhD); cell and developmental biology (PhD); ecology, evolutionary and population biology (MS, PhD), including ecology, evolutionary biology, population biology; genetics (MS, PhD); microbiology (MS, PhD); molecular biology (PhD); neurobiology (MS, PhD); plant physiology (PhD). *Faculty:* 50 full-time (13 women), 5 part-time/adjunct (1 woman). *Students:* 111 full-time (61 women), 5 part-time (0 women); includes 9 minority (1 Black or African American, non-Hispanic/Latino; 5 Asian, non-Hispanic/Latino; 3 Hispanic/Latino), 62 international. Average age 27. 170 applicants, 19% accepted, 17 enrolled. In 2013, 9 master's, 18 doctorates awarded. Terminal master's awarded for partial completion of doctoral program. *Degree requirements:* For master's, thesis (for some programs); for doctorate, thesis/dissertation, seminars, teaching experience. *Entrance requirements:* For master's, GRE General Test (minimum analytical writing score of 3.5), minimum undergraduate GPA of 3.0; for doctorate, GRE General Test (minimum analytical writing score of 3.5), minimum undergraduate GPA of 3.5. Additional exam requirements/recommendations for international students: Required—TOEFL (minimum score 600 paper-based; 107 iBT for MS, 80 iBT for PhD). *Application deadline:* For fall admission, 12/7 for domestic and international students. Applications are processed on a rolling basis. Application fee: $60 ($75 for international students). Electronic applications accepted. *Financial support:* Fellowships, research assistantships, and teaching assistantships available. Support available to part-time students. Financial award application deadline: 2/15; financial award applicants required to submit FAFSA. *Unit head:* Dr. Richard J. Kuhn, Head, 765-494-4407, E-mail: kuhnr@purdue.edu. *Application contact:* Georgina E. Rupp, Graduate Coordinator, 765-494-8142, Fax: 765-494-0876, E-mail: ruppg@purdue.edu.
Website: http://www.bio.purdue.edu/

Purdue University, Graduate School, PULSe - Purdue University Life Sciences Program, West Lafayette, IN 47907. Offers biomolecular structure and biophysics (PhD); biotechnology (PhD); chemical biology (PhD); chromatin and regulation of gene expression (PhD); integrative neuroscience (PhD); integrative plant sciences (PhD); membrane biology (PhD); microbiology (PhD); molecular evolutionary and cancer biology (PhD); molecular evolutionary genetics (PhD); molecular virology (PhD). *Students:* 154 full-time (78 women), 1 part-time (0 women); includes 23 minority (5 Black or African American, non-Hispanic/Latino; 5 Asian, non-Hispanic/Latino; 10 Hispanic/Latino; 3 Two or more races, non-Hispanic/Latino), 73 international. Average age 26. 239 applicants, 33% accepted, 40 enrolled. *Entrance requirements:* For doctorate, GRE, minimum undergraduate GPA of 3.0. Additional exam requirements/recommendations for international students: Required—TOEFL (minimum score 550 paper-based; 77 iBT). *Application deadline:* For fall admission, 1/15 priority date for domestic and international students. Applications are processed on a rolling basis. Application fee: $60 ($75 for international students). Electronic applications accepted. *Financial support:* In 2013–14, research assistantships with tuition reimbursements (averaging $22,500 per year), teaching assistantships with tuition reimbursements (averaging $22,500 per year) were awarded. *Unit head:* Dr. Christine A. Hrycyna, Head, 765-494-7322, E-mail: hrycyna@purdue.edu. *Application contact:* Colleen Gabauer, Graduate Contact, 765-494-9256, E-mail: cgabauer@purdue.edu.
Website: http://www.gradschool.purdue.edu/pulse

Queen's University at Kingston, School of Graduate Studies, Faculty of Health Sciences, Department of Anatomy and Cell Biology, Kingston, ON K7L 3N6, Canada. Offers biology of reproduction (M Sc, PhD); cancer (M Sc, PhD); cardiovascular pathophysiology (M Sc, PhD); cell and molecular biology (M Sc, PhD); drug metabolism (M Sc, PhD); endocrinology (M Sc, PhD); motor control (M Sc, PhD); neural regeneration (M Sc, PhD); neurophysiology (M Sc, PhD). Part-time programs available. *Degree requirements:* For master's, thesis; for doctorate, one foreign language, comprehensive exam, thesis/dissertation. *Entrance requirements:* Additional exam requirements/recommendations for international students: Required—TOEFL. Electronic applications accepted. *Faculty research:* Human kinetics, neuroscience, reproductive biology, cardiovascular.

Quinnipiac University, College of Arts and Sciences, Program in Molecular and Cell Biology, Hamden, CT 06518-1940. Offers MS. Part-time and evening/weekend programs available. *Faculty:* 12 full-time (6 women), 19 part-time/adjunct (8 women). *Students:* 24 full-time (11 women), 21 part-time (13 women); includes 8 minority (1 American Indian or Alaska Native, non-Hispanic/Latino; 3 Asian, non-Hispanic/Latino; 4 Hispanic/Latino), 15 international. 43 applicants, 42% accepted, 7 enrolled. In 2013, 19 master's awarded. *Degree requirements:* For master's, thesis optional. *Entrance requirements:* For master's, bachelor's degree in biological, medical, or health sciences; minimum GPA of 2.75. Additional exam requirements/recommendations for international students: Required—TOEFL (minimum score 575 paper-based; 90 iBT), IELTS (minimum score 6.5). *Application deadline:* For fall admission, 7/30 priority date for domestic students, 4/15 priority date for international students; for spring admission, 12/15 priority date for domestic students, 9/15 priority date for international students. Applications are processed on a rolling basis. Application fee: $45. Electronic applications accepted. *Expenses: Tuition:* Part-time $920 per credit. *Required fees:* $37 per credit. *Financial support:* In 2013–14, 2 students received support. Career-related internships or fieldwork, Federal Work-Study, scholarships/grants, and unspecified assistantships available. Support available to part-time students. Financial award application deadline: 6/1; financial award applicants required to submit FAFSA. *Unit head:* Dr. Michelle Geremia, Director, E-mail: michelle.geremia@quinnipiac.edu. *Application contact:* Office of Graduate Admissions, 800-462-1944, Fax: 203-582-3443, E-mail: graduate@quinnipiac.edu.
Website: http://www.quinnipiac.edu/gradmolecular

Rosalind Franklin University of Medicine and Science, School of Graduate and Postdoctoral Studies - Interdisciplinary Graduate Program in Biomedical Sciences, Department of Biochemistry and Molecular Biology, North Chicago, IL 60064-3095. Offers MS, PhD, MD/PhD. Terminal master's awarded for partial completion of doctoral program. *Degree requirements:* For master's, comprehensive exam, thesis; for doctorate, comprehensive exam, thesis/dissertation. *Entrance requirements:* For master's and doctorate, GRE General Test, minimum GPA of 3.0. Additional exam requirements/recommendations for international students: Required—TOEFL, TWE. Electronic applications accepted. *Faculty research:* Structure of control enzymes, extracellular matrix, glucose metabolism, gene expression, ATP synthesis.

Rutgers, The State University of New Jersey, Newark, Graduate School of Biomedical Sciences, Department of Biochemistry and Molecular Biology, Newark, NJ 07107. Offers MS, PhD. *Degree requirements:* For master's, thesis; for doctorate, thesis/dissertation, qualifying exam. *Entrance requirements:* For master's and doctorate, GRE General Test. Additional exam requirements/recommendations for international students: Required—TOEFL. Electronic applications accepted.

Rutgers, The State University of New Jersey, New Brunswick, Graduate School-New Brunswick, Programs in the Molecular Biosciences, Piscataway, NJ 08854-8097. Offers biochemistry (PhD); cell and developmental biology (MS, PhD); microbiology and molecular genetics (MS, PhD), including applied microbiology, clinical microbiology (MS), clinical mircobiology (PhD), computational molecular biology (PhD), immunology, microbial biochemistry, molecular genetics, virology. MS, PhD offered jointly with University of Medicine and Dentistry of New Jersey.

Rutgers, The State University of New Jersey, New Brunswick, Graduate School of Biomedical Sciences, Piscataway, NJ 08854-5635. Offers biochemistry and molecular biology (MS, PhD); biomedical engineering (MS, PhD); biomedical science (MS); cellular and molecular pharmacology (MS, PhD); clinical and translational science (MS); environmental sciences/exposure assessment (PhD); molecular genetics, microbiology and immunology (MS, PhD); neuroscience (MS, PhD); physiology and integrative biology (MS, PhD); toxicology (PhD); MD/PhD. Terminal master's awarded for partial completion of doctoral program. *Degree requirements:* For master's, thesis (for some programs), ethics training; for doctorate, comprehensive exam, thesis/dissertation, ethics training. *Entrance requirements:* For master's, GRE General Test, MCAT, DAT; for doctorate, GRE General Test. Additional exam requirements/recommendations for international students: Required—TOEFL. Electronic applications accepted.

Saint Louis University, Graduate Education and School of Medicine, Graduate Program in Biomedical Sciences and Graduate Education, Department of Biochemistry and Molecular Biology, St. Louis, MO 63103-2097. Offers PhD. *Degree requirements:* For doctorate, comprehensive exam, thesis/dissertation, departmental qualifying exams. *Entrance requirements:* For doctorate, GRE General Test, GRE Subject Test (optional), letters of recommendation, resume, interview. Additional exam requirements/recommendations for international students: Required—TOEFL (minimum score 525 paper-based). Electronic applications accepted. *Faculty research:* Transcription, chromatin modification and regulation of gene expression; structure/function of proteins and enzymes, including x-ray crystallography; inflammatory mediators in pathenogenesis of diabetes and arteriosclerosis; cellular signaling in response to growth factors, opiates and angiogenic mediators; genomics and proteomics of Cryptococcus neoformans.

San Diego State University, Graduate and Research Affairs, College of Sciences, Department of Biology, San Diego, CA 92182. Offers biology (MA, MS), including ecology (MS), molecular biology (MS), physiology (MS), systematics/evolution (MS); cell and molecular biology (PhD); ecology (MS, PhD); microbiology (MS). Terminal master's awarded for partial completion of doctoral program. *Degree requirements:* For master's, thesis; for doctorate, thesis/dissertation. *Entrance requirements:* For master's, GRE General Test, GRE Subject Test, resume or curriculum vitae, 2 letters of recommendation. Additional exam requirements/recommendations for international students: Required—TOEFL. Electronic applications accepted.

San Diego State University, Graduate and Research Affairs, College of Sciences, Molecular Biology Institute, Program in Cell and Molecular Biology, San Diego, CA 92182. Offers PhD. Program offered jointly with University of California, San Diego. *Degree requirements:* For doctorate, thesis/dissertation, oral comprehensive qualifying exam. *Entrance requirements:* For doctorate, GRE General Test, GRE Subject Test, resumé or curriculum vitae, 3 letters of recommendation. Electronic applications accepted. *Faculty research:* Structure/dynamics of protein kinesis, chromatin structure and DNA methylation membrane biochemistry, secretory protein targeting, molecular biology of cardiac myocytes.

San Francisco State University, Division of Graduate Studies, College of Science and Engineering, Department of Biology, Program in Cell and Molecular Biology, San Francisco, CA 94132-1722. Offers MS. *Application deadline:* Applications are processed on a rolling basis. *Unit head:* Dr. Diana Chu, Program Coordinator, 415-405-3487, E-mail: chud@sfsu.edu. *Application contact:* Dr. Robert Patterson, Graduate Coordinator, 415-338-1237, E-mail: patters@sfsu.edu.
Website: http://biology.sfsu.edu/programs/graduate

San Jose State University, Graduate Studies and Research, College of Science, Department of Biological Sciences, San Jose, CA 95192-0001. Offers biological sciences (MA, MS); molecular biology and microbiology (MS); organismal biology, conservation and ecology (MS); physiology (MS). Part-time programs available. *Entrance requirements:* For master's, GRE. Electronic applications accepted. *Faculty research:* Systemic physiology, molecular genetics, SEM studies, toxicology, large mammal ecology.

Seton Hall University, College of Arts and Sciences, Department of Biological Sciences, South Orange, NJ 07079-2697. Offers biology (MS); biology/business administration (MS); microbiology (MS); molecular bioscience (PhD); molecular bioscience/neuroscience (PhD). Part-time and evening/weekend programs available. *Degree requirements:* For master's, thesis optional; for doctorate, comprehensive exam, thesis/dissertation. *Entrance requirements:* For master's and doctorate, GRE or MS from accredited university in the U.S. Additional exam requirements/recommendations for international students: Required—TOEFL. Electronic applications accepted. *Faculty research:* Neurobiology, genetics, immunology, molecular biology, cellular physiology, toxicology, microbiology, bioinformatics.

Simon Fraser University, Office of Graduate Studies, Faculty of Science, Department of Molecular Biology and Biochemistry, Burnaby, BC V5A 1S6, Canada. Offers bioinformatics (Graduate Diploma); molecular biology and biochemistry (M Sc, PhD). *Faculty:* 29 full-time (10 women). *Students:* 75 full-time (40 women). 12 applicants, 75% accepted, 8 enrolled. In 2013, 13 master's, 12 doctorates awarded. *Degree requirements:* For master's, thesis; for doctorate, thesis/dissertation; for Graduate Diploma, practicum. *Entrance requirements:* For master's, minimum GPA of 3.0 (on scale of 4.33), or 3.33 based on last 60 credits of undergraduate courses; for doctorate, minimum GPA of 3.5; for Graduate Diploma, minimum GPA of 2.5 (on scale of 4.33), or 2.67 based on the last 60 credits of undergraduate courses. Additional exam requirements/recommendations for international students: Recommended—TOEFL (minimum score 580 paper-based; 100 iBT), IELTS (minimum score 7.5), TWE (minimum score 5). *Application deadline:* Applications are processed on a rolling basis. Application fee: $90 ($125 for international students). Electronic applications accepted. *Expenses: Tuition, area resident:* Full-time $5084 Canadian dollars. *Required fees:* $840 Canadian dollars. *Financial support:* In 2013–14, 45 students received support, including 48 fellowships (averaging $6,250 per year), teaching assistantships (averaging $5,608 per year); research assistantships and scholarships/grants also available.

Faculty research: Genomics and bioinformatics, cell and developmental biology, structural biology/biochemistry, immunology, nucleic acid function. *Unit head:* Dr. Michel Leroux, Graduate Chair, 778-782-6683, Fax: 778-782-5583, E-mail: mbb-grad-chair@sfu.ca. *Application contact:* Mimi Fourie, Graduate Secretary, 778-782-5631, Fax: 778-782-5583, E-mail: mbb@sfu.ca.
Website: http://www.sfu.ca/mbb

Sonoma State University, School of Science and Technology, Department of Biology, Rohnert Park, CA 94928. Offers biochemistry (MA); ecology (MS); environmental biology (MS); evolutionary biology (MS); functional morphology (MS); molecular and cell biology (MS); organismal biology (MS). Part-time programs available. *Faculty:* 9 full-time (1 woman). *Students:* 4 full-time (2 women), 21 part-time (14 women); includes 5 minority (1 American Indian or Alaska Native, non-Hispanic/Latino; 1 Asian, non-Hispanic/Latino; 2 Hispanic/Latino; 1 Two or more races, non-Hispanic/Latino), 2 international. Average age 29. 23 applicants, 65% accepted, 6 enrolled. In 2013, 6 master's awarded. *Degree requirements:* For master's, thesis or alternative, oral exam. *Entrance requirements:* For master's, GRE General Test, GRE Subject Test, minimum GPA of 3.0. Additional exam requirements/recommendations for international students: Required—TOEFL (minimum score 500 paper-based). *Application deadline:* For fall admission, 11/30 for domestic students. Applications are processed on a rolling basis. Application fee: $55. *Expenses:* Tuition, state resident: full-time $8500. Tuition, nonresident: full-time $12,964. *Required fees:* $1762. *Financial support:* In 2013–14, 1 fellowship (averaging $1,520 per year), 6 research assistantships (averaging $3,562 per year), 22 teaching assistantships (averaging $6,738 per year) were awarded; career-related internships or fieldwork, Federal Work-Study, and tuition waivers (full) also available. Financial award application deadline: 3/2; financial award applicants required to submit FAFSA. *Faculty research:* Plant physiology, comparative physiology, community ecology, restoration ecology, marine ecology, conservation genetics, primate behavior, behavioral ecology, developmental biology, plant and animal systematics. *Total annual research expenditures:* $4,400. *Unit head:* Dr. Nathan Rank, Chair, 707-664-3053, E-mail: nathan.rank@sonoma.edu. *Application contact:* Dr. Derek Girman, Graduate Adviser, 707-664-3055, E-mail: derek.girman@sonoma.edu.
Website: http://www.sonoma.edu/biology/graduate

Southern Illinois University Carbondale, Graduate School, College of Science, Program in Molecular Biology, Microbiology, and Biochemistry, Carbondale, IL 62901-4701. Offers MS, PhD. *Faculty:* 16 full-time (2 women). *Students:* 40 full-time (27 women), 39 part-time (21 women); includes 6 minority (2 Black or African American, non-Hispanic/Latino; 4 Asian, non-Hispanic/Latino), 50 international. Average age 25. 143 applicants, 6% accepted, 5 enrolled. In 2013, 5 master's, 4 doctorates awarded. *Degree requirements:* For master's, thesis; for doctorate, thesis/dissertation. *Entrance requirements:* For master's, GRE, minimum GPA of 2.7; for doctorate, GRE, minimum GPA of 3.25. Additional exam requirements/recommendations for international students: Required—TOEFL. *Application deadline:* Applications are processed on a rolling basis. Application fee: $50. *Financial support:* In 2013–14, 40 students received support, including 3 fellowships with full tuition reimbursements available, 24 research assistantships with full tuition reimbursements available, 12 teaching assistantships with full tuition reimbursements available; Federal Work-Study and institutionally sponsored loans also available. Support available to part-time students. Financial award application deadline: 3/1. *Faculty research:* Prokaryotic gene regulation and expression; eukaryotic gene regulation; microbial, phylogenetic, and metabolic diversity; immune responses to tumors, pathogens, and autoantigens; protein folding and structure. *Unit head:* Dr. Judy Davie, Director, 618-453-5002, E-mail: jdavie@siumed.edu. *Application contact:* Cindy Filla, Office Systems Specialist, 618-453-8911, E-mail: cfilla@siumed.edu.
Website: http://mbmb.siu.edu/

Southern Methodist University, Dedman College of Humanities and Sciences, Department of Biological Sciences, Dallas, TX 75275. Offers molecular and cellular biology (MA, MS, PhD). Terminal master's awarded for partial completion of doctoral program. *Degree requirements:* For master's, thesis (for MS), oral exam; for doctorate, thesis/dissertation, qualifying exam. *Entrance requirements:* For master's, GRE General Test (minimum score 1200), minimum GPA of 3.0; for doctorate, GRE General Test (minimum score: 1200), minimum GPA of 3.0. Additional exam requirements/recommendations for international students: Required—TOEFL (minimum score 550 paper-based). Electronic applications accepted. *Faculty research:* Free radicals and aging, protein structure, chromatin structure, signal processes, retroviral pathogenesis.

State University of New York Downstate Medical Center, School of Graduate Studies, Program in Molecular and Cellular Biology, Brooklyn, NY 11203-2098. Offers PhD, MD/PhD. Affiliation with a particular PhD degree-granting program is deferred to the second year. *Degree requirements:* For doctorate, comprehensive exam, thesis/dissertation. *Entrance requirements:* For doctorate, GRE General Test. Additional exam requirements/recommendations for international students: Recommended—TOEFL. *Faculty research:* Mechanism of gene regulation, molecular virology.

State University of New York Upstate Medical University, College of Graduate Studies, Program in Biochemistry and Molecular Biology, Syracuse, NY 13210-2334. Offers biochemistry (MS); biochemistry and molecular biology (PhD); MD/PhD. Terminal master's awarded for partial completion of doctoral program. *Degree requirements:* For master's, thesis; for doctorate, comprehensive exam, thesis/dissertation. *Entrance requirements:* For master's, GRE General Test, interview; for doctorate, GRE General Test, telephone interview. Additional exam requirements/recommendations for international students: Required—TOEFL. Electronic applications accepted. *Faculty research:* Enzymology, membrane structure and functions, developmental biochemistry.

Stony Brook University, State University of New York, Graduate School, College of Arts and Sciences, Department of Biochemistry and Cell Biology, Molecular and Cellular Biology Program, Stony Brook, NY 11794. Offers biochemistry and molecular biology (PhD); biological sciences (MA); immunology and pathology (PhD); molecular and cellular biology (PhD). *Faculty:* 23 full-time (7 women), 1 part-time/adjunct (0 women). *Students:* 75 full-time (42 women); includes 7 minority (5 Asian, non-Hispanic/Latino; 2 Hispanic/Latino), 46 international. Average age 30. 211 applicants, 15% accepted, 8 enrolled. In 2013, 13 master's, 15 doctorates awarded. *Degree requirements:* For doctorate, comprehensive exam, thesis/dissertation, teaching experience. *Entrance requirements:* For doctorate, GRE General Test, GRE Subject Test. Additional exam requirements/recommendations for international students: Required—TOEFL. *Application deadline:* For fall admission, 1/15 for domestic students; for spring admission, 10/1 for domestic students. Application fee: $100. *Expenses:* Tuition, state resident: full-time $9870; part-time $411 per credit. Tuition, nonresident: full-time $18,350; part-time $765 per credit. *Financial support:* In 2013–14, 22 fellowships, 18 research assistantships, 12 teaching assistantships were awarded; Federal Work-Study also available. *Unit head:* Prof. Robert Haltiwanger, Chair, 631-632-8560, E-mail: robert.haltiwanger@stonybrook.edu. *Application contact:* Joann DeLucia-Conlon, Coordinator, 631-632-8613, Fax: 631-632-9730, E-mail: joann.delucia-conlon@stonybrook.edu.

Texas A&M Health Science Center, College of Medicine, Department of Microbial and Molecular Pathogenesis, College Station, TX 77840. Offers immunology (PhD); microbiology (PhD); molecular biology (PhD); virology (PhD). *Degree requirements:* For doctorate, thesis/dissertation. *Entrance requirements:* For doctorate, GRE General Test, minimum GPA of 3.0. *Faculty research:* Molecular pathogenesis, microbial therapeutics.

Texas A&M Health Science Center, College of Medicine, Program in Cell and Molecular Biology, College Station, TX 77840. Offers PhD.

Texas Woman's University, Graduate School, College of Arts and Sciences, Department of Biology, Denton, TX 76201. Offers biology (MS); molecular biology (PhD). Part-time programs available. *Faculty:* 11 full-time (9 women), 3 part-time/adjunct (1 woman). *Students:* 9 full-time (8 women), 40 part-time (29 women); includes 9 minority (3 Black or African American, non-Hispanic/Latino; 1 American Indian or Alaska Native, non-Hispanic/Latino; 3 Asian, non-Hispanic/Latino; 2 Hispanic/Latino), 18 international. Average age 31. 17 applicants, 59% accepted, 5 enrolled. In 2013, 6 master's, 1 doctorate awarded. Terminal master's awarded for partial completion of doctoral program. *Degree requirements:* For master's, comprehensive exam, thesis; for doctorate, comprehensive exam, thesis/dissertation, residency. *Entrance requirements:* For master's, GRE General Test (preferred minimum score 149 [425 old version] verbal, 141 [425 old version] quantitative), 3 letters of reference; letter of interest; for doctorate, GRE General Test (preferred minimum score 153 [500 old version] verbal, 144 [500 old version] quantitative), 3 letters of reference, letter of interest. Additional exam requirements/recommendations for international students: Required—TOEFL (minimum score 550 paper-based; 79 iBT). *Application deadline:* For fall admission, 2/1 priority date for domestic students, 2/1 for international students. Applications are processed on a rolling basis. Application fee: $50 ($75 for international students). Electronic applications accepted. *Expenses:* Tuition, state resident: full-time $4182; part-time $233.32 per credit hour. Tuition, nonresident: full-time $10,716; part-time $595.32 per credit hour. *Financial support:* In 2013–14, 7 students received support, including 51 research assistantships (averaging $15,652 per year); career-related internships or fieldwork, Federal Work-Study, institutionally sponsored loans, scholarships/grants, traineeships, health care benefits, and unspecified assistantships also available. Support available to part-time students. Financial award application deadline: 3/1; financial award applicants required to submit FAFSA. *Faculty research:* Computational biology, protein-protein Interactions, chromatin structure and regulation, regulation of RNA synthesis, virus-host interactions, regulation of axon growth and guidance in neurons, estrogen compounds in plants, regulation of gene expression in male reproductive tissues, female gonadal hormones in the development of anxiety and depression, electron microscopy. *Total annual research expenditures:* $447,324. *Unit head:* Dr. Sarah McIntire, Chair, 940-898-2352, Fax: 940-898-2382, E-mail: smcintire@twu.edu. *Application contact:* Dr. Samuel Wheeler, Assistant Director of Admissions, 940-898-3188, Fax: 940-898-3081, E-mail: wheelersr@twu.edu.
Website: http://www.twu.edu/biology

Tufts University, Sackler School of Graduate Biomedical Sciences, Cell, Molecular, and Developmental Biology Program, Medford, MA 02155. Offers PhD. *Faculty:* 45 full-time (15 women). *Students:* 25 full-time (10 women); includes 8 minority (1 Black or African American, non-Hispanic/Latino; 5 Asian, non-Hispanic/Latino; 1 Hispanic/Latino; 1 Two or more races, non-Hispanic/Latino), 5 international. Average age 29. In 2013, 3 doctorates awarded. Terminal master's awarded for partial completion of doctoral program. *Degree requirements:* For doctorate, comprehensive exam, thesis/dissertation. *Entrance requirements:* For doctorate, GRE General Test, 3 letters of reference. Additional exam requirements/recommendations for international students: Required—TOEFL (minimum score 600 paper-based; 100 iBT). *Application deadline:* For fall admission, 12/15 for domestic and international students. Application fee: $70. Electronic applications accepted. *Financial support:* In 2013–14, 25 students received support, including 25 research assistantships with full tuition reimbursements available (averaging $31,000 per year); fellowships and health care benefits also available. *Faculty research:* Reproduction and hormone action, control of gene expression, cell-matrix and cell-cell interactions, growth control and tumorigenesis, cytoskeleton and contractile proteins. *Unit head:* Dr. John Castellot, Program Director, 617-636-0303, Fax: 617-636-0375. *Application contact:* Kellie Johnston, Associate Director of Admissions, 617-636-6767, Fax: 617-636-0375, E-mail: sackler-school@tufts.edu.
Website: http://sackler.tufts.edu/Academics/Degree-Programs/PhD-Programs/Cell-Molecular-and-Developmental-Biology

Tufts University, Sackler School of Graduate Biomedical Sciences, Molecular Microbiology Program, Medford, MA 02155. Offers PhD. *Faculty:* 17 full-time (7 women). *Students:* 33 full-time (26 women); includes 8 minority (1 Black or African American, non-Hispanic/Latino; 3 Asian, non-Hispanic/Latino; 1 Hispanic/Latino; 3 Two or more races, non-Hispanic/Latino), 2 international. Average age 27. 98 applicants, 13% accepted, 6 enrolled. In 2013, 1 doctorate awarded. Terminal master's awarded for partial completion of doctoral program. *Degree requirements:* For doctorate, comprehensive exam, thesis/dissertation. *Entrance requirements:* For doctorate, GRE General Test, 3 letters of reference. Additional exam requirements/recommendations for international students: Required—TOEFL (minimum score 600 paper-based; 100 iBT). *Application deadline:* For fall admission, 12/15 for domestic and international students. Application fee: $70. Electronic applications accepted. *Financial support:* In 2013–14, 33 students received support, including 33 research assistantships with full tuition reimbursements available (averaging $31,000 per year); traineeships and health care benefits also available. Financial award application deadline: 12/15. *Faculty research:* Mechanisms of gene regulation, interactions of microorganisms and viruses with host cells, infection response. *Unit head:* Dr. Michael Malamy, Director, 617-636-6750, Fax: 617-636-0337, E-mail: michael.malamy@tufts.edu. *Application contact:* Kellie Melchin, Associate Director of Admissions, 617-636-6767, Fax: 617-636-0375, E-mail: sackler-school@tufts.edu.
Website: http://sackler.tufts.edu/Academics/Degree-Programs/PhD-Programs/Molecular-Microbiology

Tulane University, School of Medicine and School of Liberal Arts, Graduate Programs in Biomedical Sciences, Interdisciplinary Graduate Program in Molecular and Cellular Biology, New Orleans, LA 70118-5669. Offers PhD, MD/PhD. PhD offered through the Graduate School. *Degree requirements:* For doctorate, thesis/dissertation. *Entrance requirements:* For doctorate, GRE General Test, GRE Subject Test. Additional exam requirements/recommendations for international students: Required—TOEFL. Electronic applications accepted. *Faculty research:* Developmental biology, neuroscience, virology.

Tulane University, School of Science and Engineering, Department of Cell and Molecular Biology, New Orleans, LA 70118-5669. Offers MS, PhD. Terminal master's awarded for partial completion of doctoral program. *Degree requirements:* For doctorate, thesis/dissertation. *Entrance requirements:* For master's, GRE General Test, minimum B average in undergraduate course work; for doctorate, GRE General Test. Additional exam requirements/recommendations for international students: Required—TOEFL. Electronic applications accepted.

Uniformed Services University of the Health Sciences, School of Medicine, Graduate Programs in the Biomedical Sciences and Public Health, Graduate Program in Molecular and Cell Biology, Bethesda, MD 20814-4799. Offers MS, PhD. *Faculty:* 43 full-time (11 women), 3 part-time/adjunct (0 women). *Students:* 26 full-time (13 women); includes 6 minority (2 Asian, non-Hispanic/Latino; 4 Hispanic/Latino), 11 international. Average age 26. 34 applicants, 35% accepted, 4 enrolled. In 2013, 4 doctorates

awarded. *Degree requirements:* For doctorate, comprehensive exam, thesis/dissertation, qualifying exam. *Entrance requirements:* For doctorate, GRE General Test, minimum GPA of 3.0. Additional exam requirements/recommendations for international students: Required—TOEFL. *Application deadline:* For fall admission, 1/1 priority date for domestic and international students. Applications are processed on a rolling basis. Application fee: $0. Electronic applications accepted. *Financial support:* In 2013–14, fellowships with full tuition reimbursements (averaging $27,000 per year) were awarded; scholarships/grants, health care benefits, and tuition waivers (full) also available. *Faculty research:* Immunology, biochemistry, cancer biology, stem cell biology. *Unit head:* Dr. Mary Lou Cutler, Director, 301-295-3453, Fax: 301-295-1996, E-mail: mary.cutler@usuhs.edu. *Application contact:* Tina Finley, Administrative Assistant, 301-295-3642, Fax: 301-295-1996, E-mail: netina.finley@usuhs.edu.
Website: http://www.usuhs.mil/mcb/index.html

See Display below and Close-Up on page 239.

Universidad Central del Caribe, School of Medicine, Program in Biomedical Sciences, Bayamón, PR 00960-6032. Offers anatomy and cell biology (MA, MS); biochemistry (MS); biomedical sciences (MA); cellular and molecular biology (PhD); microbiology and immunology (MA, MS); pharmacology (MS); physiology (MS).

Université de Montréal, Faculty of Medicine, Program in Molecular Biology, Montréal, QC H3C 3J7, Canada. Offers M Sc, PhD. Terminal master's awarded for partial completion of doctoral program. *Degree requirements:* For master's, thesis; for doctorate, thesis/dissertation, general exam. *Entrance requirements:* For master's and doctorate, proficiency in French, knowledge of English. Electronic applications accepted. *Faculty research:* Protein interactions, intracellular signaling, development and differentiation, hematopoiesis, stem cells.

Université Laval, Faculty of Medicine, Graduate Programs in Medicine, Programs in Cellular and Molecular Biology, Québec, QC G1K 7P4, Canada. Offers M Sc, PhD. Terminal master's awarded for partial completion of doctoral program. *Degree requirements:* For master's, thesis; for doctorate, comprehensive exam, thesis/dissertation. *Entrance requirements:* For master's and doctorate, knowledge of French, comprehension of written English. Electronic applications accepted. *Faculty research:* Oral bacterial metabolism, sugar transport.

University at Albany, State University of New York, College of Arts and Sciences, Department of Biological Sciences, Specialization in Molecular, Cellular, Developmental, and Neural Biology, Albany, NY 12222-0001. Offers MS, PhD. *Degree requirements:* For master's, one foreign language; for doctorate, one foreign language, thesis/dissertation. *Entrance requirements:* For master's and doctorate, GRE General Test.

University at Albany, State University of New York, School of Public Health, Department of Biomedical Sciences, Program in Biochemistry, Molecular Biology, and Genetics, Albany, NY 12222-0001. Offers MS, PhD. *Degree requirements:* For master's, thesis; for doctorate, thesis/dissertation. *Entrance requirements:* For master's and doctorate, GRE General Test, GRE Subject Test.

University at Buffalo, the State University of New York, Graduate School, Graduate Programs in Cancer Research and Biomedical Sciences at Roswell Park Cancer Institute, Department of Cellular and Molecular Biology at Roswell Park Cancer Institute, Buffalo, NY 14260. Offers PhD. *Faculty:* 20 full-time (2 women), 5 part-time/adjunct (1 woman). *Students:* 18 full-time (9 women); includes 3 minority (1 Black or African American, non-Hispanic/Latino; 1 Asian, non-Hispanic/Latino; 1 Hispanic/Latino), 3 international. 74 applicants, 8% accepted, 2 enrolled. In 2013, 3 doctorates awarded. *Degree requirements:* For doctorate, comprehensive exam, thesis/dissertation, oral defense of disseration. *Entrance requirements:* For doctorate, GRE General Test. Additional exam requirements/recommendations for international students: Required—TOEFL (minimum score 79 iBT). *Application deadline:* For fall admission, 1/5 priority date for domestic and international students; for winter admission, 12/30 for domestic and international students. Application fee: $75. Electronic applications accepted. *Financial support:* In 2013–14, 18 students received support, including 18 research assistantships with full tuition reimbursements available (averaging $25,000 per year); scholarships/grants, health care benefits, and unspecified assistantships also available. Financial award application deadline: 1/5. *Faculty research:* Cancer genetics, chromatin structure and replication, regulation of transcription, human gene mapping, genetic and structural approaches to regulation of gene expression. *Unit head:* Dr. Dominic J. Smiraglia, Director of Graduate Studies, 716-845-1347, Fax: 716-845-1698, E-mail: dominic.smiraglia@roswellpark.org. *Application contact:* Dr. Norman J. Karin, Associate Dean, 716-845-2339, Fax: 716-845-8178, E-mail: norman.karin@roswellpark.org.
Website: http://www.roswellpark.edu/education/phd-programs/cellular-molecular-biology

The University of Alabama at Birmingham, Graduate Programs in Joint Health Sciences, Program in Cellular and Molecular Physiology, Birmingham, AL 35294. Offers PhD. *Degree requirements:* For doctorate, comprehensive exam, thesis/dissertation.

University of Alberta, Faculty of Graduate Studies and Research, Department of Biological Sciences, Edmonton, AB T6G 2E1, Canada. Offers environmental biology and ecology (M Sc, PhD); microbiology and biotechnology (M Sc, PhD); molecular biology and genetics (M Sc, PhD); physiology and cell biology (M Sc, PhD); plant biology (M Sc, PhD); systematics and evolution (M Sc, PhD). Terminal master's awarded for partial completion of doctoral program. *Degree requirements:* For master's, thesis; for doctorate, thesis/dissertation. *Entrance requirements:* Additional exam requirements/recommendations for international students: Required—TOEFL.

University of Alberta, Faculty of Medicine and Dentistry and Faculty of Graduate Studies and Research, Graduate Programs in Medicine, Department of Cell Biology, Edmonton, AB T6G 2E1, Canada. Offers cell and molecular biology (M Sc, PhD). Terminal master's awarded for partial completion of doctoral program. *Degree requirements:* For master's, thesis; for doctorate, thesis/dissertation. *Entrance requirements:* For master's and doctorate, 3 letters of reference, curriculum vitae. Additional exam requirements/recommendations for international students: Required—TOEFL (minimum score 600 paper-based). *Faculty research:* Protein targeting, membrane trafficking, signal transduction, cell growth and division, cell-cell interaction and development.

The University of Arizona, College of Science, Department of Molecular and Cellular Biology, Tucson, AZ 85721. Offers applied biosciences (PSM); molecular and cellular biology (MS, PhD). Evening/weekend programs available. *Faculty:* 14 full-time (5 women). *Students:* 36 full-time (16 women); includes 13 minority (2 Black or African American, non-Hispanic/Latino; 2 Asian, non-Hispanic/Latino; 3 Hispanic/Latino; 6 Two or more races, non-Hispanic/Latino), 5 international. Average age 28. 34 applicants, 74% accepted, 13 enrolled. In 2013, 8 master's, 3 doctorates awarded. Terminal master's awarded for partial completion of doctoral program. *Degree requirements:* For master's, thesis; for doctorate, thesis/dissertation. *Entrance requirements:* For master's, 3 letters of recommendation; for doctorate, 3 letters of recommendation, statement of purpose. Additional exam requirements/recommendations for international students: Required—TOEFL (minimum score 600 paper-based; 90 iBT), IELTS (minimum score 7). *Application deadline:* For fall admission, 1/1 for domestic and international students. Applications are processed on a rolling basis. Application fee: $75. Electronic applications accepted. *Expenses:* Tuition, state resident: full-time $11,526. Tuition, nonresident: full-time $27,398. *Financial support:* In 2013–14, 15 research assistantships with full tuition reimbursements (averaging $24,838 per year), 5 teaching assistantships with full tuition reimbursements (averaging $22,587 per year) were

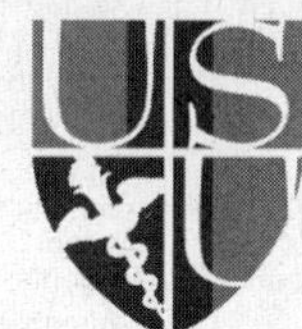

UNIFORMED SERVICES UNIVERSITY OF THE HEALTH SCIENCES

The graduate programs in biomedical sciences and public health in the USU School of Medicine are **open to civilian and military applicants.** The website, http://www.usuhs.edu/graded/index.html, provides insight into the numerous outstanding research training opportunities and the excellent faculty we have to support and challenge students.

Tuition and fees are waived for students. Civilian students do not incur service obligation to the U.S. government after the completion of their graduate studies.

For academic year 2014–15, USU-supported stipends are $27,000 for entering students and $28,000 after advancement to candidacy. University support for the stipend is for the first 3 years.

Deadline for full consideration of applications for the Fall Quarter is December 1.

*International students are considered if they earned a baccalaureate degree from a U.S. college/university.

For more information, contact:

Uniformed Services University
4301 Jones Bridge Road
Bethesda, Maryland 20814-4799
Phone: 301-295-3913 or 800-772-1747 (toll-free)
E-mail: netina.finley@usuhs.edu

http://www.usuhs.edu/graded/prospectivestudents.html

awarded; career-related internships or fieldwork, scholarships/grants, health care benefits, and unspecified assistantships also available. *Faculty research:* Plant molecular biology, cellular and molecular aspects of development, genetics of bacteria and lower eukaryotes. *Total annual research expenditures:* $5.5 million. *Unit head:* Tricia Serio, Department Head, 520-621-1519, E-mail: bmcb@email.arizona.edu. *Application contact:* 520-621-1519, E-mail: bmcb@email.arizona.edu.
Website: http://bmcb.biology.arizona.edu/

University of Arkansas, Graduate School, Interdisciplinary Program in Cell and Molecular Biology, Fayetteville, AR 72701-1201. Offers MS, PhD. *Degree requirements:* For doctorate, thesis/dissertation. Electronic applications accepted.

University of Arkansas for Medical Sciences, Graduate School, Little Rock, AR 72205. Offers biochemistry and molecular biology (MS, PhD); bioinformatics (MS, PhD); cellular physiology and molecular biophysics (MS, PhD); clinical nutrition (MS); interdisciplinary biomedical sciences (MS, PhD, Certificate); interdisciplinary toxicology (MS); microbiology and immunology (PhD); neurobiology and developmental sciences (PhD); pharmacology (PhD); MD/PhD. Bioinformatics programs hosted jointly with the University of Arkansas at Little Rock. Part-time programs available. *Faculty:* 397 full-time (205 women). *Students:* 196 full-time (126 women), 117 part-time (87 women); includes 65 minority (38 Black or African American, non-Hispanic/Latino; 1 American Indian or Alaska Native, non-Hispanic/Latino; 21 Asian, non-Hispanic/Latino; 4 Hispanic/Latino; 1 Two or more races, non-Hispanic/Latino), 57 international. 455 applicants, 27% accepted, 89 enrolled. In 2013, 41 master's, 18 doctorates, 28 other advanced degrees awarded. Terminal master's awarded for partial completion of doctoral program. *Degree requirements:* For master's, comprehensive exam (for some programs), thesis (for some programs); for doctorate, thesis/dissertation. *Entrance requirements:* For master's and doctorate, GRE. Additional exam requirements/recommendations for international students: Required—TOEFL. *Application deadline:* Applications are processed on a rolling basis. Application fee: $0. Electronic applications accepted. *Expenses:* Contact institution. *Financial support:* In 2013–14, 120 research assistantships (averaging $24,000 per year) were awarded; career-related internships or fieldwork, Federal Work-Study, and traineeships also available. Support available to part-time students. Financial award applicants required to submit FAFSA. *Unit head:* Dr. Robert E. McGehee, Jr., Dean, 501-686-5454. *Application contact:* Dr. Kristen Sterba, Assistant Dean, Office of Graduate Student Recruiting and Retention, 501-526-7396, E-mail: kmsterba@uams.edu.
Website: http://www.uams.edu/gradschool/

The University of British Columbia, Faculty of Medicine, Department of Biochemistry and Molecular Biology, Vancouver, BC V6T 1Z1, Canada. Offers M Sc, PhD. *Degree requirements:* For master's, thesis; for doctorate, comprehensive exam, thesis/dissertation. *Entrance requirements:* For master's, first class B Sc; for doctorate, master's or first class honors bachelor's degree in biochemistry. Additional exam requirements/recommendations for international students: Required—TOEFL (minimum score 625 paper-based). Electronic applications accepted. *Expenses: Tuition, area resident:* Full-time $8000 Canadian dollars. *Faculty research:* Membrane biochemistry, protein structure/function, signal transduction, biochemistry.

University of Calgary, Cumming School of Medicine and Faculty of Graduate Studies, Department of Biochemistry and Molecular Biology, Calgary, AB T2N 1N4, Canada. Offers M Sc, PhD. *Degree requirements:* For master's, thesis; for doctorate, thesis/dissertation, candidacy exam. *Entrance requirements:* For master's and doctorate, GRE General Test, minimum GPA of 3.2. Additional exam requirements/recommendations for international students: Required—TOEFL. Electronic applications accepted. *Faculty research:* Molecular and developmental genetics; molecular biology of disease; genomics, proteomics and bioinformatics; cell signaling and structure.

University of California, Berkeley, Graduate Division, College of Letters and Science, Department of Molecular and Cell Biology, Berkeley, CA 94720-1500. Offers PhD. *Faculty:* 94 full-time (28 women), 1 part-time/adjunct (0 women). *Students:* 243 full-time (126 women); includes 75 minority (5 Black or African American, non-Hispanic/Latino; 4 American Indian or Alaska Native, non-Hispanic/Latino; 29 Asian, non-Hispanic/Latino; 24 Hispanic/Latino; 4 Native Hawaiian or other Pacific Islander, non-Hispanic/Latino; 9 Two or more races, non-Hispanic/Latino), 29 international. Average age 26. 687 applicants, 16% accepted, 37 enrolled. In 2013, 37 doctorates awarded. *Degree requirements:* For doctorate, comprehensive exam, thesis/dissertation, qualifying exam, 2 semesters of teaching. *Entrance requirements:* For doctorate, GRE General Test, GRE Subject Test (recommended), minimum GPA of 3.0. Additional exam requirements/recommendations for international students: Required—TOEFL (minimum score 570 paper-based; 68 iBT), IELTS (minimum score 7). *Application deadline:* For fall admission, 12/1 for domestic and international students. Applications are processed on a rolling basis. Application fee: $80 ($100 for international students). Electronic applications accepted. *Financial support:* In 2013–14, fellowships with full tuition reimbursements (averaging $31,000 per year), research assistantships with full tuition reimbursements (averaging $31,000 per year), teaching assistantships with full tuition reimbursements (averaging $31,000 per year) were awarded; scholarships/grants, traineeships, health care benefits, tuition waivers (full), and unspecified assistantships also available. Financial award application deadline: 12/1; financial award applicants required to submit FAFSA. *Faculty research:* Biochemistry, biophysics and structural biology; cell and developmental biology; genetics, genomics and development; immunology and pathogenesis; neurobiology. *Unit head:* Tanya Sullivan, Student Services Manager, 510-642-5252. *Application contact:* Berta Parra, Graduate Student Adviser, 510-642-5252, E-mail: mcbgao@berkeley.edu.
Website: http://mcb.berkeley.edu/

University of California, Davis, Graduate Studies, Graduate Group in Biochemistry and Molecular Biology, Davis, CA 95616. Offers MS, PhD. Terminal master's awarded for partial completion of doctoral program. *Degree requirements:* For master's, comprehensive exam (for some programs), thesis (for some programs); for doctorate, thesis/dissertation. *Entrance requirements:* For master's and doctorate, GRE General Test, GRE Subject Test. Additional exam requirements/recommendations for international students: Required—TOEFL (minimum score 550 paper-based). Electronic applications accepted. *Faculty research:* Gene expression, protein structure, molecular virology, protein synthesis, enzymology, membrane transport and structural biology.

University of California, Irvine, School of Biological Sciences, Department of Molecular Biology and Biochemistry, Irvine, CA 92697. Offers biological science (MS); biological sciences (PhD); biotechnology (MS); MD/PhD. *Students:* 59 full-time (28 women), 1 part-time (0 women); includes 28 minority (1 Black or African American, non-Hispanic/Latino; 14 Asian, non-Hispanic/Latino; 12 Hispanic/Latino; 1 Native Hawaiian or other Pacific Islander, non-Hispanic/Latino), 4 international. Average age 28. In 2013, 6 master's, 10 doctorates awarded. *Degree requirements:* For doctorate, thesis/dissertation. *Entrance requirements:* For master's, GRE, minimum GPA of 3.0; for doctorate, GRE General Test, GRE Subject Test, minimum GPA of 3.0. Additional exam requirements/recommendations for international students: Required—TOEFL (minimum score 550 paper-based). *Application deadline:* For fall admission, 12/15 priority date for domestic students, 12/15 for international students. Applications are processed on a rolling basis. Application fee: $80 ($100 for international students). Electronic applications accepted. *Financial support:* Fellowships, research assistantships with full tuition reimbursements, teaching assistantships, institutionally sponsored loans, traineeships, health care benefits, and unspecified assistantships available. Financial award application deadline: 3/1; financial award applicants required to submit FAFSA. *Faculty research:* Structure and synthesis of nucleic acids and proteins, regulation, virology, biochemical genetics, gene organization. *Unit head:* Prof. Christopher Hughes, Chair, 949-824-8771, Fax: 949-824-8551, E-mail: cchughes@uci.edu. *Application contact:* Morgan Oldham, Student Affairs Assistant, 949-826-6034, Fax: 949-824-8551, E-mail: morgano@uci.edu.
Website: http://www.bio.uci.edu/

University of California, Irvine, School of Biological Sciences and School of Medicine, Interdisciplinary Graduate Program in Cellular and Molecular Biosciences, Irvine, CA 92697. Offers PhD. *Degree requirements:* For doctorate, thesis/dissertation, teaching assignment, preliminary exam. *Entrance requirements:* For doctorate, GRE General Test, three letters of recommendation, interview. Additional exam requirements/recommendations for international students: Required—TOEFL or IELTS. *Application deadline:* For fall admission, 12/8 for domestic and international students. Application fee: $60 ($80 for international students). Electronic applications accepted. *Expenses:* Contact institution. *Financial support:* Fellowships with full tuition reimbursements, institutionally sponsored loans, scholarships/grants, tuition waivers (full), unspecified assistantships, and stipends available. Financial award application deadline: 1/1; financial award applicants required to submit FAFSA. *Faculty research:* Cellular biochemistry; gene structure and expression; protein structure, function, and design; molecular genetics; pathogenesis and inherited disease. *Unit head:* Dr. David Fruman, Director, 949-824-1947, Fax: 949-824-1965, E-mail: dfruman@uci.edu. *Application contact:* Renee Frigo, Administrator, 949-824-8145, Fax: 949-824-1965, E-mail: rfrigo@uci.edu.
Website: http://cmb.uci.edu/

University of California, Los Angeles, Graduate Division, College of Letters and Science, Department of Chemistry and Biochemistry, Program in Biochemistry and Molecular Biology, Los Angeles, CA 90095. Offers MS, PhD. Terminal master's awarded for partial completion of doctoral program. *Degree requirements:* For master's, comprehensive exam or thesis; for doctorate, thesis/dissertation, oral and written qualifying exams; 3 quarters of teaching experience. *Entrance requirements:* For doctorate, GRE General Test, GRE Subject Test (recommended), bachelor's degree; minimum undergraduate GPA of 3.0 (or its equivalent if letter grade system not used). Additional exam requirements/recommendations for international students: Required—TOEFL. Electronic applications accepted.

University of California, Los Angeles, Graduate Division, College of Letters and Science, Department of Molecular, Cell and Developmental Biology, Los Angeles, CA 90095. Offers MA, PhD. Terminal master's awarded for partial completion of doctoral program. *Degree requirements:* For master's, comprehensive exam, thesis; for doctorate, thesis/dissertation, oral and written qualifying exams; 2 quarters of teaching experience. *Entrance requirements:* For doctorate, GRE General Test. Additional exam requirements/recommendations for international students: Required—TOEFL. Electronic applications accepted.

University of California, Los Angeles, Graduate Division, College of Letters and Science, Program in Molecular Biology, Los Angeles, CA 90095. Offers PhD, MD/PhD. *Degree requirements:* For doctorate, thesis/dissertation, oral and written qualifying exams. *Entrance requirements:* For doctorate, GRE General Test; GRE Subject Test (biochemistry, chemistry, biology, or physics), bachelor's degree; minimum undergraduate GPA of 3.0 (or its equivalent if letter grade system not used). Additional exam requirements/recommendations for international students: Required—TOEFL. Electronic applications accepted.

University of California, Los Angeles, Graduate Division, College of Letters and Science and David Geffen School of Medicine, UCLA ACCESS to Programs in the Molecular, Cellular and Integrative Life Sciences, Los Angeles, CA 90095. Offers biochemistry and molecular biology (PhD); biological chemistry (PhD); cellular and molecular pathology (PhD); human genetics (PhD); microbiology, immunology, and molecular genetics (PhD); molecular biology (PhD); molecular toxicology (PhD); molecular, cellular and integrative physiology (PhD); neurobiology (PhD); oral biology (PhD); physiology (PhD). *Degree requirements:* For doctorate, thesis/dissertation, oral and written qualifying exams. *Entrance requirements:* For doctorate, GRE General Test, bachelor's degree; minimum undergraduate GPA of 3.0 (or its equivalent if letter grade system not used). Additional exam requirements/recommendations for international students: Required—TOEFL. Electronic applications accepted.

University of California, Riverside, Graduate Division, Program in Cell, Molecular, and Developmental Biology, Riverside, CA 92521-0102. Offers MS, PhD. Terminal master's awarded for partial completion of doctoral program. *Degree requirements:* For master's, thesis, oral defense of thesis; for doctorate, thesis/dissertation, oral defense of thesis, qualifying exams, 2 quarters of teaching experience. *Entrance requirements:* For master's and doctorate, GRE General Test, minimum GPA of 3.2. Additional exam requirements/recommendations for international students: Required—TOEFL (minimum score 550 paper-based; 80 iBT). Electronic applications accepted.

University of California, San Francisco, Graduate Division and School of Medicine, Tetrad Graduate Program, Biochemistry and Molecular Biology Track, San Francisco, CA 94143. Offers PhD, MD/PhD. *Degree requirements:* For doctorate, thesis/dissertation. *Entrance requirements:* For doctorate, GRE General Test, GRE Subject Test. Additional exam requirements/recommendations for international students: Required—TOEFL. *Application deadline:* For fall admission, 12/1 for domestic students. Application fee: $40. *Expenses:* Contact institution. *Financial support:* Fellowships available. Financial award application deadline: 2/1. *Faculty research:* Structural biology, genetics, cell biology, cell physiology, metabolism. *Unit head:* Dr. Peter Walter, Chair, 415-476-5017. *Application contact:* Dr. Peter Walter, Chair, 415-476-5017.
Website: http://tetrad.ucsf.edu/

University of California, Santa Barbara, Graduate Division, College of Letters and Sciences, Division of Mathematics, Life, and Physical Sciences, Department of Molecular, Cellular, and Developmental Biology, Santa Barbara, CA 93106-9625. Offers molecular, cellular, and developmental biology (MA, PhD); pharmacology/biotechnology (MA); MA/PhD. *Faculty:* 29 full-time (3 women), 4 part-time/adjunct (0 women). *Students:* 48 full-time (23 women); includes 8 minority (2 Black or African American, non-Hispanic/Latino; 3 Asian, non-Hispanic/Latino; 3 Hispanic/Latino), 1 international. Average age 29. 182 applicants, 18% accepted, 11 enrolled. In 2013, 7 master's, 7 doctorates awarded. Terminal master's awarded for partial completion of doctoral program. *Degree requirements:* For master's, comprehensive exam (for some programs), thesis (for some programs); for doctorate, comprehensive exam, thesis/dissertation. *Entrance requirements:* For master's and doctorate, GRE General Test, 3 letters of recommendation, statement of purpose, personal achievements/contributions statement, resume/curriculum vitae, transcripts for post-secondary institutions attended. Additional exam requirements/recommendations for international students: Required—TOEFL (minimum score 550 paper-based; 80 iBT), IELTS (minimum score 7). *Application deadline:* For fall admission, 12/15 priority date for domestic and international students. Application fee: $80 ($100 for international students). Electronic

applications accepted. *Expenses:* Tuition, state resident: part-time $5148.26 per quarter. Tuition, nonresident: part-time $10,182.26 per quarter. *Financial support:* In 2013–14, 3 students received support, including 3 fellowships with full and partial tuition reimbursements available (averaging $22,000 per year), 40 research assistantships with full and partial tuition reimbursements available (averaging $26.250 per year), 46 teaching assistantships with partial tuition reimbursements available (averaging $17,655 per year); career-related internships or fieldwork, Federal Work-Study, institutionally sponsored loans, scholarships/grants, traineeships, health care benefits, and unspecified assistantships also available. Financial award application deadline: 3/13; financial award applicants required to submit FAFSA. *Faculty research:* Microbiology, neurobiology (including stem cell research), developmental, virology, cell biology. *Unit head:* Dr. William Smith, Chair, 805-893-7698, E-mail: wililam.smith@lifesci.ucsb.edu. *Application contact:* Nicole McCoy, Graduate Program Advisor, 805-893-8499, E-mail: nicole.mccoy@lifesci.ucsb.edu.
Website: https://www.mcdb.ucsb.edu/grad

University of California, Santa Barbara, Graduate Division, College of Letters and Sciences, Division of Mathematics, Life, and Physical Sciences, Interdepartmental Graduate Program in Biomolecular Science and Engineering, Santa Barbara, CA 93106-2014. Offers biochemistry and molecular biology (PhD), including biochemistry and molecular biology, biophysics and bioengineering. *Faculty:* 35 full-time (3 women), 3 part-time/adjunct (all women). *Students:* 26 full-time (13 women); includes 5 minority (4 Asian, non-Hispanic/Latino; 1 Hispanic/Latino), 2 international. Average age 29. 98 applicants, 17% accepted, 6 enrolled. In 2013, 6 doctorates awarded. Terminal master's awarded for partial completion of doctoral program. *Degree requirements:* For doctorate, thesis/dissertation. *Entrance requirements:* For doctorate, GRE General Test. Additional exam requirements/recommendations for international students: Required—TOEFL (minimum score 630 paper-based; 109 iBT), IELTS (minimum score 7). *Application deadline:* For fall admission, 12/15 for domestic and international students. Application fee: $80 ($100 for international students). Electronic applications accepted. *Expenses:* Tuition, state resident: part-time $5148.26 per quarter. Tuition, nonresident: part-time $10,182.26 per quarter. *Financial support:* In 2013–14, 28 students received support, including 16 fellowships with full and partial tuition reimbursements available (averaging $11,321 per year), 31 research assistantships with full and partial tuition reimbursements available (averaging $14,777 per year), 16 teaching assistantships with full and partial tuition reimbursements available (averaging $6,307 per year); Federal Work-Study, traineeships, health care benefits, tuition waivers (full and partial), and unspecified assistantships also available. Financial award application deadline: 12/15; financial award applicants required to submit FAFSA. *Faculty research:* Biochemistry and molecular biology, biophysics, biomaterials, bioengineering, systems biology. *Unit head:* Prof. Omar A. Saleh, Director/Professor, 805-893-8814, E-mail: saleh@engineering.ucsb.edu. *Application contact:* Nicole McCoy, 805-893-8499, E-mail: nicole.mccoy@lifesci.ucsb.edu.
Website: http://www.bmse.ucsb.edu/

University of California, Santa Cruz, Division of Graduate Studies, Division of Physical and Biological Sciences, Program in Molecular, Cellular, and Developmental Biology, Santa Cruz, CA 95064. Offers MA, PhD. Terminal master's awarded for partial completion of doctoral program. *Degree requirements:* For master's, thesis; for doctorate, thesis/dissertation, qualifying exam. *Entrance requirements:* For master's and doctorate, GRE General Test, 3 letters of recommendation, interview. Additional exam requirements/recommendations for international students: Required—TOEFL (minimum score 550 paper-based; 83 iBT); Recommended—IELTS (minimum score 8). Electronic applications accepted. *Faculty research:* RNA biology, chromatin and chromosome biology, neurobiology, stem cell biology and differentiation, cell structure and function.

University of Chicago, Division of Biological Sciences, Molecular Biosciences Cluster, Department of Biochemistry and Molecular Biology, Chicago, IL 60637-1513. Offers PhD, MD/PhD. *Degree requirements:* For doctorate, thesis/dissertation, ethics class, 2 teaching assistantships. *Entrance requirements:* For doctorate, GRE General Test, GRE Subject Test. Additional exam requirements/recommendations for international students: Required—TOEFL (minimum score 600 paper-based; 104 iBT), IELTS (minimum score 7). Electronic applications accepted. *Faculty research:* Molecular biology, gene expression, and DNA-protein interactions; membrane biochemistry, molecular endocrinology, and transmembrane signaling; enzyme mechanisms, physical biochemistry, and structural biology.

University of Chicago, Division of Biological Sciences, Molecular Biosciences Cluster, Graduate Program in Cell and Molecular Biology, Chicago, IL 60637-1513. Offers PhD. *Degree requirements:* For doctorate, thesis/dissertation, ethics class, 2 teaching assistantships. *Entrance requirements:* For doctorate, GRE General Test. Additional exam requirements/recommendations for international students: Required—TOEFL (minimum score 600 paper-based; 104 iBT), IELTS (minimum score 7). Electronic applications accepted. *Faculty research:* Gene expression, chromosome structure, animal viruses, plant molecular genetics.

University of Cincinnati, Graduate School, College of Medicine, Graduate Programs in Biomedical Sciences, Department of Environmental Health, Programs in Environmental Genetics and Molecular Toxicology, Cincinnati, OH 45221. Offers MS, PhD. *Degree requirements:* For doctorate, thesis/dissertation. *Entrance requirements:* For master's, GRE, minimum GPA of 3.0, 3 letters of recommendation. Additional exam requirements/recommendations for international students: Required—TOEFL (minimum score 520 paper-based).

University of Cincinnati, Graduate School, College of Medicine, Graduate Programs in Biomedical Sciences, Department of Molecular Genetics, Biochemistry and Microbiology, Cincinnati, OH 45221. Offers MS, PhD. Terminal master's awarded for partial completion of doctoral program. *Degree requirements:* For master's, thesis or alternative; for doctorate, thesis/dissertation, qualifying exam. *Entrance requirements:* For master's and doctorate, GRE General Test. Additional exam requirements/recommendations for international students: Required—TOEFL (minimum score 600 paper-based; 100 iBT), TWE. Electronic applications accepted. *Faculty research:* Cancer biology and developmental genetics, gene regulation and chromosome structure, microbiology and pathogenic mechanisms, structural biology, membrane biochemistry and signal transduction.

University of Cincinnati, Graduate School, College of Medicine, Graduate Programs in Biomedical Sciences, Department of Pediatrics, Program in Molecular and Developmental Biology, Cincinnati, OH 45221. Offers PhD. *Degree requirements:* For doctorate, thesis/dissertation, qualifying exam. *Entrance requirements:* For doctorate, GRE General Test, minimum GPA of 3.2. Additional exam requirements/recommendations for international students: Required—TOEFL (minimum score 520 paper-based). Electronic applications accepted. *Faculty research:* Cancer biology, cardiovascular biology, developmental biology, human genetics, gene therapy, genomics and bioinformatics, immunobiology, molecular medicine, neuroscience, pulmonary biology, reproductive biology, stem cell biology.

University of Colorado Boulder, Graduate School, College of Arts and Sciences, Department of Molecular, Cellular, and Developmental Biology, Boulder, CO 80309. Offers cellular structure and function (MA, PhD); developmental biology (MA, PhD); molecular biology (MA, PhD). *Faculty:* 25 full-time (7 women). *Students:* 64 full-time (36 women), 1 part-time (0 women); includes 5 minority (2 Asian, non-Hispanic/Latino; 2 Hispanic/Latino; 1 Native Hawaiian or other Pacific Islander, non-Hispanic/Latino), 9 international. Average age 27. 311 applicants, 12% accepted, 11 enrolled. In 2013, 2 master's, 11 doctorates awarded. Terminal master's awarded for partial completion of doctoral program. *Degree requirements:* For master's, comprehensive exam, thesis or alternative; for doctorate, comprehensive exam, thesis/dissertation. *Entrance requirements:* For master's, GRE General Test, GRE Subject Test, minimum undergraduate GPA of 3.0; for doctorate, GRE General Test, GRE Subject Test. *Application deadline:* For fall admission, 12/1 for domestic students, 12/15 for international students. Application fee: $50 ($60 for international students). Electronic applications accepted. *Financial support:* In 2013–14, 154 students received support, including 32 fellowships (averaging $6,403 per year), 62 research assistantships with full and partial tuition reimbursements available (averaging $30,807 per year), 11 teaching assistantships with full and partial tuition reimbursements available (averaging $27,393 per year); institutionally sponsored loans, scholarships/grants, health care benefits, and unspecified assistantships also available. Financial award application deadline: 2/1; financial award applicants required to submit FAFSA. *Faculty research:* Molecular biology, cellular biology, genetics, biological sciences, gene cloning. *Total annual research expenditures:* $14.8 million.
Website: http://mcdb.colorado.edu/

University of Colorado Denver, College of Liberal Arts and Sciences, Department of Integrative Biology, Denver, CO 80217. Offers animal behavior (MS); biology (MS); cell and developmental biology (MS); ecology (MS); evolutionary biology (MS); genetics (MS); integrative and systems biology (PhD); microbiology (MS); molecular biology (MS); neurobiology (MS); plant systematics (MS). Part-time programs available. *Faculty:* 21 full-time (7 women), 3 part-time/adjunct (2 women). *Students:* 18 full-time (11 women), 5 part-time (all women); includes 5 minority (1 Black or African American, non-Hispanic/Latino; 2 Hispanic/Latino; 2 Two or more races, non-Hispanic/Latino), 1 international. Average age 29. 25 applicants, 44% accepted, 11 enrolled. In 2013, 13 master's awarded. *Degree requirements:* For master's, comprehensive exam, thesis, 30-32 credit hours. *Entrance requirements:* For master's, GRE General Test (minimum score in 50th percentile in each section), BA/BS from accredited institution awarded within the last 10 years; minimum undergraduate GPA of 3.0; prerequisite courses: 1 year each of general biology and general chemistry; 1 semester each of general genetics, general ecology, and cell biology; and a structure/function course. Additional exam requirements/recommendations for international students: Required—TOEFL (minimum score 537 paper-based; 75 iBT); Recommended—IELTS (minimum score 6.5). *Application deadline:* For fall admission, 2/1 for domestic and international students. Application fee: $50 ($75 for international students). Electronic applications accepted. *Financial support:* In 2013–14, 8 students received support. Fellowships, research assistantships, teaching assistantships, Federal Work-Study, institutionally sponsored loans, scholarships/grants, and traineeships available. Financial award application deadline: 4/1; financial award applicants required to submit FAFSA. *Faculty research:* Molecular developmental biology; quantitative ecology, biogeography, and population dynamics; environmental signaling and endocrine disruption; speciation, the evolution of reproductive isolation, and hybrid zones; evolutionary, behavioral, and conservation ecology. *Unit head:* Dr. John Swallow, Biology Department Chair, 303-556-6154, E-mail: john.swallow@ucdenver.edu. *Application contact:* Timberley Roane, Associate Professor/Director of MS in Biology Program, 303-556-6592, E-mail: timberley.roane@ucdenver.edu.
Website: http://www.ucdenver.edu/academics/colleges/CLAS/Departments/biology/Programs/MasterofScience/Pages/BiologyMasterOfScience.aspx

University of Colorado Denver, School of Medicine, Program in Molecular Biology, Aurora, CO 80045. Offers biomolecular structure (PhD); molecular biology (PhD). *Students:* 40 full-time (27 women); includes 7 minority (1 Black or African American, non-Hispanic/Latino; 4 Asian, non-Hispanic/Latino; 2 Hispanic/Latino), 5 international. Average age 28. 30 applicants, 10% accepted, 3 enrolled. In 2013, 12 doctorates awarded. *Degree requirements:* For doctorate, comprehensive exam, thesis/dissertation, 2 years of structured didactic courses, 2-3 years of research, laboratory work, thesis project. *Entrance requirements:* For doctorate, GRE, organic chemistry (2 semesters, including 1 semester of laboratory), biology, general physics, college-level mathematics through calculus, three letters of reference. Additional exam requirements/recommendations for international students: Required—TOEFL (minimum score 550 paper-based; 80 iBT). *Application deadline:* For fall admission, 12/1 for domestic students, 11/1 for international students. Application fee: $50 ($75 for international students). Electronic applications accepted. *Expenses:* Contact institution. *Financial support:* In 2013–14, 39 students received support. Fellowships, research assistantships, teaching assistantships, institutionally sponsored loans, scholarships/grants, traineeships, health care benefits, tuition waivers (full), and unspecified assistantships available. Financial award application deadline: 3/15; financial award applicants required to submit FAFSA. *Faculty research:* Gene transcription, RNA processing, chromosome dynamics, DNA damage and repair, chromatin assembly. *Unit head:* Dr. Mark Johnston, Chair, 303-724-3203, E-mail: mark.johnston@ucdenver.edu. *Application contact:* Jennifer Miller, Program Administrator, 303-724-3245, Fax: 303-724-3247, E-mail: jennifer.e.miller@ucdenver.edu.
Website: http://www.ucdenver.edu/academics/colleges/medicalschool/programs/Molbio/Pages/MolecularBiology.aspx

University of Colorado Denver, School of Medicine, Program in Pharmacology, Aurora, CO 80045. Offers bioinformatics (PhD); biomolecular structure (PhD); pharmacology (PhD). *Students:* 15 full-time (11 women), 1 part-time (0 women); includes 2 minority (both Asian, non-Hispanic/Latino). Average age 26. 25 applicants, 8% accepted, 2 enrolled. In 2013, 5 doctorates awarded. *Degree requirements:* For doctorate, comprehensive exam, thesis/dissertation, major seminar, 3 research rotations in the first year, 30 hours each of course work and thesis. *Entrance requirements:* For doctorate, GRE General Test, three letters of recommendation, personal statement. Additional exam requirements/recommendations for international students: Required—TOEFL (minimum score 550 paper-based; 80 iBT). *Application deadline:* For fall admission, 12/15 for domestic students, 11/15 for international students. Application fee: $50 ($75 for international students). Electronic applications accepted. *Expenses:* Contact institution. *Financial support:* In 2013–14, 16 students received support. Fellowships, research assistantships, teaching assistantships, institutionally sponsored loans, scholarships/grants, traineeships, health care benefits, tuition waivers (full), and unspecified assistantships available. Financial award application deadline: 3/15; financial award applicants required to submit FAFSA. *Faculty research:* Cancer biology, drugs of abuse, neuroscience, signal transduction, structural biology. *Total annual research expenditures:* $16.7 million. *Unit head:* Dr. Andrew Thorburn, Interim Chair, 303-724-3290, Fax: 303-724-3663, E-mail: andrew.thorburn@ucdenver.edu. *Application contact:* Elizabeth Bowen, Graduate Program Coordinator, 303-724-3565, E-mail: elizabeth.bowen@ucdenver.edu.
Website: http://www.ucdenver.edu/academics/colleges/medicalschool/departments/Pharmacology/Pages/Pharmacology.aspx

University of Connecticut, Graduate School, College of Liberal Arts and Sciences, Department of Molecular and Cell Biology, Field of Microbial Systems Analysis, Storrs,

CT 06269. Offers MS, PSM. *Degree requirements:* For master's, comprehensive exam. *Entrance requirements:* For master's, GRE General Test, GRE Subject Test. Additional exam requirements/recommendations for international students: Required—TOEFL (minimum score 550 paper-based). Electronic applications accepted.

University of Connecticut Health Center, Graduate School, Programs in Biomedical Sciences, Graduate Program in Molecular Biology and Biochemistry, Farmington, CT 06030. Offers PhD, DMD/PhD, MD/PhD. *Degree requirements:* For doctorate, comprehensive exam, thesis/dissertation. *Entrance requirements:* For doctorate, GRE General Test. Additional exam requirements/recommendations for international students: Required—TOEFL (minimum score 600 paper-based). Electronic applications accepted. *Faculty research:* Molecular biology, structural biology, protein biochemistry, microbial physiology and pathogenesis.

See Display below and Close-Up on page 245.

University of Delaware, College of Arts and Sciences, Department of Biological Sciences, Newark, DE 19716. Offers biotechnology (MS); cancer biology (MS, PhD); cell and extracellular matrix biology (MS, PhD); cell and systems physiology (MS, PhD); developmental biology (MS, PhD); ecology and evolution (MS, PhD); microbiology (MS, PhD); molecular biology and genetics (MS, PhD). Terminal master's awarded for partial completion of doctoral program. *Degree requirements:* For master's, thesis, preliminary exam; for doctorate, comprehensive exam, thesis/dissertation, preliminary exam. *Entrance requirements:* For master's and doctorate, GRE General Test. Additional exam requirements/recommendations for international students: Required—TOEFL (minimum score 600 paper-based); Recommended—TWE. Electronic applications accepted. *Faculty research:* Microorganisms, bone, cancer metastasis, developmental biology, cell biology, DNA.

University of Denver, Division of Natural Sciences and Mathematics, Department of Biological Sciences, Denver, CO 80208-9010. Offers biomedical sciences (PSM); cell and molecular biology (MS, PhD); ecology and evolution (MS, PhD). Part-time programs available. *Faculty:* 23 full-time (8 women). *Students:* 1 (woman) full-time, 21 part-time (13 women); includes 3 minority (all Hispanic/Latino), 7 international. Average age 27. 50 applicants, 22% accepted, 10 enrolled. In 2013, 5 master's, 2 doctorates awarded. Terminal master's awarded for partial completion of doctoral program. *Degree requirements:* For master's, comprehensive exam (for some programs), thesis; for doctorate, one foreign language, comprehensive exam (for some programs), thesis/dissertation. *Entrance requirements:* For master's and doctorate, GRE General Test, bachelor's degree in biology or related field, transcripts, personal statement, three letters of recommendation. Additional exam requirements/recommendations for international students: Required—TOEFL (minimum score 570 paper-based; 88 iBT). *Application deadline:* For fall admission, 1/1 priority date for domestic and international students. Applications are processed on a rolling basis. Application fee: $60. Electronic applications accepted. *Financial support:* In 2013–14, 19 students received support, including 3 research assistantships with full and partial tuition reimbursements available (averaging $22,448 per year), 15 teaching assistantships with full and partial tuition reimbursements available (averaging $25,161 per year); Federal Work-Study, institutionally sponsored loans, scholarships/grants, and unspecified assistantships also available. Support available to part-time students. Financial award application deadline: 2/15; financial award applicants required to submit FAFSA. *Faculty research:* Molecular biology, cell biology, neurobiology, ecology, molecular evolution. *Unit head:* Dr. Joseph Angleson, Chair, 303-871-3463, Fax: 303-871-3471, E-mail: jangleso@du.edu. *Application contact:* Randi Flageolle, Assistant to the Chair, 303-871-3457, Fax: 303-871-3471, E-mail: rflageol@du.edu.
Website: http://www.du.edu/nsm/departments/biologicalsciences/index.html

University of Florida, College of Medicine and Graduate School, Interdisciplinary Program in Biomedical Sciences, Concentration in Biochemistry and Molecular Biology, Gainesville, FL 32611. Offers PhD. *Degree requirements:* For doctorate, thesis/dissertation. *Entrance requirements:* For doctorate, GRE General Test, minimum GPA of 3.0, biochemistry before enrollment. Additional exam requirements/recommendations for international students: Required—TOEFL. Electronic applications accepted. *Expenses:* Tuition, state resident: full-time $12,640. Tuition, nonresident: full-time $30,000. *Faculty research:* Gene expression, metabolic regulation, structural biology, enzyme mechanism, membrane transporters.

University of Florida, Graduate School, College of Agricultural and Life Sciences, Department of Animal Sciences, Interdisciplinary Concentration in Animal Molecular and Cellular Biology, Gainesville, FL 32611. Offers MS, PhD. *Students:* 13 full-time (9 women), 3 part-time (2 women); includes 2 minority (both Hispanic/Latino), 10 international. Average age 29. 7 applicants, 71% accepted, 4 enrolled. In 2013, 1 master's, 4 doctorates awarded. *Entrance requirements:* For master's and doctorate, GRE General Test, minimum GPA of 3.0. Additional exam requirements/recommendations for international students: Required—TOEFL (minimum score 550 paper-based; 80 iBT), IELTS (minimum score 6). Application fee: $30. Electronic applications accepted. *Expenses:* Tuition, state resident: full-time $12,640. Tuition, nonresident: full-time $30,000. *Financial support:* In 2013–14, 11 students received support, including 1 fellowship (averaging $12,000 per year), 11 research assistantships (averaging $18,775 per year). Financial award applicants required to submit FAFSA. *Unit head:* Geoffrey E. Dahl, PhD, Professor and Department Chair, 352-392-1981, Fax: 352-392-5595, E-mail: gdahl@ufl.edu. *Application contact:* Office of Admissions, 352-392-1365, E-mail: webrequests@admissions.ufl.edu.
Website: http://www.animal.ufl.edu/amcb/

University of Florida, Graduate School, College of Liberal Arts and Sciences, Department of Biology, Gainesville, FL 32611. Offers botany (MS, MST, PhD), including botany; zoology (MS, MST, PhD), including animal molecular and cellular biology (PhD), tropical conservation and development (MS), wetland sciences (MS), zoology. *Faculty:* 31 full-time (9 women), 26 part-time/adjunct (9 women). *Students:* 99 full-time (44 women), 6 part-time (4 women); includes 14 minority (2 Black or African American, non-Hispanic/Latino; 1 American Indian or Alaska Native, non-Hispanic/Latino; 5 Asian, non-Hispanic/Latino; 6 Hispanic/Latino), 35 international. Average age 31. 74 applicants, 32% accepted, 18 enrolled. In 2013, 4 master's, 13 doctorates awarded. *Degree requirements:* For master's, comprehensive exam (for some programs), thesis; for doctorate, comprehensive exam, thesis/dissertation. *Entrance requirements:* For master's and doctorate, GRE General Test, minimum GPA of 3.0. Additional exam requirements/recommendations for international students: Required—TOEFL (minimum score 550 paper-based; 80 iBT), IELTS (minimum score 6). *Application deadline:* For fall admission, 12/1 for domestic and international students. Applications are processed on a rolling basis. Application fee: $30. Electronic applications accepted. *Expenses:* Tuition, state resident: full-time $12,640. Tuition, nonresident: full-time $30,000. *Financial support:* In 2013–14, 98 students received support, including 7 fellowships (averaging $22,150 per year), 34 research assistantships (averaging $19,000 per year), 66 teaching assistantships (averaging $16,250 per year); unspecified assistantships also available. Financial award application deadline: 12/15; financial award applicants required to submit FAFSA. *Faculty research:* Ecology, evolution, genetics, molecular and cellular biology, physiology. *Unit head:* Craig Osenberg, PhD, Professor and Chair, 352-392-9201, Fax: 352-392-3704, E-mail: osenberg@ufl.edu. *Application contact:* William T. Barbazuk, PhD, Associate Professor/Graduate Coordinator, 352-273-8624, Fax: 352-392-3704, E-mail: bbarbazuk@ufl.edu.
Website: http://www.biology.ufl.edu/

University of Georgia, Franklin College of Arts and Sciences, Department of Biochemistry and Molecular Biology, Athens, GA 30602. Offers MS, PhD. *Degree requirements:* For master's, one foreign language, thesis; for doctorate, one foreign language, thesis/dissertation. *Entrance requirements:* For master's and doctorate, GRE General Test. Additional exam requirements/recommendations for international students: Required—TOEFL. Electronic applications accepted.

University of Guelph, Graduate Studies, College of Biological Science, Department of Molecular and Cellular Biology, Guelph, ON N1G 2W1, Canada. Offers biochemistry (M Sc, PhD); biophysics (M Sc, PhD); botany (M Sc, PhD); microbiology (M Sc, PhD); molecular biology and genetics (M Sc, PhD). *Degree requirements:* For master's, thesis, research proposal; for doctorate, comprehensive exam, thesis/dissertation, research proposal. *Entrance requirements:* For master's, minimum B-average during previous 2 years of coursework; for doctorate, minimum A-average. Additional exam requirements/recommendations for international students: Required—TOEFL (minimum score 550 paper-based), IELTS (minimum score 6.5). Electronic applications accepted. *Faculty research:* Physiology, structure, genetics, and ecology of microbes; virology and microbial technology.

University of Hawaii at Manoa, Graduate Division, College of Tropical Agriculture and Human Resources, Department of Molecular Biosciences and Bioengineering, Honolulu, HI 96822. Offers bioengineering (MS); molecular bioscience and bioengineering (MS); molecular biosciences and bioengineering (PhD). Part-time programs available. *Degree requirements:* For master's, thesis optional; for doctorate, comprehensive exam, thesis/dissertation. *Entrance requirements:* For master's and doctorate, GRE General Test. Additional exam requirements/recommendations for international students: Required—TOEFL (minimum score 550 paper-based; 79 iBT), IELTS (minimum score 5). *Faculty research:* Mechanization, agricultural systems, waste management, water management, cell culture.

University of Hawaii at Manoa, John A. Burns School of Medicine, Department of Cell and Molecular Biology, Honolulu, HI 96813. Offers MS, PhD. Part-time programs available. Terminal master's awarded for partial completion of doctoral program. *Degree requirements:* For master's, thesis optional; for doctorate, comprehensive exam, thesis/dissertation. *Entrance requirements:* For master's and doctorate, GRE General Test, minimum GPA of 3.0. Additional exam requirements/recommendations for international students: Required—TOEFL (minimum score 500 paper-based; 61 iBT), IELTS (minimum score 5).

University of Idaho, College of Graduate Studies, College of Science, Department of Biological Sciences, Moscow, ID 83844-3051. Offers biology (MS, PhD); microbiology, molecular biology and biochemistry (MS, PhD). *Faculty:* 12 full-time. *Students:* 20 full-time, 3 part-time. Average age 31. In 2013, 2 master's, 5 doctorates awarded. *Degree requirements:* For doctorate, one foreign language, thesis/dissertation. *Entrance requirements:* For master's, GRE, minimum GPA of 2.8; for doctorate, GRE, minimum undergraduate GPA of 2.8, 3.0 graduate. Additional exam requirements/recommendations for international students: Required—TOEFL. *Application deadline:* For fall admission, 8/1 for domestic students; for spring admission, 12/15 for domestic students. Applications are processed on a rolling basis. Application fee: $60. Electronic applications accepted. *Expenses:* Tuition, state resident: full-time $5596; part-time $363 per credit hour. Tuition, nonresident: full-time $18,672; part-time $1089 per credit hour. *Financial support:* Research assistantships and teaching assistantships available. Financial award applicants required to submit FAFSA. *Faculty research:* Animal behavior development, germ cell development, evolutionary biology, fish reproductive biology, molecular mechanisms. *Unit head:* Dr. James J. Nagler, Interim Department Chair, 208-885-6280, E-mail: biosci@uidaho.edu. *Application contact:* Stephanie Thomas, Graduate Recruitment Coordinator, 208-885-4001, Fax: 208-885-4406, E-mail: gadms@uidaho.edu.
Website: http://www.uidaho.edu/sci/biology

University of Illinois at Chicago, College of Medicine and Graduate College, Graduate Programs in Medicine, Department of Biochemistry and Molecular Genetics, Chicago, IL 60607-7128. Offers PhD, MD/PhD. *Faculty:* 32 full-time (11 women), 6 part-time/adjunct (1 woman). *Students:* 31 full-time (17 women), 1 (woman) part-time; includes 5 minority (4 Asian, non-Hispanic/Latino; 1 Hispanic/Latino), 16 international. Average age 29. 7 applicants, 86% accepted, 3 enrolled. In 2013, 10 doctorates awarded. Terminal master's awarded for partial completion of doctoral program. *Degree requirements:* For doctorate, thesis/dissertation. *Entrance requirements:* For doctorate, GRE General Test. Additional exam requirements/recommendations for international students: Required—TOEFL. *Application deadline:* For fall admission, 3/1 priority date for domestic students, 2/15 for international students. Applications are processed on a rolling basis. Application fee: $40 ($50 for international students). Electronic applications accepted. *Expenses:* Tuition, state resident: full-time $11,066; part-time $3689 per term. Tuition, nonresident: full-time $23,064; part-time $7688 per term. *Required fees:* $3004; $1190 per term. Tuition and fees vary according to course level and program. *Financial support:* In 2013–14, 22 students received support. Fellowships with full tuition reimbursements available, research assistantships with full tuition reimbursements available, teaching assistantships with full tuition reimbursements available, career-related internships or fieldwork, Federal Work-Study, institutionally sponsored loans, traineeships, tuition waivers (full), and unspecified assistantships available. Financial award application deadline: 3/1; financial award applicants required to submit FAFSA. *Faculty research:* Nature of cellular components, control of metabolic processes, regulation of gene expression. *Total annual research expenditures:* $6.9 million. *Unit head:* Dr. Jack Kaplan, Head, 312-355-2732, E-mail: kaplanj@uic.edu. *Application contact:* Dr. Karen Colley, Co-Director of Graduate Studies, 312-996-7756.
Website: http://www.uic.edu/com/bcmg/

The University of Iowa, Graduate College, Program in Molecular and Cellular Biology, Iowa City, IA 52242-1316. Offers PhD. *Degree requirements:* For doctorate, comprehensive exam, thesis/dissertation. *Entrance requirements:* For doctorate, GRE General Test, minimum GPA of 3.0. Additional exam requirements/recommendations for international students: Required—TOEFL (minimum score 600 paper-based; 100 iBT). Electronic applications accepted. *Faculty research:* Regulation of gene expression, inherited human genetic diseases, signal transduction mechanisms, structural biology and function.

The University of Kansas, Graduate Studies, College of Liberal Arts and Sciences, Department of Molecular Biosciences, Lawrence, KS 66045. Offers biochemistry and biophysics (MA, PhD); microbiology (MA, PhD); molecular, cellular, and developmental biology (MA, PhD). *Faculty:* 34. *Students:* 52 full-time (28 women); includes 5 minority (2 Asian, non-Hispanic/Latino; 3 Hispanic/Latino), 23 international. Average age 27. 96 applicants, 25% accepted, 13 enrolled. In 2013, 3 master's, 9 doctorates awarded. Terminal master's awarded for partial completion of doctoral program. *Degree requirements:* For master's, comprehensive exam, thesis; for doctorate, comprehensive exam, thesis/dissertation. *Entrance requirements:* For master's and doctorate, GRE General Test. Additional exam requirements/recommendations for international students: Required—TOEFL or IELTS. *Application deadline:* For fall admission, 12/15 for domestic and international students. Application fee: $55 ($65 for international students). Electronic applications accepted. *Financial support:* Fellowships with tuition reimbursements, research assistantships with tuition reimbursements, teaching assistantships with tuition reimbursements, health care benefits, and unspecified assistantships available. Financial award application deadline: 3/1. *Faculty research:* Structure and function of proteins, genetics of organism development, molecular genetics, neurophysiology, molecular virology and pathogenics, developmental biology, cell biology. *Unit head:* Dr. Mark Richter, Chair, 785-864-3334, E-mail: richter@ku.edu. *Application contact:* John Connolly, Graduate Admissions Contact, 785-864-4311, E-mail: jconnolly@ku.edu.
Website: http://www.molecularbiosciences.ku.edu/

The University of Kansas, University of Kansas Medical Center, School of Medicine, Department of Biochemistry and Molecular Biology, Kansas City, KS 66160. Offers MS, PhD, MD/PhD. *Faculty:* 18. *Students:* 9 full-time (4 women), 6 international. Average age 27. In 2013, 1 doctorate awarded. Terminal master's awarded for partial completion of doctoral program. *Degree requirements:* For master's, thesis, oral defense of thesis; for doctorate, thesis/dissertation, comprehensive oral and written exam. *Entrance requirements:* Additional exam requirements/recommendations for international students: Required—TOEFL. Application fee: $0. Electronic applications accepted. *Financial support:* Fellowships, research assistantships with partial tuition reimbursements, teaching assistantships with full and partial tuition reimbursements, traineeships, health care benefits, and unspecified assistantships available. Financial award application deadline: 3/1; financial award applicants required to submit FAFSA. *Faculty research:* Determination of portion structure, underlying bases for interaction of proteins with their target, mapping allosteric circuiting within proteins, mechanism of action of transcription factors, renal signal transduction. *Total annual research expenditures:* $2.1 million. *Unit head:* Dr. Gerald M. Carlson, Chairman, 913-588-7005, Fax: 913-588-9896, E-mail: gcarlson@kumc.edu. *Application contact:* Dr. Liskin Swint-Kruse, Associate Professor, 913-588-0399, Fax: 913-588-9896, E-mail: lswint-kruse@kumc.edu.
Website: http://www.kumc.edu/school-of-medicine/biochemistry-and-molecular-biology.html

University of Lethbridge, School of Graduate Studies, Lethbridge, AB T1K 3M4, Canada. Offers accounting (MScM); addictions counseling (M Sc); agricultural biotechnology (M Sc); agricultural studies (M Sc, MA); anthropology (MA); archaeology (M Sc, MA); art (MA, MFA); biochemistry (M Sc); biological sciences (M Sc); biomolecular science (PhD); biosystems and biodiversity (PhD); Canadian studies (MA); chemistry (M Sc); computer science (M Sc); computer science and geographical information science (M Sc); counseling (MC); counseling psychology (M Ed); dramatic arts (MA); earth, space, and physical science (PhD); economics (MA); education (MA); educational leadership (M Ed); English (MA); environmental science (M Sc); evolution and behavior (PhD); exercise science (M Sc); finance (MScM); French (MA); French/German (MA); French/Spanish (MA); general education (M Ed); general management (MScM); geography (M Sc, MA); German (MA); health sciences (M Sc); human resource management and labour relations (MScM); individualized multidisciplinary (M Sc, MA); information systems (MScM); international management (MScM); kinesiology (M Sc, MA); marketing (MScM); mathematics (M Sc); modern languages (MA); music (M Mus, MA); Native American studies (MA); neuroscience (M Sc, PhD); new media (MA, MFA); nursing (M Sc); philosophy (MA); physics (M Sc); policy and strategy (MScM); political science (MA); psychology (M Sc, MA); religious studies (MA); sociology (MA); theatre and dramatic arts (MFA); theoretical and computational science (PhD); urban and regional studies (MA); women and gender studies (MA). Part-time and evening/weekend programs available. *Degree requirements:* For doctorate, comprehensive exam, thesis/dissertation. *Entrance requirements:* For master's, GMAT (for M Sc in management), bachelor's degree in related field, minimum GPA of 3.0 during previous 20 graded semester courses, 2 years teaching or related experience (M Ed); for doctorate, master's degree, minimum graduate GPA of 3.5. Additional exam requirements/recommendations for international students: Required—TOEFL. Application fee: $60 Canadian dollars. *Financial support:* Fellowships, research assistantships, teaching assistantships, scholarships/grants, health care benefits, and unspecified assistantships available. *Faculty research:* Movement and brain plasticity, gibberellin physiology, photosynthesis, carbon cycling, molecular properties of main-group ring components. *Application contact:* School of Graduate Studies, 403-329-2793, Fax: 403-332-5239, E-mail: sgsinquiries@uleth.ca.
Website: http://www.uleth.ca/graduatestudies/

University of Louisville, School of Medicine, Department of Biochemistry and Molecular Biology, Louisville, KY 40292-0001. Offers MS, PhD, MD/PhD. *Students:* 28 full-time (13 women), 8 part-time (4 women); includes 4 minority (2 Black or African American, non-Hispanic/Latino; 1 Asian, non-Hispanic/Latino; 1 Hispanic/Latino), 9 international. Average age 30. 34 applicants, 21% accepted, 9 enrolled. In 2013, 5 master's, 4 doctorates awarded. Terminal master's awarded for partial completion of doctoral program. *Degree requirements:* For master's, thesis; for doctorate, comprehensive exam, thesis/dissertation, one first author publication. *Entrance requirements:* For master's and doctorate, GRE General Test (minimum score of 1000 verbal and quantitative), minimum GPA of 3.0. Additional exam requirements/recommendations for international students: Required—TOEFL. *Application deadline:* For fall admission, 4/15 for domestic and international students. Applications are processed on a rolling basis. Application fee: $60. Electronic applications accepted. *Expenses:* Tuition, state resident: full-time $10,788; part-time $599 per credit hour. Tuition, nonresident: full-time $22,446; part-time $1247 per credit hour. *Required fees:* $196. Tuition and fees vary according to program and reciprocity agreements. *Financial support:* In 2013–14, 12 fellowships with full tuition reimbursements (averaging $22,000 per year), 23 research assistantships with full tuition reimbursements (averaging $22,000 per year) were awarded; teaching assistantships with tuition reimbursements, scholarships/grants, traineeships, tuition waivers (full and partial), and unspecified assistantships also available. Financial award application deadline: 4/15. *Faculty research:* Genetic regulatory mechanisms, microRNAs, vesicular trafficking in cancer metastasis and angiogenesis, ribosome biogenesis and disease, regulation of foreign compound metabolism/lipid and steroid metabolism. *Unit head:* Dr. Ronald G. Gregg, Chair, 502-852-5217, Fax: 502-852-6222, E-mail: rggreg02@gwise.louisville.edu. *Application contact:* Dr. William L. Dean, Information Contact, 502-852-5227, Fax: 502-852-6222, E-mail: wldean01@gwise.louisville.edu.

University of Maine, Graduate School, College of Natural Sciences, Forestry, and Agriculture, Department of Molecular and Biomedical Sciences, Orono, ME 04469. Offers biochemistry (MPS, MS); biochemistry and molecular biology (PhD); microbiology (MPS, MS, PhD). *Faculty:* 30 full-time (6 women), 20 part-time/adjunct (4 women). *Students:* 26 full-time (17 women), 4 part-time (3 women); includes 3 minority (2 Asian, non-Hispanic/Latino; 1 Native Hawaiian or other Pacific Islander, non-Hispanic/Latino), 5 international. Average age 31. 7 applicants, 100% accepted, 5 enrolled. In 2013, 5 master's, 4 doctorates awarded. *Degree requirements:* For master's, thesis (for some programs); for doctorate, comprehensive exam, thesis/dissertation. *Entrance requirements:* For master's and doctorate, GRE General Test. Additional exam requirements/recommendations for international students: Required—TOEFL. *Application deadline:* For fall admission, 2/1 priority date for domestic students. Applications are processed on a rolling basis. Application fee: $65. Electronic applications accepted. *Expenses:* Tuition, state resident: full-time $7524. Tuition, nonresident: full-time $23,112. *Required fees:* $1970. *Financial support:* In 2013–14, 16

students received support, including 5 research assistantships with full tuition reimbursements available (averaging $22,000 per year), 10 teaching assistantships with full tuition reimbursements available (averaging $19,000 per year); tuition waivers (full and partial) also available. Financial award application deadline: 3/1. *Total annual research expenditures:* $242,844. *Unit head:* Dr. Robert Gundersen, Chair, 207-581-2802, Fax: 207-581-2801. *Application contact:* Scott G. Delcourt, Associate Dean of the Graduate School, 207-581-3291, Fax: 207-581-3232, E-mail: graduate@maine.edu.
Website: http://umaine.edu/biomed/

University of Maine, Graduate School, Graduate School of Biomedical Science and Engineering, Orono, ME 04469. Offers bioinformatics (PSM); biomedical engineering (PhD); cell and molecular biology (PhD); neuroscience (PhD); toxicology (PhD). *Faculty:* 39 full-time (10 women), 31 part-time/adjunct (8 women). *Students:* 31 full-time (18 women), 5 part-time (4 women), 11 international. Average age 30. 57 applicants, 16% accepted, 7 enrolled. In 2013, 5 doctorates awarded. *Degree requirements:* For doctorate, comprehensive exam, thesis/dissertation. *Entrance requirements:* For doctorate, GRE General Test, master's degree. Additional exam requirements/recommendations for international students: Required—TOEFL. *Application deadline:* For fall admission, 1/1 for domestic students. Application fee: $65. *Expenses:* Tuition, state resident: full-time $7524. Tuition, nonresident: full-time $23,112. *Required fees:* $1970. *Financial support:* In 2013–14, 16 students received support, including 1 fellowship with full tuition reimbursement available (averaging $18,000 per year), 13 research assistantships with full tuition reimbursements available (averaging $21,000 per year), 2 teaching assistantships (averaging $20,000 per year). *Faculty research:* Biomedical engineering, toxicology, neuroscience, cell and molecular biology, bioinformatics. *Total annual research expenditures:* $650,000. *Unit head:* Dr. David Neivandt, Director, 207-581-2803. *Application contact:* Scott G. Delcourt, Associate Dean of the Graduate School, 207-581-3291, Fax: 207-581-3232, E-mail: graduate@maine.edu.
Website: http://gsbse.umaine.edu/

The University of Manchester, Faculty of Life Sciences, Manchester, United Kingdom. Offers adaptive organismal biology (M Phil, PhD); animal biology (M Phil, PhD); biochemistry (M Phil, PhD); bioinformatics (M Phil, PhD); biomolecular sciences (M Phil, PhD); biotechnology (M Phil, PhD); cell biology (M Phil, PhD); cell matrix research (M Phil, PhD); channels and transporters (M Phil, PhD); developmental biology (M Phil, PhD); Egyptology (M Phil, PhD); environmental biology (M Phil, PhD); evolutionary biology (M Phil, PhD); gene expression (M Phil, PhD); genetics (M Phil, PhD); history of science, technology and medicine (M Phil, PhD); immunology (M Phil, PhD); integrative neurobiology and behavior (M Phil, PhD); membrane trafficking (M Phil, PhD); microbiology (M Phil, PhD); molecular and cellular neuroscience (M Phil, PhD); molecular biology (M Phil, PhD); molecular cancer studies (M Phil, PhD); neuroscience (M Phil, PhD); ophthalmology (M Phil, PhD); optometry (M Phil, PhD); organelle function (M Phil, PhD); pharmacology (M Phil, PhD); physiology (M Phil, PhD); plant sciences (M Phil, PhD); stem cell research (M Phil, PhD); structural biology (M Phil, PhD); systems neuroscience (M Phil, PhD); toxicology (M Phil, PhD).

The University of Manchester, School of Dentistry, Manchester, United Kingdom. Offers basic dental sciences (cancer studies) (M Phil, PhD); basic dental sciences (molecular genetics) (M Phil, PhD); basic dental sciences (stem cell biology) (M Phil, PhD); biomaterials sciences and dental technology (M Phil, PhD); dental public health/community dentistry (M Phil, PhD); dental science (clinical) (PhD); endodontology (M Phil, PhD); fixed and removable prosthodontics (M Phil, PhD); operative dentistry (M Phil, PhD); oral and maxillofacial surgery (M Phil, PhD); oral radiology (M Phil, PhD); orthodontics (M Phil, PhD); restorative dentistry (M Phil, PhD).

University of Maryland, Baltimore, Graduate School, Graduate Program in Life Sciences, Program in Biochemistry and Molecular Biology, Baltimore, MD 21201. Offers biochemistry (MS, PhD); MD/PhD. *Students:* 26 full-time (11 women), 3 part-time (1 woman); includes 8 minority (3 Black or African American, non-Hispanic/Latino; 1 Asian, non-Hispanic/Latino; 3 Hispanic/Latino; 1 Two or more races, non-Hispanic/Latino), 4 international. Average age 27. 47 applicants, 17% accepted, 3 enrolled. In 2013, 1 master's, 7 doctorates awarded. *Degree requirements:* For doctorate, comprehensive exam, thesis/dissertation. *Entrance requirements:* For doctorate, GRE General Test. Additional exam requirements/recommendations for international students: Required—TOEFL (minimum score 550 paper-based; 80 iBT); Recommended—IELTS (minimum score 7). *Application deadline:* For fall admission, 1/15 for domestic and international students. Application fee: $75. Electronic applications accepted. *Financial support:* In 2013–14, research assistantships with full tuition reimbursements (averaging $25,000 per year) were awarded; fellowships, health care benefits, and unspecified assistantships also available. Financial award application deadline: 3/1; financial award applicants required to submit FAFSA. *Faculty research:* Membrane transport, hormonal regulation, protein structure, molecular virology. *Unit head:* Dr. Gerald Wilson, Professor/Director, 410-706-8904. *Application contact:* Kiriaki Cozmo, Program Coordinator, 410-706-7340, Fax: 410-706-8297, E-mail: kicozmo@som.umaryland.edu.
Website: http://biochemistry.umaryland.edu

University of Maryland, Baltimore, Graduate School, Graduate Program in Life Sciences, Program in Molecular Medicine, Baltimore, MD 21201. Offers cancer biology (PhD); cell and molecular physiology (PhD); human genetics and genomic medicine (PhD); molecular medicine (MS); molecular toxicology and pharmacology (PhD); MD/PhD. *Students:* 91 full-time (49 women), 14 part-time (8 women); includes 32 minority (10 Black or African American, non-Hispanic/Latino; 12 Asian, non-Hispanic/Latino; 5 Hispanic/Latino; 5 Two or more races, non-Hispanic/Latino), 9 international. Average age 27. 180 applicants, 33% accepted, 24 enrolled. In 2013, 10 master's, 15 doctorates awarded. *Degree requirements:* For doctorate, comprehensive exam, thesis/dissertation. *Entrance requirements:* For master's and doctorate, GRE. Additional exam requirements/recommendations for international students: Required—TOEFL (minimum score 600 paper-based; 100 iBT); Recommended—IELTS (minimum score 7). *Application deadline:* For fall admission, 12/1 priority date for domestic students, 1/15 for international students. Application fee: $75. Electronic applications accepted. *Financial support:* In 2013–14, research assistantships with partial tuition reimbursements (averaging $25,000 per year) were awarded; fellowships also available. Financial award application deadline: 3/1; financial award applicants required to submit FAFSA. *Unit head:* Dr. Toni Antalis, Director, 410-706-8222, E-mail: tantalis@som.umaryland.edu. *Application contact:* Sharron Graves, Program Coordinator, 410-706-6044, Fax: 410-706-6040, E-mail: sgraves@som.umaryland.edu.
Website: http://molecularmedicine.umaryland.edu

University of Maryland, Baltimore County, Graduate School, College of Natural and Mathematical Sciences, Department of Biological Sciences, Program in Applied Molecular Biology, Baltimore, MD 21250. Offers MS. *Faculty:* 26 full-time (11 women). *Students:* 12 full-time (7 women), 2 part-time (both women); includes 6 minority (3 Black or African American, non-Hispanic/Latino; 2 Asian, non-Hispanic/Latino; 1 Two or more races, non-Hispanic/Latino), 1 international. Average age 23. 41 applicants, 37% accepted, 14 enrolled. In 2013, 9 master's awarded. *Entrance requirements:* For master's, GRE General Test, GRE Subject Test (recommended), minimum GPA of 3.0. Additional exam requirements/recommendations for international students: Required—TOEFL (minimum score 600 paper-based; 80 iBT), IELTS (minimum score 4). *Application deadline:* For fall admission, 4/1 priority date for domestic and international students. Applications are processed on a rolling basis. Application fee: $50. Electronic applications accepted. One-time fee: $200 full-time. *Financial support:* Applicants required to submit FAFSA. *Faculty research:* Structure-function of RNA, genetics and molecular biology, biological chemistry. *Unit head:* Dr. Richard E. Wolf, Director, Applied Molecular Biology Graduate Program, 410-455-3669, Fax: 410-455-3875, E-mail: biograd@umbc.edu. *Application contact:* Melody Wright, Graduate Program Coordinator, 410-455-3669, Fax: 410-455-3875, E-mail: biograd@umbc.edu.
Website: http://www.umbc.edu/biosci

University of Maryland, Baltimore County, Graduate School, College of Natural and Mathematical Sciences, Department of Biological Sciences, Program in Molecular and Cell Biology, Baltimore, MD 21250. Offers PhD. *Faculty:* 26 full-time (11 women). *Students:* 7 full-time (4 women), 1 international. Average age 29. 25 applicants, 12% accepted. In 2013, 3 doctorates awarded. *Degree requirements:* For doctorate, thesis/dissertation. *Entrance requirements:* For doctorate, GRE General Test, GRE Subject Test, minimum GPA of 3.0. Additional exam requirements/recommendations for international students: Required—TOEFL (minimum score 80 iBT). *Application deadline:* For fall admission, 1/1 priority date for domestic and international students. Application fee: $50. Electronic applications accepted. One-time fee: $200 full-time. *Financial support:* In 2013–14, 7 students received support, including 3 fellowships with full tuition reimbursements available (averaging $25,000 per year), 4 teaching assistantships with full tuition reimbursements available (averaging $22,726 per year). *Unit head:* Dr. Stephen Miller, Graduate Program Director, 410-455-3381, Fax: 410-455-3875, E-mail: biograd@umbc.edu. *Application contact:* Dr. Stephen Miller, Director, 410-455-3381, Fax: 410-455-3875, E-mail: biograd@umbc.edu.
Website: http://biology.umbc.edu

University of Maryland, College Park, Academic Affairs, College of Computer, Mathematical and Natural Sciences, Department of Biology, PhD Program in Biological Sciences, College Park, MD 20742. Offers behavior, ecology, evolution, and systematics (PhD); computational biology, bioinformatics, and genomics (PhD); molecular and cellular biology (PhD); physiological systems (PhD). *Students:* 104 full-time (59 women), 4 part-time (1 woman); includes 21 minority (2 Black or African American, non-Hispanic/Latino; 1 American Indian or Alaska Native, non-Hispanic/Latino; 9 Asian, non-Hispanic/Latino; 7 Hispanic/Latino; 2 Two or more races, non-Hispanic/Latino), 34 international. 365 applicants, 13% accepted, 20 enrolled. In 2013, 5 doctorates awarded. *Degree requirements:* For doctorate, comprehensive exam, thesis/dissertation, thesis work presentation in seminar. *Entrance requirements:* For doctorate, GRE General Test; GRE Subject Test in biology (recommended), academic transcripts, statement of purpose/research interests, 3 letters of recommendation. Additional exam requirements/recommendations for international students: Required—TOEFL. *Application deadline:* For fall admission, 12/15 for domestic and international students. Applications are processed on a rolling basis. Application fee: $75. Electronic applications accepted. *Expenses:* Tuition, state resident: full-time $10,314; part-time $573 per credit hour. Tuition, nonresident: full-time $22,248; part-time $1236 per credit. *Required fees:* $1446; $403.15 per semester. Tuition and fees vary according to program. *Financial support:* In 2013–14, 21 fellowships with full and partial tuition reimbursements (averaging $27,603 per year), 25 research assistantships (averaging $19,557 per year), 55 teaching assistantships (averaging $18,959 per year) were awarded. *Unit head:* Dr. Charles F. Delwiche, Director, 301-405-6884, E-mail: bisidirector@umd.edu. *Application contact:* Dr. Charles A. Caramello, Dean of Graduate School, 301-405-0358, Fax: 301-314-9305, E-mail: ccaramel@umd.edu.
Website: http://www.bisi.umd.edu/

University of Maryland, College Park, Academic Affairs, College of Computer, Mathematical and Natural Sciences, Department of Cell Biology and Molecular Genetics, Program in Molecular and Cellular Biology, College Park, MD 20742. Offers PhD. Part-time and evening/weekend programs available. *Students:* 18 full-time (12 women), 1 (woman) part-time; includes 5 minority (1 Black or African American, non-Hispanic/Latino; 3 Asian, non-Hispanic/Latino; 1 Hispanic/Latino), 9 international. In 2013, 3 doctorates awarded. *Degree requirements:* For doctorate, thesis/dissertation, exam, public service. *Expenses:* Tuition, state resident: full-time $10,314; part-time $573 per credit hour. Tuition, nonresident: full-time $22,248; part-time $1236 per credit. *Required fees:* $1446; $403.15 per semester. Tuition and fees vary according to program. *Financial support:* In 2013–14, 2 fellowships with full tuition reimbursements (averaging $26,421 per year), 9 research assistantships (averaging $19,782 per year), 10 teaching assistantships (averaging $19,360 per year) were awarded. Financial award applicants required to submit FAFSA. *Faculty research:* Monoclonal antibody production, oligonucleotide synthesis, macromolular processing, signal transduction, developmental biology. *Unit head:* Norma Andrews, Chair, 301-405-8418, E-mail: andrewsn@umd.edu. *Application contact:* Dr. Charles A. Caramello, Dean of Graduate School, 301-405-0358, Fax: 301-314-9305, E-mail: ccaramel@umd.edu.

University of Massachusetts Boston, Office of Graduate Studies, College of Science and Mathematics, Track in Molecular, Cellular and Organismal Biology, Boston, MA 02125-3393. Offers PhD.

University of Miami, Graduate School, Miller School of Medicine, Graduate Programs in Medicine, Department of Biochemistry and Molecular Biology, Coral Gables, FL 33124. Offers PhD, MD/PhD. *Degree requirements:* For doctorate, comprehensive exam, thesis/dissertation, proposition exams. *Faculty research:* Macromolecule metabolism, molecular genetics, protein folding and 3-D structure, regulation of gene expression and enzyme function, signal transduction and developmental biology.

University of Miami, Graduate School, Miller School of Medicine, Graduate Programs in Medicine, Department of Cell Biology and Anatomy, Coral Gables, FL 33124. Offers molecular cell and developmental biology (PhD); MD/PhD. *Degree requirements:* For doctorate, thesis/dissertation. *Entrance requirements:* For doctorate, GRE General Test, GRE Subject Test. Additional exam requirements/recommendations for international students: Required—TOEFL. Electronic applications accepted.

University of Michigan, Rackham Graduate School, College of Literature, Science, and the Arts, Department of Molecular, Cellular, and Developmental Biology, Ann Arbor, MI 48109. Offers MS, PhD. Part-time programs available. *Faculty:* 35 full-time (11 women). *Students:* 77 full-time (40 women), 2 part-time (1 woman); includes 10 minority (4 Asian, non-Hispanic/Latino; 5 Hispanic/Latino; 1 Native Hawaiian or other Pacific Islander, non-Hispanic/Latino), 42 international. Average age 27. 100 applicants, 25% accepted, 12 enrolled. In 2013, 5 master's, 7 doctorates awarded. Terminal master's awarded for partial completion of doctoral program. *Degree requirements:* For master's, 24 credits with at least 16 in molecular, cellular, and developmental biology and 4 in a cognate field; for doctorate, thesis/dissertation, preliminary exam, oral defense. *Entrance requirements:* For master's and doctorate, GRE General Test. Additional exam requirements/recommendations for international students: Required—TOEFL (minimum score 560 paper-based; 83 iBT). *Application deadline:* For fall admission, 1/5 for domestic and international students; for winter admission, 11/1 for domestic and international students; for spring admission, 4/1 for domestic and international students. Applications are processed on a rolling basis. Application fee: $75 ($90 for international students). Electronic applications accepted. Tuition and fees vary according to course level, course load, degree level, program and student level. *Financial support:* In 2013–

14, 13 fellowships with full tuition reimbursements (averaging $28,500 per year), 31 research assistantships with full tuition reimbursements (averaging $28,500 per year), 17 teaching assistantships with full tuition reimbursements (averaging $28,500 per year) were awarded; health care benefits also available. *Faculty research:* Cell biology, microbiology, neurobiology and physiology, developmental biology and plant molecular biology. *Total annual research expenditures:* $7.8 million. *Unit head:* Dr. Robert J. Denver, Department Chair, 734-764-7476, Fax: 734-615-6337, E-mail: rdenver@umich.edu. *Application contact:* Mary Carr, Graduate Coordinator, 734-615-1635, Fax: 734-764-0884, E-mail: carrmm@umich.edu.
Website: http://www.mcdb.lsa.umich.edu

University of Michigan, Rackham Graduate School, Program in Biomedical Sciences (PIBS), Interdisciplinary Program in Cellular and Molecular Biology, Ann Arbor, MI 48109. Offers PhD. *Faculty:* 169 part-time/adjunct (47 women). *Students:* 64 full-time (36 women); includes 17 minority (2 Black or African American, non-Hispanic/Latino; 1 American Indian or Alaska Native, non-Hispanic/Latino; 8 Asian, non-Hispanic/Latino; 6 Hispanic/Latino). Average age 26. In 2013, 19 doctorates awarded. *Degree requirements:* For doctorate, comprehensive exam, thesis/dissertation, preliminary exam; oral defense of dissertation. *Entrance requirements:* For doctorate, GRE General Test. *Application deadline:* For fall admission, 12/1 for domestic students. Application fee: $75 ($90 for international students). Tuition and fees vary according to course level, course load, degree level, program and student level. *Financial support:* In 2013–14, 64 students received support, including 15 fellowships with full tuition reimbursements available (averaging $28,500 per year), 41 research assistantships with full tuition reimbursements available (averaging $28,500 per year), 8 teaching assistantships with full tuition reimbursements available (averaging $28,500 per year); scholarships/grants also available. *Faculty research:* Genetics, genomics, gene regulation, models of disease, microbes. *Total annual research expenditures:* $20 million. *Unit head:* Dr. Robert S. Fuller, Director, 734-764-5428, Fax: 734-647-6232, E-mail: bfuller@umich.edu. *Application contact:* Catherine A. Mitchell, Senior Student Services Associate I, 734-764-5428, Fax: 734-647-6232, E-mail: cmbgrad@umich.edu.
Website: http://www.med.umich.edu/cmb/

University of Minnesota, Duluth, Medical School, Department of Biochemistry, Molecular Biology and Biophysics, Duluth, MN 55812-2496. Offers biochemistry, molecular biology and biophysics (MS); biology and biophysics (PhD); social, administrative, and clinical pharmacy (MS, PhD); toxicology (MS, PhD). Terminal master's awarded for partial completion of doctoral program. *Degree requirements:* For master's, comprehensive exam, thesis; for doctorate, comprehensive exam, thesis/dissertation. *Entrance requirements:* For master's and doctorate, GRE General Test. Additional exam requirements/recommendations for international students: Required—TOEFL. Electronic applications accepted. *Faculty research:* Intestinal cancer biology; hepatotoxins and mitochondriopathies; toxicology; cell cycle regulation in stem cells; neurobiology of brain development, trace metal function and blood-brain barrier; hibernation biology.

University of Minnesota, Twin Cities Campus, Graduate School, College of Biological Sciences, Biochemistry, Molecular Biology and Biophysics Graduate Program, Minneapolis, MN 55455-0213. Offers PhD. *Degree requirements:* For doctorate, thesis/dissertation. *Entrance requirements:* For doctorate, GRE, 3 letters of recommendation, more than 1 semester of laboratory experience. Additional exam requirements/recommendations for international students: Required—TOEFL (minimum score 625 paper-based; 108 iBT with writing subsection 25 and reading subsection 25) or IELTS (minimum score 7). Electronic applications accepted. *Faculty research:* Microbial biochemistry, biotechnology, molecular biology, regulatory biochemistry, structural biology and biophysics, physical biochemistry, enzymology, physiological chemistry.

University of Minnesota, Twin Cities Campus, Graduate School, Program in Molecular, Cellular, Developmental Biology and Genetics, Minneapolis, MN 55455-0213. Offers genetic counseling (MS); molecular, cellular, developmental biology and genetics (PhD). Terminal master's awarded for partial completion of doctoral program. *Degree requirements:* For master's, thesis optional; for doctorate, thesis/dissertation. *Entrance requirements:* For master's and doctorate, GRE General Test. Additional exam requirements/recommendations for international students: Required—TOEFL (minimum score 625 paper-based; 80 iBT). Electronic applications accepted. *Faculty research:* Membrane receptors and membrane transport, cell interactions, cytoskeleton and cell mobility, regulation of gene expression, plant cell and molecular biology.

University of Missouri–Kansas City, School of Biological Sciences, Program in Molecular Biology and Biochemistry, Kansas City, MO 64110-2499. Offers PhD. Offered through the School of Graduate Studies. *Faculty:* 34 full-time (9 women), 3 part-time/adjunct (all women). *Students:* 11 full-time (6 women), 7 part-time (5 women); includes 7 minority (4 Asian, non-Hispanic/Latino; 2 Hispanic/Latino; 1 Two or more races, non-Hispanic/Latino), 3 international. Average age 26. 43 applicants, 33% accepted, 10 enrolled. *Degree requirements:* For doctorate, comprehensive exam, thesis/dissertation. *Entrance requirements:* For doctorate, GRE General Test, bachelor's degree in chemistry, biology, or a related discipline; minimum GPA of 3.0. Additional exam requirements/recommendations for international students: Required—TOEFL (minimum score 550 paper-based; 80 iBT). *Application deadline:* For fall admission, 2/15 priority date for domestic and international students. Application fee: $45 ($50 for international students). *Expenses:* Tuition, state resident: full-time $6073; part-time $337.40 per credit hour. Tuition, nonresident: full-time $15,680; part-time $871.10 per credit hour. *Required fees:* $97.59 per credit hour. Full-time tuition and fees vary according to program. *Financial support:* In 2013–14, 18 research assistantships with full tuition reimbursements (averaging $23,281 per year), 14 teaching assistantships with full and partial tuition reimbursements (averaging $17,639 per year) were awarded; scholarships/grants, tuition waivers (full and partial), and unspecified assistantships also available. Financial award application deadline: 3/1; financial award applicants required to submit FAFSA. *Unit head:* Dr. Xiao-Qiang Yu, Interim Head, 816-235-6379, E-mail: yux@umkc.edu. *Application contact:* Karen Bame, Graduate Programs Officer, 816-235-2243, Fax: 816-235-5595, E-mail: bamek@umkc.edu.
Website: http://sbs.umkc.edu/

University of Missouri–St. Louis, College of Arts and Sciences, Department of Biology, St. Louis, MO 63121. Offers biotechnology (Certificate); cell and molecular biology (MS, PhD); ecology, evolution and systematics (MS, PhD); tropical biology and conservation (Certificate). Part-time programs available. *Faculty:* 33 full-time (13 women), 9 part-time/adjunct (1 woman). *Students:* 52 full-time (23 women), 58 part-time (29 women); includes 13 minority (9 Black or African American, non-Hispanic/Latino; 3 Asian, non-Hispanic/Latino; 1 Hispanic/Latino), 30 international. Average age 28. 113 applicants, 42% accepted, 22 enrolled. In 2013, 31 master's, 5 doctorates, 4 other advanced degrees awarded. *Degree requirements:* For master's, thesis or alternative; for doctorate, thesis/dissertation, 1 semester of teaching experience. *Entrance requirements:* For master's, 3 letters of recommendation; for doctorate, GRE General Test, 3 letters of recommendation. Additional exam requirements/recommendations for international students: Required—TOEFL (minimum score 79 iBT), IELTS (minimum score 6.5). *Application deadline:* For fall admission, 12/15 priority date for domestic and international students; for spring admission, 12/1 priority date for domestic and international students. Applications are processed on a rolling basis. Application fee: $50 ($40 for international students). Electronic applications accepted. *Expenses:* Tuition, state resident: full-time $7364; part-time $409.10 per credit hour. Tuition, nonresident: full-time $19,162; part-time $1008.50 per credit hour. *Financial support:* In 2013–14, 13 research assistantships with full and partial tuition reimbursements (averaging $17,000 per year), 23 teaching assistantships with full and partial tuition reimbursements (averaging $17,000 per year) were awarded; fellowships with full tuition reimbursements, career-related internships or fieldwork, and Federal Work-Study also available. Support available to part-time students. Financial award application deadline: 2/1. *Faculty research:* Molecular biology, microbial genetics, animal behavior, tropical ecology, plant systematics. *Unit head:* Dr. Teresa Thiel, Director of Graduate Studies, 314-516-6200, Fax: 314-516-6233, E-mail: thiel@umsl.edu. *Application contact:* 314-516-5458, Fax: 314-516-6996, E-mail: gradadm@umsl.edu.
Website: http://www.umsl.edu/divisions/artscience/biology/

The University of Montana, Graduate School, College of Humanities and Sciences, Division of Biological Sciences, Program in Cellular, Molecular and Microbial Biology, Missoula, MT 59812-0002. Offers cellular and developmental biology (PhD); microbial evolution and ecology (PhD); microbiology and immunology (PhD); molecular biology and biochemistry (PhD). Terminal master's awarded for partial completion of doctoral program. *Degree requirements:* For doctorate, variable foreign language requirement, thesis/dissertation. *Entrance requirements:* For doctorate, GRE General Test. *Application deadline:* For fall admission, 2/1 for domestic students. Application fee: $45. *Financial support:* In 2013–14, research assistantships with tuition reimbursements (averaging $9,400 per year), teaching assistantships with full tuition reimbursements (averaging $9,400 per year) were awarded; Federal Work-Study and tuition waivers (full and partial) also available. Financial award application deadline: 3/1; financial award applicants required to submit FAFSA. *Faculty research:* Ribosome structure, medical microbiology/pathogenesis, microbial ecology/environmental microbiology. *Unit head:* Charles Janson, Chair, 406-243-5122, E-mail: charles.janson@mso.umt.edu. *Application contact:* Information Contact, E-mail: gradschl@mso.umt.edu.
Website: http://www.biology.umt.edu/

University of Nebraska Medical Center, Department of Biochemistry and Molecular Biology, Omaha, NE 68198. Offers MS, PhD. Terminal master's awarded for partial completion of doctoral program. *Degree requirements:* For master's, comprehensive exam, thesis; for doctorate, comprehensive exam, thesis/dissertation. *Entrance requirements:* For master's and doctorate, GRE General Test. Additional exam requirements/recommendations for international students: Required—TOEFL (minimum score 550 paper-based). Electronic applications accepted. *Expenses: Required fees:* $300 per semester. Tuition and fees vary according to program. *Faculty research:* Recombinant DNA, cancer biology, diabetes and drug metabolism, biochemical endocrinology.

University of Nevada, Reno, Graduate School, Interdisciplinary Program in Cell and Molecular Biology, Reno, NV 89557. Offers MS, PhD. Terminal master's awarded for partial completion of doctoral program. *Degree requirements:* For master's, thesis; for doctorate, thesis/dissertation. *Entrance requirements:* For master's, GRE Subject Test (recommended), minimum GPA of 2.75; for doctorate, GRE Subject Test (recommended), minimum GPA of 3.0. Additional exam requirements/recommendations for international students: Required—TOEFL (minimum score 500 paper-based; 61 iBT), IELTS (minimum score 6). Electronic applications accepted. *Faculty research:* Cellular biology, biophysics, cancer, microbiology, insect biochemistry.

University of New Haven, Graduate School, College of Arts and Sciences, Program in Cellular and Molecular Biology, West Haven, CT 06516-1916. Offers MS, Graduate Certificate. Part-time and evening/weekend programs available. *Students:* 30 full-time (23 women), 9 part-time (6 women); includes 8 minority (5 Black or African American, non-Hispanic/Latino; 1 Asian, non-Hispanic/Latino; 1 Hispanic/Latino; 1 Two or more races, non-Hispanic/Latino), 16 international. 72 applicants, 68% accepted, 24 enrolled. In 2013, 19 master's, 1 other advanced degree awarded. *Degree requirements:* For master's, thesis or alternative. *Entrance requirements:* Additional exam requirements/recommendations for international students: Required—TOEFL (minimum score 80 iBT), IELTS, PTE (minimum score 53). *Application deadline:* For fall admission, 5/31 for international students; for winter admission, 10/15 for international students; for spring admission, 1/15 for international students. Applications are processed on a rolling basis. Application fee: $75. Electronic applications accepted. Application fee is waived when completed online. *Expenses: Tuition:* Full-time $21,600; part-time $800 per credit hour. *Required fees:* $45 per trimester. *Financial support:* Research assistantships with partial tuition reimbursements, teaching assistantships with partial tuition reimbursements, career-related internships or fieldwork, Federal Work-Study, scholarships/grants, and unspecified assistantships available. Support available to part-time students. Financial award application deadline: 5/1; financial award applicants required to submit FAFSA. *Unit head:* Dr. Roman Zajac, Chair, 203-932-7114, E-mail: rzajac@newhaven.edu. *Application contact:* Eloise Gormley, Director of Graduate Admissions, 203-932-7440, E-mail: gradinfo@newhaven.edu.
Website: http://www.newhaven.edu/4724/

University of New Mexico, School of Medicine, Program in Biomedical Sciences, Albuquerque, NM 87131-5196. Offers biochemistry and molecular biology (MS, PhD); cell biology and physiology (MS, PhD); clinical and translational science (Certificate); molecular genetics and microbiology (MS, PhD); neuroscience (MS, PhD); pathology (MS, PhD); toxicology (MS, PhD); university science teaching (Certificate). Part-time programs available. *Students:* 73 full-time (39 women), 14 part-time (9 women); includes 24 minority (1 Black or African American, non-Hispanic/Latino; 1 American Indian or Alaska Native, non-Hispanic/Latino; 2 Asian, non-Hispanic/Latino; 17 Hispanic/Latino; 1 Native Hawaiian or other Pacific Islander, non-Hispanic/Latino; 2 Two or more races, non-Hispanic/Latino), 16 international. Average age 29. 89 applicants, 20% accepted, 17 enrolled. In 2013, 7 master's, 17 doctorates awarded. Terminal master's awarded for partial completion of doctoral program. *Degree requirements:* For master's, thesis; for doctorate, comprehensive exam, thesis/dissertation, qualifying exam at the end of year 1/core curriculum. *Entrance requirements:* For master's and doctorate, GRE General Test, minimum undergraduate GPA of 3.0. Additional exam requirements/recommendations for international students: Required—TOEFL. *Application deadline:* For fall admission, 3/1 priority date for domestic and international students. Applications are processed on a rolling basis. Application fee: $50. Electronic applications accepted. *Financial support:* In 2013–14, 94 students received support, including 28 fellowships with full and partial tuition reimbursements available (averaging $22,000 per year), 73 research assistantships with full tuition reimbursements available (averaging $23,000 per year), 8 teaching assistantships (averaging $2,800 per year); career-related internships or fieldwork, Federal Work-Study, institutionally sponsored loans, scholarships/grants, traineeships, health care benefits, and unspecified assistantships also available. Financial award application deadline: 1/1; financial award applicants required to submit FAFSA. *Faculty research:* Infectious disease/immunity, cancer biology, cardiovascular and metabolic diseases, brain and behavioral illness, environmental health. *Unit head:* Dr. Helen J. Hathaway, Program Director, 505-272-1887, Fax: 505-272-2412, E-mail: hhathaway@salud.unm.edu. *Application contact:*

Mary Fenton, Admissions Coordinator, 505-272-1887, Fax: 505-272-2412, E-mail: mfenton@salud.unm.edu.
Website: http://hsc.unm.edu/research/brep/bsgpabout.shtm

The University of North Carolina at Chapel Hill, Graduate School, College of Arts and Sciences, Department of Biology, Chapel Hill, NC 27599. Offers botany (MA, MS, PhD); cell biology, development, and physiology (MA, MS, PhD); cell motility and cytoskeleton (PhD); ecology and behavior (MA, MS, PhD); genetics and molecular biology (MA, MS, PhD); morphology, systematics, and evolution (MA, MS, PhD). Terminal master's awarded for partial completion of doctoral program. *Degree requirements:* For master's, comprehensive exam, thesis (for some programs); for doctorate, comprehensive exam, thesis/dissertation. *Entrance requirements:* For master's, GRE General Test, GRE Subject Test, 2 semesters of calculus or statistics; 2 semesters of physics, organic chemistry; 3 semesters of biology; for doctorate, GRE General Test, GRE Subject Test, 2 semesters calculus or statistics, 2 semesters physics, organic chemistry, 3 semesters of biology. Additional exam requirements/recommendations for international students: Required—TOEFL (minimum score 550 paper-based). Electronic applications accepted. *Faculty research:* Gene expression, biomechanics, yeast genetics, plant ecology, plant molecular biology.

The University of North Carolina at Chapel Hill, School of Medicine and Graduate School, Graduate Programs in Medicine, Curriculum in Genetics and Molecular Biology, Chapel Hill, NC 27599. Offers MS, PhD. *Degree requirements:* For doctorate, comprehensive exam, thesis/dissertation. *Entrance requirements:* For doctorate, GRE, minimum GPA of 3.0. Additional exam requirements/recommendations for international students: Required—TOEFL. Electronic applications accepted. *Faculty research:* Telomere replication and germline immortality, experimental evolution in microorganisms, genetic vulnerabilities in tumor genomes, genetics of cell cycle control during Drosophila development, mammalian genetics.

University of North Dakota, Graduate School and Graduate School, Graduate Programs in Medicine, Department of Biochemistry and Molecular Biology, Grand Forks, ND 58202. Offers MS, PhD. *Degree requirements:* For master's, thesis, final exam; for doctorate, comprehensive exam, thesis/dissertation, final exam. *Entrance requirements:* For master's and doctorate, GRE General Test, minimum GPA of 3.0. Additional exam requirements/recommendations for international students: Required—TOEFL (minimum score 550 paper-based; 79 iBT), IELTS (minimum score 6.5). Electronic applications accepted. *Faculty research:* Glucose-6-phosphatase, guanine nucleotides, carbohydrate and lipid metabolism, cytoskeletal proteins, chromatin structure.

University of North Texas, Robert B. Toulouse School of Graduate Studies, Denton, TN 76203-5017. Offers accounting (MS, PhD); applied anthropology (MA, MS); applied behavior analysis (Certificate); applied technology and performance improvement (M Ed, MS, PhD); art education (MA, PhD); art history (MA); art museum education (Certificate); arts leadership (Certificate); audiology (Au D); behavior analysis (MS); biochemistry and molecular biology (MS, PhD); biology (MA, MS, PhD); business (PhD); business computer information systems (PhD); chemistry (MS, PhD); clinical psychology (PhD); communication studies (MA, MS); computer engineering (MS); computer science (MS); computer science and engineering (PhD); counseling (M Ed, MS, PhD), including clinical mental health counseling (MS), college and university counseling (M Ed, MS), elementary school counseling (M Ed, MS), secondary school counseling (M Ed, MS); counseling psychology (PhD); creative writing (MA); criminal justice (MS); curriculum and instruction (M Ed, PhD), including curriculum studies (PhD), early childhood studies (PhD), language and literacy studies (PhD); decision sciences (MBA); design (MA, MFA), including fashion design (MFA), innovation studies, interior design (MFA); early childhood studies (MS); economics (MS); educational leadership (M Ed, Ed D, PhD); educational psychology (MS), including family studies, gifted and talented (MS, PhD), human development, learning and cognition, research, measurement and evaluation; educational research (PhD), including gifted and talented (MS, PhD), human development and family studies, psychological aspects of sports and exercise, research, measurement and statistics; electrical engineering (MS); emergency management (MPA); engineering systems (MS); English (MA, PhD); environmental science (MS, PhD); experimental psychology (PhD); finance (MBA, MS, PhD); financial management (MPA); French (MA); health psychology and behavioral medicine (PhD); health services management (MBA); higher education (M Ed, Ed D, PhD); history (MA, MS, PhD), including European history (PhD), military history (PhD), United States history (PhD); hospitality management (MS); human resources management (MPA); information science (MS, PhD); information technologies (MBA); information technology and decision sciences (MS); interdisciplinary studies (MA, MS); international sustainable tourism (MS); jazz studies (MM); journalism (MA, MJ, Graduate Certificate), including interactive and virtual digital communication (Graduate Certificate), narrative journalism (Graduate Certificate), public relations (Graduate Certificate); kinesiology (MS); learning technologies (MS, PhD); library science (MS); local government management (MPA); logistics and supply chain management (MBA, PhD); long-term care, senior housing, and aging services (MA, MS); management science (PhD); marketing (MBA, PhD); materials science and engineering (MS, PhD); mathematics (MA, PhD); merchandising (MS); music (MA, MM Ed, PhD), including ethnomusicology (MA), music education (MM Ed, PhD), music theory (MA, PhD), musicology (MA, PhD), performance (MA); nonprofit management (MPA); operations and supply chain management (MBA); performance (MM, DMA); philosophy (MA, PhD); physics (MS, PhD); political science (MA, MS, PhD); public administration and management (PhD), including emergency management, nonprofit management, public financial management, urban management; radio, television and film (MA, MFA); recreation, event and sport management (MS); rehabilitation counseling (MS, Certificate); sociology (MA, MS, PhD); Spanish (MA); special education (M Ed, PhD), including autism intervention (PhD), emotional/behavioral disorders (PhD), mild/moderate disabilities (PhD); speech-language pathology (MA, MS); strategic management (MBA); studio art (MFA); taxation (MS); teaching (M Ed); MBA/MS; MS/MPH; MSES/MBA. Part-time and evening/weekend programs available. Postbaccalaureate distance learning degree programs offered. *Faculty:* 661 full-time (213 women), 240 part-time/adjunct (144 women). *Students:* 3,106 full-time (1,620 women), 3,543 part-time (2,221 women); includes 1,740 minority (533 Black or African American, non-Hispanic/Latino; 15 American Indian or Alaska Native, non-Hispanic/Latino; 286 Asian, non-Hispanic/Latino; 746 Hispanic/Latino; 3 Native Hawaiian or other Pacific Islander, non-Hispanic/Latino; 157 Two or more races, non-Hispanic/Latino), 1,145 international. Average age 32. 6,289 applicants, 43% accepted, 1751 enrolled. In 2013, 1,778 master's, 239 doctorates, 10 other advanced degrees awarded. Terminal master's awarded for partial completion of doctoral program. *Degree requirements:* For master's, variable foreign language requirement, comprehensive exam (for some programs), thesis (for some programs); for doctorate, variable foreign language requirement, comprehensive exam (for some programs), thesis/dissertation; for other advanced degree, variable foreign language requirement, comprehensive exam (for some programs). *Entrance requirements:* For master's and doctorate, GRE, GMAT. Additional exam requirements/recommendations for international students: Required—TOEFL (minimum score 550 paper-based; 79 iBT). *Application deadline:* For fall admission, 7/15 for domestic students, 3/15 for international students; for spring admission, 11/15 for domestic students, 9/15 for international students; for summer admission, 5/1 for domestic students. Applications are processed on a rolling basis. Application fee: $60. Electronic applications accepted. *Financial support:* Fellowships with partial tuition reimbursements, research assistantships with partial tuition reimbursements, teaching assistantships, career-related internships or fieldwork, Federal Work-Study, institutionally sponsored loans, scholarships/grants, health care benefits, and library assistantships available. Support available to part-time students. Financial award applicants required to submit FAFSA. *Unit head:* Mark Wardell, Dean, 940-565-2383, E-mail: mark.wardell@unt.edu. *Application contact:* Toulouse School of Graduate Studies, 940-565-2383, Fax: 940-565-2141, E-mail: gradsch@unt.edu.
Website: http://tsgs.unt.edu/

University of North Texas Health Science Center at Fort Worth, Graduate School of Biomedical Sciences, Fort Worth, TX 76107-2699. Offers anatomy and cell biology (MS, PhD); biochemistry and molecular biology (MS, PhD); biomedical sciences (MS, PhD); biotechnology (MS); forensic genetics (MS); integrative physiology (MS, PhD); medical science (MS); microbiology and immunology (MS, PhD); pharmacology (MS, PhD); science education (MS); DO/MS; DO/PhD. Terminal master's awarded for partial completion of doctoral program. *Degree requirements:* For master's, thesis; for doctorate, thesis/dissertation. *Entrance requirements:* For master's and doctorate, GRE General Test. Additional exam requirements/recommendations for international students: Required—TOEFL. *Expenses:* Contact institution. *Faculty research:* Alzheimer's disease, aging, eye diseases, cancer, cardiovascular disease.

University of Notre Dame, Graduate School, College of Science, Department of Biological Sciences, Notre Dame, IN 46556. Offers aquatic ecology, evolution and environmental biology (MS, PhD); cellular and molecular biology (MS, PhD); genetics (MS, PhD); physiology (MS, PhD); vector biology and parasitology (MS, PhD). Terminal master's awarded for partial completion of doctoral program. *Degree requirements:* For master's, comprehensive exam, thesis; for doctorate, comprehensive exam, thesis/dissertation, candidacy exam. *Entrance requirements:* For master's and doctorate, GRE General Test. Additional exam requirements/recommendations for international students: Required—TOEFL (minimum score 600 paper-based; 80 iBT). Electronic applications accepted. *Faculty research:* Tropical disease, molecular genetics, neurobiology, evolutionary biology, aquatic biology.

University of Oklahoma Health Sciences Center, College of Medicine and Graduate College, Graduate Programs in Medicine, Department of Biochemistry and Molecular Biology, Oklahoma City, OK 73190. Offers biochemistry (MS, PhD); molecular biology (MS, PhD). Part-time programs available. *Faculty:* 8 full-time (2 women). *Students:* 1 (woman) full-time, 22 part-time (12 women); includes 2 minority (1 Asian, non-Hispanic/Latino; 1 Two or more races, non-Hispanic/Latino), 9 international. Average age 28. 7 applicants, 14% accepted, 1 enrolled. In 2013, 1 master's, 5 doctorates awarded. Terminal master's awarded for partial completion of doctoral program. *Degree requirements:* For master's, thesis; for doctorate, thesis/dissertation. *Entrance requirements:* For master's, GRE General Test, 2 letters of recommendation; for doctorate, GRE General Test, 3 letters of recommendation. Additional exam requirements/recommendations for international students: Required—TOEFL. *Application deadline:* For fall admission, 1/31 for domestic students. Application fee: $50. *Expenses:* Tuition, state resident: full-time $3504; part-time $175.20 per credit hour. Tuition, nonresident: full-time $13,504; part-time $675.20 per credit hour. *Required fees:* $1545; $52.70 per credit hour. $245.25 per semester. Tuition and fees vary according to course load. *Financial support:* In 2013–14, 20 research assistantships (averaging $18,000 per year) were awarded; institutionally sponsored loans also available. Support available to part-time students. Financial award application deadline: 3/31; financial award applicants required to submit FAFSA. *Faculty research:* Gene expression, regulation of transcription, enzyme evolution, melanogenesis, signal transduction. *Unit head:* Dr. Paul H. Weigel, Chair, 405-271-2227, E-mail: paul-weigel@ouhsc.edu. *Application contact:* Dr. Gillian Air, Graduate Liaison, 405-271-2227, Fax: 405-271-3092, E-mail: gillian-air@ouhsc.edu.

University of Oregon, Graduate School, College of Arts and Sciences, Department of Biology, Eugene, OR 97403. Offers ecology and evolution (MA, MS, PhD); marine biology (MA, MS, PhD); molecular, cellular and genetic biology (PhD); neuroscience and development (PhD). Terminal master's awarded for partial completion of doctoral program. *Degree requirements:* For master's, thesis (for some programs); for doctorate, thesis/dissertation. *Entrance requirements:* For master's and doctorate, GRE General Test, minimum GPA of 3.2. Additional exam requirements/recommendations for international students: Required—TOEFL. *Faculty research:* Developmental neurobiology; evolution, population biology, and quantitative genetics; regulation of gene expression; biochemistry of marine organisms.

University of Ottawa, Faculty of Graduate and Postdoctoral Studies, Faculty of Medicine, Department of Cellular and Molecular Medicine, Ottawa, ON K1H 8M5, Canada. Offers M Sc, PhD. *Degree requirements:* For master's, thesis, seminar; for doctorate, comprehensive exam, thesis/dissertation, seminar. *Entrance requirements:* For master's, honors degree or equivalent, minimum B average; for doctorate, master's degree, minimum B+ average. Electronic applications accepted. *Faculty research:* Physiology, pharmacology, growth and development.

University of Pennsylvania, Perelman School of Medicine, Biomedical Graduate Studies, Graduate Group in Cell and Molecular Biology, Philadelphia, PA 19104. Offers cancer biology (PhD); cell biology and physiology (PhD); developmental stem cell regenerative biology (PhD); gene therapy and vaccines (PhD); genetics and gene regulation (PhD); microbiology, virology, and parasitology (PhD); MD/PhD; VMD/PhD. *Faculty:* 321. *Students:* 352 full-time (205 women); includes 99 minority (11 Black or African American, non-Hispanic/Latino; 65 Asian, non-Hispanic/Latino; 21 Hispanic/Latino; 2 Two or more races, non-Hispanic/Latino), 45 international. 488 applicants, 20% accepted, 40 enrolled. In 2013, 41 doctorates awarded. *Degree requirements:* For doctorate, thesis/dissertation. *Entrance requirements:* For doctorate, GRE General Test. Additional exam requirements/recommendations for international students: Required—TOEFL. *Application deadline:* For fall admission, 12/1 priority date for domestic and international students. Applications are processed on a rolling basis. Application fee: $80. Electronic applications accepted. *Financial support:* In 2013–14, 352 students received support. Fellowships, research assistantships, scholarships/grants, traineeships, and unspecified assistantships available. *Unit head:* Dr. Daniel Kessler, Graduate Group Chair, 215-898-1478. *Application contact:* Meagan Schofer, Coordinator, 215-898-4360.
Website: http://www.med.upenn.edu/camb/

University of Pittsburgh, Dietrich School of Arts and Sciences, Department of Biological Sciences, Program in Molecular, Cellular, and Developmental Biology, Pittsburgh, PA 15260. Offers PhD. *Faculty:* 19 full-time (4 women). *Students:* 45 full-time (24 women); includes 5 minority (1 Black or African American, non-Hispanic/Latino; 3 Asian, non-Hispanic/Latino; 1 Hispanic/Latino), 14 international. Average age 23. 180 applicants, 9% accepted, 8 enrolled. In 2013, 6 doctorates awarded. *Degree requirements:* For doctorate, comprehensive exam, thesis/dissertation, completion of research integrity module. *Entrance requirements:* For doctorate, GRE General Test, GRE Subject Test. Additional exam requirements/recommendations for international students: Required—TOEFL (minimum score 90 iBT). *Application deadline:* For fall admission, 1/3 priority date for domestic students, 12/9 priority date for international students. Applications are processed on a rolling basis. Application fee: $0 ($50 for

international students). Electronic applications accepted. *Expenses:* Tuition, state resident: full-time $19,964; part-time $807 per credit. Tuition, nonresident: full-time $32,686; part-time $1337 per credit. *Required fees:* $740; $200. Tuition and fees vary according to program. *Financial support:* In 2013–14, 26 fellowships with full tuition reimbursements (averaging $30,682 per year), 79 research assistantships with full tuition reimbursements (averaging $26,544 per year), 18 teaching assistantships with full tuition reimbursements (averaging $25,716 per year) were awarded; Federal Work-Study, scholarships/grants, traineeships, health care benefits, and tuition waivers (full) also available. *Unit head:* Dr. Jeffrey G. Lawrence, Professor, 412-624-4204, Fax: 412-624-4759, E-mail: jlawrenc@pitt.edu. *Application contact:* Cathleen M. Barr, Graduate Administrator, 412-624-4268, Fax: 412-624-4759, E-mail: cbarr@pitt.edu.
Website: http://www.biology.pitt.edu/graduate/mcdb-program

University of Pittsburgh, School of Medicine and Dietrich School of Arts and Sciences, Integrative Molecular Biology Graduate Program, Pittsburgh, PA 15260. Offers PhD. *Faculty:* 28 full-time (8 women). *Students:* 11 full-time (4 women); includes 1 minority (Asian, non-Hispanic/Latino), 6 international. Average age 26. 56 applicants, 18% accepted, 1 enrolled. In 2013, 4 doctorates awarded. *Degree requirements:* For doctorate, comprehensive exam, thesis/dissertation. *Entrance requirements:* For doctorate, GRE, minimum GPA of 3.7, 3 letters of reference. Additional exam requirements/recommendations for international students: Required—TOEFL (minimum score 650 paper-based; 114 iBT), IELTS (minimum score 7.5). *Application deadline:* For fall admission, 12/17 for domestic and international students. Application fee: $0. Electronic applications accepted. *Expenses:* Tuition, state resident: full-time $19,964; part-time $807 per credit. Tuition, nonresident: full-time $32,686; part-time $1337 per credit. *Required fees:* $740; $200. Tuition and fees vary according to program. *Financial support:* In 2013–14, 1 fellowship with full tuition reimbursement (averaging $30,000 per year), 10 research assistantships with full tuition reimbursements (averaging $26,010 per year) were awarded; institutionally sponsored loans, scholarships/grants, traineeships, and unspecified assistantships also available. *Faculty research:* Cellular, molecular, developmental biology; genomics; proteomics and gene function. *Unit head:* Dr. Jeffrey Hildebrand, Program Director, 412-648-8975, Fax: 412-648-1077, E-mail: pimbinfo@medschool.pitt.edu. *Application contact:* Susanna T. Godwin, Program Coordinator, 412-648-8957, Fax: 412-648-1077, E-mail: pimbinfo@medschool.pitt.edu.
Website: http://www.pimb.pitt.edu

University of Puerto Rico, Río Piedras Campus, College of Natural Sciences, Department of Biology, San Juan, PR 00931-3300. Offers ecology/systematics (MS, PhD); evolution/genetics (MS, PhD); molecular/cellular biology (MS, PhD); neuroscience (MS, PhD). Part-time programs available. *Degree requirements:* For master's, one foreign language, comprehensive exam, thesis; for doctorate, one foreign language, comprehensive exam, thesis/dissertation. *Entrance requirements:* For master's, GRE Subject Test, interview, minimum GPA of 3.0, letter of recommendation; for doctorate, GRE Subject Test, interview, master's degree, minimum GPA of 3.0, letter of recommendation. *Faculty research:* Environmental, poblational and systematic biology.

University of Rhode Island, Graduate School, College of the Environment and Life Sciences, Department of Cell and Molecular Biology, Kingston, RI 02881. Offers biochemistry (MS, PhD); clinical laboratory sciences (MS), including biotechnology, clinical laboratory science, cytopathology; microbiology (MS, PhD); molecular genetics (MS, PhD). Part-time programs available. *Faculty:* 17 full-time (8 women), 2 part-time/adjunct (1 woman). *Students:* 19 full-time (11 women), 40 part-time (23 women); includes 14 minority (4 Black or African American, non-Hispanic/Latino; 1 American Indian or Alaska Native, non-Hispanic/Latino; 7 Asian, non-Hispanic/Latino; 2 Hispanic/Latino), 5 international. In 2013, 20 master's, 2 doctorates awarded. *Degree requirements:* For master's, comprehensive exam (for some programs), thesis optional; for doctorate, comprehensive exam, thesis/dissertation. *Entrance requirements:* For master's and doctorate, GRE, 2 letters of recommendation. Additional exam requirements/recommendations for international students: Required—TOEFL (minimum score 550 paper-based). *Application deadline:* For fall admission, 7/15 for domestic students, 2/1 for international students; for spring admission, 11/15 for domestic students, 7/15 for international students. Application fee: $65. Electronic applications accepted. *Expenses:* Tuition, state resident: full-time $11,532; part-time $641 per credit. Tuition, nonresident: full-time $23,606; part-time $1311 per credit. *Required fees:* $1388; $36 per credit. $35 per semester. One-time fee: $130. *Financial support:* In 2013–14, 5 research assistantships with full and partial tuition reimbursements (averaging $12,078 per year), 2 teaching assistantships with full and partial tuition reimbursements (averaging $11,883 per year) were awarded. Financial award application deadline: 2/1; financial award applicants required to submit FAFSA. *Faculty research:* Genomics. *Total annual research expenditures:* $6.7 million. *Unit head:* Dr. Gongqing Sun, Chairperson, 401-874-5937, Fax: 401-874-2202, E-mail: gsun@mail.uri.edu. *Application contact:* Graduate Admissions, 401-874-2872, E-mail: gradadm@etal.uri.edu.
Website: http://cels.uri.edu/cmb/

University of Rochester, School of Medicine and Dentistry, Graduate Programs in Medicine and Dentistry, Department of Biochemistry and Biophysics, Programs in Biochemistry, Rochester, NY 14627. Offers biochemistry and molecular biology (PhD). Terminal master's awarded for partial completion of doctoral program. *Degree requirements:* For doctorate, thesis/dissertation, qualifying exam. *Entrance requirements:* For doctorate, GRE General Test. *Expenses: Tuition:* Full-time $44,580; part-time $1394 per credit hour. *Required fees:* $492.

University of South Carolina, The Graduate School, College of Arts and Sciences, Department of Biological Sciences, Graduate Training Program in Molecular, Cellular, and Developmental Biology, Columbia, SC 29208. Offers MS, PhD. *Degree requirements:* For master's, one foreign language, thesis; for doctorate, one foreign language, thesis/dissertation. *Entrance requirements:* For master's and doctorate, GRE General Test, minimum GPA of 3.0 in science. Electronic applications accepted. *Faculty research:* Marine ecology, population and evolutionary biology, molecular biology and genetics, development.

The University of South Dakota, Graduate School, School of Medicine and Graduate School, Biomedical Sciences Graduate Program, Cellular and Molecular Biology Group, Vermillion, SD 57069-2390. Offers MS, PhD. Terminal master's awarded for partial completion of doctoral program. *Degree requirements:* For master's, thesis; for doctorate, comprehensive exam, thesis/dissertation. *Entrance requirements:* For master's and doctorate, GRE General Test, GRE Subject Test, minimum GPA of 3.0. Additional exam requirements/recommendations for international students: Required—TOEFL (minimum score 550 paper-based; 80 iBT), IELTS (minimum score 6). Electronic applications accepted. *Expenses:* Contact institution. *Faculty research:* Molecular aspects of protein and DNA, neurochemistry and energy transduction, gene regulation, cellular development.

University of Southern California, Graduate School, Dana and David Dornsife College of Letters, Arts and Sciences, Department of Biological Sciences, Program in Molecular and Computational Biology, Los Angeles, CA 90089. Offers computational biology and bioinformatics (PhD); molecular biology (PhD). *Degree requirements:* For doctorate, comprehensive exam, thesis/dissertation, qualifying examination, dissertation defense. *Entrance requirements:* For doctorate, GRE, 3 letters of recommendation, personal statement, resume, minimum GPA of 3.0. Additional exam requirements/recommendations for international students: Required—TOEFL (minimum score 600 paper-based; 100 iBT). Electronic applications accepted. *Faculty research:* Biochemistry and molecular biology; genomics; computational biology and bioinformatics; cell and developmental biology, and genetics; DNA replication and repair, and cancer biology.

University of Southern California, Keck School of Medicine and Graduate School, Graduate Programs in Medicine, Department of Biochemistry and Molecular Biology, Los Angeles, CA 90089. Offers MS. *Faculty:* 22 full-time (4 women). *Students:* 30 full-time (23 women); includes 4 minority (all Asian, non-Hispanic/Latino), 26 international. Average age 24. 51 applicants, 55% accepted, 17 enrolled. In 2013, 16 master's awarded. Terminal master's awarded for partial completion of doctoral program. *Degree requirements:* For master's, thesis. *Entrance requirements:* For master's, GRE General Test, minimum GPA of 3.0. Additional exam requirements/recommendations for international students: Required—TOEFL (minimum score 600 paper-based; 100 iBT). *Application deadline:* For fall admission, 4/15 priority date for domestic and international students. Applications are processed on a rolling basis. Application fee: $85. Electronic applications accepted. *Financial support:* Application deadline: 5/4; applicants required to submit CSS PROFILE or FAFSA. *Faculty research:* Molecular genetics, gene expression, membrane biochemistry, metabolic regulation, cancer biology. *Total annual research expenditures:* $9.3 million. *Unit head:* Dr. Michael R. Stallcup, Chair, 323-442-1145, Fax: 323-442-1224, E-mail: stallcup@usc.edu. *Application contact:* Janet Stoeckert, Administrative Director, Basic Science Departments, 323-442-3568, Fax: 323-442-1610, E-mail: janet.stoeckert@usc.edu.
Website: http://www.usc.edu/medicine/biochemistry/

University of Southern California, Keck School of Medicine and Graduate School, Graduate Programs in Medicine, Department of Preventive Medicine, Division of Biostatistics, Los Angeles, CA 90089. Offers applied biostatistics and epidemiology (MS); biostatistics (MS, PhD); epidemiology (PhD); molecular epidemiology (MS). *Faculty:* 90 full-time (39 women), 4 part-time/adjunct (2 women). *Students:* 114 full-time (46 women); includes 24 minority (1 Black or African American, non-Hispanic/Latino; 1 American Indian or Alaska Native, non-Hispanic/Latino; 18 Asian, non-Hispanic/Latino; 3 Hispanic/Latino; 1 Native Hawaiian or other Pacific Islander, non-Hispanic/Latino), 69 international. Average age 29. 92 applicants, 60% accepted, 34 enrolled. In 2013, 9 master's, 10 doctorates awarded. Terminal master's awarded for partial completion of doctoral program. *Degree requirements:* For master's, thesis; for doctorate, thesis/dissertation. *Entrance requirements:* For master's, GRE General Test, GRE Subject Test, minimum GPA of 3.0; for doctorate, GRE General Test, GRE Subject Test, minimum GPA of 3.5. Additional exam requirements/recommendations for international students: Required—TOEFL (minimum score 600 paper-based; 100 iBT), IELTS (minimum score 7). *Application deadline:* For fall admission, 12/1 priority date for domestic and international students; for winter admission, 5/15 priority date for domestic and international students; for spring admission, 11/1 priority date for domestic and international students; for summer admission, 3/1 priority date for domestic and international students. Applications are processed on a rolling basis. Application fee: $85. Electronic applications accepted. *Financial support:* In 2013–14, 10 fellowships with full tuition reimbursements (averaging $30,000 per year), 49 research assistantships with full and partial tuition reimbursements (averaging $30,000 per year), 18 teaching assistantships with full and partial tuition reimbursements (averaging $30,000 per year) were awarded; career-related internships or fieldwork, Federal Work-Study, institutionally sponsored loans, scholarships/grants, traineeships, health care benefits, and unspecified assistantships also available. Financial award application deadline: 5/4; financial award applicants required to submit CSS PROFILE or FAFSA. *Faculty research:* Clinical trials in ophthalmology and cancer research, methods of analysis for epidemiological studies, genetic epidemiology. *Total annual research expenditures:* $1.3 million. *Unit head:* Dr. Kiros Berhane, Director, Graduate Programs in Biostatistics and Epidemiology, 323-442-1994, Fax: 323-442-2993, E-mail: kiros@usc.edu. *Application contact:* Mary L. Trujillo, Student Advisor, 323-442-2633, Fax: 323-442-2993, E-mail: mtrujill@usc.edu.
Website: http://keck.usc.edu/Education/Academic_Department_and_Divisions/Department_of_Preventive_Medicine/Divisions/Biostatistics.aspx

University of Southern California, Keck School of Medicine and Graduate School, Program in Genetic, Molecular and Cellular Biology, Los Angeles, CA 90089-9031. Offers PhD. *Faculty:* 236 full-time (68 women). *Students:* 114 full-time (63 women); includes 25 minority (2 Black or African American, non-Hispanic/Latino; 17 Asian, non-Hispanic/Latino; 5 Hispanic/Latino; 1 Two or more races, non-Hispanic/Latino), 57 international. Average age 29. 342 applicants, 18% accepted, 21 enrolled. In 2013, 15 doctorates awarded. *Degree requirements:* For doctorate, comprehensive exam, thesis/dissertation. *Entrance requirements:* For doctorate, GRE, minimum GPA of 3.0. Additional exam requirements/recommendations for international students: Required—TOEFL (minimum score 600 paper-based; 100 iBT). *Application deadline:* For fall admission, 12/1 priority date for domestic and international students. Application fee: $85. Electronic applications accepted. *Financial support:* In 2013–14, 114 students received support, including 11 fellowships (averaging $31,000 per year), 98 research assistantships with full tuition reimbursements available (averaging $31,000 per year), 5 teaching assistantships with full tuition reimbursements available (averaging $31,000 per year); institutionally sponsored loans, scholarships/grants, traineeships, health care benefits, and unspecified assistantships also available. Financial award application deadline: 5/4; financial award applicants required to submit FAFSA. *Unit head:* Dr. Wei Li, Director, 323-442-1475, Fax: 323-442-1199, E-mail: wli@usc.edu. *Application contact:* Dr. Joyce Perez, Manager of Student Programs, 323-442-1645, Fax: 323-442-1199, E-mail: pibbs@usc.edu.
Website: http://www.usc.edu/intbio

University of Southern Maine, College of Science, Technology, and Health, Program in Applied Medical Sciences, Portland, ME 04104-9300. Offers MS. Part-time programs available. *Faculty:* 4 full-time (0 women). *Students:* 9 full-time (8 women), 7 part-time (4 women). Average age 31. 10 applicants, 90% accepted, 4 enrolled. In 2013, 4 master's awarded. *Degree requirements:* For master's, thesis. *Entrance requirements:* For master's, GRE General Test, minimum GPA of 3.0. Additional exam requirements/recommendations for international students: Required—TOEFL. *Application deadline:* For fall admission, 5/1 priority date for domestic students; for spring admission, 11/1 for domestic students. Applications are processed on a rolling basis. Application fee: $65. Electronic applications accepted. *Expenses:* Tuition, state resident: part-time $380 per credit. Tuition, nonresident: part-time $1026 per credit. Part-time tuition and fees vary according to program. *Financial support:* Fellowships, research assistantships, teaching assistantships, career-related internships or fieldwork, and Federal Work-Study available. Support available to part-time students. Financial award application deadline: 4/1; financial award applicants required to submit FAFSA. *Faculty research:* Cancer biology, toxicology, environmental health, epidemiology, autoimmune disease, immunology, infectious disease, virology. *Application contact:* Mary Sloan, Assistant Dean of Graduate Studies and Director of Graduate Admissions, 207-780-4812, Fax: 207-780-4969, E-mail: gradstudies@usm.maine.edu.
Website: http://www.usm.maine.edu/ams/

Molecular Biology

University of Southern Mississippi, Graduate School, College of Science and Technology, Department of Biological Sciences, Hattiesburg, MS 39406-0001. Offers environmental biology (MS, PhD); marine biology (MS, PhD); microbiology (MS, PhD); molecular biology (MS, PhD). *Faculty:* 27 full-time (6 women). *Students:* 63 full-time (26 women), 4 part-time (all women); includes 4 minority (1 Black or African American, non-Hispanic/Latino; 1 Hispanic/Latino; 2 Two or more races, non-Hispanic/Latino), 17 international. Average age 32. 43 applicants, 30% accepted, 12 enrolled. In 2013, 12 master's, 9 doctorates awarded. Terminal master's awarded for partial completion of doctoral program. *Degree requirements:* For master's, comprehensive exam, thesis; for doctorate, comprehensive exam, thesis/dissertation. *Entrance requirements:* For master's, GRE General Test, minimum GPA of 3.0 on last 60 hours; for doctorate, GRE General Test, minimum GPA of 3.5. Additional exam requirements/recommendations for international students: Required—TOEFL, IELTS. *Application deadline:* For fall admission, 3/1 priority date for domestic students, 3/1 for international students; for spring admission, 1/10 priority date for domestic and international students. Applications are processed on a rolling basis. Application fee: $50. *Financial support:* In 2013–14, 25 research assistantships with full tuition reimbursements (averaging $9,700 per year), 33 teaching assistantships with full tuition reimbursements (averaging $10,600 per year) were awarded; Federal Work-Study, scholarships/grants, health care benefits, and unspecified assistantships also available. Financial award application deadline: 3/15; financial award applicants required to submit FAFSA. *Unit head:* Dr. Glenmore Shearer, Chair, 601-266-4748, Fax: 601-266-5797. *Application contact:* Dr. Jake Schaefer, Director of Graduate Studies, 601-266-4748, Fax: 601-266-5797.
Website: http://www.usm.edu/graduateschool/table.php

University of South Florida, College of Arts and Sciences, Department of Cell Biology, Microbiology, and Molecular Biology, Tampa, FL 33620-9951. Offers biology (MS), including cell and molecular biology; cancer biology (PhD); cell and molecular biology (PhD); microbiology (MS). *Faculty:* 19 full-time (5 women), 1 part-time/adjunct (0 women). *Students:* 77 full-time (46 women), 3 part-time (1 woman); includes 8 minority (5 Asian, non-Hispanic/Latino; 3 Hispanic/Latino), 19 international. Average age 27. 155 applicants, 17% accepted, 17 enrolled. In 2013, 19 master's, 12 doctorates awarded. *Degree requirements:* For master's, thesis or alternative; for doctorate, comprehensive exam, thesis/dissertation. *Entrance requirements:* For master's and doctorate, GRE General Test, minimum GPA of 3.0, extensive background in biology or chemistry. Additional exam requirements/recommendations for international students: Required—TOEFL (minimum score 550 paper-based; 79 iBT) or IELTS (minimum score 6.5). *Application deadline:* For fall admission, 2/1 for domestic students, 1/1 for international students. Application fee: $30. *Financial support:* Career-related internships or fieldwork, health care benefits, and unspecified assistantships available. Financial award application deadline: 4/1. *Faculty research:* Cell biology, microbiology and molecular biology: basic and applied science in bacterial pathogenesis, genome integrity and mechanisms of aging, structural and computational biology; cancer biology: immunology, cancer control, signal transduction, drug discovery, genomics. *Total annual research expenditures:* $1.9 million. *Unit head:* Dr. James Garey, Professor/Chair, 813-974-7103, Fax: 813-974-1614, E-mail: garey@usf.edu. *Application contact:* Dr. Kenneth Wright, Associate Professor of Cancer Biology, H. Lee Moffitt Cancer Center and Research Institute, 813-745-3918, Fax: 813-974-1614, E-mail: ken.wright@moffitt.org.
Website: http://biology.usf.edu/cmmb/

The University of Texas at Austin, Graduate School, Institute for Cellular and Molecular Biology, Austin, TX 78712-1111. Offers PhD.

The University of Texas at Dallas, School of Natural Sciences and Mathematics, Department of Biology, Richardson, TX 75080. Offers bioinformatics and computational biology (MS); biotechnology (MS); molecular and cell biology (MS, PhD). Part-time and evening/weekend programs available. *Faculty:* 20 full-time (3 women), 1 (woman) part-time/adjunct. *Students:* 99 full-time (63 women), 15 part-time (7 women); includes 10 minority (1 Black or African American, non-Hispanic/Latino; 6 Asian, non-Hispanic/Latino; 3 Hispanic/Latino), 77 international. Average age 27. 381 applicants, 23% accepted, 48 enrolled. In 2013, 49 master's, 3 doctorates awarded. *Degree requirements:* For master's, thesis optional; for doctorate, thesis/dissertation, publishable paper. *Entrance requirements:* For master's and doctorate, GRE (minimum combined score of 1000 on verbal and quantitative). Additional exam requirements/recommendations for international students: Required—TOEFL (minimum score 550 paper-based; 80 iBT). *Application deadline:* For fall admission, 7/15 for domestic students, 5/1 priority date for international students; for spring admission, 11/15 for domestic students, 9/1 priority date for international students. Applications are processed on a rolling basis. Application fee: $50 ($100 for international students). Electronic applications accepted. *Expenses:* Tuition, state resident: full-time $11,940; part-time $663.33 per credit hour. Tuition, nonresident: full-time $21,606; part-time $1200.33 per credit hour. *Financial support:* In 2013–14, 57 students received support, including 12 research assistantships with partial tuition reimbursements available (averaging $20,867 per year), 44 teaching assistantships with partial tuition reimbursements available (averaging $15,300 per year); career-related internships or fieldwork, Federal Work-Study, institutionally sponsored loans, scholarships/grants, and unspecified assistantships also available. Support available to part-time students. Financial award application deadline: 4/30; financial award applicants required to submit FAFSA. *Faculty research:* Role of mitochondria in neurodegenerative diseases, protein-DNA interactions in site-specific recombination, eukaryotic gene expression, bio-nanotechnology, sickle cell research. *Unit head:* Dr. Stephen Spiro, Department Head, 972-883-6032, Fax: 972-883-2502, E-mail: stephen.spiro@utdallas.edu. *Application contact:* Dr. Lawrence Reitzer, Graduate Advisor, 972-883-2502, Fax: 972-883-2402, E-mail: reitzer@utdallas.edu.
Website: http://www.utdallas.edu/biology/

The University of Texas at San Antonio, College of Sciences, Department of Biology, San Antonio, TX 78249-0617. Offers biology (MS); biotechnology (MS); cell and molecular biology (PhD); neurobiology (PhD). *Faculty:* 46 full-time (9 women), 15 part-time/adjunct (10 women). *Students:* 116 full-time (56 women), 62 part-time (34 women); includes 70 minority (7 Black or African American, non-Hispanic/Latino; 1 American Indian or Alaska Native, non-Hispanic/Latino; 10 Asian, non-Hispanic/Latino; 49 Hispanic/Latino; 2 Native Hawaiian or other Pacific Islander, non-Hispanic/Latino; 1 Two or more races, non-Hispanic/Latino), 34 international. Average age 29. 176 applicants, 53% accepted, 43 enrolled. In 2013, 47 master's, 6 doctorates awarded. Terminal master's awarded for partial completion of doctoral program. *Degree requirements:* For master's, comprehensive exam, thesis or alternative; for doctorate, comprehensive exam, thesis/dissertation. *Entrance requirements:* For master's, GRE General Test, bachelor's degree with 18 credit hours in field of study or in another appropriate field of study; for doctorate, GRE General Test, 3 letters of recommendation, statement of purpose, resume. Additional exam requirements/recommendations for international students: Required—TOEFL (minimum score 500 paper-based; 100 iBT), IELTS (minimum score 5). *Application deadline:* For fall admission, 7/1 for domestic students, 4/1 for international students; for spring admission, 11/1 for domestic students, 9/1 for international students. Application fee: $45 ($80 for international students). Electronic applications accepted. *Expenses:* Tuition, state resident: full-time $4671. Tuition, nonresident: full-time $8708. *International tuition:* $17,415 full-time. *Required fees:* $1924.60. Tuition and fees vary according to course load and degree level. *Financial support:* In 2013–14, 42 students received support, including 14 fellowships (averaging $26,142 per year), 19 research assistantships (averaging $24,350 per year), 9 teaching assistantships (averaging $24,350 per year). *Faculty research:* Development of human and veterinary vaccines against a fungal disease, mammalian germ cells and stem cells, dopamine neuron physiology and addiction, plant biochemistry, dendritic computation and synaptic plasticity. *Total annual research expenditures:* $2.1 million. *Unit head:* Dr. Edwin J. Barea-Rodriguez, Chair, 210-458-4511, Fax: 210-458-5658, E-mail: edwin.barea@utsa.edu. *Application contact:* Rene Munguia, Jr., Senior Program Coordinator, 210-458-4642, Fax: 210-458-5658, E-mail: rene.munguia@utsa.edu.
Website: http://bio.utsa.edu/

The University of Texas Health Science Center at Houston, Graduate School of Biomedical Sciences, Program in Biochemistry and Molecular Biology, Houston, TX 77225-0036. Offers MS, PhD, MD/PhD. Terminal master's awarded for partial completion of doctoral program. *Degree requirements:* For master's, thesis; for doctorate, thesis/dissertation. *Entrance requirements:* For master's and doctorate, GRE General Test. Additional exam requirements/recommendations for international students: Required—TOEFL. Electronic applications accepted. *Expenses:* Tuition, state resident: full-time $3474; part-time $193 per credit hour. Tuition, nonresident: full-time $13,644; part-time $758 per credit hour. *Required fees:* $226.30; $87 per credit hour. *Faculty research:* Biochemistry, membrane biology, macromolecular structure, structural biophysics, molecular models of human disease, molecular biology of the cell.

The University of Texas Health Science Center at Houston, Graduate School of Biomedical Sciences, Program in Cell and Regulatory Biology, Houston, TX 77225-0036. Offers MS, PhD, MD/PhD. Terminal master's awarded for partial completion of doctoral program. *Degree requirements:* For master's, thesis; for doctorate, thesis/dissertation. *Entrance requirements:* For master's and doctorate, GRE General Test. Additional exam requirements/recommendations for international students: Required—TOEFL. Electronic applications accepted. *Expenses:* Tuition, state resident: full-time $3474; part-time $193 per credit hour. Tuition, nonresident: full-time $13,644; part-time $758 per credit hour. *Required fees:* $226.30; $87 per credit hour. *Faculty research:* Pharmacology, cell biology, physiology, signal transduction, systems biology.

University of the Sciences, College of Graduate Studies, Misher College of Arts and Sciences, Program in Cell and Molecular Biology, Philadelphia, PA 19104-4495. Offers PhD. *Students:* 18. In 2013, 1 doctorate awarded. *Entrance requirements:* Additional exam requirements/recommendations for international students: Required—TOEFL, TWE. *Expenses: Tuition:* Part-time $1447 per credit. Tuition and fees vary according to campus/location and program. *Unit head:* Dr. Shenaz Tejani-Butt, Associate Dean, Professional Studies, 215-596-8886, Fax: 215-895-1185, E-mail: graduate@usciences.edu. *Application contact:* Christopher Miciek, Associate Director, Graduate Admissions, 215-596-8597, E-mail: c.miciek@usciences.edu.

University of Utah, School of Medicine, Program in Molecular Biology, Salt Lake City, UT 84132. Offers PhD. *Degree requirements:* For doctorate, thesis/dissertation, preliminary exams. *Entrance requirements:* For doctorate, GRE General Test, personal statement, transcripts, letters of recommendation. Additional exam requirements/recommendations for international students: Required—TOEFL (minimum score 500 paper-based; 60 iBT). Electronic applications accepted. *Expenses:* Tuition, state resident: full-time $5259. Tuition, nonresident: full-time $18,569. *Required fees:* $841. Tuition and fees vary according to course load. *Faculty research:* Biochemistry/structural biology; cancer/cell biology; genetics; developmental biology; gene expression; microbiology/immunology and neurobiology.

University of Vermont, Graduate College, Cellular, Molecular and Biomedical Sciences Program, Burlington, VT 05405. Offers MS, PhD. *Students:* 39 (13 women); includes 6 minority (1 Black or African American, non-Hispanic/Latino; 4 Asian, non-Hispanic/Latino; 1 Hispanic/Latino), 11 international. 106 applicants, 22% accepted, 5 enrolled. In 2013, 3 master's, 10 doctorates awarded. *Degree requirements:* For master's, thesis; for doctorate, thesis/dissertation. *Entrance requirements:* For master's and doctorate, GRE General Test. Additional exam requirements/recommendations for international students: Required—TOEFL (minimum score 550 paper-based; 80 iBT). *Application deadline:* For fall admission, 12/1 priority date for domestic students, 12/1 for international students. Application fee: $65. Electronic applications accepted. *Financial support:* Fellowships, research assistantships, teaching assistantships, and career-related internships or fieldwork available. Financial award application deadline: 3/1. *Unit head:* Prof. Nick Heintz, Coordinator, 802-656-9673.

University of Washington, Graduate School, School of Medicine, Graduate Programs in Medicine, Program in Molecular and Cellular Biology, Seattle, WA 98195. Offers PhD. Offered jointly with Fred Hutchinson Cancer Research Center. *Degree requirements:* For doctorate, thesis/dissertation. *Entrance requirements:* For doctorate, GRE General Test. Additional exam requirements/recommendations for international students: Required—TOEFL. Electronic applications accepted.

See Display on page 209 and Close-Up on page 247.

University of Wisconsin–La Crosse, Graduate Studies, College of Science and Health, Department of Biology, La Crosse, WI 54601-3742. Offers aquatic sciences (MS); biology (MS); cellular and molecular biology (MS); clinical microbiology (MS); microbiology (MS); nurse anesthesia (MS); physiology (MS). Part-time programs available. *Faculty:* 22 full-time (8 women), 3 part-time/adjunct (1 woman). *Students:* 21 full-time (13 women), 37 part-time (24 women); includes 7 minority (2 Asian, non-Hispanic/Latino; 4 Hispanic/Latino; 1 Two or more races, non-Hispanic/Latino), 5 international. Average age 28. 107 applicants, 26% accepted, 25 enrolled. In 2013, 16 master's awarded. *Degree requirements:* For master's, comprehensive exam, thesis. *Entrance requirements:* For master's, GRE General Test, minimum GPA of 2.85. Additional exam requirements/recommendations for international students: Required—TOEFL (minimum score 550 paper-based; 79 iBT). *Application deadline:* For fall admission, 2/1 priority date for domestic and international students; for spring admission, 1/4 priority date for domestic and international students. Applications are processed on a rolling basis. Electronic applications accepted. *Financial support:* Research assistantships with partial tuition reimbursements, Federal Work-Study, scholarships/grants, health care benefits, and tuition waivers (partial) available. Support available to part-time students. Financial award application deadline: 3/15; financial award applicants required to submit FAFSA. *Unit head:* Dr. Thomas Volk, Coordinator of Graduate Studies, 608-785-6972, Fax: 608-785-6959, E-mail: volk.thom@uwlax.edu. *Application contact:* Corey Sjoquist, Director of Admissions, 608-785-8939, E-mail: admissions@uwlax.edu.
Website: http://uwlax.edu/biology/

University of Wisconsin–Madison, Graduate School, Program in Cellular and Molecular Biology, Madison, WI 53706-1596. Offers PhD. *Degree requirements:* For doctorate, comprehensive exam, thesis/dissertation. *Entrance requirements:* For doctorate, GRE General Test, GRE Subject Test (recommended), minimum GPA of 3.0, lab experience. Additional exam requirements/recommendations for international students: Required—TOEFL (minimum score 580 paper-based; 92 iBT). Electronic applications accepted. *Expenses:* Tuition, state resident: full-time $10,728; part-time $790 per credit. Tuition, nonresident: full-time $24,054; part-time $1623 per credit.

Required fees: $1130; $119 per credit. *Faculty research:* Virology, cancer biology, transcriptional mechanisms, plant biology, immunology.

University of Wisconsin–Parkside, College of Natural and Health Sciences, Program in Applied Molecular Biology, Kenosha, WI 53141-2000. Offers MAMB. Part-time programs available. *Faculty:* 7 full-time (3 women), 1 (woman) part-time/adjunct. *Students:* 4 full-time (1 woman), 2 part-time (1 woman). Average age 25. 15 applicants, 47% accepted, 4 enrolled. In 2013, 1 master's awarded. *Degree requirements:* For master's, thesis, oral exam. *Entrance requirements:* For master's, GRE General Test, minimum GPA of 3.0; course work in biology, chemistry, math, and physics. Additional exam requirements/recommendations for international students: Required—TOEFL (minimum score 550 paper-based). *Application deadline:* For fall admission, 7/1 priority date for domestic students. Applications are processed on a rolling basis. Application fee: $65 ($110 for international students). Electronic applications accepted. *Financial support:* Career-related internships or fieldwork and Federal Work-Study available. Financial award application deadline: 7/1. *Faculty research:* Gene cloning, genome structure, cell cycle effects on gene expression, molecular biology of plant hormones, laboratory toxin production and resistance, RNA stability, pathogenicity. *Total annual research expenditures:* $200,000. *Unit head:* Dr. Traci Lee, Chair of Molecular Biology Programs, 262-595-2641, Fax: 262-595-2056, E-mail: traci.lee@uwp.edu. *Application contact:* Dr. Traci Lee, Chair of Molecular Biology Programs, 262-595-2641, Fax: 262-595-2056, E-mail: traci.lee@uwp.edu.

University of Wyoming, College of Agriculture and Natural Resources, Department of Molecular Biology, Laramie, WY 82071. Offers MA, MS, PhD. Terminal master's awarded for partial completion of doctoral program. *Degree requirements:* For master's, comprehensive exam (for some programs), thesis; for doctorate, comprehensive exam, thesis/dissertation. *Entrance requirements:* For master's and doctorate, GRE General Test, GRE Subject Test (recommended), minimum GPA of 3.0. Additional exam requirements/recommendations for international students: Required—TOEFL. Electronic applications accepted. *Faculty research:* Protein structure/function, developmental regulation, yeast genetics, bacterial pathogenesis.

University of Wyoming, Graduate Program in Molecular and Cellular Life Sciences, Laramie, WY 82071. Offers PhD. *Degree requirements:* For doctorate, thesis/dissertation, four eight-week laboratory rotations, comprehensive basic practical exam, two-part qualifying exam, seminars, symposium.

Vanderbilt University, Graduate School and School of Medicine, Department of Molecular Physiology and Biophysics, Nashville, TN 37240-1001. Offers MS, PhD, MD/PhD. *Faculty:* 35 full-time (8 women). *Students:* 42 full-time (27 women); includes 9 minority (3 Black or African American, non-Hispanic/Latino; 4 Hispanic/Latino; 2 Two or more races, non-Hispanic/Latino), 1 international. Average age 26. In 2013, 7 doctorates awarded. *Degree requirements:* For doctorate, comprehensive exam, thesis/dissertation, preliminary, qualifying, and final exams. *Entrance requirements:* For doctorate, GRE General Test, GRE Subject Test (recommended). Additional exam requirements/recommendations for international students: Required—TOEFL (minimum score 570 paper-based; 88 iBT). *Application deadline:* For fall admission, 1/15 for domestic and international students. Application fee: $0. Electronic applications accepted. *Financial support:* Fellowships with full tuition reimbursements, research assistantships with full tuition reimbursements, Federal Work-Study, institutionally sponsored loans, scholarships/grants, traineeships, health care benefits, and tuition waivers (partial) available. Financial award application deadline: 1/15; financial award applicants required to submit CSS PROFILE or FAFSA. *Faculty research:* Biophysics, cell signaling and gene regulation, human genetics, diabetes and obesity, neuroscience. *Unit head:* Prof. Roger D. Cone, Chair of the Department of Molecular Physiology and Biophysics, 615-936-7085, Fax: 615-343-0490, E-mail: roger.cone@vanderbilt.edu. *Application contact:* Walter B. Bieschke, Program Coordinator for Graduate Admissions, 615-342-0236, E-mail: walter.bieschke@vanderbilt.edu.
Website: http://www.mc.vanderbilt.edu/root/vumc.php?site-MPB

Virginia Commonwealth University, Medical College of Virginia-Professional Programs, School of Medicine, School of Medicine Graduate Programs, Department of Biochemistry, Richmond, VA 23284-9005. Offers biochemistry (MS, PhD); molecular biology (MS, PhD); MD/PhD. *Degree requirements:* For master's, thesis; for doctorate, thesis/dissertation, comprehensive oral and written exams. *Entrance requirements:* For master's and doctorate, GRE, MCAT or DAT. Electronic applications accepted. *Faculty research:* Molecular biology, peptide/protein chemistry, neurochemistry, enzyme mechanisms, macromolecular structure determination.

Virginia Commonwealth University, Medical College of Virginia-Professional Programs, School of Medicine, School of Medicine Graduate Programs, Department of Human and Molecular Genetics, Richmond, VA 23284-9005. Offers genetic counseling (MS); human genetics (PhD); molecular biology and genetics (MS, PhD); MD/PhD. *Degree requirements:* For master's, thesis; for doctorate, thesis/dissertation, comprehensive oral and written exams. *Entrance requirements:* For master's, GRE; for doctorate, GRE General Test. Additional exam requirements/recommendations for international students: Required—TOEFL (minimum score 600 paper-based; 100 iBT). Electronic applications accepted. *Faculty research:* Genetic epidemiology, biochemical genetics, quantitative genetics, human cytogenetics, molecular genetics.

Wake Forest University, School of Medicine and Graduate School of Arts and Sciences, Graduate Programs in Medicine, Molecular Genetics and Genomics Program, Winston-Salem, NC 27109. Offers PhD, MD/PhD. *Degree requirements:* For doctorate, thesis/dissertation. *Entrance requirements:* For doctorate, GRE General Test. Additional exam requirements/recommendations for international students: Required—TOEFL. Electronic applications accepted. *Faculty research:* Control of gene expression, molecular pathogenesis, protein biosynthesis, cell development, clinical cytogenetics.

Washington University in St. Louis, Graduate School of Arts and Sciences, Division of Biology and Biomedical Sciences, Program in Molecular Cell Biology, St. Louis, MO 63130-4899. Offers PhD. *Degree requirements:* For doctorate, thesis/dissertation. *Entrance requirements:* For doctorate, GRE General Test, GRE Subject Test. Electronic applications accepted.

Wayne State University, College of Liberal Arts and Sciences, Department of Biological Sciences, Detroit, MI 48202. Offers biological sciences (MA, MS); cell development and neurobiology (PhD); evolution and organismal biology (PhD); molecular biology and biotechnology (PhD); molecular biotechnology (MS). Fall application deadline for PhD is December 1. *Faculty:* 26 full-time (9 women). *Students:* 66 full-time (37 women), 8 part-time (3 women); includes 8 minority (1 Black or African American, non-Hispanic/Latino; 5 Asian, non-Hispanic/Latino; 1 Hispanic/Latino; 1 Two or more races, non-Hispanic/Latino), 41 international. Average age 29. 270 applicants, 14% accepted, 14 enrolled. In 2013, 14 master's, 8 doctorates awarded. Terminal master's awarded for partial completion of doctoral program. *Degree requirements:* For master's, thesis (for some programs); for doctorate, thesis/dissertation. *Entrance requirements:* For master's, GRE (for MS applicants), minimum GPA of 3.0; adequate preparation in biological sciences and supporting courses in chemistry, physics and mathematics; curriculum vitae; for doctorate, GRE, three letters of reference, statement of goals and career objectives, bachelor's or master's degree in biological or other science. Additional exam requirements/recommendations for international students: Required—TOEFL (minimum score 550 paper-based; 79 iBT), TWE (minimum score 5.5), Michigan English Language Assessment Battery (minimum score 85); Recommended—IELTS (minimum score 6.5). *Application deadline:* For fall admission, 4/1 for domestic students, 3/1 for international students. Applications are processed on a rolling basis. Application fee: $0. Electronic applications accepted. *Expenses:* Tuition, state resident: part-time $554.15 per credit. Tuition, nonresident: part-time $1200.35 per credit. *Required fees:* $42.15 per credit. $268.30 per semester. Tuition and fees vary according to course load and program. *Financial support:* In 2013–14, 55 students received support, including 3 fellowships with tuition reimbursements available (averaging $16,842 per year), 9 research assistantships with tuition reimbursements available (averaging $18,582 per year), 49 teaching assistantships with tuition reimbursements available (averaging $18,488 per year); institutionally sponsored loans, scholarships/grants, health care benefits, and unspecified assistantships also available. Financial award application deadline: 3/31; financial award applicants required to submit FAFSA. *Faculty research:* Transcription and chromatin remodeling, genomic and developmental evolution, community and landscape ecology and environmental degradation, microbiology and virology, cell and neurobiology. *Total annual research expenditures:* $1.7 million. *Unit head:* Dr. David Njus, Professor and Chair, 313-577-2783, Fax: 313-577-6891, E-mail: dnjus@wayne.edu. *Application contact:* Rose Mary Priest, Office Services Clerk, 313-577-6818, Fax: 313-577-6891, E-mail: rpriest@wayne.edu.
Website: http://clasweb.clas.wayne.edu/biology

Wayne State University, School of Medicine, Graduate Programs in Medicine, Department of Biochemistry and Molecular Biology, Detroit, MI 48202. Offers MS, PhD, MD/PhD. *Students:* 25 full-time (13 women); includes 5 minority (2 Black or African American, non-Hispanic/Latino; 2 Asian, non-Hispanic/Latino; 1 Two or more races, non-Hispanic/Latino), 10 international. Average age 26. 113 applicants, 18% accepted, 9 enrolled. In 2013, 7 master's, 1 doctorate awarded. Terminal master's awarded for partial completion of doctoral program. *Degree requirements:* For master's, thesis; for doctorate, thesis/dissertation. *Entrance requirements:* For master's, GRE, BA or BS in biology, chemistry, or (if approved) physics or mathematics with minimum GPA of 2.6 from accredited university; three letters of recommendation; personal statement, admission to the Graduate School; for doctorate, GRE, BA or BS in biology, chemistry or physics (preferred), undergraduate degree with minimum GPA of 3.0, admission to the Graduate School. Additional exam requirements/recommendations for international students: Required—TOEFL (minimum score 600 paper-based; 100 iBT). *Application deadline:* For fall admission, 2/1 for domestic and international students. Application fee: $0. Electronic applications accepted. *Expenses:* Contact institution. *Financial support:* In 2013–14, 11 students received support, including 3 fellowships with tuition reimbursements available (averaging $22,811 per year), 10 research assistantships with tuition reimbursements available (averaging $22,594 per year); scholarships/grants, health care benefits, and unspecified assistantships also available. Financial award application deadline: 3/31; financial award applicants required to submit FAFSA. *Faculty research:* Cancer biology, structural biology and drug design, molecular evolution, viral and fungal metabolism/resistance, cardiovascular disease, computational biology. *Unit head:* Dr. Bharati Mitra, Professor and Chair, Department of Biochemistry and Molecular Biology, 313-577-1512, Fax: 313-577-2765, E-mail: bmitra@med.wayne.edu. *Application contact:* Dr. David Evans, Graduate Program Director, 313-577-5712, E-mail: drevans@med.wayne.edu.
Website: http://gradprograms.med.wayne.edu/program-spotlight.php?id=28

Wayne State University, School of Medicine, Graduate Programs in Medicine, Program in Molecular Biology and Genetics, Detroit, MI 48201. Offers bioinformatics and computational biology (PhD); cellular neuroscience (PhD); MD/PhD. *Students:* 21 full-time (11 women), 1 part-time (0 women); includes 1 minority (Hispanic/Latino), 3 international. Average age 27. 45 applicants, 13% accepted, 4 enrolled. In 2013, 5 doctorates awarded. Terminal master's awarded for partial completion of doctoral program. *Degree requirements:* For doctorate, thesis/dissertation. *Entrance requirements:* For doctorate, GRE General Test, GRE Subject Test (chemistry or biology), minimum GPA of 3.0, strong background in one of the chemical or biological sciences, three letters of recommendation, personal statement, interview. Additional exam requirements/recommendations for international students: Required—TOEFL (minimum score 550 paper-based; 79 iBT), Michigan English Language Assessment Battery (minimum score 85); Recommended—IELTS (minimum score 6.5), TWE (minimum score 5.5). *Application deadline:* For fall admission, 3/1 for domestic students, 5/1 for international students; for winter admission, 10/1 for domestic students, 9/1 for international students; for spring admission, 2/1 for domestic students, 1/1 for international students. Applications are processed on a rolling basis. Application fee: $0. Electronic applications accepted. *Expenses:* Tuition, state resident: part-time $554.15 per credit. Tuition, nonresident: part-time $1200.35 per credit. *Required fees:* $42.15 per credit. $268.30 per semester. Tuition and fees vary according to course load and program. *Financial support:* In 2013–14, 18 students received support. Fellowships with tuition reimbursements available, research assistantships with tuition reimbursements available, teaching assistantships with tuition reimbursements available, scholarships/grants, and unspecified assistantships available. Financial award application deadline: 3/31; financial award applicants required to submit FAFSA. *Faculty research:* Human gene mapping, genome organization and sequencing, gene regulation, molecular evolution. *Total annual research expenditures:* $2.6 million. *Unit head:* Dr. Lawrence Grossman, Director, 313-577-5323, E-mail: l.grossman@wayne.edu. *Application contact:* Dr. Gregory Kapatos, Professor, Director for Education, and Graduate Officer, 313-577-5965, Fax: 313-993-4269, E-mail: gkapato@med.wayne.edu.
Website: http://genetics.wayne.edu/students/mdphd.php

Weill Cornell Medical College, Weill Cornell Graduate School of Medical Sciences, Biochemistry, Cell and Molecular Biology Allied Program, New York, NY 10065. Offers MS, PhD. Terminal master's awarded for partial completion of doctoral program. *Degree requirements:* For master's, comprehensive exam; for doctorate, thesis/dissertation, final exam. *Entrance requirements:* For doctorate, GRE General Test, background in genetics, molecular biology, chemistry, or biochemistry. Additional exam requirements/recommendations for international students: Required—TOEFL. Electronic applications accepted. *Faculty research:* Molecular structure determination, protein structure, gene structure, stem cell biology, control of gene expression, DNA replication, chromosome maintenance, RNA biosynthesis.

Wesleyan University, Graduate Studies, Department of Molecular Biology and Biochemistry, Middletown, CT 06459. Offers biochemistry (PhD); molecular biology (PhD); molecular biophysics (PhD); molecular genetics (PhD). *Degree requirements:* For doctorate, comprehensive exam, thesis/dissertation. *Entrance requirements:* For doctorate, GRE General Test, GRE Subject Test. Additional exam requirements/recommendations for international students: Required—TOEFL. Electronic applications accepted. *Faculty research:* The olfactory system and new frontiers in genome research, chromosome structure and gene expression.

West Virginia University, Eberly College of Arts and Sciences, Department of Biology, Morgantown, WV 26506. Offers cell and molecular biology (MS, PhD); environmental and evolutionary biology (MS, PhD); forensic biology (MS, PhD); genomic biology (MS, PhD); neurobiology (MS, PhD). Terminal master's awarded for partial completion of doctoral program. *Degree requirements:* For master's, thesis, final exam; for doctorate, thesis/dissertation, preliminary and final exams. *Entrance requirements:* For master's, GRE General Test, GRE Subject Test, minimum GPA of 3.0; for doctorate, GRE General Test, minimum GPA of 3.0. Additional exam requirements/recommendations for international students: Required—TOEFL. *Faculty research:* Environmental biology, genetic engineering, developmental biology, global change, biodiversity.

West Virginia University, School of Medicine, Graduate Programs at the Health Sciences Center, Interdisciplinary Graduate Programs in Biomedical Sciences, Program in Biochemistry and Molecular Biology, Morgantown, WV 26506. Offers MS, PhD, MD/PhD. *Degree requirements:* For doctorate, comprehensive exam, thesis/dissertation. *Entrance requirements:* For doctorate, GRE General Test, minimum GPA of 3.0. Additional exam requirements/recommendations for international students: Required—TOEFL. Electronic applications accepted. *Faculty research:* Regulation of gene expression, cell survival mechanisms, signal transduction, regulation of metabolism, sensory neuroscience.

Wright State University, School of Graduate Studies, College of Science and Mathematics, Department of Biochemistry and Molecular Biology, Dayton, OH 45435. Offers MS. *Degree requirements:* For master's, thesis. *Entrance requirements:* Additional exam requirements/recommendations for international students: Required—TOEFL. *Faculty research:* Regulation of gene expression, macromolecular structural function, NMR imaging, visual biochemistry.

Yale University, Graduate School of Arts and Sciences, Department of Molecular, Cellular, and Developmental Biology, Program in Biochemistry, Molecular Biology and Chemical Biology, New Haven, CT 06520. Offers PhD. *Degree requirements:* For doctorate, thesis/dissertation. *Entrance requirements:* For doctorate, GRE General Test, GRE Subject Test.

Yale University, School of Medicine and Graduate School of Arts and Sciences, Combined Program in Biological and Biomedical Sciences (BBS), Molecular Cell Biology, Genetics, and Development Track, New Haven, CT 06520. Offers PhD, MD/PhD. *Entrance requirements:* Additional exam requirements/recommendations for international students: Required—TOEFL.

Youngstown State University, Graduate School, College of Science, Technology, Engineering and Mathematics, Department of Biological Sciences, Youngstown, OH 44555-0001. Offers environmental biology (MS); molecular biology, microbiology, and genetic (MS); physiology and anatomy (MS). Part-time programs available. *Degree requirements:* For master's, comprehensive exam, thesis, oral review. *Entrance requirements:* For master's, GRE General Test, minimum GPA of 2.7. Additional exam requirements/recommendations for international students: Required—TOEFL. *Faculty research:* Cell biology, neurophysiology, molecular biology, neurobiology, gene regulation.

Molecular Medicine

Baylor College of Medicine, Graduate School of Biomedical Sciences, Program in Translational Biology and Molecular Medicine, Houston, TX 77030-3498. Offers PhD. *Degree requirements:* For doctorate, thesis/dissertation, public defense. *Entrance requirements:* For doctorate, GRE, minimum GPA of 3.0. Additional exam requirements/recommendations for international students: Required—TOEFL. Electronic applications accepted. *Faculty research:* Molecular medicine, translational biology, human disease biology and therapy.

Boston University, School of Medicine, Division of Graduate Medical Sciences, Program in Molecular Medicine, Boston, MA 02215. Offers PhD, MD/PhD. *Degree requirements:* For doctorate, thesis/dissertation. *Application deadline:* For fall admission, 1/15 for domestic students; for spring admission, 10/15 for domestic students. *Expenses: Tuition:* Full-time $43,970; part-time $1374 per credit hour. *Required fees:* $60 per semester. Tuition and fees vary according to class time, course level and program. *Unit head:* Dr. William Cruikshank, Director, 617-638-5295, E-mail: bcruiksh@bu.edu. *Application contact:* GMS Admissions Office, 617-638-5255, Fax: 617-638-5740, E-mail: natashah@bu.edu.
Website: http://www.bumc.bu.edu/gpmm

Case Western Reserve University, School of Graduate Studies, Cleveland Clinic Lerner Research Institute–Molecular Medicine PhD Program, Cleveland, OH 44106. Offers PhD. *Faculty:* 154 full-time (46 women). *Students:* 42 full-time (23 women), 2 part-time (1 woman); includes 11 minority (6 Black or African American, non-Hispanic/Latino; 4 Asian, non-Hispanic/Latino; 1 Hispanic/Latino), 9 international. Average age 27. 75 applicants, 11% accepted, 7 enrolled. In 2013, 4 doctorates awarded. *Degree requirements:* For doctorate, comprehensive exam, thesis/dissertation, seminar. *Entrance requirements:* For doctorate, GRE, 3 letters of reference, prior research experience, interview. Additional exam requirements/recommendations for international students: Required—TOEFL (minimum score 577 paper-based; 90 iBT); Recommended—IELTS (minimum score 7). *Application deadline:* For fall admission, 1/15 priority date for domestic students, 11/1 for international students. Application fee: $50. Electronic applications accepted. *Financial support:* Fellowships with full tuition reimbursements, health care benefits, and stipends available. *Faculty research:* Cancer, cardiovascular disease, neuroscience, molecular biology, genetics. *Unit head:* Dr. Marcia Tackacs Jarrett, Director of Research Education, 216-444-4860, E-mail: jarretm@ccf.org. *Application contact:* Robin Crotty, Recruiting and Development Coordinator, 216-445-4917, E-mail: crottyr@ccf.org.
Website: http://www.lerner.ccf.org/molecmed/phd/

Case Western Reserve University, School of Medicine and School of Graduate Studies, Graduate Programs in Medicine, Department of Molecular Medicine at the Lerner Research Institute, Cleveland, OH 44106. Offers PhD. *Degree requirements:* For doctorate, comprehensive exam, thesis/dissertation. *Entrance requirements:* For doctorate, GRE. Additional exam requirements/recommendations for international students: Required—TOEFL. Electronic applications accepted.

Cleveland State University, College of Graduate Studies, College of Sciences and Health Professions, Department of Chemistry, Cleveland, OH 44115. Offers analytical chemistry (MS); clinical chemistry (MS); clinical/bioanalytical chemistry (PhD), including cellular and molecular medicine, clinical chemistry, clinical/bioanalytical chemistry; environmental chemistry (MS); inorganic chemistry (MS); pharmaceutical/organic chemistry (MS); physical chemistry (MS). Part-time and evening/weekend programs available. *Faculty:* 12 full-time (0 women). *Students:* 17 full-time (10 women), 95 part-time (43 women); includes 6 minority (5 Black or African American, non-Hispanic/Latino; 1 Asian, non-Hispanic/Latino), 73 international. Average age 27. 121 applicants, 55% accepted. In 2013, 19 master's, 9 doctorates awarded. *Degree requirements:* For master's, thesis optional; for doctorate, comprehensive exam, thesis/dissertation. *Entrance requirements:* For master's and doctorate, GRE General Test. Additional exam requirements/recommendations for international students: Required—TOEFL (minimum score 525 paper-based; 65 iBT). *Application deadline:* For fall admission, 1/15 priority date for domestic and international students. Applications are processed on a rolling basis. Application fee: $30. Electronic applications accepted. *Expenses:* Tuition, state resident: full-time $8335; part-time $521 per credit hour. Tuition, nonresident: full-time $15,670; part-time $979 per credit hour. *Required fees:* $50; $25 per semester. *Financial support:* In 2013–14, 44 students received support, including 5 fellowships with full tuition reimbursements available (averaging $22,500 per year), 13 research assistantships with full tuition reimbursements available (averaging $22,500 per year), 24 teaching assistantships with full tuition reimbursements available (averaging $21,000 per year); scholarships/grants and unspecified assistantships also available. Financial award application deadline: 1/15. *Faculty research:* Bioanalytical techniques and molecular diagnostics, glycoproteomics and antithrombotic agents, drug discovery and innovation, analytical pharmacology, inflammatory disease research. *Total annual research expenditures:* $3 million. *Unit head:* Dr. David W. Ball, Chair, 216-687-2467, Fax: 216-687-9298, E-mail: d.ball@csuohio.edu. *Application contact:* Richelle P. Emery, Administrative Coordinator, 216-687-2457, Fax: 216-687-9298, E-mail: r.emery@csuohio.edu.
Website: http://www.csuohio.edu/sciences/dept/chemistry/index.html

Cornell University, Graduate School, Graduate Fields of Comparative Biomedical Sciences, Field of Comparative Biomedical Sciences, Ithaca, NY 14853-0001. Offers cellular and molecular medicine (MS, PhD); developmental and reproductive biology (MS, PhD); infectious diseases (MS, PhD); population medicine and epidemiology (MS, PhD); structural and functional biology (MS, PhD). *Faculty:* 104 full-time (32 women). *Students:* 32 full-time (22 women); includes 3 minority (1 Asian, non-Hispanic/Latino; 2 Hispanic/Latino), 12 international. Average age 29. 47 applicants, 23% accepted, 6 enrolled. In 2013, 2 master's, 12 doctorates awarded. *Degree requirements:* For master's, thesis; for doctorate, comprehensive exam, thesis/dissertation. *Entrance requirements:* For master's and doctorate, GRE General Test, 2 letters of recommendation. Additional exam requirements/recommendations for international students: Required—TOEFL (minimum score 550 paper-based; 77 iBT). *Application deadline:* For fall admission, 12/15 for domestic students. Application fee: $95. Electronic applications accepted. *Financial support:* In 2013–14, 18 students received support, including 3 fellowships with full tuition reimbursements available, 14 research assistantships with full tuition reimbursements available, 1 teaching assistantship with full tuition reimbursement available; institutionally sponsored loans, scholarships/grants, health care benefits, tuition waivers (full and partial), and unspecified assistantships also available. Financial award applicants required to submit FAFSA. *Faculty research:* Receptors and signal transduction, viral and bacterial infectious diseases, tumor metastasis, clinical sciences/nutritional disease, developmental/neurological disorders. *Unit head:* Director of Graduate Studies, 607-253-3276, Fax: 607-253-3756. *Application contact:* Graduate Field Assistant, 607-253-3276, Fax: 607-253-3756, E-mail: graduate_edcvm@cornell.edu.
Website: http://www.gradschool.cornell.edu/fields.php?id-64&a-2

Dartmouth College, Arts and Sciences Graduate Programs, Program in Experimental and Molecular Medicine, Hanover, NH 03755. Offers biomedical physiology (PhD); cancer biology and molecular therapeutics (PhD); cardiovascular diseases (PhD); molecular pharmacology, toxicology and experimental therapeutics (PhD); neuroscience (PhD); MD/PhD. *Degree requirements:* For doctorate, comprehensive exam, thesis/dissertation. *Entrance requirements:* For doctorate, GRE, 3 letters of recommendation, interview, minimum GPA of 3.0. Additional exam requirements/recommendations for international students: Required—TOEFL (minimum score 620 paper-based; 105 iBT). Electronic applications accepted.

Dartmouth College, Program in Experimental and Molecular Medicine, Hanover, NH 03755. Offers biomedical physiology (PhD); cancer biology and molecular therapeutics (PhD); cardiovascular diseases (PhD); molecular pharmacology, toxicology and experimental therapeutics (PhD); neuroscience (PhD); MD/PhD. *Degree requirements:* For doctorate, comprehensive exam, thesis/dissertation. *Entrance requirements:* For doctorate, GRE General Test, 3 letters of recommendation. Additional exam requirements/recommendations for international students: Required—TOEFL (minimum score 620 paper-based; 105 iBT). Electronic applications accepted.

Drexel University, College of Medicine, Biomedical Graduate Programs, Molecular Medicine Program, Philadelphia, PA 19104-2875. Offers MS.

Elmezzi Graduate School of Molecular Medicine, Graduate Program, Manhasset, NY 11030. Offers PhD. *Degree requirements:* For doctorate, comprehensive exam, thesis/dissertation. *Entrance requirements:* For doctorate, MD or equivalent. *Faculty research:* Cardiopulmonary disease, cancer, inflammation, genetics of complex disorders, cytokine biology.

The George Washington University, Columbian College of Arts and Sciences, Institute for Biomedical Sciences, Program in Molecular Medicine, Washington, DC 20037. Offers molecular and cellular oncology (PhD); neurosciences (PhD); pharmacology and physiology (PhD). *Students:* 6 full-time (4 women), 13 part-time (9 women); includes 3 minority (1 Black or African American, non-Hispanic/Latino; 1 Asian, non-Hispanic/Latino; 1 Hispanic/Latino), 6 international. Average age 29. In 2013, 12 doctorates awarded. *Degree requirements:* For doctorate, comprehensive exam, thesis/dissertation, general exams. *Entrance requirements:* For doctorate, GRE General Test, interview, minimum GPA of 3.0. Additional exam requirements/recommendations for international students: Required—TOEFL (minimum score 600 paper-based). *Application deadline:* For fall admission, 12/15 priority date for domestic and international students. Applications are processed on a rolling basis. Application fee: $75. Electronic applications accepted. *Financial support:* In 2013–14, 10 students received support. Fellowships with tuition reimbursements available, Federal Work-Study, institutionally sponsored loans, and tuition waivers available. Financial award application deadline: 2/1. *Unit head:* Dr. Norman Lee, Director, 202-994-2114, E-mail: beb@gwu.edu. *Application contact:* 202-994-2179, Fax: 202-994-0967, E-mail: gwibs@gwu.edu.
Website: http://www.gwumc.edu/ibs/

Georgia Regents University, The Graduate School, Program in Molecular Medicine, Augusta, GA 30912. Offers MS, PhD. *Faculty:* 50 full-time (7 women), 2 part-time/adjunct (0 women). *Students:* 19 full-time (14 women); includes 14 minority (1 Black or African American, non-Hispanic/Latino; 13 Asian, non-Hispanic/Latino), 15 international. Average age 30. In 2013, 3 doctorates awarded. *Degree requirements:* For doctorate, comprehensive exam, thesis/dissertation. *Entrance requirements:* For doctorate, GRE General Test. Additional exam requirements/recommendations for international students: Required—TOEFL (minimum score 550 paper-based; 79 iBT). *Application deadline:* For fall admission, 1/15 for domestic and international students. Application fee: $50. Electronic applications accepted. *Financial support:* In 2013–14, 4 students received support, including fellowships with partial tuition reimbursements available (averaging $26,000 per year), 17 research assistantships with partial tuition reimbursements available (averaging $23,000 per year); teaching assistantships, Federal Work-Study, institutionally sponsored loans, and scholarships/grants also available. Support available to part-time students. Financial award application deadline: 5/31; financial award applicants required to submit FAFSA. *Faculty research:* Developmental neurobiology, cancer, regenerative medicine, molecular chaperones, molecular immunology. *Total annual research expenditures:* $11.9 million. *Unit head:* Dr. Lin Mei, Director of Institute of Molecular Medicine and Genetics, 706-721-8775, Fax: 706-721-8685, E-mail: lmie@georgiahealth.edu. *Application contact:* Dr. Patricia L. Cameron, Associate Dean, 706-721-3279, E-mail: pcameron@georgiahealth.edu.
Website: http://www.gru.edu/mcg/dnrm/molecularmedicine/

Hofstra University, School of Medicine, Hempstead, NY 11549. Offers medicine (MD); molecular basis of medicine (PhD); MD/PhD. *Accreditation:* LCME/AMA.

Johns Hopkins University, School of Medicine, Graduate Programs in Medicine, Graduate Program in Cellular and Molecular Medicine, Baltimore, MD 21218-2699. Offers PhD. *Faculty:* 125 full-time (29 women). *Students:* 125 full-time (76 women); includes 49 minority (4 Black or African American, non-Hispanic/Latino; 1 American Indian or Alaska Native, non-Hispanic/Latino; 30 Asian, non-Hispanic/Latino; 8 Hispanic/Latino; 6 Two or more races, non-Hispanic/Latino), 19 international. Average age 27. 143 applicants, 39% accepted, 21 enrolled. In 2013, 25 doctorates awarded. *Degree requirements:* For doctorate, comprehensive exam, thesis/dissertation, oral exam. *Entrance requirements:* For doctorate, GRE. Additional exam requirements/recommendations for international students: Required—TOEFL. *Application deadline:* For winter admission, 1/1 for domestic students. Application fee: $85. Electronic applications accepted. *Financial support:* Fellowships, scholarships/grants, health care benefits, and tuition waivers (full) available. *Faculty research:* Cellular and molecular basis of disease. *Total annual research expenditures:* $100 million. *Unit head:* Dr. Rajini Rao, Director, 410-955-4732, Fax: 410-614-7294, E-mail: rrao@jhmi.edu. *Application contact:* Leslie Lichter-Mason, Admissions Administrator, 410-614-0391, Fax: 410-614-7294, E-mail: llichte2@jhmi.edu.
Website: http://cmm.jhmi.edu

Penn State University Park, Graduate School, Intercollege Graduate Programs, Intercollege Graduate Program in Molecular Medicine, University Park, PA 16802. Offers MS, PhD. *Unit head:* Dr. Regina Vasilatos-Younken, Interim Dean, 814-865-2516, Fax: 814-863-4627, E-mail: rxv@psu.edu. *Application contact:* Cynthia E. Nicosia, Director, Graduate Enrollment Services, 814-865-1834, Fax: 814-863-4627, E-mail: cey1@psu.edu.

Queen's University at Kingston, School of Graduate Studies, Faculty of Health Sciences, Department of Pathology and Molecular Medicine, Kingston, ON K7L 3N6, Canada. Offers M Sc, PhD. Part-time programs available. *Degree requirements:* For master's, thesis; for doctorate, comprehensive exam, thesis/dissertation. *Entrance requirements:* Additional exam requirements/recommendations for international students: Required—TOEFL. *Faculty research:* Immunopathology, cancer biology, immunology and metastases, cell differentiation, blood coagulation.

Rutgers, The State University of New Jersey, Newark, Graduate School of Biomedical Sciences, Department of Cell Biology and Molecular Medicine, Newark, NJ 07107. Offers PhD. *Degree requirements:* For doctorate, thesis/dissertation, qualifying exam. *Entrance requirements:* For doctorate, GRE General Test. Additional exam requirements/recommendations for international students: Required—TOEFL. Electronic applications accepted.

Texas A&M Health Science Center, College of Medicine, Department of Molecular and Cellular Medicine, College Station, TX 77840. Offers PhD. *Degree requirements:* For doctorate, thesis/dissertation. *Entrance requirements:* For doctorate, GRE General Test. *Faculty research:* Immunology, cell and membrane biology, protein biochemistry, molecular genetics, parasitology, vertebrate embryogenesis and microbiology.

The University of Arizona, College of Medicine, Department of Cellular and Molecular Medicine, Tucson, AZ 85721. Offers MS, PhD, Graduate Certificate. *Faculty:* 15 full-time (4 women), 1 (woman) part-time/adjunct. *Students:* 25 full-time (12 women), 2 part-time (0 women); includes 8 minority (2 Black or African American, non-Hispanic/Latino; 1 Asian, non-Hispanic/Latino; 1 Hispanic/Latino; 4 Two or more races, non-Hispanic/Latino), 4 international. Average age 28. 24 applicants, 38% accepted, 6 enrolled. In 2013, 1 master's, 3 doctorates awarded. *Degree requirements:* For doctorate, comprehensive exam. *Entrance requirements:* Additional exam requirements/recommendations for international students: Required—TOEFL, IELTS. *Application deadline:* For fall admission, 6/18 for domestic students; for spring admission, 11/15 for domestic students. Applications are processed on a rolling basis. Application fee: $75. Electronic applications accepted. *Expenses:* Tuition, state resident: full-time $11,526. Tuition, nonresident: full-time $27,398. *Financial support:* In 2013–14, 9 research assistantships with full tuition reimbursements (averaging $25,000 per year) were awarded. *Faculty research:* Heart and vascular development, neural development, cellular toxicology, immunobiology, cell biology and cancer biology. *Total annual research expenditures:* $2.6 million. *Unit head:* Dr. Carol Gregorio, Head, 520-626-6084, Fax: 520-626-2097. *Application contact:* Dr. Audrey Nickols Pallette, Associate Dean for Admissions, 520-626-6084, E-mail: apallett@email.arizona.edu.
Website: http://cmm.arizona.edu/

University of Chicago, Division of Biological Sciences, Biomedical Sciences Cluster: Cancer Biology, Immunology, Molecular Metabolism and Nutrition, Pathology, and Microbiology, Department of Pathology, Chicago, IL 60637-1513. Offers molecular pathogenesis and molecular medicine (PhD). *Degree requirements:* For doctorate, thesis/dissertation, ethics class, 2 teaching assistantships. *Entrance requirements:* For doctorate, GRE General Test. Additional exam requirements/recommendations for international students: Required—IELTS (minimum score 7); Recommended—TOEFL (minimum score 600 paper-based; 104 iBT). Electronic applications accepted. *Faculty research:* Vascular biology, apolipoproteins, cardiovascular disease, immunopathology.

University of Cincinnati, Graduate School, College of Medicine, Graduate Programs in Biomedical Sciences, Program in Pathobiology and Molecular Medicine, Cincinnati, OH 45221. Offers pathology (PhD), including anatomic pathology, laboratory medicine, pathobiology and molecular medicine. *Degree requirements:* For doctorate, thesis/dissertation, qualifying exam. *Entrance requirements:* For doctorate, GRE General Test. Additional exam requirements/recommendations for international students: Required—TOEFL (minimum score 620 paper-based). Electronic applications accepted. *Faculty research:* Cardiovascular and lipid disorders, digestive and kidney disease, endocrine and metabolic disorders, hematologic and oncogenic, immunology and infectious disease.

University of Maryland, Baltimore, Graduate School, Graduate Program in Life Sciences, Program in Molecular Medicine, Baltimore, MD 21201. Offers cancer biology (PhD); cell and molecular physiology (PhD); human genetics and genomic medicine (PhD); molecular medicine (MS); molecular toxicology and pharmacology (PhD); MD/PhD. *Students:* 91 full-time (49 women), 14 part-time (8 women); includes 32 minority (10 Black or African American, non-Hispanic/Latino; 12 Asian, non-Hispanic/Latino; 5 Hispanic/Latino; 5 Two or more races, non-Hispanic/Latino), 9 international. Average age 27. 180 applicants, 33% accepted, 24 enrolled. In 2013, 10 master's, 15 doctorates awarded. *Degree requirements:* For doctorate, comprehensive exam, thesis/dissertation. *Entrance requirements:* For master's and doctorate, GRE. Additional exam requirements/recommendations for international students: Required—TOEFL (minimum score 600 paper-based; 100 iBT); Recommended—IELTS (minimum score 7). *Application deadline:* For fall admission, 12/1 priority date for domestic students, 1/15 for international students. Application fee: $75. Electronic applications accepted. *Financial support:* In 2013–14, research assistantships with partial tuition reimbursements (averaging $25,000 per year) were awarded; fellowships also available. Financial award application deadline: 3/1; financial award applicants required to submit FAFSA. *Unit head:* Dr. Toni Antalis, Director, 410-706-8222, E-mail: tantalis@som.umaryland.edu. *Application contact:* Sharron Graves, Program Coordinator, 410-706-6044, Fax: 410-706-6040, E-mail: sgraves@som.umaryland.edu.
Website: http://molecularmedicine.umaryland.edu

University of South Florida, Morsani College of Medicine and Graduate School, Graduate Programs in Medical Sciences, Tampa, FL 33620-9951. Offers aging and neuroscience (MSMS); allergy, immunology and infectious disease (PhD); anatomy (MSMS, PhD); athletic training (MSMS); bioinformatics and computational biology (MSBCB); biotechnology (MSB); clinical and translational research (MSMS, PhD); health informatics (MSHI, MSMS); health science (MSMS); interdisciplinary medical sciences (MSMS); medical microbiology and immunology (MSMS); metabolic and nutritional medicine (MSMS); molecular medicine (MSMS, PhD); molecular pharmacology and physiology (PhD); neurology (PhD); pathology and laboratory medicine (PhD); pharmacology and therapeutics (PhD); physiology and biophysics (PhD); women's health (MSMS). *Students:* 336 full-time (182 women), 39 part-time (21 women); includes 170 minority (45 Black or African American, non-Hispanic/Latino; 54 Asian, non-Hispanic/Latino; 59 Hispanic/Latino; 2 Native Hawaiian or other Pacific Islander, non-Hispanic/Latino; 10 Two or more races, non-Hispanic/Latino), 17 international. Average age 26. 1,066 applicants, 44% accepted, 250 enrolled. In 2013, 191 master's, 12 doctorates awarded. Terminal master's awarded for partial completion of doctoral program. *Degree requirements:* For master's, comprehensive exam, thesis; for doctorate, comprehensive exam, thesis/dissertation. *Entrance requirements:* For master's, GRE General Test or GMAT, bachelor's degree or equivalent from regionally-accredited university with minimum GPA of 3.0 in upper-division sciences coursework; prerequisites in general biology, general chemistry, general physics, organic chemistry, quantitative analysis, and integral and differential calculus; for doctorate, GRE General Test (minimum score of 600 quantitative), bachelor's degree from regionally-accredited university with minimum GPA of 3.0 in upper-division sciences coursework; 3 letters of recommendation; personal interview; 1-2 page personal statement; prerequisites in biology, chemistry, physics, organic chemistry, quantitative analysis, and integral/differential calculus. Additional exam requirements/recommendations for international students: Required—TOEFL (minimum score 550 paper-based; 79 iBT) or IELTS (minimum score 6.5). *Application deadline:* For fall admission, 2/15 for domestic students, 1/2 for international students. Application fee: $30. *Expenses:* Contact institution. *Faculty research:* Anatomy, biochemistry, cancer biology, cardiovascular disease, cell biology, immunology, microbiology, molecular biology, neuroscience, pharmacology, physiology. *Unit head:* Dr. Michael Barber, Professor and Associate Dean for Graduate and Postdoctoral Affairs, 813-974-9908, Fax: 813-974-4317, E-mail: mbarber@health.usf.edu. *Application contact:* Dr. Eric Bennett, Graduate Director, PhD Program in Medical Sciences, 813-974-1545, Fax: 813-974-4317, E-mail: esbennet@health.usf.edu.
Website: http://health.usf.edu/nocms/medicine/graduatestudies/

The University of Texas Health Science Center at San Antonio, Graduate School of Biomedical Sciences, Department of Molecular Medicine, San Antonio, TX 78245-3207. Offers MS, PhD. *Faculty:* 22 full-time (6 women), 4 part-time/adjunct (1 woman). *Students:* 20 full-time (9 women), 3 part-time (1 woman); includes 1 minority (Asian, non-Hispanic/Latino), 17 international. Average age 30. In 2013, 1 master's, 3 doctorates awarded. Terminal master's awarded for partial completion of doctoral program. *Degree requirements:* For master's, comprehensive exam, thesis, written and oral qualifying exam; for doctorate, comprehensive exam, thesis/dissertation, written and oral qualifying exam. *Entrance requirements:* For master's and doctorate, GRE General Test. Additional exam requirements/recommendations for international students: Required—TOEFL (minimum score 560 paper-based; 68 iBT). *Application deadline:* For fall admission, 2/1 priority date for domestic and international students; for spring admission, 10/1 for domestic and international students. Applications are processed on a rolling basis. Application fee: $0. Electronic applications accepted. *Financial support:* Application deadline: 6/30; applicants required to submit FAFSA. *Faculty research:* DNA repair, tumor suppressor genes, vision in drosophila, gene expression (nervous system), cell-type specific gene regulation and development. *Total annual research expenditures:* $5.2 million. *Unit head:* Dr. Hui-Ming (Tim) Huang, Chair, 210-450-0025, Fax: 210-562-4161, E-mail: huangt3@uthscsa.edu. *Application contact:* Dr. Victor Jin, Committee on Graduate Studies Chair, 210-562-9209, Fax: 210-562-4161, E-mail: jinv@uthscsa.edu.
Website: http://www.molecularmedicine.uthscsa.edu/

University of Washington, Graduate School, School of Public Health, Department of Global Health, Graduate Program in Pathobiology, Seattle, WA 98195. Offers PhD. *Faculty:* 20 full-time (8 women). *Students:* 26 full-time (17 women), 8 part-time (7 women); includes 6 minority (2 Black or African American, non-Hispanic/Latino; 4 Asian, non-Hispanic/Latino), 2 international. Average age 29. 66 applicants, 17% accepted, 5 enrolled. In 2013, 6 doctorates awarded. *Degree requirements:* For doctorate, comprehensive exam, thesis/dissertation, published paper from thesis work. *Entrance requirements:* For doctorate, GRE General Test, minimum GPA of 3.0. Additional exam requirements/recommendations for international students: Required—TOEFL, IELTS. *Application deadline:* For fall admission, 12/1 for domestic and international students. Application fee: $85. Electronic applications accepted. *Financial support:* In 2013–14, 31 students received support, including 31 research assistantships with full tuition reimbursements available (averaging $28,440 per year); traineeships and unspecified assistantships also available. *Faculty research:* Malaria, immunological response to mycobacteria infections, HIV-cell interaction and the development of an anti-HIV vaccine, regulation of intercellular communication via gap junctions, genetic and nutritional regulation of proteins involved in lipid transport. *Unit head:* Dr. King K. Holmes, Chair, 206-744-3620, Fax: 206-744-3694. *Application contact:* Rachel Reichert, Program Manager, 206-543-4338, Fax: 206-543-3873, E-mail: pabio@u.washington.edu.

Molecular Medicine

Wake Forest University, School of Medicine and Graduate School of Arts and Sciences, Graduate Programs in Medicine, Molecular Genetics and Genomics Program, Winston-Salem, NC 27109. Offers PhD, MD/PhD. *Degree requirements:* For doctorate, thesis/dissertation. *Entrance requirements:* For doctorate, GRE General Test. Additional exam requirements/recommendations for international students: Required—TOEFL. Electronic applications accepted. *Faculty research:* Control of gene expression, molecular pathogenesis, protein biosynthesis, cell development, clinical cytogenetics.

Wake Forest University, School of Medicine and Graduate School of Arts and Sciences, Graduate Programs in Medicine, Program in Molecular Medicine, Winston-Salem, NC 27109. Offers MS, PhD, MD/PhD. *Degree requirements:* For master's, thesis; for doctorate, thesis/dissertation. *Entrance requirements:* For master's and doctorate, GRE General Test. Additional exam requirements/recommendations for international students: Required—TOEFL. Electronic applications accepted. *Faculty research:* Human biology and disease, scientific basis of medicine, cellular and molecular mechanisms of health and disease.

Yale University, School of Medicine and Graduate School of Arts and Sciences, Combined Program in Biological and Biomedical Sciences (BBS), Pharmacological Sciences and Molecular Medicine Track, New Haven, CT 06520. Offers PhD, MD/PhD. *Degree requirements:* For doctorate, thesis/dissertation. *Entrance requirements:* For doctorate, GRE General Test. Additional exam requirements/recommendations for international students: Required—TOEFL. Electronic applications accepted.

Structural Biology

Baylor College of Medicine, Graduate School of Biomedical Sciences, Program in Structural and Computational Biology and Molecular Biophysics, Houston, TX 77030-3498. Offers PhD, MD/PhD. MD/PhD offered jointly with Rice University and University of Houston. *Degree requirements:* For doctorate, thesis/dissertation, public defense. *Entrance requirements:* For doctorate, GRE General Test, GRE Subject Test (strongly recommended), minimum GPA of 3.0. Additional exam requirements/recommendations for international students: Required—TOEFL. Electronic applications accepted. *Faculty research:* Computational biology, structural biology, biophysics.

Carnegie Mellon University, Mellon College of Science, Department of Biological Sciences, Pittsburgh, PA 15213-3891. Offers biochemistry (PhD); biophysics (PhD); cell and developmental biology (PhD); computational biology (MS, PhD); genetics (PhD); molecular biology (PhD); neuroscience (PhD); structural biology (PhD). *Degree requirements:* For doctorate, comprehensive exam, thesis/dissertation. *Entrance requirements:* For doctorate, GRE General Test, GRE Subject Test, interview. *Application deadline:* Applications are processed on a rolling basis. Application fee: $0. Electronic applications accepted. *Financial support:* Fellowships, research assistantships, teaching assistantships, and traineeships available. *Faculty research:* Genetic structure, function, and regulation; protein structure and function; biological membranes; biological spectroscopy. *Unit head:* John L. Woolford, Acting Department Head, 412-268-3193, E-mail: jw17@andrew.cmu.edu. *Application contact:* Ena Miceli, Graduate Programs Manager, 412-268-33012, E-mail: emiceli@andrew.cmu.edu.
Website: http://www.bio.cmu.edu/

Carnegie Mellon University, Mellon College of Science, Joint Pitt + CMU Molecular Biophysics and Structural Biology Graduate Program, Pittsburgh, PA 15213-3891. Offers PhD. Program offered jointly with University of Pittsburgh. *Degree requirements:* For doctorate, comprehensive exam, thesis/dissertation. *Entrance requirements:* For doctorate, GRE General Test. Additional exam requirements/recommendations for international students: Required—TOEFL (minimum score 600 paper-based; 100 iBT), IELTS (minimum score 7). *Application deadline:* For fall admission, 12/15 priority date for domestic and international students. Application fee: $0. Electronic applications accepted. *Financial support:* Fellowships with full tuition reimbursements, research assistantships with full tuition reimbursements, institutionally sponsored loans, scholarships/grants, traineeships, and unspecified assistantships available. *Faculty research:* Structural biology, protein dynamics and folding, computational biophysics, molecular informatics, membrane biophysics and ion channels, NMR, x-ray crystallography cryaelectron microscopy. *Unit head:* Dr. Gordon Rule, Director, 412-268-1839, Fax: 412-268-7129, E-mail: rule@andrew.cmu.edu. *Application contact:* Dr. Gordon Rule, Director, 412-268-1839, Fax: 412-268-7129, E-mail: rule@andrew.cmu.edu.
Website: http://www.mbsb.pitt.edu/

Columbia University, College of Physicians and Surgeons, Integrated Program in Cellular, Molecular, Structural and Genetic Studies, New York, NY 10032. Offers PhD. Terminal master's awarded for partial completion of doctoral program. *Degree requirements:* For doctorate, thesis/dissertation. *Entrance requirements:* For doctorate, GRE General Test, GRE Subject Test. Additional exam requirements/recommendations for international students: Required—TOEFL. *Expenses:* Contact institution. *Faculty research:* Transcription, macromolecular sorting, gene expression during development, cellular interaction.

Cornell University, Graduate School, Graduate Fields of Comparative Biomedical Sciences, Field of Comparative Biomedical Sciences, Ithaca, NY 14853-0001. Offers cellular and molecular medicine (MS, PhD); developmental and reproductive biology (MS, PhD); infectious diseases (MS, PhD); population medicine and epidemiology (MS, PhD); structural and functional biology (MS, PhD). *Faculty:* 104 full-time (32 women). *Students:* 32 full-time (22 women); includes 3 minority (1 Asian, non-Hispanic/Latino; 2 Hispanic/Latino), 12 international. Average age 29. 47 applicants, 23% accepted, 6 enrolled. In 2013, 2 master's, 12 doctorates awarded. *Degree requirements:* For master's, thesis; for doctorate, comprehensive exam, thesis/dissertation. *Entrance requirements:* For master's and doctorate, GRE General Test, 2 letters of recommendation. Additional exam requirements/recommendations for international students: Required—TOEFL (minimum score 550 paper-based; 77 iBT). *Application deadline:* For fall admission, 12/15 for domestic students. Application fee: $95. Electronic applications accepted. *Financial support:* In 2013–14, 18 students received support, including 3 fellowships with full tuition reimbursements available, 14 research assistantships with full tuition reimbursements available, 1 teaching assistantship with full tuition reimbursement available; institutionally sponsored loans, scholarships/grants, health care benefits, tuition waivers (full and partial), and unspecified assistantships also available. Financial award applicants required to submit FAFSA. *Faculty research:* Receptors and signal transduction, viral and bacterial infectious diseases, tumor metastasis, clinical sciences/nutritional disease, developmental/neurological disorders. *Unit head:* Director of Graduate Studies, 607-253-3276, Fax: 607-253-3756. *Application contact:* Graduate Field Assistant, 607-253-3276, Fax: 607-253-3756, E-mail: graduate_edcvm@cornell.edu.
Website: http://www.gradschool.cornell.edu/fields.php?id-64&a-2

Duke University, Graduate School, University Program in Structural Biology and Biophysics, Durham, NC 27710. Offers Certificate. Students must be enrolled in a participating PhD program (biochemistry, cell biology, chemistry, molecular genetics, neurobiology, pharmacology). *Faculty:* 28. *Students:* 2 full-time (0 women). 32 applicants, 16% accepted, 2 enrolled. *Entrance requirements:* For degree, GRE General Test. Additional exam requirements/recommendations for international students: Required—TOEFL (minimum score 577 paper-based; 90 iBT) or IELTS (minimum score 7). *Application deadline:* For fall admission, 12/8 priority date for domestic and international students. Application fee: $80. *Financial support:* Application deadline: 12/8. *Unit head:* Harold P. Erickson, Director of Graduate Studies, 919-684-6559, Fax: 919-684-8346, E-mail: carol.richardson@duke.edu. *Application contact:* Elizabeth Hutton, Director of Admissions, 919-684-3913, Fax: 919-684-2277, E-mail: grad-admissions@duke.edu.
Website: http://sbb.duke.edu

Florida State University, The Graduate School, College of Arts and Sciences, Department of Biological Science, Specialization in Structural Biology, Tallahassee, FL 32306-4295. Offers MS, PhD. *Faculty:* 12 full-time (4 women). *Students:* 22 full-time (12 women); includes 3 minority (1 Black or African American, non-Hispanic/Latino; 2 Hispanic/Latino), 5 international. In 2013, 1 doctorate awarded. Terminal master's awarded for partial completion of doctoral program. *Degree requirements:* For master's, comprehensive exam, thesis, teaching experience, seminar presentation; for doctorate, comprehensive exam, thesis/dissertation, teaching experience, seminar presentation. *Entrance requirements:* For master's and doctorate, GRE General Test, minimum upper-division GPA of 3.0. Additional exam requirements/recommendations for international students: Required—TOEFL (minimum score 600 paper-based; 92 iBT). *Application deadline:* For fall admission, 12/1 for domestic and international students. Application fee: $30. Electronic applications accepted. *Expenses:* Tuition, state resident: part-time $403.51 per credit hour. Tuition, nonresident: part-time $1004.85 per credit hour. *Required fees:* $75.81 per credit hour. One-time fee: $20 part-time. Tuition and fees vary according to course load, campus/location and student level. *Financial support:* In 2013–14, 22 students received support, including 1 fellowship (averaging $23,000 per year), 7 research assistantships with full tuition reimbursements available (averaging $21,500 per year), 14 teaching assistantships with full tuition reimbursements available (averaging $21,500 per year); traineeships and unspecified assistantships also available. Financial award application deadline: 12/1; financial award applicants required to submit FAFSA. *Faculty research:* Molecular genetics, signal transduction and regulation of gene expression, cell and molecular biology of the cytoskeleton, olfactory signal transduction, ion channel structure-function, neuromodulation, 3-D electron microscopy and x-ray crystallography of protein complexes involved in mRNA and sulfur metabolism, olfaction, synaptic physiology and plasticity, ion channel modulation, biomechanics of cardiac and skeletal muscle, magnetic resonance of proteins. *Unit head:* Dr. Debra A. Fadool, Professor and Associate Chairman for Graduate Studies, 850-644-4775, Fax: 850-644-9829, E-mail: dfadool@bio.fsu.edu. *Application contact:* Judy Bowers, Coordinator, Graduate Affairs, 850-644-3023, Fax: 850-644-9829, E-mail: gradinfo@bio.fsu.edu.
Website: http://www.bio.fsu.edu/

Florida State University, The Graduate School, College of Arts and Sciences, Program in Molecular Biophysics, Tallahassee, FL 32306. Offers computational structural biology (PhD); molecular biophysics (PhD). *Faculty:* 34 full-time (7 women). *Students:* 25 full-time (8 women); includes 2 minority (both Hispanic/Latino), 12 international. Average age 29. 24 applicants, 33% accepted, 5 enrolled. In 2013, 4 doctorates awarded. *Degree requirements:* For doctorate, comprehensive exam, thesis/dissertation, teaching 1 term in professor's major department. *Entrance requirements:* For doctorate, GRE General Test. Additional exam requirements/recommendations for international students: Required—TOEFL (minimum score 600 paper-based; 90 iBT). *Application deadline:* For fall admission, 12/15 for domestic and international students. Applications are processed on a rolling basis. Application fee: $30. Electronic applications accepted. *Expenses:* Tuition, state resident: part-time $403.51 per credit hour. Tuition, nonresident: part-time $1004.85 per credit hour. *Required fees:* $75.81 per credit hour. One-time fee: $20 part-time. Tuition and fees vary according to course load, campus/location and student level. *Financial support:* In 2013–14, 24 students received support, including 1 fellowship with full and partial tuition reimbursement available (averaging $23,000 per year), 18 research assistantships with full and partial tuition reimbursements available (averaging $23,500 per year), 6 teaching assistantships with full and partial tuition reimbursements available (averaging $23,500 per year); scholarships/grants, health care benefits, and unspecified assistantships also available. Financial award applicants required to submit FAFSA. *Faculty research:* Protein and nucleic acid structure and function, membrane protein structure, computational biophysics, 3-D image reconstruction. *Total annual research expenditures:* $2.3 million. *Unit head:* Dr. Hong Li, Director, 850-644-6785, Fax: 850-644-7244, E-mail: hli4@fsu.edu. *Application contact:* Lyn Kittle, Academic Coordinator, Graduate Programs, 850-644-1012, Fax: 850-644-7244, E-mail: lkittle@fsu.edu.
Website: http://www.sb.fsu.edu/graduate-program

Harvard University, Graduate School of Arts and Sciences, Department of Systems Biology, Cambridge, MA 02138. Offers PhD. *Degree requirements:* For doctorate, thesis/dissertation, lab rotation, qualifying examination. *Entrance requirements:* For doctorate, GRE. Additional exam requirements/recommendations for international students: Required—TOEFL. Electronic applications accepted. *Expenses: Tuition:* Full-time $38,888. *Required fees:* $958. Tuition and fees vary according to campus/location, program and student level.

Illinois State University, Graduate School, College of Arts and Sciences, Department of Biological Sciences, Normal, IL 61790-2200. Offers animal behavior (MS); bacteriology (MS); biochemistry (MS); biological sciences (MS); biology (PhD); biophysics (MS); biotechnology (MS); botany (MS, PhD); cell biology (MS); conservation biology (MS); developmental biology (MS); ecology (MS, PhD); entomology (MS); evolutionary biology (MS); genetics (MS, PhD); immunology (MS); microbiology (MS, PhD); molecular biology (MS); molecular genetics (MS); neurobiology (MS); neuroscience (MS); parasitology (MS); physiology (MS, PhD); plant biology (MS); plant molecular biology (MS); plant sciences (MS); structural biology (MS); zoology (MS, PhD). Part-time programs available. *Degree requirements:* For master's, thesis or alternative; for doctorate, variable foreign language requirement, thesis/dissertation, 2 terms of residency. *Entrance requirements:* For master's, GRE General Test, minimum GPA of 2.6 in last 60 hours of course work; for doctorate, GRE General Test. *Faculty research:* Redoc balance and drug development in schistosoma mansoni, control of the growth of listeria monocytogenes at low temperature, regulation of cell expansion and microtubule function by SPRI, CRUI: physiology and fitness consequences of different life history phenotypes.

Iowa State University of Science and Technology, Bioinformatics and Computational Biology Program, Ames, IA 50011. Offers MS, PhD. *Degree requirements:* For doctorate, thesis/dissertation. *Entrance requirements:* For master's and doctorate, GRE General Test. Additional exam requirements/recommendations for international students: Recommended—TOEFL, IELTS. Electronic applications accepted. *Faculty research:* Functional and structural genomics, genome evolution, macromolecular structure and function, mathematical biology and biological statistics, metabolic and developmental networks.

Massachusetts Institute of Technology, School of Science, Department of Biology, Cambridge, MA 02139-4307. Offers biochemistry (PhD); biological oceanography (PhD); biology (PhD); biophysical chemistry and molecular structure (PhD); cell biology (PhD); computational and systems biology (PhD); developmental biology (PhD); genetics (PhD); immunology (PhD); microbiology (PhD); molecular biology (PhD); neurobiology (PhD). *Faculty:* 58 full-time (15 women). *Students:* 261 full-time (133 women); includes 77 minority (3 Black or African American, non-Hispanic/Latino; 1 American Indian or Alaska Native, non-Hispanic/Latino; 32 Asian, non-Hispanic/Latino; 32 Hispanic/Latino; 9 Two or more races, non-Hispanic/Latino), 46 international. Average age 26. 651 applicants, 15% accepted, 39 enrolled. In 2013, 25 doctorates awarded. *Degree requirements:* For doctorate, comprehensive exam, thesis/dissertation, two semesters as a teaching assistant. *Entrance requirements:* For doctorate, GRE General Test. Additional exam requirements/recommendations for international students: Required—TOEFL (minimum score 577 paper-based), IELTS (minimum score 6.5). *Application deadline:* For fall admission, 12/1 for domestic and international students. Application fee: $75. Electronic applications accepted. *Expenses: Tuition:* Full-time $43,210; part-time $670 per credit hour. *Required fees:* $288. *Financial support:* In 2013–14, 252 students received support, including 135 fellowships (averaging $36,800 per year), 122 research assistantships (averaging $35,500 per year), 1 teaching assistantship; Federal Work-Study, institutionally sponsored loans, scholarships/grants, traineeships, health care benefits, and unspecified assistantships also available. *Faculty research:* Cellular, developmental and molecular (plant and animal) biology; biochemistry, bioengineering, biophysics and structural biology; classical and molecular genetics, stem cell and epigenetics; immunology and microbiology; cancer biology, molecular medicine, neurobiology and human disease; computational and systems biology. *Total annual research expenditures:* $44.5 million. *Unit head:* Alan Grossman, Interim Head, 617-253-4701. *Application contact:* Biology Education Office, 617-253-3717, Fax: 617-258-9329, E-mail: gradbio@mit.edu.
Website: https://biology.mit.edu/

Mayo Graduate School, Graduate Programs in Biomedical Sciences, Programs in Biochemistry, Structural Biology, Cell Biology, and Genetics, Rochester, MN 55905. Offers biochemistry and structural biology (PhD); cell biology and genetics (PhD); molecular biology (PhD). *Degree requirements:* For doctorate, oral defense of dissertation, qualifying oral and written exam. *Entrance requirements:* For doctorate, GRE, 1 year of chemistry, biology, calculus, and physics. Additional exam requirements/recommendations for international students: Required—TOEFL. Electronic applications accepted. *Faculty research:* Gene structure and function, membranes and receptors/cytoskeleton, oncogenes and growth factors, protein structure and function, steroid hormonal action.

Miami University, College of Arts and Science, Department of Biology, Oxford, OH 45056. Offers biological sciences (MAT); biology (MS, PhD); botany (MAT, MS, PhD); cell, molecular and structural biology (MS, PhD); ecology, evolution and environmental biology (PhD); zoology (MA, MS, PhD). Part-time programs available. Postbaccalaureate distance learning degree programs offered. *Students:* 89 full-time (49 women), 612 part-time (502 women); includes 63 minority (9 Black or African American, non-Hispanic/Latino; 2 American Indian or Alaska Native, non-Hispanic/Latino; 6 Asian, non-Hispanic/Latino; 27 Hispanic/Latino; 1 Native Hawaiian or other Pacific Islander, non-Hispanic/Latino; 18 Two or more races, non-Hispanic/Latino), 35 international. Average age 34. In 2013, 133 master's, 4 doctorates awarded. *Entrance requirements:* For master's and doctorate, GRE General Test. Additional exam requirements/recommendations for international students: Recommended—TOEFL (minimum score 80 iBT), IELTS (minimum score 6.5), TSE (minimum score 54). *Application deadline:* For fall admission, 1/15 for domestic and international students. Application fee: $50. Electronic applications accepted. *Expenses:* Tuition, state resident: full-time $12,634; part-time $526 per credit hour. Tuition, nonresident: full-time $27,892; part-time $1162 per credit hour. Part-time tuition and fees vary according to course load, campus/location and program. *Financial support:* Fellowships with full tuition reimbursements, research assistantships with full tuition reimbursements, teaching assistantships with full tuition reimbursements, Federal Work-Study, health care benefits, tuition waivers (full), and unspecified assistantships available. Financial award application deadline: 1/15; financial award applicants required to submit FAFSA. *Unit head:* Dr. Douglas Meikle, Chair, 513-529-3103, E-mail: meikled@miamioh.edu.
Website: http://miamioh.edu/cas/about/biology

Michigan State University, The Graduate School, College of Natural Science, Quantitative Biology Program, East Lansing, MI 48824. Offers PhD.

New York University, School of Medicine and Graduate School of Arts and Science, Sackler Institute of Graduate Biomedical Sciences, New York, NY 10012-1019. Offers biomedical imaging (PhD); biomedical informatics (PhD); cellular and molecular biology (PhD); computational biology (PhD); developmental genetics (PhD); immunology and inflammation (PhD); microbiology (PhD); molecular biophysics (PhD); molecular oncology and tumor immunology (PhD), including immunology, molecular oncology; molecular pharmacology (PhD); neuroscience and physiology (PhD); pathobiology (PhD); stem cell biology (PhD); MD/PhD. *Faculty:* 246 full-time (57 women). *Students:* 284 full-time (164 women); includes 85 minority (18 Black or African American, non-Hispanic/Latino; 1 American Indian or Alaska Native, non-Hispanic/Latino; 35 Asian, non-Hispanic/Latino; 31 Hispanic/Latino), 85 international. Average age 27. 950 applicants, 11% accepted, 32 enrolled. In 2013, 46 doctorates awarded. *Degree requirements:* For doctorate, comprehensive exam, thesis/dissertation, qualifying exam. *Entrance requirements:* For doctorate, GRE General Test. Additional exam requirements/recommendations for international students: Required—TOEFL. *Application deadline:* For fall admission, 12/1 priority date for domestic students. Applications are processed on a rolling basis. Application fee: $85. Electronic applications accepted. *Expenses:* Contact institution. *Financial support:* In 2013–14, fellowships with tuition reimbursements (averaging $33,600 per year), research assistantships with tuition reimbursements (averaging $33,600 per year), teaching assistantships with tuition reimbursements (averaging $33,600 per year) were awarded; career-related internships or fieldwork, Federal Work-Study, institutionally sponsored loans, scholarships/grants, health care benefits, tuition waivers (full), and unspecified assistantships also available. *Unit head:* Dr. Joel D. Oppenheim, Senior Associate Dean for Graduate Studies, 212-263-8001, Fax: 212-263-7600. *Application contact:* Michael Escosia, Admissions Associate, 212-263-5648, Fax: 212-263-7600, E-mail: sackler-info@med.nyu.edu.
Website: http://sackler.med.nyu.edu/

Northwestern University, The Graduate School, Interdisciplinary Biological Sciences Program (IBiS), Evanston, IL 60208. Offers biochemistry (PhD); bioengineering and biotechnology (PhD); biotechnology (PhD); cell and molecular biology (PhD); developmental and systems biology (PhD); nanotechnology (PhD); neurobiology (PhD); structural biology and biophysics (PhD). *Degree requirements:* For doctorate, thesis/dissertation, qualifying exam. *Entrance requirements:* For doctorate, GRE General Test. Additional exam requirements/recommendations for international students: Required—TOEFL (minimum score 600 paper-based). *Application deadline:* For fall admission, 12/15 for domestic and international students. Applications are processed on a rolling basis. Application fee: $95. Electronic applications accepted. *Financial support:* Fellowships, research assistantships, teaching assistantships, career-related internships or fieldwork, institutionally sponsored loans, scholarships/grants, traineeships, health care benefits, and unspecified assistantships available. Financial award application deadline: 12/31; financial award applicants required to submit FAFSA. *Faculty research:* Biophysics/structural biology, cell/molecular biology, synthetic biology, developmental systems biology, chemical biology/nanotechnology. *Unit head:* Dr. Deborah Klos Dehring, Associate Director, 847-467-0451, E-mail: d-klos@northwestern.edu. *Application contact:* Cathy Prullage, Program Manager, 847-491-4301, E-mail: ibis@northwestern.edu.
Website: http://www.biochem.northwestern.edu/ibis/

Stanford University, School of Medicine, Graduate Programs in Medicine, Department of Structural Biology, Stanford, CA 94305-9991. Offers PhD. *Degree requirements:* For doctorate, thesis/dissertation. *Entrance requirements:* For doctorate, GRE General Test, GRE Subject Test. Additional exam requirements/recommendations for international students: Required—TOEFL. Electronic applications accepted. *Expenses: Tuition:* Full-time $42,690; part-time $949 per credit. *Required fees:* $185.

Stony Brook University, State University of New York, Graduate School, College of Arts and Sciences, Department of Biochemistry and Cell Biology, Program in Biochemistry and Structural Biology, Stony Brook, NY 11794. Offers PhD. *Students:* 32 full-time (11 women); includes 4 minority (1 Asian, non-Hispanic/Latino; 2 Hispanic/Latino; 1 Native Hawaiian or other Pacific Islander, non-Hispanic/Latino), 14 international. Average age 27. 57 applicants, 30% accepted, 13 enrolled. In 2013, 7 doctorates awarded. *Entrance requirements:* For doctorate, GRE. Additional exam requirements/recommendations for international students: Required—TOEFL. *Application deadline:* For fall admission, 1/15 for domestic students; for spring admission, 10/1 for domestic students. Application fee: $100. *Expenses:* Tuition, state resident: full-time $9870; part-time $411 per credit. Tuition, nonresident: full-time $18,350; part-time $765 per credit. *Financial support:* In 2013–14, 4 fellowships, 25 research assistantships, 5 teaching assistantships were awarded. *Unit head:* Prof. Robert Haltiwanger, Chair, 631-632-7336, Fax: 631-632-9730, E-mail: robert.haltiwanger@stonybrook.edu. *Application contact:* Joann DeLucia-Conlon, 631-632-8613, Fax: 631-632-8575, E-mail: joann.delucia-conlon@stonybrook.edu.
Website: http://www.stonybrook.edu/commcms/biochem/education/graduate/overview.html

Syracuse University, College of Arts and Sciences, Program in Structural Biology, Biochemistry and Biophysics, Syracuse, NY 13244. Offers PhD. *Students:* 3 full-time (1 woman), 1 part-time (0 women), 1 international. Average age 33. 4 applicants, 25% accepted. In 2013, 2 doctorates awarded. *Degree requirements:* For doctorate, comprehensive exam, thesis/dissertation. *Entrance requirements:* For doctorate, GRE General Test, GRE Subject Test. Additional exam requirements/recommendations for international students: Required—TOEFL (minimum score 100 iBT). *Application deadline:* For fall admission, 12/15 priority date for domestic and international students. Application fee: $75. Electronic applications accepted. *Financial support:* Fellowships with full tuition reimbursements, research assistantships with full and partial tuition reimbursements, teaching assistantships with full and partial tuition reimbursements, and tuition waivers available. Financial award application deadline: 1/1; financial award applicants required to submit FAFSA. *Unit head:* Prof. Liviu Movileanu, Director of Graduate Studies, 315-443-8078, Fax: 315-443-2012, E-mail: lmovilea@syr.edu.
Website: http://sb3.syr.edu/

Thomas Jefferson University, Jefferson Graduate School of Biomedical Sciences, PhD Program in Molecular Pharmacology and Structural Biology, Philadelphia, PA 19107. Offers PhD. *Faculty:* 39 full-time (8 women). *Students:* 18 full-time (9 women); includes 5 minority (all Asian, non-Hispanic/Latino), 5 international. 34 applicants, 18% accepted, 3 enrolled. In 2013, 1 doctorate awarded. *Degree requirements:* For doctorate, comprehensive exam, thesis/dissertation. *Entrance requirements:* For doctorate, GRE General Test, minimum GPA of 3.2. Additional exam requirements/recommendations for international students: Required—TOEFL (minimum score 100 iBT) or IELTS. *Application deadline:* For fall admission, 1/2 priority date for domestic and international students. Applications are processed on a rolling basis. Application fee: $50. Electronic applications accepted. *Financial support:* In 2013–14, 18 students received support, including 18 fellowships with full tuition reimbursements available (averaging $54,758 per year); Federal Work-Study, institutionally sponsored loans, scholarships/grants, traineeships, and stipends also available. Support available to part-time students. Financial award application deadline: 5/1; financial award applicants required to submit FAFSA. *Faculty research:* Biochemistry and cell, molecular and structural biology of cell-surface and intracellular receptors; molecular modeling; signal transduction. *Total annual research expenditures:* $22.7 million. *Unit head:* Dr. Philip Wedegaertner, Program Director, 215-503-3137, Fax: 215-923-2117, E-mail: philip.wedegaertner@mail.tju.edu. *Application contact:* Marc E. Stearns, Director of Admissions, 215-503-0155, Fax: 215-503-9920, E-mail: jcgs-info@jefferson.edu.

Tulane University, School of Medicine and School of Liberal Arts, Graduate Programs in Biomedical Sciences, Department of Structural and Cellular Biology, New Orleans, LA 70118-5669. Offers MS, PhD, MD/PhD. MS and PhD offered through the Graduate School. *Degree requirements:* For master's, one foreign language, thesis; for doctorate, 2 foreign languages, thesis/dissertation. *Entrance requirements:* For master's, GRE General Test, minimum B average in undergraduate course work; for doctorate, GRE General Test. Additional exam requirements/recommendations for international students: Required—TOEFL. Electronic applications accepted. *Faculty research:* Reproductive endocrinology, visual neuroscience, neural response to altered hormones.

University at Albany, State University of New York, School of Public Health, Department of Biomedical Sciences, Program in Cell and Molecular Structure, Albany, NY 12222-0001. Offers MS, PhD. *Degree requirements:* For master's, thesis; for doctorate, thesis/dissertation. *Entrance requirements:* For master's and doctorate, GRE General Test, GRE Subject Test.

University at Buffalo, the State University of New York, Graduate School, School of Medicine and Biomedical Sciences, Graduate Programs in Medicine and Biomedical Sciences, Department of Structural Biology, Buffalo, NY 14263. Offers MS, PhD. *Faculty:* 6 part-time/adjunct (1 woman). *Students:* 6 full-time (0 women). Average age

26. 2 applicants, 100% accepted. In 2013, 4 doctorates awarded. *Degree requirements:* For master's, comprehensive exam, thesis; for doctorate, comprehensive exam, thesis/dissertation. *Entrance requirements:* For master's, BS or BA in science, engineering, or math; for doctorate, GRE General Test, BS or BA in science, engineering, or math. Additional exam requirements/recommendations for international students: Required—TOEFL (minimum score 600 paper-based; 100 iBT). *Application deadline:* For fall admission, 2/1 priority date for domestic and international students. Applications are processed on a rolling basis. Application fee: $50. Electronic applications accepted. *Financial support:* In 2013–14, 8 research assistantships (averaging $24,000 per year) were awarded; Federal Work-Study, scholarships/grants, traineeships, and unspecified assistantships also available. Financial award application deadline: 2/1; financial award applicants required to submit FAFSA. *Faculty research:* Biomacromolecular structure and function at the level of three-dimensional atomic architecture. *Total annual research expenditures:* $3.8 million. *Unit head:* Dr. Robert H. Blessing, Interim Chair/Professor, 716-898-8613, Fax: 716-898-8660, E-mail: blessing@hwi.buffalo.edu. *Application contact:* Elizabeth A. White, Administrative Director, 716-829-3399, Fax: 716-829-2437, E-mail: bethw@buffalo.edu.
Website: http://www.hwi.buffalo.edu/graduate_studies/graduate_studies.html

University of Connecticut, Graduate School, College of Liberal Arts and Sciences, Department of Molecular and Cell Biology, Field of Biophysics and Structural Biology, Storrs, CT 06269. Offers MS, PhD. Terminal master's awarded for partial completion of doctoral program. *Degree requirements:* For master's, comprehensive exam; for doctorate, thesis/dissertation. *Entrance requirements:* For master's and doctorate, GRE General Test, GRE Subject Test. Additional exam requirements/recommendations for international students: Required—TOEFL (minimum score 550 paper-based). Electronic applications accepted.

The University of Manchester, Faculty of Life Sciences, Manchester, United Kingdom. Offers adaptive organismal biology (M Phil, PhD); animal biology (M Phil, PhD); biochemistry (M Phil, PhD); bioinformatics (M Phil, PhD); biomolecular sciences (M Phil, PhD); biotechnology (M Phil, PhD); cell biology (M Phil, PhD); cell matrix research (M Phil, PhD); channels and transporters (M Phil, PhD); developmental biology (M Phil, PhD); Egyptology (M Phil, PhD); environmental biology (M Phil, PhD); evolutionary biology (M Phil, PhD); gene expression (M Phil, PhD); genetics (M Phil, PhD); history of science, technology and medicine (M Phil, PhD); immunology (M Phil, PhD); integrative neurobiology and behavior (M Phil, PhD); membrane trafficking (M Phil, PhD); microbiology (M Phil, PhD); molecular and cellular neuroscience (M Phil, PhD); molecular biology (M Phil, PhD); molecular cancer studies (M Phil, PhD); neuroscience (M Phil, PhD); ophthalmology (M Phil, PhD); optometry (M Phil, PhD); organelle function (M Phil, PhD); pharmacology (M Phil, PhD); physiology (M Phil, PhD); plant sciences (M Phil, PhD); stem cell research (M Phil, PhD); structural biology (M Phil, PhD); systems neuroscience (M Phil, PhD); toxicology (M Phil, PhD).

University of Minnesota, Twin Cities Campus, Graduate School, College of Biological Sciences, Biochemistry, Molecular Biology and Biophysics Graduate Program, Minneapolis, MN 55455-0213. Offers PhD. *Degree requirements:* For doctorate, thesis/dissertation. *Entrance requirements:* For doctorate, GRE, 3 letters of recommendation, more than 1 semester of laboratory experience. Additional exam requirements/recommendations for international students: Required—TOEFL (minimum score 625 paper-based; 108 iBT with writing subsection 25 and reading subsection 25) or IELTS (minimum score 7). Electronic applications accepted. *Faculty research:* Microbial biochemistry, biotechnology, molecular biology, regulatory biochemistry, structural biology and biophysics, physical biochemistry, enzymology, physiological chemistry.

University of Pittsburgh, School of Medicine and Dietrich School of Arts and Sciences, Molecular Biophysics and Structural Biology Graduate Program, Pittsburgh, PA 15260. Offers PhD. PhD jointly offered by the University of Pittsburgh and Carnegie Mellon University. *Faculty:* 52 full-time (15 women). *Students:* 22 full-time (10 women); includes 3 minority (1 Asian, non-Hispanic/Latino; 1 Hispanic/Latino; 1 Native Hawaiian or other Pacific Islander, non-Hispanic/Latino), 5 international. Average age 25. 85 applicants, 8% accepted, 5 enrolled. In 2013, 2 doctorates awarded. *Degree requirements:* For doctorate, comprehensive exam, thesis/dissertation. *Entrance requirements:* For doctorate, GRE General Test. Additional exam requirements/recommendations for international students: Required—TOEFL (minimum score 600 paper-based; 100 iBT), IELTS (minimum score 7). *Application deadline:* For fall admission, 1/15 priority date for domestic and international students. Application fee: $0. Electronic applications accepted. *Expenses:* Tuition, state resident: full-time $19,964; part-time $807 per credit. Tuition, nonresident: full-time $32,686; part-time $1337 per credit. *Required fees:* $740; $200. Tuition and fees vary according to program. *Financial support:* In 2013–14, 2 fellowships with full tuition reimbursements (averaging $25,575 per year), 20 research assistantships with full tuition reimbursements (averaging $26,010 per year) were awarded; institutionally sponsored loans, scholarships/grants, traineeships, and unspecified assistantships also available. *Faculty research:* Structural biology, protein dynamics and folding, computational biophysics, molecular informatics, membrane biophysics and ion channels, x-ray crystallography cryaelectron microscopy. *Unit head:* Dr. James Conway, Director, 412-648-8957, Fax: 412-648-1077, E-mail: mbsbinfo@medschool.pitt.edu. *Application contact:* Susanna T. Godwin, Program Coordinator, 412-648-8957, Fax: 412-648-1077, E-mail: mbsbinfo@medschool.pitt.edu.
Website: http://www.mbsb.pitt.edu

University of Rochester, School of Medicine and Dentistry, Graduate Programs in Medicine and Dentistry, Department of Biochemistry and Biophysics, Programs in Biophysics, Rochester, NY 14627. Offers biophysics, structural and computational biology (PhD). Terminal master's awarded for partial completion of doctoral program. *Degree requirements:* For doctorate, thesis/dissertation, qualifying exam. *Entrance requirements:* For doctorate, GRE General Test. *Expenses: Tuition:* Full-time $44,580; part-time $1394 per credit hour. *Required fees:* $492.

The University of Texas Health Science Center at San Antonio, Graduate School of Biomedical Sciences, Department of Cellular and Structural Biology, San Antonio, TX 78229-3900. Offers MS, PhD. *Faculty:* 51 full-time (24 women), 11 part-time/adjunct (5 women). *Students:* 56 full-time (39 women), 10 part-time (7 women); includes 24 minority (3 Black or African American, non-Hispanic/Latino; 12 Asian, non-Hispanic/Latino; 9 Hispanic/Latino), 20 international. Average age 28. In 2013, 4 master's, 10 doctorates awarded. *Degree requirements:* For master's, thesis; for doctorate, comprehensive exam, thesis/dissertation. *Entrance requirements:* For master's, GRE (minimum cumulative Verbal plus Quantitative score of 1000), minimum undergraduate GPA of 3.0; for doctorate, GRE General Test, previous course work in biology, chemistry, physics, and calculus. Additional exam requirements/recommendations for international students: Required—TOEFL (minimum score 550 paper-based; 68 iBT). *Application deadline:* For fall admission, 3/1 priority date for domestic and international students. Applications are processed on a rolling basis. Application fee: $0. Electronic applications accepted. *Financial support:* In 2013–14, 7 students received support. Federal Work-Study and scholarships/grants available. Financial award application deadline: 6/30; financial award applicants required to submit FAFSA. *Faculty research:* Human/molecular genetics, endocrinology and neurobiology, cell biology, stem cell biology, cancer biology, biology of aging. *Total annual research expenditures:* $7.5 million. *Unit head:* Dr. Christi A. Walter, Department Chair, 210-567-3800, Fax: 210-567-0073, E-mail: walter@uthscsa.edu. *Application contact:* Dr. Babatunde Oyajobi, Committee on Graduate Studies Chair, 210-567-0909, Fax: 210-567-0073, E-mail: oyajobi@uthscsa.edu.
Website: http://www.uthscsa.edu/csb/

The University of Texas Medical Branch, Graduate School of Biomedical Sciences, Program in Biochemistry and Molecular Biology, Galveston, TX 77555. Offers biochemistry (PhD); bioinformatics (PhD); biophysics (PhD); cell biology (PhD); computational biology (PhD); structural biology (PhD). *Degree requirements:* For doctorate, thesis/dissertation. *Entrance requirements:* Additional exam requirements/recommendations for international students: Required—TOEFL (minimum score 550 paper-based). Electronic applications accepted.

University of Washington, Graduate School, School of Medicine, Graduate Programs in Medicine, Department of Biological Structure, Seattle, WA 98195. Offers PhD. *Degree requirements:* For doctorate, thesis/dissertation. *Faculty research:* Cellular and developmental biology, experimental immunology and hematology, molecular structure and molecular biology, neurobiology, x-rays.

Weill Cornell Medical College, Weill Cornell Graduate School of Medical Sciences, Biochemistry, Cell and Molecular Biology Allied Program, New York, NY 10065. Offers MS, PhD. Terminal master's awarded for partial completion of doctoral program. *Degree requirements:* For master's, comprehensive exam; for doctorate, thesis/dissertation, final exam. *Entrance requirements:* For doctorate, GRE General Test, background in genetics, molecular biology, chemistry, or biochemistry. Additional exam requirements/recommendations for international students: Required—TOEFL. Electronic applications accepted. *Faculty research:* Molecular structure determination, protein structure, gene structure, stem cell biology, control of gene expression, DNA replication, chromosome maintenance, RNA biosynthesis.

GERSTNER SLOAN KETTERING GRADUATE SCHOOL OF BIOMEDICAL SCIENCES

Ph.D. in Cancer Biology Program

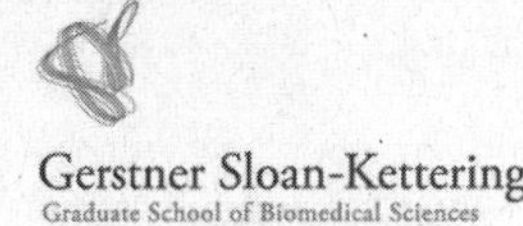

Program of Study

The Louis V. Gerstner, Jr. Graduate School of Biomedical Sciences, Memorial Sloan Kettering Cancer Center offers a doctoral program that trains laboratory scientists to work in research areas directly applicable to human disease and in particular, cancer.

Much of the recent explosion in new knowledge about normal biological functions and disease is rooted in laboratory discoveries. The unique curriculum integrates Memorial Sloan Kettering's basic science and clinical arms to maximize the potential of future basic scientists to improve human health.

During the first year, students complete a thirty-two-week core course (sixteen weeks per semester) that introduces recent findings in relevant topics through didactic lecture and discussion of research papers. Students will also complete three 5-week laboratory rotations, with each one culminating in an oral presentation of their findings; three visits with clinicians; course work in logic and critical analysis; and two semesters of the President's Research Seminar Series Journal Club, which introduces students to the published works of world-renowned speakers.

After completing the didactic portion of their education in the first year, students focus full time on thesis research at the beginning of the second year. Students are expected to present a written and oral thesis proposal by March 31 of the second year. Continuing throughout their graduate careers, students take part in the Current Topics Journal Club, along with the Graduate Student Seminar, in which students present their own research.

Students also have the opportunity to select a clinical mentor who directs the student in participating in hospital-based academic activities such as grand rounds and conferences with pathology and disease management teams.

Research Facilities

Memorial Sloan Kettering's research space totals approximately 575,000 square feet, with many cutting-edge laboratories and facilities housed within the Rockefeller Research Laboratories building and the Zuckerman Research Center, a building with open, spacious floors designed to encourage collaboration.

There are dozens of research core facilities—ranging from bioinformatics to high-throughput drug screening and x-ray crystallography—that serve both basic and clinical research needs, offering state-of-the-art instruments and technical staff support to graduate students as they train and conduct research projects. Core facilities are staffed by research experts in the technologies offered, and training is available in select cores.

The Memorial Sloan Kettering Cancer Center library subscribes to a full range of science, medical, and healthcare resources. Students have access to more than 2,800 journals, with the majority of these titles available electronically. The library's website provides access to an extensive collection of resources, including an online catalog, databases, electronic books, and electronic journals.

Financial Aid

All matriculated students receive a fellowship package that includes an annual stipend ($35,375 for 2014–15); a first-year allowance to be used for books, journals, and other school expenses; a scholarship that covers the full cost of tuition and fees; comprehensive medical and dental insurance; a laptop computer; relocation costs (up to $500); and membership in the New York Academy of Sciences.

Students may also apply for independent funding from agencies such as the National Institutes of Health and the National Science Foundation. Recipients of one of these fellowships receive an additional award of $5,000 from the school; this is in addition to any supplement necessary to bring the stipend to the common level. Travel awards are given to students who present a poster or a short talk at a scientific meeting.

Cost of Study

All tuition expenses are covered by a full fellowship, which is awarded to all students who matriculate in the school. Students are also provided with health insurance at no cost to them. Additional details are available in the Financial Aid section above.

Living and Housing Costs

Affordable housing in proximity to the research buildings is provided to all students by Memorial Sloan Kettering. Housing units are located in safe, family-oriented neighborhoods on or near Manhattan's Upper East Side. Students who have spouses or significant others can apply for family units. There is a wide range of costs, which vary depending on the size of the housing unit. The housing contract runs for the student's duration of study and is automatically renewed each year.

Student Group

Currently there are 60 full-time students (26 women, 34 men), with 16 percent minority and 35 percent international. The graduate students enrolled at Gerstner Sloan Kettering are drawn from a pool of applicants who comprise a variety of backgrounds and nationalities. Applicants are expected to hold an undergraduate degree from an accredited institution and have significant basic science research experience. College-level coursework in the following areas is required: biology, chemistry, physics, organic chemistry, mathematics, and biochemistry.

Student Outcomes

Graduates of the program are expected to enter into careers as researchers, scientists, and educators in excellent laboratories, hospitals, medical schools, and research institutions throughout the country and around the world.

Gerstner Sloan Kettering Graduate School of Biomedical Sciences

Location

The campus is located on Manhattan's Upper East Side, home to some of New York City's best shopping and dining. Several world-famous museums are within walking distance, and Central Park is a few blocks away. New York also offers theater, live music, outdoor recreation, and cultural attractions such as the Metropolitan Museum of Art, all accessible by public transportation.

The Graduate School

The Louis V. Gerstner, Jr. Graduate School of Biomedical Sciences, Memorial Sloan Kettering Cancer Center, offers the next generation of basic scientists an intensive Ph.D. program to study the biological sciences through the lens of cancer—while giving students the tools they need to put them in the vanguard of research that can be applied in any area of human disease. Students are part of a community of outstanding scientists who have extensive experience in postgraduate education and maintain a strong commitment to training and mentoring the next generation of leaders in biomedical research.

The Gerstner Sloan Kettering Graduate School of Biomedical Sciences is accredited by the New York State Board of Regents and the Commissioner of Education, located at 89 Washington Avenue, Albany, New York 12234; phone: 518-474-3852.

Applying

Prospective students must complete and submit the online application form and submit the following: official transcripts from all colleges previously attended, three letters of recommendation from advisers and/or research mentors, and official GRE scores. Official scores for the Test of English as a Foreign Language (TOEFL) exams are required for applicants who do not speak English as their first language (can be waived for those who earned their undergraduate degrees in the United States). An in-person interview is requested from those applicants being seriously considered for admission, but the requirement may be waived if geographical constraints are overwhelming and may be substituted with video interviews. The deadline to apply is December 1, and interviews take place the following January.

Correspondence and Information

Gerstner Sloan Kettering Graduate School of Biomedical Sciences
1275 York Avenue, Box 441
New York, New York 10065
Phone: 646-888-6639
Fax: 646-422-2351
E-mail: gradstudies@sloankettering.edu
Website: http://www.sloankettering.edu

THE FACULTY AND THEIR RESEARCH

Information regarding the faculty members is available online at: http://www.sloankettering.edu/research/faculty.

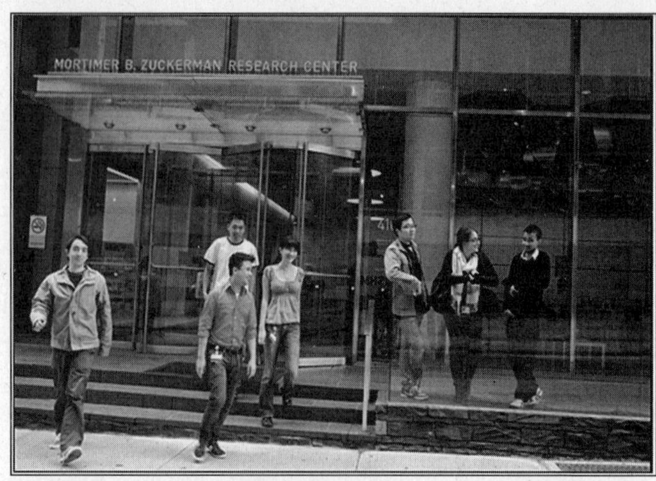

The school is located on Manhattan's Upper East Side, in the heart of a thriving biomedical research community.

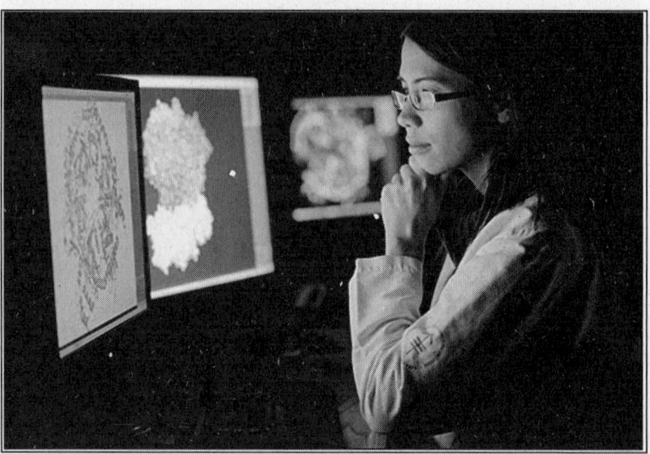

The Louis V. Gerstner, Jr. Graduate School of Biomedical Sciences, Memorial Sloan Kettering Cancer Center offers a doctoral program that trains laboratory scientists to work in research areas directly applicable to human disease, and in particular, cancer.

UNIFORMED SERVICES UNIVERSITY OF THE HEALTH SCIENCES

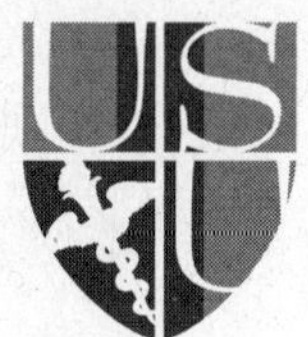

F. Edward Hébert School of Medicine Graduate Program in Molecular and Cell Biology

Program of Study

The program of study is designed for full-time students who wish to obtain a Ph.D. degree in the area of molecular and cell biology. This interdepartmental graduate program, which includes faculty members from both basic and clinical departments, offers research expertise in a wide range of areas, including bacteriology, immunology, genetics, biochemistry, regulation of gene expression, and cancer biology. The program includes core courses in molecular and cell biology that provide necessary knowledge for modern biomedical research, as well as advanced electives in areas of faculty expertise. The first-year curriculum includes courses in biochemistry, cell biology, experimental methodology, genetics, and immunology. During the first summer, students participate in laboratory rotations in two laboratories of their choice, leading to the choice of a mentor for their doctoral research. The second-year curriculum offers advanced elective courses in a variety of disciplines, including biochemistry, cell biology, immunology, molecular endocrinology, and virology, and marks the transition from classwork to original laboratory research. Throughout their graduate experience, students participate in journal clubs designed to foster interaction across disciplines and to develop the critical skills needed for data presentation and analysis. A year-round seminar series brings renowned scientists to the Uniformed Services University of the Health Sciences (USUHS) to share their results and to meet with students and faculty members. Students may also take advantage of seminars hosted by other programs and departments as well as those presented at the National Institutes of Health. Completion of the research project and preparation and successful defense of a written dissertation leads to the degree of Doctor of Philosophy.

Research Facilities

The University possesses outstanding facilities for research in molecular and cell biology. Well-equipped laboratories and extramurally funded faculty members provide an outstanding environment in which to pursue state-of-the-art research. Shared equipment in a modern biomedical instrumentation core facility includes oligonucleotide and peptide synthesizers and sequencers; a variety of imaging equipment, including laser confocal and electron microscopes; fluorescent-activated cell sorters; and an ACAS workstation. A recently added proteomics facility contains both MADLI-TOF and ESI tandem mass spectrometers. All offices, laboratories, and the Learning Resource Center are equipped with high-speed Internet connectivity and have access to an extensive online journal collection.

Financial Aid

Stipends are available for civilian applicants. Awards of stipends are competitive and may be renewed. For the 2014–15 academic year, stipends for entering students begin at $27,000. Outstanding students may be nominated for the Dean's Special Fellowship, which supports a stipend of $32,000.

Cost of Study

Graduate students are not required to pay tuition. Civilian graduate students do not incur any obligation to the United States government for service after completion of their graduate training programs. Active-duty military personnel incur an obligation for additional military service by Department of Defense regulations that govern sponsored graduate education. Students are required to maintain health insurance.

Living and Housing Costs

The University does not have housing for graduate students. However, there is an abundant supply of rental housing in the area. Living costs in the greater Washington, D.C., area are comparable to those of other East Coast metropolitan areas.

Student Group

The first graduate students in the interdisciplinary Graduate Program in Molecular and Cell Biology at USUHS were admitted in 1995. Over the last decade, the Graduate Program in Molecular and Cell Biology has grown significantly; 25 students are currently enrolled. Thirty-six Ph.D. degrees in molecular and cell biology have been awarded over the past fourteen years.

Location

Metropolitan Washington has a population of about 5 million residents in the District of Columbia and the surrounding areas of Maryland and Virginia. The region is a center of education and research and is home to five major universities, four medical schools, the National Library of Medicine and the National Institutes of Health (next to the USUHS campus), Walter Reed National Military Medical Center, the Armed Forces Institute of Pathology, the Library of Congress, the Smithsonian Institution, the National Bureau of Standards, and many other private and government research centers. Many cultural advantages of the area include the theater, a major symphony orchestra, major-league sports, and world-famous museums. The Metro subway system has a station near campus and provides a convenient connection from the University to museums and cultural attractions of downtown Washington. The University is within easy distance of three major airports: Baltimore Washington International, Reagan International, and Dulles International. Both Reagan and Dulles International airports are accessible from the University via metro subway. For outdoor activities, the Blue Ridge Mountains, the Chesapeake Bay, and the Atlantic coast beaches are all within a few hours' drive.

The University

USUHS is located just outside Washington, D.C., in Bethesda, Maryland. The campus is situated on an attractive, wooded site at the Walter Reed National Military Medical Center and is close to several major federal health research facilities. Through various affiliation agreements, these institutes provide additional resources to enhance the educational experience of graduate students at USUHS.

Applying

Both civilians and military personnel are eligible to apply for graduate study at USUHS. Before matriculation, each applicant must complete a baccalaureate degree that includes college-level courses in biology, inorganic chemistry, mathematics, organic chemistry, and physics. Advanced courses in biology, chemistry, or related fields, such as biochemistry, cell biology, genetics, immunology, microbiology, molecular biology, and physical chemistry, are desirable but not essential. Each applicant must submit a USUHS graduate training application form, complete academic transcripts of postsecondary education, GRE scores (in addition to the aptitude sections, one advanced examination is recommended), three letters of recommendation from individuals familiar with the academic achievements or research experience of the applicant, and a personal statement expressing the applicant's career objectives. Active-duty military personnel must obtain the approval and sponsorship of their parent military department in addition to acceptance from USUHS. USUHS subscribes fully to the policy of equal educational opportunity and selects students on a competitive basis without regard to race, sex, creed, or national origin. Application forms may be obtained from the website at http://www.usuhs.mil/mcb/gradapp.html#applynow. Completed applications must be received before December 1 for matriculation in August. Applications received between December 2 and June 1 may be considered if space is available.

Correspondence and Information

Associate Dean for Graduate Education
Uniformed Services University of the Health Sciences
4301 Jones Bridge Road
Bethesda, Maryland 20814
United States
Phone: 301-295-3913
800-772-1747 (toll-free)
E-mail: graduateprogram@usuhs.edu
Website: http://www.usuhs.mil/graded/

For an application and information about the molecular and cell biology program:

Dr. Mary Lou Cutler, Director
Graduate Program in Molecular and Cell Biology
Uniformed Services University of the Health Sciences
4301 Jones Bridge Road
Bethesda, Maryland 20814
United States
Phone: 301-295-3642
Fax: 301-295-1996
E-mail: netina.finley@usuhs.edu
Website: http://www.usuhs.mil/mcb/

THE FACULTY AND THEIR RESEARCH

Regina C. Armstrong, Professor; Ph.D., North Carolina at Chapel Hill, 1987. Cellular and molecular mechanisms of neural stem/progenitor cell development and regeneration in demyelinating diseases and brain injury models.

Roopa Biswas, Assistant Professor, Ph.D. Ohio State, 1997. Mechanisms of regulation of inflammation; http://www.usuhs.edu/facuty/roopabisws-apg.html.

Uniformed Services University of the Health Sciences

Jorge Blanco, Adjunct Assistant Professor; Ph.D., Buenos Aires, 1991. Receptor characterization and susceptibility of cotton rats to avian and 2009 pandemic influenza strains. *J. Virol.* 87(4):2036–45, 2013.
Christopher C. Broder, Professor and Director; Ph.D., Florida, 1989. Virus-host cell interactions; vaccines and therapeutics; HIV, Hendra and Nipah viruses, Australian bat lyssavirus.
Teodor Brumeanu, Professor; M.D., Carol Davila (Romania), 1978. Medicine.
Rolf Bünger, Professor; M.D./Ph.D., Munich, 1979. Cellular, molecular, and metabolic mechanisms of heart and brain circulation and resuscitation at various levels of organization: intact animal/isolated perfused organs/subcellular compartments of cytosol and mitochondria. *NMR Biomed.*, doi: 10.1002/nbm.1717; *Exp. Biol. Med. 234(12):1395–416, 2009; in Recent Research Developments in Physiology, Vol. 4, ed. S. G. Pandalai, 2006; Exerc. Sport Sci. Rev.* 32(4):174–9, 2004.
Barrington G. Burnett, Assistant Professor; Ph.D., Pennsylvania, 2005. The ubiquitin-proteasome system in neuronal maintenance and neurodegeneration.
Thomas P. Conrads, Ph.D., Ohio State, 1999. Discovery and validation of genomic, proteomic, and small molecule biomarkers and surrogates for enhanced cancer patient management through improved early detection, patient stratification, and monitoring for therapeutic efficacy, outcome, and recurrence.
Rachel Cox, Assistant Professor, Ph.D., North Carolina at Chapel Hill, 1998. Mitochondrial dynamics and inheritance during development. *Disease Models & Mechanisms* 2(9/10):490–9, 2009.
Mary Lou Cutler, Professor and Director; Ph.D., Hahnemann, 1980. Role of molecules that suppress transformation by the Ras oncogene; Ras signal transduction and human carcinogenesis. *Eur. J. Cell Biol.* 87:721–34, 2008; *J. Cell. Physiol.* 214:38–46, 2007; *BMC Cell Biol.* 7:34, 2006; *Exp. Cell Res.* 306:168–79, 2005.
Clifton Dalgard, Assistant Professor; Ph.D., Uniformed Services University of the Health Sciences, 2005. *Front. Mol. Neurosci.* 5:6, 2012.
Michael Daly, Professor; Ph.D., London, 1988. Pathology.
Thomas N. Darling, Professor; M.D./Ph.D., Duke, 1990. *Nat. Genet.* 44:928–33, 2012; *New Engl. J. Med.* 365:611–9, 2011; *Ann. Intern. Med.* 154:806–13, 2011; *Nat. Commun.* 2:235, 2012.
Stephen Davies, Assistant Professor; Ph.D., Cornell. Microbiology.
Regina Day, Associate Professor; Ph.D., Tufts, 1995. Mechanisms of normal tissue repair and mechanisms of fibrotic remodeling, especially radiation. *Mol. Biol. Cell* 21:4240–50, 2010; *Mol. Biol. Cell* 24:2088–07, 2013; *Mol. Pharmacol.* 85: 898–908, 2014.
Saibal Dey, Associate Professor; Ph.D., Wayne State (Michigan), 1995. Allosteric modulation of the human multidrug transporter P-glycoprotein (MDR1 or ABCB1), which confers multidrug resistance in cancer cells and alters bioavailability of many anticancer and antimicrobial agents. *J. Biol. Chem.* 281(16):10699–777, 2006; *Biochemistry* 45:2739–51, 2006; *J. Biol. Chem.* 278(20):18132–9, 2003.
Martin Doughty, Associate Professor, Department of Anatomy, Physiology, and Genetics; Ph.D. Optimizing induced pluripotent stem cells (iPSCs) for cell replacement therapy to treat traumatic brain injury (TBI); identifying transcriptional programs that function in cerebellar neurogenesis and pattern formation.
Yang Du, Assistant Professor; Ph.D., Texas Tech, 2000. Leukemia development mechanisms. *Blood* 119:6099–108, 2012.
Teresa M. Dunn, Professor; Ph.D., Brandeis, 1984. Sphingolipid synthesis and function. *J. Biol. Chem.* 277:11481–8, 2002 and 277:10194–200, 2002; *Mol. Cell Biol.* 21:109–25, 2001; *Methods Enzymol.* 312:317–30, 2000.
Gabriela S. Dveksler, Professor; Ph.D., Uniformed Services University of the Health Sciences, 1991. *J. Biol. Chem.* 286(9):7577–86, 2011; *Biol. Reprod.* 83(1):27–35, 2010.
Ying-Hong Feng, Associate Professor; Ph.D., Oxford, 1993. Pharmacology.
Thomas P. Flagg, Ph.D., Assistant Professor, Maryland, Baltimore, 2001. Cardiac ATP-sensitive potassium channel structure and function.
Zygmund Galdzicki, Assistant Professor, Ph.D., Wroclaw (Poland), 1982. Molecular and electrophysiological approach to understanding mental retardation in trisomy 21/Down syndrome.
Chou Zen Giam, Professor; Ph.D., UConn Health Center, 1983. Human T-lymphotropic viruses and Kaposi's sarcoma herpes virus; cellular senescence; cell-cycle control, I-kappa B kinases, protein ubiquitylation, cell transformation; viral oncogenesis; HTLV-1 pathogenesis; HTLV-1 latency and reactivation; transcriptional regulation. *PLoS Pathogens* 10:e1004040, 2014; *J. Virol.* 88:3496–504, 2014; *Oncogene* doi: 10.1038/onc.2013.567, 2014; *PLoS Pathogens* 7:e1002025, 2011
David A. Grahame, Professor; Ph.D., Ohio State, 1984. Metalloenzyme structure and function in bacteria and archaea. *Biochemistry* 52:1705–16, 2013; *J. Biol. Chem.* 285(20):15450–63, 2010.
Philip M. Grimley, Professor; M.D., Albany Medical College, 1961. Population studies relevant to the pathogenesis and molecular biology of ovarian and mammary epithelial cancers.
Jeffrey M. Harmon, Professor and Chair of Pharmacology; Ph.D., Rochester, 1976. Mechanism(s) that regulate sphingolipid biosynthesis and analysis of mutations in the enzyme catalyzing the rate-limiting step that result in human disease. *J. Biol. Chem.* 288(14):10144–53, 2013.
David Horowitz, Associate Professor; Ph.D., Harvard, 1986. Biochemistry of pre-mRNA splicing.
Ann E. Jerse, Associate Professor; Ph.D., Maryland, Baltimore, 1991. Estradiol-treated female mice as surrogate hosts for *Neisseria gonorrhoeae* genital-tract infections. *Front. Microbio.* 2:107, 2011, doi: 10.3389/fmicb.2011.00107.
Sharon L. Juliano, Professor; Ph.D., Pennsylvania, 1982. Mechanisms of development and plasticity in the cerebral cortex, with particular emphasis on the migration of neurons into the cortical plate; factors maintaining the function and morphology of radial glia and Cajal-Retzius cells.
Jason Lees, Assistant Professor; Ph.D., Iowa, 2004. T cell trafficking and lesion development in neuroinflammation.
Radha K. Maheshwari, Professor; Ph.D., Kanpur (India), 1974. Alphaviruses as biothreat agents: Novel approaches for the development of diagnostic biomarkers, antivirals, and vaccines; microRNA as biomarkers and therapeutic targets for traumatic brain injury and PTSD. *Vaccine* 29:953–9, 2011; *Cell Host and Microbe* 12:117–24, 2012; *J. Neurotrauma* 29:1379–87, 2012; *Antivir. Res.* 100:429–34, 2013; *J. Psychiatr. Res.* June 21, 2014.
Joseph Mattapallil, Associate Professor; Ph.D., California, Davis, 1997. Molecular and cellular mechanisms of viral pathogenesis using nonhuman primate models. *Curr. HIV Res.* 2014; *Plos One* 9(5):e98060; *J. Virol.* 87(12):7093–101, 2013; *PLos One* 8(3):e59758, 2013; *Clin. Dev. Immunol.* 2013:852418, 2013; *J. Virol.* 86(2):1069–78, 2012; *AIDS Res. Hum. Retroviruses* 27(7):763–75, 2011; *Mucosal Immunol.* 2(5): 439–49, 2009; *J. Immunol.* 182(3):1439–48, 2009; *J. Virol.* 82(22):11467–71, 2008; *Nature* 434(7037):1093–7, 2005.
Anthony T. Maurelli, Professor; Ph.D., Alabama at Birmingham, 1983. Molecular genetics of bacterial pathogens; molecular biology and pathogenesis of the intracellular pathogens *Shigella* and *Chlamydia*. *Nature* 506:507–10, 2014; *BMC Genom.* 11:272, 2010; *mBio* 2:e00051–11, 2011.
Ernest Maynard, Assistant Professor; Ph.D., Texas A&M, 2001. Zinc binding to the HCCH motif of HIV-1 virion infectivity factor induces a conformational change that mediates protein-protein interactions. *Proc. Natl. Acad. Sci. U.S.A.* 103:18475–80, 2006.
Joseph T. McCabe, Professor and Vice Chair; Ph.D., CUNY Graduate Center, 1983. Diazoxide, as a postconditioning and delayed preconditioner trigger, increases HSP25 and HSP70 in the central nervous system following combined cerebral stroke and hemorrhagic shock. *J. Neurotrauma* 24(3):532–46. 2007.
D. Scott Merrell, Associate Professor; Ph.D., Tufts, 2001. *H. pylori*, gene regulation; gastric cancer and the role of the microbiome in health and disease; http://www.usuhs.edu/faculty/douglasmerrell-mic.html. *Infect. Immun.* 78(7):3073–82, 2010.
Eleanor S. Metcalf, Professor; Ph.D., Pennsylvania, 1976. *J. Immun.*, in press; *Infect. Immun.* 80:441–9, 2012.
Alexandra C. Miller, Assistant Professor; Ph.D., SUNY, 1986. Low dose radiation and heavy metal exposure induced late effects: mechanisms and prevention. Development of models to study radiation late effects. *Rev. Environ. Health* 29(3):25–34, 2013.
Edward Mitre, Assistant Professor; M.D., Johns Hopkins, 1995. Immune modulation by parasitic helminthes; www.usuhs.mil/mic/mitre.html.
Alison D. O'Brien, Professor and Chair; Ph.D., Ohio State, 1976. The role of *E. coli* shiga toxins in the pathogenesis of hemorrhagic colitis and the hemolytic uremic syndrome; the role of toxins in the pathogenesis of *E. coli*–mediated urinary-tract infections; development of vaccines and therapeutics against *Bacillus anthracis*. *Proc. Natl. Acad. Sci. USA* 110(23):E2126–33, 2013.
Galina Petukhova, Associate Professor, Ph.D., Shemyakin & Ovchinnikov Institute of Bioorganic Chemistry, Moscow, 1994. Molecular mechanisms of genetic recombination in mammals. *Nature* 472:375–78, 2011.
Harvey Pollard, Professor and Chair; Ph.D., 1969, M.D., 1973, Chicago. Differential regulation of inflammation by inflammatory mediators in cystic fibrosis lung epithelial cells. *J. Interferon Cytokine Res.* 33:121–9, 2013.
Gerald Quinnan, Professor; M.D., Saint Louis, 1973. Understanding the significance of mutations in the envelope gene of HIV in determining the resistance of virus to neutralization; induction of neutralizing antibody responses using novel HIV-1 envelope glycoproteins and methods of administration with the goal of inducing protection against infection; attempting to understand the factors that limit B cell responses to neutralization epitopes on HIV envelope glycoproteins.
Brian C. Schaefer, Associate Professor; Ph.D., Harvard, 1995. Biology of lymphocyte activation, particularly the antigen-regulated NF-kappa B pathway; role of inflammation in traumatic brain injury; role of inflammation in cancer; imaging, biochemical, and cellular approaches to elucidate signal transduction mechanisms. *Science Signaling* 7:ra45, 2014; *Immunity* 36:947–58, 2012; *Front. Neurol.* 3:155, 2012.
Michael Shamblott, Assistant Professor; Ph.D., Johns Hopkins, 2001. Human stem cells and regenerative medicine; development of new tools for bioinformatic research. *Proc. Natl. Acad. Sci. U.S.A.* 98:113–8, 2001.
Frank Shewmaker, Assistant Professor; Ph.D., Tulane. Prions, amyloid, and protein aggregation, especially in relation to neurodegenerative disease.
Vijay K. Singh, Associate Professor, Ph.D. Preclinical development of a bridging therapy for radiation casualties. *Int. J. Radiat. Biol.* 89:334–45, 2013; *Exp. Hematol.* 40:407–17, 2012; *Exp. Hematol.* 38:61–70, 2010; *Int. J. Radiat. Biol.* 86:12–21, 2010; *Exp. Hematol.* 38(1):61–70, 2010.
Clifford M. Snapper, Professor; M.D., Albany Medical College, 1981. In vivo regulation of protein- and polysaccharide-specific humoral immunity to extracellular bacteria and development of antibacterial and antiviral vaccines. *Vaccine* 31(30):3039–45, 2013.
Andrew Snow, Assistant Professor; Ph.D., Stanford, 2005. Molecular control of human lymphocyte homeostasis via antigen receptor signaling and apoptosis; dysregulation of lymphocyte homeostasis in XLP and BENTA disease. *J. Immunol.* 192(9):4202–9, 2014. *J. Exp. Med.* 209(12):2247–61, 2012; *J. Clin. Investig.* 119(10): 2976–89, 2009.
Shiv Srivastava, Professor and Co-Director, Center for Prostate Disease Research, Department of Surgery; Ph.D., Indian Institute of Technology (New Delhi), 1980. Molecular genetics of human cancer; prostate cancer. *Clin. Chem.* 51:102–12, 2005; *Oncogene* 23:605–11, 2004; *Cancer Res.* 63:4299–304, 2003.
Tharun Sundaresan, Associate Professor; Ph.D., Centre for Cellular and Molecular Biology (India), 1995. Mechanism of eukaryotic mRNA decay, with particular focus on the role of Lsm1p-7p-Pat1p complex in the budding yeast *Saccharomyces cerevisiae*.
Viqar Syed, Associate Professor, Ph.D., Karolinska Institute, Stockholm. Progesterone inhibits endometrial cancer invasiveness by inhibiting the TGF-ß pathway *Canc. Prev. Res.* 2014.
Aviva Symes, Associate Professor; Ph.D., University College (London), 1990. Neuroinflammation, neurogenesis, and therapeutics after traumatic brain injury. *J. Neurochem.* 129:155–68, 2014; *Front. Neurol.* doi: 10.3389/fneur.2014.00082, 2014; *PLOS one* 10.1371/journal.pone.0059250, 2013
Charles S. Via, Professor; M.D., Virginia, 1973. The role of T cells in lupus and in graft-versus-host disease. *J. Immunol.* 190(9):4562–72, 2013.
Shuishu Wang, Assistant Professor, Ph.D., Purdue, 1999. Structural and functional studies of potential drug target proteins from *Mycobacterium tuberculosis* by X-ray crystallography and biochemical techniques.
Robert W. Williams, Associate Professor; Ph.D., Washington State, 1980. Inelastic neutron scattering, Raman, vibrational analysis with anharmonic corrections, and scaled quantum mechanical force field for polycrystalline L-alanine. *Chem. Phys.* 343(1):1–18, 2008.
T. John Wu, Associate Professor; Ph.D., Texas A&M, 1991. Molecular and cellular neuroendocrinology of reproduction and stress. *Mol. Endocrino.* 28:80–98, 2014, *Endocrinology* 154:783–95, 2013; *Endocrine* 42:717–25, 2012; *Endocrinology* 153:5949–60, 2012.
Xin Xiang, Professor; Ph.D., University of Medicine and Dentistry of New Jersey, 1991. HookA is a novel dynein-early endosome linker critical for cargo movement in vivo. *J. Cell Biol.* 204:1009–26, 2014.

UCONN HEALTH

Graduate Program in Cell Analysis and Modeling

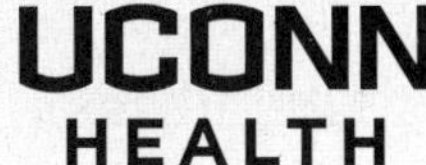

Program of Study

UConn Health's quantitative cell biology research has expanded into the area in cell analysis and modeling. Faculty members associated with this area explore complex biological systems using computational cell biology, optical imaging, and other quantitative approaches to analyze processes in living cells. The program in cell analysis and modeling is designed to train students from diverse disciplinary backgrounds in the cutting-edge research techniques that comprise the interdisciplinary research of modern cell biology. Students are provided with rigorous cross-training in areas of mathematical, physical, and computational sciences as well as biology. Students in the program take courses, attend seminars, and work on interdisciplinary research projects to broaden and strengthen their abilities to conduct quantitative cell biology research.

The cell analysis and modeling (CAM) area of concentration is based at the Richard D. Berlin Center for Cell Analysis and Modeling (CCAM) at UConn Health. Established in 1994, CCAM has emerged as a center that promotes the application of physics, chemistry, and computation to cell biology. The environment of CCAM is designed to promote interdisciplinary interactions and its cadre of physical scientists are supported and valued in a way that is unique for a medical school.

The CAM program is particularly strong in the following areas of research: cellular modeling (analysis and simulation, data integration, modeling movies boundaries, modularity and multistate complexes, molecular flux in crowded spaces, stochastic modeling and discrete particles); biophysics (biological signaling platforms, in vivo nanofabrication); optical imaging (fluorescent correlation spectroscopy, optical probe development, second harmonic generation, single-molecule imaging); cell biology (cellular tissues and development, cytoskeletal dynamics, RNA trafficking, signal transduction, molecular medicine).

Research Facilities

The program is situated at UConn Health in Farmington. This complex provides excellent physical facilities for research in both basic and clinical sciences, a computer center, and the Lyman Maynard Stowe Library. The program provides research facilities and guidance for graduate and postdoctoral work in cell biology—particularly membrane and surface function, membrane protein synthesis and turnover, cytoskeleton structure and function, stimulus-response coupling, gene expression and regulation, vascular biology, fertilization, bone biology, molecular medicine, early development, signal transduction, angiogenesis, computer modeling, and tumor biology. Facilities for training in cell culture, electron microscopy, electrophysiology, fluorescence spectroscopy, molecular biology, molecular modeling, fluorescence imaging, and intravital microscopy are available.

Financial Aid

Support for doctoral students engaged in full-time degree programs at UConn Health is provided on a competitive basis. Graduate research assistantships for 2014–15 provide a stipend of $29,000 per year, which includes a waiver of tuition/most University fees for the fall and spring semesters and the option of participating in a student health insurance plan. While financial aid is offered competitively, the UConn Health makes every possible effort to address the financial needs of all students during their period of training.

Cost of Study

For 2014–15, tuition is $12,202 per year for full-time students who are Connecticut residents and $32,258 per year for full-time students who are out-of-state residents. General University fees are added to the cost of tuition for students who do not receive a tuition waiver. These costs are usually met by traineeships or research assistantships for doctoral students.

Living and Housing Costs

There is a wide range of affordable housing options in the greater Hartford area within easy commuting distance of the campus, including an extensive complex that is adjacent to UConn Health. Costs range from $700 to $1,000 per month for a one-bedroom unit; 2 or more students sharing an apartment usually pay less. University housing is not available at on campus.

Student Group

The total number of Ph.D. students at UConn Health is approximately 150, while the medical and dental schools combined currently enroll 130 students per class.

Location

UConn Health is located in the historic town of Farmington, Connecticut. Set in the beautiful New England countryside on a hill overlooking the Farmington Valley, it is close to ski areas, hiking trails, and facilities for boating, fishing, and swimming. Connecticut's capital city of Hartford, 7 miles east of Farmington, is the center of an urban region of approximately 800,000 people. The beaches of the Long Island Sound are about 50 minutes away to the south, and the beautiful Berkshires are a short drive to the northwest. New York City and Boston can be reached within 2½ hours by car. Hartford is the home of the acclaimed Hartford Stage Company, TheatreWorks, the Hartford Symphony and Chamber orchestras, two ballet companies, an opera company, the Wadsworth Athenaeum (the oldest public art museum in the nation), the Mark Twain house, the Hartford Civic Center, and many other interesting cultural and recreational facilities. The area is also home to several branches of the University of Connecticut, Trinity College, and the University of Hartford, which includes the Hartt School of Music. Bradley International Airport (about 30 minutes from campus) serves the Hartford/Springfield area with frequent airline connections to major cities in this country and abroad. Frequent bus and rail service is also available from Hartford.

UConn Health

The Health Center

The 200-acre UConn Health campus at Farmington houses a division of the University of Connecticut Graduate School, as well as the Schools of Medicine and Dental Medicine. The campus also includes the John Dempsey Hospital, associated clinics, and extensive medical research facilities, all in a centralized facility with more than 1 million square feet of floor space. The Academic Research Building, built in 1999, is an impressive eleven-story structure providing 170,000 square feet of laboratory space. In addition, renovations are underway in the main Laboratory building, converting existing lab space to state-of-the-art open lab areas. The faculty at the center includes more than 260 full-time members. The institution has a strong commitment to graduate study within an environment that promotes social and intellectual interaction among the various educational programs. Graduate students are represented on various administrative committees concerned with curricular affairs, and the Graduate Student Organization (GSO) represents graduate students' needs and concerns to the faculty and administration, in addition to fostering social contact among graduate students in UConn Health.

Applying

Applications for admission should be submitted via the online application system and should be filed together with transcripts, three letters of recommendation, a personal statement, and recent results from the General Test of the Graduate Record Examinations. International students must take the Test of English as a Foreign Language (TOEFL) to satisfy Graduate School requirements. The deadline for completed applications and receipt of all supplemental materials is **December 1**. Please note that GRE and TOEFL exams taken after the due date will not be accepted for consideration for admission. In accordance with the laws of the state of Connecticut and of the United States, UConn Health Center does not discriminate against any person in its educational and employment activities on the grounds of race, color, creed, national origin, sex, age, or physical disability.

Correspondence and Information

Graduate Admissions Office
Ph.D. in Biomedical Science Program
UConn Health
263 Farmington Ave., MC 3906
Farmington, Connecticut 06030-3906
United States
Phone: 860-679-4509
E-mail: BiomedSciAdmissions@uchc.edu
Website: http://grad.uchc.edu/prospective/programs/phd_biosci/index.html
http://www.ccam.uchc.edu

THE FACULTY AND THEIR RESEARCH

Michael Blinov, Assistant Professor of Genetics and Developmental Biology; Ph.D., Weizmann Institute (Israel). Computational biology: modeling of signal transcription systems and protein-DNA interactions; bioinformatics: data mining and visualization; developing software tools and mathematical methods for rule-based modeling of signal transduction systems.

John H. Carson, Professor of Molecular, Microbial and Structural Biology; Ph.D., MIT. RNA transport in cells of the nervous system.

Ann E. Cowan, Professor of Molecular, Microbial, and Structural Biology; Deputy Director, Center for Biomedical Imaging Technology; Ph.D., Colorado. Research encompassing several areas of mammalian sperm development.

Greg Huber, Assistant Professor of Cell Biology; Ph.D., Boston University. Problems in biological physics, with an emphasis on the interplay of statistical mechanics, biomechanics, and fluid dynamics.

Reinhard Laubenbacher, Professor of Cell Biology; Ph.D., Northwestern. Development of mathematical algorithms and their application to problems in systems biology, in particular the modeling and simulation of molecular networks. An application area of particular interest is cancer systems biology, especially the role of iron metabolism in breast cancer.

Leslie M. Loew, Professor of Cell Biology and of Computer Science and Engineering; Ph.D., Cornell. Morphological determinants of cell physiology; image-based computational models of cellular biology; spatial variations of cell membrane electrophysiology; new optical methods for probing living cells.

Bruce J. Mayer, Professor of Genetics and Developmental Biology; Ph.D., Rockefeller. Mechanisms of signal transduction.

William A. Mohler, Ph.D., Stanford. Associate Professor of Genetics and Developmental Biology. Developmental cell fusion; *C. elegans* genetics; multidimensional imaging of developmental and cell biological processes.

Ion I. Moraru, Associate Professor of Cell Biology; M.D., Ph.D., Carol Davila (Romania). Understanding signal transduction mechanisms, in particular those related to calcium and phosphoinositides.

Vladimir Rodionov, Professor of Cell Biology; Ph.D., Moscow, 1980. Molecular mechanisms of intracellular transport; organization of microtubule cytoskeleton.

Yi Wu, Assistant Professor of Genetics and Developmental Biology; Ph.D., Northwestern. Developing quantitative imaging tools that are capable of revealing dynamics of cellular signaling at high spatial and temporal resolution (biosensors) or that enable optical control of signaling proteins at precise times and subcellular locations (optogenetics).

Ji Yu, Associate Professor of Genetics and Developmental Biology; Ph.D., Texas at Austin. Optical imaging technology; regulation mechanisms in dendritic RNA translation; cytoskeletal dynamics.

UCONN HEALTH

Graduate Program in Cell Biology

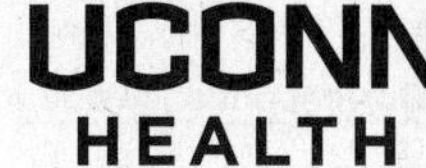

Program of Study

The program offers training leading to a Ph.D. in biomedical sciences and includes faculty members from the Department of Cell Biology as well as eight other UConn Health departments. Faculty members' research spans a broad range of interests in the areas of eukaryotic cell biology and related clinical aspects. The program is particularly strong in the following areas of research: angiogenesis, cancer biology, gene expression, molecular medicine, reproductive biology, signal transduction, vascular biology, optical methods, proteomics, and computer modeling of complex biological systems. The curriculum for the first year is tailored to the individual student and can include core courses in the basic biomedical sciences that have been specially formulated to acquaint the student with the principles and practice of modern biomedical research as well as more specialized, analytical courses. In consultation with their advisory committee, students work out a supplementary program of advanced courses, laboratory experiences, and independent study designed to prepare them for general examinations near the end of their second year. Thesis research begins in the second or third year, and research and thesis writing normally occupy the third and fourth years.

Research Facilities

The program is situated at the modern UConn Health campus in Farmington. This complex provides excellent physical facilities for research in both basic and clinical sciences, a computer center, and the Lyman Maynard Stowe Library. The program provides research facilities and guidance for graduate and postdoctoral work in cell biology—particularly membrane and surface function, membrane protein synthesis and turnover, cytoskeleton structure and function, stimulus-response coupling, gene expression and regulation, vascular biology, fertilization, bone biology, molecular medicine, early development, signal transduction, angiogenesis, computer modeling, and tumor biology. Facilities for training in cell culture, electron microscopy, electrophysiology, fluorescence spectroscopy, molecular biology, molecular modeling, fluorescence imaging, and intravital microscopy are available.

Financial Aid

Support for doctoral students engaged in full-time degree programs at UConn Health is provided on a competitive basis. Graduate research assistantships for 2014–15 provide a stipend of $29,000 per year, which includes a waiver of tuition/most University fees for the fall and spring semesters and the option of participating in a student health insurance plan. While financial aid is offered competitively, UConn Health makes every possible effort to address the financial needs of all students during their period of training.

Cost of Study

For 2014–15, tuition is $12,202 per year for full-time students who are Connecticut residents and $32,258 per year for full-time students who are out-of-state residents. General University fees are added to the cost of tuition for students who do not receive a tuition waiver. These costs are usually met by traineeships or research assistantships for doctoral students.

Living and Housing Costs

There is a wide range of affordable housing options in the greater Hartford area within easy commuting distance of the campus, including an extensive complex that is adjacent to the UConn Health. Costs range from $700 to $1,000 per month for a one-bedroom unit; 2 or more students sharing an apartment usually pay less. University housing is not available on campus.

Student Group

Currently, approximately 10 students are pursuing doctoral studies in the program. The total number of Ph.D. students at UConn Health is approximately 150, while the medical and dental schools combined currently enroll 130 students per class.

Location

UConn Health is located in the historic town of Farmington, Connecticut. Set in the beautiful New England countryside on a hill overlooking the Farmington Valley, it is close to ski areas, hiking trails, and facilities for boating, fishing, and swimming. Connecticut's capital city of Hartford, 7 miles east of Farmington, is the center of an urban region of approximately 800,000 people. The beaches of the Long Island Sound are about 50 minutes away to the south, and the beautiful Berkshires are a short drive to the northwest. New York City and Boston can be reached within 2½ hours by car. Hartford is the home of the acclaimed Hartford Stage Company, TheatreWorks, the Hartford Symphony and Chamber orchestras, two ballet companies, an opera company, the Wadsworth Athenaeum (the oldest public art museum in the nation), the Mark Twain house, the Hartford Civic Center, and many other interesting cultural and recreational facilities. The area is also home to several branches of the University of Connecticut, Trinity College, and the University of Hartford, which includes the Hartt School of Music. Bradley International Airport (about 30 minutes from campus) serves the Hartford/Springfield area with frequent airline connections to major cities in this country and abroad. Frequent bus and rail service is also available from Hartford.

The Health Center

The 200-acre UConn Health campus at Farmington houses a division of the University of Connecticut Graduate School, as well as the Schools of Medicine and Dental Medicine. The campus also includes the John Dempsey Hospital, associated clinics, and extensive medical research facilities, all in a centralized facility with more than 1 million square feet of floor space. The Academic Research Building, built in 1999, is an impressive eleven-story structure providing 170,000 square feet of laboratory space. In addition, renovations are underway in the main Laboratory building, converting existing lab space into state-of-the-art open lab areas. The faculty includes more than 260 full-time members. The institution has a strong commitment to graduate study within an environment that promotes social and intellectual interaction among the various educational programs. Graduate students are represented on various administrative committees concerned with curricular affairs, and the Graduate Student Organization (GSO) represents graduate students' needs and concerns to the faculty and administration, in addition to fostering social contact among graduate students at UConn Health.

Applying

Applications for admission should be submitted via the online application system and should be filed together with transcripts, three letters of recommendation, a personal statement, and recent results from the General Test of the Graduate Record Examinations. International students must take the Test of English as a Foreign Language (TOEFL) to satisfy Graduate School requirements. The deadline for completed applications and receipt of all supplemental materials is **December 1**. Please note that GRE and TOEFL exams taken after the due date will not be accepted for consideration for admission. In accordance with the laws of the state of Connecticut and of the United States, UConn Health does not discriminate against any person in its educational and employment activities on the grounds of race, color, creed, national origin, sex, age, or physical disability.

UConn Health

Correspondence and Information

Graduate Admissions Office
Ph.D. in Biomedical Science Program
UConn Health
263 Farmington Ave., MC 3906
Farmington, Connecticut 06030-3906
United States
Phone: 860-679-4509
E-mail: BiomedSciAdmissions@uchc.edu
Website: http://grad.uchc.edu/prospective/programs/phd_biosci/index.html

THE FACULTY AND THEIR RESEARCH

Andrew Arnold, Professor and Director, Center for Molecular Medicine; M.D., Harvard. Structure and function of the cyclin D1 oncogene and cell-cycle regulator; molecular genetics and biology of endocrine tumors; inherited endocrine neoplastic diseases.

Rashmi Bansal, Associate Professor of Neuroscience; Ph.D., Central Drug Research Institute. Developmental, cellular, and molecular biology of oligodendrocytes (OLs), the cells that synthesize myelin membrane in the central nervous system.

Gordon G. Carmichael, Professor of Microbiology; Ph.D., Harvard. Regulation of gene expression in eukaryotes.

Joan M. Caron, Assistant Professor of Cell Biology; Ph.D., Connecticut. Biochemistry and cell biology of microtubules; palmitoylation of tubulin and cell function; functional role of palmitoylation of signaling proteins.

Kevin P. Claffey, Professor of Cell Biology and Center for Vascular Biology; Ph.D., Boston University. Angiogenesis in human cancer progression and metastasis; vascular endothelial growth factor (VEGF) expression; hypoxia-mediated gene regulation.

Robert B. Clark, Professor of Medicine, Division of Rheumatic Diseases; M.D., Stanford. Basic T-lymphocyte biology, especially as it relates to autoimmune diseases, such as multiple sclerosis and rheumatoid arthritis; molecular biology and structure of the T-cell antigen receptor; T-cell function; T-cell activation.

Ann Cowan, Professor of Biochemistry and Deputy Director of the Center for Biomedical Imaging Technology; Ph.D., Colorado. Mammalian sperm development.

Anne Delany, Associate Professor of Medicine; Ph.D., Dartmouth. Function and regulation of the noncollagen matrix protein osteonectin/SPARC in bone; regulation of osteoblast gene expression by microRNAs; exploring how the extracellular matrix regulates gene expression in bone-metastatic prostate carcinoma.

Kimberly Dodge-Kafka, Associate Professor of Cell Biology, Center for Cardiology and Cardiovascular Research; Ph.D., Texas–Houston Health Science Center. Molecular mechanism of signaling pathways in the heart.

David I. Dorsky, Associate Professor of Medicine; M.D./Ph.D., Harvard. The structure and function of herpesvirus DNA polymerases and their roles in viral DNA replication.

Paul Epstein, Associate Professor of Cell Biology; Ph.D., Yeshiva (Einstein). Signal transduction in relation to leukemia and breast cancer; purification and cloning of cyclic nucleotide phosphodiesterases.

Alan Fein, Professor of Cell Biology; Ph.D., Johns Hopkins. Molecular basis of visual excitation and adaptation; signal transduction and calcium homeostasis in platelets.

Guo-Hua Fong, Associate Professor of Cell Biology and Center for Vascular Biology; Ph.D., Illinois. Cardiovascular biology.

Brenton R. Graveley, Professor, Department of Genetics and Developmental Biology; Ph.D., Vermont. Regulation of alternative splicing in the mammalian nervous system and mechanisms of alternative splicing.

David Han, Associate Professor of Cell Biology and Center for Vascular Biology; Ph.D., George Washington. Proteomic analysis of complex protein mixtures.

Arthur R. Hand, Professor of Craniofacial Sciences and Cell Biology; D.D.S., UCLA. Study of protein and gene expression in rodent salivary glands during normal growth and development and in various experimental conditions employing morphological, immunological, and biochemical methodology.

Marc Hansen, Professor of Medicine; Ph.D., Cincinnati. Analysis of genes involved in the development of the bone tumor osteosarcoma.

Greg Huber, Assistant Professor of Cell Biology; Ph.D., Boston University. Problems in biological physics, with an emphasis on the interplay of statistical mechanics, biomechanics, and fluid dynamics.

Marja Hurley, Professor of Medicine; M.D., Connecticut Health Center. Molecular mechanisms by which members of the fibroblast growth factor (FGFs) and fibroblast growth factor receptor (FGFR) families (produced by osteoblasts, osteoclasts, and stromal cells) regulate bone development, remodeling, and disorders of bone: Fgf2 knockout and Fgf2 transgenic mice are utilized in loss and gain of function experiments to elucidate the role of FGF-2 in disorders of bone, including osteoporosis.

Laurinda A. Jaffe, Professor of Cell Biology; Ph.D., UCLA. Physiology of fertilization, in particular the mechanisms by which membrane potential regulates sperm-egg fusion; transduction mechanisms coupling sperm-egg interaction to egg exocytosis; opening of ion channels in the egg membrane.

Ingela Jansson, Assistant Professor of Cell Biology; Ph.D., Stockholm. DNA-binding proteins in metallothionine induction and cytochrome P450–cytochrome b5 interactions.

Stephen M. King, Professor of Biochemistry; Ph.D., London. Cell biology; biochemistry and function of molecular motors; dynein structure and function.

Eric S. Levine, Professor of Neuroscience; Ph.D., Princeton. Synaptic physiology and plasticity; roles of nerve growth factors and endogenous cannabinoids in hippocampus and cortex.

Bruce Liang, Professor of Cardiopulmonary Medicine; M.D., Harvard. Signal transduction; cardiac and vascular cell biology; receptors; G proteins; transgenic mice.

Leslie M. Loew, Professor of Cell Biology and Director, Center for Cell Analysis and Modeling; Ph.D., Cornell. Spectroscopic methods for measuring spatial and temporal variations in membrane potential; electric field effects on cell membranes; membrane pores induced by toxins and antibiotics.

Nilanjana Maulik, Associate Professor of Surgery; Ph.D., Calcutta. Molecular and cellular signaling during myocardial ischemia and reperfusion.

Lisa Mehlmann, Assistant Professor of Cell Biology; Ph.D., Kent State. Cell signaling events that regulate oocyte maturation and fertilization; maintenance of oocyte meiotic arrest by G-protein receptors; hormonal regulation of oocyte maturation.

Ion I. Moraru, Associate Professor of Cell Biology; M.D., Ph.D., Carol Davila (Romania). Understanding signal transduction mechanisms, in particular related to calcium and phosphoinositides.

Joel Pachter, Professor of Cell Biology; Ph.D., NYU. Elucidating the mechanisms by which leukocytes and pathogens invade the central nervous system.

John J. Peluso, Professor of Cell Biology and Obstetrics and Gynecology; Ph.D., West Virginia. Cell and molecular mechanisms involving the regulating ovarian cell mitosis and apoptosis; cell-cell interaction as a regulator of ovarian cell function; identification and characterization of a putative membrane receptor for progesterone.

Carol C. Pilbeam, Professor of Medicine; M.D./Ph.D., Yale. Regulation and function of prostaglandins in bone; transcriptional regulation of cyclooxygenase-2; role of cytokines and estrogen in bone physiology and osteoporosis.

Vladimir Rodionov, Professor of Cell Biology; Ph.D., Moscow. Dynamics of cytoskeleton; self-organization of microtubule arrays; regulation of the activity of microtubule motors.

Annabelle Rodriguez-Oquendo, Professor of Cell Biology; M.D., New Jersey Medical School. Genetic link between healthy HDL cholesterol, heart disease, and infertility in women.

Daniel Rosenberg, Professor of Medicine; Ph.D., Michigan. Molecular genetics of colorectal cancer; signaling pathways in the development of tumors; toxicogenomics.

Linda H. Shapiro, Associate Professor of Cell Biology and Center for Vascular Biology; Ph.D., Michigan. Regulation and function of CD 13/aminopeptidase N in angiogenic vasculature and early myeloid cells; control of tumor and myocardial angiogenesis by peptidases; inflammatory regulation of angiogenesis.

Mark R. Terasaki, Associate Professor of Cell Biology; Ph.D., Berkeley. Structure and function of the endoplasmic reticulum; confocal microscopy.

James Watras, Associate Professor of Medicine; Ph.D., Washington State. The mechanisms by which the sarcoplasmic reticulum regulates intracellular calcium concentration in vascular smooth muscle.

Bruce A. White, Professor of Cell Biology; Ph.D., Berkeley. Regulation of prolactin gene expression by Ca and calmodulin in rat pituitary tumor cells; examination of nuclear DNA-binding proteins, nuclear calmodulin-binding proteins, and nuclear Ca-calmodulin-dependent protein kinase activity.

Catherine H. Wu, Professor of Medicine; Ph.D., CUNY, Brooklyn. Mechanisms of procollagen propeptide feedback inhibition of collagen synthesis; pretranslational control.

George Y. Wu, Professor of Medicine; M.D./Ph.D., Yeshiva (Einstein). Receptor-mediated endocytosis of glycoproteins; drug delivery by endocytic targeting; targeted gene delivery and expression.

Lixia Yue, Associate Professor of Cell Biology and Center for Cardiovascular Research; Ph.D., McGill. TRP channels and Ca^{2+} signaling mechanisms in cardiac remodeling.

UCONN HEALTH

Graduate Program in Molecular Biology and Biochemistry

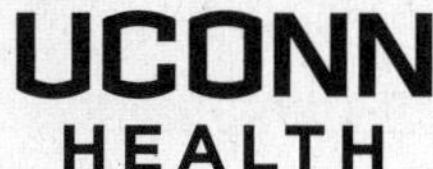

Program of Study

The Graduate Program in Molecular Biology and Biochemistry uniquely bridges modern molecular biology, microbiology, biochemistry, cell biology, and structural biology, leading to a Ph.D. in the biomedical sciences. The goals of the graduate program are to provide rigorous research training in an environment dedicated to advancing excellence in teaching and research. Whether graduates enter academic research, the biotechnology industry, liberal arts college teaching, patent law, or other disciplines, they bring to that career a solid base of knowledge, an ability to learn independently and think independently, and an enduring desire to use their full range of professional skills and experience in creative ways. Graduates are expected to have demonstrated a high degree of competence in research, as judged by publications in first-rank journals, and to have developed essential skills in identifying important research problems, planning research projects and scientific writing. In addition, students are expected to have incorporated ethical principles of scientific conduct into their professional attitudes and activities and to be sensitive to such issues throughout their careers. The success of this training approach is indicated by the high percentage of students who have developed successful independent careers in biomedical research. The current program offers an unparalleled opportunity to study a wide variety of biological problems at the biochemical, molecular, cellular, and structural levels. The interests of the faculty are summarized below.

Research Facilities

In addition to the general facilities of UConn Health, the program offers complete physical research facilities. There is research equipment, as well as expertise, for all areas of genetic, biochemical, molecular, cellular, and biophysical investigation. The department houses the UConn Health NMR Structural Biology Facility (http://structbio.uchc.edu), which includes a 400-MHz NMR spectrometer and cryoprobe-equipped 500- and 600-MHz NMR spectrometers, as well as a circular dichroism spectropolarimeter, isothermal titration calorimeter, and multi-angle laser light scattering facilities. An 800-MHz NMR spectrometer and X-ray crystallography facilities are planned. The department also houses the UConn Health Structural Biology Computational Facility, which includes a bank of Mac and Linux desktop computers connected to ultrafast servers with the latest structural biology software. Facilities are also available for electron and confocal laser scanning microscopy, low-light-level imaging microscopy (in the state-of-the-art Center for Cell Analysis and Modeling), protein purification and sequencing, cell culture, monoclonal antibody production, DNA oligonucleotide and peptide synthesis and sequencing, and gene silencing using RNAI.

Financial Aid

Support for doctoral students engaged in full-time degree programs at UConn Health is provided on a competitive basis. Graduate research assistantships for 2014–15 provide a stipend of $29,000 per year, which includes a waiver of tuition/most University fees for the fall and spring semesters and the option of participating in a student health insurance plan. While financial aid is offered competitively, UConn Health makes every possible effort to address the financial needs of all students during their period of training.

Cost of Study

For 2014–15, tuition is $12,202 per year for full-time students who are Connecticut residents and $32,258 per year for full-time out-of-state residents. General University fees are added to the cost of tuition for students who do not receive a tuition waiver. These costs are usually met by traineeships or research assistantships for doctoral students.

Living and Housing Costs

There is a wide range of affordable housing options in the greater Hartford area within easy commuting distance of the campus, including an extensive complex that is adjacent to UConn Health. Costs range from $700 to $1,000 per month for a one-bedroom unit; 2 or more students sharing an apartment usually pay less. University housing is not available on campus.

Student Group

There are approximately 20 graduate students in the molecular biology and biochemistry program. There are approximately 150 graduate students in Ph.D. programs on the UConn Health campus, and the total enrollment is about 1,000.

Location

UConn Health is located in the historic town of Farmington, Connecticut. Set in the beautiful New England countryside on a hill overlooking the Farmington Valley, it is close to ski areas, hiking trails, and facilities for boating, fishing, and swimming. Connecticut's capital city of Hartford, 7 miles east of Farmington, is the center of an urban region of approximately 800,000 people. The beaches of the Long Island Sound are about 50 minutes away to the south, and the beautiful Berkshires are a short drive to the northwest. New York City and Boston can be reached within 2½ hours by car. Hartford is the home of the acclaimed Hartford Stage Company, TheatreWorks, the Hartford Symphony and Chamber orchestras, two ballet companies, an opera company, the Wadsworth Athenaeum (the oldest public art museum in the nation), the Mark Twain house, the Hartford Civic Center, and many other interesting cultural and recreational facilities. The area is also home to several branches of the University of Connecticut, Trinity College, and the University of Hartford, which includes the Hartt School of Music. Bradley International Airport (about 30 minutes from campus) serves the Hartford/Springfield area with frequent airline connections to major cities in this country and abroad. Frequent bus and rail service is also available from Hartford.

UConn Health

The Health Center

The 200-acre UConn Health campus at Farmington houses a division of the University of Connecticut Graduate School, as well as the Schools of Medicine and Dental Medicine. The campus also includes the John Dempsey Hospital, associated clinics, and extensive medical research facilities, all in a centralized facility with more than 1 million square feet of floor space. The Academic Research Building, built in 1999, is an impressive eleven-story structure providing 170,000 square feet of laboratory space. In addition, renovations are underway in the main Laboratory building, converting existing lab space to state-of-the-art open lab areas. The faculty includes more than 260 full-time members. The institution has a strong commitment to graduate study within an environment that promotes social and intellectual interaction among the various educational programs. Graduate students are represented on various administrative committees concerned with curricular affairs, and the Graduate Student Organization (GSO) represents graduate students' needs and concerns to the faculty and administration, in addition to fostering social contact among graduate students.

Applying

Applications for admission should be submitted via the online application system and should be filed together with transcripts, three letters of recommendation, a personal statement, and recent results from the General Test of the Graduate Record Examinations. International students must take the Test of English as a Foreign Language (TOEFL) to satisfy Graduate School requirements. The deadline for completed applications and receipt of all supplemental materials is **December 1**. Please note that GRE and TOEFL exams taken after the due date will not be accepted for consideration for admission. In accordance with the laws of the state of Connecticut and of the United States, UConn Health does not discriminate against any person in its educational and employment activities on the grounds of race, color, creed, national origin, sex, age, or physical disability.

Correspondence and Information

Graduate Admissions Office
Ph.D. in Biomedical Science Program
UConn Health
263 Farmington Ave., MC 3906
Farmington, Connecticut 06030-3906
United States
Phone: 860-679-4509
E-mail: BiomedSciAdmissions@uchc.edu
Website: http://grad.uchc.edu/prospective/programs/phd_biosci/index.html

THE FACULTY AND THEIR RESEARCH

Irina Besonova, Assistant Professor of Molecular, Microbial, and Structural Biology; Ph.D., Toronto. Structural and biochemical characterization of proteins and protein complexes of p53 pathway, especially, proteins responsible for maintenance of an appropriate level of p53 in the cell.

Gordon G. Carmichael, Professor; Ph.D., Harvard. Regulation of viral gene expression and function.

John H. Carson, Professor; Ph.D., MIT. RNA transport in cells of the nervous system.

Ann Cowan, Professor; Ph.D., Colorado at Boulder. Plasma membrane proteins in sperm.

Asis Das, Professor; Ph.D., Calcutta. Gene control in bacterial adaptive response.

Kimberly Dodge-Kafka, Associate Professor of Cell Biology/Center for Cardiology and Cardiovascular Research; Ph.D., Texas Health Science Center at Houston, 1999. Molecular mechanism of signaling pathways in the heart.

Betty Eipper, Professor; Ph.D., Harvard. Biosynthesis and secretion of peptides by neurons and endocrine cells.

Michael Gryk, Associate Professor; Ph.D., Stanford. Three-dimensional structure and function of proteins involved in DNA repair.

Arthur Günzl, Professor; Ph.D., Tübingen (Germany). Transcription and antigenic variation in the mammalian parasite *Trypanosoma brucei.*

Bing Hao, Assistant Professor of Molecular, Microbial, and Structural Biology; Ph.D., Ohio State. Understanding how the cell cycle is regulated by ubiquitin-mediated proteolysis using X-ray crystallography as a primary tool.

Christopher Heinen, Associate Professor of Medicine; Ph.D., Cincinnati. Biochemical and cellular defects of the DNA mismatch repair pathway during tumorigenesis.

Jeffrey Hoch, Professor; Ph.D., Harvard. Biophysical chemistry of proteins.

Stephen M. King, Professor; Ph.D., University College, London. Structure and function of microtubule-based molecular motor proteins.

Lawrence A. Klobutcher, Professor and Associate Dean of the Graduate School; Ph.D., Yale. DNA rearrangement, programmed translational frameshifting, and phagocytosis in ciliated protozoa.

Dmitry Korzhnev, Assistant Professor, Molecular, Microbial, and Structural Biology; Ph.D., Moscow Institute of Physics and Technology. Liquid-state nuclear magnetic resonance (NMR) studies of structure and dynamics of proteins and their assemblies; multiprotein complexes involved in DNA replication and repair; protein folding.

Mark Maciejewski, Associate Professor; Ph.D., Ohio State. Enzymes of DNA replication, repair, and recombination.

Adam Schuyler, Assistant Professor of Molecular Biology and Biophysics; Ph.D., Johns Hopkins. Computational modeling of molecular dynamics and allosteric activation, nonuniform sampling techniques for multidimensional NMR experiments.

Peter Setlow, Professor; Ph.D., Brandeis. Biochemistry of bacterial spore germination.

Aziz Taghbalout, Assistant Professor of Molecular, Microbial, and Structural Biology; Ph.D., Hassan II University (Morocco). Understanding the molecular organization of the RNA degradosome, a multiprotein complex that plays essential role in the normal RNA degradation and processing in *Escherichia coli.*

Suzy V. Torti, Professor of Molecular, Microbial, and Structural Biology; Ph.D., Tufts.

Sandra K. Weller, Professor and Department Head; Ph.D., Wisconsin. Mechanisms of DNA replication and DNA encapsidation in herpes simplex virus; virus-host interactions.

UNIVERSITY OF WASHINGTON/ FRED HUTCHINSON CANCER RESEARCH CENTER

Molecular and Cellular Biology Program

W UNIVERSITY of WASHINGTON

FRED HUTCHINSON CANCER RESEARCH CENTER
A LIFE OF SCIENCE

Program of Study

The University of Washington and the Fred Hutchinson Cancer Research Center offer a program of graduate studies in molecular and cellular biology leading to the Ph.D. degree. More than 200 faculty members participate in the program and are located on the University of Washington campus in the Departments of Biochemistry, Biological Structure, Biology, Environmental Health, Genome Sciences, Immunology, Microbiology, Global Health, Pathology, Pharmacology, and Physiology and Biophysics, as well as on the Day campus at the Hutchinson Center, primarily in the Division of Basic Sciences and the Division of Human Biology. Recently, the Institute for Systems Biology (ISB), a nonprofit research institute headed by Dr. Leroy Hood, and the Seattle Biomedical Research Institute (Seattle BioMed), an infectious disease research center led by Dr. Alan Aderem, have joined the Molecular and Cellular Biology (MCB) program.

The goals of the program are to give the student a sound background in molecular and cellular biology and to provide access to the research expertise of all faculty members and laboratories working in this area. These goals are accomplished through the basic elements of the program, which include keystone courses in a student's area of interest, advanced elective courses in molecular and cellular biology, a two-quarter literature review course, one quarter of grant writing, three or more quarter-long lab rotations, two quarters of varied teaching experience, and a series of informal workshops and seminars on topics in diverse areas of molecular biology and cellular biology. Emphasis is placed on critical evaluation of the literature, exposure to current research methods, and creative thinking through independent research. Students are expected to begin active research in their first year through their lab rotations and to choose a permanent thesis adviser at the end of their first year.

Research Facilities

The program uses the research facilities of the individual departments, Hutchinson Center, ISB, and Seattle BioMed. The School of Medicine is housed in the Health Sciences Center and the South Lake Union research hub (SLU). The University Hospital and the College of Arts and Sciences are located in adjoining or nearby buildings. The Hutchinson Center's Day campus and SLU are a 15-minute shuttle ride from the University. The laboratories of participating faculty members are well equipped with the latest in research equipment and are funded by external support. The ISB and Seattle BioMed are located within easy commuting distance. Some of the other facilities available are two Howard Hughes Medical Institute research units, the Markey Molecular Medicine Center, animal quarters, shared major instrument facilities, oligonucleotide and peptide synthesis facilities, a marine biology station at Friday Harbor in the San Juan Islands, and an extensive Health Sciences Library.

Financial Aid

The program offers a salary of approximately $29,592 for twelve months. Students with satisfactory academic progress can anticipate funding that includes tuition and health insurance for the duration of their studies.

Cost of Study

Tuition, salary, and medical, dental, and vision benefits are funded for the duration of the program for students in good standing.

Living and Housing Costs

The University has a wide variety of housing available for single and married students as well as families. Students should call the University Housing Office at 206-543-4059 for further information. Private accommodations may be found within easy walking or bicycling distance.

Student Group

At the University of Washington, approximately 2,500 full-time faculty members serve a student population of 35,000 that is drawn from all over the United States and many other countries.

An average of 20 new students are admitted to the program each year. There are approximately 500 graduate students in the biological sciences at the University of Washington.

Student Outcomes

The Molecular and Cellular Biology Program received degree-granting status in 1994. The majority of students, upon earning Ph.D. degrees, secure postdoctoral research positions.

Location

All around Seattle, there is an abundance of opportunity for outdoor recreation. Unsurpassed sailing, hiking, mountain climbing, skiing, and camping are all a short distance away. Because of the saltwater expanse of the Puget Sound and the mountains both to the east and to the west, Seattle enjoys a moderate climate, with precipitation averaging 32 inches per year, mostly during the winter and early spring. The city's downtown area offers many cultural and educational advantages, including theater, museums, symphony, films, and opera, while the waterfront is home to a large marketplace, galleries, and fresh seafood restaurants. The University itself sponsors many public lectures, concerts, exhibits, film festivals, and theatrical performances.

The University

The University of Washington is located in a residential section of Seattle near the downtown area. It is bordered by two lakes and is one of the largest and most scenic institutions of higher education in the country. The University is a research-intensive institution, regularly ranking first overall among public universities in externally funded research programs. It is recognized for graduate instruction of high quality, offering more than ninety graduate and professional programs that enroll more than 7,300 graduate students on campus. The Hutchinson Center's research laboratories are located near Lake Union just north of downtown Seattle. It is the largest independent cancer research center in the country.

Applying

Applicants must have completed a baccalaureate or advanced degree by the time of matriculation; degrees emphasizing biology, physical or natural sciences, and mathematics are preferred. It is advisable to take the GRE (the General Test) by August 1 so that scores can be recorded before the deadline (code for MCB is 0206, code for UW is 4854, on the GRE registration form). New students enter the graduate program in the autumn quarter. The deadline for completion of applications is currently December 1 of the academic year preceding entrance.

Students must apply via the online application available at the MCB Program website (https://www.grad.uw.edu/applForAdmiss).

Correspondence and Information

Graduate Program Specialist
Molecular and Cellular Biology Program, Box 357275
University of Washington
Seattle, Washington 98195-7275
United States
Phone: 206-685-3155
Fax: 206-685-8174
E-mail: mcb@uw.edu
Website: http://www.mcb-seattle.edu

THE FACULTY AND THEIR RESEARCH

UNIVERSITY OF WASHINGTON

Cancer Biology

Charles Asbury, Maitreya Dunham, Douglas Fowler, Richard Gardner, Philip Greenberg, Suzanne Hoppins, Brian Iritani, Michael Lagunoff, Lawrence Loeb, Nancy Maizels, Dustin Maly, Raymond Monnat, Junko Oshima, Bradley Preston, Andrew Scharenberg, Daniel Stetson, Judit Villen, Edith Wang, Alejandro Wolf-Yadlin.

Cell Signaling and Cell/Environment Interactions

Michael Ailion, John Aitchison, Charles Asbury, Sandra Bajjalieh, Joseph Beavo, Celeste Berg, Karol Bomsztyk, Karin Bornfeldt, Mark Bothwell, Susan Brockerhoff, Steven Carlson, William Catterall, Sharon Doty, Elaine Faustman, Stanley Froehner, Richard Gardner, Sharona Gordon, E. Peter Greenberg, Ted Gross, Chris Hague, Suzanne Hoppins, James Hurley, Takato Imaizumi, Matthew Kaeberlein, David Kimelman, Michael Laflamme, John Leigh, Jaisri Lingappa, Qinghang Liu, Dustin Maly, Stanley McKnight, Alex Merz, Dana Miller, Neil Nathanson, Jennifer Nemhauser, Andrew Oberst, Leo Pallanck, Alexander Paredez, David Parichy, William Parks, Marilyn Parsons, Christine Queitsch, Hannele Ruohola-Baker, John Scott, Daniel Stetson, Daniel Storm, Rong Tian, Keiko Torii, Judit Villen, Edith Wang, Alejandro Wolf-Yadlin, Zhengui Xia, Zipora Yablonka-Reuveni, William Zagotta.

Developmental Biology, Stem Cells, and Aging
Chris Amemiya, Celeste Berg, Olivia Bermingham-McDonogh, Mark Bothwell, Steven Carlson, Jeffrey Chamberlain, Michael Chin, Vincenzo Cirulli, John Clark, Mark Cooper, Michael Cunningham, Ajay Dhaka, Christine Disteche, Marshall Horwitz, David Kimelman, Michael Laflamme, Michael MacCoss, Alex Merz, Dana Miller, William Moody, Randall Moon, Charles Murry, Leo Pallanck, David Parichy, Jay Parrish, Daniel Promislow, Peter Rabinovitch, David Raible, Thomas Reh, Hannele Ruohola-Baker, Billie Swalla, Keiko Torii, Judit Villen, Barbara Wakimoto, Robert Waterston, Zhengui Xia, Zipora Yablonka-Reuveni.

Gene Expression, Cell Cycle, and Chromosome Biology
John Aitchison, Charles Asbury, Nitin Baliga, Karol Bomsztyk, Eliot Brenowitz, Bonita Brewer, Roger Bumgarner, Daniel Campbell, Trisha Davis, Christine Disteche, Maitreya Dunham, Elaine Faustman, Stanley Fields, Takato Imaizumi, Nancy Maizels, Houra Merrikh, Raymond Monnat, Peter Myler, Shao-En Ong, Alexander Paredez, Keiko Torii, Edith Wang, Robert Waterston, Linda Wordeman, Zipora Yablonka-Reuveni.

Genetics, Genomics, and Evolution
Michael Ailion, Chris Amemiya, Nitin Baliga, Celeste Berg, Elhanan Borenstein, Bonita Brewer, Roger Bumgarner, Peter Byers, Jeffrey Chamberlain, Michael Cunningham, Trisha Davis, Christine Disteche, Aimee Dudley, Maitreya Dunham, Elaine Faustman, Stanley Fields, Douglas Fowler, Clement Furlong, Richard Gardner, Marshall Horwitz, Matthew Kaeberlein, Benjamin Kerr, Mary-Claire King, John Leigh, Mary Lidstrom, Lawrence Loeb, Nancy Maizels, Houra Merrikh, Dana Miller, Raymond Monnat, Peter Myler, Shao-En Ong, Junko Oshima, Leo Pallanck, Alexander Paredez, David Parichy, Jay Parrish, Bradley Preston, Daniel Promislow, Christine Queitsch, David Raible, Marilyn Roberts, Jay Shendure, David Sherman, Ilya Shmulevich, Daniel Stetson, Kenneth Stuart, Billie Swalla, Bruce Tempel, Rong Tian, Keiko Torii, Barbara Wakimoto, Robert Waterston, Zipora Yablonka-Reuveni.

Microbiology, Infection, and Immunity
Alan Aderem, John Aitchison, Nitin Baliga, Elhanan Borenstein, Roger Bumgarner, Daniel Campbell, Lee Ann Campbell, James Champoux, Edward Clark, Brad Cookson, Ian Nicholas Crispe, Keith Elkon, Ferric Fang, Pamela Fink, Michael Gale, Joan Goverman, E. Peter Greenberg, Philip Greenberg, Christoph Grundner, Jessica Hamerman, Caroline Harwood, Jay Heinecke, Michael Katze, Nichole Klatt, Michael Lagunoff, Jaisri Lingappa, Houra Merrikh, Alex Merz, Samuel Miller, Joseph Mougous, James Mullins, Peter Myler, Andrew Oberst, William Parks, Matthew Parsek, Marilyn Parsons, Lakshmi Rajgopal, David Rawlings Andrew Scharenberg, Jay Shendure, David Sherman, Pradeep Singh, Jason Smith, Joseph Smith, Kelly Smith, Donald Sodora, Leonidas Stamatatos, Daniel Stetson, Kenneth Stuart, Wendy Thomas, Beth Traxler, Kevin Urdahl, Wesley Van Voorhis, Joshua Woodward, Tuofu Zhu, Steven Ziegler.

Molecular Structure and Computational Biology
John Aitchison, Charles Asbury, David Baker, Elhanan Borenstein, James Champoux, Douglas Fowler, Sharona Gordon, Jay Heinecke, Rachel Klevit, Michael MacCoss, Raymond Monnat, Peter Myler, Shao-En Ong, Ram Samudrala, Ilya Shmulevich, Wendy Thomas, Gabriele Varani, Liguo Wang, Wenqing Xu, William Zagotta, Ning Zheng.

Neuroscience
Michael Ailion, Sandra Bajjalieh, Andres Barria, Joseph Beavo, Olivia Bermingham-McDonogh, Mark Bothwell, Eliot Brenowitz, Susan Brockerhoff, Steven Carlson, Jeffrey Chamberlain, Charles Chavkin, Horacio de la Iglesia, Ajay Dhaka, Sharona Gordon, Robert Hevner, James Hurley, Matthew Kaeberlein, Brian Kraemer, Stanley McKnight, William Moody, Neil Nathanson, John Neumaier, Leo Pallanck, Richard Palmiter, Jay Parrish, Paul Phillips, Nicholas Poolos, David Raible, Thomas Reh, Fred Rieke, Robert Steiner, Daniel Storm, Bruce Tempel, Rachel Wong, Zhengui Xia, William Zagotta.

FRED HUTCHINSON CANCER RESEARCH CENTER

Cancer Biology
Slobodan Beronja, Jason Bielas, Robert Bradley, William Carter, Bruce Clurman, Denise Galloway, Cyrus Ghajar, William Grady, Christopher Kemp, Hans-Peter Kiem, Paul Lampe, David MacPherson, Peter Nelson, Patrick Paddison, Susan Parkhurst, Amanda Paulovich, Peggy Porter, Martin Prlic, Nina Salama, Julian Simon, Toshiyasu Taniguchi, Stephen Tapscott, Valeri Vasioukhin, Edus Warren.

Cell Signaling and Cell/Environment Interactions
Jihong Bai, Linda Breeden, William Carter, Jonathan Cooper, Cyrus Ghajar, Daniel Gottschling, Paul Lampe, Susan Parkhurst, Amanda Paulovich, Mark Roth, Wenying Shou, Valera Vasioukhin.

Developmental Biology, Stem Cells, and Aging
Jihong Bai, Jonathan Cooper, Cyrus Ghajar, Dan Gottschling, Hans-Peter Kiem, Cecilia Moens, Patrick Paddison, Susan Parkhurst, James Priess, Akiko Shimamura, Valera Vasioukhin.

Gene Expression, Cell Cycle, and Chromosome Biology
Sue Biggins, Linda Breeden, Bruce Clurman, Adam Geballe, Daniel Gottschling, Mark Groudine, Steven Hahn, Steven Henikoff, David MacPherson, Harmit Malik, Susan Parkhurst, Amanda Paulovich, Mark Roth, Gerald Smith, Stephen Tapscott, Toshio Tsukiyama.

Genetics, Genomics, and Evolution
Trevor Bedford, Jesse Bloom, Robert Bradley, Roger Brent, Michael Emerman, Adam Geballe, Daniel Gottschling, Steven Henikoff, David MacPherson, Harmit Malik, J. Lee Nelson, Peter Nelson, Amanda Paulovich, Katie Peichel, Wenying Shou, Edus Warren.

Microbiology, Infection, and Immunity
Trevor Bedford, Jesse Bloom, William Carter, Michael Emerman, David Fredricks, Denise Galloway, Adam Geballe, Keith Jerome, Hans-Peter Kiem, Harmit Malik, Julie Overbaugh, Martin Prlic, Stanley Riddell, Harlan Robins, Nina Salama, Wenying Shou, Roland Strong, Edus Warren.

Molecular Structure and Computational Biology
Trevor Bedford, Jesse Bloom, Steven Hahn, Harlan Robins, Wenying Shou, Barry Stoddard, Roland Strong, Edus Warren.

Neuroscience
Jihong Bai, Linda Buck, Cecilia Moens, James Olson, Valera Vasioukhin.

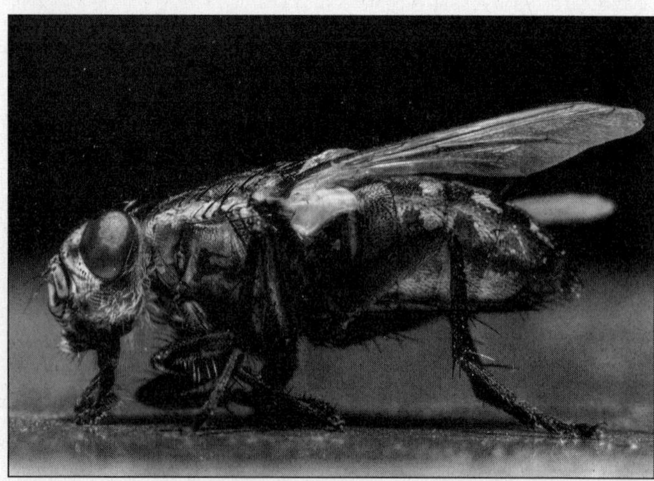

Model organism: fruit fly.

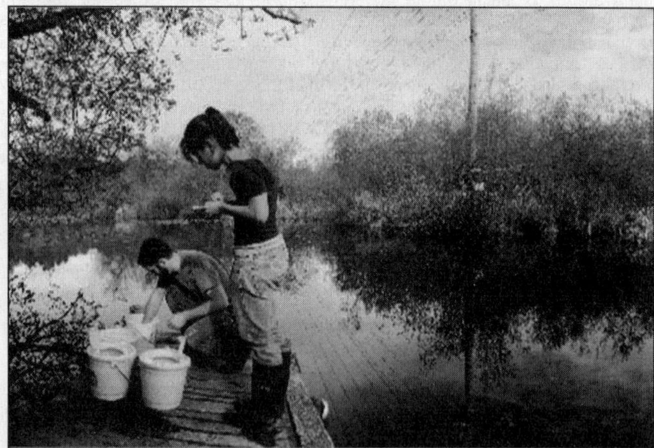

Fishing for sticklebacks.

Section 7
Computational, Systems, and Translational Biology

This section contains a directory of institutions offering graduate work in computational, systems, and translational biology. Additional information about programs listed in the directory may be obtained by writing directly to the dean of a graduate school or chair of a department at the address given in the directory.

CONTENTS

Program Directories

Computational Biology

Albert Einstein College of Medicine, Graduate Division of Biomedical Sciences, Systems and Computational Biology Program, Bronx, NY 10461. Offers PhD.

Arizona State University at the Tempe campus, College of Liberal Arts and Sciences, Department of Mathematics and Statistics, Tempe, AZ 85287-1804. Offers applied mathematics (PhD); computational biosciences (PhD); mathematics (MA, MNS, PhD); mathematics education (PhD); statistics (PhD). Part-time programs available. Terminal master's awarded for partial completion of doctoral program. *Degree requirements:* For master's, thesis or alternative, interactive Program of Study (iPOS) submitted before completing 50 percent of required credit hours; for doctorate, comprehensive exam, thesis/dissertation, interactive Program of Study (iPOS) submitted before completing 50 percent of required credit hours. *Entrance requirements:* For master's and doctorate, GRE General Test, minimum GPA of 3.0 or equivalent in last 2 years of work leading to bachelor's degree. Additional exam requirements/recommendations for international students: Required—TOEFL (minimum score 80 iBT), TOEFL, IELTS, or PTE. Electronic applications accepted. *Expenses:* Contact institution.

Baylor College of Medicine, Graduate School of Biomedical Sciences, Program in Structural and Computational Biology and Molecular Biophysics, Houston, TX 77030-3498. Offers PhD, MD/PhD. MD/PhD offered jointly with Rice University and University of Houston. *Degree requirements:* For doctorate, thesis/dissertation, public defense. *Entrance requirements:* For doctorate, GRE General Test, GRE Subject Test (strongly recommended), minimum GPA of 3.0. Additional exam requirements/recommendations for international students: Required—TOEFL. Electronic applications accepted. *Faculty research:* Computational biology, structural biology, biophysics.

Carnegie Mellon University, Joint CMU-Pitt PhD Program in Computational Biology, Pittsburgh, PA 15213-3891. Offers PhD. *Application contact:* Information Contact, 412-268-2000.

Carnegie Mellon University, Mellon College of Science, Department of Biological Sciences, Program in Computational Biology, Pittsburgh, PA 15213-3891. Offers MS. *Entrance requirements:* For master's, GRE General Test, GRE Subject Test, interview. *Application deadline:* For fall admission, 2/15 priority date for domestic students. Applications are processed on a rolling basis. Application fee: $0. *Financial support:* Fellowships, research assistantships, and traineeships available. *Unit head:* John L. Wollford, Jr., Acting Department Head, 412-268-3193, E-mail: jw17@andrew.cmu.edu. *Application contact:* Thom Gulish, Graduate Program Coordinator, 412-268-2474, E-mail: tgulish@cmu.edu.

Claremont Graduate University, Graduate Programs, Institute of Mathematical Sciences, Claremont, CA 91711-6160. Offers computational and systems biology (PhD); computational mathematics and numerical analysis (MA, MS); computational science (PhD); engineering and industrial applied mathematics (PhD); mathematics (PhD); operations research and statistics (MA, MS); physical applied mathematics (MA, MS); pure mathematics (MA, MS); scientific computing (MA, MS); systems and control theory (MA, MS). Part-time programs available. *Faculty:* 6 full-time (1 woman), 2 part-time/adjunct (0 women). *Students:* 38 full-time (11 women), 41 part-time (14 women); includes 23 minority (3 Black or African American, non-Hispanic/Latino; 11 Asian, non-Hispanic/Latino; 5 Hispanic/Latino; 1 Native Hawaiian or other Pacific Islander, non-Hispanic/Latino; 3 Two or more races, non-Hispanic/Latino), 24 international. Average age 32. In 2013, 17 master's, 16 doctorates awarded. Terminal master's awarded for partial completion of doctoral program. *Entrance requirements:* For master's and doctorate, GRE General Test. Additional exam requirements/recommendations for international students: Required—TOEFL (minimum score 550 paper-based; 80 iBT). *Application deadline:* For fall admission, 2/1 priority date for domestic and international students. Applications are processed on a rolling basis. Application fee: $80. Electronic applications accepted. *Expenses: Tuition:* Full-time $40,560; part-time $1690 per credit. *Required fees:* $275 per semester. Tuition and fees vary according to program. *Financial support:* Fellowships, research assistantships, Federal Work-Study, institutionally sponsored loans, scholarships/grants, and tuition waivers (full and partial) available. Support available to part-time students. Financial award application deadline: 2/15; financial award applicants required to submit FAFSA. *Unit head:* Allon Percus, Director, 909-607-0744, E-mail: allon.percus@cgu.edu. *Application contact:* Charlotte Ballesteros, Institute Coordinator, 909-621-8080, Fax: 909-607-8261, E-mail: charlotte.ballesteros@cgu.edu.
Website: http://www.cgu.edu/pages/168.asp

The College of William and Mary, Faculty of Arts and Sciences, Department of Applied Science, Williamsburg, VA 23187-8795. Offers accelerator science (PhD); applied mathematics (PhD); applied mechanics (PhD); applied robotics (PhD); applied science (MS); atmospheric and environmental science (PhD); computational neuroscience (PhD); interface, thin film and surface science (PhD); lasers and optics (PhD); magnetic resonance (PhD); materials science and engineering (PhD); mathematical and computational biology (PhD); medical imaging (PhD); nanotechnology (PhD); neuroscience (PhD); non-destructive evaluation (PhD); polymer chemistry (PhD); remote sensing (PhD). *Faculty:* 11 full-time (2 women). *Students:* 27 full-time (8 women), 4 part-time (2 women); includes 4 minority (2 Black or African American, non-Hispanic/Latino; 2 Asian, non-Hispanic/Latino), 14 international. Average age 28. 40 applicants, 45% accepted, 3 enrolled. In 2013, 4 master's, 8 doctorates awarded. *Median time to degree:* Of those who began their doctoral program in fall 2005, 95% received their degree in 8 years or less. *Degree requirements:* For master's, comprehensive exam, thesis; for doctorate, comprehensive exam, thesis/dissertation, 4 core courses. *Entrance requirements:* For master's and doctorate, GRE General Test, GRE Subject Test. Additional exam requirements/recommendations for international students: Required—TOEFL, TWE. *Application deadline:* For fall admission, 2/3 priority date for domestic students, 2/3 for international students; for spring admission, 10/15 priority date for domestic students, 10/14 for international students. Applications are processed on a rolling basis. Application fee: $45. Electronic applications accepted. *Expenses:* Tuition, state resident: full-time $7120; part-time $405 per credit hour. Tuition, nonresident: full-time $21,639; part-time $1050 per credit hour. *Required fees:* $4764. *Financial support:* Fellowships, research assistantships, teaching assistantships, Federal Work-Study, health care benefits, tuition waivers (full), and unspecified assistantships available. Financial award application deadline: 4/15; financial award applicants required to submit FAFSA. *Faculty research:* Computational biology, non-destructive evaluation, neurophysiology, lasers and optics. *Total annual research expenditures:* $2.3 million. *Unit head:* Dr. Christopher Del Negro, Chair, 757-221-7808, Fax: 757-221-2050, E-mail: cadeln@wm.edu. *Application contact:* Rosario Fox, Graduate Program Coordinator, 757-221-2563, Fax: 757-221-2050, E-mail: rxfoxx@wm.edu.
Website: http://www.wm.edu/as/appliedscience

Cornell University, Graduate School, Graduate Fields of Agriculture and Life Sciences, Field of Computational Biology, Ithaca, NY 14853-0001. Offers computational behavioral biology (PhD); computational biology (PhD); computational cell biology (PhD); computational ecology (PhD); computational genetics (PhD); computational macromolecular biology (PhD); computational organismal biology (PhD). *Faculty:* 37 full-time (5 women). *Students:* 26 full-time (8 women); includes 8 minority (5 Asian, non-Hispanic/Latino; 1 Hispanic/Latino; 1 Native Hawaiian or other Pacific Islander, non-Hispanic/Latino; 1 Two or more races, non-Hispanic/Latino), 8 international. Average age 25. 171 applicants, 13% accepted, 10 enrolled. *Degree requirements:* For doctorate, comprehensive exam, thesis/dissertation, 2 semesters of teaching experience. *Entrance requirements:* For doctorate, GRE General Test, GRE Subject Test (biology), 2 letters of recommendation. Additional exam requirements/recommendations for international students: Required—TOEFL (minimum score 550 paper-based; 77 iBT). *Application deadline:* For fall admission, 2/1 priority date for domestic students. Application fee: $95. Electronic applications accepted. *Financial support:* In 2013–14, 22 students received support, including 20 research assistantships with full tuition reimbursements available, 2 teaching assistantships with full tuition reimbursements available; fellowships with full tuition reimbursements available, institutionally sponsored loans, scholarships/grants, health care benefits, tuition waivers (full and partial), and unspecified assistantships also available. Financial award applicants required to submit FAFSA. *Faculty research:* Computational behavioral biology, computational biology, computational cell biology, computational ecology, computational genetics, computational macromolecular biology, computational organismal biology. *Unit head:* Dr. Andrew Clark, Director of Graduate Studies, 607-255-5488, E-mail: ac347@cornell.edu. *Application contact:* Graduate School Application Requests, 607-255-5816, E-mail: gradadmissions@cornell.edu.
Website: http://www.gradschool.cornell.edu/fields.php?id-4A

Duke University, Graduate School, Department of Computational Biology and Bioinformatics, Durham, NC 27708. Offers PhD, Certificate. *Faculty:* 57. *Students:* 44 full-time (12 women); includes 6 minority (2 Black or African American, non-Hispanic/Latino; 3 Asian, non-Hispanic/Latino; 1 Hispanic/Latino), 21 international. 95 applicants, 19% accepted, 10 enrolled. In 2013, 6 doctorates awarded. *Degree requirements:* For doctorate, thesis/dissertation. *Entrance requirements:* For doctorate, GRE General Test. Additional exam requirements/recommendations for international students: Required—TOEFL (minimum score 577 paper-based; 90 iBT) or IELTS (minimum score 7). *Application deadline:* For fall admission, 12/8 priority date for domestic and international students. Application fee: $80. Electronic applications accepted. *Financial support:* Fellowships, research assistantships, and teaching assistantships available. Financial award application deadline: 12/8. *Unit head:* Scott Schmidler, Director of Graduate Studies, 919-684-0881, Fax: 919-668-2465, E-mail: el81@duke.edu. *Application contact:* Elizabeth Hutton, Director, Graduate Admissions, 919-684-3913, Fax: 919-684-2277, E-mail: grad-admissions@duke.edu.
Website: http://www.genome.duke.edu/CBB/

Florida State University, The Graduate School, College of Arts and Sciences, Program in Molecular Biophysics, Tallahassee, FL 32306. Offers computational structural biology (PhD); molecular biophysics (PhD). *Faculty:* 34 full-time (7 women). *Students:* 25 full-time (8 women); includes 2 minority (both Hispanic/Latino), 12 international. Average age 29. 24 applicants, 33% accepted, 5 enrolled. In 2013, 4 doctorates awarded. *Degree requirements:* For doctorate, comprehensive exam, thesis/dissertation, teaching 1 term in professor's major department. *Entrance requirements:* For doctorate, GRE General Test. Additional exam requirements/recommendations for international students: Required—TOEFL (minimum score 600 paper-based; 90 iBT). *Application deadline:* For fall admission, 12/15 for domestic and international students. Applications are processed on a rolling basis. Application fee: $30. Electronic applications accepted. *Expenses:* Tuition, state resident: part-time $403.51 per credit hour. Tuition, nonresident: part-time $1004.85 per credit hour. *Required fees:* $75.81 per credit hour. One-time fee: $20 part-time. Tuition and fees vary according to course load, campus/location and student level. *Financial support:* In 2013–14, 24 students received support, including 1 fellowship with full and partial tuition reimbursement available (averaging $23,000 per year), 18 research assistantships with full and partial tuition reimbursements available (averaging $23,500 per year), 6 teaching assistantships with full and partial tuition reimbursements available (averaging $23,500 per year); scholarships/grants, health care benefits, and unspecified assistantships also available. Financial award applicants required to submit FAFSA. *Faculty research:* Protein and nucleic acid structure and function, membrane protein structure, computational biophysics, 3-D image reconstruction. *Total annual research expenditures:* $2.3 million. *Unit head:* Dr. Hong Li, Director, 850-644-6785, Fax: 850-644-7244, E-mail: hli4@fsu.edu. *Application contact:* Lyn Kittle, Academic Coordinator, Graduate Programs, 850-644-1012, Fax: 850-644-7244, E-mail: lkittle@fsu.edu.
Website: http://www.sb.fsu.edu/graduate-program

George Mason University, College of Science, School of Systems Biology, Fairfax, VA 22030. Offers bioinformatics and computational biology (MS, PhD, Graduate Certificate); biology (MS); biosciences (PhD). *Faculty:* 11 full-time (2 women), 1 part-time/adjunct (0 women). *Students:* 75 full-time (34 women), 71 part-time (35 women); includes 33 minority (5 Black or African American, non-Hispanic/Latino; 1 American Indian or Alaska Native, non-Hispanic/Latino; 22 Asian, non-Hispanic/Latino; 4 Hispanic/Latino; 1 Native Hawaiian or other Pacific Islander, non-Hispanic/Latino), 38 international. Average age 31. 153 applicants, 45% accepted, 32 enrolled. In 2013, 20 master's, 15 doctorates, 2 other advanced degrees awarded. *Degree requirements:* For master's, research project or thesis; for doctorate, comprehensive exam, thesis/dissertation. *Entrance requirements:* For master's, GRE, resume; 3 letters of recommendation; expanded goals statement; 2 copies of official transcripts; bachelor's degree in related field with minimum GPA of 3.0 in last 60 hours; for doctorate, GRE, self-assessment form; resume; 3 letters of recommendation; expanded goals statement; 2 copies of official transcripts; bachelor's degree in related field with minimum GPA of 3.0 in last 60 hours; for Graduate Certificate, resume; 2 copies of official transcripts. Additional exam requirements/recommendations for international students: Required—TOEFL (minimum score 570 paper-based; 88 iBT), IELTS (minimum score 6.5), PTE. Application fee: $65 ($80 for international students). Electronic applications accepted. *Expenses:* Tuition, state resident: full-time $9350; part-time $390 per credit. Tuition, nonresident: full-time $25,754; part-time $1073 per credit. *Required fees:* $2688; $112 per credit. *Financial support:* In 2013–14, 50 students received support, including 15 fellowships (averaging $3,801 per year), 23 research assistantships with full and partial tuition reimbursements available (averaging $14,040 per year), 33 teaching assistantships with full and partial tuition reimbursements available (averaging $14,053 per year); career-related internships or fieldwork, Federal Work-Study, scholarships/grants, unspecified assistantships, and health care benefits (for full-time research or

teaching assistantship recipients) also available. Support available to part-time students. Financial award application deadline: 3/1; financial award applicants required to submit FAFSA. *Faculty research:* Functional genomics of chronic human diseases, ecology of vector-borne infectious diseases, neurogenetics, molecular biology, computational modeling, proteomics, chronic metabolic diseases, nanotechnology. *Total annual research expenditures:* $886,819. *Unit head:* Dr. James D. Willett, Director, 703-993-8311, Fax: 703-993-8976, E-mail: jwillett@gmu.edu. *Application contact:* Diane St. Germain, Graduate Student Services Coordinator, 703-993-4263, Fax: 703-993-8976, E-mail: dstgerma@gmu.edu.
Website: http://ssb.gmu.edu/

Iowa State University of Science and Technology, Bioinformatics and Computational Biology Program, Ames, IA 50011. Offers MS, PhD. *Degree requirements:* For doctorate, thesis/dissertation. *Entrance requirements:* For master's and doctorate, GRE General Test. Additional exam requirements/recommendations for international students: Recommended—TOEFL, IELTS. Electronic applications accepted. *Faculty research:* Functional and structural genomics, genome evolution, macromolecular structure and function, mathematical biology and biological statistics, metabolic and developmental networks.

Keck Graduate Institute of Applied Life Sciences, Bioscience Program, Claremont, CA 91711. Offers applied life science (PhD); bioscience (MBS); bioscience management (Certificate); computational systems biology (PhD). *Degree requirements:* For master's, comprehensive exam, project. *Entrance requirements:* For master's, GRE General Test or MCAT. Additional exam requirements/recommendations for international students: Required—TOEFL. Electronic applications accepted. *Faculty research:* Computational biology, drug discovery and development, molecular and cellular biology, biomedical engineering, biomaterials and tissue engineering.

Massachusetts Institute of Technology, School of Engineering and School of Science, Program in Computational and Systems Biology, Cambridge, MA 02139-4307. Offers PhD. *Faculty:* 98 full-time (19 women), 8 part-time/adjunct (0 women). *Students:* 35 full-time (13 women); includes 9 minority (6 Asian, non-Hispanic/Latino; 1 Hispanic/Latino; 2 Two or more races, non-Hispanic/Latino), 10 international. Average age 26. 190 applicants, 9% accepted, 7 enrolled. In 2013, 8 doctorates awarded. *Degree requirements:* For doctorate, comprehensive exam, thesis/dissertation. *Entrance requirements:* For doctorate, GRE General Test. Additional exam requirements/recommendations for international students: Required—TOEFL (minimum score 600 paper-based; 95 iBT), IELTS (minimum score 6). *Application deadline:* For fall admission, 12/1 for domestic and international students. Application fee: $75. Electronic applications accepted. *Expenses: Tuition:* Full-time $43,210; part-time $670 per credit hour. *Required fees:* $288. *Financial support:* In 2013–14, 34 students received support, including 16 fellowships (averaging $37,200 per year), 18 research assistantships (averaging $35,200 per year), 1 teaching assistantship (averaging $35,300 per year); Federal Work-Study, institutionally sponsored loans, scholarships/grants, traineeships, health care benefits, and unspecified assistantships also available. *Faculty research:* Computational biology and bioinformatics, biological design and synthetic biology, gene and protein networks, systems biology of cancer, nanobiology and microsystems. *Unit head:* Prof. Douglas A. Lauffenburger, Director, 617-252-1629, E-mail: csbi@mit.edu. *Application contact:* Academic Office, 617-324-4144, Fax: 617-253-8699, E-mail: csbphd@mit.edu.
Website: http://csbi.mit.edu/

Massachusetts Institute of Technology, School of Science, Department of Biology, Cambridge, MA 02139-4307. Offers biochemistry (PhD); biological oceanography (PhD); biology (PhD); biophysical chemistry and molecular structure (PhD); cell biology (PhD); computational and systems biology (PhD); developmental biology (PhD); genetics (PhD); immunology (PhD); microbiology (PhD); molecular biology (PhD); neurobiology (PhD). *Faculty:* 58 full-time (15 women). *Students:* 261 full-time (133 women); includes 77 minority (3 Black or African American, non-Hispanic/Latino; 1 American Indian or Alaska Native, non-Hispanic/Latino; 32 Asian, non-Hispanic/Latino; 32 Hispanic/Latino; 9 Two or more races, non-Hispanic/Latino), 46 international. Average age 26. 651 applicants, 15% accepted, 39 enrolled. In 2013, 25 doctorates awarded. *Degree requirements:* For doctorate, comprehensive exam, thesis/dissertation, two semesters as a teaching assistant. *Entrance requirements:* For doctorate, GRE General Test. Additional exam requirements/recommendations for international students: Required—TOEFL (minimum score 577 paper-based), IELTS (minimum score 6.5). *Application deadline:* For fall admission, 12/1 for domestic and international students. Application fee: $75. Electronic applications accepted. *Expenses: Tuition:* Full-time $43,210; part-time $670 per credit hour. *Required fees:* $288. *Financial support:* In 2013–14, 252 students received support, including 135 fellowships (averaging $36,800 per year), 122 research assistantships (averaging $35,500 per year), 1 teaching assistantship; Federal Work-Study, institutionally sponsored loans, scholarships/grants, traineeships, health care benefits, and unspecified assistantships also available. *Faculty research:* Cellular, developmental and molecular (plant and animal) biology; biochemistry, bioengineering, biophysics and structural biology; classical and molecular genetics, stem cell and epigenetics; immunology and microbiology; cancer biology, molecular medicine, neurobiology and human disease; computational and systems biology. *Total annual research expenditures:* $44.5 million. *Unit head:* Alan Grossman, Interim Head, 617-253-4701. *Application contact:* Biology Education Office, 617-253-3717, Fax: 617-258-9329, E-mail: gradbio@mit.edu.
Website: https://biology.mit.edu/

New Jersey Institute of Technology, College of Science and Liberal Arts, Newark, NJ 07102. Offers applied mathematics (MS); applied physics (M Sc, PhD); applied statistics (MS); biology (MS, PhD); biostatistics (MS); chemistry (MS, PhD); computational biology (MS); environmental science (MS, PhD); history (MA, MAT); materials science and engineering (MS, PhD); mathematical and computational finance (MS); mathematics science (PhD); pharmaceutical chemistry (MS); professional and technical communications (MS). Part-time and evening/weekend programs available. *Faculty:* 150 full-time (33 women), 76 part-time/adjunct (27 women). *Students:* 245 full-time (97 women), 115 part-time (49 women); includes 75 minority (26 Black or African American, non-Hispanic/Latino; 1 American Indian or Alaska Native, non-Hispanic/Latino; 35 Asian, non-Hispanic/Latino; 12 Hispanic/Latino; 1 Native Hawaiian or other Pacific Islander, non-Hispanic/Latino), 189 international. Average age 30. 754 applicants, 59% accepted, 109 enrolled. In 2013, 104 master's, 29 doctorates awarded. Terminal master's awarded for partial completion of doctoral program. *Degree requirements:* For master's, thesis optional; for doctorate, thesis/dissertation. *Entrance requirements:* For master's, GRE General Test; for doctorate, GRE General Test, minimum graduate GPA of 3.5. Additional exam requirements/recommendations for international students: Required—TOEFL (minimum score 550 paper-based; 79 iBT). *Application deadline:* For fall admission, 6/1 priority date for domestic students, 5/1 priority date for international students; for spring admission, 11/15 priority date for domestic and international students. Applications are processed on a rolling basis. Application fee: $65. Electronic applications accepted. *Expenses:* Tuition, state resident: full-time $17,384; part-time $945 per credit. Tuition, nonresident: full-time $25,404; part-time $1341 per credit. *Required fees:* $2396; $118 per credit. *Financial support:* Fellowships with full tuition reimbursements, research assistantships with full tuition reimbursements, and teaching assistantships with full tuition reimbursements available. Financial award application deadline: 1/15. *Total annual research expenditures:* $6.9 million. *Unit head:* Dr. Fadi P. Deek, Dean, 973-596-3676, Fax: 973-565-0586, E-mail: fadi.deek@njit.edu. *Application contact:* Kathryn Kelly, Director of Admissions, 973-596-3300, Fax: 973-596-3461, E-mail: admissions@njit.edu.
Website: http://csla.njit.edu/

New York University, Graduate School of Arts and Science, Department of Biology, Program in Computational Biology, New York, NY 10012-1019. Offers PhD. *Students:* 9 full-time (6 women), 3 part-time (0 women); includes 1 minority (Asian, non-Hispanic/Latino), 5 international. Average age 29. In 2013, 3 doctorates awarded. *Entrance requirements:* For doctorate, GRE. Additional exam requirements/recommendations for international students: Required—TOEFL. *Application deadline:* For fall admission, 12/1 for domestic and international students. Application fee: $95. *Expenses: Tuition:* Full-time $35,856; part-time $1494 per unit. *Required fees:* $1408; $64 per unit. $473 per term. Tuition and fees vary according to course load and program. *Financial support:* Fellowships, research assistantships, teaching assistantships, Federal Work-Study, institutionally sponsored loans, scholarships/grants, health care benefits, and unspecified assistantships available. Financial award application deadline: 12/1. *Unit head:* Stephen Small, Chair, 212-998-8200, Fax: 212-995-4015, E-mail: biology@nyu.edu. *Application contact:* Justin Blau, Director of Graduate Studies, PhD Programs, 212-998-8200, Fax: 212-995-4015, E-mail: biology@nyu.edu.

New York University, School of Medicine and Graduate School of Arts and Science, Sackler Institute of Graduate Biomedical Sciences, Program in Computational Biology, New York, NY 10012-1019. Offers PhD. *Faculty:* 9 full-time (1 woman). *Students:* 3 full-time (2 women); includes 2 minority (both Asian, non-Hispanic/Latino), 1 international. Average age 29. *Expenses: Tuition:* Full-time $35,856; part-time $1494 per unit. *Required fees:* $1408; $64 per unit. $473 per term. Tuition and fees vary according to course load and program. *Faculty research:* Protein engineering, cheminformatics and rational drug design; bioinformatics; computational methods to analyze the transcriptional regulation of the mammalian cell cycle. *Unit head:* Dr. Joel D. Oppenheim, Senior Associate Dean for Graduate Studies, 212-263-8001, Fax: 212-263-7600. *Application contact:* Michael Escosia, Program Associate, 212-263-5648, Fax: 212-263-7600, E-mail: sackler-info@med.nyu.edu.
Website: http://cob.as.nyu.edu/page/home

Oregon Health & Science University, School of Medicine, Graduate Programs in Medicine, Department of Medical Informatics and Clinical Epidemiology, Portland, OR 97239-3098. Offers clinical informatics (MS, PhD, Certificate); computational biology (MS, PhD); health information management (Certificate). Part-time programs available. Postbaccalaureate distance learning degree programs offered (minimal on-campus study). *Faculty:* 28 full-time (17 women), 59 part-time/adjunct (24 women). *Students:* 20 full-time (11 women), 103 part-time (37 women); includes 33 minority (7 Black or African American, non-Hispanic/Latino; 17 Asian, non-Hispanic/Latino; 4 Hispanic/Latino; 5 Two or more races, non-Hispanic/Latino), 10 international. Average age 42. 125 applicants, 29% accepted, 36 enrolled. In 2013, 31 master's, 3 doctorates, 71 other advanced degrees awarded. Terminal master's awarded for partial completion of doctoral program. *Degree requirements:* For master's, thesis optional, thesis or capstone project; for doctorate, comprehensive exam, thesis/dissertation, qualifying exam. *Entrance requirements:* For master's and doctorate, GRE General Test (minimum scores: 153 Verbal/148 Quantitative/4.5 Analytical), coursework in computer programming, human anatomy and physiology. Additional exam requirements/recommendations for international students: Required—TOEFL. *Application deadline:* For fall admission, 12/1 for domestic students; for winter admission, 11/1 for domestic students; for spring admission, 2/1 for domestic students. Applications are processed on a rolling basis. Application fee: $70. Electronic applications accepted. *Expenses:* Contact institution. *Financial support:* Fellowships with full tuition reimbursements, research assistantships, Federal Work-Study, institutionally sponsored loans, scholarships/grants, health care benefits, and full tuition and stipends (for PhD students) available. Financial award application deadline: 3/1; financial award applicants required to submit FAFSA. *Faculty research:* Use of knowledge-based information by healthcare practitioners and researchers, application of text mining and machine learning techniques to the scientific literature curated databases, examining factors that affect quality of data collected in healthcare databases and the subsequent uses of that data, statistical analysis of microarray data with emphasis on time series analysis, computational biology and automatic speech recognition. *Unit head:* Dr. Allison Fryer, Associate Dean for Graduate Studies, 503-494-6222, Fax: 503-494-3400, E-mail: somgrad@ohsu.edu. *Application contact:* Lauren Ludwig, Administrative Coordinator, 503-494-2252, E-mail: informat@ohsu.edu.
Website: http://www.ohsu.edu/dmice/

Princeton University, Graduate School, Department of Molecular Biology, Princeton, NJ 08544-1019. Offers PhD. *Degree requirements:* For doctorate, thesis/dissertation. *Entrance requirements:* For doctorate, GRE General Test. Additional exam requirements/recommendations for international students: Required—TOEFL (minimum score 600 paper-based). Electronic applications accepted. *Faculty research:* Genetics, virology, biochemistry.

Rutgers, The State University of New Jersey, Camden, Graduate School of Arts and Sciences, Program in Computational and Integrative Biology, Camden, NJ 08102-1401. Offers MS, PhD. *Degree requirements:* For doctorate, original research, oral defense. *Entrance requirements:* For master's and doctorate, GRE General Test; GRE Subject Test (recommended), transcripts, personal statement, three letters of recommendation. Additional exam requirements/recommendations for international students: Required—TOEFL. Electronic applications accepted.

Rutgers, The State University of New Jersey, Newark, Graduate School, Program in Computational Biology, Newark, NJ 07102. Offers MS. Program offered jointly with New Jersey Institute of Technology. *Entrance requirements:* For master's, GRE, minimum undergraduate B average. Additional exam requirements/recommendations for international students: Required—TOEFL.

Rutgers, The State University of New Jersey, New Brunswick, Graduate School-New Brunswick, BioMaPS Institute for Quantitative Biology, Piscataway, NJ 08854-8097. Offers computational biology and molecular biophysics (PhD). *Degree requirements:* For doctorate, comprehensive exam, thesis/dissertation. *Entrance requirements:* For doctorate, GRE. Additional exam requirements/recommendations for international students: Required—TOEFL. Electronic applications accepted. *Faculty research:* Structural biology, systems biology, bioinformatics, translational medicine, genomics.

University of California, Irvine, School of Biological Sciences, Program in Mathematical, Computational and Systems Biology, Irvine, CA 92697. Offers PhD. *Students:* 11 full-time (5 women); includes 1 minority (Hispanic/Latino), 4 international. Average age 24. 80 applicants, 29% accepted, 11 enrolled. Application fee: $80 ($100 for international students). *Unit head:* Prof. Arthur D. Lander, Director, 949-824-1721, Fax: 949-824-4709, E-mail: adlander@uci.edu. *Application contact:* Aracely Dean,

Assistant Administrative Analyst, 949-824-4120, Fax: 949-824-6444, E-mail: mcsb@uci.edu.
Website: http://mcsb.bio.uci.edu/

University of Colorado Denver, College of Liberal Arts and Sciences, Department of Mathematical and Statistical Sciences, Denver, CO 80217. Offers applied mathematics (MS, PhD), including applied mathematics, applied probability (MS), applied statistics (MS), computational biology, computational mathematics (PhD), discrete mathematics, finite geometry (PhD), mathematics education (PhD), mathematics of engineering and science (MS), numerical analysis, operations research (MS), optimization and operations research (PhD), probability (PhD), statistics (PhD). Part-time programs available. *Faculty:* 20 full-time (6 women), 6 part-time/adjunct (0 women). *Students:* 41 full-time (10 women), 8 part-time (2 women); includes 10 minority (1 Black or African American, non-Hispanic/Latino; 4 Asian, non-Hispanic/Latino; 4 Hispanic/Latino; 1 Two or more races, non-Hispanic/Latino), 13 international. Average age 30. 75 applicants, 56% accepted, 9 enrolled. In 2013, 6 master's, 5 doctorates awarded. *Degree requirements:* For master's, comprehensive exam, thesis optional, 30 hours of course work with minimum GPA of 3.0; for doctorate, comprehensive exam, thesis/dissertation, 42 hours of course work with minimum GPA of 3.25. *Entrance requirements:* For master's, GRE General Test; GRE Subject Test in math (recommended), 30 hours of course work in mathematics (24 of which must be upper-division mathematics), bachelor's degree with minimum GPA of 3.0; for doctorate, GRE General Test; GRE Subject Test in math (recommended), 30 hours of course work in mathematics (24 of which must be upper-division mathematics), master's degree with minimum GPA of 3.25. Additional exam requirements/recommendations for international students: Required—TOEFL (minimum score 537 paper-based; 75 iBT); Recommended—IELTS (minimum score 6.5). *Application deadline:* For fall admission, 2/1 for domestic students, 2/1 priority date for international students; for spring admission, 10/1 for domestic students, 10/1 priority date for international students. Application fee: $50 ($75 for international students). Electronic applications accepted. *Financial support:* In 2013–14, 28 students received support. Fellowships with partial tuition reimbursements available, research assistantships with full tuition reimbursements available, teaching assistantships with full tuition reimbursements available, Federal Work-Study, institutionally sponsored loans, scholarships/grants, and traineeships available. Financial award application deadline: 4/1; financial award applicants required to submit FAFSA. *Faculty research:* Computational mathematics, computational biology, discrete mathematics and geometry, probability and statistics, optimization. *Unit head:* Dr. Jan Mandel, Professor and Chair, 303-315-1703, E-mail: jan.mandel@ucdenver.edu. *Application contact:* Margie Bopp, Graduate Program Assistant, 303-556-2341, E-mail: margie.bopp@ucdenver.edu.
Website: http://www.ucdenver.edu/academics/colleges/CLAS/Departments/math/Pages/MathStats.aspx

University of Colorado Denver, School of Medicine, Program in Computational Bioscience, Aurora, CO 80045-0511. Offers PhD. Part-time programs available. *Students:* 13 full-time (4 women); includes 2 minority (1 Black or African American, non-Hispanic/Latino; 1 Hispanic/Latino), 1 international. Average age 32. 11 applicants, 27% accepted, 3 enrolled. In 2013, 1 doctorate awarded. *Degree requirements:* For doctorate, comprehensive exam, thesis/dissertation, minimum of 30 semester credit hours of course work and 30 semester hours of dissertation research. *Entrance requirements:* For doctorate, GRE General Test, GRE Subject Test in computer science (recommended), demonstrated adequate computational and biological backgrounds, interviews. Additional exam requirements/recommendations for international students: Required—TOEFL (minimum score 550 paper-based; 80 iBT). *Application deadline:* For fall admission, 12/1 for domestic students, 11/1 for international students. Application fee: $50 ($75 for international students). Electronic applications accepted. *Expenses:* Contact institution. *Financial support:* In 2013–14, 13 students received support. Fellowships, research assistantships, teaching assistantships, Federal Work-Study, institutionally sponsored loans, scholarships/grants, traineeships, health care benefits, tuition waivers (full), and unspecified assistantships available. Financial award application deadline: 4/1; financial award applicants required to submit FAFSA. *Faculty research:* Physical simulations of biological macromolecules and their dynamics, gene expression array analysis and interpretation of expression data, natural language processing in the biomedical literature, metabolic and signaling pathway analysis, evolutionary reconstruction and disease gene finding. *Unit head:* Dr. Larry Hunter, Director, 303-724-3574, E-mail: larry.hunter@ucdenver.edu. *Application contact:* Kathleen Thomas, Administrative Coordinator, 303-724-3399, Fax: 303-724-6881, E-mail: kathy.r.thomas@ucdenver.edu.
Website: http://compbio.ucdenver.edu/

University of Idaho, College of Graduate Studies, Program in Bioinformatics and Computational Biology, Moscow, ID 83844-3051. Offers MS, PhD. *Faculty:* 14 full-time. *Students:* 16 full-time, 3 part-time. Average age 30. In 2013, 2 master's, 1 doctorate awarded. *Entrance requirements:* For master's, GRE, minimum GPA of 2.8. Additional exam requirements/recommendations for international students: Required—TOEFL. *Application deadline:* For fall admission, 8/1 for domestic students; for spring admission, 12/15 for domestic students. Applications are processed on a rolling basis. Application fee: $60. Electronic applications accepted. *Expenses:* Tuition, state resident: full-time $5596; part-time $363 per credit hour. Tuition, nonresident: full-time $18,672; part-time $1089 per credit hour. *Financial support:* Applicants required to submit FAFSA. *Unit head:* Dr. David Tank, Director, 208-885-6010, E-mail: bcb@uidaho.edu. *Application contact:* Stephanie Thomas, Graduate Recruitment Coordinator, 208-885-4001, Fax: 208-885-4406, E-mail: gadms@uidaho.edu.
Website: http://www.uidaho.edu/cogs/bcb

University of Illinois at Urbana–Champaign, Graduate College, College of Liberal Arts and Sciences, School of Molecular and Cellular Biology, Center for Biophysics and Computational Biology, Champaign, IL 61820. Offers MS, PhD. *Students:* 52 (13 women). Application fee: $75 ($90 for international students). *Unit head:* Taekjip Ha, Director, 217-265-0717, Fax: 217-244-3186, E-mail: tjha@illinois.edu. *Application contact:* Cynthia Dodds, Office Administrator, 217-333-1630, Fax: 217-244-6615, E-mail: dodds@illinois.edu.
Website: http://biophysics.illinois.edu/

The University of Iowa, Graduate College, Program in Informatics, Iowa City, IA 52242-1316. Offers bioinformatics (MS, PhD); bioinformatics and computational biology (Certificate); geoinformatics (MS, PhD, Certificate); health informatics (MS, PhD, Certificate); information science (MS, PhD, Certificate). *Degree requirements:* For master's, thesis optional; for doctorate, comprehensive exam, thesis/dissertation. *Entrance requirements:* For master's and doctorate, GRE General Test, minimum GPA of 3.0. Additional exam requirements/recommendations for international students: Required—TOEFL (minimum score 550 paper-based; 81 iBT). Electronic applications accepted.

The University of Kansas, Graduate Studies, College of Liberal Arts and Sciences, Bioinformatics Program, Lawrence, KS 66045. Offers bioinformatics and computational biology (PhD). *Faculty:* 5. *Students:* 16 full-time (6 women); includes 2 minority (both Asian, non-Hispanic/Latino), 10 international. Average age 29. 22 applicants, 14% accepted, 3 enrolled. In 2013, 2 doctorates awarded. *Entrance requirements:* For doctorate, bachelor's or master's degree in natural sciences, mathematics, engineering, or another relevant field. Additional exam requirements/recommendations for international students: Required—TOEFL. *Application deadline:* For fall admission, 12/15 for domestic and international students. Application fee: $55 ($65 for international students). *Faculty research:* Life sciences, computational modeling tools, community-wide activities in bioinformatics, education for the new generation of researchers. *Unit head:* Illya Vakser, Director, 785-864-1057, E-mail: jjray@ku.edu. *Application contact:* Jeanette Atkinson, Admissions Contact, 785-864-1057, E-mail: jean@ku.edu.
Website: http://www.bioinformatics.ku.edu/

University of Maryland, College Park, Academic Affairs, College of Computer, Mathematical and Natural Sciences, Department of Biology, PhD Program in Biological Sciences, College Park, MD 20742. Offers behavior, ecology, evolution, and systematics (PhD); computational biology, bioinformatics, and genomics (PhD); molecular and cellular biology (PhD); physiological systems (PhD). *Students:* 104 full-time (59 women), 4 part-time (1 woman); includes 21 minority (2 Black or African American, non-Hispanic/Latino; 1 American Indian or Alaska Native, non-Hispanic/Latino; 9 Asian, non-Hispanic/Latino; 7 Hispanic/Latino; 2 Two or more races, non-Hispanic/Latino), 34 international. 365 applicants, 13% accepted, 20 enrolled. In 2013, 5 doctorates awarded. *Degree requirements:* For doctorate, comprehensive exam, thesis/dissertation, thesis work presentation in seminar. *Entrance requirements:* For doctorate, GRE General Test; GRE Subject Test in biology (recommended), academic transcripts, statement of purpose/research interests, 3 letters of recommendation. Additional exam requirements/recommendations for international students: Required—TOEFL. *Application deadline:* For fall admission, 12/15 for domestic and international students. Applications are processed on a rolling basis. Application fee: $75. Electronic applications accepted. *Expenses:* Tuition, state resident: full-time $10,314; part-time $573 per credit hour. Tuition, nonresident: full-time $22,248; part-time $1236 per credit. *Required fees:* $1446; $403.15 per semester. Tuition and fees vary according to program. *Financial support:* In 2013–14, 21 fellowships with full and partial tuition reimbursements (averaging $27,603 per year), 25 research assistantships (averaging $19,557 per year), 55 teaching assistantships (averaging $18,959 per year) were awarded. *Unit head:* Dr. Charles F. Delwiche, Director, 301-405-6884, E-mail: bisidirector@umd.edu. *Application contact:* Dr. Charles A. Caramello, Dean of Graduate School, 301-405-0358, Fax: 301-314-9305, E-mail: ccaramel@umd.edu.
Website: http://www.bisi.umd.edu/

University of Massachusetts Worcester, Graduate School of Biomedical Sciences, Worcester, MA 01655-0115. Offers biochemistry and molecular pharmacology (PhD); bioinformatics and computational biology (PhD); cancer biology (PhD); cell biology (PhD); clinical and population health research (PhD); clinical investigation (MS); immunology and virology (PhD); interdisciplinary biomedical research (PhD); millennium (PhD); molecular genetics and microbiology (PhD); neuroscience (PhD); translational science (PhD); MD/PhD. *Faculty:* 1,388 full-time (521 women), 309 part-time/adjunct (198 women). *Students:* 385 full-time (210 women); includes 53 minority (13 Black or African American, non-Hispanic/Latino; 30 Asian, non-Hispanic/Latino; 10 Hispanic/Latino), 138 international. Average age 28. 491 applicants, 19% accepted, 39 enrolled. In 2013, 5 master's, 50 doctorates awarded. Terminal master's awarded for partial completion of doctoral program. *Median time to degree:* Of those who began their doctoral program in fall 2005, 67% received their degree in 8 years or less. *Degree requirements:* For master's, comprehensive exam, thesis; for doctorate, comprehensive exam, thesis/dissertation. *Entrance requirements:* For master's, MD, PhD, DVM, or PharmD; for doctorate, GRE General Test, bachelor's degree. Additional exam requirements/recommendations for international students: Required—TOEFL (minimum score 100 iBT) or IELTS (minimum score 7.5). *Application deadline:* For fall admission, 12/15 for domestic and international students; for spring admission, 5/15 for domestic students. Application fee: $80. Electronic applications accepted. *Expenses:* Contact institution. *Financial support:* In 2013–14, 431 students received support, including research assistantships with full tuition reimbursements available (averaging $29,500 per year); scholarships/grants, health care benefits, tuition waivers (full), and unspecified assistantships also available. Financial award application deadline: 5/16. *Faculty research:* RNA interference, cell/molecular/developmental biology, bioinformatics, clinical/translational research, infectious disease. *Total annual research expenditures:* $245.9 million. *Unit head:* Dr. Anthony Carruthers, Dean, 508-856-4135, E-mail: anthony.carruthers@umassmed.edu. *Application contact:* Dr. Kendall Knight, Associate Dean and Interim Director of Admissions and Recruitment, 508-856-5628, Fax: 508-856-3659, E-mail: kendall.knight@umassmed.edu.
Website: http://www.umassmed.edu/gsbs/

The University of North Carolina at Chapel Hill, School of Medicine and Graduate School, Graduate Programs in Medicine, Curriculum in Bioinformatics and Computational Biology, Chapel Hill, NC 27599. Offers PhD. *Degree requirements:* For doctorate, comprehensive exam, thesis/dissertation. *Entrance requirements:* For doctorate, GRE, minimum GPA of 3.0. Additional exam requirements/recommendations for international students: Required—TOEFL. Electronic applications accepted. *Faculty research:* Protein folding, design and evolution and molecular biophysics of disease; mathematical modeling of signaling pathways and regulatory networks; bioinformatics, medical informatics, user interface design; statistical genetics and genetic epidemiology datamining, classification and clustering analysis of gene-expression data.

University of Pennsylvania, Perelman School of Medicine, Biomedical Graduate Studies, Graduate Group in Genomics and Computational Biology, Philadelphia, PA 19104. Offers PhD, MD/PhD, VMD/PhD. *Faculty:* 70. *Students:* 35 full-time (12 women); includes 11 minority (9 Asian, non-Hispanic/Latino; 2 Hispanic/Latino), 8 international. 75 applicants, 27% accepted, 5 enrolled. In 2013, 4 doctorates awarded. *Degree requirements:* For doctorate, thesis/dissertation. *Entrance requirements:* For doctorate, GRE. Additional exam requirements/recommendations for international students: Required—TOEFL. *Application deadline:* For fall admission, 12/1 priority date for domestic and international students. Applications are processed on a rolling basis. Application fee: $80. Electronic applications accepted. *Financial support:* In 2013–14, 35 students received support. Fellowships, research assistantships, scholarships/grants, traineeships, and unspecified assistantships available. *Unit head:* Dr. Maja Bucan, Chairperson, 215-898-0020. *Application contact:* Hannah Chervitz, Graduate Coordinator, 215-746-2807.
Website: http://www.med.upenn.edu/gcb/

University of Pittsburgh, School of Medicine, Computational Biology Graduate Program, Pittsburgh, PA 15260. Offers PhD. PhD jointly offered by the University of Pittsburgh and Carnegie Mellon University. *Faculty:* 86 full-time (17 women). *Students:* 52 full-time (18 women); includes 9 minority (6 Asian, non-Hispanic/Latino; 2 Hispanic/Latino; 1 Native Hawaiian or other Pacific Islander, non-Hispanic/Latino), 20 international. Average age 25. 130 applicants, 18% accepted, 8 enrolled. In 2013, 8 doctorates awarded. Terminal master's awarded for partial completion of doctoral program. *Degree requirements:* For doctorate, comprehensive exam, thesis/dissertation, ethics training service as course assistant, seminar. *Entrance requirements:* For doctorate, GRE Subject Test (recommended), GRE General Test, 3 letters of recommendation, resume. Additional exam requirements/recommendations for international students: Required—TOEFL (minimum score 600 paper-based; 100 iBT).

Application deadline: For fall admission, 12/15 priority date for domestic and international students. Application fee: $50. Electronic applications accepted. *Expenses:* Tuition, state resident: full-time $19,964; part-time $807 per credit. Tuition, nonresident: full-time $32,686; part-time $1337 per credit. *Required fees:* $740; $200. Tuition and fees vary according to program. *Financial support:* In 2013–14, 44 students received support, including 8 fellowships with full tuition reimbursements available, 44 research assistantships with full tuition reimbursements available (averaging $26,010 per year). *Faculty research:* Computational structural biology, computational genomics, cell and systems modeling, bioimage informatics, computational neurobiology. *Unit head:* Dr. Daniel M. Zuckerman, Director, 412-648-3335, Fax: 412-648-3163, E-mail: ddmmzz@pitt.edu. *Application contact:* Kelly Gentille, Educational Programs Administrator, 412-648-8107, Fax: 412-648-3163, E-mail: kmg120@pitt.edu.
Website: http://www.compbio.pitt.edu/

University of Rochester, School of Medicine and Dentistry, Graduate Programs in Medicine and Dentistry, Department of Biochemistry and Biophysics, Programs in Biophysics, Rochester, NY 14627. Offers biophysics, structural and computational biology (PhD). Terminal master's awarded for partial completion of doctoral program. *Degree requirements:* For doctorate, thesis/dissertation, qualifying exam. *Entrance requirements:* For doctorate, GRE General Test. *Expenses: Tuition:* Full-time $44,580; part-time $1394 per credit hour. *Required fees:* $492.

University of Southern California, Graduate School, Dana and David Dornsife College of Letters, Arts and Sciences, Department of Biological Sciences, Program in Molecular and Computational Biology, Los Angeles, CA 90089. Offers computational biology and bioinformatics (PhD); molecular biology (PhD). *Degree requirements:* For doctorate, comprehensive exam, thesis/dissertation, qualifying examination, dissertation defense. *Entrance requirements:* For doctorate, GRE, 3 letters of recommendation, personal statement, resume, minimum GPA of 3.0. Additional exam requirements/recommendations for international students: Required—TOEFL (minimum score 600 paper-based; 100 iBT). Electronic applications accepted. *Faculty research:* Biochemistry and molecular biology; genomics; computational biology and bioinformatics; cell and developmental biology, and genetics; DNA replication and repair, and cancer biology.

University of South Florida, Morsani College of Medicine and Graduate School, Graduate Programs in Medical Sciences, Tampa, FL 33620-9951. Offers aging and neuroscience (MSMS); allergy, immunology and infectious disease (PhD); anatomy (MSMS, PhD); athletic training (MSMS); bioinformatics and computational biology (MSBCB); biotechnology (MSB); clinical and translational research (MSMS, PhD); health informatics (MSHI, MSMS); health science (MSMS); interdisciplinary medical sciences (MSMS); medical microbiology and immunology (MSMS); metabolic and nutritional medicine (MSMS); molecular medicine (MSMS, PhD); molecular pharmacology and physiology (PhD); neurology (PhD); pathology and laboratory medicine (PhD); pharmacology and therapeutics (PhD); physiology and biophysics (PhD); women's health (MSMS). *Students:* 336 full-time (182 women), 39 part-time (21 women); includes 170 minority (45 Black or African American, non-Hispanic/Latino; 54 Asian, non-Hispanic/Latino; 59 Hispanic/Latino; 2 Native Hawaiian or other Pacific Islander, non-Hispanic/Latino; 10 Two or more races, non-Hispanic/Latino), 17 international. Average age 26. 1,066 applicants, 44% accepted, 250 enrolled. In 2013, 191 master's, 12 doctorates awarded. Terminal master's awarded for partial completion of doctoral program. *Degree requirements:* For master's, comprehensive exam, thesis; for doctorate, comprehensive exam, thesis/dissertation. *Entrance requirements:* For master's, GRE General Test or GMAT, bachelor's degree or equivalent from regionally-accredited university with minimum GPA of 3.0 in upper-division sciences coursework; prerequisites in general biology, general chemistry, general physics, organic chemistry, quantitative analysis, and integral and differential calculus; for doctorate, GRE General Test (minimum score of 600 quantitative), bachelor's degree from regionally-accredited university with minimum GPA of 3.0 in upper-division sciences coursework; 3 letters of recommendation; personal interview; 1-2 page personal statement; prerequisites in biology, chemistry, physics, organic chemistry, quantitative analysis, and integral/differential calculus. Additional exam requirements/recommendations for international students: Required—TOEFL (minimum score 550 paper-based; 79 iBT) or IELTS (minimum score 6.5). *Application deadline:* For fall admission, 2/15 for domestic students, 1/2 for international students. Application fee: $30. *Expenses:* Contact institution. *Faculty research:* Anatomy, biochemistry, cancer biology, cardiovascular disease, cell biology, immunology, microbiology, molecular biology, neuroscience, pharmacology, physiology. *Unit head:* Dr. Michael Barber, Professor and Associate Dean for Graduate and Postdoctoral Affairs, 813-974-9908, Fax: 813-974-4317, E-mail: mbarber@health.usf.edu. *Application contact:* Dr. Eric Bennett, Graduate Director, PhD Program in Medical Sciences, 813-974-1545, Fax: 813-974-4317, E-mail: esbennet@health.usf.edu.
Website: http://health.usf.edu/nocms/medicine/graduatestudies/

The University of Texas Medical Branch, Graduate School of Biomedical Sciences, Program in Biochemistry and Molecular Biology, Galveston, TX 77555. Offers biochemistry (PhD); bioinformatics (PhD); biophysics (PhD); cell biology (PhD); computational biology (PhD); structural biology (PhD). *Degree requirements:* For doctorate, thesis/dissertation. *Entrance requirements:* Additional exam requirements/recommendations for international students: Required—TOEFL (minimum score 550 paper-based). Electronic applications accepted.

University of Wyoming, Graduate Program in Molecular and Cellular Life Sciences, Laramie, WY 82071. Offers PhD. *Degree requirements:* For doctorate, thesis/dissertation, four eight-week laboratory rotations, comprehensive basic practical exam, two-part qualifying exam, seminars, symposium.

Washington University in St. Louis, Graduate School of Arts and Sciences, Division of Biology and Biomedical Sciences, Program in Computational and Systems Biology, St. Louis, MO 63130-4899. Offers PhD. *Degree requirements:* For doctorate, thesis/dissertation. Electronic applications accepted.

Wayne State University, College of Engineering, Department of Computer Science, Detroit, MI 48202. Offers computer science (MA, MS, PhD), including bioinformatics (PhD), computational biology (PhD), computer science (PhD); scientific computing (Graduate Certificate). *Students:* 141 full-time (34 women), 48 part-time (18 women); includes 28 minority (3 Black or African American, non-Hispanic/Latino; 22 Asian, non-Hispanic/Latino; 1 Native Hawaiian or other Pacific Islander, non-Hispanic/Latino; 2 Two or more races, non-Hispanic/Latino), 137 international. Average age 28. 311 applicants, 49% accepted, 56 enrolled. In 2013, 35 master's, 9 doctorates awarded. *Degree requirements:* For master's, thesis (for some programs); for doctorate, thesis/dissertation. *Entrance requirements:* For master's, GRE (minimum scores: 450 Verbal, 750 Quantitative, 4.5 Analytical writing), minimum GPA of 3.0, three letters of recommendation, adequate preparation in computer science and mathematics courses, personal statement; for doctorate, GRE (minimum scores: 450 Verbal, 750 Quantitative, 4.5 Analytical writing), minimum GPA of 3.3 in most recent degree; three letters of recommendation; personal statement; adequate preparation in computer science and mathematics courses. Additional exam requirements/recommendations for international students: Required—TOEFL (minimum score 550 paper-based; 79 iBT), TWE (minimum score 5.5), Michigan English Language Assessment Battery (minimum score 85); Recommended—IELTS (minimum score 6.5). *Application deadline:* For fall admission, 7/1 priority date for domestic students, 5/1 priority date for international students; for winter admission, 11/1 priority date for domestic students, 9/1 priority date for international students; for spring admission, 3/15 priority date for domestic students, 1/2 priority date for international students. Applications are processed on a rolling basis. Application fee: $0. Electronic applications accepted. *Expenses:* Contact institution. *Financial support:* In 2013–14, 90 students received support, including 6 fellowships with tuition reimbursements available (averaging $15,926 per year), 26 research assistantships with tuition reimbursements available (averaging $22,229 per year), 27 teaching assistantships with tuition reimbursements available (averaging $18,071 per year); career-related internships or fieldwork, Federal Work-Study, scholarships/grants, health care benefits, and unspecified assistantships also available. Financial award application deadline: 3/31; financial award applicants required to submit FAFSA. *Faculty research:* Software engineering, databases, bioinformatics, artificial intelligence, networking, distributed and parallel computing, security, graphics, visualizations. *Total annual research expenditures:* $2.4 million. *Unit head:* Dr. Xuewen Chen, Chair, 313-577-2478, E-mail: xwchen@wayne.edu.
Website: http://engineering.wayne.edu/cs/

Wayne State University, School of Medicine, Graduate Programs in Medicine, Program in Molecular Biology and Genetics, Detroit, MI 48201. Offers bioinformatics and computational biology (PhD); cellular neuroscience (PhD); MD/PhD. *Students:* 21 full-time (11 women), 1 part-time (0 women); includes 1 minority (Hispanic/Latino), 3 international. Average age 27. 45 applicants, 13% accepted, 4 enrolled. In 2013, 5 doctorates awarded. Terminal master's awarded for partial completion of doctoral program. *Degree requirements:* For doctorate, thesis/dissertation. *Entrance requirements:* For doctorate, GRE General Test, GRE Subject Test (chemistry or biology), minimum GPA of 3.0, strong background in one of the chemical or biological sciences, three letters of recommendation, personal statement, interview. Additional exam requirements/recommendations for international students: Required—TOEFL (minimum score 550 paper-based; 79 iBT), Michigan English Language Assessment Battery (minimum score 85); Recommended—IELTS (minimum score 6.5), TWE (minimum score 5.5). *Application deadline:* For fall admission, 3/1 for domestic students, 5/1 for international students; for winter admission, 10/1 for domestic students, 9/1 for international students; for spring admission, 2/1 for domestic students, 1/1 for international students. Applications are processed on a rolling basis. Application fee: $0. Electronic applications accepted. *Expenses:* Tuition, state resident: part-time $554.15 per credit. Tuition, nonresident: part-time $1200.35 per credit. *Required fees:* $42.15 per credit. $268.30 per semester. Tuition and fees vary according to course load and program. *Financial support:* In 2013–14, 18 students received support. Fellowships with tuition reimbursements available, research assistantships with tuition reimbursements available, teaching assistantships with tuition reimbursements available, scholarships/grants, and unspecified assistantships available. Financial award application deadline: 3/31; financial award applicants required to submit FAFSA. *Faculty research:* Human gene mapping, genome organization and sequencing, gene regulation, molecular evolution. *Total annual research expenditures:* $2.6 million. *Unit head:* Dr. Lawrence Grossman, Director, 313-577-5323, E-mail: l.grossman@wayne.edu. *Application contact:* Dr. Gregory Kapatos, Professor, Director for Education, and Graduate Officer, 313-577-5965, Fax: 313-993-4269, E-mail: gkapato@med.wayne.edu.
Website: http://genetics.wayne.edu/students/mdphd.php

Weill Cornell Medical College, Weill Cornell Graduate School of Medical Sciences, Tri-Institutional Training Program in Computational Biology and Medicine, New York, NY 10065. Offers PhD. Terminal master's awarded for partial completion of doctoral program. *Degree requirements:* For doctorate, comprehensive exam, thesis/dissertation. *Entrance requirements:* For doctorate, GRE General Test, three letters of recommendation. Additional exam requirements/recommendations for international students: Required—TOEFL. Electronic applications accepted. *Faculty research:* Biophysics/structural biology, genomics/bioinformatics, modeling/systems biology, neuroscience, cancer biology.

Worcester Polytechnic Institute, Graduate Studies and Research, Program in Bioinformatics and Computational Biology, Worcester, MA 01609-2280. Offers MS, PhD. *Students:* 3 full-time (1 woman), 2 part-time (0 women), 2 international. 5 applicants, 80% accepted, 2 enrolled. *Entrance requirements:* For master's and doctorate, GRE, 3 letters of recommendation, statement of purpose. Additional exam requirements/recommendations for international students: Required—TOEFL (minimum score 563 paper-based; 84 iBT), IELTS (minimum score 7). *Application deadline:* For fall admission, 1/1 priority date for domestic and international students; for spring admission, 10/1 priority date for domestic and international students. Applications are processed on a rolling basis. Electronic applications accepted. *Financial support:* Research assistantships, teaching assistantships, and career-related internships or fieldwork available. Financial award application deadline: 1/1; financial award applicants required to submit FAFSA. *Unit head:* Elizabeth Ryder, Professor, 508-831-5543, Fax: 508-831-5936, E-mail: ryder@wpi.edu. *Application contact:* Lynne Dougherty, Administrative Assistant, 508-831-5301, Fax: 508-831-5717, E-mail: grad@wpi.edu.
Website: http://www.wpi.edu/academics/bcb/grad-programs.html

Yale University, School of Medicine and Graduate School of Arts and Sciences, Combined Program in Biological and Biomedical Sciences (BBS), Computational Biology and Bioinformatics Track, New Haven, CT 06520. Offers PhD, MD/PhD. *Entrance requirements:* Additional exam requirements/recommendations for international students: Required—TOEFL.

Systems Biology

Albert Einstein College of Medicine, Graduate Division of Biomedical Sciences, Systems and Computational Biology Program, Bronx, NY 10461. Offers PhD.

Dartmouth College, Program in Experimental and Molecular Medicine, Biomedical Physiology Track, Hanover, NH 03755. Offers PhD.

The George Washington University, Columbian College of Arts and Sciences, Institute for Biomedical Sciences, Program in Biochemistry and Systems Biology, Washington, DC 20037. Offers PhD. *Students:* 4 full-time (2 women), 3 part-time (1 woman); includes 3 minority (2 Asian, non-Hispanic/Latino; 1 Hispanic/Latino), 1 international. Average age 30. In 2013, 1 doctorate awarded. Terminal master's awarded for partial completion of doctoral program. *Degree requirements:* For doctorate, thesis/dissertation, general exam. *Entrance requirements:* For doctorate, GRE General Test, interview, minimum GPA of 3.0. Additional exam requirements/recommendations for international students: Required—TOEFL (minimum score 600 paper-based). *Application deadline:* For fall admission, 12/15 priority date for domestic and international students; for spring admission, 10/1 priority date for domestic and international students. Applications are processed on a rolling basis. Application fee: $75. Electronic applications accepted. *Financial support:* In 2013–14, 3 students received support. Fellowships, Federal Work-Study, institutionally sponsored loans, and tuition waivers available. Financial award application deadline: 2/1. *Unit head:* Dr. Eric Hoffman, Director, 202-476-6029, E-mail: ehoffman@cnmcresearch.org. *Application contact:* Information Contact, 202-994-7120, Fax: 202-994-6100, E-mail: genetics@gwu.edu.
Website: http://www.gwumc.edu/ibs/fields/biochemgenetics.html

Harvard University, Graduate School of Arts and Sciences, Department of Systems Biology, Cambridge, MA 02138. Offers PhD. *Degree requirements:* For doctorate, thesis/dissertation, lab rotation, qualifying examination. *Entrance requirements:* For doctorate, GRE. Additional exam requirements/recommendations for international students: Required—TOEFL. Electronic applications accepted. *Expenses: Tuition:* Full-time $38,888. *Required fees:* $958. Tuition and fees vary according to campus/location, program and student level.

Massachusetts Institute of Technology, School of Engineering and School of Science, Program in Computational and Systems Biology, Cambridge, MA 02139-4307. Offers PhD. *Faculty:* 98 full-time (19 women), 8 part-time/adjunct (0 women). *Students:* 35 full-time (13 women); includes 9 minority (6 Asian, non-Hispanic/Latino; 1 Hispanic/Latino; 2 Two or more races, non-Hispanic/Latino), 10 international. Average age 26. 190 applicants, 9% accepted, 7 enrolled. In 2013, 8 doctorates awarded. *Degree requirements:* For doctorate, comprehensive exam, thesis/dissertation. *Entrance requirements:* For doctorate, GRE General Test. Additional exam requirements/recommendations for international students: Required—TOEFL (minimum score 600 paper-based; 95 iBT), IELTS (minimum score 6). *Application deadline:* For fall admission, 12/1 for domestic and international students. Application fee: $75. Electronic applications accepted. *Expenses: Tuition:* Full-time $43,210; part-time $670 per credit hour. *Required fees:* $288. *Financial support:* In 2013–14, 34 students received support, including 16 fellowships (averaging $37,200 per year), 18 research assistantships (averaging $35,200 per year), 1 teaching assistantship (averaging $35,300 per year); Federal Work-Study, institutionally sponsored loans, scholarships/grants, traineeships, health care benefits, and unspecified assistantships also available. *Faculty research:* Computational biology and bioinformatics, biological design and synthetic biology, gene and protein networks, systems biology of cancer, nanobiology and microsystems. *Unit head:* Prof. Douglas A. Lauffenburger, Director, 617-252-1629, E-mail: csbi@mit.edu. *Application contact:* Academic Office, 617-324-4144, Fax: 617-253-8699, E-mail: csbphd@mit.edu.
Website: http://csbi.mit.edu/

Michigan State University, The Graduate School, College of Natural Science, Quantitative Biology Program, East Lansing, MI 48824. Offers PhD.

Northwestern University, The Graduate School, Interdisciplinary Biological Sciences Program (IBiS), Evanston, IL 60208. Offers biochemistry (PhD); bioengineering and biotechnology (PhD); biotechnology (PhD); cell and molecular biology (PhD); developmental and systems biology (PhD); nanotechnology (PhD); neurobiology (PhD); structural biology and biophysics (PhD). *Degree requirements:* For doctorate, thesis/dissertation, qualifying exam. *Entrance requirements:* For doctorate, GRE General Test. Additional exam requirements/recommendations for international students: Required—TOEFL (minimum score 600 paper-based). *Application deadline:* For fall admission, 12/15 for domestic and international students. Applications are processed on a rolling basis. Application fee: $95. Electronic applications accepted. *Financial support:* Fellowships, research assistantships, teaching assistantships, career-related internships or fieldwork, institutionally sponsored loans, scholarships/grants, traineeships, health care benefits, and unspecified assistantships available. Financial award application deadline: 12/31; financial award applicants required to submit FAFSA. *Faculty research:* Biophysics/structural biology, cell/molecular biology, synthetic biology, developmental systems biology, chemical biology/nanotechnology. *Unit head:* Dr. Deborah Klos Dehring, Associate Director, 847-467-0451, E-mail: d-klos@northwestern.edu. *Application contact:* Cathy Prullage, Program Manager, 847-491-4301, E-mail: ibis@northwestern.edu.
Website: http://www.biochem.northwestern.edu/ibis/

Purdue University, College of Pharmacy and Pharmacal Sciences and Graduate School, Graduate Programs in Pharmacy and Pharmacal Sciences, Department of Medicinal Chemistry and Molecular Pharmacology, West Lafayette, IN 47907. Offers biophysical and computational chemistry (PhD); cancer research (PhD); immunology and infectious disease (PhD); medicinal biochemistry and molecular biology (PhD); medicinal chemistry and chemical biology (PhD); molecular pharmacology (PhD); neuropharmacology, neurodegeneration, and neurotoxicity (PhD); systems biology and functional genomics (PhD). *Faculty:* 23 full-time (3 women), 6 part-time/adjunct (1 woman). *Students:* 50 full-time (21 women), 3 part-time (2 women); includes 1 minority (Asian, non-Hispanic/Latino), 30 international. Average age 26. 147 applicants, 20% accepted, 13 enrolled. In 2013, 12 doctorates awarded. *Degree requirements:* For doctorate, thesis/dissertation. *Entrance requirements:* For doctorate, GRE General Test; GRE Subject Test in biology, biochemistry, and chemistry (recommended), minimum undergraduate GPA of 3.0. Additional exam requirements/recommendations for international students: Required—TOEFL (minimum score 550 paper-based; 77 iBT); Recommended—TWE. *Application deadline:* For fall admission, 2/1 for domestic and international students. Applications are processed on a rolling basis. Application fee: $60 ($75 for international students). Electronic applications accepted. *Financial support:* Fellowships, research assistantships, teaching assistantships, and traineeships available. Support available to part-time students. Financial award applicants required to submit FAFSA. *Faculty research:* Drug design and development, cancer research, drug synthesis and analysis, chemical pharmacology, environmental toxicology. *Unit head:* Dr. Richard F. Borch, Head, 765-494-1403, E-mail: borch@purdue.edu. *Application contact:* Dr. Janine C. Mott, Graduate Contact, 765-494-1269, E-mail: jmott@purdue.edu.

Rutgers, The State University of New Jersey, New Brunswick, Graduate School-New Brunswick, BioMaPS Institute for Quantitative Biology, Piscataway, NJ 08854-8097. Offers computational biology and molecular biophysics (PhD). *Degree requirements:* For doctorate, comprehensive exam, thesis/dissertation. *Entrance requirements:* For doctorate, GRE. Additional exam requirements/recommendations for international students: Required—TOEFL. Electronic applications accepted. *Faculty research:* Structural biology, systems biology, bioinformatics, translational medicine, genomics.

Stanford University, School of Medicine, Graduate Programs in Medicine, Department of Chemical and Systems Biology, Stanford, CA 94305-9991. Offers PhD. *Degree requirements:* For doctorate, thesis/dissertation, qualifying examination. *Entrance requirements:* For doctorate, GRE General Test, GRE Subject Test. Additional exam requirements/recommendations for international students: Required—TOEFL. Electronic applications accepted. *Expenses: Tuition:* Full-time $42,690; part-time $949 per credit. *Required fees:* $185. *Faculty research:* Action of drugs such as epinephrine, cell differentiation and development, microsomal enzymes, neuropeptide gene expression.

Texas A&M Health Science Center, College of Medicine, Department of Systems Biology and Translational Medicine, College Station, TX 77840. Offers PhD. *Degree requirements:* For doctorate, thesis/dissertation. *Entrance requirements:* For doctorate, GRE General Test. *Faculty research:* Cardiovascular physiology, vascular cell and molecular biology.

University of California, Irvine, School of Biological Sciences, Program in Mathematical, Computational and Systems Biology, Irvine, CA 92697. Offers PhD. *Students:* 11 full-time (5 women); includes 1 minority (Hispanic/Latino), 4 international. Average age 24. 80 applicants, 29% accepted, 11 enrolled. Application fee: $80 ($100 for international students). *Unit head:* Prof. Arthur D. Lander, Director, 949-824-1721, Fax: 949-824-4709, E-mail: adlander@uci.edu. *Application contact:* Aracely Dean, Assistant Administrative Analyst, 949-824-4120, Fax: 949-824-6444, E-mail: mcsb@uci.edu.
Website: http://mcsb.bio.uci.edu/

University of California, Merced, Graduate Division, School of Natural Sciences, Merced, CA 95343. Offers applied mathematics (MS, PhD); chemistry and chemical biology (MS, PhD); physics (MS, PhD); quantitative and systems biology (MS, PhD). *Students:* 133 full-time (52 women); includes 48 minority (3 Black or African American, non-Hispanic/Latino; 16 Asian, non-Hispanic/Latino; 22 Hispanic/Latino; 1 Native Hawaiian or other Pacific Islander, non-Hispanic/Latino; 6 Two or more races, non-Hispanic/Latino), 29 international. Average age 28. 143 applicants, 45% accepted, 33 enrolled. In 2013, 1 master's, 8 doctorates awarded. *Degree requirements:* For master's, variable foreign language requirement, comprehensive exam, thesis (for some programs); for doctorate, variable foreign language requirement, comprehensive exam, thesis/dissertation. *Entrance requirements:* For master's and doctorate, GRE. Additional exam requirements/recommendations for international students: Required—TOEFL (minimum score 550 paper-based; 68 iBT); Recommended—IELTS. *Expenses:* Tuition, state resident: full-time $6405. Tuition, nonresident: full-time $13,956. *Financial support:* In 2013–14, 30 fellowships with full and partial tuition reimbursements (averaging $8,646 per year) were awarded; scholarships/grants also available. *Unit head:* Dr. Juan Meza, Dean, 209-228-4487, Fax: 209-228-4060, E-mail: jcmeza@ucmerced.edu. *Application contact:* Carrie King, Graduate Admissions and Academic Services Manager, 209-228-4613, Fax: 209-228-6906, E-mail: cking7@ucmerced.edu.

University of California, San Diego, Office of Graduate Studies, Program in Bioinformatics and Systems Biology, La Jolla, CA 92093. Offers biomedical informatics (PhD). Offered through the Departments of Bioengineering, Biology, Biomedical Sciences, Chemistry and Biochemistry, Computer Sciences and Engineering, Mathematics, and Physics. *Students:* 67 full-time (15 women); includes 18 minority (1 Black or African American, non-Hispanic/Latino; 15 Asian, non-Hispanic/Latino; 2 Hispanic/Latino), 12 international. 206 applicants, 17% accepted, 18 enrolled. In 2013, 7 doctorates awarded. *Degree requirements:* For doctorate, thesis/dissertation. *Entrance requirements:* For doctorate, GRE General Test. Additional exam requirements/recommendations for international students: Required—TOEFL, IELTS. *Application deadline:* For fall admission, 1/2 for domestic students. Application fee: $80 ($100 for international students). Electronic applications accepted. *Expenses:* Tuition, state resident: full-time $11,220; part-time $1870 per quarter. Tuition, nonresident: full-time $26,322; part-time $4387 per quarter. *Required fees:* $519.50 per quarter. Part-time tuition and fees vary according to course load and program. *Financial support:* Fellowships, research assistantships, scholarships/grants, and tuition waivers available. Financial award applicants required to submit FAFSA. *Faculty research:* Quantitative foundations of computational biology, comparative and population genomics, proteomics and metabolomics, epigenomics and gene expression control, genetic and molecular networks. *Unit head:* Vineet Bafna, Director, 858-534-3852, E-mail: vbafna@ucsd.edu. *Application contact:* Risa Shibata, Graduate Coordinator, 858-822-4948, E-mail: bioinfo@ucsd.edu.
Website: http://bioinformatics.ucsd.edu/

University of Chicago, Division of Biological Sciences, Molecular Biosciences Cluster, Committee on Genetics, Genomics and Systems Biology, Chicago, IL 60637-1513. Offers PhD. *Degree requirements:* For doctorate, thesis/dissertation, ethics class, 2 teaching assistantships. *Entrance requirements:* For doctorate, GRE General Test, minimum GPA of 3.0. Additional exam requirements/recommendations for international students: Required—TOEFL (minimum score 600 paper-based; 104 iBT), IELTS (minimum score 7). Electronic applications accepted. *Faculty research:* Molecular genetics, developmental genetics, population genetics, human genetics.

University of Pittsburgh, School of Medicine, Computational Biology Graduate Program, Pittsburgh, PA 15260. Offers PhD. PhD jointly offered by the University of Pittsburgh and Carnegie Mellon University. *Faculty:* 86 full-time (17 women). *Students:* 52 full-time (18 women); includes 9 minority (6 Asian, non-Hispanic/Latino; 2 Hispanic/Latino; 1 Native Hawaiian or other Pacific Islander, non-Hispanic/Latino), 20 international. Average age 25. 130 applicants, 18% accepted, 8 enrolled. In 2013, 8 doctorates awarded. Terminal master's awarded for partial completion of doctoral program. *Degree requirements:* For doctorate, comprehensive exam, thesis/dissertation, ethics training service as course assistant, seminar. *Entrance requirements:* For doctorate, GRE Subject Test (recommended), GRE General Test, 3 letters of recommendation, resume. Additional exam requirements/recommendations for

international students: Required—TOEFL (minimum score 600 paper-based; 100 iBT). *Application deadline:* For fall admission, 12/15 priority date for domestic and international students. Application fee: $50. Electronic applications accepted. *Expenses:* Tuition, state resident: full-time $19,964; part-time $807 per credit. Tuition, nonresident: full-time $32,686; part-time $1337 per credit. *Required fees:* $740; $200. Tuition and fees vary according to program. *Financial support:* In 2013–14, 44 students received support, including 8 fellowships with full tuition reimbursements available, 44 research assistantships with full tuition reimbursements available (averaging $26,010 per year). *Faculty research:* Computational structural biology, computational genomics, cell and systems modeling, bioimage informatics, computational neurobiology. *Unit head:* Dr. Daniel M. Zuckerman, Director, 412-648-3335, Fax: 412-648-3163, E-mail: ddmmzz@pitt.edu. *Application contact:* Kelly Gentille, Educational Programs Administrator, 412-648-8107, Fax: 412-648-3163, E-mail: kmg120@pitt.edu.
Website: http://www.compbio.pitt.edu/

University of Toronto, School of Graduate Studies, Faculty of Arts and Science, Department of Cell and Systems Biology, Toronto, ON M5S 1A1, Canada. Offers M Sc, PhD. *Degree requirements:* For master's, thesis, thesis defense; for doctorate, thesis/dissertation, thesis defense, oral thesis examination. *Entrance requirements:* For master's, minimum B+ average in final year, B overall, 3 letters of reference. Additional exam requirements/recommendations for international students: Required—TOEFL (minimum score 580 paper-based; 93 iBT), TWE (minimum score 5). Electronic applications accepted.

Virginia Commonwealth University, Graduate School, School of Life Sciences, Doctoral Program in Integrative Life Sciences, Richmond, VA 23284-9005. Offers PhD. *Entrance requirements:* For doctorate, GRE, minimum GPA of 3.0 in last 60 credits of undergraduate work or in graduate degree, 3 letters of recommendation. Additional exam requirements/recommendations for international students: Required—TOEFL (minimum score 600 paper-based; 100 iBT). Electronic applications accepted.

Washington University in St. Louis, Graduate School of Arts and Sciences, Division of Biology and Biomedical Sciences, Program in Computational and Systems Biology, St. Louis, MO 63130-4899. Offers PhD. *Degree requirements:* For doctorate, thesis/dissertation. Electronic applications accepted.

Weill Cornell Medical College, Weill Cornell Graduate School of Medical Sciences, Physiology, Biophysics and Systems Biology Program, New York, NY 10065. Offers MS, PhD. Terminal master's awarded for partial completion of doctoral program. *Degree requirements:* For master's, comprehensive exam; for doctorate, thesis/dissertation, final exam. *Entrance requirements:* For doctorate, GRE General Test, introductory courses in biology, inorganic and organic chemistry, physics, and mathematics. Additional exam requirements/recommendations for international students: Required—TOEFL. *Faculty research:* Receptor-mediated regulation of cell function, molecular properties of channels or receptors, bioinformatics, mathematical modeling.

Translational Biology

Baylor College of Medicine, Graduate School of Biomedical Sciences, Program in Translational Biology and Molecular Medicine, Houston, TX 77030-3498. Offers PhD. *Degree requirements:* For doctorate, thesis/dissertation, public defense. *Entrance requirements:* For doctorate, GRE, minimum GPA of 3.0. Additional exam requirements/recommendations for international students: Required—TOEFL. Electronic applications accepted. *Faculty research:* Molecular medicine, translational biology, human disease biology and therapy.

Cedars-Sinai Medical Center, Graduate Program in Biomedical Sciences and Translational Medicine, Los Angeles, CA 90048. Offers PhD. *Degree requirements:* For doctorate, comprehensive exam, thesis/dissertation. *Entrance requirements:* For doctorate, GRE, 3 letters of recommendation. Additional exam requirements/recommendations for international students: Required—TOEFL (minimum score 550 paper-based; 80 iBT), IELTS (minimum score 6.5). Electronic applications accepted. *Faculty research:* Immunology and infection, neuroscience, cardiovascular science, cancer, human genetics.

Rutgers, The State University of New Jersey, New Brunswick, Graduate School of Biomedical Sciences, Program in Clinical and Translational Science, Piscataway, NJ 08854-8097. Offers MS. Part-time programs available. *Degree requirements:* For master's, thesis.

Texas A&M Health Science Center, College of Medicine, Department of Systems Biology and Translational Medicine, College Station, TX 77840. Offers PhD. *Degree requirements:* For doctorate, thesis/dissertation. *Entrance requirements:* For doctorate, GRE General Test. *Faculty research:* Cardiovascular physiology, vascular cell and molecular biology.

The University of Iowa, Graduate College, Program in Translational Biomedicine, Iowa City, IA 52242-1316. Offers MS, PhD. Terminal master's awarded for partial completion of doctoral program. *Degree requirements:* For master's, comprehensive exam; for doctorate, comprehensive exam, thesis/dissertation. *Entrance requirements:* For master's and doctorate, minimum GPA of 3.0. Additional exam requirements/recommendations for international students: Required—TOEFL (minimum score 550 paper-based; 81 iBT). Electronic applications accepted.

University of Massachusetts Worcester, Graduate School of Biomedical Sciences, Worcester, MA 01655-0115. Offers biochemistry and molecular pharmacology (PhD); bioinformatics and computational biology (PhD); cancer biology (PhD); cell biology (PhD); clinical and population health research (PhD); clinical investigation (MS); immunology and virology (PhD); interdisciplinary biomedical research (PhD); millennium (PhD); molecular genetics and microbiology (PhD); neuroscience (PhD); translational science (PhD); MD/PhD. *Faculty:* 1,388 full-time (521 women), 309 part-time/adjunct (198 women). *Students:* 385 full-time (210 women); includes 53 minority (13 Black or African American, non-Hispanic/Latino; 30 Asian, non-Hispanic/Latino; 10 Hispanic/Latino), 138 international. Average age 28. 491 applicants, 19% accepted, 39 enrolled. In 2013, 5 master's, 50 doctorates awarded. Terminal master's awarded for partial completion of doctoral program. *Median time to degree:* Of those who began their doctoral program in fall 2005, 67% received their degree in 8 years or less. *Degree requirements:* For master's, comprehensive exam, thesis; for doctorate, comprehensive exam, thesis/dissertation. *Entrance requirements:* For master's, MD, PhD, DVM, or PharmD; for doctorate, GRE General Test, bachelor's degree. Additional exam requirements/recommendations for international students: Required—TOEFL (minimum score 100 iBT) or IELTS (minimum score 7.5). *Application deadline:* For fall admission, 12/15 for domestic and international students; for spring admission, 5/15 for domestic students. Application fee: $80. Electronic applications accepted. *Expenses:* Contact institution. *Financial support:* In 2013–14, 431 students received support, including research assistantships with full tuition reimbursements available (averaging $29,500 per year); scholarships/grants, health care benefits, tuition waivers (full), and unspecified assistantships also available. Financial award application deadline: 5/16. *Faculty research:* RNA interference, cell/molecular/developmental biology, bioinformatics, clinical/translational research, infectious disease. *Total annual research expenditures:* $245.9 million. *Unit head:* Dr. Anthony Carruthers, Dean, 508-856-4135, E-mail: anthony.carruthers@umassmed.edu. *Application contact:* Dr. Kendall Knight, Associate Dean and Interim Director of Admissions and Recruitment, 508-856-5628, Fax: 508-856-3659, E-mail: kendall.knight@umassmed.edu.
Website: http://www.umassmed.edu/gsbs/

Section 8
Ecology, Environmental Biology, and Evolutionary Biology

This section contains a directory of institutions offering graduate work in ecology, environmental biology, and evolutionary biology. Additional information about programs listed in the directory may be obtained by writing directly to the dean of a graduate school or chair of a department at the address given in the directory.

For programs offering related work, see also in this book *Biological and Biomedical Sciences; Botany and Plant Biology; Entomology; Genetics, Developmental Biology, and Reproductive Biology; Microbiological Sciences; Pharmacology and Toxicology; Public Health;* and *Zoology.* In the other guides in this series:

Graduate Programs in the Humanities, Arts & Social Sciences
See *Sociology, Anthropology, and Archaeology*

Graduate Programs in the Physical Sciences, Mathematics, Agricultural Sciences, the Environment & Natural Resources
See *Agricultural and Food Sciences, Geosciences, Marine Sciences and Oceanography,* and *Mathematical Sciences*

Graduate Programs in Engineering & Applied Sciences
See *Civil and Environmental Engineering, Management of Engineering and Technology,* and *Ocean Engineering*

CONTENTS

Program Directories

Conservation Biology

Antioch University New England, Graduate School, Department of Environmental Studies, Program in Conservation Biology, Keene, NH 03431-3552. Offers MS. *Degree requirements:* For master's, thesis or project. *Entrance requirements:* For master's, resume, 3 letters of recommendation. Additional exam requirements/recommendations for international students: Required—TOEFL (minimum score 550 paper-based). Electronic applications accepted.

California State University, Sacramento, Office of Graduate Studies, College of Natural Sciences and Mathematics, Department of Biological Sciences, Sacramento, CA 95819. Offers biological conservation (MS); marine science (MS); molecular and cellular biology (MS); stem cell (MA). Part-time programs available. *Degree requirements:* For master's, thesis, writing proficiency exam. *Entrance requirements:* For master's, GRE, bachelor's degree in biology or equivalent; minimum GPA of 3.0 in biology, 2.75 overall during last 2 years of course work. Additional exam requirements/recommendations for international students: Required—TOEFL. *Application deadline:* For fall admission, 2/1 for domestic students, 3/1 for international students; for spring admission, 9/30 for international students. Applications are processed on a rolling basis. Application fee: $55. Electronic applications accepted. *Financial support:* Research assistantships, teaching assistantships, career-related internships or fieldwork, and Federal Work-Study available. Support available to part-time students. Financial award application deadline: 3/1; financial award applicants required to submit FAFSA. *Unit head:* Jennifer Lundmark, Chair, 916-278-6535, E-mail: lundmark@csus.edu. *Application contact:* Jose Martinez, Graduate Admissions Supervisor, 916-278-7871, E-mail: martinj@skymail.csus.edu.
Website: http://www.csus.edu/bios

California State University, Stanislaus, College of Natural Sciences, Program in Ecology and Sustainability (MS), Turlock, CA 95382. Offers ecological conservation (MS); ecological economics (MS). Part-time programs available. *Degree requirements:* For master's, thesis. *Entrance requirements:* For master's, GRE, minimum GPA of 3.0, 3 letters of recommendation, personal statement. Additional exam requirements/recommendations for international students: Required—TOEFL (minimum score 550 paper-based). Electronic applications accepted.

Central Michigan University, College of Graduate Studies, College of Science and Technology, Department of Biology, Mount Pleasant, MI 48859. Offers biology (MS); conservation biology (MS). Part-time programs available. *Degree requirements:* For master's, thesis or alternative. *Entrance requirements:* For master's, GRE, bachelor's degree with a major in biological science, minimum GPA of 3.0. Electronic applications accepted. *Faculty research:* Conservation biology, morphology and taxonomy of aquatic plants, molecular biology and genetics, microbials and invertebrate ecology, vertebrates.

Colorado State University, Graduate School, Warner College of Natural Resources, Department of Fishery and Wildlife Biology, Fort Collins, CO 80523-1474. Offers fish, wildlife and conservation biology (MFWCB); fishery and wildlife biology (MFWB, MS, PhD). *Faculty:* 13 full-time (4 women), 1 part-time/adjunct (0 women). *Students:* 7 full-time (3 women), 19 part-time (7 women); includes 1 minority (Hispanic/Latino). Average age 31. 15 applicants, 27% accepted, 4 enrolled. In 2013, 2 master's, 1 doctorate awarded. Terminal master's awarded for partial completion of doctoral program. *Degree requirements:* For master's, comprehensive exam, thesis (for some programs); for doctorate, comprehensive exam, thesis/dissertation. *Entrance requirements:* For master's, GRE General Test (combined minimum score of 1200 on the Verbal and Quantitative sections), minimum GPA of 3.0, BA or BS in related field, letters of recommendation, resume, transcripts; for doctorate, GRE General Test (minimum score 1000 verbal and quantitative), minimum GPA of 3.0, MS in related field. Additional exam requirements/recommendations for international students: Required—TOEFL (minimum score 550 paper-based; 80 iBT). *Application deadline:* For fall admission, 2/15 priority date for domestic and international students. Applications are processed on a rolling basis. Application fee: $50. Electronic applications accepted. *Expenses:* Tuition, state resident: full-time $9075.40; part-time $504 per credit. Tuition, nonresident: full-time $22,248; part-time $1236 per credit. *Required fees:* $1819; $60 per credit. *Financial support:* In 2013–14, 27 students received support, including 3 fellowships with full and partial tuition reimbursements available (averaging $49,406 per year), 17 research assistantships with full and partial tuition reimbursements available (averaging $15,515 per year), 7 teaching assistantships with full and partial tuition reimbursements available (averaging $8,080 per year); career-related internships or fieldwork, scholarships/grants, tuition waivers (full and partial), and unspecified assistantships also available. Financial award application deadline: 2/15; financial award applicants required to submit FAFSA. *Faculty research:* Conservation biology, aquatic ecology, animal behavior, population modeling, habitat evaluation and management. *Total annual research expenditures:* $3.3 million. *Unit head:* Dr. Kenneth R. Wilson, Professor/Department Head, 970-491-5020, Fax: 970-491-5091, E-mail: kenneth.wilson@colostate.edu. *Application contact:* Joyce Pratt, Graduate Contact, 970-491-5020, Fax: 970-491-5091, E-mail: joyce.pratt@colostate.edu.
Website: http://warnercnr.colostate.edu/fwcb-home/

Columbia University, Graduate School of Arts and Sciences, Department of Ecology, Evolution and Environmental Biology, New York, NY 10027. Offers conservation biology (MA); ecology and evolutionary biology (PhD); evolutionary primatology (PhD). *Faculty:* 7 full-time (1 woman), 43 part-time/adjunct (15 women). *Students:* 46 full-time (36 women), 1 part-time (0 women). Average age 28. 45 applicants, 18% accepted. *Degree requirements:* For doctorate, one foreign language, thesis/dissertation, teaching experience. *Entrance requirements:* For doctorate, GRE General Test, previous course work in biology. Additional exam requirements/recommendations for international students: Required—TOEFL. Application fee: $90. Electronic applications accepted. *Financial support:* Fellowships, career-related internships or fieldwork, and institutionally sponsored loans available. Financial award application deadline: 1/5. *Faculty research:* Tropical ecology, ethnobotany, global change, systematics. *Total annual research expenditures:* $300,000. *Unit head:* Prof. Ruth DeFries, Chair, 212-851-1647, E-mail: rd2402@columbia.edu. *Application contact:* 212-854-9987.
Website: http://www.columbia.edu/cu/e3b/

Cornell University, Graduate School, Graduate Fields of Agriculture and Life Sciences, Field of Natural Resources, Ithaca, NY 14853-0001. Offers community-based natural resources management (MS, PhD); conservation biology (MS, PhD); ecosystem biology and biogeochemistry (MPS, MS, PhD); environmental management (MPS); fishery and aquatic science (MPS, MS, PhD); forest science (MPS, MS, PhD); human dimensions of natural resources management (MPS, MS, PhD); policy and institutional analysis (MS, PhD); program development and evaluation (MPS, MS, PhD); quantitative ecology (MS, PhD); wildlife science (MPS, MS, PhD). *Faculty:* 39 full-time (8 women). *Students:* 65 full-time (30 women); includes 2 minority (1 Asian, non-Hispanic/Latino; 1 Hispanic/Latino), 18 international. Average age 31. 93 applicants, 26% accepted, 20 enrolled. In 2013, 8 master's, 7 doctorates awarded. *Degree requirements:* For master's, thesis (MS), project paper (MPS); for doctorate, comprehensive exam, thesis/dissertation. *Entrance requirements:* For master's and doctorate, GRE General Test, 2 letters of recommendation. Additional exam requirements/recommendations for international students: Required—TOEFL (minimum score 550 paper-based; 77 iBT). *Application deadline:* For spring admission, 10/30 for domestic students. Applications are processed on a rolling basis. Application fee: $95. Electronic applications accepted. *Financial support:* In 2013–14, 48 students received support, including 10 fellowships with full tuition reimbursements available, 18 research assistantships with full tuition reimbursements available, 20 teaching assistantships with full tuition reimbursements available; institutionally sponsored loans, scholarships/grants, health care benefits, tuition waivers (full and partial), and unspecified assistantships also available. Financial award applicants required to submit FAFSA. *Faculty research:* Ecosystem-level dynamics, systems modeling, conservation biology/management, resource management's human dimensions, biogeochemistry. *Unit head:* Director of Graduate Studies, 607-255-2807, Fax: 607-255-0349. *Application contact:* Graduate Field Assistant, 607-255-2807, Fax: 607-255-0349, E-mail: nrgrad@cornell.edu.
Website: http://www.gradschool.cornell.edu/fields.php?id-54&a-2

Florida Institute of Technology, Graduate Programs, College of Science, Department of Biological Sciences, Melbourne, FL 32901-6975. Offers biological science (PhD); biotechnology (MS); cell and molecular biology (MS); conservation technology (MS); ecology (MS); marine biology (MS). Part-time programs available. *Faculty:* 16 full-time (1 woman), 1 (woman) part-time/adjunct. *Students:* 73 full-time (39 women), 14 part-time (11 women); includes 4 minority (1 Asian, non-Hispanic/Latino; 2 Hispanic/Latino; 1 Two or more races, non-Hispanic/Latino), 34 international. Average age 27. 204 applicants, 34% accepted, 38 enrolled. In 2013, 29 master's, 1 doctorate awarded. *Degree requirements:* For master's, thesis (for some programs), research, seminar, internship, or summer lab; for doctorate, comprehensive exam, thesis/dissertation, dissertations seminar, publications. *Entrance requirements:* For master's, GRE General Test, 3 letters of recommendation, minimum GPA of 3.0, resume, statement of objectives; for doctorate, GRE General Test, resume, 3 letters of recommendation, minimum GPA of 3.2, statement of objectives. Additional exam requirements/recommendations for international students: Required—TOEFL (minimum score 550 paper-based; 79 iBT). *Application deadline:* For fall admission, 3/1 for domestic students, 4/1 for international students; for spring admission, 9/1 for domestic and international students. Applications are processed on a rolling basis. Electronic applications accepted. *Expenses: Tuition:* Full-time $20,214; part-time $1123 per credit. Tuition and fees vary according to campus/location. *Financial support:* In 2013–14, 12 research assistantships with full and partial tuition reimbursements (averaging $11,687 per year), 22 teaching assistantships with full and partial tuition reimbursements (averaging $13,947 per year) were awarded; fellowships, career-related internships or fieldwork, institutionally sponsored loans, tuition waivers (partial), unspecified assistantships, and tuition remissions also available. Support available to part-time students. Financial award application deadline: 3/1; financial award applicants required to submit FAFSA. *Faculty research:* Initiation of protein synthesis in eukaryotic cells, fixation of radioactive carbon, changes in DNA molecule, endangered or threatened avian and mammalian species, hydroacoustics and feeding preference of the West Indian manatee. *Total annual research expenditures:* $1.4 million. *Unit head:* Dr. Richard B. Aronson, Department Head, 321-674-8034, Fax: 321-674-7238, E-mail: raronson@fit.edu. *Application contact:* Cheryl A. Brown, Associate Director of Graduate Admissions, 321-674-7581, Fax: 321-723-9468, E-mail: cbrown@fit.edu.
Website: http://cos.fit.edu/biology/

Fordham University, Graduate School of Arts and Sciences, Department of Biological Sciences, New York, NY 10458. Offers biological sciences (MS, PhD); conservation biology (Graduate Certificate). Part-time and evening/weekend programs available. *Faculty:* 18 full-time (2 women). *Students:* 56 full-time (35 women), 3 part-time (2 women); includes 2 minority (1 Asian, non-Hispanic/Latino; 1 Hispanic/Latino), 17 international. Average age 29. 99 applicants, 39% accepted, 16 enrolled. In 2013, 11 master's, 2 doctorates awarded. Terminal master's awarded for partial completion of doctoral program. *Degree requirements:* For master's, one foreign language, comprehensive exam, thesis optional; for doctorate, one foreign language, comprehensive exam, thesis/dissertation. *Entrance requirements:* For master's and doctorate, GRE General Test, GRE Subject Test (recommended). Additional exam requirements/recommendations for international students: Required—TOEFL (minimum score 550 paper-based). *Application deadline:* For fall admission, 1/4 priority date for domestic students; for spring admission, 11/1 for domestic students. Application fee: $70. Electronic applications accepted. *Financial support:* In 2013–14, 28 students received support, including 3 fellowships with full and partial tuition reimbursements available (averaging $29,000 per year), 39 teaching assistantships with full and partial tuition reimbursements available (averaging $28,319 per year); Federal Work-Study, institutionally sponsored loans, scholarships/grants, tuition waivers (full and partial), and unspecified assistantships also available. Support available to part-time students. Financial award application deadline: 1/4; financial award applicants required to submit FAFSA. *Faculty research:* Avian ecology, behavioral ecology, and conservation biology; plant, community and ecosystem responses to invasive organisms; neurobiology and ion channel disorders; biochemical, physiological and morphological basis of pattern formation; behavioral, physiological and biochemical adaptations of mammals to extreme environments; evolutionary ecology, functional morphology and ichthyology; genotypic response to biogeographic and anthropogenic factors; community-based sustainable resource use. *Total annual research expenditures:* $1.5 million. *Unit head:* Dr. James Lewis, Chair, 718-817-3642, Fax: 718-817-3645, E-mail: jdlewis@fordham.edu. *Application contact:* Bernadette Valentino-Morrison, Director of Graduate Admissions, 718-817-4419, Fax: 718-817-3566, E-mail: valentinomor@fordham.edu.

Frostburg State University, Graduate School, College of Liberal Arts and Sciences, Department of Biology, Program in Applied Ecology and Conservation Biology, Frostburg, MD 21532-1099. Offers MS. *Degree requirements:* For master's, thesis. *Entrance requirements:* For master's, GRE General Test, resume. Additional exam requirements/recommendations for international students: Required—TOEFL. Electronic applications accepted. *Expenses: Tuition, area resident:* Part-time $340 per credit hour. Tuition, state resident: part-time $340 per credit hour. Tuition, nonresident: part-time $437 per credit hour. *Faculty research:* Forest ecology, microbiology of man-made wetlands, invertebrate zoology and entomology, wildlife and carnivore ecology, aquatic pollution ecology.

Illinois State University, Graduate School, College of Arts and Sciences, Department of Biological Sciences, Normal, IL 61790-2200. Offers animal behavior (MS); bacteriology (MS); biochemistry (MS); biological sciences (MS); biology (PhD); biophysics (MS); biotechnology (MS); botany (MS, PhD); cell biology (MS); conservation biology (MS); developmental biology (MS); ecology (MS, PhD); entomology (MS); evolutionary biology (MS); genetics (MS, PhD); immunology (MS); microbiology (MS, PhD); molecular biology (MS); molecular genetics (MS); neurobiology (MS); neuroscience (MS); parasitology (MS); physiology (MS, PhD); plant biology (MS); plant molecular biology (MS); plant sciences (MS); structural biology (MS); zoology (MS, PhD). Part-time programs available. *Degree requirements:* For master's, thesis or alternative; for doctorate, variable foreign language requirement, thesis/dissertation, 2 terms of residency. *Entrance requirements:* For master's, GRE General Test, minimum GPA of 2.6 in last 60 hours of course work; for doctorate, GRE General Test. *Faculty research:* Redoc balance and drug development in schistosoma mansoni, control of the growth of listeria monocytogenes at low temperature, regulation of cell expansion and microtubule function by SPRI, CRUI: physiology and fitness consequences of different life history phenotypes.

State University of New York College of Environmental Science and Forestry, Department of Environmental and Forest Biology, Syracuse, NY 13210-2779. Offers applied ecology (MPS); chemical ecology (MPS, MS, PhD); conservation biology (MPS, MS, PhD); ecology (MPS, MS, PhD); entomology (MPS, MS, PhD); environmental interpretation (MPS, MS, PhD); environmental physiology (MPS, MS, PhD); fish and wildlife biology and management (MPS, MS, PhD); forest pathology and mycology (MPS, MS, PhD); plant biotechnology (MPS); plant science and biotechnology (MPS, MS, PhD). *Faculty:* 32 full-time (10 women). *Students:* 105 full-time (54 women), 31 part-time (16 women); includes 9 minority (2 Black or African American, non-Hispanic/Latino; 3 American Indian or Alaska Native, non-Hispanic/Latino; 2 Hispanic/Latino; 1 Native Hawaiian or other Pacific Islander, non-Hispanic/Latino; 1 Two or more races, non-Hispanic/Latino), 17 international. Average age 28. In 2013, 15 master's, 7 doctorates awarded. *Degree requirements:* For master's, thesis (for some programs), capstone seminar; for doctorate, comprehensive exam, thesis/dissertation, capstone seminar. *Entrance requirements:* For master's and doctorate, GRE General Test, minimum GPA of 3.0. Additional exam requirements/recommendations for international students: Required—TOEFL (minimum score 550 paper-based; 80 iBT), IELTS (minimum score 6). *Application deadline:* For fall admission, 2/1 priority date for domestic and international students; for spring admission, 11/1 priority date for domestic and international students. Applications are processed on a rolling basis. Application fee: $60. *Expenses:* Tuition, state resident: full-time $10,370; part-time $432 per credit hour. Tuition, nonresident: full-time $20,190; part-time $841 per credit hour. *Required fees:* $44 per credit hour. *Financial support:* In 2013–14, 4 fellowships with full and partial tuition reimbursements, 36 research assistantships with full and partial tuition reimbursements, 39 teaching assistantships with full and partial tuition reimbursements (averaging $11,490 per year) were awarded; Federal Work-Study, institutionally sponsored loans, scholarships/grants, health care benefits, and unspecified assistantships also available. Financial award application deadline: 6/30. *Faculty research:* Ecology, conservation biology, fish and wildlife biology and management, plant science, entomology. *Total annual research expenditures:* $4.1 million. *Unit head:* Dr. Donald J. Leopold, Chair, 315-470-6760, Fax: 315-470-6934, E-mail: djleopold@esf.edu. *Application contact:* Dr. Danilo D. Fernando, Director, Graduate Program/Associate Professor, 315-470-6746, Fax: 315-470-6934, E-mail: dfernando@esf.edu.
Website: http://www.esf.edu/efb/grad/default.asp

Texas State University, Graduate School, College of Science and Engineering, Department of Biology, Program in Population and Conservation Biology, San Marcos, TX 78666. Offers MS. *Faculty:* 12 full-time (3 women). *Students:* 9 full-time (8 women), 1 international. Average age 27. 5 applicants, 40% accepted, 2 enrolled. In 2013, 3 master's awarded. *Degree requirements:* For master's, thesis. *Entrance requirements:* For master's, GRE (preferred minimum combined score of 1000 Verbal and Quantitative), bachelor's degree in biology or related discipline, minimum GPA of 3.0 in last 60 hours of undergraduate course work. Additional exam requirements/recommendations for international students: Required—TOEFL (minimum score 550 paper-based; 78 iBT). *Application deadline:* For fall admission, 6/15 for domestic students, 6/1 for international students; for spring admission, 10/15 for domestic students, 10/1 for international students. Applications are processed on a rolling basis. Application fee: $40 ($90 for international students). Electronic applications accepted. *Expenses:* Tuition, state resident: full-time $6663; part-time $278 per credit hour. Tuition, nonresident: full-time $15,159; part-time $632 per credit hour. *Required fees:* $1872; $54 per credit hour. $306 per term. Tuition and fees vary according to course load. *Financial support:* In 2013–14, 6 students received support, including 1 research assistantship (averaging $11,570 per year), 7 teaching assistantships (averaging $15,371 per year); Federal Work-Study, institutionally sponsored loans, scholarships/grants, health care benefits, and unspecified assistantships also available. Support available to part-time students. Financial award application deadline: 4/1; financial award applicants required to submit FAFSA. *Unit head:* Dr. Chris Nice, Graduate Advisor, 512-245-3358, E-mail: ccnice@txstate.edu. *Application contact:* Dr. Andrea Golato, Dean of the Graduate School, 512-245-2581, Fax: 512-245-8365, E-mail: jw02@swt.edu.
Website: http://www.bio.txstate.edu/Graduate-Programs/pop-and-con-biology.html

Tropical Agriculture Research and Higher Education Center, Graduate School, Turrialba, Costa Rica. Offers agribusiness management (MS); agroforestry systems (PhD); development practices (MS); ecological agriculture (MS); environmental socioeconomics (MS); forestry in tropical and subtropical zones (PhD); integrated watershed management (MS); international sustainable tourism (MS); management and conservation of tropical rainforests and biodiversity (MS); tropical agriculture (PhD); tropical agroforestry (MS). *Entrance requirements:* For master's, GRE, 2 years of related professional experience, letters of recommendation; for doctorate, GRE, 4 letters of recommendation, letter of support from employing organization, master's degree in agronomy, biological sciences, forestry, natural resources or related field. Additional exam requirements/recommendations for international students: Required—TOEFL (minimum score 550 paper-based). Electronic applications accepted. *Faculty research:* Biodiversity in fragmented landscapes, ecosystem management, integrated pest management, environmental livestock production, biotechnology carbon balances in diverse land uses.

University at Albany, State University of New York, College of Arts and Sciences, Department of Biological Sciences, Program in Biodiversity, Conservation, and Policy, Albany, NY 12222-0001. Offers MS. *Degree requirements:* For master's, one foreign language. *Entrance requirements:* For master's, GRE General Test. *Faculty research:* Aquatic ecology, plant community ecology, biodiversity and public policy, restoration ecology, coastal and estuarine science.

University of Alberta, Faculty of Graduate Studies and Research, Department of Renewable Resources, Edmonton, AB T6G 2E1, Canada. Offers agroforestry (M Ag, M Sc, MF); conservation biology (M Sc, PhD); forest biology and management (M Sc, PhD); land reclamation and remediation (M Sc, PhD); protected areas and wildlands management (M Sc, PhD); soil science (M Ag, M Sc, PhD); water and land resources (M Ag, M Sc, PhD); wildlife ecology and management (M Sc, PhD); MBA/M Ag; MBA/MF. Part-time programs available. *Degree requirements:* For master's, thesis (for some programs); for doctorate, comprehensive exam, thesis/dissertation. *Entrance requirements:* For master's, minimum 2 years of relevant professional experiences, minimum GPA of 3.0; for doctorate, minimum GPA of 3.0. Additional exam requirements/recommendations for international students: Required—TOEFL (minimum score 550 paper-based). Electronic applications accepted. *Faculty research:* Natural and managed landscapes.

University of Central Florida, College of Sciences, Department of Biology, Orlando, FL 32816. Offers biology (MS); conservation biology (MS, PhD, Certificate). Part-time and evening/weekend programs available. *Faculty:* 22 full-time (8 women), 11 part-time/adjunct (5 women). *Students:* 58 full-time (35 women), 14 part-time (10 women); includes 8 minority (2 Asian, non-Hispanic/Latino; 5 Hispanic/Latino; 1 Two or more races, non-Hispanic/Latino), 6 international. Average age 29. 81 applicants, 38% accepted, 16 enrolled. In 2013, 9 master's, 4 doctorates, 1 other advanced degree awarded. *Degree requirements:* For master's, comprehensive exam, thesis or alternative, field exam. *Entrance requirements:* For master's, GRE General Test, minimum GPA of 3.0 in last 60 hours. Additional exam requirements/recommendations for international students: Required—TOEFL. *Application deadline:* For fall admission, 3/1 priority date for domestic students; for spring admission, 10/15 for domestic students. Application fee: $30. Electronic applications accepted. *Financial support:* In 2013–14, 53 students received support, including 16 fellowships with partial tuition reimbursements available (averaging $3,500 per year), 15 research assistantships with partial tuition reimbursements available (averaging $7,400 per year), 43 teaching assistantships with partial tuition reimbursements available (averaging $11,800 per year); career-related internships or fieldwork, Federal Work-Study, institutionally sponsored loans, tuition waivers (partial), and unspecified assistantships also available. Financial award application deadline: 3/1; financial award applicants required to submit FAFSA. *Unit head:* Dr. Laurence von Kalm, Interim Chair, 407-823-6684, Fax: 407-823-5769, E-mail: lvonkalm@ucf.edu. *Application contact:* Barbara Rodriguez Lamas, Associate Director, Admissions and Student Services, 407-823-2766, Fax: 407-823-6442, E-mail: gradadmissions@ucf.edu.
Website: http://biology.cos.ucf.edu/

University of Hawaii at Hilo, Program in Tropical Conservation Biology and Environmental Science, Hilo, HI 96720-4091. Offers MS. *Faculty:* 16 full-time (6 women), 1 (woman) part-time/adjunct. *Students:* 7 full-time (2 women), 48 part-time (32 women); includes 30 minority (5 Asian, non-Hispanic/Latino; 6 Hispanic/Latino; 3 Native Hawaiian or other Pacific Islander, non-Hispanic/Latino; 16 Two or more races, non-Hispanic/Latino). Average age 29. 34 applicants, 53% accepted, 13 enrolled. In 2013, 21 master's awarded. *Entrance requirements:* Additional exam requirements/recommendations for international students: Required—TOEFL, IELTS. *Application deadline:* For fall admission, 2/1 priority date for domestic students, 1/1 priority date for international students. Application fee: $50. Electronic applications accepted. *Expenses:* Tuition, state resident: full-time $4668. Tuition, nonresident: full-time $10,704. Tuition and fees vary according to course load and program. *Financial support:* Application deadline: 3/1; applicants required to submit FAFSA. *Unit head:* Donald Price, Director, 808-932-7506, E-mail: donaldp@hawaii.edu. *Application contact:* UH Hilo Admissions Office, 808-932-7446, Fax: 808-932-7459, E-mail: uhhadm@hawaii.edu.
Website: http://tcbes.uhh.hawaii.edu/

University of Hawaii at Manoa, Graduate Division, Interdisciplinary Specialization in Ecology, Evolution and Conservation Biology, Honolulu, HI 96822. Offers MS, PhD. *Degree requirements:* For doctorate, thesis/dissertation. *Faculty research:* Agronomy and soil science, zoology, entomology, genetics and molecular biology, botanical sciences.

University of Illinois at Urbana–Champaign, Graduate College, College of Liberal Arts and Sciences, School of Integrative Biology, Program in Ecology, Evolution and Conservation Biology, Champaign, IL 61820. Offers MS, PhD. *Students:* 28 (16 women). Application fee: $75 ($90 for international students). *Unit head:* Evan H. DeLucia, Director, 217-333-3044, Fax: 217-244-1224, E-mail: delucia@illinois.edu. *Application contact:* Kimberly Leigh, Secretary, 217-333-8208, Fax: 217-244-1224, E-mail: kaleigh@illinois.edu.
Website: http://sib.illinois.edu/peec/

University of Maryland, College Park, Academic Affairs, College of Computer, Mathematical and Natural Sciences, Department of Biology, Program in Sustainable Development and Conservation Biology, College Park, MD 20742. Offers MS. Part-time and evening/weekend programs available. *Students:* 11 full-time (8 women), 5 part-time (3 women); includes 3 minority (1 Black or African American, non-Hispanic/Latino; 1 Asian, non-Hispanic/Latino; 1 Hispanic/Latino). 61 applicants, 26% accepted, 8 enrolled. In 2013, 16 master's awarded. *Degree requirements:* For master's, internship, scholarly paper. *Entrance requirements:* For master's, GRE General Test, minimum GPA of 3.0, 3 letters of recommendation. *Application deadline:* For fall admission, 12/15 for domestic and international students. Applications are processed on a rolling basis. Application fee: $75. Electronic applications accepted. *Expenses:* Tuition, state resident: full-time $10,314; part-time $573 per credit hour. Tuition, nonresident: full-time $22,248; part-time $1236 per credit. *Required fees:* $1446; $403.15 per semester. Tuition and fees vary according to program. *Financial support:* In 2013–14, 16 teaching assistantships (averaging $18,740 per year) were awarded. Financial award application deadline: 2/1; financial award applicants required to submit FAFSA. *Faculty research:* Biodiversity, global change, conservation. *Unit head:* Dr. Karen Lips, Director, 301-405-7409, E-mail: klips@umd.edu. *Application contact:* Dr. Charles A. Caramello, Dean of Graduate School, 301-405-0358, Fax: 301-314-9305, E-mail: ccaramel@umd.edu.

University of Michigan, School of Natural Resources and Environment, Program in Natural Resources and Environment, Ann Arbor, MI 48109-1041. Offers aquatic sciences: research and management (MS); behavior, education and communication (MS); conservation biology (MS); conservation ecology (MS); environmental informatics (MS); environmental justice (MS); environmental policy and planning (MS); natural resources and environment (PhD); sustainable systems (MS); terrestrial ecosystems (MS); MS/JD; MS/MBA; MUP/MS. *Faculty:* 45 full-time, 23 part-time/adjunct. *Students:* 380 full-time (203 women); includes 59 minority (5 Black or African American, non-Hispanic/Latino; 1 American Indian or Alaska Native, non-Hispanic/Latino; 20 Asian, non-Hispanic/Latino; 21 Hispanic/Latino; 12 Two or more races, non-Hispanic/Latino), 74 international. Average age 27. 657 applicants. In 2013, 131 master's, 11 doctorates awarded. Terminal master's awarded for partial completion of doctoral program. *Degree requirements:* For master's, practicum or group project; for doctorate, comprehensive exam, thesis/dissertation, oral defense of dissertation, preliminary exam. *Entrance requirements:* For master's, GRE General Test; for doctorate, GRE General Test, master's degree. Additional exam requirements/recommendations for international students: Required—TOEFL (minimum score 560 paper-based; 84 iBT). *Application deadline:* For fall admission, 1/5 priority date for domestic and international students. Applications are processed on a rolling basis. Application fee: $65 ($75 for international students). Electronic applications accepted. Tuition and fees vary according to course level, course load, degree level, program and student level. *Financial support:* Fellowships with tuition reimbursements available. Financial award application deadline: 1/5; financial award applicants required to submit FAFSA. *Faculty research:* Stream ecology and fish biology, plant-insect interactions, environmental education, resource control and reproductive success, remote sensing, conservation ecology, sustainable systems. *Unit head:* Dr. Marie Lynn Miranda, Dean, 734-764-2550, Fax: 734-763-8965,

Conservation Biology

E-mail: mlmirand@umich.edu. *Application contact:* Sondra R. Auerbach, Director of Academic Services, 734-764-6453, Fax: 734-936-2195, E-mail: snre.admissions@umich.edu.
Website: http://www.snre.umich.edu/

University of Minnesota, Twin Cities Campus, Graduate School, College of Food, Agricultural and Natural Resource Sciences, Program in Conservation Biology, Minneapolis, MN 55455-0213. Offers MS, PhD. Part-time programs available. *Faculty:* 99 full-time (25 women), 13 part-time/adjunct (5 women). *Students:* 65 full-time (33 women); includes 4 minority (3 Asian, non-Hispanic/Latino; 1 Hispanic/Latino), 13 international. Average age 28. 58 applicants, 12% accepted, 7 enrolled. In 2013, 3 master's, 3 doctorates awarded. Terminal master's awarded for partial completion of doctoral program. *Degree requirements:* For master's, comprehensive exam, thesis; for doctorate, comprehensive exam, thesis/dissertation. *Entrance requirements:* For master's and doctorate, GRE, advanced ecology course. Additional exam requirements/recommendations for international students: Required—TOEFL (minimum score 550 paper-based; 79 iBT), IELTS (minimum score 6.5). *Application deadline:* For fall admission, 12/15 priority date for domestic and international students; for spring admission, 10/15 for domestic and international students. Applications are processed on a rolling basis. Application fee: $75 ($95 for international students). Electronic applications accepted. *Financial support:* In 2013–14, 2 students received support, including fellowships with full tuition reimbursements available (averaging $32,000 per year), research assistantships with full and partial tuition reimbursements available (averaging $32,000 per year), teaching assistantships with full and partial tuition reimbursements available (averaging $32,000 per year); scholarships/grants, health care benefits, tuition waivers, and unspecified assistantships also available. Financial award application deadline: 12/15. *Faculty research:* Wildlife conservation, fisheries and aquatic biology, invasive species, human dimensions, GIS, restoration ecology. *Unit head:* Dr. Rob Blair, Director of Graduate Studies, 612-624-2198, E-mail: blairrb@umn.edu. *Application contact:* Anup Joshi, Program Coordinator, 612-624-7751, E-mail: consbio@umn.edu.
Website: http://www.consbio.umn.edu/

University of Missouri, Graduate School, College of Agriculture, Food and Natural Resources, Department of Agricultural and Applied Economics, Columbia, MO 65211. Offers agricultural economics (MS, PhD); conservation biology (Graduate Certificate). *Faculty:* 23 full-time (3 women), 3 part-time/adjunct (1 woman). *Students:* 35 full-time (13 women), 11 part-time (4 women); includes 1 minority (Asian, non-Hispanic/Latino), 17 international. Average age 31. 57 applicants, 33% accepted, 14 enrolled. In 2013, 6 master's, 6 doctorates, 1 other advanced degree awarded. *Degree requirements:* For doctorate, comprehensive exam, thesis/dissertation. *Entrance requirements:* For master's and doctorate, GRE General Test, minimum GPA of 3.0. Additional exam requirements/recommendations for international students: Required—TOEFL (minimum score 550 paper-based; 80 iBT). *Application deadline:* For fall admission, 2/15 priority date for domestic students, 2/15 for international students; for winter admission, 9/15 for domestic and international students. Applications are processed on a rolling basis. Application fee: $55 ($75 for international students). Electronic applications accepted. *Financial support:* Fellowships, research assistantships with tuition reimbursements, teaching assistantships with tuition reimbursements, Federal Work-Study, institutionally sponsored loans, scholarships/grants, health care benefits, and unspecified assistantships available. Financial award application deadline: 3/1; financial award applicants required to submit FAFSA. *Faculty research:* Agribusiness management, contracting and strategy; collective action and cooperative theory; econometrics and price analysis; entrepreneurship; environmental and natural resource economics; food, biofuel and agricultural policy and regulation; international development; regional economics and rural development policy; science policy and innovation; sustainable agriculture and applied ethics. *Unit head:* Dr. Joe Parcell, Department Chair, 573-882-0870, E-mail: parcellj@missouri.edu. *Application contact:* Jody Pestle, Administrative Assistant, 573-882-3747, E-mail: pestlej@missouri.edu.
Website: http://dass.missouri.edu/agecon/grad/

University of Missouri, Graduate School, School of Natural Resources, Department of Fisheries and Wildlife Sciences, Columbia, MO 65211. Offers conservation biology (Certificate); fisheries and wildlife (MS, PhD). *Faculty:* 10 full-time (1 woman). *Students:* 12 full-time (5 women), 18 part-time (9 women); includes 2 minority (1 Black or African American, non-Hispanic/Latino; 1 Two or more races, non-Hispanic/Latino), 3 international. Average age 29. 15 applicants, 40% accepted, 6 enrolled. In 2013, 8 master's, 3 doctorates, 2 other advanced degrees awarded. *Degree requirements:* For doctorate, thesis/dissertation. *Entrance requirements:* For master's and doctorate, GRE General Test, minimum GPA of 3.0. Additional exam requirements/recommendations for international students: Required—TOEFL (minimum score 550 paper-based; 79 iBT). *Application deadline:* Applications are processed on a rolling basis. Application fee: $55 ($75 for international students). Electronic applications accepted. *Financial support:* Fellowships, research assistantships, teaching assistantships, institutionally sponsored loans, and scholarships/grants available. *Faculty research:* Limnology; conservation biology; landscape ecology; natural resource policy and management; rare species conservation; avian ecology; behavior and conservation; large river ecology; native fish ecology and restoration ecology; wildlife disease ecology; behavioral, population and community ecology; conservation biology; mammalian carnivores; fish bioenergetics; compensatory growth; fish population dynamics and aquaculture; endangered species recovery; wildlife stress physiology. *Unit head:* Dr. Jack Jones, Department Chair, 573-882-3543, E-mail: jonesj@missouri.edu. *Application contact:* Janice Faaborg, Academic Advisor, 573-882-9422, E-mail: faaborgj@missouri.edu.
Website: http://www.snr.missouri.edu/fw/academics/graduate-program.php

University of Missouri–St. Louis, College of Arts and Sciences, Department of Biology, St. Louis, MO 63121. Offers biotechnology (Certificate); cell and molecular biology (MS, PhD); ecology, evolution and systematics (MS, PhD); tropical biology and conservation (Certificate). Part-time programs available. *Faculty:* 33 full-time (13 women), 9 part-time/adjunct (1 woman). *Students:* 52 full-time (23 women), 58 part-time (29 women); includes 13 minority (9 Black or African American, non-Hispanic/Latino; 3 Asian, non-Hispanic/Latino; 1 Hispanic/Latino), 30 international. Average age 28. 113 applicants, 42% accepted, 22 enrolled. In 2013, 31 master's, 5 doctorates, 4 other advanced degrees awarded. *Degree requirements:* For master's, thesis or alternative; for doctorate, thesis/dissertation, 1 semester of teaching experience. *Entrance requirements:* For master's, 3 letters of recommendation; for doctorate, GRE General Test, 3 letters of recommendation. Additional exam requirements/recommendations for international students: Required—TOEFL (minimum score 79 iBT), IELTS (minimum score 6.5). *Application deadline:* For fall admission, 12/15 priority date for domestic and international students; for spring admission, 12/1 priority date for domestic and international students. Applications are processed on a rolling basis. Application fee: $50 ($40 for international students). Electronic applications accepted. *Expenses:* Tuition, state resident: full-time $7364; part-time $409.10 per credit hour. Tuition, nonresident: full-time $19,162; part-time $1008.50 per credit hour. *Financial support:* In 2013–14, 13 research assistantships with full and partial tuition reimbursements (averaging $17,000 per year), 23 teaching assistantships with full and partial tuition reimbursements (averaging $17,000 per year) were awarded; fellowships with full tuition reimbursements, career-related internships or fieldwork, and Federal Work-Study also available. Support available to part-time students. Financial award application deadline: 2/1. *Faculty research:* Molecular biology, microbial genetics, animal behavior, tropical ecology, plant systematics. *Unit head:* Dr. Teresa Thiel, Director of Graduate Studies, 314-516-6200, Fax: 314-516-6233, E-mail: thiel@umsl.edu. *Application contact:* 314-516-5458, Fax: 314-516-6996, E-mail: gradadm@umsl.edu.
Website: http://www.umsl.edu/divisions/artscience/biology/

University of Nevada, Reno, Graduate School, Interdisciplinary Program in Ecology, Evolution, and Conservation Biology, Reno, NV 89557. Offers PhD. Offered through the College of Arts and Science, the M. C. Fleischmann College of Agriculture, and the Desert Research Institute. *Degree requirements:* For doctorate, thesis/dissertation. *Entrance requirements:* For doctorate, GRE General Test, GRE Subject Test, minimum GPA of 3.0. Additional exam requirements/recommendations for international students: Required—TOEFL (minimum score 500 paper-based; 61 iBT), IELTS (minimum score 6). Electronic applications accepted. *Faculty research:* Population biology, behavioral ecology, plant response to climate change, conservation of endangered species, restoration of natural ecosystems.

University of Wisconsin–Madison, Graduate School, Gaylord Nelson Institute for Environmental Studies, Environmental Conservation Program, Madison, WI 53706-1380. Offers MS. *Faculty:* 2 full-time (0 women), 8 part-time/adjunct (2 women). *Students:* 25 full-time (20 women); includes 1 minority (American Indian or Alaska Native, non-Hispanic/Latino), 7 international. Average age 29. 44 applicants, 75% accepted, 25 enrolled. In 2013, 6 master's awarded. *Degree requirements:* For master's, thesis or alternative, spring/summer leadership (internship) experience. *Entrance requirements:* Additional exam requirements/recommendations for international students: Required—TOEFL (minimum score 550 paper-based; 80 iBT). *Application deadline:* For fall admission, 12/1 for domestic and international students; for spring admission, 10/15 for domestic and international students; for summer admission, 12/1 for domestic and international students. Applications are processed on a rolling basis. Application fee: $56. Electronic applications accepted. *Expenses:* Tuition, state resident: full-time $10,728; part-time $790 per credit. Tuition, nonresident: full-time $24,054; part-time $1623 per credit. *Required fees:* $1130; $119 per credit. *Financial support:* In 2013–14, 13 students received support, including 1 fellowship with full tuition reimbursement available (averaging $23,668 per year), 2 research assistantships with full tuition reimbursements available (averaging $21,224 per year), 8 teaching assistantships with full tuition reimbursements available (averaging $9,733 per year); career-related internships or fieldwork and scholarships/grants also available. Financial award application deadline: 12/1. *Faculty research:* Ornithology, forestry, sociology, rural sociology, plant ecology, biodiversity, sustainability, sustainable development, conservation biology. *Unit head:* Dr. Janet M. Silbernagel, Chair, 608-890-2600, Fax: 608-262-2273, E-mail: jmsilber@wisc.edu. *Application contact:* Nathan Schulfer, Student Services Coordinator, 608-890-2600, Fax: 608-262-2273, E-mail: schulfer@wisc.edu.
Website: http://nelson.wisc.edu/graduate/environmental-conservation/index.php

Ecology

Baylor University, Graduate School, College of Arts and Sciences, The Institute of Ecological, Earth and Environmental Sciences, Waco, TX 76798. Offers PhD. *Students:* 8 full-time (3 women); includes 3 minority (2 Hispanic/Latino; 1 Two or more races, non-Hispanic/Latino), 3 international. In 2013, 1 doctorate awarded. *Degree requirements:* For doctorate, variable foreign language requirement, comprehensive exam, thesis/dissertation or alternative. *Entrance requirements:* For doctorate, GRE. Additional exam requirements/recommendations for international students: Required—TOEFL (minimum score 550 paper-based; 80 iBT); Recommended—IELTS (minimum score 6.5). *Application deadline:* For fall admission, 2/15 priority date for domestic and international students; for spring admission, 11/15 for domestic and international students. Application fee: $40. Electronic applications accepted. *Expenses: Tuition:* Full-time $25,866; part-time $1437 per credit hour. *Required fees:* $2736; $152 per credit hour. Tuition and fees vary according to course load and program. *Financial support:* In 2013–14, 5 students received support, including 5 research assistantships with full and partial tuition reimbursements available (averaging $20,000 per year), 5 teaching assistantships with full and partial tuition reimbursements available (averaging $20,000 per year); career-related internships or fieldwork, scholarships/grants, traineeships, health care benefits, tuition waivers (partial), and unspecified assistantships also available. Financial award application deadline: 2/15. *Faculty research:* Ecosystem processes, environmental toxicology and risk assessment, biogeochemical cycling, chemical fate and transport, conservation management. *Unit head:* Dr. Joe C. Yelderman, Jr., Director, 254-710-2224, E-mail: joe_yelderman@baylor.edu. *Application contact:* Shannon Koehler, Administrative Associate, 254-710-2224, Fax: 254-710-2580, E-mail: shannon_koehler@baylor.edu.
Website: http://www.baylor.edu/TIEEES/

Brown University, Graduate School, Division of Biology and Medicine, Department of Ecology and Evolutionary Biology, Providence, RI 02912. Offers PhD. *Degree requirements:* For doctorate, thesis/dissertation, preliminary exam. *Entrance requirements:* For doctorate, GRE General Test, GRE Subject Test. Additional exam requirements/recommendations for international students: Required—TOEFL. Electronic applications accepted. *Faculty research:* Marine ecology, behavioral ecology, population genetics, evolutionary morphology, plant ecology.

California Institute of Integral Studies, School of Consciousness and Transformation, San Francisco, CA 94103. Offers anthropology and social change (MA, PhD); creative inquiry/interdisciplinary arts (MFA); East-West psychology (MA, PhD); philosophy and religion (MA, PhD), including Asian and comparative studies, ecology, spirituality, and religion, philosophy, cosmology, and consciousness, women's spirituality; transformative leadership (MA); transformative studies (PhD); writing and consciousness (MFA). Part-time and evening/weekend programs available.

Postbaccalaureate distance learning degree programs offered (minimal on-campus study). *Students:* 386 full-time (257 women), 127 part-time (80 women); includes 138 minority (36 Black or African American, non-Hispanic/Latino; 1 American Indian or Alaska Native, non-Hispanic/Latino; 19 Asian, non-Hispanic/Latino; 43 Hispanic/Latino; 2 Native Hawaiian or other Pacific Islander, non-Hispanic/Latino; 37 Two or more races, non-Hispanic/Latino), 46 international. Average age 38. 178 applicants, 96% accepted, 113 enrolled. In 2013, 73 master's, 50 doctorates awarded. Terminal master's awarded for partial completion of doctoral program. *Degree requirements:* For master's, thesis optional; for doctorate, comprehensive exam, thesis/dissertation, 1 foreign language (for Asian comparative studies). *Entrance requirements:* For master's, minimum GPA of 3.0, letters of recommendation, writing sample; for doctorate, master's degree, minimum GPA of 3.0, letters of recommendation, writing sample. Additional exam requirements/recommendations for international students: Required—TOEFL. *Application deadline:* For fall admission, 2/1 priority date for domestic and international students; for spring admission, 10/15 priority date for domestic and international students. Applications are processed on a rolling basis. Application fee: $65. Electronic applications accepted. *Expenses: Tuition:* Full-time $17,658; part-time $981 per credit. *Required fees:* $85 per semester. *Financial support:* In 2013–14, 285 students received support, including 5 research assistantships (averaging $800 per year), 28 teaching assistantships (averaging $825 per year); career-related internships or fieldwork, Federal Work-Study, and scholarships/grants also available. Support available to part-time students. Financial award application deadline: 4/15; financial award applicants required to submit FAFSA. *Faculty research:* Ecology and sustainability, philosophy and religion, East-West psychology, integrative health, social and cultural anthropology, transformative leadership. *Application contact:* David Townes, Senior Admissions Counselor, 415-575-6152, Fax: 415-575-1268, E-mail: admissions@ciis.edu.
Website: http://www.ciis.edu/

California State University, Stanislaus, College of Natural Sciences, Program in Ecology and Sustainability (MS), Turlock, CA 95382. Offers ecological conservation (MS); ecological economics (MS). Part-time programs available. *Degree requirements:* For master's, thesis. *Entrance requirements:* For master's, GRE, minimum GPA of 3.0, 3 letters of recommendation, personal statement. Additional exam requirements/recommendations for international students: Required—TOEFL (minimum score 550 paper-based). Electronic applications accepted.

Clemson University, Graduate School, College of Agriculture, Forestry and Life Sciences, Department of Biological Sciences, Program in Biological Sciences, Clemson, SC 29634. Offers MS, PhD. *Students:* 31 full-time (19 women), 147 part-time (101 women); includes 15 minority (4 Black or African American, non-Hispanic/Latino; 1 Asian, non-Hispanic/Latino; 5 Hispanic/Latino; 5 Two or more races, non-Hispanic/Latino), 9 international. Average age 33. 137 applicants, 70% accepted, 84 enrolled. In 2013, 6 master's, 3 doctorates awarded. *Degree requirements:* For master's, thesis optional; for doctorate, comprehensive exam, thesis/dissertation. *Entrance requirements:* For master's and doctorate, GRE General Test. Additional exam requirements/recommendations for international students: Required—TOEFL, IELTS. *Application deadline:* For fall admission, 1/15 for domestic students, 4/15 for international students. Applications are processed on a rolling basis. Application fee: $70 ($80 for international students). Electronic applications accepted. *Financial support:* In 2013–14, 27 students received support, including 3 fellowships with full and partial tuition reimbursements available (averaging $16,167 per year), 3 research assistantships with partial tuition reimbursements available (averaging $18,167 per year), 23 teaching assistantships with partial tuition reimbursements available (averaging $18,452 per year); career-related internships or fieldwork, institutionally sponsored loans, scholarships/grants, health care benefits, and unspecified assistantships also available. Support available to part-time students. Financial award application deadline: 3/15; financial award applicants required to submit FAFSA. *Unit head:* Dr. Alfred Wheeler, Department Chair, 864-656-1415, Fax: 864-656-0435, E-mail: wheeler@clemson.edu. *Application contact:* Jay Lyn Martin, Coordinator for Graduate Program, 864-656-3587, Fax: 864-656-0435, E-mail: gradbio@clemson.edu.
Website: http://www.clemson.edu/cafls/departments/biosci/

Colorado State University, Graduate School, Graduate Degree Program in Ecology, Fort Collins, CO 80523-1401. Offers MS, PhD. Part-time programs available. *Students:* 56 full-time (31 women), 114 part-time (61 women); includes 14 minority (3 Black or African American, non-Hispanic/Latino; 6 Asian, non-Hispanic/Latino; 4 Hispanic/Latino; 1 Two or more races, non-Hispanic/Latino), 16 international. Average age 31. 90 applicants, 32% accepted, 22 enrolled. In 2013, 13 master's, 13 doctorates awarded. Terminal master's awarded for partial completion of doctoral program. *Degree requirements:* For master's, comprehensive exam (for some programs), thesis; for doctorate, comprehensive exam, thesis/dissertation. *Entrance requirements:* For master's and doctorate, GRE General Test, minimum GPA of 3.0, BA/BS in related field, 3 letters of recommendation, personal statement. Additional exam requirements/recommendations for international students: Required—TOEFL (minimum score 550 paper-based; 80 iBT). *Application deadline:* For fall admission, 1/1 priority date for domestic students, 1/1 for international students; for spring admission, 10/15 priority date for domestic students, 9/15 for international students. Applications are processed on a rolling basis. Application fee: $50. Electronic applications accepted. *Expenses:* Tuition, state resident: full-time $9075.40; part-time $504 per credit. Tuition, nonresident: full-time $22,248; part-time $1236 per credit. *Required fees:* $1819; $60 per credit. *Financial support:* Teaching assistantships with full tuition reimbursements available. Financial award application deadline: 1/1; financial award applicants required to submit FAFSA. *Faculty research:* Aquatic and riparian ecology, evolutionary ecology, conservation ecology, fire ecology, community ecology. *Unit head:* Dr. N. Leroy Poff, Director, 970-491-4373, Fax: 970-491-0649, E-mail: poff@lamar.colostate.edu. *Application contact:* Jeri Morgan, Program Coordinator, 970-491-4373, Fax: 970-491-5091, E-mail: jeri.morgan@colostate.edu.
Website: http://www.ecology.colostate.edu/

Columbia University, Graduate School of Arts and Sciences, Department of Ecology, Evolution and Environmental Biology, New York, NY 10027. Offers conservation biology (MA); ecology and evolutionary biology (PhD); evolutionary primatology (PhD). *Faculty:* 7 full-time (1 woman), 43 part-time/adjunct (15 women). *Students:* 46 full-time (36 women), 1 part-time (0 women). Average age 28. 45 applicants, 18% accepted. *Degree requirements:* For doctorate, one foreign language, thesis/dissertation, teaching experience. *Entrance requirements:* For doctorate, GRE General Test, previous course work in biology. Additional exam requirements/recommendations for international students: Required—TOEFL. Application fee: $90. Electronic applications accepted. *Financial support:* Fellowships, career-related internships or fieldwork, and institutionally sponsored loans available. Financial award application deadline: 1/5. *Faculty research:* Tropical ecology, ethnobotany, global change, systematics. *Total annual research expenditures:* $300,000. *Unit head:* Prof. Ruth DeFries, Chair, 212-851-1647, E-mail: rd2402@columbia.edu. *Application contact:* 212-854-9987.
Website: http://www.columbia.edu/cu/e3b/

Cornell University, Graduate School, Graduate Fields of Agriculture and Life Sciences, Field of Computational Biology, Ithaca, NY 14853-0001. Offers computational behavioral biology (PhD); computational biology (PhD); computational cell biology (PhD); computational ecology (PhD); computational genetics (PhD); computational macromolecular biology (PhD); computational organismal biology (PhD). *Faculty:* 37 full-time (5 women). *Students:* 26 full-time (8 women); includes 8 minority (5 Asian, non-Hispanic/Latino; 1 Hispanic/Latino; 1 Native Hawaiian or other Pacific Islander, non-Hispanic/Latino; 1 Two or more races, non-Hispanic/Latino), 8 international. Average age 25. 171 applicants, 13% accepted, 10 enrolled. *Degree requirements:* For doctorate, comprehensive exam, thesis/dissertation, 2 semesters of teaching experience. *Entrance requirements:* For doctorate, GRE General Test, GRE Subject Test (biology), 2 letters of recommendation. Additional exam requirements/recommendations for international students: Required—TOEFL (minimum score 550 paper-based; 77 iBT). *Application deadline:* For fall admission, 2/1 priority date for domestic students. Application fee: $95. Electronic applications accepted. *Financial support:* In 2013–14, 22 students received support, including 20 research assistantships with full tuition reimbursements available, 2 teaching assistantships with full tuition reimbursements available; fellowships with full tuition reimbursements available, institutionally sponsored loans, scholarships/grants, health care benefits, tuition waivers (full and partial), and unspecified assistantships also available. Financial award applicants required to submit FAFSA. *Faculty research:* Computational behavioral biology, computational biology, computational cell biology, computational ecology, computational genetics, computational macromolecular biology, computational organismal biology. *Unit head:* Dr. Andrew Clark, Director of Graduate Studies, 607-255-5488, E-mail: ac347@cornell.edu. *Application contact:* Graduate School Application Requests, 607-255-5816, E-mail: gradadmissions@cornell.edu.
Website: http://www.gradschool.cornell.edu/fields.php?id-4A

Cornell University, Graduate School, Graduate Fields of Agriculture and Life Sciences, Field of Ecology and Evolutionary Biology, Ithaca, NY 14853-0001. Offers ecology (PhD), including animal ecology, applied ecology, biogeochemistry, community and ecosystem ecology, limnology, oceanography, physiological ecology, plant ecology, population ecology, theoretical ecology, vertebrate zoology; evolutionary biology (PhD), including ecological genetics, paleobiology, population biology, systematics. *Faculty:* 52 full-time (14 women). *Students:* 56 full-time (36 women); includes 8 minority (3 Asian, non-Hispanic/Latino; 3 Hispanic/Latino; 2 Two or more races, non-Hispanic/Latino), 12 international. Average age 28. 115 applicants, 13% accepted, 11 enrolled. In 2013, 10 doctorates awarded. *Degree requirements:* For doctorate, comprehensive exam, thesis/dissertation, 2 semesters of teaching experience. *Entrance requirements:* For doctorate, GRE General Test, GRE Subject Test (biology), 2 letters of recommendation. Additional exam requirements/recommendations for international students: Required—TOEFL (minimum score 550 paper-based; 77 iBT). *Application deadline:* For fall admission, 12/15 for domestic students. Application fee: $95. Electronic applications accepted. *Financial support:* In 2013–14, 43 students received support, including 14 fellowships with full tuition reimbursements available, 7 research assistantships with full tuition reimbursements available, 22 teaching assistantships with full tuition reimbursements available; institutionally sponsored loans, scholarships/grants, health care benefits, tuition waivers (full and partial), and unspecified assistantships also available. Financial award applicants required to submit FAFSA. *Faculty research:* Population and organismal biology, population and evolutionary genetics, systematics and macroevolution, biochemistry, conservation biology. *Unit head:* Director of Graduate Studies, 607-254-4230. *Application contact:* Graduate Field Assistant, 607-254-4230, E-mail: eeb_grad_req@cornell.edu.
Website: http://www.gradschool.cornell.edu/fields.php?id-46&a-2

Cornell University, Graduate School, Graduate Fields of Agriculture and Life Sciences, Field of Horticulture, Ithaca, NY 14853-0001. Offers breeding of horticultural crops (MPS); horticultural crop management systems (MPS); human-plant interactions (MPS, PhD); physiology and ecology of horticultural crops (MPS, MS, PhD). *Faculty:* 52 full-time (14 women). *Students:* 39 full-time (17 women); includes 4 minority (1 Asian, non-Hispanic/Latino; 1 Hispanic/Latino; 2 Two or more races, non-Hispanic/Latino), 12 international. Average age 30. 73 applicants, 18% accepted, 11 enrolled. In 2013, 13 master's, 1 doctorate awarded. *Degree requirements:* For master's, thesis (MS); for doctorate, comprehensive exam, thesis/dissertation. *Entrance requirements:* For master's and doctorate, GRE General Test, 3 letters of recommendation. Additional exam requirements/recommendations for international students: Required—TOEFL (minimum score 550 paper-based; 77 iBT). *Application deadline:* For fall admission, 1/15 for domestic students; for spring admission, 8/15 for domestic students. Application fee: $95. Electronic applications accepted. *Financial support:* In 2013–14, 35 students received support, including 5 fellowships with full tuition reimbursements available, 16 research assistantships with full tuition reimbursements available, 14 teaching assistantships with full tuition reimbursements available; institutionally sponsored loans, scholarships/grants, health care benefits, tuition waivers (full and partial), and unspecified assistantships also available. Financial award applicants required to submit FAFSA. *Faculty research:* Plant selection/plant materials, greenhouse management, greenhouse crop production, urban landscape management, turfgrass management. *Unit head:* Director of Graduate Studies, 607-255-4568, Fax: 607-255-0599. *Application contact:* Graduate Field Assistant, 607-255-4568, Fax: 607-255-0599, E-mail: hortgrad@cornell.edu.
Website: http://www.gradschool.cornell.edu/fields.php?id-XX&a-2

Cornell University, Graduate School, Graduate Fields of Agriculture and Life Sciences, Field of Natural Resources, Ithaca, NY 14853-0001. Offers community-based natural resources management (MS, PhD); conservation biology (MS, PhD); ecosystem biology and biogeochemistry (MPS, MS, PhD); environmental management (MPS); fishery and aquatic science (MPS, MS, PhD); forest science (MPS, MS, PhD); human dimensions of natural resources management (MPS, MS, PhD); policy and institutional analysis (MS, PhD); program development and evaluation (MPS, MS, PhD); quantitative ecology (MS, PhD); wildlife science (MPS, MS, PhD). *Faculty:* 39 full-time (8 women). *Students:* 65 full-time (30 women); includes 2 minority (1 Asian, non-Hispanic/Latino; 1 Hispanic/Latino), 18 international. Average age 31. 93 applicants, 26% accepted, 20 enrolled. In 2013, 8 master's, 7 doctorates awarded. *Degree requirements:* For master's, thesis (MS), project paper (MPS); for doctorate, comprehensive exam, thesis/dissertation. *Entrance requirements:* For master's and doctorate, GRE General Test, 2 letters of recommendation. Additional exam requirements/recommendations for international students: Required—TOEFL (minimum score 550 paper-based; 77 iBT). *Application deadline:* For spring admission, 10/30 for domestic students. Applications are processed on a rolling basis. Application fee: $95. Electronic applications accepted. *Financial support:* In 2013–14, 48 students received support, including 10 fellowships with full tuition reimbursements available, 18 research assistantships with full tuition reimbursements available, 20 teaching assistantships with full tuition reimbursements available; institutionally sponsored loans, scholarships/grants, health care benefits, tuition waivers (full and partial), and unspecified assistantships also available. Financial award applicants required to submit FAFSA. *Faculty research:* Ecosystem-level dynamics, systems modeling, conservation biology/management, resource management's human dimensions, biogeochemistry. *Unit head:* Director of Graduate Studies, 607-255-2807, Fax: 607-255-0349. *Application contact:* Graduate Field Assistant, 607-255-2807, Fax: 607-255-0349, E-mail: nrgrad@cornell.edu.
Website: http://www.gradschool.cornell.edu/fields.php?id-54&a-2

Ecology

Cornell University, Graduate School, Graduate Fields of Agriculture and Life Sciences, Field of Zoology and Wildlife Conservation, Ithaca, NY 14853-0001. Offers animal cytology (PhD); comparative and functional anatomy (PhD); developmental biology (PhD); ecology (PhD); histology (PhD); wildlife conservation (PhD). *Faculty:* 21 full-time (6 women). *Students:* 4 full-time (3 women), 1 part-time (0 women); includes 2 minority (1 Hispanic/Latino; 1 Two or more races, non-Hispanic/Latino), 1 international. Average age 26. 18 applicants, 6% accepted, 1 enrolled. In 2013, 1 doctorate awarded. *Degree requirements:* For doctorate, comprehensive exam, thesis/dissertation, 2 semesters of teaching experience. *Entrance requirements:* For doctorate, GRE General Test, GRE Subject Test (biology), 2 letters of recommendation. Additional exam requirements/recommendations for international students: Required—TOEFL (minimum score 550 paper-based; 77 iBT). *Application deadline:* For fall admission, 2/1 priority date for domestic students. Application fee: $95. Electronic applications accepted. *Financial support:* In 2013–14, 4 students received support, including 3 research assistantships with full tuition reimbursements available, 1 teaching assistantship with full tuition reimbursement available; fellowships with full tuition reimbursements available, institutionally sponsored loans, scholarships/grants, health care benefits, tuition waivers (full and partial), and unspecified assistantships also available. Financial award applicants required to submit FAFSA. *Faculty research:* Organismal biology, functional morphology, biomechanics, comparative vertebrate anatomy, comparative invertebrate anatomy, paleontology. *Unit head:* Director of Graduate Studies, 607-253-3276, Fax: 607-253-3756. *Application contact:* Graduate Field Assistant, 607-253-3276, Fax: 607-253-3756, E-mail: graduate_edcvm@cornell.edu.
Website: http://www.gradschool.cornell.edu/fields.php?id-65&a-2

Dalhousie University, Faculty of Agriculture, Halifax, NS B3H 4R2, Canada. Offers agriculture (M Sc), including air quality, animal behavior, animal molecular genetics, animal nutrition, animal technology, aquaculture, botany, crop management, crop physiology, ecology, environmental microbiology, food science, horticulture, nutrient management, pest management, physiology, plant biotechnology, plant pathology, soil chemistry, soil fertility, waste management and composting, water quality. Part-time programs available. *Degree requirements:* For master's, thesis, ATC Exam Teaching Assistantship. *Entrance requirements:* For master's, honors B Sc, minimum GPA of 3.0. Additional exam requirements/recommendations for international students: Required—TOEFL (minimum score 580 paper-based; 92 iBT), IELTS, Michigan English Language Assessment Battery, CanTEST, CAEL. *Faculty research:* Bio-product development, organic agriculture, nutrient management, air and water quality, agricultural biotechnology.

Dartmouth College, Arts and Sciences Graduate Programs, Program in Ecology and Evolutionary Biology, Hanover, NH 03755. Offers PhD. *Entrance requirements:* For doctorate, GRE General Test, GRE Subject Test in biology (highly recommended). Additional exam requirements/recommendations for international students: Required—TOEFL.

Duke University, Graduate School, Department of Ecology, Durham, NC 27708-0329. Offers PhD, Certificate. *Faculty:* 39. *Students:* 29 full-time (19 women); includes 3 minority (1 Black or African American, non-Hispanic/Latino; 1 Asian, non-Hispanic/Latino; 1 Hispanic/Latino). 48 applicants, 19% accepted, 6 enrolled. In 2013, 2 doctorates awarded. *Degree requirements:* For doctorate, thesis/dissertation. *Entrance requirements:* For doctorate, GRE General Test. Additional exam requirements/recommendations for international students: Required—TOEFL (minimum score 577 paper-based; 90 iBT) or IELTS (minimum score 7). *Application deadline:* For fall admission, 12/8 priority date for domestic and international students. Application fee: $80. Electronic applications accepted. *Financial support:* Fellowships, research assistantships, and teaching assistantships available. Financial award application deadline: 12/8. *Unit head:* Emily Bernhardt, Director of Graduate Studies, 919-613-8002, Fax: 919-613-8061, E-mail: meg.stephens@duke.edu. *Application contact:* Elizabeth Hutton, Director, Graduate Admissions, 919-684-3913, Fax: 919-684-2277, E-mail: grad-admissions@duke.edu.
Website: http://sites.duke.edu/upecology/

Eastern Kentucky University, The Graduate School, College of Arts and Sciences, Department of Biological Sciences, Richmond, KY 40475-3102. Offers biological sciences (MS); ecology (MS). Part-time programs available. *Degree requirements:* For master's, thesis. *Entrance requirements:* For master's, GRE General Test, minimum GPA of 2.5. *Faculty research:* Systematics, ecology, and biodiversity; animal behavior; protein structure and molecular genetics; biomonitoring and aquatic toxicology; pathogenesis of microbes and parasites.

Eastern Michigan University, Graduate School, College of Arts and Sciences, Department of Biology, Ypsilanti, MI 48197. Offers cell and molecular biology (MS); community college biology teaching (MS); ecology and organismal biology (MS); general biology (MS); water resources (MS). Part-time and evening/weekend programs available. Postbaccalaureate distance learning degree programs offered (minimal on-campus study). *Faculty:* 19 full-time (4 women). *Students:* 11 full-time (6 women), 31 part-time (18 women); includes 3 minority (1 Black or African American, non-Hispanic/Latino; 1 Asian, non-Hispanic/Latino; 1 Hispanic/Latino), 6 international. Average age 26. 56 applicants, 59% accepted, 20 enrolled. In 2013, 13 master's awarded. *Entrance requirements:* For master's, GRE General Test, GRE Subject Test. Additional exam requirements/recommendations for international students: Required—TOEFL. *Application deadline:* Applications are processed on a rolling basis. Application fee: $35. *Expenses:* Tuition, state resident: full-time $12,300; part-time $466 per credit hour. Tuition, nonresident: full-time $23,159; part-time $918 per credit hour. *Required fees:* $71 per credit hour. $46 per semester. One-time fee: $100. Tuition and fees vary according to course level and degree level. *Financial support:* Fellowships, research assistantships with full tuition reimbursements, teaching assistantships with full tuition reimbursements, career-related internships or fieldwork, Federal Work-Study, institutionally sponsored loans, scholarships/grants, tuition waivers (partial), and unspecified assistantships available. Support available to part-time students. Financial award applicants required to submit FAFSA. *Unit head:* Dr. Daniel Clemans, Department Head, 734-487-4242, Fax: 734-487-9235, E-mail: dclemans@emich.edu. *Application contact:* Dr. David Kass, Graduate Coordinator, 734-487-4242, Fax: 734-487-9235, E-mail: dkass@emich.edu.
Website: http://www.emich.edu/biology

Eastern New Mexico University, Graduate School, College of Liberal Arts and Sciences, Department of Biology, Portales, NM 88130. Offers applied ecology (MS); botany (MS); cell, molecular biology and biotechnology (MS); microbiology (MS); zoology (MS). Part-time programs available. *Degree requirements:* For master's, comprehensive exam, thesis optional. *Entrance requirements:* For master's, GRE, minimum GPA of 3.0, 2 letters of recommendation, statement of research interest, bachelor's degree related to field of study or proof of common knowledge. Additional exam requirements/recommendations for international students: Required—TOEFL (minimum score 550 paper-based; 79 iBT), IELTS (minimum score 6). Electronic applications accepted.

Emory University, Laney Graduate School, Division of Biological and Biomedical Sciences, Program in Population Biology, Ecology and Evolution, Atlanta, GA 30322-1100. Offers PhD. *Degree requirements:* For doctorate, comprehensive exam, thesis/dissertation. *Entrance requirements:* For doctorate, GRE General Test, minimum GPA of 3.0 in science course work (recommended). Additional exam requirements/recommendations for international students: Required—TOEFL. Electronic applications accepted. *Faculty research:* Evolution of microbes, infectious disease, the immune system, genetic disease in humans, evolution of behavior.

Florida Institute of Technology, Graduate Programs, College of Science, Department of Biological Sciences, Program in Ecology, Melbourne, FL 32901-6975. Offers MS. Part-time programs available. *Faculty:* 16 full-time (1 woman), 1 (woman) part-time/adjunct. *Students:* 5 full-time (2 women), 1 (woman) part-time; includes 1 minority (Two or more races, non-Hispanic/Latino). Average age 25. 7 applicants, 29% accepted, 2 enrolled. In 2013, 3 master's awarded. *Degree requirements:* For master's, thesis, research, seminar, internship or summer lab. *Entrance requirements:* For master's, GRE General Test, minimum GPA of 3.0, 3 letters of recommendation, statement of objectives. Additional exam requirements/recommendations for international students: Required—TOEFL (minimum score 550 paper-based; 79 iBT). *Application deadline:* For fall admission, 3/15 for domestic students; for spring admission, 10/1 for domestic students. Applications are processed on a rolling basis. Electronic applications accepted. *Expenses: Tuition:* Full-time $20,214; part-time $1123 per credit. Tuition and fees vary according to campus/location. *Financial support:* Career-related internships or fieldwork, institutionally sponsored loans, tuition waivers (partial), unspecified assistantships, and tuition remissions available. Support available to part-time students. Financial award application deadline: 3/1; financial award applicants required to submit FAFSA. *Faculty research:* Endangered or threatened avian and mammalian species, hydroacoustics and feeding preference of the West Indian manatee, habitat preference of the Florida scrub jay. *Total annual research expenditures:* $1.4 million. *Unit head:* Dr. Richard B. Aronson, Department Head, 321-674-8034, Fax: 321-674-7238, E-mail: raronson@fit.edu. *Application contact:* Cheryl A. Brown, Associate Director of Graduate Admission, 321-674-7581, Fax: 321-723-9468, E-mail: cbrown@fit.edu.
Website: http://www.fit.edu/programs/8021/ms-biological-science-ecology

Florida State University, The Graduate School, College of Arts and Sciences, Department of Biological Science, Specialization in Ecology and Evolutionary Biology, Tallahassee, FL 32306-4295. Offers MS, PhD. *Faculty:* 21 full-time (7 women). *Students:* 56 full-time (27 women); includes 4 minority (1 Black or African American, non-Hispanic/Latino; 3 Hispanic/Latino), 5 international. 120 applicants, 13% accepted, 9 enrolled. In 2013, 2 master's, 3 doctorates awarded. Terminal master's awarded for partial completion of doctoral program. *Degree requirements:* For master's, comprehensive exam, thesis, teaching experience, seminar presentation; for doctorate, comprehensive exam, thesis/dissertation, teaching experience; seminar presentation. *Entrance requirements:* For master's and doctorate, GRE General Test, minimum upper-division GPA of 3.0. Additional exam requirements/recommendations for international students: Required—TOEFL (minimum score 600 paper-based; 92 iBT). *Application deadline:* For fall admission, 12/1 for domestic and international students. Application fee: $30. Electronic applications accepted. *Expenses:* Tuition, state resident: part-time $403.51 per credit hour. Tuition, nonresident: part-time $1004.85 per credit hour. *Required fees:* $75.81 per credit hour. One-time fee: $20 part-time. Tuition and fees vary according to course load, campus/location and student level. *Financial support:* In 2013–14, 55 students received support, including 4 fellowships with tuition reimbursements available (averaging $30,000 per year), 20 research assistantships with full tuition reimbursements available (averaging $21,500 per year), 31 teaching assistantships with full tuition reimbursements available (averaging $21,500 per year); scholarships/grants and unspecified assistantships also available. Financial award application deadline: 12/1; financial award applicants required to submit FAFSA. *Faculty research:* Ecology and conservation biology; evolution; marine biology; phylogeny and systematics; theoretical, computational and mathematical biology. *Unit head:* Dr. Debra A. Fadool, Professor and Associate Chair, 850-644-4775, Fax: 850-644-9829, E-mail: dfadool@bio.fsu.edu. *Application contact:* Judy Bowers, Coordinator, Graduate Affairs, 850-644-3023, Fax: 850-644-9829, E-mail: gradinfo@bio.fsu.edu.
Website: http://www.bio.fsu.edu/

Frostburg State University, Graduate School, College of Liberal Arts and Sciences, Department of Biology, Program in Applied Ecology and Conservation Biology, Frostburg, MD 21532-1099. Offers MS. *Degree requirements:* For master's, thesis. *Entrance requirements:* For master's, GRE General Test, resume. Additional exam requirements/recommendations for international students: Required—TOEFL. Electronic applications accepted. *Expenses: Tuition, area resident:* Part-time $340 per credit hour. Tuition, state resident: part-time $340 per credit hour. Tuition, nonresident: part-time $437 per credit hour. *Faculty research:* Forest ecology, microbiology of man-made wetlands, invertebrate zoology and entomology, wildlife and carnivore ecology, aquatic pollution ecology.

Illinois State University, Graduate School, College of Arts and Sciences, Department of Biological Sciences, Normal, IL 61790-2200. Offers animal behavior (MS); bacteriology (MS); biochemistry (MS); biological sciences (MS); biology (PhD); biophysics (MS); biotechnology (MS); botany (MS, PhD); cell biology (MS); conservation biology (MS); developmental biology (MS); ecology (MS, PhD); entomology (MS); evolutionary biology (MS); genetics (MS, PhD); immunology (MS); microbiology (MS, PhD); molecular biology (MS); molecular genetics (MS); neurobiology (MS); neuroscience (MS); parasitology (MS); physiology (MS, PhD); plant biology (MS); plant molecular biology (MS); plant sciences (MS); structural biology (MS); zoology (MS, PhD). Part-time programs available. *Degree requirements:* For master's, thesis or alternative; for doctorate, variable foreign language requirement, thesis/dissertation, 2 terms of residency. *Entrance requirements:* For master's, GRE General Test, minimum GPA of 2.6 in last 60 hours of course work; for doctorate, GRE General Test. *Faculty research:* Redoc balance and drug development in schistosoma mansoni, control of the growth of listeria monocytogenes at low temperature, regulation of cell expansion and microtubule function by SPRI, CRUI: physiology and fitness consequences of different life history phenotypes.

Indiana State University, College of Graduate and Professional Studies, College of Arts and Sciences, Department of Biology, Terre Haute, IN 47809. Offers ecology (PhD); life sciences (MS); microbiology (PhD); physiology (PhD); science education (MS). *Faculty:* 23 full-time (6 women), 1 (woman) part-time/adjunct. *Students:* 73 full-time (31 women), 15 part-time (6 women); includes 7 minority (6 Asian, non-Hispanic/Latino; 1 Hispanic/Latino), 17 international. Average age 26. 63 applicants, 65% accepted, 40 enrolled. In 2013, 9 master's, 5 doctorates awarded. *Degree requirements:* For master's, thesis (for some programs); for doctorate, comprehensive exam, thesis/dissertation. *Entrance requirements:* For master's and doctorate, GRE General Test. *Application deadline:* For fall admission, 7/1 priority date for domestic students; for spring admission, 11/1 priority date for domestic students. Applications are processed on a rolling basis. Application fee: $35. Electronic applications accepted. *Financial support:* In 2013–14, 9 research assistantships with partial tuition reimbursements (averaging $7,500 per year), 19 teaching assistantships with partial tuition reimbursements (averaging $8,000 per year) were awarded; Federal Work-Study, institutionally sponsored loans, and tuition waivers (partial) also available. Financial award application deadline: 3/1; financial award applicants required to submit FAFSA. *Unit head:* Dr. Arthur M. Halpern, Interim Chairperson, 812-237-2400. *Application* *contact:* Dr. Jay Gatrell, Dean, 800-444-GRAD, Fax: 812-237-8060, E-mail: jay.gatrell@indstate.edu.

Indiana University Bloomington, School of Public and Environmental Affairs, Environmental Science Programs, Bloomington, IN 47405. Offers applied ecology (MSES); energy (MSES); environmental chemistry, toxicology, and risk assessment (MSES); environmental science (PhD); hazardous materials management (Certificate); specialized environmental science (MSES); water resources (MSES); JD/MSES; MSES/MA; MSES/MPA; MSES/MS. Part-time programs available. *Faculty:* 16 full-time (4 women), 8 part-time/adjunct (3 women). *Students:* 135 full-time (69 women), 11 part-time (7 women); includes 15 minority (1 Black or African American, non-Hispanic/Latino; 8 Asian, non-Hispanic/Latino; 6 Hispanic/Latino), 13 international. Average age 25. 171 applicants, 81% accepted, 64 enrolled. In 2013, 71 master's, 3 doctorates awarded. Terminal master's awarded for partial completion of doctoral program. *Degree requirements:* For master's, capstone or thesis; internship; for doctorate, comprehensive exam, thesis/dissertation. *Entrance requirements:* For master's, GRE General Test or GMAT, official transcripts, 3 letters of recommendation, resume, personal statement; for doctorate, GRE General Test or LSAT, official transcripts, 3 letters of recommendation, resume or curriculum vitae, statement of purpose. Additional exam requirements/recommendations for international students: Required—TOEFL (minimum score 600 paper-based; 96 iBT); Recommended—IELTS (minimum score 7). *Application deadline:* For fall admission, 2/1 priority date for domestic students, 12/1 for international students; for spring admission, 11/15 for domestic students, 9/1 for international students. Applications are processed on a rolling basis. Application fee: $55 ($65 for international students). Electronic applications accepted. *Financial support:* Fellowships with partial tuition reimbursements, research assistantships with partial tuition reimbursements, teaching assistantships with partial tuition reimbursements, career-related internships or fieldwork, Federal Work-Study, scholarships/grants, health care benefits, unspecified assistantships, and Service Corps Program; Educational Opportunity Fellowships available. Financial award application deadline: 2/1; financial award applicants required to submit FAFSA. *Faculty research:* Applied ecology, bio-geochemistry, toxicology, wetlands ecology, environmental microbiology, forest ecology, environmental chemistry. *Unit head:* Megan Siehl, Assistant Director, Admissions and Financial Aid, 812-855-9485, Fax: 812-856-3665, E-mail: speampo@indiana.edu. *Application contact:* Lane Bowman, Admissions Services Coordinator, 812-855-2840, Fax: 812-856-3665, E-mail: speaapps@indiana.edu.
Website: http://www.indiana.edu/~spea/prospective_students/masters/

Indiana University Bloomington, University Graduate School, College of Arts and Sciences, Department of Biology, Bloomington, IN 47405. Offers biology teaching (MAT); biotechnology (MA); evolution, ecology, and behavior (MA, PhD); genetics (PhD); microbiology (MA, PhD); molecular, cellular, and developmental biology (PhD); plant sciences (MA, PhD); zoology (MA, PhD). *Faculty:* 58 full-time (15 women), 21 part-time/adjunct (6 women). *Students:* 166 full-time (94 women), 2 part-time (both women); includes 22 minority (8 Black or African American, non-Hispanic/Latino; 3 Asian, non-Hispanic/Latino; 10 Hispanic/Latino; 1 Two or more races, non-Hispanic/Latino), 47 international. Average age 27. 261 applicants, 23% accepted, 32 enrolled. In 2013, 17 master's, 20 doctorates awarded. Terminal master's awarded for partial completion of doctoral program. *Degree requirements:* For master's, thesis, oral defense; for doctorate, thesis/dissertation, oral defense. *Entrance requirements:* For master's and doctorate, GRE General Test. Additional exam requirements/recommendations for international students: Required—TOEFL (minimum score 100 iBT). *Application deadline:* For fall admission, 1/5 priority date for domestic students, 12/1 priority date for international students. Application fee: $55 ($65 for international students). Electronic applications accepted. *Financial support:* In 2013–14, fellowships with tuition reimbursements (averaging $24,000 per year), research assistantships with tuition reimbursements (averaging $21,000 per year), teaching assistantships with tuition reimbursements (averaging $22,000 per year) were awarded; scholarships/grants, traineeships, health care benefits, and unspecified assistantships also available. Financial award application deadline: 1/5. *Faculty research:* Evolution, ecology and behavior; microbiology; molecular biology and genetics; plant biology. *Unit head:* Dr. Clay Fuqua, Chair, 812-856-6005, Fax: 812-855-6082, E-mail: cfuqua@indiana.edu. *Application contact:* Tracey D. Stohr, Graduate Student Recruitment Coordinator, 812-856-6303, Fax: 812-855-6082, E-mail: gradbio@indiana.edu.
Website: http://www.bio.indiana.edu/

Inter American University of Puerto Rico, Bayamón Campus, Graduate School, Bayamón, PR 00957. Offers biology (MS), including environmental sciences and ecology, molecular biotechnology; human resources (MBA). Part-time and evening/weekend programs available. *Degree requirements:* For master's, comprehensive exam, research project. *Entrance requirements:* For master's, EXADEP, GRE General Test, letters of recommendation.

Iowa State University of Science and Technology, Program in Ecology and Evolutionary Biology, Ames, IA 50011. Offers MS, PhD. *Degree requirements:* For master's, thesis or alternative; for doctorate, thesis/dissertation. *Entrance requirements:* For master's and doctorate, GRE General Test. Additional exam requirements/recommendations for international students: Required—TOEFL (minimum score 550 paper-based; 79 iBT), IELTS (minimum score 6.5). Electronic applications accepted. *Faculty research:* Landscape ecology, aquatic and method ecology, physiological ecology, population genetics and evolution, systematics.

Kent State University, College of Arts and Sciences, Department of Biological Sciences, Program in Ecology, Kent, OH 44242-0001. Offers MS, PhD. *Degree requirements:* For master's, thesis; for doctorate, thesis/dissertation. *Entrance requirements:* For master's, GRE General Test, minimum GPA of 3.0; for doctorate, GRE General Test, minimum GPA of 3.25. Additional exam requirements/recommendations for international students: Required—TOEFL (minimum score 600 paper-based). Electronic applications accepted.

Laurentian University, School of Graduate Studies and Research, Programme in Biology, Sudbury, ON P3E 2C6, Canada. Offers biology (M Sc); boreal ecology (PhD). Part-time programs available. *Degree requirements:* For master's, thesis. *Entrance requirements:* For master's, honors degree with second class or better. *Faculty research:* Recovery of acid-stressed lakes, effects of climate change, origin and maintenance of biocomplexity, radionuclide dynamics, cytogenetic studies of plants.

Lesley University, School of Education, Cambridge, MA 02138-2790. Offers arts, community, and education (M Ed); autism studies (Certificate); curriculum and instruction (M Ed, CAGS); early childhood education (M Ed); ecological teaching and learning (MS); educational studies (PhD), including adult learning, educational leadership, individually designed; elementary education (M Ed); emergent technologies for educators (Certificate); ESLArts: language learning through the arts (M Ed); high school education (M Ed); individually designed (M Ed); integrated teaching through the arts (M Ed); literacy for K-8 classroom teachers (M Ed); mathematics education (M Ed); middle school education (M Ed); moderate disabilities (M Ed); online learning (Certificate); reading (CAGS); science in education (M Ed); severe disabilities (M Ed); special needs (CAGS); specialist teacher of reading (M Ed); teacher of visual art (M Ed); technology in education (M Ed, CAGS). *Accreditation:* Teacher Education Accreditation Council. Part-time and evening/weekend programs available. Postbaccalaureate distance learning degree programs offered (no on-campus study). *Faculty:* 40 full-time (30 women), 104 part-time/adjunct (77 women). *Students:* 453 full-time (381 women), 1,672 part-time (1,435 women); includes 284 minority (139 Black or African American, non-Hispanic/Latino; 11 American Indian or Alaska Native, non-Hispanic/Latino; 38 Asian, non-Hispanic/Latino; 58 Hispanic/Latino; 5 Native Hawaiian or other Pacific Islander, non-Hispanic/Latino; 33 Two or more races, non-Hispanic/Latino), 22 international. Average age 35. In 2013, 1,137 master's, 18 doctorates, 51 other advanced degrees awarded. *Degree requirements:* For master's, practicum; for doctorate, thesis/dissertation. *Entrance requirements:* For master's, Massachusetts Tests for Educator Licensure (MTEL), transcripts, statement of purpose, recommendations; interview (for special education); for doctorate, GRE General Test, transcripts, statement of purpose, recommendations, interview, master's degree, resume; for other advanced degree, interview, master's degree. Additional exam requirements/recommendations for international students: Required—TOEFL (minimum score 550 paper-based; 80 iBT). *Application deadline:* Applications are processed on a rolling basis. Application fee: $50. Electronic applications accepted. *Expenses: Tuition:* Part-time $900 per credit. *Financial support:* In 2013–14, 15 fellowships (averaging $3,600 per year) were awarded; career-related internships or fieldwork, Federal Work-Study, scholarships/grants, tuition waivers, and unspecified assistantships also available. Financial award application deadline: 4/15; financial award applicants required to submit FAFSA. *Faculty research:* Assessment in literacy, mathematics and science; autism spectrum disorders; instructional technology and online learning; multicultural education and English language learners. *Unit head:* Dr. Jack Gillette, Dean, 617-349-8401, Fax: 617-349-8607, E-mail: jgillett@lesley.edu. *Application contact:* Martha Sheehan, Director of Admissions, 888-LESLEYU, Fax: 617-349-8313, E-mail: info@lesley.edu.
Website: http://www.lesley.edu/soe.html

Marquette University, Graduate School, College of Arts and Sciences, Department of Biology, Milwaukee, WI 53201-1881. Offers cell biology (MS, PhD); developmental biology (MS, PhD); ecology (MS, PhD); epithelial physiology (MS, PhD); genetics (MS, PhD); microbiology (MS, PhD); molecular biology (MS, PhD); muscle and exercise physiology (MS, PhD); neuroscience (PhD). *Faculty:* 21 full-time (9 women), 3 part-time/adjunct (0 women). *Students:* 34 full-time (16 women), 4 part-time (1 woman), 15 international. Average age 27. 70 applicants, 23% accepted, 5 enrolled. In 2013, 1 master's, 6 doctorates awarded. Terminal master's awarded for partial completion of doctoral program. *Degree requirements:* For master's, comprehensive exam, thesis, 1 year of teaching experience or equivalent; for doctorate, thesis/dissertation, 1 year of teaching experience or equivalent, qualifying exam. *Entrance requirements:* For master's and doctorate, GRE General Test, GRE Subject Test, official transcripts from all current and previous colleges/universities except Marquette, statement of professional goals and aspirations, three letters of recommendation. Additional exam requirements/recommendations for international students: Required—TOEFL (minimum score 530 paper-based). *Application deadline:* For fall admission, 12/15 for domestic and international students. Application fee: $50. Electronic applications accepted. *Financial support:* In 2013–14, 39 students received support, including 6 fellowships (averaging $1,208 per year), 4 research assistantships with full tuition reimbursements available (averaging $21,750 per year), 29 teaching assistantships with full tuition reimbursements available (averaging $21,750 per year); scholarships/grants, health care benefits, tuition waivers (full and partial), and unspecified assistantships also available. Support available to part-time students. Financial award application deadline: 2/15. *Faculty research:* Neurobiology, neuroendocrinology, epithelial physiology, neuropeptide interactions, synaptic transmission. *Total annual research expenditures:* $1.5 million. *Unit head:* Dr. Dale Noel, Chair and Professor, 414-288-1748. *Application contact:* Dr. Michelle Mynlieff, Professor, 414-288-1467.
Website: http://www.marquette.edu/biology/

Miami University, College of Arts and Science, Department of Biology, Oxford, OH 45056. Offers biological sciences (MAT); biology (MS, PhD); botany (MAT, MS, PhD); cell, molecular and structural biology (MS, PhD); ecology, evolution and environmental biology (PhD); zoology (MA, MS, PhD). Part-time programs available. Postbaccalaureate distance learning degree programs offered. *Students:* 89 full-time (49 women), 612 part-time (502 women); includes 63 minority (9 Black or African American, non-Hispanic/Latino; 2 American Indian or Alaska Native, non-Hispanic/Latino; 6 Asian, non-Hispanic/Latino; 27 Hispanic/Latino; 1 Native Hawaiian or other Pacific Islander, non-Hispanic/Latino; 18 Two or more races, non-Hispanic/Latino), 35 international. Average age 34. In 2013, 133 master's, 4 doctorates awarded. *Entrance requirements:* For master's and doctorate, GRE General Test. Additional exam requirements/recommendations for international students: Recommended—TOEFL (minimum score 80 iBT), IELTS (minimum score 6.5), TSE (minimum score 54). *Application deadline:* For fall admission, 1/15 for domestic and international students. Application fee: $50. Electronic applications accepted. *Expenses:* Tuition, state resident: full-time $12,634; part-time $526 per credit hour. Tuition, nonresident: full-time $27,892; part-time $1162 per credit hour. Part-time tuition and fees vary according to course load, campus/location and program. *Financial support:* Fellowships with full tuition reimbursements, research assistantships with full tuition reimbursements, teaching assistantships with full tuition reimbursements, Federal Work-Study, health care benefits, tuition waivers (full), and unspecified assistantships available. Financial award application deadline: 1/15; financial award applicants required to submit FAFSA. *Unit head:* Dr. Douglas Meikle, Chair, 513-529-3103, E-mail: meikled@miamioh.edu.
Website: http://miamioh.edu/cas/about/biology

Michigan State University, The Graduate School, College of Natural Science, Interdepartmental Program in Ecology, Evolutionary Biology and Behavior, East Lansing, MI 48824. Offers PhD. *Entrance requirements:* Additional exam requirements/recommendations for international students: Required—TOEFL. Electronic applications accepted.

Michigan Technological University, Graduate School, School of Forest Resources and Environmental Science, Houghton, MI 49931. Offers applied ecology (MS); forest ecology and management (MS); forest science (PhD); forestry (MF, MS); molecular genetics and biotechnology (MS, PhD). *Accreditation:* SAF. Part-time programs available. Terminal master's awarded for partial completion of doctoral program. *Degree requirements:* For master's, comprehensive exam (for some programs), thesis (for some programs); for doctorate, comprehensive exam, thesis/dissertation. *Entrance requirements:* For master's and doctorate, GRE (minimum scores: 500 in verbal, 500 quantitative, 3.5 in analytical), statement of purpose, official transcripts, 3 letters of recommendation, resume/curriculum vitae. Additional exam requirements/recommendations for international students: Required—TOEFL (minimum score 79 iBT) or IELTS. Electronic applications accepted. *Faculty research:* Forest molecular genetics and biotechnology, forestry, forest ecology and management, applied ecology, wood science.

Montana State University, College of Graduate Studies, College of Letters and Science, Department of Ecology, Bozeman, MT 59717. Offers ecological and environmental statistics (MS); ecology and environmental sciences (PhD); fish and wildlife biology (PhD); fish and wildlife management (MS). Part-time programs available. *Degree requirements:* For master's, comprehensive exam, thesis (for some programs);

for doctorate, comprehensive exam, thesis/dissertation. *Entrance requirements:* For master's and doctorate, GRE, minimum GPA of 3.0, letters of recommendation, essay. Additional exam requirements/recommendations for international students: Required—TOEFL (minimum score 550 paper-based). Electronic applications accepted. *Faculty research:* Community ecology, population ecology, land-use effects, management and conservation, environmental modeling.

Montclair State University, The Graduate School, College of Science and Mathematics, Department of Biology and Molecular Biology, Montclair, NJ 07043-1624. Offers biology (MS), including biological science education, biology, ecology and evolution, physiology; molecular biology (MS, Certificate). Part-time and evening/weekend programs available. *Degree requirements:* For master's, comprehensive exam, thesis or alternative. *Entrance requirements:* For master's, GRE General Test, 24 credits of course work in undergraduate biology, 2 letters of recommendation, teaching certificate (biology sciences education concentration); for Certificate, 2 letters of recommendation, essay. Additional exam requirements/recommendations for international students: Required—TOEFL (minimum score 83 iBT) or IELTS. Electronic applications accepted. *Faculty research:* Ecosystem biology, molecular biology, signal transduction, neuroscience, aquatic and coastal biology.

North Dakota State University, College of Graduate and Interdisciplinary Studies, Interdisciplinary Program in Environmental and Conservation Sciences, Fargo, ND 58108. Offers MS, PhD. *Faculty:* 4 full-time (1 woman), 1 part-time/adjunct (0 women). *Students:* 24 full-time (11 women), 13 part-time (9 women); includes 2 minority (1 Asian, non-Hispanic/Latino; 1 Hispanic/Latino), 14 international. Average age 32. 16 applicants, 38% accepted, 6 enrolled. In 2013, 6 master's, 2 doctorates awarded. *Degree requirements:* For master's, comprehensive exam, thesis. *Entrance requirements:* Additional exam requirements/recommendations for international students: Required—TOEFL (minimum score 550 paper-based; 79 iBT). *Application deadline:* For fall admission, 5/1 for international students; for spring admission, 8/1 for international students. Application fee: $35. *Unit head:* Dr. Craig Stockwell, Director, 701-231-8449, Fax: 701-231-7149, E-mail: craig.stockwell@ndsu.edu. *Application contact:* Madonna Fitzgerald, Administrative Assistant, 701-231-6456, E-mail: madonna.fitzgerald@ndsu.edu.
Website: http://www.ndsu.edu/gradschool/programs/environmental_conservation_science/

The Ohio State University, Graduate School, College of Arts and Sciences, Division of Natural and Mathematical Sciences, Department of Evolution, Ecology, and Organismal Biology, Columbus, OH 43210. Offers MS, PhD. *Faculty:* 27. *Students:* 72 full-time (32 women), 4 part-time (2 women); includes 3 minority (2 Black or African American, non-Hispanic/Latino; 1 Hispanic/Latino), 10 international. Average age 28. In 2013, 3 master's, 3 doctorates awarded. *Degree requirements:* For master's, thesis optional; for doctorate, thesis/dissertation. *Entrance requirements:* For master's and doctorate, GRE General Test. Additional exam requirements/recommendations for international students: Required—TOEFL (minimum score 600 paper-based; 100 iBT), Michigan English Language Assessment Battery (minimum score 86); Recommended—IELTS (minimum score 8). *Application deadline:* For fall admission, 12/1 priority date for domestic students, 11/30 priority date for international students; for winter admission, 12/1 for domestic students, 11/1 for international students; for spring admission, 3/1 for domestic students, 2/1 for international students. Applications are processed on a rolling basis. Application fee: $60 ($70 for international students). Electronic applications accepted. *Financial support:* Fellowships with tuition reimbursements, research assistantships with tuition reimbursements, teaching assistantships with tuition reimbursements, Federal Work-Study, and institutionally sponsored loans available. Support available to part-time students. *Unit head:* Peter S. Curtis, Chair, 614-292-8280, E-mail: curtis.7@osu.edu. *Application contact:* Graduate Admissions, 614-292-9444, Fax: 614-292-3895, E-mail: gradadmissions@osu.edu.
Website: http://eeob.osu.edu/

The Ohio State University, Graduate School, College of Food, Agricultural, and Environmental Sciences, School of Environment and Natural Resources, Columbus, OH 43210. Offers ecological restoration (MS, PhD); ecosystem science (MS, PhD); environment and natural resources (MENR); environmental social sciences (MS, PhD); fisheries and wildlife science (MS, PhD); forest science (MS, PhD); rural sociology (MS, PhD); soil science (MS, PhD). *Faculty:* 33. *Students:* 81 full-time (47 women), 17 part-time (10 women); includes 12 minority (3 Black or African American, non-Hispanic/Latino; 7 Hispanic/Latino; 2 Two or more races, non-Hispanic/Latino), 10 international. Average age 29. In 2013, 34 master's, 5 doctorates awarded. *Degree requirements:* For master's, thesis; for doctorate, thesis/dissertation. *Entrance requirements:* For master's and doctorate, GRE. Additional exam requirements/recommendations for international students: Required—TOEFL (minimum score 550 paper-based; 79 iBT), Michigan English Language Assessment Battery (minimum score 82); Recommended—IELTS (minimum score 7). *Application deadline:* Applications are processed on a rolling basis. Application fee: $60 ($70 for international students). Electronic applications accepted. *Unit head:* Ronald Hendrick, Director, 614-292-8522, E-mail: hendrick.15@osu.edu. *Application contact:* Graduate Admissions, 614-292-9444, E-mail: gradadmissions@osu.edu.
Website: http://senr.osu.edu/

Ohio University, Graduate College, College of Arts and Sciences, Department of Biological Sciences, Athens, OH 45701-2979. Offers biological sciences (MS, PhD); cell biology and physiology (MS, PhD); ecology and evolutionary biology (MS, PhD); exercise physiology and muscle biology (MS, PhD); microbiology (MS, PhD); neuroscience (MS, PhD). Terminal master's awarded for partial completion of doctoral program. *Degree requirements:* For master's, comprehensive exam, thesis, 1 quarter of teaching experience; for doctorate, comprehensive exam, thesis/dissertation, 2 quarters of teaching experience. *Entrance requirements:* For master's, GRE General Test, names of three faculty members whose research interests most closely match the applicant's interest; for doctorate, GRE General Test, essay concerning prior training, research interest and career goals, plus names of three faculty members whose research interests most closely match the applicant's interest. Additional exam requirements/recommendations for international students: Required—TOEFL (minimum score 620 paper-based; 105 iBT) or IELTS (minimum score 7.5). Electronic applications accepted. *Faculty research:* Ecology and evolutionary biology, exercise physiology and muscle biology, neurobiology, cell biology, physiology.

Old Dominion University, College of Sciences, Program in Ecological Sciences, Norfolk, VA 23529. Offers PhD. *Faculty:* 13 full-time (3 women), 41 part-time/adjunct (7 women). *Students:* 13 full-time (9 women), 9 part-time (5 women), 5 international. Average age 31. 15 applicants, 40% accepted, 4 enrolled. In 2013, 1 doctorate awarded. *Degree requirements:* For doctorate, one foreign language, comprehensive exam, thesis/dissertation. *Entrance requirements:* For doctorate, GRE General Test, 3 letters of recommendation. Additional exam requirements/recommendations for international students: Required—TOEFL (minimum score 550 paper-based; 79 iBT). *Application deadline:* For fall admission, 2/1 priority date for domestic and international students. Applications are processed on a rolling basis. Application fee: $50. Electronic applications accepted. *Expenses:* Tuition, state resident: full-time $9888; part-time $412 per credit. Tuition, nonresident: full-time $25,152; part-time $1048 per credit. *Required fees:* $59 per semester. One-time fee: $50. *Financial support:* In 2013–14, 3 fellowships with full tuition reimbursements (averaging $17,000 per year), 4 research assistantships with full tuition reimbursements (averaging $15,750 per year), 9 teaching assistantships with full tuition reimbursements (averaging $15,000 per year) were awarded; scholarships/grants also available. Financial award application deadline: 2/15; financial award applicants required to submit FAFSA. *Faculty research:* Marine ecology, physiological ecology, systematics and speciation, ecological and evolutionary processes, molecular genetics. *Total annual research expenditures:* $2 million. *Unit head:* Dr. Ian Bartol, Graduate Program Director, 757-683-4737, Fax: 757-683-5283, E-mail: ecolgpd@odu.edu. *Application contact:* William Heffelfinger, Director of Graduate Admissions, 757-683-5554, Fax: 757-683-3255, E-mail: gradadmit@odu.edu.
Website: http://sci.odu.edu/biology/academics/ecologyphd.shtml

Penn State University Park, Graduate School, Intercollege Graduate Programs, Intercollege Graduate Program in Ecology, University Park, PA 16802. Offers MS, PhD. *Unit head:* Dr. Regina Vasilatos-Younken, Interim Dean, 814-865-2516, Fax: 814-863-4627, E-mail: rxv@psu.edu. *Application contact:* Cynthia E. Nicosia, Director, Graduate Enrollment Services, 814-865-1834, Fax: 814-863-4627, E-mail: cey1@psu.edu.

Princeton University, Graduate School, Department of Ecology and Evolutionary Biology, Princeton, NJ 08544-1019. Offers PhD. *Degree requirements:* For doctorate, thesis/dissertation. *Entrance requirements:* For doctorate, GRE General Test, GRE Subject Test. Additional exam requirements/recommendations for international students: Required—TOEFL (minimum score 600 paper-based). Electronic applications accepted.

Purdue University, Graduate School, College of Agriculture, Department of Forestry and Natural Resources, West Lafayette, IN 47907. Offers fisheries and aquatic sciences (MS, MSF, PhD); forest biology (MS, MSF, PhD); natural resource social science (MS, PhD); natural resources social science (MSF); quantitative ecology (MS, MSF, PhD); wildlife science (MS, MSF, PhD); wood products and wood products manufacturing (MS, MSF, PhD). *Faculty:* 25 full-time (5 women), 14 part-time/adjunct (2 women). *Students:* 59 full-time (23 women), 8 part-time (2 women); includes 4 minority (2 American Indian or Alaska Native, non-Hispanic/Latino; 1 Hispanic/Latino; 1 Two or more races, non-Hispanic/Latino), 19 international. Average age 28. 66 applicants, 15% accepted, 10 enrolled. In 2013, 16 master's, 16 doctorates awarded. *Degree requirements:* For master's, thesis; for doctorate, thesis/dissertation. *Entrance requirements:* For master's and doctorate, GRE General Test (minimum score: verbal 50th percentile; quantitative 50th percentile; analytical writing 4.0), minimum undergraduate GPA of 3.2 or equivalent. Additional exam requirements/recommendations for international students: Required—TOEFL (minimum score 550 paper-based; 77 iBT). *Application deadline:* For fall admission, 1/5 for domestic students, 1/15 for international students; for spring admission, 9/15 for domestic and international students. Applications are processed on a rolling basis. Application fee: $60 ($75 for international students). Electronic applications accepted. *Financial support:* In 2013–14, 10 research assistantships (averaging $15,259 per year) were awarded; fellowships, teaching assistantships, career-related internships or fieldwork, and scholarships/grants also available. Support available to part-time students. Financial award application deadline: 1/5; financial award applicants required to submit FAFSA. *Faculty research:* Wildlife management, forest management, forest ecology, forest soils, limnology. *Unit head:* Dr. Robert K. Swihart, Interim Head, 765-494-3590, Fax: 765-494-9461, E-mail: rswihart@purdue.edu. *Application contact:* Kelly J. Wrede, Graduate Secretary, 765-494-3572, Fax: 765-494-9461, E-mail: kgarrett@purdue.edu.
Website: https://ag.purdue.edu/fnr

Purdue University, Graduate School, College of Science, Department of Biological Sciences, West Lafayette, IN 47907. Offers biochemistry (PhD); biophysics (PhD); cell and developmental biology (PhD); ecology, evolutionary and population biology (MS, PhD), including ecology, evolutionary biology, population biology; genetics (MS, PhD); microbiology (MS, PhD); molecular biology (PhD); neurobiology (MS, PhD); plant physiology (PhD). *Faculty:* 50 full-time (13 women), 5 part-time/adjunct (1 woman). *Students:* 111 full-time (61 women), 5 part-time (0 women); includes 9 minority (1 Black or African American, non-Hispanic/Latino; 5 Asian, non-Hispanic/Latino; 3 Hispanic/Latino), 62 international. Average age 27. 170 applicants, 19% accepted, 17 enrolled. In 2013, 9 master's, 18 doctorates awarded. Terminal master's awarded for partial completion of doctoral program. *Degree requirements:* For master's, thesis (for some programs); for doctorate, thesis/dissertation, seminars, teaching experience. *Entrance requirements:* For master's, GRE General Test (minimum analytical writing score of 3.5), minimum undergraduate GPA of 3.0; for doctorate, GRE General Test (minimum analytical writing score of 3.5), minimum undergraduate GPA of 3.5. Additional exam requirements/recommendations for international students: Required—TOEFL (minimum score 600 paper-based; 107 iBT for MS, 80 iBT for PhD). *Application deadline:* For fall admission, 12/7 for domestic and international students. Applications are processed on a rolling basis. Application fee: $60 ($75 for international students). Electronic applications accepted. *Financial support:* Fellowships, research assistantships, and teaching assistantships available. Support available to part-time students. Financial award application deadline: 2/15; financial award applicants required to submit FAFSA. *Unit head:* Dr. Richard J. Kuhn, Head, 765-494-4407, E-mail: kuhnr@purdue.edu. *Application contact:* Georgina E. Rupp, Graduate Coordinator, 765-494-8142, Fax: 765-494-0876, E-mail: ruppg@purdue.edu.
Website: http://www.bio.purdue.edu/

Purdue University, Graduate School, Interdisciplinary Graduate Program in Ecological Sciences and Engineering, West Lafayette, IN 47907. Offers MS, PhD. *Students:* 63 full-time (37 women), 9 part-time (4 women); includes 7 minority (1 American Indian or Alaska Native, non-Hispanic/Latino; 1 Asian, non-Hispanic/Latino; 1 Hispanic/Latino; 4 Two or more races, non-Hispanic/Latino), 25 international. Average age 29. 59 applicants, 59% accepted, 17 enrolled. *Degree requirements:* For master's, thesis optional; for doctorate, thesis/dissertation, written and oral preliminary exam. *Entrance requirements:* For master's and doctorate, GRE (minimum old score Verbal and Quantitative combined 1200, Analytical writing 4.0; new score 300/4.0), previous research or environmental project experience; minimum GPA of 3.3. Additional exam requirements/recommendations for international students: Required—TOEFL (minimum score 550 paper-based; 77 iBT), IELTS (minimum score 6.5); Recommended—TWE. *Application deadline:* For fall admission, 12/15 for domestic and international students. Applications are processed on a rolling basis. Application fee: $65 ($70 for international students). Electronic applications accepted. *Financial support:* Fellowships and research assistantships available. *Unit head:* Dr. Linda S. Lee, Program Head, 765-494-8612, E-mail: lslee@purdue.edu. *Application contact:* Christal Musser, Program Coordinator, 765-494-2102, E-mail: musser@purdue.edu.
Website: http://www.gradschool.purdue.edu/ese/

Rice University, Graduate Programs, Wiess School of Natural Sciences, Department of Ecology and Evolutionary Biology, Houston, TX 77251-1892. Offers MA, MS, PhD. Terminal master's awarded for partial completion of doctoral program. *Degree requirements:* For master's, comprehensive exam (for some programs), thesis (for some programs); for doctorate, comprehensive exam, thesis/dissertation. *Entrance requirements:* For master's and doctorate, GRE General Test, GRE Subject Test. Additional exam requirements/recommendations for international students: Required—

TOEFL (minimum score 600 paper-based; 90 iBT). Electronic applications accepted. *Faculty research:* Trace gas emissions, wetlands, biology, community ecology of forests and grasslands, conservation biology specialization.

Rutgers, The State University of New Jersey, New Brunswick, Graduate School-New Brunswick, Program in Ecology and Evolution, Piscataway, NJ 08854-8097. Offers MS, PhD. Part-time programs available. Terminal master's awarded for partial completion of doctoral program. *Degree requirements:* For master's, comprehensive exam; for doctorate, comprehensive exam, thesis/dissertation. *Entrance requirements:* For master's and doctorate, GRE General Test, minimum GPA of 3.0. Additional exam requirements/recommendations for international students: Required—TOEFL (minimum score 550 paper-based). Electronic applications accepted. *Faculty research:* Population and community ecology, population genetics, evolutionary biology, conservation biology, ecosystem ecology.

San Diego State University, Graduate and Research Affairs, College of Sciences, Department of Biology, Program in Ecology, San Diego, CA 92182. Offers MS, PhD. PhD offered jointly with University of California, Davis. *Degree requirements:* For master's, thesis; for doctorate, thesis/dissertation. *Entrance requirements:* For master's, GRE General Test, resumé or curriculum vitae, 2 letters of recommendation; for doctorate, GRE General Test, GRE Subject Test, resume or curriculum vitae, 3 letters of recommendation. Electronic applications accepted. *Faculty research:* Conservation and restoration ecology, coastal and marine ecology, global change and ecosystem ecology.

San Francisco State University, Division of Graduate Studies, College of Science and Engineering, Department of Biology, Program in Ecology, Evolution, and Conservation Biology, San Francisco, CA 94132-1722. Offers MS. *Application deadline:* Applications are processed on a rolling basis. *Unit head:* Dr. Robert Patterson, Program Coordinator, 415-338-1237, E-mail: patters@sfsu.edu.
Website: http://biology.sfsu.edu/graduate/ecology-evolution-and-conservation-biology-eecb-0

San Jose State University, Graduate Studies and Research, College of Science, Department of Biological Sciences, San Jose, CA 95192-0001. Offers biological sciences (MA, MS); molecular biology and microbiology (MS); organismal biology, conservation and ecology (MS); physiology (MS). Part-time programs available. *Entrance requirements:* For master's, GRE. Electronic applications accepted. *Faculty research:* Systemic physiology, molecular genetics, SEM studies, toxicology, large mammal ecology.

Sonoma State University, School of Science and Technology, Department of Biology, Rohnert Park, CA 94928. Offers biochemistry (MA); ecology (MS); environmental biology (MS); evolutionary biology (MS); functional morphology (MS); molecular and cell biology (MS); organismal biology (MS). Part-time programs available. *Faculty:* 9 full-time (1 woman). *Students:* 4 full-time (2 women), 21 part-time (14 women); includes 5 minority (1 American Indian or Alaska Native, non-Hispanic/Latino; 1 Asian, non-Hispanic/Latino; 2 Hispanic/Latino; 1 Two or more races, non-Hispanic/Latino), 2 international. Average age 29. 23 applicants, 65% accepted, 6 enrolled. In 2013, 6 master's awarded. *Degree requirements:* For master's, thesis or alternative, oral exam. *Entrance requirements:* For master's, GRE General Test, GRE Subject Test, minimum GPA of 3.0. Additional exam requirements/recommendations for international students: Required—TOEFL (minimum score 500 paper-based). *Application deadline:* For fall admission, 11/30 for domestic students. Applications are processed on a rolling basis. Application fee: $55. *Expenses:* Tuition, state resident: full-time $8500. Tuition, nonresident: full-time $12,964. *Required fees:* $1762. *Financial support:* In 2013–14, 1 fellowship (averaging $1,520 per year), 6 research assistantships (averaging $3,562 per year), 22 teaching assistantships (averaging $6,738 per year) were awarded; career-related internships or fieldwork, Federal Work-Study, and tuition waivers (full) also available. Financial award application deadline: 3/2; financial award applicants required to submit FAFSA. *Faculty research:* Plant physiology, comparative physiology, community ecology, restoration ecology, marine ecology, conservation genetics, primate behavior, behavioral ecology, developmental biology, plant and animal systematics. *Total annual research expenditures:* $4,400. *Unit head:* Dr. Nathan Rank, Chair, 707-664-3053, E-mail: nathan.rank@sonoma.edu. *Application contact:* Dr. Derek Girman, Graduate Adviser, 707-664-3055, E-mail: derek.girman@sonoma.edu.
Website: http://www.sonoma.edu/biology/graduate

Stanford University, School of Humanities and Sciences, Department of Anthropology, Stanford, CA 94305-9991. Offers archaeology (MA, PhD); culture and society (MS, PhD); ecology and environment (MA, PhD). Terminal master's awarded for partial completion of doctoral program. *Degree requirements:* For master's, thesis; for doctorate, one foreign language, thesis/dissertation. *Entrance requirements:* For master's and doctorate, GRE General Test. Additional exam requirements/recommendations for international students: Required—TOEFL. Electronic applications accepted. *Expenses: Tuition:* Full-time $42,690; part-time $949 per credit. *Required fees:* $185.

State University of New York College of Environmental Science and Forestry, Department of Environmental and Forest Biology, Syracuse, NY 13210-2779. Offers applied ecology (MPS); chemical ecology (MPS, MS, PhD); conservation biology (MPS, MS, PhD); ecology (MPS, MS, PhD); entomology (MPS, MS, PhD); environmental interpretation (MPS, MS, PhD); environmental physiology (MPS, MS, PhD); fish and wildlife biology and management (MPS, MS, PhD); forest pathology and mycology (MPS, MS, PhD); plant biotechnology (MPS); plant science and biotechnology (MPS, MS, PhD). *Faculty:* 32 full-time (10 women). *Students:* 105 full-time (54 women), 31 part-time (16 women); includes 9 minority (2 Black or African American, non-Hispanic/Latino; 3 American Indian or Alaska Native, non-Hispanic/Latino; 2 Hispanic/Latino; 1 Native Hawaiian or other Pacific Islander, non-Hispanic/Latino; 1 Two or more races, non-Hispanic/Latino), 17 international. Average age 28. In 2013, 15 master's, 7 doctorates awarded. *Degree requirements:* For master's, thesis (for some programs), capstone seminar; for doctorate, comprehensive exam, thesis/dissertation, capstone seminar. *Entrance requirements:* For master's and doctorate, GRE General Test, minimum GPA of 3.0. Additional exam requirements/recommendations for international students: Required—TOEFL (minimum score 550 paper-based; 80 iBT), IELTS (minimum score 6). *Application deadline:* For fall admission, 2/1 priority date for domestic and international students; for spring admission, 11/1 priority date for domestic and international students. Applications are processed on a rolling basis. Application fee: $60. *Expenses:* Tuition, state resident: full-time $10,370; part-time $432 per credit hour. Tuition, nonresident: full-time $20,190; part-time $841 per credit hour. *Required fees:* $44 per credit hour. *Financial support:* In 2013–14, 4 fellowships with full and partial tuition reimbursements, 36 research assistantships with full and partial tuition reimbursements, 39 teaching assistantships with full and partial tuition reimbursements (averaging $11,490 per year) were awarded; Federal Work-Study, institutionally sponsored loans, scholarships/grants, health care benefits, and unspecified assistantships also available. Financial award application deadline: 6/30. *Faculty research:* Ecology, conservation biology, fish and wildlife biology and management, plant science, entomology. *Total annual research expenditures:* $4.1 million. *Unit head:* Dr. Donald J. Leopold, Chair, 315-470-6760, Fax: 315-470-6934, E-mail: djleopold@esf.edu. *Application contact:* Dr. Danilo D. Fernando, Director, Graduate Program/Associate Professor, 315-470-6746, Fax: 315-470-6934, E-mail: dfernando@esf.edu.
Website: http://www.esf.edu/efb/grad/default.asp

State University of New York College of Environmental Science and Forestry, Department of Forest and Natural Resources Management, Syracuse, NY 13210-2779. Offers ecology and ecosystems (MPS, MS, PhD); economics, governance and human dimensions (MPS, MS, PhD); forest and natural resources management (MPS, MS, PhD); monitoring, analysis and modeling (MPS, MS, PhD). *Accreditation:* SAF. *Degree requirements:* For master's, thesis (for some programs); for doctorate, comprehensive exam, thesis/dissertation. *Entrance requirements:* For master's and doctorate, GRE General Test, minimum GPA of 3.0. Additional exam requirements/recommendations for international students: Required—TOEFL (minimum score 550 paper-based; 80 iBT), IELTS (minimum score 6). *Application deadline:* For fall admission, 2/1 priority date for domestic and international students; for spring admission, 11/1 priority date for domestic and international students. Applications are processed on a rolling basis. Application fee: $60. *Expenses:* Tuition, state resident: full-time $10,370; part-time $432 per credit hour. Tuition, nonresident: full-time $20,190; part-time $841 per credit hour. *Required fees:* $44 per credit hour. *Financial support:* Fellowships with full and partial tuition reimbursements, research assistantships with full and partial tuition reimbursements, teaching assistantships with full and partial tuition reimbursements, career-related internships or fieldwork, Federal Work-Study, institutionally sponsored loans, scholarships/grants, health care benefits, and unspecified assistantships available. Financial award application deadline: 6/30; financial award applicants required to submit FAFSA. *Faculty research:* Silviculture recreation management, tree improvement, operations management, economics. *Unit head:* Dr. David Newman, Chair, 315-470-6534, Fax: 315-470-6535. *Application contact:* Dr. Dudley J. Raynal, Dean, Instruction and Graduate Studies, 315-470-6599, Fax: 315-470-6978, E-mail: esfgrad@esf.edu.
Website: http://www.esf.edu/fnrm/

Stony Brook University, State University of New York, Graduate School, College of Arts and Sciences, Department of Ecology and Evolution, Stony Brook, NY 11794. Offers applied ecology (MA); ecology and evolution (PhD). *Faculty:* 18 full-time (7 women), 1 part-time/adjunct (0 women). *Students:* 54 full-time (29 women), 4 part-time (2 women); includes 8 minority (3 Asian, non-Hispanic/Latino; 5 Hispanic/Latino), 12 international. Average age 28. 46 applicants, 48% accepted, 9 enrolled. In 2013, 1 master's, 11 doctorates awarded. *Degree requirements:* For doctorate, one foreign language, comprehensive exam, thesis/dissertation, teaching experience. *Entrance requirements:* For doctorate, GRE General Test, GRE Subject Test. Additional exam requirements/recommendations for international students: Required—TOEFL. *Application deadline:* For fall admission, 1/15 for domestic students; for spring admission, 10/1 for domestic students. Application fee: $100. *Expenses:* Tuition, state resident: full-time $9870; part-time $411 per credit. Tuition, nonresident: full-time $18,350; part-time $765 per credit. *Financial support:* In 2013–14, 2 fellowships, 6 research assistantships, 27 teaching assistantships were awarded; Federal Work-Study also available. *Faculty research:* Theoretical and experimental population genetics, numerical taxonomy, biostatistics, population and community ecology, plant ecology. *Total annual research expenditures:* $1.7 million. *Unit head:* Dr. Walter F. Eanes, Chair, 631-632-8593, Fax: 631-632-7626, E-mail: walter.eanes@stonybrook.edu. *Application contact:* Melissa Cohen, Coordinator, 631-246-8604, Fax: 631-632-7626, E-mail: melissa.j.cohen@stonybrook.edu.
Website: http://life.bio.sunysb.edu/ee/

Tulane University, School of Science and Engineering, Department of Ecology and Evolutionary Biology, New Orleans, LA 70118-5669. Offers MS, PhD. Terminal master's awarded for partial completion of doctoral program. *Degree requirements:* For master's, thesis or alternative; for doctorate, thesis/dissertation. *Entrance requirements:* For master's, GRE General Test, minimum B average in undergraduate course work; for doctorate, GRE General Test. Additional exam requirements/recommendations for international students: Required—TOEFL. Electronic applications accepted. *Faculty research:* Ichthyology, plant systematics, crustacean endocrinology, ecotoxicology, ornithology.

Universidad Nacional Pedro Henriquez Urena, Graduate School, Santo Domingo, Dominican Republic. Offers agricultural diversity (MS), including horticultural/fruit production, tropical animal production; conservation of monuments and cultural assets (M Arch); ecology and environment (MS); environmental engineering (MEE); international relations (MA); natural resource management (MS); political science (MA); project optimization (MPM); project feasibility (MPM); project management (MPM); sanitation engineering (ME); science for teachers (MS); tropical Caribbean architecture (M Arch).

University at Albany, State University of New York, College of Arts and Sciences, Department of Biological Sciences, Specialization in Ecology, Evolution, and Behavior, Albany, NY 12222-0001. Offers MS, PhD. *Degree requirements:* For master's, one foreign language; for doctorate, one foreign language, thesis/dissertation. *Entrance requirements:* For master's and doctorate, GRE General Test.

University at Buffalo, the State University of New York, Graduate School, College of Arts and Sciences, Program in Evolution, Ecology and Behavior, Buffalo, NY 14260. Offers MS, PhD, Certificate. Terminal master's awarded for partial completion of doctoral program. *Degree requirements:* For master's, project; for doctorate, comprehensive exam, thesis/dissertation. *Entrance requirements:* For master's, GRE, minimum undergraduate GPA of 3.0; for doctorate, GRE, minimum GPA of 3.0. Additional exam requirements/recommendations for international students: Required—TOEFL (minimum score 550 paper-based; 79 iBT). Electronic applications accepted. *Faculty research:* Coral reef ecology, evolution and ecology of aquatic invertebrates, animal communication, paleobiology, primate behavior.

University of Alberta, Faculty of Graduate Studies and Research, Department of Biological Sciences, Edmonton, AB T6G 2E1, Canada. Offers environmental biology and ecology (M Sc, PhD); microbiology and biotechnology (M Sc, PhD); molecular biology and genetics (M Sc, PhD); physiology and cell biology (M Sc, PhD); plant biology (M Sc, PhD); systematics and evolution (M Sc, PhD). Terminal master's awarded for partial completion of doctoral program. *Degree requirements:* For master's, thesis; for doctorate, thesis/dissertation. *Entrance requirements:* Additional exam requirements/recommendations for international students: Required—TOEFL.

The University of Arizona, College of Science, Department of Ecology and Evolutionary Biology, Tucson, AZ 85721. Offers MS, PhD. *Faculty:* 21 full-time (5 women), 2 part-time/adjunct (0 women). *Students:* 52 full-time (23 women), 6 part-time (3 women); includes 5 minority (1 American Indian or Alaska Native, non-Hispanic/Latino; 1 Asian, non-Hispanic/Latino; 2 Hispanic/Latino; 1 Two or more races, non-Hispanic/Latino), 13 international. Average age 28. 77 applicants, 17% accepted, 9 enrolled. In 2013, 5 master's, 4 doctorates awarded. Terminal master's awarded for partial completion of doctoral program. *Degree requirements:* For master's, thesis optional; for doctorate, one foreign language, comprehensive exam, thesis/dissertation. *Entrance requirements:* For master's, GRE General Test, GRE Subject Test, statement of purpose, curriculum vitae, 3 letters of recommendation; for doctorate, GRE General Test, GRE Subject Test, curriculum vitae, 3 letters of recommendation. Additional exam

requirements/recommendations for international students: Required—TOEFL (minimum score 550 paper-based; 79 iBT). *Application deadline:* For fall admission, 12/1 for domestic students, 12/8 for international students. Application fee: $75. *Expenses:* Tuition, state resident: full-time $11,526. Tuition, nonresident: full-time $27,398. *Financial support:* In 2013–14, 10 research assistantships with full tuition reimbursements (averaging $22,896 per year), 34 teaching assistantships with full tuition reimbursements (averaging $22,896 per year) were awarded; career-related internships or fieldwork, scholarships/grants, health care benefits, and unspecified assistantships also available. *Faculty research:* Biological diversity, evolutionary history, evolutionary mechanisms, community structure. *Total annual research expenditures:* $5.6 million. *Unit head:* Dr. Richard E. Michod, Head, 520-621-7509, Fax: 520-621-9190, E-mail: michod@email.arizona.edu. *Application contact:* Carol Burleson, Administrative Associate, 520-621-9328, Fax: 520-621-9190, E-mail: oxforda@email.arizona.edu.
Website: http://eebweb.arizona.edu/

University of California, Davis, Graduate Studies, Graduate Group in Ecology, Davis, CA 95616. Offers MS, PhD. PhD offered jointly with San Diego State University. *Degree requirements:* For master's, comprehensive exam (for some programs), thesis (for some programs); for doctorate, thesis/dissertation. *Entrance requirements:* For master's and doctorate, GRE General Test. Additional exam requirements/recommendations for international students: Required—TOEFL (minimum score 550 paper-based). Electronic applications accepted. *Faculty research:* Agricultural conservation, physiological restoration, environmental policy, ecotoxicology.

University of California, Irvine, School of Biological Sciences, Department of Ecology and Evolutionary Biology, Irvine, CA 92697. Offers biological sciences (MS, PhD). *Students:* 57 full-time (31 women), 1 (woman) part-time; includes 20 minority (6 Asian, non-Hispanic/Latino; 8 Hispanic/Latino; 6 Two or more races, non-Hispanic/Latino), 3 international. Average age 27. 87 applicants, 34% accepted, 19 enrolled. In 2013, 6 doctorates awarded. *Degree requirements:* For master's, thesis; for doctorate, thesis/dissertation. *Entrance requirements:* For master's and doctorate, GRE General Test, GRE Subject Test, minimum GPA of 3.0. Additional exam requirements/recommendations for international students: Required—TOEFL (minimum score 550 paper-based). *Application deadline:* For fall admission, 1/15 priority date for domestic students, 1/15 for international students. Applications are processed on a rolling basis. Application fee: $80 ($100 for international students). Electronic applications accepted. *Financial support:* Fellowships, research assistantships with full tuition reimbursements, teaching assistantships, career-related internships or fieldwork, institutionally sponsored loans, traineeships, health care benefits, and unspecified assistantships available. Financial award application deadline: 3/1; financial award applicants required to submit FAFSA. *Faculty research:* Ecological energetics, quantitative genetics, life history evolution, plant-herbivore and plant-pollinator interactions, molecular evolution. *Unit head:* Laurence D. Mueller, Professor/Department Chair, 949-824-4744, Fax: 949-824-2181, E-mail: ldmuelle@uci.edu. *Application contact:* Pamela Mc Donald, Student Affairs Officer, 949-824-4743, Fax: 949-824-2181, E-mail: pmcdonal@uci.edu.
Website: http://ecoevo.bio.uci.edu/

University of California, Los Angeles, Graduate Division, College of Letters and Science, Department of Ecology and Evolutionary Biology, Los Angeles, CA 90095. Offers MA, PhD. Terminal master's awarded for partial completion of doctoral program. *Degree requirements:* For master's, comprehensive exam or thesis; for doctorate, thesis/dissertation, oral and written qualifying exams; 3 quarters of teaching experience. *Entrance requirements:* For master's and doctorate, GRE General Test, GRE Subject Test (biology), bachelor's degree; minimum undergraduate GPA of 3.0 (or its equivalent if letter grade system not used). Additional exam requirements/recommendations for international students: Required—TOEFL. Electronic applications accepted.

University of California, Riverside, Graduate Division, Department of Entomology, Riverside, CA 92521-0102. Offers entomology (MS, PhD); evolution and ecology (PhD). Part-time programs available. Terminal master's awarded for partial completion of doctoral program. *Degree requirements:* For master's, thesis; for doctorate, thesis/dissertation, qualifying exams. *Entrance requirements:* For master's and doctorate, GRE General Test, minimum GPA of 3.2. Additional exam requirements/recommendations for international students: Required—TOEFL (minimum score 550 paper-based; 80 iBT) or IELTS. Electronic applications accepted. *Faculty research:* Agricultural, urban, medical, and veterinary entomology; biological control; chemical ecology; insect pathogens; novel toxicants.

University of California, San Diego, Office of Graduate Studies, Division of Biological Sciences, La Jolla, CA 92093. Offers anthropogeny (PhD); bioinformatics (PhD); biology (PhD); ecology, behavior and evolution (PhD); microbiology (PhD). *Students:* 285 full-time (154 women), 8 part-time (4 women); includes 70 minority (2 Black or African American, non-Hispanic/Latino; 3 American Indian or Alaska Native, non-Hispanic/Latino; 51 Asian, non-Hispanic/Latino; 13 Hispanic/Latino; 1 Native Hawaiian or other Pacific Islander, non-Hispanic/Latino), 30 international. 626 applicants, 24% accepted, 85 enrolled. In 2013, 32 doctorates awarded. *Degree requirements:* For doctorate, thesis/dissertation, 3 quarters of teaching assistantship. *Entrance requirements:* For doctorate, GRE General Test; GRE Subject Test (recommended). Additional exam requirements/recommendations for international students: Required—TOEFL, IELTS. *Application deadline:* For fall admission, 12/4 for domestic students. Application fee: $80 ($100 for international students). Electronic applications accepted. *Expenses:* Tuition, state resident: full-time $11,220; part-time $1870 per quarter. Tuition, nonresident: full-time $26,322; part-time $4387 per quarter. *Required fees:* $519.50 per quarter. Part-time tuition and fees vary according to course load and program. *Financial support:* Fellowships, research assistantships, teaching assistantships, and scholarships/grants available. Financial award applicants required to submit FAFSA. *Faculty research:* Ecology, behavior and evolution; microbiology; bioinformatics; multi-scale biology; anthropogeny. *Unit head:* William McGinnis, Dean, 858-822-0458, E-mail: wmcginnis@ucsd.edu. *Application contact:* Cathy Pugh, Graduate Coordinator, 858-534-0181, E-mail: gradprog@biology.ucsd.edu.
Website: http://biology.ucsd.edu/

University of California, Santa Barbara, Graduate Division, College of Letters and Sciences, Division of Mathematics, Life, and Physical Sciences, Department of Ecology, Evolution, and Marine Biology, Santa Barbara, CA 93106-9620. Offers computational science and engineering (MA); computational sciences and engineering (PhD); ecology, evolution, and marine biology (MA, PhD); MA/PhD. *Faculty:* 33 full-time (8 women). *Students:* 59 full-time (33 women); includes 14 minority (1 Black or African American, non-Hispanic/Latino; 7 Asian, non-Hispanic/Latino; 6 Hispanic/Latino), 4 international. Average age 31. 120 applicants, 15% accepted, 12 enrolled. In 2013, 9 master's, 6 doctorates awarded. *Degree requirements:* For master's, comprehensive exam (for some programs), thesis (for some programs); for doctorate, comprehensive exam, thesis/dissertation. *Entrance requirements:* For master's and doctorate, GRE General Test. Additional exam requirements/recommendations for international students: Required—TOEFL (minimum score 550 paper-based; 80 iBT), IELTS. *Application deadline:* For fall admission, 12/15 for domestic and international students. Application fee: $80 ($100 for international students). Electronic applications accepted. *Expenses:* Tuition, state resident: part-time $5148.26 per quarter. Tuition, nonresident: part-time $10,182.26 per quarter. *Financial support:* In 2013–14, 50 students received support, including 55 fellowships with full and partial tuition reimbursements available (averaging $10,812 per year), 24 research assistantships with full and partial tuition reimbursements available (averaging $8,441 per year), 97 teaching assistantships with partial tuition reimbursements available (averaging $9,346 per year); Federal Work-Study, scholarships/grants, traineeships, health care benefits, and tuition waivers (full and partial) also available. Financial award application deadline: 12/15; financial award applicants required to submit FAFSA. *Faculty research:* Community ecology, evolution, marine biology, population genetics, stream ecology. *Unit head:* Dr. Craig Carlson, Chair, 805-893-2415, Fax: 805-893-5885, E-mail: eembchair@lifesci.ucsb.edu. *Application contact:* Melanie Fujii, Student Affairs Officer, 805-893-2979, Fax: 805-893-5885, E-mail: eemb-info@lifesci.ucsb.edu.
Website: http://www.lifesci.ucsb.edu/EEMB/index.html

University of California, Santa Cruz, Division of Graduate Studies, Division of Physical and Biological Sciences, Department of Ecology and Evolutionary Biology, Santa Cruz, CA 95064. Offers MA, PhD. *Degree requirements:* For master's, thesis; for doctorate, comprehensive exam, thesis/dissertation. *Entrance requirements:* For master's and doctorate, GRE General Test, GRE Subject Test, 3 letters of recommendation. Additional exam requirements/recommendations for international students: Required—TOEFL (minimum score 550 paper-based; 83 iBT); Recommended—IELTS (minimum score 8). Electronic applications accepted. *Faculty research:* Population and community ecology, evolutionary biology, physiology and behavior (marine and terrestrial), systematics and biodiversity.

University of Chicago, Division of Biological Sciences, Darwinian Sciences Cluster: Ecological, Integrative and Evolutionary Biology, Department of Ecology and Evolution, Chicago, IL 60637-1513. Offers PhD. *Degree requirements:* For doctorate, thesis/dissertation, ethics class, 2 teaching assistantships. *Entrance requirements:* For doctorate, GRE General Test. Additional exam requirements/recommendations for international students: Required—TOEFL (minimum score 600 paper-based; 104 iBT), IELTS (minimum score 7). Electronic applications accepted. *Faculty research:* Population genetics, molecular evolution, behavior.

University of Colorado Boulder, Graduate School, College of Arts and Sciences, Department of Ecology and Evolutionary Biology, Boulder, CO 80309. Offers animal behavior (MA); biology (MA, PhD); environmental biology (MA, PhD); evolutionary biology (MA, PhD); neurobiology (MA); population biology (MA); population genetics (PhD). *Faculty:* 31 full-time (12 women). *Students:* 70 full-time (30 women), 18 part-time (10 women); includes 6 minority (1 Asian, non-Hispanic/Latino; 3 Hispanic/Latino; 2 Two or more races, non-Hispanic/Latino), 5 international. Average age 30. 171 applicants, 6% accepted, 11 enrolled. In 2013, 10 master's, 11 doctorates awarded. Terminal master's awarded for partial completion of doctoral program. *Degree requirements:* For master's, comprehensive exam, thesis or alternative; for doctorate, comprehensive exam, thesis/dissertation. *Entrance requirements:* For master's, GRE General Test, GRE Subject Test, minimum undergraduate GPA of 3.0; for doctorate, GRE General Test, GRE Subject Test. *Application deadline:* For fall admission, 12/31 for domestic students, 12/1 for international students. Application fee: $50 ($60 for international students). Electronic applications accepted. *Financial support:* In 2013–14, 175 students received support, including 35 fellowships (averaging $15,283 per year), 21 research assistantships with full and partial tuition reimbursements available (averaging $29,343 per year), 48 teaching assistantships with full and partial tuition reimbursements available (averaging $31,449 per year); institutionally sponsored loans, scholarships/grants, health care benefits, and unspecified assistantships also available. Financial award applicants required to submit FAFSA. *Faculty research:* Ecology, environmental biology, evolutionary biology, biological sciences, conservation biology. *Total annual research expenditures:* $37.1 million.
Website: http://ebio.colorado.edu

University of Colorado Denver, College of Liberal Arts and Sciences, Department of Geography and Environmental Sciences, Denver, CO 80217. Offers environmental sciences (MS), including air quality, ecosystems, environmental health, environmental science education, geo-spatial analysis, hazardous waste, water quality. Part-time and evening/weekend programs available. *Faculty:* 12 full-time (4 women), 6 part-time/adjunct (1 woman). *Students:* 35 full-time (26 women), 3 part-time (2 women); includes 7 minority (1 Asian, non-Hispanic/Latino; 5 Hispanic/Latino; 1 Two or more races, non-Hispanic/Latino), 7 international. Average age 29. 34 applicants, 74% accepted, 15 enrolled. In 2013, 16 master's awarded. *Degree requirements:* For master's, thesis or alternative, 30 credits including 21 of core requirements and 9 of environmental science electives. *Entrance requirements:* For master's, GRE General Test, BA in one of the natural/physical sciences or engineering (or equivalent background); prerequisite coursework in calculus and physics (one semester each), general chemistry with lab and general biology with lab (two semesters each), three letters of recommendation. Additional exam requirements/recommendations for international students: Required—TOEFL (minimum score 537 paper-based; 75 iBT); Recommended—IELTS (minimum score 6.5). *Application deadline:* For fall admission, 4/1 for domestic and international students; for spring admission, 10/1 for domestic and international students. Application fee: $50 ($75 for international students). Electronic applications accepted. *Financial support:* In 2013–14, 7 students received support. Fellowships, research assistantships, teaching assistantships, Federal Work-Study, institutionally sponsored loans, scholarships/grants, and traineeships available. Financial award application deadline: 4/1; financial award applicants required to submit FAFSA. *Faculty research:* Air quality, environmental health, ecosystems, hazardous waste, water quality, geo-spatial analysis and environmental science education. *Unit head:* Dr. Frederick Chambers, Director of MS in Environmental Sciences Program, 303-556-2619, Fax: 303-556-6197, E-mail: frederick.chambers@ucdenver.edu. *Application contact:* Sue Eddleman, Program Assistant, 303-556-2276, E-mail: sue.eddleman@ucdenver.edu.
Website: http://www.ucdenver.edu/academics/colleges/CLAS/Departments/ges/Programs/MasterofScience/Pages/MasterofScience.aspx

University of Colorado Denver, College of Liberal Arts and Sciences, Department of Integrative Biology, Denver, CO 80217. Offers animal behavior (MS); biology (MS); cell and developmental biology (MS); ecology (MS); evolutionary biology (MS); genetics (MS); integrative and systems biology (PhD); microbiology (MS); molecular biology (MS); neurobiology (MS); plant systematics (MS). Part-time programs available. *Faculty:* 21 full-time (7 women), 3 part-time/adjunct (2 women). *Students:* 18 full-time (11 women), 5 part-time (all women); includes 5 minority (1 Black or African American, non-Hispanic/Latino; 2 Hispanic/Latino; 2 Two or more races, non-Hispanic/Latino), 1 international. Average age 29. 25 applicants, 44% accepted, 11 enrolled. In 2013, 13 master's awarded. *Degree requirements:* For master's, comprehensive exam, thesis, 30-32 credit hours. *Entrance requirements:* For master's, GRE General Test (minimum score in 50th percentile in each section), BA/BS from accredited institution awarded within the last 10 years; minimum undergraduate GPA of 3.0; prerequisite courses: 1 year each of general biology and general chemistry; 1 semester each of general genetics, general ecology, and cell biology; and a structure/function course. Additional exam requirements/recommendations for international students: Required—TOEFL (minimum score 537 paper-based; 75 iBT); Recommended—IELTS (minimum score 6.5). *Application deadline:* For fall admission, 2/1 for domestic and international

students. Application fee: $50 ($75 for international students). Electronic applications accepted. *Financial support:* In 2013–14, 8 students received support. Fellowships, research assistantships, teaching assistantships, Federal Work-Study, institutionally sponsored loans, scholarships/grants, and traineeships available. Financial award application deadline: 4/1; financial award applicants required to submit FAFSA. *Faculty research:* Molecular developmental biology; quantitative ecology, biogeography, and population dynamics; environmental signaling and endocrine disruption; speciation, the evolution of reproductive isolation, and hybrid zones; evolutionary, behavioral, and conservation ecology. *Unit head:* Dr. John Swallow, Biology Department Chair, 303-556-6154, E-mail: john.swallow@ucdenver.edu. *Application contact:* Timberley Roane, Associate Professor/Director of MS in Biology Program, 303-556-6592, E-mail: timberley.roane@ucdenver.edu.
Website: http://www.ucdenver.edu/academics/colleges/CLAS/Departments/biology/Programs/MasterofScience/Pages/BiologyMasterOfScience.aspx

University of Connecticut, Graduate School, College of Liberal Arts and Sciences, Department of Ecology and Evolutionary Biology, Storrs, CT 06269. Offers botany (MS, PhD); ecology (MS, PhD); entomology (MS, PhD); zoology (MS, PhD). Terminal master's awarded for partial completion of doctoral program. *Degree requirements:* For master's, comprehensive exam; for doctorate, thesis/dissertation. *Entrance requirements:* For master's and doctorate, GRE General Test, GRE Subject Test. Additional exam requirements/recommendations for international students: Required—TOEFL (minimum score 550 paper-based). Electronic applications accepted.

University of Connecticut, Graduate School, College of Liberal Arts and Sciences, Department of Psychology, Storrs, CT 06269. Offers behavioral neuroscience (PhD); biopsychology (PhD); clinical psychology (MA, PhD); cognition and instruction (PhD); developmental psychology (MA, PhD); ecological psychology (PhD); experimental psychology (PhD); general psychology (MA, PhD); health psychology (Graduate Certificate); industrial/organizational psychology (PhD); language and cognition (PhD); neuroscience (PhD); occupational health psychology (Graduate Certificate); social psychology (MA, PhD). *Accreditation:* APA. Terminal master's awarded for partial completion of doctoral program. *Degree requirements:* For master's, comprehensive exam; for doctorate, thesis/dissertation. *Entrance requirements:* For master's and doctorate, GRE General Test, GRE Subject Test. Additional exam requirements/recommendations for international students: Required—TOEFL (minimum score 550 paper-based). Electronic applications accepted.

University of Delaware, College of Agriculture and Natural Resources, Department of Entomology and Wildlife Ecology, Newark, DE 19716. Offers entomology and applied ecology (MS, PhD), including avian ecology, evolution and taxonomy, insect biological control, insect ecology and behavior (MS), insect genetics, pest management, plant-insect interactions, wildlife ecology and management. Part-time programs available. *Degree requirements:* For master's, comprehensive exam, thesis, oral exam, seminar; for doctorate, comprehensive exam, thesis/dissertation, qualifying exam, seminar. *Entrance requirements:* For master's, GRE General Test, minimum GPA of 3.0 in field, 2.8 overall; for doctorate, GRE General Test, GRE Subject Test (biology), minimum GPA of 3.0 in field, 2.8 overall. Additional exam requirements/recommendations for international students: Required—TOEFL. Electronic applications accepted. *Faculty research:* Ecology and evolution of plant-insect interactions, ecology of wildlife conservation management, habitat restoration, biological control, applied ecosystem management.

University of Delaware, College of Arts and Sciences, Department of Biological Sciences, Newark, DE 19716. Offers biotechnology (MS); cancer biology (MS, PhD); cell and extracellular matrix biology (MS, PhD); cell and systems physiology (MS, PhD); developmental biology (MS, PhD); ecology and evolution (MS, PhD); microbiology (MS, PhD); molecular biology and genetics (MS, PhD). Terminal master's awarded for partial completion of doctoral program. *Degree requirements:* For master's, thesis, preliminary exam; for doctorate, comprehensive exam, thesis/dissertation, preliminary exam. *Entrance requirements:* For master's and doctorate, GRE General Test. Additional exam requirements/recommendations for international students: Required—TOEFL (minimum score 600 paper-based); Recommended—TWE. Electronic applications accepted. *Faculty research:* Microorganisms, bone, cancer metastasis, developmental biology, cell biology, DNA.

University of Denver, Division of Natural Sciences and Mathematics, Department of Biological Sciences, Denver, CO 80208-9010. Offers biomedical sciences (PSM); cell and molecular biology (MS, PhD); ecology and evolution (MS, PhD). Part-time programs available. *Faculty:* 23 full-time (8 women). *Students:* 1 (woman) full-time, 21 part-time (13 women); includes 3 minority (all Hispanic/Latino), 7 international. Average age 27. 50 applicants, 22% accepted, 10 enrolled. In 2013, 5 master's, 2 doctorates awarded. Terminal master's awarded for partial completion of doctoral program. *Degree requirements:* For master's, comprehensive exam (for some programs), thesis; for doctorate, one foreign language, comprehensive exam (for some programs), thesis/dissertation. *Entrance requirements:* For master's and doctorate, GRE General Test, bachelor's degree in biology or related field, transcripts, personal statement, three letters of recommendation. Additional exam requirements/recommendations for international students: Required—TOEFL (minimum score 570 paper-based; 88 iBT). *Application deadline:* For fall admission, 1/1 priority date for domestic and international students. Applications are processed on a rolling basis. Application fee: $60. Electronic applications accepted. *Financial support:* In 2013–14, 19 students received support, including 3 research assistantships with full and partial tuition reimbursements available (averaging $22,448 per year), 15 teaching assistantships with full and partial tuition reimbursements available (averaging $25,161 per year); Federal Work-Study, institutionally sponsored loans, scholarships/grants, and unspecified assistantships also available. Support available to part-time students. Financial award application deadline: 2/15; financial award applicants required to submit FAFSA. *Faculty research:* Molecular biology, cell biology, neurobiology, ecology, molecular evolution. *Unit head:* Dr. Joseph Angleson, Chair, 303-871-3463, Fax: 303-871-3471, E-mail: jangleso@du.edu. *Application contact:* Randi Flageolle, Assistant to the Chair, 303-871-3457, Fax: 303-871-3471, E-mail: rflageol@du.edu.
Website: http://www.du.edu/nsm/departments/biologicalsciences/index.html

University of Florida, Graduate School, College of Agricultural and Life Sciences, Department of Wildlife Ecology and Conservation, Gainesville, FL 32611. Offers environmental education and communications (Certificate); wildlife ecology and conservation (MS, PhD). *Faculty:* 21 full-time (6 women), 4 part-time/adjunct (2 women). *Students:* 43 full-time (26 women), 10 part-time (3 women); includes 6 minority (4 Black or African American, non-Hispanic/Latino; 2 Hispanic/Latino), 17 international. Average age 31. 47 applicants, 13% accepted, 6 enrolled. In 2013, 7 master's, 6 doctorates awarded. *Degree requirements:* For master's, comprehensive exam, thesis optional; for doctorate, comprehensive exam, thesis/dissertation. *Entrance requirements:* For master's and doctorate, GRE General Test, minimum GPA of 3.3. Additional exam requirements/recommendations for international students: Required—TOEFL (minimum score 550 paper-based; 80 iBT), IELTS (minimum score 6). *Application deadline:* For fall admission, 6/1 priority date for domestic students; for spring admission, 12/1 for domestic students. Applications are processed on a rolling basis. Application fee: $30. Electronic applications accepted. *Expenses:* Tuition, state resident: full-time $12,640. Tuition, nonresident: full-time $30,000. *Financial support:* In 2013–14, 36 students received support, including 4 fellowships (averaging $11,235 per year), 27 research assistantships (averaging $21,960 per year), 8 teaching assistantships (averaging $16,465 per year); institutionally sponsored loans also available. Financial award applicants required to submit FAFSA. *Faculty research:* Wildlife biology and management, tropical ecology and conservation, conservation biology, landscape ecology and restoration, conservation education. *Unit head:* Eric C. Hellgren, PhD, Professor and Department Chair, 352-846-0552, E-mail: hellgren@ufl.edu. *Application contact:* Katie Sieving, PhD, Professor and Graduate Coordinator, 352-846-0569, Fax: 352-846-0841, E-mail: chucao@ufl.edu.
Website: http://www.wec.ufl.edu/

University of Florida, Graduate School, School of Natural Resources and Environment, Gainesville, FL 32611. Offers interdisciplinary ecology (MS, PhD). *Students:* 74 full-time (50 women), 27 part-time (16 women); includes 12 minority (1 Black or African American, non-Hispanic/Latino; 2 American Indian or Alaska Native, non-Hispanic/Latino; 1 Asian, non-Hispanic/Latino; 8 Hispanic/Latino), 31 international. Average age 33. 76 applicants, 32% accepted, 20 enrolled. In 2013, 14 master's, 22 doctorates awarded. *Degree requirements:* For master's, comprehensive exam, thesis; for doctorate, comprehensive exam, thesis/dissertation. *Entrance requirements:* For master's and doctorate, GRE General Test, minimum GPA of 3.0. Additional exam requirements/recommendations for international students: Required—TOEFL (minimum score 550 paper-based; 80 iBT), IELTS (minimum score 6). *Application deadline:* For fall admission, 2/1 priority date for domestic students, 2/1 for international students. Applications are processed on a rolling basis. Application fee: $30. Electronic applications accepted. *Expenses:* Tuition, state resident: full-time $12,640. Tuition, nonresident: full-time $30,000. *Financial support:* In 2013–14, 62 students received support, including 9 fellowships (averaging $26,460 per year), 59 research assistantships (averaging $14,425 per year), 20 teaching assistantships (averaging $13,630 per year). Financial award applicants required to submit FAFSA. *Faculty research:* Natural sciences, social sciences, sustainability studies, research design and methods. *Unit head:* Dr. Thomas K. Frazer, Director and Graduate Coordinator, 352-392-9230, Fax: 352-392-9748, E-mail: frazer@ufl.edu. *Application contact:* Office of Graduate Admissions, 352-392-1365, E-mail: webrequests@admissions.ufl.edu.
Website: http://www.snre.ufl.edu/

University of Georgia, School of Ecology, Athens, GA 30602. Offers conservation ecology and sustainable development (MS); ecology (MS, PhD). *Degree requirements:* For master's, thesis; for doctorate, one foreign language, thesis/dissertation. *Entrance requirements:* For master's and doctorate, GRE General Test. Electronic applications accepted.

University of Guelph, Graduate Studies, College of Biological Science, Department of Integrative Biology, Botany and Zoology, Guelph, ON N1G 2W1, Canada. Offers botany (M Sc, PhD); zoology (M Sc, PhD). Part-time programs available. *Degree requirements:* For master's, thesis, research proposal; for doctorate, thesis/dissertation, research proposal, qualifying exam. *Entrance requirements:* For master's, minimum B average during previous 2 years of course work. Additional exam requirements/recommendations for international students: Required—TOEFL (minimum score 550 paper-based), IELTS (minimum score 6.5). Electronic applications accepted. *Faculty research:* Aquatic science, environmental physiology, parasitology, wildlife biology, management.

University of Hawaii at Manoa, Graduate Division, Interdisciplinary Specialization in Ecology, Evolution and Conservation Biology, Honolulu, HI 96822. Offers MS, PhD. *Degree requirements:* For doctorate, thesis/dissertation. *Faculty research:* Agronomy and soil science, zoology, entomology, genetics and molecular biology, botanical sciences.

University of Illinois at Urbana–Champaign, Graduate College, College of Liberal Arts and Sciences, School of Integrative Biology, Department of Animal Biology, Champaign, IL 61820. Offers animal biology (ecology, ethology and evolution) (MS, PhD). *Students:* 15 (5 women). Application fee: $75 ($90 for international students). *Unit head:* Ken Paige, Head, 217-244-6606, Fax: 217-244-4565, E-mail: k-paige@illinois.edu. *Application contact:* Lisa Smith, Office Administrator, 217-333-7802, Fax: 217-244-4565, E-mail: ljsmith1@illinois.edu.
Website: http://www.life.illinois.edu/animalbiology

University of Illinois at Urbana–Champaign, Graduate College, College of Liberal Arts and Sciences, School of Integrative Biology, Program in Ecology, Evolution and Conservation Biology, Champaign, IL 61820. Offers MS, PhD. *Students:* 28 (16 women). Application fee: $75 ($90 for international students). *Unit head:* Evan H. DeLucia, Director, 217-333-3044, Fax: 217-244-1224, E-mail: delucia@illinois.edu. *Application contact:* Kimberly Leigh, Secretary, 217-333-8208, Fax: 217-244-1224, E-mail: kaleigh@illinois.edu.
Website: http://sib.illinois.edu/peec/

The University of Kansas, Graduate Studies, College of Liberal Arts and Sciences, Department of Ecology and Evolutionary Biology, Lawrence, KS 66045. Offers botany (MA, PhD); ecology and evolutionary biology (MA, PhD); entomology (MA, PhD). *Faculty:* 35. *Students:* 57 full-time (25 women); includes 3 minority (all Two or more races, non-Hispanic/Latino), 19 international. Average age 29. 48 applicants, 29% accepted, 10 enrolled. In 2013, 9 doctorates awarded. Terminal master's awarded for partial completion of doctoral program. *Degree requirements:* For master's, comprehensive exam, thesis (for some programs), 30-36 credits, thesis presentation; for doctorate, comprehensive exam, thesis/dissertation, residency, responsible scholarship and research skills, final exam, dissertation defense. *Entrance requirements:* For master's, GRE General Test, bachelor's degree with minimum undergraduate GPA of 3.0; for doctorate, GRE General Test, bachelor's degree; minimum undergraduate/graduate GPA of 3.0. Additional exam requirements/recommendations for international students: Required—TOEFL or IELTS. *Application deadline:* For fall admission, 12/1 for domestic and international students; for spring admission, 9/15 for domestic and international students. Application fee: $55 ($65 for international students). Electronic applications accepted. *Financial support:* In 2013–14, 8 fellowships with full and partial tuition reimbursements, 22 research assistantships with full and partial tuition reimbursements, 32 teaching assistantships with full and partial tuition reimbursements were awarded; scholarships/grants, traineeships, health care benefits, and unspecified assistantships also available. Financial award application deadline: 12/1. *Faculty research:* Ecology and global change, diversity and macroevolution, evolutionary mechanisms, systematics/phylogenetics, biogeography. *Unit head:* Dr. Christopher H. Haufler, Chair, 785-864-3255, Fax: 785-864-5860, E-mail: vulgare@ku.edu. *Application contact:* Aagje Ashe, Graduate Coordinator, 785-864-2362, Fax: 785-864-5860, E-mail: a4ashe@ku.edu.
Website: http://eeb.ku.edu/

University of Maine, Graduate School, College of Natural Sciences, Forestry, and Agriculture, School of Biology and Ecology, Orono, ME 04469. Offers biological sciences (PhD); botany and plant pathology (MS); ecology and environmental science (MS, PhD); entomology (MS); plant science (PhD); zoology (MS, PhD). Part-time programs available. *Faculty:* 33 full-time (13 women), 26 part-time/adjunct (5 women).

Students: 66 full-time (40 women), 4 part-time (2 women); includes 4 minority (1 American Indian or Alaska Native, non-Hispanic/Latino; 2 Asian, non-Hispanic/Latino; 1 Hispanic/Latino), 7 international. Average age 30. 97 applicants, 25% accepted, 17 enrolled. In 2013, 8 master's, 3 doctorates awarded. Terminal master's awarded for partial completion of doctoral program. *Degree requirements:* For master's, thesis (for some programs); for doctorate, comprehensive exam, thesis/dissertation. *Entrance requirements:* For master's and doctorate, GRE General Test. Additional exam requirements/recommendations for international students: Required—TOEFL. *Application deadline:* For fall admission, 2/1 priority date for domestic students. Applications are processed on a rolling basis. Application fee: $65. Electronic applications accepted. *Expenses:* Tuition, state resident: full-time $7524. Tuition, nonresident: full-time $23,112. *Required fees:* $1970. *Financial support:* In 2013–14, 66 students received support, including 3 fellowships with full tuition reimbursements available (averaging $25,000 per year), 28 research assistantships with full tuition reimbursements available (averaging $14,600 per year), 21 teaching assistantships with full tuition reimbursements available (averaging $14,600 per year); career-related internships or fieldwork, Federal Work-Study, institutionally sponsored loans, and tuition waivers (full and partial) also available. Financial award application deadline: 3/1. *Total annual research expenditures:* $569,533. *Unit head:* Dr. Ellie Groden, Director, 207-581-2551, Fax: 207-581-2537. *Application contact:* Scott G. Delcourt, Associate Dean of the Graduate School, 207-581-3291, Fax: 207-581-3232, E-mail: graduate@maine.edu.
Website: http://sbe.umaine.edu/

The University of Manchester, Faculty of Life Sciences, Manchester, United Kingdom. Offers adaptive organismal biology (M Phil, PhD); animal biology (M Phil, PhD); biochemistry (M Phil, PhD); bioinformatics (M Phil, PhD); biomolecular sciences (M Phil, PhD); biotechnology (M Phil, PhD); cell biology (M Phil, PhD); cell matrix research (M Phil, PhD); channels and transporters (M Phil, PhD); developmental biology (M Phil, PhD); Egyptology (M Phil, PhD); environmental biology (M Phil, PhD); evolutionary biology (M Phil, PhD); gene expression (M Phil, PhD); genetics (M Phil, PhD); history of science, technology and medicine (M Phil, PhD); immunology (M Phil, PhD); integrative neurobiology and behavior (M Phil, PhD); membrane trafficking (M Phil, PhD); microbiology (M Phil, PhD); molecular and cellular neuroscience (M Phil, PhD); molecular biology (M Phil, PhD); molecular cancer studies (M Phil, PhD); neuroscience (M Phil, PhD); ophthalmology (M Phil, PhD); optometry (M Phil, PhD); organelle function (M Phil, PhD); pharmacology (M Phil, PhD); physiology (M Phil, PhD); plant sciences (M Phil, PhD); stem cell research (M Phil, PhD); structural biology (M Phil, PhD); systems neuroscience (M Phil, PhD); toxicology (M Phil, PhD).

University of Manitoba, Faculty of Graduate Studies, Faculty of Science, Department of Biological Sciences, Winnipeg, MB R3T 2N2, Canada. Offers botany (M Sc, PhD); ecology (M Sc, PhD); zoology (M Sc, PhD).

University of Maryland, College Park, Academic Affairs, College of Computer, Mathematical and Natural Sciences, Department of Biology, Behavior, Ecology, Evolution, and Systematics Program, College Park, MD 20742. Offers MS, PhD. *Students:* 7 full-time (3 women), 2 part-time (1 woman); includes 2 minority (1 Asian, non-Hispanic/Latino; 1 Two or more races, non-Hispanic/Latino), 1 international. In 2013, 4 doctorates awarded. *Degree requirements:* For master's, thesis, oral defense, seminar; for doctorate, thesis/dissertation, exam, 4 seminars. *Entrance requirements:* For master's and doctorate, GRE General Test, GRE Subject Test (biology), 3 letters of recommendation. Additional exam requirements/recommendations for international students: Required—TOEFL. *Expenses:* Tuition, state resident: full-time $10,314; part-time $573 per credit hour. Tuition, nonresident: full-time $22,248; part-time $1236 per credit. *Required fees:* $1446; $403.15 per semester. Tuition and fees vary according to program. *Financial support:* In 2013–14, 3 fellowships with full tuition reimbursements (averaging $62,679 per year), 1 research assistantship (averaging $19,685 per year), 5 teaching assistantships (averaging $19,775 per year) were awarded; Federal Work-Study and scholarships/grants also available. Support available to part-time students. Financial award applicants required to submit FAFSA. *Faculty research:* Animal behavior, biostatistics, ecology, evolution, neurothology. *Unit head:* David Hawthorne, Graduate Director, 301-405-4552, E-mail: djh@umd.edu. *Application contact:* Dr. Charles A. Caramello, Dean of Graduate School, 301-405-0358, Fax: 301-314-9305, E-mail: ccaramel@umd.edu.

University of Maryland, College Park, Academic Affairs, College of Computer, Mathematical and Natural Sciences, Department of Biology, PhD Program in Biological Sciences, College Park, MD 20742. Offers behavior, ecology, evolution, and systematics (PhD); computational biology, bioinformatics, and genomics (PhD); molecular and cellular biology (PhD); physiological systems (PhD). *Students:* 104 full-time (59 women), 4 part-time (1 woman); includes 21 minority (2 Black or African American, non-Hispanic/Latino; 1 American Indian or Alaska Native, non-Hispanic/Latino; 9 Asian, non-Hispanic/Latino; 7 Hispanic/Latino; 2 Two or more races, non-Hispanic/Latino), 34 international. 365 applicants, 13% accepted, 20 enrolled. In 2013, 5 doctorates awarded. *Degree requirements:* For doctorate, comprehensive exam, thesis/dissertation, thesis work presentation in seminar. *Entrance requirements:* For doctorate, GRE General Test; GRE Subject Test in biology (recommended), academic transcripts, statement of purpose/research interests, 3 letters of recommendation. Additional exam requirements/recommendations for international students: Required—TOEFL. *Application deadline:* For fall admission, 12/15 for domestic and international students. Applications are processed on a rolling basis. Application fee: $75. Electronic applications accepted. *Expenses:* Tuition, state resident: full-time $10,314; part-time $573 per credit hour. Tuition, nonresident: full-time $22,248; part-time $1236 per credit. *Required fees:* $1446; $403.15 per semester. Tuition and fees vary according to program. *Financial support:* In 2013–14, 21 fellowships with full and partial tuition reimbursements (averaging $27,603 per year), 25 research assistantships (averaging $19,557 per year), 55 teaching assistantships (averaging $18,959 per year) were awarded. *Unit head:* Dr. Charles F. Delwiche, Director, 301-405-6884, E-mail: bisidirector@umd.edu. *Application contact:* Dr. Charles A. Caramello, Dean of Graduate School, 301-405-0358, Fax: 301-314-9305, E-mail: ccaramel@umd.edu.
Website: http://www.bisi.umd.edu/

University of Michigan, Rackham Graduate School, College of Literature, Science, and the Arts, Department of Ecology and Evolutionary Biology, Ann Arbor, MI 48109. Offers MS, PhD. Part-time programs available. Terminal master's awarded for partial completion of doctoral program. *Degree requirements:* For master's, thesis (for some programs), two seminars; for doctorate, comprehensive exam, thesis/dissertation, 2 semesters of teaching. *Entrance requirements:* For master's and doctorate, GRE. Additional exam requirements/recommendations for international students: Required—TOEFL (minimum score 560 paper-based; 84 iBT). Electronic applications accepted. Tuition and fees vary according to course level, course load, degree level, program and student level. *Faculty research:* Population and community ecology, ecosystem ecology and biogeochemistry, global change biology, biogeography and paleobiology, evolution of behavior, evolutionary genetics, phylogenetic and phylogeography, ecology and evolution of infectious disease.

University of Michigan, School of Natural Resources and Environment, Program in Natural Resources and Environment, Ann Arbor, MI 48109-1041. Offers aquatic sciences: research and management (MS); behavior, education and communication (MS); conservation biology (MS); conservation ecology (MS); environmental informatics (MS); environmental justice (MS); environmental policy and planning (MS); natural resources and environment (PhD); sustainable systems (MS); terrestrial ecosystems (MS); MS/JD; MS/MBA; MUP/MS. *Faculty:* 45 full-time, 23 part-time/adjunct. *Students:* 380 full-time (203 women); includes 59 minority (5 Black or African American, non-Hispanic/Latino; 1 American Indian or Alaska Native, non-Hispanic/Latino; 20 Asian, non-Hispanic/Latino; 21 Hispanic/Latino; 12 Two or more races, non-Hispanic/Latino), 74 international. Average age 27. 657 applicants. In 2013, 131 master's, 11 doctorates awarded. Terminal master's awarded for partial completion of doctoral program. *Degree requirements:* For master's, practicum or group project; for doctorate, comprehensive exam, thesis/dissertation, oral defense of dissertation, preliminary exam. *Entrance requirements:* For master's, GRE General Test; for doctorate, GRE General Test, master's degree. Additional exam requirements/recommendations for international students: Required—TOEFL (minimum score 560 paper-based; 84 iBT). *Application deadline:* For fall admission, 1/5 priority date for domestic and international students. Applications are processed on a rolling basis. Application fee: $65 ($75 for international students). Electronic applications accepted. Tuition and fees vary according to course level, course load, degree level, program and student level. *Financial support:* Fellowships with tuition reimbursements available. Financial award application deadline: 1/5; financial award applicants required to submit FAFSA. *Faculty research:* Stream ecology and fish biology, plant-insect interactions, environmental education, resource control and reproductive success, remote sensing, conservation ecology, sustainable systems. *Unit head:* Dr. Marie Lynn Miranda, Dean, 734-764-2550, Fax: 734-763-8965, E-mail: mlmirand@umich.edu. *Application contact:* Sondra R. Auerbach, Director of Academic Services, 734-764-6453, Fax: 734-936-2195, E-mail: snre.admissions@umich.edu.
Website: http://www.snre.umich.edu/

University of Minnesota, Twin Cities Campus, Graduate School, College of Biological Sciences, Department of Ecology, Evolution, and Behavior, St. Paul, MN 55418. Offers MS, PhD. Terminal master's awarded for partial completion of doctoral program. *Degree requirements:* For master's, comprehensive exam, thesis or projects; for doctorate, comprehensive exam, thesis/dissertation. *Entrance requirements:* For master's and doctorate, GRE General Test, minimum GPA of 3.0. Additional exam requirements/recommendations for international students: Required—TOEFL (minimum score 550 paper-based; 79 iBT), Michigan English Language Assessment Battery. Electronic applications accepted. *Faculty research:* Behavioral ecology, community ecology, community genetics, ecosystem and global change, evolution and systematics.

University of Missouri, Graduate School, College of Arts and Science, Division of Biological Sciences, Columbia, MO 65211. Offers evolutionary biology and ecology (MA, PhD); genetic, cellular and developmental biology (MA, PhD); neurobiology and behavior (MA, PhD). *Faculty:* 40 full-time (11 women), 1 part-time/adjunct (0 women). *Students:* 70 full-time (32 women), 3 part-time (2 women); includes 12 minority (4 Black or African American, non-Hispanic/Latino; 1 American Indian or Alaska Native, non-Hispanic/Latino; 2 Asian, non-Hispanic/Latino; 3 Hispanic/Latino; 2 Two or more races, non-Hispanic/Latino), 5 international. Average age 28. 46 applicants, 28% accepted, 13 enrolled. In 2013, 7 master's, 13 doctorates awarded. Terminal master's awarded for partial completion of doctoral program. *Degree requirements:* For master's, thesis; for doctorate, comprehensive exam, thesis/dissertation. *Entrance requirements:* For master's and doctorate, GRE General Test (minimum score 1200 verbal and quantitative), minimum GPA of 3.0. Additional exam requirements/recommendations for international students: Required—TOEFL (minimum score 600 paper-based; 100 iBT). *Application deadline:* For fall admission, 12/15 priority date for domestic and international students. Applications are processed on a rolling basis. Application fee: $55 ($75 for international students). Electronic applications accepted. *Financial support:* Fellowships with full tuition reimbursements, research assistantships with full tuition reimbursements, teaching assistantships with full tuition reimbursements, institutionally sponsored loans, traineeships, health care benefits, and unspecified assistantships available. *Faculty research:* Evolutionary biology, ecology and behavior; genetic, cellular, molecular and developmental biology; neurobiology and behavior; plant sciences. *Unit head:* Dr. John C. Walker, Division Director, 573-882-3583, E-mail: walkerj@missouri.edu. *Application contact:* Nila Emerich, Application Contact, 800-553-5698, E-mail: emerichn@missouri.edu.
Website: http://biology.missouri.edu/graduate-studies/

University of Missouri–St. Louis, College of Arts and Sciences, Department of Biology, St. Louis, MO 63121. Offers biotechnology (Certificate); cell and molecular biology (MS, PhD); ecology, evolution and systematics (MS, PhD); tropical biology and conservation (Certificate). Part-time programs available. *Faculty:* 33 full-time (13 women), 9 part-time/adjunct (1 woman). *Students:* 52 full-time (23 women), 58 part-time (29 women); includes 13 minority (9 Black or African American, non-Hispanic/Latino; 3 Asian, non-Hispanic/Latino; 1 Hispanic/Latino), 30 international. Average age 28. 113 applicants, 42% accepted, 22 enrolled. In 2013, 31 master's, 5 doctorates, 4 other advanced degrees awarded. *Degree requirements:* For master's, thesis or alternative; for doctorate, thesis/dissertation, 1 semester of teaching experience. *Entrance requirements:* For master's, 3 letters of recommendation; for doctorate, GRE General Test, 3 letters of recommendation. Additional exam requirements/recommendations for international students: Required—TOEFL (minimum score 79 iBT), IELTS (minimum score 6.5). *Application deadline:* For fall admission, 12/15 priority date for domestic and international students; for spring admission, 12/1 priority date for domestic and international students. Applications are processed on a rolling basis. Application fee: $50 ($40 for international students). Electronic applications accepted. *Expenses:* Tuition, state resident: full-time $7364; part-time $409.10 per credit hour. Tuition, nonresident: full-time $19,162; part-time $1008.50 per credit hour. *Financial support:* In 2013–14, 13 research assistantships with full and partial tuition reimbursements (averaging $17,000 per year), 23 teaching assistantships with full and partial tuition reimbursements (averaging $17,000 per year) were awarded; fellowships with full tuition reimbursements, career-related internships or fieldwork, and Federal Work-Study also available. Support available to part-time students. Financial award application deadline: 2/1. *Faculty research:* Molecular biology, microbial genetics, animal behavior, tropical ecology, plant systematics. *Unit head:* Dr. Teresa Thiel, Director of Graduate Studies, 314-516-6200, Fax: 314-516-6233, E-mail: thiel@umsl.edu. *Application contact:* 314-516-5458, Fax: 314-516-6996, E-mail: gradadm@umsl.edu.
Website: http://www.umsl.edu/divisions/artscience/biology/

The University of Montana, Graduate School, College of Forestry and Conservation, Missoula, MT 59812-0002. Offers fish and wildlife biology (PhD); forest and conservation sciences (PhD); forestry (MS); recreation management (MS); resource conservation (MS); systems ecology (MS, PhD); wildlife biology (MS). *Degree requirements:* For doctorate, thesis/dissertation. *Entrance requirements:* For master's and doctorate, GRE General Test. Additional exam requirements/recommendations for international students: Required—TOEFL (minimum score 575 paper-based). *Application deadline:* For fall admission, 1/31 priority date for domestic students; for spring admission, 8/31 priority date for domestic students. Applications are processed on a rolling basis. Application fee: $45. *Financial support:* Fellowships, research assistantships with tuition reimbursements, teaching assistantships with full tuition reimbursements, career-related internships or fieldwork, and Federal Work-Study

available. Financial award application deadline: 3/1; financial award applicants required to submit FAFSA. *Unit head:* James Burchfield, Dean, 406-243-6650, E-mail: james.burchfield@umontana.edu. *Application contact:* Information Contact, E-mail: gradschl@mso.umt.edu.
Website: http://www.forestry.umt.edu/

The University of Montana, Graduate School, College of Humanities and Sciences, Division of Biological Sciences, Interdisciplinary Program in Systems Ecology, Missoula, MT 59812-0002. Offers MS, PhD. *Financial support:* Traineeships as stipends (avergaing $30,000 per year plus up to $10,500 in tuition and fees) available. *Unit head:* Prof. F. Richard Hauer, Program Director, 406-243-4848, E-mail: ric.hauer@umontana.edu. *Application contact:* Sherrie Wright, Graduate Programs Coordinator, 406-243-4433, E-mail: sherrie.wright@mso.umt.edu.
Website: http://meid.dbs.umt.edu/

The University of Montana, Graduate School, College of Humanities and Sciences, Division of Biological Sciences, Program in Organismal Biology and Ecology, Missoula, MT 59812-0002. Offers MS, PhD. Terminal master's awarded for partial completion of doctoral program. *Degree requirements:* For master's, one foreign language, thesis; for doctorate, 2 foreign languages, thesis/dissertation. *Entrance requirements:* For master's and doctorate, GRE General Test. *Application deadline:* For fall admission, 2/1 for domestic students. Application fee: $45. *Financial support:* Research assistantships with full tuition reimbursements, teaching assistantships with full tuition reimbursements, and Federal Work-Study available. Financial award application deadline: 3/1; financial award applicants required to submit FAFSA. *Faculty research:* Conservation biology, ecology and behavior, evolutionary genetics, avian biology. *Unit head:* Charles Janson, Chair, 406-243-5122, E-mail: charles.janson@mso.umt.edu. *Application contact:* Information Contact, E-mail: gradschl@mso.umt.edu.
Website: http://www.biology.umt.edu/

University of Nevada, Reno, Graduate School, Interdisciplinary Program in Ecology, Evolution, and Conservation Biology, Reno, NV 89557. Offers PhD. Offered through the College of Arts and Science, the M. C. Fleischmann College of Agriculture, and the Desert Research Institute. *Degree requirements:* For doctorate, thesis/dissertation. *Entrance requirements:* For doctorate, GRE General Test, GRE Subject Test, minimum GPA of 3.0. Additional exam requirements/recommendations for international students: Required—TOEFL (minimum score 500 paper-based; 61 iBT), IELTS (minimum score 6). Electronic applications accepted. *Faculty research:* Population biology, behavioral ecology, plant response to climate change, conservation of endangered species, restoration of natural ecosystems.

University of New Haven, Graduate School, College of Arts and Sciences, Program in Environmental Sciences, West Haven, CT 06516-1916. Offers environmental ecology (MS); environmental geoscience (MS); environmental health and management (MS); environmental science (MS); environmental science education (MS); geographical information systems (MS, Certificate). Part-time and evening/weekend programs available. *Students:* 25 full-time (12 women), 20 part-time (11 women); includes 8 minority (3 Black or African American, non-Hispanic/Latino; 2 Asian, non-Hispanic/Latino; 3 Hispanic/Latino), 8 international. 42 applicants, 90% accepted, 14 enrolled. In 2013, 11 master's, 3 other advanced degrees awarded. *Degree requirements:* For master's, thesis optional, research project. *Entrance requirements:* Additional exam requirements/recommendations for international students: Required—TOEFL (minimum score 80 iBT), IELTS, PTE (minimum score 53). *Application deadline:* For fall admission, 5/31 for international students; for winter admission, 10/15 for international students; for spring admission, 1/15 for international students. Applications are processed on a rolling basis. Application fee: $75. Electronic applications accepted. Application fee is waived when completed online. *Expenses: Tuition:* Full-time $21,600; part-time $800 per credit hour. *Required fees:* $45 per trimester. *Financial support:* Research assistantships with partial tuition reimbursements, teaching assistantships with partial tuition reimbursements, career-related internships or fieldwork, Federal Work-Study, scholarships/grants, and unspecified assistantships available. Support available to part-time students. Financial award applicants required to submit FAFSA. *Faculty research:* Mapping and assessing geological and living resources in Long Island Sound, geology, San Salvador Island, Bahamas. *Unit head:* Dr. Roman Zajac, Coordinator, 203-932-7114, E-mail: rzajac@newhaven.edu. *Application contact:* Eloise Gormley, Director of Graduate Admissions, 203-932-7440, E-mail: gradinfo@newhaven.edu.
Website: http://www.newhaven.edu/4728/

The University of North Carolina at Chapel Hill, Graduate School, College of Arts and Sciences, Curriculum in Ecology, Chapel Hill, NC 27599. Offers MA, MS, PhD. *Degree requirements:* For master's, comprehensive exam, thesis (for some programs), oral defense of thesis; for doctorate, comprehensive exam, thesis/dissertation, oral exams, oral defense of dissertation. *Entrance requirements:* For master's and doctorate, GRE General Test. Additional exam requirements/recommendations for international students: Required—TOEFL (minimum score 550 paper-based). Electronic applications accepted. *Faculty research:* Community and population ecology and ecosystems, human ecology, landscape ecology, conservation ecology, marine ecology.

The University of North Carolina at Chapel Hill, Graduate School, College of Arts and Sciences, Department of Biology, Chapel Hill, NC 27599. Offers botany (MA, MS, PhD); cell biology, development, and physiology (MA, MS, PhD); cell motility and cytoskeleton (PhD); ecology and behavior (MA, MS, PhD); genetics and molecular biology (MA, MS, PhD); morphology, systematics, and evolution (MA, MS, PhD). Terminal master's awarded for partial completion of doctoral program. *Degree requirements:* For master's, comprehensive exam, thesis (for some programs); for doctorate, comprehensive exam, thesis/dissertation. *Entrance requirements:* For master's, GRE General Test, GRE Subject Test, 2 semesters of calculus or statistics; 2 semesters of physics, organic chemistry; 3 semesters of biology; for doctorate, GRE General Test, GRE Subject Test, 2 semesters calculus or statistics, 2 semesters physics, organic chemistry, 3 semesters of biology. Additional exam requirements/recommendations for international students: Required—TOEFL (minimum score 550 paper-based). Electronic applications accepted. *Faculty research:* Gene expression, biomechanics, yeast genetics, plant ecology, plant molecular biology.

University of North Dakota, Graduate School, College of Arts and Sciences, Department of Biology, Grand Forks, ND 58202. Offers botany (MS, PhD); ecology (MS, PhD); entomology (MS, PhD); environmental biology (MS, PhD); fisheries/wildlife (MS, PhD); genetics (MS, PhD); zoology (MS, PhD). Terminal master's awarded for partial completion of doctoral program. *Degree requirements:* For master's, thesis, final exam; for doctorate, comprehensive exam, thesis/dissertation, final exam. *Entrance requirements:* For master's, GRE General Test, GRE Subject Test, minimum GPA of 3.0; for doctorate, GRE General Test, GRE Subject Test, minimum GPA of 3.5. Additional exam requirements/recommendations for international students: Required—TOEFL (minimum score 550 paper-based; 79 iBT), IELTS (minimum score 6.5). Electronic applications accepted. *Faculty research:* Population biology, wildlife ecology, RNA processing, hormonal control of behavior.

University of Notre Dame, Graduate School, College of Science, Department of Biological Sciences, Notre Dame, IN 46556. Offers aquatic ecology, evolution and environmental biology (MS, PhD); cellular and molecular biology (MS, PhD); genetics (MS, PhD); physiology (MS, PhD); vector biology and parasitology (MS, PhD). Terminal master's awarded for partial completion of doctoral program. *Degree requirements:* For master's, comprehensive exam, thesis; for doctorate, comprehensive exam, thesis/dissertation, candidacy exam. *Entrance requirements:* For master's and doctorate, GRE General Test. Additional exam requirements/recommendations for international students: Required—TOEFL (minimum score 600 paper-based; 80 iBT). Electronic applications accepted. *Faculty research:* Tropical disease, molecular genetics, neurobiology, evolutionary biology, aquatic biology.

University of Oklahoma, College of Arts and Sciences, Department of Biology, Program in Ecology and Evolutionary Biology, Norman, OK 73019. Offers PhD. *Students:* 10 full-time (6 women), 12 part-time (7 women); includes 1 minority (Hispanic/Latino), 4 international. Average age 29. 6 applicants, 33% accepted, 2 enrolled. In 2013, 2 doctorates awarded. *Entrance requirements:* Additional exam requirements/recommendations for international students: Required—TOEFL (minimum score 79 iBT). *Application deadline:* For fall admission, 12/15 for domestic and international students. Application fee: $50 ($100 for international students). Electronic applications accepted. *Expenses:* Tuition, state resident: full-time $4205; part-time $175.20 per credit hour. Tuition, nonresident: full-time $16,205; part-time $675.20 per credit hour. *Required fees:* $2745; $103.85 per credit hour. $126.50 per semester. *Financial support:* In 2013–14, 22 students received support. Career-related internships or fieldwork, scholarships/grants, health care benefits, tuition waivers (partial), and unspecified assistantships available. Financial award application deadline: 6/1; financial award applicants required to submit FAFSA. *Faculty research:* Behavioral ecology, community ecology, evolutionary biology, macroecology, physiological ecology. *Unit head:* Dr. Michael Kaspari, Director, 405-325-4821, Fax: 405-325-6202, E-mail: mkaspari@ou.edu. *Application contact:* Dr. Rosemary Knapp, Director, 405-325-4389, Fax: 405-325-6202, E-mail: biologygrad@ou.edu.
Website: http://www.ou.edu/eeb

University of Oklahoma, College of Arts and Sciences, Department of Microbiology and Plant Biology, Program in Ecology and Evolutionary Biology, Norman, OK 73019. Offers PhD. *Students:* 5 full-time (1 woman), 4 part-time (0 women), 8 international. Average age 29. 6 applicants, 50% accepted, 2 enrolled. *Entrance requirements:* Additional exam requirements/recommendations for international students: Required—TOEFL (minimum score 79 iBT). *Application deadline:* For fall admission, 4/1 for domestic and international students; for spring admission, 9/1 for domestic and international students. Application fee: $50 ($100 for international students). Electronic applications accepted. *Expenses:* Tuition, state resident: full-time $4205; part-time $175.20 per credit hour. Tuition, nonresident: full-time $16,205; part-time $675.20 per credit hour. *Required fees:* $2745; $103.85 per credit hour. $126.50 per semester. *Financial support:* In 2013–14, 7 students received support. Scholarships/grants, health care benefits, tuition waivers (partial), and unspecified assistantships available. Financial award application deadline: 6/1; financial award applicants required to submit FAFSA. *Faculty research:* Behavioral ecology, community ecology, evolutionary biology, macroecology, physiological ecology. *Unit head:* Dr. Gordon Uno, Professor/Department Chair, 405-325-4321, Fax: 405-325-7619, E-mail: guno@ou.edu. *Application contact:* Adell Hopper, Staff Assistant, 405-325-4321, Fax: 405-325-7619, E-mail: ahopper@ou.edu.
Website: http://mpbio.ou.edu/

University of Oregon, Graduate School, College of Arts and Sciences, Department of Biology, Eugene, OR 97403. Offers ecology and evolution (MA, MS, PhD); marine biology (MA, MS, PhD); molecular, cellular and genetic biology (PhD); neuroscience and development (PhD). Terminal master's awarded for partial completion of doctoral program. *Degree requirements:* For master's, thesis (for some programs); for doctorate, thesis/dissertation. *Entrance requirements:* For master's and doctorate, GRE General Test, minimum GPA of 3.2. Additional exam requirements/recommendations for international students: Required—TOEFL. *Faculty research:* Developmental neurobiology; evolution, population biology, and quantitative genetics; regulation of gene expression; biochemistry of marine organisms.

University of Pittsburgh, Dietrich School of Arts and Sciences, Department of Biological Sciences, Program in Ecology and Evolution, Pittsburgh, PA 15260. Offers PhD. *Faculty:* 6 full-time (2 women). *Students:* 23 full-time (8 women); includes 4 minority (1 Black or African American, non-Hispanic/Latino; 1 American Indian or Alaska Native, non-Hispanic/Latino; 1 Asian, non-Hispanic/Latino; 1 Hispanic/Latino), 1 international. Average age 23. 34 applicants, 21% accepted, 6 enrolled. In 2013, 4 doctorates awarded. *Degree requirements:* For doctorate, comprehensive exam, thesis/dissertation, completion of research integrity module. *Entrance requirements:* For doctorate, GRE General Test, GRE Subject Test. Additional exam requirements/recommendations for international students: Required—TOEFL (minimum score 90 iBT). *Application deadline:* For fall admission, 1/3 priority date for domestic students, 12/9 priority date for international students. Applications are processed on a rolling basis. Application fee: $0 ($50 for international students). Electronic applications accepted. *Expenses:* Tuition, state resident: full-time $19,964; part-time $807 per credit. Tuition, nonresident: full-time $32,686; part-time $1337 per credit. *Required fees:* $740; $200. Tuition and fees vary according to program. *Financial support:* In 2013–14, 28 fellowships with full tuition reimbursements (averaging $30,682 per year), 14 research assistantships with full tuition reimbursements (averaging $26,775 per year), 20 teaching assistantships with full tuition reimbursements (averaging $25,610 per year) were awarded; Federal Work-Study, scholarships/grants, traineeships, health care benefits, and tuition waivers (full) also available. *Unit head:* Dr. Jeffrey G. Lawrence, Professor, 412-624-4204, Fax: 412-624-4759, E-mail: jlawrenc@pitt.edu. *Application contact:* Cathleen M. Barr, Graduate Administrator, 412-624-4268, Fax: 412-624-4759, E-mail: cbarr@pitt.edu.
Website: http://www.biology.pitt.edu/graduate/e-e-program

University of Puerto Rico, Río Piedras Campus, College of Natural Sciences, Department of Biology, San Juan, PR 00931-3300. Offers ecology/systematics (MS, PhD); evolution/genetics (MS, PhD); molecular/cellular biology (MS, PhD); neuroscience (MS, PhD). Part-time programs available. *Degree requirements:* For master's, one foreign language, comprehensive exam, thesis; for doctorate, one foreign language, comprehensive exam, thesis/dissertation. *Entrance requirements:* For master's, GRE Subject Test, interview, minimum GPA of 3.0, letter of recommendation; for doctorate, GRE Subject Test, interview, master's degree, minimum GPA of 3.0, letter of recommendation. *Faculty research:* Environmental, poblational and systematic biology.

University of South Carolina, The Graduate School, College of Arts and Sciences, Department of Biological Sciences, Graduate Training Program in Ecology, Evolution, and Organismal Biology, Columbia, SC 29208. Offers MS, PhD. *Degree requirements:* For master's, one foreign language, comprehensive exam, thesis; for doctorate, one foreign language, comprehensive exam, thesis/dissertation. *Entrance requirements:* For master's and doctorate, GRE General Test, minimum GPA of 3.0 in science. Additional exam requirements/recommendations for international students: Required—TOEFL (minimum score 570 paper-based). Electronic applications accepted.

University of South Florida, College of Arts and Sciences, Department of Integrative Biology, Tampa, FL 33620-9951. Offers biology (MS), including ecology and evolution (MS, PhD), environmental and ecological microbiology (MS, PhD), physiology and

morphology (MS, PhD); integrative biology (PhD), including ecology and evolution (MS, PhD), environmental and ecological microbiology (MS, PhD), physiology and morphology (MS, PhD). Part-time programs available. *Faculty:* 16 full-time (4 women), 1 part-time/adjunct (0 women). *Students:* 40 full-time (24 women), 7 part-time (4 women); includes 6 minority (5 Hispanic/Latino; 1 Two or more races, non-Hispanic/Latino), 3 international. Average age 29. 59 applicants, 29% accepted, 11 enrolled. In 2013, 4 master's, 5 doctorates awarded. *Degree requirements:* For master's, comprehensive exam, thesis (for some programs); for doctorate, comprehensive exam, thesis/dissertation. *Entrance requirements:* For master's and doctorate, GRE General Test (minimum preferred scores of 153 verbal, 148 quantitative, 4.5 analytical/500 verbal and 600 quantitative with 4.5 in analytical writing on old scoring), minimum GPA of 3.0 in last 60 hours of BS. Additional exam requirements/recommendations for international students: Required—TOEFL (minimum score 570 paper-based; 88 iBT). *Application deadline:* For fall admission, 2/15 priority date for domestic students, 1/2 for international students; for spring admission, 8/1 for domestic students, 6/1 for international students. Application fee: $30. Electronic applications accepted. *Financial support:* Research assistantships, teaching assistantships, and unspecified assistantships available. Financial award application deadline: 6/30; financial award applicants required to submit FAFSA. *Faculty research:* Marine ecology, ecosystem responses to urbanization, biomechanical and physiological mechanisms of animal movement, population biology and conservation, microbial ecology and public health microbiology, natural diversity of parasites and herbivores; ecosystems, vertebrates, disturbance ecology, functional and ecological morphology of feeding in fishes, rare amphibians and reptiles, genomics in ecological experiments, ecotoxicology, global carbon cycle, plant-animal interactions. *Total annual research expenditures:* $968,227. *Unit head:* Dr. Peter Stiling, Chair, Department of Integrative Biology, 813-974-6229, Fax: 813-974-3263, E-mail: pstiling@usf.edu. *Application contact:* Christine Brubaker, Graduate Program Specialist, Department of Integrative Biology, 813-974-4747, Fax: 813-974-3263, E-mail: brubaker@usf.edu.
Website: http://biology.usf.edu/ib/grad/

The University of Tennessee, Graduate School, College of Arts and Sciences, Department of Ecology and Evolutionary Biology, Knoxville, TN 37996. Offers behavior (MS, PhD); ecology (MS; PhD); evolutionary biology (MS, PhD). Part-time programs available. *Degree requirements:* For master's, thesis; for doctorate, thesis/dissertation. *Entrance requirements:* For master's and doctorate, GRE General Test, minimum GPA of 2.7. Additional exam requirements/recommendations for international students: Required—TOEFL. Electronic applications accepted. *Expenses:* Tuition, state resident: full-time $9540; part-time $531 per credit hour. Tuition, nonresident: full-time $27,728; part-time $1542 per credit hour. *Required fees:* $1404; $67 per credit hour.

The University of Tennessee, Graduate School, College of Arts and Sciences, Department of Mathematics, Knoxville, TN 37996. Offers applied mathematics (MS); mathematical ecology (PhD); mathematics (M Math, MS, PhD). Part-time programs available. *Degree requirements:* For master's, thesis or alternative; for doctorate, one foreign language, thesis/dissertation. *Entrance requirements:* For master's and doctorate, minimum GPA of 2.7. Additional exam requirements/recommendations for international students: Required—TOEFL. Electronic applications accepted. *Expenses:* Tuition, state resident: full-time $9540; part-time $531 per credit hour. Tuition, nonresident: full-time $27,728; part-time $1542 per credit hour. *Required fees:* $1404; $67 per credit hour.

The University of Texas at Austin, Graduate School, College of Natural Sciences, School of Biological Sciences, Program in Ecology, Evolution and Behavior, Austin, TX 78712-1111. Offers PhD. *Entrance requirements:* For doctorate, GRE General Test. Additional exam requirements/recommendations for international students: Required—TOEFL. Electronic applications accepted.

The University of Toledo, College of Graduate Studies, College of Natural Sciences and Mathematics, Department of Environmental Sciences, Toledo, OH 43606-3390. Offers biology (MS, PhD), including ecology; geology (MS), including earth surface processes. Part-time programs available. *Faculty:* 51. *Students:* 5 full-time (2 women), 1 (woman) part-time, 2 international. Average age 28. 2 applicants, 100% accepted, 2 enrolled. In 2013, 5 master's awarded. *Degree requirements:* For master's, thesis or alternative. *Entrance requirements:* For master's, GRE General Test, minimum cumulative point-hour ratio of 2.7 for all previous academic work, three letters of recommendation, statement of purpose, transcripts from all prior institutions attended. Additional exam requirements/recommendations for international students: Required—TOEFL (minimum score 550 paper-based; 80 iBT). *Application deadline:* For fall admission, 1/15 priority date for domestic and international students. Applications are processed on a rolling basis. Application fee: $45 ($75 for international students). Electronic applications accepted. *Financial support:* In 2013–14, 4 teaching assistantships with full and partial tuition reimbursements (averaging $10,850 per year) were awarded; Federal Work-Study, institutionally sponsored loans, scholarships/grants, tuition waivers (full), and unspecified assistantships also available. Support available to part-time students. *Faculty research:* Environmental geochemistry, geophysics, petrology and mineralogy, paleontology, geohydrology. *Unit head:* Dr. Timothy G. Fisher, Chair, 419-530-2883, E-mail: timothy.fisher@utoledo.edu. *Application contact:* Graduate School Office, 419-530-4723, Fax: 419-530-4724, E-mail: grdsch@utnet.utoledo.edu.
Website: http://www.utoledo.edu/nsm/envsciences/

University of Toronto, School of Graduate Studies, Faculty of Arts and Science, Department of Ecology and Evolutionary Biology, Toronto, ON M5S 1A1, Canada. Offers M Sc, PhD. *Degree requirements:* For master's, thesis, thesis defense; for doctorate, thesis/dissertation, thesis defense. *Entrance requirements:* For master's, minimum B average in last 2 years; knowledge of physics, chemistry, and biology. Additional exam requirements/recommendations for international students: Required—TOEFL (minimum score 580 paper-based; 93 iBT), TWE (minimum score 5). Electronic applications accepted.

University of Washington, Graduate School, College of the Environment, School of Environmental and Forest Sciences, Seattle, WA 98195. Offers bioresource science and engineering (MS, PhD); environmental horticulture (MEH); forest ecology (MS, PhD); forest management (MFR); forest soils (MS, PhD); restoration ecology (MS, PhD); restoration ecology and environmental horticulture (MS, PhD); social sciences (MS, PhD); sustainable resource management (MS, PhD); wildlife science (MS, PhD); MFR/MAIS; MPA/MS. *Accreditation:* SAF. Part-time programs available. *Degree requirements:* For master's, thesis; for doctorate, comprehensive exam (for some programs), thesis/dissertation. *Entrance requirements:* For master's and doctorate, GRE, minimum GPA of 3.0. Additional exam requirements/recommendations for international students: Required—TOEFL, GRE. Electronic applications accepted. *Faculty research:* Ecosystem analysis, silviculture and forest protection, paper science and engineering, environmental horticulture and urban forestry, natural resource policy and economics, restoration ecology and environment horticulture, conservation, human dimensions, wildlife, bioresource science and engineering.

University of Wisconsin–Madison, Graduate School, College of Agricultural and Life Sciences, Agroecology Program, Madison, WI 53706-1380. Offers MS. *Degree requirements:* For master's, thesis (for some programs). *Entrance requirements:* For master's, GRE. Additional exam requirements/recommendations for international students: Required—TOEFL (minimum score 580 paper-based; 92 iBT), IELTS (minimum score 7). Electronic applications accepted. *Expenses:* Tuition, state resident: full-time $10,728; part-time $790 per credit. Tuition, nonresident: full-time $24,054; part-time $1623 per credit. *Required fees:* $1130; $119 per credit. *Faculty research:* Multifunctional landscape, socio-ecological systems, participatory solutions to environmental problems.

University of Wyoming, Program in Ecology, Laramie, WY 82071. Offers MS, PhD. *Entrance requirements:* For master's and doctorate, GRE.

Utah State University, School of Graduate Studies, College of Natural Resources, Department of Environment and Society, Logan, UT 84322. Offers bioregional planning (MS); geography (MA, MS); human dimensions of ecosystem science and management (MS, PhD); recreation resource management (MS, PhD). *Degree requirements:* For master's, comprehensive exam, thesis (for some programs). *Entrance requirements:* For master's and doctorate, GRE General Test, minimum GPA of 3.0. Additional exam requirements/recommendations for international students: Required—TOEFL. Electronic applications accepted. *Faculty research:* Geographic information systems/geographic and environmental education, bioregional planning, natural resource and environmental policy, outdoor recreation and tourism, natural resource and environmental management.

Utah State University, School of Graduate Studies, College of Natural Resources, Department of Watershed Sciences, Logan, UT 84322. Offers ecology (MS, PhD); fisheries biology (MS, PhD); watershed science (MS, PhD). *Degree requirements:* For master's, thesis (for some programs); for doctorate, thesis/dissertation. *Entrance requirements:* For master's and doctorate, GRE General Test, minimum GPA of 3.2. Additional exam requirements/recommendations for international students: Required—TOEFL. Electronic applications accepted. *Faculty research:* Behavior, population ecology, habitat, conservation biology, restoration, aquatic ecology, fisheries management, fluvial geomorphology, remote sensing, conservation biology.

Utah State University, School of Graduate Studies, College of Natural Resources, Department of Wildland Resources, Logan, UT 84322. Offers ecology (MS, PhD); forestry (MS, PhD); range science (MS, PhD); wildlife biology (MS, PhD). Part-time programs available. *Degree requirements:* For master's, thesis; for doctorate, comprehensive exam, thesis/dissertation. *Entrance requirements:* For master's and doctorate, GRE General Test, minimum GPA of 3.0. Additional exam requirements/recommendations for international students: Required—TOEFL. *Faculty research:* Range plant ecophysiology, plant community ecology, ruminant nutrition, population ecology.

Utah State University, School of Graduate Studies, College of Science, Department of Biology, Logan, UT 84322. Offers biology (MS, PhD); ecology (MS, PhD). Part-time programs available. *Degree requirements:* For master's, thesis; for doctorate, thesis/dissertation. *Entrance requirements:* For master's and doctorate, GRE General Test, minimum GPA of 3.0. Additional exam requirements/recommendations for international students: Required—TOEFL (minimum score 575 paper-based). *Faculty research:* Plant, insect, microbial, and animal biology.

Washington University in St. Louis, Graduate School of Arts and Sciences, Division of Biology and Biomedical Sciences, Program in Evolution, Ecology and Population Biology, St. Louis, MO 63130-4899. Offers ecology (PhD); environmental biology (PhD); evolutionary biology (PhD); genetics (PhD). *Degree requirements:* For doctorate, thesis/dissertation. *Entrance requirements:* For doctorate, GRE General Test, GRE Subject Test. Electronic applications accepted.

Wesleyan University, Graduate Studies, Department of Biology, Middletown, CT 06459. Offers cell and developmental genetics (PhD); evolution and ecology (PhD); neurobiology and behavior (PhD). *Degree requirements:* For doctorate, variable foreign language requirement, thesis/dissertation. *Entrance requirements:* For doctorate, GRE. Additional exam requirements/recommendations for international students: Required—TOEFL. *Faculty research:* Microbial population genetics, genetic basis of evolutionary adaptation, genetic regulation of differentiation and pattern formation in &ITdrosophila&RO.

Yale University, Graduate School of Arts and Sciences, Department of Ecology and Evolutionary Biology, New Haven, CT 06520. Offers PhD. *Entrance requirements:* For doctorate, GRE General Test, GRE Subject Test (biology).

Environmental Biology

Baylor University, Graduate School, College of Arts and Sciences, Department of Biology, Waco, TX 76798. Offers biology (MA, MS, PhD); environmental biology (MS); limnology (MS). Part-time programs available. *Faculty:* 13 full-time (3 women). *Students:* 33 full-time (17 women), 4 part-time (all women); includes 9 minority (5 Asian, non-Hispanic/Latino; 4 Two or more races, non-Hispanic/Latino), 11 international. In 2013, 12 master's, 4 doctorates awarded. *Degree requirements:* For master's, thesis (for some programs); for doctorate, thesis/dissertation. *Entrance requirements:* For master's and doctorate, GRE General Test. Additional exam requirements/recommendations for international students: Required—TOEFL. *Application deadline:* For fall admission, 2/15 priority date for domestic and international students. Applications are processed on a rolling basis. Application fee: $25. *Expenses: Tuition:* Full-time $25,866; part-time $1437 per credit hour. *Required fees:* $2736; $152 per credit hour. Tuition and fees vary according to course load and program. *Financial support:* Research assistantships with full and partial tuition reimbursements, teaching assistantships with full and partial tuition reimbursements, career-related internships or fieldwork, Federal Work-Study, institutionally sponsored loans, and tuition waivers (full and partial) available. Support available to part-time students. Financial award application deadline: 2/28. *Faculty research:* Terrestrial ecology, aquatic ecology, genetics. *Unit head:* Dr. Ryan King,

Graduate Program Director, 254-710-2150, Fax: 254-710-2969, E-mail: ryan_s_king@baylor.edu. *Application contact:* Tamara Lehmann, Academic Support Associate, 254-710-2578, Fax: 254-710-2969, E-mail: tamara_lehmann@baylor.edu.
Website: http://www.baylor.edu/biology/

Chatham University, Program in Biology, Pittsburgh, PA 15232-2826. Offers environmental biology (MS); human biology (MS). Part-time programs available. *Faculty:* 1 (woman) part-time/adjunct. *Students:* 45 full-time (33 women), 5 part-time (all women); includes 14 minority (6 Black or African American, non-Hispanic/Latino; 3 Asian, non-Hispanic/Latino; 4 Hispanic/Latino; 1 Two or more races, non-Hispanic/Latino), 6 international. Average age 25. 83 applicants, 66% accepted, 35 enrolled. In 2013, 20 master's awarded. *Degree requirements:* For master's, thesis optional. *Entrance requirements:* For master's, 3 letters of recommendation. Additional exam requirements/recommendations for international students: Required—TOEFL (minimum score 600 paper-based; 100 iBT), IELTS (minimum score 7), TWE. *Application deadline:* For fall admission, 4/1 priority date for domestic and international students; for spring admission, 11/1 priority date for domestic students, 10/1 priority date for international students. Applications are processed on a rolling basis. Application fee: $45. Electronic applications accepted. Application fee is waived when completed online. *Expenses: Tuition:* Full-time $14,886; part-time $827 per credit hour. One-time fee: $396 full-time. *Financial support:* Applicants required to submit FAFSA. *Faculty research:* Molecular evolution of iron homeostasis, characteristics of soil bacterial communities, gene flow through seed movement, role of gonadotropins in spermatogonial proliferation, phosphatid/linositol metabolism in epithelial cells. *Unit head:* Dr. Lisa Lambert, Director, 412-365-1217, E-mail: lambert@chatham.edu. *Application contact:* Ashlee Bartko, Senior Assistant Director of Graduate Admission, 412-365-1115, Fax: 412-365-1609, E-mail: gradadmissions@chatham.edu.
Website: http://www.chatham.edu/departments/sciences/graduate/biology

Dalhousie University, Faculty of Agriculture, Halifax, NS B3H 4R2, Canada. Offers agriculture (M Sc), including air quality, animal behavior, animal molecular genetics, animal nutrition, animal technology, aquaculture, botany, crop management, crop physiology, ecology, environmental microbiology, food science, horticulture, nutrient management, pest management, physiology, plant biotechnology, plant pathology, soil chemistry, soil fertility, waste management and composting, water quality. Part-time programs available. *Degree requirements:* For master's, thesis, ATC Exam Teaching Assistantship. *Entrance requirements:* For master's, honors B Sc, minimum GPA of 3.0. Additional exam requirements/recommendations for international students: Required—TOEFL (minimum score 580 paper-based; 92 iBT), IELTS, Michigan English Language Assessment Battery, CanTEST, CAEL. *Faculty research:* Bio-product development, organic agriculture, nutrient management, air and water quality, agricultural biotechnology.

Dowling College, Programs in Arts and Sciences, Oakdale, NY 11769. Offers environmental microbiology (MS). Part-time and evening/weekend programs available. *Faculty:* 4 full-time (1 woman). *Students:* 1 (woman) full-time, 3 part-time (0 women). Average age 40. 10 applicants, 30% accepted. In 2013, 4 master's awarded. *Degree requirements:* For master's, comprehensive exam, thesis. *Entrance requirements:* For master's, minimum undergraduate GPA of 3.0, 2 letters of recommendation. Additional exam requirements/recommendations for international students: Required—TOEFL (minimum score 550 paper-based). *Application deadline:* For fall admission, 9/1 priority date for domestic students; for winter admission, 1/1 priority date for domestic students; for spring admission, 2/1 priority date for domestic students. Applications are processed on a rolling basis. Application fee: $50. Electronic applications accepted. *Expenses: Tuition:* Full-time $22,731; part-time $1029 per credit. *Required fees:* $956; $956. *Financial support:* Federal Work-Study available. Support available to part-time students. Financial award application deadline: 6/30; financial award applicants required to submit FAFSA. *Unit head:* Patricia Sandilands, Director of Operations, School of Arts and Sciences, 631-244-3237, E-mail: sandilap@dowling.edu. *Application contact:* Mary Boullianne, Director of Admissions, 631-244-3274, Fax: 631-244-1059, E-mail: boulliam@dowling.edu.
Website: http://www.dowling.edu/

Emporia State University, Department of Biological Sciences, Emporia, KS 66801-5415. Offers botany (MS); environmental biology (MS); general biology (MS); microbial and cellular biology (MS); zoology (MS). Part-time programs available. *Faculty:* 13 full-time (3 women). *Students:* 32 full-time (16 women), 7 part-time (1 woman); includes 2 minority (1 Black or African American, non-Hispanic/Latino; 1 Asian, non-Hispanic/Latino), 18 international. 25 applicants, 88% accepted, 3 enrolled. In 2013, 8 master's awarded. *Degree requirements:* For master's, comprehensive exam or thesis. *Entrance requirements:* For master's, GRE, appropriate undergraduate degree, interview, letters of reference. Additional exam requirements/recommendations for international students: Required—TOEFL (minimum score 520 paper-based; 68 iBT). *Application deadline:* For fall admission, 8/15 priority date for domestic students. Applications are processed on a rolling basis. Application fee: $30 ($75 for international students). Electronic applications accepted. *Expenses: Tuition, area resident:* Part-time $220 per credit hour. Tuition, state resident: part-time $220 per credit hour. Tuition, nonresident: part-time $685 per credit hour. *Required fees:* $73 per credit hour. *Financial support:* In 2013–14, 5 research assistantships with full tuition reimbursements (averaging $7,371 per year), 9 teaching assistantships with full tuition reimbursements (averaging $7,950 per year) were awarded; career-related internships or fieldwork, Federal Work-Study, institutionally sponsored loans, health care benefits, and unspecified assistantships also available. Financial award application deadline: 3/15; financial award applicants required to submit FAFSA. *Faculty research:* Fisheries, range, and wildlife management; aquatic, plant, grassland, vertebrate, and invertebrate ecology; mammalian and plant systematics, taxonomy, and evolution; immunology, virology, and molecular biology. *Unit head:* Dr. R. Brent Thomas, Chair, 620-341-5311, Fax: 620-341-5608, E-mail: rthomas2@emporia.edu. *Application contact:* Dr. Scott Crupper, Graduate Coordinator, 620-341-5621, Fax: 620-341-5607, E-mail: scrupper@emporia.edu.
Website: http://www.emporia.edu/info/degrees-courses/grad/biology

Georgia State University, College of Arts and Sciences, Department of Biology, Program in Applied and Environmental Microbiology, Atlanta, GA 30302-3083. Offers applied and environmental microbiology (MS, PhD); bioinformatics (MS). Part-time programs available. *Students:* Average age 30. Terminal master's awarded for partial completion of doctoral program. *Degree requirements:* For master's, comprehensive exam (for some programs), thesis optional; for doctorate, comprehensive exam, thesis/dissertation. *Entrance requirements:* For master's and doctorate, GRE. Additional exam requirements/recommendations for international students: Required—TOEFL (minimum score 550 paper-based; 82 iBT) or IELTS (minimum score 7). *Application deadline:* For fall admission, 7/1 priority date for domestic students, 6/1 priority date for international students; for spring admission, 11/15 priority date for domestic students, 10/15 priority date for international students. Applications are processed on a rolling basis. Application fee: $50. Electronic applications accepted. *Expenses: Tuition, area resident:* Full-time $4176; part-time $348 per credit hour. Tuition, state resident: full-time $14,544; part-time $1212 per credit hour. Tuition, nonresident: full-time $14,544; part-time $1212 per credit hour. Tuition and fees vary according to course load and program. *Financial support:* In 2013–14, fellowships with full tuition reimbursements (averaging $22,000 per year), research assistantships with full tuition reimbursements (averaging $20,000 per year) were awarded. Financial award application deadline: 12/3. *Faculty research:* Bioremediation, biofilms, indoor air quality control, environmental toxicology, product biosynthesis. *Unit head:* Dr. George Pierce, Professor, 404-413-5315, Fax: 404-413-5301, E-mail: gpierce@gsu.edu. *Application contact:* LaTesha Warren, Graduate Coordinator, 404-413-5314, Fax: 404-413-5301, E-mail: lwarren@gsu.edu.
Website: http://biology.gsu.edu/

Governors State University, College of Arts and Sciences, Program in Environmental Biology, University Park, IL 60484. Offers MS. Part-time and evening/weekend programs available. *Degree requirements:* For master's, thesis or alternative. *Faculty research:* Animal physiology, cell biology, animal behavior, plant physiology, plant populations.

Hampton University, Graduate College, Department of Biological Sciences, Hampton, VA 23668. Offers biology (MS); environmental science (MS); medical science (MS). Part-time and evening/weekend programs available. *Degree requirements:* For master's, thesis optional. *Entrance requirements:* For master's, GRE General Test. *Faculty research:* Marine ecology, microbial and chemical pollution, pesticide problems.

Hood College, Graduate School, Program in Environmental Biology, Frederick, MD 21701-8575. Offers MS. Part-time and evening/weekend programs available. *Faculty:* 4 full-time (1 woman), 9 part-time/adjunct (3 women). *Students:* 3 full-time (0 women), 58 part-time (33 women); includes 5 minority (2 Black or African American, non-Hispanic/Latino; 3 Hispanic/Latino), 1 international. Average age 33. 21 applicants, 76% accepted, 6 enrolled. In 2013, 5 master's awarded. *Degree requirements:* For master's, thesis or alternative. *Entrance requirements:* For master's, minimum GPA of 2.75, 1 year of undergraduate biology and chemistry, 1 semester of mathematics. Additional exam requirements/recommendations for international students: Required—TOEFL (minimum score 575 paper-based; 89 iBT), IELTS (minimum score 6.5). *Application deadline:* For fall admission, 7/15 priority date for domestic students, 7/15 for international students; for spring admission, 12/1 priority date for domestic students, 12/1 for international students. Applications are processed on a rolling basis. Application fee: $35. Electronic applications accepted. Application fee is waived when completed online. *Expenses: Tuition:* Part-time $405 per credit. *Required fees:* $100 per semester. *Financial support:* Tuition waivers (partial) and unspecified assistantships available. Financial award applicants required to submit FAFSA. *Faculty research:* Watershed ecology, invasive ecology, native insect pollinators, conservation genetics, geographic information systems (GIS). *Unit head:* Dr. April Boulton, Director, 301-696-3649, Fax: 301-694-3597, E-mail: dferrier@hood.edu. *Application contact:* Dr. Maria Green Cowles, Dean of Graduate School, 301-696-3811, Fax: 301-696-3597, E-mail: gofurther@hood.edu.
Website: http://www.hood.edu/graduate

Massachusetts Institute of Technology, School of Engineering, Department of Civil and Environmental Engineering, Cambridge, MA 02139-4309. Offers biological oceanography (PhD, Sc D); chemical oceanography (PhD, Sc D); civil and environmental engineering (M Eng, SM, PhD, Sc D); civil and environmental systems (PhD, Sc D); civil engineering (PhD, Sc D, CE); coastal engineering (PhD, Sc D); construction engineering and management (PhD, Sc D); environmental biology (PhD, Sc D); environmental chemistry (PhD, Sc D); environmental engineering (PhD, Sc D); environmental fluid mechanics (PhD, Sc D); geotechnical and geoenvironmental engineering (PhD, Sc D); hydrology (PhD, Sc D); information technology (PhD, Sc D); oceanographic engineering (PhD, Sc D); structures and materials (PhD, Sc D); transportation (PhD, Sc D); SM/MBA. *Faculty:* 33 full-time (7 women), 2 part-time/adjunct (0 women). *Students:* 220 full-time (80 women); includes 25 minority (1 Black or African American, non-Hispanic/Latino; 15 Asian, non-Hispanic/Latino; 6 Hispanic/Latino; 3 Two or more races, non-Hispanic/Latino), 120 international. Average age 26. 627 applicants, 21% accepted, 83 enrolled. In 2013, 99 master's, 13 doctorates awarded. *Degree requirements:* For master's and CE, thesis; for doctorate, comprehensive exam, thesis/dissertation. *Entrance requirements:* For master's and doctorate, GRE General Test. Additional exam requirements/recommendations for international students: Required—TOEFL (minimum score 100 iBT), IELTS (minimum score 7). *Application deadline:* For fall admission, 12/15 for domestic and international students. Application fee: $75. Electronic applications accepted. *Expenses: Tuition:* Full-time $43,210; part-time $670 per credit hour. *Required fees:* $288. *Financial support:* In 2013–14, 187 students received support, including 47 fellowships (averaging $33,200 per year), 117 research assistantships (averaging $32,200 per year), 17 teaching assistantships (averaging $33,300 per year); Federal Work-Study, institutionally sponsored loans, scholarships/grants, traineeships, health care benefits, and unspecified assistantships also available. *Faculty research:* Environmental chemistry, environmental fluid mechanics and coastal engineering, environmental microbiology, geotechnical engineering and geomechanics, hydrology and hydroclimatology, infrastructure systems, mechanics of materials and structures, transportation systems. *Total annual research expenditures:* $22.9 million. *Unit head:* Prof. Markus Buehler, Head, 617-324-6488. *Application contact:* Graduate Admissions Coordinator, 617-253-7119, E-mail: cee-admissions@mit.edu.
Website: http://cee.mit.edu/

Miami University, College of Arts and Science, Department of Biology, Oxford, OH 45056. Offers biological sciences (MAT); biology (MS, PhD); botany (MAT, MS, PhD); cell, molecular and structural biology (MS, PhD); ecology, evolution and environmental biology (PhD); zoology (MA, MS, PhD). Part-time programs available. Postbaccalaureate distance learning degree programs offered. *Students:* 89 full-time (49 women), 612 part-time (502 women); includes 63 minority (9 Black or African American, non-Hispanic/Latino; 2 American Indian or Alaska Native, non-Hispanic/Latino; 6 Asian, non-Hispanic/Latino; 27 Hispanic/Latino; 1 Native Hawaiian or other Pacific Islander, non-Hispanic/Latino; 18 Two or more races, non-Hispanic/Latino), 35 international. Average age 34. In 2013, 133 master's, 4 doctorates awarded. *Entrance requirements:* For master's and doctorate, GRE General Test. Additional exam requirements/recommendations for international students: Recommended—TOEFL (minimum score 80 iBT), IELTS (minimum score 6.5), TSE (minimum score 54). *Application deadline:* For fall admission, 1/15 for domestic and international students. Application fee: $50. Electronic applications accepted. *Expenses:* Tuition, state resident: full-time $12,634; part-time $526 per credit hour. Tuition, nonresident: full-time $27,892; part-time $1162 per credit hour. Part-time tuition and fees vary according to course load, campus/location and program. *Financial support:* Fellowships with full tuition reimbursements, research assistantships with full tuition reimbursements, teaching assistantships with full tuition reimbursements, Federal Work-Study, health care benefits, tuition waivers (full), and unspecified assistantships available. Financial award application deadline: 1/15; financial award applicants required to submit FAFSA. *Unit head:* Dr. Douglas Meikle, Chair, 513-529-3103, E-mail: meikled@miamioh.edu.
Website: http://miamioh.edu/cas/about/biology

Missouri University of Science and Technology, Graduate School, Department of Biological Sciences, Rolla, MO 65409. Offers applied and environmental biology (MS). *Entrance requirements:* For master's, GRE (minimum score 600 quantitative, 4 writing). Additional exam requirements/recommendations for international students: Required—TOEFL (minimum score 570 paper-based).

Environmental Biology

Morgan State University, School of Graduate Studies, School of Computer, Mathematical, and Natural Sciences, Department of Biology, Program in Bioenvironmental Science, Baltimore, MD 21251. Offers PhD. *Degree requirements:* For doctorate, comprehensive exam, thesis/dissertation, oral defense of dissertation. *Entrance requirements:* For doctorate, GRE General Test, GRE Subject Test (biology, chemistry, or related science), bachelor's or master's degree in biology, chemistry, physics or related field; minimum GPA of 3.0. Additional exam requirements/recommendations for international students: Required—TOEFL (minimum score 550 paper-based).

Nicholls State University, Graduate Studies, College of Arts and Sciences, Department of Biological Sciences, Thibodaux, LA 70310. Offers marine and environmental biology (MS). Part-time programs available. *Degree requirements:* For master's, comprehensive exam, thesis. *Entrance requirements:* For master's, GRE. Additional exam requirements/recommendations for international students: Required—TOEFL (minimum score 600 paper-based). *Faculty research:* Bioremediation, ecology, public health, biotechnology, physiology.

Ohio University, Graduate College, College of Arts and Sciences, Department of Environmental and Plant Biology, Athens, OH 45701-2979. Offers MS, PhD. Part-time programs available. *Degree requirements:* For master's, thesis, 2 terms of teaching experience; for doctorate, comprehensive exam, thesis/dissertation, 2 terms of teaching experience. *Entrance requirements:* For master's, GRE General Test, minimum GPA of 3.0; for doctorate, GRE General Test, minimum GPA of 3.2. Additional exam requirements/recommendations for international students: Required—TOEFL (minimum score 620 paper-based; 105 iBT) or IELTS (minimum score 7.5). Electronic applications accepted. *Faculty research:* Eastern deciduous forest ecology, evolutionary developmental plant biology, phylogenetic systematics, plant cell wall biotechnology.

Rutgers, The State University of New Jersey, New Brunswick, Graduate School-New Brunswick, Department of Environmental Sciences, Piscataway, NJ 08854-8097. Offers air pollution and resources (MS, PhD); aquatic biology (MS, PhD); aquatic chemistry (MS, PhD); atmospheric science (MS, PhD); chemistry and physics of aerosol and hydrosol systems (MS, PhD); environmental chemistry (MS, PhD); environmental microbiology (MS, PhD); environmental toxicology (PhD); exposure assessment (PhD); fate and effects of pollutants (MS, PhD); pollution prevention and control (MS, PhD); water and wastewater treatment (MS, PhD); water resources (MS, PhD). Terminal master's awarded for partial completion of doctoral program. *Degree requirements:* For master's, comprehensive exam, thesis or alternative, oral final exam; for doctorate, comprehensive exam, thesis/dissertation, thesis defense, qualifying exam. *Entrance requirements:* For master's and doctorate, GRE General Test. Additional exam requirements/recommendations for international students: Required—TOEFL. Electronic applications accepted. *Faculty research:* Biological waste treatment; contaminant fate and transport; air, soil and water quality.

Sonoma State University, School of Science and Technology, Department of Biology, Rohnert Park, CA 94928. Offers biochemistry (MA); ecology (MS); environmental biology (MS); evolutionary biology (MS); functional morphology (MS); molecular and cell biology (MS); organismal biology (MS). Part-time programs available. *Faculty:* 9 full-time (1 woman). *Students:* 4 full-time (2 women), 21 part-time (14 women); includes 5 minority (1 American Indian or Alaska Native, non-Hispanic/Latino; 1 Asian, non-Hispanic/Latino; 2 Hispanic/Latino; 1 Two or more races, non-Hispanic/Latino), 2 international. Average age 29. 23 applicants, 65% accepted, 6 enrolled. In 2013, 6 master's awarded. *Degree requirements:* For master's, thesis or alternative, oral exam. *Entrance requirements:* For master's, GRE General Test, GRE Subject Test, minimum GPA of 3.0. Additional exam requirements/recommendations for international students: Required—TOEFL (minimum score 500 paper-based). *Application deadline:* For fall admission, 11/30 for domestic students. Applications are processed on a rolling basis. Application fee: $55. *Expenses:* Tuition, state resident: full-time $8500. Tuition, nonresident: full-time $12,964. *Required fees:* $1762. *Financial support:* In 2013–14, 1 fellowship (averaging $1,520 per year), 6 research assistantships (averaging $3,562 per year), 22 teaching assistantships (averaging $6,738 per year) were awarded; career-related internships or fieldwork, Federal Work-Study, and tuition waivers (full) also available. Financial award application deadline: 3/2; financial award applicants required to submit FAFSA. *Faculty research:* Plant physiology, comparative physiology, community ecology, restoration ecology, marine ecology, conservation genetics, primate behavior, behavioral ecology, developmental biology, plant and animal systematics. *Total annual research expenditures:* $4,400. *Unit head:* Dr. Nathan Rank, Chair, 707-664-3053, E-mail: nathan.rank@sonoma.edu. *Application contact:* Dr. Derek Girman, Graduate Adviser, 707-664-3055, E-mail: derek.girman@sonoma.edu.
Website: http://www.sonoma.edu/biology/graduate

State University of New York College of Environmental Science and Forestry, Department of Environmental and Forest Biology, Syracuse, NY 13210-2779. Offers applied ecology (MPS); chemical ecology (MPS, MS, PhD); conservation biology (MPS, MS, PhD); ecology (MPS, MS, PhD); entomology (MPS, MS, PhD); environmental interpretation (MPS, MS, PhD); environmental physiology (MPS, MS, PhD); fish and wildlife biology and management (MPS, MS, PhD); forest pathology and mycology (MPS, MS, PhD); plant biotechnology (MPS); plant science and biotechnology (MPS, MS, PhD). *Faculty:* 32 full-time (10 women). *Students:* 105 full-time (54 women), 31 part-time (16 women); includes 9 minority (2 Black or African American, non-Hispanic/Latino; 3 American Indian or Alaska Native, non-Hispanic/Latino; 2 Hispanic/Latino; 1 Native Hawaiian or other Pacific Islander, non-Hispanic/Latino; 1 Two or more races, non-Hispanic/Latino), 17 international. Average age 28. In 2013, 15 master's, 7 doctorates awarded. *Degree requirements:* For master's, thesis (for some programs), capstone seminar; for doctorate, comprehensive exam, thesis/dissertation, capstone seminar. *Entrance requirements:* For master's and doctorate, GRE General Test, minimum GPA of 3.0. Additional exam requirements/recommendations for international students: Required—TOEFL (minimum score 550 paper-based; 80 iBT), IELTS (minimum score 6). *Application deadline:* For fall admission, 2/1 priority date for domestic and international students; for spring admission, 11/1 priority date for domestic and international students. Applications are processed on a rolling basis. Application fee: $60. *Expenses:* Tuition, state resident: full-time $10,370; part-time $432 per credit hour. Tuition, nonresident: full-time $20,190; part-time $841 per credit hour. *Required fees:* $44 per credit hour. *Financial support:* In 2013–14, 4 fellowships with full and partial tuition reimbursements, 36 research assistantships with full and partial tuition reimbursements, 39 teaching assistantships with full and partial tuition reimbursements (averaging $11,490 per year) were awarded; Federal Work-Study, institutionally sponsored loans, scholarships/grants, health care benefits, and unspecified assistantships also available. Financial award application deadline: 6/30. *Faculty research:* Ecology, conservation biology, fish and wildlife biology and management, plant science, entomology. *Total annual research expenditures:* $4.1 million. *Unit head:* Dr. Donald J. Leopold, Chair, 315-470-6760, Fax: 315-470-6934, E-mail: djleopold@esf.edu. *Application contact:* Dr. Danilo D. Fernando, Director, Graduate Program/Associate Professor, 315-470-6746, Fax: 315-470-6934, E-mail: dfernando@esf.edu.
Website: http://www.esf.edu/efb/grad/default.asp

Universidad del Turabo, Graduate Programs, Programs in Science and Technology, Gurabo, PR 00778-3030. Offers environmental analysis (MSE), including environmental chemistry; environmental management (MSE), including pollution management; environmental science (D Sc), including environmental biology. *Entrance requirements:* For master's, GRE, EXADEP, interview.

University of Alberta, Faculty of Graduate Studies and Research, Department of Biological Sciences, Edmonton, AB T6G 2E1, Canada. Offers environmental biology and ecology (M Sc, PhD); microbiology and biotechnology (M Sc, PhD); molecular biology and genetics (M Sc, PhD); physiology and cell biology (M Sc, PhD); plant biology (M Sc, PhD); systematics and evolution (M Sc, PhD). Terminal master's awarded for partial completion of doctoral program. *Degree requirements:* For master's, thesis; for doctorate, thesis/dissertation. *Entrance requirements:* Additional exam requirements/recommendations for international students: Required—TOEFL.

University of California, Santa Cruz, Division of Graduate Studies, Division of Physical and Biological Sciences, Environmental Toxicology Department, Santa Cruz, CA 95064. Offers MS, PhD. Terminal master's awarded for partial completion of doctoral program. *Degree requirements:* For master's, comprehensive exam, thesis; for doctorate, thesis/dissertation, qualifying exams. *Entrance requirements:* For master's and doctorate, GRE. Additional exam requirements/recommendations for international students: Required—TOEFL (minimum score 550 paper-based; 83 iBT); Recommended—IELTS (minimum score 8). Electronic applications accepted. *Faculty research:* Molecular mechanisms of reactive DNA methylation toxicity, anthropogenic perturbations of biogeochemical cycles, anaerobic microbiology and biotransformation of pollutants and toxic metals, organismal responses and therapeutic treatment of toxins, microbiology, molecular genetics, genomics.

University of Guelph, Graduate Studies, Ontario Agricultural College, Department of Environmental Biology, Guelph, ON N1G 2W1, Canada. Offers entomology (M Sc, PhD); environmental microbiology and biotechnology (M Sc, PhD); environmental toxicology (M Sc, PhD); plant and forest systems (M Sc, PhD); plant pathology (M Sc, PhD). Part-time programs available. *Degree requirements:* For master's, thesis; for doctorate, comprehensive exam, thesis/dissertation. *Entrance requirements:* For master's, minimum 75% average during previous 2 years of course work; for doctorate, minimum 75% average. Additional exam requirements/recommendations for international students: Required—TOEFL or IELTS. Electronic applications accepted. *Faculty research:* Entomology, environmental microbiology and biotechnology, environmental toxicology, forest ecology, plant pathology.

University of Louisiana at Lafayette, College of Sciences, Department of Biology, Lafayette, LA 70504. Offers biology (MS); environmental and evolutionary biology (PhD). Terminal master's awarded for partial completion of doctoral program. *Degree requirements:* For master's, thesis; for doctorate, 2 foreign languages, comprehensive exam, thesis/dissertation. *Entrance requirements:* For master's, GRE General Test, minimum GPA of 2.75; for doctorate, GRE General Test, GRE Subject Test, minimum GPA of 3.0. Additional exam requirements/recommendations for international students: Required—TOEFL (minimum score 550 paper-based). Electronic applications accepted. *Faculty research:* Structure and ultrastructure, system biology, ecology, processes, environmental physiology.

University of Louisville, Graduate School, College of Arts and Sciences, Department of Biology, Louisville, KY 40292-0001. Offers biology (MS); environmental biology (PhD). *Students:* 48 full-time (24 women), 5 part-time (2 women); includes 4 minority (2 Black or African American, non-Hispanic/Latino; 1 Asian, non-Hispanic/Latino; 1 Two or more races, non-Hispanic/Latino), 9 international. Average age 30. 43 applicants, 60% accepted, 15 enrolled. In 2013, 2 master's awarded. *Degree requirements:* For master's, thesis (for some programs); for doctorate, thesis/dissertation. *Entrance requirements:* For master's and doctorate, GRE General Test. Additional exam requirements/recommendations for international students: Required—TOEFL (minimum score 550 paper-based; 79 iBT). *Application deadline:* For fall admission, 5/1 priority date for international students; for spring admission, 11/1 priority date for international students; for summer admission, 4/1 priority date for international students. Applications are processed on a rolling basis. Application fee: $60. Electronic applications accepted. *Expenses:* Tuition, state resident: full-time $10,788; part-time $599 per credit hour. Tuition, nonresident: full-time $22,446; part-time $1247 per credit hour. *Required fees:* $196. Tuition and fees vary according to program and reciprocity agreements. *Financial support:* Fellowships, research assistantships, and teaching assistantships available. *Unit head:* Dr. Ronald Fell, Chair, 502-852-6771, Fax: 502-852-0725, E-mail: rdfell@louisville.edu. *Application contact:* Libby Leggett, Director, Graduate Admissions, 502-852-3101, Fax: 502-852-6536, E-mail: gradadm@louisville.edu.

The University of Manchester, Faculty of Life Sciences, Manchester, United Kingdom. Offers adaptive organismal biology (M Phil, PhD); animal biology (M Phil, PhD); biochemistry (M Phil, PhD); bioinformatics (M Phil, PhD); biomolecular sciences (M Phil, PhD); biotechnology (M Phil, PhD); cell biology (M Phil, PhD); cell matrix research (M Phil, PhD); channels and transporters (M Phil, PhD); developmental biology (M Phil, PhD); Egyptology (M Phil, PhD); environmental biology (M Phil, PhD); evolutionary biology (M Phil, PhD); gene expression (M Phil, PhD); genetics (M Phil, PhD); history of science, technology and medicine (M Phil, PhD); immunology (M Phil, PhD); integrative neurobiology and behavior (M Phil, PhD); membrane trafficking (M Phil, PhD); microbiology (M Phil, PhD); molecular and cellular neuroscience (M Phil, PhD); molecular biology (M Phil, PhD); molecular cancer studies (M Phil, PhD); neuroscience (M Phil, PhD); ophthalmology (M Phil, PhD); optometry (M Phil, PhD); organelle function (M Phil, PhD); pharmacology (M Phil, PhD); physiology (M Phil, PhD); plant sciences (M Phil, PhD); stem cell research (M Phil, PhD); structural biology (M Phil, PhD); systems neuroscience (M Phil, PhD); toxicology (M Phil, PhD).

University of Massachusetts Amherst, Graduate School, College of Natural Sciences, Department of Environmental Conservation, Amherst, MA 01003. Offers building systems (MS, PhD); environmental policy and human dimensions (MS, PhD); forest resources (MS, PhD); sustainability science (MS); water, wetlands and watersheds (MS, PhD); wildlife and fisheries conservation (MS, PhD). Part-time programs available. *Faculty:* 62 full-time (12 women). *Students:* 64 full-time (27 women), 40 part-time (15 women); includes 5 minority (1 Black or African American, non-Hispanic/Latino; 2 Hispanic/Latino; 2 Two or more races, non-Hispanic/Latino), 18 international. Average age 32. 105 applicants, 46% accepted, 27 enrolled. In 2013, 22 master's, 3 doctorates awarded. Terminal master's awarded for partial completion of doctoral program. *Degree requirements:* For master's, thesis or alternative; for doctorate, comprehensive exam, thesis/dissertation. *Entrance requirements:* For master's and doctorate, GRE General Test. Additional exam requirements/recommendations for international students: Required—TOEFL (minimum score 550 paper-based; 80 iBT), IELTS (minimum score 6.5). *Application deadline:* For fall admission, 2/1 for domestic and international students; for spring admission, 10/1 for domestic and international students. Applications are processed on a rolling basis. Application fee: $75. Electronic applications accepted. *Financial support:* Fellowships with full and partial tuition reimbursements, research assistantships with full and partial tuition reimbursements, teaching assistantships with full and partial tuition reimbursements, career-related internships or fieldwork, Federal Work-Study, scholarships/grants, traineeships, health care benefits, tuition waivers (full and partial), and unspecified assistantships available. Support available to part-time students. Financial award application deadline: 2/1. *Unit head:* Dr. Kevin McGarigal, Graduate Program Director, 413-545-2257, Fax: 413-545-

4358. *Application contact:* Lindsay DeSantis, Supervisor of Admissions, 413-545-0721, Fax: 413-577-0100, E-mail: gradadm@grad.umass.edu.
Website: http://eco.umass.edu/

University of Massachusetts Boston, Office of Graduate Studies, College of Science and Mathematics, Department of Environmental, Earth and Ocean Sciences, Program in Environmental Biology, Boston, MA 02125-3393. Offers PhD. Part-time and evening/weekend programs available. *Degree requirements:* For doctorate, comprehensive exam, thesis/dissertation, oral exams. *Entrance requirements:* For doctorate, GRE General Test, minimum GPA of 2.75. *Faculty research:* Polychoets biology, predator and prey relationships, population and evolutionary biology, neurobiology, biodiversity.

University of North Dakota, Graduate School, College of Arts and Sciences, Department of Biology, Grand Forks, ND 58202. Offers botany (MS, PhD); ecology (MS, PhD); entomology (MS, PhD); environmental biology (MS, PhD); fisheries/wildlife (MS, PhD); genetics (MS, PhD); zoology (MS, PhD). Terminal master's awarded for partial completion of doctoral program. *Degree requirements:* For master's, thesis, final exam; for doctorate, comprehensive exam, thesis/dissertation, final exam. *Entrance requirements:* For master's, GRE General Test, GRE Subject Test, minimum GPA of 3.0; for doctorate, GRE General Test, GRE Subject Test, minimum GPA of 3.5. Additional exam requirements/recommendations for international students: Required—TOEFL (minimum score 550 paper-based; 79 iBT), IELTS (minimum score 6.5). Electronic applications accepted. *Faculty research:* Population biology, wildlife ecology, RNA processing, hormonal control of behavior.

University of Southern California, Graduate School, Dana and David Dornsife College of Letters, Arts and Sciences, Department of Biological Sciences, Program in Marine Biology and Biological Oceanography, Los Angeles, CA 90089. Offers marine and environmental biology (MS); marine biology and biological oceanography (PhD). Terminal master's awarded for partial completion of doctoral program. *Degree requirements:* For master's, research paper; for doctorate, comprehensive exam, thesis/dissertation, qualifying examination, dissertation defense. *Entrance requirements:* For master's and doctorate, GRE, 3 letters of recommendation, personal statement, resume, minimum GPA of 3.0. Additional exam requirements/recommendations for international students: Required—TOEFL (minimum score 600 paper-based; 100 iBT). Electronic applications accepted. *Faculty research:* Microbial ecology, biogeochemistry, and geobiology; biodiversity and molecular ecology; integrative organismal biology; conservation biology; marine genomics.

University of Southern Mississippi, Graduate School, College of Science and Technology, Department of Biological Sciences, Hattiesburg, MS 39406-0001. Offers environmental biology (MS, PhD); marine biology (MS, PhD); microbiology (MS, PhD); molecular biology (MS, PhD). *Faculty:* 27 full-time (6 women). *Students:* 63 full-time (26 women), 4 part-time (all women); includes 4 minority (1 Black or African American, non-Hispanic/Latino; 1 Hispanic/Latino; 2 Two or more races, non-Hispanic/Latino), 17 international. Average age 32. 43 applicants, 30% accepted, 12 enrolled. In 2013, 12 master's, 9 doctorates awarded. Terminal master's awarded for partial completion of doctoral program. *Degree requirements:* For master's, comprehensive exam, thesis; for doctorate, comprehensive exam, thesis/dissertation. *Entrance requirements:* For master's, GRE General Test, minimum GPA of 3.0 on last 60 hours; for doctorate, GRE General Test, minimum GPA of 3.5. Additional exam requirements/recommendations for international students: Required—TOEFL, IELTS. *Application deadline:* For fall admission, 3/1 priority date for domestic students, 3/1 for international students; for spring admission, 1/10 priority date for domestic and international students. Applications are processed on a rolling basis. Application fee: $50. *Financial support:* In 2013–14, 25 research assistantships with full tuition reimbursements (averaging $9,700 per year), 33 teaching assistantships with full tuition reimbursements (averaging $10,600 per year) were awarded; Federal Work-Study, scholarships/grants, health care benefits, and unspecified assistantships also available. Financial award application deadline: 3/15; financial award applicants required to submit FAFSA. *Unit head:* Dr. Glenmore Shearer, Chair, 601-266-4748, Fax: 601-266-5797. *Application contact:* Dr. Jake Schaefer, Director of Graduate Studies, 601-266-4748, Fax: 601-266-5797.
Website: http://www.usm.edu/graduateschool/table.php

University of South Florida, College of Arts and Sciences, Department of Integrative Biology, Tampa, FL 33620-9951. Offers biology (MS), including ecology and evolution (MS, PhD), environmental and ecological microbiology (MS, PhD), physiology and morphology (MS, PhD); integrative biology (PhD), including ecology and evolution (MS, PhD), environmental and ecological microbiology (MS, PhD), physiology and morphology (MS, PhD). Part-time programs available. *Faculty:* 16 full-time (4 women), 1 part-time/adjunct (0 women). *Students:* 40 full-time (24 women), 7 part-time (4 women); includes 6 minority (5 Hispanic/Latino; 1 Two or more races, non-Hispanic/Latino), 3 international. Average age 29. 59 applicants, 29% accepted, 11 enrolled. In 2013, 4 master's, 5 doctorates awarded. *Degree requirements:* For master's, comprehensive exam, thesis (for some programs); for doctorate, comprehensive exam, thesis/dissertation. *Entrance requirements:* For master's and doctorate, GRE General Test (minimum preferred scores of 153 verbal, 148 quantitative, 4.5 analytical/500 verbal and 600 quantitative with 4.5 in analytical writing on old scoring), minimum GPA of 3.0 in last 60 hours of BS. Additional exam requirements/recommendations for international students: Required—TOEFL (minimum score 570 paper-based; 88 iBT). *Application deadline:* For fall admission, 2/15 priority date for domestic students, 1/2 for international students; for spring admission, 8/1 for domestic students, 6/1 for international students. Application fee: $30. Electronic applications accepted. *Financial support:* Research assistantships, teaching assistantships, and unspecified assistantships available. Financial award application deadline: 6/30; financial award applicants required to submit FAFSA. *Faculty research:* Marine ecology, ecosystem responses to urbanization, biomechanical and physiological mechanisms of animal movement, population biology and conservation, microbial ecology and public health microbiology, natural diversity of parasites and herbivores; ecosystems, vertebrates, disturbance ecology, functional and ecological morphology of feeding in fishes, rare amphibians and reptiles, genomics in ecological experiments, ecotoxicology, global carbon cycle, plant-animal interactions. *Total annual research expenditures:* $968,227. *Unit head:* Dr. Peter Stiling, Chair, Department of Integrative Biology, 813-974-6229, Fax: 813-974-3263, E-mail: pstiling@usf.edu. *Application contact:* Christine Brubaker, Graduate Program Specialist, Department of Integrative Biology, 813-974-4747, Fax: 813-974-3263, E-mail: brubaker@usf.edu.
Website: http://biology.usf.edu/ib/grad/

University of West Florida, College of Arts and Sciences: Sciences, School of Allied Health and Life Sciences, Department of Biology, Pensacola, FL 32514-5750. Offers biological chemistry (MS); biology (MS); biology education (MST); biotechnology (MS); coastal zone studies (MS); environmental biology (MS). *Degree requirements:* For master's, thesis. *Entrance requirements:* For master's, GRE (minimum score: verbal 450, quantitative 550), official transcripts; BS in biology or related field; letter of interest; relevant past experience; three letters of recommendation from individuals who can evaluate applicant's academic ability. Additional exam requirements/recommendations for international students: Required—TOEFL (minimum score 550 paper-based).

University of Wisconsin–Madison, School of Medicine and Public Health, Molecular and Environmental Toxicology Center, Madison, WI 53706. Offers MS, PhD. *Faculty:* 84 full-time (26 women), 1 part-time/adjunct (0 women). *Students:* 32 full-time (17 women); includes 12 minority (2 Black or African American, non-Hispanic/Latino; 3 Asian, non-Hispanic/Latino; 6 Hispanic/Latino; 1 Native Hawaiian or other Pacific Islander, non-Hispanic/Latino), 6 international. Average age 28. 38 applicants, 29% accepted, 6 enrolled. In 2013, 2 master's, 6 doctorates awarded. Terminal master's awarded for partial completion of doctoral program. *Degree requirements:* For doctorate, thesis/dissertation. *Entrance requirements:* For master's and doctorate, bachelor's degree in science-related field. Additional exam requirements/recommendations for international students: Required—TOEFL. *Application deadline:* For fall admission, 12/15 priority date for domestic and international students. Application fee: $56. Electronic applications accepted. *Expenses:* Tuition, state resident: full-time $10,728; part-time $790 per credit. Tuition, nonresident: full-time $24,054; part-time $1623 per credit. *Required fees:* $1130; $119 per credit. *Financial support:* In 2013–14, 5 research assistantships with tuition reimbursements (averaging $25,000 per year) were awarded; fellowships with tuition reimbursements, traineeships, health care benefits, and unspecified assistantships also available. *Faculty research:* Toxicology cancer, genetics, cell cycle, xenobiotic metabolism. *Unit head:* Dr. Christopher Bradfield, Director, 608-262-2024, E-mail: bradfield@oncology.wisc.edu. *Application contact:* Eileen M. Stevens, Program Administrator, 608-263-4580, Fax: 608-262-5245, E-mail: emstevens@wisc.edu.
Website: http://www.med.wisc.edu/metc/

Washington University in St. Louis, Graduate School of Arts and Sciences, Division of Biology and Biomedical Sciences, Program in Evolution, Ecology and Population Biology, St. Louis, MO 63130-4899. Offers ecology (PhD); environmental biology (PhD); evolutionary biology (PhD); genetics (PhD). *Degree requirements:* For doctorate, thesis/dissertation. *Entrance requirements:* For doctorate, GRE General Test, GRE Subject Test. Electronic applications accepted.

West Virginia University, Davis College of Agriculture, Forestry and Consumer Sciences, Division of Plant and Soil Sciences, Morgantown, WV 26506. Offers agricultural sciences (PhD), including animal and food sciences, plant and soil sciences; agronomy (MS); entomology (MS); environmental microbiology (MS); horticulture (MS); plant pathology (MS). *Degree requirements:* For master's, thesis. *Entrance requirements:* For master's, GRE, minimum GPA of 2.5. Additional exam requirements/recommendations for international students: Required—TOEFL. *Faculty research:* Water quality, reclamation of disturbed land, crop production, pest control, environmental protection.

West Virginia University, Eberly College of Arts and Sciences, Department of Biology, Morgantown, WV 26506. Offers cell and molecular biology (MS, PhD); environmental and evolutionary biology (MS, PhD); forensic biology (MS, PhD); genomic biology (MS, PhD); neurobiology (MS, PhD). Terminal master's awarded for partial completion of doctoral program. *Degree requirements:* For master's, thesis, final exam; for doctorate, thesis/dissertation, preliminary and final exams. *Entrance requirements:* For master's, GRE General Test, GRE Subject Test, minimum GPA of 3.0; for doctorate, GRE General Test, minimum GPA of 3.0. Additional exam requirements/recommendations for international students: Required—TOEFL. *Faculty research:* Environmental biology, genetic engineering, developmental biology, global change, biodiversity.

Youngstown State University, Graduate School, College of Science, Technology, Engineering and Mathematics, Department of Biological Sciences, Youngstown, OH 44555-0001. Offers environmental biology (MS); molecular biology, microbiology, and genetic (MS); physiology and anatomy (MS). Part-time programs available. *Degree requirements:* For master's, comprehensive exam, thesis, oral review. *Entrance requirements:* For master's, GRE General Test, minimum GPA of 2.7. Additional exam requirements/recommendations for international students: Required—TOEFL. *Faculty research:* Cell biology, neurophysiology, molecular biology, neurobiology, gene regulation.

Evolutionary Biology

Arizona State University at the Tempe campus, College of Liberal Arts and Sciences, School of Life Sciences, Tempe, AZ 85287-4601. Offers animal behavior (PhD); applied ethics (biomedical and health ethics) (MA); biological design (PhD); biology (MS, PhD); biology (biology and society) (MS, PhD); environmental life sciences (PhD); evolutionary biology (PhD); human and social dimensions of science and technology (PhD); microbiology (PhD); molecular and cellular biology (PhD); neuroscience (PhD); philosophy (history and philosophy of science) (MA); sustainability (PhD). Terminal master's awarded for partial completion of doctoral program. *Degree requirements:* For master's, thesis (for some programs), interactive Program of Study (iPOS) submitted before completing 50 percent of required credit hours; for doctorate, variable foreign language requirement, comprehensive exam, thesis/dissertation, interactive Program of Study (iPOS) submitted before completing 50 percent of required credit hours. *Entrance requirements:* For master's and doctorate, GRE, minimum GPA of 3.0 or equivalent in last 2 years of work leading to bachelor's degree. Additional exam requirements/recommendations for international students: Required—TOEFL (minimum score 600 paper-based; 100 iBT). Electronic applications accepted.

Brown University, Graduate School, Division of Biology and Medicine, Department of Ecology and Evolutionary Biology, Providence, RI 02912. Offers PhD. *Degree requirements:* For doctorate, thesis/dissertation, preliminary exam. *Entrance requirements:* For doctorate, GRE General Test, GRE Subject Test. Additional exam requirements/recommendations for international students: Required—TOEFL. Electronic applications accepted. *Faculty research:* Marine ecology, behavioral ecology, population genetics, evolutionary morphology, plant ecology.

Clemson University, Graduate School, College of Agriculture, Forestry and Life Sciences, Department of Biological Sciences, Program in Biological Sciences, Clemson, SC 29634. Offers MS, PhD. *Students:* 31 full-time (19 women), 147 part-time (101 women); includes 15 minority (4 Black or African American, non-Hispanic/Latino; 1

Evolutionary Biology

Asian, non-Hispanic/Latino; 5 Hispanic/Latino; 5 Two or more races, non-Hispanic/Latino), 9 international. Average age 33. 137 applicants, 70% accepted, 84 enrolled. In 2013, 6 master's, 3 doctorates awarded. *Degree requirements:* For master's, thesis optional; for doctorate, comprehensive exam, thesis/dissertation. *Entrance requirements:* For master's and doctorate, GRE General Test. Additional exam requirements/recommendations for international students: Required—TOEFL, IELTS. *Application deadline:* For fall admission, 1/15 for domestic students, 4/15 for international students. Applications are processed on a rolling basis. Application fee: $70 ($80 for international students). Electronic applications accepted. *Financial support:* In 2013–14, 27 students received support, including 3 fellowships with full and partial tuition reimbursements available (averaging $16,167 per year), 3 research assistantships with partial tuition reimbursements available (averaging $18,167 per year), 23 teaching assistantships with partial tuition reimbursements available (averaging $18,452 per year); career-related internships or fieldwork, institutionally sponsored loans, scholarships/grants, health care benefits, and unspecified assistantships also available. Support available to part-time students. Financial award application deadline: 3/15; financial award applicants required to submit FAFSA. *Unit head:* Dr. Alfred Wheeler, Department Chair, 864-656-1415, Fax: 864-656-0435, E-mail: wheeler@clemson.edu. *Application contact:* Jay Lyn Martin, Coordinator for Graduate Program, 864-656-3587, Fax: 864-656-0435, E-mail: gradbio@clemson.edu.
Website: http://www.clemson.edu/cafls/departments/biosci/

Columbia University, Graduate School of Arts and Sciences, Department of Ecology, Evolution and Environmental Biology, New York, NY 10027. Offers conservation biology (MA); ecology and evolutionary biology (PhD); evolutionary primatology (PhD). *Faculty:* 7 full-time (1 woman), 43 part-time/adjunct (15 women). *Students:* 46 full-time (36 women), 1 part-time (0 women). Average age 28. 45 applicants, 18% accepted. *Degree requirements:* For doctorate, one foreign language, thesis/dissertation, teaching experience. *Entrance requirements:* For doctorate, GRE General Test, previous course work in biology. Additional exam requirements/recommendations for international students: Required—TOEFL. Application fee: $90. Electronic applications accepted. *Financial support:* Fellowships, career-related internships or fieldwork, and institutionally sponsored loans available. Financial award application deadline: 1/5. *Faculty research:* Tropical ecology, ethnobotany, global change, systematics. *Total annual research expenditures:* $300,000. *Unit head:* Prof. Ruth DeFries, Chair, 212-851-1647, E-mail: rd2402@columbia.edu. *Application contact:* 212-854-9987.
Website: http://www.columbia.edu/cu/e3b/

Cornell University, Graduate School, Graduate Fields of Agriculture and Life Sciences, Field of Ecology and Evolutionary Biology, Ithaca, NY 14853-0001. Offers ecology (PhD), including animal ecology, applied ecology, biogeochemistry, community and ecosystem ecology, limnology, oceanography, physiological ecology, plant ecology, population ecology, theoretical ecology, vertebrate zoology; evolutionary biology (PhD), including ecological genetics, paleobiology, population biology, systematics. *Faculty:* 52 full-time (14 women). *Students:* 56 full-time (36 women); includes 8 minority (3 Asian, non-Hispanic/Latino; 3 Hispanic/Latino; 2 Two or more races, non-Hispanic/Latino), 12 international. Average age 28. 115 applicants, 13% accepted, 11 enrolled. In 2013, 10 doctorates awarded. *Degree requirements:* For doctorate, comprehensive exam, thesis/dissertation, 2 semesters of teaching experience. *Entrance requirements:* For doctorate, GRE General Test, GRE Subject Test (biology), 2 letters of recommendation. Additional exam requirements/recommendations for international students: Required—TOEFL (minimum score 550 paper-based; 77 iBT). *Application deadline:* For fall admission, 12/15 for domestic students. Application fee: $95. Electronic applications accepted. *Financial support:* In 2013–14, 43 students received support, including 14 fellowships with full tuition reimbursements available, 7 research assistantships with full tuition reimbursements available, 22 teaching assistantships with full tuition reimbursements available; institutionally sponsored loans, scholarships/grants, health care benefits, tuition waivers (full and partial), and unspecified assistantships also available. Financial award applicants required to submit FAFSA. *Faculty research:* Population and organismal biology, population and evolutionary genetics, systematics and macroevolution, biochemistry, conservation biology. *Unit head:* Director of Graduate Studies, 607-254-4230. *Application contact:* Graduate Field Assistant, 607-254-4230, E-mail: eeb_grad_req@cornell.edu.
Website: http://www.gradschool.cornell.edu/fields.php?id-46&a-2

Dartmouth College, Arts and Sciences Graduate Programs, Program in Ecology and Evolutionary Biology, Hanover, NH 03755. Offers PhD. *Entrance requirements:* For doctorate, GRE General Test, GRE Subject Test in biology (highly recommended). Additional exam requirements/recommendations for international students: Required—TOEFL.

Emory University, Laney Graduate School, Division of Biological and Biomedical Sciences, Program in Population Biology, Ecology and Evolution, Atlanta, GA 30322-1100. Offers PhD. *Degree requirements:* For doctorate, comprehensive exam, thesis/dissertation. *Entrance requirements:* For doctorate, GRE General Test, minimum GPA of 3.0 in science course work (recommended). Additional exam requirements/recommendations for international students: Required—TOEFL. Electronic applications accepted. *Faculty research:* Evolution of microbes, infectious disease, the immune system, genetic disease in humans, evolution of behavior.

Florida State University, The Graduate School, College of Arts and Sciences, Department of Biological Science, Specialization in Ecology and Evolutionary Biology, Tallahassee, FL 32306-4295. Offers MS, PhD. *Faculty:* 21 full-time (7 women). *Students:* 56 full-time (27 women); includes 4 minority (1 Black or African American, non-Hispanic/Latino; 3 Hispanic/Latino), 5 international. 120 applicants, 13% accepted, 9 enrolled. In 2013, 2 master's, 3 doctorates awarded. Terminal master's awarded for partial completion of doctoral program. *Degree requirements:* For master's, comprehensive exam, thesis, teaching experience, seminar presentation; for doctorate, comprehensive exam, thesis/dissertation, teaching experience; seminar presentation. *Entrance requirements:* For master's and doctorate, GRE General Test, minimum upper-division GPA of 3.0. Additional exam requirements/recommendations for international students: Required—TOEFL (minimum score 600 paper-based; 92 iBT). *Application deadline:* For fall admission, 12/1 for domestic and international students. Application fee: $30. Electronic applications accepted. *Expenses:* Tuition, state resident: part-time $403.51 per credit hour. Tuition, nonresident: part-time $1004.85 per credit hour. *Required fees:* $75.81 per credit hour. One-time fee: $20 part-time. Tuition and fees vary according to course load, campus/location and student level. *Financial support:* In 2013–14, 55 students received support, including 4 fellowships with tuition reimbursements available (averaging $30,000 per year), 20 research assistantships with full tuition reimbursements available (averaging $21,500 per year), 31 teaching assistantships with full tuition reimbursements available (averaging $21,500 per year); scholarships/grants and unspecified assistantships also available. Financial award application deadline: 12/1; financial award applicants required to submit FAFSA. *Faculty research:* Ecology and conservation biology; evolution; marine biology; phylogeny and systematics; theoretical, computational and mathematical biology. *Unit head:* Dr. Debra A. Fadool, Professor and Associate Chair, 850-644-4775, Fax: 850-644-9829, E-mail: dfadool@bio.fsu.edu. *Application contact:* Judy Bowers, Coordinator, Graduate Affairs, 850-644-3023, Fax: 850-644-9829, E-mail: gradinfo@bio.fsu.edu.
Website: http://www.bio.fsu.edu/

Harvard University, Graduate School of Arts and Sciences, Department of Organismic and Evolutionary Biology, Cambridge, MA 02138. Offers biology (PhD). *Degree requirements:* For doctorate, 2 foreign languages, public presentation of thesis research, exam. *Entrance requirements:* For doctorate, GRE General Test, GRE Subject Test (recommended), 7 courses in biology, chemistry, physics, mathematics, computer science, or geology. Additional exam requirements/recommendations for international students: Required—TOEFL. *Expenses: Tuition:* Full-time $38,888. *Required fees:* $958. Tuition and fees vary according to campus/location, program and student level.

Illinois State University, Graduate School, College of Arts and Sciences, Department of Biological Sciences, Normal, IL 61790-2200. Offers animal behavior (MS); bacteriology (MS); biochemistry (MS); biological sciences (MS); biology (PhD); biophysics (MS); biotechnology (MS); botany (MS, PhD); cell biology (MS); conservation biology (MS); developmental biology (MS); ecology (MS, PhD); entomology (MS); evolutionary biology (MS); genetics (MS, PhD); immunology (MS); microbiology (MS, PhD); molecular biology (MS); molecular genetics (MS); neurobiology (MS); neuroscience (MS); parasitology (MS); physiology (MS, PhD); plant biology (MS); plant molecular biology (MS); plant sciences (MS); structural biology (MS); zoology (MS, PhD). Part-time programs available. *Degree requirements:* For master's, thesis or alternative; for doctorate, variable foreign language requirement, thesis/dissertation, 2 terms of residency. *Entrance requirements:* For master's, GRE General Test, minimum GPA of 2.6 in last 60 hours of course work; for doctorate, GRE General Test. *Faculty research:* Redoc balance and drug development in schistosoma mansoni, control of the growth of listeria monocytogenes at low temperature, regulation of cell expansion and microtubule function by SPRI, CRUI: physiology and fitness consequences of different life history phenotypes.

Indiana University Bloomington, University Graduate School, College of Arts and Sciences, Department of Biology, Bloomington, IN 47405. Offers biology teaching (MAT); biotechnology (MA); evolution, ecology, and behavior (MA, PhD); genetics (PhD); microbiology (MA, PhD); molecular, cellular, and developmental biology (PhD); plant sciences (MA, PhD); zoology (MA, PhD). *Faculty:* 58 full-time (15 women), 21 part-time/adjunct (6 women). *Students:* 166 full-time (94 women), 2 part-time (both women); includes 22 minority (8 Black or African American, non-Hispanic/Latino; 3 Asian, non-Hispanic/Latino; 10 Hispanic/Latino; 1 Two or more races, non-Hispanic/Latino), 47 international. Average age 27. 261 applicants, 23% accepted, 32 enrolled. In 2013, 17 master's, 20 doctorates awarded. Terminal master's awarded for partial completion of doctoral program. *Degree requirements:* For master's, thesis, oral defense; for doctorate, thesis/dissertation, oral defense. *Entrance requirements:* For master's and doctorate, GRE General Test. Additional exam requirements/recommendations for international students: Required—TOEFL (minimum score 100 iBT). *Application deadline:* For fall admission, 1/5 priority date for domestic students, 12/1 priority date for international students. Application fee: $55 ($65 for international students). Electronic applications accepted. *Financial support:* In 2013–14, fellowships with tuition reimbursements (averaging $24,000 per year), research assistantships with tuition reimbursements (averaging $21,000 per year), teaching assistantships with tuition reimbursements (averaging $22,000 per year) were awarded; scholarships/grants, traineeships, health care benefits, and unspecified assistantships also available. Financial award application deadline: 1/5. *Faculty research:* Evolution, ecology and behavior; microbiology; molecular biology and genetics; plant biology. *Unit head:* Dr. Clay Fuqua, Chair, 812-856-6005, Fax: 812-855-6082, E-mail: cfuqua@indiana.edu. *Application contact:* Tracey D. Stohr, Graduate Student Recruitment Coordinator, 812-856-6303, Fax: 812-855-6082, E-mail: gradbio@indiana.edu.
Website: http://www.bio.indiana.edu/

Iowa State University of Science and Technology, Program in Ecology and Evolutionary Biology, Ames, IA 50011. Offers MS, PhD. *Degree requirements:* For master's, thesis or alternative; for doctorate, thesis/dissertation. *Entrance requirements:* For master's and doctorate, GRE General Test. Additional exam requirements/recommendations for international students: Required—TOEFL (minimum score 550 paper-based; 79 iBT), IELTS (minimum score 6.5). Electronic applications accepted. *Faculty research:* Landscape ecology, aquatic and method ecology, physiological ecology, population genetics and evolution, systematics.

Johns Hopkins University, School of Medicine, Graduate Programs in Medicine, Center for Functional Anatomy and Evolution, Baltimore, MD 21218-2699. Offers PhD. *Faculty:* 5 full-time (1 woman), 2 part-time/adjunct (1 woman). *Students:* 10 full-time (9 women), 3 international. Average age 26. 25 applicants, 16% accepted, 2 enrolled. In 2013, 3 doctorates awarded. *Degree requirements:* For doctorate, comprehensive exam, thesis/dissertation, oral exams. *Entrance requirements:* For doctorate, GRE. Additional exam requirements/recommendations for international students: Required—TOEFL. *Application deadline:* For fall admission, 1/10 for domestic and international students. Application fee: $85. *Financial support:* Fellowships, teaching assistantships, career-related internships or fieldwork, institutionally sponsored loans, health care benefits, and tuition waivers (full) available. *Faculty research:* Vertebrate evolution, functional anatomy, primate evolution, vertebrate paleobiology, vertebrate morphology. *Unit head:* Dr. Kenneth D. Rose, Director, 410-955-7172, Fax: 410-614-9030, E-mail: kdrose@jhmi.edu. *Application contact:* Catherine L. Will, Coordinator, Graduate Student Affairs, 410-614-3385, E-mail: grad_study@som.adm.jhu.edu.

Michigan State University, The Graduate School, College of Natural Science, Interdepartmental Program in Ecology, Evolutionary Biology and Behavior, East Lansing, MI 48824. Offers PhD. *Entrance requirements:* Additional exam requirements/recommendations for international students: Required—TOEFL. Electronic applications accepted.

Montclair State University, The Graduate School, College of Science and Mathematics, Department of Biology and Molecular Biology, Montclair, NJ 07043-1624. Offers biology (MS), including biological science education, biology, ecology and evolution, physiology; molecular biology (MS, Certificate). Part-time and evening/weekend programs available. *Degree requirements:* For master's, comprehensive exam, thesis or alternative. *Entrance requirements:* For master's, GRE General Test, 24 credits of course work in undergraduate biology, 2 letters of recommendation, teaching certificate (biology sciences education concentration); for Certificate, 2 letters of recommendation, essay. Additional exam requirements/recommendations for international students: Required—TOEFL (minimum score 83 iBT) or IELTS. Electronic applications accepted. *Faculty research:* Ecosystem biology, molecular biology, signal transduction, neuroscience, aquatic and coastal biology.

The Ohio State University, Graduate School, College of Arts and Sciences, Division of Natural and Mathematical Sciences, Department of Evolution, Ecology, and Organismal Biology, Columbus, OH 43210. Offers MS, PhD. *Faculty:* 27. *Students:* 72 full-time (32 women), 4 part-time (2 women); includes 3 minority (2 Black or African American, non-Hispanic/Latino; 1 Hispanic/Latino), 10 international. Average age 28. In 2013, 3 master's, 3 doctorates awarded. *Degree requirements:* For master's, thesis optional; for doctorate, thesis/dissertation. *Entrance requirements:* For master's and doctorate, GRE

General Test. Additional exam requirements/recommendations for international students: Required—TOEFL (minimum score 600 paper-based; 100 iBT), Michigan English Language Assessment Battery (minimum score 86); Recommended—IELTS (minimum score 8). *Application deadline:* For fall admission, 12/1 priority date for domestic students, 11/30 priority date for international students; for winter admission, 12/1 for domestic students, 11/1 for international students; for spring admission, 3/1 for domestic students, 2/1 for international students. Applications are processed on a rolling basis. Application fee: $60 ($70 for international students). Electronic applications accepted. *Financial support:* Fellowships with tuition reimbursements, research assistantships with tuition reimbursements, teaching assistantships with tuition reimbursements, Federal Work-Study, and institutionally sponsored loans available. Support available to part-time students. *Unit head:* Peter S. Curtis, Chair, 614-292-8280, E-mail: curtis.7@osu.edu. *Application contact:* Graduate Admissions, 614-292-9444, Fax: 614-292-3895, E-mail: gradadmissions@osu.edu.
Website: http://eeob.osu.edu/

Ohio University, Graduate College, College of Arts and Sciences, Department of Biological Sciences, Athens, OH 45701-2979. Offers biological sciences (MS, PhD); cell biology and physiology (MS, PhD); ecology and evolutionary biology (MS, PhD); exercise physiology and muscle biology (MS, PhD); microbiology (MS, PhD); neuroscience (MS, PhD). Terminal master's awarded for partial completion of doctoral program. *Degree requirements:* For master's, comprehensive exam, thesis, 1 quarter of teaching experience; for doctorate, comprehensive exam, thesis/dissertation, 2 quarters of teaching experience. *Entrance requirements:* For master's, GRE General Test, names of three faculty members whose research interests most closely match the applicant's interest; for doctorate, GRE General Test, essay concerning prior training, research interest and career goals, plus names of three faculty members whose research interests most closely match the applicant's interest. Additional exam requirements/recommendations for international students: Required—TOEFL (minimum score 620 paper-based; 105 iBT) or IELTS (minimum score 7.5). Electronic applications accepted. *Faculty research:* Ecology and evolutionary biology, exercise physiology and muscle biology, neurobiology, cell biology, physiology.

Princeton University, Graduate School, Department of Ecology and Evolutionary Biology, Princeton, NJ 08544-1019. Offers PhD. *Degree requirements:* For doctorate, thesis/dissertation. *Entrance requirements:* For doctorate, GRE General Test, GRE Subject Test. Additional exam requirements/recommendations for international students: Required—TOEFL (minimum score 600 paper-based). Electronic applications accepted.

Purdue University, Graduate School, College of Science, Department of Biological Sciences, West Lafayette, IN 47907. Offers biochemistry (PhD); biophysics (PhD); cell and developmental biology (PhD); ecology, evolutionary and population biology (MS, PhD), including ecology, evolutionary biology, population biology; genetics (MS, PhD); microbiology (MS, PhD); molecular biology (PhD); neurobiology (MS, PhD); plant physiology (PhD). *Faculty:* 50 full-time (13 women), 5 part-time/adjunct (1 woman). *Students:* 111 full-time (61 women), 5 part-time (0 women); includes 9 minority (1 Black or African American, non-Hispanic/Latino; 5 Asian, non-Hispanic/Latino; 3 Hispanic/Latino), 62 international. Average age 27. 170 applicants, 19% accepted, 17 enrolled. In 2013, 9 master's, 18 doctorates awarded. Terminal master's awarded for partial completion of doctoral program. *Degree requirements:* For master's, thesis (for some programs); for doctorate, thesis/dissertation, seminars, teaching experience. *Entrance requirements:* For master's, GRE General Test (minimum analytical writing score of 3.5), minimum undergraduate GPA of 3.0; for doctorate, GRE General Test (minimum analytical writing score of 3.5), minimum undergraduate GPA of 3.5. Additional exam requirements/recommendations for international students: Required—TOEFL (minimum score 600 paper-based; 107 iBT for MS, 80 iBT for PhD). *Application deadline:* For fall admission, 12/7 for domestic and international students. Applications are processed on a rolling basis. Application fee: $60 ($75 for international students). Electronic applications accepted. *Financial support:* Fellowships, research assistantships, and teaching assistantships available. Support available to part-time students. Financial award application deadline: 2/15; financial award applicants required to submit FAFSA. *Unit head:* Dr. Richard J. Kuhn, Head, 765-494-4407, E-mail: kuhnr@purdue.edu. *Application contact:* Georgina E. Rupp, Graduate Coordinator, 765-494-8142, Fax: 765-494-0876, E-mail: ruppg@purdue.edu.
Website: http://www.bio.purdue.edu/

Purdue University, Graduate School, PULSe - Purdue University Life Sciences Program, West Lafayette, IN 47907. Offers biomolecular structure and biophysics (PhD); biotechnology (PhD); chemical biology (PhD); chromatin and regulation of gene expression (PhD); integrative neuroscience (PhD); integrative plant sciences (PhD); membrane biology (PhD); microbiology (PhD); molecular evolutionary and cancer biology (PhD); molecular evolutionary genetics (PhD); molecular virology (PhD). *Students:* 154 full-time (78 women), 1 part-time (0 women); includes 23 minority (5 Black or African American, non-Hispanic/Latino; 5 Asian, non-Hispanic/Latino; 10 Hispanic/Latino; 3 Two or more races, non-Hispanic/Latino), 73 international. Average age 26. 239 applicants, 33% accepted, 40 enrolled. *Entrance requirements:* For doctorate, GRE, minimum undergraduate GPA of 3.0. Additional exam requirements/recommendations for international students: Required—TOEFL (minimum score 550 paper-based; 77 iBT). *Application deadline:* For fall admission, 1/15 priority date for domestic and international students. Applications are processed on a rolling basis. Application fee: $60 ($75 for international students). Electronic applications accepted. *Financial support:* In 2013–14, research assistantships with tuition reimbursements (averaging $22,500 per year), teaching assistantships with tuition reimbursements (averaging $22,500 per year) were awarded. *Unit head:* Dr. Christine A. Hrycyna, Head, 765-494-7322, E-mail: hrycyna@purdue.edu. *Application contact:* Colleen Gabauer, Graduate Contact, 765-494-9256, E-mail: cgabauer@purdue.edu.
Website: http://www.gradschool.purdue.edu/pulse

Rice University, Graduate Programs, Wiess School of Natural Sciences, Department of Ecology and Evolutionary Biology, Houston, TX 77251-1892. Offers MA, MS, PhD. Terminal master's awarded for partial completion of doctoral program. *Degree requirements:* For master's, comprehensive exam (for some programs), thesis (for some programs); for doctorate, comprehensive exam, thesis/dissertation. *Entrance requirements:* For master's and doctorate, GRE General Test, GRE Subject Test. Additional exam requirements/recommendations for international students: Required—TOEFL (minimum score 600 paper-based; 90 iBT). Electronic applications accepted. *Faculty research:* Trace gas emissions, wetlands, biology, community ecology of forests and grasslands, conservation biology specialization.

Rutgers, The State University of New Jersey, New Brunswick, Graduate School-New Brunswick, Program in Ecology and Evolution, Piscataway, NJ 08854-8097. Offers MS, PhD. Part-time programs available. Terminal master's awarded for partial completion of doctoral program. *Degree requirements:* For master's, comprehensive exam; for doctorate, comprehensive exam, thesis/dissertation. *Entrance requirements:* For master's and doctorate, GRE General Test, minimum GPA of 3.0. Additional exam requirements/recommendations for international students: Required—TOEFL (minimum score 550 paper-based). Electronic applications accepted. *Faculty research:* Population and community ecology, population genetics, evolutionary biology, conservation biology, ecosystem ecology.

Rutgers, The State University of New Jersey, New Brunswick, Graduate School-New Brunswick, Program in Plant Biology, Piscataway, NJ 08854-8097. Offers horticulture and plant technology (MS, PhD); molecular and cellular biology (MS, PhD); organismal and population biology (MS, PhD); plant pathology (MS, PhD). Part-time programs available. Terminal master's awarded for partial completion of doctoral program. *Degree requirements:* For master's, comprehensive exam, thesis or alternative; for doctorate, comprehensive exam, thesis/dissertation. *Entrance requirements:* For master's and doctorate, GRE General Test, GRE Subject Test (recommended). Additional exam requirements/recommendations for international students: Required—TOEFL (minimum score 600 paper-based). Electronic applications accepted. *Faculty research:* Molecular biology and biochemistry of plants, plant development and genomics, plant protection, plant improvement, plant management of horticultural and field crops.

Sonoma State University, School of Science and Technology, Department of Biology, Rohnert Park, CA 94928. Offers biochemistry (MA); ecology (MS); environmental biology (MS); evolutionary biology (MS); functional morphology (MS); molecular and cell biology (MS); organismal biology (MS). Part-time programs available. *Faculty:* 9 full-time (1 woman). *Students:* 4 full-time (2 women), 21 part-time (14 women); includes 5 minority (1 American Indian or Alaska Native, non-Hispanic/Latino; 1 Asian, non-Hispanic/Latino; 2 Hispanic/Latino; 1 Two or more races, non-Hispanic/Latino), 2 international. Average age 29. 23 applicants, 65% accepted, 6 enrolled. In 2013, 6 master's awarded. *Degree requirements:* For master's, thesis or alternative, oral exam. *Entrance requirements:* For master's, GRE General Test, GRE Subject Test, minimum GPA of 3.0. Additional exam requirements/recommendations for international students: Required—TOEFL (minimum score 500 paper-based). *Application deadline:* For fall admission, 11/30 for domestic students. Applications are processed on a rolling basis. Application fee: $55. *Expenses:* Tuition, state resident: full-time $8500. Tuition, nonresident: full-time $12,964. *Required fees:* $1762. *Financial support:* In 2013–14, 1 fellowship (averaging $1,520 per year), 6 research assistantships (averaging $3,562 per year), 22 teaching assistantships (averaging $6,738 per year) were awarded; career-related internships or fieldwork, Federal Work-Study, and tuition waivers (full) also available. Financial award application deadline: 3/2; financial award applicants required to submit FAFSA. *Faculty research:* Plant physiology, comparative physiology, community ecology, restoration ecology, marine ecology, conservation genetics, primate behavior, behavioral ecology, developmental biology, plant and animal systematics. *Total annual research expenditures:* $4,400. *Unit head:* Dr. Nathan Rank, Chair, 707-664-3053, E-mail: nathan.rank@sonoma.edu. *Application contact:* Dr. Derek Girman, Graduate Adviser, 707-664-3055, E-mail: derek.girman@sonoma.edu.
Website: http://www.sonoma.edu/biology/graduate

Stony Brook University, State University of New York, Graduate School, College of Arts and Sciences, Department of Ecology and Evolution, Stony Brook, NY 11794. Offers applied ecology (MA); ecology and evolution (PhD). *Faculty:* 18 full-time (7 women), 1 part-time/adjunct (0 women). *Students:* 54 full-time (29 women), 4 part-time (2 women); includes 8 minority (3 Asian, non-Hispanic/Latino; 5 Hispanic/Latino), 12 international. Average age 28. 46 applicants, 48% accepted, 9 enrolled. In 2013, 1 master's, 11 doctorates awarded. *Degree requirements:* For doctorate, one foreign language, comprehensive exam, thesis/dissertation, teaching experience. *Entrance requirements:* For doctorate, GRE General Test, GRE Subject Test. Additional exam requirements/recommendations for international students: Required—TOEFL. *Application deadline:* For fall admission, 1/15 for domestic students; for spring admission, 10/1 for domestic students. Application fee: $100. *Expenses:* Tuition, state resident: full-time $9870; part-time $411 per credit. Tuition, nonresident: full-time $18,350; part-time $765 per credit. *Financial support:* In 2013–14, 2 fellowships, 6 research assistantships, 27 teaching assistantships were awarded; Federal Work-Study also available. *Faculty research:* Theoretical and experimental population genetics, numerical taxonomy, biostatistics, population and community ecology, plant ecology. *Total annual research expenditures:* $1.7 million. *Unit head:* Dr. Walter F. Eanes, Chair, 631-632-8593, Fax: 631-632-7626, E-mail: walter.eanes@stonybrook.edu. *Application contact:* Melissa Cohen, Coordinator, 631-246-8604, Fax: 631-632-7626, E-mail: melissa.j.cohen@stonybrook.edu.
Website: http://life.bio.sunysb.edu/ee/

Tulane University, School of Science and Engineering, Department of Ecology and Evolutionary Biology, New Orleans, LA 70118-5669. Offers MS, PhD. Terminal master's awarded for partial completion of doctoral program. *Degree requirements:* For master's, thesis or alternative; for doctorate, thesis/dissertation. *Entrance requirements:* For master's, GRE General Test, minimum B average in undergraduate course work; for doctorate, GRE General Test. Additional exam requirements/recommendations for international students: Required—TOEFL. Electronic applications accepted. *Faculty research:* Ichthyology, plant systematics, crustacean endocrinology, ecotoxicology, ornithology.

University at Albany, State University of New York, College of Arts and Sciences, Department of Biological Sciences, Specialization in Ecology, Evolution, and Behavior, Albany, NY 12222-0001. Offers MS, PhD. *Degree requirements:* For master's, one foreign language; for doctorate, one foreign language, thesis/dissertation. *Entrance requirements:* For master's and doctorate, GRE General Test.

University at Buffalo, the State University of New York, Graduate School, College of Arts and Sciences, Program in Evolution, Ecology and Behavior, Buffalo, NY 14260. Offers MS, PhD, Certificate. Terminal master's awarded for partial completion of doctoral program. *Degree requirements:* For master's, project; for doctorate, comprehensive exam, thesis/dissertation. *Entrance requirements:* For master's, GRE, minimum undergraduate GPA of 3.0; for doctorate, GRE, minimum GPA of 3.0. Additional exam requirements/recommendations for international students: Required—TOEFL (minimum score 550 paper-based; 79 iBT). Electronic applications accepted. *Faculty research:* Coral reef ecology, evolution and ecology of aquatic invertebrates, animal communication, paleobiology, primate behavior.

University of Alberta, Faculty of Graduate Studies and Research, Department of Biological Sciences, Edmonton, AB T6G 2E1, Canada. Offers environmental biology and ecology (M Sc, PhD); microbiology and biotechnology (M Sc, PhD); molecular biology and genetics (M Sc, PhD); physiology and cell biology (M Sc, PhD); plant biology (M Sc, PhD); systematics and evolution (M Sc, PhD). Terminal master's awarded for partial completion of doctoral program. *Degree requirements:* For master's, thesis; for doctorate, thesis/dissertation. *Entrance requirements:* Additional exam requirements/recommendations for international students: Required—TOEFL.

The University of Arizona, College of Science, Department of Ecology and Evolutionary Biology, Tucson, AZ 85721. Offers MS, PhD. *Faculty:* 21 full-time (5 women), 2 part-time/adjunct (0 women). *Students:* 52 full-time (23 women), 6 part-time (3 women); includes 5 minority (1 American Indian or Alaska Native, non-Hispanic/Latino; 1 Asian, non-Hispanic/Latino; 2 Hispanic/Latino; 1 Two or more races, non-Hispanic/Latino), 13 international. Average age 28. 77 applicants, 17% accepted, 9 enrolled. In 2013, 5 master's, 4 doctorates awarded. Terminal master's awarded for

partial completion of doctoral program. *Degree requirements:* For master's, thesis optional; for doctorate, one foreign language, comprehensive exam, thesis/dissertation. *Entrance requirements:* For master's, GRE General Test, GRE Subject Test, statement of purpose, curriculum vitae, 3 letters of recommendation; for doctorate, GRE General Test, GRE Subject Test, curriculum vitae, 3 letters of recommendation. Additional exam requirements/recommendations for international students: Required—TOEFL (minimum score 550 paper-based; 79 iBT). *Application deadline:* For fall admission, 12/1 for domestic students, 12/8 for international students. Application fee: $75. *Expenses:* Tuition, state resident: full-time $11,526. Tuition, nonresident: full-time $27,398. *Financial support:* In 2013–14, 10 research assistantships with full tuition reimbursements (averaging $22,896 per year), 34 teaching assistantships with full tuition reimbursements (averaging $22,896 per year) were awarded; career-related internships or fieldwork, scholarships/grants, health care benefits, and unspecified assistantships also available. *Faculty research:* Biological diversity, evolutionary history, evolutionary mechanisms, community structure. *Total annual research expenditures:* $5.6 million. *Unit head:* Dr. Richard E. Michod, Head, 520-621-7509, Fax: 520-621-9190, E-mail: michod@email.arizona.edu. *Application contact:* Carol Burleson, Administrative Associate, 520-621-9328, Fax: 520-621-9190, E-mail: oxforda@email.arizona.edu.
Website: http://eebweb.arizona.edu/

University of California, Davis, Graduate Studies, Graduate Group in Population Biology, Davis, CA 95616. Offers PhD. *Degree requirements:* For doctorate, thesis/dissertation. *Entrance requirements:* For doctorate, GRE General Test, GRE Subject Test. Additional exam requirements/recommendations for international students: Required—TOEFL (minimum score 550 paper-based). Electronic applications accepted. *Faculty research:* Population ecology, population genetics, systematics, evolution, community ecology.

University of California, Irvine, School of Biological Sciences, Department of Ecology and Evolutionary Biology, Irvine, CA 92697. Offers biological sciences (MS, PhD). *Students:* 57 full-time (31 women), 1 (woman) part-time; includes 20 minority (6 Asian, non-Hispanic/Latino; 8 Hispanic/Latino; 6 Two or more races, non-Hispanic/Latino), 3 international. Average age 27. 87 applicants, 34% accepted, 19 enrolled. In 2013, 6 doctorates awarded. *Degree requirements:* For master's, thesis; for doctorate, thesis/dissertation. *Entrance requirements:* For master's and doctorate, GRE General Test, GRE Subject Test, minimum GPA of 3.0. Additional exam requirements/recommendations for international students: Required—TOEFL (minimum score 550 paper-based). *Application deadline:* For fall admission, 1/15 priority date for domestic students, 1/15 for international students. Applications are processed on a rolling basis. Application fee: $80 ($100 for international students). Electronic applications accepted. *Financial support:* Fellowships, research assistantships with full tuition reimbursements, teaching assistantships, career-related internships or fieldwork, institutionally sponsored loans, traineeships, health care benefits, and unspecified assistantships available. Financial award application deadline: 3/1; financial award applicants required to submit FAFSA. *Faculty research:* Ecological energetics, quantitative genetics, life history evolution, plant-herbivore and plant-pollinator interactions, molecular evolution. *Unit head:* Laurence D. Mueller, Professor/Department Chair, 949-824-4744, Fax: 949-824-2181, E-mail: ldmuelle@uci.edu. *Application contact:* Pamela Mc Donald, Student Affairs Officer, 949-824-4743, Fax: 949-824-2181, E-mail: pmcdonal@uci.edu.
Website: http://ecoevo.bio.uci.edu/

University of California, Los Angeles, Graduate Division, College of Letters and Science, Department of Ecology and Evolutionary Biology, Los Angeles, CA 90095. Offers MA, PhD. Terminal master's awarded for partial completion of doctoral program. *Degree requirements:* For master's, comprehensive exam or thesis; for doctorate, thesis/dissertation, oral and written qualifying exams; 3 quarters of teaching experience. *Entrance requirements:* For master's and doctorate, GRE General Test, GRE Subject Test (biology), bachelor's degree; minimum undergraduate GPA of 3.0 (or its equivalent if letter grade system not used). Additional exam requirements/recommendations for international students: Required—TOEFL. Electronic applications accepted.

University of California, Riverside, Graduate Division, Department of Biology, Riverside, CA 92521-0102. Offers evolution, ecology and organismal biology (MS, PhD). Terminal master's awarded for partial completion of doctoral program. *Degree requirements:* For master's, thesis, oral defense of thesis; for doctorate, thesis/dissertation, 3 quarters of teaching experience, qualifying exams. *Entrance requirements:* For master's and doctorate, GRE General Test, minimum GPA of 3.2. Additional exam requirements/recommendations for international students: Required—TOEFL (minimum score 550 paper-based, 80 iBT) or IELTS. Electronic applications accepted. *Faculty research:* Ecology, evolutionary biology, physiology, quantitative genetics, conservation biology.

University of California, Riverside, Graduate Division, Department of Entomology, Riverside, CA 92521-0102. Offers entomology (MS, PhD); evolution and ecology (PhD). Part-time programs available. Terminal master's awarded for partial completion of doctoral program. *Degree requirements:* For master's, thesis; for doctorate, thesis/dissertation, qualifying exams. *Entrance requirements:* For master's and doctorate, GRE General Test, minimum GPA of 3.2. Additional exam requirements/recommendations for international students: Required—TOEFL (minimum score 550 paper-based; 80 iBT) or IELTS. Electronic applications accepted. *Faculty research:* Agricultural, urban, medical, and veterinary entomology; biological control; chemical ecology; insect pathogens; novel toxicants.

University of California, San Diego, Office of Graduate Studies, Division of Biological Sciences, La Jolla, CA 92093. Offers anthropogeny (PhD); bioinformatics (PhD); biology (PhD); ecology, behavior and evolution (PhD); microbiology (PhD). *Students:* 285 full-time (154 women), 8 part-time (4 women); includes 70 minority (2 Black or African American, non-Hispanic/Latino; 3 American Indian or Alaska Native, non-Hispanic/Latino; 51 Asian, non-Hispanic/Latino; 13 Hispanic/Latino; 1 Native Hawaiian or other Pacific Islander, non-Hispanic/Latino), 30 international. 626 applicants, 24% accepted, 85 enrolled. In 2013, 32 doctorates awarded. *Degree requirements:* For doctorate, thesis/dissertation, 3 quarters of teaching assistantship. *Entrance requirements:* For doctorate, GRE General Test; GRE Subject Test (recommended). Additional exam requirements/recommendations for international students: Required—TOEFL, IELTS. *Application deadline:* For fall admission, 12/4 for domestic students. Application fee: $80 ($100 for international students). Electronic applications accepted. *Expenses:* Tuition, state resident: full-time $11,220; part-time $1870 per quarter. Tuition, nonresident: full-time $26,322; part-time $4387 per quarter. *Required fees:* $519.50 per quarter. Part-time tuition and fees vary according to course load and program. *Financial support:* Fellowships, research assistantships, teaching assistantships, and scholarships/grants available. Financial award applicants required to submit FAFSA. *Faculty research:* Ecology, behavior and evolution; microbiology; bioinformatics; multi-scale biology; anthropogeny. *Unit head:* William McGinnis, Dean, 858-822-0458, E-mail: wmcginnis@ucsd.edu. *Application contact:* Cathy Pugh, Graduate Coordinator, 858-534-0181, E-mail: gradprog@biology.ucsd.edu.
Website: http://biology.ucsd.edu/

University of California, Santa Barbara, Graduate Division, College of Letters and Sciences, Division of Mathematics, Life, and Physical Sciences, Department of Ecology, Evolution, and Marine Biology, Santa Barbara, CA 93106-9620. Offers computational science and engineering (MA); computational sciences and engineering (PhD); ecology, evolution, and marine biology (MA, PhD); MA/PhD. *Faculty:* 33 full-time (8 women). *Students:* 59 full-time (33 women); includes 14 minority (1 Black or African American, non-Hispanic/Latino; 7 Asian, non-Hispanic/Latino; 6 Hispanic/Latino), 4 international. Average age 31. 120 applicants, 15% accepted, 12 enrolled. In 2013, 9 master's, 6 doctorates awarded. *Degree requirements:* For master's, comprehensive exam (for some programs), thesis (for some programs); for doctorate, comprehensive exam, thesis/dissertation. *Entrance requirements:* For master's and doctorate, GRE General Test. Additional exam requirements/recommendations for international students: Required—TOEFL (minimum score 550 paper-based; 80 iBT), IELTS. *Application deadline:* For fall admission, 12/15 for domestic and international students. Application fee: $80 ($100 for international students). Electronic applications accepted. *Expenses:* Tuition, state resident: part-time $5148.26 per quarter. Tuition, nonresident: part-time $10,182.26 per quarter. *Financial support:* In 2013–14, 50 students received support, including 55 fellowships with full and partial tuition reimbursements available (averaging $10,812 per year), 24 research assistantships with full and partial tuition reimbursements available (averaging $8,441 per year), 97 teaching assistantships with partial tuition reimbursements available (averaging $9,346 per year); Federal Work-Study, scholarships/grants, traineeships, health care benefits, and tuition waivers (full and partial) also available. Financial award application deadline: 12/15; financial award applicants required to submit FAFSA. *Faculty research:* Community ecology, evolution, marine biology, population genetics, stream ecology. *Unit head:* Dr. Craig Carlson, Chair, 805-893-2415, Fax: 805-893-5885, E-mail: eembchair@lifesci.ucsb.edu. *Application contact:* Melanie Fujii, Student Affairs Officer, 805-893-2979, Fax: 805-893-5885, E-mail: eemb-info@lifesci.ucsb.edu.
Website: http://www.lifesci.ucsb.edu/EEMB/index.html

University of California, Santa Cruz, Division of Graduate Studies, Division of Physical and Biological Sciences, Department of Ecology and Evolutionary Biology, Santa Cruz, CA 95064. Offers MA, PhD. *Degree requirements:* For master's, thesis; for doctorate, comprehensive exam, thesis/dissertation. *Entrance requirements:* For master's and doctorate, GRE General Test, GRE Subject Test, 3 letters of recommendation. Additional exam requirements/recommendations for international students: Required—TOEFL (minimum score 550 paper-based; 83 iBT); Recommended—IELTS (minimum score 8). Electronic applications accepted. *Faculty research:* Population and community ecology, evolutionary biology, physiology and behavior (marine and terrestrial), systematics and biodiversity.

University of Chicago, Division of Biological Sciences, Darwinian Sciences Cluster: Ecological, Integrative and Evolutionary Biology, Committee on Evolutionary Biology, Chicago, IL 60637-1513. Offers functional and evolutionary biology (PhD). Terminal master's awarded for partial completion of doctoral program. *Degree requirements:* For doctorate, thesis/dissertation, ethics class, 2 teaching assistantships. *Entrance requirements:* For doctorate, GRE General Test. Additional exam requirements/recommendations for international students: Required—TOEFL (minimum score 600 paper-based; 104 iBT), IELTS (minimum score 7). Electronic applications accepted. *Faculty research:* Systematics and evolutionary theory, genetics, functional morphology and physiology, behavior, ecology and biogeography.

University of Colorado Boulder, Graduate School, College of Arts and Sciences, Department of Ecology and Evolutionary Biology, Boulder, CO 80309. Offers animal behavior (MA); biology (MA, PhD); environmental biology (MA, PhD); evolutionary biology (MA, PhD); neurobiology (MA); population biology (MA); population genetics (PhD). *Faculty:* 31 full-time (12 women). *Students:* 70 full-time (30 women), 18 part-time (10 women); includes 6 minority (1 Asian, non-Hispanic/Latino; 3 Hispanic/Latino; 2 Two or more races, non-Hispanic/Latino), 5 international. Average age 30. 171 applicants, 6% accepted, 11 enrolled. In 2013, 10 master's, 11 doctorates awarded. Terminal master's awarded for partial completion of doctoral program. *Degree requirements:* For master's, comprehensive exam, thesis or alternative; for doctorate, comprehensive exam, thesis/dissertation. *Entrance requirements:* For master's, GRE General Test, GRE Subject Test, minimum undergraduate GPA of 3.0; for doctorate, GRE General Test, GRE Subject Test. *Application deadline:* For fall admission, 12/31 for domestic students, 12/1 for international students. Application fee: $50 ($60 for international students). Electronic applications accepted. *Financial support:* In 2013–14, 175 students received support, including 35 fellowships (averaging $15,283 per year), 21 research assistantships with full and partial tuition reimbursements available (averaging $29,343 per year), 48 teaching assistantships with full and partial tuition reimbursements available (averaging $31,449 per year); institutionally sponsored loans, scholarships/grants, health care benefits, and unspecified assistantships also available. Financial award applicants required to submit FAFSA. *Faculty research:* Ecology, environmental biology, evolutionary biology, biological sciences, conservation biology. *Total annual research expenditures:* $37.1 million.
Website: http://ebio.colorado.edu

University of Colorado Denver, College of Liberal Arts and Sciences, Department of Integrative Biology, Denver, CO 80217. Offers animal behavior (MS); biology (MS); cell and developmental biology (MS); ecology (MS); evolutionary biology (MS); genetics (MS); integrative and systems biology (PhD); microbiology (MS); molecular biology (MS); neurobiology (MS); plant systematics (MS). Part-time programs available. *Faculty:* 21 full-time (7 women), 3 part-time/adjunct (2 women). *Students:* 18 full-time (11 women), 5 part-time (all women); includes 5 minority (1 Black or African American, non-Hispanic/Latino; 2 Hispanic/Latino; 2 Two or more races, non-Hispanic/Latino), 1 international. Average age 29. 25 applicants, 44% accepted, 11 enrolled. In 2013, 13 master's awarded. *Degree requirements:* For master's, comprehensive exam, thesis, 30-32 credit hours. *Entrance requirements:* For master's, GRE General Test (minimum score in 50th percentile in each section), BA/BS from accredited institution awarded within the last 10 years; minimum undergraduate GPA of 3.0; prerequisite courses: 1 year each of general biology and general chemistry; 1 semester each of general genetics, general ecology, and cell biology; and a structure/function course. Additional exam requirements/recommendations for international students: Required—TOEFL (minimum score 537 paper-based; 75 iBT); Recommended—IELTS (minimum score 6.5). *Application deadline:* For fall admission, 2/1 for domestic and international students. Application fee: $50 ($75 for international students). Electronic applications accepted. *Financial support:* In 2013–14, 8 students received support. Fellowships, research assistantships, teaching assistantships, Federal Work-Study, institutionally sponsored loans, scholarships/grants, and traineeships available. Financial award application deadline: 4/1; financial award applicants required to submit FAFSA. *Faculty research:* Molecular developmental biology; quantitative ecology, biogeography, and population dynamics; environmental signaling and endocrine disruption; speciation, the evolution of reproductive isolation, and hybrid zones; evolutionary, behavioral, and conservation ecology. *Unit head:* Dr. John Swallow, Biology Department Chair, 303-556-6154, E-mail: john.swallow@ucdenver.edu. *Application contact:* Timberley Roane, Associate Professor/Director of MS in Biology Program, 303-556-6592, E-mail: timberley.roane@ucdenver.edu.
Website: http://www.ucdenver.edu/academics/colleges/CLAS/Departments/biology/Programs/MasterofScience/Pages/BiologyMasterOfScience.aspx

University of Delaware, College of Arts and Sciences, Department of Biological Sciences, Newark, DE 19716. Offers biotechnology (MS); cancer biology (MS, PhD); cell and extracellular matrix biology (MS, PhD); cell and systems physiology (MS, PhD); developmental biology (MS, PhD); ecology and evolution (MS, PhD); microbiology (MS, PhD); molecular biology and genetics (MS, PhD). Terminal master's awarded for partial completion of doctoral program. *Degree requirements:* For master's, thesis, preliminary exam; for doctorate, comprehensive exam, thesis/dissertation, preliminary exam. *Entrance requirements:* For master's and doctorate, GRE General Test. Additional exam requirements/recommendations for international students: Required—TOEFL (minimum score 600 paper-based); Recommended—TWE. Electronic applications accepted. *Faculty research:* Microorganisms, bone, cancer metastasis, developmental biology, cell biology, DNA.

University of Denver, Division of Natural Sciences and Mathematics, Department of Biological Sciences, Denver, CO 80208-9010. Offers biomedical sciences (PSM); cell and molecular biology (MS, PhD); ecology and evolution (MS, PhD). Part-time programs available. *Faculty:* 23 full-time (8 women). *Students:* 1 (woman) full-time, 21 part-time (13 women); includes 3 minority (all Hispanic/Latino), 7 international. Average age 27. 50 applicants, 22% accepted, 10 enrolled. In 2013, 5 master's, 2 doctorates awarded. Terminal master's awarded for partial completion of doctoral program. *Degree requirements:* For master's, comprehensive exam (for some programs), thesis; for doctorate, one foreign language, comprehensive exam (for some programs), thesis/dissertation. *Entrance requirements:* For master's and doctorate, GRE General Test, bachelor's degree in biology or related field, transcripts, personal statement, three letters of recommendation. Additional exam requirements/recommendations for international students: Required—TOEFL (minimum score 570 paper-based; 88 iBT). *Application deadline:* For fall admission, 1/1 priority date for domestic and international students. Applications are processed on a rolling basis. Application fee: $60. Electronic applications accepted. *Financial support:* In 2013–14, 19 students received support, including 3 research assistantships with full and partial tuition reimbursements available (averaging $22,448 per year), 15 teaching assistantships with full and partial tuition reimbursements available (averaging $25,161 per year); Federal Work-Study, institutionally sponsored loans, scholarships/grants, and unspecified assistantships also available. Support available to part-time students. Financial award application deadline: 2/15; financial award applicants required to submit FAFSA. *Faculty research:* Molecular biology, cell biology, neurobiology, ecology, molecular evolution. *Unit head:* Dr. Joseph Angleson, Chair, 303-871-3463, Fax: 303-871-3471, E-mail: jangleso@du.edu. *Application contact:* Randi Flageolle, Assistant to the Chair, 303-871-3457, Fax: 303-871-3471, E-mail: rflageol@du.edu.
Website: http://www.du.edu/nsm/departments/biologicalsciences/index.html

University of Guelph, Graduate Studies, College of Biological Science, Department of Integrative Biology, Botany and Zoology, Guelph, ON N1G 2W1, Canada. Offers botany (M Sc, PhD); zoology (M Sc, PhD). Part-time programs available. *Degree requirements:* For master's, thesis, research proposal; for doctorate, thesis/dissertation, research proposal, qualifying exam. *Entrance requirements:* For master's, minimum B average during previous 2 years of course work. Additional exam requirements/recommendations for international students: Required—TOEFL (minimum score 550 paper-based), IELTS (minimum score 6.5). Electronic applications accepted. *Faculty research:* Aquatic science, environmental physiology, parasitology, wildlife biology, management.

University of Hawaii at Manoa, Graduate Division, Interdisciplinary Specialization in Ecology, Evolution and Conservation Biology, Honolulu, HI 96822. Offers MS, PhD. *Degree requirements:* For doctorate, thesis/dissertation. *Faculty research:* Agronomy and soil science, zoology, entomology, genetics and molecular biology, botanical sciences.

University of Illinois at Urbana–Champaign, Graduate College, College of Liberal Arts and Sciences, School of Integrative Biology, Department of Animal Biology, Champaign, IL 61820. Offers animal biology (ecology, ethology and evolution) (MS, PhD). *Students:* 15 (5 women). Application fee: $75 ($90 for international students). *Unit head:* Ken Paige, Head, 217-244-6606, Fax: 217-244-4565, E-mail: k-paige@illinois.edu. *Application contact:* Lisa Smith, Office Administrator, 217-333-7802, Fax: 217-244-4565, E-mail: ljsmith1@illinois.edu.
Website: http://www.life.illinois.edu/animalbiology

University of Illinois at Urbana–Champaign, Graduate College, College of Liberal Arts and Sciences, School of Integrative Biology, Program in Ecology, Evolution and Conservation Biology, Champaign, IL 61820. Offers MS, PhD. *Students:* 28 (16 women). Application fee: $75 ($90 for international students). *Unit head:* Evan H. DeLucia, Director, 217-333-3044, Fax: 217-244-1224, E-mail: delucia@illinois.edu. *Application contact:* Kimberly Leigh, Secretary, 217-333-8208, Fax: 217-244-1224, E-mail: kaleigh@illinois.edu.
Website: http://sib.illinois.edu/peec/

The University of Iowa, Graduate College, College of Liberal Arts and Sciences, Department of Biology, Iowa City, IA 52242-1324. Offers biology (MS, PhD); cell and developmental biology (MS, PhD); evolution (MS, PhD); genetics (MS, PhD); neurobiology (MS, PhD). Terminal master's awarded for partial completion of doctoral program. *Degree requirements:* For master's, thesis optional, exam; for doctorate, comprehensive exam, thesis/dissertation. *Entrance requirements:* For master's and doctorate, GRE General Test, minimum GPA of 3.0. Additional exam requirements/recommendations for international students: Required—TOEFL (minimum score 600 paper-based; 100 iBT). Electronic applications accepted. *Faculty research:* Neurobiology, evolutionary biology, genetics, cell and developmental biology.

The University of Kansas, Graduate Studies, College of Liberal Arts and Sciences, Department of Ecology and Evolutionary Biology, Lawrence, KS 66045. Offers botany (MA, PhD); ecology and evolutionary biology (MA, PhD); entomology (MA, PhD). *Faculty:* 35. *Students:* 57 full-time (25 women); includes 3 minority (all Two or more races, non-Hispanic/Latino), 19 international. Average age 29. 48 applicants, 29% accepted, 10 enrolled. In 2013, 9 doctorates awarded. Terminal master's awarded for partial completion of doctoral program. *Degree requirements:* For master's, comprehensive exam, thesis (for some programs), 30-36 credits, thesis presentation; for doctorate, comprehensive exam, thesis/dissertation, residency, responsible scholarship and research skills, final exam, dissertation defense. *Entrance requirements:* For master's, GRE General Test, bachelor's degree with minimum undergraduate GPA of 3.0; for doctorate, GRE General Test, bachelor's degree; minimum undergraduate/graduate GPA of 3.0. Additional exam requirements/recommendations for international students: Required—TOEFL or IELTS. *Application deadline:* For fall admission, 12/1 for domestic and international students; for spring admission, 9/15 for domestic and international students. Application fee: $55 ($65 for international students). Electronic applications accepted. *Financial support:* In 2013–14, 8 fellowships with full and partial tuition reimbursements, 22 research assistantships with full and partial tuition reimbursements, 32 teaching assistantships with full and partial tuition reimbursements were awarded; scholarships/grants, traineeships, health care benefits, and unspecified assistantships also available. Financial award application deadline: 12/1. *Faculty research:* Ecology and global change, diversity and macroevolution, evolutionary mechanisms, systematics/phylogenetics, biogeography. *Unit head:* Dr. Christopher H. Haufler, Chair, 785-864-3255, Fax: 785-864-5860, E-mail: vulgare@ku.edu. *Application contact:* Aagje Ashe, Graduate Coordinator, 785-864-2362, Fax: 785-864-5860, E-mail: a4ashe@ku.edu.
Website: http://eeb.ku.edu/

University of Louisiana at Lafayette, College of Sciences, Department of Biology, Lafayette, LA 70504. Offers biology (MS); environmental and evolutionary biology (PhD). Terminal master's awarded for partial completion of doctoral program. *Degree requirements:* For master's, thesis; for doctorate, 2 foreign languages, comprehensive exam, thesis/dissertation. *Entrance requirements:* For master's, GRE General Test, minimum GPA of 2.75; for doctorate, GRE General Test, GRE Subject Test, minimum GPA of 3.0. Additional exam requirements/recommendations for international students: Required—TOEFL (minimum score 550 paper-based). Electronic applications accepted. *Faculty research:* Structure and ultrastructure, system biology, ecology, processes, environmental physiology.

The University of Manchester, Faculty of Life Sciences, Manchester, United Kingdom. Offers adaptive organismal biology (M Phil, PhD); animal biology (M Phil, PhD); biochemistry (M Phil, PhD); bioinformatics (M Phil, PhD); biomolecular sciences (M Phil, PhD); biotechnology (M Phil, PhD); cell biology (M Phil, PhD); cell matrix research (M Phil, PhD); channels and transporters (M Phil, PhD); developmental biology (M Phil, PhD); Egyptology (M Phil, PhD); environmental biology (M Phil, PhD); evolutionary biology (M Phil, PhD); gene expression (M Phil, PhD); genetics (M Phil, PhD); history of science, technology and medicine (M Phil, PhD); immunology (M Phil, PhD); integrative neurobiology and behavior (M Phil, PhD); membrane trafficking (M Phil, PhD); microbiology (M Phil, PhD); molecular and cellular neuroscience (M Phil, PhD); molecular biology (M Phil, PhD); molecular cancer studies (M Phil, PhD); neuroscience (M Phil, PhD); ophthalmology (M Phil, PhD); optometry (M Phil, PhD); organelle function (M Phil, PhD); pharmacology (M Phil, PhD); physiology (M Phil, PhD); plant sciences (M Phil, PhD); stem cell research (M Phil, PhD); structural biology (M Phil, PhD); systems neuroscience (M Phil, PhD); toxicology (M Phil, PhD).

University of Maryland, College Park, Academic Affairs, College of Computer, Mathematical and Natural Sciences, Department of Biology, Behavior, Ecology, Evolution, and Systematics Program, College Park, MD 20742. Offers MS, PhD. *Students:* 7 full-time (3 women), 2 part-time (1 woman); includes 2 minority (1 Asian, non-Hispanic/Latino; 1 Two or more races, non-Hispanic/Latino), 1 international. In 2013, 4 doctorates awarded. *Degree requirements:* For master's, thesis, oral defense, seminar; for doctorate, thesis/dissertation, exam, 4 seminars. *Entrance requirements:* For master's and doctorate, GRE General Test, GRE Subject Test (biology), 3 letters of recommendation. Additional exam requirements/recommendations for international students: Required—TOEFL. *Expenses:* Tuition, state resident: full-time $10,314; part-time $573 per credit hour. Tuition, nonresident: full-time $22,248; part-time $1236 per credit. *Required fees:* $1446; $403.15 per semester. Tuition and fees vary according to program. *Financial support:* In 2013–14, 3 fellowships with full tuition reimbursements (averaging $62,679 per year), 1 research assistantship (averaging $19,685 per year), 5 teaching assistantships (averaging $19,775 per year) were awarded; Federal Work-Study and scholarships/grants also available. Support available to part-time students. Financial award applicants required to submit FAFSA. *Faculty research:* Animal behavior, biostatistics, ecology, evolution, neurothology. *Unit head:* David Hawthorne, Graduate Director, 301-405-4552, E-mail: djh@umd.edu. *Application contact:* Dr. Charles A. Caramello, Dean of Graduate School, 301-405-0358, Fax: 301-314-9305, E-mail: ccaramel@umd.edu.

University of Maryland, College Park, Academic Affairs, College of Computer, Mathematical and Natural Sciences, Department of Biology, PhD Program in Biological Sciences, College Park, MD 20742. Offers behavior, ecology, evolution, and systematics (PhD); computational biology, bioinformatics, and genomics (PhD); molecular and cellular biology (PhD); physiological systems (PhD). *Students:* 104 full-time (59 women), 4 part-time (1 woman); includes 21 minority (2 Black or African American, non-Hispanic/Latino; 1 American Indian or Alaska Native, non-Hispanic/Latino; 9 Asian, non-Hispanic/Latino; 7 Hispanic/Latino; 2 Two or more races, non-Hispanic/Latino), 34 international. 365 applicants, 13% accepted, 20 enrolled. In 2013, 5 doctorates awarded. *Degree requirements:* For doctorate, comprehensive exam, thesis/dissertation, thesis work presentation in seminar. *Entrance requirements:* For doctorate, GRE General Test; GRE Subject Test in biology (recommended), academic transcripts, statement of purpose/research interests, 3 letters of recommendation. Additional exam requirements/recommendations for international students: Required—TOEFL. *Application deadline:* For fall admission, 12/15 for domestic and international students. Applications are processed on a rolling basis. Application fee: $75. Electronic applications accepted. *Expenses:* Tuition, state resident: full-time $10,314; part-time $573 per credit hour. Tuition, nonresident: full-time $22,248; part-time $1236 per credit. *Required fees:* $1446; $403.15 per semester. Tuition and fees vary according to program. *Financial support:* In 2013–14, 21 fellowships with full and partial tuition reimbursements (averaging $27,603 per year), 25 research assistantships (averaging $19,557 per year), 55 teaching assistantships (averaging $18,959 per year) were awarded. *Unit head:* Dr. Charles F. Delwiche, Director, 301-405-6884, E-mail: bisidirector@umd.edu. *Application contact:* Dr. Charles A. Caramello, Dean of Graduate School, 301-405-0358, Fax: 301-314-9305, E-mail: ccaramel@umd.edu.
Website: http://www.bisi.umd.edu/

University of Massachusetts Amherst, Graduate School, Interdisciplinary Programs, Program in Organismic and Evolutionary Biology, Amherst, MA 01003. Offers MS, PhD. Part-time programs available. *Students:* 33 full-time (15 women), 2 part-time (1 woman); includes 4 minority (3 Hispanic/Latino; 1 Two or more races, non-Hispanic/Latino), 5 international. Average age 29. 40 applicants, 30% accepted, 8 enrolled. In 2013, 7 master's awarded. Terminal master's awarded for partial completion of doctoral program. *Degree requirements:* For master's, thesis or alternative; for doctorate, comprehensive exam, thesis/dissertation. *Entrance requirements:* For master's and doctorate, GRE General Test, 3 letters of recommendation. Additional exam requirements/recommendations for international students: Required—TOEFL (minimum score 550 paper-based; 80 iBT), IELTS (minimum score 6.5). *Application deadline:* For fall admission, 12/1 for domestic and international students. Applications are processed on a rolling basis. Application fee: $75. Electronic applications accepted. *Financial support:* Fellowships with full and partial tuition reimbursements, research assistantships with full and partial tuition reimbursements, teaching assistantships with full and partial tuition reimbursements, career-related internships or fieldwork, Federal Work-Study, scholarships/grants, traineeships, health care benefits, tuition waivers (full and partial), and unspecified assistantships available. Support available to part-time students. Financial award application deadline: 12/1; financial award applicants required to submit FAFSA. *Unit head:* Dr. Jeffrey E. Podos, Graduate Program Director, 413-545-0928, Fax: 413-545-3243, E-mail: oeb@bio.umass.edu. *Application contact:* Lindsay DeSantis, Supervisor of Admissions, 413-545-0722, Fax: 413-577-0010, E-mail: gradadm@grad.umass.edu.
Website: http://www.bio.umass.edu/oeb/

University of Massachusetts Amherst, Graduate School, Interdisciplinary Programs, Program in Plant Biology, Amherst, MA 01003. Offers biochemistry and metabolism (MS, PhD); cell biology and physiology (MS, PhD); environmental, ecological and

integrative biology (MS, PhD); genetics and evolution (MS, PhD). *Students:* 20 full-time (11 women), 9 international. Average age 28. 72 applicants, 17% accepted, 2 enrolled. In 2013, 1 master's, 2 doctorates awarded. *Degree requirements:* For master's, thesis; for doctorate, 2 foreign languages, comprehensive exam, thesis/dissertation. *Entrance requirements:* For master's and doctorate, GRE General Test. Additional exam requirements/recommendations for international students: Required—TOEFL (minimum score 550 paper-based; 80 iBT), IELTS (minimum score 6.5). *Application deadline:* For fall admission, 12/15 for domestic and international students; for spring admission, 10/1 for domestic and international students. Applications are processed on a rolling basis. Application fee: $75. Electronic applications accepted. *Financial support:* Fellowships with full and partial tuition reimbursements, research assistantships with full and partial tuition reimbursements, teaching assistantships with full and partial tuition reimbursements, career-related internships or fieldwork, Federal Work-Study, scholarships/grants, traineeships, health care benefits, tuition waivers (full and partial), and unspecified assistantships available. Support available to part-time students. Financial award application deadline: 12/15; financial award applicants required to submit FAFSA. *Unit head:* Dr. Elsbeth L. Walker, Graduate Program Director, 413-577-3217, Fax: 413-545-3243, E-mail: pb@bio.umass.edu. *Application contact:* Lindsay DeSantis, Supervisor of Admissions, 413-545-0722, Fax: 413-577-0010, E-mail: gradadm@grad.umass.edu.
Website: http://www.bio.umass.edu/plantbio/

University of Miami, Graduate School, College of Arts and Sciences, Department of Biology, Coral Gables, FL 33124. Offers biology (MS, PhD); genetics and evolution (MS, PhD). Terminal master's awarded for partial completion of doctoral program. *Degree requirements:* For master's, comprehensive exam (for some programs), thesis (for some programs); for doctorate, thesis/dissertation, oral and written qualifying exam. *Entrance requirements:* For master's, GRE General Test, 3 letters of recommendation, research papers; for doctorate, GRE General Test, 3 letters of recommendation, research papers, sponsor letter. Additional exam requirements/recommendations for international students: Required—TOEFL (minimum score 550 paper-based; 59 iBT). Electronic applications accepted. *Faculty research:* Neuroscience to ethology; plants, vertebrates and mycorrhizae; phylogenies, life histories and species interactions; molecular biology, gene expression and populations; cells, auditory neurons and vertebrate locomotion.

University of Michigan, Rackham Graduate School, College of Literature, Science, and the Arts, Department of Ecology and Evolutionary Biology, Ann Arbor, MI 48109. Offers MS, PhD. Part-time programs available. Terminal master's awarded for partial completion of doctoral program. *Degree requirements:* For master's, thesis (for some programs), two seminars; for doctorate, comprehensive exam, thesis/dissertation, 2 semesters of teaching. *Entrance requirements:* For master's and doctorate, GRE. Additional exam requirements/recommendations for international students: Required—TOEFL (minimum score 560 paper-based; 84 iBT). Electronic applications accepted. Tuition and fees vary according to course level, course load, degree level, program and student level. *Faculty research:* Population and community ecology, ecosystem ecology and biogeochemistry, global change biology, biogeography and paleobiology, evolution of behavior, evolutionary genetics, phylogenetic and phylogeography, ecology and evolution of infectious disease.

University of Minnesota, Twin Cities Campus, Graduate School, College of Biological Sciences, Department of Ecology, Evolution, and Behavior, St. Paul, MN 55418. Offers MS, PhD. Terminal master's awarded for partial completion of doctoral program. *Degree requirements:* For master's, comprehensive exam, thesis or projects; for doctorate, comprehensive exam, thesis/dissertation. *Entrance requirements:* For master's and doctorate, GRE General Test, minimum GPA of 3.0. Additional exam requirements/recommendations for international students: Required—TOEFL (minimum score 550 paper-based; 79 iBT), Michigan English Language Assessment Battery. Electronic applications accepted. *Faculty research:* Behavioral ecology, community ecology, community genetics, ecosystem and global change, evolution and systematics.

University of Missouri, Graduate School, College of Arts and Science, Division of Biological Sciences, Columbia, MO 65211. Offers evolutionary biology and ecology (MA, PhD); genetic, cellular and developmental biology (MA, PhD); neurobiology and behavior (MA, PhD). *Faculty:* 40 full-time (11 women), 1 part-time/adjunct (0 women). *Students:* 70 full-time (32 women), 3 part-time (2 women); includes 12 minority (4 Black or African American, non-Hispanic/Latino; 1 American Indian or Alaska Native, non-Hispanic/Latino; 2 Asian, non-Hispanic/Latino; 3 Hispanic/Latino; 2 Two or more races, non-Hispanic/Latino), 5 international. Average age 28. 46 applicants, 28% accepted, 13 enrolled. In 2013, 7 master's, 13 doctorates awarded. Terminal master's awarded for partial completion of doctoral program. *Degree requirements:* For master's, thesis; for doctorate, comprehensive exam, thesis/dissertation. *Entrance requirements:* For master's and doctorate, GRE General Test (minimum score 1200 verbal and quantitative), minimum GPA of 3.0. Additional exam requirements/recommendations for international students: Required—TOEFL (minimum score 600 paper-based; 100 iBT). *Application deadline:* For fall admission, 12/15 priority date for domestic and international students. Applications are processed on a rolling basis. Application fee: $55 ($75 for international students). Electronic applications accepted. *Financial support:* Fellowships with full tuition reimbursements, research assistantships with full tuition reimbursements, teaching assistantships with full tuition reimbursements, institutionally sponsored loans, traineeships, health care benefits, and unspecified assistantships available. *Faculty research:* Evolutionary biology, ecology and behavior; genetic, cellular, molecular and developmental biology; neurobiology and behavior; plant sciences. *Unit head:* Dr. John C. Walker, Division Director, 573-882-3583, E-mail: walkerj@missouri.edu. *Application contact:* Nila Emerich, Application Contact, 800-553-5698, E-mail: emerichn@missouri.edu.
Website: http://biology.missouri.edu/graduate-studies/

University of Missouri–St. Louis, College of Arts and Sciences, Department of Biology, St. Louis, MO 63121. Offers biotechnology (Certificate); cell and molecular biology (MS, PhD); ecology, evolution and systematics (MS, PhD); tropical biology and conservation (Certificate). Part-time programs available. *Faculty:* 33 full-time (13 women), 9 part-time/adjunct (1 woman). *Students:* 52 full-time (23 women), 58 part-time (29 women); includes 13 minority (9 Black or African American, non-Hispanic/Latino; 3 Asian, non-Hispanic/Latino; 1 Hispanic/Latino), 30 international. Average age 28. 113 applicants, 42% accepted, 22 enrolled. In 2013, 31 master's, 5 doctorates, 4 other advanced degrees awarded. *Degree requirements:* For master's, thesis or alternative; for doctorate, thesis/dissertation, 1 semester of teaching experience. *Entrance requirements:* For master's, 3 letters of recommendation; for doctorate, GRE General Test, 3 letters of recommendation. Additional exam requirements/recommendations for international students: Required—TOEFL (minimum score 79 iBT), IELTS (minimum score 6.5). *Application deadline:* For fall admission, 12/15 priority date for domestic and international students; for spring admission, 12/1 priority date for domestic and international students. Applications are processed on a rolling basis. Application fee: $50 ($40 for international students). Electronic applications accepted. *Expenses:* Tuition, state resident: full-time $7364; part-time $409.10 per credit hour. Tuition, nonresident: full-time $19,162; part-time $1008.50 per credit hour. *Financial support:* In 2013–14, 13 research assistantships with full and partial tuition reimbursements (averaging $17,000 per year), 23 teaching assistantships with full and partial tuition reimbursements (averaging $17,000 per year) were awarded; fellowships with full tuition reimbursements, career-related internships or fieldwork, and Federal Work-Study also available. Support available to part-time students. Financial award application deadline: 2/1. *Faculty research:* Molecular biology, microbial genetics, animal behavior, tropical ecology, plant systematics. *Unit head:* Dr. Teresa Thiel, Director of Graduate Studies, 314-516-6200, Fax: 314-516-6233, E-mail: thiel@umsl.edu. *Application contact:* 314-516-5458, Fax: 314-516-6996, E-mail: gradadm@umsl.edu.
Website: http://www.umsl.edu/divisions/artscience/biology/

University of Nevada, Reno, Graduate School, Interdisciplinary Program in Ecology, Evolution, and Conservation Biology, Reno, NV 89557. Offers PhD. Offered through the College of Arts and Science, the M. C. Fleischmann College of Agriculture, and the Desert Research Institute. *Degree requirements:* For doctorate, thesis/dissertation. *Entrance requirements:* For doctorate, GRE General Test, GRE Subject Test, minimum GPA of 3.0. Additional exam requirements/recommendations for international students: Required—TOEFL (minimum score 500 paper-based; 61 iBT), IELTS (minimum score 6). Electronic applications accepted. *Faculty research:* Population biology, behavioral ecology, plant response to climate change, conservation of endangered species, restoration of natural ecosystems.

The University of North Carolina at Chapel Hill, Graduate School, College of Arts and Sciences, Department of Biology, Chapel Hill, NC 27599. Offers botany (MA, MS, PhD); cell biology, development, and physiology (MA, MS, PhD); cell motility and cytoskeleton (PhD); ecology and behavior (MA, MS, PhD); genetics and molecular biology (MA, MS, PhD); morphology, systematics, and evolution (MA, MS, PhD). Terminal master's awarded for partial completion of doctoral program. *Degree requirements:* For master's, comprehensive exam, thesis (for some programs); for doctorate, comprehensive exam, thesis/dissertation. *Entrance requirements:* For master's, GRE General Test, GRE Subject Test, 2 semesters of calculus or statistics; 2 semesters of physics, organic chemistry; 3 semesters of biology; for doctorate, GRE General Test, GRE Subject Test, 2 semesters calculus or statistics, 2 semesters physics, organic chemistry, 3 semesters of biology. Additional exam requirements/recommendations for international students: Required—TOEFL (minimum score 550 paper-based). Electronic applications accepted. *Faculty research:* Gene expression, biomechanics, yeast genetics, plant ecology, plant molecular biology.

University of Notre Dame, Graduate School, College of Science, Department of Biological Sciences, Notre Dame, IN 46556. Offers aquatic ecology, evolution and environmental biology (MS, PhD); cellular and molecular biology (MS, PhD); genetics (MS, PhD); physiology (MS, PhD); vector biology and parasitology (MS, PhD). Terminal master's awarded for partial completion of doctoral program. *Degree requirements:* For master's, comprehensive exam, thesis; for doctorate, comprehensive exam, thesis/dissertation, candidacy exam. *Entrance requirements:* For master's and doctorate, GRE General Test. Additional exam requirements/recommendations for international students: Required—TOEFL (minimum score 600 paper-based; 80 iBT). Electronic applications accepted. *Faculty research:* Tropical disease, molecular genetics, neurobiology, evolutionary biology, aquatic biology.

University of Oklahoma, College of Arts and Sciences, Department of Biology, Program in Ecology and Evolutionary Biology, Norman, OK 73019. Offers PhD. *Students:* 10 full-time (6 women), 12 part-time (7 women); includes 1 minority (Hispanic/Latino), 4 international. Average age 29. 6 applicants, 33% accepted, 2 enrolled. In 2013, 2 doctorates awarded. *Entrance requirements:* Additional exam requirements/recommendations for international students: Required—TOEFL (minimum score 79 iBT). *Application deadline:* For fall admission, 12/15 for domestic and international students. Application fee: $50 ($100 for international students). Electronic applications accepted. *Expenses:* Tuition, state resident: full-time $4205; part-time $175.20 per credit hour. Tuition, nonresident: full-time $16,205; part-time $675.20 per credit hour. *Required fees:* $2745; $103.85 per credit hour. $126.50 per semester. *Financial support:* In 2013–14, 22 students received support. Career-related internships or fieldwork, scholarships/grants, health care benefits, tuition waivers (partial), and unspecified assistantships available. Financial award application deadline: 6/1; financial award applicants required to submit FAFSA. *Faculty research:* Behavioral ecology, community ecology, evolutionary biology, macroecology, physiological ecology. *Unit head:* Dr. Michael Kaspari, Director, 405-325-4821, Fax: 405-325-6202, E-mail: mkaspari@ou.edu. *Application contact:* Dr. Rosemary Knapp, Director, 405-325-4389, Fax: 405-325-6202, E-mail: biologygrad@ou.edu.
Website: http://www.ou.edu/eeb

University of Oklahoma, College of Arts and Sciences, Department of Microbiology and Plant Biology, Program in Ecology and Evolutionary Biology, Norman, OK 73019. Offers PhD. *Students:* 5 full-time (1 woman), 4 part-time (0 women), 8 international. Average age 29. 6 applicants, 50% accepted, 2 enrolled. *Entrance requirements:* Additional exam requirements/recommendations for international students: Required—TOEFL (minimum score 79 iBT). *Application deadline:* For fall admission, 4/1 for domestic and international students; for spring admission, 9/1 for domestic and international students. Application fee: $50 ($100 for international students). Electronic applications accepted. *Expenses:* Tuition, state resident: full-time $4205; part-time $175.20 per credit hour. Tuition, nonresident: full-time $16,205; part-time $675.20 per credit hour. *Required fees:* $2745; $103.85 per credit hour. $126.50 per semester. *Financial support:* In 2013–14, 7 students received support. Scholarships/grants, health care benefits, tuition waivers (partial), and unspecified assistantships available. Financial award application deadline: 6/1; financial award applicants required to submit FAFSA. *Faculty research:* Behavioral ecology, community ecology, evolutionary biology, macroecology, physiological ecology. *Unit head:* Dr. Gordon Uno, Professor/Department Chair, 405-325-4321, Fax: 405-325-7619, E-mail: guno@ou.edu. *Application contact:* Adell Hopper, Staff Assistant, 405-325-4321, Fax: 405-325-7619, E-mail: ahopper@ou.edu.
Website: http://mpbio.ou.edu/

University of Oregon, Graduate School, College of Arts and Sciences, Department of Biology, Eugene, OR 97403. Offers ecology and evolution (MA, MS, PhD); marine biology (MA, MS, PhD); molecular, cellular and genetic biology (PhD); neuroscience and development (PhD). Terminal master's awarded for partial completion of doctoral program. *Degree requirements:* For master's, thesis (for some programs); for doctorate, thesis/dissertation. *Entrance requirements:* For master's and doctorate, GRE General Test, minimum GPA of 3.2. Additional exam requirements/recommendations for international students: Required—TOEFL. *Faculty research:* Developmental neurobiology; evolution, population biology, and quantitative genetics; regulation of gene expression; biochemistry of marine organisms.

University of Pittsburgh, Dietrich School of Arts and Sciences, Department of Biological Sciences, Program in Ecology and Evolution, Pittsburgh, PA 15260. Offers PhD. *Faculty:* 6 full-time (2 women). *Students:* 23 full-time (8 women); includes 4 minority (1 Black or African American, non-Hispanic/Latino; 1 American Indian or Alaska Native, non-Hispanic/Latino; 1 Asian, non-Hispanic/Latino; 1 Hispanic/Latino), 1 international. Average age 23. 34 applicants, 21% accepted, 6 enrolled. In 2013, 4 doctorates awarded. *Degree requirements:* For doctorate, comprehensive exam, thesis/dissertation, completion of research integrity module. *Entrance requirements:* For doctorate, GRE General Test, GRE Subject Test. Additional exam requirements/

recommendations for international students: Required—TOEFL (minimum score 90 iBT). *Application deadline:* For fall admission, 1/3 priority date for domestic students, 12/9 priority date for international students. Applications are processed on a rolling basis. Application fee: $0 ($50 for international students). Electronic applications accepted. *Expenses:* Tuition, state resident: full-time $19,964; part-time $807 per credit. Tuition, nonresident: full-time $32,686; part-time $1337 per credit. *Required fees:* $740; $200. Tuition and fees vary according to program. *Financial support:* In 2013–14, 28 fellowships with full tuition reimbursements (averaging $30,682 per year), 14 research assistantships with full tuition reimbursements (averaging $26,775 per year), 20 teaching assistantships with full tuition reimbursements (averaging $25,610 per year) were awarded; Federal Work-Study, scholarships/grants, traineeships, health care benefits, and tuition waivers (full) also available. *Unit head:* Dr. Jeffrey G. Lawrence, Professor, 412-624-4204, Fax: 412-624-4759, E-mail: jlawrenc@pitt.edu. *Application contact:* Cathleen M. Barr, Graduate Administrator, 412-624-4268, Fax: 412-624-4759, E-mail: cbarr@pitt.edu.
Website: http://www.biology.pitt.edu/graduate/e-e-program

University of Puerto Rico, Río Piedras Campus, College of Natural Sciences, Department of Biology, San Juan, PR 00931-3300. Offers ecology/systematics (MS, PhD); evolution/genetics (MS, PhD); molecular/cellular biology (MS, PhD); neuroscience (MS, PhD). Part-time programs available. *Degree requirements:* For master's, one foreign language, comprehensive exam, thesis; for doctorate, one foreign language, comprehensive exam, thesis/dissertation. *Entrance requirements:* For master's, GRE Subject Test, interview, minimum GPA of 3.0, letter of recommendation; for doctorate, GRE Subject Test, interview, master's degree, minimum GPA of 3.0, letter of recommendation. *Faculty research:* Environmental, poblational and systematic biology.

University of South Carolina, The Graduate School, College of Arts and Sciences, Department of Biological Sciences, Graduate Training Program in Ecology, Evolution, and Organismal Biology, Columbia, SC 29208. Offers MS, PhD. *Degree requirements:* For master's, one foreign language, comprehensive exam, thesis; for doctorate, one foreign language, comprehensive exam, thesis/dissertation. *Entrance requirements:* For master's and doctorate, GRE General Test, minimum GPA of 3.0 in science. Additional exam requirements/recommendations for international students: Required—TOEFL (minimum score 570 paper-based). Electronic applications accepted.

University of Southern California, Graduate School, Dana and David Dornsife College of Letters, Arts and Sciences, Department of Biological Sciences, Program in Integrative and Evolutionary Biology, Los Angeles, CA 90089. Offers PhD. M.S. in Biology is a terminal degree only. Terminal master's awarded for partial completion of doctoral program. *Degree requirements:* For doctorate, comprehensive exam, thesis/dissertation, qualifying examination, dissertation defense. *Entrance requirements:* For doctorate, GRE, 3 letters of recommendation, personal statement, resume, minimum GPA of 3.0. Additional exam requirements/recommendations for international students: Required—TOEFL (minimum score 600 paper-based; 100 iBT). Electronic applications accepted. *Faculty research:* Organisms and their interaction with the environment, evolution and life history, integration of the control and dynamics of physiological processes, biomechanics and rehabilitation engineering, primate behavior and ecology.

University of South Florida, College of Arts and Sciences, Department of Integrative Biology, Tampa, FL 33620-9951. Offers biology (MS), including ecology and evolution (MS, PhD), environmental and ecological microbiology (MS, PhD), physiology and morphology (MS, PhD); integrative biology (PhD), including ecology and evolution (MS, PhD), environmental and ecological microbiology (MS, PhD), physiology and morphology (MS, PhD). Part-time programs available. *Faculty:* 16 full-time (4 women), 1 part-time/adjunct (0 women). *Students:* 40 full-time (24 women), 7 part-time (4 women); includes 6 minority (5 Hispanic/Latino; 1 Two or more races, non-Hispanic/Latino), 3 international. Average age 29. 59 applicants, 29% accepted, 11 enrolled. In 2013, 4 master's, 5 doctorates awarded. *Degree requirements:* For master's, comprehensive exam, thesis (for some programs); for doctorate, comprehensive exam, thesis/dissertation. *Entrance requirements:* For master's and doctorate, GRE General Test (minimum preferred scores of 153 verbal, 148 quantitative, 4.5 analytical/500 verbal and 600 quantitative with 4.5 in analytical writing on old scoring), minimum GPA of 3.0 in last 60 hours of BS. Additional exam requirements/recommendations for international students: Required—TOEFL (minimum score 570 paper-based; 88 iBT). *Application deadline:* For fall admission, 2/15 priority date for domestic students, 1/2 for international students; for spring admission, 8/1 for domestic students, 6/1 for international students. Application fee: $30. Electronic applications accepted. *Financial support:* Research assistantships, teaching assistantships, and unspecified assistantships available. Financial award application deadline: 6/30; financial award applicants required to submit FAFSA. *Faculty research:* Marine ecology, ecosystem responses to urbanization, biomechanical and physiological mechanisms of animal movement, population biology and conservation, microbial ecology and public health microbiology, natural diversity of parasites and herbivores; ecosystems, vertebrates, disturbance ecology, functional and ecological morphology of feeding in fishes, rare amphibians and reptiles, genomics in ecological experiments, ecotoxicology, global carbon cycle, plant-animal interactions. *Total annual research expenditures:* $968,227. *Unit head:* Dr. Peter Stiling, Chair, Department of Integrative Biology, 813-974-6229, Fax: 813-974-3263, E-mail: pstiling@usf.edu. *Application contact:* Christine Brubaker, Graduate Program Specialist, Department of Integrative Biology, 813-974-4747, Fax: 813-974-3263, E-mail: brubaker@usf.edu.
Website: http://biology.usf.edu/ib/grad/

The University of Tennessee, Graduate School, College of Arts and Sciences, Department of Ecology and Evolutionary Biology, Knoxville, TN 37996. Offers behavior (MS, PhD); ecology (MS, PhD); evolutionary biology (MS, PhD). Part-time programs available. *Degree requirements:* For master's, thesis; for doctorate, thesis/dissertation. *Entrance requirements:* For master's and doctorate, GRE General Test, minimum GPA of 2.7. Additional exam requirements/recommendations for international students: Required—TOEFL. Electronic applications accepted. *Expenses:* Tuition, state resident: full-time $9540; part-time $531 per credit hour. Tuition, nonresident: full-time $27,728; part-time $1542 per credit hour. *Required fees:* $1404; $67 per credit hour.

The University of Texas at Austin, Graduate School, College of Natural Sciences, School of Biological Sciences, Program in Ecology, Evolution and Behavior, Austin, TX 78712-1111. Offers PhD. *Entrance requirements:* For doctorate, GRE General Test. Additional exam requirements/recommendations for international students: Required—TOEFL. Electronic applications accepted.

University of Toronto, School of Graduate Studies, Faculty of Arts and Science, Department of Ecology and Evolutionary Biology, Toronto, ON M5S 1A1, Canada. Offers M Sc, PhD. *Degree requirements:* For master's, thesis, thesis defense; for doctorate, thesis/dissertation, thesis defense. *Entrance requirements:* For master's, minimum B average in last 2 years; knowledge of physics, chemistry, and biology. Additional exam requirements/recommendations for international students: Required—TOEFL (minimum score 580 paper-based; 93 iBT), TWE (minimum score 5). Electronic applications accepted.

Washington University in St. Louis, Graduate School of Arts and Sciences, Division of Biology and Biomedical Sciences, Program in Evolution, Ecology and Population Biology, St. Louis, MO 63130-4899. Offers ecology (PhD); environmental biology (PhD); evolutionary biology (PhD); genetics (PhD). *Degree requirements:* For doctorate, thesis/dissertation. *Entrance requirements:* For doctorate, GRE General Test, GRE Subject Test. Electronic applications accepted.

Wayne State University, College of Liberal Arts and Sciences, Department of Biological Sciences, Detroit, MI 48202. Offers biological sciences (MA, MS); cell development and neurobiology (PhD); evolution and organismal biology (PhD); molecular biology and biotechnology (PhD); molecular biotechnology (MS). Fall application deadline for PhD is December 1. *Faculty:* 26 full-time (9 women). *Students:* 66 full-time (37 women), 8 part-time (3 women); includes 8 minority (1 Black or African American, non-Hispanic/Latino; 5 Asian, non-Hispanic/Latino; 1 Hispanic/Latino; 1 Two or more races, non-Hispanic/Latino), 41 international. Average age 29. 270 applicants, 14% accepted, 14 enrolled. In 2013, 14 master's, 8 doctorates awarded. Terminal master's awarded for partial completion of doctoral program. *Degree requirements:* For master's, thesis (for some programs); for doctorate, thesis/dissertation. *Entrance requirements:* For master's, GRE (for MS applicants), minimum GPA of 3.0; adequate preparation in biological sciences and supporting courses in chemistry, physics and mathematics; curriculum vitae; for doctorate, GRE, three letters of reference, statement of goals and career objectives, bachelor's or master's degree in biological or other science. Additional exam requirements/recommendations for international students: Required—TOEFL (minimum score 550 paper-based; 79 iBT), TWE (minimum score 5.5), Michigan English Language Assessment Battery (minimum score 85); Recommended—IELTS (minimum score 6.5). *Application deadline:* For fall admission, 4/1 for domestic students, 3/1 for international students. Applications are processed on a rolling basis. Application fee: $0. Electronic applications accepted. *Expenses:* Tuition, state resident: part-time $554.15 per credit. Tuition, nonresident: part-time $1200.35 per credit. *Required fees:* $42.15 per credit. $268.30 per semester. Tuition and fees vary according to course load and program. *Financial support:* In 2013–14, 55 students received support, including 3 fellowships with tuition reimbursements available (averaging $16,842 per year), 9 research assistantships with tuition reimbursements available (averaging $18,582 per year), 49 teaching assistantships with tuition reimbursements available (averaging $18,488 per year); institutionally sponsored loans, scholarships/grants, health care benefits, and unspecified assistantships also available. Financial award application deadline: 3/31; financial award applicants required to submit FAFSA. *Faculty research:* Transcription and chromatin remodeling, genomic and developmental evolution, community and landscape ecology and environmental degradation, microbiology and virology, cell and neurobiology. *Total annual research expenditures:* $1.7 million. *Unit head:* Dr. David Njus, Professor and Chair, 313-577-2783, Fax: 313-577-6891, E-mail: dnjus@wayne.edu. *Application contact:* Rose Mary Priest, Office Services Clerk, 313-577-6818, Fax: 313-577-6891, E-mail: rpriest@wayne.edu.
Website: http://clasweb.clas.wayne.edu/biology

Wesleyan University, Graduate Studies, Department of Biology, Middletown, CT 06459. Offers cell and developmental genetics (PhD); evolution and ecology (PhD); neurobiology and behavior (PhD). *Degree requirements:* For doctorate, variable foreign language requirement, thesis/dissertation. *Entrance requirements:* For doctorate, GRE. Additional exam requirements/recommendations for international students: Required—TOEFL. *Faculty research:* Microbial population genetics, genetic basis of evolutionary adaptation, genetic regulation of differentiation and pattern formation in &ITdrosophila&RO.

West Virginia University, Eberly College of Arts and Sciences, Department of Biology, Morgantown, WV 26506. Offers cell and molecular biology (MS, PhD); environmental and evolutionary biology (MS, PhD); forensic biology (MS, PhD); genomic biology (MS, PhD); neurobiology (MS, PhD). Terminal master's awarded for partial completion of doctoral program. *Degree requirements:* For master's, thesis, final exam; for doctorate, thesis/dissertation, preliminary and final exams. *Entrance requirements:* For master's, GRE General Test, GRE Subject Test, minimum GPA of 3.0; for doctorate, GRE General Test, minimum GPA of 3.0. Additional exam requirements/recommendations for international students: Required—TOEFL. *Faculty research:* Environmental biology, genetic engineering, developmental biology, global change, biodiversity.

Yale University, Graduate School of Arts and Sciences, Department of Ecology and Evolutionary Biology, New Haven, CT 06520. Offers PhD. *Entrance requirements:* For doctorate, GRE General Test, GRE Subject Test (biology).

Section 9
Entomology

This section contains a directory of institutions offering graduate work in entomology. Additional information about programs listed in the directory may be obtained by writing directly to the dean of a graduate school or chair of a department at the address given in the directory.

For programs offering related work, see also in this book *Biochemistry; Biological and Biomedical Sciences; Botany and Plant Biology; Ecology, Environmental Biology, and Evolutionary Biology; Genetics, Developmental Biology, and Reproductive Biology; Microbiological Sciences; Physiology;* and *Zoology*. In the other guides in this series:

Graduate Programs in the Humanities, Arts & Social Sciences
See *Economics (Agricultural Economics and Agribusiness)*

Graduate Programs in the Physical Sciences, Mathematics, Agricultural Sciences, the Environment & Natural Resources
See *Agricultural and Food Sciences* and *Environmental Sciences and Management*

Graduate Programs in Engineering & Applied Sciences
See *Agricultural Engineering* and *Bioengineering*

CONTENTS

Entomology

Auburn University, Graduate School, College of Agriculture, Department of Entomology and Plant Pathology, Auburn University, AL 36849. Offers entomology (M Ag, MS, PhD); plant pathology (M Ag, MS, PhD). Part-time programs available. *Faculty:* 15 full-time (5 women). *Students:* 25 full-time (10 women), 8 part-time (3 women), 18 international. Average age 29. 23 applicants, 30% accepted, 7 enrolled. In 2013, 5 master's, 4 doctorates awarded. *Degree requirements:* For master's, thesis (for some programs); for doctorate, one foreign language, thesis/dissertation. *Entrance requirements:* For master's, GRE General Test; for doctorate, GRE General Test, GRE Subject Test, master's degree with thesis. *Application deadline:* For fall admission, 7/7 for domestic students; for spring admission, 11/24 for domestic students. Applications are processed on a rolling basis. Application fee: $50 ($60 for international students). Electronic applications accepted. *Expenses:* Tuition, state resident: full-time $8262; part-time $459 per credit hour. Tuition, nonresident: full-time $24,786; part-time $1377 per credit hour. Tuition and fees vary according to degree level and program. *Financial support:* Research assistantships, teaching assistantships, and Federal Work-Study available. Support available to part-time students. Financial award application deadline: 3/15; financial award applicants required to submit FAFSA. *Faculty research:* Pest management, biological control, systematics, medical entomology. *Unit head:* Dr. Arthur Appel, Chair, 334-844-5006. *Application contact:* Dr. George Flowers, Dean of the Graduate School, 334-844-2125.

Clemson University, Graduate School, College of Agriculture, Forestry and Life Sciences, School of Agricultural, Forest, and Environmental Sciences, Program in Entomology, Clemson, SC 29634. Offers MS, PhD. Part-time programs available. *Faculty:* 9 full-time (1 woman), 23 part-time/adjunct (2 women). *Students:* 12 full-time (7 women); includes 1 minority (Black or African American, non-Hispanic/Latino), 5 international. Average age 31. 9 applicants, 67% accepted, 3 enrolled. In 2013, 2 master's, 2 doctorates awarded. *Degree requirements:* For master's, thesis, peer-reviewed manuscript submission; conference presentation; for doctorate, comprehensive exam, thesis/dissertation, peer-reviewed manuscript submission; conference presentation; one semester of teaching. *Entrance requirements:* For master's, GRE General Test, bachelor's degree in biological science or chemistry (recommended); for doctorate, GRE General Test, master's degree in science and/or independent research experience (recommended). Additional exam requirements/recommendations for international students: Recommended—TOEFL (minimum score 550 paper-based; 90 iBT), IELTS. *Application deadline:* Applications are processed on a rolling basis. Application fee: $70 ($80 for international students). Electronic applications accepted. *Expenses:* Contact institution. *Financial support:* In 2013–14, 11 students received support, including 4 fellowships with full and partial tuition reimbursements available (averaging $6,888 per year), 8 research assistantships with partial tuition reimbursements available (averaging $13,890 per year), 2 teaching assistantships with partial tuition reimbursements available (averaging $17,000 per year); career-related internships or fieldwork, institutionally sponsored loans, scholarships/grants, health care benefits, and unspecified assistantships also available. Support available to part-time students. Financial award application deadline: 3/1. *Faculty research:* Biodiversity, urban entomology, applied ecology, agricultural entomology. *Total annual research expenditures:* $2 million. *Unit head:* Dr. Patricia Layton, School Director, 864-656-4829, Fax: 864-656-5065, E-mail: playton@clemson.edu. *Application contact:* Dr. Matthew Turnbull, Entomology Graduate Coordinator, 864-656-5038, Fax: 864-656-5065, E-mail: turnbul@clemson.edu.
Website: http://www.clemson.edu/cafls/departments/entomology_grad/

Colorado State University, Graduate School, College of Agricultural Sciences, Department of Bioagricultural Sciences and Pest Management, Fort Collins, CO 80523-1177. Offers entomology (MS, PhD); plant pathology and weed science (MS, PhD). Part-time programs available. Postbaccalaureate distance learning degree programs offered (minimal on-campus study). *Faculty:* 19 full-time (5 women). *Students:* 12 full-time (9 women), 17 part-time (6 women); includes 3 minority (1 Black or African American, non-Hispanic/Latino; 2 Hispanic/Latino), 5 international. Average age 33. 8 applicants, 63% accepted, 5 enrolled. In 2013, 5 master's, 5 doctorates awarded. *Degree requirements:* For master's, comprehensive exam, thesis; for doctorate, comprehensive exam, thesis/dissertation. *Entrance requirements:* For master's and doctorate, GRE General Test, minimum GPA of 3.0, letters of recommendation, essay, transcripts. Additional exam requirements/recommendations for international students: Required—TOEFL (minimum score 550 paper-based; 79 iBT). *Application deadline:* For fall admission, 1/15 priority date for domestic students, 1/1 priority date for international students; for spring admission, 9/1 priority date for domestic and international students. Applications are processed on a rolling basis. Application fee: $50. Electronic applications accepted. *Expenses:* Tuition, state resident: full-time $9075.40; part-time $504 per credit. Tuition, nonresident: full-time $22,248; part-time $1236 per credit. *Required fees:* $1819; $60 per credit. *Financial support:* In 2013–14, 35 students received support, including 4 fellowships with full tuition reimbursements available (averaging $47,570 per year), 20 research assistantships with full tuition reimbursements available (averaging $14,408 per year), 11 teaching assistantships with full tuition reimbursements available (averaging $13,798 per year). Financial award application deadline: 1/15; financial award applicants required to submit FAFSA. *Faculty research:* Genomics and molecular biology, ecology and biodiversity, biology and management of invasive species, integrated pest management. *Total annual research expenditures:* $3.1 million. *Unit head:* Dr. Thomas O. Holtzer, Department Head and Professor, 970-491-5261, Fax: 970-491-3862, E-mail: thomas.holtzer@colostate.edu. *Application contact:* Janet Dill, Administrative Assistant III, 970-491-0402, Fax: 970-491-3862, E-mail: janet.dill@colostate.edu.
Website: http://bspm.agsci.colostate.edu/

Cornell University, Graduate School, Graduate Fields of Agriculture and Life Sciences, Field of Entomology, Ithaca, NY 14853-0001. Offers acarology (MS, PhD); apiculture (MS, PhD); applied entomology (MS, PhD); aquatic entomology (MS, PhD); biological control (MS, PhD); insect behavior (MS, PhD); insect biochemistry (MS, PhD); insect ecology (MS, PhD); insect genetics (MS, PhD); insect morphology (MS, PhD); insect pathology (MS, PhD); insect physiology (MS, PhD); insect systematics (MS, PhD); insect toxicology and insecticide chemistry (MS, PhD); integrated pest management (MS, PhD); medical and veterinary entomology (MS, PhD). *Faculty:* 43 full-time (9 women). *Students:* 26 full-time (16 women); includes 4 minority (2 Hispanic/Latino; 2 Two or more races, non-Hispanic/Latino), 7 international. Average age 29. 37 applicants, 22% accepted, 8 enrolled. In 2013, 2 master's, 3 doctorates awarded. *Degree requirements:* For master's, thesis; for doctorate, comprehensive exam, thesis/dissertation. *Entrance requirements:* For master's and doctorate, GRE General Test, GRE Subject Test (biology), 3 letters of recommendation. Additional exam requirements/recommendations for international students: Required—TOEFL (minimum score 550 paper-based; 77 iBT). *Application deadline:* For fall admission, 12/1 for domestic students. Application fee: $95. Electronic applications accepted. *Financial support:* In 2013–14, 23 students received support, including 3 fellowships with full tuition reimbursements available, 10 research assistantships with full tuition reimbursements available, 5 teaching assistantships with full tuition reimbursements available; institutionally sponsored loans, scholarships/grants, health care benefits, tuition waivers (full and partial), and unspecified assistantships also available. Financial award applicants required to submit FAFSA. *Faculty research:* Systematics and biodiversity, integrated pest management, pathology and biological control, toxicology and physiology, ecology and behavior. *Unit head:* Director of Graduate Studies, 607-255-6198, Fax: 607-255-0939. *Application contact:* Graduate Field Assistant, 607-255-6198, Fax: 607-255-0939, E-mail: fieldofent2@cornell.edu.
Website: http://www.gradschool.cornell.edu/fields.php?id-47&a-2

Illinois State University, Graduate School, College of Arts and Sciences, Department of Biological Sciences, Normal, IL 61790-2200. Offers animal behavior (MS); bacteriology (MS); biochemistry (MS); biological sciences (MS); biology (PhD); biophysics (MS); biotechnology (MS); botany (MS, PhD); cell biology (MS); conservation biology (MS); developmental biology (MS); ecology (MS, PhD); entomology (MS); evolutionary biology (MS); genetics (MS, PhD); immunology (MS); microbiology (MS, PhD); molecular biology (MS); molecular genetics (MS); neurobiology (MS); neuroscience (MS); parasitology (MS); physiology (MS, PhD); plant biology (MS); plant molecular biology (MS); plant sciences (MS); structural biology (MS); zoology (MS, PhD). Part-time programs available. *Degree requirements:* For master's, thesis or alternative; for doctorate, variable foreign language requirement, thesis/dissertation, 2 terms of residency. *Entrance requirements:* For master's, GRE General Test, minimum GPA of 2.6 in last 60 hours of course work; for doctorate, GRE General Test. *Faculty research:* Redoc balance and drug development in schistosoma mansoni, control of the growth of listeria monocytogenes at low temperature, regulation of cell expansion and microtubule function by SPRI, CRUI: physiology and fitness consequences of different life history phenotypes.

Iowa State University of Science and Technology, Department of Entomology, Ames, IA 50011. Offers MS, PhD. *Degree requirements:* For master's, thesis; for doctorate, thesis/dissertation. *Entrance requirements:* For master's and doctorate, GRE General Test, GRE Subject Test (biology). Additional exam requirements/recommendations for international students: Required—TOEFL (minimum score 550 paper-based; 79 iBT), IELTS (minimum score 6.5). Electronic applications accepted.

Kansas State University, Graduate School, College of Agriculture, Department of Entomology, Manhattan, KS 66506. Offers MS, PhD. *Faculty:* 18 full-time (1 woman), 11 part-time/adjunct (2 women). *Students:* 29 full-time (14 women), 5 part-time (3 women); includes 4 minority (1 American Indian or Alaska Native, non-Hispanic/Latino; 3 Hispanic/Latino), 15 international. Average age 31. 17 applicants, 47% accepted, 5 enrolled. In 2013, 2 master's, 1 doctorate awarded. *Degree requirements:* For master's, thesis, oral exam; for doctorate, thesis/dissertation, written and oral exams. *Entrance requirements:* Additional exam requirements/recommendations for international students: Required—TOEFL (minimum score 550 paper-based; 79 iBT). *Application deadline:* For fall admission, 2/1 priority date for domestic and international students; for spring admission, 8/1 priority date for domestic and international students. Applications are processed on a rolling basis. Application fee: $50 ($75 for international students). Electronic applications accepted. *Financial support:* In 2013–14, 19 research assistantships (averaging $21,043 per year), 3 teaching assistantships with partial tuition reimbursements (averaging $21,520 per year) were awarded; career-related internships or fieldwork, Federal Work-Study, institutionally sponsored loans, scholarships/grants, and tuition waivers (partial) also available. Support available to part-time students. Financial award application deadline: 3/1; financial award applicants required to submit FAFSA. *Faculty research:* Molecular genetics, biologically-based pest management, host plant resistance, ecological genomics, stored product entomology. *Total annual research expenditures:* $1.7 million. *Unit head:* Dr. John Ruberson, Head, 785-532-6154, Fax: 785-532-6232, E-mail: ruberson@ksu.edu. *Application contact:* Evelyn Kennedy, Application Contact, 785-532-4702, Fax: 785-532-6232, E-mail: ekennedy@ksu.edu.
Website: http://entomology.k-state.edu

Louisiana State University and Agricultural & Mechanical College, Graduate School, College of Agriculture, Department of Entomology, Baton Rouge, LA 70803. Offers MS, PhD. *Faculty:* 14 full-time (2 women), 1 part-time/adjunct (0 women). *Students:* 24 full-time (8 women), 4 part-time (0 women); includes 2 minority (both Two or more races, non-Hispanic/Latino), 16 international. Average age 27. 13 applicants, 46% accepted, 5 enrolled. In 2013, 2 master's, 2 doctorates awarded. *Degree requirements:* For master's, thesis; for doctorate, thesis/dissertation. *Entrance requirements:* For master's and doctorate, GRE General Test, minimum GPA of 3.0. Additional exam requirements/recommendations for international students: Required—TOEFL (minimum score 550 paper-based; 79 IBT), IELTS (minimum score 6.5), or PTE (minimum score 59). *Application deadline:* For fall admission, 1/25 priority date for domestic students, 5/15 for international students; for spring admission, 10/15 for international students. Applications are processed on a rolling basis. Application fee: $50 ($70 for international students). Electronic applications accepted. *Financial support:* In 2013–14, 28 students received support, including 23 research assistantships with partial tuition reimbursements available (averaging $18,604 per year); fellowships, teaching assistantships with partial tuition reimbursements available, Federal Work-Study, institutionally sponsored loans, scholarships/grants, health care benefits, and unspecified assistantships also available. Support available to part-time students. Financial award applicants required to submit FAFSA. *Faculty research:* Conservation biology, insect systematics, insect ecology, urban entomology, agricultural pest management, insect genomics. *Total annual research expenditures:* $7,208. *Unit head:* Dr. Timothy Schowalter, Head, 225-578-1634, Fax: 225-578-2257, E-mail: tschowalter@agcenter.lsu.edu. *Application contact:* Dr. James Ottea, Graduate Coordinator, 225-578-1841, E-mail: jottea@lsu.edu.
Website: http://www.entomology.lsu.edu/

McGill University, Faculty of Graduate and Postdoctoral Studies, Faculty of Agricultural and Environmental Sciences, Department of Natural Resource Sciences, Montréal, QC H3A 2T5, Canada. Offers entomology (M Sc, PhD); environmental assessment (M Sc); forest science (M Sc, PhD); microbiology (M Sc, PhD); micrometeorology (M Sc, PhD); neotropical environment (M Sc, PhD); soil science (M Sc, PhD); wildlife biology (M Sc, PhD).

Michigan State University, The Graduate School, College of Agriculture and Natural Resources and College of Natural Science, Department of Entomology, East Lansing, MI 48824. Offers entomology (MS, PhD); integrated pest management (MS). *Entrance requirements:* Additional exam requirements/recommendations for international students: Required—TOEFL (minimum score 550 paper-based), Michigan State University ELT (minimum score 85), Michigan English Language Assessment Battery (minimum score 83). Electronic applications accepted.

Mississippi State University, College of Agriculture and Life Sciences, Department of Biochemistry, Molecular Biology, Entomology and Plant Pathology, Mississippi State, MS 39762. Offers agriculture life sciences (MS), including biochemistry (MS, PhD), entomology (MS, PhD), plant pathology (MS, PhD); life science (PhD), including biochemistry (MS, PhD), entomology (MS, PhD), plant pathology (MS, PhD); molecular biology (PhD). *Faculty:* 23 full-time (1 woman). *Students:* 43 full-time (16 women), 17 part-time (10 women); includes 5 minority (4 Black or African American, non-Hispanic/Latino; 1 Hispanic/Latino), 14 international. Average age 29. 62 applicants, 18% accepted, 10 enrolled. In 2013, 11 master's, 4 doctorates awarded. Terminal master's awarded for partial completion of doctoral program. *Degree requirements:* For master's, thesis (for some programs), final oral exam; for doctorate, thesis/dissertation, preliminary oral and written exam. *Entrance requirements:* For master's, GRE General Test, minimum GPA of 2.75; for doctorate, GRE. Additional exam requirements/recommendations for international students: Required—TOEFL (minimum score 500 paper-based; 61 iBT); Recommended—IELTS (minimum score 5.5). *Application deadline:* For fall admission, 7/1 for domestic students, 5/1 for international students; for spring admission, 11/1 for domestic students, 9/1 for international students. Applications are processed on a rolling basis. Application fee: $60. Electronic applications accepted. *Financial support:* In 2013–14, 35 research assistantships with full tuition reimbursements (averaging $16,388 per year) were awarded; Federal Work-Study, institutionally sponsored loans, and unspecified assistantships also available. Financial award application deadline: 4/1; financial award applicants required to submit FAFSA. *Faculty research:* Fish nutrition, plant and animal molecular biology, plant biochemistry, enzymology, lipid metabolism, chromatin, cell wall synthesis in rice, a model grass bioenergy species and the source of rice stover residues using reverse genetic and functional genomic and proteomic approaches. *Unit head:* Dr. Scott T. Willard, Professor and Department Head, 662-325-2640, Fax: 662-325-8664, E-mail: swilliard@ads.msstate.edu. *Application contact:* Dr. Din-Pow Ma, Professor/Graduate Coordinator, 662-325-7739, Fax: 662-325-8664, E-mail: dm1@ra.msstate.edu.
Website: http://www.biochemistry.msstate.edu

New Mexico State University, Graduate School, College of Agricultural, Consumer and Environmental Sciences, Department of Entomology, Plant Pathology and Weed Science, Las Cruces, NM 88003-8001. Offers agricultural biology (MS). Part-time programs available. *Faculty:* 10 full-time (2 women). *Students:* 7 full-time (3 women), 2 part-time (1 woman); includes 2 minority (both Hispanic/Latino), 1 international. Average age 26. 2 applicants, 100% accepted, 2 enrolled. In 2013, 4 master's awarded. *Degree requirements:* For master's, comprehensive exam, thesis. *Entrance requirements:* For master's, GRE General Test. Additional exam requirements/recommendations for international students: Required—TOEFL (minimum score 550 paper-based; 79 iBT), IELTS (minimum score 6.5). *Application deadline:* For fall admission, 7/1 priority date for domestic students; for spring admission, 11/1 priority date for domestic students. Applications are processed on a rolling basis. Application fee: $40 ($50 for international students). Electronic applications accepted. *Expenses:* Tuition, state resident: full-time $5398; part-time $224.90 per credit. Tuition, nonresident: full-time $18,821; part-time $784.20 per credit. *Required fees:* $1310; $54.60 per credit. *Financial support:* In 2013–14, 7 students received support, including 7 research assistantships (averaging $20,908 per year); career-related internships or fieldwork, Federal Work-Study, health care benefits, and unspecified assistantships also available. Financial award application deadline: 3/1. *Faculty research:* Integrated pest management; biology/ecology of plants, insects, nematodes, microorganisms; pesticide metabolism and environmental fate; urban pest management; management of pest resistance to pesticides. *Total annual research expenditures:* $2.7 million. *Unit head:* Dr. Gerald K. Sims, Interim Head, 575-646-3225, Fax: 575-646-8087, E-mail: gksims@nmsu.edu. *Application contact:* Cindy Bullard, Intermediate Administrative Assistant/Recruiting Contact, 575-646-1145, Fax: 575-646-8087, E-mail: cbullard@nmsu.edu.
Website: http://eppws.nmsu.edu/

North Carolina State University, Graduate School, College of Agriculture and Life Sciences, Department of Entomology, Raleigh, NC 27695. Offers MS, PhD. Terminal master's awarded for partial completion of doctoral program. *Degree requirements:* For master's, thesis (for some programs); for doctorate, thesis/dissertation. *Entrance requirements:* For master's and doctorate, GRE General Test. Electronic applications accepted. *Faculty research:* Physiology, biocontrol, ecology, forest entomology, apiculture.

North Dakota State University, College of Graduate and Interdisciplinary Studies, College of Agriculture, Food Systems, and Natural Resources, Department of Entomology, Fargo, ND 58108. Offers entomology (MS, PhD). Part-time programs available. *Students:* 11 full-time (7 women), 4 part-time (2 women); includes 2 minority (1 American Indian or Alaska Native, non-Hispanic/Latino; 1 Asian, non-Hispanic/Latino), 4 international. Average age 34. 4 applicants, 50% accepted, 2 enrolled. In 2013, 2 master's awarded. *Degree requirements:* For master's, thesis; for doctorate, comprehensive exam, thesis/dissertation. *Entrance requirements:* For master's and doctorate, minimum GPA of 3.0. Additional exam requirements/recommendations for international students: Required—TOEFL (minimum score 550 paper-based; 79 iBT). *Application deadline:* For fall admission, 5/1 for international students; for winter admission, 8/1 for international students. Application fee: $35. Electronic applications accepted. *Financial support:* In 2013–14, 11 research assistantships with full tuition reimbursements (averaging $13,800 per year) were awarded; Federal Work-Study, institutionally sponsored loans, and unspecified assistantships also available. Financial award application deadline: 4/15. *Faculty research:* Insect systematics, conservation biology, integrated pest management, insect behavior, insect biology. *Unit head:* Dr. Frank Casey, Chair, 701-231-7582, Fax: 701-231-8557, E-mail: francis.casey@ndsu.edu. *Application contact:* Dr. Jason Harmon, Program Leader, 701-231-7033, Fax: 701-231-8557, E-mail: jason.harmon@ndsu.edu.
Website: http://www.ndsu.edu/entomology/

The Ohio State University, Graduate School, College of Food, Agricultural, and Environmental Sciences, Department of Entomology, Columbus, OH 43210. Offers MPHM, MS, PhD. MPHM offered jointly with Department of Plant Pathology. *Faculty:* 17. *Students:* 23 full-time (10 women), 3 part-time (2 women); includes 2 minority (both Two or more races, non-Hispanic/Latino), 8 international. Average age 28. In 2013, 3 master's, 6 doctorates awarded. *Degree requirements:* For master's, variable foreign language requirement, thesis optional; for doctorate, variable foreign language requirement, thesis/dissertation. *Entrance requirements:* For master's and doctorate, GRE General Test. Additional exam requirements/recommendations for international students: Required—TOEFL (minimum score 550 paper-based; 79 iBT), Michigan English Language Assessment Battery (minimum score 82); Recommended—IELTS (minimum score 7). *Application deadline:* For fall admission, 12/13 priority date for domestic students, 11/30 priority date for international students; for spring admission, 12/6 for domestic students, 11/11 for international students; for summer admission, 4/4 for domestic students, 3/7 for international students. Applications are processed on a rolling basis. Application fee: $60 ($70 for international students). Electronic applications accepted. *Financial support:* Fellowships with tuition reimbursements, research assistantships with tuition reimbursements, teaching assistantships with tuition reimbursements, Federal Work-Study, and institutionally sponsored loans available. Support available to part-time students. *Faculty research:* Acarology, insect systematics, soil ecology, integrated pest management, chemical ecology. *Unit head:* Dr. Dan Herms, Chair, 330-202-3506, Fax: 330-263-3686, E-mail: herms.2@osu.edu. *Application contact:* Graduate Admissions Office, 614-292-9444, E-mail: gradadmissions@osu.edu.
Website: http://entomology.osu.edu/

Oklahoma State University, College of Agricultural Science and Natural Resources, Department of Entomology and Plant Pathology, Stillwater, OK 74078. Offers entomology (PhD); entomology and plant pathology (MS); plant pathology (PhD). *Faculty:* 30 full-time (11 women). *Students:* 5 full-time (3 women), 35 part-time (15 women); includes 5 minority (1 Black or African American, non-Hispanic/Latino; 1 American Indian or Alaska Native, non-Hispanic/Latino; 1 Asian, non-Hispanic/Latino; 1 Hispanic/Latino; 1 Two or more races, non-Hispanic/Latino), 15 international. Average age 30. 22 applicants, 32% accepted, 6 enrolled. In 2013, 5 master's, 4 doctorates awarded. *Degree requirements:* For master's, thesis or alternative; for doctorate, comprehensive exam, thesis/dissertation. *Entrance requirements:* For master's and doctorate, GRE or GMAT. Additional exam requirements/recommendations for international students: Required—TOEFL (minimum score 550 paper-based; 79 iBT). *Application deadline:* For fall admission, 3/1 priority date for international students; for spring admission, 8/1 priority date for international students. Applications are processed on a rolling basis. Application fee: $40 ($75 for international students). Electronic applications accepted. *Expenses:* Tuition, state resident: full-time $4272; part-time $178 per credit hour. Tuition, nonresident: full-time $17,472; part-time $709 per credit hour. *Required fees:* $2413.20; $100.55 per credit hour. One-time fee: $50 full-time. Part-time tuition and fees vary according to course load and campus/location. *Financial support:* In 2013–14, 36 research assistantships (averaging $17,554 per year), 1 teaching assistantship (averaging $18,504 per year) were awarded; career-related internships or fieldwork, Federal Work-Study, scholarships/grants, health care benefits, tuition waivers (partial), and unspecified assistantships also available. Support available to part-time students. Financial award application deadline: 3/1; financial award applicants required to submit FAFSA. *Unit head:* Dr. Phillip Mulder, Jr., Department Head, 405-744-5527, Fax: 405-744-6039, E-mail: phil.mulder@okstate.edu. *Application contact:* Dr. Brad Kard, Graduate Coordinator, 405-744-2142, Fax: 405-744-6039, E-mail: brad.kard@okstate.edu.
Website: http://entoplp.okstate.edu/

Penn State University Park, Graduate School, College of Agricultural Sciences, Department of Entomology, University Park, PA 16802. Offers MS, PhD. *Unit head:* Dr. Barbara J. Christ, Interim Dean, 814-865-2541, Fax: 814-865-3103, E-mail: ebf@psu.edu. *Application contact:* Cynthia E. Nicosia, Director of Graduate Enrollment Services, 814-865-1834, Fax: 814-863-4627, E-mail: cey1@psu.edu.
Website: http://ento.psu.edu/

Purdue University, Graduate School, College of Agriculture, Department of Entomology, West Lafayette, IN 47907. Offers MS, PhD. Part-time programs available. *Faculty:* 18 full-time (2 women), 7 part-time/adjunct (3 women). *Students:* 42 full-time (20 women), 1 (woman) part-time; includes 1 minority (Hispanic/Latino), 12 international. Average age 28. 21 applicants, 24% accepted, 5 enrolled. In 2013, 3 master's, 3 doctorates awarded. *Degree requirements:* For master's, thesis (for some programs), seminar; for doctorate, thesis/dissertation, seminar. *Entrance requirements:* For master's, GRE General Test, minimum undergraduate GPA of 3.0 or equivalent; for doctorate, GRE, minimum undergraduate GPA of 3.0 or equivalent; master's degree (highly recommended). Additional exam requirements/recommendations for international students: Required—TOEFL (minimum score 550 paper-based; 77 iBT). *Application deadline:* For fall admission, 7/1 priority date for domestic students, 3/15 for international students; for spring admission, 11/1 for domestic students, 8/15 for international students. Applications are processed on a rolling basis. Application fee: $60 ($75 for international students). Electronic applications accepted. *Financial support:* Fellowships with tuition reimbursements, research assistantships with tuition reimbursements, teaching assistantships with tuition reimbursements, and career-related internships or fieldwork available. Support available to part-time students. Financial award application deadline: 3/1; financial award applicants required to submit FAFSA. *Faculty research:* Insect biochemistry, nematology, aquatic diptera, behavioral ecology, insect physiology. *Unit head:* Dr. John S. Yaninek, Head, 765-494-4553, Fax: 765-494-0535, E-mail: steve_yaninek@purdue.edu. *Application contact:* Amanda L. Pendleton, Graduate Admissions Office, 765-494-9061, Fax: 765-494-0535, E-mail: apendle@purdue.edu.
Website: https://ag.purdue.edu/entm

Rutgers, The State University of New Jersey, New Brunswick, Graduate School-New Brunswick, Program in Entomology, Piscataway, NJ 08854-8097. Offers MS, PhD. *Degree requirements:* For master's, thesis or alternative; for doctorate, thesis/dissertation. *Entrance requirements:* For master's and doctorate, GRE General Test, GRE Subject Test (recommended). Additional exam requirements/recommendations for international students: Required—TOEFL. Electronic applications accepted. *Faculty research:* Insect toxicology, biolorial control, pathology, IPM and ecology, insect systematics.

Simon Fraser University, Office of Graduate Studies, Faculty of Science, Department of Biological Sciences, Burnaby, BC V5A 1S6, Canada. Offers bioinformatics (Graduate Diploma); biological sciences (M Sc, PhD); environmental toxicology (MET); pest management (MPM). *Faculty:* 47 full-time (15 women). *Students:* 138 full-time (70 women). 29 applicants, 59% accepted, 15 enrolled. In 2013, 27 master's, 13 doctorates awarded. *Degree requirements:* For master's, thesis; for doctorate, thesis/dissertation, candidacy exam; for Graduate Diploma, practicum. *Entrance requirements:* For master's, minimum GPA of 3.0 (on scale of 4.33), or 3.33 based on last 60 credits of undergraduate courses; for doctorate, minimum GPA of 3.5 (on scale of 4.33); for Graduate Diploma, minimum GPA of 2.5 (on scale of 4.33), or 2.67 based on the last 60 credits of undergraduate courses. Additional exam requirements/recommendations for international students: Recommended—TOEFL (minimum score 580 paper-based; 93 iBT), IELTS (minimum score 7), TWE (minimum score 5). *Application deadline:* For fall admission, 6/1 for domestic and international students; for winter admission, 10/1 for domestic and international students; for spring admission, 2/1 for domestic and international students. Applications are processed on a rolling basis. Application fee: $90 ($125 for international students). Electronic applications accepted. *Expenses: Tuition, area resident:* Full-time $5084 Canadian dollars. *Required fees:* $840 Canadian dollars. *Financial support:* In 2013–14, 68 students received support, including 77 fellowships (averaging $6,250 per year), teaching assistantships (averaging $5,608 per year); research assistantships and scholarships/grants also available. *Faculty research:* Cell biology, wildlife ecology, environmental and evolutionary physiology, environmental toxicology, pest management. *Unit head:* Dr. Julian Guttman, Graduate Chair, 778-782-4459, Fax: 778-782-3496, E-mail: bisc-grad-chair@sfu.ca. *Application contact:* Marlene

Entomology

Nguyen, Graduate Secretary, 778-782-3120, Fax: 778-782-3496, E-mail: biscgrad@sfu.ca.
Website: http://www.sfu.ca/biology

State University of New York College of Environmental Science and Forestry, Department of Environmental and Forest Biology, Syracuse, NY 13210-2779. Offers applied ecology (MPS); chemical ecology (MPS, MS, PhD); conservation biology (MPS, MS, PhD); ecology (MPS, MS, PhD); entomology (MPS, MS, PhD); environmental interpretation (MPS, MS, PhD); environmental physiology (MPS, MS, PhD); fish and wildlife biology and management (MPS, MS, PhD); forest pathology and mycology (MPS, MS, PhD); plant biotechnology (MPS); plant science and biotechnology (MPS, MS, PhD). *Faculty:* 32 full-time (10 women). *Students:* 105 full-time (54 women), 31 part-time (16 women); includes 9 minority (2 Black or African American, non-Hispanic/Latino; 3 American Indian or Alaska Native, non-Hispanic/Latino; 2 Hispanic/Latino; 1 Native Hawaiian or other Pacific Islander, non-Hispanic/Latino; 1 Two or more races, non-Hispanic/Latino), 17 international. Average age 28. In 2013, 15 master's, 7 doctorates awarded. *Degree requirements:* For master's, thesis (for some programs), capstone seminar; for doctorate, comprehensive exam, thesis/dissertation, capstone seminar. *Entrance requirements:* For master's and doctorate, GRE General Test, minimum GPA of 3.0. Additional exam requirements/recommendations for international students: Required—TOEFL (minimum score 550 paper-based; 80 iBT), IELTS (minimum score 6). *Application deadline:* For fall admission, 2/1 priority date for domestic and international students; for spring admission, 11/1 priority date for domestic and international students. Applications are processed on a rolling basis. Application fee: $60. *Expenses:* Tuition, state resident: full-time $10,370; part-time $432 per credit hour. Tuition, nonresident: full-time $20,190; part-time $841 per credit hour. *Required fees:* $44 per credit hour. *Financial support:* In 2013–14, 4 fellowships with full and partial tuition reimbursements, 36 research assistantships with full and partial tuition reimbursements, 39 teaching assistantships with full and partial tuition reimbursements (averaging $11,490 per year) were awarded; Federal Work-Study, institutionally sponsored loans, scholarships/grants, health care benefits, and unspecified assistantships also available. Financial award application deadline: 6/30. *Faculty research:* Ecology, conservation biology, fish and wildlife biology and management, plant science, entomology. *Total annual research expenditures:* $4.1 million. *Unit head:* Dr. Donald J. Leopold, Chair, 315-470-6760, Fax: 315-470-6934, E-mail: djleopold@esf.edu. *Application contact:* Dr. Danilo D. Fernando, Director, Graduate Program/Associate Professor, 315-470-6746, Fax: 315-470-6934, E-mail: dfernando@esf.edu.
Website: http://www.esf.edu/efb/grad/default.asp

Texas A&M University, College of Agriculture and Life Sciences, Department of Entomology, College Station, TX 77843. Offers MS, PhD. *Faculty:* 22. *Students:* 53 full-time (32 women), 10 part-time (2 women); includes 10 minority (1 Black or African American, non-Hispanic/Latino; 2 Asian, non-Hispanic/Latino; 7 Hispanic/Latino), 20 international. Average age 29. 20 applicants, 80% accepted, 12 enrolled. In 2013, 5 master's, 5 doctorates awarded. *Degree requirements:* For master's, comprehensive exam, thesis (for some programs); for doctorate, comprehensive exam, thesis/dissertation. *Entrance requirements:* For master's and doctorate, GRE General Test. Additional exam requirements/recommendations for international students: Required—TOEFL. *Application deadline:* For fall admission, 2/1 priority date for domestic students; for spring admission, 10/1 for domestic students. Applications are processed on a rolling basis. Application fee: $50 ($75 for international students). Electronic applications accepted. *Expenses:* Tuition, state resident: full-time $4078; part-time $226.55 per credit hour. Tuition, nonresident: full-time $10,450; part-time $580.55 per credit hour. *Required fees:* $2328; $278.50 per credit hour. $642.45 per semester. *Financial support:* In 2013–14, research assistantships with partial tuition reimbursements (averaging $16,500 per year), teaching assistantships with partial tuition reimbursements (averaging $16,500 per year) were awarded; fellowships and Federal Work-Study also available. Financial award application deadline: 3/1; financial award applicants required to submit FAFSA. *Faculty research:* Biology, biological control, integrated pest management, systematics, host plant resistance. *Unit head:* Dr. David Ragsdale, Head, 979-845-2510, Fax: 979-845-6305, E-mail: dragsdale@tamu.edu. *Application contact:* Rebecca Hapes, Senior Academic Advisor II, 979-845-9733, E-mail: rhapes@tamu.edu.
Website: http://insects.tamu.edu

The University of Arizona, Graduate Interdisciplinary Programs, Graduate Interdisciplinary Program in Entomology and Insect Science, Tucson, AZ 85721. Offers MS, PhD. Part-time programs available. *Faculty:* 8 full-time (4 women), 1 part-time/adjunct (0 women). *Students:* 23 full-time (7 women), 1 part-time (0 women); includes 8 minority (1 American Indian or Alaska Native, non-Hispanic/Latino; 1 Asian, non-Hispanic/Latino; 4 Hispanic/Latino; 2 Two or more races, non-Hispanic/Latino), 2 international. Average age 29. 20 applicants, 20% accepted, 3 enrolled. In 2013, 2 master's, 2 doctorates awarded. *Degree requirements:* For master's, thesis; for doctorate, comprehensive exam, thesis/dissertation. *Entrance requirements:* For master's, GRE General Test, GRE Subject Test, minimum GPA of 3.0, 3 letters of recommendation; for doctorate, GRE General Test, GRE Subject Test, minimum GPA of 3.0, 3 letters of recommendation, statement of purpose. Additional exam requirements/recommendations for international students: Required—TOEFL (minimum score 550 paper-based). *Application deadline:* For fall admission, 1/1 for domestic students, 12/1 for international students. Applications are processed on a rolling basis. Application fee: $75. *Expenses:* Tuition, state resident: full-time $11,526. Tuition, nonresident: full-time $27,398. *Financial support:* In 2013–14, 1 student received support, including 9 research assistantships with full and partial tuition reimbursements available (averaging $29,734 per year), 1 teaching assistantship with full and partial tuition reimbursement available (averaging $22,100 per year); fellowships, Federal Work-Study, institutionally sponsored loans, scholarships/grants, health care benefits, tuition waivers (full and partial), and unspecified assistantships also available. Financial award application deadline: 3/1. *Faculty research:* Toxicology and physiology, plant/insect relations, vector biology, insect pest management, chemical ecology. *Total annual research expenditures:* $933,509. *Unit head:* Dr. Molly E. Hunter, Professor and Head, 520-621-0847, Fax: 520-621-1150, E-mail: mhunter@ag.arizona.edu. *Application contact:* Rachel Mattull, Graduate Coordinator, 520-621-0847, Fax: 520-621-1150, E-mail: rmattull@email.arizona.edu.
Website: http://insects.arizona.edu/

University of Arkansas, Graduate School, Dale Bumpers College of Agricultural, Food and Life Sciences, Department of Entomology, Fayetteville, AR 72701-1201. Offers MS, PhD. *Degree requirements:* For master's, thesis; for doctorate, one foreign language, thesis/dissertation. *Entrance requirements:* For master's, GRE, minimum GPA of 3.0; for doctorate, GRE, minimum GPA of 3.25. Electronic applications accepted. *Faculty research:* Integrated pest management, insect virology, insect taxonomy.

University of California, Davis, Graduate Studies, Graduate Group in Integrated Pest Management, Davis, CA 95616. Offers MS. *Degree requirements:* For master's, comprehensive exam (for some programs), thesis (for some programs). *Entrance requirements:* For master's, GRE General Test, GRE Subject Test (biology), minimum GPA of 3.0. Additional exam requirements/recommendations for international students: Required—TOEFL (minimum score 550 paper-based). Electronic applications accepted.

University of California, Davis, Graduate Studies, Program in Entomology, Davis, CA 95616. Offers MS, PhD. Terminal master's awarded for partial completion of doctoral program. *Degree requirements:* For master's, comprehensive exam (for some programs), thesis (for some programs); for doctorate, thesis/dissertation. *Entrance requirements:* For master's and doctorate, GRE General Test, GRE Subject Test (biology). Additional exam requirements/recommendations for international students: Required—TOEFL (minimum score 550 paper-based). Electronic applications accepted. *Faculty research:* Bee biology, biological control, systematics, medical/veterinary entomology, pest management.

University of California, Riverside, Graduate Division, Department of Entomology, Riverside, CA 92521-0102. Offers entomology (MS, PhD); evolution and ecology (PhD). Part-time programs available. Terminal master's awarded for partial completion of doctoral program. *Degree requirements:* For master's, thesis; for doctorate, thesis/dissertation, qualifying exams. *Entrance requirements:* For master's and doctorate, GRE General Test, minimum GPA of 3.2. Additional exam requirements/recommendations for international students: Required—TOEFL (minimum score 550 paper-based; 80 iBT) or IELTS. Electronic applications accepted. *Faculty research:* Agricultural, urban, medical, and veterinary entomology; biological control; chemical ecology; insect pathogens; novel toxicants.

University of Connecticut, Graduate School, College of Liberal Arts and Sciences, Department of Ecology and Evolutionary Biology, Storrs, CT 06269. Offers botany (MS, PhD); ecology (MS, PhD); entomology (MS, PhD); zoology (MS, PhD). Terminal master's awarded for partial completion of doctoral program. *Degree requirements:* For master's, comprehensive exam; for doctorate, thesis/dissertation. *Entrance requirements:* For master's and doctorate, GRE General Test, GRE Subject Test. Additional exam requirements/recommendations for international students: Required—TOEFL (minimum score 550 paper-based). Electronic applications accepted.

University of Delaware, College of Agriculture and Natural Resources, Department of Entomology and Wildlife Ecology, Newark, DE 19716. Offers entomology and applied ecology (MS, PhD), including avian ecology, evolution and taxonomy, insect biological control, insect ecology and behavior (MS), insect genetics, pest management, plant-insect interactions, wildlife ecology and management. Part-time programs available. *Degree requirements:* For master's, comprehensive exam, thesis, oral exam, seminar; for doctorate, comprehensive exam, thesis/dissertation, qualifying exam, seminar. *Entrance requirements:* For master's, GRE General Test, minimum GPA of 3.0 in field, 2.8 overall; for doctorate, GRE General Test, GRE Subject Test (biology), minimum GPA of 3.0 in field, 2.8 overall. Additional exam requirements/recommendations for international students: Required—TOEFL. Electronic applications accepted. *Faculty research:* Ecology and evolution of plant-insect interactions, ecology of wildlife conservation management, habitat restoration, biological control, applied ecosystem management.

University of Florida, Graduate School, College of Agricultural and Life Sciences, Department of Entomology and Nematology, Gainesville, FL 32611. Offers MS, PhD. Cooperative PhD program available with Florida Agricultural and Mechanical University. Part-time and evening/weekend programs available. Postbaccalaureate distance learning degree programs offered. *Faculty:* 54 full-time (15 women), 2 part-time/adjunct (0 women). *Students:* 91 full-time (42 women), 45 part-time (20 women); includes 19 minority (1 Black or African American, non-Hispanic/Latino; 7 Asian, non-Hispanic/Latino; 11 Hispanic/Latino), 39 international. Average age 32. 63 applicants, 41% accepted, 23 enrolled. In 2013, 24 master's, 11 doctorates awarded. *Degree requirements:* For master's, comprehensive exam (for some programs), thesis (for some programs); for doctorate, comprehensive exam, thesis/dissertation. *Entrance requirements:* For master's and doctorate, GRE General Test, GRE Subject Test (biology), minimum GPA of 3.0. Additional exam requirements/recommendations for international students: Required—TOEFL (minimum score 550 paper-based; 80 iBT), IELTS (minimum score 6). *Application deadline:* For fall admission, 7/15 priority date for domestic students; for spring admission, 11/15 for domestic students. Applications are processed on a rolling basis. Application fee: $30. Electronic applications accepted. *Expenses:* Tuition, state resident: full-time $12,640. Tuition, nonresident: full-time $30,000. *Financial support:* In 2013–14, 79 students received support, including 4 fellowships (averaging $20,250 per year), 76 research assistantships (averaging $18,285 per year), 2 teaching assistantships (averaging $21,295 per year); career-related internships or fieldwork also available. Financial award applicants required to submit FAFSA. *Faculty research:* Biological control, pest management, genetics, ecology, physiology, toxicology, systematics and taxonomy, medical and veterinary entomology, urban entomology, nematology. *Unit head:* John L. Capinera, PhD, Department Chair and Professor, 352-273-3905, Fax: 352-392-0190, E-mail: capinera@ufl.edu. *Application contact:* Heather J. McAuslane, PhD, Graduate Coordinator, 352-273-3923, Fax: 352-392-0190, E-mail: hjmca@ufl.edu.
Website: http://entnemdept.ifas.ufl.edu/

University of Georgia, College of Agricultural and Environmental Sciences, Department of Entomology, Athens, GA 30602. Offers entomology (MS, PhD); plant protection and pest management (MPPPM). *Degree requirements:* For master's, thesis (MS); for doctorate, one foreign language, thesis/dissertation. *Entrance requirements:* For master's and doctorate, GRE General Test. Electronic applications accepted. *Faculty research:* Apiculture, acarology, aquatic and soil biology, ecology, systematics.

University of Guelph, Graduate Studies, Ontario Agricultural College, Department of Environmental Biology, Guelph, ON N1G 2W1, Canada. Offers entomology (M Sc, PhD); environmental microbiology and biotechnology (M Sc, PhD); environmental toxicology (M Sc, PhD); plant and forest systems (M Sc, PhD); plant pathology (M Sc, PhD). Part-time programs available. *Degree requirements:* For master's, thesis; for doctorate, comprehensive exam, thesis/dissertation. *Entrance requirements:* For master's, minimum 75% average during previous 2 years of course work; for doctorate, minimum 75% average. Additional exam requirements/recommendations for international students: Required—TOEFL or IELTS. Electronic applications accepted. *Faculty research:* Entomology, environmental microbiology and biotechnology, environmental toxicology, forest ecology, plant pathology.

University of Hawaii at Manoa, Graduate Division, College of Tropical Agriculture and Human Resources, Department of Plant and Environmental Protection Sciences, Program in Entomology, Honolulu, HI 96822. Offers MS, PhD. Part-time programs available. *Degree requirements:* For master's, thesis optional; for doctorate, comprehensive exam, thesis/dissertation. *Entrance requirements:* For master's and doctorate, GRE General Test, GRE Subject Test (biology). Additional exam requirements/recommendations for international students: Required—TOEFL (minimum score 500 paper-based; 61 iBT), IELTS (minimum score 5). *Faculty research:* Integrated pest management, biological control, urban entomology, medical/forensic entomology resistance.

University of Idaho, College of Graduate Studies, College of Agricultural and Life Sciences, Department of Plant, Soil, and Entomological Sciences, Moscow, ID 83844-2339. Offers entomology (MS, PhD); plant science (MS, PhD); soil and land resources (MS, PhD). *Faculty:* 25 full-time. *Students:* 28 full-time, 15 part-time. Average age 31. In 2013, 11 master's, 1 doctorate awarded. *Degree requirements:* For doctorate, thesis/

dissertation. *Entrance requirements:* For master's and doctorate, GRE General Test, minimum GPA of 3.0. *Application deadline:* For fall admission, 7/1 for domestic students; for spring admission, 11/1 for domestic students. Applications are processed on a rolling basis. Application fee: $60. Electronic applications accepted. *Expenses:* Tuition, state resident: full-time $5596; part-time $363 per credit hour. Tuition, nonresident: full-time $18,672; part-time $1089 per credit hour. *Financial support:* Research assistantships and teaching assistantships available. Financial award applicants required to submit FAFSA. *Faculty research:* Entomological sciences, crop and weed science, horticultural science, soil and land resources. *Unit head:* Dr. James B. Johnson, Department Head, 208-885-6274, Fax: 208-885-7760, E-mail: nthompson@uidaho.edu. *Application contact:* Stephanie Thomas, Graduate Recruitment Coordinator, 208-885-4001, Fax: 208-885-4406, E-mail: gadms@uidaho.edu.
Website: http://www.uidaho.edu/cals/pses/

University of Illinois at Urbana–Champaign, Graduate College, College of Liberal Arts and Sciences, School of Integrative Biology, Department of Entomology, Champaign, IL 61820. Offers MS, PhD. *Students:* 42 (22 women). Terminal master's awarded for partial completion of doctoral program. Application fee: $75 ($90 for international students). *Unit head:* Dr. May R. Berenbaum, Head, 217-333-7784, Fax: 217-244-3499, E-mail: maybe@illinois.edu. *Application contact:* Kimberly Leigh, Office Administrator, 217-333-2910, Fax: 217-244-3499, E-mail: kaleigh@illinois.edu.
Website: http://www.life.illinois.edu/entomology/

The University of Kansas, Graduate Studies, College of Liberal Arts and Sciences, Department of Ecology and Evolutionary Biology, Lawrence, KS 66045. Offers botany (MA, PhD); ecology and evolutionary biology (MA, PhD); entomology (MA, PhD). *Faculty:* 35. *Students:* 57 full-time (25 women); includes 3 minority (all Two or more races, non-Hispanic/Latino), 19 international. Average age 29. 48 applicants, 29% accepted, 10 enrolled. In 2013, 9 doctorates awarded. Terminal master's awarded for partial completion of doctoral program. *Degree requirements:* For master's, comprehensive exam, thesis (for some programs), 30-36 credits, thesis presentation; for doctorate, comprehensive exam, thesis/dissertation, residency, responsible scholarship and research skills, final exam, dissertation defense. *Entrance requirements:* For master's, GRE General Test, bachelor's degree with minimum undergraduate GPA of 3.0; for doctorate, GRE General Test, bachelor's degree; minimum undergraduate/graduate GPA of 3.0. Additional exam requirements/recommendations for international students: Required—TOEFL or IELTS. *Application deadline:* For fall admission, 12/1 for domestic and international students; for spring admission, 9/15 for domestic and international students. Application fee: $55 ($65 for international students). Electronic applications accepted. *Financial support:* In 2013–14, 8 fellowships with full and partial tuition reimbursements, 22 research assistantships with full and partial tuition reimbursements, 32 teaching assistantships with full and partial tuition reimbursements were awarded; scholarships/grants, traineeships, health care benefits, and unspecified assistantships also available. Financial award application deadline: 12/1. *Faculty research:* Ecology and global change, diversity and macroevolution, evolutionary mechanisms, systematics/phylogenetics, biogeography. *Unit head:* Dr. Christopher H. Haufler, Chair, 785-864-3255, Fax: 785-864-5860, E-mail: vulgare@ku.edu. *Application contact:* Aagje Ashe, Graduate Coordinator, 785-864-2362, Fax: 785-864-5860, E-mail: a4ashe@ku.edu.
Website: http://eeb.ku.edu/

University of Kentucky, Graduate School, College of Agriculture, Food and Environment, Department of Entomology, Lexington, KY 40506-0032. Offers MS, PhD. *Degree requirements:* For master's, comprehensive exam, thesis optional; for doctorate, comprehensive exam, thesis/dissertation. *Entrance requirements:* For master's, GRE General Test, minimum undergraduate GPA of 2.75; for doctorate, GRE General Test, minimum graduate GPA of 3.0. Additional exam requirements/recommendations for international students: Required—TOEFL (minimum score 550 paper-based). Electronic applications accepted. *Faculty research:* Applied entomology, behavior, insect biology and ecology, biological control, insect physiology and molecular biology.

University of Maine, Graduate School, College of Natural Sciences, Forestry, and Agriculture, School of Biology and Ecology, Orono, ME 04469. Offers biological sciences (PhD); botany and plant pathology (MS); ecology and environmental science (MS, PhD); entomology (MS); plant science (PhD); zoology (MS, PhD). Part-time programs available. *Faculty:* 33 full-time (13 women), 26 part-time/adjunct (5 women). *Students:* 66 full-time (40 women), 4 part-time (2 women); includes 4 minority (1 American Indian or Alaska Native, non-Hispanic/Latino; 2 Asian, non-Hispanic/Latino; 1 Hispanic/Latino), 7 international. Average age 30. 97 applicants, 25% accepted, 17 enrolled. In 2013, 8 master's, 3 doctorates awarded. Terminal master's awarded for partial completion of doctoral program. *Degree requirements:* For master's, thesis (for some programs); for doctorate, comprehensive exam, thesis/dissertation. *Entrance requirements:* For master's and doctorate, GRE General Test. Additional exam requirements/recommendations for international students: Required—TOEFL. *Application deadline:* For fall admission, 2/1 priority date for domestic students. Applications are processed on a rolling basis. Application fee: $65. Electronic applications accepted. *Expenses:* Tuition, state resident: full-time $7524. Tuition, nonresident: full-time $23,112. *Required fees:* $1970. *Financial support:* In 2013–14, 66 students received support, including 3 fellowships with full tuition reimbursements available (averaging $25,000 per year), 28 research assistantships with full tuition reimbursements available (averaging $14,600 per year), 21 teaching assistantships with full tuition reimbursements available (averaging $14,600 per year); career-related internships or fieldwork, Federal Work-Study, institutionally sponsored loans, and tuition waivers (full and partial) also available. Financial award application deadline: 3/1. *Total annual research expenditures:* $569,533. *Unit head:* Dr. Ellie Groden, Director, 207-581-2551, Fax: 207-581-2537. *Application contact:* Scott G. Delcourt, Associate Dean of the Graduate School, 207-581-3291, Fax: 207-581-3232, E-mail: graduate@maine.edu.
Website: http://sbe.umaine.edu/

University of Manitoba, Faculty of Graduate Studies, Faculty of Agricultural and Food Sciences, Department of Entomology, Winnipeg, MB R3T 2N2, Canada. Offers M Sc, PhD. *Degree requirements:* For master's, thesis; for doctorate, one foreign language, thesis/dissertation.

University of Maryland, College Park, Academic Affairs, College of Computer, Mathematical and Natural Sciences, Department of Entomology, College Park, MD 20742. Offers MS, PhD. Part-time and evening/weekend programs available. *Faculty:* 46 full-time (24 women), 2 part-time/adjunct (both women). *Students:* 16 full-time (9 women), 6 part-time (1 woman); includes 4 minority (1 Black or African American, non-Hispanic/Latino; 1 Asian, non-Hispanic/Latino; 1 Hispanic/Latino; 1 Two or more races, non-Hispanic/Latino), 3 international. 22 applicants, 9% accepted, 2 enrolled. In 2013, 1 master's, 1 doctorate awarded. Terminal master's awarded for partial completion of doctoral program. *Degree requirements:* For master's, thesis; for doctorate, thesis/dissertation, oral qualifying exam. *Entrance requirements:* For master's and doctorate, GRE General Test, minimum GPA of 3.0, 3 letters of recommendation. *Application deadline:* For fall admission, 12/15 for domestic and international students. Applications are processed on a rolling basis. Application fee: $75. Electronic applications accepted. *Expenses:* Tuition, state resident: full-time $10,314; part-time $573 per credit hour. Tuition, nonresident: full-time $22,248; part-time $1236 per credit. *Required fees:* $1446; $403.15 per semester. Tuition and fees vary according to program. *Financial support:* In 2013–14, 3 fellowships with full and partial tuition reimbursements (averaging $26,909 per year), 2 research assistantships (averaging $19,020 per year), 20 teaching assistantships (averaging $19,205 per year) were awarded; career-related internships or fieldwork and Federal Work-Study also available. Support available to part-time students. Financial award applicants required to submit FAFSA. *Faculty research:* Pest management, biosystematics, physiology and morphology, toxicology. *Total annual research expenditures:* $4.6 million. *Unit head:* Dr. Charles Mitter, Chair, 301-405-3912, E-mail: cmitter@umd.edu. *Application contact:* Dr. Charles A. Caramello, Dean of Graduate School, 301-405-0358, Fax: 301-314-9305, E-mail: ccaramel@umd.edu.

University of Minnesota, Twin Cities Campus, Graduate School, College of Food, Agricultural and Natural Resource Sciences, Entomology Graduate Program, Saint Paul, MN 55108. Offers MS, PhD. Part-time programs available. *Faculty:* 18 full-time (6 women), 7 part-time/adjunct (4 women). *Students:* 33 full-time (16 women), 2 part-time (both women); includes 3 minority (1 Black or African American, non-Hispanic/Latino; 2 Asian, non-Hispanic/Latino), 5 international. Average age 27. 24 applicants, 42% accepted, 10 enrolled. In 2013, 6 master's awarded. Terminal master's awarded for partial completion of doctoral program. *Degree requirements:* For master's, comprehensive exam, thesis; for doctorate, comprehensive exam, thesis/dissertation. *Entrance requirements:* For master's, GRE, minimum undergraduate GPA of 3.0; for doctorate, GRE, minimum undergraduate GPA of 3.0, graduate 3.5. Additional exam requirements/recommendations for international students: Required—TOEFL (minimum score 550 paper-based; 79 iBT), IELTS (minimum score 6.5). *Application deadline:* For fall admission, 12/15 priority date for domestic and international students; for spring admission, 10/15 priority date for domestic students, 12/15 priority date for international students. Applications are processed on a rolling basis. Application fee: $75 ($95 for international students). Electronic applications accepted. *Financial support:* In 2013–14, 1 student received support, including fellowships with full tuition reimbursements available (averaging $40,000 per year), research assistantships with full tuition reimbursements available (averaging $40,000 per year), teaching assistantships with full tuition reimbursements available (averaging $40,000 per year); scholarships/grants, traineeships, health care benefits, tuition waivers (full and partial), unspecified assistantships, and summer research assistantships also available. Financial award application deadline: 3/1. *Faculty research:* Behavior, ecology, molecular genetics, physiology, systematics and taxonomy. *Total annual research expenditures:* $4,582. *Unit head:* Dr. George Heimpel, Director of Graduate Studies, 612-624-3480, Fax: 612-625-5299, E-mail: heimp001@umn.edu. *Application contact:* Felicia Christy, Program Coordinator, 612-624-3278, Fax: 612-625-5299, E-mail: christy@umn.edu.
Website: http://www.entomology.umn.edu/

University of Missouri, Graduate School, College of Agriculture, Food and Natural Resources, Division of Plant Sciences, Columbia, MO 65211. Offers crop, soil and pest management (MS, PhD); entomology (MS, PhD); horticulture (MS, PhD); plant biology and genetics (MS, PhD); plant stress biology (MS, PhD). *Faculty:* 40 full-time (11 women). *Students:* 71 full-time (32 women), 12 part-time (3 women); includes 5 minority (2 Black or African American, non-Hispanic/Latino; 1 American Indian or Alaska Native, non-Hispanic/Latino; 1 Hispanic/Latino; 1 Two or more races, non-Hispanic/Latino), 35 international. Average age 28. 78 applicants, 27% accepted, 17 enrolled. In 2013, 10 master's, 10 doctorates awarded. Terminal master's awarded for partial completion of doctoral program. *Degree requirements:* For master's, thesis; for doctorate, comprehensive exam, thesis/dissertation. *Entrance requirements:* For master's and doctorate, GRE General Test, minimum GPA of 3.0; bachelor's degree from accredited college. Additional exam requirements/recommendations for international students: Required—TOEFL (minimum score 500 paper-based; 61 iBT), IELTS (minimum score 5.5). *Application deadline:* For fall admission, 1/15 priority date for domestic students, 1/15 for international students. Applications are processed on a rolling basis. Application fee: $55 ($75 for international students). Electronic applications accepted. *Financial support:* In 2013–14, 2 fellowships with tuition reimbursements, 59 research assistantships with tuition reimbursements, 1 teaching assistantship with tuition reimbursement were awarded; institutionally sponsored loans, scholarships/grants, health care benefits, and unspecified assistantships also available. Support available to part-time students. *Faculty research:* Crop, soil and pest management; entomology; horticulture; plant biology and genetics; plant microbiology and pathology. *Unit head:* Dr. Michael Collins, Director, 573-882-1957, E-mail: collinsm@missouri.edu. *Application contact:* Dr. James Schoelz, Director of Graduate Studies, 573-882-1185, E-mail: schoelzj@missouri.edu.
Website: http://plantsci.missouri.edu/graduate/

University of Nebraska–Lincoln, Graduate College, College of Agricultural Sciences and Natural Resources, Department of Entomology, Lincoln, NE 68588. Offers MS, PhD. Postbaccalaureate distance learning degree programs offered (no on-campus study). *Degree requirements:* For master's, thesis optional; for doctorate, comprehensive exam, thesis/dissertation. *Entrance requirements:* For master's and doctorate, GRE General Test. Additional exam requirements/recommendations for international students: Required—TOEFL (minimum score 550 paper-based). Electronic applications accepted. *Faculty research:* Ecology and behavior, insect-plant interactions, integrated pest management, genetics, urban entomology.

University of North Dakota, Graduate School, College of Arts and Sciences, Department of Biology, Grand Forks, ND 58202. Offers botany (MS, PhD); ecology (MS, PhD); entomology (MS, PhD); environmental biology (MS, PhD); fisheries/wildlife (MS, PhD); genetics (MS, PhD); zoology (MS, PhD). Terminal master's awarded for partial completion of doctoral program. *Degree requirements:* For master's, thesis, final exam; for doctorate, comprehensive exam, thesis/dissertation, final exam. *Entrance requirements:* For master's, GRE General Test, GRE Subject Test, minimum GPA of 3.0; for doctorate, GRE General Test, GRE Subject Test, minimum GPA of 3.5. Additional exam requirements/recommendations for international students: Required—TOEFL (minimum score 550 paper-based; 79 iBT), IELTS (minimum score 6.5). Electronic applications accepted. *Faculty research:* Population biology, wildlife ecology, RNA processing, hormonal control of behavior.

The University of Tennessee, Graduate School, College of Agricultural Sciences and Natural Resources, Department of Entomology and Plant Pathology, Knoxville, TN 37996. Offers entomology (MS, PhD); integrated pest management and bioactive natural products (PhD); plant pathology (MS, PhD). Part-time programs available. *Degree requirements:* For master's, thesis, seminar. *Entrance requirements:* For master's, GRE General Test, minimum GPA of 2.7, 3 reference letters, letter of intent; for doctorate, GRE General Test, minimum GPA of 2.7, 3 reference letters, letter of intent, proposed dissertation research. Additional exam requirements/recommendations for international students: Required—TOEFL. Electronic applications accepted. *Expenses:* Tuition, state resident: full-time $9540; part-time $531 per credit hour. Tuition, nonresident: full-time $27,728; part-time $1542 per credit hour. *Required fees:* $1404; $67 per credit hour.

University of Wisconsin–Madison, Graduate School, College of Agricultural and Life Sciences, Department of Entomology, Madison, WI 53706-1380. Offers MS, PhD. *Degree requirements:* For master's, thesis; for doctorate, thesis/dissertation. *Entrance* *requirements:* For master's and doctorate, GRE General Test, minimum GPA of 3.0. Additional exam requirements/recommendations for international students: Required—TOEFL. Electronic applications accepted. *Expenses:* Tuition, state resident: full-time $10,728; part-time $790 per credit. Tuition, nonresident: full-time $24,054; part-time $1623 per credit. *Required fees:* $1130; $119 per credit. *Faculty research:* Ecology, biocontrol, molecular.

University of Wyoming, College of Agriculture and Natural Resources, Department of Renewable Resources, Program in Entomology, Laramie, WY 82071. Offers MS, PhD. *Degree requirements:* For master's, thesis; for doctorate, thesis/dissertation. *Entrance requirements:* For master's and doctorate, GRE General Test, minimum GPA of 3.0. Additional exam requirements/recommendations for international students: Required—TOEFL. Electronic applications accepted. *Faculty research:* Insect pest management, taxonomy, biocontrol of weeds, forest insects, insects affecting humans and animals.

Virginia Polytechnic Institute and State University, Graduate School, College of Agriculture and Life Sciences, Blacksburg, VA 24061. Offers agricultural and applied economics (MS); agricultural and life sciences (MS); animal and poultry science (MS, PhD); crop and soil environmental sciences (MS, PhD); dairy science (MS); entomology (PhD); horticulture (MS, PhD); human nutrition, foods and exercise (MS, PhD); life sciences (MS, PhD); plant pathology, physiology and weed science (PhD). *Faculty:* 234 full-time (66 women), 1 (woman) part-time/adjunct. *Students:* 347 full-time (188 women), 80 part-time (53 women); includes 53 minority (19 Black or African American, non-Hispanic/Latino; 1 American Indian or Alaska Native, non-Hispanic/Latino; 19 Asian, non-Hispanic/Latino; 7 Hispanic/Latino; 7 Two or more races, non-Hispanic/Latino), 106 international. Average age 29. 410 applicants, 35% accepted, 111 enrolled. In 2013, 80 master's, 44 doctorates awarded. *Degree requirements:* For master's, comprehensive exam (for some programs), thesis (for some programs); for doctorate, comprehensive exam (for some programs), thesis/dissertation (for some programs). *Entrance requirements:* For master's and doctorate, GRE/GMAT (may vary by department). Additional exam requirements/recommendations for international students: Required—TOEFL (minimum score 550 paper-based). *Application deadline:* For fall admission, 8/1 for domestic students, 4/1 for international students; for spring admission, 1/1 for domestic students, 9/1 for international students. Applications are processed on a rolling basis. Application fee: $75. Electronic applications accepted. *Expenses:* Tuition, state resident: full-time $11,185; part-time $621.50 per credit hour. Tuition, nonresident: full-time $22,146; part-time $1230.25 per credit hour. *Required fees:* $2442; $449.25 per semester. Tuition and fees vary according to course load, campus/location and program. *Financial support:* In 2013–14, 1 fellowship with full tuition reimbursement (averaging $19,278 per year), 232 research assistantships with full tuition reimbursements (averaging $19,370 per year), 83 teaching assistantships with full tuition reimbursements (averaging $18,677 per year) were awarded. Financial award application deadline: 3/1; financial award applicants required to submit FAFSA. *Total annual research expenditures:* $44.3 million. *Unit head:* Dr. Alan L. Grant, Dean, 540-231-4152, Fax: 540-231-4163, E-mail: algrant@vt.edu. *Application contact:* Sheila Norman, Administrative Assistant, 540-231-4152, Fax: 540-231-4163, E-mail: snorman@vt.edu.
Website: http://www.cals.vt.edu/

Washington State University, Graduate School, College of Agricultural, Human, and Natural Resource Sciences, Department of Entomology, Pullman, WA 99164. Offers MS, PhD. Part-time programs available. Terminal master's awarded for partial completion of doctoral program. *Degree requirements:* For master's, comprehensive exam (for some programs), thesis (for some programs), oral exam; for doctorate, comprehensive exam, thesis/dissertation, oral exam, written exam. *Entrance requirements:* For master's, GRE General Test, GRE Subject Test in advanced biology (recommended), minimum GPA of 3.0, 3 letters of recommendation; for doctorate, GRE General Test, minimum GPA of 3.0, 3 letters of recommendation. Additional exam requirements/recommendations for international students: Required—TOEFL (minimum score 550 paper-based), IELTS. Electronic applications accepted. *Faculty research:* Apiculture, biological control of arthropods, integrated pest management, ecology, physiology and systematics of insects.

West Virginia University, Davis College of Agriculture, Forestry and Consumer Sciences, Division of Plant and Soil Sciences, Morgantown, WV 26506. Offers agricultural sciences (PhD), including animal and food sciences, plant and soil sciences; agronomy (MS); entomology (MS); environmental microbiology (MS); horticulture (MS); plant pathology (MS). *Degree requirements:* For master's, thesis. *Entrance requirements:* For master's, GRE, minimum GPA of 2.5. Additional exam requirements/recommendations for international students: Required—TOEFL. *Faculty research:* Water quality, reclamation of disturbed land, crop production, pest control, environmental protection.

Section 10
Genetics, Developmental Biology, and Reproductive Biology

This section contains a directory of institutions offering graduate work in genetics, developmental biology, and reproductive biology, followed by an in-depth entry submitted by an institution that chose to prepare a detailed program description. Additional information about programs listed in the directory but not augmented by an in-depth entry may be obtained by writing directly to the dean of a graduate school or chair of a department at the address given in the directory.

For programs offering related work, see also all other sections of this book. In the other guides in this series:

Graduate Programs in the Physical Sciences, Mathematics, Agricultural Sciences, the Environment & Natural Resources

See *Agricultural and Food Sciences, Chemistry,* and *Environmental Sciences and Management*

Graduate Programs in Engineering & Applied Sciences

See *Agricultural Engineering and Bioengineering* and *Biomedical Engineering and Biotechnology*

CONTENTS

Program Directories

Displays and Close-Ups

See also:

Developmental Biology

Albert Einstein College of Medicine, Graduate Division of Biomedical Sciences, Department of Anatomy and Structural Biology, Bronx, NY 10461. Offers anatomy (PhD); cell and developmental biology (PhD); MD/PhD. *Degree requirements:* For doctorate, thesis/dissertation. *Entrance requirements:* For doctorate, GRE General Test. Additional exam requirements/recommendations for international students: Required—TOEFL. Electronic applications accepted. *Faculty research:* Cell motility, cell membranes and membrane-cytoskeletal interactions as applied to processing of pancreatic hormones, mechanisms of secretion.

Albert Einstein College of Medicine, Graduate Division of Biomedical Sciences, Department of Developmental and Molecular Biology, Bronx, NY 10461. Offers PhD, MD/PhD. *Degree requirements:* For doctorate, thesis/dissertation. *Entrance requirements:* For doctorate, GRE General Test. Additional exam requirements/recommendations for international students: Required—TOEFL. *Faculty research:* DNA, RNA, and protein synthesis in prokaryotes and eukaryotes; chemical and enzymatic alteration of RNA; glycoproteins.

Baylor College of Medicine, Graduate School of Biomedical Sciences, Program in Developmental Biology, Houston, TX 77030-3498. Offers PhD, MD/PhD. *Degree requirements:* For doctorate, thesis/dissertation, public defense. *Entrance requirements:* For doctorate, GRE General Test, GRE Subject Test (strongly recommended), minimum GPA of 3.0. Additional exam requirements/recommendations for international students: Required—TOEFL. Electronic applications accepted. *Faculty research:* Stem cells, cancer, neurobiology, organogenesis, genetics of model organisms.

Brigham Young University, Graduate Studies, College of Life Sciences, Department of Physiology and Developmental Biology, Provo, UT 84602. Offers neuroscience (MS, PhD); physiology and developmental biology (MS, PhD). Part-time programs available. *Faculty:* 20 full-time (0 women). *Students:* 42 full-time (20 women); includes 12 minority (1 American Indian or Alaska Native, non-Hispanic/Latino; 7 Asian, non-Hispanic/Latino; 3 Hispanic/Latino; 1 Two or more races, non-Hispanic/Latino). Average age 28. 15 applicants, 20% accepted, 2 enrolled. In 2013, 6 master's, 5 doctorates awarded. Terminal master's awarded for partial completion of doctoral program. *Degree requirements:* For master's, thesis, oral exam; for doctorate, comprehensive exam, thesis/dissertation. *Entrance requirements:* For master's, GRE General Test, minimum GPA of 3.0 during previous 2 years; for doctorate, GRE General Test, minimum GPA of 3.0 overall. Additional exam requirements/recommendations for international students: Required—TOEFL (minimum score 580 paper-based; 85 iBT). *Application deadline:* For fall admission, 2/1 priority date for domestic and international students; for winter admission, 9/10 priority date for domestic and international students. Application fee: $50. Electronic applications accepted. *Expenses: Tuition:* Full-time $6130; part-time $340 per credit hour. Tuition and fees vary according to program and student's religious affiliation. *Financial support:* In 2013–14, 41 students received support, including 2 fellowships with partial tuition reimbursements available (averaging $7,100 per year), 20 research assistantships with full tuition reimbursements available (averaging $15,500 per year), 20 teaching assistantships with partial tuition reimbursements available (averaging $14,900 per year); career-related internships or fieldwork, institutionally sponsored loans, scholarships/grants, tuition waivers (full and partial), unspecified assistantships, and tuition awards also available. Financial award application deadline: 2/1. *Faculty research:* Sex differentiation of the brain, exercise physiology, developmental biology, membrane biophysics, neuroscience. *Total annual research expenditures:* $508,299. *Unit head:* Dr. Dixon J. Woodbury, Chair, 801-422-7562, Fax: 801-422-0700, E-mail: dixon_woodbury@byu.edu. *Application contact:* Connie L. Provost, Graduate Secretary, 801-422-3706, Fax: 801-422-0700, E-mail: connie_provost@byu.edu.
Website: http://pdbio.byu.edu

California Institute of Technology, Division of Biology, Program in Developmental Biology, Pasadena, CA 91125-0001. Offers PhD. *Degree requirements:* For doctorate, thesis/dissertation, qualifying exam. *Entrance requirements:* For doctorate, GRE General Test.

California State University, Sacramento, Office of Graduate Studies, College of Natural Sciences and Mathematics, Department of Biological Sciences, Sacramento, CA 95819. Offers biological conservation (MS); marine science (MS); molecular and cellular biology (MS); stem cell (MA). Part-time programs available. *Degree requirements:* For master's, thesis, writing proficiency exam. *Entrance requirements:* For master's, GRE, bachelor's degree in biology or equivalent; minimum GPA of 3.0 in biology, 2.75 overall during last 2 years of course work. Additional exam requirements/recommendations for international students: Required—TOEFL. *Application deadline:* For fall admission, 2/1 for domestic students, 3/1 for international students; for spring admission, 9/30 for international students. Applications are processed on a rolling basis. Application fee: $55. Electronic applications accepted. *Financial support:* Research assistantships, teaching assistantships, career-related internships or fieldwork, and Federal Work-Study available. Support available to part-time students. Financial award application deadline: 3/1; financial award applicants required to submit FAFSA. *Unit head:* Jennifer Lundmark, Chair, 916-278-6535, E-mail: lundmark@csus.edu. *Application contact:* Jose Martinez, Graduate Admissions Supervisor, 916-278-7871, E-mail: martinj@skymail.csus.edu.
Website: http://www.csus.edu/bios

Carnegie Mellon University, Mellon College of Science, Department of Biological Sciences, Pittsburgh, PA 15213-3891. Offers biochemistry (PhD); biophysics (PhD); cell and developmental biology (PhD); computational biology (MS, PhD); genetics (PhD); molecular biology (PhD); neuroscience (PhD); structural biology (PhD). *Degree requirements:* For doctorate, comprehensive exam, thesis/dissertation. *Entrance requirements:* For doctorate, GRE General Test, GRE Subject Test, interview. *Application deadline:* Applications are processed on a rolling basis. Application fee: $0. Electronic applications accepted. *Financial support:* Fellowships, research assistantships, teaching assistantships, and traineeships available. *Faculty research:* Genetic structure, function, and regulation; protein structure and function; biological membranes; biological spectroscopy. *Unit head:* John L. Woolford, Acting Department Head, 412-268-3193, E-mail: jw17@andrew.cmu.edu. *Application contact:* Ena Miceli, Graduate Programs Manager, 412-268-33012, E-mail: emiceli@andrew.cmu.edu.
Website: http://www.bio.cmu.edu/

Columbia University, College of Physicians and Surgeons, Department of Genetics and Development, New York, NY 10032. Offers genetics (M Phil, MA, PhD); MD/PhD. Only candidates for the PhD are admitted. Terminal master's awarded for partial completion of doctoral program. *Degree requirements:* For doctorate, thesis/dissertation. *Entrance requirements:* For master's and doctorate, GRE General Test. Additional exam requirements/recommendations for international students: Required—TOEFL. *Faculty research:* Mammalian cell differentiation and meiosis, developmental genetics, yeast and human genetics, chromosome structure, molecular and cellular biology.

Cornell University, Graduate School, Graduate Fields of Agriculture and Life Sciences, Field of Genetics, Genomics and Development, Ithaca, NY 14853-0001. Offers developmental biology (PhD); genetics (PhD); genomics (PhD). *Faculty:* 66 full-time (15 women). *Students:* 56 full-time (37 women); includes 7 minority (3 Black or African American, non-Hispanic/Latino; 2 Asian, non-Hispanic/Latino; 1 Hispanic/Latino; 1 Two or more races, non-Hispanic/Latino), 22 international. Average age 26. 67 applicants, 33% accepted, 12 enrolled. In 2013, 12 doctorates awarded. *Degree requirements:* For doctorate, comprehensive exam, thesis/dissertation, 2 semesters of teaching experience. *Entrance requirements:* For doctorate, GRE General Test, GRE Subject Test in biology or biochemistry (recommended), 2 letters of recommendation. Additional exam requirements/recommendations for international students: Required—TOEFL (minimum score 550 paper-based; 77 iBT). *Application deadline:* For fall admission, 1/5 for domestic students. Application fee: $95. Electronic applications accepted. *Financial support:* In 2013–14, 45 students received support, including 5 fellowships with full tuition reimbursements available, 26 research assistantships with full tuition reimbursements available, 14 teaching assistantships with full tuition reimbursements available; institutionally sponsored loans, scholarships/grants, health care benefits, tuition waivers (full and partial), and unspecified assistantships also available. Financial award applicants required to submit FAFSA. *Faculty research:* Molecular and general genetics, developmental biology and developmental genetics, evolution and population genetics, plant genetics, microbial genetics. *Unit head:* Director of Graduate Studies, 607-254-2100. *Application contact:* Graduate Field Assistant, 607-254-2100, E-mail: gendev@cornell.edu.
Website: http://www.gradschool.cornell.edu/fields.php?id-51&a-2

Cornell University, Graduate School, Graduate Fields of Agriculture and Life Sciences, Field of Zoology and Wildlife Conservation, Ithaca, NY 14853-0001. Offers animal cytology (PhD); comparative and functional anatomy (PhD); developmental biology (PhD); ecology (PhD); histology (PhD); wildlife conservation (PhD). *Faculty:* 21 full-time (6 women). *Students:* 4 full-time (3 women), 1 part-time (0 women); includes 2 minority (1 Hispanic/Latino; 1 Two or more races, non-Hispanic/Latino), 1 international. Average age 26. 18 applicants, 6% accepted, 1 enrolled. In 2013, 1 doctorate awarded. *Degree requirements:* For doctorate, comprehensive exam, thesis/dissertation, 2 semesters of teaching experience. *Entrance requirements:* For doctorate, GRE General Test, GRE Subject Test (biology), 2 letters of recommendation. Additional exam requirements/recommendations for international students: Required—TOEFL (minimum score 550 paper-based; 77 iBT). *Application deadline:* For fall admission, 2/1 priority date for domestic students. Application fee: $95. Electronic applications accepted. *Financial support:* In 2013–14, 4 students received support, including 3 research assistantships with full tuition reimbursements available, 1 teaching assistantship with full tuition reimbursement available; fellowships with full tuition reimbursements available, institutionally sponsored loans, scholarships/grants, health care benefits, tuition waivers (full and partial), and unspecified assistantships also available. Financial award applicants required to submit FAFSA. *Faculty research:* Organismal biology, functional morphology, biomechanics, comparative vertebrate anatomy, comparative invertebrate anatomy, paleontology. *Unit head:* Director of Graduate Studies, 607-253-3276, Fax: 607-253-3756. *Application contact:* Graduate Field Assistant, 607-253-3276, Fax: 607-253-3756, E-mail: graduate_edcvm@cornell.edu.
Website: http://www.gradschool.cornell.edu/fields.php?id-65&a-2

Cornell University, Graduate School, Graduate Fields of Comparative Biomedical Sciences, Field of Comparative Biomedical Sciences, Ithaca, NY 14853-0001. Offers cellular and molecular medicine (MS, PhD); developmental and reproductive biology (MS, PhD); infectious diseases (MS, PhD); population medicine and epidemiology (MS, PhD); structural and functional biology (MS, PhD). *Faculty:* 104 full-time (32 women). *Students:* 32 full-time (22 women); includes 3 minority (1 Asian, non-Hispanic/Latino; 2 Hispanic/Latino), 12 international. Average age 29. 47 applicants, 23% accepted, 6 enrolled. In 2013, 2 master's, 12 doctorates awarded. *Degree requirements:* For master's, thesis; for doctorate, comprehensive exam, thesis/dissertation. *Entrance requirements:* For master's and doctorate, GRE General Test, 2 letters of recommendation. Additional exam requirements/recommendations for international students: Required—TOEFL (minimum score 550 paper-based; 77 iBT). *Application deadline:* For fall admission, 12/15 for domestic students. Application fee: $95. Electronic applications accepted. *Financial support:* In 2013–14, 18 students received support, including 3 fellowships with full tuition reimbursements available, 14 research assistantships with full tuition reimbursements available, 1 teaching assistantship with full tuition reimbursement available; institutionally sponsored loans, scholarships/grants, health care benefits, tuition waivers (full and partial), and unspecified assistantships also available. Financial award applicants required to submit FAFSA. *Faculty research:* Receptors and signal transduction, viral and bacterial infectious diseases, tumor metastasis, clinical sciences/nutritional disease, developmental/neurological disorders. *Unit head:* Director of Graduate Studies, 607-253-3276, Fax: 607-253-3756. *Application contact:* Graduate Field Assistant, 607-253-3276, Fax: 607-253-3756, E-mail: graduate_edcvm@cornell.edu.
Website: http://www.gradschool.cornell.edu/fields.php?id-64&a-2

Duke University, Graduate School, Program in Developmental and Stem Cell Biology, Durham, NC 27710. Offers Certificate. *Faculty:* 45. *Students:* 7 full-time (4 women); includes 2 minority (both Hispanic/Latino), 1 international. 56 applicants, 25% accepted, 3 enrolled. *Entrance requirements:* For degree, GRE General Test. Additional exam requirements/recommendations for international students: Required—TOEFL (minimum score 577 paper-based; 90 iBT) or IELTS (minimum score 7). *Application deadline:* For fall admission, 12/8 priority date for domestic and international students. Application fee: $80. *Financial support:* Application deadline: 12/8. *Unit head:* David Sherwood, Head, 919-684-6629, Fax: 919-684-8346, E-mail: leslie.mavengere@duke.edu. *Application contact:* Elizabeth Hutton, Director of Admissions, 919-684-3913, Fax: 919-684-2277, E-mail: grad-admissions@duke.edu.
Website: http://devbio.duke.edu/

Emory University, Laney Graduate School, Division of Biological and Biomedical Sciences, Program in Biochemistry, Cell and Developmental Biology, Atlanta, GA 30322. Offers PhD. *Degree requirements:* For doctorate, comprehensive exam, thesis/dissertation. *Entrance requirements:* For doctorate, GRE General Test, minimum GPA of 3.0 in science course work (recommended). Additional exam requirements/recommendations for international students: Required—TOEFL. Electronic applications accepted. *Faculty research:* Signal transduction, molecular biology, enzymes and cofactors, receptor and ion channel function, membrane biology.

Illinois State University, Graduate School, College of Arts and Sciences, Department of Biological Sciences, Normal, IL 61790-2200. Offers animal behavior (MS); bacteriology (MS); biochemistry (MS); biological sciences (MS); biology (PhD); biophysics (MS); biotechnology (MS); botany (MS, PhD); cell biology (MS); conservation biology (MS); developmental biology (MS); ecology (MS, PhD); entomology (MS); evolutionary biology (MS); genetics (MS, PhD); immunology (MS); microbiology (MS, PhD); molecular biology (MS); molecular genetics (MS); neurobiology (MS); neuroscience (MS); parasitology (MS); physiology (MS, PhD); plant biology (MS); plant molecular biology (MS); plant sciences (MS); structural biology (MS); zoology (MS, PhD). Part-time programs available. *Degree requirements:* For master's, thesis or alternative; for doctorate, variable foreign language requirement, thesis/dissertation, 2 terms of residency. *Entrance requirements:* For master's, GRE General Test, minimum GPA of 2.6 in last 60 hours of course work; for doctorate, GRE General Test. *Faculty research:* Redoc balance and drug development in schistosoma mansoni, control of the growth of listeria monocytogenes at low temperature, regulation of cell expansion and microtubule function by SPRI, CRUI: physiology and fitness consequences of different life history phenotypes.

Iowa State University of Science and Technology, Program in Molecular, Cellular, and Developmental Biology, Ames, IA 50011. Offers MS, PhD. *Entrance requirements:* For master's and doctorate, GRE General Test. Additional exam requirements/recommendations for international students: Required—TOEFL (minimum score 580 paper-based; 85 iBT), IELTS (minimum score 7). Electronic applications accepted.

Johns Hopkins University, National Institutes of Health Sponsored Programs, Baltimore, MD 21218-2699. Offers biology (PhD), including biochemistry, biophysics, cell biology, developmental biology, genetic biology, molecular biology; cell, molecular, and developmental biology and biophysics (PhD). *Faculty:* 25 full-time (4 women). *Students:* 126 full-time (72 women); includes 36 minority (3 Black or African American, non-Hispanic/Latino; 1 American Indian or Alaska Native, non-Hispanic/Latino; 21 Asian, non-Hispanic/Latino; 11 Hispanic/Latino), 19 international. 282 applicants, 26% accepted, 36 enrolled. In 2013, 15 doctorates awarded. *Degree requirements:* For doctorate, comprehensive exam, thesis/dissertation. *Entrance requirements:* For doctorate, GRE General Test. Additional exam requirements/recommendations for international students: Required—TOEFL (minimum score 600 paper-based), TWE. *Application deadline:* For fall admission, 12/15 priority date for domestic students. Application fee: $60. Electronic applications accepted. *Financial support:* In 2013–14, 24 fellowships (averaging $23,000 per year), 93 research assistantships (averaging $23,000 per year), 22 teaching assistantships (averaging $23,000 per year) were awarded; Federal Work-Study, institutionally sponsored loans, scholarships/grants, traineeships, health care benefits, tuition waivers (partial), and unspecified assistantships also available. Financial award application deadline: 4/15; financial award applicants required to submit FAFSA. *Faculty research:* Protein and nucleic acid biochemistry and biophysical chemistry, molecular biology and development. *Total annual research expenditures:* $11.2 million. *Unit head:* Dr. Allen Shearn, Chair, 410-516-4693, Fax: 410-516-5213, E-mail: bio_cals@jhu.edu. *Application contact:* Joan Miller, Academic Affairs Manager, 410-516-5502, Fax: 410-516-5213, E-mail: joan@jhu.edu.

Louisiana State University Health Sciences Center, School of Graduate Studies in New Orleans, Department of Cell Biology and Anatomy, New Orleans, LA 70112-2223. Offers cell biology and anatomy (MS, PhD), including cell biology, developmental biology, neurobiology and anatomy; MD/PhD. *Degree requirements:* For master's, comprehensive exam, thesis; for doctorate, comprehensive exam, thesis/dissertation. *Entrance requirements:* For master's and doctorate, GRE General Test, GRE Subject Test, minimum undergraduate GPA of 3.0. Additional exam requirements/recommendations for international students: Required—TOEFL. *Faculty research:* Visual system organization, neural development, plasticity of sensory systems, information processing through the nervous system, visuomotor integration.

Marquette University, Graduate School, College of Arts and Sciences, Department of Biology, Milwaukee, WI 53201-1881. Offers cell biology (MS, PhD); developmental biology (MS, PhD); ecology (MS, PhD); epithelial physiology (MS, PhD); genetics (MS, PhD); microbiology (MS, PhD); molecular biology (MS, PhD); muscle and exercise physiology (MS, PhD); neuroscience (PhD). *Faculty:* 21 full-time (9 women), 3 part-time/adjunct (0 women). *Students:* 34 full-time (16 women), 4 part-time (1 woman), 15 international. Average age 27. 70 applicants, 23% accepted, 5 enrolled. In 2013, 1 master's, 6 doctorates awarded. Terminal master's awarded for partial completion of doctoral program. *Degree requirements:* For master's, comprehensive exam, thesis, 1 year of teaching experience or equivalent; for doctorate, thesis/dissertation, 1 year of teaching experience or equivalent, qualifying exam. *Entrance requirements:* For master's and doctorate, GRE General Test, GRE Subject Test, official transcripts from all current and previous colleges/universities except Marquette, statement of professional goals and aspirations, three letters of recommendation. Additional exam requirements/recommendations for international students: Required—TOEFL (minimum score 530 paper-based). *Application deadline:* For fall admission, 12/15 for domestic and international students. Application fee: $50. Electronic applications accepted. *Financial support:* In 2013–14, 39 students received support, including 6 fellowships (averaging $1,208 per year), 4 research assistantships with full tuition reimbursements available (averaging $21,750 per year), 29 teaching assistantships with full tuition reimbursements available (averaging $21,750 per year); scholarships/grants, health care benefits, tuition waivers (full and partial), and unspecified assistantships also available. Support available to part-time students. Financial award application deadline: 2/15. *Faculty research:* Neurobiology, neuroendocrinology, epithelial physiology, neuropeptide interactions, synaptic transmission. *Total annual research expenditures:* $1.5 million. *Unit head:* Dr. Dale Noel, Chair and Professor, 414-288-1748. *Application contact:* Dr. Michelle Mynlieff, Professor, 414-288-1467.
Website: http://www.marquette.edu/biology/

Massachusetts Institute of Technology, School of Science, Department of Biology, Cambridge, MA 02139-4307. Offers biochemistry (PhD); biological oceanography (PhD); biology (PhD); biophysical chemistry and molecular structure (PhD); cell biology (PhD); computational and systems biology (PhD); developmental biology (PhD); genetics (PhD); immunology (PhD); microbiology (PhD); molecular biology (PhD); neurobiology (PhD). *Faculty:* 58 full-time (15 women). *Students:* 261 full-time (133 women); includes 77 minority (3 Black or African American, non-Hispanic/Latino; 1 American Indian or Alaska Native, non-Hispanic/Latino; 32 Asian, non-Hispanic/Latino; 32 Hispanic/Latino; 9 Two or more races, non-Hispanic/Latino), 46 international. Average age 26. 651 applicants, 15% accepted, 39 enrolled. In 2013, 25 doctorates awarded. *Degree requirements:* For doctorate, comprehensive exam, thesis/dissertation, two semesters as a teaching assistant. *Entrance requirements:* For doctorate, GRE General Test. Additional exam requirements/recommendations for international students: Required—TOEFL (minimum score 577 paper-based), IELTS (minimum score 6.5). *Application deadline:* For fall admission, 12/1 for domestic and international students. Application fee: $75. Electronic applications accepted. *Expenses: Tuition:* Full-time $43,210; part-time $670 per credit hour. *Required fees:* $288. *Financial support:* In 2013–14, 252 students received support, including 135 fellowships (averaging $36,800 per year), 122 research assistantships (averaging $35,500 per year), 1 teaching assistantship; Federal Work-Study, institutionally sponsored loans, scholarships/grants, traineeships, health care benefits, and unspecified assistantships also available. *Faculty research:* Cellular, developmental and molecular (plant and animal) biology; biochemistry, bioengineering, biophysics and structural biology; classical and molecular genetics, stem cell and epigenetics; immunology and microbiology; cancer biology, molecular medicine, neurobiology and human disease; computational and systems biology. *Total annual research expenditures:* $44.5 million. *Unit head:* Alan Grossman, Interim Head, 617-253-4701. *Application contact:* Biology Education Office, 617-253-3717, Fax: 617-258-9329, E-mail: gradbio@mit.edu.
Website: https://biology.mit.edu/

Medical University of South Carolina, College of Graduate Studies, Program in Molecular and Cellular Biology and Pathobiology, Charleston, SC 29425. Offers cancer biology (PhD); cardiovascular biology (PhD); cardiovascular imaging (PhD); cell regulation (PhD); craniofacial biology (PhD); genetics and development (PhD); marine biomedicine (PhD); DMD/PhD; MD/PhD. *Degree requirements:* For doctorate, thesis/dissertation, oral and written exams. *Entrance requirements:* For doctorate, GRE General Test, interview, minimum GPA of 3.0. Additional exam requirements/recommendations for international students: Required—TOEFL (minimum score 600 paper-based; 100 iBT). Electronic applications accepted.

New York University, Graduate School of Arts and Science, Department of Biology, New York, NY 10012-1019. Offers biology (PhD); biomedical journalism (MS); cancer and molecular biology (PhD); computational biology (PhD); computers in biological research (MS); developmental genetics (PhD); general biology (MS); immunology and microbiology (PhD); molecular genetics (PhD); neurobiology (PhD); oral biology (MS); plant biology (PhD); recombinant DNA technology (MS); MS/MBA. Part-time programs available. *Faculty:* 24 full-time (5 women). *Students:* 161 full-time (88 women), 28 part-time (15 women); includes 41 minority (5 Black or African American, non-Hispanic/Latino; 23 Asian, non-Hispanic/Latino; 9 Hispanic/Latino; 4 Two or more races, non-Hispanic/Latino), 80 international. Average age 27. 412 applicants, 54% accepted, 65 enrolled. In 2013, 77 master's, 9 doctorates awarded. Terminal master's awarded for partial completion of doctoral program. *Degree requirements:* For master's, thesis or alternative, qualifying paper; for doctorate, comprehensive exam, thesis/dissertation. *Entrance requirements:* For master's and doctorate, GRE General Test. Additional exam requirements/recommendations for international students: Required—TOEFL. *Application deadline:* For fall admission, 12/1 priority date for domestic students, 12/1 for international students. Application fee: $95. *Expenses: Tuition:* Full-time $35,856; part-time $1494 per unit. *Required fees:* $1408; $64 per unit. $473 per term. Tuition and fees vary according to course load and program. *Financial support:* Fellowships with tuition reimbursements, research assistantships with tuition reimbursements, teaching assistantships with tuition reimbursements, career-related internships or fieldwork, Federal Work-Study, institutionally sponsored loans, scholarships/grants, health care benefits, and unspecified assistantships available. Financial award application deadline: 12/1; financial award applicants required to submit FAFSA. *Faculty research:* Genomics, molecular and cell biology, development and molecular genetics, molecular evolution of plants and animals. *Unit head:* Stephen Small, Chair, 212-998-8200, Fax: 212-995-4015, E-mail: biology.admissions@nyu.edu. *Application contact:* Justin Blau, Director of Graduate Studies, PhD Programs, 212-998-8200, Fax: 212-995-4015, E-mail: biology.admissions@nyu.edu.
Website: http://biology.as.nyu.edu/

New York University, School of Medicine and Graduate School of Arts and Science, Sackler Institute of Graduate Biomedical Sciences, Program in Developmental Genetics, New York, NY 10012-1019. Offers PhD. *Faculty:* 24 full-time (8 women). *Students:* 20 full-time (13 women); includes 8 minority (1 Black or African American, non-Hispanic/Latino; 1 American Indian or Alaska Native, non-Hispanic/Latino; 3 Asian, non-Hispanic/Latino; 3 Hispanic/Latino), 5 international. *Expenses: Tuition:* Full-time $35,856; part-time $1494 per unit. *Required fees:* $1408; $64 per unit. $473 per term. Tuition and fees vary according to course load and program. *Faculty research:* Developmental genetics of germline proliferation in C. elegans, maternal/fetal immune interactions, signaling mechanisms of neuromuscular synapses formation in mice. *Unit head:* Dr. Joel D. Oppenheim, Senior Associate Dean for Graduate Studies, 212-263-8001, Fax: 212-263-7600. *Application contact:* Michael Escosia, Admissions Associate, 212-263-5431, Fax: 212-263-7600, E-mail: sackler-info@med.nyu.edu.
Website: http://sackler.med.nyu.edu/graduate/developmental-genetics

New York University, School of Medicine and Graduate School of Arts and Science, Sackler Institute of Graduate Biomedical Sciences, Program in Stem Cell Biology, New York, NY 10012-1019. Offers PhD. *Faculty:* 44 full-time (16 women). *Students:* 16 full-time (7 women); includes 3 minority (1 Black or African American, non-Hispanic/Latino; 1 Asian, non-Hispanic/Latino; 1 Hispanic/Latino), 11 international. Average age 25. *Expenses: Tuition:* Full-time $35,856; part-time $1494 per unit. *Required fees:* $1408; $64 per unit. $473 per term. Tuition and fees vary according to course load and program. *Faculty research:* Stem cell self-renewal in Drosophila, electrophysiology of cardiac stem cells, developmental and physiological control of stem cells. *Unit head:* Dr. Joel D. Oppenheim, Senior Associate Dean for Graduate Studies, 212-263-8001, Fax: 212-263-7600. *Application contact:* Michael Escosia, Admissions Associate, 212-263-5648, Fax: 212-263-7600, E-mail: sackler-info@med.nyu.edu.
Website: http://sackler.med.nyu.edu/graduate/stem-cell-biology

Northwestern University, The Graduate School, Interdisciplinary Biological Sciences Program (IBiS), Evanston, IL 60208. Offers biochemistry (PhD); bioengineering and biotechnology (PhD); biotechnology (PhD); cell and molecular biology (PhD); developmental and systems biology (PhD); nanotechnology (PhD); neurobiology (PhD); structural biology and biophysics (PhD). *Degree requirements:* For doctorate, thesis/dissertation, qualifying exam. *Entrance requirements:* For doctorate, GRE General Test. Additional exam requirements/recommendations for international students: Required—TOEFL (minimum score 600 paper-based). *Application deadline:* For fall admission, 12/15 for domestic and international students. Applications are processed on a rolling basis. Application fee: $95. Electronic applications accepted. *Financial support:* Fellowships, research assistantships, teaching assistantships, career-related internships or fieldwork, institutionally sponsored loans, scholarships/grants, traineeships, health care benefits, and unspecified assistantships available. Financial award application deadline: 12/31; financial award applicants required to submit FAFSA. *Faculty research:* Biophysics/structural biology, cell/molecular biology, synthetic biology, developmental systems biology, chemical biology/nanotechnology. *Unit head:* Dr. Deborah Klos Dehring, Associate Director, 847-467-0451, E-mail: d-klos@northwestern.edu. *Application contact:* Cathy Prullage, Program Manager, 847-491-4301, E-mail: ibis@northwestern.edu.
Website: http://www.biochem.northwestern.edu/ibis/

The Ohio State University, Graduate School, College of Arts and Sciences, Division of Natural and Mathematical Sciences, Department of Molecular Genetics, Columbus, OH 43210. Offers cell and developmental biology (MS, PhD); genetics (MS, PhD); molecular biology (MS, PhD). *Faculty:* 29. *Students:* 35 full-time (15 women); includes 3 minority (1 Black or African American, non-Hispanic/Latino; 2 Asian, non-Hispanic/Latino), 16 international. Average age 26. In 2013, 1 master's, 2 doctorates awarded. *Degree requirements:* For master's, thesis; for doctorate, thesis/dissertation. *Entrance*

requirements: For doctorate, GRE General Test, GRE Subject Test in biology or chemistry (recommended). Additional exam requirements/recommendations for international students: Required—TOEFL (minimum score 550 paper-based; 79 iBT), Michigan English Language Assessment Battery (minimum score 82); Recommended—IELTS (minimum score 7). *Application deadline:* For fall admission, 12/13 priority date for domestic students, 11/30 priority date for international students; for winter admission, 12/1 for domestic students, 11/1 for international students; for spring admission, 3/1 for domestic students, 2/1 for international students. Applications are processed on a rolling basis. Application fee: $60 ($70 for international students). Electronic applications accepted. *Financial support:* Fellowships with tuition reimbursements, research assistantships with tuition reimbursements, teaching assistantships with tuition reimbursements, Federal Work-Study, and institutionally sponsored loans available. Support available to part-time students. *Unit head:* Dr. Anita Hopper, Chair, 614-688-3306, Fax: 614-292-4466, E-mail: hopper.64@osu.edu. *Application contact:* Graduate Admissions, 614-292-9444, Fax: 614-292-3895, E-mail: gradadmissions@osu.edu.
Website: https://molgen.osu.edu/

The Ohio State University, Graduate School, College of Arts and Sciences, Division of Natural and Mathematical Sciences, Program in Molecular, Cellular and Developmental Biology, Columbus, OH 43210. Offers MS, PhD. *Faculty:* 172. *Students:* 117 full-time (67 women), 5 part-time (1 woman); includes 13 minority (1 Black or African American, non-Hispanic/Latino; 6 Asian, non-Hispanic/Latino; 4 Hispanic/Latino; 2 Two or more races, non-Hispanic/Latino), 60 international. Average age 27. In 2013, 2 master's, 15 doctorates awarded. Terminal master's awarded for partial completion of doctoral program. *Degree requirements:* For master's, thesis; for doctorate, thesis/dissertation. *Entrance requirements:* For doctorate, GRE General Test, GRE Subject Test in any science (desired, preferrably biology or chemistry, biochemistry or cell and molecular biology). Additional exam requirements/recommendations for international students: Required—TOEFL (minimum score 600 paper-based; 85 iBT); Recommended—IELTS (minimum score 8). *Application deadline:* For fall admission, 12/13 priority date for domestic students, 11/30 priority date for international students; for winter admission, 12/1 for domestic students, 11/1 for international students; for spring admission, 3/1 for domestic students, 2/1 for international students. Applications are processed on a rolling basis. Application fee: $60 ($70 for international students). Electronic applications accepted. *Financial support:* Fellowships with tuition reimbursements, research assistantships with tuition reimbursements, and teaching assistantships with tuition reimbursements available. *Unit head:* David Bisaro, Director, 614-292-2804, Fax: 614-292-7817, E-mail: bisaro.1@osu.edu. *Application contact:* Graduate Admissions, 614-292-9444, Fax: 614-292-3895, E-mail: gradadmissions@osu.edu.
Website: http://mcdb.osu.edu/

Oregon Health & Science University, School of Medicine, Graduate Programs in Medicine, Program in Molecular and Cellular Biosciences, Department of Cell and Developmental Biology, Portland, OR 97239-3098. Offers PhD. *Faculty:* 8 full-time (3 women), 36 part-time/adjunct (7 women). *Students:* 16 full-time (10 women), 1 (woman) part-time; includes 2 minority (both Two or more races, non-Hispanic/Latino), 5 international. Average age 29. In 2013, 5 doctorates awarded. *Degree requirements:* For doctorate, comprehensive exam, thesis/dissertation, qualifying exam. *Entrance requirements:* For doctorate, GRE General Test (minimum scores: 153 Verbal/148 Quantitative/4.5 Analytical) or MCAT. Additional exam requirements/recommendations for international students: Required—TOEFL. *Financial support:* Health care benefits, tuition waivers (full), and full tuition and stipends available. *Faculty research:* Developmental mechanisms, molecular biology of cancer, molecular neurobiology, intracellular signaling, growth factors and development. *Unit head:* Dr. Richard Maurer, Program Director, 503-494-7811, E-mail: maurerr@ohsu.edu. *Application contact:* Lola Bichler, Program Coordinator, 503-494-5824, E-mail: bichler@ohsu.edu.
Website: http://www.ohsu.edu/cellbio

Penn State University Park, Graduate School, Intercollege Graduate Programs, Intercollege Graduate Program in Cell and Developmental Biology, University Park, PA 16802. Offers MS, PhD. *Degree requirements:* For doctorate, thesis/dissertation, laboratory rotations, research project. *Unit head:* Dr. Regina Vasilatos-Younken, Interim Dean, 814-865-2516, Fax: 814-863-4627, E-mail: rxv@psu.edu. *Application contact:* Cynthia E. Nicosia, Director, Graduate Enrollment Services, 814-865-1834, Fax: 814-863-4627, E-mail: cey1@psu.edu.

Purdue University, Graduate School, College of Science, Department of Biological Sciences, West Lafayette, IN 47907. Offers biochemistry (PhD); biophysics (PhD); cell and developmental biology (PhD); ecology, evolutionary and population biology (MS, PhD), including ecology, evolutionary biology, population biology; genetics (MS, PhD); microbiology (MS, PhD); molecular biology (PhD); neurobiology (MS, PhD); plant physiology (PhD). *Faculty:* 50 full-time (13 women), 5 part-time/adjunct (1 woman). *Students:* 111 full-time (61 women), 5 part-time (0 women); includes 9 minority (1 Black or African American, non-Hispanic/Latino; 5 Asian, non-Hispanic/Latino; 3 Hispanic/Latino), 62 international. Average age 27. 170 applicants, 19% accepted, 17 enrolled. In 2013, 9 master's, 18 doctorates awarded. Terminal master's awarded for partial completion of doctoral program. *Degree requirements:* For master's, thesis (for some programs); for doctorate, thesis/dissertation, seminars, teaching experience. *Entrance requirements:* For master's, GRE General Test (minimum analytical writing score of 3.5), minimum undergraduate GPA of 3.0; for doctorate, GRE General Test (minimum analytical writing score of 3.5), minimum undergraduate GPA of 3.5. Additional exam requirements/recommendations for international students: Required—TOEFL (minimum score 600 paper-based; 107 iBT for MS, 80 iBT for PhD). *Application deadline:* For fall admission, 12/7 for domestic and international students. Applications are processed on a rolling basis. Application fee: $60 ($75 for international students). Electronic applications accepted. *Financial support:* Fellowships, research assistantships, and teaching assistantships available. Support available to part-time students. Financial award application deadline: 2/15; financial award applicants required to submit FAFSA. *Unit head:* Dr. Richard J. Kuhn, Head, 765-494-4407, E-mail: kuhnr@purdue.edu. *Application contact:* Georgina E. Rupp, Graduate Coordinator, 765-494-8142, Fax: 765-494-0876, E-mail: ruppg@purdue.edu.
Website: http://www.bio.purdue.edu/

Rutgers, The State University of New Jersey, Newark, Graduate School of Biomedical Sciences, Newark, NJ 07107. Offers biodefense (Certificate); biomedical engineering (PhD); biomedical sciences (multidisciplinary) (PhD); cellular biology, neuroscience and physiology (PhD), including neuroscience, physiology, biophysics, cardiovascular biology, molecular pharmacology, stem cell biology; infection, immunity and inflammation (PhD), including immunology, infectious disease, microbiology, oral biology; molecular biology, genetics and cancer (PhD), including biochemistry, molecular genetics, cancer biology, radiation biology, bioinformatics; neuroscience (Certificate); pharmacological sciences (Certificate); stem cell (Certificate); DMD/PhD; MD/PhD. PhD in biomedical engineering offered jointly with New Jersey Institute of Technology. Part-time and evening/weekend programs available. Terminal master's awarded for partial completion of doctoral program. *Degree requirements:* For doctorate, thesis/dissertation, qualifying exam. *Entrance requirements:* For doctorate, GRE General Test. Additional exam requirements/recommendations for international students: Required—TOEFL. Electronic applications accepted.

Rutgers, The State University of New Jersey, New Brunswick, Graduate School-New Brunswick, Programs in the Molecular Biosciences, Program in Cell and Developmental Biology, Piscataway, NJ 08854-8097. Offers MS, PhD. MS, PhD offered jointly with University of Medicine and Dentistry of New Jersey. Part-time programs available. Terminal master's awarded for partial completion of doctoral program. *Degree requirements:* For master's, thesis; for doctorate, thesis/dissertation, written qualifying exam. *Entrance requirements:* For master's, GRE General Test; for doctorate, GRE General Test, GRE Subject Test (recommended), minimum GPA of 3.0. Additional exam requirements/recommendations for international students: Required—TOEFL. Electronic applications accepted. *Faculty research:* Signal transduction and regulation of gene expression, developmental biology, cellular biology, developmental genetics, neurobiology.

San Francisco State University, Division of Graduate Studies, College of Science and Engineering, Department of Biology, Professional Science Master's Program, San Francisco, CA 94132-1722. Offers biotechnology (PSM); stem cell science (PSM). *Unit head:* Dr. Lily Chen, Director, 415-338-6763, E-mail: lilychen@sfsu.edu. *Application contact:* Dr. Linda H. Chen, Associate Director and Program Coordinator, 415-338-1696, E-mail: psm@sfsu.edu.
Website: http://www.sfsu.edu/~psm/

Stanford University, School of Medicine, Graduate Programs in Medicine, Department of Developmental Biology, Stanford, CA 94305-9991. Offers PhD. *Degree requirements:* For doctorate, thesis/dissertation, qualifying examination. *Entrance requirements:* For doctorate, GRE General Test, GRE Subject Test. Additional exam requirements/recommendations for international students: Required—TOEFL. Electronic applications accepted. *Expenses:* Tuition: Full-time $42,690; part-time $949 per credit. *Required fees:* $185. *Faculty research:* Mammalian embryology; developmental genetics with particular emphasis on microbial systems; &ITDictyostelium&RO, &ITDrosophila&RO, the nematode, and the mouse.

Stony Brook University, State University of New York, Graduate School, College of Arts and Sciences, Department of Biochemistry and Cell Biology, Stony Brook, NY 11794. Offers biochemistry and cell biology (MS); biochemistry and structural biology (PhD); molecular and cellular biology (MA, PhD), including biochemistry and molecular biology (PhD), biological sciences (MA), cellular and developmental biology (PhD), immunology and pathology (PhD), molecular and cellular biology (PhD). *Faculty:* 23 full-time (7 women), 1 part-time/adjunct (0 women). *Students:* 132 full-time (67 women), 2 part-time (1 woman); includes 19 minority (1 Black or African American, non-Hispanic/Latino; 10 Asian, non-Hispanic/Latino; 6 Hispanic/Latino; 1 Native Hawaiian or other Pacific Islander, non-Hispanic/Latino; 1 Two or more races, non-Hispanic/Latino), 66 international. Average age 28. 409 applicants, 19% accepted, 32 enrolled. In 2013, 44 master's, 22 doctorates awarded. *Degree requirements:* For doctorate, comprehensive exam, thesis/dissertation, teaching experience. *Entrance requirements:* For doctorate, GRE General Test, GRE Subject Test. Additional exam requirements/recommendations for international students: Required—TOEFL. *Application deadline:* For fall admission, 1/15 for domestic students; for spring admission, 10/15 for domestic students. Application fee: $100. *Expenses:* Tuition, state resident: full-time $9870; part-time $411 per credit. Tuition, nonresident: full-time $18,350; part-time $765 per credit. *Financial support:* In 2013–14, 36 fellowships, 43 research assistantships, 17 teaching assistantships were awarded; Federal Work-Study also available. *Faculty research:* Genome organization and replication, cell surface dynamics, enzyme structure and mechanism, developmental and regulatory biology. *Total annual research expenditures:* $7.7 million. *Unit head:* Prof. Robert Haltiwanger, Chair, 631-632-7336, Fax: 631-632-8575, E-mail: robert.haltiwanger@stonybrook.edu. *Application contact:* Joann DeLucia-Conlon, Coordinator, 631-632-8613, Fax: 631-632-8575, E-mail: joann.delucia-conlon@stonybrook.edu.
Website: http://www.sunysb.edu/biochem/

Thomas Jefferson University, Jefferson Graduate School of Biomedical Sciences, MS Program in Cell and Developmental Biology, Philadelphia, PA 19107. Offers MS. Part-time and evening/weekend programs available. *Faculty:* 44 full-time (14 women), 27 part-time/adjunct (11 women). *Students:* 15 part-time (12 women); includes 2 minority (both Black or African American, non-Hispanic/Latino), 2 international. 12 applicants, 58% accepted, 4 enrolled. In 2013, 2 master's awarded. *Degree requirements:* For master's, thesis, clerkship. *Entrance requirements:* For master's, GRE General Test or MCAT, minimum GPA of 3.0. Additional exam requirements/recommendations for international students: Required—TOEFL (minimum score 100 iBT) or IELTS (minimum score 7). *Application deadline:* For fall admission, 8/1 priority date for domestic students, 3/1 priority date for international students; for winter admission, 12/1 priority date for domestic students, 6/1 priority date for international students; for spring admission, 4/1 priority date for domestic students. Applications are processed on a rolling basis. Application fee: $75. Electronic applications accepted. *Financial support:* Federal Work-Study and institutionally sponsored loans available. Support available to part-time students. Financial award application deadline: 5/1; financial award applicants required to submit FAFSA. *Faculty research:* Developmental biology, cell biology, planning and management, drug development. *Unit head:* Dr. Gerald B. Grunwald, Dean and Program Director, 215-503-4191, Fax: 215-503-6690, E-mail: gerald.grunwald@jefferson.edu. *Application contact:* Marc E. Stearns, Director of Admissions, 215-503-0155, Fax: 215-503-3433, E-mail: jgsbs-info@jefferson.edu.
Website: http://www.jefferson.edu/university/biomedical_sciences/programs/masters/cell-developmental-bio.html

Thomas Jefferson University, Jefferson Graduate School of Biomedical Sciences, PhD Program in Cell and Developmental Biology, Philadelphia, PA 19107. Offers PhD. *Faculty:* 75 full-time (17 women). *Students:* 29 full-time (14 women); includes 5 minority (1 Black or African American, non-Hispanic/Latino; 3 Asian, non-Hispanic/Latino; 1 Hispanic/Latino), 4 international. 40 applicants, 15% accepted, 3 enrolled. In 2013, 5 doctorates awarded. *Degree requirements:* For doctorate, comprehensive exam, thesis/dissertation. *Entrance requirements:* For doctorate, GRE General Test, minimum GPA of 3.2. Additional exam requirements/recommendations for international students: Required—TOEFL (minimum score 100 iBT). *Application deadline:* For fall admission, 1/5 priority date for domestic and international students. Applications are processed on a rolling basis. Application fee: $75. Electronic applications accepted. *Financial support:* In 2013–14, 29 students received support, including 29 fellowships with full tuition reimbursements available (averaging $56,052 per year); Federal Work-Study, institutionally sponsored loans, scholarships/grants, traineeships, and stipends also available. Support available to part-time students. Financial award application deadline: 5/1; financial award applicants required to submit FAFSA. *Unit head:* Dr. Jan B. Hoek, Program Director, 215-503-5016, Fax: 215-923-2218, E-mail: joannes.hoek@jefferson.edu. *Application contact:* Marc E. Stearns, Director of Admissions, 215-503-0155, Fax: 215-503-3433, E-mail: jgsbs-info@jefferson.edu.
Website: http://www.jefferson.edu/university/biomedical_sciences/programs/phd/cell_biology.html

Tufts University, Sackler School of Graduate Biomedical Sciences, Cell, Molecular, and Developmental Biology Program, Medford, MA 02155. Offers PhD. *Faculty:* 45 full-time (15 women). *Students:* 25 full-time (10 women); includes 8 minority (1 Black or African American, non-Hispanic/Latino; 5 Asian, non-Hispanic/Latino; 1 Hispanic/Latino;

1 Two or more races, non-Hispanic/Latino), 5 international. Average age 29. In 2013, 3 doctorates awarded. Terminal master's awarded for partial completion of doctoral program. *Degree requirements:* For doctorate, comprehensive exam, thesis/dissertation. *Entrance requirements:* For doctorate, GRE General Test, 3 letters of reference. Additional exam requirements/recommendations for international students: Required—TOEFL (minimum score 600 paper-based; 100 iBT). *Application deadline:* For fall admission, 12/15 for domestic and international students. Application fee: $70. Electronic applications accepted. *Financial support:* In 2013–14, 25 students received support, including 25 research assistantships with full tuition reimbursements available (averaging $31,000 per year); fellowships and health care benefits also available. *Faculty research:* Reproduction and hormone action, control of gene expression, cell-matrix and cell-cell interactions, growth control and tumorigenesis, cytoskeleton and contractile proteins. *Unit head:* Dr. John Castellot, Program Director, 617-636-0303, Fax: 617-636-0375. *Application contact:* Kellie Johnston, Associate Director of Admissions, 617-636-6767, Fax: 617-636-0375, E-mail: sackler-school@tufts.edu.
Website: http://sackler.tufts.edu/Academics/Degree-Programs/PhD-Programs/Cell-Molecular-and-Developmental-Biology

University at Albany, State University of New York, College of Arts and Sciences, Department of Biological Sciences, Specialization in Molecular, Cellular, Developmental, and Neural Biology, Albany, NY 12222-0001. Offers MS, PhD. *Degree requirements:* For master's, one foreign language; for doctorate, one foreign language, thesis/dissertation. *Entrance requirements:* For master's and doctorate, GRE General Test.

The University of British Columbia, Faculty of Medicine, Department of Cellular and Physiological Sciences, Vancouver, BC V6T 1Z3, Canada. Offers M Sc, PhD. *Faculty:* 29 full-time (5 women), 2 part-time/adjunct (0 women). *Students:* 69 full-time (38 women); includes 26 minority (all Asian, non-Hispanic/Latino), 17 international. 26 applicants, 35% accepted, 8 enrolled. In 2013, 4 master's, 1 doctorate awarded. *Degree requirements:* For master's, thesis, oral defense; for doctorate, comprehensive exam, thesis/dissertation, oral defense. *Entrance requirements:* For master's, minimum overall B+ average in third- and fourth-year courses; for doctorate, minimum overall B+ average in a master's degree (or equivalent) from an approved institution with clear evidence of research ability or potential. Additional exam requirements/recommendations for international students: Required—TOEFL (minimum score 550 paper-based), IELTS (minimum score 6.5). *Application deadline:* For fall admission, 4/1 priority date for domestic students, 3/9 priority date for international students. Application fee: $90 ($150 for international students). *Expenses: Tuition, area resident:* Full-time $8000 Canadian dollars. *Financial support:* In 2013–14, 9 fellowships with full tuition reimbursements (averaging $16,000 per year), 8 research assistantships with partial tuition reimbursements (averaging $17,000 per year), 18 teaching assistantships with full tuition reimbursements (averaging $7,500 per year) were awarded; Federal Work-Study, institutionally sponsored loans, scholarships/grants, traineeships, tuition waivers (full), and unspecified assistantships also available. Financial award application deadline: 9/30. *Total annual research expenditures:* $3.8 million. *Unit head:* Dr. Christian Naus, Head, 604-822-2498. *Application contact:* Vincy Yung, Student Academic Services Application Clerk, 604-822-3907, Fax: 604-822-5802, E-mail: grad.admissions@ubc.ca.
Website: http://www.cell.ubc.ca/

University of California, Davis, Graduate Studies, Graduate Group in Cell and Developmental Biology, Davis, CA 95616. Offers MS, PhD. *Degree requirements:* For master's, comprehensive exam (for some programs), thesis (for some programs); for doctorate, thesis/dissertation. *Entrance requirements:* For doctorate, GRE General Test, GRE Subject Test. Additional exam requirements/recommendations for international students: Required—TOEFL (minimum score 550 paper-based). Electronic applications accepted. *Faculty research:* Molecular basis of cell function and development.

University of California, Irvine, School of Biological Sciences, Department of Developmental and Cell Biology, Irvine, CA 92697. Offers biological sciences (MS, PhD). *Students:* 37 full-time (19 women); includes 23 minority (13 Asian, non-Hispanic/Latino; 9 Hispanic/Latino; 1 Native Hawaiian or other Pacific Islander, non-Hispanic/Latino), 1 international. Average age 29. In 2013, 4 master's, 12 doctorates awarded. *Degree requirements:* For doctorate, thesis/dissertation. *Entrance requirements:* For master's and doctorate, GRE General Test, GRE Subject Test, minimum GPA of 3.0. Additional exam requirements/recommendations for international students: Required—TOEFL (minimum score 550 paper-based). *Application deadline:* For fall admission, 12/15 priority date for domestic and international students. Application fee: $80 ($100 for international students). Electronic applications accepted. *Financial support:* Fellowships, research assistantships with full tuition reimbursements, teaching assistantships, institutionally sponsored loans, traineeships, health care benefits, and unspecified assistantships available. Financial award application deadline: 3/1; financial award applicants required to submit FAFSA. *Faculty research:* Genetics and development, oncogene signaling pathways, gene regulation, tissue regeneration and molecular genetics. *Unit head:* Prof. Diane K. O'Dowd, Department Chair, 949-824-4562, Fax: 949-824-1105, E-mail: dkodowd@uci.edu. *Application contact:* Grace Kuei, Personnel Manager, 949-824-6677, Fax: 949-824-4709, E-mail: jlmarsh@uci.edu.
Website: http://devcell.bio.uci.edu/

University of California, Los Angeles, Graduate Division, College of Letters and Science, Department of Molecular, Cell and Developmental Biology, Los Angeles, CA 90095. Offers MA, PhD. Terminal master's awarded for partial completion of doctoral program. *Degree requirements:* For master's, comprehensive exam, thesis; for doctorate, thesis/dissertation, oral and written qualifying exams; 2 quarters of teaching experience. *Entrance requirements:* For doctorate, GRE General Test. Additional exam requirements/recommendations for international students: Required—TOEFL. Electronic applications accepted.

University of California, Riverside, Graduate Division, Program in Cell, Molecular, and Developmental Biology, Riverside, CA 92521-0102. Offers MS, PhD. Terminal master's awarded for partial completion of doctoral program. *Degree requirements:* For master's, thesis, oral defense of thesis; for doctorate, thesis/dissertation, oral defense of thesis, qualifying exams, 2 quarters of teaching experience. *Entrance requirements:* For master's and doctorate, GRE General Test, minimum GPA of 3.2. Additional exam requirements/recommendations for international students: Required—TOEFL (minimum score 550 paper-based; 80 iBT). Electronic applications accepted.

University of California, San Francisco, Graduate Division and School of Medicine, Tetrad Graduate Program, San Francisco, CA 94143. Offers biochemistry and molecular biology (PhD); cell biology (PhD); developmental biology (PhD); genetics (PhD); MD/PhD. *Degree requirements:* For doctorate, thesis/dissertation. *Entrance requirements:* For doctorate, GRE General Test, GRE Subject Test. Additional exam requirements/recommendations for international students: Required—TOEFL. *Application deadline:* For fall admission, 12/1 for domestic students. Application fee: $40. *Expenses:* Contact institution. *Financial support:* Fellowships available. Financial award application deadline: 2/1. *Unit head:* Dr. Peter Walter, Chair, 415-476-5017. *Application contact:* Graduate Admissions Officer, 415-476-3941, E-mail: admissions@biochem.ucsf.edu.
Website: http://tetrad.ucsf.edu/

University of California, Santa Barbara, Graduate Division, College of Letters and Sciences, Division of Mathematics, Life, and Physical Sciences, Department of Molecular, Cellular, and Developmental Biology, Santa Barbara, CA 93106-9625. Offers molecular, cellular, and developmental biology (MA, PhD); pharmacology/biotechnology (MA); MA/PhD. *Faculty:* 29 full-time (3 women), 4 part-time/adjunct (0 women). *Students:* 48 full-time (23 women); includes 8 minority (2 Black or African American, non-Hispanic/Latino; 3 Asian, non-Hispanic/Latino; 3 Hispanic/Latino), 1 international. Average age 29. 182 applicants, 18% accepted, 11 enrolled. In 2013, 7 master's, 7 doctorates awarded. Terminal master's awarded for partial completion of doctoral program. *Degree requirements:* For master's, comprehensive exam (for some programs), thesis (for some programs); for doctorate, comprehensive exam, thesis/dissertation. *Entrance requirements:* For master's and doctorate, GRE General Test, 3 letters of recommendation, statement of purpose, personal achievements/contributions statement, resume/curriculum vitae, transcripts for post-secondary institutions attended. Additional exam requirements/recommendations for international students: Required—TOEFL (minimum score 550 paper-based; 80 iBT), IELTS (minimum score 7). *Application deadline:* For fall admission, 12/15 priority date for domestic and international students. Application fee: $80 ($100 for international students). Electronic applications accepted. *Expenses:* Tuition, state resident: part-time $5148.26 per quarter. Tuition, nonresident: part-time $10,182.26 per quarter. *Financial support:* In 2013–14, 3 students received support, including 3 fellowships with full and partial tuition reimbursements available (averaging $22,000 per year), 40 research assistantships with full and partial tuition reimbursements available (averaging $26,250 per year), 46 teaching assistantships with partial tuition reimbursements available (averaging $17,655 per year); career-related internships or fieldwork, Federal Work-Study, institutionally sponsored loans, scholarships/grants, traineeships, health care benefits, and unspecified assistantships also available. Financial award application deadline: 3/13; financial award applicants required to submit FAFSA. *Faculty research:* Microbiology, neurobiology (including stem cell research), developmental, virology, cell biology. *Unit head:* Dr. William Smith, Chair, 805-893-7698, E-mail: wililam.smith@lifesci.ucsb.edu. *Application contact:* Nicole McCoy, Graduate Program Advisor, 805-893-8499, E-mail: nicole.mccoy@lifesci.ucsb.edu.
Website: https://www.mcdb.ucsb.edu/grad

University of California, Santa Cruz, Division of Graduate Studies, Division of Physical and Biological Sciences, Program in Molecular, Cellular, and Developmental Biology, Santa Cruz, CA 95064. Offers MA, PhD. Terminal master's awarded for partial completion of doctoral program. *Degree requirements:* For master's, thesis; for doctorate, thesis/dissertation, qualifying exam. *Entrance requirements:* For master's and doctorate, GRE General Test, 3 letters of recommendation, interview. Additional exam requirements/recommendations for international students: Required—TOEFL (minimum score 550 paper-based; 83 iBT); Recommended—IELTS (minimum score 8). Electronic applications accepted. *Faculty research:* RNA biology, chromatin and chromosome biology, neurobiology, stem cell biology and differentiation, cell structure and function.

University of Chicago, Division of Biological Sciences, Molecular Biosciences Cluster, Committee on Development, Regeneration, and Stem Cell Biology, Chicago, IL 60637-1513. Offers cellular differentiation (PhD); developmental endocrinology (PhD); developmental genetics (PhD); developmental neurobiology (PhD); gene expression (PhD). *Degree requirements:* For doctorate, thesis/dissertation, ethics class, 2 teaching assistantships. *Entrance requirements:* For doctorate, GRE General Test. Additional exam requirements/recommendations for international students: Required—TOEFL (minimum score 600 paper-based; 104 iBT), IELTS (minimum score 7). Electronic applications accepted. *Faculty research:* Epidermal differentiation, neural lineages, pattern formation.

University of Cincinnati, Graduate School, College of Medicine, Graduate Programs in Biomedical Sciences, Department of Pediatrics, Program in Molecular and Developmental Biology, Cincinnati, OH 45221. Offers PhD. *Degree requirements:* For doctorate, thesis/dissertation, qualifying exam. *Entrance requirements:* For doctorate, GRE General Test, minimum GPA of 3.2. Additional exam requirements/recommendations for international students: Required—TOEFL (minimum score 520 paper-based). Electronic applications accepted. *Faculty research:* Cancer biology, cardiovascular biology, developmental biology, human genetics, gene therapy, genomics and bioinformatics, immunobiology, molecular medicine, neuroscience, pulmonary biology, reproductive biology, stem cell biology.

University of Colorado Boulder, Graduate School, College of Arts and Sciences, Department of Molecular, Cellular, and Developmental Biology, Boulder, CO 80309. Offers cellular structure and function (MA, PhD); developmental biology (MA, PhD); molecular biology (MA, PhD). *Faculty:* 25 full-time (7 women). *Students:* 64 full-time (36 women), 1 part-time (0 women); includes 5 minority (2 Asian, non-Hispanic/Latino; 2 Hispanic/Latino; 1 Native Hawaiian or other Pacific Islander, non-Hispanic/Latino), 9 international. Average age 27. 311 applicants, 12% accepted, 11 enrolled. In 2013, 2 master's, 11 doctorates awarded. Terminal master's awarded for partial completion of doctoral program. *Degree requirements:* For master's, comprehensive exam, thesis or alternative; for doctorate, comprehensive exam, thesis/dissertation. *Entrance requirements:* For master's, GRE General Test, GRE Subject Test, minimum undergraduate GPA of 3.0; for doctorate, GRE General Test, GRE Subject Test. *Application deadline:* For fall admission, 12/1 for domestic students, 12/15 for international students. Application fee: $50 ($60 for international students). Electronic applications accepted. *Financial support:* In 2013–14, 154 students received support, including 32 fellowships (averaging $6,403 per year), 62 research assistantships with full and partial tuition reimbursements available (averaging $30,807 per year), 11 teaching assistantships with full and partial tuition reimbursements available (averaging $27,393 per year); institutionally sponsored loans, scholarships/grants, health care benefits, and unspecified assistantships also available. Financial award application deadline: 2/1; financial award applicants required to submit FAFSA. *Faculty research:* Molecular biology, cellular biology, genetics, biological sciences, gene cloning. *Total annual research expenditures:* $14.8 million.
Website: http://mcdb.colorado.edu/

University of Colorado Denver, College of Liberal Arts and Sciences, Department of Integrative Biology, Denver, CO 80217. Offers animal behavior (MS); biology (MS); cell and developmental biology (MS); ecology (MS); evolutionary biology (MS); genetics (MS); integrative and systems biology (PhD); microbiology (MS); molecular biology (MS); neurobiology (MS); plant systematics (MS). Part-time programs available. *Faculty:* 21 full-time (7 women), 3 part-time/adjunct (2 women). *Students:* 18 full-time (11 women), 5 part-time (all women); includes 5 minority (1 Black or African American, non-Hispanic/Latino; 2 Hispanic/Latino; 2 Two or more races, non-Hispanic/Latino), 1 international. Average age 29. 25 applicants, 44% accepted, 11 enrolled. In 2013, 13 master's awarded. *Degree requirements:* For master's, comprehensive exam, thesis, 30-32 credit hours. *Entrance requirements:* For master's, GRE General Test (minimum score in 50th percentile in each section), BA/BS from accredited institution awarded within the last 10 years; minimum undergraduate GPA of 3.0; prerequisite courses: 1 year each of general biology and general chemistry; 1 semester each of general genetics, general ecology, and cell biology; and a structure/function course. Additional exam requirements/recommendations for international students: Required—TOEFL

(minimum score 537 paper-based; 75 iBT); Recommended—IELTS (minimum score 6.5). *Application deadline:* For fall admission, 2/1 for domestic and international students. Application fee: $50 ($75 for international students). Electronic applications accepted. *Financial support:* In 2013–14, 8 students received support. Fellowships, research assistantships, teaching assistantships, Federal Work-Study, institutionally sponsored loans, scholarships/grants, and traineeships available. Financial award application deadline: 4/1; financial award applicants required to submit FAFSA. *Faculty research:* Molecular developmental biology; quantitative ecology, biogeography, and population dynamics; environmental signaling and endocrine disruption; speciation, the evolution of reproductive isolation, and hybrid zones; evolutionary, behavioral, and conservation ecology. *Unit head:* Dr. John Swallow, Biology Department Chair, 303-556-6154, E-mail: john.swallow@ucdenver.edu. *Application contact:* Timberley Roane, Associate Professor/Director of MS in Biology Program, 303-556-6592, E-mail: timberley.roane@ucdenver.edu.
Website: http://www.ucdenver.edu/academics/colleges/CLAS/Departments/biology/Programs/MasterofScience/Pages/BiologyMasterOfScience.aspx

University of Colorado Denver, School of Medicine, Program in Cell Biology, Stem Cells, and Developmental Biology, Aurora, CO 80045. Offers cell biology, stem cells, and developmental biology (PhD); modern human anatomy (MS). *Students:* 30 full-time (16 women), 1 part-time (0 women); includes 3 minority (all Hispanic/Latino), 5 international. Average age 28. 33 applicants, 15% accepted, 5 enrolled. In 2013, 2 doctorates awarded. *Degree requirements:* For doctorate, comprehensive exam, thesis/dissertation, at least 30 credit hours of coursework and 30 credit hours of thesis research; laboratory rotations. *Entrance requirements:* For doctorate, GRE, minimum GPA of 3.0; 3 letters of reference; prerequisite coursework in organic chemistry, biology, biochemistry, physics and calculus; research experience (highly recommended). Additional exam requirements/recommendations for international students: Required—TOEFL (minimum score 550 paper-based; 80 iBT). *Application deadline:* For fall admission, 12/1 for domestic students, 11/1 priority date for international students. Application fee: $50 ($75 for international students). Electronic applications accepted. *Expenses:* Contact institution. *Financial support:* In 2013–14, 31 students received support. Fellowships, research assistantships, teaching assistantships, Federal Work-Study, institutionally sponsored loans, scholarships/grants, traineeships, health care benefits, and tuition waivers (full) available. Financial award application deadline: 3/15; financial award applicants required to submit FAFSA. *Faculty research:* Development and repair of the vertebrate nervous system; molecular, genetic and developmental mechanisms involved in the patterning of the early spinal cord (neural plate) during vertebrate embryogenesis; structural analysis of protein glycosylation using NMR and mass spectrometry; small RNAs and post-transcriptional gene regulation during nematode gametogenesis and early development; diabetes-mediated changes in cardiovascular gene expression and functional exercise capacity. *Total annual research expenditures:* $5.7 million. *Unit head:* Dr. Wendy Macklin, Department Chair, 303-724-3426, E-mail: wendy.macklin@ucdenver.edu. *Application contact:* Kenton Owsley, Program Administrator, 303-724-3468, Fax: 303-724-3420, E-mail: kenton.owsley@ucdenver.edu.
Website: http://www.ucdenver.edu/academics/colleges/medicalschool/programs/CSD/Pages/CSD.aspx

University of Connecticut, Graduate School, College of Liberal Arts and Sciences, Department of Molecular and Cell Biology, Storrs, CT 06269. Offers applied genomics (MS, PSM); biochemistry (MS, PhD); biophysics and structural biology (MS, PhD); cell and developmental biology (MS, PhD); genetics, genomics, and bioinformatics (MS, PhD); microbial systems analysis (MS, PSM); microbiology (MS, PhD); plant cell and molecular biology (MS, PhD). Terminal master's awarded for partial completion of doctoral program. *Degree requirements:* For master's, comprehensive exam; for doctorate, thesis/dissertation. *Entrance requirements:* For master's and doctorate, GRE General Test, GRE Subject Test. Additional exam requirements/recommendations for international students: Required—TOEFL (minimum score 550 paper-based). Electronic applications accepted.

University of Connecticut Health Center, Graduate School, Programs in Biomedical Sciences, Program in Genetics and Developmental Biology, Farmington, CT 06030. Offers PhD, DMD/PhD, MD/PhD. *Degree requirements:* For doctorate, comprehensive exam, thesis/dissertation. *Entrance requirements:* For doctorate, GRE General Test, GRE Subject Test. Additional exam requirements/recommendations for international students: Required—TOEFL (minimum score 600 paper-based). Electronic applications accepted. *Faculty research:* Developmental biology, genomic imprinting, RNA biology, RNA alternative splicing, human embryonic stem cells.

See Display on page 299 and Close-Up on page 313.

University of Delaware, College of Arts and Sciences, Department of Biological Sciences, Newark, DE 19716. Offers biotechnology (MS); cancer biology (MS, PhD); cell and extracellular matrix biology (MS, PhD); cell and systems physiology (MS, PhD); developmental biology (MS, PhD); ecology and evolution (MS, PhD); microbiology (MS, PhD); molecular biology and genetics (MS, PhD). Terminal master's awarded for partial completion of doctoral program. *Degree requirements:* For master's, thesis, preliminary exam; for doctorate, comprehensive exam, thesis/dissertation, preliminary exam. *Entrance requirements:* For master's and doctorate, GRE General Test. Additional exam requirements/recommendations for international students: Required—TOEFL (minimum score 600 paper-based); Recommended—TWE. Electronic applications accepted. *Faculty research:* Microorganisms, bone, cancer metastasis, developmental biology, cell biology, DNA.

University of Hawaii at Manoa, John A. Burns School of Medicine, Program in Developmental and Reproductive Biology, Honolulu, HI 96813. Offers MS, PhD. Part-time programs available. *Degree requirements:* For doctorate, thesis/dissertation. *Entrance requirements:* For doctorate, GRE General Test, GRE Subject Test. Additional exam requirements/recommendations for international students: Recommended—TOEFL (minimum score 560 paper-based), IELTS (minimum score 5). *Faculty research:* Biology of gametes and fertilization, reproductive endocrinology.

University of Illinois at Urbana–Champaign, Graduate College, College of Liberal Arts and Sciences, School of Molecular and Cellular Biology, Department of Cell and Developmental Biology, Champaign, IL 61820. Offers PhD. *Students:* 56 (31 women). Application fee: $75 ($90 for international students). *Unit head:* Jie Chen, Head, 217-265-0674, Fax: 217-244-1648, E-mail: jchen@illinois.edu. *Application contact:* Shannon J. Croft, 217-244-8116, Fax: 217-244-1648, E-mail: shannon9@illinois.edu.
Website: http://mcb.illinois.edu/departments/cdb/

The University of Kansas, Graduate Studies, College of Liberal Arts and Sciences, Department of Molecular Biosciences, Lawrence, KS 66045. Offers biochemistry and biophysics (MA, PhD); microbiology (MA, PhD); molecular, cellular, and developmental biology (MA, PhD). *Faculty:* 34. *Students:* 52 full-time (28 women); includes 5 minority (2 Asian, non-Hispanic/Latino; 3 Hispanic/Latino), 23 international. Average age 27. 96 applicants, 25% accepted, 13 enrolled. In 2013, 3 master's, 9 doctorates awarded. Terminal master's awarded for partial completion of doctoral program. *Degree requirements:* For master's, comprehensive exam, thesis; for doctorate, comprehensive exam, thesis/dissertation. *Entrance requirements:* For master's and doctorate, GRE General Test. Additional exam requirements/recommendations for international students: Required—TOEFL or IELTS. *Application deadline:* For fall admission, 12/15 for domestic and international students. Application fee: $55 ($65 for international students). Electronic applications accepted. *Financial support:* Fellowships with tuition reimbursements, research assistantships with tuition reimbursements, teaching assistantships with tuition reimbursements, health care benefits, and unspecified assistantships available. Financial award application deadline: 3/1. *Faculty research:* Structure and function of proteins, genetics of organism development, molecular genetics, neurophysiology, molecular virology and pathogenics, developmental biology, cell biology. *Unit head:* Dr. Mark Richter, Chair, 785-864-3334, E-mail: richter@ku.edu. *Application contact:* John Connolly, Graduate Admissions Contact, 785-864-4311, E-mail: jconnolly@ku.edu.
Website: http://www.molecularbiosciences.ku.edu/

The University of Manchester, Faculty of Life Sciences, Manchester, United Kingdom. Offers adaptive organismal biology (M Phil, PhD); animal biology (M Phil, PhD); biochemistry (M Phil, PhD); bioinformatics (M Phil, PhD); biomolecular sciences (M Phil, PhD); biotechnology (M Phil, PhD); cell biology (M Phil, PhD); cell matrix research (M Phil, PhD); channels and transporters (M Phil, PhD); developmental biology (M Phil, PhD); Egyptology (M Phil, PhD); environmental biology (M Phil, PhD); evolutionary biology (M Phil, PhD); gene expression (M Phil, PhD); genetics (M Phil, PhD); history of science, technology and medicine (M Phil, PhD); immunology (M Phil, PhD); integrative neurobiology and behavior (M Phil, PhD); membrane trafficking (M Phil, PhD); microbiology (M Phil, PhD); molecular and cellular neuroscience (M Phil, PhD); molecular biology (M Phil, PhD); molecular cancer studies (M Phil, PhD); neuroscience (M Phil, PhD); ophthalmology (M Phil, PhD); optometry (M Phil, PhD); organelle function (M Phil, PhD); pharmacology (M Phil, PhD); physiology (M Phil, PhD); plant sciences (M Phil, PhD); stem cell research (M Phil, PhD); structural biology (M Phil, PhD); systems neuroscience (M Phil, PhD); toxicology (M Phil, PhD).

The University of Manchester, School of Dentistry, Manchester, United Kingdom. Offers basic dental sciences (cancer studies) (M Phil, PhD); basic dental sciences (molecular genetics) (M Phil, PhD); basic dental sciences (stem cell biology) (M Phil, PhD); biomaterials sciences and dental technology (M Phil, PhD); dental public health/community dentistry (M Phil, PhD); dental science (clinical) (PhD); endodontology (M Phil, PhD); fixed and removable prosthodontics (M Phil, PhD); operative dentistry (M Phil, PhD); oral and maxillofacial surgery (M Phil, PhD); oral radiology (M Phil, PhD); orthodontics (M Phil, PhD); restorative dentistry (M Phil, PhD).

University of Massachusetts Amherst, Graduate School, Interdisciplinary Programs, Program in Molecular and Cellular Biology, Amherst, MA 01003. Offers biological chemistry and molecular biophysics (PhD); biomedicine (PhD); cellular and developmental biology (PhD). Part-time programs available. *Students:* 72 full-time (41 women); includes 15 minority (4 Black or African American, non-Hispanic/Latino; 5 Asian, non-Hispanic/Latino; 4 Hispanic/Latino; 2 Two or more races, non-Hispanic/Latino), 28 international. Average age 27. 160 applicants, 23% accepted, 20 enrolled. In 2013, 13 doctorates awarded. Terminal master's awarded for partial completion of doctoral program. *Degree requirements:* For doctorate, comprehensive exam, thesis/dissertation. *Entrance requirements:* For doctorate, GRE General Test. Additional exam requirements/recommendations for international students: Required—TOEFL (minimum score 550 paper-based; 80 iBT), IELTS (minimum score 6.5). *Application deadline:* For fall admission, 12/1 for domestic and international students. Applications are processed on a rolling basis. Application fee: $75. Electronic applications accepted. *Financial support:* Fellowships with full and partial tuition reimbursements, research assistantships with full and partial tuition reimbursements, teaching assistantships with full and partial tuition reimbursements, career-related internships or fieldwork, Federal Work-Study, scholarships/grants, traineeships, health care benefits, tuition waivers (full and partial), and unspecified assistantships available. Support available to part-time students. Financial award application deadline: 12/1; financial award applicants required to submit FAFSA. *Unit head:* Dr. Barbara Osborne, Graduate Program Director, 413-545-3246, Fax: 413-545-1812, E-mail: mcb@mcb.umass.edu. *Application contact:* Lindsay DeSantis, Supervisor of Admissions, 413-545-0722, Fax: 413-577-0010, E-mail: gradadm@grad.umass.edu.
Website: http://www.bio.umass.edu/mcb/

University of Miami, Graduate School, Miller School of Medicine, Graduate Programs in Medicine, Department of Cell Biology and Anatomy, Coral Gables, FL 33124. Offers molecular cell and developmental biology (PhD); MD/PhD. *Degree requirements:* For doctorate, thesis/dissertation. *Entrance requirements:* For doctorate, GRE General Test, GRE Subject Test. Additional exam requirements/recommendations for international students: Required—TOEFL. Electronic applications accepted.

University of Michigan, Rackham Graduate School, College of Literature, Science, and the Arts, Department of Molecular, Cellular, and Developmental Biology, Ann Arbor, MI 48109. Offers MS, PhD. Part-time programs available. *Faculty:* 35 full-time (11 women). *Students:* 77 full-time (40 women), 2 part-time (1 woman); includes 10 minority (4 Asian, non-Hispanic/Latino; 5 Hispanic/Latino; 1 Native Hawaiian or other Pacific Islander, non-Hispanic/Latino), 42 international. Average age 27. 100 applicants, 25% accepted, 12 enrolled. In 2013, 5 master's, 7 doctorates awarded. Terminal master's awarded for partial completion of doctoral program. *Degree requirements:* For master's, 24 credits with at least 16 in molecular, cellular, and developmental biology and 4 in a cognate field; for doctorate, thesis/dissertation, preliminary exam, oral defense. *Entrance requirements:* For master's and doctorate, GRE General Test. Additional exam requirements/recommendations for international students: Required—TOEFL (minimum score 560 paper-based; 83 iBT). *Application deadline:* For fall admission, 1/5 for domestic and international students; for winter admission, 11/1 for domestic and international students; for spring admission, 4/1 for domestic and international students. Applications are processed on a rolling basis. Application fee: $75 ($90 for international students). Electronic applications accepted. Tuition and fees vary according to course level, course load, degree level, program and student level. *Financial support:* In 2013–14, 13 fellowships with full tuition reimbursements (averaging $28,500 per year), 31 research assistantships with full tuition reimbursements (averaging $28,500 per year), 17 teaching assistantships with full tuition reimbursements (averaging $28,500 per year) were awarded; health care benefits also available. *Faculty research:* Cell biology, microbiology, neurobiology and physiology, developmental biology and plant molecular biology. *Total annual research expenditures:* $7.8 million. *Unit head:* Dr. Robert J. Denver, Department Chair, 734-764-7476, Fax: 734-615-6337, E-mail: rdenver@umich.edu. *Application contact:* Mary Carr, Graduate Coordinator, 734-615-1635, Fax: 734-764-0884, E-mail: carrmm@umich.edu.
Website: http://www.mcdb.lsa.umich.edu

University of Michigan, Rackham Graduate School, Program in Biomedical Sciences (PIBS), Department of Cell and Developmental Biology, Ann Arbor, MI 48109-2200. Offers PhD. *Faculty:* 39 full-time (11 women). *Students:* 16 full-time (9 women); includes 8 minority (7 Asian, non-Hispanic/Latino; 1 Hispanic/Latino). Average age 29. 57 applicants, 18% accepted, 6 enrolled. In 2013, 10 doctorates awarded. *Degree requirements:* For doctorate, thesis/dissertation, oral defense of dissertation, preliminary exam. *Entrance requirements:* For doctorate, GRE General Test, 3 letters of recommendation, research experience. Additional exam requirements/

recommendations for international students: Required—TOEFL (minimum score 84 iBT). *Application deadline:* For fall admission, 12/1 for domestic and international students. Application fee: $75 ($90 for international students). Electronic applications accepted. Tuition and fees vary according to course level, course load, degree level, program and student level. *Financial support:* In 2013–14, fellowships (averaging $28,500 per year) were awarded; scholarships/grants, health care benefits, tuition waivers (full), and unspecified assistantships also available. Financial award application deadline: 12/1. *Faculty research:* Cell signaling, stem cells, organogenesis, cell biology, developmental genetics. *Total annual research expenditures:* $4 million. *Unit head:* Dr. Deborah L. Gumucio, Professor/Interim Chair, 734-647-0172, Fax: 734-763-1166, E-mail: dgumucio@umich.edu. *Application contact:* Michelle S. Melis, Director of Student Life, 734-615-6538, Fax: 734-647-7022, E-mail: msmtegan@umich.edu.
Website: http://cdb.med.umich.edu/

University of Minnesota, Twin Cities Campus, Graduate School, Program in Molecular, Cellular, Developmental Biology and Genetics, Minneapolis, MN 55455-0213. Offers genetic counseling (MS); molecular, cellular, developmental biology and genetics (PhD). Terminal master's awarded for partial completion of doctoral program. *Degree requirements:* For master's, thesis optional; for doctorate, thesis/dissertation. *Entrance requirements:* For master's and doctorate, GRE General Test. Additional exam requirements/recommendations for international students: Required—TOEFL (minimum score 625 paper-based; 80 iBT). Electronic applications accepted. *Faculty research:* Membrane receptors and membrane transport, cell interactions, cytoskeleton and cell mobility, regulation of gene expression, plant cell and molecular biology.

University of Minnesota, Twin Cities Campus, Graduate School, Stem Cell Biology Graduate Program, Minneapolis, MN 55455-3007. Offers MS. *Degree requirements:* For master's, thesis. *Entrance requirements:* For master's, GRE, BS, BA, or foreign equivalent in biological sciences or related field; minimum undergraduate GPA of 3.2. Additional exam requirements/recommendations for international students: Required—TOEFL (minimum score 580 paper-based, with a minimum score of 4 in the TWE, or 94 Internet-based, with a minimum score of 22 on each of the reading and listening, 26 on the speaking, and 26 on the writing section. *Faculty research:* Stem cell and developmental biology; embryonic stem cells; iPS cells; muscle satellite cells; hematopoietic stem cells; neuronal stem cells; cardiovascular, kidney and limb development; regenerating systems.

The University of Montana, Graduate School, College of Humanities and Sciences, Division of Biological Sciences, Program in Cellular, Molecular and Microbial Biology, Missoula, MT 59812-0002. Offers cellular and developmental biology (PhD); microbial evolution and ecology (PhD); microbiology and immunology (PhD); molecular biology and biochemistry (PhD). Terminal master's awarded for partial completion of doctoral program. *Degree requirements:* For doctorate, variable foreign language requirement, thesis/dissertation. *Entrance requirements:* For doctorate, GRE General Test. *Application deadline:* For fall admission, 2/1 for domestic students. Application fee: $45. *Financial support:* In 2013–14, research assistantships with tuition reimbursements (averaging $9,400 per year), teaching assistantships with full tuition reimbursements (averaging $9,400 per year) were awarded; Federal Work-Study and tuition waivers (full and partial) also available. Financial award application deadline: 3/1; financial award applicants required to submit FAFSA. *Faculty research:* Ribosome structure, medical microbiology/pathogenesis, microbial ecology/environmental microbiology. *Unit head:* Charles Janson, Chair, 406-243-5122, E-mail: charles.janson@mso.umt.edu. *Application contact:* Information Contact, E-mail: gradschl@mso.umt.edu.
Website: http://www.biology.umt.edu/

The University of North Carolina at Chapel Hill, Graduate School, College of Arts and Sciences, Department of Biology, Chapel Hill, NC 27599. Offers botany (MA, MS, PhD); cell biology, development, and physiology (MA, MS, PhD); cell motility and cytoskeleton (PhD); ecology and behavior (MA, MS, PhD); genetics and molecular biology (MA, MS, PhD); morphology, systematics, and evolution (MA, MS, PhD). Terminal master's awarded for partial completion of doctoral program. *Degree requirements:* For master's, comprehensive exam, thesis (for some programs); for doctorate, comprehensive exam, thesis/dissertation. *Entrance requirements:* For master's, GRE General Test, GRE Subject Test, 2 semesters of calculus or statistics; 2 semesters of physics, organic chemistry; 3 semesters of biology; for doctorate, GRE General Test, GRE Subject Test, 2 semesters calculus or statistics, 2 semesters physics, organic chemistry, 3 semesters of biology. Additional exam requirements/recommendations for international students: Required—TOEFL (minimum score 550 paper-based). Electronic applications accepted. *Faculty research:* Gene expression, biomechanics, yeast genetics, plant ecology, plant molecular biology.

The University of North Carolina at Chapel Hill, School of Medicine and Graduate School, Graduate Programs in Medicine, Department of Cell and Developmental Biology, Chapel Hill, NC 27599. Offers PhD. *Degree requirements:* For doctorate, comprehensive exam, thesis/dissertation. *Entrance requirements:* For doctorate, GRE General Test, GRE Subject Test. Electronic applications accepted. *Faculty research:* Cell adhesion, motility and cytoskeleton; molecular analysis of signal transduction; development biology and toxicology; reproductive biology; cell and molecular imaging.

University of Pennsylvania, Perelman School of Medicine, Biomedical Graduate Studies, Graduate Group in Cell and Molecular Biology, Philadelphia, PA 19104. Offers cancer biology (PhD); cell biology and physiology (PhD); developmental stem cell regenerative biology (PhD); gene therapy and vaccines (PhD); genetics and gene regulation (PhD); microbiology, virology, and parasitology (PhD); MD/PhD; VMD/PhD. *Faculty:* 321. *Students:* 352 full-time (205 women); includes 99 minority (11 Black or African American, non-Hispanic/Latino; 65 Asian, non-Hispanic/Latino; 21 Hispanic/Latino; 2 Two or more races, non-Hispanic/Latino), 45 international. 488 applicants, 20% accepted, 40 enrolled. In 2013, 41 doctorates awarded. *Degree requirements:* For doctorate, thesis/dissertation. *Entrance requirements:* For doctorate, GRE General Test. Additional exam requirements/recommendations for international students: Required—TOEFL. *Application deadline:* For fall admission, 12/1 priority date for domestic and international students. Applications are processed on a rolling basis. Application fee: $80. Electronic applications accepted. *Financial support:* In 2013–14, 352 students received support. Fellowships, research assistantships, scholarships/grants, traineeships, and unspecified assistantships available. *Unit head:* Dr. Daniel Kessler, Graduate Group Chair, 215-898-1478. *Application contact:* Meagan Schofer, Coordinator, 215-898-4360.
Website: http://www.med.upenn.edu/camb/

University of Pittsburgh, Dietrich School of Arts and Sciences, Department of Biological Sciences, Program in Molecular, Cellular, and Developmental Biology, Pittsburgh, PA 15260. Offers PhD. *Faculty:* 19 full-time (4 women). *Students:* 45 full-time (24 women); includes 5 minority (1 Black or African American, non-Hispanic/Latino; 3 Asian, non-Hispanic/Latino; 1 Hispanic/Latino), 14 international. Average age 23. 180 applicants, 9% accepted, 8 enrolled. In 2013, 6 doctorates awarded. *Degree requirements:* For doctorate, comprehensive exam, thesis/dissertation, completion of research integrity module. *Entrance requirements:* For doctorate, GRE General Test, GRE Subject Test. Additional exam requirements/recommendations for international students: Required—TOEFL (minimum score 90 iBT). *Application deadline:* For fall admission, 1/3 priority date for domestic students, 12/9 priority date for international students. Applications are processed on a rolling basis. Application fee: $0 ($50 for international students). Electronic applications accepted. *Expenses:* Tuition, state resident: full-time $19,964; part-time $807 per credit. Tuition, nonresident: full-time $32,686; part-time $1337 per credit. *Required fees:* $740; $200. Tuition and fees vary according to program. *Financial support:* In 2013–14, 26 fellowships with full tuition reimbursements (averaging $30,682 per year), 79 research assistantships with full tuition reimbursements (averaging $26,544 per year), 18 teaching assistantships with full tuition reimbursements (averaging $25,716 per year) were awarded; Federal Work-Study, scholarships/grants, traineeships, health care benefits, and tuition waivers (full) also available. *Unit head:* Dr. Jeffrey G. Lawrence, Professor, 412-624-4204, Fax: 412-624-4759, E-mail: jlawrenc@pitt.edu. *Application contact:* Cathleen M. Barr, Graduate Administrator, 412-624-4268, Fax: 412-624-4759, E-mail: cbarr@pitt.edu.
Website: http://www.biology.pitt.edu/graduate/mcdb-program

University of Pittsburgh, School of Medicine, Graduate Programs in Medicine, Molecular Genetics and Developmental Biology Graduate Program, Pittsburgh, PA 15260. Offers PhD. *Faculty:* 49 full-time (11 women). *Students:* 12 full-time (6 women); includes 1 minority (Native Hawaiian or other Pacific Islander, non-Hispanic/Latino), 2 international. Average age 27. 517 applicants, 13% accepted, 22 enrolled. In 2013, 3 doctorates awarded. *Degree requirements:* For doctorate, comprehensive exam, thesis/dissertation. *Entrance requirements:* For doctorate, GRE General Test, GRE Subject Test, minimum QPA of 3.0. Additional exam requirements/recommendations for international students: Required—TOEFL (minimum score 600 paper-based; 100 iBT), IELTS (minimum score 7). *Application deadline:* For fall admission, 1/1 priority date for domestic and international students. Application fee: $50. Electronic applications accepted. *Expenses:* Tuition, state resident: full-time $19,964; part-time $807 per credit. Tuition, nonresident: full-time $32,686; part-time $1337 per credit. *Required fees:* $740; $200. Tuition and fees vary according to program. *Financial support:* In 2013–14, 2 fellowships with full tuition reimbursements (averaging $26,010 per year), 9 research assistantships with full tuition reimbursements (averaging $26,010 per year), 1 teaching assistantship with full tuition reimbursement (averaging $26,010 per year) were awarded; institutionally sponsored loans, scholarships/grants, traineeships, health care benefits, and unspecified assistantships also available. *Faculty research:* Developmental and stem cell biology, DNA replication and repair, gene regulation and signal transduction, oncogenes and tumor suppressor genes, protein structure and molecular dynamics. *Unit head:* Dr. Kyle E. Orwig, Graduate Program Director, 412-641-2460, Fax: 412-641-3899, E-mail: korwig@mwri.magee.edu. *Application contact:* Graduate Studies Administrator, 412-648-8957, Fax: 412-648-1077, E-mail: gradstudies@medschool.pitt.edu.
Website: http://www.gradbiomed.pitt.edu/

University of South Carolina, The Graduate School, College of Arts and Sciences, Department of Biological Sciences, Graduate Training Program in Molecular, Cellular, and Developmental Biology, Columbia, SC 29208. Offers MS, PhD. *Degree requirements:* For master's, one foreign language, thesis; for doctorate, one foreign language, thesis/dissertation. *Entrance requirements:* For master's and doctorate, GRE General Test, minimum GPA of 3.0 in science. Electronic applications accepted. *Faculty research:* Marine ecology, population and evolutionary biology, molecular biology and genetics, development.

The University of Texas Health Science Center at Houston, Graduate School of Biomedical Sciences, Program in Genes and Development, Houston, TX 77225-0036. Offers MS, PhD, MD/PhD. Terminal master's awarded for partial completion of doctoral program. *Degree requirements:* For master's, thesis; for doctorate, thesis/dissertation. *Entrance requirements:* For master's and doctorate, GRE General Test. Additional exam requirements/recommendations for international students: Required—TOEFL. Electronic applications accepted. *Expenses:* Tuition, state resident: full-time $3474; part-time $193 per credit hour. Tuition, nonresident: full-time $13,644; part-time $758 per credit hour. *Required fees:* $226.30; $87 per credit hour. *Faculty research:* Developmental biology, genetics, cell biology, structural biology, cancer.

The University of Texas Southwestern Medical Center, Southwestern Graduate School of Biomedical Sciences, Division of Basic Science, Program in Genetics and Development, Dallas, TX 75390. Offers PhD. *Faculty:* 85 full-time (16 women), 2 part-time/adjunct (0 women). *Students:* 57 full-time (28 women), 1 part-time (0 women); includes 16 minority (1 Black or African American, non-Hispanic/Latino; 1 American Indian or Alaska Native, non-Hispanic/Latino; 5 Asian, non-Hispanic/Latino; 9 Hispanic/Latino), 26 international. Average age 26. In 2013, 3 doctorates awarded. *Degree requirements:* For doctorate, thesis/dissertation, qualifying exam. *Entrance requirements:* For doctorate, GRE General Test, minimum GPA of 3.0. Additional exam requirements/recommendations for international students: Required—TOEFL. *Application deadline:* For fall admission, 12/15 priority date for domestic students. Application fee: $0. Electronic applications accepted. *Financial support:* Fellowships, research assistantships, and institutionally sponsored loans available. *Faculty research:* Human molecular genetics, chromosome structure, gene regulation, molecular biology, gene expression.
Website: http://www.utsouthwestern.edu/education/graduate-school/programs/phd-degrees/genetics-and-development/index.html

Vanderbilt University, Graduate School and School of Medicine, Department of Cell and Developmental Biology, Nashville, TN 37240-1001. Offers MS, PhD, MD/PhD. *Faculty:* 19 full-time (7 women). *Students:* 74 full-time (43 women); includes 9 minority (3 Black or African American, non-Hispanic/Latino; 3 Asian, non-Hispanic/Latino; 1 Hispanic/Latino; 1 Native Hawaiian or other Pacific Islander, non-Hispanic/Latino; 1 Two or more races, non-Hispanic/Latino), 9 international. Average age 27. In 2013, 2 master's, 9 doctorates awarded. Terminal master's awarded for partial completion of doctoral program. *Degree requirements:* For master's, thesis or alternative; for doctorate, thesis/dissertation, preliminary, qualifying, and final exams. *Entrance requirements:* For master's, GRE General Test; for doctorate, GRE General Test, GRE Subject Test (recommended). Additional exam requirements/recommendations for international students: Required—TOEFL (minimum score 570 paper-based; 88 iBT). *Application deadline:* For fall admission, 1/15 for domestic and international students. Application fee: $0. Electronic applications accepted. *Financial support:* Fellowships with full and partial tuition reimbursements, research assistantships with full and partial tuition reimbursements, career-related internships or fieldwork, Federal Work-Study, institutionally sponsored loans, scholarships/grants, traineeships, health care benefits, and tuition waivers (partial) available. Financial award application deadline: 1/15; financial award applicants required to submit CSS PROFILE or FAFSA. *Faculty research:* Cancer biology, cell cycle regulation, cell signaling, cytoskeletal biology, developmental biology, neurobiology, proteomics, stem cell biology, structural biology, reproductive biology, trafficking and transport, medical education and gross anatomy. *Unit head:* Dr. Kathleen Gould, Director of Graduate Studies, 615-343-9502, Fax: 615-343-4539, E-mail: kathy.gould@vanderbilt.edu. *Application contact:* Elaine Caine, Administrative Assistant, 615-322-2294, Fax: 615-343-4539, E-mail: elaine.caine@vanderbilt.edu.
Website: http://www.mc.vanderbilt.edu/cdb/

Washington University in St. Louis, Graduate School of Arts and Sciences, Division of Biology and Biomedical Sciences, Program in Developmental, Regenerative, and

Stem Cell Biology, St. Louis, MO 63130-4899. Offers PhD. *Degree requirements:* For doctorate, thesis/dissertation. *Entrance requirements:* For doctorate, GRE General Test, GRE Subject Test. Electronic applications accepted.

Wesleyan University, Graduate Studies, Department of Biology, Middletown, CT 06459. Offers cell and developmental genetics (PhD); evolution and ecology (PhD); neurobiology and behavior (PhD). *Degree requirements:* For doctorate, variable foreign language requirement, thesis/dissertation. *Entrance requirements:* For doctorate, GRE. Additional exam requirements/recommendations for international students: Required—TOEFL. *Faculty research:* Microbial population genetics, genetic basis of evolutionary adaptation, genetic regulation of differentiation and pattern formation in &ITdrosophila&RO.

West Virginia University, Davis College of Agriculture, Forestry and Consumer Sciences, Interdisciplinary Program in Genetics and Developmental Biology, Morgantown, WV 26506. Offers animal breeding (MS, PhD); biochemical and molecular genetics (MS, PhD); cytogenetics (MS, PhD); descriptive embryology (MS, PhD); developmental genetics (MS); experimental morphogenesis/teratology (MS); human genetics (MS, PhD); immunogenetics (MS, PhD); life cycles of animals and plants (MS, PhD); molecular aspects of development (MS, PhD); mutagenesis (MS, PhD); oncology (MS, PhD); plant genetics (MS, PhD); population and quantitative genetics (MS, PhD); regeneration (MS, PhD); teratology (PhD); toxicology (MS, PhD). *Degree requirements:* For master's, thesis; for doctorate, comprehensive exam, thesis/dissertation. *Entrance requirements:* For master's, GRE or MCAT, minimum GPA of 2.75. Additional exam requirements/recommendations for international students: Required—TOEFL.

Yale University, Graduate School of Arts and Sciences, Department of Molecular, Cellular, and Developmental Biology, New Haven, CT 06520. Offers biochemistry, molecular biology and chemical biology (PhD); cellular and developmental biology (PhD); genetics (PhD); neurobiology (PhD); plant sciences (PhD). *Degree requirements:* For doctorate, thesis/dissertation. *Entrance requirements:* For doctorate, GRE General Test, GRE Subject Test.

Genetics

Albert Einstein College of Medicine, Graduate Division of Biomedical Sciences, Department of Genetics, Bronx, NY 10461. Offers computational genetics (PhD); molecular genetics (PhD); translational genetics (PhD); MD/PhD. *Degree requirements:* For doctorate, thesis/dissertation. *Entrance requirements:* For doctorate, GRE General Test. Additional exam requirements/recommendations for international students: Required—TOEFL. *Faculty research:* Neurologic genetics in &ITdrosophila&RO, biochemical genetics of yeast, developmental genetics in the mouse.

American University of Beirut, Graduate Programs, Faculty of Medicine, Beirut, Lebanon. Offers anatomy, cell biology and human morphology (MS); biochemistry and medical genetics (MS); biomedical sciences (PhD); experimental pathology, immunology and microbiology (MS); medicine (MD); neuroscience (MS); pharmacology and toxicology (MS). Part-time programs available. *Faculty:* 259 full-time (78 women), 93 part-time/adjunct (16 women). *Students:* 364 full-time (165 women), 62 part-time (54 women). Average age 23. In 2013, 18 master's awarded. *Degree requirements:* For master's, one foreign language, comprehensive exam, thesis (for some programs); for doctorate, one foreign language, comprehensive exam, thesis/dissertation. *Entrance requirements:* For master's, letter of recommendation; for doctorate, MCAT, bachelor's degree. Additional exam requirements/recommendations for international students: Required—TOEFL (minimum score 600 paper-based; 100 iBT), IELTS (minimum score 7.5). *Application deadline:* For fall admission, 4/30 for domestic and international students; for spring admission, 11/1 for domestic and international students. Application fee: $50. *Expenses: Tuition:* Full-time $14,724; part-time $818 per credit. *Required fees:* $692. Tuition and fees vary according to course load and program. *Financial support:* In 2013–14, 242 students received support, including 60 teaching assistantships (averaging $4,000 per year); career-related internships or fieldwork, institutionally sponsored loans, scholarships/grants, health care benefits, and unspecified assistantships also available. Financial award application deadline: 2/2. *Faculty research:* Cancer research (targeted therapy, mechanisms of leukemogenesis, tumor cell extravasation and metastasis, cancer stem cells), stem cell research (regenerative medicine, drug discovery), genetic research (neurogenetics, hereditary cardiomyopathy, hemoglobinopathies, pharmacogenomics, proteomics), neuroscience research (pain, neurodegenerative disorder), metabolism (inflammation and metabolism, metabolic disorder, diabetes mellitus), vascular and renal biology, signal transduction. *Total annual research expenditures:* $2.6 million. *Unit head:* Dr. Mohamed Sayegh, Dean, 961-1350000 Ext. 4700, Fax: 961-1744464, E-mail: msayegh@aub.edu.lb. *Application contact:* Dr. Salim Kanaan, Director, Admissions Office, 961-1-350000 Ext. 2594, Fax: 96-1-1750775, E-mail: sk00@aub.edu.lb.
Website: http://www.aub.edu.lb/fm/fm_home/Pages/index.aspx

Baylor College of Medicine, Graduate School of Biomedical Sciences, Department of Molecular and Human Genetics, Houston, TX 77030-3498. Offers PhD, MD/PhD. *Degree requirements:* For doctorate, thesis/dissertation, public defense. *Entrance requirements:* For doctorate, GRE General Test, GRE Subject Test (strongly recommended), minimum GPA of 3.0. Additional exam requirements/recommendations for international students: Required—TOEFL. Electronic applications accepted. *Faculty research:* Human genetics, genome biology, epigenetics, gene therapy, model organisms.

Baylor College of Medicine, Graduate School of Biomedical Sciences, Interdepartmental Program in Cell and Molecular Biology, Houston, TX 77030-3498. Offers biochemistry (PhD); cell and molecular biology (PhD); genetics (PhD); human genetics (PhD); immunology (PhD); microbiology (PhD); virology (PhD); MD/PhD. *Degree requirements:* For doctorate, thesis/dissertation, public defense. *Entrance requirements:* For doctorate, GRE General Test, GRE Subject Test (strongly recommended), minimum GPA of 3.0. Additional exam requirements/recommendations for international students: Required—TOEFL. Electronic applications accepted. *Faculty research:* Molecular and cellular biology; cancer, aging and stem cells; genomics and proteomics; microbiome, molecular microbiology; infectious disease, immunology and translational research.

Baylor College of Medicine, Graduate School of Biomedical Sciences, Program in Developmental Biology, Houston, TX 77030-3498. Offers PhD, MD/PhD. *Degree requirements:* For doctorate, thesis/dissertation, public defense. *Entrance requirements:* For doctorate, GRE General Test, GRE Subject Test (strongly recommended), minimum GPA of 3.0. Additional exam requirements/recommendations for international students: Required—TOEFL. Electronic applications accepted. *Faculty research:* Stem cells, cancer, neurobiology, organogenesis, genetics of model organisms.

Baylor College of Medicine, Graduate School of Biomedical Sciences, Program in Translational Biology and Molecular Medicine, Houston, TX 77030-3498. Offers PhD. *Degree requirements:* For doctorate, thesis/dissertation, public defense. *Entrance requirements:* For doctorate, GRE, minimum GPA of 3.0. Additional exam requirements/recommendations for international students: Required—TOEFL. Electronic applications accepted. *Faculty research:* Molecular medicine, translational biology, human disease biology and therapy.

Boston University, School of Medicine, Division of Graduate Medical Sciences, Program in Genetics and Genomics, Boston, MA 02215. Offers PhD. *Degree requirements:* For doctorate, thesis/dissertation. *Application deadline:* For fall admission, 1/15 for domestic students; for spring admission, 10/15 for domestic students. *Expenses: Tuition:* Full-time $43,970; part-time $1374 per credit hour. *Required fees:* $60 per semester. Tuition and fees vary according to class time, course level and program. *Unit head:* Dr. Shoumita Dasgupta, Associate Professor and Director of Graduate Studies, 617-414-1580, E-mail: dasgupta@bu.edu. *Application contact:* GMS Admissions Office, 617-638-5255, Fax: 617-638-5740, E-mail: natashah@bu.edu.
Website: http://www.bumc.bu.edu/gpgg/graduate-program/

Brandeis University, Graduate School of Arts and Sciences, Program in Molecular and Cell Biology, Waltham, MA 02454-9110. Offers genetics (PhD); microbiology (PhD); molecular and cell biology (MS, PhD); molecular biology (PhD); neurobiology (PhD); quantitative biology (PhD). Terminal master's awarded for partial completion of doctoral program. *Degree requirements:* For master's, thesis or alternative, research project, research lab, or project lab; for doctorate, comprehensive exam, thesis/dissertation, journal clubs; research seminar; colloquia; qualifying exam. *Entrance requirements:* For master's, GRE General Test (or MCAT for applicants to the MS program), official transcript(s), resume, 3 letters of recommendation, statement of purpose; for doctorate, GRE General Test, official transcript(s), resume, 3 letters of recommendation, statement of purpose. Additional exam requirements/recommendations for international students: Required—TOEFL (minimum score 600 paper-based; 100 iBT), PTE (minimum score 68); Recommended—IELTS (minimum score 7). Electronic applications accepted. *Faculty research:* Structural biology; immunology; developmental biology; behavior and neurobiology; DNA replication, rearrangement, and repair; signal transduction, transcriptional regulation, and RNA processing; cancer and programmed cell death; cytoskeleton and molecular motors; nutrition.

California Institute of Technology, Division of Biology, Program in Genetics, Pasadena, CA 91125-0001. Offers PhD. *Degree requirements:* For doctorate, thesis/dissertation, qualifying exam. *Entrance requirements:* For doctorate, GRE General Test.

Carnegie Mellon University, Mellon College of Science, Department of Biological Sciences, Pittsburgh, PA 15213-3891. Offers biochemistry (PhD); biophysics (PhD); cell and developmental biology (PhD); computational biology (MS, PhD); genetics (PhD); molecular biology (PhD); neuroscience (PhD); structural biology (PhD). *Degree requirements:* For doctorate, comprehensive exam, thesis/dissertation. *Entrance requirements:* For doctorate, GRE General Test, GRE Subject Test, interview. *Application deadline:* Applications are processed on a rolling basis. Application fee: $0. Electronic applications accepted. *Financial support:* Fellowships, research assistantships, teaching assistantships, and traineeships available. *Faculty research:* Genetic structure, function, and regulation; protein structure and function; biological membranes; biological spectroscopy. *Unit head:* John L. Woolford, Acting Department Head, 412-268-3193, E-mail: jw17@andrew.cmu.edu. *Application contact:* Ena Miceli, Graduate Programs Manager, 412-268-33012, E-mail: emiceli@andrew.cmu.edu.
Website: http://www.bio.cmu.edu/

Case Western Reserve University, School of Medicine and School of Graduate Studies, Graduate Programs in Medicine, Department of Genetics, Program in Human, Molecular, and Developmental Genetics and Genomics, Cleveland, OH 44106. Offers PhD, MD/PhD. *Degree requirements:* For doctorate, comprehensive exam, thesis/dissertation. *Entrance requirements:* For doctorate, GRE General Test, GRE Subject Test. Additional exam requirements/recommendations for international students: Required—TOEFL. *Faculty research:* Regulation of gene expression, molecular control of development, genomics.

Clemson University, Graduate School, College of Agriculture, Forestry and Life Sciences, Department of Genetics and Biochemistry, Program in Genetics, Clemson, SC 29634. Offers PhD. *Students:* 13 full-time (8 women), 1 (woman) part-time; includes 1 minority (Hispanic/Latino), 4 international. Average age 26. 18 applicants, 28% accepted, 3 enrolled. In 2013, 5 doctorates awarded. *Degree requirements:* For doctorate, thesis/dissertation. *Entrance requirements:* For doctorate, GRE General Test, minimum GPA of 3.2. Additional exam requirements/recommendations for international students: Required—TOEFL, IELTS. *Application deadline:* For fall admission, 1/1 for domestic students; for spring admission, 9/1 for domestic students. Applications are processed on a rolling basis. Application fee: $70 ($80 for international students). Electronic applications accepted. *Expenses:* Contact institution. *Financial support:* In 2013–14, 13 students received support, including 4 fellowships with full and partial tuition reimbursements available (averaging $8,750 per year), 10 research assistantships with partial tuition reimbursements available (averaging $16,725 per year), 3 teaching assistantships with partial tuition reimbursements available (averaging $15,750 per year). Financial award application deadline: 3/15; financial award applicants required to submit FAFSA. *Faculty research:* Animal, plant, microbial, molecular, and biometrical genetics. *Unit head:* Dr. Keith Murphy, Chair, 864-656-6237, E-mail: kmurph2@clemson.edu. *Application contact:* Sheryl Banks, Administrative Coordinator, 866-656-6878, E-mail: sherylb@clemson.edu.
Website: http://www.clemson.edu/genbiochem

Clemson University, Graduate School, College of Health, Education, and Human Development, School of Nursing, Clemson, SC 29634. Offers healthcare genetics (PhD); nursing (MS). *Accreditation:* AACN. Part-time programs available. *Faculty:* 13 full-time (12 women). *Students:* 75 full-time (67 women), 35 part-time (30 women); includes 12 minority (4 Black or African American, non-Hispanic/Latino; 2 Asian, non-Hispanic/Latino; 2 Hispanic/Latino; 4 Two or more races, non-Hispanic/Latino), 3 international. Average age 31. 43 applicants, 63% accepted, 22 enrolled. In 2013, 38 master's, 2 doctorates awarded. Terminal master's awarded for partial completion of doctoral program. *Degree requirements:* For master's, comprehensive exam, thesis or alternative; for doctorate, comprehensive exam, thesis/dissertation. *Entrance*

requirements: For master's, GRE General Test, RN license; for doctorate, GRE General Test. Additional exam requirements/recommendations for international students: Required—TOEFL. *Application deadline:* For fall admission, 4/1 for domestic and international students; for spring admission, 10/1 for domestic and international students. Application fee: $50. Electronic applications accepted. *Expenses:* Contact institution. *Financial support:* In 2013–14, 27 students received support, including 3 fellowships with partial tuition reimbursements available (averaging $7,333 per year), 1 research assistantship with partial tuition reimbursement available (averaging $9,200 per year), 25 teaching assistantships with partial tuition reimbursements available (averaging $9,612 per year); career-related internships or fieldwork, institutionally sponsored loans, scholarships/grants, health care benefits, and unspecified assistantships also available. Financial award applicants required to submit FAFSA. *Faculty research:* Breast cancer, healthcare, genetics, international healthcare, simulation, educational innovation and technology. *Total annual research expenditures:* $381,705. *Unit head:* Dr. Rosanne Harkey Pruitt, Professor/Director, School of Nursing/ Associate Dean, College of Health, Education and Human Development, 864-656-7622, Fax: 864-656-5488, E-mail: prosan@clemson.edu. *Application contact:* Dr. Stephanie Clark Davis, Graduate Studies Coordinator, 864-656-2588, Fax: 864-656-5488, E-mail: stephad@clemson.edu.
Website: http://www.clemson.edu/nursing/

Columbia University, College of Physicians and Surgeons, Department of Genetics and Development, New York, NY 10032. Offers genetics (M Phil, MA, PhD); MD/PhD. Only candidates for the PhD are admitted. Terminal master's awarded for partial completion of doctoral program. *Degree requirements:* For doctorate, thesis/ dissertation. *Entrance requirements:* For master's and doctorate, GRE General Test. Additional exam requirements/recommendations for international students: Required—TOEFL. *Faculty research:* Mammalian cell differentiation and meiosis, developmental genetics, yeast and human genetics, chromosome structure, molecular and cellular biology.

Columbia University, College of Physicians and Surgeons, Integrated Program in Cellular, Molecular, Structural and Genetic Studies, New York, NY 10032. Offers PhD. Terminal master's awarded for partial completion of doctoral program. *Degree requirements:* For doctorate, thesis/dissertation. *Entrance requirements:* For doctorate, GRE General Test, GRE Subject Test. Additional exam requirements/recommendations for international students: Required—TOEFL. *Expenses:* Contact institution. *Faculty research:* Transcription, macromolecular sorting, gene expression during development, cellular interaction.

Cornell University, Graduate School, Graduate Fields of Agriculture and Life Sciences, Field of Computational Biology, Ithaca, NY 14853-0001. Offers computational behavioral biology (PhD); computational biology (PhD); computational cell biology (PhD); computational ecology (PhD); computational genetics (PhD); computational macromolecular biology (PhD); computational organismal biology (PhD). *Faculty:* 37 full-time (5 women). *Students:* 26 full-time (8 women); includes 8 minority (5 Asian, non-Hispanic/Latino; 1 Hispanic/Latino; 1 Native Hawaiian or other Pacific Islander, non-Hispanic/Latino; 1 Two or more races, non-Hispanic/Latino), 8 international. Average age 25. 171 applicants, 13% accepted, 10 enrolled. *Degree requirements:* For doctorate, comprehensive exam, thesis/dissertation, 2 semesters of teaching experience. *Entrance requirements:* For doctorate, GRE General Test, GRE Subject Test (biology), 2 letters of recommendation. Additional exam requirements/ recommendations for international students: Required—TOEFL (minimum score 550 paper-based; 77 iBT). *Application deadline:* For fall admission, 2/1 priority date for domestic students. Application fee: $95. Electronic applications accepted. *Financial support:* In 2013–14, 22 students received support, including 20 research assistantships with full tuition reimbursements available, 2 teaching assistantships with full tuition reimbursements available; fellowships with full tuition reimbursements available, institutionally sponsored loans, scholarships/grants, health care benefits, tuition waivers (full and partial), and unspecified assistantships also available. Financial award applicants required to submit FAFSA. *Faculty research:* Computational behavioral biology, computational biology, computational cell biology, computational ecology, computational genetics, computational macromolecular biology, computational organismal biology. *Unit head:* Dr. Andrew Clark, Director of Graduate Studies, 607-255-5488, E-mail: ac347@cornell.edu. *Application contact:* Graduate School Application Requests, 607-255-5816, E-mail: gradadmissions@cornell.edu.
Website: http://www.gradschool.cornell.edu/fields.php?id-4A

Cornell University, Graduate School, Graduate Fields of Agriculture and Life Sciences, Field of Genetics, Genomics and Development, Ithaca, NY 14853-0001. Offers developmental biology (PhD); genetics (PhD); genomics (PhD). *Faculty:* 66 full-time (15 women). *Students:* 56 full-time (37 women); includes 7 minority (3 Black or African American, non-Hispanic/Latino; 2 Asian, non-Hispanic/Latino; 1 Hispanic/Latino; 1 Two or more races, non-Hispanic/Latino), 22 international. Average age 26. 67 applicants, 33% accepted, 12 enrolled. In 2013, 12 doctorates awarded. *Degree requirements:* For doctorate, comprehensive exam, thesis/dissertation, 2 semesters of teaching experience. *Entrance requirements:* For doctorate, GRE General Test, GRE Subject Test in biology or biochemistry (recommended), 2 letters of recommendation. Additional exam requirements/recommendations for international students: Required—TOEFL (minimum score 550 paper-based; 77 iBT). *Application deadline:* For fall admission, 1/5 for domestic students. Application fee: $95. Electronic applications accepted. *Financial support:* In 2013–14, 45 students received support, including 5 fellowships with full tuition reimbursements available, 26 research assistantships with full tuition reimbursements available, 14 teaching assistantships with full tuition reimbursements available; institutionally sponsored loans, scholarships/grants, health care benefits, tuition waivers (full and partial), and unspecified assistantships also available. Financial award applicants required to submit FAFSA. *Faculty research:* Molecular and general genetics, developmental biology and developmental genetics, evolution and population genetics, plant genetics, microbial genetics. *Unit head:* Director of Graduate Studies, 607-254-2100. *Application contact:* Graduate Field Assistant, 607-254-2100, E-mail: gendev@cornell.edu.
Website: http://www.gradschool.cornell.edu/fields.php?id-51&a-2

Dartmouth College, Graduate Program in Molecular and Cellular Biology, Department of Genetics, Hanover, NH 03755. Offers PhD, MD/PhD. *Entrance requirements:* For doctorate, GRE General Test, letters of recommendation. Additional exam requirements/recommendations for international students: Required—TOEFL (minimum score 450 paper-based; 90 iBT) or IELTS (minimum score 7). Electronic applications accepted.

Drexel University, College of Medicine, Biomedical Graduate Programs, Interdisciplinary Program in Molecular and Cell Biology and Genetics, Philadelphia, PA 19104-2875. Offers MS, PhD, MD/PhD. Terminal master's awarded for partial completion of doctoral program. *Degree requirements:* For master's, comprehensive exam, thesis; for doctorate, thesis/dissertation, qualifying exam. *Entrance requirements:* For master's, GRE General Test, minimum GPA of 2.75; for doctorate, GRE General Test, minimum GPA of 3.0. Additional exam requirements/recommendations for international students: Required—TOEFL. Electronic applications accepted. *Faculty research:* Molecular anatomy, biochemistry, medical biotechnology, molecular pathology, microbiology and immunology.

Duke University, Graduate School, Department of Biochemistry, Durham, NC 27710. Offers crystallography of macromolecules (PhD); enzyme mechanisms (PhD); lipid biochemistry (PhD); membrane structure and function (PhD); molecular genetics (PhD); neurochemistry (PhD); nucleic acid structure and function (PhD); protein structure and function (PhD). *Faculty:* 30. *Students:* 63 full-time (26 women); includes 35 minority (4 Black or African American, non-Hispanic/Latino; 30 American Indian or Alaska Native, non-Hispanic/Latino; 1 Asian, non-Hispanic/Latino), 27 international. 90 applicants, 17% accepted, 5 enrolled. In 2013, 15 doctorates awarded. *Degree requirements:* For doctorate, thesis/dissertation. *Entrance requirements:* For doctorate, GRE General Test, GRE Subject Test (recommended). Additional exam requirements/recommendations for international students: Required—TOEFL (minimum score 577 paper-based; 90 iBT) or IELTS (minimum score 7). *Application deadline:* For fall admission, 12/8 priority date for domestic and international students. Application fee: $80. Electronic applications accepted. *Financial support:* Fellowships, research assistantships, teaching assistantships, and Federal Work-Study available. Financial award application deadline: 12/8. *Unit head:* Leonard Spicer, Director of Graduate Studies, 919-681-8770, Fax: 919-684-8885, E-mail: norfleet@duke.edu. *Application contact:* Elizabeth Hutton, Director of Admissions, 919-684-3913, Fax: 919-684-2277, E-mail: grad-admissions@duke.edu.
Website: http://www.biochem.duke.edu/

Duke University, Graduate School, University Program in Genetics and Genomics, Durham, NC 27710. Offers PhD. *Faculty:* 108. *Students:* 82 full-time (50 women); includes 16 minority (4 Black or African American, non-Hispanic/Latino; 7 Asian, non-Hispanic/Latino; 5 Hispanic/Latino), 15 international. 97 applicants, 15% accepted, 6 enrolled. In 2013, 21 doctorates awarded. *Degree requirements:* For doctorate, variable foreign language requirement, thesis/dissertation. *Entrance requirements:* For doctorate, GRE General Test. Additional exam requirements/recommendations for international students: Required—TOEFL (minimum score 577 paper-based; 90 iBT) or IELTS (minimum score 7). *Application deadline:* For fall admission, 12/8 priority date for domestic and international students. Application fee: $80. *Financial support:* Fellowships available. Financial award application deadline: 12/8. *Unit head:* Allison Ashley-Koch, Interim Director of Graduate Studies, 919-684-6629, Fax: 919-684-8346, E-mail: leslie.mavengere@duke.edu. *Application contact:* Elizabeth Hutton, Director of Admissions, 919-684-3913, Fax: 919-684-2277, E-mail: grad-admissions@duke.edu.
Website: http://upg.duke.edu/

Emory University, Laney Graduate School, Division of Biological and Biomedical Sciences, Program in Genetics and Molecular Biology, Atlanta, GA 30322-1100. Offers PhD. *Degree requirements:* For doctorate, comprehensive exam, thesis/dissertation. *Entrance requirements:* For doctorate, GRE General Test, minimum GPA of 3.0 in science course work (recommended). Additional exam requirements/recommendations for international students: Required—TOEFL. Electronic applications accepted. *Faculty research:* Gene regulation, genetic combination, developmental regulation.

Harvard University, Graduate School of Arts and Sciences, Division of Medical Sciences, Boston, MA 02115. Offers biological chemistry and molecular pharmacology (PhD); cell biology (PhD); genetics (PhD); microbiology and molecular genetics (PhD); pathology (PhD), including experimental pathology. *Degree requirements:* For doctorate, thesis/dissertation. *Entrance requirements:* For doctorate, GRE General Test, GRE Subject Test. Additional exam requirements/recommendations for international students: Required—TOEFL. *Expenses: Tuition:* Full-time $38,888. *Required fees:* $958. Tuition and fees vary according to campus/location, program and student level.

Illinois State University, Graduate School, College of Arts and Sciences, Department of Biological Sciences, Normal, IL 61790-2200. Offers animal behavior (MS); bacteriology (MS); biochemistry (MS); biological sciences (MS); biology (PhD); biophysics (MS); biotechnology (MS); botany (MS, PhD); cell biology (MS); conservation biology (MS); developmental biology (MS); ecology (MS, PhD); entomology (MS); evolutionary biology (MS); genetics (MS, PhD); immunology (MS); microbiology (MS, PhD); molecular biology (MS); molecular genetics (MS); neurobiology (MS); neuroscience (MS); parasitology (MS); physiology (MS, PhD); plant biology (MS); plant molecular biology (MS); plant sciences (MS); structural biology (MS); zoology (MS, PhD). Part-time programs available. *Degree requirements:* For master's, thesis or alternative; for doctorate, variable foreign language requirement, thesis/dissertation, 2 terms of residency. *Entrance requirements:* For master's, GRE General Test, minimum GPA of 2.6 in last 60 hours of course work; for doctorate, GRE General Test. *Faculty research:* Redoc balance and drug development in schistosoma mansoni, control of the growth of listeria monocytogenes at low temperature, regulation of cell expansion and microtubule function by SPRI, CRUI: physiology and fitness consequences of different life history phenotypes.

Indiana University Bloomington, University Graduate School, College of Arts and Sciences, Department of Biology, Bloomington, IN 47405. Offers biology teaching (MAT); biotechnology (MA); evolution, ecology, and behavior (MA, PhD); genetics (PhD); microbiology (MA, PhD); molecular, cellular, and developmental biology (PhD); plant sciences (MA, PhD); zoology (MA, PhD). *Faculty:* 58 full-time (15 women), 21 part-time/adjunct (6 women). *Students:* 166 full-time (94 women), 2 part-time (both women); includes 22 minority (8 Black or African American, non-Hispanic/Latino; 3 Asian, non-Hispanic/Latino; 10 Hispanic/Latino; 1 Two or more races, non-Hispanic/Latino), 47 international. Average age 27. 261 applicants, 23% accepted, 32 enrolled. In 2013, 17 master's, 20 doctorates awarded. Terminal master's awarded for partial completion of doctoral program. *Degree requirements:* For master's, thesis, oral defense; for doctorate, thesis/dissertation, oral defense. *Entrance requirements:* For master's and doctorate, GRE General Test. Additional exam requirements/recommendations for international students: Required—TOEFL (minimum score 100 iBT). *Application deadline:* For fall admission, 1/5 priority date for domestic students, 12/1 priority date for international students. Application fee: $55 ($65 for international students). Electronic applications accepted. *Financial support:* In 2013–14, fellowships with tuition reimbursements (averaging $24,000 per year), research assistantships with tuition reimbursements (averaging $21,000 per year), teaching assistantships with tuition reimbursements (averaging $22,000 per year) were awarded; scholarships/grants, traineeships, health care benefits, and unspecified assistantships also available. Financial award application deadline: 1/5. *Faculty research:* Evolution, ecology and behavior; microbiology; molecular biology and genetics; plant biology. *Unit head:* Dr. Clay Fuqua, Chair, 812-856-6005, Fax: 812-855-6082, E-mail: cfuqua@indiana.edu. *Application contact:* Tracey D. Stohr, Graduate Student Recruitment Coordinator, 812-856-6303, Fax: 812-855-6082, E-mail: gradbio@indiana.edu.
Website: http://www.bio.indiana.edu/

Iowa State University of Science and Technology, Bioinformatics and Computational Biology Program, Ames, IA 50011. Offers MS, PhD. *Degree requirements:* For doctorate, thesis/dissertation. *Entrance requirements:* For master's and doctorate, GRE General Test. Additional exam requirements/recommendations for international students: Recommended—TOEFL, IELTS. Electronic applications accepted. *Faculty research:* Functional and structural genomics, genome evolution, macromolecular structure and function, mathematical biology and biological statistics, metabolic and developmental networks.

Genetics

Iowa State University of Science and Technology, Program in Genetics, Ames, IA 50011. Offers MS, PhD. *Entrance requirements:* For master's and doctorate, GRE General Test. Additional exam requirements/recommendations for international students: Required—TOEFL (minimum score 550 paper-based; 79 iBT), IELTS (minimum score 6.5). Electronic applications accepted.

Johns Hopkins University, Bloomberg School of Public Health, Department of Epidemiology, Baltimore, MD 21205. Offers cancer etiology and prevention (MHS, Sc M, PhD, Sc D); cardiovascular diseases (MHS, Sc M, PhD, Sc D); clinical epidemiology (MHS, Sc M, PhD, Sc D); clinical trials (PhD, Sc D); epidemiology (MHS, Sc M, Dr PH, PhD, Sc D); epidemiology of aging (MHS, Sc M, PhD, Sc D); genetic epidemiology (MHS, Sc M, PhD, Sc D); infectious disease epidemiology (MHS, Sc M, PhD, Sc D); occupational and environmental epidemiology (MHS, Sc M, PhD, Sc D). Part-time programs available. *Faculty:* 80 full-time (44 women), 82 part-time/adjunct (36 women). *Students:* 141 full-time (106 women), 20 part-time (13 women); includes 32 minority (5 Black or African American, non-Hispanic/Latino; 1 American Indian or Alaska Native, non-Hispanic/Latino; 18 Asian, non-Hispanic/Latino; 6 Hispanic/Latino; 2 Two or more races, non-Hispanic/Latino), 49 international. Average age 29. 302 applicants, 35% accepted, 63 enrolled. In 2013, 26 master's, 23 doctorates awarded. *Degree requirements:* For master's, comprehensive exam, thesis, 1-year full-time residency; for doctorate, comprehensive exam, thesis/dissertation, 2 years' full-time residency, oral and written exams, student teaching. *Entrance requirements:* For master's, GRE General Test or MCAT, 3 letters of recommendation, curriculum vitae; for doctorate, GRE General Test, minimum 1 year of work experience, 3 letters of recommendation, curriculum vitae, academic records from all schools. Additional exam requirements/recommendations for international students: Required—TOEFL (minimum score 600 paper-based; 100 iBT); Recommended—IELTS (minimum score 7.5), TWE. *Application deadline:* For fall admission, 12/1 priority date for domestic students. Applications are processed on a rolling basis. Application fee: $45. Electronic applications accepted. *Financial support:* Fellowships, Federal Work-Study, institutionally sponsored loans, scholarships/grants, traineeships, tuition waivers (partial), and stipends available. Support available to part-time students. Financial award application deadline: 3/15; financial award applicants required to submit FAFSA. *Faculty research:* Cancer and congenital malformations, nutritional epidemiology, AIDS, tuberculosis, cardiovascular disease, risk assessment. *Total annual research expenditures:* $70.1 million. *Unit head:* Dr. David D. Celentano, Chair, 410-955-3286, Fax: 410-955-0863, E-mail: dcelenta@jhsph.edu. *Application contact:* Frances S. Burman, Academic Program Manager, 410-955-3926, Fax: 410-955-0863, E-mail: fburman@jhsph.edu.
Website: http://www.jhsph.edu/dept/epi/index.html

Johns Hopkins University, National Institutes of Health Sponsored Programs, Baltimore, MD 21218-2699. Offers biology (PhD), including biochemistry, biophysics, cell biology, developmental biology, genetic biology, molecular biology; cell, molecular, and developmental biology and biophysics (PhD). *Faculty:* 25 full-time (4 women). *Students:* 126 full-time (72 women); includes 36 minority (3 Black or African American, non-Hispanic/Latino; 1 American Indian or Alaska Native, non-Hispanic/Latino; 21 Asian, non-Hispanic/Latino; 11 Hispanic/Latino), 19 international. 282 applicants, 26% accepted, 36 enrolled. In 2013, 15 doctorates awarded. *Degree requirements:* For doctorate, comprehensive exam, thesis/dissertation. *Entrance requirements:* For doctorate, GRE General Test. Additional exam requirements/recommendations for international students: Required—TOEFL (minimum score 600 paper-based), TWE. *Application deadline:* For fall admission, 12/15 priority date for domestic students. Application fee: $60. Electronic applications accepted. *Financial support:* In 2013–14, 24 fellowships (averaging $23,000 per year), 93 research assistantships (averaging $23,000 per year), 22 teaching assistantships (averaging $23,000 per year) were awarded; Federal Work-Study, institutionally sponsored loans, scholarships/grants, traineeships, health care benefits, tuition waivers (partial), and unspecified assistantships also available. Financial award application deadline: 4/15; financial award applicants required to submit FAFSA. *Faculty research:* Protein and nucleic acid biochemistry and biophysical chemistry, molecular biology and development. *Total annual research expenditures:* $11.2 million. *Unit head:* Dr. Allen Shearn, Chair, 410-516-4693, Fax: 410-516-5213, E-mail: bio_cals@jhu.edu. *Application contact:* Joan Miller, Academic Affairs Manager, 410-516-5502, Fax: 410-516-5213, E-mail: joan@jhu.edu.

Kansas State University, Graduate School, College of Agriculture, Department of Plant Pathology, Manhattan, KS 66506. Offers genetics (MS, PhD); plant pathology (MS, PhD). *Faculty:* 21 full-time (5 women), 5 part-time/adjunct (0 women). *Students:* 30 full-time (10 women); includes 1 minority (Asian, non-Hispanic/Latino), 20 international. Average age 28. 27 applicants, 22% accepted, 3 enrolled. In 2013, 2 doctorates awarded. Terminal master's awarded for partial completion of doctoral program. *Degree requirements:* For master's, thesis, oral exam; for doctorate, thesis/dissertation, preliminary exams. *Entrance requirements:* For master's and doctorate, minimum undergraduate GPA of 3.0. Additional exam requirements/recommendations for international students: Required—TOEFL (minimum score 550 paper-based; 79 iBT). *Application deadline:* For fall admission, 5/15 priority date for domestic students, 11/1 priority date for international students; for spring admission, 10/15 priority date for domestic students, 6/1 priority date for international students; for summer admission, 3/1 for domestic students, 10/18 for international students. Applications are processed on a rolling basis. Application fee: $50 ($75 for international students). Electronic applications accepted. *Financial support:* In 2013–14, 30 research assistantships with full tuition reimbursements (averaging $24,600 per year) were awarded; Federal Work-Study, institutionally sponsored loans, and scholarships/grants also available. Support available to part-time students. Financial award application deadline: 3/1; financial award applicants required to submit FAFSA. *Faculty research:* Applied microbiology, microbial genetics, microbial ecology/epidemiology, integrated pest management, plant genetics/genomics/molecular biology. *Total annual research expenditures:* $6.3 million. *Unit head:* Dr. John Leslie, Head, 785-532-6176, Fax: 785-532-5692, E-mail: jfl@ksu.edu. *Application contact:* Dr. Bill Bockus, Chair of Graduate Selection Committee, 785-532-1378, Fax: 785-532-5692, E-mail: bockus@ksu.edu.
Website: http://www.plantpath.ksu.edu/p.aspx

Marquette University, Graduate School, College of Arts and Sciences, Department of Biology, Milwaukee, WI 53201-1881. Offers cell biology (MS, PhD); developmental biology (MS, PhD); ecology (MS, PhD); epithelial physiology (MS, PhD); genetics (MS, PhD); microbiology (MS, PhD); molecular biology (MS, PhD); muscle and exercise physiology (MS, PhD); neuroscience (PhD). *Faculty:* 21 full-time (9 women), 3 part-time/adjunct (0 women). *Students:* 34 full-time (16 women), 4 part-time (1 woman), 15 international. Average age 27. 70 applicants, 23% accepted, 5 enrolled. In 2013, 1 master's, 6 doctorates awarded. Terminal master's awarded for partial completion of doctoral program. *Degree requirements:* For master's, comprehensive exam, thesis, 1 year of teaching experience or equivalent; for doctorate, thesis/dissertation, 1 year of teaching experience or equivalent, qualifying exam. *Entrance requirements:* For master's and doctorate, GRE General Test, GRE Subject Test, official transcripts from all current and previous colleges/universities except Marquette, statement of professional goals and aspirations, three letters of recommendation. Additional exam requirements/recommendations for international students: Required—TOEFL (minimum score 530 paper-based). *Application deadline:* For fall admission, 12/15 for domestic and international students. Application fee: $50. Electronic applications accepted. *Financial support:* In 2013–14, 39 students received support, including 6 fellowships (averaging $1,208 per year), 4 research assistantships with full tuition reimbursements available (averaging $21,750 per year), 29 teaching assistantships with full tuition reimbursements available (averaging $21,750 per year); scholarships/grants, health care benefits, tuition waivers (full and partial), and unspecified assistantships also available. Support available to part-time students. Financial award application deadline: 2/15. *Faculty research:* Neurobiology, neuroendocrinology, epithelial physiology, neuropeptide interactions, synaptic transmission. *Total annual research expenditures:* $1.5 million. *Unit head:* Dr. Dale Noel, Chair and Professor, 414-288-1748. *Application contact:* Dr. Michelle Mynlieff, Professor, 414-288-1467.
Website: http://www.marquette.edu/biology/

Massachusetts Institute of Technology, School of Science, Department of Biology, Cambridge, MA 02139-4307. Offers biochemistry (PhD); biological oceanography (PhD); biology (PhD); biophysical chemistry and molecular structure (PhD); cell biology (PhD); computational and systems biology (PhD); developmental biology (PhD); genetics (PhD); immunology (PhD); microbiology (PhD); molecular biology (PhD); neurobiology (PhD). *Faculty:* 58 full-time (15 women). *Students:* 261 full-time (133 women); includes 77 minority (3 Black or African American, non-Hispanic/Latino; 1 American Indian or Alaska Native, non-Hispanic/Latino; 32 Asian, non-Hispanic/Latino; 32 Hispanic/Latino; 9 Two or more races, non-Hispanic/Latino), 46 international. Average age 26. 651 applicants, 15% accepted, 39 enrolled. In 2013, 25 doctorates awarded. *Degree requirements:* For doctorate, comprehensive exam, thesis/dissertation, two semesters as a teaching assistant. *Entrance requirements:* For doctorate, GRE General Test. Additional exam requirements/recommendations for international students: Required—TOEFL (minimum score 577 paper-based), IELTS (minimum score 6.5). *Application deadline:* For fall admission, 12/1 for domestic and international students. Application fee: $75. Electronic applications accepted. *Expenses: Tuition:* Full-time $43,210; part-time $670 per credit hour. *Required fees:* $288. *Financial support:* In 2013–14, 252 students received support, including 135 fellowships (averaging $36,800 per year), 122 research assistantships (averaging $35,500 per year), 1 teaching assistantship; Federal Work-Study, institutionally sponsored loans, scholarships/grants, traineeships, health care benefits, and unspecified assistantships also available. *Faculty research:* Cellular, developmental and molecular (plant and animal) biology; biochemistry, bioengineering, biophysics and structural biology; classical and molecular genetics, stem cell and epigenetics; immunology and microbiology; cancer biology, molecular medicine, neurobiology and human disease; computational and systems biology. *Total annual research expenditures:* $44.5 million. *Unit head:* Alan Grossman, Interim Head, 617-253-4701. *Application contact:* Biology Education Office, 617-253-3717, Fax: 617-258-9329, E-mail: gradbio@mit.edu.
Website: https://biology.mit.edu/

Mayo Graduate School, Graduate Programs in Biomedical Sciences, Program in Virology and Gene Therapy, Rochester, MN 55905. Offers PhD.

Mayo Graduate School, Graduate Programs in Biomedical Sciences, Programs in Biochemistry, Structural Biology, Cell Biology, and Genetics, Rochester, MN 55905. Offers biochemistry and structural biology (PhD); cell biology and genetics (PhD); molecular biology (PhD). *Degree requirements:* For doctorate, oral defense of dissertation, qualifying oral and written exam. *Entrance requirements:* For doctorate, GRE, 1 year of chemistry, biology, calculus, and physics. Additional exam requirements/recommendations for international students: Required—TOEFL. Electronic applications accepted. *Faculty research:* Gene structure and function, membranes and receptors/cytoskeleton, oncogenes and growth factors, protein structure and function, steroid hormonal action.

McMaster University, Faculty of Health Sciences and School of Graduate Studies, Program in Medical Sciences, Genetics and Cancer Area, Hamilton, ON L8S 4M2, Canada. Offers M Sc, PhD, MD/PhD. *Degree requirements:* For master's, thesis; for doctorate, comprehensive exam, thesis/dissertation. *Entrance requirements:* For master's, honors B Sc, B+ average in related field; for doctorate, M Sc, minimum B+ average, students with proven research experience and an A average may be admitted with a B Sc degree. Additional exam requirements/recommendations for international students: Required—TOEFL (minimum score 580 paper-based; 92 iBT).

Medical University of South Carolina, College of Graduate Studies, Program in Molecular and Cellular Biology and Pathobiology, Charleston, SC 29425. Offers cancer biology (PhD); cardiovascular biology (PhD); cardiovascular imaging (PhD); cell regulation (PhD); craniofacial biology (PhD); genetics and development (PhD); marine biomedicine (PhD); DMD/PhD; MD/PhD. *Degree requirements:* For doctorate, thesis/dissertation, oral and written exams. *Entrance requirements:* For doctorate, GRE General Test, interview, minimum GPA of 3.0. Additional exam requirements/recommendations for international students: Required—TOEFL (minimum score 600 paper-based; 100 iBT). Electronic applications accepted.

Michigan State University, College of Veterinary Medicine and The Graduate School, Graduate Programs in Veterinary Medicine and College of Natural Science and Graduate Programs in Human Medicine, Department of Microbiology and Molecular Genetics, East Lansing, MI 48824. Offers industrial microbiology (MS, PhD); microbiology (MS, PhD); microbiology and molecular genetics (MS, PhD); microbiology–environmental toxicology (PhD). *Entrance requirements:* For master's, GRE General Test. Additional exam requirements/recommendations for international students: Required—TOEFL (minimum score 550 paper-based), Michigan State University ELT (minimum score 85), Michigan English Language Assessment Battery (minimum score 83). Electronic applications accepted.

Michigan State University, The Graduate School, College of Agriculture and Natural Resources, MSU-DOE Plant Research Laboratory, East Lansing, MI 48824. Offers biochemistry and molecular biology (PhD); cellular and molecular biology (PhD); crop and soil sciences (PhD); genetics (PhD); microbiology and molecular genetics (PhD); plant biology (PhD); plant physiology (PhD). Offered jointly with the Department of Energy. *Degree requirements:* For doctorate, comprehensive exam, thesis/dissertation, laboratory rotation, defense of dissertation. *Entrance requirements:* For doctorate, GRE General Test, acceptance into one of the affiliated department programs; 3 letters of recommendation; bachelor's degree or equivalent in life sciences, chemistry, biochemistry, or biophysics; research experience. Electronic applications accepted. *Faculty research:* Role of hormones in the regulation of plant development and physiology, molecular mechanisms associated with signal recognition, development and application of genetic methods and materials, protein routing and function.

Michigan State University, The Graduate School, College of Natural Science, Program in Genetics, East Lansing, MI 48824. Offers genetics (MS, PhD); genetics–environmental toxicology (PhD). *Entrance requirements:* Additional exam requirements/recommendations for international students: Required—TOEFL. Electronic applications accepted.

Mississippi State University, College of Agriculture and Life Sciences, Department of Animal Dairy Sciences, Mississippi State, MS 39762. Offers agricultural life sciences (MS), including animal physiology (MS, PhD), genetics (MS, PhD); agricultural science (PhD), including animal dairy sciences, animal nutrition (MS, PhD); agriculture (MS),

including animal nutrition (MS, PhD), animal science; life sciences (PhD), including animal physiology (MS, PhD), genetics (MS, PhD). *Faculty:* 9 full-time (5 women). *Students:* 22 full-time (14 women), 7 part-time (4 women), 7 international. Average age 28. 49 applicants, 29% accepted, 9 enrolled. In 2013, 9 master's, 5 doctorates awarded. *Degree requirements:* For master's, comprehensive exam (for some programs), thesis, written proposal of intended research area; for doctorate, comprehensive exam, thesis/dissertation, written proposal of intended research area. *Entrance requirements:* For master's, GRE General Test, minimum GPA of 3.0; for doctorate, GRE General Test. Additional exam requirements/recommendations for international students: Required—TOEFL (minimum score 575 paper-based; 84 iBT), IELTS (minimum score 7). *Application deadline:* For fall admission, 7/1 for domestic students, 5/1 for international students; for spring admission, 11/1 for domestic students, 9/1 for international students. Applications are processed on a rolling basis. Application fee: $60. Electronic applications accepted. *Financial support:* In 2013–14, 10 research assistantships (averaging $11,697 per year), 1 teaching assistantship (averaging $16,360 per year) were awarded; Federal Work-Study, institutionally sponsored loans, and unspecified assistantships also available. Financial award application deadline: 4/1; financial award applicants required to submit FAFSA. *Faculty research:* Ecology and population dynamics, physiology, biochemistry and behavior, systematics. *Unit head:* Dr. John Blanton, Interim Department Head, 662-325-2802, Fax: 662-325-8873, E-mail: jblanton@ads.msstate.edu. *Application contact:* Dr. Brian Rude, Professor and Graduate Coordinator, 662-325-2802, Fax: 662-325-8873, E-mail: brude@ads.msstate.edu.
Website: http://www.ads.msstate.edu/

New York University, Graduate School of Arts and Science, Department of Biology, New York, NY 10012-1019. Offers biology (PhD); biomedical journalism (MS); cancer and molecular biology (PhD); computational biology (PhD); computers in biological research (MS); developmental genetics (PhD); general biology (MS); immunology and microbiology (PhD); molecular genetics (PhD); neurobiology (PhD); oral biology (MS); plant biology (PhD); recombinant DNA technology (MS); MS/MBA. Part-time programs available. *Faculty:* 24 full-time (5 women). *Students:* 161 full-time (88 women), 28 part-time (15 women); includes 41 minority (5 Black or African American, non-Hispanic/Latino; 23 Asian, non-Hispanic/Latino; 9 Hispanic/Latino; 4 Two or more races, non-Hispanic/Latino), 80 international. Average age 27. 412 applicants, 54% accepted, 65 enrolled. In 2013, 77 master's, 9 doctorates awarded. Terminal master's awarded for partial completion of doctoral program. *Degree requirements:* For master's, thesis or alternative, qualifying paper; for doctorate, comprehensive exam, thesis/dissertation. *Entrance requirements:* For master's and doctorate, GRE General Test. Additional exam requirements/recommendations for international students: Required—TOEFL. *Application deadline:* For fall admission, 12/1 priority date for domestic students, 12/1 for international students. Application fee: $95. *Expenses: Tuition:* Full-time $35,856; part-time $1494 per unit. *Required fees:* $1408; $64 per unit. $473 per term. Tuition and fees vary according to course load and program. *Financial support:* Fellowships with tuition reimbursements, research assistantships with tuition reimbursements, teaching assistantships with tuition reimbursements, career-related internships or fieldwork, Federal Work-Study, institutionally sponsored loans, scholarships/grants, health care benefits, and unspecified assistantships available. Financial award application deadline: 12/1; financial award applicants required to submit FAFSA. *Faculty research:* Genomics, molecular and cell biology, development and molecular genetics, molecular evolution of plants and animals. *Unit head:* Stephen Small, Chair, 212-998-8200, Fax: 212-995-4015, E-mail: biology.admissions@nyu.edu. *Application contact:* Justin Blau, Director of Graduate Studies, PhD Programs, 212-998-8200, Fax: 212-995-4015, E-mail: biology.admissions@nyu.edu.
Website: http://biology.as.nyu.edu/

North Carolina State University, Graduate School, College of Agriculture and Life Sciences, Department of Genetics, Raleigh, NC 27695. Offers MG, MS, PhD. Terminal master's awarded for partial completion of doctoral program. *Degree requirements:* For master's, thesis (for some programs); for doctorate, thesis/dissertation. *Entrance requirements:* For master's and doctorate, GRE General Test, minimum GPA of 3.0. Electronic applications accepted. *Faculty research:* Population and quantitative genetics, plant molecular genetics, developmental genetics.

The Ohio State University, College of Medicine, School of Biomedical Science, Biomedical Sciences Graduate Program, Columbus, OH 43210. Offers immunology (PhD); medical genetics (PhD); molecular virology (PhD); pharmacology (PhD). *Students:* 109 full-time (55 women), 9 part-time (6 women); includes 24 minority (5 Black or African American, non-Hispanic/Latino; 1 American Indian or Alaska Native, non-Hispanic/Latino; 10 Asian, non-Hispanic/Latino; 6 Hispanic/Latino; 1 Native Hawaiian or other Pacific Islander, non-Hispanic/Latino; 1 Two or more races, non-Hispanic/Latino), 4 international. Average age 27. In 2013, 20 doctorates awarded. *Degree requirements:* For doctorate, thesis/dissertation. *Entrance requirements:* For doctorate, GRE General Test; GRE Subject Test in biochemistry, cell and molecular biology (recommended for some programs). Additional exam requirements/recommendations for international students: Required—TOEFL (minimum score 600 paper-based; 100 iBT), Michigan English Language Assessment Battery (minimum score 86); Recommended—IELTS (minimum score 8). *Application deadline:* For fall admission, 12/13 priority date for domestic students, 11/1 priority date for international students. Applications are processed on a rolling basis. Application fee: $60 ($70 for international students). Electronic applications accepted. *Financial support:* In 2013–14, 53 students received support, including 4 fellowships with full tuition reimbursements available (averaging $19,000 per year), 49 research assistantships with full tuition reimbursements available (averaging $19,000 per year); scholarships/grants and unspecified assistantships also available. Financial award application deadline: 1/15. *Unit head:* Joanna Groden, Co-Director, 614-688-4301, Fax: 614-292-6226, E-mail: ibgp@osumc.edu. *Application contact:* Graduate Admissions, 614-292-9444, Fax: 614-292-3895, E-mail: domestic.grad@osu.edu.
Website: http://www.ibgp.org

The Ohio State University, Graduate School, College of Arts and Sciences, Division of Natural and Mathematical Sciences, Department of Molecular Genetics, Columbus, OH 43210. Offers cell and developmental biology (MS, PhD); genetics (MS, PhD); molecular biology (MS, PhD). *Faculty:* 29. *Students:* 35 full-time (15 women); includes 3 minority (1 Black or African American, non-Hispanic/Latino; 2 Asian, non-Hispanic/Latino), 16 international. Average age 26. In 2013, 1 master's, 2 doctorates awarded. *Degree requirements:* For master's, thesis; for doctorate, thesis/dissertation. *Entrance requirements:* For doctorate, GRE General Test, GRE Subject Test in biology or chemistry (recommended). Additional exam requirements/recommendations for international students: Required—TOEFL (minimum score 550 paper-based; 79 iBT), Michigan English Language Assessment Battery (minimum score 82); Recommended—IELTS (minimum score 7). *Application deadline:* For fall admission, 12/13 priority date for domestic students, 11/30 priority date for international students; for winter admission, 12/1 for domestic students, 11/1 for international students; for spring admission, 3/1 for domestic students, 2/1 for international students. Applications are processed on a rolling basis. Application fee: $60 ($70 for international students). Electronic applications accepted. *Financial support:* Fellowships with tuition reimbursements, research assistantships with tuition reimbursements, teaching assistantships with tuition reimbursements, Federal Work-Study, and institutionally sponsored loans available. Support available to part-time students. *Unit head:* Dr. Anita Hopper, Chair, 614-688-3306, Fax: 614-292-4466, E-mail: hopper.64@osu.edu. *Application contact:* Graduate Admissions, 614-292-9444, Fax: 614-292-3895, E-mail: gradadmissions@osu.edu.
Website: https://molgen.osu.edu/

Oregon Health & Science University, School of Medicine, Graduate Programs in Medicine, Program in Molecular and Cellular Biosciences, Department of Molecular and Medical Genetics, Portland, OR 97239-3098. Offers PhD. *Faculty:* 56 full-time (32 women), 8 part-time/adjunct (4 women). *Students:* 6 full-time (5 women); includes 3 minority (1 Black or African American, non-Hispanic/Latino; 2 Hispanic/Latino). Average age 28. In 2013, 2 doctorates awarded. Terminal master's awarded for partial completion of doctoral program. *Degree requirements:* For doctorate, comprehensive exam, thesis/dissertation. *Entrance requirements:* For doctorate, GRE General Test (minimum scores: 153 Verbal/148 Quantitative/4.5 Analytical) or MCAT (for some programs). Additional exam requirements/recommendations for international students: Required—TOEFL. Electronic applications accepted. *Financial support:* Health care benefits and full tuition and stipends (for PhD students) available. *Faculty research:* Biological function and molecular mechanisms of the p53 tumor suppression and c-Myc oncogenic pathways, development of liver- or muscle-directed gene transfer for the treatment of IEM, development of sequence-based testing for rare disorders, development of new rAAV vector-mediated gene and cell therapies to treat various human diseases, cellular signaling pathways involved in the generation of human cancer. *Unit head:* Dr. Susan Olson, Program Director, 503-494-7703, E-mail: olsonsu@oshsu.edu. *Application contact:* Jonna Frater, Program Coordinator, 503-494-2469, E-mail: fraterj@ohsu.edu.
Website: http://www.ohsu.edu/ohsuedu/academic/som/basicscience/genetics/

Penn State University Park, Graduate School, Intercollege Graduate Programs, Intercollege Graduate Program in Genetics, University Park, PA 16802. Offers MS, PhD. *Unit head:* Dr. Regina Vasilatos-Younken, Interim Dean, 814-865-2516, Fax: 814-863-4627, E-mail: rxv@psu.edu. *Application contact:* Cynthia E. Nicosia, Director, Graduate Enrollment Services, 814-865-1834, Fax: 814-863-4627, E-mail: cey1@psu.edu.

Purdue University, Graduate School, College of Science, Department of Biological Sciences, West Lafayette, IN 47907. Offers biochemistry (PhD); biophysics (PhD); cell and developmental biology (PhD); ecology, evolutionary and population biology (MS, PhD), including ecology, evolutionary biology, population biology; genetics (MS, PhD); microbiology (MS, PhD); molecular biology (PhD); neurobiology (MS, PhD); plant physiology (PhD). *Faculty:* 50 full-time (13 women), 5 part-time/adjunct (1 woman). *Students:* 111 full-time (61 women), 5 part-time (0 women); includes 9 minority (1 Black or African American, non-Hispanic/Latino; 5 Asian, non-Hispanic/Latino; 3 Hispanic/Latino), 62 international. Average age 27. 170 applicants, 19% accepted, 17 enrolled. In 2013, 9 master's, 18 doctorates awarded. Terminal master's awarded for partial completion of doctoral program. *Degree requirements:* For master's, thesis (for some programs); for doctorate, thesis/dissertation, seminars, teaching experience. *Entrance requirements:* For master's, GRE General Test (minimum analytical writing score of 3.5), minimum undergraduate GPA of 3.0; for doctorate, GRE General Test (minimum analytical writing score of 3.5), minimum undergraduate GPA of 3.5. Additional exam requirements/recommendations for international students: Required—TOEFL (minimum score 600 paper-based; 107 iBT for MS, 80 iBT for PhD). *Application deadline:* For fall admission, 12/7 for domestic and international students. Applications are processed on a rolling basis. Application fee: $60 ($75 for international students). Electronic applications accepted. *Financial support:* Fellowships, research assistantships, and teaching assistantships available. Support available to part-time students. Financial award application deadline: 2/15; financial award applicants required to submit FAFSA. *Unit head:* Dr. Richard J. Kuhn, Head, 765-494-4407, E-mail: kuhnr@purdue.edu. *Application contact:* Georgina E. Rupp, Graduate Coordinator, 765-494-8142, Fax: 765-494-0876, E-mail: ruppg@purdue.edu.
Website: http://www.bio.purdue.edu/

Purdue University, Graduate School, PULSe - Purdue University Life Sciences Program, West Lafayette, IN 47907. Offers biomolecular structure and biophysics (PhD); biotechnology (PhD); chemical biology (PhD); chromatin and regulation of gene expression (PhD); integrative neuroscience (PhD); integrative plant sciences (PhD); membrane biology (PhD); microbiology (PhD); molecular evolutionary and cancer biology (PhD); molecular evolutionary genetics (PhD); molecular virology (PhD). *Students:* 154 full-time (78 women), 1 part-time (0 women); includes 23 minority (5 Black or African American, non-Hispanic/Latino; 5 Asian, non-Hispanic/Latino; 10 Hispanic/Latino; 3 Two or more races, non-Hispanic/Latino), 73 international. Average age 26. 239 applicants, 33% accepted, 40 enrolled. *Entrance requirements:* For doctorate, GRE, minimum undergraduate GPA of 3.0. Additional exam requirements/recommendations for international students: Required—TOEFL (minimum score 550 paper-based; 77 iBT). *Application deadline:* For fall admission, 1/15 priority date for domestic and international students. Applications are processed on a rolling basis. Application fee: $60 ($75 for international students). Electronic applications accepted. *Financial support:* In 2013–14, research assistantships with tuition reimbursements (averaging $22,500 per year), teaching assistantships with tuition reimbursements (averaging $22,500 per year) were awarded. *Unit head:* Dr. Christine A. Hrycyna, Head, 765-494-7322, E-mail: hrycyna@purdue.edu. *Application contact:* Colleen Gabauer, Graduate Contact, 765-494-9256, E-mail: cgabauer@purdue.edu.
Website: http://www.gradschool.purdue.edu/pulse

Rutgers, The State University of New Jersey, New Brunswick, Graduate School-New Brunswick, Programs in the Molecular Biosciences, Piscataway, NJ 08854-8097. Offers biochemistry (PhD); cell and developmental biology (MS, PhD); microbiology and molecular genetics (MS, PhD), including applied microbiology, clinical microbiology (MS), clinical mircobiology (PhD), computational molecular biology (PhD), immunology, microbial biochemistry, molecular genetics, virology. MS, PhD offered jointly with University of Medicine and Dentistry of New Jersey.

Stanford University, School of Medicine, Graduate Programs in Medicine, Department of Genetics, Stanford, CA 94305-9991. Offers genetic counseling (MS); genetics (MS, PhD). *Degree requirements:* For doctorate, thesis/dissertation, qualifying examination. *Entrance requirements:* For doctorate, GRE General Test, GRE Subject Test. Additional exam requirements/recommendations for international students: Required—TOEFL. Electronic applications accepted. *Expenses: Tuition:* Full-time $42,690; part-time $949 per credit. *Required fees:* $185. *Faculty research:* Molecular biology of DNA replication in human cells, analysis of existing and search for new DNA polymorphisms in humans, molecular genetics of prokaryotic and eukaryotic genetic elements, proteins in DNA replication.

Stony Brook University, State University of New York, Graduate School, College of Arts and Sciences, Graduate Program in Genetics, Stony Brook, NY 11794. Offers PhD. *Students:* 45 full-time (23 women), 1 part-time (0 women); includes 8 minority (2 Black or African American, non-Hispanic/Latino; 3 Asian, non-Hispanic/Latino; 3 Hispanic/Latino), 16 international. Average age 27. 68 applicants, 15% accepted, 5 enrolled. In 2013, 6 doctorates awarded. *Degree requirements:* For doctorate, comprehensive exam, thesis/dissertation, teaching experience. *Entrance requirements:* For doctorate, GRE General Test, GRE Subject Test. Additional exam requirements/recommendations

for international students: Required—TOEFL. *Application deadline:* For fall admission, 1/15 for domestic students; for spring admission, 10/1 for domestic students. Application fee: $100. *Expenses:* Tuition, state resident: full-time $9870; part-time $411 per credit. Tuition, nonresident: full-time $18,350; part-time $765 per credit. *Financial support:* In 2013–14, 9 fellowships, 23 research assistantships, 6 teaching assistantships were awarded; Federal Work-Study also available. *Faculty research:* Gene structure, gene regulation. *Unit head:* Dr. Nancy Squires, Dean, 631-632-6999, Fax: 631-632-6900. *Application contact:* Melissa Jordan, Assistant Dean for Records and Admission, 631-632-9712, Fax: 631-632-7243.
Website: http://life.bio.sunysb.edu/gen/

Thomas Jefferson University, Jefferson Graduate School of Biomedical Sciences, PhD Program in Genetics, Genomics and Cancer Biology, Philadelphia, PA 19107. Offers PhD. *Faculty:* 48 full-time (16 women), 4 part-time/adjunct (3 women). *Students:* 16 full-time (8 women); includes 4 minority (2 Asian, non-Hispanic/Latino; 2 Hispanic/Latino), 1 international. 41 applicants, 24% accepted, 4 enrolled. In 2013, 5 doctorates awarded. *Degree requirements:* For doctorate, comprehensive exam, thesis/dissertation. *Entrance requirements:* For doctorate, GRE General Test, minimum GPA of 3.2. Additional exam requirements/recommendations for international students: Required—TOEFL (minimum score 100 iBT) or IELTS. *Application deadline:* For fall admission, 1/5 priority date for domestic and international students. Applications are processed on a rolling basis. Application fee: $75. Electronic applications accepted. *Financial support:* In 2013–14, 16 students received support, including 16 fellowships with full tuition reimbursements available (averaging $56,052 per year); Federal Work-Study, institutionally sponsored loans, scholarships/grants, traineeships, and stipends also available. Support available to part-time students. Financial award application deadline: 5/1; financial award applicants required to submit FAFSA. *Faculty research:* Functional genomics, cancer susceptibility, cell cycle, regulation oncogenes and tumor suppressor genes, genetics of neoplastic disease. *Unit head:* Dr. Linda D. Siracusa, Program Director, 215-503-4536, E-mail: linda.siracusa@jefferson.edu. *Application contact:* Marc E. Stearns, Director of Admissions, 215-503-0155, Fax: 215-503-3433, E-mail: jgsbs-info@jefferson.edu.
Website: http://www.jefferson.edu/university/biomedical_sciences/programs/phd/genetics.html

Tufts University, Sackler School of Graduate Biomedical Sciences, Genetics Program, Medford, MA 02155. Offers PhD. *Faculty:* 64 full-time (19 women). *Students:* 24 full-time (17 women); includes 4 minority (2 Asian, non-Hispanic/Latino; 1 Hispanic/Latino; 1 Two or more races, non-Hispanic/Latino), 5 international. Average age 28. 57 applicants, 16% accepted, 3 enrolled. In 2013, 5 doctorates awarded. Terminal master's awarded for partial completion of doctoral program. *Degree requirements:* For doctorate, comprehensive exam, thesis/dissertation. *Entrance requirements:* For doctorate, GRE General Test, 3 letters of reference. Additional exam requirements/recommendations for international students: Required—TOEFL (minimum score 600 paper-based; 100 iBT). *Application deadline:* For fall admission, 12/15 for domestic and international students. Application fee: $70. Electronic applications accepted. *Financial support:* In 2013–14, 24 students received support, including 24 research assistantships with full tuition reimbursements available (averaging $31,000 per year); traineeships and health care benefits also available. *Faculty research:* Cancer genetics, developmental and neurogenetics, microbial and yeast genetics, the genetics of bacterial and viral pathogens, Drosophila genetics, human genetics and gene discovery. *Unit head:* Dr. Rajendra Kumar-Singh, Program Director, 617-636-6836. *Application contact:* Kellie Melchin, Associate Director of Admissions, 617-636-6767, Fax: 617-636-0375.
Website: http://sackler.tufts.edu/Academics/Degree-Programs/PhD-Programs/Genetics

Université de Montréal, Faculty of Medicine, Program in Medical Genetics, Montréal, QC H3C 3J7, Canada. Offers DESS.

Université du Québec à Chicoutimi, Graduate Programs, Program in Experimental Medicine, Chicoutimi, QC G7H 2B1, Canada. Offers genetics (M Sc). *Degree requirements:* For master's, thesis. *Entrance requirements:* For master's, appropriate bachelor's degree, proficiency in French.

University at Albany, State University of New York, School of Public Health, Department of Biomedical Sciences, Program in Biochemistry, Molecular Biology, and Genetics, Albany, NY 12222-0001. Offers MS, PhD. *Degree requirements:* For master's, thesis; for doctorate, thesis/dissertation. *Entrance requirements:* For master's and doctorate, GRE General Test, GRE Subject Test.

The University of Alabama at Birmingham, Graduate Programs in Joint Health Sciences, Program in Genetics, Birmingham, AL 35294. Offers PhD. *Degree requirements:* For doctorate, comprehensive exam, thesis/dissertation. *Entrance requirements:* For doctorate, GRE General Test or MCAT, interview, evaluation forms. Electronic applications accepted. *Faculty research:* Clinical cytogenetics, cancer cytogenetics, prenatal diagnosis.

University of Alberta, Faculty of Graduate Studies and Research, Department of Biological Sciences, Edmonton, AB T6G 2E1, Canada. Offers environmental biology and ecology (M Sc, PhD); microbiology and biotechnology (M Sc, PhD); molecular biology and genetics (M Sc, PhD); physiology and cell biology (M Sc, PhD); plant biology (M Sc, PhD); systematics and evolution (M Sc, PhD). Terminal master's awarded for partial completion of doctoral program. *Degree requirements:* For master's, thesis; for doctorate, thesis/dissertation. *Entrance requirements:* Additional exam requirements/recommendations for international students: Required—TOEFL.

University of Alberta, Faculty of Medicine and Dentistry and Faculty of Graduate Studies and Research, Graduate Programs in Medicine, Department of Medical Genetics, Edmonton, AB T6G 2E1, Canada. Offers M Sc, PhD. *Degree requirements:* For master's, comprehensive exam, thesis; for doctorate, comprehensive exam, thesis/dissertation. *Entrance requirements:* For master's and doctorate, minimum GPA of 3.2. *Faculty research:* Clinical and molecular cytogenetics, ocular genetics, Prader-Willi syndrome, genomic instability, developmental genetics.

The University of Arizona, Graduate Interdisciplinary Programs, Graduate Interdisciplinary Program in Genetics, Tucson, AZ 85719. Offers MS, PhD. *Students:* 7 full-time (4 women), 2 part-time (0 women), 1 international. Average age 30. 2 applicants, 100% accepted, 1 enrolled. In 2013, 1 master's, 3 doctorates awarded. Terminal master's awarded for partial completion of doctoral program. *Degree requirements:* For master's, thesis; for doctorate, one foreign language, comprehensive exam, thesis/dissertation. *Entrance requirements:* For master's, GRE General Test, 3 letters of recommendation; for doctorate, GRE General Test, statement of purpose, 3 letters of recommendation. Additional exam requirements/recommendations for international students: Required—TOEFL (minimum score 550 paper-based; 79 iBT). *Application deadline:* For fall admission, 6/1 for domestic students, 12/1 for international students. Applications are processed on a rolling basis. Application fee: $75. Electronic applications accepted. *Expenses:* Tuition, state resident: full-time $11,526. Tuition, nonresident: full-time $27,398. *Financial support:* Career-related internships or fieldwork, scholarships/grants, health care benefits, and unspecified assistantships available. *Faculty research:* Cancer research; DNA repair; plant and animal cytogenetics; molecular, population, and ecological genetics. *Unit head:* Dr. Melanie Culver, Chair, 520-626-1452, Fax: 520-626-5097, E-mail: mculver@email.arizona.edu. *Application contact:* Angela Nelson, Program Coordinator, 520-626-1452, Fax: 520-626-5097, E-mail: cora@email.arizona.edu.
Website: http://www.genetics.arizona.edu/

The University of British Columbia, Faculty of Medicine, Department of Medical Genetics, Medical Genetics Graduate Program, Vancouver, BC V6T 1Z1, Canada. Offers M Sc, PhD. *Degree requirements:* For master's, thesis, 18 credits of coursework; for doctorate, comprehensive exam, thesis/dissertation, 18 credits of coursework. Electronic applications accepted. *Expenses: Tuition, area resident:* Full-time $8000 Canadian dollars.

The University of British Columbia, Genetics Graduate Program, Vancouver, BC V6T 1Z1, Canada. Offers M Sc, PhD. *Degree requirements:* For master's, comprehensive exam, thesis, thesis defense; for doctorate, comprehensive exam, thesis/dissertation, qualifying exam, oral and written comprehensive exams. *Entrance requirements:* Additional exam requirements/recommendations for international students: Required—TOEFL (minimum score 600 paper-based; 100 iBT). *Expenses: Tuition, area resident:* Full-time $8000 Canadian dollars. *Faculty research:* Prokaryote and eukaryote genetics.

University of Calgary, Cumming School of Medicine and Faculty of Graduate Studies, Medical Science Graduate Program, Calgary, AB T2N 1N4, Canada. Offers cancer biology (M Sc, PhD); critical care medicine (M Sc, PhD); joint injury and arthritis (M Sc, PhD); molecular and medical genetics (M Sc, PhD); mountain medicine and high altitude physiology (M Sc, PhD); pathologists' assistant (M Sc, PhD). *Degree requirements:* For master's, thesis; for doctorate, thesis/dissertation, candidacy exam. *Entrance requirements:* For master's, minimum undergraduate GPA of 3.2; for doctorate, minimum graduate GPA of 3.2. Additional exam requirements/recommendations for international students: Required—TOEFL (minimum score 600 paper-based). Electronic applications accepted. *Faculty research:* Cancer biology, immunology, joint injury and arthritis, medical education, population genomics.

University of California, Davis, Graduate Studies, Graduate Group in Genetics, Davis, CA 95616. Offers MS, PhD. Terminal master's awarded for partial completion of doctoral program. *Degree requirements:* For master's, comprehensive exam (for some programs), thesis (for some programs); for doctorate, thesis/dissertation. *Entrance requirements:* For master's and doctorate, GRE General Test, GRE Subject Test. Additional exam requirements/recommendations for international students: Required—TOEFL (minimum score 550 paper-based). Electronic applications accepted. *Faculty research:* Molecular, quantitative, and developmental genetics; cytogenetics; plant breeding.

University of California, Irvine, School of Biological Sciences and School of Medicine, Interdisciplinary Graduate Program in Cellular and Molecular Biosciences, Irvine, CA 92697. Offers PhD. *Degree requirements:* For doctorate, thesis/dissertation, teaching assignment, preliminary exam. *Entrance requirements:* For doctorate, GRE General Test, three letters of recommendation, interview. Additional exam requirements/recommendations for international students: Required—TOEFL or IELTS. *Application deadline:* For fall admission, 12/8 for domestic and international students. Application fee: $60 ($80 for international students). Electronic applications accepted. *Expenses:* Contact institution. *Financial support:* Fellowships with full tuition reimbursements, institutionally sponsored loans, scholarships/grants, tuition waivers (full), unspecified assistantships, and stipends available. Financial award application deadline: 1/1; financial award applicants required to submit FAFSA. *Faculty research:* Cellular biochemistry; gene structure and expression; protein structure, function, and design; molecular genetics; pathogenesis and inherited disease. *Unit head:* Dr. David Fruman, Director, 949-824-1947, Fax: 949-824-1965, E-mail: dfruman@uci.edu. *Application contact:* Renee Frigo, Administrator, 949-824-8145, Fax: 949-824-1965, E-mail: rfrigo@uci.edu.
Website: http://cmb.uci.edu/

University of California, Riverside, Graduate Division, Graduate Program in Genetics, Genomics, and Bioinformatics, Riverside, CA 92521-0102. Offers genomics and bioinformatics (PhD); molecular genetics (PhD); population and evolutionary genetics (PhD). *Faculty:* 72 full-time (20 women). *Students:* 32 full-time (18 women); includes 2 minority (1 Black or African American, non-Hispanic/Latino; 1 Hispanic/Latino), 15 international. Average age 30. In 2013, 2 doctorates awarded. *Degree requirements:* For doctorate, thesis/dissertation, qualifying exams, teaching experience. *Entrance requirements:* For doctorate, GRE General Test, minimum GPA of 3.2. Additional exam requirements/recommendations for international students: Required—TOEFL (minimum score 550 paper-based; 80 iBT). *Application deadline:* For fall admission, 5/1 for domestic students, 2/1 for international students; for winter admission, 9/1 for domestic students, 7/1 for international students; for spring admission, 12/1 for domestic students, 10/1 for international students. Applications are processed on a rolling basis. Application fee: $85 ($100 for international students). Electronic applications accepted. *Financial support:* In 2013–14, fellowships with tuition reimbursements (averaging $18,000 per year), research assistantships with tuition reimbursements (averaging $18,000 per year), teaching assistantships with tuition reimbursements (averaging $16,500 per year) were awarded; career-related internships or fieldwork, Federal Work-Study, institutionally sponsored loans, and tuition waivers (full and partial) also available. *Faculty research:* Molecular genetics, evolution and population genetics, genomics and bioinformatics. *Unit head:* Dr. Shizhong Xu, Director, 951-827-5898. *Application contact:* Deidra Kornfeld, Graduate Program Assistant, 800-735-0717, Fax: 951-827-5517, E-mail: genetics@ucr.edu.
Website: http://ggb.ucr.edu/

University of California, San Francisco, Graduate Division and School of Medicine, Tetrad Graduate Program, Genetics Track, San Francisco, CA 94143. Offers PhD, MD/PhD. *Degree requirements:* For doctorate, thesis/dissertation. *Entrance requirements:* For doctorate, GRE General Test, GRE Subject Test. Additional exam requirements/recommendations for international students: Required—TOEFL. *Application deadline:* For fall admission, 12/1 for domestic students. Application fee: $40. *Expenses:* Contact institution. *Financial support:* Fellowships and scholarships/grants available. Financial award application deadline: 2/1. *Faculty research:* Gene expression; chromosome structure and mechanics; medical, somatic cell, and radiation genetics. *Unit head:* Carol Gross, Co-Director, 415-476-4161, E-mail: cgross@cgl.ucsf.edu. *Application contact:* Carol Gross, Co-Director, 415-476-4161, E-mail: cgross@cgl.ucsf.edu.

University of Chicago, Division of Biological Sciences, Molecular Biosciences Cluster, Committee on Genetics, Genomics and Systems Biology, Chicago, IL 60637-1513. Offers PhD. *Degree requirements:* For doctorate, thesis/dissertation, ethics class, 2 teaching assistantships. *Entrance requirements:* For doctorate, GRE General Test, minimum GPA of 3.0. Additional exam requirements/recommendations for international students: Required—TOEFL (minimum score 600 paper-based; 104 iBT), IELTS (minimum score 7). Electronic applications accepted. *Faculty research:* Molecular genetics, developmental genetics, population genetics, human genetics.

University of Colorado Boulder, Graduate School, College of Arts and Sciences, Department of Ecology and Evolutionary Biology, Boulder, CO 80309. Offers animal behavior (MA); biology (MA, PhD); environmental biology (MA, PhD); evolutionary biology (MA, PhD); neurobiology (MA); population biology (MA); population genetics (PhD). *Faculty:* 31 full-time (12 women). *Students:* 70 full-time (30 women), 18 part-time

(10 women); includes 6 minority (1 Asian, non-Hispanic/Latino; 3 Hispanic/Latino; 2 Two or more races, non-Hispanic/Latino), 5 international. Average age 30. 171 applicants, 6% accepted, 11 enrolled. In 2013, 10 master's, 11 doctorates awarded. Terminal master's awarded for partial completion of doctoral program. *Degree requirements:* For master's, comprehensive exam, thesis or alternative; for doctorate, comprehensive exam, thesis/dissertation. *Entrance requirements:* For master's, GRE General Test, GRE Subject Test, minimum undergraduate GPA of 3.0; for doctorate, GRE General Test, GRE Subject Test. *Application deadline:* For fall admission, 12/31 for domestic students, 12/1 for international students. Application fee: $50 ($60 for international students). Electronic applications accepted. *Financial support:* In 2013–14, 175 students received support, including 35 fellowships (averaging $15,283 per year), 21 research assistantships with full and partial tuition reimbursements available (averaging $29,343 per year), 48 teaching assistantships with full and partial tuition reimbursements available (averaging $31,449 per year); institutionally sponsored loans, scholarships/grants, health care benefits, and unspecified assistantships also available. Financial award applicants required to submit FAFSA. *Faculty research:* Ecology, environmental biology, evolutionary biology, biological sciences, conservation biology. *Total annual research expenditures:* $37.1 million.
Website: http://ebio.colorado.edu

University of Colorado Denver, College of Liberal Arts and Sciences, Department of Integrative Biology, Denver, CO 80217. Offers animal behavior (MS); biology (MS); cell and developmental biology (MS); ecology (MS); evolutionary biology (MS); genetics (MS); integrative and systems biology (PhD); microbiology (MS); molecular biology (MS); neurobiology (MS); plant systematics (MS). Part-time programs available. *Faculty:* 21 full-time (7 women), 3 part-time/adjunct (2 women). *Students:* 18 full-time (11 women), 5 part-time (all women); includes 5 minority (1 Black or African American, non-Hispanic/Latino; 2 Hispanic/Latino; 2 Two or more races, non-Hispanic/Latino), 1 international. Average age 29. 25 applicants, 44% accepted, 11 enrolled. In 2013, 13 master's awarded. *Degree requirements:* For master's, comprehensive exam, thesis, 30-32 credit hours. *Entrance requirements:* For master's, GRE General Test (minimum score in 50th percentile in each section), BA/BS from accredited institution awarded within the last 10 years; minimum undergraduate GPA of 3.0; prerequisite courses: 1 year each of general biology and general chemistry; 1 semester each of general genetics, general ecology, and cell biology; and a structure/function course. Additional exam requirements/recommendations for international students: Required—TOEFL (minimum score 537 paper-based; 75 iBT); Recommended—IELTS (minimum score 6.5). *Application deadline:* For fall admission, 2/1 for domestic and international students. Application fee: $50 ($75 for international students). Electronic applications accepted. *Financial support:* In 2013–14, 8 students received support. Fellowships, research assistantships, teaching assistantships, Federal Work-Study, institutionally sponsored loans, scholarships/grants, and traineeships available. Financial award application deadline: 4/1; financial award applicants required to submit FAFSA. *Faculty research:* Molecular developmental biology; quantitative ecology, biogeography, and population dynamics; environmental signaling and endocrine disruption; speciation, the evolution of reproductive isolation, and hybrid zones; evolutionary, behavioral, and conservation ecology. *Unit head:* Dr. John Swallow, Biology Department Chair, 303-556-6154, E-mail: john.swallow@ucdenver.edu. *Application contact:* Timberley Roane, Associate Professor/Director of MS in Biology Program, 303-556-6592, E-mail: timberley.roane@ucdenver.edu.
Website: http://www.ucdenver.edu/academics/colleges/CLAS/Departments/biology/Programs/MasterofScience/Pages/BiologyMasterOfScience.aspx

University of Colorado Denver, School of Medicine, Program in Human Medical Genetics and Genomics, Aurora, CO 80045. Offers PhD. *Students:* 18 full-time (14 women); includes 2 minority (1 Black or African American, non-Hispanic/Latino; 1 Hispanic/Latino). Average age 28. 26 applicants, 12% accepted, 3 enrolled. In 2013, 1 doctorate awarded. *Degree requirements:* For doctorate, comprehensive exam, thesis/dissertation, at least 30 semester hours in course work (rotations and research courses taken prior to the completion of the comprehensive examination) and 30 semester hours of thesis/didactic credits prior to defending. *Entrance requirements:* For doctorate, GRE General Test (minimum combined score of 1205), minimum GPA of 3.0, 4 letters of recommendation; prerequisite courses in biology, chemistry (general and organic), physics, genetics, calculus, and statistics (recommended). Additional exam requirements/recommendations for international students: Required—TOEFL (minimum score 570 paper-based; 80 iBT). *Application deadline:* For fall admission, 12/1 for domestic students, 1/1 priority date for international students. Application fee: $50 ($75 for international students). Electronic applications accepted. *Expenses:* Contact institution. *Financial support:* In 2013–14, 18 students received support. Fellowships, research assistantships, teaching assistantships, Federal Work-Study, institutionally sponsored loans, scholarships/grants, traineeships, health care benefits, and unspecified assistantships available. Financial award application deadline: 3/15; financial award applicants required to submit FAFSA. *Faculty research:* Mapping, discovery, and function of disease genes affecting skin and craniofacial development and autoimmunity; genetics of colon cancer; clinical proteomics; biochemical markers of disease, including cancer; modeling human genetic diseases with patient-derived induced pluripotent stem cells; cell cycle control of DNA replication and mutagenesis in yeast and human cancer cells; mechanisms of cancer chemoprevention. *Unit head:* Dr. Richard A. Spritz, Director, 303-724-3107, E-mail: richard.spritz@ucdenver.edu. *Application contact:* M. J. Stewart, Administrator, 303-724-3102, Fax: 303-724-3100, E-mail: mj.stewart@ucdenver.edu.
Website: http://www.ucdenver.edu/academics/colleges/medicalschool/programs/HumanMedicalGenetics/Pages/Genetics.aspx

University of Connecticut, Graduate School, College of Liberal Arts and Sciences, Department of Molecular and Cell Biology, Field of Genetics, Genomics, and Bioinformatics, Storrs, CT 06269. Offers MS, PhD. Terminal master's awarded for partial completion of doctoral program. *Degree requirements:* For master's, comprehensive exam; for doctorate, thesis/dissertation. *Entrance requirements:* For master's and doctorate, GRE General Test, GRE Subject Test. Additional exam requirements/recommendations for international students: Required—TOEFL (minimum score 550 paper-based). Electronic applications accepted.

University of Connecticut Health Center, Graduate School, Programs in Biomedical Sciences, Graduate Program in Molecular Biology and Biochemistry, Farmington, CT 06030. Offers PhD, DMD/PhD, MD/PhD. *Degree requirements:* For doctorate, comprehensive exam, thesis/dissertation. *Entrance requirements:* For doctorate, GRE General Test. Additional exam requirements/recommendations for international students: Required—TOEFL (minimum score 600 paper-based). Electronic applications accepted. *Faculty research:* Molecular biology, structural biology, protein biochemistry, microbial physiology and pathogenesis.

See Display on page 224 and Close-Up on page 245.

University of Connecticut Health Center, Graduate School, Programs in Biomedical Sciences, Program in Genetics and Developmental Biology, Farmington, CT 06030. Offers PhD, DMD/PhD, MD/PhD. *Degree requirements:* For doctorate, comprehensive exam, thesis/dissertation. *Entrance requirements:* For doctorate, GRE General Test, GRE Subject Test. Additional exam requirements/recommendations for international students: Required—TOEFL (minimum score 600 paper-based). Electronic applications accepted. *Faculty research:* Developmental biology, genomic imprinting, RNA biology, RNA alternative splicing, human embryonic stem cells.

See Display below and Close-Up on page 313.

Genetics

University of Delaware, College of Arts and Sciences, Department of Biological Sciences, Newark, DE 19716. Offers biotechnology (MS); cancer biology (MS, PhD); cell and extracellular matrix biology (MS, PhD); cell and systems physiology (MS, PhD); developmental biology (MS, PhD); ecology and evolution (MS, PhD); microbiology (MS, PhD); molecular biology and genetics (MS, PhD). Terminal master's awarded for partial completion of doctoral program. *Degree requirements:* For master's, thesis, preliminary exam; for doctorate, comprehensive exam, thesis/dissertation, preliminary exam. *Entrance requirements:* For master's and doctorate, GRE General Test. Additional exam requirements/recommendations for international students: Required—TOEFL (minimum score 600 paper-based); Recommended—TWE. Electronic applications accepted. *Faculty research:* Microorganisms, bone, cancer metastasis, developmental biology, cell biology, DNA.

University of Florida, College of Medicine and Graduate School, Interdisciplinary Program in Biomedical Sciences, Concentration in Genetics, Gainesville, FL 32611. Offers PhD. *Degree requirements:* For doctorate, thesis/dissertation. *Entrance requirements:* For doctorate, GRE General Test, minimum GPA of 3.0, biochemistry before enrollment. Additional exam requirements/recommendations for international students: Required—TOEFL, IELTS. Electronic applications accepted. *Expenses:* Tuition, state resident: full-time $12,640. Tuition, nonresident: full-time $30,000.

University of Georgia, College of Agricultural and Environmental Sciences, Institute of Plant Breeding, Genetics and Genomics, Athens, GA 30602. Offers MS, PhD.

University of Georgia, Franklin College of Arts and Sciences, Department of Genetics, Athens, GA 30602. Offers MS, PhD. Terminal master's awarded for partial completion of doctoral program. *Degree requirements:* For master's, thesis; for doctorate, comprehensive exam, thesis/dissertation. *Entrance requirements:* For master's and doctorate, GRE General Test. Additional exam requirements/recommendations for international students: Required—TOEFL. Electronic applications accepted.

University of Hawaii at Manoa, John A. Burns School of Medicine, Department of Cell and Molecular Biology, Honolulu, HI 96813. Offers MS, PhD. Part-time programs available. Terminal master's awarded for partial completion of doctoral program. *Degree requirements:* For master's, thesis optional; for doctorate, comprehensive exam, thesis/dissertation. *Entrance requirements:* For master's and doctorate, GRE General Test, minimum GPA of 3.0. Additional exam requirements/recommendations for international students: Required—TOEFL (minimum score 500 paper-based; 61 iBT), IELTS (minimum score 5).

University of Illinois at Chicago, College of Medicine and Graduate College, Graduate Programs in Medicine, Department of Biochemistry and Molecular Genetics, Chicago, IL 60607-7128. Offers PhD, MD/PhD. *Faculty:* 32 full-time (11 women), 6 part-time/adjunct (1 woman). *Students:* 31 full-time (17 women), 1 (woman) part-time; includes 5 minority (4 Asian, non-Hispanic/Latino; 1 Hispanic/Latino), 16 international. Average age 29. 7 applicants, 86% accepted, 3 enrolled. In 2013, 10 doctorates awarded. Terminal master's awarded for partial completion of doctoral program. *Degree requirements:* For doctorate, thesis/dissertation. *Entrance requirements:* For doctorate, GRE General Test. Additional exam requirements/recommendations for international students: Required—TOEFL. *Application deadline:* For fall admission, 3/1 priority date for domestic students, 2/15 for international students. Applications are processed on a rolling basis. Application fee: $40 ($50 for international students). Electronic applications accepted. *Expenses:* Tuition, state resident: full-time $11,066; part-time $3689 per term. Tuition, nonresident: full-time $23,064; part-time $7688 per term. *Required fees:* $3004; $1190 per term. Tuition and fees vary according to course level and program. *Financial support:* In 2013–14, 22 students received support. Fellowships with full tuition reimbursements available, research assistantships with full tuition reimbursements available, teaching assistantships with full tuition reimbursements available, career-related internships or fieldwork, Federal Work-Study, institutionally sponsored loans, traineeships, tuition waivers (full), and unspecified assistantships available. Financial award application deadline: 3/1; financial award applicants required to submit FAFSA. *Faculty research:* Nature of cellular components, control of metabolic processes, regulation of gene expression. *Total annual research expenditures:* $6.9 million. *Unit head:* Dr. Jack Kaplan, Head, 312-355-2732, E-mail: kaplanj@uic.edu. *Application contact:* Dr. Karen Colley, Co-Director of Graduate Studies, 312-996-7756.
Website: http://www.uic.edu/com/bcmg/

The University of Iowa, Graduate College, College of Liberal Arts and Sciences, Department of Biology, Iowa City, IA 52242-1324. Offers biology (MS, PhD); cell and developmental biology (MS, PhD); evolution (MS, PhD); genetics (MS, PhD); neurobiology (MS, PhD). Terminal master's awarded for partial completion of doctoral program. *Degree requirements:* For master's, thesis optional, exam; for doctorate, comprehensive exam, thesis/dissertation. *Entrance requirements:* For master's and doctorate, GRE General Test, minimum GPA of 3.0. Additional exam requirements/recommendations for international students: Required—TOEFL (minimum score 600 paper-based; 100 iBT). Electronic applications accepted. *Faculty research:* Neurobiology, evolutionary biology, genetics, cell and developmental biology.

The University of Iowa, Graduate College, Program in Genetics, Iowa City, IA 52242-1316. Offers PhD. *Degree requirements:* For doctorate, comprehensive exam, thesis/dissertation. *Entrance requirements:* For doctorate, GRE General Test, minimum GPA of 3.0. Additional exam requirements/recommendations for international students: Required—TOEFL (minimum score 600 paper-based; 100 iBT). Electronic applications accepted. *Expenses:* Contact institution. *Faculty research:* Developmental genetics, eukaryotic gene expression, human genetics, molecular and biochemical genetics, evolutionary genetics.

The University of Iowa, Roy J. and Lucille A. Carver College of Medicine and Graduate College, Graduate Programs in Medicine, Department of Microbiology, Iowa City, IA 52242-1316. Offers general microbiology and microbial physiology (MS, PhD); immunology (MS, PhD); microbial genetics (MS, PhD); pathogenic bacteriology (MS, PhD); virology (MS, PhD). *Faculty:* 23 full-time (5 women), 10 part-time/adjunct (4 women). *Students:* 38 full-time (28 women); includes 3 minority (2 Asian, non-Hispanic/Latino; 1 Hispanic/Latino), 2 international. Average age 25. 44 applicants, 23% accepted, 8 enrolled. In 2013, 1 master's, 6 doctorates awarded. *Degree requirements:* For master's, thesis; for doctorate, comprehensive exam, thesis/dissertation. *Entrance requirements:* For master's and doctorate, GRE General Test. Additional exam requirements/recommendations for international students: Required—TOEFL (minimum score 600 paper-based). *Application deadline:* For fall admission, 1/1 for domestic and international students. Application fee: $60 ($100 for international students). Electronic applications accepted. *Financial support:* In 2013–14, 5 fellowships with full tuition reimbursements (averaging $26,000 per year), 33 research assistantships with full tuition reimbursements (averaging $26,000 per year) were awarded; institutionally sponsored loans, scholarships/grants, traineeships, and health care benefits also available. *Faculty research:* Gene regulation, processing and transport of HIV, retroviral pathogenesis, biodegradation, biofilm. *Total annual research expenditures:* $11.5 million. *Unit head:* Dr. Patrick M. Schlievert, Chair and Department Executive Officer, 319-335-7810, E-mail: grad-micro-info@uiowa.edu. *Application contact:* Kerry Yoder, Assistant Director of Graduate and Professional Evaluation, 319-335-1525, Fax: 319-335-1535, E-mail: admissions@uiowa.edu.
Website: http://www.medicine.uiowa.edu/microbiology/

The University of Manchester, Faculty of Life Sciences, Manchester, United Kingdom. Offers adaptive organismal biology (M Phil, PhD); animal biology (M Phil, PhD); biochemistry (M Phil, PhD); bioinformatics (M Phil, PhD); biomolecular sciences (M Phil, PhD); biotechnology (M Phil, PhD); cell biology (M Phil, PhD); cell matrix research (M Phil, PhD); channels and transporters (M Phil, PhD); developmental biology (M Phil, PhD); Egyptology (M Phil, PhD); environmental biology (M Phil, PhD); evolutionary biology (M Phil, PhD); gene expression (M Phil, PhD); genetics (M Phil, PhD); history of science, technology and medicine (M Phil, PhD); immunology (M Phil, PhD); integrative neurobiology and behavior (M Phil, PhD); membrane trafficking (M Phil, PhD); microbiology (M Phil, PhD); molecular and cellular neuroscience (M Phil, PhD); molecular biology (M Phil, PhD); molecular cancer studies (M Phil, PhD); neuroscience (M Phil, PhD); ophthalmology (M Phil, PhD); optometry (M Phil, PhD); organelle function (M Phil, PhD); pharmacology (M Phil, PhD); physiology (M Phil, PhD); plant sciences (M Phil, PhD); stem cell research (M Phil, PhD); structural biology (M Phil, PhD); systems neuroscience (M Phil, PhD); toxicology (M Phil, PhD).

University of Massachusetts Amherst, Graduate School, Interdisciplinary Programs, Program in Plant Biology, Amherst, MA 01003. Offers biochemistry and metabolism (MS, PhD); cell biology and physiology (MS, PhD); environmental, ecological and integrative biology (MS, PhD); genetics and evolution (MS, PhD). *Students:* 20 full-time (11 women), 9 international. Average age 28. 72 applicants, 17% accepted, 2 enrolled. In 2013, 1 master's, 2 doctorates awarded. *Degree requirements:* For master's, thesis; for doctorate, 2 foreign languages, comprehensive exam, thesis/dissertation. *Entrance requirements:* For master's and doctorate, GRE General Test. Additional exam requirements/recommendations for international students: Required—TOEFL (minimum score 550 paper-based; 80 iBT), IELTS (minimum score 6.5). *Application deadline:* For fall admission, 12/15 for domestic and international students; for spring admission, 10/1 for domestic and international students. Applications are processed on a rolling basis. Application fee: $75. Electronic applications accepted. *Financial support:* Fellowships with full and partial tuition reimbursements, research assistantships with full and partial tuition reimbursements, teaching assistantships with full and partial tuition reimbursements, career-related internships or fieldwork, Federal Work-Study, scholarships/grants, traineeships, health care benefits, tuition waivers (full and partial), and unspecified assistantships available. Support available to part-time students. Financial award application deadline: 12/15; financial award applicants required to submit FAFSA. *Unit head:* Dr. Elsbeth L. Walker, Graduate Program Director, 413-577-3217, Fax: 413-545-3243, E-mail: pb@bio.umass.edu. *Application contact:* Lindsay DeSantis, Supervisor of Admissions, 413-545-0722, Fax: 413-577-0010, E-mail: gradadm@grad.umass.edu.
Website: http://www.bio.umass.edu/plantbio/

University of Miami, Graduate School, College of Arts and Sciences, Department of Biology, Coral Gables, FL 33124. Offers biology (MS, PhD); genetics and evolution (MS, PhD). Terminal master's awarded for partial completion of doctoral program. *Degree requirements:* For master's, comprehensive exam (for some programs), thesis (for some programs); for doctorate, thesis/dissertation, oral and written qualifying exam. *Entrance requirements:* For master's, GRE General Test, 3 letters of recommendation, research papers; for doctorate, GRE General Test, 3 letters of recommendation, research papers, sponsor letter. Additional exam requirements/recommendations for international students: Required—TOEFL (minimum score 550 paper-based; 59 iBT). Electronic applications accepted. *Faculty research:* Neuroscience to ethology; plants, vertebrates and mycorrhizae; phylogenies, life histories and species interactions; molecular biology, gene expression and populations; cells, auditory neurons and vertebrate locomotion.

University of Minnesota, Twin Cities Campus, Graduate School, Program in Molecular, Cellular, Developmental Biology and Genetics, Minneapolis, MN 55455-0213. Offers genetic counseling (MS); molecular, cellular, developmental biology and genetics (PhD). Terminal master's awarded for partial completion of doctoral program. *Degree requirements:* For master's, thesis optional; for doctorate, thesis/dissertation. *Entrance requirements:* For master's and doctorate, GRE General Test. Additional exam requirements/recommendations for international students: Required—TOEFL (minimum score 625 paper-based; 80 iBT). Electronic applications accepted. *Faculty research:* Membrane receptors and membrane transport, cell interactions, cytoskeleton and cell mobility, regulation of gene expression, plant cell and molecular biology.

University of Missouri, Graduate School, College of Arts and Science, Division of Biological Sciences, Columbia, MO 65211. Offers evolutionary biology and ecology (MA, PhD); genetic, cellular and developmental biology (MA, PhD); neurobiology and behavior (MA, PhD). *Faculty:* 40 full-time (11 women), 1 part-time/adjunct (0 women). *Students:* 70 full-time (32 women), 3 part-time (2 women); includes 12 minority (4 Black or African American, non-Hispanic/Latino; 1 American Indian or Alaska Native, non-Hispanic/Latino; 2 Asian, non-Hispanic/Latino; 3 Hispanic/Latino; 2 Two or more races, non-Hispanic/Latino), 5 international. Average age 28. 46 applicants, 28% accepted, 13 enrolled. In 2013, 7 master's, 13 doctorates awarded. Terminal master's awarded for partial completion of doctoral program. *Degree requirements:* For master's, thesis; for doctorate, comprehensive exam, thesis/dissertation. *Entrance requirements:* For master's and doctorate, GRE General Test (minimum score 1200 verbal and quantitative), minimum GPA of 3.0. Additional exam requirements/recommendations for international students: Required—TOEFL (minimum score 600 paper-based; 100 iBT). *Application deadline:* For fall admission, 12/15 priority date for domestic and international students. Applications are processed on a rolling basis. Application fee: $55 ($75 for international students). Electronic applications accepted. *Financial support:* Fellowships with full tuition reimbursements, research assistantships with full tuition reimbursements, teaching assistantships with full tuition reimbursements, institutionally sponsored loans, traineeships, health care benefits, and unspecified assistantships available. *Faculty research:* Evolutionary biology, ecology and behavior; genetic, cellular, molecular and developmental biology; neurobiology and behavior; plant sciences. *Unit head:* Dr. John C. Walker, Division Director, 573-882-3583, E-mail: walkerj@missouri.edu. *Application contact:* Nila Emerich, Application Contact, 800-553-5698, E-mail: emerichn@missouri.edu.
Website: http://biology.missouri.edu/graduate-studies/

University of Missouri, Graduate School, Genetics Area Program, Columbia, MO 65211. Offers PhD. *Students:* 12 full-time (6 women), 1 part-time (0 women), 5 international. Average age 26. 8 applicants, 38% accepted, 3 enrolled. In 2013, 1 doctorate awarded. *Degree requirements:* For doctorate, comprehensive exam, thesis/dissertation. *Entrance requirements:* For doctorate, GRE General Test, minimum GPA of 3.0. Additional exam requirements/recommendations for international students: Required—TOEFL (minimum score 580 paper-based; 92 iBT). *Application deadline:* For fall admission, 1/15 priority date for domestic students, 1/15 for international students. Applications are processed on a rolling basis. Application fee: $55 ($75 for international students). Electronic applications accepted. *Financial support:* Fellowships with tuition reimbursements, research assistantships with tuition reimbursements, teaching assistantships with tuition reimbursements, institutionally sponsored loans, scholarships/grants, traineeships, health care benefits, and unspecified assistantships available.

Support available to part-time students. *Faculty research:* Aging, cancer, development, disease resistance, evolution, genomics, microbe interactions, plant molecular biology, proteomics, reproductive biology, viral genetics. *Unit head:* Dr. John F. Cannon, Director of Graduate Studies, 573-852-2780, E-mail: cannonj@missouri.edu. *Application contact:* Debbie Allen, Program Coordinator, 573-882-2816, E-mail: allendebra@missouri.edu.
Website: http://www.gap.missouri.edu/

University of Nebraska Medical Center, Department of Genetics, Cell Biology and Anatomy, Omaha, NE 68198-5805. Offers MS, PhD. Part-time programs available. Terminal master's awarded for partial completion of doctoral program. *Degree requirements:* For master's, comprehensive exam, thesis; for doctorate, comprehensive exam, thesis/dissertation. *Entrance requirements:* For master's and doctorate, GRE General Test. Additional exam requirements/recommendations for international students: Required—TOEFL (minimum score 550 paper-based). Electronic applications accepted. *Expenses: Required fees:* $300 per semester. Tuition and fees vary according to program. *Faculty research:* Hematology, immunology, developmental biology, genetics cancer biology, neuroscience.

University of New Hampshire, Graduate School, College of Life Sciences and Agriculture, Department of Molecular, Cellular and Biomedical Sciences, Program in Genetics, Durham, NH 03824. Offers MS, PhD. Part-time programs available. *Faculty:* 31 full-time. *Students:* 9 full-time (7 women), 13 part-time (8 women); includes 3 minority (1 Hispanic/Latino; 2 Two or more races, non-Hispanic/Latino), 6 international. Average age 32. 21 applicants, 24% accepted, 4 enrolled. In 2013, 1 master's, 3 doctorates awarded. *Degree requirements:* For master's, thesis; for doctorate, thesis/dissertation. *Entrance requirements:* For master's and doctorate, GRE General Test, GRE Subject Test. Additional exam requirements/recommendations for international students: Required—TOEFL (minimum score 550 paper-based; 80 iBT). *Application deadline:* For fall admission, 6/1 priority date for domestic students, 4/1 for international students; for spring admission, 12/1 for domestic students. Applications are processed on a rolling basis. Application fee: $65. Electronic applications accepted. *Expenses:* Tuition, state resident: full-time $13,500; part-time $750 per credit hour. Tuition, nonresident: full-time $26,200; part-time $1100 per credit hour. *Required fees:* $1741; $435.25 per term. Tuition and fees vary according to course level, course load, campus/location and program. *Financial support:* In 2013–14, 15 students received support, including 5 research assistantships, 10 teaching assistantships; fellowships, career-related internships or fieldwork, Federal Work-Study, and scholarships/grants also available. Support available to part-time students. Financial award application deadline: 2/15. *Unit head:* Dr. Rick Cote, Chair, 603-862-3217. *Application contact:* Flora Joyal, Administrative Assistant, 603-862-2250, E-mail: genetics.dept@unh.edu.
Website: http://genetics.unh.edu/

University of New Mexico, School of Medicine, Program in Biomedical Sciences, Albuquerque, NM 87131-5196. Offers biochemistry and molecular biology (MS, PhD); cell biology and physiology (MS, PhD); clinical and translational science (Certificate); molecular genetics and microbiology (MS, PhD); neuroscience (MS, PhD); pathology (MS, PhD); toxicology (MS, PhD); university science teaching (Certificate). Part-time programs available. *Students:* 73 full-time (39 women), 14 part-time (9 women); includes 24 minority (1 Black or African American, non-Hispanic/Latino; 1 American Indian or Alaska Native, non-Hispanic/Latino; 2 Asian, non-Hispanic/Latino; 17 Hispanic/Latino; 1 Native Hawaiian or other Pacific Islander, non-Hispanic/Latino; 2 Two or more races, non-Hispanic/Latino), 16 international. Average age 29. 89 applicants, 20% accepted, 17 enrolled. In 2013, 7 master's, 17 doctorates awarded. Terminal master's awarded for partial completion of doctoral program. *Degree requirements:* For master's, thesis; for doctorate, comprehensive exam, thesis/dissertation, qualifying exam at the end of year 1/core curriculum. *Entrance requirements:* For master's and doctorate, GRE General Test, minimum undergraduate GPA of 3.0. Additional exam requirements/recommendations for international students: Required—TOEFL. *Application deadline:* For fall admission, 3/1 priority date for domestic and international students. Applications are processed on a rolling basis. Application fee: $50. Electronic applications accepted. *Financial support:* In 2013–14, 94 students received support, including 28 fellowships with full and partial tuition reimbursements available (averaging $22,000 per year), 73 research assistantships with full tuition reimbursements available (averaging $23,000 per year), 8 teaching assistantships (averaging $2,800 per year); career-related internships or fieldwork, Federal Work-Study, institutionally sponsored loans, scholarships/grants, traineeships, health care benefits, and unspecified assistantships also available. Financial award application deadline: 1/1; financial award applicants required to submit FAFSA. *Faculty research:* Infectious disease/immunity, cancer biology, cardiovascular and metabolic diseases, brain and behavioral illness, environmental health. *Unit head:* Dr. Helen J. Hathaway, Program Director, 505-272-1887, Fax: 505-272-2412, E-mail: hhathaway@salud.unm.edu. *Application contact:* Mary Fenton, Admissions Coordinator, 505-272-1887, Fax: 505-272-2412, E-mail: mfenton@salud.unm.edu.
Website: http://hsc.unm.edu/research/brep/bsgpabout.shtm

The University of North Carolina at Chapel Hill, Graduate School, College of Arts and Sciences, Department of Biology, Chapel Hill, NC 27599. Offers botany (MA, MS, PhD); cell biology, development, and physiology (MA, MS, PhD); cell motility and cytoskeleton (PhD); ecology and behavior (MA, MS, PhD); genetics and molecular biology (MA, MS, PhD); morphology, systematics, and evolution (MA, MS, PhD). Terminal master's awarded for partial completion of doctoral program. *Degree requirements:* For master's, comprehensive exam, thesis (for some programs); for doctorate, comprehensive exam, thesis/dissertation. *Entrance requirements:* For master's, GRE General Test, GRE Subject Test, 2 semesters of calculus or statistics; 2 semesters of physics, organic chemistry; 3 semesters of biology; for doctorate, GRE General Test, GRE Subject Test, 2 semesters calculus or statistics, 2 semesters physics, organic chemistry, 3 semesters of biology. Additional exam requirements/recommendations for international students: Required—TOEFL (minimum score 550 paper-based). Electronic applications accepted. *Faculty research:* Gene expression, biomechanics, yeast genetics, plant ecology, plant molecular biology.

The University of North Carolina at Chapel Hill, School of Medicine and Graduate School, Graduate Programs in Medicine, Curriculum in Genetics and Molecular Biology, Chapel Hill, NC 27599. Offers MS, PhD. *Degree requirements:* For doctorate, comprehensive exam, thesis/dissertation. *Entrance requirements:* For doctorate, GRE, minimum GPA of 3.0. Additional exam requirements/recommendations for international students: Required—TOEFL. Electronic applications accepted. *Faculty research:* Telomere replication and germline immortality, experimental evolution in microorganisms, genetic vulnerabilities in tumor genomes, genetics of cell cycle control during Drosophila development, mammalian genetics.

University of North Dakota, Graduate School, College of Arts and Sciences, Department of Biology, Grand Forks, ND 58202. Offers botany (MS, PhD); ecology (MS, PhD); entomology (MS, PhD); environmental biology (MS, PhD); fisheries/wildlife (MS, PhD); genetics (MS, PhD); zoology (MS, PhD). Terminal master's awarded for partial completion of doctoral program. *Degree requirements:* For master's, thesis, final exam; for doctorate, comprehensive exam, thesis/dissertation, final exam. *Entrance requirements:* For master's, GRE General Test, GRE Subject Test, minimum GPA of 3.0; for doctorate, GRE General Test, GRE Subject Test, minimum GPA of 3.5. Additional exam requirements/recommendations for international students: Required—TOEFL (minimum score 550 paper-based; 79 iBT), IELTS (minimum score 6.5). Electronic applications accepted. *Faculty research:* Population biology, wildlife ecology, RNA processing, hormonal control of behavior.

University of North Texas Health Science Center at Fort Worth, Graduate School of Biomedical Sciences, Fort Worth, TX 76107-2699. Offers anatomy and cell biology (MS, PhD); biochemistry and molecular biology (MS, PhD); biomedical sciences (MS, PhD); biotechnology (MS); forensic genetics (MS); integrative physiology (MS, PhD); medical science (MS); microbiology and immunology (MS, PhD); pharmacology (MS, PhD); science education (MS); DO/MS; DO/PhD. Terminal master's awarded for partial completion of doctoral program. *Degree requirements:* For master's, thesis; for doctorate, thesis/dissertation. *Entrance requirements:* For master's and doctorate, GRE General Test. Additional exam requirements/recommendations for international students: Required—TOEFL. *Expenses:* Contact institution. *Faculty research:* Alzheimer's disease, aging, eye diseases, cancer, cardiovascular disease.

University of Notre Dame, Graduate School, College of Science, Department of Biological Sciences, Notre Dame, IN 46556. Offers aquatic ecology, evolution and environmental biology (MS, PhD); cellular and molecular biology (MS, PhD); genetics (MS, PhD); physiology (MS, PhD); vector biology and parasitology (MS, PhD). Terminal master's awarded for partial completion of doctoral program. *Degree requirements:* For master's, comprehensive exam, thesis; for doctorate, comprehensive exam, thesis/dissertation, candidacy exam. *Entrance requirements:* For master's and doctorate, GRE General Test. Additional exam requirements/recommendations for international students: Required—TOEFL (minimum score 600 paper-based; 80 iBT). Electronic applications accepted. *Faculty research:* Tropical disease, molecular genetics, neurobiology, evolutionary biology, aquatic biology.

University of Oregon, Graduate School, College of Arts and Sciences, Department of Biology, Eugene, OR 97403. Offers ecology and evolution (MA, MS, PhD); marine biology (MA, MS, PhD); molecular, cellular and genetic biology (PhD); neuroscience and development (PhD). Terminal master's awarded for partial completion of doctoral program. *Degree requirements:* For master's, thesis (for some programs); for doctorate, thesis/dissertation. *Entrance requirements:* For master's and doctorate, GRE General Test, minimum GPA of 3.2. Additional exam requirements/recommendations for international students: Required—TOEFL. *Faculty research:* Developmental neurobiology; evolution, population biology, and quantitative genetics; regulation of gene expression; biochemistry of marine organisms.

University of Pennsylvania, Perelman School of Medicine, Biomedical Graduate Studies, Graduate Group in Cell and Molecular Biology, Philadelphia, PA 19104. Offers cancer biology (PhD); cell biology and physiology (PhD); developmental stem cell regenerative biology (PhD); gene therapy and vaccines (PhD); genetics and gene regulation (PhD); microbiology, virology, and parasitology (PhD); MD/PhD; VMD/PhD. *Faculty:* 321. *Students:* 352 full-time (205 women); includes 99 minority (11 Black or African American, non-Hispanic/Latino; 65 Asian, non-Hispanic/Latino; 21 Hispanic/Latino; 2 Two or more races, non-Hispanic/Latino), 45 international. 488 applicants, 20% accepted, 40 enrolled. In 2013, 41 doctorates awarded. *Degree requirements:* For doctorate, thesis/dissertation. *Entrance requirements:* For doctorate, GRE General Test. Additional exam requirements/recommendations for international students: Required—TOEFL. *Application deadline:* For fall admission, 12/1 priority date for domestic and international students. Applications are processed on a rolling basis. Application fee: $80. Electronic applications accepted. *Financial support:* In 2013–14, 352 students received support. Fellowships, research assistantships, scholarships/grants, traineeships, and unspecified assistantships available. *Unit head:* Dr. Daniel Kessler, Graduate Group Chair, 215-898-1478. *Application contact:* Meagan Schofer, Coordinator, 215-898-4360.
Website: http://www.med.upenn.edu/camb/

University of Puerto Rico, Río Piedras Campus, College of Natural Sciences, Department of Biology, San Juan, PR 00931-3300. Offers ecology/systematics (MS, PhD); evolution/genetics (MS, PhD); molecular/cellular biology (MS, PhD); neuroscience (MS, PhD). Part-time programs available. *Degree requirements:* For master's, one foreign language, comprehensive exam, thesis; for doctorate, one foreign language, comprehensive exam, thesis/dissertation. *Entrance requirements:* For master's, GRE Subject Test, interview, minimum GPA of 3.0, letter of recommendation; for doctorate, GRE Subject Test, interview, master's degree, minimum GPA of 3.0, letter of recommendation. *Faculty research:* Environmental, poblational and systematic biology.

University of Rochester, School of Medicine and Dentistry, Graduate Programs in Medicine and Dentistry, Department of Biomedical Genetics, Rochester, NY 14627. Offers genetics, genomics and development (PhD). *Degree requirements:* For doctorate, thesis/dissertation, qualifying exam. *Entrance requirements:* For doctorate, GRE General Test. *Expenses: Tuition:* Full-time $44,580; part-time $1394 per credit hour. *Required fees:* $492.

University of Southern California, Keck School of Medicine and Graduate School, Program in Genetic, Molecular and Cellular Biology, Los Angeles, CA 90089-9031. Offers PhD. *Faculty:* 236 full-time (68 women). *Students:* 114 full-time (63 women); includes 25 minority (2 Black or African American, non-Hispanic/Latino; 17 Asian, non-Hispanic/Latino; 5 Hispanic/Latino; 1 Two or more races, non-Hispanic/Latino), 57 international. Average age 29. 342 applicants, 18% accepted, 21 enrolled. In 2013, 15 doctorates awarded. *Degree requirements:* For doctorate, comprehensive exam, thesis/dissertation. *Entrance requirements:* For doctorate, GRE, minimum GPA of 3.0. Additional exam requirements/recommendations for international students: Required—TOEFL (minimum score 600 paper-based; 100 iBT). *Application deadline:* For fall admission, 12/1 priority date for domestic and international students. Application fee: $85. Electronic applications accepted. *Financial support:* In 2013–14, 114 students received support, including 11 fellowships (averaging $31,000 per year), 98 research assistantships with full tuition reimbursements available (averaging $31,000 per year), 5 teaching assistantships with full tuition reimbursements available (averaging $31,000 per year); institutionally sponsored loans, scholarships/grants, traineeships, health care benefits, and unspecified assistantships also available. Financial award application deadline: 5/4; financial award applicants required to submit FAFSA. *Unit head:* Dr. Wei Li, Director, 323-442-1475, Fax: 323-442-1199, E-mail: wli@usc.edu. *Application contact:* Dr. Joyce Perez, Manager of Student Programs, 323-442-1645, Fax: 323-442-1199, E-mail: pibbs@usc.edu.
Website: http://www.usc.edu/intbio

The University of Tennessee, Graduate School, College of Arts and Sciences, Program in Life Sciences, Knoxville, TN 37996. Offers genome science and technology (MS, PhD); plant physiology and genetics (MS, PhD). *Degree requirements:* For doctorate, one foreign language, thesis/dissertation. *Entrance requirements:* For master's and doctorate, GRE General Test, minimum GPA of 2.7. Additional exam requirements/recommendations for international students: Required—TOEFL. Electronic applications accepted. *Expenses:* Tuition, state resident: full-time $9540; part-time $531 per credit hour. Tuition, nonresident: full-time $27,728; part-time $1542 per credit hour. *Required fees:* $1404; $67 per credit hour.

Genetics

The University of Texas Health Science Center at Houston, Graduate School of Biomedical Sciences, Program in Genes and Development, Houston, TX 77225-0036. Offers MS, PhD, MD/PhD. Terminal master's awarded for partial completion of doctoral program. *Degree requirements:* For master's, thesis; for doctorate, thesis/dissertation. *Entrance requirements:* For master's and doctorate, GRE General Test. Additional exam requirements/recommendations for international students: Required—TOEFL. Electronic applications accepted. *Expenses:* Tuition, state resident: full-time $3474; part-time $193 per credit hour. Tuition, nonresident: full-time $13,644; part-time $758 per credit hour. *Required fees:* $226.30; $87 per credit hour. *Faculty research:* Developmental biology, genetics, cell biology, structural biology, cancer.

The University of Texas Medical Branch, Graduate School of Biomedical Sciences, Program in Biochemistry and Molecular Biology, Galveston, TX 77555. Offers biochemistry (PhD); bioinformatics (PhD); biophysics (PhD); cell biology (PhD); computational biology (PhD); structural biology (PhD). *Degree requirements:* For doctorate, thesis/dissertation. *Entrance requirements:* Additional exam requirements/recommendations for international students: Required—TOEFL (minimum score 550 paper-based). Electronic applications accepted.

The University of Texas Southwestern Medical Center, Southwestern Graduate School of Biomedical Sciences, Division of Basic Science, Program in Genetics and Development, Dallas, TX 75390. Offers PhD. *Faculty:* 85 full-time (16 women), 2 part-time/adjunct (0 women). *Students:* 57 full-time (28 women), 1 part-time (0 women); includes 16 minority (1 Black or African American, non-Hispanic/Latino; 1 American Indian or Alaska Native, non-Hispanic/Latino; 5 Asian, non-Hispanic/Latino; 9 Hispanic/Latino), 26 international. Average age 26. In 2013, 3 doctorates awarded. *Degree requirements:* For doctorate, thesis/dissertation, qualifying exam. *Entrance requirements:* For doctorate, GRE General Test, minimum GPA of 3.0. Additional exam requirements/recommendations for international students: Required—TOEFL. *Application deadline:* For fall admission, 12/15 priority date for domestic students. Application fee: $0. Electronic applications accepted. *Financial support:* Fellowships, research assistantships, and institutionally sponsored loans available. *Faculty research:* Human molecular genetics, chromosome structure, gene regulation, molecular biology, gene expression.
Website: http://www.utsouthwestern.edu/education/graduate-school/programs/phd-degrees/genetics-and-development/index.html

University of Washington, Graduate School, School of Public Health, Institute for Public Health Genetics, Seattle, WA 98195. Offers genetic epidemiology (MS); public health genetics (MPH, PhD); MPH/JD. Part-time programs available. *Students:* 26 full-time (22 women), 6 part-time (5 women); includes 9 minority (7 Asian, non-Hispanic/Latino; 2 Hispanic/Latino), 3 international. Average age 30. 26 applicants, 69% accepted, 15 enrolled. In 2013, 6 master's, 2 doctorates awarded. Terminal master's awarded for partial completion of doctoral program. *Degree requirements:* For master's, thesis, practicum (MPH); for doctorate, comprehensive exam, thesis/dissertation. *Entrance requirements:* For master's, GRE General Test, experience in health sciences, bachelor's degree in related field and course in human genetics (preferred); minimum GPA of 3.0; for doctorate, GRE General Test, experience in health sciences and master's degree in related field (preferred); coursework in human genetics, minimum GPA of 3.0. Additional exam requirements/recommendations for international students: Required—TOEFL (minimum score 580 paper-based; 92 iBT). *Application deadline:* For fall admission, 12/15 for domestic students, 12/10 for international students. Application fee: $85. Electronic applications accepted. *Financial support:* In 2013–14, 4 students received support, including 3 research assistantships with full tuition reimbursements available (averaging $15,102 per year), 1 teaching assistantship with full tuition reimbursement available (averaging $15,102 per year). Financial award application deadline: 2/28; financial award applicants required to submit FAFSA. *Faculty research:* Genetic epidemiology; ethical, legal, social issues of genetics; ecogenetics; health policy. *Unit head:* Dr. Stephanie Malia Fullerton, Director, 206-616-9286. *Application contact:* Barb Snyder, Student Services Advisor, 206-616-9286, Fax: 206-685-9651, E-mail: phgen@u.washington.edu.
Website: http://depts.washington.edu/phgen

University of Wisconsin–Madison, Graduate School, College of Agricultural and Life Sciences and Graduate Programs in Medicine, Department of Genetics, Program in Genetics, Madison, WI 53706-1380. Offers PhD. *Degree requirements:* For doctorate, thesis/dissertation. *Expenses:* Tuition, state resident: full-time $10,728; part-time $790 per credit. Tuition, nonresident: full-time $24,054; part-time $1623 per credit. *Required fees:* $1130; $119 per credit.

University of Wisconsin–Madison, School of Medicine and Public Health and Graduate School, Graduate Programs in Medicine, Madison, WI 53705. Offers biomolecular chemistry (MS, PhD); cancer biology (PhD); epidemiology (MS, PhD); genetics and medical genetics (MS, PhD), including genetics (PhD), medical genetics (MS); medical physics (MS, PhD), including health physics (MS), medical physics; microbiology (PhD); molecular and cellular pharmacology (PhD); neuroscience (PhD); pathology and laboratory medicine (PhD); physiology (PhD); population health (MS, PhD), including population health; DPT/MPH; DVM/MPH; MD/MPH; MD/PhD; MPA/MPH; MS/MPH; Pharm D/MPH. Part-time programs available. Postbaccalaureate distance learning degree programs offered (minimal on-campus study). Terminal master's awarded for partial completion of doctoral program. Application fee: $45. Electronic applications accepted. *Expenses:* Contact institution. *Financial support:* Fellowships with full tuition reimbursements, research assistantships with full tuition reimbursements, teaching assistantships with full tuition reimbursements, scholarships/grants, traineeships, and tuition waivers (full) available. *Unit head:* Dr. Richard L. Moss, Senior Associate Dean for Basic Research, Biotechnology and Graduate Studies, 608-265-0523, Fax: 608-265-0522, E-mail: rlmoss@wisc.edu. *Application contact:* Information Contact, 608-262-2433, Fax: 608-262-5134, E-mail: gradadmiss@mail.bascom.wisc.edu.
Website: http://www.med.wisc.edu

University of Wyoming, Graduate Program in Molecular and Cellular Life Sciences, Laramie, WY 82071. Offers PhD. *Degree requirements:* For doctorate, thesis/dissertation, four eight-week laboratory rotations, comprehensive basic practical exam, two-part qualifying exam, seminars, symposium.

Virginia Commonwealth University, Medical College of Virginia-Professional Programs, School of Medicine, School of Medicine Graduate Programs, Department of Human and Molecular Genetics, Richmond, VA 23284-9005. Offers genetic counseling (MS); human genetics (PhD); molecular biology and genetics (MS, PhD); MD/PhD. *Degree requirements:* For master's, thesis; for doctorate, thesis/dissertation, comprehensive oral and written exams. *Entrance requirements:* For master's, GRE; for doctorate, GRE General Test. Additional exam requirements/recommendations for international students: Required—TOEFL (minimum score 600 paper-based; 100 iBT). Electronic applications accepted. *Faculty research:* Genetic epidemiology, biochemical genetics, quantitative genetics, human cytogenetics, molecular genetics.

Virginia Polytechnic Institute and State University, Graduate School, Intercollege, Blacksburg, VA 24061. Offers genetics, bioinformatics and computational biology (PhD); information technology (MIT); macromolecular science and engineering (MS, PhD). *Students:* 154 full-time (68 women), 720 part-time (261 women); includes 196 minority (61 Black or African American, non-Hispanic/Latino; 1 American Indian or Alaska Native, non-Hispanic/Latino; 80 Asian, non-Hispanic/Latino; 35 Hispanic/Latino; 19 Two or more races, non-Hispanic/Latino), 103 international. Average age 33. 700 applicants, 76% accepted, 374 enrolled. In 2013, 114 master's, 8 doctorates awarded. *Degree requirements:* For master's, comprehensive exam (for some programs), thesis (for some programs); for doctorate, comprehensive exam (for some programs), thesis/dissertation (for some programs). *Entrance requirements:* For master's and doctorate, GRE/GMAT (may vary by department). Additional exam requirements/recommendations for international students: Required—TOEFL (minimum score 550 paper-based). *Application deadline:* For fall admission, 8/1 for domestic students, 4/1 for international students; for spring admission, 1/1 for domestic students, 9/1 for international students. Applications are processed on a rolling basis. Application fee: $75. Electronic applications accepted. *Expenses:* Tuition, state resident: full-time $11,185; part-time $621.50 per credit hour. Tuition, nonresident: full-time $22,146; part-time $1230.25 per credit hour. *Required fees:* $2442; $449.25 per semester. Tuition and fees vary according to course load, campus/location and program. *Financial support:* In 2013–14, 85 research assistantships with full tuition reimbursements (averaging $22,512 per year), 16 teaching assistantships with full tuition reimbursements (averaging $18,419 per year) were awarded. Financial award application deadline: 3/1; financial award applicants required to submit FAFSA. *Unit head:* Dr. Karen P. DePauw, Vice President and Dean for Graduate Education, 540-231-7581, Fax: 540-231-1670, E-mail: kpdepauw@vt.edu. *Application contact:* Graduate Admissions and Academic Progress, 540-231-8636, Fax: 540-231-2039, E-mail: grads@vt.edu.
Website: http://www.graduateschool.vt.edu/graduate_catalog/colleges.htm

Washington University in St. Louis, Graduate School of Arts and Sciences, Division of Biology and Biomedical Sciences, Program in Evolution, Ecology and Population Biology, St. Louis, MO 63130-4899. Offers ecology (PhD); environmental biology (PhD); evolutionary biology (PhD); genetics (PhD). *Degree requirements:* For doctorate, thesis/dissertation. *Entrance requirements:* For doctorate, GRE General Test, GRE Subject Test. Electronic applications accepted.

Washington University in St. Louis, School of Medicine, Program in Clinical Investigation, St. Louis, MO 63130-4899. Offers clinical investigation (MS); genetics/genomics (MS). Part-time programs available. *Faculty:* 61 full-time (14 women), 2 part-time/adjunct (both women). *Students:* 15 full-time (5 women), 39 part-time (19 women); includes 15 minority (3 Black or African American, non-Hispanic/Latino; 8 Asian, non-Hispanic/Latino; 2 Hispanic/Latino; 2 Two or more races, non-Hispanic/Latino), 3 international. Average age 32. 34 applicants, 65% accepted, 22 enrolled. In 2013, 22 master's awarded. *Degree requirements:* For master's, thesis. *Entrance requirements:* For master's, doctoral-level degree or in process of obtaining doctoral-level degree. Additional exam requirements/recommendations for international students: Required—TOEFL. *Application deadline:* For fall admission, 5/15 for domestic students; for spring admission, 10/15 for domestic students. Application fee: $0. Electronic applications accepted. *Financial support:* In 2013–14, 6 students received support. Tuition waivers (partial) available. Financial award application deadline: 12/12. *Faculty research:* Anesthesiology, infectious diseases, neurology, obstetrics and gynecology, orthopedic surgery. *Unit head:* Dr. David Warren, Associate Professor of Medicine, 314-454-8225, Fax: 314-454-5392, E-mail: dwarren@dom.wustl.edu. *Application contact:* Angela B. Wilson, Curriculum and Evaluation Coordinator, 314-454-8936, Fax: 314-454-8279, E-mail: abwilson@dom.wustl.edu.
Website: http://crtc.wustl.edu/

Wayne State University, School of Medicine, Graduate Programs in Medicine, Program in Molecular Biology and Genetics, Detroit, MI 48201. Offers bioinformatics and computational biology (PhD); cellular neuroscience (PhD); MD/PhD. *Students:* 21 full-time (11 women), 1 part-time (0 women); includes 1 minority (Hispanic/Latino), 3 international. Average age 27. 45 applicants, 13% accepted, 4 enrolled. In 2013, 5 doctorates awarded. Terminal master's awarded for partial completion of doctoral program. *Degree requirements:* For doctorate, thesis/dissertation. *Entrance requirements:* For doctorate, GRE General Test, GRE Subject Test (chemistry or biology), minimum GPA of 3.0, strong background in one of the chemical or biological sciences, three letters of recommendation, personal statement, interview. Additional exam requirements/recommendations for international students: Required—TOEFL (minimum score 550 paper-based; 79 iBT), Michigan English Language Assessment Battery (minimum score 85); Recommended—IELTS (minimum score 6.5), TWE (minimum score 5.5). *Application deadline:* For fall admission, 3/1 for domestic students, 5/1 for international students; for winter admission, 10/1 for domestic students, 9/1 for international students; for spring admission, 2/1 for domestic students, 1/1 for international students. Applications are processed on a rolling basis. Application fee: $0. Electronic applications accepted. *Expenses:* Tuition, state resident: part-time $554.15 per credit. Tuition, nonresident: part-time $1200.35 per credit. *Required fees:* $42.15 per credit. $268.30 per semester. Tuition and fees vary according to course load and program. *Financial support:* In 2013–14, 18 students received support. Fellowships with tuition reimbursements available, research assistantships with tuition reimbursements available, teaching assistantships with tuition reimbursements available, scholarships/grants, and unspecified assistantships available. Financial award application deadline: 3/31; financial award applicants required to submit FAFSA. *Faculty research:* Human gene mapping, genome organization and sequencing, gene regulation, molecular evolution. *Total annual research expenditures:* $2.6 million. *Unit head:* Dr. Lawrence Grossman, Director, 313-577-5323, E-mail: l.grossman@wayne.edu. *Application contact:* Dr. Gregory Kapatos, Professor, Director for Education, and Graduate Officer, 313-577-5965, Fax: 313-993-4269, E-mail: gkapato@med.wayne.edu.
Website: http://genetics.wayne.edu/students/mdphd.php

Wesleyan University, Graduate Studies, Department of Biology, Middletown, CT 06459. Offers cell and developmental genetics (PhD); evolution and ecology (PhD); neurobiology and behavior (PhD). *Degree requirements:* For doctorate, variable foreign language requirement, thesis/dissertation. *Entrance requirements:* For doctorate, GRE. Additional exam requirements/recommendations for international students: Required—TOEFL. *Faculty research:* Microbial population genetics, genetic basis of evolutionary adaptation, genetic regulation of differentiation and pattern formation in &ITdrosophila&RO.

West Virginia University, Davis College of Agriculture, Forestry and Consumer Sciences, Interdisciplinary Program in Genetics and Developmental Biology, Morgantown, WV 26506. Offers animal breeding (MS, PhD); biochemical and molecular genetics (MS, PhD); cytogenetics (MS, PhD); descriptive embryology (MS, PhD); developmental genetics (MS); experimental morphogenesis/teratology (MS); human genetics (MS, PhD); immunogenetics (MS, PhD); life cycles of animals and plants (MS, PhD); molecular aspects of development (MS, PhD); mutagenesis (MS, PhD); oncology (MS, PhD); plant genetics (MS, PhD); population and quantitative genetics (MS, PhD); regeneration (MS, PhD); teratology (PhD); toxicology (MS, PhD). *Degree requirements:* For master's, thesis; for doctorate, comprehensive exam, thesis/dissertation. *Entrance requirements:* For master's, GRE or MCAT, minimum GPA of 2.75. Additional exam requirements/recommendations for international students: Required—TOEFL.

Yale University, Graduate School of Arts and Sciences, Department of Genetics, New Haven, CT 06520. Offers PhD, MD/PhD. *Degree requirements:* For doctorate, thesis/dissertation. *Entrance requirements:* For doctorate, GRE General Test, GRE Subject Test.

Yale University, Graduate School of Arts and Sciences, Department of Molecular, Cellular, and Developmental Biology, Program in Genetics, New Haven, CT 06520. Offers PhD. *Degree requirements:* For doctorate, thesis/dissertation. *Entrance requirements:* For doctorate, GRE General Test, GRE Subject Test.

Yale University, School of Medicine and Graduate School of Arts and Sciences, Combined Program in Biological and Biomedical Sciences (BBS), Molecular Cell Biology, Genetics, and Development Track, New Haven, CT 06520. Offers PhD, MD/PhD. *Entrance requirements:* Additional exam requirements/recommendations for international students: Required—TOEFL.

Genomic Sciences

Albert Einstein College of Medicine, Graduate Division of Biomedical Sciences, Department of Genetics, Bronx, NY 10461. Offers computational genetics (PhD); molecular genetics (PhD); translational genetics (PhD); MD/PhD. *Degree requirements:* For doctorate, thesis/dissertation. *Entrance requirements:* For doctorate, GRE General Test. Additional exam requirements/recommendations for international students: Required—TOEFL. *Faculty research:* Neurologic genetics in &ITDrosophila&RO, biochemical genetics of yeast, developmental genetics in the mouse.

Black Hills State University, Graduate Studies, Program in Integrative Genomics, Spearfish, SD 57799. Offers MS. *Faculty:* 9 full-time (2 women), 1 (woman) part-time/adjunct. *Students:* 10 full-time (2 women), 1 international. Average age 27. 13 applicants, 100% accepted, 4 enrolled. In 2013, 3 master's awarded. *Entrance requirements:* Additional exam requirements/recommendations for international students: Required—TOEFL (minimum score 500 paper-based; 60 iBT). *Application deadline:* For fall admission, 4/15 for domestic students. Application fee: $35. *Expenses:* Tuition, state resident: full-time $3718; part-time $201.85 per credit hour. Tuition, nonresident: full-time $7686; part-time $427.30 per credit hour. Tuition and fees vary according to course load, program and reciprocity agreements. *Financial support:* In 2013–14, 4 teaching assistantships with partial tuition reimbursements were awarded. *Unit head:* Dr. John Dixson, Coordinator, 605-642-6912, Fax: 605-642-6973, E-mail: john.dixson@bhsu.edu.

Boston University, School of Medicine, Division of Graduate Medical Sciences, Program in Genetics and Genomics, Boston, MA 02215. Offers PhD. *Degree requirements:* For doctorate, thesis/dissertation. *Application deadline:* For fall admission, 1/15 for domestic students; for spring admission, 10/15 for domestic students. *Expenses: Tuition:* Full-time $43,970; part-time $1374 per credit hour. *Required fees:* $60 per semester. Tuition and fees vary according to class time, course level and program. *Unit head:* Dr. Shoumita Dasgupta, Associate Professor and Director of Graduate Studies, 617-414-1580, E-mail: dasgupta@bu.edu. *Application contact:* GMS Admissions Office, 617-638-5255, Fax: 617-638-5740, E-mail: natashah@bu.edu.
Website: http://www.bumc.bu.edu/gpgg/graduate-program/

Case Western Reserve University, School of Medicine and School of Graduate Studies, Graduate Programs in Medicine, Department of Genetics, Program in Human, Molecular, and Developmental Genetics and Genomics, Cleveland, OH 44106. Offers PhD, MD/PhD. *Degree requirements:* For doctorate, comprehensive exam, thesis/dissertation. *Entrance requirements:* For doctorate, GRE General Test, GRE Subject Test. Additional exam requirements/recommendations for international students: Required—TOEFL. *Faculty research:* Regulation of gene expression, molecular control of development, genomics.

Concordia University, School of Graduate Studies, Faculty of Arts and Science, Department of Biology, Montréal, QC H3G 1M8, Canada. Offers biology (M Sc, PhD); biotechnology and genomics (Diploma). *Degree requirements:* For master's, thesis; for doctorate, thesis/dissertation, pedagogical training. *Entrance requirements:* For master's, honors degree in biology; for doctorate, M Sc in life science. *Faculty research:* Cell biology, animal physiology, ecology, microbiology/molecular biology, plant physiology/biochemistry and biotechnology.

Cornell University, Graduate School, Graduate Fields of Agriculture and Life Sciences, Field of Genetics, Genomics and Development, Ithaca, NY 14853-0001. Offers developmental biology (PhD); genetics (PhD); genomics (PhD). *Faculty:* 66 full-time (15 women). *Students:* 56 full-time (37 women); includes 7 minority (3 Black or African American, non-Hispanic/Latino; 2 Asian, non-Hispanic/Latino; 1 Hispanic/Latino; 1 Two or more races, non-Hispanic/Latino), 22 international. Average age 26. 67 applicants, 33% accepted, 12 enrolled. In 2013, 12 doctorates awarded. *Degree requirements:* For doctorate, comprehensive exam, thesis/dissertation, 2 semesters of teaching experience. *Entrance requirements:* For doctorate, GRE General Test, GRE Subject Test in biology or biochemistry (recommended), 2 letters of recommendation. Additional exam requirements/recommendations for international students: Required—TOEFL (minimum score 550 paper-based; 77 iBT). *Application deadline:* For fall admission, 1/5 for domestic students. Application fee: $95. Electronic applications accepted. *Financial support:* In 2013–14, 45 students received support, including 5 fellowships with full tuition reimbursements available, 26 research assistantships with full tuition reimbursements available, 14 teaching assistantships with full tuition reimbursements available; institutionally sponsored loans, scholarships/grants, health care benefits, tuition waivers (full and partial), and unspecified assistantships also available. Financial award applicants required to submit FAFSA. *Faculty research:* Molecular and general genetics, developmental biology and developmental genetics, evolution and population genetics, plant genetics, microbial genetics. *Unit head:* Director of Graduate Studies, 607-254-2100. *Application contact:* Graduate Field Assistant, 607-254-2100, E-mail: gendev@cornell.edu.
Website: http://www.gradschool.cornell.edu/fields.php?id-51&a-2

Duke University, Graduate School, University Program in Genetics and Genomics, Durham, NC 27710. Offers PhD. *Faculty:* 108. *Students:* 82 full-time (50 women); includes 16 minority (4 Black or African American, non-Hispanic/Latino; 7 Asian, non-Hispanic/Latino; 5 Hispanic/Latino), 15 international. 97 applicants, 15% accepted, 6 enrolled. In 2013, 21 doctorates awarded. *Degree requirements:* For doctorate, variable foreign language requirement, thesis/dissertation. *Entrance requirements:* For doctorate, GRE General Test. Additional exam requirements/recommendations for international students: Required—TOEFL (minimum score 577 paper-based; 90 iBT) or IELTS (minimum score 7). *Application deadline:* For fall admission, 12/8 priority date for domestic and international students. Application fee: $80. *Financial support:* Fellowships available. Financial award application deadline: 12/8. *Unit head:* Allison Ashley-Koch, Interim Director of Graduate Studies, 919-684-6629, Fax: 919-684-8346, E-mail: leslie.mavengere@duke.edu. *Application contact:* Elizabeth Hutton, Director of Admissions, 919-684-3913, Fax: 919-684-2277, E-mail: grad-admissions@duke.edu.
Website: http://upg.duke.edu/

Georgia Regents University, The Graduate School, Program in Genomic Medicine, Augusta, GA 30912. Offers MS, PhD. *Faculty:* 9 full-time (1 woman). *Students:* 5 full-time (1 woman); includes 1 minority (Asian, non-Hispanic/Latino), 3 international. Average age 27. *Degree requirements:* For doctorate, comprehensive exam, thesis/dissertation. *Entrance requirements:* For doctorate, GRE General Test. Additional exam requirements/recommendations for international students: Required—TOEFL (minimum score 550 paper-based; 79 iBT). *Application deadline:* For fall admission, 1/15 for domestic and international students. Application fee: $50. Electronic applications accepted. *Financial support:* In 2013–14, 2 research assistantships with partial tuition reimbursements (averaging $23,000 per year) were awarded; Federal Work-Study, institutionally sponsored loans, and scholarships/grants also available. Support available to part-time students. Financial award application deadline: 5/31; financial award applicants required to submit FAFSA. *Faculty research:* Genetic and genomic basis of diseases (diabetes, cancer, autoimmunity), development of diagnostic markers, bioinformatics, computational biology. *Total annual research expenditures:* $6.4 million. *Unit head:* Dr. Jin-Xiong She, Professor/Chair, 706-721-3540, E-mail: jshe@georgiahealth.edu. *Application contact:* Dr. Patricia L. Cameron, Associate Dean, 706-721-3279, Fax: 706-721-6829, E-mail: pcameron@georgiahealth.edu.
Website: http://www.cbgm.gru.edu/GraduateProgram.aspx

Harvard University, Graduate School of Arts and Sciences, Department of Systems Biology, Cambridge, MA 02138. Offers PhD. *Degree requirements:* For doctorate, thesis/dissertation, lab rotation, qualifying examination. *Entrance requirements:* For doctorate, GRE. Additional exam requirements/recommendations for international students: Required—TOEFL. Electronic applications accepted. *Expenses: Tuition:* Full-time $38,888. *Required fees:* $958. Tuition and fees vary according to campus/location, program and student level.

Massachusetts Institute of Technology, School of Engineering, Harvard-MIT Health Sciences and Technology Program, Cambridge, MA 02139-4307. Offers health sciences and technology (SM, PhD, Sc D), including bioastronautics (PhD, Sc D), bioinformatics and integrative genomics (PhD, Sc D), medical engineering and medical physics (PhD, Sc D), speech and hearing bioscience and technology (PhD, Sc D). *Students:* 281 full-time (115 women), 10 part-time (0 women); includes 84 minority (1 Black or African American, non-Hispanic/Latino; 1 American Indian or Alaska Native, non-Hispanic/Latino; 68 Asian, non-Hispanic/Latino; 11 Hispanic/Latino; 3 Two or more races, non-Hispanic/Latino), 48 international. Average age 26. 180 applicants, 17% accepted, 18 enrolled. In 2013, 7 master's, 20 doctorates awarded. Terminal master's awarded for partial completion of doctoral program. *Degree requirements:* For master's, thesis; for doctorate, comprehensive exam, thesis/dissertation. *Entrance requirements:* For doctorate, GRE General Test (for medical engineering and medical physics). Additional exam requirements/recommendations for international students: Required—TOEFL (minimum score 600 paper-based; 100 iBT), IELTS (minimum score 7). *Application deadline:* For fall admission, 12/15 for domestic and international students. Application fee: $75. Electronic applications accepted. *Expenses: Tuition:* Full-time $43,210; part-time $670 per credit hour. *Required fees:* $288. *Financial support:* In 2013–14, 144 students received support, including 66 fellowships (averaging $35,700 per year), 49 research assistantships (averaging $31,300 per year), 1 teaching assistantship (averaging $33,300 per year); Federal Work-Study, institutionally sponsored loans, scholarships/grants, traineeships, health care benefits, and unspecified assistantships also available. Financial award application deadline: 12/15. *Faculty research:* Signal processing, biomedical imaging, drug delivery, medical devices, medical diagnostics, regenerative biomedical technologies. *Unit head:* Emery N. Brown, Director, 617-452-4091. *Application contact:* Emery N. Brown, Director, 617-452-4091.
Website: http://hst.mit.edu/

North Carolina State University, Graduate School, College of Agriculture and Life Sciences, Graduate Program in Genomic Sciences, Raleigh, NC 27695. Offers MS, PhD.

North Carolina State University, Graduate School, College of Agriculture and Life Sciences, Program in Functional Genomics, Raleigh, NC 27695. Offers MFG, MS, PhD. *Degree requirements:* For master's, thesis (for some programs); for doctorate, thesis/dissertation. *Entrance requirements:* For master's and doctorate, GRE, minimum B average. Additional exam requirements/recommendations for international students: Required—TOEFL. Electronic applications accepted. *Faculty research:* Genome structure, genome expression, molecular evolution, nucleic acid structure/function, proteomics.

North Dakota State University, College of Graduate and Interdisciplinary Studies, College of Science and Mathematics, Department of Biological Sciences, Fargo, ND 58108. Offers biology (MS); botany (MS, PhD); cellular and molecular biology (PhD); genomics (PhD); zoology (MS, PhD). *Faculty:* 17 full-time (9 women), 1 part-time/adjunct (0 women). *Students:* 20 full-time (10 women), 3 part-time (all women); includes 2 minority (1 American Indian or Alaska Native, non-Hispanic/Latino; 1 Two or more races, non-Hispanic/Latino), 1 international. Average age 32. 9 applicants, 11% accepted, 1 enrolled. In 2013, 4 master's awarded. *Degree requirements:* For master's, thesis; for doctorate, thesis/dissertation. *Entrance requirements:* For master's and doctorate, GRE General Test. Additional exam requirements/recommendations for international students: Required—TOEFL. *Application deadline:* For fall admission, 1/15 for domestic students. Applications are processed on a rolling basis. Application fee: $35. Electronic applications accepted. *Financial support:* Fellowships with full tuition reimbursements, research assistantships with full tuition reimbursements, teaching assistantships with full tuition reimbursements, career-related internships or fieldwork, Federal Work-Study, institutionally sponsored loans, scholarships/grants, tuition waivers (full), and unspecified assistantships available. Support available to part-time students. Financial award application deadline: 4/15; financial award applicants required to submit FAFSA. *Faculty research:* Comparative endocrinology, physiology, behavioral ecology, plant cell biology, aquatic biology. *Unit head:* Dr. Wendy Reed, Head, 701-231-7087,

E-mail: wendy.reed@ndsu.edu. *Application contact:* Sonya Goergen, Marketing, Recruitment, and Public Relations Coordinator, 701-231-7033, Fax: 701-231-6524.
Website: http://biology.ndsu.nodak.edu/

North Dakota State University, College of Graduate and Interdisciplinary Studies, Interdisciplinary Program in Genomics and Bioinformatics, Fargo, ND 58108. Offers MS, PhD. Part-time programs available. *Students:* 9 full-time (6 women), 7 international. Average age 31. 16 applicants, 50% accepted, 7 enrolled. In 2013, 1 master's, 2 doctorates awarded. *Degree requirements:* For master's, thesis; for doctorate, comprehensive exam, thesis/dissertation. *Entrance requirements:* For master's and doctorate, minimum GPA of 3.0. Additional exam requirements/recommendations for international students: Required—TOEFL (minimum score 525 paper-based; 71 iBT). *Application deadline:* For fall admission, 5/1 for international students; for spring admission, 8/1 for international students. Applications are processed on a rolling basis. Application fee: $35. Electronic applications accepted. *Financial support:* In 2013–14, 12 research assistantships with full tuition reimbursements (averaging $15,000 per year) were awarded; unspecified assistantships also available. *Faculty research:* Genome evolution, genome mapping, genome expression, bioinformatics, data mining. *Unit head:* Dr. Phillip E. McClean, Director, 701-231-8443, Fax: 701-231-8474. *Application contact:* Sonya Goergen, Marketing, Recruitment, and Public Relations Coordinator, 701-231-7033, Fax: 701-231-6524.

Purdue University, College of Pharmacy and Pharmacal Sciences and Graduate School, Graduate Programs in Pharmacy and Pharmacal Sciences, Department of Medicinal Chemistry and Molecular Pharmacology, West Lafayette, IN 47907. Offers biophysical and computational chemistry (PhD); cancer research (PhD); immunology and infectious disease (PhD); medicinal biochemistry and molecular biology (PhD); medicinal chemistry and chemical biology (PhD); molecular pharmacology (PhD); neuropharmacology, neurodegeneration, and neurotoxicity (PhD); systems biology and functional genomics (PhD). *Faculty:* 23 full-time (3 women), 6 part-time/adjunct (1 woman). *Students:* 50 full-time (21 women), 3 part-time (2 women); includes 1 minority (Asian, non-Hispanic/Latino), 30 international. Average age 26. 147 applicants, 20% accepted, 13 enrolled. In 2013, 12 doctorates awarded. *Degree requirements:* For doctorate, thesis/dissertation. *Entrance requirements:* For doctorate, GRE General Test; GRE Subject Test in biology, biochemistry, and chemistry (recommended), minimum undergraduate GPA of 3.0. Additional exam requirements/recommendations for international students: Required—TOEFL (minimum score 550 paper-based; 77 iBT); Recommended—TWE. *Application deadline:* For fall admission, 2/1 for domestic and international students. Applications are processed on a rolling basis. Application fee: $60 ($75 for international students). Electronic applications accepted. *Financial support:* Fellowships, research assistantships, teaching assistantships, and traineeships available. Support available to part-time students. Financial award applicants required to submit FAFSA. *Faculty research:* Drug design and development, cancer research, drug synthesis and analysis, chemical pharmacology, environmental toxicology. *Unit head:* Dr. Richard F. Borch, Head, 765-494-1403, E-mail: borch@purdue.edu. *Application contact:* Dr. Janine C. Mott, Graduate Contact, 765-494-1269, E-mail: jmott@purdue.edu.

Thomas Jefferson University, Jefferson Graduate School of Biomedical Sciences, PhD Program in Genetics, Genomics and Cancer Biology, Philadelphia, PA 19107. Offers PhD. *Faculty:* 48 full-time (16 women), 4 part-time/adjunct (3 women). *Students:* 16 full-time (8 women); includes 4 minority (2 Asian, non-Hispanic/Latino; 2 Hispanic/Latino), 1 international. 41 applicants, 24% accepted, 4 enrolled. In 2013, 5 doctorates awarded. *Degree requirements:* For doctorate, comprehensive exam, thesis/dissertation. *Entrance requirements:* For doctorate, GRE General Test, minimum GPA of 3.2. Additional exam requirements/recommendations for international students: Required—TOEFL (minimum score 100 iBT) or IELTS. *Application deadline:* For fall admission, 1/5 priority date for domestic and international students. Applications are processed on a rolling basis. Application fee: $75. Electronic applications accepted. *Financial support:* In 2013–14, 16 students received support, including 16 fellowships with full tuition reimbursements available (averaging $56,052 per year); Federal Work-Study, institutionally sponsored loans, scholarships/grants, traineeships, and stipends also available. Support available to part-time students. Financial award application deadline: 5/1; financial award applicants required to submit FAFSA. *Faculty research:* Functional genomics, cancer susceptibility, cell cycle, regulation oncogenes and tumor suppressor genes, genetics of neoplastic disease. *Unit head:* Dr. Linda D. Siracusa, Program Director, 215-503-4536, E-mail: linda.siracusa@jefferson.edu. *Application contact:* Marc E. Stearns, Director of Admissions, 215-503-0155, Fax: 215-503-3433, E-mail: jgsbs-info@jefferson.edu.
Website: http://www.jefferson.edu/university/biomedical_sciences/programs/phd/genetics.html

University of California, Riverside, Graduate Division, Graduate Program in Genetics, Genomics, and Bioinformatics, Riverside, CA 92521-0102. Offers genomics and bioinformatics (PhD); molecular genetics (PhD); population and evolutionary genetics (PhD). *Faculty:* 72 full-time (20 women). *Students:* 32 full-time (18 women); includes 2 minority (1 Black or African American, non-Hispanic/Latino; 1 Hispanic/Latino), 15 international. Average age 30. In 2013, 2 doctorates awarded. *Degree requirements:* For doctorate, thesis/dissertation, qualifying exams, teaching experience. *Entrance requirements:* For doctorate, GRE General Test, minimum GPA of 3.2. Additional exam requirements/recommendations for international students: Required—TOEFL (minimum score 550 paper-based; 80 iBT). *Application deadline:* For fall admission, 5/1 for domestic students, 2/1 for international students; for winter admission, 9/1 for domestic students, 7/1 for international students; for spring admission, 12/1 for domestic students, 10/1 for international students. Applications are processed on a rolling basis. Application fee: $85 ($100 for international students). Electronic applications accepted. *Financial support:* In 2013–14, fellowships with tuition reimbursements (averaging $18,000 per year), research assistantships with tuition reimbursements (averaging $18,000 per year), teaching assistantships with tuition reimbursements (averaging $16,500 per year) were awarded; career-related internships or fieldwork, Federal Work-Study, institutionally sponsored loans, and tuition waivers (full and partial) also available. *Faculty research:* Molecular genetics, evolution and population genetics, genomics and bioinformatics. *Unit head:* Dr. Shizhong Xu, Director, 951-827-5898. *Application contact:* Deidra Kornfeld, Graduate Program Assistant, 800-735-0717, Fax: 951-827-5517, E-mail: genetics@ucr.edu.
Website: http://ggb.ucr.edu/

University of California, San Francisco, School of Pharmacy and Graduate Division, Pharmaceutical Sciences and Pharmacogenomics Program, San Francisco, CA 94158-0775. Offers PhD. *Degree requirements:* For doctorate, comprehensive exam, thesis/dissertation. *Entrance requirements:* For doctorate, GRE General Test, bachelor's degree, 3 letters of recommendation, personal statement. Additional exam requirements/recommendations for international students: Required—TOEFL. *Application deadline:* For fall admission, 12/1 for domestic and international students. Application fee: $80 ($100 for international students). Electronic applications accepted. *Expenses:* Tuition, state resident: full-time $11,220. Tuition, nonresident: full-time $26,322. *Required fees:* $5204. Full-time tuition and fees vary according to degree level and program. *Financial support:* In 2013–14, fellowships with full tuition reimbursements (averaging $32,500 per year), research assistantships with full tuition reimbursements (averaging $32,500 per year), teaching assistantships with full tuition reimbursements (averaging $32,500 per year) were awarded; career-related internships or fieldwork, institutionally sponsored loans, scholarships/grants, traineeships, tuition waivers (full), and unspecified assistantships also available. Financial award application deadline: 4/6. *Faculty research:* Drug development sciences, molecular pharmacology, therapeutic bioengineering, pharmacogenomics and functional genomics, quantitative and systems pharmacology, computational genomics. *Unit head:* Dr. Deanna L. Kroetz, Director, 415-476-1159, Fax: 415-476-6022, E-mail: deanna.kroetz@ucsf.edu. *Application contact:* Debbie Acoba-Idlebi, Administrator, 415-476-1947, Fax: 415-476-6022, E-mail: debbie.acoba@ucsf.edu.
Website: http://pspg.ucsf.edu/

University of Chicago, Division of Biological Sciences, Molecular Biosciences Cluster, Committee on Genetics, Genomics and Systems Biology, Chicago, IL 60637-1513. Offers PhD. *Degree requirements:* For doctorate, thesis/dissertation, ethics class, 2 teaching assistantships. *Entrance requirements:* For doctorate, GRE General Test, minimum GPA of 3.0. Additional exam requirements/recommendations for international students: Required—TOEFL (minimum score 600 paper-based; 104 iBT), IELTS (minimum score 7). Electronic applications accepted. *Faculty research:* Molecular genetics, developmental genetics, population genetics, human genetics.

University of Cincinnati, Graduate School, College of Medicine, Graduate Programs in Biomedical Sciences, Department of Environmental Health, Programs in Environmental Genetics and Molecular Toxicology, Cincinnati, OH 45221. Offers MS, PhD. *Degree requirements:* For doctorate, thesis/dissertation. *Entrance requirements:* For master's, GRE, minimum GPA of 3.0, 3 letters of recommendation. Additional exam requirements/recommendations for international students: Required—TOEFL (minimum score 520 paper-based).

University of Connecticut, Graduate School, College of Liberal Arts and Sciences, Department of Molecular and Cell Biology, Field of Applied Genomics, Storrs, CT 06269. Offers MS, PSM. *Degree requirements:* For master's, comprehensive exam. *Entrance requirements:* For master's, GRE General Test, GRE Subject Test. Additional exam requirements/recommendations for international students: Required—TOEFL (minimum score 550 paper-based). Electronic applications accepted.

University of Georgia, College of Agricultural and Environmental Sciences, Institute of Plant Breeding, Genetics and Genomics, Athens, GA 30602. Offers MS, PhD.

University of Maine, Graduate School, Interdisciplinary Doctoral Program, Orono, ME 04469. Offers engineering in the natural sciences (PhD); functional genomics (PhD). Part-time and evening/weekend programs available. *Students:* 38 full-time (29 women), 9 part-time (6 women); includes 4 minority (1 Black or African American, non-Hispanic/Latino; 2 American Indian or Alaska Native, non-Hispanic/Latino; 1 Hispanic/Latino), 4 international. Average age 41. 22 applicants, 55% accepted, 12 enrolled. In 2013, 2 doctorates awarded. *Degree requirements:* For doctorate, comprehensive exam, thesis/dissertation. *Entrance requirements:* For doctorate, GRE General Test, master's degree. Additional exam requirements/recommendations for international students: Required—TOEFL. *Application deadline:* For fall admission, 4/1 for domestic students; for spring admission, 11/1 for domestic students. Applications are processed on a rolling basis. Application fee: $65. Electronic applications accepted. *Expenses:* Tuition, state resident: full-time $7524. Tuition, nonresident: full-time $23,112. *Required fees:* $1970. *Financial support:* In 2013–14, 26 students received support, including 2 fellowships (averaging $17,500 per year), 5 research assistantships (averaging $14,600 per year), 7 teaching assistantships (averaging $14,600 per year). Financial award application deadline: 3/1. *Unit head:* Scott G. Delcourt, Associate Dean of the Graduate School, 207-581-3291, Fax: 207-581-3232, E-mail: graduate@maine.edu. *Application contact:* Scott G. Delcourt, Associate Dean of the Graduate School, 207-581-3291, Fax: 207-581-3232, E-mail: graduate@maine.edu.
Website: http://umaine.edu/graduate/

University of Maryland, Baltimore, School of Medicine, Department of Epidemiology and Public Health, Baltimore, MD 21201. Offers biostatistics (MS); clinical research (MS); epidemiology and preventive medicine (MPH, MS, PhD); gerontology (PhD); human genetics and genomic medicine (MS, PhD); molecular epidemiology (MS, PhD); toxicology (MS, PhD); JD/MS; MD/PhD; MS/PhD. *Accreditation:* CEPH. Part-time programs available. *Students:* 83 full-time (56 women), 76 part-time (51 women); includes 51 minority (26 Black or African American, non-Hispanic/Latino; 20 Asian, non-Hispanic/Latino; 5 Hispanic/Latino), 27 international. Average age 32. 225 applicants, 44% accepted, 37 enrolled. In 2013, 18 master's, 1 doctorate awarded. *Degree requirements:* For doctorate, comprehensive exam, thesis/dissertation. *Entrance requirements:* For master's and doctorate, GRE General Test. Additional exam requirements/recommendations for international students: Required—TOEFL (minimum score 550 paper-based; 80 iBT); Recommended—IELTS (minimum score 7). *Application deadline:* For fall admission, 1/15 for domestic and international students. Application fee: $75. Electronic applications accepted. *Expenses:* Contact institution. *Financial support:* In 2013–14, research assistantships with partial tuition reimbursements (averaging $25,000 per year) were awarded; fellowships, Federal Work-Study, scholarships/grants, and unspecified assistantships also available. Financial award application deadline: 3/1; financial award applicants required to submit FAFSA. *Unit head:* Dr. Laura Hungerford, Program Director, 410-706-8492, Fax: 410-706-4225. *Application contact:* Jessica Kelley, Program Coordinator, 410-706-8492, Fax: 410-706-4225, E-mail: jkelley@som.umaryland.edu.
Website: http://medschool.umaryland.edu/Epidemiology/

University of Maryland, College Park, Academic Affairs, College of Computer, Mathematical and Natural Sciences, Department of Biology, PhD Program in Biological Sciences, College Park, MD 20742. Offers behavior, ecology, evolution, and systematics (PhD); computational biology, bioinformatics, and genomics (PhD); molecular and cellular biology (PhD); physiological systems (PhD). *Students:* 104 full-time (59 women), 4 part-time (1 woman); includes 21 minority (2 Black or African American, non-Hispanic/Latino; 1 American Indian or Alaska Native, non-Hispanic/Latino; 9 Asian, non-Hispanic/Latino; 7 Hispanic/Latino; 2 Two or more races, non-Hispanic/Latino), 34 international. 365 applicants, 13% accepted, 20 enrolled. In 2013, 5 doctorates awarded. *Degree requirements:* For doctorate, comprehensive exam, thesis/dissertation, thesis work presentation in seminar. *Entrance requirements:* For doctorate, GRE General Test; GRE Subject Test in biology (recommended), academic transcripts, statement of purpose/research interests, 3 letters of recommendation. Additional exam requirements/recommendations for international students: Required—TOEFL. *Application deadline:* For fall admission, 12/15 for domestic and international students. Applications are processed on a rolling basis. Application fee: $75. Electronic applications accepted. *Expenses:* Tuition, state resident: full-time $10,314; part-time $573 per credit hour. Tuition, nonresident: full-time $22,248; part-time $1236 per credit. *Required fees:* $1446; $403.15 per semester. Tuition and fees vary according to program. *Financial support:* In 2013–14, 21 fellowships with full and partial tuition reimbursements (averaging $27,603 per year), 25 research assistantships (averaging $19,557 per year), 55 teaching assistantships (averaging $18,959 per year) were awarded. *Unit head:* Dr. Charles F. Delwiche, Director, 301-405-6884, E-mail:

bisidirector@umd.edu. *Application contact:* Dr. Charles A. Caramello, Dean of Graduate School, 301-405-0358, Fax: 301-314-9305, E-mail: ccaramel@umd.edu.
Website: http://www.bisi.umd.edu/

University of Pennsylvania, Perelman School of Medicine, Biomedical Graduate Studies, Graduate Group in Genomics and Computational Biology, Philadelphia, PA 19104. Offers PhD, MD/PhD, VMD/PhD. *Faculty:* 70. *Students:* 35 full-time (12 women); includes 11 minority (9 Asian, non-Hispanic/Latino; 2 Hispanic/Latino), 8 international. 75 applicants, 27% accepted, 5 enrolled. In 2013, 4 doctorates awarded. *Degree requirements:* For doctorate, thesis/dissertation. *Entrance requirements:* For doctorate, GRE. Additional exam requirements/recommendations for international students: Required—TOEFL. *Application deadline:* For fall admission, 12/1 priority date for domestic and international students. Applications are processed on a rolling basis. Application fee: $80. Electronic applications accepted. *Financial support:* In 2013–14, 35 students received support. Fellowships, research assistantships, scholarships/grants, traineeships, and unspecified assistantships available. *Unit head:* Dr. Maja Bucan, Chairperson, 215-898-0020. *Application contact:* Hannah Chervitz, Graduate Coordinator, 215-746-2807.
Website: http://www.med.upenn.edu/gcb/

University of Rochester, School of Medicine and Dentistry, Graduate Programs in Medicine and Dentistry, Department of Biomedical Genetics, Rochester, NY 14627. Offers genetics, genomics and development (PhD). *Degree requirements:* For doctorate, thesis/dissertation, qualifying exam. *Entrance requirements:* For doctorate, GRE General Test. *Expenses: Tuition:* Full-time $44,580; part-time $1394 per credit hour. *Required fees:* $492.

The University of Tennessee, Graduate School, College of Arts and Sciences, Program in Life Sciences, Knoxville, TN 37996. Offers genome science and technology (MS, PhD); plant physiology and genetics (MS, PhD). *Degree requirements:* For doctorate, one foreign language, thesis/dissertation. *Entrance requirements:* For master's and doctorate, GRE General Test, minimum GPA of 2.7. Additional exam requirements/recommendations for international students: Required—TOEFL. Electronic applications accepted. *Expenses:* Tuition, state resident: full-time $9540; part-time $531 per credit hour. Tuition, nonresident: full-time $27,728; part-time $1542 per credit hour. *Required fees:* $1404; $67 per credit hour.

The University of Tennessee–Oak Ridge National Laboratory, Graduate Program in Genome Science and Technology, Knoxville, TN 37966. Offers life sciences (MS, PhD). *Students:* Average age 30. *Degree requirements:* For master's, thesis; for doctorate, comprehensive exam, thesis/dissertation. *Entrance requirements:* For master's and doctorate, GRE General Test. Additional exam requirements/recommendations for international students: Required—TOEFL. *Application deadline:* For fall admission, 1/15 priority date for domestic students, 2/1 for international students. Electronic applications accepted. *Financial support:* Fellowships, research assistantships with full tuition reimbursements, institutionally sponsored loans, health care benefits, tuition waivers (full), and unspecified assistantships available. Financial award application deadline: 3/31. *Faculty research:* Genetics/genomics, structural biology/proteomics, computational biology/bioinformatics, bioanalytical technologies. *Unit head:* Roger Gray, Director, 865-974-9561, E-mail: rgray17@utk.edu. *Application contact:* Roger Gray, Program Resource Specialist, 865-974-9561, Fax: 865-974-5037, E-mail: rgray17@utk.edu.
Website: http://gst.tennessee.edu

The University of Toledo, College of Graduate Studies, College of Medicine and Life Sciences, Interdepartmental Programs, Toledo, OH 43606-3390. Offers bioinformatics and proteomics/genomics (MSBS); biomarkers and bioinformatics (Certificate); biomarkers and diagnostics (PSM); human donation sciences (MSBS); medical sciences (MSBS); MD/MSBS. *Faculty:* 44. *Students:* 60 full-time (27 women), 3 part-time (2 women); includes 19 minority (4 Black or African American, non-Hispanic/Latino; 13 Asian, non-Hispanic/Latino; 2 Hispanic/Latino). Average age 24. 200 applicants, 41% accepted, 57 enrolled. In 2013, 55 master's awarded. *Degree requirements:* For master's, thesis or alternative. *Entrance requirements:* For master's, GRE, minimum undergraduate GPA of 3.0, three letters of recommendation, statement of purpose, transcripts from all prior institutions attended, resume; for Certificate, minimum undergraduate GPA of 3.0, three letters of recommendation, statement of purpose, transcripts from all prior institutions attended, resume. Additional exam requirements/recommendations for international students: Required—TOEFL (minimum score 550 paper-based; 80 iBT). *Application deadline:* For fall admission, 1/15 priority date for domestic and international students. Application fee: $45 ($75 for international students). Electronic applications accepted. *Financial support:* In 2013–14, 2 research assistantships with full tuition reimbursements (averaging $10,000 per year) were awarded; scholarships/grants also available. *Unit head:* Dr. Ronald McGinnis, Interim Dean, 419-383-4243, E-mail: ronald.mcginnis@utoledo.edu. *Application contact:* Admissions Analyst, 419-383-4112, Fax: 419-383-6140.
Website: http://www.utoledo.edu/med/grad/

University of Washington, Graduate School, School of Medicine, Graduate Programs in Medicine, Department of Genome Sciences, Seattle, WA 98195. Offers PhD. *Degree requirements:* For doctorate, thesis/dissertation, general exam. *Entrance requirements:* For doctorate, GRE General Test, minimum GPA of 3.0. Additional exam requirements/recommendations for international students: Required—TOEFL. Electronic applications accepted. *Faculty research:* Model organism genetics, human and medical genetics, genomics and proteomics, computational biology.

Wake Forest University, School of Medicine and Graduate School of Arts and Sciences, Graduate Programs in Medicine, Molecular Genetics and Genomics Program, Winston-Salem, NC 27109. Offers PhD, MD/PhD. *Degree requirements:* For doctorate, thesis/dissertation. *Entrance requirements:* For doctorate, GRE General Test. Additional exam requirements/recommendations for international students: Required—TOEFL. Electronic applications accepted. *Faculty research:* Control of gene expression, molecular pathogenesis, protein biosynthesis, cell development, clinical cytogenetics.

Washington University in St. Louis, School of Medicine, Program in Clinical Investigation, St. Louis, MO 63130-4899. Offers clinical investigation (MS); genetics/genomics (MS). Part-time programs available. *Faculty:* 61 full-time (14 women), 2 part-time/adjunct (both women). *Students:* 15 full-time (5 women), 39 part-time (19 women); includes 15 minority (3 Black or African American, non-Hispanic/Latino; 8 Asian, non-Hispanic/Latino; 2 Hispanic/Latino; 2 Two or more races, non-Hispanic/Latino), 3 international. Average age 32. 34 applicants, 65% accepted, 22 enrolled. In 2013, 22 master's awarded. *Degree requirements:* For master's, thesis. *Entrance requirements:* For master's, doctoral-level degree or in process of obtaining doctoral-level degree. Additional exam requirements/recommendations for international students: Required—TOEFL. *Application deadline:* For fall admission, 5/15 for domestic students; for spring admission, 10/15 for domestic students. Application fee: $0. Electronic applications accepted. *Financial support:* In 2013–14, 6 students received support. Tuition waivers (partial) available. Financial award application deadline: 12/12. *Faculty research:* Anesthesiology, infectious diseases, neurology, obstetrics and gynecology, orthopedic surgery. *Unit head:* Dr. David Warren, Associate Professor of Medicine, 314-454-8225, Fax: 314-454-5392, E-mail: dwarren@dom.wustl.edu. *Application contact:* Angela B. Wilson, Curriculum and Evaluation Coordinator, 314-454-8936, Fax: 314-454-8279, E-mail: abwilson@dom.wustl.edu.
Website: http://crtc.wustl.edu/

West Virginia University, Eberly College of Arts and Sciences, Department of Biology, Morgantown, WV 26506. Offers cell and molecular biology (MS, PhD); environmental and evolutionary biology (MS, PhD); forensic biology (MS, PhD); genomic biology (MS, PhD); neurobiology (MS, PhD). Terminal master's awarded for partial completion of doctoral program. *Degree requirements:* For master's, thesis, final exam; for doctorate, thesis/dissertation, preliminary and final exams. *Entrance requirements:* For master's, GRE General Test, GRE Subject Test, minimum GPA of 3.0; for doctorate, GRE General Test, minimum GPA of 3.0. Additional exam requirements/recommendations for international students: Required—TOEFL. *Faculty research:* Environmental biology, genetic engineering, developmental biology, global change, biodiversity.

Yale University, School of Medicine and Graduate School of Arts and Sciences, Combined Program in Biological and Biomedical Sciences (BBS), Computational Biology and Bioinformatics Track, New Haven, CT 06520. Offers PhD, MD/PhD. *Entrance requirements:* Additional exam requirements/recommendations for international students: Required—TOEFL.

Human Genetics

Baylor College of Medicine, Graduate School of Biomedical Sciences, Department of Molecular and Human Genetics, Houston, TX 77030-3498. Offers PhD, MD/PhD. *Degree requirements:* For doctorate, thesis/dissertation, public defense. *Entrance requirements:* For doctorate, GRE General Test, GRE Subject Test (strongly recommended), minimum GPA of 3.0. Additional exam requirements/recommendations for international students: Required—TOEFL. Electronic applications accepted. *Faculty research:* Human genetics, genome biology, epigenetics, gene therapy, model organisms.

Baylor College of Medicine, Graduate School of Biomedical Sciences, Interdepartmental Program in Cell and Molecular Biology, Houston, TX 77030-3498. Offers biochemistry (PhD); cell and molecular biology (PhD); genetics (PhD); human genetics (PhD); immunology (PhD); microbiology (PhD); virology (PhD); MD/PhD. *Degree requirements:* For doctorate, thesis/dissertation, public defense. *Entrance requirements:* For doctorate, GRE General Test, GRE Subject Test (strongly recommended), minimum GPA of 3.0. Additional exam requirements/recommendations for international students: Required—TOEFL. Electronic applications accepted. *Faculty research:* Molecular and cellular biology; cancer, aging and stem cells; genomics and proteomics; microbiome, molecular microbiology; infectious disease, immunology and translational research.

Case Western Reserve University, School of Medicine and School of Graduate Studies, Graduate Programs in Medicine, Department of Genetics, Program in Human, Molecular, and Developmental Genetics and Genomics, Cleveland, OH 44106. Offers PhD, MD/PhD. *Degree requirements:* For doctorate, comprehensive exam, thesis/dissertation. *Entrance requirements:* For doctorate, GRE General Test, GRE Subject Test. Additional exam requirements/recommendations for international students: Required—TOEFL. *Faculty research:* Regulation of gene expression, molecular control of development, genomics.

Emory University, School of Medicine, Programs in Allied Health Professions, Genetic Counseling Training Program, Atlanta, GA 30322. Offers human genetics and genetic counseling (MM Sc). *Faculty:* 1 (woman) full-time, 8 part-time/adjunct (6 women). *Students:* 20 full-time (19 women); includes 2 minority (1 Asian, non-Hispanic/Latino; 1 Two or more races, non-Hispanic/Latino), 4 international. Average age 24. 45 applicants, 22% accepted, 10 enrolled. *Degree requirements:* For master's, thesis, capstone project. *Entrance requirements:* For master's, GRE General Test, minimum GPA of 3.0; prerequisites: genetics, statistics, psychology, and biochemistry. Additional exam requirements/recommendations for international students: Required—TOEFL. *Application deadline:* For winter admission, 12/15 for domestic and international students. Application fee: $50. *Financial support:* In 2013–14, 9 students received support. Stipends/scholarships (averaging $2,000-4,000 per year) available. Financial award application deadline: 4/1; financial award applicants required to submit FAFSA. *Faculty research:* Cancer genetics, lysosomal storage disease, carrier screening, public health genomics, genetic counseling, psychology, molecular genetics. *Unit head:* Dr. Cecelia Bellcross, Program Director, 404-727-3281, E-mail: cecelia.a.bellcross@emory.edu. *Application contact:* Christi Bell, Administrative Assistant, 404-727-5979, E-mail: fcbell@emory.edu.
Website: http://genetics.emory.edu/gc_training/

Johns Hopkins University, School of Medicine, Graduate Programs in Medicine, Predoctoral Training Program in Human Genetics, Baltimore, MD 21218-2699. Offers PhD, MD/PhD. *Faculty:* 59 full-time (14 women). *Students:* 71 full-time (47 women); includes 15 minority (2 Black or African American, non-Hispanic/Latino; 6 Asian, non-Hispanic/Latino; 4 Hispanic/Latino; 3 Two or more races, non-Hispanic/Latino), 14 international. Average age 27. 64 applicants, 28% accepted, 11 enrolled. In 2013, 21 doctorates awarded. Terminal master's awarded for partial completion of doctoral program. *Degree requirements:* For doctorate, comprehensive exam, thesis/dissertation. *Entrance requirements:* For doctorate, GRE General Test, GRE Subject Test. Additional exam requirements/recommendations for international students: Recommended—TOEFL. *Application deadline:* For fall admission, 1/1 priority date for domestic and international students. Application fee: $85. Electronic applications accepted. *Financial support:* Fellowships, teaching assistantships, and health care benefits available. *Faculty research:* Human, mammalian, and molecular genetics, bioinformatics, genomics. *Unit head:* Dr. David Valle, Director, 410-955-4260, Fax: 410-955-7397, E-mail: muscelli@jhmi.edu. *Application contact:* Sandy Muscelli, Administrator, 410-955-4260, Fax: 410-955-7397, E-mail: muscelli@jhmi.edu.
Website: http://humangenetics.jhmi.edu/

Human Genetics

Louisiana State University Health Sciences Center, School of Graduate Studies in New Orleans, Department of Human Genetics, New Orleans, LA 70112-2223. Offers MS, PhD, MD/PhD. Part-time programs available. Terminal master's awarded for partial completion of doctoral program. *Degree requirements:* For master's, comprehensive exam, thesis; for doctorate, comprehensive exam, thesis/dissertation. *Entrance requirements:* For master's and doctorate, GRE General Test. Additional exam requirements/recommendations for international students: Required—TOEFL. *Faculty research:* Genetic epidemiology, segregation and linkage analysis, gene mapping.

McGill University, Faculty of Graduate and Postdoctoral Studies, Faculty of Medicine, Department of Human Genetics, Montréal, QC H3A 2T5, Canada. Offers genetic counseling (M Sc); human genetics (M Sc, PhD).

Memorial University of Newfoundland, Faculty of Medicine and School of Graduate Studies, Graduate Programs in Medicine, Division of Human Genetics, St. John's, NL A1C 5S7, Canada. Offers M Sc, PhD, MD/PhD. Part-time programs available. *Degree requirements:* For master's, thesis; for doctorate, comprehensive exam, thesis/dissertation, oral defense of thesis. *Entrance requirements:* For master's, MD or B Sc; for doctorate, MD or M Sc. Additional exam requirements/recommendations for international students: Required—TOEFL. *Faculty research:* Cancer genetics, gene mapping, medical genetics, birth defects, population genetics.

Sarah Lawrence College, Graduate Studies, Joan H. Marks Graduate Program in Human Genetics, Bronxville, NY 10708-5999. Offers MS. Part-time programs available. *Faculty:* 21 part-time/adjunct (16 women). *Students:* 50 full-time (45 women), 1 (woman) part-time; includes 6 minority (4 Asian, non-Hispanic/Latino; 1 Hispanic/Latino; 1 Two or more races, non-Hispanic/Latino), 20 international. In 2013, 15 master's awarded. *Degree requirements:* For master's, thesis, fieldwork. *Entrance requirements:* For master's, previous course work in biology, chemistry, developmental biology, genetics, probability and statistics. Additional exam requirements/recommendations for international students: Required—TOEFL (minimum score 600 paper-based). *Application deadline:* For fall admission, 1/15 for domestic students. Application fee: $60. Electronic applications accepted. *Expenses:* Contact institution. *Financial support:* In 2013–14, 26 students received support, including 39 fellowships (averaging $4,870 per year); career-related internships or fieldwork, Federal Work-Study, scholarships/grants, and unspecified assistantships also available. Support available to part-time students. Financial award application deadline: 3/1; financial award applicants required to submit FAFSA. *Unit head:* Anne Greb, Director, 914-395-2371, E-mail: agreb@sarahlawrence.edu. *Application contact:* Emanual Lomax, Director of Graduate Admissions, 914-395-2371, E-mail: elomax@sarahlawrence.edu.
Website: https://www.slc.edu/genetic-counseling/

Tulane University, School of Medicine and School of Liberal Arts, Graduate Programs in Biomedical Sciences, Program in Human Genetics, New Orleans, LA 70118-5669. Offers MBS, PhD, MD/PhD. MS and PhD offered through the Graduate School. *Degree requirements:* For master's, thesis; for doctorate, thesis/dissertation. *Entrance requirements:* For master's, GRE, MCAT; for doctorate, GRE General Test. Additional exam requirements/recommendations for international students: Required—TOEFL. Electronic applications accepted. *Faculty research:* Inborn errors of metabolism, DNA methylation, gene therapy.

University of California, Los Angeles, David Geffen School of Medicine and Graduate Division, Graduate Programs in Medicine, Department of Human Genetics, Los Angeles, CA 90095. Offers MS, PhD. *Degree requirements:* For master's, thesis; for doctorate, thesis/dissertation, written and oral qualifying examination; 2 quarters of teaching experience. *Entrance requirements:* For master's and doctorate, GRE General Test; GRE Subject Test (recommended), bachelor's degree; minimum undergraduate GPA of 3.0 (or its equivalent if letter grade system not used). Additional exam requirements/recommendations for international students: Required—TOEFL. Electronic applications accepted.

University of California, Los Angeles, Graduate Division, College of Letters and Science and David Geffen School of Medicine, UCLA ACCESS to Programs in the Molecular, Cellular and Integrative Life Sciences, Los Angeles, CA 90095. Offers biochemistry and molecular biology (PhD); biological chemistry (PhD); cellular and molecular pathology (PhD); human genetics (PhD); microbiology, immunology, and molecular genetics (PhD); molecular biology (PhD); molecular toxicology (PhD); molecular, cellular and integrative physiology (PhD); neurobiology (PhD); oral biology (PhD); physiology (PhD). *Degree requirements:* For doctorate, thesis/dissertation, oral and written qualifying exams. *Entrance requirements:* For doctorate, GRE General Test, bachelor's degree; minimum undergraduate GPA of 3.0 (or its equivalent if letter grade system not used). Additional exam requirements/recommendations for international students: Required—TOEFL. Electronic applications accepted.

University of Chicago, Division of Biological Sciences, Molecular Biosciences Cluster, Department of Human Genetics, Chicago, IL 60637-1513. Offers PhD. *Degree requirements:* For doctorate, thesis/dissertation, ethics class, 2 teaching assistantships. *Entrance requirements:* For doctorate, GRE General Test. Additional exam requirements/recommendations for international students: Required—TOEFL (minimum score 600 paper-based; 104 iBT), IELTS (minimum score 7). Electronic applications accepted.

University of Manitoba, Faculty of Medicine and Faculty of Graduate Studies, Graduate Programs in Medicine, Department of Biochemistry and Medical Genetics, Winnipeg, MB R3T 2N2, Canada. Offers M Sc, PhD. Terminal master's awarded for partial completion of doctoral program. *Degree requirements:* For master's, thesis; for doctorate, thesis/dissertation. *Faculty research:* Cancer, gene expression, membrane lipids, metabolic control, genetic diseases.

University of Maryland, Baltimore, School of Medicine, Department of Epidemiology and Public Health, Baltimore, MD 21201. Offers biostatistics (MS); clinical research (MS); epidemiology and preventive medicine (MPH, MS, PhD); gerontology (PhD); human genetics and genomic medicine (MS, PhD); molecular epidemiology (MS, PhD); toxicology (MS, PhD); JD/MS; MD/PhD; MS/PhD. *Accreditation:* CEPH. Part-time programs available. *Students:* 83 full-time (56 women), 76 part-time (51 women); includes 51 minority (26 Black or African American, non-Hispanic/Latino; 20 Asian, non-Hispanic/Latino; 5 Hispanic/Latino), 27 international. Average age 32. 225 applicants, 44% accepted, 37 enrolled. In 2013, 18 master's, 1 doctorate awarded. *Degree requirements:* For doctorate, comprehensive exam, thesis/dissertation. *Entrance requirements:* For master's and doctorate, GRE General Test. Additional exam requirements/recommendations for international students: Required—TOEFL (minimum score 550 paper-based; 80 iBT); Recommended—IELTS (minimum score 7). *Application deadline:* For fall admission, 1/15 for domestic and international students. Application fee: $75. Electronic applications accepted. *Expenses:* Contact institution. *Financial support:* In 2013–14, research assistantships with partial tuition reimbursements (averaging $25,000 per year) were awarded; fellowships, Federal Work-Study, scholarships/grants, and unspecified assistantships also available. Financial award application deadline: 3/1; financial award applicants required to submit FAFSA. *Unit head:* Dr. Laura Hungerford, Program Director, 410-706-8492, Fax: 410-706-4225. *Application contact:* Jessica Kelley, Program Coordinator, 410-706-8492, Fax: 410-706-4225, E-mail: jkelley@som.umaryland.edu.
Website: http://medschool.umaryland.edu/Epidemiology/

University of Michigan, Rackham Graduate School, Program in Biomedical Sciences (PIBS), Department of Human Genetics, Ann Arbor, MI 48109. Offers genetic counseling (MS); human genetics (MS, PhD). *Faculty:* 33 full-time (16 women). *Students:* 38 full-time (25 women); includes 7 minority (1 Black or African American, non-Hispanic/Latino; 5 Asian, non-Hispanic/Latino; 1 Two or more races, non-Hispanic/Latino), 4 international. Average age 27. 192 applicants, 15% accepted, 13 enrolled. In 2013, 8 master's, 5 doctorates awarded. Terminal master's awarded for partial completion of doctoral program. *Degree requirements:* For master's, research project; for doctorate, thesis/dissertation, oral preliminary exam, oral defense of dissertation. *Entrance requirements:* For master's, GRE General Test, 3 letters of recommendation; advocacy experience (for the MS in genetic counseling); for doctorate, GRE General Test, 3 letters of recommendation. Additional exam requirements/recommendations for international students: Required—TOEFL (minimum score 84 iBT). *Application deadline:* For fall admission, 12/1 for domestic and international students; for winter admission, 1/15 for domestic and international students; for spring admission, 5/1 for domestic students, 3/15 for international students. Application fee: $75 ($90 for international students). Electronic applications accepted. Tuition and fees vary according to course level, course load, degree level, program and student level. *Financial support:* In 2013–14, 31 students received support, including 24 fellowships with full and partial tuition reimbursements available (averaging $28,500 per year), 6 research assistantships with full tuition reimbursements available (averaging $28,500 per year), 1 teaching assistantship with full and partial tuition reimbursement available (averaging $18,554 per year); Federal Work-Study, institutionally sponsored loans, scholarships/grants, traineeships, health care benefits, and unspecified assistantships also available. Financial award application deadline: 4/30; financial award applicants required to submit FAFSA. *Faculty research:* Molecular genetics, developmental genetics, disease mechanisms, translational clinical research, statistical and population genetics. *Total annual research expenditures:* $6 million. *Unit head:* Dr. Sally A. Camper, Chair, 734-763-0682, Fax: 734-763-3784, E-mail: scamper@umich.edu. *Application contact:* Michelle S. Melis, Director of Student Life, 734-615-6538, Fax: 734-647-7022, E-mail: msmtegan@umich.edu.
Website: http://www.hg.med.umich.edu/

University of Pittsburgh, Graduate School of Public Health, Department of Human Genetics, Pittsburgh, PA 15260. Offers genetic counseling (MS); human genetics (MS, PhD); public health genetics (MPH, Certificate); MD/PhD. *Faculty:* 16 full-time (7 women), 9 part-time/adjunct (3 women). *Students:* 52 full-time (34 women), 25 part-time (24 women); includes 12 minority (3 Black or African American, non-Hispanic/Latino; 5 Asian, non-Hispanic/Latino; 3 Hispanic/Latino; 1 Two or more races, non-Hispanic/Latino), 20 international. Average age 27. 119 applicants, 47% accepted, 23 enrolled. In 2013, 17 master's, 2 doctorates awarded. Terminal master's awarded for partial completion of doctoral program. *Degree requirements:* For master's, thesis (for some programs); for doctorate, thesis/dissertation. *Entrance requirements:* For master's, GRE General Test, previous course work in biochemistry, calculus, and genetics; for doctorate, GRE General Test. Additional exam requirements/recommendations for international students: Required—TOEFL (minimum score 550 paper-based; 80 iBT) or IELTS (minimum score 6.5). *Application deadline:* For fall admission, 1/15 for domestic students, 4/1 for international students; for winter admission, 9/1 for international students; for spring admission, 10/15 for domestic students, 8/1 for international students; for summer admission, 12/1 for international students. Applications are processed on a rolling basis. Application fee: $120. Electronic applications accepted. *Expenses:* Tuition, state resident: full-time $19,964; part-time $807 per credit. Tuition, nonresident: full-time $32,686; part-time $1337 per credit. *Required fees:* $740; $200. Tuition and fees vary according to program. *Financial support:* In 2013–14, 21 students received support, including 1 fellowship, 28 research assistantships (averaging $12,405 per year). *Faculty research:* Genetic mechanisms related to the transition from normal to disease states, how genes and the environment interact to affect the distribution of health and disease in human populations. *Total annual research expenditures:* $4.1 million. *Unit head:* Dr. Mohammad Kamboh, Chairman, 412-624-3066, Fax: 412-624-3020, E-mail: kamboh@pitt.edu. *Application contact:* Jeanette Norbut, Administrative Secretary, 412-624-3018, Fax: 412-624-3020, E-mail: jeanette.norbut@hgen.pitt.edu.
Website: http://www.hgen.pitt.edu

The University of Texas Health Science Center at Houston, Graduate School of Biomedical Sciences, Program in Human and Molecular Genetics, Houston, TX 77225-0036. Offers MS, PhD, MD/PhD. Terminal master's awarded for partial completion of doctoral program. *Degree requirements:* For master's, thesis; for doctorate, thesis/dissertation. *Entrance requirements:* For master's and doctorate, GRE General Test. Additional exam requirements/recommendations for international students: Required—TOEFL. Electronic applications accepted. *Expenses:* Tuition, state resident: full-time $3474; part-time $193 per credit hour. Tuition, nonresident: full-time $13,644; part-time $758 per credit hour. *Required fees:* $226.30; $87 per credit hour. *Faculty research:* Computational genomics, cancer genetics, complex disease genetics, medical genetics.

University of Utah, School of Medicine and Graduate School, Graduate Programs in Medicine, Department of Human Genetics, Salt Lake City, UT 84112-1107. Offers MS, PhD. Terminal master's awarded for partial completion of doctoral program. *Degree requirements:* For master's, comprehensive exam, thesis optional; for doctorate, comprehensive exam, thesis/dissertation. Electronic applications accepted. *Expenses:* Tuition, state resident: full-time $5259. Tuition, nonresident: full-time $18,569. *Required fees:* $841. Tuition and fees vary according to course load. *Faculty research:* RNA metabolism, drosophilia genetics, mouse genetics, protein synthesis.

Vanderbilt University, Graduate School, Program in Human Genetics, Nashville, TN 37240-1001. Offers PhD, MD/PhD. *Faculty:* 42 full-time (12 women). *Students:* 20 full-time (14 women); includes 4 minority (1 Black or African American, non-Hispanic/Latino; 1 American Indian or Alaska Native, non-Hispanic/Latino; 1 Hispanic/Latino; 1 Two or more races, non-Hispanic/Latino). Average age 29. In 2013, 2 doctorates awarded. *Degree requirements:* For doctorate, comprehensive exam, thesis/dissertation. *Entrance requirements:* For doctorate, GRE General Test. Additional exam requirements/recommendations for international students: Required—TOEFL (minimum score 570 paper-based; 88 iBT). *Application deadline:* For fall admission, 1/15 for domestic and international students. Application fee: $0. Electronic applications accepted. *Financial support:* Fellowships with full and partial tuition reimbursements, research assistantships with full and partial tuition reimbursements, Federal Work-Study, institutionally sponsored loans, traineeships, and health care benefits available. Financial award application deadline: 1/15; financial award applicants required to submit CSS PROFILE or FAFSA. *Faculty research:* Disease gene discovery, computational genomics, translational genetics. *Unit head:* Dr. Jonathan L. Haines, Director, The Center for Human Genetics Research, 615-343-5851, Fax: 615-322-1453, E-mail: jonathan.haines@vanderbilt.edu. *Application contact:* Walter B. Bieschke, Program Coordinator for Graduate Admissions, 615-342-0236, E-mail: vandygrad@vanderbilt.edu.
Website: http://chgr.mc.vanderbilt.edu/page/education

Virginia Commonwealth University, Medical College of Virginia-Professional Programs, School of Medicine, School of Medicine Graduate Programs, Department of Human and Molecular Genetics, Richmond, VA 23284-9005. Offers genetic counseling (MS); human genetics (PhD); molecular biology and genetics (MS, PhD); MD/PhD. *Degree requirements:* For master's, thesis; for doctorate, thesis/dissertation, comprehensive oral and written exams. *Entrance requirements:* For master's, GRE; for doctorate, GRE General Test. Additional exam requirements/recommendations for international students: Required—TOEFL (minimum score 600 paper-based; 100 iBT). Electronic applications accepted. *Faculty research:* Genetic epidemiology, biochemical genetics, quantitative genetics, human cytogenetics, molecular genetics.

Virginia Commonwealth University, Program in Pre-Medical Basic Health Sciences, Richmond, VA 23284-9005. Offers anatomy (CBHS); biochemistry (CBHS); human genetics (CBHS); microbiology (CBHS); pharmacology (CBHS); physiology (CBHS). *Entrance requirements:* For degree, GRE, MCAT or DAT, course work in organic chemistry, minimum undergraduate GPA of 2.8. Additional exam requirements/recommendations for international students: Required—TOEFL (minimum score 600 paper-based). Electronic applications accepted.

Wake Forest University, School of Medicine and Graduate School of Arts and Sciences, Graduate Programs in Medicine, Molecular Genetics and Genomics Program, Winston-Salem, NC 27109. Offers PhD, MD/PhD. *Degree requirements:* For doctorate, thesis/dissertation. *Entrance requirements:* For doctorate, GRE General Test. Additional exam requirements/recommendations for international students: Required—TOEFL. Electronic applications accepted. *Faculty research:* Control of gene expression, molecular pathogenesis, protein biosynthesis, cell development, clinical cytogenetics.

Washington University in St. Louis, Graduate School of Arts and Sciences, Division of Biology and Biomedical Sciences, Program in Human and Statistical Genetics, St. Louis, MO 63130-4899. Offers PhD. *Degree requirements:* For doctorate, thesis/dissertation. *Entrance requirements:* For doctorate, GRE General Test, GRE Subject Test. Electronic applications accepted.

West Virginia University, Davis College of Agriculture, Forestry and Consumer Sciences, Interdisciplinary Program in Genetics and Developmental Biology, Morgantown, WV 26506. Offers animal breeding (MS, PhD); biochemical and molecular genetics (MS, PhD); cytogenetics (MS, PhD); descriptive embryology (MS, PhD); developmental genetics (MS); experimental morphogenesis/teratology (MS); human genetics (MS, PhD); immunogenetics (MS, PhD); life cycles of animals and plants (MS, PhD); molecular aspects of development (MS, PhD); mutagenesis (MS, PhD); oncology (MS, PhD); plant genetics (MS, PhD); population and quantitative genetics (MS, PhD); regeneration (MS, PhD); teratology (PhD); toxicology (MS, PhD). *Degree requirements:* For master's, thesis; for doctorate, comprehensive exam, thesis/dissertation. *Entrance requirements:* For master's, GRE or MCAT, minimum GPA of 2.75. Additional exam requirements/recommendations for international students: Required—TOEFL.

Molecular Genetics

Albert Einstein College of Medicine, Graduate Division of Biomedical Sciences, Department of Genetics, Bronx, NY 10461. Offers computational genetics (PhD); molecular genetics (PhD); translational genetics (PhD); MD/PhD. *Degree requirements:* For doctorate, thesis/dissertation. *Entrance requirements:* For doctorate, GRE General Test. Additional exam requirements/recommendations for international students: Required—TOEFL. *Faculty research:* Neurologic genetics in &ITDrosophila&RO, biochemical genetics of yeast, developmental genetics in the mouse.

Duke University, Graduate School, Department of Molecular Genetics and Microbiology, Durham, NC 27710. Offers PhD. *Faculty:* 59. *Students:* 66 full-time (34 women); includes 11 minority (1 Black or African American, non-Hispanic/Latino; 1 American Indian or Alaska Native, non-Hispanic/Latino; 3 Asian, non-Hispanic/Latino; 6 Hispanic/Latino), 17 international. 96 applicants, 18% accepted, 12 enrolled. In 2013, 10 doctorates awarded. *Degree requirements:* For doctorate, thesis/dissertation. *Entrance requirements:* For doctorate, GRE General Test, GRE Subject Test in biology, chemistry, or biochemistry, cell and molecular biology (recommended). Additional exam requirements/recommendations for international students: Required—TOEFL (minimum score 577 paper-based; 90 iBT) or IELTS (minimum score 7). *Application deadline:* For fall admission, 12/8 priority date for domestic and international students. Application fee: $80. Electronic applications accepted. *Financial support:* Fellowships with full tuition reimbursements, research assistantships with full tuition reimbursements, and Federal Work-Study available. Financial award application deadline: 12/31. *Unit head:* Dr. Raphael Valdivia, Director of Graduate Studies, 919-684-4008, Fax: 919-684-2790, E-mail: kimberly.kobes@duke.edu. *Application contact:* Elizabeth Hutton, Director of Admissions, 919-684-3913, Fax: 919-684-2277, E-mail: grad-admissions@duke.edu.
Website: http://mgm.duke.edu/graduate/

Emory University, Laney Graduate School, Division of Biological and Biomedical Sciences, Program in Microbiology and Molecular Genetics, Atlanta, GA 30322-1100. Offers PhD. *Degree requirements:* For doctorate, comprehensive exam, thesis/dissertation. *Entrance requirements:* For doctorate, GRE General Test, minimum GPA of 3.0 in science course work (recommended). Additional exam requirements/recommendations for international students: Required—TOEFL. Electronic applications accepted. *Faculty research:* Bacterial genetics and physiology, microbial development, molecular biology of viruses and bacterial pathogens, DNA recombination.

The George Washington University, School of Medicine and Health Sciences, Department of Biochemistry and Molecular Biology, Washington, DC 20037. Offers biochemistry and molecular biology (MS); biochemistry and molecular genetics (PhD); molecular biochemistry and bioinformatics (MS). *Degree requirements:* For master's, comprehensive exam; for doctorate, thesis/dissertation, general exam. *Entrance requirements:* For master's, GRE General Test, interview, minimum GPA of 3.0; for doctorate, GRE General Test, minimum GPA of 3.0. Additional exam requirements/recommendations for international students: Required—TOEFL (minimum score 550 paper-based).

Georgia State University, College of Arts and Sciences, Department of Biology, Program in Molecular Genetics and Biochemistry, Atlanta, GA 30302-3083. Offers bioinformatics (MS); molecular genetics and biochemistry (MS, PhD). Part-time programs available. Terminal master's awarded for partial completion of doctoral program. *Degree requirements:* For master's, comprehensive exam (for some programs), thesis optional; for doctorate, comprehensive exam, thesis/dissertation. *Entrance requirements:* For master's and doctorate, GRE. Additional exam requirements/recommendations for international students: Required—TOEFL (minimum score 550 paper-based; 82 iBT) or IELTS (minimum score 7). *Application deadline:* For fall admission, 7/1 priority date for domestic students, 6/1 priority date for international students; for spring admission, 11/15 priority date for domestic students, 10/15 priority date for international students. Applications are processed on a rolling basis. Application fee: $50. Electronic applications accepted. *Expenses: Tuition, area resident:* Full-time $4176; part-time $348 per credit hour. Tuition, state resident: full-time $14,544; part-time $1212 per credit hour. Tuition, nonresident: full-time $14,544; part-time $1212 per credit hour. Tuition and fees vary according to course load and program. *Financial support:* In 2013–14, fellowships with full tuition reimbursements (averaging $22,000 per year), research assistantships with full tuition reimbursements (averaging $20,000 per year) were awarded. Financial award application deadline: 12/3. *Faculty research:* Gene regulation, microbial pathogenesis, molecular transport, protein modeling, viral pathogenesis. *Unit head:* Dr. Parjit Kaur, Professor, 404-413-5432, Fax: 404-413-5301. *Application contact:* LaTesha Warren, Graduate Coordinator, 404-413-5314, Fax: 404-413-5301, E-mail: lwarren@gsu.edu.
Website: http://biology.gsu.edu/

Harvard University, Graduate School of Arts and Sciences, Division of Medical Sciences, Boston, MA 02115. Offers biological chemistry and molecular pharmacology (PhD); cell biology (PhD); genetics (PhD); microbiology and molecular genetics (PhD); pathology (PhD), including experimental pathology. *Degree requirements:* For doctorate, thesis/dissertation. *Entrance requirements:* For doctorate, GRE General Test, GRE Subject Test. Additional exam requirements/recommendations for international students: Required—TOEFL. *Expenses: Tuition:* Full-time $38,888. *Required fees:* $958. Tuition and fees vary according to campus/location, program and student level.

Illinois State University, Graduate School, College of Arts and Sciences, Department of Biological Sciences, Normal, IL 61790-2200. Offers animal behavior (MS); bacteriology (MS); biochemistry (MS); biological sciences (MS); biology (PhD); biophysics (MS); biotechnology (MS); botany (MS, PhD); cell biology (MS); conservation biology (MS); developmental biology (MS); ecology (MS, PhD); entomology (MS); evolutionary biology (MS); genetics (MS, PhD); immunology (MS); microbiology (MS, PhD); molecular biology (MS); molecular genetics (MS); neurobiology (MS); neuroscience (MS); parasitology (MS); physiology (MS, PhD); plant biology (MS); plant molecular biology (MS); plant sciences (MS); structural biology (MS); zoology (MS, PhD). Part-time programs available. *Degree requirements:* For master's, thesis or alternative; for doctorate, variable foreign language requirement, thesis/dissertation, 2 terms of residency. *Entrance requirements:* For master's, GRE General Test, minimum GPA of 2.6 in last 60 hours of course work; for doctorate, GRE General Test. *Faculty research:* Redoc balance and drug development in schistosoma mansoni, control of the growth of listeria monocytogenes at low temperature, regulation of cell expansion and microtubule function by SPRI, CRUI: physiology and fitness consequences of different life history phenotypes.

Indiana University–Purdue University Indianapolis, Indiana University School of Medicine, Department of Medical and Molecular Genetics, Indianapolis, IN 46202-2896. Offers genetic counseling (MS); medical and molecular genetics (MS, PhD); MD/MS; MD/PhD. Part-time programs available. *Faculty:* 8 full-time (2 women). *Students:* 27 full-time (21 women), 9 part-time (8 women); includes 4 minority (3 Black or African American, non-Hispanic/Latino; 1 Asian, non-Hispanic/Latino), 8 international. Average age 26. 117 applicants, 9% accepted, 7 enrolled. In 2013, 8 master's, 2 doctorates awarded. Terminal master's awarded for partial completion of doctoral program. *Degree requirements:* For master's, thesis optional; for doctorate, thesis/dissertation, research ethics. *Entrance requirements:* For master's and doctorate, GRE General Test, minimum GPA of 3.2. *Application deadline:* For fall admission, 1/15 priority date for domestic students. Application fee: $55 ($65 for international students). *Financial support:* In 2013–14, fellowships with tuition reimbursements (averaging $12,750 per year), teaching assistantships (averaging $22,000 per year) were awarded; research assistantships with tuition reimbursements, Federal Work-Study, and institutionally sponsored loans also available. Support available to part-time students. Financial award application deadline: 1/15. *Faculty research:* Twins, human gene mapping, chromosomes and malignancy, clinical genetics. *Total annual research expenditures:* $2.1 million. *Unit head:* Dr. Joe Christian, Chair, 317-274-2241. *Application contact:* Kathleen Wilhelm, Admissions Secretary, 317-274-2241, Fax: 317-274-2387, E-mail: medgen@iupui.edu.
Website: http://genetics.medicine.iu.edu/

Iowa State University of Science and Technology, Program in Animal Breeding and Genetics, Ames, IA 50011. Offers animal breeding and genetics (MS); immunogenetics (PhD); molecular genetics (PhD); quantitative genetics (PhD). *Entrance requirements:* For master's and doctorate, GRE. Additional exam requirements/recommendations for international students: Required—TOEFL (minimum score 550 paper-based; 80 iBT), IELTS (minimum score 6.5). Electronic applications accepted.

Medical College of Wisconsin, Graduate School of Biomedical Sciences, Department of Microbiology and Molecular Genetics, Milwaukee, WI 53226-0509. Offers MS, PhD, MD/PhD. *Degree requirements:* For doctorate, comprehensive exam, thesis/dissertation. *Entrance requirements:* For master's and doctorate, GRE, official transcripts, three letters of recommendation. Additional exam requirements/recommendations for international students: Required—TOEFL. *Faculty research:* Virology, immunology, bacterial toxins, regulation of gene expression.

Michigan State University, College of Human Medicine and The Graduate School, Graduate Programs in Human Medicine, East Lansing, MI 48824. Offers biochemistry and molecular biology (MS, PhD); epidemiology (MS, PhD); microbiology (MS); microbiology and molecular genetics (PhD); pharmacology and toxicology (MS, PhD); physiology (MS, PhD); public health (MPH). *Entrance requirements:* Additional exam requirements/recommendations for international students: Required—TOEFL.

Michigan State University, College of Osteopathic Medicine and The Graduate School, Graduate Studies in Osteopathic Medicine, East Lansing, MI 48824. Offers biochemistry and molecular biology (MS, PhD); microbiology (MS); microbiology and molecular genetics (PhD); pharmacology and toxicology (MS, PhD), including integrative pharmacology (MS), pharmacology and toxicology, pharmacology and toxicology-environmental toxicology (PhD); physiology (MS, PhD).

New York University, Graduate School of Arts and Science, Department of Biology, New York, NY 10012-1019. Offers biology (PhD); biomedical journalism (MS); cancer and molecular biology (PhD); computational biology (PhD); computers in biological research (MS); developmental genetics (PhD); general biology (MS); immunology and

microbiology (PhD); molecular genetics (PhD); neurobiology (PhD); oral biology (MS); plant biology (PhD); recombinant DNA technology (MS); MS/MBA. Part-time programs available. *Faculty:* 24 full-time (5 women). *Students:* 161 full-time (88 women), 28 part-time (15 women); includes 41 minority (5 Black or African American, non-Hispanic/Latino; 23 Asian, non-Hispanic/Latino; 9 Hispanic/Latino; 4 Two or more races, non-Hispanic/Latino), 80 international. Average age 27. 412 applicants, 54% accepted, 65 enrolled. In 2013, 77 master's, 9 doctorates awarded. Terminal master's awarded for partial completion of doctoral program. *Degree requirements:* For master's, thesis or alternative, qualifying paper; for doctorate, comprehensive exam, thesis/dissertation. *Entrance requirements:* For master's and doctorate, GRE General Test. Additional exam requirements/recommendations for international students: Required—TOEFL. *Application deadline:* For fall admission, 12/1 priority date for domestic students, 12/1 for international students. Application fee: $95. *Expenses: Tuition:* Full-time $35,856; part-time $1494 per unit. *Required fees:* $1408; $64 per unit. $473 per term. Tuition and fees vary according to course load and program. *Financial support:* Fellowships with tuition reimbursements, research assistantships with tuition reimbursements, teaching assistantships with tuition reimbursements, career-related internships or fieldwork, Federal Work-Study, institutionally sponsored loans, scholarships/grants, health care benefits, and unspecified assistantships available. Financial award application deadline: 12/1; financial award applicants required to submit FAFSA. *Faculty research:* Genomics, molecular and cell biology, development and molecular genetics, molecular evolution of plants and animals. *Unit head:* Stephen Small, Chair, 212-998-8200, Fax: 212-995-4015, E-mail: biology.admissions@nyu.edu. *Application contact:* Justin Blau, Director of Graduate Studies, PhD Programs, 212-998-8200, Fax: 212-995-4015, E-mail: biology.admissions@nyu.edu.
Website: http://biology.as.nyu.edu/

The Ohio State University, Graduate School, College of Arts and Sciences, Division of Natural and Mathematical Sciences, Department of Molecular Genetics, Columbus, OH 43210. Offers cell and developmental biology (MS, PhD); genetics (MS, PhD); molecular biology (MS, PhD). *Faculty:* 29. *Students:* 35 full-time (15 women); includes 3 minority (1 Black or African American, non-Hispanic/Latino; 2 Asian, non-Hispanic/Latino), 16 international. Average age 26. In 2013, 1 master's, 2 doctorates awarded. *Degree requirements:* For master's, thesis; for doctorate, thesis/dissertation. *Entrance requirements:* For doctorate, GRE General Test, GRE Subject Test in biology or chemistry (recommended). Additional exam requirements/recommendations for international students: Required—TOEFL (minimum score 550 paper-based; 79 iBT), Michigan English Language Assessment Battery (minimum score 82); Recommended—IELTS (minimum score 7). *Application deadline:* For fall admission, 12/13 priority date for domestic students, 11/30 priority date for international students; for winter admission, 12/1 for domestic students, 11/1 for international students; for spring admission, 3/1 for domestic students, 2/1 for international students. Applications are processed on a rolling basis. Application fee: $60 ($70 for international students). Electronic applications accepted. *Financial support:* Fellowships with tuition reimbursements, research assistantships with tuition reimbursements, teaching assistantships with tuition reimbursements, Federal Work-Study, and institutionally sponsored loans available. Support available to part-time students. *Unit head:* Dr. Anita Hopper, Chair, 614-688-3306, Fax: 614-292-4466, E-mail: hopper.64@osu.edu. *Application contact:* Graduate Admissions, 614-292-9444, Fax: 614-292-3895, E-mail: gradadmissions@osu.edu.
Website: https://molgen.osu.edu/

Oklahoma State University, College of Arts and Sciences, Department of Microbiology and Molecular Genetics, Stillwater, OK 74078. Offers MS, PhD. *Faculty:* 20 full-time (5 women). *Students:* 16 full-time (10 women), 18 part-time (11 women); includes 4 minority (1 Asian, non-Hispanic/Latino; 1 Hispanic/Latino; 2 Two or more races, non-Hispanic/Latino), 17 international. Average age 28. 83 applicants, 19% accepted, 10 enrolled. In 2013, 1 master's awarded. *Degree requirements:* For master's, thesis; for doctorate, comprehensive exam, thesis/dissertation. *Entrance requirements:* For master's, GRE General Test; for doctorate, GRE General Test. Additional exam requirements/recommendations for international students: Required—TOEFL (minimum score 550 paper-based; 79 iBT). *Application deadline:* For fall admission, 3/1 priority date for international students; for spring admission, 8/1 priority date for international students. Applications are processed on a rolling basis. Application fee: $40 ($75 for international students). Electronic applications accepted. *Expenses:* Tuition, state resident: full-time $4272; part-time $178 per credit hour. Tuition, nonresident: full-time $17,472; part-time $709 per credit hour. *Required fees:* $2413.20; $100.55 per credit hour. One-time fee: $50 full-time. Part-time tuition and fees vary according to course load and campus/location. *Financial support:* In 2013–14, 16 research assistantships (averaging $21,705 per year), 14 teaching assistantships (averaging $19,632 per year) were awarded; career-related internships or fieldwork, Federal Work-Study, scholarships/grants, health care benefits, tuition waivers (partial), and unspecified assistantships also available. Support available to part-time students. Financial award application deadline: 3/1; financial award applicants required to submit FAFSA. *Faculty research:* Bioinformatics, genomics-genetics, virology, environmental microbiology, development-molecular mechanisms. *Unit head:* Dr. Bill Picking, Department Head, 405-744-6243, Fax: 405-744-6790, E-mail: william.picking@okstate.edu. *Application contact:* Dr. Wouter Hoff, Graduate Program Coordinator, 405-744-6243, Fax: 405-744-6790, E-mail: wouter.hoff@okstate.edu.
Website: http://microbiology.okstate.edu

Penn State Hershey Medical Center, College of Medicine, Graduate School Programs in the Biomedical Sciences, Graduate Program in Biomedical Sciences, Hershey, PA 17033. Offers biochemistry and molecular genetics (MS, PhD); biomedical sciences (MS, PhD); translational therapeutics (MS, PhD); virology and immunology (MS, PhD); MD/PhD; PhD/MBA. *Students:* 40 full-time (22 women); includes 7 minority (2 Black or African American, non-Hispanic/Latino; 2 Asian, non-Hispanic/Latino; 1 Hispanic/Latino; 2 Two or more races, non-Hispanic/Latino), 10 international. 215 applicants, 20% accepted, 14 enrolled. Terminal master's awarded for partial completion of doctoral program. *Degree requirements:* For master's, thesis (for some programs); for doctorate, comprehensive exam, thesis/dissertation, candidacy exam. *Entrance requirements:* For doctorate, GRE General Test. Additional exam requirements/recommendations for international students: Required—TOEFL (minimum score 550 paper-based; 80 iBT). *Application deadline:* For fall admission, 2/1 for domestic and international students. Applications are processed on a rolling basis. Application fee: $65. Electronic applications accepted. *Financial support:* In 2013–14, research assistantships (averaging $24,544 per year) were awarded; fellowships, scholarships/grants, health care benefits, and unspecified assistantships also available. Financial award applicants required to submit FAFSA. *Unit head:* Dr. Ralph L. Keil, Chair, 717-531-8595, Fax: 717-531-0388, E-mail: rlk9@psu.edu. *Application contact:* Kristin E. Smith, Enrollment Support Manager, 717-531-0003, Fax: 717-531-0388, E-mail: kec17@psu.edu.
Website: http://med.psu.edu/web/biomedical-sciences/home

Rutgers, The State University of New Jersey, Newark, Graduate School of Biomedical Sciences, Department of Microbiology and Molecular Genetics, Newark, NJ 07107. Offers PhD. *Degree requirements:* For doctorate, thesis/dissertation, qualifying exam. *Entrance requirements:* For doctorate, GRE General Test. Additional exam requirements/recommendations for international students: Required—TOEFL. Electronic applications accepted. *Faculty research:* Molecular genetics of yeast, mutagenesis and carcinogenesis of DNA, bacterial protein synthesis, mammalian cell genetics, adenovirus gene expression.

Rutgers, The State University of New Jersey, New Brunswick, Graduate School-New Brunswick, Programs in the Molecular Biosciences, Piscataway, NJ 08854-8097. Offers biochemistry (PhD); cell and developmental biology (MS, PhD); microbiology and molecular genetics (MS, PhD), including applied microbiology, clinical microbiology (MS), clinical mircobiology (PhD), computational molecular biology (PhD), immunology, microbial biochemistry, molecular genetics, virology. MS, PhD offered jointly with University of Medicine and Dentistry of New Jersey.

Rutgers, The State University of New Jersey, New Brunswick, Graduate School of Biomedical Sciences, Program in Microbiology and Molecular Genetics, Piscataway, NJ 08854-5635. Offers MS, PhD, MD/PhD. Terminal master's awarded for partial completion of doctoral program. *Degree requirements:* For master's, thesis, qualifying exam; for doctorate, thesis/dissertation, qualifying exam. *Entrance requirements:* For master's and doctorate, GRE General Test. Additional exam requirements/recommendations for international students: Required—TOEFL. Electronic applications accepted. *Faculty research:* Interferon, receptors, retrovirus evolution, Arbo virus/host cell interactions.

Stony Brook University, State University of New York, Stony Brook University Medical Center, Health Sciences Center, School of Medicine and Graduate School, Graduate Programs in Medicine, Department of Molecular Genetics and Microbiology, Stony Brook, NY 11794. Offers PhD. *Faculty:* 18 full-time (5 women), 1 (woman) part-time/adjunct. *Students:* 25 full-time (7 women); includes 7 minority (5 Asian, non-Hispanic/Latino; 2 Hispanic/Latino), 4 international. Average age 27. 56 applicants, 23% accepted, 5 enrolled. In 2013, 7 doctorates awarded. *Degree requirements:* For doctorate, comprehensive exam, thesis/dissertation. *Entrance requirements:* For doctorate, GRE General Test, GRE Subject Test, undergraduate training in biochemistry, genetics, and cell biology; recommendations; personal statement. Additional exam requirements/recommendations for international students: Required—TOEFL (minimum score 550 paper-based; 90 iBT). *Application deadline:* For fall admission, 1/15 for domestic students; for spring admission, 10/1 for domestic students. Application fee: $100. *Expenses:* Tuition, state resident: full-time $9870; part-time $411 per credit. Tuition, nonresident: full-time $18,350; part-time $765 per credit. *Financial support:* In 2013–14, 17 fellowships, 8 research assistantships were awarded; teaching assistantships and Federal Work-Study also available. Financial award application deadline: 3/15. *Faculty research:* Adenovirus molecular genetics, molecular biology of tumors, virus SV40, mechanism of tumor infection by SAV virus. *Total annual research expenditures:* $9.9 million. *Unit head:* Dr. Jorge Benach, Chair, 631-632-4225, Fax: 631-632-9797, E-mail: jorge.benach@stonybrook.edu. *Application contact:* Kathryn Bell, Graduate Program Director, 631-632-8812, Fax: 631-632-9797, E-mail: kathryn.bell@stonybrook.edu.
Website: http://www.mgm.stonybrook.edu/index.shtml

The University of Alabama at Birmingham, Graduate Programs in Joint Health Sciences, Program in Biochemistry and Molecular Genetics, Birmingham, AL 35294. Offers PhD. *Degree requirements:* For doctorate, thesis/dissertation. *Entrance requirements:* For doctorate, GRE General Test, interview, letters of recommendation, minimum GPA of 3.0. Additional exam requirements/recommendations for international students: Required—TOEFL (minimum score 600 paper-based; 100 iBT). Electronic applications accepted.

University of Calgary, Cumming School of Medicine and Faculty of Graduate Studies, Medical Science Graduate Program, Calgary, AB T2N 1N4, Canada. Offers cancer biology (M Sc, PhD); critical care medicine (M Sc, PhD); joint injury and arthritis (M Sc, PhD); molecular and medical genetics (M Sc, PhD); mountain medicine and high altitude physiology (M Sc, PhD); pathologists' assistant (M Sc, PhD). *Degree requirements:* For master's, thesis; for doctorate, thesis/dissertation, candidacy exam. *Entrance requirements:* For master's, minimum undergraduate GPA of 3.2; for doctorate, minimum graduate GPA of 3.2. Additional exam requirements/recommendations for international students: Required—TOEFL (minimum score 600 paper-based). Electronic applications accepted. *Faculty research:* Cancer biology, immunology, joint injury and arthritis, medical education, population genomics.

University of California, Irvine, School of Medicine and School of Biological Sciences, Department of Microbiology and Molecular Genetics, Irvine, CA 92697. Offers biological sciences (MS, PhD); MD/PhD. *Students:* 27 full-time (12 women); includes 18 minority (1 American Indian or Alaska Native, non-Hispanic/Latino; 11 Asian, non-Hispanic/Latino; 6 Hispanic/Latino), 1 international. Average age 28. In 2013, 1 master's, 6 doctorates awarded. *Degree requirements:* For doctorate, thesis/dissertation. *Entrance requirements:* For doctorate, GRE General Test, GRE Subject Test, minimum GPA of 3.0. Additional exam requirements/recommendations for international students: Required—TOEFL (minimum score 550 paper-based). *Application deadline:* For fall admission, 12/15 priority date for domestic students, 12/15 for international students. Application fee: $80 ($100 for international students). Electronic applications accepted. *Financial support:* Fellowships, research assistantships with full tuition reimbursements, teaching assistantships, institutionally sponsored loans, traineeships, health care benefits, and unspecified assistantships available. Financial award applicants required to submit FAFSA. *Faculty research:* Molecular biology and genetics of viruses, bacteria, and yeast; immune response; molecular biology of cultured animal cells; genetic basis of cancer; genetics and physiology of infectious agents. *Unit head:* Rozanne M. Sandri-Goldin, Chair, 949-824-7570, Fax: 949-824-8598, E-mail: rmsandri@uci.edu. *Application contact:* Renee Frigo, Program Manager, 949-824-8145, Fax: 949-824-1965, E-mail: rfrigo@uci.edu.
Website: http://www.bio.uci.edu/

University of California, Los Angeles, David Geffen School of Medicine and Graduate Division, Graduate Programs in Medicine, Department of Microbiology, Immunology and Molecular Genetics, Los Angeles, CA 90095. Offers MS, PhD. *Degree requirements:* For master's, thesis; for doctorate, thesis/dissertation, oral and written qualifying exams; 2 quarters of teaching experience. *Entrance requirements:* For master's and doctorate, GRE General Test, bachelor's degree; minimum undergraduate GPA of 3.0 (or its equivalent if letter grade system not used). Additional exam requirements/recommendations for international students: Required—TOEFL. Electronic applications accepted.

University of California, Riverside, Graduate Division, Graduate Program in Genetics, Genomics, and Bioinformatics, Riverside, CA 92521-0102. Offers genomics and bioinformatics (PhD); molecular genetics (PhD); population and evolutionary genetics (PhD). *Faculty:* 72 full-time (20 women). *Students:* 32 full-time (18 women); includes 2 minority (1 Black or African American, non-Hispanic/Latino; 1 Hispanic/Latino), 15 international. Average age 30. In 2013, 2 doctorates awarded. *Degree requirements:* For doctorate, thesis/dissertation, qualifying exams, teaching experience. *Entrance requirements:* For doctorate, GRE General Test, minimum GPA of 3.2. Additional exam requirements/recommendations for international students: Required—TOEFL (minimum score 550 paper-based; 80 iBT). *Application deadline:* For fall admission, 5/1 for domestic students, 2/1 for international students; for winter admission, 9/1 for domestic students, 7/1 for international students; for spring admission, 12/1 for domestic students,

10/1 for international students. Applications are processed on a rolling basis. Application fee: $85 ($100 for international students). Electronic applications accepted. *Financial support:* In 2013–14, fellowships with tuition reimbursements (averaging $18,000 per year), research assistantships with tuition reimbursements (averaging $18,000 per year), teaching assistantships with tuition reimbursements (averaging $16,500 per year) were awarded; career-related internships or fieldwork, Federal Work-Study, institutionally sponsored loans, and tuition waivers (full and partial) also available. *Faculty research:* Molecular genetics, evolution and population genetics, genomics and bioinformatics. *Unit head:* Dr. Shizhong Xu, Director, 951-827-5898. *Application contact:* Deidra Kornfeld, Graduate Program Assistant, 800-735-0717, Fax: 951-827-5517, E-mail: genetics@ucr.edu.
Website: http://ggb.ucr.edu/

University of Cincinnati, Graduate School, College of Medicine, Graduate Programs in Biomedical Sciences, Department of Molecular Genetics, Biochemistry and Microbiology, Cincinnati, OH 45221. Offers MS, PhD. Terminal master's awarded for partial completion of doctoral program. *Degree requirements:* For master's, thesis or alternative; for doctorate, thesis/dissertation, qualifying exam. *Entrance requirements:* For master's and doctorate, GRE General Test. Additional exam requirements/recommendations for international students: Required—TOEFL (minimum score 600 paper-based; 100 iBT), TWE. Electronic applications accepted. *Faculty research:* Cancer biology and developmental genetics, gene regulation and chromosome structure, microbiology and pathogenic mechanisms, structural biology, membrane biochemistry and signal transduction.

University of Colorado Denver, School of Medicine, Biochemistry Program, Aurora, CO 80045. Offers biochemistry (PhD); biochemistry and molecular genetics (PhD). *Students:* 14 full-time (5 women); includes 1 minority (Hispanic/Latino), 1 international. Average age 31. 2 applicants, 100% accepted, 2 enrolled. In 2013, 3 doctorates awarded. *Degree requirements:* For doctorate, comprehensive exam, thesis/dissertation, 30 credit hours each of coursework and thesis research. *Entrance requirements:* For doctorate, GRE, minimum of three letters of recommendation from qualified referees. Additional exam requirements/recommendations for international students: Required—TOEFL (minimum score 550 paper-based; 80 iBT). *Application deadline:* For fall admission, 12/1 for domestic students. Applications are processed on a rolling basis. Application fee: $50 ($75 for international students). Electronic applications accepted. *Expenses:* Contact institution. *Financial support:* In 2013–14, 14 students received support. Fellowships, research assistantships, teaching assistantships, Federal Work-Study, institutionally sponsored loans, scholarships/grants, traineeships, health care benefits, tuition waivers (full), and unspecified assistantships available. Financial award application deadline: 3/15; financial award applicants required to submit FAFSA. *Faculty research:* DNA damage, cancer and neurodegeneration, molecular mechanisms of pro-MRNA splicing, yeast RNA polymerases, DNA replication. *Total annual research expenditures:* $8.6 million. *Unit head:* Dr. Mark Johnston, Professor and Chair, 303-724-3203, Fax: 303-724-3215, E-mail: mark.johnston@ucdenver.edu. *Application contact:* Jennifer Spaulding, Administrative Assistant, 303-724-3201, Fax: 303-724-3215, E-mail: jennifer.spaulding@ucdenver.edu.
Website: http://www.ucdenver.edu/academics/colleges/medicalschool/departments/biochemistry/Pages/Home.aspx

University of Florida, College of Medicine, Department of Molecular Genetics and Microbiology, Gainesville, FL 32610-0266. Offers MS. Terminal master's awarded for partial completion of doctoral program. *Degree requirements:* For master's, thesis. *Entrance requirements:* For master's, GRE General Test, minimum GPA of 3.0. Additional exam requirements/recommendations for international students: Required—TOEFL, IELTS. Electronic applications accepted. *Expenses:* Tuition, state resident: full-time $12,640. Tuition, nonresident: full-time $30,000.

University of Guelph, Graduate Studies, College of Biological Science, Department of Molecular and Cellular Biology, Guelph, ON N1G 2W1, Canada. Offers biochemistry (M Sc, PhD); biophysics (M Sc, PhD); botany (M Sc, PhD); microbiology (M Sc, PhD); molecular biology and genetics (M Sc, PhD). *Degree requirements:* For master's, thesis, research proposal; for doctorate, comprehensive exam, thesis/dissertation, research proposal. *Entrance requirements:* For master's, minimum B-average during previous 2 years of coursework; for doctorate, minimum A-average. Additional exam requirements/recommendations for international students: Required—TOEFL (minimum score 550 paper-based), IELTS (minimum score 6.5). Electronic applications accepted. *Faculty research:* Physiology, structure, genetics, and ecology of microbes; virology and microbial technology.

University of Illinois at Chicago, College of Medicine and Graduate College, Graduate Programs in Medicine, Department of Biochemistry and Molecular Genetics, Chicago, IL 60607-7128. Offers PhD, MD/PhD. *Faculty:* 32 full-time (11 women), 6 part-time/adjunct (1 woman). *Students:* 31 full-time (17 women), 1 (woman) part-time; includes 5 minority (4 Asian, non-Hispanic/Latino; 1 Hispanic/Latino), 16 international. Average age 29. 7 applicants, 86% accepted, 3 enrolled. In 2013, 10 doctorates awarded. Terminal master's awarded for partial completion of doctoral program. *Degree requirements:* For doctorate, thesis/dissertation. *Entrance requirements:* For doctorate, GRE General Test. Additional exam requirements/recommendations for international students: Required—TOEFL. *Application deadline:* For fall admission, 3/1 priority date for domestic students, 2/15 for international students. Applications are processed on a rolling basis. Application fee: $40 ($50 for international students). Electronic applications accepted. *Expenses:* Tuition, state resident: full-time $11,066; part-time $3689 per term. Tuition, nonresident: full-time $23,064; part-time $7688 per term. *Required fees:* $3004; $1190 per term. Tuition and fees vary according to course level and program. *Financial support:* In 2013–14, 22 students received support. Fellowships with full tuition reimbursements available, research assistantships with full tuition reimbursements available, teaching assistantships with full tuition reimbursements available, career-related internships or fieldwork, Federal Work-Study, institutionally sponsored loans, traineeships, tuition waivers (full), and unspecified assistantships available. Financial award application deadline: 3/1; financial award applicants required to submit FAFSA. *Faculty research:* Nature of cellular components, control of metabolic processes, regulation of gene expression. *Total annual research expenditures:* $6.9 million. *Unit head:* Dr. Jack Kaplan, Head, 312-355-2732, E-mail: kaplanj@uic.edu. *Application contact:* Dr. Karen Colley, Co-Director of Graduate Studies, 312-996-7756.
Website: http://www.uic.edu/com/bcmg/

University of Kentucky, Graduate School, Graduate School Programs from the College of Medicine, Department of Microbiology, Immunology and Molecular Genetics, Lexington, KY 40506-0032. Offers PhD. *Degree requirements:* For doctorate, comprehensive exam, thesis/dissertation. *Entrance requirements:* For doctorate, GRE General Test, minimum undergraduate GPA of 2.75. Additional exam requirements/recommendations for international students: Required—TOEFL (minimum score 550 paper-based). Electronic applications accepted.

The University of Manchester, Faculty of Life Sciences, Manchester, United Kingdom. Offers adaptive organismal biology (M Phil, PhD); animal biology (M Phil, PhD); biochemistry (M Phil, PhD); bioinformatics (M Phil, PhD); biomolecular sciences (M Phil, PhD); biotechnology (M Phil, PhD); cell biology (M Phil, PhD); cell matrix research (M Phil, PhD); channels and transporters (M Phil, PhD); developmental biology (M Phil, PhD); Egyptology (M Phil, PhD); environmental biology (M Phil, PhD); evolutionary biology (M Phil, PhD); gene expression (M Phil, PhD); genetics (M Phil, PhD); history of science, technology and medicine (M Phil, PhD); immunology (M Phil, PhD); integrative neurobiology and behavior (M Phil, PhD); membrane trafficking (M Phil, PhD); microbiology (M Phil, PhD); molecular and cellular neuroscience (M Phil, PhD); molecular biology (M Phil, PhD); molecular cancer studies (M Phil, PhD); neuroscience (M Phil, PhD); ophthalmology (M Phil, PhD); optometry (M Phil, PhD); organelle function (M Phil, PhD); pharmacology (M Phil, PhD); physiology (M Phil, PhD); plant sciences (M Phil, PhD); stem cell research (M Phil, PhD); structural biology (M Phil, PhD); systems neuroscience (M Phil, PhD); toxicology (M Phil, PhD).

University of Maryland, College Park, Academic Affairs, College of Computer, Mathematical and Natural Sciences, Department of Cell Biology and Molecular Genetics, Program in Cell Biology and Molecular Genetics, College Park, MD 20742. Offers MS, PhD. *Students:* 24 full-time (12 women); includes 2 minority (both Asian, non-Hispanic/Latino), 8 international. In 2013, 2 master's, 11 doctorates awarded. *Degree requirements:* For master's, thesis; for doctorate, thesis/dissertation, exams. *Expenses:* Tuition, state resident: full-time $10,314; part-time $573 per credit hour. Tuition, nonresident: full-time $22,248; part-time $1236 per credit. *Required fees:* $1446; $403.15 per semester. Tuition and fees vary according to program. *Financial support:* In 2013–14, 1 fellowship with full tuition reimbursement (averaging $40,429 per year), 11 research assistantships (averaging $19,284 per year), 15 teaching assistantships (averaging $19,550 per year) were awarded. Financial award applicants required to submit FAFSA. *Faculty research:* Cytoskeletal activity, membrane biology, cell division, genetics and genomics, virology. *Unit head:* Norma Andrews, Chair, 301-405-8418, E-mail: andrewsn@umd.edu. *Application contact:* Dr. Charles A. Caramello, Dean of Graduate School, 301-405-0358, Fax: 301-314-9305, E-mail: ccaramel@umd.edu.

University of Massachusetts Worcester, Graduate School of Biomedical Sciences, Worcester, MA 01655-0115. Offers biochemistry and molecular pharmacology (PhD); bioinformatics and computational biology (PhD); cancer biology (PhD); cell biology (PhD); clinical and population health research (PhD); clinical investigation (MS); immunology and virology (PhD); interdisciplinary biomedical research (PhD); millennium (PhD); molecular genetics and microbiology (PhD); neuroscience (PhD); translational science (PhD); MD/PhD. *Faculty:* 1,388 full-time (521 women), 309 part-time/adjunct (198 women). *Students:* 385 full-time (210 women); includes 53 minority (13 Black or African American, non-Hispanic/Latino; 30 Asian, non-Hispanic/Latino; 10 Hispanic/Latino), 138 international. Average age 28. 491 applicants, 19% accepted, 39 enrolled. In 2013, 5 master's, 50 doctorates awarded. Terminal master's awarded for partial completion of doctoral program. *Median time to degree:* Of those who began their doctoral program in fall 2005, 67% received their degree in 8 years or less. *Degree requirements:* For master's, comprehensive exam, thesis; for doctorate, comprehensive exam, thesis/dissertation. *Entrance requirements:* For master's, MD, PhD, DVM, or PharmD; for doctorate, GRE General Test, bachelor's degree. Additional exam requirements/recommendations for international students: Required—TOEFL (minimum score 100 iBT) or IELTS (minimum score 7.5). *Application deadline:* For fall admission, 12/15 for domestic and international students; for spring admission, 5/15 for domestic students. Application fee: $80. Electronic applications accepted. *Expenses:* Contact institution. *Financial support:* In 2013–14, 431 students received support, including research assistantships with full tuition reimbursements available (averaging $29,500 per year); scholarships/grants, health care benefits, tuition waivers (full), and unspecified assistantships also available. Financial award application deadline: 5/16. *Faculty research:* RNA interference, cell/molecular/developmental biology, bioinformatics, clinical/translational research, infectious disease. *Total annual research expenditures:* $245.9 million. *Unit head:* Dr. Anthony Carruthers, Dean, 508-856-4135, E-mail: anthony.carruthers@umassmed.edu. *Application contact:* Dr. Kendall Knight, Associate Dean and Interim Director of Admissions and Recruitment, 508-856-5628, Fax: 508-856-3659, E-mail: kendall.knight@umassmed.edu.
Website: http://www.umassmed.edu/gsbs/

University of Pittsburgh, School of Medicine, Graduate Programs in Medicine, Molecular Genetics and Developmental Biology Graduate Program, Pittsburgh, PA 15260. Offers PhD. *Faculty:* 49 full-time (11 women). *Students:* 12 full-time (6 women); includes 1 minority (Native Hawaiian or other Pacific Islander, non-Hispanic/Latino), 2 international. Average age 27. 517 applicants, 13% accepted, 22 enrolled. In 2013, 3 doctorates awarded. *Degree requirements:* For doctorate, comprehensive exam, thesis/dissertation. *Entrance requirements:* For doctorate, GRE General Test, GRE Subject Test, minimum QPA of 3.0. Additional exam requirements/recommendations for international students: Required—TOEFL (minimum score 600 paper-based; 100 iBT), IELTS (minimum score 7). *Application deadline:* For fall admission, 1/1 priority date for domestic and international students. Application fee: $50. Electronic applications accepted. *Expenses:* Tuition, state resident: full-time $19,964; part-time $807 per credit. Tuition, nonresident: full-time $32,686; part-time $1337 per credit. *Required fees:* $740; $200. Tuition and fees vary according to program. *Financial support:* In 2013–14, 2 fellowships with full tuition reimbursements (averaging $26,010 per year), 9 research assistantships with full tuition reimbursements (averaging $26,010 per year), 1 teaching assistantship with full tuition reimbursement (averaging $26,010 per year) were awarded; institutionally sponsored loans, scholarships/grants, traineeships, health care benefits, and unspecified assistantships also available. *Faculty research:* Developmental and stem cell biology, DNA replication and repair, gene regulation and signal transduction, oncogenes and tumor suppressor genes, protein structure and molecular dynamics. *Unit head:* Dr. Kyle E. Orwig, Graduate Program Director, 412-641-2460, Fax: 412-641-3899, E-mail: korwig@mwri.magee.edu. *Application contact:* Graduate Studies Administrator, 412-648-8957, Fax: 412-648-1077, E-mail: gradstudies@medschool.pitt.edu.
Website: http://www.gradbiomed.pitt.edu/

University of Rhode Island, Graduate School, College of the Environment and Life Sciences, Department of Cell and Molecular Biology, Kingston, RI 02881. Offers biochemistry (MS, PhD); clinical laboratory sciences (MS), including biotechnology, clinical laboratory science, cytopathology; microbiology (MS, PhD); molecular genetics (MS, PhD). Part-time programs available. *Faculty:* 17 full-time (8 women), 2 part-time/adjunct (1 woman). *Students:* 19 full-time (11 women), 40 part-time (23 women); includes 14 minority (4 Black or African American, non-Hispanic/Latino; 1 American Indian or Alaska Native, non-Hispanic/Latino; 7 Asian, non-Hispanic/Latino; 2 Hispanic/Latino), 5 international. In 2013, 20 master's, 2 doctorates awarded. *Degree requirements:* For master's, comprehensive exam (for some programs), thesis optional; for doctorate, comprehensive exam, thesis/dissertation. *Entrance requirements:* For master's and doctorate, GRE, 2 letters of recommendation. Additional exam requirements/recommendations for international students: Required—TOEFL (minimum score 550 paper-based). *Application deadline:* For fall admission, 7/15 for domestic students, 2/1 for international students; for spring admission, 11/15 for domestic students, 7/15 for international students. Application fee: $65. Electronic applications accepted. *Expenses:* Tuition, state resident: full-time $11,532; part-time $641 per credit. Tuition, nonresident: full-time $23,606; part-time $1311 per credit. *Required fees:* $1388; $36 per credit. $35 per semester. One-time fee: $130. *Financial support:* In

2013–14, 5 research assistantships with full and partial tuition reimbursements (averaging $12,078 per year), 2 teaching assistantships with full and partial tuition reimbursements (averaging $11,883 per year) were awarded. Financial award application deadline: 2/1; financial award applicants required to submit FAFSA. *Faculty research:* Genomics. *Total annual research expenditures:* $6.7 million. *Unit head:* Dr. Gongqing Sun, Chairperson, 401-874-5937, Fax: 401-874-2202, E-mail: gsun@mail.uri.edu. *Application contact:* Graduate Admissions, 401-874-2872, E-mail: gradadm@etal.uri.edu.
Website: http://cels.uri.edu/cmb/

The University of Texas Health Science Center at Houston, Graduate School of Biomedical Sciences, Program in Human and Molecular Genetics, Houston, TX 77225-0036. Offers MS, PhD, MD/PhD. Terminal master's awarded for partial completion of doctoral program. *Degree requirements:* For master's, thesis; for doctorate, thesis/dissertation. *Entrance requirements:* For master's and doctorate, GRE General Test. Additional exam requirements/recommendations for international students: Required—TOEFL. Electronic applications accepted. *Expenses:* Tuition, state resident: full-time $3474; part-time $193 per credit hour. Tuition, nonresident: full-time $13,644; part-time $758 per credit hour. *Required fees:* $226.30; $87 per credit hour. *Faculty research:* Computational genomics, cancer genetics, complex disease genetics, medical genetics.

The University of Texas Health Science Center at Houston, Graduate School of Biomedical Sciences, Program in Microbiology and Molecular Genetics, Houston, TX 77225-0036. Offers MS, PhD, MD/PhD. Terminal master's awarded for partial completion of doctoral program. *Degree requirements:* For master's, thesis; for doctorate, thesis/dissertation. *Entrance requirements:* For master's and doctorate, GRE General Test. Additional exam requirements/recommendations for international students: Required—TOEFL. Electronic applications accepted. *Expenses:* Tuition, state resident: full-time $3474; part-time $193 per credit hour. Tuition, nonresident: full-time $13,644; part-time $758 per credit hour. *Required fees:* $226.30; $87 per credit hour. *Faculty research:* Disease causation, environmental signaling, gene regulation, cell growth and division, cell structure and architecture.

University of Toronto, Faculty of Medicine, Department of Molecular Genetics, Toronto, ON M5S 1A1, Canada. Offers genetic counseling (M Sc); molecular genetics (M Sc, PhD). *Degree requirements:* For master's, thesis; for doctorate, thesis/dissertation. *Entrance requirements:* For master's, B Sc or equivalent; for doctorate, M Sc or equivalent, minimum B+ average. Additional exam requirements/recommendations for international students: Required—TOEFL, IELTS (minimum score 7), Michigan English Language Assessment Battery (minimum score 85) or COPE (minimum score 4). Electronic applications accepted. *Faculty research:* Structural biology, developmental genetics, molecular medicine, genetic counseling.

University of Virginia, School of Medicine, Department of Biochemistry and Molecular Genetics, Charlottesville, VA 22903. Offers biochemistry (PhD); MD/PhD. *Faculty:* 24 full-time (3 women), 2 part-time/adjunct (both women). *Students:* 28 full-time (15 women); includes 4 minority (2 Hispanic/Latino; 2 Two or more races, non-Hispanic/Latino), 7 international. Average age 26. In 2013, 6 doctorates awarded. *Degree requirements:* For doctorate, thesis/dissertation, written research proposal and defense. *Entrance requirements:* For doctorate, GRE General Test, 3 letters of recommendation. Additional exam requirements/recommendations for international students: Recommended—TOEFL (minimum score 630 paper-based; 90 iBT). Application fee: $60. Electronic applications accepted. *Expenses:* Tuition, state resident: part-time $334 per credit hour. Tuition, nonresident: part-time $1224 per credit hour. *Financial support:* Fellowships, health care benefits, and tuition waivers (full) available. Financial award applicants required to submit FAFSA. *Unit head:* Anindya Dutta, Chair, 434-924-1940, Fax: 434-924-5069, E-mail: ad8q@virginia.edu. *Application contact:* Biomedical Sciences Graduate Studies, E-mail: bims@virginia.edu.
Website: http://www.virginia.edu/bmg/

Wake Forest University, School of Medicine and Graduate School of Arts and Sciences, Graduate Programs in Medicine, Molecular Genetics and Genomics Program, Winston-Salem, NC 27109. Offers PhD, MD/PhD. *Degree requirements:* For doctorate, thesis/dissertation. *Entrance requirements:* For doctorate, GRE General Test. Additional exam requirements/recommendations for international students: Required—TOEFL. Electronic applications accepted. *Faculty research:* Control of gene expression, molecular pathogenesis, protein biosynthesis, cell development, clinical cytogenetics.

Washington University in St. Louis, Graduate School of Arts and Sciences, Division of Biology and Biomedical Sciences, Program in Molecular Genetics and Genomics, St. Louis, MO 63130-4899. Offers PhD. *Degree requirements:* For doctorate, thesis/dissertation. *Entrance requirements:* For doctorate, GRE General Test, GRE Subject Test. Electronic applications accepted.

Wesleyan University, Graduate Studies, Department of Molecular Biology and Biochemistry, Middletown, CT 06459. Offers biochemistry (PhD); molecular biology (PhD); molecular biophysics (PhD); molecular genetics (PhD). *Degree requirements:* For doctorate, comprehensive exam, thesis/dissertation. *Entrance requirements:* For doctorate, GRE General Test, GRE Subject Test. Additional exam requirements/recommendations for international students: Required—TOEFL. Electronic applications accepted. *Faculty research:* The olfactory system and new frontiers in genome research, chromosome structure and gene expression.

Reproductive Biology

Cornell University, Graduate School, Graduate Fields of Comparative Biomedical Sciences, Field of Comparative Biomedical Sciences, Ithaca, NY 14853-0001. Offers cellular and molecular medicine (MS, PhD); developmental and reproductive biology (MS, PhD); infectious diseases (MS, PhD); population medicine and epidemiology (MS, PhD); structural and functional biology (MS, PhD). *Faculty:* 104 full-time (32 women). *Students:* 32 full-time (22 women); includes 3 minority (1 Asian, non-Hispanic/Latino; 2 Hispanic/Latino), 12 international. Average age 29. 47 applicants, 23% accepted, 6 enrolled. In 2013, 2 master's, 12 doctorates awarded. *Degree requirements:* For master's, thesis; for doctorate, comprehensive exam, thesis/dissertation. *Entrance requirements:* For master's and doctorate, GRE General Test, 2 letters of recommendation. Additional exam requirements/recommendations for international students: Required—TOEFL (minimum score 550 paper-based; 77 iBT). *Application deadline:* For fall admission, 12/15 for domestic students. Application fee: $95. Electronic applications accepted. *Financial support:* In 2013–14, 18 students received support, including 3 fellowships with full tuition reimbursements available, 14 research assistantships with full tuition reimbursements available, 1 teaching assistantship with full tuition reimbursement available; institutionally sponsored loans, scholarships/grants, health care benefits, tuition waivers (full and partial), and unspecified assistantships also available. Financial award applicants required to submit FAFSA. *Faculty research:* Receptors and signal transduction, viral and bacterial infectious diseases, tumor metastasis, clinical sciences/nutritional disease, developmental/neurological disorders. *Unit head:* Director of Graduate Studies, 607-253-3276, Fax: 607-253-3756. *Application contact:* Graduate Field Assistant, 607-253-3276, Fax: 607-253-3756, E-mail: graduate_edcvm@cornell.edu.
Website: http://www.gradschool.cornell.edu/fields.php?id-64&a-2

Eastern Virginia Medical School, Master's Program in Clinical Embryology and Andrology, Norfolk, VA 23501-1980. Offers MS. Postbaccalaureate distance learning degree programs offered (minimal on-campus study). *Faculty:* 12 full-time, 8 part-time/adjunct. *Students:* 44 full-time (35 women), 15 part-time (10 women); includes 28 minority (4 Black or African American, non-Hispanic/Latino; 21 Asian, non-Hispanic/Latino; 2 Hispanic/Latino; 1 Two or more races, non-Hispanic/Latino). 44 applicants, 27 enrolled. In 2013, 20 master's awarded. *Entrance requirements:* Additional exam requirements/recommendations for international students: Required—TOEFL (minimum score 550 paper-based; 80 iBT). *Application deadline:* For fall admission, 1/14 for domestic and international students. Applications are processed on a rolling basis. Application fee: $60. Electronic applications accepted. *Expenses:* Contact institution. *Unit head:* Dr. Jacob Mayer, Director, 757-446-5049, Fax: 757-446-5905. *Application contact:* Prof. Helena Russell, Administrator, 757-446-8482, Fax: 757-446-6179, E-mail: russelhi@evms.edu.
Website: http://evms.edu/education/masters_programs/clinical_embryology_andrology_program/

Queen's University at Kingston, School of Graduate Studies, Faculty of Health Sciences, Department of Anatomy and Cell Biology, Kingston, ON K7L 3N6, Canada. Offers biology of reproduction (M Sc, PhD); cancer (M Sc, PhD); cardiovascular pathophysiology (M Sc, PhD); cell and molecular biology (M Sc, PhD); drug metabolism (M Sc, PhD); endocrinology (M Sc, PhD); motor control (M Sc, PhD); neural regeneration (M Sc, PhD); neurophysiology (M Sc, PhD). Part-time programs available. *Degree requirements:* For master's, thesis; for doctorate, one foreign language, comprehensive exam, thesis/dissertation. *Entrance requirements:* Additional exam requirements/recommendations for international students: Required—TOEFL. Electronic applications accepted. *Faculty research:* Human kinetics, neuroscience, reproductive biology, cardiovascular.

Rutgers, The State University of New Jersey, New Brunswick, Graduate School-New Brunswick, Program in Endocrinology and Animal Biosciences, Piscataway, NJ 08854-8097. Offers MS, PhD. Terminal master's awarded for partial completion of doctoral program. *Degree requirements:* For master's, thesis; for doctorate, comprehensive exam, thesis/dissertation. *Entrance requirements:* For master's and doctorate, GRE General Test. Additional exam requirements/recommendations for international students: Required—TOEFL. Electronic applications accepted. *Faculty research:* Comparative and behavioral endocrinology, epigenetic regulation of the endocrine system, exercise physiology and immunology, fetal and neonatal developmental programming, mammary gland biology and breast cancer, neuroendocrinology and alcohol studies, reproductive and developmental toxicology.

Tufts University, Cummings School of Veterinary Medicine, North Grafton, MA 01536. Offers animals and public policy (MS); biomedical sciences (PhD), including digestive diseases, infectious diseases, neuroscience and reproductive biology, pathology; conservation medicine (MS); veterinary medicine (DVM); DVM/MPH; DVM/MS. *Accreditation:* AVMA (one or more programs are accredited). *Faculty:* 98 full-time (45 women), 13 part-time/adjunct (7 women). *Students:* 426 full-time (364 women); includes 60 minority (5 Black or African American, non-Hispanic/Latino; 1 American Indian or Alaska Native, non-Hispanic/Latino; 32 Asian, non-Hispanic/Latino; 20 Hispanic/Latino; 2 Two or more races, non-Hispanic/Latino), 4 international. Average age 25. 899 applicants, 29% accepted, 119 enrolled. In 2013, 85 master's, 2 doctorates awarded. *Degree requirements:* For master's, thesis (for some programs); for doctorate, comprehensive exam, thesis/dissertation (for some programs). *Entrance requirements:* For master's and doctorate, GRE General Test. Additional exam requirements/recommendations for international students: Required—TOEFL or IELTS. *Application deadline:* For fall admission, 11/1 for domestic and international students. Application fee: $70. Electronic applications accepted. *Expenses:* Contact institution. *Financial support:* In 2013–14, 230 students received support, including 7 research assistantships with full tuition reimbursements available (averaging $25,000 per year), 6 teaching assistantships (averaging $5,000 per year); career-related internships or fieldwork, Federal Work-Study, institutionally sponsored loans, scholarships/grants, and institutional aid awards, health care benefits for PhD students also available. Financial award application deadline: 4/15; financial award applicants required to submit FAFSA. *Faculty research:* Oncology, veterinary ethics, international veterinary medicine, veterinary genomics, pathogenesis of Clostridium difficile, wildlife fertility control. *Unit head:* Dr. Deborah T. Kochevar, Dean, 508-839-5302, Fax: 508-839-2953, E-mail: deborah.kochevar@tufts.edu. *Application contact:* Rebecca Russo, Director of Admissions, 508-839-7920, Fax: 508-887-4820, E-mail: vetadmissions@tufts.edu.
Website: http://www.tufts.edu/

The University of British Columbia, Faculty of Medicine, Department of Obstetrics and Gynecology, Program in Reproductive and Developmental Sciences, Vancouver, BC V6H 3N1, Canada. Offers M Sc, PhD. Part-time programs available. Terminal master's awarded for partial completion of doctoral program. *Degree requirements:* For master's, thesis; for doctorate, thesis/dissertation. *Entrance requirements:* For master's, B Sc or equivalent, MD, DVM, DDS; for doctorate, B Sc with first class honors, M Sc, MD, DVM, DDS. Additional exam requirements/recommendations for international students: Required—TOEFL (minimum score 580 paper-based; 80 iBT), IELTS (minimum score 7). Electronic applications accepted. *Expenses: Tuition, area resident:* Full-time $8000 Canadian dollars. *Faculty research:* Reproductive and placental endocrinology; immunology of reproductive, fertilization, and embryonic development; perinatal metabolism; neonatal development.

University of Hawaii at Manoa, John A. Burns School of Medicine, Program in Developmental and Reproductive Biology, Honolulu, HI 96813. Offers MS, PhD. Part-time programs available. *Degree requirements:* For doctorate, thesis/dissertation. *Entrance requirements:* For doctorate, GRE General Test, GRE Subject Test. Additional exam requirements/recommendations for international students: Recommended—

TOEFL (minimum score 560 paper-based), IELTS (minimum score 5). *Faculty research:* Biology of gametes and fertilization, reproductive endocrinology.

University of Saskatchewan, College of Medicine, Department of Obstetrics, Gynecology and Reproductive Services, Saskatoon, SK S7N 5A2, Canada. Offers M Sc, PhD. *Degree requirements:* For master's, thesis; for doctorate, thesis/dissertation. *Entrance requirements:* Additional exam requirements/recommendations for international students: Required—TOEFL. *Expenses: Tuition, area resident:* Full-time $3585 Canadian dollars; part-time $585 Canadian dollars per course. Tuition, nonresident: part-time $877 Canadian dollars per course. *International tuition:* $5377 Canadian dollars full-time. *Required fees:* $889.51 Canadian dollars.

University of Wyoming, College of Agriculture and Natural Resources, Department of Animal Sciences, Program in Reproductive Biology, Laramie, WY 82071. Offers MS, PhD. *Degree requirements:* For master's, thesis; for doctorate, thesis/dissertation. *Entrance requirements:* For master's, GRE General Test, minimum GPA of 3.0; for doctorate, GRE General Test, minimum GPA of 3.0 or MS degree. Additional exam requirements/recommendations for international students: Required—TOEFL. *Faculty research:* Fetal programming, chemical suppression, ovaria function, genetics.

Wayne State University, School of Medicine, Graduate Programs in Medicine, Department of Physiology, Detroit, MI 48202. Offers physiology (MS, PhD); reproductive sciences (PhD); MD/PhD. *Students:* 37 full-time (22 women), 8 part-time (6 women); includes 11 minority (3 Black or African American, non-Hispanic/Latino; 3 Asian, non-Hispanic/Latino; 3 Hispanic/Latino; 1 Native Hawaiian or other Pacific Islander, non-Hispanic/Latino; 1 Two or more races, non-Hispanic/Latino), 15 international. Average age 29. 50 applicants, 20% accepted, 8 enrolled. In 2013, 6 master's, 1 doctorate awarded. *Degree requirements:* For master's, thesis; for doctorate, thesis/dissertation. *Entrance requirements:* For master's, GRE General Test, minimum GPA of 2.75, personal statement, resume, three letters of recommendation, current curriculum vitae or resume, admission to the Graduate School; for doctorate, GRE General Test, minimum GPA of 3.0, personal statement, resume, three letters of recommendation, current curriculum vitae or resume, admission to the Graduate School. Additional exam requirements/recommendations for international students: Recommended—TOEFL (minimum score 600 paper-based; 100 iBT). *Application deadline:* For fall admission, 2/1 for domestic and international students; for winter admission, 10/1 for domestic students, 9/1 for international students; for spring admission, 2/1 for domestic students, 1/1 for international students. Application fee: $0. Electronic applications accepted. *Expenses:* Contact institution. *Financial support:* In 2013–14, 23 students received support, including 10 fellowships with tuition reimbursements available (averaging $22,521 per year), 29 research assistantships with tuition reimbursements available (averaging $22,521 per year); teaching assistantships, scholarships/grants, and unspecified assistantships also available. Support available to part-time students. Financial award application deadline: 3/31; financial award applicants required to submit FAFSA. *Faculty research:* Regulation of brain blood flow, mechanism of hormone action, regulation of pituitary hormone secretion, regulation of cellular membranes, nano biotechnology. *Unit head:* Dr. Douglas Yingst, Graduate Program Director, 313-577-1548, E-mail: dyingst@med.wayne.edu.
Website: http://physiology.med.wayne.edu/phd-physiology/index.php

West Virginia University, Davis College of Agriculture, Forestry and Consumer Sciences, Interdisciplinary Program in Genetics and Developmental Biology, Morgantown, WV 26506. Offers animal breeding (MS, PhD); biochemical and molecular genetics (MS, PhD); cytogenetics (MS, PhD); descriptive embryology (MS, PhD); developmental genetics (MS); experimental morphogenesis/teratology (MS); human genetics (MS, PhD); immunogenetics (MS, PhD); life cycles of animals and plants (MS, PhD); molecular aspects of development (MS, PhD); mutagenesis (MS, PhD); oncology (MS, PhD); plant genetics (MS, PhD); population and quantitative genetics (MS, PhD); regeneration (MS, PhD); teratology (PhD); toxicology (MS, PhD). *Degree requirements:* For master's, thesis; for doctorate, comprehensive exam, thesis/dissertation. *Entrance requirements:* For master's, GRE or MCAT, minimum GPA of 2.75. Additional exam requirements/recommendations for international students: Required—TOEFL.

Teratology

West Virginia University, Davis College of Agriculture, Forestry and Consumer Sciences, Interdisciplinary Program in Genetics and Developmental Biology, Morgantown, WV 26506. Offers animal breeding (MS, PhD); biochemical and molecular genetics (MS, PhD); cytogenetics (MS, PhD); descriptive embryology (MS, PhD); developmental genetics (MS); experimental morphogenesis/teratology (MS); human genetics (MS, PhD); immunogenetics (MS, PhD); life cycles of animals and plants (MS, PhD); molecular aspects of development (MS, PhD); mutagenesis (MS, PhD); oncology (MS, PhD); plant genetics (MS, PhD); population and quantitative genetics (MS, PhD); regeneration (MS, PhD); teratology (PhD); toxicology (MS, PhD). *Degree requirements:* For master's, thesis; for doctorate, comprehensive exam, thesis/dissertation. *Entrance requirements:* For master's, GRE or MCAT, minimum GPA of 2.75. Additional exam requirements/recommendations for international students: Required—TOEFL.

UCONN HEALTH

Graduate Program in Genetics and Developmental Biology

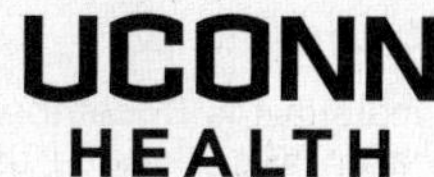

Program of Study

The genetics and developmental biology graduate program provides students with fundamental interdisciplinary training in modern molecular genetics and developmental biology, emphasizing cellular and molecular aspects as well as tissue interactions. The program is intended for students pursuing a Ph.D. degree and prepares students to compete for job opportunities in traditional medical and dental school departments as well as a productive research career in either academia or industry. Combined M.D./Ph.D. and D.M.D/Ph.D. programs are also available. Students are encouraged to obtain in-depth training through research and courses in biochemistry, molecular biology, cell biology, developmental biology, and genetics. Faculty members are from several basic science and clinical departments and study a wide range of organisms including yeast, worms, fruit flies, mice, and humans. Areas of research include the biology of human embryonic stem cells, mapping and cloning of genes responsible for human disease, RNA processing (including RNA editing, alternative splicing, antisense regulation, and RNA interference), the molecular mechanisms of aging, signal transduction pathways, microbial pathogenesis, developmental neurobiology, cell differentiation, musculoskeletal development, morphogenesis and pattern formation, reproductive biology, and endocrinology.

Research Facilities

The Department of Genetics and Developmental Biology is the academic home of the genetics and developmental biology graduate program which houses equipment and facilities for mouse transgenics, ES cell manipulation, DNA microarrays, nucleic acid sequencing, fluorescence microscopy, and digital imaging. Students also have ready access to first-rate flow cytometry and confocal microscopy facilities. Other institutional resources include a computer center and the Lyman Maynard Stowe Library which contains approximately 200,000 volumes and subscribes to more than 1,700 current periodicals. Students of the program therefore have an excellent opportunity for research and training in cutting-edge areas of genetics and developmental biology.

Financial Aid

Support for doctoral students engaged in full-time degree programs at UConn Health is provided on a competitive basis. Graduate research assistantships for 2014–15 provide a stipend of $29,000 per year, which includes a waiver of tuition/most University fees for the fall and spring semesters and the option of participating in a student health insurance plan. While financial aid is offered competitively, UConn Health makes every possible effort to address the financial needs of all students during their period of training.

Cost of Study

For 2014–15, tuition is $12,202 per year for full-time students who are Connecticut residents and $32,258 per year for full-time out-of-state residents. General University fees are added to the cost of tuition for students who do not receive a tuition waiver. These costs are usually met by traineeships or research assistantships for doctoral students.

Living and Housing Costs

There is a wide range of affordable housing options in the greater Hartford area within easy commuting distance of the campus, including an extensive complex that is adjacent to UConn Health. Costs range from $700 to $1,000 per month for a one-bedroom unit; 2 or more students sharing an apartment usually pay less. University housing is not available on campus.

Student Group

At UCHC, there are about 500 students in the Schools of Medicine and Dental Medicine, 150 Ph.D. students, and 50 postdoctoral fellows. There are no restrictions on the admission of out-of-state graduate students.

Location

UConn Health is located in the historic town of Farmington, Connecticut. Set in the beautiful New England countryside on a hill overlooking the Farmington Valley, it is close to ski areas, hiking trails, and facilities for boating, fishing, and swimming. Connecticut's capital city of Hartford, 7 miles east of Farmington, is the center of an urban region of approximately 800,000 people. The beaches of the Long Island Sound are about 50 minutes away to the south, and the beautiful Berkshires are a short drive to the northwest. New York City and Boston can be reached within 2½ hours by car. Hartford is the home of the acclaimed Hartford Stage Company, TheatreWorks, the Hartford Symphony and Chamber orchestras, two ballet companies, an opera company, the Wadsworth Athenaeum (the oldest public art museum in the nation), the Mark Twain house, the Hartford Civic Center, and many other interesting cultural and recreational facilities. The area is also home to several branches of the University of Connecticut, Trinity College, and the University of Hartford, which includes the Hartt School of Music. Bradley International Airport (about 30 minutes from campus) serves the Hartford/Springfield area with frequent airline connections to major cities in this country and abroad. Frequent bus and rail service is also available from Hartford.

The Health Center

The 200-acre UConn Health campus at Farmington houses a division of the University of Connecticut Graduate School, as well as the Schools of Medicine and Dental Medicine. The campus also includes the John Dempsey Hospital, associated clinics, and extensive medical research facilities, all in a centralized facility with more than 1 million square feet of floor space. The Academic Research Building, built in 1999, is an impressive eleven-story structure providing 170,000 square feet of laboratory space. In addition, renovations are underway in the main Laboratory building, converting existing lab space to state-of-the-art open lab areas. The faculty includes more than 260 full-time members. The institution has a strong commitment to graduate study within an environment that promotes social and intellectual interaction among the various educational programs. Graduate students are represented on various administrative committees concerned with curricular affairs, and the Graduate Student Organization (GSO) represents graduate students' needs and concerns to the faculty and administration, in addition to fostering social contact among graduate students at UConn Health.

Applying

Applications for admission should be submitted via the online application system and should be filed together with transcripts, three letters of recommendation, a personal statement, and recent results from the General Test of the Graduate Record Examinations. International students must take the Test of English as a Foreign Language (TOEFL) to satisfy Graduate School requirements. The deadline for completed applications and receipt of all supplemental materials is **December 1**. Please note that GRE and TOEFL exams taken after the due date will not be accepted for consideration for admission. In accordance with the laws of the state of Connecticut and of the United States, UConn Health does not discriminate against any person in its educational and employment activities on the grounds of race, color, creed, national origin, sex, age, or physical disability.

Correspondence and Information

Graduate Admissions Office
Ph.D. in Biomedical Science Program
UConn Health
263 Farmington Ave., MC 3906
Farmington, Connecticut 06030-3906
United States
Phone: 860-679-4509
E-mail: BiomedSciAdmissions@uchc.edu
Website: http://grad.uchc.edu/prospective/programs/phd_biosci/index.html

THE FACULTY AND THEIR RESEARCH

Hector Leonardo Aguila, Ph.D., Associate Professor of Immunology. Hematopoiesis and bone marrow microenvironment; lymphoid cell development; stem cell biology.

Andrew Arnold, M.D., Professor of Medicine and Murray-Heilig Chair in Molecular Medicine. Molecular genetic underpinnings of tumors of the endocrine glands; role of the cyclin D1 oncogene.

Michael Blinov, Ph.D., Assistant Professor of Genetics and Developmental Biology, Modeling of signal transcription systems and protein-DNA interactions; bioinformatics: data mining and visualization; developing software tools and mathematical methods for rule-based modeling of signal transduction systems.

Gordon Carmichael, Ph.D., Professor of Genetics and Developmental Biology. Regulation of gene expression in eukaryotes.

Stormy J. Chamberlain, Ph.D., Assistant Professor of Genetics and Developmental Biology. Human induced pluripotent stem (iPS) cell models to study 15q11-q13 imprinting disorders.

Jeffrey Chuang, Ph.D., Associate Professor, Genetics and Developmental Biology. Computational biology and bioinformatics; genomics, gene regulation, molecular evolution, and metabolomics; post-transcriptional regulation and cancer genomics.

Kevin Claffey, Ph.D., Assistant Professor of Cell Biology. Angiogenesis in cancer progression and metastasis; vascular endothelial growth factor (VEGF) expression; hypoxia-mediated gene regulation.

Soheil (Sam) Dadras, M.D., Ph.D., Associate Professor of Dermatology, and Genetics and Developmental Biology, Discovery of small RNAs (including microRNA) as novel biomarkers in human melanoma progression and metastasis using next generation sequencing.

Asis Das, Ph.D., Professor of Microbiology. Basic genetic and biomechanical mechanisms that govern the elongation-termination and decision in transcription.

Caroline N. Dealy, Ph.D., Associate Professor of Anatomy. Roles of various growth factors and signaling molecules, particularly IGF-I and insulin, in the regulation of chick limb development.

Paul Epstein, Ph.D., Associate Professor of Pharmacology. Receptor signal transduction, second messengers, and protein phosphorylation in control of cell growth and regulation; purification and regulation of cyclic nucleotide phosphodiesterases; role of calmodulin in mediating Ca^{2+}-dependent cell processes.

Guo-Hua Fong, Ph.D., Associate Professor of Cell Biology. Developmental biology of the vascular system, VEGF-A receptor signal transduction, embryonic stem cells, and gene knock-out in mice.

Brenton R. Graveley, Ph.D., Professor of Genetics and Developmental Biology. Regulation of alternative splicing in the mammalian nervous system and mechanisms of alternative splicing.

Arthur Günzl, Ph.D., Professor, Center for Microbial Pathogenesis. Transcription and antigenic variation in the mammalian parasite *Trypanosoma brucei*.

Marc Hansen, Ph.D., Professor of Medicine. Molecular genetics of osteosarcoma and related bone diseases.

Laura Haynes, Ph.D., Professor of Immunology. Rochester. Influence of aging on CD4 T cell function and how this impacts responses to infection and vaccination.

Laurinda Jaffe, Ph.D., Professor of Cell Biology. Physiology of fertilization.

Barbara Kream, Ph.D., Professor of Medicine. Hormonal regulation of collagen gene expression in bone.

George Kuchel, M.D., Professor of Medicine. Role of hormones and cytokines in geriatric disability. Pathogenesis of impaired detrusor contractility and urinary retention. Molecular mechanisms of bladder muscle survival.

Marc Lalande, Ph.D., Professor of Genetics and Developmental Biology. Genomic imprinting; Angelman syndrome; mechanism of tissue-specific silencing of the Angelman ubiquitin ligase in mouse and human.

James Li, Ph.D., Assistant Professor of Genetics and Developmental Biology. Identifying the molecular mechanisms underlying formation of the mammalian cerebellum.

Alexander Lichtler, Ph.D., Associate Professor of Pediatrics. Regulation of collagen gene transcription; retrovirus vectors; role of homeobox genes in limb development.

Bruce Mayer, Ph.D., Professor of Genetics and Developmental Biology. Biologically relevant Nck-interacting proteins.

Mina Mina, D.M.D., Ph.D., Associate Professor of Pediatric Dentistry. Characterization of genetic and epigenetic influences involved in pattern formation and skeletogenesis of the chick mandible and mouse tooth germ.

William Mohler, Ph.D., Associate Professor of Genetics and Developmental Biology. Molecular and cellular mechanisms of cell fusion.

John Peluso, Ph.D., Professor of Cell Biology. Control of ovarian follicle growth steroidogenesis in vitro; proto-oncogene expression and ovarian follicular growth.

Carol C. Pilbeam, Ph.D., M.D., Professor of Medicine; Mechanisms of regulation of bone formation and resorption.

Justin D. Radolf, M.D., Professor of Medicine and Genetics and Developmental Biology. Molecular pathogenesis and immunobiology of spirochetal infections.

Blanka Rogina, Ph.D., Associate Professor of Genetics and Developmental Biology. Molecular mechanism underlying aging process in *Drosophila melanogaster.*

Daniel W. Rosenberg, Ph.D., Professor of Medicine. Molecular genetics of colorectal cancer; signaling pathways in the development of tumors; toxicogenomics,

Edward F. Rossomando, D.D.S., Ph.D., Professor of BioStructure and Function. Control of gene expression in tumor and nontumor cell lines in response to stimulation by monokines; coding, transmission, and processing of environmental signals in normal and abnormal development.

Yijun Ruan, Ph.D., Professor of Genetics and Developmental Biology. Elucidating the structures and dynamics of all functional DNA elements in complex genomes through DNA sequencing analysis of genetic variations in genomes and transcriptomes.

Archana Sanjay, Ph.D., Assistant Professor of Orthopaedic Surgery, School of Medicine. Regulation of bone remodeling; examining signaling pathways that regulate osteoblast and osteoclast differentiation and function.

Mansoor Sarfarazi, Ph.D., Professor of Surgery. Positional mapping and mutation analysis of human genetic disorders; primary open angle glaucoma; primary congenital glaucoma; synpolydactyly; dyslexia; mitral valve prolapse and ascending aortic aneurysm.

Bruce White, Ph.D., Professor of Physiology. Control of prolactin gene expression at pretranslational level in GH3 cells; control of aromatase gene expression in ovarian and testicular tissues.

Ji Yu, Ph.D., Associate Professor of Genetics and Developmental Biology; Optical imaging technology; regulation mechanisms in dendritic RNA translation; cytoskeletal dynamics.

Section 11
Marine Biology

This section contains a directory of institutions offering graduate work in marine biology. Additional information about programs listed in the directory may be obtained by writing directly to the dean of a graduate school or chair of a department at the address given in the directory.

For programs offering related work, see also in this book *Biological and Biomedical Sciences* and *Zoology*. In another guide in this series:

Graduate Programs in the Physical Sciences, Mathematics, Agricultural Sciences, the Environment & Natural Resources

See *Marine Sciences and Oceanography*

CONTENTS

Program Directory

Marine Biology

College of Charleston, Graduate School, School of Sciences and Mathematics, Program in Marine Biology, Charleston, SC 29412. Offers MS. *Degree requirements:* For master's, comprehensive exam, thesis. *Entrance requirements:* For master's, GRE General Test, 3 letters of recommendation. Additional exam requirements/recommendations for international students: Required—TOEFL (minimum score 81 iBT). Electronic applications accepted. *Faculty research:* Ecology, environmental physiology, marine genomics, bioinformatics, toxicology, cell biology, population biology, fisheries science, animal physiology, biodiversity, estuarine ecology, evolution and systematics, microbial processes, plant physiology, immunology.

Florida Institute of Technology, Graduate Programs, College of Science, Department of Biological Sciences, Program in Ecology, Melbourne, FL 32901-6975. Offers MS. Part-time programs available. *Faculty:* 16 full-time (1 woman), 1 (woman) part-time/adjunct. *Students:* 5 full-time (2 women), 1 (woman) part-time; includes 1 minority (Two or more races, non-Hispanic/Latino). Average age 25. 7 applicants, 29% accepted, 2 enrolled. In 2013, 3 master's awarded. *Degree requirements:* For master's, thesis, research, seminar, internship or summer lab. *Entrance requirements:* For master's, GRE General Test, minimum GPA of 3.0, 3 letters of recommendation, statement of objectives. Additional exam requirements/recommendations for international students: Required—TOEFL (minimum score 550 paper-based; 79 iBT). *Application deadline:* For fall admission, 3/15 for domestic students; for spring admission, 10/1 for domestic students. Applications are processed on a rolling basis. Electronic applications accepted. *Expenses: Tuition:* Full-time $20,214; part-time $1123 per credit. Tuition and fees vary according to campus/location. *Financial support:* Career-related internships or fieldwork, institutionally sponsored loans, tuition waivers (partial), unspecified assistantships, and tuition remissions available. Support available to part-time students. Financial award application deadline: 3/1; financial award applicants required to submit FAFSA. *Faculty research:* Endangered or threatened avian and mammalian species, hydroacoustics and feeding preference of the West Indian manatee, habitat preference of the Florida scrub jay. *Total annual research expenditures:* $1.4 million. *Unit head:* Dr. Richard B. Aronson, Department Head, 321-674-8034, Fax: 321-674-7238, E-mail: raronson@fit.edu. *Application contact:* Cheryl A. Brown, Associate Director of Graduate Admission, 321-674-7581, Fax: 321-723-9468, E-mail: cbrown@fit.edu.
Website: http://www.fit.edu/programs/8021/ms-biological-science-ecology

Memorial University of Newfoundland, School of Graduate Studies, Department of Biology, St. John's, NL A1C 5S7, Canada. Offers biology (M Sc, PhD); marine biology (M Sc, PhD). Part-time programs available. *Degree requirements:* For master's, thesis; for doctorate, comprehensive exam, thesis/dissertation, oral defense of thesis. *Entrance requirements:* For master's, honors degree (minimum 2nd class standing) in related field. Electronic applications accepted. *Faculty research:* Northern flora and fauna, especially cold ocean and boreal environments.

Nicholls State University, Graduate Studies, College of Arts and Sciences, Department of Biological Sciences, Thibodaux, LA 70310. Offers marine and environmental biology (MS). Part-time programs available. *Degree requirements:* For master's, comprehensive exam, thesis. *Entrance requirements:* For master's, GRE. Additional exam requirements/recommendations for international students: Required—TOEFL (minimum score 600 paper-based). *Faculty research:* Bioremediation, ecology, public health, biotechnology, physiology.

Northeastern University, College of Science, Department of Biology, Boston, MA 02115-5096. Offers bioinformatics (MS, PSM); biology (MS, PhD); biotechnology (MS, PSM); marine biology (MS). Terminal master's awarded for partial completion of doctoral program. *Degree requirements:* For master's, thesis (for some programs); for doctorate, thesis/dissertation, qualifying exam. *Entrance requirements:* For master's and doctorate, GRE General Test. Additional exam requirements/recommendations for international students: Required—TOEFL (minimum score 100 iBT). Electronic applications accepted. *Faculty research:* Biochemistry, marine sciences, molecular biology, microbiology and immunology neurobiology, cellular and molecular biology, biochemistry, marine biochemistry and ecology, microbiology, neurobiology, biotechnology.

Nova Southeastern University, Oceanographic Center, Fort Lauderdale, FL 33314-7796. Offers biological sciences (MS); coastal studies (Certificate); coastal zone management (MS); marine and coastal climate change (Certificate); marine and coastal studies (MA); marine biology (MS); marine biology and oceanography (PhD), including marine biology, oceanography; marine environmental sciences (MS). Part-time and evening/weekend programs available. Postbaccalaureate distance learning degree programs offered (no on-campus study). *Faculty:* 16 full-time (2 women), 22 part-time/adjunct (11 women). *Students:* 121 full-time (74 women), 128 part-time (83 women); includes 33 minority (6 Black or African American, non-Hispanic/Latino; 1 American Indian or Alaska Native, non-Hispanic/Latino; 7 Asian, non-Hispanic/Latino; 11 Hispanic/Latino; 8 Two or more races, non-Hispanic/Latino), 5 international. Average age 29. 79 applicants, 57% accepted, 26 enrolled. In 2013, 38 master's, 8 other advanced degrees awarded. *Degree requirements:* For master's, thesis; for doctorate, comprehensive exam, thesis/dissertation, departmental qualifying exam. *Entrance requirements:* For master's, GRE General Test, 3 letters of recommendation, BS/BA in natural science (for marine biology program), BS/BA in biology (for biological sciences program), minor in the natural sciences or equivalent (for coastal zone management and marine environmental sciences); for doctorate, GRE General Test, master's degree. Additional exam requirements/recommendations for international students: Required—TOEFL (minimum score 550 paper-based). *Application deadline:* Applications are processed on a rolling basis. Application fee: $50. *Expenses:* Contact institution. *Financial support:* In 2013–14, 2 fellowships with full and partial tuition reimbursements (averaging $16,300 per year), 50 research assistantships with full and partial tuition reimbursements (averaging $19,000 per year) were awarded; teaching assistantships, career-related internships or fieldwork, Federal Work-Study, scholarships/grants, health care benefits, tuition waivers (full and partial), and unspecified assistantships also available. Support available to part-time students. Financial award applicants required to submit FAFSA. *Faculty research:* Physical, geological, chemical, and biological oceanography. *Unit head:* Dr. Richard Dodge, Dean, 954-262-3600, Fax: 954-262-4020, E-mail: dodge@nsu.nova.edu. *Application contact:* Dr. Richard Spieler, Associate Dean of Academic Programs, 954-262-3600, Fax: 954-262-4020, E-mail: spieler@nova.edu.
Website: http://www.nova.edu/ocean/

Princeton University, Graduate School, Department of Geosciences, Princeton, NJ 08544-1019. Offers atmospheric and oceanic sciences (PhD); geosciences (PhD); ocean sciences and marine biology (PhD). *Degree requirements:* For doctorate, one foreign language, thesis/dissertation. *Entrance requirements:* For doctorate, GRE General Test. Additional exam requirements/recommendations for international students: Required—TOEFL (minimum score 600 paper-based). Electronic applications accepted. *Faculty research:* Biogeochemistry, climate science, earth history, regional geology and tectonics, solid–earth geophysics.

Rutgers, The State University of New Jersey, New Brunswick, Graduate School-New Brunswick, Department of Environmental Sciences, Piscataway, NJ 08854-8097. Offers air pollution and resources (MS, PhD); aquatic biology (MS, PhD); aquatic chemistry (MS, PhD); atmospheric science (MS, PhD); chemistry and physics of aerosol and hydrosol systems (MS, PhD); environmental chemistry (MS, PhD); environmental microbiology (MS, PhD); environmental toxicology (PhD); exposure assessment (PhD); fate and effects of pollutants (MS, PhD); pollution prevention and control (MS, PhD); water and wastewater treatment (MS, PhD); water resources (MS, PhD). Terminal master's awarded for partial completion of doctoral program. *Degree requirements:* For master's, comprehensive exam, thesis or alternative, oral final exam; for doctorate, comprehensive exam, thesis/dissertation, thesis defense, qualifying exam. *Entrance requirements:* For master's and doctorate, GRE General Test. Additional exam requirements/recommendations for international students: Required—TOEFL. Electronic applications accepted. *Faculty research:* Biological waste treatment; contaminant fate and transport; air, soil and water quality.

San Francisco State University, Division of Graduate Studies, College of Science and Engineering, Department of Biology, Program in Marine Biology, San Francisco, CA 94132-1722. Offers MS. *Unit head:* Dr. Jonathon Stillman, Program Coordinator, 415-338-3790, E-mail: stillmaj@sfsu.edu. *Application contact:* Dr. Robert Patterson, Graduate Coordinator, 415-338-1237, E-mail: patters@sfsu.edu.
Website: http://biology.sfsu.edu/graduate/marine_biology

San Francisco State University, Division of Graduate Studies, College of Science and Engineering, Department of Biology, Program in Marine Science, San Francisco, CA 94132-1722. Offers MS. Program offered through the Moss Landing Marine Laboratories. *Application deadline:* Applications are processed on a rolling basis. *Unit head:* Dr. Jonathon Stillman, Program Coordinator, 415-338-3790, E-mail: stillmaj@sfsu.edu. *Application contact:* Dr. Robert Patterson, Graduate Coordinator, 415-338-1237, E-mail: patters@sfsu.edu.
Website: http://www.sfsu.edu/~bulletin/current/programs/marines.htm#282

Texas A&M University at Galveston, Department of Marine Biology, Galveston, TX 77553-1675. Offers MS, PhD. *Faculty:* 33 full-time (7 women). *Students:* 36 full-time (23 women), 7 part-time (4 women); includes 4 minority (1 Black or African American, non-Hispanic/Latino; 2 Hispanic/Latino; 1 Two or more races, non-Hispanic/Latino), 9 international. Average age 28. 42 applicants, 26% accepted, 11 enrolled. Terminal master's awarded for partial completion of doctoral program. *Degree requirements:* For master's, comprehensive exam (for some programs), thesis (for some programs); for doctorate, comprehensive exam, thesis/dissertation. *Entrance requirements:* For master's and doctorate, GRE. Additional exam requirements/recommendations for international students: Required—TOEFL (minimum score 550 paper-based; 80 iBT), IELTS (minimum score 6). *Application deadline:* For fall admission, 5/15 for domestic students, 5/1 for international students; for spring admission, 10/15 for domestic and international students. Application fee: $50 ($90 for international students). Electronic applications accepted. *Financial support:* In 2013–14, 7 research assistantships, 19 teaching assistantships were awarded; scholarships/grants, health care benefits, and unspecified assistantships also available. Financial award applicants required to submit FAFSA. *Faculty research:* Fisheries, coastal and wetland ecologies, phytoplankton, marine mammals, seafood safety, marine invertebrates and marine biospeleology. *Total annual research expenditures:* $2 million. *Unit head:* Dr. Gilbert Rowe, Professor/Chair of Marine Biology Interdisciplinary Program, 409-740-4847, E-mail: roweg@tamug.edu. *Application contact:* Nicole Kinslow, Director of Graduate Studies, 409-740-4937, Fax: 409-740-4754, E-mail: kinslown@tamug.edu.

Texas State University, Graduate School, College of Science and Engineering, Department of Biology, Program in Aquatic Resources, San Marcos, TX 78666. Offers MS, PhD. *Faculty:* 21 full-time (4 women). *Students:* 35 full-time (16 women), 5 part-time (1 woman); includes 4 minority (1 Asian, non-Hispanic/Latino; 3 Hispanic/Latino), 9 international. Average age 32. 16 applicants, 81% accepted, 5 enrolled. In 2013, 12 master's, 10 doctorates awarded. *Degree requirements:* For master's, comprehensive exam, thesis, 3 seminars. *Entrance requirements:* For master's, GRE General Test, previous course work in biology, minimum GPA of 2.75 in last 60 hours of course work; for doctorate, GRE, baccalaureate degree from regionally-accredited university; master's degree in biology, chemistry, engineering, geology, or related natural science field with minimum GPA of 3.25. Additional exam requirements/recommendations for international students: Required—TOEFL (minimum score 550 paper-based; 78 iBT). *Application deadline:* For fall admission, 6/15 priority date for domestic students, 6/1 priority date for international students; for spring admission, 10/15 priority date for domestic students, 10/1 priority date for international students. Applications are processed on a rolling basis. Application fee: $40 ($90 for international students). Electronic applications accepted. *Expenses:* Tuition, state resident: full-time $6663; part-time $278 per credit hour. Tuition, nonresident: full-time $15,159; part-time $632 per credit hour. *Required fees:* $1872; $54 per credit hour. $306 per term. Tuition and fees vary according to course load. *Financial support:* In 2013–14, 24 students received support, including 7 research assistantships (averaging $24,700 per year), 26 teaching assistantships (averaging $23,079 per year); Federal Work-Study, institutionally sponsored loans, scholarships/grants, health care benefits, and unspecified assistantships also available. Support available to part-time students. Financial award application deadline: 4/1; financial award applicants required to submit FAFSA. *Unit head:* Dr. Dittmar Hahn, PhD Advisor, 512-245-2284, Fax: 512-245-8713, E-mail: dh49@txstate.edu. *Application contact:* Dr. Andrea Golato, Dean of the Graduate School, 512-245-2581, Fax: 512-245-8365, E-mail: jw02@swt.edu.
Website: http://www.bio.txstate.edu/

University of Alaska Fairbanks, School of Fisheries and Ocean Sciences, Program in Marine Sciences and Limnology, Fairbanks, AK 99775-7220. Offers marine biology (MS, PhD); oceanography (PhD), including biological oceanography, chemical oceanography, fisheries, geological oceanography, physical oceanography. Part-time programs available. *Faculty:* 7 full-time (5 women), 1 part-time/adjunct (0 women). *Students:* 43 full-time (29 women), 15 part-time (11 women); includes 7 minority (2 Asian, non-Hispanic/Latino; 5 Hispanic/Latino), 6 international. Average age 29. 36 applicants, 17% accepted, 6 enrolled. In 2013, 5 master's, 1 doctorate awarded. *Degree requirements:* For master's, comprehensive exam, thesis, oral defense; for doctorate, comprehensive exam, thesis/dissertation, oral defense. *Entrance requirements:* For master's and doctorate, GRE General Test. Additional exam requirements/recommendations for international students: Required—TOEFL (minimum score 550 paper-based; 80 iBT). *Application deadline:* For fall admission, 6/1 for domestic students, 3/1 for international students; for spring admission, 10/15 for domestic students, 8/1 for international

students. Applications are processed on a rolling basis. Application fee: $60. Electronic applications accepted. *Expenses:* Tuition, state resident: full-time $7254; part-time $403 per credit. Tuition, nonresident: full-time $14,814; part-time $823 per credit. Tuition and fees vary according to course level, course load and reciprocity agreements. *Financial support:* In 2013–14, 26 research assistantships with tuition reimbursements (averaging $12,388 per year), 8 teaching assistantships with tuition reimbursements (averaging $9,776 per year) were awarded; fellowships with tuition reimbursements, career-related internships or fieldwork, Federal Work-Study, scholarships/grants, health care benefits, and unspecified assistantships also available. Support available to part-time students. Financial award application deadline: 7/1; financial award applicants required to submit FAFSA. *Unit head:* Katrin Iken, Co-Chair, 907-474-7289, Fax: 907-474-5863, E-mail: info@sfos.uaf.edu. *Application contact:* Libby Eddy, Registrar and Director of Admissions, 907-474-7500, Fax: 907-474-7097, E-mail: admissions@alaska.edu.
Website: https://www.sfos.uaf.edu/academics/?page_id=41

University of California, San Diego, Office of Graduate Studies, Scripps Institution of Oceanography, La Jolla, CA 92093. Offers earth sciences (MS, PhD); geophysics (PhD); marine biology (MS, PhD); oceanography (MS, PhD). PhD in geophysics is offered jointly with San Diego State University. *Students:* 258 full-time (119 women), 11 part-time (7 women); includes 46 minority (4 Black or African American, non-Hispanic/Latino; 4 American Indian or Alaska Native, non-Hispanic/Latino; 22 Asian, non-Hispanic/Latino; 16 Hispanic/Latino), 126 international. 425 applicants, 23% accepted, 56 enrolled. In 2013, 25 master's, 27 doctorates awarded. Terminal master's awarded for partial completion of doctoral program. *Degree requirements:* For master's, thesis; for doctorate, comprehensive exam, thesis/dissertation. *Entrance requirements:* For master's and doctorate, GRE General Test, GRE Subject Test. Additional exam requirements/recommendations for international students: Required—TOEFL (minimum score 550 paper-based; 80 iBT), IELTS. *Application deadline:* For fall admission, 12/16 for domestic students, 1/2 for international students. Application fee: $80 ($100 for international students). Electronic applications accepted. *Expenses:* Tuition, state resident: full-time $11,220; part-time $1870 per quarter. Tuition, nonresident: full-time $26,322; part-time $4387 per quarter. *Required fees:* $519.50 per quarter. Part-time tuition and fees vary according to course load and program. *Financial support:* Fellowships, research assistantships, teaching assistantships, scholarships/grants, and unspecified assistantships available. Financial award applicants required to submit FAFSA. *Faculty research:* Biodiversity and conservation; earth and planetary chemistry; alternative energy; global environmental monitoring; air-sea boundary, tectonic margins and the interactions between systems and environments. *Unit head:* Lisa Tauxe, Chair, 858-534-6084, E-mail: ltauxe@ucsd.edu. *Application contact:* Gilbert Bretado, Graduate Coordinator, 858-534-1694, E-mail: gbretado@ucsd.edu.
Website: https://scripps.ucsd.edu/education

University of California, Santa Barbara, Graduate Division, College of Letters and Sciences, Division of Mathematics, Life, and Physical Sciences, Department of Ecology, Evolution, and Marine Biology, Santa Barbara, CA 93106-9620. Offers computational science and engineering (MA); computational sciences and engineering (PhD); ecology, evolution, and marine biology (MA, PhD); MA/PhD. *Faculty:* 33 full-time (8 women). *Students:* 59 full-time (33 women); includes 14 minority (1 Black or African American, non-Hispanic/Latino; 7 Asian, non-Hispanic/Latino; 6 Hispanic/Latino), 4 international. Average age 31. 120 applicants, 15% accepted, 12 enrolled. In 2013, 9 master's, 6 doctorates awarded. *Degree requirements:* For master's, comprehensive exam (for some programs), thesis (for some programs); for doctorate, comprehensive exam, thesis/dissertation. *Entrance requirements:* For master's and doctorate, GRE General Test. Additional exam requirements/recommendations for international students: Required—TOEFL (minimum score 550 paper-based; 80 iBT), IELTS. *Application deadline:* For fall admission, 12/15 for domestic and international students. Application fee: $80 ($100 for international students). Electronic applications accepted. *Expenses:* Tuition, state resident: part-time $5148.26 per quarter. Tuition, nonresident: part-time $10,182.26 per quarter. *Financial support:* In 2013–14, 50 students received support, including 55 fellowships with full and partial tuition reimbursements available (averaging $10,812 per year), 24 research assistantships with full and partial tuition reimbursements available (averaging $8,441 per year), 97 teaching assistantships with partial tuition reimbursements available (averaging $9,346 per year); Federal Work-Study, scholarships/grants, traineeships, health care benefits, and tuition waivers (full and partial) also available. Financial award application deadline: 12/15; financial award applicants required to submit FAFSA. *Faculty research:* Community ecology, evolution, marine biology, population genetics, stream ecology. *Unit head:* Dr. Craig Carlson, Chair, 805-893-2415, Fax: 805-893-5885, E-mail: eembchair@lifesci.ucsb.edu. *Application contact:* Melanie Fujii, Student Affairs Officer, 805-893-2979, Fax: 805-893-5885, E-mail: eemb-info@lifesci.ucsb.edu.
Website: http://www.lifesci.ucsb.edu/EEMB/index.html

University of Colorado Boulder, Graduate School, College of Arts and Sciences, Department of Ecology and Evolutionary Biology, Boulder, CO 80309. Offers animal behavior (MA); biology (MA, PhD); environmental biology (MA, PhD); evolutionary biology (MA, PhD); neurobiology (MA); population biology (MA); population genetics (PhD). *Faculty:* 31 full-time (12 women). *Students:* 70 full-time (30 women), 18 part-time (10 women); includes 6 minority (1 Asian, non-Hispanic/Latino; 3 Hispanic/Latino; 2 Two or more races, non-Hispanic/Latino), 5 international. Average age 30. 171 applicants, 6% accepted, 11 enrolled. In 2013, 10 master's, 11 doctorates awarded. Terminal master's awarded for partial completion of doctoral program. *Degree requirements:* For master's, comprehensive exam, thesis or alternative; for doctorate, comprehensive exam, thesis/dissertation. *Entrance requirements:* For master's, GRE General Test, GRE Subject Test, minimum undergraduate GPA of 3.0; for doctorate, GRE General Test, GRE Subject Test. *Application deadline:* For fall admission, 12/31 for domestic students, 12/1 for international students. Application fee: $50 ($60 for international students). Electronic applications accepted. *Financial support:* In 2013–14, 175 students received support, including 35 fellowships (averaging $15,283 per year), 21 research assistantships with full and partial tuition reimbursements available (averaging $29,343 per year), 48 teaching assistantships with full and partial tuition reimbursements available (averaging $31,449 per year); institutionally sponsored loans, scholarships/grants, health care benefits, and unspecified assistantships also available. Financial award applicants required to submit FAFSA. *Faculty research:* Ecology, environmental biology, evolutionary biology, biological sciences, conservation biology. *Total annual research expenditures:* $37.1 million.
Website: http://ebio.colorado.edu

University of Guam, Office of Graduate Studies, College of Natural and Applied Sciences, Program in Biology, Mangilao, GU 96923. Offers tropical marine biology (MS). *Degree requirements:* For master's, comprehensive exam, thesis. *Entrance requirements:* For master's, GRE General Test, GRE Subject Test. Additional exam requirements/recommendations for international students: Required—TOEFL. *Faculty research:* Maintenance and ecology of coral reefs.

University of Hawaii at Hilo, Program in Tropical Conservation Biology and Environmental Science, Hilo, HI 96720-4091. Offers MS. *Faculty:* 16 full-time (6 women), 1 (woman) part-time/adjunct. *Students:* 7 full-time (2 women), 48 part-time (32 women); includes 30 minority (5 Asian, non-Hispanic/Latino; 6 Hispanic/Latino; 3 Native Hawaiian or other Pacific Islander, non-Hispanic/Latino; 16 Two or more races, non-Hispanic/Latino). Average age 29. 34 applicants, 53% accepted, 13 enrolled. In 2013, 21 master's awarded. *Entrance requirements:* Additional exam requirements/recommendations for international students: Required—TOEFL, IELTS. *Application deadline:* For fall admission, 2/1 priority date for domestic students, 1/1 priority date for international students. Application fee: $50. Electronic applications accepted. *Expenses:* Tuition, state resident: full-time $4668. Tuition, nonresident: full-time $10,704. Tuition and fees vary according to course load and program. *Financial support:* Application deadline: 3/1; applicants required to submit FAFSA. *Unit head:* Donald Price, Director, 808-932-7506, E-mail: donaldp@hawaii.edu. *Application contact:* UH Hilo Admissions Office, 808-932-7446, Fax: 808-932-7459, E-mail: uhhadm@hawaii.edu.
Website: http://tcbes.uhh.hawaii.edu/

University of Hawaii at Manoa, Graduate Division, School of Ocean and Earth Science and Technology, Interdisciplinary Program in Marine Biology, Honolulu, HI 96822. Offers MS, PhD. *Degree requirements:* For master's, thesis, research project; for doctorate, thesis/dissertation, research project. *Entrance requirements:* For master's and doctorate, GRE. Additional exam requirements/recommendations for international students: Required—TOEFL. *Expenses:* Contact institution. *Faculty research:* Ecology, ichthyology, behavior of marine animals, developmental biology.

University of Maine, Graduate School, College of Natural Sciences, Forestry, and Agriculture, School of Marine Sciences, Orono, ME 04469. Offers marine bio-resources (MS, PhD); marine biology (MS, PhD); marine policy (MS); oceanography (MS, PhD). Part-time programs available. *Faculty:* 40 full-time (8 women), 60 part-time/adjunct (16 women). *Students:* 49 full-time (29 women), 5 part-time (1 woman); includes 2 minority (1 American Indian or Alaska Native, non-Hispanic/Latino; 1 Hispanic/Latino), 8 international. Average age 28. 70 applicants, 14% accepted, 9 enrolled. In 2013, 11 master's, 1 doctorate awarded. *Degree requirements:* For master's, thesis; for doctorate, comprehensive exam, thesis/dissertation. *Entrance requirements:* For master's and doctorate, GRE General Test. Additional exam requirements/recommendations for international students: Required—TOEFL. *Application deadline:* For fall admission, 2/1 priority date for domestic students. Applications are processed on a rolling basis. Application fee: $65. Electronic applications accepted. *Expenses:* Tuition, state resident: full-time $7524. Tuition, nonresident: full-time $23,112. *Required fees:* $1970. *Financial support:* In 2013–14, 39 students received support, including 2 fellowships (averaging $34,500 per year), 23 research assistantships with tuition reimbursements available (averaging $14,600 per year), 9 teaching assistantships with tuition reimbursements available (averaging $14,600 per year); career-related internships or fieldwork, Federal Work-Study, and tuition waivers (full and partial) also available. Support available to part-time students. Financial award application deadline: 3/1. *Faculty research:* Coastal processes, microbial ecology, crustacean systematics. *Total annual research expenditures:* $2 million. *Unit head:* Dr. Fei Chai, Director, 207-581-3321, Fax: 207-581-4388. *Application contact:* Scott G. Delcourt, Associate Dean of the Graduate School, 207-581-3291, Fax: 207-581-3232, E-mail: graduate@maine.edu.
Website: http://www.umaine.edu/marine/

University of Massachusetts Dartmouth, Graduate School, College of Arts and Sciences, Department of Biology, North Dartmouth, MA 02747-2300. Offers biology (MS); marine biology (MS). Part-time programs available. *Faculty:* 18 full-time (6 women), 1 (woman) part-time/adjunct. *Students:* 7 full-time (all women), 13 part-time (10 women); includes 3 minority (2 Hispanic/Latino; 1 Two or more races, non-Hispanic/Latino). Average age 27. 24 applicants, 42% accepted, 4 enrolled. In 2013, 9 master's awarded. *Degree requirements:* For master's, thesis. *Entrance requirements:* For master's, GRE, statement of purpose (minimum of 300 words), resume, 3 letters of recommendation, official transcripts. Additional exam requirements/recommendations for international students: Required—TOEFL (minimum score 533 paper-based; 72 iBT). *Application deadline:* For fall admission, 2/15 priority date for domestic students, 1/15 priority date for international students. Applications are processed on a rolling basis. Application fee: $60. Electronic applications accepted. *Expenses:* Tuition, state resident: full-time $2071; part-time $86.29 per credit. Tuition, nonresident: full-time $8099; part-time $337.46 per credit. Tuition and fees vary according to course load and reciprocity agreements. *Financial support:* In 2013–14, 2 research assistantships with full tuition reimbursements (averaging $10,200 per year), 10 teaching assistantships with full tuition reimbursements (averaging $14,400 per year) were awarded; Federal Work-Study and unspecified assistantships also available. Support available to part-time students. Financial award application deadline: 3/1; financial award applicants required to submit FAFSA. *Faculty research:* Shark biology, marine mammal biology, domestication of fish, cell body, fish biology. *Total annual research expenditures:* $1.5 million. *Unit head:* Dr. Diego Bernal, Graduate Program Director, 508-999-8307, Fax: 508-999-8196, E-mail: dbernal@umassd.edu. *Application contact:* Steven Briggs, Director of Marketing and Recruitment for Graduate Studies, 508-999-8604, Fax: 508-999-8183, E-mail: graduate@umassd.edu.
Website: http://www.umassd.edu/cas/biology/

University of Miami, Graduate School, Rosenstiel School of Marine and Atmospheric Science, Division of Marine Biology and Fisheries, Coral Gables, FL 33124. Offers MA, MS, PhD. Terminal master's awarded for partial completion of doctoral program. *Degree requirements:* For master's, comprehensive exam, thesis; for doctorate, comprehensive exam, thesis/dissertation. *Entrance requirements:* For master's and doctorate, GRE General Test. Additional exam requirements/recommendations for international students: Required—TOEFL (minimum score 550 paper-based). Electronic applications accepted. *Faculty research:* Biochemistry, physiology, plankton, coral, biology.

The University of North Carolina Wilmington, College of Arts and Sciences, Department of Biology and Marine Biology, Wilmington, NC 28403-3297. Offers biology (MS); marine biology (MS, PhD). Part-time programs available. *Faculty:* 29 full-time (9 women). *Students:* 5 full-time (4 women), 67 part-time (34 women); includes 5 minority (1 Asian, non-Hispanic/Latino; 4 Hispanic/Latino), 2 international. Average age 28. 76 applicants, 25% accepted, 18 enrolled. In 2013, 13 master's, 5 doctorates awarded. *Degree requirements:* For master's, comprehensive exam, thesis; for doctorate, comprehensive exam, thesis/dissertation. *Entrance requirements:* For master's, GRE General Test, GRE Subject Test, minimum B average in undergraduate major; for doctorate, GRE General Test, minimum B average in undergraduate major and graduate courses. Additional exam requirements/recommendations for international students: Required—TOEFL (minimum score 550 paper-based; 79 iBT), IELTS (minimum score 6.5). *Application deadline:* For fall admission, 3/15 for domestic students. Applications are processed on a rolling basis. Application fee: $60. Electronic applications accepted. *Expenses:* Tuition, state resident: full-time $4163. Tuition, nonresident: full-time $16,098. *Financial support:* In 2013–14, 24 research assistantships with full and partial tuition reimbursements (averaging $14,000 per year), 36 teaching assistantships with full and partial tuition reimbursements (averaging $14,000 per year) were awarded; career-related internships or fieldwork and Federal Work-Study also available. Support available to part-time students. Financial award application deadline: 3/15. *Faculty research:* Ecology, physiology, cell and molecular biology, systematics, biomechanics. *Total annual research expenditures:* $3.1 million. *Unit head:* Dr. Chris Finelli, Chair, 910-962-3487, E-mail: finellic@uncw.edu. *Application*

Marine Biology

contact: Dr. Stephen Kinsey, Graduate Coordinator, 910-962-7398, Fax: 910-962-4066, E-mail: kinseys@uncw.edu.
Website: http://www.uncw.edu/bio/graduate.html

University of Oregon, Graduate School, College of Arts and Sciences, Department of Biology, Eugene, OR 97403. Offers ecology and evolution (MA, MS, PhD); marine biology (MA, MS, PhD); molecular, cellular and genetic biology (PhD); neuroscience and development (PhD). Terminal master's awarded for partial completion of doctoral program. *Degree requirements:* For master's, thesis (for some programs); for doctorate, thesis/dissertation. *Entrance requirements:* For master's and doctorate, GRE General Test, minimum GPA of 3.2. Additional exam requirements/recommendations for international students: Required—TOEFL. *Faculty research:* Developmental neurobiology; evolution, population biology, and quantitative genetics; regulation of gene expression; biochemistry of marine organisms.

University of Southern California, Graduate School, Dana and David Dornsife College of Letters, Arts and Sciences, Department of Biological Sciences, Program in Marine Biology and Biological Oceanography, Los Angeles, CA 90089. Offers marine and environmental biology (MS); marine biology and biological oceanography (PhD). Terminal master's awarded for partial completion of doctoral program. *Degree requirements:* For master's, research paper; for doctorate, comprehensive exam, thesis/dissertation, qualifying examination, dissertation defense. *Entrance requirements:* For master's and doctorate, GRE, 3 letters of recommendation, personal statement, resume, minimum GPA of 3.0. Additional exam requirements/recommendations for international students: Required—TOEFL (minimum score 600 paper-based; 100 iBT). Electronic applications accepted. *Faculty research:* Microbial ecology, biogeochemistry, and geobiology; biodiversity and molecular ecology; integrative organismal biology; conservation biology; marine genomics.

University of Southern Mississippi, Graduate School, College of Science and Technology, Department of Biological Sciences, Hattiesburg, MS 39406-0001. Offers environmental biology (MS, PhD); marine biology (MS, PhD); microbiology (MS, PhD); molecular biology (MS, PhD). *Faculty:* 27 full-time (6 women). *Students:* 63 full-time (26 women), 4 part-time (all women); includes 4 minority (1 Black or African American, non-Hispanic/Latino; 1 Hispanic/Latino; 2 Two or more races, non-Hispanic/Latino), 17 international. Average age 32. 43 applicants, 30% accepted, 12 enrolled. In 2013, 12 master's, 9 doctorates awarded. Terminal master's awarded for partial completion of doctoral program. *Degree requirements:* For master's, comprehensive exam, thesis; for doctorate, comprehensive exam, thesis/dissertation. *Entrance requirements:* For master's, GRE General Test, minimum GPA of 3.0 on last 60 hours; for doctorate, GRE General Test, minimum GPA of 3.5. Additional exam requirements/recommendations for international students: Required—TOEFL, IELTS. *Application deadline:* For fall admission, 3/1 priority date for domestic students, 3/1 for international students; for spring admission, 1/10 priority date for domestic and international students. Applications are processed on a rolling basis. Application fee: $50. *Financial support:* In 2013–14, 25 research assistantships with full tuition reimbursements (averaging $9,700 per year), 33 teaching assistantships with full tuition reimbursements (averaging $10,600 per year) were awarded; Federal Work-Study, scholarships/grants, health care benefits, and unspecified assistantships also available. Financial award application deadline: 3/15; financial award applicants required to submit FAFSA. *Unit head:* Dr. Glenmore Shearer, Chair, 601-266-4748, Fax: 601-266-5797. *Application contact:* Dr. Jake Schaefer, Director of Graduate Studies, 601-266-4748, Fax: 601-266-5797.
Website: http://www.usm.edu/graduateschool/table.php

University of Southern Mississippi, Graduate School, College of Science and Technology, Department of Marine Science, Stennis Space Center, MS 39529. Offers biological oceanography (MS, PhD); geological oceanography (MS, PhD); hydrographic science (MS, PhD); marine chemistry (MS, PhD); physical oceanography (MS, PhD). Part-time programs available. *Faculty:* 16 full-time (2 women). *Students:* 45 full-time (19 women), 8 part-time (3 women); includes 20 minority (6 Black or African American, non-Hispanic/Latino; 4 American Indian or Alaska Native, non-Hispanic/Latino; 10 Asian, non-Hispanic/Latino). Average age 32. 69 applicants, 55% accepted, 29 enrolled. In 2013, 13 master's, 2 doctorates awarded. *Degree requirements:* For master's, comprehensive exam, thesis, oral qualifying exam (marine science); for doctorate, 2 foreign languages, comprehensive exam, thesis/dissertation, oral qualifying exam. *Entrance requirements:* For master's, GRE General Test, minimum GPA of 3.0; for doctorate, GRE General Test, minimum GPA of 3.0 (undergraduate), 3.5 (graduate). Additional exam requirements/recommendations for international students: Required—TOEFL. *Application deadline:* For fall admission, 3/1 priority date for domestic and international students. Applications are processed on a rolling basis. Application fee: $50. Electronic applications accepted. *Financial support:* In 2013–14, 28 students received support. Research assistantships with full tuition reimbursements available, teaching assistantships with full tuition reimbursements available, Federal Work-Study, and institutionally sponsored loans available. Financial award application deadline: 3/15. *Faculty research:* Marine science; remote sensing; bio-optics; numerical modeling; hydrography, marine chemistry; biological, physical and geological oceanography. *Total annual research expenditures:* $8.2 million. *Application contact:* Linda Downs, Senior Office Support Specialist, 228-688-7097, Fax: 228-688-1121, E-mail: linda.downs@usm.edu.
Website: http://www.usm.edu/marine/

Western Illinois University, School of Graduate Studies, College of Arts and Sciences, Department of Biological Sciences, Macomb, IL 61455-1390. Offers biological sciences (MS); environmental geographic information systems (Certificate); zoo and aquarium studies (Certificate). Part-time programs available. *Students:* 52 full-time (40 women), 27 part-time (19 women); includes 3 minority (1 Black or African American, non-Hispanic/Latino; 2 Hispanic/Latino), 4 international. Average age 26. In 2013, 14 master's, 17 other advanced degrees awarded. *Degree requirements:* For master's, thesis or alternative. *Entrance requirements:* Additional exam requirements/recommendations for international students: Required—TOEFL (minimum score 550 paper-based; 80 iBT); Recommended—IELTS. *Application deadline:* Applications are processed on a rolling basis. Application fee: $30. Electronic applications accepted. *Financial support:* In 2013–14, 29 students received support, including 9 research assistantships with full tuition reimbursements available (averaging $7,544 per year), 20 teaching assistantships with full tuition reimbursements available (averaging $8,688 per year). Financial award applicants required to submit FAFSA. *Unit head:* Dr. Charles Lydeard, Chairperson, 309-298-1546. *Application contact:* Dr. Nancy Parsons, Associate Provost and Director of Graduate Studies, 309-298-1806, Fax: 309-298-2345, E-mail: grad-office@wiu.edu.
Website: http://wiu.edu/biology

Woods Hole Oceanographic Institution, MIT/WHOI Joint Program in Oceanography/Applied Ocean Science and Engineering, Woods Hole, MA 02543-1541. Offers applied ocean science and engineering (PhD); biological oceanography (PhD); chemical oceanography (PhD); marine geology and geophysics (PhD); physical oceanography (PhD). Program offered jointly with Massachusetts Institute of Technology. *Degree requirements:* For doctorate, thesis/dissertation. *Entrance requirements:* For doctorate, GRE General Test, GRE Subject Test. Additional exam requirements/recommendations for international students: Required—TOEFL. Electronic applications accepted.

Section 12
Microbiological Sciences

This section contains a directory of institutions offering graduate work in microbiological sciences, followed by in-depth entries submitted by institutions that chose to prepare detailed program descriptions. Additional information about programs listed in the directory but not augmented by an in-depth entry may be obtained by writing directly to the dean of a graduate school or chair of a department at the address given in the directory.

For programs offering related work, see also in this book *Allied Health; Biochemistry; Biological and Biomedical Sciences; Botany and Plant Biology; Cell, Molecular, and Structural Biology; Dentistry and Dental Sciences; Ecology, Environmental Biology, and Evolutionary Biology; Entomology; Genetics, Developmental Biology, and Reproductive Biology; Parasitology; Pathology and Pathobiology; Pharmacy and Pharmaceutical Sciences; Public Health; Physiology; Veterinary Medicine and Sciences;* and *Zoology*. In the other guides in this series:

Graduate Programs in the Physical Sciences, Mathematics, Agricultural Sciences, the Environment & Natural Resources

See *Agricultural and Food Sciences* and *Chemistry*

Graduate Programs in Engineering & Applied Sciences

See *Agricultural Engineering and Bioengineering* and *Biomedical Engineering and Biotechnology*

CONTENTS

Program Directories

Displays and Close-Ups

Bacteriology

Illinois State University, Graduate School, College of Arts and Sciences, Department of Biological Sciences, Normal, IL 61790-2200. Offers animal behavior (MS); bacteriology (MS); biochemistry (MS); biological sciences (MS); biology (PhD); biophysics (MS); biotechnology (MS); botany (MS, PhD); cell biology (MS); conservation biology (MS); developmental biology (MS); ecology (MS, PhD); entomology (MS); evolutionary biology (MS); genetics (MS, PhD); immunology (MS); microbiology (MS, PhD); molecular biology (MS); molecular genetics (MS); neurobiology (MS); neuroscience (MS); parasitology (MS); physiology (MS, PhD); plant biology (MS); plant molecular biology (MS); plant sciences (MS); structural biology (MS); zoology (MS, PhD). Part-time programs available. *Degree requirements:* For master's, thesis or alternative; for doctorate, variable foreign language requirement, thesis/dissertation, 2 terms of residency. *Entrance requirements:* For master's, GRE General Test, minimum GPA of 2.6 in last 60 hours of course work; for doctorate, GRE General Test. *Faculty research:* Redoc balance and drug development in schistosoma mansoni, control of the growth of listeria monocytogenes at low temperature, regulation of cell expansion and microtubule function by SPRI, CRUI: physiology and fitness consequences of different life history phenotypes.

The University of Iowa, Roy J. and Lucille A. Carver College of Medicine and Graduate College, Graduate Programs in Medicine, Department of Microbiology, Iowa City, IA 52242-1316. Offers general microbiology and microbial physiology (MS, PhD); immunology (MS, PhD); microbial genetics (MS, PhD); pathogenic bacteriology (MS, PhD); virology (MS, PhD). *Faculty:* 23 full-time (5 women), 10 part-time/adjunct (4 women). *Students:* 38 full-time (28 women); includes 3 minority (2 Asian, non-Hispanic/Latino; 1 Hispanic/Latino), 2 international. Average age 25. 44 applicants, 23% accepted, 8 enrolled. In 2013, 1 master's, 6 doctorates awarded. *Degree requirements:* For master's, thesis; for doctorate, comprehensive exam, thesis/dissertation. *Entrance requirements:* For master's and doctorate, GRE General Test. Additional exam requirements/recommendations for international students: Required—TOEFL (minimum score 600 paper-based). *Application deadline:* For fall admission, 1/1 for domestic and international students. Application fee: $60 ($100 for international students). Electronic applications accepted. *Financial support:* In 2013–14, 5 fellowships with full tuition reimbursements (averaging $26,000 per year), 33 research assistantships with full tuition reimbursements (averaging $26,000 per year) were awarded; institutionally sponsored loans, scholarships/grants, traineeships, and health care benefits also available. *Faculty research:* Gene regulation, processing and transport of HIV, retroviral pathogenesis, biodegradation, biofilm. *Total annual research expenditures:* $11.5 million. *Unit head:* Dr. Patrick M. Schlievert, Chair and Department Executive Officer, 319-335-7810, E-mail: grad-micro-info@uiowa.edu. *Application contact:* Kerry Yoder, Assistant Director of Graduate and Professional Evaluation, 319-335-1525, Fax: 319-335-1535, E-mail: admissions@uiowa.edu.
Website: http://www.medicine.uiowa.edu/microbiology/

University of Prince Edward Island, Atlantic Veterinary College, Graduate Program in Veterinary Medicine, Charlottetown, PE C1A 4P3, Canada. Offers anatomy (M Sc, PhD); bacteriology (M Sc, PhD); clinical pharmacology (M Sc, PhD); clinical sciences (M Sc, PhD); epidemiology (M Sc, PhD), including reproduction; fish health (M Sc, PhD); food animal nutrition (M Sc, PhD); immunology (M Sc, PhD); microanatomy (M Sc, PhD); parasitology (M Sc, PhD); pathology (M Sc, PhD); pharmacology (M Sc, PhD); physiology (M Sc, PhD); toxicology (M Sc, PhD); veterinary science (M Vet Sc); virology (M Sc, PhD). Part-time programs available. *Degree requirements:* For master's, thesis; for doctorate, thesis/dissertation. *Entrance requirements:* For master's, DVM, B Sc honors degree, or equivalent; for doctorate, M Sc. Additional exam requirements/recommendations for international students: Required—TOEFL (minimum score 550 paper-based; 80 iBT). *Expenses:* Contact institution. *Faculty research:* Animal health management, infectious diseases, fin fish and shellfish health, basic biomedical sciences, ecosystem health.

The University of Texas Medical Branch, Graduate School of Biomedical Sciences, Program in Emerging and Tropical Infectious Diseases, Galveston, TX 77555. Offers PhD, MD/PhD. *Degree requirements:* For doctorate, thesis/dissertation. *Entrance requirements:* For doctorate, GRE General Test. *Faculty research:* Emerging diseases, tropical diseases, parasitology, vitology and bacteriology.

University of Washington, Graduate School, School of Public Health, Department of Global Health, Graduate Program in Pathobiology, Seattle, WA 98195. Offers PhD. *Faculty:* 20 full-time (8 women). *Students:* 26 full-time (17 women), 8 part-time (7 women); includes 6 minority (2 Black or African American, non-Hispanic/Latino; 4 Asian, non-Hispanic/Latino), 2 international. Average age 29. 66 applicants, 17% accepted, 5 enrolled. In 2013, 6 doctorates awarded. *Degree requirements:* For doctorate, comprehensive exam, thesis/dissertation, published paper from thesis work. *Entrance requirements:* For doctorate, GRE General Test, minimum GPA of 3.0. Additional exam requirements/recommendations for international students: Required—TOEFL, IELTS. *Application deadline:* For fall admission, 12/1 for domestic and international students. Application fee: $85. Electronic applications accepted. *Financial support:* In 2013–14, 31 students received support, including 31 research assistantships with full tuition reimbursements available (averaging $28,440 per year); traineeships and unspecified assistantships also available. *Faculty research:* Malaria, immunological response to mycobacteria infections, HIV-cell interaction and the development of an anti-HIV vaccine, regulation of intercellular communication via gap junctions, genetic and nutritional regulation of proteins involved in lipid transport. *Unit head:* Dr. King K. Holmes, Chair, 206-744-3620, Fax: 206-744-3694. *Application contact:* Rachel Reichert, Program Manager, 206-543-4338, Fax: 206-543-3873, E-mail: pabio@u.washington.edu.

University of Wisconsin–Madison, Graduate School, College of Agricultural and Life Sciences, Department of Bacteriology, Madison, WI 53706-1380. Offers MS. Part-time programs available. *Entrance requirements:* Additional exam requirements/recommendations for international students: Required—TOEFL. Electronic applications accepted. *Expenses:* Tuition, state resident: full-time $10,728; part-time $790 per credit. Tuition, nonresident: full-time $24,054; part-time $1623 per credit. *Required fees:* $1130; $119 per credit. *Faculty research:* Microbial physiology, gene regulation, microbial ecology, plant-microbe interactions, symbiosis.

Immunology

Albany Medical College, Center for Immunology and Microbial Disease, Albany, NY 12208-3479. Offers MS, PhD. Part-time programs available. Terminal master's awarded for partial completion of doctoral program. *Degree requirements:* For master's, thesis; for doctorate, comprehensive exam, thesis/dissertation, oral qualifying exam, written preliminary exam, 1 published paper-peer review. *Entrance requirements:* For master's, GRE General Test, all transcripts, letters of recommendation; for doctorate, GRE General Test, letters of recommendation. Additional exam requirements/recommendations for international students: Required—TOEFL. *Faculty research:* Microbial and viral pathogenesis, cancer development and cell transformation, biochemical and genetic mechanisms responsible for human disease.

Albert Einstein College of Medicine, Graduate Division of Biomedical Sciences, Department of Microbiology and Immunology, Bronx, NY 10461. Offers PhD, MD/PhD. *Degree requirements:* For doctorate, thesis/dissertation. *Entrance requirements:* For doctorate, GRE General Test. Additional exam requirements/recommendations for international students: Required—TOEFL. *Faculty research:* Nature of histocompatibility antigens, lymphoid cell receptors, regulation of immune responses and mechanisms of resistance to infection.

American University of Beirut, Graduate Programs, Faculty of Medicine, Beirut, Lebanon. Offers anatomy, cell biology and human morphology (MS); biochemistry and medical genetics (MS); biomedical sciences (PhD); experimental pathology, immunology and microbiology (MS); medicine (MD); neuroscience (MS); pharmacology and toxicology (MS). Part-time programs available. *Faculty:* 259 full-time (78 women), 93 part-time/adjunct (16 women). *Students:* 364 full-time (165 women), 62 part-time (54 women). Average age 23. In 2013, 18 master's awarded. *Degree requirements:* For master's, one foreign language, comprehensive exam, thesis (for some programs); for doctorate, one foreign language, comprehensive exam, thesis/dissertation. *Entrance requirements:* For master's, letter of recommendation; for doctorate, MCAT, bachelor's degree. Additional exam requirements/recommendations for international students: Required—TOEFL (minimum score 600 paper-based; 100 iBT), IELTS (minimum score 7.5). *Application deadline:* For fall admission, 4/30 for domestic and international students; for spring admission, 11/1 for domestic and international students. Application fee: $50. *Expenses: Tuition:* Full-time $14,724; part-time $818 per credit. *Required fees:* $692. Tuition and fees vary according to course load and program. *Financial support:* In 2013–14, 242 students received support, including 60 teaching assistantships (averaging $4,000 per year); career-related internships or fieldwork, institutionally sponsored loans, scholarships/grants, health care benefits, and unspecified assistantships also available. Financial award application deadline: 2/2. *Faculty research:* Cancer research (targeted therapy, mechanisms of leukemogenesis, tumor cell extravasation and metastasis, cancer stem cells), stem cell research (regenerative medicine, drug discovery), genetic research (neurogenetics, hereditary cardiomyopathy, hemoglobinopathies, pharmacogenomics, proteomics), neuroscience research (pain, neurodegenerative disorder), metabolism (inflammation and metabolism, metabolic disorder, diabetes mellitus), vascular and renal biology, signal transduction. *Total annual research expenditures:* $2.6 million. *Unit head:* Dr. Mohamed Sayegh, Dean, 961-1350000 Ext. 4700, Fax: 961-1744464, E-mail: msayegh@aub.edu.lb. *Application contact:* Dr. Salim Kanaan, Director, Admissions Office, 961-1-350000 Ext. 2594, Fax: 96-1-1750775, E-mail: sk00@aub.edu.lb.
Website: http://www.aub.edu.lb/fm/fm_home/Pages/index.aspx

Baylor College of Medicine, Graduate School of Biomedical Sciences, Department of Immunology, Houston, TX 77030-3498. Offers PhD, MD/PhD. *Degree requirements:* For doctorate, thesis/dissertation, public defense. *Entrance requirements:* For doctorate, GRE General Test, GRE Subject Test (strongly recommended), minimum GPA of 3.0. Additional exam requirements/recommendations for international students: Required—TOEFL. Electronic applications accepted. *Faculty research:* MHC expression, inflammation and allergy, germinal center biology, HIV pathogenesis, immune responses to gene therapy.

Baylor College of Medicine, Graduate School of Biomedical Sciences, Interdepartmental Program in Cell and Molecular Biology, Houston, TX 77030-3498. Offers biochemistry (PhD); cell and molecular biology (PhD); genetics (PhD); human genetics (PhD); immunology (PhD); microbiology (PhD); virology (PhD); MD/PhD. *Degree requirements:* For doctorate, thesis/dissertation, public defense. *Entrance requirements:* For doctorate, GRE General Test, GRE Subject Test (strongly recommended), minimum GPA of 3.0. Additional exam requirements/recommendations for international students: Required—TOEFL. Electronic applications accepted. *Faculty research:* Molecular and cellular biology; cancer, aging and stem cells; genomics and proteomics; microbiome, molecular microbiology; infectious disease, immunology and translational research.

Boston University, School of Medicine, Division of Graduate Medical Sciences, Department of Microbiology, Boston, MA 02118. Offers immunology (PhD); MD/PhD. Terminal master's awarded for partial completion of doctoral program. *Degree requirements:* For doctorate, comprehensive exam, thesis/dissertation. *Entrance requirements:* Additional exam requirements/recommendations for international students: Required—TOEFL. *Application deadline:* For fall admission, 1/15 for domestic students; for spring admission, 10/15 for domestic students. *Expenses: Tuition:* Full-time $43,970; part-time $1374 per credit hour. *Required fees:* $60 per semester. Tuition and fees vary according to class time, course level and program. *Unit head:* Dr. Ronald B. Corley, Chairman, 617-638-4284, Fax: 617-638-4286, E-mail: rbcorley@bu.edu. *Application contact:* Dr. Gregory Viglianti, Graduate Director, 617-638-7790, Fax: 617-638-4286, E-mail: gviglian@bu.edu.
Website: http://www.bumc.bu.edu/microbiology/

Boston University, School of Medicine, Division of Graduate Medical Sciences, Immunology Training Program, Boston, MA 02215. Offers PhD, MD/PhD. *Degree requirements:* For doctorate, thesis/dissertation. *Application deadline:* For fall

admission, 1/15 for domestic students; for spring admission, 10/15 for domestic students. *Expenses: Tuition:* Full-time $43,970; part-time $1374 per credit hour. *Required fees:* $60 per semester. Tuition and fees vary according to class time, course level and program. *Unit head:* Dr. David Sherr, Director, 617-638-6464, E-mail: itp@bu.edu. *Application contact:* Dr. Gregory Viglianti, Associate Professor of Microbiology, 617-638-7790, E-mail: gviglian@bu.edu.
Website: http://www.bumc.bu.edu/immunology/

California Institute of Technology, Division of Biology, Program in Immunology, Pasadena, CA 91125-0001. Offers PhD. *Degree requirements:* For doctorate, thesis/dissertation, qualifying exam. *Entrance requirements:* For doctorate, GRE General Test.

Case Western Reserve University, School of Medicine and School of Graduate Studies, Graduate Programs in Medicine, Programs in Molecular and Cellular Basis of Disease/Pathology, Immunology Training Program, Cleveland, OH 44106. Offers MS, PhD, MD/PhD. *Degree requirements:* For doctorate, comprehensive exam, thesis/dissertation. *Entrance requirements:* For doctorate, GRE General Test, GRE Subject Test. Additional exam requirements/recommendations for international students: Required—TOEFL (minimum score 550 paper-based). Electronic applications accepted. *Faculty research:* Immunology, immunopathology, immunochemistry, infectious diseases.

Colorado State University, College of Veterinary Medicine and Biomedical Sciences, Department of Microbiology, Immunology and Pathology, Fort Collins, CO 80523. Offers microbiology (MS, PhD); pathology (PhD). *Faculty:* 50 full-time (22 women), 4 part-time/adjunct (1 woman). *Students:* 73 full-time (51 women), 31 part-time (24 women); includes 15 minority (1 Black or African American, non-Hispanic/Latino; 2 American Indian or Alaska Native, non-Hispanic/Latino; 3 Asian, non-Hispanic/Latino; 8 Hispanic/Latino; 1 Two or more races, non-Hispanic/Latino), 9 international. Average age 29. 135 applicants, 31% accepted, 38 enrolled. In 2013, 3 master's, 11 doctorates awarded. *Degree requirements:* For master's, thesis; for doctorate, comprehensive exam, thesis/dissertation. *Entrance requirements:* For master's, GRE General Test, minimum GPA of 3.0, BA/BS in biomedical field, reviewer evaluation forms, resume, transcripts, personal statement, 3 letters of recommendation; for doctorate, GRE General Test, minimum GPA of 3.0, BA/BS in biomedical field, reviewer evaluation forms, resume, personal statement, transcripts, 3 letters of recommendation. Additional exam requirements/recommendations for international students: Required—TOEFL (minimum score 550 paper-based). *Application deadline:* For fall admission, 1/1 priority date for domestic students; for spring admission, 10/1 priority date for domestic students. Applications are processed on a rolling basis. Application fee: $50. Electronic applications accepted. *Expenses:* Tuition, state resident: full-time $9075.40; part-time $504 per credit. Tuition, nonresident: full-time $22,248; part-time $1236 per credit. *Required fees:* $1819; $60 per credit. *Financial support:* In 2013–14, 82 students received support, including 40 fellowships with tuition reimbursements available (averaging $35,362 per year), 38 research assistantships with tuition reimbursements available (averaging $17,799 per year), 4 teaching assistantships with tuition reimbursements available (averaging $15,606 per year); Federal Work-Study, scholarships/grants, traineeships, and unspecified assistantships also available. Financial award applicants required to submit FAFSA. *Faculty research:* Medical and veterinary bacteriology, immunology, microbial physiology, pathology, vector-borne disease. *Total annual research expenditures:* $29.9 million. *Unit head:* Dr. Gregg A. Dean, Head, 970-491-6144, Fax: 970-491-1815, E-mail: gregg.dean@colostate.edu. *Application contact:* Lisa McCann, Academic Programs Coordinator, 970-491-6118, Fax: 970-491-1815, E-mail: lisa.mccann@colostate.edu.
Website: http://csu-cvmbs.colostate.edu/academics/mip/graduate/Pages/default.aspx

Cornell University, Graduate School, Graduate Fields of Comparative Biomedical Sciences, Field of Immunology, Ithaca, NY 14853-0001. Offers cellular immunology (MS, PhD); immunochemistry (MS, PhD); immunogenetics (MS, PhD); immunopathology (MS, PhD); infection and immunity (MS, PhD). *Faculty:* 33 full-time (9 women). *Students:* 12 full-time (9 women); includes 3 minority (1 Black or African American, non-Hispanic/Latino; 1 Asian, non-Hispanic/Latino; 1 Two or more races, non-Hispanic/Latino), 3 international. Average age 30. 79 applicants, 9% accepted, 2 enrolled. In 2013, 4 doctorates awarded. Terminal master's awarded for partial completion of doctoral program. *Degree requirements:* For master's, thesis; for doctorate, comprehensive exam, thesis/dissertation. *Entrance requirements:* For master's and doctorate, GRE General Test, 2 letters of recommendation. Additional exam requirements/recommendations for international students: Required—TOEFL (minimum score 550 paper-based; 77 iBT). *Application deadline:* For fall admission, 12/15 for domestic students. Application fee: $95. Electronic applications accepted. *Financial support:* In 2013–14, 8 students received support, including 1 fellowship with full tuition reimbursement available, 6 research assistantships with full tuition reimbursements available, 1 teaching assistantship with full tuition reimbursement available; institutionally sponsored loans, scholarships/grants, health care benefits, tuition waivers (full and partial), and unspecified assistantships also available. Financial award applicants required to submit FAFSA. *Faculty research:* Avian immunology, mucosal immunity, anti-parasite and anti-viral immunity, neutrophil function, reproductive immunology. *Unit head:* Director of Graduate Studies, 607-253-3276, Fax: 607-253-3756. *Application contact:* Graduate Field Assistant, 607-253-3276, Fax: 607-253-3756, E-mail: graduate_edcvm@cornell.edu.
Website: http://www.gradschool.cornell.edu/fields.php?id-52&a-2

Creighton University, School of Medicine and Graduate School, Graduate Programs in Medicine, Department of Medical Microbiology and Immunology, Omaha, NE 68178-0001. Offers MS, PhD. *Faculty:* 11 full-time (2 women). *Students:* 14 full-time (7 women); includes 1 minority (Hispanic/Latino), 3 international. Average age 26. 55 applicants, 4% accepted, 2 enrolled. In 2013, 1 master's, 3 doctorates awarded. Terminal master's awarded for partial completion of doctoral program. *Degree requirements:* For master's, comprehensive exam, thesis; for doctorate, thesis/dissertation, preliminary examination, NIH-style grant defense. *Entrance requirements:* For master's and doctorate, GRE General Test. Additional exam requirements/recommendations for international students: Required—TOEFL (minimum score 80 iBT). *Application deadline:* For fall admission, 2/1 priority date for domestic and international students. Applications are processed on a rolling basis. Application fee: $50. *Expenses: Tuition:* Full-time $13,608; part-time $756 per credit hour. *Required fees:* $149 per semester. Tuition and fees vary according to course load, campus/location, program, reciprocity agreements and student's religious affiliation. *Financial support:* In 2013–14, 6 fellowships with tuition reimbursements (averaging $22,275 per year), research assistantships with tuition reimbursements (averaging $22,275 per year) were awarded; career-related internships or fieldwork, institutionally sponsored loans, and tuition waivers (full) also available. *Faculty research:* Infectious diseases, molecular biology, genetics, antimicrobial agents and chemotherapy, virology. *Total annual research expenditures:* $2 million. *Unit head:* Dr. Richard Goering, Chair, 402-280-4091, Fax: 402-280-1875, E-mail: richardgoering@creighton.edu. *Application contact:* Dr. Patrick C. Swanson, Graduate Director, 402-280-2716, Fax: 402-280-1875, E-mail: pswanson@creighton.edu.
Website: http://mmi.creighton.edu/

Dalhousie University, Faculty of Medicine, Department of Microbiology and Immunology, Halifax, NS B3H 4R2, Canada. Offers M Sc, PhD. *Degree requirements:* For master's, thesis; for doctorate, comprehensive exam, thesis/dissertation. *Entrance requirements:* For master's, GRE General Test, honors B Sc; for doctorate, GRE General Test, honors B Sc in microbiology, M Sc in discipline or transfer after 1 year in master's program. Additional exam requirements/recommendations for international students: Required—1 of 5 approved tests: TOEFL, IELTS, CANTEST, CAEL, Michigan English Language Assessment Battery. Electronic applications accepted. *Faculty research:* Virology, molecular genetics, pathogenesis, bacteriology, immunology.

Dartmouth College, Graduate Program in Molecular and Cellular Biology, Department of Microbiology and Immunology, Program in Immunology, Hanover, NH 03755. Offers MD/PhD. *Faculty research:* Tumor immunotherapy, cell and molecular biology of connective tissue degradation in rheumatoid arthritis and cancer, immunology and immunotherapy of tumors of the central nervous system, transcriptional regulation of hematopoiesis and leukemia, bacterial pathogenesis.

Drexel University, College of Medicine, Biomedical Graduate Programs, Program in Microbiology and Immunology, Philadelphia, PA 19104-2875. Offers MS, PhD, MD/PhD. Terminal master's awarded for partial completion of doctoral program. *Degree requirements:* For master's, comprehensive exam, thesis; for doctorate, thesis/dissertation, qualifying exam. *Entrance requirements:* For master's, GRE General Test, minimum GPA of 2.75; for doctorate, GRE General Test, minimum GPA of 3.0. Additional exam requirements/recommendations for international students: Required—TOEFL. Electronic applications accepted. *Faculty research:* Immunology of malarial parasites, virology, bacteriology, molecular biology, parasitology.

Duke University, Graduate School, Department of Immunology, Durham, NC 27710. Offers PhD. *Faculty:* 23. *Students:* 36 full-time (20 women); includes 6 minority (3 Black or African American, non-Hispanic/Latino; 3 Asian, non-Hispanic/Latino), 15 international. 78 applicants, 18% accepted, 4 enrolled. In 2013, 5 doctorates awarded. *Degree requirements:* For doctorate, thesis/dissertation. *Entrance requirements:* For doctorate, GRE General Test, GRE Subject Test in biology or biochemistry, cell and molecular biology (strongly recommended). Additional exam requirements/recommendations for international students: Required—TOEFL (minimum score 577 paper-based; 90 iBT) or IELTS (minimum score 7). *Application deadline:* For fall admission, 12/8 priority date for domestic and international students. Application fee: $80. Electronic applications accepted. *Financial support:* Fellowships and research assistantships available. Financial award application deadline: 12/8. *Unit head:* Yuan Zhuang, Director of Graduate Studies, 909-613-3578, Fax: 919-684-8982, E-mail: immunologydept@mc.duke.edu. *Application contact:* Elizabeth Hutton, Director of Admissions, 919-684-3913, Fax: 919-684-2277, E-mail: grad-admissions@duke.edu.
Website: http://immunology.mc.duke.edu/

East Carolina University, Brody School of Medicine, Department of Microbiology and Immunology, Greenville, NC 27858-4353. Offers MS, MD, PhD. *Degree requirements:* For doctorate, comprehensive exam, thesis/dissertation. *Entrance requirements:* For doctorate, GRE General Test. Additional exam requirements/recommendations for international students: Required—TOEFL. *Application deadline:* For fall admission, 4/15 priority date for domestic students. Applications are processed on a rolling basis. Application fee: $50. *Expenses:* Tuition, state resident: full-time $4223. Tuition, nonresident: full-time $16,540. *Required fees:* $2184. *Financial support:* Fellowships with tuition reimbursements available. Financial award application deadline: 6/1. *Faculty research:* Molecular virology, genetics of bacteria, yeast and somatic cells, bacterial physiology and metabolism, bioterrorism. *Unit head:* Dr. Charles J. Smith, Chair, 252-744-2700, Fax: 252-744-3104, E-mail: smithcha@ecu.edu. *Application contact:* Dr. Richard A. Franklin, Director of Graduate Studies, 252-744-2705, Fax: 252-744-3104, E-mail: franklinr@ecu.edu.
Website: http://www.ecu.edu/cs-dhs/microbiology/index.cfm

Emory University, Laney Graduate School, Division of Biological and Biomedical Sciences, Program in Immunology and Molecular Pathogenesis, Atlanta, GA 30322-1100. Offers PhD. *Degree requirements:* For doctorate, comprehensive exam, thesis/dissertation. *Entrance requirements:* For doctorate, GRE General Test, minimum GPA of 3.0 in science course work (recommended). Additional exam requirements/recommendations for international students: Required—TOEFL. Electronic applications accepted. *Faculty research:* Transplantation immunology, autoimmunity, microbial pathogenesis.

Georgetown University, Graduate School of Arts and Sciences, Programs in Biomedical Sciences, Department of Microbiology and Immunology, Washington, DC 20057. Offers biohazardous threat agents and emerging infectious diseases (MS); biomedical science policy and advocacy (MS); general microbiology and immunology (MS); global infectious diseases (PhD); microbiology and immunology (PhD). Part-time programs available. *Degree requirements:* For master's, 30 credit hours of coursework; for doctorate, comprehensive exam, thesis/dissertation. *Entrance requirements:* For master's, GRE General Test, 3 letters of reference, bachelor's degree in related field; for doctorate, GRE General Test, 3 letters of reference, MS/BS in related field. Additional exam requirements/recommendations for international students: Required—TOEFL (minimum score 505 paper-based). *Application deadline:* For fall admission, 7/1 for domestic students, 6/1 priority date for international students; for winter admission, 2/2 priority date for domestic students, 1/2 priority date for international students; for spring admission, 11/1 for domestic students, 10/1 priority date for international students. Applications are processed on a rolling basis. Application fee: $75. Electronic applications accepted. *Financial support:* Fellowships with full tuition reimbursements available. *Faculty research:* Pathogenesis and basic biology of the fungus Candida albicans, molecular biology of viral immunopathological mechanisms in Multiple Sclerosis. *Unit head:* Dr. Richard A. Calderone, Chair, 202-687-1513, E-mail: calderor@georgetown.edu. *Application contact:* Kimberly Bassalian, Graduate Program Coordinator, 202-687-3422, Fax: 202-687-1800, E-mail: kdb70@georgetown.edu.
Website: http://microbiology.georgetown.edu/

The George Washington University, Columbian College of Arts and Sciences, Institute for Biomedical Sciences, Program in Microbiology and Immunology, Washington, DC 20037. Offers PhD. *Students:* 5 full-time (3 women), 17 part-time (14 women); includes 4 minority (1 American Indian or Alaska Native, non-Hispanic/Latino; 1 Asian, non-Hispanic/Latino; 1 Hispanic/Latino; 1 Two or more races, non-Hispanic/Latino), 2 international. Average age 29. In 2013, 4 doctorates awarded. *Degree requirements:* For doctorate, thesis/dissertation. *Entrance requirements:* For doctorate, GRE General Test, minimum GPA of 3.0. Additional exam requirements/recommendations for international students: Required—TOEFL (minimum score 600 paper-based). *Application deadline:* For fall admission, 12/15 priority date for domestic and international students. Applications are processed on a rolling basis. Application fee: $75. Electronic applications accepted. *Financial support:* In 2013–14, 10 students received support. Fellowships with tuition reimbursements available and tuition waivers available. *Unit head:* Dr. David Leitenberg, Director, 202-994-9475, Fax: 202-994-2913, E-mail: dleit@gwu.edu. *Application contact:* Information Contact, 202-994-3532, Fax: 202-994-2913, E-mail: mtmjxl@gwumc.edu.
Website: http://www.gwumc.edu/ibs/fields/microimmuno.html

Hood College, Graduate School, Program in Biomedical Science, Frederick, MD 21701-8575. Offers biomedical science (MS), including biotechnology/molecular

biology, microbiology/immunology/virology, regulatory compliance; regulatory compliance (Certificate). Part-time and evening/weekend programs available. *Faculty:* 3 full-time (1 woman), 14 part-time/adjunct (6 women). *Students:* 5 full-time (2 women), 91 part-time (57 women); includes 17 minority (10 Black or African American, non-Hispanic/Latino; 4 Asian, non-Hispanic/Latino; 2 Hispanic/Latino; 1 Two or more races, non-Hispanic/Latino), 6 international. Average age 31. 60 applicants, 52% accepted, 21 enrolled. In 2013, 12 master's, 4 other advanced degrees awarded. *Degree requirements:* For master's, comprehensive exam, thesis or alternative. *Entrance requirements:* For master's, bachelor's degree in biology; minimum GPA of 2.75; undergraduate course work in cell biology, chemistry, organic chemistry, and genetics. Additional exam requirements/recommendations for international students: Required—TOEFL (minimum score 575 paper-based; 89 iBT), IELTS (minimum score 6.5). *Application deadline:* For fall admission, 7/15 priority date for domestic students, 7/15 for international students; for spring admission, 12/1 priority date for domestic students, 12/1 for international students. Applications are processed on a rolling basis. Application fee: $35. Electronic applications accepted. Application fee is waived when completed online. *Expenses: Tuition:* Part-time $405 per credit. *Required fees:* $100 per semester. *Financial support:* In 2013–14, 3 students received support, including 3 research assistantships with full tuition reimbursements available (averaging $10,609 per year); tuition waivers (partial) and unspecified assistantships also available. Financial award applicants required to submit FAFSA. *Unit head:* Dr. Rachel Bagni, Director, 301-696-3650, Fax: 301-696-3597, E-mail: bagni@hood.edu. *Application contact:* Dr. Maria Green Cowles, Dean of Graduate School, 301-696-3811, Fax: 301-696-3597, E-mail: gofurther@hood.edu.
Website: http://www.hood.edu/graduate

Illinois State University, Graduate School, College of Arts and Sciences, Department of Biological Sciences, Normal, IL 61790-2200. Offers animal behavior (MS); bacteriology (MS); biochemistry (MS); biological sciences (MS); biology (PhD); biophysics (MS); biotechnology (MS); botany (MS, PhD); cell biology (MS); conservation biology (MS); developmental biology (MS); ecology (MS, PhD); entomology (MS); evolutionary biology (MS); genetics (MS, PhD); immunology (MS); microbiology (MS, PhD); molecular biology (MS); molecular genetics (MS); neurobiology (MS); neuroscience (MS); parasitology (MS); physiology (MS, PhD); plant biology (MS); plant molecular biology (MS); plant sciences (MS); structural biology (MS); zoology (MS, PhD). Part-time programs available. *Degree requirements:* For master's, thesis or alternative; for doctorate, variable foreign language requirement, thesis/dissertation, 2 terms of residency. *Entrance requirements:* For master's, GRE General Test, minimum GPA of 2.6 in last 60 hours of course work; for doctorate, GRE General Test. *Faculty research:* Redoc balance and drug development in schistosoma mansoni, control of the growth of listeria monocytogenes at low temperature, regulation of cell expansion and microtubule function by SPRI, CRUI: physiology and fitness consequences of different life history phenotypes.

Indiana University–Purdue University Indianapolis, Indiana University School of Medicine, Department of Microbiology and Immunology, Indianapolis, IN 46202-2896. Offers MS, PhD, MD/MS, MD/PhD. *Faculty:* 20 full-time (2 women). *Students:* 28 full-time (18 women), 2 part-time (1 woman); includes 7 minority (1 Black or African American, non-Hispanic/Latino; 3 Asian, non-Hispanic/Latino; 2 Hispanic/Latino; 1 Two or more races, non-Hispanic/Latino), 12 international. Average age 27. 5 applicants. In 2013, 8 doctorates awarded. Terminal master's awarded for partial completion of doctoral program. *Degree requirements:* For master's, thesis; for doctorate, thesis/dissertation. *Entrance requirements:* For master's and doctorate, GRE General Test, previous course work in calculus, cell biology, chemistry, genetics, physics, and biochemistry. *Application deadline:* For fall admission, 3/1 for domestic students. Applications are processed on a rolling basis. Application fee: $55 ($65 for international students). *Financial support:* In 2013–14, fellowships with full tuition reimbursements (averaging $8,313 per year), teaching assistantships with full tuition reimbursements (averaging $18,391 per year) were awarded; research assistantships with full tuition reimbursements, Federal Work-Study, institutionally sponsored loans, scholarships/grants, traineeships, and tuition waivers (partial) also available. Financial award application deadline: 2/1. *Faculty research:* Host-parasite interactions, molecular biology, cellular and molecular immunology and hematology, viral and bacterial pathogenesis, cancer research. *Total annual research expenditures:* $4.2 million. *Unit head:* Dr. Stanley M. Spinola, Chair, 317-274-0508, E-mail: sspinola@iu.edu. *Application contact:* 317-274-7671, Fax: 317-274-4090.
Website: http://micro.medicine.iu.edu/

Iowa State University of Science and Technology, Program in Immunobiology, Ames, IA 50011. Offers MS, PhD. *Entrance requirements:* For master's and doctorate, GRE General Test, resume. Additional exam requirements/recommendations for international students: Required—TOEFL (minimum score 600 paper-based; 85 iBT), IELTS (minimum score 7). Electronic applications accepted. *Faculty research:* Immunogenetics, cellular and molecular immunology, infectious disease, neuroimmunology.

Johns Hopkins University, Bloomberg School of Public Health, W. Harry Feinstone Department of Molecular Microbiology and Immunology, Baltimore, MD 21218-2699. Offers MHS, Sc M, PhD. *Faculty:* 41 full-time (10 women), 10 part-time/adjunct (1 woman). *Students:* 95 full-time (52 women), 2 part-time (1 woman); includes 23 minority (3 Black or African American, non-Hispanic/Latino; 13 Asian, non-Hispanic/Latino; 5 Hispanic/Latino; 2 Two or more races, non-Hispanic/Latino), 25 international. Average age 26. 192 applicants, 47% accepted, 37 enrolled. In 2013, 34 master's, 7 doctorates awarded. Terminal master's awarded for partial completion of doctoral program. *Degree requirements:* For master's, comprehensive exam, thesis (for some programs), essay, written exams; for doctorate, comprehensive exam, thesis/dissertation, 1-year full-time residency, oral and written exams. *Entrance requirements:* For master's, GRE General Test or MCAT, 3 letters of recommendation, curriculum vitae; for doctorate, GRE General Test, 3 letters of recommendation, transcripts, curriculum vitae. Additional exam requirements/recommendations for international students: Required—TOEFL (minimum score 600 paper-based). *Application deadline:* For fall admission, 1/2 priority date for domestic and international students. Applications are processed on a rolling basis. Application fee: $45. Electronic applications accepted. *Financial support:* Fellowships with full and partial tuition reimbursements, research assistantships with tuition reimbursements, Federal Work-Study, institutionally sponsored loans, scholarships/grants, and stipends available. Financial award application deadline: 3/15; financial award applicants required to submit FAFSA. *Faculty research:* Immunology, virology, bacteriology, parasitology, vector biology, disease ecology, pathogenesis of infectious disease, immune responses to infectious agents, vector-borne and tropical diseases, biochemistry and molecular biology of infectious agents, population genetics of insect vectors, genetic regulation and immune responses in insect vectors, vaccine development, hormonal effects on pathogenesis and immune responses. *Total annual research expenditures:* $14.5 million. *Unit head:* Dr. Diane E. Griffin, Chair, 410-955-3459, Fax: 410-955-0105, E-mail: dgriffin@jhsph.edu. *Application contact:* Gail O'Connor, Senior Academic Program Coordinator, 410-614-4232, Fax: 410-955-0105, E-mail: goconnor@jhsph.edu.
Website: http://www.jhsph.edu/dept/MMI/

Johns Hopkins University, School of Medicine, Graduate Programs in Medicine, Immunology Training Program, Baltimore, MD 21218-2699. Offers PhD. *Faculty:* 34 full-time (8 women). *Students:* 30 full-time (19 women); includes 12 minority (2 Black or African American, non-Hispanic/Latino; 7 Asian, non-Hispanic/Latino; 2 Hispanic/Latino; 1 Two or more races, non-Hispanic/Latino), 2 international. Average age 28. 57 applicants, 40% accepted, 4 enrolled. In 2013, 6 doctorates awarded. *Degree requirements:* For doctorate, comprehensive exam, thesis/dissertation, oral exam, final thesis seminar. *Entrance requirements:* For doctorate, GRE General Test, 2 letters of recommendation. Additional exam requirements/recommendations for international students: Required—TOEFL (minimum score 550 paper-based). *Application deadline:* For fall admission, 1/10 for domestic students. Application fee: $85. Electronic applications accepted. *Financial support:* Fellowships, research assistantships, scholarships/grants, traineeships, health care benefits, tuition waivers (full), and unspecified assistantships available. Financial award application deadline: 1/10. *Faculty research:* HIV immunity, tumor immunity, major histocompatibility complex, transplantation, genetics of antibodies and T-cell receptors; immune response to infectious agents; antigen recognition; immune regulation; autoimmune diseases; immune cell signaling. *Total annual research expenditures:* $22.9 million. *Unit head:* Dr. Mark J. Soloski, Director, 410-550-8493, Fax: 410-550-2072, E-mail: mski@jhmi.edu. *Application contact:* Angela James, Academic Program Coordinator II, 410-955-2709, Fax: 410-955-0964, E-mail: ajames@jhmi.edu.
Website: http://gradimmunology.med.som.jhmi.edu/

Long Island University–LIU Post, School of Health Professions and Nursing, Department of Biomedical Sciences, Brookville, NY 11548-1300. Offers cardiovascular perfusion (MS); clinical laboratory management (MS); medical biology (MS), including hematology, immunology, medical biology, medical chemistry, medical microbiology. Part-time and evening/weekend programs available. Postbaccalaureate distance learning degree programs offered. *Degree requirements:* For master's, thesis. *Entrance requirements:* For master's, minimum GPA of 2.75 in major. Electronic applications accepted.

Louisiana State University Health Sciences Center, School of Graduate Studies in New Orleans, Department of Microbiology, Immunology, and Parasitology, New Orleans, LA 70112-2223. Offers microbiology and immunology (MS, PhD); MD/PhD. Terminal master's awarded for partial completion of doctoral program. *Degree requirements:* For master's, comprehensive exam, thesis; for doctorate, comprehensive exam, thesis/dissertation, preliminary exam, qualifying exam. *Entrance requirements:* For master's and doctorate, GRE General Test. Additional exam requirements/recommendations for international students: Required—TOEFL. *Faculty research:* Microbial physiology, animal virology, vaccine development, AIDS drug studies, pathogenic mechanisms, molecular immunology.

Louisiana State University Health Sciences Center at Shreveport, Department of Microbiology and Immunology, Shreveport, LA 71130-3932. Offers MS, PhD, MD/PhD. *Faculty:* 17 full-time (3 women). *Students:* 24 full-time (14 women); includes 2 minority (1 American Indian or Alaska Native, non-Hispanic/Latino; 1 Asian, non-Hispanic/Latino), 2 international. Average age 23. 23 applicants, 30% accepted, 6 enrolled. In 2013, 5 doctorates awarded. Terminal master's awarded for partial completion of doctoral program. *Degree requirements:* For master's, thesis; for doctorate, thesis/dissertation. *Entrance requirements:* For master's and doctorate, GRE General Test. Additional exam requirements/recommendations for international students: Required—TOEFL. Application fee: $0. *Financial support:* In 2013–14, 4 fellowships (averaging $28,000 per year), 20 research assistantships (averaging $26,000 per year) were awarded; institutionally sponsored loans also available. Financial award application deadline: 7/1. *Faculty research:* Infectious disease, pathogenesis, molecular virology and biology. *Unit head:* Dr. Dennis J. O'Callaghan, Head, 318-675-5750, Fax: 318-675-5764. *Application contact:* Marti Glass, Coordinator, 318-675-4781, Fax: 318-675-4343, E-mail: mglass@lsuhs.edu.
Website: http://www.lsuhscmicrobiology.com

Loyola University Chicago, Graduate School, Department of Microbiology and Immunology, Maywood, IL 60153. Offers MS. *Faculty:* 15 full-time (4 women). *Students:* 31 full-time (19 women); includes 4 minority (2 Asian, non-Hispanic/Latino; 2 Hispanic/Latino), 3 international. Average age 27. 22 applicants, 32% accepted, 5 enrolled. In 2013, 2 master's awarded. Terminal master's awarded for partial completion of doctoral program. *Degree requirements:* For master's, thesis. *Entrance requirements:* For master's, GRE General Test. Additional exam requirements/recommendations for international students: Required—TOEFL. *Application deadline:* For fall admission, 3/15 for domestic and international students. Applications are processed on a rolling basis. Application fee: $0. Electronic applications accepted. *Expenses: Tuition:* Full-time $16,740; part-time $930 per credit. *Required fees:* $135 per semester. *Financial support:* In 2013–14, 5 fellowships with tuition reimbursements (averaging $27,000 per year), 24 research assistantships with tuition reimbursements (averaging $27,000 per year) were awarded; institutionally sponsored loans and scholarships/grants also available. Financial award application deadline: 1/18. *Faculty research:* Virology, microbial physiology and genetics, immune system development and regulation, signal transduction and host-pathogen interactions, biofilms. *Unit head:* Dr. Katherine L. Knight, Chair, 708-216-3385, Fax: 708-216-9574, E-mail: kknight@luc.edu. *Application contact:* Dr. Karen Visick, Graduate Program Director, 708-216-0869, Fax: 708-216-9574, E-mail: kvisick@luc.edu.

Loyola University Chicago, Graduate School, Program in Infectious Disease and Immunology, Chicago, IL 60660. Offers MS. *Faculty:* 35 full-time (12 women). *Students:* 9 full-time (8 women); includes 1 minority (Black or African American, non-Hispanic/Latino). Average age 25. 24 applicants, 33% accepted, 4 enrolled. In 2013, 3 master's awarded. *Degree requirements:* For master's, thesis. *Entrance requirements:* For master's, GRE. Additional exam requirements/recommendations for international students: Required—TOEFL. *Application deadline:* For fall admission, 6/15 for domestic and international students. Applications are processed on a rolling basis. *Expenses: Tuition:* Full-time $16,740; part-time $930 per credit. *Required fees:* $135 per semester. *Faculty research:* Immunological tolerance and memory, molecular analysis of virus assembly and entry, biofilm mediated interactions, molecular analysis of clinical isolates of C. difficile, immune system development and regulation. *Unit head:* Dr. Katherine L. Knight, Co-Director, 708-216-3385, Fax: 708-216-9574, E-mail: kknight@lumc.edu. *Application contact:* Dr. Makio Iwashima, Graduate Program Director, 708-216-5816, Fax: 708-216-9574, E-mail: miwashima@lumc.edu.

Massachusetts Institute of Technology, School of Science, Department of Biology, Cambridge, MA 02139-4307. Offers biochemistry (PhD); biological oceanography (PhD); biology (PhD); biophysical chemistry and molecular structure (PhD); cell biology (PhD); computational and systems biology (PhD); developmental biology (PhD); genetics (PhD); immunology (PhD); microbiology (PhD); molecular biology (PhD); neurobiology (PhD). *Faculty:* 58 full-time (15 women). *Students:* 261 full-time (133 women); includes 77 minority (3 Black or African American, non-Hispanic/Latino; 1 American Indian or Alaska Native, non-Hispanic/Latino; 32 Asian, non-Hispanic/Latino; 32 Hispanic/Latino; 9 Two or more races, non-Hispanic/Latino), 46 international. Average age 26. 651 applicants, 15% accepted, 39 enrolled. In 2013, 25 doctorates awarded. *Degree requirements:* For doctorate, comprehensive exam, thesis/

dissertation, two semesters as a teaching assistant. *Entrance requirements:* For doctorate, GRE General Test. Additional exam requirements/recommendations for international students: Required—TOEFL (minimum score 577 paper-based), IELTS (minimum score 6.5). *Application deadline:* For fall admission, 12/1 for domestic and international students. Application fee: $75. Electronic applications accepted. *Expenses: Tuition:* Full-time $43,210; part-time $670 per credit hour. *Required fees:* $288. *Financial support:* In 2013–14, 252 students received support, including 135 fellowships (averaging $36,800 per year), 122 research assistantships (averaging $35,500 per year), 1 teaching assistantship; Federal Work-Study, institutionally sponsored loans, scholarships/grants, traineeships, health care benefits, and unspecified assistantships also available. *Faculty research:* Cellular, developmental and molecular (plant and animal) biology; biochemistry, bioengineering, biophysics and structural biology; classical and molecular genetics, stem cell and epigenetics; immunology and microbiology; cancer biology, molecular medicine, neurobiology and human disease; computational and systems biology. *Total annual research expenditures:* $44.5 million. *Unit head:* Alan Grossman, Interim Head, 617-253-4701. *Application contact:* Biology Education Office, 617-253-3717, Fax: 617-258-9329, E-mail: gradbio@mit.edu.
Website: https://biology.mit.edu/

Mayo Graduate School, Graduate Programs in Biomedical Sciences, Program in Immunology, Rochester, MN 55905. Offers PhD. *Degree requirements:* For doctorate, oral defense of dissertation, qualifying oral and written exam. *Entrance requirements:* For doctorate, GRE, 1 year of chemistry, biology, calculus, and physics. Additional exam requirements/recommendations for international students: Required—TOEFL. Electronic applications accepted. *Faculty research:* Immunogenetics, autoimmunity, receptor signal transduction, T lymphocyte activation, transplantation.

McGill University, Faculty of Graduate and Postdoctoral Studies, Faculty of Medicine, Department of Microbiology and Immunology, Montréal, QC H3A 2T5, Canada. Offers M Sc, M Sc A, PhD.

McMaster University, Faculty of Health Sciences and School of Graduate Studies, Program in Medical Sciences, Immunity and Infection Area, Hamilton, ON L8S 4M2, Canada. Offers M Sc, PhD, MD/PhD. *Degree requirements:* For master's, thesis; for doctorate, comprehensive exam, thesis/dissertation. *Entrance requirements:* For master's, honors B Sc, B+ average in related field; for doctorate, M Sc, minimum B+ average, students with proven research experience and an A average may be admitted with a B Sc degree. Additional exam requirements/recommendations for international students: Required—TOEFL (minimum score 580 paper-based; 92 iBT).

Medical University of South Carolina, College of Graduate Studies, Department of Microbiology and Immunology, Charleston, SC 29425. Offers MS, PhD, DMD/PhD, MD/PhD. Terminal master's awarded for partial completion of doctoral program. *Degree requirements:* For master's, thesis; for doctorate, thesis/dissertation, oral and written exams. *Entrance requirements:* For master's, GRE General Test, MCAT, or DAT, minimum GPA of 3.0; for doctorate, GRE General Test, interview, minimum GPA of 3.0, research experience. Additional exam requirements/recommendations for international students: Required—TOEFL (minimum score 600 paper-based; 100 iBT). Electronic applications accepted. *Faculty research:* Inmate and adaptive immunology, gene therapy/vector development, vaccinology, proteomics of biowarfare agents, bacterial and fungal pathogenesis.

Meharry Medical College, School of Graduate Studies, Program in Biomedical Sciences, Microbiology and Immunology Emphasis, Nashville, TN 37208-9989. Offers PhD, MD/PhD. *Degree requirements:* For doctorate, comprehensive exam, thesis/dissertation. *Entrance requirements:* For doctorate, GRE General Test, GRE Subject Test, undergraduate degree in related science. *Faculty research:* Microbial and bacterial pathogenesis, viral transcription, immune response to viruses and parasites.

Memorial University of Newfoundland, Faculty of Medicine and School of Graduate Studies, Graduate Programs in Medicine, Division of Biomedical Sciences, St. John's, NL A1C 5S7, Canada. Offers cancer (M Sc, PhD); cardiovascular (M Sc, PhD); immunology (M Sc, PhD); neuroscience (M Sc, PhD). Part-time programs available. *Degree requirements:* For master's, thesis; for doctorate, comprehensive exam, thesis/dissertation, oral defense of thesis. *Entrance requirements:* For master's, MD or B Sc; for doctorate, MD or M Sc. Additional exam requirements/recommendations for international students: Required—TOEFL. *Faculty research:* Neuroscience, immunology, cardiovascular, and cancer.

Montana State University, College of Graduate Studies, College of Agriculture, Department of Immunology and Infectious Diseases, Bozeman, MT 59717. Offers MS, PhD. Part-time programs available. *Degree requirements:* For master's, comprehensive exam; for doctorate, comprehensive exam, thesis/dissertation. *Entrance requirements:* For master's and doctorate, GRE General Test. Additional exam requirements/recommendations for international students: Required—TOEFL (minimum score 550 paper-based). Electronic applications accepted. *Faculty research:* Immunology, mechanisms of infectious disease pathogenesis, mechanisms of host defense, lymphocyte development, host-pathogen interactions.

New York Medical College, Graduate School of Basic Medical Sciences, Integrated PhD Program, Valhalla, NY 10595-1691. Offers biochemistry and molecular biology (PhD); cell biology and anatomy (PhD); microbiology and immunology (PhD); pathology (PhD); pharmacology (PhD); physiology (PhD). *Faculty:* 91 full-time (16 women), 5 part-time/adjunct (2 women). *Students:* 31 full-time (21 women); includes 17 minority (4 Black or African American, non-Hispanic/Latino; 11 Asian, non-Hispanic/Latino; 2 Hispanic/Latino). Average age 27. 56 applicants, 36% accepted, 9 enrolled. In 2013, 17 doctorates awarded. *Degree requirements:* For doctorate, comprehensive exam, thesis/dissertation. *Entrance requirements:* For doctorate, GRE General Test. Additional exam requirements/recommendations for international students: Required—TOEFL. *Application deadline:* For fall admission, 1/1 priority date for domestic and international students. Applications are processed on a rolling basis. Application fee: $75 ($100 for international students). Electronic applications accepted. *Expenses: Tuition:* Full-time $49,170; part-time $910 per credit. Tuition and fees vary according to program. *Financial support:* In 2013–14, fellowships with full tuition reimbursements (averaging $25,500 per year), research assistantships with full tuition reimbursements (averaging $25,500 per year) were awarded; Federal Work-Study, scholarships/grants, traineeships, health care benefits, and tuition waivers (full) also available. Financial award applicants required to submit FAFSA. *Faculty research:* Cardiovascular sciences, infectious diseases, neuroscience, cancer and cell signaling. *Unit head:* Dr. Francis L. Belloni, Dean, 914-594-4110, Fax: 914-594-4944, E-mail: francis_belloni@nymc.edu. *Application contact:* Valerie Romeo-Messana, Director of Admissions, 914-594-4110, Fax: 914-594-4944, E-mail: v_romeomessana@nymc.edu.

New York Medical College, Graduate School of Basic Medical Sciences, Microbiology and Immunology Master's Program, Valhalla, NY 10595-1691. Offers MS, PhD, MD/PhD. Part-time and evening/weekend programs available. *Faculty:* 12 full-time (4 women). *Students:* 19 full-time (13 women); includes 10 minority (1 Black or African American, non-Hispanic/Latino; 7 Asian, non-Hispanic/Latino; 2 Hispanic/Latino). Average age 25. 20 applicants, 85% accepted, 5 enrolled. In 2013, 9 master's awarded. Terminal master's awarded for partial completion of doctoral program. *Degree requirements:* For master's, thesis; for doctorate, comprehensive exam, thesis/dissertation. *Entrance requirements:* For master's, GRE General Test, MCAT, or DAT. Additional exam requirements/recommendations for international students: Required—TOEFL. *Application deadline:* For fall admission, 7/1 priority date for domestic students, 5/1 priority date for international students; for spring admission, 12/1 for domestic students, 10/1 for international students. Applications are processed on a rolling basis. Application fee: $75 ($100 for international students). Electronic applications accepted. *Expenses: Tuition:* Full-time $49,170; part-time $910 per credit. Tuition and fees vary according to program. *Financial support:* Federal Work-Study and scholarships/grants available. Support available to part-time students. Financial award applicants required to submit FAFSA. *Faculty research:* Tumor cells, cancer vaccines, the role of stem cells in cancer, bacterial genetics pathogenesis of infectious disease and function of influenza virus antigens, molecular virology, and the biochemistry and genetics of emerging pathogens. *Unit head:* Dr. Raj Tiwari, Program Director, 914-594-4870, Fax: 914-594-4944, E-mail: raj_tiwari@nymc.edu. *Application contact:* Valerie Romeo-Messana, Director of Admissions, 914-594-4110, Fax: 914-594-4944, E-mail: v_romeomessana@nymc.edu.

New York University, Graduate School of Arts and Science, Department of Biology, New York, NY 10012-1019. Offers biology (PhD); biomedical journalism (MS); cancer and molecular biology (PhD); computational biology (PhD); computers in biological research (MS); developmental genetics (PhD); general biology (MS); immunology and microbiology (PhD); molecular genetics (PhD); neurobiology (PhD); oral biology (MS); plant biology (PhD); recombinant DNA technology (MS); MS/MBA. Part-time programs available. *Faculty:* 24 full-time (5 women). *Students:* 161 full-time (88 women), 28 part-time (15 women); includes 41 minority (5 Black or African American, non-Hispanic/Latino; 23 Asian, non-Hispanic/Latino; 9 Hispanic/Latino; 4 Two or more races, non-Hispanic/Latino), 80 international. Average age 27. 412 applicants, 54% accepted, 65 enrolled. In 2013, 77 master's, 9 doctorates awarded. Terminal master's awarded for partial completion of doctoral program. *Degree requirements:* For master's, thesis or alternative, qualifying paper; for doctorate, comprehensive exam, thesis/dissertation. *Entrance requirements:* For master's and doctorate, GRE General Test. Additional exam requirements/recommendations for international students: Required—TOEFL. *Application deadline:* For fall admission, 12/1 priority date for domestic students, 12/1 for international students. Application fee: $95. *Expenses: Tuition:* Full-time $35,856; part-time $1494 per unit. *Required fees:* $1408; $64 per unit. $473 per term. Tuition and fees vary according to course load and program. *Financial support:* Fellowships with tuition reimbursements, research assistantships with tuition reimbursements, teaching assistantships with tuition reimbursements, career-related internships or fieldwork, Federal Work-Study, institutionally sponsored loans, scholarships/grants, health care benefits, and unspecified assistantships available. Financial award application deadline: 12/1; financial award applicants required to submit FAFSA. *Faculty research:* Genomics, molecular and cell biology, development and molecular genetics, molecular evolution of plants and animals. *Unit head:* Stephen Small, Chair, 212-998-8200, Fax: 212-995-4015, E-mail: biology.admissions@nyu.edu. *Application contact:* Justin Blau, Director of Graduate Studies, PhD Programs, 212-998-8200, Fax: 212-995-4015, E-mail: biology.admissions@nyu.edu.
Website: http://biology.as.nyu.edu/

New York University, School of Medicine and Graduate School of Arts and Science, Sackler Institute of Graduate Biomedical Sciences, Program in Immunology and Inflammation, New York, NY 10012-1019. Offers PhD. *Faculty:* 33 full-time (11 women). *Students:* 15 full-time (10 women); includes 5 minority (1 Black or African American, non-Hispanic/Latino; 3 Asian, non-Hispanic/Latino; 1 Hispanic/Latino), 3 international. Average age 28. *Expenses: Tuition:* Full-time $35,856; part-time $1494 per unit. *Required fees:* $1408; $64 per unit. $473 per term. Tuition and fees vary according to course load and program. *Faculty research:* Molecular regulation of hematopoietic stem cell differentiation, immunological synapse and immunotherapy, adenosine as a regulator of inflammation. *Unit head:* Dr. Joel D. Oppenheim, Senior Associate Dean for Graduate Studies, 212-263-8001, Fax: 212-263-7600. *Application contact:* Michael Escosia, Program Associate, 212-263-5648, Fax: 212-263-7600, E-mail: sackler-info@med.nyu.edu.
Website: http://sackler.med.nyu.edu/graduate/immunology-inflammation

New York University, School of Medicine and Graduate School of Arts and Science, Sackler Institute of Graduate Biomedical Sciences, Program in Molecular Oncology and Tumor Immunology, New York, NY 10012-1019. Offers immunology (PhD); molecular oncology (PhD); MD/PhD. *Faculty:* 51 full-time (16 women). *Students:* 23 full-time (10 women); includes 5 minority (2 Black or African American, non-Hispanic/Latino; 1 Asian, non-Hispanic/Latino; 2 Hispanic/Latino), 7 international. Average age 28. In 2013, 9 doctorates awarded. *Degree requirements:* For doctorate, one foreign language, thesis/dissertation, qualifying exam. *Entrance requirements:* For doctorate, GRE General Test, GRE Subject Test. Additional exam requirements/recommendations for international students: Required—TOEFL. *Application deadline:* For fall admission, 2/1 for domestic students. Applications are processed on a rolling basis. Application fee: $85. Electronic applications accepted. *Expenses: Tuition:* Full-time $35,856; part-time $1494 per unit. *Required fees:* $1408; $64 per unit. $473 per term. Tuition and fees vary according to course load and program. *Financial support:* Tuition waivers (full) available. *Faculty research:* Stem cells, immunology, genome instability, DNA damage checkpoints. *Unit head:* Dr. Joel D. Oppenheim, Senior Associate Dean for Graduate Studies, 212-263-8001, Fax: 212-263-7600. *Application contact:* Dr. David Levy, Graduate Adviser, 212-263-8192, Fax: 212-263-8211, E-mail: david.levy@med.nyu.edu.

North Carolina State University, Graduate School, College of Agriculture and Life Sciences and College of Veterinary Medicine, Program in Immunology, Raleigh, NC 27695. Offers MS, PhD. *Degree requirements:* For master's, thesis; for doctorate, thesis/dissertation. *Entrance requirements:* For master's and doctorate, GRE General Test. Additional exam requirements/recommendations for international students: Required—TOEFL (minimum score 550 paper-based). Electronic applications accepted. *Faculty research:* Immunogenetics, immunopathology, immunotoxicology, immunoparasitology, molecular and infectious disease immunology.

The Ohio State University, College of Medicine, School of Biomedical Science, Biomedical Sciences Graduate Program, Columbus, OH 43210. Offers immunology (PhD); medical genetics (PhD); molecular virology (PhD); pharmacology (PhD). *Students:* 109 full-time (55 women), 9 part-time (6 women); includes 24 minority (5 Black or African American, non-Hispanic/Latino; 1 American Indian or Alaska Native, non-Hispanic/Latino; 10 Asian, non-Hispanic/Latino; 6 Hispanic/Latino; 1 Native Hawaiian or other Pacific Islander, non-Hispanic/Latino; 1 Two or more races, non-Hispanic/Latino), 4 international. Average age 27. In 2013, 20 doctorates awarded. *Degree requirements:* For doctorate, thesis/dissertation. *Entrance requirements:* For doctorate, GRE General Test; GRE Subject Test in biochemistry, cell and molecular biology (recommended for some programs). Additional exam requirements/recommendations for international students: Required—TOEFL (minimum score 600 paper-based; 100 iBT), Michigan English Language Assessment Battery (minimum score 86); Recommended—IELTS (minimum score 8). *Application deadline:* For fall admission, 12/13 priority date for domestic students, 11/1 priority date for international students. Applications are processed on a rolling basis. Application fee: $60 ($70 for international students). Electronic applications accepted. *Financial support:* In 2013–14, 53 students received

support, including 4 fellowships with full tuition reimbursements available (averaging $19,000 per year), 49 research assistantships with full tuition reimbursements available (averaging $19,000 per year); scholarships/grants and unspecified assistantships also available. Financial award application deadline: 1/15. *Unit head:* Joanna Groden, Co-Director, 614-688-4301, Fax: 614-292-6226, E-mail: ibgp@osumc.edu. *Application contact:* Graduate Admissions, 614-292-9444, Fax: 614-292-3895, E-mail: domestic.grad@osu.edu.
Website: http://www.ibgp.org

Oregon Health & Science University, School of Medicine, Graduate Programs in Medicine, Program in Molecular and Cellular Biosciences, Department of Molecular Microbiology and Immunology, Portland, OR 97239-3098. Offers PhD. *Faculty:* 9 full-time (3 women), 16 part-time/adjunct (2 women). *Students:* 19 full-time (12 women), 1 (woman) part-time; includes 6 minority (2 Asian, non-Hispanic/Latino; 3 Hispanic/Latino; 1 Two or more races, non-Hispanic/Latino), 2 international. Average age 29. In 2013, 5 doctorates awarded. Terminal master's awarded for partial completion of doctoral program. *Degree requirements:* For doctorate, comprehensive exam, thesis/dissertation, qualifying exam. *Entrance requirements:* For doctorate, GRE General Test (minimum scores: 153 Verbal/148 Quantitative/4.5 Analytical) or MCAT (for some programs). Additional exam requirements/recommendations for international students: Required—TOEFL. Electronic applications accepted. *Financial support:* Health care benefits and full tuition and stipends available. *Faculty research:* Molecular biology of bacterial and viral pathogens, cellular and humoral immunology, molecular biology of microbes. *Unit head:* Dr. Eric Barklis, Program Director, 503-494-7768, E-mail: mmi@ohsu.edu. *Application contact:* Lola Bichler, Program Coordinator, 503-494-5824, E-mail: bichler@ohsu.edu.
Website: http://www.ohsu.edu/microbiology

Penn State Hershey Medical Center, College of Medicine, Graduate School Programs in the Biomedical Sciences, Graduate Program in Biomedical Sciences, Hershey, PA 17033. Offers biochemistry and molecular genetics (MS, PhD); biomedical sciences (MS, PhD); translational therapeutics (MS, PhD); virology and immunology (MS, PhD); MD/PhD; PhD/MBA. *Students:* 40 full-time (22 women); includes 7 minority (2 Black or African American, non-Hispanic/Latino; 2 Asian, non-Hispanic/Latino; 1 Hispanic/Latino; 2 Two or more races, non-Hispanic/Latino), 10 international. 215 applicants, 20% accepted, 14 enrolled. Terminal master's awarded for partial completion of doctoral program. *Degree requirements:* For master's, thesis (for some programs); for doctorate, comprehensive exam, thesis/dissertation, candidacy exam. *Entrance requirements:* For doctorate, GRE General Test. Additional exam requirements/recommendations for international students: Required—TOEFL (minimum score 550 paper-based; 80 iBT). *Application deadline:* For fall admission, 2/1 for domestic and international students. Applications are processed on a rolling basis. Application fee: $65. Electronic applications accepted. *Financial support:* In 2013–14, research assistantships (averaging $24,544 per year) were awarded; fellowships, scholarships/grants, health care benefits, and unspecified assistantships also available. Financial award applicants required to submit FAFSA. *Unit head:* Dr. Ralph L. Keil, Chair, 717-531-8595, Fax: 717-531-0388, E-mail: rlk9@psu.edu. *Application contact:* Kristin E. Smith, Enrollment Support Manager, 717-531-0003, Fax: 717-531-0388, E-mail: kec17@psu.edu.
Website: http://med.psu.edu/web/biomedical-sciences/home

Penn State University Park, Graduate School, Intercollege Graduate Programs, Intercollege Graduate Program in Immunology and Infectious Diseases, University Park, PA 16802. Offers MS, PhD. *Unit head:* Dr. Regina Vasilatos-Younken, Interim Dean, 814-865-2516, Fax: 814-863-4627, E-mail: rxv@psu.edu. *Application contact:* Cynthia E. Nicosia, Director, Graduate Enrollment Services, 814-865-1834, Fax: 814-863-4627, E-mail: cey1@psu.edu.

Purdue University, College of Pharmacy and Pharmacal Sciences and Graduate School, Graduate Programs in Pharmacy and Pharmacal Sciences, Department of Medicinal Chemistry and Molecular Pharmacology, West Lafayette, IN 47907. Offers biophysical and computational chemistry (PhD); cancer research (PhD); immunology and infectious disease (PhD); medicinal biochemistry and molecular biology (PhD); medicinal chemistry and chemical biology (PhD); molecular pharmacology (PhD); neuropharmacology, neurodegeneration, and neurotoxicity (PhD); systems biology and functional genomics (PhD). *Faculty:* 23 full-time (3 women), 6 part-time/adjunct (1 woman). *Students:* 50 full-time (21 women), 3 part-time (2 women); includes 1 minority (Asian, non-Hispanic/Latino), 30 international. Average age 26. 147 applicants, 20% accepted, 13 enrolled. In 2013, 12 doctorates awarded. *Degree requirements:* For doctorate, thesis/dissertation. *Entrance requirements:* For doctorate, GRE General Test; GRE Subject Test in biology, biochemistry, and chemistry (recommended), minimum undergraduate GPA of 3.0. Additional exam requirements/recommendations for international students: Required—TOEFL (minimum score 550 paper-based; 77 iBT); Recommended—TWE. *Application deadline:* For fall admission, 2/1 for domestic and international students. Applications are processed on a rolling basis. Application fee: $60 ($75 for international students). Electronic applications accepted. *Financial support:* Fellowships, research assistantships, teaching assistantships, and traineeships available. Support available to part-time students. Financial award applicants required to submit FAFSA. *Faculty research:* Drug design and development, cancer research, drug synthesis and analysis, chemical pharmacology, environmental toxicology. *Unit head:* Dr. Richard F. Borch, Head, 765-494-1403, E-mail: borch@purdue.edu. *Application contact:* Dr. Janine C. Mott, Graduate Contact, 765-494-1269, E-mail: jmott@purdue.edu.

Purdue University, School of Veterinary Medicine and Graduate School, Graduate Programs in Veterinary Medicine, Department of Comparative Pathobiology, West Lafayette, IN 47907-2027. Offers comparative epidemiology and public health (MS); comparative epidemiology and public heath (PhD); comparative microbiology and immunology (MS, PhD); comparative pathobiology (MS, PhD); interdisciplinary studies (PhD), including microbial pathogenesis, molecular signaling and cancer biology, molecular virology; lab animal medicine (MS); veterinary anatomic pathology (MS); veterinary clinical pathology (MS). Terminal master's awarded for partial completion of doctoral program. *Degree requirements:* For master's, thesis (for some programs); for doctorate, thesis/dissertation. *Entrance requirements:* For master's and doctorate, GRE General Test. Additional exam requirements/recommendations for international students: Required—TOEFL (minimum score 575 paper-based), IELTS (minimum score 6.5), TWE (minimum score 4). Electronic applications accepted.

Queen's University at Kingston, School of Graduate Studies, Faculty of Health Sciences, Department of Microbiology and Immunology, Kingston, ON K7L 3N6, Canada. Offers M Sc, PhD. Part-time programs available. *Degree requirements:* For master's, thesis; for doctorate, comprehensive exam, thesis/dissertation. *Entrance requirements:* For master's and doctorate, minimum B+ average. Additional exam requirements/recommendations for international students: Required—TOEFL (minimum score 600 paper-based). Electronic applications accepted. *Faculty research:* Bacteriology, virology, immunology, education in microbiology and immunology, microbial pathogenesis.

Rosalind Franklin University of Medicine and Science, School of Graduate and Postdoctoral Studies - Interdisciplinary Graduate Program in Biomedical Sciences, Department of Microbiology and Immunology, North Chicago, IL 60064-3095. Offers MS, PhD, MD/PhD. Terminal master's awarded for partial completion of doctoral program. *Degree requirements:* For master's, comprehensive exam, thesis; for doctorate, comprehensive exam, thesis/dissertation. *Entrance requirements:* For master's and doctorate, GRE General Test. Additional exam requirements/recommendations for international students: Required—TOEFL, TWE. *Faculty research:* Molecular biology, parasitology, virology.

Rush University, Graduate College, Division of Immunology and Microbiology, Program in Immunology/Microbiology, Chicago, IL 60612-3832. Offers immunology (MS, PhD); virology (MS, PhD); MD/PhD. Part-time programs available. Terminal master's awarded for partial completion of doctoral program. *Degree requirements:* For master's, thesis; for doctorate, thesis/dissertation, comprehensive preliminary exam. *Entrance requirements:* For master's, GRE General Test; for doctorate, GRE General Test, interview, minimum GPA of 3.0. Additional exam requirements/recommendations for international students: Required—TOEFL. Electronic applications accepted. *Faculty research:* Human genetics, autoimmunity, tumor biology, complement, HIV immunopathology genesis.

Rutgers, The State University of New Jersey, Newark, Graduate School of Biomedical Sciences, Program in Molecular Pathology and Immunology, Newark, NJ 07107. Offers PhD. *Entrance requirements:* Additional exam requirements/recommendations for international students: Required—TOEFL. Electronic applications accepted.

Rutgers, The State University of New Jersey, New Brunswick, Graduate School-New Brunswick, Programs in the Molecular Biosciences, Piscataway, NJ 08854-8097. Offers biochemistry (PhD); cell and developmental biology (MS, PhD); microbiology and molecular genetics (MS, PhD), including applied microbiology, clinical microbiology (MS), clinical mircobiology (PhD), computational molecular biology (PhD), immunology, microbial biochemistry, molecular genetics, virology. MS, PhD offered jointly with University of Medicine and Dentistry of New Jersey.

Saint Louis University, Graduate Education and School of Medicine, Graduate Program in Biomedical Sciences, Department of Molecular Microbiology and Immunology, St. Louis, MO 63103-2097. Offers PhD. *Degree requirements:* For doctorate, comprehensive exam, thesis/dissertation, qualifying exams. *Entrance requirements:* For doctorate, GRE General Test (GRE Subject Test optional), letters of recommendation, resume, interview. Additional exam requirements/recommendations for international students: Required—TOEFL (minimum score 525 paper-based). Electronic applications accepted. *Faculty research:* Pathogenesis of hepatitis C virus, herperviruses, pox viruses, rheumatoid arthritis, antiviral drugs and vaccines in biodefense, cancer gene therapy, virology and immunology.

Stanford University, School of Medicine, Graduate Programs in Medicine, Department of Microbiology and Immunology, Stanford, CA 94305-9991. Offers PhD. *Degree requirements:* For doctorate, comprehensive exam, thesis/dissertation, 2 quarters teaching assistantship. *Entrance requirements:* For doctorate, GRE General Test, GRE Subject Test (biology or biochemistry). Additional exam requirements/recommendations for international students: Required—TOEFL. Electronic applications accepted. *Expenses: Tuition:* Full-time $42,690; part-time $949 per credit. *Required fees:* $185. *Faculty research:* Molecular pathogenesis of bacteria viruses and parasites, immune system function, autoimmunity, molecular biology.

Stanford University, School of Medicine, Graduate Programs in Medicine, Program in Immunology, Stanford, CA 94305-9991. Offers PhD. *Degree requirements:* For doctorate, thesis/dissertation, qualifying examination. *Entrance requirements:* For doctorate, GRE General Test, GRE Subject Test. Additional exam requirements/recommendations for international students: Required—TOEFL. Electronic applications accepted. *Expenses: Tuition:* Full-time $42,690; part-time $949 per credit. *Required fees:* $185.

State University of New York Upstate Medical University, College of Graduate Studies, Program in Microbiology and Immunology, Syracuse, NY 13210-2334. Offers microbiology (MS); microbiology and immunology (PhD); MD/PhD. Terminal master's awarded for partial completion of doctoral program. *Degree requirements:* For master's, thesis; for doctorate, comprehensive exam, thesis/dissertation. *Entrance requirements:* For master's, GRE General Test, interview; for doctorate, GRE General Test, telephone interview. Additional exam requirements/recommendations for international students: Required—TOEFL. Electronic applications accepted. *Faculty research:* Cancer, disorders of the nervous system, infectious diseases, diabetes/metabolic disorders/cardiovascular diseases.

Stony Brook University, State University of New York, Graduate School, College of Arts and Sciences, Department of Biochemistry and Cell Biology, Molecular and Cellular Biology Program, Stony Brook, NY 11794. Offers biochemistry and molecular biology (PhD); biological sciences (MA); immunology and pathology (PhD); molecular and cellular biology (PhD). *Faculty:* 23 full-time (7 women), 1 part-time/adjunct (0 women). *Students:* 75 full-time (42 women); includes 7 minority (5 Asian, non-Hispanic/Latino; 2 Hispanic/Latino), 46 international. Average age 30. 211 applicants, 15% accepted, 8 enrolled. In 2013, 13 master's, 15 doctorates awarded. *Degree requirements:* For doctorate, comprehensive exam, thesis/dissertation, teaching experience. *Entrance requirements:* For doctorate, GRE General Test, GRE Subject Test. Additional exam requirements/recommendations for international students: Required—TOEFL. *Application deadline:* For fall admission, 1/15 for domestic students; for spring admission, 10/1 for domestic students. Application fee: $100. *Expenses:* Tuition, state resident: full-time $9870; part-time $411 per credit. Tuition, nonresident: full-time $18,350; part-time $765 per credit. *Financial support:* In 2013–14, 22 fellowships, 18 research assistantships, 12 teaching assistantships were awarded; Federal Work-Study also available. *Unit head:* Prof. Robert Haltiwanger, Chair, 631-632-8560, E-mail: robert.haltiwanger@stonybrook.edu. *Application contact:* Joann DeLucia-Conlon, Coordinator, 631-632-8613, Fax: 631-632-9730, E-mail: joann.delucia-conlon@stonybrook.edu.

Texas A&M Health Science Center, College of Medicine, Department of Microbial and Molecular Pathogenesis, College Station, TX 77840. Offers immunology (PhD); microbiology (PhD); molecular biology (PhD); virology (PhD). *Degree requirements:* For doctorate, thesis/dissertation. *Entrance requirements:* For doctorate, GRE General Test, minimum GPA of 3.0. *Faculty research:* Molecular pathogenesis, microbial therapeutics.

Thomas Jefferson University, Jefferson Graduate School of Biomedical Sciences, PhD Program in Immunology and Microbial Pathogenesis, Philadelphia, PA 19107. Offers PhD. *Faculty:* 35 full-time (5 women), 1 part-time/adjunct (0 women). *Students:* 20 full-time (8 women); includes 3 minority (2 Asian, non-Hispanic/Latino; 1 Hispanic/Latino), 2 international. 54 applicants, 11% accepted, 2 enrolled. In 2013, 4 doctorates awarded. *Degree requirements:* For doctorate, comprehensive exam, thesis/dissertation. *Entrance requirements:* For doctorate, GRE General Test, minimum GPA of 3.2. Additional exam requirements/recommendations for international students: Required—TOEFL (minimum score 100 iBT) or IELTS. *Application deadline:* For fall admission, 1/5 priority date for domestic and international students. Applications are processed on a rolling basis. Application fee: $75. Electronic applications accepted. *Financial support:* In 2013–14, 20 students received support, including 20 fellowships with full tuition reimbursements available (averaging $56,052 per year); Federal Work-

Study, institutionally sponsored loans, scholarships/grants, traineeships, and stipends also available. Support available to part-time students. Financial award application deadline: 5/1; financial award applicants required to submit FAFSA. *Unit head:* Dr. Matthias Schnell, Program Director, 215-503-4634, Fax: 215-503-5393, E-mail: matthias.schnell@jefferson.edu. *Application contact:* Marc E. Stearns, Director of Admissions, 215-503-0155, Fax: 215-503-3433, E-mail: jgsbs-info@jefferson.edu.
Website: http://www.jefferson.edu/university/biomedical_sciences/programs/phd/immunology.html

Tufts University, Sackler School of Graduate Biomedical Sciences, Immunology Program, Medford, MA 02155. Offers PhD. *Faculty:* 25 full-time (8 women). *Students:* 26 full-time (9 women); includes 7 minority (1 Black or African American, non-Hispanic/Latino; 3 Asian, non-Hispanic/Latino; 2 Hispanic/Latino; 1 Two or more races, non-Hispanic/Latino), 2 international. Average age 29. 85 applicants, 7% accepted, 4 enrolled. In 2013, 4 doctorates awarded. Terminal master's awarded for partial completion of doctoral program. *Degree requirements:* For doctorate, comprehensive exam, thesis/dissertation. *Entrance requirements:* For doctorate, GRE General Test, 3 letters of reference. Additional exam requirements/recommendations for international students: Required—TOEFL (minimum score 600 paper-based; 100 iBT). *Application deadline:* For fall admission, 12/15 for domestic and international students. Application fee: $70. Electronic applications accepted. *Financial support:* In 2013–14, 26 students received support, including 26 research assistantships with full tuition reimbursements available (averaging $31,000 per year). *Faculty research:* Genetic regulation of the ontogeny and activation of lymphocytes, mechanisms of antigen-receptor gene rearrangement, biology and molecular biology of negative selection (tolerance) of B and T cells, activation signal pathways, gene expression and the biochemistry of apoptosis. *Unit head:* Dr. Henry H. Wortis, Director, 617-636-6836, Fax: 617-636-2990. *Application contact:* Kellie Melchin, Associate Director of Admissions, 617-636-6767, Fax: 617-636-0375, E-mail: sackler-school@tufts.edu.
Website: http://sackler.tufts.edu/Academics/Degree-Programs/PhD-Programs/Immunology

Tulane University, School of Medicine and School of Liberal Arts, Graduate Programs in Biomedical Sciences, Department of Microbiology and Immunology, New Orleans, LA 70118-5669. Offers MS, PhD, MD/PhD. MS and PhD offered through the Graduate School. *Degree requirements:* For master's, thesis; for doctorate, 2 foreign languages, thesis/dissertation. *Entrance requirements:* For master's, GRE General Test, minimum B average in undergraduate course work; for doctorate, GRE General Test, GRE Subject Test. Additional exam requirements/recommendations for international students: Required—TOEFL. Electronic applications accepted. *Faculty research:* Vaccine development, viral pathogenesis, molecular virology, bacterial pathogenesis, fungal pathogenesis.

Uniformed Services University of the Health Sciences, School of Medicine, Graduate Programs in the Biomedical Sciences and Public Health, Graduate Program in Emerging Infectious Diseases, Bethesda, MD 20814-4799. Offers PhD. *Faculty:* 35 full-time (5 women), 17 part-time/adjunct (6 women). *Students:* 33 full-time (27 women); includes 3 minority (2 Black or African American, non-Hispanic/Latino; 1 Asian, non-Hispanic/Latino), 2 international. Average age 26. 43 applicants, 44% accepted, 11 enrolled. In 2013, 7 doctorates awarded. *Degree requirements:* For doctorate, comprehensive exam, thesis/dissertation, qualifying exam. *Entrance requirements:* For doctorate, GRE General Test. Additional exam requirements/recommendations for international students: Required—TOEFL. *Application deadline:* For fall admission, 1/1 priority date for domestic and international students. Applications are processed on a rolling basis. Application fee: $0. Electronic applications accepted. *Financial support:* In 2013–14, fellowships with full tuition reimbursements (averaging $27,000 per year) were awarded; scholarships/grants, health care benefits, and tuition waivers (full) also available. *Unit head:* Dr. Christopher Broder, Director, 301-295-3401, E-mail: cbroder@usuhs.mil. *Application contact:* Patricia Grant, Program Administrative Specialist, 301-295-3400, Fax: 301-295-3773, E-mail: patricia.grant@usuhs.edu.
Website: http://www.usuhs.mil/eid

See Display on page 332 and Close-Up on page 353.

Universidad Central del Caribe, School of Medicine, Program in Biomedical Sciences, Bayamón, PR 00960-6032. Offers anatomy and cell biology (MA, MS); biochemistry (MS); biomedical sciences (MA); cellular and molecular biology (PhD); microbiology and immunology (MA, MS); pharmacology (MS); physiology (MS).

Université de Montréal, Faculty of Medicine, Department of Microbiology and Immunology, Montréal, QC H3C 3J7, Canada. Offers M Sc, PhD. Programs offered jointly with Faculty of Veterinary Medicine and Université du Québec, Institut Armand-Frappier. Terminal master's awarded for partial completion of doctoral program. *Degree requirements:* For master's, thesis; for doctorate, thesis/dissertation, general exam. *Entrance requirements:* For master's and doctorate, proficiency in French, knowledge of English. Electronic applications accepted.

Université de Montréal, Faculty of Veterinary Medicine, Program in Virology and Immunology, Montréal, QC H3C 3J7, Canada. Offers PhD. Program offered jointly with Université du Québec, Institut Armand-Frappier. *Degree requirements:* For doctorate, thesis/dissertation, general exam. *Entrance requirements:* For doctorate, proficiency in French, knowledge of English. Electronic applications accepted.

Université de Sherbrooke, Faculty of Medicine and Health Sciences, Graduate Programs in Medicine, Program in Immunology, Sherbrooke, QC J1H 5N4, Canada. Offers M Sc, PhD. Electronic applications accepted. *Faculty research:* Cytokine receptor signal transduction, lipid mediators and inflammation, TGFbeta convertases.

Université du Québec, Institut National de la Recherche Scientifique, Graduate Programs, Research Center–INRS–Institut Armand-Frappier, Laval, QC H7V 1B7, Canada. Offers applied microbiology (M Sc); biology (PhD); experimental health sciences (M Sc); virology and immunology (M Sc, PhD). Programs given in French. Part-time programs available. *Faculty:* 45 full-time. *Students:* 126 full-time (78 women), 11 part-time (7 women), 52 international. Average age 30. In 2013, 19 master's, 12 doctorates awarded. *Degree requirements:* For master's, thesis; for doctorate, thesis/dissertation. *Entrance requirements:* For master's, appropriate bachelor's degree, proficiency in French; for doctorate, appropriate master's degree, proficiency in French. *Application deadline:* For fall admission, 3/30 for domestic and international students; for winter admission, 11/1 for domestic and international students; for spring admission, 3/1 for domestic and international students. Application fee: $45 Canadian dollars. Electronic applications accepted. *Financial support:* In 2013–14, fellowships (averaging $16,500 per year) were awarded; research assistantships also available. *Faculty research:* Immunity, infection and cancer; toxicology and environmental biotechnology; molecular pharmacochemistry. *Unit head:* Charles Dozois, Director, 450-687-5010, Fax: 450-686-5566, E-mail: charles.dozois@iaf.inrs.ca. *Application contact:* Sylvie Richard, Registrar, 418-654-2518, Fax: 418-654-3858, E-mail: sylvie.richard@adm.inrs.ca.
Website: http://www.iaf.inrs.ca

Université Laval, Faculty of Medicine, Graduate Programs in Medicine, Programs in Microbiology-Immunology, Québec, QC G1K 7P4, Canada. Offers M Sc, PhD. Terminal master's awarded for partial completion of doctoral program. *Degree requirements:* For master's, thesis; for doctorate, comprehensive exam, thesis/dissertation. *Entrance requirements:* For master's and doctorate, knowledge of French, comprehension of written English. Electronic applications accepted.

University at Albany, State University of New York, School of Public Health, Department of Biomedical Sciences, Program in Immunobiology and Immunochemistry, Albany, NY 12222-0001. Offers MS, PhD. *Degree requirements:* For master's, thesis; for doctorate, thesis/dissertation. *Entrance requirements:* For master's and doctorate, GRE General Test, GRE Subject Test.

University at Buffalo, the State University of New York, Graduate School, Graduate Programs in Cancer Research and Biomedical Sciences at Roswell Park Cancer Institute, Department of Immunology at Roswell Park Cancer Institute, Buffalo, NY 14260. Offers PhD. *Faculty:* 21 full-time (7 women). *Students:* 25 full-time (14 women); includes 4 minority (3 Black or African American, non-Hispanic/Latino; 1 Asian, non-Hispanic/Latino), 3 international. 29 applicants, 24% accepted, 3 enrolled. In 2013, 2 doctorates awarded. *Degree requirements:* For doctorate, comprehensive exam, thesis/dissertation, oral defense of disseration. *Entrance requirements:* For doctorate, GRE General Test. Additional exam requirements/recommendations for international students: Required—TOEFL (minimum score 79 iBT). *Application deadline:* For fall admission, 1/5 priority date for domestic and international students. Application fee: $75. Electronic applications accepted. *Financial support:* In 2013–14, 21 students received support, including 21 research assistantships with full tuition reimbursements available (averaging $25,000 per year); scholarships/grants, health care benefits, and unspecified assistantships also available. Financial award application deadline: 1/5. *Faculty research:* Immunochemistry, immunobiology, molecular immunology, hybridoma studies, recombinant DNA studies. *Unit head:* Dr. Kelvin Lee, Chair, 716-845-4106, Fax: 716-845-2993, E-mail: kelvin.lee@roswellpark.org. *Application contact:* Dr. Norman J. Karin, Associate Dean, 716-845-4630, Fax: 716-845-8178, E-mail: norman.karin@roswellpark.org.
Website: http://www.roswellpark.edu/education/phd-programs/immunology

University at Buffalo, the State University of New York, Graduate School, School of Medicine and Biomedical Sciences, Graduate Programs in Medicine and Biomedical Sciences, Department of Microbiology and Immunology, Buffalo, NY 14260. Offers MA, PhD. *Faculty:* 14 full-time (4 women). *Students:* 23 full-time (15 women); includes 8 minority (2 Black or African American, non-Hispanic/Latino; 6 Asian, non-Hispanic/Latino), 7 international. Average age 28. 20 applicants, 15% accepted, 2 enrolled. In 2013, 1 master's, 2 doctorates awarded. *Degree requirements:* For master's, comprehensive exam; for doctorate, thesis/dissertation, departmental qualifying exam. *Entrance requirements:* For master's and doctorate, GRE General Test, 3 letters of recommendation. Additional exam requirements/recommendations for international students: Required—TOEFL (minimum score 100 iBT). *Application deadline:* For fall admission, 5/1 priority date for domestic and international students. Applications are processed on a rolling basis. Application fee: $75. Electronic applications accepted. *Financial support:* In 2013–14, 2 students received support, including 2 fellowships with tuition reimbursements available (averaging $28,000 per year), 12 research assistantships with tuition reimbursements available (averaging $25,000 per year), 1 teaching assistantship with tuition reimbursement available (averaging $25,000 per year); Federal Work-Study, institutionally sponsored loans, traineeships, health care benefits, and unspecified assistantships also available. Financial award application deadline: 2/1; financial award applicants required to submit FAFSA. *Faculty research:* Bacteriology, immunology, parasitology, virology, mycology. *Total annual research expenditures:* $2.6 million. *Unit head:* Dr. James Bangs, Chair/Professor, 716-829-2907, Fax: 716-829-2158. *Application contact:* Dr. Anders Hakansson, Director of Graduate Studies, 716-829-2176, Fax: 716-829-2158.
Website: http://www.smbs.buffalo.edu/microb/

University of Alberta, Faculty of Medicine and Dentistry and Faculty of Graduate Studies and Research, Graduate Programs in Medicine, Department of Medical Microbiology and Immunology, Edmonton, AB T6G 2E1, Canada. Offers M Sc, PhD. Terminal master's awarded for partial completion of doctoral program. *Degree requirements:* For master's, thesis; for doctorate, thesis/dissertation. *Entrance requirements:* For master's and doctorate, minimum GPA of 3.3. Additional exam requirements/recommendations for international students: Required—TOEFL (minimum score 600 paper-based; 96 iBT). *Faculty research:* Cellular and reproductive immunology, microbial pathogenesis, mechanisms of antibiotic resistance, molecular biology of mammalian viruses, antiviral chemotherapy.

The University of Arizona, College of Medicine, Department of Immunobiology, Tucson, AZ 85721. Offers MS, PhD. *Faculty:* 10 full-time (2 women). *Students:* 8 full-time (5 women); includes 1 minority (Asian, non-Hispanic/Latino), 2 international. Average age 27. 91 applicants, 66% accepted. In 2013, 1 master's, 2 doctorates awarded. *Degree requirements:* For master's, thesis; for doctorate, thesis/dissertation. *Entrance requirements:* For master's and doctorate, GRE General Test, minimum GPA of 3.0. *Application deadline:* For fall admission, 3/1 priority date for domestic students; for spring admission, 9/1 for domestic students. Application fee: $75. *Expenses:* Tuition, state resident: full-time $11,526. Tuition, nonresident: full-time $27,398. *Financial support:* In 2013–14, 4 research assistantships with full tuition reimbursements (averaging $25,000 per year) were awarded; fellowships with full tuition reimbursements, teaching assistantships with full tuition reimbursements, institutionally sponsored loans, and tuition waivers (full) also available. Financial award application deadline: 4/30. *Faculty research:* Environmental and pathogenic microbiology, molecular biology. *Total annual research expenditures:* $2.3 million. *Unit head:* Dr. Janko Nikolich-Zugich, Head, 520-626-6065, Fax: 520-626-2100, E-mail: nikolich@email.arizona.edu. *Application contact:* Dr. Richard J. Ablin, Graduate Program Chairman, 520-626-7755, E-mail: ablinrj@email.arizona.edu.
Website: http://immunobiology.arizona.edu/

University of Arkansas for Medical Sciences, Graduate School, Little Rock, AR 72205. Offers biochemistry and molecular biology (MS, PhD); bioinformatics (MS, PhD); cellular physiology and molecular biophysics (MS, PhD); clinical nutrition (MS); interdisciplinary biomedical sciences (MS, PhD, Certificate); interdisciplinary toxicology (MS); microbiology and immunology (PhD); neurobiology and developmental sciences (PhD); pharmacology (PhD); MD/PhD. Bioinformatics programs hosted jointly with the University of Arkansas at Little Rock. Part-time programs available. *Faculty:* 397 full-time (205 women). *Students:* 196 full-time (126 women), 117 part-time (87 women); includes 65 minority (38 Black or African American, non-Hispanic/Latino; 1 American Indian or Alaska Native, non-Hispanic/Latino; 21 Asian, non-Hispanic/Latino; 4 Hispanic/Latino; 1 Two or more races, non-Hispanic/Latino), 57 international. 455 applicants, 27% accepted, 89 enrolled. In 2013, 41 master's, 18 doctorates, 28 other advanced degrees awarded. Terminal master's awarded for partial completion of doctoral program. *Degree requirements:* For master's, comprehensive exam (for some programs), thesis (for some programs); for doctorate, thesis/dissertation. *Entrance requirements:* For master's and doctorate, GRE. Additional exam requirements/recommendations for international students: Required—TOEFL. *Application deadline:* Applications are processed on a rolling basis. Application fee: $0. Electronic applications accepted. *Expenses:* Contact institution. *Financial support:* In 2013–14, 120 research assistantships (averaging $24,000 per year) were awarded; career-related internships or fieldwork, Federal Work-

Immunology

Study, and traineeships also available. Support available to part-time students. Financial award applicants required to submit FAFSA. *Unit head:* Dr. Robert E. McGehee, Jr., Dean, 501-686-5454. *Application contact:* Dr. Kristen Sterba, Assistant Dean, Office of Graduate Student Recruiting and Retention, 501-526-7396, E-mail: kmsterba@uams.edu.
Website: http://www.uams.edu/gradschool/

The University of British Columbia, Faculty of Science, Department of Microbiology and Immunology, Vancouver, BC V6T 1Z1, Canada. Offers M Sc, PhD. *Degree requirements:* For master's, thesis; for doctorate, comprehensive exam, thesis/dissertation. *Entrance requirements:* For master's and doctorate, GRE General Test. Additional exam requirements/recommendations for international students: Required—TOEFL (minimum score 590 paper-based). Electronic applications accepted. *Expenses: Tuition, area resident:* Full-time $8000 Canadian dollars. *Faculty research:* Bacterial genetics, metabolism, pathogenic bacteriology, virology.

University of Calgary, Cumming School of Medicine and Faculty of Graduate Studies, Department of Microbiology, Immunology and Infectious Diseases, Calgary, AB T2N 1N4, Canada. Offers M Sc, PhD. *Degree requirements:* For master's, thesis, oral thesis exam; for doctorate, thesis/dissertation, candidacy exam, oral thesis exam. *Entrance requirements:* For master's and doctorate, minimum GPA of 3.2. Additional exam requirements/recommendations for international students: Required—TOEFL (minimum score 580 paper-based). Electronic applications accepted. *Faculty research:* Bacteriology, virology, parasitology, immunology.

University of California, Berkeley, Graduate Division, School of Public Health, Group in Infectious Diseases and Immunity, Berkeley, CA 94720-1500. Offers PhD. *Entrance requirements:* For doctorate, GRE General Test, minimum GPA of 3.0, 3 letters of recommendation.

University of California, Davis, Graduate Studies, Graduate Group in Immunology, Davis, CA 95616. Offers MS, PhD. Terminal master's awarded for partial completion of doctoral program. *Degree requirements:* For master's, comprehensive exam (for some programs), thesis (for some programs); for doctorate, thesis/dissertation. *Entrance requirements:* For master's and doctorate, GRE General Test. Additional exam requirements/recommendations for international students: Required—TOEFL (minimum score 550 paper-based). Electronic applications accepted. *Faculty research:* Immune regulation in autoimmunity, immunopathology, immunotoxicology, tumor immunology, avian immunology.

University of California, Los Angeles, David Geffen School of Medicine and Graduate Division, Graduate Programs in Medicine, Department of Microbiology, Immunology and Molecular Genetics, Los Angeles, CA 90095. Offers MS, PhD. *Degree requirements:* For master's, thesis; for doctorate, thesis/dissertation, oral and written qualifying exams; 2 quarters of teaching experience. *Entrance requirements:* For master's and doctorate, GRE General Test, bachelor's degree; minimum undergraduate GPA of 3.0 (or its equivalent if letter grade system not used). Additional exam requirements/recommendations for international students: Required—TOEFL. Electronic applications accepted.

University of California, Los Angeles, Graduate Division, College of Letters and Science and David Geffen School of Medicine, UCLA ACCESS to Programs in the Molecular, Cellular and Integrative Life Sciences, Los Angeles, CA 90095. Offers biochemistry and molecular biology (PhD); biological chemistry (PhD); cellular and molecular pathology (PhD); human genetics (PhD); microbiology, immunology, and molecular genetics (PhD); molecular biology (PhD); molecular toxicology (PhD); molecular, cellular and integrative physiology (PhD); neurobiology (PhD); oral biology (PhD); physiology (PhD). *Degree requirements:* For doctorate, thesis/dissertation, oral and written qualifying exams. *Entrance requirements:* For doctorate, GRE General Test, bachelor's degree; minimum undergraduate GPA of 3.0 (or its equivalent if letter grade system not used). Additional exam requirements/recommendations for international students: Required—TOEFL. Electronic applications accepted.

University of Chicago, Division of Biological Sciences, Biomedical Sciences Cluster: Cancer Biology, Immunology, Molecular Metabolism and Nutrition, Pathology, and Microbiology, Committee on Immunology, Chicago, IL 60637-1513. Offers PhD. *Degree requirements:* For doctorate, thesis/dissertation, ethics class, 2 teaching assistantships. *Entrance requirements:* For doctorate, GRE General Test. Additional exam requirements/recommendations for international students: Required—TOEFL (minimum score 600 paper-based; 104 iBT), IELTS (minimum score 7). Electronic applications accepted. *Faculty research:* Molecular immunology, transplantation, autoimmunology, neuroimmunology, tumor immunology.

University of Cincinnati, Graduate School, College of Medicine, Graduate Programs in Biomedical Sciences, Department of Pediatrics, Cincinnati, OH 45221. Offers immunobiology (PhD); molecular and developmental biology (PhD). *Degree requirements:* For doctorate, thesis/dissertation, qualifying exam. *Entrance requirements:* For doctorate, GRE General Test, minimum GPA of 3.0. Additional exam requirements/recommendations for international students: Required—TOEFL (minimum score 600 paper-based; 100 iBT). Electronic applications accepted. *Faculty research:* Pulmonary biology, molecular cardiovascular, developmental biology, cancer biology, genetics.

University of Cincinnati, Graduate School, College of Medicine, Graduate Programs in Biomedical Sciences, Immunobiology Training Program, Cincinnati, OH 45229-3038. Offers MS, PhD. *Degree requirements:* For master's, seminar, thesis with oral defense; for doctorate, seminar, dissertation with oral defense, written and oral candidacy exams. *Entrance requirements:* For master's and doctorate, GRE, bachelor's degree in biology-related field. Additional exam requirements/recommendations for international students: Required—TOEFL. Electronic applications accepted.

University of Colorado Denver, School of Medicine, Integrated Department of Immunology, Denver, CO 80206. Offers PhD. *Students:* 42 full-time (24 women); includes 6 minority (1 American Indian or Alaska Native, non-Hispanic/Latino; 2 Asian, non-Hispanic/Latino; 3 Hispanic/Latino). Average age 29. 45 applicants, 7% accepted, 3 enrolled. In 2013, 7 doctorates awarded. *Degree requirements:* For doctorate, thesis/dissertation, 30 credit hours of formal course work, three laboratory rotations, oral comprehensive examination, 30 credit hours of dissertation research, final defense of the dissertation. *Entrance requirements:* For doctorate, GRE, letters of recommendation, statement of purpose, interview. Additional exam requirements/recommendations for international students: Required—TOEFL (minimum score 550 paper-based; 89 iBT). *Application deadline:* For fall admission, 12/1 for domestic students, 11/1 for international students. Application fee: $50 ($75 for international students). Electronic applications accepted. *Expenses:* Contact institution. *Financial support:* In 2013–14, 42 students received support. Fellowships with full tuition reimbursements available, research assistantships, teaching assistantships, Federal Work-Study, institutionally sponsored loans, scholarships/grants, traineeships, health care benefits, tuition waivers (full), and unspecified assistantships available. Financial award application deadline: 3/15; financial award applicants required to submit FAFSA. *Faculty research:* Gene regulation, immune signaling, apoptosis, stem cells, vaccines. *Unit head:* Dr. John C. Cambier, Professor/Chairman, 303-398-1325, E-mail: john.cambier@ucdenver.edu. *Application contact:* Mellodee Phillips, Graduate Program Coordinator, 303-398-1306, Fax: 303-270-2325, E-mail: mellodee.phillips@ucdenver.edu.
Website: http://www.ucdenver.edu/academics/colleges/medicalschool/departments/immunology/Pages/Immunology.aspx

University of Colorado Denver, School of Medicine, Program in Microbiology, Aurora, CO 80045. Offers microbiology (PhD); microbiology and immunology (PhD). *Students:* 17 full-time (4 women); includes 2 minority (1 Asian, non-Hispanic/Latino; 1 Hispanic/Latino). Average age 27. 53 applicants, 4% accepted, 2 enrolled. In 2013, 1 doctorate awarded. *Degree requirements:* For doctorate, comprehensive exam, thesis/dissertation, 3 lab rotations; 30 credit hours of coursework. *Entrance requirements:* For doctorate, GRE, three letters of reference, two copies of official transcripts, minimum GPA of 3.0. Additional exam requirements/recommendations for international students: Required—TOEFL (minimum score 550 paper-based; 80 iBT). *Application deadline:* For fall admission, 12/1 for domestic students, 11/1 for international students. Application fee: $50 ($75 for international students). Electronic applications accepted. *Expenses:* Contact institution. *Financial support:* In 2013–14, 17 students received support. Fellowships with tuition reimbursements available, research assistantships, teaching assistantships, institutionally sponsored loans, scholarships/grants, traineeships, health care benefits, and tuition waivers (full) available. Financial award application deadline: 3/15; financial award applicants required to submit FAFSA. *Faculty research:* Molecular mechanisms of picornavirus replication, mechanisms of papovavirus assembly, human immune response in multiple sclerosis. *Total annual research expenditures:* $5.9 million. *Unit head:* Dr. Randall K. Holmes, Chair, 303-724-4223, E-mail: randall.holmes@ucdenver.edu. *Application contact:* Deanne Sylvester, Microbiology Graduate Program Administrator, 303-724-3244, Fax: 303-724-3247, E-mail: deanne.sylvester@ucdenver.edu.
Website: http://www.ucdenver.edu/academics/colleges/medicalschool/departments/Microbiology/Pages/microbiology.aspx

University of Connecticut Health Center, Graduate School, Programs in Biomedical Sciences, Graduate Program in Immunology, Farmington, CT 06030. Offers PhD, DMD/PhD, MD/PhD. *Degree requirements:* For doctorate, comprehensive exam, thesis/dissertation. *Entrance requirements:* For doctorate, GRE General Test. Additional exam requirements/recommendations for international students: Required—TOEFL (minimum score 600 paper-based). Electronic applications accepted. *Faculty research:* Developmental immunology, T-cell immunity, lymphoid cell development, tolerance and tumor immunity, leukocyte chemotaxis.

See Display on next page and Close-Up on page 355.

University of Florida, College of Medicine and Graduate School, Interdisciplinary Program in Biomedical Sciences, Concentration in Immunology and Microbiology, Gainesville, FL 32611. Offers PhD. *Degree requirements:* For doctorate, thesis/dissertation. *Entrance requirements:* For doctorate, GRE General Test, minimum GPA of 3.0, biochemistry before enrollment. Additional exam requirements/recommendations for international students: Required—TOEFL. Electronic applications accepted. *Expenses:* Tuition, state resident: full-time $12,640. Tuition, nonresident: full-time $30,000.

University of Guelph, Ontario Veterinary College and Graduate Studies, Graduate Programs in Veterinary Sciences, Department of Pathobiology, Guelph, ON N1G 2W1, Canada. Offers anatomic pathology (DV Sc, Diploma); clinical pathology (Diploma); comparative pathology (M Sc, PhD); immunology (M Sc, PhD); laboratory animal science (DV Sc); pathology (M Sc, PhD, Diploma); veterinary infectious diseases (M Sc, PhD); zoo animal/wildlife medicine (DV Sc). *Degree requirements:* For master's, thesis; for doctorate, thesis/dissertation. *Entrance requirements:* For master's, DVM with B average or an honours degree in biological sciences; for doctorate, DVM or MSC degree, minimum B+ average. Additional exam requirements/recommendations for international students: Required—TOEFL (minimum score 550 paper-based). *Faculty research:* Pathogenesis; diseases of animals, wildlife, fish, and laboratory animals; parasitology; immunology; veterinary infectious diseases; laboratory animal science.

University of Illinois at Chicago, College of Medicine and Graduate College, Graduate Programs in Medicine, Department of Microbiology and Immunology, Chicago, IL 60607-7128. Offers PhD, MD/PhD. *Faculty:* 13 full-time (4 women), 3 part-time/adjunct (2 women). *Students:* 14 full-time (9 women); includes 3 minority (2 Black or African American, non-Hispanic/Latino; 1 Two or more races, non-Hispanic/Latino), 6 international. Average age 30. 1 applicant, 100% accepted. In 2013, 10 doctorates awarded. *Degree requirements:* For doctorate, thesis/dissertation. *Entrance requirements:* For doctorate, GRE General Test, minimum GPA of 2.75. Additional exam requirements/recommendations for international students: Required—TOEFL. *Application deadline:* For fall admission, 3/1 priority date for domestic students, 2/15 priority date for international students. Application fee: $40 ($50 for international students). *Expenses:* Tuition, state resident: full-time $11,066; part-time $3689 per term. Tuition, nonresident: full-time $23,064; part-time $7688 per term. *Required fees:* $3004; $1190 per term. Tuition and fees vary according to course level and program. *Financial support:* In 2013–14, 5 fellowships with full tuition reimbursements were awarded; research assistantships with full tuition reimbursements, teaching assistantships with full tuition reimbursements, Federal Work-Study, scholarships/grants, traineeships, tuition waivers (full), and unspecified assistantships also available. Financial award application deadline: 3/1; financial award applicants required to submit FAFSA. *Faculty research:* Class I major histocompatibility complex molecules; proteins such as azurin with the immunoglobulin folds; T cell immunobiology relevant to disease pathogenesis, immunotherapeutics and vaccines for HIV/AIDS, tuberculosis, AIDS-related tuberculosis, and recently malaria, plague and smallpox; intracellular bacterial pathogen Listeria monocytogenes; virus infection. *Total annual research expenditures:* $6.9 million. *Unit head:* Prof. Bellur S. Prabhakar, Department Head, 312-996-4915, Fax: 312-996-6415, E-mail: bprabhkar@uic.edu. *Application contact:* Mia Johnson, Admissions and Records Officer, 312-996-9477, Fax: 312-996-6415, E-mail: mimi@uic.edu.
Website: http://www.uic.edu/depts/mcmi/index.htm

The University of Iowa, Graduate College, Program in Immunology, Iowa City, IA 52242-1316. Offers PhD. *Degree requirements:* For doctorate, comprehensive exam, thesis/dissertation. *Entrance requirements:* For doctorate, GRE General Test, minimum GPA of 3.0. Additional exam requirements/recommendations for international students: Required—TOEFL (minimum score 600 paper-based; 100 iBT). Electronic applications accepted.

The University of Iowa, Roy J. and Lucille A. Carver College of Medicine and Graduate College, Graduate Programs in Medicine, Department of Microbiology, Iowa City, IA 52242-1316. Offers general microbiology and microbial physiology (MS, PhD); immunology (MS, PhD); microbial genetics (MS, PhD); pathogenic bacteriology (MS, PhD); virology (MS, PhD). *Faculty:* 23 full-time (5 women), 10 part-time/adjunct (4 women). *Students:* 38 full-time (28 women); includes 3 minority (2 Asian, non-Hispanic/Latino; 1 Hispanic/Latino), 2 international. Average age 25. 44 applicants, 23% accepted, 8 enrolled. In 2013, 1 master's, 6 doctorates awarded. *Degree requirements:* For master's, thesis; for doctorate, comprehensive exam, thesis/dissertation. *Entrance requirements:* For master's and doctorate, GRE General Test. Additional exam

requirements/recommendations for international students: Required—TOEFL (minimum score 600 paper-based). *Application deadline:* For fall admission, 1/1 for domestic and international students. Application fee: $60 ($100 for international students). Electronic applications accepted. *Financial support:* In 2013–14, 5 fellowships with full tuition reimbursements (averaging $26,000 per year), 33 research assistantships with full tuition reimbursements (averaging $26,000 per year) were awarded; institutionally sponsored loans, scholarships/grants, traineeships, and health care benefits also available. *Faculty research:* Gene regulation, processing and transport of HIV, retroviral pathogenesis, biodegradation, biofilm. *Total annual research expenditures:* $11.5 million. *Unit head:* Dr. Patrick M. Schlievert, Chair and Department Executive Officer, 319-335-7810, E-mail: grad-micro-info@uiowa.edu. *Application contact:* Kerry Yoder, Assistant Director of Graduate and Professional Evaluation, 319-335-1525, Fax: 319-335-1535, E-mail: admissions@uiowa.edu.
Website: http://www.medicine.uiowa.edu/microbiology/

University of Kentucky, Graduate School, Graduate School Programs from the College of Medicine, Department of Microbiology, Immunology and Molecular Genetics, Lexington, KY 40506-0032. Offers PhD. *Degree requirements:* For doctorate, comprehensive exam, thesis/dissertation. *Entrance requirements:* For doctorate, GRE General Test, minimum undergraduate GPA of 2.75. Additional exam requirements/recommendations for international students: Required—TOEFL (minimum score 550 paper-based). Electronic applications accepted.

University of Louisville, School of Medicine, Department of Microbiology and Immunology, Louisville, KY 40292-0001. Offers MS, PhD, MD/PhD. *Students:* 40 full-time (24 women), 1 part-time (0 women); includes 5 minority (3 Black or African American, non-Hispanic/Latino; 1 Asian, non-Hispanic/Latino; 1 Hispanic/Latino), 12 international. Average age 29. 55 applicants, 24% accepted, 9 enrolled. In 2013, 4 master's, 4 doctorates awarded. Terminal master's awarded for partial completion of doctoral program. *Degree requirements:* For master's, thesis; for doctorate, comprehensive exam, thesis/dissertation. *Entrance requirements:* For master's and doctorate, GRE General Test (minimum score of 1000 verbal and quantitative), minimum GPA of 3.0; 1 year of course work in biology, organic chemistry, and physics; 1 semester of course work in calculus and quantitative analysis, biochemistry, or molecular biology. Additional exam requirements/recommendations for international students: Required—TOEFL. *Application deadline:* For fall admission, 2/1 priority date for domestic and international students. Applications are processed on a rolling basis. Application fee: $60. Electronic applications accepted. *Expenses:* Tuition, state resident: full-time $10,788; part-time $599 per credit hour. Tuition, nonresident: full-time $22,446; part-time $1247 per credit hour. *Required fees:* $196. Tuition and fees vary according to program and reciprocity agreements. *Financial support:* Fellowships with full tuition reimbursements and research assistantships with full tuition reimbursements available. Financial award application deadline: 4/15. *Faculty research:* Opportunistic and emerging infections; biology and regulation of the immune system; cellular and molecular bases of chronic inflammatory response; role of cytokines and chemokines in cancer, autoimmune and infectious disease; host defense and pathogenesis of viral infections. *Unit head:* Dr. Robert D. Stout, Chair, 502-852-5351, Fax: 502-852-7531, E-mail: bobstout@louisville.edu. *Application contact:* Carolyn M. Burton, Academic Coordinator, 502-852-6208, Fax: 502-852-7531, E-mail: cmburt01@gwise.louisville.edu.

The University of Manchester, Faculty of Life Sciences, Manchester, United Kingdom. Offers adaptive organismal biology (M Phil, PhD); animal biology (M Phil, PhD); biochemistry (M Phil, PhD); bioinformatics (M Phil, PhD); biomolecular sciences (M Phil, PhD); biotechnology (M Phil, PhD); cell biology (M Phil, PhD); cell matrix research (M Phil, PhD); channels and transporters (M Phil, PhD); developmental biology (M Phil, PhD); Egyptology (M Phil, PhD); environmental biology (M Phil, PhD); evolutionary biology (M Phil, PhD); gene expression (M Phil, PhD); genetics (M Phil, PhD); history of science, technology and medicine (M Phil, PhD); immunology (M Phil, PhD); integrative neurobiology and behavior (M Phil, PhD); membrane trafficking (M Phil, PhD); microbiology (M Phil, PhD); molecular and cellular neuroscience (M Phil, PhD); molecular biology (M Phil, PhD); molecular cancer studies (M Phil, PhD); neuroscience (M Phil, PhD); ophthalmology (M Phil, PhD); optometry (M Phil, PhD); organelle function (M Phil, PhD); pharmacology (M Phil, PhD); physiology (M Phil, PhD); plant sciences (M Phil, PhD); stem cell research (M Phil, PhD); structural biology (M Phil, PhD); systems neuroscience (M Phil, PhD); toxicology (M Phil, PhD).

University of Manitoba, Faculty of Medicine and Faculty of Graduate Studies, Graduate Programs in Medicine, Department of Immunology, Winnipeg, MB R3T 2N2, Canada. Offers M Sc, PhD. Terminal master's awarded for partial completion of doctoral program. *Degree requirements:* For master's, thesis; for doctorate, one foreign language, thesis/dissertation. *Faculty research:* Immediate hypersensitivity, regulation of the immune response, natural immunity, cytokines, inflammation.

University of Maryland, Baltimore, Graduate School, Graduate Program in Life Sciences, Program in Molecular Microbiology and Immunology, Baltimore, MD 21201. Offers PhD, MD/PhD. *Students:* 53 full-time (28 women), 2 part-time (0 women); includes 10 minority (2 Black or African American, non-Hispanic/Latino; 5 Asian, non-Hispanic/Latino; 1 Hispanic/Latino; 2 Two or more races, non-Hispanic/Latino), 5 international. Average age 27. 133 applicants, 14% accepted, 8 enrolled. In 2013, 5 doctorates awarded. *Degree requirements:* For doctorate, comprehensive exam, thesis/dissertation. *Entrance requirements:* For doctorate, GRE. Additional exam requirements/recommendations for international students: Required—TOEFL (minimum score 550 paper-based; 80 iBT); Recommended—IELTS (minimum score 7). *Application deadline:* For fall admission, 1/15 for domestic and international students. Application fee: $75. Electronic applications accepted. *Financial support:* In 2013–14, research assistantships with partial tuition reimbursements (averaging $25,000 per year) were awarded; fellowships also available. Financial award application deadline: 3/1; financial award applicants required to submit FAFSA. *Unit head:* Dr. Nicholas Carbonetti, Director, 410-706-7677, E-mail: ncarbone@umaryland.edu. *Application contact:* June Green, Program Coordinator, 410-706-7126, Fax: 410-706-2129, E-mail: jgreen@umaryland.edu.
Website: http://microbiology.umaryland.edu

University of Massachusetts Worcester, Graduate School of Biomedical Sciences, Worcester, MA 01655-0115. Offers biochemistry and molecular pharmacology (PhD); bioinformatics and computational biology (PhD); cancer biology (PhD); cell biology (PhD); clinical and population health research (PhD); clinical investigation (MS); immunology and virology (PhD); interdisciplinary biomedical research (PhD); millennium (PhD); molecular genetics and microbiology (PhD); neuroscience (PhD); translational science (PhD); MD/PhD. *Faculty:* 1,388 full-time (521 women), 309 part-time/adjunct (198 women). *Students:* 385 full-time (210 women); includes 53 minority (13 Black or African American, non-Hispanic/Latino; 30 Asian, non-Hispanic/Latino; 10 Hispanic/Latino), 138 international. Average age 28. 491 applicants, 19% accepted, 39 enrolled. In 2013, 5 master's, 50 doctorates awarded. Terminal master's awarded for partial completion of doctoral program. *Median time to degree:* Of those who began their doctoral program in fall 2005, 67% received their degree in 8 years or less. *Degree requirements:* For master's, comprehensive exam, thesis; for doctorate, comprehensive exam, thesis/dissertation. *Entrance requirements:* For master's, MD, PhD, DVM, or PharmD; for doctorate, GRE General Test, bachelor's degree. Additional exam requirements/recommendations for international students: Required—TOEFL (minimum score 100 iBT) or IELTS (minimum score 7.5). *Application deadline:* For fall admission, 12/15 for domestic and international students; for spring admission, 5/15 for domestic students. Application fee: $80. Electronic applications accepted. *Expenses:* Contact institution. *Financial support:* In 2013–14, 431 students received support, including

research assistantships with full tuition reimbursements available (averaging $29,500 per year); scholarships/grants, health care benefits, tuition waivers (full), and unspecified assistantships also available. Financial award application deadline: 5/16. *Faculty research:* RNA interference, cell/molecular/developmental biology, bioinformatics, clinical/translational research, infectious disease. *Total annual research expenditures:* $245.9 million. *Unit head:* Dr. Anthony Carrthers, Dean, 508-856-4135, E-mail: anthony.carruthers@umassmed.edu. *Application contact:* Dr. Kendall Knight, Associate Dean and Interim Director of Admissions and Recruitment, 508-856-5628, Fax: 508-856-3659, E-mail: kendall.knight@umassmed.edu.
Website: http://www.umassmed.edu/gsbs/

University of Miami, Graduate School, Miller School of Medicine, Graduate Programs in Medicine, Department of Microbiology and Immunology, Coral Gables, FL 33124. Offers PhD, MD/PhD. *Degree requirements:* For doctorate, thesis/dissertation, oral and written qualifying exams. *Entrance requirements:* For doctorate, GRE General Test. Additional exam requirements/recommendations for international students: Required—TOEFL. Electronic applications accepted. *Faculty research:* Cellular and molecular immunology, molecular and pathogenic virology, pathogenic bacteriology and gene therapy of cancer.

University of Michigan, Rackham Graduate School, Program in Biomedical Sciences (PIBS), Department of Microbiology and Immunology, Ann Arbor, MI 48178. Offers MS, PhD. *Faculty:* 20 full-time (10 women), 12 part-time/adjunct (4 women). *Students:* 44 full-time (28 women); includes 7 minority (1 American Indian or Alaska Native, non-Hispanic/Latino; 4 Asian, non-Hispanic/Latino; 2 Hispanic/Latino), 3 international. Average age 29. 90 applicants, 14% accepted, 13 enrolled. In 2013, 2 master's, 7 doctorates awarded. *Degree requirements:* For doctorate, thesis/dissertation, oral defense of dissertation, preliminary exam. *Entrance requirements:* For master's and doctorate, GRE General Test. Additional exam requirements/recommendations for international students: Required—TOEFL (minimum score 600 paper-based; 84 iBT), TWE. *Application deadline:* For fall admission, 12/1 for domestic and international students. Application fee: $75 ($90 for international students). Electronic applications accepted. Tuition and fees vary according to course level, course load, degree level, program and student level. *Financial support:* In 2013–14, 15 fellowships with full tuition reimbursements (averaging $28,500 per year), 20 research assistantships with full tuition reimbursements (averaging $28,500 per year) were awarded; health care benefits and tuition waivers (full) also available. Financial award application deadline: 2/1. *Faculty research:* Gene regulation, molecular biology of animal and bacterial viruses, molecular and cellular networks, pathogenesis and microbial genetics. *Total annual research expenditures:* $10.2 million. *Unit head:* Dr. Harry L. T. Mobley, Chair, 734-764-1466, Fax: 734-764-3562, E-mail: hmobley@umich.edu. *Application contact:* Heidi Thompson, Senior Student Administrative Assistant, 734-763-3532, Fax: 734-764-3562, E-mail: heiditho@umich.edu.
Website: http://www.med.umich.edu/microbio/

University of Michigan, Rackham Graduate School, Program in Biomedical Sciences (PIBS), Program in Immunology, Ann Arbor, MI 48109-0619. Offers PhD. *Faculty:* 56 full-time (16 women). *Students:* 25 full-time (14 women); includes 12 minority (1 Black or African American, non-Hispanic/Latino; 4 Asian, non-Hispanic/Latino; 5 Hispanic/Latino; 2 Native Hawaiian or other Pacific Islander, non-Hispanic/Latino). Average age 27. 34 applicants, 24% accepted, 3 enrolled. In 2013, 4 doctorates awarded. *Degree requirements:* For doctorate, thesis/dissertation, oral defense of dissertation, preliminary exam. *Entrance requirements:* For doctorate, GRE General Test, 3 letters of recommendation, research experience, personal and research statements. Additional exam requirements/recommendations for international students: Required—TOEFL (minimum score 84 iBT). *Application deadline:* For fall admission, 12/1 for domestic and international students. Application fee: $75 ($90 for international students). Electronic applications accepted. Tuition and fees vary according to course level, course load, degree level, program and student level. *Financial support:* In 2013–14, 24 students received support, including 5 fellowships with full tuition reimbursements available (averaging $28,500 per year), 20 research assistantships with full tuition reimbursements available (averaging $28,500 per year); scholarships/grants, health care benefits, tuition waivers (full), and unspecified assistantships also available. Financial award application deadline: 12/1. *Faculty research:* Cytokine networks, T and B cell activation, autoimmunity, antigen processing/ presentation, cell signaling. *Unit head:* Dr. Bethany Moore, Director, 734-647-8378, Fax: 734-615-2331, E-mail: bmoore@umich.edu. *Application contact:* Michelle S. Melis, Director of Student Life, 734-615-6538, Fax: 734-647-7022, E-mail: msmtegan@umich.edu.
Website: http://www.med.umich.edu/immprog/

University of Minnesota, Duluth, Medical School, Microbiology, Immunology and Molecular Pathobiology Section, Duluth, MN 55812-2496. Offers MS, PhD. MS, PhD offered jointly with University of Minnesota, Twin Cities Campus. Terminal master's awarded for partial completion of doctoral program. *Degree requirements:* For master's, thesis, final oral exam; for doctorate, thesis/dissertation, final exam, oral and written preliminary exams. *Entrance requirements:* For master's and doctorate, GRE General Test. Additional exam requirements/recommendations for international students: Required—TOEFL. *Faculty research:* Immunomodulation, molecular diagnosis of rabies, cytokines, cancer immunology, cytomegalovirus infection.

University of Minnesota, Twin Cities Campus, Graduate School, PhD Program in Microbiology, Immunology and Cancer Biology, Minneapolis, MN 55455-0213. Offers PhD. *Degree requirements:* For doctorate, thesis/dissertation. *Entrance requirements:* For doctorate, GRE General Test. Additional exam requirements/recommendations for international students: Required—TOEFL (minimum score 600 paper-based). Electronic applications accepted. *Faculty research:* Virology, microbiology, cancer biology, immunology.

University of Missouri, School of Medicine and Graduate School, Graduate Programs in Medicine, Department of Molecular Microbiology and Immunology, Columbia, MO 65211. Offers MS, PhD. *Faculty:* 20 full-time (4 women), 2 part-time/adjunct (0 women). *Students:* 41 full-time (21 women), 1 (woman) part-time; includes 5 minority (3 Black or African American, non-Hispanic/Latino; 1 American Indian or Alaska Native, non-Hispanic/Latino; 1 Hispanic/Latino), 15 international. Average age 29. 29 applicants, 28% accepted, 7 enrolled. In 2013, 12 doctorates awarded. Terminal master's awarded for partial completion of doctoral program. *Degree requirements:* For master's, thesis; for doctorate, thesis/dissertation. *Entrance requirements:* For master's and doctorate, GRE General Test, minimum GPA of 3.0. Additional exam requirements/recommendations for international students: Required—TOEFL (minimum score 580 paper-based; 92 iBT). *Application deadline:* For fall admission, 1/15 priority date for domestic and international students. Application fee: $55 ($75 for international students). Electronic applications accepted. *Financial support:* Fellowships, research assistantships, teaching assistantships, institutionally sponsored loans, scholarships/grants, traineeships, health care benefits, and unspecified assistantships available. Support available to part-time students. Financial award application deadline: 3/1. *Faculty research:* Molecular biology, host-parasite interactions, posttranscriptional gene regulation, molecular basis of bacterial pathogenesis, regulation of immune response, mechanism and evolution of catalysis by ribozymes, mycoplasmas, genetics of Saccharomyces cerevisiae, T-cell development/activation, application of recombinant adeno-associated virus in gene therapy, retrovirus assembly, human immune responses, HCV entry pathways, RNA processing, epigenetics. *Unit head:* Dr. Mark A. McIntosh, Department Chair, 573-882-8989, E-mail: mcintoshm@missouri.edu. *Application contact:* Jana Clark, Coordinator, 573-882-3938, E-mail: clarkjl@missouri.edu.
Website: http://mmi.missouri.edu/graduateprogram/programindex.php

The University of Montana, Graduate School, College of Humanities and Sciences, Division of Biological Sciences, Program in Cellular, Molecular and Microbial Biology, Missoula, MT 59812-0002. Offers cellular and developmental biology (PhD); microbial evolution and ecology (PhD); microbiology and immunology (PhD); molecular biology and biochemistry (PhD). Terminal master's awarded for partial completion of doctoral program. *Degree requirements:* For doctorate, variable foreign language requirement, thesis/dissertation. *Entrance requirements:* For doctorate, GRE General Test. *Application deadline:* For fall admission, 2/1 for domestic students. Application fee: $45. *Financial support:* In 2013–14, research assistantships with tuition reimbursements (averaging $9,400 per year), teaching assistantships with full tuition reimbursements (averaging $9,400 per year) were awarded; Federal Work-Study and tuition waivers (full and partial) also available. Financial award application deadline: 3/1; financial award applicants required to submit FAFSA. *Faculty research:* Ribosome structure, medical microbiology/pathogenesis, microbial ecology/environmental microbiology. *Unit head:* Charles Janson, Chair, 406-243-5122, E-mail: charles.janson@mso.umt.edu. *Application contact:* Information Contact, E-mail: gradschl@mso.umt.edu.
Website: http://www.biology.umt.edu/

The University of North Carolina at Chapel Hill, School of Medicine and Graduate School, Graduate Programs in Medicine, Department of Microbiology and Immunology, Chapel Hill, NC 27599-7290. Offers immunology (MS, PhD); microbiology (MS, PhD). Terminal master's awarded for partial completion of doctoral program. *Degree requirements:* For master's, comprehensive exam, thesis; for doctorate, comprehensive exam, thesis/dissertation. *Entrance requirements:* For master's and doctorate, GRE General Test, minimum GPA of 3.0. Electronic applications accepted. *Faculty research:* HIV pathogenesis, immune response, t-cell mediated autoimmunity, alpha-viruses, bacterial chemotaxis, francisella tularensis, pertussis, Mycobacterium tuberculosis, Burkholderia, Dengue virus.

University of North Dakota, Graduate School and Graduate School, Graduate Programs in Medicine, Department of Microbiology and Immunology, Grand Forks, ND 58202. Offers MS, PhD. *Degree requirements:* For master's, comprehensive exam, thesis or alternative; for doctorate, comprehensive exam, thesis/dissertation, final examination. *Entrance requirements:* For master's and doctorate, GRE General Test, minimum GPA of 3.0. Additional exam requirements/recommendations for international students: Required—TOEFL (minimum score 550 paper-based; 79 iBT), IELTS (minimum score 6.5). Electronic applications accepted. *Faculty research:* Genetic and immunological aspects of a murine model of human multiple sclerosis, termination of DNA replication, cell division in bacteria, yersinia pestis.

University of North Texas Health Science Center at Fort Worth, Graduate School of Biomedical Sciences, Fort Worth, TX 76107-2699. Offers anatomy and cell biology (MS, PhD); biochemistry and molecular biology (MS, PhD); biomedical sciences (MS, PhD); biotechnology (MS); forensic genetics (MS); integrative physiology (MS, PhD); medical science (MS); microbiology and immunology (MS, PhD); pharmacology (MS, PhD); science education (MS); DO/MS; DO/PhD. Terminal master's awarded for partial completion of doctoral program. *Degree requirements:* For master's, thesis; for doctorate, thesis/dissertation. *Entrance requirements:* For master's and doctorate, GRE General Test. Additional exam requirements/recommendations for international students: Required—TOEFL. *Expenses:* Contact institution. *Faculty research:* Alzheimer's disease, aging, eye diseases, cancer, cardiovascular disease.

University of Oklahoma Health Sciences Center, College of Medicine and Graduate College, Graduate Programs in Medicine, Department of Microbiology and Immunology, Oklahoma City, OK 73190. Offers immunology (MS, PhD); microbiology (MS, PhD). Part-time programs available. *Faculty:* 12 full-time (4 women), 1 part-time/adjunct (0 women). *Students:* 7 full-time (3 women), 19 part-time (9 women); includes 3 minority (1 American Indian or Alaska Native, non-Hispanic/Latino; 2 Asian, non-Hispanic/Latino), 6 international. Average age 28. 7 applicants. In 2013, 2 master's, 6 doctorates awarded. Terminal master's awarded for partial completion of doctoral program. *Degree requirements:* For master's, thesis or alternative; for doctorate, one foreign language, thesis/dissertation. *Entrance requirements:* For doctorate, GRE General Test, 3 letters of recommendation. Additional exam requirements/recommendations for international students: Required—TOEFL. *Application deadline:* For fall admission, 12/15 for domestic students. Application fee: $50. *Expenses:* Tuition, state resident: full-time $3504; part-time $175.20 per credit hour. Tuition, nonresident: full-time $13,504; part-time $675.20 per credit hour. *Required fees:* $1545; $52.70 per credit hour. $245.25 per semester. Tuition and fees vary according to course load. *Financial support:* In 2013–14, 20 research assistantships (averaging $17,000 per year) were awarded; fellowships and teaching assistantships also available. Financial award applicants required to submit FAFSA. *Faculty research:* Molecular genetics, pathogenesis, streptococcal infections, gram-positive virulence, monoclonal antibodies. *Unit head:* Dr. Jimmy Ballard, Chairman, 405-271-2133, E-mail: jimmy-ballard@ouhsc.edu. *Application contact:* Dr. Molly Hill, Graduate Liaison, 405-271-2133, E-mail: molly-hill@ouhsc.edu.

University of Ottawa, Faculty of Graduate and Postdoctoral Studies, Faculty of Medicine, Department of Biochemistry, Microbiology and Immunology, Ottawa, ON K1N 6N5, Canada. Offers biochemistry (M Sc, PhD); microbiology and immunology (M Sc, PhD). *Degree requirements:* For master's, thesis; for doctorate, comprehensive exam, thesis/dissertation, seminar. *Entrance requirements:* For master's, honors degree or equivalent, minimum B average; for doctorate, master's degree, minimum B+ average. Electronic applications accepted. *Faculty research:* General biochemistry, molecular biology, microbiology, host biology, nutrition and metabolism.

University of Pennsylvania, Perelman School of Medicine, Biomedical Graduate Studies, Graduate Group in Immunology, Philadelphia, PA 19104. Offers PhD, MD/PhD, VMD/PhD. *Faculty:* 105. *Students:* 68 full-time (37 women); includes 22 minority (2 Black or African American, non-Hispanic/Latino; 15 Asian, non-Hispanic/Latino; 2 Hispanic/Latino; 3 Two or more races, non-Hispanic/Latino), 5 international. 102 applicants, 18% accepted, 10 enrolled. In 2013, 12 doctorates awarded. *Degree requirements:* For doctorate, thesis/dissertation, 2 preliminary exams. *Entrance requirements:* For doctorate, GRE General Test, undergraduate major in natural or physical science. Additional exam requirements/recommendations for international students: Required—TOEFL. *Application deadline:* For fall admission, 12/1 priority date for domestic students, 12/1 for international students. Applications are processed on a rolling basis. Application fee: $80. Electronic applications accepted. *Financial support:* In 2013–14, 68 students received support. Fellowships, research assistantships, scholarships/grants, traineeships, and unspecified assistantships available. *Faculty research:* Immunoglobulin structure and function, cell surface receptors, lymphocyte functional transplantation immunology, cellular immunology, molecular biology of immunoglobulins. *Unit head:* Dr. Avinash Bhandoola, Chair, 215-573-0274. *Application contact:* Mary Taylor, Graduate Coordinator, 215-573-4394.
Website: http://www.med.upenn.edu/immun/

University of Pittsburgh, School of Medicine, Graduate Programs in Medicine, Immunology Graduate Program, Pittsburgh, PA 15260. Offers PhD. *Faculty:* 60 full-time (25 women). *Students:* 34 full-time (19 women); includes 4 minority (3 Black or African American, non-Hispanic/Latino; 1 Asian, non-Hispanic/Latino), 18 international. Average age 28. 517 applicants, 13% accepted, 22 enrolled. In 2013, 14 doctorates awarded. *Degree requirements:* For doctorate, comprehensive exam, thesis/dissertation. *Entrance requirements:* For doctorate, GRE General Test, GRE Subject Test, minimum QPA of 3.0. Additional exam requirements/recommendations for international students: Required—TOEFL (minimum score 600 paper-based; 100 iBT), IELTS (minimum score 7). *Application deadline:* For fall admission, 1/1 priority date for domestic and international students. Application fee: $50. Electronic applications accepted. *Expenses:* Tuition, state resident: full-time $19,964; part-time $807 per credit. Tuition, nonresident: full-time $32,686; part-time $1337 per credit. *Required fees:* $740; $200. Tuition and fees vary according to program. *Financial support:* In 2013–14, 34 research assistantships with full tuition reimbursements (averaging $26,010 per year) were awarded; institutionally sponsored loans, scholarships/grants, traineeships, health care benefits, and unspecified assistantships also available. *Faculty research:* Human T-cell biology, opportunistic infections associated with AIDS, autoimmunity, immunoglobin gene expression, tumor immunology. *Unit head:* Dr. Lawrence Kane, Graduate Program Director, 412-648-8947, Fax: 412-383-8096, E-mail: lkane@pitt.edu. *Application contact:* Graduate Studies Administrator, 412-648-8957, Fax: 412-648-1007, E-mail: gradstudies@medschool.pitt.edu.
Website: http://www.gradbiomed.pitt.edu

University of Prince Edward Island, Atlantic Veterinary College, Graduate Program in Veterinary Medicine, Charlottetown, PE C1A 4P3, Canada. Offers anatomy (M Sc, PhD); bacteriology (M Sc, PhD); clinical pharmacology (M Sc, PhD); clinical sciences (M Sc, PhD); epidemiology (M Sc, PhD), including reproduction; fish health (M Sc, PhD); food animal nutrition (M Sc, PhD); immunology (M Sc, PhD); microanatomy (M Sc, PhD); parasitology (M Sc, PhD); pathology (M Sc, PhD); pharmacology (M Sc, PhD); physiology (M Sc, PhD); toxicology (M Sc, PhD); veterinary science (M Vet Sc); virology (M Sc, PhD). Part-time programs available. *Degree requirements:* For master's, thesis; for doctorate, thesis/dissertation. *Entrance requirements:* For master's, DVM, B Sc honors degree, or equivalent; for doctorate, M Sc. Additional exam requirements/recommendations for international students: Required—TOEFL (minimum score 550 paper-based; 80 iBT). *Expenses:* Contact institution. *Faculty research:* Animal health management, infectious diseases, fin fish and shellfish health, basic biomedical sciences, ecosystem health.

University of Rochester, School of Medicine and Dentistry, Graduate Programs in Medicine and Dentistry, Department of Microbiology and Immunology, Program in Microbiology and Immunology, Rochester, NY 14627. Offers MS, PhD. *Expenses: Tuition:* Full-time $44,580; part-time $1394 per credit hour. *Required fees:* $492.

University of Saskatchewan, College of Medicine, Department of Microbiology and Immunology, Saskatoon, SK S7N 5A2, Canada. Offers M Sc, PhD. *Degree requirements:* For master's, thesis; for doctorate, thesis/dissertation. *Entrance requirements:* Additional exam requirements/recommendations for international students: Required—TOEFL. *Expenses: Tuition, area resident:* Full-time $3585 Canadian dollars; part-time $585 Canadian dollars per course. Tuition, nonresident: part-time $877 Canadian dollars per course. *International tuition:* $5377 Canadian dollars full-time. *Required fees:* $889.51 Canadian dollars.

The University of South Dakota, Graduate School, School of Medicine and Graduate School, Biomedical Sciences Graduate Program, Molecular Microbiology and Immunology Group, Vermillion, SD 57069-2390. Offers MS, PhD. Terminal master's awarded for partial completion of doctoral program. *Degree requirements:* For master's, thesis; for doctorate, comprehensive exam, thesis/dissertation. *Entrance requirements:* For master's and doctorate, GRE General Test, minimum GPA of 3.0. Additional exam requirements/recommendations for international students: Required—TOEFL (minimum score 550 paper-based; 80 iBT), IELTS (minimum score 6). Electronic applications accepted. *Expenses:* Contact institution. *Faculty research:* Structure-function membranes, plasmids, immunology, virology, pathogenesis.

University of Southern California, Keck School of Medicine and Graduate School, Graduate Programs in Medicine, Department of Molecular Microbiology and Immunology, Los Angeles, CA 90033. Offers MS. Part-time programs available. *Faculty:* 21 full-time (5 women), 1 (woman) part-time/adjunct. *Students:* 29 full-time (21 women), 1 part-time (0 women); includes 8 minority (2 Black or African American, non-Hispanic/Latino; 3 Asian, non-Hispanic/Latino; 2 Hispanic/Latino; 1 Two or more races, non-Hispanic/Latino), 16 international. Average age 25. 40 applicants, 50% accepted, 15 enrolled. In 2013, 16 master's awarded. Terminal master's awarded for partial completion of doctoral program. *Degree requirements:* For master's, comprehensive exam (for some programs), thesis optional. *Entrance requirements:* For master's, GRE General Test, minimum GPA of 3.0. Additional exam requirements/recommendations for international students: Required—TOEFL (minimum score 100 iBT), IELTS. *Application deadline:* For fall admission, 6/1 for domestic students, 5/1 for international students; for spring admission, 11/1 for domestic students, 10/1 for international students. Applications are processed on a rolling basis. Application fee: $85. Electronic applications accepted. *Financial support:* In 2013–14, 1 student received support, including 1 teaching assistantship with full tuition reimbursement available (averaging $31,000 per year); Federal Work-Study, institutionally sponsored loans, scholarships/grants, health care benefits, and unspecified assistantships also available. Financial award application deadline: 5/4; financial award applicants required to submit FAFSA. *Faculty research:* Animal virology, microbial genetics, molecular and cellular immunology, cellular differentiation control of protein synthesis, HIV. *Unit head:* Dr. Axel H. Schonthal, Associate Professor/Program Chairman, 323-442-1730, Fax: 323-442-1721, E-mail: schontha@usc.edu. *Application contact:* Silvina V. Campos, Administrative Assistant II, 323-442-1713, Fax: 323-442-1721, E-mail: scampos@usc.edu.
Website: http://www.usc.edu/schools/medicine/departments/molecularmicrobio_immunology/

University of Southern Maine, College of Science, Technology, and Health, Program in Applied Medical Sciences, Portland, ME 04104-9300. Offers MS. Part-time programs available. *Faculty:* 4 full-time (0 women). *Students:* 9 full-time (8 women), 7 part-time (4 women). Average age 31. 10 applicants, 90% accepted, 4 enrolled. In 2013, 4 master's awarded. *Degree requirements:* For master's, thesis. *Entrance requirements:* For master's, GRE General Test, minimum GPA of 3.0. Additional exam requirements/recommendations for international students: Required—TOEFL. *Application deadline:* For fall admission, 5/1 priority date for domestic students; for spring admission, 11/1 for domestic students. Applications are processed on a rolling basis. Application fee: $65. Electronic applications accepted. *Expenses:* Tuition, state resident: part-time $380 per credit. Tuition, nonresident: part-time $1026 per credit. Part-time tuition and fees vary according to program. *Financial support:* Fellowships, research assistantships, teaching assistantships, career-related internships or fieldwork, and Federal Work-Study available. Support available to part-time students. Financial award application deadline: 4/1; financial award applicants required to submit FAFSA. *Faculty research:* Cancer biology, toxicology, environmental health, epidemiology, autoimmune disease, immunology, infectious disease, virology. *Application contact:* Mary Sloan, Assistant Dean of Graduate Studies and Director of Graduate Admissions, 207-780-4812, Fax: 207-780-4969, E-mail: gradstudies@usm.maine.edu.
Website: http://www.usm.maine.edu/ams/

University of South Florida, Morsani College of Medicine and Graduate School, Graduate Programs in Medical Sciences, Tampa, FL 33620-9951. Offers aging and neuroscience (MSMS); allergy, immunology and infectious disease (PhD); anatomy (MSMS, PhD); athletic training (MSMS); bioinformatics and computational biology (MSBCB); biotechnology (MSB); clinical and translational research (MSMS, PhD); health informatics (MSHI, MSMS); health science (MSMS); interdisciplinary medical sciences (MSMS); medical microbiology and immunology (MSMS); metabolic and nutritional medicine (MSMS); molecular medicine (MSMS, PhD); molecular pharmacology and physiology (PhD); neurology (PhD); pathology and laboratory medicine (PhD); pharmacology and therapeutics (PhD); physiology and biophysics (PhD); women's health (MSMS). *Students:* 336 full-time (182 women), 39 part-time (21 women); includes 170 minority (45 Black or African American, non-Hispanic/Latino; 54 Asian, non-Hispanic/Latino; 59 Hispanic/Latino; 2 Native Hawaiian or other Pacific Islander, non-Hispanic/Latino; 10 Two or more races, non-Hispanic/Latino), 17 international. Average age 26. 1,066 applicants, 44% accepted, 250 enrolled. In 2013, 191 master's, 12 doctorates awarded. Terminal master's awarded for partial completion of doctoral program. *Degree requirements:* For master's, comprehensive exam, thesis; for doctorate, comprehensive exam, thesis/dissertation. *Entrance requirements:* For master's, GRE General Test or GMAT, bachelor's degree or equivalent from regionally-accredited university with minimum GPA of 3.0 in upper-division sciences coursework; prerequisites in general biology, general chemistry, general physics, organic chemistry, quantitative analysis, and integral and differential calculus; for doctorate, GRE General Test (minimum score of 600 quantitative), bachelor's degree from regionally-accredited university with minimum GPA of 3.0 in upper-division sciences coursework; 3 letters of recommendation; personal interview; 1-2 page personal statement; prerequisites in biology, chemistry, physics, organic chemistry, quantitative analysis, and integral/differential calculus. Additional exam requirements/recommendations for international students: Required—TOEFL (minimum score 550 paper-based; 79 iBT) or IELTS (minimum score 6.5). *Application deadline:* For fall admission, 2/15 for domestic students, 1/2 for international students. Application fee: $30. *Expenses:* Contact institution. *Faculty research:* Anatomy, biochemistry, cancer biology, cardiovascular disease, cell biology, immunology, microbiology, molecular biology, neuroscience, pharmacology, physiology. *Unit head:* Dr. Michael Barber, Professor and Associate Dean for Graduate and Postdoctoral Affairs, 813-974-9908, Fax: 813-974-4317, E-mail: mbarber@health.usf.edu. *Application contact:* Dr. Eric Bennett, Graduate Director, PhD Program in Medical Sciences, 813-974-1545, Fax: 813-974-4317, E-mail: esbennet@health.usf.edu.
Website: http://health.usf.edu/nocms/medicine/graduatestudies/

The University of Texas Health Science Center at Houston, Graduate School of Biomedical Sciences, Program in Immunology, Houston, TX 77225-0036. Offers MS, PhD, MD/PhD. Terminal master's awarded for partial completion of doctoral program. *Degree requirements:* For master's, thesis; for doctorate, thesis/dissertation. *Entrance requirements:* For master's and doctorate, GRE General Test. Additional exam requirements/recommendations for international students: Required—TOEFL. Electronic applications accepted. *Expenses:* Tuition, state resident: full-time $3474; part-time $193 per credit hour. Tuition, nonresident: full-time $13,644; part-time $758 per credit hour. *Required fees:* $226.30; $87 per credit hour. *Faculty research:* Cancer immunology, molecular immunology, immune cell signaling, immune disease, immune system development.

The University of Texas Health Science Center at San Antonio, Graduate School of Biomedical Sciences, Department of Microbiology and Immunology, San Antonio, TX 78229-3900. Offers PhD. *Faculty:* 23 full-time (5 women), 1 (woman) part-time/adjunct. *Students:* 24 full-time (15 women), 2 part-time (both women); includes 12 minority (1 Asian, non-Hispanic/Latino; 11 Hispanic/Latino), 3 international. Average age 30. In 2013, 8 doctorates awarded. *Degree requirements:* For doctorate, comprehensive exam, thesis/dissertation. *Entrance requirements:* For doctorate, GRE General Test. Additional exam requirements/recommendations for international students: Required—TOEFL (minimum score 560 paper-based; 68 iBT). *Application deadline:* For fall admission, 1/15 priority date for domestic and international students. Applications are processed on a rolling basis. Application fee: $0. Electronic applications accepted. *Financial support:* Application deadline: 6/30; applicants required to submit FAFSA. *Faculty research:* Molecular immunology, mechanisms of microbial pathogenesis, molecular genetics, vaccine and immunodiagnostic development. *Total annual research expenditures:* $5.5 million. *Unit head:* Dr. Paolo B. Casali, Chairman, 210-567-3939, Fax: 210-567-6612, E-mail: pcasali@uthscsa.edu. *Application contact:* Dr. Keith Krolick, Graduate Advisor/Committee on Graduate Studies Chair, 210-567-3968, Fax: 210-567-6612, E-mail: krolick@uthscsa.edu.
Website: http://www.uthscsa.edu/micro/

The University of Texas Medical Branch, Graduate School of Biomedical Sciences, Program in Microbiology and Immunology, Galveston, TX 77555. Offers MS, PhD. Terminal master's awarded for partial completion of doctoral program. *Degree requirements:* For master's, thesis or alternative; for doctorate, thesis/dissertation. *Entrance requirements:* For doctorate, GRE General Test, minimum GPA of 3.0. Additional exam requirements/recommendations for international students: Required—TOEFL (minimum score 550 paper-based). Electronic applications accepted.

The University of Texas Southwestern Medical Center, Southwestern Graduate School of Biomedical Sciences, Division of Basic Science, Program in Immunology, Dallas, TX 75390. Offers PhD. *Faculty:* 47 full-time (12 women), 2 part-time/adjunct (0 women). *Students:* 31 full-time (19 women), 1 part-time (0 women); includes 9 minority (1 Black or African American, non-Hispanic/Latino; 1 American Indian or Alaska Native, non-Hispanic/Latino; 1 Asian, non-Hispanic/Latino; 6 Hispanic/Latino), 7 international. Average age 26. In 2013, 3 doctorates awarded. *Degree requirements:* For doctorate, thesis/dissertation, qualifying exam. *Entrance requirements:* For doctorate, GRE General Test, minimum GPA of 3.0. Additional exam requirements/recommendations for international students: Required—TOEFL. *Application deadline:* For fall admission, 12/15 priority date for domestic students. Applications are processed on a rolling basis. Application fee: $0. Electronic applications accepted. *Financial support:* Fellowships and research assistantships available. *Faculty research:* Antibody diversity and idiotype, cytotoxic effector mechanisms, natural killer cells, biology of immunoglobulins, oncogenes. *Unit head:* Dr. Nicolai Van Oers, Chair, 214-648-1236, Fax: 214-648-1902, E-mail: nicolai.vanoers@utsouthwestern.edu.
Website: http://www.utsouthwestern.edu/education/medical-school/departments/immunology/index.html

The University of Toledo, College of Graduate Studies, College of Medicine and Life Sciences, Department of Medical Microbiology and Immunology, Toledo, OH 43606-3390. Offers infection, immunity, and transplantation (MSBS, PhD); MD/MSBS; MD/PhD. *Faculty:* 13. *Students:* 13 full-time (9 women), 3 part-time (1 woman), 9 international. Average age 28. 23 applicants, 9% accepted. In 2013, 1 doctorate awarded. Terminal master's awarded for partial completion of doctoral program. *Degree*

requirements: For master's, thesis, qualifying exam; for doctorate, thesis/dissertation, qualifying exam. *Entrance requirements:* For master's and doctorate, GRE, minimum undergraduate GPA of 3.0, three letters of recommendation, statement of purpose, transcripts from all prior institutions attended, resume. Additional exam requirements/recommendations for international students: Required—TOEFL (minimum score 550 paper-based; 80 iBT). *Application deadline:* For fall admission, 1/15 priority date for domestic and international students. Application fee: $45 ($75 for international students). Electronic applications accepted. *Financial support:* In 2013–14, 16 research assistantships with full tuition reimbursements (averaging $22,032 per year) were awarded; Federal Work-Study, institutionally sponsored loans, scholarships/grants, tuition waivers (full), and unspecified assistantships also available. *Unit head:* Dr. Akira Takashima, Chair, 419-383-5423, E-mail: akira.takashima@utoledo.edu. *Application contact:* Admissions Analyst, 419-383-4112, Fax: 419-383-6140.
Website: http://www.utoledo.edu/med/grad/

University of Toronto, Faculty of Medicine, Department of Immunology, Toronto, ON M5S 1A1, Canada. Offers M Sc, PhD, MD/PhD. *Degree requirements:* For master's, thesis, thesis defense; for doctorate, thesis/dissertation, thesis defense. *Entrance requirements:* For master's, resume, 3 letters of reference. Additional exam requirements/recommendations for international students: Required—TOEFL (minimum score 580 paper-based; 93 iBT), TWE (minimum score 5). Electronic applications accepted.

University of Washington, Graduate School, School of Medicine, Graduate Programs in Medicine, Department of Immunology, Seattle, WA 98109. Offers PhD. *Faculty:* 28 full-time (8 women). *Students:* 34 full-time (21 women); includes 13 minority (2 Black or African American, non-Hispanic/Latino; 5 Asian, non-Hispanic/Latino; 6 Hispanic/Latino), 1 international. Average age 25. 94 applicants, 13% accepted, 3 enrolled. In 2013, 6 doctorates awarded. *Degree requirements:* For doctorate, thesis/dissertation, 1st-authored paper, accepted for publication. *Entrance requirements:* For doctorate, GRE General Test, BA or BS in related field. Additional exam requirements/recommendations for international students: Required—TOEFL (minimum score 600 paper-based; 100 iBT). *Application deadline:* For fall admission, 12/7 for domestic students, 11/1 for international students. Application fee: $85. Electronic applications accepted. *Financial support:* In 2013–14, 5 students received support, including 12 fellowships with full tuition reimbursements available (averaging $28,440 per year), 21 research assistantships with full tuition reimbursements available (averaging $28,440 per year); scholarships/grants, traineeships, health care benefits, tuition waivers (full), and stipends also available. *Faculty research:* Molecular and cellular immunology, regulation of lymphocyte differentiation and responses, genetics of immune recognition genetics and pathogenesis of autoimmune diseases, signal transduction. *Total annual research expenditures:* $10.4 million. *Unit head:* Dr. Joan M. Goverman, Professor and Chair, 206-685-3956, E-mail: goverman@uw.edu. *Application contact:* Peggy A. McCune, Training Program Manager, 206-685-3955, E-mail: immgrad@u.washington.edu.
Website: http://immunology.washington.edu/

The University of Western Ontario, Faculty of Graduate Studies, Biosciences Division, Department of Microbiology and Immunology, London, ON N6A 5B8, Canada. Offers M Sc, PhD. *Degree requirements:* For master's, thesis, oral and written exam; for doctorate, thesis/dissertation, oral and written exam. *Entrance requirements:* For master's, honors degree or equivalent in microbiology, immunology, or other biological science; minimum B average; for doctorate, M Sc in microbiology and immunology. Additional exam requirements/recommendations for international students: Required—TOEFL. *Faculty research:* Virology, molecular pathogenesis, cellular immunology, molecular biology.

Vanderbilt University, Graduate School and School of Medicine, Department of Microbiology and Immunology, Nashville, TN 37240-1001. Offers MS, PhD, MD/PhD. *Faculty:* 43 full-time (13 women). *Students:* 52 full-time (35 women); includes 6 minority (1 Black or African American, non-Hispanic/Latino; 3 Asian, non-Hispanic/Latino; 1 Hispanic/Latino; 1 Two or more races, non-Hispanic/Latino), 7 international. Average age 27. In 2013, 11 doctorates awarded. Terminal master's awarded for partial completion of doctoral program. *Degree requirements:* For master's, thesis; for doctorate, thesis/dissertation, final and qualifying exams. *Entrance requirements:* For master's and doctorate, GRE General Test, GRE Subject Test (recommended). Additional exam requirements/recommendations for international students: Required—TOEFL (minimum score 570 paper-based; 88 iBT). *Application deadline:* For fall admission, 1/15 for domestic and international students. Application fee: $0. Electronic applications accepted. *Financial support:* Fellowships with full tuition reimbursements, research assistantships with full tuition reimbursements, Federal Work-Study, institutionally sponsored loans, scholarships/grants, traineeships, health care benefits, and tuition waivers (partial) available. Financial award application deadline: 1/15; financial award applicants required to submit CSS PROFILE or FAFSA. *Faculty research:* Cellular and molecular microbiology, viruses, genes, cancer, molecular pathogenesis of microbial diseases, immunobiology. *Unit head:* Prof. Samuel A. Santoro, Chair of the Department of Pathology, Microbiology and Immunology, 615-322-3234, Fax: 615-322-5551, E-mail: samuel.a.santoro@vanderbilt.edu. *Application contact:* Walter B. Bieschke, Program Coordinator for Graduate Admissions, 615-342-0236, E-mail: walter.bieschke@vanderbilt.edu.
Website: http://www.mc.vanderbilt.edu/root/vumc.php?site-vmcpathology

Virginia Commonwealth University, Medical College of Virginia-Professional Programs, School of Medicine, School of Medicine Graduate Programs, Department of Microbiology and Immunology, Richmond, VA 23284-9005. Offers microbiology and immunology (MS, PhD); MD/PhD. *Degree requirements:* For master's, thesis; for doctorate, thesis/dissertation, comprehensive oral and written exams. *Entrance requirements:* For master's and doctorate, GRE General Test or MCAT. Additional exam requirements/recommendations for international students: Required—TOEFL (minimum score 600 paper-based; 100 iBT). Electronic applications accepted. *Faculty research:* Microbial physiology and genetics, molecular biology, crystallography of biological molecules, antibiotics and chemotherapy, membrane transport.

Wake Forest University, School of Medicine and Graduate School of Arts and Sciences, Graduate Programs in Medicine, Department of Microbiology and Immunology, Winston-Salem, NC 27109. Offers PhD, MD/PhD. *Degree requirements:* For doctorate, thesis/dissertation. *Entrance requirements:* For doctorate, GRE General Test. Additional exam requirements/recommendations for international students: Required—TOEFL. Electronic applications accepted. *Faculty research:* Molecular immunology, bacterial pathogenesis and molecular genetics, viral pathogenesis, regulation of mRNA metabolism, leukocyte biology.

Washington State University, College of Veterinary Medicine, Paul G. Allen School for Global Animal Health, Pullman, WA 99164-7090. Offers immunology and infectious diseases (MS, PhD). Part-time programs available. *Faculty:* 10 full-time (4 women), 24 part-time/adjunct (9 women). *Students:* 24 full-time (11 women); includes 3 minority (1 Black or African American, non-Hispanic/Latino; 1 Asian, non-Hispanic/Latino; 1 Hispanic/Latino). Average age 31. 5 applicants, 100% accepted, 5 enrolled. In 2013, 1 master's, 2 doctorates awarded. Terminal master's awarded for partial completion of doctoral program. *Degree requirements:* For master's, thesis; for doctorate, thesis/dissertation. *Entrance requirements:* For master's and doctorate, GRE or GMAT. Additional exam requirements/recommendations for international students: Required—TOEFL, IELTS. *Application deadline:* For fall admission, 1/10 priority date for domestic and international students; for spring admission, 7/1 priority date for domestic and international students. Application fee: $75. Electronic applications accepted. *Financial support:* In 2013–14, 18 students received support, including 1 fellowship (averaging $22,860 per year), 10 research assistantships (averaging $22,194 per year), 2 teaching assistantships; health care benefits also available. Support available to part-time students. *Faculty research:* Immunology, infectious disease, virology, disease surveillance, vaccine development. *Total annual research expenditures:* $5.5 million. *Unit head:* Dr. Guy H. Palmer, Director, Paul G. Allen School for Global Animal Health, 509-335-5861, Fax: 509-335-6328, E-mail: gpalmer@vetmed.wsu.edu. *Application contact:* Jill Griffin, Administrative Manager, 509-335-5861, Fax: 509-335-6328, E-mail: griffinj@vetmed.wsu.edu.
Website: http://globalhealth.wsu.edu/

Washington State University, College of Veterinary Medicine, Program in Immunology and Infectious Diseases, Pullman, WA 99164. Offers veterinary science (MS, PhD). *Faculty:* 26 full-time (10 women), 22 part-time/adjunct (5 women). *Students:* 41 full-time (27 women); includes 2 minority (both Hispanic/Latino), 18 international. Average age 31. 52 applicants, 10% accepted, 5 enrolled. In 2013, 4 master's, 6 doctorates awarded. Terminal master's awarded for partial completion of doctoral program. *Degree requirements:* For master's, thesis, oral exam; for doctorate, thesis/dissertation, oral exam. *Entrance requirements:* For master's and doctorate, minimum GPA of 3.0. Additional exam requirements/recommendations for international students: Required—TOEFL (minimum score 550 paper-based; 80 iBT). *Application deadline:* Applications are processed on a rolling basis. Application fee: $75. Electronic applications accepted. *Financial support:* In 2013–14, 15 fellowships, 26 research assistantships were awarded; institutionally sponsored loans, scholarships/grants, traineeships, health care benefits, and unspecified assistantships also available. Financial award application deadline: 3/1. *Faculty research:* Microbial pathogenesis, veterinary and wildlife parasitology, laboratory animal pathology, immune responses to infectious diseases. *Unit head:* Dr. Michele E. Hardy, Chair, 509-335-6030, Fax: 509-335-8529, E-mail: mhardy@vetmed.wsu.edu. *Application contact:* Sue Zumwalt, Graduate Coordinator, 509-335-6027, Fax: 509-335-8529, E-mail: szumwalt@vetmed.wsu.edu.
Website: http://www.vetmed.wsu.edu/depts-vmp/graduate/MSPhD.aspx

Washington University in St. Louis, Graduate School of Arts and Sciences, Division of Biology and Biomedical Sciences, Program in Immunology, St. Louis, MO 63130-4899. Offers PhD. *Degree requirements:* For doctorate, thesis/dissertation. *Entrance requirements:* For doctorate, GRE General Test, GRE Subject Test. Electronic applications accepted.

Wayne State University, School of Medicine, Graduate Programs in Medicine, Department of Immunology and Microbiology, Detroit, MI 48202. Offers MS, PhD, MD/PhD. *Students:* 13 full-time (7 women), 1 part-time (0 women); includes 3 minority (1 Black or African American, non-Hispanic/Latino; 1 Hispanic/Latino; 1 Two or more races, non-Hispanic/Latino), 1 international. Average age 26. 78 applicants, 8% accepted, 3 enrolled. In 2013, 3 doctorates awarded. *Degree requirements:* For doctorate, thesis/dissertation. *Entrance requirements:* For master's and doctorate, GRE, minimum GPA of 3.0 in BS in biology or related scientific discipline, three letters of recommendation, statement of purpose, admission to the Graduate School. Additional exam requirements/recommendations for international students: Required—TOEFL (minimum score 100 iBT), TWE (minimum score 6). *Application deadline:* For fall admission, 2/1 priority date for domestic and international students. Application fee: $0. Electronic applications accepted. *Expenses:* Contact institution. *Financial support:* In 2013–14, 10 students received support, including 2 fellowships with tuition reimbursements available (averaging $20,309 per year), 8 research assistantships with tuition reimbursements available (averaging $22,466 per year); teaching assistantships with tuition reimbursements available, scholarships/grants, health care benefits, and unspecified assistantships also available. Financial award application deadline: 3/31; financial award applicants required to submit FAFSA. *Faculty research:* Viral replication and pathogenesis, bacterial pathogenesis, mucosal immunity, autoimmune diseases. *Unit head:* Dr. Paul C. Montgomery, Professor and Chair, 313-577-1591, Fax: 313-577-1155, E-mail: pmontgo@wayne.edu. *Application contact:* Dr. Thomas C. Holland, Associate Professor, 313-577-1455, Fax: 313-577-1155, E-mail: tholland@wayne.edu.
Website: http://www.immunomicro.med.wayne.edu/gradprogram.php

Weill Cornell Medical College, Weill Cornell Graduate School of Medical Sciences, Immunology and Microbial Pathogenesis Program, New York, NY 10065. Offers immunology (MS, PhD), including immunology, microbiology, pathology. Terminal master's awarded for partial completion of doctoral program. *Degree requirements:* For master's, comprehensive exam; for doctorate, thesis/dissertation, final exam. *Entrance requirements:* For doctorate, GRE General Test, laboratory research experience, course work in biological sciences. Additional exam requirements/recommendations for international students: Required—TOEFL. Electronic applications accepted. *Faculty research:* Microbial immunity, tumor immunology, lympholyte and leukocyte biology, auto immunity, stem cell/bone marrow transplantation.

West Virginia University, Davis College of Agriculture, Forestry and Consumer Sciences, Interdisciplinary Program in Genetics and Developmental Biology, Morgantown, WV 26506. Offers animal breeding (MS, PhD); biochemical and molecular genetics (MS, PhD); cytogenetics (MS, PhD); descriptive embryology (MS, PhD); developmental genetics (MS); experimental morphogenesis/teratology (MS); human genetics (MS, PhD); immunogenetics (MS, PhD); life cycles of animals and plants (MS, PhD); molecular aspects of development (MS, PhD); mutagenesis (MS, PhD); oncology (MS, PhD); plant genetics (MS, PhD); population and quantitative genetics (MS, PhD); regeneration (MS, PhD); teratology (PhD); toxicology (MS, PhD). *Degree requirements:* For master's, thesis; for doctorate, comprehensive exam, thesis/dissertation. *Entrance requirements:* For master's, GRE or MCAT, minimum GPA of 2.75. Additional exam requirements/recommendations for international students: Required—TOEFL.

West Virginia University, School of Medicine, Graduate Programs at the Health Sciences Center, Interdisciplinary Graduate Programs in Biomedical Sciences, Program in Immunology and Microbial Pathogenesis, Morgantown, WV 26506. Offers MS, PhD, MD/PhD. *Degree requirements:* For doctorate, comprehensive exam, thesis/dissertation. *Entrance requirements:* For doctorate, GRE General Test, minimum GPA of 3.0. Additional exam requirements/recommendations for international students: Required—TOEFL. Electronic applications accepted. *Faculty research:* Regulation of signal transduction in immune responses, immune responses in bacterial and viral diseases, peptide and DNA vaccines for contraception, inflammatory bowel disease, physiology of pathogenic microbes.

Wright State University, School of Graduate Studies, College of Science and Mathematics, Program in Microbiology and Immunology, Dayton, OH 45435. Offers MS. Part-time programs available. *Degree requirements:* For master's, thesis. *Entrance requirements:* Additional exam requirements/recommendations for international students: Required—TOEFL. *Faculty research:* Reproductive immunology, viral pathogenesis, virus-host cell interactions.

Yale University, Graduate School of Arts and Sciences, Department of Immunobiology, New Haven, CT 06520. Offers PhD. *Degree requirements:* For doctorate, thesis/dissertation. *Entrance requirements:* For doctorate, GRE General Test.

Yale University, School of Medicine and Graduate School of Arts and Sciences, Combined Program in Biological and Biomedical Sciences (BBS), Immunology Track, New Haven, CT 06520. Offers PhD, MD/PhD. *Degree requirements:* For doctorate, thesis/dissertation. *Entrance requirements:* For doctorate, GRE General Test. Additional exam requirements/recommendations for international students: Required—TOEFL. Electronic applications accepted.

Infectious Diseases

Cornell University, Graduate School, Graduate Fields of Comparative Biomedical Sciences, Field of Comparative Biomedical Sciences, Ithaca, NY 14853-0001. Offers cellular and molecular medicine (MS, PhD); developmental and reproductive biology (MS, PhD); infectious diseases (MS, PhD); population medicine and epidemiology (MS, PhD); structural and functional biology (MS, PhD). *Faculty:* 104 full-time (32 women). *Students:* 32 full-time (22 women); includes 3 minority (1 Asian, non-Hispanic/Latino; 2 Hispanic/Latino), 12 international. Average age 29. 47 applicants, 23% accepted, 6 enrolled. In 2013, 2 master's, 12 doctorates awarded. *Degree requirements:* For master's, thesis; for doctorate, comprehensive exam, thesis/dissertation. *Entrance requirements:* For master's and doctorate, GRE General Test, 2 letters of recommendation. Additional exam requirements/recommendations for international students: Required—TOEFL (minimum score 550 paper-based; 77 iBT). *Application deadline:* For fall admission, 12/15 for domestic students. Application fee: $95. Electronic applications accepted. *Financial support:* In 2013–14, 18 students received support, including 3 fellowships with full tuition reimbursements available, 14 research assistantships with full tuition reimbursements available, 1 teaching assistantship with full tuition reimbursement available; institutionally sponsored loans, scholarships/grants, health care benefits, tuition waivers (full and partial), and unspecified assistantships also available. Financial award applicants required to submit FAFSA. *Faculty research:* Receptors and signal transduction, viral and bacterial infectious diseases, tumor metastasis, clinical sciences/nutritional disease, developmental/neurological disorders. *Unit head:* Director of Graduate Studies, 607-253-3276, Fax: 607-253-3756. *Application contact:* Graduate Field Assistant, 607-253-3276, Fax: 607-253-3756, E-mail: graduate_edcvm@cornell.edu.
Website: http://www.gradschool.cornell.edu/fields.php?id-64&a-2

Georgetown University, Graduate School of Arts and Sciences, Programs in Biomedical Sciences, Department of Microbiology and Immunology, Washington, DC 20057. Offers biohazardous threat agents and emerging infectious diseases (MS); biomedical science policy and advocacy (MS); general microbiology and immunology (MS); global infectious diseases (PhD); microbiology and immunology (PhD). Part-time programs available. *Degree requirements:* For master's, 30 credit hours of coursework; for doctorate, comprehensive exam, thesis/dissertation. *Entrance requirements:* For master's, GRE General Test, 3 letters of reference, bachelor's degree in related field; for doctorate, GRE General Test, 3 letters of reference, MS/BS in related field. Additional exam requirements/recommendations for international students: Required—TOEFL (minimum score 505 paper-based). *Application deadline:* For fall admission, 7/1 for domestic students, 6/1 priority date for international students; for winter admission, 2/2 priority date for domestic students, 1/2 priority date for international students; for spring admission, 11/1 for domestic students, 10/1 priority date for international students. Applications are processed on a rolling basis. Application fee: $75. Electronic applications accepted. *Financial support:* Fellowships with full tuition reimbursements available. *Faculty research:* Pathogenesis and basic biology of the fungus Candida albicans, molecular biology of viral immunopathological mechanisms in Multiple Sclerosis. *Unit head:* Dr. Richard A. Calderone, Chair, 202-687-1513, E-mail: calderor@georgetown.edu. *Application contact:* Kimberly Bassalian, Graduate Program Coordinator, 202-687-3422, Fax: 202-687-1800, E-mail: kdb70@georgetown.edu.
Website: http://microbiology.georgetown.edu/

The George Washington University, School of Public Health and Health Services, Department of Epidemiology and Biostatistics, Washington, DC 20052. Offers biostatistics (MPH); epidemiology (MPH); microbiology and emerging infectious diseases (MSPH). *Faculty:* 29 full-time (20 women). *Students:* 54 full-time (43 women), 77 part-time (60 women); includes 37 minority (18 Black or African American, non-Hispanic/Latino; 16 Asian, non-Hispanic/Latino; 2 Hispanic/Latino; 1 Two or more races, non-Hispanic/Latino), 12 international. Average age 28. 342 applicants, 75% accepted. In 2013, 51 master's awarded. *Degree requirements:* For master's, case study or special project. *Entrance requirements:* For master's, GMAT, GRE General Test, or MCAT. Additional exam requirements/recommendations for international students: Required—TOEFL. *Application deadline:* For fall admission, 4/15 priority date for domestic students, 4/15 for international students; for spring admission, 11/1 for domestic and international students. Applications are processed on a rolling basis. Application fee: $75. *Financial support:* In 2013–14, 6 students received support. Tuition waivers available. Financial award application deadline: 2/15. *Unit head:* Dr. Alan E. Greenberg, Chair, 202-994-0612, E-mail: aeg1@gwu.edu. *Application contact:* Jane Smith, Director of Admissions, 202-994-0248, Fax: 202-994-1860, E-mail: sphhsinfo@gwumc.edu.

Johns Hopkins University, Bloomberg School of Public Health, Department of Epidemiology, Baltimore, MD 21205. Offers cancer etiology and prevention (MHS, Sc M, PhD, Sc D); cardiovascular diseases (MHS, Sc M, PhD, Sc D); clinical epidemiology (MHS, Sc M, PhD, Sc D); clinical trials (PhD, Sc D); epidemiology (MHS, Sc M, Dr PH, PhD, Sc D); epidemiology of aging (MHS, Sc M, PhD, Sc D); genetic epidemiology (MHS, Sc M, PhD, Sc D); infectious disease epidemiology (MHS, Sc M, PhD, Sc D); occupational and environmental epidemiology (MHS, Sc M, PhD, Sc D). Part-time programs available. *Faculty:* 80 full-time (44 women), 82 part-time/adjunct (36 women). *Students:* 141 full-time (106 women), 20 part-time (13 women); includes 32 minority (5 Black or African American, non-Hispanic/Latino; 1 American Indian or Alaska Native, non-Hispanic/Latino; 18 Asian, non-Hispanic/Latino; 6 Hispanic/Latino; 2 Two or more races, non-Hispanic/Latino), 49 international. Average age 29. 302 applicants, 35% accepted, 63 enrolled. In 2013, 26 master's, 23 doctorates awarded. *Degree requirements:* For master's, comprehensive exam, thesis, 1-year full-time residency; for doctorate, comprehensive exam, thesis/dissertation, 2 years' full-time residency, oral and written exams, student teaching. *Entrance requirements:* For master's, GRE General Test or MCAT, 3 letters of recommendation, curriculum vitae; for doctorate, GRE General Test, minimum 1 year of work experience, 3 letters of recommendation, curriculum vitae, academic records from all schools. Additional exam requirements/recommendations for international students: Required—TOEFL (minimum score 600 paper-based; 100 iBT); Recommended—IELTS (minimum score 7.5), TWE. *Application deadline:* For fall admission, 12/1 priority date for domestic students. Applications are processed on a rolling basis. Application fee: $45. Electronic applications accepted. *Financial support:* Fellowships, Federal Work-Study, institutionally sponsored loans, scholarships/grants, traineeships, tuition waivers (partial), and stipends available. Support available to part-time students. Financial award application deadline: 3/15; financial award applicants required to submit FAFSA. *Faculty research:* Cancer and congenital malformations, nutritional epidemiology, AIDS, tuberculosis, cardiovascular disease, risk assessment. *Total annual research expenditures:* $70.1 million. *Unit head:* Dr. David D. Celentano, Chair, 410-955-3286, Fax: 410-955-0863, E-mail: dcelenta@jhsph.edu. *Application contact:* Frances S. Burman, Academic Program Manager, 410-955-3926, Fax: 410-955-0863, E-mail: fburman@jhsph.edu.
Website: http://www.jhsph.edu/dept/epi/index.html

Loyola University Chicago, Graduate School, Marcella Niehoff School of Nursing, Population-Based Infection Control and Environmental Safety Program, Chicago, IL 60660. Offers MSN, Certificate. Part-time and evening/weekend programs available. *Faculty:* 45 full-time (44 women). *Students:* 1 (woman) full-time, 7 part-time (all women); includes 1 minority (Black or African American, non-Hispanic/Latino). Average age 38. 1 applicant, 100% accepted. In 2013, 4 master's, 1 other advanced degree awarded. *Degree requirements:* For master's, comprehensive exam. *Entrance requirements:* For master's, Illinois nursing license, 3 letters of recommendation, minimum nursing GPA of 3.0, 1000 hours of experience before starting clinical. Application fee: $50. *Expenses: Tuition:* Full-time $16,740; part-time $930 per credit. *Required fees:* $135 per semester. *Financial support:* Traineeships available. *Unit head:* Dr. Marijo Letizia, Associate Dean, MSN and DNP Programs, 708-216-9325, Fax: 708-216-9555, E-mail: meltizi@luc.edu. *Application contact:* Amy Weatherford, Enrollment Advisor, School of Nursing, 708-216-3751, Fax: 708-216-9555, E-mail: aweatherford@luc.edu.
Website: http://www.luc.edu/nursing/

Loyola University Chicago, Graduate School, Program in Infectious Disease and Immunology, Chicago, IL 60660. Offers MS. *Faculty:* 35 full-time (12 women). *Students:* 9 full-time (8 women); includes 1 minority (Black or African American, non-Hispanic/Latino). Average age 25. 24 applicants, 33% accepted, 4 enrolled. In 2013, 3 master's awarded. *Degree requirements:* For master's, thesis. *Entrance requirements:* For master's, GRE. Additional exam requirements/recommendations for international students: Required—TOEFL. *Application deadline:* For fall admission, 6/15 for domestic and international students. Applications are processed on a rolling basis. *Expenses: Tuition:* Full-time $16,740; part-time $930 per credit. *Required fees:* $135 per semester. *Faculty research:* Immunological tolerance and memory, molecular analysis of virus assembly and entry, biofilm mediated interactions, molecular analysis of clinical isolates of C. difficile, immune system development and regulation. *Unit head:* Dr. Katherine L. Knight, Co-Director, 708-216-3385, Fax: 708-216-9574, E-mail: kknight@lumc.edu. *Application contact:* Dr. Makio Iwashima, Graduate Program Director, 708-216-5816, Fax: 708-216-9574, E-mail: miwashima@lumc.edu.

Montana State University, College of Graduate Studies, College of Agriculture, Department of Immunology and Infectious Diseases, Bozeman, MT 59717. Offers MS, PhD. Part-time programs available. *Degree requirements:* For master's, comprehensive exam; for doctorate, comprehensive exam, thesis/dissertation. *Entrance requirements:* For master's and doctorate, GRE General Test. Additional exam requirements/recommendations for international students: Required—TOEFL (minimum score 550 paper-based). Electronic applications accepted. *Faculty research:* Immunology, mechanisms of infectious disease pathogenesis, mechanisms of host defense, lymphocyte development, host-pathogen interactions.

North Carolina State University, College of Veterinary Medicine, Program in Comparative Biomedical Sciences, Raleigh, NC 27695. Offers cell biology (MS, PhD); infectious disease (MS, PhD); pathology (MS, PhD); pharmacology (MS, PhD); population medicine (MS, PhD). Part-time programs available. *Degree requirements:* For master's, thesis; for doctorate, thesis/dissertation. *Entrance requirements:* For master's and doctorate, GRE General Test. Additional exam requirements/recommendations for international students: Required—TOEFL (minimum score 550 paper-based). Electronic applications accepted. *Expenses:* Contact institution. *Faculty research:* Infectious diseases, cell biology, pharmacology and toxicology, genomics, pathology and population medicine.

Penn State University Park, Graduate School, Intercollege Graduate Programs, Intercollege Graduate Program in Immunology and Infectious Diseases, University Park, PA 16802. Offers MS, PhD. *Unit head:* Dr. Regina Vasilatos-Younken, Interim Dean, 814-865-2516, Fax: 814-863-4627, E-mail: rxv@psu.edu. *Application contact:* Cynthia E. Nicosia, Director, Graduate Enrollment Services, 814-865-1834, Fax: 814-863-4627, E-mail: cey1@psu.edu.

Rutgers, The State University of New Jersey, Newark, Graduate School of Biomedical Sciences, Newark, NJ 07107. Offers biodefense (Certificate); biomedical engineering (PhD); biomedical sciences (multidisciplinary) (PhD); cellular biology, neuroscience and physiology (PhD), including neuroscience, physiology, biophysics, cardiovascular biology, molecular pharmacology, stem cell biology; infection, immunity and inflammation (PhD), including immunology, infectious disease, microbiology, oral biology; molecular biology, genetics and cancer (PhD), including biochemistry, molecular genetics, cancer biology, radiation biology, bioinformatics; neuroscience (Certificate); pharmacological sciences (Certificate); stem cell (Certificate); DMD/PhD; MD/PhD. PhD in biomedical engineering offered jointly with New Jersey Institute of Technology. Part-time and evening/weekend programs available. Terminal master's awarded for partial completion of doctoral program. *Degree requirements:* For doctorate, thesis/dissertation, qualifying exam. *Entrance requirements:* For doctorate, GRE General Test. Additional exam requirements/recommendations for international students: Required—TOEFL. Electronic applications accepted.

State University of New York Upstate Medical University, College of Graduate Studies, Major Research Areas of the College of Graduate Studies, Syracuse, NY 13210-2334.

Thomas Jefferson University, Jefferson Graduate School of Biomedical Sciences, Certificate Programs in Clinical Research, Human Clinical Investigation, and Infectious Diseases, Philadelphia, PA 19107. Offers clinical research and trials (Certificate); human clinical investigation (Certificate); infectious disease control (Certificate). *Faculty:* 44 full-time (14 women), 27 part-time/adjunct (11 women). *Students:* 15 part-time (9

women); includes 3 minority (1 Black or African American, non-Hispanic/Latino; 1 Asian, non-Hispanic/Latino; 1 Hispanic/Latino), 1 international. 8 applicants, 100% accepted, 6 enrolled. In 2013, 3 Certificates awarded. *Entrance requirements:* For degree, GRE General Test (recommended). Additional exam requirements/recommendations for international students: Required—TOEFL (minimum score 100 iBT) or IELTS (minimum score 7). *Application deadline:* For fall admission, 8/1 priority date for domestic students, 3/1 priority date for international students; for winter admission, 12/1 priority date for domestic students, 6/1 priority date for international students; for spring admission, 4/1 priority date for domestic students. Applications are processed on a rolling basis. Application fee: $75. Electronic applications accepted. *Financial support:* Federal Work-Study and institutionally sponsored loans available. Support available to part-time students. Financial award application deadline: 5/1; financial award applicants required to submit FAFSA. *Faculty research:* Epidemiology, clinical research, statistics, planning and management, disease control. *Unit head:* Dr. Dennis M. Gross, Associate Dean, 215-503-0156, Fax: 215-503-3433, E-mail: dennis.gross@jefferson.edu. *Application contact:* Marc E. Stearns, Director of Admissions, 215-503-0155, Fax: 215-503-3433, E-mail: jgsbs-info@jefferson.edu.
Website: http://www.jefferson.edu/university/biomedical_sciences/programs/certificates.html

Tufts University, Cummings School of Veterinary Medicine, North Grafton, MA 01536. Offers animals and public policy (MS); biomedical sciences (PhD), including digestive diseases, infectious diseases, neuroscience and reproductive biology, pathology; conservation medicine (MS); veterinary medicine (DVM); DVM/MPH; DVM/MS. *Accreditation:* AVMA (one or more programs are accredited). *Faculty:* 98 full-time (45 women), 13 part-time/adjunct (7 women). *Students:* 426 full-time (364 women); includes 60 minority (5 Black or African American, non-Hispanic/Latino; 1 American Indian or Alaska Native, non-Hispanic/Latino; 32 Asian, non-Hispanic/Latino; 20 Hispanic/Latino; 2 Two or more races, non-Hispanic/Latino), 4 international. Average age 25. 899 applicants, 29% accepted, 119 enrolled. In 2013, 85 master's, 2 doctorates awarded. *Degree requirements:* For master's, thesis (for some programs); for doctorate, comprehensive exam, thesis/dissertation (for some programs). *Entrance requirements:* For master's and doctorate, GRE General Test. Additional exam requirements/recommendations for international students: Required—TOEFL or IELTS. *Application deadline:* For fall admission, 11/1 for domestic and international students. Application fee: $70. Electronic applications accepted. *Expenses:* Contact institution. *Financial support:* In 2013–14, 230 students received support, including 7 research assistantships with full tuition reimbursements available (averaging $25,000 per year), 6 teaching assistantships (averaging $5,000 per year); career-related internships or fieldwork, Federal Work-Study, institutionally sponsored loans, scholarships/grants, and institutional aid awards, health care benefits for PhD students also available. Financial award application deadline: 4/15; financial award applicants required to submit FAFSA. *Faculty research:* Oncology, veterinary ethics, international veterinary medicine, veterinary genomics, pathogenesis of Clostridium difficile, wildlife fertility control. *Unit head:* Dr. Deborah T. Kochevar, Dean, 508-839-5302, Fax: 508-839-2953, E-mail: deborah.kochevar@tufts.edu. *Application contact:* Rebecca Russo, Director of Admissions, 508-839-7920, Fax: 508-887-4820, E-mail: vetadmissions@tufts.edu.
Website: http://www.tufts.edu/

Tulane University, School of Public Health and Tropical Medicine, Department of Tropical Medicine, New Orleans, LA 70118-5669. Offers clinical tropical medicine and travelers health (Diploma); parasitology (MSPH, PhD); public health and tropical medicine (MPHTM); vector borne infectious diseases (MS, PhD); MD/PhD. MS and PhD offered through the Graduate School. *Degree requirements:* For master's, thesis; for doctorate, comprehensive exam, thesis/dissertation. *Entrance requirements:* For master's, GRE General Test, minimum B average in undergraduate course work; for doctorate, GRE General Test. Additional exam requirements/recommendations for international students: Required—TOEFL.

Uniformed Services University of the Health Sciences, School of Medicine, Graduate Programs in the Biomedical Sciences and Public Health, Graduate Program in Emerging Infectious Diseases, Bethesda, MD 20814-4799. Offers PhD. *Faculty:* 35 full-time (5 women), 17 part-time/adjunct (6 women). *Students:* 33 full-time (27 women); includes 3 minority (2 Black or African American, non-Hispanic/Latino; 1 Asian, non-Hispanic/Latino), 2 international. Average age 26. 43 applicants, 44% accepted, 11 enrolled. In 2013, 7 doctorates awarded. *Degree requirements:* For doctorate, comprehensive exam, thesis/dissertation, qualifying exam. *Entrance requirements:* For doctorate, GRE General Test. Additional exam requirements/recommendations for international students: Required—TOEFL. *Application deadline:* For fall admission, 1/1 priority date for domestic and international students. Applications are processed on a rolling basis. Application fee: $0. Electronic applications accepted. *Financial support:* In 2013–14, fellowships with full tuition reimbursements (averaging $27,000 per year) were awarded; scholarships/grants, health care benefits, and tuition waivers (full) also available. *Unit head:* Dr. Christopher Broder, Director, 301-295-3401, E-mail: cbroder@usuhs.mil. *Application contact:* Patricia Grant, Program Administrative Specialist, 301-295-3400, Fax: 301-295-3773, E-mail: patricia.grant@usuhs.edu.
Website: http://www.usuhs.mil/eid

See Display below and Close-Up on page 353.

Université Laval, Faculty of Medicine, Post-Professional Programs in Medical Studies, Québec, QC G1K 7P4, Canada. Offers anatomy–pathology (DESS); anesthesiology (DESS); cardiology (DESS); care of older people (Diploma); clinical research (DESS); community health (DESS); dermatology (DESS); diagnostic radiology (DESS); emergency medicine (Diploma); family medicine (DESS); general surgery (DESS); geriatrics (DESS); hematology (DESS); internal medicine (DESS); maternal and fetal medicine (Diploma); medical biochemistry (DESS); medical microbiology and infectious diseases (DESS); medical oncology (DESS); nephrology (DESS); neurology (DESS); neurosurgery (DESS); obstetrics and gynecology (DESS); ophthalmology (DESS); orthopedic surgery (DESS); oto-rhino-laryngology (DESS); palliative medicine (Diploma); pediatrics (DESS); plastic surgery (DESS); psychiatry (DESS); pulmonary medicine (DESS); radiology–oncology (DESS); thoracic surgery (DESS); urology (DESS). *Degree requirements:* For other advanced degree, comprehensive exam. *Entrance requirements:* For degree, knowledge of French. Electronic applications accepted.

University of Calgary, Cumming School of Medicine and Faculty of Graduate Studies, Department of Microbiology, Immunology and Infectious Diseases, Calgary, AB T2N 1N4, Canada. Offers M Sc, PhD. *Degree requirements:* For master's, thesis, oral thesis exam; for doctorate, thesis/dissertation, candidacy exam, oral thesis exam. *Entrance requirements:* For master's and doctorate, minimum GPA of 3.2. Additional exam requirements/recommendations for international students: Required—TOEFL (minimum score 580 paper-based). Electronic applications accepted. *Faculty research:* Bacteriology, virology, parasitology, immunology.

University of California, Berkeley, Graduate Division, School of Public Health, Group in Epidemiology, Berkeley, CA 94720-1500. Offers epidemiology (MS, PhD); infectious diseases (MPH, PhD). *Accreditation:* CEPH (one or more programs are accredited). *Degree requirements:* For master's, comprehensive exam; for doctorate, thesis/dissertation, oral and written exam. *Entrance requirements:* For master's, GRE General Test, minimum GPA of 3.0; MD, DDS, DVM, or PhD in biomedical science (MPH); for doctorate, GRE General Test, minimum GPA of 3.0.

University of California, Berkeley, Graduate Division, School of Public Health, Group in Infectious Diseases and Immunity, Berkeley, CA 94720-1500. Offers PhD. *Entrance* *requirements:* For doctorate, GRE General Test, minimum GPA of 3.0, 3 letters of recommendation.

University of Georgia, College of Veterinary Medicine, Department of Infectious Diseases, Athens, GA 30602. Offers MS, PhD. *Degree requirements:* For master's, thesis; for doctorate, one foreign language, thesis/dissertation. *Entrance requirements:* For master's and doctorate, GRE General Test. Electronic applications accepted.

University of Guelph, Ontario Veterinary College and Graduate Studies, Graduate Programs in Veterinary Sciences, Department of Pathobiology, Guelph, ON N1G 2W1, Canada. Offers anatomic pathology (DV Sc, Diploma); clinical pathology (Diploma); comparative pathology (M Sc, PhD); immunology (M Sc, PhD); laboratory animal science (DV Sc); pathology (M Sc, PhD, Diploma); veterinary infectious diseases (M Sc, PhD); zoo animal/wildlife medicine (DV Sc). *Degree requirements:* For master's, thesis; for doctorate, thesis/dissertation. *Entrance requirements:* For master's, DVM with B average or an honours degree in biological sciences; for doctorate, DVM or MSC degree, minimum B+ average. Additional exam requirements/recommendations for international students: Required—TOEFL (minimum score 550 paper-based). *Faculty research:* Pathogenesis; diseases of animals, wildlife, fish, and laboratory animals; parasitology; immunology; veterinary infectious diseases; laboratory animal science.

University of Minnesota, Twin Cities Campus, School of Public Health, Division of Environmental Health Sciences, Area in Environmental Infectious Diseases, Minneapolis, MN 55455-0213. Offers MPH, MS, PhD. *Degree requirements:* For doctorate, thesis/dissertation. *Entrance requirements:* For master's and doctorate, GRE General Test. Electronic applications accepted.

University of Pittsburgh, Graduate School of Public Health, Department of Infectious Diseases and Microbiology, Pittsburgh, PA 15260. Offers infectious disease management, intervention, and community practice (MPH); infectious disease pathogenesis, eradication, and laboratory practice (MPH); infectious diseases and microbiology (MS, PhD). Part-time programs available. *Faculty:* 19 full-time (6 women), 4 part-time/adjunct (1 woman). *Students:* 50 full-time (42 women), 15 part-time (10 women); includes 8 minority (2 Black or African American, non-Hispanic/Latino; 4 Asian, non-Hispanic/Latino; 1 Hispanic/Latino; 1 Two or more races, non-Hispanic/Latino), 11 international. Average age 27. 155 applicants, 63% accepted, 15 enrolled. In 2013, 25 master's, 4 doctorates awarded. Terminal master's awarded for partial completion of doctoral program. *Degree requirements:* For master's, one foreign language, comprehensive exam (for some programs), thesis; for doctorate, one foreign language, comprehensive exam, thesis/dissertation. *Entrance requirements:* For master's and doctorate, GRE General Test, MCAT, or DAT. Additional exam requirements/ recommendations for international students: Required—TOEFL (minimum score 550 paper-based; 80 iBT) or IELTS (minimum score 6.5). *Application deadline:* For fall admission, 1/15 for domestic and international students; for spring admission, 10/15 for domestic students, 8/1 for international students; for summer admission, 12/1 for international students. Applications are processed on a rolling basis. Application fee: $120. Electronic applications accepted. *Expenses:* Tuition, state resident: full-time $19,964; part-time $807 per credit. Tuition, nonresident: full-time $32,686; part-time $1337 per credit. *Required fees:* $740; $200. Tuition and fees vary according to program. *Financial support:* In 2013–14, 12 research assistantships with full and partial tuition reimbursements (averaging $8,754 per year) were awarded. Financial award applicants required to submit FAFSA. *Faculty research:* HIV, Epstein-Barr virus, virology, immunology, malaria. *Total annual research expenditures:* $14.8 million. *Unit head:* Dr. Charles R. Rinaldo, Jr., Chairman, 412-624-3928, Fax: 412-624-4953, E-mail: rinaldo@pitt.edu. *Application contact:* Dr. Jeremy Martinson, Assistant Professor, 412-624-5646, Fax: 412-383-8926, E-mail: jmartins@pitt.edu.
Website: http://www.idm.pitt.edu/

University of Southern California, Keck School of Medicine and Graduate School, Program in Integrative Biology of Disease, Los Angeles, CA 90089. Offers PhD. *Faculty:* 236 full-time (68 women). *Students:* 23 full-time (13 women); includes 6 minority (4 Asian, non-Hispanic/Latino; 2 Hispanic/Latino), 6 international. Average age 30. 3 applicants, 100% accepted, 3 enrolled. In 2013, 6 doctorates awarded. *Degree requirements:* For doctorate, comprehensive exam, thesis/dissertation. *Entrance requirements:* For doctorate, GRE, minimum GPA of 3.0. Additional exam requirements/ recommendations for international students: Required—TOEFL (minimum score 600 paper-based; 100 iBT). *Application deadline:* For fall admission, 12/1 priority date for domestic and international students. Application fee: $85. Electronic applications accepted. *Financial support:* In 2013–14, 23 students received support, including 3 fellowships (averaging $31,000 per year), 19 research assistantships with full tuition reimbursements available (averaging $31,000 per year), 1 teaching assistantship with full tuition reimbursement available (averaging $31,000 per year); institutionally sponsored loans, scholarships/grants, traineeships, health care benefits, and unspecified assistantships also available. Financial award application deadline: 5/4; financial award applicants required to submit FAFSA. *Unit head:* Dr. W. Martin Kast, Director, 323-442-1475, Fax: 323-442-1199, E-mail: mkast@usc.edu. *Application contact:* Dr. Joyce Perez, Manager of Student Programs, 323-442-1645, Fax: 323-442-1199, E-mail: pibbs@usc.edu.
Website: http://www.usc.edu/intbio

The University of Texas Medical Branch, Graduate School of Biomedical Sciences, Program in Emerging and Tropical Infectious Diseases, Galveston, TX 77555. Offers PhD, MD/PhD. *Degree requirements:* For doctorate, thesis/dissertation. *Entrance requirements:* For doctorate, GRE General Test. *Faculty research:* Emerging diseases, tropical diseases, parasitology, vitology and bacteriology.

Yale University, School of Medicine and Graduate School of Arts and Sciences, Combined Program in Biological and Biomedical Sciences (BBS), Microbiology Track, New Haven, CT 06520. Offers PhD, MD/PhD. *Degree requirements:* For doctorate, thesis/dissertation. *Entrance requirements:* For doctorate, GRE General Test, GRE Subject Test. Additional exam requirements/recommendations for international students: Required—TOEFL. Electronic applications accepted.

Medical Microbiology

Creighton University, School of Medicine and Graduate School, Graduate Programs in Medicine, Department of Medical Microbiology and Immunology, Omaha, NE 68178-0001. Offers MS, PhD. *Faculty:* 11 full-time (2 women). *Students:* 14 full-time (7 women); includes 1 minority (Hispanic/Latino), 3 international. Average age 26. 55 applicants, 4% accepted, 2 enrolled. In 2013, 1 master's, 3 doctorates awarded. Terminal master's awarded for partial completion of doctoral program. *Degree requirements:* For master's, comprehensive exam, thesis; for doctorate, thesis/ dissertation, preliminary examination, NIH-style grant defense. *Entrance requirements:* For master's and doctorate, GRE General Test. Additional exam requirements/ recommendations for international students: Required—TOEFL (minimum score 80 iBT). *Application deadline:* For fall admission, 2/1 priority date for domestic and international students. Applications are processed on a rolling basis. Application fee: $50. *Expenses: Tuition:* Full-time $13,608; part-time $756 per credit hour. *Required fees:* $149 per semester. Tuition and fees vary according to course load, campus/ location, program, reciprocity agreements and student's religious affiliation. *Financial support:* In 2013–14, 6 fellowships with tuition reimbursements (averaging $22,275 per year), research assistantships with tuition reimbursements (averaging $22,275 per year) were awarded; career-related internships or fieldwork, institutionally sponsored loans, and tuition waivers (full) also available. *Faculty research:* Infectious diseases, molecular biology, genetics, antimicrobial agents and chemotherapy, virology. *Total annual research expenditures:* $2 million. *Unit head:* Dr. Richard Goering, Chair, 402-280-4091, Fax: 402-280-1875, E-mail: richardgoering@creighton.edu. *Application contact:* Dr. Patrick C. Swanson, Graduate Director, 402-280-2716, Fax: 402-280-1875, E-mail: pswanson@creighton.edu.
Website: http://mmi.creighton.edu/

Idaho State University, Office of Graduate Studies, College of Science and Engineering, Department of Biological Sciences, Pocatello, ID 83209-8007. Offers biology (MNS, MS, DA, PhD); clinical laboratory science (MS); microbiology (MS). *Accreditation:* NAACLS. Part-time programs available. *Degree requirements:* For master's, comprehensive exam, thesis; for doctorate, comprehensive exam, thesis/ dissertation, 9 credits of internship (for DA). *Entrance requirements:* For master's, GRE General Test, minimum GPA of 3.0 in all upper division classes; for doctorate, GRE General Test, GRE Subject Test (biology), diagnostic exam (DA), minimum GPA of 3.0 in all upper division classes. Additional exam requirements/recommendations for international students: Required—TOEFL (minimum score 550 paper-based; 80 iBT). Electronic applications accepted. *Faculty research:* Ecology, plant and animal physiology, plant and animal developmental biology, immunology, molecular biology, bioinfomatics.

Rutgers, The State University of New Jersey, New Brunswick, Graduate School-New Brunswick, Programs in the Molecular Biosciences, Piscataway, NJ 08854-8097. Offers biochemistry (PhD); cell and developmental biology (MS, PhD); microbiology and molecular genetics (MS, PhD), including applied microbiology, clinical microbiology (MS), clinical mircobiology (PhD), computational molecular biology (PhD), immunology, microbial biochemistry, molecular genetics, virology. MS, PhD offered jointly with University of Medicine and Dentistry of New Jersey.

Université du Québec, Institut National de la Recherche Scientifique, Graduate Programs, Research Center–INRS–Institut Armand-Frappier, Laval, QC H7V 1B7, Canada. Offers applied microbiology (M Sc); biology (PhD); experimental health sciences (M Sc); virology and immunology (M Sc, PhD). Programs given in French. Part-time programs available. *Faculty:* 45 full-time. *Students:* 126 full-time (78 women), 11 part-time (7 women), 52 international. Average age 30. In 2013, 19 master's, 12 doctorates awarded. *Degree requirements:* For master's, thesis; for doctorate, thesis/ dissertation. *Entrance requirements:* For master's, appropriate bachelor's degree, proficiency in French; for doctorate, appropriate master's degree, proficiency in French. *Application deadline:* For fall admission, 3/30 for domestic and international students; for winter admission, 11/1 for domestic and international students; for spring admission, 3/1 for domestic and international students. Application fee: $45 Canadian dollars. Electronic applications accepted. *Financial support:* In 2013–14, fellowships (averaging $16,500 per year) were awarded; research assistantships also available. *Faculty research:* Immunity, infection and cancer; toxicology and environmental biotechnology; molecular pharmacochemistry. *Unit head:* Charles Dozois, Director, 450-687-5010, Fax: 450-686-5566, E-mail: charles.dozois@iaf.inrs.ca. *Application contact:* Sylvie Richard, Registrar, 418-654-2518, Fax: 418-654-3858, E-mail: sylvie.richard@adm.inrs.ca.
Website: http://www.iaf.inrs.ca

University of Alberta, Faculty of Medicine and Dentistry and Faculty of Graduate Studies and Research, Graduate Programs in Medicine, Department of Medical Microbiology and Immunology, Edmonton, AB T6G 2E1, Canada. Offers M Sc, PhD. Terminal master's awarded for partial completion of doctoral program. *Degree requirements:* For master's, thesis; for doctorate, thesis/dissertation. *Entrance requirements:* For master's and doctorate, minimum GPA of 3.3. Additional exam requirements/recommendations for international students: Required—TOEFL (minimum score 600 paper-based; 96 iBT). *Faculty research:* Cellular and reproductive immunology, microbial pathogenesis, mechanisms of antibiotic resistance, molecular biology of mammalian viruses, antiviral chemotherapy.

University of Hawaii at Manoa, John A. Burns School of Medicine and Graduate Division, Graduate Programs in Biomedical Sciences, Department of Tropical Medicine, Medical Microbiology and Pharmacology, Honolulu, HI 96822. Offers tropical medicine (MS, PhD). Part-time programs available. Terminal master's awarded for partial completion of doctoral program. *Degree requirements:* For master's, thesis optional; for doctorate, comprehensive exam, thesis/dissertation. *Entrance requirements:* For master's and doctorate, GRE General Test. Additional exam requirements/ recommendations for international students: Required—TOEFL (minimum score 580 paper-based; 92 iBT), IELTS (minimum score 5). *Faculty research:* Immunological studies of dengue, malaria, Kawasaki's disease, lupus erythematosus, rheumatoid disease.

University of Manitoba, Faculty of Medicine and Faculty of Graduate Studies, Graduate Programs in Medicine, Department of Medical Microbiology, Winnipeg, MB R3T 2N2, Canada. Offers M Sc, PhD. Part-time programs available. Terminal master's awarded for partial completion of doctoral program. *Degree requirements:* For master's, thesis; for doctorate, one foreign language, thesis/dissertation. *Entrance requirements:* For master's and doctorate, minimum GPA of 3.0. Electronic applications accepted. *Faculty research:* HIV, bacterial adhesion, sexually transmitted diseases, virus structure/ function and assembly.

University of Minnesota, Duluth, Medical School, Microbiology, Immunology and Molecular Pathobiology Section, Duluth, MN 55812-2496. Offers MS, PhD. MS, PhD offered jointly with University of Minnesota, Twin Cities Campus. Terminal master's awarded for partial completion of doctoral program. *Degree requirements:* For master's, thesis, final oral exam; for doctorate, thesis/dissertation, final exam, oral and written preliminary exams. *Entrance requirements:* For master's and doctorate, GRE General Test. Additional exam requirements/recommendations for international students: Required—TOEFL. *Faculty research:* Immunomodulation, molecular diagnosis of rabies, cytokines, cancer immunology, cytomegalovirus infection.

University of South Florida, Morsani College of Medicine and Graduate School, Graduate Programs in Medical Sciences, Tampa, FL 33620-9951. Offers aging and neuroscience (MSMS); allergy, immunology and infectious disease (PhD); anatomy (MSMS, PhD); athletic training (MSMS); bioinformatics and computational biology (MSBCB); biotechnology (MSB); clinical and translational research (MSMS, PhD); health informatics (MSHI, MSMS); health science (MSMS); interdisciplinary medical sciences (MSMS); medical microbiology and immunology (MSMS); metabolic and nutritional medicine (MSMS); molecular medicine (MSMS, PhD); molecular pharmacology and physiology (PhD); neurology (PhD); pathology and laboratory medicine (PhD); pharmacology and therapeutics (PhD); physiology and biophysics (PhD); women's health (MSMS). *Students:* 336 full-time (182 women), 39 part-time (21 women); includes 170 minority (45 Black or African American, non-Hispanic/Latino; 54 Asian, non-Hispanic/Latino; 59 Hispanic/Latino; 2 Native Hawaiian or other Pacific Islander, non-Hispanic/Latino; 10 Two or more races, non-Hispanic/Latino), 17 international. Average age 26. 1,066 applicants, 44% accepted, 250 enrolled. In 2013, 191 master's, 12 doctorates awarded. Terminal master's awarded for partial completion of doctoral program. *Degree requirements:* For master's, comprehensive exam, thesis; for doctorate, comprehensive exam, thesis/dissertation. *Entrance requirements:* For master's, GRE General Test or GMAT, bachelor's degree or equivalent from regionally-accredited university with minimum GPA of 3.0 in upper-division sciences coursework; prerequisites in general biology, general chemistry, general physics, organic chemistry, quantitative analysis, and integral and differential calculus; for doctorate, GRE General Test (minimum score of 600 quantitative), bachelor's degree from regionally-accredited university with minimum GPA of 3.0 in upper-division sciences coursework; 3 letters of recommendation; personal interview; 1-2 page personal statement; prerequisites in biology, chemistry, physics, organic chemistry, quantitative analysis, and integral/ differential calculus. Additional exam requirements/recommendations for international students: Required—TOEFL (minimum score 550 paper-based; 79 iBT) or IELTS (minimum score 6.5). *Application deadline:* For fall admission, 2/15 for domestic students, 1/2 for international students. Application fee: $30. *Expenses:* Contact institution. *Faculty research:* Anatomy, biochemistry, cancer biology, cardiovascular disease, cell biology, immunology, microbiology, molecular biology, neuroscience, pharmacology, physiology. *Unit head:* Dr. Michael Barber, Professor and Associate Dean for Graduate and Postdoctoral Affairs, 813-974-9908, Fax: 813-974-4317, E-mail: mbarber@health.usf.edu. *Application contact:* Dr. Eric Bennett, Graduate Director, PhD Program in Medical Sciences, 813-974-1545, Fax: 813-974-4317, E-mail: esbennet@health.usf.edu.
Website: http://health.usf.edu/nocms/medicine/graduatestudies/

University of Wisconsin–La Crosse, Graduate Studies, College of Science and Health, Department of Biology, La Crosse, WI 54601-3742. Offers aquatic sciences (MS); biology (MS); cellular and molecular biology (MS); clinical microbiology (MS); microbiology (MS); nurse anesthesia (MS); physiology (MS). Part-time programs available. *Faculty:* 22 full-time (8 women), 3 part-time/adjunct (1 woman). *Students:* 21 full-time (13 women), 37 part-time (24 women); includes 7 minority (2 Asian, non-Hispanic/Latino; 4 Hispanic/Latino; 1 Two or more races, non-Hispanic/Latino), 5 international. Average age 28. 107 applicants, 26% accepted, 25 enrolled. In 2013, 16 master's awarded. *Degree requirements:* For master's, comprehensive exam, thesis. *Entrance requirements:* For master's, GRE General Test, minimum GPA of 2.85. Additional exam requirements/recommendations for international students: Required—TOEFL (minimum score 550 paper-based; 79 iBT). *Application deadline:* For fall admission, 2/1 priority date for domestic and international students; for spring admission, 1/4 priority date for domestic and international students. Applications are processed on a rolling basis. Electronic applications accepted. *Financial support:* Research assistantships with partial tuition reimbursements, Federal Work-Study, scholarships/grants, health care benefits, and tuition waivers (partial) available. Support available to part-time students. Financial award application deadline: 3/15; financial award applicants required to submit FAFSA. *Unit head:* Dr. Thomas Volk, Coordinator of Graduate Studies, 608-785-6972, Fax: 608-785-6959, E-mail: volk.thom@uwlax.edu. *Application contact:* Corey Sjoquist, Director of Admissions, 608-785-8939, E-mail: admissions@uwlax.edu.
Website: http://uwlax.edu/biology/

University of Wisconsin–Madison, School of Medicine and Public Health and Graduate School, Graduate Programs in Medicine and College of Agricultural and Life Sciences, Microbiology Doctoral Training Program, Madison, WI 53706. Offers PhD. *Faculty:* 92 full-time (31 women). *Students:* 68 full-time (41 women); includes 13 minority (2 Black or African American, non-Hispanic/Latino; 1 American Indian or Alaska Native, non-Hispanic/Latino; 1 Asian, non-Hispanic/Latino; 9 Hispanic/Latino). Average age 24. 271 applicants, 14% accepted, 13 enrolled. In 2013, 12 doctorates awarded. *Degree requirements:* For doctorate, thesis/dissertation, preliminary exam, 1 semester of teaching, professional development. *Entrance requirements:* For doctorate, GRE. Additional exam requirements/recommendations for international students: Required—TOEFL (minimum score 580 paper-based). *Application deadline:* For fall admission, 12/1 for domestic and international students. Application fee: $56. Electronic applications accepted. *Expenses:* Tuition, state resident: full-time $10,728; part-time $790 per credit. Tuition, nonresident: full-time $24,054; part-time $1623 per credit. *Required fees:* $1130; $119 per credit. *Financial support:* In 2013–14, 68 students received support, including 44 fellowships with full tuition reimbursements available (averaging $25,250 per year), 22 research assistantships with full tuition reimbursements available (averaging $25,250 per year); career-related internships or fieldwork, scholarships/grants, traineeships, health care benefits, and tuition waivers (full) also available. Financial award application deadline: 12/1. *Faculty research:* Microbial pathogenesis, gene regulation, immunology, virology, cell biology. *Total annual research expenditures:* $15.1 million. *Unit head:* Dr. John Mansfield, Director, 608-262-2596, Fax: 608-262-8418, E-mail: jmansfield@bact.wisc.edu. *Application contact:* Cathy Davis Gray, Coordinator, 608-265-0689, Fax: 608-262-8418, E-mail: cdg@bact.wisc.edu.
Website: http://www.microbiology.wisc.edu/

Microbiology

Albany Medical College, Center for Immunology and Microbial Disease, Albany, NY 12208-3479. Offers MS, PhD. Part-time programs available. Terminal master's awarded for partial completion of doctoral program. *Degree requirements:* For master's, thesis; for doctorate, comprehensive exam, thesis/dissertation, oral qualifying exam, written preliminary exam, 1 published paper-peer review. *Entrance requirements:* For master's, GRE General Test, all transcripts, letters of recommendation; for doctorate, GRE General Test, letters of recommendation. Additional exam requirements/ recommendations for international students: Required—TOEFL. *Faculty research:* Microbial and viral pathogenesis, cancer development and cell transformation, biochemical and genetic mechanisms responsible for human disease.

Albert Einstein College of Medicine, Graduate Division of Biomedical Sciences, Department of Microbiology and Immunology, Bronx, NY 10461. Offers PhD, MD/PhD. *Degree requirements:* For doctorate, thesis/dissertation. *Entrance requirements:* For doctorate, GRE General Test. Additional exam requirements/recommendations for international students: Required—TOEFL. *Faculty research:* Nature of histocompatibility antigens, lymphoid cell receptors, regulation of immune responses and mechanisms of resistance to infection.

American University of Beirut, Graduate Programs, Faculty of Medicine, Beirut, Lebanon. Offers anatomy, cell biology and human morphology (MS); biochemistry and medical genetics (MS); biomedical sciences (PhD); experimental pathology, immunology and microbiology (MS); medicine (MD); neuroscience (MS); pharmacology and toxicology (MS). Part-time programs available. *Faculty:* 259 full-time (78 women), 93 part-time/adjunct (16 women). *Students:* 364 full-time (165 women), 62 part-time (54 women). Average age 23. In 2013, 18 master's awarded. *Degree requirements:* For master's, one foreign language, comprehensive exam, thesis (for some programs); for doctorate, one foreign language, comprehensive exam, thesis/dissertation. *Entrance requirements:* For master's, letter of recommendation; for doctorate, MCAT, bachelor's degree. Additional exam requirements/recommendations for international students: Required—TOEFL (minimum score 600 paper-based; 100 iBT), IELTS (minimum score 7.5). *Application deadline:* For fall admission, 4/30 for domestic and international students; for spring admission, 11/1 for domestic and international students. Application fee: $50. *Expenses: Tuition:* Full-time $14,724; part-time $818 per credit. *Required fees:* $692. Tuition and fees vary according to course load and program. *Financial support:* In 2013–14, 242 students received support, including 60 teaching assistantships (averaging $4,000 per year); career-related internships or fieldwork, institutionally sponsored loans, scholarships/grants, health care benefits, and unspecified assistantships also available. Financial award application deadline: 2/2. *Faculty research:* Cancer research (targeted therapy, mechanisms of leukemogenesis, tumor cell extravasation and metastasis, cancer stem cells), stem cell research (regenerative medicine, drug discovery), genetic research (neurogenetics, hereditary cardiomyopathy, hemoglobinopathies, pharmacogenomics, proteomics), neuroscience research (pain, neurodegenerative disorder), metabolism (inflammation and metabolism, metabolic disorder, diabetes mellitus), vascular and renal biology, signal transduction. *Total annual research expenditures:* $2.6 million. *Unit head:* Dr. Mohamed Sayegh, Dean, 961-1350000 Ext. 4700, Fax: 961-1744464, E-mail: msayegh@aub.edu.lb. *Application contact:* Dr. Salim Kanaan, Director, Admissions Office, 961-1-350000 Ext. 2594, Fax: 96-1-1750775, E-mail: sk00@aub.edu.lb.
Website: http://www.aub.edu.lb/fm/fm_home/Pages/index.aspx

Arizona State University at the Tempe campus, College of Liberal Arts and Sciences, School of Life Sciences, Tempe, AZ 85287-4601. Offers animal behavior (PhD); applied ethics (biomedical and health ethics) (MA); biological design (PhD); biology (MS, PhD); biology (biology and society) (MS, PhD); environmental life sciences (PhD); evolutionary biology (PhD); human and social dimensions of science and technology (PhD); microbiology (PhD); molecular and cellular biology (PhD); neuroscience (PhD); philosophy (history and philosophy of science) (MA); sustainability (PhD). Terminal master's awarded for partial completion of doctoral program. *Degree requirements:* For master's, thesis (for some programs), interactive Program of Study (iPOS) submitted before completing 50 percent of required credit hours; for doctorate, variable foreign language requirement, comprehensive exam, thesis/dissertation, interactive Program of Study (iPOS) submitted before completing 50 percent of required credit hours. *Entrance requirements:* For master's and doctorate, GRE, minimum GPA of 3.0 or equivalent in last 2 years of work leading to bachelor's degree. Additional exam requirements/ recommendations for international students: Required—TOEFL (minimum score 600 paper-based; 100 iBT). Electronic applications accepted.

Auburn University, Graduate School, College of Sciences and Mathematics, Department of Biological Sciences, Auburn University, AL 36849. Offers botany (MS, PhD); microbiology (MS, PhD); zoology (MS, PhD). *Faculty:* 39 full-time (13 women), 1 (woman) part-time/adjunct. *Students:* 40 full-time (21 women), 66 part-time (26 women); includes 9 minority (2 Black or African American, non-Hispanic/Latino; 1 American Indian or Alaska Native, non-Hispanic/Latino; 4 Asian, non-Hispanic/Latino; 2 Hispanic/ Latino), 17 international. Average age 28. 99 applicants, 31% accepted, 19 enrolled. In 2013, 10 master's, 11 doctorates awarded. *Entrance requirements:* For master's and doctorate, GRE General Test. Additional exam requirements/recommendations for international students: Required—TOEFL. *Application deadline:* For fall admission, 7/7 for domestic students; for spring admission, 11/24 for domestic students. Application fee: $50 ($60 for international students). Electronic applications accepted. *Expenses:* Tuition, state resident: full-time $8262; part-time $459 per credit hour. Tuition, nonresident: full-time $24,786; part-time $1377 per credit hour. Tuition and fees vary according to degree level and program. *Financial support:* Research assistantships and teaching assistantships available. Financial award applicants required to submit FAFSA. *Unit head:* Dr. Jack W. Feminella, Chair, 334-844-3906, Fax: 334-844-1645. *Application contact:* Dr. George Flowers, Dean of the Graduate School, 334-844-2125.

Baylor College of Medicine, Graduate School of Biomedical Sciences, Department of Molecular Virology and Microbiology, Houston, TX 77030-3498. Offers PhD, MD/PhD. *Degree requirements:* For doctorate, thesis/dissertation, public defense. *Entrance requirements:* For doctorate, GRE General Test, GRE Subject Test (strongly recommended), minimum GPA of 3.0. Additional exam requirements/recommendations for international students: Required—TOEFL. Electronic applications accepted. *Faculty research:* Microbiology, viral molecular biology, bacterial molecular biology, microbial pathogenesis, microbial genomics.

Baylor College of Medicine, Graduate School of Biomedical Sciences, Interdepartmental Program in Cell and Molecular Biology, Houston, TX 77030-3498. Offers biochemistry (PhD); cell and molecular biology (PhD); genetics (PhD); human genetics (PhD); immunology (PhD); microbiology (PhD); virology (PhD); MD/PhD. *Degree requirements:* For doctorate, thesis/dissertation, public defense. *Entrance requirements:* For doctorate, GRE General Test, GRE Subject Test (strongly recommended), minimum GPA of 3.0. Additional exam requirements/recommendations for international students: Required—TOEFL. Electronic applications accepted. *Faculty research:* Molecular and cellular biology; cancer, aging and stem cells; genomics and proteomics; microbiome, molecular microbiology; infectious disease, immunology and translational research.

Brandeis University, Graduate School of Arts and Sciences, Program in Molecular and Cell Biology, Waltham, MA 02454-9110. Offers genetics (PhD); microbiology (PhD); molecular and cell biology (MS, PhD); molecular biology (PhD); neurobiology (PhD); quantitative biology (PhD). Terminal master's awarded for partial completion of doctoral program. *Degree requirements:* For master's, thesis or alternative, research project, research lab, or project lab; for doctorate, comprehensive exam, thesis/dissertation, journal clubs; research seminar; colloquia; qualifying exam. *Entrance requirements:* For master's, GRE General Test (or MCAT for applicants to the MS program), official transcript(s), resume, 3 letters of recommendation, statement of purpose; for doctorate, GRE General Test, official transcript(s), resume, 3 letters of recommendation, statement of purpose. Additional exam requirements/recommendations for international students: Required—TOEFL (minimum score 600 paper-based; 100 iBT), PTE (minimum score 68); Recommended—IELTS (minimum score 7). Electronic applications accepted. *Faculty research:* Structural biology; immunology; developmental biology; behavior and neurobiology; DNA replication, rearrangement, and repair; signal transduction, transcriptional regulation, and RNA processing; cancer and programmed cell death; cytoskeleton and molecular motors; nutrition.

Brigham Young University, Graduate Studies, College of Life Sciences, Department of Microbiology and Molecular Biology, Provo, UT 84602. Offers MS, PhD. *Faculty:* 15 full-time (3 women). *Students:* 28 full-time (11 women); includes 4 minority (3 Hispanic/Latino; 1 Native Hawaiian or other Pacific Islander, non-Hispanic/Latino), 2 international. Average age 28. 35 applicants, 34% accepted, 12 enrolled. In 2013, 4 master's awarded. Terminal master's awarded for partial completion of doctoral program. *Degree requirements:* For master's, comprehensive exam, thesis; for doctorate, comprehensive exam, thesis/dissertation. *Entrance requirements:* For master's, GRE General Test, minimum GPA of 3.0 during previous 2 years; for doctorate, GRE General Test, minimum GPA of 3.0. Additional exam requirements/recommendations for international students: Required—TOEFL (minimum score 580 paper-based; 85 iBT), IELTS (minimum score 7). *Application deadline:* For fall admission, 12/15 priority date for domestic and international students. Application fee: $50. Electronic applications accepted. *Expenses: Tuition:* Full-time $6130; part-time $340 per credit hour. Tuition and fees vary according to program and student's religious affiliation. *Financial support:* In 2013–14, 19 students received support, including 16 research assistantships with full tuition reimbursements available (averaging $21,000 per year), 2 teaching assistantships with full and partial tuition reimbursements available (averaging $18,000 per year); institutionally sponsored loans, scholarships/grants, health care benefits, and unspecified assistantships also available. Financial award application deadline: 2/1. *Faculty research:* Immunobiology, molecular genetics, molecular virology, cancer biology, pathogenic and environmental microbiology. *Total annual research expenditures:* $778,143. *Unit head:* Dr. Laura Bridgewater, Chair, 801-422-2434, Fax: 801-422-0519, E-mail: laura_bridgewater@byu.edu. *Application contact:* Dr. Joel Griffitts, Graduate Coordinator, 801-422-7997, Fax: 801-422-0519, E-mail: joel_griffitts@byu.edu.
Website: http://mmbio.byu.edu/

California State University, Long Beach, Graduate Studies, College of Natural Sciences and Mathematics, Department of Biological Sciences, Long Beach, CA 90840. Offers biology (MS); microbiology (MS). Part-time programs available. *Entrance requirements:* For master's, GRE Subject Test, minimum GPA of 3.0. Electronic applications accepted.

Case Western Reserve University, School of Medicine and School of Graduate Studies, Graduate Programs in Medicine, Department of Molecular Biology and Microbiology, Cleveland, OH 44106-4960. Offers cellular biology (PhD); microbiology (PhD); molecular biology (PhD); molecular virology (PhD); MD/PhD. Students are admitted to an integrated Biomedical Sciences Training Program involving 11 basic science programs at Case Western Reserve University. *Degree requirements:* For doctorate, thesis/dissertation. *Entrance requirements:* For doctorate, GRE General Test, GRE Subject Test. Additional exam requirements/recommendations for international students: Required—TOEFL. Electronic applications accepted. *Faculty research:* Gene expression in eukaryotic and prokaryotic systems; microbial physiology; intracellular transport and signaling; mechanisms of oncogenesis; molecular mechanisms of RNA processing, editing, and catalysis.

The Catholic University of America, School of Arts and Sciences, Department of Biology, Washington, DC 20064. Offers cell and microbial biology (MS, PhD), including cell biology, microbiology; clinical laboratory science (MS, PhD); MSLS/MS. Part-time programs available. *Faculty:* 9 full-time (4 women), 5 part-time/adjunct (4 women). *Students:* 27 full-time (19 women), 36 part-time (22 women); includes 12 minority (7 Black or African American, non-Hispanic/Latino; 2 Asian, non-Hispanic/Latino; 2 Hispanic/Latino; 1 Two or more races, non-Hispanic/Latino), 36 international. Average age 30. 66 applicants, 56% accepted, 19 enrolled. In 2013, 10 master's, 3 doctorates awarded. *Degree requirements:* For master's, comprehensive exam, thesis or alternative; for doctorate, comprehensive exam, thesis/dissertation. *Entrance requirements:* For master's and doctorate, GRE General Test, GRE Subject Test, statement of purpose, official copies of academic transcripts, three letters of recommendation. Additional exam requirements/recommendations for international students: Required—TOEFL (minimum score 580 paper-based). *Application deadline:* For fall admission, 8/1 priority date for domestic students, 7/15 for international students; for spring admission, 12/1 priority date for domestic students, 10/15 for international students. Applications are processed on a rolling basis. Application fee: $55. Electronic applications accepted. *Expenses: Tuition:* Full-time $38,500; part-time $1490 per credit hour. *Required fees:* $400; $1525 per credit hour. One-time fee: $425. Tuition and fees vary according to program. *Financial support:* Fellowships, research assistantships, teaching assistantships, Federal Work-Study, scholarships/grants, tuition waivers (full and partial), and unspecified assistantships available. Financial award application deadline: 2/1; financial award applicants required to submit FAFSA. *Faculty research:* Cell and microbiology, molecular biology of cell proliferation, cellular effects of electromagnetic radiation, biotechnology. *Total annual research expenditures:* $1.5 million. *Unit head:* Dr. Venigalla Rao, Chair, 202-319-5271, Fax: 202-319-5721, E-mail: rao@cua.edu. *Application contact:* Andrew Woodall, Director of Graduate Admissions, 202-319-5057, Fax: 202-319-6533, E-mail: cua-admissions@cua.edu.
Website: http://biology.cua.edu/

Clemson University, Graduate School, College of Agriculture, Forestry and Life Sciences, Department of Biological Sciences, Program in Microbiology, Clemson, SC 29634. Offers MS, PhD. *Students:* 21 full-time (9 women), 4 part-time (2 women); includes 1 minority (Black or African American, non-Hispanic/Latino), 7 international. Average age 26. 35 applicants, 37% accepted, 10 enrolled. In 2013, 2 master's, 2 doctorates awarded. *Degree requirements:* For master's, thesis; for doctorate, comprehensive exam, thesis/dissertation. *Entrance requirements:* For master's and doctorate, GRE General Test. Additional exam requirements/recommendations for international students: Required—TOEFL, IELTS. *Application deadline:* For fall admission, 1/15 for domestic students, 4/15 for international students. Application fee: $70 ($80 for international students). Electronic applications accepted. *Expenses:* Contact institution. *Financial support:* In 2013–14, 21 students received support, including 3 research assistantships with partial tuition reimbursements available (averaging $18,208 per year), 18 teaching assistantships with partial tuition reimbursements available (averaging $17,111 per year); fellowships with full and partial tuition reimbursements available, career-related internships or fieldwork, institutionally sponsored loans, scholarships/grants, health care benefits, and unspecified assistantships also available. Financial award application deadline: 3/1; financial award applicants required to submit FAFSA. *Faculty research:* Anaerobic microbiology, microbiology and ecology of soil and aquatic systems, microbial genetics, biofilms, nanotechnology. *Unit head:* Dr. Alfred Wheeler, Department Chair, 864-656-1415, Fax: 864-656-0435, E-mail: wheeler@clemson.edu. *Application contact:* Jay Lyn Martin, Coordinator for Graduate Program, 864-656-3587, Fax: 864-656-0435, E-mail: gradbio@clemson.edu.
Website: http://www.clemson.edu/cafls/departments/biosci/index.html

Colorado State University, College of Veterinary Medicine and Biomedical Sciences, Department of Microbiology, Immunology and Pathology, Fort Collins, CO 80523. Offers microbiology (MS, PhD); pathology (PhD). *Faculty:* 50 full-time (22 women), 4 part-time/adjunct (1 woman). *Students:* 73 full-time (51 women), 31 part-time (24 women); includes 15 minority (1 Black or African American, non-Hispanic/Latino; 2 American Indian or Alaska Native, non-Hispanic/Latino; 3 Asian, non-Hispanic/Latino; 8 Hispanic/Latino; 1 Two or more races, non-Hispanic/Latino), 9 international. Average age 29. 135 applicants, 31% accepted, 38 enrolled. In 2013, 3 master's, 11 doctorates awarded. *Degree requirements:* For master's, thesis; for doctorate, comprehensive exam, thesis/dissertation. *Entrance requirements:* For master's, GRE General Test, minimum GPA of 3.0, BA/BS in biomedical field, reviewer evaluation forms, resume, transcripts, personal statement, 3 letters of recommendation; for doctorate, GRE General Test, minimum GPA of 3.0, BA/BS in biomedical field, reviewer evaluation forms, resume, personal statement, transcripts, 3 letters of recommendation. Additional exam requirements/recommendations for international students: Required—TOEFL (minimum score 550 paper-based). *Application deadline:* For fall admission, 1/1 priority date for domestic students; for spring admission, 10/1 priority date for domestic students. Applications are processed on a rolling basis. Application fee: $50. Electronic applications accepted. *Expenses:* Tuition, state resident: full-time $9075.40; part-time $504 per credit. Tuition, nonresident: full-time $22,248; part-time $1236 per credit. *Required fees:* $1819; $60 per credit. *Financial support:* In 2013–14, 82 students received support, including 40 fellowships with tuition reimbursements available (averaging $35,362 per year), 38 research assistantships with tuition reimbursements available (averaging $17,799 per year), 4 teaching assistantships with tuition reimbursements available (averaging $15,606 per year); Federal Work-Study, scholarships/grants, traineeships, and unspecified assistantships also available. Financial award applicants required to submit FAFSA. *Faculty research:* Medical and veterinary bacteriology, immunology, microbial physiology, pathology, vector-borne disease. *Total annual research expenditures:* $29.9 million. *Unit head:* Dr. Gregg A. Dean, Head, 970-491-6144, Fax: 970-491-1815, E-mail: gregg.dean@colostate.edu. *Application contact:* Lisa McCann, Academic Programs Coordinator, 970-491-6118, Fax: 970-491-1815, E-mail: lisa.mccann@colostate.edu.
Website: http://csu-cvmbs.colostate.edu/academics/mip/graduate/Pages/default.aspx

Columbia University, College of Physicians and Surgeons, Department of Microbiology, New York, NY 10032. Offers biomedical sciences (M Phil, MA, PhD); MD/PhD. Only candidates for the PhD are admitted. Terminal master's awarded for partial completion of doctoral program. *Degree requirements:* For doctorate, thesis/dissertation. *Entrance requirements:* For master's, GRE General Test; for doctorate, GRE. Additional exam requirements/recommendations for international students: Required—TOEFL. *Faculty research:* Prokaryotic molecular biology, immunology, virology, yeast molecular genetics, regulation of gene expression.

Cornell University, Graduate School, Graduate Fields of Agriculture and Life Sciences, Field of Microbiology, Ithaca, NY 14853-0001. Offers PhD. *Faculty:* 45 full-time (13 women). *Students:* 27 full-time (18 women); includes 1 minority (Hispanic/Latino), 15 international. Average age 27. 67 applicants, 9% accepted, 4 enrolled. In 2013, 8 doctorates awarded. *Degree requirements:* For doctorate, comprehensive exam, thesis/dissertation, 2 semesters of teaching experience. *Entrance requirements:* For doctorate, GRE General Test, 3 letters of recommendation. Additional exam requirements/recommendations for international students: Required—TOEFL (minimum score 550 paper-based; 77 iBT). *Application deadline:* For fall admission, 1/15 for domestic students. Application fee: $95. Electronic applications accepted. *Financial support:* In 2013–14, 25 students received support, including 4 fellowships with full tuition reimbursements available, 13 research assistantships with full tuition reimbursements available, 8 teaching assistantships with full tuition reimbursements available; institutionally sponsored loans, scholarships/grants, health care benefits, tuition waivers (full and partial), and unspecified assistantships also available. Financial award applicants required to submit FAFSA. *Faculty research:* Microbial diversity, molecular biology, biotechnology, microbial ecology, phytobacteriology. *Unit head:* Director of Graduate Studies, 607-255-3088. *Application contact:* Graduate Field Assistant, 607-255-3088, E-mail: microfield@cornell.edu.
Website: http://www.gradschool.cornell.edu/fields.php?id-53&a-2

Dalhousie University, Faculty of Medicine, Department of Microbiology and Immunology, Halifax, NS B3H 4R2, Canada. Offers M Sc, PhD. *Degree requirements:* For master's, thesis; for doctorate, comprehensive exam, thesis/dissertation. *Entrance requirements:* For master's, GRE General Test, honors B Sc; for doctorate, GRE General Test, honors B Sc in microbiology, M Sc in discipline or transfer after 1 year in master's program. Additional exam requirements/recommendations for international students: Required—1 of 5 approved tests: TOEFL, IELTS, CANTEST, CAEL, Michigan English Language Assessment Battery. Electronic applications accepted. *Faculty research:* Virology, molecular genetics, pathogenesis, bacteriology, immunology.

Dartmouth College, Graduate Program in Molecular and Cellular Biology, Department of Microbiology and Immunology, Program in Immunology, Hanover, NH 03755. Offers MD/PhD. *Faculty research:* Tumor immunotherapy, cell and molecular biology of connective tissue degradation in rheumatoid arthritis and cancer, immunology and immunotherapy of tumors of the central nervous system, transcriptional regulation of hematopoiesis and leukemia, bacterial pathogenesis.

Dartmouth College, Graduate Program in Molecular and Cellular Biology, Department of Microbiology and Immunology, Program in Molecular Pathogenesis, Hanover, NH 03755. Offers microbiology and immunology (PhD).

Dowling College, Programs in Arts and Sciences, Oakdale, NY 11769. Offers environmental microbiology (MS). Part-time and evening/weekend programs available. *Faculty:* 4 full-time (1 woman). *Students:* 1 (woman) full-time, 3 part-time (0 women). Average age 40. 10 applicants, 30% accepted. In 2013, 4 master's awarded. *Degree requirements:* For master's, comprehensive exam, thesis. *Entrance requirements:* For master's, minimum undergraduate GPA of 3.0, 2 letters of recommendation. Additional exam requirements/recommendations for international students: Required—TOEFL (minimum score 550 paper-based). *Application deadline:* For fall admission, 9/1 priority

date for domestic students; for winter admission, 1/1 priority date for domestic students; for spring admission, 2/1 priority date for domestic students. Applications are processed on a rolling basis. Application fee: $50. Electronic applications accepted. *Expenses: Tuition:* Full-time $22,731; part-time $1029 per credit. *Required fees:* $956; $956. *Financial support:* Federal Work-Study available. Support available to part-time students. Financial award application deadline: 6/30; financial award applicants required to submit FAFSA. *Unit head:* Patricia Sandilands, Director of Operations, School of Arts and Sciences, 631-244-3237, E-mail: sandilap@dowling.edu. *Application contact:* Mary Boullianne, Director of Admissions, 631-244-3274, Fax: 631-244-1059, E-mail: boulliam@dowling.edu.
Website: http://www.dowling.edu/

Drexel University, College of Medicine, Biomedical Graduate Programs, Program in Microbiology and Immunology, Philadelphia, PA 19104-2875. Offers MS, PhD, MD/PhD. Terminal master's awarded for partial completion of doctoral program. *Degree requirements:* For master's, comprehensive exam, thesis; for doctorate, thesis/dissertation, qualifying exam. *Entrance requirements:* For master's, GRE General Test, minimum GPA of 2.75; for doctorate, GRE General Test, minimum GPA of 3.0. Additional exam requirements/recommendations for international students: Required—TOEFL. Electronic applications accepted. *Faculty research:* Immunology of malarial parasites, virology, bacteriology, molecular biology, parasitology.

Duke University, Graduate School, Department of Molecular Genetics and Microbiology, Durham, NC 27710. Offers PhD. *Faculty:* 59. *Students:* 66 full-time (34 women); includes 11 minority (1 Black or African American, non-Hispanic/Latino; 1 American Indian or Alaska Native, non-Hispanic/Latino; 3 Asian, non-Hispanic/Latino; 6 Hispanic/Latino), 17 international. 96 applicants, 18% accepted, 12 enrolled. In 2013, 10 doctorates awarded. *Degree requirements:* For doctorate, thesis/dissertation. *Entrance requirements:* For doctorate, GRE General Test, GRE Subject Test in biology, chemistry, or biochemistry, cell and molecular biology (recommended). Additional exam requirements/recommendations for international students: Required—TOEFL (minimum score 577 paper-based; 90 iBT) or IELTS (minimum score 7). *Application deadline:* For fall admission, 12/8 priority date for domestic and international students. Application fee: $80. Electronic applications accepted. *Financial support:* Fellowships with full tuition reimbursements, research assistantships with full tuition reimbursements, and Federal Work-Study available. Financial award application deadline: 12/31. *Unit head:* Dr. Raphael Valdivia, Director of Graduate Studies, 919-684-4008, Fax: 919-684-2790, E-mail: kimberly.kobes@duke.edu. *Application contact:* Elizabeth Hutton, Director of Admissions, 919-684-3913, Fax: 919-684-2277, E-mail: grad-admissions@duke.edu.
Website: http://mgm.duke.edu/graduate/

East Carolina University, Brody School of Medicine, Department of Microbiology and Immunology, Greenville, NC 27858-4353. Offers MS, MD, PhD. *Degree requirements:* For doctorate, comprehensive exam, thesis/dissertation. *Entrance requirements:* For doctorate, GRE General Test. Additional exam requirements/recommendations for international students: Required—TOEFL. *Application deadline:* For fall admission, 4/15 priority date for domestic students. Applications are processed on a rolling basis. Application fee: $50. *Expenses:* Tuition, state resident: full-time $4223. Tuition, nonresident: full-time $16,540. *Required fees:* $2184. *Financial support:* Fellowships with tuition reimbursements available. Financial award application deadline: 6/1. *Faculty research:* Molecular virology, genetics of bacteria, yeast and somatic cells, bacterial physiology and metabolism, bioterrorism. *Unit head:* Dr. Charles J. Smith, Chair, 252-744-2700, Fax: 252-744-3104, E-mail: smithcha@ecu.edu. *Application contact:* Dr. Richard A. Franklin, Director of Graduate Studies, 252-744-2705, Fax: 252-744-3104, E-mail: franklinr@ecu.edu.
Website: http://www.ecu.edu/cs-dhs/microbiology/index.cfm

Eastern New Mexico University, Graduate School, College of Liberal Arts and Sciences, Department of Biology, Portales, NM 88130. Offers applied ecology (MS); botany (MS); cell, molecular biology and biotechnology (MS); microbiology (MS); zoology (MS). Part-time programs available. *Degree requirements:* For master's, comprehensive exam, thesis optional. *Entrance requirements:* For master's, GRE, minimum GPA of 3.0, 2 letters of recommendation, statement of research interest, bachelor's degree related to field of study or proof of common knowledge. Additional exam requirements/recommendations for international students: Required—TOEFL (minimum score 550 paper-based; 79 iBT), IELTS (minimum score 6). Electronic applications accepted.

East Tennessee State University, James H. Quillen College of Medicine, Department of Biomedical Sciences, Johnson City, TN 37614. Offers anatomy (PhD); biochemistry (PhD); microbiology (PhD); pharmaceutical sciences (PhD); pharmacology (PhD); physiology (PhD); quantitative biosciences (PhD). *Faculty:* 43 full-time (11 women), 1 (woman) part-time/adjunct. *Students:* 31 full-time (17 women), 4 part-time (1 woman); includes 6 minority (2 Black or African American, non-Hispanic/Latino; 3 Asian, non-Hispanic/Latino; 1 Hispanic/Latino), 9 international. Average age 29. 53 applicants, 17% accepted, 8 enrolled. In 2013, 6 doctorates awarded. *Degree requirements:* For doctorate, thesis/dissertation, comprehensive qualifying exam. *Entrance requirements:* For doctorate, GRE General Test, GRE Subject Test. Additional exam requirements/recommendations for international students: Required—TOEFL (minimum score 550 paper-based; 79 iBT). *Application deadline:* For fall admission, 3/15 priority date for domestic students, 3/1 priority date for international students. Application fee: $35 ($45 for international students). Electronic applications accepted. *Expenses:* Contact institution. *Financial support:* In 2013–14, 30 students received support, including 30 research assistantships with full tuition reimbursements available (averaging $19,000 per year); career-related internships or fieldwork, institutionally sponsored loans, scholarships/grants, and unspecified assistantships also available. Financial award application deadline: 7/1; financial award applicants required to submit FAFSA. *Faculty research:* Cardiovascular, infectious disease, neurosciences, cancer, immunology. *Unit head:* Dr. Mitchell E. Robinson, Associate Dean/Program Director, 423-439-2031, Fax: 423-439-2140, E-mail: robinson@etsu.edu. *Application contact:* Shella Bennett, Graduate Specialist, 423-439-4708, Fax: 423-439-5624, E-mail: bennetsg@etsu.edu.
Website: http://www.etsu.edu/com/dbms/

East Tennessee State University, School of Graduate Studies, College of Arts and Sciences, Department of Biological Sciences, Johnson City, TN 37614. Offers biology (MS); biomedical sciences (MS); microbiology (MS); paleontology (MS). *Faculty:* 21 full-time (5 women), 6 part-time/adjunct (1 woman). *Students:* 36 full-time (15 women), 6 part-time (3 women); includes 2 minority (1 Black or African American, non-Hispanic/Latino; 1 Asian, non-Hispanic/Latino), 18 international. Average age 27. 64 applicants, 42% accepted, 24 enrolled. In 2013, 8 master's awarded. *Degree requirements:* For master's, comprehensive exam, thesis. *Entrance requirements:* For master's, GRE General Test or GRE Subject Test, minimum GPA of 3.0, undergraduate degree in life or physical sciences, two letters of recommendation. Additional exam requirements/recommendations for international students: Required—TOEFL (minimum score 550 paper-based; 79 iBT). *Application deadline:* For fall admission, 4/1 for domestic students, 2/1 for international students; for spring admission, 9/1 for domestic students, 7/1 for international students. Application fee: $35 ($45 for international students). Electronic applications accepted. *Expenses:* Tuition, state resident: full-time $7900; part-time $395 per credit hour. Tuition, nonresident: full-time $21,960; part-time $1098 per credit hour. *Required fees:* $1345; $84 per credit hour. *Financial support:* In 2013–14, 36 students received support, including 2 research assistantships with full tuition reimbursements available (averaging $9,000 per year), 30 teaching assistantships with full tuition reimbursements available (averaging $8,500 per year); institutionally sponsored loans, scholarships/grants, and unspecified assistantships also available. Financial award application deadline: 7/1; financial award applicants required to submit FAFSA. *Faculty research:* Neuroethology, chronobiology, molecular biology, behavioral ecology, systematics, paleobotany. *Unit head:* Dr. Darrell Moore, Interim Chair, 423-439-4329, Fax: 423-439-5958, E-mail: moored@etsu.edu. *Application contact:* Gail Powers, Graduate Specialist, 423-439-4703, Fax: 423-439-5624, E-mail: powersg@etsu.edu.

Emory University, Laney Graduate School, Division of Biological and Biomedical Sciences, Program in Microbiology and Molecular Genetics, Atlanta, GA 30322-1100. Offers PhD. *Degree requirements:* For doctorate, comprehensive exam, thesis/dissertation. *Entrance requirements:* For doctorate, GRE General Test, minimum GPA of 3.0 in science course work (recommended). Additional exam requirements/recommendations for international students: Required—TOEFL. Electronic applications accepted. *Faculty research:* Bacterial genetics and physiology, microbial development, molecular biology of viruses and bacterial pathogens, DNA recombination.

Emporia State University, Department of Biological Sciences, Emporia, KS 66801-5415. Offers botany (MS); environmental biology (MS); general biology (MS); microbial and cellular biology (MS); zoology (MS). Part-time programs available. *Faculty:* 13 full-time (3 women). *Students:* 32 full-time (16 women), 7 part-time (1 woman); includes 2 minority (1 Black or African American, non-Hispanic/Latino; 1 Asian, non-Hispanic/Latino), 18 international. 25 applicants, 88% accepted, 3 enrolled. In 2013, 8 master's awarded. *Degree requirements:* For master's, comprehensive exam or thesis. *Entrance requirements:* For master's, GRE, appropriate undergraduate degree, interview, letters of reference. Additional exam requirements/recommendations for international students: Required—TOEFL (minimum score 520 paper-based; 68 iBT). *Application deadline:* For fall admission, 8/15 priority date for domestic students. Applications are processed on a rolling basis. Application fee: $30 ($75 for international students). Electronic applications accepted. *Expenses: Tuition, area resident:* Part-time $220 per credit hour. Tuition, state resident: part-time $220 per credit hour. Tuition, nonresident: part-time $685 per credit hour. *Required fees:* $73 per credit hour. *Financial support:* In 2013–14, 5 research assistantships with full tuition reimbursements (averaging $7,371 per year), 9 teaching assistantships with full tuition reimbursements (averaging $7,950 per year) were awarded; career-related internships or fieldwork, Federal Work-Study, institutionally sponsored loans, health care benefits, and unspecified assistantships also available. Financial award application deadline: 3/15; financial award applicants required to submit FAFSA. *Faculty research:* Fisheries, range, and wildlife management; aquatic, plant, grassland, vertebrate, and invertebrate ecology; mammalian and plant systematics, taxonomy, and evolution; immunology, virology, and molecular biology. *Unit head:* Dr. R. Brent Thomas, Chair, 620-341-5311, Fax: 620-341-5608, E-mail: rthomas2@emporia.edu. *Application contact:* Dr. Scott Crupper, Graduate Coordinator, 620-341-5621, Fax: 620-341-5607, E-mail: scrupper@emporia.edu.
Website: http://www.emporia.edu/info/degrees-courses/grad/biology

Georgetown University, Graduate School of Arts and Sciences, Programs in Biomedical Sciences, Department of Microbiology and Immunology, Washington, DC 20057. Offers biohazardous threat agents and emerging infectious diseases (MS); biomedical science policy and advocacy (MS); general microbiology and immunology (MS); global infectious diseases (PhD); microbiology and immunology (PhD). Part-time programs available. *Degree requirements:* For master's, 30 credit hours of coursework; for doctorate, comprehensive exam, thesis/dissertation. *Entrance requirements:* For master's, GRE General Test, 3 letters of reference, bachelor's degree in related field; for doctorate, GRE General Test, 3 letters of reference, MS/BS in related field. Additional exam requirements/recommendations for international students: Required—TOEFL (minimum score 505 paper-based). *Application deadline:* For fall admission, 7/1 for domestic students, 6/1 priority date for international students; for winter admission, 2/2 priority date for domestic students, 1/2 priority date for international students; for spring admission, 11/1 for domestic students, 10/1 priority date for international students. Applications are processed on a rolling basis. Application fee: $75. Electronic applications accepted. *Financial support:* Fellowships with full tuition reimbursements available. *Faculty research:* Pathogenesis and basic biology of the fungus Candida albicans, molecular biology of viral immunopathological mechanisms in Multiple Sclerosis. *Unit head:* Dr. Richard A. Calderone, Chair, 202-687-1513, E-mail: calderor@georgetown.edu. *Application contact:* Kimberly Bassalian, Graduate Program Coordinator, 202-687-3422, Fax: 202-687-1800, E-mail: kdb70@georgetown.edu.
Website: http://microbiology.georgetown.edu/

The George Washington University, Columbian College of Arts and Sciences, Institute for Biomedical Sciences, Program in Microbiology and Immunology, Washington, DC 20037. Offers PhD. *Students:* 5 full-time (3 women), 17 part-time (14 women); includes 4 minority (1 American Indian or Alaska Native, non-Hispanic/Latino; 1 Asian, non-Hispanic/Latino; 1 Hispanic/Latino; 1 Two or more races, non-Hispanic/Latino), 2 international. Average age 29. In 2013, 4 doctorates awarded. *Degree requirements:* For doctorate, thesis/dissertation. *Entrance requirements:* For doctorate, GRE General Test, minimum GPA of 3.0. Additional exam requirements/recommendations for international students: Required—TOEFL (minimum score 600 paper-based). *Application deadline:* For fall admission, 12/15 priority date for domestic and international students. Applications are processed on a rolling basis. Application fee: $75. Electronic applications accepted. *Financial support:* In 2013–14, 10 students received support. Fellowships with tuition reimbursements available and tuition waivers available. *Unit head:* Dr. David Leitenberg, Director, 202-994-9475, Fax: 202-994-2913, E-mail: dleit@gwu.edu. *Application contact:* Information Contact, 202-994-3532, Fax: 202-994-2913, E-mail: mtmjxl@gwumc.edu.
Website: http://www.gwumc.edu/ibs/fields/microimmuno.html

The George Washington University, School of Medicine and Health Sciences, Health Sciences Programs, Washington, DC 20052. Offers clinical practice management (MSHS); clinical research administration (MSHS); emergency services management (MSHS); end-of-life care (MSHS); immunohematology (MSHS); physical therapy (DPT); physician assistant (MSHS); MSHS/MPH. Postbaccalaureate distance learning degree programs offered (no on-campus study). *Students:* 264 full-time (205 women), 216 part-time (162 women); includes 140 minority (54 Black or African American, non-Hispanic/Latino; 4 American Indian or Alaska Native, non-Hispanic/Latino; 48 Asian, non-Hispanic/Latino; 31 Hispanic/Latino; 3 Native Hawaiian or other Pacific Islander, non-Hispanic/Latino), 12 international. Average age 32. 1,581 applicants, 17% accepted. In 2013, 143 master's, 33 doctorates awarded. *Entrance requirements:* Additional exam requirements/recommendations for international students: Required—TOEFL (minimum score 550 paper-based). *Application deadline:* Applications are processed on a rolling basis. Application fee: $75. *Expenses:* Contact institution. *Unit head:* Jean E. Johnson, Senior Associate Dean, 202-994-3725, E-mail: jejohns@gwu.edu. *Application contact:* Joke Ogundiran, Director of Admission, 202-994-1668, Fax: 202-994-0870, E-mail: jokeogun@gwu.edu.

The George Washington University, School of Public Health and Health Services, Department of Epidemiology and Biostatistics, Washington, DC 20052. Offers biostatistics (MPH); epidemiology (MPH); microbiology and emerging infectious diseases (MSPH). *Faculty:* 29 full-time (20 women). *Students:* 54 full-time (43 women), 77 part-time (60 women); includes 37 minority (18 Black or African American, non-Hispanic/Latino; 16 Asian, non-Hispanic/Latino; 2 Hispanic/Latino; 1 Two or more races, non-Hispanic/Latino), 12 international. Average age 28. 342 applicants, 75% accepted. In 2013, 51 master's awarded. *Degree requirements:* For master's, case study or special project. *Entrance requirements:* For master's, GMAT, GRE General Test, or MCAT. Additional exam requirements/recommendations for international students: Required—TOEFL. *Application deadline:* For fall admission, 4/15 priority date for domestic students, 4/15 for international students; for spring admission, 11/1 for domestic and international students. Applications are processed on a rolling basis. Application fee: $75. *Financial support:* In 2013–14, 6 students received support. Tuition waivers available. Financial award application deadline: 2/15. *Unit head:* Dr. Alan E. Greenberg, Chair, 202-994-0612, E-mail: aeg1@gwu.edu. *Application contact:* Jane Smith, Director of Admissions, 202-994-0248, Fax: 202-994-1860, E-mail: sphhsinfo@gwumc.edu.

Georgia State University, College of Arts and Sciences, Department of Biology, Program in Applied and Environmental Microbiology, Atlanta, GA 30302-3083. Offers applied and environmental microbiology (MS, PhD); bioinformatics (MS). Part-time programs available. *Students:* Average age 30. Terminal master's awarded for partial completion of doctoral program. *Degree requirements:* For master's, comprehensive exam (for some programs), thesis optional; for doctorate, comprehensive exam, thesis/dissertation. *Entrance requirements:* For master's and doctorate, GRE. Additional exam requirements/recommendations for international students: Required—TOEFL (minimum score 550 paper-based; 82 iBT) or IELTS (minimum score 7). *Application deadline:* For fall admission, 7/1 priority date for domestic students, 6/1 priority date for international students; for spring admission, 11/15 priority date for domestic students, 10/15 priority date for international students. Applications are processed on a rolling basis. Application fee: $50. Electronic applications accepted. *Expenses: Tuition, area resident:* Full-time $4176; part-time $348 per credit hour. Tuition, state resident: full-time $14,544; part-time $1212 per credit hour. Tuition, nonresident: full-time $14,544; part-time $1212 per credit hour. Tuition and fees vary according to course load and program. *Financial support:* In 2013–14, fellowships with full tuition reimbursements (averaging $22,000 per year), research assistantships with full tuition reimbursements (averaging $20,000 per year) were awarded. Financial award application deadline: 12/3. *Faculty research:* Bioremediation, biofilms, indoor air quality control, environmental toxicology, product biosynthesis. *Unit head:* Dr. George Pierce, Professor, 404-413-5315, Fax: 404-413-5301, E-mail: gpierce@gsu.edu. *Application contact:* LaTesha Warren, Graduate Coordinator, 404-413-5314, Fax: 404-413-5301, E-mail: lwarren@gsu.edu.
Website: http://biology.gsu.edu/

Harvard University, Graduate School of Arts and Sciences, Division of Medical Sciences, Boston, MA 02115. Offers biological chemistry and molecular pharmacology (PhD); cell biology (PhD); genetics (PhD); microbiology and molecular genetics (PhD); pathology (PhD), including experimental pathology. *Degree requirements:* For doctorate, thesis/dissertation. *Entrance requirements:* For doctorate, GRE General Test, GRE Subject Test. Additional exam requirements/recommendations for international students: Required—TOEFL. *Expenses: Tuition:* Full-time $38,888. *Required fees:* $958. Tuition and fees vary according to campus/location, program and student level.

Hood College, Graduate School, Program in Biomedical Science, Frederick, MD 21701-8575. Offers biomedical science (MS), including biotechnology/molecular biology, microbiology/immunology/virology, regulatory compliance; regulatory compliance (Certificate). Part-time and evening/weekend programs available. *Faculty:* 3 full-time (1 woman), 14 part-time/adjunct (6 women). *Students:* 5 full-time (2 women), 91 part-time (57 women); includes 17 minority (10 Black or African American, non-Hispanic/Latino; 4 Asian, non-Hispanic/Latino; 2 Hispanic/Latino; 1 Two or more races, non-Hispanic/Latino), 6 international. Average age 31. 60 applicants, 52% accepted, 21 enrolled. In 2013, 12 master's, 4 other advanced degrees awarded. *Degree requirements:* For master's, comprehensive exam, thesis or alternative. *Entrance requirements:* For master's, bachelor's degree in biology; minimum GPA of 2.75; undergraduate course work in cell biology, chemistry, organic chemistry, and genetics. Additional exam requirements/recommendations for international students: Required—TOEFL (minimum score 575 paper-based; 89 iBT), IELTS (minimum score 6.5). *Application deadline:* For fall admission, 7/15 priority date for domestic students, 7/15 for international students; for spring admission, 12/1 priority date for domestic students, 12/1 for international students. Applications are processed on a rolling basis. Application fee: $35. Electronic applications accepted. Application fee is waived when completed online. *Expenses: Tuition:* Part-time $405 per credit. *Required fees:* $100 per semester. *Financial support:* In 2013–14, 3 students received support, including 3 research assistantships with full tuition reimbursements available (averaging $10,609 per year); tuition waivers (partial) and unspecified assistantships also available. Financial award applicants required to submit FAFSA. *Unit head:* Dr. Rachel Bagni, Director, 301-696-3650, Fax: 301-696-3597, E-mail: bagni@hood.edu. *Application contact:* Dr. Maria Green Cowles, Dean of Graduate School, 301-696-3811, Fax: 301-696-3597, E-mail: gofurther@hood.edu.
Website: http://www.hood.edu/graduate

Howard University, College of Medicine, Department of Microbiology, Washington, DC 20059-0002. Offers PhD. *Degree requirements:* For doctorate, one foreign language, comprehensive exam, thesis/dissertation, qualifying exam, teaching experience. *Entrance requirements:* For doctorate, GRE General Test, minimum GPA of 3.0 in sciences. Additional exam requirements/recommendations for international students: Required—TOEFL. *Faculty research:* Immunology, molecular and cellular microbiology, microbial genetics, microbial physiology, pathogenic bacteriology, medical mycology, medical parasitology, virology.

Idaho State University, Office of Graduate Studies, College of Science and Engineering, Department of Biological Sciences, Pocatello, ID 83209-8007. Offers biology (MNS, MS, DA, PhD); clinical laboratory science (MS); microbiology (MS). *Accreditation:* NAACLS. Part-time programs available. *Degree requirements:* For master's, comprehensive exam, thesis; for doctorate, comprehensive exam, thesis/dissertation, 9 credits of internship (for DA). *Entrance requirements:* For master's, GRE General Test, minimum GPA of 3.0 in all upper division classes; for doctorate, GRE General Test, GRE Subject Test (biology), diagnostic exam (DA), minimum GPA of 3.0 in all upper division classes. Additional exam requirements/recommendations for international students: Required—TOEFL (minimum score 550 paper-based; 80 iBT). Electronic applications accepted. *Faculty research:* Ecology, plant and animal physiology, plant and animal developmental biology, immunology, molecular biology, bioinfomatics.

Illinois Institute of Technology, Graduate College, College of Science and Letters, Department of Biological and Chemical Sciences, Biology Division, Chicago, IL 60616. Offers biochemistry (MBS, MS); biology (PhD); biotechnology (MBS, MS); cell and molecular biology (MBS, MS); microbiology (MB, MS); molecular biochemistry and biophysics (PhD); molecular biology and biophysics (MS). Part-time and evening/weekend programs available. Postbaccalaureate distance learning degree programs offered (minimal on-campus study). Terminal master's awarded for partial completion of doctoral program. *Degree requirements:* For master's, comprehensive exam, thesis (for some programs); for doctorate, comprehensive exam, thesis/dissertation. *Entrance requirements:* For master's, GRE General Test (minimum score 1000 Quantitative and Verbal, 2.5 Analytical Writing), minimum undergraduate GPA of 3.0; for doctorate, GRE General Test (minimum score 1200 Quantitative and Verbal, 3.0 Analytical Writing), minimum undergraduate GPA of 3.0. Additional exam requirements/recommendations for international students: Required—TOEFL (minimum score 523 paper-based; 70 iBT); Recommended—IELTS (minimum score 5.5). Electronic applications accepted. *Faculty research:* Structure and biophysics of macromolecular systems; efficacy and mechanism of action of chemopreventive agents in experimental carcinogenesis of breast, colon, lung and prostate; study of fundamental structural biochemistry problems that have direct links to the understanding and treatment of disease; spectroscopic techniques for the study of multi-domain proteins; molecular mechanisms of cancer and cancer gene therapy.

Illinois State University, Graduate School, College of Arts and Sciences, Department of Biological Sciences, Normal, IL 61790-2200. Offers animal behavior (MS); bacteriology (MS); biochemistry (MS); biological sciences (MS); biology (PhD); biophysics (MS); biotechnology (MS); botany (MS, PhD); cell biology (MS); conservation biology (MS); developmental biology (MS); ecology (MS, PhD); entomology (MS); evolutionary biology (MS); genetics (MS, PhD); immunology (MS); microbiology (MS, PhD); molecular biology (MS); molecular genetics (MS); neurobiology (MS); neuroscience (MS); parasitology (MS); physiology (MS, PhD); plant biology (MS); plant molecular biology (MS); plant sciences (MS); structural biology (MS); zoology (MS, PhD). Part-time programs available. *Degree requirements:* For master's, thesis or alternative; for doctorate, variable foreign language requirement, thesis/dissertation, 2 terms of residency. *Entrance requirements:* For master's, GRE General Test, minimum GPA of 2.6 in last 60 hours of course work; for doctorate, GRE General Test. *Faculty research:* Redoc balance and drug development in schistosoma mansoni, control of the growth of listeria monocytogenes at low temperature, regulation of cell expansion and microtubule function by SPRI, CRUI: physiology and fitness consequences of different life history phenotypes.

Indiana State University, College of Graduate and Professional Studies, College of Arts and Sciences, Department of Biology, Terre Haute, IN 47809. Offers ecology (PhD); life sciences (MS); microbiology (PhD); physiology (PhD); science education (MS). *Faculty:* 23 full-time (6 women), 1 (woman) part-time/adjunct. *Students:* 73 full-time (31 women), 15 part-time (6 women); includes 7 minority (6 Asian, non-Hispanic/Latino; 1 Hispanic/Latino), 17 international. Average age 26. 63 applicants, 65% accepted, 40 enrolled. In 2013, 9 master's, 5 doctorates awarded. *Degree requirements:* For master's, thesis (for some programs); for doctorate, comprehensive exam, thesis/dissertation. *Entrance requirements:* For master's and doctorate, GRE General Test. *Application deadline:* For fall admission, 7/1 priority date for domestic students; for spring admission, 11/1 priority date for domestic students. Applications are processed on a rolling basis. Application fee: $35. Electronic applications accepted. *Financial support:* In 2013–14, 9 research assistantships with partial tuition reimbursements (averaging $7,500 per year), 19 teaching assistantships with partial tuition reimbursements (averaging $8,000 per year) were awarded; Federal Work-Study, institutionally sponsored loans, and tuition waivers (partial) also available. Financial award application deadline: 3/1; financial award applicants required to submit FAFSA. *Unit head:* Dr. Arthur M. Halpern, Interim Chairperson, 812-237-2400. *Application contact:* Dr. Jay Gatrell, Dean, 800-444-GRAD, Fax: 812-237-8060, E-mail: jay.gatrell@indstate.edu.

Indiana University Bloomington, University Graduate School, College of Arts and Sciences, Department of Biology, Bloomington, IN 47405. Offers biology teaching (MAT); biotechnology (MA); evolution, ecology, and behavior (MA, PhD); genetics (PhD); microbiology (MA, PhD); molecular, cellular, and developmental biology (PhD); plant sciences (MA, PhD); zoology (MA, PhD). *Faculty:* 58 full-time (15 women), 21 part-time/adjunct (6 women). *Students:* 166 full-time (94 women), 2 part-time (both women); includes 22 minority (8 Black or African American, non-Hispanic/Latino; 3 Asian, non-Hispanic/Latino; 10 Hispanic/Latino; 1 Two or more races, non-Hispanic/Latino), 47 international. Average age 27. 261 applicants, 23% accepted, 32 enrolled. In 2013, 17 master's, 20 doctorates awarded. Terminal master's awarded for partial completion of doctoral program. *Degree requirements:* For master's, thesis, oral defense; for doctorate, thesis/dissertation, oral defense. *Entrance requirements:* For master's and doctorate, GRE General Test. Additional exam requirements/recommendations for international students: Required—TOEFL (minimum score 100 iBT). *Application deadline:* For fall admission, 1/5 priority date for domestic students, 12/1 priority date for international students. Application fee: $55 ($65 for international students). Electronic applications accepted. *Financial support:* In 2013–14, fellowships with tuition reimbursements (averaging $24,000 per year), research assistantships with tuition reimbursements (averaging $21,000 per year), teaching assistantships with tuition reimbursements (averaging $22,000 per year) were awarded; scholarships/grants, traineeships, health care benefits, and unspecified assistantships also available. Financial award application deadline: 1/5. *Faculty research:* Evolution, ecology and behavior; microbiology; molecular biology and genetics; plant biology. *Unit head:* Dr. Clay Fuqua, Chair, 812-856-6005, Fax: 812-855-6082, E-mail: cfuqua@indiana.edu. *Application contact:* Tracey D. Stohr, Graduate Student Recruitment Coordinator, 812-856-6303, Fax: 812-855-6082, E-mail: gradbio@indiana.edu.
Website: http://www.bio.indiana.edu/

Indiana University–Purdue University Indianapolis, Indiana University School of Medicine, Department of Microbiology and Immunology, Indianapolis, IN 46202-2896. Offers MS, PhD, MD/MS, MD/PhD. *Faculty:* 20 full-time (2 women). *Students:* 28 full-time (18 women), 2 part-time (1 woman); includes 7 minority (1 Black or African American, non-Hispanic/Latino; 3 Asian, non-Hispanic/Latino; 2 Hispanic/Latino; 1 Two or more races, non-Hispanic/Latino), 12 international. Average age 27. 5 applicants. In 2013, 8 doctorates awarded. Terminal master's awarded for partial completion of doctoral program. *Degree requirements:* For master's, thesis; for doctorate, thesis/dissertation. *Entrance requirements:* For master's and doctorate, GRE General Test, previous course work in calculus, cell biology, chemistry, genetics, physics, and biochemistry. *Application deadline:* For fall admission, 3/1 for domestic students. Applications are processed on a rolling basis. Application fee: $55 ($65 for international students). *Financial support:* In 2013–14, fellowships with full tuition reimbursements (averaging $8,313 per year), teaching assistantships with full tuition reimbursements (averaging $18,391 per year) were awarded; research assistantships with full tuition reimbursements, Federal Work-Study, institutionally sponsored loans, scholarships/grants, traineeships, and tuition waivers (partial) also available. Financial award application deadline: 2/1. *Faculty research:* Host-parasite interactions, molecular biology, cellular and molecular immunology and hematology, viral and bacterial pathogenesis, cancer research. *Total annual research expenditures:* $4.2 million. *Unit head:* Dr. Stanley M. Spinola, Chair, 317-274-0508, E-mail: sspinola@iu.edu. *Application contact:* 317-274-7671, Fax: 317-274-4090.
Website: http://micro.medicine.iu.edu/

Microbiology

Inter American University of Puerto Rico, Metropolitan Campus, Graduate Programs, Program in Medical Technology, San Juan, PR 00919-1293. Offers administration of clinical laboratories (MS); molecular microbiology (MS). *Accreditation:* NAACLS. Part-time programs available. *Degree requirements:* For master's, comprehensive exam. *Entrance requirements:* For master's, BS in medical technology, minimum GPA of 2.5. Electronic applications accepted.

Iowa State University of Science and Technology, Department of Veterinary Microbiology and Preventive Medicine, Ames, IA 50011. Offers veterinary microbiology (MS, PhD). *Entrance requirements:* For master's and doctorate, GRE General Test. Additional exam requirements/recommendations for international students: Required—TOEFL (minimum score 550 paper-based; 79 iBT), IELTS (minimum score 6.5). Electronic applications accepted. *Faculty research:* Bacteriology, immunology, virology, public health and food safety.

Iowa State University of Science and Technology, Program in Microbiology, Ames, IA 50011. Offers MS, PhD. *Entrance requirements:* For master's and doctorate, GRE General Test. Additional exam requirements/recommendations for international students: Required—TOEFL (minimum score 550 paper-based; 79 iBT), IELTS (minimum score 6.5). Electronic applications accepted.

Johns Hopkins University, Bloomberg School of Public Health, W. Harry Feinstone Department of Molecular Microbiology and Immunology, Baltimore, MD 21218-2699. Offers MHS, Sc M, PhD. *Faculty:* 41 full-time (10 women), 10 part-time/adjunct (1 woman). *Students:* 95 full-time (52 women), 2 part-time (1 woman); includes 23 minority (3 Black or African American, non-Hispanic/Latino; 13 Asian, non-Hispanic/Latino; 5 Hispanic/Latino; 2 Two or more races, non-Hispanic/Latino), 25 international. Average age 26. 192 applicants, 47% accepted, 37 enrolled. In 2013, 34 master's, 7 doctorates awarded. Terminal master's awarded for partial completion of doctoral program. *Degree requirements:* For master's, comprehensive exam, thesis (for some programs), essay, written exams; for doctorate, comprehensive exam, thesis/dissertation, 1-year full-time residency, oral and written exams. *Entrance requirements:* For master's, GRE General Test or MCAT, 3 letters of recommendation, curriculum vitae; for doctorate, GRE General Test, 3 letters of recommendation, transcripts, curriculum vitae. Additional exam requirements/recommendations for international students: Required—TOEFL (minimum score 600 paper-based). *Application deadline:* For fall admission, 1/2 priority date for domestic and international students. Applications are processed on a rolling basis. Application fee: $45. Electronic applications accepted. *Financial support:* Fellowships with full and partial tuition reimbursements, research assistantships with tuition reimbursements, Federal Work-Study, institutionally sponsored loans, scholarships/grants, and stipends available. Financial award application deadline: 3/15; financial award applicants required to submit FAFSA. *Faculty research:* Immunology, virology, bacteriology, parasitology, vector biology, disease ecology, pathogenesis of infectious disease, immune responses to infectious agents, vector-borne and tropical diseases, biochemistry and molecular biology of infectious agents, population genetics of insect vectors, genetic regulation and immune responses in insect vectors, vaccine development, hormonal effects on pathogenesis and immune responses. *Total annual research expenditures:* $14.5 million. *Unit head:* Dr. Diane E. Griffin, Chair, 410-955-3459, Fax: 410-955-0105, E-mail: dgriffin@jhsph.edu. *Application contact:* Gail O'Connor, Senior Academic Program Coordinator, 410-614-4232, Fax: 410-955-0105, E-mail: goconnor@jhsph.edu.
Website: http://www.jhsph.edu/dept/MMI/

Kansas State University, Graduate School, College of Arts and Sciences, Division of Biology, Manhattan, KS 66506. Offers biology (MS, PhD); microbiology (PhD). *Faculty:* 73 full-time (18 women), 26 part-time/adjunct (6 women). *Students:* 57 full-time (32 women), 4 part-time (2 women); includes 5 minority (1 Black or African American, non-Hispanic/Latino; 4 Hispanic/Latino), 13 international. Average age 27. 109 applicants, 7% accepted, 5 enrolled. In 2013, 4 master's, 7 doctorates awarded. Terminal master's awarded for partial completion of doctoral program. *Degree requirements:* For master's, thesis; for doctorate, thesis/dissertation. *Entrance requirements:* For master's, GRE General Test, minimum undergraduate GPA of 3.0; for doctorate, GRE General Test, minimum GPA of 3.0. Additional exam requirements/recommendations for international students: Required—TOEFL (minimum score 550 paper-based). *Application deadline:* For fall admission, 12/15 priority date for domestic and international students; for spring admission, 8/1 priority date for domestic and international students. Applications are processed on a rolling basis. Application fee: $50 ($75 for international students). Electronic applications accepted. *Financial support:* In 2013–14, 11 fellowships with full tuition reimbursements (averaging $30,000 per year), 28 research assistantships with full tuition reimbursements (averaging $20,020 per year), 27 teaching assistantships with full tuition reimbursements (averaging $20,020 per year) were awarded; institutionally sponsored loans, scholarships/grants, and health care benefits also available. Support available to part-time students. Financial award application deadline: 3/1; financial award applicants required to submit FAFSA. *Faculty research:* Ecology, genetics, developmental biology, microbiology, cell biology. *Total annual research expenditures:* $9.3 million. *Unit head:* Brian Spooner, Director/Professor, Division of Biology, 785-532-6615, Fax: 785-532-6653, E-mail: biology@ksu.edu. *Application contact:* Dave Rintoul, Graduate Program Director, 785-532-6615, Fax: 785-532-6653, E-mail: drintoul@ksu.edu.
Website: http://www.k-state.edu/biology/

Loma Linda University, School of Medicine, Department of Biochemistry/Microbiology, Loma Linda, CA 92350. Offers MS, PhD. Part-time programs available. *Degree requirements:* For master's, thesis or alternative; for doctorate, thesis/dissertation. *Entrance requirements:* For master's and doctorate, GRE General Test. Additional exam requirements/recommendations for international students: Required—TOEFL (minimum score 550 paper-based). *Faculty research:* Physical chemistry of macromolecules, biochemistry of endocrine system, biochemical mechanism of bone volume regulation.

Long Island University–LIU Post, School of Health Professions and Nursing, Department of Biomedical Sciences, Brookville, NY 11548-1300. Offers cardiovascular perfusion (MS); clinical laboratory management (MS); medical biology (MS), including hematology, immunology, medical biology, medical chemistry, medical microbiology. Part-time and evening/weekend programs available. Postbaccalaureate distance learning degree programs offered. *Degree requirements:* For master's, thesis. *Entrance requirements:* For master's, minimum GPA of 2.75 in major. Electronic applications accepted.

Louisiana State University Health Sciences Center, School of Graduate Studies in New Orleans, Department of Microbiology, Immunology, and Parasitology, New Orleans, LA 70112-2223. Offers microbiology and immunology (MS, PhD); MD/PhD. Terminal master's awarded for partial completion of doctoral program. *Degree requirements:* For master's, comprehensive exam, thesis; for doctorate, comprehensive exam, thesis/dissertation, preliminary exam, qualifying exam. *Entrance requirements:* For master's and doctorate, GRE General Test. Additional exam requirements/recommendations for international students: Required—TOEFL. *Faculty research:* Microbial physiology, animal virology, vaccine development, AIDS drug studies, pathogenic mechanisms, molecular immunology.

Louisiana State University Health Sciences Center at Shreveport, Department of Microbiology and Immunology, Shreveport, LA 71130-3932. Offers MS, PhD, MD/PhD. *Faculty:* 17 full-time (3 women). *Students:* 24 full-time (14 women); includes 2 minority (1 American Indian or Alaska Native, non-Hispanic/Latino; 1 Asian, non-Hispanic/Latino), 2 international. Average age 23. 23 applicants, 30% accepted, 6 enrolled. In 2013, 5 doctorates awarded. Terminal master's awarded for partial completion of doctoral program. *Degree requirements:* For master's, thesis; for doctorate, thesis/dissertation. *Entrance requirements:* For master's and doctorate, GRE General Test. Additional exam requirements/recommendations for international students: Required—TOEFL. Application fee: $0. *Financial support:* In 2013–14, 4 fellowships (averaging $28,000 per year), 20 research assistantships (averaging $26,000 per year) were awarded; institutionally sponsored loans also available. Financial award application deadline: 7/1. *Faculty research:* Infectious disease, pathogenesis, molecular virology and biology. *Unit head:* Dr. Dennis J. O'Callaghan, Head, 318-675-5750, Fax: 318-675-5764. *Application contact:* Marti Glass, Coordinator, 318-675-4781, Fax: 318-675-4343, E-mail: mglass@lsuhs.edu.
Website: http://www.lsuhscmicrobiology.com

Loyola University Chicago, Graduate School, Department of Microbiology and Immunology, Maywood, IL 60153. Offers MS. *Faculty:* 15 full-time (4 women). *Students:* 31 full-time (19 women); includes 4 minority (2 Asian, non-Hispanic/Latino; 2 Hispanic/Latino), 3 international. Average age 27. 22 applicants, 32% accepted, 5 enrolled. In 2013, 2 master's awarded. Terminal master's awarded for partial completion of doctoral program. *Degree requirements:* For master's, thesis. *Entrance requirements:* For master's, GRE General Test. Additional exam requirements/recommendations for international students: Required—TOEFL. *Application deadline:* For fall admission, 3/15 for domestic and international students. Applications are processed on a rolling basis. Application fee: $0. Electronic applications accepted. *Expenses: Tuition:* Full-time $16,740; part-time $930 per credit. *Required fees:* $135 per semester. *Financial support:* In 2013–14, 5 fellowships with tuition reimbursements (averaging $27,000 per year), 24 research assistantships with tuition reimbursements (averaging $27,000 per year) were awarded; institutionally sponsored loans and scholarships/grants also available. Financial award application deadline: 1/18. *Faculty research:* Virology, microbial physiology and genetics, immune system development and regulation, signal transduction and host-pathogen interactions, biofilms. *Unit head:* Dr. Katherine L. Knight, Chair, 708-216-3385, Fax: 708-216-9574, E-mail: kknight@luc.edu. *Application contact:* Dr. Karen Visick, Graduate Program Director, 708-216-0869, Fax: 708-216-9574, E-mail: kvisick@luc.edu.

Marquette University, Graduate School, College of Arts and Sciences, Department of Biology, Milwaukee, WI 53201-1881. Offers cell biology (MS, PhD); developmental biology (MS, PhD); ecology (MS, PhD); epithelial physiology (MS, PhD); genetics (MS, PhD); microbiology (MS, PhD); molecular biology (MS, PhD); muscle and exercise physiology (MS, PhD); neuroscience (PhD). *Faculty:* 21 full-time (9 women), 3 part-time/adjunct (0 women). *Students:* 34 full-time (16 women), 4 part-time (1 woman), 15 international. Average age 27. 70 applicants, 23% accepted, 5 enrolled. In 2013, 1 master's, 6 doctorates awarded. Terminal master's awarded for partial completion of doctoral program. *Degree requirements:* For master's, comprehensive exam, thesis, 1 year of teaching experience or equivalent; for doctorate, thesis/dissertation, 1 year of teaching experience or equivalent, qualifying exam. *Entrance requirements:* For master's and doctorate, GRE General Test, GRE Subject Test, official transcripts from all current and previous colleges/universities except Marquette, statement of professional goals and aspirations, three letters of recommendation. Additional exam requirements/recommendations for international students: Required—TOEFL (minimum score 530 paper-based). *Application deadline:* For fall admission, 12/15 for domestic and international students. Application fee: $50. Electronic applications accepted. *Financial support:* In 2013–14, 39 students received support, including 6 fellowships (averaging $1,208 per year), 4 research assistantships with full tuition reimbursements available (averaging $21,750 per year), 29 teaching assistantships with full tuition reimbursements available (averaging $21,750 per year); scholarships/grants, health care benefits, tuition waivers (full and partial), and unspecified assistantships also available. Support available to part-time students. Financial award application deadline: 2/15. *Faculty research:* Neurobiology, neuroendocrinology, epithelial physiology, neuropeptide interactions, synaptic transmission. *Total annual research expenditures:* $1.5 million. *Unit head:* Dr. Dale Noel, Chair and Professor, 414-288-1748. *Application contact:* Dr. Michelle Mynlieff, Professor, 414-288-1467.
Website: http://www.marquette.edu/biology/

Massachusetts Institute of Technology, School of Science, Department of Biology, Cambridge, MA 02139-4307. Offers biochemistry (PhD); biological oceanography (PhD); biology (PhD); biophysical chemistry and molecular structure (PhD); cell biology (PhD); computational and systems biology (PhD); developmental biology (PhD); genetics (PhD); immunology (PhD); microbiology (PhD); molecular biology (PhD); neurobiology (PhD). *Faculty:* 58 full-time (15 women). *Students:* 261 full-time (133 women); includes 77 minority (3 Black or African American, non-Hispanic/Latino; 1 American Indian or Alaska Native, non-Hispanic/Latino; 32 Asian, non-Hispanic/Latino; 32 Hispanic/Latino; 9 Two or more races, non-Hispanic/Latino), 46 international. Average age 26. 651 applicants, 15% accepted, 39 enrolled. In 2013, 25 doctorates awarded. *Degree requirements:* For doctorate, comprehensive exam, thesis/dissertation, two semesters as a teaching assistant. *Entrance requirements:* For doctorate, GRE General Test. Additional exam requirements/recommendations for international students: Required—TOEFL (minimum score 577 paper-based), IELTS (minimum score 6.5). *Application deadline:* For fall admission, 12/1 for domestic and international students. Application fee: $75. Electronic applications accepted. *Expenses: Tuition:* Full-time $43,210; part-time $670 per credit hour. *Required fees:* $288. *Financial support:* In 2013–14, 252 students received support, including 135 fellowships (averaging $36,800 per year), 122 research assistantships (averaging $35,500 per year), 1 teaching assistantship; Federal Work-Study, institutionally sponsored loans, scholarships/grants, traineeships, health care benefits, and unspecified assistantships also available. *Faculty research:* Cellular, developmental and molecular (plant and animal) biology; biochemistry, bioengineering, biophysics and structural biology; classical and molecular genetics, stem cell and epigenetics; immunology and microbiology; cancer biology, molecular medicine, neurobiology and human disease; computational and systems biology. *Total annual research expenditures:* $44.5 million. *Unit head:* Alan Grossman, Interim Head, 617-253-4701. *Application contact:* Biology Education Office, 617-253-3717, Fax: 617-258-9329, E-mail: gradbio@mit.edu.
Website: https://biology.mit.edu/

McGill University, Faculty of Graduate and Postdoctoral Studies, Faculty of Agricultural and Environmental Sciences, Department of Natural Resource Sciences, Montréal, QC H3A 2T5, Canada. Offers entomology (M Sc, PhD); environmental assessment (M Sc); forest science (M Sc, PhD); microbiology (M Sc, PhD); micrometeorology (M Sc, PhD); neotropical environment (M Sc, PhD); soil science (M Sc, PhD); wildlife biology (M Sc, PhD).

McGill University, Faculty of Graduate and Postdoctoral Studies, Faculty of Medicine, Department of Microbiology and Immunology, Montréal, QC H3A 2T5, Canada. Offers M Sc, M Sc A, PhD.

Medical College of Wisconsin, Graduate School of Biomedical Sciences, Department of Microbiology and Molecular Genetics, Milwaukee, WI 53226-0509. Offers MS, PhD, MD/PhD. *Degree requirements:* For doctorate, comprehensive exam, thesis/dissertation. *Entrance requirements:* For master's and doctorate, GRE, official transcripts, three letters of recommendation. Additional exam requirements/recommendations for international students: Required—TOEFL. *Faculty research:* Virology, immunology, bacterial toxins, regulation of gene expression.

Medical University of South Carolina, College of Graduate Studies, Department of Microbiology and Immunology, Charleston, SC 29425. Offers MS, PhD, DMD/PhD, MD/PhD. Terminal master's awarded for partial completion of doctoral program. *Degree requirements:* For master's, thesis; for doctorate, thesis/dissertation, oral and written exams. *Entrance requirements:* For master's, GRE General Test, MCAT, or DAT, minimum GPA of 3.0; for doctorate, GRE General Test, interview, minimum GPA of 3.0, research experience. Additional exam requirements/recommendations for international students: Required—TOEFL (minimum score 600 paper-based; 100 iBT). Electronic applications accepted. *Faculty research:* Inmate and adaptive immunology, gene therapy/vector development, vaccinology, proteomics of biowarfare agents, bacterial and fungal pathogenesis.

Meharry Medical College, School of Graduate Studies, Program in Biomedical Sciences, Microbiology and Immunology Emphasis, Nashville, TN 37208-9989. Offers PhD, MD/PhD. *Degree requirements:* For doctorate, comprehensive exam, thesis/dissertation. *Entrance requirements:* For doctorate, GRE General Test, GRE Subject Test, undergraduate degree in related science. *Faculty research:* Microbial and bacterial pathogenesis, viral transcription, immune response to viruses and parasites.

Miami University, College of Arts and Science, Department of Microbiology, Oxford, OH 45056. Offers MS, PhD. Part-time programs available. *Students:* 23 full-time (13 women); includes 1 minority (Black or African American, non-Hispanic/Latino), 5 international. Average age 27. In 2013, 4 doctorates awarded. *Entrance requirements:* For master's and doctorate, GRE General Test. Additional exam requirements/recommendations for international students: Recommended—TOEFL (minimum score 80 iBT), IELTS (minimum score 6.5), TSE (minimum score 54). *Application deadline:* For fall admission, 1/15 for domestic and international students. Application fee: $50. Electronic applications accepted. *Expenses:* Tuition, state resident: full-time $12,634; part-time $526 per credit hour. Tuition, nonresident: full-time $27,892; part-time $1162 per credit hour. Part-time tuition and fees vary according to course load, campus/location and program. *Financial support:* Fellowships with full tuition reimbursements, research assistantships with full tuition reimbursements, teaching assistantships with full tuition reimbursements, Federal Work-Study, institutionally sponsored loans, scholarships/grants, health care benefits, tuition waivers (full), and unspecified assistantships available. Financial award application deadline: 1/15; financial award applicants required to submit FAFSA. *Unit head:* Dr. Louis A. Actis, Chair, 513-529-5421, Fax: 513-529-2431, E-mail: actisla@miamioh.edu. *Application contact:* Dr. Mitchell Balish, Associate Professor and Director of Graduate Studies, 513-529-0167, E-mail: balishmf@miamioh.edu.
Website: http://microbiology.MiamiOH.edu/

Michigan State University, College of Human Medicine and The Graduate School, Graduate Programs in Human Medicine, East Lansing, MI 48824. Offers biochemistry and molecular biology (MS, PhD); epidemiology (MS, PhD); microbiology (MS); microbiology and molecular genetics (PhD); pharmacology and toxicology (MS, PhD); physiology (MS, PhD); public health (MPH). *Entrance requirements:* Additional exam requirements/recommendations for international students: Required—TOEFL.

Michigan State University, College of Osteopathic Medicine and The Graduate School, Graduate Studies in Osteopathic Medicine, East Lansing, MI 48824. Offers biochemistry and molecular biology (MS, PhD); microbiology (MS); microbiology and molecular genetics (PhD); pharmacology and toxicology (MS, PhD), including integrative pharmacology (MS), pharmacology and toxicology, pharmacology and toxicology-environmental toxicology (PhD); physiology (MS, PhD).

Michigan State University, College of Veterinary Medicine and The Graduate School, Graduate Programs in Veterinary Medicine and College of Natural Science and Graduate Programs in Human Medicine, Department of Microbiology and Molecular Genetics, East Lansing, MI 48824. Offers industrial microbiology (MS, PhD); microbiology (MS, PhD); microbiology and molecular genetics (MS, PhD); microbiology–environmental toxicology (PhD). *Entrance requirements:* For master's, GRE General Test. Additional exam requirements/recommendations for international students: Required—TOEFL (minimum score 550 paper-based), Michigan State University ELT (minimum score 85), Michigan English Language Assessment Battery (minimum score 83). Electronic applications accepted.

Michigan State University, The Graduate School, College of Agriculture and Natural Resources, MSU-DOE Plant Research Laboratory, East Lansing, MI 48824. Offers biochemistry and molecular biology (PhD); cellular and molecular biology (PhD); crop and soil sciences (PhD); genetics (PhD); microbiology and molecular genetics (PhD); plant biology (PhD); plant physiology (PhD). Offered jointly with the Department of Energy. *Degree requirements:* For doctorate, comprehensive exam, thesis/dissertation, laboratory rotation, defense of dissertation. *Entrance requirements:* For doctorate, GRE General Test, acceptance into one of the affiliated department programs; 3 letters of recommendation; bachelor's degree or equivalent in life sciences, chemistry, biochemistry, or biophysics; research experience. Electronic applications accepted. *Faculty research:* Role of hormones in the regulation of plant development and physiology, molecular mechanisms associated with signal recognition, development and application of genetic methods and materials, protein routing and function.

Montana State University, College of Graduate Studies, College of Letters and Science, Department of Microbiology, Bozeman, MT 59717. Offers MS, PhD. Part-time programs available. *Degree requirements:* For master's, comprehensive exam; for doctorate, comprehensive exam, thesis/dissertation. *Entrance requirements:* For master's and doctorate, GRE General Test. Additional exam requirements/recommendations for international students: Required—TOEFL (minimum score 550 paper-based). Electronic applications accepted. *Faculty research:* Medical microbiology, environmental microbiology, biofilms, immunology, molecular biology and bioinformatics.

New York Medical College, Graduate School of Basic Medical Sciences, Integrated PhD Program, Valhalla, NY 10595-1691. Offers biochemistry and molecular biology (PhD); cell biology and anatomy (PhD); microbiology and immunology (PhD); pathology (PhD); pharmacology (PhD); physiology (PhD). *Faculty:* 91 full-time (16 women), 5 part-time/adjunct (2 women). *Students:* 31 full-time (21 women); includes 17 minority (4 Black or African American, non-Hispanic/Latino; 11 Asian, non-Hispanic/Latino; 2 Hispanic/Latino). Average age 27. 56 applicants, 36% accepted, 9 enrolled. In 2013, 17 doctorates awarded. *Degree requirements:* For doctorate, comprehensive exam, thesis/dissertation. *Entrance requirements:* For doctorate, GRE General Test. Additional exam requirements/recommendations for international students: Required—TOEFL. *Application deadline:* For fall admission, 1/1 priority date for domestic and international students. Applications are processed on a rolling basis. Application fee: $75 ($100 for international students). Electronic applications accepted. *Expenses: Tuition:* Full-time $49,170; part-time $910 per credit. Tuition and fees vary according to program. *Financial support:* In 2013–14, fellowships with full tuition reimbursements (averaging $25,500 per year), research assistantships with full tuition reimbursements (averaging $25,500 per year) were awarded; Federal Work-Study, scholarships/grants, traineeships, health care benefits, and tuition waivers (full) also available. Financial award applicants required to submit FAFSA. *Faculty research:* Cardiovascular sciences, infectious diseases, neuroscience, cancer and cell signaling. *Unit head:* Dr. Francis L. Belloni, Dean, 914-594-4110, Fax: 914-594-4944, E-mail: francis_belloni@nymc.edu. *Application contact:* Valerie Romeo-Messana, Director of Admissions, 914-594-4110, Fax: 914-594-4944, E-mail: v_romeomessana@nymc.edu.

New York Medical College, Graduate School of Basic Medical Sciences, Microbiology and Immunology Master's Program, Valhalla, NY 10595-1691. Offers MS, PhD, MD/PhD. Part-time and evening/weekend programs available. *Faculty:* 12 full-time (4 women). *Students:* 19 full-time (13 women); includes 10 minority (1 Black or African American, non-Hispanic/Latino; 7 Asian, non-Hispanic/Latino; 2 Hispanic/Latino). Average age 25. 20 applicants, 85% accepted, 5 enrolled. In 2013, 9 master's awarded. Terminal master's awarded for partial completion of doctoral program. *Degree requirements:* For master's, thesis; for doctorate, comprehensive exam, thesis/dissertation. *Entrance requirements:* For master's, GRE General Test, MCAT, or DAT. Additional exam requirements/recommendations for international students: Required—TOEFL. *Application deadline:* For fall admission, 7/1 priority date for domestic students, 5/1 priority date for international students; for spring admission, 12/1 for domestic students, 10/1 for international students. Applications are processed on a rolling basis. Application fee: $75 ($100 for international students). Electronic applications accepted. *Expenses: Tuition:* Full-time $49,170; part-time $910 per credit. Tuition and fees vary according to program. *Financial support:* Federal Work-Study and scholarships/grants available. Support available to part-time students. Financial award applicants required to submit FAFSA. *Faculty research:* Tumor cells, cancer vaccines, the role of stem cells in cancer, bacterial genetics pathogenesis of infectious disease and function of influenza virus antigens, molecular virology, and the biochemistry and genetics of emerging pathogens. *Unit head:* Dr. Raj Tiwari, Program Director, 914-594-4870, Fax: 914-594-4944, E-mail: raj_tiwari@nymc.edu. *Application contact:* Valerie Romeo-Messana, Director of Admissions, 914-594-4110, Fax: 914-594-4944, E-mail: v_romeomessana@nymc.edu.

New York University, Graduate School of Arts and Science, Department of Biology, New York, NY 10012-1019. Offers biology (PhD); biomedical journalism (MS); cancer and molecular biology (PhD); computational biology (PhD); computers in biological research (MS); developmental genetics (PhD); general biology (MS); immunology and microbiology (PhD); molecular genetics (PhD); neurobiology (PhD); oral biology (MS); plant biology (PhD); recombinant DNA technology (MS); MS/MBA. Part-time programs available. *Faculty:* 24 full-time (5 women). *Students:* 161 full-time (88 women), 28 part-time (15 women); includes 41 minority (5 Black or African American, non-Hispanic/Latino; 23 Asian, non-Hispanic/Latino; 9 Hispanic/Latino; 4 Two or more races, non-Hispanic/Latino), 80 international. Average age 27. 412 applicants, 54% accepted, 65 enrolled. In 2013, 77 master's, 9 doctorates awarded. Terminal master's awarded for partial completion of doctoral program. *Degree requirements:* For master's, thesis or alternative, qualifying paper; for doctorate, comprehensive exam, thesis/dissertation. *Entrance requirements:* For master's and doctorate, GRE General Test. Additional exam requirements/recommendations for international students: Required—TOEFL. *Application deadline:* For fall admission, 12/1 priority date for domestic students, 12/1 for international students. Application fee: $95. *Expenses: Tuition:* Full-time $35,856; part-time $1494 per unit. *Required fees:* $1408; $64 per unit. $473 per term. Tuition and fees vary according to course load and program. *Financial support:* Fellowships with tuition reimbursements, research assistantships with tuition reimbursements, teaching assistantships with tuition reimbursements, career-related internships or fieldwork, Federal Work-Study, institutionally sponsored loans, scholarships/grants, health care benefits, and unspecified assistantships available. Financial award application deadline: 12/1; financial award applicants required to submit FAFSA. *Faculty research:* Genomics, molecular and cell biology, development and molecular genetics, molecular evolution of plants and animals. *Unit head:* Stephen Small, Chair, 212-998-8200, Fax: 212-995-4015, E-mail: biology.admissions@nyu.edu. *Application contact:* Justin Blau, Director of Graduate Studies, PhD Programs, 212-998-8200, Fax: 212-995-4015, E-mail: biology.admissions@nyu.edu.
Website: http://biology.as.nyu.edu/

New York University, School of Medicine and Graduate School of Arts and Science, Sackler Institute of Graduate Biomedical Sciences, Program in Microbiology, New York, NY 10012-1019. Offers PhD, MD/PhD. *Faculty:* 35 full-time (12 women). *Students:* 21 full-time (11 women); includes 5 minority (2 Asian, non-Hispanic/Latino; 3 Hispanic/Latino), 8 international. Average age 27. In 2013, 2 doctorates awarded. *Degree requirements:* For doctorate, one foreign language, comprehensive exam, thesis/dissertation, qualifying exam. *Entrance requirements:* For doctorate, GRE General Test, GRE Subject Test. Additional exam requirements/recommendations for international students: Required—TOEFL. *Application deadline:* For fall admission, 1/4 priority date for domestic students. Applications are processed on a rolling basis. Application fee: $85. *Expenses: Tuition:* Full-time $35,856; part-time $1494 per unit. *Required fees:* $1408; $64 per unit. $473 per term. Tuition and fees vary according to course load and program. *Financial support:* Fellowships with tuition reimbursements, research assistantships with tuition reimbursements, and teaching assistantships with tuition reimbursements available. *Faculty research:* Aspects of microbiology, parasitology, and genetics; virology. *Unit head:* Dr. Claudio Basilico, Chairman, 212-263-5341, Fax: 212-263-8276. *Application contact:* Dr. Joel Belasco, Graduate Advisor, 212-263-5409, Fax: 212-263-2150, E-mail: joel.belasco@med.nyu.edu.

North Carolina State University, Graduate School, College of Agriculture and Life Sciences, Department of Microbiology, Program in Microbiology, Raleigh, NC 27695. Offers MS, PhD. *Degree requirements:* For master's, thesis (for some programs); for doctorate, thesis/dissertation. *Entrance requirements:* For master's and doctorate, GRE. Electronic applications accepted.

North Dakota State University, College of Graduate and Interdisciplinary Studies, College of Agriculture, Food Systems, and Natural Resources, Department of Veterinary and Microbiological Sciences, Fargo, ND 58108. Offers international infectious disease (MS); microbiology (MS); molecular pathogenesis (PhD). Part-time programs available. *Faculty:* 15 full-time (8 women). *Students:* 11 full-time (6 women), 6 part-time (4 women), 5 international. Average age 30. 2 applicants, 50% accepted, 1 enrolled. In 2013, 8 master's, 1 doctorate awarded. *Degree requirements:* For master's, thesis; for doctorate, thesis/dissertation, oral and written preliminary exams. *Entrance requirements:* For master's and doctorate, GRE. Additional exam requirements/recommendations for international students: Required—TOEFL (minimum score 525 paper-based; 71 iBT). *Application deadline:* For fall admission, 2/15 priority date for domestic students. Applications are processed on a rolling basis. Application fee: $35. *Financial support:* Fellowships with full tuition reimbursements, research assistantships with full tuition reimbursements, teaching assistantships with full tuition reimbursements, Federal Work-Study, and institutionally sponsored loans available. Financial award application deadline: 4/15. *Faculty research:* Bacterial gene regulation, antibiotic

resistance, molecular virology, mechanisms of bacterial pathogenesis, immunology of animals. *Unit head:* Dr. Charlene Wolf-Hall, Head, 701-231-7667, E-mail: charlene.hall@ndsu.edu. *Application contact:* Dr. John McEvoy, Associate Professor, 701-231-8530, Fax: 701-231-7514, E-mail: eugene.berry@ndsu.edu.
Website: http://vetmicro.ndsu.nodak.edu/

The Ohio State University, Graduate School, College of Arts and Sciences, Division of Natural and Mathematical Sciences, Department of Microbiology, Columbus, OH 43210. Offers MS, PhD. *Faculty:* 15. *Students:* 44 full-time (23 women); includes 2 minority (both Asian, non-Hispanic/Latino), 16 international. Average age 26. In 2013, 2 master's, 3 doctorates awarded. Terminal master's awarded for partial completion of doctoral program. *Degree requirements:* For master's, thesis optional; for doctorate, thesis/dissertation. *Entrance requirements:* For doctorate, GRE General Test. Additional exam requirements/recommendations for international students: Required—TOEFL (minimum score 100 iBT). *Application deadline:* For fall admission, 12/13 priority date for domestic students, 11/30 priority date for international students; for winter admission, 12/1 for domestic students, 11/1 for international students; for spring admission, 3/1 for domestic students, 2/1 for international students. Applications are processed on a rolling basis. Application fee: $60 ($70 for international students). Electronic applications accepted. *Financial support:* Fellowships with tuition reimbursements, research assistantships with tuition reimbursements, teaching assistantships with tuition reimbursements, Federal Work-Study, and institutionally sponsored loans available. Support available to part-time students. *Unit head:* Dr. Tina M. Henkin, Chair, 614-688-3831, Fax: 614-292-8120, E-mail: henkin.3@osu.edu. *Application contact:* Graduate Admissions, 614-292-9444, Fax: 614-292-3895, E-mail: gradadmissions@osu.edu.
Website: http://microbiology.osu.edu/

Ohio University, Graduate College, College of Arts and Sciences, Department of Biological Sciences, Athens, OH 45701-2979. Offers biological sciences (MS, PhD); cell biology and physiology (MS, PhD); ecology and evolutionary biology (MS, PhD); exercise physiology and muscle biology (MS, PhD); microbiology (MS, PhD); neuroscience (MS, PhD). Terminal master's awarded for partial completion of doctoral program. *Degree requirements:* For master's, comprehensive exam, thesis, 1 quarter of teaching experience; for doctorate, comprehensive exam, thesis/dissertation, 2 quarters of teaching experience. *Entrance requirements:* For master's, GRE General Test, names of three faculty members whose research interests most closely match the applicant's interest; for doctorate, GRE General Test, essay concerning prior training, research interest and career goals, plus names of three faculty members whose research interests most closely match the applicant's interest. Additional exam requirements/recommendations for international students: Required—TOEFL (minimum score 620 paper-based; 105 iBT) or IELTS (minimum score 7.5). Electronic applications accepted. *Faculty research:* Ecology and evolutionary biology, exercise physiology and muscle biology, neurobiology, cell biology, physiology.

Oklahoma State University, College of Arts and Sciences, Department of Microbiology and Molecular Genetics, Stillwater, OK 74078. Offers MS, PhD. *Faculty:* 20 full-time (5 women). *Students:* 16 full-time (10 women), 18 part-time (11 women); includes 4 minority (1 Asian, non-Hispanic/Latino; 1 Hispanic/Latino; 2 Two or more races, non-Hispanic/Latino), 17 international. Average age 28. 83 applicants, 19% accepted, 10 enrolled. In 2013, 1 master's awarded. *Degree requirements:* For master's, thesis; for doctorate, comprehensive exam, thesis/dissertation. *Entrance requirements:* For master's, GRE General Test; for doctorate, GRE General Test. Additional exam requirements/recommendations for international students: Required—TOEFL (minimum score 550 paper-based; 79 iBT). *Application deadline:* For fall admission, 3/1 priority date for international students; for spring admission, 8/1 priority date for international students. Applications are processed on a rolling basis. Application fee: $40 ($75 for international students). Electronic applications accepted. *Expenses:* Tuition, state resident: full-time $4272; part-time $178 per credit hour. Tuition, nonresident: full-time $17,472; part-time $709 per credit hour. *Required fees:* $2413.20; $100.55 per credit hour. One-time fee: $50 full-time. Part-time tuition and fees vary according to course load and campus/location. *Financial support:* In 2013–14, 16 research assistantships (averaging $21,705 per year), 14 teaching assistantships (averaging $19,632 per year) were awarded; career-related internships or fieldwork, Federal Work-Study, scholarships/grants, health care benefits, tuition waivers (partial), and unspecified assistantships also available. Support available to part-time students. Financial award application deadline: 3/1; financial award applicants required to submit FAFSA. *Faculty research:* Bioinformatics, genomics-genetics, virology, environmental microbiology, development-molecular mechanisms. *Unit head:* Dr. Bill Picking, Department Head, 405-744-6243, Fax: 405-744-6790, E-mail: william.picking@okstate.edu. *Application contact:* Dr. Wouter Hoff, Graduate Program Coordinator, 405-744-6243, Fax: 405-744-6790, E-mail: wouter.hoff@okstate.edu.
Website: http://microbiology.okstate.edu

Oklahoma State University Center for Health Sciences, Graduate Program in Forensic Sciences, Tulsa, OK 74107. Offers forensic biology/DNA (MS); forensic document examination/forensic pathology (MS); forensic psychology (MS); forensic science administration (MS); microbiology (MS); trace evidence/forensic toxicology (MS). Part-time and evening/weekend programs available. Postbaccalaureate distance learning degree programs offered (no on-campus study). *Faculty:* 4 full-time (0 women), 14 part-time/adjunct (6 women). *Students:* 4 full-time (0 women), 14 part-time (6 women); includes 7 minority (4 American Indian or Alaska Native, non-Hispanic/Latino; 3 Hispanic/Latino), 3 international. Average age 31. 28 applicants, 50% accepted, 5 enrolled. In 2013, 5 master's awarded. *Degree requirements:* For master's, comprehensive exam, thesis (for some programs), creative component (for non-thesis options). *Entrance requirements:* For master's, MAT (for options in forensic science administration and forensic document examination) or GRE General Test, professional experience (for options in forensic science administration and forensic document examination). Additional exam requirements/recommendations for international students: Required—TOEFL (minimum score 100 iBT) or IELTS (minimum score 7.0). *Application deadline:* For fall admission, 3/1 for domestic and international students; for spring admission, 10/1 for domestic and international students; for summer admission, 7/1 for domestic and international students. Applications are processed on a rolling basis. Application fee: $40 ($75 for international students). Electronic applications accepted. *Expenses:* Tuition, state resident: full-time $22,127; part-time $178 per credit hour. Tuition, nonresident: full-time $43,572; part-time $728 per credit hour. *Required fees:* $910.79; $200 per semester. *Financial support:* In 2013–14, 14 students received support, including 8 research assistantships (averaging $12,000 per year); career-related internships or fieldwork, Federal Work-Study, and tuition waivers (partial) also available. Support available to part-time students. Financial award application deadline: 4/1; financial award applicants required to submit FAFSA. *Faculty research:* Studies on the variability in chromosomal DNA; development/enhancement of accessory methods useful for forensic DNA typing; development of universal methods useful for discriminating pathogenic bacteria; forensic dentistry; transmission of microbial diseases by dentures, protective athletic mouth-guards, band wind instruments, and infant pacifiers; changes in ecologies and antibiotic sensitivities of aerobic microorganisms; forensic toxicology and trace chemical method development. *Total annual research expenditures:* $58,000. *Unit head:* Dr. Robert W. Allen, Director, 918-561-1108, Fax: 918-561-8414. *Application contact:* Cathy Newsome, Coordinator, 918-561-1108, Fax: 918-561-8414, E-mail: cathy.newsome@okstate.edu.
Website: http://www.healthsciences.okstate.edu/forensic/index.cfm

Oregon Health & Science University, School of Medicine, Graduate Programs in Medicine, Program in Molecular and Cellular Biosciences, Department of Molecular Microbiology and Immunology, Portland, OR 97239-3098. Offers PhD. *Faculty:* 9 full-time (3 women), 16 part-time/adjunct (2 women). *Students:* 19 full-time (12 women), 1 (woman) part-time; includes 6 minority (2 Asian, non-Hispanic/Latino; 3 Hispanic/Latino; 1 Two or more races, non-Hispanic/Latino), 2 international. Average age 29. In 2013, 5 doctorates awarded. Terminal master's awarded for partial completion of doctoral program. *Degree requirements:* For doctorate, comprehensive exam, thesis/dissertation, qualifying exam. *Entrance requirements:* For doctorate, GRE General Test (minimum scores: 153 Verbal/148 Quantitative/4.5 Analytical) or MCAT (for some programs). Additional exam requirements/recommendations for international students: Required—TOEFL. Electronic applications accepted. *Financial support:* Health care benefits and full tuition and stipends available. *Faculty research:* Molecular biology of bacterial and viral pathogens, cellular and humoral immunology, molecular biology of microbes. *Unit head:* Dr. Eric Barklis, Program Director, 503-494-7768, E-mail: mmi@ohsu.edu. *Application contact:* Lola Bichler, Program Coordinator, 503-494-5824, E-mail: bichler@ohsu.edu.
Website: http://www.ohsu.edu/microbiology

Oregon State University, College of Science, Program in Microbiology, Corvallis, OR 97331. Offers MA, MAIS, MS, PhD. Part-time programs available. *Faculty:* 13 full-time (5 women), 2 part-time/adjunct (1 woman). *Students:* 34 full-time (17 women), 1 (woman) part-time; includes 6 minority (3 Asian, non-Hispanic/Latino; 3 Hispanic/Latino), 5 international. Average age 28. 83 applicants, 11% accepted, 6 enrolled. In 2013, 4 master's, 2 doctorates awarded. Terminal master's awarded for partial completion of doctoral program. *Degree requirements:* For master's, thesis; for doctorate, one foreign language, thesis/dissertation. *Entrance requirements:* For master's and doctorate, GRE. Additional exam requirements/recommendations for international students: Required—TOEFL (minimum score 600 paper-based; 100 iBT). *Application deadline:* For fall admission, 3/1 for domestic students. Application fee: $60. *Expenses:* Tuition, state resident: full-time $11,664; part-time $432 per credit hour. Tuition, nonresident: full-time $19,197; part-time $711 per credit hour. *Required fees:* $1446; $443 per quarter. One-time fee: $300. Tuition and fees vary according to course load and program. *Financial support:* Fellowships, research assistantships, teaching assistantships, career-related internships or fieldwork, Federal Work-Study, and institutionally sponsored loans available. Support available to part-time students. Financial award application deadline: 2/1. *Faculty research:* Genetics, physiology, biotechnology, pathogenic microbiology, plant virology. *Unit head:* Dr. Theo W. Dreher, Chair, 541-737-4441 Ext. 541, Fax: 541-737-0496, E-mail: theo.dreher@oregonstate.edu. *Application contact:* Dina Stoneman, Microbiology Advisor, 541-737-1830, E-mail: dina.stoneman@oregonstate.edu.
Website: http://microbiology.science.oregonstate.edu/

Penn State University Park, Graduate School, Eberly College of Science, Department of Biochemistry and Molecular Biology, University Park, PA 16802. Offers biochemistry, microbiology, and molecular biology (MS, PhD); biotechnology (MBIOT). *Unit head:* Dr. Daniel J. Larson, Dean, 814-865-9591, Fax: 814-865-3634, E-mail: djlarson@psu.edu. *Application contact:* Cynthia E. Nicosia, Director, Graduate Enrollment Services, 814-865-1834, Fax: 814-863-4627, E-mail: cey1@psu.edu.
Website: http://bmb.psu.edu/

Purdue University, Graduate School, College of Science, Department of Biological Sciences, West Lafayette, IN 47907. Offers biochemistry (PhD); biophysics (PhD); cell and developmental biology (PhD); ecology, evolutionary and population biology (MS, PhD), including ecology, evolutionary biology, population biology; genetics (MS, PhD); microbiology (MS, PhD); molecular biology (PhD); neurobiology (MS, PhD); plant physiology (PhD). *Faculty:* 50 full-time (13 women), 5 part-time/adjunct (1 woman). *Students:* 111 full-time (61 women), 5 part-time (0 women); includes 9 minority (1 Black or African American, non-Hispanic/Latino; 5 Asian, non-Hispanic/Latino; 3 Hispanic/Latino), 62 international. Average age 27. 170 applicants, 19% accepted, 17 enrolled. In 2013, 9 master's, 18 doctorates awarded. Terminal master's awarded for partial completion of doctoral program. *Degree requirements:* For master's, thesis (for some programs); for doctorate, thesis/dissertation, seminars, teaching experience. *Entrance requirements:* For master's, GRE General Test (minimum analytical writing score of 3.5), minimum undergraduate GPA of 3.0; for doctorate, GRE General Test (minimum analytical writing score of 3.5), minimum undergraduate GPA of 3.5. Additional exam requirements/recommendations for international students: Required—TOEFL (minimum score 600 paper-based; 107 iBT for MS, 80 iBT for PhD). *Application deadline:* For fall admission, 12/7 for domestic and international students. Applications are processed on a rolling basis. Application fee: $60 ($75 for international students). Electronic applications accepted. *Financial support:* Fellowships, research assistantships, and teaching assistantships available. Support available to part-time students. Financial award application deadline: 2/15; financial award applicants required to submit FAFSA. *Unit head:* Dr. Richard J. Kuhn, Head, 765-494-4407, E-mail: kuhnr@purdue.edu. *Application contact:* Georgina E. Rupp, Graduate Coordinator, 765-494-8142, Fax: 765-494-0876, E-mail: ruppg@purdue.edu.
Website: http://www.bio.purdue.edu/

Purdue University, Graduate School, PULSe - Purdue University Life Sciences Program, West Lafayette, IN 47907. Offers biomolecular structure and biophysics (PhD); biotechnology (PhD); chemical biology (PhD); chromatin and regulation of gene expression (PhD); integrative neuroscience (PhD); integrative plant sciences (PhD); membrane biology (PhD); microbiology (PhD); molecular evolutionary and cancer biology (PhD); molecular evolutionary genetics (PhD); molecular virology (PhD). *Students:* 154 full-time (78 women), 1 part-time (0 women); includes 23 minority (5 Black or African American, non-Hispanic/Latino; 5 Asian, non-Hispanic/Latino; 10 Hispanic/Latino; 3 Two or more races, non-Hispanic/Latino), 73 international. Average age 26. 239 applicants, 33% accepted, 40 enrolled. *Entrance requirements:* For doctorate, GRE, minimum undergraduate GPA of 3.0. Additional exam requirements/recommendations for international students: Required—TOEFL (minimum score 550 paper-based; 77 iBT). *Application deadline:* For fall admission, 1/15 priority date for domestic and international students. Applications are processed on a rolling basis. Application fee: $60 ($75 for international students). Electronic applications accepted. *Financial support:* In 2013–14, research assistantships with tuition reimbursements (averaging $22,500 per year), teaching assistantships with tuition reimbursements (averaging $22,500 per year) were awarded. *Unit head:* Dr. Christine A. Hrycyna, Head, 765-494-7322, E-mail: hrycyna@purdue.edu. *Application contact:* Colleen Gabauer, Graduate Contact, 765-494-9256, E-mail: cgabauer@purdue.edu.
Website: http://www.gradschool.purdue.edu/pulse

Purdue University, School of Veterinary Medicine and Graduate School, Graduate Programs in Veterinary Medicine, Department of Comparative Pathobiology, West Lafayette, IN 47907-2027. Offers comparative epidemiology and public health (MS); comparative epidemiology and public heath (PhD); comparative microbiology and immunology (MS, PhD); comparative pathobiology (MS, PhD); interdisciplinary studies (PhD), including microbial pathogenesis, molecular signaling and cancer biology, molecular virology; lab animal medicine (MS); veterinary anatomic pathology (MS); veterinary clinical pathology (MS). Terminal master's awarded for partial completion of doctoral program. *Degree requirements:* For master's, thesis (for some programs); for doctorate, thesis/dissertation. *Entrance requirements:* For master's and doctorate, GRE General Test. Additional exam requirements/recommendations for international students: Required—TOEFL (minimum score 575 paper-based), IELTS (minimum score 6.5), TWE (minimum score 4). Electronic applications accepted.

Queen's University at Kingston, School of Graduate Studies, Faculty of Health Sciences, Department of Microbiology and Immunology, Kingston, ON K7L 3N6, Canada. Offers M Sc, PhD. Part-time programs available. *Degree requirements:* For master's, thesis; for doctorate, comprehensive exam, thesis/dissertation. *Entrance requirements:* For master's and doctorate, minimum B+ average. Additional exam requirements/recommendations for international students: Required—TOEFL (minimum score 600 paper-based). Electronic applications accepted. *Faculty research:* Bacteriology, virology, immunology, education in microbiology and immunology, microbial pathogenesis.

Quinnipiac University, School of Health Sciences, Program in Medical Laboratory Sciences, Hamden, CT 06518-1940. Offers biomedical sciences (MHS); laboratory management (MHS); microbiology (MHS). Part-time and evening/weekend programs available. *Faculty:* 14 full-time (6 women), 20 part-time/adjunct (8 women). *Students:* 66 full-time (36 women), 30 part-time (13 women); includes 20 minority (7 Black or African American, non-Hispanic/Latino; 8 Asian, non-Hispanic/Latino; 4 Hispanic/Latino; 1 Two or more races, non-Hispanic/Latino), 41 international. 79 applicants, 73% accepted, 38 enrolled. In 2013, 47 master's awarded. *Degree requirements:* For master's, comprehensive exam, thesis optional. *Entrance requirements:* For master's, minimum GPA of 2.75; bachelor's degree in biological, medical, or health sciences. Additional exam requirements/recommendations for international students: Required—TOEFL (minimum score 575 paper-based; 90 iBT), IELTS (minimum score 6.5). *Application deadline:* For fall admission, 7/30 priority date for domestic students, 4/30 priority date for international students; for spring admission, 12/15 priority date for domestic students, 9/15 priority date for international students. Applications are processed on a rolling basis. Application fee: $45. Electronic applications accepted. *Expenses: Tuition:* Part-time $920 per credit. *Required fees:* $37 per credit. *Financial support:* In 2013–14, 7 students received support. Career-related internships or fieldwork, Federal Work-Study, scholarships/grants, and unspecified assistantships available. Support available to part-time students. Financial award application deadline: 6/1; financial award applicants required to submit FAFSA. *Faculty research:* ACL injury mechanism and running injuries and performance; transcriptional activators upstream stimulatory factor (USF); identification of novel antimicrobials; vaccines, formites and opportunistic pathogens; molecular biology of the Lyme Disease agent, Borrelia burgdorferi; molecular and microscopic techniques in host-pathogen interactions; non-invasive vascular biology, external pneumatic compression, sports performance. *Application contact:* Office of Graduate Admissions, 800-462-1944, Fax: 203-582-3443, E-mail: graduate@quinnipiac.edu.
Website: http://www.quinnipiac.edu/gradmedlab

Rosalind Franklin University of Medicine and Science, School of Graduate and Postdoctoral Studies - Interdisciplinary Graduate Program in Biomedical Sciences, Department of Microbiology and Immunology, North Chicago, IL 60064-3095. Offers MS, PhD, MD/PhD. Terminal master's awarded for partial completion of doctoral program. *Degree requirements:* For master's, comprehensive exam, thesis; for doctorate, comprehensive exam, thesis/dissertation. *Entrance requirements:* For master's and doctorate, GRE General Test. Additional exam requirements/recommendations for international students: Required—TOEFL, TWE. *Faculty research:* Molecular biology, parasitology, virology.

Rush University, Graduate College, Division of Immunology and Microbiology, Chicago, IL 60612-3832. Offers microbiology (PhD); virology (MS, PhD), including immunology, virology; MD/PhD. *Degree requirements:* For doctorate, thesis/dissertation, comprehensive preliminary exam. *Entrance requirements:* For doctorate, GRE General Test, interview, minimum GPA of 3.0. Additional exam requirements/recommendations for international students: Required—TOEFL. *Faculty research:* Immune interactions of cells and membranes, HIV immunopathogenesis, autoimmunity, tumor biology.

Rutgers, The State University of New Jersey, Newark, Graduate School of Biomedical Sciences, Department of Microbiology and Molecular Genetics, Newark, NJ 07107. Offers PhD. *Degree requirements:* For doctorate, thesis/dissertation, qualifying exam. *Entrance requirements:* For doctorate, GRE General Test. Additional exam requirements/recommendations for international students: Required—TOEFL. Electronic applications accepted. *Faculty research:* Molecular genetics of yeast, mutagenesis and carcinogenesis of DNA, bacterial protein synthesis, mammalian cell genetics, adenovirus gene expression.

Rutgers, The State University of New Jersey, New Brunswick, Graduate School-New Brunswick, Programs in the Molecular Biosciences, Piscataway, NJ 08854-8097. Offers biochemistry (PhD); cell and developmental biology (MS, PhD); microbiology and molecular genetics (MS, PhD), including applied microbiology, clinical microbiology (MS), clinical mircobiology (PhD), computational molecular biology (PhD), immunology, microbial biochemistry, molecular genetics, virology. MS, PhD offered jointly with University of Medicine and Dentistry of New Jersey.

Rutgers, The State University of New Jersey, New Brunswick, Graduate School of Biomedical Sciences, Program in Microbiology and Molecular Genetics, Piscataway, NJ 08854-5635. Offers MS, PhD, MD/PhD. Terminal master's awarded for partial completion of doctoral program. *Degree requirements:* For master's, thesis, qualifying exam; for doctorate, thesis/dissertation, qualifying exam. *Entrance requirements:* For master's and doctorate, GRE General Test. Additional exam requirements/recommendations for international students: Required—TOEFL. Electronic applications accepted. *Faculty research:* Interferon, receptors, retrovirus evolution, Arbo virus/host cell interactions.

Saint Louis University, Graduate Education and School of Medicine, Graduate Program in Biomedical Sciences, Department of Molecular Microbiology and Immunology, St. Louis, MO 63103-2097. Offers PhD. *Degree requirements:* For doctorate, comprehensive exam, thesis/dissertation, qualifying exams. *Entrance requirements:* For doctorate, GRE General Test (GRE Subject Test optional), letters of recommendation, resume, interview. Additional exam requirements/recommendations for international students: Required—TOEFL (minimum score 525 paper-based). Electronic applications accepted. *Faculty research:* Pathogenesis of hepatitis C virus, herperviruses, pox viruses, rheumatoid arthritis, antiviral drugs and vaccines in biodefense, cancer gene therapy, virology and immunology.

San Diego State University, Graduate and Research Affairs, College of Sciences, Department of Biology, Program in Microbiology, San Diego, CA 92182. Offers MS. *Degree requirements:* For master's, thesis, oral exam. *Entrance requirements:* For master's, GRE General Test, GRE Subject Test, resume or curriculum vitae, 2 letters of recommendation. Additional exam requirements/recommendations for international students: Required—TOEFL. Electronic applications accepted.

San Francisco State University, Division of Graduate Studies, College of Science and Engineering, Department of Biology, Program in Microbiology, San Francisco, CA 94132-1722. Offers MS. *Application deadline:* Applications are processed on a rolling basis. *Unit head:* Dr. Diana Chu, Program Coordinator, 415-405-3487, E-mail: chud@sfsu.edu. *Application contact:* Dr. Robert Patterson, Graduate Coordinator, 415-338-1100, E-mail: patters@sfsu.edu.
Website: http://biology.sfsu.edu/graduate/microbiology

San Jose State University, Graduate Studies and Research, College of Science, Department of Biological Sciences, San Jose, CA 95192-0001. Offers biological sciences (MA, MS); molecular biology and microbiology (MS); organismal biology, conservation and ecology (MS); physiology (MS). Part-time programs available. *Entrance requirements:* For master's, GRE. Electronic applications accepted. *Faculty research:* Systemic physiology, molecular genetics, SEM studies, toxicology, large mammal ecology.

Seton Hall University, College of Arts and Sciences, Department of Biological Sciences, South Orange, NJ 07079-2697. Offers biology (MS); biology/business administration (MS); microbiology (MS); molecular bioscience (PhD); molecular bioscience/neuroscience (PhD). Part-time and evening/weekend programs available. *Degree requirements:* For master's, thesis optional; for doctorate, comprehensive exam, thesis/dissertation. *Entrance requirements:* For master's and doctorate, GRE or MS from accredited university in the U.S. Additional exam requirements/recommendations for international students: Required—TOEFL. Electronic applications accepted. *Faculty research:* Neurobiology, genetics, immunology, molecular biology, cellular physiology, toxicology, microbiology, bioinformatics.

South Dakota State University, Graduate School, College of Agriculture and Biological Sciences, Department of Biology and Microbiology, Brookings, SD 57007. Offers biological sciences (MS, PhD). Part-time programs available. *Degree requirements:* For master's, thesis (for some programs), oral exam; for doctorate, comprehensive exam, thesis/dissertation, oral exam. *Entrance requirements:* For master's and doctorate, GRE General Test. Additional exam requirements/recommendations for international students: Required—TOEFL (minimum score 600 paper-based; 100 iBT). *Faculty research:* Ecosystem ecology; plant, animal and microbial genomics; animal infectious disease, microbial bioproducts.

Southern Illinois University Carbondale, Graduate School, College of Science, Program in Molecular Biology, Microbiology, and Biochemistry, Carbondale, IL 62901-4701. Offers MS, PhD. *Faculty:* 16 full-time (2 women). *Students:* 40 full-time (27 women), 39 part-time (21 women); includes 6 minority (2 Black or African American, non-Hispanic/Latino; 4 Asian, non-Hispanic/Latino), 50 international. Average age 25. 143 applicants, 6% accepted, 5 enrolled. In 2013, 5 master's, 4 doctorates awarded. *Degree requirements:* For master's, thesis; for doctorate, thesis/dissertation. *Entrance requirements:* For master's, GRE, minimum GPA of 2.7; for doctorate, GRE, minimum GPA of 3.25. Additional exam requirements/recommendations for international students: Required—TOEFL. *Application deadline:* Applications are processed on a rolling basis. Application fee: $50. *Financial support:* In 2013–14, 40 students received support, including 3 fellowships with full tuition reimbursements available, 24 research assistantships with full tuition reimbursements available, 12 teaching assistantships with full tuition reimbursements available; Federal Work-Study and institutionally sponsored loans also available. Support available to part-time students. Financial award application deadline: 3/1. *Faculty research:* Prokaryotic gene regulation and expression; eukaryotic gene regulation; microbial, phylogenetic, and metabolic diversity; immune responses to tumors, pathogens, and autoantigens; protein folding and structure. *Unit head:* Dr. Judy Davie, Director, 618-453-5002, E-mail: jdavie@siumed.edu. *Application contact:* Cindy Filla, Office Systems Specialist, 618-453-8911, E-mail: cfilla@siumed.edu.
Website: http://mbmb.siu.edu/

Southwestern Oklahoma State University, College of Professional and Graduate Studies, School of Behavioral Sciences and Education, Specialization in Health Sciences and Microbiology, Weatherford, OK 73096-3098. Offers M Ed.

Stanford University, School of Medicine, Graduate Programs in Medicine, Department of Microbiology and Immunology, Stanford, CA 94305-9991. Offers PhD. *Degree requirements:* For doctorate, comprehensive exam, thesis/dissertation, 2 quarters teaching assistantship. *Entrance requirements:* For doctorate, GRE General Test, GRE Subject Test (biology or biochemistry). Additional exam requirements/recommendations for international students: Required—TOEFL. Electronic applications accepted. *Expenses: Tuition:* Full-time $42,690; part-time $949 per credit. *Required fees:* $185. *Faculty research:* Molecular pathogenesis of bacteria viruses and parasites, immune system function, autoimmunity, molecular biology.

State University of New York Upstate Medical University, College of Graduate Studies, Program in Microbiology and Immunology, Syracuse, NY 13210-2334. Offers microbiology (MS); microbiology and immunology (PhD); MD/PhD. Terminal master's awarded for partial completion of doctoral program. *Degree requirements:* For master's, thesis; for doctorate, comprehensive exam, thesis/dissertation. *Entrance requirements:* For master's, GRE General Test, interview; for doctorate, GRE General Test, telephone interview. Additional exam requirements/recommendations for international students: Required—TOEFL. Electronic applications accepted. *Faculty research:* Cancer, disorders of the nervous system, infectious diseases, diabetes/metabolic disorders/cardiovascular diseases.

Stony Brook University, State University of New York, Stony Brook University Medical Center, Health Sciences Center, School of Medicine and Graduate School, Graduate Programs in Medicine, Department of Molecular Genetics and Microbiology, Stony Brook, NY 11794. Offers PhD. *Faculty:* 18 full-time (5 women), 1 (woman) part-time/adjunct. *Students:* 25 full-time (7 women); includes 7 minority (5 Asian, non-Hispanic/Latino; 2 Hispanic/Latino), 4 international. Average age 27. 56 applicants, 23% accepted, 5 enrolled. In 2013, 7 doctorates awarded. *Degree requirements:* For doctorate, comprehensive exam, thesis/dissertation. *Entrance requirements:* For doctorate, GRE General Test, GRE Subject Test, undergraduate training in biochemistry, genetics, and cell biology; recommendations; personal statement. Additional exam requirements/recommendations for international students: Required—TOEFL (minimum score 550 paper-based; 90 iBT). *Application deadline:* For fall admission, 1/15 for domestic students; for spring admission, 10/1 for domestic students. Application fee: $100. *Expenses:* Tuition, state resident: full-time $9870; part-time $411 per credit. Tuition, nonresident: full-time $18,350; part-time $765 per credit. *Financial support:* In 2013–14, 17 fellowships, 8 research assistantships were awarded; teaching assistantships and Federal Work-Study also available. Financial award application deadline: 3/15. *Faculty research:* Adenovirus molecular genetics, molecular biology of tumors, virus SV40, mechanism of tumor infection by SAV virus. *Total annual research expenditures:* $9.9 million. *Unit head:* Dr. Jorge Benach, Chair, 631-632-4225, Fax: 631-632-9797, E-mail: jorge.benach@stonybrook.edu. *Application contact:* Kathryn Bell, Graduate Program Director, 631-632-8812, Fax: 631-632-9797, E-mail: kathryn.bell@stonybrook.edu.
Website: http://www.mgm.stonybrook.edu/index.shtml

Texas A&M Health Science Center, College of Medicine, Department of Microbial and Molecular Pathogenesis, College Station, TX 77840. Offers immunology (PhD);

microbiology (PhD); molecular biology (PhD); virology (PhD). *Degree requirements:* For doctorate, thesis/dissertation. *Entrance requirements:* For doctorate, GRE General Test, minimum GPA of 3.0. *Faculty research:* Molecular pathogenesis, microbial therapeutics.

Texas A&M University, College of Science, Department of Biology, College Station, TX 77843. Offers biology (MS, PhD); botany (MS, PhD); microbiology (MS, PhD); zoology (MS, PhD). *Faculty:* 40. *Students:* 94 full-time (54 women), 7 part-time (4 women); includes 10 minority (1 Black or African American, non-Hispanic/Latino; 3 Asian, non-Hispanic/Latino; 6 Hispanic/Latino), 49 international. Average age 29. 120 applicants, 25% accepted, 19 enrolled. In 2013, 5 master's, 16 doctorates awarded. *Degree requirements:* For master's, thesis or alternative; for doctorate, comprehensive exam, thesis/dissertation. *Entrance requirements:* For master's and doctorate, GRE General Test. Additional exam requirements/recommendations for international students: Required—TOEFL. *Application deadline:* For fall admission, 1/15 for domestic students. Applications are processed on a rolling basis. Application fee: $50 ($75 for international students). Electronic applications accepted. *Expenses:* Tuition, state resident: full-time $4078; part-time $226.55 per credit hour. Tuition, nonresident: full-time $10,450; part-time $580.55 per credit hour. *Required fees:* $2328; $278.50 per credit hour. $642.45 per semester. *Financial support:* Fellowships, research assistantships, and teaching assistantships available. Financial award application deadline: 4/1; financial award applicants required to submit FAFSA. *Unit head:* Dr. Tom McKnight, Department Head, 979-845-3896, Fax: 979-845-2891, E-mail: mcknight@bio.tamu.edu. *Application contact:* Dr. Arne Lekven, Graduate Advisor, 979-458-3461, Fax: 979-845-2891, E-mail: alekven@bio.tamu.edu.
Website: http://www.bio.tamu.edu/index.html

Texas A&M University, College of Veterinary Medicine and Biomedical Sciences, Department of Veterinary Pathobiology, College Station, TX 77843. Offers veterinary microbiology (PhD); veterinary pathobiology (PhD); veterinary pathology (PhD). Part-time programs available. Postbaccalaureate distance learning degree programs offered. *Faculty:* 31. *Students:* 30 full-time (23 women), 14 part-time (12 women); includes 9 minority (2 Black or African American, non-Hispanic/Latino; 2 Asian, non-Hispanic/Latino; 4 Hispanic/Latino; 1 Two or more races, non-Hispanic/Latino), 9 international. Average age 30. 9 applicants, 100% accepted, 9 enrolled. In 2013, 4 doctorates awarded. Terminal master's awarded for partial completion of doctoral program. *Degree requirements:* For doctorate, thesis/dissertation, seminars. *Entrance requirements:* For doctorate, GRE General Test, minimum GPA of 3.0 in last 60 hours. Additional exam requirements/recommendations for international students: Required—TOEFL. *Application deadline:* For fall admission, 3/1 priority date for domestic students; for spring admission, 8/1 priority date for domestic students. Applications are processed on a rolling basis. Application fee: $50 ($75 for international students). Electronic applications accepted. *Expenses:* Tuition, state resident: full-time $4078; part-time $226.55 per credit hour. Tuition, nonresident: full-time $10,450; part-time $580.55 per credit hour. *Required fees:* $2328; $278.50 per credit hour. $642.45 per semester. *Financial support:* In 2013–14, fellowships with partial tuition reimbursements (averaging $16,000 per year), research assistantships with partial tuition reimbursements (averaging $15,400 per year), teaching assistantships with partial tuition reimbursements (averaging $16,000 per year) were awarded; Federal Work-Study, institutionally sponsored loans, scholarships/grants, traineeships, health care benefits, and unspecified assistantships also available. Support available to part-time students. Financial award applicants required to submit FAFSA. *Faculty research:* Infectious and noninfectious diseases of animals and birds, animal genetics, molecular biology, immunology, virology. *Unit head:* Dr. Linda Logan, Head, 979-862-6559, Fax: 979-845-9231, E-mail: llogan@cvm.tamu.edu. *Application contact:* Dr. Patricia Holman, Graduate Advisor, 979-845-4202, Fax: 979-845-9231, E-mail: pholman@cvm.tamu.edu.
Website: http://vetmed.tamu.edu/vtpb

Texas Tech University, Graduate School, College of Arts and Sciences, Department of Biological Sciences, Lubbock, TX 79409-3131. Offers biology (MS, PhD); environmental sustainability and natural resources management (PSM); microbiology (MS); zoology (MS, PhD). Part-time programs available. *Faculty:* 37 full-time (6 women), 1 (woman) part-time/adjunct. *Students:* 93 full-time (50 women), 10 part-time (7 women); includes 7 minority (1 Black or African American, non-Hispanic/Latino; 3 Asian, non-Hispanic/Latino; 3 Hispanic/Latino), 45 international. Average age 30. 59 applicants, 32% accepted, 7 enrolled. In 2013, 13 master's, 12 doctorates awarded. *Degree requirements:* For master's, thesis or alternative; for doctorate, thesis/dissertation. *Entrance requirements:* For master's and doctorate, GRE General Test. Additional exam requirements/recommendations for international students: Required—TOEFL (minimum score 550 paper-based; 79 iBT). *Application deadline:* For fall admission, 6/1 priority date for domestic students, 1/15 priority date for international students; for spring admission, 9/1 priority date for domestic students, 6/15 priority date for international students. Applications are processed on a rolling basis. Application fee: $60. Electronic applications accepted. *Expenses:* Tuition, state resident: full-time $6062; part-time $252.57 per credit hour. Tuition, nonresident: full-time $14,558; part-time $606.57 per credit hour. *Required fees:* $2655; $35 per credit hour. $907.50 per semester. Tuition and fees vary according to course load. *Financial support:* In 2013–14, 100 students received support, including 69 fellowships (averaging $1,404 per year), 16 research assistantships (averaging $4,232 per year), 78 teaching assistantships (averaging $4,702 per year). Financial award application deadline: 4/15; financial award applicants required to submit FAFSA. *Faculty research:* Biodiversity and evolution, climate change in arid ecosystems, plant biology and biotechnology, animal communication and behavior, zoonotic and emerging diseases. *Total annual research expenditures:* $2.1 million. *Unit head:* Dr. Llewellyn D. Densmore, Chair, 806-742-2715, Fax: 806-742-2963, E-mail: lou.densmore@ttu.edu. *Application contact:* Dr. Randall M. Jeter, Graduate Adviser, 806-742-2710 Ext. 270, Fax: 806-742-2963, E-mail: randall.jeter@ttu.edu.
Website: http://www.biol.ttu.edu/default.aspx

Thomas Jefferson University, Jefferson Graduate School of Biomedical Sciences, MS Program in Microbiology, Philadelphia, PA 19107. Offers MS. Part-time and evening/weekend programs available. *Faculty:* 44 full-time (14 women), 27 part-time/adjunct (11 women). *Students:* 41 part-time (25 women); includes 6 minority (3 Black or African American, non-Hispanic/Latino; 2 Asian, non-Hispanic/Latino; 1 Hispanic/Latino), 5 international. 28 applicants, 57% accepted, 11 enrolled. In 2013, 16 master's awarded. *Degree requirements:* For master's, thesis, clerkship. *Entrance requirements:* For master's, GRE General Test or MCAT, minimum GPA of 3.0. Additional exam requirements/recommendations for international students: Required—TOEFL (minimum score 100 iBT) or IELTS (minimum score 7). *Application deadline:* For fall admission, 8/1 priority date for domestic students, 3/1 priority date for international students; for winter admission, 12/1 priority date for domestic students, 6/1 priority date for international students; for spring admission, 4/1 priority date for domestic students. Applications are processed on a rolling basis. Application fee: $75. Electronic applications accepted. *Expenses:* Contact institution. *Financial support:* Federal Work-Study and institutionally sponsored loans available. Support available to part-time students. Financial award application deadline: 5/1; financial award applicants required to submit FAFSA. *Faculty research:* Vaccinology, epidemiology, planning and management, microbiology. *Unit head:* Dr. Gerald B. Grunwald, Dean/Program Director, 215-503-4191, Fax: 215-503-6690, E-mail: gerald.grunwald@jefferson.edu. *Application contact:* Marc E. Stearns, Director of Admissions, 215-503-0155, Fax: 215-503-3433, E-mail: jgsbs-info@jefferson.edu.
Website: http://www.jefferson.edu/university/biomedical_sciences/programs/masters/microbiology.html

Thomas Jefferson University, Jefferson Graduate School of Biomedical Sciences, PhD Program in Immunology and Microbial Pathogenesis, Philadelphia, PA 19107. Offers PhD. *Faculty:* 35 full-time (5 women), 1 part-time/adjunct (0 women). *Students:* 20 full-time (8 women); includes 3 minority (2 Asian, non-Hispanic/Latino; 1 Hispanic/Latino), 2 international. 54 applicants, 11% accepted, 2 enrolled. In 2013, 4 doctorates awarded. *Degree requirements:* For doctorate, comprehensive exam, thesis/dissertation. *Entrance requirements:* For doctorate, GRE General Test, minimum GPA of 3.2. Additional exam requirements/recommendations for international students: Required—TOEFL (minimum score 100 iBT) or IELTS. *Application deadline:* For fall admission, 1/5 priority date for domestic and international students. Applications are processed on a rolling basis. Application fee: $75. Electronic applications accepted. *Financial support:* In 2013–14, 20 students received support, including 20 fellowships with full tuition reimbursements available (averaging $56,052 per year); Federal Work-Study, institutionally sponsored loans, scholarships/grants, traineeships, and stipends also available. Support available to part-time students. Financial award application deadline: 5/1; financial award applicants required to submit FAFSA. *Unit head:* Dr. Matthias Schnell, Program Director, 215-503-4634, Fax: 215-503-5393, E-mail: matthias.schnell@jefferson.edu. *Application contact:* Marc E. Stearns, Director of Admissions, 215-503-0155, Fax: 215-503-3433, E-mail: jgsbs-info@jefferson.edu.
Website: http://www.jefferson.edu/university/biomedical_sciences/programs/phd/immunology.html

Tufts University, Sackler School of Graduate Biomedical Sciences, Molecular Microbiology Program, Medford, MA 02155. Offers PhD. *Faculty:* 17 full-time (7 women). *Students:* 33 full-time (26 women); includes 8 minority (1 Black or African American, non-Hispanic/Latino; 3 Asian, non-Hispanic/Latino; 1 Hispanic/Latino; 3 Two or more races, non-Hispanic/Latino), 2 international. Average age 27. 98 applicants, 13% accepted, 6 enrolled. In 2013, 1 doctorate awarded. Terminal master's awarded for partial completion of doctoral program. *Degree requirements:* For doctorate, comprehensive exam, thesis/dissertation. *Entrance requirements:* For doctorate, GRE General Test, 3 letters of reference. Additional exam requirements/recommendations for international students: Required—TOEFL (minimum score 600 paper-based; 100 iBT). *Application deadline:* For fall admission, 12/15 for domestic and international students. Application fee: $70. Electronic applications accepted. *Financial support:* In 2013–14, 33 students received support, including 33 research assistantships with full tuition reimbursements available (averaging $31,000 per year); traineeships and health care benefits also available. Financial award application deadline: 12/15. *Faculty research:* Mechanisms of gene regulation, interactions of microorganisms and viruses with host cells, infection response. *Unit head:* Dr. Michael Malamy, Director, 617-636-6750, Fax: 617-636-0337, E-mail: michael.malamy@tufts.edu. *Application contact:* Kellie Melchin, Associate Director of Admissions, 617-636-6767, Fax: 617-636-0375, E-mail: sackler-school@tufts.edu.
Website: http://sackler.tufts.edu/Academics/Degree-Programs/PhD-Programs/Molecular-Microbiology

Tulane University, School of Medicine and School of Liberal Arts, Graduate Programs in Biomedical Sciences, Department of Microbiology and Immunology, New Orleans, LA 70118-5669. Offers MS, PhD, MD/PhD. MS and PhD offered through the Graduate School. *Degree requirements:* For master's, thesis; for doctorate, 2 foreign languages, thesis/dissertation. *Entrance requirements:* For master's, GRE General Test, minimum B average in undergraduate course work; for doctorate, GRE General Test, GRE Subject Test. Additional exam requirements/recommendations for international students: Required—TOEFL. Electronic applications accepted. *Faculty research:* Vaccine development, viral pathogenesis, molecular virology, bacterial pathogenesis, fungal pathogenesis.

Universidad Central del Caribe, School of Medicine, Program in Biomedical Sciences, Bayamón, PR 00960-6032. Offers anatomy and cell biology (MA, MS); biochemistry (MS); biomedical sciences (MA); cellular and molecular biology (PhD); microbiology and immunology (MA, MS); pharmacology (MS); physiology (MS).

Université de Montréal, Faculty of Medicine, Department of Microbiology and Immunology, Montréal, QC H3C 3J7, Canada. Offers M Sc, PhD. Programs offered jointly with Faculty of Veterinary Medicine and Université du Québec, Institut Armand-Frappier. Terminal master's awarded for partial completion of doctoral program. *Degree requirements:* For master's, thesis; for doctorate, thesis/dissertation, general exam. *Entrance requirements:* For master's and doctorate, proficiency in French, knowledge of English. Electronic applications accepted.

Université de Sherbrooke, Faculty of Medicine and Health Sciences, Graduate Programs in Medicine, Program in Microbiology, Sherbrooke, QC J1H 5N4, Canada. Offers M Sc, PhD. Terminal master's awarded for partial completion of doctoral program. *Degree requirements:* For master's, thesis; for doctorate, thesis/dissertation. Electronic applications accepted. *Faculty research:* Oncogenes, alternative splicing mechanisms, genomics, telomerase, DNA repair, Clostridium difficile, Campylobacter jejuni.

Université du Québec, Institut National de la Recherche Scientifique, Graduate Programs, Research Center–INRS–Institut Armand-Frappier, Laval, QC H7V 1B7, Canada. Offers applied microbiology (M Sc); biology (PhD); experimental health sciences (M Sc); virology and immunology (M Sc, PhD). Programs given in French. Part-time programs available. *Faculty:* 45 full-time. *Students:* 126 full-time (78 women), 11 part-time (7 women), 52 international. Average age 30. In 2013, 19 master's, 12 doctorates awarded. *Degree requirements:* For master's, thesis; for doctorate, thesis/dissertation. *Entrance requirements:* For master's, appropriate bachelor's degree, proficiency in French; for doctorate, appropriate master's degree, proficiency in French. *Application deadline:* For fall admission, 3/30 for domestic and international students; for winter admission, 11/1 for domestic and international students; for spring admission, 3/1 for domestic and international students. Application fee: $45 Canadian dollars. Electronic applications accepted. *Financial support:* In 2013–14, fellowships (averaging $16,500 per year) were awarded; research assistantships also available. *Faculty research:* Immunity, infection and cancer; toxicology and environmental biotechnology; molecular pharmacochemistry. *Unit head:* Charles Dozois, Director, 450-687-5010, Fax: 450-686-5566, E-mail: charles.dozois@iaf.inrs.ca. *Application contact:* Sylvie Richard, Registrar, 418-654-2518, Fax: 418-654-3858, E-mail: sylvie.richard@adm.inrs.ca.
Website: http://www.iaf.inrs.ca

Université Laval, Faculty of Agricultural and Food Sciences, Program in Agricultural Microbiology, Québec, QC G1K 7P4, Canada. Offers agricultural microbiology (M Sc); agro-food microbiology (PhD). Terminal master's awarded for partial completion of doctoral program. *Degree requirements:* For master's, thesis; for doctorate, comprehensive exam, thesis/dissertation. *Entrance requirements:* For master's and doctorate, knowledge of French and English. Electronic applications accepted.

Université Laval, Faculty of Medicine, Graduate Programs in Medicine, Programs in Microbiology-Immunology, Québec, QC G1K 7P4, Canada. Offers M Sc, PhD. Terminal master's awarded for partial completion of doctoral program. *Degree requirements:* For master's, thesis; for doctorate, comprehensive exam, thesis/dissertation. *Entrance requirements:* For master's and doctorate, knowledge of French, comprehension of written English. Electronic applications accepted.

Université Laval, Faculty of Sciences and Engineering, Department of Biochemistry and Microbiology, Programs in Microbiology, Québec, QC G1K 7P4, Canada. Offers M Sc, PhD. Terminal master's awarded for partial completion of doctoral program. *Degree requirements:* For master's, thesis; for doctorate, comprehensive exam, thesis/dissertation. *Entrance requirements:* For master's and doctorate, knowledge of French, comprehension of written English. Electronic applications accepted.

University at Buffalo, the State University of New York, Graduate School, School of Medicine and Biomedical Sciences, Graduate Programs in Medicine and Biomedical Sciences, Department of Microbiology and Immunology, Buffalo, NY 14260. Offers MA, PhD. *Faculty:* 14 full-time (4 women). *Students:* 23 full-time (15 women); includes 8 minority (2 Black or African American, non-Hispanic/Latino; 6 Asian, non-Hispanic/Latino), 7 international. Average age 28. 20 applicants, 15% accepted, 2 enrolled. In 2013, 1 master's, 2 doctorates awarded. *Degree requirements:* For master's, comprehensive exam; for doctorate, thesis/dissertation, departmental qualifying exam. *Entrance requirements:* For master's and doctorate, GRE General Test, 3 letters of recommendation. Additional exam requirements/recommendations for international students: Required—TOEFL (minimum score 100 iBT). *Application deadline:* For fall admission, 5/1 priority date for domestic and international students. Applications are processed on a rolling basis. Application fee: $75. Electronic applications accepted. *Financial support:* In 2013–14, 2 students received support, including 2 fellowships with tuition reimbursements available (averaging $28,000 per year), 12 research assistantships with tuition reimbursements available (averaging $25,000 per year), 1 teaching assistantship with tuition reimbursement available (averaging $25,000 per year); Federal Work-Study, institutionally sponsored loans, traineeships, health care benefits, and unspecified assistantships also available. Financial award application deadline: 2/1; financial award applicants required to submit FAFSA. *Faculty research:* Bacteriology, immunology, parasitology, virology, mycology. *Total annual research expenditures:* $2.6 million. *Unit head:* Dr. James Bangs, Chair/Professor, 716-829-2907, Fax: 716-829-2158. *Application contact:* Dr. Anders Hakansson, Director of Graduate Studies, 716-829-2176, Fax: 716-829-2158.
Website: http://www.smbs.buffalo.edu/microb/

The University of Alabama at Birmingham, Graduate Programs in Joint Health Sciences, Program in Microbiology, Birmingham, AL 35294. Offers PhD. *Degree requirements:* For doctorate, thesis/dissertation. *Entrance requirements:* For doctorate, GRE General Test, interview, evaluations. Electronic applications accepted.

University of Alberta, Faculty of Graduate Studies and Research, Department of Biological Sciences, Edmonton, AB T6G 2E1, Canada. Offers environmental biology and ecology (M Sc, PhD); microbiology and biotechnology (M Sc, PhD); molecular biology and genetics (M Sc, PhD); physiology and cell biology (M Sc, PhD); plant biology (M Sc, PhD); systematics and evolution (M Sc, PhD). Terminal master's awarded for partial completion of doctoral program. *Degree requirements:* For master's, thesis; for doctorate, thesis/dissertation. *Entrance requirements:* Additional exam requirements/recommendations for international students: Required—TOEFL.

The University of Arizona, College of Agriculture and Life Sciences, Program in Microbiology, Tucson, AZ 85721. Offers MS, PhD. *Students:* 8 full-time (6 women), 2 part-time (1 woman); includes 4 minority (1 Asian, non-Hispanic/Latino; 2 Hispanic/Latino; 1 Two or more races, non-Hispanic/Latino), 1 international. Average age 27. 32 applicants, 13% accepted, 2 enrolled. *Degree requirements:* For master's, thesis; for doctorate, comprehensive exam, thesis/dissertation. *Entrance requirements:* For master's and doctorate, GRE, minimum GPA of 3.0, 3 letters of recommendation, letter of intent. Additional exam requirements/recommendations for international students: Required—TOEFL (minimum score 550 paper-based; 79 iBT). *Application deadline:* For fall admission, 2/28 for domestic students, 12/1 for international students. Application fee: $75. Electronic applications accepted. *Expenses:* Tuition, state resident: full-time $11,526. Tuition, nonresident: full-time $27,398. *Financial support:* In 2013–14, 8 research assistantships (averaging $14,689 per year), 7 teaching assistantships (averaging $17,255 per year) were awarded; health care benefits and unspecified assistantships also available. Financial award application deadline: 3/22. *Total annual research expenditures:* $2.7 million. *Unit head:* Dr. Charles Sterling, Head, 520-621-4580, E-mail: csterlin@email.arizona.edu. *Application contact:* Kathryn Johansen, Administrative Assistant, 520-621-4507, E-mail: millerk@email.arizona.edu.
Website: http://microvet.arizona.edu

The University of Arizona, College of Medicine, Department of Immunobiology, Tucson, AZ 85721. Offers MS, PhD. *Faculty:* 10 full-time (2 women). *Students:* 8 full-time (5 women); includes 1 minority (Asian, non-Hispanic/Latino), 2 international. Average age 27. 91 applicants, 66% accepted. In 2013, 1 master's, 2 doctorates awarded. *Degree requirements:* For master's, thesis; for doctorate, thesis/dissertation. *Entrance requirements:* For master's and doctorate, GRE General Test, minimum GPA of 3.0. *Application deadline:* For fall admission, 3/1 priority date for domestic students; for spring admission, 9/1 for domestic students. Application fee: $75. *Expenses:* Tuition, state resident: full-time $11,526. Tuition, nonresident: full-time $27,398. *Financial support:* In 2013–14, 4 research assistantships with full tuition reimbursements (averaging $25,000 per year) were awarded; fellowships with full tuition reimbursements, teaching assistantships with full tuition reimbursements, institutionally sponsored loans, and tuition waivers (full) also available. Financial award application deadline: 4/30. *Faculty research:* Environmental and pathogenic microbiology, molecular biology. *Total annual research expenditures:* $2.3 million. *Unit head:* Dr. Janko Nikolich-Zugich, Head, 520-626-6065, Fax: 520-626-2100, E-mail: nikolich@email.arizona.edu. *Application contact:* Dr. Richard J. Ablin, Graduate Program Chairman, 520-626-7755, E-mail: ablinrj@email.arizona.edu.
Website: http://immunobiology.arizona.edu/

University of Arkansas for Medical Sciences, Graduate School, Little Rock, AR 72205. Offers biochemistry and molecular biology (MS, PhD); bioinformatics (MS, PhD); cellular physiology and molecular biophysics (MS, PhD); clinical nutrition (MS); interdisciplinary biomedical sciences (MS, PhD, Certificate); interdisciplinary toxicology (MS); microbiology and immunology (PhD); neurobiology and developmental sciences (PhD); pharmacology (PhD); MD/PhD. Bioinformatics programs hosted jointly with the University of Arkansas at Little Rock. Part-time programs available. *Faculty:* 397 full-time (205 women). *Students:* 196 full-time (126 women), 117 part-time (87 women); includes 65 minority (38 Black or African American, non-Hispanic/Latino; 1 American Indian or Alaska Native, non-Hispanic/Latino; 21 Asian, non-Hispanic/Latino; 4 Hispanic/Latino; 1 Two or more races, non-Hispanic/Latino), 57 international. 455 applicants, 27% accepted, 89 enrolled. In 2013, 41 master's, 18 doctorates, 28 other advanced degrees awarded. Terminal master's awarded for partial completion of doctoral program. *Degree requirements:* For master's, comprehensive exam (for some programs), thesis (for some programs); for doctorate, thesis/dissertation. *Entrance requirements:* For master's and doctorate, GRE. Additional exam requirements/recommendations for international students: Required—TOEFL. *Application deadline:* Applications are processed on a rolling basis. Application fee: $0. Electronic applications accepted. *Expenses:* Contact institution. *Financial support:* In 2013–14, 120 research assistantships (averaging $24,000 per year) were awarded; career-related internships or fieldwork, Federal Work-Study, and traineeships also available. Support available to part-time students. Financial award applicants required to submit FAFSA. *Unit head:* Dr. Robert E. McGehee, Jr., Dean, 501-686-5454. *Application contact:* Dr. Kristen Sterba, Assistant Dean, Office of Graduate Student Recruiting and Retention, 501-526-7396, E-mail: kmsterba@uams.edu.
Website: http://www.uams.edu/gradschool/

The University of British Columbia, Faculty of Science, Department of Microbiology and Immunology, Vancouver, BC V6T 1Z1, Canada. Offers M Sc, PhD. *Degree requirements:* For master's, thesis; for doctorate, comprehensive exam, thesis/dissertation. *Entrance requirements:* For master's and doctorate, GRE General Test. Additional exam requirements/recommendations for international students: Required—TOEFL (minimum score 590 paper-based). Electronic applications accepted. *Expenses: Tuition, area resident:* Full-time $8000 Canadian dollars. *Faculty research:* Bacterial genetics, metabolism, pathogenic bacteriology, virology.

University of Calgary, Cumming School of Medicine and Faculty of Graduate Studies, Department of Microbiology, Immunology and Infectious Diseases, Calgary, AB T2N 1N4, Canada. Offers M Sc, PhD. *Degree requirements:* For master's, thesis, oral thesis exam; for doctorate, thesis/dissertation, candidacy exam, oral thesis exam. *Entrance requirements:* For master's and doctorate, minimum GPA of 3.2. Additional exam requirements/recommendations for international students: Required—TOEFL (minimum score 580 paper-based). Electronic applications accepted. *Faculty research:* Bacteriology, virology, parasitology, immunology.

University of California, Berkeley, Graduate Division, College of Natural Resources, Group in Microbiology, Berkeley, CA 94720-1500. Offers PhD. *Degree requirements:* For doctorate, thesis/dissertation. *Entrance requirements:* For doctorate, GRE General Test, minimum GPA of 3.0, 3 letters of recommendation.

University of California, Davis, Graduate Studies, Graduate Group in Microbiology, Davis, CA 95616. Offers MS, PhD. Terminal master's awarded for partial completion of doctoral program. *Degree requirements:* For master's, thesis; for doctorate, thesis/dissertation. *Entrance requirements:* For master's and doctorate, GRE General Test, minimum GPA of 3.0. Additional exam requirements/recommendations for international students: Required—TOEFL (minimum score 550 paper-based). Electronic applications accepted. *Faculty research:* Microbial physiology and genetics, microbial molecular and cellular biology, microbial ecology, microbial pathogenesis and immunology, urology.

University of California, Irvine, School of Medicine and School of Biological Sciences, Department of Microbiology and Molecular Genetics, Irvine, CA 92697. Offers biological sciences (MS, PhD); MD/PhD. *Students:* 27 full-time (12 women); includes 18 minority (1 American Indian or Alaska Native, non-Hispanic/Latino; 11 Asian, non-Hispanic/Latino; 6 Hispanic/Latino), 1 international. Average age 28. In 2013, 1 master's, 6 doctorates awarded. *Degree requirements:* For doctorate, thesis/dissertation. *Entrance requirements:* For doctorate, GRE General Test, GRE Subject Test, minimum GPA of 3.0. Additional exam requirements/recommendations for international students: Required—TOEFL (minimum score 550 paper-based). *Application deadline:* For fall admission, 12/15 priority date for domestic students, 12/15 for international students. Application fee: $80 ($100 for international students). Electronic applications accepted. *Financial support:* Fellowships, research assistantships with full tuition reimbursements, teaching assistantships, institutionally sponsored loans, traineeships, health care benefits, and unspecified assistantships available. Financial award applicants required to submit FAFSA. *Faculty research:* Molecular biology and genetics of viruses, bacteria, and yeast; immune response; molecular biology of cultured animal cells; genetic basis of cancer; genetics and physiology of infectious agents. *Unit head:* Rozanne M. Sandri-Goldin, Chair, 949-824-7570, Fax: 949-824-8598, E-mail: rmsandri@uci.edu. *Application contact:* Renee Frigo, Program Manager, 949-824-8145, Fax: 949-824-1965, E-mail: rfrigo@uci.edu.
Website: http://www.bio.uci.edu/

University of California, Los Angeles, David Geffen School of Medicine and Graduate Division, Graduate Programs in Medicine, Department of Microbiology, Immunology and Molecular Genetics, Los Angeles, CA 90095. Offers MS, PhD. *Degree requirements:* For master's, thesis; for doctorate, thesis/dissertation, oral and written qualifying exams; 2 quarters of teaching experience. *Entrance requirements:* For master's and doctorate, GRE General Test, bachelor's degree; minimum undergraduate GPA of 3.0 (or its equivalent if letter grade system not used). Additional exam requirements/recommendations for international students: Required—TOEFL. Electronic applications accepted.

University of California, Riverside, Graduate Division, Program in Microbiology, Riverside, CA 92521-0102. Offers MS, PhD. Part-time programs available. Terminal master's awarded for partial completion of doctoral program. *Degree requirements:* For master's, thesis; for doctorate, thesis/dissertation, qualifying exams. *Entrance requirements:* For master's and doctorate, GRE General Test, minimum GPA of 3.2. Additional exam requirements/recommendations for international students: Required—TOEFL (minimum score 550 paper-based; 80 iBT). Electronic applications accepted. *Faculty research:* Host-pathogen interactions; environmental microbiology; bioremediation; molecular microbiology; microbial genetics, physiology, and pathogenesis.

University of California, San Diego, Office of Graduate Studies, Division of Biological Sciences, La Jolla, CA 92093. Offers anthropogeny (PhD); bioinformatics (PhD); biology (PhD); ecology, behavior and evolution (PhD); microbiology (PhD). *Students:* 285 full-time (154 women), 8 part-time (4 women); includes 70 minority (2 Black or African American, non-Hispanic/Latino; 3 American Indian or Alaska Native, non-Hispanic/Latino; 51 Asian, non-Hispanic/Latino; 13 Hispanic/Latino; 1 Native Hawaiian or other Pacific Islander, non-Hispanic/Latino), 30 international. 626 applicants, 24% accepted, 85 enrolled. In 2013, 32 doctorates awarded. *Degree requirements:* For doctorate, thesis/dissertation, 3 quarters of teaching assistantship. *Entrance requirements:* For doctorate, GRE General Test; GRE Subject Test (recommended). Additional exam requirements/recommendations for international students: Required—TOEFL, IELTS. *Application deadline:* For fall admission, 12/4 for domestic students. Application fee: $80 ($100 for international students). Electronic applications accepted. *Expenses:* Tuition, state resident: full-time $11,220; part-time $1870 per quarter. Tuition, nonresident: full-time $26,322; part-time $4387 per quarter. *Required fees:* $519.50 per quarter. Part-time tuition and fees vary according to course load and program. *Financial support:* Fellowships, research assistantships, teaching assistantships, and scholarships/grants available. Financial award applicants required to submit FAFSA. *Faculty research:* Ecology, behavior and evolution; microbiology; bioinformatics; multi-scale biology; anthropogeny. *Unit head:* William McGinnis, Dean, 858-822-0458, E-mail: wmcginnis@ucsd.edu. *Application contact:* Cathy Pugh, Graduate Coordinator, 858-534-0181, E-mail: gradprog@biology.ucsd.edu.
Website: http://biology.ucsd.edu/

University of Chicago, Division of Biological Sciences, Biomedical Sciences Cluster: Cancer Biology, Immunology, Molecular Metabolism and Nutrition, Pathology, and Microbiology, Committee on Microbiology, Chicago, IL 60637-1513. Offers PhD. *Degree* *requirements:* For doctorate, thesis/dissertation, ethics class, 2 teaching assistantships. *Entrance requirements:* For doctorate, GRE General Test. Additional exam requirements/recommendations for international students: Required—TOEFL (minimum score 600 paper-based; 104 iBT), IELTS (minimum score 7). Electronic applications accepted. *Faculty research:* Molecular genetics, herpes virus, adipoviruses, Picarna viruses, ENS viruses.

University of Cincinnati, Graduate School, College of Medicine, Graduate Programs in Biomedical Sciences, Department of Molecular Genetics, Biochemistry and Microbiology, Cincinnati, OH 45221. Offers MS, PhD. Terminal master's awarded for partial completion of doctoral program. *Degree requirements:* For master's, thesis or alternative; for doctorate, thesis/dissertation, qualifying exam. *Entrance requirements:* For master's and doctorate, GRE General Test. Additional exam requirements/recommendations for international students: Required—TOEFL (minimum score 600 paper-based; 100 iBT), TWE. Electronic applications accepted. *Faculty research:* Cancer biology and developmental genetics, gene regulation and chromosome structure, microbiology and pathogenic mechanisms, structural biology, membrane biochemistry and signal transduction.

University of Colorado Boulder, Graduate School, College of Arts and Sciences, Department of Ecology and Evolutionary Biology, Boulder, CO 80309. Offers animal behavior (MA); biology (MA, PhD); environmental biology (MA, PhD); evolutionary biology (MA, PhD); neurobiology (MA); population biology (MA); population genetics (PhD). *Faculty:* 31 full-time (12 women). *Students:* 70 full-time (30 women), 18 part-time (10 women); includes 6 minority (1 Asian, non-Hispanic/Latino; 3 Hispanic/Latino; 2 Two or more races, non-Hispanic/Latino), 5 international. Average age 30. 171 applicants, 6% accepted, 11 enrolled. In 2013, 10 master's, 11 doctorates awarded. Terminal master's awarded for partial completion of doctoral program. *Degree requirements:* For master's, comprehensive exam, thesis or alternative; for doctorate, comprehensive exam, thesis/dissertation. *Entrance requirements:* For master's, GRE General Test, GRE Subject Test, minimum undergraduate GPA of 3.0; for doctorate, GRE General Test, GRE Subject Test. *Application deadline:* For fall admission, 12/31 for domestic students, 12/1 for international students. Application fee: $50 ($60 for international students). Electronic applications accepted. *Financial support:* In 2013–14, 175 students received support, including 35 fellowships (averaging $15,283 per year), 21 research assistantships with full and partial tuition reimbursements available (averaging $29,343 per year), 48 teaching assistantships with full and partial tuition reimbursements available (averaging $31,449 per year); institutionally sponsored loans, scholarships/grants, health care benefits, and unspecified assistantships also available. Financial award applicants required to submit FAFSA. *Faculty research:* Ecology, environmental biology, evolutionary biology, biological sciences, conservation biology. *Total annual research expenditures:* $37.1 million.
Website: http://ebio.colorado.edu

University of Colorado Denver, College of Liberal Arts and Sciences, Department of Integrative Biology, Denver, CO 80217. Offers animal behavior (MS); biology (MS); cell and developmental biology (MS); ecology (MS); evolutionary biology (MS); genetics (MS); integrative and systems biology (PhD); microbiology (MS); molecular biology (MS); neurobiology (MS); plant systematics (MS). Part-time programs available. *Faculty:* 21 full-time (7 women), 3 part-time/adjunct (2 women). *Students:* 18 full-time (11 women), 5 part-time (all women); includes 5 minority (1 Black or African American, non-Hispanic/Latino; 2 Hispanic/Latino; 2 Two or more races, non-Hispanic/Latino), 1 international. Average age 29. 25 applicants, 44% accepted, 11 enrolled. In 2013, 13 master's awarded. *Degree requirements:* For master's, comprehensive exam, thesis, 30-32 credit hours. *Entrance requirements:* For master's, GRE General Test (minimum score in 50th percentile in each section), BA/BS from accredited institution awarded within the last 10 years; minimum undergraduate GPA of 3.0; prerequisite courses: 1 year each of general biology and general chemistry; 1 semester each of general genetics, general ecology, and cell biology; and a structure/function course. Additional exam requirements/recommendations for international students: Required—TOEFL (minimum score 537 paper-based; 75 iBT); Recommended—IELTS (minimum score 6.5). *Application deadline:* For fall admission, 2/1 for domestic and international students. Application fee: $50 ($75 for international students). Electronic applications accepted. *Financial support:* In 2013–14, 8 students received support. Fellowships, research assistantships, teaching assistantships, Federal Work-Study, institutionally sponsored loans, scholarships/grants, and traineeships available. Financial award application deadline: 4/1; financial award applicants required to submit FAFSA. *Faculty research:* Molecular developmental biology; quantitative ecology, biogeography, and population dynamics; environmental signaling and endocrine disruption; speciation, the evolution of reproductive isolation, and hybrid zones; evolutionary, behavioral, and conservation ecology. *Unit head:* Dr. John Swallow, Biology Department Chair, 303-556-6154, E-mail: john.swallow@ucdenver.edu. *Application contact:* Timberley Roane, Associate Professor/Director of MS in Biology Program, 303-556-6592, E-mail: timberley.roane@ucdenver.edu.
Website: http://www.ucdenver.edu/academics/colleges/CLAS/Departments/biology/Programs/MasterofScience/Pages/BiologyMasterOfScience.aspx

University of Colorado Denver, School of Medicine, Program in Microbiology, Aurora, CO 80045. Offers microbiology (PhD); microbiology and immunology (PhD). *Students:* 17 full-time (4 women); includes 2 minority (1 Asian, non-Hispanic/Latino; 1 Hispanic/Latino). Average age 27. 53 applicants, 4% accepted, 2 enrolled. In 2013, 1 doctorate awarded. *Degree requirements:* For doctorate, comprehensive exam, thesis/dissertation, 3 lab rotations; 30 credit hours of coursework. *Entrance requirements:* For doctorate, GRE, three letters of reference, two copies of official transcripts, minimum GPA of 3.0. Additional exam requirements/recommendations for international students: Required—TOEFL (minimum score 550 paper-based; 80 iBT). *Application deadline:* For fall admission, 12/1 for domestic students, 11/1 for international students. Application fee: $50 ($75 for international students). Electronic applications accepted. *Expenses:* Contact institution. *Financial support:* In 2013–14, 17 students received support. Fellowships with tuition reimbursements available, research assistantships, teaching assistantships, institutionally sponsored loans, scholarships/grants, traineeships, health care benefits, and tuition waivers (full) available. Financial award application deadline: 3/15; financial award applicants required to submit FAFSA. *Faculty research:* Molecular mechanisms of picornavirus replication, mechanisms of papovavirus assembly, human immune response in multiple sclerosis. *Total annual research expenditures:* $5.9 million. *Unit head:* Dr. Randall K. Holmes, Chair, 303-724-4223, E-mail: randall.holmes@ucdenver.edu. *Application contact:* Deanne Sylvester, Microbiology Graduate Program Administrator, 303-724-3244, Fax: 303-724-3247, E-mail: deanne.sylvester@ucdenver.edu.
Website: http://www.ucdenver.edu/academics/colleges/medicalschool/departments/Microbiology/Pages/microbiology.aspx

University of Connecticut, Graduate School, College of Liberal Arts and Sciences, Department of Molecular and Cell Biology, Field of Microbiology, Storrs, CT 06269. Offers MS, PhD. Terminal master's awarded for partial completion of doctoral program. *Degree requirements:* For master's, comprehensive exam; for doctorate, thesis/dissertation. *Entrance requirements:* For master's and doctorate, GRE General Test, GRE Subject Test. Additional exam requirements/recommendations for international students: Required—TOEFL (minimum score 550 paper-based). Electronic applications accepted.

University of Delaware, College of Arts and Sciences, Department of Biological Sciences, Newark, DE 19716. Offers biotechnology (MS); cancer biology (MS, PhD); cell and extracellular matrix biology (MS, PhD); cell and systems physiology (MS, PhD); developmental biology (MS, PhD); ecology and evolution (MS, PhD); microbiology (MS, PhD); molecular biology and genetics (MS, PhD). Terminal master's awarded for partial completion of doctoral program. *Degree requirements:* For master's, thesis, preliminary exam; for doctorate, comprehensive exam, thesis/dissertation, preliminary exam. *Entrance requirements:* For master's and doctorate, GRE General Test. Additional exam requirements/recommendations for international students: Required—TOEFL (minimum score 600 paper-based); Recommended—TWE. Electronic applications accepted. *Faculty research:* Microorganisms, bone, cancer metastasis, developmental biology, cell biology, DNA.

University of Florida, College of Medicine, Department of Molecular Genetics and Microbiology, Gainesville, FL 32610-0266. Offers MS. Terminal master's awarded for partial completion of doctoral program. *Degree requirements:* For master's, thesis. *Entrance requirements:* For master's, GRE General Test, minimum GPA of 3.0. Additional exam requirements/recommendations for international students: Required—TOEFL, IELTS. Electronic applications accepted. *Expenses:* Tuition, state resident: full-time $12,640. Tuition, nonresident: full-time $30,000.

University of Florida, College of Medicine and Graduate School, Interdisciplinary Program in Biomedical Sciences, Concentration in Immunology and Microbiology, Gainesville, FL 32611. Offers PhD. *Degree requirements:* For doctorate, thesis/dissertation. *Entrance requirements:* For doctorate, GRE General Test, minimum GPA of 3.0, biochemistry before enrollment. Additional exam requirements/recommendations for international students: Required—TOEFL. Electronic applications accepted. *Expenses:* Tuition, state resident: full-time $12,640. Tuition, nonresident: full-time $30,000.

University of Florida, Graduate School, College of Agricultural and Life Sciences, Department of Microbiology and Cell Science, Gainesville, FL 32611. Offers MS, PhD. *Faculty:* 26 full-time (7 women), 4 part-time/adjunct (0 women). *Students:* 55 full-time (32 women), 4 part-time (2 women); includes 13 minority (5 Black or African American, non-Hispanic/Latino; 1 American Indian or Alaska Native, non-Hispanic/Latino; 2 Asian, non-Hispanic/Latino; 5 Hispanic/Latino), 26 international. Average age 28. 82 applicants, 20% accepted, 14 enrolled. In 2013, 3 master's, 4 doctorates awarded. *Degree requirements:* For master's, comprehensive exam, thesis (for some programs); for doctorate, comprehensive exam, thesis/dissertation. *Entrance requirements:* For master's, GRE General Test, minimum GPA of 3.0; for doctorate, GRE General Test, minimum GPA of 3.0. Additional exam requirements/recommendations for international students: Required—TOEFL (minimum score 550 paper-based; 80 iBT), IELTS (minimum score 6). *Application deadline:* For fall admission, 6/1 priority date for domestic students. Applications are processed on a rolling basis. Application fee: $30. Electronic applications accepted. *Expenses:* Tuition, state resident: full-time $12,640. Tuition, nonresident: full-time $30,000. *Financial support:* In 2013–14, 46 students received support, including 5 fellowships (averaging $25,325 per year), 33 research assistantships (averaging $23,830 per year), 10 teaching assistantships (averaging $22,350 per year). Financial award applicants required to submit FAFSA. *Faculty research:* Biomass conversion, membrane and cell wall chemistry, plant biochemistry and genetics. *Unit head:* Eric Triplett, PhD, Professor and Chair, 352-392-1906, Fax: 352-392-5922, E-mail: ewt@ufl.edu. *Application contact:* Tony Romeo, PhD, Graduate Coordinator, 352-392-2400, Fax: 352-392-5922, E-mail: tromeo@ufl.edu.
Website: http://microcell.ufl.edu/

University of Georgia, Franklin College of Arts and Sciences, Department of Microbiology, Athens, GA 30602. Offers MS, PhD. *Degree requirements:* For master's, thesis; for doctorate, one foreign language, thesis/dissertation. *Entrance requirements:* For master's and doctorate, GRE General Test. Additional exam requirements/recommendations for international students: Required—TOEFL (minimum score 550 paper-based). Electronic applications accepted.

University of Guelph, Graduate Studies, College of Biological Science, Department of Molecular and Cellular Biology, Guelph, ON N1G 2W1, Canada. Offers biochemistry (M Sc, PhD); biophysics (M Sc, PhD); botany (M Sc, PhD); microbiology (M Sc, PhD); molecular biology and genetics (M Sc, PhD). *Degree requirements:* For master's, thesis, research proposal; for doctorate, comprehensive exam, thesis/dissertation, research proposal. *Entrance requirements:* For master's, minimum B-average during previous 2 years of coursework; for doctorate, minimum A-average. Additional exam requirements/recommendations for international students: Required—TOEFL (minimum score 550 paper-based), IELTS (minimum score 6.5). Electronic applications accepted. *Faculty research:* Physiology, structure, genetics, and ecology of microbes; virology and microbial technology.

University of Hawaii at Manoa, Graduate Division, College of Natural Sciences, Department of Microbiology, Honolulu, HI 96822. Offers MS, PhD. Part-time programs available. *Degree requirements:* For master's, thesis optional; for doctorate, comprehensive exam, thesis/dissertation. *Entrance requirements:* For master's and doctorate, GRE General Test. Additional exam requirements/recommendations for international students: Required—TOEFL (minimum score 580 paper-based; 92 iBT), IELTS (minimum score 5). *Faculty research:* Virology, immunology, microbial physiology, medical microbiology, bacterial genetics.

University of Idaho, College of Graduate Studies, College of Science, Department of Biological Sciences, Moscow, ID 83844-3051. Offers biology (MS, PhD); microbiology, molecular biology and biochemistry (MS, PhD). *Faculty:* 12 full-time. *Students:* 20 full-time, 3 part-time. Average age 31. In 2013, 2 master's, 5 doctorates awarded. *Degree requirements:* For doctorate, one foreign language, thesis/dissertation. *Entrance requirements:* For master's, GRE, minimum GPA of 2.8; for doctorate, GRE, minimum undergraduate GPA of 2.8, 3.0 graduate. Additional exam requirements/recommendations for international students: Required—TOEFL. *Application deadline:* For fall admission, 8/1 for domestic students; for spring admission, 12/15 for domestic students. Applications are processed on a rolling basis. Application fee: $60. Electronic applications accepted. *Expenses:* Tuition, state resident: full-time $5596; part-time $363 per credit hour. Tuition, nonresident: full-time $18,672; part-time $1089 per credit hour. *Financial support:* Research assistantships and teaching assistantships available. Financial award applicants required to submit FAFSA. *Faculty research:* Animal behavior development, germ cell development, evolutionary biology, fish reproductive biology, molecular mechanisms. *Unit head:* Dr. James J. Nagler, Interim Department Chair, 208-885-6280, E-mail: biosci@uidaho.edu. *Application contact:* Stephanie Thomas, Graduate Recruitment Coordinator, 208-885-4001, Fax: 208-885-4406, E-mail: gadms@uidaho.edu.
Website: http://www.uidaho.edu/sci/biology

University of Illinois at Chicago, College of Medicine and Graduate College, Graduate Programs in Medicine, Department of Microbiology and Immunology, Chicago, IL 60607-7128. Offers PhD, MD/PhD. *Faculty:* 13 full-time (4 women), 3 part-time/adjunct (2 women). *Students:* 14 full-time (9 women); includes 3 minority (2 Black or African

American, non-Hispanic/Latino; 1 Two or more races, non-Hispanic/Latino), 6 international. Average age 30. 1 applicant, 100% accepted. In 2013, 10 doctorates awarded. *Degree requirements:* For doctorate, thesis/dissertation. *Entrance requirements:* For doctorate, GRE General Test, minimum GPA of 2.75. Additional exam requirements/recommendations for international students: Required—TOEFL. *Application deadline:* For fall admission, 3/1 priority date for domestic students, 2/15 priority date for international students. Application fee: $40 ($50 for international students). *Expenses:* Tuition, state resident: full-time $11,066; part-time $3689 per term. Tuition, nonresident: full-time $23,064; part-time $7688 per term. *Required fees:* $3004; $1190 per term. Tuition and fees vary according to course level and program. *Financial support:* In 2013–14, 5 fellowships with full tuition reimbursements were awarded; research assistantships with full tuition reimbursements, teaching assistantships with full tuition reimbursements, Federal Work-Study, scholarships/grants, traineeships, tuition waivers (full), and unspecified assistantships also available. Financial award application deadline: 3/1; financial award applicants required to submit FAFSA. *Faculty research:* Class I major histocompatibility complex molecules; proteins such as azurin with the immunoglobulin folds; T cell immunobiology relevant to disease pathogenesis, immunotherapeutics and vaccines for HIV/AIDS, tuberculosis, AIDS-related tuberculosis, and recently malaria, plague and smallpox; intracellular bacterial pathogen Listeria monocytogenes; virus infection. *Total annual research expenditures:* $6.9 million. *Unit head:* Prof. Bellur S. Prabhakar, Department Head, 312-996-4915, Fax: 312-996-6415, E-mail: bprabkhar@uic.edu. *Application contact:* Mia Johnson, Admissions and Records Officer, 312-996-9477, Fax: 312-996-6415, E-mail: mimi@uic.edu.
Website: http://www.uic.edu/depts/mcmi/index.htm

University of Illinois at Urbana–Champaign, Graduate College, College of Liberal Arts and Sciences, School of Molecular and Cellular Biology, Department of Microbiology, Champaign, IL 61820. Offers MS, PhD. *Students:* 63 (38 women). Application fee: $75 ($90 for international students). *Unit head:* John E. Cronan, Jr., Head, 217-333-7919, Fax: 217-244-6697, E-mail: jecronan@illinois.edu. *Application contact:* Shawna Smith, Coordinator of Graduate Programs, 217-244-6638, E-mail: smsmith1@illinois.edu.
Website: http://mcb.illinois.edu/departments/microbiology/

The University of Iowa, Roy J. and Lucille A. Carver College of Medicine and Graduate College, Graduate Programs in Medicine, Department of Microbiology, Iowa City, IA 52242-1316. Offers general microbiology and microbial physiology (MS, PhD); immunology (MS, PhD); microbial genetics (MS, PhD); pathogenic bacteriology (MS, PhD); virology (MS, PhD). *Faculty:* 23 full-time (5 women), 10 part-time/adjunct (4 women). *Students:* 38 full-time (28 women); includes 3 minority (2 Asian, non-Hispanic/Latino; 1 Hispanic/Latino), 2 international. Average age 25. 44 applicants, 23% accepted, 8 enrolled. In 2013, 1 master's, 6 doctorates awarded. *Degree requirements:* For master's, thesis; for doctorate, comprehensive exam, thesis/dissertation. *Entrance requirements:* For master's and doctorate, GRE General Test. Additional exam requirements/recommendations for international students: Required—TOEFL (minimum score 600 paper-based). *Application deadline:* For fall admission, 1/1 for domestic and international students. Application fee: $60 ($100 for international students). Electronic applications accepted. *Financial support:* In 2013–14, 5 fellowships with full tuition reimbursements (averaging $26,000 per year), 33 research assistantships with full tuition reimbursements (averaging $26,000 per year) were awarded; institutionally sponsored loans, scholarships/grants, traineeships, and health care benefits also available. *Faculty research:* Gene regulation, processing and transport of HIV, retroviral pathogenesis, biodegradation, biofilm. *Total annual research expenditures:* $11.5 million. *Unit head:* Dr. Patrick M. Schlievert, Chair and Department Executive Officer, 319-335-7810, E-mail: grad-micro-info@uiowa.edu. *Application contact:* Kerry Yoder, Assistant Director of Graduate and Professional Evaluation, 319-335-1525, Fax: 319-335-1535, E-mail: admissions@uiowa.edu.
Website: http://www.medicine.uiowa.edu/microbiology/

The University of Kansas, Graduate Studies, College of Liberal Arts and Sciences, Department of Molecular Biosciences, Lawrence, KS 66045. Offers biochemistry and biophysics (MA, PhD); microbiology (MA, PhD); molecular, cellular, and developmental biology (MA, PhD). *Faculty:* 34. *Students:* 52 full-time (28 women); includes 5 minority (2 Asian, non-Hispanic/Latino; 3 Hispanic/Latino), 23 international. Average age 27. 96 applicants, 25% accepted, 13 enrolled. In 2013, 3 master's, 9 doctorates awarded. Terminal master's awarded for partial completion of doctoral program. *Degree requirements:* For master's, comprehensive exam, thesis; for doctorate, comprehensive exam, thesis/dissertation. *Entrance requirements:* For master's and doctorate, GRE General Test. Additional exam requirements/recommendations for international students: Required—TOEFL or IELTS. *Application deadline:* For fall admission, 12/15 for domestic and international students. Application fee: $55 ($65 for international students). Electronic applications accepted. *Financial support:* Fellowships with tuition reimbursements, research assistantships with tuition reimbursements, teaching assistantships with tuition reimbursements, health care benefits, and unspecified assistantships available. Financial award application deadline: 3/1. *Faculty research:* Structure and function of proteins, genetics of organism development, molecular genetics, neurophysiology, molecular virology and pathogenics, developmental biology, cell biology. *Unit head:* Dr. Mark Richter, Chair, 785-864-3334, E-mail: richter@ku.edu. *Application contact:* John Connolly, Graduate Admissions Contact, 785-864-4311, E-mail: jconnolly@ku.edu.
Website: http://www.molecularbiosciences.ku.edu/

The University of Kansas, University of Kansas Medical Center, School of Medicine, Department of Microbiology, Molecular Genetics and Immunology, Kansas City, KS 66160. Offers MA, PhD, MD/PhD. *Faculty:* 12. *Students:* 11 full-time (5 women); includes 2 minority (1 Asian, non-Hispanic/Latino; 1 Two or more races, non-Hispanic/Latino), 5 international. Average age 30. In 2013, 1 master's, 3 doctorates awarded. Terminal master's awarded for partial completion of doctoral program. *Degree requirements:* For master's, thesis; for doctorate, comprehensive exam, thesis/dissertation, research skills. *Entrance requirements:* For master's and doctorate, GRE General Test, B Sc. Additional exam requirements/recommendations for international students: Required—TOEFL or IELTS. *Application deadline:* For fall admission, 1/4 priority date for domestic and international students. Applications are processed on a rolling basis. Application fee: $60. Electronic applications accepted. *Financial support:* Fellowships with full tuition reimbursements, research assistantships with full tuition reimbursements, teaching assistantships with full and partial tuition reimbursements, scholarships/grants, and unspecified assistantships available. Financial award application deadline: 3/1; financial award applicants required to submit FAFSA. *Faculty research:* Immunology, infectious disease, virology, molecular genetics, bacteriology. *Total annual research expenditures:* $4 million. *Unit head:* Dr. Michael Parmely, Chair, 913-588-7053, Fax: 913-588-7295, E-mail: mparmely@kumc.edu. *Application contact:* Dr. Indranil Biswas, Microbiology Graduate Studies Director, 913-588-7019, Fax: 913-588-7295, E-mail: ibiswas@kumc.edu.
Website: http://www.kumc.edu/school-of-medicine/microbiology-molecular-genetics-and-immunology.html

University of Kentucky, Graduate School, Graduate School Programs from the College of Medicine, Department of Microbiology, Immunology and Molecular Genetics, Lexington, KY 40506-0032. Offers PhD. *Degree requirements:* For doctorate, comprehensive exam, thesis/dissertation. *Entrance requirements:* For doctorate, GRE General Test, minimum undergraduate GPA of 2.75. Additional exam requirements/recommendations for international students: Required—TOEFL (minimum score 550 paper-based). Electronic applications accepted.

University of Louisville, School of Medicine, Department of Microbiology and Immunology, Louisville, KY 40292-0001. Offers MS, PhD, MD/PhD. *Students:* 40 full-time (24 women), 1 part-time (0 women); includes 5 minority (3 Black or African American, non-Hispanic/Latino; 1 Asian, non-Hispanic/Latino; 1 Hispanic/Latino), 12 international. Average age 29. 55 applicants, 24% accepted, 9 enrolled. In 2013, 4 master's, 4 doctorates awarded. Terminal master's awarded for partial completion of doctoral program. *Degree requirements:* For master's, thesis; for doctorate, comprehensive exam, thesis/dissertation. *Entrance requirements:* For master's and doctorate, GRE General Test (minimum score of 1000 verbal and quantitative), minimum GPA of 3.0; 1 year of course work in biology, organic chemistry, and physics; 1 semester of course work in calculus and quantitative analysis, biochemistry, or molecular biology. Additional exam requirements/recommendations for international students: Required—TOEFL. *Application deadline:* For fall admission, 2/1 priority date for domestic and international students. Applications are processed on a rolling basis. Application fee: $60. Electronic applications accepted. *Expenses:* Tuition, state resident: full-time $10,788; part-time $599 per credit hour. Tuition, nonresident: full-time $22,446; part-time $1247 per credit hour. *Required fees:* $196. Tuition and fees vary according to program and reciprocity agreements. *Financial support:* Fellowships with full tuition reimbursements and research assistantships with full tuition reimbursements available. Financial award application deadline: 4/15. *Faculty research:* Opportunistic and emerging infections; biology and regulation of the immune system; cellular and molecular bases of chronic inflammatory response; role of cytokines and chemokines in cancer, autoimmune and infectious disease; host defense and pathogenesis of viral infections. *Unit head:* Dr. Robert D. Stout, Chair, 502-852-5351, Fax: 502-852-7531, E-mail: bobstout@louisville.edu. *Application contact:* Carolyn M. Burton, Academic Coordinator, 502-852-6208, Fax: 502-852-7531, E-mail: cmburt01@gwise.louisville.edu.

University of Maine, Graduate School, College of Natural Sciences, Forestry, and Agriculture, Department of Molecular and Biomedical Sciences, Orono, ME 04469. Offers biochemistry (MPS, MS); biochemistry and molecular biology (PhD); microbiology (MPS, MS, PhD). *Faculty:* 30 full-time (6 women), 20 part-time/adjunct (4 women). *Students:* 26 full-time (17 women), 4 part-time (3 women); includes 3 minority (2 Asian, non-Hispanic/Latino; 1 Native Hawaiian or other Pacific Islander, non-Hispanic/Latino), 5 international. Average age 31. 7 applicants, 100% accepted, 5 enrolled. In 2013, 5 master's, 4 doctorates awarded. *Degree requirements:* For master's, thesis (for some programs); for doctorate, comprehensive exam, thesis/dissertation. *Entrance requirements:* For master's and doctorate, GRE General Test. Additional exam requirements/recommendations for international students: Required—TOEFL. *Application deadline:* For fall admission, 2/1 priority date for domestic students. Applications are processed on a rolling basis. Application fee: $65. Electronic applications accepted. *Expenses:* Tuition, state resident: full-time $7524. Tuition, nonresident: full-time $23,112. *Required fees:* $1970. *Financial support:* In 2013–14, 16 students received support, including 5 research assistantships with full tuition reimbursements available (averaging $22,000 per year), 10 teaching assistantships with full tuition reimbursements available (averaging $19,000 per year); tuition waivers (full and partial) also available. Financial award application deadline: 3/1. *Total annual research expenditures:* $242,844. *Unit head:* Dr. Robert Gundersen, Chair, 207-581-2802, Fax: 207-581-2801. *Application contact:* Scott G. Delcourt, Associate Dean of the Graduate School, 207-581-3291, Fax: 207-581-3232, E-mail: graduate@maine.edu.
Website: http://umaine.edu/biomed/

The University of Manchester, Faculty of Life Sciences, Manchester, United Kingdom. Offers adaptive organismal biology (M Phil, PhD); animal biology (M Phil, PhD); biochemistry (M Phil, PhD); bioinformatics (M Phil, PhD); biomolecular sciences (M Phil, PhD); biotechnology (M Phil, PhD); cell biology (M Phil, PhD); cell matrix research (M Phil, PhD); channels and transporters (M Phil, PhD); developmental biology (M Phil, PhD); Egyptology (M Phil, PhD); environmental biology (M Phil, PhD); evolutionary biology (M Phil, PhD); gene expression (M Phil, PhD); genetics (M Phil, PhD); history of science, technology and medicine (M Phil, PhD); immunology (M Phil, PhD); integrative neurobiology and behavior (M Phil, PhD); membrane trafficking (M Phil, PhD); microbiology (M Phil, PhD); molecular and cellular neuroscience (M Phil, PhD); molecular biology (M Phil, PhD); molecular cancer studies (M Phil, PhD); neuroscience (M Phil, PhD); ophthalmology (M Phil, PhD); optometry (M Phil, PhD); organelle function (M Phil, PhD); pharmacology (M Phil, PhD); physiology (M Phil, PhD); plant sciences (M Phil, PhD); stem cell research (M Phil, PhD); structural biology (M Phil, PhD); systems neuroscience (M Phil, PhD); toxicology (M Phil, PhD).

University of Manitoba, Faculty of Graduate Studies, Faculty of Science, Department of Microbiology, Winnipeg, MB R3T 2N2, Canada. Offers M Sc, PhD. *Degree requirements:* For master's, thesis; for doctorate, one foreign language, thesis/dissertation.

University of Maryland, Baltimore, Graduate School, Graduate Program in Life Sciences, Program in Molecular Microbiology and Immunology, Baltimore, MD 21201. Offers PhD, MD/PhD. *Students:* 53 full-time (28 women), 2 part-time (0 women); includes 10 minority (2 Black or African American, non-Hispanic/Latino; 5 Asian, non-Hispanic/Latino; 1 Hispanic/Latino; 2 Two or more races, non-Hispanic/Latino), 5 international. Average age 27. 133 applicants, 14% accepted, 8 enrolled. In 2013, 5 doctorates awarded. *Degree requirements:* For doctorate, comprehensive exam, thesis/dissertation. *Entrance requirements:* For doctorate, GRE. Additional exam requirements/recommendations for international students: Required—TOEFL (minimum score 550 paper-based; 80 iBT); Recommended—IELTS (minimum score 7). *Application deadline:* For fall admission, 1/15 for domestic and international students. Application fee: $75. Electronic applications accepted. *Financial support:* In 2013–14, research assistantships with partial tuition reimbursements (averaging $25,000 per year) were awarded; fellowships also available. Financial award application deadline: 3/1; financial award applicants required to submit FAFSA. *Unit head:* Dr. Nicholas Carbonetti, Director, 410-706-7677, E-mail: ncarbone@umaryland.edu. *Application contact:* June Green, Program Coordinator, 410-706-7126, Fax: 410-706-2129, E-mail: jgreen@umaryland.edu.
Website: http://microbiology.umaryland.edu

University of Massachusetts Amherst, Graduate School, College of Natural Sciences, Department of Microbiology, Amherst, MA 01003. Offers MS, PhD. Part-time programs available. *Faculty:* 14 full-time (1 woman). *Students:* 41 full-time (22 women), 6 part-time (4 women); includes 11 minority (2 Black or African American, non-Hispanic/Latino; 6 Asian, non-Hispanic/Latino; 3 Hispanic/Latino), 14 international. Average age 26. 110 applicants, 27% accepted, 20 enrolled. In 2013, 7 master's, 4 doctorates awarded. Terminal master's awarded for partial completion of doctoral program. *Degree requirements:* For master's, thesis or alternative; for doctorate, comprehensive exam, thesis/dissertation. *Entrance requirements:* For master's and doctorate, GRE General

Test. Additional exam requirements/recommendations for international students: Required—TOEFL (minimum score 550 paper-based; 80 iBT), IELTS (minimum score 6.5). *Application deadline:* For fall admission, 12/20 for domestic and international students; for spring admission, 10/1 for domestic and international students. Applications are processed on a rolling basis. Application fee: $75. Electronic applications accepted. *Financial support:* Fellowships with full and partial tuition reimbursements, research assistantships with full and partial tuition reimbursements, teaching assistantships with full and partial tuition reimbursements, career-related internships or fieldwork, Federal Work-Study, scholarships/grants, traineeships, health care benefits, tuition waivers (full and partial), and unspecified assistantships available. Support available to part-time students. Financial award application deadline: 12/20. *Unit head:* Dr. Stephen Rich, Graduate Program Director, 413-545-6675, Fax: 413-545-1578. *Application contact:* Lindsay DeSantis, Supervisor of Admissions, 413-545-0722, Fax: 413-577-0010, E-mail: gradadm@grad.umass.edu.
Website: http://www.micro.umass.edu/

See Display below and Close-Up on page 357.

University of Massachusetts Worcester, Graduate School of Biomedical Sciences, Worcester, MA 01655-0115. Offers biochemistry and molecular pharmacology (PhD); bioinformatics and computational biology (PhD); cancer biology (PhD); cell biology (PhD); clinical and population health research (PhD); clinical investigation (MS); immunology and virology (PhD); interdisciplinary biomedical research (PhD); millennium (PhD); molecular genetics and microbiology (PhD); neuroscience (PhD); translational science (PhD); MD/PhD. *Faculty:* 1,388 full-time (521 women), 309 part-time/adjunct (198 women). *Students:* 385 full-time (210 women); includes 53 minority (13 Black or African American, non-Hispanic/Latino; 30 Asian, non-Hispanic/Latino; 10 Hispanic/Latino), 138 international. Average age 28. 491 applicants, 19% accepted, 39 enrolled. In 2013, 5 master's, 50 doctorates awarded. Terminal master's awarded for partial completion of doctoral program. *Median time to degree:* Of those who began their doctoral program in fall 2005, 67% received their degree in 8 years or less. *Degree requirements:* For master's, comprehensive exam, thesis; for doctorate, comprehensive exam, thesis/dissertation. *Entrance requirements:* For master's, MD, PhD, DVM, or PharmD; for doctorate, GRE General Test, bachelor's degree. Additional exam requirements/recommendations for international students: Required—TOEFL (minimum score 100 iBT) or IELTS (minimum score 7.5). *Application deadline:* For fall admission, 12/15 for domestic and international students; for spring admission, 5/15 for domestic students. Application fee: $80. Electronic applications accepted. *Expenses:* Contact institution. *Financial support:* In 2013–14, 431 students received support, including research assistantships with full tuition reimbursements available (averaging $29,500 per year); scholarships/grants, health care benefits, tuition waivers (full), and unspecified assistantships also available. Financial award application deadline: 5/16. *Faculty research:* RNA interference, cell/molecular/developmental biology, bioinformatics, clinical/translational research, infectious disease. *Total annual research expenditures:* $245.9 million. *Unit head:* Dr. Anthony Carruthers, Dean, 508-856-4135, E-mail: anthony.carruthers@umassmed.edu. *Application contact:* Dr. Kendall Knight, Associate Dean and Interim Director of Admissions and Recruitment, 508-856-5628, Fax: 508-856-3659, E-mail: kendall.knight@umassmed.edu.
Website: http://www.umassmed.edu/gsbs/

University of Miami, Graduate School, Miller School of Medicine, Graduate Programs in Medicine, Department of Microbiology and Immunology, Coral Gables, FL 33124. Offers PhD, MD/PhD. *Degree requirements:* For doctorate, thesis/dissertation, oral and written qualifying exams. *Entrance requirements:* For doctorate, GRE General Test. Additional exam requirements/recommendations for international students: Required—TOEFL. Electronic applications accepted. *Faculty research:* Cellular and molecular immunology, molecular and pathogenic virology, pathogenic bacteriology and gene therapy of cancer.

University of Michigan, Rackham Graduate School, Program in Biomedical Sciences (PIBS), Department of Microbiology and Immunology, Ann Arbor, MI 48178. Offers MS, PhD. *Faculty:* 20 full-time (10 women), 12 part-time/adjunct (4 women). *Students:* 44 full-time (28 women); includes 7 minority (1 American Indian or Alaska Native, non-Hispanic/Latino; 4 Asian, non-Hispanic/Latino; 2 Hispanic/Latino), 3 international. Average age 29. 90 applicants, 14% accepted, 13 enrolled. In 2013, 2 master's, 7 doctorates awarded. *Degree requirements:* For doctorate, thesis/dissertation, oral defense of dissertation, preliminary exam. *Entrance requirements:* For master's and doctorate, GRE General Test. Additional exam requirements/recommendations for international students: Required—TOEFL (minimum score 600 paper-based; 84 iBT), TWE. *Application deadline:* For fall admission, 12/1 for domestic and international students. Application fee: $75 ($90 for international students). Electronic applications accepted. Tuition and fees vary according to course level, course load, degree level, program and student level. *Financial support:* In 2013–14, 15 fellowships with full tuition reimbursements (averaging $28,500 per year), 20 research assistantships with full tuition reimbursements (averaging $28,500 per year) were awarded; health care benefits and tuition waivers (full) also available. Financial award application deadline: 2/1. *Faculty research:* Gene regulation, molecular biology of animal and bacterial viruses, molecular and cellular networks, pathogenesis and microbial genetics. *Total annual research expenditures:* $10.2 million. *Unit head:* Dr. Harry L. T. Mobley, Chair, 734-764-1466, Fax: 734-764-3562, E-mail: hmobley@umich.edu. *Application contact:* Heidi Thompson, Senior Student Administrative Assistant, 734-763-3532, Fax: 734-764-3562, E-mail: heiditho@umich.edu.
Website: http://www.med.umich.edu/microbio/

University of Minnesota, Twin Cities Campus, Graduate School, PhD Program in Microbiology, Immunology and Cancer Biology, Minneapolis, MN 55455-0213. Offers PhD. *Degree requirements:* For doctorate, thesis/dissertation. *Entrance requirements:* For doctorate, GRE General Test. Additional exam requirements/recommendations for international students: Required—TOEFL (minimum score 600 paper-based). Electronic applications accepted. *Faculty research:* Virology, microbiology, cancer biology, immunology.

University of Mississippi Medical Center, School of Graduate Studies in the Health Sciences, Department of Microbiology, Jackson, MS 39216-4505. Offers PhD, MD/PhD. *Faculty:* 13 full-time (4 women), 3 part-time/adjunct (0 women). *Students:* 10 full-time (6 women), 1 (woman) part-time; includes 2 minority (1 Asian, non-Hispanic/Latino; 1 Hispanic/Latino), 1 international. Average age 28. 12 applicants, 33% accepted, 3 enrolled. In 2013, 4 doctorates awarded. *Degree requirements:* For doctorate, comprehensive exam, thesis/dissertation, first authored publication. *Entrance requirements:* For doctorate, GRE General Test (minimum score of 300), minimum GPA of 3.0. Additional exam requirements/recommendations for international students: Recommended—TOEFL (minimum score 550 paper-based; 79 iBT), IELTS (minimum score 6.5), TSE (minimum score 53). *Application deadline:* For fall admission, 12/31 priority date for domestic and international students. Applications are processed on a rolling basis. Application fee: $25. Electronic applications accepted. *Financial support:* In 2013–14, 10 students received support, including 10 research assistantships with full tuition reimbursements available (averaging $24,150 per year); scholarships/grants, health care benefits, and unspecified assistantships also available. Financial award application deadline: 12/31. *Faculty research:* Host-pathogen interaction, microbial population genetics, immunology, virology, parasitology. *Total annual research expenditures:* $1 million. *Unit head:* Dr. Richard O'Callaghan, Chairman, 601-984-1700, Fax: 601-984-1708, E-mail: rocallaghan@umc.edu. *Application contact:* Dr. Eva

Bengten, Director, Graduate Program in Microbiology, 601-984-1739, Fax: 601-984-1708, E-mail: ebengten@umc.edu.
Website: http://www.umc.edu/microbiology/

University of Missouri, School of Medicine and Graduate School, Graduate Programs in Medicine, Department of Molecular Microbiology and Immunology, Columbia, MO 65211. Offers MS, PhD. *Faculty:* 20 full-time (4 women), 2 part-time/adjunct (0 women). *Students:* 41 full-time (21 women), 1 (woman) part-time; includes 5 minority (3 Black or African American, non-Hispanic/Latino; 1 American Indian or Alaska Native, non-Hispanic/Latino; 1 Hispanic/Latino), 15 international. Average age 29. 29 applicants, 28% accepted, 7 enrolled. In 2013, 12 doctorates awarded. Terminal master's awarded for partial completion of doctoral program. *Degree requirements:* For master's, thesis; for doctorate, thesis/dissertation. *Entrance requirements:* For master's and doctorate, GRE General Test, minimum GPA of 3.0. Additional exam requirements/recommendations for international students: Required—TOEFL (minimum score 580 paper-based; 92 iBT). *Application deadline:* For fall admission, 1/15 priority date for domestic and international students. Application fee: $55 ($75 for international students). Electronic applications accepted. *Financial support:* Fellowships, research assistantships, teaching assistantships, institutionally sponsored loans, scholarships/grants, traineeships, health care benefits, and unspecified assistantships available. Support available to part-time students. Financial award application deadline: 3/1. *Faculty research:* Molecular biology, host-parasite interactions, posttranscriptional gene regulation, molecular basis of bacterial pathogenesis, regulation of immune response, mechanism and evolution of catalysis by ribozymes, mycoplasmas, genetics of Saccharomyces cerevisiae, T-cell development/activation, application of recombinant adeno-associated virus in gene therapy, retrovirus assembly, human immune responses, HCV entry pathways, RNA processing, epigenetics. *Unit head:* Dr. Mark A. McIntosh, Department Chair, 573-882-8989, E-mail: mcintoshm@missouri.edu. *Application contact:* Jana Clark, Coordinator, 573-882-3938, E-mail: clarkjl@missouri.edu.
Website: http://mmi.missouri.edu/graduateprogram/programindex.php

The University of Montana, Graduate School, College of Humanities and Sciences, Division of Biological Sciences, Program in Cellular, Molecular and Microbial Biology, Missoula, MT 59812-0002. Offers cellular and developmental biology (PhD); microbial evolution and ecology (PhD); microbiology and immunology (PhD); molecular biology and biochemistry (PhD). Terminal master's awarded for partial completion of doctoral program. *Degree requirements:* For doctorate, variable foreign language requirement, thesis/dissertation. *Entrance requirements:* For doctorate, GRE General Test. *Application deadline:* For fall admission, 2/1 for domestic students. Application fee: $45. *Financial support:* In 2013–14, research assistantships with tuition reimbursements (averaging $9,400 per year), teaching assistantships with full tuition reimbursements (averaging $9,400 per year) were awarded; Federal Work-Study and tuition waivers (full and partial) also available. Financial award application deadline: 3/1; financial award applicants required to submit FAFSA. *Faculty research:* Ribosome structure, medical microbiology/pathogenesis, microbial ecology/environmental microbiology. *Unit head:* Charles Janson, Chair, 406-243-5122, E-mail: charles.janson@mso.umt.edu. *Application contact:* Information Contact, E-mail: gradschl@mso.umt.edu.
Website: http://www.biology.umt.edu/

University of Nebraska Medical Center, Department of Pathology and Microbiology, Omaha, NE 68198-5900. Offers MS, PhD. Part-time programs available. Terminal master's awarded for partial completion of doctoral program. *Degree requirements:* For master's, comprehensive exam, thesis; for doctorate, comprehensive exam, thesis/dissertation. *Entrance requirements:* For master's, previous course work in biology, chemistry, mathematics, and physics; for doctorate, GRE General Test, previous course work in biology, chemistry, mathematics, and physics. Additional exam requirements/recommendations for international students: Required—TOEFL (minimum score 550 paper-based). Electronic applications accepted. *Expenses: Required fees:* $300 per semester. Tuition and fees vary according to program. *Faculty research:* Carcinogenesis, cancer biology, immunobiology, molecular virology, molecular genetics.

University of New Hampshire, Graduate School, College of Life Sciences and Agriculture, Department of Molecular, Cellular and Biomedical Sciences, Program in Microbiology, Durham, NH 03824. Offers MS, PhD. Part-time programs available. *Faculty:* 31 full-time. *Students:* 7 full-time (3 women), 6 part-time (3 women); includes 2 minority (1 Black or African American, non-Hispanic/Latino; 1 Hispanic/Latino), 1 international. Average age 27. 39 applicants, 13% accepted, 2 enrolled. In 2013, 5 master's, 2 doctorates awarded. Terminal master's awarded for partial completion of doctoral program. *Degree requirements:* For master's, thesis; for doctorate, thesis/dissertation. *Entrance requirements:* For master's and doctorate, GRE General Test. Additional exam requirements/recommendations for international students: Required—TOEFL (minimum score 550 paper-based; 80 iBT). *Application deadline:* For fall admission, 1/15 priority date for domestic students, 1/15 for international students; for spring admission, 11/1 for domestic students. Applications are processed on a rolling basis. Application fee: $65. Electronic applications accepted. *Expenses:* Tuition, state resident: full-time $13,500; part-time $750 per credit hour. Tuition, nonresident: full-time $26,200; part-time $1100 per credit hour. *Required fees:* $1741; $435.25 per term. Tuition and fees vary according to course level, course load, campus/location and program. *Financial support:* In 2013–14, 12 students received support, including 4 research assistantships, 8 teaching assistantships; fellowships, career-related internships or fieldwork, Federal Work-Study, scholarships/grants, and tuition waivers (full and partial) also available. Support available to part-time students. Financial award application deadline: 2/15. *Faculty research:* Bacterial host-parasite interactions, immunology, microbial structures, bacterial and bacteriophage genetics, virology. *Unit head:* Dr. Rick Cote, Chairperson, 603-862-0211. *Application contact:* Flora Joyal, Administrative Assistant, 603-862-4095, E-mail: flora.joyal@unh.edu.
Website: http://microbiology.unh.edu/

University of New Mexico, School of Medicine, Program in Biomedical Sciences, Albuquerque, NM 87131-5196. Offers biochemistry and molecular biology (MS, PhD); cell biology and physiology (MS, PhD); clinical and translational science (Certificate); molecular genetics and microbiology (MS, PhD); neuroscience (MS, PhD); pathology (MS, PhD); toxicology (MS, PhD); university science teaching (Certificate). Part-time programs available. *Students:* 73 full-time (39 women), 14 part-time (9 women); includes 24 minority (1 Black or African American, non-Hispanic/Latino; 1 American Indian or Alaska Native, non-Hispanic/Latino; 2 Asian, non-Hispanic/Latino; 17 Hispanic/Latino; 1 Native Hawaiian or other Pacific Islander, non-Hispanic/Latino; 2 Two or more races, non-Hispanic/Latino), 16 international. Average age 29. 89 applicants, 20% accepted, 17 enrolled. In 2013, 7 master's, 17 doctorates awarded. Terminal master's awarded for partial completion of doctoral program. *Degree requirements:* For master's, thesis; for doctorate, comprehensive exam, thesis/dissertation, qualifying exam at the end of year 1/core curriculum. *Entrance requirements:* For master's and doctorate, GRE General Test, minimum undergraduate GPA of 3.0. Additional exam requirements/recommendations for international students: Required—TOEFL. *Application deadline:* For fall admission, 3/1 priority date for domestic and international students. Applications are processed on a rolling basis. Application fee: $50. Electronic applications accepted. *Financial support:* In 2013–14, 94 students received support, including 28 fellowships with full and partial tuition reimbursements available (averaging $22,000 per year), 73 research assistantships with full tuition reimbursements available (averaging $23,000 per year), 8 teaching assistantships (averaging $2,800 per year); career-related internships or fieldwork, Federal Work-Study, institutionally sponsored loans, scholarships/grants, traineeships, health care benefits, and unspecified assistantships also available. Financial award application deadline: 1/1; financial award applicants required to submit FAFSA. *Faculty research:* Infectious disease/immunity, cancer biology, cardiovascular and metabolic diseases, brain and behavioral illness, environmental health. *Unit head:* Dr. Helen J. Hathaway, Program Director, 505-272-1887, Fax: 505-272-2412, E-mail: hhathaway@salud.unm.edu. *Application contact:* Mary Fenton, Admissions Coordinator, 505-272-1887, Fax: 505-272-2412, E-mail: mfenton@salud.unm.edu.
Website: http://hsc.unm.edu/research/brep/bsgpabout.shtm

The University of North Carolina at Chapel Hill, School of Medicine and Graduate School, Graduate Programs in Medicine, Department of Microbiology and Immunology, Chapel Hill, NC 27599-7290. Offers immunology (MS, PhD); microbiology (MS, PhD). Terminal master's awarded for partial completion of doctoral program. *Degree requirements:* For master's, comprehensive exam, thesis; for doctorate, comprehensive exam, thesis/dissertation. *Entrance requirements:* For master's and doctorate, GRE General Test, minimum GPA of 3.0. Electronic applications accepted. *Faculty research:* HIV pathogenesis, immune response, t-cell mediated autoimmunity, alpha-viruses, bacterial chemotaxis, francisella tularensis, pertussis, Mycobacterium tuberculosis, Burkholderia, Dengue virus.

University of North Dakota, Graduate School and Graduate School, Graduate Programs in Medicine, Department of Microbiology and Immunology, Grand Forks, ND 58202. Offers MS, PhD. *Degree requirements:* For master's, comprehensive exam, thesis or alternative; for doctorate, comprehensive exam, thesis/dissertation, final examination. *Entrance requirements:* For master's and doctorate, GRE General Test, minimum GPA of 3.0. Additional exam requirements/recommendations for international students: Required—TOEFL (minimum score 550 paper-based; 79 iBT), IELTS (minimum score 6.5). Electronic applications accepted. *Faculty research:* Genetic and immunological aspects of a murine model of human multiple sclerosis, termination of DNA replication, cell division in bacteria, yersinia pestis.

University of North Texas Health Science Center at Fort Worth, Graduate School of Biomedical Sciences, Fort Worth, TX 76107-2699. Offers anatomy and cell biology (MS, PhD); biochemistry and molecular biology (MS, PhD); biomedical sciences (MS, PhD); biotechnology (MS); forensic genetics (MS); integrative physiology (MS, PhD); medical science (MS); microbiology and immunology (MS, PhD); pharmacology (MS, PhD); science education (MS); DO/MS; DO/PhD. Terminal master's awarded for partial completion of doctoral program. *Degree requirements:* For master's, thesis; for doctorate, thesis/dissertation. *Entrance requirements:* For master's and doctorate, GRE General Test. Additional exam requirements/recommendations for international students: Required—TOEFL. *Expenses:* Contact institution. *Faculty research:* Alzheimer's disease, aging, eye diseases, cancer, cardiovascular disease.

University of Oklahoma, College of Arts and Sciences, Department of Microbiology and Plant Biology, Program in Microbiology, Norman, OK 73019. Offers MS, PhD. *Students:* 28 full-time (15 women), 23 part-time (7 women); includes 6 minority (1 Black or African American, non-Hispanic/Latino; 1 American Indian or Alaska Native, non-Hispanic/Latino; 2 Asian, non-Hispanic/Latino; 2 Two or more races, non-Hispanic/Latino), 23 international. Average age 27. 31 applicants, 35% accepted, 8 enrolled. In 2013, 3 master's, 2 doctorates awarded. Terminal master's awarded for partial completion of doctoral program. *Degree requirements:* For master's, thesis; for doctorate, one foreign language, comprehensive exam, thesis/dissertation. *Entrance requirements:* For master's and doctorate, GRE, 3 recommendation letters, letter of intent, bachelor's degree. Additional exam requirements/recommendations for international students: Required—TOEFL (minimum score 80 iBT). *Application deadline:* For fall admission, 4/1 for domestic and international students; for spring admission, 9/1 for domestic and international students. Application fee: $50 ($100 for international students). Electronic applications accepted. *Expenses:* Tuition, state resident: full-time $4205; part-time $175.20 per credit hour. Tuition, nonresident: full-time $16,205; part-time $675.20 per credit hour. *Required fees:* $2745; $103.85 per credit hour. $126.50 per semester. *Financial support:* In 2013–14, 42 students received support. Federal Work-Study, institutionally sponsored loans, scholarships/grants, health care benefits, and unspecified assistantships available. Support available to part-time students. Financial award application deadline: 6/1; financial award applicants required to submit FAFSA. *Faculty research:* Anaerobic microbiology, microbial ecology, environmental microbiology, molecular biology and genomics, microbial physiology. *Unit head:* Dr. Gordon Uno, Professor/Department Chair, 405-325-4321, Fax: 405-325-7619, E-mail: guno@ou.edu. *Application contact:* Adell Hopper, Staff Assistant, 405-325-4322, Fax: 405-325-7619, E-mail: ahopper@ou.edu.
Website: http://mpbio.ou.edu/

University of Oklahoma Health Sciences Center, College of Medicine and Graduate College, Graduate Programs in Medicine, Department of Microbiology and Immunology, Oklahoma City, OK 73190. Offers immunology (MS, PhD); microbiology (MS, PhD). Part-time programs available. *Faculty:* 12 full-time (4 women), 1 part-time/adjunct (0 women). *Students:* 7 full-time (3 women), 19 part-time (9 women); includes 3 minority (1 American Indian or Alaska Native, non-Hispanic/Latino; 2 Asian, non-Hispanic/Latino), 6 international. Average age 28. 7 applicants. In 2013, 2 master's, 6 doctorates awarded. Terminal master's awarded for partial completion of doctoral program. *Degree requirements:* For master's, thesis or alternative; for doctorate, one foreign language, thesis/dissertation. *Entrance requirements:* For doctorate, GRE General Test, 3 letters of recommendation. Additional exam requirements/recommendations for international students: Required—TOEFL. *Application deadline:* For fall admission, 12/15 for domestic students. Application fee: $50. *Expenses:* Tuition, state resident: full-time $3504; part-time $175.20 per credit hour. Tuition, nonresident: full-time $13,504; part-time $675.20 per credit hour. *Required fees:* $1545; $52.70 per credit hour. $245.25 per semester. Tuition and fees vary according to course load. *Financial support:* In 2013–14, 20 research assistantships (averaging $17,000 per year) were awarded; fellowships and teaching assistantships also available. Financial award applicants required to submit FAFSA. *Faculty research:* Molecular genetics, pathogenesis, streptococcal infections, gram-positive virulence, monoclonal antibodies. *Unit head:* Dr. Jimmy Ballard, Chairman, 405-271-2133, E-mail: jimmy-ballard@ouhsc.edu. *Application contact:* Dr. Molly Hill, Graduate Liaison, 405-271-2133, E-mail: molly-hill@ouhsc.edu.

University of Ottawa, Faculty of Graduate and Postdoctoral Studies, Faculty of Medicine, Department of Biochemistry, Microbiology and Immunology, Ottawa, ON K1N 6N5, Canada. Offers biochemistry (M Sc, PhD); microbiology and immunology (M Sc, PhD). *Degree requirements:* For master's, thesis; for doctorate, comprehensive exam, thesis/dissertation, seminar. *Entrance requirements:* For master's, honors degree or equivalent, minimum B average; for doctorate, master's degree, minimum B+ average. Electronic applications accepted. *Faculty research:* General biochemistry, molecular biology, microbiology, host biology, nutrition and metabolism.

University of Pennsylvania, Perelman School of Medicine, Biomedical Graduate Studies, Graduate Group in Cell and Molecular Biology, Philadelphia, PA 19104. Offers

cancer biology (PhD); cell biology and physiology (PhD); developmental stem cell regenerative biology (PhD); gene therapy and vaccines (PhD); genetics and gene regulation (PhD); microbiology, virology, and parasitology (PhD); MD/PhD; VMD/PhD. *Faculty:* 321. *Students:* 352 full-time (205 women); includes 99 minority (11 Black or African American, non-Hispanic/Latino; 65 Asian, non-Hispanic/Latino; 21 Hispanic/Latino; 2 Two or more races, non-Hispanic/Latino), 45 international. 488 applicants, 20% accepted, 40 enrolled. In 2013, 41 doctorates awarded. *Degree requirements:* For doctorate, thesis/dissertation. *Entrance requirements:* For doctorate, GRE General Test. Additional exam requirements/recommendations for international students: Required—TOEFL. *Application deadline:* For fall admission, 12/1 priority date for domestic and international students. Applications are processed on a rolling basis. Application fee: $80. Electronic applications accepted. *Financial support:* In 2013–14, 352 students received support. Fellowships, research assistantships, scholarships/grants, traineeships, and unspecified assistantships available. *Unit head:* Dr. Daniel Kessler, Graduate Group Chair, 215-898-1478. *Application contact:* Meagan Schofer, Coordinator, 215-898-4360.
Website: http://www.med.upenn.edu/camb/

University of Pittsburgh, Graduate School of Public Health, Department of Infectious Diseases and Microbiology, Pittsburgh, PA 15260. Offers infectious disease management, intervention, and community practice (MPH); infectious disease pathogenesis, eradication, and laboratory practice (MPH); infectious diseases and microbiology (MS, PhD). Part-time programs available. *Faculty:* 19 full-time (6 women), 4 part-time/adjunct (1 woman). *Students:* 50 full-time (42 women), 15 part-time (10 women); includes 8 minority (2 Black or African American, non-Hispanic/Latino; 4 Asian, non-Hispanic/Latino; 1 Hispanic/Latino; 1 Two or more races, non-Hispanic/Latino), 11 international. Average age 27. 155 applicants, 63% accepted, 15 enrolled. In 2013, 25 master's, 4 doctorates awarded. Terminal master's awarded for partial completion of doctoral program. *Degree requirements:* For master's, one foreign language, comprehensive exam (for some programs), thesis; for doctorate, one foreign language, comprehensive exam, thesis/dissertation. *Entrance requirements:* For master's and doctorate, GRE General Test, MCAT, or DAT. Additional exam requirements/recommendations for international students: Required—TOEFL (minimum score 550 paper-based; 80 iBT) or IELTS (minimum score 6.5). *Application deadline:* For fall admission, 1/15 for domestic and international students; for spring admission, 10/15 for domestic students, 8/1 for international students; for summer admission, 12/1 for international students. Applications are processed on a rolling basis. Application fee: $120. Electronic applications accepted. *Expenses:* Tuition, state resident: full-time $19,964; part-time $807 per credit. Tuition, nonresident: full-time $32,686; part-time $1337 per credit. *Required fees:* $740; $200. Tuition and fees vary according to program. *Financial support:* In 2013–14, 12 research assistantships with full and partial tuition reimbursements (averaging $8,754 per year) were awarded. Financial award applicants required to submit FAFSA. *Faculty research:* HIV, Epstein-Barr virus, virology, immunology, malaria. *Total annual research expenditures:* $14.8 million. *Unit head:* Dr. Charles R. Rinaldo, Jr., Chairman, 412-624-3928, Fax: 412-624-4953, E-mail: rinaldo@pitt.edu. *Application contact:* Dr. Jeremy Martinson, Assistant Professor, 412-624-5646, Fax: 412-383-8926, E-mail: jmartins@pitt.edu.
Website: http://www.idm.pitt.edu/

University of Pittsburgh, School of Medicine, Graduate Programs in Medicine, Molecular Virology and Microbiology Graduate Program, Pittsburgh, PA 15260. Offers PhD. *Faculty:* 46 full-time (13 women). *Students:* 27 full-time (12 women); includes 3 minority (1 Asian, non-Hispanic/Latino; 1 Hispanic/Latino; 1 Native Hawaiian or other Pacific Islander, non-Hispanic/Latino), 4 international. Average age 27. 517 applicants, 13% accepted, 22 enrolled. In 2013, 3 doctorates awarded. *Degree requirements:* For doctorate, comprehensive exam, thesis/dissertation. *Entrance requirements:* For doctorate, GRE General Test, GRE Subject Test, minimum QPA of 3.0. Additional exam requirements/recommendations for international students: Required—TOEFL (minimum score 600 paper-based; 100 iBT), IELTS (minimum score 7). *Application deadline:* For fall admission, 1/1 priority date for domestic and international students. Application fee: $50. Electronic applications accepted. *Expenses:* Tuition, state resident: full-time $19,964; part-time $807 per credit. Tuition, nonresident: full-time $32,686; part-time $1337 per credit. *Required fees:* $740; $200. Tuition and fees vary according to program. *Financial support:* In 2013–14, 27 research assistantships with full tuition reimbursements (averaging $26,010 per year) were awarded; institutionally sponsored loans, scholarships/grants, traineeships, health care benefits, and unspecified assistantships also available. *Faculty research:* Host-pathogen interactions, persistent microbial infections, microbial genetics and gene expression, microbial pathogenesis, anti-bacterial therapeutics. *Unit head:* Dr. Carolyn Coyne, Graduate Program Director, 412-383-5149, Fax: 412-624-1401, E-mail: ndeluca@pitt.edu. *Application contact:* Graduate Studies Administrator, 412-648-8957, Fax: 412-648-1077, E-mail: gradstudies@medschool.pitt.edu.
Website: http://www.gradbiomed.pitt.edu

University of Puerto Rico, Medical Sciences Campus, School of Medicine, Division of Graduate Studies, Department of Microbiology and Medical Zoology, San Juan, PR 00936-5067. Offers MS, PhD. *Degree requirements:* For master's, one foreign language, thesis; for doctorate, one foreign language, comprehensive exam, thesis/dissertation. *Entrance requirements:* For master's and doctorate, GRE General Test, GRE Subject Test, interview, minimum GPA of 3.0, 3 letters of recommendation. *Faculty research:* Molecular and general parasitology, immunology, development of viral vaccines and antiviral agents, antibiotic resistance, bacteriology.

University of Rhode Island, Graduate School, College of the Environment and Life Sciences, Department of Cell and Molecular Biology, Kingston, RI 02881. Offers biochemistry (MS, PhD); clinical laboratory sciences (MS), including biotechnology, clinical laboratory science, cytopathology; microbiology (MS, PhD); molecular genetics (MS, PhD). Part-time programs available. *Faculty:* 17 full-time (8 women), 2 part-time/adjunct (1 woman). *Students:* 19 full-time (11 women), 40 part-time (23 women); includes 14 minority (4 Black or African American, non-Hispanic/Latino; 1 American Indian or Alaska Native, non-Hispanic/Latino; 7 Asian, non-Hispanic/Latino; 2 Hispanic/Latino), 5 international. In 2013, 20 master's, 2 doctorates awarded. *Degree requirements:* For master's, comprehensive exam (for some programs), thesis optional; for doctorate, comprehensive exam, thesis/dissertation. *Entrance requirements:* For master's and doctorate, GRE, 2 letters of recommendation. Additional exam requirements/recommendations for international students: Required—TOEFL (minimum score 550 paper-based). *Application deadline:* For fall admission, 7/15 for domestic students, 2/1 for international students; for spring admission, 11/15 for domestic students, 7/15 for international students. Application fee: $65. Electronic applications accepted. *Expenses:* Tuition, state resident: full-time $11,532; part-time $641 per credit. Tuition, nonresident: full-time $23,606; part-time $1311 per credit. *Required fees:* $1388; $36 per credit. $35 per semester. One-time fee: $130. *Financial support:* In 2013–14, 5 research assistantships with full and partial tuition reimbursements (averaging $12,078 per year), 2 teaching assistantships with full and partial tuition reimbursements (averaging $11,883 per year) were awarded. Financial award application deadline: 2/1; financial award applicants required to submit FAFSA. *Faculty research:* Genomics. *Total annual research expenditures:* $6.7 million. *Unit head:* Dr. Gongqing Sun, Chairperson, 401-874-5937, Fax: 401-874-2202, E-mail: gsun@mail.uri.edu. *Application contact:* Graduate Admissions, 401-874-2872, E-mail: gradadm@etal.uri.edu.
Website: http://cels.uri.edu/cmb/

University of Rochester, School of Medicine and Dentistry, Graduate Programs in Medicine and Dentistry, Department of Microbiology and Immunology, Program in Medical Microbiology, Rochester, NY 14627. Offers MS, PhD. *Expenses: Tuition:* Full-time $44,580; part-time $1394 per credit hour. *Required fees:* $492.

University of Rochester, School of Medicine and Dentistry, Graduate Programs in Medicine and Dentistry, Department of Microbiology and Immunology, Program in Microbiology and Immunology, Rochester, NY 14627. Offers MS, PhD. *Expenses: Tuition:* Full-time $44,580; part-time $1394 per credit hour. *Required fees:* $492.

University of Saskatchewan, College of Medicine, Department of Microbiology and Immunology, Saskatoon, SK S7N 5A2, Canada. Offers M Sc, PhD. *Degree requirements:* For master's, thesis; for doctorate, thesis/dissertation. *Entrance requirements:* Additional exam requirements/recommendations for international students: Required—TOEFL. *Expenses: Tuition, area resident:* Full-time $3585 Canadian dollars; part-time $585 Canadian dollars per course. Tuition, nonresident: part-time $877 Canadian dollars per course. *International tuition:* $5377 Canadian dollars full-time. *Required fees:* $889.51 Canadian dollars.

University of Saskatchewan, Western College of Veterinary Medicine and College of Graduate Studies and Research, Graduate Programs in Veterinary Medicine, Department of Veterinary Microbiology, Saskatoon, SK S7N 5A2, Canada. Offers M Sc, M Vet Sc, PhD. *Degree requirements:* For master's, thesis; for doctorate, comprehensive exam (for some programs), thesis/dissertation. *Entrance requirements:* Additional exam requirements/recommendations for international students: Required—TOEFL (minimum score 80 iBT) or IELTS (minimum score 6.5). Electronic applications accepted. *Expenses: Tuition, area resident:* Full-time $3585 Canadian dollars; part-time $585 Canadian dollars per course. Tuition, nonresident: part-time $877 Canadian dollars per course. *International tuition:* $5377 Canadian dollars full-time. *Required fees:* $889.51 Canadian dollars. *Faculty research:* Immunology, vaccinology, epidemiology, virology, parasitology.

The University of South Dakota, Graduate School, School of Medicine and Graduate School, Biomedical Sciences Graduate Program, Molecular Microbiology and Immunology Group, Vermillion, SD 57069-2390. Offers MS, PhD. Terminal master's awarded for partial completion of doctoral program. *Degree requirements:* For master's, thesis; for doctorate, comprehensive exam, thesis/dissertation. *Entrance requirements:* For master's and doctorate, GRE General Test, minimum GPA of 3.0. Additional exam requirements/recommendations for international students: Required—TOEFL (minimum score 550 paper-based; 80 iBT), IELTS (minimum score 6). Electronic applications accepted. *Expenses:* Contact institution. *Faculty research:* Structure-function membranes, plasmids, immunology, virology, pathogenesis.

University of Southern California, Keck School of Medicine and Graduate School, Graduate Programs in Medicine, Department of Molecular Microbiology and Immunology, Los Angeles, CA 90033. Offers MS. Part-time programs available. *Faculty:* 21 full-time (5 women), 1 (woman) part-time/adjunct. *Students:* 29 full-time (21 women), 1 part-time (0 women); includes 8 minority (2 Black or African American, non-Hispanic/Latino; 3 Asian, non-Hispanic/Latino; 2 Hispanic/Latino; 1 Two or more races, non-Hispanic/Latino), 16 international. Average age 25. 40 applicants, 50% accepted, 15 enrolled. In 2013, 16 master's awarded. Terminal master's awarded for partial completion of doctoral program. *Degree requirements:* For master's, comprehensive exam (for some programs), thesis optional. *Entrance requirements:* For master's, GRE General Test, minimum GPA of 3.0. Additional exam requirements/recommendations for international students: Required—TOEFL (minimum score 100 iBT), IELTS. *Application deadline:* For fall admission, 6/1 for domestic students, 5/1 for international students; for spring admission, 11/1 for domestic students, 10/1 for international students. Applications are processed on a rolling basis. Application fee: $85. Electronic applications accepted. *Financial support:* In 2013–14, 1 student received support, including 1 teaching assistantship with full tuition reimbursement available (averaging $31,000 per year); Federal Work-Study, institutionally sponsored loans, scholarships/grants, health care benefits, and unspecified assistantships also available. Financial award application deadline: 5/4; financial award applicants required to submit FAFSA. *Faculty research:* Animal virology, microbial genetics, molecular and cellular immunology, cellular differentiation control of protein synthesis, HIV. *Unit head:* Dr. Axel H. Schonthal, Associate Professor/Program Chairman, 323-442-1730, Fax: 323-442-1721, E-mail: schontha@usc.edu. *Application contact:* Silvina V. Campos, Administrative Assistant II, 323-442-1713, Fax: 323-442-1721, E-mail: scampos@usc.edu.
Website: http://www.usc.edu/schools/medicine/departments/molecularmicrobio_immunology/

University of Southern Mississippi, Graduate School, College of Science and Technology, Department of Biological Sciences, Hattiesburg, MS 39406-0001. Offers environmental biology (MS, PhD); marine biology (MS, PhD); microbiology (MS, PhD); molecular biology (MS, PhD). *Faculty:* 27 full-time (6 women). *Students:* 63 full-time (26 women), 4 part-time (all women); includes 4 minority (1 Black or African American, non-Hispanic/Latino; 1 Hispanic/Latino; 2 Two or more races, non-Hispanic/Latino), 17 international. Average age 32. 43 applicants, 30% accepted, 12 enrolled. In 2013, 12 master's, 9 doctorates awarded. Terminal master's awarded for partial completion of doctoral program. *Degree requirements:* For master's, comprehensive exam, thesis; for doctorate, comprehensive exam, thesis/dissertation. *Entrance requirements:* For master's, GRE General Test, minimum GPA of 3.0 on last 60 hours; for doctorate, GRE General Test, minimum GPA of 3.5. Additional exam requirements/recommendations for international students: Required—TOEFL, IELTS. *Application deadline:* For fall admission, 3/1 priority date for domestic students, 3/1 for international students; for spring admission, 1/10 priority date for domestic and international students. Applications are processed on a rolling basis. Application fee: $50. *Financial support:* In 2013–14, 25 research assistantships with full tuition reimbursements (averaging $9,700 per year), 33 teaching assistantships with full tuition reimbursements (averaging $10,600 per year) were awarded; Federal Work-Study, scholarships/grants, health care benefits, and unspecified assistantships also available. Financial award application deadline: 3/15; financial award applicants required to submit FAFSA. *Unit head:* Dr. Glenmore Shearer, Chair, 601-266-4748, Fax: 601-266-5797. *Application contact:* Dr. Jake Schaefer, Director of Graduate Studies, 601-266-4748, Fax: 601-266-5797.
Website: http://www.usm.edu/graduateschool/table.php

University of South Florida, College of Arts and Sciences, Department of Cell Biology, Microbiology, and Molecular Biology, Tampa, FL 33620-9951. Offers biology (MS), including cell and molecular biology; cancer biology (PhD); cell and molecular biology (PhD); microbiology (MS). *Faculty:* 19 full-time (5 women), 1 part-time/adjunct (0 women). *Students:* 77 full-time (46 women), 3 part-time (1 woman); includes 8 minority (5 Asian, non-Hispanic/Latino; 3 Hispanic/Latino), 19 international. Average age 27. 155 applicants, 17% accepted, 17 enrolled. In 2013, 19 master's, 12 doctorates awarded. *Degree requirements:* For master's, thesis or alternative; for doctorate, comprehensive exam, thesis/dissertation. *Entrance requirements:* For master's and doctorate, GRE

General Test, minimum GPA of 3.0, extensive background in biology or chemistry. Additional exam requirements/recommendations for international students: Required—TOEFL (minimum score 550 paper-based; 79 iBT) or IELTS (minimum score 6.5). *Application deadline:* For fall admission, 2/1 for domestic students, 1/1 for international students. Application fee: $30. *Financial support:* Career-related internships or fieldwork, health care benefits, and unspecified assistantships available. Financial award application deadline: 4/1. *Faculty research:* Cell biology, microbiology and molecular biology: basic and applied science in bacterial pathogenesis, genome integrity and mechanisms of aging, structural and computational biology; cancer biology: immunology, cancer control, signal transduction, drug discovery, genomics. *Total annual research expenditures:* $1.9 million. *Unit head:* Dr. James Garey, Professor/Chair, 813-974-7103, Fax: 813-974-1614, E-mail: garey@usf.edu. *Application contact:* Dr. Kenneth Wright, Associate Professor of Cancer Biology, H. Lee Moffitt Cancer Center and Research Institute, 813-745-3918, Fax: 813-974-1614, E-mail: ken.wright@moffitt.org.
Website: http://biology.usf.edu/cmmb/

University of South Florida, College of Arts and Sciences, Department of Integrative Biology, Tampa, FL 33620-9951. Offers biology (MS), including ecology and evolution (MS, PhD), environmental and ecological microbiology (MS, PhD), physiology and morphology (MS, PhD); integrative biology (PhD), including ecology and evolution (MS, PhD), environmental and ecological microbiology (MS, PhD), physiology and morphology (MS, PhD). Part-time programs available. *Faculty:* 16 full-time (4 women), 1 part-time/adjunct (0 women). *Students:* 40 full-time (24 women), 7 part-time (4 women); includes 6 minority (5 Hispanic/Latino; 1 Two or more races, non-Hispanic/Latino), 3 international. Average age 29. 59 applicants, 29% accepted, 11 enrolled. In 2013, 4 master's, 5 doctorates awarded. *Degree requirements:* For master's, comprehensive exam, thesis (for some programs); for doctorate, comprehensive exam, thesis/dissertation. *Entrance requirements:* For master's and doctorate, GRE General Test (minimum preferred scores of 153 verbal, 148 quantitative, 4.5 analytical/500 verbal and 600 quantitative with 4.5 in analytical writing on old scoring), minimum GPA of 3.0 in last 60 hours of BS. Additional exam requirements/recommendations for international students: Required—TOEFL (minimum score 570 paper-based; 88 iBT). *Application deadline:* For fall admission, 2/15 priority date for domestic students, 1/2 for international students; for spring admission, 8/1 for domestic students, 6/1 for international students. Application fee: $30. Electronic applications accepted. *Financial support:* Research assistantships, teaching assistantships, and unspecified assistantships available. Financial award application deadline: 6/30; financial award applicants required to submit FAFSA. *Faculty research:* Marine ecology, ecosystem responses to urbanization, biomechanical and physiological mechanisms of animal movement, population biology and conservation, microbial ecology and public health microbiology, natural diversity of parasites and herbivores; ecosystems, vertebrates, disturbance ecology, functional and ecological morphology of feeding in fishes, rare amphibians and reptiles, genomics in ecological experiments, ecotoxicology, global carbon cycle, plant-animal interactions. *Total annual research expenditures:* $968,227. *Unit head:* Dr. Peter Stiling, Chair, Department of Integrative Biology, 813-974-6229, Fax: 813-974-3263, E-mail: pstiling@usf.edu. *Application contact:* Christine Brubaker, Graduate Program Specialist, Department of Integrative Biology, 813-974-4747, Fax: 813-974-3263, E-mail: brubaker@usf.edu.
Website: http://biology.usf.edu/ib/grad/

The University of Tennessee, Graduate School, College of Arts and Sciences, Department of Microbiology, Knoxville, TN 37996. Offers MS, PhD. Part-time programs available. *Degree requirements:* For master's, thesis; for doctorate, thesis/dissertation. *Entrance requirements:* For master's and doctorate, GRE General Test, minimum GPA of 2.7. Additional exam requirements/recommendations for international students: Required—TOEFL. Electronic applications accepted. *Expenses:* Tuition, state resident: full-time $9540; part-time $531 per credit hour. Tuition, nonresident: full-time $27,728; part-time $1542 per credit hour. *Required fees:* $1404; $67 per credit hour.

The University of Texas at Austin, Graduate School, College of Natural Sciences, School of Biological Sciences, Program in Microbiology, Austin, TX 78712-1111. Offers PhD. *Entrance requirements:* For doctorate, GRE General Test. Electronic applications accepted.

The University of Texas Health Science Center at Houston, Graduate School of Biomedical Sciences, Program in Microbiology and Molecular Genetics, Houston, TX 77225-0036. Offers MS, PhD, MD/PhD. Terminal master's awarded for partial completion of doctoral program. *Degree requirements:* For master's, thesis; for doctorate, thesis/dissertation. *Entrance requirements:* For master's and doctorate, GRE General Test. Additional exam requirements/recommendations for international students: Required—TOEFL. Electronic applications accepted. *Expenses:* Tuition, state resident: full-time $3474; part-time $193 per credit hour. Tuition, nonresident: full-time $13,644; part-time $758 per credit hour. *Required fees:* $226.30; $87 per credit hour. *Faculty research:* Disease causation, environmental signaling, gene regulation, cell growth and division, cell structure and architecture.

The University of Texas Health Science Center at San Antonio, Graduate School of Biomedical Sciences, Department of Microbiology and Immunology, San Antonio, TX 78229-3900. Offers PhD. *Faculty:* 23 full-time (5 women), 1 (woman) part-time/adjunct. *Students:* 24 full-time (15 women), 2 part-time (both women); includes 12 minority (1 Asian, non-Hispanic/Latino; 11 Hispanic/Latino), 3 international. Average age 30. In 2013, 8 doctorates awarded. *Degree requirements:* For doctorate, comprehensive exam, thesis/dissertation. *Entrance requirements:* For doctorate, GRE General Test. Additional exam requirements/recommendations for international students: Required—TOEFL (minimum score 560 paper-based; 68 iBT). *Application deadline:* For fall admission, 1/15 priority date for domestic and international students. Applications are processed on a rolling basis. Application fee: $0. Electronic applications accepted. *Financial support:* Application deadline: 6/30; applicants required to submit FAFSA. *Faculty research:* Molecular immunology, mechanisms of microbial pathogenesis, molecular genetics, vaccine and immunodiagnostic development. *Total annual research expenditures:* $5.5 million. *Unit head:* Dr. Paolo B. Casali, Chairman, 210-567-3939, Fax: 210-567-6612, E-mail: pcasali@uthscsa.edu. *Application contact:* Dr. Keith Krolick, Graduate Advisor/Committee on Graduate Studies Chair, 210-567-3968, Fax: 210-567-6612, E-mail: krolick@uthscsa.edu.
Website: http://www.uthscsa.edu/micro/

The University of Texas Medical Branch, Graduate School of Biomedical Sciences, Program in Microbiology and Immunology, Galveston, TX 77555. Offers MS, PhD. Terminal master's awarded for partial completion of doctoral program. *Degree requirements:* For master's, thesis or alternative; for doctorate, thesis/dissertation. *Entrance requirements:* For doctorate, GRE General Test, minimum GPA of 3.0. Additional exam requirements/recommendations for international students: Required—TOEFL (minimum score 550 paper-based). Electronic applications accepted.

The University of Texas Southwestern Medical Center, Southwestern Graduate School of Biomedical Sciences, Division of Basic Science, Program in Molecular Microbiology, Dallas, TX 75390. Offers PhD. *Faculty:* 34 full-time (10 women), 2 part-time/adjunct (0 women). *Students:* 24 full-time (14 women); includes 7 minority (4 Asian, non-Hispanic/Latino; 3 Hispanic/Latino), 3 international. Average age 27. In 2013, 5 doctorates awarded. *Degree requirements:* For doctorate, thesis/dissertation, oral and written exams. *Entrance requirements:* For doctorate, GRE General Test, minimum GPA of 3.0. Additional exam requirements/recommendations for international students: Required—TOEFL. *Application deadline:* For fall admission, 12/15 priority date for domestic students. Applications are processed on a rolling basis. Application fee: $0. Electronic applications accepted. *Financial support:* Fellowships, research assistantships, and institutionally sponsored loans available. *Faculty research:* Cell and molecular immunology, molecular pathogenesis of infectious disease, virology. *Unit head:* Dr. Vanessa Speraudio, Chair, 214-648-1603, Fax: 214-648-1899, E-mail: vanessa.speraudio@utsouthwestern.edu.
Website: http://www.utsouthwestern.edu/education/graduate-school/programs/phd-degrees/molecular-microbiology/index.html

University of Victoria, Faculty of Graduate Studies, Faculty of Science, Department of Biochemistry and Microbiology, Victoria, BC V8W 2Y2, Canada. Offers biochemistry (M Sc, PhD); microbiology (M Sc, PhD). *Degree requirements:* For master's, thesis, seminar; for doctorate, thesis/dissertation, seminar, candidacy exam. *Entrance requirements:* For master's, GRE General Test, minimum B+ average; for doctorate, GRE General Test, minimum B+ average, M Sc. Additional exam requirements/recommendations for international students: Required—TOEFL (minimum score 600 paper-based). Electronic applications accepted. *Faculty research:* Molecular pathogenesis, prokaryotic, eukaryotic, macromolecular interactions, microbial surfaces, virology, molecular genetics.

University of Virginia, School of Medicine, Department of Microbiology, Charlottesville, VA 22903. Offers PhD, MD/PhD. *Faculty:* 37 full-time (12 women). *Students:* 60 full-time (40 women); includes 15 minority (4 Black or African American, non-Hispanic/Latino; 1 American Indian or Alaska Native, non-Hispanic/Latino; 4 Asian, non-Hispanic/Latino; 5 Hispanic/Latino; 1 Two or more races, non-Hispanic/Latino), 2 international. Average age 27. In 2013, 10 doctorates awarded. *Degree requirements:* For doctorate, thesis/dissertation. *Entrance requirements:* For doctorate, GRE General Test, 2 or more letters of recommendation. Additional exam requirements/recommendations for international students: Required—TOEFL (minimum score 600 paper-based; 90 iBT). *Application deadline:* For fall admission, 2/1 for domestic and international students. Applications are processed on a rolling basis. Application fee: $60. Electronic applications accepted. *Expenses:* Tuition, state resident: part-time $334 per credit hour. Tuition, nonresident: part-time $1224 per credit hour. *Financial support:* Fellowships, traineeships, and unspecified assistantships available. Financial award applicants required to submit FAFSA. *Faculty research:* Virology, membrane biology and molecular genetics. *Unit head:* Kodi S. Ravichandran, Chair, 434-924-1948, Fax: 434-982-1071, E-mail: kr4h@virginia.edu. *Application contact:* Lucy Pemberton, Director of Graduate Studies, 434-243-6737, Fax: 434-924-1236, E-mail: lfp2n@virginia.edu.
Website: http://www.medicine.virginia.edu/basic-science/departments/microbiology-immunology-and-cancer-biology

University of Washington, Graduate School, School of Medicine, Graduate Programs in Medicine, Department of Microbiology, Seattle, WA 98195. Offers PhD. *Degree requirements:* For doctorate, thesis/dissertation. *Entrance requirements:* For doctorate, GRE General Test, GRE Subject Test (recommended). Electronic applications accepted. *Faculty research:* Bacterial genetics and physiology, mechanisms of bacterial and viral pathogenesis, bacterial-plant interaction.

The University of Western Ontario, Faculty of Graduate Studies, Biosciences Division, Department of Microbiology and Immunology, London, ON N6A 5B8, Canada. Offers M Sc, PhD. *Degree requirements:* For master's, thesis, oral and written exam; for doctorate, thesis/dissertation, oral and written exam. *Entrance requirements:* For master's, honors degree or equivalent in microbiology, immunology, or other biological science; minimum B average; for doctorate, M Sc in microbiology and immunology. Additional exam requirements/recommendations for international students: Required—TOEFL. *Faculty research:* Virology, molecular pathogenesis, cellular immunology, molecular biology.

University of Wisconsin–La Crosse, Graduate Studies, College of Science and Health, Department of Biology, La Crosse, WI 54601-3742. Offers aquatic sciences (MS); biology (MS); cellular and molecular biology (MS); clinical microbiology (MS); microbiology (MS); nurse anesthesia (MS); physiology (MS). Part-time programs available. *Faculty:* 22 full-time (8 women), 3 part-time/adjunct (1 woman). *Students:* 21 full-time (13 women), 37 part-time (24 women); includes 7 minority (2 Asian, non-Hispanic/Latino; 4 Hispanic/Latino; 1 Two or more races, non-Hispanic/Latino), 5 international. Average age 28. 107 applicants, 26% accepted, 25 enrolled. In 2013, 16 master's awarded. *Degree requirements:* For master's, comprehensive exam, thesis. *Entrance requirements:* For master's, GRE General Test, minimum GPA of 2.85. Additional exam requirements/recommendations for international students: Required—TOEFL (minimum score 550 paper-based; 79 iBT). *Application deadline:* For fall admission, 2/1 priority date for domestic and international students; for spring admission, 1/4 priority date for domestic and international students. Applications are processed on a rolling basis. Electronic applications accepted. *Financial support:* Research assistantships with partial tuition reimbursements, Federal Work-Study, scholarships/grants, health care benefits, and tuition waivers (partial) available. Support available to part-time students. Financial award application deadline: 3/15; financial award applicants required to submit FAFSA. *Unit head:* Dr. Thomas Volk, Coordinator of Graduate Studies, 608-785-6972, Fax: 608-785-6959, E-mail: volk.thom@uwlax.edu. *Application contact:* Corey Sjoquist, Director of Admissions, 608-785-8939, E-mail: admissions@uwlax.edu.
Website: http://uwlax.edu/biology/

University of Wisconsin–Madison, School of Medicine and Public Health and Graduate School, Graduate Programs in Medicine and College of Agricultural and Life Sciences, Microbiology Doctoral Training Program, Madison, WI 53706. Offers PhD. *Faculty:* 92 full-time (31 women). *Students:* 68 full-time (41 women); includes 13 minority (2 Black or African American, non-Hispanic/Latino; 1 American Indian or Alaska Native, non-Hispanic/Latino; 1 Asian, non-Hispanic/Latino; 9 Hispanic/Latino). Average age 24. 271 applicants, 14% accepted, 13 enrolled. In 2013, 12 doctorates awarded. *Degree requirements:* For doctorate, thesis/dissertation, preliminary exam, 1 semester of teaching, professional development. *Entrance requirements:* For doctorate, GRE. Additional exam requirements/recommendations for international students: Required—TOEFL (minimum score 580 paper-based). *Application deadline:* For fall admission, 12/1 for domestic and international students. Application fee: $56. Electronic applications accepted. *Expenses:* Tuition, state resident: full-time $10,728; part-time $790 per credit. Tuition, nonresident: full-time $24,054; part-time $1623 per credit. *Required fees:* $1130; $119 per credit. *Financial support:* In 2013–14, 68 students received support, including 44 fellowships with full tuition reimbursements available (averaging $25,250 per year), 22 research assistantships with full tuition reimbursements available (averaging $25,250 per year); career-related internships or fieldwork, scholarships/grants, traineeships, health care benefits, and tuition waivers (full) also available. Financial award application deadline: 12/1. *Faculty research:* Microbial pathogenesis, gene regulation, immunology, virology, cell biology. *Total annual research expenditures:* $15.1 million. *Unit head:* Dr. John Mansfield, Director, 608-262-2596, Fax: 608-262-

8418, E-mail: jmansfield@bact.wisc.edu. *Application contact:* Cathy Davis Gray, Coordinator, 608-265-0689, Fax: 608-262-8418, E-mail: cdg@bact.wisc.edu.
Website: http://www.microbiology.wisc.edu/

University of Wisconsin–Oshkosh, Graduate Studies, College of Letters and Science, Department of Biology and Microbiology, Oshkosh, WI 54901. Offers biology (MS), including botany, microbiology, zoology. *Degree requirements:* For master's, comprehensive exam, thesis. *Entrance requirements:* For master's, GRE General Test, minimum GPA of 3.0, BS in biology. Additional exam requirements/recommendations for international students: Required—TOEFL (minimum score 550 paper-based; 79 iBT). Electronic applications accepted.

University of Wyoming, Graduate Program in Molecular and Cellular Life Sciences, Laramie, WY 82071. Offers PhD. *Degree requirements:* For doctorate, thesis/dissertation, four eight-week laboratory rotations, comprehensive basic practical exam, two-part qualifying exam, seminars, symposium.

Vanderbilt University, Graduate School and School of Medicine, Department of Microbiology and Immunology, Nashville, TN 37240-1001. Offers MS, PhD, MD/PhD. *Faculty:* 43 full-time (13 women). *Students:* 52 full-time (35 women); includes 6 minority (1 Black or African American, non-Hispanic/Latino; 3 Asian, non-Hispanic/Latino; 1 Hispanic/Latino; 1 Two or more races, non-Hispanic/Latino), 7 international. Average age 27. In 2013, 11 doctorates awarded. Terminal master's awarded for partial completion of doctoral program. *Degree requirements:* For master's, thesis; for doctorate, thesis/dissertation, final and qualifying exams. *Entrance requirements:* For master's and doctorate, GRE General Test, GRE Subject Test (recommended). Additional exam requirements/recommendations for international students: Required—TOEFL (minimum score 570 paper-based; 88 iBT). *Application deadline:* For fall admission, 1/15 for domestic and international students. Application fee: $0. Electronic applications accepted. *Financial support:* Fellowships with full tuition reimbursements, research assistantships with full tuition reimbursements, Federal Work-Study, institutionally sponsored loans, scholarships/grants, traineeships, health care benefits, and tuition waivers (partial) available. Financial award application deadline: 1/15; financial award applicants required to submit CSS PROFILE or FAFSA. *Faculty research:* Cellular and molecular microbiology, viruses, genes, cancer, molecular pathogenesis of microbial diseases, immunobiology. *Unit head:* Prof. Samuel A. Santoro, Chair of the Department of Pathology, Microbiology and Immunology, 615-322-3234, Fax: 615-322-5551, E-mail: samuel.a.santoro@vanderbilt.edu. *Application contact:* Walter B. Bieschke, Program Coordinator for Graduate Admissions, 615-342-0236, E-mail: walter.bieschke@vanderbilt.edu.
Website: http://www.mc.vanderbilt.edu/root/vumc.php?site-vmcpathology

Virginia Commonwealth University, Medical College of Virginia-Professional Programs, School of Medicine, School of Medicine Graduate Programs, Department of Microbiology and Immunology, Richmond, VA 23284-9005. Offers microbiology and immunology (MS, PhD); MD/PhD. *Degree requirements:* For master's, thesis; for doctorate, thesis/dissertation, comprehensive oral and written exams. *Entrance requirements:* For master's and doctorate, GRE General Test or MCAT. Additional exam requirements/recommendations for international students: Required—TOEFL (minimum score 600 paper-based; 100 iBT). Electronic applications accepted. *Faculty research:* Microbial physiology and genetics, molecular biology, crystallography of biological molecules, antibiotics and chemotherapy, membrane transport.

Virginia Commonwealth University, Program in Pre-Medical Basic Health Sciences, Richmond, VA 23284-9005. Offers anatomy (CBHS); biochemistry (CBHS); human genetics (CBHS); microbiology (CBHS); pharmacology (CBHS); physiology (CBHS). *Entrance requirements:* For degree, GRE, MCAT or DAT, course work in organic chemistry, minimum undergraduate GPA of 2.8. Additional exam requirements/recommendations for international students: Required—TOEFL (minimum score 600 paper-based). Electronic applications accepted.

Wagner College, Division of Graduate Studies, Program in Microbiology, Staten Island, NY 10301-4495. Offers MS. Part-time and evening/weekend programs available. *Faculty:* 3 full-time (2 women), 3 part-time/adjunct (all women). *Students:* 28 full-time (14 women), 10 part-time (5 women); includes 6 minority (3 Black or African American, non-Hispanic/Latino; 1 Asian, non-Hispanic/Latino; 2 Two or more races, non-Hispanic/Latino). Average age 25. 28 applicants, 93% accepted, 18 enrolled. In 2013, 13 master's awarded. *Degree requirements:* For master's, comprehensive exam or thesis. *Entrance requirements:* For master's, minimum GPA of 2.6, proficiency in statistics, undergraduate major in biological science or chemistry, undergraduate microbiology course, 16 credits of chemistry including organic chemistry with lab. Additional exam requirements/recommendations for international students: Required—TOEFL (minimum score 550 paper-based; 79 iBT). *Application deadline:* For fall admission, 5/1 priority date for domestic students, 3/1 priority date for international students; for spring admission, 12/1 for domestic students, 10/1 for international students. Applications are processed on a rolling basis. Application fee: $50. *Expenses: Tuition:* Full-time $17,496; part-time $972 per credit. Tuition and fees vary according to course load. *Financial support:* In 2013–14, 19 students received support. Career-related internships or fieldwork, unspecified assistantships, and alumni fellowship grants available. Financial award applicants required to submit FAFSA. *Faculty research:* Listeria monocytogenes pathogenesis, plant extracts as anti-microbial agents, neuroimmunology. *Unit head:* Dr. Christopher Corbo, Director, 718-390-3385, E-mail: ccorbo@wagner.edu. *Application contact:* Patricia Clancy, Administrative Assistant, 718-420-4464, Fax: 718-390-3105, E-mail: patricia.clancy@wagner.edu.

Wake Forest University, School of Medicine and Graduate School of Arts and Sciences, Graduate Programs in Medicine, Department of Microbiology and Immunology, Winston-Salem, NC 27109. Offers PhD, MD/PhD. *Degree requirements:* For doctorate, thesis/dissertation. *Entrance requirements:* For doctorate, GRE General Test. Additional exam requirements/recommendations for international students: Required—TOEFL. Electronic applications accepted. *Faculty research:* Molecular immunology, bacterial pathogenesis and molecular genetics, viral pathogenesis, regulation of mRNA metabolism, leukocyte biology.

Washington University in St. Louis, Graduate School of Arts and Sciences, Division of Biology and Biomedical Sciences, Program in Molecular Microbiology and Microbial Pathogenesis, St. Louis, MO 63130-4899. Offers PhD. *Degree requirements:* For doctorate, thesis/dissertation. *Entrance requirements:* For doctorate, GRE General Test, GRE Subject Test. Electronic applications accepted.

Wayne State University, School of Medicine, Graduate Programs in Medicine, Department of Immunology and Microbiology, Detroit, MI 48202. Offers MS, PhD, MD/PhD. *Students:* 13 full-time (7 women), 1 part-time (0 women); includes 3 minority (1 Black or African American, non-Hispanic/Latino; 1 Hispanic/Latino; 1 Two or more races, non-Hispanic/Latino), 1 international. Average age 26. 78 applicants, 8% accepted, 3 enrolled. In 2013, 3 doctorates awarded. *Degree requirements:* For doctorate, thesis/dissertation. *Entrance requirements:* For master's and doctorate, GRE, minimum GPA of 3.0 in BS in biology or related scientific discipline, three letters of recommendation, statement of purpose, admission to the Graduate School. Additional exam requirements/recommendations for international students: Required—TOEFL (minimum score 100 iBT), TWE (minimum score 6). *Application deadline:* For fall admission, 2/1 priority date for domestic and international students. Application fee: $0. Electronic applications accepted. *Expenses:* Contact institution. *Financial support:* In 2013–14, 10 students received support, including 2 fellowships with tuition reimbursements available (averaging $20,309 per year), 8 research assistantships with tuition reimbursements available (averaging $22,466 per year); teaching assistantships with tuition reimbursements available, scholarships/grants, health care benefits, and unspecified assistantships also available. Financial award application deadline: 3/31; financial award applicants required to submit FAFSA. *Faculty research:* Viral replication and pathogenesis, bacterial pathogenesis, mucosal immunity, autoimmune diseases. *Unit head:* Dr. Paul C. Montgomery, Professor and Chair, 313-577-1591, Fax: 313-577-1155, E-mail: pmontgo@wayne.edu. *Application contact:* Dr. Thomas C. Holland, Associate Professor, 313-577-1455, Fax: 313-577-1155, E-mail: tholland@wayne.edu.
Website: http://www.immunomicro.med.wayne.edu/gradprogram.php

West Virginia University, School of Medicine, Graduate Programs at the Health Sciences Center, Interdisciplinary Graduate Programs in Biomedical Sciences, Program in Immunology and Microbial Pathogenesis, Morgantown, WV 26506. Offers MS, PhD, MD/PhD. *Degree requirements:* For doctorate, comprehensive exam, thesis/dissertation. *Entrance requirements:* For doctorate, GRE General Test, minimum GPA of 3.0. Additional exam requirements/recommendations for international students: Required—TOEFL. Electronic applications accepted. *Faculty research:* Regulation of signal transduction in immune responses, immune responses in bacterial and viral diseases, peptide and DNA vaccines for contraception, inflammatory bowel disease, physiology of pathogenic microbes.

Wright State University, School of Graduate Studies, College of Science and Mathematics, Program in Microbiology and Immunology, Dayton, OH 45435. Offers MS. Part-time programs available. *Degree requirements:* For master's, thesis. *Entrance requirements:* Additional exam requirements/recommendations for international students: Required—TOEFL. *Faculty research:* Reproductive immunology, viral pathogenesis, virus-host cell interactions.

Yale University, School of Medicine and Graduate School of Arts and Sciences, Combined Program in Biological and Biomedical Sciences (BBS), Microbiology Track, New Haven, CT 06520. Offers PhD, MD/PhD. *Degree requirements:* For doctorate, thesis/dissertation. *Entrance requirements:* For doctorate, GRE General Test, GRE Subject Test. Additional exam requirements/recommendations for international students: Required—TOEFL. Electronic applications accepted.

Youngstown State University, Graduate School, College of Science, Technology, Engineering and Mathematics, Department of Biological Sciences, Youngstown, OH 44555-0001. Offers environmental biology (MS); molecular biology, microbiology, and genetic (MS); physiology and anatomy (MS). Part-time programs available. *Degree requirements:* For master's, comprehensive exam, thesis, oral review. *Entrance requirements:* For master's, GRE General Test, minimum GPA of 2.7. Additional exam requirements/recommendations for international students: Required—TOEFL. *Faculty research:* Cell biology, neurophysiology, molecular biology, neurobiology, gene regulation.

Virology

Baylor College of Medicine, Graduate School of Biomedical Sciences, Department of Molecular Virology and Microbiology, Houston, TX 77030-3498. Offers PhD, MD/PhD. *Degree requirements:* For doctorate, thesis/dissertation, public defense. *Entrance requirements:* For doctorate, GRE General Test, GRE Subject Test (strongly recommended), minimum GPA of 3.0. Additional exam requirements/recommendations for international students: Required—TOEFL. Electronic applications accepted. *Faculty research:* Microbiology, viral molecular biology, bacterial molecular biology, microbial pathogenesis, microbial genomics.

Baylor College of Medicine, Graduate School of Biomedical Sciences, Interdepartmental Program in Cell and Molecular Biology, Houston, TX 77030-3498. Offers biochemistry (PhD); cell and molecular biology (PhD); genetics (PhD); human genetics (PhD); immunology (PhD); microbiology (PhD); virology (PhD); MD/PhD. *Degree requirements:* For doctorate, thesis/dissertation, public defense. *Entrance requirements:* For doctorate, GRE General Test, GRE Subject Test (strongly recommended), minimum GPA of 3.0. Additional exam requirements/recommendations for international students: Required—TOEFL. Electronic applications accepted. *Faculty research:* Molecular and cellular biology; cancer, aging and stem cells; genomics and proteomics; microbiome, molecular microbiology; infectious disease, immunology and translational research.

Case Western Reserve University, School of Medicine and School of Graduate Studies, Graduate Programs in Medicine, Department of Molecular Biology and Microbiology, Program in Molecular Virology, Cleveland, OH 44106. Offers PhD. *Entrance requirements:* Additional exam requirements/recommendations for international students: Required—TOEFL (minimum score 550 paper-based).

Mayo Graduate School, Graduate Programs in Biomedical Sciences, Program in Virology and Gene Therapy, Rochester, MN 55905. Offers PhD.

McMaster University, Faculty of Health Sciences and School of Graduate Studies, Program in Medical Sciences, Hamilton, ON L8S 4M2, Canada. Offers blood and vascular (M Sc, PhD); genetics and cancer (M Sc, PhD); immunity and infection (M Sc, PhD); metabolism and nutrition (M Sc, PhD); neurosciences and behavioral sciences (M Sc, PhD); physiology/pharmacology (M Sc, PhD); MD/PhD. *Degree requirements:* For master's, thesis; for doctorate, comprehensive exam, thesis/dissertation. *Entrance requirements:* For master's, honors B Sc, B+ average in related field; for doctorate, M Sc, minimum B+ average. Additional exam requirements/recommendations for international students: Required—TOEFL (minimum score 580 paper-based; 92 iBT).

The Ohio State University, College of Medicine, School of Biomedical Science, Biomedical Sciences Graduate Program, Columbus, OH 43210. Offers immunology (PhD); medical genetics (PhD); molecular virology (PhD); pharmacology (PhD). *Students:* 109 full-time (55 women), 9 part-time (6 women); includes 24 minority (5 Black or African American, non-Hispanic/Latino; 1 American Indian or Alaska Native, non-Hispanic/Latino; 10 Asian, non-Hispanic/Latino; 6 Hispanic/Latino; 1 Native Hawaiian or other Pacific Islander, non-Hispanic/Latino; 1 Two or more races, non-Hispanic/Latino), 4 international. Average age 27. In 2013, 20 doctorates awarded. *Degree requirements:* For doctorate, thesis/dissertation. *Entrance requirements:* For doctorate, GRE General Test; GRE Subject Test in biochemistry, cell and molecular biology (recommended for some programs). Additional exam requirements/recommendations for international students: Required—TOEFL (minimum score 600 paper-based; 100 iBT), Michigan English Language Assessment Battery (minimum score 86); Recommended—IELTS (minimum score 8). *Application deadline:* For fall admission, 12/13 priority date for domestic students, 11/1 priority date for international students. Applications are processed on a rolling basis. Application fee: $60 ($70 for international students). Electronic applications accepted. *Financial support:* In 2013–14, 53 students received support, including 4 fellowships with full tuition reimbursements available (averaging $19,000 per year), 49 research assistantships with full tuition reimbursements available (averaging $19,000 per year); scholarships/grants and unspecified assistantships also available. Financial award application deadline: 1/15. *Unit head:* Joanna Groden, Co-Director, 614-688-4301, Fax: 614-292-6226, E-mail: ibgp@osumc.edu. *Application contact:* Graduate Admissions, 614-292-9444, Fax: 614-292-3895, E-mail: domestic.grad@osu.edu.
Website: http://www.ibgp.org

Penn State Hershey Medical Center, College of Medicine, Graduate School Programs in the Biomedical Sciences, Graduate Program in Biomedical Sciences, Hershey, PA 17033. Offers biochemistry and molecular genetics (MS, PhD); biomedical sciences (MS, PhD); translational therapeutics (MS, PhD); virology and immunology (MS, PhD); MD/PhD; PhD/MBA. *Students:* 40 full-time (22 women); includes 7 minority (2 Black or African American, non-Hispanic/Latino; 2 Asian, non-Hispanic/Latino; 1 Hispanic/Latino; 2 Two or more races, non-Hispanic/Latino), 10 international. 215 applicants, 20% accepted, 14 enrolled. Terminal master's awarded for partial completion of doctoral program. *Degree requirements:* For master's, thesis (for some programs); for doctorate, comprehensive exam, thesis/dissertation, candidacy exam. *Entrance requirements:* For doctorate, GRE General Test. Additional exam requirements/recommendations for international students: Required—TOEFL (minimum score 550 paper-based; 80 iBT). *Application deadline:* For fall admission, 2/1 for domestic and international students. Applications are processed on a rolling basis. Application fee: $65. Electronic applications accepted. *Financial support:* In 2013–14, research assistantships (averaging $24,544 per year) were awarded; fellowships, scholarships/grants, health care benefits, and unspecified assistantships also available. Financial award applicants required to submit FAFSA. *Unit head:* Dr. Ralph L. Keil, Chair, 717-531-8595, Fax: 717-531-0388, E-mail: rlk9@psu.edu. *Application contact:* Kristin E. Smith, Enrollment Support Manager, 717-531-0003, Fax: 717-531-0388, E-mail: kec17@psu.edu.
Website: http://med.psu.edu/web/biomedical-sciences/home

Purdue University, Graduate School, PULSe - Purdue University Life Sciences Program, West Lafayette, IN 47907. Offers biomolecular structure and biophysics (PhD); biotechnology (PhD); chemical biology (PhD); chromatin and regulation of gene expression (PhD); integrative neuroscience (PhD); integrative plant sciences (PhD); membrane biology (PhD); microbiology (PhD); molecular evolutionary and cancer biology (PhD); molecular evolutionary genetics (PhD); molecular virology (PhD). *Students:* 154 full-time (78 women), 1 part-time (0 women); includes 23 minority (5 Black or African American, non-Hispanic/Latino; 5 Asian, non-Hispanic/Latino; 10 Hispanic/Latino; 3 Two or more races, non-Hispanic/Latino), 73 international. Average age 26. 239 applicants, 33% accepted, 40 enrolled. *Entrance requirements:* For doctorate, GRE, minimum undergraduate GPA of 3.0. Additional exam requirements/recommendations for international students: Required—TOEFL (minimum score 550 paper-based; 77 iBT). *Application deadline:* For fall admission, 1/15 priority date for domestic and international students. Applications are processed on a rolling basis. Application fee: $60 ($75 for international students). Electronic applications accepted. *Financial support:* In 2013–14, research assistantships with tuition reimbursements (averaging $22,500 per year), teaching assistantships with tuition reimbursements (averaging $22,500 per year) were awarded. *Unit head:* Dr. Christine A. Hrycyna, Head, 765-494-7322, E-mail: hrycyna@purdue.edu. *Application contact:* Colleen Gabauer, Graduate Contact, 765-494-9256, E-mail: cgabauer@purdue.edu.
Website: http://www.gradschool.purdue.edu/pulse

Purdue University, School of Veterinary Medicine and Graduate School, Graduate Programs in Veterinary Medicine, Department of Comparative Pathobiology, West Lafayette, IN 47907-2027. Offers comparative epidemiology and public health (MS); comparative epidemiology and public heath (PhD); comparative microbiology and immunology (MS, PhD); comparative pathobiology (MS, PhD); interdisciplinary studies (PhD), including microbial pathogenesis, molecular signaling and cancer biology, molecular virology; lab animal medicine (MS); veterinary anatomic pathology (MS); veterinary clinical pathology (MS). Terminal master's awarded for partial completion of doctoral program. *Degree requirements:* For master's, thesis (for some programs); for doctorate, thesis/dissertation. *Entrance requirements:* For master's and doctorate, GRE General Test. Additional exam requirements/recommendations for international students: Required—TOEFL (minimum score 575 paper-based), IELTS (minimum score 6.5), TWE (minimum score 4). Electronic applications accepted.

Rush University, Graduate College, Division of Immunology and Microbiology, Program in Immunology/Microbiology, Chicago, IL 60612-3832. Offers immunology (MS, PhD); virology (MS, PhD); MD/PhD. Part-time programs available. Terminal master's awarded for partial completion of doctoral program. *Degree requirements:* For master's, thesis; for doctorate, thesis/dissertation, comprehensive preliminary exam. *Entrance requirements:* For master's, GRE General Test; for doctorate, GRE General Test, interview, minimum GPA of 3.0. Additional exam requirements/recommendations for international students: Required—TOEFL. Electronic applications accepted. *Faculty research:* Human genetics, autoimmunity, tumor biology, complement, HIV immunopathology genesis.

Rutgers, The State University of New Jersey, New Brunswick, Graduate School-New Brunswick, Programs in the Molecular Biosciences, Piscataway, NJ 08854-8097. Offers biochemistry (PhD); cell and developmental biology (MS, PhD); microbiology and molecular genetics (MS, PhD), including applied microbiology, clinical microbiology (MS), clinical mircobiology (PhD), computational molecular biology (PhD), immunology, microbial biochemistry, molecular genetics, virology. MS, PhD offered jointly with University of Medicine and Dentistry of New Jersey.

Texas A&M Health Science Center, College of Medicine, Department of Microbial and Molecular Pathogenesis, College Station, TX 77840. Offers immunology (PhD); microbiology (PhD); molecular biology (PhD); virology (PhD). *Degree requirements:* For doctorate, thesis/dissertation. *Entrance requirements:* For doctorate, GRE General Test, minimum GPA of 3.0. *Faculty research:* Molecular pathogenesis, microbial therapeutics.

Université de Montréal, Faculty of Veterinary Medicine, Program in Virology and Immunology, Montréal, QC H3C 3J7, Canada. Offers PhD. Program offered jointly with Université du Québec, Institut Armand-Frappier. *Degree requirements:* For doctorate, thesis/dissertation, general exam. *Entrance requirements:* For doctorate, proficiency in French, knowledge of English. Electronic applications accepted.

Université du Québec, Institut National de la Recherche Scientifique, Graduate Programs, Research Center–INRS–Institut Armand-Frappier, Laval, QC H7V 1B7, Canada. Offers applied microbiology (M Sc); biology (PhD); experimental health sciences (M Sc); virology and immunology (M Sc, PhD). Programs given in French. Part-time programs available. *Faculty:* 45 full-time. *Students:* 126 full-time (78 women), 11 part-time (7 women), 52 international. Average age 30. In 2013, 19 master's, 12 doctorates awarded. *Degree requirements:* For master's, thesis; for doctorate, thesis/dissertation. *Entrance requirements:* For master's, appropriate bachelor's degree, proficiency in French; for doctorate, appropriate master's degree, proficiency in French. *Application deadline:* For fall admission, 3/30 for domestic and international students; for winter admission, 11/1 for domestic and international students; for spring admission, 3/1 for domestic and international students. Application fee: $45 Canadian dollars. Electronic applications accepted. *Financial support:* In 2013–14, fellowships (averaging $16,500 per year) were awarded; research assistantships also available. *Faculty research:* Immunity, infection and cancer; toxicology and environmental biotechnology; molecular pharmacochemistry. *Unit head:* Charles Dozois, Director, 450-687-5010, Fax: 450-686-5566, E-mail: charles.dozois@iaf.inrs.ca. *Application contact:* Sylvie Richard, Registrar, 418-654-2518, Fax: 418-654-3858, E-mail: sylvie.richard@adm.inrs.ca.
Website: http://www.iaf.inrs.ca

The University of Iowa, Roy J. and Lucille A. Carver College of Medicine and Graduate College, Graduate Programs in Medicine, Department of Microbiology, Iowa City, IA 52242-1316. Offers general microbiology and microbial physiology (MS, PhD); immunology (MS, PhD); microbial genetics (MS, PhD); pathogenic bacteriology (MS, PhD); virology (MS, PhD). *Faculty:* 23 full-time (5 women), 10 part-time/adjunct (4 women). *Students:* 38 full-time (28 women); includes 3 minority (2 Asian, non-Hispanic/Latino; 1 Hispanic/Latino), 2 international. Average age 25. 44 applicants, 23% accepted, 8 enrolled. In 2013, 1 master's, 6 doctorates awarded. *Degree requirements:* For master's, thesis; for doctorate, comprehensive exam, thesis/dissertation. *Entrance requirements:* For master's and doctorate, GRE General Test. Additional exam requirements/recommendations for international students: Required—TOEFL (minimum score 600 paper-based). *Application deadline:* For fall admission, 1/1 for domestic and international students. Application fee: $60 ($100 for international students). Electronic applications accepted. *Financial support:* In 2013–14, 5 fellowships with full tuition reimbursements (averaging $26,000 per year), 33 research assistantships with full tuition reimbursements (averaging $26,000 per year) were awarded; institutionally sponsored loans, scholarships/grants, traineeships, and health care benefits also available. *Faculty research:* Gene regulation, processing and transport of HIV, retroviral pathogenesis, biodegradation, biofilm. *Total annual research expenditures:* $11.5 million. *Unit head:* Dr. Patrick M. Schlievert, Chair and Department Executive Officer, 319-335-7810, E-mail: grad-micro-info@uiowa.edu. *Application contact:* Kerry Yoder, Assistant Director of Graduate and Professional Evaluation, 319-335-1525, Fax: 319-335-1535, E-mail: admissions@uiowa.edu.
Website: http://www.medicine.uiowa.edu/microbiology/

University of Massachusetts Worcester, Graduate School of Biomedical Sciences, Worcester, MA 01655-0115. Offers biochemistry and molecular pharmacology (PhD); bioinformatics and computational biology (PhD); cancer biology (PhD); cell biology (PhD); clinical and population health research (PhD); clinical investigation (MS); immunology and virology (PhD); interdisciplinary biomedical research (PhD); millennium (PhD); molecular genetics and microbiology (PhD); neuroscience (PhD); translational science (PhD); MD/PhD. *Faculty:* 1,388 full-time (521 women), 309 part-time/adjunct (198 women). *Students:* 385 full-time (210 women); includes 53 minority (13 Black or African American, non-Hispanic/Latino; 30 Asian, non-Hispanic/Latino; 10 Hispanic/Latino), 138 international. Average age 28. 491 applicants, 19% accepted, 39 enrolled. In 2013, 5 master's, 50 doctorates awarded. Terminal master's awarded for partial completion of doctoral program. *Median time to degree:* Of those who began their doctoral program in fall 2005, 67% received their degree in 8 years or less. *Degree requirements:* For master's, comprehensive exam, thesis; for doctorate, comprehensive exam, thesis/dissertation. *Entrance requirements:* For master's, MD, PhD, DVM, or PharmD; for doctorate, GRE General Test, bachelor's degree. Additional exam requirements/recommendations for international students: Required—TOEFL (minimum score 100 iBT) or IELTS (minimum score 7.5). *Application deadline:* For fall admission, 12/15 for domestic and international students; for spring admission, 5/15 for domestic students. Application fee: $80. Electronic applications accepted. *Expenses:* Contact institution. *Financial support:* In 2013–14, 431 students received support, including research assistantships with full tuition reimbursements available (averaging $29,500 per year); scholarships/grants, health care benefits, tuition waivers (full), and unspecified assistantships also available. Financial award application deadline: 5/16. *Faculty research:* RNA interference, cell/molecular/developmental biology, bioinformatics, clinical/translational research, infectious disease. *Total annual research expenditures:* $245.9 million. *Unit head:* Dr. Anthony Carruthers, Dean, 508-856-4135, E-mail: anthony.carruthers@umassmed.edu. *Application contact:* Dr. Kendall Knight, Associate Dean and Interim Director of Admissions and Recruitment, 508-856-5628, Fax: 508-856-3659, E-mail: kendall.knight@umassmed.edu.
Website: http://www.umassmed.edu/gsbs/

University of Minnesota, Twin Cities Campus, Graduate School, PhD Program in Microbiology, Immunology and Cancer Biology, Minneapolis, MN 55455-0213. Offers PhD. *Degree requirements:* For doctorate, thesis/dissertation. *Entrance requirements:* For doctorate, GRE General Test. Additional exam requirements/recommendations for international students: Required—TOEFL (minimum score 600 paper-based). Electronic applications accepted. *Faculty research:* Virology, microbiology, cancer biology, immunology.

University of Pennsylvania, Perelman School of Medicine, Biomedical Graduate Studies, Graduate Group in Cell and Molecular Biology, Philadelphia, PA 19104. Offers cancer biology (PhD); cell biology and physiology (PhD); developmental stem cell regenerative biology (PhD); gene therapy and vaccines (PhD); genetics and gene regulation (PhD); microbiology, virology, and parasitology (PhD); MD/PhD; VMD/PhD. *Faculty:* 321. *Students:* 352 full-time (205 women); includes 99 minority (11 Black or African American, non-Hispanic/Latino; 65 Asian, non-Hispanic/Latino; 21 Hispanic/Latino; 2 Two or more races, non-Hispanic/Latino), 45 international. 488 applicants, 20% accepted, 40 enrolled. In 2013, 41 doctorates awarded. *Degree requirements:* For doctorate, thesis/dissertation. *Entrance requirements:* For doctorate, GRE General Test. Additional exam requirements/recommendations for international students: Required—TOEFL. *Application deadline:* For fall admission, 12/1 priority date for domestic and international students. Applications are processed on a rolling basis. Application fee: $80. Electronic applications accepted. *Financial support:* In 2013–14, 352 students received support. Fellowships, research assistantships, scholarships/grants, traineeships, and unspecified assistantships available. *Unit head:* Dr. Daniel Kessler,

Virology

Graduate Group Chair, 215-898-1478. *Application contact:* Meagan Schofer, Coordinator, 215-898-4360.
Website: http://www.med.upenn.edu/camb/

University of Pittsburgh, School of Medicine, Graduate Programs in Medicine, Molecular Virology and Microbiology Graduate Program, Pittsburgh, PA 15260. Offers PhD. *Faculty:* 46 full-time (13 women). *Students:* 27 full-time (12 women); includes 3 minority (1 Asian, non-Hispanic/Latino; 1 Hispanic/Latino; 1 Native Hawaiian or other Pacific Islander, non-Hispanic/Latino), 4 international. Average age 27. 517 applicants, 13% accepted, 22 enrolled. In 2013, 3 doctorates awarded. *Degree requirements:* For doctorate, comprehensive exam, thesis/dissertation. *Entrance requirements:* For doctorate, GRE General Test, GRE Subject Test, minimum QPA of 3.0. Additional exam requirements/recommendations for international students: Required—TOEFL (minimum score 600 paper-based; 100 iBT), IELTS (minimum score 7). *Application deadline:* For fall admission, 1/1 priority date for domestic and international students. Application fee: $50. Electronic applications accepted. *Expenses:* Tuition, state resident: full-time $19,964; part-time $807 per credit. Tuition, nonresident: full-time $32,686; part-time $1337 per credit. *Required fees:* $740; $200. Tuition and fees vary according to program. *Financial support:* In 2013–14, 27 research assistantships with full tuition reimbursements (averaging $26,010 per year) were awarded; institutionally sponsored loans, scholarships/grants, traineeships, health care benefits, and unspecified assistantships also available. *Faculty research:* Host-pathogen interactions, persistent microbial infections, microbial genetics and gene expression, microbial pathogenesis, anti-bacterial therapeutics. *Unit head:* Dr. Carolyn Coyne, Graduate Program Director, 412-383-5149, Fax: 412-624-1401, E-mail: ndeluca@pitt.edu. *Application contact:* Graduate Studies Administrator, 412-648-8957, Fax: 412-648-1077, E-mail: gradstudies@medschool.pitt.edu.
Website: http://www.gradbiomed.pitt.edu

University of Prince Edward Island, Atlantic Veterinary College, Graduate Program in Veterinary Medicine, Charlottetown, PE C1A 4P3, Canada. Offers anatomy (M Sc, PhD); bacteriology (M Sc, PhD); clinical pharmacology (M Sc, PhD); clinical sciences (M Sc, PhD); epidemiology (M Sc, PhD), including reproduction; fish health (M Sc, PhD); food animal nutrition (M Sc, PhD); immunology (M Sc, PhD); microanatomy (M Sc, PhD); parasitology (M Sc, PhD); pathology (M Sc, PhD); pharmacology (M Sc, PhD); physiology (M Sc, PhD); toxicology (M Sc, PhD); veterinary science (M Vet Sc); virology (M Sc, PhD). Part-time programs available. *Degree requirements:* For master's, thesis; for doctorate, thesis/dissertation. *Entrance requirements:* For master's, DVM, B Sc honors degree, or equivalent; for doctorate, M Sc. Additional exam requirements/recommendations for international students: Required—TOEFL (minimum score 550 paper-based; 80 iBT). *Expenses:* Contact institution. *Faculty research:* Animal health management, infectious diseases, fin fish and shellfish health, basic biomedical sciences, ecosystem health.

The University of Texas Health Science Center at Houston, Graduate School of Biomedical Sciences, Program in Virology and Gene Therapy, Houston, TX 77225-0036. Offers MS, PhD, MD/PhD. Terminal master's awarded for partial completion of doctoral program. *Degree requirements:* For master's, thesis; for doctorate, thesis/dissertation. *Entrance requirements:* For master's and doctorate, GRE General Test. Additional exam requirements/recommendations for international students: Required—TOEFL. Electronic applications accepted. *Expenses:* Tuition, state resident: full-time $3474; part-time $193 per credit hour. Tuition, nonresident: full-time $13,644; part-time $758 per credit hour. *Required fees:* $226.30; $87 per credit hour. *Faculty research:* Viruses, infectious diseases, vaccines, gene therapy, cancer.

The University of Texas Medical Branch, Graduate School of Biomedical Sciences, Program in Emerging and Tropical Infectious Diseases, Galveston, TX 77555. Offers PhD, MD/PhD. *Degree requirements:* For doctorate, thesis/dissertation. *Entrance requirements:* For doctorate, GRE General Test. *Faculty research:* Emerging diseases, tropical diseases, parasitology, vitology and bacteriology.

Yale University, School of Medicine and Graduate School of Arts and Sciences, Combined Program in Biological and Biomedical Sciences (BBS), Microbiology Track, New Haven, CT 06520. Offers PhD, MD/PhD. *Degree requirements:* For doctorate, thesis/dissertation. *Entrance requirements:* For doctorate, GRE General Test, GRE Subject Test. Additional exam requirements/recommendations for international students: Required—TOEFL. Electronic applications accepted.

UNIFORMED SERVICES UNIVERSITY OF THE HEALTH SCIENCES

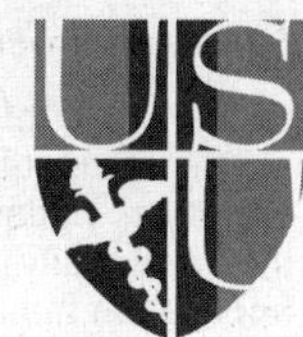

F. Edward Hébert School of Medicine
Graduate Program in Emerging Infectious Diseases

Program of Study

One of the missions of the Uniformed Services University (USU) is to provide both civilians and military students with high-quality training leading to advanced degrees in the biomedical sciences. The Graduae Program in Emerging Infectious Diseases (EID) is designed for applicants who wish to pursue an interdisciplinary program of study leading to the Ph.D. degree and was created for students who are primarily interested in the pathogenesis, host response, and epidemiology of infectious diseases. No M.S. degree program is currently offered. A broadly based core program of formal training is combined with an intensive laboratory research experience in the different disciplines encompassed by the field of infectious diseases. Courses are taught by an interdisciplinary EID faculty who hold primary appointments in the Departments of Microbiology and Immunology, Pathology, Preventive Medicine and Biometrics, Pediatrics, and Medicine. Research training emphasizes modern methods in molecular biology and cell biology, as well as interdisciplinary approaches.

During the first two years, all students are required to complete a series of broadly based core courses and laboratory rotations. Students also select one of two academic tracks in which to focus the remainder of their course work. The two tracks are Microbiology and Immunology, and Preventive Medicine and Biometrics. Advanced course work is required in each academic track. In addition, each student selects a faculty member with whom he or she would like to carry out a thesis research project. By the end of the second year, the student must complete all requirements for advancement to candidacy for the Ph.D. degree, which includes satisfactory completion of formal course work and passage of the qualifying examination. After advancement to candidacy, the student must complete an original research project and prepare and defend a written dissertation under the supervision of his or her faculty adviser and an advisory committee.

Research Facilities

Each academic department of the University is provided with laboratories for the support of a variety of research projects. Laboratories are available in most areas of study that encompass the interdisciplinary field of emerging infectious diseases, including both basic and medical aspects of bacteriology, bacterial genetics, virology, cellular and molecular immunology, parasitology, pathogenic mechanisms of disease, pathology of infectious disease, and epidemiology of infectious diseases. Resources available to students within the University include real-time PCR, microarray spotters and readers, EPICS, FACSAria and LSRII cell sorters and analyzers, Luminex 100 analyzer, automated oligonucleotide and peptide synthesizers and sequencing, MALDI-TOF Mass Spectrometer, high-resolution electron microscopes, confocal microscopes, a certified central animal facility, and state-of-the-art computer facilities. In addition, a BSL-3 biohazard containment laboratory suite is available. The library/learning resources center houses more than 521,000 bound volumes, subscribes to nearly 3,000 journals (print and online), and maintains 100 IBM and Macintosh personal computers for use by students, faculty members, and staff members. Biostatisticians serve as a resource for students and faculty members.

Financial Aid

Stipends are available for civilian applicants. Awards of stipends are competitive, are for one-year periods, and may be renewed. The 2014–15 stipend level begins at $27,000 per year. Special fellowships are also available.

Cost of Study

Graduate students in the Emerging Infectious Diseases Program are not required to pay tuition or fees. Civilian students do not incur obligations to the United States government for service after completion of their graduate training programs.

Living and Housing Costs

There is a reasonable supply of affordable rental housing in the area. The University does not have housing for graduate students. Living costs in the greater Washington, D.C., area are comparable to those of other East Coast metropolitan areas.

Student Group

The first full-time graduate students were admitted to the EID program in 2000. There are currently 30 full-time students enrolled in the EID graduate program. The University also has Ph.D. programs in departmentally based basic biomedical sciences, as well as interdisciplinary graduate programs in molecular and cell biology and in neurosciences.

Location

The greater Washington metropolitan area has a population of about 3 million that includes the District of Columbia and the surrounding areas of Maryland and Virginia. The region is a center of education and research and is home to five major universities, four medical schools, and numerous other internationally recognized private and government research centers. In addition, multiple cultural advantages exist in the area and include theaters, a major symphony orchestra, major-league sports, and world-famous museums. The Metro subway system has a station adjacent to the campus and provides a convenient connection from the University to cultural attractions and activities in downtown Washington. The international community in Washington is the source of many diverse cuisines and international cultural events. For a wide variety of outdoor activities, the Blue Ridge Mountains, Chesapeake Bay, and Atlantic coast beaches are all within a 1- to 3-hour drive. Many national and local parks serve the area for weekend hikes, bicycling, and picnics.

The University

USU is located just outside Washington, D.C., in Bethesda, Maryland. The campus is situated in an attractive, park-like setting on the grounds of the Walter Reed National Military Medical Center (WRNMMC) and across the street from the National Institutes of Health (NIH). Wooded areas with jogging and biking trails surround the University. NIH and other research institutes in the area provide additional resources to enhance the education experience of graduate students at USU. Students can visit the USUHS website at http://www.usuhs.edu/eid.

Applying

The Admissions Committee, in consultation with other faculty members, evaluates applications to the program. Each applicant must submit an application form, complete academic transcripts of postsecondary education, and results of the Graduate Record Examinations. No GRE Subject Test is required. In addition, three letters of recommendation from individuals familiar with the academic achievements and/or research experience of the applicant are required, as well as a personal statement that expresses the applicant's career objectives. USU subscribes fully to the policy of equal educational opportunity and selects students on a competitive basis without regard to race, color, gender, creed, or national origin. Application forms may be obtained from the University website (available at http://www.usuhs.mil/graded/application.html). Completed applications should be received on or before December 1.

Both civilians and military personnel are eligible to apply. Prior to acceptance, each applicant must complete a baccalaureate degree that includes required courses in mathematics, biology, physics, and chemistry (inorganic, organic, and biochemistry). Advanced-level courses in microbiology, molecular biology, genetics, and cell biology are very strongly recommended. All students are expected to have a reasonable level of computer literacy. Active-duty military applicants must obtain the approval and sponsorship of their parent military service, in addition to acceptance into the EID graduate program.

Correspondence and Information

Dr. Gregory Mueller
Associate Dean for Graduate Education (Acting)
Uniformed Services University
4301 Jones Bridge Road
Bethesda, Maryland 20814-4755
United States
Phone: 800-772-1747 (toll-free)
Website: http://www.usuhs.mil

Dr. Christopher C. Broder, Director
Graduate Program in Emerging Infectious Diseases
Uniformed Services University
4301 Jones Bridge Road
Bethesda, Maryland 20814-4755
United States
Phone: 301-295-5749
Fax: 301-295-9861
E-mail: christopher.broder@usuhs.edu
Website: http://www.usuhs.edu/eid

THE FACULTY

The interdisciplinary graduate programs at USU are superimposed on the departmental structure. Therefore, all faculty members in the interdisciplinary Graduate Program in Emerging Infectious Diseases (EID) have primary appointments in either a basic science or a clinical department and secondary appointments in EID. The faculty is derived primarily from the Departments of Microbiology and Immunology, Pathology, Preventive Medicine and Biometrics, Pediatrics, and Medicine. Thus, the faculty in EID includes the experts in infectious diseases, regardless of department. For additional information, students should visit the USU Academic Department website at http://www.usuhs.mil/academic.html. To address e-mail to specific faculty members at USU, students should use the first name, a period, the last name, and @usuhs.edu as the address; for example, to send e-mail to John Doe, the address would be john.doe@usuhs.edu.

Richard G. Andre, Ph.D.; Professor, Preventive Medicine and Biometrics.
Naomi E. Aronson, M.D.; Professor, Medicine.
Kimberly A. Bishop-Lilly, Ph.D.; Adjunct Assistant Professor, Navy Medical Research Center.
Christopher C. Broder, Ph.D.; Professor, Microbiology and Immunology.
Timothy H. Burgess, M.D., M.P.H.; Assistant Professor, Medicine.
Drusilla L. Burns, Ph.D.; Adjunct Assistant Professor, CBER, FDA.
David F. Cruess, Ph.D.; Professor, Preventive Medicine and Biometrics.
Stephen J. Davies, Ph.D.; Associate Professor, Microbiology and Immunology.
Saibal Dey, Ph.D.; Adjunct Assistant Professor, Biochemistry.
Michael W. Ellis, M.D.; Assistant Professor, Medicine.
Chou-Zen Giam, Ph.D.; Professor, Microbiology and Immunology.
Scott W. Gordon, Ph.D.; Adjunct Assistant Professor, Preventive Medicine and Biometrics.
John Grieco, Ph.D.; Assistant Professor, Preventive Medicine and Biometrics.
Patricia Guerry, Ph.D.; Assistant Professor, Immunology, NMRC.
Val G. Hemming, M.D.; Professor, Pediatrics.
Ann E. Jerse, Ph.D.; Professor, Microbiology and Immunology.
Elliott Kagan, M.D.; Professor, Pathology.
Barbara Knollman-Ritschel, M.D.; Professor, Pathology.
Philip R. Krause, M.D.; Assistant Professor, CBER, FDA.
Larry W. Laughlin, M.D., Ph.D.; Professor, Preventive Medicine and Biometrics.
Radha K. Maheshwari, Ph.D.; Professor, Pathology.
Joseph Mattapallil, Ph.D.; Associate Professor, Microbiology and Immunology.
Anthony T. Maurelli, Ph.D.; Professor, Microbiology and Immunology.
Ernest L. Maynard, Ph.D.; Assistant Professor, Biochemistry and Molecular Biology.
D. Scotty Merrell, Ph.D.; Professor, Microbiology and Immunology.
Eleanor S. Metcalf, Ph.D.; Professor, Microbiology and Immunology.
Nelson L. Michael, M.D., Ph.D.; Adjunct Assistant Professor, Medicine.
Edward Mitre, M.D.; Associate Professor, Microbiology and Immunology.
Alison D. O'Brien, Ph.D.; Professor, Microbiology and Immunology.
Christian F. Ockenhouse, M.D., Ph.D.; Adjunct Assistant Professor, Infectious Diseases, WRAIR.
Martin G. Ottolini, M.D.; Associate Professor, Pediatrics.
Julie A. Pavlin, M.D., Ph.D.; Associate Professor, Preventive Medicine and Biometrics.
Gerald V. Quinnan Jr., M.D.; Professor, Preventive Medicine and Biometrics.
Allen L. Richards, Ph.D.; Associate Professor, Preventive Medicine and Biometrics.
Capt. Stephen J. Savarino, M.D.; Adjunct Assistant Professor, Infectious Diseases, NMRC.
Brian C. Schaefer, Ph.D.; Associate Professor, Microbiology and Immunology.
Connie S. Schmaljohn, Ph.D.; Adjunct Assistant Professor, USAMRIID.
Frank P. Shewmaker, Ph.D.; Assistant Professor, Pharmacology.
David W. Scott, Ph.D.; Professor, Medicine.
Clifford M. Snapper, M.D.; Professor, Pathology.
Andrew L. Snow, Ph.D.; Assistant Professor, Pharmacology.
Shanmuga Sozhamannan, Ph.D.; Adjunct Assistant Professor, Biological Defense Research, NMRC.
V. Ann Stewart, D.V.M., Ph.D.; Associate Professor, Preventive Medicine and Biometrics.
J. Thomas Stocker, M.D.; Professor, Pathology.
Hendrick Streeck, M.D., Ph.D.; Adjunct Assistant Professor, Immunology, WRAIR.
Terrill L. Tops, M.D., Assistant Professor, Pathology.
Charles Via, M.D.; Assistant Professor, Pathology.
Shuishu Wang, Ph.D.; Assistant Professor, Biochemistry.
Lt. Col. Glenn W. Wortmann, M.D.; Adjunct Assistant Professor. Infectious Diseases, WRAIR.
Shuenn-Jue L. Wu, Ph.D.; Adjunct Associate Professor, Immunology, NMRC.
Pengfei Zhang, Ph.D.; Research Associate Professor, Preventive Medicine and Biometrics.

UCONN HEALTH

Graduate Program in Immunology

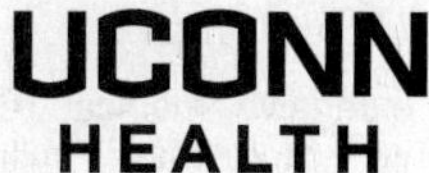

Program of Study

A Ph.D. in immunology is offered through an interdepartmental program consisting of approximately 15 faculty members. The immunology faculty members also participate in training students in the combined M.D./Ph.D. and D.M.D./Ph.D. programs. The central focus of the program is to train students to become independent investigators who will provide meaningful research and educational contributions to the areas of basic, applied, or clinical immunology. This goal is achieved by lectures, seminars, laboratory rotations, research presentations, and a concentration on laboratory research. In addition to basic and advanced immunology courses, students are given a strong foundation in biomedical sciences through the core curriculum in biochemistry, genetics, molecular biology, and cell biology. Research laboratory training aims to provide a foundation in modern laboratory techniques and concentrates on hypothesis-based analysis of problems. Research in the program is focused on the cellular and molecular aspects of immune system structure and function in animal models and in humans. Areas of emphasis include molecular immunology (mechanisms of antigen presentation, major histocompatibility complex genetics and function, cytokines and cytokine receptors, and tumor antigens), cellular immunology (biochemical mechanisms and biological aspects of signal transduction of lymphocytes and granulocytes; cellular and molecular requirements for thymic T-lymphocyte development, selection, and activation; cytokines in B- and T-cell development; regulation of antitumor immunity; immunoparasitology, including parasite genetics and immune recognition of parasite antigens; and mechanisms of inflammation), organ-based immunology (immune effector mechanisms of the intestine, lymphocyte interactions in the lung, and immune regulation of the eye), immunity to infectious agents (viruses, bacteria, parasites, including vector-borne organisms), and autoimmunity (animal models of autoimmune disease and effector mechanisms in human autoimmunity).

Research Facilities

The Graduate Program in Immunology is interdepartmental, and therefore provides a broad base of training possibilities as well as ample shared facilities. State-of-the-art equipment is available in individual laboratories for analysis of molecular and cellular parameters of immune system structure and function. In addition, UConn Health–supported facilities provide equipment and expertise in areas of advanced data acquisition and analysis. These facilities include the Center for Cell Analysis and Modeling, the Fluorescence Flow Cytometry Facility, the Gene Targeting and Transgenic Facility, the Molecular Core Facility, the Microarray Facility, the Gregory P. Mullen Structural Biology Facility, and the Electron Microscopy Facility. The Lyman Maynard Stowe Library is well equipped with extensive journal and book holdings and rapid electronic access to database searching, Internet, and library holdings. A computer center is also housed in the library for student use and training.

Financial Aid

Support for doctoral students engaged in full-time degree programs at UConn Health is provided on a competitive basis. Graduate research assistantships for 2014–15 provide a stipend of $29,000 per year, which includes a waiver of tuition/most University fees for the fall and spring semesters and the option of participating in a student health insurance plan. While financial aid is offered competitively, UConn Health makes every possible effort to address the financial needs of all students.

Cost of Study

For 2014–15, tuition is $12,202 per year for full-time students who are Connecticut residents and $32,258 per year for full-time out-of-state residents. General University fees are added to the cost of tuition for students who do not receive a tuition waiver. These costs are usually met by traineeships or research assistantships for doctoral students.

Living and Housing Costs

There is a wide range of affordable housing options in the greater Hartford area within easy commuting distance of the campus, including an extensive complex that is adjacent to UConn Health. Costs range from $700 to $1,000 per month for a one-bedroom unit; 2 or more students sharing an apartment usually pay less. University housing is not available.

Student Group

At present, there are approximately 15 students in the Graduate Program in Immunology. There are 150 students in the various Ph.D. programs on the UConn Health campus.

Student Outcomes

Graduates have traditionally been accepted into high-quality laboratories for postdoctoral training. Following their training, graduates have accepted a wide range of positions in research in universities, colleges, research institutes, and industry, including the biotechnology sector.

Location

UConn Health is located in the historic town of Farmington, Connecticut. Set in the beautiful New England countryside on a hill overlooking the Farmington Valley, it is close to ski areas, hiking trails, and facilities for boating, fishing, and swimming. Connecticut's capital city of Hartford, 7 miles east of Farmington, is the center of an urban region of approximately 800,000 people. The beaches of the Long Island Sound are about 50 minutes away to the south, and the beautiful Berkshires are a short drive to the northwest. New York City and Boston can be reached within 2½ hours by car. Hartford is the home of the acclaimed Hartford Stage Company, TheatreWorks, the Hartford Symphony and Chamber orchestras, two ballet companies, an opera company, the Wadsworth Athenaeum (the oldest public art museum in the nation), the Mark Twain house, the Hartford Civic Center, and many other interesting cultural and recreational facilities. The area is also home to several branches of the University of Connecticut, Trinity College, and the University of Hartford, which includes the Hartt School of Music. Bradley International Airport (about 30 minutes from campus) serves the Hartford/Springfield area with frequent airline connections to major cities in this country and abroad. Frequent bus and rail service is also available from Hartford.

The Health Center

The 200-acre UConn Health campus at Farmington houses a division of the University of Connecticut Graduate School, as well as the Schools of Medicine and Dental Medicine. The campus also includes the John Dempsey Hospital, associated clinics, and extensive medical research facilities, all in a centralized facility with more than 1 million square feet of floor space. The Academic Research Building, built in 1999, is an impressive eleven-story structure providing 170,000 square feet of laboratory space. In addition, renovations are underway in the main laboratory building, converting existing lab space to state-of-the-art open lab areas. The faculty includes more than 260 full-time members. The institution has a strong commitment to graduate study within an environment that promotes social and intellectual interaction among the various educational programs. Graduate students are represented on various administrative committees concerned with curricular affairs, and the Graduate Student Organization (GSO) represents graduate students' needs and concerns to the faculty and administration, in addition to fostering social contact among graduate students at UConn Health.

Applying

Applications for admission should be submitted via the online application system and should be filed together with transcripts, three letters of recommendation, a personal statement, and recent results from the General Test of the Graduate Record Examinations. International students must take the Test of English as a Foreign Language (TOEFL) to satisfy Graduate School requirements. The deadline for completed applications and receipt of all supplemental materials is **December 1**. Please note that GRE and TOEFL exams taken after the due date will not be accepted for consideration for admission. In accordance with the laws of the state of Connecticut and of the United States, UConn Health does not discriminate against any person in its educational and employment activities on the grounds of race, color, creed, national origin, sex, age, or physical disability.

Correspondence and Information

Graduate Admissions Office
Ph.D. in Biomedical Science Program
UConn Health
263 Farmington Ave., MC 3906
Farmington, Connecticut 06030-3906
United States
Phone: 860-679-4509
E-mail: BiomedSciAdmissions@uchc.edu
Website:
http://grad.uchc.edu/prospective/programs/phd_biosci/index.html

THE FACULTY AND THEIR RESEARCH

Adam J. Adler, Professor of Immunology; Ph.D., Columbia. Mechanisms of T-cell tolerance induction to peripheral self- and tumor-antigens; immunological properties of prostate cancer.

Hector L. Aguila, Associate Professor of Immunology; Ph.D., Yeshiva (Einstein). Hematopoiesis and bone marrow microenvironment; lymphoid cell development; stem cell biology.

Linda Cauley, Assistant Professor of Immunology; D.Phil., Oxford. T-cell memory and respiratory virus infections.

Robert B. Clark, Professor of Immunology; M.D., Stanford. Autoimmunity; immune regulation; regulatory T cells.

Laura Haynes, Professor of Immunology, Ph.D., Rochester. Influence of aging on CD4 T cell function and how this impacts responses to infection and vaccination.

Kamal Khanna, Assistant Professor of Immunology, Ph.D., Pittsburgh. Identifying the factors and the role they play in controlling the anatomy of a primary and secondary immune response in the hopes of explicating the underlying mechanisms that guide the complex movement of T cells during infection and recall responses in lymphoid and non-lymphoid tissues.

Joseph A. Lorenzo, Professor of Medicine; M.D., SUNY Downstate Medical Center. Relationships between bone-absorbing osteoclasts and immune cells.

Andrei Medvedev, Associate Professor of Immunology; Ph.D., Gabrichevsky Institute of Epidemiology and Microbiology (Moscow). How distorted control of TLR signaling underlies immune pathologies.

Lynn Puddington, Associate Professor of Immunology; Ph.D., Wake Forest. Allergic asthma; neonatal immunity and tolerance; developmental immunology.

Justin D. Radolf, Professor of Medicine and Center for Microbial Pathogenesis; M.D., California, San Francisco. Molecular pathogenesis and immunobiology of spirochetal infections.

Juan C. Salazar, Professor of Pediatrics; M.D., Universidad Javeriana (Bogatá, Columbia). Analysis of the immunologic interactions between syphilis and HIV and the pathogenesis of spirochetal diseases including Lyme disease.

Lauren Sansing, Assistant Professor of Neurology; M.D., Stony Brook, SUNY.

Pramod K. Srivastava, Professor of Medicine; Ph.D., Hyderabad (India). Heat shock proteins as peptide chaperones; roles in antigen presentation and applications in immunotherapy of cancer, infectious diseases, and autoimmune disorders.

Anthony T. Vella, Professor of Immunology; Ph.D., Cornell. T-cell immunity; costimulation; adjuvants and cytokines.

Richard A. Zeff, Professor of Immunology; Ph.D., Rush. Major histocompatibility complex; antigen processing and presentation.

UNIVERSITY OF MASSACHUSETTS AMHERST

Department of Microbiology

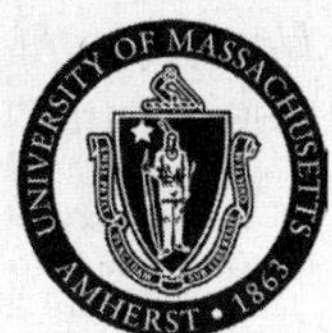

Programs of Study

The Department of Microbiology at the University of Massachusetts Amherst (UMass) offers programs of graduate study leading to the M.S. and Ph.D. degrees in microbiology. Postdoctoral training is also available. Courses covering various areas in the field of microbiology are offered by the Departmental faculty members, listed in the Faculty and Their Research section.

In the Ph.D. program, formal course work is completed during the first two years. From the start, a large portion of a student's time is dedicated to research. Students actively participate in ongoing research during two 1-semester rotations and then select dissertation problems from the wide spectrum of research areas pursued by the faculty. The following research fields are represented: microbial physiology, genetics, immunology, parasitology, pathogenic bacteriology, molecular biology, microbial ecology, and environmental microbiology. In the second year, Ph.D. candidates must pass a comprehensive preliminary examination. Degree requirements are completed by submission and defense of a dissertation. There is no foreign language requirement. Completion of the Ph.D. program generally takes four years beyond the bachelor's degree.

Research Facilities

The Department of Microbiology occupies space in the Morrill Science Center, Life Science Laboratories, and Fernald Hall. Laboratories are spacious and well equipped for research and teaching. State-of-the-art equipment necessary for investigation into all aspects of microbiology is available within the Department. The Department's facilities include tissue- and cell-culture laboratories, animal quarters, and various instrument rooms containing preparative and analytical ultracentrifuges, scintillation counters, fermentors, anaerobic chambers, equipment for chromatographic and electrophoretic procedures, photography, and other standard laboratory procedures. Centralized facilities provide state-of-the-art equipment and expertise to support research projects, such as the Central Microscopy Facility, Genomics and Bioinformatics Facility, High Field NMR Facility, and Mass Spectrometry Facility.

Financial Aid

Financial aid is available in the form of University fellowships and teaching assistantships. Research assistantships are available for advanced graduate students. All assistantships include a waiver of tuition.

Cost of Study

In academic year 2014–15, annual tuition for in-state residents is $110 per credit; nonresident tuition is $414 per credit. Full-time students register for at least 9 credits per semester. The mandatory fees and tuition assessed for full-time graduate students (9 credits) is $6,695 per semester for in-state residents and $13,030 for nonresidents. Note: These fees include tuition and curriculum fees, which are waived with eligible graduate assistantships. Fees are subject to change. More information on fees is available in the Bursar's Office fee schedule online at http://www.umass.edu/bursar.

Living and Housing Costs

Graduate student housing is available in several twelve-month campus residence halls through University Housing Services. The University owns and manages unfurnished apartments of various sizes for family housing on or near the campus. Off-campus housing is available; rents vary widely and depend on factors such as size and location. A free bus system connects UMass with all neighboring communities.

Student Group

The Department has approximately 40 graduate and 175 undergraduate students as well as 10 postdoctoral fellows. Enrollment at the Amherst campus is about 26,000, including 4,000 graduate students.

Location

The 1,450-acre campus of the University provides a rich cultural environment in a rural setting. Amherst is situated in the picturesque Pioneer Valley in historic western Massachusetts. The area is renowned for its natural beauty. Green open land framed by the outline of the Holyoke Range, clear streams, country roads, forests, grazing cattle, and shade trees are characteristic of the region. A broad spectrum of cultural activities and extensive recreational facilities are available within the University and at four neighboring colleges—Smith, Amherst, Mount Holyoke, and Hampshire. Opportunities for outdoor winter sports are exceptional. Amherst is 90 miles west of Boston and 175 miles north of New York City, and Cape Cod is a 3½-hour drive away.

The University

The University of Massachusetts is the state university of the Commonwealth of Massachusetts and is the flagship campus of the five-campus UMass system. Departments affiliated with the ten colleges and schools of the University offer a variety of graduate degrees through the Graduate School. The Amherst campus consists of approximately 150 buildings, including the twenty-eight-story W. E. B. DuBois Library, which is the largest at a state-supported institution in New England. The library features more than 5.8 million items and is home to a state-of-the-art learning commons equipped with computer workstations and high-speed network access.

Applying

The secure online application is available on the University of Massachusetts Graduate School website: http://www.umass.edu/gradschool. Prospective students are required to take the Graduate Record Examination. Applications for admission should be received by the Graduate Admissions Office by December 20 for September enrollment. Applications received after this date are considered only if space is available.

Correspondence and Information

Graduate Program Director
Department of Microbiology
Morrill IV, N203
639 North Pleasant Street
University of Massachusetts Amherst
Amherst, Massachusetts 01003-9298
United States
Phone: 413-545-2051
Fax: 413-545-1578
E-mail: microbio-dept@microbio.umass.edu
Website: http://www.micro.umass.edu

University of Massachusetts Amherst

THE FACULTY AND THEIR RESEARCH

J. M. Lopes, Professor and Department Head; Ph.D., South Carolina. Regulation of gene expression in eukaryotes. *Genes, Genomes & Genomics* 4:761–7, 2014; *J. Mol. Biol.* 425:457–65, 2013; *Mol. Microbiol.* 83:395–407, 2012.

J. P. Burand, Professor; Ph.D., Washington State. Biology and molecular biology of insect pathogenic viruses, particularly nonoccluded insect viruses and bee viruses, with emphasis on virus-host interactions that affect the virulence and persistence of these viruses in insects. *Viruses* 4:28–61, 2012; *J. Invertebr. Pathol.* 108:217–9, 2011; *Appl. Environ. Micro.* 75:7862–5, 2009; *Virol. Sin.* 24:428–35, 2009; *Arch. Virol.* 154:909–18, 2009.

P. Chien, Adjunct Assistant Professor; Ph.D., California, San Francisco. Protein degradation during bacterial cell-cycle progression. *Proc. Natl. Acad. Sci. Unit. States Am.* Nov 5:110(45):18138–43, 2013; *Cell* 154:623–36, 2013. *Mol. Microbiol.* 88(6):1083–92, 2013; *Mol. Microbiol.* 87(6):1277–89, 2013; *Mol. Cell* 43(4):550–60, 2013; *Structure* 20(7):1223–32, 2012.

D. R. Cooley, Adjunct Associate Professor; Ph.D., Massachusetts. Ecology of diseases; plant pathogenic fungi and bacteria; plant disease management; integrated pest management; development of sustainable agricultural systems.

K. M. DeAngelis, Assistant Professor; Ph.D., Berkeley. Microbial ecology of carbon cycling in soils; microbial feedbacks to climate change; lignocellulosic biofuels. *Front. Microbiol.* 4:280, 2013; *Soil Biol. Biochem.* 66:60–8, 2013; *PLos One* 6(4):e19306, 2011; *Environ. Microbiol.* 12(12):3137–49, 2010.

S. Goodwin, Dean, College of Natural Sciences; Ph.D., Wisconsin.

K. L. Griffith, Assistant Professor; Ph.D., Maryland. Cell-cell signaling in bacteria; development of tools for studying regulatory networks. *J. Mol. Bio.* 381:261–75, 2008; *Mol. Microbiol.* 70:1012–25, 2008.

J. F. Holden, Associate Professor; Ph.D., Washington (Seattle). Physiology of hyperthermophilic archaea; geomicrobiology; hydrothermal vents; agricultural waste remediation and bioenergy using thermophiles. *Proc. Natl. Acad. Sci. Unit. States Am.*, in press; *Oceanography* 25:196–208, 2012; *Appl. Environ. Microbiol.* 77:3169–73, 2011.

M. M. Klingbeil, Associate Professor and Graduate Program Director; Ph.D., Toledo. Molecular and biochemical parasitology, replication and repair of mitochondrial DNA (kinetoplast DNA) and nuclear DNA replication initiation in African trypanosomes. *Mol. Microbiol.* 87:196–210, 2013; *Eukaryot. Cell* 11:844–55, 2012; *Eukaryot. Cell* 10:734–43, 2011; *Mol. Biochem. Parasitol.* 175:68–75, 2011; *Mol. Microbiol.* 75:1414–25, 2010; *Mol. Cell* 5:398–400, 2009; *Eukaryot. Cell* 7:2141–6, 2008; *Science* 309:409–15, 2005; *Proc. Natl. Acad. Sci. U.S.A.* 101:4333–4, 2004; *J. Biol. Chem.* 278:49095–101, 2003; *Mol. Cell* 10:175–86, 2002; *Protist* 152:255–62, 2001.

D. R. Lovley, Distinguished University Professor; Ph.D., Michigan State. Genome-enabled study of the physiology, ecology, and evolution of novel anaerobic microorganisms; microbe-electrode interactions with a focus on novel bioenergy solutions; biological computing and sensing; direct electron exchange between microorganisms; bioremediation of metal and organic contamination; life in extreme environments. *Curr. Opin. Biotechnol.* 24:385–90, 2013; *Nature Nanotechnology* 6:573–9, 2011; *Adv. Microb. Physiol.* 59:1–100, 2011; *Nat. Rev. Microbiol.* 9:39–50, 2011; *Science* 330:1413–5, 2010; *Nature* 435:1098–101, 2005; *Science* 301:934, 2003; *Nature* 416:767–9, 2002; *Science* 295:483–5, 2002; *Nature* 415:312–6, 2002.

W. J. Manning, Adjunct Professor; Ph.D., Delaware. Effects of ozone on plants and associated mycoflora; plants as bioindicators of ozone; effects of ozone and other air pollutants on plants in urban environments; managing invasive plants with fungal pathogens. *Environ. Pollut.* 126:73–81, 2003.

Y. S. Morita, Assistant Professor; Ph.D., Johns Hopkins. Biosynthesis of lipids and glycans and the pathogenesis of mycobacterial diseases. *mBio* 4:e00472–512, 2013; *J. Biol. Chem.* 285:16643–50, 2010; *J. Biol. Chem.* 285:13326–36, 2010.

S. Nugen, Adjunct Assistant Professor; Ph.D., Cornell. Food and water pathogen detection; rapid biosensor technology; microfluidic assay development; nanofabrication; diagnostics for low resource settings. *Nanotechnology* 25:225101, 2014; *Analyst* 139(12):3002–8, 2014; *Microfluidics and Nanofluidics* 16(5):879–86, 2014; *Analyst,* 2013, doi:10.1039/C3AN01114C; *Biomedical Microdevices,* 2013, doi:10.1007/s10544-013-9760-1; *Microsystem Technologies,* 2013, doi:10.1007/s00542-013-1742-y; *Mater. Lett.* 92:17–20, 2013; *Colloid Surface Physicochem Eng. Aspect* 414:251–8, 2012.

K. Nüsslein, Professor; Ph.D., Michigan State. Microbial ecology of terrestrial and aquatic environments; relating the stress of environmental influences to community structure and function, with emphasis on understanding interactions among bacterial communities. *The ISME Journal* 8:1548–50, 2014; *Mol. Ecol.* 23:2988–99, 2014; *Appl. Environ. Microbiol.* 80:281–8, 2014; *PNAS* 110:988–93, 2013; *Appl. Microbio. Biotechnol.,* 2013, doi: 10.1007/s00253-013-4963-1; *Front. Extr. Microbiol.* 3:175, 2012; *Bioresource Technology* 123:207–13, 2012; *Appl. Microbiol. Biotechnol.* 2:6, 2012; *Biointerfaces* 87(1):109–15, 2011; *Water Res.* 44:4970–9, 2010; *Curr. Opin. Biotechnol.* 21:339–45, 2010; *Geomicrobiology* 26:9–20, 2009; *Geology* 36:139–42, 2008.

S. T. Petsch, Adjunct Associate Professor; Ph.D., Yale. Transport, transformation, and biodegradation of natural organic matter in sediments, soils, and sedimentary rocks. *Geology,* 36:139–42, 2008; *Appl. Environ. Microbiol.* 73:4171–9, 2007; *Geochim. Cosmochim. Acta* 71:4233–50, 2007; *SEPM* 5:5–9, 2007; *Am. J. Sci.* 306:575–615, 2006; *Palaeogeogr. Palaeoclim. Palaeoecol.* 219:157–70, 2005; *Gas Technol. Inst.* GRI-05/0023, 2004; *Am. J. Sci.* 304:234–49, 2004; *Org. Geochem.* 34:731–43, 2003.

S. M. Rich, Professor; Ph.D. California, Irvine. Population genetics and evolution of vectorborne and zoonotic diseases. *Proc. Natl. Acad. Sci. Unit. States Am.* 106:14902–7; *Emerg. Infect. Dis.* 15:585–7; *Gene* 304:65–75; *Proc. Natl. Acad. Sci. Unit. States Am.* 98:15038–43; *J. Clin. Microbiol.* 39:494–7; *Proc. Natl. Acad. Sci. Unit. States Am.* 95:4425–30; *Proc. Natl. Acad. Sci. Unit. States Am.* 94:13040–45; *Insect Mol. Biol.* 6:123–9; *Proc. Natl. Acad. Sci. Unit. States Am.* 92:6284–8.

S. J. Sandler, Professor; Ph.D., Berkeley. Molecular genetics of recombination; DNA replication and DNA repair in bacteria. *Mol. Microbiol.* 57:1074, 2005; *Mol. Microbiol.* 53:1343, 2004.

D. A. Sela, Adjunct Assistant Professor; Ph.D., California, Davis. Dietary influences on the human microbiome; nutritional microbiology; comparative microbial genomics; next generation probiotics/prebiotics; food fermentations; biotechnology. *Am. J. Clin. Nutr.* PMID:24452239, 2014; *Appl. Environ. Microbiol.* PMID:22138995, 2013; *J. Biol. Chem.* PMID:21288901, 2011; *Trends Microbiol.* PMID:20409714, 2010; *Proc. Natl. Acad. Sci. Unit. States. Am.* PMID:19033196, 2008.

W. Webley, Associate Professor; Ph.D., Massachusetts. Immunology and pathogenic bacteriology; understanding the role and mechanism of *Chlamydia* involvement in chronic severe asthma; design and development of a novel multi-subunit vaccine display/delivery system for *Chlamydia;* design of a point-of-care diagnostic test for Chlamydia infections in farm animals. *PLos One* 8(12), 2013; *Biology of AIDS*, 2nd edition, Kendall/Hunt Publishing; *Vaccine* 30(41):5942–8, 2012; *Plos One* 7(4), 2012; *Resp. Res.* 13(1):32, 2012; *Eur. Respir. J.* 38(4)994–5, 2011; *Respirology* 16(7):1081–7, 2011; *Pediatr. Infect. Dis. J.,* 29(12):1093–8, 2010; *Eur. Respir. J.,* 33:1–8, 2009; *Biology of AIDS,* 2nd ed., Dubuque, Iowa: Kendall/Hunt Publishing Company, 2008; *CHEST* 134(suppl.), 2008; *CHEST* 132(4):607, 2007; *J. Clin. Apheresis* 3, 2006; *BMC Infect. Dis.* 6:23, 2006; *Am. J. Respir. Crit. Care Med.* 171(10):1083–8, 2005; *BMC Infect. Dis.* 4(1):23, 2004 (with Stuart and Norkin); *Curr. Microbiol.* 49(1):13–21, 2004; *Am. J. Respir. Crit. Care Med.* 169(7):A586, 2004; *J. Clin. Apheresis* 18(2), 2003; *Exp. Cell Res.* 287(1):67–78, 2003.

H. Xiao, Adjunct Associate Professor; Ph.D., Wisconsin–Madison. Cancer preventive dietary components; diet-based strategy for cancer prevention; enhancement of biological activity of dietary components by combination regimen; food processing, and nanotechnology.

Section 13
Neuroscience and Neurobiology

This section contains a directory of institutions offering graduate work in neuroscience and neurobiology, followed by in-depth entries submitted by institutions that chose to prepare detailed program descriptions. Additional information about programs listed in the directory but not augmented by an in-depth entry may be obtained by writing directly to the dean of a graduate school or chair of a department at the address given in the directory.

For programs offering related work, see also in this book *Anatomy; Biochemistry; Biological and Biomedical Sciences; Biophysics; Cell, Molecular, and Structural Biology; Genetics, Developmental Biology, and Reproductive Biology; Optometry and Vision Sciences; Pathology and Pathobiology; Pharmacology and Toxicology; Physiology;* and *Zoology*. In another guide in this series:

Graduate Programs in the Humanities, Arts & Social Sciences
See *Psychology and Counseling*

CONTENTS

Biopsychology

Adler School of Professional Psychology, Programs in Psychology, Chicago, IL 60602. Offers advanced Adlerian psychotherapy (Certificate); art therapy (MA); clinical neuropsychology (Certificate); clinical psychology (Psy D); community psychology (MA); counseling and organizational psychology (MA); counseling psychology (MA); criminology (MA); emergency management leadership (MA); forensic psychology (MA); marriage and family counseling (MA); marriage and family therapy (Certificate); military psychology (MA); nonprofit management (MA); organizational psychology (MA); police psychology (MA); public policy and administration (MA); rehabilitation counseling (MA); sport and health psychology (MA); substance abuse counseling (Certificate); Psy D/Certificate; Psy D/MACAT; Psy D/MACP; Psy D/MAMFC; Psy D/MASAC. *Accreditation:* APA. Part-time and evening/weekend programs available. Postbaccalaureate distance learning degree programs offered (minimal on-campus study). Terminal master's awarded for partial completion of doctoral program. *Degree requirements:* For master's, thesis or alternative, oral exam, practicum; for doctorate, thesis/dissertation, clinical exam, internship, oral exam, practicum, written qualifying exam. *Entrance requirements:* For master's, 12 semester hours in psychology, minimum GPA of 3.0; for doctorate, 18 semester hours in psychology, minimum GPA of 3.25; for Certificate, appropriate master's or doctoral degree. Additional exam requirements/recommendations for international students: Required—TOEFL (minimum score 550 paper-based; 79 iBT). Electronic applications accepted.

American University, College of Arts and Sciences, Washington, DC 20016-8012. Offers addiction and addictive behavior (Certificate); anthropology (PhD); applied microeconomics (Certificate); applied statistics (Certificate); art history (MA); arts management (MA, Certificate); Asian studies (Certificate); audio production (Certificate); audio technology (MA); behavior, cognition, and neuroscience (PhD); bilingual education (MA, Certificate); biology (MA, MS); chemistry (MS); clinical psychology (PhD); computer science (MS, Certificate); creative writing (MFA); curriculum and instruction (M Ed, Certificate); economics (MA, PhD); environmental assessment (Certificate); environmental science (MS); ethics, peace, and global affairs (MA); gender analysis in economics (Certificate); health promotion management (MS); history (MA, PhD); international arts management (Certificate); international economic relations (Certificate); international economics (MA); international training and education (MA); literature (MA); mathematics (MA); North American studies (Certificate); nutrition education (MS, Certificate); philosophy (MA); professional science: biotechnology (MS); professional science: environmental assessment (MS); professional science: quantitative analysis (MS); psychobiology of healing (Certificate); psychology (MA); psychology: general (PhD); public anthropology (MA, Certificate); public sociology (Certificate); social research (Certificate); sociology (MA); Spanish: Latin American studies (MA); special education: learning disabilities (MA); statistics (MS); studio art (MFA); teaching (MAT); teaching English as a foreign language (MA); teaching: early childhood (Certificate); teaching: elementary (Certificate); teaching: ESOL (Certificate); teaching: secondary (Certificate); technology in arts management (Certificate); TESOL (MA); translation: French (Certificate); translation: Russian (Certificate); translation: Spanish (Certificate); women's, gender, and sexuality studies (Certificate). Part-time and evening/weekend programs available. Postbaccalaureate distance learning degree programs offered (no on-campus study). *Faculty:* 358 full-time (187 women), 254 part-time/adjunct (127 women). *Students:* 627 full-time (411 women), 416 part-time (300 women); includes 206 minority (91 Black or African American, non-Hispanic/Latino; 5 American Indian or Alaska Native, non-Hispanic/Latino; 32 Asian, non-Hispanic/Latino; 64 Hispanic/Latino; 1 Native Hawaiian or other Pacific Islander, non-Hispanic/Latino; 13 Two or more races, non-Hispanic/Latino), 124 international. Average age 29. 1,672 applicants, 52% accepted, 361 enrolled. In 2013, 382 master's, 38 doctorates, 33 other advanced degrees awarded. Terminal master's awarded for partial completion of doctoral program. *Degree requirements:* For master's, comprehensive exam (for some programs), thesis (for some programs); for doctorate, comprehensive exam (for some programs), thesis/dissertation. *Entrance requirements:* For master's, GRE, minimum GPA of 3.0 in last 60 credit hours, letter of recommendation, statement of purpose, resume, unofficial transcript; for doctorate, GRE, minimum GPA of 3.0 for all graduate work, letter of recommendation, statement of purpose, resume, unofficial transcript. Additional exam requirements/recommendations for international students: Required—TOEFL (minimum score 600 paper-based; 100 iBT), IELTS (minimum score 7). *Application deadline:* For fall admission, 2/1 for domestic students; for spring admission, 10/1 for domestic students. Applications are processed on a rolling basis. Application fee: $55. Electronic applications accepted. *Expenses: Tuition:* Full-time $25,920; part-time $1482 per credit hour. *Required fees:* $430. Tuition and fees vary according to course load and program. *Financial support:* Fellowships, research assistantships with full and partial tuition reimbursements, teaching assistantships with full and partial tuition reimbursements, career-related internships or fieldwork, Federal Work-Study, institutionally sponsored loans, scholarships/grants, traineeships, tuition waivers (full and partial), and unspecified assistantships available. Support available to part-time students. Financial award applicants required to submit FAFSA. *Unit head:* Dr. Peter Starr, Dean, 202-885-2446, Fax: 202-885-2429, E-mail: pstarr@american.edu. *Application contact:* Kathleen Clowery, Associate Director, Graduate Enrollment Management, 202-885-3621, Fax: 202-885-1505, E-mail: clowery@american.edu.
Website: http://www.american.edu/cas/

Argosy University, Atlanta, College of Psychology and Behavioral Sciences, Atlanta, GA 30328. Offers clinical psychology (MA, Psy D, Postdoctoral Respecialization Certificate), including child and family psychology (Psy D), general adult clinical (Psy D), health psychology (Psy D), neuropsychology/geropsychology (Psy D); community counseling (MA), including marriage and family therapy; counselor education and supervision (Ed D); forensic psychology (MA); industrial organizational psychology (MA); marriage and family therapy (Certificate); sport-exercise psychology (MA). *Accreditation:* APA.

Argosy University, Twin Cities, College of Psychology and Behavioral Sciences, Eagan, MN 55121. Offers clinical psychology (MA, Psy D), including child and family psychology (Psy D), forensic psychology (Psy D), health and neuropsychology (Psy D), trauma (Psy D); forensic counseling (Post-Graduate Certificate); forensic psychology (MA); industrial organizational psychology (MA); marriage and family therapy (MA, DMFT), including forensic counseling (MA). *Accreditation:* AAMFT; AAMFT/COAMFTE; APA.

Binghamton University, State University of New York, Graduate School, School of Arts and Sciences, Department of Psychology, Specialization in Behavioral Neuroscience, Vestal, NY 13850. Offers PhD. *Students:* 16 full-time (9 women), 6 part-time (5 women); includes 5 minority (2 Black or African American, non-Hispanic/Latino; 1 American Indian or Alaska Native, non-Hispanic/Latino; 2 Asian, non-Hispanic/Latino). Average age 27. 30 applicants, 20% accepted, 2 enrolled. In 2013, 3 doctorates awarded. *Degree requirements:* For doctorate, thesis/dissertation, departmental qualifying exam. *Entrance requirements:* For doctorate, GRE General Test, GRE Subject Test. Additional exam requirements/recommendations for international students: Required—TOEFL (minimum score 550 paper-based; 80 iBT). *Application deadline:* For fall admission, 1/15 priority date for domestic and international students. Applications are processed on a rolling basis. Application fee: $75. Electronic applications accepted. *Financial support:* In 2013–14, 21 students received support, including 5 research assistantships with full tuition reimbursements available (averaging $18,500 per year), 11 teaching assistantships with full tuition reimbursements available (averaging $18,500 per year); career-related internships or fieldwork, Federal Work-Study, institutionally sponsored loans, scholarships/grants, health care benefits, tuition waivers (full and partial), and unspecified assistantships also available. Financial award application deadline: 2/15; financial award applicants required to submit FAFSA. *Unit head:* Dr. Peter Gerhardstein, Graduate Coordinator, 607-777-4383, E-mail: gerhard@binghamton.edu. *Application contact:* Kishan Zuber, Recruiting and Admissions Coordinator, 607-777-2151, Fax: 607-777-2501, E-mail: kzuber@binghamton.edu.

Boston University, School of Medicine, Division of Graduate Medical Sciences, Program in Mental Health Counseling and Behavioral Medicine, Boston, MA 02215. Offers MA. *Expenses: Tuition:* Full-time $43,970; part-time $1374 per credit hour. *Required fees:* $60 per semester. Tuition and fees vary according to class time, course level and program. *Faculty research:* HIV/AIDS, trauma, behavioral medicine (obesity, breast cancer), neurosciences, autism, serious mental illness, sports psychology. *Unit head:* Dr. Stephen Brady, Director, 617-414-2320, Fax: 617-414-2323, E-mail: sbrady@bu.edu. *Application contact:* Bernice Mark, Administrative Assistant, 617-414-2328, E-mail: nicey@bu.edu.
Website: http://www.bumc.bu.edu/mhbm/

Carnegie Mellon University, College of Humanities and Social Sciences, Department of Psychology, Area of Cognitive Neuroscience, Pittsburgh, PA 15213-3891. Offers PhD. *Degree requirements:* For doctorate, comprehensive exam, thesis/dissertation. *Entrance requirements:* For doctorate, GRE General Test. Additional exam requirements/recommendations for international students: Required—TOEFL. *Application deadline:* For fall admission, 1/2 for domestic students. Application fee: $45. *Unit head:* Dr. Roberta L. Klatzky, Head, 412-268-3151, Fax: 412-268-2781, E-mail: klatzky@cmu.edu. *Application contact:* Dr. Roberta L. Klatzky, Head, 412-268-3151, Fax: 412-268-2781, E-mail: klatzky@cmu.edu.

Connecticut College, Department of Psychology, New London, CT 06320-4196. Offers behavioral medicine/health psychology (MA); clinical psychology (MA); neuroscience/psychobiology (MA); social/personality psychology (MA). Part-time programs available. *Students:* 4 full-time (1 woman), 3 part-time (2 women); includes 1 minority (Black or African American, non-Hispanic/Latino). Average age 33. 11 applicants, 45% accepted, 3 enrolled. *Degree requirements:* For master's, thesis. *Entrance requirements:* For master's, GRE General Test, statistics course. Additional exam requirements/recommendations for international students: Required—TOEFL (minimum score 600 paper-based). *Application deadline:* For fall admission, 2/1 for domestic and international students. Application fee: $60. *Expenses: Tuition:* Full-time $11,700; part-time $1950 per course. *Financial support:* Tuition remission available. Financial award application deadline: 2/1; financial award applicants required to submit CSS PROFILE or FAFSA. *Unit head:* Dr. Ruth Grahn, Chair, 860-439-2387, Fax: 860-439-5300, E-mail: ruth.grahn@conncoll.edu. *Application contact:* Nancy M. MacLeod, Academic Department Assistant, 860-439-2330, Fax: 860-439-5300, E-mail: nancy.macleod@conncoll.edu.

Cornell University, Graduate School, Graduate Fields of Arts and Sciences, Field of Psychology, Ithaca, NY 14853-0001. Offers biopsychology (PhD); human experimental psychology (PhD); personality and social psychology (PhD). *Faculty:* 41 full-time (17 women). *Students:* 38 full-time (21 women); includes 6 minority (1 Black or African American, non-Hispanic/Latino; 2 Asian, non-Hispanic/Latino; 2 Hispanic/Latino; 1 Two or more races, non-Hispanic/Latino), 9 international. Average age 28. 232 applicants, 5% accepted, 8 enrolled. In 2013, 8 doctorates awarded. *Degree requirements:* For doctorate, comprehensive exam, thesis/dissertation, 2 semesters of teaching experience. *Entrance requirements:* For doctorate, GRE General Test, 3 letters of recommendation. Additional exam requirements/recommendations for international students: Required—TOEFL (minimum score 550 paper-based; 77 iBT). *Application deadline:* For fall admission, 12/15 for domestic students. Application fee: $95. Electronic applications accepted. *Financial support:* In 2013–14, 30 students received support, including 6 fellowships with full tuition reimbursements available, 24 teaching assistantships with full tuition reimbursements available; research assistantships with full tuition reimbursements available, institutionally sponsored loans, scholarships/grants, health care benefits, tuition waivers (full and partial), and unspecified assistantships also available. Financial award applicants required to submit FAFSA. *Faculty research:* Sensory and perceptual systems, social cognition, cognitive development, quantitative and computational modeling, behavioral neuroscience. *Unit head:* Director of Graduate Studies, 607-255-6364, Fax: 607-255-8433. *Application contact:* Graduate Field Assistant, 607-255-3834, Fax: 607-255-8433, E-mail: psychapp@cornell.edu.
Website: http://www.gradschool.cornell.edu/fields.php?id-62&a-2

Drexel University, College of Arts and Sciences, Department of Psychology, Philadelphia, PA 19104-2875. Offers clinical psychology (PhD), including clinical psychology, forensic psychology, health psychology, neuropsychology; law-psychology (PhD); psychology (MS); JD/PhD. *Accreditation:* APA (one or more programs are accredited). *Degree requirements:* For doctorate, thesis/dissertation, internship. *Entrance requirements:* For doctorate, GRE General Test. Additional exam requirements/recommendations for international students: Required—TOEFL. Electronic applications accepted. *Expenses:* Contact institution. *Faculty research:* Neurosciences, rehabilitation psychology, cognitive science, neurological assessment.

Duke University, Graduate School, Department of Psychology and Neuroscience, Durham, NC 27708. Offers biological psychology (PhD); clinical psychology (PhD); cognitive psychology (PhD); developmental psychology (PhD); experimental psychology (PhD); health psychology (PhD); human social development (PhD); JD/MA. *Accreditation:* APA (one or more programs are accredited). *Faculty:* 40. *Students:* 94 full-time (71 women); includes 16 minority (3 Black or African American, non-Hispanic/Latino; 7 Asian, non-Hispanic/Latino; 6 Hispanic/Latino), 10 international. 557 applicants, 3% accepted, 9 enrolled. In 2013, 12 doctorates awarded. *Degree requirements:* For doctorate, thesis/dissertation. *Entrance requirements:* For doctorate, GRE General Test. Additional exam requirements/recommendations for international students: Required—TOEFL (minimum score 577 paper-based; 90 iBT) or IELTS (minimum score 7). *Application deadline:* For fall admission, 12/8 priority date for domestic and international students. Application fee: $80. Electronic applications

accepted. *Financial support:* Fellowships, research assistantships, teaching assistantships, career-related internships or fieldwork, and Federal Work-Study available. Financial award application deadline: 12/8. *Unit head:* Melanie Bonner, Director of Graduate Studies, 919-660-5715, Fax: 919-660-5726, E-mail: morrell@duke.edu. *Application contact:* Elizabeth Hutton, Director of Admissions, 919-684-3913, Fax: 919-684-2277, E-mail: grad-admissions@duke.edu.
Website: http://psychandneuro.duke.edu/graduate

The Graduate Center, City University of New York, Graduate Studies, Program in Psychology, New York, NY 10016-4039. Offers basic applied neurocognition (PhD); biopsychology (PhD); clinical psychology (PhD); developmental psychology (PhD); environmental psychology (PhD); experimental psychology (PhD); industrial psychology (PhD); learning processes (PhD); neuropsychology (PhD); psychology (PhD); social personality (PhD). *Degree requirements:* For doctorate, one foreign language, thesis/dissertation. *Entrance requirements:* For doctorate, GRE General Test. Additional exam requirements/recommendations for international students: Required—TOEFL. Electronic applications accepted.

Harvard University, Graduate School of Arts and Sciences, Department of Psychology, Cambridge, MA 02138. Offers psychology (PhD), including behavior and decision analysis, cognition, developmental psychology, experimental psychology, personality, psychobiology, psychopathology; social psychology (PhD). *Accreditation:* APA. *Degree requirements:* For doctorate, thesis/dissertation, general exams. *Entrance requirements:* For doctorate, GRE General Test. Additional exam requirements/recommendations for international students: Required—TOEFL. *Expenses: Tuition:* Full-time $38,888. *Required fees:* $958. Tuition and fees vary according to campus/location, program and student level.

Howard University, Graduate School, Department of Psychology, Washington, DC 20059-0002. Offers clinical psychology (PhD); developmental psychology (PhD); experimental psychology (PhD); neuropsychology (PhD); personality psychology (PhD); psychology (MS); social psychology (PhD). *Accreditation:* APA (one or more programs are accredited). Part-time programs available. *Degree requirements:* For master's, thesis; for doctorate, comprehensive exam, thesis/dissertation, qualifying exam. *Entrance requirements:* For master's, GRE General Test, minimum GPA of 2.5, bachelor's degree in psychology or related field; for doctorate, GRE General Test, minimum GPA of 3.0. *Faculty research:* Personality and psychophysiology, educational and social development of African-American children, child and adult psychopathology.

Indiana University–Purdue University Indianapolis, School of Science, Department of Psychology, Indianapolis, IN 46202-3275. Offers clinical psychology (MS); industrial/organizational psychology (MS); psychobiology of addictions (PhD). *Accreditation:* APA (one or more programs are accredited). *Faculty:* 25 full-time (13 women), 2 part-time/adjunct (both women). *Students:* 46 full-time (35 women), 12 part-time (8 women); includes 9 minority (3 Black or African American, non-Hispanic/Latino; 3 Asian, non-Hispanic/Latino; 2 Hispanic/Latino; 1 Two or more races, non-Hispanic/Latino), 3 international. Average age 28. 165 applicants, 8% accepted, 12 enrolled. In 2013, 13 master's, 2 doctorates awarded. Terminal master's awarded for partial completion of doctoral program. *Degree requirements:* For master's, thesis; for doctorate, thesis/dissertation. *Entrance requirements:* For master's, GRE General Test, minimum undergraduate GPA of 3.0; for doctorate, GRE General Test, GRE Subject Test (clinical psychology), minimum undergraduate GPA of 3.2. Additional exam requirements/recommendations for international students: Required—TOEFL (minimum score 567 paper-based; 86 iBT). *Application deadline:* For fall admission, 12/1 priority date for domestic and international students. Electronic applications accepted. *Financial support:* In 2013–14, 3 fellowships with partial tuition reimbursements (averaging $22,500 per year) were awarded; research assistantships with partial tuition reimbursements, teaching assistantships with partial tuition reimbursements, career-related internships or fieldwork, Federal Work-Study, institutionally sponsored loans, traineeships, health care benefits, and unspecified assistantships also available. Financial award application deadline: 3/1; financial award applicants required to submit FAFSA. *Faculty research:* Severe mental illness, health psychology, neurological research, alcoholism and psychopathology, functional activities within organizations. *Unit head:* Dr. Peggy S. Stockdale, Chair, 317-278-3838, E-mail: pstockda@iupui.edu. *Application contact:* Heather Sissons, Office Manager and Graduate Coordinator, 317-274-6945, E-mail: hsissons@iupui.edu.
Website: http://www.psych.iupui.edu/

Louisiana State University and Agricultural & Mechanical College, Graduate School, College of Humanities and Social Sciences, Department of Psychology, Baton Rouge, LA 70803. Offers biological psychology (MA, PhD); clinical psychology (MA, PhD); cognitive psychology (MA, PhD); developmental psychology (MA, PhD); school psychology (MA, PhD). PhD programs offered jointly with Southeastern Louisiana University. *Accreditation:* APA (one or more programs are accredited). *Faculty:* 23 full-time (11 women). *Students:* 70 full-time (50 women), 28 part-time (23 women); includes 9 minority (2 Black or African American, non-Hispanic/Latino; 1 American Indian or Alaska Native, non-Hispanic/Latino; 2 Asian, non-Hispanic/Latino; 2 Hispanic/Latino; 2 Two or more races, non-Hispanic/Latino), 2 international. Average age 27. 219 applicants, 6% accepted, 12 enrolled. In 2013, 13 master's, 8 doctorates awarded. Terminal master's awarded for partial completion of doctoral program. *Degree requirements:* For master's, thesis; for doctorate, thesis/dissertation, 1-year internship. *Entrance requirements:* For master's and doctorate, GRE General Test, minimum GPA of 3.0. Additional exam requirements/recommendations for international students: Required—TOEFL (minimum score 550 paper-based; 79 IBT), IELTS (minimum score 6.5), or PTE (minimum score 59). *Application deadline:* For fall admission, 1/15 for domestic and international students. Applications are processed on a rolling basis. Application fee: $50 ($70 for international students). Electronic applications accepted. *Financial support:* In 2013–14, 94 students received support, including 2 fellowships (averaging $29,130 per year), 10 research assistantships with partial tuition reimbursements available (averaging $14,600 per year), 51 teaching assistantships with partial tuition reimbursements available (averaging $12,654 per year); career-related internships or fieldwork, Federal Work-Study, institutionally sponsored loans, scholarships/grants, health care benefits, and tuition waivers (full and partial) also available. Financial award applicants required to submit FAFSA. *Faculty research:* Clinical psychology, autism, anxiety, addition, neuropsychology, school psychology, cognitive psychology, experimental psychology. *Total annual research expenditures:* $940,667. *Unit head:* Dr. Robert Matthews, Chair, 225-578-8745, Fax: 225-578-4125, E-mail: psmath@lsu.edu. *Application contact:* Dr. Jason Hicks, Coordinator of Graduate Studies, 225-578-4109, Fax: 225-578-4125, E-mail: jhicks@lsu.edu.
Website: http://www.lsu.edu/psychology/graduate.html

Memorial University of Newfoundland, School of Graduate Studies, Interdisciplinary Program in Cognitive and Behavioral Ecology, St. John's, NL A1C 5S7, Canada. Offers M Sc, PhD. *Degree requirements:* For master's, thesis, public lecture; for doctorate, comprehensive exam, thesis/dissertation, oral defense of dissertation. *Entrance requirements:* For master's, honors degree (minimum 2nd class standing) in related field; for doctorate, master's degree. Electronic applications accepted. *Faculty research:* Seabird feeding ecology, marine mammal and seabird energetics, systems of fish, seabird/seal/fisheries interaction.

Northwestern University, The Graduate School, Judd A. and Marjorie Weinberg College of Arts and Sciences, Department of Psychology, Evanston, IL 60208. Offers brain, behavior and cognition (PhD); clinical psychology (PhD); cognitive psychology (PhD); personality psychology (PhD); social psychology (PhD); JD/PhD. Admissions and degrees offered through The Graduate School. *Accreditation:* APA (one or more programs are accredited). Part-time programs available. *Degree requirements:* For doctorate, thesis/dissertation. *Entrance requirements:* For doctorate, GRE General Test, GRE Subject Test. Additional exam requirements/recommendations for international students: Required—TOEFL. Electronic applications accepted. *Faculty research:* Memory and higher order cognition, anxiety and depression, effectiveness of psychotherapy, social cognition, molecular basis of memory.

Northwestern University, The Graduate School and Fienberg School of Medicine, Program in Clinical Psychology, Evanston, IL 60208. Offers clinical psychology (PhD), including clinical neuropsychology. Admissions and degree offered through The Graduate School. *Accreditation:* APA. *Degree requirements:* For doctorate, thesis/dissertation, clinical internship. *Entrance requirements:* For doctorate, GRE General Test, GRE Subject Test, minimum GPA of 3.2, course work in psychology. Additional exam requirements/recommendations for international students: Required—TOEFL. *Faculty research:* Cancer and cardiovascular risk reduction, evaluation of mental health services and policy, neuropsychological assessment, outcome of psychotherapy, cognitive therapy, pediatric and clinical child psychology.

Oregon Health & Science University, School of Medicine, Graduate Programs in Medicine, Department of Behavioral Neuroscience, Portland, OR 97239-3098. Offers PhD. *Faculty:* 34 full-time (14 women). *Students:* 28 full-time (15 women), 1 (woman) part-time; includes 6 minority (1 Asian, non-Hispanic/Latino; 3 Hispanic/Latino; 2 Two or more races, non-Hispanic/Latino). Average age 28. 105 applicants, 4% accepted, 4 enrolled. In 2013, 5 doctorates awarded. Terminal master's awarded for partial completion of doctoral program. *Degree requirements:* For doctorate, comprehensive exam, thesis/dissertation, qualifying exam. *Entrance requirements:* For doctorate, GRE General Test (minimum scores: 153 Verbal/148 Quantitative/4.5 Analytical), undergraduate coursework in biopsychology and other basic science areas. Additional exam requirements/recommendations for international students: Required—TOEFL. *Application deadline:* For fall admission, 12/1 for domestic students. Application fee: $70. Electronic applications accepted. *Financial support:* Fellowships, research assistantships, health care benefits, tuition waivers (full), and stipends (for PhD students) available. *Faculty research:* Behavioral neuroscience, behavioral genomics, biological basis of drug and alcohol abuse, cognitive neuroscience, neuropharmacology and neuroendocrinology. *Unit head:* Dr. Suzanne Mitchell, Program Director, 503-494-1650, E-mail: mitchesu@ohsu.edu. *Application contact:* Kris Thomason, Graduate Program Manager, 503-494-8464, E-mail: thomason@ohsu.edu.
Website: http://www.ohsu.edu/som-BehNeuro/

Palo Alto University, PGSP-Stanford Psy D Consortium Program, Palo Alto, CA 94303-4232. Offers Psy D. Program offered jointly with Stanford University. *Accreditation:* APA. *Degree requirements:* For doctorate, thesis/dissertation. *Entrance requirements:* For doctorate, GRE, BA or MA in psychology or related area, minimum undergraduate GPA of 3.0, minimum graduate GPA of 3.3. Additional exam requirements/recommendations for international students: Required—TOEFL. Electronic applications accepted. *Faculty research:* Biopsychosocial research, neurobiology, psychopharmacology.

Penn State University Park, Graduate School, College of Health and Human Development, Department of Biobehavioral Health, University Park, PA 16802. Offers MS, PhD. *Unit head:* Dr. Ann C. Crouter, Dean, 814-865-1420, Fax: 814-865-3282, E-mail: ac1@psu.edu. *Application contact:* Cynthia E. Nicosia, Director, Graduate Enrollment Services, 814-865-1834, Fax: 814-863-4627, E-mail: cey1@psu.edu.
Website: http://bbh.hhdev.psu.edu/

Philadelphia College of Osteopathic Medicine, Graduate and Professional Programs, Department of Psychology, Philadephia, PA 19131. Offers applied behavior analysis (Certificate); clinical health psychology (Post-Doctoral Certificate); clinical neuropsychology (Post-Doctoral Certificate); clinical psychology (Psy D); mental health counseling (MS); organizational development and leadership (MS); psychology (Certificate); school psychology (MS, Psy D, Ed S). *Accreditation:* APA. *Faculty:* 19 full-time (11 women), 122 part-time/adjunct (58 women). *Students:* 403 (311 women); includes 75 minority (49 Black or African American, non-Hispanic/Latino; 12 Asian, non-Hispanic/Latino; 9 Hispanic/Latino; 5 Two or more races, non-Hispanic/Latino). 357 applicants, 53% accepted, 132 enrolled. In 2013, 68 master's, 38 doctorates, 17 other advanced degrees awarded. Terminal master's awarded for partial completion of doctoral program. *Degree requirements:* For master's, comprehensive exam (for some programs), thesis (for some programs); for doctorate, comprehensive exam, thesis/dissertation. *Entrance requirements:* For master's, GRE or MAT, minimum GPA of 3.0; bachelor's degree from regionally-accredited college or university; for doctorate, PRAXIS II (for PsyD in school psychology), minimum undergraduate GPA of 3.0; for other advanced degree, GRE (for Ed S). Additional exam requirements/recommendations for international students: Required—TOEFL (minimum score 79 iBT). *Application deadline:* For fall admission, 3/1 priority date for domestic students. Applications are processed on a rolling basis. Application fee: $50. Electronic applications accepted. *Financial support:* In 2013–14, 28 teaching assistantships were awarded; Federal Work-Study, institutionally sponsored loans, and scholarships/grants also available. Financial award application deadline: 3/15; financial award applicants required to submit FAFSA. *Faculty research:* Adult and childhood anxiety and ADHD; coping with chronic illness; primary care psychology/integrated health care; applied behavior analysis; psychological, educational, and neuropsychological assessment. *Total annual research expenditures:* $533,489. *Unit head:* Dr. Robert DiTomasso, Chairman, 215-871-6442, Fax: 215-871-6458, E-mail: robertd@pcom.edu. *Application contact:* Kari A. Shotwell, Director of Admissions, 215-871-6700, Fax: 215-871-6719, E-mail: karis@pcom.edu.

Rutgers, The State University of New Jersey, Newark, Graduate School, Program in Psychology, Newark, NJ 07102. Offers cognitive neuroscience (PhD); cognitive science (PhD); perception (PhD); psychobiology (PhD); social cognition (PhD). *Degree requirements:* For doctorate, comprehensive exam, thesis/dissertation. *Entrance requirements:* For doctorate, GRE General Test, GRE Subject Test, minimum undergraduate B average. Electronic applications accepted. *Faculty research:* Visual perception (luminance, motion), neuroendocrine mechanisms in behavior (reproduction, pain), attachment theory, connectionist modeling of cognition.

Rutgers, The State University of New Jersey, New Brunswick, Graduate School-New Brunswick, Program in Psychology, Piscataway, NJ 08854-8097. Offers behavioral neuroscience (PhD); clinical psychology (PhD); cognitive psychology (PhD); interdisciplinary health psychology (PhD); social psychology (PhD). *Accreditation:* APA. *Degree requirements:* For doctorate, comprehensive exam, thesis/dissertation. *Entrance requirements:* For doctorate, GRE General Test, 3 letters of recommendation. Additional exam requirements/recommendations for international students: Required—TOEFL (minimum score 577 paper-based). Electronic applications accepted. *Faculty research:* Learning and memory, behavioral ecology, hormones and behavior, psychopharmacology, anxiety disorders.

Biopsychology

Texas A&M University, College of Liberal Arts, Department of Psychology, College Station, TX 77843. Offers behavioral and cellular neuroscience (PhD); clinical psychology (PhD); cognitive psychology (PhD); developmental psychology (PhD); industrial/organizational psychology (PhD); psychology (MS); social psychology (PhD). *Accreditation:* APA (one or more programs are accredited). *Faculty:* 37. *Students:* 95 full-time (55 women), 11 part-time (9 women); includes 27 minority (4 Black or African American, non-Hispanic/Latino; 6 Asian, non-Hispanic/Latino; 17 Hispanic/Latino), 16 international. Average age 28. 393 applicants, 3% accepted, 8 enrolled. In 2013, 5 master's, 7 doctorates awarded. *Degree requirements:* For doctorate, comprehensive exam (for some programs), thesis/dissertation. *Entrance requirements:* For doctorate, GRE General Test. Additional exam requirements/recommendations for international students: Required—TOEFL. *Application deadline:* For fall admission, 1/5 for domestic and international students. Application fee: $50 ($75 for international students). Electronic applications accepted. *Expenses:* Tuition, state resident: full-time $4078; part-time $226.55 per credit hour. Tuition, nonresident: full-time $10,450; part-time $580.55 per credit hour. *Required fees:* $2328; $278.50 per credit hour. $642.45 per semester. *Financial support:* Fellowships with partial tuition reimbursements, research assistantships with partial tuition reimbursements, teaching assistantships with partial tuition reimbursements, career-related internships or fieldwork, institutionally sponsored loans, health care benefits, and unspecified assistantships available. Financial award application deadline: 1/5; financial award applicants required to submit FAFSA. *Unit head:* Dr. Doug Woods, Head, 979-845-2540, E-mail: dowoods@tamu.edu. *Application contact:* Dr. Charles D. Samuelson, Director of Graduate Studies, 979-845-0880, Fax: 979-845-4727, E-mail: c-samuelson@tamu.edu.
Website: http://psychology.tamu.edu

University at Albany, State University of New York, College of Arts and Sciences, Department of Psychology, Albany, NY 12222-0001. Offers autism (Certificate); biopsychology (PhD); clinical psychology (PhD); general/experimental psychology (PhD); industrial/organizational psychology (PhD); psychology (MA); social/personality psychology (PhD). *Accreditation:* APA (one or more programs are accredited). *Degree requirements:* For doctorate, thesis/dissertation. *Entrance requirements:* For doctorate, GRE General Test, GRE Subject Test. Additional exam requirements/recommendations for international students: Required—TOEFL (minimum score 550 paper-based). Electronic applications accepted.

The University of British Columbia, Faculty of Arts and Faculty of Graduate Studies, Department of Psychology, Vancouver, BC V6T 1Z4, Canada. Offers behavioral neuroscience (MA, PhD); clinical psychology (MA, PhD); cognitive science (MA, PhD); developmental psychology (MA, PhD); health psychology (MA, PhD); quantitative methods (MA, PhD); social/personality psychology (MA, PhD). *Accreditation:* APA (one or more programs are accredited). Terminal master's awarded for partial completion of doctoral program. *Degree requirements:* For master's, thesis; for doctorate, comprehensive exam, thesis/dissertation. *Entrance requirements:* For master's and doctorate, GRE General Test. Additional exam requirements/recommendations for international students: Required—TOEFL (minimum score 550 paper-based; 80 iBT). Electronic applications accepted. *Expenses: Tuition, area resident:* Full-time $8000 Canadian dollars. *Faculty research:* Clinical, developmental, social/personality, cognition, behavioral neuroscience.

University of Connecticut, Graduate School, College of Liberal Arts and Sciences, Department of Psychology, Storrs, CT 06269. Offers behavioral neuroscience (PhD); biopsychology (PhD); clinical psychology (MA, PhD); cognition and instruction (PhD); developmental psychology (MA, PhD); ecological psychology (PhD); experimental psychology (PhD); general psychology (MA, PhD); health psychology (Graduate Certificate); industrial/organizational psychology (PhD); language and cognition (PhD); neuroscience (PhD); occupational health psychology (Graduate Certificate); social psychology (MA, PhD). *Accreditation:* APA. Terminal master's awarded for partial completion of doctoral program. *Degree requirements:* For master's, comprehensive exam; for doctorate, thesis/dissertation. *Entrance requirements:* For master's and doctorate, GRE General Test, GRE Subject Test. Additional exam requirements/recommendations for international students: Required—TOEFL (minimum score 550 paper-based). Electronic applications accepted.

University of Michigan, Rackham Graduate School, College of Literature, Science, and the Arts, Department of Psychology, Ann Arbor, MI 48109. Offers biopsychology (PhD); clinical science (PhD); cognition and cognitive neuroscience (PhD); developmental psychology (PhD); personality and social contexts (PhD); social psychology (PhD). *Accreditation:* APA. *Faculty:* 80 full-time (36 women), 32 part-time/adjunct (21 women). *Students:* 138 full-time (94 women); includes 62 minority (16 Black or African American, non-Hispanic/Latino; 2 American Indian or Alaska Native, non-Hispanic/Latino; 17 Asian, non-Hispanic/Latino; 25 Hispanic/Latino; 2 Two or more races, non-Hispanic/Latino), 12 international. Average age 27. 611 applicants, 6% accepted, 16 enrolled. In 2013, 29 doctorates awarded. *Degree requirements:* For doctorate, comprehensive exam, thesis/dissertation, oral defense of dissertation, preliminary exam. *Entrance requirements:* For doctorate, GRE General Test. Additional exam requirements/recommendations for international students: Required—TOEFL. *Application deadline:* For fall admission, 12/1 for domestic and international students. Application fee: $75 ($90 for international students). Electronic applications accepted. Tuition and fees vary according to course level, course load, degree level, program and student level. *Financial support:* In 2013–14, 82 students received support, including 45 fellowships with full tuition reimbursements available (averaging $20,900 per year), 16 research assistantships with full tuition reimbursements available (averaging $27,900 per year), 50 teaching assistantships with full tuition reimbursements available (averaging $24,000 per year); career-related internships or fieldwork also available. Financial award application deadline: 4/15. *Unit head:* Prof. Stephanie Rowley, Interim Chair, 734-764-7429. *Application contact:* Danielle Joanette, Psychology Student Academic Affairs, 731-764-2580, Fax: 734-615-7584, E-mail: psych.saa@umich.edu.
Website: http://www.lsa.umich.edu/psych/

University of Minnesota, Twin Cities Campus, Graduate School, College of Liberal Arts, Department of Psychology, Program in Cognitive and Biological Psychology, Minneapolis, MN 55455-0213. Offers PhD. *Degree requirements:* For doctorate, comprehensive exam, thesis/dissertation. *Entrance requirements:* For doctorate, GRE General Test, GRE Subject Test (recommended), 12 credits of upper-level psychology courses, including a course in statistics or psychological measurement. Additional exam requirements/recommendations for international students: Required—TOEFL (minimum score 550 paper-based; 79 iBT).

University of Nebraska–Lincoln, Graduate College, College of Arts and Sciences, Department of Psychology, Lincoln, NE 68588. Offers biopsychology (PhD); clinical psychology (PhD); cognitive psychology (PhD); developmental psychology (PhD); psychology (MA); social/personality psychology (PhD); JD/MA; JD/PhD. *Accreditation:* APA (one or more programs are accredited). *Degree requirements:* For master's, thesis optional; for doctorate, comprehensive exam, thesis/dissertation. *Entrance requirements:* For master's and doctorate, GRE General Test. Additional exam requirements/recommendations for international students: Required—TOEFL (minimum score 550 paper-based). Electronic applications accepted. *Faculty research:* Law and psychology, rural mental health, chronic mental illness, neuropsychology, child clinical psychology.

The University of North Carolina at Chapel Hill, Graduate School, College of Arts and Sciences, Department of Psychology, Chapel Hill, NC 27599-3270. Offers behavioral neuroscience psychology (PhD); clinical psychology (PhD); cognitive psychology (PhD); developmental psychology (PhD); quantitative psychology (PhD); social psychology (PhD). *Accreditation:* APA. *Degree requirements:* For doctorate, comprehensive exam, thesis/dissertation. *Entrance requirements:* For doctorate, GRE General Test, minimum GPA of 3.0. Additional exam requirements/recommendations for international students: Required—TOEFL (minimum score 550 paper-based; 79 iBT), IELTS (minimum score 7). Electronic applications accepted. *Faculty research:* Expressed emotion, cognitive development, social cognitive neuroscience, human memory personality.

University of Oklahoma Health Sciences Center, College of Medicine and Graduate College, Graduate Programs in Medicine, Department of Psychiatry and Behavioral Sciences, Oklahoma City, OK 73190. Offers biological psychology (MS, PhD). *Faculty:* 4 full-time (all women). *Degree requirements:* For master's, thesis; for doctorate, thesis/dissertation. *Entrance requirements:* For doctorate, GRE General Test, 3 letters of recommendation. Additional exam requirements/recommendations for international students: Required—TOEFL. *Application deadline:* For fall admission, 1/31 for domestic students. Application fee: $50. *Expenses:* Tuition, state resident: full-time $3504; part-time $175.20 per credit hour. Tuition, nonresident: full-time $13,504; part-time $675.20 per credit hour. *Required fees:* $1545; $52.70 per credit hour. $245.25 per semester. Tuition and fees vary according to course load. *Financial support:* In 2013–14, research assistantships (averaging $18,000 per year) were awarded; fellowships, career-related internships or fieldwork, institutionally sponsored loans, and tuition waivers (full and partial) also available. Support available to part-time students. *Faculty research:* Behavioral neuroscience, human neuropsychology, psychophysiology, behavioral medicine, health psychology. *Unit head:* Dr. Frank Holloway, Director, 405-271-2011, E-mail: frank-holloway@ouhsc.edu. *Application contact:* Dr. Larry Gonzalez, Graduate Liaison, 405-271-2011, E-mail: larry-gonzalez@ouhsc.edu.

University of Oregon, Graduate School, College of Arts and Sciences, Department of Psychology, Eugene, OR 97403. Offers clinical psychology (PhD); cognitive psychology (MA, MS, PhD); developmental psychology (MA, MS, PhD); physiological psychology (MA, MS, PhD); psychology (MA, MS, PhD); social/personality psychology (MA, MS, PhD). *Accreditation:* APA (one or more programs are accredited). Terminal master's awarded for partial completion of doctoral program. *Degree requirements:* For doctorate, thesis/dissertation. *Entrance requirements:* For master's, GRE General Test, minimum GPA of 3.0; for doctorate, GRE General Test. Additional exam requirements/recommendations for international students: Required—TOEFL.

The University of Texas at Austin, Graduate School, The Institute for Neuroscience, Austin, TX 78712-1111. Offers PhD, MD/PhD. Terminal master's awarded for partial completion of doctoral program. *Degree requirements:* For doctorate, thesis/dissertation. *Entrance requirements:* For doctorate, GRE. Electronic applications accepted. *Faculty research:* Cellular/molecular biology, neurobiology, pharmacology, behavioral neuroscience.

University of Windsor, Faculty of Graduate Studies, Faculty of Arts and Social Sciences, Department of Psychology, Windsor, ON N9B 3P4, Canada. Offers adult clinical (MA, PhD); applied social psychology (MA, PhD); child clinical (MA, PhD); clinical neuropsychology (MA, PhD). *Accreditation:* APA (one or more programs are accredited). *Degree requirements:* For master's, thesis; for doctorate, comprehensive exam, thesis/dissertation. *Entrance requirements:* For master's, GRE General Test, GRE Subject Test in psychology, minimum B average; for doctorate, GRE General Test, GRE Subject Test in psychology, master's degree. Additional exam requirements/recommendations for international students: Required—TOEFL (minimum score 600 paper-based). Electronic applications accepted. *Faculty research:* Gambling, suicidology, emotional competence, psychotherapy and trauma.

University of Wisconsin–Madison, Graduate School, College of Letters and Science, Department of Psychology, Program in Biology of Brain and Behavior, Madison, WI 53706-1380. Offers PhD. *Degree requirements:* For doctorate, comprehensive exam, thesis/dissertation. *Entrance requirements:* For doctorate, GRE General Test, minimum undergraduate GPA of 3.0. Additional exam requirements/recommendations for international students: Required—TOEFL. Electronic applications accepted. *Expenses:* Tuition, state resident: full-time $10,728; part-time $790 per credit. Tuition, nonresident: full-time $24,054; part-time $1623 per credit. *Required fees:* $1130; $119 per credit.

Virginia Commonwealth University, Graduate School, College of Humanities and Sciences, Department of Psychology, Program in General Psychology, Richmond, VA 23284-9005. Offers biopsychology (PhD); developmental psychology (PhD); social psychology (PhD). *Degree requirements:* For doctorate, thesis/dissertation. *Entrance requirements:* For doctorate, GRE General Test. Additional exam requirements/recommendations for international students: Required—TOEFL (minimum score 600 paper-based; 100 iBT); Recommended—IELTS (minimum score 6.5). Electronic applications accepted. *Faculty research:* Biopsychology, developmental and social psychology.

Wayne State University, School of Medicine, Graduate Programs in Medicine, Department of Psychiatry and Behavioral Neurosciences, Detroit, MI 48202. Offers psychiatry (MS); translational neuroscience (PhD). *Students:* 9 full-time (5 women); includes 2 minority (1 Asian, non-Hispanic/Latino; 1 Two or more races, non-Hispanic/Latino), 1 international. Average age 28. 40 applicants, 5% accepted. *Degree requirements:* For master's, thesis, oral thesis defense; for doctorate, thesis/dissertation. *Entrance requirements:* For master's and doctorate, GRE, minimum undergradute GPA of 3.0, bachelor's degree from accredited institution, coursework in biological sciences and other scientific disciplines, personal statement, three letters of recommendation. Additional exam requirements/recommendations for international students: Required—TOEFL (minimum score 600 paper-based; 100 iBT). *Application deadline:* For fall admission, 12/15 for domestic and international students. Application fee: $0. Electronic applications accepted. *Expenses:* Contact institution. *Financial support:* In 2013–14, 8 students received support, including 2 fellowships with tuition reimbursements available (averaging $24,700 per year), 6 research assistantships with tuition reimbursements available (averaging $25,617 per year); scholarships/grants, health care benefits, and unspecified assistantships also available. Financial award application deadline: 3/31; financial award applicants required to submit FAFSA. *Faculty research:* Substance abuse, brain imaging, schizophrenia, child psychopathy, child development, neurobiology of monoamine systems. *Unit head:* Dr. David R. Rosenberg, Chair, 313-577-9000, E-mail: drosen@med.wayne.edu. *Application contact:* Dr. Jeffery Stanely, Graduate Program Director, 313-577-9090, E-mail: jstanley@med.wayne.edu.
Website: http://psychiatry.med.wayne.edu/

Neurobiology

Albert Einstein College of Medicine, Graduate Division of Biomedical Sciences, Department of Neuroscience, Bronx, NY 10461. Offers PhD, MD/PhD. *Degree requirements:* For doctorate, thesis/dissertation. *Entrance requirements:* For doctorate, GRE General Test. Additional exam requirements/recommendations for international students: Required—TOEFL. *Faculty research:* Structure-function relations at chemical and electrical synapses, mechanisms of electrogenesis, analysis of neuronal subsystems.

Boston University, School of Medicine, Division of Graduate Medical Sciences, Department of Anatomy and Neurobiology, Boston, MA 02118. Offers MA, PhD, MD/PhD. Part-time programs available. Terminal master's awarded for partial completion of doctoral program. *Degree requirements:* For master's, thesis; for doctorate, thesis/dissertation. *Application deadline:* For fall admission, 1/15 for domestic students; for spring admission, 10/15 for domestic students. *Expenses: Tuition:* Full-time $43,970; part-time $1374 per credit hour. *Required fees:* $60 per semester. Tuition and fees vary according to class time, course level and program. *Unit head:* Dr. Mark Moss, Chairman, 617-638-4200, Fax: 617-638-4216. *Application contact:* Patricia Jones, Financial Coordinator, 617-414-2315, E-mail: psterlin@bu.edu.
Website: http://www.bumc.bu.edu/anatneuro/

Brandeis University, Graduate School of Arts and Sciences, Program in Molecular and Cell Biology, Waltham, MA 02454-9110. Offers genetics (PhD); microbiology (PhD); molecular and cell biology (MS, PhD); molecular biology (PhD); neurobiology (PhD); quantitative biology (PhD). Terminal master's awarded for partial completion of doctoral program. *Degree requirements:* For master's, thesis or alternative, research project, research lab, or project lab; for doctorate, comprehensive exam, thesis/dissertation, journal clubs; research seminar; colloquia; qualifying exam. *Entrance requirements:* For master's, GRE General Test (or MCAT for applicants to the MS program), official transcript(s), resume, 3 letters of recommendation, statement of purpose; for doctorate, GRE General Test, official transcript(s), resume, 3 letters of recommendation, statement of purpose. Additional exam requirements/recommendations for international students: Required—TOEFL (minimum score 600 paper-based; 100 iBT), PTE (minimum score 68); Recommended—IELTS (minimum score 7). Electronic applications accepted. *Faculty research:* Structural biology; immunology; developmental biology; behavior and neurobiology; DNA replication, rearrangement, and repair; signal transduction, transcriptional regulation, and RNA processing; cancer and programmed cell death; cytoskeleton and molecular motors; nutrition.

California Institute of Technology, Division of Biology, Program in Neurobiology, Pasadena, CA 91125-0001. Offers PhD. *Degree requirements:* For doctorate, thesis/dissertation, qualifying exam. *Entrance requirements:* For doctorate, GRE General Test.

Carnegie Mellon University, Mellon College of Science, Department of Biological Sciences, Pittsburgh, PA 15213-3891. Offers biochemistry (PhD); biophysics (PhD); cell and developmental biology (PhD); computational biology (MS, PhD); genetics (PhD); molecular biology (PhD); neuroscience (PhD); structural biology (PhD). *Degree requirements:* For doctorate, comprehensive exam, thesis/dissertation. *Entrance requirements:* For doctorate, GRE General Test, GRE Subject Test, interview. *Application deadline:* Applications are processed on a rolling basis. Application fee: $0. Electronic applications accepted. *Financial support:* Fellowships, research assistantships, teaching assistantships, and traineeships available. *Faculty research:* Genetic structure, function, and regulation; protein structure and function; biological membranes; biological spectroscopy. *Unit head:* John L. Woolford, Acting Department Head, 412-268-3193, E-mail: jw17@andrew.cmu.edu. *Application contact:* Ena Miceli, Graduate Programs Manager, 412-268-33012, E-mail: emiceli@andrew.cmu.edu.
Website: http://www.bio.cmu.edu/

Case Western Reserve University, School of Medicine and School of Graduate Studies, Graduate Programs in Medicine, Department of Neurosciences, Cleveland, OH 44106. Offers neurobiology (PhD); neuroscience (PhD); MD/PhD. *Degree requirements:* For doctorate, thesis/dissertation. *Entrance requirements:* For doctorate, GRE General Test, 3 letters of recommendation. Additional exam requirements/recommendations for international students: Required—TOEFL. Electronic applications accepted. *Faculty research:* Neurotropic factors, synapse formation, regeneration, determination of cell fate, cellular neuroscience.

Columbia University, College of Physicians and Surgeons, Program in Neurobiology and Behavior, New York, NY 10032. Offers PhD. Only candidates for the PhD are admitted. *Degree requirements:* For doctorate, thesis/dissertation. *Entrance requirements:* For doctorate, GRE General Test. Additional exam requirements/recommendations for international students: Required—TOEFL. *Expenses:* Contact institution. *Faculty research:* Cellular and molecular mechanisms of neural development, neuropathology, neuropharmacology.

Cornell University, Graduate School, Graduate Fields of Agriculture and Life Sciences, Field of Neurobiology and Behavior, Ithaca, NY 14853-0001. Offers behavioral biology (PhD), including behavioral ecology, chemical ecology, ethology, neuroethology, sociobiology; neurobiology (PhD), including cellular and molecular neurobiology, neuroanatomy, neurochemistry, neuropharmacology, neurophysiology, sensory physiology. *Faculty:* 49 full-time (9 women). *Students:* 34 full-time (11 women); includes 6 minority (1 Black or African American, non-Hispanic/Latino; 1 Asian, non-Hispanic/Latino; 3 Hispanic/Latino; 1 Two or more races, non-Hispanic/Latino), 3 international. Average age 28. 92 applicants, 11% accepted, 5 enrolled. In 2013, 3 doctorates awarded. *Degree requirements:* For doctorate, comprehensive exam, thesis/dissertation, 1 year of teaching experience, seminar presentation. *Entrance requirements:* For doctorate, GRE General Test, GRE Subject Test (biology), 3 letters of recommendation. Additional exam requirements/recommendations for international students: Required—TOEFL (minimum score 550 paper-based; 77 iBT). *Application deadline:* For fall admission, 12/1 for domestic students. Application fee: $95. Electronic applications accepted. *Financial support:* In 2013–14, 28 students received support, including 7 fellowships with full tuition reimbursements available, 3 research assistantships with full tuition reimbursements available, 18 teaching assistantships with full tuition reimbursements available; institutionally sponsored loans, scholarships/grants, health care benefits, tuition waivers (full and partial), and unspecified assistantships also available. Financial award applicants required to submit FAFSA. *Faculty research:* Cellular neurobiology and neuropharmacology, integrative neurobiology, social behavior, chemical ecology, neuroethology. *Unit head:* Director of Graduate Studies, 607-254-4340, Fax: 607-254-4340. *Application contact:* Graduate Field Assistant, 607-254-4340, Fax: 607-254-4340, E-mail: nbb_field@cornell.edu.
Website: http://www.gradschool.cornell.edu/fields.php?id-55&a-2

Dalhousie University, Faculty of Graduate Studies and Faculty of Medicine, Graduate Programs in Medicine, Department of Anatomy and Neurobiology, Halifax, NS B3H 4R2, Canada. Offers M Sc, PhD. *Degree requirements:* For master's, thesis; for doctorate, thesis/dissertation. *Entrance requirements:* For master's and doctorate, GRE (recommended), minimum A- average. Additional exam requirements/recommendations for international students: Required—1 of 5 approved tests: TOEFL, IELTS, CANTEST, CAEL, Michigan English Language Assessment Battery. Electronic applications accepted. *Faculty research:* Neuroscience histology, cell biology, neuroendocrinology, evolutionary biology.

Duke University, Graduate School, Department of Evolutionary Anthropology, Durham, NC 27708. Offers cellular and molecular biology (PhD); gross anatomy and physical anthropology (PhD), including comparative morphology of human and non-human primates, primate social behavior, vertebrate paleontology; neuroanatomy (PhD). *Faculty:* 12. *Students:* 16 full-time (9 women); includes 5 minority (2 Black or African American, non-Hispanic/Latino; 1 Asian, non-Hispanic/Latino; 2 Hispanic/Latino). 69 applicants, 6% accepted, 3 enrolled. In 2013, 1 degree awarded. *Median time to degree:* Of those who began their doctoral program in fall 2005, 87% received their degree in 8 years or less. *Degree requirements:* For doctorate, one foreign language, thesis/dissertation. *Entrance requirements:* For doctorate, GRE General Test. Additional exam requirements/recommendations for international students: Required—TOEFL (minimum score 577 paper-based; 90 iBT) or IELTS (minimum score 7). *Application deadline:* For fall admission, 12/8 priority date for domestic and international students. Application fee: $80. Electronic applications accepted. *Financial support:* Fellowships, teaching assistantships, and Federal Work-Study available. Financial award application deadline: 12/31. *Unit head:* Richard Kay, Director of Graduate Studies, 919-684-4124, Fax: 919-684-8542, E-mail: mlsquire@duke.edu. *Application contact:* Elizabeth Hutton, Director of Admissions, 919-684-3913, Fax: 919-684-2277, E-mail: grad-admissions@duke.edu.
Website: http://evolutionaryanthropology.duke.edu/

Duke University, Graduate School, Department of Neurobiology, Durham, NC 27710. Offers PhD. *Faculty:* 45. *Students:* 47 full-time (18 women); includes 15 minority (1 Black or African American, non-Hispanic/Latino; 1 American Indian or Alaska Native, non-Hispanic/Latino; 6 Asian, non-Hispanic/Latino; 7 Hispanic/Latino), 13 international. 167 applicants, 14% accepted, 10 enrolled. In 2013, 3 doctorates awarded. *Degree requirements:* For doctorate, variable foreign language requirement, thesis/dissertation. *Entrance requirements:* For doctorate, GRE General Test. Additional exam requirements/recommendations for international students: Required—TOEFL (minimum score 577 paper-based; 90 iBT) or IELTS (minimum score 7). *Application deadline:* For fall admission, 12/8 priority date for domestic and international students. Application fee: $80. Electronic applications accepted. *Financial support:* Fellowships, research assistantships, teaching assistantships, and Federal Work-Study available. Financial award application deadline: 12/8. *Unit head:* Richard Mooney, Director, 919-681-4243, Fax: 919-684-4431, E-mail: beth.peloquin@duke.edu. *Application contact:* Elizabeth Hutton, Director of Admissions, 919-684-3913, Fax: 919-684-2277, E-mail: grad-admissions@duke.edu.
Website: http://www.neuro.duke.edu/

Georgia State University, College of Arts and Sciences, Department of Biology, Program in Neurobiology and Behavior, Atlanta, GA 30302-3083. Offers bioinformatics (MS); neurobiology and behavior (MS, PhD). Part-time programs available. Terminal master's awarded for partial completion of doctoral program. *Degree requirements:* For master's, comprehensive exam (for some programs), thesis optional; for doctorate, comprehensive exam, thesis/dissertation. *Entrance requirements:* For master's and doctorate, GRE. Additional exam requirements/recommendations for international students: Required—TOEFL (minimum score 550 paper-based; 82 iBT) or IELTS (minimum score 7). *Application deadline:* For fall admission, 7/1 priority date for domestic students, 6/1 priority date for international students; for spring admission, 11/15 priority date for domestic students, 10/15 priority date for international students. Applications are processed on a rolling basis. Application fee: $50. Electronic applications accepted. *Expenses: Tuition, area resident:* Full-time $4176; part-time $348 per credit hour. Tuition, state resident: full-time $14,544; part-time $1212 per credit hour. Tuition, nonresident: full-time $14,544; part-time $1212 per credit hour. Tuition and fees vary according to course load and program. *Financial support:* In 2013–14, fellowships with full tuition reimbursements (averaging $22,000 per year), research assistantships with full tuition reimbursements (averaging $20,000 per year) were awarded. Financial award application deadline: 12/3. *Faculty research:* Behavior, Circadian and Circa-annual rhythms, developmental genetics, neuroendocrinology, cytoskeletal dynamics. *Unit head:* Dr. Vincent Rehder, Professor, 404-413-5307, Fax: 404-413-5301, E-mail: vrehder@gsu.edu. *Application contact:* LaTesha Warren, Graduate Coordinator, 404-413-5314, Fax: 404-413-5301, E-mail: lwarren@gsu.edu.
Website: http://biology.gsu.edu/

Harvard University, Graduate School of Arts and Sciences, Program in Neuroscience, Boston, MA 02115. Offers neurobiology (PhD). *Degree requirements:* For doctorate, thesis/dissertation, qualifying exam. *Entrance requirements:* For doctorate, GRE General Test, GRE Subject Test. Additional exam requirements/recommendations for international students: Required—TOEFL. *Expenses: Tuition:* Full-time $38,888. *Required fees:* $958. Tuition and fees vary according to campus/location, program and student level. *Faculty research:* Relationship between diseases of the nervous system and basic science.

Illinois State University, Graduate School, College of Arts and Sciences, Department of Biological Sciences, Normal, IL 61790-2200. Offers animal behavior (MS); bacteriology (MS); biochemistry (MS); biological sciences (MS); biology (PhD); biophysics (MS); biotechnology (MS); botany (MS, PhD); cell biology (MS); conservation biology (MS); developmental biology (MS); ecology (MS, PhD); entomology (MS); evolutionary biology (MS); genetics (MS, PhD); immunology (MS); microbiology (MS, PhD); molecular biology (MS); molecular genetics (MS); neurobiology (MS); neuroscience (MS); parasitology (MS); physiology (MS, PhD); plant biology (MS); plant molecular biology (MS); plant sciences (MS); structural biology (MS); zoology (MS, PhD). Part-time programs available. *Degree requirements:* For master's, thesis or alternative; for doctorate, variable foreign language requirement, thesis/dissertation, 2 terms of residency. *Entrance requirements:* For master's, GRE General Test, minimum GPA of 2.6 in last 60 hours of course work; for doctorate, GRE General Test. *Faculty research:* Redoc balance and drug development in schistosoma mansoni, control of the growth of listeria monocytogenes at low temperature, regulation of cell expansion and microtubule function by SPRI, CRUI: physiology and fitness consequences of different life history phenotypes.

Indiana University–Purdue University Indianapolis, Indiana University School of Medicine, Stark Neurosciences Research Institute, Indianapolis, IN 46202-2896. Offers PhD. *Students:* 21 full-time (15 women); includes 5 minority (1 Black or African American, non-Hispanic/Latino; 1 Asian, non-Hispanic/Latino; 3 Hispanic/Latino), 7 international. Average age 33. In 2013, 4 doctorates awarded. *Degree requirements:* For

doctorate, thesis/dissertation. *Entrance requirements:* For doctorate, GRE General Test, previous course work in calculus, organic chemistry, and physics. *Application deadline:* For fall admission, 2/1 for domestic students; for spring admission, 9/15 for domestic students. Applications are processed on a rolling basis. Application fee: $55 ($65 for international students). *Financial support:* Fellowships with full tuition reimbursements, research assistantships with full tuition reimbursements, teaching assistantships with full tuition reimbursements, career-related internships or fieldwork, Federal Work-Study, institutionally sponsored loans, scholarships/grants, traineeships, tuition waivers (partial), and unspecified assistantships available. Financial award application deadline: 2/1. *Faculty research:* Neurobiology from molecular level to complex behavioral interactions. *Total annual research expenditures:* $5.3 million. *Unit head:* Dr. Gerry S. Oxford, Executive Director, 317-278-5808. *Application contact:* Director of Admissions, 317-274-3772, E-mail: inmedadm@iupui.edu.
Website: http://snri.iusm.iu.edu/

Louisiana State University Health Sciences Center, School of Graduate Studies in New Orleans, Department of Cell Biology and Anatomy, New Orleans, LA 70112-2223. Offers cell biology and anatomy (MS, PhD), including cell biology, developmental biology, neurobiology and anatomy; MD/PhD. *Degree requirements:* For master's, comprehensive exam, thesis; for doctorate, comprehensive exam, thesis/dissertation. *Entrance requirements:* For master's and doctorate, GRE General Test, GRE Subject Test, minimum undergraduate GPA of 3.0. Additional exam requirements/recommendations for international students: Required—TOEFL. *Faculty research:* Visual system organization, neural development, plasticity of sensory systems, information processing through the nervous system, visuomotor integration.

Loyola University Chicago, Graduate School, Department of Cell Biology, Neurobiology and Anatomy, Chicago, IL 60660. Offers MS, PhD. Part-time programs available. *Faculty:* 16 full-time (6 women), 9 part-time/adjunct (4 women). *Students:* 16 full-time (6 women); includes 3 minority (2 Black or African American, non-Hispanic/Latino; 1 Hispanic/Latino), 1 international. Average age 27. 17 applicants, 24% accepted. In 2013, 1 master's, 6 doctorates awarded. Terminal master's awarded for partial completion of doctoral program. *Degree requirements:* For master's, thesis; for doctorate, comprehensive exam, thesis/dissertation. *Entrance requirements:* For master's, GRE General Test, minimum GPA of 3.0; for doctorate, GRE General Test, GRE Subject Test (biology), minimum GPA of 3.0. Additional exam requirements/recommendations for international students: Required—TOEFL (minimum score 600 paper-based). *Application deadline:* For fall admission, 5/1 priority date for domestic and international students. Applications are processed on a rolling basis. Application fee: $50. Electronic applications accepted. *Expenses: Tuition:* Full-time $16,740; part-time $930 per credit. *Required fees:* $135 per semester. *Financial support:* In 2013–14, 5 fellowships with full tuition reimbursements (averaging $23,000 per year), 5 research assistantships with full tuition reimbursements (averaging $23,000 per year) were awarded; Federal Work-Study and unspecified assistantships also available. Financial award application deadline: 5/1; financial award applicants required to submit FAFSA. *Faculty research:* Brain steroids, immunology, neuroregeneration, cytokines. *Total annual research expenditures:* $1 million. *Unit head:* Dr. Phong Le, Head, 708-216-3603, Fax: 708-216-3913, E-mail: ple@lumc.edu. *Application contact:* Ginny Hayes, Graduate Program Secretary, 708-216-3353, Fax: 708-216-3913, E-mail: vhayes@lumc.edu.

Massachusetts Institute of Technology, School of Science, Department of Biology, Cambridge, MA 02139-4307. Offers biochemistry (PhD); biological oceanography (PhD); biology (PhD); biophysical chemistry and molecular structure (PhD); cell biology (PhD); computational and systems biology (PhD); developmental biology (PhD); genetics (PhD); immunology (PhD); microbiology (PhD); molecular biology (PhD); neurobiology (PhD). *Faculty:* 58 full-time (15 women). *Students:* 261 full-time (133 women); includes 77 minority (3 Black or African American, non-Hispanic/Latino; 1 American Indian or Alaska Native, non-Hispanic/Latino; 32 Asian, non-Hispanic/Latino; 32 Hispanic/Latino; 9 Two or more races, non-Hispanic/Latino), 46 international. Average age 26. 651 applicants, 15% accepted, 39 enrolled. In 2013, 25 doctorates awarded. *Degree requirements:* For doctorate, comprehensive exam, thesis/dissertation, two semesters as a teaching assistant. *Entrance requirements:* For doctorate, GRE General Test. Additional exam requirements/recommendations for international students: Required—TOEFL (minimum score 577 paper-based), IELTS (minimum score 6.5). *Application deadline:* For fall admission, 12/1 for domestic and international students. Application fee: $75. Electronic applications accepted. *Expenses: Tuition:* Full-time $43,210; part-time $670 per credit hour. *Required fees:* $288. *Financial support:* In 2013–14, 252 students received support, including 135 fellowships (averaging $36,800 per year), 122 research assistantships (averaging $35,500 per year), 1 teaching assistantship; Federal Work-Study, institutionally sponsored loans, scholarships/grants, traineeships, health care benefits, and unspecified assistantships also available. *Faculty research:* Cellular, developmental and molecular (plant and animal) biology; biochemistry, bioengineering, biophysics and structural biology; classical and molecular genetics, stem cell and epigenetics; immunology and microbiology; cancer biology, molecular medicine, neurobiology and human disease; computational and systems biology. *Total annual research expenditures:* $44.5 million. *Unit head:* Alan Grossman, Interim Head, 617-253-4701. *Application contact:* Biology Education Office, 617-253-3717, Fax: 617-258-9329, E-mail: gradbio@mit.edu.
Website: https://biology.mit.edu/

New York University, Graduate School of Arts and Science, Department of Biology, New York, NY 10012-1019. Offers biology (PhD); biomedical journalism (MS); cancer and molecular biology (PhD); computational biology (PhD); computers in biological research (MS); developmental genetics (PhD); general biology (MS); immunology and microbiology (PhD); molecular genetics (PhD); neurobiology (PhD); oral biology (MS); plant biology (PhD); recombinant DNA technology (MS); MS/MBA. Part-time programs available. *Faculty:* 24 full-time (5 women). *Students:* 161 full-time (88 women), 28 part-time (15 women); includes 41 minority (5 Black or African American, non-Hispanic/Latino; 23 Asian, non-Hispanic/Latino; 9 Hispanic/Latino; 4 Two or more races, non-Hispanic/Latino), 80 international. Average age 27. 412 applicants, 54% accepted, 65 enrolled. In 2013, 77 master's, 9 doctorates awarded. Terminal master's awarded for partial completion of doctoral program. *Degree requirements:* For master's, thesis or alternative, qualifying paper; for doctorate, comprehensive exam, thesis/dissertation. *Entrance requirements:* For master's and doctorate, GRE General Test. Additional exam requirements/recommendations for international students: Required—TOEFL. *Application deadline:* For fall admission, 12/1 priority date for domestic students, 12/1 for international students. Application fee: $95. *Expenses: Tuition:* Full-time $35,856; part-time $1494 per unit. *Required fees:* $1408; $64 per unit. $473 per term. Tuition and fees vary according to course load and program. *Financial support:* Fellowships with tuition reimbursements, research assistantships with tuition reimbursements, teaching assistantships with tuition reimbursements, career-related internships or fieldwork, Federal Work-Study, institutionally sponsored loans, scholarships/grants, health care benefits, and unspecified assistantships available. Financial award application deadline: 12/1; financial award applicants required to submit FAFSA. *Faculty research:* Genomics, molecular and cell biology, development and molecular genetics, molecular evolution of plants and animals. *Unit head:* Stephen Small, Chair, 212-998-8200, Fax: 212-995-4015, E-mail: biology.admissions@nyu.edu. *Application contact:* Justin Blau, Director of Graduate Studies, PhD Programs, 212-998-8200, Fax: 212-995-4015, E-mail: biology.admissions@nyu.edu.
Website: http://biology.as.nyu.edu/

Northwestern University, The Graduate School, Interdisciplinary Biological Sciences Program (IBiS), Evanston, IL 60208. Offers biochemistry (PhD); bioengineering and biotechnology (PhD); biotechnology (PhD); cell and molecular biology (PhD); developmental and systems biology (PhD); nanotechnology (PhD); neurobiology (PhD); structural biology and biophysics (PhD). *Degree requirements:* For doctorate, thesis/dissertation, qualifying exam. *Entrance requirements:* For doctorate, GRE General Test. Additional exam requirements/recommendations for international students: Required—TOEFL (minimum score 600 paper-based). *Application deadline:* For fall admission, 12/15 for domestic and international students. Applications are processed on a rolling basis. Application fee: $95. Electronic applications accepted. *Financial support:* Fellowships, research assistantships, teaching assistantships, career-related internships or fieldwork, institutionally sponsored loans, scholarships/grants, traineeships, health care benefits, and unspecified assistantships available. Financial award application deadline: 12/31; financial award applicants required to submit FAFSA. *Faculty research:* Biophysics/structural biology, cell/molecular biology, synthetic biology, developmental systems biology, chemical biology/nanotechnology. *Unit head:* Dr. Deborah Klos Dehring, Associate Director, 847-467-0451, E-mail: d-klos@northwestern.edu. *Application contact:* Cathy Prullage, Program Manager, 847-491-4301, E-mail: ibis@northwestern.edu.
Website: http://www.biochem.northwestern.edu/ibis/

Northwestern University, The Graduate School, Judd A. and Marjorie Weinberg College of Arts and Sciences, Department of Neurobiology, Evanston, IL 60208. Offers neurobiology and physiology (MS). Admissions and degrees offered through The Graduate School. Part-time programs available. *Degree requirements:* For master's, thesis. *Entrance requirements:* For master's, GRE General Test and MCAT (strongly recommended). Additional exam requirements/recommendations for international students: Required—TOEFL. Electronic applications accepted. *Expenses:* Contact institution. *Faculty research:* Sensory neurobiology and neuroendocrinology, reproductive biology, vision physiology and psychophysics, cell and developmental biology.

Purdue University, Graduate School, College of Science, Department of Biological Sciences, West Lafayette, IN 47907. Offers biochemistry (PhD); biophysics (PhD); cell and developmental biology (PhD); ecology, evolutionary and population biology (MS, PhD), including ecology, evolutionary biology, population biology; genetics (MS, PhD); microbiology (MS, PhD); molecular biology (PhD); neurobiology (MS, PhD); plant physiology (PhD). *Faculty:* 50 full-time (13 women), 5 part-time/adjunct (1 woman). *Students:* 111 full-time (61 women), 5 part-time (0 women); includes 9 minority (1 Black or African American, non-Hispanic/Latino; 5 Asian, non-Hispanic/Latino; 3 Hispanic/Latino), 62 international. Average age 27. 170 applicants, 19% accepted, 17 enrolled. In 2013, 9 master's, 18 doctorates awarded. Terminal master's awarded for partial completion of doctoral program. *Degree requirements:* For master's, thesis (for some programs); for doctorate, thesis/dissertation, seminars, teaching experience. *Entrance requirements:* For master's, GRE General Test (minimum analytical writing score of 3.5), minimum undergraduate GPA of 3.0; for doctorate, GRE General Test (minimum analytical writing score of 3.5), minimum undergraduate GPA of 3.5. Additional exam requirements/recommendations for international students: Required—TOEFL (minimum score 600 paper-based; 107 iBT for MS, 80 iBT for PhD). *Application deadline:* For fall admission, 12/7 for domestic and international students. Applications are processed on a rolling basis. Application fee: $60 ($75 for international students). Electronic applications accepted. *Financial support:* Fellowships, research assistantships, and teaching assistantships available. Support available to part-time students. Financial award application deadline: 2/15; financial award applicants required to submit FAFSA. *Unit head:* Dr. Richard J. Kuhn, Head, 765-494-4407, E-mail: kuhnr@purdue.edu. *Application contact:* Georgina E. Rupp, Graduate Coordinator, 765-494-8142, Fax: 765-494-0876, E-mail: ruppg@purdue.edu.
Website: http://www.bio.purdue.edu/

Queen's University at Kingston, School of Graduate Studies, Faculty of Health Sciences, Department of Anatomy and Cell Biology, Kingston, ON K7L 3N6, Canada. Offers biology of reproduction (M Sc, PhD); cancer (M Sc, PhD); cardiovascular pathophysiology (M Sc, PhD); cell and molecular biology (M Sc, PhD); drug metabolism (M Sc, PhD); endocrinology (M Sc, PhD); motor control (M Sc, PhD); neural regeneration (M Sc, PhD); neurophysiology (M Sc, PhD). Part-time programs available. *Degree requirements:* For master's, thesis; for doctorate, one foreign language, comprehensive exam, thesis/dissertation. *Entrance requirements:* Additional exam requirements/recommendations for international students: Required—TOEFL. Electronic applications accepted. *Faculty research:* Human kinetics, neuroscience, reproductive biology, cardiovascular.

Université Laval, Faculty of Medicine, Graduate Programs in Medicine, Programs in Neurobiology, Québec, QC G1K 7P4, Canada. Offers M Sc, PhD. Terminal master's awarded for partial completion of doctoral program. *Degree requirements:* For master's, thesis; for doctorate, comprehensive exam, thesis/dissertation. *Entrance requirements:* For master's and doctorate, knowledge of French and English. Electronic applications accepted.

University at Albany, State University of New York, College of Arts and Sciences, Department of Biological Sciences, Specialization in Molecular, Cellular, Developmental, and Neural Biology, Albany, NY 12222-0001. Offers MS, PhD. *Degree requirements:* For master's, one foreign language; for doctorate, one foreign language, thesis/dissertation. *Entrance requirements:* For master's and doctorate, GRE General Test.

The University of Alabama at Birmingham, Graduate Programs in Joint Health Sciences, Program in Neurobiology, Birmingham, AL 35294. Offers PhD. *Degree requirements:* For doctorate, thesis/dissertation. *Entrance requirements:* For doctorate, GRE or MCAT, interview, evaluation forms. Electronic applications accepted.

University of Arkansas for Medical Sciences, Graduate School, Little Rock, AR 72205. Offers biochemistry and molecular biology (MS, PhD); bioinformatics (MS, PhD); cellular physiology and molecular biophysics (MS, PhD); clinical nutrition (MS); interdisciplinary biomedical sciences (MS, PhD, Certificate); interdisciplinary toxicology (MS); microbiology and immunology (PhD); neurobiology and developmental sciences (PhD); pharmacology (PhD); MD/PhD. Bioinformatics programs hosted jointly with the University of Arkansas at Little Rock. Part-time programs available. *Faculty:* 397 full-time (205 women). *Students:* 196 full-time (126 women), 117 part-time (87 women); includes 65 minority (38 Black or African American, non-Hispanic/Latino; 1 American Indian or Alaska Native, non-Hispanic/Latino; 21 Asian, non-Hispanic/Latino; 4 Hispanic/Latino; 1 Two or more races, non-Hispanic/Latino), 57 international. 455 applicants, 27% accepted, 89 enrolled. In 2013, 41 master's, 18 doctorates, 28 other advanced degrees awarded. Terminal master's awarded for partial completion of doctoral program. *Degree requirements:* For master's, comprehensive exam (for some programs), thesis (for some programs); for doctorate, thesis/dissertation. *Entrance requirements:* For master's and doctorate, GRE. Additional exam requirements/recommendations for international

students: Required—TOEFL. *Application deadline:* Applications are processed on a rolling basis. Application fee: $0. Electronic applications accepted. *Expenses:* Contact institution. *Financial support:* In 2013–14, 120 research assistantships (averaging $24,000 per year) were awarded; career-related internships or fieldwork, Federal Work-Study, and traineeships also available. Support available to part-time students. Financial award applicants required to submit FAFSA. *Unit head:* Dr. Robert E. McGehee, Jr., Dean, 501-686-5454. *Application contact:* Dr. Kristen Sterba, Assistant Dean, Office of Graduate Student Recruiting and Retention, 501-526-7396, E-mail: kmsterba@uams.edu.
Website: http://www.uams.edu/gradschool/

University of California, Irvine, School of Biological Sciences, Department of Neurobiology and Behavior, Irvine, CA 92697. Offers biological sciences (MS, PhD); MD/PhD. *Students:* 33 full-time (20 women); includes 7 minority (5 Asian, non-Hispanic/Latino; 2 Hispanic/Latino). Average age 28. In 2013, 1 master's, 12 doctorates awarded. *Degree requirements:* For doctorate, thesis/dissertation. *Entrance requirements:* For master's and doctorate, GRE General Test, GRE Subject Test, minimum GPA of 3.0. Additional exam requirements/recommendations for international students: Required—TOEFL (minimum score 550 paper-based). *Application deadline:* For fall admission, 1/15 priority date for domestic students, 1/15 for international students. Applications are processed on a rolling basis. Application fee: $80 ($100 for international students). Electronic applications accepted. *Financial support:* Fellowships, research assistantships with full tuition reimbursements, teaching assistantships, institutionally sponsored loans, traineeships, health care benefits, and unspecified assistantships available. Financial award application deadline: 3/1; financial award applicants required to submit FAFSA. *Faculty research:* Synaptic processes, neurophysiology, neuroendocrinology, neuroanatomy, molecular neurobiology. *Unit head:* Prof. Frank LaFerla, Chair, 949-824-1232, Fax: 949-824-7356, E-mail: laferla@uci.edu. *Application contact:* Naima Louridi, Student Affairs Officer, 949-824-8519, Fax: 949-824-2447, E-mail: nlouridi@uci.edu.
Website: http://neurobiology.uci.edu/

University of California, Irvine, School of Medicine and School of Biological Sciences, Department of Anatomy and Neurobiology, Irvine, CA 92697. Offers biological sciences (MS, PhD); MD/PhD. *Faculty:* 26 full-time (13 women), 2 part-time/adjunct (1 woman). *Students:* 26 full-time (13 women), 2 part-time (1 woman); includes 10 minority (9 Asian, non-Hispanic/Latino; 1 Hispanic/Latino), 4 international. Average age 27. In 2013, 1 master's, 7 doctorates awarded. *Degree requirements:* For doctorate, thesis/dissertation. *Entrance requirements:* For master's and doctorate, GRE General Test, GRE Subject Test. Additional exam requirements/recommendations for international students: Required—TOEFL (minimum score 550 paper-based). *Application deadline:* For fall admission, 1/15 priority date for domestic students, 1/15 for international students. Applications are processed on a rolling basis. Application fee: $80 ($100 for international students). Electronic applications accepted. *Financial support:* Fellowships, research assistantships with full tuition reimbursements, teaching assistantships, institutionally sponsored loans, traineeships, health care benefits, and unspecified assistantships available. Financial award application deadline: 3/1; financial award applicants required to submit FAFSA. *Faculty research:* Neurotransmitter immunocytochemistry, intracellular physiology, molecular neurobiology, forebrain organization and development, structure and function of sensory and motor systems. *Unit head:* Prof. Ivan Soltesz, Professor and Chair, 949-824-3957, Fax: 949-824-9860, E-mail: isoltesz@uci.edu. *Application contact:* Sara Johnson, Chief Administrative Officer, 949-824-6340, Fax: 949-824-8549, E-mail: sara.johnson@uci.edu.

University of California, Los Angeles, David Geffen School of Medicine and Graduate Division, Graduate Programs in Medicine, Department of Neurobiology, Los Angeles, CA 90095. Offers MS, PhD. Terminal master's awarded for partial completion of doctoral program. *Degree requirements:* For master's, comprehensive exam; for doctorate, thesis/dissertation, oral and written qualifying exams; 2 quarters of teaching experience. *Entrance requirements:* For doctorate, GRE General Test; GRE Subject Test, bachelor's degree; minimum undergraduate GPA of 3.0 (or its equivalent if letter grade system not used). Additional exam requirements/recommendations for international students: Required—TOEFL. Electronic applications accepted.

University of California, Los Angeles, Graduate Division, College of Letters and Science and David Geffen School of Medicine, UCLA ACCESS to Programs in the Molecular, Cellular and Integrative Life Sciences, Los Angeles, CA 90095. Offers biochemistry and molecular biology (PhD); biological chemistry (PhD); cellular and molecular pathology (PhD); human genetics (PhD); microbiology, immunology, and molecular genetics (PhD); molecular biology (PhD); molecular toxicology (PhD); molecular, cellular and integrative physiology (PhD); neurobiology (PhD); oral biology (PhD); physiology (PhD). *Degree requirements:* For doctorate, thesis/dissertation, oral and written qualifying exams. *Entrance requirements:* For doctorate, GRE General Test, bachelor's degree; minimum undergraduate GPA of 3.0 (or its equivalent if letter grade system not used). Additional exam requirements/recommendations for international students: Required—TOEFL. Electronic applications accepted.

University of Chicago, Division of Biological Sciences, Neuroscience Graduate Programs, Committee on Neurobiology, Chicago, IL 60637-1513. Offers PhD. *Degree requirements:* For doctorate, thesis/dissertation, ethics class, 2 teaching assistantships. *Entrance requirements:* For doctorate, GRE General Test. Additional exam requirements/recommendations for international students: Required—TOEFL (minimum score 600 paper-based; 104 iBT), IELTS (minimum score 7). Electronic applications accepted. *Faculty research:* Immunogenetic aspects of neurologic disease.

University of Colorado Boulder, Graduate School, College of Arts and Sciences, Department of Ecology and Evolutionary Biology, Boulder, CO 80309. Offers animal behavior (MA); biology (MA, PhD); environmental biology (MA, PhD); evolutionary biology (MA, PhD); neurobiology (MA); population biology (MA); population genetics (PhD). *Faculty:* 31 full-time (12 women). *Students:* 70 full-time (30 women), 18 part-time (10 women); includes 6 minority (1 Asian, non-Hispanic/Latino; 3 Hispanic/Latino; 2 Two or more races, non-Hispanic/Latino), 5 international. Average age 30. 171 applicants, 6% accepted, 11 enrolled. In 2013, 10 master's, 11 doctorates awarded. Terminal master's awarded for partial completion of doctoral program. *Degree requirements:* For master's, comprehensive exam, thesis or alternative; for doctorate, comprehensive exam, thesis/dissertation. *Entrance requirements:* For master's, GRE General Test, GRE Subject Test, minimum undergraduate GPA of 3.0; for doctorate, GRE General Test, GRE Subject Test. *Application deadline:* For fall admission, 12/31 for domestic students, 12/1 for international students. Application fee: $50 ($60 for international students). Electronic applications accepted. *Financial support:* In 2013–14, 175 students received support, including 35 fellowships (averaging $15,283 per year), 21 research assistantships with full and partial tuition reimbursements available (averaging $29,343 per year), 48 teaching assistantships with full and partial tuition reimbursements available (averaging $31,449 per year); institutionally sponsored loans, scholarships/grants, health care benefits, and unspecified assistantships also available. Financial award applicants required to submit FAFSA. *Faculty research:* Ecology, environmental biology, evolutionary biology, biological sciences, conservation biology. *Total annual research expenditures:* $37.1 million.
Website: http://ebio.colorado.edu

University of Colorado Denver, College of Liberal Arts and Sciences, Department of Integrative Biology, Denver, CO 80217. Offers animal behavior (MS); biology (MS); cell and developmental biology (MS); ecology (MS); evolutionary biology (MS); genetics (MS); integrative and systems biology (PhD); microbiology (MS); molecular biology (MS); neurobiology (MS); plant systematics (MS). Part-time programs available. *Faculty:* 21 full-time (7 women), 3 part-time/adjunct (2 women). *Students:* 18 full-time (11 women), 5 part-time (all women); includes 5 minority (1 Black or African American, non-Hispanic/Latino; 2 Hispanic/Latino; 2 Two or more races, non-Hispanic/Latino), 1 international. Average age 29. 25 applicants, 44% accepted, 11 enrolled. In 2013, 13 master's awarded. *Degree requirements:* For master's, comprehensive exam, thesis, 30-32 credit hours. *Entrance requirements:* For master's, GRE General Test (minimum score in 50th percentile in each section), BA/BS from accredited institution awarded within the last 10 years; minimum undergraduate GPA of 3.0; prerequisite courses: 1 year each of general biology and general chemistry; 1 semester each of general genetics, general ecology, and cell biology; and a structure/function course. Additional exam requirements/recommendations for international students: Required—TOEFL (minimum score 537 paper-based; 75 iBT); Recommended—IELTS (minimum score 6.5). *Application deadline:* For fall admission, 2/1 for domestic and international students. Application fee: $50 ($75 for international students). Electronic applications accepted. *Financial support:* In 2013–14, 8 students received support. Fellowships, research assistantships, teaching assistantships, Federal Work-Study, institutionally sponsored loans, scholarships/grants, and traineeships available. Financial award application deadline: 4/1; financial award applicants required to submit FAFSA. *Faculty research:* Molecular developmental biology; quantitative ecology, biogeography, and population dynamics; environmental signaling and endocrine disruption; speciation, the evolution of reproductive isolation, and hybrid zones; evolutionary, behavioral, and conservation ecology. *Unit head:* Dr. John Swallow, Biology Department Chair, 303-556-6154, E-mail: john.swallow@ucdenver.edu. *Application contact:* Timberley Roane, Associate Professor/Director of MS in Biology Program, 303-556-6592, E-mail: timberley.roane@ucdenver.edu.
Website: http://www.ucdenver.edu/academics/colleges/CLAS/Departments/biology/Programs/MasterofScience/Pages/BiologyMasterOfScience.aspx

University of Connecticut, Graduate School, College of Liberal Arts and Sciences, Department of Physiology and Neurobiology, Storrs, CT 06269-3156. Offers comparative physiology (MS, PhD); endocrinology (MS, PhD), including comparative physiology (MS), neurobiology (MS); neurobiology (MS, PhD). Terminal master's awarded for partial completion of doctoral program. *Degree requirements:* For master's, comprehensive exam; for doctorate, thesis/dissertation. *Entrance requirements:* For master's and doctorate, GRE General Test, GRE Subject Test. Additional exam requirements/recommendations for international students: Required—TOEFL (minimum score 550 paper-based). Electronic applications accepted. *Faculty research:* Adult stem cells and brain repair, neural development and brain disorders, autism, epilepsy and stroke, mental and neurological disorders, multiple sclerosis, obstructive sleep apnea.

See Display on page 455 and Close-Up on page 461.

The University of Iowa, Graduate College, College of Liberal Arts and Sciences, Department of Biology, Iowa City, IA 52242-1324. Offers biology (MS, PhD); cell and developmental biology (MS, PhD); evolution (MS, PhD); genetics (MS, PhD); neurobiology (MS, PhD). Terminal master's awarded for partial completion of doctoral program. *Degree requirements:* For master's, thesis optional, exam; for doctorate, comprehensive exam, thesis/dissertation. *Entrance requirements:* For master's and doctorate, GRE General Test, minimum GPA of 3.0. Additional exam requirements/recommendations for international students: Required—TOEFL (minimum score 600 paper-based; 100 iBT). Electronic applications accepted. *Faculty research:* Neurobiology, evolutionary biology, genetics, cell and developmental biology.

University of Kentucky, Graduate School, Graduate School Programs from the College of Medicine, Department of Anatomy and Neurobiology, Lexington, KY 40506-0032. Offers PhD. *Degree requirements:* For doctorate, comprehensive exam, thesis/dissertation. *Entrance requirements:* For doctorate, GRE General Test, minimum undergraduate GPA of 2.75. Additional exam requirements/recommendations for international students: Required—TOEFL (minimum score 550 paper-based). Electronic applications accepted. *Faculty research:* Neuroendocrinology, developmental neurobiology, neurotrophic substances, neural plasticity and trauma, neurobiology of aging.

University of Louisville, School of Medicine, Department of Anatomical Sciences and Neurobiology, Louisville, KY 40292-0001. Offers MS, PhD, MD/PhD. *Students:* 25 full-time (16 women), 9 part-time (4 women); includes 9 minority (1 Black or African American, non-Hispanic/Latino; 3 Asian, non-Hispanic/Latino; 1 Hispanic/Latino; 4 Two or more races, non-Hispanic/Latino), 8 international. Average age 29. 39 applicants, 31% accepted, 9 enrolled. In 2013, 3 master's, 2 doctorates awarded. Terminal master's awarded for partial completion of doctoral program. *Degree requirements:* For master's, thesis; for doctorate, comprehensive exam, thesis/dissertation. *Entrance requirements:* For master's and doctorate, GRE General Test (minimum score of 1000 verbal and quantitative), minimum GPA of 3.0. Additional exam requirements/recommendations for international students: Required—TOEFL. *Application deadline:* For fall admission, 1/15 priority date for domestic students; for spring admission, 4/15 priority date for domestic and international students. Applications are processed on a rolling basis. Application fee: $60. Electronic applications accepted. *Expenses:* Tuition, state resident: full-time $10,788; part-time $599 per credit hour. Tuition, nonresident: full-time $22,446; part-time $1247 per credit hour. *Required fees:* $196. Tuition and fees vary according to program and reciprocity agreements. *Financial support:* Fellowships with full tuition reimbursements, research assistantships with full tuition reimbursements, health care benefits, and unspecified assistantships available. Financial award application deadline: 4/15. *Faculty research:* Human adult neural stem cells, development and plasticity of the nervous system, organization of the dorsal thalamus, electrophysiology/neuroanatomy of central neurons mediating control of reproductive and pelvic organs, normal neural mechanisms and plasticity following injury and/or chronic pain, differentiation and regeneration of motor neurons and oligodendrocytes. *Total annual research expenditures:* $4 million. *Unit head:* Dr. Fred J. Roisen, Chair, 502-852-5165, Fax: 502-852-6228, E-mail: fjrois01@gwise.louisville.edu. *Application contact:* Dr. Charles Hubscher, Director of Graduate Studies, 502-852-3058, Fax: 502-852-6228, E-mail: chhub01@louisville.edu.

The University of Manchester, Faculty of Life Sciences, Manchester, United Kingdom. Offers adaptive organismal biology (M Phil, PhD); animal biology (M Phil, PhD); biochemistry (M Phil, PhD); bioinformatics (M Phil, PhD); biomolecular sciences (M Phil, PhD); biotechnology (M Phil, PhD); cell biology (M Phil, PhD); cell matrix research (M Phil, PhD); channels and transporters (M Phil, PhD); developmental biology (M Phil, PhD); Egyptology (M Phil, PhD); environmental biology (M Phil, PhD); evolutionary biology (M Phil, PhD); gene expression (M Phil, PhD); genetics (M Phil, PhD); history of science, technology and medicine (M Phil, PhD); immunology (M Phil, PhD); integrative neurobiology and behavior (M Phil, PhD); membrane trafficking (M Phil, PhD); microbiology (M Phil, PhD); molecular and cellular neuroscience (M Phil, PhD); molecular biology (M Phil, PhD); molecular cancer studies (M Phil, PhD); neuroscience (M Phil, PhD); ophthalmology (M Phil, PhD); optometry (M Phil, PhD); organelle function

(M Phil, PhD); pharmacology (M Phil, PhD); physiology (M Phil, PhD); plant sciences (M Phil, PhD); stem cell research (M Phil, PhD); structural biology (M Phil, PhD); systems neuroscience (M Phil, PhD); toxicology (M Phil, PhD).

University of Maryland, Baltimore, Graduate School, Graduate Program in Life Sciences, Program in Neuroscience, Baltimore, MD 21201. Offers PhD, MD/PhD. Part-time programs available. *Students:* 48 full-time (25 women), 5 part-time (2 women); includes 10 minority (1 Black or African American, non-Hispanic/Latino; 5 Asian, non-Hispanic/Latino; 2 Hispanic/Latino; 2 Two or more races, non-Hispanic/Latino), 3 international. Average age 27. 85 applicants, 9% accepted, 7 enrolled. In 2013, 9 doctorates awarded. *Degree requirements:* For doctorate, comprehensive exam, thesis/dissertation. *Entrance requirements:* For doctorate, GRE General Test, minimum GPA of 3.0. Additional exam requirements/recommendations for international students: Required—TOEFL (minimum score 550 paper-based; 80 iBT); Recommended—IELTS (minimum score 7). *Application deadline:* For fall admission, 12/1 for domestic students, 1/15 for international students. Application fee: $75. Electronic applications accepted. *Financial support:* In 2013–14, research assistantships with partial tuition reimbursements (averaging $25,000 per year) were awarded; fellowships, health care benefits, and unspecified assistantships also available. Financial award application deadline: 3/1; financial award applicants required to submit FAFSA. *Faculty research:* Molecular, biochemical, and cellular pharmacology; membrane biophysics; synaptology; developmental neurobiology. *Unit head:* Dr. Jessica Mong, Director, 410-706-4295, E-mail: jmong@umaryland.edu. *Application contact:* Rachael Holms, Coordinator, 410-706-4701, Fax: 410-706-4724, E-mail: neurosci@umaryland.edu.
Website: http://neuroscience.umaryland.edu

University of Minnesota, Twin Cities Campus, Graduate School, Graduate Program in Neuroscience, Minneapolis, MN 55455-0213. Offers MS, PhD. Terminal master's awarded for partial completion of doctoral program. *Degree requirements:* For master's, thesis; for doctorate, thesis/dissertation. *Entrance requirements:* For doctorate, GRE. Additional exam requirements/recommendations for international students: Required—TOEFL. Electronic applications accepted. *Faculty research:* Cellular and molecular neuroscience, behavioral neuroscience, developmental neuroscience, neurodegenerative diseases, pain, addiction, motor control.

University of Missouri, Graduate School, College of Arts and Science, Division of Biological Sciences, Columbia, MO 65211. Offers evolutionary biology and ecology (MA, PhD); genetic, cellular and developmental biology (MA, PhD); neurobiology and behavior (MA, PhD). *Faculty:* 40 full-time (11 women), 1 part-time/adjunct (0 women). *Students:* 70 full-time (32 women), 3 part-time (2 women); includes 12 minority (4 Black or African American, non-Hispanic/Latino; 1 American Indian or Alaska Native, non-Hispanic/Latino; 2 Asian, non-Hispanic/Latino; 3 Hispanic/Latino; 2 Two or more races, non-Hispanic/Latino), 5 international. Average age 28. 46 applicants, 28% accepted, 13 enrolled. In 2013, 7 master's, 13 doctorates awarded. Terminal master's awarded for partial completion of doctoral program. *Degree requirements:* For master's, thesis; for doctorate, comprehensive exam, thesis/dissertation. *Entrance requirements:* For master's and doctorate, GRE General Test (minimum score 1200 verbal and quantitative), minimum GPA of 3.0. Additional exam requirements/recommendations for international students: Required—TOEFL (minimum score 600 paper-based; 100 iBT). *Application deadline:* For fall admission, 12/15 priority date for domestic and international students. Applications are processed on a rolling basis. Application fee: $55 ($75 for international students). Electronic applications accepted. *Financial support:* Fellowships with full tuition reimbursements, research assistantships with full tuition reimbursements, teaching assistantships with full tuition reimbursements, institutionally sponsored loans, traineeships, health care benefits, and unspecified assistantships available. *Faculty research:* Evolutionary biology, ecology and behavior; genetic, cellular, molecular and developmental biology; neurobiology and behavior; plant sciences. *Unit head:* Dr. John C. Walker, Division Director, 573-882-3583, E-mail: walkerj@missouri.edu. *Application contact:* Nila Emerich, Application Contact, 800-553-5698, E-mail: emerichn@missouri.edu.
Website: http://biology.missouri.edu/graduate-studies/

The University of North Carolina at Chapel Hill, School of Medicine and Graduate School, Graduate Programs in Medicine, Curriculum in Neurobiology, Chapel Hill, NC 27599. Offers PhD. *Degree requirements:* For doctorate, comprehensive exam, thesis/dissertation. *Entrance requirements:* For doctorate, GRE General Test, minimum GPA of 3.0. Electronic applications accepted.

University of Oklahoma, College of Arts and Sciences, Department of Biology and School of Aerospace and Mechanical Engineering and Department of Chemistry and Biochemistry, Program in Cellular and Behavioral Neurobiology, Norman, OK 73019. Offers PhD. *Students:* 1 (woman) full-time, 3 part-time (1 woman), 3 international. Average age 28. 2 applicants. *Degree requirements:* For doctorate, comprehensive exam, thesis/dissertation, lab rotations. *Entrance requirements:* For doctorate, GRE, transcripts, 3 letters of recommendation, personal statement. Additional exam requirements/recommendations for international students: Required—TOEFL (minimum score 79 iBT). *Application deadline:* For fall admission, 12/15 for domestic and international students. Application fee: $50 ($100 for international students). Electronic applications accepted. *Expenses:* Tuition, state resident: full-time $4205; part-time $175.20 per credit hour. Tuition, nonresident: full-time $16,205; part-time $675.20 per credit hour. *Required fees:* $2745; $103.85 per credit hour. $126.50 per semester. *Financial support:* In 2013–14, 4 students received support. Scholarships/grants and assistantships (with tuition waivers and health insurance) available. Financial award application deadline: 6/1; financial award applicants required to submit FAFSA. *Faculty research:* Behavioral neurobiology, cellular neurobiology, molecular neurobiology, developmental neurobiology, cell signaling. *Unit head:* Dr. Ari Berkowitz, Director, 405-325-3492, Fax: 405-325-6202, E-mail: cbn@ou.edu. *Application contact:* Dr. Rosemary Knapp, Associate Professor and Director of Graduate Studies, 405-325-4389, Fax: 405-325-6202, E-mail: biologygrad@ou.edu.
Website: http://www.ou.edu/cbn

University of Rochester, School of Medicine and Dentistry, Graduate Programs in Medicine and Dentistry, Department of Neurobiology and Anatomy, Programs in Neurobiology and Anatomy, Rochester, NY 14627. Offers PhD, MD/MS. *Degree requirements:* For doctorate, thesis/dissertation, qualifying exam. *Entrance requirements:* For doctorate, GRE General Test. *Expenses: Tuition:* Full-time $44,580; part-time $1394 per credit hour. *Required fees:* $492.

University of Southern California, Graduate School, Dana and David Dornsife College of Letters, Arts and Sciences, Department of Biological Sciences, Program in Neurobiology, Los Angeles, CA 90089. Offers PhD. M.S. is terminal degree only. Terminal master's awarded for partial completion of doctoral program. *Degree requirements:* For doctorate, comprehensive exam, thesis/dissertation, qualifying examination, dissertation defense. *Entrance requirements:* For doctorate, GRE, 3 letters of recommendation, personal statement, resume, minimum GPA of 3.0. Additional exam requirements/recommendations for international students: Required—TOEFL (minimum score 600 paper-based; 100 iBT). Electronic applications accepted. *Faculty research:* Neural basis of emotion and motivation, learning and memory, cell biology and physiology of neuronal signaling, sensory processing, development and aging.

The University of Texas at Austin, Graduate School, The Institute for Neuroscience, Austin, TX 78712-1111. Offers PhD, MD/PhD. Terminal master's awarded for partial completion of doctoral program. *Degree requirements:* For doctorate, thesis/dissertation. *Entrance requirements:* For doctorate, GRE. Electronic applications accepted. *Faculty research:* Cellular/molecular biology, neurobiology, pharmacology, behavioral neuroscience.

The University of Texas at San Antonio, College of Sciences, Department of Biology, San Antonio, TX 78249-0617. Offers biology (MS); biotechnology (MS); cell and molecular biology (PhD); neurobiology (PhD). *Faculty:* 46 full-time (9 women), 15 part-time/adjunct (10 women). *Students:* 116 full-time (56 women), 62 part-time (34 women); includes 70 minority (7 Black or African American, non-Hispanic/Latino; 1 American Indian or Alaska Native, non-Hispanic/Latino; 10 Asian, non-Hispanic/Latino; 49 Hispanic/Latino; 2 Native Hawaiian or other Pacific Islander, non-Hispanic/Latino; 1 Two or more races, non-Hispanic/Latino), 34 international. Average age 29. 176 applicants, 53% accepted, 43 enrolled. In 2013, 47 master's, 6 doctorates awarded. Terminal master's awarded for partial completion of doctoral program. *Degree requirements:* For master's, comprehensive exam, thesis or alternative; for doctorate, comprehensive exam, thesis/dissertation. *Entrance requirements:* For master's, GRE General Test, bachelor's degree with 18 credit hours in field of study or in another appropriate field of study; for doctorate, GRE General Test, 3 letters of recommendation, statement of purpose, resume. Additional exam requirements/recommendations for international students: Required—TOEFL (minimum score 500 paper-based; 100 iBT), IELTS (minimum score 5). *Application deadline:* For fall admission, 7/1 for domestic students, 4/1 for international students; for spring admission, 11/1 for domestic students, 9/1 for international students. Application fee: $45 ($80 for international students). Electronic applications accepted. *Expenses:* Tuition, state resident: full-time $4671. Tuition, nonresident: full-time $8708. *International tuition:* $17,415 full-time. *Required fees:* $1924.60. Tuition and fees vary according to course load and degree level. *Financial support:* In 2013–14, 42 students received support, including 14 fellowships (averaging $26,142 per year), 19 research assistantships (averaging $24,350 per year), 9 teaching assistantships (averaging $24,350 per year). *Faculty research:* Development of human and veterinary vaccines against a fungal disease, mammalian germ cells and stem cells, dopamine neuron physiology and addiction, plant biochemistry, dendritic computation and synaptic plasticity. *Total annual research expenditures:* $2.1 million. *Unit head:* Dr. Edwin J. Barea-Rodriguez, Chair, 210-458-4511, Fax: 210-458-5658, E-mail: edwin.barea@utsa.edu. *Application contact:* Rene Munguia, Jr., Senior Program Coordinator, 210-458-4642, Fax: 210-458-5658, E-mail: rene.munguia@utsa.edu.
Website: http://bio.utsa.edu/

University of Utah, School of Medicine and Graduate School, Graduate Programs in Medicine, Department of Neurobiology and Anatomy, Salt Lake City, UT 84112-1107. Offers PhD. Part-time programs available. Terminal master's awarded for partial completion of doctoral program. *Degree requirements:* For doctorate, comprehensive exam, thesis/dissertation. *Entrance requirements:* For doctorate, GRE General Test. Additional exam requirements/recommendations for international students: Required—TOEFL. *Expenses:* Tuition, state resident: full-time $5259. Tuition, nonresident: full-time $18,569. *Required fees:* $841. Tuition and fees vary according to course load. *Faculty research:* Neuroscience, neuroanatomy, developmental neurobiology, neurogenetics.

University of Washington, Graduate School, School of Medicine, Graduate Programs in Medicine, Graduate Program in Neurobiology and Behavior, Seattle, WA 98195. Offers PhD. *Degree requirements:* For doctorate, thesis/dissertation. *Entrance requirements:* For doctorate, GRE. Additional exam requirements/recommendations for international students: Required—TOEFL. Electronic applications accepted. *Faculty research:* Motor, sensory systems, neuroplasticity, animal behavior, neuroendocrinology, computational neuroscience.

University of Wisconsin–Madison, School of Medicine and Public Health and Graduate School, Graduate Programs in Medicine, Madison, WI 53705. Offers biomolecular chemistry (MS, PhD); cancer biology (PhD); epidemiology (MS, PhD); genetics and medical genetics (MS, PhD), including genetics (PhD), medical genetics (MS); medical physics (MS, PhD), including health physics (MS), medical physics; microbiology (PhD); molecular and cellular pharmacology (PhD); neuroscience (PhD); pathology and laboratory medicine (PhD); physiology (PhD); population health (MS, PhD), including population health; DPT/MPH; DVM/MPH; MD/MPH; MD/PhD; MPA/MPH; MS/MPH; Pharm D/MPH. Part-time programs available. Postbaccalaureate distance learning degree programs offered (minimal on-campus study). Terminal master's awarded for partial completion of doctoral program. Application fee: $45. Electronic applications accepted. *Expenses:* Contact institution. *Financial support:* Fellowships with full tuition reimbursements, research assistantships with full tuition reimbursements, teaching assistantships with full tuition reimbursements, scholarships/grants, traineeships, and tuition waivers (full) available. *Unit head:* Dr. Richard L. Moss, Senior Associate Dean for Basic Research, Biotechnology and Graduate Studies, 608-265-0523, Fax: 608-265-0522, E-mail: rlmoss@wisc.edu. *Application contact:* Information Contact, 608-262-2433, Fax: 608-262-5134, E-mail: gradadmiss@mail.bascom.wisc.edu.
Website: http://www.med.wisc.edu

Virginia Commonwealth University, Medical College of Virginia-Professional Programs, School of Medicine, School of Medicine Graduate Programs, Department of Anatomy and Neurobiology, Program in Anatomy and Neurobiology, Richmond, VA 23284-9005. Offers PhD. *Accreditation:* APTA. *Degree requirements:* For doctorate, thesis/dissertation. *Entrance requirements:* For doctorate, GRE, MCAT or DAT. Electronic applications accepted.

Wake Forest University, School of Medicine and Graduate School of Arts and Sciences, Graduate Programs in Medicine, Department of Neurobiology and Anatomy, Winston-Salem, NC 27109. Offers PhD, MD/PhD. *Degree requirements:* For doctorate, thesis/dissertation. *Entrance requirements:* For doctorate, GRE General Test. Additional exam requirements/recommendations for international students: Required—TOEFL. Electronic applications accepted. *Faculty research:* Sensory neurobiology, reproductive endocrinology, regulatory processes in cell biology.

Wayne State University, College of Liberal Arts and Sciences, Department of Biological Sciences, Detroit, MI 48202. Offers biological sciences (MA, MS); cell development and neurobiology (PhD); evolution and organismal biology (PhD); molecular biology and biotechnology (PhD); molecular biotechnology (MS). Fall application deadline for PhD is December 1. *Faculty:* 26 full-time (9 women). *Students:* 66 full-time (37 women), 8 part-time (3 women); includes 8 minority (1 Black or African American, non-Hispanic/Latino; 5 Asian, non-Hispanic/Latino; 1 Hispanic/Latino; 1 Two or more races, non-Hispanic/Latino), 41 international. Average age 29. 270 applicants, 14% accepted, 14 enrolled. In 2013, 14 master's, 8 doctorates awarded. Terminal master's awarded for partial completion of doctoral program. *Degree requirements:* For master's, thesis (for some programs); for doctorate, thesis/dissertation. *Entrance requirements:* For master's, GRE (for MS applicants), minimum GPA of 3.0; adequate preparation in biological sciences and supporting courses in chemistry, physics and mathematics; curriculum vitae; for doctorate, GRE, three letters of reference, statement of goals and career objectives, bachelor's or master's degree in biological or other

science. Additional exam requirements/recommendations for international students: Required—TOEFL (minimum score 550 paper-based; 79 iBT), TWE (minimum score 5.5), Michigan English Language Assessment Battery (minimum score 85); Recommended—IELTS (minimum score 6.5). *Application deadline:* For fall admission, 4/1 for domestic students, 3/1 for international students. Applications are processed on a rolling basis. Application fee: $0. Electronic applications accepted. *Expenses:* Tuition, state resident: part-time $554.15 per credit. Tuition, nonresident: part-time $1200.35 per credit. *Required fees:* $42.15 per credit. $268.30 per semester. Tuition and fees vary according to course load and program. *Financial support:* In 2013–14, 55 students received support, including 3 fellowships with tuition reimbursements available (averaging $16,842 per year), 9 research assistantships with tuition reimbursements available (averaging $18,582 per year), 49 teaching assistantships with tuition reimbursements available (averaging $18,488 per year); institutionally sponsored loans, scholarships/grants, health care benefits, and unspecified assistantships also available. Financial award application deadline: 3/31; financial award applicants required to submit FAFSA. *Faculty research:* Transcription and chromatin remodeling, genomic and developmental evolution, community and landscape ecology and environmental degradation, microbiology and virology, cell and neurobiology. *Total annual research expenditures:* $1.7 million. *Unit head:* Dr. David Njus, Professor and Chair, 313-577-2783, Fax: 313-577-6891, E-mail: dnjus@wayne.edu. *Application contact:* Rose Mary Priest, Office Services Clerk, 313-577-6818, Fax: 313-577-6891, E-mail: rpriest@wayne.edu.
Website: http://clasweb.clas.wayne.edu/biology

Wesleyan University, Graduate Studies, Department of Biology, Middletown, CT 06459. Offers cell and developmental genetics (PhD); evolution and ecology (PhD); neurobiology and behavior (PhD). *Degree requirements:* For doctorate, variable foreign language requirement, thesis/dissertation. *Entrance requirements:* For doctorate, GRE. Additional exam requirements/recommendations for international students: Required—TOEFL. *Faculty research:* Microbial population genetics, genetic basis of evolutionary adaptation, genetic regulation of differentiation and pattern formation in &ITdrosophila&RO.

West Virginia University, Eberly College of Arts and Sciences, Department of Biology, Morgantown, WV 26506. Offers cell and molecular biology (MS, PhD); environmental and evolutionary biology (MS, PhD); forensic biology (MS, PhD); genomic biology (MS, PhD); neurobiology (MS, PhD). Terminal master's awarded for partial completion of doctoral program. *Degree requirements:* For master's, thesis, final exam; for doctorate, thesis/dissertation, preliminary and final exams. *Entrance requirements:* For master's, GRE General Test, GRE Subject Test, minimum GPA of 3.0; for doctorate, GRE General Test, minimum GPA of 3.0. Additional exam requirements/recommendations for international students: Required—TOEFL. *Faculty research:* Environmental biology, genetic engineering, developmental biology, global change, biodiversity.

Yale University, Graduate School of Arts and Sciences, Department of Molecular, Cellular, and Developmental Biology, Program in Neurobiology, New Haven, CT 06520. Offers PhD. *Degree requirements:* For doctorate, thesis/dissertation. *Entrance requirements:* For doctorate, GRE General Test, GRE Subject Test.

Yale University, School of Medicine and Graduate School of Arts and Sciences, Combined Program in Biological and Biomedical Sciences (BBS), Department of Neurobiology, New Haven, CT 06520. Offers PhD. *Degree requirements:* For doctorate, thesis/dissertation. *Entrance requirements:* For doctorate, GRE General Test, GRE Subject Test.

Neuroscience

Albany Medical College, Center for Neuropharmacology and Neuroscience, Albany, NY 12208-3479. Offers MS, PhD. Terminal master's awarded for partial completion of doctoral program. *Degree requirements:* For master's, thesis; for doctorate, comprehensive exam, thesis/dissertation. *Entrance requirements:* For master's, GRE General Test, all transcripts, letters of recommendation; for doctorate, GRE General Test, letters of recommendation. Additional exam requirements/recommendations for international students: Required—TOEFL. *Faculty research:* Molecular and cellular neuroscience, neuronal development, addiction.

Alliant International University–San Diego, Shirley M. Hufstedler School of Education, Educational Psychology Programs, San Diego, CA 92131-1799. Offers educational psychology (Psy D); pupil personnel services (Credential); school neuropsychology (Certificate); school psychology (MA); school-based mental health (Certificate). Part-time programs available. *Faculty:* 1 full-time (0 women), 14 part-time/adjunct (9 women). *Students:* 20 full-time (19 women), 13 part-time (all women); includes 16 minority (2 Black or African American, non-Hispanic/Latino; 13 Hispanic/Latino; 1 Two or more races, non-Hispanic/Latino), 1 international. Average age 30. 23 applicants, 87% accepted, 15 enrolled. In 2013, 8 master's, 6 doctorates awarded. *Degree requirements:* For doctorate, comprehensive exam, thesis/dissertation, internship. *Entrance requirements:* For master's, minimum GPA of 2.5, letters of recommendation; for doctorate, minimum GPA of 3.0, letters of recommendation. Additional exam requirements/recommendations for international students: Required—TOEFL (minimum score 550 paper-based; 80 iBT), TWE (minimum score 5). *Application deadline:* For fall admission, 4/15 priority date for domestic and international students; for spring admission, 11/3 priority date for domestic and international students. Applications are processed on a rolling basis. Application fee: $65. Electronic applications accepted. *Financial support:* Career-related internships or fieldwork, Federal Work-Study, institutionally sponsored loans, and scholarships/grants available. Financial award application deadline: 2/15; financial award applicants required to submit FAFSA. *Faculty research:* School-based mental health, pupil personnel services, childhood mood, school-based assessment. *Unit head:* Dr. Steve Fisher, Program Director, 828-635-4825, Fax: 858-635-4739, E-mail: admissions@alliant.edu. *Application contact:* Alliant International University Central Contact Center, 866-U-ALLIANT, Fax: 858-635-4555, E-mail: admissions@alliant.edu.
Website: http://www.alliant.edu/hsoe

American University, College of Arts and Sciences, Washington, DC 20016-8012. Offers addiction and addictive behavior (Certificate); anthropology (PhD); applied microeconomics (Certificate); applied statistics (Certificate); art history (MA); arts management (MA, Certificate); Asian studies (Certificate); audio production (Certificate); audio technology (MA); behavior, cognition, and neuroscience (PhD); bilingual education (MA, Certificate); biology (MA, MS); chemistry (MS); clinical psychology (PhD); computer science (MS, Certificate); creative writing (MFA); curriculum and instruction (M Ed, Certificate); economics (MA, PhD); environmental assessment (Certificate); environmental science (MS); ethics, peace, and global affairs (MA); gender analysis in economics (Certificate); health promotion management (MS); history (MA, PhD); international arts management (Certificate); international economic relations (Certificate); international economics (MA); international training and education (MA); literature (MA); mathematics (MA); North American studies (Certificate); nutrition education (MS, Certificate); philosophy (MA); professional science: biotechnology (MS); professional science: environmental assessment (MS); professional science: quantitative analysis (MS); psychobiology of healing (Certificate); psychology (MA); psychology: general (PhD); public anthropology (MA, Certificate); public sociology (Certificate); social research (Certificate); sociology (MA); Spanish: Latin American studies (MA); special education: learning disabilities (MA); statistics (MS); studio art (MFA); teaching (MAT); teaching English as a foreign language (MA); teaching: early childhood (Certificate); teaching: elementary (Certificate); teaching: ESOL (Certificate); teaching: secondary (Certificate); technology in arts management (Certificate); TESOL (MA); translation: French (Certificate); translation: Russian (Certificate); translation: Spanish (Certificate); women's, gender, and sexuality studies (Certificate). Part-time and evening/weekend programs available. Postbaccalaureate distance learning degree programs offered (no on-campus study). *Faculty:* 358 full-time (187 women), 254 part-time/adjunct (127 women). *Students:* 627 full-time (411 women), 416 part-time (300 women); includes 206 minority (91 Black or African American, non-Hispanic/Latino; 5 American Indian or Alaska Native, non-Hispanic/Latino; 32 Asian, non-Hispanic/Latino; 64 Hispanic/Latino; 1 Native Hawaiian or other Pacific Islander, non-Hispanic/Latino; 13 Two or more races, non-Hispanic/Latino), 124 international. Average age 29. 1,672 applicants, 52% accepted, 361 enrolled. In 2013, 382 master's, 38 doctorates, 33 other advanced degrees awarded. Terminal master's awarded for partial completion of doctoral program. *Degree requirements:* For master's, comprehensive exam (for some programs), thesis (for some programs); for doctorate, comprehensive exam (for some programs), thesis/dissertation. *Entrance requirements:* For master's, GRE, minimum GPA of 3.0 in last 60 credit hours, letter of recommendation, statement of purpose, resume, unofficial transcript; for doctorate, GRE, minimum GPA of 3.0 for all graduate work, letter of recommendation, statement of purpose, resume, unofficial transcript. Additional exam requirements/recommendations for international students: Required—TOEFL (minimum score 600 paper-based; 100 iBT), IELTS (minimum score 7). *Application deadline:* For fall admission, 2/1 for domestic students; for spring admission, 10/1 for domestic students. Applications are processed on a rolling basis. Application fee: $55. Electronic applications accepted. *Expenses: Tuition:* Full-time $25,920; part-time $1482 per credit hour. *Required fees:* $430. Tuition and fees vary according to course load and program. *Financial support:* Fellowships, research assistantships with full and partial tuition reimbursements, teaching assistantships with full and partial tuition reimbursements, career-related internships or fieldwork, Federal Work-Study, institutionally sponsored loans, scholarships/grants, traineeships, tuition waivers (full and partial), and unspecified assistantships available. Support available to part-time students. Financial award applicants required to submit FAFSA. *Unit head:* Dr. Peter Starr, Dean, 202-885-2446, Fax: 202-885-2429, E-mail: pstarr@american.edu. *Application contact:* Kathleen Clowery, Associate Director, Graduate Enrollment Management, 202-885-3621, Fax: 202-885-1505, E-mail: clowery@american.edu.
Website: http://www.american.edu/cas/

American University of Beirut, Graduate Programs, Faculty of Medicine, Beirut, Lebanon. Offers anatomy, cell biology and human morphology (MS); biochemistry and medical genetics (MS); biomedical sciences (PhD); experimental pathology, immunology and microbiology (MS); medicine (MD); neuroscience (MS); pharmacology and toxicology (MS). Part-time programs available. *Faculty:* 259 full-time (78 women), 93 part-time/adjunct (16 women). *Students:* 364 full-time (165 women), 62 part-time (54 women). Average age 23. In 2013, 18 master's awarded. *Degree requirements:* For master's, one foreign language, comprehensive exam, thesis (for some programs); for doctorate, one foreign language, comprehensive exam, thesis/dissertation. *Entrance requirements:* For master's, letter of recommendation; for doctorate, MCAT, bachelor's degree. Additional exam requirements/recommendations for international students: Required—TOEFL (minimum score 600 paper-based; 100 iBT), IELTS (minimum score 7.5). *Application deadline:* For fall admission, 4/30 for domestic and international students; for spring admission, 11/1 for domestic and international students. Application fee: $50. *Expenses: Tuition:* Full-time $14,724; part-time $818 per credit. *Required fees:* $692. Tuition and fees vary according to course load and program. *Financial support:* In 2013–14, 242 students received support, including 60 teaching assistantships (averaging $4,000 per year); career-related internships or fieldwork, institutionally sponsored loans, scholarships/grants, health care benefits, and unspecified assistantships also available. Financial award application deadline: 2/2. *Faculty research:* Cancer research (targeted therapy, mechanisms of leukemogenesis, tumor cell extravasation and metastasis, cancer stem cells), stem cell research (regenerative medicine, drug discovery), genetic research (neurogenetics, hereditary cardiomyopathy, hemoglobinopathies, pharmacogenomics, proteomics), neuroscience research (pain, neurodegenerative disorder), metabolism (inflammation and metabolism, metabolic disorder, diabetes mellitus), vascular and renal biology, signal transduction. *Total annual research expenditures:* $2.6 million. *Unit head:* Dr. Mohamed Sayegh, Dean, 961-1350000 Ext. 4700, Fax: 961-1744464, E-mail: msayegh@aub.edu.lb. *Application contact:* Dr. Salim Kanaan, Director, Admissions Office, 961-1-350000 Ext. 2594, Fax: 96-1-1750775, E-mail: sk00@aub.edu.lb.
Website: http://www.aub.edu.lb/fm/fm_home/Pages/index.aspx

Argosy University, Chicago, College of Psychology and Behavioral Sciences, Doctoral Program in Clinical Psychology, Chicago, IL 60601. Offers child and adolescent psychology (Psy D); client-centered and experiential psychotherapies (Psy D); diversity and multicultural psychology (Psy D); family psychology (Psy D); forensic psychology (Psy D); health psychology (Psy D); neuropsychology (Psy D); organizational consulting (Psy D); psychoanalytic psychology (Psy D); psychology and spirituality (Psy D). *Accreditation:* APA.

Argosy University, Phoenix, College of Psychology and Behavioral Sciences, Program in Clinical Psychology, Phoenix, AZ 85021. Offers clinical psychology (MA); neuropsychology (Psy D); sports-exercise psychology (Psy D). *Accreditation:* APA (one or more programs are accredited).

Argosy University, Phoenix, College of Psychology and Behavioral Sciences, Program in Neuropsychology, Phoenix, AZ 85021. Offers Psy D.

Argosy University, Schaumburg, College of Psychology and Behavioral Sciences, Schaumburg, IL 60173-5403. Offers clinical health psychology (Post-Graduate

Certificate); clinical psychology (MA, Psy D), including child and family psychology (Psy D), clinical health psychology (Psy D), diversity and multicultural psychology (Psy D), forensic psychology (Psy D), neuropsychology (Psy D); community counseling (MA); counseling psychology (Ed D), including counselor education and supervision; counselor education and supervision (Ed D); forensic psychology (Post-Graduate Certificate); industrial organizational psychology (MA). *Accreditation:* ACA; APA.

Argosy University, Tampa, College of Psychology and Behavioral Sciences, Program in Clinical Psychology, Tampa, FL 33607. Offers clinical psychology (MA, Psy D), including child and adolescent psychology (Psy D), geropsychology (Psy D), marriage/couples and family therapy (Psy D), neuropsychology (Psy D). *Accreditation:* APA.

Arizona State University at the Tempe campus, College of Liberal Arts and Sciences, Department of Psychology, Tempe, AZ 85287-1104. Offers behavioral neuroscience (PhD); clinical psychology (PhD); cognition, action and perception (PhD); developmental psychology (PhD); quantitative psychology (PhD); social psychology (PhD). *Accreditation:* APA. *Degree requirements:* For doctorate, comprehensive exam, thesis/dissertation, interactive Program of Study (iPOS) submitted before completing 50 percent of required credit hours. *Entrance requirements:* For doctorate, GRE General Test, GRE Subject Test, minimum GPA of 3.0 or equivalent in last 2 years of work leading to bachelor's degree. Additional exam requirements/recommendations for international students: Required—TOEFL (minimum score 80 iBT), TOEFL, IELTS, or PTE. Electronic applications accepted.

Arizona State University at the Tempe campus, College of Liberal Arts and Sciences, School of Life Sciences, Tempe, AZ 85287-4601. Offers animal behavior (PhD); applied ethics (biomedical and health ethics) (MA); biological design (PhD); biology (MS, PhD); biology (biology and society) (MS, PhD); environmental life sciences (PhD); evolutionary biology (PhD); human and social dimensions of science and technology (PhD); microbiology (PhD); molecular and cellular biology (PhD); neuroscience (PhD); philosophy (history and philosophy of science) (MA); sustainability (PhD). Terminal master's awarded for partial completion of doctoral program. *Degree requirements:* For master's, thesis (for some programs), interactive Program of Study (iPOS) submitted before completing 50 percent of required credit hours; for doctorate, variable foreign language requirement, comprehensive exam, thesis/dissertation, interactive Program of Study (iPOS) submitted before completing 50 percent of required credit hours. *Entrance requirements:* For master's and doctorate, GRE, minimum GPA of 3.0 or equivalent in last 2 years of work leading to bachelor's degree. Additional exam requirements/recommendations for international students: Required—TOEFL (minimum score 600 paper-based; 100 iBT). Electronic applications accepted.

Arizona State University at the Tempe campus, Graduate College, Interdisciplinary Graduate Program in Neuroscience, Tempe, AZ 85287-1003. Offers PhD. Terminal master's awarded for partial completion of doctoral program. *Degree requirements:* For doctorate, comprehensive exam, thesis/dissertation, All students must submit an interactive Program of Study (iPOS) before completing 50 percent of the credit hours required for their degree program. A student is not eligible to apply for the Foreign Language Examination (if appl), comprehensive exams, dissertation proposal/prospectus or dissertation defense (if appl) without an approved iPOS. *Entrance requirements:* For doctorate, GRE, GPA of 3.0 or better in the last 2 years of work leading to the bachelor's degree, 3 letters of recommendation, statement of research interests and goals, CV or resume, and the completed Interdisciplinary Neuroscience Academic Record form. See program web page for additional information. Additional exam requirements/recommendations for international students: Required—TOEFL (minimum score 550 paper-based; 80 iBT), IELTS (minimum score 6.5). Electronic applications accepted.

Baylor College of Medicine, Graduate School of Biomedical Sciences, Department of Neuroscience, Houston, TX 77030-3498. Offers PhD, MD/PhD. *Degree requirements:* For doctorate, thesis/dissertation, public defense. *Entrance requirements:* For doctorate, GRE General Test, GRE Subject Test (strongly recommended), minimum GPA of 3.0. Additional exam requirements/recommendations for international students: Required—TOEFL. Electronic applications accepted. *Faculty research:* Neurodegenerative, neurodevelopment, neurophysiology, addiction, learning and memory.

Baylor College of Medicine, Graduate School of Biomedical Sciences, Program in Developmental Biology, Houston, TX 77030-3498. Offers PhD, MD/PhD. *Degree requirements:* For doctorate, thesis/dissertation, public defense. *Entrance requirements:* For doctorate, GRE General Test, GRE Subject Test (strongly recommended), minimum GPA of 3.0. Additional exam requirements/recommendations for international students: Required—TOEFL. Electronic applications accepted. *Faculty research:* Stem cells, cancer, neurobiology, organogenesis, genetics of model organisms.

Boston University, School of Medicine, Division of Graduate Medical Sciences, Graduate Program for Neuroscience, Boston, MA 02215. Offers PhD, MD/PhD. *Degree requirements:* For doctorate, thesis/dissertation. *Expenses: Tuition:* Full-time $43,970; part-time $1374 per credit hour. *Required fees:* $60 per semester. Tuition and fees vary according to class time, course level and program. *Unit head:* Dr. Shelley Russek, Director, 617-638-4319, E-mail: srussek@bu.edu. *Application contact:* GMS Admissions Office, 617-638-5255, Fax: 617-638-5740, E-mail: natashah@bu.edu.
Website: http://www.bu.edu/neuro/graduate/

Boston University, School of Medicine, Division of Graduate Medical Sciences, Program in Behavioral Neuroscience, Boston, MA 02215. Offers PhD, MD/PhD. Part-time programs available. *Degree requirements:* For doctorate, thesis/dissertation. *Application deadline:* For fall admission, 1/15 for domestic students; for spring admission, 10/15 for domestic students. *Expenses: Tuition:* Full-time $43,970; part-time $1374 per credit hour. *Required fees:* $60 per semester. Tuition and fees vary according to class time, course level and program. *Financial support:* Federal Work-Study, scholarships/grants, and traineeships available. *Unit head:* Dr. Marlene Oscar Berman, Director, 617-638-4803, Fax: 617-638-4806, E-mail: oscar@bu.edu. *Application contact:* Rose Razzino, Administrative Manager, 617-638-4803.
Website: http://www.bumc.bu.edu/busm-bns/

Brandeis University, Graduate School of Arts and Sciences, Department of Psychology, Waltham, MA 02454-9110. Offers brain, body and behavior (PhD); cognitive neuroscience (PhD); general psychology (MA); social/developmental psychology (PhD). Part-time programs available. Terminal master's awarded for partial completion of doctoral program. *Degree requirements:* For master's, thesis; for doctorate, thesis/dissertation, research reports. *Entrance requirements:* For master's and doctorate, GRE General Test; GRE Subject Test (recommended), 3 letters of recommendation, statement of purpose, transcript(s), resume. Additional exam requirements/recommendations for international students: Required—TOEFL (minimum score 600 paper-based; 100 iBT), PTE (minimum score 68); Recommended—IELTS (minimum score 7). Electronic applications accepted. *Faculty research:* Cognitive neuroscience, social developmental psychology, motor control, visual perception, taste physiology and psychophysics, memory, learning, aging, child development, aggression, emotion, personality and cognition in adulthood and old age, social relations and health, stereotypes, nonverbal communication.

Brandeis University, Graduate School of Arts and Sciences, Program in Neuroscience, Waltham, MA 02454-9110. Offers neuroscience (MS, PhD); quantitative biology (PhD). Terminal master's awarded for partial completion of doctoral program. *Degree requirements:* For master's, thesis optional, research project; for doctorate, comprehensive exam, thesis/dissertation, qualifying exams, teaching experience, journal club, research seminars. *Entrance requirements:* For master's and doctorate, GRE General Test, official transcript(s), statement of purpose, resume, 3 letters of recommendation. Additional exam requirements/recommendations for international students: Required—TOEFL (minimum score 600 paper-based; 100 iBT), PTE (minimum score 68); Recommended—IELTS (minimum score 7). Electronic applications accepted. *Faculty research:* Behavioral neuroscience, cellular and molecular neuroscience, cognitive neuroscience, computational and integrative neuroscience, systems neuroscience.

Brigham Young University, Graduate Studies, College of Family, Home, and Social Sciences, Department of Psychology, Provo, UT 84602. Offers clinical psychology (PhD); general psychology (MS); psychology (PhD), including applied social psychology, behavioral neuroscience. *Accreditation:* APA (one or more programs are accredited). *Faculty:* 31 full-time (6 women). *Students:* 63 full-time (33 women); includes 11 minority (1 Black or African American, non-Hispanic/Latino; 1 American Indian or Alaska Native, non-Hispanic/Latino; 6 Asian, non-Hispanic/Latino; 3 Hispanic/Latino), 3 international. Average age 26. 61 applicants, 25% accepted, 13 enrolled. In 2013, 4 master's, 13 doctorates awarded. *Degree requirements:* For master's, thesis; for doctorate, comprehensive exam, thesis/dissertation, publishable paper. *Entrance requirements:* For master's and doctorate, GRE General Test, minimum GPA of 3.0 in last 60 hours of upper-division course work. Additional exam requirements/recommendations for international students: Required—TOEFL. *Application deadline:* For fall admission, 12/15 for domestic students. Application fee: $50. Electronic applications accepted. *Expenses: Tuition:* Full-time $6130; part-time $340 per credit hour. Tuition and fees vary according to program and student's religious affiliation. *Financial support:* In 2013–14, 43 students received support, including 22 research assistantships with partial tuition reimbursements available (averaging $10,000 per year), 11 teaching assistantships with partial tuition reimbursements available (averaging $10,000 per year); fellowships, career-related internships or fieldwork, scholarships/grants, tuition waivers (partial), and unspecified assistantships also available. Financial award application deadline: 5/31. *Faculty research:* Psychotherapy process, Alzheimer's disease/dementia, psychology and law, health, psychology, developmental. *Total annual research expenditures:* $1 million. *Unit head:* Dr. Dawson Hedges, Chair, 801-422-6357, Fax: 801-422-0602, E-mail: dawson_hedges@byu.edu. *Application contact:* Leesa D. Scott, Coordinator of Student Programs, 801-422-4560, Fax: 801-422-0602, E-mail: leesa_scott@byu.edu.
Website: http://psychology.byu.edu/

Brigham Young University, Graduate Studies, College of Life Sciences, Department of Physiology and Developmental Biology, Provo, UT 84602. Offers neuroscience (MS, PhD); physiology and developmental biology (MS, PhD). Part-time programs available. *Faculty:* 20 full-time (0 women). *Students:* 42 full-time (20 women); includes 12 minority (1 American Indian or Alaska Native, non-Hispanic/Latino; 7 Asian, non-Hispanic/Latino; 3 Hispanic/Latino; 1 Two or more races, non-Hispanic/Latino). Average age 28. 15 applicants, 20% accepted, 2 enrolled. In 2013, 6 master's, 5 doctorates awarded. Terminal master's awarded for partial completion of doctoral program. *Degree requirements:* For master's, thesis, oral exam; for doctorate, comprehensive exam, thesis/dissertation. *Entrance requirements:* For master's, GRE General Test, minimum GPA of 3.0 during previous 2 years; for doctorate, GRE General Test, minimum GPA of 3.0 overall. Additional exam requirements/recommendations for international students: Required—TOEFL (minimum score 580 paper-based; 85 iBT). *Application deadline:* For fall admission, 2/1 priority date for domestic and international students; for winter admission, 9/10 priority date for domestic and international students. Application fee: $50. Electronic applications accepted. *Expenses: Tuition:* Full-time $6130; part-time $340 per credit hour. Tuition and fees vary according to program and student's religious affiliation. *Financial support:* In 2013–14, 41 students received support, including 2 fellowships with partial tuition reimbursements available (averaging $7,100 per year), 20 research assistantships with full tuition reimbursements available (averaging $15,500 per year), 20 teaching assistantships with partial tuition reimbursements available (averaging $14,900 per year); career-related internships or fieldwork, institutionally sponsored loans, scholarships/grants, tuition waivers (full and partial), unspecified assistantships, and tuition awards also available. Financial award application deadline: 2/1. *Faculty research:* Sex differentiation of the brain, exercise physiology, developmental biology, membrane biophysics, neuroscience. *Total annual research expenditures:* $508,299. *Unit head:* Dr. Dixon J. Woodbury, Chair, 801-422-7562, Fax: 801-422-0700, E-mail: dixon_woodbury@byu.edu. *Application contact:* Connie L. Provost, Graduate Secretary, 801-422-3706, Fax: 801-422-0700, E-mail: connie_provost@byu.edu.
Website: http://pdbio.byu.edu

Brock University, Faculty of Graduate Studies, Faculty of Social Sciences, Program in Psychology, St. Catharines, ON L2S 3A1, Canada. Offers behavioral neuroscience (MA, PhD); life span development (MA, PhD); social personality (MA, PhD). Part-time programs available. *Degree requirements:* For master's, thesis; for doctorate, thesis/dissertation. *Entrance requirements:* For master's, GRE, honors degree; for doctorate, GRE, master's degree. Additional exam requirements/recommendations for international students: Required—TOEFL (minimum score 550 paper-based; 80 iBT), IELTS (minimum score 6.5), TWE (minimum score 4). Electronic applications accepted. *Faculty research:* Social personality, behavioral neuroscience, life-span development.

Brown University, Graduate School, Division of Biology and Medicine, Department of Neuroscience, Providence, RI 02912. Offers PhD. *Degree requirements:* For doctorate, thesis/dissertation, preliminary exam. *Entrance requirements:* For doctorate, GRE General Test, GRE Subject Test. Additional exam requirements/recommendations for international students: Required—TOEFL. Electronic applications accepted. *Faculty research:* Neurophysiology, systems neuroscience, membrane biophysics, neuropharmacology, sensory systems.

Brown University, National Institutes of Health Sponsored Programs, Providence, RI 02912. Offers neuroscience (PhD).

California Institute of Technology, Division of Engineering and Applied Science, Option in Computation and Neural Systems, Pasadena, CA 91125-0001. Offers MS, PhD. Terminal master's awarded for partial completion of doctoral program. *Degree requirements:* For doctorate, thesis/dissertation, qualifying exam. *Entrance requirements:* For doctorate, GRE General Test. *Faculty research:* Biological and artificial computational devices, modeling of sensory processes and learning, theory of collective computation.

Carleton University, Faculty of Graduate Studies, Faculty of Arts and Social Sciences, Department of Psychology, Ottawa, ON K1S 5B6, Canada. Offers neuroscience (M Sc); psychology (MA, PhD). Part-time programs available. *Degree requirements:* For master's, thesis; for doctorate, comprehensive exam, thesis/dissertation. *Entrance requirements:* For master's, honors degree; for doctorate, GRE, master's degree. Additional exam requirements/recommendations for international students: Required—TOEFL. *Faculty research:* Behavioral neuroscience, social and personality psychology, cognitive/perception, developmental psychology, computer user research and evaluation, forensic psychology, health psychology.

Carnegie Mellon University, Center for the Neural Basis of Cognition, Pittsburgh, PA 15213-3891. Offers PhD. *Application contact:* Information Contact, 412-268-2000.

Case Western Reserve University, School of Medicine and School of Graduate Studies, Graduate Programs in Medicine, Department of Neurosciences, Cleveland, OH 44106. Offers neurobiology (PhD); neuroscience (PhD); MD/PhD. *Degree requirements:* For doctorate, thesis/dissertation. *Entrance requirements:* For doctorate, GRE General Test, 3 letters of recommendation. Additional exam requirements/recommendations for international students: Required—TOEFL. Electronic applications accepted. *Faculty research:* Neurotropic factors, synapse formation, regeneration, determination of cell fate, cellular neuroscience.

Central Michigan University, College of Graduate Studies, College of Humanities and Social and Behavioral Sciences, Department of Psychology, Program in Neuroscience, Mount Pleasant, MI 48859. Offers MS, PhD. *Degree requirements:* For master's, comprehensive exam, thesis or alternative; for doctorate, thesis/dissertation. *Entrance requirements:* For master's and doctorate, GRE. Electronic applications accepted.

College of Staten Island of the City University of New York, Graduate Programs, Program in Neuroscience, Mental Retardation and Developmental Disabilities, Staten Island, NY 10314-6600. Offers MS. Part-time and evening/weekend programs available. *Faculty:* 7 full-time (1 woman), 2 part-time/adjunct (1 woman). *Students:* 35 (22 women). Average age 31. 30 applicants, 53% accepted, 11 enrolled. In 2013, 11 master's awarded. Terminal master's awarded for partial completion of doctoral program. *Degree requirements:* For master's, thesis, oral preliminary exam, thesis defense. *Entrance requirements:* For master's, 3 letters of recommendation; minimum GPA of 3.0 in undergraduate biology, mathematics, psychology or other science courses; interview. Additional exam requirements/recommendations for international students: Required—TOEFL (minimum score 550 paper-based; 79 iBT), IELTS (minimum score 6.5). *Application deadline:* For fall admission, 4/22 priority date for domestic and international students; for spring admission, 11/19 priority date for domestic and international students. Applications are processed on a rolling basis. Application fee: $125. Electronic applications accepted. *Expenses:* Tuition, state resident: full-time $9240; part-time $385 per credit hour. Tuition, nonresident: full-time $17,040; part-time $710 per credit hour. *Required fees:* $428; $128 per term. *Financial support:* In 2013–14, 2 students received support. Career-related internships or fieldwork, Federal Work-Study, and scholarships/grants available. Support available to part-time students. Financial award applicants required to submit FAFSA. *Unit head:* Dr. Alejandra Alonso, Graduate Program Coordinator, 718-982-4153, Fax: 718-982-3953, E-mail: alejandra.alonso@csi.cuny.edu. *Application contact:* Sasha Spence, Assistant Director for Graduate Admissions, 718-982-2019, Fax: 718-982-2500, E-mail: sasha.spence@csi.cuny.edu.
Website: http://www.csi.cuny.edu/catalog/graduate/master-of-science-in-neuroscience-mental-retardation-and-developmental-disabilities-ms.htm

The College of William and Mary, Faculty of Arts and Sciences, Department of Applied Science, Williamsburg, VA 23187-8795. Offers accelerator science (PhD); applied mathematics (PhD); applied mechanics (PhD); applied robotics (PhD); applied science (MS); atmospheric and environmental science (PhD); computational neuroscience (PhD); interface, thin film and surface science (PhD); lasers and optics (PhD); magnetic resonance (PhD); materials science and engineering (PhD); mathematical and computational biology (PhD); medical imaging (PhD); nanotechnology (PhD); neuroscience (PhD); non-destructive evaluation (PhD); polymer chemistry (PhD); remote sensing (PhD). *Faculty:* 11 full-time (2 women). *Students:* 27 full-time (8 women), 4 part-time (2 women); includes 4 minority (2 Black or African American, non-Hispanic/Latino; 2 Asian, non-Hispanic/Latino), 14 international. Average age 28. 40 applicants, 45% accepted, 3 enrolled. In 2013, 4 master's, 8 doctorates awarded. *Median time to degree:* Of those who began their doctoral program in fall 2005, 95% received their degree in 8 years or less. *Degree requirements:* For master's, comprehensive exam, thesis; for doctorate, comprehensive exam, thesis/dissertation, 4 core courses. *Entrance requirements:* For master's and doctorate, GRE General Test, GRE Subject Test. Additional exam requirements/recommendations for international students: Required—TOEFL, TWE. *Application deadline:* For fall admission, 2/3 priority date for domestic students, 2/3 for international students; for spring admission, 10/15 priority date for domestic students, 10/14 for international students. Applications are processed on a rolling basis. Application fee: $45. Electronic applications accepted. *Expenses:* Tuition, state resident: full-time $7120; part-time $405 per credit hour. Tuition, nonresident: full-time $21,639; part-time $1050 per credit hour. *Required fees:* $4764. *Financial support:* Fellowships, research assistantships, teaching assistantships, Federal Work-Study, health care benefits, tuition waivers (full), and unspecified assistantships available. Financial award application deadline: 4/15; financial award applicants required to submit FAFSA. *Faculty research:* Computational biology, non-destructive evaluation, neurophysiology, lasers and optics. *Total annual research expenditures:* $2.3 million. *Unit head:* Dr. Christopher Del Negro, Chair, 757-221-7808, Fax: 757-221-2050, E-mail: cadeln@wm.edu. *Application contact:* Rosario Fox, Graduate Program Coordinator, 757-221-2563, Fax: 757-221-2050, E-mail: rxfoxx@wm.edu.
Website: http://www.wm.edu/as/appliedscience

Colorado State University, Graduate School, Program in Molecular, Cellular and Integrative Neurosciences, Fort Collins, CO 80523-1617. Offers PhD. *Students:* 3 full-time (0 women), 1 international. Average age 26. 30 applicants, 10% accepted, 3 enrolled. *Degree requirements:* For doctorate, comprehensive exam (for some programs), thesis/dissertation (for some programs). *Entrance requirements:* For doctorate, GRE, minimum GPA of 3.0. Additional exam requirements/recommendations for international students: Required—TOEFL (minimum score 630 paper-based; 109 iBT). *Application deadline:* For fall admission, 12/15 priority date for domestic and international students. Application fee: $50. Electronic applications accepted. *Expenses:* Tuition, state resident: full-time $9075.40; part-time $504 per credit. Tuition, nonresident: full-time $22,248; part-time $1236 per credit. *Required fees:* $1819; $60 per credit. *Financial support:* In 2013–14, 2 students received support, including 2 research assistantships with partial tuition reimbursements available (averaging $13,037 per year); fellowships, teaching assistantships with partial tuition reimbursements available, scholarships/grants, health care benefits, and unspecified assistantships also available. Financial award application deadline: 1/1; financial award applicants required to submit FAFSA. *Faculty research:* Ion channels and trafficking, neurotransmission and plasticity cognition and perception, sensory neurobiology, neurodegenerative and prion diseases. *Unit head:* Dr. Kathryn Partin, Professor and Director, 970-491-2263, Fax: 970-491-7907, E-mail: kathy.partin@colostate.edu. *Application contact:* Nancy Graham, Administrative Assistant, 970-491-0425, Fax: 970-491-7907, E-mail: nancy.graham@colostate.edu.
Website: http://mcin.colostate.edu/

Connecticut College, Department of Psychology, New London, CT 06320-4196. Offers behavioral medicine/health psychology (MA); clinical psychology (MA); neuroscience/psychobiology (MA); social/personality psychology (MA). Part-time programs available. *Students:* 4 full-time (1 woman), 3 part-time (2 women); includes 1 minority (Black or African American, non-Hispanic/Latino). Average age 33. 11 applicants, 45% accepted, 3 enrolled. *Degree requirements:* For master's, thesis. *Entrance requirements:* For master's, GRE General Test, statistics course. Additional exam requirements/recommendations for international students: Required—TOEFL (minimum score 600 paper-based). *Application deadline:* For fall admission, 2/1 for domestic and international students. Application fee: $60. *Expenses: Tuition:* Full-time $11,700; part-time $1950 per course. *Financial support:* Tuition remission available. Financial award application deadline: 2/1; financial award applicants required to submit CSS PROFILE or FAFSA. *Unit head:* Dr. Ruth Grahn, Chair, 860-439-2387, Fax: 860-439-5300, E-mail: ruth.grahn@conncoll.edu. *Application contact:* Nancy M. MacLeod, Academic Department Assistant, 860-439-2330, Fax: 860-439-5300, E-mail: nancy.macleod@conncoll.edu.

Dalhousie University, Faculty of Graduate Studies, Neuroscience Institute, Halifax, NS B3H 4H7, Canada. Offers M Sc, PhD. *Degree requirements:* For doctorate, thesis/dissertation. *Entrance requirements:* For master's and doctorate, 4 year honors degree or equivalent, minimum A- average. Additional exam requirements/recommendations for international students: Required—1 of 5 approved tests: TOEFL, IELTS, CANTEST, CAEL, Michigan English Language Assessment Battery. Electronic applications accepted. *Faculty research:* Molecular, cellular, systems, behavioral and clinical neuroscience.

Dalhousie University, Faculty of Science, Department of Psychology, Halifax, NS B3H 4R2, Canada. Offers clinical psychology (PhD); psychology (M Sc, PhD); psychology/neuroscience (M Sc, PhD). *Degree requirements:* For master's, thesis; for doctorate, thesis/dissertation. *Entrance requirements:* For doctorate, GRE General Test. Additional exam requirements/recommendations for international students: Required—TOEFL, IELTS, CANTEST, CAEL, or Michigan English Language Assessment Battery. Electronic applications accepted. *Faculty research:* Physiological psychology, psychology of learning, learning and behavior, forensic clinical health psychology, development perception and cognition.

Dartmouth College, Arts and Sciences Graduate Programs, Department of Psychological and Brain Sciences, Hanover, NH 03755. Offers cognitive neuroscience (PhD); psychology (PhD). *Degree requirements:* For doctorate, thesis/dissertation. *Entrance requirements:* For doctorate, GRE General Test, GRE Subject Test. Additional exam requirements/recommendations for international students: Required—TOEFL. *Faculty research:* Behavioral neuroscience, cognitive neuroscience, cognitive science, social/personality psychology.

Dartmouth College, Arts and Sciences Graduate Programs, Program in Experimental and Molecular Medicine, The Neuroscience Center, Hanover, NH 03755. Offers PhD, MD/PhD. Degrees awarded through participating programs. *Entrance requirements:* Additional exam requirements/recommendations for international students: Required—TOEFL (minimum score 620 paper-based; 105 iBT). Electronic applications accepted.

Dartmouth College, Program in Experimental and Molecular Medicine, Neuroscience Track, Hanover, NH 03755. Offers PhD.

Delaware State University, Graduate Programs, Department of Biological Sciences, Dover, DE 19901-2277. Offers biological sciences (MA, MS); biology education (MS); molecular and cellular neuroscience (MS); neuroscience (PhD). Part-time and evening/weekend programs available. *Degree requirements:* For master's, thesis (for some programs). *Entrance requirements:* For master's, GRE, minimum GPA of 3.0 in major, 2.75 overall. Additional exam requirements/recommendations for international students: Required—TOEFL (minimum score 550 paper-based). Electronic applications accepted. *Faculty research:* Cell biology, immunology, microbiology, genetics, ecology.

Drexel University, College of Arts and Sciences, Department of Psychology, Clinical Psychology Program, Philadelphia, PA 19104-2875. Offers clinical psychology (PhD); forensic psychology (PhD); health psychology (PhD); neuropsychology (PhD). *Accreditation:* APA. Terminal master's awarded for partial completion of doctoral program. *Degree requirements:* For doctorate, thesis/dissertation, qualifying exam. *Entrance requirements:* For doctorate, GRE General Test, GRE Subject Test, minimum GPA of 3.0. Electronic applications accepted. *Expenses:* Contact institution. *Faculty research:* Cognitive behavioral therapy, stress and coping, eating disorders, substance abuse, developmental disabilities.

Drexel University, College of Medicine, Biomedical Graduate Programs, Program in Neuroscience, Philadelphia, PA 19104-2875. Offers MS, PhD, MD/PhD. *Degree requirements:* For doctorate, thesis/dissertation, qualifying exam. *Entrance requirements:* For doctorate, GRE General Test, or MCAT, minimum GPA of 2.75. Additional exam requirements/recommendations for international students: Required—TOEFL. Electronic applications accepted. *Faculty research:* Central monoamine systems, drugs of abuse, anatomy/physiology of sensory systems, neurodegenerative disorders and recovery of function, neuromodulation and synaptic plasticity.

Duke University, Graduate School, Cognitive Neuroscience Admitting Program, Durham, NC 27708. Offers PhD, Certificate. PhD offered through one of the participating departments: Neurobiology, Psychology and Neuroscience, Biomedical Engineering, Computer Science, Evolutionary Anthropology, or Philosophy. *Faculty:* 43. *Students:* 11 full-time (6 women); includes 2 minority (1 Black or African American, non-Hispanic/Latino; 1 Asian, non-Hispanic/Latino), 1 international. 109 applicants, 10% accepted, 5 enrolled. *Degree requirements:* For doctorate, thesis/dissertation. *Entrance requirements:* For doctorate, GRE General Test. Additional exam requirements/recommendations for international students: Required—TOEFL (minimum score 577 paper-based; 90 iBT) or IELTS (minimum score 7). *Application deadline:* For fall admission, 12/8 priority date for domestic and international students. Application fee: $80. Electronic applications accepted. *Financial support:* Fellowships, research assistantships, and teaching assistantships available. Financial award application deadline: 12/8. *Unit head:* Elizabeth Brannon, Director of Graduate Studies, 919-684-3422, Fax: 919-684-3475, E-mail: tanya.schreiber@duke.edu. *Application contact:* Elizabeth Hutton, Director of Admissions, 919-684-3913, Fax: 919-684-2277, E-mail: grad-admissions@duke.edu.
Website: http://dibs.duke.edu/education/graduate/cogneuro-ap

Emory University, Laney Graduate School, Department of Psychology, Atlanta, GA 30322-1100. Offers clinical psychology (PhD); cognition and development (PhD); neuroscience and animal behavior (PhD). *Accreditation:* APA. *Degree requirements:* For doctorate, comprehensive exam, thesis/dissertation. *Entrance requirements:* For doctorate, GRE General Test, minimum GPA of 3.25. Additional exam requirements/recommendations for international students: Required—TOEFL. Electronic applications accepted. *Faculty research:* Neuroscience and animal behavior; adult and child psychopathology, cognition development assessment.

Emory University, Laney Graduate School, Division of Biological and Biomedical Sciences, Program in Neuroscience, Atlanta, GA 30322-1100. Offers PhD. *Degree requirements:* For doctorate, comprehensive exam, thesis/dissertation. *Entrance requirements:* For doctorate, GRE General Test, minimum GPA of 3.0 in science course work (recommended). Additional exam requirements/recommendations for international students: Required—TOEFL. Electronic applications accepted. *Faculty research:* Cell and molecular biology, development, behavior, neurodegenerative disease.

Fielding Graduate University, Graduate Programs, School of Psychology, Santa Barbara, CA 93105-3814. Offers clinical psychology (PhD, Graduate Certificate), including forensic psychology (PhD), health psychology (PhD), neuropsychology (PhD),

parent-infant mental health (PhD), violence prevention and control (PhD); clinical psychology respecialization (Post-Doctoral Certificate); media psychology (MA, PhD), including forensic psychology (PhD); neuropsychology (Post-Doctoral Certificate). *Accreditation:* APA. Postbaccalaureate distance learning degree programs offered (minimal on-campus study). *Faculty:* 30 full-time (17 women), 36 part-time/adjunct (19 women). *Students:* 467 full-time (344 women), 86 part-time (60 women); includes 153 minority (58 Black or African American, non-Hispanic/Latino; 7 American Indian or Alaska Native, non-Hispanic/Latino; 23 Asian, non-Hispanic/Latino; 51 Hispanic/Latino; 14 Two or more races, non-Hispanic/Latino), 2 international. Average age 42. 162 applicants, 60% accepted, 68 enrolled. In 2013, 17 master's, 43 doctorates, 14 other advanced degrees awarded. Terminal master's awarded for partial completion of doctoral program. *Degree requirements:* For master's, thesis or alternative, capstone project; for doctorate, comprehensive exam, thesis/dissertation. *Entrance requirements:* For master's, BA from regionally accredited institution or equivalent, minimum GPA of 2.5; for doctorate, BA or MA from regionally-accredited institution or equivalent, writing sample, minimum GPA of 3.0. *Application deadline:* For fall admission, 2/25 for domestic and international students; for spring admission, 8/25 for domestic and international students. Application fee: $75. Electronic applications accepted. *Expenses:* Contact institution. *Financial support:* In 2013–14, 108 students received support, including 7 teaching assistantships (averaging $1,600 per year); scholarships/grants, health care benefits, and unspecified assistantships also available. Support available to part-time students. *Unit head:* Dr. Mario Borunda, Interim Provost, 805-898-2940, E-mail: mborunda@fielding.edu. *Application contact:* Kathy Wells, Admission Counselor, 800-340-1099 Ext. 4098, Fax: 805-687-9793, E-mail: psyadmissions@fielding.edu.
Website: http://www.fielding.edu/programs/psy/default.aspx

Florida Atlantic University, Charles E. Schmidt College of Science, Center for Complex Systems and Brain Sciences, Boca Raton, FL 33431-0991. Offers PhD. *Faculty:* 5 full-time (1 woman). *Students:* 10 full-time (5 women), 4 part-time (1 woman); includes 3 minority (1 Black or African American, non-Hispanic/Latino; 2 Hispanic/Latino), 2 international. Average age 30. 24 applicants, 17% accepted, 4 enrolled. In 2013, 1 doctorate awarded. *Degree requirements:* For doctorate, thesis/dissertation. *Entrance requirements:* For doctorate, GRE General Test, minimum GPA of 3.0 in last 60 hours of undergraduate course work. Additional exam requirements/recommendations for international students: Required—TOEFL (minimum score 500 paper-based; 61 iBT), IELTS (minimum score 6). *Application deadline:* For fall admission, 1/15 priority date for domestic and international students. Application fee: $30. *Expenses:* Tuition, state resident: full-time $6660; part-time $370 per credit hour. Tuition, nonresident: full-time $18,450; part-time $1025 per credit hour. Tuition and fees vary according to course load. *Financial support:* In 2013–14, 12 students received support. Fellowships with full tuition reimbursements available, research assistantships with partial tuition reimbursements available, teaching assistantships with partial tuition reimbursements available, Federal Work-Study, traineeships, and unspecified assistantships available. *Faculty research:* Motor behavior, speech perception, nonlinear dynamics and fractals, behavioral neuroscience, cellular and molecular neuroscience. *Unit head:* Dr. Janet Blanks, Director, 561-297-2229, Fax: 561-297-3634, E-mail: blanks@ccs.fau.edu. *Application contact:* Rhona Frankel, Associate Director, 561-297-2230, E-mail: frankel@fau.edu.
Website: http://www.ccs.fau.edu/

Florida State University, College of Medicine, Department of Biomedical Sciences, Tallahassee, FL 32306-4300. Offers biomedical sciences (PhD); neuroscience (PhD). *Faculty:* 27 full-time (7 women). *Students:* 34 full-time (20 women); includes 13 minority (2 Black or African American, non-Hispanic/Latino; 7 Asian, non-Hispanic/Latino; 4 Hispanic/Latino), 6 international. Average age 27. 51 applicants, 10% accepted, 5 enrolled. In 2013, 4 doctorates awarded. *Degree requirements:* For doctorate, thesis/dissertation. *Entrance requirements:* For doctorate, GRE. Additional exam requirements/recommendations for international students: Required—TOEFL (minimum score 550 paper-based; 80 iBT). *Application deadline:* For fall admission, 12/15 for domestic and international students. Application fee: $30. *Expenses:* Tuition, state resident: part-time $403.51 per credit hour. Tuition, nonresident: part-time $1004.85 per credit hour. *Required fees:* $75.81 per credit hour. One-time fee: $20 part-time. Tuition and fees vary according to course load, campus/location and student level. *Financial support:* In 2013–14, 34 research assistantships with full tuition reimbursements (averaging $23,000 per year) were awarded. Financial award applicants required to submit FAFSA. *Unit head:* Dr. Richard S. Nowakowski, Professor/Chair, 850-644-7963, Fax: 850-644-5781, E-mail: richard.nowakowski@med.fsu.edu. *Application contact:* Lilly Lewis, Academic Program Specialist, 850-645-6420, Fax: 850-644-5781, E-mail: lilly.lewis@med.fsu.edu.

Florida State University, The Graduate School, College of Arts and Sciences, Department of Psychology, Interdisciplinary Program in Neuroscience, Tallahassee, FL 32306. Offers PhD. *Faculty:* 8 full-time (3 women). *Students:* 23 full-time (11 women); includes 4 minority (1 Black or African American, non-Hispanic/Latino; 1 Asian, non-Hispanic/Latino; 2 Hispanic/Latino). Average age 26. 36 applicants, 17% accepted, 5 enrolled. In 2013, 2 doctorates awarded. *Degree requirements:* For doctorate, thesis/dissertation, preliminary exam. *Entrance requirements:* For doctorate, GRE General Test (suggested minimum GRE score above 60th percentile on both verbal and quantitative sections), minimum GPA of 3.0, research experience, letters of recommendation. Additional exam requirements/recommendations for international students: Required—TOEFL (minimum score 550 paper-based; 80 iBT). *Application deadline:* For fall admission, 12/1 for domestic and international students. Application fee: $30. Electronic applications accepted. *Expenses:* Tuition, state resident: part-time $403.51 per credit hour. Tuition, nonresident: part-time $1004.85 per credit hour. *Required fees:* $75.81 per credit hour. One-time fee: $20 part-time. Tuition and fees vary according to course load, campus/location and student level. *Financial support:* In 2013–14, 23 students received support, including 5 fellowships with full tuition reimbursements available (averaging $22,000 per year), 6 research assistantships with full tuition reimbursements available (averaging $21,500 per year), 12 teaching assistantships with full tuition reimbursements available (averaging $21,500 per year); Federal Work-Study, institutionally sponsored loans, scholarships/grants, traineeships, health care benefits, and unspecified assistantships also available. Financial award application deadline: 12/1; financial award applicants required to submit FAFSA. *Faculty research:* Sensory processes, neural development and plasticity, circadian rhythms, behavioral and molecular genetics, hormonal control of behavior. *Total annual research expenditures:* $3 million. *Unit head:* Dr. Richard Hyson, Director, 850-644-3076, Fax: 850-645-0349, E-mail: hyson@psy.fsu.edu. *Application contact:* Cherie P. Miller, Graduate Program Assistant, 850-644-2499, Fax: 850-644-7739, E-mail: grad-info@psy.fsu.edu.
Website: http://www.neuro.fsu.edu

Gallaudet University, The Graduate School, Washington, DC 20002-3625. Offers ASL/English bilingual early childhood education: birth to 5 (Certificate); audiology (Au D); clinical psychology (PhD); critical studies in the education of deaf learners (PhD); deaf and hard of hearing infants, toddlers, and their families (Certificate); deaf education (Ed S); deaf education: advanced studies (MA); deaf education: special programs (MA); deaf history (Certificate); deaf studies (MA, Certificate); educating deaf students with disabilities (Certificate); education: teacher preparation (MA), including deaf education, early childhood education and deaf education, elementary education and deaf education, secondary education and deaf education; educational neuroscience (PhD); hearing, speech and language sciences (MS, PhD); international development (MA); interpretation (MA, PhD), including combined interpreting practice and research (MA), interpreting research (MA); linguistics (MA, PhD); mental health counseling (MA); peer mentoring (Certificate); public administration (MPA); school counseling (MA); school psychology (Psy S); sign language teaching (MA); social work (MSW); speech-language pathology (MS). Part-time programs available. *Faculty:* 55 full-time (37 women). *Students:* 361 full-time (279 women), 108 part-time (73 women); includes 98 minority (39 Black or African American, non-Hispanic/Latino; 1 American Indian or Alaska Native, non-Hispanic/Latino; 12 Asian, non-Hispanic/Latino; 36 Hispanic/Latino; 1 Native Hawaiian or other Pacific Islander, non-Hispanic/Latino; 9 Two or more races, non-Hispanic/Latino), 31 international. Average age 30. 602 applicants, 49% accepted, 177 enrolled. In 2013, 140 master's, 32 doctorates, 11 other advanced degrees awarded. Terminal master's awarded for partial completion of doctoral program. *Degree requirements:* For master's, comprehensive exam (for some programs), thesis optional; for doctorate, comprehensive exam, thesis/dissertation. *Entrance requirements:* For master's and doctorate, GRE General Test or MAT, letters of recommendation, interviews, goals statement, ASL proficiency interview, written English competency. Additional exam requirements/recommendations for international students: Required—TOEFL. *Application deadline:* For fall admission, 2/15 for domestic students. Applications are processed on a rolling basis. Application fee: $75. Electronic applications accepted. *Expenses: Tuition:* Full-time $14,774; part-time $821 per credit. *Required fees:* $198 per semester. *Financial support:* In 2013–14, 325 students received support. Fellowships, research assistantships, teaching assistantships, career-related internships or fieldwork, Federal Work-Study, scholarships/grants, tuition waivers (partial), and unspecified assistantships available. Support available to part-time students. Financial award applicants required to submit FAFSA. *Faculty research:* Bimodal bilingualism development, cochlear implants, telecommunications access, cancer genetics, linguistics, visual language and visual learning, advancement of avatar and robotics translation, algal productivity and physiology in the Anacostia River. *Unit head:* Dr. Carol J. Erting, Dean, Research, Graduate School, Continuing Studies, and International Programs, 202-651-5520, Fax: 202-651-5027, E-mail: carol.erting@gallaudet.edu. *Application contact:* Wednesday Luria, Coordinator of Prospective Graduate Student Services, 202-651-5400, Fax: 202-651-5295, E-mail: graduate.school@gallaudet.edu.
Website: http://www.gallaudet.edu/x26696.xml

George Mason University, College of Science, Program in Neuroscience, Fairfax, VA 22030. Offers PhD. *Faculty:* 27 full-time (8 women), 1 part-time/adjunct (0 women). *Students:* 21 full-time (10 women), 5 part-time (3 women); includes 5 minority (4 Asian, non-Hispanic/Latino; 1 Hispanic/Latino), 4 international. Average age 33. 20 applicants, 30% accepted, 5 enrolled. In 2013, 3 doctorates awarded. *Degree requirements:* For doctorate, comprehensive exam, thesis/dissertation, at least one publication in a refereed journal (print or press). *Entrance requirements:* For doctorate, GRE, bachelor's degree in related field with minimum GPA of 3.25; expanded goals statement; 2 copies of official transcripts; 3 letters of recommendation. Additional exam requirements/recommendations for international students: Required—TOEFL (minimum score 570 paper-based; 88 iBT), IELTS (minimum score 6.5), PTE. *Application deadline:* For fall admission, 4/15 priority date for domestic students. Application fee: $65 ($80 for international students). Electronic applications accepted. *Expenses:* Tuition, state resident: full-time $9350; part-time $390 per credit. Tuition, nonresident: full-time $25,754; part-time $1073 per credit. *Required fees:* $2688; $112 per credit. *Financial support:* In 2013–14, 21 students received support, including 2 fellowships (averaging $10,667 per year), 18 research assistantships with full and partial tuition reimbursements available (averaging $20,389 per year), 2 teaching assistantships with full and partial tuition reimbursements available (averaging $13,250 per year); career-related internships or fieldwork, Federal Work-Study, scholarships/grants, unspecified assistantships, and health care benefits (for full-time research or teaching assistantship recipients) also available. Support available to part-time students. Financial award application deadline: 3/1; financial award applicants required to submit FAFSA. *Faculty research:* Complexity of the human brain; research in behavior, anatomy, physiology, biochemistry; computational modeling, informatics. *Total annual research expenditures:* $101,075. *Unit head:* James L. Olds, Director and Chief Academic Unit Officer, 703-993-4333, Fax: 703-993-4325, E-mail: jolds@gmu.edu. *Application contact:* Kim (Avrama) L. Blackwell, Director of PhD Program, 703-993-4381, Fax: 703-993-4325, E-mail: avrama@gmu.edu.
Website: http://neuroscience.gmu.edu/

Georgetown University, Graduate School of Arts and Sciences, Programs in Biomedical Sciences, Program in Neuroscience, Washington, DC 20057. Offers PhD, MD/PhD. *Degree requirements:* For doctorate, thesis/dissertation. *Entrance requirements:* For doctorate, GRE General Test. Additional exam requirements/recommendations for international students: Required—TOEFL. *Application deadline:* For fall admission, 1/15 priority date for domestic students. Application fee: $50 ($55 for international students). *Unit head:* Dr. Barbara M. Bayer, Chair, 202-687-0617. *Application contact:* Graduate School Admissions Office, 202-687-5568.

Georgia Regents University, The Graduate School, Program in Neuroscience, Augusta, GA 30912. Offers MS, PhD. *Students:* 15 full-time (7 women); includes 8 minority (7 Asian, non-Hispanic/Latino; 1 Two or more races, non-Hispanic/Latino), 6 international. Average age 27. In 2013, 1 doctorate awarded. *Degree requirements:* For doctorate, comprehensive exam, thesis/dissertation. *Entrance requirements:* For doctorate, GRE General Test. Additional exam requirements/recommendations for international students: Required—TOEFL (minimum score 550 paper-based; 79 iBT). *Application deadline:* For fall admission, 1/15 for domestic and international students. Application fee: $50. Electronic applications accepted. *Financial support:* In 2013–14, 2 students received support, including 13 research assistantships with partial tuition reimbursements available (averaging $23,000 per year); Federal Work-Study also available. Support available to part-time students. Financial award application deadline: 5/31. *Faculty research:* Learning and memory, neuronal migration, synapse formation, regeneration, developmental neurobiology, neurodegeneration and neural repair. *Total annual research expenditures:* $1.2 million. *Unit head:* Dr. Lin Mei, Director of Institute of Molecular Medicine and Genetics, 706-721-8775, Fax: 706-721-7915, E-mail: lmei@georgiahealth.edu. *Application contact:* Dr. Patricia L. Cameron, Acting Vice Dean, 706-721-3279, E-mail: pcameron@georgiahealth.edu.
Website: http://www.gru.edu/mcg/dnrm/neuroscience/

Georgia State University, College of Arts and Sciences, Department of Psychology, Atlanta, GA 30302-3083. Offers clinical (PhD); cognitive sciences (PhD); community (PhD); developmental (PhD); neuropsychology and behavioral neuroscience (PhD). *Accreditation:* APA. *Faculty:* 32 full-time (19 women). *Students:* 102 full-time (86 women), 6 part-time (5 women); includes 30 minority (10 Black or African American, non-Hispanic/Latino; 9 Asian, non-Hispanic/Latino; 5 Hispanic/Latino; 6 Two or more races, non-Hispanic/Latino), 8 international. Average age 28. 531 applicants, 6% accepted, 20 enrolled. In 2013, 17 doctorates awarded. *Degree requirements:* For doctorate, comprehensive exam, thesis/dissertation, residency year (for clinical only). *Entrance requirements:* For doctorate, GRE. Additional exam requirements/

recommendations for international students: Required—TOEFL (minimum score 550 paper-based; 80 iBT). *Application deadline:* For fall admission, 12/1 for domestic and international students. Application fee: $50. Electronic applications accepted. *Expenses: Tuition, area resident:* Full-time $4176; part-time $348 per credit hour. Tuition, state resident: full-time $14,544; part-time $1212 per credit hour. Tuition, nonresident: full-time $14,544; part-time $1212 per credit hour. Tuition and fees vary according to course load and program. *Financial support:* In 2013–14, fellowships with full tuition reimbursements (averaging $19,282 per year), research assistantships with full tuition reimbursements (averaging $5,173 per year), teaching assistantships with full tuition reimbursements (averaging $6,389 per year) were awarded; scholarships/grants, traineeships, health care benefits, and unspecified assistantships also available. *Faculty research:* Clinical psychology, developmental psychology, community psychology, neuropsychology and behavioral neuroscience, cognitive sciences. *Unit head:* Dr. Lisa Armistead, Chair, 404-413-6205, Fax: 404-413-6207, E-mail: lparmistead@gsu.edu. *Application contact:* Dr. Lindsey Cohen, Director of Graduate Studies, 404-413-6263, Fax: 404-413-6207, E-mail: llcohen@gsu.edu.
Website: http://www2.gsu.edu/~wwwpsy/graduate_programs.html

Georgia State University, College of Arts and Sciences, Neuroscience Institute, Atlanta, GA 30302-3083. Offers PhD. *Faculty:* 20 full-time (7 women). *Students:* 40 full-time (23 women); includes 5 minority (1 Black or African American, non-Hispanic/Latino; 1 Asian, non-Hispanic/Latino; 3 Two or more races, non-Hispanic/Latino), 5 international. Average age 28. 71 applicants, 15% accepted, 7 enrolled. In 2013, 3 doctorates awarded. Terminal master's awarded for partial completion of doctoral program. *Degree requirements:* For doctorate, comprehensive exam, thesis/dissertation. *Entrance requirements:* For doctorate, GRE. Additional exam requirements/recommendations for international students: Required—TOEFL. *Application deadline:* For fall admission, 12/10 for domestic and international students. Application fee: $50. Electronic applications accepted. *Expenses: Tuition, area resident:* Full-time $4176; part-time $348 per credit hour. Tuition, state resident: full-time $14,544; part-time $1212 per credit hour. Tuition, nonresident: full-time $14,544; part-time $1212 per credit hour. Tuition and fees vary according to course load and program. *Financial support:* In 2013–14, fellowships (averaging $22,000 per year), research assistantships (averaging $22,000 per year) were awarded. *Faculty research:* Neuroendocrinology; computational neuroscience; brain plasticity; neuromodulation of social behavior; neurobiology of learning and memory, drugs of abuse, and motor and sensory systems. *Unit head:* Prof. Walter Wilczynski, Director, 404-413-6307, E-mail: wwilczynski@gsu.edu. *Application contact:* Dr. Laura L. Carruth, Director of Graduate Studies, 404-413-5340, E-mail: lcarruth@gsu.edu.
Website: http://www.neuroscience.gsu.edu/

The Graduate Center, City University of New York, Graduate Studies, Program in Psychology, New York, NY 10016-4039. Offers basic applied neurocognition (PhD); biopsychology (PhD); clinical psychology (PhD); developmental psychology (PhD); environmental psychology (PhD); experimental psychology (PhD); industrial psychology (PhD); learning processes (PhD); neuropsychology (PhD); psychology (PhD); social personality (PhD). *Degree requirements:* For doctorate, one foreign language, thesis/dissertation. *Entrance requirements:* For doctorate, GRE General Test. Additional exam requirements/recommendations for international students: Required—TOEFL. Electronic applications accepted.

Harvard University, Graduate School of Arts and Sciences, Program in Neuroscience, Boston, MA 02115. Offers neurobiology (PhD). *Degree requirements:* For doctorate, thesis/dissertation, qualifying exam. *Entrance requirements:* For doctorate, GRE General Test, GRE Subject Test. Additional exam requirements/recommendations for international students: Required—TOEFL. *Expenses: Tuition:* Full-time $38,888. *Required fees:* $958. Tuition and fees vary according to campus/location, program and student level. *Faculty research:* Relationship between diseases of the nervous system and basic science.

Icahn School of Medicine at Mount Sinai, Graduate School of Biological Sciences, New York, NY 10029-6504. Offers biomedical sciences (MS, PhD); clinical research education (MS, PhD); community medicine (MPH); genetic counseling (MS); neurosciences (PhD); MD/PhD. Terminal master's awarded for partial completion of doctoral program. *Degree requirements:* For master's, thesis; for doctorate, comprehensive exam, thesis/dissertation. *Entrance requirements:* For master's, GRE General Test; for doctorate, GRE General Test, GRE Subject Test, 3 years of college pre-med course work. Additional exam requirements/recommendations for international students: Required—TOEFL. Electronic applications accepted. *Faculty research:* Cancer, genetics and genomics, immunology, neuroscience, developmental and stem cell biology, translational research.

Illinois State University, Graduate School, College of Arts and Sciences, Department of Biological Sciences, Normal, IL 61790-2200. Offers animal behavior (MS); bacteriology (MS); biochemistry (MS); biological sciences (MS); biology (PhD); biophysics (MS); biotechnology (MS); botany (MS, PhD); cell biology (MS); conservation biology (MS); developmental biology (MS); ecology (MS, PhD); entomology (MS); evolutionary biology (MS); genetics (MS, PhD); immunology (MS); microbiology (MS, PhD); molecular biology (MS); molecular genetics (MS); neurobiology (MS); neuroscience (MS); parasitology (MS); physiology (MS, PhD); plant biology (MS); plant molecular biology (MS); plant sciences (MS); structural biology (MS); zoology (MS, PhD). Part-time programs available. *Degree requirements:* For master's, thesis or alternative; for doctorate, variable foreign language requirement, thesis/dissertation, 2 terms of residency. *Entrance requirements:* For master's, GRE General Test, minimum GPA of 2.6 in last 60 hours of course work; for doctorate, GRE General Test. *Faculty research:* Redoc balance and drug development in schistosoma mansoni, control of the growth of listeria monocytogenes at low temperature, regulation of cell expansion and microtubule function by SPRI, CRUI: physiology and fitness consequences of different life history phenotypes.

Immaculata University, College of Graduate Studies, Department of Psychology, Immaculata, PA 19345. Offers clinical mental health couneling (MA); clinical psychology (Psy D); forensic psychology (Graduate Certificate); integrative psychotherapy (Graduate Certificate); neuropsychology (Graduate Certificate); psychodynamic psychotherapy (Graduate Certificate); psychological testing (Graduate Certificate); school counseling (MA, Graduate Certificate); school psychology (MA). *Accreditation:* APA. Part-time and evening/weekend programs available. Terminal master's awarded for partial completion of doctoral program. *Degree requirements:* For master's, comprehensive exam, thesis optional; for doctorate, comprehensive exam, thesis/dissertation. *Entrance requirements:* For master's, GRE General Test or MAT, minimum GPA of 3.0; for doctorate, GRE General Test or MAT, minimum GPA of 3.5. Additional exam requirements/recommendations for international students: Required—TOEFL, IELTS. *Application deadline:* Applications are processed on a rolling basis. Application fee: $50. Electronic applications accepted. *Expenses: Tuition:* Part-time $660 per credit. Part-time tuition and fees vary according to degree level and program. *Financial support:* Application deadline: 5/1. *Faculty research:* Supervision ethics, psychology of teaching, gender. *Unit head:* Dr. Jed A. Yalof, Chair, 610-647-4400 Ext. 3503, Fax: 610-993-8550, E-mail: jyalof@immaculata.edu. *Application contact:* Office of Graduate Admission, 610-647-4400 Ext. 3211, Fax: 610-993-8550, E-mail: graduate@immaculata.edu.
Website: http://www.immaculata.edu

Indiana University Bloomington, University Graduate School, College of Arts and Sciences, Department of Psychological and Brain Sciences, Bloomington, IN 47405. Offers clinical science (PhD); cognitive neuroscience (PhD); cognitive psychology (PhD); developmental psychology (PhD); methods of behavior (PhD); molecular systems neuroscience (PhD); social psychology (PhD). *Accreditation:* APA. *Faculty:* 54 full-time (15 women). *Students:* 92 full-time (54 women); includes 17 minority (4 Black or African American, non-Hispanic/Latino; 5 Asian, non-Hispanic/Latino; 6 Hispanic/Latino; 2 Two or more races, non-Hispanic/Latino), 17 international. Average age 24. 383 applicants, 8% accepted, 20 enrolled. In 2013, 20 doctorates awarded. *Degree requirements:* For doctorate, comprehensive exam, 90 credit hours, 2 advanced statistics/methods courses, 2 written research projects, the teaching of psychology course, teaching 1 semester of undergraduate methods course, qualifying examination, minor or a second major, first-year research seminar course, dissertation defense, written dissertation. *Entrance requirements:* For doctorate, GRE. Additional exam requirements/recommendations for international students: Required—TOEFL (minimum score 550 paper-based; 79 iBT). *Application deadline:* For fall admission, 12/1 for domestic and international students. Application fee: $55 ($65 for international students). Electronic applications accepted. *Financial support:* In 2013–14, 26 fellowships with full tuition reimbursements (averaging $25,000 per year), research assistantships with full tuition reimbursements (averaging $19,000 per year), teaching assistantships with full tuition reimbursements (averaging $19,000 per year) were awarded; career-related internships or fieldwork, scholarships/grants, traineeships, health care benefits, and unspecified assistantships also available. *Faculty research:* Clinical science, cognitive neuroscience, cognitive psychology, developmental psychology, mechanisms of behavior, molecular and systems neuroscience, social psychology. *Unit head:* Dr. William Hetrick, Chair, 812-855-2012, Fax: 812-855-4691, E-mail: whetrick@indiana.edu. *Application contact:* Dale Sengelaub, Graduate Admissions, 812-855-9149, Fax: 812-855-4691, E-mail: psychgrd@indiana.edu.
Website: http://www.psych.indiana.edu

Indiana University Bloomington, University Graduate School, College of Arts and Sciences, Program in Neuroscience, Bloomington, IN 47405. Offers PhD. *Faculty:* 25 full-time (13 women). *Students:* 14 full-time (6 women); includes 1 minority (Black or African American, non-Hispanic/Latino), 3 international. Average age 28. 50 applicants, 8% accepted, 2 enrolled. In 2013, 5 doctorates awarded. *Degree requirements:* For doctorate, comprehensive exam, thesis/dissertation, qualifying exam. *Entrance requirements:* For doctorate, GRE, bachelor's degree. Additional exam requirements/recommendations for international students: Required—TOEFL (minimum score 200 paper-based). *Application deadline:* For fall admission, 12/1 for domestic and international students. Applications are processed on a rolling basis. Application fee: $55 ($65 for international students). Electronic applications accepted. *Financial support:* In 2013–14, 3 fellowships with full and partial tuition reimbursements (averaging $20,000 per year), 4 teaching assistantships with full and partial tuition reimbursements (averaging $19,474 per year) were awarded. Financial award application deadline: 12/1. *Faculty research:* Cellular and molecular neuroscience, cognitive neuroscience, developmental neuroscience, disorders of the nervous system, sensory and motor processes. *Unit head:* Dr. George V. Rebec, Director of Graduate Studies, 812-855-4832, Fax: 812-855-4520, E-mail: rebec@indiana.edu. *Application contact:* Faye Caylor, Administrative Assistant, 812-855-7756, Fax: 812-855-4520, E-mail: fcaylor@indiana.edu.
Website: http://www.indiana.edu/~neurosci/

Iowa State University of Science and Technology, Program in Neuroscience, Ames, IA 50011. Offers MS, PhD. *Degree requirements:* For master's, thesis; for doctorate, thesis/dissertation. *Entrance requirements:* For master's and doctorate, GRE General Test, resume. Additional exam requirements/recommendations for international students: Required—TOEFL (minimum score 580 paper-based; 85 iBT), IELTS (minimum score 7). Electronic applications accepted. *Faculty research:* Behavioral pharmacology and immunology, developmental neurobiology, neuroendocrinology, neuroregulatory mechanisms at the cellular level, signal transduction in neurons.

Johns Hopkins University, School of Medicine, Graduate Programs in Medicine, Neuroscience Training Program, Baltimore, MD 21218-2699. Offers PhD. *Faculty:* 66 full-time (10 women). *Students:* 90 full-time (50 women); includes 25 minority (4 Black or African American, non-Hispanic/Latino; 13 Asian, non-Hispanic/Latino; 6 Hispanic/Latino; 2 Two or more races, non-Hispanic/Latino), 35 international. Average age 26. 212 applicants, 14% accepted, 13 enrolled. In 2013, 11 doctorates awarded. *Degree requirements:* For doctorate, comprehensive exam, thesis/dissertation, thesis defense. *Entrance requirements:* For doctorate, GRE General Test, bachelor's degree in science or mathematics. Additional exam requirements/recommendations for international students: Required—TOEFL. *Application deadline:* For winter admission, 12/7 for domestic and international students. Application fee: $85. Electronic applications accepted. *Financial support:* Fellowships, scholarships/grants, and tuition waivers (full and partial) available. Financial award application deadline: 1/1. *Faculty research:* Neurophysiology, neurochemistry, neuroanatomy, pharmacology, development. *Total annual research expenditures:* $15.5 million. *Unit head:* Dr. David D. Ginty, Professor and Director of Graduate Studies, 410-614-9494, Fax: 410-614-6249, E-mail: dginty@jhmi.edu. *Application contact:* Rita G. Ragan, Graduate Program Manager, 410-955-7947, Fax: 410-614-6249, E-mail: rgragan@jhmi.edu.
Website: http://www.neuroscience.jhu.edu/

Kent State University, School of Biomedical Sciences, Program in Neuroscience, Kent, OH 44242-0001. Offers MS, PhD. Offered in cooperation with Northeastern Ohio Universities College of Medicine. Terminal master's awarded for partial completion of doctoral program. *Degree requirements:* For master's, thesis; for doctorate, thesis/dissertation. *Entrance requirements:* For master's and doctorate, GRE General Test, minimum GPA of 3.0. Additional exam requirements/recommendations for international students: Required—TOEFL. Electronic applications accepted. *Faculty research:* Plasticity of the nervous system, learning and memory processes–neural correlates, neuroendocrinology of cyclic behavior, synaptic neurochemistry.

Lehigh University, College of Arts and Sciences, Department of Biological Sciences, Bethlehem, PA 18015. Offers biochemistry (PhD); cell and molecular biology (PhD); integrative biology and neuroscience (PhD); molecular biology (MS). Part-time programs available. Postbaccalaureate distance learning degree programs offered (no on-campus study). *Faculty:* 18 full-time (9 women). *Students:* 38 full-time (20 women), 30 part-time (23 women); includes 8 minority (4 Black or African American, non-Hispanic/Latino; 2 Asian, non-Hispanic/Latino; 2 Hispanic/Latino), 5 international. Average age 29. 54 applicants, 41% accepted, 11 enrolled. In 2013, 8 master's, 5 doctorates awarded. Terminal master's awarded for partial completion of doctoral program. *Degree requirements:* For master's, research report; for doctorate, comprehensive exam, thesis/dissertation. *Entrance requirements:* For doctorate, GRE General Test. Additional exam requirements/recommendations for international students: Required—TOEFL. *Application deadline:* For fall admission, 12/15 for domestic and international students. Applications are processed on a rolling basis. Application fee: $75. Electronic

applications accepted. *Financial support:* In 2013–14, 2 fellowships with full tuition reimbursements (averaging $24,500 per year), 8 research assistantships with full tuition reimbursements (averaging $23,750 per year), 20 teaching assistantships with full tuition reimbursements (averaging $23,750 per year) were awarded; scholarships/grants and unspecified assistantships also available. Financial award application deadline: 12/15. *Faculty research:* Gene expression, cytoskeleton and cell structure, cell cycle and growth regulation, neuroscience, animal behavior, microbiology. *Total annual research expenditures:* $1.7 million. *Unit head:* Dr. Murray Itzkowitz, Chairperson, 610-758-3680, Fax: 610-758-4004, E-mail: mi00@lehigh.edu. *Application contact:* Dr. Mary Kathryn Iovine, Graduate Coordinator, 610-758-6981, Fax: 610-758-4004, E-mail: mki3@lehigh.edu.
Website: http://www.lehigh.edu/~inbios/

Louisiana State University Health Sciences Center, School of Graduate Studies in New Orleans, Interdisciplinary Neuroscience Graduate Program, New Orleans, LA 70112-2223. Offers MS, PhD, MD/PhD. *Degree requirements:* For master's, comprehensive exam, thesis; for doctorate, comprehensive exam, thesis/dissertation. *Entrance requirements:* For master's, GRE; for doctorate, GRE General Test, GRE Subject Test, previous course work in chemistry, mathematics, physics, and computer science. Additional exam requirements/recommendations for international students: Required—TOEFL. *Faculty research:* Visual system, second messengers, drugs and behavior, signal transduction, plasticity and development.

Loyola University Chicago, Graduate School, Program in Neuroscience, Maywood, IL 60153. Offers MS, PhD. *Faculty:* 22 full-time (9 women). *Students:* 7 full-time (2 women); includes 1 minority (Asian, non-Hispanic/Latino). Average age 25. 14 applicants, 29% accepted, 1 enrolled. In 2013, 2 master's, 2 doctorates awarded. Terminal master's awarded for partial completion of doctoral program. *Degree requirements:* For master's, comprehensive exam, thesis; for doctorate, comprehensive exam, thesis/dissertation. *Entrance requirements:* For master's, GRE or MCAT; for doctorate, GRE General Test. Additional exam requirements/recommendations for international students: Required—TOEFL (minimum score 600 paper-based). *Application deadline:* For fall admission, 3/15 priority date for domestic and international students. Applications are processed on a rolling basis. Application fee: $50. Electronic applications accepted. *Expenses: Tuition:* Full-time $16,740; part-time $930 per credit. *Required fees:* $135 per semester. *Financial support:* In 2013–14, 3 fellowships with full tuition reimbursements (averaging $25,000 per year) were awarded; Federal Work-Study, scholarships/grants, and health care benefits also available. Financial award application deadline: 3/15; financial award applicants required to submit FAFSA. *Faculty research:* Parkinson's disease, drugs of abuse, neuroendocrinology, neuroimmunology, neurotoxicity. *Total annual research expenditures:* $3.5 million. *Unit head:* Dr. Edward J. Neafsey, Director, 708-216-3355, Fax: 708-216-6823, E-mail: eneafse@lumc.edu. *Application contact:* Kim Stubbs, Administrative Secretary, 708-216-3361, Fax: 708-216-3913, E-mail: kstubbs@lumc.edu.

Marquette University, Graduate School, College of Arts and Sciences, Department of Biology, Milwaukee, WI 53201-1881. Offers cell biology (MS, PhD); developmental biology (MS, PhD); ecology (MS, PhD); epithelial physiology (MS, PhD); genetics (MS, PhD); microbiology (MS, PhD); molecular biology (MS, PhD); muscle and exercise physiology (MS, PhD); neuroscience (PhD). *Faculty:* 21 full-time (9 women), 3 part-time/adjunct (0 women). *Students:* 34 full-time (16 women), 4 part-time (1 woman), 15 international. Average age 27. 70 applicants, 23% accepted, 5 enrolled. In 2013, 1 master's, 6 doctorates awarded. Terminal master's awarded for partial completion of doctoral program. *Degree requirements:* For master's, comprehensive exam, thesis, 1 year of teaching experience or equivalent; for doctorate, thesis/dissertation, 1 year of teaching experience or equivalent, qualifying exam. *Entrance requirements:* For master's and doctorate, GRE General Test, GRE Subject Test, official transcripts from all current and previous colleges/universities except Marquette, statement of professional goals and aspirations, three letters of recommendation. Additional exam requirements/recommendations for international students: Required—TOEFL (minimum score 530 paper-based). *Application deadline:* For fall admission, 12/15 for domestic and international students. Application fee: $50. Electronic applications accepted. *Financial support:* In 2013–14, 39 students received support, including 6 fellowships (averaging $1,208 per year), 4 research assistantships with full tuition reimbursements available (averaging $21,750 per year), 29 teaching assistantships with full tuition reimbursements available (averaging $21,750 per year); scholarships/grants, health care benefits, tuition waivers (full and partial), and unspecified assistantships also available. Support available to part-time students. Financial award application deadline: 2/15. *Faculty research:* Neurobiology, neuroendocrinology, epithelial physiology, neuropeptide interactions, synaptic transmission. *Total annual research expenditures:* $1.5 million. *Unit head:* Dr. Dale Noel, Chair and Professor, 414-288-1748. *Application contact:* Dr. Michelle Mynlieff, Professor, 414-288-1467.
Website: http://www.marquette.edu/biology/

Massachusetts Institute of Technology, School of Science, Department of Brain and Cognitive Sciences, Cambridge, MA 02139-4307. Offers cognitive science (PhD); neuroscience (PhD). *Faculty:* 37 full-time (14 women), 1 (woman) part-time/adjunct. *Students:* 102 full-time (25 women); includes 22 minority (2 Black or African American, non-Hispanic/Latino; 1 American Indian or Alaska Native, non-Hispanic/Latino; 6 Asian, non-Hispanic/Latino; 8 Hispanic/Latino; 5 Two or more races, non-Hispanic/Latino), 24 international. Average age 28. 542 applicants, 4% accepted, 11 enrolled. In 2013, 13 doctorates awarded. *Degree requirements:* For doctorate, comprehensive exam, thesis/dissertation. *Entrance requirements:* For doctorate, GRE General Test. Additional exam requirements/recommendations for international students: Required—TOEFL (minimum score 577 paper-based; 90 iBT), IELTS (minimum score 7). *Application deadline:* For fall admission, 12/1 for domestic and international students. Application fee: $75. Electronic applications accepted. *Expenses: Tuition:* Full-time $43,210; part-time $670 per credit hour. *Required fees:* $288. *Financial support:* In 2013–14, 95 students received support, including 73 fellowships (averaging $30,900 per year), 22 research assistantships (averaging $34,600 per year), 6 teaching assistantships (averaging $36,100 per year); Federal Work-Study, institutionally sponsored loans, scholarships/grants, traineeships, health care benefits, and unspecified assistantships also available. *Faculty research:* Vision, audition, and other perceptual systems: physiology and computation; learning, memory, and executive control: molecular and systems approaches; sensorimotor systems: physiology and computation; neural and cognitive development and plasticity; language and high-level cognition: learning, acquisition, and computation. *Total annual research expenditures:* $30.7 million. *Unit head:* Prof. James Dicarlo, Head, 617-253-5748, Fax: 617-258-9126, E-mail: bcs-info@mit.edu. *Application contact:* Academic Office, 617-253-7403, Fax: 617-253-9767, E-mail: bcs-admissions@mit.edu.
Website: http://bcs.mit.edu/

Mayo Graduate School, Graduate Programs in Biomedical Sciences, Program in Molecular Neuroscience, Rochester, MN 55905. Offers PhD. Program also offered in Jacksonville, FL. *Degree requirements:* For doctorate, oral defense of dissertation, qualifying oral and written exam. *Entrance requirements:* For doctorate, GRE, 1 year of chemistry, biology, calculus, and physics. Additional exam requirements/recommendations for international students: Required—TOEFL. Electronic applications accepted. *Faculty research:* Cholinergic receptor/Alzheimer's; molecular biology, channels, receptors, and mental disease; neuronal cytoskeleton; growth factors; gene regulation.

McGill University, Faculty of Graduate and Postdoctoral Studies, Faculty of Medicine, Department of Neurology and Neurosurgery, Montréal, QC H3A 2T5, Canada. Offers M Sc, PhD.

McMaster University, Faculty of Health Sciences and School of Graduate Studies, Program in Medical Sciences, Neurosciences and Behavioral Sciences Area, Hamilton, ON L8S 4M2, Canada. Offers M Sc, PhD, MD/PhD. *Degree requirements:* For master's, thesis; for doctorate, comprehensive exam, thesis/dissertation. *Entrance requirements:* For master's, honors B Sc, B+ average in related field; for doctorate, M Sc, minimum B+ average, students with proven research experience and an A average may be admitted with a B Sc degree. Additional exam requirements/recommendations for international students: Required—TOEFL (minimum score 580 paper-based).

Medical College of Wisconsin, Graduate School of Biomedical Sciences, Neuroscience Doctoral Program, Milwaukee, WI 53226-0509. Offers PhD, MD/PhD. *Degree requirements:* For doctorate, comprehensive exam, thesis/dissertation. *Entrance requirements:* For doctorate, GRE, official transcripts, three letters of recommendation. Additional exam requirements/recommendations for international students: Required—TOEFL. *Faculty research:* Neurobiology, development, neuroscience, teratology.

Medical University of South Carolina, College of Graduate Studies, Department of Neurosciences, Charleston, SC 29425. Offers MS, PhD, DMD/PhD, MD/PhD. Terminal master's awarded for partial completion of doctoral program. *Degree requirements:* For master's, thesis; for doctorate, thesis/dissertation, oral and written exams. *Entrance requirements:* For master's, GRE General Test; for doctorate, GRE General Test, interview, minimum GPA of 3.0. Additional exam requirements/recommendations for international students: Required—TOEFL (minimum score 600 paper-based; 100 iBT). Electronic applications accepted. *Faculty research:* Addiction, aging, movement disorders, membrane physiology, neurotransmission and behavior.

Meharry Medical College, School of Graduate Studies, Program in Biomedical Sciences, Neuroscience Emphasis, Nashville, TN 37208-9989. Offers PhD, MD/PhD. *Degree requirements:* For doctorate, comprehensive exam, thesis/dissertation. *Entrance requirements:* For doctorate, GRE. *Faculty research:* Neurochemistry, pain, smooth muscle tone, HP axis and peptides neural plasticity.

Memorial University of Newfoundland, Faculty of Medicine and School of Graduate Studies, Graduate Programs in Medicine, Division of Biomedical Sciences, St. John's, NL A1C 5S7, Canada. Offers cancer (M Sc, PhD); cardiovascular (M Sc, PhD); immunology (M Sc, PhD); neuroscience (M Sc, PhD). Part-time programs available. *Degree requirements:* For master's, thesis; for doctorate, comprehensive exam, thesis/dissertation, oral defense of thesis. *Entrance requirements:* For master's, MD or B Sc; for doctorate, MD or M Sc. Additional exam requirements/recommendations for international students: Required—TOEFL. *Faculty research:* Neuroscience, immunology, cardiovascular, and cancer.

Michigan State University, The Graduate School, College of Natural Science, Program in Neuroscience, East Lansing, MI 48824. Offers MS, PhD. *Entrance requirements:* Additional exam requirements/recommendations for international students: Required—TOEFL. Electronic applications accepted.

Montana State University, College of Graduate Studies, College of Letters and Science, Department of Cell Biology and Neuroscience, Bozeman, MT 59717. Offers biological sciences (PhD); neuroscience (MS, PhD). Part-time programs available. *Degree requirements:* For master's, comprehensive exam; for doctorate, comprehensive exam, thesis/dissertation. *Entrance requirements:* For master's and doctorate, GRE General Test. Additional exam requirements/recommendations for international students: Required—TOEFL (minimum score 550 paper-based). Electronic applications accepted. *Faculty research:* Development of the nervous system, neuronal mechanisms of visual perception, ion channel biophysics, mechanisms of sensory coding, neuroinformatics.

New York University, Graduate School of Arts and Science, Center for Neural Science, New York, NY 10012-1019. Offers PhD. *Faculty:* 15 full-time (3 women). *Students:* 45 full-time (23 women); includes 8 minority (1 Black or African American, non-Hispanic/Latino; 5 Asian, non-Hispanic/Latino; 1 Hispanic/Latino; 1 Two or more races, non-Hispanic/Latino), 12 international. Average age 28. 250 applicants, 10% accepted, 11 enrolled. In 2013, 10 doctorates awarded. *Degree requirements:* For doctorate, one foreign language, thesis/dissertation. *Entrance requirements:* For doctorate, GRE, interview. Additional exam requirements/recommendations for international students: Required—TOEFL. *Application deadline:* For fall admission, 12/12 for domestic and international students. Application fee: $95. *Expenses: Tuition:* Full-time $35,856; part-time $1494 per unit. *Required fees:* $1408; $64 per unit. $473 per term. Tuition and fees vary according to course load and program. *Financial support:* Fellowships with tuition reimbursements, research assistantships with tuition reimbursements, career-related internships or fieldwork, Federal Work-Study, institutionally sponsored loans, scholarships/grants, health care benefits, and unspecified assistantships available. Financial award application deadline: 12/12; financial award applicants required to submit FAFSA. *Faculty research:* Systems and integrative neuroscience; combining biology, cognition, computation, and theory. *Unit head:* J. Anthony Movshon, Chair, 212-998-7780, Fax: 212-995-4011, E-mail: admissions@cns.nyu.edu. *Application contact:* Alex Reyes, Director of Graduate Studies, 212-998-7780, Fax: 212-995-4011, E-mail: admissions@cns.nyu.edu.
Website: http://www.cns.nyu.edu/

New York University, School of Medicine and Graduate School of Arts and Science, Sackler Institute of Graduate Biomedical Sciences, Program in Neuroscience and Physiology, New York, NY 10012-1019. Offers PhD, MD/PhD. *Faculty:* 54 full-time (6 women). *Students:* 54 full-time (32 women); includes 12 minority (3 Black or African American, non-Hispanic/Latino; 4 Asian, non-Hispanic/Latino; 5 Hispanic/Latino), 13 international. Average age 28. In 2013, 7 doctorates awarded. *Degree requirements:* For doctorate, one foreign language, comprehensive exam, thesis/dissertation, qualifying exam. *Entrance requirements:* For doctorate, GRE General Test. Additional exam requirements/recommendations for international students: Required—TOEFL. *Application deadline:* For fall admission, 1/4 priority date for domestic students. Applications are processed on a rolling basis. Application fee: $85. *Expenses: Tuition:* Full-time $35,856; part-time $1494 per unit. *Required fees:* $1408; $64 per unit. $473 per term. Tuition and fees vary according to course load and program. *Financial support:* Fellowships with tuition reimbursements, research assistantships with tuition reimbursements, and teaching assistantships with tuition reimbursements available. *Faculty research:* Rhythms in neural networks, genetic basis of neural circuit formation and function, behavior and memory formation in mouse models of neurodevelopmental disorders. *Unit head:* Dr. Gordon Fishell, Graduate Program Director, 212-263-7691, E-mail: gordon.fishell@med.nyu.edu. *Application contact:* Dr. Annette Gray, Graduate Program Manager, 212-263-9134, E-mail: annette.gray@nyumc.org.

Northwestern University, Fienberg School of Medicine, Department of Physical Therapy and Human Movement Sciences, Chicago, IL 60611-2814. Offers neuroscience (PhD), including movement and rehabilitation science; physical therapy (DPT); DPT/PhD. *Accreditation:* APTA. *Degree requirements:* For doctorate, synthesis research project. *Entrance requirements:* For doctorate, GRE General Test (for DPT), baccalaureate degree with minimum GPA of 3.0 in required course work (DPT). Additional exam requirements/recommendations for international students: Required—TOEFL. Electronic applications accepted. *Expenses:* Contact institution. *Faculty research:* Motor control, robotics, neuromuscular imaging, student performance (academic/professional), clinical outcomes.

Northwestern University, The Graduate School, Interdepartmental Neuroscience Program, Evanston, IL 60208. Offers PhD. Admissions and degree offered through The Graduate School. *Degree requirements:* For doctorate, thesis/dissertation. *Entrance requirements:* For doctorate, GRE General Test. Additional exam requirements/ recommendations for international students: Required—TOEFL. *Faculty research:* Circadian rhythms, synaptic neurotransmissions, cognitive neuroscience, sensory/motor systems, cell biology and structure/function, neurobiology of disease.

The Ohio State University, Graduate School, College of Arts and Sciences, Division of Natural and Mathematical Sciences, Neuroscience Graduate Studies Program, Columbus, OH 43210. Offers PhD. *Students:* 19 full-time (6 women), 17 part-time (9 women); includes 2 minority (1 Asian, non-Hispanic/Latino; 1 Two or more races, non-Hispanic/Latino), 3 international. Average age 28. In 2013, 4 doctorates awarded. *Degree requirements:* For doctorate, comprehensive exam, thesis/dissertation. *Entrance requirements:* For doctorate, GRE General Test, GRE Subject Test in biology, psychology, biochemistry, or cell and molecular biology (recommended). Additional exam requirements/recommendations for international students: Required—TOEFL (minimum score 600 paper-based; 100 iBT); Recommended—IELTS (minimum score 8). *Application deadline:* For fall admission, 12/1 for domestic students, 11/30 for international students. Applications are processed on a rolling basis. Application fee: $40 ($50 for international students). Electronic applications accepted. *Financial support:* Fellowships with tuition reimbursements, research assistantships with tuition reimbursements, and unspecified assistantships available. *Faculty research:* Neurotrauma and disease, behavioral neuroscience, systems neuroscience, stress and neuroimmunology, molecular and cellular neuroscience. *Unit head:* Randy Nelson, Chair, 614-688-8327, E-mail: nelson.427@osu.edu. *Application contact:* Neuroscience Graduate Studies Program, 614-292-2379, Fax: 614-292-0490, E-mail: ngsp@osu.edu.
Website: http://www.ngsp.osu.edu/

The Ohio State University, Graduate School, College of Arts and Sciences, Division of Social and Behavioral Sciences, Department of Psychology, Columbus, OH 43210. Offers behavioral neuroscience (PhD); clinical psychology (PhD); cognitive psychology (PhD); developmental psychology (PhD); intellectual and developmental disabilities psychology (PhD); quantitative psychology (PhD); social psychology (PhD). *Accreditation:* APA. *Faculty:* 57. *Students:* 145 full-time (87 women), 2 part-time (both women); includes 24 minority (7 Black or African American, non-Hispanic/Latino; 1 American Indian or Alaska Native, non-Hispanic/Latino; 6 Asian, non-Hispanic/Latino; 7 Hispanic/Latino; 3 Two or more races, non-Hispanic/Latino), 16 international. Average age 27. In 2013, 13 doctorates awarded. *Degree requirements:* For doctorate, thesis/ dissertation. *Entrance requirements:* For doctorate, GRE General Test. Additional exam requirements/recommendations for international students: Required—TOEFL (minimum score 600 paper-based; 100 iBT); Recommended—IELTS (minimum score 8). *Application deadline:* For fall admission, 12/1 priority date for domestic students, 11/30 priority date for international students. Applications are processed on a rolling basis. Application fee: $60 ($70 for international students). Electronic applications accepted. *Financial support:* Fellowships with tuition reimbursements, research assistantships with tuition reimbursements, and teaching assistantships with tuition reimbursements available. *Unit head:* Dr. Richard Petty, Chair, 614-292-1640, E-mail: petty.1@osu.edu. *Application contact:* Graduate Admissions, 614-292-9444, Fax: 614-292-3895, E-mail: gradadmissions@osu.edu.
Website: http://www.psy.ohio-state.edu/

Ohio University, Graduate College, College of Arts and Sciences, Department of Biological Sciences, Athens, OH 45701-2979. Offers biological sciences (MS, PhD); cell biology and physiology (MS, PhD); ecology and evolutionary biology (MS, PhD); exercise physiology and muscle biology (MS, PhD); microbiology (MS, PhD); neuroscience (MS, PhD). Terminal master's awarded for partial completion of doctoral program. *Degree requirements:* For master's, comprehensive exam, thesis, 1 quarter of teaching experience; for doctorate, comprehensive exam, thesis/dissertation, 2 quarters of teaching experience. *Entrance requirements:* For master's, GRE General Test, names of three faculty members whose research interests most closely match the applicant's interest; for doctorate, GRE General Test, essay concerning prior training, research interest and career goals, plus names of three faculty members whose research interests most closely match the applicant's interest. Additional exam requirements/recommendations for international students: Required—TOEFL (minimum score 620 paper-based; 105 iBT) or IELTS (minimum score 7.5). Electronic applications accepted. *Faculty research:* Ecology and evolutionary biology, exercise physiology and muscle biology, neurobiology, cell biology, physiology.

Oregon Health & Science University, School of Medicine, Graduate Programs in Medicine, Department of Behavioral Neuroscience, Portland, OR 97239-3098. Offers PhD. *Faculty:* 34 full-time (14 women). *Students:* 28 full-time (15 women), 1 (woman) part-time; includes 6 minority (1 Asian, non-Hispanic/Latino; 3 Hispanic/Latino; 2 Two or more races, non-Hispanic/Latino). Average age 28. 105 applicants, 4% accepted, 4 enrolled. In 2013, 5 doctorates awarded. Terminal master's awarded for partial completion of doctoral program. *Degree requirements:* For doctorate, comprehensive exam, thesis/dissertation, qualifying exam. *Entrance requirements:* For doctorate, GRE General Test (minimum scores: 153 Verbal/148 Quantitative/4.5 Analytical), undergraduate coursework in biopsychology and other basic science areas. Additional exam requirements/recommendations for international students: Required—TOEFL. *Application deadline:* For fall admission, 12/1 for domestic students. Application fee: $70. Electronic applications accepted. *Financial support:* Fellowships, research assistantships, health care benefits, tuition waivers (full), and stipends (for PhD students) available. *Faculty research:* Behavioral neuroscience, behavioral genomics, biological basis of drug and alcohol abuse, cognitive neuroscience, neuropharmacology and neuroendocrinology. *Unit head:* Dr. Suzanne Mitchell, Program Director, 503-494-1650, E-mail: mitchesu@ohsu.edu. *Application contact:* Kris Thomason, Graduate Program Manager, 503-494-8464, E-mail: thomason@ohsu.edu.
Website: http://www.ohsu.edu/som-BehNeuro/

Oregon Health & Science University, School of Medicine, Graduate Programs in Medicine, Neuroscience Graduate Program, Portland, OR 97239-3098. Offers PhD. *Faculty:* 145 full-time (45 women). *Students:* 45 full-time (26 women), 2 part-time (both women); includes 5 minority (2 Asian, non-Hispanic/Latino; 2 Hispanic/Latino; 1 Two or more races, non-Hispanic/Latino), 6 international. Average age 29. 93 applicants, 9% accepted, 8 enrolled. In 2013, 10 doctorates awarded. Terminal master's awarded for partial completion of doctoral program. *Degree requirements:* For doctorate, comprehensive exam, thesis/dissertation, qualifying exam. *Entrance requirements:* For doctorate, GRE General Test (minimum scores: 153 Verbal/148 Quantitative/4.5 Analytical) or MCAT (for some programs). Additional exam requirements/ recommendations for international students: Required—TOEFL. *Application deadline:* For fall admission, 12/15 for domestic students. Application fee: $70. Electronic applications accepted. *Financial support:* Health care benefits and full tuition and stipends (for PhD students) available. *Faculty research:* Development, neurobiology of disease, molecular, systems, behavioral, cellular, biophysics of channels and transporters, gene regulation, neuronal signaling, synapses and circuits, sensory systems, neuroendocrinology, neurobiology of disease. *Unit head:* Dr. Gary Westbrook, Program Director, 503-494-6932, E-mail: ngp@ohsu.edu. *Application contact:* Liz Lawson-Weber, Program Coordinator, 503-494-6932, E-mail: ngp@ohsu.edu.
Website: http://www.ohsu.edu/xd/education/schools/school-of-medicine/academic-programs/neuroscience-graduate-program/?WT_rank-1

Penn State Hershey Medical Center, College of Medicine, Graduate School Programs in the Biomedical Sciences, The Huck Institutes of the Life Sciences, Intercollege Graduate Program in Neuroscience, Hershey, PA 17033. Offers MS, PhD, MD/PhD. *Students:* 18 full-time (11 women); includes 3 minority (1 Black or African American, non-Hispanic/Latino; 2 Asian, non-Hispanic/Latino). 32 applicants, 16% accepted, 4 enrolled. Terminal master's awarded for partial completion of doctoral program. *Degree requirements:* For master's, thesis or alternative; for doctorate, comprehensive exam, thesis/dissertation, oral exam. *Entrance requirements:* For master's, GRE General Test; for doctorate, GRE General Test, minimum GPA of 3.0. Additional exam requirements/ recommendations for international students: Required—TOEFL (minimum score 500 paper-based). *Application deadline:* For fall admission, 12/31 for domestic and international students. Applications are processed on a rolling basis. Application fee: $65. Electronic applications accepted. *Financial support:* In 2013–14, research assistantships with full tuition reimbursements (averaging $24,544 per year) were awarded; fellowships with full tuition reimbursements, career-related internships or fieldwork, institutionally sponsored loans, scholarships/grants, health care benefits, and unspecified assistantships also available. Financial award applicants required to submit FAFSA. *Faculty research:* Behavioral neuroscience, growth factors and neuropeptides, molecular neurobiology and neurogenetics, neuronal aging and brain metabolism, neuronal and glial development. *Unit head:* Dr. Colin Barnstable, Program Director, 717-531-8982, Fax: 717-531-0786, E-mail: neuro-grad-hmc@psu.edu. *Application contact:* Kathy Shuey, Program Assistant, 717-531-8982, Fax: 717-531-0786, E-mail: neuro-grad-hmc@psu.edu.
Website: http://www2.med.psu.edu/neurograd/

Princeton University, Graduate School, Department of Psychology, Princeton, NJ 08544-1019. Offers neuroscience (PhD); psychology (PhD). *Degree requirements:* For doctorate, thesis/dissertation. *Entrance requirements:* For doctorate, GRE General Test, GRE Subject Test. Additional exam requirements/recommendations for international students: Required—TOEFL (minimum score 550 paper-based). Electronic applications accepted.

Princeton University, Princeton Neuroscience Institute, Princeton, NJ 08544-1019. Offers PhD. Electronic applications accepted.

Purdue University, College of Pharmacy and Pharmacal Sciences and Graduate School, Graduate Programs in Pharmacy and Pharmacal Sciences, Department of Medicinal Chemistry and Molecular Pharmacology, West Lafayette, IN 47907. Offers biophysical and computational chemistry (PhD); cancer research (PhD); immunology and infectious disease (PhD); medicinal biochemistry and molecular biology (PhD); medicinal chemistry and chemical biology (PhD); molecular pharmacology (PhD); neuropharmacology, neurodegeneration, and neurotoxicity (PhD); systems biology and functional genomics (PhD). *Faculty:* 23 full-time (3 women), 6 part-time/adjunct (1 woman). *Students:* 50 full-time (21 women), 3 part-time (2 women); includes 1 minority (Asian, non-Hispanic/Latino), 30 international. Average age 26. 147 applicants, 20% accepted, 13 enrolled. In 2013, 12 doctorates awarded. *Degree requirements:* For doctorate, thesis/dissertation. *Entrance requirements:* For doctorate, GRE General Test; GRE Subject Test in biology, biochemistry, and chemistry (recommended), minimum undergraduate GPA of 3.0. Additional exam requirements/recommendations for international students: Required—TOEFL (minimum score 550 paper-based; 77 iBT); Recommended—TWE. *Application deadline:* For fall admission, 2/1 for domestic and international students. Applications are processed on a rolling basis. Application fee: $60 ($75 for international students). Electronic applications accepted. *Financial support:* Fellowships, research assistantships, teaching assistantships, and traineeships available. Support available to part-time students. Financial award applicants required to submit FAFSA. *Faculty research:* Drug design and development, cancer research, drug synthesis and analysis, chemical pharmacology, environmental toxicology. *Unit head:* Dr. Richard F. Borch, Head, 765-494-1403, E-mail: borch@purdue.edu. *Application contact:* Dr. Janine C. Mott, Graduate Contact, 765-494-1269, E-mail: jmott@purdue.edu.

Purdue University, Graduate School, College of Health and Human Sciences, Department of Psychological Sciences, West Lafayette, IN 47907. Offers behavioral neuroscience (PhD); clinical psychology (PhD); cognitive psychology (PhD); industrial/ organizational psychology (PhD); mathematical and computational cognitive science (PhD). *Accreditation:* APA. *Faculty:* 44 full-time (15 women), 15 part-time/adjunct (6 women). *Students:* 67 full-time (43 women), 2 part-time (both women); includes 9 minority (2 Black or African American, non-Hispanic/Latino; 4 Asian, non-Hispanic/ Latino; 2 Hispanic/Latino; 1 Two or more races, non-Hispanic/Latino), 14 international. Average age 26. 388 applicants, 7% accepted, 16 enrolled. In 2013, 13 doctorates awarded. Terminal master's awarded for partial completion of doctoral program. *Degree requirements:* For doctorate, thesis/dissertation. *Entrance requirements:* For doctorate, GRE General Test, minimum undergraduate GPA of 3.0 or equivalent. Additional exam requirements/recommendations for international students: Required—TOEFL (minimum score 550 paper-based; 77 iBT); Recommended—TWE. *Application deadline:* For fall admission, 12/3 for domestic and international students. Applications are processed on a rolling basis. Application fee: $60 ($75 for international students). Electronic applications accepted. *Financial support:* Fellowships with partial tuition reimbursements, research assistantships with partial tuition reimbursements, teaching assistantships with partial tuition reimbursements, and career-related internships or fieldwork available. Support available to part-time students. Financial award applicants required to submit FAFSA. *Faculty research:* Career development of women in science, development of friendships during childhood and adolescence, social competence, human information processing. *Unit head:* Dr. Christopher R. Agnew, Head, 765-494-6061, Fax: 765-496-1264, E-mail: agnew@psych.purdue.edu. *Application contact:* Nancy A. O'Brien, Graduate Contact, 765-494-6067, Fax: 765-496-1264, E-mail: nobrien@psych.pardue.edu.
Website: http://www.psych.purdue.edu/

Purdue University, Graduate School, PULSe - Purdue University Life Sciences Program, West Lafayette, IN 47907. Offers biomolecular structure and biophysics (PhD); biotechnology (PhD); chemical biology (PhD); chromatin and regulation of gene expression (PhD); integrative neuroscience (PhD); integrative plant sciences (PhD); membrane biology (PhD); microbiology (PhD); molecular evolutionary and cancer biology (PhD); molecular evolutionary genetics (PhD); molecular virology (PhD).

Neuroscience

Students: 154 full-time (78 women), 1 part-time (0 women); includes 23 minority (5 Black or African American, non-Hispanic/Latino; 5 Asian, non-Hispanic/Latino; 10 Hispanic/Latino; 3 Two or more races, non-Hispanic/Latino), 73 international. Average age 26. 239 applicants, 33% accepted, 40 enrolled. *Entrance requirements:* For doctorate, GRE, minimum undergraduate GPA of 3.0. Additional exam requirements/recommendations for international students: Required—TOEFL (minimum score 550 paper-based; 77 iBT). *Application deadline:* For fall admission, 1/15 priority date for domestic and international students. Applications are processed on a rolling basis. Application fee: $60 ($75 for international students). Electronic applications accepted. *Financial support:* In 2013–14, research assistantships with tuition reimbursements (averaging $22,500 per year), teaching assistantships with tuition reimbursements (averaging $22,500 per year) were awarded. *Unit head:* Dr. Christine A. Hrycyna, Head, 765-494-7322, E-mail: hrycyna@purdue.edu. *Application contact:* Colleen Gabauer, Graduate Contact, 765-494-9256, E-mail: cgabauer@purdue.edu.
Website: http://www.gradschool.purdue.edu/pulse

Queen's University at Kingston, School of Graduate Studies, Faculty of Health Sciences, Department of Anatomy and Cell Biology, Kingston, ON K7L 3N6, Canada. Offers biology of reproduction (M Sc, PhD); cancer (M Sc, PhD); cardiovascular pathophysiology (M Sc, PhD); cell and molecular biology (M Sc, PhD); drug metabolism (M Sc, PhD); endocrinology (M Sc, PhD); motor control (M Sc, PhD); neural regeneration (M Sc, PhD); neurophysiology (M Sc, PhD). Part-time programs available. *Degree requirements:* For master's, thesis; for doctorate, one foreign language, comprehensive exam, thesis/dissertation. *Entrance requirements:* Additional exam requirements/recommendations for international students: Required—TOEFL. Electronic applications accepted. *Faculty research:* Human kinetics, neuroscience, reproductive biology, cardiovascular.

Rosalind Franklin University of Medicine and Science, School of Graduate and Postdoctoral Studies - Interdisciplinary Graduate Program in Biomedical Sciences, Department of Neuroscience, North Chicago, IL 60064-3095. Offers PhD, MD/PhD. *Degree requirements:* For doctorate, comprehensive exam, thesis/dissertation, original research project. *Entrance requirements:* For doctorate, GRE General Test. Additional exam requirements/recommendations for international students: Required—TOEFL, TWE.

Rush University, Graduate College, Division of Neuroscience, Chicago, IL 60612-3832. Offers MS, PhD. Terminal master's awarded for partial completion of doctoral program. *Degree requirements:* For master's, thesis; for doctorate, thesis/dissertation. *Entrance requirements:* For master's and doctorate, GRE General Test. Additional exam requirements/recommendations for international students: Required—TOEFL. Electronic applications accepted. *Faculty research:* Neurodegenerative disorders, neurobiology of memory, aging, pathology and genetics of Alzheimer's disease.

Rutgers, The State University of New Jersey, Newark, Graduate School of Biomedical Sciences, Program in Integrative Neuroscience, Newark, NJ 07107. Offers PhD. Program offered jointly with Rutgers, The State University of New Jersey, New Brunswick. *Degree requirements:* For doctorate, thesis/dissertation, qualifying exam. *Entrance requirements:* For doctorate, GRE General Test, minimum GPA of 3.5. Additional exam requirements/recommendations for international students: Required—TOEFL. Electronic applications accepted.

Rutgers, The State University of New Jersey, Newark, Graduate School, Program in Psychology, Newark, NJ 07102. Offers cognitive neuroscience (PhD); cognitive science (PhD); perception (PhD); psychobiology (PhD); social cognition (PhD). *Degree requirements:* For doctorate, comprehensive exam, thesis/dissertation. *Entrance requirements:* For doctorate, GRE General Test, GRE Subject Test, minimum undergraduate B average. Electronic applications accepted. *Faculty research:* Visual perception (luminance, motion), neuroendocrine mechanisms in behavior (reproduction, pain), attachment theory, connectionist modeling of cognition.

Rutgers, The State University of New Jersey, New Brunswick, Graduate School-New Brunswick, Program in Endocrinology and Animal Biosciences, Piscataway, NJ 08854-8097. Offers MS, PhD. Terminal master's awarded for partial completion of doctoral program. *Degree requirements:* For master's, thesis; for doctorate, comprehensive exam, thesis/dissertation. *Entrance requirements:* For master's and doctorate, GRE General Test. Additional exam requirements/recommendations for international students: Required—TOEFL. Electronic applications accepted. *Faculty research:* Comparative and behavioral endocrinology, epigenetic regulation of the endocrine system, exercise physiology and immunology, fetal and neonatal developmental programming, mammary gland biology and breast cancer, neuroendocrinology and alcohol studies, reproductive and developmental toxicology.

Rutgers, The State University of New Jersey, New Brunswick, Graduate School of Biomedical Sciences, Program in Neuroscience, Piscataway, NJ 08854-5635. Offers MS, PhD, MD/PhD. *Degree requirements:* For master's, thesis, qualifying exam; for doctorate, thesis/dissertation, qualifying exam. *Entrance requirements:* Additional exam requirements/recommendations for international students: Required—TOEFL. Electronic applications accepted.

Seton Hall University, College of Arts and Sciences, Department of Biological Sciences, South Orange, NJ 07079-2697. Offers biology (MS); biology/business administration (MS); microbiology (MS); molecular bioscience (PhD); molecular bioscience/neuroscience (PhD). Part-time and evening/weekend programs available. *Degree requirements:* For master's, thesis optional; for doctorate, comprehensive exam, thesis/dissertation. *Entrance requirements:* For master's and doctorate, GRE or MS from accredited university in the U.S. Additional exam requirements/recommendations for international students: Required—TOEFL. Electronic applications accepted. *Faculty research:* Neurobiology, genetics, immunology, molecular biology, cellular physiology, toxicology, microbiology, bioinformatics.

Seton Hall University, College of Arts and Sciences, Department of Psychology, South Orange, NJ 07079-2697. Offers experimental psychology (MS), including behavioral neuroscience. Part-time and evening/weekend programs available. *Entrance requirements:* For master's, GRE. Additional exam requirements/recommendations for international students: Required—TOEFL. Electronic applications accepted. *Faculty research:* Behavioral neuroscience, cognitive psychology, social psychology, perception/motor skills, memory, depression, anxiety.

Stanford University, School of Medicine, Graduate Programs in Medicine, Neurosciences Program, Stanford, CA 94305-9991. Offers PhD. *Degree requirements:* For doctorate, thesis/dissertation. *Entrance requirements:* For doctorate, GRE General Test, GRE Subject Test. Additional exam requirements/recommendations for international students: Required—TOEFL. Electronic applications accepted. *Expenses: Tuition:* Full-time $42,690; part-time $949 per credit. *Required fees:* $185.

State University of New York Downstate Medical Center, School of Graduate Studies, Program in Neural and Behavioral Science, Brooklyn, NY 11203-2098. Offers PhD, MD/PhD. *Degree requirements:* For doctorate, comprehensive exam, thesis/dissertation. *Entrance requirements:* For doctorate, GRE. Additional exam requirements/recommendations for international students: Recommended—TOEFL. *Faculty research:* Molecular neuroscience, cellular neuroscience, systems neuroscience, behavioral neuroscience, behavior.

State University of New York Upstate Medical University, College of Graduate Studies, Program in Neuroscience, Syracuse, NY 13210-2334. Offers PhD. *Degree requirements:* For doctorate, comprehensive exam, thesis/dissertation. *Entrance requirements:* For doctorate, GRE General Test, telephone interview. Additional exam requirements/recommendations for international students: Required—TOEFL. Electronic applications accepted. *Faculty research:* Cancer, disorders of the nervous system, infectious diseases, diabetes/metabolic disorders/cardiovascular diseases.

Stony Brook University, State University of New York, Graduate School, College of Arts and Sciences, Department of Neurobiology and Behavior, Stony Brook, NY 11794. Offers neuroscience (MS, PhD). *Faculty:* 18 full-time (5 women), 2 part-time/adjunct (0 women). *Students:* 39 full-time (18 women), 1 part-time (0 women); includes 11 minority (3 Black or African American, non-Hispanic/Latino; 5 Asian, non-Hispanic/Latino; 2 Hispanic/Latino; 1 Two or more races, non-Hispanic/Latino), 11 international. Average age 27. 90 applicants, 17% accepted, 4 enrolled. In 2013, 1 master's, 3 doctorates awarded. *Degree requirements:* For doctorate, comprehensive exam, thesis/dissertation, teaching experience. *Entrance requirements:* For doctorate, GRE General Test, GRE Subject Test, minimum GPA of 3.0. Additional exam requirements/recommendations for international students: Required—TOEFL. *Application deadline:* For fall admission, 1/15 for domestic students; for spring admission, 10/1 for domestic students. Application fee: $100. *Expenses:* Tuition, state resident: full-time $9870; part-time $411 per credit. Tuition, nonresident: full-time $18,350; part-time $765 per credit. *Financial support:* In 2013–14, 13 fellowships, 24 research assistantships, 7 teaching assistantships were awarded; Federal Work-Study also available. *Faculty research:* Biophysics; neurochemistry; cellular, developmental, and integrative neurobiology. *Total annual research expenditures:* $5.1 million. *Unit head:* Dr. Lorna Role, Director, PhD Program, 631-632-8616, Fax: 631-632-6661, E-mail: lorna.role@stonybrook.edu. *Application contact:* Odalis Hernandez, Coordinator, 631-632-8078, Fax: 631-632-6661, E-mail: odalis.hernandez@stonybrook.edu.
Website: http://medicine.stonybrookmedicine.edu/neurobiology/

Stony Brook University, State University of New York, Graduate School, College of Arts and Sciences, Department of Psychology, Program in Integrative Neuroscience, Stony Brook, NY 11794. Offers PhD. *Students:* 16 full-time (11 women); includes 2 minority (1 Black or African American, non-Hispanic/Latino; 1 Asian, non-Hispanic/Latino), 3 international. Average age 28. 29 applicants, 14% accepted, 4 enrolled. In 2013, 3 doctorates awarded. *Degree requirements:* For doctorate, thesis/dissertation. *Entrance requirements:* For doctorate, GRE General Test, GRE Subject Test. Additional exam requirements/recommendations for international students: Required—TOEFL. *Application deadline:* For fall admission, 1/15 for domestic students; for spring admission, 10/1 for domestic students. Application fee: $100. *Expenses:* Tuition, state resident: full-time $9870; part-time $411 per credit. Tuition, nonresident: full-time $18,350; part-time $765 per credit. *Unit head:* Dr. Daniel Klein, Head, 631-632-7792, Fax: 632-7876, E-mail: daniel.klein@stonybrook.edu. *Application contact:* Marilynn Wollmuth, Coordinator, 631-632-7855, Fax: 631-632-7876, E-mail: marilyn.wollmuth@stonybrook.edu.

Teachers College, Columbia University, Graduate Faculty of Education, Department of Biobehavioral Studies, Program in Neuroscience and Education, New York, NY 10027. Offers MA. *Faculty:* 1 full-time. *Students:* 10 full-time (all women), 46 part-time (33 women); includes 23 minority (6 Black or African American, non-Hispanic/Latino; 10 Asian, non-Hispanic/Latino; 4 Hispanic/Latino; 3 Two or more races, non-Hispanic/Latino), 9 international. Average age 30. 42 applicants, 88% accepted, 23 enrolled. In 2013, 25 master's awarded. *Degree requirements:* For master's, integrative project, practicum, research experience. *Application deadline:* For fall admission, 1/15 priority date for domestic students; for spring admission, 11/1 for domestic students. Applications are processed on a rolling basis. Application fee: $65. Electronic applications accepted. *Financial support:* Career-related internships or fieldwork, Federal Work-Study, institutionally sponsored loans, and tuition waivers (full and partial) available. Support available to part-time students. Financial award application deadline: 2/1. *Faculty research:* Neuropsychological diagnosis and intervention. *Unit head:* Prof. Peter Gordon, Program Coordinator, 212-678-8162, E-mail: pgordon@tc.edu. *Application contact:* Debbie Lesperance, Assistant Director of Admission, 212-678-3710, Fax: 212-678-4171.
Website: http://www.tc.edu/bbs/NeuroSci/

Texas A&M Health Science Center, College of Medicine, Department of Neuroscience and Experimental Therapeutics, College Station, TX 77840. Offers PhD.

Texas A&M University, College of Liberal Arts, Department of Psychology, College Station, TX 77843. Offers behavioral and cellular neuroscience (PhD); clinical psychology (PhD); cognitive psychology (PhD); developmental psychology (PhD); industrial/organizational psychology (PhD); psychology (MS); social psychology (PhD). *Accreditation:* APA (one or more programs are accredited). *Faculty:* 37. *Students:* 95 full-time (55 women), 11 part-time (9 women); includes 27 minority (4 Black or African American, non-Hispanic/Latino; 6 Asian, non-Hispanic/Latino; 17 Hispanic/Latino), 16 international. Average age 28. 393 applicants, 3% accepted, 8 enrolled. In 2013, 5 master's, 7 doctorates awarded. *Degree requirements:* For doctorate, comprehensive exam (for some programs), thesis/dissertation. *Entrance requirements:* For doctorate, GRE General Test. Additional exam requirements/recommendations for international students: Required—TOEFL. *Application deadline:* For fall admission, 1/5 for domestic and international students. Application fee: $50 ($75 for international students). Electronic applications accepted. *Expenses:* Tuition, state resident: full-time $4078; part-time $226.55 per credit hour. Tuition, nonresident: full-time $10,450; part-time $580.55 per credit hour. *Required fees:* $2328; $278.50 per credit hour. $642.45 per semester. *Financial support:* Fellowships with partial tuition reimbursements, research assistantships with partial tuition reimbursements, teaching assistantships with partial tuition reimbursements, career-related internships or fieldwork, institutionally sponsored loans, health care benefits, and unspecified assistantships available. Financial award application deadline: 1/5; financial award applicants required to submit FAFSA. *Unit head:* Dr. Doug Woods, Head, 979-845-2540, E-mail: dowoods@tamu.edu. *Application contact:* Dr. Charles D. Samuelson, Director of Graduate Studies, 979-845-0880, Fax: 979-845-4727, E-mail: c-samuelson@tamu.edu.
Website: http://psychology.tamu.edu

Texas Christian University, College of Science and Engineering, Department of Psychology, Fort Worth, TX 76129-0002. Offers developmental trauma (MS); experimental psychology (PhD), including behavioral neuroscience, cognition, learning, social; psychology (MA, MS). *Faculty:* 11 full-time (4 women), 1 part-time/adjunct (0 women). *Students:* 7 full-time (5 women), 21 part-time (9 women); includes 1 minority (Hispanic/Latino), 4 international. Average age 27. 35 applicants, 29% accepted, 9 enrolled. In 2013, 9 master's, 3 doctorates awarded. Terminal master's awarded for partial completion of doctoral program. *Degree requirements:* For master's, thesis; for doctorate, thesis/dissertation. *Entrance requirements:* For master's and doctorate, GRE General Test. Additional exam requirements/recommendations for international students: Recommended—TOEFL. *Application deadline:* For fall admission, 12/30 for domestic and international students; for spring admission, 12/1 for domestic students.

Application fee: $60. Electronic applications accepted. *Expenses:* Contact institution. *Financial support:* In 2013–14, 28 students received support. Teaching assistantships with full tuition reimbursements available and unspecified assistantships available. Financial award application deadline: 12/30. *Faculty research:* Neural and behavioral mechanisms mediating after damage to the brain, neural immune interactions, physiological psychology, learning, bird song, qualitative methods, parenting and attachment. *Unit head:* Dr. Charles Lord, Director of Graduate Studies, 817-257-6425, Fax: 817-257-7681, E-mail: c.lord@tcu.edu. *Application contact:* Cindy Hayes, Administrative Assistant, 817-257-7410, Fax: 817-257-7681, E-mail: c.hayes@tcu.edu.
Website: http://www.psy.tcu.edu/gradpro.html

Thomas Jefferson University, Jefferson Graduate School of Biomedical Sciences, PhD Program in Neuroscience, Philadelphia, PA 19107. Offers PhD. Offered jointly with the Farber Institute for Neuroscience. *Faculty:* 37 full-time (12 women). *Students:* 20 full-time (8 women); includes 1 minority (Asian, non-Hispanic/Latino), 4 international. 57 applicants, 12% accepted, 3 enrolled. In 2013, 1 doctorate awarded. *Degree requirements:* For doctorate, comprehensive exam, thesis/dissertation. *Entrance requirements:* For doctorate, GRE General Test, strong background in the sciences, interview, previous research experience. Additional exam requirements/recommendations for international students: Required—TOEFL (minimum score 100 iBT) or IELTS. *Application deadline:* For fall admission, 1/5 priority date for domestic and international students. Application fee: $75. *Financial support:* In 2013–14, 20 students received support, including 20 fellowships with full tuition reimbursements available (averaging $56,052 per year); institutionally sponsored loans, scholarships/grants, and stipends also available. Financial award application deadline: 5/1. *Unit head:* Dr. Manuel L. Covarrubias, Program Director, 215-503-4340, Fax: 215-955-4949, E-mail: manuel.covarrubias@jefferson.edu. *Application contact:* Marc E. Stearns, Director of Admissions and Recruitment, 215-503-4400, Fax: 215-503-3433, E-mail: jgsbs-info@jefferson.edu.
Website: http://www.jefferson.edu/Biomedical_Sciences/programs/phd/Neuroscience/

Tufts University, Cummings School of Veterinary Medicine, North Grafton, MA 01536. Offers animals and public policy (MS); biomedical sciences (PhD), including digestive diseases, infectious diseases, neuroscience and reproductive biology, pathology; conservation medicine (MS); veterinary medicine (DVM); DVM/MPH; DVM/MS. *Accreditation:* AVMA (one or more programs are accredited). *Faculty:* 98 full-time (45 women), 13 part-time/adjunct (7 women). *Students:* 426 full-time (364 women); includes 60 minority (5 Black or African American, non-Hispanic/Latino; 1 American Indian or Alaska Native, non-Hispanic/Latino; 32 Asian, non-Hispanic/Latino; 20 Hispanic/Latino; 2 Two or more races, non-Hispanic/Latino), 4 international. Average age 25. 899 applicants, 29% accepted, 119 enrolled. In 2013, 85 master's, 2 doctorates awarded. *Degree requirements:* For master's, thesis (for some programs); for doctorate, comprehensive exam, thesis/dissertation (for some programs). *Entrance requirements:* For master's and doctorate, GRE General Test. Additional exam requirements/recommendations for international students: Required—TOEFL or IELTS. *Application deadline:* For fall admission, 11/1 for domestic and international students. Application fee: $70. Electronic applications accepted. *Expenses:* Contact institution. *Financial support:* In 2013–14, 230 students received support, including 7 research assistantships with full tuition reimbursements available (averaging $25,000 per year), 6 teaching assistantships (averaging $5,000 per year); career-related internships or fieldwork, Federal Work-Study, institutionally sponsored loans, scholarships/grants, and institutional aid awards, health care benefits for PhD students also available. Financial award application deadline: 4/15; financial award applicants required to submit FAFSA. *Faculty research:* Oncology, veterinary ethics, international veterinary medicine, veterinary genomics, pathogenesis of Clostridium difficile, wildlife fertility control. *Unit head:* Dr. Deborah T. Kochevar, Dean, 508-839-5302, Fax: 508-839-2953, E-mail: deborah.kochevar@tufts.edu. *Application contact:* Rebecca Russo, Director of Admissions, 508-839-7920, Fax: 508-887-4820, E-mail: vetadmissions@tufts.edu.
Website: http://www.tufts.edu/

Tufts University, Sackler School of Graduate Biomedical Sciences, Neuroscience Program, Medford, MA 02155. Offers PhD. *Faculty:* 32 full-time (14 women). *Students:* 28 full-time (18 women); includes 10 minority (1 Black or African American, non-Hispanic/Latino; 6 Asian, non-Hispanic/Latino; 1 Hispanic/Latino; 2 Two or more races, non-Hispanic/Latino), 1 international. Average age 29. 130 applicants, 9% accepted, 5 enrolled. In 2013, 1 doctorate awarded. Terminal master's awarded for partial completion of doctoral program. *Degree requirements:* For doctorate, comprehensive exam, thesis/dissertation. *Entrance requirements:* For doctorate, GRE General Test, 3 letters of reference. Additional exam requirements/recommendations for international students: Required—TOEFL (minimum score 600 paper-based; 100 iBT). *Application deadline:* For fall admission, 12/15 for domestic and international students. Application fee: $70. Electronic applications accepted. *Financial support:* In 2013–14, 28 students received support, including 28 research assistantships with full tuition reimbursements available (averaging $31,000 per year); health care benefits also available. *Faculty research:* Molecular, cellular, and systems analyses of synapses and circuits and their implications for neurological disease. *Unit head:* Dr. F. Rob Jackson, Director, 617-636-3796, E-mail: rob.jackson@tufts.edu. *Application contact:* Kellie Melchin, Associate Director of Admissions, 617-636-6767, Fax: 617-636-0375, E-mail: sackler-school@tufts.edu.
Website: http://sackler.tufts.edu/Academics/Degree-Programs/PhD-Programs/Neuroscience

Tulane University, School of Medicine and School of Liberal Arts, Graduate Programs in Biomedical Sciences, Program in Neuroscience, New Orleans, LA 70118-5669. Offers MS, PhD, MD/PhD. MS and PhD offered through the Graduate School. *Degree requirements:* For doctorate, thesis/dissertation, qualifying exam. *Entrance requirements:* For doctorate, GRE General Test. Additional exam requirements/recommendations for international students: Required—TOEFL. Electronic applications accepted. *Faculty research:* Neuroendocrinology, ion channels, neuropeptides.

Tulane University, School of Science and Engineering, Neuroscience Program, New Orleans, LA 70118-5669. Offers MS, PhD.

Uniformed Services University of the Health Sciences, School of Medicine, Graduate Programs in the Biomedical Sciences and Public Health, Graduate Program in Neuroscience, Bethesda, MD 20814-4799. Offers PhD. *Faculty:* 54 full-time (18 women), 2 part-time/adjunct (1 woman). *Students:* 34 full-time (17 women); includes 7 minority (2 Black or African American, non-Hispanic/Latino; 5 Asian, non-Hispanic/Latino), 5 international. Average age 26. 34 applicants, 32% accepted, 8 enrolled. In 2013, 3 doctorates awarded. *Degree requirements:* For doctorate, comprehensive exam, thesis/dissertation, qualifying exams. *Entrance requirements:* For doctorate, GRE General Test, minimum GPA of 3.0; course work in biology, general chemistry, organic chemistry. Additional exam requirements/recommendations for international students: Required—TOEFL. *Application deadline:* For fall admission, 1/1 priority date for domestic and international students. Applications are processed on a rolling basis. Application fee: $0. Electronic applications accepted. *Financial support:* In 2013–14, fellowships with full tuition reimbursements (averaging $27,000 per year) were awarded; scholarships/grants, health care benefits, and tuition waivers (full) also available. *Faculty research:* Neuronal development and plasticity, molecular neurobiology, environmental adaptations, stress and injury. *Unit head:* Dr. Sharon Juliano, Director, 301-295-3673, Fax: 301-295-1996, E-mail: sjuliano@usuhs.mil. *Application contact:* Tina Finley, Administrative Assistant, 301-295-3642, Fax: 301-295-1996, E-mail: netina.finley@usuhs.edu.
Website: http://www.usuhs.mil/nes/index.html

See Display on next page and Close-Up on page 385.

Universidad de Iberoamerica, Graduate School, San Jose, Costa Rica. Offers clinical neuropsychology (PhD); clinical psychology (M Psych); educational psychology (M Psych); forensic psychology (M Psych); hospital management (MHA); intensive care nursing (MN); medicine (MD).

Université de Montréal, Faculty of Medicine, Department of Physiology, Program in Neurological Sciences, Montréal, QC H3C 3J7, Canada. Offers M Sc, PhD. Terminal master's awarded for partial completion of doctoral program. *Degree requirements:* For master's, thesis; for doctorate, thesis/dissertation, general exam. *Entrance requirements:* For master's and doctorate, proficiency in French, knowledge of English. Electronic applications accepted.

University at Albany, State University of New York, School of Public Health, Department of Biomedical Sciences, Program in Neuroscience, Albany, NY 12222-0001. Offers MS, PhD. *Degree requirements:* For master's, thesis; for doctorate, thesis/dissertation. *Entrance requirements:* For master's and doctorate, GRE General Test, GRE Subject Test.

University at Buffalo, the State University of New York, Graduate School, School of Medicine and Biomedical Sciences, Graduate Programs in Medicine and Biomedical Sciences, Neuroscience Program, Buffalo, NY 14263. Offers MS, PhD. *Faculty:* 33 full-time (11 women). *Students:* 43 full-time (26 women); includes 17 minority (all Asian, non-Hispanic/Latino). Average age 23. 22 applicants, 55% accepted, 10 enrolled. In 2013, 6 master's, 2 doctorates awarded. Terminal master's awarded for partial completion of doctoral program. *Degree requirements:* For master's, thesis (for some programs); for doctorate, comprehensive exam, thesis/dissertation. *Entrance requirements:* For master's, GRE General Test, 3 letters of recommendation, transcripts. Additional exam requirements/recommendations for international students: Required—TOEFL (minimum score 100 iBT). *Application deadline:* For fall admission, 7/15 priority date for domestic and international students. Applications are processed on a rolling basis. Application fee: $75. Electronic applications accepted. *Financial support:* In 2013–14, 17 students received support, including 17 research assistantships with full tuition reimbursements available (averaging $25,000 per year). Financial award application deadline: 9/1. *Faculty research:* Neural plasticity, development, synapse, neurodisease, genetics of neuropathology. *Total annual research expenditures:* $6 million. *Unit head:* Dr. Malcolm Slaughter, Professor, 716-829-3240, E-mail: mslaught@buffalo.edu. *Application contact:* Kristen Kahi, Program Administrator, 716-829-2419, E-mail: kkms@buffalo.edu.
Website: http://wings.buffalo.edu/neuroscience/

The University of Alabama at Birmingham, College of Arts and Sciences, Program in Psychology, Birmingham, AL 35294-1170. Offers behavioral neuroscience (PhD); lifespan development psychology (PhD); medical clinical psychology (PhD); psychology (MA). *Accreditation:* APA (one or more programs are accredited). Electronic applications accepted. *Faculty research:* Biological basis of behavior structure, function of the nervous system.

University of Alberta, Faculty of Medicine and Dentistry and Faculty of Graduate Studies and Research, Graduate Programs in Medicine, Centre for Neuroscience, Edmonton, AB T6G 2E1, Canada. Offers M Sc, PhD. Terminal master's awarded for partial completion of doctoral program. *Degree requirements:* For master's, thesis; for doctorate, thesis/dissertation. *Entrance requirements:* For master's and doctorate, minimum GPA of 3.3. Additional exam requirements/recommendations for international students: Required—TOEFL (minimum score 600 paper-based). Electronic applications accepted. *Faculty research:* Sensory and motor mechanisms, neural growth and regeneration, molecular neurobiology, synaptic mechanisms, behavioral and psychiatric neuroscience.

The University of Arizona, Graduate Interdisciplinary Programs, Graduate Interdisciplinary Program in Neuroscience, Tucson, AZ 85719. Offers PhD. *Faculty:* 7 full-time (2 women). *Students:* 23 full-time (12 women); includes 4 minority (1 Black or African American, non-Hispanic/Latino; 2 Hispanic/Latino; 1 Two or more races, non-Hispanic/Latino), 1 international. Average age 29. 51 applicants, 14% accepted, 7 enrolled. In 2013, 5 doctorates awarded. *Degree requirements:* For doctorate, thesis/dissertation. *Entrance requirements:* For doctorate, GRE (minimum score 1100), minimum GPA of 3.5, 3 letters of recommendation. Additional exam requirements/recommendations for international students: Required—TOEFL (minimum score 550 paper-based; 79 iBT). *Application deadline:* For fall admission, 12/1 for domestic and international students. Application fee: $75. Electronic applications accepted. *Expenses:* Tuition, state resident: full-time $11,526. Tuition, nonresident: full-time $27,398. *Financial support:* In 2013–14, 3 research assistantships with full tuition reimbursements (averaging $23,000 per year), 1 teaching assistantship with full tuition reimbursement (averaging $22,000 per year) were awarded; health care benefits, tuition waivers (full), and unspecified assistantships also available. Financial award application deadline: 12/1. *Faculty research:* Cognitive neuroscience, developmental neurobiology, speech and hearing, motor control, insect neurobiology. *Total annual research expenditures:* $2 million. *Unit head:* Dr. Konrad E. Zinsmaier, Chairman, 520-621-1343, Fax: 520-621-8282, E-mail: kez@neurobio.arizona.edu. *Application contact:* Kristen Grabo, Graduate Coordinator, 520-621-8380, Fax: 520-626-2618, E-mail: nrsc@u.arizona.edu.
Website: http://www.neuroscience.arizona.edu/

The University of British Columbia, Faculty of Arts and Faculty of Graduate Studies, Department of Psychology, Vancouver, BC V6T 1Z4, Canada. Offers behavioral neuroscience (MA, PhD); clinical psychology (MA, PhD); cognitive science (MA, PhD); developmental psychology (MA, PhD); health psychology (MA, PhD); quantitative methods (MA, PhD); social/personality psychology (MA, PhD). *Accreditation:* APA (one or more programs are accredited). Terminal master's awarded for partial completion of doctoral program. *Degree requirements:* For master's, thesis; for doctorate, comprehensive exam, thesis/dissertation. *Entrance requirements:* For master's and doctorate, GRE General Test. Additional exam requirements/recommendations for international students: Required—TOEFL (minimum score 550 paper-based; 80 iBT). Electronic applications accepted. *Expenses: Tuition, area resident:* Full-time $8000 Canadian dollars. *Faculty research:* Clinical, developmental, social/personality, cognition, behavioral neuroscience.

University of Calgary, Cumming School of Medicine and Faculty of Graduate Studies, Department of Neuroscience, Calgary, AB T2N 1N4, Canada. Offers M Sc, PhD. *Degree requirements:* For master's, thesis, oral thesis exam; for doctorate, thesis/dissertation, candidacy exam, oral thesis exam. *Entrance requirements:* For master's and doctorate, minimum GPA of 3.2 during previous 2 years. Additional exam requirements/recommendations for international students: Required—TOEFL (minimum score 580 paper-based). Electronic applications accepted. *Faculty research:* Cellular pharmacology and neurotoxicology, developmental neurobiology, molecular basis of neurodegenerative diseases, neural systems, ion channels.

University of California, Berkeley, Graduate Division, Neuroscience Graduate Program, Berkeley, CA 94720-3370. Offers PhD. *Degree requirements:* For doctorate, qualifying exam, teaching, research thesis/dissertation. *Entrance requirements:* For doctorate, GRE General Test, minimum GPA of 3.0, 3 letters of recommendation, at least one year of laboratory experience. Additional exam requirements/ recommendations for international students: Required—TOEFL or IELTS. Electronic applications accepted. *Faculty research:* Analysis of ion channels, signal transduction mechanisms, and gene regulation; development of neurons, synapses, and circuits; synapse function and plasticity; mechanisms of sensory processing; principles of function of cerebral cortex; neural basis for learning, attention, and sleep; neural basis for human emotion, language, motor control, and other high-level cognitive processes.

University of California, Davis, Graduate Studies, Graduate Group in Neuroscience, Davis, CA 95616. Offers PhD. *Degree requirements:* For doctorate, thesis/dissertation. *Entrance requirements:* For doctorate, GRE General Test, GRE Subject Test. Additional exam requirements/recommendations for international students: Required—TOEFL (minimum score 550 paper-based). Electronic applications accepted. *Faculty research:* Neuroethology, cognitive neurosciences, cortical neurophysics, cellular and molecular neurobiology.

University of California, Irvine, School of Biological Sciences, Interdepartmental Neuroscience Program, Irvine, CA 92697. Offers PhD. *Students:* 10 full-time (7 women); includes 3 minority (1 Asian, non-Hispanic/Latino; 1 Hispanic/Latino; 1 Two or more races, non-Hispanic/Latino). Average age 25. 168 applicants, 17% accepted, 10 enrolled. *Application deadline:* For fall admission, 12/2 for domestic students. Application fee: $80 ($100 for international students). Electronic applications accepted. *Unit head:* Prof. Albert F. Bennett, Dean, 949-824-5315, Fax: 949-824-3035, E-mail: abennett@uci.edu. *Application contact:* Gary R. Roman, Program Administrator, 949-824-6226, Fax: 949-824-4150, E-mail: gary.roman@uci.edu.
Website: http://www.inp.uci.edu/

University of California, Los Angeles, David Geffen School of Medicine and Graduate Division, Graduate Programs in Medicine, Interdepartmental Program in Neuroscience, Los Angeles, CA 90095. Offers PhD. *Degree requirements:* For doctorate, thesis/ dissertation, oral and written qualifying exams; 1 quarter of teaching experience. *Entrance requirements:* For doctorate, GRE General Test or MCAT, bachelor's degree; minimum undergraduate GPA of 3.0 (or its equivalent if letter grade system not used). Additional exam requirements/recommendations for international students: Required—TOEFL. Electronic applications accepted.

University of California, Riverside, Graduate Division, Program in Neuroscience, Riverside, CA 92521-0102. Offers PhD. *Degree requirements:* For doctorate, comprehensive exam, thesis/dissertation, 2 quarters of teaching experience, qualifying exams. *Entrance requirements:* For doctorate, GRE General Test, minimum GPA of 3.2. Additional exam requirements/recommendations for international students: Required—TOEFL (minimum score 550 paper-based; 80 iBT). Electronic applications accepted. *Faculty research:* Cellular and molecular neuroscience, development and plasticity, systems neuroscience and behavior, computational neuroscience, cognitive neuroscience, medical neuroscience.

University of California, San Diego, Office of Graduate Studies, Department of Structural Engineering, La Jolla, CA 92093. Offers computational neuroscience (PhD); health monitoring, prognosis, and validated simulations (MS); structural engineering (MS, PhD). *Students:* 151 full-time (29 women), 2 part-time (0 women); includes 49 minority (3 Black or African American, non-Hispanic/Latino; 39 Asian, non-Hispanic/ Latino; 7 Hispanic/Latino), 38 international. 437 applicants, 36% accepted, 47 enrolled. In 2013, 33 master's, 11 doctorates awarded. *Degree requirements:* For master's, comprehensive exam or thesis; for doctorate, comprehensive exam, thesis/dissertation, candidacy exam; 1-quarter teaching assistantship. *Entrance requirements:* For master's, GRE General Test, minimum GPA of 3.0; for doctorate, GRE General Test. Additional exam requirements/recommendations for international students: Required—TOEFL (minimum score 550 paper-based; 80 iBT), IELTS. *Application deadline:* For fall admission, 1/6 for domestic students. Application fee: $80 ($100 for international students). Electronic applications accepted. *Expenses:* Tuition, state resident: full-time $11,220; part-time $1870 per quarter. Tuition, nonresident: full-time $26,322; part-time $4387 per quarter. *Required fees:* $519.50 per quarter. Part-time tuition and fees vary according to course load and program. *Financial support:* Fellowships, research assistantships, teaching assistantships, and scholarships/grants available. Financial award application deadline: 3/2; financial award applicants required to submit FAFSA. *Faculty research:* Civil structures, aerospace (composite structures), renewal of structures, earthquake engineering, structural dynamic/vibration modeling and analysis. *Unit head:* J. E. Luco, Chair, 858-534-4338, E-mail: jeluco@ucsd.edu. *Application contact:* Yvonne C. Wilson, Graduate Coordinator, 858-822-1421, E-mail: ywilson@ ucsd.edu.
Website: http://www.structures.ucsd.edu/

University of California, San Diego, Office of Graduate Studies, Interdisciplinary PhD Program in Cognitive Science, La Jolla, CA 92093. Offers cognitive science and anthropology (PhD); cognitive science and communication (PhD); cognitive science and computer science and engineering (PhD); cognitive science and linguistics (PhD); cognitive science and neuroscience (PhD); cognitive science and philosophy (PhD); cognitive science and psychology (PhD); cognitive science and sociology (PhD). Admissions offered through affiliated departments. *Students:* 39 full-time (13 women); includes 7 minority (1 Black or African American, non-Hispanic/Latino; 3 Asian, non-Hispanic/Latino; 3 Hispanic/Latino), 6 international. 152 applicants, 9% accepted, 7 enrolled. In 2013, 3 doctorates awarded. *Degree requirements:* For doctorate, thesis/ dissertation, demonstrated proficiency in another language or 1 quarter of study in approved language course; 1-quarter teaching assistantship for each academic year in residence. *Entrance requirements:* For doctorate, GRE General Test, minimum GPA of 3.0. Additional exam requirements/recommendations for international students: Required—TOEFL (minimum score 550 paper-based; 80 iBT), IELTS. *Application deadline:* For fall admission, 12/2 for domestic students. Application fee: $80 ($100 for international students). Electronic applications accepted. *Expenses:* Tuition, state resident: full-time $11,220; part-time $1870 per quarter. Tuition, nonresident: full-time $26,322; part-time $4387 per quarter. *Required fees:* $519.50 per quarter. Part-time tuition and fees vary according to course load and program. *Financial support:* Fellowships and scholarships/grants available. Financial award applicants required to submit FAFSA. *Faculty research:* Normal development of spatial analytic processing, flexible problem solving, specific language impairment, empirical analysis of change in scientific culture, co-evolutionary analysis of drug resistance in HIV. *Unit head:* Marta Kutas, Chair, 858-534-7141, E-mail: mkutas@ucsd.edu. *Application contact:* Beverley Walton, Graduate Coordinator, 858-534-7141, E-mail: gradinfo@cogsci.ucsd.edu.
Website: http://www.cogsci.ucsd.edu/graduate-study/idp/

University of California, San Diego, School of Medicine and Office of Graduate Studies, Program in Neurosciences, La Jolla, CA 92093. Offers PhD. *Students:* 79 full-time (38 women), 1 (woman) part-time; includes 32 minority (2 Black or African American, non-Hispanic/Latino; 3 American Indian or Alaska Native, non-Hispanic/ Latino; 17 Asian, non-Hispanic/Latino; 10 Hispanic/Latino), 5 international. 499 applicants, 11% accepted, 18 enrolled. In 2013, 14 doctorates awarded. *Degree requirements:* For doctorate, thesis/dissertation, 1-quarter teaching assistantship. *Entrance requirements:* For doctorate, GRE General Test. Additional exam

requirements/recommendations for international students: Required—TOEFL, IELTS. *Application deadline:* For fall admission, 12/1 for domestic students. Application fee: $80 ($100 for international students). Electronic applications accepted. *Expenses:* Tuition, state resident: full-time $11,220; part-time $1870 per quarter. Tuition, nonresident: full-time $26,322; part-time $4387 per quarter. *Required fees:* $519.50 per quarter. Part-time tuition and fees vary according to course load and program. *Financial support:* Fellowships, research assistantships, teaching assistantships, scholarships/grants, tuition waivers, unspecified assistantships, and readerships available. Financial award application deadline: 1/15; financial award applicants required to submit FAFSA. *Faculty research:* Cellular and developmental; biochemistry and molecular; cognitive, behavioral and psychopharmacology; clinical; computational. *Unit head:* Timothy Gentner, Chair, 858-822-6763, E-mail: tgentner@ucsd.edu. *Application contact:* Erin Gilbert, Program Administrator, 858-534-3377, E-mail: neurograd@ucsd.edu.
Website: http://healthsciences.ucsd.edu/education/neurograd/pages/default.aspx

University of California, San Francisco, Graduate Division, Program in Neuroscience, San Francisco, CA 94143. Offers PhD. *Degree requirements:* For doctorate, thesis/dissertation. *Entrance requirements:* For doctorate, GRE General Test or MCAT, official transcripts, two letters of recommendation. Additional exam requirements/recommendations for international students: Required—TOEFL. *Application deadline:* For fall admission, 12/1 for domestic students. Application fee: $40. Electronic applications accepted. *Expenses:* Tuition, state resident: full-time $11,220. Tuition, nonresident: full-time $26,322. *Required fees:* $5204. Full-time tuition and fees vary according to degree level and program. *Financial support:* Application deadline: 1/10. *Faculty research:* Molecular neurobiology, synaptic plasticity, mechanisms of motor learning. *Unit head:* Dr. Roger Nicoll, Director, 415-476-2018, E-mail: roger.nicoll@ucst.edu. *Application contact:* Pat Veitch, Program Administrator, 415-476-2248, Fax: 415-476-2098, E-mail: neuroscience@phy.ucst.edu.
Website: http://www.neuroscience.ucsf.edu/neurograd/

University of California, Santa Barbara, Graduate Division, College of Letters and Sciences, Division of Mathematics, Life, and Physical Sciences, Interdepartmental Graduate Program in Dynamical Neuroscience, Santa Barbara, CA 93106-2014. Offers PhD. *Expenses:* Tuition, state resident: part-time $5148.26 per quarter. Tuition, nonresident: part-time $10,182.26 per quarter. *Unit head:* Prof. Gregory Ashby, Department Chair, 805-893-7909, E-mail: ashby@psych.ucsb.edu. *Application contact:* Graduate Admissions Coordinator, 805-893-2104, Fax: 805-893-8259, E-mail: gradadmissions@graddiv.ucsb.edu.
Website: http://www.dyns.ucsb.edu/program.html

University of Chicago, Division of Biological Sciences, Neuroscience Graduate Programs, Committee on Computational Neuroscience, Chicago, IL 60637-1513. Offers PhD. *Degree requirements:* For doctorate, thesis/dissertation, ethics class, 2 teaching assistantships. *Entrance requirements:* For doctorate, GRE General Test. Additional exam requirements/recommendations for international students: Required—TOEFL (minimum score 600 paper-based; 104 iBT), IELTS (minimum score 7). Electronic applications accepted.

University of Chicago, Division of Biological Sciences, Neuroscience Graduate Programs, Committee on Integrative Neuroscience, Chicago, IL 60637-1513. Offers cell physiology (PhD); pharmacological and physiological sciences (PhD). *Degree requirements:* For doctorate, thesis/dissertation, preliminary exam. *Entrance requirements:* For doctorate, GRE General Test. Additional exam requirements/recommendations for international students: Required—TOEFL. Electronic applications accepted. *Faculty research:* Psychopharmacology, neuropharmacology.

University of Cincinnati, Graduate School, Interdisciplinary PhD Study Program in Neuroscience, Cincinnati, OH 45221. Offers PhD. *Degree requirements:* For doctorate, thesis/dissertation, qualifying exam. *Entrance requirements:* For doctorate, GRE General Test. Additional exam requirements/recommendations for international students: Required—TOEFL. Electronic applications accepted. *Faculty research:* Developmental neurobiology, membrane and channel biophysics, molecular neurobiology, neuroendocrinology, neuronal cell biology.

University of Colorado Denver, School of Medicine, Program in Neuroscience, Aurora, CO 80045. Offers PhD. *Students:* 36 full-time (15 women); includes 4 minority (1 Black or African American, non-Hispanic/Latino; 1 Asian, non-Hispanic/Latino; 1 Hispanic/Latino; 1 Two or more races, non-Hispanic/Latino), 1 international. Average age 28. 27 applicants, 7% accepted, 2 enrolled. In 2013, 3 doctorates awarded. *Degree requirements:* For doctorate, comprehensive exam, thesis/dissertation, structured class schedule each year paired with lab rotations. *Entrance requirements:* For doctorate, GRE, baccalaureate degree in a biological science, chemistry, physics or engineering (recommended); minimum GPA of 3.2. Additional exam requirements/recommendations for international students: Required—TOEFL (minimum score 550 paper-based; 80 iBT). *Application deadline:* For fall admission, 12/1 for domestic students, 11/1 priority date for international students. Application fee: $50 ($75 for international students). Electronic applications accepted. *Expenses:* Contact institution. *Financial support:* In 2013–14, 36 students received support. Fellowships, research assistantships, teaching assistantships, Federal Work-Study, institutionally sponsored loans, scholarships/grants, traineeships, health care benefits, tuition waivers (full), and unspecified assistantships available. Financial award application deadline: 3/15; financial award applicants required to submit FAFSA. *Faculty research:* Neurobiology of olfaction, ion channels, schizophrenia, spinal cord regeneration, neurotransplantation. *Unit head:* Dr. Wendy Macklin, Professor and Chair, 303-724-3426, Fax: 303-724-3420, E-mail: wendy.macklin@ucdenver.edu. *Application contact:* Emily Dailey, Program Administrator, 303-724-3120, Fax: 303-724-3121, E-mail: emily.dailey@ucdenver.edu.
Website: http://www.ucdenver.edu/academics/colleges/medicalschool/programs/Neuroscience/Pages/Neuroscience.aspx

University of Connecticut, Graduate School, College of Liberal Arts and Sciences, Department of Psychology, Storrs, CT 06269. Offers behavioral neuroscience (PhD); biopsychology (PhD); clinical psychology (MA, PhD); cognition and instruction (PhD); developmental psychology (MA, PhD); ecological psychology (PhD); experimental psychology (PhD); general psychology (MA, PhD); health psychology (Graduate Certificate); industrial/organizational psychology (PhD); language and cognition (PhD); neuroscience (PhD); occupational health psychology (Graduate Certificate); social psychology (MA, PhD). *Accreditation:* APA. Terminal master's awarded for partial completion of doctoral program. *Degree requirements:* For master's, comprehensive exam; for doctorate, thesis/dissertation. *Entrance requirements:* For master's and doctorate, GRE General Test, GRE Subject Test. Additional exam requirements/recommendations for international students: Required—TOEFL (minimum score 550 paper-based). Electronic applications accepted.

University of Connecticut Health Center, Graduate School, Programs in Biomedical Sciences, Program in Neuroscience, Farmington, CT 06030. Offers PhD, DMD/PhD, MD/PhD. *Degree requirements:* For doctorate, comprehensive exam, thesis/dissertation. *Entrance requirements:* For doctorate, GRE General Test, interview (recommended). Additional exam requirements/recommendations for international students: Required—TOEFL (minimum score 600 paper-based). Electronic applications accepted. *Faculty research:* Molecular and systems neuroscience, neuroanatomy, neurophysiology, neurochemistry, neuropathology.

See Display below and Close-Up on page 387.

University of Delaware, College of Arts and Sciences, Department of Psychology, Newark, DE 19716. Offers behavioral neuroscience (PhD); clinical psychology (PhD);

cognitive psychology (PhD); social psychology (PhD). *Accreditation:* APA. *Degree requirements:* For doctorate, thesis/dissertation. *Entrance requirements:* For doctorate, GRE General Test. Additional exam requirements/recommendations for international students: Required—TOEFL (minimum score 600 paper-based). Electronic applications accepted. *Faculty research:* Emotion development, neural and cognitive aspects of memory, neural control of feeding, intergroup relations, social cognition and communication.

University of Denver, Division of Arts, Humanities and Social Sciences, Department of Psychology, Denver, CO 80208. Offers affective/social psychology (PhD); clinical child psychology (PhD); cognitive psychology (PhD); developmental cognitive neuroscience (PhD); developmental psychology (PhD). *Accreditation:* APA. *Faculty:* 24 full-time (11 women), 2 part-time/adjunct (both women). *Students:* 21 full-time (20 women), 7 part-time (all women); includes 6 minority (2 Black or African American, non-Hispanic/Latino; 3 Asian, non-Hispanic/Latino; 1 Hispanic/Latino), 2 international. Average age 27. 367 applicants, 3% accepted, 7 enrolled. In 2013, 5 doctorates awarded. Terminal master's awarded for partial completion of doctoral program. *Degree requirements:* For doctorate, variable foreign language requirement, comprehensive exam (for some programs), thesis/dissertation. *Entrance requirements:* For doctorate, GRE General Test, master's degree, transcripts, biographical statement, three letters of recommendation. Additional exam requirements/recommendations for international students: Required—TOEFL (minimum score 550 paper-based; 80 iBT). *Application deadline:* For fall admission, 12/1 priority date for domestic and international students. Application fee: $65. Electronic applications accepted. *Financial support:* In 2013–14, 28 students received support, including 14 research assistantships with full and partial tuition reimbursements available (averaging $23,026 per year), 22 teaching assistantships with full and partial tuition reimbursements available (averaging $26,647 per year); Federal Work-Study, institutionally sponsored loans, scholarships/grants, and unspecified assistantships also available. Support available to part-time students. Financial award application deadline: 2/15; financial award applicants required to submit FAFSA. *Faculty research:* Developmental cognitive neuroscience, social and emotional processes, child and adolescent development, clinical child psychology. *Total annual research expenditures:* $3.5 million. *Unit head:* Dr. Daniel McIntosh, Chair, 303-871-3712, Fax: 303-871-4747, E-mail: daniel.mcintosh@du.edu. *Application contact:* Paula Houghtaling, Graduate Program Administrator, 303-871-3803, Fax: 303-871-4747, E-mail: phoughta@du.edu.
Website: http://www.du.edu/ahss/psychology/index.html

University of Florida, College of Medicine and Graduate School, Interdisciplinary Program in Biomedical Sciences, Concentration in Neuroscience, Gainesville, FL 32611. Offers PhD. *Degree requirements:* For doctorate, thesis/dissertation. *Entrance requirements:* For doctorate, GRE General Test, minimum GPA of 3.0, biochemistry before enrollment. Additional exam requirements/recommendations for international students: Required—TOEFL. Electronic applications accepted. *Expenses:* Tuition, state resident: full-time $12,640. Tuition, nonresident: full-time $30,000. *Faculty research:* Neural injury and repair, neurophysiology, neurotoxicology, cellular and molecular neurobiology, neuroimmunology and endocrinology.

University of Georgia, Biomedical and Health Sciences Institute, Athens, GA 30602. Offers neuroscience (PhD). *Entrance requirements:* For doctorate, GRE, official transcripts, 3 letters of recommendation, statement of interest. Additional exam requirements/recommendations for international students: Required—TOEFL.

University of Guelph, Ontario Veterinary College and Graduate Studies, Graduate Programs in Veterinary Sciences, Department of Biomedical Sciences, Guelph, ON N1G 2W1, Canada. Offers morphology (M Sc, DV Sc, PhD); neuroscience (M Sc, DV Sc, PhD); pharmacology (M Sc, DV Sc, PhD); physiology (M Sc, DV Sc, PhD); toxicology (M Sc, DV Sc, PhD). Part-time programs available. *Degree requirements:* For master's, thesis; for doctorate, comprehensive exam, thesis/dissertation. *Entrance requirements:* For master's, honors B Sc, minimum 75% average in last 20 courses; for doctorate, M Sc with thesis from accredited institution. Additional exam requirements/recommendations for international students: Required—TOEFL (minimum score 550 paper-based; 89 iBT). Electronic applications accepted. *Faculty research:* Cellular morphology; endocrine, vascular and reproductive physiology; clinical pharmacology; veterinary toxicology; developmental biology, neuroscience.

University of Guelph, Ontario Veterinary College and Graduate Studies, Graduate Programs in Veterinary Sciences, Department of Clinical Studies, Guelph, ON N1G 2W1, Canada. Offers anesthesiology (M Sc, DV Sc); cardiology (DV Sc, Diploma); clinical studies (Diploma); dermatology (M Sc); diagnostic imaging (M Sc, DV Sc); emergency/critical care (M Sc, DV Sc, Diploma); medicine (M Sc, DV Sc); neurology (M Sc, DV Sc); ophthalmology (M Sc, DV Sc); surgery (M Sc, DV Sc). *Degree requirements:* For master's, thesis; for doctorate, comprehensive exam, thesis/dissertation. *Entrance requirements:* Additional exam requirements/recommendations for international students: Required—TOEFL (minimum score 550 paper-based), IELTS (minimum score 6.5). Electronic applications accepted. *Faculty research:* Orthopedics, respirology, oncology, exercise physiology, cardiology.

University of Hartford, College of Arts and Sciences, Department of Biology, Program in Neuroscience, West Hartford, CT 06117-1599. Offers MS. Part-time and evening/weekend programs available. *Degree requirements:* For master's, comprehensive exam, thesis optional, oral exams. *Entrance requirements:* For master's, GRE General Test, GRE Subject Test, MCAT. Additional exam requirements/recommendations for international students: Required—TOEFL (minimum score 550 paper-based). Electronic applications accepted. *Faculty research:* Neurobiology of aging, central actions of neural steroids, neuroendocrine control of reproduction, retinopathies in sharks, plasticity in the central nervous system.

University of Idaho, College of Graduate Studies, Program in Neuroscience, Moscow, ID 83844-3051. Offers MS, PhD. *Faculty:* 6 full-time, 1 part-time/adjunct. *Students:* 7 full-time, 2 part-time. Average age 28. *Entrance requirements:* Additional exam requirements/recommendations for international students: Required—TOEFL. *Application deadline:* For fall admission, 2/15 for domestic students. Applications are processed on a rolling basis. Application fee: $60. Electronic applications accepted. *Expenses:* Tuition, state resident: full-time $5596; part-time $363 per credit hour. Tuition, nonresident: full-time $18,672; part-time $1089 per credit hour. *Financial support:* Applicants required to submit FAFSA. *Unit head:* Dr. Steffen Werner, Director, 208-885-6010, Fax: 208-885-6198, E-mail: neuro@uidaho.edu. *Application contact:* Stephane Thomas, Graduate Recruitment Coordinator, 208-885-4001, Fax: 208-885-4406, E-mail: gadms@uidaho.edu.
Website: http://www.uidaho.edu/cogs/neuroscience

University of Illinois at Chicago, Graduate College, Program in Neuroscience, Chicago, IL 60612. Offers cellular and systems neuroscience and cell biology (PhD); neuroscience (MS). *Students:* 17 full-time (9 women); includes 3 minority (1 Asian, non-Hispanic/Latino; 1 Hispanic/Latino; 1 Two or more races, non-Hispanic/Latino), 3 international. Average age 28. 63 applicants, 13% accepted, 6 enrolled. In 2013, 5 doctorates awarded. *Expenses:* Tuition, state resident: full-time $11,066; part-time $3689 per term. Tuition, nonresident: full-time $23,064; part-time $7688 per term. *Required fees:* $3004; $1190 per term. Tuition and fees vary according to course level and program. *Unit head:* Dr. Daniel Corcos, Program Chair, 312-355-1708, Fax: 312-423-3699, E-mail: dcorcos@uic.edu. *Application contact:* Perry Clark, Program Coordinator, 312-413-0185, Fax: 312-413-0354, E-mail: pclark5@uic.edu.
Website: http://www.uic.edu/depts/neurosci/

University of Illinois at Urbana–Champaign, Graduate College, College of Liberal Arts and Sciences, School of Molecular and Cellular Biology, Neuroscience Program, Champaign, IL 61820. Offers PhD. *Students:* 60 (34 women). Application fee: $75 ($90 for international students). *Unit head:* Neal J. Cohen, Director, 217-244-4339, Fax: 217-244-4339, E-mail: njc@illinois.edu. *Application contact:* Sam Beshers, Program Coordinator, 217-333-4971, Fax: 217-244-3499, E-mail: beshers@illinois.edu.
Website: http://neuroscience.illinois.edu/

The University of Iowa, Graduate College, Program in Neuroscience, Iowa City, IA 52242-1316. Offers PhD. *Degree requirements:* For doctorate, comprehensive exam, thesis/dissertation. *Entrance requirements:* For doctorate, GRE General Test, minimum GPA of 3.0. Additional exam requirements/recommendations for international students: Required—TOEFL (minimum score 600 paper-based; 100 iBT). Electronic applications accepted. *Faculty research:* Molecular, cellular, and developmental systems; behavioral neurosciences.

The University of Kansas, Graduate Studies, School of Pharmacy, Department of Pharmacology and Toxicology, Lawrence, KS 66045. Offers neurosciences (MS, PhD); pharmacology and toxicology (MS, PhD). *Faculty:* 12. *Students:* 24 full-time (20 women); includes 1 minority (Two or more races, non-Hispanic/Latino), 12 international. Average age 26. 64 applicants, 9% accepted, 4 enrolled. In 2013, 3 master's, 4 doctorates awarded. Terminal master's awarded for partial completion of doctoral program. *Degree requirements:* For master's, comprehensive exam; for doctorate, comprehensive exam, thesis/dissertation. *Entrance requirements:* For master's and doctorate, GRE General Test, bachelor's degree in related field, 3 letters of recommendation, resume or curriculum vitae, official transcripts, 1-2 page personal statement. Additional exam requirements/recommendations for international students: Required—TOEFL (minimum score 600 paper-based; 100 iBT). *Application deadline:* For fall admission, 1/1 priority date for domestic students, 1/15 priority date for international students. Application fee: $55 ($65 for international students). Electronic applications accepted. *Financial support:* Fellowships with full tuition reimbursements, research assistantships with full tuition reimbursements, and teaching assistantships available. Financial award application deadline: 2/1. *Faculty research:* Molecular neurobiology, gene regulation, neurotransmitter receptors, drug metabolism. *Unit head:* Nancy Muma, Chair, 785-864-4002, Fax: 785-864-5219, E-mail: nmuma@ku.edu. *Application contact:* Debbie Thompson, Senior Administrative Associate, 785-864-4002, Fax: 785-864-1010, E-mail: djthompson@ku.edu.
Website: http://pharmtox.ku.edu/

The University of Kansas, Graduate Studies, School of Pharmacy, Program in Neurosciences, Lawrence, KS 66047. Offers MS, PhD. *Faculty:* 12. *Students:* 10 full-time (6 women); includes 1 minority (Two or more races, non-Hispanic/Latino), 1 international. Average age 28. 23 applicants. In 2013, 2 doctorates awarded. *Degree requirements:* For master's, comprehensive exam, thesis; for doctorate, comprehensive exam, thesis/dissertation. *Entrance requirements:* For master's, GRE, BA or BS in neuroscience or a related study, three letters of recommendation, personal statement, minimum GPA of 3.0; for doctorate, GRE. Additional exam requirements/recommendations for international students: Required—TOEFL. *Application deadline:* For fall admission, 1/15 priority date for domestic and international students. Applications are processed on a rolling basis. Application fee: $55 ($65 for international students). Electronic applications accepted. *Financial support:* Fellowships with partial tuition reimbursements, research assistantships with full tuition reimbursements, and teaching assistantships with full tuition reimbursements available. Financial award application deadline: 1/15. *Unit head:* Ruth Anne Atchley, Professor/Director, 785-864-4131, E-mail: ratchley@ku.edu. *Application contact:* Susan D. Wakefield, Program Assistant, 785-864-7339, Fax: 785-864-5738, E-mail: swakefield@ku.edu.
Website: http://www.neuroscience.ku.edu/

The University of Kansas, University of Kansas Medical Center, School of Medicine, Department of Molecular and Integrative Physiology, Neuroscience Graduate Program, Kansas City, KS 66045-7582. Offers MS, PhD. *Students:* 5 full-time (3 women); includes 1 minority (Two or more races, non-Hispanic/Latino). Average age 27. *Degree requirements:* For master's, thesis; for doctorate, comprehensive exam, thesis/dissertation. *Entrance requirements:* For master's and doctorate, GRE. Additional exam requirements/recommendations for international students: Required—TOEFL. *Financial support:* Fellowships with partial tuition reimbursements, research assistantships with full tuition reimbursements, and teaching assistantships with full tuition reimbursements available. Financial award application deadline: 3/1; financial award applicants required to submit FAFSA. *Unit head:* Dr. Paul D. Cheney, Chair of Molecular and Integrative Physiology, 913-588-7400, Fax: 913-588-7430, E-mail: pcheney@kumc.edu. *Application contact:* Marcia Jones, Director of Graduate Studies, 913-588-1238, Fax: 913-588-5242, E-mail: mjones@kumc.edu.
Website: http://www.neuroscience.ku.edu/

University of Lethbridge, School of Graduate Studies, Lethbridge, AB T1K 3M4, Canada. Offers accounting (MScM); addictions counseling (M Sc); agricultural biotechnology (M Sc); agricultural studies (M Sc, MA); anthropology (MA); archaeology (M Sc, MA); art (MA, MFA); biochemistry (M Sc); biological sciences (M Sc); biomolecular science (PhD); biosystems and biodiversity (PhD); Canadian studies (MA); chemistry (M Sc); computer science (M Sc); computer science and geographical information science (M Sc); counseling (MC); counseling psychology (M Ed); dramatic arts (MA); earth, space, and physical science (PhD); economics (MA); education (MA); educational leadership (M Ed); English (MA); environmental science (M Sc); evolution and behavior (PhD); exercise science (M Sc); finance (MScM); French (MA); French/German (MA); French/Spanish (MA); general education (M Ed); general management (MScM); geography (M Sc, MA); German (MA); health sciences (M Sc); human resource management and labour relations (MScM); individualized multidisciplinary (M Sc, MA); information systems (MScM); international management (MScM); kinesiology (M Sc, MA); marketing (MScM); mathematics (M Sc); modern languages (MA); music (M Mus, MA); Native American studies (MA); neuroscience (M Sc, PhD); new media (MA, MFA); nursing (M Sc); philosophy (MA); physics (M Sc); policy and strategy (MScM); political science (MA); psychology (M Sc, MA); religious studies (MA); sociology (MA); theatre and dramatic arts (MFA); theoretical and computational science (PhD); urban and regional studies (MA); women and gender studies (MA). Part-time and evening/weekend programs available. *Degree requirements:* For doctorate, comprehensive exam, thesis/dissertation. *Entrance requirements:* For master's, GMAT (for M Sc in management), bachelor's degree in related field, minimum GPA of 3.0 during previous 20 graded semester courses, 2 years teaching or related experience (M Ed); for doctorate, master's degree, minimum graduate GPA of 3.5. Additional exam requirements/recommendations for international students: Required—TOEFL. Application fee: $60 Canadian dollars. *Financial support:* Fellowships, research assistantships, teaching assistantships, scholarships/grants, health care benefits, and unspecified assistantships available. *Faculty research:* Movement and brain plasticity, gibberellin physiology, photosynthesis, carbon cycling, molecular properties of main-

group ring components. *Application contact:* School of Graduate Studies, 403-329-2793, Fax: 403-332-5239, E-mail: sgsinquiries@uleth.ca.
Website: http://www.uleth.ca/graduatestudies/

University of Maine, Graduate School, Graduate School of Biomedical Science and Engineering, Orono, ME 04469. Offers bioinformatics (PSM); biomedical engineering (PhD); cell and molecular biology (PhD); neuroscience (PhD); toxicology (PhD). *Faculty:* 39 full-time (10 women), 31 part-time/adjunct (8 women). *Students:* 31 full-time (18 women), 5 part-time (4 women), 11 international. Average age 30. 57 applicants, 16% accepted, 7 enrolled. In 2013, 5 doctorates awarded. *Degree requirements:* For doctorate, comprehensive exam, thesis/dissertation. *Entrance requirements:* For doctorate, GRE General Test, master's degree. Additional exam requirements/recommendations for international students: Required—TOEFL. *Application deadline:* For fall admission, 1/1 for domestic students. Application fee: $65. *Expenses:* Tuition, state resident: full-time $7524. Tuition, nonresident: full-time $23,112. *Required fees:* $1970. *Financial support:* In 2013–14, 16 students received support, including 1 fellowship with full tuition reimbursement available (averaging $18,000 per year), 13 research assistantships with full tuition reimbursements available (averaging $21,000 per year), 2 teaching assistantships (averaging $20,000 per year). *Faculty research:* Biomedical engineering, toxicology, neuroscience, cell and molecular biology, bioinformatics. *Total annual research expenditures:* $650,000. *Unit head:* Dr. David Neivandt, Director, 207-581-2803. *Application contact:* Scott G. Delcourt, Associate Dean of the Graduate School, 207-581-3291, Fax: 207-581-3232, E-mail: graduate@maine.edu.
Website: http://gsbse.umaine.edu/

The University of Manchester, Faculty of Life Sciences, Manchester, United Kingdom. Offers adaptive organismal biology (M Phil, PhD); animal biology (M Phil, PhD); biochemistry (M Phil, PhD); bioinformatics (M Phil, PhD); biomolecular sciences (M Phil, PhD); biotechnology (M Phil, PhD); cell biology (M Phil, PhD); cell matrix research (M Phil, PhD); channels and transporters (M Phil, PhD); developmental biology (M Phil, PhD); Egyptology (M Phil, PhD); environmental biology (M Phil, PhD); evolutionary biology (M Phil, PhD); gene expression (M Phil, PhD); genetics (M Phil, PhD); history of science, technology and medicine (M Phil, PhD); immunology (M Phil, PhD); integrative neurobiology and behavior (M Phil, PhD); membrane trafficking (M Phil, PhD); microbiology (M Phil, PhD); molecular and cellular neuroscience (M Phil, PhD); molecular biology (M Phil, PhD); molecular cancer studies (M Phil, PhD); neuroscience (M Phil, PhD); ophthalmology (M Phil, PhD); optometry (M Phil, PhD); organelle function (M Phil, PhD); pharmacology (M Phil, PhD); physiology (M Phil, PhD); plant sciences (M Phil, PhD); stem cell research (M Phil, PhD); structural biology (M Phil, PhD); systems neuroscience (M Phil, PhD); toxicology (M Phil, PhD).

University of Maryland, Baltimore, Graduate School, Graduate Program in Life Sciences, Program in Neuroscience, Baltimore, MD 21201. Offers PhD, MD/PhD. Part-time programs available. *Students:* 48 full-time (25 women), 5 part-time (2 women); includes 10 minority (1 Black or African American, non-Hispanic/Latino; 5 Asian, non-Hispanic/Latino; 2 Hispanic/Latino; 2 Two or more races, non-Hispanic/Latino), 3 international. Average age 27. 85 applicants, 9% accepted, 7 enrolled. In 2013, 9 doctorates awarded. *Degree requirements:* For doctorate, comprehensive exam, thesis/dissertation. *Entrance requirements:* For doctorate, GRE General Test, minimum GPA of 3.0. Additional exam requirements/recommendations for international students: Required—TOEFL (minimum score 550 paper-based; 80 iBT); Recommended—IELTS (minimum score 7). *Application deadline:* For fall admission, 12/1 for domestic students, 1/15 for international students. Application fee: $75. Electronic applications accepted. *Financial support:* In 2013–14, research assistantships with partial tuition reimbursements (averaging $25,000 per year) were awarded; fellowships, health care benefits, and unspecified assistantships also available. Financial award application deadline: 3/1; financial award applicants required to submit FAFSA. *Faculty research:* Molecular, biochemical, and cellular pharmacology; membrane biophysics; synaptology; developmental neurobiology. *Unit head:* Dr. Jessica Mong, Director, 410-706-4295, E-mail: jmong@umaryland.edu. *Application contact:* Rachael Holms, Coordinator, 410-706-4701, Fax: 410-706-4724, E-mail: neurosci@umaryland.edu.
Website: http://neuroscience.umaryland.edu

University of Maryland, Baltimore County, Graduate School, College of Natural and Mathematical Sciences, Department of Biological Sciences, Program in Neuroscience and Cognitive Sciences, Baltimore, MD 21250. Offers PhD. *Faculty:* 5 full-time (3 women). *Students:* 2 full-time (1 woman); includes 1 minority (Black or African American, non-Hispanic/Latino), 1 international. Average age 24. 13 applicants, 8% accepted, 1 enrolled. In 2013, 1 doctorate awarded. *Degree requirements:* For doctorate, thesis/dissertation. *Entrance requirements:* For doctorate, GRE General Test, minimum GPA of 3.0. Additional exam requirements/recommendations for international students: Required—TOEFL (minimum score 80 iBT). *Application deadline:* For fall admission, 1/1 priority date for domestic and international students. Application fee: $50. Electronic applications accepted. One-time fee: $200 full-time. *Financial support:* In 2013–14, 2 students received support, including 1 fellowship with full tuition reimbursement available (averaging $22,000 per year), 1 research assistantship with full tuition reimbursement available (averaging $22,726 per year). *Unit head:* Dr. Stephen Miller, Graduate Program Director, 410-455-3669, Fax: 410-455-3875, E-mail: biograd@umbc.edu. *Application contact:* Dr. Stephen Miller, Director, 410-455-3381, Fax: 410-455-3875, E-mail: biograd@umbc.edu.
Website: http://biology.umbc.edu

University of Maryland, College Park, Academic Affairs, College of Behavioral and Social Sciences, Department of Hearing and Speech Sciences, College Park, MD 20742. Offers audiology (MA, PhD); hearing and speech sciences (Au D); language pathology (MA, PhD); neuroscience (PhD); speech (MA, PhD). *Accreditation:* ASHA (one or more programs are accredited). *Faculty:* 19 full-time (18 women), 14 part-time/adjunct (12 women). *Students:* 70 full-time (65 women), 24 part-time (22 women); includes 11 minority (3 Black or African American, non-Hispanic/Latino; 2 Asian, non-Hispanic/Latino; 3 Hispanic/Latino; 3 Two or more races, non-Hispanic/Latino), 1 international. 385 applicants, 19% accepted, 21 enrolled. In 2013, 19 master's, 5 doctorates awarded. *Degree requirements:* For master's, thesis optional; for doctorate, thesis/dissertation, written and oral exams. *Entrance requirements:* For master's, GRE General Test, minimum GPA of 3.5, 3 letters of recommendation; for doctorate, GRE General Test, minimum GPA of 3.5. Additional exam requirements/recommendations for international students: Required—TOEFL. *Application deadline:* For fall admission, 1/15 for domestic and international students. Applications are processed on a rolling basis. Application fee: $75. Electronic applications accepted. *Expenses:* Tuition, state resident: full-time $10,314; part-time $573 per credit hour. Tuition, nonresident: full-time $22,248; part-time $1236 per credit. *Required fees:* $1446; $403.15 per semester. Tuition and fees vary according to program. *Financial support:* In 2013–14, 2 fellowships with full tuition reimbursements (averaging $37,014 per year), 1 research assistantship (averaging $15,266 per year), 2 teaching assistantships (averaging $15,355 per year) were awarded; career-related internships or fieldwork, Federal Work-Study, scholarships/grants, and health care benefits also available. Support available to part-time students. Financial award applicants required to submit FAFSA. *Faculty research:* Speech perception, language acquisition, bilingualism, hearing loss. *Total annual research expenditures:* $734,130. *Unit head:* Dr. Nan B. Bernstein-Ratner, Chair, 301-405-4217, Fax: 301-314-2023, E-mail: nratner@umd.edu. *Application contact:* Dr. Charles A. Caramello, Dean of Graduate School, 301-405-0358, Fax: 301-314-9305.

University of Maryland, College Park, Academic Affairs, College of Behavioral and Social Sciences, Program in Neurosciences and Cognitive Sciences, College Park, MD 20742. Offers PhD. *Faculty:* 6 full-time (3 women). *Students:* 48 full-time (21 women), 4 part-time (3 women); includes 7 minority (4 Black or African American, non-Hispanic/Latino; 2 Asian, non-Hispanic/Latino; 1 Two or more races, non-Hispanic/Latino), 12 international. 114 applicants, 8% accepted, 4 enrolled. In 2013, 5 doctorates awarded. *Degree requirements:* For doctorate, comprehensive exam, thesis/dissertation. *Entrance requirements:* For doctorate, GRE General Test, 3 letters of recommendation. Additional exam requirements/recommendations for international students: Required—TOEFL. *Application deadline:* For fall admission, 12/1 for domestic and international students. Applications are processed on a rolling basis. Application fee: $75. Electronic applications accepted. *Expenses:* Tuition, state resident: full-time $10,314; part-time $573 per credit hour. Tuition, nonresident: full-time $22,248; part-time $1236 per credit. *Required fees:* $1446; $403.15 per semester. Tuition and fees vary according to program. *Financial support:* In 2013–14, 18 fellowships with full and partial tuition reimbursements (averaging $24,189 per year), 15 research assistantships (averaging $18,110 per year), 27 teaching assistantships (averaging $17,417 per year) were awarded; Federal Work-Study and scholarships/grants also available. Support available to part-time students. Financial award applicants required to submit FAFSA. *Faculty research:* Molecular neurobiology, cognition, neural and behavioral systems language, memory, human development. *Unit head:* Robert Dooling, Director, 301-405-5925, Fax: 301-405-7104, E-mail: rdooling@umd.edu. *Application contact:* Dr. Charles A. Caramello, Dean of Graduate School, 301-405-0358, Fax: 301-314-9305, E-mail: ccaramel@umd.edu.

University of Massachusetts Amherst, Graduate School, Interdisciplinary Programs, Program in Neuroscience and Behavior, Amherst, MA 01003. Offers animal behavior and learning (PhD); molecular and cellular neuroscience (PhD); neural and behavioral development (PhD); neuroendocrinology (PhD); neuroscience and behavior (MS); sensorimotor, cognitive, and computational neuroscience (PhD). *Students:* 27 full-time (19 women), 2 part-time (0 women); includes 4 minority (1 Asian, non-Hispanic/Latino; 3 Hispanic/Latino), 4 international. Average age 27. 129 applicants, 11% accepted, 8 enrolled. In 2013, 3 master's awarded. Terminal master's awarded for partial completion of doctoral program. *Degree requirements:* For master's, thesis or alternative; for doctorate, comprehensive exam, thesis/dissertation. *Entrance requirements:* For master's, GRE General Test; for doctorate, GRE General Test; GRE Subect Test in psychology, biology, or mathematics (recommended). Additional exam requirements/recommendations for international students: Required—TOEFL (minimum score 550 paper-based; 80 iBT), IELTS (minimum score 6.5). *Application deadline:* For fall admission, 12/15 for domestic and international students. Applications are processed on a rolling basis. Application fee: $75. Electronic applications accepted. *Financial support:* Fellowships with full and partial tuition reimbursements, research assistantships with full and partial tuition reimbursements, teaching assistantships with full and partial tuition reimbursements, career-related internships or fieldwork, Federal Work-Study, scholarships/grants, traineeships, health care benefits, tuition waivers (full and partial), and unspecified assistantships available. Support available to part-time students. Financial award application deadline: 12/14; financial award applicants required to submit FAFSA. *Unit head:* Dr. Jeffrey D. Blaustein, Graduate Program Director, 413-545-2046, Fax: 413-545-3243, E-mail: nsb@bio.umass.edu. *Application contact:* Lindsay DeSantis, Supervisor of Admissions, 413-545-0722, Fax: 413-577-0010, E-mail: gradadm@grad.umass.edu.
Website: http://www.umass.edu/neuro/

University of Massachusetts Worcester, Graduate School of Biomedical Sciences, Worcester, MA 01655-0115. Offers biochemistry and molecular pharmacology (PhD); bioinformatics and computational biology (PhD); cancer biology (PhD); cell biology (PhD); clinical and population health research (PhD); clinical investigation (MS); immunology and virology (PhD); interdisciplinary biomedical research (PhD); millennium (PhD); molecular genetics and microbiology (PhD); neuroscience (PhD); translational science (PhD); MD/PhD. *Faculty:* 1,388 full-time (521 women), 309 part-time/adjunct (198 women). *Students:* 385 full-time (210 women); includes 53 minority (13 Black or African American, non-Hispanic/Latino; 30 Asian, non-Hispanic/Latino; 10 Hispanic/Latino), 138 international. Average age 28. 491 applicants, 19% accepted, 39 enrolled. In 2013, 5 master's, 50 doctorates awarded. Terminal master's awarded for partial completion of doctoral program. *Median time to degree:* Of those who began their doctoral program in fall 2005, 67% received their degree in 8 years or less. *Degree requirements:* For master's, comprehensive exam, thesis; for doctorate, comprehensive exam, thesis/dissertation. *Entrance requirements:* For master's, MD, PhD, DVM, or PharmD; for doctorate, GRE General Test, bachelor's degree. Additional exam requirements/recommendations for international students: Required—TOEFL (minimum score 100 iBT) or IELTS (minimum score 7.5). *Application deadline:* For fall admission, 12/15 for domestic and international students; for spring admission, 5/15 for domestic students. Application fee: $80. Electronic applications accepted. *Expenses:* Contact institution. *Financial support:* In 2013–14, 431 students received support, including research assistantships with full tuition reimbursements available (averaging $29,500 per year); scholarships/grants, health care benefits, tuition waivers (full), and unspecified assistantships also available. Financial award application deadline: 5/16. *Faculty research:* RNA interference, cell/molecular/developmental biology, bioinformatics, clinical/translational research, infectious disease. *Total annual research expenditures:* $245.9 million. *Unit head:* Dr. Anthony Carruthers, Dean, 508-856-4135, E-mail: anthony.carruthers@umassmed.edu. *Application contact:* Dr. Kendall Knight, Associate Dean and Interim Director of Admissions and Recruitment, 508-856-5628, Fax: 508-856-3659, E-mail: kendall.knight@umassmed.edu.
Website: http://www.umassmed.edu/gsbs/

University of Miami, Graduate School, College of Arts and Sciences, Department of Psychology, Coral Gables, FL 33124. Offers adult clinical (PhD); behavioral neuroscience (PhD); child clinical (PhD); developmental psychology (PhD); health clinical (PhD); psychology (MS). *Accreditation:* APA (one or more programs are accredited). *Degree requirements:* For doctorate, comprehensive exam, thesis/dissertation. *Entrance requirements:* For doctorate, GRE General Test, minimum GPA of 3.5. Additional exam requirements/recommendations for international students: Required—TOEFL. Electronic applications accepted. *Faculty research:* Behavioral factors in cardiovascular disease and cancer adult psychopathology, developmental disabilities, social and emotional development, mechanisms of coping.

University of Miami, Graduate School, Miller School of Medicine, Graduate Programs in Medicine, Neuroscience Program, Coral Gables, FL 33124. Offers PhD, MD/PhD. *Degree requirements:* For doctorate, thesis/dissertation, qualifying exam. *Entrance requirements:* For doctorate, GRE General Test. Additional exam requirements/recommendations for international students: Required—TOEFL (minimum score 550 paper-based). Electronic applications accepted. *Faculty research:* Cellular and molecular biology, transduction, nerve regeneration and embryonic development, membrane biophysics.

Neuroscience

University of Michigan, Rackham Graduate School, College of Literature, Science, and the Arts, Department of Psychology, Ann Arbor, MI 48109. Offers biopsychology (PhD); clinical science (PhD); cognition and cognitive neuroscience (PhD); developmental psychology (PhD); personality and social contexts (PhD); social psychology (PhD). *Accreditation:* APA. *Faculty:* 80 full-time (36 women), 32 part-time/adjunct (21 women). *Students:* 138 full-time (94 women); includes 62 minority (16 Black or African American, non-Hispanic/Latino; 2 American Indian or Alaska Native, non-Hispanic/Latino; 17 Asian, non-Hispanic/Latino; 25 Hispanic/Latino; 2 Two or more races, non-Hispanic/Latino), 12 international. Average age 27. 611 applicants, 6% accepted, 16 enrolled. In 2013, 29 doctorates awarded. *Degree requirements:* For doctorate, comprehensive exam, thesis/dissertation, oral defense of dissertation, preliminary exam. *Entrance requirements:* For doctorate, GRE General Test. Additional exam requirements/recommendations for international students: Required—TOEFL. *Application deadline:* For fall admission, 12/1 for domestic and international students. Application fee: $75 ($90 for international students). Electronic applications accepted. Tuition and fees vary according to course level, course load, degree level, program and student level. *Financial support:* In 2013–14, 82 students received support, including 45 fellowships with full tuition reimbursements available (averaging $20,900 per year), 16 research assistantships with full tuition reimbursements available (averaging $27,900 per year), 50 teaching assistantships with full tuition reimbursements available (averaging $24,000 per year); career-related internships or fieldwork also available. Financial award application deadline: 4/15. *Unit head:* Prof. Stephanie Rowley, Interim Chair, 734-764-7429. *Application contact:* Danielle Joanette, Psychology Student Academic Affairs, 731-764-2580, Fax: 734-615-7584, E-mail: psych.saa@umich.edu.
Website: http://www.lsa.umich.edu/psych/

University of Michigan, Rackham Graduate School, Program in Biomedical Sciences (PIBS), Neuroscience Graduate Program, Ann Arbor, MI 48072-2215. Offers PhD. *Faculty:* 130 full-time (38 women). *Students:* 61 full-time (30 women); includes 26 minority (5 Black or African American, non-Hispanic/Latino; 1 American Indian or Alaska Native, non-Hispanic/Latino; 6 Asian, non-Hispanic/Latino; 12 Hispanic/Latino; 2 Native Hawaiian or other Pacific Islander, non-Hispanic/Latino), 3 international. Average age 27. 122 applicants, 12% accepted, 2 enrolled. In 2013, 7 doctorates awarded. *Degree requirements:* For doctorate, thesis/dissertation, oral defense of dissertation, preliminary exam. *Entrance requirements:* For doctorate, GRE General Test, 3 letters of recommendation, research experience. Additional exam requirements/recommendations for international students: Required—TOEFL (minimum score 84 iBT). *Application deadline:* For fall admission, 12/1 for domestic and international students. Application fee: $75 ($90 for international students). Electronic applications accepted. Tuition and fees vary according to course level, course load, degree level, program and student level. *Financial support:* In 2013–14, 61 students received support, including 61 fellowships with full tuition reimbursements available (averaging $28,500 per year); scholarships/grants, health care benefits, tuition waivers (full), and unspecified assistantships also available. Financial award application deadline: 12/1. *Faculty research:* Developmental neurobiology, cellular and molecular neurobiology, cognitive neuroscience, sensory neuroscience, behavioral neuroscience. *Unit head:* Dr. Edward Stuenkel, Director, 734-763-9638, Fax: 734-647-0717, E-mail: esterm@umich.edu. *Application contact:* Rachel F. Flaten, Student Services Administrator, 734-763-9638, Fax: 734-647-0717, E-mail: rachelfk@umich.edu.
Website: http://neuroscience.med.umich.edu/

University of Minnesota, Twin Cities Campus, Graduate School, Graduate Program in Neuroscience, Minneapolis, MN 55455-0213. Offers MS, PhD. Terminal master's awarded for partial completion of doctoral program. *Degree requirements:* For master's, thesis; for doctorate, thesis/dissertation. *Entrance requirements:* For doctorate, GRE. Additional exam requirements/recommendations for international students: Required—TOEFL. Electronic applications accepted. *Faculty research:* Cellular and molecular neuroscience, behavioral neuroscience, developmental neuroscience, neurodegenerative diseases, pain, addiction, motor control.

University of Mississippi Medical Center, School of Graduate Studies in the Health Sciences, Program in Neuroscience, Jackson, MS 39216-4505. Offers PhD. *Faculty:* 43 full-time (11 women). *Students:* 14 full-time (6 women), 2 international. Average age 29. 17 applicants, 18% accepted, 3 enrolled. In 2013, 2 doctorates awarded. *Degree requirements:* For doctorate, comprehensive exam, thesis/dissertation, 1st authored publication. *Entrance requirements:* For doctorate, GRE, BA, BS. Additional exam requirements/recommendations for international students: Required—TOEFL (minimum score 550 paper-based, 79 iBT), IELTS (minimum score 6.5), or PTE (minimum score 53). *Application deadline:* For fall admission, 12/31 priority date for domestic and international students. Application fee: $25. Electronic applications accepted. *Financial support:* In 2013–14, 9 students received support, including 9 fellowships with full tuition reimbursements available (averaging $24,100 per year), 5 research assistantships with full tuition reimbursements available (averaging $24,100 per year); health care benefits and unspecified assistantships also available. Financial award application deadline: 12/31. *Faculty research:* Neuroendocrinology, drugs of abuse, psychiatric neuroscience, sensory neuroscience, circadian rhythms. *Total annual research expenditures:* $5 million. *Unit head:* Dr. Ian A. Paul, Director, 601-984-5898, E-mail: ipaul@umc.edu. *Application contact:* Barbara Westerfield, Director, Student Records/Registrar, 601-984-1080, Fax: 601-984-1079, E-mail: bwesterfield@umc.edu.
Website: http://www.umc.edu/neuroscience/

University of Missouri, Graduate School, Interdisciplinary Neuroscience Program, Columbia, MO 65211. Offers MS, PhD. *Students:* 8 full-time (3 women), 1 part-time (0 women), 2 international. Average age 28. 22 applicants, 5% accepted, 1 enrolled. In 2013, 1 master's, 1 doctorate awarded. *Entrance requirements:* For master's and doctorate, GRE (minimum score: Verbal and Quantitative 1200), bachelor's degree or its equivalent. Additional exam requirements/recommendations for international students: Required—TOEFL (minimum score 600 paper-based; 100 iBT). *Application deadline:* For fall admission, 1/15 priority date for domestic and international students. Application fee: $55 ($75 for international students). Electronic applications accepted. *Financial support:* Scholarships/grants, health care benefits, and unspecified assistantships available. Support available to part-time students. *Faculty research:* Molecular and cellular organization of the nervous system, structure and function of neural systems (including vision and hearing), behaviors generated by the nervous system, neurological diseases and disorders. *Unit head:* Dr. Andrew McClellan, Director, 573-882-1447, E-mail: mcclellana@missouri.edu. *Application contact:* Nila Emerich, Senior Secretary, 573-882-1847, E-mail: emerichn@missouri.edu.
Website: http://neuroscience.missouri.edu/graduate-studies/

University of Missouri–St. Louis, College of Arts and Sciences, Department of Psychology, St. Louis, MO 63121. Offers behavioral neuroscience (PhD); clinical community psychology (PhD); clinical psychology respecialization (Certificate); general psychology (MA); industrial/organizational psychology (PhD); trauma studies (Certificate). *Accreditation:* APA (one or more programs are accredited). Evening/weekend programs available. *Faculty:* 17 full-time (9 women), 9 part-time/adjunct (2 women). *Students:* 63 full-time (46 women), 12 part-time (9 women); includes 8 minority (2 Black or African American, non-Hispanic/Latino; 1 American Indian or Alaska Native, non-Hispanic/Latino; 3 Asian, non-Hispanic/Latino; 2 Hispanic/Latino). Average age 27. 232 applicants, 7% accepted, 15 enrolled. In 2013, 19 master's, 7 doctorates awarded. Terminal master's awarded for partial completion of doctoral program. *Degree requirements:* For master's, thesis; for doctorate, thesis/dissertation. *Entrance requirements:* For master's, GRE General Test, 3 letters of recommendation; for doctorate, GRE General Test, GRE Subject Test, 3 letters of recommendation. Additional exam requirements/recommendations for international students: Required—TOEFL (minimum score 550 paper-based; 79 iBT), IELTS (minimum score 6.5). *Application deadline:* For fall admission, 12/15 for domestic and international students. Application fee: $50 ($40 for international students). Electronic applications accepted. *Expenses:* Tuition, state resident: full-time $7364; part-time $409.10 per credit hour. Tuition, nonresident: full-time $19,162; part-time $1008.50 per credit hour. *Financial support:* In 2013–14, 7 research assistantships with full and partial tuition reimbursements (averaging $10,714 per year), 29 teaching assistantships with full and partial tuition reimbursements (averaging $9,210 per year) were awarded; fellowships with full tuition reimbursements also available. Financial award applicants required to submit FAFSA. *Faculty research:* Bereavement and loss, neuroscience, post-traumatic stress disorder, conflict and negotiation, social psychology. *Unit head:* Dr. Ann Steffen, Chair, 314-516-5391, Fax: 314-516-5392, E-mail: umslpsychology@msx.umsl.edu. *Application contact:* 314-516-5458, Fax: 314-516-6996, E-mail: gradadm@umsl.edu.
Website: http://www.umsl.edu/divisions/artscience/psychology/

The University of Montana, Graduate School, College of Health Professions and Biomedical Sciences, Skaggs School of Pharmacy, Department of Biomedical and Pharmaceutical Sciences, Missoula, MT 59812-0002. Offers biomedical sciences (PhD); medicinal chemistry (MS, PhD); molecular and cellular toxicology (MS, PhD); neuroscience (PhD); pharmaceutical sciences (MS). *Accreditation:* ACPE. *Degree requirements:* For master's, oral defense of thesis; for doctorate, research dissertation defense. *Entrance requirements:* For master's and doctorate, GRE General Test. Additional exam requirements/recommendations for international students: Required—TOEFL (minimum score 540 paper-based). *Application deadline:* For fall admission, 3/1 priority date for domestic and international students. Applications are processed on a rolling basis. Application fee: $45. Electronic applications accepted. *Financial support:* Teaching assistantships with full and partial tuition reimbursements, Federal Work-Study, scholarships/grants, and tuition waivers (full and partial) available. Financial award application deadline: 3/1. *Faculty research:* Cardiovascular pharmacology, medicinal chemistry, neurosciences, environmental toxicology, pharmacogenetics, cancer. *Unit head:* Dr. Richard Bridges, Chair, 406-243-4972, E-mail: richard.bridges@umontana.edu. *Application contact:* Information Contact, E-mail: gradschl@mso.umt.edu.
Website: http://www.umt.edu/pharmsci/

University of Nebraska Medical Center, Department of Pharmacology and Experimental Neuroscience, Omaha, NE 68198-5800. Offers neuroscience (MS, PhD); pharmacology (MS, PhD). Terminal master's awarded for partial completion of doctoral program. *Degree requirements:* For master's, comprehensive exam, thesis; for doctorate, comprehensive exam, thesis/dissertation. *Entrance requirements:* For master's and doctorate, GRE General Test. Additional exam requirements/recommendations for international students: Required—TOEFL (minimum score 600 paper-based). Electronic applications accepted. *Expenses: Required fees:* $300 per semester. Tuition and fees vary according to program. *Faculty research:* Neuropharmacology, molecular pharmacology, toxicology, molecular biology, neuroscience.

University of New Mexico, Graduate School, College of Arts and Sciences, Department of Psychology, Albuquerque, NM 87131-2039. Offers behavioral neuroscience (PhD); clinical psychology (PhD); cognitive neuroimaging (PhD); developmental psychology (PhD); evolution (PhD); health psychology (PhD); quantitative methodology (PhD). *Faculty:* 24 full-time (9 women), 2 part-time/adjunct (both women). *Students:* 67 full-time (42 women), 8 part-time (6 women); includes 20 minority (1 American Indian or Alaska Native, non-Hispanic/Latino; 4 Asian, non-Hispanic/Latino; 14 Hispanic/Latino; 1 Two or more races, non-Hispanic/Latino), 1 international. Average age 33. 123 applicants, 17% accepted, 12 enrolled. In 2013, 9 doctorates awarded. *Degree requirements:* For doctorate, comprehensive exam, thesis/dissertation. *Entrance requirements:* For doctorate, GRE General Test, GRE Subject Test (psychology), minimum GPA of 3.0. Additional exam requirements/recommendations for international students: Required—TOEFL (minimum score 550 paper-based; 79 iBT), IELTS (minimum score 6.5). *Application deadline:* For fall admission, 12/15 priority date for domestic and international students. Applications are processed on a rolling basis. Application fee: $50. Electronic applications accepted. *Financial support:* In 2013–14, 62 students received support, including 8 fellowships (averaging $13,124 per year), 37 research assistantships with full and partial tuition reimbursements available (averaging $11,655 per year), 67 teaching assistantships with full and partial tuition reimbursements available (averaging $13,600 per year); career-related internships or fieldwork, Federal Work-Study, institutionally sponsored loans, scholarships/grants, health care benefits, tuition waivers (partial), and unspecified assistantships also available. Financial award application deadline: 3/1; financial award applicants required to submit FAFSA. *Faculty research:* Addiction, cognition, brain and behavior, developmental, evolutionary, functioning neuroimaging, health psychology, learning and memory, neuroscience. *Unit head:* Dr. Jane Ellen Smith, Department Chair, 505-277-4121, Fax: 505-277-1394. *Application contact:* Rikk Murphy, Graduate Program Coordinator, 505-277-5009, Fax: 505-277-1394, E-mail: advising@unm.edu.
Website: http://psych.unm.edu

University of New Mexico, School of Medicine, Program in Biomedical Sciences, Albuquerque, NM 87131-5196. Offers biochemistry and molecular biology (MS, PhD); cell biology and physiology (MS, PhD); clinical and translational science (Certificate); molecular genetics and microbiology (MS, PhD); neuroscience (MS, PhD); pathology (MS, PhD); toxicology (MS, PhD); university science teaching (Certificate). Part-time programs available. *Students:* 73 full-time (39 women), 14 part-time (9 women); includes 24 minority (1 Black or African American, non-Hispanic/Latino; 1 American Indian or Alaska Native, non-Hispanic/Latino; 2 Asian, non-Hispanic/Latino; 17 Hispanic/Latino; 1 Native Hawaiian or other Pacific Islander, non-Hispanic/Latino; 2 Two or more races, non-Hispanic/Latino), 16 international. Average age 29. 89 applicants, 20% accepted, 17 enrolled. In 2013, 7 master's, 17 doctorates awarded. Terminal master's awarded for partial completion of doctoral program. *Degree requirements:* For master's, thesis; for doctorate, comprehensive exam, thesis/dissertation, qualifying exam at the end of year 1/core curriculum. *Entrance requirements:* For master's and doctorate, GRE General Test, minimum undergraduate GPA of 3.0. Additional exam requirements/recommendations for international students: Required—TOEFL. *Application deadline:* For fall admission, 3/1 priority date for domestic and international students. Applications are processed on a rolling basis. Application fee: $50. Electronic applications accepted. *Financial support:* In 2013–14, 94 students received support, including 28 fellowships with full and partial tuition reimbursements available (averaging $22,000 per year), 73 research assistantships with full tuition reimbursements available (averaging $23,000 per year), 8 teaching assistantships (averaging $2,800 per year); career-related internships or fieldwork, Federal Work-Study, institutionally sponsored loans, scholarships/grants, traineeships, health care benefits, and unspecified assistantships also available. Financial award application deadline: 1/1; financial award applicants

required to submit FAFSA. *Faculty research:* Infectious disease/immunity, cancer biology, cardiovascular and metabolic diseases, brain and behavioral illness, environmental health. *Unit head:* Dr. Helen J. Hathaway, Program Director, 505-272-1887, Fax: 505-272-2412, E-mail: hhathaway@salud.unm.edu. *Application contact:* Mary Fenton, Admissions Coordinator, 505-272-1887, Fax: 505-272-2412, E-mail: mfenton@salud.unm.edu.
Website: http://hsc.unm.edu/research/brep/bsgpabout.shtm

The University of North Carolina at Chapel Hill, Graduate School, College of Arts and Sciences, Department of Psychology, Chapel Hill, NC 27599-3270. Offers behavioral neuroscience psychology (PhD); clinical psychology (PhD); cognitive psychology (PhD); developmental psychology (PhD); quantitative psychology (PhD); social psychology (PhD). *Accreditation:* APA. *Degree requirements:* For doctorate, comprehensive exam, thesis/dissertation. *Entrance requirements:* For doctorate, GRE General Test, minimum GPA of 3.0. Additional exam requirements/recommendations for international students: Required—TOEFL (minimum score 550 paper-based; 79 iBT), IELTS (minimum score 7). Electronic applications accepted. *Faculty research:* Expressed emotion, cognitive development, social cognitive neuroscience, human memory personality.

University of Oklahoma Health Sciences Center, College of Medicine and Graduate College, Graduate Programs in Medicine, Department of Neuroscience, Oklahoma City, OK 73190. Offers MS, PhD. *Faculty:* 8 full-time (1 woman), 1 (woman) part-time/adjunct. *Students:* 3 full-time (0 women), 7 part-time (4 women); includes 1 minority (Black or African American, non-Hispanic/Latino), 3 international. Average age 26. 10 applicants. In 2013, 1 doctorate awarded. *Degree requirements:* For doctorate, thesis/dissertation. *Entrance requirements:* For master's and doctorate, GRE General Test, 3 letters of recommendation. Additional exam requirements/recommendations for international students: Required—TOEFL. *Application deadline:* For fall admission, 12/1 for domestic students. Application fee: $50. *Expenses:* Tuition, state resident: full-time $3504; part-time $175.20 per credit hour. Tuition, nonresident: full-time $13,504; part-time $675.20 per credit hour. *Required fees:* $1545; $52.70 per credit hour. $245.25 per semester. Tuition and fees vary according to course load. *Financial support:* In 2013–14, 3 research assistantships (averaging $18,000 per year) were awarded. *Unit head:* Dr. Beverley Greenwood, Director, 405-271-6267, E-mail: beverley.greenwood@ouhsc.edu. *Application contact:* Anthony Johnson, Graduate Liaison, 405-271-8244, Fax: 405-271-3552, E-mail: anthony.johnson@ouhsc.edu.

University of Oregon, Graduate School, College of Arts and Sciences, Department of Biology, Eugene, OR 97403. Offers ecology and evolution (MA, MS, PhD); marine biology (MA, MS, PhD); molecular, cellular and genetic biology (PhD); neuroscience and development (PhD). Terminal master's awarded for partial completion of doctoral program. *Degree requirements:* For master's, thesis (for some programs); for doctorate, thesis/dissertation. *Entrance requirements:* For master's and doctorate, GRE General Test, minimum GPA of 3.2. Additional exam requirements/recommendations for international students: Required—TOEFL. *Faculty research:* Developmental neurobiology; evolution, population biology, and quantitative genetics; regulation of gene expression; biochemistry of marine organisms.

University of Pennsylvania, Perelman School of Medicine, Biomedical Graduate Studies, Graduate Group in Neuroscience, Philadelphia, PA 19104. Offers PhD, MD/PhD, VMD/PhD. *Faculty:* 135. *Students:* 121 full-time (62 women); includes 33 minority (4 Black or African American, non-Hispanic/Latino; 2 American Indian or Alaska Native, non-Hispanic/Latino; 23 Asian, non-Hispanic/Latino; 4 Hispanic/Latino), 9 international. 236 applicants, 17% accepted, 9 enrolled. In 2013, 19 doctorates awarded. *Degree requirements:* For doctorate, thesis/dissertation. *Entrance requirements:* For doctorate, GRE General Test. Additional exam requirements/recommendations for international students: Required—TOEFL. *Application deadline:* For fall admission, 12/1 priority date for domestic and international students. Applications are processed on a rolling basis. Application fee: $80. Electronic applications accepted. *Financial support:* In 2013–14, 121 students received support. Fellowships, research assistantships, teaching assistantships, scholarships/grants, traineeships, and unspecified assistantships available. *Faculty research:* Molecular and cellular neuroscience, behavioral neuroscience, developmental neurobiology, systems neuroscience and neurophysiology, neurochemistry. *Unit head:* Dr. Joshua Gold, Chair, 215-746-0028. *Application contact:* Jane Hoshi, Coordinator, 215-898-8048.
Website: http://www.med.upenn.edu/ngg

University of Pittsburgh, Dietrich School of Arts and Sciences and School of Medicine, Center for Neuroscience, Pittsburgh, PA 15260. Offers neurobiology (PhD); neuroscience (PhD). Program held jointly with School of Medicine. *Faculty:* 107 full-time (36 women). *Students:* 73 full-time (37 women); includes 10 minority (1 Black or African American, non-Hispanic/Latino; 7 Asian, non-Hispanic/Latino; 2 Hispanic/Latino), 12 international. Average age 25. 175 applicants, 20% accepted, 12 enrolled. In 2013, 9 doctorates awarded. *Degree requirements:* For doctorate, comprehensive exam, thesis/dissertation. *Entrance requirements:* For doctorate, GRE, interview. Additional exam requirements/recommendations for international students: Required—TOEFL (minimum score 600 paper-based; 100 iBT). *Application deadline:* For fall admission, 12/1 priority date for domestic and international students. Application fee: $50. Electronic applications accepted. *Expenses:* Contact institution. *Financial support:* In 2013–14, 67 students received support, including 23 fellowships with full tuition reimbursements available (averaging $26,010 per year), 43 research assistantships with full tuition reimbursements available (averaging $26,010 per year), 1 teaching assistantship with full tuition reimbursement available (averaging $26,010 per year); traineeships, health care benefits, and unspecified assistantships also available. Financial award application deadline: 12/1. *Faculty research:* Behavioral/systems/cognitive, cell and molecular, development/plasticity/repair, neurobiology of disease. *Unit head:* Dr. Alan Sved, Co-Director, 412-624-6996, Fax: 412-624-9198. *Application contact:* Joan M. Blaney, Administrator, 412-624-5043, Fax: 412-624-9198, E-mail: jblaney@pitt.edu.
Website: http://cnup.neurobio.pitt.edu/

University of Puerto Rico, Río Piedras Campus, College of Natural Sciences, Department of Biology, San Juan, PR 00931-3300. Offers ecology/systematics (MS, PhD); evolution/genetics (MS, PhD); molecular/cellular biology (MS, PhD); neuroscience (MS, PhD). Part-time programs available. *Degree requirements:* For master's, one foreign language, comprehensive exam, thesis; for doctorate, one foreign language, comprehensive exam, thesis/dissertation. *Entrance requirements:* For master's, GRE Subject Test, interview, minimum GPA of 3.0, letter of recommendation; for doctorate, GRE Subject Test, interview, master's degree, minimum GPA of 3.0, letter of recommendation. *Faculty research:* Environmental, poblational and systematic biology.

University of Rochester, School of Medicine and Dentistry, Graduate Programs in Medicine and Dentistry, Department of Neurobiology and Anatomy, Interdepartmental Programs in Neuroscience, Rochester, NY 14627. Offers PhD. Terminal master's awarded for partial completion of doctoral program. *Degree requirements:* For doctorate, one foreign language, thesis/dissertation, qualifying exam. *Entrance requirements:* For doctorate, GRE General Test. *Expenses: Tuition:* Full-time $44,580; part-time $1394 per credit hour. *Required fees:* $492.

The University of South Dakota, Graduate School, School of Medicine and Graduate School, Biomedical Sciences Graduate Program, Program in Neuroscience, Vermillion, SD 57069-2390. Offers MS, PhD. Terminal master's awarded for partial completion of doctoral program. *Degree requirements:* For master's, thesis; for doctorate, comprehensive exam, thesis/dissertation. *Entrance requirements:* For master's and doctorate, GRE General Test, minimum GPA of 3.0. Additional exam requirements/recommendations for international students: Required—TOEFL (minimum score 550 paper-based; 80 iBT), IELTS (minimum score 6). Electronic applications accepted. *Expenses:* Contact institution. *Faculty research:* Central nervous system learning, neural plasticity, respiratory control.

University of Southern California, Graduate School, Dana and David Dornsife College of Letters, Arts and Sciences, Program in Neuroscience, Los Angeles, CA 90089. Offers MS, PhD. M.S. degree is terminal degree only. Terminal master's awarded for partial completion of doctoral program. *Degree requirements:* For master's, research paper; for doctorate, comprehensive exam, thesis/dissertation, qualifying examination, dissertation defense. *Entrance requirements:* For doctorate, GRE, 3 letters of recommendation, personal statement, resume. Additional exam requirements/recommendations for international students: Required—TOEFL (minimum score 600 paper-based; 100 iBT). Electronic applications accepted. *Faculty research:* Cellular and molecular neurobiology, behavioral and systems neurobiology, cognitive neuroscience, computation neuroscience and neural engineering, neuroscience of aging.

University of South Florida, College of Arts and Sciences, Department of Psychology, Tampa, FL 33620-9951. Offers clinical psychology (PhD); cognitive and neural sciences (PhD); industrial-organizational psychology (PhD). *Accreditation:* APA. *Faculty:* 33 full-time (15 women), 5 part-time/adjunct (4 women). *Students:* 91 full-time (58 women), 22 part-time (11 women); includes 24 minority (2 Black or African American, non-Hispanic/Latino; 11 Asian, non-Hispanic/Latino; 9 Hispanic/Latino; 2 Two or more races, non-Hispanic/Latino), 11 international. Average age 28. 464 applicants, 4% accepted, 16 enrolled. In 2013, 18 doctorates awarded. *Degree requirements:* For doctorate, comprehensive exam, thesis/dissertation, internship. *Entrance requirements:* For doctorate, GRE General Test (minimum recommended verbal and quantitative scores each above the 50th percentile), minimum upper-division GPA of 3.4, three letters of recommendation, personal goals statement. Additional exam requirements/recommendations for international students: Required—TOEFL (minimum score 550 paper-based; 79 iBT) or IELTS (minimum score 6.5). *Application deadline:* For fall admission, 12/1 for domestic and international students. Application fee: $30. Electronic applications accepted. *Expenses:* Contact institution. *Financial support:* In 2013–14, 75 students received support, including 18 research assistantships with tuition reimbursements available (averaging $14,727 per year), 57 teaching assistantships with tuition reimbursements available (averaging $14,543 per year); tuition waivers (partial) and unspecified assistantships also available. Financial award applicants required to submit FAFSA. *Faculty research:* Clinical, cognitive, neuroscience, social, and industrial/organizational. *Total annual research expenditures:* $2 million. *Unit head:* Michael Brannick, Chairperson, 813-974-0478, Fax: 813-974-4617, E-mail: mbrannick@usf.edu. *Application contact:* Dr. Stephen Stark, Associate Professor and Graduate Program Director, 813-974-8015, Fax: 813-974-4617, E-mail: sestark@usf.edu.
Website: http://psychology.usf.edu/

University of South Florida, Innovative Education Graduate Certificate Programs, Tampa, FL 33620-9951. *Unit head:* Kathy Barnes, Interdisciplinary Programs Coordinator, 813-974-8031, Fax: 813-974-7061, E-mail: barnesk@usf.edu. *Application contact:* Karen Tylinski, Metro Initiatives, 813-974-9943, Fax: 813-974-7061, E-mail: ktylinsk@usf.edu.
Website: http://www.usf.edu/innovative-education/

University of South Florida, Morsani College of Medicine and Graduate School, Graduate Programs in Medical Sciences, Tampa, FL 33620-9951. Offers aging and neuroscience (MSMS); allergy, immunology and infectious disease (PhD); anatomy (MSMS, PhD); athletic training (MSMS); bioinformatics and computational biology (MSBCB); biotechnology (MSB); clinical and translational research (MSMS, PhD); health informatics (MSHI, MSMS); health science (MSMS); interdisciplinary medical sciences (MSMS); medical microbiology and immunology (MSMS); metabolic and nutritional medicine (MSMS); molecular medicine (MSMS, PhD); molecular pharmacology and physiology (PhD); neurology (PhD); pathology and laboratory medicine (PhD); pharmacology and therapeutics (PhD); physiology and biophysics (PhD); women's health (MSMS). *Students:* 336 full-time (182 women), 39 part-time (21 women); includes 170 minority (45 Black or African American, non-Hispanic/Latino; 54 Asian, non-Hispanic/Latino; 59 Hispanic/Latino; 2 Native Hawaiian or other Pacific Islander, non-Hispanic/Latino; 10 Two or more races, non-Hispanic/Latino), 17 international. Average age 26. 1,066 applicants, 44% accepted, 250 enrolled. In 2013, 191 master's, 12 doctorates awarded. Terminal master's awarded for partial completion of doctoral program. *Degree requirements:* For master's, comprehensive exam, thesis; for doctorate, comprehensive exam, thesis/dissertation. *Entrance requirements:* For master's, GRE General Test or GMAT, bachelor's degree or equivalent from regionally-accredited university with minimum GPA of 3.0 in upper-division sciences coursework; prerequisites in general biology, general chemistry, general physics, organic chemistry, quantitative analysis, and integral and differential calculus; for doctorate, GRE General Test (minimum score of 600 quantitative), bachelor's degree from regionally-accredited university with minimum GPA of 3.0 in upper-division sciences coursework; 3 letters of recommendation; personal interview; 1-2 page personal statement; prerequisites in biology, chemistry, physics, organic chemistry, quantitative analysis, and integral/differential calculus. Additional exam requirements/recommendations for international students: Required—TOEFL (minimum score 550 paper-based; 79 iBT) or IELTS (minimum score 6.5). *Application deadline:* For fall admission, 2/15 for domestic students, 1/2 for international students. Application fee: $30. *Expenses:* Contact institution. *Faculty research:* Anatomy, biochemistry, cancer biology, cardiovascular disease, cell biology, immunology, microbiology, molecular biology, neuroscience, pharmacology, physiology. *Unit head:* Dr. Michael Barber, Professor and Associate Dean for Graduate and Postdoctoral Affairs, 813-974-9908, Fax: 813-974-4317, E-mail: mbarber@health.usf.edu. *Application contact:* Dr. Eric Bennett, Graduate Director, PhD Program in Medical Sciences, 813-974-1545, Fax: 813-974-4317, E-mail: esbennet@health.usf.edu.
Website: http://health.usf.edu/nocms/medicine/graduatestudies/

The University of Texas at Austin, Graduate School, College of Liberal Arts, Department of Psychology, Austin, TX 78712-1111. Offers behavioral neuroscience (PhD); clinical psychology (PhD); cognitive systems (PhD); developmental psychology (PhD); individual differences and evolutionary psychology (PhD); perceptual systems (PhD); social psychology (PhD). *Accreditation:* APA. *Degree requirements:* For doctorate, thesis/dissertation. *Entrance requirements:* For doctorate, GRE General Test. Electronic applications accepted. *Faculty research:* Behavioral neuroscience, sensory neuroscience, evolutionary psychology, cognitive processes in psychopathology, cognitive processes and their development.

The University of Texas at Austin, Graduate School, The Institute for Neuroscience, Austin, TX 78712-1111. Offers PhD, MD/PhD. Terminal master's awarded for partial completion of doctoral program. *Degree requirements:* For doctorate, thesis/dissertation. *Entrance requirements:* For doctorate, GRE. Electronic applications accepted. *Faculty research:* Cellular/molecular biology, neurobiology, pharmacology, behavioral neuroscience.

The University of Texas at Dallas, School of Behavioral and Brain Sciences, Program in Cognition and Neuroscience, Richardson, TX 75080. Offers applied cognition and neuroscience (MS); cognition and neuroscience (PhD). Part-time and evening/weekend programs available. *Faculty:* 27 full-time (10 women). *Students:* 147 full-time (83 women), 33 part-time (21 women); includes 49 minority (9 Black or African American, non-Hispanic/Latino; 1 American Indian or Alaska Native, non-Hispanic/Latino; 16 Asian, non-Hispanic/Latino; 19 Hispanic/Latino; 4 Two or more races, non-Hispanic/Latino), 37 international. Average age 29. 148 applicants, 53% accepted, 65 enrolled. In 2013, 42 master's, 7 doctorates awarded. *Degree requirements:* For master's, internship; for doctorate, thesis/dissertation. *Entrance requirements:* For master's and doctorate, GRE General Test, minimum GPA of 3.0 in upper-level coursework in field. Additional exam requirements/recommendations for international students: Required—TOEFL (minimum score 550 paper-based). *Application deadline:* For fall admission, 7/15 for domestic students, 5/1 priority date for international students; for spring admission, 11/15 for domestic students, 9/1 priority date for international students. Applications are processed on a rolling basis. Application fee: $50 ($100 for international students). Electronic applications accepted. *Expenses:* Tuition, state resident: full-time $11,940; part-time $663.33 per credit hour. Tuition, nonresident: full-time $21,606; part-time $1200.33 per credit hour. *Financial support:* In 2013–14, 110 students received support, including 21 research assistantships with partial tuition reimbursements available (averaging $24,978 per year), 30 teaching assistantships with partial tuition reimbursements available (averaging $14,860 per year); career-related internships or fieldwork, Federal Work-Study, institutionally sponsored loans, scholarships/grants, and unspecified assistantships also available. Support available to part-time students. Financial award application deadline: 4/30; financial award applicants required to submit FAFSA. *Faculty research:* Neural plasticity, neuroimaging, face recognition, cognitive and neurobiological mechanisms of human memory, treatment interventions for semantic memory retrieval problems. *Unit head:* Dr. James C. Bartlett, Program Head, 972-883-2079, Fax: 972-883-2491, E-mail: jbartlet@utdallas.edu. *Application contact:* Dr. Christa McIntyre, Associate Program Head, 972-883-2235, Fax: 972-883-2491, E-mail: christa.mcintyre@utdallas.edu.
Website: http://bbs.utdallas.edu/cogneuro/

The University of Texas Health Science Center at Houston, Graduate School of Biomedical Sciences, Program in Neuroscience, Houston, TX 77225-0036. Offers MS, PhD, MD/PhD. Terminal master's awarded for partial completion of doctoral program. *Degree requirements:* For master's, thesis; for doctorate, thesis/dissertation. *Entrance requirements:* For master's and doctorate, GRE General Test. Additional exam requirements/recommendations for international students: Required—TOEFL. Electronic applications accepted. *Expenses:* Tuition, state resident: full-time $3474; part-time $193 per credit hour. Tuition, nonresident: full-time $13,644; part-time $758 per credit hour. *Required fees:* $226.30; $87 per credit hour. *Faculty research:* Behavior, cognitive, computational, neuroimaging, substance abuse.

The University of Texas Health Science Center at San Antonio, Graduate School of Biomedical Sciences, Department of Pharmacology, San Antonio, TX 78229-3900. Offers neuroscience (PhD). *Faculty:* 41 full-time (14 women), 10 part-time/adjunct (1 woman). *Students:* 29 full-time (18 women), 4 part-time (2 women); includes 12 minority (1 Black or African American, non-Hispanic/Latino; 1 Asian, non-Hispanic/Latino; 10 Hispanic/Latino), 6 international. Average age 29. In 2013, 4 doctorates awarded. *Degree requirements:* For doctorate, comprehensive exam, thesis/dissertation. *Entrance requirements:* For doctorate, GRE General Test, minimum GPA of 3.0. Additional exam requirements/recommendations for international students: Required—TOEFL (minimum score 560 paper-based; 68 iBT). *Application deadline:* For fall admission, 1/15 priority date for domestic and international students. Applications are processed on a rolling basis. Application fee: $0. Electronic applications accepted. *Financial support:* Application deadline: 6/30; applicants required to submit FAFSA. *Faculty research:* Neuropharmacology, autonomic and endocrine homeostasis, aging, cancer biology. *Total annual research expenditures:* $9.4 million. *Unit head:* Dr. Alan Frazer, Department Chair, 210-567-4205, Fax: 210-567-4300, E-mail: frazer@uthscsa.edu. *Application contact:* Dr. Julie Hensler, Graduate Advisor/Committee on Graduate Studies Chair, 210-567-4236, Fax: 210-567-4300, E-mail: hensler@uthscsa.edu.
Website: http://pharmacology.uthscsa.edu

The University of Texas Medical Branch, Graduate School of Biomedical Sciences, Program in Neuroscience, Galveston, TX 77555. Offers PhD. *Degree requirements:* For doctorate, thesis/dissertation. *Entrance requirements:* For doctorate, GRE General Test. Additional exam requirements/recommendations for international students: Required—TOEFL (minimum score 550 paper-based). Electronic applications accepted.

The University of Texas Southwestern Medical Center, Southwestern Graduate School of Biomedical Sciences, Division of Basic Science, Program in Neuroscience, Dallas, TX 75390. Offers PhD. *Faculty:* 35 full-time (5 women). *Students:* 48 full-time (28 women), 1 part-time (0 women); includes 11 minority (2 Black or African American, non-Hispanic/Latino; 3 Asian, non-Hispanic/Latino; 6 Hispanic/Latino), 7 international. Average age 28. In 2013, 11 doctorates awarded. *Degree requirements:* For doctorate, thesis/dissertation, qualifying exam. *Entrance requirements:* For doctorate, GRE General Test, minimum GPA of 3.0. Additional exam requirements/recommendations for international students: Required—TOEFL. *Application deadline:* For fall admission, 12/15 priority date for domestic students. Applications are processed on a rolling basis. Application fee: $0. Electronic applications accepted. *Financial support:* Fellowships and research assistantships available. *Faculty research:* Ion channels, sensory transduction, membrane excitability and biophysics, synaptic transmission, developmental neurogenetics.
Website: http://www.utsouthwestern.edu/education/graduate-school/programs/phd-degrees/neuroscience/index.html

The University of Toledo, College of Graduate Studies, College of Medicine and Life Sciences, Department of Neurosciences, Toledo, OH 43606-3390. Offers MSBS, PhD, MD/MSBS, MD/PhD. *Faculty:* 14. *Students:* 11 full-time (3 women); includes 1 minority (Hispanic/Latino), 4 international. Average age 25. 18 applicants, 28% accepted, 3 enrolled. In 2013, 2 doctorates awarded. Terminal master's awarded for partial completion of doctoral program. *Degree requirements:* For master's, thesis, qualifying exam; for doctorate, thesis/dissertation, qualifying exam. *Entrance requirements:* For master's and doctorate, GRE, minimum undergraduate GPA of 3.0, three letters of recommendation, statement of purpose, transcripts from all prior institutions attended, resume. Additional exam requirements/recommendations for international students: Required—TOEFL (minimum score 550 paper-based; 80 iBT). *Application deadline:* For fall admission, 1/15 priority date for domestic and international students. Application fee: $45 ($75 for international students). Electronic applications accepted. *Financial support:* In 2013–14, 11 research assistantships with full tuition reimbursements (averaging $22,032 per year) were awarded; Federal Work-Study, institutionally sponsored loans, scholarships/grants, tuition waivers (full), and unspecified assistantships also available. *Unit head:* Dr. Bryan Yamamoto, Chair, 419-383-3346, E-mail: bryan.yamamoto@utoledo.edu. *Application contact:* Admissions Analyst, 419-383-4112, Fax: 419-383-6140.
Website: http://www.utoledo.edu/med/grad/

University of Utah, School of Medicine and Graduate School, Graduate Programs in Medicine, Program in Neuroscience, Salt Lake City, UT 84112-1107. Offers PhD. *Degree requirements:* For doctorate, thesis/dissertation. *Entrance requirements:* For doctorate, GRE General Test, minimum GPA of 3.0. Additional exam requirements/recommendations for international students: Required—TOEFL (minimum score 500 paper-based); Recommended—TWE (minimum score 6). Electronic applications accepted. *Expenses:* Tuition, state resident: full-time $5259. Tuition, nonresident: full-time $18,569. *Required fees:* $841. Tuition and fees vary according to course load. *Faculty research:* Brain and behavioral neuroscience, cellular neuroscience, molecular neuroscience, neurobiology of disease, developmental neuroscience.

University of Vermont, College of Medicine and Graduate College, Graduate Programs in Medicine, Graduate Program in Neuroscience, Burlington, VT 05405. Offers PhD. *Students:* 25 (11 women); includes 5 minority (1 Black or African American, non-Hispanic/Latino; 4 Hispanic/Latino), 2 international. 42 applicants, 26% accepted, 4 enrolled. In 2013, 6 doctorates awarded. *Degree requirements:* For doctorate, thesis/dissertation. *Entrance requirements:* For doctorate, GRE General Test. Additional exam requirements/recommendations for international students: Required—TOEFL (minimum score 550 paper-based; 80 iBT). *Application deadline:* For fall admission, 12/1 priority date for domestic students, 12/1 for international students. Application fee: $65. Electronic applications accepted. *Financial support:* Research assistantships and teaching assistantships available. Financial award application deadline: 3/1. *Unit head:* Dr. Rae Nishi, Director, 802-656-2230, E-mail: rae.nishi@uvm.edu. *Application contact:* E-mail: graduate.admissions@uvm.edu.

University of Virginia, School of Medicine, Department of Neuroscience, Charlottesville, VA 22903. Offers PhD, MD/PhD. *Faculty:* 10 full-time (3 women). *Students:* 35 full-time (17 women); includes 5 minority (2 Black or African American, non-Hispanic/Latino; 2 Asian, non-Hispanic/Latino; 1 Hispanic/Latino), 5 international. Average age 27. In 2013, 6 doctorates awarded. *Degree requirements:* For doctorate, thesis/dissertation. *Entrance requirements:* For doctorate, GRE General Test, 2 letters of recommendation. Additional exam requirements/recommendations for international students: Required—TOEFL. *Application deadline:* For fall admission, 4/15 for domestic and international students. Applications are processed on a rolling basis. Application fee: $60. Electronic applications accepted. *Expenses:* Tuition, state resident: part-time $334 per credit hour. Tuition, nonresident: part-time $1224 per credit hour. *Financial support:* Application deadline: 1/15; applicants required to submit FAFSA. *Unit head:* Dr. Manoj Patel, Director, 434-924-5528, Fax: 434-982-4380, E-mail: uva-ngp@virginia.edu. *Application contact:* Nadia Badr Cempre, Graduate Program Coordinator, 434-982-4285, Fax: 434-982-4380, E-mail: nab4g@virginia.edu.
Website: http://www.healthsystem.virginia.edu/internet/neuroscience/home.cfm

The University of Western Ontario, Faculty of Graduate Studies, Biosciences Division, Department of Clinical Neurological Sciences, London, ON N6A 5B8, Canada. Offers M Sc, PhD. Terminal master's awarded for partial completion of doctoral program. *Degree requirements:* For master's, thesis; for doctorate, thesis/dissertation. *Entrance requirements:* For master's, honors degree or equivalent, minimum B+ average; for doctorate, master's degree, minimum B+ average. *Faculty research:* Behavioral neuroscience, neural regeneration and degeneration, visual development, human motor function.

University of Wisconsin–Madison, Graduate School, College of Letters and Science, Department of Psychology, Program in Cognitive Neurosciences, Madison, WI 53706-1380. Offers PhD. *Degree requirements:* For doctorate, comprehensive exam, thesis/dissertation. *Entrance requirements:* For doctorate, GRE General Test, minimum undergraduate GPA of 3.0. Additional exam requirements/recommendations for international students: Required—TOEFL. Electronic applications accepted. *Expenses:* Tuition, state resident: full-time $10,728; part-time $790 per credit. Tuition, nonresident: full-time $24,054; part-time $1623 per credit. *Required fees:* $1130; $119 per credit.

University of Wisconsin–Madison, School of Medicine and Public Health and Graduate School, Graduate Programs in Medicine, Madison, WI 53705. Offers biomolecular chemistry (MS, PhD); cancer biology (PhD); epidemiology (MS, PhD); genetics and medical genetics (MS, PhD), including genetics (PhD), medical genetics (MS); medical physics (MS, PhD), including health physics (MS), medical physics; microbiology (PhD); molecular and cellular pharmacology (PhD); neuroscience (PhD); pathology and laboratory medicine (PhD); physiology (PhD); population health (MS, PhD), including population health; DPT/MPH; DVM/MPH; MD/MPH; MD/PhD; MPA/MPH; MS/MPH; Pharm D/MPH. Part-time programs available. Postbaccalaureate distance learning degree programs offered (minimal on-campus study). Terminal master's awarded for partial completion of doctoral program. Application fee: $45. Electronic applications accepted. *Expenses:* Contact institution. *Financial support:* Fellowships with full tuition reimbursements, research assistantships with full tuition reimbursements, teaching assistantships with full tuition reimbursements, scholarships/grants, traineeships, and tuition waivers (full) available. *Unit head:* Dr. Richard L. Moss, Senior Associate Dean for Basic Research, Biotechnology and Graduate Studies, 608-265-0523, Fax: 608-265-0522, E-mail: rlmoss@wisc.edu. *Application contact:* Information Contact, 608-262-2433, Fax: 608-262-5134, E-mail: gradadmiss@mail.bascom.wisc.edu.
Website: http://www.med.wisc.edu

Virginia Commonwealth University, Medical College of Virginia-Professional Programs, School of Medicine, Graduate Program in Neuroscience, Richmond, VA 23284-9005. Offers PhD. Program offered with Departments of Anatomy, Biochemistry and Molecular Biophysics, Pharmacology and Toxicology, and Physiology. *Entrance requirements:* For doctorate, GRE or MCAT. Additional exam requirements/recommendations for international students: Required—TOEFL (minimum score 600 paper-based; 100 iBT). Electronic applications accepted.

Virginia Commonwealth University, Medical College of Virginia-Professional Programs, School of Medicine, School of Medicine Graduate Programs, Department of Anatomy and Neurobiology, Richmond, VA 23284-9005. Offers anatomy (MS); anatomy and neurobiology (PhD); neurobiology (MS); neuroscience (MS); MD/PhD. *Degree requirements:* For master's, thesis; for doctorate, thesis/dissertation, comprehensive oral and written exams. *Entrance requirements:* For master's and doctorate, GRE, MCAT or DAT. Electronic applications accepted.

Virginia Commonwealth University, Medical College of Virginia-Professional Programs, School of Medicine, School of Medicine Graduate Programs, Department of Pharmacology and Toxicology, Richmond, VA 23284-9005. Offers neuroscience (PhD); pharmacology (Certificate); pharmacology and toxicology (MS, PhD); MD/PhD. Terminal master's awarded for partial completion of doctoral program. *Degree requirements:* For master's, thesis; for doctorate, thesis/dissertation, comprehensive oral and written exams. *Entrance requirements:* For master's and doctorate, GRE or MCAT. Additional exam requirements/recommendations for international students: Required—TOEFL (minimum score 600 paper-based; 100 iBT). Electronic applications accepted. *Faculty* *research:* Drug abuse, drug metabolism, pharmacodynamics, peptide synthesis, receptor mechanisms.

Wake Forest University, School of Medicine and Graduate School of Arts and Sciences, Graduate Programs in Medicine, Interdisciplinary Program in Neuroscience, Winston-Salem, NC 27109. Offers PhD, MD/PhD. *Degree requirements:* For doctorate, thesis/dissertation. *Entrance requirements:* For doctorate, GRE General Test. Additional exam requirements/recommendations for international students: Required—TOEFL. Electronic applications accepted. *Faculty research:* Neurobiology of substance abuse, learning and memory, aging, sensory neurobiology, nervous system development.

Washington State University, College of Veterinary Medicine, Program in Neuroscience, Pullman, WA 99164-7620. Offers MS, PhD. Part-time programs available. *Faculty:* 48 full-time (15 women). *Students:* 30 full-time (13 women); includes 3 minority (2 Asian, non-Hispanic/Latino; 1 Hispanic/Latino), 7 international. Average age 28. 50 applicants, 20% accepted, 9 enrolled. In 2013, 6 doctorates awarded. Terminal master's awarded for partial completion of doctoral program. *Degree requirements:* For master's, thesis, written exam; for doctorate, thesis/dissertation, written exam, oral exam. *Entrance requirements:* For master's and doctorate, GRE General Test, MCAT, minimum GPA of 3.0. Additional exam requirements/ recommendations for international students: Required—TOEFL (minimum score 550 paper-based; 88 iBT). *Application deadline:* For fall admission, 12/31 for domestic and international students; for spring admission, 8/1 for domestic and international students. Applications are processed on a rolling basis. Application fee: $50. Electronic applications accepted. *Financial support:* In 2013–14, 22 students received support, including 14 research assistantships with full tuition reimbursements available (averaging $22,422 per year), 9 teaching assistantships with full tuition reimbursements available (averaging $22,422 per year); fellowships, scholarships/grants, health care benefits, and unspecified assistantships also available. Financial award application deadline: 4/15. *Faculty research:* Addiction, sleep and performance, body weight and energy balance, emotion and well being, learning and memory, reproduction, vision, movement. *Total annual research expenditures:* $5.2 million. *Unit head:* Dr. Steve Simasko, Chair, 509-335-6624, Fax: 509-335-4650, E-mail: simasko@vetmed.wsu.edu. *Application contact:* Bobbi Sauer, Program Assistant, 509-335-7675, Fax: 509-335-4650, E-mail: grad.neuro@vetmed.wsu.edu.
Website: http://www.vetmed.wsu.edu/Neuroscience/

Washington University in St. Louis, Graduate School of Arts and Sciences, Department of Philosophy, Program in Philosophy-Neuroscience-Psychology, St. Louis, MO 63130-4899. Offers PhD. *Students:* 18 full-time (6 women), 4 international. 60 applicants, 15% accepted, 4 enrolled. In 2013, 1 doctorate awarded. *Degree requirements:* For doctorate, thesis/dissertation. *Entrance requirements:* For doctorate, GRE General Test, sample of written work. Additional exam requirements/ recommendations for international students: Required—TOEFL. *Application deadline:* For fall admission, 12/31 for domestic students. Application fee: $45. Electronic applications accepted. *Financial support:* Fellowships and tuition waivers (full and partial) available. Financial award application deadline: 1/15. *Faculty research:* Philosophy of mind and language with a special emphasis on the philosophical dimensions of psychology, neuroscience, and linguistics. *Unit head:* Dr. Ron Mallon, Chair, 314-935-6670.
Website: http://pnp.artsci.wustl.edu/

Washington University in St. Louis, Graduate School of Arts and Sciences, Division of Biology and Biomedical Sciences, Program in Neurosciences, St. Louis, MO 63130-4899. Offers PhD. *Degree requirements:* For doctorate, thesis/dissertation. *Entrance requirements:* For doctorate, GRE General Test, GRE Subject Test. Electronic applications accepted.

Wayne State University, College of Liberal Arts and Sciences, Department of Psychology, Detroit, MI 48202. Offers behavioral and cognitive neuroscience (PhD); clinical psychology (PhD); cognitive, developmental and social psychology (PhD); industrial and organizational psychology (MA, PhD); social psychology (PhD). Fall application deadline for PhD is December 15. *Accreditation:* APA (one or more programs are accredited). *Faculty:* 37 full-time (13 women), 8 part-time/adjunct (4 women). *Students:* 106 full-time (71 women), 28 part-time (17 women); includes 19 minority (7 Black or African American, non-Hispanic/Latino; 4 Asian, non-Hispanic/ Latino; 6 Hispanic/Latino; 2 Two or more races, non-Hispanic/Latino), 12 international. Average age 28. 420 applicants, 11% accepted, 24 enrolled. In 2013, 32 master's, 18 doctorates awarded. Terminal master's awarded for partial completion of doctoral program. *Degree requirements:* For master's, thesis (for some programs); for doctorate, thesis/dissertation, training assignments. *Entrance requirements:* For master's, GRE General Test, admission to Graduate School, minimum undergraduate upper-division cumulative GPA of 3.0, courses in introductory psychology and statistics (for industrial and organizational psychology; for doctorate, GRE General Test, admission to Graduate School; bachelor's, master's, or other advanced degree; at least three letters of recommendation; statement of purpose. Additional exam requirements/ recommendations for international students: Required—TOEFL (minimum score 550 paper-based; 79 iBT), TWE (minimum score 5.5), Michigan English Language Assessment Battery (minimum score 85); Recommended—IELTS (minimum score 6.5). *Application deadline:* For fall admission, 6/15 for domestic students, 5/1 for international students; for winter admission, 10/15 for domestic students, 9/1 for international students; for spring admission, 3/15 for domestic students, 1/1 for international students. Application fee: $0. Electronic applications accepted. *Expenses:* Tuition, state resident: part-time $554.15 per credit. Tuition, nonresident: part-time $1200.35 per credit. *Required fees:* $42.15 per credit. $268.30 per semester. Tuition and fees vary according to course load and program. *Financial support:* In 2013–14, 90 students received support, including 9 fellowships with tuition reimbursements available (averaging $19,808 per year), 13 research assistantships with tuition reimbursements available (averaging $17,430 per year), 50 teaching assistantships with tuition reimbursements available (averaging $16,508 per year); career-related internships or fieldwork, scholarships/grants, health care benefits, and unspecified assistantships also available. Financial award application deadline: 3/31; financial award applicants required to submit FAFSA. *Faculty research:* Neuroscience, including functional cognitive imaging, neural physiology, behavioral pharmacology, and neurobehavioral teratology, cognitive and neurochemical processes associated with aging, drug addiction and neurological disorders to studies of the neural circuits that underlie learning, emotion, and weight regulation, the life-long developmental plasticity of the neurobiological processes of behavior, neuropsychology, child clinical psychology, health psychology, community psychology. *Total annual research expenditures:* $2.3 million. *Unit head:* Boris Baltes, PhD, Acting Chair/Professor, 313-577-2800, Fax: 313-577-7636, E-mail: b.baltes@wayne.edu. *Application contact:* Alia Allen, Academic Services Officer, 313-577-2823, E-mail: aallen@wayne.edu.
Website: http://clasweb.clas.wayne.edu/psychology

Wayne State University, School of Medicine, Graduate Programs in Medicine, Department of Psychiatry and Behavioral Neurosciences, Detroit, MI 48202. Offers psychiatry (MS); translational neuroscience (PhD). *Students:* 9 full-time (5 women); includes 2 minority (1 Asian, non-Hispanic/Latino; 1 Two or more races, non-Hispanic/ Latino), 1 international. Average age 28. 40 applicants, 5% accepted. *Degree requirements:* For master's, thesis, oral thesis defense; for doctorate, thesis/dissertation. *Entrance requirements:* For master's and doctorate, GRE, minimum undergradute GPA of 3.0, bachelor's degree from accredited institution, coursework in biological sciences and other scientific disciplines, personal statement, three letters of recommendation. Additional exam requirements/recommendations for international students: Required—TOEFL (minimum score 600 paper-based; 100 iBT). *Application deadline:* For fall admission, 12/15 for domestic and international students. Application fee: $0. Electronic applications accepted. *Expenses:* Contact institution. *Financial support:* In 2013–14, 8 students received support, including 2 fellowships with tuition reimbursements available (averaging $24,700 per year), 6 research assistantships with tuition reimbursements available (averaging $25,617 per year); scholarships/grants, health care benefits, and unspecified assistantships also available. Financial award application deadline: 3/31; financial award applicants required to submit FAFSA. *Faculty research:* Substance abuse, brain imaging, schizophrenia, child psychopathy, child development, neurobiology of monoamine systems. *Unit head:* Dr. David R. Rosenberg, Chair, 313-577-9000, E-mail: drosen@med.wayne.edu. *Application contact:* Dr. Jeffery Stanely, Graduate Program Director, 313-577-9090, E-mail: jstanley@med.wayne.edu.
Website: http://psychiatry.med.wayne.edu/

Wayne State University, School of Medicine, Graduate Programs in Medicine, Program in Molecular Biology and Genetics, Detroit, MI 48201. Offers bioinformatics and computational biology (PhD); cellular neuroscience (PhD); MD/PhD. *Students:* 21 full-time (11 women), 1 part-time (0 women); includes 1 minority (Hispanic/Latino), 3 international. Average age 27. 45 applicants, 13% accepted, 4 enrolled. In 2013, 5 doctorates awarded. Terminal master's awarded for partial completion of doctoral program. *Degree requirements:* For doctorate, thesis/dissertation. *Entrance requirements:* For doctorate, GRE General Test, GRE Subject Test (chemistry or biology), minimum GPA of 3.0, strong background in one of the chemical or biological sciences, three letters of recommendation, personal statement, interview. Additional exam requirements/recommendations for international students: Required—TOEFL (minimum score 550 paper-based; 79 iBT), Michigan English Language Assessment Battery (minimum score 85); Recommended—IELTS (minimum score 6.5), TWE (minimum score 5.5). *Application deadline:* For fall admission, 3/1 for domestic students, 5/1 for international students; for winter admission, 10/1 for domestic students, 9/1 for international students; for spring admission, 2/1 for domestic students, 1/1 for international students. Applications are processed on a rolling basis. Application fee: $0. Electronic applications accepted. *Expenses:* Tuition, state resident: part-time $554.15 per credit. Tuition, nonresident: part-time $1200.35 per credit. *Required fees:* $42.15 per credit. $268.30 per semester. Tuition and fees vary according to course load and program. *Financial support:* In 2013–14, 18 students received support. Fellowships with tuition reimbursements available, research assistantships with tuition reimbursements available, teaching assistantships with tuition reimbursements available, scholarships/ grants, and unspecified assistantships available. Financial award application deadline: 3/31; financial award applicants required to submit FAFSA. *Faculty research:* Human gene mapping, genome organization and sequencing, gene regulation, molecular evolution. *Total annual research expenditures:* $2.6 million. *Unit head:* Dr. Lawrence Grossman, Director, 313-577-5323, E-mail: l.grossman@wayne.edu. *Application contact:* Dr. Gregory Kapatos, Professor, Director for Education, and Graduate Officer, 313-577-5965, Fax: 313-993-4269, E-mail: gkapato@med.wayne.edu.
Website: http://genetics.wayne.edu/students/mdphd.php

Weill Cornell Medical College, Weill Cornell Graduate School of Medical Sciences, Neuroscience Program, New York, NY 10065. Offers MS, PhD. Terminal master's awarded for partial completion of doctoral program. *Degree requirements:* For master's, comprehensive exam; for doctorate, thesis/dissertation, final exam. *Entrance requirements:* For doctorate, GRE General Test, undergraduate training in biology, organic chemistry, physics, and mathematics. Additional exam requirements/ recommendations for international students: Required—TOEFL. Electronic applications accepted. *Faculty research:* Regulation of neuronal development, neuronal stem cells, information processing, behavior, neuronal plasticity.

West Virginia University, School of Medicine, Graduate Programs at the Health Sciences Center, Interdisciplinary Graduate Programs in Biomedical Sciences, Program in Neuroscience, Morgantown, WV 26506. Offers PhD, MD/PhD. *Degree requirements:* For doctorate, comprehensive exam, thesis/dissertation. *Entrance requirements:* For doctorate, GRE General Test, minimum GPA of 3.0. Additional exam requirements/ recommendations for international students: Required—TOEFL. Electronic applications accepted. *Faculty research:* Sensory neuroscience, cognitive neuroscience, neural injury, homeostasis, behavioral neuroscience.

Wilfrid Laurier University, Faculty of Graduate and Postdoctoral Studies, Faculty of Science, Department of Psychology, Waterloo, ON N2L 3C5, Canada. Offers behavioral neuroscience (M Sc, PhD); cognitive neuroscience (M Sc, PhD); community psychology (MA, PhD); social and developmental psychology (MA, PhD). Part-time programs available. *Degree requirements:* For master's, thesis; for doctorate, thesis/dissertation. *Entrance requirements:* For master's, GRE General Test, honors BA or the equivalent in psychology, minimum B average in undergraduate course work; for doctorate, GRE General Test, master's degree, minimum A- average. Additional exam requirements/ recommendations for international students: Required—TOEFL (minimum score 89 iBT). Electronic applications accepted. *Faculty research:* Brain and cognition, community psychology, social and developmental psychology.

Yale University, Graduate School of Arts and Sciences, Department of Psychology, New Haven, CT 06520. Offers behavioral neuroscience (PhD); clinical psychology (PhD); cognitive psychology (PhD); developmental psychology (PhD); social/personality psychology (PhD). *Accreditation:* APA. *Degree requirements:* For doctorate, thesis/ dissertation. *Entrance requirements:* For doctorate, GRE General Test.

Yale University, Graduate School of Arts and Sciences, Interdepartmental Neuroscience Program, New Haven, CT 06520. Offers PhD. *Degree requirements:* For doctorate, thesis/dissertation. *Entrance requirements:* For doctorate, GRE General Test. *Expenses:* Contact institution.

Yale University, School of Medicine and Graduate School of Arts and Sciences, Combined Program in Biological and Biomedical Sciences (BBS), Neuroscience Track, New Haven, CT 06520. Offers PhD, MD/PhD. *Degree requirements:* For doctorate, thesis/dissertation. *Entrance requirements:* For doctorate, GRE General Test. Additional exam requirements/recommendations for international students: Required—TOEFL. Electronic applications accepted.

UNIFORMED SERVICES UNIVERSITY OF THE HEALTH SCIENCES

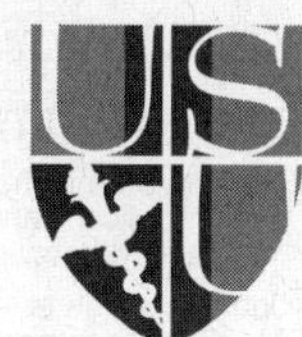

F. Edward Hébert School of Medicine Graduate Program in Neuroscience

Program of Study

The Uniformed Services University of the Health Sciences (USUHS) offers the Graduate Program in Neuroscience, a broadly based interdisciplinary program leading to the Ph.D. degree in neuroscience. Courses and research training are provided by the neuroscience faculty members, who hold primary appointments in the Departments of Anatomy, Physiology, and Genetics; Biochemistry; Medical and Clinical Psychology; Microbiology and Immunology; Neurology; Pathology; Pediatrics; Pharmacology; and Psychiatry at the University. The program permits considerable flexibility in the choice of courses and research areas; training programs are tailored to meet the individual requirements of each student. The program is designed for students with strong undergraduate training in the physical sciences, biology, or psychology who wish to pursue a professional career in neuroscience research. Integrated instruction in the development, structure, function, and pathology of the nervous system and its interaction with the environment is provided. Students in the program conduct their research under the direction of neuroscience faculty members in laboratories that are located in the medical school. During the first year of study, students begin formal course work. Each student is required to take laboratory training rotations in the research laboratories of program faculty members. By the end of the first year, students select a research area and a faculty thesis adviser. During the second year, students complete requirements for advancement to candidacy, including required course work and passage of the qualifying examination. After advancement to candidacy, each student develops an original research project and prepares and defends a written dissertation under the guidance of his or her faculty adviser and advisory committee.

Research Facilities

Each academic department at the University is provided with laboratories for the support of a variety of research projects. Neuroscience research laboratories available to students are suitable for research in most areas of neuroscience, including behavioral studies, electrophysiology, molecular and cellular neurobiology, neuroanatomy, neurochemistry, neuropathology, neuropharmacology, and neurophysiology. High-resolution electron microscopes, confocal microscopes, two photon microscopes, deconvolution wide-field fluorescence microscopes, a central resource facility providing custom synthesis of oligonucleotides and peptides and DNA sequencing, centralized animal facilities, computer support, a medical library, and a learning resources center are available within the University.

Financial Aid

Stipends are available on a competitive basis. Awards are made on a yearly basis and are renewable. For the 2014–15 academic year, stipends for entering students begin at $27,000. Outstanding students may be nominated for the Dean's Special Fellowship or other special fellowships, which support a stipend of $32,000.

Cost of Study

Graduate students in the neuroscience program are not required to pay tuition or fees. Civilian students incur no obligation to the United States government for service after completion of their graduate training program. Students are required to carry health insurance.

Living and Housing Costs

There is a reasonable supply of affordable rental housing in the area. The University does not have housing for graduate students. Students are responsible for making their own arrangements for accommodations. Costs in the Washington, D.C., area are comparable to those in other major metropolitan areas.

Student Group

The neuroscience graduate program is an active and growing graduate program; approximately 27 students are enrolled. The Uniformed Services University (USU) also has Ph.D. programs in departmentally based basic biomedical sciences, as well as interdisciplinary graduate programs in molecular and cell biology and in emerging infectious diseases. In addition to the graduate and medical programs in the medical school, the nursing school has graduate programs for nurse practitioners and nurse anesthetists.

Student Outcomes

Graduates hold faculty, research associate, postdoctoral, science policy, and other positions in universities, medical schools, government, and industrial research institutions. Thirty-seven Ph.D.'s have been awarded since 1998. Currently 3 USU neuroscience graduates hold faculty positions within the Neuroscience Graduate Program.

Location

Metropolitan Washington has a population of about 5 million residents in the District of Columbia and the surrounding areas of Maryland and Virginia. The region is a center of education and research and is home to five major universities, four medical schools, the National Library of Medicine and the National Institutes of Health (next to the USUHS campus), Walter Reed National Military Medical Center, the Armed Forces Institute of Pathology, the Library of Congress, the Smithsonian Institution, the National Bureau of Standards, and many other private and government research centers. Many cultural advantages of the area include the theater, a major symphony orchestra, major league sports, and world-famous museums. The Metro subway system has a station near campus and provides a convenient connection from the University to museums and cultural attractions of downtown Washington. The University is within an easy distance of three major airports, Baltimore Washington International, Reagan International, and Dulles International. Both Reagan and Dulles International airports are accessible from the campus via Metro subway. For outdoor activities, the Blue Ridge Mountains, the Chesapeake Bay, and the Atlantic coast beaches are all within a few hours of driving distance.

The University

The University was established by Congress in 1972 to provide a comprehensive education in medicine to those who demonstrate potential for careers as Medical Corps officers in the uniformed services. Graduate programs in the basic medical sciences are offered to both civilian and military students and are an essential part of the academic environment at the University. The University is located in proximity to major research facilities, including the National Institutes of Health (NIH), the National Library of Medicine, Walter Reed Army Medical Center at the National Naval Medical Center, the Armed Forces Institute of Pathology, the National Institute of Standards and Technology, and numerous biotechnology companies.

Uniformed Services University subscribes fully to the policy of equal educational opportunity and accepts students on a competitive basis without regard to race, color, sex, age, or creed.

Applying

Civilian applicants are accepted as full-time students only. Each applicant must have a bachelor's degree from an accredited academic institution. A strong background in science with courses in several of the following disciplines—biochemistry, biology, chemistry, mathematics, physics, physiology, and psychology—is desirable. Applicants must arrange for official transcripts of all prior college-level courses taken and their GRE scores (taken within the last two years) to be sent to the Office of Graduate Education. Students may elect to submit scores obtained in one or more GRE Subject Tests (from the subject areas listed above) in support of their application. Applicants must also arrange for letters of recommendation from 3 people who are familiar with their academic work to be sent to the University. For full consideration and evaluation for stipend support, completed applications should be received before December 1 for matriculation in late August. Late applications are evaluated on a space-available basis. There is no application fee. Application forms may be obtained from the website at http://www.usuhs.mil/nes/progdescription.html#app.

Correspondence and Information

For applications:

Associate Dean for Graduate Education
Uniformed Services University
4301 Jones Bridge Road
Bethesda, Maryland 20814-4799
United States
Phone: 301-295-3913
800-772-1747 (toll-free)
E-mail: netina.finley@usuhs.edu
Website: http://www.usuhs.mil/graded/

For information about the neuroscience program:

Sharon Juliano, Ph.D.
Director, Graduate Program in Neuroscience
Uniformed Services University
4301 Jones Bridge Road
Bethesda, Maryland 20814-4799
United States
Phone: 301-295-3642
Fax: 301-295-1996
E-mail: netina.finley@usuhs.edu
Website: http://www.usuhs.mil/nes/index.html

Uniformed Services University of the Health Sciences

THE FACULTY AND THEIR RESEARCH

Denes V. Agoston, M.D., Ph.D., Professor, Department of Anatomy, Physiology, and Genetics. Traumatic brain injury; disease mechanism, diagnosis, and prognosis using biomarkers.

Juanita Anders, Ph.D., Professor, Department of Anatomy, Physiology, and Genetics. Innovative therapies for neuronal regeneration of injured central and peripheral nervous systems; light-cellular interaction.

Regina Armstrong, Ph.D., Professor, Department of Anatomy, Physiology, and Genetics, and Director, Center for Neuroscience and Regenerative Medicine. Cellular and molecular mechanisms of neural stem/progenitor cell development and regeneration in demyelinating diseases and brain injury models.

Suzanne B. Bausch, Ph.D., Associate Professor, Department of Pharmacology. Synaptic plasticity in traumatic brain injury and epileptogenesis; and therapies to prevent posttraumatic epilepsy.

David Benedek, M.D., Professor, Department of Psychiatry.

Diane E. Borst, Ph.D., Research Assistant Professor, Department of Anatomy, Physiology, and Genetics. Molecular mechanisms of retinal gene regulation and function.

Maria F. Braga, D.D.S., Ph.D., Professor, Department of Anatomy, Physiology, and Genetics. Cellular and molecular mechanisms regulating neuronal excitability in the amygdala; pathophysiology of anxiety disorders and epilepsy.

Barrington G. Burnett, Ph.D., Assistant Professor, Department of Anatomy, Physiology, and Genetics. The ubiquitin-proteasome system in neuronal maintenance and neurodegeneration.

Howard Bryant, Ph.D., Associate Professor, Department of Anatomy, Physiology, and Genetics. Electrophysiology of vascular smooth muscle.

Kimberly Byrnes, Ph.D., Assistant Professor, Department of Anatomy, Physiology, and Genetics. Microglial and macrophage-based chronic inflammation after traumatic brain and spinal cord injury; noninvasive imaging of post-injury metabolic and inflammatory events.

Col. William W. Campbell, USA, MC; M.D., M.S.H.A.; Professor and Chair, Department of Neurology, and Professor, Department of Neuroscience. Neuromuscular disease and clinical neurophysiology.

Kwang Choi, Ph.D., Assistant Professor, Department of Psychiatry. Pre-clinical research on anxiety disorders and substance abuse using animal models including intravenous drug self-administration, Pavlovian fear conditioning, elevated plus maze, and locomotor sensitization.

Jeffrey Cole, Ph.D., Assistant Professor, Department of Neurology. Translational research on traumatic brain injury, focusing on branched chain amino acids and metabolomics.

De-Maw Chuang, Ph.D., Adjunct Professor, Department of Psychiatry. Molecular and cellular of actions of mood stabilizers: neuroprotection against excitotoxicity-related neurodegeneration.

Thomas Côté, Ph.D., Associate Professor, Department of Pharmacology. Mu opioid receptor interaction with GTP-binding proteins and RGS proteins.

Brian Cox, Ph.D., Professor, Department of Pharmacology. Opiate drugs, endogenous opioids, neuropeptides; mechanisms underlying synaptic plasticity, drug tolerance and dependence, and responses to brain injury.

Clifton Dalgard, Ph.D., Assistant Professor, Department of Anatomy, Physiology, and Genetics. Molecular mechanisms of damage-associated inflammation.

Patricia A. Deuster, Ph.D., M.P.H., Professor, Department of Military and Emergency Medicine. Mechanisms of neuroendocrine and immune activation with stress.

Martin Doughty, Ph.D., Associate Professor, Department of Anatomy, Physiology, and Genetics. Optimizing induced pluripotent stem cells (iPSCs) for cell replacement therapy to treat traumatic brain injury (TBI); identifying transcriptional programs that function in cerebellar neurogenesis and pattern formation.

Ying-Hong Feng, Associate Professor, M.D., Ph.D. Angiotensin receptor and signal transduction.

Zygmunt Galdzicki, Ph.D., Professor, Department of Anatomy, Physiology, and Genetics. Molecular and electrophysiological approach to understand mental retardation in Down syndrome; neuroepigenetics and role of stress and brain trauma in neurodegenerative disorders

Neil Grunberg, Ph.D., Professor, Department of Medical and Clinical Psychology. Nicotine and tobacco; drug abuse; stress; traumatic brain injury; PTSD.

Carl Gunderson, M.D., Professor, Department of Neurology. Education of medical students; history of military neurology.

Harry Holloway, M.D., Professor, Department of Psychiatry. Clinical psychiatry; alcohol and drug misuse; posttraumatic stress; neurobiology of psychiatric disorders; clinical psychopharmacology.

David Jacobowitz, Ph.D., Professor, Department of Anatomy, Physiology, and Genetics. Gene and protein discovery in the diseased and developing brain.

Martha Johnson, Ph.D., Associate Professor, Department of Anatomy, Physiology, and Genetics. Education of first-year medical and graduate students in the anatomical and physiological sciences.

Sharon Juliano, Ph.D., Professor, Department of Anatomy, Physiology, and Genetics. Mechanisms of development and plasticity in the cerebral cortex, with particular emphasis on the migration of neurons into the cortical plate and factors maintaining the function and morphology of radial glia and Cajal-Retzius cells.

Fabio Leonessa, M.D., Research Assistant Professor, Department of Neurology. Pathobiology and biomarkers of traumatic brain injury and posttraumatic stress disorder.

He Li, M.D., Ph.D., Associate Professor, Department of Psychiatry. Neurobiological basis of post-traumatic stress disorder: synaptic plasticity and neuronal signaling in the amygdala circuitry.

Geoffrey Ling, M.D., Ph.D., Professor, Departments of Anesthesiology, Neurology, and Surgery. Novel therapeutics and diagnostic tools for traumatic brain injury and hemorrhagic shock; mechanisms of cellular injury and edema formation in traumatic brain injury.

Ann M. Marini, Ph.D., M.D., Professor, Department of Neurology. Molecular and cellular mechanisms of intrinsic survival pathways to protect against neurodegenerative disorders.

Joseph McCabe, Ph.D., Professor and Vice Chair, Department of Anatomy, Physiology, and Genetics. Traumatic brain injury and modeling; neuroprotection.

Debra McLaughlin, Ph.D., Research Assistant Professor, Department of Anatomy, Physiology, and Genetics. Sensory processing and cortical neurophysiology.

David Mears, Ph.D., Associate Professor, Department of Anatomy, Physiology, and Genetics. Electrophysiology and calcium signaling in neuroendocrine cells.

Chantal Moratz, Ph.D, Assistant Professor, Department of Medicine. Mechanisms of inflammation regulation in systemic lupus erythematosus, neuroinflammation in mild traumatic brain injury.

Gregory Mueller, Ph.D., Professor, Department of Anatomy, Physiology, and Genetics. Neuroimmunology; brain autoantibodies; brain injury biomarkers and the proteomics of brain injury.

Aryan Namboodiri, Ph.D., Associate Professor, Department of Anatomy, Physiology, and Genetics. Neurobiology of N-acetylaspartate (NAA); pathogenesis and treatment of Canavan disease and intranasal brain delivery of neuroprotectants.

Feresh Nugent, Ph.D., Assistant Professor, Department of Pharmacology. Synaptic plasticity and drug addiction.

J. Timothy O'Neill, Ph.D., Associate Professor, Departments of Pediatrics and Anatomy, Physiology, and Genetics. Effects of perinatal carbon monoxide and nicotine on cortical development and behavior; mechanisms of control of newborn and developmental cerebral blood and oxygen supply.

Paul Pasquina, M.D., Chairman, Department of Physical Medicine and Rehabilitation, and Director, Center for Rehabilitation Sciences Research. Clinical studies on advanced prosthetics, neurorehabilitation, traumatic brain injury, and pain management.

Harvey B. Pollard, M.D., Ph.D., Professor and Chair, Department of Anatomy, Physiology, and Genetics. Molecular biology of secretory processes.

Sylvie Poluch, Ph.D., Research Assistant Professor, Department of Anatomy, Physiology, and Genetics. Development of the cerebral cortex.

Brian Schaefer, Ph.D., Associate Professor, Department of Microbiology and Immunology. Biology of lymphocyte activation, particularly the antigen-regulated NF-kappaB pathway; role of inflammation in traumatic brain injury; imaging, biochemical, and cellular approaches to elucidate signal transduction mechanisms.

Jeremy T. Smyth, Ph.D., Assistant Professor, Department of Anatomy, Physiology, and Genetics. Physiology of the endoplasmic reticulum in developmental and neurodegenerative processes; intracellular calcium signaling; Drosophila developmental genetics.

Aviva Symes, Ph.D., Associate Professor, Department of Pharmacology. Glial response to traumatic brain and spinal cord injury; mechanism of cytokine action in the CNS after injury.

E. Fuller Torrey, M.D., Professor, Department of Psychiatry. Infectious agents as causes of schizophrenia and bipolar disorder.

Jack W. Tsao, M.D., Ph.D., Professor, Departments of Neurology and Physical Medicine and Rehabilitation. Clinical studies on phantom limb pain and traumatic brain injury; basic science studies on cellular and developmental mechanisms governing nerve degeneration.

Robert J. Ursano, M.D., Professor and Chairman, Department of Psychiatry, and Director, Center for the Study of Traumatic Stress. Posttraumatic stress disorder.

Capt. Will Watson, M.D., Ph.D., Associate Professor, Department of Neurology and Neuroscience Graduate Program. Local and systemic inflammatory response to traumatic brain injury; energy metabolism post brain injury, especially responses of the aspartate malate shuttle, pyruvate dehydrogenase complex, and coupling of glucose and calcium.

Maree J. Webster, Ph.D., Assistant Professor, Department of Psychiatry. Neuropathology of severe mental illness; schizophrenia and bipolar disorder.

T. John Wu, Ph.D., Associate Professor, Department of Obstetrics and Gynecology. Neuroendocrine regulation of reproduction and stress.

Lei Zhang, M.D., Associate Professor, Department of Psychiatry. PTSD and biomarkers.

Yumin Zhang, M.D., Ph.D., Associate Professor, Department of Anatomy, Physiology, and Genetics. Cellular and molecular mechanisms of oligodendroglial and neuronal toxicity.

UCONN HEALTH

Graduate Program in Neuroscience

UCONN HEALTH

Program of Study

The neuroscience graduate program at UConnecticut Health offers an interdisciplinary training environment that is committed to preparing students for research and teaching careers in both academic and industrial settings. The curriculum and research are dedicated to understanding the normal function and disorders of the nervous system.

All course requirements are fulfilled within the first two years of the program. Introductory core courses establish a strong foundation in molecular, cellular, and systems-level neurobiology.

A wide selection of advanced elective courses on such topics as physiology of excitable tissue, computational neuroscience, neuropharmacology, neuroimmunology, neurobiology of disease, microscopy, biochemistry, immunology, genetics, and cell biology allows tailoring of the curriculum to accommodate the specific needs and diverse interests of students. Participation in weekly journal clubs provides a broad perspective of cutting-edge research in the field.

During the first year of the program, three research rotation projects are performed in laboratories of the student's choice and a laboratory is identified for the dissertation research project by the beginning of the second year. Experimental training opportunities ranging from recombinant DNA to human studies are available. The breadth of these opportunities is shown in a survey of the areas of faculty research, which include regulation of gene expression, signal transduction, and intracellular trafficking in neurons and glia; function of voltage-sensitive ion channels and neurotransmitter receptors; biology of neuropeptides; synaptic transmission and neuroplasticity; development of neurons and glia; synaptic organization and stimulus coding; and sensory perception, behavior, and human psychophysics. Research pertaining to specific maladies of the nervous system includes neuroinflammation, autoimmunity, and neurodegeneration; substance abuse; stroke; epilepsy; multiple sclerosis; and deafness. Approaches employed include genetic engineering; cell and brain slice cultures; stem cells; electrophysiology; confocal microscopy and other imaging; neuroanatomical, virtual cell and mathematical modeling; and behavioral and transgenic animal models.

Research Facilities

Because of the interdepartmental format, the students have access to all of the facilities of modern biomedical research at UConn Health, including those in clinical and basic science departments. Most of the neuroscience faculty members are housed in the same building on adjoining floors, providing for a congenial atmosphere of informal scientific exchange and collaborations between laboratories. The Center for Cell Analysis and Modeling (CCAM) has state-of-the-art facilities for confocal and two-photon microscopy and image analysis and is available to members of the Program in Neuroscience. The Lyman Maynard Stowe Library has an extensive collection of periodicals and monographs as well as subscriptions to journals of current interest in the field of neuroscience.

Financial Aid

Support for doctoral students engaged in full-time degree programs at UConn Health is provided on a competitive basis. Graduate research assistantships for 2014–15 provide a stipend of $29,000 per year, which includes a waiver of tuition/most University fees for the fall and spring semesters and the option of participating in a student health insurance plan. While financial aid is offered competitively, UConn Health makes every possible effort to address the financial needs of all students.

Cost of Study

For 2014–15, tuition is $12,202 per year for full-time students who are Connecticut residents and $32,258 per year for full-time students who are out-of-state residents. General University fees are added to the cost of tuition for students who do not receive a tuition waiver. These costs are usually met by traineeships or research assistantships for doctoral students.

Living and Housing Costs

There is a wide range of affordable housing options in the greater Hartford area within easy commuting distance of the campus, including an extensive complex that is adjacent to UConn Health. Costs range from $700 to $1,000 per month for a one-bedroom unit; 2 or more students sharing an apartment usually pay less. University housing is not available.

Student Group

Seventeen students are registered in the Ph.D. program in the Neuroscience Program (including combined-degree students). The total number of master's and Ph.D. students at UConn Health is approximately 400, and there are about 125 medical and dental students per class.

Location

UConn Health is located in the historic town of Farmington, Connecticut. Set in the beautiful New England countryside on a hill overlooking the Farmington Valley, it is close to ski areas, hiking trails, and facilities for boating, fishing, and swimming. Connecticut's capital city of Hartford, 7 miles east of Farmington, is the center of an urban region of approximately 800,000 people. The beaches of the Long Island Sound are about 50 minutes away to the south, and the beautiful Berkshires are a short drive to the northwest. New York City and Boston can be reached within 2½ hours by car. Hartford is the home of the acclaimed Hartford Stage Company, TheatreWorks, the Hartford Symphony and Chamber orchestras, two ballet companies, an opera company, the Wadsworth Athenaeum (the oldest public art museum in the nation), the Mark Twain house, the Hartford Civic Center, and many other interesting cultural and recreational facilities. The area is also home to several branches of the University of Connecticut, Trinity College, and the University of Hartford, which includes the Hartt School of Music. Bradley International Airport (about 30 minutes from campus) serves the Hartford/Springfield area with frequent airline connections to major cities in this country and abroad. Frequent bus and rail service is also available from Hartford.

The Health Center

The 200-acre UConn Health campus at Farmington houses a division of the University of Connecticut Graduate School, as well as the School of Medicine and Dental Medicine. The campus also includes the John Dempsey Hospital, associated clinics, and extensive medical research facilities, all in a centralized facility with more than 1 million square feet of floor space. The Academic Research Building, built in 1999, is an impressive eleven-story structure providing 170,000 square feet of laboratory space. In addition, renovations are underway in the main Laboratory building, converting existing lab space to state-of-the-art open lab areas. The faculty includes more than 260 full-time members. The institution has a strong commitment to graduate study within an environment that promotes social and intellectual interaction among the various educational programs. Graduate students are represented on various administrative committees concerned with curricular affairs, and the Graduate Student Organization (GSO) represents graduate students' needs and concerns to the faculty and administration, in addition to fostering social contact among graduate students at UConn Health.

Applying

Applications for admission should be submitted via the online application system and should be filed together with transcripts, three letters of recommendation, a personal statement, and recent results from the General Test of the Graduate Record Examinations. International students must take the Test of English as a Foreign Language (TOEFL) to satisfy Graduate School requirements. The deadline for completed applications and receipt of all supplemental materials is **December 1**. Please note that GRE and TOEFL exams taken after the due date will not be accepted for consideration for admission. Applicants should have had undergraduate instruction in chemistry and biology. In accordance with the laws of the state of Connecticut and of the United States, UConn Health does not discriminate against any person in its educational and employment activities on the grounds of race, color, creed, national origin, sex, age, or physical disability.

Correspondence and Information

Graduate Admissions Office
Ph.D. in Biomedical Science Program
UConn Health
263 Farmington Ave., MC 3906
Farmington, Connecticut 06030-3906
United States
Phone: 860-679-4509
E-mail: BiomedSciAdmissions@uchc.edu
Website: http://grad.uchc.edu/prospective/programs/phd_biosci/index.html

THE FACULTY AND THEIR RESEARCH

Srdjan Antic, Associate Professor of Neuroscience; M.D., Belgrade. Dendritic integration of synaptic inputs; dopaminergic modulation of dendritic excitability.

Rashmi Bansal, Professor of Neuroscience; Ph.D., Central Drug Research Institute. Developmental, cellular, and molecular biology of oligodendrocytes; growth-factor regulation of development and function and its relationship to neurodegenerative disease, including multiple sclerosis.

Elisa Barbarese, Professor of Neuroscience and Neurology; Ph.D. McGill. Molecular and cellular biology of neural cells, with emphasis on RNA trafficking.

Leslie R. Bernstein, Professor of Neuroscience; Ph.D., Illinois. Behavioral neuroscience: psychoacoustics, binaural hearing.

John H. Carson, Professor of Molecular, Microbial, and Structural Biology; Ph.D., MIT. Molecular and developmental neurobiology; myelination; intracellular RNA trafficking.

Jonathan Covault, Professor of Psychiatry; M.D., Ph.D., Iowa. Genetic correlates of alcohol use disorders; role of neuroactive steroids in the effects of alcohol.

Stephen Crocker, Assistant Professor of Neuroscience; Ph.D., Ottawa. Brain injury and repair in neurodegenerative diseases, with a focus on neuroinflammation; myelin injury; neural stem cell differentiation; signal transduction; glia; matrix metalloproteinases and their tissue inhibitors.

Betty Eipper, Professor of Neuroscience; Ph.D., Harvard. Cell biology, biochemistry, and physiology of peptide synthesis, storage, and secretion in neurons and endocrine cells.

Marion E. Frank, Professor of BioStructure and Function and Director, Connecticut Chemosensory Clinical Research Center; Ph.D., Brown. Gustatory neurophysiology, neuroanatomy, behavior, and disorders; chemosensory information processing; clinical testing of oral chemosensory function in humans.

Duck O. Kim, Professor of Neuroscience and Biological Engineering Program; D.Sc., Washington (St. Louis). Neurobiology and biophysics of the auditory system; computational neuroscience of single neurons and neural systems; experimental otolaryngology; biomedical engineering.

Shigeyuki Kuwada, Professor of Neuroscience; Ph.D., Cincinnati. Neurophysiology and anatomy of mammalian auditory system; principles of binaural signal processing, electrical audiometry in infants.

Eric S. Levine, Professor of Neuroscience; Ph.D., Princeton. Synapse plasticity and role of neuromodulators in brain development and learning, focusing on neurotrophins and endocannabinoids.

James Li, Associate Professor of Genetics and Developmental Biology; Ph.D., Texas. Development of the central nervous system, with an emphasis on the cellular and molecular mechanisms underlying formation of the mammalian cerebellum.

Jun Li, Assistant Professor of Neuroscience; Ph.D., Dublin—Trinity.

Xue-Jun Li, Assistant Professor of Neuroscience; Ph.D., Fudan (China). Stem cell biology: mechanisms and pathways underlying the development and degeneration of human motor neurons, using human stem cells as an experimental system.

Leslie Loew, Professor of Cell Biology; Ph.D., Cornell. Morphological determinants of cell physiology; image-based computational models of cellular biology; spatial variations of cell membrane electrophysiology; new optical methods for probing living cells.

Xin-Ming Ma, Assistant Professor of Neuroscience; Ph.D., Beijing. Synaptogenesis and spine plasticity in hippocampal neurons; estrogen hormones and synaptic plasticity; stress and neuronal plasticity.

Richard Mains, Professor and Chair of Neuroscience; Ph.D., Harvard. Pituitary; neuronal tissue culture; peptides, vesicles; enzymes; drug abuse; development.

Louise McCullough, Professor of Neurology and Neuroscience; M.D., Ph.D., Connecticut. Effects of estrogens on stroke.

Douglas L. Oliver, Professor of Neuroscience and Biomedical Engineering; Ph.D., Duke. Synaptic organization; parallel information processing in CNS; role of ionic currents, channel expression in information processing; neurocytology, morphology, cellular physiology of CNS sensory systems; biology of hearing and deafness.

Joel S. Pachter, Professor of Cell Biology; Ph.D., NYU. Mechanisms regulating pathogenesis of CNS infectious/inflammatory disease.

Lauren Sansing, Assistant Professor of Neurology; M.D., Stony Brook, SUNY.

Henry Smilowitz, Professor of Radiology, Ph.D., MIT. Development of novel therapies for experimental advanced, imminently lethal, malignant brain tumors in rats and mice; use of gold nanoparticles to develop a new form of radiation therapy (gold-enhanced radiation therapy) and novel approaches to both tumor and vascular imaging.

David M. Waitzman, Associate Professor of Neurology; M.D./Ph.D., CUNY, Mount Sinai. Neurophysiology; oculomotor system; gaze control system; modeling of CNS.

Zhaowen Wang, Associate Professor of Neuroscience; Ph.D., Michigan State. Molecular mechanisms of synaptic transmission, focusing on neurotransmitter release and mechanisms of potassium channel localization, using *C. elegans* as a model organism.

Ji Yu, Associate Professor of Genetics and Developmental Biology; Ph.D., Texas. Optical imaging technology; regulatory mechanisms in dendritic RNA translation; cytoskeletal dynamics.

Nada Zecevic, Professor of Neuroscience; M.D., Ph.D., Belgrade. Cellular and molecular aspects of CNS development; primate cerebral cortex; oligodendrocyte progenitors, stem cells, microglia; multiple sclerosis.

Section 14
Nutrition

This section contains a directory of institutions offering graduate work in nutrition. Additional information about programs listed in the directory but not augmented by an in-depth entry may be obtained by writing directly to the dean of a graduate school or chair of a department at the address given in the directory.

For programs offering related work, see also in this book *Allied Health, Biochemistry, Biological and Biomedical Sciences, Botany and Plant Biology, Microbiological Sciences, Pathology and Pathobiology, Pharmacology and Toxicology, Physiology, Public Health,* and *Veterinary Medicine and Sciences.* In the other guides in this series:

Graduate Programs in the Humanities, Arts & Social Sciences

See *Economics (Agricultural Economics and Agribusiness)* and *Family and Consumer Sciences*

Graduate Programs in the Physical Sciences, Mathematics, Agricultural Sciences, the Environment & Natural Resources

See *Agricultural and Food Sciences* and *Chemistry*

Graduate Programs in Engineering & Applied Sciences

See *Agricultural Engineering and Bioengineering* and *Biomedical Engineering and Biotechnology*

CONTENTS

Program Directory

Display and Close-Up

See:

Nutrition

Adelphi University, College of Nursing and Public Health, Garden City, NY 11530. Offers adult/geriatric nurse practitioner (MS); health information technology (Advanced Certificate); nurse practitioner in adult health nursing (Certificate); nursing (PhD); nursing administration (MS, Certificate); nursing education (MS, Certificate); nutrition (MS); public health (MPH). *Accreditation:* AACN. Part-time and evening/weekend programs available. *Faculty:* 40 full-time (34 women), 176 part-time/adjunct (169 women). *Students:* 9 full-time (7 women), 178 part-time (158 women); includes 107 minority (57 Black or African American, non-Hispanic/Latino; 1 American Indian or Alaska Native, non-Hispanic/Latino; 28 Asian, non-Hispanic/Latino; 13 Hispanic/Latino; 1 Native Hawaiian or other Pacific Islander, non-Hispanic/Latino; 7 Two or more races, non-Hispanic/Latino). Average age 40. 221 applicants, 52% accepted, 74 enrolled. In 2013, 25 master's, 3 doctorates, 1 other advanced degree awarded. *Degree requirements:* For master's, thesis or alternative. *Entrance requirements:* For master's, BSN, clinical experience, 1 course in basic statistics, minimum GPA of 3.0, 2 letters of recommendation, resume or curriculum vitae; for doctorate, GRE, licensure as RN in New York, professional writing sample (scholarly writing), 3 letters of recommendation, resume or curriculum vitae; for other advanced degree, MSN. Additional exam requirements/recommendations for international students: Required—TOEFL (minimum score 550 paper-based; 80 iBT). *Application deadline:* For fall admission, 3/15 for domestic students, 4/1 for international students; for spring admission, 11/1 for international students. Application fee: $50. Electronic applications accepted. *Expenses: Tuition:* Full-time $32,530; part-time $1010 per credit. *Required fees:* $1150. Tuition and fees vary according to degree level and program. *Financial support:* In 2013–14, 13 research assistantships (averaging $4,217 per year) were awarded; career-related internships or fieldwork, tuition waivers (partial), unspecified assistantships, and achievement awards also available. Support available to part-time students. Financial award application deadline: 2/15; financial award applicants required to submit FAFSA. *Faculty research:* Social practices in healthcare, bereavement, family grief, historiography, gerontology. *Unit head:* Dr. Patrick Coonan, Dean, 516-877-4511, E-mail: coonan@adelphi.edu. *Application contact:* Christine Murphy, Director of Admissions, 516-877-3050, Fax: 516-877-3039, E-mail: graduateadmissions@adelphi.edu.

Website: http://nursing.adelphi.edu/

See Display on page 624 and Close-Up on page 813.

American College of Healthcare Sciences, Graduate Programs, Portland, OR 97239-3719. Offers aromatherapy (Graduate Certificate); complementary alternative medicine (MS, Graduate Certificate); herbal medicine (Graduate Certificate); nutrition (Graduate Certificate). Part-time and evening/weekend programs available. Postbaccalaureate distance learning degree programs offered (no on-campus study). *Degree requirements:* For master's, capstone project. *Entrance requirements:* For master's, interview, letters of recommendation, essay.

American University, College of Arts and Sciences, Washington, DC 20016-8012. Offers addiction and addictive behavior (Certificate); anthropology (PhD); applied microeconomics (Certificate); applied statistics (Certificate); art history (MA); arts management (MA, Certificate); Asian studies (Certificate); audio production (Certificate); audio technology (MA); behavior, cognition, and neuroscience (PhD); bilingual education (MA, Certificate); biology (MA, MS); chemistry (MS); clinical psychology (PhD); computer science (MS, Certificate); creative writing (MFA); curriculum and instruction (M Ed, Certificate); economics (MA, PhD); environmental assessment (Certificate); environmental science (MS); ethics, peace, and global affairs (MA); gender analysis in economics (Certificate); health promotion management (MS); history (MA, PhD); international arts management (Certificate); international economic relations (Certificate); international economics (MA); international training and education (MA); literature (MA); mathematics (MA); North American studies (Certificate); nutrition education (MS, Certificate); philosophy (MA); professional science: biotechnology (MS); professional science: environmental assessment (MS); professional science: quantitative analysis (MS); psychobiology of healing (Certificate); psychology (MA); psychology: general (PhD); public anthropology (MA, Certificate); public sociology (Certificate); social research (Certificate); sociology (MA); Spanish: Latin American studies (MA); special education: learning disabilities (MA); statistics (MS); studio art (MFA); teaching (MAT); teaching English as a foreign language (MA); teaching: early childhood (Certificate); teaching: elementary (Certificate); teaching: ESOL (Certificate); teaching: secondary (Certificate); technology in arts management (Certificate); TESOL (MA); translation: French (Certificate); translation: Russian (Certificate); translation: Spanish (Certificate); women's, gender, and sexuality studies (Certificate). Part-time and evening/weekend programs available. Postbaccalaureate distance learning degree programs offered (no on-campus study). *Faculty:* 358 full-time (187 women), 254 part-time/adjunct (127 women). *Students:* 627 full-time (411 women), 416 part-time (300 women); includes 206 minority (91 Black or African American, non-Hispanic/Latino; 5 American Indian or Alaska Native, non-Hispanic/Latino; 32 Asian, non-Hispanic/Latino; 64 Hispanic/Latino; 1 Native Hawaiian or other Pacific Islander, non-Hispanic/Latino; 13 Two or more races, non-Hispanic/Latino), 124 international. Average age 29. 1,672 applicants, 52% accepted, 361 enrolled. In 2013, 382 master's, 38 doctorates, 33 other advanced degrees awarded. Terminal master's awarded for partial completion of doctoral program. *Degree requirements:* For master's, comprehensive exam (for some programs), thesis (for some programs); for doctorate, comprehensive exam (for some programs), thesis/dissertation. *Entrance requirements:* For master's, GRE, minimum GPA of 3.0 in last 60 credit hours, letter of recommendation, statement of purpose, resume, unofficial transcript; for doctorate, GRE, minimum GPA of 3.0 for all graduate work, letter of recommendation, statement of purpose, resume, unofficial transcript. Additional exam requirements/recommendations for international students: Required—TOEFL (minimum score 600 paper-based; 100 iBT), IELTS (minimum score 7). *Application deadline:* For fall admission, 2/1 for domestic students; for spring admission, 10/1 for domestic students. Applications are processed on a rolling basis. Application fee: $55. Electronic applications accepted. *Expenses: Tuition:* Full-time $25,920; part-time $1482 per credit hour. *Required fees:* $430. Tuition and fees vary according to course load and program. *Financial support:* Fellowships, research assistantships with full and partial tuition reimbursements, teaching assistantships with full and partial tuition reimbursements, career-related internships or fieldwork, Federal Work-Study, institutionally sponsored loans, scholarships/grants, traineeships, tuition waivers (full and partial), and unspecified assistantships available. Support available to part-time students. Financial award applicants required to submit FAFSA. *Unit head:* Dr. Peter Starr, Dean, 202-885-2446, Fax: 202-885-2429, E-mail: pstarr@american.edu. *Application contact:* Kathleen Clowery, Associate Director, Graduate Enrollment Management, 202-885-3621, Fax: 202-885-1505, E-mail: clowery@american.edu.

Website: http://www.american.edu/cas/

American University of Beirut, Graduate Programs, Faculty of Agricultural and Food Sciences, Beirut, Lebanon. Offers agricultural economics (MS); animal sciences (MS); ecosystem management (MSES); food technology (MS); irrigation (MS); nutrition (MS); plant protection (MS); plant science (MS); poultry science (MS); rural community development (MS). Part-time programs available. *Faculty:* 21 full-time (6 women), 1 part-time/adjunct (0 women). *Students:* 10 full-time (8 women), 70 part-time (55 women). Average age 26. 75 applicants, 68% accepted, 9 enrolled. In 2013, 32 master's awarded. *Degree requirements:* For master's, one foreign language, comprehensive exam, thesis (for some programs). *Entrance requirements:* Additional exam requirements/recommendations for international students: Required—TOEFL (minimum score 600 paper-based; 100 iBT), IELTS (minimum score 7.5). *Application deadline:* For fall admission, 2/7 for domestic and international students; for spring admission, 11/1 for domestic and international students. Application fee: $50. Electronic applications accepted. *Expenses: Tuition:* Full-time $14,724; part-time $818 per credit. *Required fees:* $692. Tuition and fees vary according to course load and program. *Financial support:* In 2013–14, 3 research assistantships with partial tuition reimbursements (averaging $4,000 per year), 27 teaching assistantships with full and partial tuition reimbursements (averaging $800 per year) were awarded; scholarships/grants, health care benefits, and unspecified assistantships also available. Financial award application deadline: 2/2. *Faculty research:* Evidence-based nutrition intervention, regional knowledge management and knowledge sharing network, micronutrient nutrition landscaping, production of biodiesel from algae, landscape character development for natural heritage conservation. *Total annual research expenditures:* $415,339. *Unit head:* Prof. Nahla Hwalla, Dean, 961-1343002 Ext. 4400, Fax: 961-1744460, E-mail: nahla@aub.edu.lb. *Application contact:* Dr. Rabih Talhouk, Director, Graduate Council, 961-1-350000 Ext. 4386, Fax: 96-1-1374374, E-mail: graduate.council@aub.edu.lb.

Website: http://www.aub.edu.lb/fafs/fafs_home/Pages/index.aspx

Andrews University, School of Health Professions, Department of Nutrition, Berrien Springs, MI 49104. Offers MS. Part-time programs available. *Faculty:* 5 full-time (3 women). *Students:* 3 full-time (all women), 25 part-time (20 women); includes 10 minority (3 Black or African American, non-Hispanic/Latino; 3 Asian, non-Hispanic/Latino; 4 Hispanic/Latino), 5 international. Average age 32. 38 applicants, 79% accepted, 21 enrolled. In 2013, 1 master's awarded. *Entrance requirements:* For master's, GRE. Additional exam requirements/recommendations for international students: Required—TOEFL (minimum score 550 paper-based). *Application deadline:* Applications are processed on a rolling basis. Application fee: $40. *Unit head:* Dr. Winston Craig, Chairperson, 269-471-3370. *Application contact:* Monica Wringer, Supervisor of Graduate Admission, 800-253-2874, Fax: 269-471-6321, E-mail: graduate@andrews.edu.

Website: http://www.andrews.edu/shp/nutrition/

Appalachian State University, Cratis D. Williams Graduate School, Department of Nutrition and Health Care Management, Boone, NC 28608. Offers nutrition (MS). Part-time programs available. Electronic applications accepted. *Faculty research:* Food antioxidants and nutrition.

Arizona State University at the Tempe campus, College of Nursing and Health Innovation, Phoenix, AZ 85004. Offers advanced nursing practice (DNP); child/family mental health nurse practitioner (Graduate Certificate); clinical research management (MS); community and public health practice (Graduate Certificate); community health (MS); exercise and wellness (MS), including exercise and wellness; family nurse practitioner (Graduate Certificate); healthcare innovation (MHI); international health for healthcare (Graduate Certificate); kinesiology (MS, PhD); nursing (MS, Graduate Certificate); nursing and healthcare innovation (PhD); nutrition (MS); physical activity nutrition and wellness (PhD), including physical activity, nutrition and wellness; public health (MPH); regulatory science and health safety (MS). *Accreditation:* AACN. Postbaccalaureate distance learning degree programs offered (minimal on-campus study). *Degree requirements:* For master's, comprehensive exam (for some programs), thesis (for some programs), interactive Program of Study (iPOS) submitted before completing 50 percent of required credit hours; for doctorate, comprehensive exam, thesis/dissertation, interactive Program of Study (iPOS) submitted before completing 50 percent of required credit hours. *Entrance requirements:* For master's and doctorate, GRE, minimum GPA of 3.0 or equivalent in last 2 years of work leading to bachelor's degree. Additional exam requirements/recommendations for international students: Required—TOEFL (minimum score 80 iBT), TOEFL, IELTS, or PTE. Electronic applications accepted. *Expenses:* Contact institution.

Auburn University, Graduate School, College of Human Sciences, Department of Nutrition and Food Science, Auburn University, AL 36849. Offers global hospitality and retailing (Graduate Certificate); nutrition (MS, PhD). Part-time programs available. *Faculty:* 13 full-time (5 women). *Students:* 28 full-time (18 women), 18 part-time (10 women); includes 9 minority (6 Black or African American, non-Hispanic/Latino; 3 Asian, non-Hispanic/Latino), 17 international. Average age 30. 55 applicants, 44% accepted, 10 enrolled. In 2013, 16 master's, 2 doctorates awarded. *Degree requirements:* For master's, thesis (for some programs); for doctorate, thesis/dissertation. *Entrance requirements:* For master's and doctorate, GRE General Test. *Application deadline:* For fall admission, 7/7 for domestic students; for spring admission, 11/24 for domestic students. Applications are processed on a rolling basis. Application fee: $50 ($60 for international students). Electronic applications accepted. *Expenses:* Tuition, state resident: full-time $8262; part-time $459 per credit hour. Tuition, nonresident: full-time $24,786; part-time $1377 per credit hour. Tuition and fees vary according to degree level and program. *Financial support:* Research assistantships, teaching assistantships, career-related internships or fieldwork, and Federal Work-Study available. Support available to part-time students. Financial award application deadline: 3/15; financial award applicants required to submit FAFSA. *Faculty research:* Food quality and safety, diet, food supply, physical activity in maintenance of health, prevention of selected chronic disease states. *Unit head:* Dr. Martin O'Neill, Head, 334-844-3266. *Application contact:* Dr. George Flowers, Dean of the Graduate School, 334-844-2125.

Website: http://www.humsci.auburn.edu/nufs/

Bastyr University, School of Natural Health Arts and Sciences, Kenmore, WA 98028-4966. Offers counseling psychology (MA); holistic landscape design (Certificate); midwifery (MS); nutrition (MS); nutrition and clinical health psychology (MS). *Accreditation:* AND. Part-time programs available. *Students:* 328 full-time (295 women), 40 part-time (38 women); includes 74 minority (5 Black or African American, non-Hispanic/Latino; 1 American Indian or Alaska Native, non-Hispanic/Latino; 28 Asian, non-Hispanic/Latino; 13 Hispanic/Latino; 27 Two or more races, non-Hispanic/Latino), 21 international. Average age 30. *Degree requirements:* For master's, thesis optional. *Entrance requirements:* For master's, 1-2 years' basic sciences course work (depending on program). Additional exam requirements/recommendations for international students: Required—TOEFL (minimum score 550 paper-based; 79 iBT). *Application deadline:* For

fall admission, 3/15 priority date for domestic and international students. Applications are processed on a rolling basis. Application fee: $75. *Financial support:* In 2013–14, 47 students received support. Career-related internships or fieldwork, Federal Work-Study, and scholarships/grants available. Support available to part-time students. Financial award application deadline: 4/15; financial award applicants required to submit FAFSA. *Faculty research:* Whole-food nutrition for type 2 diabetes; meditation in end-of-life care; stress management; Qi Gong, Tai Chi and yoga for older adults; Echinacea and immunology. *Unit head:* Dr. Timothy Callahan, Vice President and Provost, 425-602-3110, Fax: 425-823-6222. *Application contact:* Admissions Office, 425-602-3330, Fax: 425-602-3090, E-mail: admissions@bastyr.edu.
Website: http://www.bastyr.edu/academics/schools-departments/school-natural-health-arts-sciences

Baylor University, Graduate School, Military Programs, Program in Nutrition, Waco, TX 76798. Offers MS. *Faculty:* 7 full-time (6 women), 6 part-time/adjunct (all women). *Students:* 26 full-time (23 women); includes 2 minority (1 Hispanic/Latino; 1 Native Hawaiian or other Pacific Islander, non-Hispanic/Latino). Average age 26. 25 applicants, 48% accepted, 12 enrolled. In 2013, 13 master's awarded. *Degree requirements:* For master's, comprehensive exam, thesis. *Entrance requirements:* For master's, GRE. *Application deadline:* Applications are processed on a rolling basis. Electronic applications accepted. *Expenses: Tuition:* Full-time $25,866; part-time $1437 per credit hour. *Required fees:* $2736; $152 per credit hour. Tuition and fees vary according to course load and program. *Faculty research:* Weight control, critical care nutrition, breast feeding, intuitive eating. *Unit head:* Col. LesLee Funderburk, Graduate Program Director, 210-221-6274, Fax: 210-221-7363, E-mail: leslee.k.funderburk.mil@mail.mil. *Application contact:* Sgt. Malinda Moody-Williams, Administrative Assistant, 210-295-6274, E-mail: malinda.l.moodywilliams@mail.mil.
Website: http://www.baylor.edu/graduate/nutrition/

Benedictine University, Graduate Programs, Program in Nutrition and Wellness, Lisle, IL 60532-0900. Offers MS. *Students:* 29 full-time (28 women), 44 part-time (42 women); includes 13 minority (4 Black or African American, non-Hispanic/Latino; 6 Asian, non-Hispanic/Latino; 3 Hispanic/Latino). 49 applicants, 67% accepted, 25 enrolled. In 2013, 22 master's awarded. *Entrance requirements:* Additional exam requirements/recommendations for international students: Required—TOEFL (minimum score 550 paper-based). *Application deadline:* For fall admission, 9/1 for domestic students; for winter admission, 12/1 for domestic students; for spring admission, 2/15 for domestic students. Applications are processed on a rolling basis. Application fee: $40. Electronic applications accepted. *Expenses: Tuition:* Part-time $590 per credit hour. *Financial support:* Career-related internships or fieldwork and health care benefits available. Support available to part-time students. *Faculty research:* Community and corporate wellness risk assessment, health behavior change, self-efficacy, evaluation of health program impact and effectiveness. *Total annual research expenditures:* $8,335. *Unit head:* Catherine Arnold, Director, 630-829-6534, E-mail: carnold@ben.edu. *Application contact:* Kari Gibbons, Associate Vice President, Enrollment Center, 630-829-6200, Fax: 630-829-6584, E-mail: kgibbons@ben.edu.

Benedictine University, Graduate Programs, Program in Public Health, Lisle, IL 60532-0900. Offers administration of health care institutions (MPH); dietetics (MPH); disaster management (MPH); health education (MPH); health information systems (MPH); MBA/MPH; MPH/MS. Part-time and evening/weekend programs available. Postbaccalaureate distance learning degree programs offered. *Students:* 78 full-time (62 women), 340 part-time (254 women); includes 159 minority (97 Black or African American, non-Hispanic/Latino; 3 American Indian or Alaska Native, non-Hispanic/Latino; 47 Asian, non-Hispanic/Latino; 11 Hispanic/Latino; 1 Native Hawaiian or other Pacific Islander, non-Hispanic/Latino), 14 international. Average age 33. 195 applicants, 86% accepted, 143 enrolled. In 2013, 207 master's awarded. *Entrance requirements:* For master's, MAT, GRE, or GMAT. Additional exam requirements/recommendations for international students: Required—TOEFL (minimum score 550 paper-based). *Application deadline:* For fall admission, 9/1 for domestic students; for winter admission, 12/1 for domestic students; for spring admission, 2/15 for domestic students. Application fee: $40. *Expenses: Tuition:* Part-time $590 per credit hour. *Financial support:* Career-related internships or fieldwork and health care benefits available. Support available to part-time students. *Unit head:* Dr. Georgeen Polyak, Director, 630-829-6217, E-mail: gpolyak@ben.edu. *Application contact:* Kari Gibbons, Associate Vice President, Enrollment Center, 630-829-6200, Fax: 630-829-6584, E-mail: kgibbons@ben.edu.

Boston University, College of Health and Rehabilitation Sciences: Sargent College, Department of Health Sciences, Program in Nutrition, Boston, MA 02215. Offers MS. *Faculty:* 10 full-time (9 women), 5 part-time/adjunct (3 women). *Students:* 46 full-time (44 women), 2 part-time (both women); includes 3 minority (all Asian, non-Hispanic/Latino), 1 international. Average age 27. 83 applicants, 51% accepted, 17 enrolled. In 2013, 23 master's awarded. *Entrance requirements:* For master's, GRE General Test, minimum GPA of 3.0. Additional exam requirements/recommendations for international students: Required—TOEFL (minimum score 550 paper-based; 84 iBT). *Application deadline:* For fall admission, 2/15 priority date for domestic and international students; for spring admission, 10/1 for domestic and international students. Applications are processed on a rolling basis. Application fee: $80. Electronic applications accepted. *Expenses: Tuition:* Full-time $43,970; part-time $1374 per credit hour. *Required fees:* $60 per semester. Tuition and fees vary according to class time, course level and program. *Financial support:* In 2013–14, 39 students received support, including 42 fellowships (averaging $12,450 per year), 4 teaching assistantships; career-related internships or fieldwork, Federal Work-Study, institutionally sponsored loans, scholarships/grants, and tuition waivers (partial) also available. Support available to part-time students. Financial award application deadline: 4/15; financial award applicants required to submit FAFSA. *Faculty research:* Metabolism, health promotion, obesity, epidemiology. *Unit head:* Dr. Kathleen Morgan, Chair, 617-353-2717, E-mail: kmorgan@bu.edu. *Application contact:* Sharon Sankey, Director, Student Services, 617-353-2713, Fax: 617-353-7500, E-mail: ssankey@bu.edu.

Boston University, School of Medicine, Division of Graduate Medical Sciences, Programs in Medical Nutrition Sciences, Boston, MA 02215. Offers MA, PhD. *Degree requirements:* For master's, thesis; for doctorate, thesis/dissertation. *Application deadline:* For fall admission, 1/15 for domestic students; for spring admission, 10/15 for domestic students. *Expenses: Tuition:* Full-time $43,970; part-time $1374 per credit hour. *Required fees:* $60 per semester. Tuition and fees vary according to class time, course level and program. *Unit head:* Dr. Susan K. Fried, Director, 617-638-7110, E-mail: skfried@bu.edu. *Application contact:* Dr. Lynn Moore, Program Director, 617-638-8088, E-mail: llmoore@bu.edu.
Website: http://www.bumc.bu.edu/gms/nutrition-metabolism/

Bowling Green State University, Graduate College, College of Education and Human Development, School of Family and Consumer Sciences, Bowling Green, OH 43403. Offers food and nutrition (MFCS); human development and family studies (MFCS). Part-time programs available. *Degree requirements:* For master's, thesis. *Entrance requirements:* For master's, GRE General Test, minimum GPA of 3.0. Additional exam requirements/recommendations for international students: Required—TOEFL. Electronic applications accepted. *Faculty research:* Public health, wellness, social issues and policies, ethnic foods, nutrition and aging.

Brigham Young University, Graduate Studies, College of Life Sciences, Department of Nutrition, Dietetics and Food Science, Provo, UT 84602. Offers food science (MS); nutrition (MS). *Faculty:* 12 full-time (5 women). *Students:* 8 full-time (6 women); includes 1 minority (Asian, non-Hispanic/Latino). Average age 24. 3 applicants, 67% accepted, 2 enrolled. In 2013, 3 master's awarded. *Degree requirements:* For master's, comprehensive exam, thesis. *Entrance requirements:* For master's, GRE General Test. Additional exam requirements/recommendations for international students: Required—TOEFL. *Application deadline:* For fall admission, 2/1 for domestic students, 2/1 priority date for international students; for winter admission, 6/30 for domestic students, 6/30 priority date for international students. Application fee: $50. Electronic applications accepted. *Expenses: Tuition:* Full-time $6130; part-time $340 per credit hour. Tuition and fees vary according to program and student's religious affiliation. *Financial support:* In 2013–14, 9 students received support, including 5 research assistantships (averaging $20,325 per year), 3 teaching assistantships (averaging $20,325 per year); career-related internships or fieldwork, institutionally sponsored loans, and scholarships/grants also available. Financial award application deadline: 4/1. *Faculty research:* Dairy foods, lipid oxidation, food processes, magnesium and selenium nutrition, nutrient effect on gene expression. *Total annual research expenditures:* $382,427. *Unit head:* Dr. Michael L. Dunn, Chair, 801-422-6670, Fax: 801-422-0258, E-mail: michael_dunn@byu.edu. *Application contact:* Dr. Susan Fullmer, Graduate Coordinator, 801-422-3349, Fax: 801-422-0258, E-mail: susan_fullmer@byu.edu.

Brooklyn College of the City University of New York, School of Natural and Behavioral Sciences, Department of Health and Nutrition Sciences, Program in Nutrition, Brooklyn, NY 11210-2889. Offers MS. Part-time programs available. *Degree requirements:* For master's, thesis or comprehensive exam. *Entrance requirements:* For master's, 18 credits in health-related areas, 2 letters of recommendation, essay. Additional exam requirements/recommendations for international students: Required—TOEFL. *Application deadline:* For fall admission, 3/1 priority date for domestic students, 2/1 priority date for international students; for spring admission, 11/1 priority date for domestic students, 10/1 priority date for international students. Applications are processed on a rolling basis. Application fee: $125. Electronic applications accepted. *Expenses: Tuition, area resident:* Full-time $4585; part-time $385 per credit. Tuition, state resident: full-time $4585; part-time $385 per credit. Tuition, nonresident: part-time $710 per credit. *Required fees:* $430; $153 per semester. Tuition and fees vary according to course load. *Financial support:* Federal Work-Study, institutionally sponsored loans, and scholarships/grants available. Support available to part-time students. Financial award application deadline: 5/1; financial award applicants required to submit FAFSA. *Faculty research:* Medical ethics, AIDS, history of public health, diet restriction, palliative care, risk reduction/disease prevention, metabolism, diabetes. *Unit head:* Dr. Kathleen Axen, Graduate Deputy Chairperson, 718-951-5909, Fax: 718-951-4670, E-mail: kaxen@brooklyn.cuny.edu. *Application contact:* Dr. Kathleen Axen, Graduate Deputy Chairperson, 718-951-5909, Fax: 718-951-4670, E-mail: kaxen@brooklyn.cuny.edu.

California Baptist University, Program in Public Health, Riverside, CA 92504-3206. Offers food, nutrition and health (MPH); health policy and administration (MPH); physical activity (MPH). Part-time and evening/weekend programs available. *Degree requirements:* For master's, capstone project; practicum. *Entrance requirements:* For master's, minimum undergraduate GPA of 2.75, bachelor's degree transcripts, three recommendations, 500-word essay, resume, interview. Additional exam requirements/recommendations for international students: Required—TOEFL (minimum score 80 iBT). *Application deadline:* For fall admission, 8/1 priority date for domestic students, 7/1 for international students; for spring admission, 12/1 priority date for domestic students, 11/1 for international students. Applications are processed on a rolling basis. Application fee: $45. Electronic applications accepted. *Expenses:* Contact institution. *Financial support:* Applicants required to submit CSS PROFILE or FAFSA. *Unit head:* Dr. Chuck Sands, Dean, College of Allied Health, 951-343-4619, E-mail: csands@calbaptist.edu. *Application contact:* Dr. Wayne Fletcher, Chair, Department of Health Sciences, 951-552-8724, E-mail: wfletcher@calbaptist.edu.
Website: http://www.calbaptist.edu/explore-cbu/schools-colleges/college-allied-health/health-sciences/master-public-health/

California State University, Chico, Office of Graduate Studies, College of Natural Sciences, Department of Nutrition and Food Science, Chico, CA 95929-0722. Offers general nutritional science (MS); nutrition education (MS). Part-time programs available. *Degree requirements:* For master's, thesis, professional paper, or oral defense. *Entrance requirements:* For master's, GRE General Test, two letters of recommendation, statement of purpose, resume. Additional exam requirements/recommendations for international students: Required—TOEFL (minimum score 550 paper-based; 80 iBT), IELTS (minimum score 6.5), PTE (minimum score 59). Electronic applications accepted.

California State University, Long Beach, Graduate Studies, College of Health and Human Services, Department of Family and Consumer Sciences, Master of Science in Nutritional Science Program, Long Beach, CA 90840. Offers food science (MS); hospitality foodservice and hotel management (MS); nutritional science (MS). Part-time programs available. *Degree requirements:* For master's, thesis, oral presentation of thesis or directed project. *Entrance requirements:* For master's, GRE, minimum GPA of 2.5 in last 60 units. Electronic applications accepted. *Faculty research:* Protein and water-soluble vitamins, sensory evaluation of foods, mineral deficiencies in humans, child nutrition, minerals and blood pressure.

California State University, Long Beach, Graduate Studies, College of Health and Human Services, Department of Kinesiology, Long Beach, CA 90840. Offers adapted physical education (MA); coaching and student athlete development (MA); exercise physiology and nutrition (MS); exercise science (MS); individualized studies (MA); kinesiology (MA); pedagogical studies (MA); sport and exercise psychology (MS); sport management (MA); sports medicine and injury studies (MS). Part-time programs available. *Degree requirements:* For master's, oral and written comprehensive exams or thesis. *Entrance requirements:* For master's, GRE General Test, minimum GPA of 2.75 during previous 2 years of course work. Electronic applications accepted. *Faculty research:* Pulmonary functioning, feedback and practice structure, strength training, history and politics of sports, special population research issues.

California State University, Los Angeles, Graduate Studies, College of Health and Human Services, Department of Kinesiology and Nutritional Sciences, Los Angeles, CA 90032-8530. Offers nutritional science (MS); physical education and kinesiology (MA, MS). *Accreditation:* AND. Part-time and evening/weekend programs available. *Faculty:* 6 full-time (3 women), 1 part-time/adjunct (0 women). *Students:* 69 full-time (65 women), 50 part-time (36 women); includes 64 minority (3 Black or African American, non-Hispanic/Latino; 30 Asian, non-Hispanic/Latino; 25 Hispanic/Latino; 1 Native Hawaiian or other Pacific Islander, non-Hispanic/Latino; 5 Two or more races, non-Hispanic/Latino), 8 international. Average age 31. 138 applicants, 24% accepted, 23 enrolled. In 2013, 60 master's awarded. *Degree requirements:* For master's, comprehensive exam, project or thesis. *Entrance requirements:* For master's, minimum GPA of 2.75. Additional exam requirements/recommendations for international students: Required—TOEFL (minimum score 500 paper-based). *Application deadline:* For fall admission, 5/1 for domestic and international students. Applications are processed on a rolling basis.

Application fee: $55. *Financial support:* Federal Work-Study available. Support available to part-time students. Financial award application deadline: 3/1. *Unit head:* Dr. Nazareth Khodiguian, Chair, 323-343-4650, Fax: 323-343-6482, E-mail: nkhodig@calstatela.edu. *Application contact:* Dr. Larry Fritz, Dean of Graduate Studies, 323-343-3820, Fax: 323-343-5653, E-mail: lfritz@calstatela.edu.
Website: http://www.calstatela.edu/dept/pe/

Canisius College, Graduate Division, School of Education and Human Services, Office of Professional Studies, Buffalo, NY 14208-1098. Offers applied nutrition (MS, Certificate); community and school health (MS); health and human performance (MS); health information technology (MS); respiratory care (MS). Postbaccalaureate distance learning degree programs offered (no on-campus study). *Faculty:* 17 part-time/adjunct (11 women). *Students:* 51 full-time (35 women), 37 part-time (26 women); includes 16 minority (8 Black or African American, non-Hispanic/Latino; 1 American Indian or Alaska Native, non-Hispanic/Latino; 7 Hispanic/Latino), 2 international. Average age 32. 98 applicants, 57% accepted, 24 enrolled. In 2013, 29 master's awarded. *Entrance requirements:* Additional exam requirements/recommendations for international students: Required—TOEFL (minimum score 550 paper-based, 80 iBT), IELTS (minimum score 6.5), or CAEL (minimum score 70). *Application deadline:* Applications are processed on a rolling basis. Application fee: $25. Electronic applications accepted. Application fee is waived when completed online. *Expenses: Tuition:* Part-time $750 per credit hour. *Financial support:* Career-related internships or fieldwork, Federal Work-Study, scholarships/grants, and unspecified assistantships available. Support available to part-time students. Financial award application deadline: 4/30; financial award applicants required to submit FAFSA. *Faculty research:* Nutrition, community and school health; community and health; health and human performance applied; nutrition and respiratory care. *Unit head:* Dr. Khalid Bibi, Executive Director, 716-888-8296. *Application contact:* Julie A. Zulewski, Director of Graduate Admission, 716-888-2548, Fax: 716-888-3195, E-mail: zulewskj@canisius.edu.
Website: http://www.canisius.edu/graduate/

Case Western Reserve University, School of Medicine and School of Graduate Studies, Graduate Programs in Medicine, Department of Nutrition, Cleveland, OH 44106. Offers dietetics (MS); nutrition (MS, PhD), including molecular nutrition (PhD), nutrition and biochemistry (PhD); public health nutrition (MS). Part-time programs available. Terminal master's awarded for partial completion of doctoral program. *Degree requirements:* For master's, thesis (for some programs); for doctorate, thesis/dissertation. *Entrance requirements:* For master's, GRE General Test; for doctorate, GRE General Test, GRE Subject Test. Additional exam requirements/recommendations for international students: Required—TOEFL. *Faculty research:* Fatty acid metabolism, application of gene therapy to nutritional problems, dietary intake methodology, nutrition and physical fitness, metabolism during infancy and pregnancy.

Cedar Crest College, Dietetic Internship Certificate Program, Allentown, PA 18104-6196. Offers Graduate Certificate. Postbaccalaureate distance learning degree programs offered (no on-campus study). *Faculty:* 2 full-time (both women), 2 part-time/adjunct (1 woman). *Students:* 25 part-time (all women); includes 1 minority (Asian, non-Hispanic/Latino). Average age 26. In 2013, 25 Graduate Certificates awarded. *Entrance requirements:* For degree, two semesters of medical nutrition therapy coursework completed no more than four years prior to application; one biochemistry course completed no more than five years prior to application. *Expenses: Tuition:* Part-time $661 per credit. *Unit head:* Kati Fosselius, Director, 610-606-4666 Ext. 3445, E-mail: kdfossel@cedarcrest.edu. *Application contact:* Mary Ellen Hickes, Director of School of Adult and Graduate Education, 610-437-4471, E-mail: sage@cedarcrest.edu.
Website: http://sage.cedarcrest.edu/graduate/dietetic-internship/

Central Michigan University, Central Michigan University Global Campus, Program in Health Administration, Mount Pleasant, MI 48859. Offers health administration (DHA); international health (Certificate); nutrition and dietetics (MS). Part-time and evening/weekend programs available. Postbaccalaureate distance learning degree programs offered (minimal on-campus study). Electronic applications accepted. *Financial support:* Scholarships/grants available. Support available to part-time students. Financial award applicants required to submit FAFSA. *Unit head:* Dr. Steven D. Berkshire, Director, 989-774-1640, E-mail: berks1sd@cmich.edu. *Application contact:* Off-Campus Programs Call Center, 877-268-4636, E-mail: cmuoffcampus@cmich.edu.

Central Michigan University, College of Graduate Studies, College of Education and Human Services, Department of Human Environmental Studies, Mount Pleasant, MI 48859. Offers apparel product development and merchandising technology (MS); gerontology (Graduate Certificate); human development and family studies (MA); nutrition and dietetics (MS). Part-time and evening/weekend programs available. *Degree requirements:* For master's, thesis or alternative. Electronic applications accepted. *Faculty research:* Human growth and development, family studies and human sexuality, human nutrition and dietetics, apparel and textile retailing, computer-aided design for apparel.

Central Washington University, Graduate Studies and Research, College of Education and Professional Studies, Department of Nutrition, Exercise and Health Services, Ellensburg, WA 98926. Offers exercise science (MS); nutrition (MS). Part-time programs available. *Degree requirements:* For master's, thesis or alternative. *Entrance requirements:* For master's, GRE, minimum GPA of 3.0; writing sample (for exercise students). Additional exam requirements/recommendations for international students: Required—TOEFL (minimum score 550 paper-based; 79 iBT). Electronic applications accepted.

Chapman University, Schmid College of Science and Technology, Food Science Program, Orange, CA 92866. Offers MS, MBA/MS. Part-time and evening/weekend programs available. *Faculty:* 4 full-time (3 women), 4 part-time/adjunct (all women). *Students:* 29 full-time (20 women), 28 part-time (21 women); includes 22 minority (2 Black or African American, non-Hispanic/Latino; 14 Asian, non-Hispanic/Latino; 4 Hispanic/Latino; 2 Native Hawaiian or other Pacific Islander, non-Hispanic/Latino), 17 international. Average age 26. 54 applicants, 74% accepted, 26 enrolled. In 2013, 14 master's awarded. *Degree requirements:* For master's, comprehensive exam, thesis optional. *Entrance requirements:* For master's, GRE or GMAT, minimum undergraduate GPA of 3.0. Additional exam requirements/recommendations for international students: Required—TOEFL (minimum score 550 paper-based; 80 iBT). *Application deadline:* For fall admission, 5/2 priority date for domestic students; for spring admission, 11/1 priority date for domestic students. Application fee: $60. Electronic applications accepted. Tuition and fees vary according to program. *Financial support:* Fellowships, Federal Work-Study, and scholarships/grants available. Financial award applicants required to submit FAFSA. *Unit head:* Dr. Anuradha Prakash, Program Director, 714-744-7895, E-mail: prakash@chapman.edu. *Application contact:* Derek Robinson, Graduate Admission Counselor, 714-997-6711, E-mail: drobinso@chapman.edu.

Clemson University, Graduate School, College of Agriculture, Forestry and Life Sciences, Department of Food, Nutrition and Packaging Sciences, Program in Food, Nutrition, and Culinary Science, Clemson, SC 29634. Offers MS. *Students:* 29 full-time (22 women), 9 part-time (7 women); includes 4 minority (2 Black or African American, non-Hispanic/Latino; 1 Asian, non-Hispanic/Latino; 1 Hispanic/Latino), 13 international. Average age 25. 64 applicants, 27% accepted, 15 enrolled. In 2013, 15 master's awarded. *Degree requirements:* For master's, thesis. *Entrance requirements:* For master's, GRE General Test. Additional exam requirements/recommendations for international students: Required—TOEFL, IELTS. *Application deadline:* For fall admission, 6/1 for domestic students, 4/15 for international students; for spring admission, 9/15 for international students. Applications are processed on a rolling basis. Application fee: $70 ($80 for international students). Electronic applications accepted. *Expenses:* Contact institution. *Financial support:* In 2013–14, 15 students received support, including 1 fellowship with full and partial tuition reimbursement available (averaging $10,000 per year), 9 research assistantships with partial tuition reimbursements available (averaging $12,077 per year), 5 teaching assistantships with partial tuition reimbursements available (averaging $14,400 per year); career-related internships or fieldwork, institutionally sponsored loans, scholarships/grants, health care benefits, and unspecified assistantships also available. Support available to part-time students. Financial award applicants required to submit FAFSA. *Unit head:* Dr. Anthony Pometto, III, Chair, 864-656-4382, Fax: 864-656-3131, E-mail: pometto@clemson.edu. *Application contact:* Dr. Paul Dawson, Coordinator, 864-656-1138, Fax: 864-656-3131, E-mail: pdawson@clemson.edu.
Website: http://www.clemson.edu/foodscience

College of Saint Elizabeth, Department of Foods and Nutrition, Morristown, NJ 07960-6989. Offers dietetic internship (Certificate); dietetics verification (Certificate); nutrition (MS); sports nutrition and wellness (Certificate). *Accreditation:* AND. Part-time programs available. *Faculty:* 3 full-time (all women), 1 (woman) part-time/adjunct. *Students:* 7 full-time (6 women), 42 part-time (39 women); includes 5 minority (1 Asian, non-Hispanic/Latino; 4 Hispanic/Latino). Average age 30. In 2013, 11 master's, 18 other advanced degrees awarded. *Entrance requirements:* For master's, minimum cumulative undergraduate GPA of 3.0. Additional exam requirements/recommendations for international students: Required—TOEFL. *Application deadline:* Applications are processed on a rolling basis. Application fee: $35. Electronic applications accepted. *Expenses: Tuition:* Full-time $19,152; part-time $1064 per credit. *Financial support:* Tuition waivers (partial) and unspecified assistantships available. Support available to part-time students. Financial award application deadline: 3/15; financial award applicants required to submit FAFSA. *Faculty research:* Medical nutrition intervention, public policy, obesity, hunger and food security, osteoporosis, nutrition and exercise. *Unit head:* Dr. Marie Boyle, Program Chair, 973-290-4127, Fax: 973-290-4167, E-mail: mboyle01@cse.edu. *Application contact:* Deborah S. Cobo, Associate Director of Graduate Admission, 973-290-4194, Fax: 973-290-4710, E-mail: dscobo@cse.edu.

Colorado State University, Graduate School, College of Health and Human Sciences, Department of Food Science and Human Nutrition, Fort Collins, CO 80523-1571. Offers MS, PhD. *Accreditation:* AND. Part-time programs available. Postbaccalaureate distance learning degree programs offered (no on-campus study). *Faculty:* 16 full-time (9 women). *Students:* 41 full-time (35 women), 54 part-time (43 women); includes 7 minority (1 Black or African American, non-Hispanic/Latino; 1 Asian, non-Hispanic/Latino; 4 Hispanic/Latino; 1 Two or more races, non-Hispanic/Latino), 4 international. Average age 32. 103 applicants, 22% accepted, 15 enrolled. In 2013, 24 master's, 1 doctorate awarded. Terminal master's awarded for partial completion of doctoral program. *Degree requirements:* For master's, thesis; for doctorate, thesis/dissertation. *Entrance requirements:* For master's and doctorate, GRE (minimum 50th percentile), minimum GPA of 3.0 overall and in science, resume, 3 letters of recommendation, 2 transcripts from each educational institution (college/university). Additional exam requirements/recommendations for international students: Required—TOEFL (minimum score 550 paper-based; 80 iBT), IELTS. *Application deadline:* For fall admission, 2/1 priority date for domestic and international students; for spring admission, 8/1 priority date for domestic and international students. Application fee: $50. Electronic applications accepted. *Expenses:* Tuition, state resident: full-time $9075.40; part-time $504 per credit. Tuition, nonresident: full-time $22,248; part-time $1236 per credit. *Required fees:* $1819; $60 per credit. *Financial support:* In 2013–14, 28 students received support, including 19 research assistantships with tuition reimbursements available (averaging $10,137 per year), 9 teaching assistantships with tuition reimbursements available (averaging $11,576 per year); Federal Work-Study, scholarships/grants, and unspecified assistantships also available. Financial award application deadline: 2/1; financial award applicants required to submit FAFSA. *Faculty research:* Community nutrition, bioactive compounds, nutrition and obesity, nutrition and health disparities, fatty acids and pregnancy, nutrition and obesity-related disorders. *Total annual research expenditures:* $2.2 million. *Unit head:* Dr. Michael Pagliassotti, Department Head, 970-491-1390, Fax: 970-491-7252, E-mail: michael.pagliassotti@colostate.edu. *Application contact:* Paula Coleman, Administrative Assistant, 970-491-3819, Fax: 970-491-3875, E-mail: paula.coleman@colostate.edu.
Website: http://www.fshn.chhs.colostate.edu/

Colorado State University, Graduate School, College of Health and Human Sciences, Department of Health and Exercise Science, Fort Collins, CO 80523-1582. Offers exercise science and nutrition (MS); health and exercise science (MS); human bioenergetics (PhD). *Faculty:* 14 full-time (3 women). *Students:* 29 full-time (18 women), 10 part-time (3 women), 1 international. Average age 29. 27 applicants, 48% accepted, 11 enrolled. In 2013, 4 master's, 1 doctorate awarded. *Degree requirements:* For master's, thesis; for doctorate, comprehensive exam, thesis/dissertation, mentored teaching. *Entrance requirements:* For master's and doctorate, GRE General Test, minimum GPA of 3.0. *Application deadline:* For fall admission, 1/31 priority date for domestic and international students; for spring admission, 9/30 priority date for domestic and international students. Application fee: $50. Electronic applications accepted. *Expenses:* Tuition, state resident: full-time $9075.40; part-time $504 per credit. Tuition, nonresident: full-time $22,248; part-time $1236 per credit. *Required fees:* $1819; $60 per credit. *Financial support:* In 2013–14, 30 students received support, including 1 fellowship (averaging $19,632 per year), 8 research assistantships with full tuition reimbursements available (averaging $14,263 per year), 21 teaching assistantships with full tuition reimbursements available (averaging $12,951 per year). Financial award application deadline: 1/31; financial award applicants required to submit FAFSA. *Faculty research:* Chronic disease, aging, neuromuscular function, cardiovascular function. *Total annual research expenditures:* $1.7 million. *Unit head:* Dr. Richard Gay Israel, Department Head, 970-491-3785, Fax: 970-491-0216, E-mail: richard.israel@colostate.edu. *Application contact:* Dr. Matthew Hickey, Department Operations, 970-491-5727, Fax: 970-491-0445, E-mail: matthew.hickey@colostate.edu.
Website: http://www.hes.chhs.colostate.edu/

Columbia University, College of Physicians and Surgeons, Institute of Human Nutrition, MS Program in Nutrition, New York, NY 10032. Offers MS, MPH/MS. Part-time and evening/weekend programs available. *Degree requirements:* For master's, thesis. *Entrance requirements:* For master's, GRE General Test, TOEFL, MCAT. Additional exam requirements/recommendations for international students: Required—TOEFL.

Columbia University, College of Physicians and Surgeons, Institute of Human Nutrition and Graduate School of Arts and Sciences at the College of Physicians and Surgeons, PhD Program in Nutrition, New York, NY 10032. Offers PhD. *Degree requirements:* For doctorate, thesis/dissertation. *Entrance requirements:* For doctorate, GRE General Test. Additional exam requirements/recommendations for international students: Required—TOEFL. *Faculty research:* Growth and development, nutrition and metabolism.

Cornell University, Graduate School, Graduate Fields of Agriculture and Life Sciences, Field of Global Development, Ithaca, NY 14853-0001. Offers development policy (MPS); international agriculture and development (MPS); international development (MPS); international nutrition (MPS); international planning (MPS); international population (MPS); science and technology policy (MPS). *Faculty:* 97 full-time (29 women). *Students:* 25 full-time (20 women); includes 2 minority (1 Black or African American, non-Hispanic/Latino; 1 Asian, non-Hispanic/Latino), 11 international. Average age 27. 46 applicants, 65% accepted, 22 enrolled. In 2013, 13 master's awarded. *Degree requirements:* For master's, project paper. *Entrance requirements:* For master's, GRE General Test (recommended), 2 years of development experience, 2 letters of recommendation. Additional exam requirements/recommendations for international students: Required—TOEFL (minimum score 550 paper-based; 77 iBT). *Application deadline:* For fall admission, 3/1 for domestic students. Application fee: $95. Electronic applications accepted. *Financial support:* In 2013–14, 3 students received support, including 1 research assistantship with full tuition reimbursement available, 2 teaching assistantships with full tuition reimbursements available; fellowships with full tuition reimbursements available, institutionally sponsored loans, scholarships/grants, health care benefits, tuition waivers (full and partial), and unspecified assistantships also available. Financial award applicants required to submit FAFSA. *Unit head:* Director of Graduate Studies, 607-255-3037, Fax: 607-255-1005. *Application contact:* Graduate Field Assistant, 607-255-3035, Fax: 607-255-1005, E-mail: mpsiard@cornell.edu. Website: http://gradschool.cornell.edu/academics/fields-study/catalog/?fid-87

Cornell University, Graduate School, Graduate Fields of Agriculture and Life Sciences and Graduate Fields of Human Ecology, Field of Nutrition, Ithaca, NY 14853-0001. Offers animal nutrition (MPS, PhD); community nutrition (MPS, PhD); human nutrition (MPS, PhD); international nutrition (MPS, PhD); molecular biochemistry (MPS, PhD). *Faculty:* 55 full-time (29 women). *Students:* 64 full-time (57 women); includes 16 minority (6 Black or African American, non-Hispanic/Latino; 4 Asian, non-Hispanic/Latino; 3 Hispanic/Latino; 3 Two or more races, non-Hispanic/Latino), 19 international. Average age 28. 112 applicants, 12% accepted, 10 enrolled. In 2013, 1 master's, 9 doctorates awarded. *Degree requirements:* For master's, thesis (MS), project papers (MPS); for doctorate, comprehensive exam, thesis/dissertation. *Entrance requirements:* For master's and doctorate, GRE General Test, previous course work in organic chemistry (with laboratory) and biochemistry; 2 letters of recommendation. Additional exam requirements/recommendations for international students: Required—TOEFL (minimum score 550 paper-based; 77 iBT). *Application deadline:* For fall admission, 1/10 priority date for domestic students; for spring admission, 10/1 for domestic students. Application fee: $95. Electronic applications accepted. *Financial support:* In 2013–14, 41 students received support, including 9 fellowships with full tuition reimbursements available, 6 research assistantships with full tuition reimbursements available, 26 teaching assistantships with full tuition reimbursements available; institutionally sponsored loans, scholarships/grants, health care benefits, tuition waivers (full and partial), and unspecified assistantships also available. Financial award applicants required to submit FAFSA. *Faculty research:* Nutritional biochemistry, experimental human and animal nutrition, international nutrition, community nutrition. *Unit head:* Director of Graduate Studies, 607-255-2528, Fax: 607-255-0178. *Application contact:* Graduate Field Assistant, 607-255-2628, Fax: 607-225-0178, E-mail: nutrition_gfr@cornell.edu. Website: http://www.gradschool.cornell.edu/fields.php?id-56&a-2

Drexel University, College of Arts and Sciences, Department of Biology, Program in Human Nutrition, Philadelphia, PA 19104-2875. Offers MS. *Accreditation:* AND. Part-time programs available. Terminal master's awarded for partial completion of doctoral program. *Degree requirements:* For master's, thesis. *Entrance requirements:* For master's, GRE General Test. Additional exam requirements/recommendations for international students: Required—TOEFL. Electronic applications accepted. *Faculty research:* Metabolism of lipids, W-3 fatty acids, obesity, diabetes and heart disease, mineral metabolism.

D'Youville College, Department of Dietetics, Buffalo, NY 14201-1084. Offers MS. Five-year program begins at freshman entry. *Accreditation:* AND. *Students:* 88 full-time (83 women), 9 part-time (8 women); includes 10 minority (2 Black or African American, non-Hispanic/Latino; 4 Asian, non-Hispanic/Latino; 4 Two or more races, non-Hispanic/Latino), 10 international. Average age 24. 130 applicants, 58% accepted, 47 enrolled. In 2013, 14 master's awarded. *Degree requirements:* For master's, thesis. *Entrance requirements:* Additional exam requirements/recommendations for international students: Required—TOEFL (minimum score 500 paper-based). *Application deadline:* For fall admission, 5/1 priority date for international students; for spring admission, 9/1 priority date for international students. Applications are processed on a rolling basis. Application fee: $25. Electronic applications accepted. *Faculty research:* Nutrition education, clinical nutrition, herbal supplements, obesity. *Unit head:* Dr. Charlotte Baumgart, Chair, 716-829-7752, Fax: 716-829-8137. *Application contact:* Dr. Steven Smith, Director of Admissions, 716-829-7600, Fax: 716-829-7900, E-mail: admissons@dyc.edu.

East Carolina University, Graduate School, College of Human Ecology, Department of Nutrition Science, Greenville, NC 27858-4353. Offers MS. Part-time programs available. *Degree requirements:* For master's, comprehensive exam, thesis optional. *Entrance requirements:* For master's, GRE. Additional exam requirements/recommendations for international students: Required—TOEFL. *Application deadline:* For fall admission, 6/1 priority date for domestic students. Applications are processed on a rolling basis. Application fee: $50. *Expenses:* Tuition, state resident: full-time $4223. Tuition, nonresident: full-time $16,540. *Required fees:* $2184. *Financial support:* Fellowships, teaching assistantships with partial tuition reimbursements, Federal Work-Study, institutionally sponsored loans, scholarships/grants, and unspecified assistantships available. Support available to part-time students. Financial award application deadline: 6/1. *Faculty research:* Lifecycle nutrition, nutrition and disease, nutrition for fish species, food service management. *Unit head:* Dr. Melani Duffrin, Interim Chair, 252-328-5698, E-mail: duffrinm@ecu.edu. *Application contact:* Dean of Graduate School, 252-328-6012, Fax: 252-328-6071, E-mail: gradschool@ecu.edu.

Eastern Illinois University, Graduate School, Lumpkin College of Business and Applied Sciences, School of Family and Consumer Sciences, Charleston, IL 61920-3099. Offers dietetics (MS); family and consumer sciences (MS). Part-time programs available. *Degree requirements:* For master's, comprehensive exam. *Expenses: Tuition, area resident:* Part-time $283 per credit hour. Tuition, state resident: part-time $283 per credit hour. Tuition, nonresident: part-time $679 per credit hour.

Eastern Kentucky University, The Graduate School, College of Health Sciences, Department of Family and Consumer Sciences, Richmond, KY 40475-3102. Offers community nutrition (MS). Part-time programs available. *Entrance requirements:* For master's, GRE General Test, minimum GPA of 2.5.

Eastern Michigan University, Graduate School, College of Health and Human Services, School of Health Sciences, Programs in Dietetics and Human Nutrition, Ypsilanti, MI 48197. Offers human nutrition (MS). *Accreditation:* AND. Part-time and evening/weekend programs available. Postbaccalaureate distance learning degree programs offered (minimal on-campus study). *Students:* 31 full-time (29 women), 57 part-time (51 women); includes 15 minority (4 Black or African American, non-Hispanic/Latino; 1 American Indian or Alaska Native, non-Hispanic/Latino; 7 Asian, non-Hispanic/Latino; 2 Hispanic/Latino; 1 Native Hawaiian or other Pacific Islander, non-Hispanic/Latino), 2 international. Average age 34. 39 applicants, 69% accepted, 21 enrolled. In 2013, 29 master's awarded. *Entrance requirements:* Additional exam requirements/recommendations for international students: Required—TOEFL. *Application deadline:* Applications are processed on a rolling basis. Application fee: $35. *Expenses:* Tuition, state resident: full-time $12,300; part-time $466 per credit hour. Tuition, nonresident: full-time $23,159; part-time $918 per credit hour. *Required fees:* $71 per credit hour. $46 per semester. One-time fee: $100. Tuition and fees vary according to course level and degree level. *Financial support:* Fellowships, research assistantships with full tuition reimbursements, teaching assistantships with full tuition reimbursements, career-related internships or fieldwork, Federal Work-Study, institutionally sponsored loans, scholarships/grants, tuition waivers (partial), and unspecified assistantships available. Support available to part-time students. Financial award applicants required to submit FAFSA. *Unit head:* Dr. Colleen Croxall, Director, 734-487-4096, Fax: 734-487-4095, E-mail: ccroxall@emich.edu. *Application contact:* Lydia Kret, Program Director, 734-487-7862, Fax: 734-487-4095, E-mail: lydia.kret@emich.edu.

East Tennessee State University, School of Graduate Studies, College of Clinical and Rehabilitative Health Sciences, Department of Allied Health Science, Johnson City, TN 37614. Offers allied health (MSAH); clinical nutrition (MS). Part-time programs available. Postbaccalaureate distance learning degree programs offered (no on-campus study). *Faculty:* 15 full-time (11 women), 1 part-time/adjunct (0 women). *Students:* 21 full-time (20 women), 29 part-time (25 women); includes 5 minority (2 Black or African American, non-Hispanic/Latino; 2 Hispanic/Latino; 1 Two or more races, non-Hispanic/Latino). Average age 31. 9 applicants, 22% accepted, 2 enrolled. In 2013, 15 master's awarded. *Degree requirements:* For master's, comprehensive exam, thesis optional, advanced practice seminar (for MSAH non-thesis option); internship (for clinical nutrition). *Entrance requirements:* For master's, GRE General Test, professional license in allied health discipline, minimum GPA of 2.75 (MSAH); bachelor's degree from undergraduate didactic program in dietetics with minimum GPA of 3.0 in DPD coursework (clinical nutrition). Additional exam requirements/recommendations for international students: Required—TOEFL (minimum score 550 paper-based; 79 iBT). *Application deadline:* For fall admission, 2/15 for domestic and international students; for spring admission, 11/1 for domestic students, 9/30 for international students. Application fee: $35 ($45 for international students). Electronic applications accepted. *Expenses:* Tuition, state resident: full-time $7900; part-time $395 per credit hour. Tuition, nonresident: full-time $21,960; part-time $1098 per credit hour. *Required fees:* $1345; $84 per credit hour. *Financial support:* In 2013–14, 18 students received support, including 3 research assistantships with full tuition reimbursements available (averaging $6,000 per year), 4 teaching assistantships with full tuition reimbursements available (averaging $6,000 per year); career-related internships or fieldwork, institutionally sponsored loans, scholarships/grants, and unspecified assistantships also available. Financial award application deadline: 7/1; financial award applicants required to submit FAFSA. *Faculty research:* Recruitment and retention of allied health professionals, relationship between APACHEE II scores and the need for a tracheotomy, health care workers, patient care, occupational stress, radiofrequency lesioning, absorption of lipophilic compounds, Vitamin D status in college-age students, childhood and adolescence obesity, nutrition education/interventions. *Unit head:* Dr. Charles Faust, Chair, 423-439-7888, Fax: 423-547-4900, E-mail: faust@etsu.edu. *Application contact:* Mary Duncan, Graduate Specialist, 423-439-4302, Fax: 423-439-5624, E-mail: duncanm@etsu.edu. Website: http://www.etsu.edu/crhs/alliedhealth/msah/

Emory University, Laney Graduate School, Division of Biological and Biomedical Sciences, Program in Nutrition and Health Sciences, Atlanta, GA 30322-1100. Offers PhD. *Degree requirements:* For doctorate, comprehensive exam, thesis/dissertation. *Entrance requirements:* For doctorate, GRE General Test, minimum GPA of 3.0 in science course work (recommended). Additional exam requirements/recommendations for international students: Required—TOEFL. Electronic applications accepted. *Faculty research:* Biochemistry, molecular and cell biology, clinical nutrition, community and preventive health, nutritional epidemiology.

Emory University, Rollins School of Public Health, Hubert Department of Global Health, Atlanta, GA 30322-1100. Offers global health (MPH); public nutrition (MSPH). *Accreditation:* CEPH. *Degree requirements:* For master's, thesis, practicum. *Entrance requirements:* For master's, GRE General Test. Additional exam requirements/recommendations for international students: Required—TOEFL (minimum score 550 paper-based; 80 iBT). Electronic applications accepted.

Florida International University, Robert Stempel College of Public Health and Social Work, Department of Dietetics and Nutrition, Miami, FL 33199. Offers MS, PhD. Part-time programs available. *Degree requirements:* For master's, thesis; for doctorate, comprehensive exam, thesis/dissertation. *Entrance requirements:* For master's, minimum GPA of 3.0; for doctorate, GRE General Test, minimum GPA of 3.0, resume, letters of recommendation, faculty sponsor. Additional exam requirements/recommendations for international students: Required—TOEFL (minimum score 550 paper-based; 80 iBT). Electronic applications accepted. *Faculty research:* Clinical nutrition, cultural food habits, pediatric nutrition, diabetes, dietetic education.

Florida State University, The Graduate School, College of Human Sciences, Department of Nutrition, Food and Exercise Sciences, Tallahassee, FL 32306-1493. Offers exercise physiology (MS, PhD); nutrition and food science (MS, PhD), including clinical nutrition (MS), food science, human nutrition (PhD), nutrition education and health promotion (MS), nutrition science (MS); sports nutrition (MS); sports sciences (MS). Part-time programs available. *Faculty:* 19 full-time (12 women). *Students:* 102 full-time (55 women), 17 part-time (13 women); includes 21 minority (7 Black or African American, non-Hispanic/Latino; 3 Asian, non-Hispanic/Latino; 2 Hispanic/Latino; 9 Two or more races, non-Hispanic/Latino), 24 international. Average age 26. 168 applicants, 51% accepted, 43 enrolled. In 2013, 29 master's, 3 doctorates awarded. *Degree requirements:* For master's, comprehensive exam (for some programs), thesis optional; for doctorate, thesis/dissertation. *Entrance requirements:* For master's, GRE General Test, minimum upper-division GPA of 3.0; for doctorate, GRE General Test, minimum upper-division GPA of 3.0, MS. Additional exam requirements/recommendations for international students: Required—TOEFL (minimum score 550 paper-based; 80 iBT). *Application deadline:* For fall admission, 7/1 for domestic and international students; for spring admission, 11/1 for domestic and international students. Applications are processed on a rolling basis. Application fee: $30. Electronic applications accepted. *Expenses:* Tuition, state resident: part-time $403.51 per credit hour. Tuition, nonresident: part-time $1004.85 per credit hour. *Required fees:* $75.81 per credit hour. One-time fee: $20 part-time. Tuition and fees vary according to course load, campus/location and student level. *Financial support:* In 2013–14, 54 students received support, including 3 fellowships with partial tuition reimbursements available (averaging $2,362 per year), 21 research assistantships with full tuition reimbursements available (averaging $3,902 per year), 42 teaching assistantships with full tuition reimbursements available (averaging $10,993 per year); career-related internships or fieldwork, Federal Work-Study, institutionally sponsored loans, scholarships/grants, and unspecified assistantships also available. Financial award application deadline: 2/1; financial award applicants required to submit FAFSA. *Faculty research:* Body composition, functional food, chronic disease and aging response; food safety, food allergy, and safety/quality

detection methods; sports nutrition, energy and human performance; strength training, functional performance, cardiovascular physiology, sarcopenia. *Total annual research expenditures:* $497,515. *Unit head:* Dr. Bahram H. Arjmandi, Professor/Chair, 850-645-1517, Fax: 850-645-5000, E-mail: barjmandi@fsu.edu. *Application contact:* Ann R. Smith, Office Administrator, 850-644-1828, Fax: 850-645-5000, E-mail: asmith@fsu.edu.
Website: http://www.chs.fsu.edu/Departments/Nutrition-Food-Exercise-Sciences

Framingham State University, Continuing Education, Programs in Food and Nutrition, Coordinated Program in Dietetics, Framingham, MA 01701-9101. Offers MS.

Framingham State University, Continuing Education, Programs in Food and Nutrition, Food Science and Nutrition Science Program, Framingham, MA 01701-9101. Offers MS. Part-time and evening/weekend programs available. *Entrance requirements:* For master's, GRE General Test.

Framingham State University, Continuing Education, Programs in Food and Nutrition, Program in Human Nutrition: Education and Media Technologies, Framingham, MA 01701-9101. Offers MS.

George Mason University, College of Health and Human Services, Program in Health Science, Fairfax, VA 22030. Offers food security (Certificate); nutrition (MS, Certificate). *Faculty:* 5 full-time (all women), 5 part-time/adjunct (all women). *Students:* 16 full-time (12 women), 27 part-time (24 women); includes 11 minority (3 Black or African American, non-Hispanic/Latino; 7 Hispanic/Latino; 1 Two or more races, non-Hispanic/Latino), 1 international. Average age 32. 60 applicants, 83% accepted, 41 enrolled. In 2013, 2 other advanced degrees awarded. *Degree requirements:* For master's, comprehensive exam, thesis optional. *Entrance requirements:* For master's, resume, 3 letters of recommendation, expanded goal statement. Additional exam requirements/recommendations for international students: Required—TOEFL (minimum score 570 paper-based; 88 iBT), IELTS (minimum score 6.5), PTE. *Application deadline:* For fall admission, 4/1 for domestic students. Application fee: $65 ($80 for international students). *Expenses:* Tuition, state resident: full-time $9350; part-time $390 per credit. Tuition, nonresident: full-time $25,754; part-time $1073 per credit. *Required fees:* $2688; $112 per credit. *Financial support:* In 2013–14, 1 student received support, including 1 research assistantship (averaging $18,000 per year); career-related internships or fieldwork, Federal Work-Study, and health care benefits (for full-time research or teaching assistantship recipients) also available. Support available to part-time students. Financial award applicants required to submit FAFSA. *Faculty research:* Childhood obesity, maternal and child health, and vulnerable, underserved and disadvantaged groups. *Total annual research expenditures:* $98,739. *Unit head:* Dr. Lisa Pawloski, Chair, 703-993-4628, Fax: 703-934-2193, E-mail: lpawlosk@gmu.edu. *Application contact:* Joe Wilson, Manager, Department of Food and Nutrition, 703-993-9709, Fax: 703-993-2193, E-mail: jwilso25@gmu.edu.
Website: http://chhs.gmu.edu/nfs/

Georgia State University, Byrdine F. Lewis School of Nursing, Division of Nutrition, Atlanta, GA 30302-3083. Offers MS. *Accreditation:* AND. Part-time programs available. *Faculty:* 6 full-time (4 women), 9 part-time/adjunct (0 women). *Students:* 43 full-time (41 women), 5 part-time (all women); includes 10 minority (3 Black or African American, non-Hispanic/Latino; 2 Asian, non-Hispanic/Latino; 2 Hispanic/Latino; 3 Two or more races, non-Hispanic/Latino). Average age 28. 44 applicants, 45% accepted, 17 enrolled. In 2013, 22 master's awarded. *Degree requirements:* For master's, portfolio or thesis. *Entrance requirements:* For master's, GRE, prerequisite courses in inorganic chemistry (1 semester), organic chemistry (1 semester), and human anatomy and physiology (2 semesters); transcripts; resume; statement of goals; letters of recommendation. Additional exam requirements/recommendations for international students: Required—TOEFL (minimum score 550 paper-based; 80 iBT). *Application deadline:* For fall admission, 5/15 for domestic and international students; for spring admission, 10/1 for domestic and international students. Application fee: $50. Electronic applications accepted. *Expenses: Tuition, area resident:* Full-time $4176; part-time $348 per credit hour. Tuition, state resident: full-time $14,544; part-time $1212 per credit hour. Tuition, nonresident: full-time $14,544; part-time $1212 per credit hour. Tuition and fees vary according to course load and program. *Financial support:* In 2013–14, research assistantships with full and partial tuition reimbursements (averaging $1,647 per year), teaching assistantships with full tuition reimbursements (averaging $2,666 per year) were awarded. Financial award application deadline: 4/1. *Faculty research:* Energy balance and body composition, nutrition and HIV in Kenya, lipid peroxidation, energy requirements in obese children, diet and incidence of type I diabetes. *Unit head:* Dr. Anita Nucci, Department Head, 404-413-1225, Fax: 404-413-1230. *Application contact:* Bill Andrews, Academic Advisor, 404-413-1000, Fax: 404-413-1001, E-mail: wandrews@gsu.edu.
Website: http://nutrition.gsu.edu/

Harvard University, Harvard School of Public Health, Department of Nutrition, Boston, MA 02115-6096. Offers nutrition (PhD, SD); nutritional epidemiology (SD); public health nutrition (SD). *Faculty:* 11 full-time (5 women), 22 part-time/adjunct (6 women). *Students:* 29 full-time, 2 part-time; includes 6 minority (1 Asian, non-Hispanic/Latino; 2 Hispanic/Latino; 3 Two or more races, non-Hispanic/Latino), 17 international. Average age 29. 51 applicants, 16% accepted, 8 enrolled. In 2013, 6 doctorates awarded. *Degree requirements:* For doctorate, thesis/dissertation, qualifying exam. *Entrance requirements:* For doctorate, GRE. Additional exam requirements/recommendations for international students: Required—TOEFL (minimum score 600 paper-based; 100 iBT); Recommended—IELTS (minimum score 7). *Application deadline:* For fall admission, 12/15 for domestic and international students. Application fee: $120. Electronic applications accepted. *Expenses: Tuition:* Full-time $38,888. *Required fees:* $958. Tuition and fees vary according to campus/location, program and student level. *Financial support:* Fellowships, research assistantships, teaching assistantships, Federal Work-Study, scholarships/grants, traineeships, and unspecified assistantships available. Support available to part-time students. Financial award application deadline: 2/15; financial award applicants required to submit FAFSA. *Faculty research:* Dietary and genetic factors affecting heart diseases in humans; interactions among nutrition, immunity, and infection; role of diet and lifestyle in preventing macrovascular complications in diabetics. *Unit head:* Dr. Walter Willett, Chair, 617-432-1333, Fax: 617-432-2435, E-mail: walter.willett@channing.harvard.edu. *Application contact:* Vincent W. James, Director of Admissions, 617-432-1031, Fax: 617-432-7080, E-mail: admissions@hsph.harvard.edu.
Website: http://www.hsph.harvard.edu/nutrition/

Howard University, Graduate School, Department of Nutritional Sciences, Washington, DC 20059-0002. Offers nutrition (MS, PhD). Part-time and evening/weekend programs available. *Degree requirements:* For master's, comprehensive exam, thesis; for doctorate, comprehensive exam, thesis/dissertation. *Entrance requirements:* For master's and doctorate, minimum GPA of 3.0, general chemistry, organic chemistry, biochemistry, nutrition. Additional exam requirements/recommendations for international students: Required—TOEFL. Electronic applications accepted. *Faculty research:* Dietary fiber, phytate, trace minerals, cardio-vascular diseases, overweight/obesity.

Hunter College of the City University of New York, Graduate School, Schools of the Health Professions, School of Health Sciences, Programs in Urban Public Health, Program in Nutrition, New York, NY 10065-5085. Offers MPH. *Accreditation:* AND. Part-time and evening/weekend programs available. *Faculty:* 2 full-time (both women), 2 part-time/adjunct (both women). *Students:* 19 full-time (14 women), 26 part-time (all women); includes 9 minority (2 Black or African American, non-Hispanic/Latino; 1 American Indian or Alaska Native, non-Hispanic/Latino; 4 Asian, non-Hispanic/Latino; 2 Hispanic/Latino), 3 international. Average age 30. 97 applicants, 33% accepted, 25 enrolled. In 2013, 33 master's awarded. *Degree requirements:* For master's, comprehensive exam, thesis optional, internship. *Entrance requirements:* For master's, GRE General Test, previous course work in calculus and statistics. Additional exam requirements/recommendations for international students: Required—TOEFL. *Application deadline:* For fall admission, 4/1 for domestic students; for spring admission, 11/1 for domestic students. Application fee: $125. *Financial support:* In 2013–14, 6 fellowships were awarded; career-related internships or fieldwork, Federal Work-Study, institutionally sponsored loans, and tuition waivers (partial) also available. Support available to part-time students. *Unit head:* Prof. Krusheed Navder, Program Director, 212-396-7775, Fax: 212-481-5260, E-mail: knavder@hunter.cuny.edu. *Application contact:* Milena Solo, Director of Graduate Admissions, 212-772-4288, E-mail: milena.solo@hunter.cuny.edu.
Website: http://cuny.edu/site/sph/hunter-college/a-programs/graduate/nutrition/nutrition-msdpd.html

Huntington College of Health Sciences, Program in Nutrition, Knoxville, TN 37918. Offers clinical nutrition (DHS); nutrition (MS); personalized option (DHS). Part-time and evening/weekend programs available. Postbaccalaureate distance learning degree programs offered (no on-campus study). *Faculty:* 1 (woman) full-time, 9 part-time/adjunct (7 women). *Students:* 1 (woman) full-time, 48 part-time (38 women); includes 5 minority (all Black or African American, non-Hispanic/Latino), 7 international. Average age 32. 40 applicants, 73% accepted, 19 enrolled. In 2013, 6 master's awarded. *Degree requirements:* For doctorate, comprehensive exam, thesis/dissertation. *Entrance requirements:* For master's, bachelor's degree, essay, resume/curriculum vitae; for doctorate, master's degree, essay, references, interview, resume/curriculum vitae. Additional exam requirements/recommendations for international students: Required—TOEFL (minimum score 550 paper-based; 80 iBT); Recommended—IELTS. Application fee: $75. Electronic applications accepted. *Expenses: Tuition:* Full-time $6714; part-time $368 per credit hour. One-time fee: $200. *Unit head:* Dr. Denise Wood, Dean of Graduate Studies, 865-524-8079 Ext. 4. *Application contact:* Kim Galyon, Director of Admissions, 865-524-8079 Ext. 1.
Website: http://www.hchs.edu

Idaho State University, Office of Graduate Studies, Kasiska College of Health Professions, Department of Health and Nutrition Sciences, Pocatello, ID 83209-8109. Offers dietetics (Certificate); health education (MHE); public health (MPH). Part-time programs available. *Degree requirements:* For master's, comprehensive exam, internship, thesis or project. *Entrance requirements:* For master's, GRE General Test or GPA greater than 3.5, minimum GPA of 3.0 for upper division classes, 2 letters of recommendation. Additional exam requirements/recommendations for international students: Required—TOEFL (minimum score 600 paper-based). Electronic applications accepted. *Faculty research:* Epidemiology, environmental health, nutrition and aging, dietetics.

Immaculata University, College of Graduate Studies, Program in Nutrition Education, Immaculata, PA 19345. Offers nutrition education for the registered dietitian (MA); nutrition education with dietetic internship (MA); nutrition education with wellness promotion (MA). Part-time and evening/weekend programs available. *Degree requirements:* For master's, comprehensive exam, thesis optional. *Entrance requirements:* For master's, GRE or MAT, minimum GPA of 3.0. Additional exam requirements/recommendations for international students: Required—TOEFL. *Application deadline:* Applications are processed on a rolling basis. Application fee: $50. Electronic applications accepted. *Expenses: Tuition:* Part-time $660 per credit. Part-time tuition and fees vary according to degree level and program. *Financial support:* Application deadline: 5/1; applicants required to submit FAFSA. *Faculty research:* Sports nutrition, pediatric nutrition, changes in food consumption patterns in weight loss, nutritional counseling. *Unit head:* Dr. Laura Frank, Chair, 610-647-4400 Ext. 3482, E-mail: lfrank@immaculata.edu.

Indiana State University, College of Graduate and Professional Studies, College of Arts and Sciences, Department of Family and Consumer Sciences, Terre Haute, IN 47809. Offers dietetics (MS); family and consumer sciences education (MS); inter-area option (MS). *Accreditation:* AND. Part-time programs available. *Faculty:* 5 full-time (4 women). *Students:* 12 full-time (all women), 7 part-time (6 women); includes 4 minority (3 Black or African American, non-Hispanic/Latino; 1 Asian, non-Hispanic/Latino), 2 international. Average age 33. 13 applicants, 100% accepted, 5 enrolled. In 2013, 9 master's awarded. *Degree requirements:* For master's, thesis optional. *Application deadline:* For fall admission, 7/1 priority date for domestic students; for spring admission, 11/1 priority date for domestic students. Applications are processed on a rolling basis. Application fee: $35. Electronic applications accepted. *Financial support:* In 2013–14, 2 research assistantships with partial tuition reimbursements (averaging $7,000 per year) were awarded; teaching assistantships and tuition waivers (partial) also available. Financial award application deadline: 3/1; financial award applicants required to submit FAFSA. *Unit head:* Dr. Frederica Kramer, Chairperson, 812-237-3297. *Application contact:* Dr. Jay Gatrell, Dean, 800-444-GRAD, Fax: 812-237-8060, E-mail: jay.gatrell@indstate.edu.

Indiana University Bloomington, School of Public Health, Department of Applied Health Science, Bloomington, IN 47405. Offers behavioral, social, and community health (MPH); family health (MPH); health behavior (PhD); nutrition science (MS); professional health education (MPH); public health administration (MPH); safety management (MS); school and college health education (MS). *Accreditation:* CEPH (one or more programs are accredited). *Faculty:* 30 full-time (19 women). *Students:* 144 full-time (104 women), 26 part-time (16 women); includes 46 minority (23 Black or African American, non-Hispanic/Latino; 1 American Indian or Alaska Native, non-Hispanic/Latino; 8 Asian, non-Hispanic/Latino; 10 Hispanic/Latino; 4 Two or more races, non-Hispanic/Latino), 32 international. Average age 30. 129 applicants, 71% accepted, 58 enrolled. In 2013, 53 master's, 6 doctorates awarded. *Degree requirements:* For master's, thesis optional; for doctorate, comprehensive exam, thesis/dissertation. *Entrance requirements:* For master's, GRE (for MS in nutrition science), 3 recommendations; for doctorate, GRE, 3 recommendations. Additional exam requirements/recommendations for international students: Required—TOEFL (minimum score 550 paper-based; 80 iBT). *Application deadline:* For fall admission, 2/1 priority date for domestic students, 12/1 priority date for international students; for spring admission, 11/15 priority date for domestic students, 9/1 priority date for international students. Application fee: $55 ($65 for international students). Electronic applications accepted. *Financial support:* Fellowships, research assistantships with full and partial tuition reimbursements, teaching assistantships with full and partial tuition reimbursements, career-related internships or fieldwork, Federal Work-Study, institutionally sponsored loans, scholarships/grants, health care benefits, tuition waivers (partial), unspecified assistantships, and fee remissions available. Financial award application deadline: 3/1; financial award applicants required to submit FAFSA. *Faculty research:* Cancer education, HIV/AIDS and drug education, public

health, parent-child interactions, safety education, obesity, public health policy, public health administration, school health, health education, human development, nutrition, human sexuality, chronic disease, early childhood health. *Total annual research expenditures:* $1.4 million. *Unit head:* Dr. David K. Lohrmann, Chair, 812-856-5101, Fax: 812-855-3936, E-mail: dlohrman@indiana.edu. *Application contact:* Dr. Susan Middlestadt, Associate Professor and Graduate Coordinator, 812-856-5768, Fax: 812-855-3936, E-mail: semiddle@indiana.edu.
Website: http://www.publichealth.indiana.edu/departments/applied-health-science/index.shtml

Indiana University of Pennsylvania, School of Graduate Studies and Research, College of Health and Human Services, Department of Food and Nutrition, Program in Food and Nutrition, Indiana, PA 15705-1087. Offers MS. Part-time programs available. *Faculty:* 5 full-time (all women). *Students:* 6 full-time (5 women), 25 part-time (24 women); includes 1 minority (Asian, non-Hispanic/Latino). Average age 25. 35 applicants, 66% accepted, 19 enrolled. In 2013, 9 master's awarded. *Degree requirements:* For master's, thesis optional. *Entrance requirements:* For master's, GRE General Test, 2 letters of recommendation. Additional exam requirements/recommendations for international students: Required—TOEFL (minimum score 540 paper-based). *Application deadline:* Applications are processed on a rolling basis. Application fee: $50. Electronic applications accepted. *Expenses:* Tuition, state resident: full-time $3978; part-time $442 per credit. Tuition, nonresident: full-time $5967; part-time $663 per credit. *Required fees:* $2080; $115.55 per credit. $93 per semester. Tuition and fees vary according to degree level and program. *Financial support:* In 2013–14, 5 research assistantships with full and partial tuition reimbursements (averaging $5,058 per year) were awarded. Financial award application deadline: 4/15; financial award applicants required to submit FAFSA. *Unit head:* Dr. Stephanie Taylor-Davis, Graduate Coordinator, 724-357-7733, E-mail: stdavis@iup.edu.

Indiana University–Purdue University Indianapolis, School of Health and Rehabilitation Sciences, Indianapolis, IN 46202. Offers health and rehabilitation sciences (PhD); health sciences (MS); nutrition and dietetics (MS); occupational therapy (MS); physical therapy (DPT); physician assistant (MPAS). Part-time and evening/weekend programs available. *Faculty:* 4 full-time (3 women). *Students:* 266 full-time (201 women), 13 part-time (12 women); includes 21 minority (6 Black or African American, non-Hispanic/Latino; 7 Asian, non-Hispanic/Latino; 4 Hispanic/Latino; 1 Native Hawaiian or other Pacific Islander, non-Hispanic/Latino; 3 Two or more races, non-Hispanic/Latino), 11 international. Average age 26. 381 applicants, 23% accepted, 77 enrolled. In 2013, 33 master's, 39 doctorates awarded. *Degree requirements:* For master's, thesis (for some programs). *Entrance requirements:* For master's, GRE General Test, minimum GPA of 3.0 (for MS in health sciences, nutrition and dietetics), 3.2 (for MS in occupational therapy), 3.0 cumulative and prerequisite math/science (for MPAS); for doctorate, GRE, minimum cumulative and prerequisite math/science GPA of 3.2. Additional exam requirements/recommendations for international students: Required—TOEFL (minimum score 550 paper-based; 79 iBT), IELTS (minimum score 6.5), PTE (minimum score 54). *Application deadline:* For fall admission, 10/1 for domestic students; for spring admission, 10/15 for domestic students. Electronic applications accepted. *Expenses:* Contact institution. *Financial support:* Fellowships, research assistantships, Federal Work-Study, institutionally sponsored loans, and scholarships/grants available. Support available to part-time students. Financial award applicants required to submit FAFSA. *Faculty research:* Function and mobility across the lifespan, pediatric nutrition, driving and mobility rehabilitation, neurorehabilitation and biomechanics, rehabilitation and integrative therapy. *Total annual research expenditures:* $1.1 million. *Unit head:* Dr. Augustine Agho, Dean, 317-274-4704, E-mail: aagho@iu.edu. *Application contact:* Kim Crockett, Student Data Coordinator, 317-278-6744, E-mail: kimecroc@iu.edu.
Website: http://shrs.iupui.edu/

Instituto Tecnologico de Santo Domingo, Graduate School, Area of Health Sciences, Santo Domingo, Dominican Republic. Offers bioethics (M Bioethics); clinical bioethics (Certificate); clinical nutrition (Certificate); comprehensive health and the adolescent (Certificate); comrehensive adloescent health (MS); health and social security (M Mgmt).

Iowa State University of Science and Technology, Program in Diet and Exercise, Ames, IA 50011. Offers MS. *Entrance requirements:* For master's, GRE, minimum GPA of 3.5, 3 letters of recommendation. Additional exam requirements/recommendations for international students: Required—TOEFL (minimum score 550 paper-based; 79 iBT), IELTS (minimum score 6.5). Electronic applications accepted.

Iowa State University of Science and Technology, Program in Nutritional Sciences, Ames, IA 50011. Offers MS, PhD. *Entrance requirements:* For master's and doctorate, GRE General Test. Additional exam requirements/recommendations for international students: Required—TOEFL (minimum score 550 paper-based; 79 iBT), IELTS (minimum score 6.5). Electronic applications accepted.

Johns Hopkins University, Bloomberg School of Public Health, Department of International Health, Baltimore, MD 21205. Offers global disease epidemiology and control (MHS, PhD); health systems (MHS, PhD); human nutrition (MHS, PhD); international health (MSPH, Dr PH); registered dietician (MSPH); social and behavioral interventions (MHS, PhD). *Faculty:* 137 full-time (82 women), 185 part-time/adjunct (63 women). *Students:* 284 full-time (212 women), 4 part-time (3 women); includes 70 minority (11 Black or African American, non-Hispanic/Latino; 1 American Indian or Alaska Native, non-Hispanic/Latino; 41 Asian, non-Hispanic/Latino; 6 Hispanic/Latino; 11 Two or more races, non-Hispanic/Latino), 73 international. Average age 28. 515 applicants, 44% accepted, 104 enrolled. In 2013, 78 master's, 24 doctorates awarded. *Degree requirements:* For master's, comprehensive exam, thesis (for some programs), 1-year full-time residency, 4-9 month internship; for doctorate, comprehensive exam, thesis/dissertation or alternative, 1.5 years' full-time residency, oral and written exams. *Entrance requirements:* For master's, GRE General Test or MCAT, 3 letters of recommendation, resume; for doctorate, GRE General Test or MCAT, 3 letters of recommendation, resume, transcripts. Additional exam requirements/recommendations for international students: Required—TOEFL (minimum score 600 paper-based; 100 iBT); Recommended—IELTS (minimum score 7). *Application deadline:* For fall admission, 1/2 priority date for domestic and international students. Applications are processed on a rolling basis. Application fee: $45. Electronic applications accepted. *Financial support:* Fellowships, Federal Work-Study, institutionally sponsored loans, scholarships/grants, traineeships, and stipends available. Financial award application deadline: 1/2. *Faculty research:* Nutrition, infectious diseases, health systems, health economics, humanitarian emergencies. *Total annual research expenditures:* $72 million. *Unit head:* Dr. David Peters, Chair, 410-955-3928, Fax: 410-955-7159, E-mail: dpeters@jhsph.edu. *Application contact:* Cristina G. Salazar, Academic Program Manager, 410-955-3734, Fax: 410-955-7159, E-mail: csalazar@jhsph.edu.
Website: http://www.jhsph.edu/dept/IH/

Kansas State University, Graduate School, College of Human Ecology, Department of Human Nutrition, Manhattan, KS 66506. Offers human nutrition (MS, PhD); nutritional sciences (PhD); public health nutrition (PhD); public health physical activity (PhD); sensory analysis and consumer behavior (PhD). Part-time programs available. *Faculty:* 17 full-time (10 women), 11 part-time/adjunct (3 women). *Students:* 19 full-time (11 women), 5 part-time (3 women); includes 3 minority (2 Asian, non-Hispanic/Latino; 1 Hispanic/Latino), 13 international. Average age 30. 34 applicants, 21% accepted, 5 enrolled. In 2013, 3 doctorates awarded. *Degree requirements:* For master's, thesis or alternative, residency; for doctorate, thesis/dissertation, residency. *Entrance requirements:* For master's, GRE General Test, minimum undergraduate GPA of 3.0; for doctorate, GRE General Test, minimum graduate GPA of 3.0. Additional exam requirements/recommendations for international students: Required—TOEFL (minimum score 550 paper-based; 79 iBT), IELTS (minimum score 6.5). *Application deadline:* For fall admission, 2/1 priority date for domestic and international students; for spring admission, 8/1 priority date for domestic and international students. Applications are processed on a rolling basis. Application fee: $50 ($75 for international students). Electronic applications accepted. *Financial support:* In 2013–14, 15 students received support, including 18 research assistantships (averaging $20,000 per year), 4 teaching assistantships with tuition reimbursements available (averaging $11,671 per year); career-related internships or fieldwork, Federal Work-Study, institutionally sponsored loans, scholarships/grants, health care benefits, and tuition waivers (full) also available. Support available to part-time students. Financial award application deadline: 3/1; financial award applicants required to submit FAFSA. *Faculty research:* Biochemical and molecular nutrition, public health nutrition, human and clinical nutrition, sensory analysis and consumer behavior. *Total annual research expenditures:* $809,805. *Unit head:* Dr. Mark Haub, Head, 785-532-5508, Fax: 785-532-3132, E-mail: nutrgrad@ksu.edu. *Application contact:* Janet Finney, Senior Administrative Specialist, 785-532-5508, Fax: 785-532-3132, E-mail: nutrgrad@ksu.edu.
Website: http://www.he.k-state.edu/hn/

Kent State University, Graduate School of Education, Health, and Human Services, School of Health Sciences, Program in Nutrition, Kent, OH 44242-0001. Offers MS. *Faculty:* 6 full-time (all women), 2 part-time/adjunct (both women). *Students:* 39 full-time (33 women), 8 part-time (7 women); includes 3 minority (2 Black or African American, non-Hispanic/Latino; 1 Native Hawaiian or other Pacific Islander, non-Hispanic/Latino), 8 international. 67 applicants, 58% accepted. In 2013, 16 master's awarded. *Degree requirements:* For master's, thesis optional. *Entrance requirements:* For master's, 3 letters of reference, goals statement, minimum GPA of 3.0. Additional exam requirements/recommendations for international students: Required—TOEFL (minimum score 550 paper-based; 80 iBT). Application fee: $30 ($60 for international students). *Financial support:* In 2013–14, 5 research assistantships (averaging $8,500 per year) were awarded; Federal Work-Study also available. *Unit head:* Karen Gordon, Coordinator, 330-672-2248, E-mail: klowry@kent.edu. *Application contact:* Nancy Miller, Academic Program Director, Office of Graduate Student Services, 330-672-2576, Fax: 330-672-9162.
Website: http://www.kent.edu/ehhs/nutr/

Lehman College of the City University of New York, School of Natural and Social Sciences, Department of Health Sciences, Program in Nutrition, Bronx, NY 10468-1589. Offers clinical nutrition (MS); community nutrition (MS); dietetic internship (MS). *Degree requirements:* For master's, thesis or alternative.

Liberty University, School of Health Sciences, Lynchburg, VA 24515. Offers biomedical sciences (MS); clinical mental health counseling (MA); global health (MPH); health promotion (MPH); human services (MA), including addictions and recovery, business, Christian ministry, criminal justice, crisis response and trauma, executive leadership, health and wellness, life coaching, marriage and family, military resilience; marriage and family therapy (MA); nurse educator (MS); nursing (MSN); nursing administration (MSN); nutrition (MPH); pastoral care and counseling (PhD); professional counseling (MA, PhD). *Students:* 2,830 full-time (2,293 women), 6,275 part-time (5,051 women); includes 1,677 minority (1,178 Black or African American, non-Hispanic/Latino; 19 American Indian or Alaska Native, non-Hispanic/Latino; 36 Asian, non-Hispanic/Latino; 278 Hispanic/Latino; 7 Native Hawaiian or other Pacific Islander, non-Hispanic/Latino; 159 Two or more races, non-Hispanic/Latino), 177 international. Average age 37. 9,147 applicants, 50% accepted, 2939 enrolled. In 2013, 2,618 master's, 11 doctorates awarded. *Degree requirements:* For master's, thesis (for some programs); for doctorate, thesis/dissertation. *Entrance requirements:* For doctorate, MAT or GRE, minimum GPA of 3.25 in master's program, 2-3 recommendations, writing samples (for some programs), letter of intent, professional vitae. Additional exam requirements/recommendations for international students: Required—TOEFL (minimum score 600 paper-based; 100 iBT). Application fee: $50. *Expenses: Tuition:* Full-time $9630; part-time $535 per credit hour. *Required fees:* $175 per term. One-time fee: $50. Tuition and fees vary according to course load, degree level, campus/location and program. *Application contact:* Jay Bridge, Director of Admissions, 800-424-9595, Fax: 800-628-7977, E-mail: gradadmissions@liberty.edu.

Life University, Program in Sport Health Science, Marietta, GA 30060-2903. Offers chiropractic sport science (MS); clinical nutrition (MS); exercise sport science (MS); nutrition and sport health science (MS); sport coaching (MS); sport injury management (MS). Part-time programs available. *Degree requirements:* For master's, comprehensive exam (for some programs), thesis optional. *Entrance requirements:* For master's, GRE General Test or MAT, minimum GPA of 3.0, 3 letters of recommendation. Additional exam requirements/recommendations for international students: Required—TOEFL (minimum score 500 paper-based). Electronic applications accepted.

Lipscomb University, Program in Exercise and Nutrition Science, Nashville, TN 37204-3951. Offers MS. Part-time and evening/weekend programs available. *Faculty:* 5 full-time (3 women). *Students:* 22 full-time (17 women), 32 part-time (24 women); includes 6 minority (5 Black or African American, non-Hispanic/Latino; 1 Asian, non-Hispanic/Latino), 3 international. Average age 27. 31 applicants, 52% accepted, 14 enrolled. In 2013, 11 master's awarded. *Degree requirements:* For master's, comprehensive exam (for some programs), thesis optional. *Entrance requirements:* For master's, GRE (minimum score of 800), minimum GPA of 2.75 on all undergraduate work; 2 letters of recommendation; resume. Additional exam requirements/recommendations for international students: Required—TOEFL (minimum score 570 paper-based). *Application deadline:* For fall admission, 6/1 for domestic students; for spring admission, 12/1 for domestic students. Applications are processed on a rolling basis. Application fee: $50 ($75 for international students). Electronic applications accepted. *Expenses: Tuition:* Full-time $15,570; part-time $865 per credit hour. Tuition and fees vary according to degree level and program. *Financial support:* Unspecified assistantships available. Financial award applicants required to submit FAFSA. *Unit head:* Dr. Karen Robichaud, Director, 615-966-5602, E-mail: karen.robichaud@lipscomb.edu. *Application contact:* Barbara Blackman, Coordinator of Graduate Studies, 615-966-6287, Fax: 615-966-7619, E-mail: graduatestudies@lipscomb.edu.
Website: http://www.lipscomb.edu/kinesiology/graduate-programs

Logan University, College of Health Sciences, Chesterfield, MO 63017. Offers nutrition and human performance (MS); sports science and rehabilitation (MS). Part-time programs available. Postbaccalaureate distance learning degree programs offered (no on-campus study). *Faculty:* 10 full-time (3 women), 15 part-time/adjunct (8 women). *Students:* 19 full-time (9 women), 63 part-time (31 women); includes 12 minority (2 Black or African American, non-Hispanic/Latino; 5 Asian, non-Hispanic/Latino; 3 Hispanic/Latino; 2 Two or more races, non-Hispanic/Latino), 1 international. Average age 32. In 2013, 82 master's awarded. *Degree requirements:* For master's, comprehensive exam.

Nutrition

Entrance requirements: For master's, GRE or National Board of Chiropractic Examiners test, minimum GPA of 2.5; specific undergraduate coursework based on program of interest. Additional exam requirements/recommendations for international students: Required—TOEFL (minimum score 79 iBT). *Application deadline:* For fall admission, 7/15 priority date for domestic and international students; for winter admission, 11/15 priority date for domestic and international students; for spring admission, 3/15 priority date for domestic students, 3/15 for international students. Applications are processed on a rolling basis. Application fee: $50. Electronic applications accepted. *Expenses:* Contact institution. *Financial support:* Federal Work-Study and scholarships/grants available. Support available to part-time students. Financial award applicants required to submit FAFSA. *Faculty research:* Ankle injury prevention in high school athletes, low back pain in college football players, short arc banding and low back pain, the effects of enzymes on inflammatory blood markers, gait analysis in high school and college athletes. *Unit head:* Dr. Sherri Cole, Vice President, Academic Affairs, 636-227-2100 Ext. 2702, Fax: 636-207-2431, E-mail: sherri.cole@logan.edu. *Application contact:* Stacey Till, Director of Admissions, 636-227-2100 Ext. 1749, Fax: 636-207-2425, E-mail: admissions@logan.edu.
Website: http://www.logan.edu

Loma Linda University, School of Public Health, Department of Nutrition, Loma Linda, CA 92350. Offers public health nutrition (MPH, Dr PH). *Accreditation:* AND. *Degree requirements:* For doctorate, thesis/dissertation. *Entrance requirements:* For doctorate, GRE General Test. Additional exam requirements/recommendations for international students: Required—Michigan English Language Assessment Battery or TOEFL. *Faculty research:* Sports nutrition in minorities, dietary determinance of chronic disease, protein adequacy in vegetarian diets, relationship of dietary intake to hormone level.

Long Island University–LIU Post, School of Health Professions and Nursing, Department of Nutrition, Brookville, NY 11548-1300. Offers dietetic internship (Certificate); nutrition (MS). Part-time and evening/weekend programs available. *Degree requirements:* For master's, thesis. *Entrance requirements:* For master's, minimum GPA of 2.75 in major. Electronic applications accepted. *Faculty research:* Hematopoiesis, interleukins in allergy, growth factors effect in metastasis affecting behavioral change for nutrition.

Louisiana Tech University, Graduate School, College of Applied and Natural Sciences, School of Human Ecology, Ruston, LA 71272. Offers nutrition and dietetics (MS). Part-time programs available. *Degree requirements:* For master's, thesis or alternative, Registered Dietician Exam eligibility. *Entrance requirements:* For master's, GRE General Test. *Application deadline:* For fall admission, 7/29 priority date for domestic students; for spring admission, 2/3 for domestic students. Applications are processed on a rolling basis. Application fee: $20 ($30 for international students). *Financial support:* Fellowships, research assistantships, career-related internships or fieldwork, and Federal Work-Study available. Financial award application deadline: 2/1. *Unit head:* Dr. Amy Yates, Director, 318-257-3727, Fax: 318-257-4014. *Application contact:* Dr. William Campbell, Director of Graduate Studies, 318-257-4287, Fax: 318-257-5060, E-mail: campbell@latech.edu.
Website: http://ans.latech.edu/human-ecology.html

Loyola University Chicago, Graduate School, Marcella Niehoff School of Nursing, Dietetics Program, Chicago, IL 60660. Offers MS, Certificate. *Faculty:* 45 full-time (44 women). *Students:* 19 full-time (18 women), 10 part-time (all women); includes 4 minority (1 Black or African American, non-Hispanic/Latino; 2 Asian, non-Hispanic/Latino; 1 Hispanic/Latino). Average age 24. 12 applicants, 83% accepted, 10 enrolled. In 2013, 10 master's, 11 other advanced degrees awarded. *Degree requirements:* For master's, comprehensive exam. *Expenses: Tuition:* Full-time $16,740; part-time $930 per credit. *Required fees:* $135 per semester. *Unit head:* Dr. Joanne Kouba, Assistant Professor, 708-216-4132, Fax: 708-216-9555, E-mail: jkouba@luc.edu. *Application contact:* Amy Weatherford, Enrollment Advisor, School of Nursing, 708-216-3751, Fax: 708-216-9555, E-mail: aweatherford@luc.edu.
Website: http://www.luc.edu/nursing/

Marshall University, Academic Affairs Division, College of Health Professions, Department of Dietetics, Huntington, WV 25755. Offers MS. *Students:* 10 full-time (8 women), 2 part-time (both women). Average age 27. In 2013, 10 master's awarded. *Unit head:* Dr. Kelli Williams, Chairperson, 304-696-4336, E-mail: williamsk@marshall.edu. *Application contact:* Information Contact, 304-746-1900, Fax: 304-746-1902, E-mail: services@marshall.edu.

Marywood University, Academic Affairs, College of Health and Human Services, Department of Nutrition and Dietetics, Program in Dietetic Internship, Scranton, PA 18509-1598. Offers Certificate. *Entrance requirements:* Additional exam requirements/recommendations for international students: Required—TOEFL (minimum score 550 paper-based; 79 iBT). Application fee: $35. Electronic applications accepted. *Expenses: Tuition:* Part-time $775 per credit. Tuition and fees vary according to degree level. *Financial support:* Research assistantships, career-related internships or fieldwork, scholarships/grants, and unspecified assistantships available. Support available to part-time students. Financial award application deadline: 6/30; financial award applicants required to submit FAFSA. *Unit head:* Maureen Dunne-Touhey, Director, 570-961-4751, E-mail: dunnetouhey@marywood.edu. *Application contact:* Tammy Manka, Assistant Director of Graduate Admissions, 866-279-9663, E-mail: tmanka@marywood.edu.
Website: http://www.marywood.edu/nutrition/internship/

Marywood University, Academic Affairs, College of Health and Human Services, Department of Nutrition and Dietetics, Program in Nutrition, Scranton, PA 18509-1598. Offers MS. *Entrance requirements:* Additional exam requirements/recommendations for international students: Required—TOEFL (minimum score 550 paper-based; 79 iBT). *Application deadline:* For fall admission, 4/1 priority date for domestic students, 3/31 priority date for international students; for spring admission, 11/1 priority date for domestic students, 8/31 priority date for international students. Applications are processed on a rolling basis. Application fee: $35. Electronic applications accepted. *Expenses: Tuition:* Part-time $775 per credit. Tuition and fees vary according to degree level. *Financial support:* Career-related internships or fieldwork, scholarships/grants, and unspecified assistantships available. Support available to part-time students. Financial award application deadline: 6/30; financial award applicants required to submit FAFSA. *Faculty research:* Obesity and childhood nutrition, dietary supplements (Resveratrol). *Unit head:* Dr. Lee Harrison, Chairperson, 570-348-6211 Ext. 2303, E-mail: harrisonl@marywood.edu. *Application contact:* Tammy Manka, Assistant Director of Graduate Admissions, 866-279-9663, E-mail: tmanka@marywood.edu.
Website: http://www.marywood.edu/nutrition/graduate-programs/nutrition/

Marywood University, Academic Affairs, College of Health and Human Services, Department of Nutrition and Dietetics, Program in Sports Nutrition and Exercise Science, Scranton, PA 18509-1598. Offers MS. *Entrance requirements:* Additional exam requirements/recommendations for international students: Required—TOEFL (minimum score 550 paper-based; 79 iBT). *Application deadline:* For fall admission, 4/1 priority date for domestic students, 3/31 priority date for international students; for spring admission, 11/1 priority date for domestic students, 8/31 priority date for international students. Applications are processed on a rolling basis. Application fee: $35. Electronic applications accepted. *Expenses: Tuition:* Part-time $775 per credit. Tuition and fees vary according to degree level. *Financial support:* Career-related internships or fieldwork, scholarships/grants, and unspecified assistantships available. Support available to part-time students. Financial award application deadline: 6/30; financial award applicants required to submit FAFSA. *Faculty research:* Lung function studies (pulmonary diffusing capacity of nitric oxide). *Unit head:* Dr. Lee Harrison, Chairperson, 570-348-6211 Ext. 2303, E-mail: harrisonl@marywood.edu. *Application contact:* Tammy Manka, Assistant Director of Graduate Admissions, 866-279-9663, E-mail: tmanka@marywood.edu.
Website: http://www.marywood.edu/nutrition/graduate-programs/sports-nutrition/

McGill University, Faculty of Graduate and Postdoctoral Studies, Faculty of Agricultural and Environmental Sciences, School of Dietetics and Human Nutrition, Montréal, QC H3A 2T5, Canada. Offers dietetics (M Sc A, Graduate Diploma); human nutrition (M Sc, M Sc A, PhD).

McMaster University, Faculty of Health Sciences and School of Graduate Studies, Program in Medical Sciences, Metabolism and Nutrition Area, Hamilton, ON L8S 4M2, Canada. Offers M Sc, PhD, MD/PhD. *Degree requirements:* For master's, thesis; for doctorate, comprehensive exam, thesis/dissertation. *Entrance requirements:* For master's, honors B Sc, B+ average in related field; for doctorate, M Sc, minimum B+ average, students with proven research experience and an A average may be admitted with a B Sc degree. Additional exam requirements/recommendations for international students: Required—TOEFL (minimum score 580 paper-based; 92 iBT).

McNeese State University, Doré School of Graduate Studies, Burton College of Education, Department of Health and Human Performance, Lake Charles, LA 70609. Offers exercise physiology (MS); health promotion (MS); nutrition and wellness (MS). *Accreditation:* NCATE. Evening/weekend programs available. *Entrance requirements:* For master's, GRE, undergraduate major or minor in health and human performance or related field of study.

Meredith College, John E. Weems Graduate School, Department of Human Environmental Sciences, Raleigh, NC 27607-5298. Offers dietetic internship (Postbaccalaureate Certificate); nutrition (MS). *Degree requirements:* For master's, thesis optional. *Entrance requirements:* For master's, GRE, recommendations, interview. Additional exam requirements/recommendations for international students: Required—TOEFL. Electronic applications accepted. *Expenses:* Contact institution.

Michigan State University, The Graduate School, College of Agriculture and Natural Resources and College of Natural Science, Department of Food Science and Human Nutrition, East Lansing, MI 48824. Offers food science (MS, PhD); food science - environmental toxicology (PhD); human nutrition (MS, PhD); human nutrition-environmental toxicology (PhD). *Entrance requirements:* Additional exam requirements/recommendations for international students: Required—TOEFL (minimum score 550 paper-based), Michigan State University ELT (minimum score 85), Michigan English Language Assessment Battery (minimum score 83). Electronic applications accepted.

Mississippi State University, College of Agriculture and Life Sciences, Department of Food Science, Nutrition and Health Promotion, Mississippi State, MS 39762. Offers food science and technology (MS, PhD); health promotion (MS); nutrition (MS, PhD). Postbaccalaureate distance learning degree programs offered (no on-campus study). *Faculty:* 7 full-time (1 woman). *Students:* 61 full-time (43 women), 40 part-time (32 women); includes 16 minority (10 Black or African American, non-Hispanic/Latino; 2 American Indian or Alaska Native, non-Hispanic/Latino; 1 Asian, non-Hispanic/Latino; 3 Hispanic/Latino), 20 international. Average age 29. 174 applicants, 30% accepted, 38 enrolled. In 2013, 30 master's, 2 doctorates awarded. *Degree requirements:* For master's, comprehensive exam, thesis; for doctorate, comprehensive exam, thesis/dissertation. *Entrance requirements:* For master's, GRE General Test, minimum GPA of 2.75; for doctorate, GRE General Test, minimum GPA of 2.75 undergraduate, 3.0 graduate. Additional exam requirements/recommendations for international students: Required—TOEFL (minimum score 550 paper-based; 79 iBT); Recommended—IELTS (minimum score 6.5). *Application deadline:* For fall admission, 7/1 for domestic students, 5/1 for international students; for spring admission, 11/1 for domestic students, 9/1 for international students. Applications are processed on a rolling basis. Application fee: $60. Electronic applications accepted. *Financial support:* In 2013–14, 12 research assistantships with full tuition reimbursements (averaging $15,205 per year), 5 teaching assistantships with full tuition reimbursements (averaging $11,591 per year) were awarded; Federal Work-Study, institutionally sponsored loans, scholarships/grants, and unspecified assistantships also available. Financial award application deadline: 4/1; financial award applicants required to submit FAFSA. *Faculty research:* Food preservation, food chemistry, food safety, food processing, product development. *Unit head:* Dr. Sam Chang, Professor and Head, 662-325-3200, Fax: 662-325-8728, E-mail: sc1690@msstate.edu. *Application contact:* Dr. Zee Haque, Graduate Coordinator, 662-325-3200, Fax: 662-325-8728, E-mail: haque@ra.msstate.edu.
Website: http://www.fsnhp.msstate.edu

Montclair State University, The Graduate School, College of Education and Human Services, Department of Exercise Science and Physical Education, Nutrition and Exercise Science Certificate Program, Montclair, NJ 07043-1624. Offers Certificate. Electronic applications accepted.

Montclair State University, The Graduate School, College of Education and Human Services, Department of Health and Nutrition Sciences, Post Baccalaureate Didactic Program in Dietetics Certificate, Montclair, NJ 07043-1624. Offers Postbaccalaureate Certificate. Part-time and evening/weekend programs available. *Entrance requirements:* Additional exam requirements/recommendations for international students: Required—TOEFL (minimum score 65 iBT), IELTS. Electronic applications accepted.

Montclair State University, The Graduate School, College of Education and Human Services, Department of Health and Nutrition Sciences, Program in Nutrition and Food Science, Montclair, NJ 07043-1624. Offers MS. Part-time and evening/weekend programs available. *Degree requirements:* For master's, comprehensive exam, thesis or alternative. *Entrance requirements:* For master's, GRE General Test, essay, 2 letters of recommendation. Additional exam requirements/recommendations for international students: Required—TOEFL (minimum score 83 iBT), IELTS (minimum score 6.5). Electronic applications accepted.

Mount Mary University, Graduate Division, Program in Dietetics, Milwaukee, WI 53222-4597. Offers administrative dietetics (MS); clinical dietetics (MS); nutrition education (MS). Part-time and evening/weekend programs available. *Faculty:* 3 full-time (all women), 1 part-time/adjunct (0 women). *Students:* 13 full-time (all women), 20 part-time (all women); includes 1 minority (Hispanic/Latino), 1 international. Average age 29. 91 applicants, 18% accepted, 13 enrolled. In 2013, 10 master's awarded. *Degree requirements:* For master's, thesis or alternative. *Entrance requirements:* For master's, minimum GPA of 2.75, completion of ADA and DPD requirements. Additional exam requirements/recommendations for international students: Required—TOEFL (minimum score 80 iBT) or IELTS (minimum score 6.5). *Application deadline:* For fall admission, 8/1 for domestic and international students; for spring admission, 12/1 for domestic and international students. Applications are processed on a rolling basis. Application fee: $45 ($100 for international students). Electronic applications accepted. *Expenses:* Contact institution. *Financial support:* Career-related internships or fieldwork and Federal Work-Study available. Support available to part-time students. Financial award

application deadline: 5/1; financial award applicants required to submit FAFSA. *Unit head:* Lisa Stark, Director, 414-258-4810 Ext. 398, E-mail: starkl@mtmary.edu. *Application contact:* Dr. Douglas J. Mickelson, Dean for Graduate Education, 414-256-1252, Fax: 414-256-0167, E-mail: mickelsd@mtmary.edu.
Website: http://www.mtmary.edu/majors-programs/graduate/dietetics/index.html

Mount Saint Vincent University, Graduate Programs, Department of Applied Human Nutrition, Halifax, NS B3M 2J6, Canada. Offers M Sc AHN, MAHN. Part-time and evening/weekend programs available. *Degree requirements:* For master's, thesis (for some programs). *Entrance requirements:* For master's, bachelor's degree in related field, minimum GPA of 3.0, professional experience. Electronic applications accepted.

New Mexico State University, Graduate School, College of Agricultural, Consumer and Environmental Sciences, Department of Family and Consumer Sciences, Las Cruces, NM 88003. Offers family and child science (MS); family and consumer science education (MS); food science and technology (MS); marriage and family therapy (MS); nutrition and dietetic science (MS). Part-time programs available. *Faculty:* 12 full-time (10 women). *Students:* 32 full-time (27 women), 10 part-time (9 women); includes 28 minority (all Hispanic/Latino), 1 international. Average age 30. 16 applicants, 81% accepted, 12 enrolled. In 2013, 12 master's awarded. *Degree requirements:* For master's, comprehensive exam (for some programs), thesis (for some programs), oral exam. *Entrance requirements:* For master's, GRE, 3 letters of reference, resume, letter of interest. Additional exam requirements/recommendations for international students: Required—TOEFL (minimum score 550 paper-based; 79 iBT), IELTS (minimum score 6.5). *Application deadline:* For fall admission, 3/1 priority date for domestic and international students; for spring admission, 11/30 for domestic and international students. Applications are processed on a rolling basis. Application fee: $40 ($50 for international students). Electronic applications accepted. *Expenses:* Tuition, state resident: full-time $5398; part-time $224.90 per credit. Tuition, nonresident: full-time $18,821; part-time $784.20 per credit. *Required fees:* $1310; $54.60 per credit. *Financial support:* In 2013–14, 26 students received support, including 1 research assistantship (averaging $18,972 per year), 5 teaching assistantships (averaging $9,943 per year); career-related internships or fieldwork, Federal Work-Study, scholarships/grants, health care benefits, and unspecified assistantships also available. Support available to part-time students. Financial award application deadline: 3/1; financial award applicants required to submit FAFSA. *Faculty research:* Food product analysis, childhood obesity, couple relationship education, military families, Latino college students. *Total annual research expenditures:* $429,265. *Unit head:* Dr. Esther Lynn Devall, Head, 575-646-3936, Fax: 575-646-1889, E-mail: edevall@nmsu.edu. *Application contact:* Dr. Ann Bock, Coordinator, 575-646-1178, Fax: 575-646-1889, E-mail: abock@nmsu.edu.
Website: http://fcs.nmsu.edu

New York Chiropractic College, Program in Applied Clinical Nutrition, Seneca Falls, NY 13148-0800. Offers MS. Part-time and evening/weekend programs available. *Entrance requirements:* For master's, minimum GPA of 2.5, transcripts, writing sample. Additional exam requirements/recommendations for international students: Recommended—TOEFL. *Application deadline:* Applications are processed on a rolling basis. Application fee: $60. Electronic applications accepted. *Financial support:* Federal Work-Study and scholarships/grants available. Financial award applicants required to submit FAFSA. *Unit head:* Dr. Peter Nickless, Director, 315-568-3310. *Application contact:* Kimberly McCrea, Senior Admissions Counselor for Online Programs, 717-387-3146, E-mail: kmccrea@nycc.edu.
Website: http://www.nycc.edu/AcademicPrograms_MSACNprogram.htm

New York Institute of Technology, School of Health Professions, Department of Interdisciplinary Health Sciences, Old Westbury, NY 11568-8000. Offers alcohol and substance abuse counseling (AC); clinical nutrition (MS). Part-time and evening/weekend programs available. Postbaccalaureate distance learning degree programs offered (minimal on-campus study). *Faculty:* 4 full-time (3 women), 8 part-time/adjunct (7 women). *Students:* 5 full-time (4 women), 39 part-time (33 women); includes 15 minority (1 Black or African American, non-Hispanic/Latino; 6 Asian, non-Hispanic/Latino; 7 Hispanic/Latino; 1 Two or more races, non-Hispanic/Latino), 1 international. Average age 31. 35 applicants, 71% accepted, 16 enrolled. In 2013, 24 master's, 5 other advanced degrees awarded. *Degree requirements:* For master's, comprehensive exam, thesis (for some programs). *Entrance requirements:* For master's, minimum QPA of 2.85. Additional exam requirements/recommendations for international students: Required—TOEFL (minimum score 550 paper-based; 79 iBT), IELTS (minimum score 6). *Application deadline:* For fall admission, 7/1 priority date for domestic students, 6/1 for international students; for spring admission, 12/1 priority date for domestic students, 12/1 for international students. Applications are processed on a rolling basis. Application fee: $50. Electronic applications accepted. *Expenses: Tuition:* Full-time $18,900; part-time $1050 per credit. *Financial support:* Research assistantships with partial tuition reimbursements, career-related internships or fieldwork, scholarships/grants, health care benefits, tuition waivers (full and partial), and unspecified assistantships available. Support available to part-time students. Financial award applicants required to submit FAFSA. *Faculty research:* Diabetes prevention and treatment, college students' health behavior, online education in health sciences, autism, mental health and aging. *Unit head:* Dr. Mindy Haar, Director, 516-686-3818, Fax: 516-686-3795, E-mail: mhaar@nyit.edu. *Application contact:* Alice Dolitsky, Director, Graduate Admissions, 516-686-7520, Fax: 516-686-1116, E-mail: nyitgrad@nyit.edu.
Website: http://www.nyit.edu/interdisciplinary_health_sciences

New York University, Steinhardt School of Culture, Education, and Human Development, Department of Nutrition, Food Studies, and Public Health, Program in Nutrition and Dietetics, New York, NY 10003. Offers nutrition and dietetics (MS, PhD), including clinical nutrition (MS), food and nutrition (MS), nutrition and dietetics (MS). Part-time programs available. *Faculty:* 9 full-time (8 women). *Students:* 85 full-time (80 women), 94 part-time (89 women); includes 29 minority (6 Black or African American, non-Hispanic/Latino; 8 Asian, non-Hispanic/Latino; 12 Hispanic/Latino; 3 Two or more races, non-Hispanic/Latino), 15 international. Average age 28. 231 applicants, 23% accepted, 30 enrolled. In 2013, 60 master's, 1 doctorate awarded. *Degree requirements:* For master's, thesis (for some programs); for doctorate, thesis/dissertation. *Entrance requirements:* For doctorate, GRE General Test, interview. Additional exam requirements/recommendations for international students: Required—TOEFL (minimum score 100 iBT). *Application deadline:* For fall admission, 12/1 priority date for domestic students, 12/15 for international students; for spring admission, 10/1 for domestic and international students. Applications are processed on a rolling basis. Application fee: $75. Electronic applications accepted. *Expenses: Tuition:* Full-time $35,856; part-time $1494 per unit. *Required fees:* $1408; $64 per unit. $473 per term. Tuition and fees vary according to course load and program. *Financial support:* Fellowships with full and partial tuition reimbursements, career-related internships or fieldwork, Federal Work-Study, institutionally sponsored loans, scholarships/grants, tuition waivers (partial), and unspecified assistantships available. Financial award application deadline: 2/1; financial award applicants required to submit FAFSA. *Faculty research:* Nutrition and race, childhood obesity and other eating disorders, nutritional epidemiology, nutrition policy, nutrition and health promotion. *Unit head:* Dr. Krishnendu Ray, Associate Professor of Food Studies/Department Chair, 212-998-5580, Fax: 212-995-4194, E-mail: krishnendu.ray@nyu.edu. *Application contact:* 212-998-5030, Fax: 212-995-4328, E-mail: steinhardt.gradadmissions@nyu.edu.
Website: http://steinhardt.nyu.edu/nutrition/dietetics

New York University, Steinhardt School of Culture, Education, and Human Development, Department of Nutrition, Food Studies, and Public Health, Program in Public Health, New York, NY 10003. Offers community and international health (MPH); global health leadership (MPH); public health nutrition (MPH). *Accreditation:* CEPH. Part-time programs available. *Faculty:* 7 full-time (5 women). *Students:* 6 full-time (all women), 2 part-time (both women); includes 3 minority (2 Asian, non-Hispanic/Latino; 1 Hispanic/Latino). Average age 32. 44 applicants, 7% accepted, 2 enrolled. In 2013, 1 degree awarded. *Degree requirements:* For master's, thesis (for some programs). *Entrance requirements:* For master's, GRE General Test. Additional exam requirements/recommendations for international students: Required—TOEFL. *Application deadline:* For fall admission, 12/1 priority date for domestic and international students; for spring admission, 11/1 for domestic and international students. Applications are processed on a rolling basis. Application fee: $75. Electronic applications accepted. *Expenses: Tuition:* Full-time $35,856; part-time $1494 per unit. *Required fees:* $1408; $64 per unit. $473 per term. Tuition and fees vary according to course load and program. *Financial support:* Fellowships with full and partial tuition reimbursements, career-related internships or fieldwork, Federal Work-Study, institutionally sponsored loans, scholarships/grants, and tuition waivers (partial) available. Support available to part-time students. Financial award application deadline: 2/1; financial award applicants required to submit FAFSA. *Faculty research:* Social epidemiology, primary health care, global health, immigrants and health, infectious disease prevention, HIV/AIDS. *Unit head:* Prof. James Macinko, Director, 212-998-5592, Fax: 212-995-4192, E-mail: james.macinko@nyu.edu. *Application contact:* 212-998-5030, Fax: 212-995-4328, E-mail: steinhardt.gradadmissions@nyu.edu.
Website: http://steinhardt.nyu.edu/nutrition/public_health

North Carolina Agricultural and Technical State University, School of Graduate Studies, School of Agriculture and Environmental Sciences, Department of Family and Consumer Sciences, Greensboro, NC 27411. Offers child development early education and family studies (MAT); family and consumer sciences (MAT); food and nutrition (MS). Part-time and evening/weekend programs available. *Degree requirements:* For master's, comprehensive exam, thesis or alternative, qualifying exam. *Entrance requirements:* For master's, GRE General Test, minimum GPA of 2.6.

North Carolina State University, Graduate School, College of Agriculture and Life Sciences and College of Veterinary Medicine, Program in Nutrition, Raleigh, NC 27695. Offers MN, MS, PhD. Part-time programs available. *Degree requirements:* For master's, thesis (for some programs); for doctorate, thesis/dissertation. *Entrance requirements:* For master's and doctorate, GRE General Test. Additional exam requirements/recommendations for international students: Required—TOEFL (minimum score 550 paper-based). Electronic applications accepted. *Faculty research:* Effects of food/feed ingredients and components on health and growth, community nutrition, waste management and reduction, experimental animal nutrition.

North Dakota State University, College of Graduate and Interdisciplinary Studies, College of Human Development and Education, Department of Health, Nutrition, and Exercise Sciences, Fargo, ND 58108. Offers athletic training (MS); dietetics (MS); exercise science (MS); nutrition science (MS); sport pedagogy (MS); sports recreation management (MS). Part-time and evening/weekend programs available. Postbaccalaureate distance learning degree programs offered (no on-campus study). *Faculty:* 17 full-time (14 women). *Students:* 54 full-time (30 women), 18 part-time (8 women); includes 5 minority (2 Hispanic/Latino; 3 Two or more races, non-Hispanic/Latino), 2 international. Average age 28. 27 applicants, 78% accepted, 16 enrolled. In 2013, 23 master's awarded. *Degree requirements:* For master's, thesis (for some programs). *Entrance requirements:* For master's, minimum GPA of 3.0. Additional exam requirements/recommendations for international students: Required—TOEFL (minimum score 525 paper-based; 71 iBT). *Application deadline:* For fall admission, 3/1 priority date for domestic and international students. Applications are processed on a rolling basis. Application fee: $35. Electronic applications accepted. *Financial support:* In 2013–14, 18 teaching assistantships with full tuition reimbursements (averaging $6,500 per year) were awarded. Financial award application deadline: 3/31. *Faculty research:* Biomechanics, sport specialization, recreation, nutrition, athletic training. *Unit head:* Dr. Margaret Fitzgerald, Head, 701-231-7474, Fax: 701-231-8872, E-mail: margaret.fitzgerald@ndsu.edu. *Application contact:* Dr. Gary Liguori, Graduate Coordinator, 701-231-7474, Fax: 701-231-6524.
Website: http://www.ndsu.edu/hnes/

Northeastern University, College of Professional Studies, Boston, MA 02115-5096. Offers applied nutrition (MS); commerce and economic development (MS); corporate and organizational communication (MS); digital media (MPS); geographic information technology (MPS); global studies and international affairs (MS); homeland security (MA); human services (MS); informatics (MPS); leadership (MS); nonprofit management (MS); project management (MS); regulatory affairs for drugs, biologics, and medical devices (MS); regulatory affairs of food and food industries (MS); respiratory care leadership (MS); technical communication (MS). Postbaccalaureate distance learning degree programs offered (no on-campus study).

Northern Illinois University, Graduate School, College of Health and Human Sciences, School of Family, Consumer and Nutrition Sciences, De Kalb, IL 60115-2854. Offers applied family and child studies (MS); nutrition and dietetics (MS). *Accreditation:* AAMFT/COAMFTE. Part-time programs available. *Faculty:* 16 full-time (14 women), 2 part-time/adjunct (1 woman). *Students:* 71 full-time (65 women), 15 part-time (all women); includes 18 minority (2 Black or African American, non-Hispanic/Latino; 1 American Indian or Alaska Native, non-Hispanic/Latino; 1 Asian, non-Hispanic/Latino; 11 Hispanic/Latino; 3 Two or more races, non-Hispanic/Latino), 4 international. Average age 26. 85 applicants, 54% accepted, 20 enrolled. In 2013, 32 master's awarded. *Degree requirements:* For master's, comprehensive exam, internship, thesis (nutrition and dietetics). *Entrance requirements:* For master's, GRE General Test, minimum GPA of 2.75. Additional exam requirements/recommendations for international students: Required—TOEFL (minimum score 550 paper-based). *Application deadline:* For fall admission, 6/1 for domestic students, 5/1 for international students; for spring admission, 11/1 for domestic students, 10/1 for international students. Applications are processed on a rolling basis. Application fee: $40. Electronic applications accepted. *Financial support:* In 2013–14, 9 research assistantships with full tuition reimbursements, 33 teaching assistantships with full tuition reimbursements were awarded; fellowships with full tuition reimbursements, career-related internships or fieldwork, Federal Work-Study, scholarships/grants, tuition waivers (full), and staff assistantships also available. Support available to part-time students. Financial award applicants required to submit FAFSA. *Faculty research:* Preliminary child development, hospitality administration in Asia, sports nutrition, eating disorders. *Unit head:* Dr. Thomas Pavkov, Chair, 815-753-6342, Fax: 815-753-1321, E-mail: tpavkov@niu.edu. *Application contact:* Graduate School Office, 815-753-0395, E-mail: gradsch@niu.edu.
Website: http://www.fcns.niu.edu/

The Ohio State University, Graduate School, College of Education and Human Ecology, Department of Human Sciences, Columbus, OH 43210. Offers consumer

sciences (MS, PhD); human development and family science (PhD); human nutrition (MS, PhD); kinesiology (MA, PhD). Part-time programs available. *Faculty:* 65. *Students:* 97 full-time (77 women), 4 part-time (3 women); includes 14 minority (5 Black or African American, non-Hispanic/Latino; 6 Asian, non-Hispanic/Latino; 3 Hispanic/Latino), 40 international. Average age 29. In 2013, 13 master's, 21 doctorates awarded. *Degree requirements:* For master's, thesis optional; for doctorate, thesis/dissertation. *Entrance requirements:* For master's and doctorate, GRE. Additional exam requirements/recommendations for international students: Required—TOEFL (minimum score 550 paper-based; 79 iBT), Michigan English Language Assessment Battery (minimum score 82); Recommended—IELTS (minimum score 7). *Application deadline:* For fall admission, 12/1 priority date for domestic and international students; for winter admission, 12/1 for domestic students, 11/1 for international students; for spring admission, 3/1 for domestic students, 2/1 for international students. Applications are processed on a rolling basis. Application fee: $60 ($70 for international students). Electronic applications accepted. *Financial support:* Fellowships with tuition reimbursements, research assistantships with tuition reimbursements, teaching assistantships with tuition reimbursements, Federal Work-Study, and institutionally sponsored loans available. Support available to part-time students. *Unit head:* Earl Harrison, Chair, 614-292-8189, E-mail: harrison.304@osu.edu. *Application contact:* Graduate Admissions, 614-292-6031, Fax: 614-292-3656, E-mail: gradadmissions@osu.edu.
Website: http://ehe.osu.edu/human-sciences/

The Ohio State University, Graduate School, College of Education and Human Ecology, Human Nutrition Program, Columbus, OH 43210. Offers PhD. Offered jointly with College of Food, Agricultural, and Environmental Sciences, College of Medicine, and College of Veterinary Medicine. *Faculty:* 49. *Students:* 24 full-time (18 women); includes 2 minority (1 Asian, non-Hispanic/Latino; 1 Hispanic/Latino), 13 international. Average age 28. *Degree requirements:* For doctorate, thesis/dissertation. *Entrance requirements:* For doctorate, GRE. Additional exam requirements/recommendations for international students: Required—TOEFL (minimum score 600 paper-based; 100 iBT); Recommended—IELTS (minimum score 8). *Application deadline:* For fall admission, 12/13 priority date for domestic students, 11/30 priority date for international students; for spring admission, 12/6 for domestic students, 11/11 for international students; for summer admission, 4/4 for domestic students, 3/7 for international students. Applications are processed on a rolling basis. Application fee: $60 ($70 for international students). Electronic applications accepted. *Financial support:* Applicants required to submit FAFSA. *Unit head:* Dr. Jeff Firkins, Director, 614-292-9957, E-mail: osun@osu.edu. *Application contact:* Graduate Admissions, 614-292-9444, Fax: 614-292-3895, E-mail: gradadmissions@osu.edu.
Website: http://osun.osu.edu/

Ohio University, Graduate College, College of Health Sciences and Professions, School of Applied Health Sciences and Wellness, Program in Food and Nutrition, Athens, OH 45701-2979. Offers human and consumer sciences (MS).

Oklahoma State University, College of Human Sciences, Department of Nutritional Sciences, Stillwater, OK 74078. Offers MS, PhD. Postbaccalaureate distance learning degree programs offered. *Faculty:* 18 full-time (15 women), 1 (woman) part-time/adjunct. *Students:* 36 full-time (34 women), 37 part-time (31 women); includes 18 minority (4 Black or African American, non-Hispanic/Latino; 4 American Indian or Alaska Native, non-Hispanic/Latino; 2 Asian, non-Hispanic/Latino; 3 Hispanic/Latino; 5 Two or more races, non-Hispanic/Latino), 10 international. Average age 29. 51 applicants, 59% accepted, 20 enrolled. In 2013, 16 master's, 3 doctorates awarded. *Degree requirements:* For master's, thesis (for some programs); for doctorate, comprehensive exam, thesis/dissertation. *Entrance requirements:* For master's and doctorate, GRE or GMAT. Additional exam requirements/recommendations for international students: Required—TOEFL (minimum score 550 paper-based; 79 iBT). *Application deadline:* For fall admission, 3/1 priority date for international students; for spring admission, 8/1 priority date for international students. Applications are processed on a rolling basis. Application fee: $40 ($75 for international students). Electronic applications accepted. *Expenses:* Tuition, state resident: full-time $4272; part-time $178 per credit hour. Tuition, nonresident: full-time $17,472; part-time $709 per credit hour. *Required fees:* $2413.20; $100.55 per credit hour. One-time fee: $50 full-time. Part-time tuition and fees vary according to course load and campus/location. *Financial support:* In 2013–14, 22 research assistantships (averaging $10,182 per year), 15 teaching assistantships (averaging $9,550 per year) were awarded; career-related internships or fieldwork, Federal Work-Study, scholarships/grants, health care benefits, tuition waivers (partial), and unspecified assistantships also available. Support available to part-time students. Financial award application deadline: 3/1; financial award applicants required to submit FAFSA. *Faculty research:* Nutritional sciences, micronutrients and chronic disease, phytochemicals, nutrition education, osteoporosis, food service administration. *Unit head:* Dr. Nancy M. Betts, Department Head, 405-744-5040, Fax: 405-744-1357, E-mail: nancy.betts@okstate.edu. *Application contact:* Dr. Gail Gates, Graduate Coordinator, 405-744-3845, Fax: 405-744-1357, E-mail: gail.gates@okstate.edu.
Website: http://humansciences.okstate.edu/nsci/

Oregon Health & Science University, School of Medicine, Graduate Programs in Medicine, Program in Clinical Nutrition, Portland, OR 97239-3098. Offers MS, Certificate. Part-time programs available. *Faculty:* 2 full-time (both women), 9 part-time/adjunct (7 women). *Students:* 26 full-time (24 women), 2 part-time (both women); includes 5 minority (2 Asian, non-Hispanic/Latino; 3 Hispanic/Latino). Average age 26. 67 applicants, 34% accepted, 23 enrolled. In 2013, 8 master's, 24 other advanced degrees awarded. *Degree requirements:* For master's, thesis optional. *Entrance requirements:* For master's, GRE General Test (minimum scores: 153 Verbal/148 Quantitative/4.5 Analytical). *Application deadline:* For fall admission, 1/1 for domestic students. Application fee: $120. *Financial support:* Health care benefits available. *Unit head:* Dr. Diane Stadler, Program Director. *Application contact:* Jeri Greenberg, 503-494-0745.

Oregon State University, College of Public Health and Human Sciences, Program in Nutrition, Corvallis, OR 97331. Offers MS, PhD. Part-time programs available. *Faculty:* 8 full-time (5 women). *Students:* 10 full-time (9 women); includes 1 minority (Asian, non-Hispanic/Latino), 2 international. Average age 26. 31 applicants, 13% accepted, 4 enrolled. In 2013, 2 master's, 3 doctorates awarded. *Degree requirements:* For master's, thesis; for doctorate, thesis/dissertation. *Entrance requirements:* For master's and doctorate, GRE, minimum GPA of 3.0 in last 90 hours of course work. Additional exam requirements/recommendations for international students: Required—TOEFL (minimum score 80 iBT), IELTS (minimum score 6.5). *Application deadline:* For fall admission, 12/1 for domestic students. Applications are processed on a rolling basis. Application fee: $60. *Expenses:* Tuition, state resident: full-time $11,664; part-time $432 per credit hour. Tuition, nonresident: full-time $19,197; part-time $711 per credit hour. *Required fees:* $1446; $443 per quarter. One-time fee: $300. Tuition and fees vary according to course load and program. *Financial support:* Fellowships, research assistantships, teaching assistantships, career-related internships or fieldwork, Federal Work-Study, and institutionally sponsored loans available. Support available to part-time students. Financial award application deadline: 2/1. *Faculty research:* Human metabolic studies, trace minerals, food science, food management. *Unit head:* Dr. Donald B. Jump, Professor and Director, Nutrition Graduate Program, 541-737-4007, Fax: 541-737-6914, E-mail: donald.jump@oregonstate.edu. *Application contact:* Debi Rothermund, Nutrition Advisor, 541-737-3324, Fax: 541-737-6914, E-mail: debi.rothermund@oregonstate.edu.
Website: http://health.oregonstate.edu/degrees/graduate/nutrition

Penn State University Park, Graduate School, College of Health and Human Development, Department of Nutritional Sciences, University Park, PA 16802. Offers MS, PhD. *Unit head:* Dr. Ann C. Crouter, Dean, 814-865-1420, Fax: 814-865-3282, E-mail: ac1@psu.edu. *Application contact:* Cynthia E. Nicosia, Director, Graduate Enrollment Services, 814-865-1834, Fax: 814-863-4627, E-mail: cey1@psu.edu.
Website: http://nutrition.hhd.psu.edu/

Purdue University, Graduate School, College of Health and Human Sciences, Department of Nutrition Science, West Lafayette, IN 47907. Offers animal health (MS, PhD); biochemical and molecular nutrition (MS, PhD); growth and development (MS, PhD); human and clinical nutrition (MS, PhD); public health and education (MS, PhD). *Faculty:* 22 full-time (14 women), 10 part-time/adjunct (all women). *Students:* 44 full-time (37 women), 2 part-time (both women); includes 5 minority (2 Black or African American, non-Hispanic/Latino; 1 Asian, non-Hispanic/Latino; 1 Hispanic/Latino; 1 Two or more races, non-Hispanic/Latino), 20 international. Average age 27. 78 applicants, 21% accepted, 10 enrolled. In 2013, 2 master's, 4 doctorates awarded. *Degree requirements:* For master's, thesis; for doctorate, thesis/dissertation. *Entrance requirements:* For master's and doctorate, GRE General Test (minimum scores in verbal and quantitative areas of 1000 or 300 on new scoring), minimum undergraduate GPA of 3.0 or equivalent. Additional exam requirements/recommendations for international students: Required—TOEFL (minimum score 600 paper-based; 77 iBT). *Application deadline:* For fall admission, 1/10 for domestic and international students. Applications are processed on a rolling basis. Application fee: $60 ($75 for international students). Electronic applications accepted. *Financial support:* Fellowships, research assistantships, and teaching assistantships available. Support available to part-time students. Financial award applicants required to submit FAFSA. *Faculty research:* Nutrient requirements, nutrient metabolism, nutrition and disease prevention. *Unit head:* Dr. Connie M. Weaver, Head, 765-494-8237, Fax: 765-494-0674, E-mail: weavercm@purdue.edu. *Application contact:* James C. Smith, Chair of the Graduate Committee, 765-494-0302, E-mail: fleet@purdue.edu.
Website: http://www.cfs.purdue.edu/fn/

Rosalind Franklin University of Medicine and Science, College of Health Professions, Department of Nutrition, North Chicago, IL 60064-3095. Offers clinical nutrition (MS); nutrition education (MS). Part-time and evening/weekend programs available. Postbaccalaureate distance learning degree programs offered (no on-campus study). *Degree requirements:* For master's, thesis optional, portfolio. *Entrance requirements:* For master's, minimum GPA of 2.75, registered dietitian (RD), professional certificate or license. Additional exam requirements/recommendations for international students: Required—TOEFL. *Expenses:* Contact institution. *Faculty research:* Nutrition education, distance learning, computer-based graduate education, childhood obesity, nutrition medical education.

Rush University, College of Health Sciences, Department of Clinical Nutrition, Chicago, IL 60612. Offers MS. Part-time programs available. *Degree requirements:* For master's, thesis. *Entrance requirements:* For master's, GRE General Test, minimum GPA of 3.0, course work in statistics, undergraduate didactic program approved by the American Dietetic Association. Additional exam requirements/recommendations for international students: Required—TOEFL. *Faculty research:* Food service management, chronic disease prevention/treatment, obesity, Alzheimer's.

Rutgers, The State University of New Jersey, Newark, School of Health Related Professions, Department of Nutritional Sciences, Dietetic Internship Program, Newark, NJ 07102. Offers Certificate. Postbaccalaureate distance learning degree programs offered (minimal on-campus study). *Entrance requirements:* For degree, bachelor's degree in dietetics, nutrition, or related field; interview; minimum GPA of 2.9. Additional exam requirements/recommendations for international students: Required—TOEFL (minimum score 500 paper-based; 79 iBT). Electronic applications accepted.

Rutgers, The State University of New Jersey, Newark, School of Health Related Professions, Department of Nutritional Sciences, Program in Clinical Nutrition, Newark, NJ 07102. Offers MS, DCN. Part-time and evening/weekend programs available. Postbaccalaureate distance learning degree programs offered (minimal on-campus study). *Entrance requirements:* For master's, statement of career goals, minimum GPA of 3.2, proof of registered dietician status, interview, transcript of highest degree, bachelor's degree, 1 reference letter; for doctorate, minimum GPA of 3.4, transcript of highest degree, statement of career goals, interview, master's degree, 1 reference letter. Additional exam requirements/recommendations for international students: Required—TOEFL (minimum score 500 paper-based; 79 iBT). Electronic applications accepted.

Rutgers, The State University of New Jersey, New Brunswick, Graduate School-New Brunswick, Program in Nutritional Sciences, Piscataway, NJ 08854-8097. Offers MS, PhD. Part-time programs available. Terminal master's awarded for partial completion of doctoral program. *Degree requirements:* For master's, thesis; for doctorate, thesis/dissertation, written qualifying exam. *Entrance requirements:* For master's and doctorate, GRE General Test, 3 letters of recommendation. Additional exam requirements/recommendations for international students: Required—TOEFL (minimum score 560 paper-based; 83 iBT). Electronic applications accepted. *Faculty research:* Nutrition and gene expression, nutrition and disease (obesity, diabetes, cancer, osteoporosis, alcohol), community nutrition and nutrition education, cellular lipid transport and metabolism.

Sage Graduate School, School of Health Sciences, Program in Nutrition, Troy, NY 12180-4115. Offers applied nutrition (MS); dietetic internship (Certificate); nutrition (Certificate). Part-time and evening/weekend programs available. *Faculty:* 2 full-time (both women), 2 part-time/adjunct (1 woman). *Students:* 60 full-time (52 women), 22 part-time (20 women); includes 10 minority (2 Black or African American, non-Hispanic/Latino; 1 American Indian or Alaska Native, non-Hispanic/Latino; 2 Asian, non-Hispanic/Latino; 3 Hispanic/Latino; 2 Two or more races, non-Hispanic/Latino), 2 international. Average age 29. 167 applicants, 39% accepted, 38 enrolled. In 2013, 8 master's, 24 other advanced degrees awarded. *Entrance requirements:* For master's, minimum GPA of 2.75, resume, 2 letters of recommendation, interview with director. Additional exam requirements/recommendations for international students: Required—TOEFL (minimum score 550 paper-based). *Application deadline:* Applications are processed on a rolling basis. Application fee: $40. *Expenses: Tuition:* Full-time $11,880; part-time $660 per credit hour. *Financial support:* Fellowships, research assistantships, Federal Work-Study, scholarships/grants, and unspecified assistantships available. Support available to part-time students. *Unit head:* Dr. Esther Haskevitz, Dean, School of Health Sciences, 518-244-2296, Fax: 518-244-4571, E-mail: haskve@sage.edu. *Application contact:* Rayane AbuSabha, Director of Didactic Program in Dietetics, 518-244-2396, Fax: 518-244-4586, E-mail: abusar@sage.edu.

Sage Graduate School, School of Management, Program in Health Services Administration, Troy, NY 12180-4115. Offers dietetic internship (Certificate); gerontology (MS). Part-time and evening/weekend programs available. *Faculty:* 2 full-time (both women), 28 part-time/adjunct (21 women). *Students:* 3 full-time (all women), 38 part-time (27 women); includes 6 minority (3 Black or African American, non-Hispanic/Latino; 3 Asian, non-Hispanic/Latino). Average age 33. 46 applicants, 41% accepted, 13 enrolled. In 2013, 8 master's awarded. *Entrance requirements:* For master's, minimum GPA of 2.75, resume, 2 letters of recommendation. Additional exam requirements/recommendations for international students: Required—TOEFL (minimum score 550 paper-based). Application fee: $40. *Expenses: Tuition:* Full-time $11,880; part-time $660 per credit hour. *Financial support:* Fellowships, research assistantships, Federal Work-Study, scholarships/grants, and unspecified assistantships available. Support available to part-time students. Financial award application deadline: 3/1; financial award applicants required to submit FAFSA. *Unit head:* Dr. Kimberly Fredricks, Associate Dean, School of Management, 518-292-1700, Fax: 518-292-1964, E-mail: fredek1@sage.edu. *Application contact:* Wendy D. Diefendorf, Director of Graduate and Adult Admission, 518-244-2443, Fax: 518-244-6880, E-mail: diefew@sage.edu.

Saint Louis University, Graduate Education, Doisy College of Health Sciences and Graduate Education, Department of Nutrition and Dietetics, St. Louis, MO 63103-2097. Offers medical dietetics (MS); nutrition and physical performance (MS). Part-time programs available. *Degree requirements:* For master's, comprehensive exam (for some programs). *Entrance requirements:* For master's, GRE General Test, letters of recommendation, resume, interview. Additional exam requirements/recommendations for international students: Required—TOEFL (minimum score 525 paper-based). Electronic applications accepted. *Faculty research:* Sustainable food systems, nutrition education, public health nutrition, culinary nutrition and physical performance.

Sam Houston State University, College of Humanities and Social Sciences, Department of Family and Consumer Sciences, Huntsville, TX 77341. Offers dietetics (MS); family and consumer sciences (MS). Part-time and evening/weekend programs available. *Faculty:* 4 full-time (3 women). *Students:* 22 full-time (21 women), 7 part-time (all women); includes 5 minority (1 Black or African American, non-Hispanic/Latino; 1 Asian, non-Hispanic/Latino; 3 Hispanic/Latino), 1 international. Average age 28. 25 applicants, 92% accepted, 13 enrolled. In 2013, 10 master's awarded. *Degree requirements:* For master's, comprehensive exam, thesis optional. *Entrance requirements:* For master's, GRE General Test, minimum GPA of 2.5. Additional exam requirements/recommendations for international students: Required—TOEFL (minimum score 550 paper-based; 79 iBT), IELTS (minimum score 6.5). *Application deadline:* For fall admission, 8/1 for domestic students, 6/25 for international students; for spring admission, 12/1 for domestic students, 11/12 for international students. Applications are processed on a rolling basis. Application fee: $45 ($75 for international students). Electronic applications accepted. *Financial support:* In 2013–14, 2 teaching assistantships (averaging $1,915 per year) were awarded; career-related internships or fieldwork, Federal Work-Study, institutionally sponsored loans, scholarships/grants, and unspecified assistantships also available. Support available to part-time students. Financial award application deadline: 5/31; financial award applicants required to submit FAFSA. *Unit head:* Dr. Janis White, Chair, 936-294-1242, Fax: 936-294-4204, E-mail: jwhite@shsu.edu. *Application contact:* Dr. Paula Tripp, Graduate Director, 936-294-4129, E-mail: pjtripp@shsu.edu.
Website: http://www.shsu.edu/~hec_www/

San Diego State University, Graduate and Research Affairs, College of Health and Human Services, School of Exercise and Nutritional Sciences, Program in Nutritional Sciences, San Diego, CA 92182. Offers MS, MS/MS. *Degree requirements:* For master's, thesis. *Entrance requirements:* For master's, GRE General Test, 2 letters of reference. Additional exam requirements/recommendations for international students: Required—TOEFL. Electronic applications accepted.

San Jose State University, Graduate Studies and Research, College of Applied Sciences and Arts, Department of Nutrition, Food Science, and Packaging, San Jose, CA 95192-0001. Offers nutritional science (MS). Electronic applications accepted.

Saybrook University, School of Mind-Body Medicine, San Francisco, CA 94111-1920. Offers MS, PhD, Certificate. *Entrance requirements:* Additional exam requirements/recommendations for international students: Required—TOEFL (minimum score 580 paper-based; 93 iBT). Electronic applications accepted. *Expenses: Tuition:* Full-time $22,560. *Required fees:* $2200; $1000 per credit. $2200 per year. One-time fee: $450.

Simmons College, School of Nursing and Health Sciences, Boston, MA 02115. Offers didactic dietetics (Certificate); dietetic internship (Certificate); health professions education (CAGS); nursing (MS); nursing practice (DNP); nutrition and health promotion (MS); physical therapy (DPT); sports nutrition (Certificate). Part-time programs available. Postbaccalaureate distance learning degree programs offered (minimal on-campus study). *Students:* 143 full-time (129 women), 347 part-time (329 women); includes 72 minority (31 Black or African American, non-Hispanic/Latino; 17 Asian, non-Hispanic/Latino; 15 Hispanic/Latino; 9 Two or more races, non-Hispanic/Latino), 4 international. 196 applicants, 56% accepted, 88 enrolled. In 2013, 70 master's, 45 doctorates awarded. *Entrance requirements:* For doctorate, GRE. Additional exam requirements/recommendations for international students: Required—TOEFL (minimum score 570 paper-based; 88 iBT). *Application deadline:* For fall admission, 6/1 for international students. Application fee: $50. Electronic applications accepted. *Financial support:* In 2013–14, 33 students received support, including 24 teaching assistantships (averaging $6,000 per year); scholarships/grants and unspecified assistantships also available. *Unit head:* Dr. Judy Beal, Dean, 617-521-2139. *Application contact:* Carmen Fortin, Assistant Dean/Director of Admission, 617-521-2651, Fax: 617-521-3137, E-mail: gshsadm@simmons.edu.
Website: http://www.simmons.edu/snhs/

South Carolina State University, School of Graduate and Professional Studies, Department of Family and Consumer Sciences, Orangeburg, SC 29117-0001. Offers individual and family development (MS); nutritional sciences (MS). Part-time and evening/weekend programs available. *Faculty:* 4 full-time (3 women), 1 (woman) part-time/adjunct. *Students:* 8 full-time (all women), 10 part-time (9 women); includes 17 minority (16 Black or African American, non-Hispanic/Latino; 1 Asian, non-Hispanic/Latino). Average age 29. 10 applicants, 80% accepted, 3 enrolled. In 2013, 8 master's awarded. *Degree requirements:* For master's, comprehensive exam, thesis optional, departmental qualifying exam. *Entrance requirements:* For master's, GRE, MAT, or NTE, minimum GPA of 2.7. *Application deadline:* For fall admission, 6/15 priority date for domestic students, 6/15 for international students; for spring admission, 11/1 for domestic and international students. Applications are processed on a rolling basis. Application fee: $25. Electronic applications accepted. *Expenses:* Tuition, state resident: full-time $8906; part-time $543 per credit hour. Tuition, nonresident: full-time $18,040; part-time $1051 per credit hour. *Financial support:* Fellowships and institutionally sponsored loans available. Financial award application deadline: 6/1. *Faculty research:* Societal competence, relationship of parent-child interaction to adult, quality of well-being of rural elders. *Unit head:* Dr. Ethel G. Jones, Chair, 803-536-8958, Fax: 803-533-3268, E-mail: egjones@scsu.edu. *Application contact:* Curtis Foskey, Coordinator of Graduate Admission, 803-536-8419, Fax: 803-536-8812, E-mail: cfoskey@scsu.edu.

South Dakota State University, Graduate School, College of Education and Human Sciences, Department of Nutrition, Food Science and Hospitality, Brookings, SD 57007. Offers dietetics (MS); nutrition, food science and hospitality (MFCS); nutritional sciences (MS, PhD). Part-time programs available. *Degree requirements:* For master's, comprehensive exam (for some programs), thesis (for some programs), oral exam. *Entrance requirements:* Additional exam requirements/recommendations for international students: Required—TOEFL (minimum score 525 paper-based). *Faculty research:* Food chemistry, bone density, functional food, nutrition education, nutrition biochemistry.

Southeast Missouri State University, School of Graduate Studies, Department of Health, Human Performance and Recreation, Cape Girardeau, MO 63701-4799. Offers nutrition and exercise science (MS). Part-time and evening/weekend programs available. *Faculty:* 6 full-time (2 women), 2 part-time/adjunct (0 women). *Students:* 23 full-time (12 women), 7 part-time (6 women); includes 2 minority (1 Black or African American, non-Hispanic/Latino; 1 Hispanic/Latino), 12 international. Average age 24. 29 applicants, 86% accepted, 15 enrolled. In 2013, 4 master's awarded. *Degree requirements:* For master's, comprehensive exam, thesis optional, internship. *Entrance requirements:* For master's, GRE General Test (minimum combined score of 950), minimum undergraduate GPA of 3.0, minimum B grade in prerequisite courses. Additional exam requirements/recommendations for international students: Required—TOEFL (minimum score 550 paper-based; 79 iBT), IELTS (minimum score 6), PTE (minimum score 53). *Application deadline:* For fall admission, 8/1 for domestic students, 5/1 for international students; for spring admission, 11/21 for domestic students, 10/1 for international students; for summer admission, 5/15 for domestic students. Applications are processed on a rolling basis. Application fee: $30 ($40 for international students). Electronic applications accepted. *Expenses:* Tuition, state resident: full-time $5139; part-time $285.50 per credit hour. Tuition, nonresident: full-time $9099; part-time $505.50 per credit hour. *Financial support:* In 2013–14, 18 students received support. Career-related internships or fieldwork, Federal Work-Study, scholarships/grants, traineeships, tuition waivers (full), and unspecified assistantships available. Financial award application deadline: 6/30; financial award applicants required to submit FAFSA. *Faculty research:* Blood lipids, body composition assessment, exercise testing, perceptual responses to physical activity, sport governance, youth sports participation. *Unit head:* Dr. Joe Pujol, Chairperson, 573-651-2664, E-mail: jpujol@semo.edu. *Application contact:* Alisa Aleen McFerron, Assistant Director of Admissions for Operations, 573-651-5937, E-mail: amcferron@semo.edu.
Website: http://www.semo.edu/health/

Southern Illinois University Carbondale, Graduate School, College of Agriculture, Department of Animal Science, Food and Nutrition, Program in Food and Nutrition, Carbondale, IL 62901-4701. Offers MS. *Faculty:* 12 full-time (4 women). *Students:* 17 full-time (15 women), 8 part-time (all women); includes 1 minority (Black or African American, non-Hispanic/Latino), 1 international. Average age 29. 23 applicants, 39% accepted, 8 enrolled. In 2013, 8 master's awarded. *Degree requirements:* For master's, thesis or alternative. *Entrance requirements:* For master's, GRE, minimum GPA of 2.7. Additional exam requirements/recommendations for international students: Required—TOEFL (minimum score 550 paper-based; 80 iBT). *Application deadline:* For fall admission, 1/1 for domestic students. Application fee: $50. Electronic applications accepted. *Financial support:* In 2013–14, 12 students received support. Fellowships, research assistantships, teaching assistantships, career-related internships or fieldwork, Federal Work-Study, institutionally sponsored loans, and tuition waivers (full) available. Support available to part-time students. *Faculty research:* Public health nutrition, nutrition physiology, soybean utilization, nutrition education. *Total annual research expenditures:* $100,000. *Unit head:* Dr. William Banz, Chair, 618-453-1763, E-mail: banz@siu.edu. *Application contact:* Terry Richardson, Office Support Specialist, 618-453-1762, E-mail: cerebus@siu.edu.
Website: http://coas.siu.edu/academics/departments/animal-science-food-nutrition/index.html

State University of New York College at Oneonta, Graduate Education, Department of Human Ecology, Oneonta, NY 13820-4015. Offers nutrition and dietetics (MS). Postbaccalaureate distance learning degree programs offered (no on-campus study).

Stony Brook University, State University of New York, Stony Brook University Medical Center, Health Sciences Center, School of Medicine and Graduate School, Graduate Programs in Medicine, Department of Family Medicine, Stony Brook, NY 11794. Offers nutrition (MS, Advanced Certificate). Postbaccalaureate distance learning degree programs offered (no on-campus study). *Faculty:* 17 full-time (10 women), 4 part-time/adjunct (3 women). *Students:* 2 full-time (both women), 21 part-time (18 women); includes 3 minority (2 Asian, non-Hispanic/Latino; 1 Hispanic/Latino). 24 applicants, 79% accepted, 18 enrolled. *Application deadline:* For fall admission, 7/1 for domestic students; for summer admission, 4/1 for domestic students. Electronic applications accepted. *Expenses:* Tuition, state resident: full-time $9870; part-time $411 per credit. Tuition, nonresident: full-time $18,350; part-time $765 per credit. *Total annual research expenditures:* $1.2 million. *Unit head:* Dr. Josephine Connelly-Schoonen, Executive Director, Stony Brook Medicine Nutrition Division, 631-444-2111. *Application contact:* Sharon Schmidt, 631-638-2132, E-mail: sharon.schmidt@stonybrookmedicine.edu.
Website: http://medicine.stonybrookmedicine.edu/gradnutrition

Syracuse University, Falk College of Sport and Human Dynamics, Program in Nutrition Science, Syracuse, NY 13244. Offers MA, MS. *Accreditation:* AND. Part-time programs available. *Students:* 23 full-time (22 women), 3 part-time (all women); includes 2 minority (1 Asian, non-Hispanic/Latino; 1 Hispanic/Latino), 6 international. Average age 28. 31 applicants, 52% accepted, 7 enrolled. In 2013, 11 master's awarded. *Degree requirements:* For master's, comprehensive exam, thesis. *Entrance requirements:* For master's, GRE General Test. Additional exam requirements/recommendations for international students: Required—TOEFL (minimum score 100 iBT). *Application deadline:* For fall admission, 3/15 priority date for domestic and international students; for spring admission, 11/1 priority date for domestic and international students. Applications are processed on a rolling basis. Application fee: $75. Electronic applications accepted. *Financial support:* Fellowships with full tuition reimbursements, research assistantships with full and partial tuition reimbursements, teaching assistantships with full and partial tuition reimbursements, and tuition waivers available. Financial award application deadline: 1/1; financial award applicants required to submit FAFSA. *Unit head:* Dr. Sudha Raj, Program Director, 315-443-2386, Fax: 315-443-2562, E-mail: inquire@hshp.syr.edu. *Application contact:* Felicia Otero, Information Contact, 315-443-5555, E-mail: inquire@hshp.syr.edu.
Website: http://falk.syr.edu/NutritionScienceDietetics/Default.aspx

Teachers College, Columbia University, Graduate Faculty of Education, Department of Health and Behavioral Studies, Program in Nutrition, New York, NY 10027. Offers nutrition education (Ed M, MS, Ed D); nutrition education and public health nutrition (Ed M, MS, Ed D), including community nutrition education (Ed M), nutrition and public health (MS, Ed D), nutrition education (MS, Ed D). Part-time and evening/weekend programs available. *Faculty:* 8 full-time, 5 part-time/adjunct. *Students:* 20 full-time (19 women), 69 part-time (63 women); includes 16 minority (5 Black or African American, non-Hispanic/Latino; 9 Asian, non-Hispanic/Latino; 1 Hispanic/Latino; 1 Two or more races, non-Hispanic/Latino), 8 international. Average age 32. 55 applicants, 73% accepted, 18 enrolled. In 2013, 28 master's, 8 doctorates awarded. Terminal master's awarded for partial completion of doctoral program. *Degree requirements:* For master's,

thesis optional, integrative project; for doctorate, thesis/dissertation. *Entrance requirements:* For master's, GRE General Test; for doctorate, GRE General Test, sample of written work. *Application deadline:* For fall admission, 1/15 for domestic students; for spring admission, 11/1 for domestic students. Applications are processed on a rolling basis. Application fee: $65. Electronic applications accepted. *Financial support:* Fellowships, research assistantships, career-related internships or fieldwork, Federal Work-Study, institutionally sponsored loans, and tuition waivers (full and partial) available. Support available to part-time students. Financial award application deadline: 2/1; financial award applicants required to submit FAFSA. *Faculty research:* Psychosocial determinants of eating behavior, food supply and environmental education, development and evaluation of nutrition education. *Unit head:* Prof. Isobel R. Contento, Program Coordinator, 212-678-3949, E-mail: contento@tc.edu. *Application contact:* Peter Shon, Assistant Director of Admission, 212-678-3305, Fax: 212-678-4171, E-mail: shon@exchange.tc.columbia.edu.
Website: http://www.tc.columbia.edu/hbs/Nutrition

Texas A&M University, College of Agriculture and Life Sciences, Department of Nutrition and Food Science, College Station, TX 77843. Offers food science and technology (M Agr); nutrition (MS, PhD). *Faculty:* 11. *Students:* 50 full-time (40 women), 9 part-time (7 women); includes 9 minority (1 Black or African American, non-Hispanic/Latino; 1 Asian, non-Hispanic/Latino; 6 Hispanic/Latino; 1 Two or more races, non-Hispanic/Latino), 25 international. Average age 27. 152 applicants, 15% accepted, 19 enrolled. In 2013, 2 master's, 2 doctorates awarded. *Degree requirements:* For master's, thesis; for doctorate, thesis/dissertation. *Entrance requirements:* For master's and doctorate, GRE General Test. Additional exam requirements/recommendations for international students: Required—TOEFL. *Application deadline:* For fall admission, 2/1 priority date for domestic students; for spring admission, 10/1 priority date for domestic students. Applications are processed on a rolling basis. Application fee: $50 ($75 for international students). *Expenses:* Tuition, state resident: full-time $4078; part-time $226.55 per credit hour. Tuition, nonresident: full-time $10,450; part-time $580.55 per credit hour. *Required fees:* $2328; $278.50 per credit hour. $642.45 per semester. *Financial support:* Fellowships, research assistantships, teaching assistantships, career-related internships or fieldwork, and scholarships/grants available. *Faculty research:* Food safety, microbiology, product development. *Unit head:* Dr. Jimmy T. Keeton, Department Head, 979-458-3428, E-mail: jkeeton@tamu.edu. *Application contact:* Graduate Admissions, 979-845-1044, E-mail: admissions@tamu.edu.
Website: http://nfs.tamu.edu

Texas State University, Graduate School, College of Applied Arts, School of Family and Consumer Sciences, San Marcos, TX 78666. Offers family and child studies (MS); human nutrition (MS); merchandising and consumer studies (MS). Part-time programs available. *Faculty:* 15 full-time (13 women), 1 (woman) part-time/adjunct. *Students:* 93 full-time (74 women), 35 part-time (28 women); includes 30 minority (3 Black or African American, non-Hispanic/Latino; 1 American Indian or Alaska Native, non-Hispanic/Latino; 3 Asian, non-Hispanic/Latino; 21 Hispanic/Latino; 2 Two or more races, non-Hispanic/Latino), 9 international. Average age 27. 99 applicants, 68% accepted, 58 enrolled. In 2013, 29 master's awarded. *Degree requirements:* For master's, comprehensive exam, thesis (for some programs). *Entrance requirements:* For master's, GRE General Test (preferred), minimum GPA of 3.0 in last 60 hours of course work. Additional exam requirements/recommendations for international students: Required—TOEFL (minimum score 550 paper-based; 78 iBT). *Application deadline:* For fall admission, 6/15 priority date for domestic students, 6/1 for international students; for spring admission, 10/15 priority date for domestic students, 10/1 for international students. Applications are processed on a rolling basis. Application fee: $40 ($90 for international students). Electronic applications accepted. *Expenses:* Tuition, state resident: full-time $6663; part-time $278 per credit hour. Tuition, nonresident: full-time $15,159; part-time $632 per credit hour. *Required fees:* $1872; $54 per credit hour. $306 per term. Tuition and fees vary according to course load. *Financial support:* In 2013–14, 43 students received support, including 10 research assistantships (averaging $9,363 per year), 23 teaching assistantships (averaging $10,932 per year). Financial award application deadline: 4/1; financial award applicants required to submit FAFSA. *Faculty research:* Healthy marriages, best food fits, hair fiber products, retinol and cancer met, light/color assessment, interactive vitamin A, testing of ALKA-V6, dietary herbs. *Total annual research expenditures:* $746,640. *Unit head:* Dr. Maria E. Canabal, Chair, 512-245-2155, Fax: 512-245-3829, E-mail: mc57@txstate.edu. *Application contact:* Dr. Andrea Golato, Dean of the Graduate College, 512-245-2581, Fax: 512-245-8365, E-mail: gradcollege@txstate.edu.
Website: http://www.fcs.txstate.edu/

Texas Tech University, Graduate School, College of Human Sciences, Department of Nutrition, Hospitality, and Retailing, Lubbock, TX 79409-1240. Offers hospitality administration (PhD); hospitality and retail management (MS); nutritional sciences (MS, PhD). Part-time and evening/weekend programs available. *Faculty:* 24 full-time (14 women). *Students:* 90 full-time (66 women), 16 part-time (10 women); includes 11 minority (1 Black or African American, non-Hispanic/Latino; 4 Asian, non-Hispanic/Latino; 6 Hispanic/Latino), 41 international. Average age 29. 74 applicants, 64% accepted, 33 enrolled. In 2013, 23 master's, 17 doctorates awarded. Terminal master's awarded for partial completion of doctoral program. *Degree requirements:* For master's, thesis or alternative; for doctorate, thesis/dissertation. *Entrance requirements:* For master's, GRE, professional experience (restaurant, hotel, and institutional management); for doctorate, GRE General Test. Additional exam requirements/recommendations for international students: Required—TOEFL (minimum score 550 paper-based; 79 iBT). *Application deadline:* For fall admission, 6/1 priority date for domestic students, 1/15 priority date for international students; for spring admission, 9/1 priority date for domestic students, 6/15 priority date for international students. Applications are processed on a rolling basis. Application fee: $60. Electronic applications accepted. *Expenses:* Tuition, state resident: full-time $6062; part-time $252.57 per credit hour. Tuition, nonresident: full-time $14,558; part-time $606.57 per credit hour. *Required fees:* $2655; $35 per credit hour. $907.50 per semester. Tuition and fees vary according to course load. *Financial support:* In 2013–14, 80 students received support, including 61 fellowships (averaging $2,868 per year), 11 research assistantships (averaging $5,042 per year), 43 teaching assistantships (averaging $5,073 per year). Financial award application deadline: 4/15; financial award applicants required to submit FAFSA. *Faculty research:* Selenium, obesity prevention, wine marketing, food safety, cross-border retailing. *Total annual research expenditures:* $305,963. *Unit head:* Dr. Shane Blum, Chair, 806-742-3068 Ext. 253, Fax: 806-742-3042, E-mail: shane.blum@ttu.edu. *Application contact:* Dr. Debra Reed, Graduate Advisor, Nutritional Sciences, 806-742-3068 Ext. 251, Fax: 806-742-3042, E-mail: debra.reed@ttu.edu.
Website: http://www.depts.ttu.edu/hs/nhr

Texas Woman's University, Graduate School, College of Health Sciences, Department of Nutrition and Food Sciences, Program in Exercise and Sports Nutrition, Denton, TX 76201. Offers MS. Part-time programs available. *Students:* 8 full-time (6 women), 2 part-time (both women); includes 4 minority (1 Black or African American, non-Hispanic/Latino; 1 Asian, non-Hispanic/Latino; 2 Hispanic/Latino). Average age 27. 2 applicants, 50% accepted, 1 enrolled. In 2013, 3 master's awarded. *Degree requirements:* For master's, comprehensive exam, thesis or alternative. *Entrance requirements:* For master's, GRE General Test (preferred minimum score 153 [500 old version] Verbal, 140 [400 old version] Quantitative), 9 hours each of chemistry, nutrition, and kinesiology; 3 hours of human physiology; minimum GPA of 3.0 in last 60 hours; resume; 2 letters of recommendation. Additional exam requirements/recommendations for international students: Required—TOEFL (minimum score 550 paper-based; 79 iBT). *Application deadline:* For fall admission, 7/1 priority date for domestic students, 3/1 for international students; for spring admission, 11/1 priority date for domestic students, 7/1 for international students. Applications are processed on a rolling basis. Application fee: $50 ($75 for international students). Electronic applications accepted. *Expenses:* Tuition, state resident: full-time $4182; part-time $233.32 per credit hour. Tuition, nonresident: full-time $10,716; part-time $595.32 per credit hour. *Financial support:* In 2013–14, 8 students received support, including 6 research assistantships (averaging $11,520 per year), teaching assistantships (averaging $11,520 per year); career-related internships or fieldwork, Federal Work-Study, institutionally sponsored loans, scholarships/grants, traineeships, health care benefits, and unspecified assistantships also available. Support available to part-time students. Financial award application deadline: 3/1; financial award applicants required to submit FAFSA. *Faculty research:* Metabolism of lipoproteins, bone metabolism, osteoporosis, adult and childhood obesity. *Unit head:* Dr. Gay James, Interim Program Director, 940-898-2636, Fax: 940-898-2634, E-mail: nutrfdsci@twu.edu. *Application contact:* Dr. Samuel Wheeler, Assistant Director of Admissions, 940-898-3188, Fax: 940-898-3081, E-mail: wheelersr@twu.edu.
Website: http://www.twu.edu/nutrition-food-sciences/

Tufts University, The Gerald J. and Dorothy R. Friedman School of Nutrition Science and Policy, Boston, MA 02111. Offers agriculture, food and environment (MS, PhD); biochemical and molecular nutrition (PhD); dietetic internship (MS); food policy and applied nutrition (MS, PhD); humanitarian assistance (MAHA); nutrition (MS, PhD); nutrition communication (MS); nutritional epidemiology (MS, PhD). Part-time programs available. *Degree requirements:* For doctorate, comprehensive exam, thesis/dissertation. *Entrance requirements:* For master's and doctorate, GRE General Test. Additional exam requirements/recommendations for international students: Required—TOEFL. Electronic applications accepted. *Expenses:* Contact institution. *Faculty research:* Nutritional biochemistry and metabolism, cell and molecular biochemistry, epidemiology, policy/planning, applied nutrition.

Tulane University, School of Public Health and Tropical Medicine, Department of Community Health Sciences, Program in Nutrition, New Orleans, LA 70118-5669. Offers MPH. *Degree requirements:* For master's, comprehensive exam. *Entrance requirements:* For master's, GRE General Test. Additional exam requirements/recommendations for international students: Required—TOEFL.

Tuskegee University, Graduate Programs, College of Agriculture, Environment and Nutrition Sciences, Department of Food and Nutritional Sciences, Tuskegee, AL 36088. Offers MS. *Degree requirements:* For master's, thesis. *Entrance requirements:* For master's, GRE General Test. Additional exam requirements/recommendations for international students: Required—TOEFL (minimum score 500 paper-based). *Application deadline:* For fall admission, 7/15 for domestic students. Applications are processed on a rolling basis. Application fee: $25 ($35 for international students). *Financial support:* Application deadline: 4/15. *Unit head:* Dr. Ralphenia Pace, Head, 334-727-8162. *Application contact:* Dr. Cynthia Sellers-Simon, Vice President for Student Affairs and Enrollment Management, 334-724-4746, Fax: 334-727-5750, E-mail: sellersc@mytu.tuskegee.edu.
Website: http://www.tuskegee.edu/academics/colleges/caens/food_nutritional_sci.aspx

Université de Moncton, School of Food Science, Nutrition and Family Studies, Moncton, NB E1A 3E9, Canada. Offers foods/nutrition (M Sc). Part-time programs available. *Degree requirements:* For master's, one foreign language, thesis. *Entrance requirements:* For master's, previous course work in statistics. Electronic applications accepted. *Faculty research:* Clinic nutrition (anemia, elderly, osteoporosis), applied nutrition, metabolic activities of lactic bacteria, solubility of low density lipoproteins, bile acids.

Université de Montréal, Faculty of Medicine, Department of Nutrition, Montréal, QC H3C 3J7, Canada. Offers M Sc, PhD, DESS. Terminal master's awarded for partial completion of doctoral program. *Degree requirements:* For master's, thesis; for doctorate, thesis/dissertation, general exam. *Entrance requirements:* For master's, MD, B Sc in nutrition or equivalent, proficiency in French; for doctorate, M Sc in nutrition or equivalent, proficiency in French. Electronic applications accepted. *Faculty research:* Nutritional aspects of diabetes, obesity, anorexia nervosa, lipid metabolism, hepatic function.

Université Laval, Faculty of Agricultural and Food Sciences, Department of Food Sciences and Nutrition, Programs in Nutrition, Québec, QC G1K 7P4, Canada. Offers M Sc, PhD. Terminal master's awarded for partial completion of doctoral program. *Degree requirements:* For master's, thesis; for doctorate, comprehensive exam, thesis/dissertation. *Entrance requirements:* For master's and doctorate, knowledge of French and English. Electronic applications accepted.

University at Buffalo, the State University of New York, Graduate School, School of Public Health and Health Professions, Department of Exercise and Nutrition Sciences, Buffalo, NY 14260. Offers exercise science (MS, PhD); nutrition (MS, Advanced Certificate). Part-time programs available. *Faculty:* 11 full-time (2 women), 3 part-time/adjunct (2 women). *Students:* 72 full-time (45 women), 2 part-time (1 woman); includes 13 minority (2 Black or African American, non-Hispanic/Latino; 11 Asian, non-Hispanic/Latino), 17 international. Average age 24. 136 applicants, 45% accepted, 33 enrolled. In 2013, 35 master's, 3 doctorates, 17 other advanced degrees awarded. *Degree requirements:* For master's, comprehensive exam or thesis; for doctorate, comprehensive exam, thesis/dissertation. *Entrance requirements:* For master's, doctorate, and Advanced Certificate, GRE General Test, minimum GPA of 3.0. Additional exam requirements/recommendations for international students: Required—TOEFL (minimum score 550 paper-based; 79 iBT), IELTS (minimum score 6.5). *Application deadline:* For fall admission, 4/1 for domestic students, 3/1 for international students; for spring admission, 8/15 for international students. Applications are processed on a rolling basis. Application fee: $50. Electronic applications accepted. *Financial support:* In 2013–14, 14 students received support, including 1 research assistantship with full tuition reimbursement available (averaging $15,000 per year), 11 teaching assistantships with full and partial tuition reimbursements available (averaging $6,980 per year); tuition waivers (full) and Fulbright Scholarship also available. Financial award application deadline: 3/15; financial award applicants required to submit FAFSA. *Faculty research:* Cardiovascular disease-diet and exercise, respiratory control and muscle function, plasticity of connective and neural tissue, exercise nutrition, diet and cancer. *Unit head:* Dr. Gaspar Farkas, Interim Chair, 716-829-6756, Fax: 716-829-2428, E-mail: farkas@buffalo.edu. *Application contact:* Dr. John Wilson, Director of Graduate Studies, 716-829-5596, Fax: 716-829-2428, E-mail: phhpadv@buffalo.edu.
Website: http://sphhp.buffalo.edu/exercise-and-nutrition-sciences.html

The University of Akron, Graduate School, College of Health Professions, School of Nutrition and Dietetics, Akron, OH 44325. Offers MS. *Faculty:* 5 full-time (all women), 5 part-time/adjunct (all women). *Students:* 4 full-time (0 women), 1 part-time (0 women), 1 international. Average age 28. 6 applicants, 67% accepted, 3 enrolled. In 2013, 4

master's awarded. *Degree requirements:* For master's, comprehensive exam, thesis or project. *Entrance requirements:* For master's, GRE, minimum GPA of 2.75, three letters of recommendation, statement of purpose, resume. Additional exam requirements/ recommendations for international students: Required—TOEFL (minimum score 550 paper-based; 79 iBT). *Application deadline:* For fall admission, 3/1 for domestic and international students; for spring admission, 10/1 for domestic and international students. Application fee: $40 ($60 for international students). Electronic applications accepted. *Expenses:* Tuition, state resident: full-time $7430; part-time $412.80 per credit hour. Tuition, nonresident: full-time $12,722; part-time $706.80 per credit hour. *Required fees:* $53 per credit hour. $12 per semester. Tuition and fees vary according to course load and program. *Financial support:* In 2013–14, 1 teaching assistantship with full tuition reimbursement was awarded. *Unit head:* Dr. Sandra Hudak, Director, 330-972-6043, E-mail: slhudak@uakron.edu. *Application contact:* Dr. Deborah Marino, Program Coordinator, 330-972-6322, E-mail: debora7@uakron.edu.
Website: http://www.uakron.edu/nutritiondietetics/index.dot

The University of Alabama, Graduate School, College of Human Environmental Sciences, Department of Human Nutrition and Hospitality Management, Tuscaloosa, AL 35487. Offers MSHES. Part-time programs available. Postbaccalaureate distance learning degree programs offered (no on-campus study). *Faculty:* 11 full-time (10 women). *Students:* 14 full-time (all women), 70 part-time (68 women); includes 8 minority (2 Black or African American, non-Hispanic/Latino; 1 Asian, non-Hispanic/ Latino; 5 Hispanic/Latino), 1 international. Average age 31. 68 applicants, 54% accepted, 28 enrolled. In 2013, 36 master's awarded. *Degree requirements:* For master's, comprehensive exam, thesis optional. *Entrance requirements:* For master's, minimum GPA of 3.0. Additional exam requirements/recommendations for international students: Required—TOEFL, IELTS. *Application deadline:* For fall admission, 7/1 for domestic students; for spring admission, 11/1 for domestic students. Applications are processed on a rolling basis. Application fee: $50 ($60 for international students). Electronic applications accepted. *Expenses:* Tuition, state resident: full-time $9450. Tuition, nonresident: full-time $23,950. *Financial support:* In 2013–14, 4 students received support, including 2 research assistantships (averaging $8,100 per year), 4 teaching assistantships (averaging $8,100 per year); career-related internships or fieldwork also available. Financial award application deadline: 3/15. *Faculty research:* Maternal and child nutrition, childhood obesity, community nutrition interventions, geriatric nutrition, family eating patterns, food chemistry, phytochemicals, dietary antioxidants. *Unit head:* Dr. Mary K. Meyer, Chair/Professor, 205-348-6150, Fax: 205-348-3789, E-mail: mkmeyer@ches.ua.edu. *Application contact:* Patrick D. Fuller, Admissions Officer, 205-348-5923, Fax: 205-348-0400, E-mail: patrick.d.fuller@ua.edu.
Website: http://www.ches.ua.edu/

The University of Alabama at Birmingham, School of Health Professions, Program in Nutrition Sciences, Birmingham, AL 35294. Offers clinical nutrition (MS); nutrition sciences (PhD). *Degree requirements:* For doctorate, thesis/dissertation. *Entrance requirements:* For doctorate, GRE General Test. *Faculty research:* Energy metabolism, obesity, body composition, cancer prevention, bone metabolism.

University of Alaska Fairbanks, School of Fisheries and Ocean Sciences, Fairbanks, AK 99775-7220. Offers fisheries (MS, PhD); marine sciences and limnology (MS, PhD), including marine biology, oceanography (PhD); seafood science and nutrition (MS, PhD). Part-time programs available. *Faculty:* 61 full-time (27 women), 4 part-time/ adjunct (1 woman). *Students:* 86 full-time (54 women), 41 part-time (23 women); includes 15 minority (4 Asian, non-Hispanic/Latino; 10 Hispanic/Latino; 1 Two or more races, non-Hispanic/Latino), 7 international. Average age 30. 58 applicants, 26% accepted, 15 enrolled. In 2013, 16 master's, 6 doctorates awarded. Terminal master's awarded for partial completion of doctoral program. *Degree requirements:* For master's, comprehensive exam, thesis or alternative; for doctorate, comprehensive exam, thesis/ dissertation, oral defense. *Entrance requirements:* For master's and doctorate, GRE General Test. Additional exam requirements/recommendations for international students: Required—TOEFL (minimum score 550 paper-based; 80 iBT). *Application deadline:* For fall admission, 6/1 for domestic students, 3/1 for international students; for spring admission, 10/15 for domestic students, 9/1 for international students. Applications are processed on a rolling basis. Application fee: $60. Electronic applications accepted. *Expenses:* Tuition, state resident: full-time $7254; part-time $403 per credit. Tuition, nonresident: full-time $14,814; part-time $823 per credit. Tuition and fees vary according to course level, course load and reciprocity agreements. *Financial support:* In 2013–14, 51 research assistantships with tuition reimbursements (averaging $13,209 per year), 13 teaching assistantships with tuition reimbursements (averaging $9,005 per year) were awarded; fellowships with tuition reimbursements, career-related internships or fieldwork, Federal Work-Study, scholarships/grants, health care benefits, and unspecified assistantships also available. Support available to part-time students. Financial award application deadline: 2/15; financial award applicants required to submit FAFSA. *Faculty research:* Marine mammals, hydrology, sea ice, harmful algal blooms, polar ecology. *Total annual research expenditures:* $18.7 million. *Unit head:* Michael Castellini, Dean, 907-474-7824, Fax: 907-474-7204, E-mail: info@sfos.uaf.edu. *Application contact:* Christina Neumann, Academic Manager, 907-474-7289, Fax: 907-474-5863, E-mail: clneumann@alaska.edu.
Website: http://www.sfos.uaf.edu/

The University of Arizona, College of Agriculture and Life Sciences, Department of Nutritional Sciences, Tucson, AZ 85721. Offers MS, PhD. *Faculty:* 3 full-time (2 women), 3 part-time/adjunct (all women). *Students:* 11 full-time (10 women); includes 2 minority (both Two or more races, non-Hispanic/Latino). Average age 28. 21 applicants, 33% accepted, 3 enrolled. In 2013, 4 master's, 5 doctorates awarded. *Entrance requirements:* For master's, GRE, minimum GPA of 3.0, 2 letters of recommendation; for doctorate, GRE, minimum GPA of 3.0, 2 letters of recommendation, statement of purpose. Additional exam requirements/recommendations for international students: Required—TOEFL (minimum score 550 paper-based; 79 iBT). *Application deadline:* For fall admission, 12/15 for domestic and international students. Applications are processed on a rolling basis. Application fee: $75. Electronic applications accepted. *Expenses:* Tuition, state resident: full-time $11,526. Tuition, nonresident: full-time $27,398. *Financial support:* In 2013–14, 1 research assistantship with full and partial tuition reimbursement (averaging $20,185 per year), 6 teaching assistantships with full and partial tuition reimbursements (averaging $17,441 per year) were awarded; fellowships, scholarships/grants, health care benefits, tuition waivers (full and partial), and unspecified assistantships also available. *Faculty research:* Bioactive compounds, nutrients and lifestyle: relationships to cancer; metabolic and behavior factors influencing body composition; diabetes, obesity, musculoskeletal and cardiovascular diseases. *Total annual research expenditures:* $3.3 million. *Unit head:* Dr. Scott Going, Department Head, 520-621-4705, Fax: 520-621-9446, E-mail: going@email.arizona.edu. *Application contact:* Nancy Driscoll, Information Contact, 520-626-0970, Fax: 520-621-9446, E-mail: nancya@email.arizona.edu.

University of Arkansas for Medical Sciences, Graduate School, Little Rock, AR 72205. Offers biochemistry and molecular biology (MS, PhD); bioinformatics (MS, PhD); cellular physiology and molecular biophysics (MS, PhD); clinical nutrition (MS); interdisciplinary biomedical sciences (MS, PhD, Certificate); interdisciplinary toxicology (MS); microbiology and immunology (PhD); neurobiology and developmental sciences (PhD); pharmacology (PhD); MD/PhD. Bioinformatics programs hosted jointly with the University of Arkansas at Little Rock. Part-time programs available. *Faculty:* 397 full-time (205 women). *Students:* 196 full-time (126 women), 117 part-time (87 women); includes 65 minority (38 Black or African American, non-Hispanic/Latino; 1 American Indian or Alaska Native, non-Hispanic/Latino; 21 Asian, non-Hispanic/Latino; 4 Hispanic/Latino; 1 Two or more races, non-Hispanic/Latino), 57 international. 455 applicants, 27% accepted, 89 enrolled. In 2013, 41 master's, 18 doctorates, 28 other advanced degrees awarded. Terminal master's awarded for partial completion of doctoral program. *Degree requirements:* For master's, comprehensive exam (for some programs), thesis (for some programs); for doctorate, thesis/dissertation. *Entrance requirements:* For master's and doctorate, GRE. Additional exam requirements/recommendations for international students: Required—TOEFL. *Application deadline:* Applications are processed on a rolling basis. Application fee: $0. Electronic applications accepted. *Expenses:* Contact institution. *Financial support:* In 2013–14, 120 research assistantships (averaging $24,000 per year) were awarded; career-related internships or fieldwork, Federal Work-Study, and traineeships also available. Support available to part-time students. Financial award applicants required to submit FAFSA. *Unit head:* Dr. Robert E. McGehee, Jr., Dean, 501-686-5454. *Application contact:* Dr. Kristen Sterba, Assistant Dean, Office of Graduate Student Recruiting and Retention, 501-526-7396, E-mail: kmsterba@uams.edu.
Website: http://www.uams.edu/gradschool/

University of Bridgeport, Nutrition Institute, Bridgeport, CT 06604. Offers human nutrition (MS). Part-time and evening/weekend programs available. Postbaccalaureate distance learning degree programs offered (no on-campus study). *Faculty:* 2 full-time (0 women), 12 part-time/adjunct (6 women). *Students:* 247 part-time (197 women); includes 41 minority (16 Black or African American, non-Hispanic/Latino; 9 Asian, non-Hispanic/Latino; 12 Hispanic/Latino; 4 Two or more races, non-Hispanic/Latino), 4 international. Average age 37. 265 applicants, 69% accepted, 42 enrolled. In 2013, 114 master's awarded. *Degree requirements:* For master's, thesis, research project. *Entrance requirements:* For master's, previous course work in anatomy, biochemistry, organic chemistry, or physiology. Additional exam requirements/recommendations for international students: Recommended—TOEFL (minimum score 550 paper-based; 80 iBT), IELTS (minimum score 6.5). *Application deadline:* For fall admission, 8/1 priority date for domestic and international students; for spring admission, 12/1 priority date for domestic and international students. Applications are processed on a rolling basis. Application fee: $50. Electronic applications accepted. *Expenses:* Contact institution. *Financial support:* In 2013–14, 33 students received support. Available to part-time students. Application deadline: 6/1; applicants required to submit FAFSA. *Unit head:* Dr. David M. Brady, Director, 203-576-4667, Fax: 203-576-4591, E-mail: dbrady@bridgeport.edu. *Application contact:* Leanne Proctor, Director of Health Science Admission, 203-576-4352, Fax: 203-576-4941, E-mail: nutrition@bridgeport.edu.

The University of British Columbia, Faculty of Land and Food Systems, Human Nutrition Program, Vancouver, BC V6T 1Z1, Canada. Offers M Sc, PhD. Part-time programs available. *Faculty:* 7 full-time (5 women), 3 part-time/adjunct (all women). *Students:* 26 full-time (23 women). Average age 28. 35 applicants, 14% accepted, 4 enrolled. In 2013, 6 master's awarded. Terminal master's awarded for partial completion of doctoral program. *Degree requirements:* For master's, thesis; for doctorate, comprehensive exam, thesis/dissertation. *Entrance requirements:* Additional exam requirements/recommendations for international students: Required—TOEFL (minimum score 577 paper-based; 90 iBT), IELTS (minimum score 6.5). *Application deadline:* For fall admission, 1/1 for domestic and international students; for winter admission, 6/1 for domestic and international students; for spring admission, 9/1 for domestic and international students. Applications are processed on a rolling basis. Application fee: $95 Canadian dollars ($153 Canadian dollars for international students). Electronic applications accepted. *Expenses: Tuition, area resident:* Full-time $8000 Canadian dollars. *Financial support:* Fellowships, research assistantships, teaching assistantships, institutionally sponsored loans, scholarships/grants, and unspecified assistantships available. *Faculty research:* Basic nutrition, clinical nutrition, community nutrition, women's health, pediatric nutrition. *Total annual research expenditures:* $655,645. *Unit head:* Dr. Tim Green, Graduate Advisor, 604-822-0421, E-mail: tim.green@ubc.ca. *Application contact:* Lia Maria Dragan, Graduate Programs Assistant, 604-822-8373, Fax: 604-822-4400, E-mail: gradapp@interchange.ubc.ca.
Website: http://www.landfood.ubc.ca

University of California, Berkeley, Graduate Division, College of Natural Resources, Group in Molecular and Biochemical Nutrition, Berkeley, CA 94720-1500. Offers PhD. *Degree requirements:* For doctorate, thesis/dissertation, qualifying exam. *Entrance requirements:* For doctorate, GRE General Test, minimum GPA of 3.0, 3 letters of recommendation. Additional exam requirements/recommendations for international students: Required—TOEFL. Electronic applications accepted. *Faculty research:* Regulation of metabolism; nutritional genomics and nutrient-gene interactions; transport, metabolism and function of minerals; carcinogenesis and dietary anti-carcinogens.

University of California, Davis, Graduate Studies, Graduate Group in Nutritional Biology, Davis, CA 95616. Offers MS, PhD. *Degree requirements:* For master's, thesis; for doctorate, thesis/dissertation. *Entrance requirements:* For master's and doctorate, GRE General Test, minimum GPA of 3.0. Additional exam requirements/ recommendations for international students: Required—TOEFL (minimum score 550 paper-based). Electronic applications accepted. *Faculty research:* Human/animal nutrition.

University of California, Davis, Graduate Studies, Program in Maternal and Child Nutrition, Davis, CA 95616. Offers MAS. *Degree requirements:* For master's, comprehensive exam. *Entrance requirements:* Additional exam requirements/ recommendations for international students: Required—TOEFL (minimum score 550 paper-based).

University of Central Oklahoma, The Jackson College of Graduate Studies, College of Education and Professional Studies, Department of Human Environmental Sciences, Edmond, OK 73034-5209. Offers family and child studies (MS), including family life education, infant/child specialist, marriage and family therapy; nutrition-food management (MS). Part-time programs available. *Faculty:* 4 full-time (3 women), 12 part-time/adjunct (9 women). *Students:* 42 full-time (36 women), 96 part-time (92 women); includes 50 minority (34 Black or African American, non-Hispanic/Latino; 4 American Indian or Alaska Native, non-Hispanic/Latino; 2 Asian, non-Hispanic/Latino; 5 Hispanic/Latino; 5 Two or more races, non-Hispanic/Latino), 9 international. Average age 32. 60 applicants, 68% accepted, 29 enrolled. In 2013, 36 master's awarded. *Degree requirements:* For master's, comprehensive exam (for some programs), thesis (for some programs). *Entrance requirements:* For master's, GRE, essay, physical, CPR and First Aid training. Additional exam requirements/recommendations for international students: Required—TOEFL (minimum score 550 paper-based; 79 iBT), IELTS (minimum score 6.5). *Application deadline:* For fall admission, 7/1 for international students; for spring admission, 11/1 for international students. Applications are processed on a rolling basis. Application fee: $50. Electronic applications accepted. *Expenses:* Tuition, state resident: full-time $4137; part-time $206.85 per credit hour. Tuition, nonresident: full-time $10,359; part-time $517.95 per credit hour. *Required fees:* $481. Tuition and fees vary according to course load and program. *Financial support:* In

2013–14, 11 students received support, including 3 research assistantships with partial tuition reimbursements available (averaging $2,958 per year); teaching assistantships with partial tuition reimbursements available, career-related internships or fieldwork, scholarships/grants, tuition waivers (partial), and unspecified assistantships also available. Financial award application deadline: 3/31; financial award applicants required to submit FAFSA. *Unit head:* Dr. Kaye Sears, Chair, 405-974-5786, Fax: 405-974-3851, E-mail: ksears@uco.edu. *Application contact:* Dr. Richard Bernard, Dean, Graduate College, 405-974-3493, Fax: 405-974-3852, E-mail: gradcoll@uco.edu.

University of Chicago, Division of Biological Sciences, Biomedical Sciences Cluster: Cancer Biology, Immunology, Molecular Metabolism and Nutrition, Pathology, and Microbiology, Committee on Molecular Metabolism and Nutrition, Chicago, IL 60637-1513. Offers PhD. *Degree requirements:* For doctorate, thesis/dissertation, ethics class, 2 teaching assistantships. *Entrance requirements:* For doctorate, GRE General Test. Additional exam requirements/recommendations for international students: Required—TOEFL (minimum score 600 paper-based; 104 iBT), IELTS (minimum score 7). Electronic applications accepted. *Faculty research:* Regulation of lipoprotein metabolism, cellular vitamin metabolism, obesity and body composition, adipocyte differentiation.

University of Cincinnati, Graduate School, College of Allied Health Sciences, Department of Nutritional Sciences, Cincinnati, OH 45221. Offers MS. Part-time programs available. *Degree requirements:* For master's, thesis. *Entrance requirements:* For master's, GRE General Test. Additional exam requirements/recommendations for international students: Required—TOEFL (minimum score 550 paper-based). Electronic applications accepted. *Faculty research:* Phytochemicals-osteoarthritis, pediatric hypertension and hypercholesterol, cancer prevention/Type II diabetes.

University of Colorado Colorado Springs, College of Letters, Arts and Sciences, Master of Sciences Program, Colorado Springs, CO 80933-7150. Offers biology (M Sc); chemistry (M Sc); health promotion (M Sc); mathematics (M Sc); physics (M Sc); sports medicine (M Sc), including strength and conditioning; sports nutrition (M Sc). Part-time programs available. *Students:* 50 full-time (36 women), 35 part-time (23 women); includes 12 minority (1 Black or African American, non-Hispanic/Latino; 1 American Indian or Alaska Native, non-Hispanic/Latino; 3 Asian, non-Hispanic/Latino; 5 Hispanic/Latino; 2 Two or more races, non-Hispanic/Latino), 11 international. Average age 29. 122 applicants, 47% accepted, 36 enrolled. In 2013, 37 master's awarded. *Degree requirements:* For master's, thesis or alternative. *Entrance requirements:* For master's, minimum GPA of 2.75. Additional exam requirements/recommendations for international students: Required—TOEFL (minimum score 525 paper-based). *Application deadline:* For fall admission, 3/1 priority date for domestic students; for spring admission, 12/1 for domestic students. Applications are processed on a rolling basis. Application fee: $60 ($75 for international students). Electronic applications accepted. *Expenses:* Contact institution. *Financial support:* In 2013–14, 21 students received support, including 21 fellowships (averaging $2,600 per year); research assistantships, teaching assistantships, career-related internships or fieldwork, Federal Work-Study, and scholarships/grants also available. Support available to part-time students. Financial award application deadline: 3/1; financial award applicants required to submit FAFSA. *Faculty research:* Biomechanics and physiology of elite athletic training, genetic engineering in yeast and bacteria including phage display and DNA repair, immunology and cell biology, synthetic organic chemistry. *Total annual research expenditures:* $38,075. *Unit head:* Dr. Peter A. Braza, Dean, 719-255-4550, Fax: 719-255-4200, E-mail: pbraza@uccs.edu. *Application contact:* Taryn Bailey, Graduate Recruitment Specialist, 719-255-3702, Fax: 719-255-3037, E-mail: gradinfo@uccs.edu.

University of Connecticut, Graduate School, College of Agriculture and Natural Resources, Department of Nutritional Sciences, Storrs, CT 06269. Offers MS, PhD. Terminal master's awarded for partial completion of doctoral program. *Degree requirements:* For master's, comprehensive exam, thesis; for doctorate, thesis/dissertation. *Entrance requirements:* For master's and doctorate, GRE General Test. Additional exam requirements/recommendations for international students: Required—TOEFL (minimum score 550 paper-based). Electronic applications accepted.

University of Delaware, College of Health Sciences, Department of Behavioral Health and Nutrition, Newark, DE 19716. Offers health promotion (MS); human nutrition (MS). Part-time programs available. *Degree requirements:* For master's, thesis. *Entrance requirements:* For master's, GRE General Test, interview, minimum GPA of 3.0. Additional exam requirements/recommendations for international students: Required—TOEFL (minimum score 550 paper-based). Electronic applications accepted. *Faculty research:* Sport biomechanics, rehabilitation biomechanics, vascular dynamics.

University of Florida, Graduate School, College of Agricultural and Life Sciences, Department of Food Science and Human Nutrition, Gainesville, FL 32611. Offers food science (PhD); food science and human nutrition (MS); nutritional sciences (MS, PhD). *Faculty:* 25 full-time (12 women), 4 part-time/adjunct (3 women). *Students:* 45 full-time (36 women), 17 part-time (8 women); includes 6 minority (2 Black or African American, non-Hispanic/Latino; 2 Asian, non-Hispanic/Latino; 2 Hispanic/Latino), 28 international. Average age 27. 193 applicants, 15% accepted, 21 enrolled. In 2013, 21 master's, 13 doctorates awarded. *Degree requirements:* For master's, thesis optional; for doctorate, thesis/dissertation. *Entrance requirements:* For master's and doctorate, GRE General Test, minimum GPA of 3.0. Additional exam requirements/recommendations for international students: Required—TOEFL. *Application deadline:* For fall admission, 6/1 priority date for domestic students. Applications are processed on a rolling basis. Application fee: $30. Electronic applications accepted. *Expenses:* Tuition, state resident: full-time $12,640. Tuition, nonresident: full-time $30,000. *Financial support:* In 2013–14, 45 students received support, including 1 fellowship (averaging $12,000 per year), 28 research assistantships (averaging $16,005 per year), 21 teaching assistantships (averaging $13,490 per year); career-related internships or fieldwork also available. Financial award applicants required to submit FAFSA. *Faculty research:* Pesticide research, nutritional biochemistry and microbiology, food safety and toxicology assessment and dietetics, food chemistry. *Unit head:* Susan S. Percival, PhD, Chair and Professor, 352-392-1991 Ext. 202, Fax: 352-392-1991, E-mail: percival@ufl.edu.
Website: http://fshn.ifas.ufl.edu/

University of Georgia, College of Family and Consumer Sciences, Department of Foods and Nutrition, Athens, GA 30602. Offers MFCS, MS, PhD. *Degree requirements:* For master's, thesis (MS); for doctorate, thesis/dissertation. *Entrance requirements:* For master's, GRE General Test, minimum GPA of 3.0, course work in biochemistry and physiology; for doctorate, GRE General Test, master's degree, minimum GPA of 3.0. Electronic applications accepted.

University of Guelph, Graduate Studies, College of Biological Science, Department of Human Health and Nutritional Sciences, Guelph, ON N1G 2W1, Canada. Offers nutritional sciences (M Sc, PhD). Part-time programs available. *Degree requirements:* For master's, thesis (for some programs); for doctorate, comprehensive exam, thesis/dissertation. *Entrance requirements:* For master's, minimum B-average during previous 2 years of coursework; for doctorate, minimum A-average. Additional exam requirements/recommendations for international students: Required—TOEFL (minimum score 550 paper-based). Electronic applications accepted. *Faculty research:* Nutrition and biochemistry, exercise metabolism and physiology, toxicology, gene expression, biomechanics and ergonomics.

University of Guelph, Graduate Studies, College of Social and Applied Human Sciences, Department of Family Relations and Applied Nutrition, Guelph, ON N1G 2W1, Canada. Offers applied nutrition (MAN); family relations and human development (M Sc, PhD), including applied human nutrition, couple and family therapy (M Sc), family relations and human development. *Accreditation:* AAMFT/COAMFTE (one or more programs are accredited). Part-time programs available. *Degree requirements:* For master's, thesis (for some programs); for doctorate, comprehensive exam, thesis/dissertation. *Entrance requirements:* For master's, minimum B+ average; for doctorate, master's degree in family relations and human development or related field with a minimum B+ average or master's degree in applied human nutrition. Additional exam requirements/recommendations for international students: Required—TOEFL (minimum score 600 paper-based). Electronic applications accepted. *Faculty research:* Child and adolescent development, social gerontology, family roles and relations, couple and family therapy, applied human nutrition.

University of Hawaii at Manoa, Graduate Division, College of Tropical Agriculture and Human Resources, Department of Human Nutrition, Food and Animal Sciences, Program in Nutrition, Honolulu, HI 96822. Offers PhD. Part-time programs available. *Degree requirements:* For doctorate, comprehensive exam, thesis/dissertation. *Entrance requirements:* For doctorate, GRE General Test. Additional exam requirements/recommendations for international students: Required—TOEFL (minimum score 580 paper-based; 92 iBT), IELTS (minimum score 5).

University of Hawaii at Manoa, Graduate Division, College of Tropical Agriculture and Human Resources, Department of Human Nutrition, Food and Animal Sciences, Program in Nutritional Sciences, Honolulu, HI 96822. Offers MS, PhD. Part-time programs available. *Degree requirements:* For master's, thesis optional; for doctorate, comprehensive exam, thesis/dissertation. *Entrance requirements:* For master's and doctorate, GRE General Test. Additional exam requirements/recommendations for international students: Required—TOEFL (minimum score 580 paper-based; 92 iBT), IELTS (minimum score 5). *Faculty research:* Nutritional biochemistry, human nutrition, nutrition education, international nutrition, nutritional epidemiology.

University of Houston, College of Liberal Arts and Social Sciences, Department of Health and Human Performance, Houston, TX 77204. Offers exercise science (MS); human nutrition (MS); human space exploration sciences (MS); kinesiology (PhD); physical education (M Ed). *Accreditation:* NCATE (one or more programs are accredited). Part-time and evening/weekend programs available. *Degree requirements:* For master's, comprehensive exam (for some programs), thesis (for some programs); for doctorate, comprehensive exam, thesis/dissertation, qualifying exam, candidacy paper. *Entrance requirements:* For master's, GRE (minimum 35th percentile on each section), minimum cumulative GPA of 3.0; for doctorate, GRE (minimum 35th percentile on each section), minimum cumulative GPA of 3.3. Additional exam requirements/recommendations for international students: Required—TOEFL (minimum score 550 paper-based; 79 iBT). Electronic applications accepted. *Faculty research:* Biomechanics, exercise physiology, obesity, nutrition, space exploration science.

University of Illinois at Chicago, Graduate College, College of Applied Health Sciences, Program in Nutrition, Chicago, IL 60607-7128. Offers MS, PhD. *Accreditation:* AND. *Students:* 60 full-time (57 women), 7 part-time (6 women); includes 15 minority (5 Black or African American, non-Hispanic/Latino; 4 Asian, non-Hispanic/Latino; 3 Hispanic/Latino; 3 Two or more races, non-Hispanic/Latino), 5 international. Average age 30. 85 applicants, 38% accepted, 20 enrolled. In 2013, 19 master's awarded. *Degree requirements:* For master's, thesis; for doctorate, thesis/dissertation. *Entrance requirements:* For master's and doctorate, GRE General Test, minimum GPA of 2.75. Additional exam requirements/recommendations for international students: Required—TOEFL. *Application deadline:* For fall admission, 12/13 priority date for domestic and international students. Application fee: $40 ($50 for international students). Electronic applications accepted. *Expenses:* Tuition, state resident: full-time $11,066; part-time $3689 per term. Tuition, nonresident: full-time $23,064; part-time $7688 per term. *Required fees:* $3004; $1190 per term. Tuition and fees vary according to course level and program. *Financial support:* Fellowships with full tuition reimbursements, research assistantships with full tuition reimbursements, teaching assistantships with full tuition reimbursements, career-related internships or fieldwork, Federal Work-Study, institutionally sponsored loans, traineeships, tuition waivers (full), and unspecified assistantships available. Financial award application deadline: 3/1; financial award applicants required to submit FAFSA. *Faculty research:* Nutrition for the elderly, inborn errors of metabolism, nutrition and cancer, lipid metabolism, dietary fat markers. *Total annual research expenditures:* $4 million. *Unit head:* Charles B. Walter, Department Head, 312-413-0319, Fax: 312-355-1713, E-mail: cbwalter@uic.edu. *Application contact:* Receptionist, 312-413-2550, E-mail: gradcoll@uic.edu.
Website: http://www.ahs.uic.edu/kn/academics/msncp/

University of Illinois at Urbana–Champaign, Graduate College, College of Agricultural, Consumer and Environmental Sciences, Department of Food Science and Human Nutrition, Champaign, IL 61820. Offers food science (MS); food science and human nutrition (MS, PhD), including professional science (MS); human nutrition (MS). Part-time programs available. Postbaccalaureate distance learning degree programs offered (no on-campus study). *Students:* 137 (95 women). Application fee: $75 ($90 for international students). *Unit head:* Sharon M. Nickols-Richardson, Head, 217-244-4498, Fax: 217-265-0925, E-mail: nickrich@illinois.edu. *Application contact:* Terri Cummings, Director of Student Services, 217-244-4405, Fax: 217-265-0925, E-mail: tcumming@illinois.edu.
Website: http://fshn.illinois.edu/

University of Illinois at Urbana–Champaign, Graduate College, College of Agricultural, Consumer and Environmental Sciences, Division of Nutritional Sciences, Champaign, IL 61820. Offers MS, PhD, PhD/MPH. *Students:* 41 (27 women). Application fee: $75 ($90 for international students). *Unit head:* Rodney W. Johnson, Director, 217-333-2118, Fax: 217-333-9368, E-mail: rwjohn@illinois.edu. *Application contact:* Jessica L. Hartke, Program Coordinator, 217-333-4177, Fax: 217-333-9368, E-mail: jessh@illinois.edu.
Website: http://nutrsci.illinois.edu/

The University of Kansas, University of Kansas Medical Center, School of Health Professions, Department of Dietetics and Nutrition, Lawrence, KS 66045. Offers dietetic internship (Graduate Certificate); dietetics and integrative medicine (Graduate Certificate); dietetics and nutrition (MS); medical nutrition science (PhD). Part-time programs available. Postbaccalaureate distance learning degree programs offered (no on-campus study). *Faculty:* 17. *Students:* 41 full-time (37 women), 17 part-time (16 women); includes 2 minority (both Asian, non-Hispanic/Latino), 3 international. Average age 28. 90 applicants, 28% accepted, 24 enrolled. In 2013, 21 master's, 1 doctorate, 16 other advanced degrees awarded. *Degree requirements:* For master's, thesis optional, oral exam; for doctorate, comprehensive exam, thesis/dissertation, oral exam. *Entrance requirements:* For master's, GRE, prerequisite courses in nutrition, biochemistry, and physiology; for doctorate, GRE; for Graduate Certificate, GRE, minimum cumulative GPA of 3.0. Additional exam requirements/recommendations for international students:

Required—TOEFL. *Application deadline:* For fall admission, 7/1 for domestic students, 6/1 for international students; for winter admission, 12/1 for domestic students, 11/1 for international students; for spring admission, 11/1 for domestic students, 10/1 for international students; for summer admission, 4/1 for domestic students, 3/1 for international students. Applications are processed on a rolling basis. Application fee: $60. Electronic applications accepted. *Financial support:* Fellowships, research assistantships with full tuition reimbursements, teaching assistantships with full tuition reimbursements, career-related internships or fieldwork, Federal Work-Study, institutionally sponsored loans, scholarships/grants, traineeships, tuition waivers, and unspecified assistantships available. Support available to part-time students. Financial award application deadline: 3/1; financial award applicants required to submit FAFSA. *Faculty research:* Obesity prevention and treatment, omega-3 fatty acids impact on infant development and immunity, vitamin D and bone metabolism in osteosarcoma cells, cancer prevention and recovery maternal diet intake and weight gain impact on infant body composition and development. *Total annual research expenditures:* $838,000. *Unit head:* Dr. Debra Kay Sullivan, Chairperson, 913-588-5357, Fax: 913-588-8946, E-mail: dsulliva@kumc.edu. *Application contact:* Dr. Heather Gibbs, Graduate Director, 913-945-9138.
Website: http://www.kumc.edu/school-of-health-professions/dietetics-and-nutrition.html

University of Kentucky, Graduate School, College of Agriculture, Food and Environment, Program in Hospitality and Dietetics Administration, Lexington, KY 40506-0032. Offers MS. *Degree requirements:* For master's, comprehensive exam, thesis optional. *Entrance requirements:* For master's, GRE General Test, minimum undergraduate GPA of 2.75. Additional exam requirements/recommendations for international students: Required—TOEFL (minimum score 550 paper-based). Electronic applications accepted.

University of Kentucky, Graduate School, Graduate Center for Nutritional Sciences, Lexington, KY 40506-0032. Offers MSNS, PhD. *Degree requirements:* For doctorate, comprehensive exam, thesis/dissertation. *Entrance requirements:* For master's, GRE General Test, minimum undergraduate GPA of 2.75; for doctorate, GRE General Test, minimum graduate GPA of 3.0. Additional exam requirements/recommendations for international students: Required—TOEFL (minimum score 550 paper-based). Electronic applications accepted. *Faculty research:* Nutrition and AIDS, nutrition and alcoholism, nutrition and cardiovascular disease, nutrition and cancer, nutrition and diabetes.

University of Maine, Graduate School, College of Natural Sciences, Forestry, and Agriculture, School of Food and Agriculture, Orono, ME 04469. Offers animal sciences (MPS, MS); food and nutrition sciences (PhD); food science and human nutrition (MS); foods and nutrition (CGS); horticulture (MS); plant, soil and environmental sciences (MS). Part-time programs available. *Faculty:* 31 full-time (13 women), 1 part-time/adjunct (0 women). *Students:* 45 full-time (30 women), 14 part-time (9 women); includes 3 minority (all American Indian or Alaska Native, non-Hispanic/Latino), 6 international. Average age 28. 78 applicants, 41% accepted, 16 enrolled. In 2013, 17 master's, 2 doctorates awarded. *Degree requirements:* For master's, thesis (for some programs); for doctorate, comprehensive exam, thesis/dissertation. *Entrance requirements:* For master's and doctorate, GRE General Test. Additional exam requirements/recommendations for international students: Required—TOEFL. *Application deadline:* For fall admission, 2/1 priority date for domestic students. Applications are processed on a rolling basis. Application fee: $65. Electronic applications accepted. *Expenses:* Tuition, state resident: full-time $7524. Tuition, nonresident: full-time $23,112. *Required fees:* $1970. *Financial support:* In 2013–14, 36 students received support, including 2 fellowships (averaging $14,600 per year), 18 research assistantships with full tuition reimbursements available (averaging $14,600 per year), 4 teaching assistantships with full tuition reimbursements available (averaging $14,600 per year); Federal Work-Study, institutionally sponsored loans, and tuition waivers (full and partial) also available. Financial award application deadline: 3/1. *Faculty research:* Soil organic matter, sustainable agriculture, crop ecology and management, horticulture, plant pathology, phytochemicals, nutrition education, analytical methods development, food processing, developing healthy foods, nutrients and cardiovascular disease, reproduction, nutrition, cattle, horses, aquaculture. *Unit head:* Dr. Sue Erich, Chair, 207-581-2947, Fax: 207-581-2770. *Application contact:* Scott G. Delcourt, Associate Dean of the Graduate School, 207-581-3291, Fax: 207-581-3232, E-mail: graduate@maine.edu.
Website: http://umaine.edu/foodandagriculture

University of Manitoba, Faculty of Graduate Studies, Faculty of Agricultural and Food Sciences, Department of Food Science, Winnipeg, MB R3T 2N2, Canada. Offers food and nutritional sciences (PhD); food science (M Sc); foods and nutrition (M Sc). *Degree requirements:* For master's, thesis.

University of Manitoba, Faculty of Graduate Studies, Faculty of Human Ecology, Department of Human Nutritional Sciences, Winnipeg, MB R3T 2N2, Canada. Offers M Sc. *Degree requirements:* For master's, thesis.

University of Maryland, College Park, Academic Affairs, College of Agriculture and Natural Resources, Department of Nutrition and Food Science, Program in Nutrition, College Park, MD 20742. Offers MS, PhD. *Students:* 26 full-time (21 women), 2 part-time (both women); includes 7 minority (2 Black or African American, non-Hispanic/Latino; 4 Asian, non-Hispanic/Latino; 1 Hispanic/Latino), 11 international. 26 applicants, 19% accepted, 5 enrolled. In 2013, 3 master's awarded. *Degree requirements:* For master's, thesis; for doctorate, comprehensive exam, thesis/dissertation, candidacy exam. *Entrance requirements:* For master's, GRE General Test, minimum GPA of 3.0, 3 letters of recommendation; for doctorate, GRE General Test, minimum GPA of 3.0. Additional exam requirements/recommendations for international students: Required—TOEFL. *Application deadline:* For fall admission, 12/15 for domestic and international students; for spring admission, 6/1 for domestic and international students. Applications are processed on a rolling basis. Application fee: $75. Electronic applications accepted. *Expenses:* Tuition, state resident: full-time $10,314; part-time $573 per credit hour. Tuition, nonresident: full-time $22,248; part-time $1236 per credit. *Required fees:* $1446; $403.15 per semester. Tuition and fees vary according to program. *Financial support:* In 2013–14, 3 fellowships with partial tuition reimbursements (averaging $10,050 per year), 3 research assistantships (averaging $15,367 per year), 13 teaching assistantships (averaging $15,646 per year) were awarded. Financial award applicants required to submit FAFSA. *Faculty research:* Nutrition education, carbohydrates and physical activity. *Unit head:* Dr. Robert Jackson, Acting Chair, 301-405-0773, Fax: 301-314-3313, E-mail: bojack@umd.edu. *Application contact:* Dr. Charles A. Caramello, Dean of Graduate School, 301-405-0358, Fax: 301-314-9305, E-mail: ccaramel@umd.edu.

University of Massachusetts Amherst, Graduate School, School of Public Health and Health Sciences, Department of Nutrition, Amherst, MA 01003. Offers community nutrition (MS); nutrition science (MS). Part-time and evening/weekend programs available. Postbaccalaureate distance learning degree programs offered (no on-campus study). *Faculty:* 15 full-time (9 women). *Students:* 11 full-time (10 women), 3 part-time (2 women); includes 1 minority (Two or more races, non-Hispanic/Latino), 5 international. Average age 27. 36 applicants, 19% accepted, 3 enrolled. In 2013, 2 master's awarded. Terminal master's awarded for partial completion of doctoral program. *Degree requirements:* For master's, thesis or alternative. *Entrance requirements:* For master's, GRE General Test. Additional exam requirements/recommendations for international students: Required—TOEFL (minimum score 550 paper-based; 80 iBT), IELTS (minimum score 6.5). *Application deadline:* For fall admission, 2/1 for domestic and international students; for spring admission, 10/1 for domestic and international students. Applications are processed on a rolling basis. Application fee: $75. Electronic applications accepted. *Financial support:* Fellowships with full and partial tuition reimbursements, research assistantships with full and partial tuition reimbursements, teaching assistantships with full and partial tuition reimbursements, career-related internships or fieldwork, Federal Work-Study, scholarships/grants, traineeships, health care benefits, tuition waivers (full and partial), and unspecified assistantships available. Support available to part-time students. Financial award application deadline: 2/1; financial award applicants required to submit FAFSA. *Unit head:* Dr. Elena T. Carbone, Graduate Program Director, 413-545-0740, Fax: 413-545-1074. *Application contact:* Lindsay DeSantis, Supervisor of Admissions, 413-545-0722, Fax: 413-577-0010, E-mail: gradadm@grad.umass.edu.
Website: http://www.umass.edu/sphhs/nutrition/

University of Massachusetts Amherst, Graduate School, School of Public Health and Health Sciences, Department of Public Health, Amherst, MA 01003. Offers biostatistics (MPH, MS, PhD); community health education (MPH, MS, PhD); environmental health sciences (MPH, MS, PhD); epidemiology (MPH, MS, PhD); health policy and management (MPH, MS, PhD); nutrition (MPH, PhD); public health practice (MPH); MPH/MPPA. *Accreditation:* CEPH (one or more programs are accredited). Part-time and evening/weekend programs available. Postbaccalaureate distance learning degree programs offered (no on-campus study). *Faculty:* 53 full-time (29 women). *Students:* 117 full-time (83 women), 271 part-time (213 women); includes 89 minority (34 Black or African American, non-Hispanic/Latino; 23 Asian, non-Hispanic/Latino; 25 Hispanic/Latino; 7 Two or more races, non-Hispanic/Latino), 45 international. Average age 36. 359 applicants, 69% accepted, 94 enrolled. In 2013, 120 master's, 1 doctorate awarded. Terminal master's awarded for partial completion of doctoral program. *Degree requirements:* For master's, thesis (for some programs); for doctorate, comprehensive exam, thesis/dissertation. *Entrance requirements:* For master's and doctorate, GRE General Test. Additional exam requirements/recommendations for international students: Required—TOEFL (minimum score 550 paper-based; 80 iBT), IELTS (minimum score 6.5). *Application deadline:* For fall admission, 2/1 for domestic and international students. Applications are processed on a rolling basis. Application fee: $75. Electronic applications accepted. *Financial support:* Fellowships with full and partial tuition reimbursements, research assistantships with full and partial tuition reimbursements, teaching assistantships with full and partial tuition reimbursements, career-related internships or fieldwork, Federal Work-Study, scholarships/grants, traineeships, health care benefits, tuition waivers (full and partial), and unspecified assistantships available. Support available to part-time students. Financial award application deadline: 2/1; financial award applicants required to submit FAFSA. *Unit head:* Dr. Paula Stamps, Graduate Program Director, 413-545-2861, Fax: 413-545-1645. *Application contact:* Lindsay DeSantis, Supervisor of Admissions, 413-545-0722, Fax: 413-577-0010, E-mail: gradadm@grad.umass.edu.
Website: http://www.umass.edu/sphhs/public_health/

University of Massachusetts Lowell, College of Health Sciences, Department of Clinical Laboratory and Nutritional Sciences, Lowell, MA 01854-2881. Offers clinical laboratory sciences (MS); clinical pathology (Graduate Certificate); nutritional sciences (Graduate Certificate); public health laboratory sciences (Graduate Certificate). *Accreditation:* NAACLS. Part-time programs available. Postbaccalaureate distance learning degree programs offered. *Degree requirements:* For master's, thesis optional. *Entrance requirements:* For master's, GRE General Test, minimum GPA of 3.0, letters of recommendation. *Faculty research:* Cardiovascular disease, lipoprotein metabolism, micronutrient evaluation, alcohol metabolism, mycobacterial drug resistance.

University of Memphis, Graduate School, College of Education, Department of Health and Sport Sciences, Memphis, TN 38152. Offers clinical nutrition (MS); exercise and sport science (MS); health promotion (MS); physical education teacher education (MS), including teacher education; sport and leisure commerce (MS). Part-time and evening/weekend programs available. *Faculty:* 22 full-time (8 women), 3 part-time/adjunct (2 women). *Students:* 83 full-time (51 women), 28 part-time (23 women); includes 37 minority (29 Black or African American, non-Hispanic/Latino; 6 Asian, non-Hispanic/Latino; 2 Two or more races, non-Hispanic/Latino), 7 international. Average age 27. 86 applicants, 67% accepted, 29 enrolled. In 2013, 35 master's awarded. *Degree requirements:* For master's, comprehensive exam, thesis. *Entrance requirements:* For master's, GRE General Test or GMAT (for sport and leisure commerce). *Application deadline:* For fall admission, 5/1 priority date for domestic students; for spring admission, 11/1 for domestic students. Applications are processed on a rolling basis. Application fee: $35 ($60 for international students). *Financial support:* In 2013–14, 59 students received support. Research assistantships with full tuition reimbursements available, teaching assistantships with full tuition reimbursements available, career-related internships or fieldwork, Federal Work-Study, scholarships/grants, tuition waivers (partial), and unspecified assistantships available. Financial award application deadline: 2/15; financial award applicants required to submit FAFSA. *Faculty research:* Sport marketing and consumer analysis, health psychology, smoking cessation, psychosocial aspects of cardiovascular disease, global health promotion. *Unit head:* Linda H. Clemens, Interim Chair, 901-678-2324, Fax: 901-678-3591, E-mail: lhclemns@memphis.edu. *Application contact:* Dr. Kenneth Ward, Graduate Studies Coordinator, 901-678-1714, E-mail: kdward@memphis.edu.
Website: http://coe.memphis.edu/hss/

University of Miami, Graduate School, School of Education and Human Development, Department of Kinesiology and Sport Sciences, Program in Nutrition for Health and Human Performance, Coral Gables, FL 33124. Offers MS Ed. *Faculty:* 3 full-time (1 woman), 4 part-time/adjunct (3 women). *Students:* 1 applicant. *Degree requirements:* For master's, comprehensive examination or research project. *Entrance requirements:* For master's, GRE. Additional exam requirements/recommendations for international students: Required—TOEFL (minimum score 550 paper-based; 80 iBT). *Application deadline:* For fall admission, 10/1 for international students. Application fee: $65. *Financial support:* Application deadline: 3/1; applicants required to submit FAFSA. *Unit head:* Dr. Wesley Smith, Assistant Professor and Program Director, 305-284-5756, Fax: 305-284-5168, E-mail: wes@miami.edu. *Application contact:* Lois Heffernan, Graduate Admissions Coordinator, 305-284-2167, Fax: 305-284-9395, E-mail: lheffernan@miami.edu.
Website: http://www.education.miami.edu/program/Programs.asp?Program_ID=147&Src=Graduate

University of Michigan, School of Public Health, Department of Environmental Health Sciences, Ann Arbor, MI 48109. Offers environmental health sciences (MS, PhD); environmental quality and health (MPH); human nutrition (MPH); industrial hygiene (MPH, MS); nutritional sciences (MS); occupational and environmental epidemiology (MPH); toxicology (MPH, MS, PhD). *Accreditation:* CEPH (one or more programs are accredited). Part-time programs available. Terminal master's awarded for partial completion of doctoral program. *Degree requirements:* For master's, thesis (for some programs); for doctorate, thesis/dissertation, preliminary exam, oral defense of dissertation. *Entrance requirements:* For master's and doctorate, GRE General Test and/or MCAT. Additional exam requirements/recommendations for international students: Required—TOEFL (minimum score 560 paper-based; 100 iBT). Electronic applications accepted. Tuition and fees vary according to course level, course load, degree level, program and student level. *Faculty research:* Toxicology, occupational hygiene, nutrition, environmental exposure sciences, environmental epidemiology.

University of Minnesota, Twin Cities Campus, Graduate School, College of Food, Agricultural and Natural Resource Sciences, Program in Nutrition, St. Paul, MN 55108. Offers MS, PhD. Part-time programs available. *Faculty:* 51 full-time (33 women). *Students:* 56 full-time (45 women); includes 8 minority (1 Black or African American, non-Hispanic/Latino; 2 American Indian or Alaska Native, non-Hispanic/Latino; 3 Asian, non-Hispanic/Latino; 2 Hispanic/Latino), 15 international. Average age 30. 47 applicants, 23% accepted, 10 enrolled. In 2013, 9 master's, 7 doctorates awarded. Terminal master's awarded for partial completion of doctoral program. *Degree requirements:* For master's, comprehensive exam, thesis; for doctorate, comprehensive exam, thesis/dissertation. *Entrance requirements:* For master's, GRE General Test, previous course work in general chemistry, organic chemistry, physiology, biology, biochemistry, statistics; minimum GPA of 3.0 (preferred); for doctorate, GRE General Test, previous course work in general chemistry, organic chemistry, calculus, biology, physics, physiology, biochemistry, statistics; minimum GPA of 3.0 (preferred). Additional exam requirements/recommendations for international students: Required—TOEFL (minimum score 550 paper-based; 79 iBT), IELTS (minimum score 6.5). *Application deadline:* For fall admission, 12/15 for domestic and international students; for spring admission, 10/15 for domestic and international students. Applications are processed on a rolling basis. Application fee: $75 ($95 for international students). Electronic applications accepted. *Financial support:* In 2013–14, fellowships with full tuition reimbursements (averaging $40,000 per year), research assistantships with full and partial tuition reimbursements (averaging $40,000 per year), teaching assistantships with full and partial tuition reimbursements (averaging $40,000 per year) were awarded; career-related internships or fieldwork, scholarships/grants, traineeships, health care benefits, tuition waivers, and unspecified assistantships also available. Support available to part-time students. *Faculty research:* Diet and chronic disease: from basic biological and molecular biology approaches to a public health/intervention/ epidemiology perspective. *Total annual research expenditures:* $3 million. *Unit head:* Dr. Marla Reicks, Director of Graduate Studies, 612-624-4735, Fax: 612-625-5272, E-mail: mreicks@umn.edu. *Application contact:* Nancy L. Toedt, Program Coordinator, 612-624-6753, Fax: 612-625-5272, E-mail: sviker@umn.edu.
Website: http://fscn.cfans.umn.edu/graduate_programs/nutritiongraduate/index.htm

University of Minnesota, Twin Cities Campus, School of Public Health, Major in Public Health Nutrition, Minneapolis, MN 55455-0213. Offers MPH. *Accreditation:* AND. Part-time programs available. *Degree requirements:* For master's, fieldwork, project. *Entrance requirements:* For master's, GRE General Test. Additional exam requirements/ recommendations for international students: Required—TOEFL. Electronic applications accepted. *Expenses:* Contact institution. *Faculty research:* Nutrition and pregnancy outcomes, nutrition and women's health, child growth and nutrition, child and adolescent nutrition and eating behaviors, obesity and eating disorder prevention.

University of Mississippi, Graduate School, School of Applied Sciences, Department of Nutrition and Hospitality Management, University, MS 38677. Offers food and nutrition services (MS). *Faculty:* 12 full-time (10 women), 3 part-time/adjunct (1 woman). *Students:* 17 full-time (15 women), 10 part-time (8 women); includes 4 minority (2 Black or African American, non-Hispanic/Latino; 2 Hispanic/Latino). In 2013, 14 master's awarded. Application fee: $40. *Unit head:* Dr. Kathy B. Knight, Interim Chair, 662-915-7371, E-mail: nhm@olemiss.edu. *Application contact:* Dr. Christy M. Wyandt, Associate Dean of Graduate School, 662-915-7474, Fax: 662-915-7577, E-mail: cwyandt@olemiss.edu.

University of Missouri, Graduate School, College of Agriculture, Food and Natural Resources, Department of Food Science, Columbia, MO 65211. Offers food science (MS, PhD); foods and food systems management (MS); human nutrition (MS). *Faculty:* 12 full-time (4 women), 2 part-time/adjunct (0 women). *Students:* 24 full-time (14 women), 25 part-time (14 women); includes 2 minority (1 Hispanic/Latino; 1 Two or more races, non-Hispanic/Latino), 33 international. Average age 28. 79 applicants, 15% accepted, 10 enrolled. In 2013, 5 master's, 3 doctorates awarded. Terminal master's awarded for partial completion of doctoral program. *Degree requirements:* For doctorate, comprehensive exam, thesis/dissertation. *Entrance requirements:* For master's, GRE General Test (minimum score: Verbal and Quantitative 1000 with neither section below 400, 297 combined under new scoring; Analytical 3.5), minimum GPA of 3.0; BS in food science from accredited university; for doctorate, GRE General Test (minimum score: Verbal and Quantitative 1000 with neither section below 400, Analytical 3.5), minimum GPA of 3.0; BS and MS in food science from accredited university. Additional exam requirements/recommendations for international students: Required—TOEFL (minimum score 550 paper-based; 79 iBT). *Application deadline:* For fall admission, 4/1 priority date for domestic students; for winter admission, 10/31 priority date for domestic students. Application fee: $55 ($75 for international students). Electronic applications accepted. *Financial support:* Fellowships, research assistantships with tuition reimbursements, teaching assistantships with tuition reimbursements, institutionally sponsored loans, scholarships/grants, health care benefits, and unspecified assistantships available. Support available to part-time students. *Faculty research:* Food chemistry, food analysis, food microbiology, food engineering and process control, functional foods, meat science and processing technology. *Unit head:* Dr. Jinglu Tan, Department Chair, 573-882-2369, E-mail: tanj@missouri.edu. *Application contact:* Starsha Ferguson, Office Support Assistant IV, 573-882-4113, E-mail: fergusonsd@missouri.edu.
Website: http://foodscience.missouri.edu/graduate/

University of Missouri, Graduate School, College of Human Environmental Sciences, Department of Nutrition and Exercise Physiology, Columbia, MO 65211. Offers exercise physiology (MA, PhD); nutritional sciences (MS, PhD). *Faculty:* 10 full-time (7 women). *Students:* 8 full-time (4 women), 11 part-time (6 women), 3 international. Average age 27. 20 applicants, 25% accepted, 1 enrolled. In 2013, 6 master's awarded. *Degree requirements:* For doctorate, thesis/dissertation. *Entrance requirements:* For master's and doctorate, GRE General Test, minimum GPA of 3.0. Additional exam requirements/ recommendations for international students: Required—TOEFL (minimum score 500 paper-based; 61 iBT). *Application deadline:* For fall admission, 12/31 priority date for domestic and international students. Applications are processed on a rolling basis. Application fee: $55 ($75 for international students). Electronic applications accepted. *Financial support:* Fellowships with full and partial tuition reimbursements, research assistantships with full and partial tuition reimbursements, teaching assistantships with full and partial tuition reimbursements, institutionally sponsored loans, scholarships/ grants, health care benefits, and unspecified assistantships available. Support available to part-time students. *Faculty research:* Fitness and wellness; body composition research; child care provider workforce development; childhood overweight: etiology and outcomes; development during infancy and early childhood; regulation and organization of glycolysis; metabolomics; diabetes and smooth muscle metabolism; lipid metabolism and lipotoxicity - mitochondrial dysfunction in diabetes, atherosclerosis, and cell phenotype transformation; magnetic resonance measures of cellular metabolism; smooth muscle physiology/pathophysiology. *Unit head:* Dr. Chris Hardin, Department Chair, 573-882-4288, E-mail: hardinc@missouri.edu. *Application contact:* Tammy Conrad, Academic Advisor, 573-882-1144, E-mail: conradt@missouri.edu.
Website: http://ns.missouri.edu/

University of Nebraska–Lincoln, Graduate College, College of Agricultural Sciences and Natural Resources, Interdepartmental Area of Nutrition, Lincoln, NE 68588. Offers MS, PhD. *Degree requirements:* For master's, thesis optional; for doctorate, comprehensive exam, thesis/dissertation. *Entrance requirements:* For master's and doctorate, GRE General Test. Additional exam requirements/recommendations for international students: Required—TOEFL (minimum score 550 paper-based). Electronic applications accepted. *Faculty research:* Human nutrition and metabolism, animal nutrition and metabolism, biochemistry, community and clinical nutrition.

University of Nebraska–Lincoln, Graduate College, College of Education and Human Sciences, Department of Nutrition and Health Sciences, Lincoln, NE 68588. Offers community nutrition and health promotion (MS); nutrition (MS, PhD); nutrition and exercise (MS); nutrition and health sciences (MS, PhD). *Degree requirements:* For master's, thesis optional. *Entrance requirements:* For master's, GRE General Test. Additional exam requirements/recommendations for international students: Required—TOEFL (minimum score 550 paper-based). Electronic applications accepted. *Faculty research:* Foods/food service administration, community nutrition science, diet-health relationships.

University of Nebraska Medical Center, School of Allied Health Professions and College of Medicine, UNMC Dietetic Internship Program (Medical Nutrition Education Division), Omaha, NE 68198. Offers Certificate. *Entrance requirements:* Additional exam requirements/recommendations for international students: Required—TOEFL. *Expenses: Required fees:* $300 per semester. Tuition and fees vary according to program. *Faculty research:* Nutrition intervention outcomes.

University of Nevada, Reno, Graduate School, College of Agriculture, Biotechnology and Natural Resources, Department of Nutrition, Reno, NV 89557. Offers MS. *Degree requirements:* For master's, thesis optional. *Entrance requirements:* For master's, GRE, minimum GPA of 2.75. Additional exam requirements/recommendations for international students: Required—TOEFL (minimum score 500 paper-based; 61 iBT), IELTS (minimum score 6). Electronic applications accepted. *Faculty research:* Nutritional education, food technology, therapeutic human nutrition, human nutritional requirements, diet and disease.

University of New Hampshire, Graduate School, College of Life Sciences and Agriculture, Department of Molecular, Cellular and Biomedical Sciences, Program in Animal and Nutritional Sciences, Durham, NH 03824. Offers PhD. Part-time programs available. *Faculty:* 31 full-time. *Students:* 4 full-time (all women), 3 part-time (2 women); includes 2 minority (both Hispanic/Latino), 1 international. Average age 31. 4 applicants, 25% accepted, 1 enrolled. In 2013, 3 doctorates awarded. *Entrance requirements:* For doctorate, GRE. Additional exam requirements/recommendations for international students: Required—TOEFL (minimum score 550 paper-based; 80 iBT). *Application deadline:* For fall admission, 6/1 priority date for domestic students, 4/1 priority date for international students; for spring admission, 12/1 for domestic students. Applications are processed on a rolling basis. Application fee: $65. Electronic applications accepted. *Expenses:* Tuition, state resident: full-time $13,500; part-time $750 per credit hour. Tuition, nonresident: full-time $26,200; part-time $1100 per credit hour. *Required fees:* $1741; $435.25 per term. Tuition and fees vary according to course level, course load, campus/location and program. *Financial support:* In 2013–14, 4 students received support, including 1 fellowship, 1 research assistantship, 2 teaching assistantships; scholarships/grants, traineeships, and unspecified assistantships also available. Support available to part-time students. *Unit head:* Dr. Rick Cote, Chairperson, 603-862-2458. *Application contact:* Flora Joyal, Administrative Assistant, 603-862-4095, E-mail: ansc.grad.program.info@unh.edu.
Website: http://www.biolsci.unh.edu/

University of New Hampshire, Graduate School, College of Life Sciences and Agriculture, Department of Molecular, Cellular and Biomedical Sciences, Program in Nutritional Sciences, Durham, NH 03824. Offers MS. Part-time programs available. *Faculty:* 31 full-time. *Students:* 1 (woman) full-time. Average age 48. 10 applicants, 10% accepted, 1 enrolled. In 2013, 1 master's awarded. *Degree requirements:* For master's, thesis. *Entrance requirements:* Additional exam requirements/recommendations for international students: Required—TOEFL (minimum score 550 paper-based; 80 iBT). *Application deadline:* For fall admission, 4/1 priority date for domestic students, 4/1 for international students; for spring admission, 12/1 for domestic students. Applications are processed on a rolling basis. Application fee: $65. Electronic applications accepted. *Expenses:* Tuition, state resident: full-time $13,500; part-time $750 per credit hour. Tuition, nonresident: full-time $26,200; part-time $1100 per credit hour. *Required fees:* $1741; $435.25 per term. Tuition and fees vary according to course level, course load, campus/location and program. *Financial support:* In 2013–14, 1 student received support, including 1 teaching assistantship; fellowships, research assistantships, career-related internships or fieldwork, Federal Work-Study, and scholarships/grants also available. Support available to part-time students. Financial award application deadline: 2/15. *Unit head:* Dr. Rick Cote, Chair, 603-862-2458. *Application contact:* Flora Joyal, Administrative Assistant, 603-862-4095.
Website: http://www.msnutrition.unh.edu/

University of New Haven, Graduate School, College of Arts and Sciences, Program in Human Nutrition, West Haven, CT 06516-1916. Offers MS. Part-time and evening/ weekend programs available. *Students:* 8 full-time (all women), 13 part-time (10 women); includes 2 minority (1 Black or African American, non-Hispanic/Latino; 1 Asian, non-Hispanic/Latino), 5 international. 33 applicants, 70% accepted, 9 enrolled. In 2013, 8 master's awarded. *Degree requirements:* For master's, internship. *Entrance requirements:* Additional exam requirements/recommendations for international students: Required—TOEFL (minimum score 80 iBT), IELTS, PTE (minimum score 53). *Application deadline:* For fall admission, 5/31 for international students; for winter admission, 10/15 for international students; for spring admission, 1/15 for international students. Applications are processed on a rolling basis. Application fee: $75. Electronic applications accepted. Application fee is waived when completed online. *Expenses: Tuition:* Full-time $21,600; part-time $800 per credit hour. *Required fees:* $45 per trimester. *Financial support:* Research assistantships with partial tuition reimbursements, teaching assistantships with partial tuition reimbursements, career-related internships or fieldwork, Federal Work-Study, scholarships/grants, tuition waivers, and unspecified assistantships available. Support available to part-time students. Financial award applicants required to submit FAFSA. *Unit head:* Dr. Rosa A. Mo, Interim Assistant Dean, 203-932-7040, E-mail: rmo@newhaven.edu. *Application contact:* Eloise Gormley, Director of Graduate Admissions, 203-932-7440, E-mail: gradinfo@newhaven.edu.
Website: http://www.newhaven.edu/4729/

University of New Mexico, Graduate School, College of Education, Department of Individual, Family and Community Education, Program in Nutrition, Albuquerque, NM 87131. Offers MS. Part-time programs available. *Faculty:* 3 full-time (2 women), 2 part-time/adjunct (0 women). *Students:* 13 full-time (12 women), 9 part-time (all women);

includes 6 minority (all Hispanic/Latino), 2 international. Average age 31. 13 applicants, 62% accepted, 8 enrolled. In 2013, 5 master's awarded. *Degree requirements:* For master's, comprehensive exam or thesis. *Entrance requirements:* For master's, GRE. Additional exam requirements/recommendations for international students: Required—TOEFL. *Application deadline:* For fall admission, 2/1 priority date for domestic students, 2/1 for international students; for spring admission, 11/1 priority date for domestic students, 11/1 for international students. Application fee: $50. Electronic applications accepted. *Financial support:* In 2013–14, 12 students received support, including 1 teaching assistantship (averaging $6,722 per year); unspecified assistantships also available. Financial award application deadline: 3/1; financial award applicants required to submit FAFSA. *Faculty research:* Nutritional needs of children, obesity prevention, phytochemicals, international nutrition. *Unit head:* Dr. Carole Conn, Graduate Coordinator, 505-277-8185, Fax: 505-277-8361, E-mail: cconn@unm.edu. *Application contact:* Cynthia Salas, Program Office, 505-277-4535, Fax: 505-277-8361, E-mail: casalas@unm.edu.
Website: http://coe.unm.edu/departments/ifce/nutrition-and-dietetics/nutrition-ms.html

The University of North Carolina at Chapel Hill, Graduate School, Gillings School of Global Public Health, Department of Nutrition, Chapel Hill, NC 27599. Offers nutrition (MPH, PhD); nutritional biochemistry (MS). *Accreditation:* AND. *Degree requirements:* For master's, comprehensive exam, thesis, major paper; for doctorate, comprehensive exam, thesis/dissertation. *Entrance requirements:* For master's and doctorate, GRE General Test, minimum GPA of 3.0 (recommended). Additional exam requirements/recommendations for international students: Required—TOEFL. Electronic applications accepted. *Faculty research:* Nutrition policy, management and leadership development, lipid and carbohydrate metabolism, dietary trends and determinants, transmembrane signal transduction and carcinogenesis, maternal and child nutrition.

The University of North Carolina at Greensboro, Graduate School, School of Human Environmental Sciences, Department of Nutrition, Greensboro, NC 27412-5001. Offers MS, PhD. *Degree requirements:* For master's, thesis; for doctorate, thesis/dissertation. *Entrance requirements:* For master's and doctorate, GRE General Test. Additional exam requirements/recommendations for international students: Required—TOEFL. Electronic applications accepted.

University of North Florida, Brooks College of Health, Department of Nutrition and Dietetics, Jacksonville, FL 32224. Offers MSH. Part-time programs available. *Faculty:* 7 full-time (6 women). *Students:* 33 full-time (29 women), 10 part-time (all women); includes 8 minority (2 Black or African American, non-Hispanic/Latino; 5 Hispanic/Latino; 1 Two or more races, non-Hispanic/Latino), 1 international. Average age 26. 50 applicants, 46% accepted, 21 enrolled. In 2013, 14 master's awarded. *Entrance requirements:* For master's, GRE General Test, minimum GPA of 3.0 in last 60 hours. Additional exam requirements/recommendations for international students: Required—TOEFL (minimum score 500 paper-based; 61 iBT). *Application deadline:* For fall admission, 7/1 for domestic students, 5/1 for international students; for spring admission, 11/1 for domestic students, 10/1 for international students. Application fee: $30. Electronic applications accepted. *Expenses:* Tuition, state resident: full-time $9794; part-time $408.10 per credit hour. Tuition, nonresident: full-time $22,383; part-time $932.61 per credit hour. *Required fees:* $2020; $84.20 per credit hour. Tuition and fees vary according to course load and program. *Financial support:* In 2013–14, 12 students received support, including 2 teaching assistantships (averaging $1,500 per year); research assistantships, career-related internships or fieldwork, Federal Work-Study, scholarships/grants, and tuition waivers (partial) also available. Financial award application deadline: 4/1; financial award applicants required to submit FAFSA. *Total annual research expenditures:* $3,171. *Unit head:* Dr. Judy Rodriguez, Chair, 904-620-1298, E-mail: jrodrigu@unf.edu. *Application contact:* Dr. Catherine Christie, Program Director, 904-620-1423, Fax: 904-620-1942, E-mail: c.christie@unf.edu.
Website: http://www.unf.edu/brooks/nutrition

University of Oklahoma Health Sciences Center, Graduate College, College of Allied Health, Department of Nutritional Sciences, Oklahoma City, OK 73190. Offers MS. *Accreditation:* AND. *Faculty:* 5 full-time (4 women). *Students:* 20 full-time (16 women), 12 part-time (10 women); includes 11 minority (1 Black or African American, non-Hispanic/Latino; 2 Asian, non-Hispanic/Latino; 5 Hispanic/Latino; 3 Two or more races, non-Hispanic/Latino), 2 international. Average age 28. 41 applicants, 80% accepted, 16 enrolled. In 2013, 10 master's awarded. *Degree requirements:* For master's, comprehensive exam, thesis optional. *Entrance requirements:* For master's, GRE General Test, interview, 3 letters of reference. Additional exam requirements/recommendations for international students: Required—TOEFL (minimum score 550 paper-based). *Application deadline:* For fall admission, 7/1 for domestic students; for winter admission, 5/1 for domestic students; for spring admission, 12/1 for domestic students. Application fee: $50. *Expenses:* Tuition, state resident: full-time $3504; part-time $175.20 per credit hour. Tuition, nonresident: full-time $13,504; part-time $675.20 per credit hour. *Required fees:* $1545; $52.70 per credit hour. $245.25 per semester. Tuition and fees vary according to course load. *Unit head:* Dr. Allen Kneehans, Chair, 405-271-2113, E-mail: allen-kneehans@ouhsc.edu. *Application contact:* Associate Dean, Academic and Student Affairs.

University of Pittsburgh, School of Health and Rehabilitation Sciences, Coordinated Master's in Nutrition and Dietetics Program, Pittsburgh, PA 15260. Offers MS. *Accreditation:* AND. Part-time and evening/weekend programs available. *Faculty:* 4 full-time (all women), 3 part-time/adjunct (all women). *Students:* 35 full-time (32 women), 2 international. Average age 26. 26 applicants, 81% accepted, 19 enrolled. In 2013, 16 master's awarded. *Entrance requirements:* For master's, GRE. Additional exam requirements/recommendations for international students: Required—TOEFL (minimum score 550 paper-based; 80 iBT), IELTS (minimum score 6.5). *Application deadline:* For fall admission, 3/15 for domestic and international students. Application fee: $50. Electronic applications accepted. *Expenses:* Contact institution. *Faculty research:* Targeted approaches to weight control, pediatric obesity treatment, effect of tart cherry juice on muscles. *Total annual research expenditures:* $35,080. *Unit head:* Dr. Scott Lephart, Department Chair and Associate Professor, 412-383-6530, Fax: 412-383-6527, E-mail: lephart@pitt.edu. *Application contact:* Jessica Maguire, Director of Admissions, 412-383-6557, Fax: 412-383-6535, E-mail: maguire@pitt.edu.
Website: http://www.shrs.pitt.edu/cmd/

University of Puerto Rico, Medical Sciences Campus, Graduate School of Public Health, Department of Human Development, Program in Nutrition, San Juan, PR 00936-5067. Offers MS. Part-time programs available. *Degree requirements:* For master's, thesis. *Entrance requirements:* For master's, GRE, previous course work in algebra, biochemistry, biology, chemistry, and social sciences.

University of Puerto Rico, Medical Sciences Campus, School of Health Professions, Program in Dietetics Internship, San Juan, PR 00936-5067. Offers Certificate. *Degree requirements:* For Certificate, one foreign language, clinical practice. *Entrance requirements:* For degree, minimum GPA of 2.5, interview, participation in the computer matching process by the American Dietetic Association.

University of Puerto Rico, Medical Sciences Campus, School of Medicine, Division of Graduate Studies, Department of Biochemistry, San Juan, PR 00936-5067. Offers MS, PhD. *Degree requirements:* For master's, thesis; for doctorate, comprehensive exam, thesis/dissertation. *Entrance requirements:* For master's and doctorate, GRE General Test, GRE Subject Test, interview, minimum GPA of 3.0. Electronic applications accepted. *Faculty research:* Genetics, cell and molecular biology, cancer biology, protein structure/function, glycosilation of proteins.

University of Puerto Rico, Río Piedras Campus, College of Education, Program in Family Ecology and Nutrition, San Juan, PR 00931-3300. Offers M Ed. Part-time programs available. *Degree requirements:* For master's, thesis. *Entrance requirements:* For master's, PAEG or GRE, minimum GPA of 3.0, letter of recommendation.

University of Rhode Island, Graduate School, College of the Environment and Life Sciences, Department of Nutrition and Food Sciences, Kingston, RI 02881. Offers dietetic internship (MS); nutrition (MS, PhD). Part-time programs available. *Faculty:* 7 full-time (5 women), 1 (woman) part-time/adjunct. *Students:* 12 full-time (9 women), 10 part-time (7 women); includes 2 minority (1 Asian, non-Hispanic/Latino; 1 Hispanic/Latino), 1 international. In 2013, 9 master's awarded. *Degree requirements:* For master's, comprehensive exam (for some programs), thesis optional; for doctorate, thesis/dissertation. *Entrance requirements:* For master's, GRE, 2 letters of recommendation (3 for MS in dietetic internship); for doctorate, GRE, 2 letters of recommendation. Additional exam requirements/recommendations for international students: Required—TOEFL (minimum score 550 paper-based). *Application deadline:* For fall admission, 2/15 for domestic students, 2/1 for international students; for spring admission, 11/15 for domestic students, 7/15 for international students. Application fee: $65. Electronic applications accepted. *Expenses:* Tuition, state resident: full-time $11,532; part-time $641 per credit. Tuition, nonresident: full-time $23,606; part-time $1311 per credit. *Required fees:* $1388; $36 per credit. $35 per semester. One-time fee: $130. *Financial support:* In 2013–14, 3 teaching assistantships with full and partial tuition reimbursements (averaging $13,203 per year) were awarded; research assistantships also available. Financial award application deadline: 2/15; financial award applicants required to submit FAFSA. *Faculty research:* Food safety and quality, marine resource utilization, nutrition in underserved populations, eating behavior, lipid metabolism. *Total annual research expenditures:* $1.6 million. *Unit head:* Dr. Geoffrey Greene, Chair, 401-874-4028, Fax: 401-874-5974, E-mail: gwg@uri.edu. *Application contact:* Graduate Admissions, 401-874-2872, E-mail: gradadm@etal.uri.edu.
Website: http://cels.uri.edu/nfs/

University of Saint Joseph, Department of Nutrition and Dietetics, West Hartford, CT 06117-2700. Offers nutrition (MS). Part-time and evening/weekend programs available. Postbaccalaureate distance learning degree programs offered. *Entrance requirements:* For master's, 2 letters of recommendation, letter of intent. *Application deadline:* Applications are processed on a rolling basis. Application fee: $50. Electronic applications accepted. Application fee is waived when completed online. *Financial support:* Career-related internships or fieldwork and unspecified assistantships available. Support available to part-time students. Financial award applicants required to submit FAFSA. *Application contact:* Graduate Admissions Office, 860-231-5261, E-mail: graduate@usj.edu.
Website: http://www.usj.edu/academics/schools/school-of-health-natural-sciences/nutrition-dietetics/

University of Southern Mississippi, Graduate School, College of Health, Department of Community Health Sciences, Hattiesburg, MS 39406-0001. Offers epidemiology and biostatistics (MPH); health education (MPH); health policy/administration (MPH); occupational/environmental health (MPH); public health nutrition (MPH). *Accreditation:* CEPH. Part-time and evening/weekend programs available. *Faculty:* 8 full-time (4 women), 1 part-time/adjunct (0 women). *Students:* 92 full-time (60 women), 9 part-time (4 women); includes 38 minority (29 Black or African American, non-Hispanic/Latino; 1 American Indian or Alaska Native, non-Hispanic/Latino; 2 Asian, non-Hispanic/Latino; 6 Two or more races, non-Hispanic/Latino), 13 international. Average age 34. 71 applicants, 93% accepted, 45 enrolled. *Degree requirements:* For master's, comprehensive exam, thesis (for some programs). *Entrance requirements:* For master's, GRE General Test, minimum GPA of 2.75 in last 60 hours. Additional exam requirements/recommendations for international students: Required—TOEFL, IELTS. *Application deadline:* For fall admission, 3/1 priority date for domestic and international students; for spring admission, 1/10 priority date for domestic and international students. Applications are processed on a rolling basis. Application fee: $50. Electronic applications accepted. *Financial support:* In 2013–14, 5 research assistantships with full tuition reimbursements (averaging $7,000 per year), 1 teaching assistantship with full tuition reimbursement (averaging $8,263 per year) were awarded; career-related internships or fieldwork, Federal Work-Study, institutionally sponsored loans, scholarships/grants, health care benefits, and unspecified assistantships also available. Financial award application deadline: 3/15; financial award applicants required to submit FAFSA. *Faculty research:* Rural health care delivery, school health, nutrition of pregnant teens, risk factor reduction, sexually transmitted diseases. *Unit head:* Dr. Ray Newman, Interim Chair, 601-266-5437, Fax: 601-266-5043. *Application contact:* Shonna Breland, Manager of Graduate Admissions, 601-266-6563, Fax: 601-266-5138.
Website: http://www.usm.edu/chs

University of Southern Mississippi, Graduate School, College of Health, Department of Nutrition and Food Systems, Hattiesburg, MS 39406-0001. Offers nutrition (MS, PhD). Part-time programs available. *Faculty:* 6 full-time (5 women). *Students:* 14 full-time (12 women), 34 part-time (29 women); includes 3 minority (all Black or African American, non-Hispanic/Latino), 3 international. Average age 28. 8 applicants, 63% accepted, 3 enrolled. In 2013, 15 master's, 1 doctorate awarded. *Degree requirements:* For master's, comprehensive exam, thesis (for some programs); for doctorate, comprehensive exam, thesis/dissertation. *Entrance requirements:* For master's, GRE General Test, minimum GPA of 2.75 on last 60 hours; for doctorate, GRE General Test, minimum GPA of 3.5. Additional exam requirements/recommendations for international students: Required—TOEFL, IELTS. *Application deadline:* For fall admission, 3/1 for domestic and international students; for spring admission, 1/10 priority date for domestic and international students. Application fee: $50. *Financial support:* In 2013–14, 2 research assistantships with full tuition reimbursements (averaging $12,069 per year), 6 teaching assistantships with full tuition reimbursements (averaging $7,676 per year) were awarded; career-related internships or fieldwork, Federal Work-Study, institutionally sponsored loans, scholarships/grants, traineeships, health care benefits, and unspecified assistantships also available. Financial award applicants required to submit FAFSA. *Unit head:* Dr. Kathleen Yadrick, Chair, 601-266-5377, Fax: 601-266-6343. *Application contact:* Belynda Brock, Graduate Admission Secretary, 601-266-5377, Fax: 601-266-5138.
Website: http://www.usm.edu/graduateschool/table.php

University of South Florida, Innovative Education Graduate Certificate Programs, Tampa, FL 33620-9951. *Unit head:* Kathy Barnes, Interdisciplinary Programs Coordinator, 813-974-8031, Fax: 813-974-7061, E-mail: barnesk@usf.edu. *Application contact:* Karen Tylinski, Metro Initiatives, 813-974-9943, Fax: 813-974-7061, E-mail: ktylinsk@usf.edu.
Website: http://www.usf.edu/innovative-education/

University of South Florida, Morsani College of Medicine and Graduate School, Graduate Programs in Medical Sciences, Tampa, FL 33620-9951. Offers aging and neuroscience (MSMS); allergy, immunology and infectious disease (PhD); anatomy

(MSMS, PhD); athletic training (MSMS); bioinformatics and computational biology (MSBCB); biotechnology (MSB); clinical and translational research (MSMS, PhD); health informatics (MSHI, MSMS); health science (MSMS); interdisciplinary medical sciences (MSMS); medical microbiology and immunology (MSMS); metabolic and nutritional medicine (MSMS); molecular medicine (MSMS, PhD); molecular pharmacology and physiology (PhD); neurology (PhD); pathology and laboratory medicine (PhD); pharmacology and therapeutics (PhD); physiology and biophysics (PhD); women's health (MSMS). *Students:* 336 full-time (182 women), 39 part-time (21 women); includes 170 minority (45 Black or African American, non-Hispanic/Latino; 54 Asian, non-Hispanic/Latino; 59 Hispanic/Latino; 2 Native Hawaiian or other Pacific Islander, non-Hispanic/Latino; 10 Two or more races, non-Hispanic/Latino), 17 international. Average age 26. 1,066 applicants, 44% accepted, 250 enrolled. In 2013, 191 master's, 12 doctorates awarded. Terminal master's awarded for partial completion of doctoral program. *Degree requirements:* For master's, comprehensive exam, thesis; for doctorate, comprehensive exam, thesis/dissertation. *Entrance requirements:* For master's, GRE General Test or GMAT, bachelor's degree or equivalent from regionally-accredited university with minimum GPA of 3.0 in upper-division sciences coursework; prerequisites in general biology, general chemistry, general physics, organic chemistry, quantitative analysis, and integral and differential calculus; for doctorate, GRE General Test (minimum score of 600 quantitative), bachelor's degree from regionally-accredited university with minimum GPA of 3.0 in upper-division sciences coursework; 3 letters of recommendation; personal interview; 1-2 page personal statement; prerequisites in biology, chemistry, physics, organic chemistry, quantitative analysis, and integral/differential calculus. Additional exam requirements/recommendations for international students: Required—TOEFL (minimum score 550 paper-based; 79 iBT) or IELTS (minimum score 6.5). *Application deadline:* For fall admission, 2/15 for domestic students, 1/2 for international students. Application fee: $30. *Expenses:* Contact institution. *Faculty research:* Anatomy, biochemistry, cancer biology, cardiovascular disease, cell biology, immunology, microbiology, molecular biology, neuroscience, pharmacology, physiology. *Unit head:* Dr. Michael Barber, Professor and Associate Dean for Graduate and Postdoctoral Affairs, 813-974-9908, Fax: 813-974-4317, E-mail: mbarber@health.usf.edu. *Application contact:* Dr. Eric Bennett, Graduate Director, PhD Program in Medical Sciences, 813-974-1545, Fax: 813-974-4317, E-mail: esbennet@health.usf.edu.
Website: http://health.usf.edu/nocms/medicine/graduatestudies/

The University of Tennessee, Graduate School, College of Education, Health and Human Sciences, Department of Nutrition, Knoxville, TN 37996. Offers nutrition (MS), including nutrition science, public health nutrition; MS/MPH. Part-time programs available. *Degree requirements:* For master's, thesis or alternative. *Entrance requirements:* For master's, GRE General Test, minimum GPA of 2.7. Additional exam requirements/recommendations for international students: Required—TOEFL. Electronic applications accepted. *Expenses:* Tuition, state resident: full-time $9540; part-time $531 per credit hour. Tuition, nonresident: full-time $27,728; part-time $1542 per credit hour. *Required fees:* $1404; $67 per credit hour.

The University of Tennessee at Martin, Graduate Programs, College of Agriculture and Applied Sciences, Department of Family and Consumer Sciences, Martin, TN 38238-1000. Offers dietetics (MSFCS); general family and consumer sciences (MSFCS). Part-time programs available. *Faculty:* 7. *Students:* 27 part-time (26 women); includes 7 minority (4 Black or African American, non-Hispanic/Latino; 1 Hispanic/Latino; 2 Two or more races, non-Hispanic/Latino). 13 applicants, 62% accepted, 6 enrolled. In 2013, 11 master's awarded. *Degree requirements:* For master's, comprehensive exam, thesis optional. *Entrance requirements:* For master's, GRE General Test, minimum GPA of 2.5. Additional exam requirements/recommendations for international students: Required—TOEFL (minimum score 525 paper-based; 71 iBT). *Application deadline:* For fall admission, 7/29 priority date for domestic and international students; for spring admission, 12/12 priority date for domestic and international students. Applications are processed on a rolling basis. Application fee: $30 ($130 for international students). Electronic applications accepted. *Financial support:* Teaching assistantships with full tuition reimbursements, scholarships/grants, and unspecified assistantships available. Support available to part-time students. Financial award application deadline: 2/15; financial award applicants required to submit FAFSA. *Faculty research:* Children with developmental disabilities, regional food product development and marketing, parent education. *Unit head:* Dr. Lisa LeBleu, Coordinator, 731-881-7116, Fax: 731-881-7106, E-mail: llebleu@utm.edu. *Application contact:* Jolene L. Cunningham, Student Services Specialist, 731-881-7012, Fax: 731-881-7499, E-mail: jcunningham@utm.edu.
Website: http://www.utm.edu/departments/caas/fcs/index.php

The University of Texas at Austin, Graduate School, College of Natural Sciences, School of Human Ecology, Program in Nutritional Sciences, Austin, TX 78712-1111. Offers nutrition (MA); nutritional sciences (PhD). *Degree requirements:* For master's, thesis; for doctorate, thesis/dissertation. *Entrance requirements:* For master's and doctorate, GRE General Test. Additional exam requirements/recommendations for international students: Required—TOEFL. Electronic applications accepted. *Faculty research:* Nutritional biochemistry, nutrient health assessment, obesity, nutrition education, molecular/cellular aspects of nutrient functions.

The University of Texas at San Antonio, College of Education and Human Development, Department of Kinesiology, Health, and Nutrition, San Antonio, TX 78249-0617. Offers dietetics studies (MSD); health and kinesiology (MS). Part-time and evening/weekend programs available. *Faculty:* 17 full-time (7 women), 1 part-time/adjunct (0 women). *Students:* 65 full-time (38 women), 66 part-time (29 women); includes 88 minority (12 Black or African American, non-Hispanic/Latino; 4 Asian, non-Hispanic/Latino; 71 Hispanic/Latino; 1 Two or more races, non-Hispanic/Latino), 9 international. Average age 28. 79 applicants, 95% accepted, 45 enrolled. In 2013, 48 master's awarded. *Degree requirements:* For master's, comprehensive exam, thesis optional. *Entrance requirements:* For master's, bachelor's degree with minimum GPA of 3.0 in last 60 hours of coursework; resume; statement of purpose; two letters of recommendation. Additional exam requirements/recommendations for international students: Required—TOEFL (minimum score 550 paper-based; 79 iBT), IELTS (minimum score 6.5). *Application deadline:* For fall admission, 7/1 for domestic students, 4/1 for international students; for spring admission, 11/1 for domestic students, 9/1 for international students; for summer admission, 4/1 for domestic students, 3/1 for international students. Applications are processed on a rolling basis. Application fee: $45 ($80 for international students). Electronic applications accepted. *Expenses:* Tuition, state resident: full-time $4671. Tuition, nonresident: full-time $8708. *International tuition:* $17,415 full-time. *Required fees:* $1924.60. Tuition and fees vary according to course load and degree level. *Faculty research:* Motor behavior, motor skills, exercise and nutrition, athlete efficacy, diabetes prevention. *Unit head:* Dr. Wan Xiang Yao, Chair, 210-458-6224, Fax: 210-452-5873, E-mail: wanxiang.yao@utsa.edu. *Application contact:* Dr. Alberto Cordova, Graduate Advisor of Record, 210-458-6226, Fax: 210-458-5873, E-mail: alberto.cordova@utsa.edu.
Website: http://education.utsa.edu/health_and_kinesiology

The University of Texas Southwestern Medical Center, Southwestern School of Health Professions, Clinical Nutrition Program, Dallas, TX 75390. Offers MCN. *Accreditation:* AND. *Students:* 32 full-time (29 women); includes 14 minority (2 Black or African American, non-Hispanic/Latino; 5 Asian, non-Hispanic/Latino; 7 Hispanic/Latino), 1 international. Average age 25. 43 applicants, 51% accepted, 17 enrolled. *Unit head:* Dr. Raul Caetano, Dean, 214-648-1500. *Application contact:* Anne Mclane, Associate Director of Admissions, 214-648-6708, Fax: 214-648-2102, E-mail: admissions@utsouthwestern.edu.

University of the District of Columbia, College of Arts and Sciences, Department of Biological and Environmental Sciences, Program in Nutrition and Dietetics, Washington, DC 20008-1175. Offers MS. *Degree requirements:* For master's, thesis. *Entrance requirements:* For master's, GRE, 3 letters of recommendation, personal interview. *Expenses: Tuition, area resident:* Full-time $7883.28; part-time $437.96 per credit hour. Tuition, state resident: full-time $8923.14. Tuition, nonresident: full-time $15,163; part-time $842.40 per credit hour. *Required fees:* $620; $30 per credit hour.

University of the Incarnate Word, School of Graduate Studies and Research, H-E-B School of Business and Administration, Programs in Administration, San Antonio, TX 78209-6397. Offers adult education (MAA); communication arts (MAA); healthcare administration (MAA); instructional technology (MAA); nutrition (MAA); organizational development (MAA); sports management (MAA). Part-time and evening/weekend programs available. Postbaccalaureate distance learning degree programs offered (no on-campus study). *Faculty:* 20 full-time (10 women), 14 part-time/adjunct (6 women). *Students:* 31 full-time (22 women), 54 part-time (36 women); includes 61 minority (14 Black or African American, non-Hispanic/Latino; 1 Asian, non-Hispanic/Latino; 46 Hispanic/Latino), 6 international. Average age 31. 63 applicants, 68% accepted, 21 enrolled. In 2013, 35 master's awarded. *Degree requirements:* For master's, capstone. *Entrance requirements:* For master's, GRE, GMAT, undergraduate degree, minimum GPA of 2.5. Additional exam requirements/recommendations for international students: Required—TOEFL (minimum score 560 paper-based; 83 iBT). *Application deadline:* Applications are processed on a rolling basis. Application fee: $20. Electronic applications accepted. *Expenses: Tuition:* Part-time $815 per credit hour. *Required fees:* $86 per credit hour. One-time fee: $40 part-time. Tuition and fees vary according to degree level and program. *Financial support:* Federal Work-Study and scholarships/grants available. Financial award applicants required to submit FAFSA. *Unit head:* Dr. Mark Teachout, MAA Programs Director, 210-829-3177, Fax: 210-805-3564, E-mail: teachout@uiwtx.edu. *Application contact:* Andrea Cyterski-Acosta, Dean of Enrollment, 210-829-6005, Fax: 210-829-3921, E-mail: admis@uiwtx.edu.
Website: http://www.uiw.edu/maa/

University of the Incarnate Word, School of Graduate Studies and Research, School of Mathematics, Science, and Engineering, Program in Nutrition, San Antonio, TX 78209-6397. Offers administration (MS); nutrition education and health promotion (MS). Part-time and evening/weekend programs available. *Faculty:* 3 full-time (2 women), 2 part-time/adjunct (both women). *Students:* 10 full-time (8 women), 19 part-time (16 women); includes 16 minority (1 Black or African American, non-Hispanic/Latino; 1 Asian, non-Hispanic/Latino; 14 Hispanic/Latino), 1 international. Average age 26. 59 applicants, 63% accepted, 17 enrolled. In 2013, 5 master's awarded. *Degree requirements:* For master's, comprehensive exam, thesis or alternative. *Entrance requirements:* For master's, two letters of recommendation. Additional exam requirements/recommendations for international students: Required—TOEFL (minimum score 560 paper-based; 83 iBT). *Application deadline:* Applications are processed on a rolling basis. Application fee: $20. Electronic applications accepted. *Expenses: Tuition:* Part-time $815 per credit hour. *Required fees:* $86 per credit hour. One-time fee: $40 part-time. Tuition and fees vary according to degree level and program. *Financial support:* In 2013–14, research assistantships (averaging $5,000 per year) were awarded; Federal Work-Study and scholarships/grants also available. Financial award applicants required to submit FAFSA. *Faculty research:* Nutrition. *Total annual research expenditures:* $109,000. *Unit head:* Dr. Beth Senne-Duff, Associate Professor, 210-829-3165, Fax: 210-829-3153, E-mail: beths@uiwtx.edu. *Application contact:* Andrea Cyterski-Acosta, Dean of Enrollment, 210-829-6005, Fax: 210-829-3921, E-mail: admis@uiwtx.edu.
Website: http://www.uiw.edu/nutrition/nutrition3.htm

The University of Toledo, College of Graduate Studies, College of Medicine and Life Sciences, Department of Public Health and Preventative Medicine, Toledo, OH 43606-3390. Offers biostatistics and epidemiology (Certificate); contemporary gerontological practice (Certificate); environmental and occupational health and safety (MPH); epidemiology (Certificate); global public health (Certificate); health promotion and education (MPH); industrial hygiene (MSOH); medical and health science teaching and learning (Certificate); occupational health (Certificate); public health administration (MPH); public health and emergency response (Certificate); public health epidemiology (MPH); public health nutrition (MPH); MD/MPH. Part-time and evening/weekend programs available. *Faculty:* 9. *Students:* 69 full-time (50 women), 88 part-time (66 women); includes 50 minority (35 Black or African American, non-Hispanic/Latino; 10 Asian, non-Hispanic/Latino; 4 Hispanic/Latino; 1 Two or more races, non-Hispanic/Latino), 6 international. Average age 30. 92 applicants, 80% accepted, 52 enrolled. In 2013, 59 master's, 15 other advanced degrees awarded. *Degree requirements:* For master's, thesis or alternative. *Entrance requirements:* For master's, GRE, minimum undergraduate GPA of 3.0, three letters of recommendation, statement of purpose, transcripts from all prior institutions attended, resume; for Certificate, minimum undergraduate GPA of 3.0, three letters of recommendation, statement of purpose, transcripts from all prior institutions attended, resume. Additional exam requirements/recommendations for international students: Required—TOEFL (minimum score 550 paper-based; 80 iBT), IELTS (minimum score 6.5). *Application deadline:* For fall admission, 6/15 for domestic students, 3/15 priority date for international students; for spring admission, 10/15 for domestic students, 6/15 for international students; for summer admission, 3/15 for domestic students, 10/15 for international students. Applications are processed on a rolling basis. Application fee: $45 ($75 for international students). Electronic applications accepted. *Financial support:* In 2013–14, 4 research assistantships with full tuition reimbursements (averaging $10,000 per year) were awarded; Federal Work-Study, institutionally sponsored loans, scholarships/grants, tuition waivers (full and partial), and unspecified assistantships also available. *Unit head:* Dr. Sheryl A. Milz, Chair, 419-383-3976, Fax: 419-383-6140, E-mail: sheryl.milz@utoledo.edu. *Application contact:* Admissions Analyst, 419-383-4112, Fax: 419-383-6140.
Website: http://nocphmph.org/

University of Toronto, Faculty of Medicine, Department of Nutritional Sciences, Toronto, ON M5S 1A1, Canada. Offers M Sc, PhD. Part-time programs available. *Degree requirements:* For master's, thesis, oral thesis defense; for doctorate, comprehensive exam, thesis/dissertation, departmental examination, oral examination. *Entrance requirements:* For master's, minimum B average, background in nutrition or an area of biological or health sciences, 2 letters of reference; for doctorate, minimum B+ average in final 2 years, background in nutrition or an area of biological or health sciences, 2 letters of reference. Additional exam requirements/recommendations for international students: Required—TOEFL (580 paper-based), TWE (5), IELTS (7), Michigan English Language Assessment Battery (85), or COPE (4). Electronic applications accepted.

University of Utah, Graduate School, College of Health, Division of Nutrition, Salt Lake City, UT 84112. Offers MS. *Accreditation:* AND. *Faculty:* 4 full-time (2 women), 14 part-time/adjunct (12 women). *Students:* 30 full-time (27 women); includes 3 minority (1 Asian, non-Hispanic/Latino; 2 Hispanic/Latino), 4 international. Average age 25. 65 applicants, 23% accepted, 15 enrolled. In 2013, 18 master's awarded. *Degree requirements:* For master's, comprehensive exam, thesis. *Entrance requirements:* For master's, GRE General Test, minimum undergraduate GPA of 3.0. Additional exam requirements/recommendations for international students: Required—TOEFL (minimum score 500 paper-based). *Application deadline:* For fall admission, 2/15 for domestic and international students. Application fee: $55 ($65 for international students). Electronic applications accepted. *Expenses:* Contact institution. *Financial support:* In 2013–14, 29 students received support, including 1 research assistantship with partial tuition reimbursement available (averaging $6,500 per year), 11 teaching assistantships with partial tuition reimbursements available (averaging $6,500 per year); career-related internships or fieldwork, scholarships/grants, and unspecified assistantships also available. Financial award application deadline: 2/15; financial award applicants required to submit FAFSA. *Faculty research:* Cholesterol metabolism, sport nutrition education, metabolic and critical care, cardiovascular nutrition, wilderness nutrition, pediatric nutrition. *Total annual research expenditures:* $20,000. *Unit head:* Dr. Julie Metos, Director, 801-587-3024, Fax: 801-585-3874, E-mail: julie.metos@hsc.utah.edu. *Application contact:* Jean Zancanella, Academic Adviser, 801-581-5280, Fax: 801-585-3874, E-mail: jean.zancanella@health.utah.edu.
Website: http://www.health.utah.edu/fdnu/

University of Vermont, Graduate College, College of Agriculture and Life Sciences, Department of Nutrition and Food Sciences, Program in Dietetics, Burlington, VT 05405. Offers MSD. *Students:* 12 (all women); includes 1 minority (Asian, non-Hispanic/Latino). 11 applicants, 55% accepted, 6 enrolled. In 2013, 6 master's awarded. *Entrance requirements:* For master's, GRE General Test. Additional exam requirements/recommendations for international students: Required—TOEFL (minimum score 550 paper-based; 80 iBT). *Application deadline:* For fall admission, 12/15 priority date for domestic and international students. Application fee: $65. Electronic applications accepted. *Unit head:* Prof. Amy Nickerson, Director, 802-656-3374.

University of Vermont, Graduate College, College of Agriculture and Life Sciences, Program in Animal, Nutrition and Food Sciences, Burlington, VT 05405. Offers PhD. *Students:* 20 (10 women); includes 1 minority (Asian, non-Hispanic/Latino), 10 international. 16 applicants, 25% accepted. In 2013, 2 doctorates awarded. *Degree requirements:* For doctorate, one foreign language, thesis/dissertation. *Entrance requirements:* For doctorate, GRE General Test. Additional exam requirements/recommendations for international students: Required—TOEFL (minimum score 550 paper-based; 80 iBT). *Application deadline:* For fall admission, 4/1 priority date for domestic students, 4/1 for international students. Applications are processed on a rolling basis. Application fee: $65. Electronic applications accepted. *Financial support:* Application deadline: 3/1. *Unit head:* Dr. Andre-Denis Wright, Chairperson, 802-656-2070. *Application contact:* Dr. David Kerr, Coordinator, 802-656-2070.

University of Washington, Graduate School, School of Public Health, Nutritional Sciences Program, Seattle, WA 98195. Offers MPH, MS, PhD. *Accreditation:* AND. Part-time programs available. *Students:* 32 full-time (30 women), 13 part-time (11 women); includes 8 minority (1 American Indian or Alaska Native, non-Hispanic/Latino; 7 Asian, non-Hispanic/Latino), 4 international. Average age 28. 147 applicants, 30% accepted, 16 enrolled. In 2013, 15 master's, 2 doctorates awarded. Terminal master's awarded for partial completion of doctoral program. *Degree requirements:* For master's, thesis, practicum (MPH); for doctorate, thesis/dissertation. *Entrance requirements:* For master's, GRE General Test; for doctorate, GRE General Test, master's degree, minimum GPA of 3.0. Additional exam requirements/recommendations for international students: Required—TOEFL (minimum score 580 paper-based; 92 iBT), IELTS (minimum score 7). *Application deadline:* For fall admission, 12/1 for domestic and international students. Application fee: $85. Electronic applications accepted. *Financial support:* In 2013–14, 18 students received support, including 1 fellowship (averaging $5,000 per year), 2 research assistantships (averaging $15,000 per year), 15 teaching assistantships with partial tuition reimbursements available (averaging $5,034 per year); scholarships/grants also available. *Faculty research:* Dietary behavior, dietary supplements, obesity, clinical nutrition, addictive behaviors. *Unit head:* Dr. Adam Drewnowski, Director, 206-543-8016. *Application contact:* Graduate Student Services Coordinator, 206-543-1730, Fax: 206-685-1696, E-mail: nutr@u.washington.edu.
Website: http://depts.washington.edu/nutr/

University of Wisconsin–Madison, Graduate School, College of Agricultural and Life Sciences, Department of Nutritional Sciences, Madison, WI 53706. Offers MS, PhD. Terminal master's awarded for partial completion of doctoral program. *Degree requirements:* For master's, thesis or research report; for doctorate, comprehensive exam, thesis/dissertation. *Entrance requirements:* For master's and doctorate, GRE General Test. Additional exam requirements/recommendations for international students: Required—TOEFL (minimum score 550 paper-based; 80 iBT). Electronic applications accepted. *Expenses:* Tuition, state resident: full-time $10,728; part-time $790 per credit. Tuition, nonresident: full-time $24,054; part-time $1623 per credit. *Required fees:* $1130; $119 per credit. *Faculty research:* Human and animal nutrition, nutrition epidemiology, nutrition education, biochemical and molecular nutrition.

University of Wisconsin–Stevens Point, College of Professional Studies, School of Health Promotion and Human Development, Program in Nutritional Sciences, Stevens Point, WI 54481-3897. Offers MS. Part-time programs available. *Degree requirements:* For master's, thesis or alternative. *Entrance requirements:* For master's, minimum GPA of 2.75.

University of Wisconsin–Stout, Graduate School, College of Human Development, Program in Food and Nutritional Sciences, Menomonie, WI 54751. Offers MS. Part-time programs available. *Degree requirements:* For master's, thesis. *Entrance requirements:* For master's, minimum GPA of 3.0. Additional exam requirements/recommendations for international students: Required—TOEFL (minimum score 500 paper-based; 61 iBT). Electronic applications accepted. *Faculty research:* Disease states and nutrition, childhood obesity, nutraceuticals, food safety, nanotechnology.

University of Wyoming, College of Agriculture and Natural Resources, Department of Animal Sciences, Program in Food Science and Human Nutrition, Laramie, WY 82071. Offers MS. *Degree requirements:* For master's, thesis. *Entrance requirements:* For master's, GRE General Test, minimum GPA of 3.0. Additional exam requirements/recommendations for international students: Required—TOEFL (minimum score 525 paper-based). Electronic applications accepted. *Faculty research:* Protein and lipid metabolism, food microbiology, food safety, meat science.

Utah State University, School of Graduate Studies, College of Agriculture, Department of Nutrition, Dietetics, and Food Sciences, Logan, UT 84322. Offers dietetic administration (MDA); nutrition and food sciences (MS, PhD). Postbaccalaureate distance learning degree programs offered. *Degree requirements:* For master's, thesis; for doctorate, comprehensive exam, thesis/dissertation, teaching experience. *Entrance requirements:* For master's, GRE General Test, minimum GPA of 3.0, course work in chemistry, biochemistry, physics, math, bacteriology, physiology; for doctorate, GRE General Test, minimum GPA of 3.2, course work in chemistry, MS or manuscript in referred journal. Additional exam requirements/recommendations for international students: Required—TOEFL (minimum score 550 paper-based). Electronic applications accepted. *Faculty research:* Mineral balance, meat microbiology and nitrate interactions, milk ultrafiltration, lactic culture, milk coagulation.

Virginia Polytechnic Institute and State University, Graduate School, College of Agriculture and Life Sciences, Blacksburg, VA 24061. Offers agricultural and applied economics (MS); agricultural and life sciences (MS); animal and poultry science (MS, PhD); crop and soil environmental sciences (MS, PhD); dairy science (MS); entomology (PhD); horticulture (MS, PhD); human nutrition, foods and exercise (MS, PhD); life sciences (MS, PhD); plant pathology, physiology and weed science (PhD). *Faculty:* 234 full-time (66 women), 1 (woman) part-time/adjunct. *Students:* 347 full-time (188 women), 80 part-time (53 women); includes 53 minority (19 Black or African American, non-Hispanic/Latino; 1 American Indian or Alaska Native, non-Hispanic/Latino; 19 Asian, non-Hispanic/Latino; 7 Hispanic/Latino; 7 Two or more races, non-Hispanic/Latino), 106 international. Average age 29. 410 applicants, 35% accepted, 111 enrolled. In 2013, 80 master's, 44 doctorates awarded. *Degree requirements:* For master's, comprehensive exam (for some programs), thesis (for some programs); for doctorate, comprehensive exam (for some programs), thesis/dissertation (for some programs). *Entrance requirements:* For master's and doctorate, GRE/GMAT (may vary by department). Additional exam requirements/recommendations for international students: Required—TOEFL (minimum score 550 paper-based). *Application deadline:* For fall admission, 8/1 for domestic students, 4/1 for international students; for spring admission, 1/1 for domestic students, 9/1 for international students. Applications are processed on a rolling basis. Application fee: $75. Electronic applications accepted. *Expenses:* Tuition, state resident: full-time $11,185; part-time $621.50 per credit hour. Tuition, nonresident: full-time $22,146; part-time $1230.25 per credit hour. *Required fees:* $2442; $449.25 per semester. Tuition and fees vary according to course load, campus/location and program. *Financial support:* In 2013–14, 1 fellowship with full tuition reimbursement (averaging $19,278 per year), 232 research assistantships with full tuition reimbursements (averaging $19,370 per year), 83 teaching assistantships with full tuition reimbursements (averaging $18,677 per year) were awarded. Financial award application deadline: 3/1; financial award applicants required to submit FAFSA. *Total annual research expenditures:* $44.3 million. *Unit head:* Dr. Alan L. Grant, Dean, 540-231-4152, Fax: 540-231-4163, E-mail: algrant@vt.edu. *Application contact:* Sheila Norman, Administrative Assistant, 540-231-4152, Fax: 540-231-4163, E-mail: snorman@vt.edu.
Website: http://www.cals.vt.edu/

Washington State University, Graduate School, College of Pharmacy, Pullman, WA 99164. Offers dietetics, nutrition, and exercise physiology (MS); pharmacy (PhD, Pharm D). *Accreditation:* ACPE (one or more programs are accredited). *Degree requirements:* For master's, comprehensive exam, thesis, oral exam; for doctorate, comprehensive exam, thesis/dissertation, oral exam (for PhD). *Entrance requirements:* For master's, GRE General Test, minimum GPA of 3.0, interview; for doctorate, GRE General Test, minimum GPA of 3.0, interview, minimum 60 hours of documented pharmacy experience. *Faculty research:* Hormonal carcinogenesis, drug metabolism/transport, toxicology of chlorinated compounds, alcohol effects on immune system, effects of cocaine on neuronal function.

Washington State University Spokane, Master of Science Coordinated Program in Dietetics Nutrition and Exercise Physiology, Spokane, WA 99210-1495. Offers dietetics and nutrition (MS). *Degree requirements:* For master's, internship. *Entrance requirements:* For master's, BS in nutrition and exercise physiology, exercise science, human nutrition, or related degree; interview.

Wayne State University, College of Liberal Arts and Sciences, Department of Nutrition and Food Science, Detroit, MI 48202. Offers MA, MS, PhD. *Faculty:* 10 full-time (7 women), 6 part-time/adjunct (3 women). *Students:* 57 full-time (45 women), 9 part-time (all women); includes 5 minority (2 Black or African American, non-Hispanic/Latino; 2 Asian, non-Hispanic/Latino; 1 Two or more races, non-Hispanic/Latino), 26 international. Average age 30. 98 applicants, 27% accepted, 14 enrolled. In 2013, 18 master's, 1 doctorate awarded. *Degree requirements:* For master's, thesis (for some programs), essay (for MA); for doctorate, thesis/dissertation. *Entrance requirements:* For master's, GRE General Test, admission to Graduate School, minimum GPA of 3.0, undergraduate degree with major in science, courses in human nutrition and metabolism, food chemistry, introductory microbiology, anatomy and physiology, organic chemistry; for doctorate, GRE General Test, admission to Graduate School; MS (in exceptional cases, an outstanding undergraduate record); two letters of recommendation; personal statement. Additional exam requirements/recommendations for international students: Required—TOEFL (minimum score 550 paper-based; 79 iBT), TWE (minimum score 5.5), Michigan English Language Assessment Battery (minimum score 85); Recommended—IELTS (minimum score 6.5). *Application deadline:* For fall admission, 6/1 priority date for domestic students, 5/1 priority date for international students; for winter admission, 10/1 priority date for domestic students, 9/1 priority date for international students; for spring admission, 2/1 priority date for domestic students, 1/1 priority date for international students. Applications are processed on a rolling basis. Application fee: $0. Electronic applications accepted. *Expenses:* Tuition, state resident: part-time $554.15 per credit. Tuition, nonresident: part-time $1200.35 per credit. *Required fees:* $42.15 per credit. $268.30 per semester. Tuition and fees vary according to course load and program. *Financial support:* In 2013–14, 22 students received support, including 1 fellowship with tuition reimbursement available (averaging $16,842 per year), 3 research assistantships with tuition reimbursements available (averaging $15,949 per year), 9 teaching assistantships with tuition reimbursements available (averaging $18,071 per year); scholarships/grants, health care benefits, and unspecified assistantships also available. Financial award application deadline: 3/31; financial award applicants required to submit FAFSA. *Faculty research:* Nutrition cancer; mechanisms by which aging increases cancer risk; nutrition and exercise, nutrition, cancer and metabolomics; diet-induced obesity and diabetes; cholesterol and lipoprotein metabolism; dietetics; food microbiology, antimicrobial resistance, microbial detection; food and nutraceutical chemistry. *Total annual research expenditures:* $414,755. *Unit head:* Dr. Ahmad R. Hydari, Interim Chair, 313-577-2500, E-mail: ahmad.heydari@wayne.edu. *Application contact:* Dr. Pramod Khosla, Graduate Director, 313-577-0448, Fax: 313-577-8616, E-mail: aa0987@wayne.edu.
Website: http://clasweb.clas.wayne.edu/nfs

West Chester University of Pennsylvania, College of Health Sciences, Department of Health, West Chester, PA 19383. Offers community health (MPH); emergency preparedness (Certificate); environmental health (MPH); health care management (MPH, Certificate); integrative health (MPH, Certificate); nutrition (MPH); school health (M Ed). *Accreditation:* CEPH. Part-time and evening/weekend programs available. *Faculty:* 17 full-time (13 women), 3 part-time/adjunct (all women). *Students:* 115 full-time (85 women), 95 part-time (73 women); includes 79 minority (66 Black or African American, non-Hispanic/Latino; 1 American Indian or Alaska Native, non-Hispanic/Latino; 5 Asian, non-Hispanic/Latino; 3 Hispanic/Latino; 4 Two or more races, non-Hispanic/Latino), 15 international. Average age 31. 156 applicants, 83% accepted, 76 enrolled. In 2013, 101 master's, 18 other advanced degrees awarded. *Degree*

Nutrition

requirements: For master's, thesis or alternative, minimum GPA of 3.0; research report (for M Ed); major project and practicum (for MPH); for Certificate, minimum GPA of 3.0. *Entrance requirements:* For master's, goal statement, two letters of recommendation, undergraduate Introduction to Statistics course. Additional exam requirements/recommendations for international students: Required—TOEFL (minimum score 550 paper-based; 80 iBT). *Application deadline:* For fall admission, 4/15 priority date for domestic students, 3/15 for international students; for spring admission, 10/15 priority date for domestic students, 9/1 for international students. Applications are processed on a rolling basis. Application fee: $45. Electronic applications accepted. *Expenses:* Tuition, state resident: full-time $7956; part-time $442 per credit. Tuition, nonresident: full-time $11,934; part-time $663 per credit. *Required fees:* $2134.20; $106.24 per credit. Tuition and fees vary according to campus/location and program. *Financial support:* Unspecified assistantships available. Support available to part-time students. Financial award application deadline: 2/15; financial award applicants required to submit FAFSA. *Faculty research:* Healthy school communities, community health issues and evidence-based programs, environment and health, nutrition and health, integrative health. *Unit head:* Dr. Bethann Cinelli, Chair, 610-436-2267, E-mail: bcinelli@wcupa.edu. *Application contact:* Dr. Lynn Carson, Graduate Coordinator, 610-436-2138, E-mail: lcarson@wcupa.edu.

Website: http://www.wcupa.edu/_ACADEMICS/HealthSciences/health/

West Virginia University, Davis College of Agriculture, Forestry and Consumer Sciences, Division of Animal and Nutritional Sciences, Program in Animal and Nutritional Sciences, Morgantown, WV 26506. Offers breeding (MS); food sciences (MS); nutrition (MS); physiology (MS); production management (MS); reproduction (MS). Part-time programs available. *Degree requirements:* For master's, thesis, oral and written exams. *Entrance requirements:* For master's, GRE, minimum GPA of 2.5. Additional exam requirements/recommendations for international students: Required—TOEFL. *Faculty research:* Animal nutrition, reproductive physiology, food science.

Winthrop University, College of Arts and Sciences, Department of Human Nutrition, Rock Hill, SC 29733. Offers MS. Part-time programs available. *Degree requirements:* For master's, thesis optional. *Entrance requirements:* For master's, GRE General Test, PRAXIS, or MAT, interview, minimum GPA of 3.0. Electronic applications accepted.

Section 15
Parasitology

This section contains a directory of institutions offering graduate work in parasitology. Additional information about programs listed in the directory may be obtained by writing directly to the dean of a graduate school or chair of a department at the address given in the directory.

For programs offering related work, see also in this book *Allied Health, Biological and Biomedical Sciences, Microbiological Sciences,* and *Public Health.*

CONTENTS

Program Directory

Parasitology

Illinois State University, Graduate School, College of Arts and Sciences, Department of Biological Sciences, Normal, IL 61790-2200. Offers animal behavior (MS); bacteriology (MS); biochemistry (MS); biological sciences (MS); biology (PhD); biophysics (MS); biotechnology (MS); botany (MS, PhD); cell biology (MS); conservation biology (MS); developmental biology (MS); ecology (MS, PhD); entomology (MS); evolutionary biology (MS); genetics (MS, PhD); immunology (MS); microbiology (MS, PhD); molecular biology (MS); molecular genetics (MS); neurobiology (MS); neuroscience (MS); parasitology (MS); physiology (MS, PhD); plant biology (MS); plant molecular biology (MS); plant sciences (MS); structural biology (MS); zoology (MS, PhD). Part-time programs available. *Degree requirements:* For master's, thesis or alternative; for doctorate, variable foreign language requirement, thesis/dissertation, 2 terms of residency. *Entrance requirements:* For master's, GRE General Test, minimum GPA of 2.6 in last 60 hours of course work; for doctorate, GRE General Test. *Faculty research:* Redoc balance and drug development in schistosoma mansoni, control of the growth of listeria monocytogenes at low temperature, regulation of cell expansion and microtubule function by SPRI, CRUI: physiology and fitness consequences of different life history phenotypes.

Louisiana State University Health Sciences Center, School of Graduate Studies in New Orleans, Department of Microbiology, Immunology, and Parasitology, New Orleans, LA 70112-2223. Offers microbiology and immunology (MS, PhD); MD/PhD. Terminal master's awarded for partial completion of doctoral program. *Degree requirements:* For master's, comprehensive exam, thesis; for doctorate, comprehensive exam, thesis/dissertation, preliminary exam, qualifying exam. *Entrance requirements:* For master's and doctorate, GRE General Test. Additional exam requirements/ recommendations for international students: Required—TOEFL. *Faculty research:* Microbial physiology, animal virology, vaccine development, AIDS drug studies, pathogenic mechanisms, molecular immunology.

McGill University, Faculty of Graduate and Postdoctoral Studies, Faculty of Agricultural and Environmental Sciences, Institute of Parasitology, Montréal, QC H3A 2T5, Canada. Offers biotechnology (M Sc A, Certificate); parasitology (M Sc, PhD).

Tulane University, School of Public Health and Tropical Medicine, Department of Tropical Medicine, New Orleans, LA 70118-5669. Offers clinical tropical medicine and travelers health (Diploma); parasitology (MSPH, PhD); public health and tropical medicine (MPHTM); vector borne infectious diseases (MS, PhD); MD/PhD. MS and PhD offered through the Graduate School. *Degree requirements:* For master's, thesis; for doctorate, comprehensive exam, thesis/dissertation. *Entrance requirements:* For master's, GRE General Test, minimum B average in undergraduate course work; for doctorate, GRE General Test. Additional exam requirements/recommendations for international students: Required—TOEFL.

University of Notre Dame, Graduate School, College of Science, Department of Biological Sciences, Notre Dame, IN 46556. Offers aquatic ecology, evolution and environmental biology (MS, PhD); cellular and molecular biology (MS, PhD); genetics (MS, PhD); physiology (MS, PhD); vector biology and parasitology (MS, PhD). Terminal master's awarded for partial completion of doctoral program. *Degree requirements:* For master's, comprehensive exam, thesis; for doctorate, comprehensive exam, thesis/ dissertation, candidacy exam. *Entrance requirements:* For master's and doctorate, GRE General Test. Additional exam requirements/recommendations for international students: Required—TOEFL (minimum score 600 paper-based; 80 iBT). Electronic applications accepted. *Faculty research:* Tropical disease, molecular genetics, neurobiology, evolutionary biology, aquatic biology.

University of Prince Edward Island, Atlantic Veterinary College, Graduate Program in Veterinary Medicine, Charlottetown, PE C1A 4P3, Canada. Offers anatomy (M Sc, PhD); bacteriology (M Sc, PhD); clinical pharmacology (M Sc, PhD); clinical sciences (M Sc, PhD); epidemiology (M Sc, PhD), including reproduction; fish health (M Sc, PhD); food animal nutrition (M Sc, PhD); immunology (M Sc, PhD); microanatomy (M Sc, PhD); parasitology (M Sc, PhD); pathology (M Sc, PhD); pharmacology (M Sc, PhD); physiology (M Sc, PhD); toxicology (M Sc, PhD); veterinary science (M Vet Sc); virology (M Sc, PhD). Part-time programs available. *Degree requirements:* For master's, thesis; for doctorate, thesis/dissertation. *Entrance requirements:* For master's, DVM, B Sc honors degree, or equivalent; for doctorate, M Sc. Additional exam requirements/ recommendations for international students: Required—TOEFL (minimum score 550 paper-based; 80 iBT). *Expenses:* Contact institution. *Faculty research:* Animal health management, infectious diseases, fin fish and shellfish health, basic biomedical sciences, ecosystem health.

University of Washington, Graduate School, School of Public Health, Department of Global Health, Graduate Program in Pathobiology, Seattle, WA 98195. Offers PhD. *Faculty:* 20 full-time (8 women). *Students:* 26 full-time (17 women), 8 part-time (7 women); includes 6 minority (2 Black or African American, non-Hispanic/Latino; 4 Asian, non-Hispanic/Latino), 2 international. Average age 29. 66 applicants, 17% accepted, 5 enrolled. In 2013, 6 doctorates awarded. *Degree requirements:* For doctorate, comprehensive exam, thesis/dissertation, published paper from thesis work. *Entrance requirements:* For doctorate, GRE General Test, minimum GPA of 3.0. Additional exam requirements/recommendations for international students: Required—TOEFL, IELTS. *Application deadline:* For fall admission, 12/1 for domestic and international students. Application fee: $85. Electronic applications accepted. *Financial support:* In 2013–14, 31 students received support, including 31 research assistantships with full tuition reimbursements available (averaging $28,440 per year); traineeships and unspecified assistantships also available. *Faculty research:* Malaria, immunological response to mycobacteria infections, HIV-cell interaction and the development of an anti-HIV vaccine, regulation of intercellular communication via gap junctions, genetic and nutritional regulation of proteins involved in lipid transport. *Unit head:* Dr. King K. Holmes, Chair, 206-744-3620, Fax: 206-744-3694. *Application contact:* Rachel Reichert, Program Manager, 206-543-4338, Fax: 206-543-3873, E-mail: pabio@u.washington.edu.

Section 16
Pathology and Pathobiology

This section contains a directory of institutions offering graduate work in pathology and pathobiology, followed by an in-depth entry submitted by an institution that chose to submit a detailed program description. Additional information about programs listed in the directory but not augmented by an in-depth entry may be obtained by writing directly to the dean of a graduate school or chair of a department at the address given in the directory.

For programs offering related work, see also in this book *Allied Health; Anatomy; Biochemistry; Biological and Biomedical Sciences; Cell, Molecular, and Structural Biology; Genetics, Developmental Biology, and Reproductive Biology; Microbiological Sciences; Pharmacology and Toxicology; Physiology, Public Health,* and *Veterinary Medicine and Sciences.*

CONTENTS

Program Directories

Close-Up

Molecular Pathogenesis

Dartmouth College, Graduate Program in Molecular and Cellular Biology, Department of Microbiology and Immunology, Program in Molecular Pathogenesis, Hanover, NH 03755. Offers microbiology and immunology (PhD).

Emory University, Laney Graduate School, Division of Biological and Biomedical Sciences, Program in Immunology and Molecular Pathogenesis, Atlanta, GA 30322-1100. Offers PhD. *Degree requirements:* For doctorate, comprehensive exam, thesis/dissertation. *Entrance requirements:* For doctorate, GRE General Test, minimum GPA of 3.0 in science course work (recommended). Additional exam requirements/recommendations for international students: Required—TOEFL. Electronic applications accepted. *Faculty research:* Transplantation immunology, autoimmunity, microbial pathogenesis.

North Dakota State University, College of Graduate and Interdisciplinary Studies, College of Agriculture, Food Systems, and Natural Resources, Department of Veterinary and Microbiological Sciences, Fargo, ND 58108. Offers international infectious disease (MS); microbiology (MS); molecular pathogenesis (PhD). Part-time programs available. *Faculty:* 15 full-time (8 women). *Students:* 11 full-time (6 women), 6 part-time (4 women), 5 international. Average age 30. 2 applicants, 50% accepted, 1 enrolled. In 2013, 8 master's, 1 doctorate awarded. *Degree requirements:* For master's, thesis; for doctorate, thesis/dissertation, oral and written preliminary exams. *Entrance requirements:* For master's and doctorate, GRE. Additional exam requirements/recommendations for international students: Required—TOEFL (minimum score 525 paper-based; 71 iBT). *Application deadline:* For fall admission, 2/15 priority date for domestic students. Applications are processed on a rolling basis. Application fee: $35. *Financial support:* Fellowships with full tuition reimbursements, research assistantships with full tuition reimbursements, teaching assistantships with full tuition reimbursements, Federal Work-Study, and institutionally sponsored loans available. Financial award application deadline: 4/15. *Faculty research:* Bacterial gene regulation, antibiotic resistance, molecular virology, mechanisms of bacterial pathogenesis, immunology of animals. *Unit head:* Dr. Charlene Wolf-Hall, Head, 701-231-7667, E-mail: charlene.hall@ndsu.edu. *Application contact:* Dr. John McEvoy, Associate Professor, 701-231-8530, Fax: 701-231-7514, E-mail: eugene.berry@ndsu.edu.
Website: http://vetmicro.ndsu.nodak.edu/

Texas A&M Health Science Center, College of Medicine, Department of Microbial and Molecular Pathogenesis, College Station, TX 77840. Offers immunology (PhD); microbiology (PhD); molecular biology (PhD); virology (PhD). *Degree requirements:* For doctorate, thesis/dissertation. *Entrance requirements:* For doctorate, GRE General Test, minimum GPA of 3.0. *Faculty research:* Molecular pathogenesis, microbial therapeutics.

University at Albany, State University of New York, School of Public Health, Department of Biomedical Sciences, Program in Molecular Pathogenesis, Albany, NY 12222-0001. Offers MS, PhD. *Degree requirements:* For master's, thesis; for doctorate, thesis/dissertation. *Entrance requirements:* For master's and doctorate, GRE General Test, GRE Subject Test.

University of Chicago, Division of Biological Sciences, Biomedical Sciences Cluster: Cancer Biology, Immunology, Molecular Metabolism and Nutrition, Pathology, and Microbiology, Department of Pathology, Chicago, IL 60637-1513. Offers molecular pathogenesis and molecular medicine (PhD). *Degree requirements:* For doctorate, thesis/dissertation, ethics class, 2 teaching assistantships. *Entrance requirements:* For doctorate, GRE General Test. Additional exam requirements/recommendations for international students: Required—IELTS (minimum score 7); Recommended—TOEFL (minimum score 600 paper-based; 104 iBT). Electronic applications accepted. *Faculty research:* Vascular biology, apolipoproteins, cardiovascular disease, immunopathology.

Washington University in St. Louis, Graduate School of Arts and Sciences, Division of Biology and Biomedical Sciences, Program in Molecular Microbiology and Microbial Pathogenesis, St. Louis, MO 63130-4899. Offers PhD. *Degree requirements:* For doctorate, thesis/dissertation. *Entrance requirements:* For doctorate, GRE General Test, GRE Subject Test. Electronic applications accepted.

Molecular Pathology

Rutgers, The State University of New Jersey, Newark, Graduate School of Biomedical Sciences, Program in Molecular Pathology and Immunology, Newark, NJ 07107. Offers PhD. *Entrance requirements:* Additional exam requirements/recommendations for international students: Required—TOEFL. Electronic applications accepted.

Texas Tech University Health Sciences Center, School of Allied Health Sciences, Program in Molecular Pathology, Lubbock, TX 79430. Offers MS. *Faculty:* 9 full-time (7 women). *Students:* 19 full-time (6 women); includes 8 minority (2 Black or African American, non-Hispanic/Latino; 2 Asian, non-Hispanic/Latino; 4 Hispanic/Latino). Average age 28. 45 applicants, 49% accepted, 22 enrolled. In 2013, 21 master's awarded. *Entrance requirements:* Additional exam requirements/recommendations for international students: Required—TOEFL, IELTS. *Application deadline:* For spring admission, 2/1 priority date for domestic students. Applications are processed on a rolling basis. Application fee: $40. Electronic applications accepted. *Financial support:* Career-related internships or fieldwork, institutionally sponsored loans, and scholarships/grants available. Financial award applicants required to submit FAFSA. *Unit head:* Ericka Hendrix, Program Director, 806-743-4015 Ext. 272, E-mail: ericka.hendrix@ttuhsc.edu. *Application contact:* Lindsay Johnson, Associate Dean for Admissions and Student Affairs, 806-743-3220, Fax: 806-743-2994, E-mail: lindsay.johnson@ttuhsc.edu.
Website: http://www.ttuhsc.edu/sah/msmp/

University of Michigan, Rackham Graduate School, Program in Biomedical Sciences (PIBS), Program in Molecular and Cellular Pathology, Ann Arbor, MI 48109. Offers PhD. *Faculty:* 34 full-time (9 women). *Students:* 25 full-time (15 women); includes 7 minority (1 Black or African American, non-Hispanic/Latino; 5 Asian, non-Hispanic/Latino; 1 Hispanic/Latino), 5 international. Average age 28. 48 applicants, 13% accepted, 4 enrolled. In 2013, 6 doctorates awarded. *Degree requirements:* For doctorate, comprehensive exam, thesis/dissertation. *Entrance requirements:* For doctorate, GRE General Test, 3 letters of recommendation, research experience. Additional exam requirements/recommendations for international students: Required—TOEFL (minimum score 84 iBT). *Application deadline:* For fall admission, 12/1 for domestic and international students. Application fee: $75 ($90 for international students). Electronic applications accepted. Tuition and fees vary according to course level, course load, degree level, program and student level. *Financial support:* In 2013–14, research assistantships with full tuition reimbursements (averaging $28,500 per year) were awarded; scholarships/grants, traineeships, health care benefits, and unspecified assistantships also available. *Faculty research:* Cancer biology, stem cell and developmental biology, immunopathology and inflammatory disease, epigenetics and gene regulation, cell death and regulation. *Unit head:* Dr. Zaneta Nikolovska-Coleska, Assistant Professor of Pathology/Director, 734-763-6454, Fax: 734-615-2331, E-mail: pathgradprog@med.umich.edu. *Application contact:* Laura A. Labut, Administrative Specialist, 734-763-6454, Fax: 734-615-2331, E-mail: laszczem@med.umich.edu.
Website: http://www.pathology.med.umich.edu/

University of Pittsburgh, School of Medicine, Graduate Programs in Medicine, Cellular and Molecular Pathology Graduate Program, Pittsburgh, PA 15260. Offers PhD. *Faculty:* 67 full-time (22 women). *Students:* 31 full-time (15 women); includes 6 minority (2 Black or African American, non-Hispanic/Latino; 2 Asian, non-Hispanic/Latino; 2 Hispanic/Latino), 7 international. Average age 28. 517 applicants, 13% accepted, 22 enrolled. In 2013, 8 doctorates awarded. *Degree requirements:* For doctorate, comprehensive exam, thesis/dissertation. *Entrance requirements:* For doctorate, GRE General Test, GRE Subject Test, minimum QPA of 3.0. Additional exam requirements/recommendations for international students: Required—TOEFL (minimum score 600 paper-based; 100 iBT), IELTS (minimum score 7). *Application deadline:* For fall admission, 1/1 priority date for domestic and international students. Application fee: $50. Electronic applications accepted. *Expenses:* Tuition, state resident: full-time $19,964; part-time $807 per credit. Tuition, nonresident: full-time $32,686; part-time $1337 per credit. *Required fees:* $740; $200. Tuition and fees vary according to program. *Financial support:* In 2013–14, 10 fellowships with full tuition reimbursements (averaging $26,010 per year), 21 research assistantships with full tuition reimbursements (averaging $26,010 per year) were awarded; institutionally sponsored loans, scholarships/grants, traineeships, health care benefits, and unspecified assistantships also available. *Faculty research:* Liver growth and differentiation, pathogenesis of neurodegeneration, cancer research. *Unit head:* Dr. Wendy Mars, Graduate Program Director, 412-648-9690, Fax: 412-648-9846, E-mail: wmars@pitt.edu. *Application contact:* Graduate Studies Administrator, 412-648-8957, Fax: 412-648-1077, E-mail: gradstudies@medschool.pitt.edu.
Website: http://www.gradbiomed.pitt.edu

The University of Texas Health Science Center at Houston, Graduate School of Biomedical Sciences, Program in Molecular Pathology, Houston, TX 77225-0036. Offers MS, PhD, MD/PhD. Terminal master's awarded for partial completion of doctoral program. *Degree requirements:* For master's, thesis; for doctorate, thesis/dissertation. *Entrance requirements:* For master's and doctorate, GRE General Test. Additional exam requirements/recommendations for international students: Required—TOEFL. Electronic applications accepted. *Expenses:* Tuition, state resident: full-time $3474; part-time $193 per credit hour. Tuition, nonresident: full-time $13,644; part-time $758 per credit hour. *Required fees:* $226.30; $87 per credit hour. *Faculty research:* Infectious disease, carcinogenesis, structural biology, cell biology.

Yale University, School of Medicine and Graduate School of Arts and Sciences, Combined Program in Biological and Biomedical Sciences (BBS), Pharmacological Sciences and Molecular Medicine Track, New Haven, CT 06520. Offers PhD, MD/PhD. *Degree requirements:* For doctorate, thesis/dissertation. *Entrance requirements:* For doctorate, GRE General Test. Additional exam requirements/recommendations for international students: Required—TOEFL. Electronic applications accepted.

Pathobiology

Auburn University, College of Veterinary Medicine and Graduate School, Graduate Programs in Veterinary Medicine, Auburn University, AL 36849. Offers biomedical sciences (MS, PhD), including anatomy, physiology and pharmacology (MS), biomedical sciences (PhD), clinical sciences (MS), large animal surgery and medicine (MS), pathobiology (MS), radiology (MS), small animal surgery and medicine (MS); DVM/MS. Part-time programs available. *Faculty:* 100 full-time (41 women), 4 part-time/adjunct (1 woman). *Students:* 24 full-time (16 women), 38 part-time (25 women); includes 5 minority (1 Black or African American, non-Hispanic/Latino; 1 American Indian or Alaska

Native, non-Hispanic/Latino; 2 Asian, non-Hispanic/Latino; 1 Hispanic/Latino), 22 international. Average age 30. 36 applicants, 44% accepted, 13 enrolled. In 2013, 12 master's, 8 doctorates awarded. *Degree requirements:* For doctorate, thesis/dissertation. *Entrance requirements:* For master's, GRE General Test; for doctorate, GRE General Test, GRE Subject Test. *Application deadline:* For fall admission, 7/7 for domestic students; for spring admission, 11/24 for domestic students. Applications are processed on a rolling basis. Application fee: $50 ($60 for international students). Electronic applications accepted. *Expenses:* Tuition, state resident: full-time $8262; part-time $459 per credit hour. Tuition, nonresident: full-time $24,786; part-time $1377 per credit hour. Tuition and fees vary according to degree level and program. *Financial support:* Research assistantships, teaching assistantships, and Federal Work-Study available. Support available to part-time students. Financial award application deadline: 3/15; financial award applicants required to submit FAFSA. *Unit head:* Dr. Calvin Johnson, Acting Dean, 334-844-2650. *Application contact:* Dr. George Flowers, Dean of the Graduate School, 334-844-2125.

Brown University, Graduate School, Division of Biology and Medicine, Department of Pathology and Laboratory Medicine, Providence, RI 02912. Offers Sc M, PhD, MD/PhD. Terminal master's awarded for partial completion of doctoral program. *Degree requirements:* For doctorate, thesis/dissertation, preliminary exam. *Entrance requirements:* For master's and doctorate, GRE General Test, GRE Subject Test. Additional exam requirements/recommendations for international students: Required—TOEFL. Electronic applications accepted. *Faculty research:* Environmental pathology, carcinogenesis, immunopathology, signal transduction, innate immunity.

Columbia University, College of Physicians and Surgeons, Department of Pathology, New York, NY 10032. Offers pathobiology (M Phil, MA, PhD); MD/PhD. Only candidates for the PhD are admitted. Terminal master's awarded for partial completion of doctoral program. *Degree requirements:* For doctorate, thesis/dissertation. *Entrance requirements:* For master's and doctorate, GRE General Test. Additional exam requirements/recommendations for international students: Required—TOEFL. *Faculty research:* Virology, molecular biology, cell biology, neurobiology, immunology.

Drexel University, College of Medicine, Biomedical Graduate Programs, Interdisciplinary Program in Molecular Pathobiology, Philadelphia, PA 19104-2875. Offers MS, PhD, MD/PhD. *Degree requirements:* For doctorate, comprehensive exam, thesis/dissertation, qualifying exams. *Entrance requirements:* For doctorate, GRE General Test, minimum GPA of 3.0. Additional exam requirements/recommendations for international students: Required—TOEFL. Electronic applications accepted. *Faculty research:* Cell and molecular immunology, tumor immunology, molecular genetics, immunopathology, immunology of aging.

Johns Hopkins University, School of Medicine, Graduate Programs in Medicine, Department of Pathology, Baltimore, MD 21218-2699. Offers pathobiology (PhD). *Faculty:* 68 full-time (14 women). *Students:* 47 full-time (28 women); includes 7 minority (1 Black or African American, non-Hispanic/Latino; 4 Asian, non-Hispanic/Latino; 1 Hispanic/Latino; 1 Two or more races, non-Hispanic/Latino), 23 international. Average age 28. 47 applicants, 21% accepted, 6 enrolled. In 2013, 7 doctorates awarded. *Degree requirements:* For doctorate, thesis/dissertation, qualifying oral exam. *Entrance requirements:* For doctorate, GRE General Test, previous course work with laboratory in organic and inorganic chemistry, general biology, calculus; interview. Additional exam requirements/recommendations for international students: Required—TOEFL. *Application deadline:* For winter admission, 1/10 for domestic students. Application fee: $85. Electronic applications accepted. *Financial support:* Fellowships and scholarships/grants available. *Faculty research:* Role of mutant proteins in Alzheimer's disease, nuclear protein function in breast and prostate cancer, medically important fungi, glycoproteins in HIV pathogenesis. *Total annual research expenditures:* $38.6 million. *Unit head:* Dr. J. Brooks Jackson, Chair, 410-955-9790, Fax: 410-955-0394. *Application contact:* Wilhelmena M. Braswell, Senior Academic Program Coordinator, 443-287-3163, Fax: 410-614-3548, E-mail: wbraswel@jhmi.edu.
Website: http://www.pathology.jhu.edu/

Kansas State University, College of Veterinary Medicine, Department of Diagnostic Medicine/Pathobiology, Manhattan, KS 66506. Offers biomedical science (MS); diagnostic medicine/pathobiology (PhD). *Faculty:* 23 full-time (6 women), 5 part-time/adjunct (3 women). *Students:* 30 full-time (11 women), 7 part-time (4 women); includes 3 minority (1 Black or African American, non-Hispanic/Latino; 1 Hispanic/Latino; 1 Native Hawaiian or other Pacific Islander, non-Hispanic/Latino), 15 international. Average age 32. 14 applicants, 29% accepted, 3 enrolled. In 2013, 1 doctorate awarded. Terminal master's awarded for partial completion of doctoral program. *Degree requirements:* For doctorate, thesis/dissertation. *Entrance requirements:* For master's and doctorate, interviews. Additional exam requirements/recommendations for international students: Required—TOEFL (minimum score 550 paper-based). *Application deadline:* For fall admission, 2/1 priority date for domestic and international students; for spring admission, 8/1 priority date for domestic and international students. Applications are processed on a rolling basis. Application fee: $50 ($75 for international students). Electronic applications accepted. *Financial support:* In 2013–14, 22 research assistantships (averaging $21,849 per year) were awarded; Federal Work-Study, institutionally sponsored loans, and scholarships/grants also available. Financial award application deadline: 3/1; financial award applicants required to submit FAFSA. *Faculty research:* Infectious disease of animals, food safety and security, epidemiology and public health, toxicology, pathology. *Total annual research expenditures:* $9.2 million. *Unit head:* M. M. Chengappa, Head, 785-532-4403, E-mail: chengap@ksu.edu. *Application contact:* T. G. Nagaraja, Director, 785-532-1214, E-mail: tnagaraj@ksu.edu.
Website: http://www.vet.k-state.edu/education/dmp/

Medical University of South Carolina, College of Graduate Studies, Program in Molecular and Cellular Biology and Pathobiology, Charleston, SC 29425. Offers cancer biology (PhD); cardiovascular biology (PhD); cardiovascular imaging (PhD); cell regulation (PhD); craniofacial biology (PhD); genetics and development (PhD); marine biomedicine (PhD); DMD/PhD; MD/PhD. *Degree requirements:* For doctorate, thesis/dissertation, oral and written exams. *Entrance requirements:* For doctorate, GRE General Test, interview, minimum GPA of 3.0. Additional exam requirements/recommendations for international students: Required—TOEFL (minimum score 600 paper-based; 100 iBT). Electronic applications accepted.

Michigan State University, College of Veterinary Medicine and The Graduate School, Graduate Programs in Veterinary Medicine, Department of Pathobiology and Diagnostic Investigation, East Lansing, MI 48824. Offers pathology (MS, PhD); pathology–environmental toxicology (PhD). *Entrance requirements:* Additional exam requirements/recommendations for international students: Required—TOEFL. Electronic applications accepted.

New York University, School of Medicine and Graduate School of Arts and Science, Sackler Institute of Graduate Biomedical Sciences, Program in Pathobiology, New York, NY 10012-1019. Offers PhD. *Faculty:* 28 full-time (6 women). *Students:* 20 full-time (16 women); includes 7 minority (2 Black or African American, non-Hispanic/Latino; 1 Asian, non-Hispanic/Latino; 4 Hispanic/Latino), 2 international. Average age 26. In 2013, 4 doctorates awarded. *Expenses: Tuition:* Full-time $35,856; part-time $1494 per unit. *Required fees:* $1408; $64 per unit. $473 per term. Tuition and fees vary according to course load and program. *Faculty research:* Identification of new targets for treatment in melanoma and pre-clinical drug testing, respiratory syncytial virus and pediatric infectious diseases, immunotherapy of cancer. *Unit head:* Dr. Joel D. Oppenheim, Senior Associate Dean for Graduate Studies, 212-263-8001, Fax: 212-263-7600. *Application contact:* Michael Escosia, Admissions Associate, 212-263-5648, Fax: 212-263-7600, E-mail: sackler-info@med.nyu.edu.

The Ohio State University, College of Medicine, Department of Pathology, Columbus, OH 43210. Offers experimental pathobiology (MS); pathology assistant (MS). *Accreditation:* NAACLS. *Faculty:* 62. *Students:* 1 (woman) full-time. In 2013, 3 master's awarded. *Degree requirements:* For master's, comprehensive exam (for some programs), thesis. *Entrance requirements:* For master's, GRE General Test. Additional exam requirements/recommendations for international students: Required—TOEFL (minimum score 550 paper-based; 79 iBT), IELTS (minimum score 7) or Michigan English Language Assessment Battery (minimum score 82). *Application deadline:* For fall admission, 12/13 priority date for domestic students, 11/30 priority date for international students. Applications are processed on a rolling basis. Application fee: $60 ($70 for international students). Electronic applications accepted. *Financial support:* In 2013–14, fellowships with full tuition reimbursements (averaging $19,008 per year), research assistantships with full tuition reimbursements (averaging $19,008 per year) were awarded; Federal Work-Study and institutionally sponsored loans also available. *Faculty research:* Clinical pathology, transplantation pathology, cancer research, neuropathology, vascular pathology. *Total annual research expenditures:* $4.1 million. *Unit head:* W. James Waldman, Graduate Studies Committee Chair, 614-292-2064, Fax: 614-292-7072, E-mail: waldman.1@osu.edu. *Application contact:* Graduate Admissions, 614-292-9444, Fax: 614-292-3895, E-mail: gradadmissions@osu.edu.
Website: http://www.pathology.osu.edu/

Penn State University Park, Graduate School, College of Agricultural Sciences, Department of Veterinary and Biomedical Sciences, University Park, PA 16802. Offers pathobiology (MS, PhD). *Unit head:* Dr. Barbara J. Christ, Interim Dean, 814-865-2541, Fax: 814-865-3103, E-mail: ebf@psu.edu. *Application contact:* Cynthia E. Nicosia, Director of Graduate Enrollment Services, 814-865-1834, Fax: 814-863-4627, E-mail: cey1@psu.edu.
Website: http://vbs.psu.edu/

Purdue University, School of Veterinary Medicine and Graduate School, Graduate Programs in Veterinary Medicine, Department of Comparative Pathobiology, West Lafayette, IN 47907-2027. Offers comparative epidemiology and public health (MS); comparative epidemiology and public heath (PhD); comparative microbiology and immunology (MS, PhD); comparative pathobiology (MS, PhD); interdisciplinary studies (PhD), including microbial pathogenesis, molecular signaling and cancer biology, molecular virology; lab animal medicine (MS); veterinary anatomic pathology (MS); veterinary clinical pathology (MS). Terminal master's awarded for partial completion of doctoral program. *Degree requirements:* For master's, thesis (for some programs); for doctorate, thesis/dissertation. *Entrance requirements:* For master's and doctorate, GRE General Test. Additional exam requirements/recommendations for international students: Required—TOEFL (minimum score 575 paper-based), IELTS (minimum score 6.5), TWE (minimum score 4). Electronic applications accepted.

Texas A&M University, College of Veterinary Medicine and Biomedical Sciences, Department of Veterinary Pathobiology, College Station, TX 77843. Offers veterinary microbiology (PhD); veterinary pathobiology (PhD); veterinary pathology (PhD). Part-time programs available. Postbaccalaureate distance learning degree programs offered. *Faculty:* 31. *Students:* 30 full-time (23 women), 14 part-time (12 women); includes 9 minority (2 Black or African American, non-Hispanic/Latino; 2 Asian, non-Hispanic/Latino; 4 Hispanic/Latino; 1 Two or more races, non-Hispanic/Latino), 9 international. Average age 30. 9 applicants, 100% accepted, 9 enrolled. In 2013, 4 doctorates awarded. Terminal master's awarded for partial completion of doctoral program. *Degree requirements:* For doctorate, thesis/dissertation, seminars. *Entrance requirements:* For doctorate, GRE General Test, minimum GPA of 3.0 in last 60 hours. Additional exam requirements/recommendations for international students: Required—TOEFL. *Application deadline:* For fall admission, 3/1 priority date for domestic students; for spring admission, 8/1 priority date for domestic students. Applications are processed on a rolling basis. Application fee: $50 ($75 for international students). Electronic applications accepted. *Expenses:* Tuition, state resident: full-time $4078; part-time $226.55 per credit hour. Tuition, nonresident: full-time $10,450; part-time $580.55 per credit hour. *Required fees:* $2328; $278.50 per credit hour. $642.45 per semester. *Financial support:* In 2013–14, fellowships with partial tuition reimbursements (averaging $16,000 per year), research assistantships with partial tuition reimbursements (averaging $15,400 per year), teaching assistantships with partial tuition reimbursements (averaging $16,000 per year) were awarded; Federal Work-Study, institutionally sponsored loans, scholarships/grants, traineeships, health care benefits, and unspecified assistantships also available. Support available to part-time students. Financial award applicants required to submit FAFSA. *Faculty research:* Infectious and noninfectious diseases of animals and birds, animal genetics, molecular biology, immunology, virology. *Unit head:* Dr. Linda Logan, Head, 979-862-6559, Fax: 979-845-9231, E-mail: llogan@cvm.tamu.edu. *Application contact:* Dr. Patricia Holman, Graduate Advisor, 979-845-4202, Fax: 979-845-9231, E-mail: pholman@cvm.tamu.edu.
Website: http://vetmed.tamu.edu/vtpb

University of Cincinnati, Graduate School, College of Medicine, Graduate Programs in Biomedical Sciences, Program in Pathobiology and Molecular Medicine, Cincinnati, OH 45221. Offers pathology (PhD), including anatomic pathology, laboratory medicine, pathobiology and molecular medicine. *Degree requirements:* For doctorate, thesis/dissertation, qualifying exam. *Entrance requirements:* For doctorate, GRE General Test. Additional exam requirements/recommendations for international students: Required—TOEFL (minimum score 620 paper-based). Electronic applications accepted. *Faculty research:* Cardiovascular and lipid disorders, digestive and kidney disease, endocrine and metabolic disorders, hematologic and oncogenic, immunology and infectious disease.

University of Connecticut, Graduate School, College of Agriculture and Natural Resources, Department of Pathobiology and Veterinary Science, Storrs, CT 06269. Offers pathobiology (MS, PhD). Terminal master's awarded for partial completion of doctoral program. *Degree requirements:* For master's, comprehensive exam; for doctorate, thesis/dissertation. *Entrance requirements:* For master's and doctorate, GRE General Test, GRE Subject Test. Additional exam requirements/recommendations for international students: Required—TOEFL (minimum score 550 paper-based). Electronic applications accepted.

University of Illinois at Urbana–Champaign, College of Veterinary Medicine, Department of Pathobiology, Urbana, IL 61802. Offers MS, PhD, DVM/PhD. *Students:* 21 (8 women). Terminal master's awarded for partial completion of doctoral program. *Degree requirements:* For doctorate, thesis/dissertation. Application fee: $75 ($90 for international students). *Unit head:* Mark S. Kuhlenschmidt, Head, 217-333-9039, Fax: 217-244-7421, E-mail: kuhlensc@illinois.edu. *Application contact:* Paula Moxley, Administrative Aide, 217-244-8924, Fax: 217-244-7421, E-mail: pkm@illinois.edu.
Website: http://vetmed.illinois.edu/path/

University of Missouri, College of Veterinary Medicine and Graduate School, Graduate Programs in Veterinary Medicine, Department of Veterinary Pathobiology, Columbia, MO 65211. Offers comparative medicine (MS); pathobiology (MS, PhD). *Faculty:* 41 full-time (14 women), 5 part-time/adjunct (2 women). *Students:* 30 full-time (18 women), 17 part-time (12 women); includes 7 minority (1 Black or African American, non-Hispanic/Latino; 2 Asian, non-Hispanic/Latino; 3 Hispanic/Latino; 1 Two or more races, non-Hispanic/Latino), 7 international. Average age 31. 37 applicants, 46% accepted, 13 enrolled. In 2013, 5 doctorates awarded. *Degree requirements:* For master's, thesis; for doctorate, 2 foreign languages, thesis/dissertation. *Entrance requirements:* For master's and doctorate, GRE General Test, minimum GPA of 3.0. Additional exam requirements/recommendations for international students: Required—TOEFL (minimum score 500 paper-based; 61 iBT). *Application deadline:* For fall admission, 1/15 for domestic students; for spring admission, 9/1 for domestic students. Application fee: $55 ($75 for international students). Electronic applications accepted. *Financial support:* Research assistantships with full tuition reimbursements, teaching assistantships with full tuition reimbursements, institutionally sponsored loans, scholarships/grants, traineeships, health care benefits, and unspecified assistantships available. Support available to part-time students. *Faculty research:* Bacteriology, cell biology, clinical pathology, comparative medicine, cytoskeletal regulation, gene expression and control, gene therapy, immunology, infectious disease, inflammatory diseases, microbiology, microscopy, molecular diagnostics, molecular genetics and genomic analysis. *Unit head:* Dr. George C. Stewart, Department Chair, 573-884-2866, E-mail: stewartgc@missouri.edu. *Application contact:* Anne Chegwidden, Grants and Contracts Specialist, 573-884-2444, E-mail: chegwiddena@missouri.edu.
Website: http://vpbio.missouri.edu/

University of Southern California, Keck School of Medicine and Graduate School, Graduate Programs in Medicine, Department of Pathology, Los Angeles, CA 90033. Offers experimental and molecular pathology (MS); pathobiology (PhD). *Faculty:* 33 full-time (5 women), 1 part-time/adjunct (0 women). *Students:* 17 full-time (11 women); includes 4 minority (1 Black or African American, non-Hispanic/Latino; 2 Asian, non-Hispanic/Latino; 1 Hispanic/Latino), 7 international. Average age 26. 8 applicants, 75% accepted, 4 enrolled. In 2013, 6 master's, 5 doctorates awarded. *Degree requirements:* For master's, experiment-based thesis or theory-based scholarly review; for doctorate, thesis/dissertation. *Entrance requirements:* For master's, GRE General Test, minimum GPA of 3.0; for doctorate, GRE General Test, minimum GPA of 3.0, BS in natural sciences. Additional exam requirements/recommendations for international students: Required—TOEFL (minimum score 600 paper-based; 100 iBT). *Application deadline:* For fall admission, 6/15 for domestic students, 6/15 priority date for international students; for spring admission, 12/1 for domestic students, 12/1 priority date for international students. Application fee: $85. Electronic applications accepted. *Financial support:* In 2013–14, 11 students received support, including 1 fellowship (averaging $31,000 per year), 10 research assistantships (averaging $31,000 per year); Federal Work-Study, institutionally sponsored loans, scholarships/grants, health care benefits, and unspecified assistantships also available. Financial award application deadline: 5/4. *Faculty research:* Cellular and molecular biology of cancer; chemical carcinogenesis; virology; stem cell and developmental pathology; liver and pulmonary diseases; environmental pathology; circulatory, endocrine, and neurodegenerative diseases. *Total annual research expenditures:* $7.5 million. *Unit head:* Dr. Michael E. Selsted, Chair, 323-442-1179, Fax: 323-442-3049, E-mail: selsted@usc.edu. *Application contact:* Lisa A. Doumak, Student Services Assistant, 323-442-1168, Fax: 323-442-3049, E-mail: doumak@usc.edu.
Website: http://www.usc.edu/hsc/medicine/pathology/

University of Toronto, Faculty of Medicine, Department of Laboratory Medicine and Pathobiology, Toronto, ON M5S 1A1, Canada. Offers M Sc, PhD. *Degree requirements:* For master's, thesis; for doctorate, thesis/dissertation, oral défense of thesis. *Entrance requirements:* For master's, minimum B+ average in final 2 years, research experience, 2 letters of recommendation, resume, interview; for doctorate, minimum A- average, 2 letters of recommendation, research experience, resume, interview. Additional exam requirements/recommendations for international students: Required—TOEFL (600 paper-based), TWE (5) or IELTS (7). Electronic applications accepted.

University of Washington, Graduate School, School of Public Health, Department of Global Health, Graduate Program in Pathobiology, Seattle, WA 98195. Offers PhD. *Faculty:* 20 full-time (8 women). *Students:* 26 full-time (17 women), 8 part-time (7 women); includes 6 minority (2 Black or African American, non-Hispanic/Latino; 4 Asian, non-Hispanic/Latino), 2 international. Average age 29. 66 applicants, 17% accepted, 5 enrolled. In 2013, 6 doctorates awarded. *Degree requirements:* For doctorate, comprehensive exam, thesis/dissertation, published paper from thesis work. *Entrance requirements:* For doctorate, GRE General Test, minimum GPA of 3.0. Additional exam requirements/recommendations for international students: Required—TOEFL, IELTS. *Application deadline:* For fall admission, 12/1 for domestic and international students. Application fee: $85. Electronic applications accepted. *Financial support:* In 2013–14, 31 students received support, including 31 research assistantships with full tuition reimbursements available (averaging $28,440 per year); traineeships and unspecified assistantships also available. *Faculty research:* Malaria, immunological response to mycobacteria infections, HIV-cell interaction and the development of an anti-HIV vaccine, regulation of intercellular communication via gap junctions, genetic and nutritional regulation of proteins involved in lipid transport. *Unit head:* Dr. King K. Holmes, Chair, 206-744-3620, Fax: 206-744-3694. *Application contact:* Rachel Reichert, Program Manager, 206-543-4338, Fax: 206-543-3873, E-mail: pabio@u.washington.edu.

University of Wyoming, College of Agriculture and Natural Resources, Department of Veterinary Sciences, Laramie, WY 82071. Offers pathobiology (MS). *Degree requirements:* For master's, thesis. *Entrance requirements:* For master's, GRE General Test, minimum GPA of 3.0. Additional exam requirements/recommendations for international students: Required—TOEFL. *Faculty research:* Infectious diseases, pathology, toxicology, immunology, microbiology.

Wake Forest University, School of Medicine and Graduate School of Arts and Sciences, Graduate Programs in Medicine, Program in Molecular and Cellular Pathobiology, Winston-Salem, NC 27109. Offers MS, PhD, MD/PhD. *Degree requirements:* For master's, thesis; for doctorate, thesis/dissertation. *Entrance requirements:* For master's and doctorate, GRE General Test. Additional exam requirements/recommendations for international students: Required—TOEFL. Electronic applications accepted. *Faculty research:* Atherosclerosis, lipoproteins, arterial wall metabolism.

Yale University, School of Medicine and Graduate School of Arts and Sciences, Combined Program in Biological and Biomedical Sciences (BBS), Pharmacological Sciences and Molecular Medicine Track, New Haven, CT 06520. Offers PhD, MD/PhD. *Degree requirements:* For doctorate, thesis/dissertation. *Entrance requirements:* For doctorate, GRE General Test. Additional exam requirements/recommendations for international students: Required—TOEFL. Electronic applications accepted.

Pathology

Albert Einstein College of Medicine, Graduate Division of Biomedical Sciences, Department of Pathology, Bronx, NY 10467. Offers PhD, MD/PhD. *Degree requirements:* For doctorate, thesis/dissertation. *Entrance requirements:* For doctorate, GRE General Test. Additional exam requirements/recommendations for international students: Required—TOEFL. *Faculty research:* Clinical and disease-related research at tissue, cellular, and subcellular levels; biochemistry and morphology of enzyme and lysosome disorders.

Baylor College of Medicine, Graduate School of Biomedical Sciences, Program in Developmental Biology, Houston, TX 77030-3498. Offers PhD, MD/PhD. *Degree requirements:* For doctorate, thesis/dissertation, public defense. *Entrance requirements:* For doctorate, GRE General Test, GRE Subject Test (strongly recommended), minimum GPA of 3.0. Additional exam requirements/recommendations for international students: Required—TOEFL. Electronic applications accepted. *Faculty research:* Stem cells, cancer, neurobiology, organogenesis, genetics of model organisms.

Boston University, School of Medicine, Division of Graduate Medical Sciences, Department of Pathology and Laboratory Medicine, Boston, MA 02118. Offers PhD, MD/PhD. Part-time programs available. *Degree requirements:* For doctorate, thesis/dissertation. *Entrance requirements:* Additional exam requirements/recommendations for international students: Required—TOEFL. *Application deadline:* For fall admission, 1/15 for domestic students; for spring admission, 10/15 for domestic students. *Expenses: Tuition:* Full-time $43,970; part-time $1374 per credit hour. *Required fees:* $60 per semester. Tuition and fees vary according to class time, course level and program. *Financial support:* Scholarships/grants and traineeships available. Financial award applicants required to submit FAFSA. *Unit head:* Dr. Daniel G. Remick, Chairman, 617-414-7043, E-mail: remickd@bu.edu. *Application contact:* Debra Kiley, Assistant to the Chair, 617-414-7914, E-mail: dekiley@bu.edu.
Website: http://www.bumc.bu.edu/busm-pathology/

Case Western Reserve University, School of Medicine and School of Graduate Studies, Graduate Programs in Medicine, Programs in Molecular and Cellular Basis of Disease/Pathology, Cleveland, OH 44106. Offers cancer biology (PhD); cell biology (MS, PhD); immunology (MS, PhD); pathology (MS, PhD); MD/PhD. Terminal master's awarded for partial completion of doctoral program. *Degree requirements:* For master's, thesis; for doctorate, thesis/dissertation. *Entrance requirements:* For master's and doctorate, GRE General Test, GRE Subject Test. Additional exam requirements/recommendations for international students: Required—TOEFL (minimum score 550 paper-based). Electronic applications accepted. *Faculty research:* Neurobiology, molecular biology, cancer biology, biomaterials, biocompatibility.

Colorado State University, College of Veterinary Medicine and Biomedical Sciences, Department of Microbiology, Immunology and Pathology, Fort Collins, CO 80523. Offers microbiology (MS, PhD); pathology (PhD). *Faculty:* 50 full-time (22 women), 4 part-time/adjunct (1 woman). *Students:* 73 full-time (51 women), 31 part-time (24 women); includes 15 minority (1 Black or African American, non-Hispanic/Latino; 2 American Indian or Alaska Native, non-Hispanic/Latino; 3 Asian, non-Hispanic/Latino; 8 Hispanic/Latino; 1 Two or more races, non-Hispanic/Latino), 9 international. Average age 29. 135 applicants, 31% accepted, 38 enrolled. In 2013, 3 master's, 11 doctorates awarded. *Degree requirements:* For master's, thesis; for doctorate, comprehensive exam, thesis/dissertation. *Entrance requirements:* For master's, GRE General Test, minimum GPA of 3.0, BA/BS in biomedical field, reviewer evaluation forms, resume, transcripts, personal statement, 3 letters of recommendation; for doctorate, GRE General Test, minimum GPA of 3.0, BA/BS in biomedical field, reviewer evaluation forms, resume, personal statement, transcripts, 3 letters of recommendation. Additional exam requirements/recommendations for international students: Required—TOEFL (minimum score 550 paper-based). *Application deadline:* For fall admission, 1/1 priority date for domestic students; for spring admission, 10/1 priority date for domestic students. Applications are processed on a rolling basis. Application fee: $50. Electronic applications accepted. *Expenses:* Tuition, state resident: full-time $9075.40; part-time $504 per credit. Tuition, nonresident: full-time $22,248; part-time $1236 per credit. *Required fees:* $1819; $60 per credit. *Financial support:* In 2013–14, 82 students received support, including 40 fellowships with tuition reimbursements available (averaging $35,362 per year), 38 research assistantships with tuition reimbursements available (averaging $17,799 per year), 4 teaching assistantships with tuition reimbursements available (averaging $15,606 per year); Federal Work-Study, scholarships/grants, traineeships, and unspecified assistantships also available. Financial award applicants required to submit FAFSA. *Faculty research:* Medical and veterinary bacteriology, immunology, microbial physiology, pathology, vector-borne disease. *Total annual research expenditures:* $29.9 million. *Unit head:* Dr. Gregg A. Dean, Head, 970-491-6144, Fax: 970-491-1815, E-mail: gregg.dean@colostate.edu. *Application contact:* Lisa McCann, Academic Programs Coordinator, 970-491-6118, Fax: 970-491-1815, E-mail: lisa.mccann@colostate.edu.
Website: http://csu-cvmbs.colostate.edu/academics/mip/graduate/Pages/default.aspx

Columbia University, College of Physicians and Surgeons, Department of Pathology, New York, NY 10032. Offers pathobiology (M Phil, MA, PhD); MD/PhD. Only candidates for the PhD are admitted. Terminal master's awarded for partial completion of doctoral program. *Degree requirements:* For doctorate, thesis/dissertation. *Entrance requirements:* For master's and doctorate, GRE General Test. Additional exam requirements/recommendations for international students: Required—TOEFL. *Faculty research:* Virology, molecular biology, cell biology, neurobiology, immunology.

Dalhousie University, Faculty of Graduate Studies and Faculty of Medicine, Graduate Programs in Medicine, Department of Pathology, Halifax, NS B3H 4R2, Canada. Offers M Sc, PhD. *Degree requirements:* For master's, oral defense of thesis. *Entrance requirements:* Additional exam requirements/recommendations for international students: Required—1 of 5 approved tests: TOEFL, IELTS, CANTEST, CAEL, Michigan English Language Assessment Battery. Electronic applications accepted. *Faculty* *research:* Tumor immunology, molecular oncology, clinical chemistry, hematology, molecular genetics/oncology.

Duke University, Graduate School, Department of Pathology, Durham, NC 27710. Offers PhD. *Accreditation:* NAACLS. *Faculty:* 37. *Students:* 19 full-time (6 women); includes 5 minority (3 Black or African American, non-Hispanic/Latino; 2 Asian, non-Hispanic/Latino), 9 international. 29 applicants, 14% accepted, 1 enrolled. In 2013, 6 doctorates awarded. *Degree requirements:* For doctorate, thesis/dissertation. *Entrance requirements:* For doctorate, GRE General Test, GRE Subject Test (recommended). Additional exam requirements/recommendations for international students: Required—TOEFL (minimum score 577 paper-based; 90 iBT) or IELTS (minimum score 7). *Application deadline:* For fall admission, 12/8 priority date for domestic and international students. Application fee: $80. Electronic applications accepted. *Financial support:* Fellowships, research assistantships, and Federal Work-Study available. Financial award application deadline: 12/8. *Unit head:* Soman Abraham, Director of Graduate Studies, 919-684-9929, Fax: 919-681-8868, E-mail: harri232@mc.duke.edu. *Application contact:* Elizabeth Hutton, Director of Admissions, 919-684-3913, Fax: 919-684-2277, E-mail: grad-admissions@duke.edu.
Website: http://pathology.duke.edu/home

Duke University, School of Medicine, Pathologists' Assistant Program, Durham, NC 27708-0586. Offers MHS. *Accreditation:* NAACLS. *Faculty:* 1 (woman) full-time, 45 part-time/adjunct (23 women). *Students:* 16 full-time (13 women); includes 5 minority (1 Black or African American, non-Hispanic/Latino; 3 Asian, non-Hispanic/Latino; 1 Hispanic/Latino). Average age 26. 64 applicants, 14% accepted, 8 enrolled. In 2013, 8 master's awarded. *Degree requirements:* For master's, comprehensive exam. *Entrance requirements:* For master's, GRE. Additional exam requirements/recommendations for international students: Required—TOEFL, IELTS. *Application deadline:* For fall admission, 1/31 priority date for domestic students. Application fee: $55. *Expenses:* Contact institution. *Financial support:* In 2013–14, 7 students received support. Fellowships, research assistantships, teaching assistantships, and scholarships/grants available. Financial award application deadline: 5/1; financial award applicants required to submit FAFSA. *Unit head:* Dr. Rex C. Bentley, Program Director, 919-684-6423, Fax: 919-681-7634, E-mail: bentl003@mc.duke.edu. *Application contact:* Pamela Vollmer, Associate Director, 919-684-2159, Fax: 919-684-8693, E-mail: pamela.vollmer@duke.edu.
Website: http://pathology.mc.duke.edu/website/webform.aspx?id-AP_PATHASSISTMAIN

East Carolina University, Brody School of Medicine, Department of Pathology and Laboratory Medicine, Greenville, NC 27858-4353. Offers PhD. *Degree requirements:* For doctorate, comprehensive exam, thesis/dissertation. *Entrance requirements:* For doctorate, GRE General Test, bachelor's degree in biological chemistry or physical science. *Application deadline:* For fall admission, 6/1 priority date for domestic students. Application fee: $50. *Expenses:* Tuition, state resident: full-time $4223. Tuition, nonresident: full-time $16,540. *Required fees:* $2184. *Financial support:* Fellowships available. Financial award application deadline: 6/1. *Unit head:* Dr. Peter J. Kragel, Chair, 252-744-2803, E-mail: kragelp@ecu.edu. *Application contact:* Contact Center, 252-744-1020.
Website: http://www.pathology.ecu.edu/Public/graduate/phdinfo_new.htm

Harvard University, Graduate School of Arts and Sciences, Division of Medical Sciences, Boston, MA 02115. Offers biological chemistry and molecular pharmacology (PhD); cell biology (PhD); genetics (PhD); microbiology and molecular genetics (PhD); pathology (PhD), including experimental pathology. *Degree requirements:* For doctorate, thesis/dissertation. *Entrance requirements:* For doctorate, GRE General Test, GRE Subject Test. Additional exam requirements/recommendations for international students: Required—TOEFL. *Expenses: Tuition:* Full-time $38,888. *Required fees:* $958. Tuition and fees vary according to campus/location, program and student level.

Indiana University–Purdue University Indianapolis, Indiana University School of Medicine, Department of Pathology and Laboratory Medicine, Indianapolis, IN 46202-2896. Offers MS, PhD, MD/PhD. *Faculty:* 27 full-time (4 women). *Students:* 5 full-time (3 women), 4 part-time (3 women); includes 1 minority (Hispanic/Latino), 1 international. Average age 26. 65 applicants, 6% accepted, 4 enrolled. In 2013, 5 master's awarded. *Degree requirements:* For master's, thesis; for doctorate, thesis/dissertation. *Entrance requirements:* For master's and doctorate, GRE General Test. Additional exam requirements/recommendations for international students: Required—TOEFL. *Application deadline:* For fall admission, 1/15 priority date for domestic students. Applications are processed on a rolling basis. Application fee: $55 ($65 for international students). *Financial support:* Fellowships, research assistantships with full tuition reimbursements, teaching assistantships with full tuition reimbursements, and institutionally sponsored loans available. Financial award application deadline: 2/1. *Faculty research:* Intestinal microecology and anaerobes, molecular pathogenesis of infectious diseases, AIDS, pneumocystis, sports medicine toxicology, neuropathology of aging. *Unit head:* Dr. John Eble, Chairman, 317-274-4806. *Application contact:* Dr. Diane S. Leland, Graduate Adviser, 317-274-0148.
Website: http://www.pathology.iupui.edu

Iowa State University of Science and Technology, Department of Veterinary Pathology, Ames, IA 50011. Offers MS, PhD. *Entrance requirements:* For master's and doctorate, GRE General Test. Additional exam requirements/recommendations for international students: Recommended—TOEFL (minimum score 550 paper-based; 79 iBT), IELTS (minimum score 6.5). Electronic applications accepted.

Johns Hopkins University, School of Medicine, Graduate Programs in Medicine, Department of Pathology, Baltimore, MD 21218-2699. Offers pathobiology (PhD). *Faculty:* 68 full-time (14 women). *Students:* 47 full-time (28 women); includes 7 minority (1 Black or African American, non-Hispanic/Latino; 4 Asian, non-Hispanic/Latino; 1 Hispanic/Latino; 1 Two or more races, non-Hispanic/Latino), 23 international. Average age 28. 47 applicants, 21% accepted, 6 enrolled. In 2013, 7 doctorates awarded. *Degree requirements:* For doctorate, thesis/dissertation, qualifying oral exam. *Entrance requirements:* For doctorate, GRE General Test, previous course work with laboratory in organic and inorganic chemistry, general biology, calculus; interview. Additional exam requirements/recommendations for international students: Required—TOEFL. *Application deadline:* For winter admission, 1/10 for domestic students. Application fee: $85. Electronic applications accepted. *Financial support:* Fellowships and scholarships/grants available. *Faculty research:* Role of mutant proteins in Alzheimer's disease, nuclear protein function in breast and prostate cancer, medically important fungi, glycoproteins in HIV pathogenesis. *Total annual research expenditures:* $38.6 million. *Unit head:* Dr. J. Brooks Jackson, Chair, 410-955-9790, Fax: 410-955-0394. *Application contact:* Wilhelmena M. Braswell, Senior Academic Program Coordinator, 443-287-3163, Fax: 410-614-3548, E-mail: wbraswel@jhmi.edu.
Website: http://www.pathology.jhu.edu/

Loma Linda University, School of Medicine, Department of Pathology and Human Anatomy, Loma Linda, CA 92350. Offers MS, PhD. Part-time programs available. Terminal master's awarded for partial completion of doctoral program. *Degree requirements:* For master's, thesis; for doctorate, 2 foreign languages, thesis/dissertation. *Entrance requirements:* For master's and doctorate, GRE General Test. Additional exam requirements/recommendations for international students: Required—TOEFL (minimum score 550 paper-based). *Faculty research:* Neuroendocrine system, histochemistry and image analysis, effect of age and diabetes on PNS, electron microscopy, histology.

McGill University, Faculty of Graduate and Postdoctoral Studies, Faculty of Medicine, Department of Pathology, Montréal, QC H3A 2T5, Canada. Offers M Sc, PhD.

Medical University of South Carolina, College of Graduate Studies, Department of Pathology and Laboratory Medicine, Charleston, SC 29425. Offers MS, PhD, DMD/PhD, MD/PhD. Terminal master's awarded for partial completion of doctoral program. *Degree requirements:* For master's, thesis; for doctorate, thesis/dissertation, oral and written exams. *Entrance requirements:* For master's, GRE General Test; for doctorate, GRE General Test, interview, minimum GPA of 3.0. Additional exam requirements/recommendations for international students: Required—TOEFL (minimum score 600 paper-based; 100 iBT). Electronic applications accepted. *Faculty research:* Neurobiology of hearing loss; inner ear ion homeostasis; cancer biology, genetics and stem cell biology; cellular defense mechanisms.

Michigan State University, College of Veterinary Medicine and The Graduate School, Graduate Programs in Veterinary Medicine, Department of Pathobiology and Diagnostic Investigation, East Lansing, MI 48824. Offers pathology (MS, PhD); pathology–environmental toxicology (PhD). *Entrance requirements:* Additional exam requirements/recommendations for international students: Required—TOEFL. Electronic applications accepted.

New York Medical College, Graduate School of Basic Medical Sciences, Integrated PhD Program, Valhalla, NY 10595-1691. Offers biochemistry and molecular biology (PhD); cell biology and anatomy (PhD); microbiology and immunology (PhD); pathology (PhD); pharmacology (PhD); physiology (PhD). *Faculty:* 91 full-time (16 women), 5 part-time/adjunct (2 women). *Students:* 31 full-time (21 women); includes 17 minority (4 Black or African American, non-Hispanic/Latino; 11 Asian, non-Hispanic/Latino; 2 Hispanic/Latino). Average age 27. 56 applicants, 36% accepted, 9 enrolled. In 2013, 17 doctorates awarded. *Degree requirements:* For doctorate, comprehensive exam, thesis/dissertation. *Entrance requirements:* For doctorate, GRE General Test. Additional exam requirements/recommendations for international students: Required—TOEFL. *Application deadline:* For fall admission, 1/1 priority date for domestic and international students. Applications are processed on a rolling basis. Application fee: $75 ($100 for international students). Electronic applications accepted. *Expenses: Tuition:* Full-time $49,170; part-time $910 per credit. Tuition and fees vary according to program. *Financial support:* In 2013–14, fellowships with full tuition reimbursements (averaging $25,500 per year), research assistantships with full tuition reimbursements (averaging $25,500 per year) were awarded; Federal Work-Study, scholarships/grants, traineeships, health care benefits, and tuition waivers (full) also available. Financial award applicants required to submit FAFSA. *Faculty research:* Cardiovascular sciences, infectious diseases, neuroscience, cancer and cell signaling. *Unit head:* Dr. Francis L. Belloni, Dean, 914-594-4110, Fax: 914-594-4944, E-mail: francis_belloni@nymc.edu. *Application contact:* Valerie Romeo-Messana, Director of Admissions, 914-594-4110, Fax: 914-594-4944, E-mail: v_romeomessana@nymc.edu.

New York Medical College, Graduate School of Basic Medical Sciences, Pathology Master's Program, Valhalla, NY 10595-1691. Offers MS, PhD, MD/PhD. Part-time and evening/weekend programs available. *Faculty:* 19 full-time (2 women). *Students:* 11 full-time (7 women); includes 4 minority (2 Asian, non-Hispanic/Latino; 2 Hispanic/Latino). Average age 25. 6 applicants, 83% accepted, 2 enrolled. In 2013, 1 master's awarded. Terminal master's awarded for partial completion of doctoral program. *Degree requirements:* For master's, thesis; for doctorate, comprehensive exam, thesis/dissertation. *Entrance requirements:* For master's, GRE General Test, MCAT, or DAT. Additional exam requirements/recommendations for international students: Required—TOEFL. *Application deadline:* For fall admission, 7/1 priority date for domestic students, 5/1 priority date for international students; for spring admission, 12/1 priority date for domestic students, 9/15 priority date for international students. Applications are processed on a rolling basis. Application fee: $75 ($100 for international students). Electronic applications accepted. *Expenses: Tuition:* Full-time $49,170; part-time $910 per credit. Tuition and fees vary according to program. *Financial support:* Federal Work-Study and scholarships/grants available. Support available to part-time students. Financial award applicants required to submit FAFSA. *Faculty research:* Examination of the underlying mechanisms involved in biochemical toxicology, cancer cell biology, cell-cycle regulation and apoptosis, chemical carcinogenesis and tissue engineering. *Unit head:* Dr. Fred Moy, Program Director, 914-594-4174, Fax: 914-594-4944, E-mail: fred_moy@nymc.edu. *Application contact:* Valerie Romeo-Messana, Director of Admissions, 914-594-4110, Fax: 914-594-4944, E-mail: v_romeomessana@nymc.edu.

North Carolina State University, College of Veterinary Medicine, Program in Comparative Biomedical Sciences, Raleigh, NC 27695. Offers cell biology (MS, PhD); infectious disease (MS, PhD); pathology (MS, PhD); pharmacology (MS, PhD); population medicine (MS, PhD). Part-time programs available. *Degree requirements:* For master's, thesis; for doctorate, thesis/dissertation. *Entrance requirements:* For master's and doctorate, GRE General Test. Additional exam requirements/recommendations for international students: Required—TOEFL (minimum score 550 paper-based). Electronic applications accepted. *Expenses:* Contact institution. *Faculty research:* Infectious diseases, cell biology, pharmacology and toxicology, genomics, pathology and population medicine.

North Dakota State University, College of Graduate and Interdisciplinary Studies, College of Agriculture, Food Systems, and Natural Resources, Department of Veterinary and Microbiological Sciences, Fargo, ND 58108. Offers international infectious disease (MS); microbiology (MS); molecular pathogenesis (PhD). Part-time programs available. *Faculty:* 15 full-time (8 women). *Students:* 11 full-time (6 women), 6 part-time (4 women), 5 international. Average age 30. 2 applicants, 50% accepted, 1 enrolled. In 2013, 8 master's, 1 doctorate awarded. *Degree requirements:* For master's, thesis; for doctorate, thesis/dissertation, oral and written preliminary exams. *Entrance requirements:* For master's and doctorate, GRE. Additional exam requirements/recommendations for international students: Required—TOEFL (minimum score 525 paper-based; 71 iBT). *Application deadline:* For fall admission, 2/15 priority date for domestic students. Applications are processed on a rolling basis. Application fee: $35. *Financial support:* Fellowships with full tuition reimbursements, research assistantships with full tuition reimbursements, teaching assistantships with full tuition reimbursements, Federal Work-Study, and institutionally sponsored loans available. Financial award application deadline: 4/15. *Faculty research:* Bacterial gene regulation, antibiotic resistance, molecular virology, mechanisms of bacterial pathogenesis, immunology of animals. *Unit head:* Dr. Charlene Wolf-Hall, Head, 701-231-7667, E-mail: charlene.hall@ndsu.edu. *Application contact:* Dr. John McEvoy, Associate Professor, 701-231-8530, Fax: 701-231-7514, E-mail: eugene.berry@ndsu.edu.
Website: http://vetmicro.ndsu.nodak.edu/

The Ohio State University, College of Medicine, Department of Pathology, Columbus, OH 43210. Offers experimental pathobiology (MS); pathology assistant (MS). *Accreditation:* NAACLS. *Faculty:* 62. *Students:* 1 (woman) full-time. In 2013, 3 master's awarded. *Degree requirements:* For master's, comprehensive exam (for some

programs), thesis. *Entrance requirements:* For master's, GRE General Test. Additional exam requirements/recommendations for international students: Required—TOEFL (minimum score 550 paper-based; 79 iBT), IELTS (minimum score 7) or Michigan English Language Assessment Battery (minimum score 82). *Application deadline:* For fall admission, 12/13 priority date for domestic students, 11/30 priority date for international students. Applications are processed on a rolling basis. Application fee: $60 ($70 for international students). Electronic applications accepted. *Financial support:* In 2013–14, fellowships with full tuition reimbursements (averaging $19,008 per year), research assistantships with full tuition reimbursements (averaging $19,008 per year) were awarded; Federal Work-Study and institutionally sponsored loans also available. *Faculty research:* Clinical pathology, transplantation pathology, cancer research, neuropathology, vascular pathology. *Total annual research expenditures:* $4.1 million. *Unit head:* W. James Waldman, Graduate Studies Committee Chair, 614-292-2064, Fax: 614-292-7072, E-mail: waldman.1@osu.edu. *Application contact:* Graduate Admissions, 614-292-9444, Fax: 614-292-3895, E-mail: gradadmissions@osu.edu.
Website: http://www.pathology.osu.edu/

Oklahoma State University Center for Health Sciences, Graduate Program in Forensic Sciences, Tulsa, OK 74107. Offers forensic biology/DNA (MS); forensic document examination/forensic pathology (MS); forensic psychology (MS); forensic science administration (MS); microbiology (MS); trace evidence/forensic toxicology (MS). Part-time and evening/weekend programs available. Postbaccalaureate distance learning degree programs offered (no on-campus study). *Faculty:* 4 full-time (0 women), 14 part-time/adjunct (6 women). *Students:* 4 full-time (0 women), 14 part-time (6 women); includes 7 minority (4 American Indian or Alaska Native, non-Hispanic/Latino; 3 Hispanic/Latino), 3 international. Average age 31. 28 applicants, 50% accepted, 5 enrolled. In 2013, 5 master's awarded. *Degree requirements:* For master's, comprehensive exam, thesis (for some programs), creative component (for non-thesis options). *Entrance requirements:* For master's, MAT (for options in forensic science administration and forensic document examination) or GRE General Test, professional experience (for options in forensic science administration and forensic document examination). Additional exam requirements/recommendations for international students: Required—TOEFL (minimum score 100 iBT) or IELTS (minimum score 7.0). *Application deadline:* For fall admission, 3/1 for domestic and international students; for spring admission, 10/1 for domestic and international students; for summer admission, 7/1 for domestic and international students. Applications are processed on a rolling basis. Application fee: $40 ($75 for international students). Electronic applications accepted. *Expenses:* Tuition, state resident: full-time $22,127; part-time $178 per credit hour. Tuition, nonresident: full-time $43,572; part-time $728 per credit hour. *Required fees:* $910.79; $200 per semester. *Financial support:* In 2013–14, 14 students received support, including 8 research assistantships (averaging $12,000 per year); career-related internships or fieldwork, Federal Work-Study, and tuition waivers (partial) also available. Support available to part-time students. Financial award application deadline: 4/1; financial award applicants required to submit FAFSA. *Faculty research:* Studies on the variability in chromosomal DNA; development/enhancement of accessory methods useful for forensic DNA typing; development of universal methods useful for discriminating pathogenic bacteria; forensic dentistry; transmission of microbial diseases by dentures, protective athletic mouth-guards, band wind instruments, and infant pacifiers; changes in ecologies and antibiotic sensitivities of aerobic microorganisms; forensic toxicology and trace chemical method development. *Total annual research expenditures:* $58,000. *Unit head:* Dr. Robert W. Allen, Director, 918-561-1108, Fax: 918-561-8414. *Application contact:* Cathy Newsome, Coordinator, 918-561-1108, Fax: 918-561-8414, E-mail: cathy.newsome@okstate.edu.
Website: http://www.healthsciences.okstate.edu/forensic/index.cfm

Purdue University, School of Veterinary Medicine and Graduate School, Graduate Programs in Veterinary Medicine, Department of Comparative Pathobiology, West Lafayette, IN 47907-2027. Offers comparative epidemiology and public health (MS); comparative epidemiology and public heath (PhD); comparative microbiology and immunology (MS, PhD); comparative pathobiology (MS, PhD); interdisciplinary studies (PhD), including microbial pathogenesis, molecular signaling and cancer biology, molecular virology; lab animal medicine (MS); veterinary anatomic pathology (MS); veterinary clinical pathology (MS). Terminal master's awarded for partial completion of doctoral program. *Degree requirements:* For master's, thesis (for some programs); for doctorate, thesis/dissertation. *Entrance requirements:* For master's and doctorate, GRE General Test. Additional exam requirements/recommendations for international students: Required—TOEFL (minimum score 575 paper-based), IELTS (minimum score 6.5), TWE (minimum score 4). Electronic applications accepted.

Queen's University at Kingston, School of Graduate Studies, Faculty of Health Sciences, Department of Pathology and Molecular Medicine, Kingston, ON K7L 3N6, Canada. Offers M Sc, PhD. Part-time programs available. *Degree requirements:* For master's, thesis; for doctorate, comprehensive exam, thesis/dissertation. *Entrance requirements:* Additional exam requirements/recommendations for international students: Required—TOEFL. *Faculty research:* Immunopathology, cancer biology, immunology and metastases, cell differentiation, blood coagulation.

Quinnipiac University, School of Health Sciences, Program for Pathologists' Assistant, Hamden, CT 06518-1940. Offers MHS. *Accreditation:* NAACLS. *Faculty:* 1 full-time (0 women), 4 part-time/adjunct (3 women). *Students:* 39 full-time (27 women); includes 9 minority (4 Black or African American, non-Hispanic/Latino; 2 Asian, non-Hispanic/Latino; 3 Hispanic/Latino). 150 applicants, 18% accepted, 22 enrolled. In 2013, 18 master's awarded. *Degree requirements:* For master's, residency. *Entrance requirements:* For master's, interview, coursework in biological and health sciences, minimum GPA of 2.8. *Application deadline:* For fall admission, 11/1 for domestic students; for summer admission, 10/1 for domestic students. Applications are processed on a rolling basis. Application fee: $45. Electronic applications accepted. *Expenses: Tuition:* Part-time $920 per credit. *Required fees:* $37 per credit. *Financial support:* In 2013–14, 8 students received support. Career-related internships or fieldwork, scholarships/grants, and unspecified assistantships available. Support available to part-time students. Financial award application deadline: 6/1; financial award applicants required to submit FAFSA. *Faculty research:* ACL injury mechanism and running injuries and performance; transcriptional activators upstream stimulatory factor (USF); identification of novel antimicrobials; vaccines, formites and opportunistic pathogens; molecular biology of the Lyme Disease agent, Borrelia burgdorferi; molecular and microscopic techniques in host-pathogen interactions; non-invasive vascular biology, external pneumatic compression, sports performance. *Unit head:* Dr. Kenneth Kaloustian, Director, E-mail: kenneth.kaloustian@quinnipiac.edu. *Application contact:* Office of Graduate Admissions, 800-462-1944, Fax: 203-582-3443, E-mail: paadmissions@quinnipiac.edu.
Website: http://www.quinnipiac.edu/gradpathologists

Rosalind Franklin University of Medicine and Science, College of Health Professions, Pathologists' Assistant Department, North Chicago, IL 60064-3095. Offers MS. *Accreditation:* NAACLS. *Entrance requirements:* For master's, bachelor's degree from an accredited college or university, minimum cumulative GPA of 3.0. Additional exam requirements/recommendations for international students: Required—TOEFL. *Faculty research:* Adaptation of ACGME/ADASP pathology resident training competencies to pathologists' assistant clinical education, utilization of structural portfolios in pathologists' assistant clinical education.

Rutgers, The State University of New Jersey, Newark, Graduate School of Biomedical Sciences, Program in Molecular Pathology and Immunology, Newark, NJ 07107. Offers PhD. *Entrance requirements:* Additional exam requirements/recommendations for international students: Required—TOEFL. Electronic applications accepted.

Saint Louis University, Graduate Education and School of Medicine, Graduate Program in Biomedical Sciences and Graduate Education, Department of Pathology, St. Louis, MO 63103-2097. Offers PhD. *Degree requirements:* For doctorate, comprehensive exam, thesis/dissertation, oral and written preliminary exams, oral defense of dissertation. *Entrance requirements:* For doctorate, GRE General Test (GRE Subject Test optional), letters of recommendation, resume, interview. Additional exam requirements/recommendations for international students: Required—TOEFL (minimum score 525 paper-based). Electronic applications accepted. *Faculty research:* Cancer research, hepatitis C virology, cell imaging, liver disease.

Stony Brook University, State University of New York, Graduate School, College of Arts and Sciences, Department of Biochemistry and Cell Biology, Molecular and Cellular Biology Program, Stony Brook, NY 11794. Offers biochemistry and molecular biology (PhD); biological sciences (MA); immunology and pathology (PhD); molecular and cellular biology (PhD). *Faculty:* 23 full-time (7 women), 1 part-time/adjunct (0 women). *Students:* 75 full-time (42 women); includes 7 minority (5 Asian, non-Hispanic/Latino; 2 Hispanic/Latino), 46 international. Average age 30. 211 applicants, 15% accepted, 8 enrolled. In 2013, 13 master's, 15 doctorates awarded. *Degree requirements:* For doctorate, comprehensive exam, thesis/dissertation, teaching experience. *Entrance requirements:* For doctorate, GRE General Test, GRE Subject Test. Additional exam requirements/recommendations for international students: Required—TOEFL. *Application deadline:* For fall admission, 1/15 for domestic students; for spring admission, 10/1 for domestic students. Application fee: $100. *Expenses:* Tuition, state resident: full-time $9870; part-time $411 per credit. Tuition, nonresident: full-time $18,350; part-time $765 per credit. *Financial support:* In 2013–14, 22 fellowships, 18 research assistantships, 12 teaching assistantships were awarded; Federal Work-Study also available. *Unit head:* Prof. Robert Haltiwanger, Chair, 631-632-8560, E-mail: robert.haltiwanger@stonybrook.edu. *Application contact:* Joann DeLucia-Conlon, Coordinator, 631-632-8613, Fax: 631-632-9730, E-mail: joann.delucia-conlon@stonybrook.edu.

Texas A&M University, College of Veterinary Medicine and Biomedical Sciences, Department of Veterinary Pathobiology, College Station, TX 77843. Offers veterinary microbiology (PhD); veterinary pathobiology (PhD); veterinary pathology (PhD). Part-time programs available. Postbaccalaureate distance learning degree programs offered. *Faculty:* 31. *Students:* 30 full-time (23 women), 14 part-time (12 women); includes 9 minority (2 Black or African American, non-Hispanic/Latino; 2 Asian, non-Hispanic/Latino; 4 Hispanic/Latino; 1 Two or more races, non-Hispanic/Latino), 9 international. Average age 30. 9 applicants, 100% accepted, 9 enrolled. In 2013, 4 doctorates awarded. Terminal master's awarded for partial completion of doctoral program. *Degree requirements:* For doctorate, thesis/dissertation, seminars. *Entrance requirements:* For doctorate, GRE General Test, minimum GPA of 3.0 in last 60 hours. Additional exam requirements/recommendations for international students: Required—TOEFL. *Application deadline:* For fall admission, 3/1 priority date for domestic students; for spring admission, 8/1 priority date for domestic students. Applications are processed on a rolling basis. Application fee: $50 ($75 for international students). Electronic applications accepted. *Expenses:* Tuition, state resident: full-time $4078; part-time $226.55 per credit hour. Tuition, nonresident: full-time $10,450; part-time $580.55 per credit hour. *Required fees:* $2328; $278.50 per credit hour. $642.45 per semester. *Financial support:* In 2013–14, fellowships with partial tuition reimbursements (averaging $16,000 per year), research assistantships with partial tuition reimbursements (averaging $15,400 per year), teaching assistantships with partial tuition reimbursements (averaging $16,000 per year) were awarded; Federal Work-Study, institutionally sponsored loans, scholarships/grants, traineeships, health care benefits, and unspecified assistantships also available. Support available to part-time students. Financial award applicants required to submit FAFSA. *Faculty research:* Infectious and noninfectious diseases of animals and birds, animal genetics, molecular biology, immunology, virology. *Unit head:* Dr. Linda Logan, Head, 979-862-6559, Fax: 979-845-9231, E-mail: llogan@cvm.tamu.edu. *Application contact:* Dr. Patricia Holman, Graduate Advisor, 979-845-4202, Fax: 979-845-9231, E-mail: pholman@cvm.tamu.edu.
Website: http://vetmed.tamu.edu/vtpb

Tufts University, Cummings School of Veterinary Medicine, North Grafton, MA 01536. Offers animals and public policy (MS); biomedical sciences (PhD), including digestive diseases, infectious diseases, neuroscience and reproductive biology, pathology; conservation medicine (MS); veterinary medicine (DVM); DVM/MPH; DVM/MS. *Accreditation:* AVMA (one or more programs are accredited). *Faculty:* 98 full-time (45 women), 13 part-time/adjunct (7 women). *Students:* 426 full-time (364 women); includes 60 minority (5 Black or African American, non-Hispanic/Latino; 1 American Indian or Alaska Native, non-Hispanic/Latino; 32 Asian, non-Hispanic/Latino; 20 Hispanic/Latino; 2 Two or more races, non-Hispanic/Latino), 4 international. Average age 25. 899 applicants, 29% accepted, 119 enrolled. In 2013, 85 master's, 2 doctorates awarded. *Degree requirements:* For master's, thesis (for some programs); for doctorate, comprehensive exam, thesis/dissertation (for some programs). *Entrance requirements:* For master's and doctorate, GRE General Test. Additional exam requirements/recommendations for international students: Required—TOEFL or IELTS. *Application deadline:* For fall admission, 11/1 for domestic and international students. Application fee: $70. Electronic applications accepted. *Expenses:* Contact institution. *Financial support:* In 2013–14, 230 students received support, including 7 research assistantships with full tuition reimbursements available (averaging $25,000 per year), 6 teaching assistantships (averaging $5,000 per year); career-related internships or fieldwork, Federal Work-Study, institutionally sponsored loans, scholarships/grants, and institutional aid awards, health care benefits for PhD students also available. Financial award application deadline: 4/15; financial award applicants required to submit FAFSA. *Faculty research:* Oncology, veterinary ethics, international veterinary medicine, veterinary genomics, pathogenesis of Clostridium difficile, wildlife fertility control. *Unit head:* Dr. Deborah T. Kochevar, Dean, 508-839-5302, Fax: 508-839-2953, E-mail: deborah.kochevar@tufts.edu. *Application contact:* Rebecca Russo, Director of Admissions, 508-839-7920, Fax: 508-887-4820, E-mail: vetadmissions@tufts.edu.
Website: http://www.tufts.edu/

Université de Montréal, Faculty of Medicine, Department of Pathology and Cellular Biology, Montréal, QC H3C 3J7, Canada. Offers M Sc, PhD. Terminal master's awarded for partial completion of doctoral program. *Degree requirements:* For master's, thesis; for doctorate, thesis/dissertation, general exam. *Entrance requirements:* For master's and doctorate, proficiency in French, knowledge of English. Electronic applications accepted. *Faculty research:* Immunopathology, cardiovascular pathology, oncogenetics, cellular neurocytology, muscular dystrophy.

Université Laval, Faculty of Medicine, Post-Professional Programs in Medical Studies, Québec, QC G1K 7P4, Canada. Offers anatomy–pathology (DESS); anesthesiology

(DESS); cardiology (DESS); care of older people (Diploma); clinical research (DESS); community health (DESS); dermatology (DESS); diagnostic radiology (DESS); emergency medicine (Diploma); family medicine (DESS); general surgery (DESS); geriatrics (DESS); hematology (DESS); internal medicine (DESS); maternal and fetal medicine (Diploma); medical biochemistry (DESS); medical microbiology and infectious diseases (DESS); medical oncology (DESS); nephrology (DESS); neurology (DESS); neurosurgery (DESS); obstetrics and gynecology (DESS); ophthalmology (DESS); orthopedic surgery (DESS); oto-rhino-laryngology (DESS); palliative medicine (Diploma); pediatrics (DESS); plastic surgery (DESS); psychiatry (DESS); pulmonary medicine (DESS); radiology–oncology (DESS); thoracic surgery (DESS); urology (DESS). *Degree requirements:* For other advanced degree, comprehensive exam. *Entrance requirements:* For degree, knowledge of French. Electronic applications accepted.

University at Buffalo, the State University of New York, Graduate School, Graduate Programs in Cancer Research and Biomedical Sciences at Roswell Park Cancer Institute, Department of Cancer Pathology and Prevention at Roswell Park Cancer Institute, Buffalo, NY 14260. Offers PhD. *Faculty:* 32 full-time (14 women). *Students:* 11 full-time (8 women); includes 2 minority (both Black or African American, non-Hispanic/Latino), 2 international. 44 applicants, 14% accepted, 4 enrolled. In 2013, 2 doctorates awarded. *Degree requirements:* For doctorate, comprehensive exam, thesis/dissertation, oral defense of disseration. *Entrance requirements:* For doctorate, GRE General Test. Additional exam requirements/recommendations for international students: Required—TOEFL (minimum score 79 iBT). *Application deadline:* For fall admission, 1/5 priority date for domestic and international students. Application fee: $75. Electronic applications accepted. *Financial support:* In 2013–14, 11 students received support, including 11 research assistantships with full tuition reimbursements available (averaging $25,000 per year); scholarships/grants, health care benefits, and unspecified assistantships also available. Financial award application deadline: 1/5. *Faculty research:* Molecular pathology of cancer, chemoprevention of cancer, genomic instability, molecular diagnosis and prognosis of cancer, molecular epidemiology. *Unit head:* Dr. Kirsten Moysich, Chairman, 716-845-8004, Fax: 716-845-1126, E-mail: kirsten.moysich@roswellpark.org. *Application contact:* Dr. Norman J. Karin, Associate Dean, 716-845-2339, Fax: 716-845-8178, E-mail: norman.karin@roswellpark.org.
Website: http://www.roswellpark.edu/education/phd-programs/cancer-pathology-and-prevention

University at Buffalo, the State University of New York, Graduate School, School of Medicine and Biomedical Sciences, Graduate Programs in Medicine and Biomedical Sciences, Department of Pathology and Anatomical Sciences, Buffalo, NY 14214. Offers anatomical sciences (MA, PhD); pathology (MA, PhD). Part-time programs available. *Faculty:* 16 full-time (5 women). *Students:* 6 full-time (1 woman). Average age 29. 18 applicants, 17% accepted, 3 enrolled. In 2013, 2 master's, 2 doctorates awarded. *Degree requirements:* For master's, thesis; for doctorate, comprehensive exam, thesis/dissertation. *Entrance requirements:* For master's and doctorate, GRE, MCAT, or DAT, 3 letters of recommendation. Additional exam requirements/recommendations for international students: Required—TOEFL (minimum score 600 paper-based; 100 iBT). *Application deadline:* For fall admission, 3/1 priority date for domestic and international students. Application fee: $75. *Financial support:* In 2013–14, 2 students received support, including 1 research assistantship with full tuition reimbursement available (averaging $24,900 per year), 1 teaching assistantship with full tuition reimbursement available (averaging $24,900 per year); health care benefits also available. Financial award application deadline: 2/1; financial award applicants required to submit FAFSA. *Faculty research:* Immunopathology-immunobiology, experimental hypertension, neuromuscular disease, molecular pathology, cell motility and cytoskeleton. *Unit head:* Dr. John E. Tomaszewski, Department Chair, 716-829-2846, Fax: 716-829-2911, E-mail: johntoma@buffalo.edu. *Application contact:* Graduate Program Coordinator, 716-829-2846, Fax: 716-829-2911, E-mail: ubpathad@buffalo.edu.
Website: http://wings.buffalo.edu/smbs/path/

The University of Alabama at Birmingham, Graduate Programs in Joint Health Sciences, Program in Pathology, Birmingham, AL 35294. Offers PhD. *Degree requirements:* For doctorate, thesis/dissertation. *Entrance requirements:* For doctorate, GRE General Test, interview, evaluations. Additional exam requirements/recommendations for international students: Required—TOEFL, TWE. Electronic applications accepted. *Faculty research:* AIDS vaccine development and T-cell biology of HIV infection and pathogenesis of AIDS; metabolic bone disease and cellular signaling and death; extracellular matrix control of normal and cancerous cell movement and growth; mechanisms of neuronal cell death and neoplasia; tumor invasion, tumor markers, and cancer genetics; bacterial and mycotic infections; mechanisms of insulin and growth hormone action.

University of Alberta, Faculty of Medicine and Dentistry and Faculty of Graduate Studies and Research, Graduate Programs in Medicine, Department of Laboratory Medicine and Pathology, Edmonton, AB T6G 2E1, Canada. Offers medical sciences (M Sc, PhD). Part-time programs available. Terminal master's awarded for partial completion of doctoral program. *Degree requirements:* For master's, thesis; for doctorate, thesis/dissertation, candidacy exam. *Entrance requirements:* For master's and doctorate, 3 letters of recommendation, minimum GPA of 3.0. Additional exam requirements/recommendations for international students: Required—TOEFL. *Faculty research:* Transplantation, renal pathology, molecular mechanisms of diseases, cryobiology, immunodiagnostics, informatics/cyber medicine, neuroimmunology, microbiology.

The University of British Columbia, Faculty of Medicine, Department of Pathology and Laboratory Medicine, Vancouver, BC V5Z 1M9, Canada. Offers experimental pathology (M Sc, PhD). *Degree requirements:* For master's, thesis; for doctorate, comprehensive exam, thesis/dissertation, internal oral defense. *Entrance requirements:* For master's, GRE, upper-level course work in biochemistry and physiology; for doctorate, GRE. Additional exam requirements/recommendations for international students: Required—TOEFL (minimum score 550 paper-based), IELTS (minimum score 6.5). Electronic applications accepted. *Expenses: Tuition, area resident:* Full-time $8000 Canadian dollars. *Faculty research:* Molecular biology of disease processes, cancer, hematopathology, atherosclerosis, pulmonary and cardiovascular pathophysiology.

University of Calgary, Cumming School of Medicine and Faculty of Graduate Studies, Medical Science Graduate Program, Calgary, AB T2N 1N4, Canada. Offers cancer biology (M Sc, PhD); critical care medicine (M Sc, PhD); joint injury and arthritis (M Sc, PhD); molecular and medical genetics (M Sc, PhD); mountain medicine and high altitude physiology (M Sc, PhD); pathologists' assistant (M Sc, PhD). *Degree requirements:* For master's, thesis; for doctorate, thesis/dissertation, candidacy exam. *Entrance requirements:* For master's, minimum undergraduate GPA of 3.2; for doctorate, minimum graduate GPA of 3.2. Additional exam requirements/recommendations for international students: Required—TOEFL (minimum score 600 paper-based). Electronic applications accepted. *Faculty research:* Cancer biology, immunology, joint injury and arthritis, medical education, population genomics.

University of California, Davis, Graduate Studies, Graduate Group in Comparative Pathology, Davis, CA 95616. Offers MS, PhD. *Accreditation:* NAACLS. Terminal master's awarded for partial completion of doctoral program. *Degree requirements:* For master's, comprehensive exam (for some programs), thesis (for some programs); for doctorate, thesis/dissertation. *Entrance requirements:* For master's and doctorate, GRE General Test. Additional exam requirements/recommendations for international students: Required—TOEFL (minimum score 550 paper-based). Electronic applications accepted. *Faculty research:* Immunopathology, toxicological and environmental pathology, reproductive pathology, pathology of infectious diseases.

University of California, Irvine, School of Medicine, Department of Pathology and Laboratory Medicine, Irvine, CA 92697. Offers experimental pathology (PhD). *Accreditation:* NAACLS. *Students:* 4 full-time (0 women); includes 3 minority (1 Asian, non-Hispanic/Latino; 2 Hispanic/Latino). Average age 29. In 2013, 2 doctorates awarded. Application fee: $80 ($100 for international students). *Unit head:* Dr. Edwin S. Monuki, Interim Chairman, 949-824-9604, Fax: 949-824-2160, E-mail: emonuki@uci.edu. *Application contact:* Prof. F. Allan Hubbell, Associate Dean, 949-824-3975, Fax: 949-824-2676, E-mail: fahubbel@uci.edu.
Website: http://www.pathology.uci.edu/

University of California, Los Angeles, David Geffen School of Medicine and Graduate Division, Graduate Programs in Medicine, Program in Cellular and Molecular Pathology, Los Angeles, CA 90095. Offers MS, PhD. Terminal master's awarded for partial completion of doctoral program. *Degree requirements:* For master's, thesis; for doctorate, thesis/dissertation, written and oral qualifying examinations; 2 quarters of teaching experience. *Entrance requirements:* For doctorate, GRE General Test, bachelor's degree; minimum undergraduate GPA of 3.0 (or its equivalent if letter grade system not used). Additional exam requirements/recommendations for international students: Required—TOEFL. Electronic applications accepted.

University of California, Los Angeles, David Geffen School of Medicine and Graduate Division, Graduate Programs in Medicine, Program in Experimental Pathology, Los Angeles, CA 90095. Offers MS, PhD. *Degree requirements:* For doctorate, thesis/dissertation, oral and written qualifying exams. *Entrance requirements:* For master's, GRE General Test; for doctorate, GRE General Test, previous course work in physical chemistry and physics.

University of California, Los Angeles, Graduate Division, College of Letters and Science and David Geffen School of Medicine, UCLA ACCESS to Programs in the Molecular, Cellular and Integrative Life Sciences, Los Angeles, CA 90095. Offers biochemistry and molecular biology (PhD); biological chemistry (PhD); cellular and molecular pathology (PhD); human genetics (PhD); microbiology, immunology, and molecular genetics (PhD); molecular biology (PhD); molecular toxicology (PhD); molecular, cellular and integrative physiology (PhD); neurobiology (PhD); oral biology (PhD); physiology (PhD). *Degree requirements:* For doctorate, thesis/dissertation, oral and written qualifying exams. *Entrance requirements:* For doctorate, GRE General Test, bachelor's degree; minimum undergraduate GPA of 3.0 (or its equivalent if letter grade system not used). Additional exam requirements/recommendations for international students: Required—TOEFL. Electronic applications accepted.

University of Chicago, Division of Biological Sciences, Biomedical Sciences Cluster: Cancer Biology, Immunology, Molecular Metabolism and Nutrition, Pathology, and Microbiology, Department of Pathology, Chicago, IL 60637-1513. Offers molecular pathogenesis and molecular medicine (PhD). *Degree requirements:* For doctorate, thesis/dissertation, ethics class, 2 teaching assistantships. *Entrance requirements:* For doctorate, GRE General Test. Additional exam requirements/recommendations for international students: Required—IELTS (minimum score 7); Recommended—TOEFL (minimum score 600 paper-based; 104 iBT). Electronic applications accepted. *Faculty research:* Vascular biology, apolipoproteins, cardiovascular disease, immunopathology.

University of Cincinnati, Graduate School, College of Medicine, Graduate Programs in Biomedical Sciences, Program in Pathobiology and Molecular Medicine, Cincinnati, OH 45221. Offers pathology (PhD), including anatomic pathology, laboratory medicine, pathobiology and molecular medicine. *Degree requirements:* For doctorate, thesis/dissertation, qualifying exam. *Entrance requirements:* For doctorate, GRE General Test. Additional exam requirements/recommendations for international students: Required—TOEFL (minimum score 620 paper-based). Electronic applications accepted. *Faculty research:* Cardiovascular and lipid disorders, digestive and kidney disease, endocrine and metabolic disorders, hematologic and oncogenic, immunology and infectious disease.

University of Georgia, College of Veterinary Medicine, Department of Pathology, Athens, GA 30602. Offers MS, PhD. *Degree requirements:* For master's, thesis; for doctorate, one foreign language, thesis/dissertation. *Entrance requirements:* For master's and doctorate, GRE General Test. Electronic applications accepted.

University of Guelph, Ontario Veterinary College and Graduate Studies, Graduate Programs in Veterinary Sciences, Department of Pathobiology, Guelph, ON N1G 2W1, Canada. Offers anatomic pathology (DV Sc, Diploma); clinical pathology (Diploma); comparative pathology (M Sc, PhD); immunology (M Sc, PhD); laboratory animal science (DV Sc); pathology (M Sc, PhD, Diploma); veterinary infectious diseases (M Sc, PhD); zoo animal/wildlife medicine (DV Sc). *Degree requirements:* For master's, thesis; for doctorate, thesis/dissertation. *Entrance requirements:* For master's, DVM with B average or an honours degree in biological sciences; for doctorate, DVM or MSC degree, minimum B+ average. Additional exam requirements/recommendations for international students: Required—TOEFL (minimum score 550 paper-based). *Faculty research:* Pathogenesis; diseases of animals, wildlife, fish, and laboratory animals; parasitology; immunology; veterinary infectious diseases; laboratory animal science.

The University of Iowa, Roy J. and Lucille A. Carver College of Medicine and Graduate College, Graduate Programs in Medicine, Department of Pathology, Iowa City, IA 52242-1316. Offers MS. *Faculty:* 24 full-time (4 women). *Students:* 5 full-time (1 woman); includes 1 minority (Two or more races, non-Hispanic/Latino). Average age 25. 12 applicants, 8% accepted, 1 enrolled. In 2013, 3 master's awarded. *Degree requirements:* For master's, thesis. *Entrance requirements:* For master's, GRE, minimum GPA of 3.0. Additional exam requirements/recommendations for international students: Required—TOEFL. *Application deadline:* For fall admission, 2/15 priority date for domestic students, 1/15 priority date for international students. Applications are processed on a rolling basis. Application fee: $60 ($100 for international students). Electronic applications accepted. *Financial support:* In 2013–14, 5 students received support, including 5 research assistantships with full tuition reimbursements available (averaging $26,000 per year); health care benefits also available. *Faculty research:* Oncology, microbiology, vascular biology, immunology, neuroscience, stem cells, virology, signaling and cell death. *Total annual research expenditures:* $5.3 million. *Unit head:* Dr. Nitin Karandikar, Chair and Department Executive Officer, 319-384-9609, Fax: 319-335-8348, E-mail: nitin-karandikar@uiowa.edu. *Application contact:* Dr. Thomas J. Waldschmidt, Graduate Program Director, 319-335-8223, Fax: 319-335-8453, E-mail: thomas-waldschmidt@uiowa.edu.
Website: http://www.medicine.uiowa.edu/pathology/

The University of Kansas, University of Kansas Medical Center, School of Medicine, Department of Pathology and Laboratory Medicine, Kansas City, KS 66160. Offers MA, PhD, MD/PhD. *Faculty:* 17. *Students:* 18 full-time (11 women); includes 1 minority (Hispanic/Latino), 11 international. Average age 28. In 2013, 1 master's, 3 doctorates awarded. Terminal master's awarded for partial completion of doctoral program. *Degree*

requirements: For master's, one foreign language, comprehensive exam (for some programs), thesis; for doctorate, one foreign language, comprehensive exam, thesis/dissertation. *Entrance requirements:* For master's, GRE, curriculum vitae, 3 reference letters; for doctorate, GRE, curriculum vitae, statement of research and career interests, official transcripts for all undergraduate and graduate coursework, 3 reference letters. Additional exam requirements/recommendations for international students: Required—TOEFL (preferred) or IELTS. *Application deadline:* For fall admission, 1/15 priority date for domestic and international students. Applications are processed on a rolling basis. Application fee: $60. *Financial support:* In 2013–14, 1 student received support. Fellowships, research assistantships with full tuition reimbursements available, teaching assistantships with full and partial tuition reimbursements available, Federal Work-Study, scholarships/grants, traineeships, tuition waivers (full), and unspecified assistantships available. Financial award application deadline: 3/1; financial award applicants required to submit FAFSA. *Faculty research:* Cancer biology, developmental biology and cell differentiation, stem cell biology, microbial and viral pathogenesis. *Total annual research expenditures:* $7.4 million. *Unit head:* Dr. Soumen Paul, Director, Pathology Graduate Program, 913-588-7236, Fax: 913-588-5242, E-mail: spaul2@kumc.edu. *Application contact:* Graduate Studies, 785-864-8040, Fax: 785-864-7209, E-mail: graduate@ku.edu.
Website: http://www.kumc.edu/school-of-medicine/pathology.html

University of Manitoba, Faculty of Medicine and Faculty of Graduate Studies, Graduate Programs in Medicine, Department of Pathology, Winnipeg, MB R3E 3P5, Canada. Offers M Sc. *Degree requirements:* For master's, thesis. *Entrance requirements:* For master's, B Sc honours degree. Additional exam requirements/recommendations for international students: Required—TOEFL (minimum score 550 paper-based; 80 iBT), IELTS (minimum score 6.5). *Faculty research:* Experimental hydrocephalus; brain development; stroke; developmental neurobiology; myelination in Rett Syndrome; glial migration during cortical development; growth factors and breast cancer; transgenic models of breast cancer; molecular genetics and cancer diagnosis; graft-vs-host disease; biology of natural killer cells; transplantation immunology.

University of Maryland, Baltimore, School of Medicine, Department of Pathology, Baltimore, MD 21201. Offers pathologists' assistant (MS). *Accreditation:* NAACLS. *Students:* 21 full-time (20 women); includes 3 minority (2 Asian, non-Hispanic/Latino; 1 Hispanic/Latino). Average age 25. 72 applicants, 17% accepted, 11 enrolled. In 2013, 10 master's awarded. *Entrance requirements:* For master's, GRE General Test. Additional exam requirements/recommendations for international students: Required—TOEFL (minimum score 600 paper-based; 100 iBT); Recommended—IELTS (minimum score 7). *Application deadline:* For fall admission, 2/1 for domestic and international students. Application fee: $75. Electronic applications accepted. *Expenses:* Contact institution. *Financial support:* Application deadline: 3/1; applicants required to submit FAFSA. *Unit head:* Dr. Rudy Castellani, Program Director, 410-328-5555, Fax: 410-706-8414, E-mail: rcastellani@som.umaryland.edu. *Application contact:* Carlen Miller, Associate Director, 410-328-5555, Fax: 410-706-8414, E-mail: cmiller@som.umaryland.edu.
Website: http://medschool.umaryland.edu/pathology/

University of Massachusetts Lowell, College of Health Sciences, Department of Clinical Laboratory and Nutritional Sciences, Lowell, MA 01854-2881. Offers clinical laboratory sciences (MS); clinical pathology (Graduate Certificate); nutritional sciences (Graduate Certificate); public health laboratory sciences (Graduate Certificate). *Accreditation:* NAACLS. Part-time programs available. Postbaccalaureate distance learning degree programs offered. *Degree requirements:* For master's, thesis optional. *Entrance requirements:* For master's, GRE General Test, minimum GPA of 3.0, letters of recommendation. *Faculty research:* Cardiovascular disease, lipoprotein metabolism, micronutrient evaluation, alcohol metabolism, mycobacterial drug resistance.

University of Michigan, Rackham Graduate School, Program in Biomedical Sciences (PIBS), Program in Molecular and Cellular Pathology, Ann Arbor, MI 48109. Offers PhD. *Faculty:* 34 full-time (9 women). *Students:* 25 full-time (15 women); includes 7 minority (1 Black or African American, non-Hispanic/Latino; 5 Asian, non-Hispanic/Latino; 1 Hispanic/Latino), 5 international. Average age 28. 48 applicants, 13% accepted, 4 enrolled. In 2013, 6 doctorates awarded. *Degree requirements:* For doctorate, comprehensive exam, thesis/dissertation. *Entrance requirements:* For doctorate, GRE General Test, 3 letters of recommendation, research experience. Additional exam requirements/recommendations for international students: Required—TOEFL (minimum score 84 iBT). *Application deadline:* For fall admission, 12/1 for domestic and international students. Application fee: $75 ($90 for international students). Electronic applications accepted. Tuition and fees vary according to course level, course load, degree level, program and student level. *Financial support:* In 2013–14, research assistantships with full tuition reimbursements (averaging $28,500 per year) were awarded; scholarships/grants, traineeships, health care benefits, and unspecified assistantships also available. *Faculty research:* Cancer biology, stem cell and developmental biology, immunopathology and inflammatory disease, epigenetics and gene regulation, cell death and regulation. *Unit head:* Dr. Zaneta Nikolovska-Coleska, Assistant Professor of Pathology/Director, 734-763-6454, Fax: 734-615-2331, E-mail: pathgradprog@med.umich.edu. *Application contact:* Laura A. Labut, Administrative Specialist, 734-763-6454, Fax: 734-615-2331, E-mail: laszczem@med.umich.edu.
Website: http://www.pathology.med.umich.edu/

University of Mississippi Medical Center, School of Graduate Studies in the Health Sciences, Department of Pathology, Jackson, MS 39216-4505. Offers PhD, MD/PhD. *Faculty:* 7 full-time (2 women). *Students:* 2 full-time (0 women); includes 1 minority (Asian, non-Hispanic/Latino), 1 international. Average age 36. 7 applicants, 57% accepted, 2 enrolled. In 2013, 2 doctorates awarded. *Degree requirements:* For doctorate, thesis/dissertation, first authored publication in peer-reviewed journal. *Entrance requirements:* For doctorate, GRE General Test, GRE Subject Test, minimum GPA of 3.0. Additional exam requirements/recommendations for international students: Required—TOEFL. *Application deadline:* For fall admission, 7/1 for domestic students. Applications are processed on a rolling basis. Application fee: $25. *Financial support:* In 2013–14, 3 students received support, including 1 research assistantship (averaging $24,150 per year). Financial award application deadline: 3/31. *Faculty research:* Toll-like receptor expression and function in metastatic breast cancer patients, innate immunity, circulating tumor cells, natural killer cells, pro-inflammatory T cell transcriptional profile during progression of HIV-1 infection, renal allografts hinges on microvascular endothelium response, immunoregulatory gene expression affecting regulatory cells. *Unit head:* Dr. Julius M. Cruse, Director of Pathology PhD Program, 601-984-1565, Fax: 601-984-1835, E-mail: sbigler@pathology.umsmed.edu. *Application contact:* Dr. Julius M. Cruse, Director, 601-984-1561, Fax: 601-984-1835, E-mail: jcruse@pathology.umsmed.edu.
Website: http://www.umc.edu/Education/Schools/Medicine/Clinical_Science/Pathology/Academics(Pathology)/Graduate_Program_in_Pathology.aspx

University of Missouri, School of Medicine and Graduate School, Graduate Programs in Medicine, Department of Pathology and Anatomical Sciences, Columbia, MO 65211. Offers MS. *Faculty:* 22 full-time (8 women), 7 part-time/adjunct (3 women). *Students:* 2 applicants. *Entrance requirements:* For master's, GRE (minimum Verbal and Analytical score of 1250), letters of recommendation, minimum GPA of 3.5. Additional exam requirements/recommendations for international students: Required—TOEFL. Application fee: $55 ($75 for international students). Electronic applications accepted. *Faculty research:* Anatomic pathology, cancer biology, diabetes, integrative anatomy, laboratory medicine, neurobiology, tissue procurement core. *Unit head:* Dr. Lester Layfield, Chair, 573-882-8915, E-mail: layfieldl@missouri.edu. *Application contact:* Dr. Carol V. Ward, Director of Graduate Studies, 573-884-7303, E-mail: wardcv@missouri.edu.
Website: http://pathology-anatomy.missouri.edu/

University of Nebraska Medical Center, Department of Pathology and Microbiology, Omaha, NE 68198-5900. Offers MS, PhD. Part-time programs available. Terminal master's awarded for partial completion of doctoral program. *Degree requirements:* For master's, comprehensive exam, thesis; for doctorate, comprehensive exam, thesis/dissertation. *Entrance requirements:* For master's, previous course work in biology, chemistry, mathematics, and physics; for doctorate, GRE General Test, previous course work in biology, chemistry, mathematics, and physics. Additional exam requirements/recommendations for international students: Required—TOEFL (minimum score 550 paper-based). Electronic applications accepted. *Expenses: Required fees:* $300 per semester. Tuition and fees vary according to program. *Faculty research:* Carcinogenesis, cancer biology, immunobiology, molecular virology, molecular genetics.

University of New Mexico, School of Medicine, Program in Biomedical Sciences, Albuquerque, NM 87131-5196. Offers biochemistry and molecular biology (MS, PhD); cell biology and physiology (MS, PhD); clinical and translational science (Certificate); molecular genetics and microbiology (MS, PhD); neuroscience (MS, PhD); pathology (MS, PhD); toxicology (MS, PhD); university science teaching (Certificate). Part-time programs available. *Students:* 73 full-time (39 women), 14 part-time (9 women); includes 24 minority (1 Black or African American, non-Hispanic/Latino; 1 American Indian or Alaska Native, non-Hispanic/Latino; 2 Asian, non-Hispanic/Latino; 17 Hispanic/Latino; 1 Native Hawaiian or other Pacific Islander, non-Hispanic/Latino; 2 Two or more races, non-Hispanic/Latino), 16 international. Average age 29. 89 applicants, 20% accepted, 17 enrolled. In 2013, 7 master's, 17 doctorates awarded. Terminal master's awarded for partial completion of doctoral program. *Degree requirements:* For master's, thesis; for doctorate, comprehensive exam, thesis/dissertation, qualifying exam at the end of year 1/core curriculum. *Entrance requirements:* For master's and doctorate, GRE General Test, minimum undergraduate GPA of 3.0. Additional exam requirements/recommendations for international students: Required—TOEFL. *Application deadline:* For fall admission, 3/1 priority date for domestic and international students. Applications are processed on a rolling basis. Application fee: $50. Electronic applications accepted. *Financial support:* In 2013–14, 94 students received support, including 28 fellowships with full and partial tuition reimbursements available (averaging $22,000 per year), 73 research assistantships with full tuition reimbursements available (averaging $23,000 per year), 8 teaching assistantships (averaging $2,800 per year); career-related internships or fieldwork, Federal Work-Study, institutionally sponsored loans, scholarships/grants, traineeships, health care benefits, and unspecified assistantships also available. Financial award application deadline: 1/1; financial award applicants required to submit FAFSA. *Faculty research:* Infectious disease/immunity, cancer biology, cardiovascular and metabolic diseases, brain and behavioral illness, environmental health. *Unit head:* Dr. Helen J. Hathaway, Program Director, 505-272-1887, Fax: 505-272-2412, E-mail: hhathaway@salud.unm.edu. *Application contact:* Mary Fenton, Admissions Coordinator, 505-272-1887, Fax: 505-272-2412, E-mail: mfenton@salud.unm.edu.
Website: http://hsc.unm.edu/research/brep/bsgpabout.shtm

The University of North Carolina at Chapel Hill, School of Medicine and Graduate School, Graduate Programs in Medicine, Department of Pathology and Laboratory Medicine, Chapel Hill, NC 27599-7525. Offers experimental pathology (PhD). *Accreditation:* NAACLS. *Degree requirements:* For doctorate, comprehensive exam, thesis/dissertation, oral exam, proposal defense. *Entrance requirements:* For doctorate, GRE General Test. Additional exam requirements/recommendations for international students: Required—TOEFL (minimum score 550 paper-based). Electronic applications accepted. *Faculty research:* Carcinogenesis, mutagenesis and cancer biology; molecular biology, genetics and animal models of human disease; cardiovascular biology, hemostasis, and thrombosis; immunology and infectious disease; progenitor cell research.

University of Oklahoma Health Sciences Center, College of Medicine and Graduate College, Graduate Programs in Medicine, Department of Pathology, Oklahoma City, OK 73190. Offers PhD. *Faculty:* 6 full-time (0 women), 3 part-time/adjunct (1 woman). *Students:* 2 full-time (both women), 7 part-time (3 women); includes 1 minority (Asian, non-Hispanic/Latino), 5 international. Average age 29. 4 applicants. In 2013, 3 doctorates awarded. *Degree requirements:* For doctorate, thesis/dissertation. *Entrance requirements:* For doctorate, GRE General Test, 3 letters of recommendation. Additional exam requirements/recommendations for international students: Required—TOEFL. *Application deadline:* For fall admission, 12/15 for domestic students. Application fee: $50. *Expenses:* Tuition, state resident: full-time $3504; part-time $175.20 per credit hour. Tuition, nonresident: full-time $13,504; part-time $675.20 per credit hour. *Required fees:* $1545; $52.70 per credit hour. $245.25 per semester. Tuition and fees vary according to course load. *Financial support:* In 2013–14, 3 research assistantships (averaging $17,000 per year) were awarded; Federal Work-Study, institutionally sponsored loans, and tuition waivers (full) also available. *Faculty research:* Molecular pathology, tissue response in disease, anatomic pathology, immunopathology, histocytochemistry. *Unit head:* Dr. Michael Talbert, Chair, 405-271-2422, E-mail: michael-talbert@ouhsc.edu. *Application contact:* Dr. Joe Zhao, Graduate Liaison, 405-271-2422, E-mail: joe-zhao@ouhsc.edu.

University of Pittsburgh, School of Medicine, Graduate Programs in Medicine, Cellular and Molecular Pathology Graduate Program, Pittsburgh, PA 15260. Offers PhD. *Faculty:* 67 full-time (22 women). *Students:* 31 full-time (15 women); includes 6 minority (2 Black or African American, non-Hispanic/Latino; 2 Asian, non-Hispanic/Latino; 2 Hispanic/Latino), 7 international. Average age 28. 517 applicants, 13% accepted, 22 enrolled. In 2013, 8 doctorates awarded. *Degree requirements:* For doctorate, comprehensive exam, thesis/dissertation. *Entrance requirements:* For doctorate, GRE General Test, GRE Subject Test, minimum QPA of 3.0. Additional exam requirements/recommendations for international students: Required—TOEFL (minimum score 600 paper-based; 100 iBT), IELTS (minimum score 7). *Application deadline:* For fall admission, 1/1 priority date for domestic and international students. Application fee: $50. Electronic applications accepted. *Expenses:* Tuition, state resident: full-time $19,964; part-time $807 per credit. Tuition, nonresident: full-time $32,686; part-time $1337 per credit. *Required fees:* $740; $200. Tuition and fees vary according to program. *Financial support:* In 2013–14, 10 fellowships with full tuition reimbursements (averaging $26,010 per year), 21 research assistantships with full tuition reimbursements (averaging $26,010 per year) were awarded; institutionally sponsored loans, scholarships/grants, traineeships, health care benefits, and unspecified assistantships also available. *Faculty research:* Liver growth and differentiation, pathogenesis of neurodegeneration, cancer research. *Unit head:* Dr. Wendy Mars, Graduate Program Director, 412-648-9690, Fax: 412-648-9846, E-mail: wmars@pitt.edu. *Application contact:* Graduate

Studies Administrator, 412-648-8957, Fax: 412-648-1077, E-mail: gradstudies@medschool.pitt.edu.
Website: http://www.gradbiomed.pitt.edu

University of Prince Edward Island, Atlantic Veterinary College, Graduate Program in Veterinary Medicine, Charlottetown, PE C1A 4P3, Canada. Offers anatomy (M Sc, PhD); bacteriology (M Sc, PhD); clinical pharmacology (M Sc, PhD); clinical sciences (M Sc, PhD); epidemiology (M Sc, PhD), including reproduction; fish health (M Sc, PhD); food animal nutrition (M Sc, PhD); immunology (M Sc, PhD); microanatomy (M Sc, PhD); parasitology (M Sc, PhD); pathology (M Sc, PhD); pharmacology (M Sc, PhD); physiology (M Sc, PhD); toxicology (M Sc, PhD); veterinary science (M Vet Sc); virology (M Sc, PhD). Part-time programs available. *Degree requirements:* For master's, thesis; for doctorate, thesis/dissertation. *Entrance requirements:* For master's, DVM, B Sc honors degree, or equivalent; for doctorate, M Sc. Additional exam requirements/recommendations for international students: Required—TOEFL (minimum score 550 paper-based; 80 iBT). *Expenses:* Contact institution. *Faculty research:* Animal health management, infectious diseases, fin fish and shellfish health, basic biomedical sciences, ecosystem health.

University of Rochester, School of Medicine and Dentistry, Graduate Programs in Medicine and Dentistry, Department of Pathology and Laboratory Medicine, Rochester, NY 14627. Offers pathology (PhD). *Degree requirements:* For doctorate, variable foreign language requirement, thesis/dissertation, qualifying exam. *Entrance requirements:* For doctorate, GRE General Test, GRE Subject Test. *Expenses: Tuition:* Full-time $44,580; part-time $1394 per credit hour. *Required fees:* $492.

University of Saskatchewan, College of Medicine, Department of Pathology, Saskatoon, SK S7N 5A2, Canada. Offers M Sc, PhD. *Degree requirements:* For master's, thesis; for doctorate, thesis/dissertation. *Entrance requirements:* Additional exam requirements/recommendations for international students: Required—TOEFL. *Expenses: Tuition, area resident:* Full-time $3585 Canadian dollars; part-time $585 Canadian dollars per course. Tuition, nonresident: part-time $877 Canadian dollars per course. *International tuition:* $5377 Canadian dollars full-time. *Required fees:* $889.51 Canadian dollars.

University of Saskatchewan, Western College of Veterinary Medicine and College of Graduate Studies and Research, Graduate Programs in Veterinary Medicine, Department of Veterinary Pathology, Saskatoon, SK S7N 5A2, Canada. Offers M Sc, M Vet Sc, PhD. *Degree requirements:* For master's, thesis; for doctorate, comprehensive exam (for some programs), thesis/dissertation. *Entrance requirements:* Additional exam requirements/recommendations for international students: Required—TOEFL or IELTS (minimum score 6.5). Electronic applications accepted. *Expenses: Tuition, area resident:* Full-time $3585 Canadian dollars; part-time $585 Canadian dollars per course. Tuition, nonresident: part-time $877 Canadian dollars per course. *International tuition:* $5377 Canadian dollars full-time. *Required fees:* $889.51 Canadian dollars. *Faculty research:* Thyroid, oncology, immunology/infectious diseases, vaccinology.

University of Southern California, Keck School of Medicine and Graduate School, Graduate Programs in Medicine, Department of Pathology, Los Angeles, CA 90033. Offers experimental and molecular pathology (MS); pathobiology (PhD). *Faculty:* 33 full-time (5 women), 1 part-time/adjunct (0 women). *Students:* 17 full-time (11 women); includes 4 minority (1 Black or African American, non-Hispanic/Latino; 2 Asian, non-Hispanic/Latino; 1 Hispanic/Latino), 7 international. Average age 26. 8 applicants, 75% accepted, 4 enrolled. In 2013, 6 master's, 5 doctorates awarded. *Degree requirements:* For master's, experiment-based thesis or theory-based scholarly review; for doctorate, thesis/dissertation. *Entrance requirements:* For master's, GRE General Test, minimum GPA of 3.0; for doctorate, GRE General Test, minimum GPA of 3.0, BS in natural sciences. Additional exam requirements/recommendations for international students: Required—TOEFL (minimum score 600 paper-based; 100 iBT). *Application deadline:* For fall admission, 6/15 for domestic students, 6/15 priority date for international students; for spring admission, 12/1 for domestic students, 12/1 priority date for international students. Application fee: $85. Electronic applications accepted. *Financial support:* In 2013–14, 11 students received support, including 1 fellowship (averaging $31,000 per year), 10 research assistantships (averaging $31,000 per year); Federal Work-Study, institutionally sponsored loans, scholarships/grants, health care benefits, and unspecified assistantships also available. Financial award application deadline: 5/4. *Faculty research:* Cellular and molecular biology of cancer; chemical carcinogenesis; virology; stem cell and developmental pathology; liver and pulmonary diseases; environmental pathology; circulatory, endocrine, and neurodegenerative diseases. *Total annual research expenditures:* $7.5 million. *Unit head:* Dr. Michael E. Selsted, Chair, 323-442-1179, Fax: 323-442-3049, E-mail: selsted@usc.edu. *Application contact:* Lisa A. Doumak, Student Services Assistant, 323-442-1168, Fax: 323-442-3049, E-mail: doumak@usc.edu.
Website: http://www.usc.edu/hsc/medicine/pathology/

University of South Florida, Morsani College of Medicine and Graduate School, Graduate Programs in Medical Sciences, Tampa, FL 33620-9951. Offers aging and neuroscience (MSMS); allergy, immunology and infectious disease (PhD); anatomy (MSMS, PhD); athletic training (MSMS); bioinformatics and computational biology (MSBCB); biotechnology (MSB); clinical and translational research (MSMS, PhD); health informatics (MSHI, MSMS); health science (MSMS); interdisciplinary medical sciences (MSMS); medical microbiology and immunology (MSMS); metabolic and nutritional medicine (MSMS); molecular medicine (MSMS, PhD); molecular pharmacology and physiology (PhD); neurology (PhD); pathology and laboratory medicine (PhD); pharmacology and therapeutics (PhD); physiology and biophysics (PhD); women's health (MSMS). *Students:* 336 full-time (182 women), 39 part-time (21 women); includes 170 minority (45 Black or African American, non-Hispanic/Latino; 54 Asian, non-Hispanic/Latino; 59 Hispanic/Latino; 2 Native Hawaiian or other Pacific Islander, non-Hispanic/Latino; 10 Two or more races, non-Hispanic/Latino), 17 international. Average age 26. 1,066 applicants, 44% accepted, 250 enrolled. In 2013, 191 master's, 12 doctorates awarded. Terminal master's awarded for partial completion of doctoral program. *Degree requirements:* For master's, comprehensive exam, thesis; for doctorate, comprehensive exam, thesis/dissertation. *Entrance requirements:* For master's, GRE General Test or GMAT, bachelor's degree or equivalent from regionally-accredited university with minimum GPA of 3.0 in upper-division sciences coursework; prerequisites in general biology, general chemistry, general physics, organic chemistry, quantitative analysis, and integral and differential calculus; for doctorate, GRE General Test (minimum score of 600 quantitative), bachelor's degree from regionally-accredited university with minimum GPA of 3.0 in upper-division sciences coursework; 3 letters of recommendation; personal interview; 1-2 page personal statement; prerequisites in biology, chemistry, physics, organic chemistry, quantitative analysis, and integral/differential calculus. Additional exam requirements/recommendations for international students: Required—TOEFL (minimum score 550 paper-based; 79 iBT) or IELTS (minimum score 6.5). *Application deadline:* For fall admission, 2/15 for domestic students, 1/2 for international students. Application fee: $30. *Expenses:* Contact institution. *Faculty research:* Anatomy, biochemistry, cancer biology, cardiovascular disease, cell biology, immunology, microbiology, molecular biology, neuroscience, pharmacology, physiology. *Unit head:* Dr. Michael Barber, Professor and Associate Dean for Graduate and Postdoctoral Affairs, 813-974-9908, Fax: 813-974-4317, E-mail: mbarber@health.usf.edu. *Application contact:* Dr. Eric Bennett, Graduate Director, PhD Program in Medical Sciences, 813-974-1545, Fax: 813-974-4317, E-mail: esbennet@health.usf.edu.
Website: http://health.usf.edu/nocms/medicine/graduatestudies/

The University of Tennessee Health Science Center, College of Health Professions, Memphis, TN 38163-0002. Offers audiology (MS, Au D); clinical laboratory science (MSCLS); cytopathology practice (MCP); health informatics and information management (MHIIM); occupational therapy (MOT); physical therapy (DPT, ScDPT); physician assistant (MMS); speech-language pathology (MS). *Accreditation:* AOTA; APTA. Part-time and evening/weekend programs available. Postbaccalaureate distance learning degree programs offered (minimal on-campus study). Terminal master's awarded for partial completion of doctoral program. *Degree requirements:* For master's, comprehensive exam, thesis; for doctorate, comprehensive exam, residency. *Entrance requirements:* For master's, GRE (MOT, MSCLS), minimum GPA of 3.0, 3 letters of reference, national accreditation (MSCLS), GRE if GPA is less than 3.0 (MCP); for doctorate, GRE. Additional exam requirements/recommendations for international students: Required—TOEFL (minimum score 550 paper-based; 80 iBT). *Application deadline:* For fall admission, 1/30 priority date for domestic students; for winter admission, 10/1 priority date for domestic students. Application fee: $50. Electronic applications accepted. *Expenses:* Contact institution. *Financial support:* Teaching assistantships, Federal Work-Study, institutionally sponsored loans, and scholarships/grants available. Support available to part-time students. Financial award application deadline: 2/15; financial award applicants required to submit FAFSA. *Faculty research:* Gait deviation, muscular dystrophy and strength, hemophilia and exercise, pediatric neurology, self-efficacy. *Unit head:* Dr. Noma Anderson, Dean, 901-528-5588, Fax: 901-528-7545, E-mail: nander13@uthsc.edu. *Application contact:* Dr. Noma Anderson, Dean, 901-528-5588, Fax: 901-528-7545, E-mail: nander13@uthsc.edu.
Website: http://www.uthsc.edu/health-professions/

The University of Texas Medical Branch, Graduate School of Biomedical Sciences, Program in Experimental Pathology, Galveston, TX 77555. Offers PhD. *Degree requirements:* For doctorate, thesis/dissertation. *Entrance requirements:* For doctorate, GRE General Test. Additional exam requirements/recommendations for international students: Required—TOEFL (minimum score 550 paper-based). Electronic applications accepted.

The University of Toledo, College of Graduate Studies, College of Medicine and Life Sciences, Department of Pathology, Toledo, OH 43606-3390. Offers pathology (Certificate); pathology assistant (MSBS). *Faculty:* 5. *Students:* 1 full-time (0 women), 4 part-time (3 women); includes 2 minority (both Asian, non-Hispanic/Latino). Average age 28. 3 applicants, 67% accepted, 2 enrolled. In 2013, 3 Certificates awarded. *Entrance requirements:* For degree, second-year medical student in good academic standing with recommendation by UT Medical School. Application fee: $45 ($75 for international students). Electronic applications accepted. *Financial support:* In 2013–14, 3 fellowships with full tuition reimbursements were awarded; tuition waivers (full and partial) also available. *Unit head:* Dr. Amira Gohara, Chair, 419-383-3469, E-mail: robert.mrak@utoledo.edu. *Application contact:* Cathie Harman, Assistant to the Chair, 419-383-3469, E-mail: cathie.harman@utoledo.edu.
Website: http://www.utoledo.edu/med/grad/

University of Utah, School of Medicine and Graduate School, Graduate Programs in Medicine, Department of Pathology, Salt Lake City, UT 84112-1107. Offers experimental pathology (PhD); laboratory medicine and biomedical science (MS). PhD offered after acceptance into the combined Program in Molecular Biology. *Degree requirements:* For doctorate, comprehensive exam, thesis/dissertation. *Entrance requirements:* For doctorate, GRE, minimum GPA of 3.0. *Expenses:* Tuition, state resident: full-time $5259. Tuition, nonresident: full-time $18,569. *Required fees:* $841. Tuition and fees vary according to course load. *Faculty research:* Immunology, cell biology, signal transduction, gene regulation, receptor biology.

University of Vermont, College of Medicine and Graduate College, Graduate Programs in Medicine, Department of Pathology, Burlington, VT 05405. Offers MS. *Students:* 4 (3 women); includes 1 minority (Hispanic/Latino), 1 international. 12 applicants, 8% accepted, 1 enrolled. In 2013, 1 master's awarded. *Degree requirements:* For master's, thesis. *Entrance requirements:* For master's, GRE General Test. Additional exam requirements/recommendations for international students: Required—TOEFL (minimum score 550 paper-based; 80 iBT). *Application deadline:* For fall admission, 3/1 priority date for domestic students, 3/1 for international students. Applications are processed on a rolling basis. Application fee: $65. Electronic applications accepted. *Financial support:* Fellowships, research assistantships, and traineeships available. Financial award application deadline: 3/1. *Unit head:* Debra Leonard, Chairperson, 802-656-3606. *Application contact:* Arti Shukla, Coordinator, 802-656-2132.

University of Virginia, School of Medicine, Program in Experimental Pathology, Charlottesville, VA 22903. Offers PhD. *Students:* 17 full-time (10 women); includes 2 minority (both Black or African American, non-Hispanic/Latino), 2 international. Average age 27. In 2013, 4 doctorates awarded. *Degree requirements:* For doctorate, thesis/dissertation, oral defense of thesis. *Entrance requirements:* For doctorate, GRE General Test; GRE Subject Test (recommended), 2 letters of recommendation. Additional exam requirements/recommendations for international students: Required—TOEFL. *Application deadline:* For fall admission, 1/15 for domestic and international students. *Expenses:* Tuition, state resident: part-time $334 per credit hour. Tuition, nonresident: part-time $1224 per credit hour. *Financial support:* Application deadline: 1/15. *Unit head:* Janet V. Cross, Program Director, 434-924-7185, E-mail: molmed@virginia.edu. *Application contact:* Michael Kidd, Coordinator, 434-924-9446, E-mail: mcbd@virginia.edu.
Website: http://www.medicine.virginia.edu/clinical/departments/pathology/Education/mcbd

University of Washington, Graduate School, School of Medicine, Graduate Programs in Medicine, Department of Pathology, Seattle, WA 98195. Offers experimental and molecular pathology (PhD). *Degree requirements:* For doctorate, thesis/dissertation. *Entrance requirements:* For doctorate, GRE General Test. *Faculty research:* Viral oncogenesis, aging, mutagenesis and repair, extracellular matrix biology, vascular biology.

The University of Western Ontario, Faculty of Graduate Studies, Biosciences Division, Department of Pathology, London, ON N6A 5B8, Canada. Offers M Sc, PhD. *Degree requirements:* For master's, thesis; for doctorate, comprehensive exam, thesis/dissertation. *Entrance requirements:* For master's and doctorate, minimum B+ average, honors degree. Additional exam requirements/recommendations for international students: Required—TOEFL. *Faculty research:* Heavy metal toxicology, transplant pathology, immunopathology, immunological cancers, neurochemistry, aging and dementia, cancer pathology.

University of Wisconsin–Madison, School of Medicine and Public Health and Graduate School, Graduate Programs in Medicine, Department of Pathology and Laboratory Medicine, Madison, WI 53706-1380. Offers PhD. *Accreditation:* NAACLS.

Faculty: 83 full-time (23 women). *Students:* 47 full-time (24 women); includes 16 minority (2 Black or African American, non-Hispanic/Latino; 1 American Indian or Alaska Native, non-Hispanic/Latino; 2 Asian, non-Hispanic/Latino; 11 Hispanic/Latino), 5 international. Average age 25. 112 applicants, 13% accepted, 9 enrolled. In 2013, 3 doctorates awarded. *Degree requirements:* For doctorate, thesis/dissertation. *Entrance requirements:* For doctorate, GRE, minimum GPA of 3.0. Additional exam requirements/recommendations for international students: Required—TOEFL (minimum score 580 paper-based; 92 iBT). *Application deadline:* For fall admission, 12/1 priority date for domestic and international students. Applications are processed on a rolling basis. Application fee: $56. Electronic applications accepted. *Expenses:* Tuition, state resident: full-time $10,728; part-time $790 per credit. Tuition, nonresident: full-time $24,054; part-time $1623 per credit. *Required fees:* $1130; $119 per credit. *Financial support:* In 2013–14, 47 students received support, including 8 fellowships with full tuition reimbursements available (averaging $25,000 per year), 39 research assistantships with full tuition reimbursements available (averaging $25,000 per year); health care benefits also available. Financial award application deadline: 12/1. *Faculty research:* Cellular and molecular pathology: immunology/immunopathology, cancer biology, neuroscience/neuropathology, growth factor/matrix biology, developmental pathology. *Unit head:* Dr. Andreas Friedl, Chair, 608-265-4262, Fax: 608-265-3301, E-mail: krasmusson@wisc.edu. *Application contact:* Joanne Thornton, Student Services Coordinator, 608-262-2665, Fax: 608-265-3301, E-mail: gradinfo@pathology.wisc.edu. Website: http://www.cmp.wisc.edu/

See Close-Up on page 421.

Vanderbilt University, Graduate School and School of Medicine, Department of Pathology, Nashville, TN 37240-1001. Offers PhD, MD/PhD. *Faculty:* 43 full-time (13 women). *Students:* 20 full-time (11 women); includes 5 minority (2 Black or African American, non-Hispanic/Latino; 3 Hispanic/Latino), 6 international. Average age 28. In 2013, 2 doctorates awarded. *Degree requirements:* For doctorate, thesis/dissertation, qualifying and final exams. *Entrance requirements:* For doctorate, GRE General Test. Additional exam requirements/recommendations for international students: Required—TOEFL (minimum score 570 paper-based; 88 iBT). *Application deadline:* For fall admission, 1/15 for domestic and international students. Application fee: $0. Electronic applications accepted. *Financial support:* Fellowships with full tuition reimbursements, research assistantships with full tuition reimbursements, Federal Work-Study, institutionally sponsored loans, traineeships, health care benefits, and tuition waivers (partial) available. Financial award application deadline: 1/15; financial award applicants required to submit CSS PROFILE or FAFSA. *Faculty research:* Vascular biology and biochemistry, tumor pathology, the immune response, inflammation and repair, the biology of the extracellular matrix in response to disease processes, the pathogenesis of infectious agents, the regulation of gene expression in disease. *Unit head:* Lorie Franklin, Administrative Assistant/Director of Graduate Studies Assistant, 615-343-4882, Fax: 615-322-0576, E-mail: lorie.franklin@vanderbilt.edu. *Application contact:* Walter B. Bieschke, Program Coordinator for Graduate Admissions, 615-342-0236, E-mail: vandygrad@vanderbilt.edu.
Website: http://www.mc.vanderbilt.edu/root/vumc.php?site-vmcpathology

Virginia Commonwealth University, Medical College of Virginia-Professional Programs, School of Medicine, School of Medicine Graduate Programs, Department of Pathology, Richmond, VA 23284-9005. Offers PhD, MD/PhD. Part-time programs available. Terminal master's awarded for partial completion of doctoral program. *Degree requirements:* For doctorate, thesis/dissertation, comprehensive oral and written exams. *Entrance requirements:* For doctorate, GRE General Test, MCAT. *Faculty research:* Biochemical and clinical applications of enzyme and protein immobilization, clinical enzymology.

Wayne State University, School of Medicine, Graduate Programs in Medicine, Department of Pathology, Detroit, MI 48202. Offers PhD. *Accreditation:* NAACLS. *Students:* 4 full-time (3 women). Average age 27. 28 applicants, 7% accepted, 2 enrolled. In 2013, 2 doctorates awarded. *Degree requirements:* For doctorate, thesis/dissertation. *Entrance requirements:* For doctorate, GRE General Test, personal statement, three letters of recommendation, admission to the Graduate School. Additional exam requirements/recommendations for international students: Required—TOEFL (minimum score 100 iBT). *Application deadline:* For fall admission, 2/1 for domestic and international students. Application fee: $0. Electronic applications accepted. *Expenses:* Contact institution. *Financial support:* In 2013–14, 3 students received support, including 4 fellowships with tuition reimbursements available (averaging $18,088 per year), 3 research assistantships with tuition reimbursements available (averaging $22,049 per year); teaching assistantships with tuition reimbursements available, scholarships/grants, health care benefits, and unspecified assistantships also available. Financial award application deadline: 3/31; financial award applicants required to submit FAFSA. *Faculty research:* Cancer, tumor microenvironment, metaloproteases, metabolism, diabetes and obesity. *Unit head:* Dr. Todd Leff, Program Director, 313-577-3006, E-mail: tleff@med.wayne.edu.
Website: http://pathology.med.wayne.edu/grad_program.php

Yale University, Graduate School of Arts and Sciences, Department of Experimental Pathology, New Haven, CT 06520. Offers MS, PhD. *Degree requirements:* For doctorate, thesis/dissertation, qualifying exam. *Entrance requirements:* For doctorate, GRE General Test.

Yale University, School of Medicine and Graduate School of Arts and Sciences, Combined Program in Biological and Biomedical Sciences (BBS), Pharmacological Sciences and Molecular Medicine Track, New Haven, CT 06520. Offers PhD, MD/PhD. *Degree requirements:* For doctorate, thesis/dissertation. *Entrance requirements:* For doctorate, GRE General Test. Additional exam requirements/recommendations for international students: Required—TOEFL. Electronic applications accepted.

UNIVERSITY OF WISCONSIN–MADISON

Department of Pathology and Laboratory Medicine

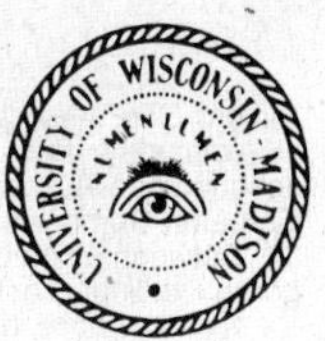

Program of Study

The Cellular and Molecular Pathology (CMP) graduate training program originated more than fifty years ago as a program focused on general pathology research and education. Through the years, much of the training involved examination of pathological specimens, and graduates were highly valued for their skills by health institutions and industry. Ten years ago, the graduate program was restructured to emphasize the pathogenesis of human disease, and the program faculty was expanded. Today, the faculty of the CMP program includes 83 National Institutes of Health/National Science Foundation or similarly funded investigators focusing on research programs in immunology, cancer biology, neuropathology, and signal transduction. These investigators come from twenty different basic science, preclinical, and clinical departments. Of these trainers, 50 hold Ph.D. degrees and 33 hold M.D. or M.D./Ph.D. degrees, and carry out both patient care and basic research. The Department of Pathology serves as a core for the CMP graduate program, integrating these faculty and trainers from across campus into a unified, multidisciplinary graduate training program focused on the pathogenesis of human diseases.

The primary objective of the CMP program is to prepare graduates for productive careers in scientific research and education and to position them to make significant contributions toward the nation's health-related research needs.

The CMP program focuses on the integration of medical knowledge into graduate education, and the Department of Pathology offers a "translational bridge" between basic and clinical sciences by offering an interdisciplinary curriculum focused on the concepts of human disease pathogenesis and translational research.

Research Facilities

The Department is housed in the Medical School complex at the center of the Madison campus and at the Clinical Sciences Center on the west side of campus. The Department has modern research facilities including centralized support facilities. In addition, the Integrated Microscopy Resource on the Madison campus is a national microscopy center that provides equipment and support for scanning and transmission of electron microscopy and video-enhanced fluorescence microscopy. Extensive library facilities, including Departmental collections, the Medical School Library, and extensive holdings at other science libraries on the Madison campus, are available.

Financial Aid

It is the intention of the program that students receive stipend support during the duration of their graduate study. Support for students is offered through a variety of sources, including Department research and teaching assistantships, research assistantships from individual faculty research grants, project assistantships, fellowships, the thesis adviser's research funds, or other campus sources. In addition, students compete for University fellowships and research assistantships on several training grants on the Madison campus. For the 2014–15 school year, the stipend rate for graduate students in the Department of Pathology and Laboratory Medicine is $25,000, with an increase of approximately 4 percent annually. In addition, assistantship recipients qualify for full remission of nonresident and resident tuition and subsidized enrollment in the Graduate Assistant Health Insurance program.

Cost of Study

As discussed in the Financial Aid section, students receive stipend support throughout their graduate study. In the fall of 2014, tuition and fees are $5,932.20 per semester for Wisconsin residents and $12,595.64 per semester for nonresidents.

Living and Housing Costs

For single graduate students, the University maintains graduate student apartments that offer one- and two-bedroom units; rents range from $660 to $1079 per month in 2014–15. University Student Apartments, better known as Eagle Heights, offers one- to three-bedroom unfurnished apartments; rents range from $730 to $1,058 per month in 2014–15. There may be a waiting list for the Eagle Heights units, and priority is given to students with dependent children.

For more details, students should visit the Division of University Housing website at http://www.housing.wisc.edu. Most students live off campus; costs for off-campus housing vary depending on size and location. Additional information about off-campus housing is available at the UW–Madison Campus Information, Assistance, and Orientation website at http://www.wisc.edu/cac/housing/.

Student Group

The Madison campus is the flagship of the University of Wisconsin, with an enrollment of more than 40,000 students, including 9,000 graduate students. In the sciences, the graduate students belong to individual department graduate programs or are members of interdepartmental training programs, such as the CMP program.

Student Outcomes

Students in this program have successfully pursued a number of options after obtaining their Ph.D. degrees. They have received postdoctoral training and obtained faculty positions in academic institutions, taken research positions in industry, or continued on to medical school and secured faculty positions in medical institutions.

Location

Madison, recently ranked as one of the top American cities to live in, is the capital of the state, with a metropolitan population of approximately 240,000. The city, situated on four picturesque lakes, is approximately 150 miles northwest of Chicago. The city and the University offer a wide variety of educational, cultural, and recreational opportunities. Superb facilities are available for summer and winter sports, such as sailing, camping, hiking, ice skating, skiing, and bicycling.

The University

The University, founded in 1848, is one of the Big Ten schools and has a rich tradition of excellence in research. The University System includes the main campus in Madison plus twelve other comprehensive universities, thirteen freshman/sophomore campuses (UW Colleges), and the UW–Extension Program.

Applying

Applicants should have a bachelor's degree and an undergraduate minimum grade point average of 3.0 (on a 4.0 scale). Applicants should have a strong background in organic and physical chemistry, biochemistry, biology (including genetics), and mathematics through calculus. Completed application forms, Graduate Record Examinations (GRE) scores, transcripts, a resume, statement of purpose, and a minimum of three letters of recommendation are required for an admission decision. The application submission deadline for fall admission is December 1.

Correspondence and Information

CMP Program Coordinator
Department of Pathology and Laboratory Medicine
3170-10K/L Medical Foundation Centennial Building
University of Wisconsin–Madison
1685 Highland Avenue
Madison, Wisconsin 53705
United States
Phone: 608-262-2665
Fax: 608-265-3301
E-mail: gradinfo@pathology.wisc.edu
Website: http://www.cmp.wisc.edu

THE FACULTY AND THEIR RESEARCH

Nihal Ahmad, Professor, Dermatology. Cancer biology; prevention and experimental therapeutics of cancer.

Caroline Alexander, Associate Professor, Oncology. Role of breast stem cells in tumor induction; multiple functions of Wnt signaling in the regulation of mammary epithelial cell growth; changes in tumor susceptibility that are effected by alterations of normal development.

B. Lynn Allen-Hoffmann, Professor, Pathology. Keratinocytes; cancer biology; extracellular matrices.

David Andes, Associate Professor, Medicine. Identification of strategies to combat antimicrobial (especially antifungal) drug resistance.

Fotis Asimakopoulos, Assistant Professor, Medicine. Myeloma research; phase I experimental therapeutics.

Alan Attie, Professor, Biochemistry. Identify genes and pathways involved in obesity-induced type 2 diabetes.

Craig S. Atwood, Associate Professor, Medicine. Hormonal regulation of aging and neurodegenerative diseases.

Barbara Bendlin, Assistant Professor, Medicine. Aging; Alzheimer's disease, neurobiology of disease, behavior, and cognition.

Emery H. Bresnick, Professor, Pharmacology. Regulation of transcription, hematopoiesis, and leukemogenesis.

Karl W. Broman, Professor, Biostatistics and Medical Informatics. Signal transduction; statistical problems in genetics, genomics, and molecular biology.

Corina Burger, Associate Professor, Neurology. Molecular neuroscience; Behavior: cognition and aging; neurobiology of disease; synaptic plasticity.

Mark Burkard, Assistant Professor, Medicine. Breast cancer and drug development.

William J. Burlingham, Professor, Surgery. Mechanisms of transplant tolerance and rejection.

Wade Bushman, Urology. Prostate cancer.

Christian Capitini, Assistant Professor, Pediatrics. Allogeneic blood and marrow transplantation models; prevention of graft-versus-host disease and maximize graft-versus-tumor effects.

Michael Carrithers, Associate Professor, Neurology. Novel immune-mediated repair mechanisms relevant to the pathogenesis of multiple sclerosis and other inflammatory diseases.

Herbert Chen, Professor, Surgery. Development, progression, and treatment of endocrine tumors including gastrointestinal carcinoids; thyroid cancer, adrenal cancer, and pancreatic islet cell tumors.

University of Wisconsin–Madison

Clifford Cho, Associate Professor, Surgery. Influence of cancer on the integrity of the immune system.
Joshua Coon, Associate Professor, Chemistry. Bioanalytical chemistry; mass spectrometry.
Cameron Currie, Associate Professor, Bacteriology. Evolution of symbiotic associations between animals and microbes.
Loren Denlinger, Associate Professor, Medicine. Host-pathogen interactions; the role of macrophages in immunity to intracellular pathogens.
Arjang Djamali, Associate Professor, Medicine. The mechanisms of disease progression in kidney disease.
Marina Emborg, Assistant Professor, Medical Physics. Solutions for neurodegenerative disorders, in particular Parkinson's disease.
Zsuzsa Fabry, Professor, Pathology. Immunopathology; neuroimmunology; multiple sclerosis.
John Fleming, Professor, Neurology. Multiple sclerosis.
Andreas Friedl, Professor, Pathology. Heparan sulfate proteoglycans as modulators of growth factors in human disease; tumor angiogenesis.
Thomas Friedrich, Assistant Professor, Pathobiological Sciences. Viral immunity; pathogenesis.
Ying Ge, Assistant Professor, Cell and Regenerative Biology. Ultra high-resolution mass spectrometry-based proteomics and metabolomics technology for biomedical research.
James Gern, Professor, Pediatrics. Interactions between host and viral factors.
Daniel Greenspan, Professor, Pathology. Extracellular controls of cell behavior.
Jenny Gumperz, Associate Professor, Medical Microbiology and Immunology. Autoreactivity.
Richard Halberg, Assistant Professor,Medicine. Interactions among initiated clones/colon cancer.
Jeff Hardin, Professor, Zoology. Morphogenesis and pattern formation during early development.
Peiman Hematti, Associate Professor, Medicine. Characterization and study of mesenchymal stromal cells derived from human embryonic stem cells; development of a preclinical rhesus macaque model.
Anna Huttenlocher, Associate Professor, Medical Microbiology and Immunology. Cell migration and chemotaxis; adhesive mechanisms that regulate cell migration; the role of integrin signaling.
Nizar Jarjour, Professor, Medicine. Asthma; circadian rhythm; investigative bronchoscopy.
Juan Jaume, Associate Professor, Medicine. Endocrine autoimmunity, type 1 diabetes, and thyroid diseases.
Shannon Kenney, Professor, Medicine. Epstein-Barr virus pathogenesis and treatment.
K. C. Kent, Professor, Surgery. Molecular and cellular mechanisms underlying vascular disease.
Judith Kimble, Professor, Biochemisty. Immunology/Immunopatholgoy; Germline stem cells and their control.
Michelle Kimple, Assistant Professor. How beta cells of the pancreas respond to nutrient and hormonal stimulation to affect biological changes.
Bruce Klein, Professor, Pediatrics. Microbial immunology and pathogenesis.
John Kuo, Associate Professor, Neurosurgery. Brain tumor stem cells; molecular mechanisms of tumorigenesis.
Aparna Lakkaraju, Assistant Professor, Ophthalmology and Visual Services. Cellular basis of retinal degenerative diseases.
Youngsook Lee, Associate Professor, Anatomy. Transcriptional control of cardiovascular development and mechanisms of cardiac-specific gene regulation.
Peter W. Lewis, Assistant Professor, Biomolecular Chemistry. Epigenetic mechanisms in development and cancer.
Bo Liu, Associate Professor, Surgery. Vascular diseases, cell apoptosis, inflammation, signaling, adult progenitor cells, gene therapy.
Riccardo Lloyd, Professor, Department of Pathology and Laboratory Medicine.
Dan Loeb, Professor, Department of Oncology. Molecular biology of the hepatitis B viruses.
Albee Messing, Professor, Pathobiological Sciences. Transgenic mice; developmental neuropathology; molecular neurobiology.
Joshua Mezrich, Assistant Professor, Surgery. Transplant tolerance.
Deane F. Mosher, Professor, Medicine. Extracellular matrix and cell adhesion.
Robert Nickells, Professor, Ophthalmology and Visual Sciences. Glaucoma; neurodegeneration; complex genetics; neuronal apoptosis.
David O'Connor, Professor, Pathology. HIV/AIDS pathogenesis.
Shelby O'Connor, Assistant Professor, Pathology and Laboratory Medicine. Host and vaccine-elicited immune responses to SIV/HIV.
Caitlin Pepperell, Assistant Professor, Medicine. Bacterial pathogenesis.
Donna P. Peters, Professor, Pathology. Cell-matrix signaling in the human eye; glaucoma.
Luigi Puglielli, Associate Professor, Medicine. Aging of the brain; Alzheimer's disease; neurodegeneration; lipid signaling; protein signaling; post-translational modification; membrane transport; translational research.
Alan Rapraeger, Professor, Pathology. Mechanisms by which the syndecan family of cell-surface receptors regulate cell growth, adhesion, and migration.
Kurt Reed, Professor, Pathology. Infectious disease; molecular ecology and transmission of zoonotic and environmental pathogens.
Lixin Rui, Assistant Professor, Medicine. Signaling pathway in lymphoid malignancies.
Matyas Sandor, Professor, Pathology. Immune responses to infectious disease.
John-Demain (JD) Sauer, Medical Microbiology and Immunology. Bacterial pathogenesis, innate immunity, cell mediated immunity.
Christine M. Seroogy, Associate Professor, Pediatrics. Biological role of a novel E3 ubiquitin ligase called GRAIL in T-cell function and hematopoietic tissue development.
John Sheehan, Associate Professor, Medicine. Blood coagulation; intrinsic tenase regulation; coagulation factor IX.
Nader Sheibani, Professor, Ophthalmology and Visual Sciences. Cell adhesion and signaling in vascular cells; diabetic retinopathy.
Miriam Shelef, Assistant Professor, Medicine. Rheumatoid arthritis; peptidylarginine; autoimmunity; inflammation; autoantibodies; neutrophils.
Igor Slukvin, Associate Professor, Pathology. Hematopoietic differentiation of human embryonic stem cells; immune-privileged properties of embryonic and fetal tissues.
Judith Smith, Assistant Professor, Pediatrics, Regulation of type I IFN production in macrophages.
Paul M. Sondel, Professor, Pediatrics. Immune-mediated recognition and destruction of neoplasms.
Rupa Sridharan, Assistant Professor, Cell and Regenerative Biology. Epigenetics of cell fate change.
M. Suresh, Professor, Pathobiological Sciences. Molecular and cellular basis of T-cell memory; $CD8^+$ T-cell responses in chronic viral infections.
Masatoshi Suzuki, Assistant Professor, Comparative Biosciences. Application of stem cells to developmental modeling and cell-based therapy.
John Svaren, Professor, Comparative Biosciences. Role of EGR and NAB proteins in peripheral nerve myelination; genomic analysis of physiological regulation; role of chromatin structure in gene regulation.
Adel Talaat, Associate Professor, Pathobiological Sciences. Genomic and functional analyses of tuberculosis and paratuberculosis to understand pathogenesis and develop novel vaccines.
Robert Thorne, Assistant Professor, Pharmacy. Using biopharmaceuticals to treat neurological disorders (e.g., Alzheimer's disease, Parkinson's disease, and stroke); intranasal targeting of drugs to the brain, spinal cord, and cervical lymph nodes.
Raghu Vemuganti, Associate Professor, Neurosurgery. Traumatic brain injury.
Deric Wheeler, Assistant Professor, Human Oncology. Mechanisms of resistance to targeted therapies.
Timothy Yoshino, Professor, Pathobiological Sciences. Physiological interactions between parasites and their invertebrate hosts.
Su-Chun Zhang, Professor, Neuroscience. Stem cell approaches to neural degeneration and regeneration.
Xinyu Zhao, Associate Professor, Neuroscience. Using molecular mechanisms that regulate neural stem cells and neurodevelopment to treat neurological disorders and injuries.
Weixiong Zhong, Associate Professor, Pathology. Redox effects of selenium in human prostate cancer chemoprevention.

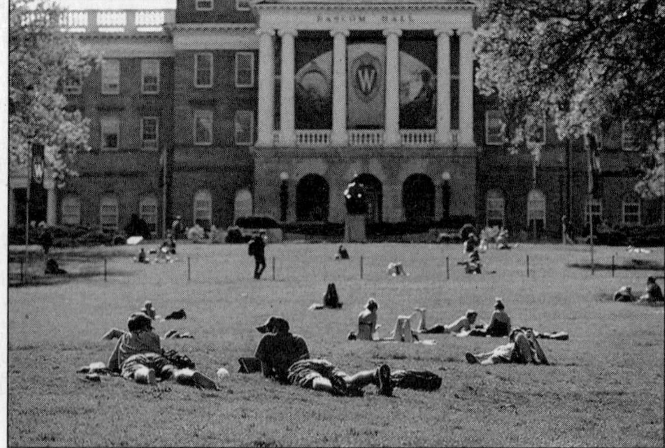

Bascom Hill on the UW–Madison campus.

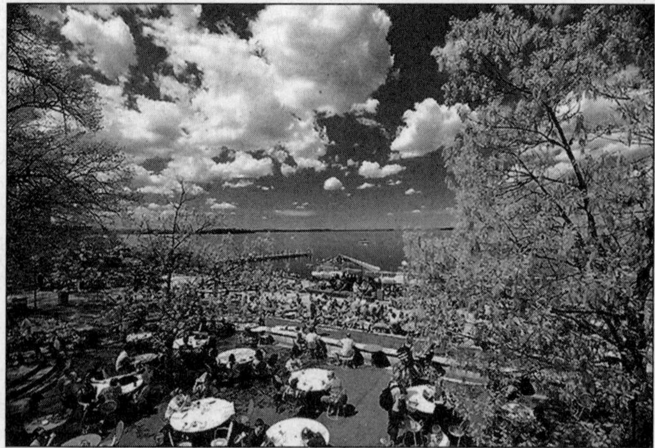

Memorial Student Union terrace.

Section 17
Pharmacology and Toxicology

This section contains a directory of institutions offering graduate work in pharmacology and toxicology. Additional information about programs listed in the directory may be obtained by writing directly to the dean of a graduate school or chair of a department at the address given in the directory.

For programs offering related work, see also in this book *Biochemistry; Biological and Biomedical Sciences; Cell, Molecular, and Structural Biology; Ecology, Environmental Biology, and Evolutionary Biology; Genetics, Developmental Biology, and Reproductive Biology; Neuroscience and Neurobiology; Nutrition; Pathology and Pathobiology; Pharmacy and Pharmaceutical Sciences; Physiology; Public Health;* and *Veterinary Medicine and Sciences.* In the other guides in this series:

Graduate Programs in the Humanities, Arts & Social Sciences
See *Psychology and Counseling*

Graduate Programs in the Physical Sciences, Mathematics, Agricultural Sciences, the Environment & Natural Resources
See *Chemistry* and *Environmental Sciences and Management*

Graduate Programs in Engineering & Applied Sciences
See *Chemical Engineering* and *Civil and Environmental Engineering*

CONTENTS

Program Directories

Molecular Pharmacology

Albert Einstein College of Medicine, Graduate Division of Biomedical Sciences, Department of Molecular Pharmacology, Bronx, NY 10461. Offers PhD, MD/PhD. *Degree requirements:* For doctorate, thesis/dissertation. *Entrance requirements:* For doctorate, GRE General Test. Additional exam requirements/recommendations for international students: Required—TOEFL. *Faculty research:* Effects of drugs on macromolecules, enzyme systems, cell morphology and function.

Brown University, Graduate School, Division of Biology and Medicine, Department of Molecular Pharmacology, Physiology and Biotechnology, Providence, RI 02912. Offers biomedical engineering (Sc M, PhD); biotechnology (PhD); molecular pharmacology and physiology (PhD); MD/PhD. *Degree requirements:* For doctorate, thesis/dissertation, preliminary exam. *Entrance requirements:* For master's and doctorate, GRE General Test, GRE Subject Test. Additional exam requirements/recommendations for international students: Required—TOEFL. Electronic applications accepted. *Faculty research:* Structural biology, antiplatelet drugs, nicotinic receptor structure/function.

Dartmouth College, Program in Experimental and Molecular Medicine, Molecular Pharmacology, Toxicology and Experimental Therapeutics Track, Hanover, NH 03755. Offers PhD.

Harvard University, Graduate School of Arts and Sciences, Division of Medical Sciences, Boston, MA 02115. Offers biological chemistry and molecular pharmacology (PhD); cell biology (PhD); genetics (PhD); microbiology and molecular genetics (PhD); pathology (PhD), including experimental pathology. *Degree requirements:* For doctorate, thesis/dissertation. *Entrance requirements:* For doctorate, GRE General Test, GRE Subject Test. Additional exam requirements/recommendations for international students: Required—TOEFL. *Expenses: Tuition:* Full-time $38,888. *Required fees:* $958. Tuition and fees vary according to campus/location, program and student level.

Mayo Graduate School, Graduate Programs in Biomedical Sciences, Program in Molecular Pharmacology and Experimental Therapeutics, Rochester, MN 55905. Offers PhD. *Degree requirements:* For doctorate, oral defense of dissertation, qualifying oral and written exam. *Entrance requirements:* For doctorate, GRE, 1 year of chemistry, biology, calculus, and physics. Additional exam requirements/recommendations for international students: Required—TOEFL. Electronic applications accepted. *Faculty research:* Patch clamping, G-proteins, pharmacogenetics, receptor-induced transcriptional events, cholinesterase biology.

Medical University of South Carolina, College of Graduate Studies, Program in Cell and Molecular Pharmacology and Experimental Therapeutics, Charleston, SC 29425. Offers MS, PhD, DMD/PhD, MD/PhD. Terminal master's awarded for partial completion of doctoral program. *Degree requirements:* For master's, thesis; for doctorate, comprehensive exam, thesis/dissertation, oral and written exams. *Entrance requirements:* For master's, GRE General Test; for doctorate, GRE General Test, interview, minimum GPA of 3.0. Additional exam requirements/recommendations for international students: Required—TOEFL (minimum score 600 paper-based; 100 iBT). Electronic applications accepted. *Faculty research:* Cancer drug discovery and development, growth factor receptor signaling, regulation of G-protein signaling, redox signal transduction, proteomics and mass spectrometry.

New York University, School of Medicine and Graduate School of Arts and Science, Sackler Institute of Graduate Biomedical Sciences, Program in Molecular Pharmacology, New York, NY 10012-1019. Offers PhD, MD/PhD. *Faculty:* 52 full-time (10 women). *Students:* 20 full-time (14 women); includes 11 minority (6 Black or African American, non-Hispanic/Latino; 3 Asian, non-Hispanic/Latino; 2 Hispanic/Latino), 4 international. Average age 26. In 2013, 5 doctorates awarded. *Degree requirements:* For doctorate, comprehensive exam, thesis/dissertation, qualifying exam. *Entrance requirements:* For doctorate, GRE General Test. Additional exam requirements/recommendations for international students: Required—TOEFL. *Application deadline:* For fall admission, 1/4 priority date for domestic students. Applications are processed on a rolling basis. Application fee: $85. *Expenses: Tuition:* Full-time $35,856; part-time $1494 per unit. *Required fees:* $1408; $64 per unit. $473 per term. Tuition and fees vary according to course load and program. *Financial support:* Fellowships with tuition reimbursements, research assistantships with tuition reimbursements, teaching assistantships with tuition reimbursements, and tuition waivers (full) available. *Faculty research:* Pharmacology and neurobiology, neuropeptides, receptor biochemistry, cytoskeleton, endocrinology. *Unit head:* Dr. Erika Bach, Chair, 212-263-5963, E-mail: erika.bach@nyu.edu. *Application contact:* Michael Escosia, Program Associate, 212-263-5648, E-mail: sackler-info@med.nyu.edu.

Purdue University, College of Pharmacy and Pharmacal Sciences and Graduate School, Graduate Programs in Pharmacy and Pharmacal Sciences, Department of Medicinal Chemistry and Molecular Pharmacology, West Lafayette, IN 47907. Offers biophysical and computational chemistry (PhD); cancer research (PhD); immunology and infectious disease (PhD); medicinal biochemistry and molecular biology (PhD); medicinal chemistry and chemical biology (PhD); molecular pharmacology (PhD); neuropharmacology, neurodegeneration, and neurotoxicity (PhD); systems biology and functional genomics (PhD). *Faculty:* 23 full-time (3 women), 6 part-time/adjunct (1 woman). *Students:* 50 full-time (21 women), 3 part-time (2 women); includes 1 minority (Asian, non-Hispanic/Latino), 30 international. Average age 26. 147 applicants, 20% accepted, 13 enrolled. In 2013, 12 doctorates awarded. *Degree requirements:* For doctorate, thesis/dissertation. *Entrance requirements:* For doctorate, GRE General Test; GRE Subject Test in biology, biochemistry, and chemistry (recommended), minimum undergraduate GPA of 3.0. Additional exam requirements/recommendations for international students: Required—TOEFL (minimum score 550 paper-based; 77 iBT); Recommended—TWE. *Application deadline:* For fall admission, 2/1 for domestic and international students. Applications are processed on a rolling basis. Application fee: $60 ($75 for international students). Electronic applications accepted. *Financial support:* Fellowships, research assistantships, teaching assistantships, and traineeships available. Support available to part-time students. Financial award applicants required to submit FAFSA. *Faculty research:* Drug design and development, cancer research, drug synthesis and analysis, chemical pharmacology, environmental toxicology. *Unit head:* Dr. Richard F. Borch, Head, 765-494-1403, E-mail: borch@purdue.edu. *Application contact:* Dr. Janine C. Mott, Graduate Contact, 765-494-1269, E-mail: jmott@purdue.edu.

Rosalind Franklin University of Medicine and Science, School of Graduate and Postdoctoral Studies - Interdisciplinary Graduate Program in Biomedical Sciences, Department of Cellular and Molecular Pharmacology, North Chicago, IL 60064-3095. Offers MS, PhD, MD/PhD. Terminal master's awarded for partial completion of doctoral program. *Degree requirements:* For master's, comprehensive exam, thesis; for doctorate, comprehensive exam, thesis/dissertation. *Entrance requirements:* For master's and doctorate, GRE General Test. Additional exam requirements/recommendations for international students: Required—TOEFL, TWE. Electronic applications accepted. *Faculty research:* Control of gene expression in higher organisms, molecular mechanism of action of growth factors and hormones, hormonal regulation in brain neuropsychopharmacology.

Rutgers, The State University of New Jersey, New Brunswick, Graduate School of Biomedical Sciences, Program in Cellular and Molecular Pharmacology, Piscataway, NJ 08854-5635. Offers MS, PhD, MD/PhD. *Degree requirements:* For master's, thesis, qualifying exam; for doctorate, thesis/dissertation, qualifying exam. *Entrance requirements:* Additional exam requirements/recommendations for international students: Required—TOEFL. Electronic applications accepted.

Thomas Jefferson University, Jefferson Graduate School of Biomedical Sciences, PhD Program in Biochemistry and Molecular Pharmacology, Philadelphia, PA 19107. Offers PhD. *Faculty:* 68 full-time (19 women), 1 (woman) part-time/adjunct. *Students:* 36 full-time (21 women); includes 9 minority (all Asian, non-Hispanic/Latino), 9 international. Average age 24. 64 applicants, 34% accepted, 6 enrolled. In 2013, 4 doctorates awarded. *Degree requirements:* For doctorate, comprehensive exam, thesis/dissertation. *Entrance requirements:* For doctorate, GRE General Test or MCAT, minimum GPA of 3.2. Additional exam requirements/recommendations for international students: Required—TOEFL (minimum score 100 iBT) or IELTS. *Application deadline:* For fall admission, 1/2 priority date for domestic and international students. Applications are processed on a rolling basis. Application fee: $75. Electronic applications accepted. *Financial support:* In 2013–14, 36 students received support, including 36 fellowships with full tuition reimbursements available (averaging $56,052 per year); Federal Work-Study, institutionally sponsored loans, scholarships/grants, traineeships, and stipends also available. Financial award application deadline: 5/1; financial award applicants required to submit FAFSA. *Faculty research:* Signal transduction and molecular genetics, translational biochemistry, human mitochondrial genetics, molecular biology of protein-RNA interaction, mammalian mitochondrial biogenesis and function. *Unit head:* Dr. Michael J. Root, Program Director, 215-503-4564, Fax: 215-923-2117, E-mail: michael.root@jefferson.edu. *Application contact:* Marc E. Stearns, Director of Admissions, 215-503-0155, Fax: 215-503-3433, E-mail: jgsbs-info@jefferson.edu. Website: http://www.jefferson.edu/university/biomedical_sciences/programs/phd/biochemistry_pharmacology.html

Thomas Jefferson University, Jefferson Graduate School of Biomedical Sciences, PhD Program in Molecular Pharmacology and Structural Biology, Philadelphia, PA 19107. Offers PhD. *Faculty:* 39 full-time (8 women). *Students:* 18 full-time (9 women); includes 5 minority (all Asian, non-Hispanic/Latino), 5 international. 34 applicants, 18% accepted, 3 enrolled. In 2013, 1 doctorate awarded. *Degree requirements:* For doctorate, comprehensive exam, thesis/dissertation. *Entrance requirements:* For doctorate, GRE General Test, minimum GPA of 3.2. Additional exam requirements/recommendations for international students: Required—TOEFL (minimum score 100 iBT) or IELTS. *Application deadline:* For fall admission, 1/2 priority date for domestic and international students. Applications are processed on a rolling basis. Application fee: $50. Electronic applications accepted. *Financial support:* In 2013–14, 18 students received support, including 18 fellowships with full tuition reimbursements available (averaging $54,758 per year); Federal Work-Study, institutionally sponsored loans, scholarships/grants, traineeships, and stipends also available. Support available to part-time students. Financial award application deadline: 5/1; financial award applicants required to submit FAFSA. *Faculty research:* Biochemistry and cell, molecular and structural biology of cell-surface and intracellular receptors; molecular modeling; signal transduction. *Total annual research expenditures:* $22.7 million. *Unit head:* Dr. Philip Wedegaertner, Program Director, 215-503-3137, Fax: 215-923-2117, E-mail: philip.wedegaertner@mail.tju.edu. *Application contact:* Marc E. Stearns, Director of Admissions, 215-503-0155, Fax: 215-503-9920, E-mail: jcgs-info@jefferson.edu.

University of Massachusetts Worcester, Graduate School of Biomedical Sciences, Worcester, MA 01655-0115. Offers biochemistry and molecular pharmacology (PhD); bioinformatics and computational biology (PhD); cancer biology (PhD); cell biology (PhD); clinical and population health research (PhD); clinical investigation (MS); immunology and virology (PhD); interdisciplinary biomedical research (PhD); millennium (PhD); molecular genetics and microbiology (PhD); neuroscience (PhD); translational science (PhD); MD/PhD. *Faculty:* 1,388 full-time (521 women), 309 part-time/adjunct (198 women). *Students:* 385 full-time (210 women); includes 53 minority (13 Black or African American, non-Hispanic/Latino; 30 Asian, non-Hispanic/Latino; 10 Hispanic/Latino), 138 international. Average age 28. 491 applicants, 19% accepted, 39 enrolled. In 2013, 5 master's, 50 doctorates awarded. Terminal master's awarded for partial completion of doctoral program. *Median time to degree:* Of those who began their doctoral program in fall 2005, 67% received their degree in 8 years or less. *Degree requirements:* For master's, comprehensive exam, thesis; for doctorate, comprehensive exam, thesis/dissertation. *Entrance requirements:* For master's, MD, PhD, DVM, or PharmD; for doctorate, GRE General Test, bachelor's degree. Additional exam requirements/recommendations for international students: Required—TOEFL (minimum score 100 iBT) or IELTS (minimum score 7.5). *Application deadline:* For fall admission, 12/15 for domestic and international students; for spring admission, 5/15 for domestic students. Application fee: $80. Electronic applications accepted. *Expenses:* Contact institution. *Financial support:* In 2013–14, 431 students received support, including research assistantships with full tuition reimbursements available (averaging $29,500 per year); scholarships/grants, health care benefits, tuition waivers (full), and unspecified assistantships also available. Financial award application deadline: 5/16. *Faculty research:* RNA interference, cell/molecular/developmental biology, bioinformatics, clinical/translational research, infectious disease. *Total annual research expenditures:* $245.9 million. *Unit head:* Dr. Anthony Carruthers, Dean, 508-856-4135, E-mail: anthony.carruthers@umassmed.edu. *Application contact:* Dr. Kendall Knight, Associate Dean and Interim Director of Admissions and Recruitment, 508-856-5628, Fax: 508-856-3659, E-mail: kendall.knight@umassmed.edu.
Website: http://www.umassmed.edu/gsbs/

University of Nevada, Reno, Graduate School, Interdisciplinary Program in Cellular and Molecular Pharmacology and Physiology, Reno, NV 89557. Offers PhD. *Degree requirements:* For doctorate, one foreign language, thesis/dissertation. *Entrance requirements:* For doctorate, GRE General Test or MCAT, minimum GPA of 3.0. Additional exam requirements/recommendations for international students: Required—TOEFL (minimum score 500 paper-based; 61 iBT), IELTS (minimum score 6). Electronic applications accepted. *Faculty research:* Neuropharmacology, toxicology, cardiovascular pharmacology, neuromuscular pharmacology.

University of Pittsburgh, School of Medicine, Graduate Programs in Medicine, Molecular Pharmacology Graduate Program, Pittsburgh, PA 15260. Offers PhD. *Faculty:* 61 full-time (11 women). *Students:* 21 full-time (10 women); includes 6 minority (2 Black or African American, non-Hispanic/Latino; 3 Asian, non-Hispanic/Latino; 1

Hispanic/Latino), 2 international. Average age 27. 517 applicants, 13% accepted, 22 enrolled. In 2013, 6 doctorates awarded. *Degree requirements:* For doctorate, comprehensive exam, thesis/dissertation. *Entrance requirements:* For doctorate, GRE General Test, GRE Subject Test, minimum QPA of 3.0. Additional exam requirements/ recommendations for international students: Required—TOEFL (minimum score 600 paper-based; 100 iBT), IELTS (minimum score 7). *Application deadline:* For fall admission, 1/1 priority date for domestic and international students. Application fee: $50. Electronic applications accepted. *Expenses:* Tuition, state resident: full-time $19,964; part-time $807 per credit. Tuition, nonresident: full-time $32,686; part-time $1337 per credit. *Required fees:* $740; $200. Tuition and fees vary according to program. *Financial support:* In 2013–14, 1 fellowship with full tuition reimbursement (averaging $26,010 per year), 20 research assistantships with full tuition reimbursements (averaging $26,010 per year) were awarded; institutionally sponsored loans, scholarships/grants, traineeships, health care benefits, tuition waivers (full), and unspecified assistantships also available. *Faculty research:* Drug discovery, signal transduction, cancer therapeutics, neuropharmacology, cardiovascular and renal pharmacology. *Unit head:* Dr. Patrick Pagano, Graduate Program Director, 412-383-6505, Fax: 412-648-9009, E-mail: pagano@pitt.edu. *Application contact:* Graduate Studies Administrator, 412-648-8957, Fax: 412-648-1007, E-mail: gradstudies@medschool.pitt.edu.
Website: http://www.gradbiomed.pitt.edu/

University of Southern California, Graduate School, School of Pharmacy, Graduate Programs in Molecular Pharmacology and Toxicology, Los Angeles, CA 90033. Offers pharmacology and pharmaceutical sciences (MS, PhD). Terminal master's awarded for partial completion of doctoral program. *Degree requirements:* For master's, comprehensive exam, thesis, 24 units of formal course work, excluding research and seminar courses; for doctorate, comprehensive exam, thesis/dissertation, 24 units of formal course work, excluding research and seminar courses. *Entrance requirements:* For master's and doctorate, GRE. Additional exam requirements/recommendations for international students: Required—TOEFL (minimum score 603 paper-based; 100 iBT). Electronic applications accepted. *Expenses:* Contact institution. *Faculty research:* Degenerative diseases, toxicology of drugs.

University of South Florida, Morsani College of Medicine and Graduate School, Graduate Programs in Medical Sciences, Tampa, FL 33620-9951. Offers aging and neuroscience (MSMS); allergy, immunology and infectious disease (PhD); anatomy (MSMS, PhD); athletic training (MSMS); bioinformatics and computational biology (MSBCB); biotechnology (MSB); clinical and translational research (MSMS, PhD); health informatics (MSHI, MSMS); health science (MSMS); interdisciplinary medical sciences (MSMS); medical microbiology and immunology (MSMS); metabolic and nutritional medicine (MSMS); molecular medicine (MSMS, PhD); molecular pharmacology and physiology (PhD); neurology (PhD); pathology and laboratory medicine (PhD); pharmacology and therapeutics (PhD); physiology and biophysics (PhD); women's health (MSMS). *Students:* 336 full-time (182 women), 39 part-time (21 women); includes 170 minority (45 Black or African American, non-Hispanic/Latino; 54 Asian, non-Hispanic/Latino; 59 Hispanic/Latino; 2 Native Hawaiian or other Pacific Islander, non-Hispanic/Latino; 10 Two or more races, non-Hispanic/Latino), 17 international. Average age 26. 1,066 applicants, 44% accepted, 250 enrolled. In 2013, 191 master's, 12 doctorates awarded. Terminal master's awarded for partial completion of doctoral program. *Degree requirements:* For master's, comprehensive exam, thesis; for doctorate, comprehensive exam, thesis/dissertation. *Entrance requirements:* For master's, GRE General Test or GMAT, bachelor's degree or equivalent from regionally-accredited university with minimum GPA of 3.0 in upper-division sciences coursework; prerequisites in general biology, general chemistry, general physics, organic chemistry, quantitative analysis, and integral and differential calculus; for doctorate, GRE General Test (minimum score of 600 quantitative), bachelor's degree from regionally-accredited university with minimum GPA of 3.0 in upper-division sciences coursework; 3 letters of recommendation; personal interview; 1-2 page personal statement; prerequisites in biology, chemistry, physics, organic chemistry, quantitative analysis, and integral/ differential calculus. Additional exam requirements/recommendations for international students: Required—TOEFL (minimum score 550 paper-based; 79 iBT) or IELTS (minimum score 6.5). *Application deadline:* For fall admission, 2/15 for domestic students, 1/2 for international students. Application fee: $30. *Expenses:* Contact institution. *Faculty research:* Anatomy, biochemistry, cancer biology, cardiovascular disease, cell biology, immunology, microbiology, molecular biology, neuroscience, pharmacology, physiology. *Unit head:* Dr. Michael Barber, Professor and Associate Dean for Graduate and Postdoctoral Affairs, 813-974-9908, Fax: 813-974-4317, E-mail: mbarber@health.usf.edu. *Application contact:* Dr. Eric Bennett, Graduate Director, PhD Program in Medical Sciences, 813-974-1545, Fax: 813-974-4317, E-mail: esbennet@ health.usf.edu.
Website: http://health.usf.edu/nocms/medicine/graduatestudies/

Molecular Toxicology

Massachusetts Institute of Technology, School of Science, Department of Biology, Cambridge, MA 02139-4307. Offers biochemistry (PhD); biological oceanography (PhD); biology (PhD); biophysical chemistry and molecular structure (PhD); cell biology (PhD); computational and systems biology (PhD); developmental biology (PhD); genetics (PhD); immunology (PhD); microbiology (PhD); molecular biology (PhD); neurobiology (PhD). *Faculty:* 58 full-time (15 women). *Students:* 261 full-time (133 women); includes 77 minority (3 Black or African American, non-Hispanic/Latino; 1 American Indian or Alaska Native, non-Hispanic/Latino; 32 Asian, non-Hispanic/Latino; 32 Hispanic/Latino; 9 Two or more races, non-Hispanic/Latino), 46 international. Average age 26. 651 applicants, 15% accepted, 39 enrolled. In 2013, 25 doctorates awarded. *Degree requirements:* For doctorate, comprehensive exam, thesis/ dissertation, two semesters as a teaching assistant. *Entrance requirements:* For doctorate, GRE General Test. Additional exam requirements/recommendations for international students: Required—TOEFL (minimum score 577 paper-based), IELTS (minimum score 6.5). *Application deadline:* For fall admission, 12/1 for domestic and international students. Application fee: $75. Electronic applications accepted. *Expenses: Tuition:* Full-time $43,210; part-time $670 per credit hour. *Required fees:* $288. *Financial support:* In 2013–14, 252 students received support, including 135 fellowships (averaging $36,800 per year), 122 research assistantships (averaging $35,500 per year), 1 teaching assistantship; Federal Work-Study, institutionally sponsored loans, scholarships/grants, traineeships, health care benefits, and unspecified assistantships also available. *Faculty research:* Cellular, developmental and molecular (plant and animal) biology; biochemistry, bioengineering, biophysics and structural biology; classical and molecular genetics, stem cell and epigenetics; immunology and microbiology; cancer biology, molecular medicine, neurobiology and human disease; computational and systems biology. *Total annual research expenditures:* $44.5 million. *Unit head:* Alan Grossman, Interim Head, 617-253-4701. *Application contact:* Biology Education Office, 617-253-3717, Fax: 617-258-9329, E-mail: gradbio@mit.edu.
Website: https://biology.mit.edu/

New York University, Graduate School of Arts and Science, Department of Environmental Medicine, New York, NY 10012-1019. Offers environmental health sciences (MS, PhD), including biostatistics (PhD), environmental hygiene (MS), epidemiology (PhD), ergonomics and biomechanics (PhD), exposure assessment and health effects (PhD), molecular toxicology/carcinogenesis (PhD), toxicology. Part-time programs available. *Faculty:* 26 full-time (7 women). *Students:* 55 full-time (34 women), 13 part-time (3 women); includes 16 minority (1 Black or African American, non-Hispanic/Latino; 8 Asian, non-Hispanic/Latino; 6 Hispanic/Latino; 1 Two or more races, non-Hispanic/Latino), 23 international. Average age 31. 69 applicants, 55% accepted, 18 enrolled. In 2013, 14 master's, 7 doctorates awarded. Terminal master's awarded for partial completion of doctoral program. *Degree requirements:* For master's, thesis or alternative; for doctorate, one foreign language, thesis/dissertation, oral and written exams. *Entrance requirements:* For master's and doctorate, GRE General Test, minimum GPA of 3.0; bachelor's degree in biological, physical, or engineering science. Additional exam requirements/recommendations for international students: Required—TOEFL. *Application deadline:* For fall admission, 12/18 for domestic and international students. Application fee: $95. *Expenses: Tuition:* Full-time $35,856; part-time $1494 per unit. *Required fees:* $1408; $64 per unit. $473 per term. Tuition and fees vary according to course load and program. *Financial support:* Fellowships with tuition reimbursements, teaching assistantships with tuition reimbursements, career-related internships or fieldwork, Federal Work-Study, institutionally sponsored loans, and health care benefits available. Financial award application deadline: 12/18; financial award applicants required to submit FAFSA. *Unit head:* Dr. Max Costa, Chair, 845-731-3661, Fax: 845-351-2058, E-mail: ehs@env.med.nyu.edu. *Application contact:* Dr. Jerome J. Solomon, Director of Graduate Studies, 845-731-3661, Fax: 845-351-2058, E-mail: ehs@env.med.nyu.edu.
Website: http://environmental-medicine.med.nyu.edu/

North Carolina State University, Graduate School, College of Agriculture and Life Sciences and College of Veterinary Medicine, Department of Environmental and Molecular Toxicology, Raleigh, NC 27695. Offers M Tox, MS, PhD. Terminal master's awarded for partial completion of doctoral program. *Degree requirements:* For master's, thesis (for some programs); for doctorate, thesis/dissertation. *Entrance requirements:* For master's and doctorate, GRE General Test, minimum GPA of 3.0. Electronic applications accepted. *Faculty research:* Chemical fate, carcinogenesis, developmental and endocrine toxicity, xenobiotic metabolism, signal transduction.

University of California, Berkeley, Graduate Division, College of Natural Resources, Group in Molecular Toxicology, Berkeley, CA 94720-1500. Offers PhD. *Entrance requirements:* For doctorate, GRE General Test, 3 letters of recommendation.

University of California, Los Angeles, Graduate Division, School of Public Health, Department of Environmental Health Sciences, Interdepartmental Program in Molecular Toxicology, Los Angeles, CA 90095. Offers PhD. *Degree requirements:* For doctorate, thesis/dissertation, oral and written qualifying exams. *Entrance requirements:* For doctorate, GRE General Test. Electronic applications accepted.

University of Cincinnati, Graduate School, College of Medicine, Graduate Programs in Biomedical Sciences, Department of Environmental Health, Programs in Environmental Genetics and Molecular Toxicology, Cincinnati, OH 45221. Offers MS, PhD. *Degree requirements:* For doctorate, thesis/dissertation. *Entrance requirements:* For master's, GRE, minimum GPA of 3.0, 3 letters of recommendation. Additional exam requirements/ recommendations for international students: Required—TOEFL (minimum score 520 paper-based).

Pharmacology

Albany College of Pharmacy and Health Sciences, School of Pharmacy and Pharmaceutical Sciences, Albany, NY 12208. Offers health outcomes research (MS); pharmaceutical sciences (MS), including pharmaceutics, pharmacology; pharmacy (Pharm D). *Accreditation:* ACPE. *Students:* 527 full-time (308 women), 15 part-time (10 women); includes 138 minority (19 Black or African American, non-Hispanic/Latino; 95 Asian, non-Hispanic/Latino; 13 Hispanic/Latino; 1 Native Hawaiian or other Pacific Islander, non-Hispanic/Latino; 10 Two or more races, non-Hispanic/Latino), 64 international. Average age 24. 1,209 applicants, 15% accepted, 78 enrolled. In 2013, 6 master's, 283 doctorates awarded. *Degree requirements:* For master's, thesis; for doctorate, practice experience. *Entrance requirements:* For master's, GRE, minimum GPA of 3.0; for doctorate, PCAT, minimum GPA of 2.5. Additional exam requirements/ recommendations for international students: Required—TOEFL (minimum score 84 iBT). *Application deadline:* For fall admission, 3/1 for domestic and international students. Applications are processed on a rolling basis. Application fee: $75. Electronic applications accepted. *Financial support:* In 2013–14, 20 students received support. Federal Work-Study and scholarships/grants available. Support available to part-time

students. Financial award application deadline: 3/1; financial award applicants required to submit FAFSA. *Faculty research:* Therapeutic use of drugs, pharmacokinetics, drug delivery and design. *Unit head:* Dr. Angela Dominelli, Dean, School of Pharmacy and Pharmaceutical Sciences, 518-694-7333. *Application contact:* Ann Bruno, Coordinator, Graduate Programs, 518-694-7130, E-mail: graduate@acphs.edu.
Website: http://www.acphs.edu/academics/schools-departments/school-pharmacy-pharmaceutical-sciences

Albany Medical College, Center for Neuropharmacology and Neuroscience, Albany, NY 12208-3479. Offers MS, PhD. Terminal master's awarded for partial completion of doctoral program. *Degree requirements:* For master's, thesis; for doctorate, comprehensive exam, thesis/dissertation. *Entrance requirements:* For master's, GRE General Test, all transcripts, letters of recommendation; for doctorate, GRE General Test, letters of recommendation. Additional exam requirements/recommendations for international students: Required—TOEFL. *Faculty research:* Molecular and cellular neuroscience, neuronal development, addiction.

Alliant International University–San Francisco, California School of Professional Psychology, Program in Psychopharmacology, San Francisco, CA 94133-1221. Offers Post-Doctoral MS. Part-time programs available. Postbaccalaureate distance learning degree programs offered. *Faculty:* 1 full-time (0 women), 9 part-time/adjunct (1 woman). *Students:* 1 (woman) full-time, 34 part-time (22 women); includes 12 minority (4 Black or African American, non-Hispanic/Latino; 2 American Indian or Alaska Native, non-Hispanic/Latino; 1 Asian, non-Hispanic/Latino; 1 Hispanic/Latino; 1 Native Hawaiian or other Pacific Islander, non-Hispanic/Latino; 3 Two or more races, non-Hispanic/Latino), 2 international. Average age 42. In 2013, 25 master's awarded. *Entrance requirements:* For master's, doctorate in clinical psychology. Additional exam requirements/recommendations for international students: Required—TOEFL (minimum score 550 paper-based; 80 iBT), TWE (minimum score 5). *Application deadline:* For fall admission, 4/1 priority date for domestic and international students. Applications are processed on a rolling basis. Application fee: $65. Electronic applications accepted. *Financial support:* Federal Work-Study available. Financial award application deadline: 2/15; financial award applicants required to submit FAFSA. *Unit head:* Dr. Alan Lincoln, Director, 858-635-4768, E-mail: admissions@alliant.edu. *Application contact:* Alliant International University Central Contact Center, 866-U-ALLIANT, Fax: 858-635-4555, E-mail: admissions@alliant.edu.

American University of Beirut, Graduate Programs, Faculty of Medicine, Beirut, Lebanon. Offers anatomy, cell biology and human morphology (MS); biochemistry and medical genetics (MS); biomedical sciences (PhD); experimental pathology, immunology and microbiology (MS); medicine (MD); neuroscience (MS); pharmacology and toxicology (MS). Part-time programs available. *Faculty:* 259 full-time (78 women), 93 part-time/adjunct (16 women). *Students:* 364 full-time (165 women), 62 part-time (54 women). Average age 23. In 2013, 18 master's awarded. *Degree requirements:* For master's, one foreign language, comprehensive exam, thesis (for some programs); for doctorate, one foreign language, comprehensive exam, thesis/dissertation. *Entrance requirements:* For master's, letter of recommendation; for doctorate, MCAT, bachelor's degree. Additional exam requirements/recommendations for international students: Required—TOEFL (minimum score 600 paper-based; 100 iBT), IELTS (minimum score 7.5). *Application deadline:* For fall admission, 4/30 for domestic and international students; for spring admission, 11/1 for domestic and international students. Application fee: $50. *Expenses: Tuition:* Full-time $14,724; part-time $818 per credit. *Required fees:* $692. Tuition and fees vary according to course load and program. *Financial support:* In 2013–14, 242 students received support, including 60 teaching assistantships (averaging $4,000 per year); career-related internships or fieldwork, institutionally sponsored loans, scholarships/grants, health care benefits, and unspecified assistantships also available. Financial award application deadline: 2/2. *Faculty research:* Cancer research (targeted therapy, mechanisms of leukemogenesis, tumor cell extravasation and metastasis, cancer stem cells), stem cell research (regenerative medicine, drug discovery), genetic research (neurogenetics, hereditary cardiomyopathy, hemoglobinopathies, pharmacogenomics, proteomics), neuroscience research (pain, neurodegenerative disorder), metabolism (inflammation and metabolism, metabolic disorder, diabetes mellitus), vascular and renal biology, signal transduction. *Total annual research expenditures:* $2.6 million. *Unit head:* Dr. Mohamed Sayegh, Dean, 961-1350000 Ext. 4700, Fax: 961-1744464, E-mail: msayegh@aub.edu.lb. *Application contact:* Dr. Salim Kanaan, Director, Admissions Office, 961-1-350000 Ext. 2594, Fax: 96-1-1750775, E-mail: sk00@aub.edu.lb.
Website: http://www.aub.edu.lb/fm/fm_home/Pages/index.aspx

Argosy University, Hawai`i, College of Psychology and Behavioral Sciences, Program in Psychopharmacology, Honolulu, HI 96813. Offers MS, Certificate.

Auburn University, College of Veterinary Medicine and Graduate School, Graduate Programs in Veterinary Medicine, Auburn University, AL 36849. Offers biomedical sciences (MS, PhD), including anatomy, physiology and pharmacology (MS), biomedical sciences (PhD), clinical sciences (MS), large animal surgery and medicine (MS), pathobiology (MS), radiology (MS), small animal surgery and medicine (MS); DVM/MS. Part-time programs available. *Faculty:* 100 full-time (41 women), 4 part-time/adjunct (1 woman). *Students:* 24 full-time (16 women), 38 part-time (25 women); includes 5 minority (1 Black or African American, non-Hispanic/Latino; 1 American Indian or Alaska Native, non-Hispanic/Latino; 2 Asian, non-Hispanic/Latino; 1 Hispanic/Latino), 22 international. Average age 30. 36 applicants, 44% accepted, 13 enrolled. In 2013, 12 master's, 8 doctorates awarded. *Degree requirements:* For doctorate, thesis/dissertation. *Entrance requirements:* For master's, GRE General Test; for doctorate, GRE General Test, GRE Subject Test. *Application deadline:* For fall admission, 7/7 for domestic students; for spring admission, 11/24 for domestic students. Applications are processed on a rolling basis. Application fee: $50 ($60 for international students). Electronic applications accepted. *Expenses:* Tuition, state resident: full-time $8262; part-time $459 per credit hour. Tuition, nonresident: full-time $24,786; part-time $1377 per credit hour. Tuition and fees vary according to degree level and program. *Financial support:* Research assistantships, teaching assistantships, and Federal Work-Study available. Support available to part-time students. Financial award application deadline: 3/15; financial award applicants required to submit FAFSA. *Unit head:* Dr. Calvin Johnson, Acting Dean, 334-844-2650. *Application contact:* Dr. George Flowers, Dean of the Graduate School, 334-844-2125.

Baylor College of Medicine, Graduate School of Biomedical Sciences, Department of Pharmacology, Houston, TX 77030-3498. Offers PhD, MD/PhD. *Degree requirements:* For doctorate, thesis/dissertation, public defense. *Entrance requirements:* For doctorate, GRE General Test, GRE Subject Test (strongly recommended), minimum GPA of 3.0. Additional exam requirements/recommendations for international students: Required—TOEFL. Electronic applications accepted. *Faculty research:* Drug discovery, antibiotics, antitumor, computational drug design, signal transduction complex.

Boston University, School of Medicine, Division of Graduate Medical Sciences, Department of Pharmacology and Experimental Therapeutics, Boston, MA 02118. Offers MA, PhD, MD/PhD. Terminal master's awarded for partial completion of doctoral program. *Degree requirements:* For master's, thesis; for doctorate, thesis/dissertation. *Application deadline:* For fall admission, 1/15 for domestic students; for spring admission, 10/15 for domestic students. *Expenses: Tuition:* Full-time $43,970; part-time $1374 per credit hour. *Required fees:* $60 per semester. Tuition and fees vary according to class time, course level and program. *Unit head:* Dr. David H. Farb, Chairman, 617-638-4300, Fax: 617-638-4329, E-mail: dfarb@bu.edu. *Application contact:* Dr. Carol T. Walsh, Graduate Director, 617-638-4326, Fax: 617-638-4329, E-mail: ctwalsh@bu.edu.
Website: http://www.bumc.bu.edu/busm-pm/

Boston University, School of Medicine, Division of Graduate Medical Sciences, Program in Clinical Investigation, Boston, MA 02215. Offers MA. *Degree requirements:* For master's, thesis. *Application deadline:* For spring admission, 10/15 for domestic students. *Expenses: Tuition:* Full-time $43,970; part-time $1374 per credit hour. *Required fees:* $60 per semester. Tuition and fees vary according to class time, course level and program. *Unit head:* Dr. Susan S. Fish, Director, 617-638-7715, E-mail: sfish@bu.edu. *Application contact:* Stacey Hess Pino, Assistant Director, 617-638-5211, Fax: 617-638-5740, E-mail: sahess@bu.edu.
Website: http://www.bumc.bu.edu/gms/maci/

Case Western Reserve University, School of Medicine and School of Graduate Studies, Graduate Programs in Medicine, Department of Pharmacology, Cleveland, OH 44106. Offers PhD, MD/PhD. Terminal master's awarded for partial completion of doctoral program. *Degree requirements:* For doctorate, comprehensive exam, thesis/dissertation. *Entrance requirements:* For doctorate, GRE General Test, GRE Subject Test, or MCAT. Additional exam requirements/recommendations for international students: Required—TOEFL. Electronic applications accepted. *Faculty research:* Aspects of cellular, molecular, and clinical pharmacology; neuroendocrine pharmacology; drug metabolism.

Columbia University, College of Physicians and Surgeons, Department of Pharmacology, New York, NY 10032. Offers pharmacology (M Phil, MA, PhD); pharmacology-toxicology (M Phil, MA, PhD); MD/PhD. Only candidates for the PhD are admitted. Terminal master's awarded for partial completion of doctoral program. *Degree requirements:* For doctorate, thesis/dissertation. *Entrance requirements:* For master's and doctorate, GRE General Test. Additional exam requirements/recommendations for international students: Required—TOEFL. *Faculty research:* Cardiovascular pharmacology, receptor pharmacology, neuropharmacology, membrane biophysics, eicosanoids.

Cornell University, Graduate School, Graduate Fields of Comparative Biomedical Sciences, Field of Pharmacology, Ithaca, NY 14853-0001. Offers MS, PhD. *Faculty:* 32 full-time (9 women). *Students:* 11 full-time (6 women); includes 3 minority (1 Asian, non-Hispanic/Latino; 1 Hispanic/Latino; 1 Native Hawaiian or other Pacific Islander, non-Hispanic/Latino), 2 international. Average age 27. 17 applicants, 6% accepted, 1 enrolled. In 2013, 1 doctorate awarded. *Degree requirements:* For master's, thesis; for doctorate, comprehensive exam, thesis/dissertation. *Entrance requirements:* For master's and doctorate, GRE General Test, 3 letters of recommendation. Additional exam requirements/recommendations for international students: Required—TOEFL (minimum score 550 paper-based; 77 iBT). *Application deadline:* For fall admission, 12/5 for domestic students. Application fee: $95. Electronic applications accepted. *Financial support:* In 2013–14, 7 students received support, including 1 fellowship with full tuition reimbursement available, 6 research assistantships with full tuition reimbursements available; teaching assistantships with full tuition reimbursements available, institutionally sponsored loans, scholarships/grants, health care benefits, tuition waivers (full and partial), and unspecified assistantships also available. Financial award applicants required to submit FAFSA. *Faculty research:* Signal transduction, ion channels, calcium signaling, G proteins, cancer cell biology. *Unit head:* Director of Graduate Studies, 607-253-3276, Fax: 607-253-3756. *Application contact:* Graduate Field Assistant, 607-253-3276, Fax: 607-253-3756, E-mail: graduate_edcvm@cornell.edu.
Website: http://www.gradschool.cornell.edu/fields.php?id-66&a-2

Creighton University, School of Medicine and Graduate School, Graduate Programs in Medicine, Department of Pharmacology, Omaha, NE 68178-0001. Offers pharmaceutical sciences (MS); pharmacology (MS, PhD); Pharm D/MS. *Faculty:* 10 full-time (3 women). *Students:* 7 full-time (4 women); includes 1 minority (Asian, non-Hispanic/Latino), 2 international. Average age 25. 20 applicants, 10% accepted, 2 enrolled. In 2013, 1 doctorate awarded. Terminal master's awarded for partial completion of doctoral program. *Degree requirements:* For master's, comprehensive exam, thesis; for doctorate, comprehensive exam, thesis/dissertation, oral and written preliminary exams. *Entrance requirements:* For master's and doctorate, GRE General Test, minimum GPA of 3.0, undergraduate degree in sciences. Additional exam requirements/recommendations for international students: Required—TOEFL. *Application deadline:* For spring admission, 4/1 priority date for domestic and international students. Applications are processed on a rolling basis. Application fee: $35. Electronic applications accepted. *Expenses: Tuition:* Full-time $13,608; part-time $756 per credit hour. *Required fees:* $149 per semester. Tuition and fees vary according to course load, campus/location, program, reciprocity agreements and student's religious affiliation. *Financial support:* In 2013–14, 6 fellowships with full tuition reimbursements (averaging $23,868 per year) were awarded; institutionally sponsored loans and tuition waivers (full and partial) also available. Financial award application deadline: 4/1. *Faculty research:* Pharmacology secretion, cardiovascular-renal pharmacology, adrenergic receptors, signal transduction, genetic regulation of receptors. *Total annual research expenditures:* $2.3 million. *Unit head:* Dr. Thomas F. Murray, Chair, 402-280-2983, Fax: 402-280-2142, E-mail: tfmurray@creighton.edu. *Application contact:* Dr. Margaret A. Scofield, Associate Professor, 402-280-2245, Fax: 402-280-2142, E-mail: mscof@creighton.edu.
Website: http://medschool.creighton.edu/medicine/departments/pharmacology/

Dalhousie University, Faculty of Graduate Studies and Faculty of Medicine, Graduate Programs in Medicine, Department of Pharmacology, Halifax, NS B3H 4R2, Canada. Offers M Sc, PhD. *Degree requirements:* For master's, thesis; for doctorate, comprehensive exam, thesis/dissertation. *Entrance requirements:* Additional exam requirements/recommendations for international students: Required—1 of 5 approved tests: TOEFL, IELTS, CANTEST, CAEL, Michigan English Language Assessment Battery. Electronic applications accepted. *Faculty research:* Electrophysiology and neurochemistry; endocrinology, immunology and cancer research; molecular biology; cardiovascular and autonomic; drug biotransformation and metabolism; ocular pharmacology.

Dartmouth College, Arts and Sciences Graduate Programs, Department of Pharmacology and Toxicology, Hanover, NH 03755. Offers PhD, MD/PhD. *Degree requirements:* For doctorate, thesis/dissertation. *Entrance requirements:* For doctorate, GRE General Test, GRE Subject Test, bachelor's degree in biological, chemical, or physical science. Additional exam requirements/recommendations for international students: Required—TOEFL. Electronic applications accepted. *Faculty research:* Molecular biology of carcinogenesis, DNA repair and gene expression, biochemical and environmental toxicology, protein receptor ligand interactions.

Drexel University, College of Medicine, Biomedical Graduate Programs, Pharmacology and Physiology Program, Philadelphia, PA 19104-2875. Offers MS, PhD, MD/PhD. Part-time programs available. Terminal master's awarded for partial completion of doctoral program. *Degree requirements:* For master's, comprehensive exam; for doctorate, thesis/dissertation, qualifying exam. *Entrance requirements:* For master's, GRE General Test, minimum GPA of 2.75; for doctorate, GRE General Test, minimum GPA of 3.0. Additional exam requirements/recommendations for international students: Required—TOEFL. Electronic applications accepted. *Faculty research:* Cardiovascular pharmacology, drugs of abuse, neurotransmitter mechanisms.

Duke University, Graduate School, Department of Pharmacology and Cancer Biology, Durham, NC 27710. Offers pharmacology (PhD). *Faculty:* 50 full-time. *Students:* 62 full-time (31 women). Average age 23. 72 applicants, 14% accepted, 6 enrolled. In 2013, 8 doctorates awarded. *Degree requirements:* For doctorate, thesis/dissertation. *Entrance requirements:* For doctorate, GRE General Test, minimum GPA of 3.0. Additional exam requirements/recommendations for international students: Required—TOEFL or IELTS. *Application deadline:* For fall admission, 12/8 priority date for domestic and international students. Application fee: $80. Electronic applications accepted. *Financial support:* In 2013–14, 10 fellowships with tuition reimbursements (averaging $29,420 per year), 52 research assistantships with tuition reimbursements (averaging $29,420 per year) were awarded; scholarships/grants, traineeships, health care benefits, and unspecified assistantships also available. Financial award application deadline: 12/8. *Faculty research:* Developmental pharmacology, neuropharmacology, molecular pharmacology, toxicology, cell growth and metabolism. *Unit head:* Dr. Jeffrey Rathmell, Director of Graduate Studies, 919-681-1084, Fax: 919-684-8922, E-mail: jeff.rathmell@duke.edu. *Application contact:* Jamie Baize-Smith, Assistant Director of Graduate Studies, 919-613-8600, Fax: 919-681-7139, E-mail: baize@duke.edu.
Website: http://pharmacology.mc.duke.edu/

Duquesne University, Mylan School of Pharmacy, Graduate School of Pharmaceutical Sciences, Program in Pharmacology, Pittsburgh, PA 15282-0001. Offers MS, PhD. *Faculty:* 6 full-time (4 women). *Students:* 13 full-time (9 women); includes 1 minority (Black or African American, non-Hispanic/Latino), 6 international. Average age 27. 56 applicants, 4% accepted, 2 enrolled. In 2013, 2 master's, 1 doctorate awarded. *Degree requirements:* For master's, thesis; for doctorate, comprehensive exam, thesis/dissertation. *Entrance requirements:* For master's and doctorate, GRE General Test. Additional exam requirements/recommendations for international students: Required—TOEFL or IELTS (minimum score 7). *Application deadline:* For fall admission, 2/1 priority date for domestic and international students; for spring admission, 10/1 priority date for domestic and international students. Applications are processed on a rolling basis. Application fee: $50. Electronic applications accepted. *Expenses: Tuition:* Full-time $18,162; part-time $1009 per credit. *Required fees:* $1728; $96 per credit. Tuition and fees vary according to program. *Financial support:* In 2013–14, 11 students received support, including 11 teaching assistantships with full tuition reimbursements available; research assistantships with full tuition reimbursements available also available. *Unit head:* Dr. Christopher K. Surratt, Head, 412-396-5007. *Application contact:* Information Contact, 412-396-1172, E-mail: gsps-adm@duq.edu.
Website: http://www.duq.edu/academics/schools/pharmacy/graduate-school-of-pharmaceutical-sciences

East Carolina University, Brody School of Medicine, Department of Pharmacology and Toxicology, Greenville, NC 27858-4353. Offers PhD, MD/PhD. *Degree requirements:* For doctorate, comprehensive exam, thesis/dissertation. *Entrance requirements:* For doctorate, GRE General Test, GRE Subject Test. Additional exam requirements/recommendations for international students: Required—TOEFL. *Application deadline:* For fall admission, 6/15 priority date for domestic students. Applications are processed on a rolling basis. Application fee: $50. *Expenses:* Tuition, state resident: full-time $4223. Tuition, nonresident: full-time $16,540. *Required fees:* $2184. *Financial support:* Fellowships with full tuition reimbursements available. Financial award application deadline: 6/1. *Faculty research:* GNS/behavioral pharmacology, cardiovascular pharmacology, cell signaling and second messenger, effects of calcium channel blockers. *Unit head:* Dr. David A. Taylor, Chairman, 252-744-2734, Fax: 252-744-3203, E-mail: taylorda@ecu.edu. *Application contact:* Contact Center, 252-744-1020.
Website: http://www.ecu.edu/cs-dhs/pharmacology/Graduate-Program09.cfm

East Tennessee State University, James H. Quillen College of Medicine, Department of Biomedical Sciences, Johnson City, TN 37614. Offers anatomy (PhD); biochemistry (PhD); microbiology (PhD); pharmaceutical sciences (PhD); pharmacology (PhD); physiology (PhD); quantitative biosciences (PhD). *Faculty:* 43 full-time (11 women), 1 (woman) part-time/adjunct. *Students:* 31 full-time (17 women), 4 part-time (1 woman); includes 6 minority (2 Black or African American, non-Hispanic/Latino; 3 Asian, non-Hispanic/Latino; 1 Hispanic/Latino), 9 international. Average age 29. 53 applicants, 17% accepted, 8 enrolled. In 2013, 6 doctorates awarded. *Degree requirements:* For doctorate, thesis/dissertation, comprehensive qualifying exam. *Entrance requirements:* For doctorate, GRE General Test, GRE Subject Test. Additional exam requirements/recommendations for international students: Required—TOEFL (minimum score 550 paper-based; 79 iBT). *Application deadline:* For fall admission, 3/15 priority date for domestic students, 3/1 priority date for international students. Application fee: $35 ($45 for international students). Electronic applications accepted. *Expenses:* Contact institution. *Financial support:* In 2013–14, 30 students received support, including 30 research assistantships with full tuition reimbursements available (averaging $19,000 per year); career-related internships or fieldwork, institutionally sponsored loans, scholarships/grants, and unspecified assistantships also available. Financial award application deadline: 7/1; financial award applicants required to submit FAFSA. *Faculty research:* Cardiovascular, infectious disease, neurosciences, cancer, immunology. *Unit head:* Dr. Mitchell E. Robinson, Associate Dean/Program Director, 423-439-2031, Fax: 423-439-2140, E-mail: robinson@etsu.edu. *Application contact:* Shella Bennett, Graduate Specialist, 423-439-4708, Fax: 423-439-5624, E-mail: bennetsg@etsu.edu.
Website: http://www.etsu.edu/com/dbms/

Emory University, Laney Graduate School, Division of Biological and Biomedical Sciences, Program in Molecular and Systems Pharmacology, Atlanta, GA 30322-1100. Offers PhD. *Degree requirements:* For doctorate, comprehensive exam, thesis/dissertation. *Entrance requirements:* For doctorate, GRE General Test, minimum GPA of 3.0 in science course work (recommended). Additional exam requirements/recommendations for international students: Required—TOEFL. Electronic applications accepted. *Faculty research:* Transmembrane signaling, neuropharmacology, neurophysiology and neurodegeneration, metabolism and molecular toxicology, cell and developmental biology.

Fairleigh Dickinson University, College at Florham, Silberman College of Business, Program in Pharmaceutical Studies, Madison, NJ 07940-1099. Offers MBA, Certificate.

Florida Agricultural and Mechanical University, Division of Graduate Studies, Research, and Continuing Education, College of Pharmacy and Pharmaceutical Sciences, Graduate Programs in Pharmaceutical Sciences, Tallahassee, FL 32307-3200. Offers environmental toxicology (PhD); medicinal chemistry (MS, PhD); pharmaceutics (MS, PhD); pharmacology/toxicology (MS, PhD); pharmacy administration (MS). *Accreditation:* CEPH. *Degree requirements:* For master's, comprehensive exam, thesis, publishable paper; for doctorate, comprehensive exam, thesis/dissertation, publishable paper. *Entrance requirements:* For master's and doctorate, GRE General Test, minimum GPA of 3.0 in last 60 hours. Additional exam requirements/recommendations for international students: Required—TOEFL. *Faculty research:* Anticancer agents, anti-inflammatory drugs, chronopharmacology, neuroendocrinology, microbiology.

Georgetown University, Graduate School of Arts and Sciences, Programs in Biomedical Sciences, Department of Pharmacology, Washington, DC 20057. Offers MS, PhD, MD/PhD, MS/PhD. *Degree requirements:* For doctorate, comprehensive exam, thesis/dissertation. *Entrance requirements:* For doctorate, GRE General Test, previous course work in biology and chemistry. Additional exam requirements/recommendations for international students: Required—TOEFL. Application fee: $50 ($55 for international students). *Faculty research:* Neuropharmacology, techniques in biochemistry and tissue culture. *Unit head:* Dr. Kenneth L. Dretchen, Chair, 202-687-7007. *Application contact:* Graduate School Admissions Office, 202-687-5568.

Georgia Regents University, The Graduate School, Program in Pharmacology, Augusta, GA 30912. Offers MS, PhD. *Faculty:* 13 full-time (2 women), 1 (woman) part-time/adjunct. *Students:* 6 full-time (2 women); includes 5 minority (1 Black or African American, non-Hispanic/Latino; 4 Asian, non-Hispanic/Latino), 4 international. Average age 30. In 2013, 1 doctorate awarded. *Degree requirements:* For doctorate, comprehensive exam, thesis/dissertation. *Entrance requirements:* For doctorate, GRE General Test. Additional exam requirements/recommendations for international students: Required—TOEFL (minimum score 550 paper-based; 79 iBT). *Application deadline:* For fall admission, 1/15 for domestic and international students. Application fee: $50. Electronic applications accepted. *Financial support:* In 2013–14, 3 students received support, including 8 research assistantships with partial tuition reimbursements available (averaging $23,000 per year); fellowships with partial tuition reimbursements available, Federal Work-Study, institutionally sponsored loans, and scholarships/grants also available. Support available to part-time students. Financial award application deadline: 5/31; financial award applicants required to submit FAFSA. *Faculty research:* Protein signaling, neural development, cardiovascular pharmacology, endothelial cell function, neuropharmacology. *Total annual research expenditures:* $3.5 million. *Unit head:* Dr. R. William Caldwell, Chair, 706-721-3383, Fax: 706-721-6059, E-mail: wcaldwell@georgiahealth.edu. *Application contact:* Dr. Patricia L. Cameron, Acting Vice Dean, 706-721-3279, E-mail: pcameron@georgiahealth.edu.
Website: http://www.gru.edu/mcg/phmtox/phtx_graduate.php

Howard University, College of Medicine, Department of Pharmacology, Washington, DC 20059-0002. Offers MS, PhD, MD/PhD. Part-time programs available. *Degree requirements:* For master's, comprehensive exam, thesis; for doctorate, one foreign language, comprehensive exam, thesis/dissertation, qualifying exam. *Entrance requirements:* For master's, GRE General Test, minimum GPA of 3.2, BS in chemistry, biology, pharmacy, psychology or related field; for doctorate, GRE General Test, minimum graduate GPA of 3.2. Additional exam requirements/recommendations for international students: Recommended—TOEFL. *Faculty research:* Biochemical pharmacology, molecular pharmacology, neuropharmacology, drug metabolism, cancer research.

Idaho State University, Office of Graduate Studies, College of Pharmacy, Department of Biomedical and Pharmaceutical Sciences, Pocatello, ID 83209-8334. Offers biopharmaceutical analysis (PhD); drug delivery (PhD); medicinal chemistry (PhD); pharmaceutical sciences (MS); pharmacology (PhD). Part-time programs available. *Degree requirements:* For master's, one foreign language, comprehensive exam, thesis, thesis research, classes in speech and technical writing; for doctorate, comprehensive exam, thesis/dissertation, written and oral exams, classes in speech and technical writing. *Entrance requirements:* For master's, GRE General Test, minimum GPA of 3.0, 3 letters of recommendation; for doctorate, GRE General Test, BS in pharmacy or related field, minimum GPA of 3.0, 3 letters of recommendation. Additional exam requirements/recommendations for international students: Required—TOEFL (minimum score 550 paper-based; 80 iBT). Electronic applications accepted. *Expenses:* Contact institution. *Faculty research:* Metabolic toxicity of heavy metals, neuroendocrine pharmacology, cardiovascular pharmacology, cancer biology, immunopharmacology.

Indiana University–Purdue University Indianapolis, Indiana University School of Medicine, Department of Pharmacology and Toxicology, Indianapolis, IN 46202-2896. Offers pharmacology (MS, PhD); toxicology (MS, PhD); MD/PhD. *Faculty:* 11 full-time (2 women). *Students:* 28 full-time (22 women); includes 5 minority (2 Black or African American, non-Hispanic/Latino; 2 Asian, non-Hispanic/Latino; 1 Hispanic/Latino), 9 international. Average age 27. 1 applicant, 100% accepted, 1 enrolled. In 2013, 1 doctorate awarded. Terminal master's awarded for partial completion of doctoral program. *Degree requirements:* For master's, thesis; for doctorate, thesis/dissertation. *Entrance requirements:* For master's and doctorate, GRE General Test, GRE Subject Test, minimum GPA of 3.0. *Application deadline:* For fall admission, 1/15 priority date for domestic students. Applications are processed on a rolling basis. Application fee: $55 ($65 for international students). *Financial support:* In 2013–14, teaching assistantships (averaging $20,940 per year) were awarded; fellowships with partial tuition reimbursements, research assistantships with partial tuition reimbursements, Federal Work-Study, institutionally sponsored loans, and tuition waivers (partial) also available. Financial award application deadline: 1/15. *Faculty research:* Neuropharmacology, cardiovascular biopharmacology, chemotherapy, oncogenesis. *Unit head:* Dr. Theodore R. Cummins, Interim Chairman, 317-274-9342. *Application contact:* Director of Graduate Studies, 317-274-1564, Fax: 317-274-7714, E-mail: inmedadm@iupui.edu.
Website: http://pharmtox.iusm.iu.edu/

Johns Hopkins University, School of Medicine, Graduate Programs in Medicine, Department of Pharmacology and Molecular Sciences, Baltimore, MD 21205. Offers PhD. *Faculty:* 42 full-time (8 women). *Students:* 52 full-time (27 women); includes 15 minority (3 Black or African American, non-Hispanic/Latino; 9 Asian, non-Hispanic/Latino; 2 Hispanic/Latino; 1 Two or more races, non-Hispanic/Latino), 10 international. Average age 26. 76 applicants, 17% accepted, 9 enrolled. In 2013, 6 doctorates awarded. *Degree requirements:* For doctorate, comprehensive exam, thesis/dissertation, departmental seminar. *Entrance requirements:* For doctorate, GRE General Test. Additional exam requirements/recommendations for international students: Required—TOEFL. *Application deadline:* For fall admission, 1/10 for domestic and international students. Application fee: $85. Electronic applications accepted. *Unit head:* Dr. Philip A. Cole, Chairman, 410-614-0540, Fax: 410-614-7717, E-mail: pcole@jhmi.edu. *Application contact:* Dr. James T. Stivers, Director of Admissions, 410-955-7117, Fax: 410-955-3023, E-mail: jstivers@jhmi.edu.
Website: http://www.hopkinsmedicine.org/pharmacology/

Kent State University, School of Biomedical Sciences, Program in Pharmacology, Kent, OH 44242-0001. Offers MS, PhD. Offered in cooperation with Northeastern Ohio Universities College of Medicine. Terminal master's awarded for partial completion of doctoral program. *Degree requirements:* For master's, thesis; for doctorate, thesis/dissertation. *Entrance requirements:* For master's and doctorate, GRE General Test, minimum GPA of 3.0, 3 letters of recommendation. Additional exam requirements/recommendations for international students: Required—TOEFL. Electronic applications accepted. *Faculty research:* Neuropharmacology, psychotherapeutics and substance abuse, molecular biology of substance abuse, toxicology.

Loma Linda University, School of Medicine, Department of Physiology/Pharmacology, Loma Linda, CA 92350. Offers MS, PhD. Part-time programs available. *Degree* *requirements:* For master's, thesis or alternative; for doctorate, 2 foreign languages, thesis/dissertation. *Entrance requirements:* For master's and doctorate, GRE General Test. *Faculty research:* Drug metabolism, biochemical pharmacology, structure and function of cell membranes, neuropharmacology.

Long Island University–LIU Brooklyn, Arnold and Marie Schwartz College of Pharmacy and Health Sciences, Graduate Programs in Pharmacy, Division of Pharmaceutical Sciences, Brooklyn, NY 11201-8423. Offers cosmetic science (MS); industrial pharmacy (MS); pharmaceutics (PhD); pharmacology/toxicology (MS). Part-time and evening/weekend programs available. Terminal master's awarded for partial completion of doctoral program. *Degree requirements:* For master's, thesis optional; for doctorate, thesis/dissertation, candidacy exam. *Entrance requirements:* For master's and doctorate, minimum GPA of 3.0.

Louisiana State University Health Sciences Center, School of Graduate Studies in New Orleans, Department of Pharmacology and Experimental Therapeutics, New Orleans, LA 70112-2223. Offers MS, PhD, MD/PhD. Terminal master's awarded for partial completion of doctoral program. *Degree requirements:* For master's, comprehensive exam, thesis; for doctorate, comprehensive exam, thesis/dissertation. *Entrance requirements:* For master's, GRE; for doctorate, GRE General Test. Additional exam requirements/recommendations for international students: Required—TOEFL. *Faculty research:* Neuropharmacology, gastrointestinal pharmacology, drug metabolism, behavioral pharmacology, cardiovascular pharmacology.

Louisiana State University Health Sciences Center at Shreveport, Department of Pharmacology, Toxicology and Neuroscience, Shreveport, LA 71130-3932. Offers pharmacology (PhD); MD/PhD. *Faculty:* 9 full-time (2 women), 5 part-time/adjunct (2 women). *Students:* 12 full-time (all women); includes 4 minority (2 Black or African American, non-Hispanic/Latino; 1 Asian, non-Hispanic/Latino; 1 Hispanic/Latino), 1 international. Average age 25. 16 applicants, 25% accepted, 3 enrolled. In 2013, 1 doctorate awarded. Terminal master's awarded for partial completion of doctoral program. *Degree requirements:* For doctorate, thesis/dissertation. *Entrance requirements:* For doctorate, GRE General Test, minimum GPA of 3.0. Additional exam requirements/recommendations for international students: Required—TOEFL. *Application deadline:* For fall admission, 12/1 priority date for domestic students. Application fee: $0. *Financial support:* In 2013–14, 3 fellowships (averaging $28,000 per year), 9 research assistantships (averaging $24,000 per year) were awarded; teaching assistantships and institutionally sponsored loans also available. Financial award application deadline: 5/1. *Faculty research:* Behavioral, cardiovascular, clinical, and gastrointestinal pharmacology; neuropharmacology; psychopharmacology; drug abuse; pharmacokinetics; neuroendocrinology, psychoneuroimmunology, and stress; toxicology. *Unit head:* Dr. Nicholas E. Goeders, Head, 318-675-7850, Fax: 318-675-7857, E-mail: ngoede@lsuhsc.edu. *Application contact:* Dr. Mike Salvatore, Associate Professor, 318-675-7874, Fax: 318-675-7857, E-mail: msalva@lsuhsc.edu.
Website: http://www.lsuhscshreveport.edu/pharmacologytoxicologyandneuroscience/pharmacologytoxicologyandneurosciencehome.aspx

Loyola University Chicago, Graduate School, Department of Molecular Pharmacology and Therapeutics, Chicago, IL 60626. Offers MS. *Faculty:* 18 full-time (4 women), 11 part-time/adjunct (2 women). *Students:* 14 full-time (8 women), 5 international. Average age 26. 21 applicants, 10% accepted, 2 enrolled. In 2013, 1 master's awarded. Terminal master's awarded for partial completion of doctoral program. *Degree requirements:* For master's, comprehensive exam, thesis. *Entrance requirements:* For master's, GRE General Test, minimum GPA of 3.0. Additional exam requirements/recommendations for international students: Required—TOEFL. *Application deadline:* For fall admission, 2/1 for domestic and international students. Application fee: $50. Electronic applications accepted. *Expenses: Tuition:* Full-time $16,740; part-time $930 per credit. *Required fees:* $135 per semester. *Financial support:* In 2013–14, 2 fellowships with full tuition reimbursements (averaging $32,165 per year), 7 research assistantships with full tuition reimbursements (averaging $25,000 per year), 1 teaching assistantship with full tuition reimbursement (averaging $36,000 per year) were awarded; career-related internships or fieldwork and Federal Work-Study also available. Financial award application deadline: 2/1; financial award applicants required to submit FAFSA. *Faculty research:* Neuropharmacology, molecular pharmacology, neuroendocrinology, hematopharmacology, neurodegeneration. *Unit head:* Dr. Tarun Patel, Chair, 708-216-5773, Fax: 708-216-6956. *Application contact:* Dr. Kenneth L. Byron, Graduate Program Director, 708-327-2819, Fax: 708-216-6596, E-mail: kbyron@luc.edu.
Website: http://www.stritch.luc.edu/pharmacology/

McGill University, Faculty of Graduate and Postdoctoral Studies, Faculty of Medicine, Department of Pharmacology and Therapeutics, Montréal, QC H3A 2T5, Canada. Offers M Sc, PhD.

McMaster University, Faculty of Health Sciences and School of Graduate Studies, Program in Medical Sciences, Physiology/Pharmacology Area, Hamilton, ON L8S 4M2, Canada. Offers M Sc, PhD, MD/PhD. *Degree requirements:* For master's, thesis; for doctorate, comprehensive exam, thesis/dissertation. *Entrance requirements:* For master's, honors B Sc, B+ average in related field; for doctorate, M Sc, minimum B+ average, students with proven research experience and an A average may be admitted with a B Sc degree. Additional exam requirements/recommendations for international students: Required—TOEFL (minimum score 580 paper-based; 92 iBT).

MCPHS University, Graduate Studies, Program in Pharmacology, Boston, MA 02115-5896. Offers MS, PhD. *Accreditation:* ACPE (one or more programs are accredited). Terminal master's awarded for partial completion of doctoral program. *Degree requirements:* For master's, oral defense of thesis; for doctorate, one foreign language, oral defense of dissertation, qualifying exam. *Entrance requirements:* For master's and doctorate, GRE General Test, minimum QPA of 3.0. Additional exam requirements/recommendations for international students: Required—TOEFL (minimum score 550 paper-based; 79 iBT). *Faculty research:* Neuropharmacology, cardiovascular pharmacology, nutritional pharmacology, pulmonary physiology, drug metabolism.

Medical College of Wisconsin, Graduate School of Biomedical Sciences, Department of Pharmacology and Toxicology, Milwaukee, WI 53226-0509. Offers PhD, MD/PhD. *Degree requirements:* For doctorate, comprehensive exam, thesis/dissertation, oral and written qualifying exams. *Entrance requirements:* For doctorate, GRE, official transcripts, three letters of recommendation. Additional exam requirements/recommendations for international students: Required—TOEFL. Electronic applications accepted. *Faculty research:* Cardiovascular physiology and pharmacology, drugs of abuse, environmental and aquatic toxicology, central nervous system and biochemical pharmacology, signal transduction.

Meharry Medical College, School of Graduate Studies, Program in Biomedical Sciences, Pharmacology Emphasis, Nashville, TN 37208-9989. Offers PhD, MD/PhD. *Degree requirements:* For doctorate, comprehensive exam, thesis/dissertation. *Entrance requirements:* For doctorate, GRE. *Faculty research:* Neuropharmacology, cardiovascular pharmacology, behavioral pharmacology, molecular pharmacology, drug metabolism, anticancer.

Michigan State University, College of Human Medicine and The Graduate School, Graduate Programs in Human Medicine, East Lansing, MI 48824. Offers biochemistry and molecular biology (MS, PhD); epidemiology (MS, PhD); microbiology (MS); microbiology and molecular genetics (PhD); pharmacology and toxicology (MS, PhD); physiology (MS, PhD); public health (MPH). *Entrance requirements:* Additional exam requirements/recommendations for international students: Required—TOEFL.

Michigan State University, College of Osteopathic Medicine and The Graduate School, Graduate Studies in Osteopathic Medicine and Graduate Programs in Human Medicine and Graduate Programs in Veterinary Medicine, Department of Pharmacology and Toxicology, East Lansing, MI 48824. Offers integrative pharmacology (MS); pharmacology and toxicology (MS, PhD); pharmacology and toxicology-environmental toxicology (PhD). *Entrance requirements:* Additional exam requirements/recommendations for international students: Required—TOEFL (minimum score 600 paper-based). Electronic applications accepted.

Michigan State University, College of Veterinary Medicine and The Graduate School, Graduate Programs in Veterinary Medicine, East Lansing, MI 48824. Offers comparative medicine and integrative biology (MS, PhD), including comparative medicine and integrative biology, comparative medicine and integrative biology–environmental toxicology (PhD); food safety and toxicology (MS), including food safety; integrative toxicology (PhD), including animal science–environmental toxicology, biochemistry and molecular biology–environmental toxicology, chemistry–environmental toxicology, crop and soil sciences–environmental toxicology, environmental engineering–environmental toxicology, environmental geosciences–environmental toxicology, fisheries and wildlife–environmental toxicology, food science–environmental toxicology, forestry–environmental toxicology, genetics–environmental toxicology, human nutrition–environmental toxicology, microbiology–environmental toxicology, pharmacology and toxicology–environmental toxicology, zoology–environmental toxicology; large animal clinical sciences (MS, PhD); microbiology and molecular genetics (MS, PhD), including industrial microbiology, microbiology, microbiology and molecular genetics, microbiology–environmental toxicology (PhD); pathobiology and diagnostic investigation (MS, PhD), including pathology, pathology–environmental toxicology (PhD); pharmacology and toxicology (MS, PhD); pharmacology and toxicology–environmental toxicology (PhD); physiology (MS, PhD); small animal clinical sciences (MS). Electronic applications accepted. *Faculty research:* Molecular genetics, food safety/toxicology, comparative orthopedics, airway disease, population medicine.

Montclair State University, The Graduate School, College of Science and Mathematics, Department of Chemistry and Biochemistry, Program in Pharmaceutical Biochemistry, Montclair, NJ 07043-1624. Offers MS. Part-time and evening/weekend programs available. *Entrance requirements:* For master's, GRE General Test, 24 undergraduate credits in chemistry, 2 letters of recommendation, essay. Electronic applications accepted. *Faculty research:* Enzyme kinetics, enzyme expression, pharmaceutical biochemistry, medicinal chemistry, biophysical chemistry.

New Jersey Institute of Technology, Newark College of Engineering, Newark, NJ 07102. Offers biomedical engineering (MS, PhD); chemical engineering (MS, PhD); computer engineering (MS, PhD); electrical engineering (MS, PhD); engineering management (MS); healthcare systems management (MS); industrial engineering (MS, PhD); Internet engineering (MS); manufacturing engineering (MS); mechanical engineering (MS, PhD); occupational safety and health engineering (MS); pharmaceutical bioprocessing (MS); pharmaceutical engineering (MS); pharmaceutical systems management (MS); power and energy systems (MS); telecommunications (MS); transportation (MS, PhD). Part-time and evening/weekend programs available. *Faculty:* 133 full-time (18 women), 101 part-time/adjunct (14 women). *Students:* 823 full-time (222 women), 535 part-time (130 women); includes 361 minority (92 Black or African American, non-Hispanic/Latino; 4 American Indian or Alaska Native, non-Hispanic/Latino; 142 Asian, non-Hispanic/Latino; 123 Hispanic/Latino), 605 international. Average age 29. 2,800 applicants, 68% accepted, 523 enrolled. In 2013, 471 master's, 32 doctorates awarded. Terminal master's awarded for partial completion of doctoral program. *Degree requirements:* For master's, thesis optional; for doctorate, thesis/dissertation. *Entrance requirements:* For master's, GRE General Test; for doctorate, GRE General Test, minimum graduate GPA of 3.5. Additional exam requirements/recommendations for international students: Required—TOEFL (minimum score 550 paper-based; 79 iBT). *Application deadline:* For fall admission, 6/1 priority date for domestic students, 5/1 priority date for international students; for spring admission, 11/15 priority date for domestic and international students. Applications are processed on a rolling basis. Application fee: $65. Electronic applications accepted. *Expenses:* Tuition, state resident: full-time $17,384; part-time $945 per credit. Tuition, nonresident: full-time $25,404; part-time $1341 per credit. *Required fees:* $2396; $118 per credit. *Financial support:* Fellowships with full and partial tuition reimbursements, research assistantships with full and partial tuition reimbursements, and teaching assistantships with full and partial tuition reimbursements available. Financial award application deadline: 1/15. *Total annual research expenditures:* $16 million. *Unit head:* Dr. Basil Baltzis, Dean, 973-596-3000, E-mail: sunil.saigal@njit.edu. *Application contact:* Stephen Eck, Director of Admissions, 973-596-3300, Fax: 973-596-3461, E-mail: admissions@njit.edu.
Website: http://engineering.njit.edu/

New York Medical College, Graduate School of Basic Medical Sciences, Integrated PhD Program, Valhalla, NY 10595-1691. Offers biochemistry and molecular biology (PhD); cell biology and anatomy (PhD); microbiology and immunology (PhD); pathology (PhD); pharmacology (PhD); physiology (PhD). *Faculty:* 91 full-time (16 women), 5 part-time/adjunct (2 women). *Students:* 31 full-time (21 women); includes 17 minority (4 Black or African American, non-Hispanic/Latino; 11 Asian, non-Hispanic/Latino; 2 Hispanic/Latino). Average age 27. 56 applicants, 36% accepted, 9 enrolled. In 2013, 17 doctorates awarded. *Degree requirements:* For doctorate, comprehensive exam, thesis/dissertation. *Entrance requirements:* For doctorate, GRE General Test. Additional exam requirements/recommendations for international students: Required—TOEFL. *Application deadline:* For fall admission, 1/1 priority date for domestic and international students. Applications are processed on a rolling basis. Application fee: $75 ($100 for international students). Electronic applications accepted. *Expenses: Tuition:* Full-time $49,170; part-time $910 per credit. Tuition and fees vary according to program. *Financial support:* In 2013–14, fellowships with full tuition reimbursements (averaging $25,500 per year), research assistantships with full tuition reimbursements (averaging $25,500 per year) were awarded; Federal Work-Study, scholarships/grants, traineeships, health care benefits, and tuition waivers (full) also available. Financial award applicants required to submit FAFSA. *Faculty research:* Cardiovascular sciences, infectious diseases, neuroscience, cancer and cell signaling. *Unit head:* Dr. Francis L. Belloni, Dean, 914-594-4110, Fax: 914-594-4944, E-mail: francis_belloni@nymc.edu. *Application contact:* Valerie Romeo-Messana, Director of Admissions, 914-594-4110, Fax: 914-594-4944, E-mail: v_romeomessana@nymc.edu.

New York Medical College, Graduate School of Basic Medical Sciences, Pharmacology Master's Program, Valhalla, NY 10595-1691. Offers MS, PhD, MD/PhD. Part-time and evening/weekend programs available. *Faculty:* 13 full-time (2 women). *Students:* 5 full-time (3 women); includes 2 minority (both Asian, non-Hispanic/Latino). Average age 27. 16 applicants, 44% accepted, 2 enrolled. In 2013, 8 master's awarded. Terminal master's awarded for partial completion of doctoral program. *Degree requirements:* For master's, thesis; for doctorate, comprehensive exam, thesis/dissertation. *Entrance requirements:* For master's, GRE General Test, MCAT, or DAT.

Additional exam requirements/recommendations for international students: Required—TOEFL. *Application deadline:* For fall admission, 7/1 priority date for domestic students, 5/1 priority date for international students; for spring admission, 12/1 for domestic students, 10/1 for international students. Applications are processed on a rolling basis. Application fee: $75 ($100 for international students). Electronic applications accepted. *Expenses: Tuition:* Full-time $49,170; part-time $910 per credit. Tuition and fees vary according to program. *Financial support:* Federal Work-Study and scholarships/grants available. Support available to part-time students. Financial award applicants required to submit FAFSA. *Faculty research:* Investigation into the therapeutic and pathophysiologic role of bioactive lipids (eicosanoids) in cancer, ophthalmology, and cardiovascular diseases including hypertension, kidney disease, stroke, diabetes, atherosclerosis and inflammatory conditions; cytochrome P-450 function and control; patch-clamp analysis of ion transport; the roles of vasoactive hormones and inflammatory cytokines in hypertension, end-organ damage and cardiovascular function. *Unit head:* Dr. Charles Stier, Program Director, 914-594-4138, Fax: 914-594-4944, E-mail: charles_stier@nymc.edu. *Application contact:* Valerie Romeo-Messana, Director of Admissions, 914-594-4110, Fax: 914-594-4944, E-mail: v_romeomessana@nymc.edu.

North Carolina State University, College of Veterinary Medicine, Program in Comparative Biomedical Sciences, Raleigh, NC 27695. Offers cell biology (MS, PhD); infectious disease (MS, PhD); pathology (MS, PhD); pharmacology (MS, PhD); population medicine (MS, PhD). Part-time programs available. *Degree requirements:* For master's, thesis; for doctorate, thesis/dissertation. *Entrance requirements:* For master's and doctorate, GRE General Test. Additional exam requirements/recommendations for international students: Required—TOEFL (minimum score 550 paper-based). Electronic applications accepted. *Expenses:* Contact institution. *Faculty research:* Infectious diseases, cell biology, pharmacology and toxicology, genomics, pathology and population medicine.

Northeastern University, Bouvé College of Health Sciences, Boston, MA 02115-5096. Offers audiology (Au D); biotechnology (MS); counseling psychology (MS, PhD, CAGS); counseling/school psychology (PhD); exercise physiology (MS), including exercise physiology, public health; health informatics (MS); nursing (MS, PhD, CAGS), including acute care (MS), administration (MS), anesthesia (MS), primary care (MS), psychiatric mental health (MS); pharmaceutical sciences (PhD); pharmaceutics and drug delivery systems (MS); pharmacology (MS); physical therapy (DPT); physician assistant (MS); school psychology (PhD, CAGS); school/counseling psychology (PhD); speech language pathology (MS); urban public health (MPH); MS/MBA. *Accreditation:* ACPE (one or more programs are accredited). Part-time and evening/weekend programs available. *Degree requirements:* For doctorate, thesis/dissertation (for some programs); for CAGS, comprehensive exam.

Nova Southeastern University, Center for Psychological Studies, Fort Lauderdale, FL 33314-7796. Offers clinical psychology (PhD, Psy D); clinical psychopharmacology (MS); counseling (MS); forensic psychology (MS); general psychology (MS); mental health counseling (MS); school counseling (MS); school psychology (Psy D, Psy S). *Accreditation:* APA (one or more programs are accredited). Postbaccalaureate distance learning degree programs offered. *Faculty:* 41 full-time (15 women), 134 part-time/adjunct (80 women). *Students:* 1,820 (1,568 women); includes 832 minority (289 Black or African American, non-Hispanic/Latino; 4 American Indian or Alaska Native, non-Hispanic/Latino; 46 Asian, non-Hispanic/Latino; 464 Hispanic/Latino; 29 Two or more races, non-Hispanic/Latino), 38 international. Average age 31. 1,185 applicants, 52% accepted, 403 enrolled. In 2013, 462 master's, 73 doctorates, 16 other advanced degrees awarded. Terminal master's awarded for partial completion of doctoral program. *Degree requirements:* For master's, comprehensive exam, 3 practica; for doctorate, thesis/dissertation, clinical internship, competency exam; for Psy S, comprehensive exam, internship. *Entrance requirements:* For doctorate, GRE General Test, GRE Subject Test (recommended), minimum undergraduate GPA of 3.0; for Psy S, GRE General Test. Additional exam requirements/recommendations for international students: Required—TOEFL (minimum score 550 paper-based). *Application deadline:* Applications are processed on a rolling basis. Application fee: $50. Electronic applications accepted. *Expenses:* Contact institution. *Financial support:* In 2013–14, 5 research assistantships, 34 teaching assistantships (averaging $1,000 per year) were awarded; career-related internships or fieldwork, Federal Work-Study, institutionally sponsored loans, scholarships/grants, and unspecified assistantships also available. Support available to part-time students. Financial award application deadline: 4/1. *Faculty research:* Clinical and child clinical psychology, geriatrics, interpersonal violence. *Unit head:* Karen Grosby, EdD, Dean, 954-262-5701, Fax: 954-262-3859, E-mail: grosby@nova.edu. *Application contact:* Carlos Perez, Enrollment Management, 954-262-5790, Fax: 954-262-3893, E-mail: cpsinfo@cps.nova.edu.
Website: http://www.cps.nova.edu/

The Ohio State University, College of Medicine, School of Biomedical Science, Biomedical Sciences Graduate Program, Columbus, OH 43210. Offers immunology (PhD); medical genetics (PhD); molecular virology (PhD); pharmacology (PhD). *Students:* 109 full-time (55 women), 9 part-time (6 women); includes 24 minority (5 Black or African American, non-Hispanic/Latino; 1 American Indian or Alaska Native, non-Hispanic/Latino; 10 Asian, non-Hispanic/Latino; 6 Hispanic/Latino; 1 Native Hawaiian or other Pacific Islander, non-Hispanic/Latino; 1 Two or more races, non-Hispanic/Latino), 4 international. Average age 27. In 2013, 20 doctorates awarded. *Degree requirements:* For doctorate, thesis/dissertation. *Entrance requirements:* For doctorate, GRE General Test; GRE Subject Test in biochemistry, cell and molecular biology (recommended for some programs). Additional exam requirements/recommendations for international students: Required—TOEFL (minimum score 600 paper-based; 100 iBT), Michigan English Language Assessment Battery (minimum score 86); Recommended—IELTS (minimum score 8). *Application deadline:* For fall admission, 12/13 priority date for domestic students, 11/1 priority date for international students. Applications are processed on a rolling basis. Application fee: $60 ($70 for international students). Electronic applications accepted. *Financial support:* In 2013–14, 53 students received support, including 4 fellowships with full tuition reimbursements available (averaging $19,000 per year), 49 research assistantships with full tuition reimbursements available (averaging $19,000 per year); scholarships/grants and unspecified assistantships also available. Financial award application deadline: 1/15. *Unit head:* Joanna Groden, Co-Director, 614-688-4301, Fax: 614-292-6226, E-mail: ibgp@osumc.edu. *Application contact:* Graduate Admissions, 614-292-9444, Fax: 614-292-3895, E-mail: domestic.grad@osu.edu.
Website: http://www.ibgp.org

The Ohio State University, College of Pharmacy, Columbus, OH 43210. Offers MS, PhD, Pharm D, Pharm D/MBA, Pharm D/MPH. *Accreditation:* ACPE (one or more programs are accredited). Part-time programs available. *Faculty:* 44. *Students:* 561 full-time (336 women), 3 part-time (1 woman); includes 136 minority (20 Black or African American, non-Hispanic/Latino; 1 American Indian or Alaska Native, non-Hispanic/Latino; 97 Asian, non-Hispanic/Latino; 14 Hispanic/Latino; 4 Two or more races, non-Hispanic/Latino), 56 international. Average age 25. In 2013, 12 master's, 133 doctorates awarded. *Degree requirements:* For doctorate, thesis/dissertation (for some programs). *Entrance requirements:* For master's, GRE General Test, minimum GPA of 3.0; for doctorate, GRE General Test; PCAT (for Pharm D), minimum GPA of 3.0. Additional exam requirements/recommendations for international students: Required—TOEFL (minimum score 600 paper-based; 100 iBT), Michigan English Language Assessment Battery (minimum score 84). *Application deadline:* For fall admission, 12/15 priority date for domestic students, 12/15 for international students. Application fee: $60 ($70 for international students). Electronic applications accepted. *Expenses:* Contact institution. *Financial support:* Fellowships with full tuition reimbursements, research assistantships with full tuition reimbursements, teaching assistantships with full tuition reimbursements, career-related internships or fieldwork, Federal Work-Study, institutionally sponsored loans, scholarships/grants, and traineeships available. *Unit head:* Dr. Henry J. Mann, Dean, 614-292-5711, Fax: 614-292-2588, E-mail: odmail@pharmacy.ohio-state.edu. *Application contact:* Mary Kivel, Graduate Program Coordinator, 614-292-6822, Fax: 614-292-2588, E-mail: gradprogram@pharmacy.ohio-state.edu.
Website: http://www.pharmacy.osu.edu

Oregon Health & Science University, School of Medicine, Graduate Programs in Medicine, Program in Molecular and Cellular Biosciences, Department of Physiology and Pharmacology, Portland, OR 97239-3098. Offers PhD. *Faculty:* 22 full-time (9 women). *Students:* 9 full-time (6 women). Average age 28. In 2013, 1 doctorate awarded. *Degree requirements:* For doctorate, comprehensive exam, thesis/dissertation. *Entrance requirements:* For doctorate, GRE General Test (minimum scores: 153 Verbal/148 Quantitative/4.5 Analytical) or MCAT (for some programs). Additional exam requirements/recommendations for international students: Required—TOEFL. Electronic applications accepted. *Financial support:* Full tuition and stipends available. *Faculty research:* Ion conduction and gating in K+ channels, autonomic neuron plasticity, neurotransmitter/receptor expression, fetal/neonatal pharmacology, molecular pharmacology. *Unit head:* Dr. Beth Habecker, Program Director, 503-494-6252, E-mail: habecker@ohsu.edu. *Application contact:* Julie Walvatne, Program Coordinator, 503-494-6252.

Purdue University, College of Pharmacy and Pharmacal Sciences and Graduate School, Graduate Programs in Pharmacy and Pharmacal Sciences, Department of Medicinal Chemistry and Molecular Pharmacology, West Lafayette, IN 47907. Offers biophysical and computational chemistry (PhD); cancer research (PhD); immunology and infectious disease (PhD); medicinal biochemistry and molecular biology (PhD); medicinal chemistry and chemical biology (PhD); molecular pharmacology (PhD); neuropharmacology, neurodegeneration, and neurotoxicity (PhD); systems biology and functional genomics (PhD). *Faculty:* 23 full-time (3 women), 6 part-time/adjunct (1 woman). *Students:* 50 full-time (21 women), 3 part-time (2 women); includes 1 minority (Asian, non-Hispanic/Latino), 30 international. Average age 26. 147 applicants, 20% accepted, 13 enrolled. In 2013, 12 doctorates awarded. *Degree requirements:* For doctorate, thesis/dissertation. *Entrance requirements:* For doctorate, GRE General Test; GRE Subject Test in biology, biochemistry, and chemistry (recommended), minimum undergraduate GPA of 3.0. Additional exam requirements/recommendations for international students: Required—TOEFL (minimum score 550 paper-based; 77 iBT); Recommended—TWE. *Application deadline:* For fall admission, 2/1 for domestic and international students. Applications are processed on a rolling basis. Application fee: $60 ($75 for international students). Electronic applications accepted. *Financial support:* Fellowships, research assistantships, teaching assistantships, and traineeships available. Support available to part-time students. Financial award applicants required to submit FAFSA. *Faculty research:* Drug design and development, cancer research, drug synthesis and analysis, chemical pharmacology, environmental toxicology. *Unit head:* Dr. Richard F. Borch, Head, 765-494-1403, E-mail: borch@purdue.edu. *Application contact:* Dr. Janine C. Mott, Graduate Contact, 765-494-1269, E-mail: jmott@purdue.edu.

Purdue University, School of Veterinary Medicine and Graduate School, Graduate Programs in Veterinary Medicine, Department of Basic Medical Sciences, West Lafayette, IN 47907. Offers anatomy (MS, PhD); pharmacology (MS, PhD); physiology (MS, PhD). Part-time programs available. Terminal master's awarded for partial completion of doctoral program. *Degree requirements:* For master's, thesis; for doctorate, thesis/dissertation. *Entrance requirements:* For master's and doctorate, GRE General Test. Additional exam requirements/recommendations for international students: Required—TOEFL. Electronic applications accepted. *Faculty research:* Development and regeneration, tissue injury and shock, biomedical engineering, ovarian function, bone and cartilage biology, cell and molecular biology.

Queen's University at Kingston, School of Graduate Studies, Faculty of Health Sciences, Department of Pharmacology and Toxicology, Kingston, ON K7L 3N6, Canada. Offers M Sc, PhD. *Degree requirements:* For master's, thesis; for doctorate, comprehensive exam, thesis/dissertation. *Entrance requirements:* For master's, minimum 2nd class standing, honors bachelor of science degree (life sciences, health sciences, or equivalent); for doctorate, masters of science degree or outstanding performance in honors bachelor of science program. Additional exam requirements/recommendations for international students: Required—TOEFL (minimum score 600 paper-based). Electronic applications accepted. *Faculty research:* Biochemical toxicology, cardiovascular pharmacology and neuropharmacology.

Rush University, Graduate College, Division of Pharmacology, Chicago, IL 60612-3832. Offers clinical research (MS); pharmacology (MS, PhD); MD/PhD. Terminal master's awarded for partial completion of doctoral program. *Degree requirements:* For master's, thesis; for doctorate, thesis/dissertation. *Entrance requirements:* For master's and doctorate, GRE General Test, interview. Additional exam requirements/recommendations for international students: Required—TOEFL (minimum score 550 paper-based). *Faculty research:* Dopamine neurobiology and Parkinson's disease; cardiac electrophysiology and clinical pharmacology; neutrophil motility, apoptosis, and adhesion; angiogenesis; pulmonary vascular physiology.

Rutgers, The State University of New Jersey, Newark, Graduate School of Biomedical Sciences, Department of Pharmacology and Physiology, Newark, NJ 07107. Offers PhD. *Degree requirements:* For doctorate, thesis/dissertation, qualifying exam. *Entrance requirements:* For doctorate, GRE General Test. Additional exam requirements/recommendations for international students: Required—TOEFL. Electronic applications accepted.

Saint Louis University, Graduate Education and School of Medicine, Graduate Program in Biomedical Sciences and Graduate Education, Department of Pharmacological and Physiological Science, St. Louis, MO 63103-2097. Offers PhD. *Degree requirements:* For doctorate, comprehensive exam, thesis/dissertation, departmental qualifying exams. *Entrance requirements:* For doctorate, GRE General Test (GRE Subject Test optional), letters of recommendation, resume, interview. Additional exam requirements/recommendations for international students: Required—TOEFL (minimum score 525 paper-based). Electronic applications accepted. *Faculty research:* Molecular endocrinology, neuropharmacology, cardiovascular science, drug abuse, neurotransmitter and hormonal signaling mechanisms.

Southern Illinois University Carbondale, Graduate School, Graduate Program in Medicine, Program in Pharmacology, Springfield, IL 62794-9629. Offers MS, PhD. *Faculty:* 13 full-time (1 woman). *Students:* 17 full-time (9 women), 1 (woman) part-time, 12 international. Average age 30. 25 applicants, 16% accepted, 4 enrolled. In 2013, 3 doctorates awarded. *Degree requirements:* For master's, thesis; for doctorate, thesis/

dissertation. *Entrance requirements:* For master's, minimum GPA of 3.0; for doctorate, minimum GPA of 3.25. Additional exam requirements/recommendations for international students: Required—TOEFL. *Application deadline:* For fall admission, 2/15 for domestic students; for spring admission, 12/31 for domestic students. Applications are processed on a rolling basis. Application fee: $50. *Financial support:* Fellowships with full tuition reimbursements and tuition waivers (full) available. *Faculty research:* Autonomic nervous system pharmacology, biochemical pharmacology, neuropharmacology, toxicology, cardiovascular pharmacology. *Unit head:* Dr. Carl L. Faingold, Chairman, 217-545-2185, Fax: 217-524-0145, E-mail: cfaingold@siumed.edu. *Application contact:* Linda Moss, Secretary, 217-545-2875, E-mail: lmoss@siumed.edu.
Website: http://www.siumed.edu/pharm/home.html

State University of New York Upstate Medical University, College of Graduate Studies, Program in Pharmacology, Syracuse, NY 13210-2334. Offers PhD, MD/PhD. Terminal master's awarded for partial completion of doctoral program. *Degree requirements:* For doctorate, comprehensive exam, thesis/dissertation. *Entrance requirements:* For doctorate, GRE General Test, telephone interview. Additional exam requirements/recommendations for international students: Required—TOEFL. Electronic applications accepted. *Faculty research:* Cancer, disorders of the nervous system, infectious diseases, diabetes/metabolic disorders/cardiovascular diseases.

Stony Brook University, State University of New York, Stony Brook University Medical Center, Health Sciences Center, School of Medicine and Graduate School, Graduate Programs in Medicine, Department of Pharmacological Sciences, Graduate Program in Molecular and Cellular Pharmacology, Stony Brook, NY 11794. Offers PhD. *Faculty:* 17 full-time (3 women). *Students:* 40 full-time (21 women), 1 (woman) part-time; includes 14 minority (3 Black or African American, non-Hispanic/Latino; 5 Asian, non-Hispanic/Latino; 6 Hispanic/Latino), 7 international. Average age 28. 75 applicants, 21% accepted, 8 enrolled. In 2013, 7 doctorates awarded. *Degree requirements:* For doctorate, thesis/dissertation, departmental qualifying exam. *Entrance requirements:* For doctorate, GRE General Test. Additional exam requirements/recommendations for international students: Required—TOEFL. *Application deadline:* For fall admission, 1/15 priority date for domestic students; for spring admission, 10/1 for domestic students. Applications are processed on a rolling basis. Application fee: $100. Electronic applications accepted. *Expenses:* Tuition, state resident: full-time $9870; part-time $411 per credit. Tuition, nonresident: full-time $18,350; part-time $765 per credit. *Financial support:* In 2013–14, 14 fellowships, 10 research assistantships, 2 teaching assistantships were awarded; Federal Work-Study also available. Financial award application deadline: 3/15; financial award applicants required to submit FAFSA. *Faculty research:* Toxicology, molecular and cellular biochemistry. *Total annual research expenditures:* $6.1 million. *Unit head:* Dr. Michael A. Frohman, Chair, 631-444-3050, Fax: 631-444-9749, E-mail: michael.frohman@stonybrook.edu. *Application contact:* Odalis Hernandez, Coordinator, 631-444-3057, Fax: 631-444-9749, E-mail: odalis.hernandez@stonybrook.edu.
Website: http://www.pharm.stonybrook.edu/about-graduate-program

Thomas Jefferson University, Jefferson Graduate School of Biomedical Sciences, MS Program in Pharmacology, Philadelphia, PA 19107. Offers MS. Part-time and evening/weekend programs available. *Faculty:* 44 full-time (14 women), 27 part-time/adjunct (11 women). *Students:* 19 part-time (10 women); includes 5 minority (1 Black or African American, non-Hispanic/Latino; 4 Asian, non-Hispanic/Latino), 3 international. 12 applicants, 33% accepted, 2 enrolled. In 2013, 8 master's awarded. *Degree requirements:* For master's, thesis, clerkship. *Entrance requirements:* For master's, GRE General Test or MCAT, minimum GPA of 3.0. Additional exam requirements/recommendations for international students: Required—TOEFL (minimum score 100 iBT) or IELTS (minimum score 7). *Application deadline:* For fall admission, 8/1 priority date for domestic students, 3/1 priority date for international students; for winter admission, 12/1 priority date for domestic students, 6/1 priority date for international students; for spring admission, 4/1 priority date for domestic students. Applications are processed on a rolling basis. Application fee: $75. Electronic applications accepted. *Expenses:* Contact institution. *Financial support:* Federal Work-Study and institutionally sponsored loans available. Support available to part-time students. Financial award application deadline: 5/1; financial award applicants required to submit FAFSA. *Faculty research:* Pharmacology, drug development, planning and management, biostatistics. *Unit head:* Dr. Carol L. Beck, Assistant Dean/Director, 215-503-6539, Fax: 215-503-3433, E-mail: carol.beck@jefferson.edu. *Application contact:* Marc E. Stearns, Director of Admissions, 215-503-0155, Fax: 215-503-3433, E-mail: jgsbs-info@jefferson.edu.
Website: http://www.jefferson.edu/university/biomedical_sciences/programs/masters/pharmacology.html

Tufts University, Sackler School of Graduate Biomedical Sciences, Pharmacology and Experimental Therapeutics Program, Medford, MA 02155. Offers pharmacology and drug development (MS); pharmacology and experimental therapeutics (PhD). *Faculty:* 22 full-time (5 women). *Students:* 22 full-time (16 women); includes 3 minority (all Asian, non-Hispanic/Latino), 12 international. Average age 30. 59 applicants, 34% accepted, 9 enrolled. In 2013, 2 doctorates awarded. Terminal master's awarded for partial completion of doctoral program. *Degree requirements:* For master's, thesis; for doctorate, comprehensive exam, thesis/dissertation. *Entrance requirements:* For master's and doctorate, GRE General Test, 3 letters of reference. Additional exam requirements/recommendations for international students: Required—TOEFL (minimum score 600 paper-based; 100 iBT). *Application deadline:* For fall admission, 12/15 for domestic and international students. Application fee: $70. Electronic applications accepted. *Expenses:* Contact institution. *Financial support:* In 2013–14, 12 students received support, including 12 research assistantships with full tuition reimbursements available (averaging $31,000 per year); health care benefits also available. Financial award application deadline: 1/15. *Faculty research:* Biochemical mechanisms of narcotic addiction, clinical psychopharmacology, pharmacokinetics, neurotransmitter receptors, neuropeptides. *Unit head:* Dr. Emmanuel Pothos, Director, 617-636-6940, E-mail: emmanuel.pothos@tufts.edu. *Application contact:* Kellie Melchin, Associate Director of Admissions, 617-636-6767, Fax: 617-636-0375, E-mail: sackler-school@tufts.edu.
Website: http://sackler.tufts.edu/Academics/Degree-Programs/PhD-Programs/Pharmacology-and-Experimental-Therapeutics

Tulane University, School of Medicine and School of Liberal Arts, Graduate Programs in Biomedical Sciences, Department of Pharmacology, New Orleans, LA 70118-5669. Offers MS, PhD, MD/MS, MD/PhD. MS and PhD offered through the Graduate School. *Degree requirements:* For master's, one foreign language, thesis; for doctorate, 2 foreign languages, thesis/dissertation. *Entrance requirements:* For master's, GRE General Test, minimum B average in undergraduate course work; for doctorate, GRE General Test. Additional exam requirements/recommendations for international students: Required—TOEFL. Electronic applications accepted.

Universidad Central del Caribe, School of Medicine, Program in Biomedical Sciences, Bayamón, PR 00960-6032. Offers anatomy and cell biology (MA, MS); biochemistry (MS); biomedical sciences (MA); cellular and molecular biology (PhD); microbiology and immunology (MA, MS); pharmacology (MS); physiology (MS).

Université de Montréal, Faculty of Medicine, Department of Pharmacology, Montréal, QC H3C 3J7, Canada. Offers M Sc, PhD. Terminal master's awarded for partial completion of doctoral program. *Degree requirements:* For master's, thesis; for doctorate, thesis/dissertation, general exam. *Entrance requirements:* For master's, proficiency in French, knowledge of English; for doctorate, master's degree, proficiency in French. Electronic applications accepted. *Faculty research:* Molecular, clinical, and cardiovascular pharmacology; pharmacokinetics; mechanisms of drug interactions and toxicity; neuropharmacology and receptology.

Université de Sherbrooke, Faculty of Medicine and Health Sciences, Graduate Programs in Medicine, Department of Pharmacology, Sherbrooke, QC J1H 5N4, Canada. Offers M Sc, PhD. Terminal master's awarded for partial completion of doctoral program. *Degree requirements:* For master's, thesis; for doctorate, thesis/dissertation. Electronic applications accepted. *Faculty research:* Pharmacology of peptide hormones, pharmacology of lipid mediators, protein-protein interactions, medicinal pharmacology.

University at Buffalo, the State University of New York, Graduate School, School of Medicine and Biomedical Sciences, Graduate Programs in Medicine and Biomedical Sciences, Department of Pharmacology and Toxicology, Buffalo, NY 14260. Offers pharmacology (MS, PhD); MD/PhD. *Faculty:* 22 full-time (3 women), 1 part-time/adjunct (0 women). *Students:* 23 full-time (11 women); includes 11 minority (5 Black or African American, non-Hispanic/Latino; 1 American Indian or Alaska Native, non-Hispanic/Latino; 4 Asian, non-Hispanic/Latino; 1 Hispanic/Latino), 3 international. Average age 25. 76 applicants, 22% accepted, 8 enrolled. In 2013, 9 master's, 2 doctorates awarded. Terminal master's awarded for partial completion of doctoral program. *Degree requirements:* For master's, thesis; for doctorate, thesis/dissertation. *Entrance requirements:* For master's and doctorate, GRE General Test, 3 letters of recommendation. Additional exam requirements/recommendations for international students: Required—TOEFL (minimum score 79 iBT). *Application deadline:* For fall admission, 2/14 priority date for domestic and international students. Applications are processed on a rolling basis. Application fee: $75. Electronic applications accepted. *Financial support:* In 2013–14, 1 student received support, including 2 fellowships with full tuition reimbursements available (averaging $30,000 per year), 14 research assistantships with full tuition reimbursements available (averaging $25,000 per year); teaching assistantships, Federal Work-Study, scholarships/grants, health care benefits, and unspecified assistantships also available. Financial award application deadline: 2/14; financial award applicants required to submit FAFSA. *Faculty research:* Neuropharmacology, toxicology, signal transduction, molecular pharmacology, behavioral pharmacology. *Total annual research expenditures:* $3.5 million. *Unit head:* Dr. Margarita L. Dubocovich, Professor and Chair, 716-829-3048, Fax: 716-829-2801, E-mail: mdubo@buffalo.edu. *Application contact:* Linda LeRoy, Admissions Assistant, 716-829-2800, Fax: 716-829-2801, E-mail: pmygrad@buffalo.edu.
Website: http://medicine.buffalo.edu/pharmtox

The University of Alabama at Birmingham, Graduate Programs in Joint Health Sciences, Program in Pharmacology and Toxicology, Birmingham, AL 35294. Offers PhD. *Degree requirements:* For doctorate, thesis/dissertation. *Entrance requirements:* For doctorate, GRE General Test; GRE Subject Test (recommended), interview, three evaluations. Additional exam requirements/recommendations for international students: Required—TOEFL, TWE. Electronic applications accepted. *Expenses:* Contact institution. *Faculty research:* Anticancer and antiviral chemotherapy, with emphasis on drugs used in the management of AIDS and related opportunistic infections; metabolism and biliary excretion of drugs (and metabolites) as well as the mechanisms of drug toxicity.

University of Alberta, Faculty of Graduate Studies and Research, Department of Pharmacology, Edmonton, AB T6G 2E1, Canada. Offers M Sc, PhD. Terminal master's awarded for partial completion of doctoral program. *Degree requirements:* For master's, thesis; for doctorate, thesis/dissertation. *Entrance requirements:* For master's, B Sc, minimum GPA of 3.3; for doctorate, M Sc in pharmacology or closely related field, honors B Sc in pharmacology. *Faculty research:* Cardiovascular pharmacology, neuropharmacology, cancer pharmacology, molecular pharmacology, toxicology.

The University of Arizona, College of Pharmacy, Department of Pharmacology and Toxicology, Graduate Program in Medical Pharmacology, Tucson, AZ 85721. Offers medical pharmacology (PhD); perfusion science (MS). *Faculty:* 11 full-time (3 women). *Students:* 24 full-time (18 women); includes 11 minority (2 Black or African American, non-Hispanic/Latino; 4 Asian, non-Hispanic/Latino; 3 Hispanic/Latino; 2 Two or more races, non-Hispanic/Latino), 3 international. Average age 27. 34 applicants, 18% accepted, 5 enrolled. In 2013, 3 master's, 3 doctorates awarded. *Degree requirements:* For master's, thesis; for doctorate, comprehensive exam, thesis/dissertation. *Entrance requirements:* For master's, GRE General Test, 3 letters of recommendation; for doctorate, GRE General Test, personal statement, 3 letters of recommendation. Additional exam requirements/recommendations for international students: Required—TOEFL (minimum score 550 paper-based; 79 iBT). *Application deadline:* For fall admission, 1/1 for domestic and international students. Applications are processed on a rolling basis. Application fee: $75. Electronic applications accepted. *Expenses:* Tuition, state resident: full-time $11,526. Tuition, nonresident: full-time $27,398. *Financial support:* In 2013–14, 17 research assistantships with full tuition reimbursements (averaging $23,929 per year) were awarded; institutionally sponsored loans and tuition waivers (partial) also available. Financial award applicants required to submit FAFSA. *Faculty research:* Immunopharmacology, pharmacogenetics, pharmacogenomics, clinical pharmacology, ocularpharmacology and neuropharmacology. *Unit head:* Dr. I. Glenn Sipes, Head, 520-626-7123, Fax: 520-626-2204, E-mail: sipes@email.arizona.edu. *Application contact:* Vicki Healey, Coordinator, 520-626-7218, Fax: 520-626-2204, E-mail: stanley@email.arizona.edu.
Website: http://www.pharmacology.arizona.edu/

University of Arkansas for Medical Sciences, Graduate School, Little Rock, AR 72205. Offers biochemistry and molecular biology (MS, PhD); bioinformatics (MS, PhD); cellular physiology and molecular biophysics (MS, PhD); clinical nutrition (MS); interdisciplinary biomedical sciences (MS, PhD, Certificate); interdisciplinary toxicology (MS); microbiology and immunology (PhD); neurobiology and developmental sciences (PhD); pharmacology (PhD); MD/PhD. Bioinformatics programs hosted jointly with the University of Arkansas at Little Rock. Part-time programs available. *Faculty:* 397 full-time (205 women). *Students:* 196 full-time (126 women), 117 part-time (87 women); includes 65 minority (38 Black or African American, non-Hispanic/Latino; 1 American Indian or Alaska Native, non-Hispanic/Latino; 21 Asian, non-Hispanic/Latino; 4 Hispanic/Latino; 1 Two or more races, non-Hispanic/Latino), 57 international. 455 applicants, 27% accepted, 89 enrolled. In 2013, 41 master's, 18 doctorates, 28 other advanced degrees awarded. Terminal master's awarded for partial completion of doctoral program. *Degree requirements:* For master's, comprehensive exam (for some programs), thesis (for some programs); for doctorate, thesis/dissertation. *Entrance requirements:* For master's and doctorate, GRE. Additional exam requirements/recommendations for international students: Required—TOEFL. *Application deadline:* Applications are processed on a rolling basis. Application fee: $0. Electronic applications accepted. *Expenses:* Contact institution. *Financial support:* In 2013–14, 120 research assistantships (averaging $24,000 per year) were awarded; career-related internships or fieldwork, Federal Work-Study, and traineeships also available. Support available to part-time students. Financial award applicants required to submit FAFSA. *Unit head:* Dr. Robert E. McGehee, Jr., Dean, 501-686-5454. *Application contact:* Dr. Kristen Sterba, Assistant Dean, Office of

Graduate Student Recruiting and Retention, 501-526-7396, E-mail: kmsterba@uams.edu.
Website: http://www.uams.edu/gradschool/

The University of British Columbia, Faculty of Medicine, Department of Anesthesiology, Pharmacology and Therapeutics, Vancouver, BC V6T 1Z3, Canada. Offers M Sc, PhD. *Faculty:* 20 full-time (4 women), 2 part-time/adjunct (0 women). *Students:* 29 full-time (12 women); includes 11 minority (10 Asian, non-Hispanic/Latino; 1 Hispanic/Latino), 8 international. Average age 28. 29 applicants, 17% accepted, 5 enrolled. In 2013, 2 master's, 1 doctorate awarded. Terminal master's awarded for partial completion of doctoral program. *Degree requirements:* For master's, thesis; for doctorate, comprehensive exam, thesis/dissertation. *Entrance requirements:* For master's, MD or appropriate bachelor's degree; for doctorate, MD or M Sc. Additional exam requirements/recommendations for international students: Required—TOEFL (minimum score 600 paper-based; 100 iBT). *Application deadline:* For fall admission, 4/1 for domestic students, 3/1 for international students; for winter admission, 8/1 for domestic students, 7/1 for international students; for spring admission, 12/1 for domestic students, 11/1 for international students. Application fee: $90 Canadian dollars ($150 Canadian dollars for international students). Electronic applications accepted. *Expenses: Tuition, area resident:* Full-time $8000 Canadian dollars. *Financial support:* In 2013–14, 10 students received support, including 10 fellowships (averaging $21,409 per year), 16 research assistantships with full and partial tuition reimbursements available (averaging $20,576 per year); institutionally sponsored loans, scholarships/grants, and unspecified assistantships also available. Financial award application deadline: 10/15. *Faculty research:* Cellular, biochemical, autonomic, and cardiovascular pharmacology; neuropharmacology and pulmonary pharmacology. *Total annual research expenditures:* $406,074 Canadian dollars. *Unit head:* Dr. C. B. Warriner, Head, 604-822-2575, Fax: 604-822-2281, E-mail: brian.warriner@vch.ca. *Application contact:* Wynne Leung, Graduate Secretary, 604-827-3289, Fax: 604-822-6012, E-mail: wynne.leung@ubc.ca.
Website: http://www.apt.ubc.ca/

University of California, Davis, Graduate Studies, Graduate Group in Pharmacology and Toxicology, Davis, CA 95616. Offers MS, PhD. Terminal master's awarded for partial completion of doctoral program. *Degree requirements:* For master's, comprehensive exam or thesis; for doctorate, thesis/dissertation, qualifying exam. *Entrance requirements:* For master's and doctorate, GRE General Test, minimum GPA of 3.0, course work in biochemistry and/or physiology. Additional exam requirements/recommendations for international students: Required—TOEFL (minimum score 550 paper-based). Electronic applications accepted. *Faculty research:* Respiratory, neurochemical, molecular, genetic, and ecological toxicology.

University of California, Los Angeles, David Geffen School of Medicine and Graduate Division, Graduate Programs in Medicine, Department of Molecular and Medical Pharmacology, Los Angeles, CA 90095. Offers MS, PhD. *Degree requirements:* For master's, thesis; for doctorate, thesis/dissertation, written and oral qualifying exams; 2 quarters of teaching experience. *Entrance requirements:* For doctorate, GRE General Test, bachelor's degree; minimum undergraduate GPA of 3.0 (or its equivalent if letter grade system not used). Additional exam requirements/recommendations for international students: Required—TOEFL. Electronic applications accepted.

University of California, San Francisco, School of Pharmacy and Graduate Division, Pharmaceutical Sciences and Pharmacogenomics Program, San Francisco, CA 94158-0775. Offers PhD. *Degree requirements:* For doctorate, comprehensive exam, thesis/dissertation. *Entrance requirements:* For doctorate, GRE General Test, bachelor's degree, 3 letters of recommendation, personal statement. Additional exam requirements/recommendations for international students: Required—TOEFL. *Application deadline:* For fall admission, 12/1 for domestic and international students. Application fee: $80 ($100 for international students). Electronic applications accepted. *Expenses:* Tuition, state resident: full-time $11,220. Tuition, nonresident: full-time $26,322. *Required fees:* $5204. Full-time tuition and fees vary according to degree level and program. *Financial support:* In 2013–14, fellowships with full tuition reimbursements (averaging $32,500 per year), research assistantships with full tuition reimbursements (averaging $32,500 per year), teaching assistantships with full tuition reimbursements (averaging $32,500 per year) were awarded; career-related internships or fieldwork, institutionally sponsored loans, scholarships/grants, traineeships, tuition waivers (full), and unspecified assistantships also available. Financial award application deadline: 4/6. *Faculty research:* Drug development sciences, molecular pharmacology, therapeutic bioengineering, pharmacogenomics and functional genomics, quantitative and systems pharmacology, computational genomics. *Unit head:* Dr. Deanna L. Kroetz, Director, 415-476-1159, Fax: 415-476-6022, E-mail: deanna.kroetz@ucsf.edu. *Application contact:* Debbie Acoba-Idlebi, Administrator, 415-476-1947, Fax: 415-476-6022, E-mail: debbie.acoba@ucsf.edu.
Website: http://pspg.ucsf.edu/

University of California, Santa Barbara, Graduate Division, College of Letters and Sciences, Division of Mathematics, Life, and Physical Sciences, Department of Molecular, Cellular, and Developmental Biology, Santa Barbara, CA 93106-9625. Offers molecular, cellular, and developmental biology (MA, PhD); pharmacology/biotechnology (MA); MA/PhD. *Faculty:* 29 full-time (3 women), 4 part-time/adjunct (0 women). *Students:* 48 full-time (23 women); includes 8 minority (2 Black or African American, non-Hispanic/Latino; 3 Asian, non-Hispanic/Latino; 3 Hispanic/Latino), 1 international. Average age 29. 182 applicants, 18% accepted, 11 enrolled. In 2013, 7 master's, 7 doctorates awarded. Terminal master's awarded for partial completion of doctoral program. *Degree requirements:* For master's, comprehensive exam (for some programs), thesis (for some programs); for doctorate, comprehensive exam, thesis/dissertation. *Entrance requirements:* For master's and doctorate, GRE General Test, 3 letters of recommendation, statement of purpose, personal achievements/contributions statement, resume/curriculum vitae, transcripts for post-secondary institutions attended. Additional exam requirements/recommendations for international students: Required—TOEFL (minimum score 550 paper-based; 80 iBT), IELTS (minimum score 7). *Application deadline:* For fall admission, 12/15 priority date for domestic and international students. Application fee: $80 ($100 for international students). Electronic applications accepted. *Expenses:* Tuition, state resident: part-time $5148.26 per quarter. Tuition, nonresident: part-time $10,182.26 per quarter. *Financial support:* In 2013–14, 3 students received support, including 3 fellowships with full and partial tuition reimbursements available (averaging $22,000 per year), 40 research assistantships with full and partial tuition reimbursements available (averaging $26,250 per year), 46 teaching assistantships with partial tuition reimbursements available (averaging $17,655 per year); career-related internships or fieldwork, Federal Work-Study, institutionally sponsored loans, scholarships/grants, traineeships, health care benefits, and unspecified assistantships also available. Financial award application deadline: 3/13; financial award applicants required to submit FAFSA. *Faculty research:* Microbiology, neurobiology (including stem cell research), developmental, virology, cell biology. *Unit head:* Dr. William Smith, Chair, 805-893-7698, E-mail: wililam.smith@lifesci.ucsb.edu. *Application contact:* Nicole McCoy, Graduate Program Advisor, 805-893-8499, E-mail: nicole.mccoy@lifesci.ucsb.edu.
Website: https://www.mcdb.ucsb.edu/grad

University of Chicago, Division of Biological Sciences, Neuroscience Graduate Programs, Committee on Integrative Neuroscience, Chicago, IL 60637-1513. Offers cell physiology (PhD); pharmacological and physiological sciences (PhD). *Degree requirements:* For doctorate, thesis/dissertation, preliminary exam. *Entrance requirements:* For doctorate, GRE General Test. Additional exam requirements/recommendations for international students: Required—TOEFL. Electronic applications accepted. *Faculty research:* Psychopharmacology, neuropharmacology.

University of Cincinnati, Graduate School, College of Medicine, Graduate Programs in Biomedical Sciences, Department of Pharmacology and Cell Biophysics, Cincinnati, OH 45221. Offers cell biophysics (PhD); pharmacology (PhD). *Degree requirements:* For doctorate, thesis/dissertation, qualifying exam. *Entrance requirements:* For doctorate, GRE General Test. Additional exam requirements/recommendations for international students: Required—TOEFL. Electronic applications accepted. *Faculty research:* Lipoprotein research, enzyme regulation, electrophysiology, gene actuation.

University of Colorado Denver, School of Medicine, Program in Pharmacology, Aurora, CO 80045. Offers bioinformatics (PhD); biomolecular structure (PhD); pharmacology (PhD). *Students:* 15 full-time (11 women), 1 part-time (0 women); includes 2 minority (both Asian, non-Hispanic/Latino). Average age 26. 25 applicants, 8% accepted, 2 enrolled. In 2013, 5 doctorates awarded. *Degree requirements:* For doctorate, comprehensive exam, thesis/dissertation, major seminar, 3 research rotations in the first year, 30 hours each of course work and thesis. *Entrance requirements:* For doctorate, GRE General Test, three letters of recommendation, personal statement. Additional exam requirements/recommendations for international students: Required—TOEFL (minimum score 550 paper-based; 80 iBT). *Application deadline:* For fall admission, 12/15 for domestic students, 11/15 for international students. Application fee: $50 ($75 for international students). Electronic applications accepted. *Expenses:* Contact institution. *Financial support:* In 2013–14, 16 students received support. Fellowships, research assistantships, teaching assistantships, institutionally sponsored loans, scholarships/grants, traineeships, health care benefits, tuition waivers (full), and unspecified assistantships available. Financial award application deadline: 3/15; financial award applicants required to submit FAFSA. *Faculty research:* Cancer biology, drugs of abuse, neuroscience, signal transduction, structural biology. *Total annual research expenditures:* $16.7 million. *Unit head:* Dr. Andrew Thorburn, Interim Chair, 303-724-3290, Fax: 303-724-3663, E-mail: andrew.thorburn@ucdenver.edu. *Application contact:* Elizabeth Bowen, Graduate Program Coordinator, 303-724-3565, E-mail: elizabeth.bowen@ucdenver.edu.
Website: http://www.ucdenver.edu/academics/colleges/medicalschool/departments/Pharmacology/Pages/Pharmacology.aspx

University of Connecticut, Graduate School, School of Pharmacy, Department of Pharmaceutical Sciences, Graduate Program in Pharmacology and Toxicology, Storrs, CT 06269. Offers pharmacology (MS, PhD); toxicology (MS, PhD). Terminal master's awarded for partial completion of doctoral program. *Degree requirements:* For master's, comprehensive exam, thesis; for doctorate, thesis/dissertation. *Entrance requirements:* For master's and doctorate, GRE General Test. Additional exam requirements/recommendations for international students: Required—TOEFL (minimum score 550 paper-based). Electronic applications accepted.

University of Florida, College of Medicine and Graduate School, Interdisciplinary Program in Biomedical Sciences, Concentration in Physiology and Pharmacology, Gainesville, FL 32611. Offers PhD. *Degree requirements:* For doctorate, thesis/dissertation. *Entrance requirements:* For doctorate, GRE General Test, minimum GPA of 3.0, biochemistry before enrollment. Electronic applications accepted. *Expenses:* Tuition, state resident: full-time $12,640. Tuition, nonresident: full-time $30,000.

University of Florida, Graduate School, College of Pharmacy and Graduate School, Graduate Programs in Pharmacy, Department of Pharmacodynamics, Gainesville, FL 32610. Offers MSP, PhD, Pharm D/PhD. *Faculty:* 7 full-time (2 women). *Students:* 10 full-time (3 women), 5 international. Average age 29. 9 applicants. In 2013, 3 doctorates awarded. *Degree requirements:* For doctorate, comprehensive exam, thesis/dissertation. *Entrance requirements:* For master's and doctorate, GRE General Test, minimum GPA of 3.0. Additional exam requirements/recommendations for international students: Required—TOEFL (minimum score 550 paper-based; 80 iBT), IELTS (minimum score 6). *Application deadline:* For fall admission, 2/15 priority date for domestic students, 2/15 for international students. Applications are processed on a rolling basis. Application fee: $30. Electronic applications accepted. *Expenses:* Tuition, state resident: full-time $12,640. Tuition, nonresident: full-time $30,000. *Financial support:* In 2013–14, 10 students received support, including 1 research assistantship (averaging $26,100 per year), 10 teaching assistantships (averaging $18,350 per year); institutionally sponsored loans and unspecified assistantships also available. Support available to part-time students. Financial award application deadline: 2/15; financial award applicants required to submit FAFSA. *Faculty research:* Neurochemistry and neurologic pathways involved in addiction and stress; cellular and molecular neurobiology of epilepsy, dementia and Parkinson's; hypertension and cardiac hypertrophy; stress hormone effects on fetal and neonatal development; cellular mechanism of glaucoma. *Unit head:* Maureen Keller-Wood, PhD, Professor and Chair, 352-273-7687, Fax: 352-273-7705, E-mail: kellerwd@cop.ufl.edu. *Application contact:* Charles J. Frazier, PhD, Associate Professor and Graduate Coordinator, 352-273-7686, Fax: 352-273-7705, E-mail: frazier@cop.ufl.edu.
Website: http://pharmacy.ufl.edu/pd/

University of Georgia, College of Veterinary Medicine, Department of Physiology and Pharmacology, Athens, GA 30602. Offers pharmacology (MS, PhD); physiology (MS, PhD). *Degree requirements:* For master's, thesis; for doctorate, one foreign language, thesis/dissertation. *Entrance requirements:* For master's and doctorate, GRE General Test. Electronic applications accepted.

University of Guelph, Ontario Veterinary College and Graduate Studies, Graduate Programs in Veterinary Sciences, Department of Biomedical Sciences, Guelph, ON N1G 2W1, Canada. Offers morphology (M Sc, DV Sc, PhD); neuroscience (M Sc, DV Sc, PhD); pharmacology (M Sc, DV Sc, PhD); physiology (M Sc, DV Sc, PhD); toxicology (M Sc, DV Sc, PhD). Part-time programs available. *Degree requirements:* For master's, thesis; for doctorate, comprehensive exam, thesis/dissertation. *Entrance requirements:* For master's, honors B Sc, minimum 75% average in last 20 courses; for doctorate, M Sc with thesis from accredited institution. Additional exam requirements/recommendations for international students: Required—TOEFL (minimum score 550 paper-based; 89 iBT). Electronic applications accepted. *Faculty research:* Cellular morphology; endocrine, vascular and reproductive physiology; clinical pharmacology; veterinary toxicology; developmental biology, neuroscience.

University of Hawaii at Hilo, Program in Clinical Psychopharmacology, Hilo, HI 96720-4091. Offers MS. *Students:* 2 full-time (1 woman), 4 part-time (2 women); includes 3 minority (1 Asian, non-Hispanic/Latino; 2 Two or more races, non-Hispanic/Latino). Average age 34. *Entrance requirements:* Additional exam requirements/recommendations for international students: Required—TOEFL, IELTS. *Application deadline:* For fall admission, 2/1 priority date for domestic students, 1/1 priority date for international students. Application fee: $50. Electronic applications accepted. *Expenses:* Tuition, state resident: full-time $4668. Tuition, nonresident: full-time $10,704. Tuition

and fees vary according to course load and program. *Financial support:* Application deadline: 3/1; applicants required to submit FAFSA. *Unit head:* Edward Fisher, Program Director, 808-932-7697, Fax: 808-933-2974, E-mail: pharmacy@hawaii.edu.
Website: http://hilo.hawaii.edu/catalog/ms-clinincal-psychopharmacology.html

University of Houston, College of Pharmacy, Houston, TX 77204. Offers pharmaceutics (MSPHR, PhD); pharmacology (MSPHR, PhD); pharmacy (Pharm D); pharmacy administration (MSPHR, PhD). *Accreditation:* ACPE. Part-time programs available. Terminal master's awarded for partial completion of doctoral program. *Entrance requirements:* For doctorate, PCAT (for Pharm D). Additional exam requirements/recommendations for international students: Required—TOEFL. Electronic applications accepted. *Faculty research:* Drug screening and design, cardiovascular pharmacology, infectious disease, asthma research, herbal medicine.

University of Illinois at Chicago, College of Medicine and Graduate College, Graduate Programs in Medicine, Department of Pharmacology, Chicago, IL 60612. Offers PhD, MD/PhD. *Faculty:* 43 full-time (11 women), 6 part-time/adjunct (1 woman). *Students:* 30 full-time (17 women), 1 part-time (0 women); includes 8 minority (1 Black or African American, non-Hispanic/Latino; 3 Asian, non-Hispanic/Latino; 3 Hispanic/Latino; 1 Two or more races, non-Hispanic/Latino), 8 international. Average age 27. 9 applicants, 89% accepted, 5 enrolled. In 2013, 8 doctorates awarded. *Degree requirements:* For doctorate, thesis/dissertation. *Entrance requirements:* For doctorate, GRE General Test. Additional exam requirements/recommendations for international students: Required—TOEFL. *Application deadline:* For fall admission, 1/15 priority date for domestic students, 2/15 for international students. Application fee: $50 ($60 for international students). *Expenses:* Tuition, state resident: full-time $11,066; part-time $3689 per term. Tuition, nonresident: full-time $23,064; part-time $7688 per term. *Required fees:* $3004; $1190 per term. Tuition and fees vary according to course level and program. *Financial support:* In 2013–14, 4 fellowships with full tuition reimbursements were awarded; research assistantships with full tuition reimbursements, tuition waivers (full), and unspecified assistantships also available. *Faculty research:* Cardiovascular and lung biology, cell signaling, molecular pharmacology of G-proteins, immunopharmacology, molecular and cellular basis of inflammation, neuroscience. *Total annual research expenditures:* $16 million. *Unit head:* Prof. Asrar B. Malik, Department Head, 312-996-7635, Fax: 312-996-1225, E-mail: abmalik@uic.edu. *Application contact:* Jackie Perry, Graduate College Receptionist, 312-413-2550, Fax: 312-413-0185, E-mail: gradcoll@uic.edu.
Website: http://mcph.uic.edu/home

The University of Iowa, Roy J. and Lucille A. Carver College of Medicine and Graduate College, Graduate Programs in Medicine, Department of Pharmacology, Iowa City, IA 52242-1316. Offers MS, PhD. *Faculty:* 17 full-time (3 women), 12 part-time/adjunct (4 women). *Students:* 17 full-time (10 women); includes 4 minority (2 Black or African American, non-Hispanic/Latino; 1 Asian, non-Hispanic/Latino; 1 Hispanic/Latino), 2 international. Average age 28. In 2013, 4 doctorates awarded. *Degree requirements:* For master's, thesis. *Entrance requirements:* For master's, GRE General Test. Additional exam requirements/recommendations for international students: Required—TOEFL (minimum score 600 paper-based). *Application deadline:* For fall admission, 2/1 priority date for domestic and international students. Applications are processed on a rolling basis. Application fee: $60 ($100 for international students). Electronic applications accepted. *Financial support:* In 2013–14, 17 research assistantships with full tuition reimbursements (averaging $26,000 per year) were awarded; scholarships/grants, traineeships, and unspecified assistantships also available. *Faculty research:* Cancer and cell cycle, hormones and growth factors, nervous system function and dysfunction, receptors and signal transduction, stroke and hypertension. *Total annual research expenditures:* $5.2 million. *Unit head:* Dr. Curt Sigmund, Chair and Department Executive Officer, 319-335-7946, Fax: 319-335-8930, E-mail: curt-sigmund@uiowa.edu. *Application contact:* Dr. Frederick Quelle, Director, Graduate Admissions, 319-335-8539, Fax: 319-335-8930, E-mail: pharmacology-admissions@uiowa.edu.
Website: http://www.medicine.uiowa.edu/pharmacology/

The University of Kansas, Graduate Studies, School of Pharmacy, Department of Pharmacology and Toxicology, Program in Pharmacology and Toxicology, Lawrence, KS 66045. Offers MS, PhD. *Faculty:* 12. *Students:* 14 full-time (all women), 11 international. Average age 24. 41 applicants, 15% accepted, 4 enrolled. In 2013, 4 doctorates awarded. Terminal master's awarded for partial completion of doctoral program. *Degree requirements:* For master's, comprehensive exam, thesis; for doctorate, comprehensive exam, thesis/dissertation. *Entrance requirements:* For master's, GRE, bachelor's degree in related field, 3 letters of recommendation, resume or curriculum vitae, official transcripts, 1-2 page personal statement; for doctorate, GRE (minimum score: 600 verbal, 600 quantitative, 4.5 analytical), bachelor's degree in related field, 3 letters of recommendation, resume or curriculum vitae, official transcripts, 1-2 page personal statement. Additional exam requirements/recommendations for international students: Required—TOEFL (minimum score 600 paper-based; 100 iBT). *Application deadline:* For fall admission, 1/15 for domestic students, 2/1 for international students. Applications are processed on a rolling basis. Application fee: $55 ($65 for international students). Electronic applications accepted. *Financial support:* Fellowships with full tuition reimbursements and research assistantships with full tuition reimbursements available. Financial award application deadline: 2/1. *Faculty research:* Neurodegeneration, diabetes, neurological disorders, neuropharmacology, drug metabolism. *Unit head:* Nancy Muma, Chair, 785-864-4002, Fax: 785-864-5219, E-mail: nmuma@ku.edu. *Application contact:* Debbie Thompson, Administrative Associate, 785-864-4002, E-mail: djthompson@ku.edu.
Website: http://www.pharmtox.pharm.ku.edu

The University of Kansas, University of Kansas Medical Center, School of Medicine, Department of Pharmacology, Toxicology and Therapeutics, Kansas City, KS 66160. Offers pharmacology (MA, MS, PhD); toxicology (MS, PhD); MD/MS; MD/PhD. *Faculty:* 18. *Students:* 26 full-time (12 women); includes 3 minority (1 Black or African American, non-Hispanic/Latino; 2 Two or more races, non-Hispanic/Latino), 12 international. Average age 29. In 2013, 6 doctorates awarded. Terminal master's awarded for partial completion of doctoral program. *Degree requirements:* For master's, comprehensive exam, thesis; for doctorate, one foreign language, comprehensive exam, thesis/dissertation. *Entrance requirements:* For master's and doctorate, GRE General Test. Additional exam requirements/recommendations for international students: Required—TOEFL. *Application deadline:* For fall admission, 1/15 priority date for domestic students. Applications are processed on a rolling basis. Application fee: $0. Electronic applications accepted. *Financial support:* Fellowships with full tuition reimbursements, research assistantships with full tuition reimbursements, teaching assistantships with full tuition reimbursements, Federal Work-Study, scholarships/grants, traineeships, and unspecified assistantships available. Support available to part-time students. Financial award application deadline: 3/1; financial award applicants required to submit FAFSA. *Faculty research:* Liver nuclear receptors, hepatobiliary transporters, pharmacogenomics, estrogen-induced carcinogenesis, neuropharmacology of pain and depression. *Total annual research expenditures:* $6.3 million. *Unit head:* Dr. Hartmut Jaeschke, Professor and Chair, 913-588-7969, Fax: 913-588-7501, E-mail: hjaeschke@kumc.edu. *Application contact:* Chair, Departmental Graduate Committee, 913-588-7140, Fax: 913-588-7501.
Website: http://www.kumc.edu/school-of-medicine/pharmacology-toxicology-and-therapeutics.html

University of Kentucky, Graduate School, Graduate School Programs from the College of Medicine, Program in Molecular and Biomedical Pharmacology, Lexington, KY 40506-0032. Offers PhD, MD/PhD. *Degree requirements:* For doctorate, comprehensive exam, thesis/dissertation. *Entrance requirements:* For doctorate, GRE General Test, minimum undergraduate GPA of 2.75, graduate 3.0. Additional exam requirements/recommendations for international students: Required—TOEFL (minimum score 550 paper-based). Electronic applications accepted.

University of Louisville, School of Medicine, Department of Pharmacology and Toxicology, Louisville, KY 40292-0001. Offers MS, PhD, MD/PhD. *Students:* 26 full-time (16 women), 15 part-time (2 women); includes 5 minority (4 Black or African American, non-Hispanic/Latino; 1 Asian, non-Hispanic/Latino), 10 international. Average age 28. 63 applicants, 21% accepted, 10 enrolled. In 2013, 2 master's awarded. Terminal master's awarded for partial completion of doctoral program. *Degree requirements:* For master's, thesis; for doctorate, comprehensive exam, thesis/dissertation. *Entrance requirements:* For master's and doctorate, GRE General Test (minimum score of 1000 verbal and quantitative), minimum GPA of 3.0. Additional exam requirements/recommendations for international students: Required—TOEFL. *Application deadline:* For fall admission, 1/15 priority date for domestic and international students. Applications are processed on a rolling basis. Application fee: $60. Electronic applications accepted. *Expenses:* Tuition, state resident: full-time $10,788; part-time $599 per credit hour. Tuition, nonresident: full-time $22,446; part-time $1247 per credit hour. *Required fees:* $196. Tuition and fees vary according to program and reciprocity agreements. *Financial support:* Fellowships with full tuition reimbursements and research assistantships with full tuition reimbursements available. Financial award application deadline: 4/15. *Faculty research:* Molecular pharmacogenetics; epidemiology; functional genomics; genetic predisposition to chemical carcinogenesis and drug toxicity; mechanisms of oxidative stress; alcohol-induced hepatitis, pancreatitis, and hepatocellular carcinoma; molecular and cardiac toxicology; molecular biology and genetics of DNA damage and repair in humans; mechanisms of chemoresistance; arsenic toxicity and cell cycle disruption; molecular pharmacology of novel G protein-coupled receptors. *Unit head:* Dr. David W. Hein, Chair, 502-852-5141, Fax: 502-852-7868, E-mail: dhein@louisville.edu. *Application contact:* Heddy R. Rubin, Information Contact, 502-852-5741, Fax: 502-852-7868, E-mail: hrrubi01@gwise.louisville.edu.

The University of Manchester, Faculty of Life Sciences, Manchester, United Kingdom. Offers adaptive organismal biology (M Phil, PhD); animal biology (M Phil, PhD); biochemistry (M Phil, PhD); bioinformatics (M Phil, PhD); biomolecular sciences (M Phil, PhD); biotechnology (M Phil, PhD); cell biology (M Phil, PhD); cell matrix research (M Phil, PhD); channels and transporters (M Phil, PhD); developmental biology (M Phil, PhD); Egyptology (M Phil, PhD); environmental biology (M Phil, PhD); evolutionary biology (M Phil, PhD); gene expression (M Phil, PhD); genetics (M Phil, PhD); history of science, technology and medicine (M Phil, PhD); immunology (M Phil, PhD); integrative neurobiology and behavior (M Phil, PhD); membrane trafficking (M Phil, PhD); microbiology (M Phil, PhD); molecular and cellular neuroscience (M Phil, PhD); molecular biology (M Phil, PhD); molecular cancer studies (M Phil, PhD); neuroscience (M Phil, PhD); ophthalmology (M Phil, PhD); optometry (M Phil, PhD); organelle function (M Phil, PhD); pharmacology (M Phil, PhD); physiology (M Phil, PhD); plant sciences (M Phil, PhD); stem cell research (M Phil, PhD); structural biology (M Phil, PhD); systems neuroscience (M Phil, PhD); toxicology (M Phil, PhD).

University of Manitoba, Faculty of Medicine and Faculty of Graduate Studies, Graduate Programs in Medicine, Department of Pharmacology and Therapeutics, Winnipeg, MB R3T 2N2, Canada. Offers M Sc, PhD. Part-time programs available. Terminal master's awarded for partial completion of doctoral program. *Degree requirements:* For master's, thesis; for doctorate, thesis/dissertation. *Entrance requirements:* For master's and doctorate, GRE. Additional exam requirements/recommendations for international students: Required—TOEFL. *Faculty research:* Clinical pharmacology; neuropharmacology; cardiac, hepatic, and renal pharmacology.

University of Maryland, Baltimore, Graduate School, Graduate Program in Life Sciences, Program in Molecular Medicine, Baltimore, MD 21201. Offers cancer biology (PhD); cell and molecular physiology (PhD); human genetics and genomic medicine (PhD); molecular medicine (MS); molecular toxicology and pharmacology (PhD); MD/PhD. *Students:* 91 full-time (49 women), 14 part-time (8 women); includes 32 minority (10 Black or African American, non-Hispanic/Latino; 12 Asian, non-Hispanic/Latino; 5 Hispanic/Latino; 5 Two or more races, non-Hispanic/Latino), 9 international. Average age 27. 180 applicants, 33% accepted, 24 enrolled. In 2013, 10 master's, 15 doctorates awarded. *Degree requirements:* For doctorate, comprehensive exam, thesis/dissertation. *Entrance requirements:* For master's and doctorate, GRE. Additional exam requirements/recommendations for international students: Required—TOEFL (minimum score 600 paper-based; 100 iBT); Recommended—IELTS (minimum score 7). *Application deadline:* For fall admission, 12/1 priority date for domestic students, 1/15 for international students. Application fee: $75. Electronic applications accepted. *Financial support:* In 2013–14, research assistantships with partial tuition reimbursements (averaging $25,000 per year) were awarded; fellowships also available. Financial award application deadline: 3/1; financial award applicants required to submit FAFSA. *Unit head:* Dr. Toni Antalis, Director, 410-706-8222, E-mail: tantalis@som.umaryland.edu. *Application contact:* Sharron Graves, Program Coordinator, 410-706-6044, Fax: 410-706-6040, E-mail: sgraves@som.umaryland.edu.
Website: http://molecularmedicine.umaryland.edu

University of Maryland, Baltimore, Graduate School, Graduate Programs in Pharmacy, Program in Pharmacometrics, Baltimore, MD 21201. Offers MS.

University of Miami, Graduate School, Miller School of Medicine, Graduate Programs in Medicine, Department of Molecular and Cellular Pharmacology, Coral Gables, FL 33124. Offers PhD, MD/PhD. *Degree requirements:* For doctorate, thesis/dissertation, dissertation defense, laboratory rotations, qualifying exam. *Entrance requirements:* For doctorate, GRE General Test. Additional exam requirements/recommendations for international students: Required—TOEFL (minimum score 550 paper-based). *Faculty research:* Membrane and cardiovascular pharmacology, muscle contraction, hormone action signal transduction, nuclear transport.

University of Michigan, Rackham Graduate School, Program in Biomedical Sciences (PIBS), Department of Pharmacology, Ann Arbor, MI 48109-5632. Offers MS, PhD. *Faculty:* 25 full-time (5 women). *Students:* 26 full-time (13 women); includes 2 minority (1 Black or African American, non-Hispanic/Latino; 1 Asian, non-Hispanic/Latino), 3 international. Average age 26. 45 applicants, 20% accepted, 4 enrolled. In 2013, 3 master's, 4 doctorates awarded. Terminal master's awarded for partial completion of doctoral program. *Degree requirements:* For master's, thesis, oral presentation; for doctorate, thesis/dissertation, oral preliminary exam, oral defense of dissertation. *Entrance requirements:* For master's, 3 letters of recommendation, research experience, all undergraduate transcripts; for doctorate, GRE General Test, 3 letters of

recommendation, research experience, all undergraduate transcripts. Additional exam requirements/recommendations for international students: Required—TOEFL (minimum score 84 iBT). *Application deadline:* For fall admission, 12/1 for domestic students. Applications are processed on a rolling basis. Application fee: $75 ($90 for international students). Electronic applications accepted. Tuition and fees vary according to course level, course load, degree level, program and student level. *Financial support:* In 2013–14, 25 students received support, including 15 fellowships with full tuition reimbursements available (averaging $28,500 per year), 10 research assistantships with full tuition reimbursements available (averaging $28,500 per year); scholarships/grants, traineeships, health care benefits, and unspecified assistantships also available. Financial award application deadline: 12/1. *Faculty research:* Signal transduction, addiction research, cancer pharmacology, drug metabolism and pharmacogenetics. *Total annual research expenditures:* $6.8 million. *Unit head:* Dr. Paul F. Hollenberg, Professor/Chair of Pharmacology, 734-764-8166, Fax: 734-763-5387, E-mail: phollen@umich.edu. *Application contact:* Michelle S. Melis, Director of Student Life, 734-615-6538, Fax: 734-647-7022, E-mail: msmtegan@umich.edu.
Website: http://www.pharmacology.med.umich.edu/Pharmacology/Home.html

University of Minnesota, Duluth, Medical School, Program in Pharmacology, Duluth, MN 55812-2496. Offers MS, PhD. MS, PhD offered jointly with University of Minnesota, Twin Cities Campus. Terminal master's awarded for partial completion of doctoral program. *Degree requirements:* For master's, thesis, final oral exam; for doctorate, thesis/dissertation, final oral exam, oral and written preliminary exams. *Entrance requirements:* For master's and doctorate, GRE General Test. Additional exam requirements/recommendations for international students: Required—TOEFL. *Faculty research:* Drug addiction, alcohol and hypertension, neurotransmission, allergic airway disease, auditory neuroscience.

University of Minnesota, Twin Cities Campus, College of Pharmacy and Graduate School, Graduate Programs in Pharmacy, Graduate Program in Experimental and Clinical Pharmacology, Minneapolis, MN 55455-0213. Offers MS, PhD. *Degree requirements:* For doctorate, thesis/dissertation.

University of Minnesota, Twin Cities Campus, Medical School, Department of Pharmacology, Minneapolis, MN 55455. Offers MS, PhD. *Faculty:* 46 full-time (9 women). *Students:* 36 full-time (20 women); includes 5 minority (1 Black or African American, non-Hispanic/Latino; 3 Asian, non-Hispanic/Latino; 1 Hispanic/Latino), 13 international. Average age 26. 36 applicants, 44% accepted, 14 enrolled. In 2013, 2 master's, 9 doctorates awarded. Terminal master's awarded for partial completion of doctoral program. *Degree requirements:* For master's, thesis (for some programs); for doctorate, thesis/dissertation. *Entrance requirements:* For master's and doctorate, GRE General Test. Additional exam requirements/recommendations for international students: Required—TOEFL (minimum score 603 paper-based; 100 iBT). *Application deadline:* For fall admission, 12/1 for domestic and international students. Applications are processed on a rolling basis. Application fee: $75 ($95 for international students). Electronic applications accepted. *Financial support:* In 2013–14, 29 students received support, including 9 fellowships with full tuition reimbursements available (averaging $25,000 per year), 20 research assistantships with full tuition reimbursements available (averaging $25,000 per year); scholarships/grants, traineeships, and unspecified assistantships also available. Financial award application deadline: 4/15. *Faculty research:* Molecular pharmacology, cancer chemotherapy, neuropharmacology, biochemical pharmacology, behavioral pharmacology. *Total annual research expenditures:* $4.9 million. *Unit head:* Dr. Jill Siegfried, Head, 612-625-9997, Fax: 612-625-8408, E-mail: jsiegfri@umn.edu. *Application contact:* Graduate Program Assistant, 612-625-9997, Fax: 612-625-8408, E-mail: phclgrad@umn.edu.
Website: http://www.pharmacology.med.umn.edu/

University of Mississippi, Graduate School, School of Pharmacy, Graduate Programs in Pharmacy, University, MS 38677. Offers medicinal chemistry (PhD); pharmaceutical sciences (MS); pharmaceutics (PhD); pharmacognosy (PhD); pharmacology (PhD); pharmacy administration (PhD). *Faculty:* 41 full-time (17 women), 14 part-time/adjunct (7 women). *Students:* 81 full-time (27 women), 8 part-time (5 women); includes 4 minority (2 Black or African American, non-Hispanic/Latino; 2 Asian, non-Hispanic/Latino), 61 international. In 2013, 5 master's, 16 doctorates awarded. Application fee: $40. *Unit head:* Dr. David Allen, Dean, 662-915-7267, Fax: 662-915-5118, E-mail: sop@olemiss.edu. *Application contact:* Dr. Christy M. Wyandt, Associate Dean, 662-915-7474, Fax: 662-915-7577, E-mail: cwyandt@olemiss.edu.

University of Mississippi Medical Center, School of Graduate Studies in the Health Sciences, Department of Pharmacology and Toxicology, Jackson, MS 39216-4505. Offers PhD. *Faculty:* 18 full-time (3 women). *Students:* 13 full-time (8 women); includes 2 minority (both Black or African American, non-Hispanic/Latino), 5 international. Average age 28. 11 applicants, 18% accepted, 2 enrolled. In 2013, 3 doctorates awarded. *Degree requirements:* For doctorate, comprehensive exam, thesis/dissertation, first authored publication. *Entrance requirements:* For doctorate, GRE General Test, minimum GPA of 3.0. Additional exam requirements/recommendations for international students: Required—TOEFL (minimum score 550 paper-based, 79 iBT), IELTS or PTE. *Application deadline:* For fall admission, 2/17 priority date for domestic and international students. Application fee: $25. Electronic applications accepted. *Financial support:* In 2013–14, 11 research assistantships (averaging $24,150 per year) were awarded; health care benefits also available. Financial award application deadline: 4/1. *Faculty research:* Renal and cardiovascular pharmacology, genetic basis of cardio-renal diseases, diabetes, obesity, metabolic diseases, cancer chemotherapy. *Total annual research expenditures:* $4.3 million. *Unit head:* Dr. Richard J. Roman, Chair, 601-984-1600, Fax: 601-984-1602, E-mail: rroman@umc.edu. *Application contact:* Barbara Westerfield, Director, Student Records/Registrar, 601-984-1080, Fax: 601-984-1079, E-mail: bwesterfield@umc.edu.
Website: http://www.umc.edu/Education/Schools/Medicine/Basic_Science/Pharmacology_and_Toxicology/Academics(Pharmacology_and_Toxicology)/Academics_Home.aspx

University of Missouri, School of Medicine and Graduate School, Graduate Programs in Medicine, Department of Medical Pharmacology and Physiology, Columbia, MO 65211. Offers MS, PhD. *Faculty:* 29 full-time (4 women), 3 part-time/adjunct (1 woman). *Students:* 14 full-time (9 women), 2 part-time (both women); includes 1 minority (Black or African American, non-Hispanic/Latino), 10 international. Average age 28. 42 applicants, 10% accepted, 4 enrolled. In 2013, 1 master's, 1 doctorate awarded. *Degree requirements:* For master's, thesis; for doctorate, thesis/dissertation. *Entrance requirements:* For master's and doctorate, GRE General Test, minimum GPA of 3.0. Additional exam requirements/recommendations for international students: Required—TOEFL (minimum score 500 paper-based; 61 iBT). *Application deadline:* For fall admission, 1/10 priority date for domestic and international students; for winter admission, 10/10 priority date for domestic and international students. Applications are processed on a rolling basis. Application fee: $55 ($75 for international students). Electronic applications accepted. *Financial support:* Fellowships, research assistantships, teaching assistantships, institutionally sponsored loans, scholarships/grants, health care benefits, and unspecified assistantships available. Support available to part-time students. *Faculty research:* Endocrine and metabolic pharmacology, biochemical pharmacology, neuropharmacology, receptors and transmembrane signaling. *Unit head:* Dr. Ron Korthuis, Department Chair, 573-882-8029, E-mail: korthuisr@missouri.edu. *Application contact:* Melinda Nichols, Administrative Assistant, 573-882-8432, E-mail: nicholsmk@missouri.edu.
Website: http://mpp.missouri.edu/

University of Missouri–Kansas City, School of Pharmacy, Kansas City, MO 64110-2499. Offers pharmaceutical sciences (PhD); pharmacology and toxicology (PhD); pharmacy (Pharm D). PhD offered through School of Graduate Studies. *Accreditation:* ACPE (one or more programs are accredited). Postbaccalaureate distance learning degree programs offered (minimal on-campus study). *Faculty:* 54 full-time (26 women), 6 part-time/adjunct (3 women). *Students:* 424 full-time (252 women); includes 77 minority (14 Black or African American, non-Hispanic/Latino; 2 American Indian or Alaska Native, non-Hispanic/Latino; 43 Asian, non-Hispanic/Latino; 10 Hispanic/Latino; 1 Native Hawaiian or other Pacific Islander, non-Hispanic/Latino; 7 Two or more races, non-Hispanic/Latino), 1 international. Average age 26. 365 applicants, 37% accepted, 136 enrolled. In 2013, 122 doctorates awarded. *Degree requirements:* For doctorate, comprehensive exam (for some programs), thesis/dissertation (for some programs). *Entrance requirements:* For doctorate, PCAT (for Pharm D). Additional exam requirements/recommendations for international students: Required—TOEFL (minimum score 550 paper-based; 80 iBT). *Application deadline:* For fall admission, 3/1 for domestic and international students. Applications are processed on a rolling basis. Application fee: $45 ($50 for international students). Electronic applications accepted. *Expenses:* Contact institution. *Financial support:* In 2013–14, 26 research assistantships with full and partial tuition reimbursements (averaging $11,585 per year), 26 teaching assistantships with full tuition reimbursements (averaging $14,213 per year) were awarded; career-related internships or fieldwork, Federal Work-Study, institutionally sponsored loans, tuition waivers (full and partial), and unspecified assistantships also available. Financial award application deadline: 3/1; financial award applicants required to submit FAFSA. *Faculty research:* Bio-organic and medicinal chemistry, drug delivery, pharmaceutics, molecular neurobiology, neurology. *Unit head:* Dr. Russell B. Melchert, Dean, 816-235-1609, Fax: 816-235-5190, E-mail: melchertr@umkc.edu. *Application contact:* Shelly M. Janasz, Director, Student Services, 816-235-2400, Fax: 816-235-5190, E-mail: janaszs@umkc.edu.
Website: http://pharmacy.umkc.edu/

University of Nebraska Medical Center, Department of Pharmacology and Experimental Neuroscience, Omaha, NE 68198-5800. Offers neuroscience (MS, PhD); pharmacology (MS, PhD). Terminal master's awarded for partial completion of doctoral program. *Degree requirements:* For master's, comprehensive exam, thesis; for doctorate, comprehensive exam, thesis/dissertation. *Entrance requirements:* For master's and doctorate, GRE General Test. Additional exam requirements/recommendations for international students: Required—TOEFL (minimum score 600 paper-based). Electronic applications accepted. *Expenses: Required fees:* $300 per semester. Tuition and fees vary according to program. *Faculty research:* Neuropharmacology, molecular pharmacology, toxicology, molecular biology, neuroscience.

The University of North Carolina at Chapel Hill, School of Medicine and Graduate School, Graduate Programs in Medicine, Department of Pharmacology, Chapel Hill, NC 27599-7365. Offers PhD. *Degree requirements:* For doctorate, comprehensive exam, thesis/dissertation. *Entrance requirements:* For doctorate, GRE General Test, minimum GPA of 3.0. Additional exam requirements/recommendations for international students: Required—TOEFL. Electronic applications accepted. *Faculty research:* Signal transduction, cell adhesion, receptors, ion channels.

University of North Dakota, Graduate School and Graduate School, Graduate Programs in Medicine, Department of Pharmacology, Physiology, and Therapeutics, Grand Forks, ND 58202. Offers pharmacology (MS, PhD); physiology (MS, PhD). *Degree requirements:* For master's, comprehensive exam, thesis; for doctorate, thesis/dissertation, written and oral exams. *Entrance requirements:* For master's, GRE General Test or MCAT, minimum GPA of 3.0; for doctorate, GRE General Test, minimum GPA of 3.5. Additional exam requirements/recommendations for international students: Required—TOEFL (minimum score 550 paper-based; 79 iBT), IELTS (minimum score 6.5). Electronic applications accepted.

University of North Texas Health Science Center at Fort Worth, Graduate School of Biomedical Sciences, Fort Worth, TX 76107-2699. Offers anatomy and cell biology (MS, PhD); biochemistry and molecular biology (MS, PhD); biomedical sciences (MS, PhD); biotechnology (MS); forensic genetics (MS); integrative physiology (MS, PhD); medical science (MS); microbiology and immunology (MS, PhD); pharmacology (MS, PhD); science education (MS); DO/MS; DO/PhD. Terminal master's awarded for partial completion of doctoral program. *Degree requirements:* For master's, thesis; for doctorate, thesis/dissertation. *Entrance requirements:* For master's and doctorate, GRE General Test. Additional exam requirements/recommendations for international students: Required—TOEFL. *Expenses:* Contact institution. *Faculty research:* Alzheimer's disease, aging, eye diseases, cancer, cardiovascular disease.

University of Pennsylvania, Perelman School of Medicine, Biomedical Graduate Studies, Graduate Group in Pharmacology, Philadelphia, PA 19104. Offers PhD, MD/PhD, VMD/PhD. *Faculty:* 95. *Students:* 64 full-time (36 women); includes 21 minority (5 Black or African American, non-Hispanic/Latino; 14 Asian, non-Hispanic/Latino; 2 Hispanic/Latino), 6 international. 59 applicants, 24% accepted, 8 enrolled. In 2013, 9 doctorates awarded. *Degree requirements:* For doctorate, thesis/dissertation. *Entrance requirements:* For doctorate, GRE General Test, previous course work in physical or natural science. Additional exam requirements/recommendations for international students: Required—TOEFL. *Application deadline:* For fall admission, 12/1 priority date for domestic and international students. Applications are processed on a rolling basis. Application fee: $80. Electronic applications accepted. *Financial support:* In 2013–14, 64 students received support. Fellowships, research assistantships, scholarships/grants, traineeships, and unspecified assistantships available. *Faculty research:* Properties and regulation of receptors for biogenic amines, molecular aspects of transduction, mechanisms of biosynthesis, biological mechanisms of depression, developmental events in the nervous system. *Unit head:* Dr. Julie Blendy, Chair, 215-898-0730. *Application contact:* Sarah Squire, Admissions Coordinator, 215-898-1790.
Website: http://www.med.upenn.edu/ggps

University of Prince Edward Island, Atlantic Veterinary College, Graduate Program in Veterinary Medicine, Charlottetown, PE C1A 4P3, Canada. Offers anatomy (M Sc, PhD); bacteriology (M Sc, PhD); clinical pharmacology (M Sc, PhD); clinical sciences (M Sc, PhD); epidemiology (M Sc, PhD), including reproduction; fish health (M Sc, PhD); food animal nutrition (M Sc, PhD); immunology (M Sc, PhD); microanatomy (M Sc, PhD); parasitology (M Sc, PhD); pathology (M Sc, PhD); pharmacology (M Sc, PhD); physiology (M Sc, PhD); toxicology (M Sc, PhD); veterinary science (M Vet Sc); virology (M Sc, PhD). Part-time programs available. *Degree requirements:* For master's, thesis; for doctorate, thesis/dissertation. *Entrance requirements:* For master's, DVM, B Sc honors degree, or equivalent; for doctorate, M Sc. Additional exam requirements/recommendations for international students: Required—TOEFL (minimum score 550 paper-based; 80 iBT). *Expenses:* Contact institution. *Faculty research:* Animal health management, infectious diseases, fin fish and shellfish health, basic biomedical sciences, ecosystem health.

Pharmacology

University of Puerto Rico, Medical Sciences Campus, School of Medicine, Division of Graduate Studies, Department of Pharmacology and Toxicology, San Juan, PR 00936-5067. Offers MS, PhD. *Degree requirements:* For master's, one foreign language, thesis; for doctorate, one foreign language, comprehensive exam, thesis/dissertation. *Entrance requirements:* For master's and doctorate, GRE General Test, GRE Subject Test, interview, minimum GPA of 3.0, 3 letters of recommendation. Electronic applications accepted. *Faculty research:* Cardiovascular, central nervous system, and endocrine pharmacology; anti-cancer drugs; sodium pump; mitochondrial DNA repair; Huntington's disease.

University of Rhode Island, Graduate School, College of Pharmacy, Department of Biomedical and Pharmaceutical Sciences, Kingston, RI 02881. Offers medicinal chemistry and pharmacognosy (MS, PhD); pharmaceutics and pharmacokinetics (MS, PhD); pharmacology and toxicology (MS, PhD). Part-time programs available. *Faculty:* 21 full-time (7 women). *Students:* 37 full-time (14 women), 15 part-time (7 women); includes 3 minority (1 Black or African American, non-Hispanic/Latino; 1 Asian, non-Hispanic/Latino; 1 Two or more races, non-Hispanic/Latino), 29 international. In 2013, 3 master's, 18 doctorates awarded. *Entrance requirements:* For master's and doctorate, GRE (minimum new/old format scores: Verbal 350/143; Quantitative 550/146; Analytical, 3.0), 2 letters of recommendation. Additional exam requirements/recommendations for international students: Required—TOEFL (minimum score 550 paper-based). *Application deadline:* For fall admission, 7/15 for domestic students, 2/1 for international students. Application fee: $65. Electronic applications accepted. *Expenses:* Tuition, state resident: full-time $11,532; part-time $641 per credit. Tuition, nonresident: full-time $23,606; part-time $1311 per credit. *Required fees:* $1388; $36 per credit. $35 per semester. One-time fee: $130. *Financial support:* In 2013–14, 8 research assistantships with full and partial tuition reimbursements (averaging $12,147 per year), 13 teaching assistantships with full and partial tuition reimbursements (averaging $13,579 per year) were awarded. Financial award application deadline: 2/1; financial award applicants required to submit FAFSA. *Faculty research:* Chemical carcinogenesis with a major emphasis on the structural and synthetic aspects of DNA-adduct formation, drug-drug/herb interaction, drug-genetic interaction, signaling of nuclear receptors, transcriptional regulation, oncogenesis. *Total annual research expenditures:* $5.8 million. *Unit head:* Dr. Bingfang Yan, Chair, 401-874-5032, Fax: 401-874-2181, E-mail: byan@uri.edu. *Application contact:* Graduate Admissions, 401-874-2872, E-mail: gradadm@etal.uri.edu.
Website: http://www.uri.edu/pharmacy/departments/bps/index.shtml

University of Rochester, School of Medicine and Dentistry, Graduate Programs in Medicine and Dentistry, Department of Pharmacology and Physiology, Programs in Pharmacology, Rochester, NY 14627. Offers MS, PhD. Terminal master's awarded for partial completion of doctoral program. *Degree requirements:* For master's, thesis; for doctorate, thesis/dissertation, qualifying exam. *Entrance requirements:* For master's and doctorate, GRE General Test. *Expenses: Tuition:* Full-time $44,580; part-time $1394 per credit hour. *Required fees:* $492.

University of Saskatchewan, College of Medicine, Department of Pharmacology, Saskatoon, SK S7N 5A2, Canada. Offers M Sc, PhD. *Degree requirements:* For master's, thesis; for doctorate, thesis/dissertation. *Entrance requirements:* Additional exam requirements/recommendations for international students: Required—TOEFL. *Expenses: Tuition, area resident:* Full-time $3585 Canadian dollars; part-time $585 Canadian dollars per course. Tuition, nonresident: part-time $877 Canadian dollars per course. *International tuition:* $5377 Canadian dollars full-time. *Required fees:* $889.51 Canadian dollars. *Faculty research:* Neuropharmacology, mechanisms of action of anticancer drugs, clinical pharmacology, cardiovascular pharmacology, toxicology: alcohol-related changes in fetal brain development.

The University of South Dakota, Graduate School, School of Medicine and Graduate School, Biomedical Sciences Graduate Program, Physiology and Pharmacology Group, Vermillion, SD 57069-2390. Offers MS, PhD. Terminal master's awarded for partial completion of doctoral program. *Degree requirements:* For master's, thesis; for doctorate, comprehensive exam, thesis/dissertation. *Entrance requirements:* For master's and doctorate, GRE General Test, minimum GPA of 3.0. Additional exam requirements/recommendations for international students: Required—TOEFL (minimum score 550 paper-based; 80 iBT), IELTS (minimum score 6). Electronic applications accepted. *Expenses:* Contact institution. *Faculty research:* Pulmonary physiology and pharmacology, drug abuse, reproduction, signal transduction, cardiovascular physiology and pharmacology.

University of South Florida, Morsani College of Medicine and Graduate School, Graduate Programs in Medical Sciences, Tampa, FL 33620-9951. Offers aging and neuroscience (MSMS); allergy, immunology and infectious disease (PhD); anatomy (MSMS, PhD); athletic training (MSMS); bioinformatics and computational biology (MSBCB); biotechnology (MSB); clinical and translational research (MSMS, PhD); health informatics (MSHI, MSMS); health science (MSMS); interdisciplinary medical sciences (MSMS); medical microbiology and immunology (MSMS); metabolic and nutritional medicine (MSMS); molecular medicine (MSMS, PhD); molecular pharmacology and physiology (PhD); neurology (PhD); pathology and laboratory medicine (PhD); pharmacology and therapeutics (PhD); physiology and biophysics (PhD); women's health (MSMS). *Students:* 336 full-time (182 women), 39 part-time (21 women); includes 170 minority (45 Black or African American, non-Hispanic/Latino; 54 Asian, non-Hispanic/Latino; 59 Hispanic/Latino; 2 Native Hawaiian or other Pacific Islander, non-Hispanic/Latino; 10 Two or more races, non-Hispanic/Latino), 17 international. Average age 26. 1,066 applicants, 44% accepted, 250 enrolled. In 2013, 191 master's, 12 doctorates awarded. Terminal master's awarded for partial completion of doctoral program. *Degree requirements:* For master's, comprehensive exam, thesis; for doctorate, comprehensive exam, thesis/dissertation. *Entrance requirements:* For master's, GRE General Test or GMAT, bachelor's degree or equivalent from regionally-accredited university with minimum GPA of 3.0 in upper-division sciences coursework; prerequisites in general biology, general chemistry, general physics, organic chemistry, quantitative analysis, and integral and differential calculus; for doctorate, GRE General Test (minimum score of 600 quantitative), bachelor's degree from regionally-accredited university with minimum GPA of 3.0 in upper-division sciences coursework; 3 letters of recommendation; personal interview; 1-2 page personal statement; prerequisites in biology, chemistry, physics, organic chemistry, quantitative analysis, and integral/differential calculus. Additional exam requirements/recommendations for international students: Required—TOEFL (minimum score 550 paper-based; 79 iBT) or IELTS (minimum score 6.5). *Application deadline:* For fall admission, 2/15 for domestic students, 1/2 for international students. Application fee: $30. *Expenses:* Contact institution. *Faculty research:* Anatomy, biochemistry, cancer biology, cardiovascular disease, cell biology, immunology, microbiology, molecular biology, neuroscience, pharmacology, physiology. *Unit head:* Dr. Michael Barber, Professor and Associate Dean for Graduate and Postdoctoral Affairs, 813-974-9908, Fax: 813-974-4317, E-mail: mbarber@health.usf.edu. *Application contact:* Dr. Eric Bennett, Graduate Director, PhD Program in Medical Sciences, 813-974-1545, Fax: 813-974-4317, E-mail: esbennet@health.usf.edu.
Website: http://health.usf.edu/nocms/medicine/graduatestudies/

The University of Tennessee Health Science Center, College of Graduate Health Sciences, Memphis, TN 38163-0002. Offers biomedical engineering (MS, PhD); biomedical sciences (PhD); dental sciences (MDS); epidemiology (MS); health outcomes and policy research (PhD); laboratory research and management (MS); nursing science (PhD); pharmaceutical sciences (PhD); pharmacology (MS); speech and hearing science (PhD); DDS/PhD; DNP/PhD; MD/PhD; Pharm D/PhD. *Faculty:* 318 full-time (92 women), 59 part-time/adjunct (16 women). *Students:* 220 full-time (102 women), 22 part-time (13 women); includes 194 minority (22 Black or African American, non-Hispanic/Latino; 161 Asian, non-Hispanic/Latino; 7 Hispanic/Latino; 3 Native Hawaiian or other Pacific Islander, non-Hispanic/Latino; 1 Two or more races, non-Hispanic/Latino), 106 international. Average age 25. 404 applicants, 17% accepted, 64 enrolled. In 2013, 13 master's, 25 doctorates awarded. Terminal master's awarded for partial completion of doctoral program. *Degree requirements:* For master's, comprehensive exam, thesis; for doctorate, comprehensive exam, thesis/dissertation, oral and written preliminary and comprehensive exams. *Entrance requirements:* For master's and doctorate, GRE General Test, minimum GPA of 3.0. Additional exam requirements/recommendations for international students: Required—TOEFL (minimum score 79 iBT); Recommended—IELTS (minimum score 6.5). *Application deadline:* For fall admission, 5/15 priority date for domestic students. Applications are processed on a rolling basis. Application fee: $0. Electronic applications accepted. *Financial support:* In 2013–14, 125 students received support, including 125 research assistantships (averaging $23,000 per year); career-related internships or fieldwork, Federal Work-Study, institutionally sponsored loans, and tuition waivers (full and partial) also available. Support available to part-time students. Financial award application deadline: 2/25; financial award applicants required to submit FAFSA. *Unit head:* Dr. Donald B. Thomason, Dean, 901-448-5538, E-mail: dthomaso@uthsc.edu. *Application contact:* William Carter, Director for Admissions, 901-448-1687, E-mail: wcarte17@uthsc.edu.
Website: http://www.uthsc.edu/grad/

The University of Texas at Austin, Graduate School, College of Pharmacy, Graduate Programs in Pharmacy, Austin, TX 78712-1111. Offers health outcomes and pharmacy practice (PhD); health outcomes and pharmacy practice (MS); medicinal chemistry (PhD); pharmaceutics (PhD); pharmacology and toxicology (PhD); pharmacotherapy (MS, PhD); translational science (PhD). PhD in translational science offered jointly with The University of Texas Health Science Center at San Antonio and The University of Texas at San Antonio. *Degree requirements:* For master's, thesis; for doctorate, thesis/dissertation. *Entrance requirements:* For master's and doctorate, GRE General Test. Electronic applications accepted. *Faculty research:* Synthetic medical chemistry, synthetic molecular biology, bio-organic chemistry, pharmacoeconomics, pharmacy practice.

The University of Texas Health Science Center at San Antonio, Graduate School of Biomedical Sciences, Department of Pharmacology, San Antonio, TX 78229-3900. Offers neuroscience (PhD). *Faculty:* 41 full-time (14 women), 10 part-time/adjunct (1 woman). *Students:* 29 full-time (18 women), 4 part-time (2 women); includes 12 minority (1 Black or African American, non-Hispanic/Latino; 1 Asian, non-Hispanic/Latino; 10 Hispanic/Latino), 6 international. Average age 29. In 2013, 4 doctorates awarded. *Degree requirements:* For doctorate, comprehensive exam, thesis/dissertation. *Entrance requirements:* For doctorate, GRE General Test, minimum GPA of 3.0. Additional exam requirements/recommendations for international students: Required—TOEFL (minimum score 560 paper-based; 68 iBT). *Application deadline:* For fall admission, 1/15 priority date for domestic and international students. Applications are processed on a rolling basis. Application fee: $0. Electronic applications accepted. *Financial support:* Application deadline: 6/30; applicants required to submit FAFSA. *Faculty research:* Neuropharmacology, autonomic and endocrine homeostasis, aging, cancer biology. *Total annual research expenditures:* $9.4 million. *Unit head:* Dr. Alan Frazer, Department Chair, 210-567-4205, Fax: 210-567-4300, E-mail: frazer@uthscsa.edu. *Application contact:* Dr. Julie Hensler, Graduate Advisor/Committee on Graduate Studies Chair, 210-567-4236, Fax: 210-567-4300, E-mail: hensler@uthscsa.edu.
Website: http://pharmacology.uthscsa.edu

The University of Texas Medical Branch, Graduate School of Biomedical Sciences, Program in Pharmacology and Toxicology, Galveston, TX 77555. Offers pharmacology (MS); pharmacology and toxicology (PhD). *Degree requirements:* For master's, thesis or alternative; for doctorate, thesis/dissertation. *Entrance requirements:* For master's and doctorate, GRE General Test. Additional exam requirements/recommendations for international students: Required—TOEFL (minimum score 550 paper-based).

University of the Sciences, College of Graduate Studies, Program in Chemistry, Biochemistry and Pharmacognosy, Philadelphia, PA 19104-4495. Offers biochemistry (MS, PhD); chemistry (MS, PhD); pharmacognosy (MS, PhD). Part-time programs available. *Faculty:* 10 full-time (1 woman), 1 part-time/adjunct (0 women). *Students:* 30 full-time (15 women), 15 part-time (10 women); includes 7 minority (4 Black or African American, non-Hispanic/Latino; 3 Asian, non-Hispanic/Latino), 6 international. Average age 28. 52 applicants, 83% accepted, 9 enrolled. In 2013, 4 master's, 2 doctorates awarded. *Degree requirements:* For master's, thesis, qualifying exams; for doctorate, comprehensive exam, thesis/dissertation, qualifying exams. *Entrance requirements:* For master's and doctorate, GRE General Test, GRE Subject Test. Additional exam requirements/recommendations for international students: Required—TOEFL, TWE. *Application deadline:* For fall admission, 5/1 for international students; for winter admission, 10/1 for international students; for spring admission, 3/1 for international students. Applications are processed on a rolling basis. Application fee: $50. *Expenses:* Contact institution. *Financial support:* In 2013–14, 17 students received support, including 1 fellowship with full tuition reimbursement available, 2 research assistantships with full tuition reimbursements available (averaging $13,884 per year), 11 teaching assistantships with full tuition reimbursements available (averaging $18,836 per year); institutionally sponsored loans, scholarships/grants, and tuition waivers (full) also available. Financial award application deadline: 5/1. *Faculty research:* Organic and medicinal synthesis, mass spectroscopy use in protein analysis, study of analogues of taxol, cholesteryl esters. *Unit head:* Dr. Shenaz Tejani-Butt, Associate Dean, Graduate Studies, E-mail: graduate@usciences.edu. *Application contact:* Christopher Miciek, Associate Director, Graduate Admissions, 215-596-8597, E-mail: c.miciek@usciences.edu.

University of the Sciences, College of Graduate Studies, Program in Pharmacology and Toxicology, Philadelphia, PA 19104-4495. Offers pharmacology (MS, PhD); toxicology (MS, PhD). *Faculty:* 5 full-time (0 women). *Students:* 10 full-time (6 women), 11 part-time (7 women); includes 2 minority (1 Asian, non-Hispanic/Latino; 1 Hispanic/Latino), 5 international. Average age 30. 14 applicants, 29% accepted, 3 enrolled. In 2013, 1 master's, 1 doctorate awarded. Terminal master's awarded for partial completion of doctoral program. *Degree requirements:* For master's, thesis; for doctorate, comprehensive exam, thesis/dissertation. *Entrance requirements:* For master's and doctorate, GRE General Test. Additional exam requirements/recommendations for international students: Required—TOEFL, TWE. *Application deadline:* For fall admission, 5/1 for international students; for winter admission, 10/1 for international students; for spring admission, 3/1 for international students. Applications are processed on a rolling basis. Application fee: $50. *Expenses:* Contact institution.

Financial support: In 2013–14, 14 students received support, including 8 teaching assistantships with tuition reimbursements available (averaging $21,694 per year); institutionally sponsored loans and tuition waivers (partial) also available. Financial award application deadline: 5/1. *Faculty research:* Autonomic, cardiovascular, cellular, and molecular pharmacology; mechanisms of carcinogenesis; drug metabolism. *Unit head:* Dr. Shenaz Tejani-Butt, Associate Dean, Graduate Studies, 215-596-8597, E-mail: graduate@usciences.edu. *Application contact:* Christopher Miciek, Associate Director, Graduate Studies, 215-596-8597, E-mail: c.miciek@usciences.edu.

The University of Toledo, College of Graduate Studies, College of Pharmacy and Pharmaceutical Sciences, Program in Experimental Therapeutics, Toledo, OH 43606-3390. Offers PhD. *Entrance requirements:* For doctorate, GRE, bachelors degree in chemistry, biology, pharmaceutical sciences, pharmacy or a related discipline. Additional exam requirements/recommendations for international students: Required—TOEFL.

The University of Toledo, College of Graduate Studies, College of Pharmacy and Pharmaceutical Sciences, Program in Pharmaceutical Sciences, Toledo, OH 43606-3390. Offers administrative pharmacy (MSPS); industrial pharmacy (MSPS); pharmacology toxicology (MSPS). *Degree requirements:* For master's, thesis. *Entrance requirements:* For master's, GRE General Test. Additional exam requirements/recommendations for international students: Required—TOEFL (minimum score 550 paper-based; 80 iBT). Electronic applications accepted.

University of Toronto, Faculty of Medicine, Department of Pharmacology and Toxicology, Toronto, ON M5S 1A1, Canada. Offers pharmacology (M Sc, PhD). Part-time programs available. *Degree requirements:* For master's, thesis; for doctorate, thesis/dissertation. *Entrance requirements:* For master's, B Sc or equivalent; background in pharmacology, biochemistry, and physiology; minimum B+ earned in at least 4 senior level classes; for doctorate, minimum B+ average. Additional exam requirements/recommendations for international students: Required—TOEFL (minimum score 580 paper-based; 93 iBT), TWE (minimum score 5). Electronic applications accepted.

University of Utah, Graduate School, College of Pharmacy, Department of Pharmacology and Toxicology, Salt Lake City, UT 84112. Offers PhD. *Faculty:* 14 full-time (4 women), 6 part-time/adjunct (2 women). *Students:* 9 full-time (6 women), 4 international. Average age 28. 34 applicants. In 2013, 3 doctorates awarded. Terminal master's awarded for partial completion of doctoral program. *Degree requirements:* For doctorate, comprehensive exam, thesis/dissertation, final exam. *Entrance requirements:* For doctorate, GRE General Test, BS in biology, chemistry, neuroscience. Additional exam requirements/recommendations for international students: Required—TOEFL (minimum score 550 paper-based; 80 iBT), IELTS (minimum score 6.5). *Application deadline:* For fall admission, 12/15 for domestic and international students. Application fee: $55 ($65 for international students). Electronic applications accepted. *Expenses:* Tuition, state resident: full-time $5259. Tuition, nonresident: full-time $18,569. *Required fees:* $841. Tuition and fees vary according to course load. *Financial support:* In 2013–14, 13 students received support, including fellowships with full tuition reimbursements available (averaging $25,000 per year), research assistantships with full tuition reimbursements available (averaging $25,000 per year); tuition waivers (full) also available. Financial award application deadline: 1/15. *Faculty research:* Neuropharmacology of anti-seizure drugs and drugs of abuse, drug metabolism, signal transduction pathways and oncogenic processes, drug analyses in biological samples, natural products drug discovery. *Total annual research expenditures:* $5.4 million. *Unit head:* Dr. William R. Crowley, Chairman, 801-581-6287, Fax: 801-585-5111, E-mail: william.crowley@deans.pharm.utah.edu. *Application contact:* Linda Wright, Program Assistant, 801-581-6281, Fax: 801-585-5111, E-mail: linda.wright@utah.edu.
Website: http://www.pharmacy.utah.edu/pharmtox/

University of Vermont, College of Medicine and Graduate College, Graduate Programs in Medicine, Department of Pharmacology, Burlington, VT 05405. Offers MS. *Faculty:* 12 full-time (1 woman). *Students:* 4 (1 woman); includes 1 minority (Hispanic/Latino), 2 international. 5 applicants, 20% accepted. *Degree requirements:* For master's, thesis. *Entrance requirements:* For master's, GRE General Test. Additional exam requirements/recommendations for international students: Required—TOEFL (minimum score 550 paper-based; 80 iBT). *Application deadline:* For fall admission, 1/15 priority date for domestic students, 1/15 for international students. Applications are processed on a rolling basis. Application fee: $65. Electronic applications accepted. *Financial support:* Fellowships, research assistantships, and teaching assistantships available. Financial award application deadline: 3/1. *Faculty research:* Cardiovascular drugs, anticancer drugs. *Unit head:* Dr. M. Nelson, Chairperson, 802-656-2500. *Application contact:* Dr. Anthony Morielli, Director of Graduate Studies, 802-656-2500.

University of Virginia, School of Medicine, Department of Pharmacology, Charlottesville, VA 22903. Offers PhD, MD/PhD. *Faculty:* 26 full-time (7 women), 1 part-time/adjunct (0 women). *Students:* 18 full-time (11 women), 1 international. Average age 26. In 2013, 1 doctorate awarded. *Degree requirements:* For doctorate, thesis/dissertation. *Entrance requirements:* For doctorate, GRE General Test, GRE Subject Test (recommended), 2 letters of recommendation. Additional exam requirements/recommendations for international students: Required—TOEFL. *Application deadline:* For fall admission, 1/15 for domestic and international students. Applications are processed on a rolling basis. Application fee: $60. Electronic applications accepted. *Expenses:* Tuition, state resident: part-time $334 per credit hour. Tuition, nonresident: part-time $1224 per credit hour. *Financial support:* Fellowships, research assistantships, and teaching assistantships available. Financial award applicants required to submit FAFSA. *Unit head:* Dr. Douglas A. Bayliss, Chairman, 434-924-1919, Fax: 434-982-3878, E-mail: dab3y@virginia.edu. *Application contact:* Dr. Paula Barrett, Graduate Advisor, 434-924-5454, E-mail: pqb4b@virginia.edu.
Website: http://www.healthsystem.virginia.edu/internet/pharmacology/

University of Washington, Graduate School, School of Medicine, Graduate Programs in Medicine, Department of Pharmacology, Seattle, WA 98195. Offers PhD. *Degree requirements:* For doctorate, thesis/dissertation. *Entrance requirements:* For doctorate, GRE General Test, minimum GPA of 3.0. *Faculty research:* Neuroscience, cell physiology, molecular biology, regulation of metabolism, signal transduction.

University of Wisconsin–Madison, School of Medicine and Public Health and Graduate School, Graduate Programs in Medicine, Molecular and Cellular Pharmacology Program, Madison, WI 53706. Offers PhD. *Faculty:* 67 full-time (19 women). *Students:* 36 full-time (17 women); includes 9 minority (2 Black or African American, non-Hispanic/Latino; 5 Asian, non-Hispanic/Latino; 1 Hispanic/Latino; 1 Native Hawaiian or other Pacific Islander, non-Hispanic/Latino), 7 international. Average age 26. 87 applicants, 17% accepted, 3 enrolled. In 2013, 4 doctorates awarded. *Degree requirements:* For doctorate, comprehensive exam, thesis/dissertation. *Entrance requirements:* For doctorate, GRE. Additional exam requirements/recommendations for international students: Required—TOEFL (minimum score 550 paper-based; 80 iBT). *Application deadline:* For fall admission, 12/1 priority date for domestic and international students. Applications are processed on a rolling basis. Application fee: $56. Electronic applications accepted. *Expenses:* Tuition, state resident: full-time $10,728; part-time $790 per credit. Tuition, nonresident: full-time $24,054; part-time $1623 per credit. *Required fees:* $1130; $119 per credit. *Financial support:* In 2013–14, 36 students received support, including 5 fellowships with full tuition reimbursements available (averaging $25,000 per year), 31 research assistantships with full tuition reimbursements available (averaging $25,000 per year), teaching assistantships with full tuition reimbursements available (averaging $24,500 per year); scholarships/grants, traineeships, health care benefits, and unspecified assistantships also available. *Faculty research:* Protein kinases, signaling pathways, neurotransmitters, molecular recognition, receptors and transporters. *Unit head:* Dr. Anjon Audhya, Director, 608-262-3761, E-mail: audhya@wisc.edu. *Application contact:* Lynn Louise Squire, Student Services Coordinator, 608-262-9826, E-mail: lsquire@wisc.edu.
Website: http://molpharm.wisc.edu/

Vanderbilt University, Graduate School and School of Medicine, Department of Pharmacology, Nashville, TN 37240-1001. Offers PhD, MD/PhD. *Faculty:* 26 full-time (7 women). *Students:* 53 full-time (24 women); includes 12 minority (4 Black or African American, non-Hispanic/Latino; 4 Asian, non-Hispanic/Latino; 2 Hispanic/Latino; 2 Two or more races, non-Hispanic/Latino), 7 international. Average age 27. In 2013, 8 doctorates awarded. *Degree requirements:* For doctorate, comprehensive exam, thesis/dissertation, preliminary, qualifying, and final exams. *Entrance requirements:* For doctorate, GRE General Test, GRE Subject Test (recommended). Additional exam requirements/recommendations for international students: Required—TOEFL (minimum score 570 paper-based; 88 iBT). *Application deadline:* For fall admission, 1/15 for domestic and international students. Application fee: $0. Electronic applications accepted. *Financial support:* Fellowships with full tuition reimbursements, research assistantships with full tuition reimbursements, Federal Work-Study, institutionally sponsored loans, scholarships/grants, traineeships, health care benefits, and tuition waivers (partial) available. Financial award application deadline: 1/15; financial award applicants required to submit CSS PROFILE or FAFSA. *Faculty research:* Molecular pharmacology, neuropharmacology, drug disposition and toxicology, genetic mechanics, cell regulation. *Unit head:* Dr. Karen Gieg, Educational Programs Coordinator, 615-322-1182, Fax: 615-936-3910, E-mail: karen.gieg@vanderbilt.edu.
Website: http://medschool.vanderbilt.edu/pharmacology/

Virginia Commonwealth University, Medical College of Virginia-Professional Programs, School of Medicine, School of Medicine Graduate Programs, Department of Pharmacology and Toxicology, Richmond, VA 23284-9005. Offers neuroscience (PhD); pharmacology (Certificate); pharmacology and toxicology (MS, PhD); MD/PhD. Terminal master's awarded for partial completion of doctoral program. *Degree requirements:* For master's, thesis; for doctorate, thesis/dissertation, comprehensive oral and written exams. *Entrance requirements:* For master's and doctorate, GRE or MCAT. Additional exam requirements/recommendations for international students: Required—TOEFL (minimum score 600 paper-based; 100 iBT). Electronic applications accepted. *Faculty research:* Drug abuse, drug metabolism, pharmacodynamics, peptide synthesis, receptor mechanisms.

Virginia Commonwealth University, Program in Pre-Medical Basic Health Sciences, Richmond, VA 23284-9005. Offers anatomy (CBHS); biochemistry (CBHS); human genetics (CBHS); microbiology (CBHS); pharmacology (CBHS); physiology (CBHS). *Entrance requirements:* For degree, GRE, MCAT or DAT, course work in organic chemistry, minimum undergraduate GPA of 2.8. Additional exam requirements/recommendations for international students: Required—TOEFL (minimum score 600 paper-based). Electronic applications accepted.

Wake Forest University, School of Medicine and Graduate School of Arts and Sciences, Graduate Programs in Medicine, Program in Physiology and Pharmacology, Winston-Salem, NC 27109. Offers pharmacology (PhD); physiology (PhD); MD/PhD. *Degree requirements:* For doctorate, thesis/dissertation. *Entrance requirements:* For doctorate, GRE General Test. Additional exam requirements/recommendations for international students: Required—TOEFL. Electronic applications accepted. *Faculty research:* Aging, substance abuse, cardiovascular control, endocrine systems, toxicology.

Wayne State University, Eugene Applebaum College of Pharmacy and Health Sciences, Department of Pharmaceutical Sciences, Detroit, MI 48202. Offers medicinal chemistry (MS, PhD); pharmaceutics (MS, PhD); pharmacology/toxicology (MS, PhD). *Accreditation:* ACPE (one or more programs are accredited). Part-time programs available. *Faculty:* 17 full-time (3 women). *Students:* 33 full-time (15 women), 2 part-time (1 woman); includes 3 minority (1 American Indian or Alaska Native, non-Hispanic/Latino; 2 Asian, non-Hispanic/Latino), 29 international. Average age 25. 205 applicants, 8% accepted, 9 enrolled. In 2013, 1 master's, 3 doctorates awarded. *Degree requirements:* For master's, thesis; for doctorate, thesis/dissertation. *Entrance requirements:* For master's, GRE General Test, admission to the Graduate School, bachelor's degree, three letters of recommendation, personal statement; for doctorate, GRE General Test, admission to the Graduate School; bachelor's or master's degree in one of the behavioral, biological, pharmaceutical or physical sciences; minimum undergraduate GPA of 3.0; three letters of recommendation. Additional exam requirements/recommendations for international students: Required—TOEFL (minimum score 550 paper-based; 79 iBT), Michigan English Language Assessment Battery (minimum score 85); Recommended—IELTS (minimum score 6.5), TWE (minimum score 5.5). *Application deadline:* For fall admission, 3/1 for domestic and international students. Application fee: $0. Electronic applications accepted. *Expenses:* Contact institution. *Financial support:* In 2013–14, 13 students received support, including 2 fellowships with tuition reimbursements available (averaging $24,272 per year), 11 research assistantships with full tuition reimbursements available (averaging $24,565 per year); scholarships/grants, health care benefits, and unspecified assistantships also available. Financial award application deadline: 3/31; financial award applicants required to submit FAFSA. *Faculty research:* Mechanisms of resistance of bacteria to anti-microbial agents, drug metabolism and disposition in children, treatment strategies for stroke/neurovascular disease, prevalence and treatment of diabetes in Arab-Americans, ethnic variability in development of osteoporosis. *Unit head:* Dr. George Corcoran, Chair and Professor, 313-577-1737, E-mail: corcoran@wayne.edu. *Application contact:* 313-577-1047, E-mail: pscgrad@wayne.edu.
Website: http://www.cphs.wayne.edu/psc/index.php

Wayne State University, School of Medicine, Graduate Programs in Medicine, Department of Pharmacology, Detroit, MI 48202. Offers molecular and environmental toxicology (PhD); pharmacology (MS); MD/PhD. *Students:* 8 full-time (6 women); includes 2 minority (both Hispanic/Latino), 2 international. Average age 26. 58 applicants, 3% accepted, 2 enrolled. In 2013, 1 doctorate awarded. Terminal master's awarded for partial completion of doctoral program. *Degree requirements:* For master's, thesis; for doctorate, thesis/dissertation. *Entrance requirements:* For doctorate, GRE General Test, minimum undergraduate GPA of 3.0 for upper-division course work, personal statement, three letters of recommendation, background in chemical or biological sciences, admission to Graduate School. Additional exam requirements/recommendations for international students: Required—TOEFL (minimum score 600 paper-based; 100 iBT), TWE (minimum score 6). *Application deadline:* For fall admission, 4/15 for domestic and international students. Application fee: $0. Electronic applications accepted. *Expenses:* Contact institution. *Financial support:* In 2013–14, 5

students received support, including 1 fellowship with tuition reimbursement available (averaging $21,716 per year), 8 research assistantships with tuition reimbursements available (averaging $22,341 per year); teaching assistantships, scholarships/grants, health care benefits, and unspecified assistantships also available. *Faculty research:* Molecular and cellular biology of cancer and anti-cancer therapies; molecular and cellular biology of protein trafficking, signal transduction and aging; environmental toxicology and drug metabolism; functional cellular and in vivo imaging; neuroscience. *Unit head:* Dr. Roy McCauley, Graduate Program Director, 313-577-6737, E-mail: rmccaul@med.wayne.edu. *Application contact:* Dr. Hai-Young Wu, Chairman, Graduate Admissions Committee, 313-577-1584, Fax: 313-577-6739, E-mail: haiwu@med.wayne.edu.
Website: http://www.med.wayne.edu/pharmacology/index.asp

Weill Cornell Medical College, Weill Cornell Graduate School of Medical Sciences, Pharmacology Program, New York, NY 10065. Offers MS, PhD. Terminal master's awarded for partial completion of doctoral program. *Degree requirements:* For master's, comprehensive exam; for doctorate, thesis/dissertation, final exam. *Entrance requirements:* For doctorate, GRE General Test, previous course work in natural and/or health sciences. Additional exam requirements/recommendations for international students: Required—TOEFL. *Faculty research:* Modulation of gene expression by drugs, signal transduction, nitric oxide signaling RNA trafficking, neuropharmacology of opiates.

West Virginia University, School of Medicine, Graduate Programs at the Health Sciences Center, Interdisciplinary Graduate Programs in Biomedical Sciences, Program in Pharmaceutical and Pharmacological Sciences, Morgantown, WV 26506. Offers MS, PhD, MD/PhD. *Degree requirements:* For doctorate, comprehensive exam, thesis/dissertation. *Entrance requirements:* For doctorate, GRE General Test, minimum GPA of 3.0. Additional exam requirements/recommendations for international students: Required—TOEFL. Electronic applications accepted. *Faculty research:* Medicinal chemistry, pharmacokinetics, nano-pharmaceutics, polymer-based drug delivery, molecular therapeutics.

Wright State University, School of Medicine, Program in Pharmacology and Toxicology, Dayton, OH 45435. Offers MS. *Degree requirements:* For master's, thesis optional.

Yale University, School of Medicine and Graduate School of Arts and Sciences, Combined Program in Biological and Biomedical Sciences (BBS), Department of Pharmacology, New Haven, CT 06520. Offers PhD. *Degree requirements:* For doctorate, thesis/dissertation. *Entrance requirements:* For doctorate, GRE General Test. Additional exam requirements/recommendations for international students: Required—TOEFL. *Expenses:* Contact institution.

Yale University, School of Medicine and Graduate School of Arts and Sciences, Combined Program in Biological and Biomedical Sciences (BBS), Pharmacological Sciences and Molecular Medicine Track, New Haven, CT 06520. Offers PhD, MD/PhD. *Degree requirements:* For doctorate, thesis/dissertation. *Entrance requirements:* For doctorate, GRE General Test. Additional exam requirements/recommendations for international students: Required—TOEFL. Electronic applications accepted.

Toxicology

American University of Beirut, Graduate Programs, Faculty of Medicine, Beirut, Lebanon. Offers anatomy, cell biology and human morphology (MS); biochemistry and medical genetics (MS); biomedical sciences (PhD); experimental pathology, immunology and microbiology (MS); medicine (MD); neuroscience (MS); pharmacology and toxicology (MS). Part-time programs available. *Faculty:* 259 full-time (78 women), 93 part-time/adjunct (16 women). *Students:* 364 full-time (165 women), 62 part-time (54 women). Average age 23. In 2013, 18 master's awarded. *Degree requirements:* For master's, one foreign language, comprehensive exam, thesis (for some programs); for doctorate, one foreign language, comprehensive exam, thesis/dissertation. *Entrance requirements:* For master's, letter of recommendation; for doctorate, MCAT, bachelor's degree. Additional exam requirements/recommendations for international students: Required—TOEFL (minimum score 600 paper-based; 100 iBT), IELTS (minimum score 7.5). *Application deadline:* For fall admission, 4/30 for domestic and international students; for spring admission, 11/1 for domestic and international students. Application fee: $50. *Expenses: Tuition:* Full-time $14,724; part-time $818 per credit. *Required fees:* $692. Tuition and fees vary according to course load and program. *Financial support:* In 2013–14, 242 students received support, including 60 teaching assistantships (averaging $4,000 per year); career-related internships or fieldwork, institutionally sponsored loans, scholarships/grants, health care benefits, and unspecified assistantships also available. Financial award application deadline: 2/2. *Faculty research:* Cancer research (targeted therapy, mechanisms of leukemogenesis, tumor cell extravasation and metastasis, cancer stem cells), stem cell research (regenerative medicine, drug discovery), genetic research (neurogenetics, hereditary cardiomyopathy, hemoglobinopathies, pharmacogenomics, proteomics), neuroscience research (pain, neurodegenerative disorder), metabolism (inflammation and metabolism, metabolic disorder, diabetes mellitus), vascular and renal biology, signal transduction. *Total annual research expenditures:* $2.6 million. *Unit head:* Dr. Mohamed Sayegh, Dean, 961-1350000 Ext. 4700, Fax: 961-1744464, E-mail: msayegh@aub.edu.lb. *Application contact:* Dr. Salim Kanaan, Director, Admissions Office, 961-1-350000 Ext. 2594, Fax: 96-1-1750775, E-mail: sk00@aub.edu.lb.
Website: http://www.aub.edu.lb/fm/fm_home/Pages/index.aspx

Columbia University, College of Physicians and Surgeons, Department of Pharmacology, New York, NY 10032. Offers pharmacology (M Phil, MA, PhD); pharmacology-toxicology (M Phil, MA, PhD); MD/PhD. Only candidates for the PhD are admitted. Terminal master's awarded for partial completion of doctoral program. *Degree requirements:* For doctorate, thesis/dissertation. *Entrance requirements:* For master's and doctorate, GRE General Test. Additional exam requirements/recommendations for international students: Required—TOEFL. *Faculty research:* Cardiovascular pharmacology, receptor pharmacology, neuropharmacology, membrane biophysics, eicosanoids.

Cornell University, Graduate School, Graduate Fields of Agriculture and Life Sciences, Field of Environmental Toxicology, Ithaca, NY 14853-0001. Offers cellular and molecular toxicology (MS, PhD); ecotoxicology and environmental chemistry (MS, PhD); nutritional and food toxicology (MS, PhD); risk assessment, management and public policy (MS, PhD). *Faculty:* 37 full-time (11 women). *Students:* 6 full-time (1 woman), 2 international. Average age 27. 13 applicants, 8% accepted, 1 enrolled. In 2013, 2 doctorates awarded. *Degree requirements:* For master's, thesis; for doctorate, comprehensive exam, thesis/dissertation. *Entrance requirements:* For master's and doctorate, GRE General Test, GRE Subject Test (biology or chemistry recommended), 2 letters of recommendation. Additional exam requirements/recommendations for international students: Required—TOEFL (minimum score 600 paper-based; 77 iBT). *Application deadline:* For fall admission, 1/15 for domestic students. Application fee: $95. Electronic applications accepted. *Financial support:* In 2013–14, 4 students received support, including 1 fellowship with full tuition reimbursement available, 2 research assistantships with full tuition reimbursements available, 1 teaching assistantship with full tuition reimbursement available; institutionally sponsored loans, scholarships/grants, health care benefits, tuition waivers (full and partial), and unspecified assistantships also available. Financial award applicants required to submit FAFSA. *Faculty research:* Cellular and molecular toxicology, cancer toxicology, bioremediation, ecotoxicology, nutritional and food toxicology, reproductive toxicology. *Unit head:* Director of Graduate Studies, 607-255-8008, Fax: 607-755-0238. *Application contact:* Graduate Field Assistant, 607-255-8008, Fax: 607-255-0238, E-mail: envtox@cornell.edu.
Website: http://www.gradschool.cornell.edu/fields.php?id-48&a-2

Dartmouth College, Arts and Sciences Graduate Programs, Department of Pharmacology and Toxicology, Hanover, NH 03755. Offers PhD, MD/PhD. *Degree requirements:* For doctorate, thesis/dissertation. *Entrance requirements:* For doctorate, GRE General Test, GRE Subject Test, bachelor's degree in biological, chemical, or physical science. Additional exam requirements/recommendations for international students: Required—TOEFL. Electronic applications accepted. *Faculty research:* Molecular biology of carcinogenesis, DNA repair and gene expression, biochemical and environmental toxicology, protein receptor ligand interactions.

Dartmouth College, Program in Experimental and Molecular Medicine, Molecular Pharmacology, Toxicology and Experimental Therapeutics Track, Hanover, NH 03755. Offers PhD.

Duke University, Graduate School, Integrated Toxicology and Environmental Health Program, Durham, NC 27708. Offers Certificate. *Faculty:* 33. *Students:* 5 full-time (3 women); includes 1 minority (Black or African American, non-Hispanic/Latino), 1 international. 23 applicants, 13% accepted, 2 enrolled. *Entrance requirements:* Additional exam requirements/recommendations for international students: Required—TOEFL (minimum score 577 paper-based; 90 iBT) or IELTS (minimum score 7). *Application deadline:* For fall admission, 12/8 priority date for domestic and international students. Application fee: $80. Electronic applications accepted. *Financial support:* Fellowships available. Financial award application deadline: 12/8. *Unit head:* Cynthia Kuhn, Director, 919-613-8078, Fax: 919-668-1799, E-mail: emarion@duke.edu. *Application contact:* Elizabeth Hutton, Director of Admissions, 919-684-3913, Fax: 919-684-2277, E-mail: grad-admissions@duke.edu.
Website: http://sites.nicholas.duke.edu/envhealth/

Florida Agricultural and Mechanical University, Division of Graduate Studies, Research, and Continuing Education, College of Pharmacy and Pharmaceutical Sciences, Graduate Programs in Pharmaceutical Sciences, Tallahassee, FL 32307-3200. Offers environmental toxicology (PhD); medicinal chemistry (MS, PhD); pharmaceutics (MS, PhD); pharmacology/toxicology (MS, PhD); pharmacy administration (MS). *Accreditation:* CEPH. *Degree requirements:* For master's, comprehensive exam, thesis, publishable paper; for doctorate, comprehensive exam, thesis/dissertation, publishable paper. *Entrance requirements:* For master's and doctorate, GRE General Test, minimum GPA of 3.0 in last 60 hours. Additional exam requirements/recommendations for international students: Required—TOEFL. *Faculty research:* Anticancer agents, anti-inflammatory drugs, chronopharmacology, neuroendocrinology, microbiology.

The George Washington University, Columbian College of Arts and Sciences, Department of Forensic Sciences, Washington, DC 20052. Offers crime scene investigation (MFS); forensic chemistry (MFS); forensic molecular biology (MFS); forensic toxicology (MFS); high-technology crime investigation (MFS); security management (MFS). High-technology crime investigation and security management programs offered in Arlington, VA. Part-time and evening/weekend programs available. *Faculty:* 8 full-time (1 woman). *Students:* 69 full-time (61 women), 50 part-time (34 women); includes 35 minority (15 Black or African American, non-Hispanic/Latino; 2 American Indian or Alaska Native, non-Hispanic/Latino; 6 Asian, non-Hispanic/Latino; 10 Hispanic/Latino; 2 Two or more races, non-Hispanic/Latino), 11 international. Average age 26. 148 applicants, 76% accepted, 59 enrolled. In 2013, 56 master's awarded. *Degree requirements:* For master's, comprehensive exam. *Entrance requirements:* For master's, GRE General Test, minimum GPA of 3.0. Additional exam requirements/recommendations for international students: Required—TOEFL (minimum score 550 paper-based; 80 iBT). *Application deadline:* For fall admission, 1/16 priority date for international students; for spring admission, 10/1 priority date for domestic students, 9/1 priority date for international students. Applications are processed on a rolling basis. Application fee: $75. Electronic applications accepted. *Financial support:* In 2013–14, 19 students received support. Fellowships with partial tuition reimbursements available, Federal Work-Study, and tuition waivers available. *Unit head:* Dr. Victor Weedn, Chair, 202-994-6977, E-mail: vweedn@gwu.edu. *Application contact:* 202-994-6210, Fax: 202-994-6213, E-mail: askccas@gwu.edu.
Website: http://www.gwu.edu/~forensic/

Indiana University Bloomington, School of Public and Environmental Affairs, Environmental Science Programs, Bloomington, IN 47405. Offers applied ecology (MSES); energy (MSES); environmental chemistry, toxicology, and risk assessment (MSES); environmental science (PhD); hazardous materials management (Certificate); specialized environmental science (MSES); water resources (MSES); JD/MSES; MSES/MA; MSES/MPA; MSES/MS. Part-time programs available. *Faculty:* 16 full-time (4 women), 8 part-time/adjunct (3 women). *Students:* 135 full-time (69 women), 11 part-time (7 women); includes 15 minority (1 Black or African American, non-Hispanic/Latino; 8 Asian, non-Hispanic/Latino; 6 Hispanic/Latino), 13 international. Average age 25. 171 applicants, 81% accepted, 64 enrolled. In 2013, 71 master's, 3 doctorates awarded. Terminal master's awarded for partial completion of doctoral program. *Degree requirements:* For master's, capstone or thesis; internship; for doctorate, comprehensive exam, thesis/dissertation. *Entrance requirements:* For master's, GRE General Test or GMAT, official transcripts, 3 letters of recommendation, resume, personal statement; for doctorate, GRE General Test or LSAT, official transcripts, 3 letters of recommendation, resume or curriculum vitae, statement of purpose. Additional exam requirements/

recommendations for international students: Required—TOEFL (minimum score 600 paper-based; 96 iBT); Recommended—IELTS (minimum score 7). *Application deadline:* For fall admission, 2/1 priority date for domestic students, 12/1 for international students; for spring admission, 11/15 for domestic students, 9/1 for international students. Applications are processed on a rolling basis. Application fee: $55 ($65 for international students). Electronic applications accepted. *Financial support:* Fellowships with partial tuition reimbursements, research assistantships with partial tuition reimbursements, teaching assistantships with partial tuition reimbursements, career-related internships or fieldwork, Federal Work-Study, scholarships/grants, health care benefits, unspecified assistantships, and Service Corps Program; Educational Opportunity Fellowships available. Financial award application deadline: 2/1; financial award applicants required to submit FAFSA. *Faculty research:* Applied ecology, bio-geochemistry, toxicology, wetlands ecology, environmental microbiology, forest ecology, environmental chemistry. *Unit head:* Megan Siehl, Assistant Director, Admissions and Financial Aid, 812-855-9485, Fax: 812-856-3665, E-mail: speampo@indiana.edu. *Application contact:* Lane Bowman, Admissions Services Coordinator, 812-855-2840, Fax: 812-856-3665, E-mail: speapps@indiana.edu.
Website: http://www.indiana.edu/~spea/prospective_students/masters/

Indiana University–Purdue University Indianapolis, Indiana University School of Medicine, Department of Pharmacology and Toxicology, Indianapolis, IN 46202-2896. Offers pharmacology (MS, PhD); toxicology (MS, PhD); MD/PhD. *Faculty:* 11 full-time (2 women). *Students:* 28 full-time (22 women); includes 5 minority (2 Black or African American, non-Hispanic/Latino; 2 Asian, non-Hispanic/Latino; 1 Hispanic/Latino), 9 international. Average age 27. 1 applicant, 100% accepted, 1 enrolled. In 2013, 1 doctorate awarded. Terminal master's awarded for partial completion of doctoral program. *Degree requirements:* For master's, thesis; for doctorate, thesis/dissertation. *Entrance requirements:* For master's and doctorate, GRE General Test, GRE Subject Test, minimum GPA of 3.0. *Application deadline:* For fall admission, 1/15 priority date for domestic students. Applications are processed on a rolling basis. Application fee: $55 ($65 for international students). *Financial support:* In 2013–14, teaching assistantships (averaging $20,940 per year) were awarded; fellowships with partial tuition reimbursements, research assistantships with partial tuition reimbursements, Federal Work-Study, institutionally sponsored loans, and tuition waivers (partial) also available. Financial award application deadline: 1/15. *Faculty research:* Neuropharmacology, cardiovascular biopharmacology, chemotherapy, oncogenesis. *Unit head:* Dr. Theodore R. Cummins, Interim Chairman, 317-274-9342. *Application contact:* Director of Graduate Studies, 317-274-1564, Fax: 317-274-7714, E-mail: inmedadm@iupui.edu.
Website: http://pharmtox.iusm.iu.edu/

Iowa State University of Science and Technology, Program in Toxicology, Ames, IA 50011. Offers MS, PhD. *Entrance requirements:* For master's and doctorate, GRE General Test. Additional exam requirements/recommendations for international students: Required—TOEFL (minimum score 550 paper-based; 79 iBT), IELTS (minimum score 6.5). Electronic applications accepted.

Johns Hopkins University, Bloomberg School of Public Health, Department of Environmental Health Sciences, Baltimore, MD 21218-2699. Offers environmental health engineering (PhD); environmental health sciences (MHS, Dr PH); occupational and environmental health (PhD); occupational and environmental hygiene (MHS, MHS); physiology (PhD); toxicology (PhD). Postbaccalaureate distance learning degree programs offered (minimal on-campus study). *Faculty:* 71 full-time (27 women), 58 part-time/adjunct (26 women). *Students:* 67 full-time (42 women), 22 part-time (17 women); includes 30 minority (8 Black or African American, non-Hispanic/Latino; 14 Asian, non-Hispanic/Latino; 5 Hispanic/Latino; 3 Two or more races, non-Hispanic/Latino), 13 international. Average age 29. 112 applicants, 54% accepted, 40 enrolled. In 2013, 23 master's, 11 doctorates awarded. *Degree requirements:* For master's, essay, presentation; for doctorate, comprehensive exam, thesis/dissertation, 1-year full-time residency, oral and written exams. *Entrance requirements:* For master's, GRE General Test or MCAT, 3 letters of recommendation, transcripts; for doctorate, GRE General Test or MCAT, 3 letters of recommendation. Additional exam requirements/recommendations for international students: Required—TOEFL (minimum score 600 paper-based). *Application deadline:* For fall admission, 12/15 priority date for domestic and international students. Applications are processed on a rolling basis. Application fee: $45. Electronic applications accepted. *Financial support:* Fellowships with full tuition reimbursements, Federal Work-Study, institutionally sponsored loans, scholarships/grants, traineeships, health care benefits, and stipends available. Support available to part-time students. Financial award application deadline: 3/15; financial award applicants required to submit FAFSA. *Faculty research:* Chemical carcinogenesis/toxicology, lung disease, occupational and environmental health, nuclear imaging, molecular epidemiology. *Total annual research expenditures:* $23.7 million. *Unit head:* Dr. John Davis Groopman, Chair, 410-955-3720, Fax: 410-955-0617, E-mail: jgroopma@jhsph.edu. *Application contact:* Nina J. Kulacki, Academic Program Manager, 410-955-2212, Fax: 410-955-0617, E-mail: nkulacki@jhsph.edu.
Website: http://www.jhsph.edu/Dept/EHS/

Long Island University–LIU Brooklyn, Arnold and Marie Schwartz College of Pharmacy and Health Sciences, Graduate Programs in Pharmacy, Division of Pharmaceutical Sciences, Brooklyn, NY 11201-8423. Offers cosmetic science (MS); industrial pharmacy (MS); pharmaceutics (PhD); pharmacology/toxicology (MS). Part-time and evening/weekend programs available. Terminal master's awarded for partial completion of doctoral program. *Degree requirements:* For master's, thesis optional; for doctorate, thesis/dissertation, candidacy exam. *Entrance requirements:* For master's and doctorate, minimum GPA of 3.0.

Louisiana State University and Agricultural & Mechanical College, Graduate School, School of the Coast and Environment, Department of Environmental Sciences, Baton Rouge, LA 70803. Offers environmental planning and management (MS); environmental science (PhD); environmental toxicology (MS). *Faculty:* 8 full-time (3 women), 1 part-time/adjunct (0 women). *Students:* 29 full-time (19 women), 13 part-time (7 women); includes 4 minority (2 Black or African American, non-Hispanic/Latino; 2 Hispanic/Latino), 5 international. Average age 28. 21 applicants, 57% accepted, 8 enrolled. In 2013, 18 master's awarded. *Degree requirements:* For master's, thesis (for some programs). *Entrance requirements:* For master's, GRE General Test, minimum GPA of 3.0. Additional exam requirements/recommendations for international students: Required—TOEFL (minimum score 550 paper-based; 79 IBT), IELTS (minimum score 6.5), or PTE (minimum score 59). *Application deadline:* For fall admission, 1/25 priority date for domestic students, 5/15 for international students; for spring admission, 10/15 for international students. Applications are processed on a rolling basis. Application fee: $50 ($70 for international students). Electronic applications accepted. *Financial support:* In 2013–14, 33 students received support, including 15 research assistantships with full and partial tuition reimbursements available (averaging $17,440 per year), 11 teaching assistantships with full and partial tuition reimbursements available (averaging $13,500 per year); fellowships with full and partial tuition reimbursements available, career-related internships or fieldwork, Federal Work-Study, institutionally sponsored loans, scholarships/grants, health care benefits, and unspecified assistantships also available. Support available to part-time students. Financial award applicants required to submit FAFSA. *Faculty research:* Environmental toxicology, environmental policy and law, microbial ecology, bioremediation, genetic toxicology. *Total annual research expenditures:* $1.9 million. *Unit head:* Dr. Lawrence Rouse, Chair, 225-578-8521, Fax: 225-578-4286, E-mail: lrouse@lsu.edu. *Application contact:* Dr. Aixin Hou, Graduate Coordinator, 225-578-4294, Fax: 225-578-4286, E-mail: ahou@lsu.edu.
Website: http://www.environmental.lsu.edu/

Massachusetts Institute of Technology, School of Engineering, Department of Biological Engineering, Cambridge, MA 02139-4307. Offers applied biosciences (PhD, Sc D); bioengineering (PhD, Sc D); biological engineering (PhD, Sc D); biomedical engineering (M Eng); toxicology (SM); SM/MBA. *Faculty:* 33 full-time (6 women). *Students:* 128 full-time (52 women); includes 42 minority (3 Black or African American, non-Hispanic/Latino; 27 Asian, non-Hispanic/Latino; 8 Hispanic/Latino; 4 Two or more races, non-Hispanic/Latino), 37 international. Average age 26. 401 applicants, 9% accepted, 23 enrolled. In 2013, 4 master's, 21 doctorates awarded. Terminal master's awarded for partial completion of doctoral program. *Degree requirements:* For master's, thesis; for doctorate, comprehensive exam, thesis/dissertation. *Entrance requirements:* For master's and doctorate, GRE General Test. Additional exam requirements/recommendations for international students: Required—IELTS (minimum score 7). *Application deadline:* For fall admission, 12/15 for domestic and international students. Application fee: $75. Electronic applications accepted. *Expenses: Tuition:* Full-time $43,210; part-time $670 per credit hour. *Required fees:* $288. *Financial support:* In 2013–14, 123 students received support, including 55 fellowships (averaging $37,500 per year), 67 research assistantships (averaging $36,000 per year); teaching assistantships, Federal Work-Study, institutionally sponsored loans, scholarships/grants, traineeships, health care benefits, and unspecified assistantships also available. *Faculty research:* Biomaterials; biophysics; cell and tissue engineering; computational modeling of biological and physiological systems; discovery and delivery of molecular therapeutics; new tools for genomics; functional genomics; proteomics and glycomics; macromolecular biochemistry and biophysics; molecular, cell and tissue biomechanics; synthetic biology; systems biology. *Total annual research expenditures:* $47.5 million. *Unit head:* Prof. Douglas A. Lauffenburger, Head, 617-253-1712, E-mail: be-acad@mit.edu. *Application contact:* Graduate Admissions, 617-253-1712, Fax: 617-258-8676, E-mail: be-acad@mit.edu.
Website: http://web.mit.edu/be/

Medical College of Wisconsin, Graduate School of Biomedical Sciences, Department of Pharmacology and Toxicology, Milwaukee, WI 53226-0509. Offers PhD, MD/PhD. *Degree requirements:* For doctorate, comprehensive exam, thesis/dissertation, oral and written qualifying exams. *Entrance requirements:* For doctorate, GRE, official transcripts, three letters of recommendation. Additional exam requirements/recommendations for international students: Required—TOEFL. Electronic applications accepted. *Faculty research:* Cardiovascular physiology and pharmacology, drugs of abuse, environmental and aquatic toxicology, central nervous system and biochemical pharmacology, signal transduction.

Medical University of South Carolina, College of Graduate Studies, Department of Pharmaceutical and Biomedical Sciences, Charleston, SC 29425. Offers cell injury and repair (PhD); drug discovery (PhD); medicinal chemistry (PhD); toxicology (PhD); DMD/PhD; MD/PhD; Pharm D/PhD. *Degree requirements:* For doctorate, thesis/dissertation, oral and written exams, teaching and research seminar. *Entrance requirements:* For doctorate, GRE General Test, interview, minimum GPA of 3.0. Additional exam requirements/recommendations for international students: Required—TOEFL (minimum score 600 paper-based; 100 iBT). Electronic applications accepted. *Faculty research:* Drug discovery, toxicology, metabolomics, cell stress and injury.

Michigan State University, College of Human Medicine and The Graduate School, Graduate Programs in Human Medicine, East Lansing, MI 48824. Offers biochemistry and molecular biology (MS, PhD); epidemiology (MS, PhD); microbiology (MS); microbiology and molecular genetics (PhD); pharmacology and toxicology (MS, PhD); physiology (MS, PhD); public health (MPH). *Entrance requirements:* Additional exam requirements/recommendations for international students: Required—TOEFL.

Michigan State University, College of Osteopathic Medicine and The Graduate School, Graduate Studies in Osteopathic Medicine and Graduate Programs in Human Medicine and Graduate Programs in Veterinary Medicine, Department of Pharmacology and Toxicology, East Lansing, MI 48824. Offers integrative pharmacology (MS); pharmacology and toxicology (MS, PhD); pharmacology and toxicology-environmental toxicology (PhD). *Entrance requirements:* Additional exam requirements/recommendations for international students: Required—TOEFL (minimum score 600 paper-based). Electronic applications accepted.

Michigan State University, College of Veterinary Medicine and The Graduate School, Graduate Programs in Veterinary Medicine, Center for Integrative Toxicology, East Lansing, MI 48824. Offers animal science–environmental toxicology (PhD); biochemistry and molecular biology–environmental toxicology (PhD); chemistry–environmental toxicology (PhD); crop and soil sciences–environmental toxicology (PhD); environmental engineering–environmental toxicology (PhD); environmental geosciences–environmental toxicology (PhD); fisheries and wildlife–environmental toxicology (PhD); food science–environmental toxicology (PhD); forestry–environmental toxicology (PhD); genetics–environmental toxicology (PhD); human nutrition–environmental toxicology (PhD); microbiology–environmental toxicology (PhD); pharmacology and toxicology–environmental toxicology (PhD); zoology–environmental toxicology (PhD). *Entrance requirements:* Additional exam requirements/recommendations for international students: Required—TOEFL (minimum score 550 paper-based), Michigan State University ELT (minimum score 85), Michigan English Language Assessment Battery (minimum score 83). Electronic applications accepted. *Faculty research:* Environmental risk assessment, toxicogenomics, phytoremediation, storage and disposal of hazardous waste, environmental regulation.

Michigan State University, College of Veterinary Medicine and The Graduate School, Graduate Programs in Veterinary Medicine and College of Natural Science and Graduate Programs in Human Medicine, Department of Microbiology and Molecular Genetics, East Lansing, MI 48824. Offers industrial microbiology (MS, PhD); microbiology (MS, PhD); microbiology and molecular genetics (MS, PhD); microbiology–environmental toxicology (PhD). *Entrance requirements:* For master's, GRE General Test. Additional exam requirements/recommendations for international students: Required—TOEFL (minimum score 550 paper-based), Michigan State University ELT (minimum score 85), Michigan English Language Assessment Battery (minimum score 83). Electronic applications accepted.

Michigan State University, The Graduate School, College of Agriculture and Natural Resources, Department of Animal Science, East Lansing, MI 48824. Offers animal science (MS, PhD); animal science-environmental toxicology (PhD). *Entrance requirements:* Additional exam requirements/recommendations for international students: Required—TOEFL (minimum score 550 paper-based), Michigan State University ELT (minimum score 85), Michigan English Language Assessment Battery (minimum score 83). Electronic applications accepted.

Michigan State University, The Graduate School, College of Agriculture and Natural Resources, Department of Crop and Soil Sciences, East Lansing, MI 48824. Offers crop and soil sciences (MS, PhD); crop and soil sciences-environmental toxicology (PhD);

plant breeding and genetics-crop and soil sciences (MS); plant breeding, genetics and biotechnology-crop and soil sciences (PhD). *Entrance requirements:* Additional exam requirements/recommendations for international students: Required—TOEFL (minimum score 550 paper-based), Michigan State University ELT (minimum score 85), Michigan Michigan English Language Assessment Battery (minimum score 83). Electronic applications accepted.

Michigan State University, The Graduate School, College of Agriculture and Natural Resources and College of Natural Science, Department of Food Science and Human Nutrition, East Lansing, MI 48824. Offers food science (MS, PhD); food science - environmental toxicology (PhD); human nutrition (MS, PhD); human nutrition-environmental toxicology (PhD). *Entrance requirements:* Additional exam requirements/recommendations for international students: Required—TOEFL (minimum score 550 paper-based), Michigan State University ELT (minimum score 85), Michigan English Language Assessment Battery (minimum score 83). Electronic applications accepted.

Michigan State University, The Graduate School, College of Engineering, Department of Civil and Environmental Engineering, East Lansing, MI 48824. Offers civil engineering (MS, PhD); environmental engineering (MS, PhD); environmental engineering-environmental toxicology (PhD). Part-time programs available. *Entrance requirements:* Additional exam requirements/recommendations for international students: Required—TOEFL. Electronic applications accepted.

Michigan State University, The Graduate School, College of Natural Science and Graduate Programs in Human Medicine and Graduate Studies in Osteopathic Medicine, Department of Biochemistry and Molecular Biology, East Lansing, MI 48824. Offers biochemistry and molecular biology (MS, PhD); biochemistry and molecular biology/environmental toxicology (PhD). *Entrance requirements:* Additional exam requirements/recommendations for international students: Required—TOEFL. Electronic applications accepted.

Michigan State University, The Graduate School, College of Natural Science, Department of Chemistry, East Lansing, MI 48824. Offers chemical physics (PhD); chemistry (MS, PhD); chemistry-environmental toxicology (PhD); computational chemistry (MS). *Entrance requirements:* Additional exam requirements/recommendations for international students: Required—TOEFL. Electronic applications accepted. *Faculty research:* Analytical chemistry, inorganic and organic chemistry, nuclear chemistry, physical chemistry, theoretical and computational chemistry.

Michigan State University, The Graduate School, College of Natural Science, Department of Geological Sciences, East Lansing, MI 48824. Offers environmental geosciences (MS, PhD); environmental geosciences-environmental toxicology (PhD); geological sciences (MS, PhD). *Degree requirements:* For master's, thesis (for those without prior thesis work); for doctorate, thesis/dissertation. *Entrance requirements:* For master's, GRE General Test, minimum GPA of 3.0, course work in geoscience, 3 letters of recommendation; for doctorate, GRE General Test, 3 letters of recommendation. Additional exam requirements/recommendations for international students: Required—TOEFL (minimum score 550 paper-based), Michigan State University ELT (minimum score 85), Michigan English Language Assessment Battery (minimum score 83). Electronic applications accepted. *Faculty research:* Water in the environment, global and biological change, crystal dynamics.

Michigan State University, The Graduate School, College of Natural Science, Program in Genetics, East Lansing, MI 48824. Offers genetics (MS, PhD); genetics–environmental toxicology (PhD). *Entrance requirements:* Additional exam requirements/recommendations for international students: Required—TOEFL. Electronic applications accepted.

New York University, Graduate School of Arts and Science, Department of Environmental Medicine, New York, NY 10012-1019. Offers environmental health sciences (MS, PhD), including biostatistics (PhD), environmental hygiene (MS), epidemiology (PhD), ergonomics and biomechanics (PhD), exposure assessment and health effects (PhD), molecular toxicology/carcinogenesis (PhD), toxicology. Part-time programs available. *Faculty:* 26 full-time (7 women). *Students:* 55 full-time (34 women), 13 part-time (3 women); includes 16 minority (1 Black or African American, non-Hispanic/Latino; 8 Asian, non-Hispanic/Latino; 6 Hispanic/Latino; 1 Two or more races, non-Hispanic/Latino), 23 international. Average age 31. 69 applicants, 55% accepted, 18 enrolled. In 2013, 14 master's, 7 doctorates awarded. Terminal master's awarded for partial completion of doctoral program. *Degree requirements:* For master's, thesis or alternative; for doctorate, one foreign language, thesis/dissertation, oral and written exams. *Entrance requirements:* For master's and doctorate, GRE General Test, minimum GPA of 3.0; bachelor's degree in biological, physical, or engineering science. Additional exam requirements/recommendations for international students: Required—TOEFL. *Application deadline:* For fall admission, 12/18 for domestic and international students. Application fee: $95. *Expenses: Tuition:* Full-time $35,856; part-time $1494 per unit. *Required fees:* $1408; $64 per unit. $473 per term. Tuition and fees vary according to course load and program. *Financial support:* Fellowships with tuition reimbursements, teaching assistantships with tuition reimbursements, career-related internships or fieldwork, Federal Work-Study, institutionally sponsored loans, and health care benefits available. Financial award application deadline: 12/18; financial award applicants required to submit FAFSA. *Unit head:* Dr. Max Costa, Chair, 845-731-3661, Fax: 845-351-2058, E-mail: ehs@env.med.nyu.edu. *Application contact:* Dr. Jerome J. Solomon, Director of Graduate Studies, 845-731-3661, Fax: 845-351-2058, E-mail: ehs@env.med.nyu.edu.
Website: http://environmental-medicine.med.nyu.edu/

North Carolina State University, Graduate School, College of Agriculture and Life Sciences and College of Veterinary Medicine, Department of Environmental and Molecular Toxicology, Raleigh, NC 27695. Offers M Tox, MS, PhD. Terminal master's awarded for partial completion of doctoral program. *Degree requirements:* For master's, thesis (for some programs); for doctorate, thesis/dissertation. *Entrance requirements:* For master's and doctorate, GRE General Test, minimum GPA of 3.0. Electronic applications accepted. *Faculty research:* Chemical fate, carcinogenesis, developmental and endocrine toxicity, xenobiotic metabolism, signal transduction.

Oklahoma State University, Graduate College, Stillwater, OK 74078. Offers aerospace security (Graduate Certificate); bioenergy and sustainable technology (Graduate Certificate); bioinformatics (Graduate Certificate); business data mining (Graduate Certificate); business sustainability (Graduate Certificate); engineering and technology management (Graduate Certificate); entrepreneurship (Graduate Certificate); environmental science (MS); global issues (Graduate Certificate); grassland management (Graduate Certificate); information assurance (Graduate Certificate); interdisciplinary sciences (MS); interdisciplinary toxicology (Graduate Certificate); international studies (MS); non-profit management (Graduate Certificate); online teaching (Graduate Certificate); photonics (PhD); plant science (PhD); teaching English to speakers of other languages (Graduate Certificate); telecommunications management (MS). Programs are interdisciplinary. *Faculty:* 4 full-time (2 women), 2 part-time/adjunct (1 woman). *Students:* 74 full-time (58 women), 147 part-time (74 women); includes 44 minority (12 Black or African American, non-Hispanic/Latino; 8 American Indian or Alaska Native, non-Hispanic/Latino; 10 Asian, non-Hispanic/Latino; 6 Hispanic/Latino; 8 Two or more races, non-Hispanic/Latino), 43 international. Average age 32. 495 applicants, 70% accepted, 75 enrolled. In 2013, 55 master's, 11 doctorates awarded. *Degree requirements:* For master's, thesis (for some programs); for doctorate, comprehensive exam, thesis/dissertation. *Entrance requirements:* For master's and doctorate, GRE or GMAT. Additional exam requirements/recommendations for international students: Required—TOEFL (minimum score 550 paper-based; 79 iBT). *Application deadline:* For fall admission, 3/1 priority date for international students; for spring admission, 8/1 priority date for international students. Applications are processed on a rolling basis. Application fee: $40 ($75 for international students). Electronic applications accepted. *Expenses:* Tuition, state resident: full-time $4272; part-time $178 per credit hour. Tuition, nonresident: full-time $17,472; part-time $709 per credit hour. *Required fees:* $2413.20; $100.55 per credit hour. One-time fee: $50 full-time. Part-time tuition and fees vary according to course load and campus/location. *Financial support:* Career-related internships or fieldwork, Federal Work-Study, scholarships/grants, health care benefits, tuition waivers (partial), and unspecified assistantships available. Support available to part-time students. Financial award application deadline: 3/1; financial award applicants required to submit FAFSA. *Unit head:* Dr. Sheryl Tucker, Dean, 405-744-7099, Fax: 405-744-0355, E-mail: grad-i@okstate.edu. *Application contact:* Dr. Susan Mathew, Coordinator of Admissions, 405-744-6368, Fax: 405-744-0355, E-mail: grad-i@okstate.edu.
Website: http://gradcollege.okstate.edu/

Oklahoma State University Center for Health Sciences, Graduate Program in Forensic Sciences, Tulsa, OK 74107. Offers forensic biology/DNA (MS); forensic document examination/forensic pathology (MS); forensic psychology (MS); forensic science administration (MS); microbiology (MS); trace evidence/forensic toxicology (MS). Part-time and evening/weekend programs available. Postbaccalaureate distance learning degree programs offered (no on-campus study). *Faculty:* 4 full-time (0 women), 14 part-time/adjunct (6 women). *Students:* 4 full-time (0 women), 14 part-time (6 women); includes 7 minority (4 American Indian or Alaska Native, non-Hispanic/Latino; 3 Hispanic/Latino), 3 international. Average age 31. 28 applicants, 50% accepted, 5 enrolled. In 2013, 5 master's awarded. *Degree requirements:* For master's, comprehensive exam, thesis (for some programs), creative component (for non-thesis options). *Entrance requirements:* For master's, MAT (for options in forensic science administration and forensic document examination) or GRE General Test, professional experience (for options in forensic science administration and forensic document examination). Additional exam requirements/recommendations for international students: Required—TOEFL (minimum score 100 iBT) or IELTS (minimum score 7.0). *Application deadline:* For fall admission, 3/1 for domestic and international students; for spring admission, 10/1 for domestic and international students; for summer admission, 7/1 for domestic and international students. Applications are processed on a rolling basis. Application fee: $40 ($75 for international students). Electronic applications accepted. *Expenses:* Tuition, state resident: full-time $22,127; part-time $178 per credit hour. Tuition, nonresident: full-time $43,572; part-time $728 per credit hour. *Required fees:* $910.79; $200 per semester. *Financial support:* In 2013–14, 14 students received support, including 8 research assistantships (averaging $12,000 per year); career-related internships or fieldwork, Federal Work-Study, and tuition waivers (partial) also available. Support available to part-time students. Financial award application deadline: 4/1; financial award applicants required to submit FAFSA. *Faculty research:* Studies on the variability in chromosomal DNA; development/enhancement of accessory methods useful for forensic DNA typing; development of universal methods useful for discriminating pathogenic bacteria; forensic dentistry; transmission of microbial diseases by dentures, protective athletic mouth-guards, band wind instruments, and infant pacifiers; changes in ecologies and antibiotic sensitivities of aerobic microorganisms; forensic toxicology and trace chemical method development. *Total annual research expenditures:* $58,000. *Unit head:* Dr. Robert W. Allen, Director, 918-561-1108, Fax: 918-561-8414. *Application contact:* Cathy Newsome, Coordinator, 918-561-1108, Fax: 918-561-8414, E-mail: cathy.newsome@okstate.edu.
Website: http://www.healthsciences.okstate.edu/forensic/index.cfm

Oregon State University, College of Agricultural Sciences, Program in Toxicology, Corvallis, OR 97331. Offers M Ag, MS, PhD. *Faculty:* 13 full-time (5 women), 3 part-time/adjunct (1 woman). *Students:* 21 full-time (10 women), 1 part-time (0 women), 2 international. Average age 28. 33 applicants, 15% accepted, 4 enrolled. In 2013, 2 master's, 7 doctorates awarded. *Median time to degree:* Of those who began their doctoral program in fall 2005, 40% received their degree in 8 years or less. *Degree requirements:* For master's, thesis; for doctorate, thesis/dissertation. *Entrance requirements:* For master's and doctorate, GRE, bachelor's degree in chemistry or biological sciences, minimum GPA of 3.0 in last 90 hours of course work. Additional exam requirements/recommendations for international students: Required—TOEFL (minimum score 80 iBT), IELTS (minimum score 6.5). *Application deadline:* For fall admission, 12/31 for domestic students. Application fee: $60. *Expenses:* Tuition, state resident: full-time $11,664; part-time $432 per credit hour. Tuition, nonresident: full-time $19,197; part-time $711 per credit hour. *Required fees:* $1446; $443 per quarter. One-time fee: $300. Tuition and fees vary according to course load and program. *Financial support:* Fellowships, research assistantships, Federal Work-Study, and institutionally sponsored loans available. Support available to part-time students. Financial award application deadline: 2/1. *Faculty research:* Biochemical mechanisms for toxicology; analytical, comparative, aquatic, and food toxicology; aquaculture of salmonids; immunotoxicology; fish toxicology. *Unit head:* Dr. Craig Marcus, Department Head, 541-737-1808, E-mail: craig.marcus@oregonstate.edu. *Application contact:* Mary Mucia, Toxicology Advisor, 541-737-9079, E-mail: mary.mucia@oregonstate.edu.
Website: http://emt.oregonstate.edu/prospectivegrads

Prairie View A&M University, College of Arts and Sciences, Department of Biology, Prairie View, TX 77446-0519. Offers bio-environmental toxicology (MS); biology (MS). Part-time and evening/weekend programs available. *Faculty:* 5 full-time (2 women). *Students:* 1 (woman) part-time; minority (Black or African American, non-Hispanic/Latino). Average age 25. In 2013, 8 master's awarded. *Degree requirements:* For master's, comprehensive exam, thesis optional. *Entrance requirements:* For master's, GRE General Test. Additional exam requirements/recommendations for international students: Required—TOEFL. *Application deadline:* For fall admission, 7/1 for domestic and international students; for spring admission, 11/1 for domestic and international students. Applications are processed on a rolling basis. Application fee: $50. Electronic applications accepted. *Expenses:* Tuition, state resident: full-time $3776; part-time $209.77 per credit hour. Tuition, nonresident: full-time $10,183; part-time $565.77 per credit hour. *Required fees:* $2037; $446.50 per credit hour. *Financial support:* In 2013–14, 3 students received support, including 3 teaching assistantships (averaging $13,440 per year); Federal Work-Study and unspecified assistantships also available. Financial award application deadline: 4/1; financial award applicants required to submit FAFSA. *Faculty research:* Genomics, hypertension, control of gene express, proteins, ligands that interact with hormone receptors, prostate cancer, renin-angiotensin yeast metabolism. *Unit head:* Dr. Harriette Howard-Lee-Block, Head, 936-261-3160, Fax: 936-261-3179, E-mail: hlblock@pvamu.edu. *Application contact:* Dr. Seab A. Smith, Associate Professor, 936-261-3169, Fax: 936-261-3179, E-mail: sasmith@pvamu.edu.

Purdue University, Graduate School, College of Health and Human Sciences, School of Health Sciences, West Lafayette, IN 47907. Offers health physics (MS, PhD); medical physics (MS, PhD); occupational and environmental health science (MS, PhD), including

aerosol deposition and lung disease, ergonomics, exposure and risk assessment, indoor air quality and bioaerosols (PhD), liver/lung toxicology; radiation biology (PhD); toxicology (PhD); MS/PhD. Part-time programs available. *Faculty:* 11 full-time (5 women), 28 part-time/adjunct (5 women). *Students:* 28 full-time (8 women), 10 part-time (3 women); includes 6 minority (1 Black or African American, non-Hispanic/Latino; 3 Asian, non-Hispanic/Latino; 1 Hispanic/Latino; 1 Two or more races, non-Hispanic/Latino), 10 international. Average age 28. 77 applicants, 42% accepted, 13 enrolled. In 2013, 6 master's, 6 doctorates awarded. *Degree requirements:* For master's, thesis optional; for doctorate, one foreign language, thesis/dissertation. *Entrance requirements:* For master's and doctorate, GRE General Test, minimum undergraduate GPA of 3.0 or equivalent. Additional exam requirements/recommendations for international students: Required—TOEFL (minimum score 550 paper-based; 77 iBT); Recommended—TWE. *Application deadline:* For fall admission, 5/15 for domestic and international students; for spring admission, 10/15 for domestic and international students. Applications are processed on a rolling basis. Application fee: $60 ($75 for international students). Electronic applications accepted. *Financial support:* In 2013–14, fellowships with tuition reimbursements (averaging $14,400 per year), research assistantships with tuition reimbursements (averaging $12,000 per year), teaching assistantships with tuition reimbursements (averaging $12,000 per year) were awarded; career-related internships or fieldwork and traineeships also available. Support available to part-time students. Financial award applicants required to submit FAFSA. *Faculty research:* Environmental toxicology, industrial hygiene, radiation dosimetry. *Unit head:* Dr. Wei Zheng, Head, 765-494-1419, E-mail: wz18@purdue.edu. *Application contact:* Jennifer S. Franklin, Graduate Contact, 765-494-0248, E-mail: jfranklin@purdue.edu.
Website: http://www.healthsciences.purdue.edu/

Queen's University at Kingston, School of Graduate Studies, Faculty of Health Sciences, Department of Pharmacology and Toxicology, Kingston, ON K7L 3N6, Canada. Offers M Sc, PhD. *Degree requirements:* For master's, thesis; for doctorate, comprehensive exam, thesis/dissertation. *Entrance requirements:* For master's, minimum 2nd class standing, honors bachelor of science degree (life sciences, health sciences, or equivalent); for doctorate, masters of science degree or outstanding performance in honors bachelor of science program. Additional exam requirements/recommendations for international students: Required—TOEFL (minimum score 600 paper-based). Electronic applications accepted. *Faculty research:* Biochemical toxicology, cardiovascular pharmacology and neuropharmacology.

Rutgers, The State University of New Jersey, New Brunswick, Graduate School-New Brunswick, Department of Environmental Sciences, Piscataway, NJ 08854-8097. Offers air pollution and resources (MS, PhD); aquatic biology (MS, PhD); aquatic chemistry (MS, PhD); atmospheric science (MS, PhD); chemistry and physics of aerosol and hydrosol systems (MS, PhD); environmental chemistry (MS, PhD); environmental microbiology (MS, PhD); environmental toxicology (PhD); exposure assessment (PhD); fate and effects of pollutants (MS, PhD); pollution prevention and control (MS, PhD); water and wastewater treatment (MS, PhD); water resources (MS, PhD). Terminal master's awarded for partial completion of doctoral program. *Degree requirements:* For master's, comprehensive exam, thesis or alternative, oral final exam; for doctorate, comprehensive exam, thesis/dissertation, thesis defense, qualifying exam. *Entrance requirements:* For master's and doctorate, GRE General Test. Additional exam requirements/recommendations for international students: Required—TOEFL. Electronic applications accepted. *Faculty research:* Biological waste treatment; contaminant fate and transport; air, soil and water quality.

Rutgers, The State University of New Jersey, New Brunswick, Graduate School-New Brunswick, Joint Program in Toxicology, Piscataway, NJ 08854-8097. Offers environmental toxicology (MS, PhD); industrial-occupational toxicology (MS, PhD); nutritional toxicology (MS, PhD); pharmaceutical toxicology (MS, PhD). MS, PhD offered jointly with University of Medicine and Dentistry of New Jersey. *Degree requirements:* For master's, thesis; for doctorate, comprehensive exam, thesis/dissertation, qualifying exams (written and oral). *Entrance requirements:* For master's and doctorate, GRE General Test. Additional exam requirements/recommendations for international students: Required—TOEFL. Electronic applications accepted. *Faculty research:* Neurotoxicants, immunotoxicology, carcinogenesis and chemoprevention, molecular toxicology, xenobiotic metabolism.

Rutgers, The State University of New Jersey, New Brunswick, Graduate School of Biomedical Sciences, Piscataway, NJ 08854-5635. Offers biochemistry and molecular biology (MS, PhD); biomedical engineering (MS, PhD); biomedical science (MS); cellular and molecular pharmacology (MS, PhD); clinical and translational science (MS); environmental sciences/exposure assessment (PhD); molecular genetics, microbiology and immunology (MS, PhD); neuroscience (MS, PhD); physiology and integrative biology (MS, PhD); toxicology (PhD); MD/PhD. Terminal master's awarded for partial completion of doctoral program. *Degree requirements:* For master's, thesis (for some programs), ethics training; for doctorate, comprehensive exam, thesis/dissertation, ethics training. *Entrance requirements:* For master's, GRE General Test, MCAT, DAT; for doctorate, GRE General Test. Additional exam requirements/recommendations for international students: Required—TOEFL. Electronic applications accepted.

St. John's University, College of Pharmacy and Health Sciences, Graduate Programs in Pharmaceutical Sciences, Program in Toxicology, Queens, NY 11439. Offers MS. Part-time and evening/weekend programs available. *Students:* 12 full-time (9 women), 8 part-time (4 women); includes 9 minority (3 Asian, non-Hispanic/Latino; 5 Hispanic/Latino; 1 Two or more races, non-Hispanic/Latino), 4 international. Average age 25. 19 applicants, 58% accepted, 6 enrolled. In 2013, 4 master's awarded. *Degree requirements:* For master's, comprehensive exam, thesis optional, one-year residency. *Entrance requirements:* For master's, GRE General Test, minimum GPA of 3.0; 2 letters of recommendation, bachelor's degree in related area. Additional exam requirements/recommendations for international students: Required—TOEFL (minimum score 600 paper-based; 100 iBT), IELTS (minimum score 5.5). *Application deadline:* For fall admission, 3/1 priority date for domestic students, 5/1 priority date for international students; for spring admission, 11/1 priority date for domestic and international students. Applications are processed on a rolling basis. Application fee: $70. Electronic applications accepted. *Expenses:* Contact institution. *Financial support:* Fellowships, research assistantships, career-related internships or fieldwork, and scholarships/grants available. Support available to part-time students. Financial award application deadline: 3/1; financial award applicants required to submit FAFSA. *Faculty research:* Neurotoxicology, renal toxicology, toxicology of metals, regulatory toxicology. *Unit head:* Dr. Louis Trombetta, Chair, 718-990-6025, E-mail: trombetl@stjohns.edu. *Application contact:* Robert Medrano, Director of Graduate Admission, 718-990-1601, Fax: 718-990-5686, E-mail: gradhelp@stjohns.edu.
Website: http://www.stjohns.edu//academics/schools-and-colleges/college-pharmacy-and-health-sciences/programs-and-majors/toxicology-master-science

San Diego State University, Graduate and Research Affairs, College of Health and Human Services, Graduate School of Public Health, San Diego, CA 92182. Offers environmental health (MPH); epidemiology (MPH, PhD), including biostatistics (MPH); global emergency preparedness and response (MS); global health (PhD); health behavior (PhD); health promotion (MPH); health services administration (MPH); toxicology (MS); MPH/MA; MSW/MPH. *Accreditation:* CAHME (one or more programs are accredited); CEPH (one or more programs are accredited). Part-time programs available. *Degree requirements:* For master's, comprehensive exam (for some programs), thesis (for some programs); for doctorate, thesis/dissertation. *Entrance requirements:* For master's, GMAT (MPH in health services administration), GRE General Test; for doctorate, GRE General Test. Additional exam requirements/recommendations for international students: Required—TOEFL. *Faculty research:* Evaluation of tobacco, AIDS prevalence and prevention, mammography, infant death project, Alzheimer's in elderly Chinese.

Simon Fraser University, Office of Graduate Studies, Faculty of Science, Department of Biological Sciences, Burnaby, BC V5A 1S6, Canada. Offers bioinformatics (Graduate Diploma); biological sciences (M Sc, PhD); environmental toxicology (MET); pest management (MPM). *Faculty:* 47 full-time (15 women). *Students:* 138 full-time (70 women). 29 applicants, 59% accepted, 15 enrolled. In 2013, 27 master's, 13 doctorates awarded. *Degree requirements:* For master's, thesis; for doctorate, thesis/dissertation, candidacy exam; for Graduate Diploma, practicum. *Entrance requirements:* For master's, minimum GPA of 3.0 (on scale of 4.33), or 3.33 based on last 60 credits of undergraduate courses; for doctorate, minimum GPA of 3.5 (on scale of 4.33); for Graduate Diploma, minimum GPA of 2.5 (on scale of 4.33), or 2.67 based on the last 60 credits of undergraduate courses. Additional exam requirements/recommendations for international students: Recommended—TOEFL (minimum score 580 paper-based; 93 iBT), IELTS (minimum score 7), TWE (minimum score 5). *Application deadline:* For fall admission, 6/1 for domestic and international students; for winter admission, 10/1 for domestic and international students; for spring admission, 2/1 for domestic and international students. Applications are processed on a rolling basis. Application fee: $90 ($125 for international students). Electronic applications accepted. *Expenses: Tuition, area resident:* Full-time $5084 Canadian dollars. *Required fees:* $840 Canadian dollars. *Financial support:* In 2013–14, 68 students received support, including 77 fellowships (averaging $6,250 per year), teaching assistantships (averaging $5,608 per year); research assistantships and scholarships/grants also available. *Faculty research:* Cell biology, wildlife ecology, environmental and evolutionary physiology, environmental toxicology, pest management. *Unit head:* Dr. Julian Guttman, Graduate Chair, 778-782-4459, Fax: 778-782-3496, E-mail: bisc-grad-chair@sfu.ca. *Application contact:* Marlene Nguyen, Graduate Secretary, 778-782-3120, Fax: 778-782-3496, E-mail: biscgrad@sfu.ca.
Website: http://www.sfu.ca/biology

Texas A&M University, College of Veterinary Medicine and Biomedical Sciences, Department of Veterinary Physiology and Pharmacology, College Station, TX 77843. Offers biomedical science (MS, PhD); toxicology (PhD). *Faculty:* 16. *Students:* 25 full-time (13 women), 3 part-time (2 women); includes 6 minority (1 Black or African American, non-Hispanic/Latino; 2 Asian, non-Hispanic/Latino; 2 Hispanic/Latino; 1 Two or more races, non-Hispanic/Latino), 9 international. Average age 28. 6 applicants, 100% accepted, 6 enrolled. In 2013, 6 master's, 3 doctorates awarded. *Entrance requirements:* For master's and doctorate, GRE General Test. Additional exam requirements/recommendations for international students: Required—TOEFL. Application fee: $50 ($75 for international students). *Expenses:* Tuition, state resident: full-time $4078; part-time $226.55 per credit hour. Tuition, nonresident: full-time $10,450; part-time $580.55 per credit hour. *Required fees:* $2328; $278.50 per credit hour. $642.45 per semester. *Financial support:* Fellowships, research assistantships, and teaching assistantships available. Financial award application deadline: 4/1; financial award applicants required to submit FAFSA. *Faculty research:* Gamete and embryo physiology, endocrinology, equine laminitis. *Unit head:* Dr. John Stallone, Head, 979-862-3065, E-mail: john-n-stallone@exchange.tamu.edu. *Application contact:* Graduate Admissions, 979-845-1044, E-mail: admissions@tamu.edu.
Website: http://vetmed.tamu.edu/vtpp

Texas Southern University, School of Science and Technology, Program in Environmental Toxicology, Houston, TX 77004-4584. Offers MS, PhD. Part-time programs available. *Faculty:* 6 full-time (1 woman), 2 part-time/adjunct (0 women). *Students:* 32 full-time (21 women), 22 part-time (10 women); includes 46 minority (34 Black or African American, non-Hispanic/Latino; 10 Asian, non-Hispanic/Latino; 2 Hispanic/Latino), 2 international. Average age 35. 36 applicants, 58% accepted, 12 enrolled. In 2013, 9 master's, 4 doctorates awarded. *Degree requirements:* For master's, thesis; for doctorate, thesis/dissertation. *Entrance requirements:* For master's, minimum GPA of 2.75; for doctorate, GRE, minimum GPA of 2.75. *Application deadline:* For fall admission, 7/1 for domestic and international students; for spring admission, 11/1 for domestic and international students. Applications are processed on a rolling basis. Application fee: $35 ($75 for international students). Electronic applications accepted. *Expenses:* Contact institution. *Financial support:* In 2013–14, 3 research assistantships (averaging $10,167 per year), 6 teaching assistantships (averaging $4,133 per year) were awarded; fellowships, institutionally sponsored loans, scholarships/grants, tuition waivers (partial), and unspecified assistantships also available. Financial award application deadline: 5/1; financial award applicants required to submit FAFSA. *Faculty research:* Air quality, water quality, soil remediation, computer modeling. *Unit head:* Dr. Lei Yu, Interim Chair, 713-313-7282, E-mail: yu_lx@tsu.edu. *Application contact:* Charlotte Whaley, Administrative Assistant, 713-313-7009, E-mail: whaley_cs@tsu.edu.

Texas Tech University, Graduate School, College of Arts and Sciences, Department of Environmental Toxicology, Lubbock, TX 79409-1163. Offers MS, PhD, JD/MS, MBA/MS, MPA/MS. Part-time programs available. *Faculty:* 15 full-time (2 women). *Students:* 48 full-time (29 women), 1 part-time (0 women); includes 4 minority (1 Black or African American, non-Hispanic/Latino; 2 Hispanic/Latino; 1 Two or more races, non-Hispanic/Latino), 13 international. Average age 28. 25 applicants, 60% accepted, 12 enrolled. In 2013, 6 master's, 6 doctorates awarded. Terminal master's awarded for partial completion of doctoral program. *Degree requirements:* For master's, thesis; for doctorate, comprehensive exam, thesis/dissertation. *Entrance requirements:* For master's and doctorate, GRE. Additional exam requirements/recommendations for international students: Required—TOEFL (minimum score 550 paper-based; 79 iBT); Recommended—IELTS (minimum score 6.5), TSE (minimum score 60). *Application deadline:* For fall admission, 6/1 priority date for domestic students, 1/15 priority date for international students; for spring admission, 9/1 priority date for domestic students, 6/15 priority date for international students. Applications are processed on a rolling basis. Application fee: $60. Electronic applications accepted. *Expenses:* Tuition, state resident: full-time $6062; part-time $252.57 per credit hour. Tuition, nonresident: full-time $14,558; part-time $606.57 per credit hour. *Required fees:* $2655; $35 per credit hour. $907.50 per semester. Tuition and fees vary according to course load. *Financial support:* In 2013–14, 48 students received support, including 30 fellowships (averaging $2,465 per year), 41 research assistantships (averaging $4,386 per year), 5 teaching assistantships (averaging $3,658 per year); Federal Work-Study, institutionally sponsored loans, scholarships/grants, and health care benefits also available. Financial award application deadline: 4/15; financial award applicants required to submit FAFSA. *Faculty research:* Wildlife toxicology; molecular epidemiology and genomics; endangered species toxicology; reproductive, molecular, and developmental toxicology; environmental chemistry. *Total annual research expenditures:* $1.1 million. *Unit head:* Dr. Todd Anderson, Chair, 806-834-1587, E-mail: todd.anderson@ttu.edu. *Application*

contact: Dr. Christopher Salice, Graduate Officer, 806-834-8102, E-mail: chris.salice@ttu.edu.
Website: http://www.tiehh.ttu.edu/

Université de Montréal, Faculty of Medicine, Program in Toxicology and Risk Analysis, Montréal, QC H3C 3J7, Canada. Offers DESS. Electronic applications accepted.

University at Albany, State University of New York, School of Public Health, Department of Environmental Health Sciences, Albany, NY 12222-0001. Offers environmental and analytical chemistry (MS, PhD); environmental and occupational health (MS, PhD); toxicology (MS, PhD). *Degree requirements:* For master's, thesis; for doctorate, comprehensive exam, thesis/dissertation. *Entrance requirements:* For master's and doctorate, GRE General Test, GRE Subject Test, 3 letters of reference. Additional exam requirements/recommendations for international students: Required—TOEFL (minimum score 600 paper-based). Electronic applications accepted. *Faculty research:* Xenobiotic metabolism, neurotoxicity of halogenated hydrocarbons, pharmac/toxicogenomics, environmental analytical chemistry.

University at Buffalo, the State University of New York, Graduate School, School of Medicine and Biomedical Sciences, Graduate Programs in Medicine and Biomedical Sciences, Department of Pharmacology and Toxicology, Buffalo, NY 14260. Offers pharmacology (MS, PhD); MD/PhD. *Faculty:* 22 full-time (3 women), 1 part-time/adjunct (0 women). *Students:* 23 full-time (11 women); includes 11 minority (5 Black or African American, non-Hispanic/Latino; 1 American Indian or Alaska Native, non-Hispanic/Latino; 4 Asian, non-Hispanic/Latino; 1 Hispanic/Latino), 3 international. Average age 25. 76 applicants, 22% accepted, 8 enrolled. In 2013, 9 master's, 2 doctorates awarded. Terminal master's awarded for partial completion of doctoral program. *Degree requirements:* For master's, thesis; for doctorate, thesis/dissertation. *Entrance requirements:* For master's and doctorate, GRE General Test, 3 letters of recommendation. Additional exam requirements/recommendations for international students: Required—TOEFL (minimum score 79 iBT). *Application deadline:* For fall admission, 2/14 priority date for domestic and international students. Applications are processed on a rolling basis. Application fee: $75. Electronic applications accepted. *Financial support:* In 2013–14, 1 student received support, including 2 fellowships with full tuition reimbursements available (averaging $30,000 per year), 14 research assistantships with full tuition reimbursements available (averaging $25,000 per year); teaching assistantships, Federal Work-Study, scholarships/grants, health care benefits, and unspecified assistantships also available. Financial award application deadline: 2/14; financial award applicants required to submit FAFSA. *Faculty research:* Neuropharmacology, toxicology, signal transduction, molecular pharmacology, behavioral pharmacology. *Total annual research expenditures:* $3.5 million. *Unit head:* Dr. Margarita L. Dubocovich, Professor and Chair, 716-829-3048, Fax: 716-829-2801, E-mail: mdubo@buffalo.edu. *Application contact:* Linda LeRoy, Admissions Assistant, 716-829-2800, Fax: 716-829-2801, E-mail: pmygrad@buffalo.edu.
Website: http://medicine.buffalo.edu/pharmtox

The University of Alabama at Birmingham, Graduate Programs in Joint Health Sciences, Program in Pharmacology and Toxicology, Birmingham, AL 35294. Offers PhD. *Degree requirements:* For doctorate, thesis/dissertation. *Entrance requirements:* For doctorate, GRE General Test; GRE Subject Test (recommended), interview, three evaluations. Additional exam requirements/recommendations for international students: Required—TOEFL, TWE. Electronic applications accepted. *Expenses:* Contact institution. *Faculty research:* Anticancer and antiviral chemotherapy, with emphasis on drugs used in the management of AIDS and related opportunistic infections; metabolism and biliary excretion of drugs (and metabolites) as well as the mechanisms of drug toxicity.

The University of Alabama at Birmingham, School of Public Health, Program in Public Health, Birmingham, AL 35294. Offers accelerated industrial hygiene (MPH); applied epidemiology (MSPH); biostatistics (MPH); clinical and translational science (MSPH); environmental health (MPH); environmental health and toxicology (MSPH); epidemiology (MPH); general theory and practice (MPH); health behavior (MPH); health care organization (MPH); health policy quantitative policy analysis (MPH); industrial hygiene (MPH, MSPH); maternal and child health policy (Dr PH); maternal and child health policy and leadership (MPH); occupational health and safety (MPH); outcomes research (MSPH, Dr PH); pharmacoepidemiology and comparative effectiveness research (MSPH); public health (PhD); public health management (Dr PH); public health preparedness management (MPH). *Accreditation:* CEPH. *Entrance requirements:* For master's and doctorate, GRE, evaluations. Additional exam requirements/recommendations for international students: Recommended—TOEFL (minimum score 550 paper-based; 79 iBT), IELTS (minimum score 6.5).

University of Arkansas for Medical Sciences, Graduate School, Little Rock, AR 72205. Offers biochemistry and molecular biology (MS, PhD); bioinformatics (MS, PhD); cellular physiology and molecular biophysics (MS, PhD); clinical nutrition (MS); interdisciplinary biomedical sciences (MS, PhD, Certificate); interdisciplinary toxicology (MS); microbiology and immunology (PhD); neurobiology and developmental sciences (PhD); pharmacology (PhD); MD/PhD. Bioinformatics programs hosted jointly with the University of Arkansas at Little Rock. Part-time programs available. *Faculty:* 397 full-time (205 women). *Students:* 196 full-time (126 women), 117 part-time (87 women); includes 65 minority (38 Black or African American, non-Hispanic/Latino; 1 American Indian or Alaska Native, non-Hispanic/Latino; 21 Asian, non-Hispanic/Latino; 4 Hispanic/Latino; 1 Two or more races, non-Hispanic/Latino), 57 international. 455 applicants, 27% accepted, 89 enrolled. In 2013, 41 master's, 18 doctorates, 28 other advanced degrees awarded. Terminal master's awarded for partial completion of doctoral program. *Degree requirements:* For master's, comprehensive exam (for some programs), thesis (for some programs); for doctorate, thesis/dissertation. *Entrance requirements:* For master's and doctorate, GRE. Additional exam requirements/recommendations for international students: Required—TOEFL. *Application deadline:* Applications are processed on a rolling basis. Application fee: $0. Electronic applications accepted. *Expenses:* Contact institution. *Financial support:* In 2013–14, 120 research assistantships (averaging $24,000 per year) were awarded; career-related internships or fieldwork, Federal Work-Study, and traineeships also available. Support available to part-time students. Financial award applicants required to submit FAFSA. *Unit head:* Dr. Robert E. McGehee, Jr., Dean, 501-686-5454. *Application contact:* Dr. Kristen Sterba, Assistant Dean, Office of Graduate Student Recruiting and Retention, 501-526-7396, E-mail: kmsterba@uams.edu.
Website: http://www.uams.edu/gradschool/

University of California, Davis, Graduate Studies, Graduate Group in Pharmacology and Toxicology, Davis, CA 95616. Offers MS, PhD. Terminal master's awarded for partial completion of doctoral program. *Degree requirements:* For master's, comprehensive exam or thesis; for doctorate, thesis/dissertation, qualifying exam. *Entrance requirements:* For master's and doctorate, GRE General Test, minimum GPA of 3.0, course work in biochemistry and/or physiology. Additional exam requirements/recommendations for international students: Required—TOEFL (minimum score 550 paper-based). Electronic applications accepted. *Faculty research:* Respiratory, neurochemical, molecular, genetic, and ecological toxicology.

University of California, Irvine, School of Medicine, Department of Pharmacology, Program in Pharmacology and Toxicology, Irvine, CA 92697. Offers MS, PhD, MD/PhD. *Students:* 29 full-time (8 women), 1 part-time (0 women); includes 15 minority (10 Asian, non-Hispanic/Latino; 3 Hispanic/Latino; 2 Two or more races, non-Hispanic/Latino), 6 international. Average age 28. 40 applicants, 40% accepted, 5 enrolled. In 2013, 5 master's, 6 doctorates awarded. *Degree requirements:* For doctorate, thesis/dissertation. *Entrance requirements:* For master's, GRE, minimum GPA of 3.0; for doctorate, GRE General Test, GRE Subject Test, minimum GPA of 3.0. Additional exam requirements/recommendations for international students: Required—TOEFL (minimum score 550 paper-based). *Application deadline:* For fall admission, 1/15 priority date for domestic students, 1/15 for international students. Applications are processed on a rolling basis. Application fee: $80 ($100 for international students). Electronic applications accepted. *Financial support:* Fellowships, research assistantships, teaching assistantships, institutionally sponsored loans, traineeships, and unspecified assistantships available. Financial award application deadline: 3/1; financial award applicants required to submit FAFSA. *Unit head:* Dr. Olivier Civelli, Chair, 949-924-2522, Fax: 949-824-4855, E-mail: ocivelli@uci.edu. *Application contact:* Dale Lee, Chief Administrative Officer, 949-824-6772, Fax: 949-824-4855, E-mail: dtly@uci.edu.

University of California, Los Angeles, Graduate Division, College of Letters and Science and David Geffen School of Medicine, UCLA ACCESS to Programs in the Molecular, Cellular and Integrative Life Sciences, Los Angeles, CA 90095. Offers biochemistry and molecular biology (PhD); biological chemistry (PhD); cellular and molecular pathology (PhD); human genetics (PhD); microbiology, immunology, and molecular genetics (PhD); molecular biology (PhD); molecular toxicology (PhD); molecular, cellular and integrative physiology (PhD); neurobiology (PhD); oral biology (PhD); physiology (PhD). *Degree requirements:* For doctorate, thesis/dissertation, oral and written qualifying exams. *Entrance requirements:* For doctorate, GRE General Test, bachelor's degree; minimum undergraduate GPA of 3.0 (or its equivalent if letter grade system not used). Additional exam requirements/recommendations for international students: Required—TOEFL. Electronic applications accepted.

University of California, Riverside, Graduate Division, Program in Environmental Toxicology, Riverside, CA 92521-0102. Offers MS, PhD. Terminal master's awarded for partial completion of doctoral program. *Degree requirements:* For master's, thesis; for doctorate, comprehensive exam, thesis/dissertation, qualifying exams. *Entrance requirements:* For master's and doctorate, GRE General Test, minimum GPA of 3.25. Additional exam requirements/recommendations for international students: Required—TOEFL (minimum score 550 paper-based; 80 iBT). Electronic applications accepted. *Faculty research:* Cellular/molecular toxicology, atmospheric chemistry, bioremediation, carcinogenesis, mechanism of toxicity.

University of California, Santa Cruz, Division of Graduate Studies, Division of Physical and Biological Sciences, Environmental Toxicology Department, Santa Cruz, CA 95064. Offers MS, PhD. Terminal master's awarded for partial completion of doctoral program. *Degree requirements:* For master's, comprehensive exam, thesis; for doctorate, thesis/dissertation, qualifying exams. *Entrance requirements:* For master's and doctorate, GRE. Additional exam requirements/recommendations for international students: Required—TOEFL (minimum score 550 paper-based; 83 iBT); Recommended—IELTS (minimum score 8). Electronic applications accepted. *Faculty research:* Molecular mechanisms of reactive DNA methylation toxicity, anthropogenic perturbations of biogeochemical cycles, anaerobic microbiology and biotransformation of pollutants and toxic metals, organismal responses and therapeutic treatment of toxins, microbiology, molecular genetics, genomics.

University of Colorado Denver, School of Pharmacy, Program in Toxicology, Aurora, CO 80045. Offers PhD. *Students:* 23 full-time (12 women); includes 4 minority (1 Black or African American, non-Hispanic/Latino; 1 Asian, non-Hispanic/Latino; 2 Hispanic/Latino), 8 international. Average age 28. 20 applicants, 20% accepted, 4 enrolled. In 2013, 6 doctorates awarded. *Degree requirements:* For doctorate, comprehensive exam, thesis/dissertation, 60 credit hours (30 in upper-level course work and 30 in thesis research hours). *Entrance requirements:* For doctorate, GRE, minimum undergraduate GPA of 3.0; prior coursework in general chemistry, organic chemistry, calculus, biology, and physics. Additional exam requirements/recommendations for international students: Required—TOEFL (minimum score 550 paper-based; 80 iBT). *Application deadline:* For fall admission, 1/15 for domestic students, 12/15 for international students. Application fee: $50 ($75 for international students). Electronic applications accepted. *Expenses:* Contact institution. *Financial support:* In 2013–14, 23 students received support. Fellowships, research assistantships, teaching assistantships, Federal Work-Study, institutionally sponsored loans, scholarships/grants, traineeships, and unspecified assistantships available. Financial award application deadline: 3/15; financial award applicants required to submit FAFSA. *Faculty research:* Regulation of apoptotic cell death; cancer chemoprevention; innate immunity and hepatotoxicity; role of chronic inflammation in cancer; Parkinson's disease, epilepsy and oxidative stress. *Unit head:* Dr. David Ross, Chair/Professor of Toxicology, 303-724-7265, Fax: 303-724-7266, E-mail: david.ross@ucdenver.edu. *Application contact:* Jackie Milowski, Information Contact, 303-724-7263, E-mail: jackie.milowski@ucdenver.edu.
Website: http://www.ucdenver.edu/academics/colleges/pharmacy/AcademicPrograms/PhDPrograms/PhDToxicology/Pages/PhDToxicology.aspx

University of Connecticut, Graduate School, School of Pharmacy, Department of Pharmaceutical Sciences, Graduate Program in Pharmacology and Toxicology, Storrs, CT 06269. Offers pharmacology (MS, PhD); toxicology (MS, PhD). Terminal master's awarded for partial completion of doctoral program. *Degree requirements:* For master's, comprehensive exam, thesis; for doctorate, thesis/dissertation. *Entrance requirements:* For master's and doctorate, GRE General Test. Additional exam requirements/recommendations for international students: Required—TOEFL (minimum score 550 paper-based). Electronic applications accepted.

University of Florida, College of Veterinary Medicine, Graduate Program in Veterinary Medical Sciences, Gainesville, FL 32611. Offers forensic toxicology (Certificate); veterinary medical sciences (MS, PhD), including forensic toxicology (MS). Postbaccalaureate distance learning degree programs offered (no on-campus study). Terminal master's awarded for partial completion of doctoral program. *Degree requirements:* For master's, thesis; for doctorate, thesis/dissertation. *Entrance requirements:* For master's and doctorate, GRE General Test, minimum GPA of 3.0. Additional exam requirements/recommendations for international students: Required—TOEFL (minimum score 550 paper-based). Electronic applications accepted. *Expenses:* Contact institution.

University of Florida, Graduate School, College of Pharmacy, Programs in Forensic Science, Gainesville, FL 32611. Offers clinical toxicology (Certificate); drug chemistry (Certificate); environmental forensics (Certificate); forensic death investigation (Certificate); forensic DNA and serology (MSP, Certificate); forensic drug chemistry (MSP); forensic science (MSP); forensic toxicology (Certificate). Part-time and evening/weekend programs available. Postbaccalaureate distance learning degree programs offered (no on-campus study). *Faculty:* 13 full-time (3 women). *Students:* 23 full-time (18 women), 184 part-time (142 women); includes 36 minority (18 Black or African American, non-Hispanic/Latino; 2 American Indian or Alaska Native, non-Hispanic/Latino; 4 Asian, non-Hispanic/Latino; 12 Hispanic/Latino), 10 international. Average age

32. In 2013, 100 master's awarded. *Degree requirements:* For master's, comprehensive exam. *Entrance requirements:* For master's, GRE General Test, minimum GPA of 3.0. Additional exam requirements/recommendations for international students: Required—TOEFL (minimum score 550 paper-based; 80 iBT), IELTS (minimum score 6). Application fee: $30. *Expenses:* Tuition, state resident: full-time $12,640. Tuition, nonresident: full-time $30,000. *Financial support:* Applicants required to submit FAFSA. *Unit head:* Dr. Ian Tibbett, Director, 352-273-6871, Fax: 352-273-8716, E-mail: itebbett@ufl.edu. *Application contact:* Dr. Ian Tibbett, Director, 352-273-6871, Fax: 352-273-8716, E-mail: itebbett@ufl.edu.
Website: http://www.forensicscience.ufl.edu/

University of Guelph, Graduate Studies, Ontario Agricultural College, Department of Environmental Biology, Guelph, ON N1G 2W1, Canada. Offers entomology (M Sc, PhD); environmental microbiology and biotechnology (M Sc, PhD); environmental toxicology (M Sc, PhD); plant and forest systems (M Sc, PhD); plant pathology (M Sc, PhD). Part-time programs available. *Degree requirements:* For master's, thesis; for doctorate, comprehensive exam, thesis/dissertation. *Entrance requirements:* For master's, minimum 75% average during previous 2 years of course work; for doctorate, minimum 75% average. Additional exam requirements/recommendations for international students: Required—TOEFL or IELTS. Electronic applications accepted. *Faculty research:* Entomology, environmental microbiology and biotechnology, environmental toxicology, forest ecology, plant pathology.

University of Guelph, Ontario Veterinary College and Graduate Studies, Graduate Programs in Veterinary Sciences, Department of Biomedical Sciences, Guelph, ON N1G 2W1, Canada. Offers morphology (M Sc, DV Sc, PhD); neuroscience (M Sc, DV Sc, PhD); pharmacology (M Sc, DV Sc, PhD); physiology (M Sc, DV Sc, PhD); toxicology (M Sc, DV Sc, PhD). Part-time programs available. *Degree requirements:* For master's, thesis; for doctorate, comprehensive exam, thesis/dissertation. *Entrance requirements:* For master's, honors B Sc, minimum 75% average in last 20 courses; for doctorate, M Sc with thesis from accredited institution. Additional exam requirements/recommendations for international students: Required—TOEFL (minimum score 550 paper-based; 89 iBT). Electronic applications accepted. *Faculty research:* Cellular morphology; endocrine, vascular and reproductive physiology; clinical pharmacology; veterinary toxicology; developmental biology, neuroscience.

University of Guelph, Ontario Veterinary College, Interdepartmental Program in Toxicology, Guelph, ON N1G 2W1, Canada. Offers M Sc, PhD. Part-time programs available. *Degree requirements:* For master's, thesis (for some programs); for doctorate, comprehensive exam, thesis/dissertation. *Entrance requirements:* For master's, B Sc; for doctorate, M Sc. Additional exam requirements/recommendations for international students: Required—TOEFL (minimum score 550 paper-based; 89 iBT).

University of Illinois at Chicago, College of Pharmacy and Graduate College, Graduate Programs in Pharmacy, Program in Forensic Science, Chicago, IL 60607-7128. Offers forensic toxicology (MS). *Students:* 7 full-time (4 women); includes 2 minority (1 Black or African American, non-Hispanic/Latino; 1 Asian, non-Hispanic/Latino). Average age 30. 39 applicants, 33% accepted, 4 enrolled. In 2013, 4 master's awarded. *Degree requirements:* For master's, thesis. *Entrance requirements:* For master's, GRE General Test. Additional exam requirements/recommendations for international students: Required—TOEFL. *Application deadline:* For fall admission, 1/1 for domestic students, 2/15 for international students. Application fee: $40 ($50 for international students). *Expenses:* Tuition, state resident: full-time $11,066; part-time $3689 per term. Tuition, nonresident: full-time $23,064; part-time $7688 per term. *Required fees:* $3004; $1190 per term. Tuition and fees vary according to course level and program. *Financial support:* In 2013–14, 13 students received support. Fellowships with full tuition reimbursements available, research assistantships with full tuition reimbursements available, teaching assistantships with full tuition reimbursements available, career-related internships or fieldwork, Federal Work-Study, institutionally sponsored loans, and tuition waivers (full) available. Financial award application deadline: 2/1; financial award applicants required to submit FAFSA. *Faculty research:* Interpretation of physical evidence, utilization of physical evidence, analytical toxicology of controlled substances, automated fingerprint systems, dye and ink characterizations. *Unit head:* Prof. Albert Karl Larsen, Director, Forensic Science Graduate Studies, 312-996-2250, E-mail: forensicdgs@uic.edu. *Application contact:* Jackie Perry, Graduate College Receptionist, 312-413-2550, Fax: 312-413-0185, E-mail: gradcoll@uic.edu.
Website: http://www.uic.edu/pharmacy/depts/Forensic_Science/

The University of Iowa, Graduate College, Program in Human Toxicology, Iowa City, IA 52242-1316. Offers MS, PhD. *Degree requirements:* For master's, thesis; for doctorate, comprehensive exam, thesis/dissertation. *Entrance requirements:* For master's and doctorate, GRE General Test, minimum GPA of 3.0. Additional exam requirements/recommendations for international students: Required—TOEFL (minimum score 600 paper-based; 100 iBT). Electronic applications accepted.

The University of Kansas, Graduate Studies, School of Pharmacy, Department of Pharmacology and Toxicology, Program in Pharmacology and Toxicology, Lawrence, KS 66045. Offers MS, PhD. *Faculty:* 12. *Students:* 14 full-time (all women), 11 international. Average age 24. 41 applicants, 15% accepted, 4 enrolled. In 2013, 4 doctorates awarded. Terminal master's awarded for partial completion of doctoral program. *Degree requirements:* For master's, comprehensive exam, thesis; for doctorate, comprehensive exam, thesis/dissertation. *Entrance requirements:* For master's, GRE, bachelor's degree in related field, 3 letters of recommendation, resume or curriculum vitae, official transcripts, 1-2 page personal statement; for doctorate, GRE (minimum score: 600 verbal, 600 quantitative, 4.5 analytical), bachelor's degree in related field, 3 letters of recommendation, resume or curriculum vitae, official transcripts, 1-2 page personal statement. Additional exam requirements/recommendations for international students: Required—TOEFL (minimum score 600 paper-based; 100 iBT). *Application deadline:* For fall admission, 1/15 for domestic students, 2/1 for international students. Applications are processed on a rolling basis. Application fee: $55 ($65 for international students). Electronic applications accepted. *Financial support:* Fellowships with full tuition reimbursements and research assistantships with full tuition reimbursements available. Financial award application deadline: 2/1. *Faculty research:* Neurodegeneration, diabetes, neurological disorders, neuropharmacology, drug metabolism. *Unit head:* Nancy Muma, Chair, 785-864-4002, Fax: 785-864-5219, E-mail: nmuma@ku.edu. *Application contact:* Debbie Thompson, Administrative Associate, 785-864-4002, E-mail: djthompson@ku.edu.
Website: http://www.pharmtox.pharm.ku.edu

The University of Kansas, University of Kansas Medical Center, School of Medicine, Department of Pharmacology, Toxicology and Therapeutics, Kansas City, KS 66160. Offers pharmacology (MA, MS, PhD); toxicology (MS, PhD); MD/MS; MD/PhD. *Faculty:* 18. *Students:* 26 full-time (12 women); includes 3 minority (1 Black or African American, non-Hispanic/Latino; 2 Two or more races, non-Hispanic/Latino), 12 international. Average age 29. In 2013, 6 doctorates awarded. Terminal master's awarded for partial completion of doctoral program. *Degree requirements:* For master's, comprehensive exam, thesis; for doctorate, one foreign language, comprehensive exam, thesis/dissertation. *Entrance requirements:* For master's and doctorate, GRE General Test. Additional exam requirements/recommendations for international students: Required—TOEFL. *Application deadline:* For fall admission, 1/15 priority date for domestic students. Applications are processed on a rolling basis. Application fee: $0. Electronic applications accepted. *Financial support:* Fellowships with full tuition reimbursements, research assistantships with full tuition reimbursements, teaching assistantships with full tuition reimbursements, Federal Work-Study, scholarships/grants, traineeships, and unspecified assistantships available. Support available to part-time students. Financial award application deadline: 3/1; financial award applicants required to submit FAFSA. *Faculty research:* Liver nuclear receptors, hepatobiliary transporters, pharmacogenomics, estrogen-induced carcinogenesis, neuropharmacology of pain and depression. *Total annual research expenditures:* $6.3 million. *Unit head:* Dr. Hartmut Jaeschke, Professor and Chair, 913-588-7969, Fax: 913-588-7501, E-mail: hjaeschke@kumc.edu. *Application contact:* Chair, Departmental Graduate Committee, 913-588-7140, Fax: 913-588-7501.
Website: http://www.kumc.edu/school-of-medicine/pharmacology-toxicology-and-therapeutics.html

University of Kentucky, Graduate School, Graduate School Programs from the College of Medicine, Program in Toxicology, Lexington, KY 40506-0032. Offers MS, PhD. Terminal master's awarded for partial completion of doctoral program. *Degree requirements:* For master's, comprehensive exam, thesis optional; for doctorate, comprehensive exam, thesis/dissertation. *Entrance requirements:* For master's, GRE General Test, minimum undergraduate GPA of 2.75; for doctorate, GRE General Test, minimum graduate GPA of 3.0. Additional exam requirements/recommendations for international students: Required—TOEFL (minimum score 550 paper-based). Electronic applications accepted. *Faculty research:* Chemical carcinogenesis, immunotoxicology, neurotoxicology, metabolism and disposition, gene regulation.

University of Louisiana at Monroe, Graduate School, College of Health and Pharmaceutical Sciences, School of Pharmacy, Monroe, LA 71209-0001. Offers pharmacy (PhD); toxicology (PhD). *Accreditation:* ACPE. *Degree requirements:* For doctorate, comprehensive exam, thesis/dissertation. *Entrance requirements:* For doctorate, GRE General Test, minimum undergraduate GPA of 2.5. Additional exam requirements/recommendations for international students: Required—TOEFL (minimum score 500 paper-based; 61 iBT). *Application deadline:* For fall admission, 3/1 for domestic and international students; for winter admission, 12/14 for domestic students; for spring admission, 9/1 for domestic and international students. Applications are processed on a rolling basis. Application fee: $20 ($30 for international students). Electronic applications accepted. *Expenses:* Tuition, state resident: full-time $6607. Tuition, nonresident: full-time $17,179. Full-time tuition and fees vary according to program. *Financial support:* Research assistantships, Federal Work-Study, and unspecified assistantships available. Financial award application deadline: 4/1; financial award applicants required to submit FAFSA. *Unit head:* Dr. Benny L. Blaylock, Dean, 318-342-1603, E-mail: blaylock@ulm.edu. *Application contact:* Dr. Paul W. Sylvester, Director, Research and Graduate Studies, 318-342-1958, Fax: 318-342-1606, E-mail: sylvester@ulm.edu.
Website: http://www.ulm.edu/pharmacy/

University of Louisville, School of Medicine, Department of Pharmacology and Toxicology, Louisville, KY 40292-0001. Offers MS, PhD, MD/PhD. *Students:* 26 full-time (16 women), 15 part-time (2 women); includes 5 minority (4 Black or African American, non-Hispanic/Latino; 1 Asian, non-Hispanic/Latino), 10 international. Average age 28. 63 applicants, 21% accepted, 10 enrolled. In 2013, 2 master's awarded. Terminal master's awarded for partial completion of doctoral program. *Degree requirements:* For master's, thesis; for doctorate, comprehensive exam, thesis/dissertation. *Entrance requirements:* For master's and doctorate, GRE General Test (minimum score of 1000 verbal and quantitative), minimum GPA of 3.0. Additional exam requirements/recommendations for international students: Required—TOEFL. *Application deadline:* For fall admission, 1/15 priority date for domestic and international students. Applications are processed on a rolling basis. Application fee: $60. Electronic applications accepted. *Expenses:* Tuition, state resident: full-time $10,788; part-time $599 per credit hour. Tuition, nonresident: full-time $22,446; part-time $1247 per credit hour. *Required fees:* $196. Tuition and fees vary according to program and reciprocity agreements. *Financial support:* Fellowships with full tuition reimbursements and research assistantships with full tuition reimbursements available. Financial award application deadline: 4/15. *Faculty research:* Molecular pharmacogenetics; epidemiology; functional genomics; genetic predisposition to chemical carcinogenesis and drug toxicity; mechanisms of oxidative stress; alcohol-induced hepatitis, pancreatitis, and hepatocellular carcinoma; molecular and cardiac toxicology; molecular biology and genetics of DNA damage and repair in humans; mechanisms of chemoresistance; arsenic toxicity and cell cycle disruption; molecular pharmacology of novel G protein-coupled receptors. *Unit head:* Dr. David W. Hein, Chair, 502-852-5141, Fax: 502-852-7868, E-mail: dhein@louisville.edu. *Application contact:* Heddy R. Rubin, Information Contact, 502-852-5741, Fax: 502-852-7868, E-mail: hrrubi01@gwise.louisville.edu.

University of Maine, Graduate School, Graduate School of Biomedical Science and Engineering, Orono, ME 04469. Offers bioinformatics (PSM); biomedical engineering (PhD); cell and molecular biology (PhD); neuroscience (PhD); toxicology (PhD). *Faculty:* 39 full-time (10 women), 31 part-time/adjunct (8 women). *Students:* 31 full-time (18 women), 5 part-time (4 women), 11 international. Average age 30. 57 applicants, 16% accepted, 7 enrolled. In 2013, 5 doctorates awarded. *Degree requirements:* For doctorate, comprehensive exam, thesis/dissertation. *Entrance requirements:* For doctorate, GRE General Test, master's degree. Additional exam requirements/recommendations for international students: Required—TOEFL. *Application deadline:* For fall admission, 1/1 for domestic students. Application fee: $65. *Expenses:* Tuition, state resident: full-time $7524. Tuition, nonresident: full-time $23,112. *Required fees:* $1970. *Financial support:* In 2013–14, 16 students received support, including 1 fellowship with full tuition reimbursement available (averaging $18,000 per year), 13 research assistantships with full tuition reimbursements available (averaging $21,000 per year), 2 teaching assistantships (averaging $20,000 per year). *Faculty research:* Biomedical engineering, toxicology, neuroscience, cell and molecular biology, bioinformatics. *Total annual research expenditures:* $650,000. *Unit head:* Dr. David Neivandt, Director, 207-581-2803. *Application contact:* Scott G. Delcourt, Associate Dean of the Graduate School, 207-581-3291, Fax: 207-581-3232, E-mail: graduate@maine.edu.
Website: http://gsbse.umaine.edu/

The University of Manchester, Faculty of Life Sciences, Manchester, United Kingdom. Offers adaptive organismal biology (M Phil, PhD); animal biology (M Phil, PhD); biochemistry (M Phil, PhD); bioinformatics (M Phil, PhD); biomolecular sciences (M Phil, PhD); biotechnology (M Phil, PhD); cell biology (M Phil, PhD); cell matrix research (M Phil, PhD); channels and transporters (M Phil, PhD); developmental biology (M Phil, PhD); Egyptology (M Phil, PhD); environmental biology (M Phil, PhD); evolutionary biology (M Phil, PhD); gene expression (M Phil, PhD); genetics (M Phil, PhD); history of science, technology and medicine (M Phil, PhD); immunology (M Phil, PhD); integrative neurobiology and behavior (M Phil, PhD); membrane trafficking (M Phil, PhD); microbiology (M Phil, PhD); molecular and cellular neuroscience (M Phil, PhD); molecular biology (M Phil, PhD); molecular cancer studies (M Phil, PhD); neuroscience (M Phil, PhD); ophthalmology (M Phil, PhD); optometry (M Phil, PhD); organelle function

(M Phil, PhD); pharmacology (M Phil, PhD); physiology (M Phil, PhD); plant sciences (M Phil, PhD); stem cell research (M Phil, PhD); structural biology (M Phil, PhD); systems neuroscience (M Phil, PhD); toxicology (M Phil, PhD).

University of Maryland, Baltimore, Graduate School, Graduate Program in Life Sciences, Program in Toxicology, Baltimore, MD 21201. Offers MS, PhD, MD/MS, MD/PhD. Part-time programs available. *Students:* 24 full-time (14 women), 8 part-time (4 women); includes 5 minority (2 Black or African American, non-Hispanic/Latino; 3 Asian, non-Hispanic/Latino), 12 international. Average age 29. 42 applicants, 24% accepted, 1 enrolled. In 2013, 3 master's, 2 doctorates awarded. *Degree requirements:* For doctorate, comprehensive exam, thesis/dissertation. *Entrance requirements:* For master's and doctorate, GRE General Test, GRE Subject Test, minimum GPA of 3.0. Additional exam requirements/recommendations for international students: Required—TOEFL (minimum score 550 paper-based; 80 iBT); Recommended—IELTS (minimum score 7). *Application deadline:* For fall admission, 2/1 for domestic students, 1/15 for international students. Application fee: $75. Electronic applications accepted. *Financial support:* In 2013–14, research assistantships with partial tuition reimbursements (averaging $25,000 per year) were awarded; fellowships also available. Financial award application deadline: 3/1; financial award applicants required to submit FAFSA. *Unit head:* Dr. Katherine S. Squibb, Director, 410-706-8196, E-mail: ksquibb@umaryland.edu. *Application contact:* Linda Horne, Program Coordinator, 410-706-5422, E-mail: lhorne@som.umaryland.edu.
Website: http://toxicology.umaryland.edu

University of Maryland, Baltimore, School of Medicine, Department of Epidemiology and Public Health, Baltimore, MD 21201. Offers biostatistics (MS); clinical research (MS); epidemiology and preventive medicine (MPH, MS, PhD); gerontology (PhD); human genetics and genomic medicine (MS, PhD); molecular epidemiology (MS, PhD); toxicology (MS, PhD); JD/MS; MD/PhD; MS/PhD. *Accreditation:* CEPH. Part-time programs available. *Students:* 83 full-time (56 women), 76 part-time (51 women); includes 51 minority (26 Black or African American, non-Hispanic/Latino; 20 Asian, non-Hispanic/Latino; 5 Hispanic/Latino), 27 international. Average age 32. 225 applicants, 44% accepted, 37 enrolled. In 2013, 18 master's, 1 doctorate awarded. *Degree requirements:* For doctorate, comprehensive exam, thesis/dissertation. *Entrance requirements:* For master's and doctorate, GRE General Test. Additional exam requirements/recommendations for international students: Required—TOEFL (minimum score 550 paper-based; 80 iBT); Recommended—IELTS (minimum score 7). *Application deadline:* For fall admission, 1/15 for domestic and international students. Application fee: $75. Electronic applications accepted. *Expenses:* Contact institution. *Financial support:* In 2013–14, research assistantships with partial tuition reimbursements (averaging $25,000 per year) were awarded; fellowships, Federal Work-Study, scholarships/grants, and unspecified assistantships also available. Financial award application deadline: 3/1; financial award applicants required to submit FAFSA. *Unit head:* Dr. Laura Hungerford, Program Director, 410-706-8492, Fax: 410-706-4225. *Application contact:* Jessica Kelley, Program Coordinator, 410-706-8492, Fax: 410-706-4225, E-mail: jkelley@som.umaryland.edu.
Website: http://medschool.umaryland.edu/Epidemiology/

University of Maryland Eastern Shore, Graduate Programs, Department of Natural Sciences, Program in Toxicology, Princess Anne, MD 21853-1299. Offers MS, PhD.

University of Michigan, School of Public Health, Department of Environmental Health Sciences, Ann Arbor, MI 48109. Offers environmental health sciences (MS, PhD); environmental quality and health (MPH); human nutrition (MPH); industrial hygiene (MPH, MS); nutritional sciences (MS); occupational and environmental epidemiology (MPH); toxicology (MPH, MS, PhD). *Accreditation:* CEPH (one or more programs are accredited). Part-time programs available. Terminal master's awarded for partial completion of doctoral program. *Degree requirements:* For master's, thesis (for some programs); for doctorate, thesis/dissertation, preliminary exam, oral defense of dissertation. *Entrance requirements:* For master's and doctorate, GRE General Test and/or MCAT. Additional exam requirements/recommendations for international students: Required—TOEFL (minimum score 560 paper-based; 100 iBT). Electronic applications accepted. Tuition and fees vary according to course level, course load, degree level, program and student level. *Faculty research:* Toxicology, occupational hygiene, nutrition, environmental exposure sciences, environmental epidemiology.

University of Minnesota, Duluth, Graduate School, Program in Toxicology, Duluth, MN 55812-2496. Offers MS, PhD. MS, PhD offered jointly with University of Minnesota, Twin Cities Campus. Terminal master's awarded for partial completion of doctoral program. *Degree requirements:* For master's, thesis; for doctorate, comprehensive exam, thesis/dissertation, written and oral preliminary and final exams. *Entrance requirements:* For master's and doctorate, GRE General Test, BS in basic science; full year each of biology, chemistry, and physics; mathematics coursework through calculus. Additional exam requirements/recommendations for international students: Required—TOEFL (minimum score 550 paper-based; 79 iBT). Electronic applications accepted. *Faculty research:* Structure activity correlations, neurotoxicity, aquatic toxicology, biochemical mechanisms, immunotoxicology.

University of Minnesota, Duluth, Medical School, Department of Biochemistry, Molecular Biology and Biophysics, Duluth, MN 55812-2496. Offers biochemistry, molecular biology and biophysics (MS); biology and biophysics (PhD); social, administrative, and clinical pharmacy (MS, PhD); toxicology (MS, PhD). Terminal master's awarded for partial completion of doctoral program. *Degree requirements:* For master's, comprehensive exam, thesis; for doctorate, comprehensive exam, thesis/dissertation. *Entrance requirements:* For master's and doctorate, GRE General Test. Additional exam requirements/recommendations for international students: Required—TOEFL. Electronic applications accepted. *Faculty research:* Intestinal cancer biology; hepatotoxins and mitochondriopathies; toxicology; cell cycle regulation in stem cells; neurobiology of brain development, trace metal function and blood-brain barrier; hibernation biology.

University of Minnesota, Twin Cities Campus, School of Public Health, Division of Environmental Health Sciences, Area in Environmental Toxicology, Minneapolis, MN 55455-0213. Offers MPH, MS, PhD. *Degree requirements:* For doctorate, thesis/dissertation. *Entrance requirements:* For master's and doctorate, GRE General Test. Electronic applications accepted.

University of Mississippi Medical Center, School of Graduate Studies in the Health Sciences, Department of Pharmacology and Toxicology, Jackson, MS 39216-4505. Offers PhD. *Faculty:* 18 full-time (3 women). *Students:* 13 full-time (8 women); includes 2 minority (both Black or African American, non-Hispanic/Latino), 5 international. Average age 28. 11 applicants, 18% accepted, 2 enrolled. In 2013, 3 doctorates awarded. *Degree requirements:* For doctorate, comprehensive exam, thesis/dissertation, first authored publication. *Entrance requirements:* For doctorate, GRE General Test, minimum GPA of 3.0. Additional exam requirements/recommendations for international students: Required—TOEFL (minimum score 550 paper-based, 79 iBT), IELTS or PTE. *Application deadline:* For fall admission, 2/17 priority date for domestic and international students. Application fee: $25. Electronic applications accepted. *Financial support:* In 2013–14, 11 research assistantships (averaging $24,150 per year) were awarded; health care benefits also available. Financial award application deadline: 4/1. *Faculty research:* Renal and cardiovascular pharmacology, genetic basis of cardio-renal diseases, diabetes, obesity, metabolic diseases, cancer chemotherapy. *Total annual research expenditures:* $4.3 million. *Unit head:* Dr. Richard J. Roman, Chair, 601-984-1600, Fax: 601-984-1602, E-mail: rroman@umc.edu. *Application contact:* Barbara Westerfield, Director, Student Records/Registrar, 601-984-1080, Fax: 601-984-1079, E-mail: bwesterfield@umc.edu.
Website: http://www.umc.edu/Education/Schools/Medicine/Basic_Science/Pharmacology_and_Toxicology/Academics(Pharmacology_and_Toxicology)/Academics_Home.aspx

University of Missouri–Kansas City, School of Pharmacy, Kansas City, MO 64110-2499. Offers pharmaceutical sciences (PhD); pharmacology and toxicology (PhD); pharmacy (Pharm D). PhD offered through School of Graduate Studies. *Accreditation:* ACPE (one or more programs are accredited). Postbaccalaureate distance learning degree programs offered (minimal on-campus study). *Faculty:* 54 full-time (26 women), 6 part-time/adjunct (3 women). *Students:* 424 full-time (252 women); includes 77 minority (14 Black or African American, non-Hispanic/Latino; 2 American Indian or Alaska Native, non-Hispanic/Latino; 43 Asian, non-Hispanic/Latino; 10 Hispanic/Latino; 1 Native Hawaiian or other Pacific Islander, non-Hispanic/Latino; 7 Two or more races, non-Hispanic/Latino), 1 international. Average age 26. 365 applicants, 37% accepted, 136 enrolled. In 2013, 122 doctorates awarded. *Degree requirements:* For doctorate, comprehensive exam (for some programs), thesis/dissertation (for some programs). *Entrance requirements:* For doctorate, PCAT (for Pharm D). Additional exam requirements/recommendations for international students: Required—TOEFL (minimum score 550 paper-based; 80 iBT). *Application deadline:* For fall admission, 3/1 for domestic and international students. Applications are processed on a rolling basis. Application fee: $45 ($50 for international students). Electronic applications accepted. *Expenses:* Contact institution. *Financial support:* In 2013–14, 26 research assistantships with full and partial tuition reimbursements (averaging $11,585 per year), 26 teaching assistantships with full tuition reimbursements (averaging $14,213 per year) were awarded; career-related internships or fieldwork, Federal Work-Study, institutionally sponsored loans, tuition waivers (full and partial), and unspecified assistantships also available. Financial award application deadline: 3/1; financial award applicants required to submit FAFSA. *Faculty research:* Bio-organic and medicinal chemistry, drug delivery, pharmaceutics, molecular neurobiology, neurology. *Unit head:* Dr. Russell B. Melchert, Dean, 816-235-1609, Fax: 816-235-5190, E-mail: melchertr@umkc.edu. *Application contact:* Shelly M. Janasz, Director, Student Services, 816-235-2400, Fax: 816-235-5190, E-mail: janaszs@umkc.edu.
Website: http://pharmacy.umkc.edu/

The University of Montana, Graduate School, College of Health Professions and Biomedical Sciences, Skaggs School of Pharmacy, Department of Biomedical and Pharmaceutical Sciences, Missoula, MT 59812-0002. Offers biomedical sciences (PhD); medicinal chemistry (MS, PhD); molecular and cellular toxicology (MS, PhD); neuroscience (PhD); pharmaceutical sciences (MS). *Accreditation:* ACPE. *Degree requirements:* For master's, oral defense of thesis; for doctorate, research dissertation defense. *Entrance requirements:* For master's and doctorate, GRE General Test. Additional exam requirements/recommendations for international students: Required—TOEFL (minimum score 540 paper-based). *Application deadline:* For fall admission, 3/1 priority date for domestic and international students. Applications are processed on a rolling basis. Application fee: $45. Electronic applications accepted. *Financial support:* Teaching assistantships with full and partial tuition reimbursements, Federal Work-Study, scholarships/grants, and tuition waivers (full and partial) available. Financial award application deadline: 3/1. *Faculty research:* Cardiovascular pharmacology, medicinal chemistry, neurosciences, environmental toxicology, pharmacogenetics, cancer. *Unit head:* Dr. Richard Bridges, Chair, 406-243-4972, E-mail: richard.bridges@umontana.edu. *Application contact:* Information Contact, E-mail: gradschl@mso.umt.edu.
Website: http://www.umt.edu/pharmsci/

University of Nebraska–Lincoln, Graduate College, Interdepartmental Area of Environmental Health, Occupational Health and Toxicology, Lincoln, NE 68588. Offers MS, PhD. MS, PhD offered jointly with University of Nebraska Medical Center. *Entrance requirements:* Additional exam requirements/recommendations for international students: Required—TOEFL (minimum score 550 paper-based). Electronic applications accepted.

University of New Mexico, School of Medicine, Program in Biomedical Sciences, Albuquerque, NM 87131-5196. Offers biochemistry and molecular biology (MS, PhD); cell biology and physiology (MS, PhD); clinical and translational science (Certificate); molecular genetics and microbiology (MS, PhD); neuroscience (MS, PhD); pathology (MS, PhD); toxicology (MS, PhD); university science teaching (Certificate). Part-time programs available. *Students:* 73 full-time (39 women), 14 part-time (9 women); includes 24 minority (1 Black or African American, non-Hispanic/Latino; 1 American Indian or Alaska Native, non-Hispanic/Latino; 2 Asian, non-Hispanic/Latino; 17 Hispanic/Latino; 1 Native Hawaiian or other Pacific Islander, non-Hispanic/Latino; 2 Two or more races, non-Hispanic/Latino), 16 international. Average age 29. 89 applicants, 20% accepted, 17 enrolled. In 2013, 7 master's, 17 doctorates awarded. Terminal master's awarded for partial completion of doctoral program. *Degree requirements:* For master's, thesis; for doctorate, comprehensive exam, thesis/dissertation, qualifying exam at the end of year 1/core curriculum. *Entrance requirements:* For master's and doctorate, GRE General Test, minimum undergraduate GPA of 3.0. Additional exam requirements/recommendations for international students: Required—TOEFL. *Application deadline:* For fall admission, 3/1 priority date for domestic and international students. Applications are processed on a rolling basis. Application fee: $50. Electronic applications accepted. *Financial support:* In 2013–14, 94 students received support, including 28 fellowships with full and partial tuition reimbursements available (averaging $22,000 per year), 73 research assistantships with full tuition reimbursements available (averaging $23,000 per year), 8 teaching assistantships (averaging $2,800 per year); career-related internships or fieldwork, Federal Work-Study, institutionally sponsored loans, scholarships/grants, traineeships, health care benefits, and unspecified assistantships also available. Financial award application deadline: 1/1; financial award applicants required to submit FAFSA. *Faculty research:* Infectious disease/immunity, cancer biology, cardiovascular and metabolic diseases, brain and behavioral illness, environmental health. *Unit head:* Dr. Helen J. Hathaway, Program Director, 505-272-1887, Fax: 505-272-2412, E-mail: hhathaway@salud.unm.edu. *Application contact:* Mary Fenton, Admissions Coordinator, 505-272-1887, Fax: 505-272-2412, E-mail: mfenton@salud.unm.edu.
Website: http://hsc.unm.edu/research/brep/bsgpabout.shtm

The University of North Carolina at Chapel Hill, School of Medicine, Curriculum in Toxicology, Chapel Hill, NC 27599. Offers MS, PhD. Terminal master's awarded for partial completion of doctoral program. *Degree requirements:* For master's, comprehensive exam, thesis; for doctorate, comprehensive exam, thesis/dissertation. *Entrance requirements:* For doctorate, GRE General Test. Electronic applications accepted. *Faculty research:* Molecular and cellular toxicology, carcinogenesis, neurotoxicology, pulmonary toxicology, developmental toxicology.

University of Prince Edward Island, Atlantic Veterinary College, Graduate Program in Veterinary Medicine, Charlottetown, PE C1A 4P3, Canada. Offers anatomy (M Sc, PhD); bacteriology (M Sc, PhD); clinical pharmacology (M Sc, PhD); clinical sciences (M Sc, PhD); epidemiology (M Sc, PhD), including reproduction; fish health (M Sc, PhD); food animal nutrition (M Sc, PhD); immunology (M Sc, PhD); microanatomy (M Sc, PhD); parasitology (M Sc, PhD); pathology (M Sc, PhD); pharmacology (M Sc, PhD); physiology (M Sc, PhD); toxicology (M Sc, PhD); veterinary science (M Vet Sc); virology (M Sc, PhD). Part-time programs available. *Degree requirements:* For master's, thesis; for doctorate, thesis/dissertation. *Entrance requirements:* For master's, DVM, B Sc honors degree, or equivalent; for doctorate, M Sc. Additional exam requirements/recommendations for international students: Required—TOEFL (minimum score 550 paper-based; 80 iBT). *Expenses:* Contact institution. *Faculty research:* Animal health management, infectious diseases, fin fish and shellfish health, basic biomedical sciences, ecosystem health.

University of Puerto Rico, Medical Sciences Campus, School of Medicine, Division of Graduate Studies, Department of Pharmacology and Toxicology, San Juan, PR 00936-5067. Offers MS, PhD. *Degree requirements:* For master's, one foreign language, thesis; for doctorate, one foreign language, comprehensive exam, thesis/dissertation. *Entrance requirements:* For master's and doctorate, GRE General Test, GRE Subject Test, interview, minimum GPA of 3.0, 3 letters of recommendation. Electronic applications accepted. *Faculty research:* Cardiovascular, central nervous system, and endocrine pharmacology; anti-cancer drugs; sodium pump; mitochondrial DNA repair; Huntington's disease.

University of Rhode Island, Graduate School, College of Pharmacy, Department of Biomedical and Pharmaceutical Sciences, Kingston, RI 02881. Offers medicinal chemistry and pharmacognosy (MS, PhD); pharmaceutics and pharmacokinetics (MS, PhD); pharmacology and toxicology (MS, PhD). Part-time programs available. *Faculty:* 21 full-time (7 women). *Students:* 37 full-time (14 women), 15 part-time (7 women); includes 3 minority (1 Black or African American, non-Hispanic/Latino; 1 Asian, non-Hispanic/Latino; 1 Two or more races, non-Hispanic/Latino), 29 international. In 2013, 3 master's, 18 doctorates awarded. *Entrance requirements:* For master's and doctorate, GRE (minimum new/old format scores: Verbal 350/143; Quantitative 550/146; Analytical, 3.0), 2 letters of recommendation. Additional exam requirements/recommendations for international students: Required—TOEFL (minimum score 550 paper-based). *Application deadline:* For fall admission, 7/15 for domestic students, 2/1 for international students. Application fee: $65. Electronic applications accepted. *Expenses:* Tuition, state resident: full-time $11,532; part-time $641 per credit. Tuition, nonresident: full-time $23,606; part-time $1311 per credit. *Required fees:* $1388; $36 per credit. $35 per semester. One-time fee: $130. *Financial support:* In 2013–14, 8 research assistantships with full and partial tuition reimbursements (averaging $12,147 per year), 13 teaching assistantships with full and partial tuition reimbursements (averaging $13,579 per year) were awarded. Financial award application deadline: 2/1; financial award applicants required to submit FAFSA. *Faculty research:* Chemical carcinogenesis with a major emphasis on the structural and synthetic aspects of DNA-adduct formation, drug-drug/herb interaction, drug-genetic interaction, signaling of nuclear receptors, transcriptional regulation, oncogenesis. *Total annual research expenditures:* $5.8 million. *Unit head:* Dr. Bingfang Yan, Chair, 401-874-5032, Fax: 401-874-2181, E-mail: byan@uri.edu. *Application contact:* Graduate Admissions, 401-874-2872, E-mail: gradadm@etal.uri.edu.
Website: http://www.uri.edu/pharmacy/departments/bps/index.shtml

University of Rochester, School of Medicine and Dentistry, Graduate Programs in Medicine and Dentistry, Department of Environmental Medicine, Programs in Toxicology, Rochester, NY 14627. Offers PhD. *Degree requirements:* For doctorate, thesis/dissertation, qualifying exam. *Entrance requirements:* For doctorate, GRE General Test. *Expenses: Tuition:* Full-time $44,580; part-time $1394 per credit hour. *Required fees:* $492.

University of Saskatchewan, College of Graduate Studies and Research, Toxicology Centre, Saskatoon, SK S7N 5A2, Canada. Offers M Sc, PhD, Diploma. *Degree requirements:* For master's, thesis; for doctorate, thesis/dissertation. *Entrance requirements:* Additional exam requirements/recommendations for international students: Required—TOEFL. *Expenses: Tuition, area resident:* Full-time $3585 Canadian dollars; part-time $585 Canadian dollars per course. Tuition, nonresident: part-time $877 Canadian dollars per course. *International tuition:* $5377 Canadian dollars full-time. *Required fees:* $889.51 Canadian dollars.

University of South Alabama, Graduate School, Program in Environmental Toxicology, Mobile, AL 36688-0002. Offers MS. *Faculty:* 1 full-time (0 women). *Students:* 15 full-time (10 women), 4 part-time (1 woman); includes 2 minority (both Black or African American, non-Hispanic/Latino), 3 international. 12 applicants, 50% accepted, 6 enrolled. In 2013, 6 master's awarded. *Degree requirements:* For master's, thesis. *Entrance requirements:* For master's, GRE. *Application deadline:* For fall admission, 7/15 for domestic students, 6/15 for international students; for spring admission, 12/1 for domestic students, 11/1 for international students. Application fee: $35. *Expenses:* Tuition, state resident: full-time $8976; part-time $374 per credit hour. Tuition, nonresident: full-time $17,952; part-time $748 per credit hour. *Unit head:* Dr. B. Keith Harrison, Dean of the Graduate School, 251-460-6310, E-mail: kharrison@southalabama.edu. *Application contact:* Dr. David Forbes, Director of Graduate Studies, 251-460-6181, E-mail: dforbes@southalabama.edu.

University of Southern California, Graduate School, School of Pharmacy, Graduate Programs in Molecular Pharmacology and Toxicology, Los Angeles, CA 90033. Offers pharmacology and pharmaceutical sciences (MS, PhD). Terminal master's awarded for partial completion of doctoral program. *Degree requirements:* For master's, comprehensive exam, thesis, 24 units of formal course work, excluding research and seminar courses; for doctorate, comprehensive exam, thesis/dissertation, 24 units of formal course work, excluding research and seminar courses. *Entrance requirements:* For master's and doctorate, GRE. Additional exam requirements/recommendations for international students: Required—TOEFL (minimum score 603 paper-based; 100 iBT). Electronic applications accepted. *Expenses:* Contact institution. *Faculty research:* Degenerative diseases, toxicology of drugs.

The University of Texas at Austin, Graduate School, College of Pharmacy, Graduate Programs in Pharmacy, Austin, TX 78712-1111. Offers health outcomes and pharmacy practice (PhD); health outcomes and pharmacy practice (MS); medicinal chemistry (PhD); pharmaceutics (PhD); pharmacology and toxicology (PhD); pharmacotherapy (MS, PhD); translational science (PhD). PhD in translational science offered jointly with The University of Texas Health Science Center at San Antonio and The University of Texas at San Antonio. *Degree requirements:* For master's, thesis; for doctorate, thesis/dissertation. *Entrance requirements:* For master's and doctorate, GRE General Test. Electronic applications accepted. *Faculty research:* Synthetic medical chemistry, synthetic molecular biology, bio-organic chemistry, pharmacoeconomics, pharmacy practice.

The University of Texas Health Science Center at San Antonio, School of Health Professions, San Antonio, TX 78229-3900. Offers occupational therapy (MOT); physical therapy (DPT); physician assistant studies (MS); toxicology (MS). *Accreditation:* AOTA; APTA; ARC-PA. *Faculty:* 75 full-time (31 women), 49 part-time/adjunct (19 women). *Students:* 353 full-time (258 women), 2 part-time (1 woman); includes 180 minority (15 Black or African American, non-Hispanic/Latino; 29 Asian, non-Hispanic/Latino; 129 Hispanic/Latino; 1 Native Hawaiian or other Pacific Islander, non-Hispanic/Latino; 6 Two or more races, non-Hispanic/Latino), 3 international. Average age 28. 605 applicants, 21% accepted, 125 enrolled. In 2013, 73 master's, 63 doctorates awarded. *Degree requirements:* For master's, comprehensive exam, thesis (for some programs); for doctorate, comprehensive exam. *Entrance requirements:* For master's, GRE (for toxicology), minimum GPA of 3.0 and bachelor's degree in clinical laboratory science or closely-related science discipline (for MS in toxicology); minimum GPA of 3.0, bachelor's degree, PA shadowing, and community service (for MS in physician assistant); for doctorate, GRE, minimum GPA of 3.0, bachelor's degree, PT shadowing, observation hours. Additional exam requirements/recommendations for international students: Required—TOEFL (minimum score 560 paper-based). *Application deadline:* For fall admission, 6/1 for domestic and international students; for spring admission, 10/1 for domestic and international students. Application fee: $60. Electronic applications accepted. *Financial support:* In 2013–14, 219 students received support. Federal Work-Study, scholarships/grants, and stipends, department payments available. Financial award application deadline: 6/30; financial award applicants required to submit FAFSA. *Total annual research expenditures:* $760,563. *Unit head:* Dr. Susan Dollar, Assistant Dean, 210-567-4837, Fax: 210-567-4828, E-mail: dollar@uthscsa.edu. *Application contact:* Dr. David L. Henzi, Assistant Dean for Admissions, 210-567-4818, Fax: 210-567-4828, E-mail: henzi@uthscsa.edu.
Website: http://www.uthscsa.edu/shp/

The University of Texas Medical Branch, Graduate School of Biomedical Sciences, Program in Pharmacology and Toxicology, Galveston, TX 77555. Offers pharmacology (MS); pharmacology and toxicology (PhD). *Degree requirements:* For master's, thesis or alternative; for doctorate, thesis/dissertation. *Entrance requirements:* For master's and doctorate, GRE General Test. Additional exam requirements/recommendations for international students: Required—TOEFL (minimum score 550 paper-based).

University of the Sciences, College of Graduate Studies, Program in Pharmacology and Toxicology, Philadelphia, PA 19104-4495. Offers pharmacology (MS, PhD); toxicology (MS, PhD). *Faculty:* 5 full-time (0 women). *Students:* 10 full-time (6 women), 11 part-time (7 women); includes 2 minority (1 Asian, non-Hispanic/Latino; 1 Hispanic/Latino), 5 international. Average age 30. 14 applicants, 29% accepted, 3 enrolled. In 2013, 1 master's, 1 doctorate awarded. Terminal master's awarded for partial completion of doctoral program. *Degree requirements:* For master's, thesis; for doctorate, comprehensive exam, thesis/dissertation. *Entrance requirements:* For master's and doctorate, GRE General Test. Additional exam requirements/recommendations for international students: Required—TOEFL, TWE. *Application deadline:* For fall admission, 5/1 for international students; for winter admission, 10/1 for international students; for spring admission, 3/1 for international students. Applications are processed on a rolling basis. Application fee: $50. *Expenses:* Contact institution. *Financial support:* In 2013–14, 14 students received support, including 8 teaching assistantships with tuition reimbursements available (averaging $21,694 per year); institutionally sponsored loans and tuition waivers (partial) also available. Financial award application deadline: 5/1. *Faculty research:* Autonomic, cardiovascular, cellular, and molecular pharmacology; mechanisms of carcinogenesis; drug metabolism. *Unit head:* Dr. Shenaz Tejani-Butt, Associate Dean, Graduate Studies, 215-596-8597, E-mail: graduate@usciences.edu. *Application contact:* Christopher Miciek, Associate Director, Graduate Studies, 215-596-8597, E-mail: c.miciek@usciences.edu.

University of Utah, Graduate School, College of Pharmacy, Department of Pharmacology and Toxicology, Salt Lake City, UT 84112. Offers PhD. *Faculty:* 14 full-time (4 women), 6 part-time/adjunct (2 women). *Students:* 9 full-time (6 women), 4 international. Average age 28. 34 applicants. In 2013, 3 doctorates awarded. Terminal master's awarded for partial completion of doctoral program. *Degree requirements:* For doctorate, comprehensive exam, thesis/dissertation, final exam. *Entrance requirements:* For doctorate, GRE General Test, BS in biology, chemistry, neuroscience. Additional exam requirements/recommendations for international students: Required—TOEFL (minimum score 550 paper-based; 80 iBT), IELTS (minimum score 6.5). *Application deadline:* For fall admission, 12/15 for domestic and international students. Application fee: $55 ($65 for international students). Electronic applications accepted. *Expenses:* Tuition, state resident: full-time $5259. Tuition, nonresident: full-time $18,569. *Required fees:* $841. Tuition and fees vary according to course load. *Financial support:* In 2013–14, 13 students received support, including fellowships with full tuition reimbursements available (averaging $25,000 per year), research assistantships with full tuition reimbursements available (averaging $25,000 per year); tuition waivers (full) also available. Financial award application deadline: 1/15. *Faculty research:* Neuropharmacology of anti-seizure drugs and drugs of abuse, drug metabolism, signal transduction pathways and oncogenic processes, drug analyses in biological samples, natural products drug discovery. *Total annual research expenditures:* $5.4 million. *Unit head:* Dr. William R. Crowley, Chairman, 801-581-6287, Fax: 801-585-5111, E-mail: william.crowley@deans.pharm.utah.edu. *Application contact:* Linda Wright, Program Assistant, 801-581-6281, Fax: 801-585-5111, E-mail: linda.wright@utah.edu.
Website: http://www.pharmacy.utah.edu/pharmtox/

University of Washington, Graduate School, School of Public Health, Department of Environmental and Occupational Health Sciences, Seattle, WA 98195. Offers environmental and occupational health (MPH); environmental and occupational hygiene (PhD); environmental health (MS); occupational and environmental exposure sciences (MS); occupational and environmental medicine (MPH); toxicology (MS, PhD); MPH/MPA; MS/MPA. Part-time programs available. *Faculty:* 34 full-time (9 women), 7 part-time/adjunct (3 women). *Students:* 65 full-time (42 women), 9 part-time (6 women); includes 22 minority (3 Black or African American, non-Hispanic/Latino; 3 American Indian or Alaska Native, non-Hispanic/Latino; 16 Asian, non-Hispanic/Latino), 6 international. Average age 30. 114 applicants, 32% accepted, 22 enrolled. In 2013, 16 master's, 6 doctorates awarded. Terminal master's awarded for partial completion of doctoral program. *Degree requirements:* For master's, comprehensive exam, thesis (for some programs), project or thesis; for doctorate, comprehensive exam, thesis/dissertation. *Entrance requirements:* For master's, GRE General Test, one year each of physics, general chemistry, and biology; two quarters of organic chemistry; one quarter of calculus; for doctorate, GRE General Test, minimum GPA of 3.0, prerequisite course work in biology, chemistry, physics, calculus. Additional exam requirements/recommendations for international students: Required—TOEFL (minimum score 580 paper-based; 92 iBT). *Application deadline:* For fall admission, 12/1 for domestic and international students. Application fee: $85. Electronic applications accepted. *Financial support:* In 2013–14, 70 students received support, including 65 fellowships with full tuition reimbursements available (averaging $42,000 per year), 111 research assistantships with full tuition reimbursements available (averaging $42,000 per year), 19 teaching assistantships with full tuition reimbursements available (averaging $42,000 per year); career-related internships or fieldwork, institutionally sponsored loans, scholarships/grants, traineeships, health care benefits, and unspecified assistantships also available. Financial award application deadline: 12/1. *Faculty research:* Developmental and behavioral toxicology, biochemical toxicology, exposure assessment, hazardous waste, industrial chemistry. *Unit head:* Dr. David Kalman, Chair,

206-543-6991, Fax: 206-543-0477. *Application contact:* Rory A. Murphy, Manager, Student Services, 206-543-6991, Fax: 206-543-0477, E-mail: ehgrad@u.washington.edu.
Website: http://depts.washington.edu/envhlth/

University of Wisconsin–Madison, School of Medicine and Public Health, Molecular and Environmental Toxicology Center, Madison, WI 53706. Offers MS, PhD. *Faculty:* 84 full-time (26 women), 1 part-time/adjunct (0 women). *Students:* 32 full-time (17 women); includes 12 minority (2 Black or African American, non-Hispanic/Latino; 3 Asian, non-Hispanic/Latino; 6 Hispanic/Latino; 1 Native Hawaiian or other Pacific Islander, non-Hispanic/Latino), 6 international. Average age 28. 38 applicants, 29% accepted, 6 enrolled. In 2013, 2 master's, 6 doctorates awarded. Terminal master's awarded for partial completion of doctoral program. *Degree requirements:* For doctorate, thesis/dissertation. *Entrance requirements:* For master's and doctorate, bachelor's degree in science-related field. Additional exam requirements/recommendations for international students: Required—TOEFL. *Application deadline:* For fall admission, 12/15 priority date for domestic and international students. Application fee: $56. Electronic applications accepted. *Expenses:* Tuition, state resident: full-time $10,728; part-time $790 per credit. Tuition, nonresident: full-time $24,054; part-time $1623 per credit. *Required fees:* $1130; $119 per credit. *Financial support:* In 2013–14, 5 research assistantships with tuition reimbursements (averaging $25,000 per year) were awarded; fellowships with tuition reimbursements, traineeships, health care benefits, and unspecified assistantships also available. *Faculty research:* Toxicology cancer, genetics, cell cycle, xenobiotic metabolism. *Unit head:* Dr. Christopher Bradfield, Director, 608-262-2024, E-mail: bradfield@oncology.wisc.edu. *Application contact:* Eileen M. Stevens, Program Administrator, 608-263-4580, Fax: 608-262-5245, E-mail: emstevens@wisc.edu.
Website: http://www.med.wisc.edu/metc/

Utah State University, School of Graduate Studies, College of Agriculture, Program in Toxicology, Logan, UT 84322. Offers MS, PhD. Terminal master's awarded for partial completion of doctoral program. *Degree requirements:* For master's, thesis; for doctorate, thesis/dissertation. *Entrance requirements:* For master's and doctorate, GRE General Test, minimum GPA of 3.0. Additional exam requirements/recommendations for international students: Required—TOEFL. *Faculty research:* Free-radical mechanisms, toxicity of iron, carcinogenesis of natural compounds, molecular mechanisms of retinoid toxicity, aflatoxins.

Virginia Commonwealth University, Graduate School, College of Humanities and Sciences, Department of Forensic Science, Richmond, VA 23284-9005. Offers forensic biology (MS); forensic chemistry/drugs and toxicology (MS); forensic chemistry/trace (MS); forensic physical evidence (MS). Part-time programs available. *Entrance requirements:* For master's, GRE General Test, bachelor's degree in a natural science discipline, including forensic science, or a degree with equivalent work. Additional exam requirements/recommendations for international students: Required—TOEFL (minimum score 600 paper-based; 100 iBT) or IELTS (minimum score 6.5). Electronic applications accepted.

Virginia Commonwealth University, Medical College of Virginia-Professional Programs, School of Medicine, School of Medicine Graduate Programs, Department of Pharmacology and Toxicology, Richmond, VA 23284-9005. Offers neuroscience (PhD); pharmacology (Certificate); pharmacology and toxicology (MS, PhD); MD/PhD. Terminal master's awarded for partial completion of doctoral program. *Degree requirements:* For master's, thesis; for doctorate, thesis/dissertation, comprehensive oral and written exams. *Entrance requirements:* For master's and doctorate, GRE or MCAT. Additional exam requirements/recommendations for international students: Required—TOEFL (minimum score 600 paper-based; 100 iBT). Electronic applications accepted. *Faculty research:* Drug abuse, drug metabolism, pharmacodynamics, peptide synthesis, receptor mechanisms.

Wayne State University, Eugene Applebaum College of Pharmacy and Health Sciences, Department of Pharmaceutical Sciences, Detroit, MI 48202. Offers medicinal chemistry (MS, PhD); pharmaceutics (MS, PhD); pharmacology/toxicology (MS, PhD). *Accreditation:* ACPE (one or more programs are accredited). Part-time programs available. *Faculty:* 17 full-time (3 women). *Students:* 33 full-time (15 women), 2 part-time (1 woman); includes 3 minority (1 American Indian or Alaska Native, non-Hispanic/Latino; 2 Asian, non-Hispanic/Latino), 29 international. Average age 25. 205 applicants, 8% accepted, 9 enrolled. In 2013, 1 master's, 3 doctorates awarded. *Degree requirements:* For master's, thesis; for doctorate, thesis/dissertation. *Entrance requirements:* For master's, GRE General Test, admission to the Graduate School, bachelor's degree, three letters of recommendation, personal statement; for doctorate, GRE General Test, admission to the Graduate School; bachelor's or master's degree in one of the behavioral, biological, pharmaceutical or physical sciences; minimum undergraduate GPA of 3.0; three letters of recommendation. Additional exam requirements/recommendations for international students: Required—TOEFL (minimum score 550 paper-based; 79 iBT), Michigan English Language Assessment Battery (minimum score 85); Recommended—IELTS (minimum score 6.5), TWE (minimum score 5.5). *Application deadline:* For fall admission, 3/1 for domestic and international students. Application fee: $0. Electronic applications accepted. *Expenses:* Contact institution. *Financial support:* In 2013–14, 13 students received support, including 2 fellowships with tuition reimbursements available (averaging $24,272 per year), 11 research assistantships with full tuition reimbursements available (averaging $24,565 per year); scholarships/grants, health care benefits, and unspecified assistantships also available. Financial award application deadline: 3/31; financial award applicants required to submit FAFSA. *Faculty research:* Mechanisms of resistance of bacteria to anti-microbial agents, drug metabolism and disposition in children, treatment strategies for stroke/neurovascular disease, prevalence and treatment of diabetes in Arab-Americans, ethnic variability in development of osteoporosis. *Unit head:* Dr. George Corcoran, Chair and Professor, 313-577-1737, E-mail: corcoran@wayne.edu. *Application contact:* 313-577-1047, E-mail: pscgrad@wayne.edu.
Website: http://www.cphs.wayne.edu/psc/index.php

Wayne State University, Graduate School, Interdisciplinary Program in Molecular and Cellular Toxicology, Detroit, MI 48201-2427. Offers MS, PhD. *Students:* 5 full-time (3 women), 4 international. Average age 26. 17 applicants, 12% accepted, 2 enrolled. *Degree requirements:* For doctorate, thesis/dissertation. *Entrance requirements:* For master's, recommendation by thesis adviser or graduate program director; for doctorate, GRE, bachelor's degree from accredited college, preferably with a background in the basic sciences; minimum undergraduate GPA of 3.0. Additional exam requirements/recommendations for international students: Required—TOEFL (minimum score 550 paper-based); Recommended—TWE (minimum score 6). *Application deadline:* For fall admission, 6/1 priority date for domestic students, 5/1 priority date for international students; for winter admission, 10/1 priority date for domestic students, 9/1 priority date for international students; for spring admission, 2/1 priority date for domestic students, 1/1 priority date for international students. Applications are processed on a rolling basis. Application fee: $50. Electronic applications accepted. *Expenses:* Tuition, state resident: part-time $554.15 per credit. Tuition, nonresident: part-time $1200.35 per credit. *Required fees:* $42.15 per credit. $268.30 per semester. Tuition and fees vary according to course load and program. *Financial support:* Fellowships with tuition reimbursements, research assistantships with tuition reimbursements, teaching assistantships with tuition reimbursements, institutionally sponsored loans, scholarships/grants, and unspecified assistantships available. Financial award application deadline: 2/1. *Faculty research:* Molecular and cellular mechanisms of chemically-induced cell injury and death; effect of xenobiotics on cell growth, proliferation, transformation and differentiation; regulation of gene expression; cell signaling; global gene expression profiling. *Unit head:* Dr. Melissa Runge-Morris, Professor and Director, Institute of Environmental Health Sciences, 313-577-5598, E-mail: m.runge-morris@wayne.edu. *Application contact:* Graduate Admissions Office, 313-577-2170, Fax: 313-577-2903, E-mail: gradschool@wayne.edu.
Website: http://iehs.wayne.edu/education.php

West Virginia University, Davis College of Agriculture, Forestry and Consumer Sciences, Interdisciplinary Program in Genetics and Developmental Biology, Morgantown, WV 26506. Offers animal breeding (MS, PhD); biochemical and molecular genetics (MS, PhD); cytogenetics (MS, PhD); descriptive embryology (MS, PhD); developmental genetics (MS); experimental morphogenesis/teratology (MS); human genetics (MS, PhD); immunogenetics (MS, PhD); life cycles of animals and plants (MS, PhD); molecular aspects of development (MS, PhD); mutagenesis (MS, PhD); oncology (MS, PhD); plant genetics (MS, PhD); population and quantitative genetics (MS, PhD); regeneration (MS, PhD); teratology (PhD); toxicology (MS, PhD). *Degree requirements:* For master's, thesis; for doctorate, comprehensive exam, thesis/dissertation. *Entrance requirements:* For master's, GRE or MCAT, minimum GPA of 2.75. Additional exam requirements/recommendations for international students: Required—TOEFL.

West Virginia University, School of Pharmacy, Program in Pharmaceutical and Pharmacological Sciences, Morgantown, WV 26506. Offers administrative pharmacy (PhD); behavioral pharmacy (MS, PhD); biopharmaceutics/pharmacokinetics (MS, PhD); industrial pharmacy (MS); medicinal chemistry (MS, PhD); pharmaceutical chemistry (MS, PhD); pharmaceutics (MS, PhD); pharmacology and toxicology (MS); pharmacy (MS); pharmacy administration (MS). Part-time programs available. Terminal master's awarded for partial completion of doctoral program. *Degree requirements:* For master's, thesis; for doctorate, one foreign language, comprehensive exam, thesis/dissertation. *Entrance requirements:* For master's and doctorate, GRE General Test, minimum GPA of 2.75. Additional exam requirements/recommendations for international students: Required—TOEFL; Recommended—TWE. Electronic applications accepted. *Expenses:* Contact institution. *Faculty research:* Pharmaceutics, medicinal chemistry, biopharmaceutics/pharmacokinetics, health outcomes research.

Wright State University, School of Medicine, Program in Pharmacology and Toxicology, Dayton, OH 45435. Offers MS. *Degree requirements:* For master's, thesis optional.

Section 18
Physiology

This section contains a directory of institutions offering graduate work in physiology, followed by an in-depth entry submitted by an institution that chose to prepare a detailed program description. Additional information about programs listed in the directory but not augmented by an in-depth entry may be obtained by writing directly to the dean of a graduate school or chair of a department at the address given in the directory.

For programs offering related work, see also all other sections in this book. In the other guides in this series:

Graduate Programs in the Physical Sciences, Mathematics, Agricultural Sciences, the Environment & Natural Resources

See *Agricultural and Food Sciences, Chemistry,* and *Marine Sciences and Oceanography*

Graduate Programs in Engineering & Applied Sciences

See *Agricultural Engineering and Bioengineering, Biomedical Engineering and Biotechnology, Electrical and Computer Engineering,* and *Mechanical Engineering and Mechanics*

CONTENTS

Program Directories

Display and Close-Up

Cardiovascular Sciences

Albany Medical College, Center for Cardiovascular Sciences, Albany, NY 12208-3479. Offers MS, PhD. Part-time programs available. Terminal master's awarded for partial completion of doctoral program. *Degree requirements:* For master's, thesis; for doctorate, comprehensive exam, thesis/dissertation, candidacy exam, written preliminary exam, 1 published paper-peer review. *Entrance requirements:* For master's, GRE General Test, letters of recommendation; for doctorate, GRE General Test, all transcripts, letters of recommendation. Additional exam requirements/recommendations for international students: Required—TOEFL. *Faculty research:* Vascular smooth muscle, endothelial cell biology, molecular and genetic bases underlying cardiac disease, reactive oxygen and nitrogen species biology, fatty acid trafficking and fatty acid mediated transcription control.

Baylor College of Medicine, Graduate School of Biomedical Sciences, Department of Molecular Physiology and Biophysics, Houston, TX 77030-3498. Offers cardiovascular sciences (PhD); molecular physiology and biophysics (PhD); MD/PhD. *Degree requirements:* For doctorate, thesis/dissertation, public defense. *Entrance requirements:* For doctorate, GRE General Test, GRE Subject Test (strongly recommended), minimum GPA of 3.0. Additional exam requirements/recommendations for international students: Required—TOEFL. Electronic applications accepted. *Faculty research:* Cardiovascular disease; skeletal muscle disease (myasthenia gravis, muscular dystrophy, malignant hyperthermia, central core disease); cancer; Alzheimer's disease; developmental diseases of the nervous system, eye and heart; diabetes; motor neuron disease (amyotrophic lateral sclerosis and spinal muscular atrophy); asthma; autoimmune diseases.

Dartmouth College, Program in Experimental and Molecular Medicine, Cardiovascular Diseases Track, Hanover, NH 03755. Offers PhD.

Geneva College, Master of Science in Cardiovascular Science Program, Beaver Falls, PA 15010-3599. Offers MS. *Faculty:* 1 full-time (0 women), 4 part-time/adjunct (2 women). *Students:* 4 full-time (1 woman); includes 2 minority (both Asian, non-Hispanic/Latino). Average age 24. 2 applicants, 100% accepted, 2 enrolled. In 2013, 1 master's awarded. *Degree requirements:* For master's, six semesters (includes 2 summers), RCIS and RCES registry exams. *Entrance requirements:* For master's, GRE, BS in biology or related field, minimum undergraduate GPA of 3.0, two letters of reference, one-day orientation at the cardiac catheterization labs at INOVA Heart and Vascular Institute campus. Additional exam requirements/recommendations for international students: Required—TOEFL. *Application deadline:* For fall admission, 5/30 for domestic students. Applications are processed on a rolling basis. Electronic applications accepted. *Expenses:* Contact institution. *Financial support:* Application deadline: 8/1; applicants required to submit FAFSA. *Unit head:* Dr. David A. Essig, Program Coordinator, 724-847-6900, E-mail: dessig@geneva.edu. *Application contact:* Dr. David Essig, Program Coordinator, 724-847-6900, E-mail: dessig@geneva.edu.
Website: http://www.geneva.edu/object/cvt

Georgia Regents University, The Graduate School, Program in Vascular Biology, Augusta, GA 30912. Offers MS, PhD. *Faculty:* 20 full-time (4 women), 1 (woman) part-time/adjunct. *Students:* 9 full-time (7 women); includes 7 minority (1 Black or African American, non-Hispanic/Latino; 6 Asian, non-Hispanic/Latino), 7 international. Average age 26. In 2013, 3 doctorates awarded. *Degree requirements:* For doctorate, comprehensive exam, thesis/dissertation. *Entrance requirements:* For doctorate, GRE General Test. Additional exam requirements/recommendations for international students: Required—TOEFL (minimum score 550 paper-based; 79 iBT). *Application deadline:* For fall admission, 1/15 for domestic and international students. Application fee: $50. Electronic applications accepted. *Financial support:* In 2013–14, 5 fellowships with partial tuition reimbursements (averaging $26,000 per year), 19 research assistantships with partial tuition reimbursements (averaging $23,000 per year) were awarded; Federal Work-Study, institutionally sponsored loans, scholarships/grants, and traineeships also available. Support available to part-time students. Financial award application deadline: 5/31. *Faculty research:* Hypertension and renal disease, diabetes and obesity, peripheral vascular disease, acute lung injury, signal transduction. *Total annual research expenditures:* $8.3 million. *Unit head:* Dr. John D. Catravas, Professor/Director of Vascular Biology Center, 706-721-6338, Fax: 706-721-8545, E-mail: jcatrava@mail.mcg.edu. *Application contact:* Dr. Patricia L. Cameron, Acting Vice Dean, 706-721-3279, E-mail: pcameron@georgiahealth.edu.
Website: http://www.gru.edu/centers/vbc/grad_prog.php

Johns Hopkins University, Bloomberg School of Public Health, Department of Epidemiology, Baltimore, MD 21205. Offers cancer etiology and prevention (MHS, Sc M, PhD, Sc D); cardiovascular diseases (MHS, Sc M, PhD, Sc D); clinical epidemiology (MHS, Sc M, PhD, Sc D); clinical trials (PhD, Sc D); epidemiology (MHS, Sc M, Dr PH, PhD, Sc D); epidemiology of aging (MHS, Sc M, PhD, Sc D); genetic epidemiology (MHS, Sc M, PhD, Sc D); infectious disease epidemiology (MHS, Sc M, PhD, Sc D); occupational and environmental epidemiology (MHS, Sc M, PhD, Sc D). Part-time programs available. *Faculty:* 80 full-time (44 women), 82 part-time/adjunct (36 women). *Students:* 141 full-time (106 women), 20 part-time (13 women); includes 32 minority (5 Black or African American, non-Hispanic/Latino; 1 American Indian or Alaska Native, non-Hispanic/Latino; 18 Asian, non-Hispanic/Latino; 6 Hispanic/Latino; 2 Two or more races, non-Hispanic/Latino), 49 international. Average age 29. 302 applicants, 35% accepted, 63 enrolled. In 2013, 26 master's, 23 doctorates awarded. *Degree requirements:* For master's, comprehensive exam, thesis, 1-year full-time residency; for doctorate, comprehensive exam, thesis/dissertation, 2 years' full-time residency, oral and written exams, student teaching. *Entrance requirements:* For master's, GRE General Test or MCAT, 3 letters of recommendation, curriculum vitae; for doctorate, GRE General Test, minimum 1 year of work experience, 3 letters of recommendation, curriculum vitae, academic records from all schools. Additional exam requirements/recommendations for international students: Required—TOEFL (minimum score 600 paper-based; 100 iBT); Recommended—IELTS (minimum score 7.5), TWE. *Application deadline:* For fall admission, 12/1 priority date for domestic students. Applications are processed on a rolling basis. Application fee: $45. Electronic applications accepted. *Financial support:* Fellowships, Federal Work-Study, institutionally sponsored loans, scholarships/grants, traineeships, tuition waivers (partial), and stipends available. Support available to part-time students. Financial award application deadline: 3/15; financial award applicants required to submit FAFSA. *Faculty research:* Cancer and congenital malformations, nutritional epidemiology, AIDS, tuberculosis, cardiovascular disease, risk assessment. *Total annual research expenditures:* $70.1 million. *Unit head:* Dr. David D. Celentano, Chair, 410-955-3286, Fax: 410-955-0863, E-mail: dcelenta@jhsph.edu. *Application contact:* Frances S. Burman, Academic Program Manager, 410-955-3926, Fax: 410-955-0863, E-mail: fburman@jhsph.edu.
Website: http://www.jhsph.edu/dept/epi/index.html

Long Island University–LIU Post, School of Health Professions and Nursing, Department of Biomedical Sciences, Brookville, NY 11548-1300. Offers cardiovascular perfusion (MS); clinical laboratory management (MS); medical biology (MS), including hematology, immunology, medical biology, medical chemistry, medical microbiology. Part-time and evening/weekend programs available. Postbaccalaureate distance learning degree programs offered. *Degree requirements:* For master's, thesis. *Entrance requirements:* For master's, minimum GPA of 2.75 in major. Electronic applications accepted.

Loyola University Chicago, Graduate School, Marcella Niehoff School of Nursing, Adult Nurse Practitioner Program, Chicago, IL 60660. Offers adult clinical nurse practitioner (MSN); adult health (Certificate); adult nurse practitioner (MSN); cardiovascular nursing (Certificate). *Accreditation:* AACN. Part-time and evening/weekend programs available. Postbaccalaureate distance learning degree programs offered (minimal on-campus study). *Students:* 6 full-time (all women), 34 part-time (31 women); includes 8 minority (2 Black or African American, non-Hispanic/Latino; 5 Asian, non-Hispanic/Latino; 1 Hispanic/Latino). Average age 33. 41 applicants, 68% accepted, 21 enrolled. In 2013, 8 master's awarded. *Degree requirements:* For master's, comprehensive exam or oral thesis defense. *Entrance requirements:* For master's, BSN, minimum nursing GPA of 3.0, Illinois nursing license, 3 letters of recommendation, 1000 hours of experience before starting clinical. *Application deadline:* Applications are processed on a rolling basis. Application fee: $50. Electronic applications accepted. *Expenses: Tuition:* Full-time $16,740; part-time $930 per credit. *Required fees:* $135 per semester. *Financial support:* Traineeships available. *Faculty research:* Menopause. *Unit head:* Dr. Marijo Letizia, Associate Dean, 708-216-9325, Fax: 708-216-9555, E-mail: mletizi@luc.edu. *Application contact:* Amy Weatherford, Enrollment Advisor, School of Nursing, 773-508-3249, Fax: 773-508-3241, E-mail: aweatherford@luc.edu.
Website: http://www.luc.edu/nursing/index.shtml

Marquette University, Graduate School, Program in Transfusion Medicine, Milwaukee, WI 53201-1881. Offers MSTM. Program is held in collaboration with BloodCenter of Wisconsin. Part-time programs available. *Students:* 1 (woman) full-time, 3 part-time (2 women), 1 international. Average age 34. 7 applicants, 14% accepted, 1 enrolled. In 2013, 2 master's awarded. *Entrance requirements:* For master's, official transcripts from all current and previous colleges, three letters of recommendation. Additional exam requirements/recommendations for international students: Required—TOEFL. *Application deadline:* For fall admission, 4/1 for domestic and international students. Application fee: $50.
Website: http://www.bcw.edu/bcw/education/sbbprogram/mstm/index.htm

McMaster University, Faculty of Health Sciences and School of Graduate Studies, Program in Medical Sciences, Blood and Vascular Area, Hamilton, ON L8S 4M2, Canada. Offers M Sc, PhD, MD/PhD. *Degree requirements:* For master's, thesis; for doctorate, comprehensive exam, thesis/dissertation. *Entrance requirements:* For master's, honors B Sc, B+ average in related field; for doctorate, M Sc, minimum B+ average, students with proven research experience and an A average may be admitted with a B Sc degree. Additional exam requirements/recommendations for international students: Required—TOEFL (minimum score 580 paper-based; 92 iBT).

Medical University of South Carolina, College of Graduate Studies, Program in Molecular and Cellular Biology and Pathobiology, Charleston, SC 29425. Offers cancer biology (PhD); cardiovascular biology (PhD); cardiovascular imaging (PhD); cell regulation (PhD); craniofacial biology (PhD); genetics and development (PhD); marine biomedicine (PhD); DMD/PhD; MD/PhD. *Degree requirements:* For doctorate, thesis/dissertation, oral and written exams. *Entrance requirements:* For doctorate, GRE General Test, interview, minimum GPA of 3.0. Additional exam requirements/recommendations for international students: Required—TOEFL (minimum score 600 paper-based; 100 iBT). Electronic applications accepted.

Memorial University of Newfoundland, Faculty of Medicine and School of Graduate Studies, Graduate Programs in Medicine, Division of Biomedical Sciences, St. John's, NL A1C 5S7, Canada. Offers cancer (M Sc, PhD); cardiovascular (M Sc, PhD); immunology (M Sc, PhD); neuroscience (M Sc, PhD). Part-time programs available. *Degree requirements:* For master's, thesis; for doctorate, comprehensive exam, thesis/dissertation, oral defense of thesis. *Entrance requirements:* For master's, MD or B Sc; for doctorate, MD or M Sc. Additional exam requirements/recommendations for international students: Required—TOEFL. *Faculty research:* Neuroscience, immunology, cardiovascular, and cancer.

Midwestern University, Glendale Campus, College of Health Sciences, Arizona Campus, Program in Cardiovascular Science, Glendale, AZ 85308. Offers MCVS. *Expenses:* Contact institution.

Milwaukee School of Engineering, Department of Electrical Engineering and Computer Science, Program in Perfusion, Milwaukee, WI 53202-3109. Offers MS. Part-time and evening/weekend programs available. *Faculty:* 1 full-time (0 women), 8 part-time/adjunct (3 women). *Students:* 12 full-time (4 women). Average age 33. 46 applicants, 15% accepted, 7 enrolled. In 2013, 4 master's awarded. *Degree requirements:* For master's, comprehensive exam, thesis, exam. *Entrance requirements:* For master's, GRE General Test or GMAT (percentiles must average 50% or better), BS in appropriate discipline (biomedical engineering, biology, biomedical sciences, etc.), 3 letters of recommendation, personal interview, observation of 2 perfusion clinical cases. Additional exam requirements/recommendations for international students: Required—TOEFL (minimum score 79 iBT), IELTS (minimum score 6.5). *Application deadline:* Applications are processed on a rolling basis. Application fee: $0. Electronic applications accepted. Application fee is waived when completed online. *Expenses: Tuition:* Full-time $6939; part-time $771 per credit. *Financial support:* Career-related internships or fieldwork, institutionally sponsored loans, and scholarships/grants available. Financial award application deadline: 3/15; financial award applicants required to submit FAFSA. *Faculty research:* Heart medicine. *Unit head:* Dr. Ronald Gerrits, Director, 414-277-7561, Fax: 414-277-7494, E-mail: gerrits@msoe.edu. *Application contact:* Katie Weinschenk, Graduate Program Associate, 800-321-6763, Fax: 414-277-7208, E-mail: weinschenk@msoe.edu.
Website: http://www.msoe.edu/academics/academic_departments/eecs/msp/

Queen's University at Kingston, School of Graduate Studies, Faculty of Health Sciences, Department of Anatomy and Cell Biology, Kingston, ON K7L 3N6, Canada. Offers biology of reproduction (M Sc, PhD); cancer (M Sc, PhD); cardiovascular pathophysiology (M Sc, PhD); cell and molecular biology (M Sc, PhD); drug metabolism (M Sc, PhD); endocrinology (M Sc, PhD); motor control (M Sc, PhD); neural regeneration (M Sc, PhD); neurophysiology (M Sc, PhD). Part-time programs available. *Degree requirements:* For master's, thesis; for doctorate, one foreign language, comprehensive exam, thesis/dissertation. *Entrance requirements:* Additional exam requirements/recommendations for international students: Required—TOEFL.

Electronic applications accepted. *Faculty research:* Human kinetics, neuroscience, reproductive biology, cardiovascular.

Quinnipiac University, School of Health Sciences, Program in Cardiovascular Perfusion, Hamden, CT 06518-1940. Offers MHS. *Faculty:* 1 full-time (0 women), 3 part-time/adjunct (0 women). *Students:* 14 full-time (10 women); includes 3 minority (2 Black or African American, non-Hispanic/Latino; 1 Asian, non-Hispanic/Latino). 34 applicants, 38% accepted, 9 enrolled. In 2013, 3 master's awarded. *Entrance requirements:* For master's, bachelor's degree in science or health-related discipline from an accredited American or Canadian college or university; 2 years of health care work experience; interview. *Application deadline:* For fall admission, 2/1 priority date for domestic students, 4/30 for international students. Applications are processed on a rolling basis. Application fee: $45. Electronic applications accepted. *Expenses: Tuition:* Part-time $920 per credit. *Required fees:* $37 per credit. *Financial support:* In 2013–14, 5 students received support. Career-related internships or fieldwork, Federal Work-Study, scholarships/grants, and unspecified assistantships available. Support available to part-time students. Financial award application deadline: 6/1; financial award applicants required to submit FAFSA. *Faculty research:* Methods of preventing systemic inflammatory response syndrome (SIRS) during extracorporeal circulation of blood, investigations into the role of P-selectin in causing monocyte-platelet interaction, effect of simulated cardiopulmonary bypass on platelets and other formed elements in the blood. *Unit head:* Dr. Michael Smith, Director, 203-582-3427, E-mail: michael.smith@quinnipiac.edu. *Application contact:* Office of Graduate Admissions, 800-462-1944, Fax: 208-582-3443, E-mail: graduate@quinnipiac.edu.
Website: http://www.quinnipiac.edu/gradperfusion

State University of New York Upstate Medical University, College of Graduate Studies, Major Research Areas of the College of Graduate Studies, Syracuse, NY 13210-2334.

Université Laval, Faculty of Medicine, Post-Professional Programs in Medical Studies, Québec, QC G1K 7P4, Canada. Offers anatomy–pathology (DESS); anesthesiology (DESS); cardiology (DESS); care of older people (Diploma); clinical research (DESS); community health (DESS); dermatology (DESS); diagnostic radiology (DESS); emergency medicine (Diploma); family medicine (DESS); general surgery (DESS); geriatrics (DESS); hematology (DESS); internal medicine (DESS); maternal and fetal medicine (Diploma); medical biochemistry (DESS); medical microbiology and infectious diseases (DESS); medical oncology (DESS); nephrology (DESS); neurology (DESS); neurosurgery (DESS); obstetrics and gynecology (DESS); ophthalmology (DESS); orthopedic surgery (DESS); oto-rhino-laryngology (DESS); palliative medicine (Diploma); pediatrics (DESS); plastic surgery (DESS); psychiatry (DESS); pulmonary medicine (DESS); radiology–oncology (DESS); thoracic surgery (DESS); urology (DESS). *Degree requirements:* For other advanced degree, comprehensive exam. *Entrance requirements:* For degree, knowledge of French. Electronic applications accepted.

University of Calgary, Cumming School of Medicine and Faculty of Graduate Studies, Program in Cardiovascular and Respiratory Sciences, Calgary, AB T2N 1N4, Canada. Offers M Sc, PhD. *Degree requirements:* For master's, thesis; for doctorate, thesis/dissertation, candidacy exam. *Entrance requirements:* For master's and doctorate, minimum GPA of 3.2. Additional exam requirements/recommendations for international students: Required—TOEFL (minimum score 600 paper-based). Electronic applications accepted. *Faculty research:* Cardiac mechanics, physiology and pharmacology; lung mechanics, physiology and pathophysiology; smooth muscle biochemistry; physiology and pharmacology.

University of Guelph, Ontario Veterinary College and Graduate Studies, Graduate Programs in Veterinary Sciences, Department of Clinical Studies, Guelph, ON N1G 2W1, Canada. Offers anesthesiology (M Sc, DV Sc); cardiology (DV Sc, Diploma); clinical studies (Diploma); dermatology (M Sc); diagnostic imaging (M Sc, DV Sc); emergency/critical care (M Sc, DV Sc, Diploma); medicine (M Sc, DV Sc); neurology (M Sc, DV Sc); ophthalmology (M Sc, DV Sc); surgery (M Sc, DV Sc). *Degree requirements:* For master's, thesis; for doctorate, comprehensive exam, thesis/dissertation. *Entrance requirements:* Additional exam requirements/recommendations for international students: Required—TOEFL (minimum score 550 paper-based), IELTS (minimum score 6.5). Electronic applications accepted. *Faculty research:* Orthopedics, respirology, oncology, exercise physiology, cardiology.

University of Mary, School of Health Sciences, Program in Respiratory Therapy, Bismarck, ND 58504-9652. Offers MS. *Entrance requirements:* For master's, minimum GPA of 3.0, 3 letters of reference, interview. Additional exam requirements/recommendations for international students: Required—TOEFL (minimum score 500 paper-based; 71 iBT). Electronic applications accepted.

The University of South Dakota, Graduate School, School of Medicine and Graduate School, Biomedical Sciences Graduate Program, Cardiovascular Research Program, Vermillion, SD 57069-2390. Offers MS, PhD. Terminal master's awarded for partial completion of doctoral program. *Degree requirements:* For master's, thesis; for doctorate, comprehensive exam, thesis/dissertation. *Entrance requirements:* For master's and doctorate, GRE General Test, minimum GPA of 3.0. Additional exam requirements/recommendations for international students: Required—TOEFL (minimum score 550 paper-based; 80 iBT), IELTS (minimum score 6). Electronic applications accepted. *Expenses:* Contact institution. *Faculty research:* Cardiovascular disease.

University of South Florida, Innovative Education Graduate Certificate Programs, Tampa, FL 33620-9951. *Unit head:* Kathy Barnes, Interdisciplinary Programs Coordinator, 813-974-8031, Fax: 813-974-7061, E-mail: barnesk@usf.edu. *Application contact:* Karen Tylinski, Metro Initiatives, 813-974-9943, Fax: 813-974-7061, E-mail: ktylinsk@usf.edu.
Website: http://www.usf.edu/innovative-education/

The University of Toledo, College of Graduate Studies, College of Medicine and Life Sciences, Department of Physiology and Pharmacology, Toledo, OH 43606-3390. Offers cardiovascular and metabolic diseases (MSBS, PhD); MD/MSBS; MD/PhD. *Faculty:* 21. *Students:* 21 full-time (8 women), 5 part-time (2 women); includes 1 minority (Black or African American, non-Hispanic/Latino), 21 international. Average age 28. 16 applicants, 69% accepted, 6 enrolled. In 2013, 6 doctorates awarded. Terminal master's awarded for partial completion of doctoral program. *Degree requirements:* For master's, thesis, qualifying exam; for doctorate, thesis/dissertation, qualifying exam. *Entrance requirements:* For master's and doctorate, GRE, minimum undergraduate GPA of 3.0, three letters of recommendation, statement of purpose, transcripts from all prior institutions attended, resume. Additional exam requirements/recommendations for international students: Required—TOEFL (minimum score 550 paper-based; 80 iBT). *Application deadline:* For fall admission, 1/15 priority date for domestic and international students. Application fee: $45 ($75 for international students). Electronic applications accepted. *Financial support:* In 2013–14, 25 research assistantships with full tuition reimbursements (averaging $22,032 per year) were awarded; Federal Work-Study, institutionally sponsored loans, scholarships/grants, tuition waivers (full), and unspecified assistantships also available. *Unit head:* Dr. Andrew Beavis, Chair, 419-383-4396, E-mail: andrew.beavis@utoledo.edu. *Application contact:* Admissions Analyst, 419-383-4112, Fax: 419-383-6140.
Website: http://www.utoledo.edu/med/grad/

Molecular Physiology

Baylor College of Medicine, Graduate School of Biomedical Sciences, Department of Molecular Physiology and Biophysics, Houston, TX 77030-3498. Offers cardiovascular sciences (PhD); molecular physiology and biophysics (PhD); MD/PhD. *Degree requirements:* For doctorate, thesis/dissertation, public defense. *Entrance requirements:* For doctorate, GRE General Test, GRE Subject Test (strongly recommended), minimum GPA of 3.0. Additional exam requirements/recommendations for international students: Required—TOEFL. Electronic applications accepted. *Faculty research:* Cardiovascular disease; skeletal muscle disease (myasthenia gravis, muscular dystrophy, malignant hyperthermia, central core disease); cancer; Alzheimer's disease; developmental diseases of the nervous system, eye and heart; diabetes; motor neuron disease (amyotrophic lateral sclerosis and spinal muscular atrophy); asthma; autoimmune diseases.

Case Western Reserve University, School of Medicine and School of Graduate Studies, Graduate Programs in Medicine, Department of Physiology and Biophysics, Cleveland, OH 44106. Offers cell and molecular physiology (MS); cell physiology (PhD); molecular/cellular biophysics (PhD); physiology and biophysics (PhD); systems physiology (PhD); MD/PhD. Terminal master's awarded for partial completion of doctoral program. *Degree requirements:* For master's, thesis; for doctorate, thesis/dissertation. *Entrance requirements:* For master's, GRE General Test, minimum GPA of 3.28; for doctorate, GRE General Test, minimum GPA of 3.6. Additional exam requirements/recommendations for international students: Required—TOEFL. Electronic applications accepted. *Faculty research:* Cardiovascular physiology, calcium metabolism, epithelial cell biology.

Loyola University Chicago, Graduate School, Programs in Cell and Molecular Physiology, Chicago, IL 60660. Offers MS, PhD. *Faculty:* 14 full-time (4 women), 19 part-time/adjunct (4 women). *Students:* 34 full-time (5 women); includes 9 minority (2 Black or African American, non-Hispanic/Latino; 3 Asian, non-Hispanic/Latino; 1 Hispanic/Latino; 3 Two or more races, non-Hispanic/Latino). Average age 24. 239 applicants, 24% accepted, 28 enrolled. In 2013, 17 master's, 3 doctorates awarded. *Degree requirements:* For master's, thesis; for doctorate, comprehensive exam, thesis/dissertation. *Entrance requirements:* For master's, GRE General Test or MCAT; for doctorate, GRE General Test. Additional exam requirements/recommendations for international students: Required—TOEFL. *Application deadline:* For fall admission, 5/15 for domestic and international students. Application fee: $0. Electronic applications accepted. *Expenses: Tuition:* Full-time $16,740; part-time $930 per credit. *Required fees:* $135 per semester. *Financial support:* In 2013–14, 5 fellowships with tuition reimbursements (averaging $23,000 per year), 9 research assistantships with tuition reimbursements (averaging $23,000 per year) were awarded. *Faculty research:* Cardiovascular system: neural and metabolic control of circulation, ion channels, excitation contraction coupling, molecular cloning; neuroscience: neuroendocrine, neuronal excitability studies. *Unit head:* Dr. Pieter P. deTombe, Chair, 708-216-6305, Fax: 708-216-6308, E-mail: pdetombe@luc.edu. *Application contact:* Dr. Erika S. Piedras-Renteria, Graduate Program Director, 708-216-9508, Fax: 708-216-6308, E-mail: rmestri@luc.edu.

Rutgers, The State University of New Jersey, New Brunswick, Graduate School-New Brunswick, Program in Endocrinology and Animal Biosciences, Piscataway, NJ 08854-8097. Offers MS, PhD. Terminal master's awarded for partial completion of doctoral program. *Degree requirements:* For master's, thesis; for doctorate, comprehensive exam, thesis/dissertation. *Entrance requirements:* For master's and doctorate, GRE General Test. Additional exam requirements/recommendations for international students: Required—TOEFL. Electronic applications accepted. *Faculty research:* Comparative and behavioral endocrinology, epigenetic regulation of the endocrine system, exercise physiology and immunology, fetal and neonatal developmental programming, mammary gland biology and breast cancer, neuroendocrinology and alcohol studies, reproductive and developmental toxicology.

Stony Brook University, State University of New York, Stony Brook University Medical Center, Health Sciences Center, School of Medicine and Graduate School, Graduate Programs in Medicine, Department of Physiology and Biophysics, Stony Brook, NY 11794. Offers PhD. *Faculty:* 17 full-time (6 women). *Students:* 27 full-time (16 women), 2 part-time (both women); includes 16 minority (11 Black or African American, non-Hispanic/Latino; 2 Asian, non-Hispanic/Latino; 3 Hispanic/Latino), 3 international. Average age 29. 4 applicants, 25% accepted, 1 enrolled. In 2013, 1 doctorate awarded. *Degree requirements:* For doctorate, comprehensive exam, thesis/dissertation. *Entrance requirements:* For doctorate, GRE General Test, GRE Subject Test, BS in related field, minimum GPA of 3.0, recommendation. Additional exam requirements/recommendations for international students: Required—TOEFL (minimum score 550 paper-based). *Application deadline:* For fall admission, 1/15 for domestic students; for spring admission, 10/1 for domestic students. Application fee: $100. *Expenses:* Tuition, state resident: full-time $9870; part-time $411 per credit. Tuition, nonresident: full-time $18,350; part-time $765 per credit. *Financial support:* In 2013–14, 4 fellowships, 10 research assistantships were awarded; teaching assistantships and Federal Work-Study also available. Financial award application deadline: 3/15. *Faculty research:* Cellular electrophysiology, membrane permeation and transport, metabolic endocrinology. *Total annual research expenditures:* $7.3 million. *Unit head:* Dr. Peter Brink, Chair, 631-444-3124, Fax: 631-444-3432, E-mail: peter.brink@stonybrook.edu. *Application contact:* Odalis Hernandez, Coordinator, 631-444-3057, Fax: 631-444-3432, E-mail: odalis.hernandez@stonybrook.edu.
Website: http://pnb.informatics.stonybrook.edu/

Thomas Jefferson University, Jefferson Graduate School of Biomedical Sciences, Program in Molecular Physiology and Biophysics, Philadelphia, PA 19107. Offers PhD. *Faculty:* 10 full-time (5 women). *Students:* 1 full-time (0 women). *Degree requirements:*

Molecular Physiology

For doctorate, comprehensive exam, thesis/dissertation. *Entrance requirements:* For doctorate, GRE General Test, minimum GPA of 3.2. Additional exam requirements/recommendations for international students: Required—TOEFL (minimum score 100 iBT). *Application deadline:* For fall admission, 1/15 for domestic and international students. *Financial support:* In 2013–14, 1 fellowship with full tuition reimbursement (averaging $56,052 per year) was awarded; Federal Work-Study, institutionally sponsored loans, scholarships/grants, traineeships, and stipends also available. Support available to part-time students. Financial award application deadline: 5/1; financial award applicants required to submit FAFSA. *Faculty research:* Cardiovascular physiology, smooth muscle physiology, pathophysiology of myocardial ischemia, endothelial cell physiology, molecular biology of ion channel physiology. *Total annual research expenditures:* $893,526. *Unit head:* Dr. Thomas M. Butler, Program Director, 215-503-6583, E-mail: thomas.butler@jefferson.edu. *Application contact:* Marc E. Stearns, Director of Admissions, 215-503-0155, Fax: 215-503-3433, E-mail: jgsbs-info@jefferson.edu.
Website: http://www.jefferson.edu/jmc/departments/physiology.html

Tufts University, Sackler School of Graduate Biomedical Sciences, Cellular and Molecular Physiology Program, Medford, MA 02155. Offers PhD. *Faculty:* 24 full-time (7 women). *Students:* 15 full-time (6 women); includes 2 minority (1 Asian, non-Hispanic/Latino; 1 Hispanic/Latino), 4 international. Average age 28. In 2013, 1 doctorate awarded. Terminal master's awarded for partial completion of doctoral program. *Degree requirements:* For doctorate, comprehensive exam, thesis/dissertation. *Entrance requirements:* For doctorate, GRE General Test, 3 letters of reference. Additional exam requirements/recommendations for international students: Required—TOEFL (minimum score 600 paper-based; 100 iBT). *Application deadline:* For fall admission, 12/15 for domestic and international students. Application fee: $70. Electronic applications accepted. *Financial support:* In 2013–14, 15 students received support, including 15 research assistantships with full tuition reimbursements available (averaging $31,000 per year); health care benefits also available. *Faculty research:* Molecular signaling networks controlling cell growth and motility, molecular and cellular dissection of protein- and lipid-based trafficking pathways, signaling within and among neurons and glia. *Unit head:* Dr. Ira Herman, Director, 617-636-0291. *Application contact:* Kellie Melchin, Associate Director of Admissions, 617-636-6767, Fax: 617-636-0375, E-mail: sackler-school@tufts.edu.
Website: http://sackler.tufts.edu/Academics/Degree-Programs/PhD-Programs/Cellular-and-Molecular-Physiology

The University of Alabama at Birmingham, Graduate Programs in Joint Health Sciences, Program in Cellular and Molecular Physiology, Birmingham, AL 35294. Offers PhD. *Degree requirements:* For doctorate, comprehensive exam, thesis/dissertation.

University of California, Los Angeles, Graduate Division, College of Letters and Science, Program in Molecular, Cellular and Integrative Physiology, Los Angeles, CA 90095. Offers PhD. *Degree requirements:* For doctorate, thesis/dissertation, oral and written qualifying exams. *Entrance requirements:* For doctorate, GRE General Test; GRE Subject Test (biology or applicant's undergraduate major), bachelor's degree; minimum undergraduate GPA of 3.0 (or its equivalent if letter grade system not used); interview. Additional exam requirements/recommendations for international students: Required—TOEFL. Electronic applications accepted.

University of Chicago, Division of Biological Sciences, Neuroscience Graduate Programs, Chicago, IL 60637-1513. Offers cellular and molecular physiology (PhD); computational neuroscience (PhD); integrative neuroscience (PhD), including cell physiology, pharmacological and physiological sciences; neurobiology (PhD). *Degree requirements:* For doctorate, thesis/dissertation, ethics class, 2 teaching assistantships. *Entrance requirements:* For doctorate, GRE General Test. Additional exam requirements/recommendations for international students: Required—TOEFL (minimum score 600 paper-based; 104 iBT), IELTS (minimum score 7). Electronic applications accepted.

University of Chicago, Division of Biological Sciences, Program in Cellular and Molecular Physiology, Chicago, IL 60637-1513. Offers PhD. *Degree requirements:* For doctorate, thesis/dissertation, ethics class, 2 teaching assistantships. *Entrance requirements:* For doctorate, GRE General Test. Additional exam requirements/recommendations for international students: Required—TOEFL (minimum score 600 paper-based; 104 iBT), IELTS (minimum score 7). Electronic applications accepted. *Faculty research:* Molecular genetics, biochemical biological and physical approaches to cell physiology.

University of Illinois at Urbana–Champaign, Graduate College, College of Liberal Arts and Sciences, School of Molecular and Cellular Biology, Department of Molecular and Integrative Physiology, Champaign, IL 61820. Offers MS, PhD. *Students:* 28 (12 women). Application fee: $75 ($90 for international students). *Unit head:* Milan Bagchi, Head, 217-333-1735, Fax: 217-333-1133, E-mail: mbagchi@illinois.edu. *Application contact:* Shawna Smith, Office Manager, 217-244-6638, Fax: 217-333-1133, E-mail: smsmith1@illinois.edu.
Website: http://mcb.illinois.edu/departments/mip/

The University of North Carolina at Chapel Hill, School of Medicine and Graduate School, Graduate Programs in Medicine, Department of Cell and Molecular Physiology, Chapel Hill, NC 27599. Offers PhD. Terminal master's awarded for partial completion of doctoral program. *Degree requirements:* For doctorate, comprehensive exam, thesis/dissertation, ethics training. *Entrance requirements:* For doctorate, GRE General Test. Electronic applications accepted. *Faculty research:* Signal transduction; growth factors; cardiovascular diseases; neurobiology; hormones, receptors, ion channels.

University of Pittsburgh, School of Medicine, Graduate Programs in Medicine, Cell Biology and Molecular Physiology Graduate Program, Pittsburgh, PA 15260. Offers PhD. *Faculty:* 45 full-time (10 women). *Students:* 3 full-time (2 women). Average age 30. 517 applicants, 13% accepted, 22 enrolled. In 2013, 3 doctorates awarded. *Degree requirements:* For doctorate, comprehensive exam, thesis/dissertation. *Entrance requirements:* For doctorate, GRE General Test, GRE Subject Test, minimum QPA of 3.0. Additional exam requirements/recommendations for international students: Required—TOEFL (minimum score 600 paper-based; 100 iBT), IELTS (minimum score 7). *Application deadline:* For fall admission, 1/1 priority date for domestic and international students. Application fee: $50. Electronic applications accepted. *Expenses:* Tuition, state resident: full-time $19,964; part-time $807 per credit. Tuition, nonresident: full-time $32,686; part-time $1337 per credit. *Required fees:* $740; $200. Tuition and fees vary according to program. *Financial support:* In 2013–14, 1 research assistantship with full tuition reimbursement (averaging $26,010 per year), 2 teaching assistantships with full tuition reimbursements (averaging $26,010 per year) were awarded; institutionally sponsored loans, scholarships/grants, traineeships, health care benefits, and unspecified assistantships also available. *Faculty research:* Genetic disorders of ion channels, regulation of gene expression/development, membrane traffic of proteins and lipids, reproductive biology, signal transduction in diabetes and metabolism. *Unit head:* Dr. Donna B. Stolz, Graduate Program Director, 412-383-7283, Fax: 412-648-2927, E-mail: dstolz@pitt.edu. *Application contact:* Graduate Studies Administrator, 412-648-8957, Fax: 412-648-1077, E-mail: gradstudies@medschool.pitt.edu.
Website: http://www.gradbiomed.pitt.edu

University of Virginia, School of Medicine, Department of Molecular Physiology and Biological Physics, Charlottesville, VA 22903. Offers biological and physical sciences (MS); physiology (PhD); MD/PhD. *Faculty:* 27 full-time (6 women), 1 part-time/adjunct (0 women). *Students:* 5 full-time (3 women). Average age 27. In 2013, 23 master's, 6 doctorates awarded. *Entrance requirements:* For doctorate, GRE General Test, GRE Subject Test. Additional exam requirements/recommendations for international students: Required—TOEFL. *Application deadline:* For fall admission, 2/15 for domestic and international students. Applications are processed on a rolling basis. Application fee: $60. Electronic applications accepted. *Expenses:* Tuition, state resident: part-time $334 per credit hour. Tuition, nonresident: part-time $1224 per credit hour. *Financial support:* Fellowships, research assistantships, and teaching assistantships available. Financial award applicants required to submit FAFSA. *Unit head:* Dr. Mark Yeager, Chair, 434-924-5108, Fax: 434-982-1616, E-mail: my3r@virginia.edu. *Application contact:* Director of Graduate Studies, E-mail: physiograd@virginia.edu.
Website: http://www.healthsystem.virginia.edu/internet/physio/

Vanderbilt University, Graduate School and School of Medicine, Department of Molecular Physiology and Biophysics, Nashville, TN 37240-1001. Offers MS, PhD, MD/PhD. *Faculty:* 35 full-time (8 women). *Students:* 42 full-time (27 women); includes 9 minority (3 Black or African American, non-Hispanic/Latino; 4 Hispanic/Latino; 2 Two or more races, non-Hispanic/Latino), 1 international. Average age 26. In 2013, 7 doctorates awarded. *Degree requirements:* For doctorate, comprehensive exam, thesis/dissertation, preliminary, qualifying, and final exams. *Entrance requirements:* For doctorate, GRE General Test, GRE Subject Test (recommended). Additional exam requirements/recommendations for international students: Required—TOEFL (minimum score 570 paper-based; 88 iBT). *Application deadline:* For fall admission, 1/15 for domestic and international students. Application fee: $0. Electronic applications accepted. *Financial support:* Fellowships with full tuition reimbursements, research assistantships with full tuition reimbursements, Federal Work-Study, institutionally sponsored loans, scholarships/grants, traineeships, health care benefits, and tuition waivers (partial) available. Financial award application deadline: 1/15; financial award applicants required to submit CSS PROFILE or FAFSA. *Faculty research:* Biophysics, cell signaling and gene regulation, human genetics, diabetes and obesity, neuroscience. *Unit head:* Prof. Roger D. Cone, Chair of the Department of Molecular Physiology and Biophysics, 615-936-7085, Fax: 615-343-0490, E-mail: roger.cone@vanderbilt.edu. *Application contact:* Walter B. Bieschke, Program Coordinator for Graduate Admissions, 615-342-0236, E-mail: walter.bieschke@vanderbilt.edu.
Website: http://www.mc.vanderbilt.edu/root/vumc.php?site-MPB

Yale University, Graduate School of Arts and Sciences, Department of Cellular and Molecular Physiology, New Haven, CT 06520. Offers PhD. *Degree requirements:* For doctorate, thesis/dissertation. *Entrance requirements:* For doctorate, GRE General Test, GRE Subject Test.

Physiology

Albert Einstein College of Medicine, Graduate Division of Biomedical Sciences, Department of Physiology and Biophysics, Bronx, NY 10461. Offers PhD, MD/PhD. *Degree requirements:* For doctorate, thesis/dissertation. *Entrance requirements:* For doctorate, GRE General Test. Additional exam requirements/recommendations for international students: Required—TOEFL. *Faculty research:* Biophysical and biochemical basis of body function at the subcellular, cellular, organ, and whole-body level.

Ball State University, Graduate School, College of Sciences and Humanities, Department of Physiology and Health Science, Program in Physiology, Muncie, IN 47306-1099. Offers MA, MS. *Students:* 18 full-time (5 women), 4 part-time (1 woman); includes 3 minority (1 Black or African American, non-Hispanic/Latino; 1 Asian, non-Hispanic/Latino; 1 Hispanic/Latino), 10 international. Average age 22. 28 applicants, 68% accepted, 3 enrolled. In 2013, 16 master's awarded. Application fee: $50. *Financial support:* In 2013–14, 11 students received support. Application deadline: 3/1. *Unit head:* Dr. Jeffrey K. Clark, Director, 765-285-1502, Fax: 765-285-3210, E-mail: jclark@bsu.edu. *Application contact:* Dr. Marianna Tucker, Director of Graduate Programs, 765-285-5961, Fax: 765-285-3210, E-mail: jclark@bsu.edu.
Website: http://www.bsu.edu/chs/phs/

Boston University, College of Health and Rehabilitation Sciences: Sargent College, Department of Health Sciences, Programs in Human Physiology, Boston, MA 02215. Offers MS, PhD. *Faculty:* 10 full-time (9 women), 5 part-time/adjunct (2 women). *Students:* 7 full-time (6 women), 4 part-time (2 women); includes 5 minority (2 Black or African American, non-Hispanic/Latino; 2 Asian, non-Hispanic/Latino; 1 Hispanic/Latino). Average age 25. 40 applicants, 48% accepted, 6 enrolled. In 2013, 5 master's, 5 doctorates awarded. Terminal master's awarded for partial completion of doctoral program. *Degree requirements:* For master's, thesis or alternative; for doctorate, comprehensive exam, thesis/dissertation. *Entrance requirements:* For master's, GRE General Test, minimum GPA of 3.0; for doctorate, GRE General Test. Additional exam requirements/recommendations for international students: Required—TOEFL (minimum score 550 paper-based; 84 iBT). *Application deadline:* For fall admission, 1/15 priority date for domestic and international students; for spring admission, 10/1 for domestic and international students. Applications are processed on a rolling basis. Application fee: $80. Electronic applications accepted. *Expenses: Tuition:* Full-time $43,970; part-time $1374 per credit hour. *Required fees:* $60 per semester. Tuition and fees vary according to class time, course level and program. *Financial support:* In 2013–14, 1 fellowship with full tuition reimbursement (averaging $20,000 per year), 1 research assistantship with full tuition reimbursement (averaging $18,000 per year) were awarded; teaching assistantships, career-related internships or fieldwork, Federal Work-Study, institutionally sponsored loans, scholarships/grants, and tuition waivers (partial) also available. Support available to part-time students. Financial award application deadline: 4/15; financial award applicants required to submit FAFSA. *Faculty research:* Skeletal muscle, neural systems, smooth muscle, muscular dystrophy. *Total annual research expenditures:* $1.3 million. *Unit head:* Dr. Kathleen Morgan, Chair, 617-353-2717, E-mail: kmorgan@bu.edu. *Application contact:* Sharon Sankey, Director, Student Services, 617-353-2713, Fax: 617-353-7500, E-mail: ssankey@bu.edu.

Boston University, School of Medicine, Division of Graduate Medical Sciences, Department of Physiology and Biophysics, Boston, MA 02118. Offers MA, PhD, MD/PhD. Part-time programs available. Terminal master's awarded for partial completion of doctoral program. *Degree requirements:* For master's, thesis; for doctorate, thesis/dissertation. *Application deadline:* For fall admission, 1/15 for domestic students; for spring admission, 10/15 for domestic students. *Expenses: Tuition:* Full-time $43,970; part-time $1374 per credit hour. *Required fees:* $60 per semester. Tuition and fees vary according to class time, course level and program. *Faculty research:* X-ray scattering, NMR spectroscopy, protein crystallography, structural electron. *Unit head:* Dr. David Atkinson, Chairman, 617-638-4015, Fax: 617-638-4041, E-mail: atkinson@bu.edu. *Application contact:* Dr. Esther Bullitt, Associate Professor, 617-638-5037, E-mail: bullitt@bu.edu.
Website: http://www.bumc.bu.edu/phys-biophys/

Brigham Young University, Graduate Studies, College of Life Sciences, Department of Physiology and Developmental Biology, Provo, UT 84602. Offers neuroscience (MS, PhD); physiology and developmental biology (MS, PhD). Part-time programs available. *Faculty:* 20 full-time (0 women). *Students:* 42 full-time (20 women); includes 12 minority (1 American Indian or Alaska Native, non-Hispanic/Latino; 7 Asian, non-Hispanic/Latino; 3 Hispanic/Latino; 1 Two or more races, non-Hispanic/Latino). Average age 28. 15 applicants, 20% accepted, 2 enrolled. In 2013, 6 master's, 5 doctorates awarded. Terminal master's awarded for partial completion of doctoral program. *Degree requirements:* For master's, thesis, oral exam; for doctorate, comprehensive exam, thesis/dissertation. *Entrance requirements:* For master's, GRE General Test, minimum GPA of 3.0 during previous 2 years; for doctorate, GRE General Test, minimum GPA of 3.0 overall. Additional exam requirements/recommendations for international students: Required—TOEFL (minimum score 580 paper-based; 85 iBT). *Application deadline:* For fall admission, 2/1 priority date for domestic and international students; for winter admission, 9/10 priority date for domestic and international students. Application fee: $50. Electronic applications accepted. *Expenses: Tuition:* Full-time $6130; part-time $340 per credit hour. Tuition and fees vary according to program and student's religious affiliation. *Financial support:* In 2013–14, 41 students received support, including 2 fellowships with partial tuition reimbursements available (averaging $7,100 per year), 20 research assistantships with full tuition reimbursements available (averaging $15,500 per year), 20 teaching assistantships with partial tuition reimbursements available (averaging $14,900 per year); career-related internships or fieldwork, institutionally sponsored loans, scholarships/grants, tuition waivers (full and partial), unspecified assistantships, and tuition awards also available. Financial award application deadline: 2/1. *Faculty research:* Sex differentiation of the brain, exercise physiology, developmental biology, membrane biophysics, neuroscience. *Total annual research expenditures:* $508,299. *Unit head:* Dr. Dixon J. Woodbury, Chair, 801-422-7562, Fax: 801-422-0700, E-mail: dixon_woodbury@byu.edu. *Application contact:* Connie L. Provost, Graduate Secretary, 801-422-3706, Fax: 801-422-0700, E-mail: connie_provost@byu.edu.
Website: http://pdbio.byu.edu

Brown University, Graduate School, Division of Biology and Medicine, Department of Molecular Pharmacology, Physiology and Biotechnology, Providence, RI 02912. Offers biomedical engineering (Sc M, PhD); biotechnology (PhD); molecular pharmacology and physiology (PhD); MD/PhD. *Degree requirements:* For doctorate, thesis/dissertation, preliminary exam. *Entrance requirements:* For master's and doctorate, GRE General Test, GRE Subject Test. Additional exam requirements/recommendations for international students: Required—TOEFL. Electronic applications accepted. *Faculty research:* Structural biology, antiplatelet drugs, nicotinic receptor structure/function.

Case Western Reserve University, School of Medicine and School of Graduate Studies, Graduate Programs in Medicine, Department of Physiology and Biophysics, Cleveland, OH 44106. Offers cell and molecular physiology (MS); cell physiology (PhD); molecular/cellular biophysics (PhD); physiology and biophysics (PhD); systems physiology (PhD); MD/PhD. Terminal master's awarded for partial completion of doctoral program. *Degree requirements:* For master's, thesis; for doctorate, thesis/dissertation. *Entrance requirements:* For master's, GRE General Test, minimum GPA of 3.28; for doctorate, GRE General Test, minimum GPA of 3.6. Additional exam requirements/recommendations for international students: Required—TOEFL. Electronic applications accepted. *Faculty research:* Cardiovascular physiology, calcium metabolism, epithelial cell biology.

Columbia University, College of Physicians and Surgeons, Department of Physiology and Cellular Biophysics, New York, NY 10032. Offers M Phil, MA, PhD, MD/PhD. Only candidates for the PhD are admitted. Terminal master's awarded for partial completion of doctoral program. *Degree requirements:* For doctorate, thesis/dissertation. *Entrance requirements:* For master's and doctorate, GRE General Test. Additional exam requirements/recommendations for international students: Required—TOEFL. *Faculty research:* Membrane physiology, cellular biology, cardiovascular physiology, neurophysiology.

Cornell University, Graduate School, Graduate Fields of Agriculture and Life Sciences, Field of Horticulture, Ithaca, NY 14853-0001. Offers breeding of horticultural crops (MPS); horticultural crop management systems (MPS); human-plant interactions (MPS, PhD); physiology and ecology of horticultural crops (MPS, MS, PhD). *Faculty:* 52 full-time (14 women). *Students:* 39 full-time (17 women); includes 4 minority (1 Asian, non-Hispanic/Latino; 1 Hispanic/Latino; 2 Two or more races, non-Hispanic/Latino), 12 international. Average age 30. 73 applicants, 18% accepted, 11 enrolled. In 2013, 13 master's, 1 doctorate awarded. *Degree requirements:* For master's, thesis (MS); for doctorate, comprehensive exam, thesis/dissertation. *Entrance requirements:* For master's and doctorate, GRE General Test, 3 letters of recommendation. Additional exam requirements/recommendations for international students: Required—TOEFL (minimum score 550 paper-based; 77 iBT). *Application deadline:* For fall admission, 1/15 for domestic students; for spring admission, 8/15 for domestic students. Application fee: $95. Electronic applications accepted. *Financial support:* In 2013–14, 35 students received support, including 5 fellowships with full tuition reimbursements available, 16 research assistantships with full tuition reimbursements available, 14 teaching assistantships with full tuition reimbursements available; institutionally sponsored loans, scholarships/grants, health care benefits, tuition waivers (full and partial), and unspecified assistantships also available. Financial award applicants required to submit FAFSA. *Faculty research:* Plant selection/plant materials, greenhouse management, greenhouse crop production, urban landscape management, turfgrass management. *Unit head:* Director of Graduate Studies, 607-255-4568, Fax: 607-255-0599. *Application contact:* Graduate Field Assistant, 607-255-4568, Fax: 607-255-0599, E-mail: hortgrad@cornell.edu.
Website: http://www.gradschool.cornell.edu/fields.php?id-XX&a-2

Cornell University, Graduate School, Graduate Fields of Comparative Biomedical Sciences, Field of Molecular and Integrative Physiology, Ithaca, NY 14853-0001. Offers behavioral physiology (MS, PhD); cardiovascular and respiratory physiology (MS, PhD); endocrinology (MS, PhD); environmental and comparative physiology (MS, PhD); gastrointestinal and metabolic physiology (MS, PhD); membrane and epithelial physiology (MS, PhD); molecular and cellular physiology (MS, PhD); neural and sensory physiology (MS, PhD); physiological genomics (MS, PhD); reproductive physiology (MS, PhD). *Faculty:* 45 full-time (19 women). *Students:* 8 full-time (6 women); includes 1 minority (Hispanic/Latino), 3 international. Average age 27. 7 applicants, 14% accepted, 1 enrolled. In 2013, 5 doctorates awarded. *Degree requirements:* For master's, thesis; for doctorate, comprehensive exam, thesis/dissertation, 1 semester of teaching experience, seminar presentation. *Entrance requirements:* For master's and doctorate, GRE General Test, GRE Subject Test (biochemistry, cell and molecular biology, biology, or chemistry), 2 letters of recommendation. Additional exam requirements/recommendations for international students: Required—TOEFL (minimum score 550 paper-based; 77 iBT). *Application deadline:* For fall admission, 12/15 for domestic students. Application fee: $95. Electronic applications accepted. *Financial support:* In 2013–14, 7 students received support, including 2 fellowships with full tuition reimbursements available, 4 research assistantships with full tuition reimbursements available, 1 teaching assistantship with full tuition reimbursement available; institutionally sponsored loans, scholarships/grants, health care benefits, tuition waivers (full and partial), and unspecified assistantships also available. Financial award applicants required to submit FAFSA. *Faculty research:* Endocrinology and reproductive physiology, cardiovascular and respiratory physiology, gastrointestinal and metabolic physiology, molecular and cellular physiology, physiological genomics. *Unit head:* Director of Graduate Studies, 607-253-3276, Fax: 607-253-3756. *Application contact:* Graduate Field Assistant, 607-253-3276, Fax: 607-253-3756, E-mail: graduate_edcvm@cornell.edu.
Website: http://www.gradschool.cornell.edu/fields.php?id-57&a-2

Dalhousie University, Faculty of Agriculture, Halifax, NS B3H 4R2, Canada. Offers agriculture (M Sc), including air quality, animal behavior, animal molecular genetics, animal nutrition, animal technology, aquaculture, botany, crop management, crop physiology, ecology, environmental microbiology, food science, horticulture, nutrient management, pest management, physiology, plant biotechnology, plant pathology, soil chemistry, soil fertility, waste management and composting, water quality. Part-time programs available. *Degree requirements:* For master's, thesis, ATC Exam Teaching Assistantship. *Entrance requirements:* For master's, honors B Sc, minimum GPA of 3.0. Additional exam requirements/recommendations for international students: Required—TOEFL (minimum score 580 paper-based; 92 iBT), IELTS, Michigan English Language Assessment Battery, CanTEST, CAEL. *Faculty research:* Bio-product development, organic agriculture, nutrient management, air and water quality, agricultural biotechnology.

Dalhousie University, Faculty of Medicine, Department of Physiology and Biophysics, Halifax, NS B3H 1X5, Canada. Offers M Sc, PhD, M Sc/PhD. *Degree requirements:* For master's, thesis; for doctorate, thesis/dissertation. *Entrance requirements:* For master's and doctorate, GRE Subject Test (for international students). Additional exam requirements/recommendations for international students: Required—1 of 5 approved tests: TOEFL, IELTS, CANTEST, CAEL, Michigan English Language Assessment Battery. Electronic applications accepted. *Faculty research:* Computer modeling, reproductive and endocrine physiology, cardiovascular physiology, neurophysiology, membrane biophysics.

Dartmouth College, Arts and Sciences Graduate Programs, Department of Physiology, Lebanon, NH 03756. Offers PhD, MD/PhD. *Degree requirements:* For doctorate, thesis/dissertation. *Entrance requirements:* For doctorate, GRE General Test, GRE Subject Test. Additional exam requirements/recommendations for international students: Required—TOEFL. *Faculty research:* Respiratory control, endocrinology of reproduction and immunology, regulation of receptors and channels, electrophysiology of membranes, renal function.

East Carolina University, Brody School of Medicine, Department of Physiology, Greenville, NC 27858-4353. Offers PhD. *Degree requirements:* For doctorate, comprehensive exam, thesis/dissertation. *Entrance requirements:* For doctorate, GRE General Test. Additional exam requirements/recommendations for international students: Required—TOEFL. *Application deadline:* For fall admission, 6/1 priority date for domestic students. Applications are processed on a rolling basis. Application fee: $50. *Expenses:* Tuition, state resident: full-time $4223. Tuition, nonresident: full-time $16,540. *Required fees:* $2184. *Financial support:* Fellowships with full and partial tuition reimbursements available. Financial award application deadline: 6/1. *Faculty research:* Cell and nerve biophysics; neurophysiology; cardiovascular, renal, endocrine, and gastrointestinal physiology; pulmonary/asthma. *Unit head:* Dr. Robert Lust, Chairman, 252-744-2762, Fax: 252-744-3460, E-mail: lustr@ecu.edu. *Application contact:* Dr. Mike Van Scott, Graduate Director, 252-744-3654, Fax: 252-744-3460, E-mail: vanscottmi@ecu.edu.
Website: http://www.ecu.edu/physiology/

Eastern Michigan University, Graduate School, College of Health and Human Services, School of Health Promotion and Human Performance, Programs in Exercise Physiology, Ypsilanti, MI 48197. Offers exercise physiology (MS); sports medicine-biomechanics (MS); sports medicine-corporate adult fitness (MS); sports medicine-exercise physiology (MS). Part-time and evening/weekend programs available. *Students:* 13 full-time (9 women), 36 part-time (12 women); includes 12 minority (5 Black or African American, non-Hispanic/Latino; 1 American Indian or Alaska Native, non-Hispanic/Latino; 2 Asian, non-Hispanic/Latino; 2 Hispanic/Latino; 2 Two or more races, non-Hispanic/Latino), 3 international. Average age 29. 46 applicants, 74% accepted, 18 enrolled. In 2013, 29 master's awarded. *Degree requirements:* For master's, comprehensive exam, thesis or 450-hour internship. *Entrance requirements:* Additional exam requirements/recommendations for international students: Required—TOEFL. *Application deadline:* For fall admission, 8/1 for domestic students, 5/1 for international students; for winter admission, 12/1 for domestic students, 10/1 for international students; for spring admission, 3/15 for domestic students, 3/1 for international students. Application fee: $35. *Expenses:* Tuition, state resident: full-time $12,300; part-time $466 per credit hour. Tuition, nonresident: full-time $23,159; part-time $918 per credit hour. *Required fees:* $71 per credit hour. $46 per semester. One-time fee: $100. Tuition and fees vary according to course level and degree level. *Unit head:* Dr. Christopher Herman, Director, 734-487-2815, Fax: 734-487-2024, E-mail: cherman2@emich.edu. *Application contact:* Dr. Stephen McGregor, Program Coordinator, 734-487-2820, Fax: 734-487-2024, E-mail: stephen.mcgregor@emich.edu.

East Tennessee State University, James H. Quillen College of Medicine, Department of Biomedical Sciences, Johnson City, TN 37614. Offers anatomy (PhD); biochemistry (PhD); microbiology (PhD); pharmaceutical sciences (PhD); pharmacology (PhD); physiology (PhD); quantitative biosciences (PhD). *Faculty:* 43 full-time (11 women), 1 (woman) part-time/adjunct. *Students:* 31 full-time (17 women), 4 part-time (1 woman); includes 6 minority (2 Black or African American, non-Hispanic/Latino; 3 Asian, non-Hispanic/Latino; 1 Hispanic/Latino), 9 international. Average age 29. 53 applicants, 17% accepted, 8 enrolled. In 2013, 6 doctorates awarded. *Degree requirements:* For doctorate, thesis/dissertation, comprehensive qualifying exam. *Entrance requirements:* For doctorate, GRE General Test, GRE Subject Test. Additional exam requirements/recommendations for international students: Required—TOEFL (minimum score 550

paper-based; 79 iBT). *Application deadline:* For fall admission, 3/15 priority date for domestic students, 3/1 priority date for international students. Application fee: $35 ($45 for international students). Electronic applications accepted. *Expenses:* Contact institution. *Financial support:* In 2013–14, 30 students received support, including 30 research assistantships with full tuition reimbursements available (averaging $19,000 per year); career-related internships or fieldwork, institutionally sponsored loans, scholarships/grants, and unspecified assistantships also available. Financial award application deadline: 7/1; financial award applicants required to submit FAFSA. *Faculty research:* Cardiovascular, infectious disease, neurosciences, cancer, immunology. *Unit head:* Dr. Mitchell E. Robinson, Associate Dean/Program Director, 423-439-2031, Fax: 423-439-2140, E-mail: robinson@etsu.edu. *Application contact:* Shella Bennett, Graduate Specialist, 423-439-4708, Fax: 423-439-5624, E-mail: bennetsg@etsu.edu.
Website: http://www.etsu.edu/com/dbms/

Georgia Institute of Technology, Graduate Studies and Research, College of Sciences, School of Applied Physiology, Program in Prosthetics and Orthotics, Atlanta, GA 30332-0001. Offers MS.

Georgia Regents University, The Graduate School, Program in Physiology, Augusta, GA 30912. Offers MS, PhD. *Faculty:* 10 full-time (4 women), 2 part-time/adjunct (both women). *Students:* 20 full-time (13 women); includes 10 minority (3 Black or African American, non-Hispanic/Latino; 7 Asian, non-Hispanic/Latino), 11 international. Average age 29. In 2013, 5 doctorates awarded. *Degree requirements:* For doctorate, comprehensive exam, thesis/dissertation. *Entrance requirements:* For doctorate, GRE General Test. Additional exam requirements/recommendations for international students: Required—TOEFL (minimum score 550 paper-based; 79 iBT). *Application deadline:* For fall admission, 1/15 for domestic and international students. Application fee: $50. Electronic applications accepted. *Financial support:* In 2013–14, 1 student received support, including 4 fellowships with partial tuition reimbursements available (averaging $26,000 per year), 7 research assistantships with partial tuition reimbursements available (averaging $23,000 per year); Federal Work-Study, institutionally sponsored loans, scholarships/grants, and traineeships also available. Support available to part-time students. Financial award application deadline: 5/31; financial award applicants required to submit FAFSA. *Faculty research:* Cardiovascular and renal physiology, behavioral neuroscience and genetics, neurophysiology, adrenal steroid endocrinology and genetics, inflammatory mediators and cardiovascular disease, hypertension, diabetes and stroke. *Total annual research expenditures:* $4.8 million. *Unit head:* Dr. Clinton Webb, Chair and Professor, 706-721-7742, Fax: 706-721-7299, E-mail: cwebb@georgiahealth.edu. *Application contact:* Dr. Patricia L. Cameron, Acting Vice Dean, 706-721-3279, E-mail: pcameron@georgiahealth.edu.
Website: http://www.gru.edu/mcg/phy/phys_graduate.php

Georgia State University, College of Arts and Sciences, Department of Biology, Program in Cellular and Molecular Biology and Physiology, Atlanta, GA 30302-3083. Offers bioinformatics (MS); cellular and molecular biology and physiology (MS, PhD). Part-time programs available. Terminal master's awarded for partial completion of doctoral program. *Degree requirements:* For master's, comprehensive exam (for some programs), thesis optional; for doctorate, comprehensive exam, thesis/dissertation. *Entrance requirements:* For master's and doctorate, GRE. Additional exam requirements/recommendations for international students: Required—TOEFL (minimum score 550 paper-based; 82 iBT) or IELTS (minimum score 7). *Application deadline:* For fall admission, 7/1 priority date for domestic students, 6/1 priority date for international students; for spring admission, 11/15 priority date for domestic students, 10/15 priority date for international students. Applications are processed on a rolling basis. Application fee: $50. Electronic applications accepted. *Expenses: Tuition, area resident:* Full-time $4176; part-time $348 per credit hour. Tuition, state resident: full-time $14,544; part-time $1212 per credit hour. Tuition, nonresident: full-time $14,544; part-time $1212 per credit hour. Tuition and fees vary according to course load and program. *Financial support:* In 2013–14, fellowships with full tuition reimbursements (averaging $22,000 per year), research assistantships with full tuition reimbursements (averaging $20,000 per year) were awarded. Financial award application deadline: 12/3. *Faculty research:* Membrane transport, viral infection, molecular immunology, protein modeling, gene regulation. *Unit head:* Dr. Julia Hilliard, Professor, 404-413-6560, Fax: 404-413-5301, E-mail: jhilliard@gsu.edu. *Application contact:* LaTesha Warren, Graduate Coordinator, 404-413-5314, Fax: 404-413-5301, E-mail: lwarren@gsu.edu.
Website: http://biology.gsu.edu/

Harvard University, Graduate School of Arts and Sciences, Department of Systems Biology, Cambridge, MA 02138. Offers PhD. *Degree requirements:* For doctorate, thesis/dissertation, lab rotation, qualifying examination. *Entrance requirements:* For doctorate, GRE. Additional exam requirements/recommendations for international students: Required—TOEFL. Electronic applications accepted. *Expenses: Tuition:* Full-time $38,888. *Required fees:* $958. Tuition and fees vary according to campus/location, program and student level.

Harvard University, Harvard School of Public Health, Department of Environmental Health, Boston, MA 02115-6096. Offers environmental health (SM, PhD, SD); exposure, epidemiology, and risk (SM, SD); occupational health (SM, SD); physiology (PhD, SD). Part-time programs available. *Faculty:* 24 full-time (3 women), 41 part-time/adjunct (10 women). *Students:* 86 full-time (55 women), 1 part-time (0 women); includes 15 minority (2 Black or African American, non-Hispanic/Latino; 8 Asian, non-Hispanic/Latino; 4 Hispanic/Latino; 1 Two or more races, non-Hispanic/Latino), 51 international. Average age 26. 86 applicants, 45% accepted, 25 enrolled. In 2013, 14 master's, 12 doctorates awarded. *Degree requirements:* For doctorate, thesis/dissertation, qualifying exam. *Entrance requirements:* For master's, GRE, MCAT; for doctorate, GRE. Additional exam requirements/recommendations for international students: Required—TOEFL (minimum score 600 paper-based; 100 iBT); Recommended—IELTS (minimum score 7). *Application deadline:* For fall admission, 12/15 for domestic and international students. Application fee: $120. Electronic applications accepted. *Expenses: Tuition:* Full-time $38,888. *Required fees:* $958. Tuition and fees vary according to campus/location, program and student level. *Financial support:* Fellowships, research assistantships, teaching assistantships, career-related internships or fieldwork, Federal Work-Study, scholarships/grants, traineeships, and unspecified assistantships available. Support available to part-time students. Financial award application deadline: 2/15; financial award applicants required to submit FAFSA. *Faculty research:* Exposure assessment, epidemiology, risk assessment, environmental epidemiology, ergonomics and safety, environmental exposure assessment, occupational hygiene, industrial hygiene and occupational safety, population genetics, indoor and outdoor air pollution, cell and molecular biology of the lungs, infectious diseases. *Unit head:* Dr. Douglas Dockery, Chairman, 617-432-1270, Fax: 617-432-6913. *Application contact:* Vincent W. James, Director of Admissions, 617-432-1031, Fax: 617-432-7080, E-mail: admissions@hsph.harvard.edu.
Website: http://www.hsph.harvard.edu/environmental-health/

Howard University, Graduate School, Department of Physiology and Biophysics, Washington, DC 20059-0002. Offers biophysics (PhD); physiology (PhD). *Degree requirements:* For doctorate, comprehensive exam, thesis/dissertation. *Entrance requirements:* For doctorate, GRE General Test, minimum B average in field. *Faculty research:* Cardiovascular physiology, pulmonary physiology, renal physiology, neurophysiology, endocrinology.

Illinois State University, Graduate School, College of Arts and Sciences, Department of Biological Sciences, Normal, IL 61790-2200. Offers animal behavior (MS); bacteriology (MS); biochemistry (MS); biological sciences (MS); biology (PhD); biophysics (MS); biotechnology (MS); botany (MS, PhD); cell biology (MS); conservation biology (MS); developmental biology (MS); ecology (MS, PhD); entomology (MS); evolutionary biology (MS); genetics (MS, PhD); immunology (MS); microbiology (MS, PhD); molecular biology (MS); molecular genetics (MS); neurobiology (MS); neuroscience (MS); parasitology (MS); physiology (MS, PhD); plant biology (MS); plant molecular biology (MS); plant sciences (MS); structural biology (MS); zoology (MS, PhD). Part-time programs available. *Degree requirements:* For master's, thesis or alternative; for doctorate, variable foreign language requirement, thesis/dissertation, 2 terms of residency. *Entrance requirements:* For master's, GRE General Test, minimum GPA of 2.6 in last 60 hours of course work; for doctorate, GRE General Test. *Faculty research:* Redoc balance and drug development in schistosoma mansoni, control of the growth of listeria monocytogenes at low temperature, regulation of cell expansion and microtubule function by SPRI, CRUI: physiology and fitness consequences of different life history phenotypes.

Indiana State University, College of Graduate and Professional Studies, College of Arts and Sciences, Department of Biology, Terre Haute, IN 47809. Offers ecology (PhD); life sciences (MS); microbiology (PhD); physiology (PhD); science education (MS). *Faculty:* 23 full-time (6 women), 1 (woman) part-time/adjunct. *Students:* 73 full-time (31 women), 15 part-time (6 women); includes 7 minority (6 Asian, non-Hispanic/Latino; 1 Hispanic/Latino), 17 international. Average age 26. 63 applicants, 65% accepted, 40 enrolled. In 2013, 9 master's, 5 doctorates awarded. *Degree requirements:* For master's, thesis (for some programs); for doctorate, comprehensive exam, thesis/dissertation. *Entrance requirements:* For master's and doctorate, GRE General Test. *Application deadline:* For fall admission, 7/1 priority date for domestic students; for spring admission, 11/1 priority date for domestic students. Applications are processed on a rolling basis. Application fee: $35. Electronic applications accepted. *Financial support:* In 2013–14, 9 research assistantships with partial tuition reimbursements (averaging $7,500 per year), 19 teaching assistantships with partial tuition reimbursements (averaging $8,000 per year) were awarded; Federal Work-Study, institutionally sponsored loans, and tuition waivers (partial) also available. Financial award application deadline: 3/1; financial award applicants required to submit FAFSA. *Unit head:* Dr. Arthur M. Halpern, Interim Chairperson, 812-237-2400. *Application contact:* Dr. Jay Gatrell, Dean, 800-444-GRAD, Fax: 812-237-8060, E-mail: jay.gatrell@indstate.edu.

Johns Hopkins University, Bloomberg School of Public Health, Department of Environmental Health Sciences, Baltimore, MD 21218-2699. Offers environmental health engineering (PhD); environmental health sciences (MHS, Dr PH); occupational and environmental health (PhD); occupational and environmental hygiene (MHS, MHS); physiology (PhD); toxicology (PhD). Postbaccalaureate distance learning degree programs offered (minimal on-campus study). *Faculty:* 71 full-time (27 women), 58 part-time/adjunct (26 women). *Students:* 67 full-time (42 women), 22 part-time (17 women); includes 30 minority (8 Black or African American, non-Hispanic/Latino; 14 Asian, non-Hispanic/Latino; 5 Hispanic/Latino; 3 Two or more races, non-Hispanic/Latino), 13 international. Average age 29. 112 applicants, 54% accepted, 40 enrolled. In 2013, 23 master's, 11 doctorates awarded. *Degree requirements:* For master's, essay, presentation; for doctorate, comprehensive exam, thesis/dissertation, 1-year full-time residency, oral and written exams. *Entrance requirements:* For master's, GRE General Test or MCAT, 3 letters of recommendation, transcripts; for doctorate, GRE General Test or MCAT, 3 letters of recommendation. Additional exam requirements/recommendations for international students: Required—TOEFL (minimum score 600 paper-based). *Application deadline:* For fall admission, 12/15 priority date for domestic and international students. Applications are processed on a rolling basis. Application fee: $45. Electronic applications accepted. *Financial support:* Fellowships with full tuition reimbursements, Federal Work-Study, institutionally sponsored loans, scholarships/grants, traineeships, health care benefits, and stipends available. Support available to part-time students. Financial award application deadline: 3/15; financial award applicants required to submit FAFSA. *Faculty research:* Chemical carcinogenesis/toxicology, lung disease, occupational and environmental health, nuclear imaging, molecular epidemiology. *Total annual research expenditures:* $23.7 million. *Unit head:* Dr. John Davis Groopman, Chair, 410-955-3720, Fax: 410-955-0617, E-mail: jgroopma@jhsph.edu. *Application contact:* Nina J. Kulacki, Academic Program Manager, 410-955-2212, Fax: 410-955-0617, E-mail: nkulacki@jhsph.edu.
Website: http://www.jhsph.edu/Dept/EHS/

Johns Hopkins University, School of Medicine, Graduate Programs in Medicine, Department of Physiology, Baltimore, MD 21205. Offers cellular and molecular physiology (PhD); physiology (PhD). *Faculty:* 19 full-time (6 women). *Students:* 19 full-time (9 women); includes 2 minority (both Black or African American, non-Hispanic/Latino), 13 international. Average age 23. 8 applicants, 50% accepted, 3 enrolled. In 2013, 3 doctorates awarded. *Degree requirements:* For doctorate, thesis/dissertation, oral and qualifying exams. *Entrance requirements:* For doctorate, GRE General Test, previous course work in biology, calculus, chemistry, and physics. Additional exam requirements/recommendations for international students: Required—TOEFL. *Application deadline:* For fall admission, 1/10 for domestic and international students. Application fee: $85. Electronic applications accepted. *Financial support:* Fellowships, research assistantships, teaching assistantships, scholarships/grants, traineeships, tuition waivers (full), unspecified assistantships, and stipends available. Financial award application deadline: 1/10. *Faculty research:* Membrane biochemistry and biophysics; signal transduction; developmental genetics and physiology; physiology and biochemistry; transporters, carriers, and ion channels. *Unit head:* Dr. William B. Guggino, Director, 410-955-7166, Fax: 410-955-0461. *Application contact:* Madeline J. McLaughlin, Academic Program Manager, 410-955-8333, Fax: 410-955-0461, E-mail: mmclaugh@jhmi.edu.
Website: http://physiology.bs.jhmi.edu/Pages/default.aspx#

Kansas State University, College of Veterinary Medicine, Department of Anatomy and Physiology, Manhattan, KS 66506. Offers physiology (PhD). *Faculty:* 28 full-time (8 women), 7 part-time/adjunct (3 women). *Students:* 10 full-time (6 women), 3 part-time (1 woman), 7 international. Average age 30. 4 applicants, 50% accepted, 1 enrolled. In 2013, 3 doctorates awarded. Terminal master's awarded for partial completion of doctoral program. *Entrance requirements:* For doctorate, GRE. Additional exam requirements/recommendations for international students: Required—TOEFL. *Application deadline:* For fall admission, 2/1 priority date for international students; for spring admission, 8/1 priority date for international students; for summer admission, 12/1 priority date for international students. Applications are processed on a rolling basis. Application fee: $50 ($75 for international students). Electronic applications accepted. *Financial support:* In 2013–14, 46 research assistantships (averaging $23,772 per year) were awarded; fellowships, Federal Work-Study, institutionally sponsored loans, and scholarships/grants also available. Financial award application deadline: 3/1. *Faculty research:* Cardiovascular and pulmonary, immunophysiology, neuroscience,

pharmacology, epithelial. *Total annual research expenditures:* $3.5 million. *Unit head:* Michael J. Kenney, Head, 785-532-4513, Fax: 785-532-4557, E-mail: mkenny@vet.ksu.edu. *Application contact:* Mark Weiss, Director, 785-532-4520, Fax: 785-532-4557, E-mail: mweiss@vet.k-state.edu.
Website: http://www.vet.k-state.edu/depts/ap/

Kent State University, College of Arts and Sciences, Department of Biological Sciences, Program in Physiology, Kent, OH 44242-0001. Offers MS, PhD. *Degree requirements:* For master's, thesis; for doctorate, thesis/dissertation. *Entrance requirements:* For master's, GRE General Test, minimum GPA of 3.0; for doctorate, GRE General Test, minimum GPA of 3.25. Additional exam requirements/recommendations for international students: Required—TOEFL (minimum score 600 paper-based).

Kent State University, School of Biomedical Sciences, Program in Physiology, Kent, OH 44242-0001. Offers MS, PhD. *Degree requirements:* For master's, thesis; for doctorate, thesis/dissertation. *Entrance requirements:* For master's and doctorate, GRE General Test, minimum GPA of 3.0, 3 letters of recommendation. Additional exam requirements/recommendations for international students: Required—TOEFL (minimum score 600 paper-based). Electronic applications accepted.

Loma Linda University, School of Medicine, Department of Physiology/Pharmacology, Loma Linda, CA 92350. Offers MS, PhD. Part-time programs available. *Degree requirements:* For master's, thesis or alternative; for doctorate, 2 foreign languages, thesis/dissertation. *Entrance requirements:* For master's and doctorate, GRE General Test. *Faculty research:* Drug metabolism, biochemical pharmacology, structure and function of cell membranes, neuropharmacology.

Louisiana State University Health Sciences Center, School of Graduate Studies in New Orleans, Department of Physiology, New Orleans, LA 70112-2223. Offers MS, PhD, MD/PhD. Terminal master's awarded for partial completion of doctoral program. *Degree requirements:* For master's, comprehensive exam, thesis; for doctorate, comprehensive exam, thesis/dissertation. *Entrance requirements:* For master's and doctorate, GRE General Test. Additional exam requirements/recommendations for international students: Required—TOEFL. *Faculty research:* Host defense, lipoprotein metabolism, regulation of cardiopulmonary function, alcohol and drug abuse, cell to cell communication, cytokinesis, physiologic functions of nitric oxide.

Louisiana State University Health Sciences Center at Shreveport, Department of Molecular and Cellular Physiology, Shreveport, LA 71130-3932. Offers physiology (MS, PhD); MD/PhD. *Faculty:* 10 full-time (4 women), 5 part-time/adjunct (0 women). *Students:* 10 full-time (6 women); includes 6 minority (all Asian, non-Hispanic/Latino), 8 international. Average age 28. 7 applicants, 43% accepted, 3 enrolled. In 2013, 1 master's, 1 doctorate awarded. *Degree requirements:* For master's, thesis; for doctorate, thesis/dissertation. *Entrance requirements:* For master's and doctorate, GRE General Test. Additional exam requirements/recommendations for international students: Required—TOEFL, IELTS. *Application deadline:* For fall admission, 1/31 priority date for domestic students. *Financial support:* In 2013–14, 5 students received support, including 2 fellowships with full tuition reimbursements available (averaging $28,000 per year), 8 research assistantships with full tuition reimbursements available (averaging $24,000 per year); institutionally sponsored loans also available. *Faculty research:* Cardiovascular, gastrointestinal, renal, and neutrophil function; cellular detoxification systems; hypoxia and mitochondria function. *Unit head:* Dr. D. Neil Grainger, Head, 318-675-6011. *Application contact:* Deborah Fausto, Coordinator, 318-675-6011, Fax: 318-675-4156, E-mail: dfaust1@lsuhsc.edu.
Website: http://www.shreveportphysiology.com

Loyola University Chicago, Graduate School, Programs in Cell and Molecular Physiology, Chicago, IL 60660. Offers MS, PhD. *Faculty:* 14 full-time (4 women), 19 part-time/adjunct (4 women). *Students:* 34 full-time (5 women); includes 9 minority (2 Black or African American, non-Hispanic/Latino; 3 Asian, non-Hispanic/Latino; 1 Hispanic/Latino; 3 Two or more races, non-Hispanic/Latino). Average age 24. 239 applicants, 24% accepted, 28 enrolled. In 2013, 17 master's, 3 doctorates awarded. *Degree requirements:* For master's, thesis; for doctorate, comprehensive exam, thesis/dissertation. *Entrance requirements:* For master's, GRE General Test or MCAT; for doctorate, GRE General Test. Additional exam requirements/recommendations for international students: Required—TOEFL. *Application deadline:* For fall admission, 5/15 for domestic and international students. Application fee: $0. Electronic applications accepted. *Expenses: Tuition:* Full-time $16,740; part-time $930 per credit. *Required fees:* $135 per semester. *Financial support:* In 2013–14, 5 fellowships with tuition reimbursements (averaging $23,000 per year), 9 research assistantships with tuition reimbursements (averaging $23,000 per year) were awarded. *Faculty research:* Cardiovascular system: neural and metabolic control of circulation, ion channels, excitation contraction coupling, molecular cloning; neuroscience: neuroendocrine, neuronal excitability studies. *Unit head:* Dr. Pieter P. deTombe, Chair, 708-216-6305, Fax: 708-216-6308, E-mail: pdetombe@luc.edu. *Application contact:* Dr. Erika S. Piedras-Renteria, Graduate Program Director, 708-216-9508, Fax: 708-216-6308, E-mail: rmestri@luc.edu.

Marquette University, Graduate School, College of Arts and Sciences, Department of Biology, Milwaukee, WI 53201-1881. Offers cell biology (MS, PhD); developmental biology (MS, PhD); ecology (MS, PhD); epithelial physiology (MS, PhD); genetics (MS, PhD); microbiology (MS, PhD); molecular biology (MS, PhD); muscle and exercise physiology (MS, PhD); neuroscience (PhD). *Faculty:* 21 full-time (9 women), 3 part-time/adjunct (0 women). *Students:* 34 full-time (16 women), 4 part-time (1 woman), 15 international. Average age 27. 70 applicants, 23% accepted, 5 enrolled. In 2013, 1 master's, 6 doctorates awarded. Terminal master's awarded for partial completion of doctoral program. *Degree requirements:* For master's, comprehensive exam, thesis, 1 year of teaching experience or equivalent; for doctorate, thesis/dissertation, 1 year of teaching experience or equivalent, qualifying exam. *Entrance requirements:* For master's and doctorate, GRE General Test, GRE Subject Test, official transcripts from all current and previous colleges/universities except Marquette, statement of professional goals and aspirations, three letters of recommendation. Additional exam requirements/recommendations for international students: Required—TOEFL (minimum score 530 paper-based). *Application deadline:* For fall admission, 12/15 for domestic and international students. Application fee: $50. Electronic applications accepted. *Financial support:* In 2013–14, 39 students received support, including 6 fellowships (averaging $1,208 per year), 4 research assistantships with full tuition reimbursements available (averaging $21,750 per year), 29 teaching assistantships with full tuition reimbursements available (averaging $21,750 per year); scholarships/grants, health care benefits, tuition waivers (full and partial), and unspecified assistantships also available. Support available to part-time students. Financial award application deadline: 2/15. *Faculty research:* Neurobiology, neuroendocrinology, epithelial physiology, neuropeptide interactions, synaptic transmission. *Total annual research expenditures:* $1.5 million. *Unit head:* Dr. Dale Noel, Chair and Professor, 414-288-1748. *Application contact:* Dr. Michelle Mynlieff, Professor, 414-288-1467.
Website: http://www.marquette.edu/biology/

McGill University, Faculty of Graduate and Postdoctoral Studies, Faculty of Medicine, Department of Physiology, Montréal, QC H3A 2T5, Canada. Offers M Sc, PhD.

McMaster University, Faculty of Health Sciences and School of Graduate Studies, Program in Medical Sciences, Physiology/Pharmacology Area, Hamilton, ON L8S 4M2, Canada. Offers M Sc, PhD, MD/PhD. *Degree requirements:* For master's, thesis; for doctorate, comprehensive exam, thesis/dissertation. *Entrance requirements:* For master's, honors B Sc, B+ average in related field; for doctorate, M Sc, minimum B+ average, students with proven research experience and an A average may be admitted with a B Sc degree. Additional exam requirements/recommendations for international students: Required—TOEFL (minimum score 580 paper-based; 92 iBT).

Medical College of Wisconsin, Graduate School of Biomedical Sciences, Department of Physiology, Milwaukee, WI 53226-0509. Offers PhD, MD/PhD. *Degree requirements:* For doctorate, comprehensive exam, thesis/dissertation. *Entrance requirements:* For doctorate, GRE, official transcripts, three letters of recommendation. Additional exam requirements/recommendations for international students: Required—TOEFL. *Faculty research:* Cardiovascular, respiratory, renal, and exercise physiology; mathematical modeling; molecular and cellular biology.

Michigan State University, College of Human Medicine and The Graduate School, Graduate Programs in Human Medicine, East Lansing, MI 48824. Offers biochemistry and molecular biology (MS, PhD); epidemiology (MS, PhD); microbiology (MS); microbiology and molecular genetics (PhD); pharmacology and toxicology (MS, PhD); physiology (MS, PhD); public health (MPH). *Entrance requirements:* Additional exam requirements/recommendations for international students: Required—TOEFL.

Michigan State University, College of Osteopathic Medicine and The Graduate School, Graduate Studies in Osteopathic Medicine, East Lansing, MI 48824. Offers biochemistry and molecular biology (MS, PhD); microbiology (MS); microbiology and molecular genetics (PhD); pharmacology and toxicology (MS, PhD), including integrative pharmacology (MS), pharmacology and toxicology, pharmacology and toxicology-environmental toxicology (PhD); physiology (MS, PhD).

Michigan State University, College of Veterinary Medicine and The Graduate School, Graduate Programs in Veterinary Medicine, East Lansing, MI 48824. Offers comparative medicine and integrative biology (MS, PhD), including comparative medicine and integrative biology, comparative medicine and integrative biology–environmental toxicology (PhD); food safety and toxicology (MS), including food safety; integrative toxicology (PhD), including animal science–environmental toxicology, biochemistry and molecular biology–environmental toxicology, chemistry–environmental toxicology, crop and soil sciences–environmental toxicology, environmental engineering–environmental toxicology, environmental geosciences–environmental toxicology, fisheries and wildlife–environmental toxicology, food science–environmental toxicology, forestry–environmental toxicology, genetics–environmental toxicology, human nutrition–environmental toxicology, microbiology–environmental toxicology, pharmacology and toxicology–environmental toxicology, zoology–environmental toxicology; large animal clinical sciences (MS, PhD); microbiology and molecular genetics (MS, PhD), including industrial microbiology, microbiology, microbiology and molecular genetics, microbiology–environmental toxicology (PhD); pathobiology and diagnostic investigation (MS, PhD), including pathology, pathology–environmental toxicology (PhD); pharmacology and toxicology (MS, PhD); pharmacology and toxicology–environmental toxicology (PhD); physiology (MS, PhD); small animal clinical sciences (MS). Electronic applications accepted. *Faculty research:* Molecular genetics, food safety/toxicology, comparative orthopedics, airway disease, population medicine.

Michigan State University, The Graduate School, College of Natural Science and Graduate Programs in Human Medicine and Graduate Studies in Osteopathic Medicine, Department of Physiology, East Lansing, MI 48824. Offers MS, PhD. *Entrance requirements:* Additional exam requirements/recommendations for international students: Required—TOEFL (minimum score 600 paper-based). Electronic applications accepted.

Montclair State University, The Graduate School, College of Science and Mathematics, Department of Biology and Molecular Biology, Montclair, NJ 07043-1624. Offers biology (MS), including biological science education, biology, ecology and evolution, physiology; molecular biology (MS, Certificate). Part-time and evening/weekend programs available. *Degree requirements:* For master's, comprehensive exam, thesis or alternative. *Entrance requirements:* For master's, GRE General Test, 24 credits of course work in undergraduate biology, 2 letters of recommendation, teaching certificate (biology sciences education concentration); for Certificate, 2 letters of recommendation, essay. Additional exam requirements/recommendations for international students: Required—TOEFL (minimum score 83 iBT) or IELTS. Electronic applications accepted. *Faculty research:* Ecosystem biology, molecular biology, signal transduction, neuroscience, aquatic and coastal biology.

New York Medical College, Graduate School of Basic Medical Sciences, Integrated PhD Program, Valhalla, NY 10595-1691. Offers biochemistry and molecular biology (PhD); cell biology and anatomy (PhD); microbiology and immunology (PhD); pathology (PhD); pharmacology (PhD); physiology (PhD). *Faculty:* 91 full-time (16 women), 5 part-time/adjunct (2 women). *Students:* 31 full-time (21 women); includes 17 minority (4 Black or African American, non-Hispanic/Latino; 11 Asian, non-Hispanic/Latino; 2 Hispanic/Latino). Average age 27. 56 applicants, 36% accepted, 9 enrolled. In 2013, 17 doctorates awarded. *Degree requirements:* For doctorate, comprehensive exam, thesis/dissertation. *Entrance requirements:* For doctorate, GRE General Test. Additional exam requirements/recommendations for international students: Required—TOEFL. *Application deadline:* For fall admission, 1/1 priority date for domestic and international students. Applications are processed on a rolling basis. Application fee: $75 ($100 for international students). Electronic applications accepted. *Expenses: Tuition:* Full-time $49,170; part-time $910 per credit. Tuition and fees vary according to program. *Financial support:* In 2013–14, fellowships with full tuition reimbursements (averaging $25,500 per year), research assistantships with full tuition reimbursements (averaging $25,500 per year) were awarded; Federal Work-Study, scholarships/grants, traineeships, health care benefits, and tuition waivers (full) also available. Financial award applicants required to submit FAFSA. *Faculty research:* Cardiovascular sciences, infectious diseases, neuroscience, cancer and cell signaling. *Unit head:* Dr. Francis L. Belloni, Dean, 914-594-4110, Fax: 914-594-4944, E-mail: francis_belloni@nymc.edu. *Application contact:* Valerie Romeo-Messana, Director of Admissions, 914-594-4110, Fax: 914-594-4944, E-mail: v_romeomessana@nymc.edu.

New York Medical College, Graduate School of Basic Medical Sciences, Physiology Master's Program, Valhalla, NY 10595-1691. Offers MS, PhD, MD/PhD. Part-time and evening/weekend programs available. *Faculty:* 22 full-time (2 women), 1 (woman) part-time/adjunct. *Students:* 12 full-time (7 women); includes 5 minority (4 Asian, non-Hispanic/Latino; 1 Hispanic/Latino). Average age 27. 7 applicants, 86% accepted, 5 enrolled. In 2013, 5 master's awarded. Terminal master's awarded for partial completion of doctoral program. *Degree requirements:* For master's, thesis; for doctorate, comprehensive exam, thesis/dissertation. *Entrance requirements:* For master's, GRE General Test, DAT, or MCAT. Additional exam requirements/recommendations for international students: Required—TOEFL. *Application deadline:* For fall admission, 7/1 priority date for domestic students, 5/1 priority date for international students; for spring admission, 12/1 priority date for domestic students, 9/15 priority date for international students. Applications are processed on a rolling basis. Application fee: $75 ($100 for international students). Electronic applications accepted. *Expenses: Tuition:* Full-time $49,170; part-time $910 per credit. Tuition and fees vary according to program. *Financial support:* Federal Work-Study and scholarships/grants available. Support available to part-time students. Financial award applicants required to submit FAFSA. *Faculty research:* Cellular neurophysiology, regulation of sleep and awake states, neural and endocrine control of the heart and circulation microcirculation, the physiology of gene expression, heart failure and the physiological effects of oxygen metabolites. *Unit head:* Dr. Carl I. Thompson, Program Director, 914-594-4106, Fax: 914-594-4944, E-mail: carl_thompson@nymc.edu. *Application contact:* Valerie Romeo-Messana, Director of Admissions, 914-594-4110, Fax: 914-594-4944, E-mail: v_romeomessana@nymc.edu.

New York University, School of Medicine and Graduate School of Arts and Science, Sackler Institute of Graduate Biomedical Sciences, Program in Neuroscience and Physiology, New York, NY 10012-1019. Offers PhD, MD/PhD. *Faculty:* 54 full-time (6 women). *Students:* 54 full-time (32 women); includes 12 minority (3 Black or African American, non-Hispanic/Latino; 4 Asian, non-Hispanic/Latino; 5 Hispanic/Latino), 13 international. Average age 28. In 2013, 7 doctorates awarded. *Degree requirements:* For doctorate, one foreign language, comprehensive exam, thesis/dissertation, qualifying exam. *Entrance requirements:* For doctorate, GRE General Test. Additional exam requirements/recommendations for international students: Required—TOEFL. *Application deadline:* For fall admission, 1/4 priority date for domestic students. Applications are processed on a rolling basis. Application fee: $85. *Expenses: Tuition:* Full-time $35,856; part-time $1494 per unit. *Required fees:* $1408; $64 per unit. $473 per term. Tuition and fees vary according to course load and program. *Financial support:* Fellowships with tuition reimbursements, research assistantships with tuition reimbursements, and teaching assistantships with tuition reimbursements available. *Faculty research:* Rhythms in neural networks, genetic basis of neural circuit formation and function, behavior and memory formation in mouse models of neurodevelopmental disorders. *Unit head:* Dr. Gordon Fishell, Graduate Program Director, 212-263-7691, E-mail: gordon.fishell@med.nyu.edu. *Application contact:* Dr. Annette Gray, Graduate Program Manager, 212-263-9134, E-mail: annette.gray@nyumc.org.

North Carolina State University, Graduate School, College of Agriculture and Life Sciences and College of Veterinary Medicine, Program in Physiology, Raleigh, NC 27695. Offers MP, MS, PhD. *Degree requirements:* For master's, thesis (for some programs); for doctorate, thesis/dissertation. *Entrance requirements:* For master's and doctorate, GRE General Test. Electronic applications accepted. *Faculty research:* Neurophysiology, gastrointestinal physiology, reproductive physiology, environmental/stress physiology, cardiovascular physiology.

Northwestern University, The Graduate School, Judd A. and Marjorie Weinberg College of Arts and Sciences, Department of Neurobiology, Evanston, IL 60208. Offers neurobiology and physiology (MS). Admissions and degrees offered through The Graduate School. Part-time programs available. *Degree requirements:* For master's, thesis. *Entrance requirements:* For master's, GRE General Test and MCAT (strongly recommended). Additional exam requirements/recommendations for international students: Required—TOEFL. Electronic applications accepted. *Expenses:* Contact institution. *Faculty research:* Sensory neurobiology and neuroendocrinology, reproductive biology, vision physiology and psychophysics, cell and developmental biology.

Ohio University, Graduate College, College of Arts and Sciences, Department of Biological Sciences, Athens, OH 45701-2979. Offers biological sciences (MS, PhD); cell biology and physiology (MS, PhD); ecology and evolutionary biology (MS, PhD); exercise physiology and muscle biology (MS, PhD); microbiology (MS, PhD); neuroscience (MS, PhD). Terminal master's awarded for partial completion of doctoral program. *Degree requirements:* For master's, comprehensive exam, thesis, 1 quarter of teaching experience; for doctorate, comprehensive exam, thesis/dissertation, 2 quarters of teaching experience. *Entrance requirements:* For master's, GRE General Test, names of three faculty members whose research interests most closely match the applicant's interest; for doctorate, GRE General Test, essay concerning prior training, research interest and career goals, plus names of three faculty members whose research interests most closely match the applicant's interest. Additional exam requirements/recommendations for international students: Required—TOEFL (minimum score 620 paper-based; 105 iBT) or IELTS (minimum score 7.5). Electronic applications accepted. *Faculty research:* Ecology and evolutionary biology, exercise physiology and muscle biology, neurobiology, cell biology, physiology.

Oregon Health & Science University, School of Medicine, Graduate Programs in Medicine, Program in Molecular and Cellular Biosciences, Department of Physiology and Pharmacology, Portland, OR 97239-3098. Offers PhD. *Faculty:* 22 full-time (9 women). *Students:* 9 full-time (6 women). Average age 28. In 2013, 1 doctorate awarded. *Degree requirements:* For doctorate, comprehensive exam, thesis/dissertation. *Entrance requirements:* For doctorate, GRE General Test (minimum scores: 153 Verbal/148 Quantitative/4.5 Analytical) or MCAT (for some programs). Additional exam requirements/recommendations for international students: Required—TOEFL. Electronic applications accepted. *Financial support:* Full tuition and stipends available. *Faculty research:* Ion conduction and gating in K+ channels, autonomic neuron plasticity, neurotransmitter/receptor expression, fetal/neonatal pharmacology, molecular pharmacology. *Unit head:* Dr. Beth Habecker, Program Director, 503-494-6252, E-mail: habecker@ohsu.edu. *Application contact:* Julie Walvatne, Program Coordinator, 503-494-6252.

Penn State University Park, Graduate School, Intercollege Graduate Programs, Intercollege Graduate Program in Physiology, University Park, PA 16802. Offers MS, PhD. *Unit head:* Dr. Regina Vasilatos-Younken, Interim Dean, 814-531-8567, Fax: 814-865-4627, E-mail: rxv@psu.edu. *Application contact:* Cynthia E. Nicosia, Director, Graduate Enrollment Services, 814-865-1834, Fax: 814-863-4627, E-mail: cey1@psu.edu.

Purdue University, School of Veterinary Medicine and Graduate School, Graduate Programs in Veterinary Medicine, Department of Basic Medical Sciences, West Lafayette, IN 47907. Offers anatomy (MS, PhD); pharmacology (MS, PhD); physiology (MS, PhD). Part-time programs available. Terminal master's awarded for partial completion of doctoral program. *Degree requirements:* For master's, thesis; for doctorate, thesis/dissertation. *Entrance requirements:* For master's and doctorate, GRE General Test. Additional exam requirements/recommendations for international students: Required—TOEFL. Electronic applications accepted. *Faculty research:* Development and regeneration, tissue injury and shock, biomedical engineering, ovarian function, bone and cartilage biology, cell and molecular biology.

Queen's University at Kingston, School of Graduate Studies, Faculty of Health Sciences, Department of Physiology, Kingston, ON K7L 3N6, Canada. Offers M Sc, PhD. *Degree requirements:* For master's, thesis; for doctorate, comprehensive exam, thesis/dissertation. *Entrance requirements:* For master's, minimum upper B average. Additional exam requirements/recommendations for international students: Required—TOEFL. *Faculty research:* Cardiovascular and respiratory physiology, exercise, gastrointestinal physiology, neuroscience.

Rocky Mountain University of Health Professions, Doctor of Science Program in Clinical Electrophysiology, Provo, UT 84606. Offers D Sc. Postbaccalaureate distance learning degree programs offered (minimal on-campus study). *Students:* 10 part-time (1 woman); includes 1 minority (Black or African American, non-Hispanic/Latino). Average age 43. *Degree requirements:* For doctorate, thesis/dissertation. *Entrance requirements:* For doctorate, clinical entry-level master's or doctorate degree; professional licensure as a chiropractor, nurse practitioner, occupational therapist, physical therapist, physician or physician assistant; minimum of 100 hours experience in electroneuromyography. *Application deadline:* For fall admission, 3/23 for domestic students. *Unit head:* Dr. Arthur J. Nitz, Director, 801-375-5125. *Application contact:* Bryce Greenberg, Director of Admissions, 801-734-6832, Fax: 801-734-6833, E-mail: bgreenberg@rmuohp.edu. Website: http://rmuohp.edu/academics/dsc_clinical_electrophysiology/

Rosalind Franklin University of Medicine and Science, School of Graduate and Postdoctoral Studies - Interdisciplinary Graduate Program in Biomedical Sciences, Department of Physiology and Biophysics, North Chicago, IL 60064-3095. Offers MS, PhD, MD/PhD. Terminal master's awarded for partial completion of doctoral program. *Degree requirements:* For master's, comprehensive exam, thesis; for doctorate, comprehensive exam, thesis/dissertation. *Entrance requirements:* For master's and doctorate, GRE General Test. Additional exam requirements/recommendations for international students: Required—TOEFL, TWE. *Faculty research:* Membrane transport, mechanisms of cellular regulation, brain metabolism, peptide metabolism.

Rush University, Graduate College, Department of Molecular Biophysics and Physiology, Chicago, IL 60612-3832. Offers physiology (PhD); MD/PhD. *Degree requirements:* For doctorate, thesis/dissertation. *Entrance requirements:* For doctorate, GRE General Test. Additional exam requirements/recommendations for international students: Required—TOEFL. *Faculty research:* Physiological exocytosis, raft formation and growth, voltage-gated proton channels, molecular biophysics and physiology.

Rutgers, The State University of New Jersey, Newark, Graduate School of Biomedical Sciences, Department of Pharmacology and Physiology, Newark, NJ 07107. Offers PhD. *Degree requirements:* For doctorate, thesis/dissertation, qualifying exam. *Entrance requirements:* For doctorate, GRE General Test. Additional exam requirements/recommendations for international students: Required—TOEFL. Electronic applications accepted.

Rutgers, The State University of New Jersey, New Brunswick, Graduate School-New Brunswick, Program in Endocrinology and Animal Biosciences, Piscataway, NJ 08854-8097. Offers MS, PhD. Terminal master's awarded for partial completion of doctoral program. *Degree requirements:* For master's, thesis; for doctorate, comprehensive exam, thesis/dissertation. *Entrance requirements:* For master's and doctorate, GRE General Test. Additional exam requirements/recommendations for international students: Required—TOEFL. Electronic applications accepted. *Faculty research:* Comparative and behavioral endocrinology, epigenetic regulation of the endocrine system, exercise physiology and immunology, fetal and neonatal developmental programming, mammary gland biology and breast cancer, neuroendocrinology and alcohol studies, reproductive and developmental toxicology.

Rutgers, The State University of New Jersey, New Brunswick, Graduate School of Biomedical Sciences, Program in Physiology and Integrative Biology, Piscataway, NJ 08854-5635. Offers MS, PhD, MD/PhD. *Entrance requirements:* Additional exam requirements/recommendations for international students: Required—TOEFL. Electronic applications accepted.

Saint Louis University, Graduate Education and School of Medicine, Graduate Program in Biomedical Sciences and Graduate Education, Department of Pharmacological and Physiological Science, St. Louis, MO 63103-2097. Offers PhD. *Degree requirements:* For doctorate, comprehensive exam, thesis/dissertation, departmental qualifying exams. *Entrance requirements:* For doctorate, GRE General Test (GRE Subject Test optional), letters of recommendation, resume, interview. Additional exam requirements/recommendations for international students: Required—TOEFL (minimum score 525 paper-based). Electronic applications accepted. *Faculty research:* Molecular endocrinology, neuropharmacology, cardiovascular science, drug abuse, neurotransmitter and hormonal signaling mechanisms.

Salisbury University, Program in Applied Health Physiology, Salisbury, MD 21801-6837. Offers MS. Part-time programs available. *Faculty:* 4 full-time (0 women), 1 part-time/adjunct (0 women). *Students:* 24 full-time (13 women), 18 part-time (10 women); includes 4 minority (2 Black or African American, non-Hispanic/Latino; 1 Asian, non-Hispanic/Latino; 1 Hispanic/Latino). Average age 25. 23 applicants, 65% accepted, 15 enrolled. In 2013, 25 master's awarded. *Entrance requirements:* For master's, minimum GPA of 3.0, 2 recommendations, personal statement, completion of undergraduate course work in human anatomy, physiology and exercise physiology. Additional exam requirements/recommendations for international students: Required—TOEFL (minimum score 550 paper-based; 79 iBT), IELTS (minimum score 6.5). *Application deadline:* For fall admission, 8/7 priority date for domestic and international students; for winter admission, 12/7 priority date for domestic and international students; for spring admission, 1/7 priority date for domestic and international students; for summer admission, 5/7 priority date for domestic and international students. Applications are processed on a rolling basis. Application fee: $50. Electronic applications accepted. *Expenses:* Tuition, state resident: part-time $342 per credit hour. Tuition, nonresident: part-time $631 per credit hour. *Required fees:* $76 per credit hour. Tuition and fees vary according to program. *Financial support:* In 2013–14, 22 teaching assistantships with full tuition reimbursements (averaging $4,920 per year) were awarded; career-related internships or fieldwork, institutionally sponsored loans, scholarships/grants, and unspecified assistantships also available. Support available to part-time students. Financial award application deadline: 3/1; financial award applicants required to submit FAFSA. *Faculty research:* Cardiovascular physiology, clinical physiology, exercise physiology, applied strength and conditioning. *Unit head:* Dr. Sidney Schneider, Director of Graduate Program in Applied Health Physiology, 410-543-6409, E-mail: srschneider@salisbury.edu. *Application contact:* Sue Harman, Program Management Specialist, 410-543-6365, E-mail: seharman@salisbury.edu.
Website: http://www.salisbury.edu/ahph

San Francisco State University, Division of Graduate Studies, College of Science and Engineering, Department of Biology, Program in Physiology and Behavioral Biology, San Francisco, CA 94132-1722. Offers MS. *Application deadline:* Applications are processed on a rolling basis. *Unit head:* Dr. Megumi Fuse, Coordinator, 415-405-0728, E-mail: fuse@sfsu.edu. *Application contact:* Dr. Robert Patterson, Graduate Coordinator, 415-338-1237, E-mail: patters@sfsu.edu.
Website: http://biology.sfsu.edu/graduate/physiology_and_behavior

San Jose State University, Graduate Studies and Research, College of Science, Department of Biological Sciences, San Jose, CA 95192-0001. Offers biological sciences (MA, MS); molecular biology and microbiology (MS); organismal biology, conservation and ecology (MS); physiology (MS). Part-time programs available. *Entrance requirements:* For master's, GRE. Electronic applications accepted. *Faculty research:* Systemic physiology, molecular genetics, SEM studies, toxicology, large mammal ecology.

Southern Illinois University Carbondale, Graduate School, Graduate Program in Medicine, Department of Physiology, Carbondale, IL 62901-4701. Offers MS, PhD. *Faculty:* 18 full-time (4 women). Terminal master's awarded for partial completion of doctoral program. *Degree requirements:* For master's, thesis; for doctorate, thesis/dissertation. *Entrance requirements:* For master's, GRE General Test, minimum GPA of 3.0; for doctorate, GRE General Test, minimum GPA of 3.25. Additional exam requirements/recommendations for international students: Required—TOEFL. *Application deadline:* For fall admission, 6/1 priority date for domestic students. Applications are processed on a rolling basis. Application fee: $0. *Financial support:* In 2013–14, 3 fellowships with full tuition reimbursements, 1 research assistantship with full tuition reimbursement, 10 teaching assistantships with full tuition reimbursements were awarded; institutionally sponsored loans and tuition waivers (full) also available. *Faculty research:* Hormones, neurotransmitters, cell biology, membrane protein, membranes transport. *Unit head:* Richard Steger, Chair, 618-453-1512, Fax: 618-453-1517, E-mail: rsteger@siumed.edu. *Application contact:* Graduate Program Committee, 618-453-1544, Fax: 618-453-1517.

Southern Illinois University Carbondale, Graduate School, Graduate Program in Medicine, Program in Molecular, Cellular and Systemic Physiology, Carbondale, IL 62901-4701. Offers MS. *Students:* 4 full-time (2 women), 16 part-time (12 women); includes 1 minority (Asian, non-Hispanic/Latino), 10 international. 17 applicants, 12% accepted, 2 enrolled. In 2013, 3 master's awarded. Application fee: $50. *Unit head:* Dr. Prema Narayan, Director of Graduate Studies, 618-453-1567, Fax: 618-453-1517, E-mail: pnarayan@siumed.edu. *Application contact:* Pamela Jacobini, Office Manager, 618-453-1512, Fax: 618-453-1517, E-mail: pjacobini@siumed.edu.

Southern Methodist University, Annette Caldwell Simmons School of Education and Human Development, Department of Allied Physiology and Wellness, Dallas, TX 75275. Offers sport management (MS). Program offered jointly with Cox School of Business. *Entrance requirements:* For master's, GMAT, resume, essays, transcripts from all colleges and universities attended, two references. Additional exam requirements/recommendations for international students: Required—TOEFL or PTE.

Stanford University, School of Medicine, Graduate Programs in Medicine, Department of Molecular and Cellular Physiology, Stanford, CA 94305-9991. Offers PhD. *Degree requirements:* For doctorate, thesis/dissertation, qualifying exams. *Entrance requirements:* For doctorate, GRE General Test, GRE Subject Test. Additional exam requirements/recommendations for international students: Required—TOEFL. Electronic applications accepted. *Expenses: Tuition:* Full-time $42,690; part-time $949 per credit. *Required fees:* $185. *Faculty research:* Signal transduction, ion channels, intracellular calcium, synaptic transmission.

State University of New York Upstate Medical University, College of Graduate Studies, Program in Physiology, Syracuse, NY 13210-2334. Offers MS, PhD, MD/PhD. Terminal master's awarded for partial completion of doctoral program. *Degree requirements:* For master's, thesis; for doctorate, comprehensive exam, thesis/dissertation. *Entrance requirements:* For master's, GRE General Test, interview; for doctorate, GRE General Test, telephone interview. Additional exam requirements/recommendations for international students: Required—TOEFL. Electronic applications accepted.

Stony Brook University, State University of New York, Stony Brook University Medical Center, Health Sciences Center, School of Medicine and Graduate School, Graduate Programs in Medicine, Department of Physiology and Biophysics, Stony Brook, NY 11794. Offers PhD. *Faculty:* 17 full-time (6 women). *Students:* 27 full-time (16 women), 2 part-time (both women); includes 16 minority (11 Black or African American, non-Hispanic/Latino; 2 Asian, non-Hispanic/Latino; 3 Hispanic/Latino), 3 international. Average age 29. 4 applicants, 25% accepted, 1 enrolled. In 2013, 1 doctorate awarded. *Degree requirements:* For doctorate, comprehensive exam, thesis/dissertation. *Entrance requirements:* For doctorate, GRE General Test, GRE Subject Test, BS in related field, minimum GPA of 3.0, recommendation. Additional exam requirements/recommendations for international students: Required—TOEFL (minimum score 550 paper-based). *Application deadline:* For fall admission, 1/15 for domestic students; for spring admission, 10/1 for domestic students. Application fee: $100. *Expenses:* Tuition, state resident: full-time $9870; part-time $411 per credit. Tuition, nonresident: full-time $18,350; part-time $765 per credit. *Financial support:* In 2013–14, 4 fellowships, 10 research assistantships were awarded; teaching assistantships and Federal Work-Study also available. Financial award application deadline: 3/15. *Faculty research:* Cellular electrophysiology, membrane permeation and transport, metabolic endocrinology. *Total annual research expenditures:* $7.3 million. *Unit head:* Dr. Peter Brink, Chair, 631-444-3124, Fax: 631-444-3432, E-mail: peter.brink@stonybrook.edu. *Application contact:* Odalis Hernandez, Coordinator, 631-444-3057, Fax: 631-444-3432, E-mail: odalis.hernandez@stonybrook.edu.
Website: http://pnb.informatics.stonybrook.edu/

Teachers College, Columbia University, Graduate Faculty of Education, Department of Biobehavioral Studies, Program in Applied Physiology, New York, NY 10027. Offers Ed M, MA, Ed D. *Faculty:* 2 full-time, 2 part-time/adjunct. *Students:* 11 full-time (9 women), 28 part-time (25 women); includes 8 minority (1 Black or African American, non-Hispanic/Latino; 3 Asian, non-Hispanic/Latino; 4 Hispanic/Latino), 2 international. Average age 28. 33 applicants, 67% accepted, 11 enrolled. In 2013, 16 master's awarded. *Degree requirements:* For master's, final project; for doctorate, comprehensive exam (for some programs), thesis/dissertation. *Application deadline:* For fall admission, 1/15 priority date for domestic students; for spring admission, 11/15 for domestic students. Applications are processed on a rolling basis. Application fee: $65. Electronic applications accepted. *Faculty research:* Modulators of autonomic outflow, the effects of aerobic improvements on autonomic and blood pressure regulation, the role of physical activity in the prevention and treatment of chronic diseases, rehabilitation and cerebral palsy. *Unit head:* Prof. Carol Ewing Garber, Program Coordinator, 212-678-3891, E-mail: garber@tc.columbia.edu. *Application contact:* Morgan Oakes, Admissions Counselor, 212-678-6613, E-mail: meo2142@columbia.edu.
Website: http://www.tc.columbia.edu/bbs/Movement/index.asp?Id=Specializations&Info=Applied+Exercise+Physiology

Texas A&M University, College of Veterinary Medicine and Biomedical Sciences, Department of Veterinary Physiology and Pharmacology, College Station, TX 77843. Offers biomedical science (MS, PhD); toxicology (PhD). *Faculty:* 16. *Students:* 25 full-time (13 women), 3 part-time (2 women); includes 6 minority (1 Black or African American, non-Hispanic/Latino; 2 Asian, non-Hispanic/Latino; 2 Hispanic/Latino; 1 Two or more races, non-Hispanic/Latino), 9 international. Average age 28. 6 applicants, 100% accepted, 6 enrolled. In 2013, 6 master's, 3 doctorates awarded. *Entrance requirements:* For master's and doctorate, GRE General Test. Additional exam requirements/recommendations for international students: Required—TOEFL. Application fee: $50 ($75 for international students). *Expenses:* Tuition, state resident: full-time $4078; part-time $226.55 per credit hour. Tuition, nonresident: full-time $10,450; part-time $580.55 per credit hour. *Required fees:* $2328; $278.50 per credit hour. $642.45 per semester. *Financial support:* Fellowships, research assistantships, and teaching assistantships available. Financial award application deadline: 4/1; financial award applicants required to submit FAFSA. *Faculty research:* Gamete and embryo physiology, endocrinology, equine laminitis. *Unit head:* Dr. John Stallone, Head, 979-862-3065, E-mail: john-n-stallone@exchange.tamu.edu. *Application contact:* Graduate Admissions, 979-845-1044, E-mail: admissions@tamu.edu.
Website: http://vetmed.tamu.edu/vtpp

Tulane University, School of Medicine and School of Liberal Arts, Graduate Programs in Biomedical Sciences, Department of Physiology, New Orleans, LA 70118-5669. Offers MS, PhD, MD/PhD. MS and PhD offered through the Graduate School. *Degree requirements:* For master's, one foreign language, thesis; for doctorate, 2 foreign languages, thesis/dissertation. *Entrance requirements:* For master's, GRE General Test, minimum B average in undergraduate course work; for doctorate, GRE General Test. Additional exam requirements/recommendations for international students: Required—TOEFL. Electronic applications accepted. *Faculty research:* Renal microcirculation, neurophysiology, NA+ transport, renin/angio tensin system, cell and molecular endocrinology.

Universidad Central del Caribe, School of Medicine, Program in Biomedical Sciences, Bayamón, PR 00960-6032. Offers anatomy and cell biology (MA, MS); biochemistry (MS); biomedical sciences (MA); cellular and molecular biology (PhD); microbiology and immunology (MA, MS); pharmacology (MS); physiology (MS).

Université de Montréal, Faculty of Medicine, Department of Physiology, Montréal, QC H3C 3J7, Canada. Offers neurological sciences (M Sc, PhD); physiology (M Sc, PhD). Terminal master's awarded for partial completion of doctoral program. *Degree requirements:* For master's, thesis; for doctorate, thesis/dissertation, general exam. *Entrance requirements:* For master's and doctorate, proficiency in French, knowledge of English. Electronic applications accepted. *Faculty research:* Cardiovascular, neuropeptides, membrane transport and biophysics, signaling pathways.

Université de Sherbrooke, Faculty of Medicine and Health Sciences, Graduate Programs in Medicine, Department of Physiology and Biophysics, Sherbrooke, QC J1H 5N4, Canada. Offers M Sc, PhD. Terminal master's awarded for partial completion of doctoral program. *Degree requirements:* For master's, thesis; for doctorate, thesis/dissertation. Electronic applications accepted. *Faculty research:* Ion channels, neurological basis of pain, insulin resistance, obesity.

Université Laval, Faculty of Medicine, Graduate Programs in Medicine, Programs in Physiology-Endocrinology, Québec, QC G1K 7P4, Canada. Offers M Sc, PhD. Terminal master's awarded for partial completion of doctoral program. *Degree requirements:* For master's, thesis; for doctorate, comprehensive exam, thesis/dissertation. Electronic applications accepted.

University at Buffalo, the State University of New York, Graduate School, School of Medicine and Biomedical Sciences, Graduate Programs in Medicine and Biomedical Sciences, Department of Physiology and Biophysics, Buffalo, NY 14214. Offers biophysics (MS, PhD); physiology (MA, PhD). *Faculty:* 19 full-time (4 women). *Students:* 25 full-time (5 women); includes 9 minority (all Asian, non-Hispanic/Latino). Average age 29. 59 applicants, 46% accepted, 10 enrolled. In 2013, 2 master's, 2 doctorates awarded. Terminal master's awarded for partial completion of doctoral program. *Degree requirements:* For master's, thesis, oral exam, project; for doctorate, thesis/dissertation, oral and written qualifying exam or 2 research proposals. *Entrance requirements:* For master's and doctorate, GRE General Test, unofficial transcripts, 3 letters of recommendation, personal statement, curriculum vitae. Additional exam requirements/recommendations for international students: Required—TOEFL (minimum score 600 paper-based; 100 iBT). *Application deadline:* For fall admission, 2/1 priority date for domestic and international students. Applications are processed on a rolling basis. Application fee: $75. Electronic applications accepted. *Financial support:* In 2013–14, 1 student received support, including 12 research assistantships with full and partial tuition reimbursements available (averaging $25,000 per year); Federal Work-Study, institutionally sponsored loans, health care benefits, and unspecified assistantships also available. Financial award application deadline: 2/1; financial award applicants required to submit FAFSA. *Faculty research:* Neurosciences, ion channels, cardiac physiology, renal/epithelial transport, cardiopulmonary exercise. *Total annual research expenditures:* $2.4 million. *Unit head:* Dr. Perry M. Hogan, Chair, 716-829-2738, Fax: 716-829-2344, E-mail: phogan@buffalo.edu. *Application contact:* Samantha A. Greenwood, Faculty Support Coordinator, 716-829-2738, Fax: 716-829-2344, E-mail: sagreenw@buffalo.edu.
Website: http://www.smbs.buffalo.edu/phb/

University of Alberta, Faculty of Graduate Studies and Research, Department of Biological Sciences, Edmonton, AB T6G 2E1, Canada. Offers environmental biology and ecology (M Sc, PhD); microbiology and biotechnology (M Sc, PhD); molecular biology and genetics (M Sc, PhD); physiology and cell biology (M Sc, PhD); plant biology (M Sc, PhD); systematics and evolution (M Sc, PhD). Terminal master's awarded for partial completion of doctoral program. *Degree requirements:* For master's, thesis; for doctorate, thesis/dissertation. *Entrance requirements:* Additional exam requirements/recommendations for international students: Required—TOEFL.

University of Alberta, Faculty of Medicine and Dentistry and Faculty of Graduate Studies and Research, Graduate Programs in Medicine, Department of Physiology, Edmonton, AB T6G 2E1, Canada. Offers M Sc, PhD. Terminal master's awarded for partial completion of doctoral program. *Degree requirements:* For master's, thesis; for doctorate, thesis/dissertation. *Entrance requirements:* For master's and doctorate, minimum GPA of 3.0. Additional exam requirements/recommendations for international students: Required—TOEFL (minimum score 580 paper-based). Electronic applications accepted. *Faculty research:* Membrane transport, cell biology, perinatal endocrinology, neurophysiology, cardiovascular.

The University of Arizona, Graduate Interdisciplinary Programs, Graduate Interdisciplinary Program in Physiological Sciences, Tucson, AZ 85721. Offers MS, PhD. *Faculty:* 14 full-time (7 women), 1 part-time/adjunct (0 women). *Students:* 42 full-time (21 women), 7 part-time (3 women); includes 17 minority (2 Black or African American, non-Hispanic/Latino; 6 Hispanic/Latino; 9 Two or more races, non-Hispanic/Latino), 6 international. Average age 27. 40 applicants, 45% accepted, 11 enrolled. In 2013, 17 master's, 4 doctorates awarded. *Degree requirements:* For doctorate, thesis/dissertation. *Entrance requirements:* For master's, GRE General Test, 3 letters of recommendation, statement of purpose; for doctorate, GRE General Test, 3 letters of recommendation. Additional exam requirements/recommendations for international students: Required—TOEFL (minimum score 600 paper-based). *Application deadline:* For fall admission, 3/15 for domestic and international students. Applications are processed on a rolling basis. Application fee: $75. Electronic applications accepted. *Expenses:* Tuition, state resident: full-time $11,526. Tuition, nonresident: full-time $27,398. *Financial support:* In 2013–14, 7 research assistantships with full tuition reimbursements (averaging $22,656 per year), 16 teaching assistantships with full tuition reimbursements (averaging $23,553 per year) were awarded; health care benefits and unspecified assistantships also available. *Faculty research:* Cellular transport and signaling, receptor and messenger modulation, neural interaction and biomechanics, fluid network regulation, environmental adaptation. *Total annual research expenditures:* $5.4 million. *Unit head:* Dr. Ronald Lynch, Department Chair, 520-626-2472, E-mail: rlynch@u.arizona.edu. *Application contact:* Holly Lopez, Information Contact, 520-626-2898, Fax: 520-626-2382, E-mail: hollyl@email.arizona.edu.
Website: http://physiological-sciences.arizona.edu/

Physiology

University of Arkansas for Medical Sciences, Graduate School, Little Rock, AR 72205. Offers biochemistry and molecular biology (MS, PhD); bioinformatics (MS, PhD); cellular physiology and molecular biophysics (MS, PhD); clinical nutrition (MS); interdisciplinary biomedical sciences (MS, PhD, Certificate); interdisciplinary toxicology (MS); microbiology and immunology (PhD); neurobiology and developmental sciences (PhD); pharmacology (PhD); MD/PhD. Bioinformatics programs hosted jointly with the University of Arkansas at Little Rock. Part-time programs available. *Faculty:* 397 full-time (205 women). *Students:* 196 full-time (126 women), 117 part-time (87 women); includes 65 minority (38 Black or African American, non-Hispanic/Latino; 1 American Indian or Alaska Native, non-Hispanic/Latino; 21 Asian, non-Hispanic/Latino; 4 Hispanic/Latino; 1 Two or more races, non-Hispanic/Latino), 57 international. 455 applicants, 27% accepted, 89 enrolled. In 2013, 41 master's, 18 doctorates, 28 other advanced degrees awarded. Terminal master's awarded for partial completion of doctoral program. *Degree requirements:* For master's, comprehensive exam (for some programs), thesis (for some programs); for doctorate, thesis/dissertation. *Entrance requirements:* For master's and doctorate, GRE. Additional exam requirements/recommendations for international students: Required—TOEFL. *Application deadline:* Applications are processed on a rolling basis. Application fee: $0. Electronic applications accepted. *Expenses:* Contact institution. *Financial support:* In 2013–14, 120 research assistantships (averaging $24,000 per year) were awarded; career-related internships or fieldwork, Federal Work-Study, and traineeships also available. Support available to part-time students. Financial award applicants required to submit FAFSA. *Unit head:* Dr. Robert E. McGehee, Jr., Dean, 501-686-5454. *Application contact:* Dr. Kristen Sterba, Assistant Dean, Office of Graduate Student Recruiting and Retention, 501-526-7396, E-mail: kmsterba@uams.edu.
Website: http://www.uams.edu/gradschool/

University of Calgary, Cumming School of Medicine and Faculty of Graduate Studies, Medical Science Graduate Program, Calgary, AB T2N 1N4, Canada. Offers cancer biology (M Sc, PhD); critical care medicine (M Sc, PhD); joint injury and arthritis (M Sc, PhD); molecular and medical genetics (M Sc, PhD); mountain medicine and high altitude physiology (M Sc, PhD); pathologists' assistant (M Sc, PhD). *Degree requirements:* For master's, thesis; for doctorate, thesis/dissertation, candidacy exam. *Entrance requirements:* For master's, minimum undergraduate GPA of 3.2; for doctorate, minimum graduate GPA of 3.2. Additional exam requirements/recommendations for international students: Required—TOEFL (minimum score 600 paper-based). Electronic applications accepted. *Faculty research:* Cancer biology, immunology, joint injury and arthritis, medical education, population genomics.

University of Calgary, Cumming School of Medicine and Faculty of Graduate Studies, Program in Gastrointestinal Sciences, Calgary, AB T2N 1N4, Canada. Offers M Sc, PhD. *Degree requirements:* For master's, thesis; for doctorate, thesis/dissertation, candidacy exam. *Entrance requirements:* For master's and doctorate, minimum GPA of 3.2 during previous 2 years. Additional exam requirements/recommendations for international students: Required—TOEFL. Electronic applications accepted. *Faculty research:* Physiology, biochemistry, molecular biology, pharmacology, immunology.

University of California, Berkeley, Graduate Division, College of Letters and Science, Group in Endocrinology, Berkeley, CA 94720-1500. Offers MA, PhD. *Degree requirements:* For doctorate, thesis/dissertation, oral qualifying exam. *Entrance requirements:* For master's, GRE General Test or the equivalent (MCAT), minimum GPA of 3.0, 3 letters of recommendation; for doctorate, GRE General Test or the equivalent (MCAT), minimum GPA of 3.4, 3 letters of recommendation. Additional exam requirements/recommendations for international students: Required—TOEFL.

University of California, Davis, Graduate Studies, Molecular, Cellular and Integrative Physiology Graduate Group, Davis, CA 95616. Offers MS, PhD. *Degree requirements:* For master's, comprehensive exam (for some programs), thesis (for some programs); for doctorate, thesis/dissertation. *Entrance requirements:* For master's and doctorate, GRE General Test. Additional exam requirements/recommendations for international students: Required—TOEFL (minimum score 550 paper-based). Electronic applications accepted. *Faculty research:* Systemic physiology, cellular physiology, neurophysiology, cardiovascular physiology, endocrinology.

University of California, Irvine, School of Medicine and School of Biological Sciences, Department of Physiology and Biophysics, Irvine, CA 92697. Offers biological sciences (PhD); MD/PhD. *Students:* 11 full-time (5 women); includes 5 minority (3 Asian, non-Hispanic/Latino; 1 Hispanic/Latino; 1 Native Hawaiian or other Pacific Islander, non-Hispanic/Latino), 1 international. Average age 28. In 2013, 4 doctorates awarded. *Degree requirements:* For doctorate, thesis/dissertation. *Entrance requirements:* For doctorate, GRE General Test, GRE Subject Test, minimum GPA of 3.0. Additional exam requirements/recommendations for international students: Required—TOEFL (minimum score 550 paper-based). *Application deadline:* For fall admission, 1/15 priority date for domestic students, 1/15 for international students. Application fee: $80 ($100 for international students). Electronic applications accepted. *Financial support:* Fellowships, research assistantships with full tuition reimbursements, teaching assistantships, institutionally sponsored loans, traineeships, health care benefits, and unspecified assistantships available. Financial award application deadline: 3/1; financial award applicants required to submit FAFSA. *Faculty research:* Membrane physiology, exercise physiology, regulation of hormone biosynthesis and action, endocrinology, ion channels and signal transduction. *Unit head:* Prof. Michael Cahalan, Chairman, 949-824-7776, Fax: 949-824-3143, E-mail: mcahalan@uci.edu. *Application contact:* Jamie K. Matsuno-Rich, Assistant Director, 949-824-3484, Fax: 949-824-2636, E-mail: jmrich@uci.edu.
Website: http://www.physiology.uci.edu/

University of California, Los Angeles, David Geffen School of Medicine and Graduate Division, Graduate Programs in Medicine, Department of Physiology, Los Angeles, CA 90095. Offers PhD. *Degree requirements:* For doctorate, thesis/dissertation, oral and written qualifying exams. *Entrance requirements:* For doctorate, GRE General Test, GRE Subject Test. *Faculty research:* Membrane physiology, cell physiology, muscle physiology, neurophysiology, cardiopulmonary physiology.

University of California, Los Angeles, Graduate Division, College of Letters and Science, Department of Integrative Biology and Physiology, Los Angeles, CA 90095. Offers physiological science (MS). *Degree requirements:* For master's, thesis. *Entrance requirements:* For master's, GRE General Test or MCAT, bachelor's degree; minimum undergraduate GPA of 3.0 (or its equivalent if letter grade system not used). Additional exam requirements/recommendations for international students: Required—TOEFL. Electronic applications accepted.

University of California, Los Angeles, Graduate Division, College of Letters and Science and David Geffen School of Medicine, UCLA ACCESS to Programs in the Molecular, Cellular and Integrative Life Sciences, Los Angeles, CA 90095. Offers biochemistry and molecular biology (PhD); biological chemistry (PhD); cellular and molecular pathology (PhD); human genetics (PhD); microbiology, immunology, and molecular genetics (PhD); molecular biology (PhD); molecular toxicology (PhD); molecular, cellular and integrative physiology (PhD); neurobiology (PhD); oral biology (PhD); physiology (PhD). *Degree requirements:* For doctorate, thesis/dissertation, oral and written qualifying exams. *Entrance requirements:* For doctorate, GRE General Test, bachelor's degree; minimum undergraduate GPA of 3.0 (or its equivalent if letter grade system not used). Additional exam requirements/recommendations for international students: Required—TOEFL. Electronic applications accepted.

University of Chicago, Division of Biological Sciences, Neuroscience Graduate Programs, Committee on Integrative Neuroscience, Chicago, IL 60637-1513. Offers cell physiology (PhD); pharmacological and physiological sciences (PhD). *Degree requirements:* For doctorate, thesis/dissertation, preliminary exam. *Entrance requirements:* For doctorate, GRE General Test. Additional exam requirements/recommendations for international students: Required—TOEFL. Electronic applications accepted. *Faculty research:* Psychopharmacology, neuropharmacology.

University of Cincinnati, Graduate School, College of Medicine, Graduate Programs in Biomedical Sciences, Department of Molecular and Cellular Physiology, Cincinnati, OH 45221. Offers physiology (PhD). *Degree requirements:* For doctorate, comprehensive exam, thesis/dissertation, publication. *Entrance requirements:* For doctorate, GRE General Test, GRE Subject Test. Additional exam requirements/recommendations for international students: Required—TOEFL (minimum score 560 paper-based). Electronic applications accepted. *Faculty research:* Endocrinology, cardiovascular physiology, muscle physiology, neurophysiology, transgenic mouse physiology.

University of Colorado Boulder, Graduate School, College of Arts and Sciences, Department of Integrative Physiology, Boulder, CO 80309. Offers MS, PhD. *Faculty:* 23 full-time (8 women). *Students:* 68 full-time (35 women), 6 part-time (1 woman); includes 12 minority (3 Asian, non-Hispanic/Latino; 7 Hispanic/Latino; 2 Two or more races, non-Hispanic/Latino), 2 international. Average age 26. 83 applicants, 28% accepted, 20 enrolled. In 2013, 24 master's, 7 doctorates awarded. Terminal master's awarded for partial completion of doctoral program. *Degree requirements:* For master's, comprehensive exam, thesis or alternative; for doctorate, thesis/dissertation. *Entrance requirements:* For master's, GRE General Test, minimum undergraduate GPA of 2.75. *Application deadline:* For fall admission, 1/15 for domestic students, 12/15 for international students. Applications are processed on a rolling basis. Application fee: $50 ($60 for international students). Electronic applications accepted. *Financial support:* In 2013–14, 184 students received support, including 28 fellowships (averaging $8,335 per year), 38 research assistantships with full and partial tuition reimbursements available (averaging $17,566 per year), 47 teaching assistantships with full and partial tuition reimbursements available (averaging $26,509 per year); institutionally sponsored loans, scholarships/grants, health care benefits, and unspecified assistantships also available. Financial award application deadline: 2/1; financial award applicants required to submit FAFSA. *Faculty research:* Aging/gerontology, human physiology, nervous system, neurophysiology, physiological controls and systems. *Total annual research expenditures:* $7.6 million.
Website: http://www.colorado.edu/intphys/

University of Colorado Denver, School of Medicine, Program in Physiology, Aurora, CO 80045. Offers PhD. *Students:* 30 full-time (19 women); includes 9 minority (1 Black or African American, non-Hispanic/Latino; 3 Asian, non-Hispanic/Latino; 2 Hispanic/Latino; 3 Two or more races, non-Hispanic/Latino), 2 international. Average age 28. 47 applicants, 40% accepted, 19 enrolled. In 2013, 1 doctorate awarded. *Degree requirements:* For doctorate, comprehensive exam, 30 semester credit hours each of coursework and thesis, 3 lab rotations within 1st year. *Entrance requirements:* For doctorate, GRE General Test, 2 transcripts, 4 letters of recommendation, minimum GPA of 3.2, completion of college-level mathematics through calculus, one year each of organic chemistry, physical chemistry, and physics, two years of biology. Additional exam requirements/recommendations for international students: Required—TOEFL (minimum score 550 paper-based; 80 iBT). *Application deadline:* For fall admission, 1/1 for domestic students, 12/1 for international students. Application fee: $50 ($75 for international students). Electronic applications accepted. *Expenses:* Contact institution. *Financial support:* In 2013–14, 6 students received support, including 1 fellowship with full tuition reimbursement available (averaging $25,000 per year); research assistantships, teaching assistantships, Federal Work-Study, institutionally sponsored loans, scholarships/grants, traineeships, health care benefits, tuition waivers (full), and unspecified assistantships also available. Financial award application deadline: 3/15; financial award applicants required to submit FAFSA. *Faculty research:* Nicotinic receptors, immunity, molecular structure, function and regulation of ion channels, calcium influx in the function of cytotoxic T lymphocytes. *Unit head:* Dr. Sukumar Vijayaraghavan, Director, 303-724-4531, E-mail: sukumar.v@ucdenver.edu. *Application contact:* Robby Rigby, Program Administrator, 303-724-4500, Fax: 303-724-4501, E-mail: robby.rigby@ucdenver.edu.
Website: http://www.ucdenver.edu/academics/colleges/medicalschool/departments/physiology/Pages/home.aspx

University of Connecticut, Graduate School, College of Liberal Arts and Sciences, Department of Physiology and Neurobiology, Storrs, CT 06269-3156. Offers comparative physiology (MS, PhD); endocrinology (MS, PhD), including comparative physiology (MS), neurobiology (MS); neurobiology (MS, PhD). Terminal master's awarded for partial completion of doctoral program. *Degree requirements:* For master's, comprehensive exam; for doctorate, thesis/dissertation. *Entrance requirements:* For master's and doctorate, GRE General Test, GRE Subject Test. Additional exam requirements/recommendations for international students: Required—TOEFL (minimum score 550 paper-based). Electronic applications accepted. *Faculty research:* Adult stem cells and brain repair, neural development and brain disorders, autism, epilepsy and stroke, mental and neurological disorders, multiple sclerosis, obstructive sleep apnea.

See Display on next page and Close-Up on page 461.

University of Delaware, College of Arts and Sciences, Department of Biological Sciences, Newark, DE 19716. Offers biotechnology (MS); cancer biology (MS, PhD); cell and extracellular matrix biology (MS, PhD); cell and systems physiology (MS, PhD); developmental biology (MS, PhD); ecology and evolution (MS, PhD); microbiology (MS, PhD); molecular biology and genetics (MS, PhD). Terminal master's awarded for partial completion of doctoral program. *Degree requirements:* For master's, thesis, preliminary exam; for doctorate, comprehensive exam, thesis/dissertation, preliminary exam. *Entrance requirements:* For master's and doctorate, GRE General Test. Additional exam requirements/recommendations for international students: Required—TOEFL (minimum score 600 paper-based); Recommended—TWE. Electronic applications accepted. *Faculty research:* Microorganisms, bone, cancer metastasis, developmental biology, cell biology, DNA.

University of Delaware, College of Health Sciences, Department of Kinesiology and Applied Physiology, Newark, DE 19716. Offers MS, PhD.

University of Florida, College of Medicine and Graduate School, Interdisciplinary Program in Biomedical Sciences, Concentration in Physiology and Pharmacology, Gainesville, FL 32611. Offers PhD. *Degree requirements:* For doctorate, thesis/dissertation. *Entrance requirements:* For doctorate, GRE General Test, minimum GPA of 3.0, biochemistry before enrollment. Electronic applications accepted. *Expenses:* Tuition, state resident: full-time $12,640. Tuition, nonresident: full-time $30,000.

University of Florida, Graduate School, College of Health and Human Performance, Department of Applied Physiology and Kinesiology, Gainesville, FL 32611. Offers

athletic training/sport medicine (MS); biobehavioral science (MS); clinical exercise physiology (MS); health and human performance (PhD), including applied physiology and kinesiology, biobehavioral science, exercise physiology; human performance (MS). *Faculty:* 18 full-time (3 women), 3 part-time/adjunct (1 woman). *Students:* 73 full-time (32 women), 6 part-time (3 women); includes 9 minority (1 Black or African American, non-Hispanic/Latino; 3 Asian, non-Hispanic/Latino; 5 Hispanic/Latino), 18 international. Average age 27. 163 applicants, 23% accepted, 21 enrolled. In 2013, 23 master's, 8 doctorates awarded. *Degree requirements:* For master's, comprehensive exam, thesis (for some programs); for doctorate, comprehensive exam, thesis/dissertation. *Entrance requirements:* For master's and doctorate, GRE General Test, minimum GPA of 3.0. Additional exam requirements/recommendations for international students: Required—TOEFL (minimum score 550 paper-based; 80 iBT), IELTS (minimum score 6). *Application deadline:* For fall admission, 6/1 priority date for domestic students, 6/1 for international students; for spring admission, 9/15 for domestic and international students. Applications are processed on a rolling basis. Application fee: $30. Electronic applications accepted. *Expenses:* Tuition, state resident: full-time $12,640. Tuition, nonresident: full-time $30,000. *Financial support:* In 2013–14, 55 students received support, including 18 research assistantships (averaging $17,260 per year), 41 teaching assistantships (averaging $12,166 per year); unspecified assistantships also available. Financial award application deadline: 2/1; financial award applicants required to submit FAFSA. *Faculty research:* Cardiovascular disease; basic mechanisms that underlie exercise-induced changes in the body at the organ, tissue, cellular and molecular level; development of rehabilitation techniques for regaining motor control after stroke or as a consequence of Parkinson's disease; maintaining optimal health and delaying age-related declines in physiological function; psychomotor mechanisms impacting health and performance across the life span. *Unit head:* Michael Delp, PhD, Professor and Chair, 352-392-0584 Ext. 1338, E-mail: mdelp@hhp.ufl.edu. *Application contact:* Evangelos A. Christou, PhD, Associate Professor and Graduate Coordinator, 352-294-1719 Ext. 1270, E-mail: eachristou@hhp.ufl.edu.
Website: http://apk.hhp.ufl.edu/

University of Georgia, College of Veterinary Medicine, Department of Physiology and Pharmacology, Athens, GA 30602. Offers pharmacology (MS, PhD); physiology (MS, PhD). *Degree requirements:* For master's, thesis; for doctorate, one foreign language, thesis/dissertation. *Entrance requirements:* For master's and doctorate, GRE General Test. Electronic applications accepted.

University of Guelph, Ontario Veterinary College and Graduate Studies, Graduate Programs in Veterinary Sciences, Department of Biomedical Sciences, Guelph, ON N1G 2W1, Canada. Offers morphology (M Sc, DV Sc, PhD); neuroscience (M Sc, DV Sc, PhD); pharmacology (M Sc, DV Sc, PhD); physiology (M Sc, DV Sc, PhD); toxicology (M Sc, DV Sc, PhD). Part-time programs available. *Degree requirements:* For master's, thesis; for doctorate, comprehensive exam, thesis/dissertation. *Entrance requirements:* For master's, honors B Sc, minimum 75% average in last 20 courses; for doctorate, M Sc with thesis from accredited institution. Additional exam requirements/recommendations for international students: Required—TOEFL (minimum score 550 paper-based; 89 iBT). Electronic applications accepted. *Faculty research:* Cellular morphology; endocrine, vascular and reproductive physiology; clinical pharmacology; veterinary toxicology; developmental biology, neuroscience.

University of Hawaii at Manoa, John A. Burns School of Medicine, Program in Developmental and Reproductive Biology, Honolulu, HI 96813. Offers MS, PhD. Part-time programs available. *Degree requirements:* For doctorate, thesis/dissertation. *Entrance requirements:* For doctorate, GRE General Test, GRE Subject Test. Additional exam requirements/recommendations for international students: Recommended—TOEFL (minimum score 560 paper-based), IELTS (minimum score 5). *Faculty research:* Biology of gametes and fertilization, reproductive endocrinology.

University of Illinois at Chicago, College of Medicine and Graduate College, Graduate Programs in Medicine, Department of Physiology and Biophysics, Chicago, IL 60607-7128. Offers MS, PhD. *Faculty:* 19 full-time (5 women), 3 part-time/adjunct (1 woman). *Students:* 14 full-time (6 women); includes 4 minority (1 Asian, non-Hispanic/Latino; 3 Hispanic/Latino), 3 international. Average age 28. 12 applicants, 42% accepted, 3 enrolled. In 2013, 3 master's, 4 doctorates awarded. Terminal master's awarded for partial completion of doctoral program. *Degree requirements:* For master's, thesis; for doctorate, thesis/dissertation. *Entrance requirements:* For master's and doctorate, GRE General Test. Additional exam requirements/recommendations for international students: Required—TOEFL. *Application deadline:* For fall admission, 1/15 priority date for domestic students, 2/15 for international students. Applications are processed on a rolling basis. Application fee: $40 ($50 for international students). Electronic applications accepted. *Expenses:* Tuition, state resident: full-time $11,066; part-time $3689 per term. Tuition, nonresident: full-time $23,064; part-time $7688 per term. *Required fees:* $3004; $1190 per term. Tuition and fees vary according to course level and program. *Financial support:* In 2013–14, 5 fellowships with full tuition reimbursements were awarded; research assistantships with full tuition reimbursements, teaching assistantships with full tuition reimbursements, Federal Work-Study, traineeships, and tuition waivers (full) also available. Financial award application deadline: 3/1; financial award applicants required to submit FAFSA. *Faculty research:* Neuroscience, endocrinology and reproduction, cell physiology, exercise physiology, NMR, cardiovascular physiology and metabolism, cytoskeleton and vascular biology, gastrointestinal and epithelial cell biology, reproductive and endocrine sciences. *Total annual research expenditures:* $7.5 million. *Unit head:* Prof. R. John Solaro, Department Head, 312-996-7620, Fax: 312-996-1414, E-mail: solarorj@uic.edu. *Application contact:* Jackie Perry, Graduate College Receptionist, 312-413-2550, Fax: 312-413-0185, E-mail: gradcoll@uic.edu.
Website: http://www.physiology.uic.edu/

University of Illinois at Urbana–Champaign, Graduate College, College of Liberal Arts and Sciences, School of Integrative Biology, Program in Physiological and Molecular Plant Biology, Champaign, IL 61820. Offers PhD. *Students:* 3 full-time (1 woman), 2 international. Application fee: $75 ($90 for international students). *Unit head:* Stephen Moose, Director, 217-244-6308, Fax: 217-244-1224, E-mail: smoose@illinois.edu. *Application contact:* Kimberly Leigh, Office Manager, 217-333-8208, Fax: 217-244-1224, E-mail: kaleigh@illinois.edu.
Website: http://www.life.illinois.edu/plantbio/pmpb/

University of Illinois at Urbana–Champaign, Graduate College, College of Liberal Arts and Sciences, School of Molecular and Cellular Biology, Department of Molecular and Integrative Physiology, Champaign, IL 61820. Offers MS, PhD. *Students:* 28 (12 women). Application fee: $75 ($90 for international students). *Unit head:* Milan Bagchi, Head, 217-333-1735, Fax: 217-333-1133, E-mail: mbagchi@illinois.edu. *Application contact:* Shawna Smith, Office Manager, 217-244-6638, Fax: 217-333-1133, E-mail: smsmith1@illinois.edu.
Website: http://mcb.illinois.edu/departments/mip/

The University of Iowa, Roy J. and Lucille A. Carver College of Medicine and Graduate College, Graduate Programs in Medicine, Department of Molecular Physiology and Biophysics, Iowa City, IA 52240. Offers MS, PhD. *Faculty:* 17 full-time (3 women), 17 part-time/adjunct (2 women). *Students:* 19 full-time (4 women); includes 4 minority (all Asian, non-Hispanic/Latino), 3 international. Average age 25. In 2013, 1 master's, 1 doctorate awarded. *Degree requirements:* For master's, comprehensive exam; for doctorate, comprehensive exam, thesis/dissertation. *Entrance requirements:* For master's, GRE General Test; for doctorate, GRE. Additional exam requirements/recommendations for international students: Required—TOEFL. *Application deadline:* For fall admission, 4/1 for domestic students, 3/1 for international students; for spring

admission, 10/1 for domestic students, 9/1 for international students. Applications are processed on a rolling basis. Application fee: $60 ($80 for international students). Electronic applications accepted. *Financial support:* In 2013–14, 1 fellowship with full tuition reimbursement (averaging $25,500 per year), 17 research assistantships with full tuition reimbursements (averaging $25,500 per year) were awarded; traineeships also available. Financial award application deadline: 4/1. *Faculty research:* Cellular and molecular endocrinology, membrane structure and function, cardiac cell electrophysiology, regulation of gene expression, neurophysiology. *Unit head:* Dr. Kevin P. Campbell, Chair and Department Executive Officer, 319-335-7800, Fax: 319-335-7330, E-mail: kevin-campbell@uiowa.edu. *Application contact:* Dr. Mark Stamnes, Director of Graduate Studies, 319-335-7858, Fax: 319-335-7330, E-mail: mark-stamnes@uiowa.edu.
Website: http://www.physiology.uiowa.edu/

The University of Kansas, University of Kansas Medical Center, School of Medicine, Department of Molecular and Integrative Physiology, Kansas City, KS 66160. Offers molecular and integrative physiology (MS, PhD); neuroscience (MS, PhD); MD/PhD. *Faculty:* 45. *Students:* 21 full-time (13 women), 1 part-time (0 women), 15 international. Average age 27. In 2013, 10 doctorates awarded. Terminal master's awarded for partial completion of doctoral program. *Degree requirements:* For master's, thesis; for doctorate, comprehensive exam, thesis/dissertation. *Entrance requirements:* For doctorate, GRE. Additional exam requirements/recommendations for international students: Required—TOEFL. *Application deadline:* For fall admission, 1/15 priority date for domestic and international students. Applications are processed on a rolling basis. Application fee: $10. Electronic applications accepted. *Financial support:* Research assistantships with partial tuition reimbursements, teaching assistantships with full and partial tuition reimbursements, scholarships/grants, and unspecified assistantships available. Financial award application deadline: 3/1; financial award applicants required to submit FAFSA. *Faculty research:* Male reproductive physiology and contraception, ovarian development and regulation by pituitary and hypothalamus, neural control of movement and stroke recovery, cardio-pulmonary physiology and hypoxia, plasticity of the autonomic nervous system, renal physiology. *Total annual research expenditures:* $7.7 million. *Unit head:* Dr. Paul D. Cheney, Chairman, 913-588-7400, Fax: 913-588-7430, E-mail: pcheney@kumc.edu. *Application contact:* Dr. Michael W. Wolfe, Director of Graduate Studies, 913-588-7418, Fax: 913-588-7430, E-mail: mwolfe2@kumc.edu.
Website: http://www.kumc.edu/school-of-medicine/molecular-and-integrative-physiology.html

University of Kentucky, Graduate School, Graduate School Programs from the College of Medicine, Program in Physiology, Lexington, KY 40506-0032. Offers PhD. *Degree requirements:* For doctorate, comprehensive exam, thesis/dissertation. *Entrance requirements:* For doctorate, GRE General Test, minimum undergraduate GPA of 2.75, graduate 3.0. Additional exam requirements/recommendations for international students: Required—TOEFL (minimum score 550 paper-based). Electronic applications accepted.

University of Louisville, School of Medicine, Department of Physiology and Biophysics, Louisville, KY 40292-0001. Offers MS, PhD, MD/PhD. *Students:* 31 full-time (9 women), 7 part-time (5 women); includes 8 minority (3 Black or African American, non-Hispanic/Latino; 4 Asian, non-Hispanic/Latino; 1 Two or more races, non-Hispanic/Latino), 7 international. Average age 28. 25 applicants, 52% accepted, 10 enrolled. In 2013, 13 master's, 6 doctorates awarded. Terminal master's awarded for partial completion of doctoral program. *Degree requirements:* For master's, thesis; for doctorate, comprehensive exam, thesis/dissertation. *Entrance requirements:* For master's and doctorate, GRE General Test (minimum score of 1000 verbal and quantitative), minimum GPA of 3.0. Additional exam requirements/recommendations for international students: Required—TOEFL. *Application deadline:* For fall admission, 1/15 priority date for domestic students. Applications are processed on a rolling basis. Application fee: $60. Electronic applications accepted. *Expenses:* Tuition, state resident: full-time $10,788; part-time $599 per credit hour. Tuition, nonresident: full-time $22,446; part-time $1247 per credit hour. *Required fees:* $196. Tuition and fees vary according to program and reciprocity agreements. *Financial support:* Fellowships with full tuition reimbursements and research assistantships with full tuition reimbursements available. Financial award application deadline: 4/15. *Faculty research:* Control of microvascular function during normal and disease states; mechanisms of cellular adhesive interactions on endothelial cells lining blood vessels; changes in blood rheological properties and mechanisms associated with increased blood fibrinogen content; role of nutrition in microvascular control mechanisms; mechanism of cardiovascular-renal remodeling in hypertension, diabetes, and heart failure. *Unit head:* Dr. Irving G. Joshua, Chair, 502-852-5371, Fax: 502-852-6239, E-mail: igjosh01@gwise.louisville.edu. *Application contact:* Dr. William Wead, Director of Admissions, 502-852-7571, Fax: 502-852-6849, E-mail: wbwead01@gwise.louisville.edu.
Website: http://louisville.edu/medschool/physiology/

The University of Manchester, Faculty of Life Sciences, Manchester, United Kingdom. Offers adaptive organismal biology (M Phil, PhD); animal biology (M Phil, PhD); biochemistry (M Phil, PhD); bioinformatics (M Phil, PhD); biomolecular sciences (M Phil, PhD); biotechnology (M Phil, PhD); cell biology (M Phil, PhD); cell matrix research (M Phil, PhD); channels and transporters (M Phil, PhD); developmental biology (M Phil, PhD); Egyptology (M Phil, PhD); environmental biology (M Phil, PhD); evolutionary biology (M Phil, PhD); gene expression (M Phil, PhD); genetics (M Phil, PhD); history of science, technology and medicine (M Phil, PhD); immunology (M Phil, PhD); integrative neurobiology and behavior (M Phil, PhD); membrane trafficking (M Phil, PhD); microbiology (M Phil, PhD); molecular and cellular neuroscience (M Phil, PhD); molecular biology (M Phil, PhD); molecular cancer studies (M Phil, PhD); neuroscience (M Phil, PhD); ophthalmology (M Phil, PhD); optometry (M Phil, PhD); organelle function (M Phil, PhD); pharmacology (M Phil, PhD); physiology (M Phil, PhD); plant sciences (M Phil, PhD); stem cell research (M Phil, PhD); structural biology (M Phil, PhD); systems neuroscience (M Phil, PhD); toxicology (M Phil, PhD).

University of Manitoba, Faculty of Medicine and Faculty of Graduate Studies, Graduate Programs in Medicine, Department of Physiology, Winnipeg, MB R3T 2N2, Canada. Offers M Sc, PhD, MD/PhD. Terminal master's awarded for partial completion of doctoral program. *Degree requirements:* For master's, one foreign language, thesis; for doctorate, one foreign language, thesis/dissertation. *Entrance requirements:* For master's, minimum GPA of 3.5; for doctorate, minimum GPA of 3.5, M Sc. *Faculty research:* Cardiovascular research, gene technology, cell biology, neuroscience, respiration.

University of Massachusetts Amherst, Graduate School, Interdisciplinary Programs, Program in Plant Biology, Amherst, MA 01003. Offers biochemistry and metabolism (MS, PhD); cell biology and physiology (MS, PhD); environmental, ecological and integrative biology (MS, PhD); genetics and evolution (MS, PhD). *Students:* 20 full-time (11 women), 9 international. Average age 28. 72 applicants, 17% accepted, 2 enrolled. In 2013, 1 master's, 2 doctorates awarded. *Degree requirements:* For master's, thesis; for doctorate, 2 foreign languages, comprehensive exam, thesis/dissertation. *Entrance requirements:* For master's and doctorate, GRE General Test. Additional exam requirements/recommendations for international students: Required—TOEFL (minimum score 550 paper-based; 80 iBT), IELTS (minimum score 6.5). *Application deadline:* For fall admission, 12/15 for domestic and international students; for spring admission, 10/1 for domestic and international students. Applications are processed on a rolling basis. Application fee: $75. Electronic applications accepted. *Financial support:* Fellowships with full and partial tuition reimbursements, research assistantships with full and partial tuition reimbursements, teaching assistantships with full and partial tuition reimbursements, career-related internships or fieldwork, Federal Work-Study, scholarships/grants, traineeships, health care benefits, tuition waivers (full and partial), and unspecified assistantships available. Support available to part-time students. Financial award application deadline: 12/15; financial award applicants required to submit FAFSA. *Unit head:* Dr. Elsbeth L. Walker, Graduate Program Director, 413-577-3217, Fax: 413-545-3243, E-mail: pb@bio.umass.edu. *Application contact:* Lindsay DeSantis, Supervisor of Admissions, 413-545-0722, Fax: 413-577-0010, E-mail: gradadm@grad.umass.edu.
Website: http://www.bio.umass.edu/plantbio/

University of Miami, Graduate School, Miller School of Medicine, Graduate Programs in Medicine, Department of Physiology and Biophysics, Coral Gables, FL 33124. Offers PhD, MD/PhD. *Degree requirements:* For doctorate, thesis/dissertation, qualifying exam. *Entrance requirements:* For doctorate, GRE General Test, minimum GPA of 3.0 in sciences. Additional exam requirements/recommendations for international students: Required—TOEFL. *Faculty research:* Cell and membrane physiology, cell-to-cell communication, molecular neurobiology, neuroimmunology, neural development.

University of Michigan, Rackham Graduate School, Program in Biomedical Sciences (PIBS), Department of Molecular and Integrative Physiology, Ann Arbor, MI 48109. Offers MS, PhD. *Faculty:* 33 full-time (11 women), 6 part-time/adjunct (2 women). *Students:* 57 full-time (32 women); includes 15 minority (2 Black or African American, non-Hispanic/Latino; 10 Asian, non-Hispanic/Latino; 1 Hispanic/Latino; 2 Two or more races, non-Hispanic/Latino). Average age 25. 137 applicants, 40% accepted, 28 enrolled. In 2013, 23 master's, 7 doctorates awarded. *Degree requirements:* For master's, thesis (for some programs), capstone project (for some programs); for doctorate, thesis/dissertation, oral defense of dissertation, preliminary exam. *Entrance requirements:* For master's, GRE, MCAT, DAT or PCAT, minimum science and overall GPA of 3.0; for doctorate, GRE General Test, 3 letters of recommendation, research experience. Additional exam requirements/recommendations for international students: Required—TOEFL (minimum score 84 iBT) or Michigan English Language Assessment Battery. *Application deadline:* For fall admission, 12/1 for domestic and international students. Application fee: $75 ($90 for international students). Electronic applications accepted. Tuition and fees vary according to course level, course load, degree level, program and student level. *Financial support:* In 2013–14, 26 students received support, including 26 fellowships with full tuition reimbursements available (averaging $28,500 per year); scholarships/grants, health care benefits, tuition waivers (full), and unspecified assistantships also available. Financial award application deadline: 12/1. *Faculty research:* Ion transport, cardiovascular physiology, gene expression, hormone action, gastrointestinal physiology, endocrinology, muscle, signal transduction. *Unit head:* Dr. Bishr Omary, Chair, 734-764-4376, Fax: 734-936-8813, E-mail: mbishr@umich.edu. *Application contact:* Michelle S. Melis, Director of Student Life, 734-615-6538, Fax: 734-647-7022, E-mail: msmtegan@umich.edu.
Website: http://medicine.umich.edu/dept/molecular-integrative-physiology

University of Minnesota, Duluth, Medical School, Graduate Program in Physiology, Duluth, MN 55812-2496. Offers MS, PhD. MS, PhD offered jointly with University of Minnesota, Twin Cities Campus. Terminal master's awarded for partial completion of doctoral program. *Degree requirements:* For master's, thesis; for doctorate, thesis/dissertation. *Entrance requirements:* For master's, GRE or MCAT; for doctorate, GRE or MCAT, 1 year of course work in each calculus, physics, and biology; 2 years of course work in chemistry; minimum GPA of 3.0 in science. Additional exam requirements/recommendations for international students: Required—TOEFL. *Faculty research:* Neural control of posture and locomotion, transport and metabolic phenomena in biological systems, control of organ blood flow, intracellular means of communication.

University of Minnesota, Twin Cities Campus, Graduate School, Department of Integrative Biology and Physiology, Minneapolis, MN 55455-0213. Offers PhD. Part-time programs available. *Degree requirements:* For doctorate, comprehensive exam, thesis/dissertation. *Entrance requirements:* For doctorate, GRE General Test. Electronic applications accepted. *Faculty research:* Cardiovascular physiology.

University of Mississippi Medical Center, School of Graduate Studies in the Health Sciences, Department of Physiology and Biophysics, Jackson, MS 39216-4505. Offers PhD, MD/PhD. *Faculty:* 20 full-time (5 women). *Students:* 7 full-time (2 women); includes 2 minority (1 Black or African American, non-Hispanic/Latino; 1 Asian, non-Hispanic/Latino). Average age 25. 10 applicants, 30% accepted, 3 enrolled. *Degree requirements:* For doctorate, thesis/dissertation, first authored publication. *Entrance requirements:* For doctorate, GRE General Test, minimum GPA of 3.0. *Application deadline:* For fall admission, 8/1 for domestic students. Applications are processed on a rolling basis. Application fee: $10. *Financial support:* In 2013–14, 7 students received support, including 7 research assistantships with full tuition reimbursements available (averaging $24,150 per year); health care benefits also available. Financial award application deadline: 4/1. *Faculty research:* Cardiovascular, renal, endocrine, and cellular neurophysiology; molecular physiology. *Unit head:* Dr. John E. Hall, Chairman, 601-984-1801, Fax: 601-984-1817. *Application contact:* Dr. Michael J. Ryan, Director, 601-984-1801, Fax: 601-984-1817, E-mail: mjryan@umc.edu.
Website: http://www.umc.edu/Education/Schools/Medicine/Basic_Science/Physiology_and_Biophysics/Graduate_Program%28Physiology%29/Academics.aspx

University of Missouri, School of Medicine and Graduate School, Graduate Programs in Medicine, Department of Medical Pharmacology and Physiology, Columbia, MO 65211. Offers MS, PhD. *Faculty:* 29 full-time (4 women), 3 part-time/adjunct (1 woman). *Students:* 14 full-time (9 women), 2 part-time (both women); includes 1 minority (Black or African American, non-Hispanic/Latino), 10 international. Average age 28. 42 applicants, 10% accepted, 4 enrolled. In 2013, 1 master's, 1 doctorate awarded. *Degree requirements:* For master's, thesis; for doctorate, thesis/dissertation. *Entrance requirements:* For master's and doctorate, GRE General Test, minimum GPA of 3.0. Additional exam requirements/recommendations for international students: Required—TOEFL (minimum score 500 paper-based; 61 iBT). *Application deadline:* For fall admission, 1/10 priority date for domestic and international students; for winter admission, 10/10 priority date for domestic and international students. Applications are processed on a rolling basis. Application fee: $55 ($75 for international students). Electronic applications accepted. *Financial support:* Fellowships, research assistantships, teaching assistantships, institutionally sponsored loans, scholarships/grants, health care benefits, and unspecified assistantships available. Support available to part-time students. *Faculty research:* Endocrine and metabolic pharmacology, biochemical pharmacology, neuropharmacology, receptors and transmembrane signaling. *Unit head:* Dr. Ron Korthuis, Department Chair, 573-882-8029, E-mail: korthuisr@missouri.edu. *Application contact:* Melinda Nichols, Administrative Assistant, 573-882-8432, E-mail: nicholsmk@missouri.edu.
Website: http://mpp.missouri.edu/

University of Nebraska Medical Center, Department of Cellular and Integrative Physiology, Omaha, NE 68198-5850. Offers physiology (MS, PhD). Terminal master's awarded for partial completion of doctoral program. *Degree requirements:* For master's, comprehensive exam, thesis optional; for doctorate, comprehensive exam, thesis/dissertation, at least one first-author research publication. *Entrance requirements:* For master's and doctorate, GRE General Test or MCAT, course work in biology, chemistry, mathematics, and physics. Additional exam requirements/recommendations for international students: Required—TOEFL (minimum score 600 paper-based; 100 iBT). Electronic applications accepted. *Expenses: Required fees:* $300 per semester. Tuition and fees vary according to program. *Faculty research:* Cardiovascular, renal and visual physiology, neuroscience, reproductive endocrinology.

University of Nevada, Reno, Graduate School, Interdisciplinary Program in Cellular and Molecular Pharmacology and Physiology, Reno, NV 89557. Offers PhD. *Degree requirements:* For doctorate, one foreign language, thesis/dissertation. *Entrance requirements:* For doctorate, GRE General Test or MCAT, minimum GPA of 3.0. Additional exam requirements/recommendations for international students: Required—TOEFL (minimum score 500 paper-based; 61 iBT), IELTS (minimum score 6). Electronic applications accepted. *Faculty research:* Neuropharmacology, toxicology, cardiovascular pharmacology, neuromuscular pharmacology.

University of New Mexico, School of Medicine, Program in Biomedical Sciences, Albuquerque, NM 87131-5196. Offers biochemistry and molecular biology (MS, PhD); cell biology and physiology (MS, PhD); clinical and translational science (Certificate); molecular genetics and microbiology (MS, PhD); neuroscience (MS, PhD); pathology (MS, PhD); toxicology (MS, PhD); university science teaching (Certificate). Part-time programs available. *Students:* 73 full-time (39 women), 14 part-time (9 women); includes 24 minority (1 Black or African American, non-Hispanic/Latino; 1 American Indian or Alaska Native, non-Hispanic/Latino; 2 Asian, non-Hispanic/Latino; 17 Hispanic/Latino; 1 Native Hawaiian or other Pacific Islander, non-Hispanic/Latino; 2 Two or more races, non-Hispanic/Latino), 16 international. Average age 29. 89 applicants, 20% accepted, 17 enrolled. In 2013, 7 master's, 17 doctorates awarded. Terminal master's awarded for partial completion of doctoral program. *Degree requirements:* For master's, thesis; for doctorate, comprehensive exam, thesis/dissertation, qualifying exam at the end of year 1/core curriculum. *Entrance requirements:* For master's and doctorate, GRE General Test, minimum undergraduate GPA of 3.0. Additional exam requirements/recommendations for international students: Required—TOEFL. *Application deadline:* For fall admission, 3/1 priority date for domestic and international students. Applications are processed on a rolling basis. Application fee: $50. Electronic applications accepted. *Financial support:* In 2013–14, 94 students received support, including 28 fellowships with full and partial tuition reimbursements available (averaging $22,000 per year), 73 research assistantships with full tuition reimbursements available (averaging $23,000 per year), 8 teaching assistantships (averaging $2,800 per year); career-related internships or fieldwork, Federal Work-Study, institutionally sponsored loans, scholarships/grants, traineeships, health care benefits, and unspecified assistantships also available. Financial award application deadline: 1/1; financial award applicants required to submit FAFSA. *Faculty research:* Infectious disease/immunity, cancer biology, cardiovascular and metabolic diseases, brain and behavioral illness, environmental health. *Unit head:* Dr. Helen J. Hathaway, Program Director, 505-272-1887, Fax: 505-272-2412, E-mail: hhathaway@salud.unm.edu. *Application contact:* Mary Fenton, Admissions Coordinator, 505-272-1887, Fax: 505-272-2412, E-mail: mfenton@salud.unm.edu.
Website: http://hsc.unm.edu/research/brep/bsgpabout.shtm

University of North Dakota, Graduate School and Graduate School, Graduate Programs in Medicine, Department of Pharmacology, Physiology, and Therapeutics, Grand Forks, ND 58202. Offers pharmacology (MS, PhD); physiology (MS, PhD). *Degree requirements:* For master's, comprehensive exam, thesis; for doctorate, thesis/dissertation, written and oral exams. *Entrance requirements:* For master's, GRE General Test or MCAT, minimum GPA of 3.0; for doctorate, GRE General Test, minimum GPA of 3.5. Additional exam requirements/recommendations for international students: Required—TOEFL (minimum score 550 paper-based; 79 iBT), IELTS (minimum score 6.5). Electronic applications accepted.

University of North Texas Health Science Center at Fort Worth, Graduate School of Biomedical Sciences, Fort Worth, TX 76107-2699. Offers anatomy and cell biology (MS, PhD); biochemistry and molecular biology (MS, PhD); biomedical sciences (MS, PhD); biotechnology (MS); forensic genetics (MS); integrative physiology (MS, PhD); medical science (MS); microbiology and immunology (MS, PhD); pharmacology (MS, PhD); science education (MS); DO/MS; DO/PhD. Terminal master's awarded for partial completion of doctoral program. *Degree requirements:* For master's, thesis; for doctorate, thesis/dissertation. *Entrance requirements:* For master's and doctorate, GRE General Test. Additional exam requirements/recommendations for international students: Required—TOEFL. *Expenses:* Contact institution. *Faculty research:* Alzheimer's disease, aging, eye diseases, cancer, cardiovascular disease.

University of Notre Dame, Graduate School, College of Science, Department of Biological Sciences, Notre Dame, IN 46556. Offers aquatic ecology, evolution and environmental biology (MS, PhD); cellular and molecular biology (MS, PhD); genetics (MS, PhD); physiology (MS, PhD); vector biology and parasitology (MS, PhD). Terminal master's awarded for partial completion of doctoral program. *Degree requirements:* For master's, comprehensive exam, thesis; for doctorate, comprehensive exam, thesis/dissertation, candidacy exam. *Entrance requirements:* For master's and doctorate, GRE General Test. Additional exam requirements/recommendations for international students: Required—TOEFL (minimum score 600 paper-based; 80 iBT). Electronic applications accepted. *Faculty research:* Tropical disease, molecular genetics, neurobiology, evolutionary biology, aquatic biology.

University of Oklahoma Health Sciences Center, College of Medicine and Graduate College, Graduate Programs in Medicine, Department of Physiology, Oklahoma City, OK 73190. Offers MS, PhD. Part-time programs available. *Faculty:* 5 full-time (1 woman), 1 part-time/adjunct (0 women). *Students:* 10 full-time (7 women), 1 part-time (0 women), 9 international. Average age 29. 9 applicants, 33% accepted, 3 enrolled. In 2013, 2 master's, 1 doctorate awarded. Terminal master's awarded for partial completion of doctoral program. *Degree requirements:* For master's, thesis (for some programs); for doctorate, thesis/dissertation. *Entrance requirements:* For master's, GRE General Test, statement of career goals, 3 letters of recommendation; for doctorate, GRE General Test, 3 letters of recommendation. Additional exam requirements/recommendations for international students: Required—TOEFL. *Application deadline:* For fall admission, 12/15 for domestic students. Application fee: $25 ($50 for international students). *Expenses:* Tuition, state resident: full-time $3504; part-time $175.20 per credit hour. Tuition, nonresident: full-time $13,504; part-time $675.20 per credit hour. *Required fees:* $1545; $52.70 per credit hour. $245.25 per semester. Tuition and fees vary according to course load. *Financial support:* In 2013–14, 4 research assistantships (averaging $18,000 per year) were awarded; fellowships, teaching assistantships, and career-related internships or fieldwork also available. *Faculty research:* Cardiopulmonary physiology, neurophysiology, exercise physiology, cell and molecular physiology. *Unit head:* Dr. Jay Ma, Chair, 405-271-2226, E-mail: jay-ma@ouhsc.edu. *Application contact:* Dr. Sinya Benyajati, Graduate Liaison, 405-271-2284, Fax: 405-271-3181, E-mail: sinya-benyajati@ouhsc.edu.

University of Oregon, Graduate School, College of Arts and Sciences, Department of Human Physiology, Eugene, OR 97403. Offers MS, PhD. *Degree requirements:* For master's, thesis optional; for doctorate, one foreign language, thesis/dissertation. *Entrance requirements:* For master's, GRE General Test, minimum GPA of 2.75 in undergraduate course work; for doctorate, GRE General Test. *Faculty research:* Balance control, muscle fatigue, lower extremity function, knee control.

University of Pennsylvania, Perelman School of Medicine, Biomedical Graduate Studies, Graduate Group in Cell and Molecular Biology, Philadelphia, PA 19104. Offers cancer biology (PhD); cell biology and physiology (PhD); developmental stem cell regenerative biology (PhD); gene therapy and vaccines (PhD); genetics and gene regulation (PhD); microbiology, virology, and parasitology (PhD); MD/PhD; VMD/PhD. *Faculty:* 321. *Students:* 352 full-time (205 women); includes 99 minority (11 Black or African American, non-Hispanic/Latino; 65 Asian, non-Hispanic/Latino; 21 Hispanic/Latino; 2 Two or more races, non-Hispanic/Latino), 45 international. 488 applicants, 20% accepted, 40 enrolled. In 2013, 41 doctorates awarded. *Degree requirements:* For doctorate, thesis/dissertation. *Entrance requirements:* For doctorate, GRE General Test. Additional exam requirements/recommendations for international students: Required—TOEFL. *Application deadline:* For fall admission, 12/1 priority date for domestic and international students. Applications are processed on a rolling basis. Application fee: $80. Electronic applications accepted. *Financial support:* In 2013–14, 352 students received support. Fellowships, research assistantships, scholarships/grants, traineeships, and unspecified assistantships available. *Unit head:* Dr. Daniel Kessler, Graduate Group Chair, 215-898-1478. *Application contact:* Meagan Schofer, Coordinator, 215-898-4360.
Website: http://www.med.upenn.edu/camb/

University of Prince Edward Island, Atlantic Veterinary College, Graduate Program in Veterinary Medicine, Charlottetown, PE C1A 4P3, Canada. Offers anatomy (M Sc, PhD); bacteriology (M Sc, PhD); clinical pharmacology (M Sc, PhD); clinical sciences (M Sc, PhD); epidemiology (M Sc, PhD), including reproduction; fish health (M Sc, PhD); food animal nutrition (M Sc, PhD); immunology (M Sc, PhD); microanatomy (M Sc, PhD); parasitology (M Sc, PhD); pathology (M Sc, PhD); pharmacology (M Sc, PhD); physiology (M Sc, PhD); toxicology (M Sc, PhD); veterinary science (M Vet Sc); virology (M Sc, PhD). Part-time programs available. *Degree requirements:* For master's, thesis; for doctorate, thesis/dissertation. *Entrance requirements:* For master's, DVM, B Sc honors degree, or equivalent; for doctorate, M Sc. Additional exam requirements/recommendations for international students: Required—TOEFL (minimum score 550 paper-based; 80 iBT). *Expenses:* Contact institution. *Faculty research:* Animal health management, infectious diseases, fin fish and shellfish health, basic biomedical sciences, ecosystem health.

University of Puerto Rico, Medical Sciences Campus, School of Medicine, Division of Graduate Studies, Department of Physiology, San Juan, PR 00936-5067. Offers MS, PhD. Terminal master's awarded for partial completion of doctoral program. *Degree requirements:* For master's, one foreign language, thesis; for doctorate, one foreign language, comprehensive exam, thesis/dissertation. *Entrance requirements:* For master's and doctorate, GRE General Test, GRE Subject Test, interview; course work in biology, chemistry and physics; minimum GPA of 3.0; 3 letters of recommendation. Electronic applications accepted. *Faculty research:* Respiration, neuroendocrinology, cellular and molecular physiology, cardiovascular, exercise physiology and neurobiology.

University of Rochester, School of Medicine and Dentistry, Graduate Programs in Medicine and Dentistry, Department of Pharmacology and Physiology, Programs in Physiology, Rochester, NY 14627. Offers MS, PhD. Terminal master's awarded for partial completion of doctoral program. *Degree requirements:* For master's, thesis; for doctorate, thesis/dissertation, qualifying exam. *Entrance requirements:* For master's and doctorate, GRE General Test. *Expenses: Tuition:* Full-time $44,580; part-time $1394 per credit hour. *Required fees:* $492.

University of Saskatchewan, College of Medicine, Department of Physiology, Saskatoon, SK S7N 5A2, Canada. Offers M Sc, PhD. *Degree requirements:* For master's, thesis; for doctorate, thesis/dissertation. *Entrance requirements:* Additional exam requirements/recommendations for international students: Required—TOEFL. *Expenses: Tuition, area resident:* Full-time $3585 Canadian dollars; part-time $585 Canadian dollars per course. Tuition, nonresident: part-time $877 Canadian dollars per course. *International tuition:* $5377 Canadian dollars full-time. *Required fees:* $889.51 Canadian dollars.

University of Saskatchewan, Western College of Veterinary Medicine and College of Graduate Studies and Research, Graduate Programs in Veterinary Medicine, Department of Veterinary Biomedical Sciences, Saskatoon, SK S7N 5A2, Canada. Offers veterinary anatomy (M Sc); veterinary biomedical sciences (M Vet Sc); veterinary physiological sciences (M Sc, PhD). *Degree requirements:* For master's, thesis; for doctorate, comprehensive exam (for some programs), thesis/dissertation. *Entrance requirements:* Additional exam requirements/recommendations for international students: Required—TOEFL (minimum score 80 iBT); Recommended—IELTS (minimum score 6.5). Electronic applications accepted. *Expenses: Tuition, area resident:* Full-time $3585 Canadian dollars; part-time $585 Canadian dollars per course. Tuition, nonresident: part-time $877 Canadian dollars per course. *International tuition:* $5377 Canadian dollars full-time. *Required fees:* $889.51 Canadian dollars. *Faculty research:* Toxicology, animal reproduction, pharmacology, chloride channels, pulmonary pathobiology.

The University of South Dakota, Graduate School, School of Medicine and Graduate School, Biomedical Sciences Graduate Program, Physiology and Pharmacology Group, Vermillion, SD 57069-2390. Offers MS, PhD. Terminal master's awarded for partial completion of doctoral program. *Degree requirements:* For master's, thesis; for doctorate, comprehensive exam, thesis/dissertation. *Entrance requirements:* For master's and doctorate, GRE General Test, minimum GPA of 3.0. Additional exam requirements/recommendations for international students: Required—TOEFL (minimum score 550 paper-based; 80 iBT), IELTS (minimum score 6). Electronic applications accepted. *Expenses:* Contact institution. *Faculty research:* Pulmonary physiology and pharmacology, drug abuse, reproduction, signal transduction, cardiovascular physiology and pharmacology.

University of Southern California, Keck School of Medicine and Graduate School, Graduate Programs in Medicine, Department of Physiology and Biophysics, Los Angeles, CA 90089. Offers MS. *Faculty:* 13 full-time (2 women). *Students:* 6 full-time (2 women), 4 international. Average age 27. 6 applicants, 17% accepted, 1 enrolled. In 2013, 2 master's awarded. *Degree requirements:* For master's, thesis optional. *Entrance requirements:* For master's, GRE General Test, minimum GPA of 3.0. Additional exam requirements/recommendations for international students: Required—TOEFL (minimum score 600 paper-based; 100 iBT). *Application deadline:* For fall admission, 12/1 priority date for domestic and international students. Application fee: $85. Electronic applications accepted. *Financial support:* Federal Work-Study, institutionally sponsored loans, scholarships/grants, traineeships, health care benefits, and unspecified assistantships available. Financial award application deadline: 5/4. *Faculty research:* Endocrinology and metabolism, neurophysiology, mathematical modeling, cell transport, autoimmunity and cancer immunotherapy. *Total annual research expenditures:* $4.5 million. *Unit head:* Dr. Berislav Zlokavic, Chair, 323-442-2566, Fax: 323-442-2230, E-mail: zlokovic@usc.edu. *Application contact:* Janet Stoeckert, Administrative Director, Basic Sciences Departments, 323-442-3568, Fax: 323-442-1610, E-mail: janet.stoeckert@usc.edu.

University of South Florida, College of Arts and Sciences, Department of Integrative Biology, Tampa, FL 33620-9951. Offers biology (MS), including ecology and evolution (MS, PhD), environmental and ecological microbiology (MS, PhD), physiology and morphology (MS, PhD); integrative biology (PhD), including ecology and evolution (MS, PhD), environmental and ecological microbiology (MS, PhD), physiology and morphology (MS, PhD). Part-time programs available. *Faculty:* 16 full-time (4 women), 1 part-time/adjunct (0 women). *Students:* 40 full-time (24 women), 7 part-time (4 women); includes 6 minority (5 Hispanic/Latino; 1 Two or more races, non-Hispanic/Latino), 3 international. Average age 29. 59 applicants, 29% accepted, 11 enrolled. In 2013, 4 master's, 5 doctorates awarded. *Degree requirements:* For master's, comprehensive exam, thesis (for some programs); for doctorate, comprehensive exam, thesis/dissertation. *Entrance requirements:* For master's and doctorate, GRE General Test (minimum preferred scores of 153 verbal, 148 quantitative, 4.5 analytical/500 verbal and 600 quantitative with 4.5 in analytical writing on old scoring), minimum GPA of 3.0 in last 60 hours of BS. Additional exam requirements/recommendations for international students: Required—TOEFL (minimum score 570 paper-based; 88 iBT). *Application deadline:* For fall admission, 2/15 priority date for domestic students, 1/2 for international students; for spring admission, 8/1 for domestic students, 6/1 for international students. Application fee: $30. Electronic applications accepted. *Financial support:* Research assistantships, teaching assistantships, and unspecified assistantships available. Financial award application deadline: 6/30; financial award applicants required to submit FAFSA. *Faculty research:* Marine ecology, ecosystem responses to urbanization, biomechanical and physiological mechanisms of animal movement, population biology and conservation, microbial ecology and public health microbiology, natural diversity of parasites and herbivores; ecosystems, vertebrates, disturbance ecology, functional and ecological morphology of feeding in fishes, rare amphibians and reptiles, genomics in ecological experiments, ecotoxicology, global carbon cycle, plant-animal interactions. *Total annual research expenditures:* $968,227. *Unit head:* Dr. Peter Stiling, Chair, Department of Integrative Biology, 813-974-6229, Fax: 813-974-3263, E-mail: pstiling@usf.edu. *Application contact:* Christine Brubaker, Graduate Program Specialist, Department of Integrative Biology, 813-974-4747, Fax: 813-974-3263, E-mail: brubaker@usf.edu.
Website: http://biology.usf.edu/ib/grad/

University of South Florida, Morsani College of Medicine and Graduate School, Graduate Programs in Medical Sciences, Tampa, FL 33620-9951. Offers aging and neuroscience (MSMS); allergy, immunology and infectious disease (PhD); anatomy (MSMS, PhD); athletic training (MSMS); bioinformatics and computational biology (MSBCB); biotechnology (MSB); clinical and translational research (MSMS, PhD); health informatics (MSHI, MSMS); health science (MSMS); interdisciplinary medical sciences (MSMS); medical microbiology and immunology (MSMS); metabolic and nutritional medicine (MSMS); molecular medicine (MSMS, PhD); molecular pharmacology and physiology (PhD); neurology (PhD); pathology and laboratory medicine (PhD); pharmacology and therapeutics (PhD); physiology and biophysics (PhD); women's health (MSMS). *Students:* 336 full-time (182 women), 39 part-time (21 women); includes 170 minority (45 Black or African American, non-Hispanic/Latino; 54 Asian, non-Hispanic/Latino; 59 Hispanic/Latino; 2 Native Hawaiian or other Pacific Islander, non-Hispanic/Latino; 10 Two or more races, non-Hispanic/Latino), 17 international. Average age 26. 1,066 applicants, 44% accepted, 250 enrolled. In 2013, 191 master's, 12 doctorates awarded. Terminal master's awarded for partial completion of doctoral program. *Degree requirements:* For master's, comprehensive exam, thesis; for doctorate, comprehensive exam, thesis/dissertation. *Entrance requirements:* For master's, GRE General Test or GMAT, bachelor's degree or equivalent from regionally-accredited university with minimum GPA of 3.0 in upper-division sciences coursework; prerequisites in general biology, general chemistry, general physics, organic chemistry, quantitative analysis, and integral and differential calculus; for doctorate, GRE General Test (minimum score of 600 quantitative), bachelor's degree from regionally-accredited university with minimum GPA of 3.0 in upper-division sciences coursework; 3 letters of recommendation; personal interview; 1-2 page personal statement; prerequisites in biology, chemistry, physics, organic chemistry, quantitative analysis, and integral/differential calculus. Additional exam requirements/recommendations for international students: Required—TOEFL (minimum score 550 paper-based; 79 iBT) or IELTS (minimum score 6.5). *Application deadline:* For fall admission, 2/15 for domestic students, 1/2 for international students. Application fee: $30. *Expenses:* Contact institution. *Faculty research:* Anatomy, biochemistry, cancer biology, cardiovascular disease, cell biology, immunology, microbiology, molecular biology, neuroscience, pharmacology, physiology. *Unit head:* Dr. Michael Barber, Professor and Associate Dean for Graduate and Postdoctoral Affairs, 813-974-9908, Fax: 813-974-4317, E-mail: mbarber@health.usf.edu. *Application contact:* Dr. Eric Bennett, Graduate Director, PhD Program in Medical Sciences, 813-974-1545, Fax: 813-974-4317, E-mail: esbennet@health.usf.edu.
Website: http://health.usf.edu/nocms/medicine/graduatestudies/

The University of Tennessee, Graduate School, College of Agricultural Sciences and Natural Resources, Department of Animal Science, Knoxville, TN 37996. Offers animal anatomy (PhD); breeding (MS, PhD); management (MS, PhD); nutrition (MS, PhD); physiology (MS, PhD). Part-time programs available. *Degree requirements:* For master's, thesis; for doctorate, thesis/dissertation. *Entrance requirements:* For master's and doctorate, GRE General Test, minimum GPA of 2.7. Additional exam requirements/recommendations for international students: Required—TOEFL. Electronic applications accepted. *Expenses:* Tuition, state resident: full-time $9540; part-time $531 per credit hour. Tuition, nonresident: full-time $27,728; part-time $1542 per credit hour. *Required fees:* $1404; $67 per credit hour.

The University of Texas Health Science Center at San Antonio, Graduate School of Biomedical Sciences, Department of Physiology, San Antonio, TX 78229-3900. Offers MS, PhD. *Faculty:* 36 full-time (8 women), 6 part-time/adjunct (2 women). *Students:* 15 full-time (9 women), 2 part-time (1 woman); includes 2 minority (1 Black or African American, non-Hispanic/Latino; 1 Hispanic/Latino), 8 international. Average age 30. In 2013, 1 master's, 4 doctorates awarded. *Degree requirements:* For master's, thesis; for doctorate, comprehensive exam, thesis/dissertation. *Entrance requirements:* For master's, GRE General Test, MAT; for doctorate, GRE General Test. Additional exam requirements/recommendations for international students: Required—TOEFL (minimum score 560 paper-based; 68 iBT). *Application deadline:* For fall admission, 1/15 priority date for domestic and international students. Applications are processed on a rolling basis. Application fee: $0. Electronic applications accepted. *Financial support:* Application deadline: 6/30; applicants required to submit FAFSA. *Faculty research:* Ion channels, cardiovascular function, neuroscience and aging. *Total annual research expenditures:* $6.8 million. *Unit head:* Dr. Manzoor Bhat, Department Chair, 210-567-4327, Fax: 210-567-4410, E-mail: bhatm@uthscsa.edu. *Application contact:* Dr. Mark Shapiro, Applicant Advisor/Committee on Graduate Studies Chair, 210-567-4045, Fax: 210-567-4410, E-mail: shapirom@uthscsa.edu.
Website: http://physiology.uthscsa.edu/

The University of Texas Medical Branch, Graduate School of Biomedical Sciences, Program in Cellular Physiology and Molecular Biophysics, Galveston, TX 77555. Offers MS, PhD. *Degree requirements:* For master's, thesis or alternative; for doctorate, thesis/dissertation. *Entrance requirements:* For master's and doctorate, GRE General Test. Additional exam requirements/recommendations for international students: Required—TOEFL (minimum score 550 paper-based). Electronic applications accepted.

University of Toronto, Faculty of Medicine, Department of Physiology, Toronto, ON M5S 1A1, Canada. Offers M Sc, PhD, MD/PhD. *Degree requirements:* For master's, thesis; for doctorate, thesis/dissertation. *Entrance requirements:* For master's and doctorate, minimum B+ average in final year, 2 letters of reference. Additional exam requirements/recommendations for international students: Required—TOEFL (600 paper-based), Michigan English Language Assessment Battery (95), IELTS (8) or COPE (5). Electronic applications accepted.

University of Utah, School of Medicine and Graduate School, Graduate Programs in Medicine, Department of Physiology, Salt Lake City, UT 84112-1107. Offers PhD. *Degree requirements:* For doctorate, thesis/dissertation, comprehensive qualifying exam, preliminary exam. *Entrance requirements:* For doctorate, GRE General Test, GRE Subject Test, minimum GPA of 3.0. Additional exam requirements/recommendations for international students: Required—TOEFL (minimum score 650 paper-based; 100 iBT); Recommended—TWE (minimum score 6). Electronic applications accepted. *Expenses:* Tuition, state resident: full-time $5259. Tuition, nonresident: full-time $18,569. *Required fees:* $841. Tuition and fees vary according to course load. *Faculty research:* Cell neurobiology, chemosensory systems, cardiovascular and kidney physiology, endocrinology.

University of Virginia, School of Medicine, Department of Molecular Physiology and Biological Physics, Program in Physiology, Charlottesville, VA 22903. Offers PhD, MD/PhD. *Students:* 5 full-time (3 women). Average age 27. In 2013, 6 doctorates awarded. *Entrance requirements:* For doctorate, GRE General Test, 2 letters of recommendation. Additional exam requirements/recommendations for international students: Required—TOEFL. *Application deadline:* For fall admission, 1/15 for domestic and international students. Applications are processed on a rolling basis. Application fee: $60. Electronic applications accepted. *Expenses:* Tuition, state resident: part-time $334 per credit hour. Tuition, nonresident: part-time $1224 per credit hour. *Financial support:* Fellowships, research assistantships, and teaching assistantships available. Financial award applicants required to submit FAFSA. *Unit head:* Dr. Mark Yeager, Chair, 434-924-5108, Fax: 434-982-1616, E-mail: my3r@virginia.edu. *Application contact:* E-mail: physiograd@virginia.edu.
Website: http://www.healthsystem.virginia.edu/internet/physio/

University of Washington, Graduate School, School of Medicine, Graduate Programs in Medicine, Department of Physiology and Biophysics, Seattle, WA 98195. Offers PhD. *Degree requirements:* For doctorate, thesis/dissertation. *Entrance requirements:* For doctorate, GRE General Test. Additional exam requirements/recommendations for international students: Required—TOEFL (minimum score 580 paper-based; 70 iBT). *Faculty research:* Membrane and cell biophysics, neuroendocrinology, cardiovascular and respiratory physiology, systems neurophysiology and behavior, molecular physiology.

The University of Western Ontario, Faculty of Graduate Studies, Biosciences Division, Department of Physiology and Pharmacology, London, ON N6A 5B8, Canada. Offers M Sc, PhD. *Degree requirements:* For master's, thesis, seminar course; for doctorate, comprehensive exam, thesis/dissertation. *Entrance requirements:* For master's, minimum B average, honors degree; for doctorate, minimum B average, honors degree, M Sc. *Faculty research:* Reproductive and endocrine physiology, neurophysiology, cardiovascular and renal physiology, cell physiology, gastrointestinal and metabolic physiology.

University of Wisconsin–La Crosse, Graduate Studies, College of Science and Health, Department of Biology, La Crosse, WI 54601-3742. Offers aquatic sciences (MS); biology (MS); cellular and molecular biology (MS); clinical microbiology (MS); microbiology (MS); nurse anesthesia (MS); physiology (MS). Part-time programs available. *Faculty:* 22 full-time (8 women), 3 part-time/adjunct (1 woman). *Students:* 21 full-time (13 women), 37 part-time (24 women); includes 7 minority (2 Asian, non-Hispanic/Latino; 4 Hispanic/Latino; 1 Two or more races, non-Hispanic/Latino), 5 international. Average age 28. 107 applicants, 26% accepted, 25 enrolled. In 2013, 16 master's awarded. *Degree requirements:* For master's, comprehensive exam, thesis. *Entrance requirements:* For master's, GRE General Test, minimum GPA of 2.85. Additional exam requirements/recommendations for international students: Required—TOEFL (minimum score 550 paper-based; 79 iBT). *Application deadline:* For fall admission, 2/1 priority date for domestic and international students; for spring admission, 1/4 priority date for domestic and international students. Applications are processed on a rolling basis. Electronic applications accepted. *Financial support:* Research assistantships with partial tuition reimbursements, Federal Work-Study, scholarships/grants, health care benefits, and tuition waivers (partial) available. Support available to part-time students. Financial award application deadline: 3/15; financial award applicants required to submit FAFSA. *Unit head:* Dr. Thomas Volk, Coordinator of Graduate Studies, 608-785-6972, Fax: 608-785-6959, E-mail: volk.thom@uwlax.edu. *Application contact:* Corey Sjoquist, Director of Admissions, 608-785-8939, E-mail: admissions@uwlax.edu.
Website: http://uwlax.edu/biology/

University of Wisconsin–Madison, School of Medicine and Public Health, Endocrinology and Reproductive Physiology Program, Madison, WI 53706. Offers MS, PhD. *Faculty:* 43 full-time (16 women). *Students:* 29 full-time (15 women), 3 part-time (0 women); includes 10 minority (3 Black or African American, non-Hispanic/Latino; 2 Asian, non-Hispanic/Latino; 4 Hispanic/Latino; 1 Native Hawaiian or other Pacific Islander, non-Hispanic/Latino), 9 international. Average age 30. 42 applicants, 24% accepted, 7 enrolled. In 2013, 2 master's, 4 doctorates awarded. Terminal master's awarded for partial completion of doctoral program. *Degree requirements:* For master's, comprehensive exam, thesis, oral defense of thesis; for doctorate, comprehensive exam, thesis/dissertation, oral defense of dissertation. *Entrance requirements:* For master's and doctorate, GRE, resume, 3 letters of recommendation. Additional exam requirements/recommendations for international students: Required—TOEFL (minimum score 580 paper-based; 92 iBT), IELTS (minimum score 7). *Application deadline:* For fall admission, 12/1 for domestic and international students. Application fee: $56. Electronic applications accepted. *Expenses:* Tuition, state resident: full-time $10,728; part-time $790 per credit. Tuition, nonresident: full-time $24,054; part-time $1623 per credit. *Required fees:* $1130; $119 per credit. *Financial support:* In 2013–14, 4 fellowships with full tuition reimbursements (averaging $25,000 per year), 19 research assistantships with full and partial tuition reimbursements (averaging $25,000 per year) were awarded; scholarships/grants, traineeships, health care benefits, and unspecified assistantships also available. *Faculty research:* Ovarian physiology and endocrinology, fertilization and gamete biology, hormone action and cell signaling, placental function and pregnancy,

embryo and fetal development. *Unit head:* Dr. Ian M. Bird, Director, 608-262-7456, E-mail: imbird@wisc.edu. *Application contact:* Grace Jensen, Student Services Coordinator, 608-265-5838, E-mail: gjensen2@wisc.edu.
Website: http://www.erp.wisc.edu/

University of Wisconsin–Madison, School of Medicine and Public Health and Graduate School, Graduate Programs in Medicine, Madison, WI 53705. Offers biomolecular chemistry (MS, PhD); cancer biology (PhD); epidemiology (MS, PhD); genetics and medical genetics (MS, PhD), including genetics (PhD), medical genetics (MS); medical physics (MS, PhD), including health physics (MS), medical physics; microbiology (PhD); molecular and cellular pharmacology (PhD); neuroscience (PhD); pathology and laboratory medicine (PhD); physiology (PhD); population health (MS, PhD), including population health; DPT/MPH; DVM/MPH; MD/MPH; MD/PhD; MPA/MPH; MS/MPH; Pharm D/MPH. Part-time programs available. Postbaccalaureate distance learning degree programs offered (minimal on-campus study). Terminal master's awarded for partial completion of doctoral program. Application fee: $45. Electronic applications accepted. *Expenses:* Contact institution. *Financial support:* Fellowships with full tuition reimbursements, research assistantships with full tuition reimbursements, teaching assistantships with full tuition reimbursements, scholarships/grants, traineeships, and tuition waivers (full) available. *Unit head:* Dr. Richard L. Moss, Senior Associate Dean for Basic Research, Biotechnology and Graduate Studies, 608-265-0523, Fax: 608-265-0522, E-mail: rlmoss@wisc.edu. *Application contact:* Information Contact, 608-262-2433, Fax: 608-262-5134, E-mail: gradadmiss@mail.bascom.wisc.edu.
Website: http://www.med.wisc.edu

University of Wisconsin–Madison, School of Medicine and Public Health, Physiology Graduate Training Program, Madison, WI 53706. Offers PhD. *Faculty:* 62 full-time (20 women). *Students:* 17 full-time (7 women); includes 1 minority (Black or African American, non-Hispanic/Latino), 11 international. Average age 25. 31 applicants, 16% accepted, 2 enrolled. *Degree requirements:* For doctorate, comprehensive exam, thesis/dissertation, written exams. *Entrance requirements:* For doctorate, GRE, minimum GPA of 3.0. Additional exam requirements/recommendations for international students: Required—TOEFL. *Application deadline:* For fall admission, 12/15 priority date for domestic and international students. Applications are processed on a rolling basis. Application fee: $56. Electronic applications accepted. *Expenses:* Tuition, state resident: full-time $10,728; part-time $790 per credit. Tuition, nonresident: full-time $24,054; part-time $1623 per credit. *Required fees:* $1130; $119 per credit. *Financial support:* In 2013–14, research assistantships with tuition reimbursements (averaging $25,000 per year) were awarded; fellowships with tuition reimbursements and teaching assistantships with tuition reimbursements also available. *Faculty research:* Studies in molecular cellular systems, cardiovascular, neuroscience. *Unit head:* Dr. Donata Oertel, Director, 608-263-6281, E-mail: doertel@wisc.edu. *Application contact:* Eileen M. Stevens, Administrator, 608-263-7380, Fax: 608-262-5245, E-mail: emstevens@wisc.edu.
Website: http://www.pgtp.wisc.edu/

University of Wyoming, College of Arts and Sciences, Department of Zoology and Physiology, Laramie, WY 82071. Offers MS, PhD. Part-time programs available. *Degree requirements:* For master's, comprehensive exam (for some programs), thesis; for doctorate, comprehensive exam (for some programs), thesis/dissertation. *Entrance requirements:* For master's and doctorate, GRE General Test, minimum GPA of 3.0. Additional exam requirements/recommendations for international students: Required—TOEFL. Electronic applications accepted. *Faculty research:* Cell biology, ecology/wildlife, organismal physiology, zoology.

Virginia Commonwealth University, Graduate School, School of Allied Health Professions, Department of Physical Therapy, Richmond, VA 23284-9005. Offers advanced physical therapy (DPT); entry-level physical therapy (DPT); health related sciences (PhD); physiology/physical therapy (PhD). *Accreditation:* APTA (one or more programs are accredited). *Degree requirements:* For doctorate, thesis/dissertation. *Entrance requirements:* For doctorate, GRE General Test, Physical Therapist Centralized Application Service (PTCAS). Additional exam requirements/recommendations for international students: Required—TOEFL (minimum score 600 paper-based; 100 iBT). Electronic applications accepted. *Faculty research:* Eye movement, bilabyrinthectomy on ferret muscle fiber typing, neck disability index, cost-effective care, training effect on muscle.

Virginia Commonwealth University, Medical College of Virginia-Professional Programs, School of Medicine, School of Medicine Graduate Programs, Department of Physiology and Biophysics, Richmond, VA 23284-9005. Offers physical therapy (PhD); physiology (MS, PhD); MD/PhD. Terminal master's awarded for partial completion of doctoral program. *Degree requirements:* For master's, thesis; for doctorate, thesis/dissertation, comprehensive oral and written exams. *Entrance requirements:* For master's, GRE General Test, MCAT, or DAT; for doctorate, GRE, MCAT or DAT. Additional exam requirements/recommendations for international students: Required—TOEFL (minimum score 600 paper-based; 100 iBT). Electronic applications accepted.

Virginia Commonwealth University, Program in Pre-Medical Basic Health Sciences, Richmond, VA 23284-9005. Offers anatomy (CBHS); biochemistry (CBHS); human genetics (CBHS); microbiology (CBHS); pharmacology (CBHS); physiology (CBHS). *Entrance requirements:* For degree, GRE, MCAT or DAT, course work in organic chemistry, minimum undergraduate GPA of 2.8. Additional exam requirements/recommendations for international students: Required—TOEFL (minimum score 600 paper-based). Electronic applications accepted.

Wake Forest University, School of Medicine and Graduate School of Arts and Sciences, Graduate Programs in Medicine, Program in Physiology and Pharmacology, Winston-Salem, NC 27109. Offers pharmacology (PhD); physiology (PhD); MD/PhD. *Degree requirements:* For doctorate, thesis/dissertation. *Entrance requirements:* For doctorate, GRE General Test. Additional exam requirements/recommendations for international students: Required—TOEFL. Electronic applications accepted. *Faculty research:* Aging, substance abuse, cardiovascular control, endocrine systems, toxicology.

Wayne State University, School of Medicine, Graduate Programs in Medicine, Department of Physiology, Detroit, MI 48202. Offers physiology (MS, PhD); reproductive sciences (PhD); MD/PhD. *Students:* 37 full-time (22 women), 8 part-time (6 women); includes 11 minority (3 Black or African American, non-Hispanic/Latino; 3 Asian, non-Hispanic/Latino; 3 Hispanic/Latino; 1 Native Hawaiian or other Pacific Islander, non-Hispanic/Latino; 1 Two or more races, non-Hispanic/Latino), 15 international. Average age 29. 50 applicants, 20% accepted, 8 enrolled. In 2013, 6 master's, 1 doctorate awarded. *Degree requirements:* For master's, thesis; for doctorate, thesis/dissertation. *Entrance requirements:* For master's, GRE General Test, minimum GPA of 2.75, personal statement, resume, three letters of recommendation, current curriculum vitae or resume, admission to the Graduate School; for doctorate, GRE General Test, minimum GPA of 3.0, personal statement, resume, three letters of recommendation, current curriculum vitae or resume, admission to the Graduate School. Additional exam requirements/recommendations for international students: Recommended—TOEFL (minimum score 600 paper-based; 100 iBT). *Application deadline:* For fall admission, 2/1 for domestic and international students; for winter admission, 10/1 for domestic students, 9/1 for international students; for spring admission, 2/1 for domestic students, 1/1 for international students. Application fee: $0. Electronic applications accepted. *Expenses:* Contact institution. *Financial support:* In 2013–14, 23 students received support, including 10 fellowships with tuition reimbursements available (averaging $22,521 per year), 29 research assistantships with tuition reimbursements available (averaging $22,521 per year); teaching assistantships, scholarships/grants, and unspecified assistantships also available. Support available to part-time students. Financial award application deadline: 3/31; financial award applicants required to submit FAFSA. *Faculty research:* Regulation of brain blood flow, mechanism of hormone action, regulation of pituitary hormone secretion, regulation of cellular membranes, nano biotechnology. *Unit head:* Dr. Douglas Yingst, Graduate Program Director, 313-577-1548, E-mail: dyingst@med.wayne.edu.
Website: http://physiology.med.wayne.edu/phd-physiology/index.php

Weill Cornell Medical College, Weill Cornell Graduate School of Medical Sciences, Physiology, Biophysics and Systems Biology Program, New York, NY 10065. Offers MS, PhD. Terminal master's awarded for partial completion of doctoral program. *Degree requirements:* For master's, comprehensive exam; for doctorate, thesis/dissertation, final exam. *Entrance requirements:* For doctorate, GRE General Test, introductory courses in biology, inorganic and organic chemistry, physics, and mathematics. Additional exam requirements/recommendations for international students: Required—TOEFL. *Faculty research:* Receptor-mediated regulation of cell function, molecular properties of channels or receptors, bioinformatics, mathematical modeling.

Western Michigan University, Graduate College, College of Education and Human Development, Department of Health, Physical Education and Recreation, Kalamazoo, MI 49008. Offers exercise and sports medicine (MS), including athletic training, exercise physiology; physical education (MA), including coaching sport performance, pedagogy, special physical education, sport management.

West Virginia University, Davis College of Agriculture, Forestry and Consumer Sciences, Division of Animal and Nutritional Sciences, Program in Animal and Nutritional Sciences, Morgantown, WV 26506. Offers breeding (MS); food sciences (MS); nutrition (MS); physiology (MS); production management (MS); reproduction (MS). Part-time programs available. *Degree requirements:* For master's, thesis, oral and written exams. *Entrance requirements:* For master's, GRE, minimum GPA of 2.5. Additional exam requirements/recommendations for international students: Required—TOEFL. *Faculty research:* Animal nutrition, reproductive physiology, food science.

West Virginia University, Davis College of Agriculture, Forestry and Consumer Sciences, Interdisciplinary Program in Reproductive Physiology, Morgantown, WV 26506. Offers MS, PhD. Part-time programs available. Terminal master's awarded for partial completion of doctoral program. *Degree requirements:* For master's, thesis; for doctorate, comprehensive exam, thesis/dissertation. *Entrance requirements:* For master's, minimum GPA of 2.75; for doctorate, minimum GPA of 3.0. Additional exam requirements/recommendations for international students: Required—TOEFL. Electronic applications accepted. *Faculty research:* Uterine prostaglandins, luteal function, neural control of luteinizing hormone and follicle-stimulating hormone, follicular development, embryonic and fetal loss.

West Virginia University, School of Medicine, Graduate Programs at the Health Sciences Center, Interdisciplinary Graduate Programs in Biomedical Sciences, Program in Cellular and Integrative Physiology, Morgantown, WV 26506. Offers MS, PhD, MD/PhD. *Degree requirements:* For doctorate, comprehensive exam, thesis/dissertation. *Entrance requirements:* For doctorate, GRE General Test, minimum GPA of 3.0. Additional exam requirements/recommendations for international students: Required—TOEFL. Electronic applications accepted. *Faculty research:* Cell signaling and development of the microvasculature, neural control of reproduction, learning and memory, airway responsiveness and remodeling.

Wright State University, School of Graduate Studies, College of Science and Mathematics, Department of Neuroscience, Cell Biology, and Physiology, Dayton, OH 45435. Offers anatomy (MS); physiology and biophysics (MS). *Degree requirements:* For master's, thesis optional. *Entrance requirements:* Additional exam requirements/recommendations for international students: Required—TOEFL. *Faculty research:* Reproductive cell biology, neurobiology of pain, neurohistochemistry.

Yale University, School of Medicine and Graduate School of Arts and Sciences, Combined Program in Biological and Biomedical Sciences (BBS), Physiology and Integrative Medical Biology Track, New Haven, CT 06520. Offers PhD, MD/PhD. *Entrance requirements:* Additional exam requirements/recommendations for international students: Required—TOEFL.

Youngstown State University, Graduate School, College of Science, Technology, Engineering and Mathematics, Department of Biological Sciences, Youngstown, OH 44555-0001. Offers environmental biology (MS); molecular biology, microbiology, and genetic (MS); physiology and anatomy (MS). Part-time programs available. *Degree requirements:* For master's, comprehensive exam, thesis, oral review. *Entrance requirements:* For master's, GRE General Test, minimum GPA of 2.7. Additional exam requirements/recommendations for international students: Required—TOEFL. *Faculty research:* Cell biology, neurophysiology, molecular biology, neurobiology, gene regulation.

UNIVERSITY OF CONNECTICUT

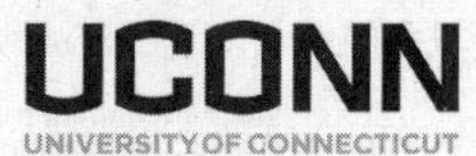

College of Liberal Arts and Sciences
Department of Physiology and Neurobiology

Programs of Study

The Department offers course work and research programs leading to M.S. and Ph.D. degrees in physiology and neurobiology with concentrations in the areas of neurobiology, endocrinology, and comparative physiology. In addition, the Department of Molecular and Cell Biology, the Department of Ecology and Evolutionary Biology, and the Biotechnology Center provide the opportunity for students to obtain a comprehensive background in biological sciences and offer the possibility of collaborative research. Graduate programs are designed to fit the individual student's background and scientific interests. In the first year, students take two courses on the foundations of physiology and neurobiology. Through the first two years, and occasionally into the third year of training, students select from a number of additional seminars and courses in their area of major interest and related areas. By the end of the first year, the student selects the area of dissertation research, and a committee consisting of a major adviser and 3 associate advisers is formed. Students may begin dissertation research during the first year.

Research Facilities

The Department of Physiology and Neurobiology (PNB) is located primarily in the new state-of-the-art Pharmacy/Biology Building. The Department houses both shared and individual laboratories for behavioral, cellular, electrophysiological, and molecular research in physiology. The Department also houses the University's electron microscopy facility, which contains equipment for scanning and transmission EM as well as electron probe analysis. Departmental faculty members also utilize the Marine Research Laboratories at Noank and Avery Point, Connecticut.

Financial Aid

Several types of financial support are available to graduate students. Most students are supported either on teaching assistantships or research assistantships from faculty grants. For the 2014–15, academic year, full-time teaching assistantships (nine months) pay $20,966 for beginning graduate students, $22,061 for those with an M.S. or the equivalent, and $24,527 for those who have passed the Ph.D. general examination. Both half and full graduate assistantships come with a tuition waiver, and students may purchase health-care coverage, subsidized by the University of Connecticut. In addition, the Graduate School provides the Outstanding Scholar Award to as many as 10 incoming Ph.D. candidates during the first year of study. Several additional research fellowships and University fellowships are awarded on a competitive basis. Many labs also provide additional funding for summer research (up to $6,000–$7,000).

Cost of Study

Tuition is waived for full-time graduate assistants; however, they pay the full-time University fees of approximately $1,200 per semester. Tuition is prorated for graduate assistants registering for fewer than 9 credits per semester.

Living and Housing Costs

Privately owned apartments are available near the campus at moderate rents. Houses and apartments for rent may also be found in the surrounding communities. More information is available online at http://www.reslife.uconn.edu/graduate_housing.html.

Student Group

Approximately 18,000 undergraduates and 8,000 graduate students are enrolled at the main campus at Storrs. Eighty-one percent of the undergraduate students and 70 percent of the graduate students are from Connecticut. The rest of the students come from forty-three states and more than 100 countries. The Department of Physiology and Neurobiology has about 40 graduate students (https://uconn.edu/pdf/UConn_Facts_2014.pdf).

Location

The University is located in a scenic countryside setting of small villages, streams, and rolling hills. There is easy access by car and bus to major urban and cultural centers, including Hartford, New Haven, Boston, and New York, and to other educational institutions, such as Yale, Harvard, and MIT. Recreational opportunities include skiing, fishing, sailing, hiking, ice-skating, and athletic events. The University of Connecticut offers a range of culturally—and gastronomically—rich attractions. Students can visit diverse and distinct museums; attend world-class performances in music, theater, and the performing arts; and frequent nearby Storrs Downtown, a vibrant town square featuring cafés, restaurants, and shopping galore. There are also several large shopping centers nearby.

The University

The University of Connecticut at Storrs is the state's flagship public research university and is in the midst of a $2.3 billion transformation, ensuring its place as one of the premier public research universities in the country. Perennially ranked the top public university in New England, the University of Connecticut now stands among the best public institutions in the nation. The University was founded in 1881 and is a state-supported institution. The 1,800-acre main campus at Storrs is the site of vigorous undergraduate and graduate programs in agriculture, liberal arts and sciences, fine arts, engineering, education, business administration, human development and family relations, physical education, pharmacy, nursing, and physical therapy. Extensive cultural and recreational programs and athletic facilities are available.

Applying

For admission to the fall semester, it is suggested (but not required) that applications be submitted by January 15. To be considered for financial support, students should submit applications by March 15 for admission the following August. U.S. applicants must submit scores on the General Test of the Graduate Record Examinations (or MCATs) and must have maintained at least a 3.0 quality point ratio (GPA) for admission as graduate students with regular status. Although there is no official deadline, applications and credentials from international students should be received by March 1 for admission in the fall semester or by October 1 for the spring semester and must include TOEFL scores. The University does not discriminate in admission on the basis of race, gender, age, or national origin. Students can apply online at http://www.grad.uconn.edu/applications.html. Prospective students are asked to fill out the PNB Department's preliminary questionnaire online at http://www.pnb.uconn.edu/PNB_Base/graduate/questionnaire.html.

Correspondence and Information

Graduate Admissions Committee
Department of Physiology and Neurobiology
University of Connecticut
Box U-3156
Storrs, Connecticut 06269-3156
United States
E-mail: kathleen.kelleher@uconn.edu
Website: http://www.pnb.uconn.edu

THE FACULTY AND THEIR RESEARCH

Marie E. Cantino, Associate Professor; Ph.D., Washington (Seattle). Research in this laboratory is directed toward understanding the mechanisms of contraction in striated muscle. In particular, the lab is using electron microscopy and biochemical and mechanical assays to study the structure and organization of proteins in the contractile filaments and the mechanisms by which calcium regulates the interactions of these proteins.

William D. Chapple, Professor; Ph.D., Stanford. Primary interest is in the neuronal mechanisms employed in postural control in arthropods. Study involves how the last two pairs of thoracic legs in hermit crabs lift and control the position of the shell in which they live. These legs are innervated by motoneurons from the last thoracic ganglion and receive sensory signals from afferents in the legs. Electrophysiological records from the neurons involved will provide the basis for a control system model that incorporates neuronal and biomechanical elements.

Joanne Conover, Associate Professor; Ph.D., Bath (England). Research in the laboratory focuses on stem cell niche dynamics supporting neurogenesis and other reparative functions in the adult mouse brain. A combination of techniques, including cell culture of neural and embryonic stem cells, RT-PCR–based gene expression analysis, and examination of mouse genetic models for neurodegenerative diseases and mild traumatic brain injury aid us in understanding the potential for stem cell–mediated contributions for repair and replacement in human disease and aging.

Joseph F. Crivello, Professor (joint appointment in Marine Sciences); Ph.D., Wisconsin. Research is centered in two areas. One area examines the impact of pollution on marine organisms at a biochemical and genetic level. The other area examines pollution as a selective pressure altering the genetic diversity of marine organisms.

Angel L. de Blas, Professor; Ph.D., Indiana. Research mainly focuses on the brain receptors for the inhibitory transmitter GABA. Studies are being conducted on elucidating the molecular structure of GABA receptors with other synaptic proteins that determine the synaptic localization of the GABA receptors. Techniques include recombinant DNA, transgenic expression of proteins; mRNA; protein regulation; monoclonal antibodies; cell culture; and light, electron, and laser confocal microscopy.

Robert V. Gallo, Professor; Ph.D., Purdue. The objective of the research program is to understand the neuroendocrine mechanisms regulating luteinizing hormone release during different physiological conditions. In particular, the research examines the involvement of CNS neurotransmitters and endogenous opioid peptides in this process.

Alexander C. Jackson, Assistant Professor; Ph.D. Harvard. Research in the laboratory is focused on the cellular and synaptic neurophysiology of neural circuits in the mammalian hypothalamus that regulate fundamental behavioral states such as sleep, arousal and feeding. Techniques are centered on using patch-clamp electrophysiology and pharmacology in brain slices in order to elucidate the cellular and synaptic properties of specific hypothalamic cell-types and their local and long-range synaptic connectivity. This approach is carried out in concert with a toolbox of neuroanatomical methods and optogenetic strategies to manipulate the excitability of genetically targeted neurons.

Rahul N. Kanadia, Assistant Professor, Ph.D., Florida. Research is focused on deciphering the role of alternative splicing in neural development. The neural mouse retina is employed as a model system to investigate this question. Various techniques such as in situ hybridizations and molecular biology techniques are used to detect different forms of RNA. Since this is studied in development, live imaging is also used to document changes in splice pattern and its impact on cell fate determination and differentiation.

Joseph J. LoTurco, Professor; Ph.D., Stanford. Research in the laboratory focuses on understanding mechanisms that direct development of the neocortex. Currently, a combination of molecular genetics, patch clamp electrophysiology, and cell culture are being used to study the mechanisms that regulate neurogenesis in the cerebral cortex.

Andrew Moiseff, Professor and Associate Dean for Life Sciences, CLAS; Ph.D., Cornell. The laboratory is interested in the extraction and processing of sensory information by the nervous system. We are currently focused on identifying generalizable principles of visual system organization by employing behavioral and electrophysiological techniques to study flash signaling in fireflies.

Daniel K. Mulkey, Associate Professor; Ph.D., Wright State. Research focuses on the cellular and molecular mechanisms by which the brain controls breathing, in particular, understanding the molecular mechanism by which respiratory chemoreceptors sense changes in pH to drive breathing and the cellular mechanisms that modulate activity of these cells. Another interest is the role of nitric oxide on state-dependent modulation of respiratory motor neurons for a better understanding of the mechanisms underlying respiratory control, leading to new therapeutic approaches for the treatment of disorders such as sudden infant death syndrome and sleep apnea. Techniques include cellular electrophysiology in brain slices, cell culture, and single-cell RT-PCR.

Akiko Nishiyama, Professor; M.D., Nippon Medical School; Ph.D., Niigata (Japan). Research focuses on the lineage and function of oligodendrocyte progenitor cells (NG2 cells) in the central nervous system in normal and pathological states. Current studies apply immunohistochemical, tissue culture, biochemical, and molecular biological analyses on various mouse genetic models to understand the mechanisms that regulate proliferation and differentiation of these glial cells and to explore their role in the neural network.

J. Larry Renfro, Professor and Department Head; Ph.D., Oklahoma. Currently we are studying the mechanisms and regulation of epithelial transport of phosphate and xenobiotics by tissues isolated from a variety of vertebrates, including rats, birds, and fishes. Work has concentrated on ion transport and its regulation in primary monolayer cultures of renal epithelium and choroid plexus. The laboratory also studies transport by renal tubule brush border and basolateral membrane vesicles.

Daniel Schwartz, Assistant Professor; Ph.D., Harvard. Research is focused on computational and experimental techniques to discover, catalog, and functionally understand short linear protein motifs. Specific projects include: (1) the continued improvement of the motif-x and scan-x web-tools, (2) the development of experimental methodologies to uncover kinase motifs, and (3) the analysis of motif signatures on viral protein primary structure toward the goal of elucidating mechanisms of viral propagation and developing therapeutic agents.

Jianjun Sun, Assistant Professor; Ph.D., Florida State. Research in the laboratory focuses on reproductive physiology and ovarian cancer. Powerful genetic tools in *Drosophila* will be applied to decipher the formation and physiological function of the secretory cells in the female reproductive tract, the cells of origin of ovarian cancer. Another focus in the lab is to decipher the intrinsic mechanism controlling follicle rupture and ovulation, a process positively linked to ovarian cancer risk. The conserved molecular mechanisms will be further verified in mice with conditional knock-out models, which will ultimately aid in understanding the basic biology of the female reproductive system and their contributions to ovarian cancer.

Anastasios Tzingounis, Associate Professor; Ph.D., Oregon Health & Science. Research in the laboratory concentrates on the cellular and molecular mechanisms that control neuronal excitability in the mammalian brain. To study the molecules and signaling networks that tune the brain's innate ability to prevent epilepsy, a multidisciplinary approach is used that combines molecular and genetic techniques with optical imaging and electrophysiology.

Randall S. Walikonis, Associate Professor; Ph.D., Mayo. Research is directed at studying the postsynaptic signal transduction systems of excitatory synapses. The laboratory uses biochemical and molecular biological techniques to identify proteins associated with NMDA receptors and to determine their specific roles in the function of excitatory synapses. The lab also studies the role of growth factors in modifying excitatory synapses.

Li Wang, Associate Professor; Ph.D., Research in this laboratory is focused on several related areas centered on nuclear receptor regulation of chronic liver diseases: 1) transcriptional and translational regulation of non-coding RNA (microRNA and lncRNA) in bile acid metabolism and cholestatic liver fibrosis; 2) nutrient mediated mTOR and metabolic signaling in the epigenetic control of liver cancer; 3) circadian clock control of ER stress signaling and homocysteine metabolism in alcoholic fatty liver. Our approach makes full use of system biology, molecular biology, biochemistry, and genome-wide high throughput transcriptomics (RNA-seq) and metabolomics (GC-MS). Both in vitro cell culture and in vivo single- and double-knockout mouse models are employed for our studies.

AFFILIATED FACULTY

Lawrence E. Armstrong, Professor (primary appointment in Kinesiology); Ph.D., Ball State. Research focuses on human physiological responses to mild dehydration, exercise, dietary intervention (i.e., caffeine, low-salt diet, glucose-electrolyte solutions, amino acid supplementation), pharmacological agents, heat tolerance, and acclimatization to heat. Laboratory measurements of metabolic, ventilatory, cardiovascular, fluid-electrolyte, and strength perturbations are complemented by field observations. This research includes illnesses that arise in association with exercise in hot environments.

Thomas T. Chen, Professor (primary appointment in Molecular and Cell Biology); Ph.D., Alberta; postdoctoral study at Queen's. Structure, evolution, regulation, and molecular actions of growth hormone and insulin-like growth factor genes; regulation of foreign genes in transgenic fish; development of model transgenic fish.

William J. Kraemer, Professor (primary appointment in Kinesiology); Ph.D., Wyoming. Research focus is directed at the neuroendocrine responses and adaptations with exercise as it relates to target tissues of muscle, bone, and immune cells. Current studies utilize receptor techniques and hormonal immunoassays and bioassays to better understand androgen, adrenal, and pituitary hormone interactions with target cells and their relationship to outcome variables of physiological function and physical performance.

Louise D. McCullough, Professor of Neurology and Neuroscience; M.D./Ph.D., Connecticut. Specific interest is in the basic mechanisms involved in cerebral ischemia with a major focus on examining how the male and female brain differ in their response to ischemia. Clinical academic interests have been the development of emergent therapies for acute ischemic and hemorrhagic stroke and neurology residency education in stroke care.

Linda S. Pescatello, Distinguished Professor of Kinesiology; Ph.D., FACSM, FAHA, Connecticut. Research focus is on the interaction between the environment, neurohormones, and genetics on the exercise response in order to determine for whom exercise works best as a therapeutic modality. Current projects examine humoral, nutritional, and genetic explanations for the blood pressure response to exercise, the influence of genetics on the muscle strength and hypertrophy response to resistance exercise training, overweight and obesity, and habitual physical activity levels, and the response of acute phase reactants associated with adverse cardiovascular events before and after exercise training among firefighters.

Steven A. Zinn, Associate Professor (primary appointment in Animal Science); Ph.D., Michigan State. The laboratory is interested in the somatotropic axis and its influence on growth and lactation. The laboratory is investigating the influence of poor maternal nutrition during gestation on muscle and adipose development In the offspring. The long-term goal is to understand changes in tissue-specific expression of growth factors that result in the impaired development of these offspring.

Adam Zweifach, Professor (primary appointment in Molecular and Cell Biology); Ph.D., Yale. Research focuses on the physiology of cytotoxic T lymphocytes (CTLs) and natural killer cells (NKs), cells that kill virus-infected cells, tumor cells, and transplanted tissues. The long-term goal is to understand signal transduction in these cells, which play critical roles in the immune response to viruses and cancers, and which are also involved in transplant rejection and the etiology of many autoimmune diseases.

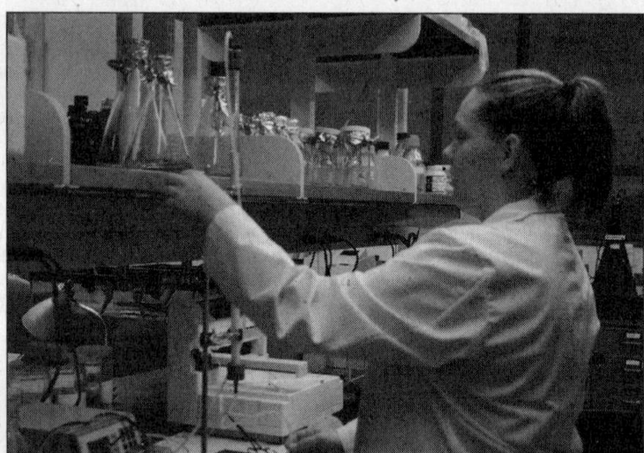

PNB graduate student conducting experiments in the Crivello Lab in the UConn PNB Department.

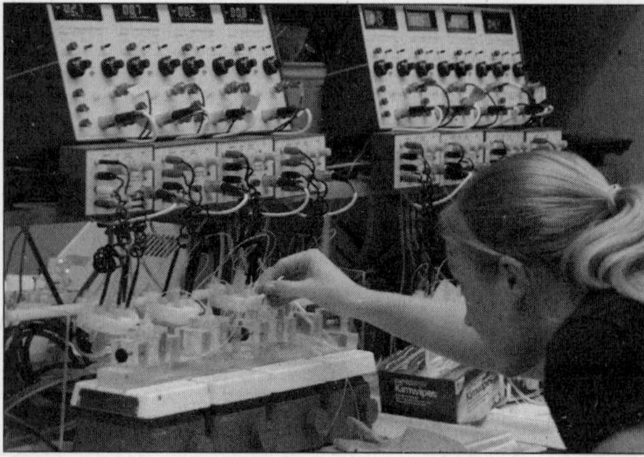

PNB graduate student conducting experiments in the Renfro Lab in the UConn PNB Department.

Section 19
Zoology

This section contains a directory of institutions offering graduate work in zoology. Additional information about programs listed in the directory may be obtained by writing directly to the dean of a graduate school or chair of a department at the address given in the directory.

For programs offering related work, see also in this book *Anatomy; Biochemistry; Biological and Biomedical Sciences; Cell, Molecular, and Structural Biology; Ecology, Environmental Biology, and Evolutionary Biology; Entomology; Genetics, Developmental Biology, and Reproductive Biology; Microbiological Sciences; Neuroscience and Neurobiology; Neurobiology; Physiology;* and *Veterinary Medicine and Sciences.* In the other guides in this series:

Graduate Programs in the Physical Sciences, Mathematics, Agricultural Sciences, the Environment & Natural Resources

See *Agricultural and Food Sciences, Environmental Sciences and Management,* and *Marine Sciences and Oceanography*

Graduate Programs in Engineering & Applied Sciences

See *Agricultural Engineering and Bioengineering* and *Ocean Engineering*

CONTENTS

Program Directories

Animal Behavior

Arizona State University at the Tempe campus, College of Liberal Arts and Sciences, School of Life Sciences, Tempe, AZ 85287-4601. Offers animal behavior (PhD); applied ethics (biomedical and health ethics) (MA); biological design (PhD); biology (MS, PhD); biology (biology and society) (MS, PhD); environmental life sciences (PhD); evolutionary biology (PhD); human and social dimensions of science and technology (PhD); microbiology (PhD); molecular and cellular biology (PhD); neuroscience (PhD); philosophy (history and philosophy of science) (MA); sustainability (PhD). Terminal master's awarded for partial completion of doctoral program. *Degree requirements:* For master's, thesis (for some programs), interactive Program of Study (iPOS) submitted before completing 50 percent of required credit hours; for doctorate, variable foreign language requirement, comprehensive exam, thesis/dissertation, interactive Program of Study (iPOS) submitted before completing 50 percent of required credit hours. *Entrance requirements:* For master's and doctorate, GRE, minimum GPA of 3.0 or equivalent in last 2 years of work leading to bachelor's degree. Additional exam requirements/recommendations for international students: Required—TOEFL (minimum score 600 paper-based; 100 iBT). Electronic applications accepted.

Bucknell University, Graduate Studies, College of Arts and Sciences, Department of Animal Behavior, Lewisburg, PA 17837. Offers MS. *Degree requirements:* For master's, thesis. *Entrance requirements:* For master's, GRE General Test, GRE Subject Test, minimum GPA of 3.0. Additional exam requirements/recommendations for international students: Required—TOEFL (minimum score 600 paper-based).

Cornell University, Graduate School, Graduate Fields of Agriculture and Life Sciences, Field of Neurobiology and Behavior, Ithaca, NY 14853-0001. Offers behavioral biology (PhD), including behavioral ecology, chemical ecology, ethology, neuroethology, sociobiology; neurobiology (PhD), including cellular and molecular neurobiology, neuroanatomy, neurochemistry, neuropharmacology, neurophysiology, sensory physiology. *Faculty:* 49 full-time (9 women). *Students:* 34 full-time (11 women); includes 6 minority (1 Black or African American, non-Hispanic/Latino; 1 Asian, non-Hispanic/Latino; 3 Hispanic/Latino; 1 Two or more races, non-Hispanic/Latino), 3 international. Average age 28. 92 applicants, 11% accepted, 5 enrolled. In 2013, 3 doctorates awarded. *Degree requirements:* For doctorate, comprehensive exam, thesis/dissertation, 1 year of teaching experience, seminar presentation. *Entrance requirements:* For doctorate, GRE General Test, GRE Subject Test (biology), 3 letters of recommendation. Additional exam requirements/recommendations for international students: Required—TOEFL (minimum score 550 paper-based; 77 iBT). *Application deadline:* For fall admission, 12/1 for domestic students. Application fee: $95. Electronic applications accepted. *Financial support:* In 2013–14, 28 students received support, including 7 fellowships with full tuition reimbursements available, 3 research assistantships with full tuition reimbursements available, 18 teaching assistantships with full tuition reimbursements available; institutionally sponsored loans, scholarships/grants, health care benefits, tuition waivers (full and partial), and unspecified assistantships also available. Financial award applicants required to submit FAFSA. *Faculty research:* Cellular neurobiology and neuropharmacology, integrative neurobiology, social behavior, chemical ecology, neuroethology. *Unit head:* Director of Graduate Studies, 607-254-4340, Fax: 607-254-4340. *Application contact:* Graduate Field Assistant, 607-254-4340, Fax: 607-254-4340, E-mail: nbb_field@cornell.edu.
Website: http://www.gradschool.cornell.edu/fields.php?id-55&a-2

Emory University, Laney Graduate School, Department of Psychology, Atlanta, GA 30322-1100. Offers clinical psychology (PhD); cognition and development (PhD); neuroscience and animal behavior (PhD). *Accreditation:* APA. *Degree requirements:* For doctorate, comprehensive exam, thesis/dissertation. *Entrance requirements:* For doctorate, GRE General Test, minimum GPA of 3.25. Additional exam requirements/recommendations for international students: Required—TOEFL. Electronic applications accepted. *Faculty research:* Neuroscience and animal behavior; adult and child psychopathology, cognition development assessment.

Illinois State University, Graduate School, College of Arts and Sciences, Department of Biological Sciences, Normal, IL 61790-2200. Offers animal behavior (MS); bacteriology (MS); biochemistry (MS); biological sciences (MS); biology (PhD); biophysics (MS); biotechnology (MS); botany (MS, PhD); cell biology (MS); conservation biology (MS); developmental biology (MS); ecology (MS, PhD); entomology (MS); evolutionary biology (MS); genetics (MS, PhD); immunology (MS); microbiology (MS, PhD); molecular biology (MS); molecular genetics (MS); neurobiology (MS); neuroscience (MS); parasitology (MS); physiology (MS, PhD); plant biology (MS); plant molecular biology (MS); plant sciences (MS); structural biology (MS); zoology (MS, PhD). Part-time programs available. *Degree requirements:* For master's, thesis or alternative; for doctorate, variable foreign language requirement, thesis/dissertation, 2 terms of residency. *Entrance requirements:* For master's, GRE General Test, minimum GPA of 2.6 in last 60 hours of course work; for doctorate, GRE General Test. *Faculty research:* Redoc balance and drug development in schistosoma mansoni, control of the growth of listeria monocytogenes at low temperature, regulation of cell expansion and microtubule function by SPRI, CRUI: physiology and fitness consequences of different life history phenotypes.

University of California, Davis, Graduate Studies, Graduate Group in Animal Behavior, Davis, CA 95616. Offers PhD. *Degree requirements:* For doctorate, thesis/dissertation. *Entrance requirements:* For doctorate, GRE General Test. Additional exam requirements/recommendations for international students: Required—TOEFL (minimum score 550 paper-based), IELTS (minimum score 7). Electronic applications accepted. *Faculty research:* Wildlife behavior, conservation biology, companion animal behavior, behavioral endocrinology, animal communication.

University of Colorado Boulder, Graduate School, College of Arts and Sciences, Department of Ecology and Evolutionary Biology, Boulder, CO 80309. Offers animal behavior (MA); biology (MA, PhD); environmental biology (MA, PhD); evolutionary biology (MA, PhD); neurobiology (MA); population biology (MA); population genetics (PhD). *Faculty:* 31 full-time (12 women). *Students:* 70 full-time (30 women), 18 part-time (10 women); includes 6 minority (1 Asian, non-Hispanic/Latino; 3 Hispanic/Latino; 2 Two or more races, non-Hispanic/Latino), 5 international. Average age 30. 171 applicants, 6% accepted, 11 enrolled. In 2013, 10 master's, 11 doctorates awarded. Terminal master's awarded for partial completion of doctoral program. *Degree requirements:* For master's, comprehensive exam, thesis or alternative; for doctorate, comprehensive exam, thesis/dissertation. *Entrance requirements:* For master's, GRE General Test, GRE Subject Test, minimum undergraduate GPA of 3.0; for doctorate, GRE General Test, GRE Subject Test. *Application deadline:* For fall admission, 12/31 for domestic students, 12/1 for international students. Application fee: $50 ($60 for international students). Electronic applications accepted. *Financial support:* In 2013–14, 175 students received support, including 35 fellowships (averaging $15,283 per year), 21 research assistantships with full and partial tuition reimbursements available (averaging $29,343 per year), 48 teaching assistantships with full and partial tuition reimbursements available (averaging $31,449 per year); institutionally sponsored loans, scholarships/grants, health care benefits, and unspecified assistantships also available. Financial award applicants required to submit FAFSA. *Faculty research:* Ecology, environmental biology, evolutionary biology, biological sciences, conservation biology. *Total annual research expenditures:* $37.1 million.
Website: http://ebio.colorado.edu

University of Colorado Denver, College of Liberal Arts and Sciences, Department of Integrative Biology, Denver, CO 80217. Offers animal behavior (MS); biology (MS); cell and developmental biology (MS); ecology (MS); evolutionary biology (MS); genetics (MS); integrative and systems biology (PhD); microbiology (MS); molecular biology (MS); neurobiology (MS); plant systematics (MS). Part-time programs available. *Faculty:* 21 full-time (7 women), 3 part-time/adjunct (2 women). *Students:* 18 full-time (11 women), 5 part-time (all women); includes 5 minority (1 Black or African American, non-Hispanic/Latino; 2 Hispanic/Latino; 2 Two or more races, non-Hispanic/Latino), 1 international. Average age 29. 25 applicants, 44% accepted, 11 enrolled. In 2013, 13 master's awarded. *Degree requirements:* For master's, comprehensive exam, thesis, 30-32 credit hours. *Entrance requirements:* For master's, GRE General Test (minimum score in 50th percentile in each section), BA/BS from accredited institution awarded within the last 10 years; minimum undergraduate GPA of 3.0; prerequisite courses: 1 year each of general biology and general chemistry; 1 semester each of general genetics, general ecology, and cell biology; and a structure/function course. Additional exam requirements/recommendations for international students: Required—TOEFL (minimum score 537 paper-based; 75 iBT); Recommended—IELTS (minimum score 6.5). *Application deadline:* For fall admission, 2/1 for domestic and international students. Application fee: $50 ($75 for international students). Electronic applications accepted. *Financial support:* In 2013–14, 8 students received support. Fellowships, research assistantships, teaching assistantships, Federal Work-Study, institutionally sponsored loans, scholarships/grants, and traineeships available. Financial award application deadline: 4/1; financial award applicants required to submit FAFSA. *Faculty research:* Molecular developmental biology; quantitative ecology, biogeography, and population dynamics; environmental signaling and endocrine disruption; speciation, the evolution of reproductive isolation, and hybrid zones; evolutionary, behavioral, and conservation ecology. *Unit head:* Dr. John Swallow, Biology Department Chair, 303-556-6154, E-mail: john.swallow@ucdenver.edu. *Application contact:* Timberley Roane, Associate Professor/Director of MS in Biology Program, 303-556-6592, E-mail: timberley.roane@ucdenver.edu.
Website: http://www.ucdenver.edu/academics/colleges/CLAS/Departments/biology/Programs/MasterofScience/Pages/BiologyMasterOfScience.aspx

University of Massachusetts Amherst, Graduate School, Interdisciplinary Programs, Program in Neuroscience and Behavior, Amherst, MA 01003. Offers animal behavior and learning (PhD); molecular and cellular neuroscience (PhD); neural and behavioral development (PhD); neuroendocrinology (PhD); neuroscience and behavior (MS); sensorimotor, cognitive, and computational neuroscience (PhD). *Students:* 27 full-time (19 women), 2 part-time (0 women); includes 4 minority (1 Asian, non-Hispanic/Latino; 3 Hispanic/Latino), 4 international. Average age 27. 129 applicants, 11% accepted, 8 enrolled. In 2013, 3 master's awarded. Terminal master's awarded for partial completion of doctoral program. *Degree requirements:* For master's, thesis or alternative; for doctorate, comprehensive exam, thesis/dissertation. *Entrance requirements:* For master's, GRE General Test; for doctorate, GRE General Test; GRE Subect Test in psychology, biology, or mathematics (recommended). Additional exam requirements/recommendations for international students: Required—TOEFL (minimum score 550 paper-based; 80 iBT), IELTS (minimum score 6.5). *Application deadline:* For fall admission, 12/15 for domestic and international students. Applications are processed on a rolling basis. Application fee: $75. Electronic applications accepted. *Financial support:* Fellowships with full and partial tuition reimbursements, research assistantships with full and partial tuition reimbursements, teaching assistantships with full and partial tuition reimbursements, career-related internships or fieldwork, Federal Work-Study, scholarships/grants, traineeships, health care benefits, tuition waivers (full and partial), and unspecified assistantships available. Support available to part-time students. Financial award application deadline: 12/14; financial award applicants required to submit FAFSA. *Unit head:* Dr. Jeffrey D. Blaustein, Graduate Program Director, 413-545-2046, Fax: 413-545-3243, E-mail: nsb@bio.umass.edu. *Application contact:* Lindsay DeSantis, Supervisor of Admissions, 413-545-0722, Fax: 413-577-0010, E-mail: gradadm@grad.umass.edu.
Website: http://www.umass.edu/neuro/

University of Minnesota, Twin Cities Campus, Graduate School, College of Biological Sciences, Department of Ecology, Evolution, and Behavior, St. Paul, MN 55418. Offers MS, PhD. Terminal master's awarded for partial completion of doctoral program. *Degree requirements:* For master's, comprehensive exam, thesis or projects; for doctorate, comprehensive exam, thesis/dissertation. *Entrance requirements:* For master's and doctorate, GRE General Test, minimum GPA of 3.0. Additional exam requirements/recommendations for international students: Required—TOEFL (minimum score 550 paper-based; 79 iBT), Michigan English Language Assessment Battery. Electronic applications accepted. *Faculty research:* Behavioral ecology, community ecology, community genetics, ecosystem and global change, evolution and systematics.

The University of Montana, Graduate School, College of Humanities and Sciences, Department of Psychology, Missoula, MT 59812-0002. Offers clinical psychology (PhD); experimental psychology (PhD), including animal behavior psychology, developmental psychology; school psychology (MA, PhD, Ed S). *Accreditation:* APA (one or more programs are accredited). Terminal master's awarded for partial completion of doctoral program. *Degree requirements:* For master's, thesis; for doctorate, thesis/dissertation. *Entrance requirements:* For master's, doctorate, and Ed S, GRE General Test. Additional exam requirements/recommendations for international students: Required—TOEFL. *Application deadline:* For fall admission, 1/15 for domestic students. Application fee: $45. *Financial support:* Teaching assistantships with full tuition reimbursements, career-related internships or fieldwork, Federal Work-Study, scholarships/grants, traineeships, and unspecified assistantships available. Financial award application deadline: 3/1; financial award applicants required to submit FAFSA. *Unit head:* Christine Fiore, Chair, 406-243-4521, E-mail: christine.fiore@umontana.edu. *Application contact:* Information Contact, E-mail: gradschl@mso.umt.edu.
Website: http://psychweb.psy.umt.edu/

The University of Tennessee, Graduate School, College of Arts and Sciences, Department of Ecology and Evolutionary Biology, Knoxville, TN 37996. Offers behavior (MS, PhD); ecology (MS, PhD); evolutionary biology (MS, PhD). Part-time programs available. *Degree requirements:* For master's, thesis; for doctorate, thesis/dissertation. *Entrance requirements:* For master's and doctorate, GRE General Test, minimum GPA of 2.7. Additional exam requirements/recommendations for international students: Required—TOEFL. Electronic applications accepted. *Expenses:* Tuition, state resident: full-time $9540; part-time $531 per credit hour. Tuition, nonresident: full-time $27,728; part-time $1542 per credit hour. *Required fees:* $1404; $67 per credit hour.

The University of Texas at Austin, Graduate School, College of Natural Sciences, School of Biological Sciences, Program in Ecology, Evolution and Behavior, Austin, TX 78712-1111. Offers PhD. *Entrance requirements:* For doctorate, GRE General Test. Additional exam requirements/recommendations for international students: Required—TOEFL. Electronic applications accepted.

University of Washington, Graduate School, College of Arts and Sciences, Department of Psychology, Seattle, WA 98195. Offers animal behavior (PhD); child psychology (PhD); clinical psychology (PhD); cognition and perception (PhD); developmental psychology (PhD); quantitative psychology (PhD); social psychology and personality (PhD). *Accreditation:* APA. *Degree requirements:* For doctorate, thesis/dissertation. *Entrance requirements:* For doctorate, GRE General Test, minimum GPA of 3.0. Electronic applications accepted. *Faculty research:* Addictive behaviors, artificial intelligence, child psychopathology, mechanisms and development of vision, physiology of ingestive behaviors.

Zoology

Auburn University, Graduate School, College of Sciences and Mathematics, Department of Biological Sciences, Auburn University, AL 36849. Offers botany (MS, PhD); microbiology (MS, PhD); zoology (MS, PhD). *Faculty:* 39 full-time (13 women), 1 (woman) part-time/adjunct. *Students:* 40 full-time (21 women), 66 part-time (26 women); includes 9 minority (2 Black or African American, non-Hispanic/Latino; 1 American Indian or Alaska Native, non-Hispanic/Latino; 4 Asian, non-Hispanic/Latino; 2 Hispanic/Latino), 17 international. Average age 28. 99 applicants, 31% accepted, 19 enrolled. In 2013, 10 master's, 11 doctorates awarded. *Entrance requirements:* For master's and doctorate, GRE General Test. Additional exam requirements/recommendations for international students: Required—TOEFL. *Application deadline:* For fall admission, 7/7 for domestic students; for spring admission, 11/24 for domestic students. Application fee: $50 ($60 for international students). Electronic applications accepted. *Expenses:* Tuition, state resident: full-time $8262; part-time $459 per credit hour. Tuition, nonresident: full-time $24,786; part-time $1377 per credit hour. Tuition and fees vary according to degree level and program. *Financial support:* Research assistantships and teaching assistantships available. Financial award applicants required to submit FAFSA. *Unit head:* Dr. Jack W. Feminella, Chair, 334-844-3906, Fax: 334-844-1645. *Application contact:* Dr. George Flowers, Dean of the Graduate School, 334-844-2125.

Canisius College, Graduate Division, College of Arts and Sciences, Department of Animal Behavior, Ecology and Conservation, Buffalo, NY 14208-1098. Offers anthrozoology (MS). Applicants accepted in Fall only. Part-time programs available. Postbaccalaureate distance learning degree programs offered (minimal on-campus study). *Faculty:* 4 full-time (2 women), 3 part-time/adjunct (2 women). *Students:* 23 full-time (20 women), 24 part-time (22 women); includes 5 minority (1 American Indian or Alaska Native, non-Hispanic/Latino; 2 Hispanic/Latino; 2 Two or more races, non-Hispanic/Latino), 2 international. Average age 34. 107 applicants, 23% accepted, 20 enrolled. In 2013, 13 master's awarded. *Entrance requirements:* For master's, official transcript of all college work; bachelor's degree. Additional exam requirements/recommendations for international students: Required—TOEFL (minimum score 550 paper-based, 80 iBT), IELTS (minimum score 6.5), or CAEL (minimum score 70). *Application deadline:* For fall admission, 3/1 for domestic and international students. Applications are processed on a rolling basis. Application fee: $25. Electronic applications accepted. Application fee is waived when completed online. *Expenses: Tuition:* Part-time $750 per credit hour. *Financial support:* Scholarships/grants available. Financial award application deadline: 4/30; financial award applicants required to submit FAFSA. *Unit head:* Dr. Michael Noonan, Program Director, 716-888-2770, E-mail: noonan@canisius.edu. *Application contact:* Julie A. Zulewski, Director, Graduate Admissions, 716-888-2548, Fax: 716-888-3195, E-mail: zulewskj@canisius.edu.
Website: http://www.canisius.edu/abec/

Colorado State University, Graduate School, College of Natural Sciences, Department of Biology, Fort Collins, CO 80523-1878. Offers botany (MS, PhD); zoology (MS, PhD). *Faculty:* 25 full-time (10 women), 1 part-time/adjunct (0 women). *Students:* 18 full-time (11 women), 25 part-time (15 women); includes 6 minority (4 Asian, non-Hispanic/Latino; 2 Hispanic/Latino), 6 international. Average age 30. 45 applicants, 27% accepted, 10 enrolled. In 2013, 5 master's, 7 doctorates awarded. Terminal master's awarded for partial completion of doctoral program. *Degree requirements:* For master's, comprehensive exam, thesis; for doctorate, comprehensive exam, thesis/dissertation. *Entrance requirements:* For master's and doctorate, GRE General Test (minimum scores above 70th percentile), 2 transcripts, 3 letters of recommendation, statement of educational goals/research interests, minimum GPA of 3.0. Additional exam requirements/recommendations for international students: Required—TOEFL (minimum score 550 paper-based; 80 iBT), IELTS (minimum score 6.5). *Application deadline:* For fall admission, 1/15 priority date for domestic and international students; for spring admission, 11/1 priority date for domestic and international students. Applications are processed on a rolling basis. Application fee: $50. Electronic applications accepted. *Expenses:* Tuition, state resident: full-time $9075.40; part-time $504 per credit. Tuition, nonresident: full-time $22,248; part-time $1236 per credit. *Required fees:* $1819; $60 per credit. *Financial support:* In 2013–14, 106 students received support, including 19 fellowships (averaging $31,747 per year), 22 research assistantships with full tuition reimbursements available (averaging $10,909 per year), 65 teaching assistantships with full tuition reimbursements available (averaging $13,683 per year); career-related internships or fieldwork, Federal Work-Study, institutionally sponsored loans, scholarships/grants, traineeships, health care benefits, and unspecified assistantships also available. Financial award application deadline: 3/1; financial award applicants required to submit FAFSA. *Faculty research:* Organismal interactions in infectious disease, stream ecology, muscle protein structure, molecular evolution, plant biotechnology. *Total annual research expenditures:* $9.7 million. *Unit head:* Dr. Michael Antolin, Professor and Interim Chair, 970-491-1911, Fax: 970-491-0649, E-mail: michael.antolin@colostate.edu. *Application contact:* Dorothy Ramirez, Graduate Coordinator, 970-491-1923, Fax: 970-491-0649, E-mail: dorothy.ramirez@colostate.edu.
Website: http://www.biology.colostate.edu/

Cornell University, Graduate School, Graduate Fields of Agriculture and Life Sciences, Field of Zoology and Wildlife Conservation, Ithaca, NY 14853-0001. Offers animal cytology (PhD); comparative and functional anatomy (PhD); developmental biology (PhD); ecology (PhD); histology (PhD); wildlife conservation (PhD). *Faculty:* 21 full-time (6 women). *Students:* 4 full-time (3 women), 1 part-time (0 women); includes 2 minority (1 Hispanic/Latino; 1 Two or more races, non-Hispanic/Latino), 1 international. Average age 26. 18 applicants, 6% accepted, 1 enrolled. In 2013, 1 doctorate awarded. *Degree requirements:* For doctorate, comprehensive exam, thesis/dissertation, 2 semesters of teaching experience. *Entrance requirements:* For doctorate, GRE General Test, GRE Subject Test (biology), 2 letters of recommendation. Additional exam requirements/recommendations for international students: Required—TOEFL (minimum score 550 paper-based; 77 iBT). *Application deadline:* For fall admission, 2/1 priority date for domestic students. Application fee: $95. Electronic applications accepted. *Financial support:* In 2013–14, 4 students received support, including 3 research assistantships with full tuition reimbursements available, 1 teaching assistantship with full tuition reimbursement available; fellowships with full tuition reimbursements available, institutionally sponsored loans, scholarships/grants, health care benefits, tuition waivers (full and partial), and unspecified assistantships also available. Financial award applicants required to submit FAFSA. *Faculty research:* Organismal biology, functional morphology, biomechanics, comparative vertebrate anatomy, comparative invertebrate anatomy, paleontology. *Unit head:* Director of Graduate Studies, 607-253-3276, Fax: 607-253-3756. *Application contact:* Graduate Field Assistant, 607-253-3276, Fax: 607-253-3756, E-mail: graduate_edcvm@cornell.edu.
Website: http://www.gradschool.cornell.edu/fields.php?id-65&a-2

Eastern New Mexico University, Graduate School, College of Liberal Arts and Sciences, Department of Biology, Portales, NM 88130. Offers applied ecology (MS); botany (MS); cell, molecular biology and biotechnology (MS); microbiology (MS); zoology (MS). Part-time programs available. *Degree requirements:* For master's, comprehensive exam, thesis optional. *Entrance requirements:* For master's, GRE, minimum GPA of 3.0, 2 letters of recommendation, statement of research interest, bachelor's degree related to field of study or proof of common knowledge. Additional exam requirements/recommendations for international students: Required—TOEFL (minimum score 550 paper-based; 79 iBT), IELTS (minimum score 6). Electronic applications accepted.

Emporia State University, Department of Biological Sciences, Emporia, KS 66801-5415. Offers botany (MS); environmental biology (MS); general biology (MS); microbial and cellular biology (MS); zoology (MS). Part-time programs available. *Faculty:* 13 full-time (3 women). *Students:* 32 full-time (16 women), 7 part-time (1 woman); includes 2 minority (1 Black or African American, non-Hispanic/Latino; 1 Asian, non-Hispanic/Latino), 18 international. 25 applicants, 88% accepted, 3 enrolled. In 2013, 8 master's awarded. *Degree requirements:* For master's, comprehensive exam or thesis. *Entrance requirements:* For master's, GRE, appropriate undergraduate degree, interview, letters of reference. Additional exam requirements/recommendations for international students: Required—TOEFL (minimum score 520 paper-based; 68 iBT). *Application deadline:* For fall admission, 8/15 priority date for domestic students. Applications are processed on a rolling basis. Application fee: $30 ($75 for international students). Electronic applications accepted. *Expenses: Tuition, area resident:* Part-time $220 per credit hour. Tuition, state resident: part-time $220 per credit hour. Tuition, nonresident: part-time $685 per credit hour. *Required fees:* $73 per credit hour. *Financial support:* In 2013–14, 5 research assistantships with full tuition reimbursements (averaging $7,371 per year), 9 teaching assistantships with full tuition reimbursements (averaging $7,950 per year) were awarded; career-related internships or fieldwork, Federal Work-Study, institutionally sponsored loans, health care benefits, and unspecified assistantships also available. Financial award application deadline: 3/15; financial award applicants required to submit FAFSA. *Faculty research:* Fisheries, range, and wildlife management; aquatic, plant, grassland, vertebrate, and invertebrate ecology; mammalian and plant systematics, taxonomy, and evolution; immunology, virology, and molecular biology. *Unit head:* Dr. R. Brent Thomas, Chair, 620-341-5311, Fax: 620-341-5608, E-mail: rthomas2@emporia.edu. *Application contact:* Dr. Scott Crupper, Graduate Coordinator, 620-341-5621, Fax: 620-341-5607, E-mail: scrupper@emporia.edu.
Website: http://www.emporia.edu/info/degrees-courses/grad/biology

Illinois State University, Graduate School, College of Arts and Sciences, Department of Biological Sciences, Normal, IL 61790-2200. Offers animal behavior (MS); bacteriology (MS); biochemistry (MS); biological sciences (MS); biology (PhD); biophysics (MS); biotechnology (MS); botany (MS, PhD); cell biology (MS); conservation biology (MS); developmental biology (MS); ecology (MS, PhD); entomology (MS); evolutionary biology (MS); genetics (MS, PhD); immunology (MS); microbiology (MS, PhD); molecular biology (MS); molecular genetics (MS); neurobiology (MS); neuroscience (MS); parasitology (MS); physiology (MS, PhD); plant biology (MS); plant molecular biology (MS); plant sciences (MS); structural biology (MS); zoology (MS, PhD). Part-time programs available. *Degree requirements:* For master's, thesis or alternative; for doctorate, variable foreign language requirement, thesis/dissertation, 2 terms of residency. *Entrance requirements:* For master's, GRE General Test, minimum GPA of 2.6 in last 60 hours of course work; for doctorate, GRE General Test. *Faculty research:* Redoc balance and drug development in schistosoma mansoni, control of the growth of listeria monocytogenes at low temperature, regulation of cell expansion and microtubule function by SPRI, CRUI: physiology and fitness consequences of different life history phenotypes.

Indiana University Bloomington, University Graduate School, College of Arts and Sciences, Department of Biology, Bloomington, IN 47405. Offers biology teaching (MAT); biotechnology (MA); evolution, ecology, and behavior (MA, PhD); genetics (PhD); microbiology (MA, PhD); molecular, cellular, and developmental biology (PhD); plant sciences (MA, PhD); zoology (MA, PhD). *Faculty:* 58 full-time (15 women), 21 part-time/adjunct (6 women). *Students:* 166 full-time (94 women), 2 part-time (both women); includes 22 minority (8 Black or African American, non-Hispanic/Latino; 3 Asian, non-Hispanic/Latino; 10 Hispanic/Latino; 1 Two or more races, non-Hispanic/Latino), 47 international. Average age 27. 261 applicants, 23% accepted, 32 enrolled. In 2013, 17 master's, 20 doctorates awarded. Terminal master's awarded for partial completion of doctoral program. *Degree requirements:* For master's, thesis, oral defense; for doctorate, thesis/dissertation, oral defense. *Entrance requirements:* For master's and doctorate, GRE General Test. Additional exam requirements/recommendations for international students: Required—TOEFL (minimum score 100 iBT). *Application deadline:* For fall admission, 1/5 priority date for domestic students, 12/1 priority date for international students. Application fee: $55 ($65 for international students). Electronic applications accepted. *Financial support:* In 2013–14, fellowships with tuition reimbursements (averaging $24,000 per year), research assistantships with tuition

reimbursements (averaging $21,000 per year), teaching assistantships with tuition reimbursements (averaging $22,000 per year) were awarded; scholarships/grants, traineeships, health care benefits, and unspecified assistantships also available. Financial award application deadline: 1/5. *Faculty research:* Evolution, ecology and behavior; microbiology; molecular biology and genetics; plant biology. *Unit head:* Dr. Clay Fuqua, Chair, 812-856-6005, Fax: 812-855-6082, E-mail: cfuqua@indiana.edu. *Application contact:* Tracey D. Stohr, Graduate Student Recruitment Coordinator, 812-856-6303, Fax: 812-855-6082, E-mail: gradbio@indiana.edu.
Website: http://www.bio.indiana.edu/

Miami University, College of Arts and Science, Department of Biology, Oxford, OH 45056. Offers biological sciences (MAT); biology (MS, PhD); botany (MAT, MS, PhD); cell, molecular and structural biology (MS, PhD); ecology, evolution and environmental biology (PhD); zoology (MA, MS, PhD). Part-time programs available. Postbaccalaureate distance learning degree programs offered. *Students:* 89 full-time (49 women), 612 part-time (502 women); includes 63 minority (9 Black or African American, non-Hispanic/Latino; 2 American Indian or Alaska Native, non-Hispanic/Latino; 6 Asian, non-Hispanic/Latino; 27 Hispanic/Latino; 1 Native Hawaiian or other Pacific Islander, non-Hispanic/Latino; 18 Two or more races, non-Hispanic/Latino), 35 international. Average age 34. In 2013, 133 master's, 4 doctorates awarded. *Entrance requirements:* For master's and doctorate, GRE General Test. Additional exam requirements/recommendations for international students: Recommended—TOEFL (minimum score 80 iBT), IELTS (minimum score 6.5), TSE (minimum score 54). *Application deadline:* For fall admission, 1/15 for domestic and international students. Application fee: $50. Electronic applications accepted. *Expenses:* Tuition, state resident: full-time $12,634; part-time $526 per credit hour. Tuition, nonresident: full-time $27,892; part-time $1162 per credit hour. Part-time tuition and fees vary according to course load, campus/location and program. *Financial support:* Fellowships with full tuition reimbursements, research assistantships with full tuition reimbursements, teaching assistantships with full tuition reimbursements, Federal Work-Study, health care benefits, tuition waivers (full), and unspecified assistantships available. Financial award application deadline: 1/15; financial award applicants required to submit FAFSA. *Unit head:* Dr. Douglas Meikle, Chair, 513-529-3103, E-mail: meikled@miamioh.edu.
Website: http://miamioh.edu/cas/about/biology

Michigan State University, The Graduate School, College of Natural Science, Department of Zoology, East Lansing, MI 48824. Offers zoo and aquarium management (MS); zoology (MS, PhD); zoology-environmental toxicology (PhD). *Entrance requirements:* Additional exam requirements/recommendations for international students: Required—TOEFL. Electronic applications accepted.

North Carolina State University, Graduate School, College of Agriculture and Life Sciences, Department of Zoology, Raleigh, NC 27695. Offers MS, MZS, PhD. Terminal master's awarded for partial completion of doctoral program. *Degree requirements:* For master's, thesis (for some programs), oral exam; for doctorate, thesis/dissertation, oral and written exams. *Entrance requirements:* For master's and doctorate, GRE General Test, minimum GPA of 3.0. Additional exam requirements/recommendations for international students: Required—TOEFL. Electronic applications accepted. *Faculty research:* Acquatic and terrestrial ecology, herpetology, behavioral biology, neurobiology, avian ecology.

North Dakota State University, College of Graduate and Interdisciplinary Studies, College of Science and Mathematics, Department of Biological Sciences, Fargo, ND 58108. Offers biology (MS); botany (MS, PhD); cellular and molecular biology (PhD); genomics (PhD); zoology (MS, PhD). *Faculty:* 17 full-time (9 women), 1 part-time/adjunct (0 women). *Students:* 20 full-time (10 women), 3 part-time (all women); includes 2 minority (1 American Indian or Alaska Native, non-Hispanic/Latino; 1 Two or more races, non-Hispanic/Latino), 1 international. Average age 32. 9 applicants, 11% accepted, 1 enrolled. In 2013, 4 master's awarded. *Degree requirements:* For master's, thesis; for doctorate, thesis/dissertation. *Entrance requirements:* For master's and doctorate, GRE General Test. Additional exam requirements/recommendations for international students: Required—TOEFL. *Application deadline:* For fall admission, 1/15 for domestic students. Applications are processed on a rolling basis. Application fee: $35. Electronic applications accepted. *Financial support:* Fellowships with full tuition reimbursements, research assistantships with full tuition reimbursements, teaching assistantships with full tuition reimbursements, career-related internships or fieldwork, Federal Work-Study, institutionally sponsored loans, scholarships/grants, tuition waivers (full), and unspecified assistantships available. Support available to part-time students. Financial award application deadline: 4/15; financial award applicants required to submit FAFSA. *Faculty research:* Comparative endocrinology, physiology, behavioral ecology, plant cell biology, aquatic biology. *Unit head:* Dr. Wendy Reed, Head, 701-231-7087, E-mail: wendy.reed@ndsu.edu. *Application contact:* Sonya Goergen, Marketing, Recruitment, and Public Relations Coordinator, 701-231-7033, Fax: 701-231-6524.
Website: http://biology.ndsu.nodak.edu/

Oklahoma State University, College of Arts and Sciences, Department of Zoology, Stillwater, OK 74078. Offers MS, PhD. *Faculty:* 25 full-time (14 women), 1 (woman) part-time/adjunct. *Students:* 7 full-time (3 women), 60 part-time (33 women); includes 11 minority (1 Black or African American, non-Hispanic/Latino; 2 Asian, non-Hispanic/Latino; 4 Hispanic/Latino; 4 Two or more races, non-Hispanic/Latino), 8 international. Average age 28. 445 applicants, 6% accepted, 17 enrolled. In 2013, 7 master's, 5 doctorates awarded. *Degree requirements:* For master's, thesis; for doctorate, comprehensive exam, thesis/dissertation. *Entrance requirements:* For master's and doctorate, GRE General Test. Additional exam requirements/recommendations for international students: Required—TOEFL (minimum score 550 paper-based; 79 iBT). *Application deadline:* For fall admission, 3/1 priority date for international students; for spring admission, 8/1 priority date for international students. Applications are processed on a rolling basis. Application fee: $40 ($75 for international students). Electronic applications accepted. *Expenses:* Tuition, state resident: full-time $4272; part-time $178 per credit hour. Tuition, nonresident: full-time $17,472; part-time $709 per credit hour. *Required fees:* $2413.20; $100.55 per credit hour. One-time fee: $50 full-time. Part-time tuition and fees vary according to course load and campus/location. *Financial support:* In 2013–14, 11 research assistantships (averaging $20,416 per year), 51 teaching assistantships (averaging $19,952 per year) were awarded; career-related internships or fieldwork, Federal Work-Study, scholarships/grants, health care benefits, tuition waivers (partial), and unspecified assistantships also available. Support available to part-time students. Financial award application deadline: 3/1; financial award applicants required to submit FAFSA. *Unit head:* Dr. Loren Smith, Department Head, 405-744-5555, Fax: 405-744-7824, E-mail: loren.smith@okstate.edu.
Website: http://zoology.okstate.edu

Oregon State University, College of Science, Program in Integrative Biology, Corvallis, OR 97331. Offers MA, MAIS, MS, PhD. *Faculty:* 23 full-time (7 women), 2 part-time/adjunct (0 women). *Students:* 49 full-time (34 women); includes 9 minority (1 Black or African American, non-Hispanic/Latino; 1 American Indian or Alaska Native, non-Hispanic/Latino; 6 Asian, non-Hispanic/Latino; 1 Two or more races, non-Hispanic/Latino), 3 international. Average age 28. 73 applicants, 16% accepted, 11 enrolled. In 2013, 7 doctorates awarded. Terminal master's awarded for partial completion of doctoral program. *Degree requirements:* For doctorate, thesis/dissertation. *Entrance requirements:* For master's and doctorate, GRE. Additional exam requirements/recommendations for international students: Required—TOEFL (minimum score 80 iBT), IELTS (minimum score 6.5). *Application deadline:* For fall admission, 12/15 for domestic students. Application fee: $60. *Expenses:* Tuition, state resident: full-time $11,664; part-time $432 per credit hour. Tuition, nonresident: full-time $19,197; part-time $711 per credit hour. *Required fees:* $1446; $443 per quarter. One-time fee: $300. Tuition and fees vary according to course load and program. *Financial support:* Fellowships, research assistantships, teaching assistantships, Federal Work-Study, and institutionally sponsored loans available. Support available to part-time students. Financial award application deadline: 2/1. *Faculty research:* Ecology and evolutionary biology, physiology and behavior, development and cell biology. *Unit head:* Dr. Virginia M. Weis, Professor and Chair of Integrative Biology, 541-737-4359, E-mail: weisv@science.oregonstate.edu. *Application contact:* Traci Durrell-Khalife, Graduate Admissions Coordinator, 541-737-5335, E-mail: durrellt@science.oregonstate.edu.
Website: http://ib.oregonstate.edu/

Southern Illinois University Carbondale, Graduate School, College of Science, Department of Zoology, Carbondale, IL 62901-4701. Offers MS, PhD. *Faculty:* 25 full-time (1 woman). *Students:* 23 full-time (8 women), 61 part-time (31 women); includes 2 minority (1 Asian, non-Hispanic/Latino; 1 Hispanic/Latino), 8 international. Average age 25. 36 applicants, 33% accepted, 11 enrolled. In 2013, 18 master's, 2 doctorates awarded. *Degree requirements:* For master's, thesis; for doctorate, thesis/dissertation. *Entrance requirements:* For master's, GRE, minimum GPA of 2.7; for doctorate, GRE, minimum GPA of 3.25. Additional exam requirements/recommendations for international students: Required—TOEFL. *Application deadline:* Applications are processed on a rolling basis. Application fee: $50. *Financial support:* In 2013–14, 5 fellowships with full tuition reimbursements, 45 research assistantships with full tuition reimbursements, 20 teaching assistantships with full tuition reimbursements were awarded; Federal Work-Study, institutionally sponsored loans, and tuition waivers (full) also available. Support available to part-time students. *Faculty research:* Ecology, fisheries and wildlife, systematics, behavior, vertebrate and invertebrate biology. *Unit head:* Dr. Carey Krajewski, Chairperson, 618-453-4128, E-mail: careyk@siu.edu. *Application contact:* William G. Dyer, Associate Dean, 618-536-6666.

Texas A&M University, College of Science, Department of Biology, College Station, TX 77843. Offers biology (MS, PhD); botany (MS, PhD); microbiology (MS, PhD); zoology (MS, PhD). *Faculty:* 40. *Students:* 94 full-time (54 women), 7 part-time (4 women); includes 10 minority (1 Black or African American, non-Hispanic/Latino; 3 Asian, non-Hispanic/Latino; 6 Hispanic/Latino), 49 international. Average age 29. 120 applicants, 25% accepted, 19 enrolled. In 2013, 5 master's, 16 doctorates awarded. *Degree requirements:* For master's, thesis or alternative; for doctorate, comprehensive exam, thesis/dissertation. *Entrance requirements:* For master's and doctorate, GRE General Test. Additional exam requirements/recommendations for international students: Required—TOEFL. *Application deadline:* For fall admission, 1/15 for domestic students. Applications are processed on a rolling basis. Application fee: $50 ($75 for international students). Electronic applications accepted. *Expenses:* Tuition, state resident: full-time $4078; part-time $226.55 per credit hour. Tuition, nonresident: full-time $10,450; part-time $580.55 per credit hour. *Required fees:* $2328; $278.50 per credit hour. $642.45 per semester. *Financial support:* Fellowships, research assistantships, and teaching assistantships available. Financial award application deadline: 4/1; financial award applicants required to submit FAFSA. *Unit head:* Dr. Tom McKnight, Department Head, 979-845-3896, Fax: 979-845-2891, E-mail: mcknight@bio.tamu.edu. *Application contact:* Dr. Arne Lekven, Graduate Advisor, 979-458-3461, Fax: 979-845-2891, E-mail: alekven@bio.tamu.edu.
Website: http://www.bio.tamu.edu/index.html

Texas Tech University, Graduate School, College of Arts and Sciences, Department of Biological Sciences, Lubbock, TX 79409-3131. Offers biology (MS, PhD); environmental sustainability and natural resources management (PSM); microbiology (MS); zoology (MS, PhD). Part-time programs available. *Faculty:* 37 full-time (6 women), 1 (woman) part-time/adjunct. *Students:* 93 full-time (50 women), 10 part-time (7 women); includes 7 minority (1 Black or African American, non-Hispanic/Latino; 3 Asian, non-Hispanic/Latino; 3 Hispanic/Latino), 45 international. Average age 30. 59 applicants, 32% accepted, 7 enrolled. In 2013, 13 master's, 12 doctorates awarded. *Degree requirements:* For master's, thesis or alternative; for doctorate, thesis/dissertation. *Entrance requirements:* For master's and doctorate, GRE General Test. Additional exam requirements/recommendations for international students: Required—TOEFL (minimum score 550 paper-based; 79 iBT). *Application deadline:* For fall admission, 6/1 priority date for domestic students, 1/15 priority date for international students; for spring admission, 9/1 priority date for domestic students, 6/15 priority date for international students. Applications are processed on a rolling basis. Application fee: $60. Electronic applications accepted. *Expenses:* Tuition, state resident: full-time $6062; part-time $252.57 per credit hour. Tuition, nonresident: full-time $14,558; part-time $606.57 per credit hour. *Required fees:* $2655; $35 per credit hour. $907.50 per semester. Tuition and fees vary according to course load. *Financial support:* In 2013–14, 100 students received support, including 69 fellowships (averaging $1,404 per year), 16 research assistantships (averaging $4,232 per year), 78 teaching assistantships (averaging $4,702 per year). Financial award application deadline: 4/15; financial award applicants required to submit FAFSA. *Faculty research:* Biodiversity and evolution, climate change in arid ecosystems, plant biology and biotechnology, animal communication and behavior, zoonotic and emerging diseases. *Total annual research expenditures:* $2.1 million. *Unit head:* Dr. Llewellyn D. Densmore, Chair, 806-742-2715, Fax: 806-742-2963, E-mail: lou.densmore@ttu.edu. *Application contact:* Dr. Randall M. Jeter, Graduate Adviser, 806-742-2710 Ext. 270, Fax: 806-742-2963, E-mail: randall.jeter@ttu.edu.
Website: http://www.biol.ttu.edu/default.aspx

Uniformed Services University of the Health Sciences, School of Medicine, Graduate Programs in the Biomedical Sciences and Public Health, Bethesda, MD 20814. Offers emerging infectious diseases (PhD); medical and clinical psychology (PhD), including clinical psychology, medical psychology; molecular and cell biology (MS, PhD); neuroscience (PhD); preventive medicine and biometrics (MPH, MS, MSPH, MTMH, Dr PH, PhD), including environmental health sciences (PhD), healthcare administration and policy (MS), medical zoology (PhD), public health (MPH, MSPH, Dr PH), tropical medicine and hygiene (MTMH). *Faculty:* 372 full-time (119 women), 4,044 part-time/adjunct (908 women). *Students:* 240 full-time (133 women); includes 40 minority (15 Black or African American, non-Hispanic/Latino; 13 Asian, non-Hispanic/Latino; 12 Hispanic/Latino), 30 international. Average age 25. 598 applicants, 17% accepted, 77 enrolled. In 2013, 19 master's, 50 doctorates awarded. Terminal master's awarded for partial completion of doctoral program. *Degree requirements:* For master's, comprehensive exam, thesis or alternative; for doctorate, comprehensive exam, thesis/dissertation, qualifying exam. *Entrance requirements:* For master's, GRE General Test; for doctorate, GRE General Test, minimum GPA of 3.0. Additional exam requirements/recommendations for international students: Required—TOEFL. *Application deadline:* For fall admission, 1/1 priority date for domestic and international students. Applications are processed on a rolling basis. Application fee: $0. Electronic applications accepted. *Financial support:* In 2013–14, fellowships with full tuition reimbursements (averaging $27,000 per year), research assistantships with full tuition reimbursements (averaging

$27,000 per year) were awarded; career-related internships or fieldwork, scholarships/grants, health care benefits, and tuition waivers (full) also available. *Unit head:* Dr. Eleanor S. Metcalf, Associate Dean, 301-295-1104, E-mail: emetcalf@usuhs.edu. *Application contact:* Tina Finley, Administrative Officer, 301-295-3642, Fax: 301-295-6772, E-mail: netina.finley@usuhs.edu.
Website: http://www.usuhs.mil/graded

Uniformed Services University of the Health Sciences, School of Medicine, Graduate Programs in the Biomedical Sciences and Public Health, Department of Preventive Medicine and Biometrics, Program in Medical Zoology, Bethesda, MD 20814-4799. Offers PhD. *Degree requirements:* For doctorate, comprehensive exam, thesis/dissertation, qualifying exam. *Entrance requirements:* For doctorate, GRE General Test, GRE Subject Test, minimum GPA of 3.0, U.S. citizenship. Additional exam requirements/recommendations for international students: Required—TOEFL. *Application deadline:* For fall admission, 1/1 priority date for domestic students. Applications are processed on a rolling basis. Application fee: $0. *Financial support:* Fellowships with full tuition reimbursements, scholarships/grants, health care benefits, and tuition waivers (full) available. *Faculty research:* Epidemiology, biostatistics, tropical public health, parasitology, vector biology. *Unit head:* Dr. David Cruess, Director, 301-295-3465, Fax: 301-295-1933, E-mail: dcruess@usuhs.edu. *Application contact:* Elena Marina Sherman, Program Administrative Specialist, 301-295-3913, Fax: 301-295-6772, E-mail: elena.sherman@usuhs.edu.
Website: http://www.usuhs.mil/pmb

University of Alaska Fairbanks, College of Natural Sciences and Mathematics, Department of Biology and Wildlife, Fairbanks, AK 99775-6100. Offers biological sciences (MS, PhD), including biology, botany, wildlife biology (PhD), zoology; biology (MAT, MS); wildlife biology (MS). Part-time programs available. *Faculty:* 21 full-time (9 women). *Students:* 73 full-time (39 women), 29 part-time (17 women); includes 7 minority (1 Asian, non-Hispanic/Latino; 4 Hispanic/Latino; 2 Two or more races, non-Hispanic/Latino), 5 international. Average age 31. 47 applicants, 21% accepted, 10 enrolled. In 2013, 12 master's, 8 doctorates awarded. *Degree requirements:* For master's, comprehensive exam, thesis, oral exam, oral defense; for doctorate, comprehensive exam, thesis/dissertation, oral exam, oral defense. *Entrance requirements:* For master's and doctorate, GRE General Test, GRE Subject Test (biology). Additional exam requirements/recommendations for international students: Required—TOEFL (minimum score 550 paper-based; 80 iBT), TWE. *Application deadline:* For fall admission, 6/1 for domestic students, 3/1 for international students; for spring admission, 10/15 for domestic students, 9/1 for international students. Applications are processed on a rolling basis. Application fee: $60. Electronic applications accepted. *Expenses:* Tuition, state resident: full-time $7254; part-time $403 per credit. Tuition, nonresident: full-time $14,814; part-time $823 per credit. Tuition and fees vary according to course level, course load and reciprocity agreements. *Financial support:* In 2013–14, 33 research assistantships with tuition reimbursements (averaging $15,138 per year), 21 teaching assistantships with tuition reimbursements (averaging $8,654 per year) were awarded; fellowships with tuition reimbursements, career-related internships or fieldwork, Federal Work-Study, scholarships/grants, health care benefits, and unspecified assistantships also available. Support available to part-time students. Financial award application deadline: 7/1; financial award applicants required to submit FAFSA. *Faculty research:* Plant-herbivore interactions, plant metabolic defenses, insect manufacture of glycerol, ice nucleators, structure and functions of arctic and subarctic freshwater ecosystems. *Unit head:* Diane Wagner, Department Chair, 907-474-7671, Fax: 907-474-6716, E-mail: uaf-bw-dept@alaska.edu. *Application contact:* Libby Eddy, Registrar and Director of Admissions, 907-474-7500, Fax: 907-474-7097, E-mail: admissions@uaf.edu.
Website: http://www.bw.uaf.edu

The University of British Columbia, Faculty of Science, Department of Zoology, Vancouver, BC V6T 1Z1, Canada. Offers M Sc, PhD. *Degree requirements:* For master's, thesis, final defense; for doctorate, comprehensive exam, thesis/dissertation, final defense. *Entrance requirements:* For master's and doctorate, faculty support. Additional exam requirements/recommendations for international students: Required—TOEFL. Electronic applications accepted. *Expenses: Tuition, area resident:* Full-time $8000 Canadian dollars. *Faculty research:* Cell and developmental biology; community, environmental, and population biology; comparative physiology and biochemistry; fisheries; ecology and evolutionary biology.

University of California, Davis, Graduate Studies, Graduate Group in Avian Sciences, Davis, CA 95616. Offers MS. *Degree requirements:* For master's, comprehensive exam (for some programs), thesis (for some programs). *Entrance requirements:* For master's, GRE General Test, minimum GPA of 3.0. Additional exam requirements/recommendations for international students: Required—TOEFL (minimum score 550 paper-based). Electronic applications accepted. *Faculty research:* Reproduction, nutrition, toxicology, food products, ecology of avian species.

University of Chicago, Division of Biological Sciences, Darwinian Sciences Cluster: Ecological, Integrative and Evolutionary Biology, Department of Organismal Biology and Anatomy, Chicago, IL 60637-1513. Offers integrative biology (PhD). *Degree requirements:* For doctorate, thesis/dissertation, ethics class, 2 teaching assistantships. *Entrance requirements:* For doctorate, GRE General Test. Additional exam requirements/recommendations for international students: Required—TOEFL (minimum score 600 paper-based; 104 iBT), IELTS (minimum score 7). Electronic applications accepted. *Faculty research:* Ecological physiology, evolution of fossil reptiles, vertebrate paleontology.

University of Connecticut, Graduate School, College of Liberal Arts and Sciences, Department of Ecology and Evolutionary Biology, Storrs, CT 06269. Offers botany (MS, PhD); ecology (MS, PhD); entomology (MS, PhD); zoology (MS, PhD). Terminal master's awarded for partial completion of doctoral program. *Degree requirements:* For master's, comprehensive exam; for doctorate, thesis/dissertation. *Entrance requirements:* For master's and doctorate, GRE General Test, GRE Subject Test. Additional exam requirements/recommendations for international students: Required—TOEFL (minimum score 550 paper-based). Electronic applications accepted.

University of Florida, Graduate School, College of Liberal Arts and Sciences, Department of Biology, Gainesville, FL 32611. Offers botany (MS, MST, PhD), including botany; zoology (MS, MST, PhD), including animal molecular and cellular biology (PhD), tropical conservation and development (MS), wetland sciences (MS), zoology. *Faculty:* 31 full-time (9 women), 26 part-time/adjunct (9 women). *Students:* 99 full-time (44 women), 6 part-time (4 women); includes 14 minority (2 Black or African American, non-Hispanic/Latino; 1 American Indian or Alaska Native, non-Hispanic/Latino; 5 Asian, non-Hispanic/Latino; 6 Hispanic/Latino), 35 international. Average age 31. 74 applicants, 32% accepted, 18 enrolled. In 2013, 4 master's, 13 doctorates awarded. *Degree requirements:* For master's, comprehensive exam (for some programs), thesis; for doctorate, comprehensive exam, thesis/dissertation. *Entrance requirements:* For master's and doctorate, GRE General Test, minimum GPA of 3.0. Additional exam requirements/recommendations for international students: Required—TOEFL (minimum score 550 paper-based; 80 iBT), IELTS (minimum score 6). *Application deadline:* For fall admission, 12/1 for domestic and international students. Applications are processed on a rolling basis. Application fee: $30. Electronic applications accepted. *Expenses:* Tuition, state resident: full-time $12,640. Tuition, nonresident: full-time $30,000. *Financial support:* In 2013–14, 98 students received support, including 7 fellowships (averaging $22,150 per year), 34 research assistantships (averaging $19,000 per year), 66 teaching assistantships (averaging $16,250 per year); unspecified assistantships also available. Financial award application deadline: 12/15; financial award applicants required to submit FAFSA. *Faculty research:* Ecology, evolution, genetics, molecular and cellular biology, physiology. *Unit head:* Craig Osenberg, PhD, Professor and Chair, 352-392-9201, Fax: 352-392-3704, E-mail: osenberg@ufl.edu. *Application contact:* William T. Barbazuk, PhD, Associate Professor/Graduate Coordinator, 352-273-8624, Fax: 352-392-3704, E-mail: bbarbazuk@ufl.edu.
Website: http://www.biology.ufl.edu/

University of Guelph, Graduate Studies, College of Biological Science, Department of Integrative Biology, Botany and Zoology, Guelph, ON N1G 2W1, Canada. Offers botany (M Sc, PhD); zoology (M Sc, PhD). Part-time programs available. *Degree requirements:* For master's, thesis, research proposal; for doctorate, thesis/dissertation, research proposal, qualifying exam. *Entrance requirements:* For master's, minimum B average during previous 2 years of course work. Additional exam requirements/recommendations for international students: Required—TOEFL (minimum score 550 paper-based), IELTS (minimum score 6.5). Electronic applications accepted. *Faculty research:* Aquatic science, environmental physiology, parasitology, wildlife biology, management.

University of Hawaii at Manoa, Graduate Division, College of Natural Sciences, Department of Zoology, Honolulu, HI 96822. Offers MS, PhD. Part-time programs available. *Degree requirements:* For master's, one foreign language, thesis optional; for doctorate, one foreign language, comprehensive exam, thesis/dissertation, seminar. *Entrance requirements:* For master's and doctorate, GRE General Test, GRE Subject Test. Additional exam requirements/recommendations for international students: Required—TOEFL (minimum score 600 paper-based; 100 iBT), IELTS (minimum score 7). *Faculty research:* Molecular evolution, reproductive biology, animal behavior, conservation biology, avian biology.

University of Illinois at Urbana–Champaign, Graduate College, College of Liberal Arts and Sciences, School of Integrative Biology, Department of Animal Biology, Champaign, IL 61820. Offers animal biology (ecology, ethology and evolution) (MS, PhD). *Students:* 15 (5 women). Application fee: $75 ($90 for international students). *Unit head:* Ken Paige, Head, 217-244-6606, Fax: 217-244-4565, E-mail: k-paige@illinois.edu. *Application contact:* Lisa Smith, Office Administrator, 217-333-7802, Fax: 217-244-4565, E-mail: ljsmith1@illinois.edu.
Website: http://www.life.illinois.edu/animalbiology

University of Maine, Graduate School, College of Natural Sciences, Forestry, and Agriculture, School of Biology and Ecology, Orono, ME 04469. Offers biological sciences (PhD); botany and plant pathology (MS); ecology and environmental science (MS, PhD); entomology (MS); plant science (PhD); zoology (MS, PhD). Part-time programs available. *Faculty:* 33 full-time (13 women), 26 part-time/adjunct (5 women). *Students:* 66 full-time (40 women), 4 part-time (2 women); includes 4 minority (1 American Indian or Alaska Native, non-Hispanic/Latino; 2 Asian, non-Hispanic/Latino; 1 Hispanic/Latino), 7 international. Average age 30. 97 applicants, 25% accepted, 17 enrolled. In 2013, 8 master's, 3 doctorates awarded. Terminal master's awarded for partial completion of doctoral program. *Degree requirements:* For master's, thesis (for some programs); for doctorate, comprehensive exam, thesis/dissertation. *Entrance requirements:* For master's and doctorate, GRE General Test. Additional exam requirements/recommendations for international students: Required—TOEFL. *Application deadline:* For fall admission, 2/1 priority date for domestic students. Applications are processed on a rolling basis. Application fee: $65. Electronic applications accepted. *Expenses:* Tuition, state resident: full-time $7524. Tuition, nonresident: full-time $23,112. *Required fees:* $1970. *Financial support:* In 2013–14, 66 students received support, including 3 fellowships with full tuition reimbursements available (averaging $25,000 per year), 28 research assistantships with full tuition reimbursements available (averaging $14,600 per year), 21 teaching assistantships with full tuition reimbursements available (averaging $14,600 per year); career-related internships or fieldwork, Federal Work-Study, institutionally sponsored loans, and tuition waivers (full and partial) also available. Financial award application deadline: 3/1. *Total annual research expenditures:* $569,533. *Unit head:* Dr. Ellie Groden, Director, 207-581-2551, Fax: 207-581-2537. *Application contact:* Scott G. Delcourt, Associate Dean of the Graduate School, 207-581-3291, Fax: 207-581-3232, E-mail: graduate@maine.edu.
Website: http://sbe.umaine.edu/

University of Manitoba, Faculty of Graduate Studies, Faculty of Science, Department of Biological Sciences, Winnipeg, MB R3T 2N2, Canada. Offers botany (M Sc, PhD); ecology (M Sc, PhD); zoology (M Sc, PhD).

The University of Montana, Graduate School, College of Humanities and Sciences, Division of Biological Sciences, Program in Organismal Biology and Ecology, Missoula, MT 59812-0002. Offers MS, PhD. Terminal master's awarded for partial completion of doctoral program. *Degree requirements:* For master's, one foreign language, thesis; for doctorate, 2 foreign languages, thesis/dissertation. *Entrance requirements:* For master's and doctorate, GRE General Test. *Application deadline:* For fall admission, 2/1 for domestic students. Application fee: $45. *Financial support:* Research assistantships with full tuition reimbursements, teaching assistantships with full tuition reimbursements, and Federal Work-Study available. Financial award application deadline: 3/1; financial award applicants required to submit FAFSA. *Faculty research:* Conservation biology, ecology and behavior, evolutionary genetics, avian biology. *Unit head:* Charles Janson, Chair, 406-243-5122, E-mail: charles.janson@mso.umt.edu. *Application contact:* Information Contact, E-mail: gradschl@mso.umt.edu.
Website: http://www.biology.umt.edu/

University of New Hampshire, Graduate School, College of Life Sciences and Agriculture, Department of Biological Sciences, Program in Zoology, Durham, NH 03824. Offers MS, PhD. Part-time programs available. *Faculty:* 27 full-time. *Students:* 8 full-time (4 women), 21 part-time (13 women); includes 2 minority (1 Asian, non-Hispanic/Latino; 1 Two or more races, non-Hispanic/Latino), 1 international. Average age 31. 35 applicants, 20% accepted, 6 enrolled. In 2013, 12 master's, 8 doctorates awarded. Terminal master's awarded for partial completion of doctoral program. *Degree requirements:* For master's, thesis; for doctorate, one foreign language, thesis/dissertation. *Entrance requirements:* For master's and doctorate, GRE General Test, GRE Subject Test. Additional exam requirements/recommendations for international students: Required—TOEFL (minimum score 550 paper-based; 80 iBT). *Application deadline:* For fall admission, 6/1 priority date for domestic students, 4/1 for international students; for spring admission, 12/1 for domestic students. Applications are processed on a rolling basis. Application fee: $65. Electronic applications accepted. *Expenses:* Tuition, state resident: full-time $13,500; part-time $750 per credit hour. Tuition, nonresident: full-time $26,200; part-time $1100 per credit hour. *Required fees:* $1741; $435.25 per term. Tuition and fees vary according to course level, course load, campus/location and program. *Financial support:* In 2013–14, 18 students received support, including 1 fellowship, 6 research assistantships, 10 teaching assistantships; career-related internships or fieldwork, Federal Work-Study, scholarships/grants, and tuition waivers (full and partial) also available. Support available to part-time students. Financial

award application deadline: 2/15. *Faculty research:* Behavior development, ecology, endocrinology, fisheries, invertebrates. *Unit head:* Dr. Larry Harris, Chairperson, 603-862-3897. *Application contact:* Diane Lavalliere, Administrative Assistant, 603-862-2100, E-mail: zoology.dept@unh.edu.
Website: http://zoology.unh.edu/

University of North Dakota, Graduate School, College of Arts and Sciences, Department of Biology, Grand Forks, ND 58202. Offers botany (MS, PhD); ecology (MS, PhD); entomology (MS, PhD); environmental biology (MS, PhD); fisheries/wildlife (MS, PhD); genetics (MS, PhD); zoology (MS, PhD). Terminal master's awarded for partial completion of doctoral program. *Degree requirements:* For master's, thesis, final exam; for doctorate, comprehensive exam, thesis/dissertation, final exam. *Entrance requirements:* For master's, GRE General Test, GRE Subject Test, minimum GPA of 3.0; for doctorate, GRE General Test, GRE Subject Test, minimum GPA of 3.5. Additional exam requirements/recommendations for international students: Required—TOEFL (minimum score 550 paper-based; 79 iBT), IELTS (minimum score 6.5). Electronic applications accepted. *Faculty research:* Population biology, wildlife ecology, RNA processing, hormonal control of behavior.

University of Wisconsin–Madison, Graduate School, College of Letters and Science, Department of Zoology, Madison, WI 53706-1380. Offers MA, MS, PhD. Part-time programs available. *Degree requirements:* For master's, thesis; for doctorate, one foreign language, thesis/dissertation. *Entrance requirements:* For master's and doctorate, GRE General Test. Additional exam requirements/recommendations for international students: Required—TOEFL. Electronic applications accepted. *Expenses:* Tuition, state resident: full-time $10,728; part-time $790 per credit. Tuition, nonresident: full-time $24,054; part-time $1623 per credit. *Required fees:* $1130; $119 per credit. *Faculty research:* Developmental biology, ecology, neurobiology, aquatic ecology, animal behavior.

University of Wisconsin–Oshkosh, Graduate Studies, College of Letters and Science, Department of Biology and Microbiology, Oshkosh, WI 54901. Offers biology (MS), including botany, microbiology, zoology. *Degree requirements:* For master's, comprehensive exam, thesis. *Entrance requirements:* For master's, GRE General Test, minimum GPA of 3.0, BS in biology. Additional exam requirements/recommendations for international students: Required—TOEFL (minimum score 550 paper-based; 79 iBT). Electronic applications accepted.

University of Wyoming, College of Arts and Sciences, Department of Zoology and Physiology, Laramie, WY 82071. Offers MS, PhD. Part-time programs available. *Degree requirements:* For master's, comprehensive exam (for some programs), thesis; for doctorate, comprehensive exam (for some programs), thesis/dissertation. *Entrance requirements:* For master's and doctorate, GRE General Test, minimum GPA of 3.0. Additional exam requirements/recommendations for international students: Required—TOEFL. Electronic applications accepted. *Faculty research:* Cell biology, ecology/wildlife, organismal physiology, zoology.

Washington State University, Graduate School, College of Arts and Sciences, Program in Zoology, Pullman, WA 99164-4236. Offers MS, PhD. *Degree requirements:* For master's, comprehensive exam (for some programs), thesis, oral exam; for doctorate, comprehensive exam, thesis/dissertation, oral exam, proposal defense. *Entrance requirements:* For master's and doctorate, GRE General Test, GRE Subject Test, three letters of recommendation, official transcripts from each university-level school attended, minimum GPA of 3.0. Additional exam requirements/recommendations for international students: Required—TOEFL, IELTS. *Faculty research:* Evolutionary biology, evolutionary ecology, population genetics, ecological genomics, disease ecology, population ecology, animal physiology.

Western Illinois University, School of Graduate Studies, College of Arts and Sciences, Department of Biological Sciences, Macomb, IL 61455-1390. Offers biological sciences (MS); environmental geographic information systems (Certificate); zoo and aquarium studies (Certificate). Part-time programs available. *Students:* 52 full-time (40 women), 27 part-time (19 women); includes 3 minority (1 Black or African American, non-Hispanic/Latino; 2 Hispanic/Latino), 4 international. Average age 26. In 2013, 14 master's, 17 other advanced degrees awarded. *Degree requirements:* For master's, thesis or alternative. *Entrance requirements:* Additional exam requirements/recommendations for international students: Required—TOEFL (minimum score 550 paper-based; 80 iBT); Recommended—IELTS. *Application deadline:* Applications are processed on a rolling basis. Application fee: $30. Electronic applications accepted. *Financial support:* In 2013–14, 29 students received support, including 9 research assistantships with full tuition reimbursements available (averaging $7,544 per year), 20 teaching assistantships with full tuition reimbursements available (averaging $8,688 per year). Financial award applicants required to submit FAFSA. *Unit head:* Dr. Charles Lydeard, Chairperson, 309-298-1546. *Application contact:* Dr. Nancy Parsons, Associate Provost and Director of Graduate Studies, 309-298-1806, Fax: 309-298-2345, E-mail: grad-office@wiu.edu.
Website: http://wiu.edu/biology

ACADEMIC AND PROFESSIONAL PROGRAMS IN HEALTH-RELATED PROFESSIONS

Section 20
Allied Health

This section contains a directory of institutions offering graduate work in allied health, followed by an in-depth entry submitted by an institution that chose to prepare a detailed program description. Additional information about programs listed in the directory but not augmented by an in-depth entry may be obtained by writing directly to the dean of a graduate school or chair of a department at the address given in the directory.

For programs offering related work, see also in this book *Anatomy, Biophysics, Dentistry and Dental Sciences, Health Services, Microbiological Sciences, Pathology and Pathobiology, Physiology,* and *Public Health.* In the other guides in this series:

Graduate Programs in the Humanities, Arts & Social Sciences

See *Art and Art History (Art Therapy), Family and Consumer Sciences (Gerontology), Performing Arts (Therapies),* and *Psychology and Counseling'*

Graduate Programs in the Physical Sciences, Mathematics, Agricultural Sciences, the Environment & Natural Resources

See *Physics (Acoustics)*

Graduate Programs in Engineering & Applied Sciences

See *Agricultural Engineering and Bioengineering (Bioengineering), Biomedical Engineering and Biotechnology,* and *Energy and Power Engineering (Nuclear Engineering)*

Graduate Programs in Business, Education, Information Studies, Law & Social Work

See *Administration, Instruction, and Theory (Educational Psychology); Special Focus (Education of the Multiply Handicapped); Social Work;* and *Subject Areas (Counselor Education)*

CONTENTS

Program Directories

Display and Close-Up

Allied Health—General

Alabama State University, College of Health Sciences, Montgomery, AL 36101-0271. Offers MRC, MS, DPT. *Faculty:* 7 full-time (5 women). *Students:* 163 full-time (109 women), 33 part-time (24 women); includes 106 minority (94 Black or African American, non-Hispanic/Latino; 4 American Indian or Alaska Native, non-Hispanic/Latino; 3 Asian, non-Hispanic/Latino; 4 Hispanic/Latino; 1 Two or more races, non-Hispanic/Latino), 1 international. Average age 28. 232 applicants, 35% accepted, 81 enrolled. In 2013, 25 master's, 31 doctorates awarded. *Entrance requirements:* Additional exam requirements/recommendations for international students: Required—TOEFL (minimum score 500 paper-based). *Application deadline:* For fall admission, 7/15 for domestic students; for spring admission, 12/15 for domestic students. Applications are processed on a rolling basis. Application fee: $25. *Expenses:* Tuition, state resident: full-time $7958; part-time $343 per credit hour. Tuition, nonresident: full-time $14,132; part-time $686 per credit hour. *Required fees:* $446 per term. One-time fee: $1784 full-time; $892 part-time. Tuition and fees vary according to course load. *Financial support:* In 2013–14, 4 research assistantships (averaging $9,450 per year) were awarded. *Unit head:* Dr. Steven B. Chesbro, Dean, 334-229-5053, E-mail: schesbro@alasu.edu. *Application contact:* Dr. William Person, Dean of Graduate Studies, 334-229-4274, Fax: 334-229-4928, E-mail: wperson@alasu.edu.
Website: http://www.alasu.edu/academics/colleges—departments/health-sciences/index.aspx

American College of Healthcare Sciences, Graduate Programs, Portland, OR 97239-3719. Offers aromatherapy (Graduate Certificate); complementary alternative medicine (MS, Graduate Certificate); herbal medicine (Graduate Certificate); nutrition (Graduate Certificate). Part-time and evening/weekend programs available. Postbaccalaureate distance learning degree programs offered (no on-campus study). *Degree requirements:* For master's, capstone project. *Entrance requirements:* For master's, interview, letters of recommendation, essay.

Andrews University, School of Health Professions, Department of Medical Laboratory Sciences, Berrien Springs, MI 49104. Offers MSMLS. *Accreditation:* APTA. *Faculty:* 5 full-time (3 women). *Students:* 4 full-time (3 women), 1 part-time (0 women); includes 1 minority (Hispanic/Latino), 3 international. Average age 31. 8 applicants, 63% accepted, 3 enrolled. *Entrance requirements:* For master's, GRE. Additional exam requirements/recommendations for international students: Required—TOEFL (minimum score 550 paper-based). *Application deadline:* Applications are processed on a rolling basis. Application fee: $40. *Unit head:* Dr. Marcia A. Kilsby, Chair, 269-471-3336. *Application contact:* Monica Wringer, Supervisor of Graduate Admission, 800-253-2874, Fax: 269-471-6321, E-mail: graduate@andrews.edu.
Website: http://www.andrews.edu/shp/mls/

Athabasca University, Centre for Nursing and Health Studies, Athabasca, AB T9S 3A3, Canada. Offers advanced nursing practice (MN, Advanced Diploma); generalist (MN); health studies-leadership (MHS). Part-time programs available. Postbaccalaureate distance learning degree programs offered. *Degree requirements:* For master's, comprehensive exam (for some programs). *Entrance requirements:* For master's, bachelor's degree in health-related field, 2 years professional health service experience (MHS), bachelor's degree in nursing, 2 years nursing experience (MN), minimum GPA of 3.0 in final 30 credits; for Advanced Diploma, RN license, 2 years health care experience. Electronic applications accepted. *Expenses:* Contact institution.

A.T. Still University, Arizona School of Health Sciences, Mesa, AZ 85206. Offers advanced occupational therapy (MS); advanced physician assistant studies (MS); athletic training (MS); audiology (Au D); health sciences (DHSc); human movement (MS); occupational therapy (MS, DOT); physical therapy (DPT); physician assistant (MS); transitional audiology (Au D); transitional physical therapy (DPT). *Accreditation:* AOTA (one or more programs are accredited); ASHA. Part-time and evening/weekend programs available. Postbaccalaureate distance learning degree programs offered (minimal on-campus study). *Faculty:* 47 full-time (27 women), 279 part-time/adjunct (173 women). *Students:* 531 full-time (354 women), 865 part-time (547 women); includes 315 minority (79 Black or African American, non-Hispanic/Latino; 10 American Indian or Alaska Native, non-Hispanic/Latino; 114 Asian, non-Hispanic/Latino; 83 Hispanic/Latino; 6 Native Hawaiian or other Pacific Islander, non-Hispanic/Latino; 23 Two or more races, non-Hispanic/Latino), 82 international. Average age 36. 3,325 applicants, 14% accepted, 329 enrolled. In 2013, 252 master's, 370 doctorates awarded. *Degree requirements:* For master's, thesis (for some programs); for doctorate, thesis/dissertation (for some programs). *Entrance requirements:* For master's, GRE General Test; for doctorate, GRE, Evaluation of Practicing Audiologists Capabilities (Au D), Physical Therapist Evaluation Tool (DPT), current state licensure, master's degree or equivalent (Au D). Additional exam requirements/recommendations for international students: Required—TOEFL (minimum score 550 paper-based; 80 iBT). *Application deadline:* For fall admission, 8/1 for domestic and international students. Applications are processed on a rolling basis. Application fee: $70. Electronic applications accepted. *Expenses:* Contact institution. *Financial support:* In 2013–14, 151 students received support. Federal Work-Study and scholarships/grants available. Financial award application deadline: 5/1; financial award applicants required to submit FAFSA. *Faculty research:* Pediatric sport-related concussion, adolescent athlete health-related quality of life; geriatric and pediatric well-being, pain management for participation, practice-based research network, BMI and dental caries. *Total annual research expenditures:* $174,826. *Unit head:* Dr. Randy Danielsen, Dean, 480-219-6000, Fax: 480-219-6110, E-mail: rdanielsen@atsu.edu. *Application contact:* Donna Sparks, Associate Director, Admissions Processing, 660-626-2117, Fax: 660-626-2969, E-mail: admissions@atsu.edu.
Website: http://www.atsu.edu/ashs

Baylor University, Graduate School, Military Programs, Waco, TX 76798. Offers MHA, MS, D Sc, D Sc PA, DPT. *Accreditation:* APTA (one or more programs are accredited). *Students:* 220 full-time (83 women); includes 18 minority (5 Black or African American, non-Hispanic/Latino; 3 Asian, non-Hispanic/Latino; 8 Hispanic/Latino; 1 Native Hawaiian or other Pacific Islander, non-Hispanic/Latino; 1 Two or more races, non-Hispanic/Latino). In 2013, 67 master's, 49 doctorates awarded. *Entrance requirements:* For master's, GRE General Test or GMAT; for doctorate, GRE General Test. *Application deadline:* Applications are processed on a rolling basis. *Expenses:* Contact institution. *Unit head:* Col. Josef Moore, Dean, 210-221-6457, Fax: 210-221-6457, E-mail: josef.h.moore.mil@mail.mil. *Application contact:* Lori McNamara, Admissions Coordinator, 254-710-3588, Fax: 254-710-3870.

Belmont University, Gordon E. Inman College of Health Sciences and Nursing, Nashville, TN 37212-3757. Offers nursing (MSN, DNP); occupational therapy (MSOT, OTD); physical therapy (DPT). Part-time programs available. Postbaccalaureate distance learning degree programs offered (minimal on-campus study). *Students:* 290 full-time (172 women), 1 part-time (0 women); includes 43 minority (12 Black or African American, non-Hispanic/Latino; 22 Asian, non-Hispanic/Latino; 8 Hispanic/Latino; 1 Two or more races, non-Hispanic/Latino), 3 international. Average age 26. *Degree requirements:* For master's, comprehensive exam, thesis; for doctorate, comprehensive exam. *Entrance requirements:* For master's, GRE, BSN, minimum GPA of 3.0. Additional exam requirements/recommendations for international students: Required—TOEFL (minimum score 550 paper-based). *Application deadline:* Applications are processed on a rolling basis. Application fee: $50. Electronic applications accepted. *Expenses:* Contact institution. *Financial support:* Teaching assistantships with full tuition reimbursements, career-related internships or fieldwork, scholarships/grants, and traineeships available. Financial award application deadline: 3/1; financial award applicants required to submit FAFSA. *Unit head:* Dean, 615-460-6916, Fax: 615-460-6750. *Application contact:* David Mee, Dean of Enrollment Services, 615-460-6785, Fax: 615-460-5434, E-mail: david.mee@belmont.edu.
Website: http://www.belmont.edu/healthsciences/

Bennington College, Graduate Programs, Postbaccalaureate Premedical Program, Bennington, VT 05201. Offers allied and health sciences (Certificate). *Expenses:* Contact institution. *Faculty research:* Cellular functions of Hsp90, foundations of quantum mechanics, history and philosophy of physics, cytosolic quality control, forest ecology, plate tectonics of rift systems, amphibian evolutionary physiology, photochemistry of gold complexes.

Boston University, College of Health and Rehabilitation Sciences: Sargent College, Boston, MA 02215. Offers MS, MSOT, DPT, OTD, PhD. *Accreditation:* APTA (one or more programs are accredited). Postbaccalaureate distance learning degree programs offered (minimal on-campus study). *Faculty:* 54 full-time (42 women), 44 part-time/adjunct (28 women). *Students:* 406 full-time (348 women), 41 part-time (34 women); includes 59 minority (3 Black or African American, non-Hispanic/Latino; 33 Asian, non-Hispanic/Latino; 16 Hispanic/Latino; 7 Two or more races, non-Hispanic/Latino), 16 international. Average age 26. 1,729 applicants, 26% accepted, 139 enrolled. In 2013, 122 master's, 81 doctorates awarded. Terminal master's awarded for partial completion of doctoral program. *Degree requirements:* For master's, comprehensive exam (for some programs), thesis optional; for doctorate, variable foreign language requirement, comprehensive exam (for some programs), thesis/dissertation. *Entrance requirements:* For master's and doctorate, GRE General Test. Additional exam requirements/recommendations for international students: Required—TOEFL (minimum score 550 paper-based). *Application deadline:* For fall admission, 2/1 priority date for domestic and international students. Applications are processed on a rolling basis. Application fee: $80. Electronic applications accepted. *Expenses: Tuition:* Full-time $43,970; part-time $1374 per credit hour. *Required fees:* $60 per semester. Tuition and fees vary according to class time, course level and program. *Financial support:* In 2013–14, 275 students received support, including 237 fellowships (averaging $12,000 per year), 18 research assistantships with full tuition reimbursements available (averaging $20,000 per year), 20 teaching assistantships (averaging $5,000 per year); career-related internships or fieldwork, Federal Work-Study, institutionally sponsored loans, scholarships/grants, and health care benefits also available. Support available to part-time students. Financial award application deadline: 4/15; financial award applicants required to submit FAFSA. *Faculty research:* Outcome measurement, gerontology, neuroanatomy, aphasia, autism, Parkinson's Disease, psychiatric rehabilitation, obesity prevention, speech production and imaging. *Total annual research expenditures:* $9.2 million. *Unit head:* Dr. Kathleen Morgan, Interim Dean, 617-353-2704, Fax: 617-353-7500, E-mail: kmorgan@bu.edu. *Application contact:* Sharon Sankey, Director, Student Services, 617-353-2713, Fax: 617-353-7500, E-mail: ssankey@bu.edu.
Website: http://www.bu.edu/sargent/

Brock University, Faculty of Graduate Studies, Faculty of Applied Health Sciences, St. Catharines, ON L2S 3A1, Canada. Offers M Sc, MA, PhD. *Degree requirements:* For master's, thesis. *Entrance requirements:* For master's, honors degree, BA and/or B Sc. Additional exam requirements/recommendations for international students: Required—TOEFL (minimum score 550 paper-based; 80 iBT), IELTS (minimum score 6.5), TWE (minimum score 4). Electronic applications accepted. *Faculty research:* Health and physical activity, aging and health, health advocacy, exercise psychology, community development.

Canisius College, Graduate Division, School of Education and Human Services, Office of Professional Studies, Buffalo, NY 14208-1098. Offers applied nutrition (MS, Certificate); community and school health (MS); health and human performance (MS); health information technology (MS); respiratory care (MS). Postbaccalaureate distance learning degree programs offered (no on-campus study). *Faculty:* 17 part-time/adjunct (11 women). *Students:* 51 full-time (35 women), 37 part-time (26 women); includes 16 minority (8 Black or African American, non-Hispanic/Latino; 1 American Indian or Alaska Native, non-Hispanic/Latino; 7 Hispanic/Latino), 2 international. Average age 32. 98 applicants, 57% accepted, 24 enrolled. In 2013, 29 master's awarded. *Entrance requirements:* Additional exam requirements/recommendations for international students: Required—TOEFL (minimum score 550 paper-based, 80 iBT), IELTS (minimum score 6.5), or CAEL (minimum score 70). *Application deadline:* Applications are processed on a rolling basis. Application fee: $25. Electronic applications accepted. Application fee is waived when completed online. *Expenses: Tuition:* Part-time $750 per credit hour. *Financial support:* Career-related internships or fieldwork, Federal Work-Study, scholarships/grants, and unspecified assistantships available. Support available to part-time students. Financial award application deadline: 4/30; financial award applicants required to submit FAFSA. *Faculty research:* Nutrition, community and school health; community and health; health and human performance applied; nutrition and respiratory care. *Unit head:* Dr. Khalid Bibi, Executive Director, 716-888-8296. *Application contact:* Julie A. Zulewski, Director of Graduate Admission, 716-888-2548, Fax: 716-888-3195, E-mail: zulewskj@canisius.edu.
Website: http://www.canisius.edu/graduate/

Cleveland State University, College of Graduate Studies, College of Sciences and Health Professions, School of Health Sciences, Program in Health Sciences, Cleveland, OH 44115. Offers MS. Part-time and evening/weekend programs available. Postbaccalaureate distance learning degree programs offered (no on-campus study). *Faculty:* 20 full-time (14 women), 16 part-time/adjunct (11 women). *Students:* 67 full-time (51 women), 76 part-time (57 women); includes 23 minority (13 Black or African American, non-Hispanic/Latino; 7 Asian, non-Hispanic/Latino; 1 Hispanic/Latino; 2 Two or more races, non-Hispanic/Latino), 4 international. Average age 31. 85 applicants, 73% accepted, 50 enrolled. In 2013, 50 master's awarded. *Degree requirements:* For master's, thesis. *Application deadline:* For fall admission, 5/15 for international students; for winter admission, 4/1 for international students; for spring admission, 11/1 for international students. *Expenses:* Tuition, state resident: full-time $8335; part-time $521 per credit hour. Tuition, nonresident: full-time $15,670; part-time $979 per credit hour. *Required fees:* $50; $25 per semester. *Financial support:* Research assistantships

available. *Faculty research:* Assisted technologies, biomechanics, clinical administration, cultural health, gerontology. *Unit head:* Dr. Myrita Sipp Wilhite, Director, 216-687-3808, E-mail: m.wilhite@csuohio.edu. *Application contact:* Karen Armstrong, Secretary, 216-687-3567, Fax: 216-687-9316, E-mail: k.bradley@csuohio.edu.
Website: http://www.csuohio.edu/sciences/dept/healthsciences/graduate/index.html

The Commonwealth Medical College, Professional Program in Medicine, Scranton, PA 18509. Offers MD, MD/MHA, MD/MPH. *Students:* 309 full-time (143 women). *Expenses: Tuition:* Full-time $50,000. *Required fees:* $6112. Tuition and fees vary according to degree level, program and student level. *Application contact:* Jillian Golaszewski, Enrollment Management Recruiter, 570-504-7000, Fax: 570-504-2794, E-mail: jgolaszewski@tcmedc.org.
Website: http://www.tcmc.edu/md

Creighton University, School of Pharmacy and Health Professions, Omaha, NE 68178-0001. Offers MS, DPT, OTD, Pharm D, Pharm D/MS. *Accreditation:* ACPE (one or more programs are accredited). Postbaccalaureate distance learning degree programs offered (minimal on-campus study). *Entrance requirements:* For doctorate, PCAT (for Pharm D); GRE (for DPT). Electronic applications accepted. *Expenses:* Contact institution. *Faculty research:* Patient safety in health services research, health information technology and health services research, interdisciplinary educational research in the health professions, outcomes research in the health professions, cross-cultural care in the health professions.

Dominican College, Division of Allied Health, Orangeburg, NY 10962-1210. Offers MS, DPT. Part-time and evening/weekend programs available. Postbaccalaureate distance learning degree programs offered (minimal on-campus study). *Faculty:* 9 full-time (6 women), 27 part-time/adjunct (14 women). *Students:* 138 full-time (96 women), 191 part-time (98 women). Average age 37. In 2013, 27 master's, 126 doctorates awarded. *Application deadline:* Applications are processed on a rolling basis. *Expenses: Tuition:* Part-time $815 per credit. *Required fees:* $180 per semester. *Unit head:* Dr. Sandra Countee, Division Director, 845-848-6039, Fax: 845-398-4893, E-mail: sandra.countee@dc.edu. *Application contact:* Joyce Elbe, Director of Admissions, 845-848-7896 Ext. 15, Fax: 845-365-3150, E-mail: admissions@dc.edu.

Drexel University, College of Nursing and Health Professions, Philadelphia, PA 19104-2875. Offers MA, MFT, MHS, MS, MSN, DPT, Dr NP, PPDPT, PhD, Certificate, PMC. Part-time and evening/weekend programs available. Terminal master's awarded for partial completion of doctoral program. *Degree requirements:* For master's, comprehensive exam, thesis (for some programs); for doctorate, thesis/dissertation, qualifying exam. *Entrance requirements:* For doctorate, GRE General Test. Electronic applications accepted.

Duquesne University, John G. Rangos, Sr. School of Health Sciences, Pittsburgh, PA 15282-0001. Offers health management systems (MHMS); occupational therapy (MS, OTD); physical therapy (DPT); physician assistant studies (MPAS); rehabilitation science (MS, PhD); speech-language pathology (MS); MBA/MHMS. *Accreditation:* AOTA (one or more programs are accredited); APTA (one or more programs are accredited); ASHA. Postbaccalaureate distance learning degree programs offered (minimal on-campus study). *Faculty:* 41 full-time (29 women), 32 part-time/adjunct (15 women). *Students:* 232 full-time (174 women), 14 part-time (7 women); includes 12 minority (2 Black or African American, non-Hispanic/Latino; 7 Asian, non-Hispanic/Latino; 1 Hispanic/Latino; 2 Two or more races, non-Hispanic/Latino), 7 international. Average age 23. 951 applicants, 11% accepted, 35 enrolled. In 2013, 119 master's, 40 doctorates awarded. *Degree requirements:* For doctorate, comprehensive exam (for some programs), thesis/dissertation (for some programs). *Entrance requirements:* For master's, GRE General Test (speech-language pathology), 3 letters of recommendation; minimum GPA of 2.75 (health management systems), 3.0 (speech-language pathology); for doctorate, GRE General Test (for physical therapy and rehabilitation science), 3 letters of recommendation, minimum GPA of 3.0, personal interview. Additional exam requirements/recommendations for international students: Required—TOEFL (minimum score 550 paper-based; 90 iBT). *Application deadline:* For fall admission, 2/1 for domestic and international students; for spring admission, 7/1 for domestic and international students. Applications are processed on a rolling basis. Electronic applications accepted. *Expenses:* Contact institution. *Financial support:* Federal Work-Study available. Financial award applicants required to submit FAFSA. *Faculty research:* Neuronal processing, electrical stimulation on peripheral neuropathy, central nervous system (CNS) stimulatory and inhibitory signals, behavioral genetic methodologies to development disorders of speech, neurogenic communication disorders. *Total annual research expenditures:* $83,650. *Unit head:* Dr. Gregory H. Frazer, Dean, 412-396-5303, Fax: 412-396-5554, E-mail: frazer@duq.edu. *Application contact:* Christopher R. Hilf, Recruiter/Academic Advisor, 412-396-5653, Fax: 412-396-5554, E-mail: hilfc@duq.edu.
Website: http://www.duq.edu/academics/schools/health-sciences

East Carolina University, Graduate School, School of Allied Health Sciences, Greenville, NC 27858-4353. Offers MS, MSOT, DPT, PhD, Certificate, Au D/PhD. Part-time and evening/weekend programs available. Postbaccalaureate distance learning degree programs offered (no on-campus study). *Degree requirements:* For master's, comprehensive exam. *Entrance requirements:* For master's, GRE General Test. Additional exam requirements/recommendations for international students: Required—TOEFL. Application fee: $50. *Expenses:* Tuition, state resident: full-time $4223. Tuition, nonresident: full-time $16,540. *Required fees:* $2184. *Financial support:* Research assistantships with partial tuition reimbursements, teaching assistantships with partial tuition reimbursements, career-related internships or fieldwork, Federal Work-Study, and scholarships/grants available. Support available to part-time students. Financial award application deadline: 6/1; financial award applicants required to submit FAFSA. *Faculty research:* Hearing, stuttering, therapeutic activities, ACL injury. *Unit head:* Dr. Stephen Thomas, Dean, 252-744-6010, E-mail: thomass@ecu.edu. *Application contact:* Dean of Graduate School, 252-328-6012, Fax: 252-328-6071, E-mail: gradschool@ecu.edu.
Website: http://www.ecu.edu/cs-dhs/ah/

Eastern Kentucky University, The Graduate School, College of Health Sciences, Richmond, KY 40475-3102. Offers MPH, MS, MSN. Part-time programs available. *Entrance requirements:* For master's, GRE General Test, minimum GPA of 2.75.

East Tennessee State University, School of Graduate Studies, College of Clinical and Rehabilitative Health Sciences, Department of Allied Health Science, Johnson City, TN 37614. Offers allied health (MSAH); clinical nutrition (MS). Part-time programs available. Postbaccalaureate distance learning degree programs offered (no on-campus study). *Faculty:* 15 full-time (11 women), 1 part-time/adjunct (0 women). *Students:* 21 full-time (20 women), 29 part-time (25 women); includes 5 minority (2 Black or African American, non-Hispanic/Latino; 2 Hispanic/Latino; 1 Two or more races, non-Hispanic/Latino). Average age 31. 9 applicants, 22% accepted, 2 enrolled. In 2013, 15 master's awarded. *Degree requirements:* For master's, comprehensive exam, thesis optional, advanced practice seminar (for MSAH non-thesis option); internship (for clinical nutrition). *Entrance requirements:* For master's, GRE General Test, professional license in allied health discipline, minimum GPA of 2.75 (MSAH); bachelor's degree from undergraduate didactic program in dietetics with minimum GPA of 3.0 in DPD coursework (clinical nutrition). Additional exam requirements/recommendations for international students: Required—TOEFL (minimum score 550 paper-based; 79 iBT). *Application deadline:* For fall admission, 2/15 for domestic and international students; for spring admission, 11/1 for domestic students, 9/30 for international students. Application fee: $35 ($45 for international students). Electronic applications accepted. *Expenses:* Tuition, state resident: full-time $7900; part-time $395 per credit hour. Tuition, nonresident: full-time $21,960; part-time $1098 per credit hour. *Required fees:* $1345; $84 per credit hour. *Financial support:* In 2013–14, 18 students received support, including 3 research assistantships with full tuition reimbursements available (averaging $6,000 per year), 4 teaching assistantships with full tuition reimbursements available (averaging $6,000 per year); career-related internships or fieldwork, institutionally sponsored loans, scholarships/grants, and unspecified assistantships also available. Financial award application deadline: 7/1; financial award applicants required to submit FAFSA. *Faculty research:* Recruitment and retention of allied health professionals, relationship between APACHEE II scores and the need for a tracheotomy, health care workers, patient care, occupational stress, radiofrequency lesioning, absorption of lipopholic compounds, Vitamin D status in college-age students, childhood and adolescence obesity, nutrition education/interventions. *Unit head:* Dr. Charles Faust, Chair, 423-439-7888, Fax: 423-547-4900, E-mail: faust@etsu.edu. *Application contact:* Mary Duncan, Graduate Specialist, 423-439-4302, Fax: 423-439-5624, E-mail: duncanm@etsu.edu.
Website: http://www.etsu.edu/crhs/alliedhealth/msah/

East Tennessee State University, School of Graduate Studies, College of Public Health, Johnson City, TN 37614. Offers MPH, MSEH, DPH, PhD, Postbaccalaureate Certificate. Part-time and evening/weekend programs available. *Faculty:* 37 full-time (10 women), 9 part-time/adjunct (4 women). *Students:* 65 full-time (47 women), 52 part-time (37 women); includes 16 minority (11 Black or African American, non-Hispanic/Latino; 3 Asian, non-Hispanic/Latino; 2 Two or more races, non-Hispanic/Latino), 11 international. Average age 30. 116 applicants, 64% accepted, 57 enrolled. In 2013, 25 master's, 7 doctorates, 1 other advanced degree awarded. *Expenses:* Tuition, state resident: full-time $7900; part-time $395 per credit hour. Tuition, nonresident: full-time $21,960; part-time $1098 per credit hour. *Required fees:* $1345; $84 per credit hour. *Financial support:* In 2013–14, 56 students received support, including 33 research assistantships with full and partial tuition reimbursements available (averaging $9,000 per year), 3 teaching assistantships with full and partial tuition reimbursements available (averaging $10,000 per year). Financial award application deadline: 7/1; financial award applicants required to submit FAFSA. *Unit head:* Dr. Randy Wykoff, Dean, 423-439-4243, Fax: 423-439-5238, E-mail: wykoff@etsu.edu. *Application contact:* Mary Duncan, Graduate Specialist, 423-439-4302, Fax: 423-439-5624, E-mail: duncanm@etsu.edu.
Website: http://www.etsu.edu/cph/

Emory University, School of Medicine, Programs in Allied Health Professions, Atlanta, GA 30322-1100. Offers anesthesiology assistant (MM Sc); genetic counseling (MM Sc), including human genetics and genetic counseling; physical therapy (DPT); physician assistant (MM Sc). *Faculty:* 25 full-time (19 women), 34 part-time/adjunct (19 women). *Students:* 462 full-time (318 women); includes 88 minority (28 Black or African American, non-Hispanic/Latino; 1 American Indian or Alaska Native, non-Hispanic/Latino; 31 Asian, non-Hispanic/Latino; 17 Hispanic/Latino; 11 Two or more races, non-Hispanic/Latino), 7 international. Average age 27. 2,165 applicants, 12% accepted, 168 enrolled. In 2013, 87 master's, 63 doctorates awarded. *Entrance requirements:* For master's, GRE or MCAT; for doctorate, GRE. *Application deadline:* Applications are processed on a rolling basis. Electronic applications accepted. *Expenses:* Contact institution. *Financial support:* In 2013–14, 160 students received support. Institutionally sponsored loans and scholarships/grants available. Financial award application deadline: 3/1; financial award applicants required to submit FAFSA. *Unit head:* Dr. John William Eley, Executive Associate Dean, Medical Education and Student Affairs, 404-727-5655, Fax: 404-727-0045, E-mail: jeley@emory.edu. *Application contact:* Mary Kaye Garcia, Associate Director of Registration and Student Affairs, 404-712-9921, Fax: 404-727-0045, E-mail: mkgarci@emory.edu.

Ferris State University, College of Health Professions, Big Rapids, MI 49307. Offers MSN. Part-time and evening/weekend programs available. Postbaccalaureate distance learning degree programs offered (no on-campus study). *Faculty:* 5 full-time (all women), 1 (woman) part-time/adjunct. *Students:* 1 (woman) full-time, 103 part-time (91 women); includes 5 minority (2 Black or African American, non-Hispanic/Latino; 1 American Indian or Alaska Native, non-Hispanic/Latino; 1 Native Hawaiian or other Pacific Islander, non-Hispanic/Latino; 1 Two or more races, non-Hispanic/Latino). Average age 41. 25 applicants, 92% accepted, 21 enrolled. In 2013, 20 master's awarded. *Degree requirements:* For master's, comprehensive exam, practicum, practicum project. *Entrance requirements:* For master's, BS in nursing or bachelor's degree in related field with registered nurse license; minimum GPA of 3.0; writing sample; 3 professional references. Additional exam requirements/recommendations for international students: Required—TOEFL (minimum score 500 paper-based; 61 iBT). *Application deadline:* For fall admission, 4/15 priority date for domestic students; for spring admission, 10/5 for domestic students. Applications are processed on a rolling basis. Application fee: $30. Electronic applications accepted. Application fee is waived when completed online. *Financial support:* In 2013–14, 3 students received support. Career-related internships or fieldwork and scholarships/grants available. Financial award application deadline: 4/15; financial award applicants required to submit FAFSA. *Unit head:* Dr. Susan Owens, Interim MSN Program Coordinator, 231-591-2267, Fax: 231-591-3788, E-mail: owenss3@ferris.edu. *Application contact:* Debby Buck, Off-Campus Student Support, 231-591-2094, Fax: 231-591-3788, E-mail: buckd@ferris.edu.
Website: http://www.ferris.edu/htmls/colleges/alliedhe/

Florida Agricultural and Mechanical University, Division of Graduate Studies, Research, and Continuing Education, School of Allied Health Sciences, Tallahassee, FL 32307-3200. Offers health administration (MS); occupational therapy (MOT); physical therapy (MPT). *Degree requirements:* For master's, thesis (for some programs). *Entrance requirements:* For master's, GRE General Test or GMAT, minimum GPA of 3.0. Additional exam requirements/recommendations for international students: Required—TOEFL (minimum score 550 paper-based).

Florida Gulf Coast University, College of Health Professions, Fort Myers, FL 33965-6565. Offers MS, MSN, DPT. *Accreditation:* AOTA. Part-time and evening/weekend programs available. Postbaccalaureate distance learning degree programs offered (minimal on-campus study). *Degree requirements:* For master's, thesis or alternative. *Entrance requirements:* For master's, GRE General Test or MAT, minimum GPA of 3.0. Additional exam requirements/recommendations for international students: Required—TOEFL (minimum score 550 paper-based). Electronic applications accepted. *Faculty research:* Gerontology, health care policy, health administration, community-based services.

Georgia Regents University, The Graduate School, Program in Allied Health Sciences, Augusta, GA 30912. Offers dental hygiene (MS). Part-time programs available. Postbaccalaureate distance learning degree programs offered (no on-campus study). *Degree requirements:* For master's, thesis. *Entrance requirements:* For master's, GRE General Test. Additional exam requirements/recommendations for international students: Required—TOEFL (minimum score 550 paper-based; 79 iBT). Electronic applications accepted. *Faculty research:* Patient- and family-centered care, public health informatics, vascular health promotion through physical activity, improving air quality for school children, movement therapies for Parkinson's Disease.

Georgia Southern University, Jack N. Averitt College of Graduate Studies, College of Health and Human Sciences, Statesboro, GA 30460. Offers MS, MSN, DNP. Part-time and evening/weekend programs available. Postbaccalaureate distance learning degree programs offered (no on-campus study). *Faculty:* 57 full-time (36 women), 2 part-time/adjunct (both women). *Students:* 99 full-time (67 women), 132 part-time (77 women); includes 38 minority (24 Black or African American, non-Hispanic/Latino; 1 American Indian or Alaska Native, non-Hispanic/Latino; 3 Asian, non-Hispanic/Latino; 4 Hispanic/Latino; 6 Two or more races, non-Hispanic/Latino), 5 international. Average age 30. 244 applicants, 46% accepted, 65 enrolled. In 2013, 91 master's, 6 doctorates awarded. *Degree requirements:* For master's, comprehensive exam (for some programs), thesis (for some programs), exams; for doctorate, comprehensive exam, practicum. *Entrance requirements:* For master's, GRE General Test, MAT or GMAT; for doctorate, GRE or MAT. Additional exam requirements/recommendations for international students: Required—TOEFL (minimum score 550 paper-based; 80 iBT), IELTS (minimum score 6). *Application deadline:* For fall admission, 3/1 priority date for domestic students, 3/1 for international students; for spring admission, 10/1 priority date for domestic students, 10/1 for international students. Applications are processed on a rolling basis. Application fee: $50. Electronic applications accepted. *Expenses:* Tuition, state resident: full-time $7068; part-time $270 per semester hour. Tuition, nonresident: full-time $26,446; part-time $1077 per semester hour. *Required fees:* $2092. *Financial support:* In 2013–14, 56 students received support, including 57 research assistantships with partial tuition reimbursements available (averaging $7,200 per year), teaching assistantships with partial tuition reimbursements available (averaging $7,200 per year); career-related internships or fieldwork, Federal Work-Study, scholarships/grants, traineeships, tuition waivers (partial), and unspecified assistantships also available. Support available to part-time students. Financial award application deadline: 4/15; financial award applicants required to submit FAFSA. *Total annual research expenditures:* $99,590. *Unit head:* Dr. Barry Joyner, Dean, 912-478-5322, Fax: 912-478-5349, E-mail: joyner@georgiasouthern.edu. *Application contact:* Amanda Gilliland, Coordinator for Graduate Student Recruitment, 912-478-5384, Fax: 912-478-0740, E-mail: gradadmissions@georgiasouthern.edu.
Website: http://chhs.georgiasouthern.edu/

Georgia State University, Byrdine F. Lewis School of Nursing, Division of Respiratory Therapy, Atlanta, GA 30302-3083. Offers MS. *Faculty:* 3 full-time (2 women). *Students:* 25 full-time (13 women), 5 part-time (2 women); includes 9 minority (5 Black or African American, non-Hispanic/Latino; 2 Asian, non-Hispanic/Latino; 2 Two or more races, non-Hispanic/Latino), 12 international. Average age 27. 38 applicants, 74% accepted, 23 enrolled. In 2013, 9 master's awarded. *Degree requirements:* For master's, thesis. *Entrance requirements:* For master's, GRE, transcripts, resume, statement of goals, letters of recommendation. Additional exam requirements/recommendations for international students: Required—TOEFL (minimum score 550 paper-based; 80 iBT). *Application deadline:* For fall admission, 5/1 for domestic and international students; for spring admission, 9/15 for domestic and international students. Application fee: $50. Electronic applications accepted. *Expenses: Tuition, area resident:* Full-time $4176; part-time $348 per credit hour. Tuition, state resident: full-time $14,544; part-time $1212 per credit hour. Tuition, nonresident: full-time $14,544; part-time $1212 per credit hour. Tuition and fees vary according to course load and program. *Financial support:* In 2013–14, research assistantships with full tuition reimbursements (averaging $2,000 per year), teaching assistantships with full tuition reimbursements (averaging $2,000 per year) were awarded; scholarships/grants and unspecified assistantships also available. Financial award application deadline: 6/1; financial award applicants required to submit FAFSA. *Faculty research:* Aerosol delivery methods, aerosol devices, smoking cessation, continuing and professional respiratory therapy education, chronic lung disease management. *Unit head:* Dr. Robert Harwood, Department Head, 404-413-1225, Fax: 404-413-1230. *Application contact:* Vanessa Thomas-Meikle, Academic Advisor, 404-413-1000, Fax: 404-413-1001, E-mail: vthomas@gsu.edu.
Website: http://respiratorytherapy.gsu.edu/

Grand Valley State University, College of Health Professions, Allendale, MI 49401-9403. Offers MPAS, MS, DPT. *Entrance requirements:* For master's, volunteer work, interview, minimum GPA of 3.0, writing sample; for doctorate, GRE, 50 hours of volunteer work, interview, minimum GPA of 3.0 in last 60 hours and in prerequisites, writing sample. Additional exam requirements/recommendations for international students: Required—TOEFL (minimum score 610 paper-based). Electronic applications accepted. *Faculty research:* Skeletal muscle structure, blood platelets, thrombospondin activity, FES exercise for quadriplegics, balance.

Harding University, College of Allied Health, Searcy, AR 72149-0001. Offers MS, DPT. *Faculty:* 24 full-time (13 women), 6 part-time/adjunct (4 women). *Students:* 220 full-time (147 women); includes 13 minority (3 Black or African American, non-Hispanic/Latino; 2 American Indian or Alaska Native, non-Hispanic/Latino; 1 Asian, non-Hispanic/Latino; 6 Hispanic/Latino; 1 Two or more races, non-Hispanic/Latino). Average age 27. 805 applicants, 13% accepted, 84 enrolled. In 2013, 49 master's awarded. *Expenses: Tuition:* Full-time $11,574; part-time $643 per credit hour. *Required fees:* $432; $24 per credit hour. Tuition and fees vary according to course load, degree level and program. *Financial support:* In 2013–14, 6 students received support. *Application contact:* Dr. Cheri Yecke, Dean of Graduate Programs, 501-279-4335, Fax: 501-279-5192, E-mail: cyecke@harding.edu.
Website: http://www.harding.edu/gradprogram/

Idaho State University, Office of Graduate Studies, Kasiska College of Health Professions, Pocatello, ID 83209-8090. Offers M Coun, MHE, MOT, MPAS, MPH, MS, Au D, DPT, PhD, Certificate, Ed S, Post-Doctoral Certificate, Post-Master's Certificate, Postbaccalaureate Certificate. *Accreditation:* APTA (one or more programs are accredited). Part-time programs available. *Degree requirements:* For master's, comprehensive exam, thesis (for some programs), 8-week externship; for doctorate, comprehensive exam, thesis/dissertation, clinical rotation (for some programs); for other advanced degree, comprehensive exam, thesis, case study, oral exam. *Entrance requirements:* For master's, GRE General Test or MAT, minimum GPA of 3.0, 3 letters of recommendation; for doctorate, GRE General Test or MAT, minimum GPA of 3.0, counseling license, professional research, interview, work experience, 3 letters of recommendation; for other advanced degree, GRE General Test or MAT, master's degree in similar field of study, 3 letters of recommendation, 2 years of work experience. Additional exam requirements/recommendations for international students: Required—TOEFL (minimum score 600 paper-based; 80 iBT). Electronic applications accepted. *Expenses:* Contact institution. *Faculty research:* Mental health, information technology, dental health, nursing.

Ithaca College, School of Health Sciences and Human Performance, Ithaca, NY 14850. Offers MS, DPT. Part-time programs available. *Faculty:* 53 full-time (35 women). *Students:* 302 full-time (244 women), 16 part-time (12 women); includes 38 minority (4 Black or African American, non-Hispanic/Latino; 6 Asian, non-Hispanic/Latino; 21 Hispanic/Latino; 7 Two or more races, non-Hispanic/Latino), 12 international. Average age 23. In 2013, 122 master's, 63 doctorates awarded. Terminal master's awarded for partial completion of doctoral program. *Degree requirements:* For master's, comprehensive exam (for some programs), thesis optional; for doctorate, thesis/dissertation optional. *Entrance requirements:* Additional exam requirements/recommendations for international students: Required—TOEFL (minimum score 550 paper-based; 80 iBT). *Application deadline:* Applications are processed on a rolling basis. Application fee: $40. Electronic applications accepted. *Expenses:* Contact institution. *Financial support:* In 2013–14, 223 students received support, including 72 teaching assistantships (averaging $10,565 per year); career-related internships or fieldwork, Federal Work-Study, scholarships/grants, and unspecified assistantships also available. Support available to part-time students. Financial award applicants required to submit CSS PROFILE or FAFSA. *Unit head:* Dr. Linda Petrosino, Dean, 607-274-3143, Fax: 607-274-1263, E-mail: gps@ithaca.edu. *Application contact:* Gerard Turbide, Director, Office of Admission, 607-274-3143, Fax: 607-274-1263, E-mail: gps@ithaca.edu.
Website: http://www.ithaca.edu/hshp

Loma Linda University, School of Allied Health Professions, Loma Linda, CA 92350. Offers MHIS, MOT, MPT, MS, D Sc, DPT, DPTSc, OTD. *Accreditation:* AOTA; APTA. *Entrance requirements:* For master's, minimum GPA of 2.0; for doctorate, minimum 2.0 GPA, associate degree in physical therapy. Additional exam requirements/recommendations for international students: Required—TOEFL (minimum score 550 paper-based). Electronic applications accepted.

Long Island University–LIU Post, School of Health Professions and Nursing, Brookville, NY 11548-1300. Offers MS, MSW, Certificate. Part-time and evening/weekend programs available. Postbaccalaureate distance learning degree programs offered. *Degree requirements:* For master's, thesis. Electronic applications accepted. *Faculty research:* PCR techniques, breast CA-mammography compliance, smoking patterns.

Marymount University, School of Health Professions, Arlington, VA 22207-4299. Offers MS, MSN, DNP, DPT, Certificate. Part-time and evening/weekend programs available. *Faculty:* 16 full-time (13 women), 4 part-time/adjunct (all women). *Students:* 123 full-time (91 women), 71 part-time (65 women); includes 59 minority (26 Black or African American, non-Hispanic/Latino; 2 American Indian or Alaska Native, non-Hispanic/Latino; 16 Asian, non-Hispanic/Latino; 10 Hispanic/Latino; 2 Native Hawaiian or other Pacific Islander, non-Hispanic/Latino; 3 Two or more races, non-Hispanic/Latino), 7 international. Average age 31. 686 applicants, 32% accepted, 61 enrolled. In 2013, 40 master's, 30 doctorates, 1 other advanced degree awarded. *Degree requirements:* For master's, thesis or alternative. *Entrance requirements:* For master's, GRE, MAT, 2 letters of recommendation, interview, resume; for doctorate, GRE, 2 letters of recommendation, resume; for Certificate, interview. Additional exam requirements/recommendations for international students: Required—TOEFL (minimum score 600 paper-based; 96 iBT), IELTS (minimum score 6.5). *Application deadline:* For fall admission, 7/1 for international students; for spring admission, 10/15 for international students. Applications are processed on a rolling basis. Application fee: $40. Electronic applications accepted. *Expenses: Tuition:* Part-time $850 per credit. *Required fees:* $10 per credit. One-time fee: $200 part-time. Tuition and fees vary according to program. *Financial support:* In 2013–14, 20 students received support, including 3 research assistantships with full and partial tuition reimbursements available, 7 teaching assistantships with full and partial tuition reimbursements available; career-related internships or fieldwork, Federal Work-Study, scholarships/grants, and unspecified assistantships also available. Support available to part-time students. Financial award applicants required to submit FAFSA. *Unit head:* Dr. Tess Cappello, Dean, 703-284-1580, Fax: 703-284-3819, E-mail: tess.cappello@marymount.edu. *Application contact:* Francesca Reed, Director, Graduate Admissions, 703-284-5901, Fax: 703-527-3815, E-mail: grad.admissions@marymount.edu.
Website: http://www.marymount.edu/academics/schools/shp

Maryville University of Saint Louis, College of Health Professions, St. Louis, MO 63141-7299. Offers MARC, MMT, MOT, MSN, DNP, DPT, CAGS. *Accreditation:* CORE. Part-time and evening/weekend programs available. *Faculty:* 29 full-time (22 women), 88 part-time/adjunct (80 women). *Students:* 129 full-time (104 women), 1,646 part-time (1,500 women); includes 373 minority (187 Black or African American, non-Hispanic/Latino; 17 American Indian or Alaska Native, non-Hispanic/Latino; 61 Asian, non-Hispanic/Latino; 73 Hispanic/Latino; 5 Native Hawaiian or other Pacific Islander, non-Hispanic/Latino; 30 Two or more races, non-Hispanic/Latino), 4 international. Average age 35. In 2013, 85 master's, 33 doctorates awarded. *Entrance requirements:* Additional exam requirements/recommendations for international students: Required—TOEFL (minimum score 550 paper-based). *Application deadline:* Applications are processed on a rolling basis. Application fee: $40 ($60 for international students). Electronic applications accepted. Application fee is waived when completed online. *Expenses: Tuition:* Full-time $23,812; part-time $728 per credit hour. *Required fees:* $395 per year. Tuition and fees vary according to course load, degree level and program. *Financial support:* Career-related internships or fieldwork, Federal Work-Study, and campus employment available. Financial award application deadline: 3/1; financial award applicants required to submit FAFSA. *Faculty research:* Disability work transition, assessment, reducing work-related musculoskeletal injuries, women's health/AIDS. *Unit head:* Dr. Charles Gulas, Dean, 314-529-9625, Fax: 314-529-9495, E-mail: hlthprofessions@maryville.edu. *Application contact:* Crystal Jacobsmeyer, Assistant Director, Graduate Enrollment Advising, 314-529-9654, Fax: 314-529-9927, E-mail: cjacobsmeyer@maryville.edu.
Website: http://www.maryville.edu/hp/

Medical University of South Carolina, College of Health Professions, Charleston, SC 29425. Offers MHA, MS, MSNA, MSOT, DHA, DPT, PhD. *Accreditation:* CAHME (one or more programs are accredited). Part-time programs available. *Degree requirements:* For doctorate, comprehensive exam, thesis/dissertation. *Entrance requirements:* For master's, GRE. Additional exam requirements/recommendations for international students: Required—TOEFL (minimum score 600 paper-based). Electronic applications accepted. *Expenses:* Contact institution. *Faculty research:* Spinal cord injury, geriatrics, rehabilitation sciences, behavioral medicine.

Mercy College, School of Health and Natural Sciences, Dobbs Ferry, NY 10522-1189. Offers communication disorders (MS); nursing (MS), including nursing administration, nursing education; occupational therapy (MS); physical therapy (DPT); physician assistant studies (MS). Part-time and evening/weekend programs available. Postbaccalaureate distance learning degree programs offered (minimal on-campus study). *Students:* 345 full-time (262 women), 245 part-time (211 women); includes 240 minority (105 Black or African American, non-Hispanic/Latino; 1 American Indian or Alaska Native, non-Hispanic/Latino; 70 Asian, non-Hispanic/Latino; 53 Hispanic/Latino; 6 Native Hawaiian or other Pacific Islander, non-Hispanic/Latino; 5 Two or more races, non-Hispanic/Latino), 10 international. Average age 33. 1,028 applicants, 20% accepted, 144 enrolled. In 2013, 145 master's, 24 doctorates awarded. *Degree requirements:* For master's, comprehensive exam (for some programs), thesis (for some programs). *Entrance requirements:* For master's and doctorate, essay, interview, resume, letters of recommendation, undergraduate transcripts. Additional exam requirements/recommendations for international students: Required—TOEFL (minimum score 600 paper-based; 79 iBT), IELTS (minimum score 8). *Application deadline:* For fall

admission, 8/1 for international students. Applications are processed on a rolling basis. Application fee: $40. Electronic applications accepted. *Expenses:* Contact institution. *Financial support:* Career-related internships or fieldwork, Federal Work-Study, scholarships/grants, and unspecified assistantships available. Support available to part-time students. Financial award applicants required to submit FAFSA. *Unit head:* Dr. Joan Toglia, Interim Dean, 914-674-7837, E-mail: jtoglia@mercy.edu. *Application contact:* Allison Gurdineer, Senior Director of Admissions, 877-637-2946, Fax: 914-674-7382, E-mail: admissions@mercy.edu.
Website: https://www.mercy.edu/academics/school-of-health-and-natural-sciences/

Midwestern University, Downers Grove Campus, College of Health Sciences, Illinois Campus, Doctor of Health Science Program, Downers Grove, IL 60515-1235. Offers DHS. Part-time programs available. *Entrance requirements:* For doctorate, master's or bachelor's degree, minimum cumulative GPA of 3.0.

Midwestern University, Glendale Campus, College of Health Sciences, Arizona Campus, Glendale, AZ 85308. Offers MA, MBS, MCVS, MMS, MOT, MS, DPM, DPT, Psy D. Part-time programs available. *Expenses:* Contact institution.

Minnesota State University Mankato, College of Graduate Studies and Research, College of Allied Health and Nursing, Mankato, MN 56001. Offers MA, MS, MSN, DNP, Postbaccalaureate Certificate. Part-time programs available. *Students:* 117 full-time (80 women), 128 part-time (98 women). *Degree requirements:* For master's, comprehensive exam; for Postbaccalaureate Certificate, thesis. *Entrance requirements:* For master's, GRE (for some programs), minimum GPA of 3.0 during previous 2 years; for Postbaccalaureate Certificate, GRE General Test, minimum GPA of 3.0. *Application deadline:* Applications are processed on a rolling basis. Application fee: $40. Electronic applications accepted. *Financial support:* Research assistantships with full tuition reimbursements, teaching assistantships with full tuition reimbursements, career-related internships or fieldwork, Federal Work-Study, institutionally sponsored loans, and unspecified assistantships available. Support available to part-time students. Financial award application deadline: 3/15; financial award applicants required to submit FAFSA. *Unit head:* Dr. Harry Krampf, Interim Dean, 507-389-6315. *Application contact:* 507-389-2321, E-mail: grad@mnsu.edu.
Website: http://ahn.mnsu.edu/

Misericordia University, College of Health Sciences, Dallas, PA 18612-1098. Offers MSN, MSOT, MSSLP, DPT, OTD. Part-time and evening/weekend programs available. *Faculty:* 24 full-time (17 women), 27 part-time/adjunct (21 women). *Students:* 206 full-time (153 women), 162 part-time (141 women); includes 24 minority (4 Black or African American, non-Hispanic/Latino; 1 American Indian or Alaska Native, non-Hispanic/Latino; 4 Asian, non-Hispanic/Latino; 11 Hispanic/Latino; 4 Two or more races, non-Hispanic/Latino), 3 international. Average age 28. In 2013, 100 master's, 26 doctorates awarded. *Entrance requirements:* For doctorate, interview, references. Additional exam requirements/recommendations for international students: Required—TOEFL. *Application deadline:* Applications are processed on a rolling basis. Application fee: $35. Electronic applications accepted. *Expenses: Tuition:* Full-time $14,450; part-time $680 per credit. Tuition and fees vary according to degree level. *Financial support:* In 2013–14, 237 students received support. Teaching assistantships, career-related internships or fieldwork, Federal Work-Study, scholarships/grants, traineeships, and tuition waivers (partial) available. Support available to part-time students. Financial award application deadline: 6/30; financial award applicants required to submit FAFSA. *Unit head:* Dr. Glen Tellis, Interim Dean of the College of Health Sciences, 570-674-6159, E-mail: gtellis@misericordia.edu. *Application contact:* Maureen Sheridan, Assistant Director of Admissions, Part-Time Undergraduate and Graduate Programs, 570-674-6451, Fax: 570-674-6232, E-mail: msherida@misericordia.edu.
Website: http://www.misericordia.edu/misericordia_pg.cfm?page_id=404&subcat_id=157

Moravian College, Moravian College Comenius Center, Business and Management Programs, Bethlehem, PA 18018-6650. Offers accounting (MBA); business analytics (MBA); general management (MBA); health administration (MHA); healthcare management (MBA); human resource management (MBA); leadership (MSHRM); learning and performance management (MSHRM); supply chain management (MBA). Part-time and evening/weekend programs available. *Entrance requirements:* For master's, GMAT. Additional exam requirements/recommendations for international students: Required—TOEFL (minimum score 550 paper-based; 90 iBT). Application fee is waived when completed online. *Expenses:* Contact institution. *Faculty research:* Leadership, change management, human resources.

New Jersey City University, Graduate Studies and Continuing Education, College of Professional Studies, Department of Health Sciences, Jersey City, NJ 07305-1597. Offers community health education (MS); health administration (MS); school health education (MS). Part-time and evening/weekend programs available. *Faculty:* 5 full-time (all women), 7 part-time/adjunct (2 women). *Students:* 10 full-time (7 women), 58 part-time (50 women); includes 32 minority (15 Black or African American, non-Hispanic/Latino; 7 Asian, non-Hispanic/Latino; 10 Hispanic/Latino), 2 international. Average age 40. In 2013, 18 master's awarded. *Degree requirements:* For master's, thesis or alternative, internship. *Entrance requirements:* Additional exam requirements/recommendations for international students: Required—TOEFL (minimum score 61 iBT). *Application deadline:* For fall admission, 8/1 priority date for domestic students; for spring admission, 12/1 for domestic students. Applications are processed on a rolling basis. Application fee: $0. *Expenses: Tuition, area resident:* Part-time $527.90 per credit. Tuition, nonresident: part-time $947.75 per credit. *Financial support:* Career-related internships or fieldwork and unspecified assistantships available. *Unit head:* Dr. Lilliam Rosado, Chairperson, 201-200-3431, E-mail: lrosado@njcu.edu. *Application contact:* Dr. William Bajor, Dean of Graduate Studies, 201-200-3409, Fax: 201-200-3411, E-mail: wbajor@njcu.edu.

Northeastern University, Bouvé College of Health Sciences, Boston, MA 02115-5096. Offers audiology (Au D); biotechnology (MS); counseling psychology (MS, PhD, CAGS); counseling/school psychology (PhD); exercise physiology (MS), including exercise physiology, public health; health informatics (MS); nursing (MS, PhD, CAGS), including acute care (MS), administration (MS), anesthesia (MS), primary care (MS), psychiatric mental health (MS); pharmaceutical sciences (PhD); pharmaceutics and drug delivery systems (MS); pharmacology (MS); physical therapy (DPT); physician assistant (MS); school psychology (PhD, CAGS); school/counseling psychology (PhD); speech language pathology (MS); urban public health (MPH); MS/MBA. *Accreditation:* ACPE (one or more programs are accredited). Part-time and evening/weekend programs available. *Degree requirements:* For doctorate, thesis/dissertation (for some programs); for CAGS, comprehensive exam.

Northern Arizona University, Graduate College, College of Health and Human Services, Flagstaff, AZ 86011. Offers MPAS, MS, MSN, DNP, DPT, Certificate. *Accreditation:* APTA (one or more programs are accredited). Part-time programs available. *Faculty:* 69 full-time (55 women), 21 part-time/adjunct (18 women). *Students:* 328 full-time (212 women), 217 part-time (196 women); includes 111 minority (4 Black or African American, non-Hispanic/Latino; 8 American Indian or Alaska Native, non-Hispanic/Latino; 19 Asian, non-Hispanic/Latino; 68 Hispanic/Latino; 1 Native Hawaiian or other Pacific Islander, non-Hispanic/Latino; 11 Two or more races, non-Hispanic/Latino), 3 international. Average age 32. 1,612 applicants, 12% accepted, 168 enrolled. In 2013, 98 master's, 47 doctorates, 5 other advanced degrees awarded. Application fee: $65. *Financial support:* In 2013–14, 3 research assistantships (averaging $9,100 per year) were awarded; tuition waivers (full and partial) also available. Financial award applicants required to submit FAFSA. *Unit head:* Leslie Schulz, Executive Dean, 928-523-4331, E-mail: leslie.schulz@nau.edu. *Application contact:* April Sandoval, Coordinator, 928-523-4348, Fax: 928-523-8950, E-mail: april.sandoval@nau.edu.
Website: http://nau.edu/chhs/

Nova Southeastern University, College of Health Care Sciences, Fort Lauderdale, FL 33314-7796. Offers audiology (Au D); health science (MH Sc, DHSc, PhD); occupational therapy (MOT, OTD, PhD); physical therapy (DPT, PhD, TDPT); physician assistant (MMS). Postbaccalaureate distance learning degree programs offered (minimal on-campus study). *Faculty:* 117 full-time (68 women), 110 part-time/adjunct (57 women). *Students:* 1,187 full-time (844 women), 509 part-time (340 women); includes 560 minority (184 Black or African American, non-Hispanic/Latino; 2 American Indian or Alaska Native, non-Hispanic/Latino; 120 Asian, non-Hispanic/Latino; 218 Hispanic/Latino; 36 Two or more races, non-Hispanic/Latino), 20 international. Average age 31. 5,996 applicants, 14% accepted, 548 enrolled. In 2013, 374 master's, 132 doctorates awarded. *Degree requirements:* For master's, thesis; for doctorate, comprehensive exam, thesis/dissertation. *Entrance requirements:* For master's and doctorate, GRE General Test. *Application deadline:* Applications are processed on a rolling basis. Application fee: $50. Electronic applications accepted. *Expenses:* Contact institution. *Financial support:* In 2013–14, 10 students received support, including 2 research assistantships (averaging $3,500 per year); institutionally sponsored loans and unspecified assistantships also available. *Unit head:* Dr. Stanley Wilson, Dean, 954-262-1203, E-mail: swilson@nova.edu. *Application contact:* Joey Jankie, Admissions Counselor, 954-262-7249, E-mail: joey@nova.edu.
Website: http://www.nova.edu/chcs/

Oakland University, Graduate Study and Lifelong Learning, School of Health Sciences, Rochester, MI 48309-4401. Offers MS, MSPT, DPT, Dr Sc PT, Certificate. *Accreditation:* APTA (one or more programs are accredited). *Faculty:* 17 full-time (12 women), 5 part-time/adjunct (2 women). *Students:* 179 full-time (118 women), 84 part-time (50 women); includes 26 minority (12 Black or African American, non-Hispanic/Latino; 1 American Indian or Alaska Native, non-Hispanic/Latino; 7 Asian, non-Hispanic/Latino; 5 Hispanic/Latino; 1 Two or more races, non-Hispanic/Latino), 8 international. Average age 27. 517 applicants, 17% accepted, 85 enrolled. In 2013, 12 master's, 38 doctorates, 28 other advanced degrees awarded. *Entrance requirements:* For master's, minimum GPA of 3.0; for doctorate, GRE General Test. Additional exam requirements/recommendations for international students: Required—TOEFL (minimum score 550 paper-based). *Application deadline:* For fall admission, 10/15 for domestic and international students. Applications are processed on a rolling basis. Application fee: $0. Electronic applications accepted. *Expenses:* Contact institution. *Financial support:* Fellowships, Federal Work-Study, institutionally sponsored loans, and tuition waivers (full) available. Financial award application deadline: 3/1; financial award applicants required to submit FAFSA. *Unit head:* Dr. Kenneth R. Hightower, Dean, 248-370-3562, Fax: 248-370-4227, E-mail: hightower@oakland.edu. *Application contact:* Christina J. Grabowski, Associate Director of Graduate Study and Lifelong Learning, 248-370-3167, Fax: 248-370-4114, E-mail: grabowsk@oakland.edu.

The Ohio State University, College of Medicine, School of Health and Rehabilitation Sciences, Program in Allied Health, Columbus, OH 43210. Offers MS. *Students:* 26 full-time (22 women), 12 part-time (all women); includes 3 minority (1 American Indian or Alaska Native, non-Hispanic/Latino; 1 Asian, non-Hispanic/Latino; 1 Two or more races, non-Hispanic/Latino), 1 international. Average age 27. In 2013, 22 master's awarded. *Application deadline:* Applications are processed on a rolling basis. Application fee: $60 ($70 for international students). Electronic applications accepted. *Unit head:* Dr. Kay Wolf, Graduate Studies Committee Chair, 614-292-8131, E-mail: wolf.4@osu.edu.

Old Dominion University, College of Health Sciences, Norfolk, VA 23529. Offers MS, MSN, DNP, DPT, PhD. Part-time and evening/weekend programs available. Postbaccalaureate distance learning degree programs offered (minimal on-campus study). *Students:* 260 full-time (202 women), 145 part-time (127 women); includes 85 minority (46 Black or African American, non-Hispanic/Latino; 18 Asian, non-Hispanic/Latino; 12 Hispanic/Latino; 9 Two or more races, non-Hispanic/Latino), 7 international. Average age 34. 1,263 applicants, 30% accepted, 296 enrolled. In 2013, 73 master's, 76 doctorates awarded. *Degree requirements:* For master's and doctorate, comprehensive exam. *Entrance requirements:* Additional exam requirements/recommendations for international students: Required—TOEFL. *Application deadline:* Applications are processed on a rolling basis. Application fee: $50. Electronic applications accepted. *Expenses:* Tuition, state resident: full-time $9888; part-time $412 per credit. Tuition, nonresident: full-time $25,152; part-time $1048 per credit. *Required fees:* $59 per semester. One-time fee: $50. *Financial support:* In 2013–14, 210 students received support, including 9 fellowships with full tuition reimbursements available (averaging $15,000 per year), 6 research assistantships with tuition reimbursements available (averaging $10,000 per year), 10 teaching assistantships with tuition reimbursements available (averaging $11,000 per year); career-related internships or fieldwork, institutionally sponsored loans, scholarships/grants, traineeships, tuition waivers (partial), and unspecified assistantships also available. Support available to part-time students. Financial award application deadline: 2/15; financial award applicants required to submit FAFSA. *Faculty research:* Health promotion and wellness, health care ethics, health policy, health services, cultural competency. *Total annual research expenditures:* $2.7 million. *Unit head:* Dr. Shelley Mishoe, Dean, 757-683-4960, Fax: 757-683-3674, E-mail: smishoe@odu.edu. *Application contact:* William Heffelfinger, Director of Graduate Admissions, 757-683-5554, Fax: 757-683-3255, E-mail: gradadmit@odu.edu.
Website: http://hs.odu.edu/

Oregon State University, Interdisciplinary/Institutional Programs, Program in Comparative Health Sciences, Corvallis, OR 97331. Offers MS, PhD. *Entrance requirements:* For master's and doctorate, GRE. Additional exam requirements/recommendations for international students: Required—TOEFL (minimum score 80 iBT), IELTS (minimum score 6.5). *Application deadline:* For fall admission, 6/1 for domestic students. Application fee: $60. *Expenses:* Tuition, state resident: full-time $11,664; part-time $432 per credit hour. Tuition, nonresident: full-time $19,197; part-time $711 per credit hour. *Required fees:* $1446; $443 per quarter. One-time fee: $300. Tuition and fees vary according to course load and program. *Unit head:* Dr. Luiz E. Bermudez, Department Head/Professor, 541-737-6538. *Application contact:* Beth Chamblin, 541-737-3206, E-mail: beth.chamblin@oregonstate.edu.

Purdue University, Graduate School, College of Health and Human Sciences, School of Health Sciences, West Lafayette, IN 47907. Offers health physics (MS, PhD); medical physics (MS, PhD); occupational and environmental health science (MS, PhD), including aerosol deposition and lung disease, ergonomics, exposure and risk assessment, indoor air quality and bioaerosols (PhD), liver/lung toxicology; radiation biology (PhD); toxicology (PhD); MS/PhD. Part-time programs available. *Faculty:* 11 full-time (5 women), 28 part-time/adjunct (5 women). *Students:* 28 full-time (8 women), 10 part-time (3 women); includes 6 minority (1 Black or African American, non-Hispanic/Latino; 3 Asian, non-Hispanic/Latino; 1 Hispanic/Latino; 1 Two or more races, non-Hispanic/

Latino), 10 international. Average age 28. 77 applicants, 42% accepted, 13 enrolled. In 2013, 6 master's, 6 doctorates awarded. *Degree requirements:* For master's, thesis optional; for doctorate, one foreign language, thesis/dissertation. *Entrance requirements:* For master's and doctorate, GRE General Test, minimum undergraduate GPA of 3.0 or equivalent. Additional exam requirements/recommendations for international students: Required—TOEFL (minimum score 550 paper-based; 77 iBT); Recommended—TWE. *Application deadline:* For fall admission, 5/15 for domestic and international students; for spring admission, 10/15 for domestic and international students. Applications are processed on a rolling basis. Application fee: $60 ($75 for international students). Electronic applications accepted. *Financial support:* In 2013–14, fellowships with tuition reimbursements (averaging $14,400 per year), research assistantships with tuition reimbursements (averaging $12,000 per year), teaching assistantships with tuition reimbursements (averaging $12,000 per year) were awarded; career-related internships or fieldwork and traineeships also available. Support available to part-time students. Financial award applicants required to submit FAFSA. *Faculty research:* Environmental toxicology, industrial hygiene, radiation dosimetry. *Unit head:* Dr. Wei Zheng, Head, 765-494-1419, E-mail: wz18@purdue.edu. *Application contact:* Jennifer S. Franklin, Graduate Contact, 765-494-0248, E-mail: jfranklin@purdue.edu.
Website: http://www.healthsciences.purdue.edu/

Quinnipiac University, School of Health Sciences, Hamden, CT 06518-1940. Offers MHS, MHS, MOT, DPT. *Accreditation:* AOTA. *Faculty:* 65 full-time (41 women), 94 part-time/adjunct (47 women). *Students:* 634 full-time (479 women), 51 part-time (29 women); includes 86 minority (20 Black or African American, non-Hispanic/Latino; 2 American Indian or Alaska Native, non-Hispanic/Latino; 39 Asian, non-Hispanic/Latino; 23 Hispanic/Latino; 2 Two or more races, non-Hispanic/Latino), 42 international. 2,016 applicants, 17% accepted, 271 enrolled. In 2013, 202 master's, 69 doctorates awarded. *Entrance requirements:* Additional exam requirements/recommendations for international students: Required—TOEFL (minimum score 575 paper-based; 90 iBT), IELTS (minimum score 6.5). *Application deadline:* For fall admission, 4/30 priority date for international students; for spring admission, 9/15 priority date for international students. Applications are processed on a rolling basis. Application fee: $45. Electronic applications accepted. *Expenses: Tuition:* Part-time $920 per credit. *Required fees:* $37 per credit. *Financial support:* In 2013–14, 359 students received support. Career-related internships or fieldwork, Federal Work-Study, scholarships/grants, and unspecified assistantships available. Support available to part-time students. Financial award application deadline: 4/15; financial award applicants required to submit FAFSA. *Application contact:* Office of Graduate Admissions, 800-462-1944, Fax: 203-582-3443, E-mail: graduate@quinnipiac.edu.
Website: http://www.quinnipiac.edu/gradprograms

Regis University, Rueckert-Hartman College for Health Professions, Denver, CO 80221-1099. Offers MA, MS, MSN, DNP, DPT, Pharm D, Post-Graduate Certificate, Postbaccalaureate Certificate. Part-time and evening/weekend programs available. Postbaccalaureate distance learning degree programs offered (no on-campus study). *Faculty:* 89 full-time (64 women), 88 part-time/adjunct (70 women). *Students:* 1,118 full-time (856 women), 285 part-time (249 women); includes 340 minority (60 Black or African American, non-Hispanic/Latino; 12 American Indian or Alaska Native, non-Hispanic/Latino; 104 Asian, non-Hispanic/Latino; 113 Hispanic/Latino; 2 Native Hawaiian or other Pacific Islander, non-Hispanic/Latino; 49 Two or more races, non-Hispanic/Latino), 8 international. Average age 44. 2,475 applicants, 41% accepted, 545 enrolled. In 2013, 250 master's, 197 doctorates awarded. *Degree requirements:* For master's, thesis (for some programs), internship. *Entrance requirements:* For master's, official transcript reflecting baccalaureate degree awarded from regionally-accredited college or university. Additional exam requirements/recommendations for international students: Required—TOEFL (minimum score 550 paper-based; 82 iBT). Application fee: $75. Electronic applications accepted. *Expenses:* Contact institution. *Financial support:* In 2013–14, 82 students received support. Federal Work-Study and scholarships/grants available. Financial award application deadline: 4/15; financial award applicants required to submit FAFSA. *Faculty research:* Normal and pathological balance and gait research, normal/pathological upper limb motor control/biomechanics, exercise energy/metabolism research, optical treatment protocols for therapeutic modalities. *Unit head:* Dr. Janet Houser, Academic Dean, 303-458-4174, E-mail: jhouser@regis.edu. *Application contact:* Sarah Engel, Director of Admissions, 303-458-4900, Fax: 303-964-5534, E-mail: regisadm@regis.edu.
Website: http://www.regis.edu/RHCHP.aspx

Rosalind Franklin University of Medicine and Science, College of Health Professions, North Chicago, IL 60064-3095. Offers MS, D Sc, DPT, PhD, TDPT, Certificate. Part-time programs available. Postbaccalaureate distance learning degree programs offered (minimal on-campus study). Terminal master's awarded for partial completion of doctoral program.

Rutgers, The State University of New Jersey, Newark, School of Health Related Professions, Newark, NJ 07102. Offers MS, DCN, DPT, PhD, Certificate, DMD/MS, MD/MS. *Accreditation:* APTA (one or more programs are accredited); NAACLS. Part-time programs available. *Degree requirements:* For master's, thesis (for some programs). *Entrance requirements:* Additional exam requirements/recommendations for international students: Required—TOEFL. Electronic applications accepted. *Expenses:* Contact institution. *Faculty research:* Clinical outcomes.

Saint Louis University, Graduate Education, Doisy College of Health Sciences, St. Louis, MO 63103-2097. Offers MAT, MMS, MOT, MS, MSN, DNP, DPT, PhD, Certificate. Part-time programs available. *Degree requirements:* For master's, comprehensive exam. *Entrance requirements:* Additional exam requirements/recommendations for international students: Required—TOEFL (minimum score 525 paper-based).

Sam Houston State University, College of Health Sciences, Huntsville, TX 77341. Offers MA. *Faculty:* 11 full-time (5 women). *Students:* 34 full-time (14 women), 29 part-time (19 women); includes 18 minority (10 Black or African American, non-Hispanic/Latino; 1 Asian, non-Hispanic/Latino; 7 Hispanic/Latino), 12 international. Average age 28. 48 applicants, 98% accepted, 23 enrolled. In 2013, 28 master's awarded. Application fee: $45 ($75 for international students). *Financial support:* In 2013–14, 1 research assistantship, 2 teaching assistantships were awarded. *Unit head:* Dr. Michael Lacourse, Dean, 936-294-2300, E-mail: mlacourse@shsu.edu. *Application contact:* Dr. Kandi Tayebi, Dean of Graduate Studies/Associate Vice President for Academic Affairs, 936-294-1971, Fax: 936-294-1271, E-mail: graduate@shsu.edu.
Website: http://www.shsu.edu/academics/health-sciences/

Seton Hall University, School of Health and Medical Sciences, Program in Health Sciences, South Orange, NJ 07079-2697. Offers PhD. Part-time and evening/weekend programs available. *Degree requirements:* For doctorate, comprehensive exam (for some programs), thesis/dissertation, candidacy exam, practicum, research projects. *Entrance requirements:* For doctorate, GRE (preferred), interview, minimum GPA of 3.0, letters of recommendation. Additional exam requirements/recommendations for international students: Required—TOEFL. Electronic applications accepted. *Faculty research:* Movement science, motor learning, dual tasks, clinical decision making, online education, teaching strategies.

Shenandoah University, School of Health Professions, Winchester, VA 22601-5195. Offers MS, MSN, DNP, DPT, Certificate. Part-time programs available. Postbaccalaureate distance learning degree programs offered. *Faculty:* 25 full-time (22 women), 14 part-time/adjunct (9 women). *Students:* 323 full-time (254 women), 124 part-time (96 women); includes 66 minority (14 Black or African American, non-Hispanic/Latino; 2 American Indian or Alaska Native, non-Hispanic/Latino; 27 Asian, non-Hispanic/Latino; 22 Hispanic/Latino; 1 Two or more races, non-Hispanic/Latino), 6 international. Average age 29. 1,747 applicants, 14% accepted, 137 enrolled. In 2013, 64 master's, 94 doctorates, 1 other advanced degree awarded. *Entrance requirements:* For master's, GRE, college transcripts; thorough background in sciences, humanities and mathematics; for doctorate, GRE, PCAT. Additional exam requirements/recommendations for international students: Required—TOEFL (minimum score 550 paper-based; 79 iBT), IELTS (minimum score 6.5), Sakae Institute of Study Abroad (SISA) test (minimum score 15). *Application deadline:* For fall admission, 7/31 for domestic and international students; for summer admission, 1/15 for domestic and international students. Application fee: $30. Electronic applications accepted. *Expenses: Tuition:* Full-time $19,176; part-time $799 per credit. *Required fees:* $365 per term. Tuition and fees vary according to course level, course load and program. *Financial support:* In 2013–14, 48 students received support, including 3 teaching assistantships with partial tuition reimbursements available (averaging $4,912 per year); career-related internships or fieldwork, scholarships/grants, and unspecified assistantships also available. Support available to part-time students. Financial award application deadline: 3/15; financial award applicants required to submit FAFSA. *Application contact:* Andrew Woodall, Executive Director of Recruitment and Admissions, 540-665-4581, Fax: 540-665-4627, E-mail: admit@su.edu.
Website: http://www.health.su.edu/

South Carolina State University, School of Graduate and Professional Studies, Department of Health Sciences, Orangeburg, SC 29117-0001. Offers speech pathology and audiology (MA). *Accreditation:* ASHA. Part-time and evening/weekend programs available. *Faculty:* 7 full-time (5 women). *Students:* 48 full-time (45 women), 47 part-time (46 women); includes 50 minority (49 Black or African American, non-Hispanic/Latino; 1 Asian, non-Hispanic/Latino), 1 international. Average age 27. 103 applicants, 46% accepted, 38 enrolled. In 2013, 34 master's awarded. *Degree requirements:* For master's, thesis optional, departmental qualifying exam. *Entrance requirements:* For master's, GRE or NTE, minimum GPA of 3.0. *Application deadline:* For fall admission, 6/15 for domestic and international students; for spring admission, 11/1 for domestic and international students. Application fee: $25. Electronic applications accepted. *Expenses:* Tuition, state resident: full-time $8906; part-time $543 per credit hour. Tuition, nonresident: full-time $18,040; part-time $1051 per credit hour. *Financial support:* Fellowships, career-related internships or fieldwork, Federal Work-Study, and institutionally sponsored loans available. Financial award application deadline: 6/1. *Unit head:* Dr. Cecelia Jeffries, Interim Chair, 803-536-8074, Fax: 803-536-8593, E-mail: cjeffrie@scsu.edu. *Application contact:* Curtis Foskey, Coordinator of Graduate Admission, 803-536-8419, Fax: 803-536-8812, E-mail: cfoskey@scsu.edu.

Southwestern Oklahoma State University, College of Professional and Graduate Studies, School of Behavioral Sciences and Education, Specialization in Health Sciences and Microbiology, Weatherford, OK 73096-3098. Offers M Ed.

Temple University, College of Health Professions and Social Work, Philadelphia, PA 19140. Offers Ed M, MA, MOT, MPH, MS, MSN, MSW, DNP, DOT, DPT, PhD. *Accreditation:* APTA (one or more programs are accredited). Part-time and evening/weekend programs available. Postbaccalaureate distance learning degree programs offered (minimal on-campus study). *Faculty:* 133 full-time (86 women), 3 part-time/adjunct (all women). *Students:* 770 full-time (615 women), 486 part-time (388 women); includes 368 minority (201 Black or African American, non-Hispanic/Latino; 1 American Indian or Alaska Native, non-Hispanic/Latino; 69 Asian, non-Hispanic/Latino; 69 Hispanic/Latino; 2 Native Hawaiian or other Pacific Islander, non-Hispanic/Latino; 26 Two or more races, non-Hispanic/Latino), 24 international. 1,701 applicants, 23% accepted, 322 enrolled. In 2013, 502 master's, 258 doctorates awarded. *Degree requirements:* For doctorate, thesis/dissertation. *Entrance requirements:* Additional exam requirements/recommendations for international students: Required—TOEFL (minimum score 550 paper-based; 79 iBT). Application fee: $60. *Financial support:* Fellowships, research assistantships, teaching assistantships with full tuition reimbursements, career-related internships or fieldwork, Federal Work-Study, institutionally sponsored loans, traineeships, and tuition waivers (partial) available. Support available to part-time students. Financial award application deadline: 1/15. *Total annual research expenditures:* $10.1 million. *Unit head:* Dr. Laura Siminoff, Dean, 215-707-4802, Fax: 215-707-7819.
Website: http://chpsw.temple.edu/

Tennessee State University, The School of Graduate Studies and Research, College of Health Sciences, Nashville, TN 37209-1561. Offers MOT, MPH, MS, DPT. *Accreditation:* ASHA (one or more programs are accredited). Part-time and evening/weekend programs available. *Entrance requirements:* For master's, GRE General Test, MAT, minimum GPA of 3.5. Electronic applications accepted. *Faculty research:* Community problems of the elderly, language disorders in children, aphasia, sickle cell disturbances, regional and foreign dialects.

Texas Christian University, Harris College of Nursing and Health Sciences, Fort Worth, TX 76129-0002. Offers MS, MSN, MSNA, DNP, DNP-A. Postbaccalaureate distance learning degree programs offered. *Faculty:* 39 full-time (27 women), 2 part-time/adjunct (both women). *Students:* Average age 33. 417 applicants, 23% accepted, 68 enrolled. *Degree requirements:* For master's and doctorate, professional project. *Entrance requirements:* For master's, GRE General Test, 3 letters of reference; for doctorate, APRN recognition (national certification) or master's and experience in nursing administration. Additional exam requirements/recommendations for international students: Required—TOEFL. *Application deadline:* For fall admission, 11/15 for domestic students; for winter admission, 7/4 for domestic students. Application fee: $60. *Expenses: Tuition:* Part-time $1270 per credit hour. Tuition and fees vary according to course load and program. *Financial support:* Teaching assistantships available. Financial award applicants required to submit FAFSA. *Unit head:* Dr. Paulette Burns, Dean, 817-257-6742, Fax: 817-257-6751, E-mail: p.burns@tcu.edu. *Application contact:* Sybil White, Assistant to the Dean of Graduate Studies, 817-257-6750, Fax: 817-257-6751, E-mail: s.white@tcu.edu.
Website: http://www.harriscollege.tcu.edu/

Texas State University, Graduate School, College of Health Professions, San Marcos, TX 78666. Offers MA, MHA, MS, MSCD, DPT. Part-time and evening/weekend programs available. *Faculty:* 37 full-time (21 women), 6 part-time/adjunct (0 women). *Students:* 248 full-time (170 women), 19 part-time (14 women); includes 102 minority (14 Black or African American, non-Hispanic/Latino; 1 American Indian or Alaska Native, non-Hispanic/Latino; 14 Asian, non-Hispanic/Latino; 64 Hispanic/Latino; 9 Two or more races, non-Hispanic/Latino), 4 international. Average age 28. 738 applicants, 16% accepted, 85 enrolled. In 2013, 62 master's awarded. *Degree requirements:* For master's, comprehensive exam. *Entrance requirements:* For master's, GRE General Test (for some programs); for doctorate, GRE (minimum score of 1000 Verbal and Quantitative), bachelor's degree in physical therapy. Additional exam requirements/

recommendations for international students: Required—TOEFL (minimum score 550 paper-based; 78 iBT). *Application deadline:* For fall admission, 6/15 for domestic students, 6/1 for international students; for spring admission, 10/15 priority date for domestic students, 10/1 for international students. Applications are processed on a rolling basis. Application fee: $40 ($90 for international students). Electronic applications accepted. *Expenses:* Tuition, state resident: full-time $6663; part-time $278 per credit hour. Tuition, nonresident: full-time $15,159; part-time $632 per credit hour. *Required fees:* $1872; $54 per credit hour. $306 per term. Tuition and fees vary according to course load. *Financial support:* In 2013–14, 78 students received support, including 7 research assistantships (averaging $7,199 per year), 25 teaching assistantships (averaging $7,887 per year); fellowships, career-related internships or fieldwork, Federal Work-Study, institutionally sponsored loans, scholarships/grants, unspecified assistantships, and stipends also available. Support available to part-time students. Financial award application deadline: 4/1; financial award applicants required to submit FAFSA. *Faculty research:* Health information, health information technology, cognitive impairment, hand-held cell phone use. *Total annual research expenditures:* $2.4 million. *Unit head:* Dr. Ruth Welborn, Dean, 512-245-3300, Fax: 512-245-3791, E-mail: mw01@txstate.edu. *Application contact:* Dr. Andrea Golato, Dean of Graduate School, 512-245-2581, Fax: 512-245-8365, E-mail: gradcollege@txstate.edu.
Website: http://www.health.txstate.edu/

Texas Tech University Health Sciences Center, School of Allied Health Sciences, Lubbock, TX 79430. Offers MAT, MOT, MPAS, MRC, MS, Au D, DPT, PhD, Sc D, TDPT. *Accreditation:* APTA (one or more programs are accredited). *Faculty:* 68 full-time (26 women), 2 part-time/adjunct (0 women). *Students:* 658 full-time (470 women), 337 part-time (214 women); includes 325 minority (70 Black or African American, non-Hispanic/Latino; 12 American Indian or Alaska Native, non-Hispanic/Latino; 77 Asian, non-Hispanic/Latino; 121 Hispanic/Latino; 3 Native Hawaiian or other Pacific Islander, non-Hispanic/Latino; 42 Two or more races, non-Hispanic/Latino), 6 international. Average age 30. 2,670 applicants, 17% accepted, 464 enrolled. In 2013, 254 master's, 130 doctorates awarded. *Entrance requirements:* Additional exam requirements/recommendations for international students: Required—TOEFL (minimum score 550 paper-based), IELTS. *Application deadline:* Applications are processed on a rolling basis. Application fee: $40. Electronic applications accepted. *Financial support:* Fellowships, research assistantships, teaching assistantships, institutionally sponsored loans, and scholarships/grants available. Financial award application deadline: 9/1; financial award applicants required to submit FAFSA. *Unit head:* Lindsay R. Johnson, Associate Dean for Admissions and Student Affairs, 806-743-3220, Fax: 806-743-2994, E-mail: lindsay.johnson@ttuhsc.edu. *Application contact:* Lindsay Johnson, Associate Dean for Admissions and Student Affairs, 806-743-3220, Fax: 806-743-2994, E-mail: lindsay.johnson@ttuhsc.edu.
Website: http://www.ttuhsc.edu/sah/

Texas Woman's University, Graduate School, College of Health Sciences, Denton, TX 76201. Offers MA, MHA, MOT, MS, DPT, Ed D, PhD. Part-time and evening/weekend programs available. Postbaccalaureate distance learning degree programs offered. *Faculty:* 100 full-time (77 women), 28 part-time/adjunct (20 women). *Students:* 1,056 full-time (919 women), 464 part-time (382 women); includes 488 minority (136 Black or African American, non-Hispanic/Latino; 17 American Indian or Alaska Native, non-Hispanic/Latino; 127 Asian, non-Hispanic/Latino; 207 Hispanic/Latino; 1 Native Hawaiian or other Pacific Islander, non-Hispanic/Latino), 42 international. Average age 30. 1,629 applicants, 28% accepted, 332 enrolled. In 2013, 407 master's, 115 doctorates awarded. Terminal master's awarded for partial completion of doctoral program. *Degree requirements:* For master's, comprehensive exam (for some programs), thesis (for some programs); for doctorate, comprehensive exam, thesis/dissertation, qualifying exam. *Entrance requirements:* For master's and doctorate, minimum GPA of 3.0. Additional exam requirements/recommendations for international students: Required—TOEFL (minimum score 550 paper-based; 79 iBT). *Application deadline:* For fall admission, 7/1 priority date for domestic students, 3/1 for international students; for spring admission, 12/1 priority date for domestic students, 7/1 for international students. Applications are processed on a rolling basis. Application fee: $50 ($75 for international students). Electronic applications accepted. *Expenses:* Tuition, state resident: full-time $4182; part-time $233.32 per credit hour. Tuition, nonresident: full-time $10,716; part-time $595.32 per credit hour. *Financial support:* In 2013–14, 747 students received support, including 59 research assistantships (averaging $11,499 per year), 15 teaching assistantships (averaging $11,499 per year); career-related internships or fieldwork, Federal Work-Study, institutionally sponsored loans, scholarships/grants, traineeships, health care benefits, and unspecified assistantships also available. Support available to part-time students. Financial award application deadline: 3/1; financial award applicants required to submit FAFSA. *Total annual research expenditures:* $690,244. *Unit head:* Dr. Jimmy Ishee, Dean, 940-898-2852, Fax: 940-898-2853, E-mail: jishee@twu.edu. *Application contact:* Dr. Samuel Wheeler, Assistant Director of Admissions, 940-898-3188, Fax: 940-898-3081, E-mail: wheelersr@twu.edu.
Website: http://www.twu.edu/college-health-sciences/

Towson University, Program in Health Science, Towson, MD 21252-0001. Offers MS. Part-time and evening/weekend programs available. *Students:* 25 full-time (21 women), 104 part-time (83 women); includes 64 minority (54 Black or African American, non-Hispanic/Latino; 1 American Indian or Alaska Native, non-Hispanic/Latino; 3 Asian, non-Hispanic/Latino; 2 Hispanic/Latino; 4 Two or more races, non-Hispanic/Latino), 9 international. *Degree requirements:* For master's, thesis optional. *Entrance requirements:* For master's, undergraduate degree in a health science field or substantial upper-division course work in those fields, or experience in those same areas; minimum B grade in previous statistics course; minimum GPA of 3.0. *Application deadline:* Applications are processed on a rolling basis. Application fee: $45. Electronic applications accepted. *Financial support:* Application deadline: 4/1. *Unit head:* Dr. Susan Radius, Graduate Program Director, 410-704-4216, E-mail: sradius@towson.edu. *Application contact:* Alicia Arkell-Kleis, Information Contact, 410-704-6004, E-mail: grads@towson.edu.
Website: http://grad.towson.edu/program/master/hlth-ms/

University at Buffalo, the State University of New York, Graduate School, School of Public Health and Health Professions, Buffalo, NY 14260. Offers MA, MPH, MS, DPT, PhD, Advanced Certificate, Certificate. Part-time programs available. *Faculty:* 60 full-time (27 women), 12 part-time/adjunct (5 women). *Students:* 440 full-time (277 women), 31 part-time (19 women); includes 63 minority (16 Black or African American, non-Hispanic/Latino; 1 American Indian or Alaska Native, non-Hispanic/Latino; 41 Asian, non-Hispanic/Latino; 4 Hispanic/Latino; 1 Native Hawaiian or other Pacific Islander, non-Hispanic/Latino), 67 international. Average age 27. 745 applicants, 51% accepted, 189 enrolled. In 2013, 122 master's, 53 doctorates, 20 other advanced degrees awarded. Terminal master's awarded for partial completion of doctoral program. *Degree requirements:* For master's, comprehensive exam (for some programs), thesis (for some programs); for doctorate, comprehensive exam, thesis/dissertation. *Entrance requirements:* For master's and doctorate, GRE General Test. Additional exam requirements/recommendations for international students: Required—TOEFL (minimum score 79 iBT). *Application deadline:* For fall admission, 2/1 priority date for domestic and international students. Application fee: $50. Electronic applications accepted. *Financial support:* In 2013–14, 47 students received support, including 8 fellowships with full tuition reimbursements available (averaging $2,500 per year), 15 research assistantships with full tuition reimbursements available (averaging $15,000 per year), 16 teaching assistantships with full tuition reimbursements available (averaging $8,500 per year); career-related internships or fieldwork, Federal Work-Study, institutionally sponsored loans, scholarships/grants, tuition waivers (full and partial), and unspecified assistantships also available. Financial award application deadline: 3/15; financial award applicants required to submit FAFSA. *Faculty research:* Public health, epidemiology, rehabilitation, assistive technology, exercise and nutrition science. *Total annual research expenditures:* $6 million. *Unit head:* Dr. Lynn Kozlowski, Dean, 716-829-6951, Fax: 716-829-6040, E-mail: lk22@buffalo.edu. *Application contact:* Cassandra Walker-Whiteside, Office of Academic and Student Affairs, 716-829-6769, Fax: 716-829-2034, E-mail: phhp.mph@buffalo.edu.
Website: http://sphhp.buffalo.edu/

The University of Alabama at Birmingham, School of Health Professions, Birmingham, AL 35294. Offers MS, MSHA, MSHI, MSPAS, D Sc, DPT, PhD. *Accreditation:* AANA/CANAEP (one or more programs are accredited); APTA (one or more programs are accredited); CAHME (one or more programs are accredited). Part-time programs available. *Degree requirements:* For doctorate, thesis/dissertation. Electronic applications accepted. *Expenses:* Contact institution.

University of Arkansas at Little Rock, Graduate School, College of Professional Studies, Department of Health Sciences, Little Rock, AR 72204-1099. Offers MS. Part-time and evening/weekend programs available. *Degree requirements:* For master's, directed study or residency. *Entrance requirements:* For master's, GMAT or GRE General Test, interview, minimum GPA of 2.75. *Expenses:* Tuition, state resident: full-time $5690; part-time $284.50 per credit hour. Tuition, nonresident: full-time $13,030; part-time $651.50 per credit hour. *Required fees:* $1121; $672 per term. One-time fee: $40 full-time.

University of Connecticut, Graduate School, College of Agriculture and Natural Resources, Department of Allied Health Sciences, Storrs, CT 06269. Offers MS. *Accreditation:* APTA. *Degree requirements:* For master's, comprehensive exam. *Entrance requirements:* For master's, GRE General Test. Additional exam requirements/recommendations for international students: Required—TOEFL (minimum score 550 paper-based). Electronic applications accepted.

University of Detroit Mercy, College of Health Professions, Detroit, MI 48221. Offers MHSA, MS, MSN, Certificate. *Entrance requirements:* For master's, GRE General Test, minimum GPA of 3.0. *Faculty research:* Research design, respiratory physiology, AIDS prevention, adolescent health, community, low income health education.

University of Florida, Graduate School, College of Public Health and Health Professions, Gainesville, FL 32611. Offers MA, MHA, MHS, MHS, MOT, MPH, MS, Au D, DPT, PhD, Certificate, DPT/MPH, DVM/MPH, JD/MPH, MBA/MHA, MD/MPH, PhD/MPH, Pharm D/MPH. *Accreditation:* CAHME (one or more programs are accredited). Part-time programs available. *Faculty:* 91 full-time (48 women), 78 part-time/adjunct (46 women). *Students:* 620 full-time (465 women), 160 part-time (114 women); includes 194 minority (55 Black or African American, non-Hispanic/Latino; 5 American Indian or Alaska Native, non-Hispanic/Latino; 50 Asian, non-Hispanic/Latino; 84 Hispanic/Latino), 105 international. Average age 29. 1,519 applicants, 25% accepted, 193 enrolled. In 2013, 200 master's, 31 doctorates, 50 other advanced degrees awarded. Terminal master's awarded for partial completion of doctoral program. *Degree requirements:* For master's, thesis (for some programs); for doctorate, comprehensive exam, thesis/dissertation. *Entrance requirements:* For master's and doctorate, GRE General Test, minimum GPA of 3.0. Additional exam requirements/recommendations for international students: Required—TOEFL (minimum score 550 paper-based; 80 iBT), IELTS (minimum score 6). *Application deadline:* Applications are processed on a rolling basis. Application fee: $30. Electronic applications accepted. *Expenses:* Tuition, state resident: full-time $12,640. Tuition, nonresident: full-time $30,000. *Financial support:* In 2013–14, 195 students received support, including 27 fellowships (averaging $15,980 per year), 99 research assistantships (averaging $15,200 per year), 91 teaching assistantships (averaging $13,705 per year); career-related internships or fieldwork, Federal Work-Study, institutionally sponsored loans, and unspecified assistantships also available. Support available to part-time students. Financial award applicants required to submit FAFSA. *Unit head:* Dr. Michael G. Perri, Dean, 352-273-6214, Fax: 352-273-6199, E-mail: mperri@phhp.ufl.edu. *Application contact:* Office of Admissions, 352-392-1365, E-mail: webrequests@admissions.ufl.edu.
Website: http://www.phhp.ufl.edu/

University of Illinois at Chicago, Graduate College, College of Applied Health Sciences, Chicago, IL 60607-7128. Offers MS, DPT, OTD, PhD, CAS, Certificate. *Accreditation:* AOTA. Part-time programs available. *Faculty:* 80 full-time (48 women), 65 part-time/adjunct (43 women). *Students:* 471 full-time (361 women), 538 part-time (385 women); includes 348 minority (120 Black or African American, non-Hispanic/Latino; 2 American Indian or Alaska Native, non-Hispanic/Latino; 132 Asian, non-Hispanic/Latino; 60 Hispanic/Latino; 7 Native Hawaiian or other Pacific Islander, non-Hispanic/Latino; 27 Two or more races, non-Hispanic/Latino), 56 international. Average age 35. 977 applicants, 37% accepted, 287 enrolled. In 2013, 188 master's, 62 doctorates, 30 other advanced degrees awarded. *Degree requirements:* For doctorate, thesis/dissertation. *Entrance requirements:* For master's, GRE General Test, minimum GPA of 2.75. Additional exam requirements/recommendations for international students: Required—TOEFL. *Application deadline:* For fall admission, 3/15 for domestic students, 2/15 for international students; for spring admission, 11/1 for domestic students. Applications are processed on a rolling basis. Application fee: $40 ($50 for international students). Electronic applications accepted. *Expenses:* Tuition, state resident: full-time $11,066; part-time $3689 per term. Tuition, nonresident: full-time $23,064; part-time $7688 per term. *Required fees:* $3004; $1190 per term. Tuition and fees vary according to course level and program. *Financial support:* In 2013–14, 2 fellowships with full tuition reimbursements were awarded; research assistantships with full tuition reimbursements, teaching assistantships with full tuition reimbursements, career-related internships or fieldwork, Federal Work-Study, institutionally sponsored loans, traineeships, tuition waivers (full and partial), and unspecified assistantships also available. Financial award application deadline: 3/1; financial award applicants required to submit FAFSA. *Faculty research:* Care of the elderly, nutritional status for various diseases, immunohematology, computer-aided graphics. *Total annual research expenditures:* $13.1 million. *Unit head:* Bo Fernhall, Dean, 312-996-6695, E-mail: fernhall@uic.edu. *Application contact:* Receptionist, 312-413-2550, E-mail: gradcoll@uic.edu.
Website: http://www.ahs.uic.edu/

The University of Kansas, University of Kansas Medical Center, School of Health Professions, Kansas City, KS 66160. Offers MOT, MS, Au D, DNP, DPT, OTD, PhD, Graduate Certificate. *Faculty:* 120. *Students:* 347 full-time (267 women), 68 part-time (58 women); includes 33 minority (12 Black or African American, non-Hispanic/Latino; 1 American Indian or Alaska Native, non-Hispanic/Latino; 7 Asian, non-Hispanic/Latino; 8 Hispanic/Latino; 5 Two or more races, non-Hispanic/Latino), 27 international. Average age 28. 695 applicants, 29% accepted, 155 enrolled. In 2013, 76 master's, 58 doctorates, 16 other advanced degrees awarded. *Total annual research expenditures:* $2.2 million. *Unit head:* Dr. Karen L. Miller, Dean, 913-588-5235, Fax: 913-588-5254,

E-mail: kmiller@kumc.edu. *Application contact:* Moffett Ferguson, Student Affairs Coordinator, 913-588-5275, Fax: 913-588-5254, E-mail: mfergus1@kumc.edu.
Website: http://www.kumc.edu/school-of-health-professions.html

University of Kentucky, Graduate School, College of Health Sciences, Lexington, KY 40506-0032. Offers MS, MSCD, MSHP, MSPAS, MSPT, MSRMP, DS, PhD. Part-time programs available. *Degree requirements:* For master's, comprehensive exam, thesis (for some programs). *Entrance requirements:* For master's, GRE General Test, minimum undergraduate GPA of 2.75; for doctorate, GRE General Test, minimum undergraduate GPA of 3.0. Additional exam requirements/recommendations for international students: Required—TOEFL (minimum score 550 paper-based). Electronic applications accepted.

University of Massachusetts Lowell, College of Health Sciences, Lowell, MA 01854-2881. Offers MS, DPT, PhD, Sc D, Certificate, Graduate Certificate. *Accreditation:* APTA (one or more programs are accredited). Part-time programs available. *Degree requirements:* For master's, thesis optional; for doctorate, thesis/dissertation. *Entrance requirements:* For master's and doctorate, GRE General Test.

University of Mississippi Medical Center, School of Health Related Professions, Jackson, MS 39216-4505. Offers MOT, MPT. *Accreditation:* AOTA; NAACLS. Part-time programs available.

University of Nebraska Medical Center, School of Allied Health Professions, Omaha, NE 68198-4000. Offers MPAS, MPS, DPT, Certificate. *Accreditation:* APTA (one or more programs are accredited). *Entrance requirements:* For master's and doctorate, GRE. Additional exam requirements/recommendations for international students: Required—TOEFL. *Expenses: Required fees:* $300 per semester. Tuition and fees vary according to program.

University of Nevada, Las Vegas, Graduate College, School of Allied Health Sciences, Las Vegas, NV 89154-3018. Offers MS, DPT, PhD. Part-time programs available. *Faculty:* 18 full-time (5 women), 4 part-time/adjunct (all women). *Students:* 137 full-time (66 women), 19 part-time (9 women); includes 38 minority (2 Black or African American, non-Hispanic/Latino; 10 Asian, non-Hispanic/Latino; 11 Hispanic/Latino; 15 Two or more races, non-Hispanic/Latino), 3 international. Average age 28. 63 applicants, 75% accepted, 24 enrolled. In 2013, 20 master's, 28 doctorates awarded. *Degree requirements:* For master's, thesis optional. *Entrance requirements:* Additional exam requirements/recommendations for international students: Required—TOEFL (minimum score 550 paper-based; 80 iBT), IELTS (minimum score 7). *Application deadline:* For fall admission, 5/1 for international students; for spring admission, 10/1 for international students. Application fee: $60 ($95 for international students). Electronic applications accepted. *Expenses:* Tuition, state resident: full-time $4752; part-time $264 per credit. Tuition, nonresident: full-time $18,662; part-time $554.50 per credit. *International tuition:* $18,952 full-time. *Required fees:* $532; $12 per credit. $266 per semester. One-time fee: $35. Tuition and fees vary according to course load and program. *Financial support:* In 2013–14, 47 students received support, including 20 research assistantships with partial tuition reimbursements available (averaging $11,129 per year), 27 teaching assistantships with partial tuition reimbursements available (averaging $9,205 per year); institutionally sponsored loans, scholarships/grants, health care benefits, and unspecified assistantships also available. Financial award application deadline: 3/1. *Total annual research expenditures:* $727,053. *Unit head:* Dr. Carolyn Yucha, Interim Dean, 702-895-3906, Fax: 702-895-5050, E-mail: carolyn.yucha@unlv.edu. *Application contact:* Graduate College Admissions Evaluator, 702-895-3320, Fax: 702-895-4180, E-mail: gradcollege@unlv.edu.
Website: http://healthsciences.unlv.edu/

The University of North Carolina at Chapel Hill, School of Medicine and Graduate School, Graduate Programs in Medicine, Department of Allied Health Sciences, Chapel Hill, NC 27599. Offers human movement science (PhD); occupational science (MS, PhD), including occupational science; physical therapy (DPT), including physical therapy - off campus, physical therapy - on campus; rehabilitation counseling and psychology (MS); speech and hearing sciences (MS, Au D, PhD), including audiology (Au D), speech and hearing sciences (MS, PhD). *Accreditation:* APTA (one or more programs are accredited). Postbaccalaureate distance learning degree programs offered. *Entrance requirements:* For master's, GRE General Test; for doctorate, GRE General Test, minimum GPA of 3.0. Additional exam requirements/recommendations for international students: Required—TOEFL (minimum score 550 paper-based), TWE. Electronic applications accepted.

University of North Florida, Brooks College of Health, Jacksonville, FL 32224. Offers MHA, MPH, MS, MSH, MSN, DNP, DPT, Certificate. Part-time and evening/weekend programs available. *Faculty:* 67 full-time (47 women), 9 part-time/adjunct (4 women). *Students:* 332 full-time (229 women), 153 part-time (115 women); includes 118 minority (38 Black or African American, non-Hispanic/Latino; 3 American Indian or Alaska Native, non-Hispanic/Latino; 18 Asian, non-Hispanic/Latino; 47 Hispanic/Latino; 12 Two or more races, non-Hispanic/Latino), 9 international. Average age 30. 492 applicants, 43% accepted, 138 enrolled. In 2013, 116 master's, 31 doctorates awarded. *Entrance requirements:* For master's, GRE General Test, minimum GPA of 3.0 in last 60 hours. Additional exam requirements/recommendations for international students: Required—TOEFL (minimum score 500 paper-based; 61 iBT). *Application deadline:* For fall admission, 7/1 priority date for domestic students, 5/1 for international students; for spring admission, 11/1 priority date for domestic students, 10/1 for international students. Applications are processed on a rolling basis. Application fee: $30. Electronic applications accepted. *Expenses:* Contact institution. *Financial support:* In 2013–14, 106 students received support, including 6 teaching assistantships (averaging $2,750 per year); research assistantships, career-related internships or fieldwork, Federal Work-Study, scholarships/grants, and tuition waivers (partial) also available. Support available to part-time students. Financial award application deadline: 4/1; financial award applicants required to submit FAFSA. *Faculty research:* Adolescent substance abuse, detection of bacterial agents, spirituality and health, non-vitamin and non-mineral supplements, analyzing ticks and their ability to transfer diseases to humans. *Total annual research expenditures:* $248,157. *Unit head:* Dr. Pamela Chally, Dean, 904-620-2810, Fax: 904-620-1030, E-mail: pchally@unf.edu. *Application contact:* Dr. Heather Kenney, Director of Advising, 904-620-2810, Fax: 904-620-1030, E-mail: heather.kenney@unf.edu.
Website: http://www.unf.edu/brooks

University of Oklahoma Health Sciences Center, College of Medicine, Program in Physician Associate, Oklahoma City, OK 73190. Offers MHS. *Faculty:* 10 full-time (8 women). *Students:* 230 full-time (184 women), 2 part-time (1 woman); includes 50 minority (4 Black or African American, non-Hispanic/Latino; 4 American Indian or Alaska Native, non-Hispanic/Latino; 15 Asian, non-Hispanic/Latino; 11 Hispanic/Latino; 16 Two or more races, non-Hispanic/Latino), 2 international. Average age 27. 590 applicants, 17% accepted, 75 enrolled. In 2013, 76 master's awarded. *Expenses:* Tuition, state resident: full-time $3504; part-time $175.20 per credit hour. Tuition, nonresident: full-time $13,504; part-time $675.20 per credit hour. *Required fees:* $1545; $52.70 per credit hour. $245.25 per semester. Tuition and fees vary according to course load. *Unit head:* Dr. David Brand, Program Director, 405-271-8183, E-mail: james-brand@ouhsc.edu. *Application contact:* James Albertson, Dean of the Graduate College, 405-271-2316, Fax: 405-271-1155, E-mail: james-albertson@ouhsc.edu.

University of Oklahoma Health Sciences Center, Graduate College, College of Allied Health, Oklahoma City, OK 73190. Offers MOT, MPT, MS, Au D, PhD, Certificate. *Accreditation:* AOTA; APTA. Part-time programs available. *Faculty:* 38 full-time (31 women), 1 part-time/adjunct (0 women). *Students:* 342 full-time (266 women), 65 part-time (55 women); includes 85 minority (9 Black or African American, non-Hispanic/Latino; 14 American Indian or Alaska Native, non-Hispanic/Latino; 15 Asian, non-Hispanic/Latino; 21 Hispanic/Latino; 26 Two or more races, non-Hispanic/Latino), 3 international. Average age 26. 658 applicants, 37% accepted, 143 enrolled. In 2013, 65 master's, 3 doctorates, 29 other advanced degrees awarded. Terminal master's awarded for partial completion of doctoral program. *Degree requirements:* For master's, comprehensive exam, thesis optional; for doctorate, one foreign language, comprehensive exam, thesis/dissertation. *Entrance requirements:* For master's and doctorate, GRE General Test, 3 letters of recommendation. Additional exam requirements/recommendations for international students: Required—TOEFL. *Application deadline:* For fall admission, 7/1 priority date for domestic students; for winter admission, 5/1 for domestic students; for spring admission, 12/1 for domestic students. Application fee: $50. *Expenses:* Tuition, state resident: full-time $3504; part-time $175.20 per credit hour. Tuition, nonresident: full-time $13,504; part-time $675.20 per credit hour. *Required fees:* $1545; $52.70 per credit hour. $245.25 per semester. Tuition and fees vary according to course load. *Financial support:* Fellowships, career-related internships or fieldwork, Federal Work-Study, institutionally sponsored loans, and traineeships available. Support available to part-time students. *Unit head:* Dr. Kevin Rudeen, Dean, 405-271-2288, Fax: 405-271-1190, E-mail: kevin-rudeen@ouhsc.edu. *Application contact:* Susan Tucker, Associate Dean, Academic and Student Affairs, 405-271-6588, Fax: 405-271-3120, E-mail: susan-tucker@ouhsc.edu.

University of Phoenix–Las Vegas Campus, College of Human Services, Las Vegas, NV 89135. Offers marriage, family, and child therapy (MSC); mental health counseling (MSC); school counseling (MSC). Postbaccalaureate distance learning degree programs offered. *Entrance requirements:* For master's, minimum undergraduate GPA of 2.5, 3 years of work experience. Additional exam requirements/recommendations for international students: Required—TOEFL (minimum score 550 paper-based; 79 iBT). Electronic applications accepted.

University of Puerto Rico, Medical Sciences Campus, School of Health Professions, San Juan, PR 00936-5067. Offers MS, Au D, Certificate. *Degree requirements:* For master's, one foreign language, thesis (for some programs). *Entrance requirements:* For master's, GRE or EXADEP, interview; for doctorate, EXADEP; for Certificate, Allied Health Professions Admissions Test, minimum GPA of 2.5, interview. Electronic applications accepted. *Faculty research:* Infantile autism, aphasia, language problems, toxicology, immunohematology, medical record documentation and quality.

University of South Alabama, Graduate School, College of Allied Health Professions, Mobile, AL 36688-0002. Offers MHS, MS, Au D, DPT, PhD. *Faculty:* 29 full-time (21 women), 1 part-time/adjunct (0 women). *Students:* 346 full-time (266 women), 1 (woman) part-time; includes 27 minority (8 Black or African American, non-Hispanic/Latino; 2 American Indian or Alaska Native, non-Hispanic/Latino; 4 Asian, non-Hispanic/Latino; 8 Hispanic/Latino; 1 Native Hawaiian or other Pacific Islander, non-Hispanic/Latino; 4 Two or more races, non-Hispanic/Latino), 2 international. 646 applicants, 33% accepted, 90 enrolled. In 2013, 85 master's, 39 doctorates awarded. *Degree requirements:* For master's, thesis optional, externship; for doctorate, thesis/dissertation, clinical internship. *Entrance requirements:* For master's, GRE General Test; for doctorate, GRE (for Au D). Additional exam requirements/recommendations for international students: Required—TOEFL (minimum score 525 paper-based). *Application deadline:* For fall admission, 7/15 priority date for domestic students, 6/15 for international students; for spring admission, 12/1 for domestic students, 11/1 for international students. Applications are processed on a rolling basis. Application fee: $35. *Expenses:* Tuition, state resident: full-time $8976; part-time $374 per credit hour. Tuition, nonresident: full-time $17,952; part-time $748 per credit hour. *Financial support:* Fellowships, research assistantships, and career-related internships or fieldwork available. Support available to part-time students. Financial award application deadline: 4/1. *Unit head:* Dr. Richard Talbott, Dean, 251-445-9250. *Application contact:* Dr. Julio Turrens, Director of Graduate Studies, 251-445-9250.
Website: http://www.southalabama.edu/alliedhealth

The University of South Dakota, Graduate School, School of Health Sciences, Vermillion, SD 57069-2390. Offers addiction studies (MA); alcohol and drug studies (Graduate Certificate); occupational therapy (MS); physical therapy (DPT); physician assistant studies (MS); social work (MSW). Part-time programs available. *Entrance requirements:* For master's, GRE General Test, GRE Subject Test. *Faculty research:* Occupational therapy, physical therapy, vision, pediatrics, geriatrics.

The University of Tennessee Health Science Center, College of Graduate Health Sciences, Memphis, TN 38163-0002. Offers biomedical engineering (MS, PhD); biomedical sciences (PhD); dental sciences (MDS); epidemiology (MS); health outcomes and policy research (PhD); laboratory research and management (MS); nursing science (PhD); pharmaceutical sciences (PhD); pharmacology (MS); speech and hearing science (PhD); DDS/PhD; DNP/PhD; MD/PhD; Pharm D/PhD. *Faculty:* 318 full-time (92 women), 59 part-time/adjunct (16 women). *Students:* 220 full-time (102 women), 22 part-time (13 women); includes 194 minority (22 Black or African American, non-Hispanic/Latino; 161 Asian, non-Hispanic/Latino; 7 Hispanic/Latino; 3 Native Hawaiian or other Pacific Islander, non-Hispanic/Latino; 1 Two or more races, non-Hispanic/Latino), 106 international. Average age 25. 404 applicants, 17% accepted, 64 enrolled. In 2013, 13 master's, 25 doctorates awarded. Terminal master's awarded for partial completion of doctoral program. *Degree requirements:* For master's, comprehensive exam, thesis; for doctorate, comprehensive exam, thesis/dissertation, oral and written preliminary and comprehensive exams. *Entrance requirements:* For master's and doctorate, GRE General Test, minimum GPA of 3.0. Additional exam requirements/recommendations for international students: Required—TOEFL (minimum score 79 iBT); Recommended—IELTS (minimum score 6.5). *Application deadline:* For fall admission, 5/15 priority date for domestic students. Applications are processed on a rolling basis. Application fee: $0. Electronic applications accepted. *Financial support:* In 2013–14, 125 students received support, including 125 research assistantships (averaging $23,000 per year); career-related internships or fieldwork, Federal Work-Study, institutionally sponsored loans, and tuition waivers (full and partial) also available. Support available to part-time students. Financial award application deadline: 2/25; financial award applicants required to submit FAFSA. *Unit head:* Dr. Donald B. Thomason, Dean, 901-448-5538, E-mail: dthomaso@uthsc.edu. *Application contact:* William Carter, Director for Admissions, 901-448-1687, E-mail: wcarte17@uthsc.edu.
Website: http://www.uthsc.edu/grad/

The University of Tennessee Health Science Center, College of Health Professions, Memphis, TN 38163-0002. Offers audiology (MS, Au D); clinical laboratory science (MSCLS); cytopathology practice (MCP); health informatics and information management (MHIIM); occupational therapy (MOT); physical therapy (DPT, ScDPT); physician assistant (MMS); speech-language pathology (MS). *Accreditation:* AOTA; APTA. Part-time and evening/weekend programs available. Postbaccalaureate distance

learning degree programs offered (minimal on-campus study). Terminal master's awarded for partial completion of doctoral program. *Degree requirements:* For master's, comprehensive exam, thesis; for doctorate, comprehensive exam, residency. *Entrance requirements:* For master's, GRE (MOT, MSCLS), minimum GPA of 3.0, 3 letters of reference, national accreditation (MSCLS), GRE if GPA is less than 3.0 (MCP); for doctorate, GRE. Additional exam requirements/recommendations for international students: Required—TOEFL (minimum score 550 paper-based; 80 iBT). *Application deadline:* For fall admission, 1/30 priority date for domestic students; for winter admission, 10/1 priority date for domestic students. Application fee: $50. Electronic applications accepted. *Expenses:* Contact institution. *Financial support:* Teaching assistantships, Federal Work-Study, institutionally sponsored loans, and scholarships/grants available. Support available to part-time students. Financial award application deadline: 2/15; financial award applicants required to submit FAFSA. *Faculty research:* Gait deviation, muscular dystrophy and strength, hemophilia and exercise, pediatric neurology, self-efficacy. *Unit head:* Dr. Noma Anderson, Dean, 901-528-5588, Fax: 901-528-7545, E-mail: nander13@uthsc.edu. *Application contact:* Dr. Noma Anderson, Dean, 901-528-5588, Fax: 901-528-7545, E-mail: nander13@uthsc.edu.
Website: http://www.uthsc.edu/health-professions/

The University of Texas at El Paso, Graduate School, College of Health Sciences, Program in Interdisciplinary Health Sciences, El Paso, TX 79968-0001. Offers PhD. *Degree requirements:* For doctorate, thesis/dissertation. *Entrance requirements:* For doctorate, GRE, three letters of reference, relevant personal/professional experience, evidence of a master's degree (MS or MA) or other terminal degree, official transcripts. Additional exam requirements/recommendations for international students: Required—TOEFL (minimum score 550 paper-based); Recommended—IELTS. Electronic applications accepted.

The University of Texas Medical Branch, School of Health Professions, Galveston, TX 77555. Offers MOT, MPAS, MPT, DPT. *Degree requirements:* For master's, thesis or alternative; for doctorate, thesis/dissertation or alternative. *Entrance requirements:* For master's, GRE, experience in field, minimum GPA of 3.0; for doctorate, GRE, documentation of 40 hours experience. Additional exam requirements/recommendations for international students: Required—TOEFL (minimum score 550 paper-based). Electronic applications accepted.

University of Vermont, Graduate College, College of Nursing and Health Sciences, Burlington, VT 05405. Offers MS, DNP, DPT. *Students:* 205 (166 women); includes 12 minority (3 Black or African American, non-Hispanic/Latino; 2 Asian, non-Hispanic/Latino; 6 Hispanic/Latino; 1 Two or more races, non-Hispanic/Latino), 3 international. 617 applicants, 28% accepted, 38 enrolled. In 2013, 44 master's, 38 doctorates awarded. *Degree requirements:* For master's, thesis. *Entrance requirements:* For master's and doctorate, GRE General Test. Additional exam requirements/recommendations for international students: Required—TOEFL (minimum score 550 paper-based; 80 iBT). *Application deadline:* For fall admission, 4/1 priority date for domestic students. Applications are processed on a rolling basis. Application fee: $65. Electronic applications accepted. *Financial support:* Fellowships, research assistantships, teaching assistantships, and Federal Work-Study available. Financial award application deadline: 3/1. *Unit head:* Dr. Patricia Prelock, Dean, 802-656-3830.

University of Wisconsin–Milwaukee, Graduate School, College of Health Sciences, Milwaukee, WI 53211. Offers MS, DPT, PhD, Certificate. Part-time programs available. *Faculty:* 42 full-time (24 women), 4 part-time/adjunct (2 women). *Students:* 215 full-time (162 women), 32 part-time (21 women); includes 23 minority (13 Asian, non-Hispanic/Latino; 10 Two or more races, non-Hispanic/Latino), 14 international. Average age 28. 258 applicants, 33% accepted, 61 enrolled. In 2013, 75 master's, 7 doctorates awarded. *Degree requirements:* For master's, thesis; for doctorate, comprehensive exam, thesis/dissertation. *Entrance requirements:* For doctorate, GRE General Test, master's degree. Additional exam requirements/recommendations for international students: Required—TOEFL (minimum score 600 paper-based), IELTS (minimum score 6.5). *Application deadline:* For fall admission, 1/1 priority date for domestic students; for spring admission, 9/1 for domestic students. Applications are processed on a rolling basis. Application fee: $56 ($96 for international students). *Expenses:* Contact institution. *Financial support:* In 2013–14, 6 research assistantships, 12 teaching assistantships were awarded; career-related internships or fieldwork, Federal Work-Study, and unspecified assistantships also available. Support available to part-time students. Financial award application deadline: 4/15. *Total annual research expenditures:* $2.5 million. *Unit head:* Chukuka S. Enwemeka, Dean, 414-229-4712, E-mail: enwemeka@uwm.edu. *Application contact:* Roger O. Smith, General Information Contact, 414-229-6697, Fax: 414-229-6697, E-mail: smithro@uwm.edu.
Website: http://www4.uwm.edu/chs/

Virginia Commonwealth University, Graduate School, School of Allied Health Professions, Doctoral Program in Health Related Sciences, Richmond, VA 23284-9005. Offers clinical laboratory sciences (PhD); gerontology (PhD); health administration (PhD); nurse anesthesia (PhD); occupational therapy (PhD); physical therapy (PhD); radiation sciences (PhD); rehabilitation leadership (PhD). *Entrance requirements:* For doctorate, GRE General Test or MAT, minimum GPA of 3.3 in master's degree. Additional exam requirements/recommendations for international students: Required—TOEFL (minimum score 600 paper-based; 100 iBT); Recommended—IELTS (minimum score 6.5). Electronic applications accepted.

Western University of Health Sciences, College of Allied Health Professions, Pomona, CA 91766-1854. Offers MS, DPT. *Accreditation:* APTA (one or more programs are accredited). *Faculty:* 21 full-time (14 women), 5 part-time/adjunct (4 women). *Students:* 364 full-time (249 women), 43 part-time (29 women); includes 183 minority (12 Black or African American, non-Hispanic/Latino; 100 Asian, non-Hispanic/Latino; 51 Hispanic/Latino; 20 Two or more races, non-Hispanic/Latino), 5 international. Average age 28. 2,502 applicants, 10% accepted, 152 enrolled. In 2013, 109 master's, 60 doctorates awarded. *Entrance requirements:* For master's, GRE, minimum GPA of 2.5, letters of recommendation; for doctorate, GRE General Test, minimum GPA of 2.8, letters of recommendation, interview, bachelor's degree. Additional exam requirements/recommendations for international students: Required—TOEFL. *Application deadline:* For fall admission, 12/1 for domestic students. Electronic applications accepted. *Expenses:* Contact institution. *Financial support:* Institutionally sponsored loans and scholarships/grants available. Financial award application deadline: 3/2; financial award applicants required to submit FAFSA. *Unit head:* Dr. Stephanie Bowlin, Dean, 909-469-5390, Fax: 909-469-5438, E-mail: sbowlin@westernu.edu. *Application contact:* Karen Hutton-Lopez, Director of Admissions, 909-469-5335, Fax: 909-469-5570, E-mail: admissions@westernu.edu.
Website: http://www.westernu.edu/allied-health/

Wichita State University, Graduate School, College of Health Professions, Wichita, KS 67260. Offers MA, MPA, MSN, Au D, DNP, DPT, PhD. *Accreditation:* APTA (one or more programs are accredited). Part-time programs available. *Unit head:* Dr. Keith Pickus, Interim Dean, 316-978-3600, Fax: 316-978-3025, E-mail: keith.pickus@wichita.edu. *Application contact:* Jordan Oleson, Admissions Coordinator, 316-978-3095, Fax: 316-978-3253, E-mail: jordan.oleson@wichita.edu.
Website: http://www.wichita.edu/chp

Anesthesiologist Assistant Studies

Case Western Reserve University, School of Medicine and School of Graduate Studies, Graduate Programs in Medicine, Department of Anesthesiology, Cleveland, OH 44106. Offers MS. *Accreditation:* AANA/CANAEP. *Degree requirements:* For master's, thesis. *Entrance requirements:* For master's, MCAT. Additional exam requirements/recommendations for international students: Required—TOEFL. Electronic applications accepted. *Faculty research:* Metabolism of bioamines, cerebral metabolism, cardiovascular hemodynamics, genetics.

Emory University, School of Medicine, Programs in Allied Health Professions, Anesthesiology Assistant Program, Atlanta, GA 30322. Offers MM Sc. *Faculty:* 13 part-time/adjunct (5 women). *Students:* 78 full-time (40 women); includes 9 minority (6 Black or African American, non-Hispanic/Latino; 3 Asian, non-Hispanic/Latino), 2 international. Average age 28. 222 applicants, 18% accepted, 35 enrolled. In 2013, 38 master's awarded. *Entrance requirements:* For master's, GRE General Test, MCAT. Additional exam requirements/recommendations for international students: Required—TOEFL (minimum score 600 paper-based; 94 iBT). *Application deadline:* For fall admission, 11/15 for domestic and international students. Application fee: $60. Electronic applications accepted. *Expenses:* Contact institution. *Financial support:* In 2013–14, 44 students received support. Institutionally sponsored loans and scholarships/grants available. Financial award application deadline: 3/1; financial award applicants required to submit FAFSA. *Unit head:* Dr. Richard G. Brouillard, Director of Academic Affairs, 404-727-5910, Fax: 404-727-3021, E-mail: rbrouil@emory.edu. *Application contact:* Jerri J. Elder, Director of Admissions, 404-727-7125, Fax: 404-727-3021, E-mail: jjelder@emory.edu.
Website: http://www.anesthesiology.emory.edu/

Quinnipiac University, School of Health Sciences, Program for Anesthesiologist Assistant, Hamden, CT 06518-1940. Offers MHS. *Faculty:* 3 full-time (1 woman), 1 part-time/adjunct (0 women). *Students:* 4 full-time (3 women); includes 1 minority (Black or African American, non-Hispanic/Latino). 12 applicants, 42% accepted, 4 enrolled. *Entrance requirements:* For master's, GRE or MCAT, bachelor's degree; official transcripts of all undergraduate and graduate course work; two letters of recommendation; essay; interview; criminal background check. *Application deadline:* For summer admission, 1/15 for domestic students. Application fee: $45. *Expenses: Tuition:* Part-time $920 per credit. *Required fees:* $37 per credit. *Financial support:* In 2013–14, 1 student received support. Career-related internships or fieldwork, Federal Work-Study, scholarships/grants, and unspecified assistantships available. Support available to part-time students. Financial award application deadline: 6/1; financial award applicants required to submit FAFSA. *Unit head:* William Paulsen, Program Director, E-mail: aaprogram@quinnipiac.edu. *Application contact:* Victoria Pavasaris, Coordinator, E-mail: aaprogram@quinnipiac.edu.
Website: http://www.quinnipiac.edu/school-of-medicine/academics/anesthesiologist-assistant-program/

South University, Graduate Programs, College of Health Professions, Program in Anesthesiologist Assistant, Savannah, GA 31406. Offers MM Sc.

Université Laval, Faculty of Medicine, Post-Professional Programs in Medical Studies, Québec, QC G1K 7P4, Canada. Offers anatomy–pathology (DESS); anesthesiology (DESS); cardiology (DESS); care of older people (Diploma); clinical research (DESS); community health (DESS); dermatology (DESS); diagnostic radiology (DESS); emergency medicine (Diploma); family medicine (DESS); general surgery (DESS); geriatrics (DESS); hematology (DESS); internal medicine (DESS); maternal and fetal medicine (Diploma); medical biochemistry (DESS); medical microbiology and infectious diseases (DESS); medical oncology (DESS); nephrology (DESS); neurology (DESS); neurosurgery (DESS); obstetrics and gynecology (DESS); ophthalmology (DESS); orthopedic surgery (DESS); oto-rhino-laryngology (DESS); palliative medicine (Diploma); pediatrics (DESS); plastic surgery (DESS); psychiatry (DESS); pulmonary medicine (DESS); radiology–oncology (DESS); thoracic surgery (DESS); urology (DESS). *Degree requirements:* For other advanced degree, comprehensive exam. *Entrance requirements:* For degree, knowledge of French. Electronic applications accepted.

University of Colorado Denver, School of Medicine, Program in Anesthesiology, Denver, CO 80217-3364. Offers MS. *Students:* 7 full-time (3 women). Average age 25. 8 applicants, 100% accepted, 7 enrolled. *Degree requirements:* For master's, seven-semester curriculum, including several rounds of anesthesiology clinical practice. *Entrance requirements:* For master's, GRE or MCAT, three letters of recommendation; curriculum vitae or resume; statement of purpose. Additional exam requirements/recommendations for international students: Required—TOEFL (minimum score 26 iBT). *Financial support:* Career-related internships or fieldwork, Federal Work-Study, institutionally sponsored loans, scholarships/grants, and traineeships available. *Unit head:* Dr. Thomas Henthorn, 303-372-6341, E-mail: thomas.henthorn@ucdenver.edu. *Application contact:* Office of Admissions, 303-724-8025, E-mail: somadmin@ucdenver.edu.
Website: http://www.ucdenver.edu/academics/colleges/medicalschool/departments/Anesthesiology/Pages/Anesthesiology.aspx

University of Guelph, Ontario Veterinary College and Graduate Studies, Graduate Programs in Veterinary Sciences, Department of Clinical Studies, Guelph, ON N1G 2W1, Canada. Offers anesthesiology (M Sc, DV Sc); cardiology (DV Sc, Diploma); clinical studies (Diploma); dermatology (M Sc); diagnostic imaging (M Sc, DV Sc); emergency/critical care (M Sc, DV Sc, Diploma); medicine (M Sc, DV Sc); neurology (M Sc, DV Sc); ophthalmology (M Sc, DV Sc); surgery (M Sc, DV Sc). *Degree requirements:* For master's, thesis; for doctorate, comprehensive exam, thesis/dissertation. *Entrance requirements:* Additional exam requirements/recommendations for international students: Required—TOEFL (minimum score 550 paper-based), IELTS (minimum score 6.5). Electronic applications accepted. *Faculty research:* Orthopedics, respirology, oncology, exercise physiology, cardiology.

University of Missouri–Kansas City, School of Medicine, Kansas City, MO 64110-2499. Offers anesthesia (MS); bioinformatics (MS); health professions education (MS); medicine (MD); physician assistant (MMS); MD/PhD. *Accreditation:* LCME/AMA. *Faculty:* 49 full-time (20 women), 13 part-time/adjunct (6 women). *Students:* 462 full-time (241 women), 16 part-time (8 women); includes 253 minority (33 Black or African American, non-Hispanic/Latino; 2 American Indian or Alaska Native, non-Hispanic/Latino; 196 Asian, non-Hispanic/Latino; 14 Hispanic/Latino; 1 Native Hawaiian or other Pacific Islander, non-Hispanic/Latino; 7 Two or more races, non-Hispanic/Latino), 3 international. Average age 24. 1,070 applicants, 11% accepted, 94 enrolled. In 2013, 12 master's, 88 doctorates awarded. *Degree requirements:* For doctorate, one foreign language, United States Medical Licensing Exam Step 1 and 2. *Entrance requirements:* For doctorate, interview. *Application deadline:* For fall admission, 11/15 for domestic and international students. Application fee: $50. *Expenses:* Contact institution. *Financial support:* In 2013–14, 4 fellowships (averaging $38,964 per year), 4 research assistantships (averaging $17,373 per year) were awarded; career-related internships or fieldwork, Federal Work-Study, institutionally sponsored loans, scholarships/grants, and tuition waivers (partial) also available. Financial award application deadline: 3/1; financial award applicants required to submit FAFSA. *Faculty research:* Cardiovascular disease, women's and children's health, trauma and infectious diseases, neurological, metabolic disease. *Unit head:* Dr. Betty Drees, Dean, 816-235-1808, E-mail: dreesb@umkc.edu. *Application contact:* Janine Kluckhohn, Admissions Coordinator, 816-235-1870, Fax: 816-235-6579, E-mail: kluckhohnj@umkc.edu.
Website: http://www.med.umkc.edu/

Clinical Laboratory Sciences/Medical Technology

Albany College of Pharmacy and Health Sciences, School of Health Sciences, Albany, NY 12208. Offers clinical laboratory sciences (MS); cytotechnology and molecular cytology (MS); molecular biosciences (MS). *Students:* 14 full-time (10 women), 5 part-time (2 women), 7 international. Average age 25. 53 applicants, 64% accepted, 13 enrolled. In 2013, 20 master's awarded. *Degree requirements:* For master's, thesis. *Entrance requirements:* For master's, GRE, minimum GPA of 3.0. Additional exam requirements/recommendations for international students: Required—TOEFL (minimum score 84 iBT). *Application deadline:* For fall admission, 4/15 for domestic and international students. Applications are processed on a rolling basis. Application fee: $75. Electronic applications accepted. *Financial support:* Federal Work-Study and scholarships/grants available. Support available to part-time students. Financial award application deadline: 3/1; financial award applicants required to submit FAFSA. *Unit head:* Dr. Martha Hass, Dean of Graduate Studies, 518-694-7238. *Application contact:* Ann Bruno, Coordinator, Graduate Programs, 518-694-7130, E-mail: graduate@acphs.edu.
Website: http://acphs.edu/academics/schools-departments/school-arts-and-sciences

Austin Peay State University, College of Graduate Studies, College of Science and Mathematics, Department of Biology, Clarksville, TN 37044. Offers clinical laboratory science (MS); radiologic science (MS). Part-time programs available. *Faculty:* 12 full-time (5 women). *Students:* 5 full-time (4 women), 28 part-time (15 women); includes 3 minority (2 Black or African American, non-Hispanic/Latino; 1 Two or more races, non-Hispanic/Latino), 2 international. Average age 27. 15 applicants, 100% accepted, 12 enrolled. In 2013, 10 master's awarded. *Degree requirements:* For master's, comprehensive exam, thesis optional. *Entrance requirements:* For master's, GRE General Test, 3 letters of recommendation, minimum undergraduate GPA of 2.5. Additional exam requirements/recommendations for international students: Required—TOEFL (minimum score 500 paper-based). *Application deadline:* For fall admission, 8/5 priority date for domestic students. Applications are processed on a rolling basis. Application fee: $25. Electronic applications accepted. *Expenses:* Tuition, state resident: full-time $7500; part-time $375 per credit hour. Tuition, nonresident: full-time $20,800; part-time $1040 per credit hour. *Required fees:* $1284; $64.20 per credit hour. *Financial support:* In 2013–14, research assistantships with full tuition reimbursements (averaging $6,500 per year) were awarded; career-related internships or fieldwork, Federal Work-Study, institutionally sponsored loans, scholarships/grants, and unspecified assistantships also available. Support available to part-time students. Financial award application deadline: 3/1. *Faculty research:* Non-paint source pollution, amphibian biomonitoring, aquatic toxicology, biological indicators of water quality, taxonomy. *Unit head:* Dr. Don Dailey, Chair, 931-221-7781, Fax: 931-221-6323, E-mail: daileyd@apsu.edu. *Application contact:* June D. Lee, Graduate Coordinator, 800-859-4723, Fax: 931-221-7641, E-mail: gradadmissions@apsu.edu.
Website: http://www.apsu.edu/biology

Baylor College of Medicine, Graduate School of Biomedical Sciences, Program in Clinical Scientist Training, Houston, TX 77030-3498. Offers MS, PhD. Terminal master's awarded for partial completion of doctoral program. *Degree requirements:* For master's, thesis; for doctorate, thesis/dissertation, public defense. Electronic applications accepted. *Faculty research:* Cardiology, pulmonary, HIV, rheumatology, cancer.

The Catholic University of America, School of Arts and Sciences, Department of Biology, Washington, DC 20064. Offers cell and microbial biology (MS, PhD), including cell biology, microbiology; clinical laboratory science (MS, PhD); MSLS/MS. Part-time programs available. *Faculty:* 9 full-time (4 women), 5 part-time/adjunct (4 women). *Students:* 27 full-time (19 women), 36 part-time (22 women); includes 12 minority (7 Black or African American, non-Hispanic/Latino; 2 Asian, non-Hispanic/Latino; 2 Hispanic/Latino; 1 Two or more races, non-Hispanic/Latino), 36 international. Average age 30. 66 applicants, 56% accepted, 19 enrolled. In 2013, 10 master's, 3 doctorates awarded. *Degree requirements:* For master's, comprehensive exam, thesis or alternative; for doctorate, comprehensive exam, thesis/dissertation. *Entrance requirements:* For master's and doctorate, GRE General Test, GRE Subject Test, statement of purpose, official copies of academic transcripts, three letters of recommendation. Additional exam requirements/recommendations for international students: Required—TOEFL (minimum score 580 paper-based). *Application deadline:* For fall admission, 8/1 priority date for domestic students, 7/15 for international students; for spring admission, 12/1 priority date for domestic students, 10/15 for international students. Applications are processed on a rolling basis. Application fee: $55. Electronic applications accepted. *Expenses: Tuition:* Full-time $38,500; part-time $1490 per credit hour. *Required fees:* $400; $1525 per credit hour. One-time fee: $425. Tuition and fees vary according to program. *Financial support:* Fellowships, research assistantships, teaching assistantships, Federal Work-Study, scholarships/grants, tuition waivers (full and partial), and unspecified assistantships available. Financial award application deadline: 2/1; financial award applicants required to submit FAFSA. *Faculty research:* Cell and microbiology, molecular biology of cell proliferation, cellular effects of electromagnetic radiation, biotechnology. *Total annual research expenditures:* $1.5 million. *Unit head:* Dr. Venigalla Rao, Chair, 202-319-5271, Fax: 202-319-5721, E-mail: rao@cua.edu. *Application contact:* Andrew Woodall, Director of Graduate Admissions, 202-319-5057, Fax: 202-319-6533, E-mail: cua-admissions@cua.edu.
Website: http://biology.cua.edu/

Dominican University of California, School of Health and Natural Sciences, Program in Clinical Laboratory Sciences, San Rafael, CA 94901-2298. Offers MS. Evening/weekend programs available. *Faculty:* 2 part-time/adjunct (1 woman). *Students:* 11 part-time (8 women); includes 5 minority (1 Black or African American, non-Hispanic/Latino; 4 Asian, non-Hispanic/Latino). Average age 44. 20 applicants, 65% accepted, 11 enrolled. *Unit head:* Dr. Randall Hall. *Application contact:* Shannon Lovelace-White, Director, 415-485-3287, Fax: 415-485-3214, E-mail: shannon.lovelace-white@dominican.edu.

Duke University, School of Medicine, Clinical Leadership Program, Durham, NC 27701. Offers MHS. *Faculty:* 9 part-time/adjunct (3 women). In 2013, 5 master's awarded. *Degree requirements:* For master's, project. *Entrance requirements:* For master's, GRE. *Application deadline:* For fall admission, 5/1 priority date for domestic students; for spring admission, 9/1 priority date for domestic students. Applications are processed on a rolling basis. Application fee: $100. *Financial support:* Fellowships, research assistantships, and teaching assistantships available. Financial award application deadline: 5/1; financial award applicants required to submit FAFSA. *Unit head:* Dr. Anh N. Tran, Assistant Professor, 919-681-5724, Fax: 919-613-6899, E-mail: anh.tran@duke.edu. *Application contact:* Claudia Graham, Project Coordinator, 919-681-5724, Fax: 919-681-6899, E-mail: claudia.graham@duke.edu.
Website: http://clinical-leadership.mc.duke.edu

Fairleigh Dickinson University, Metropolitan Campus, University College: Arts, Sciences, and Professional Studies, Henry P. Becton School of Nursing and Allied Health, Program in Medical Technology, Teaneck, NJ 07666-1914. Offers MS.

Inter American University of Puerto Rico, Metropolitan Campus, Graduate Programs, Program in Medical Technology, San Juan, PR 00919-1293. Offers administration of clinical laboratories (MS); molecular microbiology (MS). *Accreditation:* NAACLS. Part-time programs available. *Degree requirements:* For master's, comprehensive exam. *Entrance requirements:* For master's, BS in medical technology, minimum GPA of 2.5. Electronic applications accepted.

Long Island University–LIU Post, School of Health Professions and Nursing, Department of Biomedical Sciences, Brookville, NY 11548-1300. Offers cardiovascular perfusion (MS); clinical laboratory management (MS); medical biology (MS), including hematology, immunology, medical biology, medical chemistry, medical microbiology. Part-time and evening/weekend programs available. Postbaccalaureate distance learning degree programs offered. *Degree requirements:* For master's, thesis. *Entrance requirements:* For master's, minimum GPA of 2.75 in major. Electronic applications accepted.

Medical College of Wisconsin, Graduate School of Biomedical Sciences, Program in Clinical and Translational Science, Milwaukee, WI 53226-0509. Offers MS. Program offered in collaboration with the Clinical and Translational Science Institute (CTSI) of Southeast Wisconsin. *Entrance requirements:* For master's, GRE, official transcripts, three letters of recommendation. Additional exam requirements/recommendations for international students: Required—TOEFL.

Medical College of Wisconsin, Graduate School of Biomedical Sciences, Program in Health Care Technologies Management, Milwaukee, WI 53226-0509. Offers MS. *Entrance requirements:* For master's, GRE, official transcripts, three letters of recommendation. Additional exam requirements/recommendations for international students: Required—TOEFL.

Medical College of Wisconsin, Graduate School of Biomedical Sciences, Program in Translational Science, Milwaukee, WI 53226-0509. Offers PhD. *Entrance requirements:* For doctorate, GRE, official transcripts, three letters of recommendation. Additional exam requirements/recommendations for international students: Required—TOEFL.

Michigan State University, The Graduate School, College of Natural Science, Biomedical Laboratory Diagnostics Program, East Lansing, MI 48824. Offers biomedical laboratory operations (MS); clinical laboratory sciences (MS). *Entrance requirements:* Additional exam requirements/recommendations for international students: Required—TOEFL. Electronic applications accepted.

Milwaukee School of Engineering, Department of Electrical Engineering and Computer Science, Program in Perfusion, Milwaukee, WI 53202-3109. Offers MS. Part-time and evening/weekend programs available. *Faculty:* 1 full-time (0 women), 8 part-time/adjunct (3 women). *Students:* 12 full-time (4 women). Average age 33. 46 applicants, 15% accepted, 7 enrolled. In 2013, 4 master's awarded. *Degree requirements:* For master's, comprehensive exam, thesis, exam. *Entrance requirements:* For master's, GRE General Test or GMAT (percentiles must average 50% or better), BS in appropriate discipline (biomedical engineering, biology, biomedical sciences, etc.), 3 letters of recommendation, personal interview, observation of 2 perfusion clinical cases. Additional exam requirements/recommendations for international students: Required—TOEFL (minimum score 79 iBT), IELTS (minimum score 6.5). *Application deadline:* Applications are processed on a rolling basis. Application fee: $0. Electronic applications accepted. Application fee is waived when completed online. *Expenses: Tuition:* Full-time $6939; part-time $771 per credit. *Financial support:* Career-related internships or fieldwork, institutionally sponsored loans, and scholarships/grants available. Financial award application deadline: 3/15; financial award applicants required to submit FAFSA. *Faculty research:* Heart medicine. *Unit head:* Dr. Ronald Gerrits, Director, 414-277-7561, Fax: 414-277-7494, E-mail: gerrits@msoe.edu. *Application contact:* Katie Weinschenk, Graduate Program Associate, 800-321-6763, Fax: 414-277-7208, E-mail: weinschenk@msoe.edu.
Website: http://www.msoe.edu/academics/academic_departments/eecs/msp/

Northwestern University, School of Professional Studies, Program in Regulatory Compliance, Evanston, IL 60208. Offers clinical research (MS); healthcare compliance (MS); quality systems (MS). Offered in partnership with Northwestern University's Clinical and Translational Sciences Institute.

Pontifical Catholic University of Puerto Rico, College of Sciences, School of Medical Technology, Ponce, PR 00717-0777. Offers Certificate. *Entrance requirements:* For degree, letters of recommendation, interview, minimum GPA of 2.75.

Quinnipiac University, School of Health Sciences, Program for Pathologists' Assistant, Hamden, CT 06518-1940. Offers MHS. *Accreditation:* NAACLS. *Faculty:* 1 full-time (0 women), 4 part-time/adjunct (3 women). *Students:* 39 full-time (27 women); includes 9 minority (4 Black or African American, non-Hispanic/Latino; 2 Asian, non-Hispanic/Latino; 3 Hispanic/Latino). 150 applicants, 18% accepted, 22 enrolled. In 2013, 18 master's awarded. *Degree requirements:* For master's, residency. *Entrance requirements:* For master's, interview, coursework in biological and health sciences, minimum GPA of 2.8. *Application deadline:* For fall admission, 11/1 for domestic students; for summer admission, 10/1 for domestic students. Applications are processed on a rolling basis. Application fee: $45. Electronic applications accepted. *Expenses: Tuition:* Part-time $920 per credit. *Required fees:* $37 per credit. *Financial support:* In 2013–14, 8 students received support. Career-related internships or fieldwork, scholarships/grants, and unspecified assistantships available. Support available to part-time students. Financial award application deadline: 6/1; financial award applicants required to submit FAFSA. *Faculty research:* ACL injury mechanism and running injuries and performance; transcriptional activators upstream stimulatory factor (USF); identification of novel antimicrobials; vaccines, fomites and opportunistic pathogens; molecular biology of the Lyme Disease agent, Borrelia burgdorferi; molecular and microscopic techniques in host-pathogen interactions; non-invasive vascular biology, external pneumatic compression, sports performance. *Unit head:* Dr. Kenneth Kaloustian, Director, E-mail: kenneth.kaloustian@quinnipiac.edu. *Application contact:* Office of Graduate Admissions, 800-462-1944, Fax: 203-582-3443, E-mail: paadmissions@quinnipiac.edu.
Website: http://www.quinnipiac.edu/gradpathologists

Quinnipiac University, School of Health Sciences, Program in Medical Laboratory Sciences, Hamden, CT 06518-1940. Offers biomedical sciences (MHS); laboratory management (MHS); microbiology (MHS). Part-time and evening/weekend programs available. *Faculty:* 14 full-time (6 women), 20 part-time/adjunct (8 women). *Students:* 66 full-time (36 women), 30 part-time (13 women); includes 20 minority (7 Black or African American, non-Hispanic/Latino; 8 Asian, non-Hispanic/Latino; 4 Hispanic/Latino; 1 Two or more races, non-Hispanic/Latino), 41 international. 79 applicants, 73% accepted, 38 enrolled. In 2013, 47 master's awarded. *Degree requirements:* For master's, comprehensive exam, thesis optional. *Entrance requirements:* For master's, minimum GPA of 2.75; bachelor's degree in biological, medical, or health sciences. Additional exam requirements/recommendations for international students: Required—TOEFL (minimum score 575 paper-based; 90 iBT), IELTS (minimum score 6.5). *Application deadline:* For fall admission, 7/30 priority date for domestic students, 4/30 priority date for international students; for spring admission, 12/15 priority date for domestic students, 9/15 priority date for international students. Applications are processed on a rolling basis. Application fee: $45. Electronic applications accepted. *Expenses: Tuition:* Part-time $920 per credit. *Required fees:* $37 per credit. *Financial support:* In 2013–14, 7 students received support. Career-related internships or fieldwork, Federal Work-Study, scholarships/grants, and unspecified assistantships available. Support available to part-time students. Financial award application deadline: 6/1; financial award applicants required to submit FAFSA. *Faculty research:* ACL injury mechanism and running injuries and performance; transcriptional activators upstream stimulatory factor (USF); identification of novel antimicrobials; vaccines, fomites and opportunistic pathogens; molecular biology of the Lyme Disease agent, Borrelia burgdorferi; molecular and microscopic techniques in host-pathogen interactions; non-invasive vascular biology, external pneumatic compression, sports performance. *Application contact:* Office of Graduate Admissions, 800-462-1944, Fax: 203-582-3443, E-mail: graduate@quinnipiac.edu.
Website: http://www.quinnipiac.edu/gradmedlab

Rush University, College of Health Sciences, Department of Clinical Laboratory Sciences, Chicago, IL 60612-3832. Offers clinical laboratory management (MS); clinical laboratory science (MS). *Accreditation:* NAACLS. Part-time programs available. *Degree requirements:* For master's, comprehensive exam, graduate project. *Entrance requirements:* For master's, 16 semester hours of chemistry, 12 semester hours of biology, 3 semester hours of mathematics, interview. Additional exam requirements/recommendations for international students: Required—TOEFL. Electronic applications accepted. *Faculty research:* Hematopoietic disorders, molecular techniques, biochemistry, microbial susceptibility, immunology.

Rutgers, The State University of New Jersey, Newark, School of Health Related Professions, Department of Clinical Laboratory Sciences, Newark, NJ 07102. Offers MS. Part-time programs available. Postbaccalaureate distance learning degree programs offered (no on-campus study). *Degree requirements:* For master's, project. *Entrance requirements:* For master's, two recommendations, personal statement, current resume or curriculum vita, minimum GPA of 2.75. Additional exam requirements/recommendations for international students: Required—TOEFL.

Rutgers, The State University of New Jersey, New Brunswick, Graduate School of Biomedical Sciences, Program in Clinical and Translational Science, Piscataway, NJ 08854-8097. Offers MS. Part-time programs available. *Degree requirements:* For master's, thesis.

State University of New York Upstate Medical University, Program in Medical Technology, Syracuse, NY 13210-2334. Offers MS. *Accreditation:* NAACLS. *Degree requirements:* For master's, thesis. *Entrance requirements:* For master's, GRE General Test, GRE Subject Test, 2 years of medical technology experience.

Tarleton State University, College of Graduate Studies, College of Science and Technology, Department of Medical Laboratory Sciences, Stephenville, TX 76402. Offers MS. Part-time and evening/weekend programs available. *Faculty:* 6 full-time (4 women), 1 (woman) part-time/adjunct. *Students:* 5 full-time (4 women), 10 part-time (8 women); includes 6 minority (1 Asian, non-Hispanic/Latino; 5 Hispanic/Latino), 3 international. Average age 29. 6 applicants, 83% accepted, 3 enrolled. In 2013, 1 master's awarded. *Degree requirements:* For master's, comprehensive exam, thesis optional. *Entrance requirements:* For master's, GRE, minimum GPA of 3.0. Additional exam requirements/recommendations for international students: Required—TOEFL (minimum score 550 paper-based; 80 iBT). *Application deadline:* For fall admission, 8/15 for domestic students; for spring admission, 1/7 for domestic students. Applications are processed on a rolling basis. Application fee: $35. Electronic applications accepted. *Expenses:* Tuition, state resident: full-time $3312; part-time $184 per credit hour. Tuition, nonresident: full-time $9144; part-time $508 per credit hour. *Required fees:* $1916. Tuition and fees vary according to course load and campus/location. *Financial support:* Career-related internships or fieldwork, Federal Work-Study, and scholarships/grants available. Support available to part-time students. Financial award application deadline: 5/1; financial award applicants required to submit FAFSA. *Unit head:* Sally Lewis, Head, 817-926-1101, E-mail: slewis@tarleton.edu. *Application contact:* Information Contact, 254-968-9104, Fax: 254-968-9670, E-mail: gradoffice@tarleton.edu.
Website: http://www.tarleton.edu/COSTWEB/medicallab/

Thomas Jefferson University, Jefferson School of Health Professions, Department of Bioscience Technologies, Philadelphia, PA 19107. Offers MS. Part-time and evening/weekend programs available. *Faculty:* 4 full-time (3 women), 3 part-time/adjunct (0 women). *Students:* 40 full-time (25 women), 9 part-time (5 women); includes 21 minority (11 Black or African American, non-Hispanic/Latino; 9 Asian, non-Hispanic/Latino; 1 Hispanic/Latino), 5 international. Average age 27. 79 applicants, 59% accepted, 35 enrolled. In 2013, 34 master's awarded. *Entrance requirements:* Additional exam requirements/recommendations for international students: Required—TOEFL. *Application deadline:* For fall admission, 7/15 for domestic students, 6/15 for international students; for winter admission, 12/1 for domestic students, 9/1 for international students; for spring admission, 4/1 for domestic students. Applications are processed on a rolling basis. Application fee: $95. Electronic applications accepted. *Financial support:* In 2013–14, 22 students received support. Federal Work-Study, institutionally sponsored loans, scholarships/grants, and unspecified assistantships available. Support available to part-time students. Financial award application deadline: 4/1; financial award applicants required to submit FAFSA. *Faculty research:* Molecular biology of BCR-ABL in chronic myeloid leukemia, diagnostic cytogenetics, ATP binding cassette (ABC), gene family, education outcome studies. *Total annual research expenditures:* $51,210. *Unit head:* Shirley Greening, Chair, 215-503-8561, Fax: 215-503-2189, E-mail: shirley.greening@jefferson.edu. *Application contact:* Jennifer Raab, Assistant Director of Admissions, 215-503-1046, Fax: 215-503-7241, E-mail: jshpadmissions@jefferson.edu.
Website: http://www.jefferson.edu/health_professions/departments/bioscience_technologies

Universidad de las Américas Puebla, Division of Graduate Studies, School of Sciences, Program in Clinical Analysis (Biomedicine), Puebla, Mexico. Offers MS. Part-time and evening/weekend programs available. *Degree requirements:* For master's, one foreign language, thesis. *Faculty research:* Clinical techniques, clinical research.

Université de Sherbrooke, Faculty of Medicine and Health Sciences, Graduate Programs in Medicine, Program in Clinical Sciences, Sherbrooke, QC J1H 5N4, Canada. Offers M Sc, PhD. Part-time programs available. Terminal master's awarded for partial completion of doctoral program. *Degree requirements:* For master's, thesis; for doctorate, thesis/dissertation. Electronic applications accepted. *Faculty research:* Population health, health services, ethics, clinical research.

University at Buffalo, the State University of New York, Graduate School, School of Medicine and Biomedical Sciences, Graduate Programs in Medicine and Biomedical Sciences, Department of Biotechnical and Clinical Laboratory Sciences, Buffalo, NY 14214. Offers biotechnology (MS). *Accreditation:* NAACLS. Part-time programs available. *Faculty:* 7 full-time (3 women). *Students:* 13 full-time (8 women); includes 2 minority (1 Asian, non-Hispanic/Latino; 1 Hispanic/Latino), 9 international. 95 applicants, 15% accepted, 4 enrolled. In 2013, 13 master's awarded. *Degree requirements:* For master's, thesis. *Entrance requirements:* For master's, GRE General Test (minimum 50th percentile), minimum GPA of 3.0. Additional exam requirements/recommendations for international students: Required—TOEFL (minimum score 79 iBT). *Application deadline:* For fall admission, 3/1 priority date for domestic students, 2/1 priority date for international students. Applications are processed on a rolling basis. Application fee: $75. Electronic applications accepted. *Financial support:* In 2013–14, 5 students received support, including 5 teaching assistantships with full tuition reimbursements available (averaging $10,000 per year); unspecified assistantships also available. Financial award application deadline: 3/1. *Faculty research:* Immunology, cancer biology, toxicology, clinical chemistry, hematology, chemistry. *Total annual research expenditures:* $741,728. *Unit head:* Dr. Paul J. Kostyniak, Chair, 716-829-5188, Fax: 716-829-3601, E-mail: pjkost@buffalo.edu. *Application contact:* Dr. Stephen T. Koury, Director of Graduate Studies, 716-829-5188, Fax: 716-829-3601, E-mail: stvkoury@buffalo.edu.
Website: http://www.smbs.buffalo.edu/cls/biotech-ms.html

The University of Alabama at Birmingham, School of Health Professions, Program in Clinical Laboratory Science, Birmingham, AL 35294. Offers MS. *Accreditation:* NAACLS. *Degree requirements:* For master's, thesis optional. *Entrance requirements:* For master's, GRE General Test, interview. Additional exam requirements/recommendations for international students: Required—TOEFL, TWE. Electronic applications accepted. *Faculty research:* Computer-enhanced instruction, antiphospholipid antibodies, alternate site testing, technology assessment.

The University of Alabama at Birmingham, School of Public Health, Program in Public Health, Birmingham, AL 35294. Offers accelerated industrial hygiene (MPH); applied epidemiology (MSPH); biostatistics (MPH); clinical and translational science (MSPH); environmental health (MPH); environmental health and toxicology (MSPH); epidemiology (MPH); general theory and practice (MPH); health behavior (MPH); health care organization (MPH); health policy quantitative policy analysis (MPH); industrial hygiene (MPH, MSPH); maternal and child health policy (Dr PH); maternal and child health policy and leadership (MPH); occupational health and safety (MPH); outcomes research (MSPH, Dr PH); pharmacoepidemiology and comparative effectiveness research (MSPH); public health (PhD); public health management (Dr PH); public health preparedness management (MPH). *Accreditation:* CEPH. *Entrance requirements:* For master's and doctorate, GRE, evaluations. Additional exam requirements/recommendations for international students: Recommended—TOEFL (minimum score 550 paper-based; 79 iBT), IELTS (minimum score 6.5).

University of Alberta, Faculty of Medicine and Dentistry and Faculty of Graduate Studies and Research, Graduate Programs in Medicine, Department of Laboratory Medicine and Pathology, Edmonton, AB T6G 2E1, Canada. Offers medical sciences (M Sc, PhD). Part-time programs available. Terminal master's awarded for partial completion of doctoral program. *Degree requirements:* For master's, thesis; for doctorate, thesis/dissertation, candidacy exam. *Entrance requirements:* For master's and doctorate, 3 letters of recommendation, minimum GPA of 3.0. Additional exam requirements/recommendations for international students: Required—TOEFL. *Faculty research:* Transplantation, renal pathology, molecular mechanisms of diseases, cryobiology, immunodiagnostics, informatics/cyber medicine, neuroimmunology, microbiology.

University of California, San Diego, Office of Graduate Studies, Department of Electrical and Computer Engineering, La Jolla, CA 92093. Offers applied ocean science (MS, PhD); applied physics (MS, PhD); communication theory and systems (MS, PhD); computer engineering (MS, PhD); electronic circuits and systems (MS, PhD); engineering sciences/electrical and computer engineering (PhD); intelligent systems, robotics and control (MS, PhD); medical devices and systems (MS, PhD); nanoscale devices and systems (MS, PhD); photonics (MS, PhD); signal and image processing (MS, PhD). PhD in engineering sciences/electrical and computer engineering is offered jointly with San Diego State University. Applicants must apply through SDSU. *Students:* 411 full-time (78 women), 37 part-time (6 women); includes 73 minority (3 Black or African American, non-Hispanic/Latino; 1 American Indian or Alaska Native, non-Hispanic/Latino; 63 Asian, non-Hispanic/Latino; 6 Hispanic/Latino), 293 international. 2,640 applicants, 20% accepted, 134 enrolled. In 2013, 100 master's, 36 doctorates awarded. *Degree requirements:* For master's, thesis or written exam; for doctorate, thesis/dissertation. *Entrance requirements:* For master's and doctorate, GRE General

Test, minimum GPA of 3.0. Additional exam requirements/recommendations for international students: Required—TOEFL (minimum score 550 paper-based; 80 iBT), IELTS. *Application deadline:* For fall admission, 12/16 for domestic students. Application fee: $80 ($100 for international students). Electronic applications accepted. *Expenses:* Tuition, state resident: full-time $11,220; part-time $1870 per quarter. Tuition, nonresident: full-time $26,322; part-time $4387 per quarter. *Required fees:* $519.50 per quarter. Part-time tuition and fees vary according to course load and program. *Financial support:* Fellowships, research assistantships, teaching assistantships, and scholarships/grants available. Financial award applicants required to submit FAFSA. *Faculty research:* High speed transistors, telecommunications, opto-electronics, algorithms for automatic detection and classification. *Unit head:* Shaya Fainman, Chair, 858-534-8987, E-mail: yfainman@ece.ucsd.edu. *Application contact:* Shana Slebioda, Graduate Coordinator, 858-822-2513, E-mail: ecegradapps@ece.ucsd.edu.
Website: http://ece.ucsd.edu/

University of California, San Diego, Office of Graduate Studies, Program in Medical Device Engineering, La Jolla, CA 92093. Offers MAS. *Students:* 29 part-time (22 women); includes 9 minority (1 Black or African American, non-Hispanic/Latino; 6 Asian, non-Hispanic/Latino; 2 Hispanic/Latino), 4 international. 30 applicants, 70% accepted, 18 enrolled. In 2013, 5 master's awarded. *Degree requirements:* For master's, capstone project. *Entrance requirements:* For master's, 3 letters of recommendation; statement of purpose; bachelor's degree in engineering, science, or mathematics; minimum undergraduate GPA of 3.0 in final two years of study; two years of relevant work experience; curriculum vitae/resume. Additional exam requirements/recommendations for international students: Required—TOEFL or IELTS. *Application deadline:* For fall admission, 7/31 priority date for domestic students. Application fee: $80 ($100 for international students). Electronic applications accepted. *Expenses:* Tuition, state resident: full-time $11,220; part-time $1870 per quarter. Tuition, nonresident: full-time $26,322; part-time $4387 per quarter. *Required fees:* $519.50 per quarter. Part-time tuition and fees vary according to course load and program. *Financial support:* Applicants required to submit FAFSA. *Unit head:* Juan C. Lasheras, Chair, 858-822-0162, E-mail: jlasheras@ucsd.edu. *Application contact:* Linda McKamey, Program Coordinator, 858-534-4065, E-mail: lmckamey@ucsd.edu.
Website: http://maseng.ucsd.edu/mde/

University of Colorado Denver, School of Medicine, Clinical Science Graduate Program, Aurora, CO 80045. Offers clinical investigation (PhD); clinical sciences (MS); health information technology (PhD); health services research (PhD). *Students:* 25 full-time (17 women), 29 part-time (15 women); includes 10 minority (2 Black or African American, non-Hispanic/Latino; 2 Asian, non-Hispanic/Latino; 2 Hispanic/Latino; 1 Native Hawaiian or other Pacific Islander, non-Hispanic/Latino; 3 Two or more races, non-Hispanic/Latino), 1 international. Average age 34. 16 applicants, 81% accepted, 13 enrolled. In 2013, 11 master's, 7 doctorates awarded. *Degree requirements:* For master's, thesis, minimum of 30 credit hours, defense/final exam of thesis or publishable paper; for doctorate, comprehensive exam, thesis/dissertation, at least 30 credit hours of thesis work. *Entrance requirements:* For master's, GRE General Test or MCAT (waived if candidate has earned MS/MA or PhD from accredited U.S. school), minimum undergraduate GPA of 3.0, 3-4 letters of recommendation; for doctorate, GRE General Test or MCAT (waived if candidate has earned MS/MA or PhD from accredited U.S. school), health care graduate, professional degree, or graduate degree related to health sciences; minimum GPA of 3.0, 3-4 letters of recommendation. Additional exam requirements/recommendations for international students: Required—TOEFL (minimum score 550 paper-based; 80 iBT). *Application deadline:* For fall admission, 2/1 for domestic students, 1/15 priority date for international students; for spring admission, 10/1 for domestic students. Application fee: $50 ($75 for international students). Electronic applications accepted. *Expenses:* Contact institution. *Financial support:* In 2013–14, 18 students received support. Fellowships, research assistantships, teaching assistantships, Federal Work-Study, institutionally sponsored loans, scholarships/grants, traineeships, and unspecified assistantships available. Financial award application deadline: 3/15; financial award applicants required to submit FAFSA. *Unit head:* Dr. Ronald Sokol, Program Director, 720-777-6669, E-mail: ronald.sokol@childrenscolorado.org. *Application contact:* Galit Mankin, Program Administrator, 720-848-6249, Fax: 303-848-7381, E-mail: galit.mankin@ucdenver.edu.
Website: http://cctsi.ucdenver.edu/training-and-education/CLSC/Pages/default.aspx

University of Florida, Graduate School, College of Engineering, Department of Materials Science and Engineering, Gainesville, FL 32611. Offers material science and engineering (MS), including clinical and translational science; nuclear engineering (ME, PhD), including imaging science and technology (PhD), nuclear engineering sciences (ME, MS, PhD); nuclear engineering (MS), including nuclear engineering sciences (ME, MS, PhD); JD/MS. Part-time programs available. Postbaccalaureate distance learning degree programs offered. *Faculty:* 32 full-time (5 women), 32 part-time/adjunct (9 women). *Students:* 263 full-time (57 women), 41 part-time (12 women); includes 44 minority (9 Black or African American, non-Hispanic/Latino; 21 Asian, non-Hispanic/Latino; 14 Hispanic/Latino), 173 international. Average age 27. 555 applicants, 61% accepted, 75 enrolled. In 2013, 64 master's, 23 doctorates awarded. Terminal master's awarded for partial completion of doctoral program. *Degree requirements:* For master's, comprehensive exam, thesis; for doctorate, comprehensive exam, thesis/dissertation; for Engr, thesis optional. *Entrance requirements:* For master's and doctorate, minimum GPA of 3.0; for Engr, GRE General Test. Additional exam requirements/recommendations for international students: Required—TOEFL (minimum score 550 paper-based; 80 iBT), IELTS (minimum score 6). *Application deadline:* For fall admission, 7/1 priority date for domestic students, 5/1 for international students; for spring admission, 11/1 for domestic students, 9/1 for international students. Applications are processed on a rolling basis. Application fee: $30. Electronic applications accepted. *Expenses:* Tuition, state resident: full-time $12,640. Tuition, nonresident: full-time $30,000. *Financial support:* In 2013–14, 103 students received support, including 6 fellowships (averaging $20,925 per year), 105 research assistantships (averaging $19,015 per year), 3 teaching assistantships (averaging $10,111 per year). Financial award applicants required to submit FAFSA. *Faculty research:* Polymeric system, biomaterials and biomimetics; inorganic and organic electronic materials; functional ceramic materials for energy systems and microelectronic applications; advanced metallic systems for aerospace, transportation and biological applications; nuclear materials. *Unit head:* Simon R. Phillpot, PhD, Chair, 352-846-3782, Fax: 352-392-7219, E-mail: sphil@mse.ufl.edu. *Application contact:* Dr. Jack Mecholsky, Jr., Graduate Coordinator, 352-846-3306, Fax: 352-846-1182, E-mail: jmech@mse.ufl.edu.
Website: http://www.mse.ufl.edu/

University of Florida, Graduate School, College of Nursing, Gainesville, FL 32611. Offers clinical and translational science (PhD); nursing (MSN); nursing sciences (DNP). *Accreditation:* AACN; ACNM/ACME (one or more programs are accredited). Part-time programs available. *Faculty:* 13 full-time (11 women), 5 part-time/adjunct (3 women). *Students:* 72 full-time (64 women), 55 part-time (49 women); includes 20 minority (5 Black or African American, non-Hispanic/Latino; 4 Asian, non-Hispanic/Latino; 11 Hispanic/Latino), 4 international. Average age 36. 51 applicants, 27% accepted, 13 enrolled. In 2013, 79 master's, 5 doctorates awarded. *Degree requirements:* For master's, thesis optional; for doctorate, thesis/dissertation. *Entrance requirements:* For master's and doctorate, GRE General Test, minimum GPA of 3.0. Additional exam requirements/recommendations for international students: Required—TOEFL (minimum score 550 paper-based; 80 iBT), IELTS (minimum score 6). *Application deadline:* For fall admission, 3/15 priority date for domestic students, 3/15 for international students. Applications are processed on a rolling basis. Application fee: $30. Electronic applications accepted. *Expenses:* Tuition, state resident: full-time $12,640. Tuition, nonresident: full-time $30,000. *Financial support:* In 2013–14, 5 students received support, including 5 fellowships with partial tuition reimbursements available (averaging $24,000 per year); career-related internships or fieldwork and Federal Work-Study also available. Support available to part-time students. Financial award applicants required to submit FAFSA. *Faculty research:* Aging and health: cancer survivorship, interventions to promote healthy aging, and symptom management; women's health, fetal and infant development; biobehavioral interventions: interrelationships among the biological, behavioral, psychological, social and spiritual factors that influence wellness and disease; health policy: influence of local and national policy on physical and psychological health. *Unit head:* Anna M. McDaniel, PhD, Dean, College of Nursing, 352-273-6324, Fax: 352-273-6505, E-mail: annammcdaniel@ufl.edu. *Application contact:* Bridgette Hart-Sams, Coordinator, Student Academic Services, 352-273-6331, Fax: 352-273-6440, E-mail: bhart@ufl.edu.
Website: http://nursing.ufl.edu/

University of Florida, Graduate School, College of Pharmacy and Graduate School, Graduate Programs in Pharmacy, Department of Pharmaceutics, Gainesville, FL 32610. Offers clinical and translational sciences (PhD); pharmaceutical sciences (MSP, PhD); pharmacy (MSP, PhD). *Faculty:* 11 full-time (2 women), 10 part-time/adjunct (1 woman). *Students:* 18 full-time (9 women), 2 part-time (1 woman); includes 1 minority (Asian, non-Hispanic/Latino), 17 international. Average age 30. 234 applicants, 48% accepted, 86 enrolled. In 2013, 1 master's, 9 doctorates awarded. *Degree requirements:* For doctorate, comprehensive exam, thesis/dissertation. *Entrance requirements:* For master's and doctorate, GRE General Test, minimum GPA of 3.0. Additional exam requirements/recommendations for international students: Required—TOEFL (minimum score 550 paper-based; 80 iBT), IELTS (minimum score 6). *Application deadline:* For fall admission, 2/1 priority date for domestic students, 2/1 for international students; for spring admission, 9/1 for domestic students, 10/1 for international students. Applications are processed on a rolling basis. Application fee: $30. Electronic applications accepted. *Expenses:* Tuition, state resident: full-time $12,640. Tuition, nonresident: full-time $30,000. *Financial support:* In 2013–14, 18 students received support, including 4 research assistantships (averaging $13,785 per year), 16 teaching assistantships (averaging $15,745 per year); tuition waivers (full) and unspecified assistantships also available. Financial award applicants required to submit FAFSA. *Faculty research:* Basic, applied, and clinical investigations in pharmacokinetics/biopharmaceutics; pharmaceutical analysis, pharmaceutical biotechnology and drug delivery; herbal medicine. *Unit head:* Hartmut Derendorf, PhD, Professor and Chair, 352-273-7856, Fax: 352-392-4447, E-mail: hartmut@ufl.edu. *Application contact:* Dr. Anthony Palmieri, III, Graduate Coordinator, 352-273-7868, E-mail: palmieri@cop.ufl.edu.
Website: http://www.cop.ufl.edu/pc/

University of Florida, Graduate School, College of Public Health and Health Professions, Department of Clinical and Health Psychology, Gainesville, FL 32610. Offers clinical and health psychology (PhD); clinical and translational science (PhD); psychology (MA, MS). *Accreditation:* APA (one or more programs are accredited). *Faculty:* 22 full-time (10 women), 12 part-time/adjunct (4 women). *Students:* 96 full-time (67 women), 4 part-time (3 women); includes 26 minority (7 Black or African American, non-Hispanic/Latino; 1 American Indian or Alaska Native, non-Hispanic/Latino; 4 Asian, non-Hispanic/Latino; 14 Hispanic/Latino), 2 international. Average age 27. 278 applicants, 5% accepted, 11 enrolled. In 2013, 13 master's, 12 doctorates awarded. *Degree requirements:* For doctorate, comprehensive exam, thesis/dissertation, pre-doctoral internship. *Entrance requirements:* For master's and doctorate, GRE General Test, minimum GPA of 3.0. Additional exam requirements/recommendations for international students: Required—TOEFL (minimum score 550 paper-based; 80 iBT), IELTS (minimum score 6). *Application deadline:* For fall admission, 12/1 for domestic and international students. Application fee: $30. Electronic applications accepted. *Expenses:* Tuition, state resident: full-time $12,640. Tuition, nonresident: full-time $30,000. *Financial support:* In 2013–14, 62 students received support, including 15 fellowships with partial tuition reimbursements available (averaging $15,225 per year), 54 research assistantships with partial tuition reimbursements available (averaging $18,310 per year), 4 teaching assistantships (averaging $9,585 per year); career-related internships or fieldwork, Federal Work-Study, institutionally sponsored loans, scholarships/grants, and unspecified assistantships also available. Financial award application deadline: 12/1; financial award applicants required to submit FAFSA. *Faculty research:* Clinical child and pediatric psychology, medical psychology, neuropsychology, health promotion and aging. *Unit head:* Wlliam W. Latimer, PhD, Professor and Chair, 352-273-6556, Fax: 352-273-6156, E-mail: wwlatimer@phhp.ufl.edu. *Application contact:* Office of Admissions, 352-392-1365, E-mail: webrequests@admissions.ufl.edu.
Website: http://www.phhp.ufl.edu/chp/

University of Florida, Graduate School, College of Public Health and Health Professions, Department of Epidemiology, Gainesville, FL 32610. Offers clinical and translational science (PhD); epidemiology (MS, PhD). *Faculty:* 10 full-time (5 women). *Students:* 23 full-time (13 women), 3 part-time (1 woman); includes 5 minority (2 Black or African American, non-Hispanic/Latino; 2 Asian, non-Hispanic/Latino; 1 Hispanic/Latino), 10 international. Average age 30. 50 applicants, 8% accepted, 4 enrolled. In 2013, 2 doctorates awarded. *Degree requirements:* For master's, thesis; for doctorate, thesis/dissertation. *Entrance requirements:* For master's and doctorate, GRE, minimum GPA of 3.0. Additional exam requirements/recommendations for international students: Required—TOEFL (minimum score 550 paper-based; 80 iBT), IELTS (minimum score 6). *Application deadline:* For fall admission, 2/1 for domestic students. Application fee: $30. *Expenses:* Tuition, state resident: full-time $12,640. Tuition, nonresident: full-time $30,000. *Financial support:* In 2013–14, 18 students received support, including 3 fellowships (averaging $18,695 per year), 8 research assistantships (averaging $15,010 per year), 10 teaching assistantships (averaging $19,220 per year). Financial award applicants required to submit FAFSA. *Unit head:* Linda Cottler, PhD, Chair, 352-273-5468, E-mail: lbcottler@ufl.edu. *Application contact:* Betsy Jones, Program Assistant, 352-273-5961, E-mail: bjcop@ufl.edu.
Website: http://epidemiology.phhp.ufl.edu/

University of Florida, Graduate School, College of Public Health and Health Professions, Program in Rehabilitation Science, Gainesville, FL 32610. Offers clinical and translational science (PhD); rehabilitation science (PhD); PhD/MPH. *Faculty:* 10 full-time (6 women). *Students:* 27 full-time (13 women), 6 part-time (4 women); includes 6 minority (2 Black or African American, non-Hispanic/Latino; 2 Asian, non-Hispanic/Latino; 2 Hispanic/Latino), 17 international. Average age 33. 18 applicants, 39% accepted, 7 enrolled. In 2013, 6 doctorates awarded. *Degree requirements:* For doctorate, comprehensive exam, thesis/dissertation. *Entrance requirements:* For doctorate, GRE General Test, minimum GPA of 3.0. Additional exam requirements/recommendations for international students: Required—TOEFL (minimum score 550 paper-based; 80 iBT), IELTS (minimum score 6). *Application deadline:* For fall admission, 3/15 for domestic and international students; for spring admission, 7/15 for domestic and international students. Applications are processed on a rolling basis.

Application fee: $30. Electronic applications accepted. *Expenses:* Tuition, state resident: full-time $12,640. Tuition, nonresident: full-time $30,000. *Financial support:* In 2013–14, 24 students received support, including 3 fellowships (averaging $18,695 per year), 18 research assistantships (averaging $19,795 per year), 5 teaching assistantships (averaging $17,555 per year). Financial award application deadline: 4/1; financial award applicants required to submit FAFSA. *Faculty research:* Movement science, applied neuroscience, community mobility, rehabilitation outcomes, assistive technology/environmental interventions. *Unit head:* David Fuller, PhD, Professor and Program Director, 352-273-6634, Fax: 352-273-6109, E-mail: ddf@phhp.ufl.edu. *Application contact:* Amy Ladendorf, Rehabilitation Science Program Admissions, 352-273-6507, E-mail: gradinfo@ufl.edu.
Website: http://rehabsci.phhp.ufl.edu/

University of Maryland, Baltimore, Graduate School, Department of Medical and Research Technology, Baltimore, MD 21201. Offers MS. *Accreditation:* NAACLS. Part-time programs available. *Students:* 4 full-time (3 women), 6 part-time (4 women); includes 2 minority (1 Black or African American, non-Hispanic/Latino; 1 Asian, non-Hispanic/Latino), 6 international. Average age 31. 4 applicants, 75% accepted, 2 enrolled. In 2013, 4 master's awarded. *Degree requirements:* For master's, thesis or management project. *Entrance requirements:* For master's, GRE General Test, minimum GPA of 3.0. Additional exam requirements/recommendations for international students: Required—TOEFL (minimum score 550 paper-based; 80 iBT) or IELTS (minimum score 7). *Application deadline:* For fall admission, 5/1 priority date for domestic students, 1/15 for international students; for spring admission, 11/30 priority date for domestic students. Application fee: $75. Electronic applications accepted. *Financial support:* Fellowships and research assistantships available. Financial award application deadline: 3/1; financial award applicants required to submit FAFSA. *Faculty research:* Clinical microbiology, immunology, immunohematology, hematology, clinical chemistry, molecular biology. *Unit head:* Dr. Sanford Stass, Chair, 410-328-1237. *Application contact:* Dr. Ivana Vucenik, Graduate Program Director, 410-706-1832, E-mail: ivucenik@som.umaryland.edu.

University of Massachusetts Dartmouth, Graduate School, College of Engineering, Program in Biomedical Engineering and Biotechnology, North Dartmouth, MA 02747-2300. Offers bioengineering (PhD); biology (PhD); biomedical engineering/biotechnology (MS, PhD); chemistry (PhD); civil engineering (PhD); computer and information science (PhD); electrical/computer engineering (PhD); mathematics (PhD); mechanical engineering (PhD); medical laboratory science (PhD); physics (PhD). Part-time programs available. *Students:* 8 full-time (4 women), 18 part-time (10 women); includes 1 minority (Hispanic/Latino), 14 international. Average age 31. 28 applicants, 29% accepted, 3 enrolled. In 2013, 2 master's, 1 doctorate awarded. *Degree requirements:* For doctorate, comprehensive exam, thesis/dissertation. *Entrance requirements:* For master's and doctorate, GRE, statement of purpose (minimum of 300 words), resume, 3 letters of recommendation, official transcripts. Additional exam requirements/recommendations for international students: Required—TOEFL (minimum score 550 paper-based). *Application deadline:* For fall admission, 2/15 priority date for domestic students, 1/15 priority date for international students; for spring admission, 11/15 priority date for domestic students, 10/15 priority date for international students. Applications are processed on a rolling basis. Application fee: $60. Electronic applications accepted. *Expenses:* Tuition, state resident: full-time $2071; part-time $86.29 per credit. Tuition, nonresident: full-time $8099; part-time $337.46 per credit. Tuition and fees vary according to course load and reciprocity agreements. *Financial support:* In 2013–14, 1 fellowship with full tuition reimbursement (averaging $8,308 per year), 4 research assistantships with full tuition reimbursements (averaging $13,748 per year), 4 teaching assistantships with full tuition reimbursements (averaging $15,000 per year) were awarded; Federal Work-Study and unspecified assistantships also available. Support available to part-time students. Financial award application deadline: 3/1; financial award applicants required to submit FAFSA. *Faculty research:* Comparative immunology, vaccine design, biosensors, biomimetic materials, polymer science, soft electronics, hydrogels, regenerative biological materials. *Total annual research expenditures:* $894,000. *Unit head:* Sanka Bhowmick, Graduate Program Director for Engineering Options, 508-999-8619, Fax: 508-999-8881, E-mail: sbhowmick@umassd.edu. *Application contact:* Steven Briggs, Director of Marketing and Recruitment for Graduate Studies, 508-999-8604, Fax: 508-999-8183, E-mail: graduate@umassd.edu.
Website: http://www.umassd.edu/engineering/graduate/doctoraldegreeprograms/biomedicalengineeringandbiotechnology/

University of Massachusetts Lowell, College of Health Sciences, Department of Clinical Laboratory and Nutritional Sciences, Lowell, MA 01854-2881. Offers clinical laboratory sciences (MS); clinical pathology (Graduate Certificate); nutritional sciences (Graduate Certificate); public health laboratory sciences (Graduate Certificate). *Accreditation:* NAACLS. Part-time programs available. Postbaccalaureate distance learning degree programs offered. *Degree requirements:* For master's, thesis optional. *Entrance requirements:* For master's, GRE General Test, minimum GPA of 3.0, letters of recommendation. *Faculty research:* Cardiovascular disease, lipoprotein metabolism, micronutrient evaluation, alcohol metabolism, mycobacterial drug resistance.

University of Minnesota, Twin Cities Campus, College of Science and Engineering, Technological Leadership Institute, Program in Medical Device Innovation, Minneapolis, MN 55455-0213. Offers MS. *Faculty:* 8. *Students:* 18 (5 women); includes 1 minority (Black or African American, non-Hispanic/Latino), 3 international. *Entrance requirements:* Additional exam requirements/recommendations for international students: Required—TOEFL. Application fee: $75 ($95 for international students). Electronic applications accepted. *Faculty research:* Dynamics of medical device innovation, including technology innovation, project and business management, intellectual property, regulatory affairs, and public policy. *Unit head:* Dr. Massoud Amin, Director, 612-624-5747, Fax: 612-624-7510. *Application contact:* MDI Program, E-mail: mdi@umn.edu.
Website: http://tli.umn.edu/graduate/mdi

University of Nebraska Medical Center, School of Allied Health Professions, Program in Clinical Perfusion Education, Omaha, NE 68198-4144. Offers distance education perfusion education (MPS); perfusion science (MPS). *Accreditation:* NAACLS. Postbaccalaureate distance learning degree programs offered. *Degree requirements:* For master's, comprehensive exam, thesis. *Entrance requirements:* For master's, GRE. Electronic applications accepted. *Expenses: Required fees:* $300 per semester. Tuition and fees vary according to program. *Faculty research:* Platelet gel, hemoconcentrators.

University of Nebraska Medical Center, School of Allied Health Professions, Program in Cytotechnology, Omaha, NE 68198. Offers Certificate. *Accreditation:* NAACLS. Postbaccalaureate distance learning degree programs offered (minimal on-campus study). Electronic applications accepted. *Expenses: Required fees:* $300 per semester. Tuition and fees vary according to program. *Faculty research:* HPV vaccine.

University of New Mexico, School of Medicine, Master's Program in Clinical Laboratory Science, Albuquerque, NM 87131. Offers education (MS); laboratory management (MS); research and development (MS). Part-time programs available. *Faculty:* 1 full-time (0 women). *Students:* 1 full-time (0 women), 1 part-time (0 women); both minorities (both Hispanic/Latino). Average age 30. 1 applicant. In 2013, 1 master's awarded. *Degree requirements:* For master's, project thesis; presentation at national meeting. *Entrance requirements:* For master's, ASCP Board of Certification Exam. Additional exam requirements/recommendations for international students: Required—TOEFL. *Application deadline:* For fall admission, 7/15 priority date for domestic students, 6/15 priority date for international students. Application fee: $50. Electronic applications accepted. *Financial support:* In 2013–14, 1 student received support. Career-related internships or fieldwork available. Financial award application deadline: 7/15; financial award applicants required to submit FAFSA. *Faculty research:* Prostate cancer, educational techniques, online training, molecular diagnostics, laboratory medicine, laboratory management, laboratory test assessment. *Unit head:* Dr. Paul B. Roth, Dean, 505-272-8273, Fax: 505-272-6857. *Application contact:* Dr. Roberto Gomez, Associate Dean of Students, 505-272-3414, Fax: 505-272-6857, E-mail: rgomez@unm.edu.
Website: http://pathology.unm.edu/medical-laboratory-sciences/program/graduate-m.s.-degree-program.html

University of New Mexico, School of Medicine, Program in Biomedical Sciences, Program in Clinical and Translational Science, Albuquerque, NM 87131-2039. Offers Certificate. *Faculty:* 1 full-time (0 women). *Students:* 5 part-time (3 women); includes 2 minority (1 Asian, non-Hispanic/Latino; 1 Hispanic/Latino). Average age 38. 2 applicants, 50% accepted. In 2013, 3 Certificates awarded. *Unit head:* Dr. Helen J. Hathaway, Program Director, 505-272-1469, E-mail: hhathaway@salud.unm.edu. *Application contact:* Angel Cooke-Jackson, Coordinator, 505-272-1887, Fax: 505-272-8738, E-mail: acooke-jackson@salud.unm.edu.

University of North Dakota, Graduate School and Graduate School, Graduate Programs in Medicine, Department of Clinical Laboratory Science, Grand Forks, ND 58202. Offers MS. *Accreditation:* NAACLS. Postbaccalaureate distance learning degree programs offered (minimal on-campus study). *Degree requirements:* For master's, comprehensive exam, thesis or alternative. *Entrance requirements:* For master's, minimum GPA of 3.0. Additional exam requirements/recommendations for international students: Required—TOEFL (minimum score 550 paper-based; 79 iBT), IELTS (minimum score 5.5). Electronic applications accepted.

University of Pennsylvania, Perelman School of Medicine, Master's Program in Translational Research, Philadelphia, PA 19104-4283. Offers translational therapeutics (MTR); MD/MTR. *Faculty:* 45 full-time (14 women), 13 part-time/adjunct (5 women). *Students:* 15 full-time (8 women); includes 10 minority (3 Black or African American, non-Hispanic/Latino; 6 Asian, non-Hispanic/Latino; 1 Hispanic/Latino), 1 international. Average age 32. 22 applicants, 73% accepted, 15 enrolled. In 2013, 17 master's awarded. *Degree requirements:* For master's, thesis. *Entrance requirements:* For master's, curriculum vitae, personal statement, research plan, three recommendation letters including one from department chair or division chief and one from primary mentor. *Application deadline:* For fall admission, 4/1 priority date for domestic and international students. Applications are processed on a rolling basis. Application fee: $45. Electronic applications accepted. *Expenses:* Contact institution. *Financial support:* In 2013–14, 14 students received support, including 14 fellowships with full tuition reimbursements available. Financial award application deadline: 10/30. *Faculty research:* Treatment of acute kidney injury, functional neurosurgery, immune-based cancer therapy, treatment of metastatic melanoma, pediatric nephrology. *Unit head:* Dr. Emma A. Meagher, MD, Director, Translational Research Programs, 215-662-2174, Fax: 215-614-0378, E-mail: mtrpor@mail.med.upenn.edu. *Application contact:* Marti Dandridge, Coordinator, 215-349-8627, Fax: 215-614-0378, E-mail: mtrpor@mail.med.upenn.edu.
Website: http://www.itmat.upenn.edu/ctsa/mtr/index.shtml

University of Pittsburgh, School of Medicine, Clinical and Translational Science Graduate Program, Pittsburgh, PA 15260. Offers PhD. Part-time programs available. *Faculty:* 44 full-time (26 women). *Students:* 11 part-time (4 women); includes 5 minority (3 Black or African American, non-Hispanic/Latino; 1 Asian, non-Hispanic/Latino; 1 Hispanic/Latino), 1 international. Average age 36. 9 applicants, 44% accepted, 4 enrolled. In 2013, 2 doctorates awarded. *Degree requirements:* For doctorate, comprehensive exam, thesis/dissertation. *Entrance requirements:* For doctorate, MCAT, GRE, GMAT or PCAT. Additional exam requirements/recommendations for international students: Required—TOEFL (minimum score 600 paper-based; 100 iBT). *Application deadline:* For spring admission, 4/15 priority date for domestic and international students. Electronic applications accepted. *Expenses:* Tuition, state resident: full-time $19,964; part-time $807 per credit. Tuition, nonresident: full-time $32,686; part-time $1337 per credit. *Required fees:* $740; $200. Tuition and fees vary according to program. *Faculty research:* Research design and methodology, healthcare outcomes and process assessment, organ and tissue donation and transplantation, measuring and improving function in patients with chronic kidney disease. *Unit head:* Dr. Wishwa Kapoor, Program Director, 412-586-9670, Fax: 412-586-9672, E-mail: kapoorwn@upmc.edu. *Application contact:* Jennifer Holliman, Program Coordinator, 412-586-9673, Fax: 412-586-9672, E-mail: hollimanjm@upmc.edu.
Website: http://www.icre.pitt.edu/phd/index.html

University of Puerto Rico, Medical Sciences Campus, School of Health Professions, Program in Clinical Laboratory Science, San Juan, PR 00936-5067. Offers MS. *Accreditation:* NAACLS. Part-time and evening/weekend programs available. *Degree requirements:* For master's, one foreign language, thesis or alternative. *Entrance requirements:* For master's, EXADEP or GRE General Test, minimum GPA of 2.75, bachelor's degree in medical technology, 1 year lab experience, interview. *Faculty research:* Toxicology, virology, biochemistry, immunohematology, nervous system regeneration.

University of Puerto Rico, Medical Sciences Campus, School of Health Professions, Program in Cytotechnology, San Juan, PR 00936-5067. Offers Certificate. *Degree requirements:* For Certificate, one foreign language, research project. *Entrance requirements:* For degree, minimum GPA of 2.5, interview.

University of Puerto Rico, Medical Sciences Campus, School of Health Professions, Program in Medical Technology, San Juan, PR 00936-5067. Offers Certificate. Part-time programs available. *Degree requirements:* For Certificate, one foreign language, clinical practice. *Entrance requirements:* For degree, bachelor's degree in science, minimum GPA of 2.5.

University of Rhode Island, Graduate School, College of the Environment and Life Sciences, Department of Cell and Molecular Biology, Kingston, RI 02881. Offers biochemistry (MS, PhD); clinical laboratory sciences (MS), including biotechnology, clinical laboratory science, cytopathology; microbiology (MS, PhD); molecular genetics (MS, PhD). Part-time programs available. *Faculty:* 17 full-time (8 women), 2 part-time/adjunct (1 woman). *Students:* 19 full-time (11 women), 40 part-time (23 women); includes 14 minority (4 Black or African American, non-Hispanic/Latino; 1 American Indian or Alaska Native, non-Hispanic/Latino; 7 Asian, non-Hispanic/Latino; 2 Hispanic/Latino), 5 international. In 2013, 20 master's, 2 doctorates awarded. *Degree requirements:* For master's, comprehensive exam (for some programs), thesis optional; for doctorate, comprehensive exam, thesis/dissertation. *Entrance requirements:* For master's and doctorate, GRE, 2 letters of recommendation. Additional exam requirements/recommendations for international students: Required—TOEFL (minimum score 550 paper-based). *Application deadline:* For fall admission, 7/15 for domestic

students, 2/1 for international students; for spring admission, 11/15 for domestic students, 7/15 for international students. Application fee: $65. Electronic applications accepted. *Expenses:* Tuition, state resident: full-time $11,532; part-time $641 per credit. Tuition, nonresident: full-time $23,606; part-time $1311 per credit. *Required fees:* $1388; $36 per credit. $35 per semester. One-time fee: $130. *Financial support:* In 2013–14, 5 research assistantships with full and partial tuition reimbursements (averaging $12,078 per year), 2 teaching assistantships with full and partial tuition reimbursements (averaging $11,883 per year) were awarded. Financial award application deadline: 2/1; financial award applicants required to submit FAFSA. *Faculty research:* Genomics. *Total annual research expenditures:* $6.7 million. *Unit head:* Dr. Gongqing Sun, Chairperson, 401-874-5937, Fax: 401-874-2202, E-mail: gsun@mail.uri.edu. *Application contact:* Graduate Admissions, 401-874-2872, E-mail: gradadm@etal.uri.edu.
Website: http://cels.uri.edu/cmb/

University of Southern Mississippi, Graduate School, College of Health, Department of Medical Technology, Hattiesburg, MS 39406-0001. Offers MS. *Accreditation:* NAACLS. Part-time programs available. Postbaccalaureate distance learning degree programs offered. *Faculty:* 5 full-time (all women). *Students:* 13 full-time (8 women), 11 part-time (9 women); includes 4 minority (3 Black or African American, non-Hispanic/Latino; 1 Asian, non-Hispanic/Latino), 2 international. Average age 33. 5 applicants, 80% accepted, 2 enrolled. In 2013, 6 master's awarded. *Degree requirements:* For master's, comprehensive exam, thesis (for some programs). *Entrance requirements:* For master's, GRE General Test, minimum GPA of 2.75. Additional exam requirements/recommendations for international students: Required—TOEFL, IELTS. *Application deadline:* For fall admission, 3/1 priority date for domestic students, 3/1 for international students; for spring admission, 1/10 priority date for domestic and international students. Application fee: $50. Electronic applications accepted. *Financial support:* In 2013–14, 3 teaching assistantships with full tuition reimbursements (averaging $7,200 per year) were awarded; research assistantships, career-related internships or fieldwork, Federal Work-Study, institutionally sponsored loans, scholarships/grants, health care benefits, and unspecified assistantships also available. Financial award application deadline: 3/15; financial award applicants required to submit FAFSA. *Faculty research:* Clinical chemistry, clinical microbiology, hematology, clinical management and education, immunohematology. *Unit head:* Dr. Mary Lux, Chair, 601-266-4908. *Application contact:* Shonna Breland, Manager of Graduate Admissions, 601-266-6563, Fax: 601-266-5138.
Website: http://www.usm.edu/graduateschool/table.php

The University of Tennessee Health Science Center, College of Graduate Health Sciences, Memphis, TN 38163-0002. Offers biomedical engineering (MS, PhD); biomedical sciences (PhD); dental sciences (MDS); epidemiology (MS); health outcomes and policy research (PhD); laboratory research and management (MS); nursing science (PhD); pharmaceutical sciences (PhD); pharmacology (MS); speech and hearing science (PhD); DDS/PhD; DNP/PhD; MD/PhD; Pharm D/PhD. *Faculty:* 318 full-time (92 women), 59 part-time/adjunct (16 women). *Students:* 220 full-time (102 women), 22 part-time (13 women); includes 194 minority (22 Black or African American, non-Hispanic/Latino; 161 Asian, non-Hispanic/Latino; 7 Hispanic/Latino; 3 Native Hawaiian or other Pacific Islander, non-Hispanic/Latino; 1 Two or more races, non-Hispanic/Latino), 106 international. Average age 25. 404 applicants, 17% accepted, 64 enrolled. In 2013, 13 master's, 25 doctorates awarded. Terminal master's awarded for partial completion of doctoral program. *Degree requirements:* For master's, comprehensive exam, thesis; for doctorate, comprehensive exam, thesis/dissertation, oral and written preliminary and comprehensive exams. *Entrance requirements:* For master's and doctorate, GRE General Test, minimum GPA of 3.0. Additional exam requirements/recommendations for international students: Required—TOEFL (minimum score 79 iBT); Recommended—IELTS (minimum score 6.5). *Application deadline:* For fall admission, 5/15 priority date for domestic students. Applications are processed on a rolling basis. Application fee: $0. Electronic applications accepted. *Financial support:* In 2013–14, 125 students received support, including 125 research assistantships (averaging $23,000 per year); career-related internships or fieldwork, Federal Work-Study, institutionally sponsored loans, and tuition waivers (full and partial) also available. Support available to part-time students. Financial award application deadline: 2/25; financial award applicants required to submit FAFSA. *Unit head:* Dr. Donald B. Thomason, Dean, 901-448-5538, E-mail: dthomaso@uthsc.edu. *Application contact:* William Carter, Director for Admissions, 901-448-1687, E-mail: wcarte17@uthsc.edu.
Website: http://www.uthsc.edu/grad/

The University of Tennessee Health Science Center, College of Health Professions, Memphis, TN 38163-0002. Offers audiology (MS, Au D); clinical laboratory science (MSCLS); cytopathology practice (MCP); health informatics and information management (MHIIM); occupational therapy (MOT); physical therapy (DPT, ScDPT); physician assistant (MMS); speech-language pathology (MS). *Accreditation:* AOTA; APTA. Part-time and evening/weekend programs available. Postbaccalaureate distance learning degree programs offered (minimal on-campus study). Terminal master's awarded for partial completion of doctoral program. *Degree requirements:* For master's, comprehensive exam, thesis; for doctorate, comprehensive exam, residency. *Entrance requirements:* For master's, GRE (MOT, MSCLS), minimum GPA of 3.0, 3 letters of reference, national accreditation (MSCLS), GRE if GPA is less than 3.0 (MCP); for doctorate, GRE. Additional exam requirements/recommendations for international students: Required—TOEFL (minimum score 550 paper-based; 80 iBT). *Application deadline:* For fall admission, 1/30 priority date for domestic students; for winter admission, 10/1 priority date for domestic students. Application fee: $50. Electronic applications accepted. *Expenses:* Contact institution. *Financial support:* Teaching assistantships, Federal Work-Study, institutionally sponsored loans, and scholarships/grants available. Support available to part-time students. Financial award application deadline: 2/15; financial award applicants required to submit FAFSA. *Faculty research:* Gait deviation, muscular dystrophy and strength, hemophilia and exercise, pediatric neurology, self-efficacy. *Unit head:* Dr. Noma Anderson, Dean, 901-528-5588, Fax: 901-528-7545, E-mail: nander13@uthsc.edu. *Application contact:* Dr. Noma Anderson, Dean, 901-528-5588, Fax: 901-528-7545, E-mail: nander13@uthsc.edu.
Website: http://www.uthsc.edu/health-professions/

The University of Texas at Austin, Graduate School, College of Pharmacy, Graduate Programs in Pharmacy, Austin, TX 78712-1111. Offers health outcomes and pharmacy practice (PhD); health outcomes and pharmacy practice (MS); medicinal chemistry (PhD); pharmaceutics (PhD); pharmacology and toxicology (PhD); pharmacotherapy (MS, PhD); translational science (PhD). PhD in translational science offered jointly with The University of Texas Health Science Center at San Antonio and The University of Texas at San Antonio. *Degree requirements:* For master's, thesis; for doctorate, thesis/dissertation. *Entrance requirements:* For master's and doctorate, GRE General Test. Electronic applications accepted. *Faculty research:* Synthetic medical chemistry, synthetic molecular biology, bio-organic chemistry, pharmacoeconomics, pharmacy practice.

The University of Texas Health Science Center at San Antonio, Graduate School of Biomedical Sciences, Translational Science Program, San Antonio, TX 78229-3900. Offers PhD. Part-time programs available. *Faculty:* 8 part-time/adjunct (3 women). *Students:* 9 part-time (7 women); includes 4 minority (2 Asian, non-Hispanic/Latino; 2 Hispanic/Latino), 1 international. Average age 40. 32 applicants, 16% accepted, 2 enrolled. *Degree requirements:* For doctorate, comprehensive exam, thesis/dissertation. *Entrance requirements:* For doctorate, GRE if minimum educational requirement is less than a doctoral degree; waived if student has a graduate degree from a participating university. Additional exam requirements/recommendations for international students: Required—TOEFL or IELTS. *Application deadline:* For fall admission, 12/1 for domestic and international students. Application fee: $0. Electronic applications accepted. *Financial support:* In 2013–14, 2 research assistantships (averaging $26,000 per year) were awarded. *Faculty research:* Inflammation - tissue injury, regeneration, disease; antibiotic resistance among Gram-positive bacteria; comparative effectiveness research; patient centered outcomes research; schistosomiasis pathogenesis; epilepsy; role of oxidative and nitrative stress in placental function; integrated systems computational biology - kinetic modeling of metabolic and cell signaling pathways. *Unit head:* Dr. Michael J. Lichtenstein, Professor in Internal Medicine/Director, Translational Science PhD Program, 210-567-4304, Fax: 210-567-4301, E-mail: lichtenstei@uthscsa.edu. *Application contact:* Susan Stappenbeck, Senior Project Coordinator, 210-567-4304, Fax: 210-567-4301, E-mail: stappenbeck@uthscsa.edu.
Website: http://iims.uthscsa.edu/ed_trans_sci_phd.html

The University of Texas Medical Branch, Graduate School of Biomedical Sciences, Program in Clinical Science, Galveston, TX 77555. Offers MS, PhD.

University of Utah, School of Medicine and Graduate School, Graduate Programs in Medicine, Department of Pathology, Program in Laboratory Medicine and Biomedical Science, Salt Lake City, UT 84112-1107. Offers MS. Part-time programs available. *Degree requirements:* For master's, comprehensive exam, thesis, thesis research. *Entrance requirements:* For master's, minimum GPA of 3.0 during last 2 years of undergraduate course work, BS in medical laboratory science or related field. Additional exam requirements/recommendations for international students: Required—TOEFL (minimum score 550 paper-based). *Expenses:* Tuition, state resident: full-time $5259. Tuition, nonresident: full-time $18,569. *Required fees:* $841. Tuition and fees vary according to course load. *Faculty research:* Clinical chemistry, hematology, diagnostic microbiology, immunohematology, cell biology, immunology.

University of Vermont, College of Medicine and Graduate College, Graduate Programs in Medicine, Program in Clinical and Translational Science, Burlington, VT 05405. Offers MS, PhD. *Students:* 13 (6 women), 2 international. 5 applicants, 20% accepted, 1 enrolled. In 2013, 2 master's, 3 doctorates awarded. *Entrance requirements:* For master's and doctorate, GRE. Additional exam requirements/recommendations for international students: Recommended—TOEFL (minimum score 550 paper-based; 80 iBT). *Application deadline:* For fall admission, 5/1 for domestic and international students. Applications are processed on a rolling basis. Application fee: $65. Electronic applications accepted. *Financial support:* Teaching assistantships available. *Unit head:* Dr. Alan Rubin, Director, 802-656-8228, E-mail: alan.rubin@uvm.edu.

University of Washington, Graduate School, School of Medicine, Graduate Programs in Medicine, Department of Laboratory Medicine, Seattle, WA 98195. Offers MS. *Accreditation:* NAACLS. Part-time programs available. *Degree requirements:* For master's, thesis. *Entrance requirements:* For master's, GRE General Test, medical technology certification or specialist in an area of laboratory medicine.

Virginia Commonwealth University, Graduate School, School of Allied Health Professions, Department of Clinical Laboratory Sciences, Richmond, VA 23284-9005. Offers MS. *Accreditation:* NAACLS. *Degree requirements:* For master's, one foreign language, thesis. *Entrance requirements:* For master's, GRE General Test, major in clinical laboratory sciences, biology, or chemistry; minimum GPA of 2.7. Additional exam requirements/recommendations for international students: Required—TOEFL (minimum score 600 paper-based; 100 iBT); Recommended—IELTS (minimum score 6.5). Electronic applications accepted. *Faculty research:* Educational outcomes assessment, virtual instrumentation development, cost-effective treatment of bacteremia using third generation cephalosporins.

Virginia Commonwealth University, Graduate School, School of Allied Health Professions, Doctoral Program in Health Related Sciences, Richmond, VA 23284-9005. Offers clinical laboratory sciences (PhD); gerontology (PhD); health administration (PhD); nurse anesthesia (PhD); occupational therapy (PhD); physical therapy (PhD); radiation sciences (PhD); rehabilitation leadership (PhD). *Entrance requirements:* For doctorate, GRE General Test or MAT, minimum GPA of 3.3 in master's degree. Additional exam requirements/recommendations for international students: Required—TOEFL (minimum score 600 paper-based; 100 iBT); Recommended—IELTS (minimum score 6.5). Electronic applications accepted.

Clinical Research

Albert Einstein College of Medicine, Graduate Division of Biomedical Sciences, Clinical Investigation Program, Bronx, NY 10461. Offers PhD.

American University of Health Sciences, School of Clinical Research, Signal Hill, CA 90755. Offers MSCR.

Boston University, School of Medicine, Division of Graduate Medical Sciences, Program in Clinical Investigation, Boston, MA 02215. Offers MA. *Degree requirements:* For master's, thesis. *Application deadline:* For spring admission, 10/15 for domestic students. *Expenses:* *Tuition:* Full-time $43,970; part-time $1374 per credit hour. *Required fees:* $60 per semester. Tuition and fees vary according to class time, course level and program. *Unit head:* Dr. Susan S. Fish, Director, 617-638-7715, E-mail: sfish@bu.edu. *Application contact:* Stacey Hess Pino, Assistant Director, 617-638-5211, Fax: 617-638-5740, E-mail: sahess@bu.edu.
Website: http://www.bumc.bu.edu/gms/maci/

Case Western Reserve University, School of Medicine, Clinical Research Scholars Program, Cleveland, OH 44106. Offers MS.

Duke University, School of Medicine, Clinical Research Program, Durham, NC 27708-0586. Offers MHS. Part-time programs available. *Faculty:* 23 part-time/adjunct (6 women). *Students:* 15 full-time (10 women), 98 part-time (60 women); includes 31 minority (7 Black or African American, non-Hispanic/Latino; 22 Asian, non-Hispanic/Latino; 2 Hispanic/Latino), 14 international. 73 applicants, 96% accepted, 70 enrolled. In 2013, 43 master's awarded. *Degree requirements:* For master's, research project. *Entrance requirements:* For master's, GRE. Additional exam requirements/recommendations for international students: Required—TOEFL. *Application deadline:* For fall admission, 5/15 for domestic students. *Expenses:* Contact institution. *Financial support:* Fellowships, research assistantships, teaching assistantships, and scholarships/grants available. Financial award application deadline: 5/1; financial award applicants required to submit FAFSA. *Unit head:* Dr. Steven C. Grambow, Director, 919-286-0411, Fax: 919-681-4569, E-mail: steven.grambow@duke.edu. *Application contact:* Gail Ladd, Program Coordinator, 919-681-4560, Fax: 919-681-4569, E-mail: gail.ladd@duke.edu.
Website: http://crtp.mc.duke.edu/

Eastern Michigan University, Graduate School, College of Health and Human Services, School of Health Sciences, Program in Clinical Research Administration, Ypsilanti, MI 48197. Offers MS, Graduate Certificate. Part-time and evening/weekend programs available. Postbaccalaureate distance learning degree programs offered (minimal on-campus study). *Students:* 14 full-time (8 women), 21 part-time (14 women); includes 4 minority (2 Black or African American, non-Hispanic/Latino; 2 Two or more races, non-Hispanic/Latino), 17 international. Average age 30. 51 applicants, 53% accepted, 17 enrolled. In 2013, 18 master's, 2 other advanced degrees awarded. *Entrance requirements:* Additional exam requirements/recommendations for international students: Required—TOEFL. *Application deadline:* Applications are processed on a rolling basis. Application fee: $35. *Expenses:* Tuition, state resident: full-time $12,300; part-time $466 per credit hour. Tuition, nonresident: full-time $23,159; part-time $918 per credit hour. *Required fees:* $71 per credit hour. $46 per semester. One-time fee: $100. Tuition and fees vary according to course level and degree level. *Financial support:* Fellowships, research assistantships with full tuition reimbursements, teaching assistantships with full tuition reimbursements, career-related internships or fieldwork, Federal Work-Study, institutionally sponsored loans, scholarships/grants, tuition waivers (partial), and unspecified assistantships available. Support available to part-time students. Financial award applicants required to submit FAFSA. *Unit head:* Dr. Colleen Croxall, Director, 734-487-4096, Fax: 734-487-4095, E-mail: ccroxall@emich.edu. *Application contact:* Dr. Stephen Sonstein, Program Director, 734-487-1238, Fax: 734-487-4095, E-mail: stephen.sonstein@emich.edu.

Emory University, Laney Graduate School, Program in Clinical Research, Atlanta, GA 30322-1100. Offers MS. *Degree requirements:* For master's, thesis. *Entrance requirements:* Additional exam requirements/recommendations for international students: Recommended—TOEFL. Electronic applications accepted.

Georgia Regents University, The Graduate School, Program in Clinical and Translational Science, Augusta, GA 30912. Offers MCTS, CCTS.

Icahn School of Medicine at Mount Sinai, Graduate School of Biological Sciences, New York, NY 10029-6504. Offers biomedical sciences (MS, PhD); clinical research education (MS, PhD); community medicine (MPH); genetic counseling (MS); neurosciences (PhD); MD/PhD. Terminal master's awarded for partial completion of doctoral program. *Degree requirements:* For master's, thesis; for doctorate, comprehensive exam, thesis/dissertation. *Entrance requirements:* For master's, GRE General Test; for doctorate, GRE General Test, GRE Subject Test, 3 years of college pre-med course work. Additional exam requirements/recommendations for international students: Required—TOEFL. Electronic applications accepted. *Faculty research:* Cancer, genetics and genomics, immunology, neuroscience, developmental and stem cell biology, translational research.

Johns Hopkins University, Bloomberg School of Public Health, Graduate Training Program in Clinical Investigation, Baltimore, MD 21287. Offers MHS, Sc M, PhD. *Faculty:* 18 full-time (5 women). *Students:* 14 full-time (11 women), 29 part-time (18 women); includes 17 minority (4 Black or African American, non-Hispanic/Latino; 8 Asian, non-Hispanic/Latino; 2 Hispanic/Latino; 3 Two or more races, non-Hispanic/Latino), 4 international. Average age 35. 30 applicants, 87% accepted, 15 enrolled. In 2013, 11 master's, 8 doctorates awarded. *Degree requirements:* For master's, comprehensive exam, thesis; for doctorate, comprehensive exam, thesis/dissertation. *Entrance requirements:* For master's, GRE or MCAT; United States Medical Licensing Exam, 2 letters of recommendation, curriculum vitae, transcripts, statement of purpose; for doctorate, GRE or MCAT; United States Medical Licensing Exam, 2 letters of recommendation, curriculum vitae. Additional exam requirements/recommendations for international students: Required—TOEFL (minimum score 600 paper-based). *Application deadline:* For spring admission, 3/1 for domestic and international students. Applications are processed on a rolling basis. Application fee: $45. Electronic applications accepted. *Financial support:* Fellowships with partial tuition reimbursements, institutionally sponsored loans, scholarships/grants, and stipends available. Support available to part-time students. Financial award application deadline: 3/15; financial award applicants required to submit FAFSA. *Faculty research:* Ethical issues, biomedical writing, grant writing, epidemiology, biostatistics. *Unit head:* Dr. N. Franklin Adkinson, Jr., Director, 410-550-2051, Fax: 410-550-2055, E-mail: fadkinso@jhmi.edu. *Application contact:* Kristi Baschnagel, Senior Academic Coordinator, 410-502-6965, Fax: 410-502-6966, E-mail: gtpci@jhsph.edu.
Website: http://www.jhsph.edu/gtpci/

Loyola University Chicago, Graduate School, Program in Clinical Research Methods, Chicago, IL 60660. Offers MS. Part-time programs available. *Faculty:* 5 full-time (2 women). *Students:* 5 part-time (4 women); includes 2 minority (both Asian, non-Hispanic/Latino). Average age 33. 10 applicants, 20% accepted, 2 enrolled. In 2013, 8 master's awarded. *Degree requirements:* For master's, research project. *Entrance requirements:* For master's, MCAT; GRE. *Application deadline:* For fall admission, 5/15 for domestic students, 5/1 for international students; for spring admission, 12/15 for domestic students, 12/1 for international students. Applications are processed on a rolling basis. Electronic applications accepted. Application fee is waived when completed online. *Expenses: Tuition:* Full-time $16,740; part-time $930 per credit. *Required fees:* $135 per semester. *Financial support:* Applicants required to submit FAFSA. *Faculty research:* Genetics of hypertension and obesity, Vitamin D metabolism, kidney diseases. *Unit head:* Dr. Samuel Attoh, Dean, 773-508-3459, Fax: 773-508-2460, E-mail: sattoh@luc.edu. *Application contact:* Ron Martin, Assistant Director of Enrollment Management, 312-915-8950, Fax: 312-915-8905, E-mail: gradapp@luc.edu.

Medical College of Wisconsin, Graduate School of Biomedical Sciences, Medical Scientist Training Program, Milwaukee, WI 53226-0509. Offers MD/PhD. *Entrance requirements:* Additional exam requirements/recommendations for international students: Required—TOEFL.

Medical University of South Carolina, College of Graduate Studies, South Carolina Clinical and Translational Research Institute, Charleston, SC 29425-5010. Offers MS. Postbaccalaureate distance learning degree programs offered (no on-campus study). *Degree requirements:* For master's, thesis, oral dissertation of grant proposal. *Entrance requirements:* For master's, essay, letter of support. Additional exam requirements/recommendations for international students: Required—TOEFL (minimum score 600 paper-based; 100 iBT). Electronic applications accepted. *Faculty research:* Cardiovascular epidemiology/hypertension, cystic fibrosis, comparative effectivenessstudies, community-engaged research.

Memorial University of Newfoundland, Faculty of Medicine and School of Graduate Studies, Graduate Programs in Medicine, Division of Applied Health Services Research, St. John's, NL A1C 5S7, Canada. Offers M Sc.

Morehouse School of Medicine, Master of Science in Clinical Research Program, Atlanta, GA 30310-1495. Offers MS. Part-time programs available. *Students:* 8 full-time (6 women), 1 (woman) part-time; includes 3 minority (2 Black or African American, non-Hispanic/Latino; 1 Hispanic/Latino), 1 international. *Degree requirements:* For master's, thesis. *Application deadline:* For fall admission, 4/6 for domestic and international students. Application fee: $0. Electronic applications accepted. *Expenses: Tuition:* Full-time $36,903; part-time $523 per credit hour. *Required fees:* $6470; $5650 per year. Tuition and fees vary according to course load, degree level, program and student level. *Financial support:* Applicants required to submit FAFSA. *Unit head:* Dr. Elizabeth Ofili, Director, 404-756-5051, E-mail: eofili@msm.edu. *Application contact:* Brandon Hunter, Director of Admissions, 404-752-1650, Fax: 404-752-1512, E-mail: bhunter@msm.edu.
Website: http://www.msm.edu/Education/GEBS/MSinClinicalResearch.php

New York University, College of Dentistry, Program in Clinical Research, New York, NY 10010. Offers MS. Part-time programs available. *Faculty:* 242 full-time (85 women), 689 part-time/adjunct (186 women). *Students:* 21 full-time (16 women); includes 4 minority (3 Asian, non-Hispanic/Latino; 1 Hispanic/Latino), 14 international. Average age 29. 49 applicants, 47% accepted, 16 enrolled. In 2013, 10 master's awarded. *Entrance requirements:* For master's, GRE. Additional exam requirements/recommendations for international students: Required—TOEFL (minimum score 570 paper-based; 90 iBT). *Application deadline:* For fall admission, 2/28 for domestic and international students. Application fee: $100. Electronic applications accepted. *Expenses: Tuition:* Full-time $35,856; part-time $1494 per unit. *Required fees:* $1408; $64 per unit. $473 per term. Tuition and fees vary according to course load and program. *Financial support:* Application deadline: 3/1. *Unit head:* Dr. Ananda Dasanayake, Program Director, 212-998-9631, Fax: 212-998-9766, E-mail: ad75@nyu.edu. *Application contact:* Julianna Cools, Administrative Aide, 212-998-9934, Fax: 212-995-4317, E-mail: jc1290@nyu.edu.
Website: http://dental.nyu.edu/academicprograms/masters-degree-programs/clinical-research.html

Northwestern University, Fienberg School of Medicine, Program in Clinical Investigation, Evanston, IL 60208. Offers MSCI. Part-time and evening/weekend programs available. *Entrance requirements:* For master's, GRE or MCAT, doctoral degree in healthcare-related field. Additional exam requirements/recommendations for international students: Required—TOEFL. Electronic applications accepted. *Faculty research:* Clinical research.

Northwestern University, The Graduate School, Program in Clinical Investigation, Evanston, IL 60208. Offers MSCI, Certificate. Part-time and evening/weekend programs available.

Northwestern University, School of Professional Studies, Program in Regulatory Compliance, Evanston, IL 60208. Offers clinical research (MS); healthcare compliance (MS); quality systems (MS). Offered in partnership with Northwestern Univesity's Clinical and Translational Sciences Institute.

Oregon Health & Science University, School of Medicine, Graduate Programs in Medicine, Human Investigations Program, Portland, OR 97239-3098. Offers clinical research (MCR, Certificate). MCR program only open to those currently enrolled in the certificate program. Part-time programs available. *Faculty:* 14 part-time/adjunct (9 women). *Students:* 95 part-time (53 women); includes 26 minority (2 Black or African American, non-Hispanic/Latino; 20 Asian, non-Hispanic/Latino; 3 Hispanic/Latino; 1 Two or more races, non-Hispanic/Latino), 9 international. Average age 36. 46 applicants, 78% accepted, 36 enrolled. In 2013, 13 master's, 13 Certificates awarded. *Entrance requirements:* For master's and Certificate, MD, MD/PhD, DO, DDS, DMD, DC, Pharm D, OD, ND or PhD with clinical responsibilities or patient-oriented research; faculty or staff member, clinical or post-doctoral fellows and graduate students at OHSU, Kaiser Permanente, Portland VA Medical Center or other health care facilities in Oregon or the Northwest. *Application deadline:* For fall admission, 7/15 for domestic students; for winter admission, 12/15 for domestic students; for spring admission, 3/15 for domestic students. Applications are processed on a rolling basis. Electronic applications accepted. *Unit head:* Dr. Cynthia Morris, Director, 503-494-3095, Fax: 503-494-5128, E-mail: morrisc@ohsu.edu. *Application contact:* Karen McCracken, Education Program Coordinator, 503-494-3095, Fax: 503-494-5128, E-mail: hip@ohsu.edu.
Website: http://www.ohsu.edu/hip

Palmer College of Chiropractic, Division of Graduate Studies, Davenport, IA 52803-5287. Offers clinical research (MS). *Degree requirements:* For master's, 2 mentored practicum projects. *Entrance requirements:* For master's, GRE General Test, minimum GPA of 2.5, bachelor's and doctoral-level health professions degrees. Additional exam requirements/recommendations for international students: Required—TOEFL. Electronic applications accepted. *Expenses:* Contact institution. *Faculty research:* Chiropractic clinical research.

Temple University, College of Health Professions and Social Work, Department of Public Health, Philadelphia, PA 19122. Offers clinical research and translational medicine (MS); environmental health (MPH); epidemiology (MS); epidemiology and biostatistics (MPH); health policy (PhD); health policy and management (MPH); school health education (Ed M); social and behavioral sciences (MPH, PhD). *Accreditation:* CEPH (one or more programs are accredited). Part-time and evening/weekend programs available. *Faculty:* 27 full-time (18 women). *Students:* 47 full-time (30 women), 45 part-time (37 women); includes 27 minority (9 Black or African American, non-Hispanic/Latino; 10 Asian, non-Hispanic/Latino; 7 Hispanic/Latino; 1 Two or more races, non-Hispanic/Latino), 9 international. 188 applicants, 45% accepted, 29 enrolled. In 2013, 29 master's, 3 doctorates awarded. Terminal master's awarded for partial completion of doctoral program. *Degree requirements:* For master's, thesis (for some programs), capstone project; for doctorate, comprehensive exam, thesis/dissertation. *Entrance requirements:* For master's, GRE General Test (for MS only); DAT, GMAT, MCAT, OAT, PCAT (alternates for MPH, Ed M), minimum undergraduate GPA of 3.0, letters of reference, statement of goals, writing sample, resume, interview (only for MS); for doctorate, GRE General Test, minimum undergraduate GPA of 3.0, 3 letters of reference, statement of goals, writing sample, resume. Additional exam requirements/recommendations for international students: Required—TOEFL (minimum score 550 paper-based; 79 iBT). *Application deadline:* For fall admission, 3/1 for domestic students, 2/1 for international students; for spring admission, 10/15 for domestic students, 8/1 for international students. Applications are processed on a rolling basis. Application fee: $60. Electronic applications accepted. *Financial support:* In 2013–14, 1 fellowship with tuition reimbursement, 4 research assistantships with tuition reimbursements, 8 teaching assistantships with tuition reimbursements were awarded; career-related internships or fieldwork, Federal Work-Study, scholarships/grants, tuition

waivers (partial), and unspecified assistantships also available. Financial award application deadline: 1/15. *Faculty research:* Smoking cessation, obesity prevention, tobacco policy, community engagement, health communication. *Total annual research expenditures:* $3.9 million. *Unit head:* Dr. Alice J. Hausman, Chair, 215-204-5112, Fax: 215-204-1854, E-mail: hausman@temple.edu. *Application contact:* Joyce Hankins, 215-204-7213, E-mail: joyce.hankins@temple.edu.
Website: http://chpsw.temple.edu/publichealth/home

Thomas Jefferson University, Jefferson Graduate School of Biomedical Sciences, Certificate Programs in Clinical Research, Human Clinical Investigation, and Infectious Diseases, Philadelphia, PA 19107. Offers clinical research and trials (Certificate); human clinical investigation (Certificate); infectious disease control (Certificate). *Faculty:* 44 full-time (14 women), 27 part-time/adjunct (11 women). *Students:* 15 part-time (9 women); includes 3 minority (1 Black or African American, non-Hispanic/Latino; 1 Asian, non-Hispanic/Latino; 1 Hispanic/Latino), 1 international. 8 applicants, 100% accepted, 6 enrolled. In 2013, 3 Certificates awarded. *Entrance requirements:* For degree, GRE General Test (recommended). Additional exam requirements/recommendations for international students: Required—TOEFL (minimum score 100 iBT) or IELTS (minimum score 7). *Application deadline:* For fall admission, 8/1 priority date for domestic students, 3/1 priority date for international students; for winter admission, 12/1 priority date for domestic students, 6/1 priority date for international students; for spring admission, 4/1 priority date for domestic students. Applications are processed on a rolling basis. Application fee: $75. Electronic applications accepted. *Financial support:* Federal Work-Study and institutionally sponsored loans available. Support available to part-time students. Financial award application deadline: 5/1; financial award applicants required to submit FAFSA. *Faculty research:* Epidemiology, clinical research, statistics, planning and management, disease control. *Unit head:* Dr. Dennis M. Gross, Associate Dean, 215-503-0156, Fax: 215-503-3433, E-mail: dennis.gross@jefferson.edu. *Application contact:* Marc E. Stearns, Director of Admissions, 215-503-0155, Fax: 215-503-3433, E-mail: jgsbs-info@jefferson.edu.
Website: http://www.jefferson.edu/university/biomedical_sciences/programs/certificates.html

Trident University International, College of Health Sciences, Program in Health Sciences, Cypress, CA 90630. Offers clinical research administration (MS, Certificate); emergency and disaster management (MS, Certificate); environmental health science (Certificate); health care administration (PhD); health care management (MS), including health informatics; health education (MS, Certificate); health informatics (Certificate); health sciences (PhD); international health (MS); international health: educator or researcher option (PhD); international health: practitioner option (PhD); law and expert witness studies (MS, Certificate); public health (MS); quality assurance (Certificate). Part-time and evening/weekend programs available. Postbaccalaureate distance learning degree programs offered (no on-campus study). *Degree requirements:* For doctorate, comprehensive exam, thesis/dissertation, defense of dissertation. *Entrance requirements:* For master's, minimum GPA of 2.5 (students with GPA 3.0 or greater may transfer up to 30% of graduate level credits); for doctorate, minimum GPA of 3.4, curriculum vitae, course work in research methods or statistics. Additional exam requirements/recommendations for international students: Required—TOEFL. Electronic applications accepted.

Tufts University, Sackler School of Graduate Biomedical Sciences, Clinical and Translational Science Program, Medford, MA 02155. Offers MS, PhD. *Faculty:* 34 full-time (10 women). *Students:* 24 full-time (11 women), 3 part-time (2 women); includes 3 minority (all Asian, non-Hispanic/Latino), 8 international. Average age 37. 20 applicants, 65% accepted, 10 enrolled. In 2013, 13 master's, 1 doctorate awarded. Terminal master's awarded for partial completion of doctoral program. *Degree requirements:* For master's, thesis; for doctorate, comprehensive exam, thesis/dissertation. *Entrance requirements:* For master's, MD or PhD, strong clinical research background. Additional exam requirements/recommendations for international students: Required—TOEFL (minimum score 600 paper-based; 100 iBT). *Application deadline:* For fall admission, 12/15 for domestic and international students. Application fee: $70. Electronic applications accepted. *Financial support:* Application deadline: 12/15. *Faculty research:* Clinical study design, mathematical modeling, meta analysis, epidemiologic research, coronary heart disease. *Unit head:* Dr. David Kent, Program Director, 617-636-3234, Fax: 617-636-8023, E-mail: dkent@tuftsmedicalcenter.edu. *Application contact:* Kellie Melchin, Associate Director of Admissions, 617-636-6767, Fax: 617-636-0375, E-mail: sackler-school@tufts.edu.
Website: http://sackler.tufts.edu/Academics/Degree-Programs/PhD-Programs/Clinical-and-Translational-Science

University of California, Berkeley, UC Berkeley Extension, Certificate Programs in Sciences, Biotechnology and Mathematics, Berkeley, CA 94720-1500. Offers clinical research conduct and management (Certificate). Postbaccalaureate distance learning degree programs offered.

University of California, Davis, Graduate Studies, Graduate Group in Clinical Research, Davis, CA 95616. Offers MAS. *Degree requirements:* For master's, comprehensive exam. *Entrance requirements:* Additional exam requirements/recommendations for international students: Required—TOEFL (minimum score 550 paper-based).

University of California, Los Angeles, David Geffen School of Medicine and Graduate Division, Graduate Programs in Medicine, Department of Biomathematics, Program in Clinical Research, Los Angeles, CA 90095. Offers MS. *Degree requirements:* For master's, thesis. *Entrance requirements:* For master's, GRE General Test, bachelor's degree; minimum undergraduate GPA of 3.0 (or its equivalent if letter grade system not used). Additional exam requirements/recommendations for international students: Required—TOEFL. Electronic applications accepted.

University of California, San Diego, School of Medicine, Program in Clinical Research, La Jolla, CA 92093. Offers MAS. Part-time programs available. *Students:* 4 full-time (2 women), 41 part-time (22 women); includes 12 minority (2 Black or African American, non-Hispanic/Latino; 6 Asian, non-Hispanic/Latino; 4 Hispanic/Latino), 22 international. 21 applicants, 100% accepted, 19 enrolled. In 2013, 33 master's awarded. *Degree requirements:* For master's, independent study project. *Entrance requirements:* For master's, minimum GPA of 3.0. Additional exam requirements/recommendations for international students: Required—TOEFL (minimum score 80 iBT), IELTS. *Application deadline:* For winter admission, 10/1 for domestic students; for summer admission, 4/29 for domestic students. Application fee: $80 ($100 for international students). Electronic applications accepted. *Expenses:* Tuition, state resident: full-time $11,220; part-time $1870 per quarter. Tuition, nonresident: full-time $26,322; part-time $4387 per quarter. *Required fees:* $519.50 per quarter. Part-time tuition and fees vary according to course load and program. *Financial support:* Scholarships/grants available. Financial award applicants required to submit FAFSA. *Unit head:* Ravindra Mehta, Program Director, 619-543-7310, E-mail: rmehta@ucsd.edu. *Application contact:* Hailey Marshall, Program Coordinator, 858-534-9164, E-mail: clre@ucsd.edu.
Website: http://clre.ucsd.edu/

University of Colorado Denver, School of Medicine, Clinical Science Graduate Program, Aurora, CO 80045. Offers clinical investigation (PhD); clinical sciences (MS); health information technology (PhD); health services research (PhD). *Students:* 25 full-time (17 women), 29 part-time (15 women); includes 10 minority (2 Black or African American, non-Hispanic/Latino; 2 Asian, non-Hispanic/Latino; 2 Hispanic/Latino; 1 Native Hawaiian or other Pacific Islander, non-Hispanic/Latino; 3 Two or more races, non-Hispanic/Latino), 1 international. Average age 34. 16 applicants, 81% accepted, 13 enrolled. In 2013, 11 master's, 7 doctorates awarded. *Degree requirements:* For master's, thesis, minimum of 30 credit hours, defense/final exam of thesis or publishable paper; for doctorate, comprehensive exam, thesis/dissertation, at least 30 credit hours of thesis work. *Entrance requirements:* For master's, GRE General Test or MCAT (waived if candidate has earned MS/MA or PhD from accredited U.S. school), minimum undergraduate GPA of 3.0, 3-4 letters of recommendation; for doctorate, GRE General Test or MCAT (waived if candidate has earned MS/MA or PhD from accredited U.S. school), health care graduate, professional degree, or graduate degree related to health sciences; minimum GPA of 3.0, 3-4 letters of recommendation. Additional exam requirements/recommendations for international students: Required—TOEFL (minimum score 550 paper-based; 80 iBT). *Application deadline:* For fall admission, 2/1 for domestic students, 1/15 priority date for international students; for spring admission, 10/1 for domestic students. Application fee: $50 ($75 for international students). Electronic applications accepted. *Expenses:* Contact institution. *Financial support:* In 2013–14, 18 students received support. Fellowships, research assistantships, teaching assistantships, Federal Work-Study, institutionally sponsored loans, scholarships/grants, traineeships, and unspecified assistantships available. Financial award application deadline: 3/15; financial award applicants required to submit FAFSA. *Unit head:* Dr. Ronald Sokol, Program Director, 720-777-6669, E-mail: ronald.sokol@childrenscolorado.org. *Application contact:* Galit Mankin, Program Administrator, 720-848-6249, Fax: 303-848-7381, E-mail: galit.mankin@ucdenver.edu.
Website: http://cctsi.ucdenver.edu/training-and-education/CLSC/Pages/default.aspx

University of Connecticut, Graduate School, University of Connecticut Health Center, Field of Clinical and Translational Research, Storrs, CT 06269. Offers MS. *Degree requirements:* For master's, comprehensive exam. *Entrance requirements:* Additional exam requirements/recommendations for international students: Required—TOEFL (minimum score 550 paper-based). Electronic applications accepted.

University of Connecticut Health Center, Graduate School, Program in Clinical and Translational Research, Farmington, CT 06030. Offers MS. Part-time programs available. *Entrance requirements:* For master's, GRE. Additional exam requirements/recommendations for international students: Required—TOEFL (minimum score 600 paper-based).

University of Florida, College of Medicine, Program in Clinical Investigation, Gainesville, FL 32611. Offers clinical investigation (MS); epidemiology (MS); public health (MPH). Part-time programs available. *Entrance requirements:* For master's, GRE, MD, PhD, DMD/DDS or Pharm D. *Expenses:* Tuition, state resident: full-time $12,640. Tuition, nonresident: full-time $30,000.

University of Florida, Graduate School, College of Engineering, Department of Biomedical Engineering, Gainesville, FL 32611. Offers biomedical engineering (ME, MS, PhD, Certificate); clinical and translational science (PhD); medical physics (MS, PhD); MD/PhD. *Faculty:* 26 full-time (5 women), 25 part-time/adjunct (6 women). *Students:* 119 full-time (48 women), 15 part-time (6 women); includes 24 minority (1 Black or African American, non-Hispanic/Latino; 8 Asian, non-Hispanic/Latino; 15 Hispanic/Latino), 49 international. Average age 27. 227 applicants, 26% accepted, 26 enrolled. In 2013, 31 master's, 18 doctorates awarded. Terminal master's awarded for partial completion of doctoral program. *Degree requirements:* For master's, comprehensive exam (for some programs), thesis (for some programs); for doctorate, comprehensive exam (for some programs), thesis/dissertation (for some programs). *Entrance requirements:* For master's and doctorate, minimum GPA of 3.0. Additional exam requirements/recommendations for international students: Required—TOEFL (minimum score 550 paper-based; 80 iBT), IELTS (minimum score 6). *Application deadline:* For fall admission, 12/15 priority date for domestic students, 12/15 for international students; for spring admission, 7/31 for domestic and international students. Applications are processed on a rolling basis. Application fee: $30. Electronic applications accepted. *Expenses:* Tuition, state resident: full-time $12,640. Tuition, nonresident: full-time $30,000. *Financial support:* In 2013–14, 65 students received support, including 2 fellowships with full tuition reimbursements available (averaging $31,000 per year), 66 research assistantships with full tuition reimbursements available (averaging $21,340 per year), 1 teaching assistantship (averaging $2,610 per year). Financial award application deadline: 12/31; financial award applicants required to submit FAFSA. *Faculty research:* Neural engineering, tissue engineering, biomedical imaging. *Unit head:* Christine E. Schmidt, PhD, Chair, 352-273-9222, Fax: 352-392-9791, E-mail: schmidt@bme.ufl.edu. *Application contact:* Hans Van Oostrom, PhD, Associate Professor/Associate Chair/Graduate Coordinator, 352-273-9315, Fax: 352-392-9221, E-mail: oostrom@ufl.edu.
Website: http://www.bme.ufl.edu/

The University of Iowa, Graduate College, College of Public Health, Department of Epidemiology, Iowa City, IA 52242-1316. Offers clinical investigation (MS); epidemiology (MPH, MS, PhD). *Accreditation:* CEPH. *Degree requirements:* For master's, thesis optional, exam; for doctorate, comprehensive exam, thesis/dissertation. *Entrance requirements:* For master's and doctorate, GRE General Test, minimum GPA of 3.0. Additional exam requirements/recommendations for international students: Required—TOEFL (minimum score 600 paper-based; 100 iBT). Electronic applications accepted.

The University of Kansas, University of Kansas Medical Center, School of Medicine, Department of Preventive Medicine and Public Health, Kansas City, KS 66160. Offers clinical research (MS); environmental health sciences (MPH); epidemiology (MPH); public health management (MPH); social and behavioral health (MPH); MD/MPH; PhD/MPH. Part-time programs available. *Faculty:* 69. *Students:* 30 full-time (23 women), 60 part-time (41 women); includes 27 minority (6 Black or African American, non-Hispanic/Latino; 2 American Indian or Alaska Native, non-Hispanic/Latino; 11 Asian, non-Hispanic/Latino; 3 Hispanic/Latino; 5 Two or more races, non-Hispanic/Latino), 7 international. Average age 34. 62 applicants, 52% accepted, 24 enrolled. In 2013, 37 master's awarded. *Degree requirements:* For master's, thesis, capstone practicum defense. *Entrance requirements:* For master's, GRE, MCAT, LSAT, GMAT or other equivalent graduate professional exam. Additional exam requirements/recommendations for international students: Required—TOEFL. *Application deadline:* For fall admission, 3/1 for domestic and international students. Applications are processed on a rolling basis. Application fee: $60. Electronic applications accepted. *Financial support:* Research assistantships, career-related internships or fieldwork, Federal Work-Study, scholarships/grants, and unspecified assistantships available. Financial award application deadline: 3/1; financial award applicants required to submit FAFSA. *Faculty research:* Cancer screening and prevention, smoking cessation, obesity and physical activity, health services/outcomes research, health disparities. *Total annual research expenditures:* $6.9 million. *Unit head:* Dr. Edward F. Ellerbeck, Chairman, 913-588-2774, Fax: 913-588-2780, E-mail: eellerbe@kumc.edu. *Application contact:* Tanya

Honderick, MPH Director, 913-588-2720, Fax: 913-588-8505, E-mail: thonderick@kumc.edu.
Website: http://www.kumc.edu/school-of-medicine/preventive-medicine-and-public-health.html

University of Kentucky, Graduate School, College of Public Health, Program in Clinical Research Design, Lexington, KY 40506-0032. Offers MS.

University of Louisville, Graduate School, School of Public Health and Information Sciences, Louisville, KY 40292-0001. Offers bioinformatics and biostatistics (MS, PhD), including biostatistics (MPH, MS, PhD), decision science (MS); clinical investigation sciences (M Sc, Certificate); environmental and occupational health sciences (PhD), including public health; epidemiology and population health (MS), including epidemiology (MPH, MS, PhD); epidemiology and public health (MPH, PhD), including biostatistics (MPH, MS, PhD), environmental and occupational health sciences (MPH), epidemiology (MPH, MS, PhD), health management, health promotion and behavior (MPH); health management and systems sciences (PhD), including public health sciences - health management; health promotion and behavioral sciences (PhD), including health promotion; public health sciences (PhD), including environmental health, epidemiology (MPH, MS, PhD), health management (MPH, PhD), health promotion. Part-time and evening/weekend programs available. *Students:* 125 full-time (82 women), 47 part-time (30 women); includes 39 minority (14 Black or African American, non-Hispanic/Latino; 14 Asian, non-Hispanic/Latino; 6 Hispanic/Latino; 5 Two or more races, non-Hispanic/Latino), 31 international. Average age 32. 174 applicants, 69% accepted, 62 enrolled. In 2013, 36 master's, 5 doctorates awarded. *Degree requirements:* For master's, thesis; for doctorate, comprehensive exam, thesis/dissertation. *Entrance requirements:* For master's, GRE General Test, GMAT, DAT, MCAT, official transcripts, statement of purpose, resume/curriculum vitae, letters of recommendation; for doctorate, GRE General Test, official transcripts, statement of purpose, resume/curriculum vitae, letters of recommendation. Additional exam requirements/recommendations for international students: Required—TOEFL (minimum score 600 paper-based; 100 iBT). *Application deadline:* For fall admission, 2/1 for domestic and international students. Applications are processed on a rolling basis. Application fee: $60. Electronic applications accepted. *Expenses:* Tuition, state resident: full-time $10,788; part-time $599 per credit hour. Tuition, nonresident: full-time $22,446; part-time $1247 per credit hour. *Required fees:* $196. Tuition and fees vary according to program and reciprocity agreements. *Financial support:* Research assistantships with full tuition reimbursements, scholarships/grants, health care benefits, and unspecified assistantships available. Financial award application deadline: 5/1; financial award applicants required to submit FAFSA. *Faculty research:* Breast cancer, controlled clinical trials, environmental hazards, chlorine toxicity mitigation, public health preparedness. *Total annual research expenditures:* $6.5 million. *Unit head:* Dr. Craig Blakely, Associate Dean for Academic Affairs, 502-852-3297, Fax: 502-852-3291, E-mail: craig.blakely@louisville.edu. *Application contact:* Vicki Lewis, Administrative Assistant, 502-852-1798, Fax: 502-852-3294, E-mail: vicki.lewis@louisville.edu.
Website: http://louisville.edu/sphis

University of Maryland, Baltimore, Graduate School, Clinical Research Certificate Program, Baltimore, MD 21201. Offers Postbaccalaureate Certificate. *Students:* 2 part-time (0 women); includes 1 minority (Hispanic/Latino). Average age 37. 9 applicants, 33% accepted. *Unit head:* Dr. Bruce E. Jarrell, Chief Academic and Research Officer, 410-706-2304, Fax: 410-706-0500, E-mail: bjarrell@som.umaryland.edu. *Application contact:* Keith T. Brooks, Assistant Dean, 410-706-7131, Fax: 410-706-3473, E-mail: kbrooks@umaryland.edu.

University of Maryland, Baltimore, School of Medicine, Department of Epidemiology and Public Health, Baltimore, MD 21201. Offers biostatistics (MS); clinical research (MS); epidemiology and preventive medicine (MPH, MS, PhD); gerontology (PhD); human genetics and genomic medicine (MS, PhD); molecular epidemiology (MS, PhD); toxicology (MS, PhD); JD/MS; MD/PhD; MS/PhD. *Accreditation:* CEPH. Part-time programs available. *Students:* 83 full-time (56 women), 76 part-time (51 women); includes 51 minority (26 Black or African American, non-Hispanic/Latino; 20 Asian, non-Hispanic/Latino; 5 Hispanic/Latino), 27 international. Average age 32. 225 applicants, 44% accepted, 37 enrolled. In 2013, 18 master's, 1 doctorate awarded. *Degree requirements:* For doctorate, comprehensive exam, thesis/dissertation. *Entrance requirements:* For master's and doctorate, GRE General Test. Additional exam requirements/recommendations for international students: Required—TOEFL (minimum score 550 paper-based; 80 iBT); Recommended—IELTS (minimum score 7). *Application deadline:* For fall admission, 1/15 for domestic and international students. Application fee: $75. Electronic applications accepted. *Expenses:* Contact institution. *Financial support:* In 2013–14, research assistantships with partial tuition reimbursements (averaging $25,000 per year) were awarded; fellowships, Federal Work-Study, scholarships/grants, and unspecified assistantships also available. Financial award application deadline: 3/1; financial award applicants required to submit FAFSA. *Unit head:* Dr. Laura Hungerford, Program Director, 410-706-8492, Fax: 410-706-4225. *Application contact:* Jessica Kelley, Program Coordinator, 410-706-8492, Fax: 410-706-4225, E-mail: jkelley@som.umaryland.edu.
Website: http://medschool.umaryland.edu/Epidemiology/

University of Massachusetts Worcester, Graduate School of Biomedical Sciences, Worcester, MA 01655-0115. Offers biochemistry and molecular pharmacology (PhD); bioinformatics and computational biology (PhD); cancer biology (PhD); cell biology (PhD); clinical and population health research (PhD); clinical investigation (MS); immunology and virology (PhD); interdisciplinary biomedical research (PhD); millennium (PhD); molecular genetics and microbiology (PhD); neuroscience (PhD); translational science (PhD); MD/PhD. *Faculty:* 1,388 full-time (521 women), 309 part-time/adjunct (198 women). *Students:* 385 full-time (210 women); includes 53 minority (13 Black or African American, non-Hispanic/Latino; 30 Asian, non-Hispanic/Latino; 10 Hispanic/Latino), 138 international. Average age 28. 491 applicants, 19% accepted, 39 enrolled. In 2013, 5 master's, 50 doctorates awarded. Terminal master's awarded for partial completion of doctoral program. *Median time to degree:* Of those who began their doctoral program in fall 2005, 67% received their degree in 8 years or less. *Degree requirements:* For master's, comprehensive exam, thesis; for doctorate, comprehensive exam, thesis/dissertation. *Entrance requirements:* For master's, MD, PhD, DVM, or PharmD; for doctorate, GRE General Test, bachelor's degree. Additional exam requirements/recommendations for international students: Required—TOEFL (minimum score 100 iBT) or IELTS (minimum score 7.5). *Application deadline:* For fall admission, 12/15 for domestic and international students; for spring admission, 5/15 for domestic students. Application fee: $80. Electronic applications accepted. *Expenses:* Contact institution. *Financial support:* In 2013–14, 431 students received support, including research assistantships with full tuition reimbursements available (averaging $29,500 per year); scholarships/grants, health care benefits, tuition waivers (full), and unspecified assistantships also available. Financial award application deadline: 5/16. *Faculty research:* RNA interference, cell/molecular/developmental biology, bioinformatics, clinical/translational research, infectious disease. *Total annual research expenditures:* $245.9 million. *Unit head:* Dr. Anthony Carruthers, Dean, 508-856-4135, E-mail: anthony.carruthers@umassmed.edu. *Application contact:* Dr. Kendall Knight, Associate Dean and Interim Director of Admissions and Recruitment, 508-856-5628, Fax: 508-856-3659, E-mail: kendall.knight@umassmed.edu.
Website: http://www.umassmed.edu/gsbs/

University of Michigan, School of Public Health, Program in Clinical Research Design and Statistical Analysis, Ann Arbor, MI 48109. Offers MS. Offered through the Horace H. Rackham School of Graduate Studies; program admits applicants in odd-numbered calendar years only. Evening/weekend programs available. *Degree requirements:* For master's, comprehensive exam. *Entrance requirements:* For master's, GRE General Test or MCAT. Additional exam requirements/recommendations for international students: Recommended—TOEFL (minimum score 560 paper-based; 100 iBT). Electronic applications accepted. *Expenses:* Contact institution. *Faculty research:* Survival analysis, missing data, Bayesian inference, health economics, quality of life.

University of Minnesota, Twin Cities Campus, School of Public Health, Major in Clinical Research, Minneapolis, MN 55455-0213. Offers MS. Part-time programs available. *Degree requirements:* For master's, thesis. *Entrance requirements:* For master's, advanced health professional degree. Additional exam requirements/recommendations for international students: Required—TOEFL. Electronic applications accepted. *Faculty research:* Osteoporosis prevention; heart disease prevention; role of inflammatory dental disease in the genesis of atherosclerosis; interventional research into AIDS and cancer.

The University of North Carolina Wilmington, School of Nursing, Wilmington, NC 28403-5995. Offers clinical research and product development (MS); family nurse practitioner (MSN). *Faculty:* 10 full-time (9 women), 1 (woman) part-time/adjunct. *Students:* 59 full-time (54 women), 61 part-time (53 women); includes 17 minority (6 Black or African American, non-Hispanic/Latino; 5 American Indian or Alaska Native, non-Hispanic/Latino; 5 Hispanic/Latino; 1 Two or more races, non-Hispanic/Latino). Average age 32. 134 applicants, 44% accepted, 43 enrolled. In 2013, 13 master's awarded. *Degree requirements:* For master's, comprehensive exam, thesis or project. *Entrance requirements:* For master's, GRE General Test, bachelor's degree in nursing. Additional exam requirements/recommendations for international students: Required—TOEFL (minimum score 550 paper-based; 79 iBT), IELTS (minimum score 6.5). *Application deadline:* For fall admission, 3/1 for domestic students. Applications are processed on a rolling basis. Application fee: $60. Electronic applications accepted. *Expenses:* Tuition, state resident: full-time $4163. Tuition, nonresident: full-time $16,098. *Financial support:* In 2013–14, 2 teaching assistantships with full and partial tuition reimbursements (averaging $9,500 per year) were awarded. Financial award application deadline: 3/15. *Unit head:* Dr. Deborah Pollard, Interim Director, 910-962-7410, E-mail: pollardd@uncw.edu. *Application contact:* Dr. Julie Taylor, Graduate Coordinator, 910-962-7927, E-mail: taylorjs@uncw.edu.
Website: http://www.uncw.edu/son/

University of Pittsburgh, School of Medicine, Clinical Research Graduate Programs, Pittsburgh, PA 15260. Offers MS, Certificate. Part-time programs available. *Faculty:* 44 full-time (26 women). *Students:* 75 part-time (48 women); includes 18 minority (5 Black or African American, non-Hispanic/Latino; 12 Asian, non-Hispanic/Latino; 1 Hispanic/Latino), 20 international. Average age 33. 46 applicants, 87% accepted, 40 enrolled. In 2013, 10 master's, 23 other advanced degrees awarded. *Degree requirements:* For master's, thesis. *Entrance requirements:* For master's, MCAT, GRE, GMAT, or PCAT. Additional exam requirements/recommendations for international students: Required—TOEFL (minimum score 600 paper-based; 100 iBT). *Application deadline:* For fall admission, 10/31 priority date for domestic and international students; for spring admission, 4/15 priority date for domestic and international students. Electronic applications accepted. *Expenses:* Tuition, state resident: full-time $19,964; part-time $807 per credit. Tuition, nonresident: full-time $32,686; part-time $1337 per credit. *Required fees:* $740; $200. Tuition and fees vary according to program. *Financial support:* Tuition waivers (partial) available. *Faculty research:* Quality of life, mood disorders in children, pediatric palliative care, female pelvic medicines, antibiotic use and racial variations, medication use. *Unit head:* Dr. Wishwa Kapoor, Program Director, 412-692-2686, Fax: 412-586-9672, E-mail: kapoorwn@upmc.edu. *Application contact:* Jennifer Holliman, Program Coordinator, 412-586-9673, Fax: 412-586-9672, E-mail: hollimanjm@upmc.edu.
Website: http://www.icre.pitt.edu/degrees/degrees.html

University of Puerto Rico, Medical Sciences Campus, School of Health Professions, Program in Clinical Research, San Juan, PR 00936-5067. Offers MS, Graduate Certificate.

University of Rochester, School of Medicine and Dentistry, Graduate Programs in Medicine and Dentistry, Department of Community and Preventive Medicine, Programs in Public Health and Clinical Investigation, Rochester, NY 14627. Offers clinical investigation (MS); public health (MPH); MBA/MPH; MD/MPH; MPH/MS; MPH/PhD. *Accreditation:* CEPH. *Entrance requirements:* For master's, GRE General Test. *Expenses: Tuition:* Full-time $44,580; part-time $1394 per credit hour. *Required fees:* $492.

University of Rochester, School of Medicine and Dentistry, Graduate Programs in Medicine and Dentistry, Interdepartmental Program in Clinical Translational Research, Rochester, NY 14627. Offers MS. *Expenses: Tuition:* Full-time $44,580; part-time $1394 per credit hour. *Required fees:* $492.

University of Rochester, School of Nursing, Rochester, NY 14642. Offers acute care nurse practitioner (MS); adult nurse practitioner (MS); adult/geriatric nurse practitioner (MS); clinical nurse leader (MS); clinical research coordinator (MS); family nurse practitioner (MS); family psychiatric mental health nurse practitioner (MS); health care organization management and leadership (MS); health practice research (PhD); nursing (DNP); pediatric nurse practitioner (MS); pediatric nurse practitioner/neonatal nurse practitioner (MS). *Accreditation:* AACN. Part-time programs available. Postbaccalaureate distance learning degree programs offered (minimal on-campus study). *Faculty:* 60 full-time (52 women), 61 part-time/adjunct (47 women). *Students:* 33 full-time (29 women), 213 part-time (195 women); includes 32 minority (8 Black or African American, non-Hispanic/Latino; 10 Asian, non-Hispanic/Latino; 8 Hispanic/Latino; 6 Two or more races, non-Hispanic/Latino), 4 international. Average age 34. 41 applicants, 54% accepted, 16 enrolled. In 2013, 58 master's, 11 doctorates awarded. Terminal master's awarded for partial completion of doctoral program. *Degree requirements:* For master's, comprehensive exam (for some programs); for doctorate, thesis/dissertation. *Entrance requirements:* For master's, BS in nursing, minimum GPA of 3.0, course work in statistics; for doctorate, GRE General Test, MS in nursing, minimum GPA of 3.5. Additional exam requirements/recommendations for international students: Required—TOEFL (minimum score 560 paper-based; 88 iBT) or IELTS (minimum score 6.5) recommended. *Application deadline:* For fall admission, 4/1 for domestic and international students; for spring admission, 9/1 for domestic and international students; for summer admission, 1/2 for domestic and international students. Application fee: $50. Electronic applications accepted. *Expenses: Tuition:* Full-time $44,580; part-time $1394 per credit hour. *Required fees:* $492. *Financial support:* In 2013–14, 41 students received support, including 2 fellowships with full and partial tuition reimbursements available (averaging $30,200 per year); scholarships/grants, traineeships, health care benefits, tuition waivers (partial), and unspecified

assistantships also available. Support available to part-time students. Financial award application deadline: 6/30. *Faculty research:* Symptom assessment and self-management, illness prevention, nursing intervention research with vulnerable populations, palliative care, aging. *Total annual research expenditures:* $3.5 million. *Unit head:* Dr. Kathy H. Rideout, Dean, 585-273-8902, Fax: 585-273-1268, E-mail: kathy_rideout@urmc.rochester.edu. *Application contact:* Elaine Andolina, Director of Admissions, 585-275-2375, Fax: 585-756-8299, E-mail: elaine_andolina@urmc.rochester.edu.
Website: http://www.son.rochester.edu

University of Southern California, Graduate School, School of Pharmacy, Regulatory Science Programs, Los Angeles, CA 90089. Offers clinical research design and management (Graduate Certificate); food safety (Graduate Certificate); patient and product safety (Graduate Certificate); preclinical drug development (Graduate Certificate); regulatory and clinical affairs (Graduate Certificate); regulatory science (MS, DRSc). Part-time and evening/weekend programs available. Postbaccalaureate distance learning degree programs offered (minimal on-campus study). Terminal master's awarded for partial completion of doctoral program. *Degree requirements:* For master's, thesis optional; for doctorate, comprehensive exam, thesis/dissertation. *Entrance requirements:* For master's, GRE. Additional exam requirements/recommendations for international students: Required—TOEFL (minimum score 603 paper-based; 100 iBT). Electronic applications accepted.

University of South Florida, Innovative Education Graduate Certificate Programs, Tampa, FL 33620-9951. *Unit head:* Kathy Barnes, Interdisciplinary Programs Coordinator, 813-974-8031, Fax: 813-974-7061, E-mail: barnesk@usf.edu. *Application contact:* Karen Tylinski, Metro Initiatives, 813-974-9943, Fax: 813-974-7061, E-mail: ktylinsk@usf.edu.
Website: http://www.usf.edu/innovative-education/

University of South Florida, Morsani College of Medicine and Graduate School, Graduate Programs in Medical Sciences, Tampa, FL 33620-9951. Offers aging and neuroscience (MSMS); allergy, immunology and infectious disease (PhD); anatomy (MSMS, PhD); athletic training (MSMS); bioinformatics and computational biology (MSBCB); biotechnology (MSB); clinical and translational research (MSMS, PhD); health informatics (MSHI, MSMS); health science (MSMS); interdisciplinary medical sciences (MSMS); medical microbiology and immunology (MSMS); metabolic and nutritional medicine (MSMS); molecular medicine (MSMS, PhD); molecular pharmacology and physiology (PhD); neurology (PhD); pathology and laboratory medicine (PhD); pharmacology and therapeutics (PhD); physiology and biophysics (PhD); women's health (MSMS). *Students:* 336 full-time (182 women), 39 part-time (21 women); includes 170 minority (45 Black or African American, non-Hispanic/Latino; 54 Asian, non-Hispanic/Latino; 59 Hispanic/Latino; 2 Native Hawaiian or other Pacific Islander, non-Hispanic/Latino; 10 Two or more races, non-Hispanic/Latino), 17 international. Average age 26. 1,066 applicants, 44% accepted, 250 enrolled. In 2013, 191 master's, 12 doctorates awarded. Terminal master's awarded for partial completion of doctoral program. *Degree requirements:* For master's, comprehensive exam, thesis; for doctorate, comprehensive exam, thesis/dissertation. *Entrance requirements:* For master's, GRE General Test or GMAT, bachelor's degree or equivalent from regionally-accredited university with minimum GPA of 3.0 in upper-division sciences coursework; prerequisites in general biology, general chemistry, general physics, organic chemistry, quantitative analysis, and integral and differential calculus; for doctorate, GRE General Test (minimum score of 600 quantitative), bachelor's degree from regionally-accredited university with minimum GPA of 3.0 in upper-division sciences coursework; 3 letters of recommendation; personal interview; 1-2 page personal statement; prerequisites in biology, chemistry, physics, organic chemistry, quantitative analysis, and integral/differential calculus. Additional exam requirements/recommendations for international students: Required—TOEFL (minimum score 550 paper-based; 79 iBT) or IELTS (minimum score 6.5). *Application deadline:* For fall admission, 2/15 for domestic students, 1/2 for international students. Application fee: $30. *Expenses:* Contact institution. *Faculty research:* Anatomy biochemistry, cancer biology, cardiovascular disease, cell biology, immunology, microbiology, molecular biology, neuroscience, pharmacology, physiology. *Unit head:* Dr. Michael Barber, Professor and Associate Dean for Graduate and Postdoctoral Affairs, 813-974-9908, Fax: 813-974-4317, E-mail: mbarber@health.usf.edu. *Application contact:* Dr. Eric Bennett, Graduate Director, PhD Program in Medical Sciences, 813-974-1545, Fax: 813-974-4317, E-mail: esbennet@health.usf.edu.
Website: http://health.usf.edu/nocms/medicine/graduatestudies/

The University of Texas Health Science Center at San Antonio, Graduate School of Biomedical Sciences, Master's in Clinical Investigation Program, San Antonio, TX 78229-3900. Offers MS. Part-time programs available. *Faculty:* 98 part-time/adjunct (30 women). *Students:* 1 (woman) full-time, 17 part-time (10 women); includes 12 minority (9 Asian, non-Hispanic/Latino; 2 Hispanic/Latino; 1 Native Hawaiian or other Pacific Islander, non-Hispanic/Latino), 2 international. Average age 42. 14 applicants, 21% accepted, 3 enrolled. In 2013, 8 master's awarded. *Degree requirements:* For master's, comprehensive exam, submission of one full-length research manuscript to peer-reviewed scientific or medical journal. *Entrance requirements:* Additional exam requirements/recommendations for international students: Required—TOEFL (minimum score 550 paper-based) or IELTS (minimum score 6.5). *Application deadline:* For fall admission, 6/1 for domestic students, 4/1 for international students; for spring admission, 10/1 for domestic students. Applications are processed on a rolling basis. Application fee: $0. Electronic applications accepted. *Faculty research:* Evaluation and medical management of elders; inflammation in tissue injury, regeneration, and disease; mammalian TOR in aging and cancer; psychometrics; Type 2 diabetes; metabolic studies. *Unit head:* Dr. Michael J. Lichtenstein, Interim Dean, 210-567-0034, Fax: 210-567-4301, E-mail: lichtenstei@uthscsa.edu. *Application contact:* Lora Tumlinson, Academic Programs Coordinator, 210-567-4631, Fax: 210-567-4301, E-mail: tumlinson@uthscsa.edu.
Website: http://gsbs.uthscsa.edu/main/academics/graduprograms/ms/clinicalinvestigation.asp

University of Virginia, School of Medicine, Department of Public Health Sciences, Program in Clinical Research, Charlottesville, VA 22903. Offers clinical investigation and patient-oriented research (MS); informatics in medicine (MS). Part-time programs available. *Students:* 3 full-time (1 woman), 5 part-time (3 women). Average age 35. 17 applicants, 29% accepted, 4 enrolled. In 2013, 12 master's awarded. *Degree requirements:* For master's, thesis (for some programs). *Entrance requirements:* For master's, 2 letters of recommendation. Additional exam requirements/recommendations for international students: Required—TOEFL (minimum score 600 paper-based; 90 iBT). *Application deadline:* For fall admission, 3/1 priority date for domestic and international students. Application fee: $60. Electronic applications accepted. *Expenses:* Tuition, state resident: part-time $334 per credit hour. Tuition, nonresident: part-time $1224 per credit hour. *Financial support:* Career-related internships or fieldwork available. Financial award applicants required to submit FAFSA. *Unit head:* Dr. Jean Eby, Program Director, 434-924-8430, Fax: 434-924-8437, E-mail: jmg5b@virginia.edu. *Application contact:* Tracey L. Brookman, Academic Programs Administrator, 434-924-8430, Fax: 434-924-8437, E-mail: phsdegrees@virginia.edu.
Website: http://www.healthsystem.virginia.edu/internet/phs/ms/mshome.cfm

University of Washington, Graduate School, School of Public Health, Department of Biostatistics, Seattle, WA 98195. Offers biostatistics (MPH, MS, PhD); clinical research (MS), including biostatistics; statistical genetics (PhD). Part-time programs available. *Faculty:* 41 full-time (17 women), 5 part-time/adjunct (3 women). *Students:* 82 full-time (42 women), 7 part-time (3 women); includes 1 minority (Black or African American, non-Hispanic/Latino), 25 international. Average age 28. 257 applicants, 23% accepted, 23 enrolled. In 2013, 6 master's, 10 doctorates awarded. Terminal master's awarded for partial completion of doctoral program. *Degree requirements:* For master's, comprehensive exam, thesis, practicum (MPH); for doctorate, comprehensive exam, thesis/dissertation. *Entrance requirements:* For master's and doctorate, GRE General Test, coursework on multivariate calculus, linear algebra and probability; minimum GPA of 3.0. Additional exam requirements/recommendations for international students: Required—TOEFL. *Application deadline:* For fall admission, 12/1 for domestic students. Application fee: $85. Electronic applications accepted. *Financial support:* In 2013–14, 75 research assistantships with full tuition reimbursements (averaging $21,000 per year), 28 teaching assistantships with full tuition reimbursements (averaging $21,000 per year) were awarded; scholarships/grants, traineeships, health care benefits, and tuition waivers (partial) also available. *Faculty research:* Statistical methods for survival data analysis, clinical trials, epidemiological case control and cohort studies, statistical genetics. *Unit head:* Dr. Bruce Weir, Department Chair, 206-543-1044. *Application contact:* Alex MacKenzie, Curriculum Coordinator, 206-543-1044, Fax: 206-543-3286, E-mail: alexam@u.washington.edu.
Website: http://www.biostat.washington.edu/

University of Washington, Graduate School, School of Public Health, Department of Epidemiology, Seattle, WA 98195. Offers clinical research (MS); epidemiology (MPH, MS, PhD); global health (MPH); maternal/child health (MPH); MPH/MPA. *Accreditation:* CEPH (one or more programs are accredited). *Faculty:* 65 full-time (38 women), 39 part-time/adjunct (17 women). *Students:* 120 full-time (84 women), 30 part-time (20 women); includes 19 minority (3 Black or African American, non-Hispanic/Latino; 2 American Indian or Alaska Native, non-Hispanic/Latino; 14 Asian, non-Hispanic/Latino), 12 international. Average age 32. 234 applicants, 37% accepted, 40 enrolled. In 2013, 41 master's, 18 doctorates awarded. *Degree requirements:* For master's, comprehensive exam (for some programs), thesis; for doctorate, comprehensive exam, thesis/dissertation, general exam, dissertation proposal, final exam (dissertation defense). *Entrance requirements:* For master's, GRE (except for those holding PhD, MD, DDS, DVM, DO or equivalent from U.S. institutions); for doctorate, GRE. Additional exam requirements/recommendations for international students: Required—TOEFL (minimum score 580 paper-based, 92 iBT), IELTS (minimum score 7), or PTE (minimum score of 65). *Application deadline:* For fall admission, 12/1 for domestic students, 11/1 for international students. Application fee: $85. Electronic applications accepted. *Expenses:* Contact institution. *Financial support:* In 2013–14, 138 students received support, including 70 fellowships with partial tuition reimbursements available, 40 research assistantships with partial tuition reimbursements available, 12 teaching assistantships with partial tuition reimbursements available; career-related internships or fieldwork, Federal Work-Study, traineeships, health care benefits, tuition waivers, and unspecified assistantships also available. Support available to part-time students. Financial award application deadline: 12/1; financial award applicants required to submit FAFSA. *Faculty research:* Chronic disease, health disparities and social determinants of health, aging and neuroepidemiology, maternal and child health, molecular and genetic epidemiology. *Unit head:* Dr. Scott Davis, Chair, 206-543-1065, E-mail: epiapply@uw.edu. *Application contact:* Kate O'Brien, Student Services Manager, 206-543-1065, E-mail: epiapply@uw.edu.
Website: http://depts.washington.edu/epidem/

University of Washington, Graduate School, School of Public Health, Department of Health Services, Seattle, WA 98195. Offers clinical research (MS); community-oriented public health practice (MPH); evaluative sciences and statistics (PhD); health behavior and social determinants of health (PhD); health economics (PhD); health informatics and health information management (MHIHIM); health services (MS, PhD); health services administration (EMHA, MHA); health systems and policy (MPH); health systems research (PhD); maternal and child health (MPH); social and behavioral sciences (MPH); JD/MHA; MHA/MBA; MHA/MD; MHA/MPA; MPH/JD; MPH/MD; MPH/MN; MPH/MPA; MPH/MS; MPH/MSD; MPH/MSW; MPH/PhD. *Faculty:* 63 full-time (30 women), 56 part-time/adjunct (25 women). *Students:* 121 full-time (101 women), 19 part-time (11 women); includes 28 minority (3 Black or African American, non-Hispanic/Latino; 2 American Indian or Alaska Native, non-Hispanic/Latino; 23 Asian, non-Hispanic/Latino), 5 international. Average age 30. 242 applicants, 48% accepted, 36 enrolled. In 2013, 43 master's, 9 doctorates awarded. Terminal master's awarded for partial completion of doctoral program. *Degree requirements:* For master's, thesis (for some programs), practicum (MPH); for doctorate, comprehensive exam, thesis/dissertation. *Entrance requirements:* For master's and doctorate, GRE General Test, minimum GPA of 3.0. Additional exam requirements/recommendations for international students: Required—TOEFL (minimum score 580 paper-based; 92 iBT), IELTS (minimum score 7). *Application deadline:* For fall admission, 1/1 for domestic students, 11/1 for international students. Application fee: 85 Albanian leks. Electronic applications accepted. *Financial support:* In 2013–14, 45 students received support, including 12 fellowships with full and partial tuition reimbursements available (averaging $22,000 per year), 9 research assistantships with full and partial tuition reimbursements available (averaging $18,700 per year), 9 teaching assistantships with full and partial tuition reimbursements available (averaging $4,575 per year); institutionally sponsored loans, traineeships, and health care benefits also available. Financial award application deadline: 2/28; financial award applicants required to submit FAFSA. *Faculty research:* Public health practice, health promotion and disease prevention, maternal and child health, organizational behavior and culture, health policy. *Unit head:* Dr. Larry Kessler, Chair, 206-543-2930. *Application contact:* Kitty A. Andert, MPH/MS/PhD Programs Manager, 206-616-2926, Fax: 206-543-3964, E-mail: hservmph@u.washington.edu.
Website: http://depts.washington.edu/hserv/

Vanderbilt University, School of Medicine, Clinical Investigation Program, Nashville, TN 37240-1001. Offers MS. *Entrance requirements:* Additional exam requirements/recommendations for international students: Required—TOEFL.

Walden University, Graduate Programs, School of Health Sciences, Minneapolis, MN 55401. Offers clinical research administration (MS, Graduate Certificate); health education and promotion (MS); health informatics (MS); health services (PhD), including community health, healthcare administration, leadership, public health policy, self-designed; healthcare administration (MHA); public health (MPH, Dr PH, PhD), including community health and education (PhD), epidemiology (PhD). Part-time and evening/weekend programs available. Postbaccalaureate distance learning degree programs offered (minimal on-campus study). *Faculty:* 18 full-time (12 women), 236 part-time/adjunct (120 women). *Students:* 2,563 full-time (1,867 women), 1,775 part-time (1,233 women); includes 2,532 minority (1,963 Black or African American, non-Hispanic/Latino; 29 American Indian or Alaska Native, non-Hispanic/Latino; 212 Asian, non-Hispanic/

Latino; 238 Hispanic/Latino; 15 Native Hawaiian or other Pacific Islander, non-Hispanic/Latino; 75 Two or more races, non-Hispanic/Latino), 97 international. Average age 39. 1,191 applicants, 94% accepted, 861 enrolled. In 2013, 723 master's, 121 doctorates, 17 other advanced degrees awarded. *Degree requirements:* For doctorate, thesis/dissertation, residency. *Entrance requirements:* For master's, bachelor's degree or higher; minimum GPA of 2.5; official transcripts; goal statement (for some programs); access to computer and Internet; for doctorate, master's degree or higher; three years of related professional or academic experience (preferred); minimum GPA of 3.0; goal statement and current resume (select programs); official transcripts; access to computer and Internet; for Graduate Certificate, relevant work experience; access to computer and Internet. Additional exam requirements/recommendations for international students: Required—TOEFL (minimum score 550 paper-based; 79 iBT), IELTS (minimum score 6.5), Michigan English Language Assessment Battery (minimum score 82), or PTE. *Application deadline:* Applications are processed on a rolling basis. Application fee: $0. Electronic applications accepted. *Expenses: Tuition:* Full-time $11,813.55; part-time $500 per credit. *Required fees:* $618.76. *Financial support:* Fellowships, Federal Work-Study, scholarships/grants, unspecified assistantships, and family tuition reduction, active duty/veteran tuition reduction, group tuition reduction, interest-free payment plans, employee tuition reduction available. Support available to part-time students. Financial award applicants required to submit FAFSA. *Unit head:* Dr. Jorg Westermann, Associate Dean, 800-925-3368. *Application contact:* Jennifer Hall, Vice President of Enrollment Management, 866-4-WALDEN, E-mail: info@waldenu.edu.
Website: http://www.waldenu.edu/colleges-schools/school-of-health-sciences

Washington University in St. Louis, School of Medicine, Program in Clinical Investigation, St. Louis, MO 63130-4899. Offers clinical investigation (MS); genetics/genomics (MS). Part-time programs available. *Faculty:* 61 full-time (14 women), 2 part-time/adjunct (both women). *Students:* 15 full-time (5 women), 39 part-time (19 women); includes 15 minority (3 Black or African American, non-Hispanic/Latino; 8 Asian, non-Hispanic/Latino; 2 Hispanic/Latino; 2 Two or more races, non-Hispanic/Latino), 3 international. Average age 32. 34 applicants, 65% accepted, 22 enrolled. In 2013, 22 master's awarded. *Degree requirements:* For master's, thesis. *Entrance requirements:* For master's, doctoral-level degree or in process of obtaining doctoral-level degree. Additional exam requirements/recommendations for international students: Required—TOEFL. *Application deadline:* For fall admission, 5/15 for domestic students; for spring admission, 10/15 for domestic students. Application fee: $0. Electronic applications accepted. *Financial support:* In 2013–14, 6 students received support. Tuition waivers (partial) available. Financial award application deadline: 12/12. *Faculty research:* Anesthesiology, infectious diseases, neurology, obstetrics and gynecology, orthopedic surgery. *Unit head:* Dr. David Warren, Associate Professor of Medicine, 314-454-8225, Fax: 314-454-5392, E-mail: dwarren@dom.wustl.edu. *Application contact:* Angela B. Wilson, Curriculum and Evaluation Coordinator, 314-454-8936, Fax: 314-454-8279, E-mail: abwilson@dom.wustl.edu.
Website: http://crtc.wustl.edu/

Communication Disorders

Abilene Christian University, Graduate School, College of Education and Human Services, Department of Communication Sciences and Disorders, Abilene, TX 79699-9100. Offers MS. *Accreditation:* ASHA. *Faculty:* 6 part-time/adjunct (5 women). *Students:* 43 full-time (41 women); includes 8 minority (1 American Indian or Alaska Native, non-Hispanic/Latino; 5 Hispanic/Latino; 2 Two or more races, non-Hispanic/Latino), 2 international. 154 applicants, 24% accepted, 22 enrolled. In 2013, 15 master's awarded. *Degree requirements:* For master's, one foreign language, comprehensive exam. *Entrance requirements:* For master's, GRE General Test. Additional exam requirements/recommendations for international students: Required—TOEFL (minimum score 550 paper-based; 90 iBT), IELTS (minimum score 6.5), PTE. *Application deadline:* For fall admission, 2/1 priority date for domestic students. Applications are processed on a rolling basis. Application fee: $50. Electronic applications accepted. *Expenses: Tuition:* Full-time $17,100; part-time $950 per credit hour. *Financial support:* In 2013–14, 17 students received support. Research assistantships and scholarships/grants available. Financial award application deadline: 4/1; financial award applicants required to submit FAFSA. *Unit head:* Dr. Terry Baggs, Graduate Director, 325-674-4819, Fax: 325-674-2552, E-mail: terry.baggs@acu.edu. *Application contact:* Corey Patterson, Director of Graduate Admission and Recruiting, 325-674-6566, Fax: 325-674-6717, E-mail: gradinfo@acu.edu.

Adelphi University, Ruth S. Ammon School of Education, Program in Communication Sciences and Disorders, Garden City, NY 11530-0701. Offers audiology (MS, DA); speech-language pathology (MS, DA). *Accreditation:* ASHA. Part-time programs available. *Students:* 220 full-time (213 women), 5 part-time (all women); includes 29 minority (5 Black or African American, non-Hispanic/Latino; 5 Asian, non-Hispanic/Latino; 15 Hispanic/Latino; 4 Two or more races, non-Hispanic/Latino). Average age 25. In 2013, 103 master's, 5 doctorates awarded. *Degree requirements:* For master's, comprehensive exam, clinical practice; for doctorate, one foreign language, comprehensive exam, thesis/dissertation. *Entrance requirements:* For master's, GRE General Test, writing exam, 3 letters of recommendation, interview, resume, 19 credits of prerequisite course work or communications disorders training; for doctorate, GRE General Test, 3 letters of recommendation, interview. Additional exam requirements/recommendations for international students: Required—TOEFL (minimum score 550 paper-based; 80 iBT). *Application deadline:* For fall admission, 3/1 priority date for domestic students, 3/1 for international students; for spring admission, 10/1 priority date for domestic students, 10/1 for international students. Applications are processed on a rolling basis. Application fee: $50. Electronic applications accepted. *Expenses: Tuition:* Full-time $32,530; part-time $1010 per credit. *Required fees:* $1150. Tuition and fees vary according to degree level and program. *Financial support:* Research assistantships, career-related internships or fieldwork, Federal Work-Study, institutionally sponsored loans, tuition waivers, and unspecified assistantships available. Support available to part-time students. Financial award application deadline: 2/15; financial award applicants required to submit FAFSA. *Faculty research:* Pediatric audiology, child speech perception with hearing loss, auditory deprivation, fluency, cultural diversity. *Unit head:* Dr. Robert Goldfarb, Chairperson, 516-877-4785, E-mail: goldfarb2@adelphi.edu. *Application contact:* Christine Murphy, Director of Admissions, 516-877-3050, Fax: 516-877-3039, E-mail: graduateadmissions@adelphi.edu.

Alabama Agricultural and Mechanical University, School of Graduate Studies, School of Education, Department of Counseling and Special Education, Area in Communicative Disorders, Huntsville, AL 35811. Offers M Ed, MS. *Accreditation:* ASHA. Part-time programs available. *Degree requirements:* For master's, comprehensive exam. *Entrance requirements:* For master's, GRE General Test, minimum GPA of 2.5. Additional exam requirements/recommendations for international students: Required—TOEFL (minimum score 500 paper-based; 61 iBT). Electronic applications accepted. *Faculty research:* Alternative methods of teaching speech and language to handicapped individuals.

Appalachian State University, Cratis D. Williams Graduate School, Department of Communication Sciences and Disorders, Boone, NC 28608. Offers speech-language pathology (MS). *Accreditation:* ASHA. Part-time programs available. *Degree requirements:* For master's, comprehensive exam, thesis optional. *Entrance requirements:* For master's, GRE General Test, 3 letters of recommendation. Additional exam requirements/recommendations for international students: Required—TOEFL (minimum score 570 paper-based), IELTS (minimum score 6.5). Electronic applications accepted. *Faculty research:* Clinical service delivery, voice disorders, language disorders, fluency disorders, neurogenic disorders.

Arizona State University at the Tempe campus, College of Liberal Arts and Sciences, Department of Speech and Hearing Science, Tempe, AZ 85287-0102. Offers audiology (Au D); communication disorders (MS); speech and hearing science (PhD). *Accreditation:* ASHA (one or more programs are accredited). *Degree requirements:* For master's, comprehensive exam (for some programs), thesis optional, interactive Program of Study (iPOS) submitted before completing 50 percent of required credit hours; for doctorate, comprehensive exam, thesis/dissertation (for some programs), academic/practicum components (Au D); interactive Program of Study (iPOS) submitted before completing 50 percent of required credit hours. *Entrance requirements:* For master's and doctorate, GRE, minimum GPA of 3.0 or equivalent in last 2 years of work leading to bachelor's degree. Additional exam requirements/recommendations for international students: Required—TOEFL (minimum score 80 iBT), TOEFL, IELTS, or PTE. *Expenses:* Contact institution.

Arkansas State University, Graduate School, College of Nursing and Health Professions, Department of Communication Disorders, State University, AR 72467. Offers MCD. *Accreditation:* ASHA. Part-time programs available. *Faculty:* 5 full-time (3 women). *Students:* 52 full-time (50 women); includes 3 minority (1 Black or African American, non-Hispanic/Latino; 1 Asian, non-Hispanic/Latino; 1 Hispanic/Latino). Average age 25. 71 applicants, 37% accepted, 26 enrolled. In 2013, 23 master's awarded. *Degree requirements:* For master's, comprehensive exam, thesis or alternative. *Entrance requirements:* For master's, GRE General Test, appropriate bachelor's degree, letters of recommendation, official transcripts, immunization records. Additional exam requirements/recommendations for international students: Required—TOEFL (minimum score 550 paper-based; 79 iBT), IELTS (minimum score 6), PTE (minimum score 56). *Application deadline:* For fall admission, 2/15 for domestic and international students. Applications are processed on a rolling basis. Application fee: $30 ($40 for international students). Electronic applications accepted. *Expenses:* Contact institution. *Financial support:* In 2013–14, 14 students received support. Career-related internships or fieldwork, scholarships/grants, and unspecified assistantships available. Financial award application deadline: 7/1; financial award applicants required to submit FAFSA. *Unit head:* Dr. Richard Neeley, Director, 870-972-3106, Fax: 870-972-3788, E-mail: rneeley@astate.edu. *Application contact:* Vickey Ring, Graduate Admissions Coordinator, 870-972-3029, Fax: 870-972-3857, E-mail: vickeyring@astate.edu.
Website: http://www.astate.edu/college/conhp/departments/communication-disorders

Armstrong State University, School of Graduate Studies, Program in Communication Sciences, Savannah, GA 31419-1997. Offers MS. *Accreditation:* ASHA. Part-time and evening/weekend programs available. *Faculty:* 3 full-time (all women), 1 (woman) part-time/adjunct. *Students:* 43 full-time (42 women), 1 (woman) part-time; includes 4 minority (all Black or African American, non-Hispanic/Latino), 1 international. Average age 24. 157 applicants, 16% accepted, 25 enrolled. In 2013, 12 master's awarded. *Degree requirements:* For master's, comprehensive exam, 400 client contact hours, PRAXIS II, minimum B average. *Entrance requirements:* For master's, GRE, criminal background check and drug screen, CPR certification, clinical observation hours, minimum GPA of 3.0, letter of intent, college transcript. Additional exam requirements/recommendations for international students: Required—TOEFL (minimum score 523 paper-based). *Application deadline:* For fall admission, 1/15 for domestic and international students. Application fee: $30. Electronic applications accepted. *Expenses:* Tuition, state resident: part-time $201 per credit hour. Tuition, nonresident: part-time $745 per credit hour. *Required fees:* $310 per semester. Tuition and fees vary according to course load, campus/location and program. *Financial support:* In 2013–14, research assistantships with full tuition reimbursements (averaging $5,000 per year) were awarded; Federal Work-Study, scholarships/grants, and unspecified assistantships also available. Support available to part-time students. Financial award application deadline: 3/15; financial award applicants required to submit FAFSA. *Faculty research:* Cognitive impairment and traumatic brain injury, cultural and linguistic differences, aphasia and quality of life. *Unit head:* Maya Clark, Program Coordinator and Professor, 912-344-2606, Fax: 912-344-3439, E-mail: maya.clark@armstrong.edu. *Application contact:* Jill Bell, Director, Graduate Enrollment Services, 912-344-2798, Fax: 912-344-3477, E-mail: graduate@armstrong.edu.
Website: http://www.armstrong.edu/Health_Professions/rehabilitation_sciences/rehab_sci_ms_communication_sciences

A.T. Still University, Arizona School of Health Sciences, Mesa, AZ 85206. Offers advanced occupational therapy (MS); advanced physician assistant studies (MS); athletic training (MS); audiology (Au D); health sciences (DHSc); human movement (MS); occupational therapy (MS, DOT); physical therapy (DPT); physician assistant (MS); transitional audiology (Au D); transitional physical therapy (DPT). *Accreditation:* AOTA (one or more programs are accredited); ASHA. Part-time and evening/weekend programs available. Postbaccalaureate distance learning degree programs offered (minimal on-campus study). *Faculty:* 47 full-time (27 women), 279 part-time/adjunct (173 women). *Students:* 531 full-time (354 women), 865 part-time (547 women); includes 315 minority (79 Black or African American, non-Hispanic/Latino; 10 American Indian or Alaska Native, non-Hispanic/Latino; 114 Asian, non-Hispanic/Latino; 83 Hispanic/Latino; 6 Native Hawaiian or other Pacific Islander, non-Hispanic/Latino; 23 Two or more races, non-Hispanic/Latino), 82 international. Average age 36. 3,325 applicants, 14% accepted, 329 enrolled. In 2013, 252 master's, 370 doctorates awarded. *Degree requirements:* For master's, thesis (for some programs); for doctorate, thesis/

dissertation (for some programs). *Entrance requirements:* For master's, GRE General Test; for doctorate, GRE, Evaluation of Practicing Audiologists Capabilities (Au D), Physical Therapist Evaluation Tool (DPT), current state licensure, master's degree or equivalent (Au D). Additional exam requirements/recommendations for international students: Required—TOEFL (minimum score 550 paper-based; 80 iBT). *Application deadline:* For fall admission, 8/1 for domestic and international students. Applications are processed on a rolling basis. Application fee: $70. Electronic applications accepted. *Expenses:* Contact institution. *Financial support:* In 2013–14, 151 students received support. Federal Work-Study and scholarships/grants available. Financial award application deadline: 5/1; financial award applicants required to submit FAFSA. *Faculty research:* Pediatric sport-related concussion, adolescent athlete health-related quality of life; geriatric and pediatric well-being, pain management for participation, practice-based research network, BMI and dental caries. *Total annual research expenditures:* $174,826. *Unit head:* Dr. Randy Danielsen, Dean, 480-219-6000, Fax: 480-219-6110, E-mail: rdanielsen@atsu.edu. *Application contact:* Donna Sparks, Associate Director, Admissions Processing, 660-626-2117, Fax: 660-626-2969, E-mail: admissions@atsu.edu.
Website: http://www.atsu.edu/ashs

Auburn University, Graduate School, College of Liberal Arts, Department of Communication Disorders, Auburn University, AL 36849. Offers audiology (MCD, MS, Au D); speech pathology (MCD, MS). *Accreditation:* ASHA (one or more programs are accredited). Part-time programs available. *Faculty:* 15 full-time (12 women), 3 part-time/adjunct (all women). *Students:* 68 full-time (66 women), 6 part-time (4 women); includes 6 minority (4 Black or African American, non-Hispanic/Latino; 2 Hispanic/Latino). Average age 24. 286 applicants, 18% accepted, 28 enrolled. In 2013, 24 master's, 8 doctorates awarded. *Degree requirements:* For master's, comprehensive exam (MCD), thesis (MS). *Entrance requirements:* For master's, GRE General Test. *Application deadline:* For fall admission, 7/7 for domestic students; for spring admission, 11/24 for domestic students. Applications are processed on a rolling basis. Application fee: $50 ($60 for international students). Electronic applications accepted. *Expenses:* Tuition, state resident: full-time $8262; part-time $459 per credit hour. Tuition, nonresident: full-time $24,786; part-time $1377 per credit hour. Tuition and fees vary according to degree level and program. *Financial support:* Research assistantships, teaching assistantships, and Federal Work-Study available. Support available to part-time students. Financial award application deadline: 3/15; financial award applicants required to submit FAFSA. *Unit head:* Dr. Rebekah H. Pindzola, Chair, 334-844-7916. *Application contact:* Dr. George Flowers, Dean of the Graduate School, 334-844-2125.
Website: http://www.cla.auburn.edu/communicationdisorders/

Ball State University, Graduate School, College of Sciences and Humanities, Department of Speech Pathology and Audiology, Muncie, IN 47306-1099. Offers MA, Au D. *Accreditation:* ASHA. *Faculty:* 11 full-time (9 women), 2 part-time/adjunct (1 woman). *Students:* 93 full-time (89 women), 22 part-time (21 women); includes 5 minority (1 Black or African American, non-Hispanic/Latino; 2 Asian, non-Hispanic/Latino; 1 Hispanic/Latino; 1 Native Hawaiian or other Pacific Islander, non-Hispanic/Latino). Average age 25. 273 applicants, 21% accepted, 8 enrolled. In 2013, 41 master's, 9 doctorates awarded. *Entrance requirements:* For master's, GRE General Test; for doctorate, GRE General Test, interview. Application fee: $50. *Financial support:* In 2013–14, 37 students received support, including 25 teaching assistantships with full and partial tuition reimbursements available (averaging $10,821 per year); career-related internships or fieldwork also available. Financial award application deadline: 3/1. *Faculty research:* Adult neurological disorders, stuttering, tinnitus masking, brain stem responses. *Unit head:* Dr. Mary Jo Germani, Chairman, 765-285-8162, Fax: 765-285-5623, E-mail: mgermani@bsu.edu. *Application contact:* Dr. Robert Morris, Associate Provost for Research and Dean of the Graduate School, 765-285-1300, E-mail: rmorris@bsu.edu.
Website: http://www.bsu.edu/csh/spa/

Barry University, School of Education, Program in Education for Teachers of Students with Hearing Impairments, Miami Shores, FL 33161-6695. Offers MS.

Baylor University, Graduate School, College of Arts and Sciences, Department of Communication Sciences and Disorders, Waco, TX 76798-7332. Offers MA, MSCSD. *Accreditation:* ASHA (one or more programs are accredited). *Faculty:* 11 full-time (8 women), 1 (woman) part-time/adjunct. *Students:* 41 full-time (39 women), 2 part-time (both women); includes 12 minority (1 Asian, non-Hispanic/Latino; 6 Hispanic/Latino; 5 Two or more races, non-Hispanic/Latino). Average age 24. 177 applicants, 23% accepted, 9 enrolled. In 2013, 35 master's awarded. *Degree requirements:* For master's, comprehensive exam (for some programs), thesis (for some programs). *Entrance requirements:* For master's, GRE General Test. Additional exam requirements/recommendations for international students: Required—TOEFL. *Application deadline:* For fall admission, 2/15 for domestic and international students; for spring admission, 9/15 for domestic and international students; for summer admission, 2/15 for domestic and international students. Electronic applications accepted. *Expenses:* Contact institution. *Financial support:* In 2013–14, 25 students received support, including 54 fellowships with full and partial tuition reimbursements available (averaging $29,999 per year), 3 research assistantships (averaging $1,800 per year), 14 teaching assistantships (averaging $1,800 per year); Federal Work-Study, institutionally sponsored loans, and tuition waivers (partial) also available. Financial award application deadline: 5/1. *Faculty research:* Nasality, language impairment, stuttering, Spanish speech perception, language literacy. *Unit head:* Dr. David Garrett, Program Director, 254-710-2567, Fax: 254-710-2590. *Application contact:* Kathryn Fadal Williams, Manager, 254-710-2571, Fax: 254-710-2590, E-mail: kathryn_williams@baylor.edu.
Website: http://www.baylor.edu/communication_disorders/

Bloomsburg University of Pennsylvania, School of Graduate Studies, College of Education, Department of Exceptionality Programs, Program in Education of the Deaf/Hard of Hearing, Bloomsburg, PA 17815-1301. Offers MS. *Faculty:* 2 full-time (both women). *Students:* 1 (woman) full-time, 5 part-time (all women); includes 1 minority (Asian, non-Hispanic/Latino). Average age 24. 10 applicants, 50% accepted, 2 enrolled. In 2013, 8 master's awarded. *Degree requirements:* For master's, thesis, minimum QPA of 3.0, practicum. *Entrance requirements:* For master's, PRAXIS, GRE, minimum QPA of 3.0, letter of intent, 3 letters of recommendation, interview. Additional exam requirements/recommendations for international students: Required—TOEFL (minimum score 550 paper-based). *Application deadline:* For fall admission, 3/15 for domestic students. Application fee: $35 ($60 for international students). Electronic applications accepted. *Expenses:* Tuition, state resident: full-time $7956; part-time $442 per credit. Tuition, nonresident: full-time $11,934; part-time $663 per credit. *Required fees:* $95.50 per credit. $55 per semester. Tuition and fees vary according to course load. *Financial support:* Unspecified assistantships available. *Unit head:* Dr. Tegan Kotarski, College of Education Graduate Coordinator, 570-389-3883, Fax: 570-389-5049, E-mail: tkotarsk@bloomu.edu. *Application contact:* Jennifer Richard, Administrative Assistant, 570-389-4015, Fax: 570-389-3054, E-mail: jrichard@bloomu.edu.
Website: http://www.bloomu.edu/gradschool/deaf-education

Bloomsburg University of Pennsylvania, School of Graduate Studies, College of Science and Technology, Department of Audiology and Speech Pathology, Program in Audiology, Bloomsburg, PA 17815-1301. Offers Au D. *Accreditation:* ASHA. *Faculty:* 9 full-time (3 women), 9 part-time/adjunct (8 women). *Students:* 18 full-time (13 women), 43 part-time (34 women); includes 6 minority (1 Black or African American, non-Hispanic/Latino; 2 Asian, non-Hispanic/Latino; 3 Hispanic/Latino), 4 international. Average age 26. 24 applicants, 96% accepted, 9 enrolled. In 2013, 5 doctorates awarded. *Degree requirements:* For doctorate, comprehensive exam, thesis/dissertation, minimum QPA of 3.0, practicum. *Entrance requirements:* For doctorate, GRE, 3 letters of recommendation, interview, personal statement, minimum QPA of 3.0. Additional exam requirements/recommendations for international students: Required—TOEFL. *Application deadline:* For fall admission, 3/15 for domestic students. Application fee: $35 ($60 for international students). Electronic applications accepted. *Expenses:* Tuition, state resident: full-time $7956; part-time $442 per credit. Tuition, nonresident: full-time $11,934; part-time $663 per credit. *Required fees:* $95.50 per credit. $55 per semester. Tuition and fees vary according to course load. *Financial support:* Unspecified assistantships available. *Unit head:* Dr. Jorge Gonzalez, Chair/Clinical Director, 570-389-5370, Fax: 570-389-2035, E-mail: jgonzale@bloomu.edu. *Application contact:* Jennifer Richard, Administrative Assistant, 570-389-4015, Fax: 570-389-3054, E-mail: jrichard@bloomu.edu.
Website: http://www.bloomu.edu/gradschool/audiology

Bloomsburg University of Pennsylvania, School of Graduate Studies, College of Science and Technology, Department of Audiology and Speech Pathology, Program in Speech Pathology, Bloomsburg, PA 17815-1301. Offers school-based speech-language pathology (M Ed); speech-language pathology (MS). *Accreditation:* ASHA. *Faculty:* 10 full-time (4 women), 14 part-time/adjunct (13 women). *Students:* 40 full-time (39 women), 56 part-time (52 women); includes 2 minority (1 Black or African American, non-Hispanic/Latino; 1 Hispanic/Latino), 2 international. Average age 25. 84 applicants, 85% accepted, 44 enrolled. In 2013, 43 master's awarded. *Degree requirements:* For master's, thesis optional, minimum QPA of 3.0, clinical experience. *Entrance requirements:* For master's, GRE, minimum QPA of 3.0, 3 letters of recommendation, personal statement. Additional exam requirements/recommendations for international students: Required—TOEFL (minimum score 550 paper-based). *Application deadline:* For fall admission, 2/15 for domestic students. Application fee: $35 ($60 for international students). Electronic applications accepted. *Expenses:* Tuition, state resident: full-time $7956; part-time $442 per credit. Tuition, nonresident: full-time $11,934; part-time $663 per credit. *Required fees:* $95.50 per credit. $55 per semester. Tuition and fees vary according to course load. *Financial support:* Unspecified assistantships available. *Unit head:* Dr. Shaheen Awan, Coordinator, 570-389-4443, Fax: 570-389-2035, E-mail: sawan@bloomu.edu. *Application contact:* Jennifer Richard, Administrative Assistant, 570-389-4015, Fax: 570-389-3054, E-mail: jrichard@bloomu.edu.
Website: http://www.bloomu.edu/gradschool/impress

Boston University, College of Health and Rehabilitation Sciences: Sargent College, Department of Speech, Language and Hearing Sciences, Boston, MA 02215. Offers speech, language and hearing sciences (PhD); speech-language pathology (MS). *Accreditation:* ASHA. *Faculty:* 12 full-time (10 women), 12 part-time/adjunct (5 women). *Students:* 85 full-time (82 women); includes 4 minority (1 Black or African American, non-Hispanic/Latino; 2 Asian, non-Hispanic/Latino; 1 Hispanic/Latino), 4 international. Average age 25. 456 applicants, 34% accepted, 49 enrolled. In 2013, 45 master's awarded. Terminal master's awarded for partial completion of doctoral program. *Degree requirements:* For master's, comprehensive exam, thesis optional; for doctorate, comprehensive exam, thesis/dissertation. *Entrance requirements:* For master's and doctorate, GRE General Test. Additional exam requirements/recommendations for international students: Required—TOEFL (minimum score 550 paper-based). *Application deadline:* For fall admission, 1/1 priority date for domestic and international students. Applications are processed on a rolling basis. Application fee: $100. Electronic applications accepted. *Expenses: Tuition:* Full-time $43,970; part-time $1374 per credit hour. *Required fees:* $60 per semester. Tuition and fees vary according to class time, course level and program. *Financial support:* In 2013–14, 60 students received support, including 48 fellowships (averaging $11,300 per year), 7 research assistantships with full tuition reimbursements available (averaging $20,000 per year), 7 teaching assistantships (averaging $3,000 per year); career-related internships or fieldwork, Federal Work-Study, institutionally sponsored loans, scholarships/grants, and tuition waivers (partial) also available. Financial award application deadline: 4/15; financial award applicants required to submit FAFSA. *Faculty research:* Child language, fluency, autism, speech science, perception of complex sounds. *Total annual research expenditures:* $3.9 million. *Unit head:* Dr. Melanie Matthies, Chair, 617-353-3188, E-mail: slhs@bu.edu. *Application contact:* Sharon Sankey, Director, Student Services, 617-353-2713, Fax: 617-353-7500, E-mail: ssankey@bu.edu.
Website: http://www.bu.edu/sargent/

Bowling Green State University, Graduate College, College of Education and Human Development, School of Education and Intervention Services, Intervention Services Division, Program in Special Education, Bowling Green, OH 43403. Offers assistive technology (M Ed); early childhood intervention (M Ed); gifted education (M Ed); hearing impaired intervention (M Ed); mild/moderate intervention (M Ed); moderate/intensive intervention (M Ed). *Accreditation:* NCATE. Part-time programs available. *Degree requirements:* For master's, thesis or alternative. *Entrance requirements:* For master's, GRE General Test. Additional exam requirements/recommendations for international students: Required—TOEFL. Electronic applications accepted. *Faculty research:* Reading and special populations, deafness, early childhood, gifted and talented, behavior disorders.

Bowling Green State University, Graduate College, College of Health and Human Services, Department of Communication Disorders, Bowling Green, OH 43403. Offers communication disorders (PhD); speech-language pathology (MS). *Accreditation:* ASHA (one or more programs are accredited). *Degree requirements:* For master's, thesis or alternative; for doctorate, comprehensive exam, thesis/dissertation, foreign language or research tool. *Entrance requirements:* For master's, GRE General Test, minimum GPA of 3.0; for doctorate, GRE General Test, minimum GPA of 3.2. Additional exam requirements/recommendations for international students: Required—TOEFL. Electronic applications accepted. *Faculty research:* Rehabilitation and mental disorders, forensic rehabilitation, rehabilitation and substance abuse, private rehabilitation and disability management, adjustment to disability.

Brigham Young University, Graduate Studies, David O. McKay School of Education, Department of Communication Disorders, Provo, UT 84602-1001. Offers MS. *Accreditation:* ASHA. *Faculty:* 11 full-time (5 women), 5 part-time/adjunct (all women). *Students:* 44 full-time (43 women); includes 2 minority (1 Asian, non-Hispanic/Latino; 1 Hispanic/Latino). Average age 26. 82 applicants, 41% accepted, 24 enrolled. In 2013, 25 master's awarded. *Degree requirements:* For master's, comprehensive exam, thesis, exit interview, PRAXIS. *Entrance requirements:* For master's, GRE General Test, 3 letters of recommendation, statement of intent. Additional exam requirements/recommendations for international students: Required—TOEFL (minimum score 580 paper-based; 85 iBT). *Application deadline:* For fall admission, 2/1 for domestic and international students. Application fee: $50. Electronic applications accepted. *Expenses: Tuition:* Full-time $6130; part-time $340 per credit hour. Tuition and fees vary according to program and student's religious affiliation. *Financial support:* In 2013–14, 40 students received support, including 20 research assistantships (averaging $1,701 per year), 18

teaching assistantships (averaging $2,786 per year); fellowships, institutionally sponsored loans, and scholarships/grants also available. Financial award application deadline: 2/1. *Faculty research:* Foreign language speech audiometry materials; language sample analysis, language measurement; speech motor control physiology; aerodynamic and kinematic analysis of speech production; social skills and outcomes of children with language impairment. *Unit head:* Dr. Christopher Dromey, Chair, 801-422-6461, Fax: 801-422-0197, E-mail: christopher_dromey@byu.edu. *Application contact:* Sandy Alger, Department Secretary, 801-422-5117, Fax: 801-422-0197, E-mail: sandy_alger@byu.edu.
Website: http://education.byu.edu/comd/

Brooklyn College of the City University of New York, School of Humanities and Social Sciences, Department of Speech Communication Arts and Sciences, Brooklyn, NY 11210-2889. Offers audiology (Au D); speech (MA), including public communication; speech-language pathology (MS). Au D offered jointly with Hunter College of the City University of New York. *Accreditation:* ASHA (one or more programs are accredited). Part-time programs available. Terminal master's awarded for partial completion of doctoral program. *Degree requirements:* For master's, comprehensive exam, NTE. *Entrance requirements:* For master's, GRE, minimum GPA of 3.0, interview, essay. Additional exam requirements/recommendations for international students: Required—TOEFL (minimum score 500 paper-based; 61 iBT). *Application deadline:* For fall admission, 2/1 priority date for domestic and international students. Applications are processed on a rolling basis. Electronic applications accepted. *Expenses: Tuition, area resident:* Full-time $4585; part-time $385 per credit. Tuition, state resident: full-time $4585; part-time $385 per credit. Tuition, nonresident: part-time $710 per credit. *Required fees:* $430; $153 per semester. Tuition and fees vary according to course load. *Financial support:* Career-related internships or fieldwork, Federal Work-Study, institutionally sponsored loans, scholarships/grants, and traineeships available. Support available to part-time students. Financial award application deadline: 5/1; financial award applicants required to submit FAFSA. *Faculty research:* Language and learning disorders, aphasia, auditory disorders, public and business communication, voice and fluency disorders. *Unit head:* Michele Emmer, Chairperson, 718-951-5225, Fax: 718-951-4167. *Application contact:* Michele Emmer, Chairperson, 718-951-5225, Fax: 718-951-4167.

Buffalo State College, State University of New York, The Graduate School, Faculty of Applied Science and Education, Department of Speech-Language Pathology, Buffalo, NY 14222-1095. Offers MS Ed. *Accreditation:* ASHA. Part-time and evening/weekend programs available. *Degree requirements:* For master's, thesis or alternative, project. *Entrance requirements:* For master's, minimum GPA of 3.0 in last 60 hours, 22 hours in communication disorders. Additional exam requirements/recommendations for international students: Required—TOEFL (minimum score 550 paper-based).

California State University, Chico, Office of Graduate Studies, College of Communication and Education, Department of Communication Arts and Sciences, Program in Communication Sciences and Disorders, Chico, CA 95929-0722. Offers MA. *Accreditation:* ASHA. *Degree requirements:* For master's, thesis or project. *Entrance requirements:* For master's, GRE General Test, 3 letters of recommendation, statement of purpose, resume. Additional exam requirements/recommendations for international students: Required—TOEFL (minimum score 550 paper-based; 80 iBT), IELTS (minimum score 6.5), PTE (minimum score 59). Electronic applications accepted.

California State University, East Bay, Office of Academic Programs and Graduate Studies, College of Letters, Arts, and Social Sciences, Department of Communicative Sciences and Disorders, Hayward, CA 94542-3000. Offers speech-language pathology (MS). *Accreditation:* ASHA. Part-time programs available. *Degree requirements:* For master's, comprehensive exam, internship or thesis. *Entrance requirements:* For master's, minimum GPA of 3.0 in last 2 years of course work; baccalaureate degree in speech pathology and audiology; minimum of 60 hours supervised clinical practice. Additional exam requirements/recommendations for international students: Required—TOEFL (minimum score 550 paper-based). Electronic applications accepted. *Faculty research:* Aphasia, autism, dementia, diversity, voice.

California State University, Fresno, Division of Graduate Studies, College of Health and Human Services, Department of Communicative Disorders, Fresno, CA 93740-8027. Offers communicative disorders (MA), including deaf education, speech/language pathology. *Accreditation:* ASHA. Part-time programs available. *Degree requirements:* For master's, thesis or alternative. *Entrance requirements:* For master's, GRE General Test, minimum GPA of 3.0. Additional exam requirements/recommendations for international students: Required—TOEFL. Electronic applications accepted. *Faculty research:* Disabilities education, technology, writing skills at multiple levels, stuttering treatment.

California State University, Fullerton, Graduate Studies, College of Communications, Department of Human Communications, Fullerton, CA 92834-9480. Offers communication studies (MA); communicative disorders (MA). *Accreditation:* ASHA. Part-time programs available. *Students:* 65 full-time (56 women), 35 part-time (25 women); includes 52 minority (2 Black or African American, non-Hispanic/Latino; 23 Asian, non-Hispanic/Latino; 25 Hispanic/Latino; 2 Two or more races, non-Hispanic/Latino), 4 international. Average age 31. 401 applicants, 7% accepted, 12 enrolled. In 2013, 42 master's awarded. *Degree requirements:* For master's, comprehensive exam, thesis or alternative. *Entrance requirements:* For master's, minimum GPA of 3.0 in major. Application fee: $55. *Financial support:* Teaching assistantships, career-related internships or fieldwork, Federal Work-Study, institutionally sponsored loans, and scholarships/grants available. Support available to part-time students. Financial award application deadline: 3/1; financial award applicants required to submit FAFSA. *Faculty research:* Speech therapy. *Unit head:* Dr. John Reinard, Chair, 657-278-3617. *Application contact:* Admissions/Applications, 657-278-2371.

California State University, Fullerton, Graduate Studies, College of Humanities and Social Sciences, Program in Linguistics, Fullerton, CA 92834-9480. Offers analysis of specific language structures (MA); anthropological linguistics (MA); applied linguistics (MA); communication and semantics (MA); disorders of communication (MA); experimental phonetics (MA). Part-time programs available. *Students:* 29 full-time (17 women), 17 part-time (9 women); includes 11 minority (5 Asian, non-Hispanic/Latino; 5 Hispanic/Latino; 1 Two or more races, non-Hispanic/Latino), 23 international. Average age 30. 47 applicants, 47% accepted, 14 enrolled. In 2013, 6 master's awarded. *Degree requirements:* For master's, one foreign language, thesis or alternative, project. *Entrance requirements:* For master's, minimum GPA of 3.0, undergraduate major in linguistics or related field. Application fee: $55. *Financial support:* Career-related internships or fieldwork, Federal Work-Study, institutionally sponsored loans, and scholarships/grants available. Support available to part-time students. Financial award application deadline: 3/1; financial award applicants required to submit FAFSA. *Unit head:* Dr. Franz Muller-Gotama, Adviser, 657-278-2441. *Application contact:* Admissions/Applications, 657-278-2371.

California State University, Long Beach, Graduate Studies, College of Health and Human Services, Department of Communicative Disorders, Long Beach, CA 90840. Offers MA. *Accreditation:* ASHA. Part-time programs available. *Degree requirements:* For master's, comprehensive exam or thesis. *Entrance requirements:* For master's, GRE, minimum GPA of 3.0 in last 60 units. Electronic applications accepted.

California State University, Los Angeles, Graduate Studies, College of Health and Human Services, Department of Communication Disorders, Los Angeles, CA 90032-8530. Offers speech and hearing (MA); speech-language pathology (MA). *Accreditation:* ASHA. Part-time and evening/weekend programs available. *Faculty:* 8 full-time (5 women), 6 part-time/adjunct (5 women). *Students:* 62 full-time (57 women), 35 part-time (31 women); includes 56 minority (1 Black or African American, non-Hispanic/Latino; 20 Asian, non-Hispanic/Latino; 30 Hispanic/Latino; 1 Native Hawaiian or other Pacific Islander, non-Hispanic/Latino; 4 Two or more races, non-Hispanic/Latino), 2 international. Average age 30. 292 applicants, 15% accepted, 34 enrolled. In 2013, 19 master's awarded. *Degree requirements:* For master's, comprehensive exam. *Entrance requirements:* For master's, undergraduate major in communication disorders or related area, minimum GPA of 2.75 in last 90 units. Additional exam requirements/recommendations for international students: Required—TOEFL (minimum score 500 paper-based). *Application deadline:* For fall admission, 5/1 for domestic and international students. Applications are processed on a rolling basis. Application fee: $55. *Financial support:* Career-related internships or fieldwork and Federal Work-Study available. Support available to part-time students. Financial award application deadline: 3/1. *Faculty research:* Language disabilities, minority child language learning. *Unit head:* Dr. Edward Klein, Chair, 323-343-4690, Fax: 323-343-4698, E-mail: eklein@cslanet.calstatela.edu. *Application contact:* Dr. Larry Fritz, Dean of Graduate Studies, 323-343-3820, Fax: 323-343-5653, E-mail: lfritz@calstatela.edu.
Website: http://www.calstatela.edu/dept/com_dis/

California State University, Northridge, Graduate Studies, College of Health and Human Development, Department of Communication Disorders and Sciences, Northridge, CA 91330. Offers audiology (MS); speech language pathology (MS). *Accreditation:* ASHA. *Degree requirements:* For master's, PRAXIS. *Entrance requirements:* For master's, GRE or minimum GPA of 3.5. Additional exam requirements/recommendations for international students: Required—TOEFL. *Faculty research:* Infant stimulation, early intervention program.

California State University, Sacramento, Office of Graduate Studies, College of Health and Human Services, Department of Speech Pathology and Audiology, Sacramento, CA 95819. Offers speech pathology (MS). *Accreditation:* ASHA. *Degree requirements:* For master's, thesis, project, or comprehensive exam; writing proficiency exam. *Entrance requirements:* For master's, GRE General Test, appropriate bachelor's degree, minimum GPA of 3.0 in last 2 years of course work. Additional exam requirements/recommendations for international students: Required—TOEFL. *Application deadline:* For fall admission, 2/15 for domestic students, 3/1 for international students; for spring admission, 9/30 for international students. Applications are processed on a rolling basis. Application fee: $55. Electronic applications accepted. *Financial support:* Career-related internships or fieldwork and Federal Work-Study available. Support available to part-time students. Financial award application deadline: 3/1; financial award applicants required to submit FAFSA. *Unit head:* Ann Blanton, Chair, 916-278-6679, E-mail: blantona@saclink.csus.edu. *Application contact:* Jose Martinez, Graduate Admissions Supervisor, 916-278-7871, E-mail: martinj@skymail.csus.edu.
Website: http://www.csus.edu/hhs/spa

California University of Pennsylvania, School of Graduate Studies and Research, College of Education and Human Services, Department of Communication Disorders, California, PA 15419-1394. Offers MS. *Accreditation:* ASHA. Part-time and evening/weekend programs available. *Degree requirements:* For master's, comprehensive exam, thesis optional. *Entrance requirements:* For master's, GRE General Test, minimum GPA of 3.0, references. Additional exam requirements/recommendations for international students: Required—TOEFL (minimum score 550 paper-based; 80 iBT). Electronic applications accepted. *Faculty research:* Normative voice database, communication disorders and health.

Canisius College, Graduate Division, School of Education and Human Services, Department of Graduate Education and Leadership, Buffalo, NY 14208-1098. Offers business and marketing education (MS Ed); college student personnel (MS Ed); deaf education (MS Ed); deaf/adolescent education, grades 7-12 (MS Ed); deaf/childhood education, grades 1-6 (MS Ed); differentiated instruction (MS Ed); education administration (MS); educational administration (MS Ed); educational technologies (Certificate); gifted education extension (Certificate); literacy (MS Ed); reading (Certificate); school building leadership (MS Ed, Certificate); school district leadership (Certificate); teacher leader (Certificate); TESOL (MS Ed). *Accreditation:* NCATE. Part-time and evening/weekend programs available. Postbaccalaureate distance learning degree programs offered (minimal on-campus study). *Faculty:* 6 full-time (5 women), 33 part-time/adjunct (20 women). *Students:* 134 full-time (106 women), 267 part-time (213 women); includes 36 minority (22 Black or African American, non-Hispanic/Latino; 1 American Indian or Alaska Native, non-Hispanic/Latino; 3 Asian, non-Hispanic/Latino; 8 Hispanic/Latino; 2 Two or more races, non-Hispanic/Latino), 2 international. Average age 30. 282 applicants, 80% accepted, 120 enrolled. In 2013, 178 master's awarded. *Entrance requirements:* For master's, GRE if cumulative GPA less than 2.7, transcripts, two letters of recommendation. Additional exam requirements/recommendations for international students: Required—TOEFL (minimum score 550 paper-based, 80 iBT), IELTS (minimum score 6.5), or CAEL (minimum score 70). *Application deadline:* Applications are processed on a rolling basis. Application fee: $25. Electronic applications accepted. Application fee is waived when completed online. *Expenses: Tuition:* Part-time $750 per credit hour. *Financial support:* Career-related internships or fieldwork, Federal Work-Study, scholarships/grants, tuition waivers (partial), and unspecified assistantships available. Support available to part-time students. Financial award application deadline: 4/30; financial award applicants required to submit FAFSA. *Faculty research:* Asperger's disease, autism, private higher education, reading strategies. *Unit head:* Dr. Rosemary K. Murray, Chair/Associate Professor of Graduate Education and Leadership, 716-888-3723, E-mail: murray1@canisius.edu. *Application contact:* Julie A. Zulewski, Director of Graduate Admissions, 716-888-2548, Fax: 716-888-3195, E-mail: zulewskj@canisius.edu.
Website: http://www.canisius.edu/graduate/

Carlos Albizu University, Graduate Programs, San Juan, PR 00901. Offers clinical psychology (MS, PhD, Psy D); general psychology (PhD); industrial/organizational psychology (MS, PhD); speech and language pathology (MS). *Accreditation:* APA (one or more programs are accredited). Part-time and evening/weekend programs available. Terminal master's awarded for partial completion of doctoral program. *Degree requirements:* For master's, one foreign language, comprehensive exam, thesis; for doctorate, one foreign language, comprehensive exam, thesis/dissertation, written qualifying exams. *Entrance requirements:* For master's, GRE General Test or EXADEP, interview; minimum GPA of 2.8 (industrial/organizational psychology); for doctorate, GRE General Test or EXADEP, interview; minimum GPA of 3.0 (PhD in industrial/organizational psychology and clinical psychology), 3.25 (Psy D). *Faculty research:* Psychotherapeutic techniques for Hispanics, psychology of the aged, school dropouts, stress, violence.

Communication Disorders

Case Western Reserve University, School of Graduate Studies, Psychological Sciences Department, Program in Communication Sciences, Cleveland, OH 44106. Offers speech-language pathology (MA, PhD). *Accreditation:* ASHA (one or more programs are accredited). Part-time programs available. *Faculty:* 5 full-time (all women), 4 part-time/adjunct (2 women). *Students:* 15 full-time (14 women), 4 part-time (all women); includes 2 minority (1 Black or African American, non-Hispanic/Latino; 1 Two or more races, non-Hispanic/Latino), 1 international. Average age 25. 68 applicants, 18% accepted, 10 enrolled. In 2013, 8 master's awarded. Terminal master's awarded for partial completion of doctoral program. *Degree requirements:* For master's, comprehensive exam, thesis optional; for doctorate, thesis/dissertation. *Entrance requirements:* For master's and doctorate, GRE General Test, 3 letters of recommendation; interview. Additional exam requirements/recommendations for international students: Required—TOEFL (minimum score 577 paper-based; 90 iBT); Recommended—IELTS (minimum score 7). *Application deadline:* For fall admission, 1/31 for domestic students. Application fee: $50. Electronic applications accepted. *Financial support:* Research assistantships, tuition waivers (partial), and unspecified assistantships available. Financial award application deadline: 1/31; financial award applicants required to submit FAFSA. *Faculty research:* Traumatic brain injury, phonological disorders, child language disorders, communication problems in the aged and Alzheimer's patients, cleft palate, voice disorders. *Unit head:* Dr. Lee Thompson, Chair, 216-368-6477, Fax: 216-368-6078, E-mail: lee.thompson@case.edu. *Application contact:* Patricia Maar, Assistant, 216-368-2470, Fax: 216-368-6078, E-mail: cosigrad@case.edu.
Website: http://www.case.edu/artsci/cosi/

Central Michigan University, College of Graduate Studies, The Herbert H. and Grace A. Dow College of Health Professions, Department of Communication Disorders, Doctor of Audiology Program, Mount Pleasant, MI 48859. Offers Au D. *Accreditation:* ASHA. *Degree requirements:* For doctorate, comprehensive exam, thesis/dissertation or alternative. *Entrance requirements:* For doctorate, GRE, interview. Electronic applications accepted. *Faculty research:* Auditory electrophysiology, auditory process disorders, neuroanatomy, pediatric audiology, rehabilitative audiology.

Central Michigan University, College of Graduate Studies, The Herbert H. and Grace A. Dow College of Health Professions, Department of Communication Disorders, Program in Speech-Language Pathology, Mount Pleasant, MI 48859. Offers MA. *Accreditation:* ASHA. *Degree requirements:* For master's, thesis or alternative. Electronic applications accepted. *Expenses:* Contact institution. *Faculty research:* Traumatic brain injury, neuro-linguistics, multidisciplinary and transdisciplinary therapy, speech audiometry, phonological disorders.

Chapman University, College of Educational Studies, Orange, CA 92866. Offers communication sciences and disorders (MS); counseling (MA), including school counseling (MA, Credential); education (PhD), including cultural and curricular studies, disability studies, leadership studies, school psychology (PhD, Credential); educational psychology (MA); leadership development (MA); pupil personnel services (Credential), including school counseling (MA, Credential), school psychology (PhD, Credential); school psychology (Ed S); single subject (Credential); special education (MA, Credential), including mild/moderate (Credential), moderate/severe (Credential); speech language pathology (Credential); teaching (MA), including elementary education, secondary education. *Accreditation:* Teacher Education Accreditation Council. Part-time and evening/weekend programs available. *Faculty:* 29 full-time (18 women), 56 part-time/adjunct (38 women). *Students:* 251 full-time (208 women), 194 part-time (150 women); includes 185 minority (13 Black or African American, non-Hispanic/Latino; 61 Asian, non-Hispanic/Latino; 97 Hispanic/Latino; 1 Native Hawaiian or other Pacific Islander, non-Hispanic/Latino; 13 Two or more races, non-Hispanic/Latino), 7 international. Average age 29. 580 applicants, 42% accepted, 166 enrolled. In 2013, 140 master's, 10 doctorates awarded. *Entrance requirements:* Additional exam requirements/recommendations for international students: Required—TOEFL (minimum score 550 paper-based; 80 iBT). *Application deadline:* Applications are processed on a rolling basis. Application fee: $60. Electronic applications accepted. Tuition and fees vary according to program. *Financial support:* Fellowships and scholarships/grants available. Financial award application deadline: 6/30; financial award applicants required to submit FAFSA. *Unit head:* Dr. Don Cardinal, Dean, 714-997-6781, E-mail: cardinal@chapman.edu. *Application contact:* Admissions Coordinator, 714-997-6714.
Website: http://www.chapman.edu/CES/

Clarion University of Pennsylvania, Office of Transfer, Adult and Graduate Admissions, On-Campus Master's Programs, Clarion, PA 16214. Offers rehabilitative sciences (MS); special education (MS); speech language pathology (MS). *Accreditation:* ASHA. Part-time programs available. Postbaccalaureate distance learning degree programs offered (no on-campus study). *Faculty:* 23 full-time (16 women). *Students:* 113 full-time (97 women), 42 part-time (33 women); includes 4 minority (2 Black or African American, non-Hispanic/Latino; 1 American Indian or Alaska Native, non-Hispanic/Latino; 1 Hispanic/Latino). Average age 24. 297 applicants, 18% accepted, 44 enrolled. In 2013, 68 master's awarded. *Degree requirements:* For master's, comprehensive exam (for some programs), thesis or alternative. *Entrance requirements:* For master's, GRE, minimum QPA of 3.0. Additional exam requirements/recommendations for international students: Required—TOEFL (minimum score 600 paper-based; 89 iBT), IELTS (minimum score 7.5). *Application deadline:* For fall admission, 1/31 for domestic and international students. Applications are processed on a rolling basis. Application fee: $40. Electronic applications accepted. *Expenses:* Tuition, state resident: part-time $442 per credit. Tuition, nonresident: part-time $451 per credit. *Required fees:* $142.40 per semester. One-time fee: $150 part-time. *Financial support:* In 2013–14, 21 research assistantships with full and partial tuition reimbursements (averaging $9,240 per year) were awarded; career-related internships or fieldwork also available. Support available to part-time students. Financial award application deadline: 3/1. *Unit head:* Dr. Colleen McAleer, Chair, 814-393-2581, Fax: 814-393-2206, E-mail: cmcaleer@clarion.edu. *Application contact:* Michelle Ritzler, Assistant Director, Graduate Programs, 814-393-2337, Fax: 814-393-2722, E-mail: gradstudies@clarion.edu.
Website: http://www.clarion.edu/991/

Cleveland State University, College of Graduate Studies, College of Sciences and Health Professions, School of Health Sciences, Program in Speech Pathology and Audiology, Cleveland, OH 44115. Offers MA. *Accreditation:* ASHA. *Faculty:* 7 full-time (6 women), 5 part-time/adjunct (all women). *Students:* 51 full-time (49 women), 3 part-time (all women); includes 2 minority (1 Asian, non-Hispanic/Latino; 1 Hispanic/Latino). Average age 26. 296 applicants, 39% accepted, 24 enrolled. In 2013, 31 master's awarded. *Degree requirements:* For master's, comprehensive exam, thesis optional. *Entrance requirements:* For master's, GRE. Additional exam requirements/recommendations for international students: Required—TOEFL. *Application deadline:* For fall admission, 2/1 priority date for domestic and international students. Application fee: $30. Electronic applications accepted. *Expenses:* Tuition, state resident: full-time $8335; part-time $521 per credit hour. Tuition, nonresident: full-time $15,670; part-time $979 per credit hour. *Required fees:* $50; $25 per semester. *Financial support:* In 2013–14, 9 students received support, including 9 teaching assistantships with partial tuition reimbursements available; career-related internships or fieldwork, Federal Work-Study, and unspecified assistantships also available. Financial award application deadline: 2/1; financial award applicants required to submit FAFSA. *Faculty research:* Child language and literacy development, cultural diversity, variant dialects, voice disorders, neurogenic communication disorders. *Unit head:* Dr. Monica Gordon Pershey, Program Director, 216-687-4534, Fax: 216-687-6993, E-mail: m.pershey@csuohio.edu. *Application contact:* Donna Helwig, Administrative Coordinator to the Chairperson, 216-687-3807, Fax: 216-687-6993, E-mail: d.helwig@csuohio.edu.
Website: http://www.csuohio.edu/sciences/dept/healthsciences/graduate/SPH/index.html

The College of Saint Rose, Graduate Studies, School of Education, Department of Communication Sciences and Disorders, Albany, NY 12203-1419. Offers MS Ed. *Accreditation:* ASHA. Part-time and evening/weekend programs available. *Degree requirements:* For master's, comprehensive exam or thesis. *Entrance requirements:* For master's, minimum undergraduate GPA of 3.0, on-campus interview, 32 undergraduate credits if undergraduate degree is not in communication disorders. Additional exam requirements/recommendations for international students: Required—TOEFL (minimum score 550 paper-based). Electronic applications accepted.

Dalhousie University, Faculty of Health Professions, School of Human Communication Disorders, Halifax, NS B3H 1R2, Canada. Offers audiology (M Sc); speech-language pathology (M Sc). *Degree requirements:* For master's, thesis or alternative. *Entrance requirements:* Additional exam requirements/recommendations for international students: Required—TOEFL, IELTS, CANTEST, CAEL, or Michigan English Language Assessment Battery. Electronic applications accepted. *Expenses:* Contact institution. *Faculty research:* Audiology, hearing aids, speech and voice disorders, language development and disorders, treatment efficacy.

Duquesne University, John G. Rangos, Sr. School of Health Sciences, Pittsburgh, PA 15282-0001. Offers health management systems (MHMS); occupational therapy (MS, OTD); physical therapy (DPT); physician assistant studies (MPAS); rehabilitation science (MS, PhD); speech-language pathology (MS); MBA/MHMS. *Accreditation:* AOTA (one or more programs are accredited); APTA (one or more programs are accredited); ASHA. Postbaccalaureate distance learning degree programs offered (minimal on-campus study). *Faculty:* 41 full-time (29 women), 32 part-time/adjunct (15 women). *Students:* 232 full-time (174 women), 14 part-time (7 women); includes 12 minority (2 Black or African American, non-Hispanic/Latino; 7 Asian, non-Hispanic/Latino; 1 Hispanic/Latino; 2 Two or more races, non-Hispanic/Latino), 7 international. Average age 23. 951 applicants, 11% accepted, 35 enrolled. In 2013, 119 master's, 40 doctorates awarded. *Degree requirements:* For doctorate, comprehensive exam (for some programs), thesis/dissertation (for some programs). *Entrance requirements:* For master's, GRE General Test (speech-language pathology), 3 letters of recommendation; minimum GPA of 2.75 (health management systems), 3.0 (speech-language pathology); for doctorate, GRE General Test (for physical therapy and rehabilitation science), 3 letters of recommendation, minimum GPA of 3.0, personal interview. Additional exam requirements/recommendations for international students: Required—TOEFL (minimum score 550 paper-based; 90 iBT). *Application deadline:* For fall admission, 2/1 for domestic and international students; for spring admission, 7/1 for domestic and international students. Applications are processed on a rolling basis. Electronic applications accepted. *Expenses:* Contact institution. *Financial support:* Federal Work-Study available. Financial award applicants required to submit FAFSA. *Faculty research:* Neuronal processing, electrical stimulation on peripheral neuropathy, central nervous system (CNS) stimulatory and inhibitory signals, behavioral genetic methodologies to development disorders of speech, neurogenic communication disorders. *Total annual research expenditures:* $83,650. *Unit head:* Dr. Gregory H. Frazer, Dean, 412-396-5303, Fax: 412-396-5554, E-mail: frazer@duq.edu. *Application contact:* Christopher R. Hilf, Recruiter/Academic Advisor, 412-396-5653, Fax: 412-396-5554, E-mail: hilfc@duq.edu.
Website: http://www.duq.edu/academics/schools/health-sciences

East Carolina University, Graduate School, School of Allied Health Sciences, Department of Communication Sciences and Disorders, Greenville, NC 27858-4353. Offers MS, PhD, Au D/PhD. *Accreditation:* ASHA (one or more programs are accredited). Postbaccalaureate distance learning degree programs offered (no on-campus study). *Degree requirements:* For master's, comprehensive exam, thesis or alternative; for doctorate, comprehensive exam, thesis/dissertation. *Entrance requirements:* For master's and doctorate, GRE General Test. Additional exam requirements/recommendations for international students: Required—TOEFL. *Application deadline:* For fall admission, 4/1 for domestic students. Application fee: $50. *Expenses:* Tuition, state resident: full-time $4223. Tuition, nonresident: full-time $16,540. *Required fees:* $2184. *Financial support:* Research assistantships with partial tuition reimbursements, teaching assistantships with partial tuition reimbursements, and unspecified assistantships available. Financial award application deadline: 6/1. *Faculty research:* Hearing, language disorders, stuttering, reading disorder. *Unit head:* Dr. Kathleen Cox, Interim Chair, 252-744-6095, E-mail: coxka@ecu.edu. *Application contact:* Graduate School, 252-328-6012, Fax: 252-328-6071, E-mail: gradschool@ecu.edu.
Website: http://www.ecu.edu/cs-dhs/csd/index.cfm

Eastern Illinois University, Graduate School, College of Sciences, Department of Communication Disorders and Sciences, Charleston, IL 61920-3099. Offers MS. *Accreditation:* ASHA. *Degree requirements:* For master's, comprehensive exam. *Expenses: Tuition, area resident:* Part-time $283 per credit hour. Tuition, state resident: part-time $283 per credit hour. Tuition, nonresident: part-time $679 per credit hour.

Eastern Kentucky University, The Graduate School, College of Education, Department of Special Education, Program in Communication Disorders, Richmond, KY 40475-3102. Offers MA Ed. *Accreditation:* ASHA. *Degree requirements:* For master's, comprehensive exam, thesis optional, 375 clinical clock hours. *Entrance requirements:* For master's, GRE General Test, minimum GPA of 3.0. *Faculty research:* Distance learning, fluency, phonemic awareness, technology, autism.

Eastern Michigan University, Graduate School, College of Education, Department of Special Education, Program in Hearing Impairment, Ypsilanti, MI 48197. Offers MA. *Students:* 2 full-time (both women); both minorities (both Black or African American, non-Hispanic/Latino). Average age 27. Application fee: $35. *Expenses:* Tuition, state resident: full-time $12,300; part-time $466 per credit hour. Tuition, nonresident: full-time $23,159; part-time $918 per credit hour. *Required fees:* $71 per credit hour. $46 per semester. One-time fee: $100. Tuition and fees vary according to course level and degree level. *Unit head:* Dr. Janet Fisher, Interim Department Head, 734-487-3300, Fax: 734-487-2473, E-mail: psmith16@emich.edu. *Application contact:* Linda Polter, Coordinator, 734-487-3300, Fax: 734-487-2473, E-mail: lpolter1@emich.edu.

Eastern Michigan University, Graduate School, College of Education, Department of Special Education, Program in Speech-Language Pathology, Ypsilanti, MI 48197. Offers MA. *Accreditation:* ASHA. Part-time and evening/weekend programs available. Postbaccalaureate distance learning degree programs offered (minimal on-campus study). *Students:* 78 full-time (72 women), 32 part-time (30 women); includes 4 minority (1 Black or African American, non-Hispanic/Latino; 2 Asian, non-Hispanic/Latino; 1 Hispanic/Latino), 3 international. Average age 27. 311 applicants, 37% accepted, 25 enrolled. In 2013, 38 master's awarded. *Entrance requirements:* For master's, GRE

General Test. Additional exam requirements/recommendations for international students: Required—TOEFL. *Application deadline:* Applications are processed on a rolling basis. Application fee: $35. *Expenses:* Tuition, state resident: full-time $12,300; part-time $466 per credit hour. Tuition, nonresident: full-time $23,159; part-time $918 per credit hour. *Required fees:* $71 per credit hour. $46 per semester. One-time fee: $100. Tuition and fees vary according to course level and degree level. *Financial support:* Fellowships, research assistantships with full tuition reimbursements, teaching assistantships with full tuition reimbursements, career-related internships or fieldwork, Federal Work-Study, institutionally sponsored loans, scholarships/grants, tuition waivers (partial), and unspecified assistantships available. Support available to part-time students. Financial award applicants required to submit FAFSA. *Unit head:* Dr. Janet Fisher, Interim Department Head, 734-487-2716, Fax: 734-487-2473, E-mail: jfisher3@emich.edu. *Application contact:* Dr. Lizbeth Stevens, Advisor, 734-487-3300, Fax: 734-487-2473, E-mail: lstevens@emich.edu.
Website: http://www.emich.edu/coe/slp/

Eastern New Mexico University, Graduate School, College of Liberal Arts and Sciences, Department of Health and Human Services, Portales, NM 88130. Offers nursing (MSN); speech pathology and audiology (MS). *Accreditation:* ASHA. Part-time programs available. Postbaccalaureate distance learning degree programs offered (minimal on-campus study). *Degree requirements:* For master's, thesis optional, oral and written comprehensive exam, oral presentation of professional portfolio. *Entrance requirements:* For master's, GRE, three letters of recommendation, resume, two essays. Additional exam requirements/recommendations for international students: Required—TOEFL (minimum score 550 paper-based; 79 iBT), IELTS (minimum score 6). Electronic applications accepted.

Eastern Washington University, Graduate Studies, College of Science, Health and Engineering, Department of Communication Disorders, Cheney, WA 99004-2431. Offers MS. *Accreditation:* ASHA. *Faculty:* 12 full-time (9 women). *Students:* 53 full-time (46 women); includes 2 minority (1 American Indian or Alaska Native, non-Hispanic/Latino; 1 Two or more races, non-Hispanic/Latino). Average age 30. 257 applicants, 8% accepted, 21 enrolled. In 2013, 25 master's awarded. *Degree requirements:* For master's, comprehensive exam, thesis or alternative. *Entrance requirements:* For master's, GRE General Test, minimum GPA of 3.0. *Application deadline:* For fall admission, 3/1 for domestic students. Applications are processed on a rolling basis. Application fee: $60. *Financial support:* In 2013–14, 12 teaching assistantships with partial tuition reimbursements (averaging $7,000 per year) were awarded; career-related internships or fieldwork, Federal Work-Study, institutionally sponsored loans, scholarships/grants, health care benefits, tuition waivers (partial), and unspecified assistantships also available. Support available to part-time students. Financial award application deadline: 2/1; financial award applicants required to submit FAFSA. *Unit head:* Dr. Judd A. Case, Dean, 509-359-2532, E-mail: jcase@mail.ewu.edu. *Application contact:* Dr. Roberta Jackson, Advisor, 509-359-6622, Fax: 509-359-6802.
Website: http://www.ewu.edu/CSHE/Programs/Communication-Disorders/ComD-Degrees/MSCD.xml

East Stroudsburg University of Pennsylvania, Graduate College, College of Health Sciences, Department of Speech Pathology and Audiology, East Stroudsburg, PA 18301-2999. Offers MS. *Accreditation:* ASHA. Part-time and evening/weekend programs available. Postbaccalaureate distance learning degree programs offered. *Faculty:* 6 full-time (5 women), 2 part-time/adjunct (both women). *Students:* 53 full-time (49 women), 1 (woman) part-time; includes 6 minority (1 American Indian or Alaska Native, non-Hispanic/Latino; 1 Asian, non-Hispanic/Latino; 2 Hispanic/Latino; 2 Two or more races, non-Hispanic/Latino). Average age 24. 246 applicants, 21% accepted, 25 enrolled. In 2013, 25 master's awarded. *Degree requirements:* For master's, comprehensive exam, portfolio. *Entrance requirements:* For master's, GRE General Test, minimum undergraduate QPA of 3.0 overall and in major, 3 letters of recommendation. Additional exam requirements/recommendations for international students: Required—TOEFL (minimum score 560 paper-based; 83 iBT) or IELTS. *Application deadline:* For fall admission, 2/1 priority date for domestic and international students; for spring admission, 11/30 for domestic and international students. Applications are processed on a rolling basis. Application fee: $50. Electronic applications accepted. *Expenses:* Tuition, state resident: full-time $7956; part-time $442 per credit. Tuition, nonresident: full-time $11,934; part-time $663 per credit. *Required fees:* $2129; $118 per credit. *Financial support:* Research assistantships with full and partial tuition reimbursements, Federal Work-Study, and institutionally sponsored loans available. Financial award application deadline: 3/1; financial award applicants required to submit FAFSA. *Faculty research:* Computer-assisted classroom instruction. *Unit head:* Dr. Robert Ackerman, Graduate Coordinator, 570-422-3247, Fax: 570-422-3506, E-mail: rackerman@po-box.esu.edu. *Application contact:* Kevin Quintero, Graduate Admissions Coordinator, 570-422-3536, Fax: 570-422-2711, E-mail: kquintero@esu.edu.

East Tennessee State University, School of Graduate Studies, College of Clinical and Rehabilitative Health Sciences, Department of Audiology and Speech-Language Pathology, Johnson City, TN 37614-1710. Offers audiology (Au D); communicative disorders (MS), including speech pathology. *Accreditation:* ASHA (one or more programs are accredited). *Faculty:* 15 full-time (11 women), 14 part-time/adjunct (8 women). *Students:* 85 full-time (80 women), 9 part-time (all women); includes 4 minority (1 Black or African American, non-Hispanic/Latino; 1 Hispanic/Latino; 2 Two or more races, non-Hispanic/Latino), 1 international. Average age 26. 292 applicants, 28% accepted, 36 enrolled. In 2013, 25 master's, 5 doctorates awarded. *Degree requirements:* For master's, comprehensive exam, case study or thesis; for doctorate, comprehensive exam, externship. *Entrance requirements:* For master's, GRE General Test, minimum GPA of 3.0, three letters of recommendation, resume; for doctorate, GRE General Test, minimum GPA of 3.0, three letters of recommendation. Additional exam requirements/recommendations for international students: Required—TOEFL (minimum score 550 paper-based; 79 iBT). *Application deadline:* For fall admission, 2/1 for domestic and international students. Application fee: $35 ($45 for international students). Electronic applications accepted. *Expenses:* Tuition, state resident: full-time $7900; part-time $395 per credit hour. Tuition, nonresident: full-time $21,960; part-time $1098 per credit hour. *Required fees:* $1345; $84 per credit hour. *Financial support:* In 2013–14, 62 students received support, including 20 research assistantships with full and partial tuition reimbursements available (averaging $3,200 per year), 3 teaching assistantships with full tuition reimbursements available (averaging $6,000 per year); career-related internships or fieldwork, institutionally sponsored loans, scholarships/grants, and unspecified assistantships also available. Financial award application deadline: 7/1; financial award applicants required to submit FAFSA. *Faculty research:* Vestibular assessment and management, tinnitus management, speech perception, hearing amplification, early speech and language intervention for children with cleft palate, assessment and management of speech sound disorders, pediatric language intervention, voice disorders and vocal fatigue. *Unit head:* Dr. Brenda Louw, Chair, 423-439-4272, Fax: 423-439-4350, E-mail: louwb1@etsu.edu. *Application contact:* Shella Bennett, Graduate Specialist, 423-439-4708, Fax: 423-439-5624, E-mail: bennetsg@etsu.edu.
Website: http://www.etsu.edu/crhs/aslp/

Edinboro University of Pennsylvania, Department of Speech, Language and Hearing, Edinboro, PA 16444. Offers speech-language pathology (MA). *Accreditation:* ASHA. Part-time and evening/weekend programs available. *Degree requirements:* For master's, thesis or alternative, competency exam. *Entrance requirements:* For master's, GRE or MAT, minimum QPA of 2.5. *Application deadline:* Applications are processed on a rolling basis. Application fee: $30. Electronic applications accepted. *Expenses:* Tuition, state resident: part-time $454 per credit hour. Tuition, nonresident: part-time $681 per credit hour. *Required fees:* $143.55 per credit hour. Part-time tuition and fees vary according to campus/location and program. *Financial support:* Research assistantships with full and partial tuition reimbursements, career-related internships or fieldwork, Federal Work-Study, scholarships/grants, and unspecified assistantships available. Support available to part-time students. Financial award application deadline: 2/15; financial award applicants required to submit FAFSA. *Unit head:* Dr. Roy Shinn, Coordinator, 814-732-2730, E-mail: shinn@edinboro.edu. *Application contact:* Dr. Roy Shinn, Coordinator, 814-732-2730, E-mail: shinn@edinboro.edu.

Elmhurst College, Graduate Programs, Program in Communication Sciences and Disorders, Elmhurst, IL 60126-3296. Offers MS. *Faculty:* 4 full-time (3 women), 1 (woman) part-time/adjunct. *Students:* 16 full-time (15 women); includes 1 minority (Hispanic/Latino), 1 international. Average age 23. 28 applicants, 96% accepted, 16 enrolled. *Degree requirements:* For master's, clinical practicum. *Entrance requirements:* For master's, GRE General Test, 3 recommendations, resume, statement of purpose. Additional exam requirements/recommendations for international students: Required—TOEFL (minimum score 550 paper-based; 79 iBT). *Application deadline:* Applications are processed on a rolling basis. Application fee: $0. Electronic applications accepted. *Expenses:* Contact institution. *Financial support:* In 2013–14, 10 students received support. Federal Work-Study and scholarships/grants available. Financial award application deadline: 2/1; financial award applicants required to submit FAFSA. *Application contact:* Timothy J. Panfil, Director of Enrollment Management, School for Professional Studies, 630-617-3300 Ext. 3256, Fax: 630-617-6471, E-mail: panfilt@elmhurst.edu.
Website: http://public.elmhurst.edu/masters_communication_sciences_disorders

Elms College, Division of Communication Sciences and Disorders, Chicopee, MA 01013-2839. Offers autism spectrum disorders (MS, CAGS); autism spectrum disorders with practicum (MS, CAGS); communication sciences and disorders (CAGS). Part-time programs available. *Entrance requirements:* For degree, minimum GPA of 3.0. Additional exam requirements/recommendations for international students: Required—TOEFL.

Emerson College, Graduate Studies, School of Communication, Department of Communication Sciences and Disorders, Program in Communication Disorders, Boston, MA 02116-4624. Offers MS. *Accreditation:* ASHA. *Faculty:* 13 full-time (6 women), 4 part-time/adjunct (3 women). *Students:* 90 full-time (84 women), 2 part-time (both women); includes 8 minority (2 Black or African American, non-Hispanic/Latino; 2 Asian, non-Hispanic/Latino; 4 Hispanic/Latino), 2 international. Average age 23. 675 applicants, 23% accepted, 47 enrolled. In 2013, 47 degrees awarded. *Degree requirements:* For master's, comprehensive exam, thesis or alternative. *Entrance requirements:* For master's, GRE General Test. Additional exam requirements/recommendations for international students: Required—TOEFL (minimum score 550 paper-based; 80 iBT), IELTS (minimum score 6.5). *Application deadline:* For fall admission, 2/15 priority date for domestic and international students. Applications are processed on a rolling basis. Application fee: $60 ($75 for international students). Electronic applications accepted. *Expenses: Tuition:* Part-time $1145 per credit. *Financial support:* In 2013–14, 25 students received support, including 19 fellowships with partial tuition reimbursements available (averaging $10,230 per year), 16 research assistantships with partial tuition reimbursements available (averaging $12,000 per year); Federal Work-Study, scholarships/grants, and unspecified assistantships also available. Financial award application deadline: 2/15; financial award applicants required to submit FAFSA. *Unit head:* Dr. Sandra Cohn Thau, Graduate Program Director, 617-824-8730, E-mail: cynthia_bartlett@emerson.edu. *Application contact:* Sean Ganas, Office of Graduate Admission, 617-824-8610, Fax: 617-824-8614, E-mail: gradapp@emerson.edu.
Website: http://www.emerson.edu/graduate_admission

Florida Atlantic University, College of Education, Department of Communication Sciences and Disorders, Boca Raton, FL 33431-0991. Offers speech-language pathology (MS). *Accreditation:* ASHA. *Faculty:* 7 full-time (5 women), 5 part-time/adjunct (0 women). *Students:* 45 full-time (43 women), 7 part-time (6 women); includes 16 minority (2 Black or African American, non-Hispanic/Latino; 2 American Indian or Alaska Native, non-Hispanic/Latino; 3 Asian, non-Hispanic/Latino; 8 Hispanic/Latino; 1 Two or more races, non-Hispanic/Latino). Average age 25. 259 applicants, 22% accepted, 25 enrolled. In 2013, 15 master's awarded. *Degree requirements:* For master's, thesis optional. *Entrance requirements:* For master's, GRE General Test, minimum undergraduate GPA of 3.0 in last 60 hours of course work or graduate 3.5. Additional exam requirements/recommendations for international students: Required—TOEFL (minimum score 500 paper-based; 61 iBT), IELTS (minimum score 6). *Application deadline:* For fall admission, 2/1 for domestic and international students. Application fee: $30. *Expenses:* Tuition, state resident: full-time $6660; part-time $370 per credit hour. Tuition, nonresident: full-time $18,450; part-time $1025 per credit hour. Tuition and fees vary according to course load. *Financial support:* Career-related internships or fieldwork available. *Faculty research;* Fluency disorders, auditory processing, child language, adult language and cognition, multicultural speech and language issues. *Unit head:* Dr. Deena Louise Wener, Chair, 561-297-2258, Fax: 561-297-2268, E-mail: wener@fau.edu. *Application contact:* Dr. Eliah Watlington, Associate Dean, 561-296-8520, Fax: 261-297-2991, E-mail: ewatling@fau.edu.
Website: http://www.coe.fau.edu/academicdepartments/csd/

Florida International University, College of Nursing and Health Sciences, Department of Communication Sciences and Disorders, Miami, FL 33199. Offers speech-language pathology (MS). *Accreditation:* ASHA. Part-time and evening/weekend programs available. *Degree requirements:* For master's, thesis optional. *Entrance requirements:* For master's, minimum undergraduate GPA of 3.0 in upper-level coursework; letter of intent; 2 letters of recommendation. Additional exam requirements/recommendations for international students: Required—TOEFL (minimum score 550 paper-based; 80 iBT). Electronic applications accepted.

Florida State University, The Graduate School, College of Communication and Information, School of Communication Science and Disorders, Tallahassee, FL 32306-1200. Offers MS, PhD. *Accreditation:* ASHA (one or more programs are accredited). Part-time programs available. Postbaccalaureate distance learning degree programs offered (minimal on-campus study). *Faculty:* 17 full-time (13 women), 13 part-time/adjunct (all women). *Students:* 79 full-time (77 women), 128 part-time (122 women); includes 28 minority (9 Black or African American, non-Hispanic/Latino; 1 Asian, non-Hispanic/Latino; 15 Hispanic/Latino; 3 Two or more races, non-Hispanic/Latino). Average age 25. 399 applicants, 29% accepted, 84 enrolled. In 2013, 57 master's, 5 doctorates awarded. *Degree requirements:* For master's, thesis optional; for doctorate, thesis/dissertation. *Entrance requirements:* For master's, GRE General Test, minimum GPA of 3.0; for doctorate, GRE General Test, minimum GPA of 3.0 (undergraduate), 3.5

(graduate). Additional exam requirements/recommendations for international students: Required—TOEFL (minimum score 550 paper-based; 80 iBT). *Application deadline:* For fall admission, 1/15 for domestic and international students. Application fee: $30. Electronic applications accepted. *Expenses:* Tuition, state resident: part-time $403.51 per credit hour. Tuition, nonresident: part-time $1004.85 per credit hour. *Required fees:* $75.81 per credit hour. One-time fee: $20 part-time. Tuition and fees vary according to course load, campus/location and student level. *Financial support:* In 2013–14, 63 students received support, including 1 fellowship with full tuition reimbursement available (averaging $11,000 per year), 28 research assistantships with partial tuition reimbursements available (averaging $6,000 per year), 34 teaching assistantships with partial tuition reimbursements available (averaging $9,000 per year); career-related internships or fieldwork, Federal Work-Study, institutionally sponsored loans, scholarships/grants, tuition waivers (partial), and unspecified assistantships also available. Financial award application deadline: 1/1; financial award applicants required to submit FAFSA. *Faculty research:* Autism, neurogenic disorders, early intervention, child language disorders, literacy development and disorders, augmentative communication, dialectal influences on language development, speech development. *Total annual research expenditures:* $1.3 million. *Unit head:* Dr. Hugh W. Catts, Director, 850-644-6566, Fax: 850-645-8994, E-mail: hugh.catts@cci.fsu.edu. *Application contact:* Jennifer Boss Kekelis, Academic Program Specialist, 850-644-2253, Fax: 850-644-8994, E-mail: jennifer.kekelis@cci.fsu.edu.
Website: http://www.commdisorders.cci.fsu.edu/

Fontbonne University, Graduate Programs, Department of Communication Disorders and Deaf Education, Studies in Early Intervention in Deaf Education, St. Louis, MO 63105-3098. Offers MA. *Entrance requirements:* For master's, minimum GPA of 3.0. *Expenses: Tuition:* Full-time $11,646; part-time $647 per credit hour. *Required fees:* $324; $18 per credit hour. Tuition and fees vary according to course load and program.

Fontbonne University, Graduate Programs, Department of Communication Disorders and Deaf Education, Studies in Speech-Language Pathology, St. Louis, MO 63105-3098. Offers MS. *Accreditation:* ASHA. *Entrance requirements:* For master's, minimum GPA of 3.0. *Expenses: Tuition:* Full-time $11,646; part-time $647 per credit hour. *Required fees:* $324; $18 per credit hour. Tuition and fees vary according to course load and program.

Fort Hays State University, Graduate School, College of Health and Life Sciences, Department of Communication Disorders, Hays, KS 67601-4099. Offers speech-language pathology (MS). *Accreditation:* ASHA. Part-time programs available. *Degree requirements:* For master's, comprehensive exam, thesis optional. *Entrance requirements:* For master's, GRE General Test. Additional exam requirements/recommendations for international students: Required—TOEFL (minimum score 550 paper-based). Electronic applications accepted. *Faculty research:* Aural rehabilitation, phonological and articulation skills, middle ear diseases, output capability of stereo cassette units, language development.

Gallaudet University, The Graduate School, Washington, DC 20002-3625. Offers ASL/English bilingual early childhood education: birth to 5 (Certificate); audiology (Au D); clinical psychology (PhD); critical studies in the education of deaf learners (PhD); deaf and hard of hearing infants, toddlers, and their families (Certificate); deaf education (Ed S); deaf education: advanced studies (MA); deaf education: special programs (MA); deaf history (Certificate); deaf studies (MA, Certificate); educating deaf students with disabilities (Certificate); education: teacher preparation (MA), including deaf education, early childhood education and deaf education, elementary education and deaf education, secondary education and deaf education; educational neuroscience (PhD); hearing, speech and language sciences (MS, PhD); international development (MA); interpretation (MA, PhD), including combined interpreting practice and research (MA), interpreting research (MA); linguistics (MA, PhD); mental health counseling (MA); peer mentoring (Certificate); public administration (MPA); school counseling (MA); school psychology (Psy S); sign language teaching (MA); social work (MSW); speech-language pathology (MS). Part-time programs available. *Faculty:* 55 full-time (37 women). *Students:* 361 full-time (279 women), 108 part-time (73 women); includes 98 minority (39 Black or African American, non-Hispanic/Latino; 1 American Indian or Alaska Native, non-Hispanic/Latino; 12 Asian, non-Hispanic/Latino; 36 Hispanic/Latino; 1 Native Hawaiian or other Pacific Islander, non-Hispanic/Latino; 9 Two or more races, non-Hispanic/Latino), 31 international. Average age 30. 602 applicants, 49% accepted, 177 enrolled. In 2013, 140 master's, 32 doctorates, 11 other advanced degrees awarded. Terminal master's awarded for partial completion of doctoral program. *Degree requirements:* For master's, comprehensive exam (for some programs), thesis optional; for doctorate, comprehensive exam, thesis/dissertation. *Entrance requirements:* For master's and doctorate, GRE General Test or MAT, letters of recommendation, interviews, goals statement, ASL proficiency interview, written English competency. Additional exam requirements/recommendations for international students: Required—TOEFL. *Application deadline:* For fall admission, 2/15 for domestic students. Applications are processed on a rolling basis. Application fee: $75. Electronic applications accepted. *Expenses: Tuition:* Full-time $14,774; part-time $821 per credit. *Required fees:* $198 per semester. *Financial support:* In 2013–14, 325 students received support. Fellowships, research assistantships, teaching assistantships, career-related internships or fieldwork, Federal Work-Study, scholarships/grants, tuition waivers (partial), and unspecified assistantships available. Support available to part-time students. Financial award applicants required to submit FAFSA. *Faculty research:* Bimodal bilingualism development, cochlear implants, telecommunications access, cancer genetics, linguistics, visual language and visual learning, advancement of avatar and robotics translation, algal productivity and physiology in the Anacostia River. *Unit head:* Dr. Carol J. Erting, Dean, Research, Graduate School, Continuing Studies, and International Programs, 202-651-5520, Fax: 202-651-5027, E-mail: carol.erting@gallaudet.edu. *Application contact:* Wednesday Luria, Coordinator of Prospective Graduate Student Services, 202-651-5400, Fax: 202-651-5295, E-mail: graduate.school@gallaudet.edu.
Website: http://www.gallaudet.edu/x26696.xml

The George Washington University, Columbian College of Arts and Sciences, Department of Speech and Hearing Sciences, Washington, DC 20052. Offers speech-language pathology (MA). *Accreditation:* ASHA. *Faculty:* 12 full-time (8 women). *Students:* 68 full-time (66 women), 12 part-time (all women); includes 13 minority (5 Black or African American, non-Hispanic/Latino; 2 Asian, non-Hispanic/Latino; 5 Hispanic/Latino; 1 Two or more races, non-Hispanic/Latino). Average age 25. 399 applicants, 19% accepted, 37 enrolled. In 2013, 29 master's awarded. *Degree requirements:* For master's, comprehensive exam, thesis or alternative. *Entrance requirements:* For master's, GRE General Test, interview, minimum GPA of 3.0. Additional exam requirements/recommendations for international students: Required—TOEFL (minimum score 550 paper-based; 80 iBT). *Application deadline:* For fall admission, 2/1 priority date for domestic students, 1/15 priority date for international students. Applications are processed on a rolling basis. Application fee: $75. Electronic applications accepted. *Financial support:* In 2013–14, 16 students received support. Fellowships with tuition reimbursements available, teaching assistantships with tuition reimbursements available, career-related internships or fieldwork, Federal Work-Study, and tuition waivers available. Financial award application deadline: 1/15. *Unit head:* James Mahshie, Chair, 202-994-2052, E-mail: jmahshie@gwu.edu. *Application contact:* Information Contact, 202-994-7362, Fax: 202-994-2589, E-mail: gwusphr@gwu.edu.
Website: http://www.gwu.edu/~sphr/

Georgia State University, College of Education, Department of Educational Psychology, Special Education, and Communication Disorders, Program in Communication Disorders, Atlanta, GA 30302-3083. Offers M Ed. *Accreditation:* ASHA; NCATE. *Entrance requirements:* For master's, GRE, minimum undergraduate GPA of 3.0. Additional exam requirements/recommendations for international students: Required—TOEFL (minimum score 550 paper-based; 79 iBT), IELTS (minimum score 6.5). *Application deadline:* For fall admission, 1/15 for domestic and international students. Application fee: $50. Electronic applications accepted. *Expenses: Tuition, area resident:* Full-time $4176; part-time $348 per credit hour. Tuition, state resident: full-time $14,544; part-time $1212 per credit hour. Tuition, nonresident: full-time $14,544; part-time $1212 per credit hour. Tuition and fees vary according to course load and program. *Faculty research:* Dialect, aphasia, motor speech disorders, child language development, high risk populations. *Unit head:* Dr. Jacqueline Sue Laures-Gore, Program Coordinator, 404-413-8299, E-mail: jlaures@gsu.edu. *Application contact:* Sandy Vaughn, Senior Administrative Coordinator, 404-413-8318, Fax: 404-413-8043, E-mail: svaughn@gsu.edu.
Website: http://education.gsu.edu/EPSE/4717.html

Georgia State University, College of Education, Department of Educational Psychology, Special Education, and Communication Disorders, Program in Education of Students with Exceptionalities, Atlanta, GA 30302-3083. Offers autism spectrum disorders (PhD); behavior disorders (PhD); communication disorders (PhD); early childhood special education (PhD); learning disabilities (PhD); mental retardation (PhD); orthopedic impairments (PhD); sensory impairments (PhD). *Accreditation:* NCATE. Part-time and evening/weekend programs available. *Degree requirements:* For doctorate, comprehensive exam, thesis/dissertation. *Entrance requirements:* Additional exam requirements/recommendations for international students: Required—TOEFL (minimum score 550 paper-based; 79 iBT) or IELTS (minimum score 6.5). *Application deadline:* For fall admission, 6/1 for domestic and international students; for winter admission, 11/1 for domestic and international students; for spring admission, 5/1 for domestic and international students. Application fee: $50. Electronic applications accepted. *Expenses: Tuition, area resident:* Full-time $4176; part-time $348 per credit hour. Tuition, state resident: full-time $14,544; part-time $1212 per credit hour. Tuition, nonresident: full-time $14,544; part-time $1212 per credit hour. Tuition and fees vary according to course load and program. *Financial support:* In 2013–14, fellowships with full tuition reimbursements (averaging $28,000 per year), research assistantships with full tuition reimbursements (averaging $2,000 per year) were awarded; scholarships/grants, health care benefits, and unspecified assistantships also available. *Faculty research:* Academic and behavioral supports for students with emotional/behavior disorders; academic interventions for learning disabilities; cultural, socioeconomic, and linguistic diversity; language and literacy development, disorders, and instruction. *Unit head:* Dr. Kristine Jolivette, Associate Professor, 404-413-8040, Fax: 404-413-8043, E-mail: kjolivette@gsu.edu. *Application contact:* Sandy Vaughn, Senior Administrative Coordinator, 404-413-8318, Fax: 404-413-8043, E-mail: svaughn@gsu.edu.
Website: http://education.gsu.edu/EPSE/4922.html

Georgia State University, College of Education, Department of Educational Psychology, Special Education, and Communication Disorders, Program in Multiple and Severe Disabilities, Atlanta, GA 30302-3083. Offers early childhood special education (M Ed); special education adapted curriculum (intellectual disabilities) (M Ed); special education deaf education (M Ed); special education general and adapted curriculum (autism spectrum disorders) (M Ed); special education physical and health disabilities (orthopedic impairments) (M Ed). *Accreditation:* NCATE. Part-time programs available. *Degree requirements:* For master's, variable foreign language requirement, comprehensive exam, thesis (for some programs). *Entrance requirements:* For master's, GRE. Additional exam requirements/recommendations for international students: Required—TOEFL (minimum score 550 paper-based; 79 iBT) or IELTS (minimum score 6.5). *Application deadline:* For fall admission, 6/1 for domestic and international students; for winter admission, 11/1 for domestic and international students; for spring admission, 5/1 for domestic and international students. Application fee: $50. Electronic applications accepted. *Expenses: Tuition, area resident:* Full-time $4176; part-time $348 per credit hour. Tuition, state resident: full-time $14,544; part-time $1212 per credit hour. Tuition, nonresident: full-time $14,544; part-time $1212 per credit hour. Tuition and fees vary according to course load and program. *Financial support:* In 2013–14, fellowships with full tuition reimbursements (averaging $25,000 per year), research assistantships with full tuition reimbursements (averaging $2,000 per year) were awarded; teaching assistantships with full tuition reimbursements, scholarships/grants, health care benefits, and unspecified assistantships also available. *Faculty research:* Literacy, language, behavioral supports. *Unit head:* Dr. Kathryn Wolff Heller, Professor, 404-413-8040, E-mail: kheller@gsu.edu. *Application contact:* Sandy Vaughn, Senior Administrative Coordinator, 404-413-8318, Fax: 404-413-8043, E-mail: svaughn@gsu.edu.
Website: http://education.gsu.edu/EPSE/4637.html

Governors State University, College of Health Professions, Program in Communication Disorders, University Park, IL 60484. Offers MHS. *Accreditation:* ASHA. Part-time and evening/weekend programs available. *Degree requirements:* For master's, comprehensive exam, thesis or alternative, practicum. *Entrance requirements:* For master's, minimum GPA of 3.3. *Faculty research:* Speech perception of hearing-impaired, effects of binaural listening, communication assessment of infants, voice characteristics of head-neck cancer patients.

The Graduate Center, City University of New York, Graduate Studies, Program in Audiology, New York, NY 10016-4039. Offers Au D. *Entrance requirements:* For doctorate, GRE General Test. Additional exam requirements/recommendations for international students: Required—TOEFL. Electronic applications accepted.

The Graduate Center, City University of New York, Graduate Studies, Program in Speech and Hearing Sciences, New York, NY 10016-4039. Offers PhD. *Accreditation:* ASHA. *Degree requirements:* For doctorate, one foreign language, thesis/dissertation. *Entrance requirements:* For doctorate, GRE General Test. Additional exam requirements/recommendations for international students: Required—TOEFL. Electronic applications accepted.

Hampton University, Graduate College, Department of Communicative Sciences and Disorders, Hampton, VA 23668. Offers speech-language pathology (MA). *Accreditation:* ASHA. Part-time and evening/weekend programs available. *Entrance requirements:* For master's, GRE General Test. *Faculty research:* Language development, language pathology.

Harding University, College of Allied Health, Program in Communication Sciences and Disorders, Searcy, AR 72149-0001. Offers MS. *Accreditation:* ASHA. *Faculty:* 9 full-time (7 women), 4 part-time/adjunct (3 women). *Students:* 27 full-time (26 women). Average age 24. 112 applicants, 13% accepted, 13 enrolled. In 2013, 14 master's awarded. *Application deadline:* For fall admission, 3/1 for domestic and international students. Application fee: $40. *Expenses: Tuition:* Full-time $11,574; part-time $643 per credit

hour. *Required fees:* $432; $24 per credit hour. Tuition and fees vary according to course load, degree level and program. *Financial support:* In 2013–14, 6 students received support. Application deadline: 3/1. *Unit head:* Dr. Dan Tullos, Professor and Chair, 501-279-4633, Fax: 501-279-4325, E-mail: tullos@harding.edu. *Application contact:* Dr. Cheri Yecke, Dean of Graduate Programs, 501-279-4335, Fax: 501-279-5192, E-mail: cyecke@harding.edu.
Website: http://www.harding.edu/csd/Graduate.html

Hofstra University, School of Health Sciences and Human Services, Programs in Speech Language Pathology and Audiology, Hempstead, NY 11549. Offers audiology (Au D); speech-language pathology (MA). *Accreditation:* ASHA (one or more programs are accredited).

Howard University, School of Communications, Department of Communication Sciences and Disorders, Washington, DC 20059-0002. Offers communication sciences (PhD); speech pathology (MS). Offered through the Graduate School of Arts and Sciences. *Accreditation:* ASHA (one or more programs are accredited). Part-time programs available. *Degree requirements:* For master's, comprehensive exam, thesis or alternative; for doctorate, one foreign language, comprehensive exam, thesis/dissertation. *Entrance requirements:* For master's, GRE General Test, minimum GPA of 3.2; for doctorate, GRE General Test, minimum GPA of 3.5. Additional exam requirements/recommendations for international students: Required—TOEFL. Electronic applications accepted. *Faculty research:* Multiculturalism, augmentative communication, adult neurological disorders, child language disorders.

Hunter College of the City University of New York, Graduate School, Schools of the Health Professions, School of Health Sciences, Communication Sciences Program, New York, NY 10065-5085. Offers speech-language pathology (MS). *Accreditation:* ASHA. Part-time programs available. *Faculty:* 5 full-time (4 women), 12 part-time/adjunct (all women). *Students:* 6 full-time (5 women), 1 (woman) part-time; includes 1 minority (Asian, non-Hispanic/Latino). Average age 25. 111 applicants, 53% accepted, 28 enrolled. In 2013, 19 master's awarded. *Degree requirements:* For master's, comprehensive exam (for some programs), NTE, research project. *Entrance requirements:* For master's, GRE, letters of reference. Additional exam requirements/recommendations for international students: Required—TOEFL. *Application deadline:* For fall admission, 4/1 for domestic students, 2/1 for international students; for spring admission, 11/1 for domestic students, 9/1 for international students. Application fee: $125. *Financial support:* In 2013–14, 11 students received support, including 3 fellowships with partial tuition reimbursements available (averaging $1,000 per year), 6 research assistantships; career-related internships or fieldwork, Federal Work-Study, institutionally sponsored loans, scholarships/grants, and tuition waivers (full and partial) also available. Support available to part-time students. Financial award application deadline: 3/1. *Faculty research:* Aging and communication disorders, fluency, speech science, diagnostic audiology, amplification. *Total annual research expenditures:* $600,000. *Unit head:* Dr. Paul Cascella, Department Chair, 212-481-3273, Fax: 212-481-4458, E-mail: paul.cascella@hunter.cuny.edu. *Application contact:* Milena Solo, Director for Graduate Admissions, 212-772-4288, E-mail: admissions@hunter.cuny.edu.
Website: http://www.hunter.cuny.edu/schoolhp/comsc/index.htm

Idaho State University, Office of Graduate Studies, Kasiska College of Health Professions, Department of Communication Sciences and Disorders and Education of the Deaf, Pocatello, ID 83209-8116. Offers audiology (MS, Au D); communication sciences and disorders (Postbaccalaureate Certificate); communication sciences and disorders and education of the deaf (Certificate); deaf education (MS); speech language pathology (MS). *Accreditation:* ASHA (one or more programs are accredited). Part-time programs available. *Degree requirements:* For master's, thesis optional, written and oral comprehensive exams; for doctorate, comprehensive exam, thesis/dissertation optional, externship, 1 year full time clinical practicum, 3rd year spent in Boise. *Entrance requirements:* For master's, GRE General Test, minimum GPA of 3.0, 3 letters of recommendation; for doctorate, GRE General Test (at least 2 scores minimum 40th percentile), minimum GPA of 3.0, 3 letters of recommendation, bachelor's degree. Additional exam requirements/recommendations for international students: Required—TOEFL (minimum score 600 paper-based; 80 iBT). Electronic applications accepted. *Faculty research:* Neurogenic disorders, central auditory processing disorders, vestibular disorders, cochlear implants, language disorders, professional burnout, swallowing disorders.

Illinois State University, Graduate School, College of Arts and Sciences, Department of Communication Sciences and Disorders, Normal, IL 61790-2200. Offers MA, MS. *Accreditation:* ASHA. *Degree requirements:* For master's, thesis or alternative, 1 term of residency, 2 practica. *Entrance requirements:* For master's, GRE General Test, minimum GPA of 3.0 in last 60 hours.

Indiana University Bloomington, University Graduate School, College of Arts and Sciences, Department of Speech and Hearing Sciences, Clinical Program in Audiology, Bloomington, IN 47405-7000. Offers Au D. *Accreditation:* ASHA. *Students:* 28 full-time (25 women), 1 part-time (0 women); includes 4 minority (1 Black or African American, non-Hispanic/Latino; 1 Asian, non-Hispanic/Latino; 2 Hispanic/Latino), 1 international. Average age 27. 86 applicants, 52% accepted, 9 enrolled. In 2013, 6 doctorates awarded. Application fee: $55 ($65 for international students). *Unit head:* Larry Humes, Chairperson, 812-855-3507, E-mail: humes@indiana.edu. *Application contact:* Jennifer J. Lentz, Graduate Advisor, 812-855-8945, E-mail: jjlentz@indiana.edu.
Website: http://www.indiana.edu/~sphs/academics/aud/

Indiana University Bloomington, University Graduate School, College of Arts and Sciences, Department of Speech and Hearing Sciences, Program in Speech and Hearing Sciences, Bloomington, IN 47405-7000. Offers auditory sciences (Au D, PhD); language sciences (PhD); speech and voice sciences (PhD); speech-language pathology (MA). *Accreditation:* ASHA. *Faculty:* 34 full-time (25 women), 11 part-time/adjunct (8 women). *Students:* 84 full-time (83 women), 11 part-time (10 women); includes 13 minority (3 Black or African American, non-Hispanic/Latino; 2 Asian, non-Hispanic/Latino; 7 Hispanic/Latino; 1 Two or more races, non-Hispanic/Latino), 6 international. Average age 26. 280 applicants, 34% accepted, 33 enrolled. In 2013, 35 master's, 1 doctorate awarded. *Application deadline:* For fall admission, 1/15 priority date for domestic students, 12/1 priority date for international students. Application fee: $55 ($65 for international students). *Financial support:* In 2013–14, 4 fellowships (averaging $22,000 per year), 3 research assistantships (averaging $15,750 per year), 4 teaching assistantships (averaging $15,750 per year) were awarded. *Unit head:* Larry Humes, Chair, 812-855-3507, E-mail: humes@indiana.edu. *Application contact:* Kimberly Elkins, Graduate Secretary, 812-855-4202, E-mail: kelkins@indiana.edu.
Website: http://www.indiana.edu/~sphs/home/

Indiana University of Pennsylvania, School of Graduate Studies and Research, College of Education and Educational Technology, Department of Special Education and Clinical Services, Program in Speech-Language Pathology, Indiana, PA 15705-1087. Offers MS. *Accreditation:* ASHA. Part-time programs available. *Faculty:* 9 full-time (8 women), 2 part-time/adjunct (both women). *Students:* 43 full-time (42 women), 1 (woman) part-time. Average age 24. 220 applicants, 10% accepted, 22 enrolled. In 2013, 23 master's awarded. *Degree requirements:* For master's, comprehensive exam, thesis optional. *Entrance requirements:* For master's, GRE, 2 letters of recommendation, minimum undergraduate GPA of 3.0. Additional exam requirements/recommendations for international students: Required—TOEFL. *Application deadline:* For fall admission, 2/15 priority date for domestic students. Application fee: $50. Electronic applications accepted. *Expenses:* Tuition, state resident: full-time $3978; part-time $442 per credit. Tuition, nonresident: full-time $5967; part-time $663 per credit. *Required fees:* $2080; $115.55 per credit. $93 per semester. Tuition and fees vary according to degree level and program. *Financial support:* In 2013–14, 21 research assistantships with full and partial tuition reimbursements (averaging $2,545 per year) were awarded; fellowships, career-related internships or fieldwork, Federal Work-Study, scholarships/grants, and unspecified assistantships also available. Support available to part-time students. Financial award application deadline: 4/15; financial award applicants required to submit FAFSA. *Unit head:* Dr. David Stein, Graduate Coordinator, 724-357-7841, E-mail: david.stein@iup.edu. *Application contact:* Paula Stossel, Assistant Dean for Administration, 724-357-4511, Fax: 724-357-4862, E-mail: graduate-admissions@iup.edu.
Website: http://www.iup.edu/grad/speechlanguage/default.aspx

Indiana University–Purdue University Fort Wayne, College of Arts and Sciences, Department of Communication Sciences and Disorders, Fort Wayne, IN 46805-1499. Offers speech and language pathology (MA). *Unit head:* Dr. Jonathan Dalby, Interim Chair/Associate Professor, 260-481-6409, Fax: 260-481-6985, E-mail: dalbyj@ipfw.edu. *Application contact:* Susan Humphrey, Graduate Applications Coordinator, 260-481-6145, Fax: 260-481-6880, E-mail: ask@ipfw.edu.

Ithaca College, School of Health Sciences and Human Performance, Program in Speech-Language Pathology and Audiology, Ithaca, NY 14850. Offers speech-language pathology (MS). *Accreditation:* ASHA. *Faculty:* 9 full-time (6 women). *Students:* 49 full-time (47 women), 4 part-time (all women); includes 6 minority (5 Hispanic/Latino; 1 Two or more races, non-Hispanic/Latino), 5 international. Average age 25. 241 applicants, 35% accepted, 22 enrolled. In 2013, 29 master's awarded. *Degree requirements:* For master's, comprehensive exam, thesis optional. *Entrance requirements:* For master's, GRE General Test, minimum GPA of 3.0. Additional exam requirements/recommendations for international students: Required—TOEFL (minimum score 550 paper-based; 80 iBT). *Application deadline:* For fall admission, 2/1 priority date for domestic and international students. Applications are processed on a rolling basis. Application fee: $40. Electronic applications accepted. Tuition and fees vary according to program. *Financial support:* In 2013–14, 27 students received support, including 26 teaching assistantships (averaging $10,265 per year); career-related internships or fieldwork, Federal Work-Study, scholarships/grants, and unspecified assistantships also available. Support available to part-time students. Financial award application deadline: 2/1; financial award applicants required to submit CSS PROFILE or FAFSA. *Faculty research:* Learning enhancement in higher education, augmentative/alternative communication, cultural and linguistic variables in communication, language and literacy acquisition. *Unit head:* Dr. Richard Schissel, Graduate Chair, 607-274-3143, Fax: 607-274-1263, E-mail: gps@ithaca.edu. *Application contact:* Gerard Turbide, Director, Office of Admission, 607-274-3143, Fax: 607-274-1263, E-mail: gps@ithaca.edu.
Website: http://www.ithaca.edu/gps/gradprograms/slpa

Jackson State University, Graduate School, College of Public Service, Department of Communicative Disorders, Jackson, MS 39217. Offers MS. *Accreditation:* ASHA. *Degree requirements:* For master's, comprehensive exam. *Entrance requirements:* For master's, GRE General Test. Additional exam requirements/recommendations for international students: Required—TOEFL (minimum score 520 paper-based; 67 iBT).

James Madison University, The Graduate School, College of Health and Behavioral Studies, Department of Communication Sciences and Disorders, Program in Audiology, Harrisonburg, VA 22807. Offers Au D. *Accreditation:* ASHA. Part-time programs available. *Students:* 21 full-time (20 women). Average age 27. In 2013, 7 doctorates awarded. *Entrance requirements:* For doctorate, 3 letters of recommendation, interview. Additional exam requirements/recommendations for international students: Required—TOEFL. *Application deadline:* For fall admission, 2/1 for domestic students. Applications are processed on a rolling basis. Application fee: $55. Electronic applications accepted. *Financial support:* In 2013–14, 20 students received support. 6 graduate assistantships (averaging $7530), 14 doctoral assistantships available. Financial award application deadline: 3/1. *Unit head:* Dr. Cynthia R. O'Donoghue, Interim Department Head, 540-568-6440, E-mail: odonogcr@jmu.edu. *Application contact:* Lynette M. Bible, Director of Graduate Admissions, 540-568-6395, Fax: 540-568-7860, E-mail: biblem@jmu.edu.

James Madison University, The Graduate School, College of Health and Behavioral Studies, Department of Communication Sciences and Disorders, Program in Speech-Language Pathology, Harrisonburg, VA 22807. Offers audiology (PhD); clinical audiology (PhD); speech-language pathology (MS, PhD). *Accreditation:* ASHA. Part-time programs available. *Students:* 61 full-time (59 women), 33 part-time (31 women); includes 12 minority (5 Black or African American, non-Hispanic/Latino; 3 Asian, non-Hispanic/Latino; 2 Hispanic/Latino; 1 Native Hawaiian or other Pacific Islander, non-Hispanic/Latino; 1 Two or more races, non-Hispanic/Latino), 1 international. Average age 27. In 2013, 33 master's awarded. *Degree requirements:* For master's, thesis. *Entrance requirements:* For master's, GRE General Test, 2 letters of recommendation; for doctorate, GRE, 3 letters of recommendation, interview. Additional exam requirements/recommendations for international students: Required—TOEFL. *Application deadline:* For fall admission, 5/1 priority date for domestic students. Applications are processed on a rolling basis. Application fee: $55. Electronic applications accepted. *Financial support:* In 2013–14, 28 students received support. Federal Work-Study and 24 graduate assistantships (averaging $7530), 4 doctoral assistantships available. Financial award application deadline: 3/1; financial award applicants required to submit FAFSA. *Unit head:* Dr. Cynthia R. O'Donoghue, Interim Academic Unit Head, 540-568-6440, E-mail: odonogcr@jmu.edu. *Application contact:* Lynette M. Bible, Director of Graduate Admissions, 540-568-6395, Fax: 540-568-7860, E-mail: biblem@jmu.edu.

Kansas State University, Graduate School, College of Human Ecology, School of Family Studies and Human Services, Manhattan, KS 66506. Offers communication sciences and disorders (MS); conflict resolution (Graduate Certificate); early childhood education (MS); family and community services (MS); family studies (MS, PhD); life span human development (MS, PhD); marriage and family therapy (MS, PhD); personal financial planning (MS, PhD, Graduate Certificate); youth development (MS, Graduate Certificate). *Accreditation:* AAMFT/COAMFTE; ASHA. Part-time programs available. Postbaccalaureate distance learning degree programs offered (no on-campus study). *Faculty:* 34 full-time (22 women), 11 part-time/adjunct (8 women). *Students:* 68 full-time (56 women), 131 part-time (86 women); includes 42 minority (19 Black or African American, non-Hispanic/Latino; 2 American Indian or Alaska Native, non-Hispanic/Latino; 4 Asian, non-Hispanic/Latino; 14 Hispanic/Latino; 1 Native Hawaiian or other Pacific Islander, non-Hispanic/Latino; 2 Two or more races, non-Hispanic/Latino), 3 international. Average age 31. 248 applicants, 29% accepted, 48 enrolled. In 2013, 35 master's, 7 doctorates awarded. *Degree requirements:* For master's, thesis or alternative. *Entrance requirements:* For master's, GRE, minimum GPA of 3.0 in last 2 years of undergraduate study; for doctorate, GRE. Additional exam requirements/recommendations for international students: Required—TOEFL (minimum score 600 paper-based). *Application deadline:* For fall admission, 2/1 priority date for domestic

students, 1/1 priority date for international students; for spring admission, 10/1 priority date for domestic students, 8/1 priority date for international students; for summer admission, 2/1 priority date for domestic students, 12/1 priority date for international students. Applications are processed on a rolling basis. Application fee: $50 ($75 for international students). Electronic applications accepted. *Financial support:* In 2013–14, 63 students received support, including 45 research assistantships (averaging $13,500 per year), 18 teaching assistantships with full tuition reimbursements available (averaging $11,000 per year). Financial award application deadline: 3/1. *Faculty research:* Health and security of military families, personal and family risk assessment and evaluation, disorders of communication and swallowing, families and health. *Total annual research expenditures:* $14.9 million. *Unit head:* Dr. Maurice MacDonald, Director, 785-532-5510, Fax: 785-532-5505, E-mail: morey@ksu.edu. *Application contact:* Connie Fechter, Administrative Specialist, 785-532-5510, Fax: 785-532-5505, E-mail: fechter@ksu.edu.
Website: http://www.he.k-state.edu/fshs/

Kean University, College of Education, Program in Speech Language Pathology, Union, NJ 07083. Offers MA. *Accreditation:* ASHA. Part-time programs available. *Faculty:* 9 full-time (7 women). *Students:* 141 full-time (132 women), 35 part-time (34 women); includes 39 minority (8 Black or African American, non-Hispanic/Latino; 7 Asian, non-Hispanic/Latino; 22 Hispanic/Latino; 2 Two or more races, non-Hispanic/Latino), 1 international. Average age 26. 356 applicants, 39% accepted, 89 enrolled. In 2013, 64 master's awarded. *Degree requirements:* For master's, comprehensive exam, thesis, practicum, clinical. *Entrance requirements:* For master's, GRE General Test, minimum cumulative GPA of 3.2, official transcripts from all institutions attended, personal statement, three letters of recommendation, professional resume/curriculum vitae. Additional exam requirements/recommendations for international students: Required—TOEFL (minimum score 550 paper-based; 79 iBT). *Application deadline:* For fall admission, 2/1 for domestic and international students. Application fee: $75 ($150 for international students). Electronic applications accepted. *Expenses:* Tuition, state resident: full-time $12,099; part-time $589 per credit. Tuition, nonresident: full-time $16,399; part-time $722 per credit. *Required fees:* $3050; $139 per credit. Part-time tuition and fees vary according to course level, course load, degree level and program. *Financial support:* In 2013–14, 30 research assistantships with full tuition reimbursements (averaging $3,713 per year) were awarded; unspecified assistantships also available. Financial award applicants required to submit FAFSA. *Unit head:* Dr. Barbara D. Glazewski, Program Coordinator, 908-737-5807, E-mail: bglazews@kean.edu. *Application contact:* Steven Koch, Admissions Counselor, 908-737-5924, Fax: 908-737-5925, E-mail: skoch@kean.edu.
Website: http://grad.kean.edu/slp

Kent State University, Graduate School of Education, Health, and Human Services, School of Health Sciences, Program in Audiology, Kent, OH 44242-0001. Offers Au D, PhD. *Faculty:* 4 full-time (2 women), 1 part-time/adjunct (0 women). *Students:* 43 full-time (40 women); includes 4 minority (all Black or African American, non-Hispanic/Latino). 49 applicants, 45% accepted. In 2013, 1 doctorate awarded. *Entrance requirements:* For doctorate, GRE, 3 letters of reference, goals statement. Additional exam requirements/recommendations for international students: Required—TOEFL (minimum score 550 paper-based; 80 iBT). Application fee: $30 ($60 for international students). *Financial support:* In 2013–14, 2 research assistantships (averaging $12,000 per year) were awarded; teaching assistantships, Federal Work-Study, scholarships/grants, unspecified assistantships, and 1 administrative assistantship (averaging $12,000 per year) also available. *Unit head:* Lynne Rowan, Coordinator, 330-672-9785, Fax: 330-672-2643, E-mail: lrowan@kent.edu. *Application contact:* Nancy Miller, Academic Program Director, Office of Graduate Student Services, 330-672-2576, Fax: 330-672-9162, E-mail: ogs@kent.edu.

Kent State University, Graduate School of Education, Health, and Human Services, School of Health Sciences, Program in Speech Language Pathology, Kent, OH 44242-0001. Offers MA, PhD. *Accreditation:* ASHA. *Faculty:* 12 full-time (all women). *Students:* 78 full-time (75 women), 3 part-time (all women); includes 4 minority (1 Black or African American, non-Hispanic/Latino; 1 American Indian or Alaska Native, non-Hispanic/Latino; 2 Native Hawaiian or other Pacific Islander, non-Hispanic/Latino). 246 applicants, 28% accepted. In 2013, 33 master's, 1 doctorate awarded. *Degree requirements:* For doctorate, comprehensive exam, thesis/dissertation. *Entrance requirements:* For master's and doctorate, GRE, 3 letters of reference, goals statement. Additional exam requirements/recommendations for international students: Required—TOEFL (minimum score 550 paper-based; 80 iBT). Application fee: $30 ($60 for international students). *Financial support:* In 2013–14, 7 research assistantships (averaging $9,500 per year) were awarded; teaching assistantships, Federal Work-Study, institutionally sponsored loans, and unspecified assistantships also available. *Unit head:* Lynne Rowan, Coordinator, 330-672-9785, E-mail: lrowan@kent.edu. *Application contact:* Nancy Miller, Academic Program Director, Office of Graduate Student Services, 330-672-2576, Fax: 330-672-9162, E-mail: ogs@kent.edu.

Kent State University, Graduate School of Education, Health, and Human Services, School of Lifespan Development and Educational Sciences, Program in Special Education, Kent, OH 44242-0001. Offers deaf education (M Ed); early childhood education (M Ed); educational interpreter K-12 (M Ed); general special education (M Ed); gifted education (M Ed); mild/moderate intervention (M Ed); special education (PhD, Ed S); transition to work (M Ed). *Accreditation:* NCATE. *Faculty:* 11 full-time (6 women), 12 part-time/adjunct (all women). *Students:* 75 full-time (61 women), 59 part-time (50 women); includes 15 minority (12 Black or African American, non-Hispanic/Latino; 1 Asian, non-Hispanic/Latino; 2 Native Hawaiian or other Pacific Islander, non-Hispanic/Latino), 8 international. 80 applicants, 35% accepted. In 2013, 44 master's, 4 doctorates awarded. *Degree requirements:* For doctorate, comprehensive exam, thesis/dissertation. *Entrance requirements:* For master's, minimum undergraduate GPA of 2.75, moral character form, 2 letters of reference, goals statement; for doctorate and Ed S, GRE General Test, goals statement, 2 letters of reference, interview, resume. Additional exam requirements/recommendations for international students: Required—TOEFL (minimum score 550 paper-based; 80 iBT). *Application deadline:* Applications are processed on a rolling basis. Application fee: $30 ($60 for international students). Electronic applications accepted. *Financial support:* In 2013–14, 6 research assistantships with full tuition reimbursements (averaging $9,667 per year), 1 teaching assistantship with full tuition reimbursement (averaging $12,000 per year) were awarded; career-related internships or fieldwork, Federal Work-Study, institutionally sponsored loans, scholarships/grants, health care benefits, and unspecified assistantships also available. Support available to part-time students. Financial award application deadline: 4/1; financial award applicants required to submit FAFSA. *Faculty research:* Social/emotional needs of gifted, inclusion transition services, early intervention/ecobehavioral assessments, applied behavioral analysis. *Unit head:* Sonya Wisdom, Coordinator, 330-672-0578, E-mail: swisdom@kent.edu. *Application contact:* Nancy Miller, Academic Program Director, Office of Graduate Student Services, 330-672-2576, Fax: 330-672-9162, E-mail: ogs@kent.edu.
Website: http://www.kent.edu/ehhs/sped/

Lamar University, College of Graduate Studies, College of Fine Arts and Communication, Department of Speech and Hearing Science, Beaumont, TX 77710. Offers audiology (MS, Au D); speech language pathology (MS). *Degree requirements:* For master's, thesis optional; for doctorate, thesis/dissertation. *Entrance requirements:* For master's, GRE General Test, performance IQ score of 115 (for deaf students), minimum GPA of 2.5; for doctorate, GRE General Test, performance IQ score of 115 (for deaf students). Additional exam requirements/recommendations for international students: Required—TOEFL.

La Salle University, School of Nursing and Health Sciences, Program in Speech-Language-Hearing Science, Philadelphia, PA 19141-1199. Offers MS. *Accreditation:* ASHA. *Faculty:* 5 full-time (3 women), 5 part-time/adjunct (4 women). *Students:* 60 full-time (57 women), 2 part-time (both women); includes 2 minority (both Asian, non-Hispanic/Latino). Average age 25. 274 applicants, 11% accepted, 26 enrolled. In 2013, 40 master's awarded. *Degree requirements:* For master's, comprehensive exam, capstone project, which includes a written manuscript suitable for publication in a scholarly journal. *Entrance requirements:* For master's, GRE, personal essay; 3 letters of recommendation; CSDCAS centralized application. Additional exam requirements/recommendations for international students: Required—TOEFL. *Application deadline:* For fall admission, 2/1 for domestic and international students. Application fee: $100. *Expenses:* Contact institution. *Financial support:* In 2013–14, 18 students received support. Federal Work-Study and scholarships/grants available. Financial award application deadline: 8/31; financial award applicants required to submit FAFSA. *Unit head:* Dr. Barbara Amster, Director, 215-951-1986, Fax: 215-951-5171, E-mail: slh@lasalle.edu. *Application contact:* Paul J. Reilly, Assistant Vice President, Enrollment Services, 215-951-1946, Fax: 215-951-1462, E-mail: reilly@lasalle.edu.
Website: http://www.lasalle.edu/grad/index.php?section-snhs&group-slhs&page-index

Lehman College of the City University of New York, Division of Arts and Humanities, Department of Speech–Language–Hearing Sciences, Bronx, NY 10468-1589. Offers speech-language pathology and audiology (MA). *Accreditation:* ASHA. Part-time and evening/weekend programs available. *Degree requirements:* For master's, thesis or alternative.

Lewis & Clark College, Graduate School of Education and Counseling, Department of Teacher Education, Program in Special Education, Portland, OR 97219-7899. Offers M Ed. *Accreditation:* NCATE. Part-time and evening/weekend programs available. *Entrance requirements:* For master's, minimum GPA of 2.75. Additional exam requirements/recommendations for international students: Required—TOEFL (minimum score 575 paper-based). Electronic applications accepted.

Loma Linda University, School of Allied Health Professions, Department of Speech-Language Pathology and Audiology, Loma Linda, CA 92350. Offers MS. *Accreditation:* ASHA. Part-time programs available. *Degree requirements:* For master's, thesis or alternative. *Entrance requirements:* For master's, GRE General Test. Additional exam requirements/recommendations for international students: Required—TOEFL (minimum score 550 paper-based). Electronic applications accepted.

Long Island University–LIU Brooklyn, Richard L. Conolly College of Liberal Arts and Sciences, Department of Communication Sciences and Disorders, Brooklyn, NY 11201-8423. Offers speech-language pathology (MS). *Accreditation:* ASHA. *Entrance requirements:* For master's, 2 letters of recommendation. Additional exam requirements/recommendations for international students: Required—TOEFL (minimum score 500 paper-based). Electronic applications accepted.

Long Island University–LIU Post, School of Education, Department of Communication Sciences and Disorders, Brookville, NY 11548-1300. Offers speech language pathology (MA). *Accreditation:* ASHA. Part-time and evening/weekend programs available. *Degree requirements:* For master's, comprehensive exam or thesis. *Entrance requirements:* For master's, minimum GPA of 3.0, bachelor's degree in communication sciences and disorders. Electronic applications accepted. *Faculty research:* Aural rehabilitation, spouses' perceptions of speech therapy with their ephasic partners, establish norms associated with swallowing.

Longwood University, College of Graduate and Professional Studies, College of Education and Human Services, Department of Social Work and Communication Sciences and Disorders, Farmville, VA 23909. Offers communication sciences and disorders (MS). *Accreditation:* ASHA. *Faculty:* 6 full-time (all women), 2 part-time/adjunct (0 women). *Students:* 41 full-time (38 women), 12 part-time (11 women); includes 8 minority (2 Black or African American, non-Hispanic/Latino; 1 American Indian or Alaska Native, non-Hispanic/Latino; 1 Asian, non-Hispanic/Latino; 3 Hispanic/Latino; 1 Native Hawaiian or other Pacific Islander, non-Hispanic/Latino). 156 applicants, 28% accepted, 22 enrolled. In 2013, 17 master's awarded. *Degree requirements:* For master's, comprehensive exam, thesis optional. *Entrance requirements:* For master's, GRE, bachelor's degree from regionally-accredited institution, minimum GPA of 3.0, CSDCAS application. Additional exam requirements/recommendations for international students: Required—TOEFL (minimum score 570 paper-based), IELTS (minimum score 6.5). *Application deadline:* For fall admission, 2/1 for domestic students. Application fee: $50. Electronic applications accepted. *Expenses:* Tuition, state resident: full-time $7506; part-time $327 per credit hour. Tuition, nonresident: full-time $17,100; part-time $837 per credit hour. Tuition and fees vary according to course load and campus/location. *Unit head:* Dr. Lissa A. Power-deFur, Graduate Program Coordinator, 434-395-2369, E-mail: powerdefurea@longwood.edu. *Application contact:* College of Graduate and Professional Studies, 434-395-2380, Fax: 434-395-2750, E-mail: graduate@longwood.edu.
Website: http://www.longwood.edu/socialworkcsds/

Louisiana State University and Agricultural & Mechanical College, Graduate School, College of Humanities and Social Sciences, Department of Communication Sciences and Disorders, Baton Rouge, LA 70803. Offers MA, PhD. *Accreditation:* ASHA (one or more programs are accredited). *Faculty:* 14 full-time (11 women). *Students:* 62 full-time (58 women), 2 part-time (both women); includes 6 minority (5 Black or African American, non-Hispanic/Latino; 1 Asian, non-Hispanic/Latino), 6 international. Average age 24. 149 applicants, 23% accepted, 25 enrolled. In 2013, 24 master's, 1 doctorate awarded. *Degree requirements:* For doctorate, thesis/dissertation. *Entrance requirements:* For master's and doctorate, GRE General Test, minimum GPA of 3.0. Additional exam requirements/recommendations for international students: Required—TOEFL (minimum score 550 paper-based; 79 IBT), IELTS (minimum score 6.5), or PTE (minimum score 59). *Application deadline:* For fall admission, 1/25 priority date for domestic students, 5/15 for international students; for spring admission, 10/15 for international students. Application fee: $25. Electronic applications accepted. *Financial support:* In 2013–14, 50 students received support, including 2 fellowships with full tuition reimbursements available (averaging $28,335 per year), 10 research assistantships with partial tuition reimbursements available (averaging $10,680 per year), 8 teaching assistantships with partial tuition reimbursements available (averaging $12,400 per year); Federal Work-Study, institutionally sponsored loans, health care benefits, and unspecified assistantships also available. Financial award application deadline: 4/1; financial award applicants required to submit FAFSA. *Faculty research:* Language development, language intervention, aphasia, language of the deaf. *Total annual research expenditures:* $614,772. *Unit head:* Dr. Paul R. Hoffman, Chair, 225-

578-2545, Fax: 225-578-2995, E-mail: cdhoff@lsu.edu. *Application contact:* Dr. Janna Oetting, Graduate Adviser, 225-578-3932, Fax: 225-578-2995, E-mail: cdjana@lsu.edu. Website: http://appl003.lsu.edu/artsci/comd.nsf/index

Louisiana State University Health Sciences Center, School of Allied Health Professions, Department of Communication Disorders, New Orleans, LA 70112-2223. Offers audiology (Au D); speech pathology (MCD). *Accreditation:* ASHA (one or more programs are accredited). *Faculty:* 11 full-time (7 women), 4 part-time/adjunct (all women). *Students:* 100 full-time (90 women); includes 12 minority (2 Black or African American, non-Hispanic/Latino; 1 American Indian or Alaska Native, non-Hispanic/Latino; 2 Asian, non-Hispanic/Latino; 7 Hispanic/Latino). Average age 24. 214 applicants, 17% accepted, 37 enrolled. In 2013, 26 master's, 10 doctorates awarded. *Degree requirements:* For master's, comprehensive exam or thesis. *Entrance requirements:* For master's, GRE General Test (minimum 297 combined score), minimum undergraduate GPA of 3.0, 3 letters of recommendation; for doctorate, GRE General Test (minimum 300 combined score), 3 letters of recommendation, minimum undergraduate GPA of 3.0. *Application deadline:* For fall admission, 2/15 for domestic students; for summer admission, 2/15 for domestic students. Application fee: $50. *Financial support:* In 2013–14, 43 students received support. Scholarships/grants, traineeships, and work assistantships available. Financial award application deadline: 4/15. *Faculty research:* Hearing aids, clinical audiology, swallowing respiration, language acquisition, speech science. *Total annual research expenditures:* $42,500. *Unit head:* Dr. Sylvia Davis, Interim Head, 504-568-4338, Fax: 504-568-4352, E-mail: sdavis2@lsuhsc.edu. *Application contact:* Yudialys Delgado, Student Affairs Director, 504-568-4253, Fax: 504-568-3185, E-mail: ydelga@lsuhsc.edu.
Website: http://alliedhealth.lsuhsc.edu/cd/

Louisiana Tech University, Graduate School, College of Liberal Arts, Department of Speech, Ruston, LA 71272. Offers audiology (Au D); speech-language pathology (MA); speech: theatre (MA). *Accreditation:* ASHA (one or more programs are accredited). *Degree requirements:* For master's, thesis or alternative. *Entrance requirements:* For master's, GRE General Test. *Application deadline:* For fall admission, 1/15 for domestic students; for spring admission, 2/3 for domestic students. Application fee: $40. *Financial support:* Fellowships, career-related internships or fieldwork, Federal Work-Study, institutionally sponsored loans, and unspecified assistantships available. Financial award application deadline: 2/1. *Unit head:* Dr. Brenda L. Heiman, Interim Head, 318-257-4764, Fax: 318-257-4492. *Application contact:* Marilyn J. Robinson, Assistant to the Dean of the Graduate School, 318-257-2924, Fax: 318-257-4487.
Website: http://www.latech.edu/speech/

Loyola University Maryland, Graduate Programs, Loyola College of Arts and Sciences, Department of Speech-Language Pathology, Baltimore, MD 21210-2699. Offers speech-language pathology/audiology (MS). *Accreditation:* ASHA. *Degree requirements:* For master's, comprehensive exam, thesis. *Entrance requirements:* Additional exam requirements/recommendations for international students: Required—TOEFL (minimum score 550 paper-based). Electronic applications accepted.

Marquette University, Graduate School, College of Health Sciences, Department of Speech Pathology and Audiology, Milwaukee, WI 53201-1881. Offers bilingual English/Spanish (Certificate); speech-language pathology (MS). *Accreditation:* ASHA (one or more programs are accredited). Part-time programs available. *Faculty:* 10 full-time (6 women), 5 part-time/adjunct (all women). *Students:* 46 full-time (45 women), 12 part-time (all women); includes 6 minority (2 Asian, non-Hispanic/Latino; 3 Hispanic/Latino; 1 Two or more races, non-Hispanic/Latino), 1 international. Average age 24. 300 applicants, 27% accepted, 25 enrolled. In 2013, 21 master's awarded. *Degree requirements:* For master's, comprehensive exam, thesis (for some programs). *Entrance requirements:* For master's, GRE General Test, official transcripts from all current and previous colleges/universities except Marquette, three letters of recommendation, personal statement. Additional exam requirements/recommendations for international students: Required—TOEFL (minimum score 530 paper-based). *Application deadline:* For fall admission, 1/15 for domestic students. Application fee: $50. Electronic applications accepted. *Financial support:* In 2013–14, 30 students received support, including 1 fellowship with full tuition reimbursement available (averaging $20,000 per year), 4 research assistantships with full tuition reimbursements available (averaging $13,285 per year); career-related internships or fieldwork, scholarships/grants, health care benefits, tuition waivers (partial), and unspecified assistantships also available. Support available to part-time students. Financial award application deadline: 2/15. *Faculty research:* Language processing in the brain, vocal aging, early language development, birth-to-three intervention, computer applications. *Total annual research expenditures:* $23,438. *Unit head:* Dr. Edward Korabic, Chair, 414-288-5665, Fax: 414-288-3980, E-mail: edward.korabic@marquette.edu. *Application contact:* Dr. Steven Long, Professor, 414-288-3215.
Website: http://www.marquette.edu/chs/speech/graduate.shtml

Marshall University, Academic Affairs Division, College of Health Professions, Department of Communication Disorders, Huntington, WV 25755. Offers MS. *Accreditation:* ASHA. *Students:* 39 full-time (36 women), 6 part-time (all women); includes 1 minority (Hispanic/Latino). Average age 25. In 2013, 25 master's awarded. *Degree requirements:* For master's, thesis optional. *Entrance requirements:* For master's, GRE General Test. Application fee: $40. *Financial support:* Fellowships available. *Unit head:* Karen McNealy, Chairperson, 304-696-3634, E-mail: mcnealy@marshall.edu. *Application contact:* Information Contact, 304-746-1900, Fax: 304-746-1902, E-mail: services@marshall.edu.

Marywood University, Academic Affairs, Reap College of Education and Human Development, Department of Communication Sciences and Disorders, Scranton, PA 18509-1598. Offers speech-language pathology (MS). *Accreditation:* ASHA. *Entrance requirements:* Additional exam requirements/recommendations for international students: Required—TOEFL (minimum score 550 paper-based; 79 iBT). Application fee: $35. Electronic applications accepted. *Expenses: Tuition:* Part-time $775 per credit. Tuition and fees vary according to degree level. *Financial support:* Career-related internships or fieldwork, scholarships/grants, and unspecified assistantships available. Support available to part-time students. Financial award application deadline: 6/30; financial award applicants required to submit FAFSA. *Faculty research:* Augmentative/alternative communication. *Unit head:* Andrea M. Novak, Chair, 570-348-6211 Ext. 2363, E-mail: novak@marywood.edu. *Application contact:* Tammy Manka, Assistant Director of Graduate Admissions, 570-348-6211 Ext. 2322, E-mail: tmanka@marywood.edu.
Website: http://www.marywood.edu/csd/

Massachusetts Institute of Technology, School of Engineering, Harvard-MIT Health Sciences and Technology Program, Cambridge, MA 02139-4307. Offers health sciences and technology (SM, PhD, Sc D), including bioastronautics (PhD, Sc D), bioinformatics and integrative genomics (PhD, Sc D), medical engineering and medical physics (PhD, Sc D), speech and hearing bioscience and technology (PhD, Sc D). *Students:* 281 full-time (115 women), 10 part-time (0 women); includes 84 minority (1 Black or African American, non-Hispanic/Latino; 1 American Indian or Alaska Native, non-Hispanic/Latino; 68 Asian, non-Hispanic/Latino; 11 Hispanic/Latino; 3 Two or more races, non-Hispanic/Latino), 48 international. Average age 26. 180 applicants, 17% accepted, 18 enrolled. In 2013, 7 master's, 20 doctorates awarded. Terminal master's awarded for partial completion of doctoral program. *Degree requirements:* For master's, thesis; for doctorate, comprehensive exam, thesis/dissertation. *Entrance requirements:* For doctorate, GRE General Test (for medical engineering and medical physics). Additional exam requirements/recommendations for international students: Required—TOEFL (minimum score 600 paper-based; 100 iBT), IELTS (minimum score 7). *Application deadline:* For fall admission, 12/15 for domestic and international students. Application fee: $75. Electronic applications accepted. *Expenses: Tuition:* Full-time $43,210; part-time $670 per credit hour. *Required fees:* $288. *Financial support:* In 2013–14, 144 students received support, including 66 fellowships (averaging $35,700 per year), 49 research assistantships (averaging $31,300 per year), 1 teaching assistantship (averaging $33,300 per year); Federal Work-Study, institutionally sponsored loans, scholarships/grants, traineeships, health care benefits, and unspecified assistantships also available. Financial award application deadline: 12/15. *Faculty research:* Signal processing, biomedical imaging, drug delivery, medical devices, medical diagnostics, regenerative biomedical technologies. *Unit head:* Emery N. Brown, Director, 617-452-4091. *Application contact:* Emery N. Brown, Director, 617-452-4091.
Website: http://hst.mit.edu/

McGill University, Faculty of Graduate and Postdoctoral Studies, Faculty of Medicine, School of Communication Sciences and Disorders, Montréal, QC H3A 2T5, Canada. Offers communication science and disorders (M Sc); communication sciences and disorders (PhD); speech-language pathology (M Sc A). *Accreditation:* ASHA.

Mercy College, School of Health and Natural Sciences, Program in Communication Disorders, Dobbs Ferry, NY 10522-1189. Offers MS. *Accreditation:* ASHA. Part-time and evening/weekend programs available. *Students:* 88 full-time (84 women), 15 part-time (all women); includes 20 minority (6 Black or African American, non-Hispanic/Latino; 5 Asian, non-Hispanic/Latino; 8 Hispanic/Latino; 1 Two or more races, non-Hispanic/Latino), 1 international. Average age 33. 468 applicants, 12% accepted, 45 enrolled. In 2013, 43 master's awarded. *Entrance requirements:* For master's, essay, interview, resume, 2 letters of recommendation, undergraduate transcripts. Additional exam requirements/recommendations for international students: Required—TOEFL (minimum score 600 paper-based; 100 iBT), IELTS (minimum score 8). *Application deadline:* Applications are processed on a rolling basis. Application fee: $62. Electronic applications accepted. *Expenses:* Contact institution. *Financial support:* Career-related internships or fieldwork, Federal Work-Study, scholarships/grants, and unspecified assistantships available. Support available to part-time students. Financial award applicants required to submit FAFSA. *Faculty research:* Phonology, articulation, hearing deficits, fluency, attention. *Unit head:* Dr. Joan Toglia, Dean, School of Health and Natural Sciences, 914-674-7837, E-mail: jtoglia@mercy.edu. *Application contact:* Allison Gurdineer, Senior Director of Admissions, 877-637-2946, Fax: 914-674-7382, E-mail: admissions@mercy.edu.
Website: https://www.mercy.edu/academics/school-of-health-and-natural-sciences/department-of-health-professions/ms-in-communication-disorders/

MGH Institute of Health Professions, School of Health and Rehabilitation Sciences, Department of Communication Sciences and Disorders, Boston, MA 02129. Offers reading (Certificate); speech-language pathology (MS). *Accreditation:* ASHA (one or more programs are accredited). Part-time programs available. *Faculty:* 12 full-time (9 women), 2 part-time/adjunct (1 woman). *Students:* 111 full-time (104 women), 10 part-time (9 women); includes 37 minority (9 Black or African American, non-Hispanic/Latino; 18 Asian, non-Hispanic/Latino; 10 Hispanic/Latino). Average age 28. 527 applicants, 35% accepted, 82 enrolled. In 2013, 55 master's, 26 other advanced degrees awarded. *Degree requirements:* For master's, thesis or alternative, research proposal. *Entrance requirements:* For master's, GRE General Test, bachelor's degree from regionally-accredited college or university. Additional exam requirements/recommendations for international students: Required—TOEFL (minimum score 550 paper-based; 80 iBT). *Application deadline:* For fall admission, 1/1 for domestic and international students. Applications are processed on a rolling basis. Electronic applications accepted. *Expenses: Tuition:* Part-time $1114 per credit. *Required fees:* $620 per term. One-time fee: $475 part-time. *Financial support:* In 2013–14, 45 students received support, including 8 research assistantships (averaging $1,200 per year), 4 teaching assistantships (averaging $1,200 per year); career-related internships or fieldwork, scholarships/grants, and unspecified assistantships also available. Support available to part-time students. Financial award application deadline: 4/1; financial award applicants required to submit FAFSA. *Faculty research:* Children's language disorders, reading, speech disorders, voice disorders, augmentative communication, autism. *Unit head:* Dr. Gregory L. Lof, Department Chair, 617-724-6313, E-mail: glot@mghihp.edu. *Application contact:* Catherine Hamilton, Assistant Director of Admission and Multicultural Recruitment, 617-726-3140, Fax: 617-726-8010, E-mail: admissions@mghihp.edu.
Website: http://www.mghihp.edu/academics/communication-sciences-and-disorders/

Miami University, College of Arts and Science, Department of Speech Pathology and Audiology, Oxford, OH 45056. Offers MA, MS. *Accreditation:* ASHA. Part-time programs available. *Students:* 57 full-time (54 women), 2 part-time (both women); includes 4 minority (2 Hispanic/Latino; 2 Two or more races, non-Hispanic/Latino). Average age 24. In 2013, 23 master's awarded. *Entrance requirements:* For master's, GRE. Additional exam requirements/recommendations for international students: Recommended—TOEFL (minimum score 80 iBT), IELTS (minimum score 6.5), TSE (minimum score 54). *Application deadline:* For fall admission, 1/1 for domestic and international students. Application fee: $50. Electronic applications accepted. *Expenses:* Tuition, state resident: full-time $12,634; part-time $526 per credit hour. Tuition, nonresident: full-time $27,892; part-time $1162 per credit hour. Part-time tuition and fees vary according to course load, campus/location and program. *Financial support:* Fellowships with full and partial tuition reimbursements, research assistantships with full and partial tuition reimbursements, teaching assistantships with full and partial tuition reimbursements, career-related internships or fieldwork, Federal Work-Study, health care benefits, and unspecified assistantships available. Financial award application deadline: 2/15; financial award applicants required to submit FAFSA. *Unit head:* Dr. Susan Baker Brehm, Chair, 513-529-2500, E-mail: spa@miamioh.edu. *Application contact:* Dr. Donna Scarborough, Director of Graduate Studies, 513-529-2500, E-mail: spa@miamioh.edu.
Website: http://www.MiamiOH.edu/spa/

Michigan State University, The Graduate School, College of Communication Arts and Sciences, Department of Communicative Sciences and Disorders, East Lansing, MI 48824. Offers MA, PhD. *Accreditation:* ASHA (one or more programs are accredited). *Entrance requirements:* Additional exam requirements/recommendations for international students: Required—TOEFL. Electronic applications accepted.

Minnesota State University Mankato, College of Graduate Studies and Research, College of Allied Health and Nursing, Program in Communication Disorders, Mankato, MN 56001. Offers MS. *Accreditation:* ASHA. Part-time programs available. *Students:* 41 full-time (40 women), 3 part-time (all women). *Degree requirements:* For master's, comprehensive exam, thesis or alternative. *Entrance requirements:* For master's, GRE General Test, minimum GPA of 3.0 during previous 2 years, references, writing sample. Additional exam requirements/recommendations for international students: Required—TOEFL. *Application deadline:* For fall admission, 2/1 priority date for domestic students, 2/1 for international students. Applications are processed on a rolling basis. Application

fee: $40. *Financial support:* Research assistantships with full tuition reimbursements, teaching assistantships with full tuition reimbursements, career-related internships or fieldwork, Federal Work-Study, and institutionally sponsored loans available. Support available to part-time students. Financial award application deadline: 3/15; financial award applicants required to submit FAFSA. *Faculty research:* Internet/technology issues related to speech-language pathology. *Unit head:* Dr. Renee Shellum, Graduate Coordinator, 507-389-5842. *Application contact:* 507-389-2321, E-mail: grad@mnsu.edu.
Website: http://ahn.mnsu.edu/cd/graduate/

Minnesota State University Moorhead, Graduate Studies, College of Education and Human Services, Program in Speech-Language Pathology, Moorhead, MN 56563-0002. Offers MS. *Accreditation:* ASHA. *Degree requirements:* For master's, comprehensive exam, final oral exam, project or thesis. *Entrance requirements:* For master's, GRE General Test, minimum GPA of 2.75, undergraduate major in speech/language/hearing sciences, 3 letters of recommendation. Additional exam requirements/recommendations for international students: Required—TOEFL (minimum score 550 paper-based). Electronic applications accepted.

Minot State University, Graduate School, Department of Communication Disorders, Minot, ND 58707-0002. Offers audiology (MS); speech-language pathology (MS). *Accreditation:* ASHA. *Degree requirements:* For master's, comprehensive exam (for some programs), thesis (for some programs). *Entrance requirements:* For master's, GRE General Test, minimum GPA of 3.0. Additional exam requirements/recommendations for international students: Required—TOEFL. *Faculty research:* Auditory evoked potentials, pathologies of auditory system, newborn hearing screening, cleft palate research, intervention, the diagnostic process, early language, the pedagogy of clinical teaching, phonology, geriatric communication problems, dysphagia, and brain functioning after injury.

Misericordia University, College of Health Sciences, Department of Speech-Language Pathology, Dallas, PA 18612-1098. Offers MSSLP. *Accreditation:* ASHA. *Faculty:* 5 full-time (3 women), 5 part-time/adjunct (4 women). *Students:* 39 full-time (37 women), 2 part-time (both women); includes 4 minority (all Hispanic/Latino), 1 international. Average age 25. In 2013, 30 master's awarded. *Entrance requirements:* For master's, GRE, minimum undergraduate GPA of 3.5. Additional exam requirements/recommendations for international students: Required—TOEFL. *Application deadline:* For fall admission, 2/1 priority date for domestic students. Application fee: $35. *Expenses: Tuition:* Full-time $14,450; part-time $680 per credit. Tuition and fees vary according to degree level. *Financial support:* In 2013–14, 38 students received support. Scholarships/grants available. Support available to part-time students. Financial award application deadline: 6/30; financial award applicants required to submit FAFSA. *Unit head:* Dr. Glen Tellis, Chair, 570-674-6471, E-mail: gtellis@misericordia.edu. *Application contact:* Maureen Sheridan, Assistant Director of Admissions, 570-674-6255, Fax: 570-674-6232, E-mail: msherida@misericordia.edu.
Website: http://www.misericordia.edu/slp

Mississippi University for Women, Graduate School, College of Nursing and Speech Language Pathology, Columbus, MS 39701-9998. Offers nursing (MSN, PMC); speech-language pathology (MS). *Accreditation:* AACN. Part-time programs available. *Degree requirements:* For master's, comprehensive exam, thesis. *Entrance requirements:* For master's, GRE General Test, bachelor's degree in nursing, previous course work in statistics, proficiency in English.

Missouri State University, Graduate College, College of Health and Human Services, Department of Communication Sciences and Disorders, Springfield, MO 65897. Offers audiology (Au D); communication sciences and disorders (MS), including education of deaf/hard of hearing, speech-language pathology. *Accreditation:* ASHA (one or more programs are accredited). *Faculty:* 18 full-time (15 women), 11 part-time/adjunct (2 women). *Students:* 101 full-time (91 women), 2 part-time (1 woman); includes 8 minority (2 Black or African American, non-Hispanic/Latino; 1 American Indian or Alaska Native, non-Hispanic/Latino; 2 Asian, non-Hispanic/Latino; 2 Hispanic/Latino; 1 Two or more races, non-Hispanic/Latino), 4 international. Average age 25. 20 applicants, 95% accepted, 19 enrolled. In 2013, 33 master's, 12 doctorates awarded. *Degree requirements:* For master's, comprehensive exam, thesis or alternative; for doctorate, comprehensive exam, thesis/dissertation or alternative, clinical externship. *Entrance requirements:* For master's and doctorate, GRE, minimum GPA of 3.0. Additional exam requirements/recommendations for international students: Required—TOEFL (minimum score 550 paper-based; 79 iBT). *Application deadline:* For fall admission, 2/1 for domestic and international students. Application fee: $35 ($50 for international students). Electronic applications accepted. *Expenses:* Tuition, state resident: full-time $4500; part-time $250 per credit hour. Tuition, nonresident: full-time $9018; part-time $501 per credit hour. *Required fees:* $361 per semester. Tuition and fees vary according to course level, course load and program. *Financial support:* In 2013–14, 3 research assistantships with full tuition reimbursements (averaging $8,324 per year) were awarded; career-related internships or fieldwork, Federal Work-Study, scholarships/grants, and unspecified assistantships also available. Support available to part-time students. Financial award application deadline: 3/31; financial award applicants required to submit FAFSA. *Faculty research:* Dysphagia, phonological intervention, elderly adult aural rehabilitation, vestibular disorders. *Unit head:* Dr. Letitia White, Head, 417-836-5368, Fax: 417-836-4242, E-mail: csd@missouristate.edu. *Application contact:* Misty Stewart, Coordinator of Graduate Recruitment, 417-836-6079, Fax: 417-836-6200, E-mail: mistystewart@missouristate.edu.
Website: http://www.missouristate.edu/CSD/

Molloy College, Program in Speech Language Pathology, Rockville Centre, NY 11571-5002. Offers MS. *Faculty:* 5 full-time (all women), 3 part-time/adjunct (1 woman). *Students:* 39 full-time (all women); includes 4 minority (3 Asian, non-Hispanic/Latino; 1 Hispanic/Latino). Average age 24. 248 applicants, 23% accepted, 20 enrolled. In 2013, 7 master's awarded. Application fee: $60. *Expenses: Tuition:* Full-time $16,920; part-time $940 per credit. *Required fees:* $880. *Faculty research:* Voice in Parkinson's Disease, neurophysiology of language, cultural competency, motor speech intervention. *Unit head:* Dr. Barbara Schmidt, Associate Dean of Speech-Language Pathology, 516-323-3519, E-mail: bschmidt@molloy.edu. *Application contact:* Alina Haitz, Assistant Director of Graduate Admissions, 516-323-4008, E-mail: ahaitz@molloy.edu.

Monmouth University, The Graduate School, School of Education, West Long Branch, NJ 07764-1898. Offers applied behavioral analysis (Certificate); autism (Certificate); initial certification (MAT), including elementary level, K-12, secondary level; principal (MS Ed); principal/school administrator (MS Ed); reading specialist (MS Ed); school counseling (MS Ed); special education (MS Ed), including autism, learning disabilities teacher-consultant, teacher of students with disabilities, teaching in inclusive settings; speech-language pathology (MS Ed); student affairs and college counseling (MS Ed); teaching English to speakers of other languages (TESOL) (Certificate). *Accreditation:* NCATE. Part-time and evening/weekend programs available. *Faculty:* 15 full-time (11 women), 19 part-time/adjunct (17 women). *Students:* 125 full-time (97 women), 168 part-time (146 women); includes 38 minority (12 Black or African American, non-Hispanic/Latino; 5 Asian, non-Hispanic/Latino; 16 Hispanic/Latino; 5 Two or more races, non-Hispanic/Latino). Average age 28. 176 applicants, 90% accepted, 112 enrolled. In 2013, 147 master's awarded. *Entrance requirements:* For master's, GRE within last 5 years (for MS Ed in speech-language pathology), minimum GPA of 3.0 in major; 2 letters of recommendation (for some programs), resume, personal statement or essay (depending on degree program). Additional exam requirements/recommendations for international students: Required—TOEFL (minimum score 550 paper-based; 79 iBT), IELTS (minimum score 6), Michigan English Language Assessment Battery (minimum score 77). *Application deadline:* For fall admission, 7/15 priority date for domestic students, 7/1 for international students; for spring admission, 11/15 priority date for domestic students, 11/1 for international students. Applications are processed on a rolling basis. Application fee: $50. Electronic applications accepted. *Expenses: Tuition:* Part-time $1004 per credit hour. *Required fees:* $157 per semester. *Financial support:* In 2013–14, 191 students received support, including 159 fellowships (averaging $2,786 per year), 30 research assistantships (averaging $8,755 per year); career-related internships or fieldwork, scholarships/grants, and unspecified assistantships also available. Support available to part-time students. Financial award applicants required to submit FAFSA. *Faculty research:* Multicultural literacy, science and mathematics teaching strategies, teacher as reflective practitioner, children with disabilities. *Unit head:* Dr. Jason Barr, Program Director, 732-263-5238, Fax: 732-263-5277, E-mail: jbarr@monmouth.edu. *Application contact:* Lauren Vento-Cifelli, Associate Vice President of Undergraduate and Graduate Admission, 732-571-3452, Fax: 732-263-5123, E-mail: gradadm@monmouth.edu.
Website: http://www.monmouth.edu/academics/schools/education/default.asp

Montclair State University, The Graduate School, College of Humanities and Social Sciences, Department of Communication Sciences and Disorders, Doctoral Program in Audiology, Montclair, NJ 07043-1624. Offers Sc D. Part-time and evening/weekend programs available. *Degree requirements:* For doctorate, comprehensive exam (for some programs), thesis/dissertation (for some programs). *Entrance requirements:* For doctorate, GRE General Test, essay, 2 letters of recommendation. Additional exam requirements/recommendations for international students: Required—TOEFL (minimum score 83 iBT), IELTS (minimum score 6.5). Electronic applications accepted. *Faculty research:* Child language development and disorders, word finding in discourse of aphasica and non-aphasics, phonological assessment and remediation, behavioral and electrophysiological measures of aging and spatial hearing, behavioral and electrophysiological measures of bilingual speech perception.

Montclair State University, The Graduate School, College of Humanities and Social Sciences, Department of Communication Sciences and Disorders, Program in Audiology, Montclair, NJ 07043-1624. Offers Au D. Part-time and evening/weekend programs available. *Degree requirements:* For doctorate, comprehensive exam (for some programs), thesis/dissertation (for some programs). *Entrance requirements:* For doctorate, GRE General Test, 3 letters of recommendation, essay. Additional exam requirements/recommendations for international students: Required—TOEFL (minimum score 83 iBT), IELTS (minimum score 6.5). Electronic applications accepted. *Faculty research:* Child language development and disorders, word finding in discourse of aphasica and non-aphasics, phonological assessment and remediation, behavioral and electrophysiological measures of aging and spatial hearing, behavioral and electrophysiological measures of bilingual speech perception.

Montclair State University, The Graduate School, College of Humanities and Social Sciences, Department of Communication Sciences and Disorders, Program in Communication Sciences and Disorders, Montclair, NJ 07043-1624. Offers MA. Part-time and evening/weekend programs available. *Degree requirements:* For master's, comprehensive exam, thesis (for some programs). *Entrance requirements:* For master's, GRE General Test, 2 letters of recommendation, essay. Additional exam requirements/recommendations for international students: Required—TOEFL (minimum score 83 iBT), IELTS (minimum score 6.5). Electronic applications accepted. *Faculty research:* Child language development and disorders, word-finding in discourse of aphasica and non-aphasics, phonological assessment and remediation, behavioral and electrophysiological measures of aging and spatial hearing, behavioral and electrophysiological measures of bilingual speech perception.

Murray State University, College of Health Sciences and Human Services, Department of Wellness and Therapeutic Sciences, Program in Speech-Language Pathology, Murray, KY 42071. Offers MS. *Accreditation:* ASHA. Part-time programs available. *Degree requirements:* For master's, comprehensive exam, thesis optional. *Entrance requirements:* For master's, GRE General Test or MAT, minimum GPA of 3.0. Additional exam requirements/recommendations for international students: Required—TOEFL.

National University, Academic Affairs, School of Education, La Jolla, CA 92037-1011. Offers applied behavior analysis (Certificate); applied school leadership (MS); autism (Certificate); best practices (Certificate); e-teaching and learning (Certificate); early childhood education (Certificate); education (MA), including best practices (M Ed, MA), e-teaching and learning (M Ed, MA), education technology, teacher leadership (M Ed, MA), teaching and learning in a global society (M Ed, MA), teaching mathematics (M Ed, MA); education with preliminary multiple or single subject (M Ed), including best practices (M Ed, MA), e-teaching and learning (M Ed, MA), educational technology (M Ed, MA), teacher leadership (M Ed, MA), teaching and learning in a global society (M Ed, MA), teaching mathematics (M Ed, MA); educational administration (MS); educational and instructional technology (MS); educational counseling (MS); educational technology (Certificate); higher education administration (MS); innovative school leadership (MS); instructional leadership (MS); juvenile justice special education (MS); reading (Certificate); school psychology (MS); special education (MS), including deaf and hard-of-hearing, mild/moderate disabilities, moderate/severe disabilities; teacher leadership (Certificate); teaching (MA), including applied behavioral analysis, autism, best practices (M Ed, MA), e-teaching and learning (M Ed, MA), early childhood education, educational technology (M Ed, MA), reading, special education, teacher leadership (M Ed, MA), teaching and learning in a global society (M Ed, MA), teaching mathematics (M Ed, MA); teaching mathematics (Certificate). Part-time and evening/weekend programs available. Postbaccalaureate distance learning degree programs offered (no on-campus study). *Faculty:* 72 full-time (43 women), 287 part-time/adjunct (170 women). *Students:* 2,433 full-time (1,744 women), 2,017 part-time (1,371 women); includes 1,834 minority (358 Black or African American, non-Hispanic/Latino; 15 American Indian or Alaska Native, non-Hispanic/Latino; 250 Asian, non-Hispanic/Latino; 1,056 Hispanic/Latino; 29 Native Hawaiian or other Pacific Islander, non-Hispanic/Latino; 126 Two or more races, non-Hispanic/Latino), 1 international. Average age 34. 1,339 applicants, 100% accepted, 1035 enrolled. In 2013, 1,662 master's awarded. *Degree requirements:* For master's, thesis (for some programs). *Entrance requirements:* For master's, interview, minimum GPA of 2.5. Additional exam requirements/recommendations for international students: Required—TOEFL (minimum score 550 paper-based; 79 iBT), IELTS (minimum score 6). *Application deadline:* Applications are processed on a rolling basis. Application fee: $60 ($65 for international students). Electronic applications accepted. *Expenses: Tuition:* Full-time $13,824; part-time $1728 per course. One-time fee: $160. *Financial support:* Career-related internships or fieldwork, institutionally sponsored loans, scholarships/grants, and tuition waivers (partial) available. Support available to part-time students. Financial award application deadline: 6/30. *Faculty research:* Teacher education, special education, educational effectiveness, teaching abroad, school counseling. *Unit head:* School of Education, 800-

628-8648, E-mail: soe@nu.edu. *Application contact:* Louis Cruz, Interim Vice President for Enrollment Services, 800-628-8648, E-mail: advisor@nu.edu.
Website: http://www.nu.edu/OurPrograms/SchoolOfEducation.html

Nazareth College of Rochester, Graduate Studies, Department of Speech-Language Pathology, Communication Sciences and Disorders Program, Rochester, NY 14618-3790. Offers MS. *Accreditation:* ASHA. Part-time programs available. Postbaccalaureate distance learning degree programs offered. *Degree requirements:* For master's, comprehensive exam. *Entrance requirements:* For master's, GRE General Test, minimum GPA of 3.0.

New Mexico State University, Graduate School, College of Education, Department of Special Education and Communication Disorders, Las Cruces, NM 88003-8001. Offers bilingual/multicultural special education (Ed D, PhD); communication disorders (MA); special education (MA, Ed D, PhD). *Accreditation:* ASHA (one or more programs are accredited); NCATE. Part-time and evening/weekend programs available. Postbaccalaureate distance learning degree programs offered. *Faculty:* 15 full-time (13 women), 2 part-time/adjunct (1 woman). *Students:* 87 full-time (80 women), 53 part-time (40 women); includes 75 minority (3 Asian, non-Hispanic/Latino; 68 Hispanic/Latino; 4 Two or more races, non-Hispanic/Latino), 6 international. Average age 33. 157 applicants, 27% accepted, 35 enrolled. In 2013, 47 master's, 3 doctorates awarded. *Degree requirements:* For master's, comprehensive exam, thesis optional; for doctorate, comprehensive exam, thesis/dissertation. *Entrance requirements:* For master's, GRE General Test or MAT. Additional exam requirements/recommendations for international students: Required—TOEFL (minimum score 550 paper-based; 79 iBT), IELTS (minimum score 6.5). *Application deadline:* For fall admission, 2/1 priority date for domestic students. Applications are processed on a rolling basis. Application fee: $40 ($50 for international students). Electronic applications accepted. *Expenses:* Tuition, state resident: full-time $5398; part-time $224.90 per credit. Tuition, nonresident: full-time $18,821; part-time $784.20 per credit. *Required fees:* $1310; $54.60 per credit. *Financial support:* In 2013–14, 65 students received support, including 1 research assistantship (averaging $18,261 per year), 25 teaching assistantships (averaging $8,389 per year); career-related internships or fieldwork, Federal Work-Study, health care benefits, and unspecified assistantships also available. Support available to part-time students. Financial award application deadline: 3/1; financial award applicants required to submit FAFSA. *Faculty research:* Multicultural special education, multicultural communication disorders, mild disability, multicultural assessment, deaf education, early childhood, bilingual special education. *Total annual research expenditures:* $289,421. *Unit head:* Dr. Eric Joseph Lopez, Interim Department Head, 575-646-2402, Fax: 575-646-7712, E-mail: leric@nmsu.edu. *Application contact:* Coordinator, 575-646-2736, Fax: 575-646-7721, E-mail: gradinfo@nmsu.edu.
Website: http://education.nmsu.edu/spedcd/

New York Medical College, School of Health Sciences and Practice, Department of Speech-Language Pathology, Valhalla, NY 10595-1691. Offers MS. *Accreditation:* ASHA. *Faculty:* 5 full-time, 15 part-time/adjunct. *Students:* 28 full-time. Average age 27. 140 applicants, 36% accepted, 28 enrolled. In 2013, 28 master's awarded. *Degree requirements:* For master's, comprehensive exam, thesis or alternative. *Entrance requirements:* For master's, GRE, minimum GPA of 3.5. Additional exam requirements/recommendations for international students: Required—TOEFL (minimum score 637 paper-based; 117 iBT), IELTS (minimum score 7). *Application deadline:* For fall admission, 3/1 for domestic and international students; for winter admission, 2/3 for domestic and international students. Applications are processed on a rolling basis. Application fee: $75 ($100 for international students). Electronic applications accepted. *Expenses: Tuition:* Full-time $49,170; part-time $910 per credit. Tuition and fees vary according to program. *Financial support:* Applicants required to submit FAFSA. *Unit head:* Dr. Kate Franklin, Chair, 914-594-4239, Fax: 914-594-4239, E-mail: kate_franklin@nymc.edu. *Application contact:* Pamela Suett, Director of Recruitment, 914-594-4510, Fax: 914-594-4292, E-mail: shsp_admissions@nymc.edu.
Website: http://nymc.edu./slp

New York University, Steinhardt School of Culture, Education, and Human Development, Department of Communication Sciences and Disorders, New York, NY 10003-6860. Offers MS, PhD. *Accreditation:* ASHA. Part-time programs available. *Faculty:* 14 full-time (12 women), 19 part-time/adjunct (18 women). *Students:* 116 full-time (112 women), 29 part-time (all women); includes 31 minority (3 Black or African American, non-Hispanic/Latino; 15 Asian, non-Hispanic/Latino; 10 Hispanic/Latino; 3 Two or more races, non-Hispanic/Latino), 5 international. Average age 28. 476 applicants, 34% accepted, 41 enrolled. In 2013, 70 master's, 1 doctorate awarded. *Degree requirements:* For master's, thesis (for some programs); for doctorate, thesis/dissertation. *Entrance requirements:* For master's, GRE General Test; for doctorate, GRE General Test, interview. Additional exam requirements/recommendations for international students: Required—TOEFL (minimum score 100 iBT). *Application deadline:* For fall admission, 12/1 priority date for domestic and international students. Applications are processed on a rolling basis. Application fee: $75. Electronic applications accepted. *Expenses: Tuition:* Full-time $35,856; part-time $1494 per unit. *Required fees:* $1408; $64 per unit. $473 per term. Tuition and fees vary according to course load and program. *Financial support:* Fellowships with full and partial tuition reimbursements, research assistantships with full and partial tuition reimbursements, career-related internships or fieldwork, Federal Work-Study, institutionally sponsored loans, scholarships/grants, tuition waivers (partial), and unspecified assistantships available. Support available to part-time students. Financial award application deadline: 2/1; financial award applicants required to submit FAFSA. *Faculty research:* Evidence-based practice, phonological acquisition, dysphagia, child language acquisition and disorders, neuromotor disorders. *Unit head:* Prof. Christina Rueterskiold, Chairperson, 212-998-5637, E-mail: ecw4@nyu.edu. *Application contact:* 212-998-5030, Fax: 212-995-4328, E-mail: steinhardt.gradadmissions@nyu.edu.
Website: http://steinhardt.nyu.edu/csd

North Carolina Central University, School of Education, Department of Communication Disorders, Durham, NC 27707-3129. Offers M Ed. *Accreditation:* ASHA. Part-time and evening/weekend programs available. *Degree requirements:* For master's, comprehensive exam, thesis or alternative. *Entrance requirements:* For master's, GRE, minimum GPA of 3.0 in major, 2.5 overall. Additional exam requirements/recommendations for international students: Required—TOEFL. *Faculty research:* Vocational programs for special needs learners.

Northeastern State University, College of Science and Health Professions, Department of Health Professions, Program in Speech-Language Pathology, Tahlequah, OK 74464-2399. Offers MS. *Accreditation:* ASHA. Part-time and evening/weekend programs available. *Faculty:* 6 full-time (4 women). *Students:* 64 full-time (58 women), 2 part-time (both women); includes 23 minority (1 Black or African American, non-Hispanic/Latino; 10 American Indian or Alaska Native, non-Hispanic/Latino; 2 Asian, non-Hispanic/Latino; 4 Hispanic/Latino; 6 Two or more races, non-Hispanic/Latino), 1 international. Average age 27. In 2013, 30 master's awarded. *Degree requirements:* For master's, thesis, capstone experience. *Entrance requirements:* For master's, GRE, minimum GPA of 2.75. Additional exam requirements/recommendations for international students: Required—TOEFL. *Application deadline:* For fall admission, 6/1 priority date for domestic students. Applications are processed on a rolling basis. Application fee: $25. Electronic applications accepted. *Expenses:* Tuition, state resident: full-time $3029; part-time $168.25 per credit hour. Tuition, nonresident: full-time $7709; part-time $428.25 per credit hour. *Required fees:* $35.90 per credit hour. *Financial support:* Teaching assistantships, career-related internships or fieldwork, and Federal Work-Study available. Financial award application deadline: 3/1. *Unit head:* Dr. Karen Patterson, Chair, 918-456-5111 Ext. 3778, Fax: 918-458-2351. *Application contact:* Margie Railey, Administrative Assistant, 918-456-5511 Ext. 2093, Fax: 918-458-2061, E-mail: railey@nsouk.edu.
Website: http://academics.nsuok.edu/healthprofessions/DegreePrograms/Graduate/SpeechLanguagePathologyMS.aspx

Northeastern University, Bouvé College of Health Sciences, Boston, MA 02115-5096. Offers audiology (Au D); biotechnology (MS); counseling psychology (MS, PhD, CAGS); counseling/school psychology (PhD); exercise physiology (MS), including exercise physiology, public health; health informatics (MS); nursing (MS, PhD, CAGS), including acute care (MS), administration (MS), anesthesia (MS), primary care (MS), psychiatric mental health (MS); pharmaceutical sciences (PhD); pharmaceutics and drug delivery systems (MS); pharmacology (MS); physical therapy (DPT); physician assistant (MS); school psychology (PhD, CAGS); school/counseling psychology (PhD); speech language pathology (MS); urban public health (MPH); MS/MBA. *Accreditation:* ACPE (one or more programs are accredited). Part-time and evening/weekend programs available. *Degree requirements:* For doctorate, thesis/dissertation (for some programs); for CAGS, comprehensive exam.

Northern Arizona University, Graduate College, College of Health and Human Services, Department of Communication Sciences and Disorders, Flagstaff, AZ 86011. Offers clinical speech pathology (MS). *Accreditation:* ASHA. Part-time programs available. *Faculty:* 9 full-time (8 women), 5 part-time/adjunct (all women). *Students:* 56 full-time (51 women), 109 part-time (101 women); includes 31 minority (4 Asian, non-Hispanic/Latino; 26 Hispanic/Latino; 1 Two or more races, non-Hispanic/Latino), 3 international. Average age 29. 247 applicants, 9% accepted, 19 enrolled. In 2013, 64 master's awarded. *Entrance requirements:* For master's, GRE General Test, minimum GPA of 3.0. Additional exam requirements/recommendations for international students: Required—TOEFL (minimum score 550 paper-based; 80 iBT), IELTS (minimum score 7). *Application deadline:* For fall admission, 1/31 priority date for domestic students, 1/31 for international students. Application fee: $65. Electronic applications accepted. *Financial support:* In 2013–14, 3 research assistantships (averaging $9,100 per year) were awarded; career-related internships or fieldwork, Federal Work-Study, scholarships/grants, health care benefits, tuition waivers (full and partial), and unspecified assistantships also available. Financial award applicants required to submit FAFSA. *Faculty research:* Meta-analysis of language, laryngeal speech, aphasia. *Unit head:* Dr. Elise Lindstedt, Chair, 928-523-2969, E-mail: elise.lindstedt@nau.edu. *Application contact:* Joan Brakefield, Program Coordinator, 928-523-7444, Fax: 928-523-0034, E-mail: speech@nau.edu.
Website: http://nau.edu/chhs/csd/

Northern Illinois University, Graduate School, College of Health and Human Sciences, School of Allied Health and Communicative Disorders, Program in Communicative Disorders, De Kalb, IL 60115-2854. Offers MA, Au D. *Accreditation:* ASHA (one or more programs are accredited); CORE. *Faculty:* 9 full-time (6 women), 2 part-time/adjunct (1 woman). *Students:* 85 full-time (71 women), 6 part-time (4 women); includes 11 minority (2 Black or African American, non-Hispanic/Latino; 1 Asian, non-Hispanic/Latino; 6 Hispanic/Latino; 2 Two or more races, non-Hispanic/Latino). Average age 27. 369 applicants, 27% accepted, 28 enrolled. In 2013, 48 master's, 13 doctorates awarded. *Degree requirements:* For master's, comprehensive exam, thesis optional, practicum; for doctorate, practicum, research project. *Entrance requirements:* For master's, GRE General Test, minimum undergraduate GPA of 3.0; for doctorate, GRE General Test, minimum undergraduate GPA of 3.2. Additional exam requirements/recommendations for international students: Required—TOEFL (minimum score 550 paper-based). *Application deadline:* For fall admission, 2/1 priority date for domestic students, 5/1 for international students; for spring admission, 9/1 priority date for domestic students, 10/1 for international students. Applications are processed on a rolling basis. Application fee: $40. Electronic applications accepted. *Financial support:* Fellowships with full tuition reimbursements, research assistantships with full tuition reimbursements, teaching assistantships with full tuition reimbursements, career-related internships or fieldwork, Federal Work-Study, scholarships/grants, tuition waivers (full), and unspecified assistantships available. Support available to part-time students. Financial award applicants required to submit FAFSA. *Faculty research:* Impact of disability employment, deaf education, American Sign Language, autism, bilingualism. *Unit head:* Dr. Sherrill Morris, Chair, 815-753-1484, Fax: 815-753-9123, E-mail: ahcd@niu.edu. *Application contact:* Graduate School Office, 815-753-0395, E-mail: gradsch@niu.edu.
Website: http://www.chhs.niu.edu/slp/graduate/index.shtml

Northwestern University, The Graduate School, School of Communication, The Roxelyn and Richard Pepper Department of Communication Sciences and Disorders, Evanston, IL 60208. Offers audiology (Au D); communication sciences and disorders (PhD); speech, language, and learning (MS). Admissions and degrees offered through The Graduate School. *Accreditation:* ASHA (one or more programs are accredited). Terminal master's awarded for partial completion of doctoral program. *Degree requirements:* For master's, seminar paper; for doctorate, thesis/dissertation, pre-dissertation research project, qualifying exam. *Entrance requirements:* For master's and doctorate, GRE General Test, letters of recommendation. Additional exam requirements/recommendations for international students: Required—TOEFL. *Faculty research:* Swallow behavior, verb structure in aphasia, language decline in dementia, cognitive processing in children, word-finding defects in children.

Nova Southeastern University, Abraham S. Fischler School of Education, North Miami Beach, FL 33162. Offers education (MS, Ed D, Ed S); instructional design and diversity education (MS); instructional technology and distance education (MS); speech language pathology (MS, SLPD); teaching and learning (MA). Part-time and evening/weekend programs available. Postbaccalaureate distance learning degree programs offered. *Faculty:* 120 full-time (73 women), 279 part-time/adjunct (208 women). *Students:* 2,970 full-time (2,377 women), 3,619 part-time (2,946 women); includes 3,896 minority (2,352 Black or African American, non-Hispanic/Latino; 21 American Indian or Alaska Native, non-Hispanic/Latino; 90 Asian, non-Hispanic/Latino; 1,348 Hispanic/Latino; 6 Native Hawaiian or other Pacific Islander, non-Hispanic/Latino; 79 Two or more races, non-Hispanic/Latino), 39 international. Average age 40. 2,794 applicants, 53% accepted, 968 enrolled. In 2013, 1,103 master's, 426 doctorates, 349 other advanced degrees awarded. *Degree requirements:* For master's, practicum, internship; for doctorate, thesis/dissertation; for Ed S, thesis, practicum, internship. *Entrance requirements:* For master's, MAT or GRE (for some programs), CLAST, PRAXIS I, CBEST, General Knowledge Test, teaching certification, minimum GPA of 2.5, verification of teaching, BS; for doctorate, MAT or GRE, master's degree, minimum cumulative GPA of 3.0; for Ed S, MAT or GRE, master's degree, teaching certificate; minimum GPA of 3.0. Additional exam requirements/recommendations for international students: Recommended—TOEFL (minimum score 550 paper-based; 80 iBT), IELTS (minimum score 6). *Application deadline:* Applications are processed on a rolling basis. Application

fee: $50. Electronic applications accepted. *Financial support:* In 2013–14, 68 students received support. Career-related internships or fieldwork and Federal Work-Study available. Support available to part-time students. Financial award application deadline: 4/15; financial award applicants required to submit FAFSA. *Faculty research:* Instructional technology and distance education, educational leadership, speech language pathology, quality of life. *Total annual research expenditures:* $1.8 million. *Unit head:* Dr. H. Wells Singleton, Provost/Dean, 954-262-8730, Fax: 954-262-3894, E-mail: singlew@nova.edu. *Application contact:* Dr. Timothy Shields, Dean of Student Affairs, 800-986-3223 Ext. 8500, E-mail: shieldsd@nova.edu.
Website: http://www.fischlerschool.nova.edu/

Nova Southeastern University, College of Health Care Sciences, Fort Lauderdale, FL 33314-7796. Offers audiology (Au D); health science (MH Sc, DHSc, PhD); occupational therapy (MOT, OTD, PhD); physical therapy (DPT, PhD, TDPT); physician assistant (MMS). Postbaccalaureate distance learning degree programs offered (minimal on-campus study). *Faculty:* 117 full-time (68 women), 110 part-time/adjunct (57 women). *Students:* 1,187 full-time (844 women), 509 part-time (340 women); includes 560 minority (184 Black or African American, non-Hispanic/Latino; 2 American Indian or Alaska Native, non-Hispanic/Latino; 120 Asian, non-Hispanic/Latino; 218 Hispanic/Latino; 36 Two or more races, non-Hispanic/Latino), 20 international. Average age 31. 5,996 applicants, 14% accepted, 548 enrolled. In 2013, 374 master's, 132 doctorates awarded. *Degree requirements:* For master's, thesis; for doctorate, comprehensive exam, thesis/dissertation. *Entrance requirements:* For master's and doctorate, GRE General Test. *Application deadline:* Applications are processed on a rolling basis. Application fee: $50. Electronic applications accepted. *Expenses:* Contact institution. *Financial support:* In 2013–14, 10 students received support, including 2 research assistantships (averaging $3,500 per year); institutionally sponsored loans and unspecified assistantships also available. *Unit head:* Dr. Stanley Wilson, Dean, 954-262-1203, E-mail: swilson@nova.edu. *Application contact:* Joey Jankie, Admissions Counselor, 954-262-7249, E-mail: joey@nova.edu.
Website: http://www.nova.edu/chcs/

The Ohio State University, Graduate School, College of Arts and Sciences, Division of Social and Behavioral Sciences, Department of Speech and Hearing Science, Columbus, OH 43210. Offers audiology (Au D, PhD); hearing science (PhD); speech hearing science (MA); speech-language pathology (MA, PhD); speech-language science (PhD). *Accreditation:* ASHA (one or more programs are accredited). *Faculty:* 13. *Students:* 106 full-time (98 women), 4 part-time (3 women); includes 8 minority (2 American Indian or Alaska Native, non-Hispanic/Latino; 3 Asian, non-Hispanic/Latino; 3 Hispanic/Latino), 3 international. Average age 26. In 2013, 19 master's, 11 doctorates awarded. *Degree requirements:* For master's, thesis optional; for doctorate, thesis/dissertation. *Entrance requirements:* For master's and doctorate, GRE General Test. Additional exam requirements/recommendations for international students: Required—TOEFL (minimum score 600 paper-based; 100 iBT); Recommended—IELTS (minimum score 9). *Application deadline:* For fall admission, 12/1 priority date for domestic students, 11/30 priority date for international students; for winter admission, 12/1 for domestic students, 11/1 for international students; for spring admission, 3/1 for domestic students, 2/1 for international students. Applications are processed on a rolling basis. Application fee: $60 ($70 for international students). Electronic applications accepted. *Financial support:* Fellowships with tuition reimbursements, research assistantships with tuition reimbursements, teaching assistantships with tuition reimbursements, Federal Work-Study, and institutionally sponsored loans available. Support available to part-time students. *Unit head:* Robert A. Fox, Chair, 614-292-1628, E-mail: fox.2@osu.edu. *Application contact:* Vikki Back, Graduate Program Coordinator, 614-292-4673, Fax: 614-292-7504, E-mail: back.3@osu.edu.
Website: http://sphs.osu.edu/

Ohio University, Graduate College, College of Health Sciences and Professions, School of Rehabilitation and Communication Sciences, Division of Communication Sciences and Disorders, Athens, OH 45701-2979. Offers clinical audiology (Au D); hearing science (PhD); speech language pathology (MA); speech language science (PhD).

Oklahoma State University, College of Arts and Sciences, Department of Communications Sciences and Disorders, Stillwater, OK 74078. Offers MS. *Accreditation:* ASHA. *Faculty:* 11 full-time (8 women), 8 part-time/adjunct (all women). *Students:* 56 full-time (55 women), 1 (woman) part-time; includes 8 minority (2 Hispanic/Latino; 6 Two or more races, non-Hispanic/Latino). Average age 25. 149 applicants, 28% accepted, 22 enrolled. In 2013, 25 master's awarded. *Degree requirements:* For master's, thesis or creative research project, clinical practicum experience. *Entrance requirements:* For master's, GRE, minimum GPA of 3.0 in undergraduate major. Additional exam requirements/recommendations for international students: Required—TOEFL (minimum score 550 paper-based; 79 iBT). *Application deadline:* For fall admission, 3/1 priority date for international students; for spring admission, 8/1 priority date for international students. Applications are processed on a rolling basis. Application fee: $40 ($75 for international students). Electronic applications accepted. *Expenses:* Tuition, state resident: full-time $4272; part-time $178 per credit hour. Tuition, nonresident: full-time $17,472; part-time $709 per credit hour. *Required fees:* $2413.20; $100.55 per credit hour. One-time fee: $50 full-time. Part-time tuition and fees vary according to course load and campus/location. *Financial support:* In 2013–14, 15 teaching assistantships (averaging $6,180 per year) were awarded; career-related internships or fieldwork, Federal Work-Study, scholarships/grants, health care benefits, tuition waivers (partial), and unspecified assistantships also available. Support available to part-time students. Financial award application deadline: 3/1; financial award applicants required to submit FAFSA. *Faculty research:* Speech communications. *Unit head:* Dr. Cheryl Giddens, Department Head, 405-744-6021, E-mail: cheryl.giddens@okstate.edu. *Application contact:* Dr. Kaye Aulgur, Dean, 405-744-2996, E-mail: kaye.strom@okstate.edu.
Website: http://cdis.okstate.edu/

Old Dominion University, Darden College of Education, Program in Speech-Language Pathology, Norfolk, VA 23529. Offers MS Ed. *Accreditation:* ASHA. *Faculty:* 8 full-time (all women), 6 part-time/adjunct (5 women). *Students:* 58 full-time (57 women), 5 part-time (all women); includes 10 minority (6 Black or African American, non-Hispanic/Latino; 1 Asian, non-Hispanic/Latino; 2 Hispanic/Latino; 1 Native Hawaiian or other Pacific Islander, non-Hispanic/Latino). Average age 25. 112 applicants, 21% accepted, 24 enrolled. In 2013, 19 master's awarded. *Degree requirements:* For master's, comprehensive exam, thesis, written exams, practica. *Entrance requirements:* For master's, GRE General Test, minimum GPA of 3.0 in major, 2.8 overall. *Application deadline:* For fall admission, 2/1 for domestic students; for spring admission, 11/1 for domestic students. Application fee: $50. Electronic applications accepted. *Expenses:* Tuition, state resident: full-time $9888; part-time $412 per credit. Tuition, nonresident: full-time $25,152; part-time $1048 per credit. *Required fees:* $59 per semester. One-time fee: $50. *Financial support:* In 2013–14, 14 students received support, including 6 fellowships (averaging $6,000 per year), 1 research assistantship; teaching assistantships, career-related internships or fieldwork, scholarships/grants, and tuition waivers (partial) also available. Financial award application deadline: 2/1; financial award applicants required to submit CSS PROFILE or FAFSA. *Faculty research:* Childhood language disorders, phonological disorders, stuttering, aphasia, hearing aid outcomes. *Total annual research expenditures:* $10,000. *Unit head:* Dr. Anastasia M. Raymer, Graduate Program Director, 757-683-4117, Fax: 757-683-5593, E-mail: sraymer@odu.edu. *Application contact:* William Heffelfinger, Director of Graduate Admissions, 757-683-5554, Fax: 757-683-3255, E-mail: gradadmit@odu.edu.
Website: http://www.odu.edu/cdse

Our Lady of the Lake University of San Antonio, School of Professional Studies, Program in Communication and Learning Disorders, San Antonio, TX 78207-4689. Offers MA. *Accreditation:* ASHA. Part-time and evening/weekend programs available. *Faculty:* 6 full-time (all women), 1 (woman) part-time/adjunct. *Students:* 48 full-time (47 women), 4 part-time (all women); includes 32 minority (4 Black or African American, non-Hispanic/Latino; 1 Asian, non-Hispanic/Latino; 27 Hispanic/Latino). Average age 26. 284 applicants, 10% accepted, 24 enrolled. In 2013, 18 master's awarded. *Degree requirements:* For master's, thesis optional, comprehensive clinical practicum. *Entrance requirements:* For master's, GRE General Test or MAT. Additional exam requirements/recommendations for international students: Required—TOEFL. *Application deadline:* For fall admission, 2/1 priority date for domestic students, 2/1 for international students. Application fee: $25 ($50 for international students). Electronic applications accepted. *Expenses: Tuition:* Full-time $9120; part-time $760 per credit. *Required fees:* $698; $334 per trimester. Tuition and fees vary according to course load, degree level, campus/location and program. *Financial support:* Research assistantships, teaching assistantships, and career-related internships or fieldwork available. Support available to part-time students. Financial award application deadline: 3/15. *Faculty research:* Multicultural issues, neurogenic disorders, neural networks, equivalence learning. *Unit head:* Dr. Evangeline Nwokah, Head, 210-434-6711 Ext. 2608, E-mail: eenwokah@lake.ollusa.edu. *Application contact:* Graduate Admission, 210-431-3961, Fax: 210-431-4013, E-mail: gradadm@lake.ollusa.edu.
Website: http://www.ollusa.edu/s/1190/ollu.aspx?sid=1190&gid=1&pgid=990

Penn State University Park, Graduate School, College of Health and Human Development, Department of Communication Sciences and Disorders, University Park, PA 16802. Offers MS, PhD, Certificate. *Accreditation:* ASHA (one or more programs are accredited). *Unit head:* Dr. Ann C. Crouter, Dean, 814-865-1420, Fax: 814-865-3282, E-mail: ac1@psu.edu. *Application contact:* Cynthia E. Nicosia, Director, Graduate Enrollment Services, 814-865-1834, Fax: 814-863-4627, E-mail: cey1@psu.edu.
Website: http://csd.hhd.psu.edu/

Portland State University, Graduate Studies, College of Liberal Arts and Sciences, Department of Speech and Hearing Sciences, Portland, OR 97207-0751. Offers speech-language pathology (MA, MS). *Accreditation:* ASHA (one or more programs are accredited). *Faculty:* 13 full-time (10 women), 11 part-time/adjunct (8 women). *Students:* 100 full-time (93 women), 6 part-time (all women); includes 11 minority (5 Asian, non-Hispanic/Latino; 5 Hispanic/Latino; 1 Two or more races, non-Hispanic/Latino), 4 international. Average age 31. 96 applicants, 54% accepted, 52 enrolled. In 2013, 47 master's awarded. *Degree requirements:* For master's, variable foreign language requirement, thesis or alternative, oral exam. *Entrance requirements:* For master's, GRE General Test, minimum GPA of 3.0 in upper-division course work or 2.75 overall, BA/BS in speech and hearing sciences. Additional exam requirements/recommendations for international students: Required—TOEFL (minimum score 550 paper-based). *Application deadline:* For fall admission, 2/1 for domestic and international students. Application fee: $50. *Expenses:* Tuition, state resident: full-time $9207; part-time $341 per credit. Tuition, nonresident: full-time $14,391; part-time $533 per credit. *Required fees:* $1263; $22 per credit. $98 per quarter. One-time fee: $150. Tuition and fees vary according to program. *Financial support:* In 2013–14, 2 research assistantships with full tuition reimbursements (averaging $6,691 per year), 3 teaching assistantships with full tuition reimbursements (averaging $5,622 per year) were awarded; career-related internships or fieldwork, Federal Work-Study, and institutionally sponsored loans also available. Support available to part-time students. Financial award application deadline: 3/1; financial award applicants required to submit FAFSA. *Faculty research:* Adolescents with clefts, spectral analysis of stuttering, communication in late talkers, speech intelligibility, brainstem response in fitting hearing aids. *Total annual research expenditures:* $156,870. *Unit head:* Christina Gildersleeve Neumann, PhD, Chair, 503-725-3230, Fax: 503-725-5385, E-mail: cegn@pdx.edu. *Application contact:* Rebecca Field, Office Coordinator, 503-725-5380, E-mail: sphr@pdx.edu.
Website: http://www.sphr.pdx.edu/overview/

Purdue University, Graduate School, College of Health and Human Sciences, Department of Speech, Language, and Hearing Sciences, West Lafayette, IN 47907. Offers audiology clinic (MS, Au D, PhD); linguistics (MS, PhD); speech and hearing science (MS, PhD); speech-language pathology (MS, PhD). *Accreditation:* ASHA. *Faculty:* 23 full-time (11 women), 5 part-time/adjunct (3 women). *Students:* 81 full-time (76 women), 15 part-time (13 women); includes 6 minority (1 Black or African American, non-Hispanic/Latino; 3 Asian, non-Hispanic/Latino; 1 Hispanic/Latino; 1 Two or more races, non-Hispanic/Latino), 9 international. Average age 25. 282 applicants, 32% accepted, 32 enrolled. In 2013, 24 master's, 9 doctorates awarded. *Degree requirements:* For master's, comprehensive exam (for some programs), thesis optional; for doctorate, comprehensive exam, thesis/dissertation. *Entrance requirements:* For master's and doctorate, GRE General Test, minimum undergraduate GPA of 3.0 or equivalent. Additional exam requirements/recommendations for international students: Required—TOEFL (minimum score 77 iBT). *Application deadline:* For fall admission, 1/1 priority date for domestic and international students; for spring admission, 8/1 priority date for domestic and international students. Applications are processed on a rolling basis. Application fee: $60 ($75 for international students). Electronic applications accepted. *Financial support:* Fellowships with full tuition reimbursements, research assistantships with full tuition reimbursements, teaching assistantships with full tuition reimbursements, career-related internships or fieldwork, and scholarships/grants available. Support available to part-time students. Financial award application deadline: 2/1; financial award applicants required to submit FAFSA. *Faculty research:* Psychoacoustics, speech perception, speech physiology, stuttering, child language. *Unit head:* Dr. Keith R. Kluender, Head, 765-494-3788, Fax: 765-494-0771, E-mail: kkluender@purdue.edu. *Application contact:* Vickie L. Parker-Black, Graduate Contact, 765-494-3786, Fax: 765-494-0771, E-mail: vpblack@purdue.edu.
Website: http://www.purdue.edu/hhs/slhs/

Queens College of the City University of New York, Division of Graduate Studies, Arts and Humanities Division, Department of Linguistics and Communication Disorders, Program in Speech Pathology, Flushing, NY 11367-1597. Offers MA. *Accreditation:* ASHA. *Degree requirements:* For master's, thesis optional, clinical internships. *Entrance requirements:* For master's, GRE General Test, minimum GPA of 3.0. Additional exam requirements/recommendations for international students: Required—TOEFL.

Radford University, College of Graduate and Professional Studies, Waldron College of Health and Human Services, Department of Communication Sciences and Disorders, Radford, VA 24142. Offers speech-language pathology (MA, MS). *Accreditation:* ASHA (one or more programs are accredited). Part-time programs available. *Faculty:* 7 full-time (6 women), 8 part-time/adjunct (6 women). *Students:* 61 full-time (59 women), 1 (woman) part-time; includes 1 minority (Asian, non-Hispanic/Latino), 1 international. Average age 25. 235 applicants, 27% accepted, 28 enrolled. In 2013, 24 master's

awarded. *Degree requirements:* For master's, comprehensive exam, thesis (for some programs). *Entrance requirements:* For master's, GRE, minimum GPA of 3.0; completed CSDCAS application with 3 letters of reference; personal essay; resume. Additional exam requirements/recommendations for international students: Required—TOEFL (minimum score 550 paper-based; 79 iBT). *Application deadline:* For fall admission, 2/1 priority date for domestic students, 12/1 for international students; for spring admission, 7/1 for international students. Applications are processed on a rolling basis. Application fee: $50. Electronic applications accepted. *Expenses:* Tuition, state resident: full-time $6800; part-time $283 per credit hour. Tuition, nonresident: full-time $15,610; part-time $627 per credit hour. *Required fees:* $2944; $123 per credit hour. Tuition and fees vary according to program. *Financial support:* In 2013–14, 30 students received support, including 27 research assistantships with partial tuition reimbursements available (averaging $4,741 per year), 3 teaching assistantships with partial tuition reimbursements available (averaging $7,000 per year); career-related internships or fieldwork, Federal Work-Study, institutionally sponsored loans, scholarships/grants, and unspecified assistantships also available. Financial award application deadline: 3/1; financial award applicants required to submit FAFSA. *Unit head:* Dr. Diane C. Millar, Chair, 540-831-7635, Fax: 540-831-7699, E-mail: dcmillar@radford.edu. *Application contact:* Rebecca Conner, Director, Graduate Enrollment, 540-831-6296, Fax: 540-831-6061, E-mail: gradcollege@radford.edu.
Website: http://www.radford.edu/content/wchs/home/cosd.html

The Richard Stockton College of New Jersey, School of Graduate and Continuing Studies, Program in Communication Disorders, Galloway, NJ 08205-9441. Offers MS. *Accreditation:* ASHA. *Faculty:* 6 full-time (5 women), 6 part-time/adjunct (4 women). *Students:* 80 full-time (74 women), 19 part-time (16 women); includes 12 minority (1 Black or African American, non-Hispanic/Latino; 1 American Indian or Alaska Native, non-Hispanic/Latino; 2 Asian, non-Hispanic/Latino; 5 Hispanic/Latino; 3 Two or more races, non-Hispanic/Latino). Average age 27. 223 applicants, 30% accepted, 37 enrolled. *Degree requirements:* For master's, comprehensive exam (for some programs), thesis optional. *Entrance requirements:* For master's, GRE, 3 letters of recommendation, official transcripts from all colleges/universities attended, minimum undergraduate cumulative GPA of 3.2. *Application deadline:* For fall admission, 2/1 for domestic students. Electronic applications accepted. *Expenses: Tuition, area resident:* Part-time $559 per credit. Tuition, state resident: part-time $559 per credit. Tuition, nonresident: part-time $861 per credit. *Required fees:* $168.23 per credit. $75 per semester. Tuition and fees vary according to course load and degree level. *Financial support:* In 2013–14, 16 research assistantships with partial tuition reimbursements were awarded; fellowships, career-related internships or fieldwork, Federal Work-Study, scholarships/grants, and unspecified assistantships also available. Support available to part-time students. Financial award application deadline: 3/1. *Unit head:* Dr. Amy Hadley, Program Director, 609-626-3640, E-mail: graduatestudies@stockton.edu. *Application contact:* Tara Williams, Assistant Director of Enrollment Management, 609-626-3640, Fax: 609-626-6050, E-mail: gradschool@stockton.edu.

Rockhurst University, School of Graduate and Professional Studies, Program in Communication Sciences and Disorders, Kansas City, MO 64110-2561. Offers MS. *Accreditation:* ASHA. Part-time and evening/weekend programs available. *Faculty:* 3 full-time (all women), 5 part-time/adjunct (4 women). *Students:* 71 full-time (69 women), 2 part-time (both women); includes 5 minority (2 Asian, non-Hispanic/Latino; 2 Hispanic/Latino; 1 Two or more races, non-Hispanic/Latino). Average age 24. 194 applicants, 42% accepted, 28 enrolled. In 2013, 33 master's awarded. *Entrance requirements:* For master's, GRE General Test, interview, minimum GPA of 3.0, letters of recommendation. Additional exam requirements/recommendations for international students: Required—TOEFL (minimum score 550 paper-based; 79 iBT). *Application deadline:* Applications are processed on a rolling basis. Application fee: $25. Electronic applications accepted. Application fee is waived when completed online. Tuition and fees vary according to program. *Financial support:* Career-related internships or fieldwork, institutionally sponsored loans, and unspecified assistantships available. Financial award applicants required to submit FAFSA. *Faculty research:* Bioacoustics, physiology, applied speech science, pediatric nutrition/dysphagia, communication/cognition. *Unit head:* Kathy Ermgodts, Chair, 816-501-4505, Fax: 816-501-4169, E-mail: kathy.ermgodts@rockhurst.edu. *Application contact:* Cheryl Hooper, Director of Graduate Admission, 816-501-4097, Fax: 816-501-4241, E-mail: cherly.hooper@rockhurst.edu.
Website: http://www.rockhurst.edu/academic/csd/index.asp

Rush University, College of Health Sciences, Department of Communication Disorders and Sciences, Chicago, IL 60612-3832. Offers audiology (Au D); speech-language pathology (MS). *Accreditation:* ASHA (one or more programs are accredited). Part-time programs available. *Degree requirements:* For master's, comprehensive exam, thesis optional; for doctorate, comprehensive exam, investigative project. *Entrance requirements:* For master's and doctorate, GRE General Test, minimum GPA of 3.0. Additional exam requirements/recommendations for international students: Required—TOEFL. Electronic applications accepted. *Expenses:* Contact institution. *Faculty research:* Electrostimulation of subthalamic nucleus, sensory feedback in speech modulation, sentence complexity in children's writing, velopharyngeal function, adult neurology.

St. Ambrose University, College of Education and Health Sciences, Program in Speech-Language Pathology, Davenport, IA 52803-2898. Offers MSLP. Part-time and evening/weekend programs available. *Entrance requirements:* Additional exam requirements/recommendations for international students: Required—TOEFL. Electronic applications accepted.

St. Cloud State University, School of Graduate Studies, School of Health and Human Services, Department of Communication Sciences and Disorders, St. Cloud, MN 56301-4498. Offers MS. *Accreditation:* ASHA. *Degree requirements:* For master's, comprehensive exam (for some programs), thesis or alternative. *Entrance requirements:* For master's, GRE General Test, minimum GPA of 2.75. Additional exam requirements/recommendations for international students: Required—Michigan English Language Assessment Battery; Recommended—TOEFL (minimum score 550 paper-based), IELTS (minimum score 6.5). Electronic applications accepted.

St. John's University, St. John's College of Liberal Arts and Sciences, Department of Communication Sciences and Disorders, Queens, NY 11439. Offers MA, Au D. *Accreditation:* ASHA. Evening/weekend programs available. *Students:* 100 full-time (97 women), 42 part-time (37 women); includes 38 minority (1 Black or African American, non-Hispanic/Latino; 12 Asian, non-Hispanic/Latino; 23 Hispanic/Latino; 2 Two or more races, non-Hispanic/Latino). Average age 24. 554 applicants, 18% accepted, 44 enrolled. In 2013, 52 master's, 4 doctorates awarded. *Degree requirements:* For master's, comprehensive exam, thesis, practicum, residency ; for doctorate, practicum. *Entrance requirements:* For master's, GRE, minimum GPA of 3.0, 3 letters of recommendation, statement of goals, bachelor's degree; for doctorate, GRE, official transcript from all schools attended, minimum GPA of 3.0, 3 letters of recommendation, essay, interview. Additional exam requirements/recommendations for international students: Required—TOEFL (minimum score 600 paper-based; 100 iBT), IELTS (minimum score 5.5). *Application deadline:* For fall admission, 2/1 for domestic students, 2/1 priority date for international students; for spring admission, 10/1 for domestic students, 10/1 priority date for international students. Applications are processed on a rolling basis. Application fee: $70. Electronic applications accepted. *Expenses:* Contact institution. *Financial support:* Research assistantships, career-related internships or fieldwork, and scholarships/grants available. Support available to part-time students. Financial award application deadline: 3/1; financial award applicants required to submit FAFSA. *Faculty research:* Bilingualism and adult and child language disorders, neural processing of speech, dysphagia, speech motor control, electrophysiological measurement of hearing, central auditory processing disorders, scholarship of teaching and learning, evidence-based education, developmental dyslexia. *Total annual research expenditures:* $24,000. *Unit head:* Dr. Tina Jupiter, Chair, 718-990-6450, E-mail: jupitert@stjohns.edu. *Application contact:* Robert Medrano, Director of Graduate Admission, 718-990-1601, Fax: 718-990-5686, E-mail: gradhelp@stjohns.edu.

Saint Louis University, Graduate Education, College of Arts and Sciences and Graduate Education, Department of Communication Sciences and Disorders, St. Louis, MO 63103-2097. Offers MA, MA-R. *Accreditation:* ASHA (one or more programs are accredited). *Degree requirements:* For master's, thesis optional, comprehensive oral and written exams. *Entrance requirements:* For master's, GRE General Test, letters of recommendation, resume. Additional exam requirements/recommendations for international students: Required—TOEFL (minimum score 525 paper-based). Electronic applications accepted. *Faculty research:* Communication disorders in culturally and linguistically diverse populations, disability study-specific to World Health Organization classifications, early intervention in communication disorders and literacy skills, communication difficulties in internationally adopted children, voice and swallowing disorders secondary to cancer treatments.

Saint Xavier University, Graduate Studies, College of Arts and Sciences, Department of Communication Sciences and Disorders, Chicago, IL 60655-3105. Offers speech-language pathology (MS). *Accreditation:* ASHA. *Entrance requirements:* For master's, GRE General Test, minimum GPA of 3.0, undergraduate course work in speech. *Expenses:* Contact institution.

Salus University, George S. Osborne College of Audiology, Elkins Park, PA 19027-1598. Offers Au D. *Accreditation:* ASHA. *Entrance requirements:* Additional exam requirements/recommendations for international students: Required—TOEFL. Electronic applications accepted.

San Diego State University, Graduate and Research Affairs, College of Health and Human Services, School of Speech, Language, and Hearing Sciences, San Diego, CA 92182. Offers audiology (Au D); communicative disorders (MA); language and communicative disorders (PhD). PhD offered jointly with University of California, San Diego. *Accreditation:* ASHA (one or more programs are accredited). Part-time programs available. *Degree requirements:* For master's, comprehensive exam (for some programs), thesis (for some programs); for doctorate, thesis/dissertation. *Entrance requirements:* For master's and doctorate, GRE General Test. Additional exam requirements/recommendations for international students: Required—TOEFL. Electronic applications accepted. *Faculty research:* Brain/behavior relationships in language development, grammatical processing and language disorders, interdisciplinary training of bilingual speech pathologists.

San Francisco State University, Division of Graduate Studies, College of Education, Department of Special Education, Program in Communicative Disorders, San Francisco, CA 94132-1722. Offers MS. *Accreditation:* ASHA. *Unit head:* Dr. Nancy B. Robinson, Interim Chair, 415-338-1001, E-mail: cdinfo@sfsu.edu. *Application contact:* Dr. Laura Epstein, Program Coordinator, 415-338-1001, E-mail: lepstein@sfsu.edu.
Website: http://www.sfsu.edu/~comdis/

San Jose State University, Graduate Studies and Research, Connie L. Lurie College of Education, Department of Communicative Disorders and Sciences, San Jose, CA 95192-0001. Offers speech-language pathology (MA). *Accreditation:* ASHA. Evening/weekend programs available. *Entrance requirements:* For master's, MAT. Electronic applications accepted.

Seton Hall University, School of Health and Medical Sciences, Program in Speech-Language Pathology, South Orange, NJ 07079-2697. Offers MS. *Accreditation:* ASHA. *Entrance requirements:* For master's, GRE, bachelor's degree, clinical experience; minimum GPA of 3.0, undergraduate preprofessional coursework in communication sciences and disorders. Additional exam requirements/recommendations for international students: Recommended—TOEFL. Electronic applications accepted. *Faculty research:* Child language disorders, motor speech control, voice disorders, dysphagia, early intervention/teaming.

South Carolina State University, School of Graduate and Professional Studies, Department of Health Sciences, Orangeburg, SC 29117-0001. Offers speech pathology and audiology (MA). *Accreditation:* ASHA. Part-time and evening/weekend programs available. *Faculty:* 7 full-time (5 women). *Students:* 48 full-time (45 women), 47 part-time (46 women); includes 50 minority (49 Black or African American, non-Hispanic/Latino; 1 Asian, non-Hispanic/Latino), 1 international. Average age 27. 103 applicants, 46% accepted, 38 enrolled. In 2013, 34 master's awarded. *Degree requirements:* For master's, thesis optional, departmental qualifying exam. *Entrance requirements:* For master's, GRE or NTE, minimum GPA of 3.0. *Application deadline:* For fall admission, 6/15 for domestic and international students; for spring admission, 11/1 for domestic and international students. Application fee: $25. Electronic applications accepted. *Expenses:* Tuition, state resident: full-time $8906; part-time $543 per credit hour. Tuition, nonresident: full-time $18,040; part-time $1051 per credit hour. *Financial support:* Fellowships, career-related internships or fieldwork, Federal Work-Study, and institutionally sponsored loans available. Financial award application deadline: 6/1. *Unit head:* Dr. Cecelia Jeffries, Interim Chair, 803-536-8074, Fax: 803-536-8593, E-mail: cjeffrie@scsu.edu. *Application contact:* Curtis Foskey, Coordinator of Graduate Admission, 803-536-8419, Fax: 803-536-8812, E-mail: cfoskey@scsu.edu.

Southeastern Louisiana University, College of Nursing and Health Sciences, Department of Health and Human Sciences, Hammond, LA 70402. Offers communication sciences and disorders (MS); counselor education (M Ed). *Accreditation:* ASHA; NCATE. *Faculty:* 15 full-time (all women), 1 (woman) part-time/adjunct. *Students:* 87 full-time (83 women), 70 part-time (60 women); includes 35 minority (24 Black or African American, non-Hispanic/Latino; 7 Hispanic/Latino; 4 Two or more races, non-Hispanic/Latino). Average age 26. 221 applicants, 64% accepted, 26 enrolled. In 2013, 33 master's awarded. *Degree requirements:* For master's, comprehensive exam, thesis optional, 25 clock hours of clinical observation. *Entrance requirements:* For master's, GRE (verbal and quantitative), minimum GPA of 2.75; undergraduate degree; three letters of reference; favorable criminal background check. Additional exam requirements/recommendations for international students: Required—TOEFL (minimum score 500 paper-based; 61 iBT). *Application deadline:* For fall admission, 3/1 priority date for domestic students, 6/1 priority date for international students; for spring admission, 10/1 priority date for domestic and international students. Applications are processed on a rolling basis. Application fee: $20 ($30 for international students). Electronic applications accepted. *Expenses:* Tuition, state resident: full-time $5047. Tuition, nonresident: full-time $17,066. *Required fees:* $1213. Tuition and fees vary according to degree level. *Financial support:* In 2013–14, 1 research assistantship (averaging $9,000 per year) was awarded; career-related internships or fieldwork,

Federal Work-Study, institutionally sponsored loans, scholarships/grants, and unspecified assistantships also available. Support available to part-time students. Financial award application deadline: 5/1; financial award applicants required to submit FAFSA. *Faculty research:* Aphasia, autism spectrum disorders, child language and literacy, language and dementia, clinical supervision. *Unit head:* Dr. Jacqueline Guendouzi, Interim Department Head, 985-549-2309, Fax: 985-549-5030, E-mail: jguendouzi@selu.edu. *Application contact:* Sandra Meyers, Graduate Admissions Analyst, 985-549-5620, Fax: 985-549-5632, E-mail: admissions@selu.edu.
Website: http://www.southeastern.edu/acad_research/depts/hhs/

Southeast Missouri State University, School of Graduate Studies, Department of Communication Disorders, Cape Girardeau, MO 63701-4799. Offers MA. *Accreditation:* ASHA. *Faculty:* 7 full-time (5 women), 2 part-time/adjunct (both women). *Students:* 30 full-time (all women), 5 part-time (all women). Average age 26. 146 applicants, 10% accepted, 15 enrolled. In 2013, 15 master's awarded. *Degree requirements:* For master's, comprehensive exam, thesis optional, research project. *Entrance requirements:* For master's, GRE General Test, minimum undergraduate GPA of 3.0; 2 letters of recommendation; undergraduate degree in field or prerequisite coursework. Additional exam requirements/recommendations for international students: Required—TOEFL (minimum score 550 paper-based; 79 iBT), IELTS (minimum score 6), PTE (minimum score 53). *Application deadline:* For fall admission, 2/1 for domestic and international students. Applications are processed on a rolling basis. Application fee: $30 ($40 for international students). Electronic applications accepted. *Expenses:* Tuition, state resident: full-time $5139; part-time $285.50 per credit hour. Tuition, nonresident: full-time $9099; part-time $505.50 per credit hour. *Financial support:* In 2013–14, 11 students received support, including 6 teaching assistantships with full tuition reimbursements available (averaging $8,144 per year); career-related internships or fieldwork, Federal Work-Study, scholarships/grants, traineeships, tuition waivers (full), and unspecified assistantships also available. Financial award application deadline: 6/30; financial award applicants required to submit FAFSA. *Faculty research:* Dysphagia, fluency disorders, voice disorders, language disorders, speech disorders. *Unit head:* Dr. Thomas Linares, Department of Communication Disorders Chair, 573-651-2488, E-mail: tlinares@semo.edu.
Website: http://www5.semo.edu/commdisorders/

Southern Connecticut State University, School of Graduate Studies, School of Health and Human Services, Department of Communication Disorders, New Haven, CT 06515-1355. Offers speech pathology (MS). *Accreditation:* ASHA. Part-time programs available. *Degree requirements:* For master's, thesis or alternative, clinical experience. *Entrance requirements:* For master's, GRE, interview, minimum QPA of 3.0. Electronic applications accepted.

Southern Illinois University Carbondale, Graduate School, College of Education and Human Services, Department of Communication Disorders and Sciences, Carbondale, IL 62901-4701. Offers MS. *Accreditation:* ASHA. *Faculty:* 4 full-time (2 women). *Students:* 53 full-time (52 women), 7 part-time (6 women); includes 7 minority (4 Black or African American, non-Hispanic/Latino; 1 Asian, non-Hispanic/Latino; 2 Hispanic/Latino). Average age 29. 179 applicants, 11% accepted, 20 enrolled. In 2013, 24 master's awarded. *Degree requirements:* For master's, thesis. *Entrance requirements:* For master's, GRE, minimum GPA of 3.0. Additional exam requirements/recommendations for international students: Required—TOEFL. *Application deadline:* For fall admission, 2/1 for domestic students. Application fee: $50. *Financial support:* In 2013–14, 17 students received support, including 1 fellowship with full tuition reimbursement available, 7 research assistantships with full tuition reimbursements available; teaching assistantships with full tuition reimbursements available, career-related internships or fieldwork, Federal Work-Study, institutionally sponsored loans, tuition waivers (full), and unspecified assistantships also available. *Faculty research:* Neurolinguistics, language processing, child language, fluency, phonology. *Unit head:* Dr. Carl Flowers, Director, 618-453-8280, E-mail: cflowers@siu.edu. *Application contact:* Sheila Dingrando, Office Support Specialist, 618-453-8262, E-mail: sding@siu.edu.

Southern Illinois University Edwardsville, Graduate School, School of Education, Department of Special Education and Communication Disorders, Program in Speech-Language Pathology, Edwardsville, IL 62026. Offers MS. *Accreditation:* ASHA. Part-time and evening/weekend programs available. *Students:* 56 full-time (53 women), 1 (woman) part-time; includes 3 minority (1 Asian, non-Hispanic/Latino; 1 Hispanic/Latino; 1 Two or more races, non-Hispanic/Latino). 242 applicants, 41% accepted. In 2013, 30 master's awarded. *Degree requirements:* For master's, thesis (for some programs), final exam. *Entrance requirements:* For master's, GRE, minimum GPA of 3.0. Additional exam requirements/recommendations for international students: Required—TOEFL (minimum score 550 paper-based, 79 iBT), IELTS (minimum score 6.5), Michigan Test of English Language Proficiency or PTE. *Application deadline:* For fall admission, 1/15 for domestic and international students. Application fee: $30. Electronic applications accepted. *Expenses:* Tuition, state resident: full-time $3551. Tuition, nonresident: full-time $8378. *Financial support:* In 2013–14, 2 fellowships with full tuition reimbursements (averaging $8,370 per year), 2 research assistantships with full tuition reimbursements (averaging $9,585 per year), 15 teaching assistantships with full tuition reimbursements (averaging $9,585 per year) were awarded; institutionally sponsored loans, scholarships/grants, and unspecified assistantships also available. Financial award application deadline: 3/1; financial award applicants required to submit FAFSA. *Unit head:* Dr. Steffany Chleboun, Chair, 618-650-3677, E-mail: schlebo@siue.edu. *Application contact:* Melissa K. Mace, Assistant Director of Graduate and International Recruitment, 618-650-2756, Fax: 618-650-3618, E-mail: mmace@siue.edu.
Website: http://www.siue.edu/education/secd/

State University of New York at Fredonia, Graduate Studies, Department of Speech Pathology and Audiology, Fredonia, NY 14063-1136. Offers MS, MS Ed. *Accreditation:* ASHA. Part-time and evening/weekend programs available. *Degree requirements:* For master's, thesis optional, clinical practice. *Expenses:* Tuition, state resident: full-time $7398; part-time $411 per credit hour. Tuition, nonresident: full-time $13,770; part-time $765 per credit hour. *Required fees:* $1143.90; $63.55 per credit hour. Tuition and fees vary according to course load.

State University of New York at New Paltz, Graduate School, School of Liberal Arts and Sciences, Department of Communication Disorders, New Paltz, NY 12561. Offers communication disorders (MS), including speech-language disabilities, speech-language pathology. *Accreditation:* ASHA. Part-time and evening/weekend programs available. *Faculty:* 9 full-time (all women), 5 part-time/adjunct (all women). *Students:* 61 full-time (59 women), 2 part-time (both women); includes 9 minority (1 Black or African American, non-Hispanic/Latino; 3 Asian, non-Hispanic/Latino; 4 Hispanic/Latino; 1 Two or more races, non-Hispanic/Latino). Average age 27. 197 applicants, 22% accepted, 23 enrolled. In 2013, 18 master's awarded. *Degree requirements:* For master's, comprehensive exam, thesis. *Entrance requirements:* For master's, GRE General Test or MAT, minimum GPA of 3.0. Additional exam requirements/recommendations for international students: Required—TOEFL (minimum score 550 paper-based; 80 iBT), IELTS (minimum score 6.5). *Application deadline:* For fall admission, 3/1 for domestic and international students. Application fee: $50. Electronic applications accepted. *Expenses:* Tuition, state resident: full-time $9870; part-time $411 per credit. Tuition, nonresident: full-time $18,350; part-time $765 per credit. *Required fees:* $1213. Tuition and fees vary according to program. *Financial support:* In 2013–14, 4 teaching assistantships with partial tuition reimbursements (averaging $5,000 per year) were awarded. Financial award application deadline: 8/1. *Unit head:* Prof. Wendy Bower, Department Chair, 845-257-3620, E-mail: commdis@newpaltz.edu. *Application contact:* Dr. Anne Balant, Graduate Coordinator, 845-257-3453, E-mail: balanta@newpaltz.edu.
Website: http://www.newpaltz.edu/commdis/

State University of New York at Plattsburgh, Division of Education, Health, and Human Services, Department of Communication Disorders, Plattsburgh, NY 12901-2681. Offers speech-language pathology (MA). *Accreditation:* ASHA. Part-time programs available. *Students:* 38 full-time (37 women); includes 2 minority (1 Black or African American, non-Hispanic/Latino; 1 Two or more races, non-Hispanic/Latino), 2 international. Average age 25. *Entrance requirements:* For master's, GRE General Test, minimum GPA of 3.0. Additional exam requirements/recommendations for international students: Required—TOEFL. *Application deadline:* For fall admission, 2/15 priority date for domestic students. Applications are processed on a rolling basis. Application fee: $75. *Financial support:* Career-related internships or fieldwork and Federal Work-Study available. Support available to part-time students. Financial award application deadline: 4/15; financial award applicants required to submit FAFSA. *Faculty research:* Autotoxins and noise effects on hearing, language impairment in Alzheimer's disease, attitudes on stuttering, diagnostic audiology. *Unit head:* Dr. Raymond Domenico, Chair, 518-564-3154, E-mail: domenira@plattsburgh.edu. *Application contact:* Betsy Kane, Director, Graduate Admissions, 518-564-4723, Fax: 518-564-4722, E-mail: bkane002@plattsburgh.edu.

Stephen F. Austin State University, Graduate School, College of Education, Department of Human Services, Nacogdoches, TX 75962. Offers counseling (MA); school psychology (MA); special education (M Ed); speech pathology (MS). *Accreditation:* ACA (one or more programs are accredited); ASHA (one or more programs are accredited); CORE; NCATE. *Degree requirements:* For master's, comprehensive exam, thesis (for some programs). *Entrance requirements:* For master's, GRE General Test, minimum GPA of 2.8. Additional exam requirements/recommendations for international students: Required—TOEFL.

Syracuse University, College of Arts and Sciences, Program in Audiology, Syracuse, NY 13244. Offers Au D, PhD. *Accreditation:* ASHA. Part-time programs available. *Students:* 26 full-time (20 women), 3 part-time (all women); includes 1 minority (Hispanic/Latino), 4 international. Average age 25. 41 applicants, 85% accepted, 10 enrolled. In 2013, 7 doctorates awarded. *Degree requirements:* For doctorate, thesis/dissertation, internship. *Entrance requirements:* For doctorate, GRE General Test. Additional exam requirements/recommendations for international students: Required—TOEFL (minimum score 100 iBT). *Application deadline:* For fall admission, 2/1 priority date for domestic and international students. Application fee: $75. Electronic applications accepted. *Financial support:* Fellowships with full and partial tuition reimbursements, research assistantships with full and partial tuition reimbursements, and teaching assistantships with full and partial tuition reimbursements available. Financial award application deadline: 1/1. *Unit head:* Dr. Linda Milosky, Department Chair, 315-443-9637. *Application contact:* Jennifer Steigerwald, Information Contact, 315-443-9615, E-mail: jssteige@syr.edu.
Website: http://csd.syr.edu/

Syracuse University, College of Arts and Sciences, Program in Speech Language Pathology, Syracuse, NY 13244. Offers MS, PhD. *Accreditation:* ASHA. Part-time programs available. *Students:* 71 full-time (67 women); includes 5 minority (1 Black or African American, non-Hispanic/Latino; 1 Asian, non-Hispanic/Latino; 3 Hispanic/Latino), 7 international. Average age 24. 141 applicants, 78% accepted, 32 enrolled. In 2013, 39 master's awarded. *Degree requirements:* For master's, thesis or alternative; for doctorate, thesis/dissertation. *Entrance requirements:* For master's and doctorate, GRE. Additional exam requirements/recommendations for international students: Required—TOEFL (minimum score 100 iBT). *Application deadline:* For fall admission, 2/1 priority date for domestic and international students. Application fee: $45. Electronic applications accepted. *Financial support:* Fellowships with full tuition reimbursements, research assistantships with full and partial tuition reimbursements, and teaching assistantships with full and partial tuition reimbursements available. Financial award application deadline: 1/1; financial award applicants required to submit FAFSA. *Unit head:* Dr. Linda Milosky, Chair, 315-443-9637, E-mail: csd@syr.edu. *Application contact:* Jennifer Steigerwald, Information Contact, 315-443-9615.
Website: http://csd.syr.edu/

Teachers College, Columbia University, Graduate Faculty of Education, Department of Biobehavioral Studies, Program in Speech-Language Pathology, New York, NY 10027-6696. Offers Ed M, MS, Ed D, PhD. *Accreditation:* ASHA. *Faculty:* 8 full-time, 4 part-time/adjunct. *Students:* 97 full-time (89 women), 53 part-time (49 women); includes 59 minority (11 Black or African American, non-Hispanic/Latino; 29 Asian, non-Hispanic/Latino; 16 Hispanic/Latino; 3 Two or more races, non-Hispanic/Latino), 10 international. Average age 27. 878 applicants, 14% accepted, 53 enrolled. In 2013, 67 master's, 1 doctorate awarded. Terminal master's awarded for partial completion of doctoral program. *Degree requirements:* For doctorate, thesis/dissertation. *Entrance requirements:* For doctorate, professional master's degree in communication sciences and disorders. *Application deadline:* For fall admission, 1/2 priority date for domestic students. Applications are processed on a rolling basis. Application fee: $75. *Financial support:* Fellowships, teaching assistantships, career-related internships or fieldwork, Federal Work-Study, institutionally sponsored loans, and tuition waivers (full and partial) available. Support available to part-time students. Financial award application deadline: 2/1. *Faculty research:* Neuropathology of speech, stuttering, language disorders in children and adults, motor speech. *Unit head:* Prof. John Saxman, Program Coordinator, 212-678-3895, E-mail: saxman@tc.edu. *Application contact:* Morgan Oakes, Admission Counselor, 212-678-6613, E-mail: meo2142@columbia.edu.

Teachers College, Columbia University, Graduate Faculty of Education, Department of Health and Behavioral Studies, Program in Deaf and Hard of Hearing, New York, NY 10027-6696. Offers MA, Ed D. *Faculty:* 7 full-time, 13 part-time/adjunct. *Students:* 11 full-time (all women), 12 part-time (11 women); includes 9 minority (3 Black or African American, non-Hispanic/Latino; 2 Asian, non-Hispanic/Latino; 2 Hispanic/Latino; 2 Two or more races, non-Hispanic/Latino), 1 international. Average age 25. 16 applicants, 81% accepted, 7 enrolled. In 2013, 26 master's awarded. *Degree requirements:* For master's, comprehensive exam (for some programs), project; for doctorate, thesis/dissertation. *Application deadline:* For fall admission, 1/15 priority date for domestic students; for spring admission, 11/1 for domestic students. Applications are processed on a rolling basis. Application fee: $65. Electronic applications accepted. *Financial support:* Fellowships, career-related internships or fieldwork, Federal Work-Study, institutionally sponsored loans, and tuition waivers (full and partial) available. Support available to part-time students. Financial award application deadline: 2/1; financial award applicants required to submit FAFSA. *Faculty research:* Language development, reading/writing, cognitive abilities, text analysis, auditory streaming. *Unit head:* Prof. Robert Kretschmer, Program Coordinator, 212-678-3867, E-mail: kretschmer@tc.edu. *Application contact:* Elizabeth Puleio, Assistant Director of Admission, 212-678-3710, Fax: 212-678-4171, E-mail: tcinfo@tc.edu.

Teachers College, Columbia University, Graduate Faculty of Education, Department of Health and Behavioral Studies, Program in Teaching of Sign Language, New York, NY 10027-6696. Offers MA. *Accreditation:* NCATE. *Faculty:* 7 full-time, 13 part-time/adjunct. *Students:* 5 part-time (4 women); includes 2 minority (both Hispanic/Latino). Average age 27. 1 applicant. In 2013, 3 master's awarded. *Degree requirements:* For master's, comprehensive exam, project. *Entrance requirements:* For master's, demonstrated proficiency in American Sign Language. *Application deadline:* For fall admission, 1/15 for domestic students; for spring admission, 11/1 for domestic students. Application fee: $65. *Financial support:* Applicants required to submit FAFSA. *Faculty research:* Teaching of the deaf and hard of hearing; linguistics of English and American Sign Language (ASL); literacy development; text structure; school psychology; auditory streaming; sociology, anthropology, and history of deaf community and culture; American Sign Language; second language acquisition, curriculum, and instruction; disability studies. *Unit head:* Prof. Russell S. Rosen, Program Coordinator, 212-678-3880, E-mail: rrosen@tc.edu. *Application contact:* Elizabeth Puleio, Assistant Director of Admission, 212-678-3710, Fax: 212-678-4171, E-mail: eap2136@tc.columbia.edu.
Website: http://www.tc.columbia.edu/hbs/ASL/index.asp

Temple University, College of Health Professions and Social Work, Department of Communication Sciences and Disorders, Philadelphia, PA 19122. Offers communication sciences (PhD); speech-language-hearing (MA). *Accreditation:* ASHA. *Faculty:* 16 full-time (12 women). *Students:* 60 full-time (58 women), 6 part-time (all women); includes 12 minority (1 Black or African American, non-Hispanic/Latino; 3 Asian, non-Hispanic/Latino; 5 Hispanic/Latino; 3 Two or more races, non-Hispanic/Latino). 429 applicants, 13% accepted, 26 enrolled. In 2013, 31 master's awarded. *Degree requirements:* For master's, comprehensive exam; for doctorate, comprehensive exam, thesis/dissertation. *Entrance requirements:* For master's, GRE General Test, minimum GPA of 3.0, 2 letters of reference, statement of goals; for doctorate, GRE General Test, minimum GPA of 3.0, 3 letters of reference, statement of goals, writing sample, resume. Additional exam requirements/recommendations for international students: Required—TOEFL (minimum score 550 paper-based; 79 iBT). *Application deadline:* For fall admission, 1/1 for domestic and international students; for spring admission, 11/1 for domestic students, 10/1 for international students. Application fee: $60. Electronic applications accepted. *Financial support:* Federal Work-Study, institutionally sponsored loans, and unspecified assistantships available. Financial award application deadline: 1/15. *Faculty research:* Bilingualism, biliteracy, adult neurogenic language disorders including aphasia, dementia, school readiness. *Total annual research expenditures:* $1.1 million. *Unit head:* Dr. Carol Scheffner Hammer, Interim Chair, 215-204-7543, E-mail: cjhammer@temple.edu. *Application contact:* Dawn Dandridge, Coordinator of Outreach, 215-204-9005, E-mail: ddandrid@temple.edu.
Website: http://chpsw.temple.edu/commsci/home

Tennessee State University, The School of Graduate Studies and Research, College of Health Sciences, Department of Speech Pathology and Audiology, Nashville, TN 37209-1561. Offers speech and hearing science (MS). Part-time programs available. Postbaccalaureate distance learning degree programs offered (minimal on-campus study). *Degree requirements:* For master's, comprehensive exam, thesis optional. *Entrance requirements:* For master's, GRE General Test or MAT, minimum GPA of 3.5. Additional exam requirements/recommendations for international students: Required—TOEFL. *Faculty research:* Assessment and management of dysphagia, early intervention language disorders, multicultural diversity.

Texas A&M University–Kingsville, College of Graduate Studies, College of Arts and Sciences, Department of Clinical Health Sciences, Kingsville, TX 78363. Offers communication sciences and disorders (MS). *Faculty:* 5 full-time (0 women), 1 part-time/adjunct (0 women). *Students:* 39 full-time (36 women), 2 part-time (both women); includes 18 minority (1 Black or African American, non-Hispanic/Latino; 17 Hispanic/Latino), 1 international. Average age 27. 118 applicants, 14% accepted, 14 enrolled. In 2013, 20 master's awarded. *Degree requirements:* For master's, comprehensive exam, thesis or alternative. *Entrance requirements:* For master's, GRE General Test, minimum GPA of 3.0. Additional exam requirements/recommendations for international students: Required—TOEFL. *Application deadline:* Applications are processed on a rolling basis. Application fee: $35 ($50 for international students). Electronic applications accepted. *Financial support:* Career-related internships or fieldwork and Federal Work-Study available. Support available to part-time students. Financial award applicants required to submit FAFSA. *Unit head:* Dr. James Pierce, Chair, 361-593-3803, E-mail: kfjrp00@tamuk.edu. *Application contact:* Director of Admissions, 361-593-2315.

Texas Christian University, Harris College of Nursing and Health Sciences, Department of Communication Sciences and Disorders, Fort Worth, TX 76129. Offers speech-language pathology (MS). *Accreditation:* ASHA. *Faculty:* 5 full-time (4 women). *Students:* 30 full-time (29 women), 5 part-time (all women); includes 8 minority (7 Hispanic/Latino; 1 Two or more races, non-Hispanic/Latino). Average age 23. 207 applicants, 10% accepted, 20 enrolled. In 2013, 14 master's awarded. *Degree requirements:* For master's, comprehensive exam, thesis optional. *Entrance requirements:* For master's, GRE General Test, previous course work in speech-language pathology. Additional exam requirements/recommendations for international students: Required—TOEFL. *Application deadline:* For fall admission, 1/15 for domestic students. Application fee: $60. Electronic applications accepted. *Expenses: Tuition:* Part-time $1270 per credit hour. Tuition and fees vary according to course load and program. *Financial support:* In 2013–14, 28 students received support, including 28 teaching assistantships with tuition reimbursements available; unspecified assistantships also available. Financial award application deadline: 1/15; financial award applicants required to submit FAFSA. *Unit head:* Dr. Christopher Watts, Chairperson, 817-257-7621, E-mail: c.watts@tcu.edu. *Application contact:* Sybil White, Admissions, TCU Graduate Studies Office, 817-257-7515, Fax: 817-257-7484, E-mail: frogmail@tcu.edu.
Website: http://csd.tcu.edu/

Texas State University, Graduate School, College of Health Professions, Program in Communication Disorders, San Marcos, TX 78666. Offers MA, MSCD. *Accreditation:* ASHA (one or more programs are accredited). Part-time programs available. *Faculty:* 10 full-time (8 women). *Students:* 57 full-time (54 women); includes 25 minority (2 Black or African American, non-Hispanic/Latino; 1 Asian, non-Hispanic/Latino; 21 Hispanic/Latino; 1 Two or more races, non-Hispanic/Latino). Average age 24. 541 applicants, 6% accepted, 30 enrolled. In 2013, 27 master's awarded. *Degree requirements:* For master's, comprehensive exam, thesis (for some programs), practicum. *Entrance requirements:* For master's, minimum GPA of 3.0 in communications disorders and in last 60 hours of course work; 25 hours of observation; 2 letters of recommendation from professors in previous major; resume on form provided by department. Additional exam requirements/recommendations for international students: Required—TOEFL (minimum score 550 paper-based; 78 iBT). *Application deadline:* For fall admission, 2/1 for domestic and international students. Applications are processed on a rolling basis. Application fee: $40 ($90 for international students). Electronic applications accepted. *Expenses:* Tuition, state resident: full-time $6663; part-time $278 per credit hour. Tuition, nonresident: full-time $15,159; part-time $632 per credit hour. *Required fees:* $1872; $54 per credit hour. $306 per term. Tuition and fees vary according to course load. *Financial support:* In 2013–14, 14 students received support, including 5 research assistantships (averaging $5,690 per year), 9 teaching assistantships (averaging $5,683 per year); fellowships, career-related internships or fieldwork, Federal Work-Study, institutionally sponsored loans, scholarships/grants, and unspecified assistantships also available. Support available to part-time students. Financial award application deadline: 4/1; financial award applicants required to submit FAFSA. *Faculty research:* Cognitive impairment. *Total annual research expenditures:* $16,415. *Unit head:* Dr. Valarie Fleming, Graduate Advisor, 512-245-2330, Fax: 512-245-2029, E-mail: vf13@txstate.edu. *Application contact:* Dr. Andrea Golato, Dean of Graduate School, 512-245-2581, Fax: 512-245-8365, E-mail: gradcollege@txstate.edu.
Website: http://www.health.txstate.edu/CDIS/

Texas Tech University Health Sciences Center, School of Allied Health Sciences, Program in Speech, Language and Hearing Sciences, Lubbock, TX 79430. Offers MS, Au D, PhD. *Accreditation:* ASHA (one or more programs are accredited). *Faculty:* 21 full-time (14 women), 2 part-time/adjunct (0 women). *Students:* 114 full-time (105 women), 11 part-time (8 women); includes 22 minority (1 Black or African American, non-Hispanic/Latino; 2 American Indian or Alaska Native, non-Hispanic/Latino; 3 Asian, non-Hispanic/Latino; 13 Hispanic/Latino; 1 Native Hawaiian or other Pacific Islander, non-Hispanic/Latino; 2 Two or more races, non-Hispanic/Latino). Average age 27. 272 applicants, 19% accepted, 51 enrolled. In 2013, 34 master's, 10 doctorates awarded. *Degree requirements:* For master's, comprehensive exam, thesis optional; for doctorate, comprehensive exam, thesis/dissertation. *Entrance requirements:* For master's, GRE General Test, GRE Writing Test; for doctorate, GRE. Additional exam requirements/recommendations for international students: Required—TOEFL, IELTS. *Application deadline:* For fall admission, 11/1 for domestic students; for spring admission, 1/15 for domestic students. Applications are processed on a rolling basis. Application fee: $40. Electronic applications accepted. *Financial support:* In 2013–14, 3 research assistantships (averaging $5,000 per year), 7 teaching assistantships were awarded; institutionally sponsored loans and scholarships/grants also available. Financial award application deadline: 9/1; financial award applicants required to submit FAFSA. *Unit head:* Dr. Rajinder Koul, Chairperson, 806-743-5660 Ext. 227, Fax: 806-743-5670, E-mail: rajinder.koul@ttuhsc.edu. *Application contact:* Lindsay Johnson, Associate Dean for Admissions and Student Affairs, 806-743-3220, Fax: 806-742-2994, E-mail: lindsay.johnson@ttuhsc.edu.
Website: http://www.ttuhsc.edu/sah/cdu/

Texas Woman's University, Graduate School, College of Health Sciences, Department of Communication Sciences and Disorders, Denton, TX 76201. Offers education of the deaf (MS); speech/language pathology (MS). *Accreditation:* ASHA. Part-time programs available. Postbaccalaureate distance learning degree programs offered (no on-campus study). *Faculty:* 17 full-time (16 women), 6 part-time/adjunct (all women). *Students:* 198 full-time (191 women), 21 part-time (20 women); includes 76 minority (10 Black or African American, non-Hispanic/Latino; 1 American Indian or Alaska Native, non-Hispanic/Latino; 11 Asian, non-Hispanic/Latino; 54 Hispanic/Latino). Average age 31. 262 applicants, 7% accepted, 13 enrolled. In 2013, 146 master's awarded. *Degree requirements:* For master's, comprehensive exam, thesis (for some programs). *Entrance requirements:* For master's, GRE General Test (preferred minimum score 156 [550 old version] Verbal, 140 [400 old version] Quantitative), 2 letters of reference (3 for speech/language pathology), personal essay. Additional exam requirements/recommendations for international students: Required—TOEFL (minimum score 550 paper-based; 79 iBT). *Application deadline:* For fall admission, 2/1 priority date for domestic students, 2/1 for international students. Applications are processed on a rolling basis. Application fee: $50 ($75 for international students). Electronic applications accepted. *Expenses:* Tuition, state resident: full-time $4182; part-time $233.32 per credit hour. Tuition, nonresident: full-time $10,716; part-time $595.32 per credit hour. *Financial support:* In 2013–14, 94 students received support, including 9 research assistantships (averaging $9,684 per year); career-related internships or fieldwork, Federal Work-Study, institutionally sponsored loans, scholarships/grants, traineeships, health care benefits, and unspecified assistantships also available. Support available to part-time students. Financial award application deadline: 3/1; financial award applicants required to submit FAFSA. *Faculty research:* Stroke, language assessment auditory processing and relationship between speech and language, effectiveness of distance education learning, neuromodulation of recovery of aphasia. *Total annual research expenditures:* $11,160. *Unit head:* Dr. Erika Armstrong, Interim Co-Chair, 940-898-2025, Fax: 940-898-2070, E-mail: coms@twu.edu. *Application contact:* Dr. Samuel Wheeler, Assistant Director of Admissions, 940-898-3188, Fax: 940-898-3081, E-mail: wheelersr@twu.edu.
Website: http://www.twu.edu/communication-sciences/

Touro College, School of Health Sciences, Bay Shore, NY 11706. Offers occupational therapy (MS); physical therapy (DPT); physicians assistant (MS); speech-language pathology (MS). *Faculty:* 20 full-time, 94 part-time/adjunct. *Students:* 975 full-time (710 women), 160 part-time (114 women); includes 271 minority (58 Black or African American, non-Hispanic/Latino; 1 American Indian or Alaska Native, non-Hispanic/Latino; 132 Asian, non-Hispanic/Latino; 60 Hispanic/Latino; 4 Native Hawaiian or other Pacific Islander, non-Hispanic/Latino; 16 Two or more races, non-Hispanic/Latino), 10 international. *Expenses:* Contact institution. *Financial support:* Fellowships available. *Unit head:* Dr. Louis Primavera, Dean, School of Health Sciences, 516-673-3200, E-mail: louis.primavera@touro.edu. *Application contact:* Brian J. Diele, Associate Director of Central Admissions, 631-665-1600 Ext. 6311, E-mail: brian.diele@touro.edu.

Towson University, Program in Audiology, Towson, MD 21252-0001. Offers Au D. *Accreditation:* ASHA. *Students:* 54 full-time (48 women), 1 (woman) part-time; includes 9 minority (2 Black or African American, non-Hispanic/Latino; 3 Asian, non-Hispanic/Latino; 3 Hispanic/Latino; 1 Two or more races, non-Hispanic/Latino). *Entrance requirements:* For doctorate, GRE, 3 letters of recommendation, minimum GPA of 3.0, interview, essay. Additional exam requirements/recommendations for international students: Required—TOEFL (minimum score 600 paper-based). *Application deadline:* For fall admission, 2/1 for domestic students. Application fee: $45. Electronic applications accepted. *Financial support:* Application deadline: 4/1. *Unit head:* Dr. Peggy Korczak, Graduate Program Director, 410-704-5903, E-mail: pkorczak@towson.edu. *Application contact:* Alicia Arkell-Kleis, Information Contact, 410-704-6004, E-mail: grads@towson.edu.
Website: http://grad.towson.edu/program/doctoral/acsd-aud/

Towson University, Program in Speech-Language Pathology, Towson, MD 21252-0001. Offers MS. *Accreditation:* ASHA. *Students:* 81 full-time (all women); includes 9 minority (3 Black or African American, non-Hispanic/Latino; 2 Asian, non-Hispanic/Latino; 3 Hispanic/Latino; 1 Two or more races, non-Hispanic/Latino). *Degree requirements:* For master's, thesis (for some programs). *Entrance requirements:* For master's, GRE, bachelor's degree in speech-language pathology and audiology; CLEP or advanced placement (AP) examination credits in biological sciences, physical sciences, social/behavioral sciences and statistics; minimum GPA of 3.0 in major; 3 letters of recommendation; essay. Additional exam requirements/recommendations for international students: Required—TOEFL (minimum score 600 paper-based). *Application deadline:* For fall admission, 1/15 for domestic students. Applications are processed on a rolling basis. Application fee: $45. Electronic applications accepted. *Financial support:* Application deadline: 4/1. *Unit head:* Dr. Karen Fallon, Graduate

Program Director, 410-704-2449, E-mail: kfallon@towson.edu. *Application contact:* Alicia Arkell-Kleis, Information Contact, 410-704-6004, E-mail: grads@towson.edu.
Website: http://grad.towson.edu/program/master/sppa-ms/

Truman State University, Graduate School, School of Health Sciences and Education, Program in Communication Disorders, Kirksville, MO 63501-4221. Offers MA. *Accreditation:* ASHA. *Degree requirements:* For master's, comprehensive exam, thesis optional. *Entrance requirements:* For master's, GRE General Test, minimum GPA of 3.0. Additional exam requirements/recommendations for international students: Required—TOEFL (minimum score 550 paper-based). Electronic applications accepted.

Universidad del Turabo, Graduate Programs, School of Health Sciences, Program in Speech and Language Pathology, Gurabo, PR 00778-3030. Offers MS.

Université de Montréal, Faculty of Medicine, School of Speech Therapy and Audiology, Montréal, QC H3C 3J7, Canada. Offers audiology (PMS); speech therapy (PMS, DESS). *Degree requirements:* For master's, thesis. *Entrance requirements:* For master's, B Sc in speech-language pathology and audiology, proficiency in French. Electronic applications accepted. *Faculty research:* Aphasia in adults, dysarthria, speech and hearing-impaired children, noise-induced hearing impairment, computerized audiometry.

Université Laval, Faculty of Medicine, Graduate Programs in Medicine, Program in Speech Therapy, Québec, QC G1K 7P4, Canada. Offers M Sc. *Entrance requirements:* For master's, knowledge of French, interview. Electronic applications accepted.

University at Buffalo, the State University of New York, Graduate School, College of Arts and Sciences, Department of Communicative Disorders and Sciences, Buffalo, NY 14260. Offers audiology (Au D); communicative disorders and sciences (MA, PhD). *Accreditation:* ASHA (one or more programs are accredited). *Faculty:* 18 full-time (13 women), 1 (woman) part-time/adjunct. *Students:* 116 full-time (107 women); includes 12 minority (2 Black or African American, non-Hispanic/Latino; 7 Asian, non-Hispanic/Latino; 3 Hispanic/Latino). 316 applicants, 22% accepted, 40 enrolled. In 2013, 27 master's, 6 doctorates awarded. *Degree requirements:* For master's, thesis or alternative, exam; for doctorate, thesis/dissertation, exams. *Entrance requirements:* For master's and doctorate, GRE General Test, minimum GPA of 3.0. Additional exam requirements/recommendations for international students: Required—TOEFL (minimum score 550 paper-based; 79 iBT). *Application deadline:* For fall admission, 1/1 priority date for domestic and international students. Application fee: $75. Electronic applications accepted. *Financial support:* In 2013–14, 20 students received support, including 2 fellowships (averaging $10,800 per year), 3 research assistantships with full and partial tuition reimbursements available (averaging $13,000 per year), 19 teaching assistantships with full and partial tuition reimbursements available (averaging $7,000 per year); career-related internships or fieldwork, Federal Work-Study, institutionally sponsored loans, scholarships/grants, health care benefits, tuition waivers (partial), and unspecified assistantships also available. Financial award applicants required to submit FAFSA. *Faculty research:* Hearing and speech science, child and adult language disorders, augmentative communication, cochlear implants, tinnitus. *Total annual research expenditures:* $2.6 million. *Unit head:* Dr. Joan Sussman, Chairperson, 716-829-5551, Fax: 716-829-3979, E-mail: jsussman@buffalo.edu. *Application contact:* Virginia L. Majewski, Graduate Coordinator, 716-829-5570, Fax: 716-829-3979, E-mail: vmajewsk@buffalo.edu.
Website: http://cdswebserver.med.buffalo.edu/drupal/

The University of Akron, Graduate School, College of Health Professions, School of Speech-Language Pathology and Audiology, Program in Audiology, Akron, OH 44325. Offers Au D. *Accreditation:* ASHA. *Students:* 43 full-time (36 women); includes 3 minority (2 Black or African American, non-Hispanic/Latino; 1 Hispanic/Latino). Average age 25. 74 applicants, 35% accepted, 16 enrolled. In 2013, 10 doctorates awarded. *Degree requirements:* For doctorate, 2000 clock hours of clinical experience, academic and clinical competency-based exams. *Entrance requirements:* For doctorate, GRE, minimum GPA of 3.0, letters of recommendation, statement of purpose. Additional exam requirements/recommendations for international students: Required—TOEFL (minimum score 550 paper-based; 79 iBT). *Application deadline:* For fall admission, 2/1 for domestic and international students. Application fee: $40 ($60 for international students). Electronic applications accepted. *Expenses:* Tuition, state resident: full-time $7430; part-time $412.80 per credit hour. Tuition, nonresident: full-time $12,722; part-time $706.80 per credit hour. *Required fees:* $53 per credit hour. $12 per semester. Tuition and fees vary according to course load and program. *Unit head:* Dr. Roberta DePompei, School Director, 330-972-6803, E-mail: rdepom1@uakron.edu. *Application contact:* Dr. James Steiger, Program Coordinator, 330-972-8190, E-mail: steiger@uakron.edu.

The University of Akron, Graduate School, College of Health Professions, School of Speech-Language Pathology and Audiology, Program in Speech-Language Pathology, Akron, OH 44325. Offers MA. *Accreditation:* ASHA. *Students:* 85 full-time (80 women), 15 part-time (all women); includes 7 minority (3 Black or African American, non-Hispanic/Latino; 2 Asian, non-Hispanic/Latino; 2 Hispanic/Latino). Average age 26. 223 applicants, 20% accepted, 41 enrolled. In 2013, 60 master's awarded. *Degree requirements:* For master's, thesis optional. *Entrance requirements:* For master's, GRE, baccalaureate degree in speech-language pathology, minimum GPA of 2.75, three letters of recommendation, statement of purpose, resume. Additional exam requirements/recommendations for international students: Required—TOEFL (minimum score 550 paper-based; 79 iBT). *Application deadline:* For fall admission, 1/1 for domestic and international students. Application fee: $40 ($60 for international students). Electronic applications accepted. *Expenses:* Tuition, state resident: full-time $7430; part-time $412.80 per credit hour. Tuition, nonresident: full-time $12,722; part-time $706.80 per credit hour. *Required fees:* $53 per credit hour. $12 per semester. Tuition and fees vary according to course load and program. *Unit head:* Dr. Roberta DePompei, Director, 330-972-6114, E-mail: rdepom1@uakron.edu. *Application contact:* Dr. Mark Tausig, Associate Dean, 330-972-6266, Fax: 330-972-6475, E-mail: mtausig@uakron.edu.

The University of Alabama, Graduate School, College of Arts and Sciences, Department of Communicative Disorders, Tuscaloosa, AL 35487. Offers speech language pathology (MS). *Accreditation:* ASHA. *Faculty:* 9 full-time (7 women). *Students:* 76 full-time (75 women), 1 (woman) part-time; includes 4 minority (1 Black or African American, non-Hispanic/Latino; 1 Asian, non-Hispanic/Latino; 1 Hispanic/Latino; 1 Two or more races, non-Hispanic/Latino), 1 international. Average age 24. 256 applicants, 27% accepted, 42 enrolled. In 2013, 27 master's awarded. *Degree requirements:* For master's, comprehensive exam, thesis optional. *Entrance requirements:* For master's, GRE or MAT, minimum GPA of 3.0. Additional exam requirements/recommendations for international students: Required—TOEFL. *Application deadline:* For fall and spring admission, 1/15 for domestic and international students. Application fee: $50 ($60 for international students). Electronic applications accepted. *Expenses:* Tuition, state resident: full-time $9450. Tuition, nonresident: full-time $23,950. *Financial support:* In 2013–14, 12 students received support, including 3 fellowships with full and partial tuition reimbursements available (averaging $10,500 per year), 20 teaching assistantships with partial tuition reimbursements available (averaging $6,462 per year); career-related internships or fieldwork, Federal Work-Study, scholarships/grants, traineeships, health care benefits, and unspecified assistantships also available. Financial award application deadline: 1/15. *Faculty research:* Aphasia, cochlear implants, autism, voice, balance, multicultural, fluency, dysphagia. *Total annual research expenditures:* $3.3 million. *Unit head:* Dr. Marcia Jean Hay-McCutcheon, Associate Professor and Chair, 205-348-7131, Fax: 205-348-1845, E-mail: marcia.hay-mccutcheon@ua.edu. *Application contact:* Patrick D. Fuller, Senior Graduate Admissions Counselor, 205-348-5923, Fax: 205-348-0400, E-mail: patrick.d.fuller@ua.edu.
Website: http://cd.ua.edu/

University of Alberta, Faculty of Graduate Studies and Research, Department of Speech Pathology and Audiology, Edmonton, AB T6G 2E1, Canada. Offers speech pathology and audiology (PhD); speech-language pathology (M Sc). *Degree requirements:* For master's, thesis (for some programs), clinical practicum (MSLP). *Entrance requirements:* For master's, GRE, minimum GPA of 6.5 on a 9.0 scale. Additional exam requirements/recommendations for international students: Required—TOEFL. *Faculty research:* Clinical education, hearing conservation, motor speech disorders, child language, voice resonance.

The University of Arizona, College of Science, Department of Speech, Language, and Hearing Sciences, Tucson, AZ 85721. Offers MS, Au D, PhD. *Accreditation:* ASHA (one or more programs are accredited). *Faculty:* 14 full-time (9 women). *Students:* 90 full-time (79 women), 5 part-time (all women); includes 19 minority (1 Black or African American, non-Hispanic/Latino; 3 Asian, non-Hispanic/Latino; 8 Hispanic/Latino; 7 Two or more races, non-Hispanic/Latino), 1 international. Average age 28. 276 applicants, 12% accepted, 31 enrolled. In 2013, 24 master's, 6 doctorates awarded. *Degree requirements:* For master's, thesis optional; for doctorate, thesis/dissertation. *Entrance requirements:* For master's, GRE General Test, 3 letters of recommendation; for doctorate, GRE General Test, 3 letters of recommendation, personal statement, writing sample. Additional exam requirements/recommendations for international students: Required—TOEFL (minimum score 550 paper-based; 79 iBT). *Application deadline:* Applications are processed on a rolling basis. Application fee: $75. Electronic applications accepted. *Expenses:* Tuition, state resident: full-time $11,526. Tuition, nonresident: full-time $27,398. *Financial support:* In 2013–14, 16 research assistantships with full tuition reimbursements (averaging $21,933 per year), 19 teaching assistantships with full tuition reimbursements (averaging $19,856 per year) were awarded; career-related internships or fieldwork, Federal Work-Study, institutionally sponsored loans, scholarships/grants, health care benefits, tuition waivers (full and partial), and unspecified assistantships also available. Financial award application deadline: 2/1. *Faculty research:* Alzheimer's disease, speech motor control, auditory-evoked potentials, analyzing pathological speech. *Total annual research expenditures:* $2.2 million. *Unit head:* Dr. Pelagie Beeson, Head, 520-621-9879, Fax: 520-621-9901, E-mail: pelagie@email.arizona.edu. *Application contact:* Denise Minipoli, Information Contact, 520-621-1192, E-mail: minopold@email.arizona.edu.
Website: http://slhs.arizona.edu/

University of Arkansas, Graduate School, College of Education and Health Professions, Department of Rehabilitation, Human Resources and Communication Disorders, Program in Communication Disorders, Fayetteville, AR 72701-1201. Offers MS. *Accreditation:* ASHA. Part-time programs available. *Degree requirements:* For master's, thesis optional, 8-week externship. *Entrance requirements:* For master's, GRE General Test. Electronic applications accepted.

University of Arkansas for Medical Sciences, College of Health Professions, Little Rock, AR 72205-7199. Offers audiology (Au D); communication sciences and disorders (MS, PhD); genetic counseling (MS); nuclear medicine advanced associate (MIS); physician assistant studies (MPAS); radiologist assistant (MIS). PhD offered through consortium with University of Arkansas at Little Rock and University of Central Arkansas. Part-time programs available. Postbaccalaureate distance learning degree programs offered (minimal on-campus study). *Faculty:* 54 full-time (34 women), 16 part-time/adjunct (11 women). *Students:* 55 full-time (43 women), 32 part-time (24 women); includes 9 minority (3 Black or African American, non-Hispanic/Latino; 1 American Indian or Alaska Native, non-Hispanic/Latino; 1 Asian, non-Hispanic/Latino; 3 Hispanic/Latino; 1 Two or more races, non-Hispanic/Latino). In 2013, 10 master's, 8 doctorates awarded. *Degree requirements:* For master's, thesis (for some programs); for doctorate, comprehensive exam (for some programs), thesis/dissertation (for some programs). *Entrance requirements:* For master's, GRE. Additional exam requirements/recommendations for international students: Required—TOEFL (minimum score 550 paper-based; 79 iBT). Application fee: $40. Electronic applications accepted. *Expenses:* Contact institution. *Financial support:* Unspecified assistantships available. Financial award application deadline: 6/15; financial award applicants required to submit FAFSA. *Faculty research:* Auditory-based intervention, soy diet, nutrition and cancer. *Unit head:* Dr. Douglas L. Murphy, Dean, 501-686-5730. *Application contact:* Phyllis Fields, Assistant Dean, Student Affairs, 501-686-5730, E-mail: pafields@uams.edu.
Website: http://healthprofessions.uams.edu/

The University of British Columbia, Faculty of Medicine, School of Audiology and Speech Sciences, Vancouver, BC V6T 1Z3, Canada. Offers M Sc, PhD. *Accreditation:* ASHA. *Faculty:* 12 full-time (8 women), 4 part-time/adjunct (all women). *Students:* 69 full-time (60 women); includes 16 minority (all Asian, non-Hispanic/Latino). Average age 25. 152 applicants, 28% accepted, 36 enrolled. In 2013, 24 master's, 1 doctorate awarded. *Degree requirements:* For master's, thesis or alternative, externship; for doctorate, comprehensive exam, thesis/dissertation. *Entrance requirements:* For master's, 4-year undergraduate degree; for doctorate, master's degree, research proposal. Additional exam requirements/recommendations for international students: Required—TOEFL (minimum score 600 paper-based; 100 iBT), IELTS (minimum score 7). *Application deadline:* For fall admission, 2/1 for domestic and international students. Applications are processed on a rolling basis. Application fee: $93 Canadian dollars ($153 Canadian dollars for international students). Electronic applications accepted. *Expenses: Tuition, area resident:* Full-time $8000 Canadian dollars. *Financial support:* In 2013–14, 16 students received support, including 1 fellowship (averaging $17,000 per year), 6 research assistantships; teaching assistantships, career-related internships or fieldwork, Federal Work-Study, institutionally sponsored loans, scholarships/grants, and unspecified assistantships also available. Financial award application deadline: 1/15. *Faculty research:* Language development, experimental phonetics, linguistic aphasiology, amplification, auditory physiology. *Unit head:* Dr. Valter Ciocca, Director, 604-822-5795, Fax: 604-822-6569, E-mail: director@audiospeech.ubc.ca. *Application contact:* Sue Madura Bryant, Graduate Program Assistant, 604-827-5920, Fax: 604-822-6569, E-mail: inquiry@audiospeech.ubc.ca.
Website: http://www.audiospeech.ubc.ca/

University of California, San Diego, Office of Graduate Studies, Interdisciplinary Program in Language and Communicative Disorders, La Jolla, CA 92093. Offers PhD. Program offered jointly with San Diego State University. *Accreditation:* ASHA. *Students:* 14 (11 women); includes 4 minority (1 Black or African American, non-Hispanic/Latino; 2 Asian, non-Hispanic/Latino; 1 Hispanic/Latino). In 2013, 3 doctorates awarded. *Degree requirements:* For doctorate, thesis/dissertation, teaching assistantship. *Entrance requirements:* For doctorate, GRE General Test. Additional exam requirements/recommendations for international students: Required—TOEFL, IELTS. *Application*

deadline: For fall admission, 1/20 for domestic students. Electronic applications accepted. *Expenses:* Tuition, state resident: full-time $11,220; part-time $1870 per quarter. Tuition, nonresident: full-time $26,322; part-time $4387 per quarter. *Required fees:* $519.50 per quarter. Part-time tuition and fees vary according to course load and program. *Financial support:* Applicants required to submit FAFSA. *Faculty research:* Bilingualism, underlying neural mechanisms involved in language development and comprehension, language development in disorders, American Sign Language. *Unit head:* Rachael Mayberry, Program Director, 858-534-2929, E-mail: rmayberry@ucsd.edu. *Application contact:* Margaret Paulson, Graduate Coordinator, 858-534-0714, E-mail: mpaulson@ucsd.edu.
Website: http://slhs.sdsu.edu/programs/phd/

University of California, San Diego, School of Medicine, Program in Audiology, La Jolla, CA 92093-0970. Offers Au D. Program offered jointly with San Diego State University. *Students:* 8 full-time (5 women), 3 part-time (all women); includes 3 minority (all Asian, non-Hispanic/Latino). In 2013, 6 doctorates awarded. *Degree requirements:* For doctorate, comprehensive exam, thesis/dissertation, 2,950 clinic hours; externship. *Entrance requirements:* For doctorate, GRE General Test, minimum GPA of 3.0; at least one course in each of the following areas: statistics, biological science, physical science, and American Sign Language; additional courses in behavioral/social sciences and biological or physical sciences. Additional exam requirements/recommendations for international students: Required—TOEFL, IELTS. *Application deadline:* For fall admission, 1/9 for domestic students. Electronic applications accepted. *Expenses:* Tuition, state resident: full-time $11,220; part-time $1870 per quarter. Tuition, nonresident: full-time $26,322; part-time $4387 per quarter. *Required fees:* $519.50 per quarter. Part-time tuition and fees vary according to course load and program. *Financial support:* Fellowships, scholarships/grants, and unspecified assistantships available. Financial award applicants required to submit FAFSA. *Faculty research:* Peripheral auditory physiology, auditory evoked potentials, psychoacoustics, epidemiology of age-related hearing loss, aural rehabilitation. *Unit head:* Erika Zettner, Head and Program Co-Director, 858-657-8057, E-mail: ezettner@ucsd.edu.
Website: http://slhs.sdsu.edu/programs/aud/overview/

University of Central Arkansas, Graduate School, College of Health and Behavioral Sciences, Department of Communication Sciences and Disorders, Conway, AR 72035-0001. Offers communication sciences and disorders (PhD); speech-language pathology (MS). *Accreditation:* ASHA (one or more programs are accredited). *Degree requirements:* For master's, comprehensive exam, thesis optional, portfolio, internship. *Entrance requirements:* For master's, GRE General Test, NTE, minimum GPA of 2.7. Additional exam requirements/recommendations for international students: Required—TOEFL (minimum score 550 paper-based). Electronic applications accepted. *Expenses:* Contact institution.

University of Central Florida, College of Education and Human Performance, Education Doctoral Programs, Orlando, FL 32816. Offers communication sciences and disorders (PhD); counselor education (PhD); early childhood education (PhD); education (Ed D); elementary education (PhD); exceptional education (PhD); exercise physiology (PhD); higher education (PhD); hospitality education (PhD); instructional technology (PhD); mathematics education (PhD); reading education (PhD); science education (PhD); social science education (PhD); TESOL (PhD). *Students:* 137 full-time (94 women), 86 part-time (64 women); includes 45 minority (24 Black or African American, non-Hispanic/Latino; 5 Asian, non-Hispanic/Latino; 13 Hispanic/Latino; 3 Two or more races, non-Hispanic/Latino), 22 international. Average age 39. 132 applicants, 54% accepted, 54 enrolled. In 2013, 38 doctorates awarded. Application fee: $30. Electronic applications accepted. *Financial support:* In 2013–14, 84 students received support, including 38 fellowships with partial tuition reimbursements available (averaging $6,600 per year), 41 research assistantships with partial tuition reimbursements available (averaging $7,800 per year), 53 teaching assistantships with partial tuition reimbursements available (averaging $7,700 per year). *Unit head:* Dr. Edward Robinson, Director of Doctoral Programs, 407-823-6106, E-mail: edward.robinson@ucf.edu. *Application contact:* Barbara Rodriguez Lamas, Associate Director, Admissions and Student Services, 407-823-2766, Fax: 407-823-6442, E-mail: gradadmissions@ucf.edu.
Website: http://education.ucf.edu/departments.cfm

University of Central Florida, College of Health and Public Affairs, Department of Communication Sciences and Disorders, Orlando, FL 32816. Offers communication sciences and disorders (MA); medical speech-language pathology (Certificate). *Accreditation:* ASHA (one or more programs are accredited). Part-time and evening/weekend programs available. *Faculty:* 24 full-time (17 women), 21 part-time/adjunct (16 women). *Students:* 180 full-time (169 women), 11 part-time (10 women); includes 51 minority (8 Black or African American, non-Hispanic/Latino; 4 Asian, non-Hispanic/Latino; 35 Hispanic/Latino; 4 Two or more races, non-Hispanic/Latino), 4 international. Average age 25. 357 applicants, 22% accepted, 23 enrolled. In 2013, 88 master's, 1 other advanced degree awarded. *Degree requirements:* For master's, comprehensive exam, thesis or alternative. *Entrance requirements:* For master's, GRE General Test, minimum GPA of 3.0 in last 60 hours. Additional exam requirements/recommendations for international students: Required—TOEFL. *Application deadline:* For fall admission, 4/1 for domestic students; for spring admission, 11/1 for domestic students. Electronic applications accepted. *Financial support:* In 2013–14, 11 students received support, including 2 research assistantships with partial tuition reimbursements available (averaging $3,900 per year), 9 teaching assistantships with partial tuition reimbursements available (averaging $5,100 per year); career-related internships or fieldwork, Federal Work-Study, institutionally sponsored loans, and unspecified assistantships also available. Financial award application deadline: 3/1; financial award applicants required to submit FAFSA. *Unit head:* Dr. Dawn Oetjen, Interim Chair, 407-823-5668, E-mail: dawn.oetjen@ucf.edu. *Application contact:* Barbara Rodriguez Lamas, Director, Admissions and Student Services, 407-823-2766, Fax: 407-823-6442, E-mail: gradadmissions@ucf.edu.
Website: http://www.cohpa.ucf.edu/comdis/

University of Central Missouri, The Graduate School, Warrensburg, MO 6409. Offers accountancy (MA); accounting (MBA); applied mathematics (MS); aviation safety (MA); biology (MS); business administration (MBA); career and technical education leadership (MS); college student personnel administration (MS); communication (MA); computer science (MS); counseling (MS); criminal justice (MS); educational leadership (Ed D); educational technology (MS); elementary and early childhood education (MSE); English (MA); environmental studies (MA); finance (MBA); history (MA); human services/educational technology (Ed S); human services/learning resources (Ed S); human services/professional counseling (Ed S); industrial hygiene (MS); industrial management (MS); information systems (MBA); information technology (MS); kinesiology (MS); library science and information services (MS); literacy education (MSE); marketing (MBA); mathematics (MS); music (MA); occupational safety management (MS); psychology (MS); rural family nursing (MS); school administration (MSE); social gerontology (MS); sociology (MA); special education (MSE); speech language pathology (MS); superintendency (Ed S); teaching (MAT); teaching English as a second language (MA); technology (MS); technology management (PhD); theatre (MA). Part-time programs available. *Faculty:* 233. *Students:* 890 full-time (396 women), 1,486 part-time (1,001 women); includes 192 minority (97 Black or African American, non-Hispanic/Latino; 9 American Indian or Alaska Native, non-Hispanic/Latino; 32 Asian, non-Hispanic/Latino; 40 Hispanic/Latino; 3 Native Hawaiian or other Pacific Islander, non-Hispanic/Latino; 11 Two or more races, non-Hispanic/Latino), 539 international. Average age 31. 1,953 applicants, 75% accepted. In 2013, 719 master's, 58 other advanced degrees awarded. *Degree requirements:* For master's and Ed S, comprehensive exam (for some programs), thesis (for some programs). *Entrance requirements:* Additional exam requirements/recommendations for international students: Required—TOEFL (minimum score 550 paper-based; 79 iBT). *Application deadline:* For fall admission, 6/1 for domestic students; for spring admission, 10/1 for domestic and international students. Applications are processed on a rolling basis. Application fee: $30 ($75 for international students). Electronic applications accepted. *Expenses:* Tuition, state resident: full-time $7326; part-time $276.25 per credit hour. Tuition, nonresident: full-time $13,956; part-time $552.50 per credit hour. *Required fees:* $29 per credit hour. *Financial support:* In 2013–14, 118 students received support, including 271 research assistantships with full and partial tuition reimbursements available (averaging $7,500 per year), 109 teaching assistantships with full and partial tuition reimbursements available (averaging $7,500 per year); career-related internships or fieldwork, Federal Work-Study, scholarships/grants, and administrative and laboratory assistantships also available. Support available to part-time students. Financial award application deadline: 3/1; financial award applicants required to submit FAFSA. *Unit head:* Dr. Joseph Vaughn, Assistant Provost for Research/Dean, 660-543-4092, Fax: 660-543-4778, E-mail: vaughn@ucmo.edu. *Application contact:* Brittany Lawrence, Graduate Student Services Coordinator, 660-543-4621, Fax: 660-543-4778, E-mail: gradinfo@ucmo.edu.
Website: http://www.ucmo.edu/graduate/

University of Central Oklahoma, The Jackson College of Graduate Studies, College of Education and Professional Studies, Department of Advanced Professional and Special Services, Edmond, OK 73034-5209. Offers educational leadership (M Ed); library media education (M Ed); reading (M Ed); school counseling (M Ed); special education (M Ed), including mild/moderate disabilities, severe-profound/multiple disabilities, special education; speech-language pathology (MS). Part-time programs available. *Faculty:* 14 full-time (9 women), 16 part-time/adjunct (8 women). *Students:* 87 full-time (80 women), 298 part-time (251 women); includes 77 minority (32 Black or African American, non-Hispanic/Latino; 10 American Indian or Alaska Native, non-Hispanic/Latino; 2 Asian, non-Hispanic/Latino; 15 Hispanic/Latino; 18 Two or more races, non-Hispanic/Latino), 9 international. Average age 34. 147 applicants, 94% accepted, 89 enrolled. In 2013, 163 master's awarded. *Degree requirements:* For master's, comprehensive exam (for some programs), thesis (for some programs). *Entrance requirements:* For master's, GRE. Additional exam requirements/recommendations for international students: Required—TOEFL (minimum score 550 paper-based; 79 iBT), IELTS (minimum score 6.5). *Application deadline:* For fall admission, 7/1 for international students; for spring admission, 7/1 for international students. Applications are processed on a rolling basis. Application fee: $50. Electronic applications accepted. *Expenses:* Tuition, state resident: full-time $4137; part-time $206.85 per credit hour. Tuition, nonresident: full-time $10,359; part-time $517.95 per credit hour. *Required fees:* $481. Tuition and fees vary according to course load and program. *Financial support:* In 2013–14, 93 students received support, including 4 research assistantships with partial tuition reimbursements available (averaging $8,133 per year); teaching assistantships with partial tuition reimbursements available, career-related internships or fieldwork, scholarships/grants, tuition waivers (partial), and unspecified assistantships also available. Financial award application deadline: 3/31; financial award applicants required to submit FAFSA. *Faculty research:* Intellectual freedom, fair use copyright, technology integration, young adult literature, distance learning. *Unit head:* Dr. Patsy Couts, Chair, 405-974-3888, Fax: 405-974-3857, E-mail: pcouts@uco.edu. *Application contact:* Dr. Richard Bernard, Dean, Graduate College, 405-974-3493, Fax: 405-974-3852, E-mail: gradcoll@uco.edu.
Website: http://www.uco.edu/ceps/dept/apss/

University of Cincinnati, Graduate School, College of Allied Health Sciences, Department of Communication Sciences and Disorders, Cincinnati, OH 45221. Offers MA, Au D, PhD. *Accreditation:* ASHA (one or more programs are accredited). *Degree requirements:* For master's, thesis optional; for doctorate, comprehensive exam, thesis/dissertation. *Entrance requirements:* For master's and doctorate, GRE General Test, minimum GPA of 3.0. Additional exam requirements/recommendations for international students: Required—TOEFL (minimum score 600 paper-based). Electronic applications accepted. *Faculty research:* Neurogenic speech and language disorders, speech science, linguistics, swallowing disorders, speech-language pathology.

University of Cincinnati, Graduate School, College of Education, Criminal Justice, and Human Services, Division of Teacher Education, Cincinnati, OH 45221. Offers curriculum and instruction (M Ed, Ed D); deaf studies (Certificate); early childhood education (M Ed); middle childhood education (M Ed); postsecondary literacy instruction (Certificate); reading/literacy (M Ed, Ed D); secondary education (M Ed); special education (M Ed, Ed D); teaching English as a second language (M Ed, Ed D, Certificate); teaching science (MS). Part-time programs available. *Degree requirements:* For doctorate, thesis/dissertation. *Entrance requirements:* For master's, GRE General Test. Additional exam requirements/recommendations for international students: Required—TOEFL (minimum score 550 paper-based). Electronic applications accepted.

University of Colorado Boulder, Graduate School, College of Arts and Sciences, Department of Speech, Language and Hearing Sciences, Boulder, CO 80309. Offers audiology (Au D, PhD); clinical research and practice in audiology (PhD); speech, language and hearing sciences (MA, PhD); speech-language pathology (MA, PhD). *Accreditation:* ASHA (one or more programs are accredited). *Faculty:* 10 full-time (8 women). *Students:* 113 full-time (102 women), 2 part-time (both women); includes 15 minority (3 Asian, non-Hispanic/Latino; 9 Hispanic/Latino; 3 Two or more races, non-Hispanic/Latino), 2 international. Average age 28. 592 applicants, 17% accepted, 47 enrolled. In 2013, 35 master's, 9 doctorates awarded. Terminal master's awarded for partial completion of doctoral program. *Degree requirements:* For master's, comprehensive exam, thesis or alternative; for doctorate, one foreign language, thesis/dissertation. *Entrance requirements:* For master's, GRE General Test, minimum undergraduate GPA of 3.25; for doctorate, GRE General Test. *Application deadline:* For fall admission, 1/15 for domestic students, 12/1 for international students. Applications are processed on a rolling basis. Application fee: $50 ($60 for international students). Electronic applications accepted. *Financial support:* In 2013–14, 134 students received support, including 93 fellowships (averaging $2,727 per year), 11 teaching assistantships with full and partial tuition reimbursements available (averaging $28,396 per year); institutionally sponsored loans, scholarships/grants, health care benefits, and unspecified assistantships also available. Financial award application deadline: 2/1; financial award applicants required to submit FAFSA. *Faculty research:* Cognitive development/processes, language acquisition and development, speech communicative disorders. *Total annual research expenditures:* $1 million.
Website: http://slhs.colorado.edu

University of Connecticut, Graduate School, College of Liberal Arts and Sciences, Department of Communication Sciences, Program in Audiology, Storrs, CT 06269. Offers Au D, PhD, Au D/PhD. *Accreditation:* ASHA. *Degree requirements:* For doctorate, thesis/dissertation. *Entrance requirements:* For doctorate, GRE General Test. Additional exam requirements/recommendations for international students: Required—TOEFL (minimum score 550 paper-based). Electronic applications accepted.

University of Connecticut, Graduate School, College of Liberal Arts and Sciences, Department of Communication Sciences, Program in Speech-Language Pathology, Storrs, CT 06269. Offers MA, PhD. *Accreditation:* ASHA. Terminal master's awarded for partial completion of doctoral program. *Degree requirements:* For master's, comprehensive exam, thesis optional; for doctorate, thesis/dissertation. *Entrance requirements:* For master's and doctorate, GRE General Test. Additional exam requirements/recommendations for international students: Required—TOEFL (minimum score 550 paper-based). Electronic applications accepted.

University of Florida, Graduate School, College of Public Health and Health Professions, Department of Speech, Language and Hearing Sciences, Gainesville, FL 32611. Offers audiology (Au D); communication sciences and disorders (MA). *Accreditation:* ASHA (one or more programs are accredited). *Faculty:* 8 full-time (4 women), 12 part-time/adjunct (7 women). *Students:* 160 full-time (136 women), 40 part-time (35 women); includes 35 minority (10 Black or African American, non-Hispanic/Latino; 6 Asian, non-Hispanic/Latino; 19 Hispanic/Latino), 27 international. Average age 31. 418 applicants, 24% accepted, 56 enrolled. In 2013, 30 master's, 2 doctorates awarded. *Degree requirements:* For master's, thesis optional; for doctorate, comprehensive exam, thesis/dissertation. *Entrance requirements:* For master's and doctorate, GRE General Test, minimum GPA of 3.0. Additional exam requirements/recommendations for international students: Required—TOEFL (minimum score 550 paper-based; 80 iBT), IELTS (minimum score 6). *Application deadline:* For fall admission, 1/15 priority date for domestic students, 1/15 for international students. Applications are processed on a rolling basis. Application fee: $30. Electronic applications accepted. *Expenses:* Tuition, state resident: full-time $12,640. Tuition, nonresident: full-time $30,000. *Financial support:* In 2013–14, 35 students received support, including 4 fellowships (averaging $10,250 per year), 2 research assistantships (averaging $7,375 per year), 33 teaching assistantships (averaging $10,550 per year); career-related internships or fieldwork and unspecified assistantships also available. Financial award application deadline: 1/15; financial award applicants required to submit FAFSA. *Faculty research:* Phonetic science, cochlear implant, dyslexia, auditory development, voice. *Unit head:* Scott Griffiths, PhD, Associate Professor and Chair, 352-273-3725, E-mail: sgriff@ufl.edu. *Application contact:* Office of Admissions, 352-392-1365, E-mail: webrequests@admissions.ufl.edu.
Website: http://slhs.phhp.ufl.edu/

University of Georgia, College of Education, Department of Communication Sciences and Special Education, Athens, GA 30602. Offers communication science and disorders (M Ed, MA, PhD, Ed S); special education (M Ed, Ed D, PhD, Ed S). *Accreditation:* ASHA (one or more programs are accredited). Terminal master's awarded for partial completion of doctoral program. *Degree requirements:* For master's, comprehensive exam (for some programs), thesis (for some programs); for doctorate, thesis/dissertation. *Entrance requirements:* For master's, doctorate, and Ed S, GRE General Test. Additional exam requirements/recommendations for international students: Required—TOEFL. Electronic applications accepted.

University of Hawaii at Manoa, John A. Burns School of Medicine, Department of Communication Sciences and Disorders, Honolulu, HI 96822. Offers MS. *Accreditation:* ASHA. Part-time programs available. *Degree requirements:* For master's, thesis optional. *Entrance requirements:* For master's, GRE General Test, minimum GPA of 3.0. Additional exam requirements/recommendations for international students: Required—TOEFL (minimum score 580 paper-based; 92 iBT), IELTS (minimum score 5). *Faculty research:* Emerging language (child phonology and special populations), central auditory function, developmental phonology, processing in the aging.

University of Houston, College of Liberal Arts and Social Sciences, Department of Communication Sciences and Disorders, Houston, TX 77204. Offers MA. *Accreditation:* ASHA. Part-time programs available. *Degree requirements:* For master's, comprehensive exam, thesis optional. *Entrance requirements:* For master's, GRE General Test, minimum GPA of 3.0 in last 60 hours. Additional exam requirements/recommendations for international students: Required—TOEFL (minimum score 550 paper-based; 79 iBT). *Faculty research:* Stuttering, voice disorders, language disorders, phonological processing, cognition.

University of Illinois at Urbana–Champaign, Graduate College, College of Applied Health Sciences, Department of Speech and Hearing Science, Champaign, IL 61820. Offers audiology (Au D); speech and hearing science (MA, PhD). *Accreditation:* ASHA (one or more programs are accredited). *Students:* 82 (75 women). Application fee: $75 ($90 for international students). *Unit head:* Karen Kirk, Head, 217-244-8241, Fax: 217-244-2235, E-mail: kikirk@illinois.edu. *Application contact:* J. Thomas Fleener, Office Support, 217-333-2230, Fax: 217-244-2235, E-mail: jfleener@illinois.edu.
Website: http://www.shs.illinois.edu/

The University of Iowa, Graduate College, College of Liberal Arts and Sciences, Department of Communication Sciences and Disorders, Iowa City, IA 52242-1316. Offers MA, Au D, PhD, Au D/PhD. *Accreditation:* ASHA. *Degree requirements:* For master's, thesis optional, exam; for doctorate, comprehensive exam (for some programs), thesis/dissertation (for some programs). *Entrance requirements:* For master's and doctorate, GRE General Test, minimum GPA of 3.0. Additional exam requirements/recommendations for international students: Required—TOEFL (minimum score 550 paper-based; 81 iBT). Electronic applications accepted.

The University of Kansas, Graduate Studies, College of Liberal Arts and Sciences, Intercampus Program in Communicative Disorders, Lawrence, KS 66045. Offers audiology (PhD); speech-language pathology (MA, PhD). Offered jointly with the Department of Hearing and Speech at the Kansas City campus. *Accreditation:* ASHA. Part-time programs available. *Faculty:* 12. *Students:* 76 full-time (all women), 5 part-time (all women); includes 9 minority (2 American Indian or Alaska Native, non-Hispanic/Latino; 1 Asian, non-Hispanic/Latino; 2 Hispanic/Latino; 4 Two or more races, non-Hispanic/Latino), 9 international. Average age 29. 222 applicants, 36% accepted, 31 enrolled. In 2013, 27 master's, 2 doctorates awarded. Terminal master's awarded for partial completion of doctoral program. *Degree requirements:* For master's, comprehensive exam, thesis optional; for doctorate, comprehensive exam, thesis/dissertation. *Entrance requirements:* For master's and doctorate, GRE General Test, minimum GPA of 3.0, bachelor's degree. Additional exam requirements/recommendations for international students: Required—TOEFL. *Application deadline:* For fall admission, 1/15 priority date for domestic and international students; for spring admission, 10/1 for domestic and international students. Application fee: $55 ($75 for international students). Electronic applications accepted. *Financial support:* In 2013–14, 11 students received support. Research assistantships, teaching assistantships, career-related internships or fieldwork, Federal Work-Study, institutionally sponsored loans, scholarships/grants, traineeships, and unspecified assistantships available. Support available to part-time students. Financial award application deadline: 3/1; financial award applicants required to submit FAFSA. *Faculty research:* Reading disorders, language acquisition, auditory electrophysiology, genetics of language, phonological development. *Total annual research expenditures:* $3 million. *Unit head:* Holly L. Storkel, Chair, 785-864-0630, Fax: 785-864-3974, E-mail: hstorkel@ku.edu. *Application contact:* Angela Carrasco, Admissions Coordinator, 913-588-5935, Fax: 913-588-5923, E-mail: hearingspeech@kumc.edu.
Website: http://splh.ku.edu/ipcd/

The University of Kansas, University of Kansas Medical Center, School of Health Professions, Intercampus Program in Communicative Disorders, Lawrence, KS 66045. Offers audiology (Au D). *Faculty:* 32. *Students:* 24 full-time (22 women), 6 part-time (5 women); includes 4 minority (2 Asian, non-Hispanic/Latino; 1 Hispanic/Latino; 1 Two or more races, non-Hispanic/Latino), 2 international. Average age 25. 54 applicants, 41% accepted, 12 enrolled. In 2013, 9 doctorates awarded. Terminal master's awarded for partial completion of doctoral program. *Degree requirements:* For doctorate, comprehensive exam, thesis/dissertation. *Entrance requirements:* For doctorate, GRE, bachelor's degree, minimum GPA of 3.25. Additional exam requirements/recommendations for international students: Required—TOEFL. *Application deadline:* For fall admission, 1/15 for domestic and international students. Application fee: $60. Electronic applications accepted. *Financial support:* Research assistantships with partial tuition reimbursements, teaching assistantships with partial tuition reimbursements, institutionally sponsored loans, scholarships/grants, traineeships, and unspecified assistantships available. Financial award application deadline: 3/1; financial award applicants required to submit FAFSA. *Faculty research:* Child language development, diagnosis and treatment of language disorders; newborn/pediatric hearing testing and treatment of hearing loss in children; voice disorders; auditory physiology and applied electrophysiology; diagnosis and treatment for adult speech and language disorders. *Total annual research expenditures:* $649,000. *Unit head:* Dr. John A. Ferraro, Chair, Department of Hearing and Speech/Co-Director, 913-588-5937, Fax: 913-588-5923, E-mail: jferraro@kumc.edu. *Application contact:* Angela Carrasco, Admissions Coordinator, 913-588-5935, Fax: 913-588-5923, E-mail: hearingspeech@kumc.edu.
Website: http://splh.ku.edu/ipcd/

University of Kentucky, Graduate School, College of Health Sciences, Program in Speech-Language Pathology, Lexington, KY 40506-0032. Offers MS. *Accreditation:* ASHA. *Degree requirements:* For master's, comprehensive exam. *Entrance requirements:* For master's, GRE General Test, minimum undergraduate GPA of 2.75. Additional exam requirements/recommendations for international students: Required—TOEFL (minimum score 550 paper-based). Electronic applications accepted. *Faculty research:* Swallowing disorders, infant speech development, child language intervention, augmentative communication.

University of Louisiana at Lafayette, College of Liberal Arts, Department of Communicative Disorders, Lafayette, LA 70504. Offers MS, PhD. *Accreditation:* ASHA (one or more programs are accredited). *Degree requirements:* For master's, thesis or alternative. *Entrance requirements:* For master's, GRE General Test, minimum GPA of 2.75. Additional exam requirements/recommendations for international students: Required—TOEFL (minimum score 550 paper-based).

University of Louisiana at Monroe, Graduate School, College of Health and Pharmaceutical Sciences, Department of Speech-Language Pathology, Monroe, LA 71209-0001. Offers MS. *Accreditation:* ASHA. *Degree requirements:* For master's, thesis. *Entrance requirements:* For master's, GRE, minimum GPA of 2.5. Additional exam requirements/recommendations for international students: Required—TOEFL (minimum score 500 paper-based; 61 iBT). *Application deadline:* For fall admission, 8/24 priority date for domestic students, 7/1 for international students; for winter admission, 12/14 priority date for domestic students; for spring admission, 1/19 for domestic students, 11/1 for international students. Applications are processed on a rolling basis. Application fee: $20 ($30 for international students). Electronic applications accepted. *Expenses:* Tuition, state resident: full-time $6607. Tuition, nonresident: full-time $17,179. Full-time tuition and fees vary according to program. *Financial support:* Research assistantships, career-related internships or fieldwork, Federal Work-Study, and unspecified assistantships available. Financial award application deadline: 4/1; financial award applicants required to submit FAFSA. *Faculty research:* Child language, stuttering, multicultural issues, ethics. *Unit head:* Dr. Johanna Boult, Head, 318-342-3190, Fax: 318-342-1687, E-mail: boult@ulm.edu. *Application contact:* Dr. Johanna Boult, Head, 318-342-3190, Fax: 318-342-1687, E-mail: boult@ulm.edu.
Website: http://www.ulm.edu/slp/

University of Louisville, School of Medicine, Department of Surgery, Louisville, KY 40292-0001. Offers audiology (Au D); communicative disorders (MS). *Students:* 82 full-time (76 women), 2 part-time (1 woman); includes 5 minority (1 Asian, non-Hispanic/Latino; 2 Hispanic/Latino; 2 Two or more races, non-Hispanic/Latino). Average age 26. 209 applicants, 47% accepted, 37 enrolled. In 2013, 21 master's, 7 doctorates awarded. Application fee: $60. *Expenses:* Tuition, state resident: full-time $10,788; part-time $599 per credit hour. Tuition, nonresident: full-time $22,446; part-time $1247 per credit hour. *Required fees:* $196. Tuition and fees vary according to program and reciprocity agreements. *Unit head:* Dr. Edward C. Halperin, Dean, 502-852-1499, Fax: 502-852-1484, E-mail: edward.halperin@louisville.edu. *Application contact:* Director of Admissions, 502-852-5793, Fax: 502-852-6849.

University of Maine, Graduate School, College of Natural Sciences, Forestry, and Agriculture, Department of Communication Sciences and Disorders, Orono, ME 04469. Offers MA. *Accreditation:* ASHA. *Faculty:* 6 full-time (4 women), 6 part-time/adjunct (5 women). *Students:* 33 full-time (30 women), 1 (woman) part-time, 7 international. Average age 27. 106 applicants, 31% accepted, 16 enrolled. In 2013, 17 master's awarded. *Degree requirements:* For master's, comprehensive exam. *Entrance requirements:* For master's, GRE General Test. Additional exam requirements/recommendations for international students: Required—TOEFL. *Application deadline:* For fall admission, 12/31 priority date for domestic students. Applications are processed on a rolling basis. Application fee: $65. Electronic applications accepted. *Expenses:* Tuition, state resident: full-time $7524. Tuition, nonresident: full-time $23,112. *Required fees:* $1970. *Financial support:* In 2013–14, 12 students received support, including 3 research assistantships (averaging $7,300 per year), 3 teaching assistantships with partial tuition reimbursements available (averaging $5,000 per year); career-related internships or fieldwork, Federal Work-Study, institutionally sponsored loans, and tuition waivers (full and partial) also available. Support available to part-time students. Financial award application deadline: 3/1. *Faculty research:* Interpersonal communication between supervisor and supervised, clinicians and clients; language and voice impairments; children's pragmatics. *Total annual research expenditures:* $719. *Unit head:* Dr. Allan Smith, Chair, 207-581-2006, Fax: 207-581-1953. *Application contact:* Scott G. Delcourt, Associate Dean of the Graduate School, 207-581-3291, Fax: 207-581-3232, E-mail: graduate@maine.edu.
Website: http://umaine.edu/comscidis/

The University of Manchester, School of Psychological Sciences, Manchester, United Kingdom. Offers audiology (M Phil, PhD); clinical psychology (M Phil, PhD, Psy D); psychology (M Phil, PhD).

University of Maryland, College Park, Academic Affairs, College of Behavioral and Social Sciences, Department of Hearing and Speech Sciences, College Park, MD 20742. Offers audiology (MA, PhD); hearing and speech sciences (Au D); language pathology (MA, PhD); neuroscience (PhD); speech (MA, PhD). *Accreditation:* ASHA (one or more programs are accredited). *Faculty:* 19 full-time (18 women), 14 part-time/adjunct (12 women). *Students:* 70 full-time (65 women), 24 part-time (22 women); includes 11 minority (3 Black or African American, non-Hispanic/Latino; 2 Asian, non-Hispanic/Latino; 3 Hispanic/Latino; 3 Two or more races, non-Hispanic/Latino), 1 international. 385 applicants, 19% accepted, 21 enrolled. In 2013, 19 master's, 5 doctorates awarded. *Degree requirements:* For master's, thesis optional; for doctorate, thesis/dissertation, written and oral exams. *Entrance requirements:* For master's, GRE General Test, minimum GPA of 3.5, 3 letters of recommendation; for doctorate, GRE General Test, minimum GPA of 3.5. Additional exam requirements/recommendations for international students: Required—TOEFL. *Application deadline:* For fall admission, 1/15 for domestic and international students. Applications are processed on a rolling basis. Application fee: $75. Electronic applications accepted. *Expenses:* Tuition, state resident: full-time $10,314; part-time $573 per credit hour. Tuition, nonresident: full-time $22,248; part-time $1236 per credit. *Required fees:* $1446; $403.15 per semester. Tuition and fees vary according to program. *Financial support:* In 2013–14, 2 fellowships with full tuition reimbursements (averaging $37,014 per year), 1 research assistantship (averaging $15,266 per year), 2 teaching assistantships (averaging $15,355 per year) were awarded; career-related internships or fieldwork, Federal Work-Study, scholarships/grants, and health care benefits also available. Support available to part-time students. Financial award applicants required to submit FAFSA. *Faculty research:* Speech perception, language acquisition, bilingualism, hearing loss. *Total annual research expenditures:* $734,130. *Unit head:* Dr. Nan B. Bernstein-Ratner, Chair, 301-405-4217, Fax: 301-314-2023, E-mail: nratner@umd.edu. *Application contact:* Dr. Charles A. Caramello, Dean of Graduate School, 301-405-0358, Fax: 301-314-9305.

University of Massachusetts Amherst, Graduate School, School of Public Health and Health Sciences, Department of Communication Disorders, Amherst, MA 01003. Offers audiology (Au D, PhD); clinical audiology (PhD); speech-language pathology (MA, PhD). *Accreditation:* ASHA (one or more programs are accredited). Part-time programs available. *Faculty:* 17 full-time (15 women). *Students:* 75 full-time (68 women), 3 part-time (all women); includes 9 minority (1 Black or African American, non-Hispanic/Latino; 4 Asian, non-Hispanic/Latino; 2 Hispanic/Latino; 2 Two or more races, non-Hispanic/Latino). Average age 27. 311 applicants, 25% accepted, 33 enrolled. In 2013, 30 master's, 12 doctorates awarded. Terminal master's awarded for partial completion of doctoral program. *Degree requirements:* For master's, thesis optional; for doctorate, comprehensive exam, thesis/dissertation. *Entrance requirements:* For master's and doctorate, GRE General Test. Additional exam requirements/recommendations for international students: Required—TOEFL (minimum score 550 paper-based; 80 iBT), IELTS (minimum score 6.5). *Application deadline:* For fall admission, 2/1 for domestic and international students; for spring admission, 10/1 for domestic and international students. Applications are processed on a rolling basis. Application fee: $75. Electronic applications accepted. *Financial support:* Fellowships with full and partial tuition reimbursements, research assistantships with full and partial tuition reimbursements, teaching assistantships with full and partial tuition reimbursements, career-related internships or fieldwork, Federal Work-Study, scholarships/grants, traineeships, health care benefits, tuition waivers (full and partial), and unspecified assistantships available. Support available to part-time students. Financial award application deadline: 2/1; financial award applicants required to submit FAFSA. *Unit head:* Dr. Karen S. Helfer, Graduate Program Director, 413-545-0131, Fax: 413-545-0803. *Application contact:* Lindsay DeSantis, Supervisor of Admissions, 413-545-0722, Fax: 413-577-0010, E-mail: gradadm@grad.umass.edu.
Website: http://www.umass.edu/sphhs/comdis/

University of Memphis, Graduate School, School of Audiology and Speech-Language Pathology, Memphis, TN 38152. Offers MA, Au D, PhD. *Accreditation:* ASHA. Part-time programs available. *Faculty:* 13 full-time (5 women), 3 part-time/adjunct (2 women). *Students:* 12 full-time (11 women), 7 part-time (5 women); includes 1 minority (Asian, non-Hispanic/Latino), 1 international. Average age 26. 290 applicants, 31% accepted, 35 enrolled. In 2013, 22 master's, 2 doctorates awarded. Terminal master's awarded for partial completion of doctoral program. *Degree requirements:* For master's, comprehensive exam, thesis or alternative; for doctorate, thesis/dissertation, qualifying exam. *Entrance requirements:* For master's, GRE General Test or MAT, minimum GPA of 3.0, ASHA certification; for doctorate, GRE General Test, minimum GPA of 3.5, letters of recommendation. *Application deadline:* For fall admission, 2/1 for domestic students. Application fee: $35 ($60 for international students). *Financial support:* In 2013–14, 64 students received support. Research assistantships with full tuition reimbursements available, Federal Work-Study, scholarships/grants, and unspecified assistantships available. Financial award application deadline: 2/15; financial award applicants required to submit FAFSA. *Faculty research:* Hearing aid characteristic selection, language acquisition, speech disorders, characteristics of the aging voice, hearing science. *Total annual research expenditures:* $1.5 million. *Unit head:* Dr. Maurice Mendel, Dean, 901-678-5800, Fax: 901-525-1282, E-mail: dlluna@memphis.edu. *Application contact:* Dr. David J. Wark, Coordinator of Graduate Studies, 901-678-5891, E-mail: dwark@memphis.edu.
Website: http://www.memphis.edu/ausp

University of Minnesota, Duluth, Graduate School, College of Education and Human Service Professions, Department of Communication Sciences and Disorders, Duluth, MN 55812-2496. Offers MA. *Accreditation:* ASHA. Part-time programs available. *Degree requirements:* For master's, research project, oral exam. *Entrance requirements:* For master's, minimum GPA of 3.0, undergraduate degree in communication sciences and disorders. Additional exam requirements/recommendations for international students: Required—TOEFL (minimum score 550 paper-based). *Faculty research:* Clinical supervision, augmentative communication, speech understanding, fluency, developmental apraxia of speech.

University of Minnesota, Twin Cities Campus, Graduate School, College of Liberal Arts, Department of Speech-Language-Hearing Sciences, Minneapolis, MN 55455. Offers audiology (Au D); speech-language pathology (MA); speech-language-hearing sciences (PhD). *Accreditation:* ASHA (one or more programs are accredited). Terminal master's awarded for partial completion of doctoral program. *Degree requirements:* For master's, thesis, 375 client contact hours; for doctorate, comprehensive exam, thesis/dissertation. *Entrance requirements:* For master's and doctorate, GRE General Test, minimum GPA of 3.0. Additional exam requirements/recommendations for international students: Required—TOEFL. Electronic applications accepted. *Faculty research:* Normal and disordered child phonology, specific language impairment, bilingual and multicultural aspects of language, TBI, AAC.

University of Mississippi, Graduate School, School of Applied Sciences, Department of Communicative Disorders, University, MS 38677. Offers MS. *Accreditation:* ASHA. *Faculty:* 6 full-time (4 women), 3 part-time/adjunct (all women). *Students:* 58 full-time (57 women), 12 part-time (all women); includes 15 minority (12 Black or African American, non-Hispanic/Latino; 1 Asian, non-Hispanic/Latino; 1 Hispanic/Latino; 1 Two or more races, non-Hispanic/Latino). In 2013, 22 master's awarded. *Entrance requirements:* For master's, GRE General Test, minimum GPA of 3.0. Additional exam requirements/recommendations for international students: Required—TOEFL. *Application deadline:* For fall admission, 2/1 for domestic students; for spring admission, 10/1 for domestic students. Applications are processed on a rolling basis. Application fee: $40. Electronic applications accepted. *Financial support:* Scholarships/grants available. Financial award application deadline: 3/1; financial award applicants required to submit FAFSA. *Unit head:* Dr. Lennette J. Ivy, Interim Chair, 662-915-7652, Fax: 662-915-5717, E-mail: csd@olemiss.edu. *Application contact:* Dr. Christy M. Wyandt, Associate Dean, 662-915-7474, Fax: 662-915-7577, E-mail: cwyandt@olemiss.edu.

University of Missouri, School of Health Professions, Program in Communication Science and Disorders, Columbia, MO 65211. Offers MHS, PhD. *Accreditation:* ASHA (one or more programs are accredited). *Faculty:* 8 full-time (7 women), 2 part-time/adjunct (1 woman). *Students:* 42 full-time (41 women); includes 1 minority (Asian, non-Hispanic/Latino), 1 international. Average age 25. 112 applicants, 16% accepted, 17 enrolled. In 2013, 18 master's awarded. *Entrance requirements:* For master's, GRE General Test, minimum GPA of 3.0. Additional exam requirements/recommendations for international students: Required—TOEFL (minimum score 600 paper-based; 100 iBT). *Application deadline:* For fall admission, 1/15 priority date for domestic and international students; for winter admission, 10/15 priority date for domestic students, 10/15 for international students. Applications are processed on a rolling basis. Application fee: $55 ($75 for international students). Electronic applications accepted. *Financial support:* Research assistantships, teaching assistantships, and institutionally sponsored loans available. *Faculty research:* Cognitive mechanisms that underlie vocabulary and grammar acquisition (child language lab); infant vocalization and language emergence; language and fluency examination, transcription, coding and analysis; investigations of the interaction of memory and language across lifespan and in aphasia. *Unit head:* Dr. Judith Goodman, Department Chair, 573-882-8407, E-mail: goodmanjc@health.missouri.edu. *Application contact:* Dr. Barbara McLay, Director of Graduate Studies, 573-882-8409, E-mail: mclayb@missouri.edu.
Website: http://shp.missouri.edu/csd/

University of Montevallo, College of Arts and Sciences, Department of Communication Science and Disorders, Montevallo, AL 35115. Offers speech-language pathology (MS). *Accreditation:* ASHA. *Students:* 50 full-time (49 women), 1 (woman) part-time; includes 5 minority (2 Black or African American, non-Hispanic/Latino; 1 Asian, non-Hispanic/Latino; 1 Hispanic/Latino; 1 Native Hawaiian or other Pacific Islander, non-Hispanic/Latino). In 2013, 23 master's awarded. *Degree requirements:* For master's, comprehensive exam. *Entrance requirements:* For master's, GRE General Test, MAT. Additional exam requirements/recommendations for international students: Required—TOEFL (minimum score 550 paper-based). *Application deadline:* For fall admission, 7/15 for domestic students; for spring admission, 11/15 for domestic students. Application fee: $25. *Financial support:* Federal Work-Study, scholarships/grants, and unspecified assistantships available. *Unit head:* Dr. Claire Edwards, Chair, 205-665-6724, E-mail: edwardsc@montevallo.edu. *Application contact:* Kevin Thornthwaite, Acting Director, Graduate Admissions and Records, 205-665-6350, E-mail: graduate@montevallo.edu.
Website: http://www.montevallo.edu/csd/

University of Nebraska at Kearney, Graduate Programs, College of Education, Department of Communication Disorders, Kearney, NE 68849-0001. Offers speech/language pathology (MS Ed). *Accreditation:* ASHA. Part-time programs available. *Entrance requirements:* For master's, GRE General Test, personal statement, letters of recommendation. Additional exam requirements/recommendations for international students: Required—TOEFL (minimum score: 550 paper-based, 79 iBT) or IELTS (6.5). Electronic applications accepted. *Faculty research:* Neurogenic, communication disorders in adults, phonological development and disorders, orofacial anomalies, audiologic rehabilitation of the elderly.

University of Nebraska at Omaha, Graduate Studies, College of Education, Department of Special Education and Communication Disorders, Omaha, NE 68182. Offers special education (MA, MS); speech-language pathology (MS). *Accreditation:* ASHA (one or more programs are accredited); NCATE. Part-time and evening/weekend programs available. *Faculty:* 12 full-time (8 women). *Students:* 36 full-time (33 women), 59 part-time (52 women); includes 9 minority (1 American Indian or Alaska Native, non-Hispanic/Latino; 1 Asian, non-Hispanic/Latino; 4 Hispanic/Latino; 3 Two or more races, non-Hispanic/Latino), 2 international. Average age 31. 183 applicants, 26% accepted, 21 enrolled. In 2013, 29 master's awarded. *Degree requirements:* For master's, comprehensive exam, thesis (for some programs). *Entrance requirements:* For master's, minimum GPA of 3.0, statement of purpose, 2 letters of recommendation, copy of teaching certificate. Additional exam requirements/recommendations for international students: Required—TOEFL, IELTS, PTE. *Application deadline:* For fall admission, 8/1 for domestic students; for spring admission, 12/1 for domestic students; for summer admission, 5/1 for domestic students. Applications are processed on a rolling basis. Application fee: $45. Electronic applications accepted. *Financial support:* In 2013–14, 6 students received support, including 4 research assistantships with tuition reimbursements available, 2 teaching assistantships with tuition reimbursements available; fellowships, career-related internships or fieldwork, Federal Work-Study, institutionally sponsored loans, scholarships/grants, tuition waivers (partial), and unspecified assistantships also available. Support available to part-time students. Financial award application deadline: 3/1; financial award applicants required to submit FAFSA. *Unit head:* Dr. Kristine Swain, Chairperson, 402-554-2201. *Application contact:* Dr. Philip Nordness, Graduate Program Chair, 402-554-3582, E-mail: graduate@unomaha.edu.

University of Nebraska–Lincoln, Graduate College, College of Education and Human Sciences, Department of Special Education and Communication Disorders, Program in Speech-Language Pathology and Audiology, Lincoln, NE 68588. Offers audiology and hearing science (Au D); speech-language pathology and audiology (MS). *Accreditation:* ASHA. *Degree requirements:* For master's, thesis optional. *Entrance requirements:* For master's, GRE. Additional exam requirements/recommendations for international students: Required—TOEFL (minimum score 500 paper-based). Electronic applications accepted.

University of Nevada, Reno, Graduate School, Division of Health Sciences, Department of Speech Pathology and Audiology, Reno, NV 89557. Offers speech pathology (PhD); speech pathology and audiology (MS). *Accreditation:* ASHA (one or more programs are accredited). Terminal master's awarded for partial completion of doctoral program. *Degree requirements:* For master's, thesis optional; for doctorate, thesis/dissertation. *Entrance requirements:* For master's, GRE General Test, minimum GPA of 2.75; for doctorate, GRE General Test, minimum GPA of 3.0. Additional exam requirements/recommendations for international students: Required—TOEFL (minimum score 500 paper-based; 61 iBT), IELTS (minimum score 6). Electronic applications accepted. *Faculty research:* Language impairment in children, voice disorders, stuttering.

University of New Hampshire, Graduate School, School of Health and Human Services, Department of Communication Sciences and Disorders, Durham, NH 03824. Offers communication sciences and disorders (MS); early childhood intervention (MS); language and literature disabilities (MS). Program offered in fall only. *Accreditation:* ASHA. Part-time programs available. *Faculty:* 6 full-time (3 women). *Students:* 33 full-time (29 women), 4 part-time (all women); includes 1 minority (Asian, non-Hispanic/Latino), 1 international. Average age 26. 144 applicants, 26% accepted, 15 enrolled. In 2013, 20 master's awarded. *Degree requirements:* For master's, thesis or alternative. *Entrance requirements:* For master's, GRE General Test or MAT. Additional exam

requirements/recommendations for international students: Required—TOEFL (minimum score 550 paper-based; 80 iBT). *Application deadline:* For fall admission, 1/15 priority date for domestic students, 4/1 for international students. Applications are processed on a rolling basis. Application fee: $65. Electronic applications accepted. *Expenses:* Tuition, state resident: full-time $13,500; part-time $750 per credit hour. Tuition, nonresident: full-time $26,200; part-time $1100 per credit hour. *Required fees:* $1741; $435.25 per term. Tuition and fees vary according to course level, course load, campus/location and program. *Financial support:* In 2013–14, 9 students received support, including 5 teaching assistantships; fellowships, research assistantships, career-related internships or fieldwork, Federal Work-Study, scholarships/grants, and tuition waivers (full and partial) also available. Support available to part-time students. Financial award application deadline: 2/15. *Faculty research:* Speech pathology. *Unit head:* Penelope Webster, Chairperson, 603-862-2125. *Application contact:* Maria Russell, Administrative Assistant, 603-862-0144, E-mail: communication.disorders@unh.edu.
Website: http://chhs.unh.edu/csd/index

University of New Mexico, Graduate School, College of Arts and Sciences, Department of Speech and Hearing Sciences, Albuquerque, NM 87131. Offers speech-language pathology (MS). *Accreditation:* ASHA. *Faculty:* 6 full-time (4 women), 4 part-time/adjunct (2 women). *Students:* 57 full-time (50 women), 2 part-time (both women); includes 21 minority (1 American Indian or Alaska Native, non-Hispanic/Latino; 3 Asian, non-Hispanic/Latino; 17 Hispanic/Latino). Average age 30. 102 applicants, 59% accepted, 32 enrolled. In 2013, 16 master's awarded. *Degree requirements:* For master's, comprehensive exam, thesis optional. *Entrance requirements:* For master's, GRE General Test, minimum GPA of 3.4 in speech and hearing sciences coursework. Additional exam requirements/recommendations for international students: Required—TOEFL (minimum score 550 paper-based; 80 iBT). *Application deadline:* For fall admission, 2/1 for domestic students, 1/1 for international students. Application fee: $50. Electronic applications accepted. *Financial support:* In 2013–14, 24 students received support, including 10 research assistantships with partial tuition reimbursements available (averaging $6,235 per year); career-related internships or fieldwork, Federal Work-Study, scholarships/grants, health care benefits, and unspecified assistantships also available. Financial award application deadline: 2/1; financial award applicants required to submit FAFSA. *Faculty research:* Augmentative and alternative communication (AAC), behavioral genetic studies of language, child language assessment, bilingual language acquisition, bilingual phonology, speech perception, swallowing disorders, transition from oral language to literacy. *Total annual research expenditures:* $114,602. *Unit head:* Dr. Barbara Rodriguez, Chair, 505-277-9728, Fax: 505-277-0968, E-mail: brodrig@unm.edu. *Application contact:* Tracy Wenzl, Department Administrator, 505-277-4453, Fax: 505-277-0968, E-mail: twenzl@unm.edu.
Website: http://shs.unm.edu

The University of North Carolina at Chapel Hill, School of Medicine and Graduate School, Graduate Programs in Medicine, Chapel Hill, NC 27599. Offers allied health sciences (MPT, MS, Au D, DPT, PhD), including human movement science (MS, PhD), occupational science (MS, PhD), physical therapy (MPT, MS, DPT), rehabilitation counseling and psychology (MS), speech and hearing sciences (MS, Au D, PhD); biochemistry and biophysics (MS, PhD); bioinformatics and computational biology (PhD); biomedical engineering (MS, PhD); cell and developmental biology (PhD); cell and molecular physiology (PhD); genetics and molecular biology (PhD); microbiology and immunology (MS, PhD), including immunology, microbiology; neurobiology (PhD); pathology and laboratory medicine (PhD), including experimental pathology; pharmacology (PhD); MD/PhD. Postbaccalaureate distance learning degree programs offered. Terminal master's awarded for partial completion of doctoral program. *Degree requirements:* For master's, comprehensive exam; for doctorate, thesis/dissertation. Electronic applications accepted. *Expenses:* Contact institution.

The University of North Carolina at Chapel Hill, School of Medicine and Graduate School, Graduate Programs in Medicine, Department of Allied Health Sciences, Division of Speech and Hearing Sciences, Chapel Hill, NC 27599. Offers audiology (Au D); speech and hearing sciences (MS, PhD). *Accreditation:* ASHA (one or more programs are accredited). Postbaccalaureate distance learning degree programs offered (no on-campus study). *Degree requirements:* For master's, comprehensive exam, thesis optional; for doctorate, comprehensive exam, thesis/dissertation. *Entrance requirements:* For master's, GRE General Test, minimum GPA of 3.0; for doctorate, GRE, minimum GPA of 3.0. Additional exam requirements/recommendations for international students: Required—TOEFL (minimum score 550 paper-based). Electronic applications accepted. *Faculty research:* Child language and literacy, family participation in early intervention, child and adult hearing loss and treatment, vocal characteristics of African-American speakers and aging populations, adult apraxia of speech.

The University of North Carolina at Greensboro, Graduate School, School of Health and Human Performance, Department of Communication Sciences and Disorders, Greensboro, NC 27412-5001. Offers speech language pathology (PhD); speech pathology and audiology (MA). *Accreditation:* ASHA. *Degree requirements:* For master's, thesis or alternative. *Entrance requirements:* For master's, GRE General Test. Additional exam requirements/recommendations for international students: Required—TOEFL. Electronic applications accepted.

University of North Dakota, Graduate School, College of Arts and Sciences, Department of Communication Sciences and Disorders, Grand Forks, ND 58202. Offers communication sciences and disorders (PhD); speech-language pathology (MS). *Accreditation:* ASHA (one or more programs are accredited). Part-time programs available. *Degree requirements:* For master's, comprehensive exam, thesis or alternative; for doctorate, comprehensive exam, thesis/dissertation, final exam. *Entrance requirements:* For master's and doctorate, GRE General Test, minimum GPA of 3.0. Additional exam requirements/recommendations for international students: Required—TOEFL (minimum score 550 paper-based; 79 iBT), IELTS (minimum score 6.5). Electronic applications accepted. *Faculty research:* Mass communications, journalism, community law, international communications, cultural studies.

University of Northern Colorado, Graduate School, College of Natural and Health Sciences, School of Human Sciences, Program in Audiology and Speech Language Sciences, Greeley, CO 80639. Offers audiology (Au D); speech language pathology (MA). *Accreditation:* ASHA (one or more programs are accredited). Part-time and evening/weekend programs available. Postbaccalaureate distance learning degree programs offered (no on-campus study). *Degree requirements:* For master's, comprehensive exam, thesis or alternative; for doctorate, comprehensive exam, thesis/dissertation. *Entrance requirements:* For master's and doctorate, GRE General Test. Electronic applications accepted.

University of Northern Iowa, Graduate College, College of Humanities, Arts and Sciences, Department of Communicative Sciences and Disorders, Cedar Falls, IA 50614. Offers speech-language pathology (MA). *Accreditation:* ASHA. Part-time and evening/weekend programs available. *Students:* 82 full-time (80 women), 2 part-time (both women); includes 6 minority (1 Black or African American, non-Hispanic/Latino; 1 Asian, non-Hispanic/Latino; 3 Hispanic/Latino; 1 Two or more races, non-Hispanic/Latino), 1 international. 151 applicants, 19% accepted, 28 enrolled. In 2013, 38 master's awarded. *Degree requirements:* For master's, comprehensive exam, thesis or alternative. *Entrance requirements:* For master's, GRE, minimum GPA of 3.0. Additional exam requirements/recommendations for international students: Required—TOEFL (minimum score 500 paper-based; 61 iBT). *Application deadline:* For fall admission, 8/1 priority date for domestic students. Applications are processed on a rolling basis. Application fee: $50 ($70 for international students). *Financial support:* Career-related internships or fieldwork, Federal Work-Study, scholarships/grants, and tuition waivers (full and partial) available. Financial award application deadline: 2/1. *Unit head:* Dr. Carlin Hageman, Department Head/Professor, 319-273-2497, Fax: 319-273-6384, E-mail: carlin.hageman@uni.edu. *Application contact:* Laurie S. Russell, Record Analyst, 319-273-2623, Fax: 319-273-2885, E-mail: laurie.russell@uni.edu.
Website: http://www.uni.edu/comdis/

University of North Florida, College of Education and Human Services, Department of Exceptional Student and Deaf Education, Jacksonville, FL 32224. Offers American Sign Language/English interpreting (M Ed); applied behavior analysis (M Ed); autism (M Ed); deaf education (M Ed); disability services (M Ed); exceptional student education (M Ed). *Accreditation:* NCATE. Part-time and evening/weekend programs available. *Faculty:* 11 full-time (9 women), 4 part-time/adjunct (all women). *Students:* 26 full-time (21 women), 52 part-time (44 women); includes 15 minority (9 Black or African American, non-Hispanic/Latino; 2 Asian, non-Hispanic/Latino; 3 Hispanic/Latino; 1 Two or more races, non-Hispanic/Latino), 2 international. Average age 32. 39 applicants, 51% accepted, 15 enrolled. In 2013, 51 master's awarded. *Entrance requirements:* For master's, GRE General Test, minimum GPA of 3.0 in last 60 hours, interview, 3 letters of recommendation. Additional exam requirements/recommendations for international students: Required—TOEFL (minimum score 500 paper-based). *Application deadline:* For fall admission, 7/1 priority date for domestic students, 5/1 for international students; for spring admission, 11/1 priority date for domestic students, 10/1 for international students. Application fee: $30. Electronic applications accepted. *Expenses:* Tuition, state resident: full-time $9794; part-time $408.10 per credit hour. Tuition, nonresident: full-time $22,383; part-time $932.61 per credit hour. *Required fees:* $2020; $84.20 per credit hour. Tuition and fees vary according to course load and program. *Financial support:* In 2013–14, 19 students received support, including 1 research assistantship (averaging $4,524 per year); teaching assistantships, career-related internships or fieldwork, Federal Work-Study, scholarships/grants, tuition waivers (partial), and unspecified assistantships also available. Support available to part-time students. Financial award application deadline: 4/1; financial award applicants required to submit FAFSA. *Faculty research:* Transition, integrating technology into teacher education, written language development, professional school development, learning strategies. *Total annual research expenditures:* $816,202. *Unit head:* Dr. Karen Patterson, Chair, 904-620-2930, Fax: 904-620-3895, E-mail: karen.patterson@unf.edu. *Application contact:* Dr. Amanda Pascale, Director, The Graduate School, 904-620-1360, Fax: 904-620-1362, E-mail: graduateschool@unf.edu.
Website: http://www.unf.edu/coehs/edie/

University of North Texas, Robert B. Toulouse School of Graduate Studies, Denton, TN 76203-5017. Offers accounting (MS, PhD); applied anthropology (MA, MS); applied behavior analysis (Certificate); applied technology and performance improvement (M Ed, MS, PhD); art education (MA, PhD); art history (MA); art museum education (Certificate); arts leadership (Certificate); audiology (Au D); behavior analysis (MS); biochemistry and molecular biology (MS, PhD); biology (MA, MS, PhD); business (PhD); business computer information systems (PhD); chemistry (MS, PhD); clinical psychology (PhD); communication studies (MA, MS); computer engineering (MS); computer science (MS); computer science and engineering (PhD); counseling (M Ed, MS, PhD), including clinical mental health counseling (MS), college and university counseling (M Ed, MS), elementary school counseling (M Ed, MS), secondary school counseling (M Ed, MS); counseling psychology (PhD); creative writing (MA); criminal justice (MS); curriculum and instruction (M Ed, PhD), including curriculum studies (PhD), early childhood studies (PhD), language and literacy studies (PhD); decision sciences (MBA); design (MA, MFA), including fashion design (MFA), innovation studies, interior design (MFA); early childhood studies (MS); economics (MS); educational leadership (M Ed, Ed D, PhD); educational psychology (MS), including family studies, gifted and talented (MS, PhD), human development, learning and cognition, research, measurement and evaluation; educational research (PhD), including gifted and talented (MS, PhD), human development and family studies, psychological aspects of sports and exercise, research, measurement and statistics; electrical engineering (MS); emergency management (MPA); engineering systems (MS); English (MA, PhD); environmental science (MS, PhD); experimental psychology (PhD); finance (MBA, MS, PhD); financial management (MPA); French (MA); health psychology and behavioral medicine (PhD); health services management (MBA); higher education (M Ed, Ed D, PhD); history (MA, MS, PhD), including European history (PhD), military history (PhD), United States history (PhD); hospitality management (MS); human resources management (MPA); information science (MS, PhD); information technologies (MBA); information technology and decision sciences (MS); interdisciplinary studies (MA, MS); international sustainable tourism (MS); jazz studies (MM); journalism (MA, MJ, Graduate Certificate), including interactive and virtual digital communication (Graduate Certificate), narrative journalism (Graduate Certificate), public relations (Graduate Certificate); kinesiology (MS); learning technologies (MS, PhD); library science (MS); local government management (MPA); logistics and supply chain management (MBA, PhD); long-term care, senior housing, and aging services (MA, MS); management science (PhD); marketing (MBA, PhD); materials science and engineering (MS, PhD); mathematics (MA, PhD); merchandising (MS); music (MA, MM Ed, PhD), including ethnomusicology (MA), music education (MM Ed, PhD), music theory (MA, PhD), musicology (MA, PhD), performance (MA); nonprofit management (MPA); operations and supply chain management (MBA); performance (MM, DMA); philosophy (MA, PhD); physics (MS, PhD); political science (MA, MS, PhD); public administration and management (PhD), including emergency management, nonprofit management, public financial management, urban management; radio, television and film (MA, MFA); recreation, event and sport management (MS); rehabilitation counseling (MS, Certificate); sociology (MA, MS, PhD); Spanish (MA); special education (M Ed, PhD), including autism intervention (PhD), emotional/behavioral disorders (PhD), mild/moderate disabilities (PhD); speech-language pathology (MA, MS); strategic management (MBA); studio art (MFA); taxation (MS); teaching (M Ed); MBA/MS; MS/MPH; MSES/MBA. Part-time and evening/weekend programs available. Postbaccalaureate distance learning degree programs offered. *Faculty:* 661 full-time (213 women), 240 part-time/adjunct (144 women). *Students:* 3,106 full-time (1,620 women), 3,543 part-time (2,221 women); includes 1,740 minority (533 Black or African American, non-Hispanic/Latino; 15 American Indian or Alaska Native, non-Hispanic/Latino; 286 Asian, non-Hispanic/Latino; 746 Hispanic/Latino; 3 Native Hawaiian or other Pacific Islander, non-Hispanic/Latino; 157 Two or more races, non-Hispanic/Latino), 1,145 international. Average age 32. 6,289 applicants, 43% accepted, 1751 enrolled. In 2013, 1,778 master's, 239 doctorates, 10 other advanced degrees awarded. Terminal master's awarded for partial completion of doctoral program. *Degree requirements:* For master's, variable foreign language requirement, comprehensive exam (for some programs), thesis (for some programs); for doctorate, variable foreign language requirement, comprehensive exam (for some programs), thesis/dissertation; for other advanced degree, variable foreign language requirement, comprehensive exam (for some programs). *Entrance requirements:* For master's and doctorate, GRE, GMAT. Additional exam requirements/recommendations

for international students: Required—TOEFL (minimum score 550 paper-based; 79 iBT). *Application deadline:* For fall admission, 7/15 for domestic students, 3/15 for international students; for spring admission, 11/15 for domestic students, 9/15 for international students; for summer admission, 5/1 for domestic students. Applications are processed on a rolling basis. Application fee: $60. Electronic applications accepted. *Financial support:* Fellowships with partial tuition reimbursements, research assistantships with partial tuition reimbursements, teaching assistantships, career-related internships or fieldwork, Federal Work-Study, institutionally sponsored loans, scholarships/grants, health care benefits, and library assistantships available. Support available to part-time students. Financial award applicants required to submit FAFSA. *Unit head:* Mark Wardell, Dean, 940-565-2383, E-mail: mark.wardell@unt.edu. *Application contact:* Toulouse School of Graduate Studies, 940-565-2383, Fax: 940-565-2141, E-mail: gradsch@unt.edu.
Website: http://tsgs.unt.edu/

University of Oklahoma Health Sciences Center, Graduate College, College of Allied Health, Department of Communication Sciences and Disorders, Oklahoma City, OK 73190. Offers audiology (MS, Au D, PhD); communication sciences and disorders (Certificate), including reading, speech-language pathology; education of the deaf (MS); speech-language pathology (MS, PhD). *Accreditation:* ASHA (one or more programs are accredited). Part-time programs available. *Faculty:* 15 full-time (12 women). *Students:* 72 full-time (67 women), 5 part-time (4 women); includes 12 minority (3 Asian, non-Hispanic/Latino; 1 Hispanic/Latino; 8 Two or more races, non-Hispanic/Latino). Average age 26. 181 applicants, 45% accepted, 30 enrolled. In 2013, 19 master's, 3 doctorates awarded. Terminal master's awarded for partial completion of doctoral program. *Degree requirements:* For master's, comprehensive exam, thesis optional; for doctorate, one foreign language, comprehensive exam, thesis/dissertation. *Entrance requirements:* For master's and doctorate, GRE General Test, 3 letters of recommendation. Additional exam requirements/recommendations for international students: Required—TOEFL (minimum score 550 paper-based). *Application deadline:* For fall admission, 2/1 for domestic students. Applications are processed on a rolling basis. Application fee: $50. *Expenses:* Tuition, state resident: full-time $3504; part-time $175.20 per credit hour. Tuition, nonresident: full-time $13,504; part-time $675.20 per credit hour. *Required fees:* $1545; $52.70 per credit hour. $245.25 per semester. Tuition and fees vary according to course load. *Financial support:* In 2013–14, 8 research assistantships (averaging $16,000 per year) were awarded; fellowships, career-related internships or fieldwork, Federal Work-Study, institutionally sponsored loans, and traineeships also available. Support available to part-time students. *Faculty research:* Event-related potentials, cleft palate, fluency disorders, language disorders, hearing and speech science. *Unit head:* Dr. Stephen Painton, Chair, 405-271-4214, E-mail: stephen-painton@ouhsc.edu. *Application contact:* Dr. Sarah Buckinghan, Graduate Liaison, 405-271-4214, Fax: 405-271-1153, E-mail: sarah-buckingham@ouhsc.edu.

University of Ottawa, Faculty of Graduate and Postdoctoral Studies, Faculty of Health Sciences, School of Rehabilitation Sciences, Ottawa, ON K1N 6N5, Canada. Offers audiology (M Sc); orthophony (M Sc). Part-time and evening/weekend programs available. *Entrance requirements:* For master's, honors degree or equivalent, minimum B average. Electronic applications accepted.

University of Pittsburgh, School of Health and Rehabilitation Sciences, Department of Communication Science and Disorders, Pittsburgh, PA 15260. Offers MA, MS, Au D, CScD, PhD. *Accreditation:* ASHA (one or more programs are accredited). *Faculty:* 17 full-time (13 women), 8 part-time/adjunct (6 women). *Students:* 139 full-time (127 women), 18 part-time (14 women); includes 13 minority (1 Black or African American, non-Hispanic/Latino; 6 Asian, non-Hispanic/Latino; 6 Hispanic/Latino), 12 international. Average age 28. 582 applicants, 34% accepted, 63 enrolled. In 2013, 42 master's, 16 doctorates awarded. *Degree requirements:* For master's, comprehensive exam, thesis (for some programs); for doctorate, comprehensive exam, thesis/dissertation. *Entrance requirements:* For master's and doctorate, GRE General Test. Additional exam requirements/recommendations for international students: Required—TOEFL (minimum score 550 paper-based; 80 iBT), IELTS (minimum score 6.5). *Application deadline:* For fall admission, 12/15 for domestic and international students. Applications are processed on a rolling basis. Application fee: $100. Electronic applications accepted. *Expenses:* Contact institution. *Financial support:* In 2013–14, 18 students received support, including 6 research assistantships with full and partial tuition reimbursements available (averaging $18,187 per year), 3 teaching assistantships with full tuition reimbursements available (averaging $16,300 per year); career-related internships or fieldwork, Federal Work-Study, scholarships/grants, and traineeships also available. Financial award applicants required to submit FAFSA. *Faculty research:* Pediatric and geriatric neurogenic speech and language, pediatric hearing disorders, hearing aids, language development, speech motor control. *Total annual research expenditures:* $2.6 million. *Unit head:* Dr. Malcolm R. McNeil, Chairman, 412-383-6541, Fax: 412-383-6555, E-mail: mcneil@pitt.edu. *Application contact:* Pamela Morocco, Administrator, 412-383-6540, Fax: 412-383-6555, E-mail: pjm79@pitt.edu.
Website: http://www.shrs.pitt.edu/csd/

University of Puerto Rico, Medical Sciences Campus, School of Health Professions, Program in Audiology, San Juan, PR 00936-5067. Offers Au D. *Faculty research:* Hearing, auditory brainstem responses, otoacoustic emissions.

University of Puerto Rico, Medical Sciences Campus, School of Health Professions, Program in Speech-Language Pathology, San Juan, PR 00936-5067. Offers MS. *Accreditation:* ASHA. *Degree requirements:* For master's, one foreign language, comprehensive exam, thesis or alternative. *Entrance requirements:* For master's, EXADEP, interview; previous course work in linguistics, statistics, human development, and basic concepts in speech-language pathology; minimum GPA of 2.5. *Faculty research:* Aphasia, autism, language, aphasia, assistive technology.

University of Redlands, College of Arts and Sciences, Department of Communicative Disorders, Redlands, CA 92373-0999. Offers MS. *Accreditation:* ASHA. *Degree requirements:* For master's, final exam. *Entrance requirements:* For master's, GMAT or GRE, minimum GPA of 3.0, 3 letters of recommendation. Additional exam requirements/recommendations for international students: Required—TOEFL (minimum score 550 paper-based). Electronic applications accepted. *Expenses:* Contact institution. *Faculty research:* Neuropathy.

University of Rhode Island, Graduate School, College of Human Science and Services, Department of Communicative Disorders, Kingston, RI 02881. Offers speech-language pathology (MS). *Accreditation:* ASHA. Part-time programs available. *Faculty:* 8 full-time (6 women). *Students:* 41 full-time (39 women), 7 part-time (all women); includes 4 minority (1 American Indian or Alaska Native, non-Hispanic/Latino; 1 Asian, non-Hispanic/Latino; 1 Hispanic/Latino; 1 Native Hawaiian or other Pacific Islander, non-Hispanic/Latino). In 2013, 21 master's awarded. *Degree requirements:* For master's, comprehensive exam (for some programs), thesis optional. *Entrance requirements:* For master's, GRE or MAT, 2 letters of recommendation (3 recommended). Additional exam requirements/recommendations for international students: Required—TOEFL (minimum score 550 paper-based). *Application deadline:* For fall admission, 3/1 for domestic students, 2/1 for international students; for spring admission, 10/15 for domestic students, 7/15 for international students. Application fee: $65. Electronic applications accepted. *Expenses:* Tuition, state resident: full-time $11,532; part-time $641 per credit. Tuition, nonresident: full-time $23,606; part-time $1311 per credit. *Required fees:* $1388; $36 per credit. $35 per semester. One-time fee: $130. *Financial support:* In 2013–14, 3 teaching assistantships with full and partial tuition reimbursements (averaging $7,922 per year) were awarded. Financial award application deadline: 2/1; financial award applicants required to submit FAFSA. *Faculty research:* Efficacy of treatment for acquired alexia in individuals with aphasia, application of principles of neuroplasticity to individuals with motor speech disorders secondary to neurological deficits, study of the conversation factors that promote fluency or exacerbate stuttering in young children. *Unit head:* Dr. Dana Kovarsky, Chair, 401-874-2735, Fax: 401-874-4404, E-mail: dana@uri.edu. *Application contact:* Dr. Ann Weiss, Graduate Program Coordinator, 401-874-9071, Fax: 401-874-5787, E-mail: alw@uri.edu.
Website: http://www.uri.edu/hss/cmd/

University of San Diego, School of Leadership and Education Sciences, Department of Learning and Teaching, San Diego, CA 92110-2492. Offers curriculum and instruction (M Ed); special education (M Ed); special education with deaf and hard of hearing (M Ed); teaching (MAT); TESOL, literacy and culture (M Ed). Part-time and evening/weekend programs available. *Faculty:* 10 full-time (6 women), 46 part-time/adjunct (38 women). *Students:* 132 full-time (100 women), 52 part-time (43 women); includes 141 minority (1 Black or African American, non-Hispanic/Latino; 16 American Indian or Alaska Native, non-Hispanic/Latino; 30 Asian, non-Hispanic/Latino; 79 Hispanic/Latino; 1 Native Hawaiian or other Pacific Islander, non-Hispanic/Latino; 14 Two or more races, non-Hispanic/Latino), 4 international. Average age 29. 253 applicants, 85% accepted, 108 enrolled. In 2013, 94 master's awarded. *Degree requirements:* For master's, thesis (for some programs), international experience. *Entrance requirements:* For master's, California Basic Educational Skills Test, minimum GPA of 3.0. Additional exam requirements/recommendations for international students: Required—TOEFL (minimum score 580 paper-based; 83 iBT), TWE. *Application deadline:* For fall admission, 3/1 priority date for domestic and international students; for spring admission, 10/15 priority date for domestic and international students. Applications are processed on a rolling basis. Application fee: $45. Electronic applications accepted. *Expenses: Tuition:* Full-time $23,580; part-time $1310 per credit. *Required fees:* $350. *Financial support:* In 2013–14, 52 students received support. Career-related internships or fieldwork, Federal Work-Study, institutionally sponsored loans, and stipends available. Support available to part-time students. Financial award application deadline: 4/1; financial award applicants required to submit FAFSA. *Faculty research:* Action research methodology, cultural studies, instructional theories and practices, second language acquisition, school reform. *Unit head:* Dr. Heather Lattimer, Director, 619-260-7616, Fax: 619-260-8159, E-mail: hlattimer@sandiego.edu. *Application contact:* Monica Mahon, Associate Director of Graduate Admissions, 619-260-4524, Fax: 619-260-4158, E-mail: grads@sandiego.edu.
Website: http://www.sandiego.edu/soles/departments/learning-and-teaching/

University of South Alabama, Graduate School, College of Allied Health Professions, Department of Speech Pathology and Audiology, Mobile, AL 36688-0002. Offers audiology (Au D); communication sciences and disorders (PhD); speech and hearing sciences (MS). *Accreditation:* ASHA. *Faculty:* 11 full-time (7 women). *Students:* 87 full-time (83 women), 1 (woman) part-time; includes 4 minority (2 Black or African American, non-Hispanic/Latino; 1 Asian, non-Hispanic/Latino; 1 Hispanic/Latino). 235 applicants, 32% accepted, 35 enrolled. In 2013, 21 master's, 5 doctorates awarded. *Degree requirements:* For master's, thesis optional, externship; for doctorate, thesis/dissertation, clinical internship; minimum of 11 full-time semesters of academic study. *Entrance requirements:* For master's, GRE, bachelor's degree in communication sciences and disorders; for doctorate, GRE, minimum GPA of 3.0. Additional exam requirements/recommendations for international students: Required—TOEFL. *Application deadline:* For fall admission, 2/1 priority date for domestic students. Applications are processed on a rolling basis. Application fee: $35. *Expenses:* Tuition, state resident: full-time $8976; part-time $374 per credit hour. Tuition, nonresident: full-time $17,952; part-time $748 per credit hour. *Financial support:* Fellowships, research assistantships, and career-related internships or fieldwork available. Support available to part-time students. Financial award application deadline: 4/1. *Faculty research:* Computer applications to speech and hearing science, telecommunications and clinical research in articulation and languages. *Unit head:* Dr. Robert Moore, Chair, 251-445-9378, E-mail: rmoore@usouthal.edu. *Application contact:* Dr. Julio Turrens, Director of Graduate Studies, 251-445-9250.
Website: http://www.southalabama.edu/alliedhealth/speechandhearing

University of South Carolina, The Graduate School, Arnold School of Public Health, Department of Communication Sciences and Disorders, Columbia, SC 29208. Offers MCD, MSP, PhD. *Accreditation:* ASHA (one or more programs are accredited). Postbaccalaureate distance learning degree programs offered. *Degree requirements:* For master's, thesis optional; for doctorate, comprehensive exam, thesis/dissertation. *Entrance requirements:* For master's, GRE General Test, minimum GPA of 3.0; for doctorate, GRE General Test. Electronic applications accepted. *Faculty research:* Noise-induced hearing loss, recurrent laryngeal nerve regeneration, cleft palate, child language-phonology, epidemiology of craniofacial anomalies.

The University of South Dakota, Graduate School, College of Arts and Sciences, Department of Communication Disorders, Vermillion, SD 57069-2390. Offers audiology (Au D); speech-language pathology (MA). *Accreditation:* ASHA (one or more programs are accredited). Part-time programs available. *Degree requirements:* For master's, comprehensive exam; for doctorate, comprehensive exam, thesis/dissertation. *Entrance requirements:* For master's, GRE General Test, minimum GPA of 3.0. Additional exam requirements/recommendations for international students: Required—TOEFL (minimum score 550 paper-based; 79 iBT). Electronic applications accepted. *Faculty research:* Craniofacial anomalies, central auditory processing, phonological disorders.

University of Southern Mississippi, Graduate School, College of Health, Department of Speech and Hearing Sciences, Hattiesburg, MS 39406-0001. Offers audiology (Au D); speech language pathology (MA, MS), including deaf education (MS). *Accreditation:* ASHA (one or more programs are accredited). *Faculty:* 10 full-time (4 women). *Students:* 84 full-time (79 women), 1 part-time (0 women); includes 8 minority (4 Black or African American, non-Hispanic/Latino; 2 Asian, non-Hispanic/Latino; 1 Hispanic/Latino; 1 Two or more races, non-Hispanic/Latino), 3 international. Average age 25. 138 applicants, 34% accepted, 24 enrolled. In 2013, 31 master's, 5 doctorates awarded. *Degree requirements:* For master's, comprehensive exam, thesis or alternative; for doctorate, comprehensive exam, thesis/dissertation. *Entrance requirements:* For master's, GRE General Test, minimum GPA of 3.0 in field of study, 2.75 in last 60 hours; for doctorate, GRE General Test, minimum GPA of 3.5. Additional exam requirements/recommendations for international students: Required—TOEFL, IELTS. *Application deadline:* For fall admission, 3/1 for domestic and international students; for spring admission, 1/10 priority date for domestic and international students. Application fee: $50. Electronic applications accepted. *Financial support:* In 2013–14, 9 research assistantships with full and partial tuition reimbursements (averaging $7,200 per year), teaching assistantships with full and partial tuition reimbursements (averaging $7,200 per year) were awarded; career-related internships or fieldwork, Federal Work-Study, institutionally sponsored loans, scholarships/grants, health care benefits, and unspecified assistantships also available. Financial award application deadline: 3/15;

financial award applicants required to submit FAFSA. *Faculty research:* Voice disorders, auditory-evoked responses, acoustic analysis of speech, child language, parent-child interaction. *Unit head:* Dr. Steve Cloud, Interim Chair, 601-266-5217. *Application contact:* Shonna Breland, Manager of Graduate Admissions, 601-266-6563, Fax: 601-266-5138.
Website: http://www.usm.edu/graduateschool/table.php

University of South Florida, College of Behavioral and Community Sciences, Department of Communication Sciences and Disorders, Tampa, FL 33620. Offers audiology (Au D); hearing science (PhD); language and speech science (PhD); neurocommunicative science (PhD); speech-language pathology (MS). *Accreditation:* ASHA (one or more programs are accredited). Part-time and evening/weekend programs available. Postbaccalaureate distance learning degree programs offered (minimal on-campus study). *Faculty:* 29 full-time (22 women), 13 part-time/adjunct (10 women). *Students:* 157 full-time (145 women), 61 part-time (56 women); includes 39 minority (6 Black or African American, non-Hispanic/Latino; 3 Asian, non-Hispanic/Latino; 29 Hispanic/Latino; 1 Two or more races, non-Hispanic/Latino), 4 international. Average age 26. 596 applicants, 16% accepted, 86 enrolled. In 2013, 65 master's, 12 doctorates awarded. *Degree requirements:* For doctorate, comprehensive exam, thesis/dissertation. *Entrance requirements:* For master's, GRE General Test (for MS in speech language pathology and audiology), demonstrated competency in communication skills, 3 letters of recommendation, and letter of intent; minimum GPA of 3.2 in upper-division undergraduate course work and resume (for speech language pathology); minimum GPA of 3.0 for last 60 hours of bachelor's degree (for audiology); for doctorate, GRE General Test (minimum verbal and quantitative scores in the 33rd percentile or above and analytical writing score of 4.0), minimum GPA of 3.5 during bachelor's, master's, and/or graduate study (for PhD), 3.0 during last 60 hours of bachelor's degree (for AuD); three letters of recommendation; letter of intent. Additional exam requirements/recommendations for international students: Required—TOEFL (minimum score 550 paper-based; 79 iBT) or IELTS (minimum score 6.5). *Application deadline:* For fall admission, 12/1 for domestic and international students; for spring admission, 2/1 for domestic and international students. Application fee: $30. Electronic applications accepted. *Financial support:* In 2013–14, 25 students received support, including 1 research assistantship with tuition reimbursement available (averaging $10,920 per year), 15 teaching assistantships with full and partial tuition reimbursements available (averaging $10,881 per year); career-related internships or fieldwork, traineeships, health care benefits, and unspecified assistantships also available. Financial award application deadline: 2/1; financial award applicants required to submit FAFSA. *Faculty research:* Auditory perception and intervention; language and literacy; neurophysiology of hearing, speech, and language; adult neurogenics; bilingualism and language variation; language processing and intervention; speech and voice production; speech perception; translational science. *Total annual research expenditures:* $931,493. *Unit head:* Dr. Theresa Chisolm, Chair and Professor, 813-974-9826, Fax: 813-974-0822, E-mail: chisolm@usf.edu. *Application contact:* Dr. Jean Krause, PhD Program Director/Associate Professor, 813-974-9798, Fax: 813-974-0822, E-mail: jeankrause@usf.edu.
Website: http://csd.cbcs.usf.edu/

University of South Florida, Innovative Education Graduate Certificate Programs, Tampa, FL 33620-9951. *Unit head:* Kathy Barnes, Interdisciplinary Programs Coordinator, 813-974-8031, Fax: 813-974-7061, E-mail: barnesk@usf.edu. *Application contact:* Karen Tylinski, Metro Initiatives, 813-974-9943, Fax: 813-974-7061, E-mail: ktylinsk@usf.edu.
Website: http://www.usf.edu/innovative-education/

The University of Tennessee, Graduate School, College of Arts and Sciences, Department of Audiology and Speech Pathology, Program in Audiology, Knoxville, TN 37996. Offers MA. *Accreditation:* ASHA. *Degree requirements:* For master's, thesis or alternative. *Entrance requirements:* For master's, GRE General Test, minimum GPA of 2.7. Additional exam requirements/recommendations for international students: Required—TOEFL. Electronic applications accepted. *Expenses:* Tuition, state resident: full-time $9540; part-time $531 per credit hour. Tuition, nonresident: full-time $27,728; part-time $1542 per credit hour. *Required fees:* $1404; $67 per credit hour.

The University of Tennessee, Graduate School, College of Arts and Sciences, Department of Audiology and Speech Pathology, Program in Speech and Hearing Science, Knoxville, TN 37996. Offers audiology (PhD); hearing science (PhD); speech and language pathology (PhD); speech and language science (PhD). *Accreditation:* ASHA. *Degree requirements:* For doctorate, thesis/dissertation. *Entrance requirements:* For doctorate, GRE General Test, minimum GPA of 2.7. Additional exam requirements/recommendations for international students: Required—TOEFL. Electronic applications accepted. *Expenses:* Tuition, state resident: full-time $9540; part-time $531 per credit hour. Tuition, nonresident: full-time $27,728; part-time $1542 per credit hour. *Required fees:* $1404; $67 per credit hour.

The University of Tennessee, Graduate School, College of Arts and Sciences, Department of Audiology and Speech Pathology, Program in Speech Pathology, Knoxville, TN 37996. Offers MA. *Accreditation:* ASHA. *Degree requirements:* For master's, thesis or alternative. *Entrance requirements:* For master's, GRE General Test, minimum GPA of 2.7. Additional exam requirements/recommendations for international students: Required—TOEFL. Electronic applications accepted. *Expenses:* Tuition, state resident: full-time $9540; part-time $531 per credit hour. Tuition, nonresident: full-time $27,728; part-time $1542 per credit hour. *Required fees:* $1404; $67 per credit hour.

The University of Tennessee, Graduate School, College of Education, Health and Human Sciences, Program in Education, Knoxville, TN 37996. Offers art education (MS); counseling education (PhD); cultural studies in education (PhD); curriculum (MS, Ed S); curriculum, educational research and evaluation (Ed D, PhD); early childhood education (PhD); early childhood special education (MS); education of deaf and hard of hearing (MS); educational administration and policy studies (Ed D, PhD); educational administration and supervision (Ed S); educational psychology (Ed D, PhD); elementary education (MS, Ed S); elementary teaching (MS); English education (MS, Ed S); exercise science (PhD); foreign language/ESL education (MS, Ed S); instructional technology (MS, Ed D, PhD, Ed S); literacy, language and ESL education (PhD); literacy, language education, and ESL education (Ed D); mathematics education (MS, Ed S); modified and comprehensive special education (MS); reading education (MS, Ed S); school counseling (Ed S); school psychology (PhD, Ed S); science education (MS, Ed S); secondary teaching (MS); social foundations (MS); social science education (MS, Ed S); socio-cultural foundations of sports and education (PhD); special education (Ed S); teacher education (Ed D, PhD). *Accreditation:* NCATE. Part-time and evening/weekend programs available. *Degree requirements:* For master's and Ed S, thesis optional; for doctorate, variable foreign language requirement, thesis/dissertation. *Entrance requirements:* For master's, minimum GPA of 2.7; for doctorate and Ed S, GRE General Test, minimum GPA of 2.7. Additional exam requirements/recommendations for international students: Required—TOEFL. Electronic applications accepted. *Expenses:* Tuition, state resident: full-time $9540; part-time $531 per credit hour. Tuition, nonresident: full-time $27,728; part-time $1542 per credit hour. *Required fees:* $1404; $67 per credit hour.

The University of Tennessee Health Science Center, College of Graduate Health Sciences, Memphis, TN 38163-0002. Offers biomedical engineering (MS, PhD); biomedical sciences (PhD); dental sciences (MDS); epidemiology (MS); health outcomes and policy research (PhD); laboratory research and management (MS); nursing science (PhD); pharmaceutical sciences (PhD); pharmacology (MS); speech and hearing science (PhD); DDS/PhD; DNP/PhD; MD/PhD; Pharm D/PhD. *Faculty:* 318 full-time (92 women), 59 part-time/adjunct (16 women). *Students:* 220 full-time (102 women), 22 part-time (13 women); includes 194 minority (22 Black or African American, non-Hispanic/Latino; 161 Asian, non-Hispanic/Latino; 7 Hispanic/Latino; 3 Native Hawaiian or other Pacific Islander, non-Hispanic/Latino; 1 Two or more races, non-Hispanic/Latino), 106 international. Average age 25. 404 applicants, 17% accepted, 64 enrolled. In 2013, 13 master's, 25 doctorates awarded. Terminal master's awarded for partial completion of doctoral program. *Degree requirements:* For master's, comprehensive exam, thesis; for doctorate, comprehensive exam, thesis/dissertation, oral and written preliminary and comprehensive exams. *Entrance requirements:* For master's and doctorate, GRE General Test, minimum GPA of 3.0. Additional exam requirements/recommendations for international students: Required—TOEFL (minimum score 79 iBT); Recommended—IELTS (minimum score 6.5). *Application deadline:* For fall admission, 5/15 priority date for domestic students. Applications are processed on a rolling basis. Application fee: $0. Electronic applications accepted. *Financial support:* In 2013–14, 125 students received support, including 125 research assistantships (averaging $23,000 per year); career-related internships or fieldwork, Federal Work-Study, institutionally sponsored loans, and tuition waivers (full and partial) also available. Support available to part-time students. Financial award application deadline: 2/25; financial award applicants required to submit FAFSA. *Unit head:* Dr. Donald B. Thomason, Dean, 901-448-5538, E-mail: dthomaso@uthsc.edu. *Application contact:* William Carter, Director for Admissions, 901-448-1687, E-mail: wcarte17@uthsc.edu.
Website: http://www.uthsc.edu/grad/

The University of Tennessee Health Science Center, College of Health Professions, Memphis, TN 38163-0002. Offers audiology (MS, Au D); clinical laboratory science (MSCLS); cytopathology practice (MCP); health informatics and information management (MHIIM); occupational therapy (MOT); physical therapy (DPT, ScDPT); physician assistant (MMS); speech-language pathology (MS). *Accreditation:* AOTA; APTA. Part-time and evening/weekend programs available. Postbaccalaureate distance learning degree programs offered (minimal on-campus study). Terminal master's awarded for partial completion of doctoral program. *Degree requirements:* For master's, comprehensive exam, thesis; for doctorate, comprehensive exam, residency. *Entrance requirements:* For master's, GRE (MOT, MSCLS), minimum GPA of 3.0, 3 letters of reference, national accreditation (MSCLS), GRE if GPA is less than 3.0 (MCP); for doctorate, GRE. Additional exam requirements/recommendations for international students: Required—TOEFL (minimum score 550 paper-based; 80 iBT). *Application deadline:* For fall admission, 1/30 priority date for domestic students; for winter admission, 10/1 priority date for domestic students. Application fee: $50. Electronic applications accepted. *Expenses:* Contact institution. *Financial support:* Teaching assistantships, Federal Work-Study, institutionally sponsored loans, and scholarships/grants available. Support available to part-time students. Financial award application deadline: 2/15; financial award applicants required to submit FAFSA. *Faculty research:* Gait deviation, muscular dystrophy and strength, hemophilia and exercise, pediatric neurology, self-efficacy. *Unit head:* Dr. Noma Anderson, Dean, 901-528-5588, Fax: 901-528-7545, E-mail: nander13@uthsc.edu. *Application contact:* Dr. Noma Anderson, Dean, 901-528-5588, Fax: 901-528-7545, E-mail: nander13@uthsc.edu.
Website: http://www.uthsc.edu/health-professions/

The University of Texas at Austin, Graduate School, College of Communication, Department of Communication Sciences and Disorders, Austin, TX 78712-1111. Offers audiology (Au D); communication sciences and disorders (PhD); speech language pathology (MA). *Accreditation:* ASHA (one or more programs are accredited). *Entrance requirements:* For master's and doctorate, GRE General Test.

The University of Texas at Dallas, School of Behavioral and Brain Sciences, Program in Audiology, Dallas, TX 75080. Offers Au D. *Accreditation:* ASHA. *Faculty:* 9 full-time (4 women), 3 part-time/adjunct (2 women). *Students:* 34 full-time (29 women), 8 part-time (all women); includes 10 minority (1 Black or African American, non-Hispanic/Latino; 5 Asian, non-Hispanic/Latino; 2 Hispanic/Latino; 2 Two or more races, non-Hispanic/Latino), 1 international. Average age 26. 111 applicants, 9% accepted, 10 enrolled. In 2013, 11 doctorates awarded. *Degree requirements:* For doctorate, research project. *Entrance requirements:* For doctorate, GRE. Additional exam requirements/recommendations for international students: Required—TOEFL (minimum score 550 paper-based). *Application deadline:* For fall admission, 7/15 for domestic students, 5/1 priority date for international students; for spring admission, 11/15 for domestic students, 9/1 priority date for international students. Applications are processed on a rolling basis. Application fee: $50 ($100 for international students). Electronic applications accepted. *Expenses:* Tuition, state resident: full-time $11,940; part-time $663.33 per credit hour. Tuition, nonresident: full-time $21,606; part-time $1200.33 per credit hour. *Financial support:* In 2013–14, 42 students received support. Research assistantships with partial tuition reimbursements available, teaching assistantships with partial tuition reimbursements available, career-related internships or fieldwork, Federal Work-Study, institutionally sponsored loans, scholarships/grants, and unspecified assistantships available. Support available to part-time students. Financial award application deadline: 4/30; financial award applicants required to submit FAFSA. *Faculty research:* Hearing disorders, amplification of hearing aids, cochlear implants and aural habilitation. *Unit head:* Dr. Ross Roeser, Program Head, 214-905-3002, E-mail: roeser@callier.utdallas.edu. *Application contact:* Cathy Bittner, Program Assistant, 214-905-3116, E-mail: cbittner@utdallas.edu.
Website: http://bbs.utdallas.edu/aud

The University of Texas at Dallas, School of Behavioral and Brain Sciences, Program in Communication Sciences and Disorders, Richardson, TX 75080. Offers communication disorders (MS); communication science and disorders (PhD). Part-time and evening/weekend programs available. *Faculty:* 13 full-time (9 women), 9 part-time/adjunct (all women). *Students:* 240 full-time (236 women), 11 part-time (all women); includes 55 minority (4 Black or African American, non-Hispanic/Latino; 14 Asian, non-Hispanic/Latino; 28 Hispanic/Latino; 9 Two or more races, non-Hispanic/Latino), 8 international. Average age 25. 560 applicants, 16% accepted, 68 enrolled. In 2013, 129 master's, 1 doctorate awarded. *Degree requirements:* For doctorate, thesis/dissertation. *Entrance requirements:* For master's and doctorate, GRE General Test, minimum GPA of 3.0 in upper-level course work in field. Additional exam requirements/recommendations for international students: Required—TOEFL (minimum score 550 paper-based). *Application deadline:* For fall admission, 7/15 for domestic students, 5/1 priority date for international students; for spring admission, 11/15 for domestic students, 9/1 priority date for international students. Applications are processed on a rolling basis. Application fee: $50 ($100 for international students). Electronic applications accepted. *Expenses:* Tuition, state resident: full-time $11,940; part-time $663.33 per credit hour. Tuition, nonresident: full-time $21,606; part-time $1200.33 per credit hour. *Financial support:* In 2013–14, 188 students received support, including 3 research assistantships with partial tuition reimbursements available (averaging $25,221 per year), 14 teaching assistantships with partial tuition reimbursements available (averaging $14,850 per year); fellowships, Federal Work-Study, institutionally sponsored loans, scholarships/grants, and unspecified assistantships also available. Support

available to part-time students. Financial award application deadline: 4/30; financial award applicants required to submit FAFSA. *Faculty research:* Developmental neurolinguistics, brain plasticity and biofeedback treatment, autism spectrum disorders, speech production, neurogenic speech and language disorders. *Unit head:* Dr. Robert D. Stillman, Program Head, 214-905-3106, Fax: 972-883-3022, E-mail: stillman@utdallas.edu. *Application contact:* 972-883-3106, Fax: 972-883-3022, E-mail: commsciphd@utdallas.edu.
Website: http://bbs.utdallas.edu/csd/

The University of Texas at El Paso, Graduate School, College of Health Sciences, Department of Speech-Language Pathology, El Paso, TX 79968-0001. Offers MS. *Accreditation:* ASHA. *Degree requirements:* For master's, comprehensive exam, thesis optional. *Entrance requirements:* For master's, GRE, minimum GPA of 3.0, resume, letters of recommendation, writing sample, interview. Additional exam requirements/recommendations for international students: Required—TOEFL; Recommended—IELTS. Electronic applications accepted. *Faculty research:* Bilingual language disorders, clinical supervision, hearing loss, traumatic brain injury, aphasia, policy, augmentative communication.

The University of Texas Health Science Center at San Antonio, School of Medicine, San Antonio, TX 78229-3900. Offers deaf education and hearing (MS); medicine (MD); MPH/MD. *Accreditation:* LCME/AMA. *Faculty:* 838 full-time (348 women), 394 part-time/adjunct (142 women). *Students:* 876 full-time (420 women), 20 part-time (all women); includes 392 minority (41 Black or African American, non-Hispanic/Latino; 152 Asian, non-Hispanic/Latino; 179 Hispanic/Latino; 20 Two or more races, non-Hispanic/Latino), 1 international. Average age 26. 4,100 applicants, 17% accepted, 220 enrolled. In 2013, 12 master's, 228 doctorates awarded. *Degree requirements:* For master's, comprehensive exam, practicum assignments. *Entrance requirements:* For master's, minimum GPA of 3.0, interview, 3 professional letters of recommendation; for doctorate, MCAT. *Application deadline:* For fall admission, 10/1 for domestic and international students. Applications are processed on a rolling basis. Application fee: $140. Electronic applications accepted. *Expenses:* Contact institution. *Financial support:* In 2013–14, 599 students received support. Federal Work-Study, institutionally sponsored loans, tuition waivers (full and partial), and stipends, department payments available. Financial award application deadline: 6/1; financial award applicants required to submit FAFSA. *Faculty research:* Geriatrics, diabetes, cancer, AIDS, obesity. *Total annual research expenditures:* $117.4 million. *Unit head:* Dr. Francisco Gonzalez-Scarano, Dean, 210-567-4432, Fax: 210-567-3435, E-mail: scarano@uthscsa.edu. *Application contact:* Dr. David J. Jones, Senior Associate Dean for Admissions, 210-567-6080, Fax: 210-567-6962, E-mail: jonesd@uthscsa.edu.
Website: som.uthscsa.edu

The University of Texas–Pan American, College of Health Sciences and Human Services, Department of Communication Sciences and Disorders, Edinburg, TX 78539. Offers MS. *Accreditation:* ASHA. *Degree requirements:* For master's, comprehensive exam, thesis optional, NESPA exam. *Entrance requirements:* For master's, GRE General Test, minimum GPA of 3.0 in major, 3 letters of recommendation, resume. Additional exam requirements/recommendations for international students: Required—TOEFL (minimum score 550 paper-based). Electronic applications accepted. *Expenses:* Tuition, state resident: full-time $5986; part-time $333 per credit hour. Tuition, nonresident: full-time $12,358; part-time $687 per credit hour. *Required fees:* $782. Tuition and fees vary according to program. *Faculty research:* Bilingual/bicultural language development/disorders, elementary-age language disorders, voice disorders.

University of the District of Columbia, College of Arts and Sciences, Department of Language and Communication Disorders, Program in Speech and Language Pathology, Washington, DC 20008-1175. Offers MS. *Accreditation:* ASHA. Part-time programs available. *Degree requirements:* For master's, comprehensive exam, thesis optional. *Entrance requirements:* For master's, GRE General Test, writing proficiency exam. *Expenses: Tuition, area resident:* Full-time $7883.28; part-time $437.96 per credit hour. Tuition, state resident: full-time $8923.14. Tuition, nonresident: full-time $15,163; part-time $842.40 per credit hour. *Required fees:* $620; $30 per credit hour. *Faculty research:* Child language, dialect variation, English as a second language.

University of the Pacific, Thomas J. Long School of Pharmacy and Health Sciences, Department of Speech-Language Pathology, Stockton, CA 95211-0197. Offers MS. *Accreditation:* ASHA. *Faculty:* 8 full-time (5 women), 14 part-time/adjunct (13 women). *Students:* 55 full-time (50 women), 1 (woman) part-time; includes 21 minority (9 Asian, non-Hispanic/Latino; 11 Hispanic/Latino; 1 Two or more races, non-Hispanic/Latino). Average age 25. 318 applicants, 16% accepted, 29 enrolled. In 2013, 44 master's awarded. *Entrance requirements:* For master's, GRE General Test. Additional exam requirements/recommendations for international students: Required—TOEFL (minimum score 475 paper-based). *Application deadline:* For fall admission, 2/1 for domestic students. Application fee: $75. *Financial support:* Institutionally sponsored loans available. Support available to part-time students. Financial award application deadline: 2/1; financial award applicants required to submit FAFSA. *Unit head:* Dr. Robert Hanyak, Chairman, 209-946-3223, E-mail: rhanyak@pacific.edu. *Application contact:* Ron Espejo, Recruitment Specialist, 209-946-3957, Fax: 209-946-3147, E-mail: respejo@pacific.edu.

The University of Toledo, College of Graduate Studies, College of Health Sciences, Department of Rehabilitation Sciences, Toledo, OH 43606-3390. Offers occupational therapy (OTD); physical therapy (DPT); speech-language pathology (MA). *Faculty:* 30. *Students:* 180 full-time (148 women), 31 part-time (29 women); includes 11 minority (2 Black or African American, non-Hispanic/Latino; 3 Asian, non-Hispanic/Latino; 2 Hispanic/Latino; 4 Two or more races, non-Hispanic/Latino). Average age 25. 230 applicants, 58% accepted, 61 enrolled. In 2013, 25 master's, 43 doctorates awarded. *Degree requirements:* For master's, comprehensive exam, thesis; for doctorate, thesis/dissertation or alternative. *Entrance requirements:* For master's, GRE, minimum cumulative GPA of 2.7 for all previous academic work, letters of recommendation; for doctorate, GRE, minimum cumulative GPA of 3.0 for all previous academic work, letters of recommendation; OTCAS or PTCAS application and UT supplemental application (for OTD and DPT). Additional exam requirements/recommendations for international students: Required—TOEFL (minimum score 550 paper-based; 80 iBT). *Application deadline:* For fall admission, 11/1 for domestic and international students. Application fee: $45 ($75 for international students). Electronic applications accepted. *Financial support:* In 2013–14, 16 teaching assistantships with full and partial tuition reimbursements (averaging $5,002 per year) were awarded; Federal Work-Study, scholarships/grants, tuition waivers (full and partial), unspecified assistantships, and administrative assistantships also available. Financial award applicants required to submit FAFSA. *Unit head:* Dr. Michelle Masterson, Chair, 419-530-6671, Fax: 419-530-4780, E-mail: michelle.masterson@utoledo.edu. *Application contact:* College of Graduate Studies, 419-383-4112, Fax: 419-383-6140, E-mail: grdsch@utnet.utoledo.edu.
Website: http://www.utoledo.edu/eduhshs/

University of Toronto, Faculty of Medicine, Department of Speech-Language Pathology, Toronto, ON M5S 1A1, Canada. Offers M Sc, MH Sc, PhD. Part-time programs available. *Degree requirements:* For master's, thesis (for some programs), clinical internship (MH Sc), oral thesis defense (M Sc); for doctorate, comprehensive exam, thesis/dissertation, oral thesis defense. *Entrance requirements:* For master's, minimum B+ average in last 2 years (MH Sc), B average in final year (M Sc); volunteer/work experience in a clinical setting (MH Sc); for doctorate, previous research experience or thesis, resume, 3 writing samples, 3 letters of recommendation. Electronic applications accepted.

The University of Tulsa, Graduate School, College of Arts and Sciences, Program in Speech-Language Pathology, Tulsa, OK 74104-3189. Offers MS. *Accreditation:* ASHA. Part-time programs available. *Faculty:* 8 full-time (all women). *Students:* 40 full-time (all women); includes 10 minority (1 Black or African American, non-Hispanic/Latino; 6 American Indian or Alaska Native, non-Hispanic/Latino; 1 Asian, non-Hispanic/Latino; 2 Hispanic/Latino), 2 international. Average age 24. 103 applicants, 34% accepted, 19 enrolled. In 2013, 22 master's awarded. *Degree requirements:* For master's, thesis optional. *Entrance requirements:* For master's, GRE General Test. Additional exam requirements/recommendations for international students: Required—TOEFL (minimum score 577 paper-based; 90 iBT), IELTS (minimum score 6.5). *Application deadline:* For fall admission, 2/1 priority date for domestic students. Application fee: $40. Electronic applications accepted. *Expenses: Tuition:* Full-time $19,566; part-time $1087 per credit hour. *Required fees:* $1690; $5 per credit hour. $160 per semester. Tuition and fees vary according to course load. *Financial support:* In 2013–14, 15 students received support, including 1 fellowship with full and partial tuition reimbursement available (averaging $15,250 per year), 14 teaching assistantships with full and partial tuition reimbursements available (averaging $9,458 per year); career-related internships or fieldwork, Federal Work-Study, scholarships/grants, traineeships, health care benefits, tuition waivers (full and partial), and unspecified assistantships also available. Support available to part-time students. Financial award application deadline: 2/1; financial award applicants required to submit FAFSA. *Faculty research:* Disorders of fluency, delayed language and literacy, aphasia, voice, speech articulation, swallowing, cognition. *Total annual research expenditures:* $38,000. *Unit head:* Dr. Kalpana Misra, Dean, 918-631-2222, Fax: 918-631-3721, E-mail: kalpana-misra@utulsa.edu. *Application contact:* Dr. Paula Cadogan, Adviser, 918-631-2897, Fax: 918-631-3668, E-mail: paula-cadogan@utulsa.edu.

University of Utah, Graduate School, College of Education, Department of Special Education, Salt Lake City, UT 84112. Offers deaf and hard of hearing (M Ed, MS); deaf/blind (M Ed); early childhood special education (M Ed, MS, PhD); early childhood vision impairments (M Ed, MS); mild/moderate disabilities (M Ed, MS, PhD); severe disabilities (M Ed, MS, PhD); visual impairment (M Ed, MS). Part-time and evening/weekend programs available. Postbaccalaureate distance learning degree programs offered (no on-campus study). *Faculty:* 9 full-time (6 women), 8 part-time/adjunct (7 women). *Students:* 28 full-time (23 women), 12 part-time (10 women); includes 7 minority (2 Black or African American, non-Hispanic/Latino; 3 Hispanic/Latino; 1 Native Hawaiian or other Pacific Islander, non-Hispanic/Latino; 1 Two or more races, non-Hispanic/Latino), 1 international. Average age 33. 15 applicants, 93% accepted, 13 enrolled. In 2013, 36 master's, 4 doctorates awarded. Terminal master's awarded for partial completion of doctoral program. *Degree requirements:* For master's, comprehensive exam, thesis (for some programs), qualifying exam; for doctorate, thesis/dissertation, qualifying exam. *Entrance requirements:* For master's, GRE or Analytical Writing portion of GRE plus PRAXIS I, minimum GPA of 3.0; for doctorate, GRE General Test (minimum scores: Verbal 600; Quantitative 600; Analytical/Writing 4), minimum GPA of 3.0 (3.5 recommended). Additional exam requirements/recommendations for international students: Required—TOEFL (minimum score 600 paper-based; 100 iBT); Recommended—IELTS (minimum score 7). *Application deadline:* For fall admission, 3/1 for domestic and international students; for spring admission, 11/1 for domestic and international students. Application fee: $55 ($65 for international students). Electronic applications accepted. *Expenses:* Contact institution. *Financial support:* In 2013–14, 27 students received support, including 27 fellowships with full and partial tuition reimbursements available (averaging $5,015 per year), 4 teaching assistantships with full tuition reimbursements available (averaging $17,175 per year); research assistantships and career-related internships or fieldwork also available. Support available to part-time students. Financial award application deadline: 3/1; financial award applicants required to submit FAFSA. *Faculty research:* Inclusive education, positive behavior support, reading, instruction and intervention strategies. *Total annual research expenditures:* $5,926. *Unit head:* Dr. Robert E. O'Neill, Chair, 801-581-8121, Fax: 801-585-6476, E-mail: rob.oneill@utah.edu. *Application contact:* Patty Davis, Academic Advisor, 801-581-4764, Fax: 801-585-6476, E-mail: patty.davis@utah.edu.
Website: http://www.ed.utah.edu/sped/

University of Utah, Graduate School, College of Health, Department of Communication Sciences and Disorders, Salt Lake City, UT 84112. Offers audiology (Au D, PhD); speech-language pathology (MA, MS, PhD). *Accreditation:* ASHA (one or more programs are accredited). *Faculty:* 8 full-time (3 women), 10 part-time/adjunct (9 women). *Students:* 126 full-time (106 women), 3 part-time (1 woman); includes 7 minority (2 Asian, non-Hispanic/Latino; 4 Hispanic/Latino; 1 Two or more races, non-Hispanic/Latino), 5 international. Average age 27. 243 applicants, 49% accepted, 63 enrolled. In 2013, 36 master's, 9 doctorates awarded. Terminal master's awarded for partial completion of doctoral program. *Degree requirements:* For master's, thesis optional, written exam; for doctorate, thesis/dissertation, written and oral exams. *Entrance requirements:* For master's and doctorate, GRE General Test, minimum GPA of 3.0. Additional exam requirements/recommendations for international students: Required—TOEFL (minimum score 600 paper-based; 100 iBT). *Application deadline:* For fall admission, 1/15 for domestic and international students. Application fee: $55 ($65 for international students). Electronic applications accepted. *Expenses:* Contact institution. *Financial support:* In 2013–14, 19 students received support, including 25 research assistantships with partial tuition reimbursements available (averaging $9,000 per year), 1 teaching assistantship with full tuition reimbursement available (averaging $18,000 per year); career-related internships or fieldwork, Federal Work-Study, scholarships/grants, tuition waivers (partial), and unspecified assistantships also available. Financial award application deadline: 2/15; financial award applicants required to submit FAFSA. *Faculty research:* Motor speech disorders, fluency disorders, language disorders, voice disorders, speech perception. *Unit head:* Dr. Michael Blomgren, Department Chair, 801-581-6725, Fax: 801-581-7955, E-mail: michael.blomgren@hsc.utah.edu. *Application contact:* Dr. Kathy Chapman, Director of Graduate Studies, 801-581-6725, Fax: 801-581-7955, E-mail: kathy.chapman@hsc.utah.edu.
Website: http://www.health.utah.edu/csd

University of Vermont, Graduate College, College of Nursing and Health Sciences, Department of Communication Sciences and Disorders, Burlington, VT 05405. Offers MS. *Accreditation:* ASHA. *Students:* 30 (28 women); includes 1 minority (Asian, non-Hispanic/Latino), 2 international. 130 applicants, 32% accepted, 15 enrolled. In 2013, 24 master's awarded. *Entrance requirements:* For master's, GRE General Test. Additional exam requirements/recommendations for international students: Required—TOEFL (minimum score 550 paper-based; 80 iBT). *Application deadline:* For fall admission, 1/1 for domestic and international students. Application fee: $65. Electronic applications accepted. *Financial support:* Fellowships available. Financial award application deadline: 3/1. *Unit head:* Prof. Shelley Velleman, Chair and Coordinator, 802-656-3858.

Communication Disorders

University of Virginia, Curry School of Education, Department of Human Services, Program in Communication Disorders, Charlottesville, VA 22903. Offers M Ed. *Accreditation:* ASHA. *Students:* 60 full-time (57 women), 2 part-time (both women); includes 10 minority (2 Black or African American, non-Hispanic/Latino; 4 Asian, non-Hispanic/Latino; 3 Hispanic/Latino; 1 Two or more races, non-Hispanic/Latino). Average age 24. 340 applicants, 19% accepted, 23 enrolled. In 2013, 24 master's awarded. *Entrance requirements:* For master's, GRE General Test, 2 letters of recommendation. Additional exam requirements/recommendations for international students: Required—TOEFL (minimum score 600 paper-based; 90 iBT), IELTS (minimum score 7). *Application deadline:* Applications are processed on a rolling basis. Application fee: $60. Electronic applications accepted. *Expenses:* Tuition, state resident: part-time $334 per credit hour. Tuition, nonresident: part-time $1224 per credit hour. *Financial support:* Applicants required to submit FAFSA. *Unit head:* Randall R. Robey, Director, 434-924-6351, E-mail: robey@virginia.edu. *Application contact:* Vicki Thomas, Information Contact, 434-924-7472, E-mail: vat3w@virginia.edu.
Website: http://curry.virginia.edu/academics/areas-of-study/speech-pathology-audiology

University of Washington, Graduate School, College of Arts and Sciences, Department of Speech and Hearing Sciences, Seattle, WA 98195. Offers audiology (Au D); speech and hearing sciences (PhD); speech-language pathology (MS). *Accreditation:* ASHA (one or more programs are accredited). *Degree requirements:* For master's, comprehensive exam, thesis or alternative; for doctorate, thesis/dissertation. *Entrance requirements:* For master's and doctorate, GRE, minimum GPA of 3.0. Additional exam requirements/recommendations for international students: Required—TOEFL. Electronic applications accepted. *Faculty research:* Treatment of communication disorders across the life span, speech physiology, auditory perception, behavioral and physiologic audiology.

The University of Western Ontario, Faculty of Graduate Studies, Health Sciences Division, School of Communication Sciences and Disorders, London, ON N6A 5B8, Canada. Offers audiology (M Cl Sc, M Sc); speech-language pathology (M Cl Sc, M Sc). *Degree requirements:* For master's, thesis (for some programs), supervised clinical practicum. *Entrance requirements:* For master's, 14 hours volunteer experience in field of study, minimum B average during last 2 years, previous course work in developmental psychology and statistics, 4 year honors degree. Additional exam requirements/recommendations for international students: Required—TOEFL (minimum score 620 paper-based). *Faculty research:* Child language, voice, neurogenics; auditory function, stuttering.

University of West Georgia, College of Education, Department of Clinical and Professional Studies, Carrollton, GA 30118. Offers professional counseling (M Ed, Ed S), including clinical mental health counseling, college student affairs, school counseling; professional counseling and supervision (Ed D); speech pathology (M Ed). Part-time and evening/weekend programs available. *Faculty:* 10 full-time (6 women), 1 (woman) part-time/adjunct. *Students:* 212 full-time (177 women), 89 part-time (83 women); includes 106 minority (84 Black or African American, non-Hispanic/Latino; 6 Asian, non-Hispanic/Latino; 7 Hispanic/Latino; 9 Two or more races, non-Hispanic/Latino), 3 international. Average age 29. 167 applicants, 89% accepted, 92 enrolled. In 2013, 82 master's, 6 doctorates, 10 other advanced degrees awarded. *Degree requirements:* For master's, comprehensive exam; for Ed S, research project. *Entrance requirements:* For master's, GRE, GACE basic skills (for school counseling M Ed area), minimum GPA of 2.7; for Ed S, GRE, master's degree, minimum graduate GPA of 2.7. Additional exam requirements/recommendations for international students: Required—TOEFL (minimum score 523 paper-based; 69 iBT); Recommended—IELTS (minimum score 6). *Application deadline:* For fall admission, 6/3 for domestic students, 6/1 for international students; for spring admission, 10/7 for domestic students, 10/15 for international students. Applications are processed on a rolling basis. Application fee: $40. Electronic applications accepted. *Expenses:* Tuition, state resident: full-time $4600; part-time $192 per semester hour. Tuition, nonresident: full-time $17,880; part-time $745 per semester hour. *Required fees:* $1858; $46.34 per semester hour. $512 per semester. Tuition and fees vary according to course load, degree level, campus/location and program. *Financial support:* In 2013–14, 15 students received support, including 5 research assistantships with full tuition reimbursements available (averaging $3,000 per year); career-related internships or fieldwork and scholarships/grants also available. Support available to part-time students. Financial award application deadline: 4/1; financial award applicants required to submit FAFSA. *Total annual research expenditures:* $134,000. *Unit head:* Dr. Mark S. Parrish, Chair, 678-839-6117, Fax: 678-839-6162, E-mail: mparrish@westga.edu. *Application contact:* Deanna Richards, Coordinator, Graduate Studies, 678-839-5946, E-mail: drichard@westga.edu.
Website: http://www.westga.edu/coecps/

University of Wisconsin–Eau Claire, College of Education and Human Sciences, Program in Communication Sciences and Disorders, Eau Claire, WI 54702-4004. Offers MS. *Accreditation:* ASHA. Part-time programs available. *Faculty:* 7 full-time (5 women), 1 (woman) part-time/adjunct. *Students:* 37 full-time (35 women); includes 1 minority (Hispanic/Latino). Average age 27. 162 applicants, 12% accepted, 18 enrolled. In 2013, 19 master's awarded. *Degree requirements:* For master's, comprehensive exam, thesis optional, written or oral exam with thesis, externship. *Entrance requirements:* For master's, GRE, Wisconsin residency; minimum GPA of 3.0 in communication disorders, 2.75 overall. Additional exam requirements/recommendations for international students: Required—TOEFL (minimum score 79 iBT). *Application deadline:* For fall admission, 2/1 priority date for domestic and international students. Applications are processed on a rolling basis. Application fee: $56. *Expenses:* Tuition, state resident: full-time $7640; part-time $424.47 per credit. Tuition, nonresident: full-time $16,771; part-time $931.74 per credit. *Required fees:* $1146; $63.65 per credit. *Financial support:* In 2013–14, 10 students received support. Federal Work-Study and unspecified assistantships available. Financial award application deadline: 3/1; financial award applicants required to submit FAFSA. *Unit head:* Dr. Marie Stadler, Chair, 715-836-4861, Fax: 715-836-4846, E-mail: stadlema@uwec.edu. *Application contact:* Dr. Vicki Samelson, Graduate Program Coordinator, 715-836-4846, E-mail: samelsvm@uwec.edu.
Website: http://www.uwec.edu/csd/

University of Wisconsin–Madison, Graduate School, College of Letters and Science, Department of Communicative Disorders, Madison, WI 53706-1380. Offers normal aspects of speech, language and hearing (MS, PhD); speech-language pathology (MS, PhD); MS/PhD. *Accreditation:* ASHA (one or more programs are accredited). *Degree requirements:* For doctorate, thesis/dissertation. *Entrance requirements:* For master's and doctorate, GRE. Electronic applications accepted. *Expenses:* Tuition, state resident: full-time $10,728; part-time $790 per credit. Tuition, nonresident: full-time $24,054; part-time $1623 per credit. *Required fees:* $1130; $119 per credit. *Faculty research:* Language disorders in children and adults, disorders of speech production, intelligibility, fluency, hearing impairment, deafness.

University of Wisconsin–Milwaukee, Graduate School, College of Health Sciences, Department of Communication Sciences and Disorders, Milwaukee, WI 53211. Offers MS, Certificate. *Accreditation:* ASHA (one or more programs are accredited). Part-time programs available. *Faculty:* 6 full-time (5 women), 1 (woman) part-time/adjunct. *Students:* 53 full-time (51 women), 1 (woman) part-time; includes 4 minority (3 Asian, non-Hispanic/Latino; 1 Two or more races, non-Hispanic/Latino). Average age 28. 84 applicants, 32% accepted, 25 enrolled. In 2013, 22 master's awarded. *Degree requirements:* For master's, comprehensive exam, thesis optional. *Entrance requirements:* For master's, GRE General Test, minimum GPA of 3.0. Additional exam requirements/recommendations for international students: Required—TOEFL (minimum score 550 paper-based; 79 iBT), IELTS (minimum score 6.5). *Application deadline:* For fall admission, 1/1 priority date for domestic students; for spring admission, 9/1 for domestic students. Applications are processed on a rolling basis. Application fee: $56 ($96 for international students). *Financial support:* In 2013–14, 1 teaching assistantship was awarded; fellowships, research assistantships, career-related internships or fieldwork, unspecified assistantships, and project assistantships also available. Support available to part-time students. Financial award application deadline: 4/15. *Unit head:* Marylou Gelfer, Department Chair, 414-229-6465, E-mail: gelfer@uwm.edu. *Application contact:* General Information Contact, 414-229-4982, Fax: 414-229-6967, E-mail: gradschool@uwm.edu.
Website: http://www4.uwm.edu/chs/academics/comm_sci_disorders/

University of Wisconsin–River Falls, Outreach and Graduate Studies, College of Education and Professional Studies, Department of Communicative Disorders, River Falls, WI 54022. Offers communicative disorders (MS); secondary education-communicative disorders (MSE). *Accreditation:* ASHA (one or more programs are accredited). Part-time programs available. *Degree requirements:* For master's, comprehensive exam. *Entrance requirements:* For master's, minimum GPA of 2.75, 3 letters of reference. Additional exam requirements/recommendations for international students: Required—TOEFL (minimum score 500 paper-based; 65 iBT), IELTS (minimum score 5.5). *Faculty research:* Voice, language, audiology.

University of Wisconsin–Stevens Point, College of Professional Studies, School of Communicative Disorders, Stevens Point, WI 54481-3897. Offers audiology (Au D); speech-language pathology (MS). *Accreditation:* ASHA (one or more programs are accredited). *Degree requirements:* For master's, thesis optional, clinical semester and capstone project; for doctorate, capstone project, full-time clinical externship. *Entrance requirements:* For master's, completion of specific course contents and practicum experiences at the undergraduate level.

University of Wisconsin–Whitewater, School of Graduate Studies, College of Education and Professional Studies, Program in Communication Sciences and Disorders, Whitewater, WI 53190-1790. Offers MS. *Accreditation:* ASHA. Part-time and evening/weekend programs available. Postbaccalaureate distance learning degree programs offered (no on-campus study). *Degree requirements:* For master's, comprehensive exam. *Entrance requirements:* For master's, 2 letters of recommendation. Additional exam requirements/recommendations for international students: Required—TOEFL (minimum score 550 paper-based; 80 iBT), IELTS (minimum score 6). Electronic applications accepted. *Faculty research:* Occupational hearing conservation.

University of Wyoming, College of Health Sciences, Division of Communication Disorders, Laramie, WY 82071. Offers speech-language pathology (MS). *Accreditation:* ASHA. Part-time programs available. Postbaccalaureate distance learning degree programs offered (minimal on-campus study). *Entrance requirements:* For master's, GRE General Test, minimum GPA of 3.0. Additional exam requirements/recommendations for international students: Required—TOEFL. Electronic applications accepted. *Faculty research:* Child language, visual reinforcement audiometry, voice, auditory brain response, TBI.

Utah State University, School of Graduate Studies, Emma Eccles Jones College of Education and Human Services, Department of Communicative Disorders and Deaf Education, Logan, UT 84322. Offers audiology (Au D, Ed S); communication disorders and deaf education (M Ed); communicative disorders and deaf education (MA, MS). *Accreditation:* ASHA (one or more programs are accredited). Evening/weekend programs available. Postbaccalaureate distance learning degree programs offered (minimal on-campus study). *Degree requirements:* For master's, thesis optional; for Ed S, thesis or alternative. *Entrance requirements:* For master's, GRE General Test, minimum GPA of 3.0, 3 recommendations; for doctorate, GRE General Test, interview, minimum GPA of 3.25. Additional exam requirements/recommendations for international students: Required—TOEFL. *Expenses:* Contact institution. *Faculty research:* Parent-infant intervention with hearing-impaired infants, voice disorders, language development and disorders, oto-accoustic emissions, deaf or hard-of-hearing infants.

Vanderbilt University, School of Medicine, Department of Hearing and Speech Sciences, Nashville, TN 37240-1001. Offers audiology (Au D, PhD); deaf education (MED); speech-language pathology (MS). *Degree requirements:* For master's, thesis optional; for doctorate, thesis/dissertation, final and qualifying exams. *Entrance requirements:* For master's and doctorate, GRE General Test. Additional exam requirements/recommendations for international students: Required—TOEFL. Electronic applications accepted. *Faculty research:* Child language.

Washington State University Spokane, Graduate Programs, Program in Speech and Hearing Sciences, Spokane, WA 99210. Offers MA. *Degree requirements:* For master's, comprehensive exam, thesis (for some programs). *Entrance requirements:* For master's, GRE, minimum GPA of 3.0, 3 letters of recommendation. Additional exam requirements/recommendations for international students: Required—TOEFL (minimum score 550 paper-based). Electronic applications accepted. *Faculty research:* Autism spectrum disorder, childhood apraxia of speech, cleft palate and craniofacial disorders, motor speech disorders in patients with neurodegenerative disease and galactosemia, early language and literacy in multicultural populations.

Washington University in St. Louis, School of Medicine, Program in Audiology and Communication Sciences, Saint Louis, MO 63110. Offers audiology (Au D); deaf education (MS); speech and hearing sciences (PhD). *Accreditation:* ASHA (one or more programs are accredited). *Faculty:* 22 full-time (12 women), 18 part-time/adjunct (12 women). *Students:* 73 full-time (71 women). Average age 24. 136 applicants, 29% accepted, 27 enrolled. In 2013, 10 master's, 11 doctorates awarded. *Degree requirements:* For master's, comprehensive exam, thesis, independent study project, oral exam; for doctorate, comprehensive exam, thesis/dissertation, capstone project. *Entrance requirements:* For master's and doctorate, GRE General Test, minimum B average in previous college/university coursework (recommended). Additional exam requirements/recommendations for international students: Required—TOEFL (minimum score 100 iBT). *Application deadline:* For fall admission, 2/15 for domestic and international students. Application fee: $60 ($80 for international students). Electronic applications accepted. *Expenses:* Contact institution. *Financial support:* In 2013–14, 72 students received support, including 73 fellowships with full and partial tuition reimbursements available (averaging $15,000 per year), 6 teaching assistantships with partial tuition reimbursements available (averaging $1,000 per year); career-related internships or fieldwork, Federal Work-Study, institutionally sponsored loans, scholarships/grants, traineeships, health care benefits, tuition waivers (partial), and unspecified assistantships also available. Financial award application deadline: 2/15; financial award applicants required to submit FAFSA. *Faculty research:* Audiology, deaf education, speech and hearing sciences, sensory neuroscience. *Unit head:* Dr. William W. Clark, Program Director, 314-747-0104, Fax: 314-747-0105. *Application contact:*

Elizabeth A. Elliott, Director, Finance and Student Academic Affairs, 314-747-0104, Fax: 314-747-0105, E-mail: elliottb@wustl.edu.
Website: http://pacs.wustl.edu/

Wayne State University, College of Liberal Arts and Sciences, Department of Communications Disorders and Sciences, Detroit, MI 48202. Offers audiology (Au D); communication disorders and science (PhD); speech-language pathology (MA). *Accreditation:* ASHA (one or more programs are accredited). *Faculty:* 11 full-time (8 women), 13 part-time/adjunct (6 women). *Students:* 114 full-time (101 women), 3 part-time (all women); includes 9 minority (1 Black or African American, non-Hispanic/Latino; 4 Asian, non-Hispanic/Latino; 4 Hispanic/Latino), 22 international. Average age 27. 393 applicants, 12% accepted, 44 enrolled. In 2013, 34 master's, 11 doctorates awarded. *Degree requirements:* For master's, comprehensive exam (for some programs), thesis (for some programs); for doctorate, thesis/dissertation (for some programs), 121-125 credits in the major plus written and/or oral comprehensive examinations. *Entrance requirements:* For master's, GRE, letters of recommendation, minimum GPA of 3.0, three letters of recommendation, written statement of intent, official transcripts, CSDCAS Centralized Application Service; for doctorate, GRE, minimum GPA of 3.0, three letters of recommendation, written statement of intent, official transcripts, CSDCAS Centralized Application Service (for audiology applicants). Additional exam requirements/recommendations for international students: Required—TOEFL (minimum score 550 paper-based; 79 iBT), TWE (minimum score 5.5), Michigan English Language Assessment Battery (minimum score 85); Recommended—IELTS (minimum score 6.5). *Application deadline:* For fall admission, 1/15 for domestic and international students. Application fee: $0. Electronic applications accepted. *Expenses:* Tuition, state resident: part-time $554.15 per credit. Tuition, nonresident: part-time $1200.35 per credit. *Required fees:* $42.15 per credit. $268.30 per semester. Tuition and fees vary according to course load and program. *Financial support:* In 2013–14, 23 students received support, including 1 fellowship with tuition reimbursement available (averaging $16,842 per year), 1 research assistantship with tuition reimbursement available (averaging $16,215 per year); teaching assistantships, career-related internships or fieldwork, scholarships/grants, health care benefits, and unspecified assistantships also available. Financial award application deadline: 3/31; financial award applicants required to submit FAFSA. *Faculty research:* Aphasia, stuttering/fluency, speech and auditory genetics, neuroscience, tinnitus. *Unit head:* Dr. Jean Andruski, Chair, 313-577-3339, E-mail: ag0611@wayne.edu. *Application contact:* Dr. Li Hsieh, Associate Professor, 313-577-3339, E-mail: csdadmissions@wayne.edu.
Website: http://clasweb.clas.wayne.edu/csd

West Chester University of Pennsylvania, College of Health Sciences, Department of Communication Sciences and Disorders, West Chester, PA 19383. Offers communicative disorders (MA); speech correction (Teaching Certificate). *Accreditation:* ASHA (one or more programs are accredited). Part-time and evening/weekend programs available. *Faculty:* 5 full-time (all women), 7 part-time/adjunct (all women). *Students:* 50 full-time (45 women), 10 part-time (all women); includes 2 minority (1 Black or African American, non-Hispanic/Latino; 1 Two or more races, non-Hispanic/Latino). Average age 28. 336 applicants, 17% accepted, 28 enrolled. In 2013, 28 master's awarded. *Degree requirements:* For master's, comprehensive exam, thesis optional, 62 semester credit hours. *Entrance requirements:* For master's, GRE, two letters of recommendation, personal statement of academic and professional goals, logs of clinical observation, practicum hours, structured vita, minimum cumulative and major GPA of 3.0; for Teaching Certificate, bachelor's degree in speech language pathology. Additional exam requirements/recommendations for international students: Required—TOEFL (minimum score 550 paper-based; 80 iBT). *Application deadline:* For fall admission, 4/15 priority date for domestic students, 3/15 for international students; for spring admission, 10/15 priority date for domestic students, 9/1 for international students. Applications are processed on a rolling basis. Application fee: $45. Electronic applications accepted. *Expenses:* Tuition, state resident: full-time $7956; part-time $442 per credit. Tuition, nonresident: full-time $11,934; part-time $663 per credit. *Required fees:* $2134.20; $106.24 per credit. Tuition and fees vary according to campus/location and program. *Financial support:* Unspecified assistantships available. Support available to part-time students. Financial award application deadline: 2/15; financial award applicants required to submit FAFSA. *Faculty research:* Identification/interaction with students with communicative disorders, voice therapy, autism, bilingual assessment and intervention, critical thinking, literacy development, fluency. *Unit head:* Dr. Cheryl Gunter, Chair, 610-436-3401, Fax: 610-436-3388, E-mail: cgunter@wcupa.edu. *Application contact:* Dr. Mareile Koenig, Graduate Coordinator, 610-436-3218, Fax: 610-436-3388, E-mail: mkoenig@wcupa.edu.
Website: http://www.wcupa.edu/_ACADEMICS/HealthSciences/commdisorder/

Western Carolina University, Graduate School, College of Health and Human Sciences, Department of Communication Sciences and Disorders, Cullowhee, NC 28723. Offers MS. *Accreditation:* ASHA. Part-time programs available. *Degree requirements:* For master's, comprehensive exam, thesis or alternative. *Entrance requirements:* For master's, GRE, appropriate undergraduate degree with minimum GPA of 3.0, 3 letters of recommendation. Additional exam requirements/recommendations for international students: Required—TOEFL (minimum score 550 paper-based; 79 iBT). *Faculty research:* Early assessment and intervention in language, stuttering, school-family partnerships, voice and organic disorders, accent reduction.

Western Illinois University, School of Graduate Studies, College of Fine Arts and Communication, Department of Communication Sciences and Disorders, Macomb, IL 61455-1390. Offers MS. *Accreditation:* ASHA. Part-time programs available. *Students:* 37 full-time (36 women), 1 part-time (0 women); includes 4 minority (2 Black or African American, non-Hispanic/Latino; 2 Hispanic/Latino), 1 international. Average age 24. In 2013, 16 master's awarded. *Degree requirements:* For master's, comprehensive exam, thesis or alternative. *Entrance requirements:* For master's, GRE, minimum GPA of 3.0. Additional exam requirements/recommendations for international students: Required—TOEFL (minimum score 550 paper-based; 80 iBT). *Application deadline:* For fall admission, 2/1 priority date for domestic students. Applications are processed on a rolling basis. Application fee: $30. Electronic applications accepted. *Financial support:* In 2013–14, 12 students received support, including 11 research assistantships with full tuition reimbursements available (averaging $7,544 per year), 1 teaching assistantship with full tuition reimbursement available (averaging $8,688 per year). Financial award applicants required to submit FAFSA. *Unit head:* Dr. Stacy Betz, Chairperson, 309-298-1955. *Application contact:* Dr. Nancy Parsons, Associate Provost and Director of Graduate Studies, 309-298-1806, Fax: 309-298-2345, E-mail: grad-office@wiu.edu.
Website: http://wiu.edu/csd

Western Kentucky University, Graduate Studies, College of Health and Human Services, Department of Communication Disorders, Bowling Green, KY 42101. Offers MS. *Accreditation:* ASHA. Part-time and evening/weekend programs available. Postbaccalaureate distance learning degree programs offered (no on-campus study). *Degree requirements:* For master's, comprehensive exam, written exam. *Entrance requirements:* For master's, GRE General Test, 3 letters of recommendation. Additional exam requirements/recommendations for international students: Required—TOEFL (minimum score 555 paper-based; 79 iBT).

Western Michigan University, Graduate College, College of Health and Human Services, Department of Speech Pathology and Audiology, Kalamazoo, MI 49008. Offers audiology (Au D); speech-language pathology (MA). *Accreditation:* ASHA. *Degree requirements:* For master's, thesis optional, clinical practicum. *Entrance requirements:* For master's, GRE General Test.

Western Washington University, Graduate School, College of Humanities and Social Sciences, Department of Communication Sciences and Disorders, Bellingham, WA 98225-5996. Offers MA. *Accreditation:* ASHA. Part-time programs available. *Degree requirements:* For master's, comprehensive exam, thesis optional. *Entrance requirements:* For master's, GRE General Test, minimum GPA of 3.0 in last 60 semester hours or last 90 quarter hours. Additional exam requirements/recommendations for international students: Required—TOEFL (minimum score 567 paper-based). Electronic applications accepted. *Faculty research:* Autism, stroke and stroke perception, aural rehabilitation and cochlear implants, auditory processing, speech in individuals with Parkinson's disease.

West Texas A&M University, College of Nursing and Health Sciences, Department of Communication Disorders, Canyon, TX 79016-0001. Offers MS. *Accreditation:* ASHA. Part-time programs available. *Degree requirements:* For master's, comprehensive exam, thesis optional. *Entrance requirements:* For master's, GRE General Test, minimum B average in all clinical courses, liability insurance, first aid card, immunizations. Additional exam requirements/recommendations for international students: Required—TOEFL (minimum score 550 paper-based).

West Virginia University, College of Human Resources and Education, Department of Speech Pathology and Audiology, Morgantown, WV 26506. Offers audiology (Au D); speech-language pathology (MS). *Accreditation:* ASHA. *Degree requirements:* For master's, thesis optional, PRAXIS; for doctorate, thesis/dissertation or alternative, PRAXIS. *Entrance requirements:* For master's, GRE General Test, minimum GPA of 3.0, letter of recommendation; for doctorate, GRE General Test, letters of recommendation, minimum GPA of 3.0. Additional exam requirements/recommendations for international students: Required—TOEFL. Electronic applications accepted. *Faculty research:* Speech perception, language disorders in children, auditory skills, fluency disorders, phonological disorders in children.

Wichita State University, Graduate School, College of Health Professions, Department of Communication Sciences and Disorders, Wichita, KS 67260. Offers MA, Au D, PhD. *Accreditation:* ASHA (one or more programs are accredited). *Financial support:* Teaching assistantships available. *Unit head:* Dr. Kathy Coufal, Chairperson, 316-978-3240, Fax: 316-978-3302, E-mail: kathy.coufal@wichita.edu. *Application contact:* Jordan Oleson, Admissions Coordinator, 316-978-3095, Fax: 316-978-3253, E-mail: jordan.oleson@wichita.edu.
Website: http://www.wichita.edu/

William Paterson University of New Jersey, College of Science and Health, Wayne, NJ 07470-8420. Offers biotechnology (MS); communication disorders (MS); exercise and sports studies (MS); general biology (MS); nursing (MSN); nursing practice (DNP). Part-time and evening/weekend programs available. *Faculty:* 29 full-time (10 women), 10 part-time/adjunct (1 woman). *Students:* 67 full-time (56 women), 160 part-time (138 women); includes 76 minority (19 Black or African American, non-Hispanic/Latino; 26 Asian, non-Hispanic/Latino; 29 Hispanic/Latino; 2 Two or more races, non-Hispanic/Latino). Average age 35. 490 applicants, 33% accepted, 83 enrolled. In 2013, 51 master's awarded. *Degree requirements:* For master's, comprehensive exam (for some programs), thesis (for some programs), non-thesis internship/practicum (for some programs). *Entrance requirements:* For master's, GRE/MAT, minimum GPA of 2.75; for doctorate, GRE/MAT, minimum GPA of 3.3. Additional exam requirements/recommendations for international students: Required—TOEFL (minimum score 550 paper-based; 79 iBT), IELTS (minimum score 6). *Application deadline:* For fall admission, 6/1 for domestic students, 5/1 for international students; for spring admission, 11/1 for domestic students, 10/1 for international students. Applications are processed on a rolling basis. Application fee: $50. Electronic applications accepted. *Financial support:* Research assistantships with full tuition reimbursements, career-related internships or fieldwork, and unspecified assistantships available. Support available to part-time students. Financial award application deadline: 4/1; financial award applicants required to submit FAFSA. *Faculty research:* Human biomechanics, autism, nanomaterials, health and environment, red-tide causing algae. *Unit head:* Dr. Kenneth Wolf, Dean, 973-720-2194, E-mail: wolfk@wpunj.edu. *Application contact:* Christina Aiello, Assistant Director, Graduate Admissions, 973-720-2506, Fax: 973-720-2035, E-mail: aielloc@wpunj.edu.
Website: http://www.wpunj.edu/cosh

Worcester State University, Graduate Studies, Program in Speech-Language Pathology, Worcester, MA 01602-2597. Offers MS. *Accreditation:* ASHA. Part-time and evening/weekend programs available. *Faculty:* 6 full-time (5 women), 3 part-time/adjunct (all women). *Students:* 54 full-time (all women), 30 part-time (29 women); includes 3 minority (2 Asian, non-Hispanic/Latino; 1 Two or more races, non-Hispanic/Latino). Average age 25. 237 applicants, 24% accepted, 23 enrolled. In 2013, 32 master's awarded. *Degree requirements:* For master's, comprehensive exam, thesis, national licensing exam. *Entrance requirements:* For master's, GRE General Test or MAT, 15 credits of course work in human communication. Additional exam requirements/recommendations for international students: Required—TOEFL (minimum score 500 paper-based; 61 iBT). *Application deadline:* For fall admission, 2/1 for domestic and international students. Applications are processed on a rolling basis. Application fee: $40. Electronic applications accepted. *Expenses:* Contact institution. *Financial support:* In 2013–14, 12 students received support, including 12 research assistantships with full tuition reimbursements available (averaging $4,800 per year); career-related internships or fieldwork, scholarships/grants, and unspecified assistantships also available. Financial award application deadline: 3/1; financial award applicants required to submit FAFSA. *Faculty research:* Hearing threshold norms, language learning disabilities. *Unit head:* Dr. Sharon Antonucci, Coordinator, 508-929-8567, Fax: 508-929-8475, E-mail: sharon.antonucci@worcester.edu. *Application contact:* Sara Grady, Assistant Dean of Graduate and Continuing Education, 508-929-8787, Fax: 508-929-8100, E-mail: sara.grady@worcester.edu.

Dental Hygiene

Boston University, Henry M. Goldman School of Dental Medicine, Boston, MA 02118. Offers advanced general dentistry (CAGS); dental public health (MS, MSD, D Sc D, CAGS); dentistry (DMD); endodontics (MSD, D Sc D, CAGS); operative dentistry (MSD, D Sc D, CAGS); oral and maxillofacial surgery (MSD, D Sc D, CAGS); oral biology (MSD, D Sc, D Sc D, PhD); orthodontics (MSD, D Sc D, CAGS); pediatric dentistry (MSD, D Sc D, CAGS); periodontology (MSD, D Sc D, CAGS); prosthodontics (MSD, D Sc D, CAGS). *Accreditation:* ADA (one or more programs are accredited). *Faculty:* 119 full-time (53 women), 83 part-time/adjunct (24 women). *Students:* 818 full-time (423 women); includes 158 minority (8 Black or African American, non-Hispanic/Latino; 1 American Indian or Alaska Native, non-Hispanic/Latino; 102 Asian, non-Hispanic/Latino; 40 Hispanic/Latino; 7 Two or more races, non-Hispanic/Latino), 359 international. Average age 28. 6,681 applicants, 8% accepted, 263 enrolled. In 2013, 14 master's, 199 doctorates, 55 other advanced degrees awarded. *Degree requirements:* For master's and CAGS, thesis; for doctorate, thesis/dissertation (for some programs). *Entrance requirements:* For doctorate, DAT (for DMD), minimum recommended GPA of 3.0 (for DMD); for CAGS, National Board Dental Exam Part 1, dental degree. Additional exam requirements/recommendations for international students: Required—TOEFL. *Application deadline:* For fall admission, 12/1 for domestic and international students. Applications are processed on a rolling basis. Application fee: $75 ($105 for international students). Electronic applications accepted. *Expenses:* Contact institution. *Financial support:* In 2013–14, 480 students received support. Career-related internships or fieldwork, institutionally sponsored loans, and stipends and scholarships (for Advanced Education in General Dentistry and Oral and Maxillofacial Surgery residents) available. Financial award application deadline: 4/15; financial award applicants required to submit FAFSA. *Faculty research:* Defense mechanisms, bone-cell regulation, protein biochemistry, molecular biology, biomaterials. *Unit head:* Dr. Jeffrey W. Hutter, Dean, 617-638-4780. *Application contact:* Admissions Representative, 617-638-4787, Fax: 617-638-4798, E-mail: sdmadmis@bu.edu.
Website: http://www.bu.edu/dental

Eastern Washington University, Graduate Studies, College of Science, Health and Engineering, Department of Dental Hygiene, Cheney, WA 99004-2431. Offers MS. *Students:* 6 full-time (all women), 7 part-time (all women); includes 3 minority (all Asian, non-Hispanic/Latino). 6 applicants, 67% accepted, 4 enrolled. In 2013, 6 master's awarded. Application fee: $50. *Financial support:* In 2013–14, 3 teaching assistantships (averaging $7,000 per year) were awarded. *Unit head:* Rebecca Stolberg, Chair, 509-368-6528, Fax: 509-368-6514, E-mail: rstolberg@mail.ewu.edu. *Application contact:* Julie Marr, Advisor/Recruiter for Graduate Studies, 509-359-6297, Fax: 509-359-6044, E-mail: gradprograms@ewu.edu.
Website: http://www.ewu.edu/cshe/programs/dental-hygiene.xml

Georgia Regents University, The Graduate School, Program in Allied Health Sciences, Augusta, GA 30912. Offers dental hygiene (MS). Part-time programs available. Postbaccalaureate distance learning degree programs offered (no on-campus study). *Degree requirements:* For master's, thesis. *Entrance requirements:* For master's, GRE General Test. Additional exam requirements/recommendations for international students: Required—TOEFL (minimum score 550 paper-based; 79 iBT). Electronic applications accepted. *Faculty research:* Patient- and family-centered care, public health informatics, vascular health promotion through physical activity, improving air quality for school children, movement therapies for Parkinson's Disease.

Idaho State University, Office of Graduate Studies, Kasiska College of Health Professions, Department of Dental Hygiene, Pocatello, ID 83209-8048. Offers MS. Part-time programs available. *Degree requirements:* For master's, comprehensive exam, thesis, thesis defense, practicum experience, oral exam. *Entrance requirements:* For master's, GRE, MAT, baccalaureate degree in dental hygiene, minimum GPA of 3.0 in upper-division and dental hygiene coursework, current dental hygiene licensure in good standing. Additional exam requirements/recommendations for international students: Required—TOEFL (minimum score 600 paper-based; 80 iBT). Electronic applications accepted.

Missouri Southern State University, Program in Dental Hygiene, Joplin, MO 64801-1595. Offers MS. Program offered jointly with University of Missouri–Kansas City. Part-time programs available. *Degree requirements:* For master's, project. *Entrance requirements:* For master's, copy of current dental hygiene license. Electronic applications accepted.

The Ohio State University, College of Dentistry, Columbus, OH 43210. Offers dental anesthesiology (MS); dental hygiene (MDH); dentistry (DDS); endodontics (MS); oral and maxillofacial pathology (MS); oral and maxillofacial surgery (MS); oral biology (PhD); orthodontics (MS); pediatric dentistry (MS); periodontology (MS); prosthodontics (MS); DDS/PhD. *Accreditation:* ADA (one or more programs are accredited). *Faculty:* 75. *Students:* 510 full-time (220 women), 7 part-time (4 women); includes 89 minority (12 Black or African American, non-Hispanic/Latino; 51 Asian, non-Hispanic/Latino; 16 Hispanic/Latino; 10 Two or more races, non-Hispanic/Latino), 26 international. Average age 26. In 2013, 17 master's, 105 doctorates awarded. Terminal master's awarded for partial completion of doctoral program. *Degree requirements:* For master's, thesis; for doctorate, thesis/dissertation (for some programs). *Entrance requirements:* For master's, GRE General Test (for all applicants with cumulative GPA below 3.0); for doctorate, DAT (for DDS); GRE General Test, GRE Subject Test in biology recommended (for PhD). Additional exam requirements/recommendations for international students: Required—TOEFL (minimum score 550 paper-based; 79 iBT), Michigan English Language Assessment Battery (minimum score 82), IELTS (minimum score 7) for MS and PhD; TOEFL (minimum score 577 paper-based; 90 iBT), Michigan English Language Assessment Battery (minimum score 84), IELTS (minimum score 7.5) for DDS. *Application deadline:* Applications are processed on a rolling basis. Electronic applications accepted. *Expenses:* Contact institution. *Financial support:* Fellowships with tuition reimbursements, research assistantships with tuition reimbursements, teaching assistantships with tuition reimbursements, Federal Work-Study, and institutionally sponsored loans available. Financial award application deadline: 2/15. *Faculty research:* Neurobiology, inflammation and immunity, materials science, bone biology. *Total annual research expenditures:* $3.4 million. *Unit head:* Dr. Patrick M. Lloyd, Dean, 614-292-9755, E-mail: lloyd.256@osu.edu. *Application contact:* Graduate and Professional Admissions, 614-292-9444, Fax: 614-292-3656.
Website: http://www.dent.osu.edu/

Old Dominion University, College of Health Sciences, School of Dental Hygiene, Norfolk, VA 23529. Offers MS. Part-time and evening/weekend programs available. Postbaccalaureate distance learning degree programs offered (no on-campus study). *Faculty:* 9 full-time (8 women). *Students:* 3 full-time (all women), 10 part-time (9 women); includes 2 minority (1 Asian, non-Hispanic/Latino; 1 Two or more races, non-Hispanic/Latino), 2 international. Average age 31. 12 applicants, 25% accepted, 2 enrolled. In 2013, 10 master's awarded. *Degree requirements:* For master's, comprehensive exam, thesis optional, writing proficiency exam. *Entrance requirements:* For master's, Dental Hygiene National Board Examination, BS or certificate in dental hygiene or related area, minimum GPA of 2.8 (3.0 in major), letters of recommendation. Additional exam requirements/recommendations for international students: Required—TOEFL (minimum score 550 paper-based; 79 iBT). *Application deadline:* For fall admission, 7/1 for domestic students, 4/15 for international students; for spring admission, 12/1 for domestic students, 10/1 for international students. Applications are processed on a rolling basis. Application fee: $50. Electronic applications accepted. *Expenses:* Tuition, state resident: full-time $9888; part-time $412 per credit. Tuition, nonresident: full-time $25,152; part-time $1048 per credit. *Required fees:* $59 per semester. One-time fee: $50. *Financial support:* In 2013–14, 4 students received support, including 2 teaching assistantships with partial tuition reimbursements available (averaging $10,000 per year); fellowships, research assistantships, career-related internships or fieldwork, scholarships/grants, tuition waivers, and unspecified assistantships also available. Support available to part-time students. Financial award application deadline: 2/15; financial award applicants required to submit CSS PROFILE or FAFSA. *Faculty research:* Clinical dental hygiene, dental hygiene client health behaviors, dental hygiene education interventions, oral product testing, cold plasma. *Total annual research expenditures:* $524,962. *Unit head:* Prof. Gayle B. McCombs, Graduate Program Director, 757-683-3338, Fax: 757-683-5329, E-mail: gmccombs@odu.edu. *Application contact:* William Heffelfinger, Director of Graduate Admissions, 757-683-5554, Fax: 757-683-3255, E-mail: gradadmit@odu.edu.
Website: http://hs.odu.edu/dental/academics/ms/about.shtml

Texas A&M Health Science Center, Baylor College of Dentistry, Caruth School of Dental Hygiene, College Station, TX 77840. Offers MS. Part-time programs available. *Degree requirements:* For master's, thesis (for some programs). *Entrance requirements:* For master's, GRE General Test, National Dental Hygiene Board Examination, minimum GPA of 3.0 in dental hygiene course work, 2.7 overall. *Faculty research:* Assessment of outcomes, dental materials, educational research, HIV patients, underserved patient populations, handicapped patients.

Université de Montréal, Faculty of Dental Medicine, Program in Stomatology Residency, Montréal, QC H3C 3J7, Canada. Offers Certificate.

University of Alberta, Faculty of Medicine and Dentistry, Department of Dentistry, Program in Dental Hygiene, Edmonton, AB T6G 2E1, Canada. Offers Diploma. Electronic applications accepted.

University of Bridgeport, Fones School of Dental Hygiene, Bridgeport, CT 06604. Offers MS. Part-time and evening/weekend programs available. Postbaccalaureate distance learning degree programs offered (no on-campus study). *Faculty:* 3 full-time (all women), 3 part-time/adjunct (all women). *Students:* 1 (woman) full-time, 55 part-time (54 women); includes 13 minority (3 Black or African American, non-Hispanic/Latino; 4 Asian, non-Hispanic/Latino; 3 Hispanic/Latino; 3 Two or more races, non-Hispanic/Latino). Average age 36. 12 applicants, 8% accepted. In 2013, 6 master's awarded. *Degree requirements:* For master's, thesis. *Entrance requirements:* For master's, Dental Hygiene National Board Examination. Additional exam requirements/recommendations for international students: Recommended—TOEFL (minimum score 550 paper-based; 80 iBT), IELTS (minimum score 6.5). *Application deadline:* For fall admission, 8/1 priority date for domestic and international students; for spring admission, 12/1 priority date for domestic and international students. Application fee: $50. *Expenses:* Contact institution. *Financial support:* Applicants required to submit FAFSA. *Unit head:* Dr. Marcia H. Lorentzen, Dean, 203-576-4138, Fax: 203-576-4220, E-mail: marcia@bridgeport.edu. *Application contact:* Leanne Proctor, Director of Health Science Admissions, 203-576-4352, Fax: 203-576-4941, E-mail: fones@bridgeport.edu.

University of Maryland, Baltimore, Graduate School, Graduate Programs in Dentistry, Department of Dental Hygiene, Baltimore, MD 21201. Offers MS. *Students:* 8 applicants. In 2013, 12 master's awarded. *Degree requirements:* For master's, thesis or alternative. *Entrance requirements:* For master's, minimum GPA of 3.0. Additional exam requirements/recommendations for international students: Required—TOEFL (minimum score 550 paper-based; 80 iBT) or IELTS (minimum score 7). *Application deadline:* For fall admission, 6/30 for domestic students, 1/15 for international students; for spring admission, 11/30 for domestic students. Application fee: $50. Electronic applications accepted. *Financial support:* Fellowships available. Support available to part-time students. Financial award application deadline: 2/15; financial award applicants required to submit FAFSA. *Faculty research:* Dental hygiene education, health care management, health system theory and policy development, hospital dental hygiene, clinical practice. *Unit head:* Jacqueline Fried, Chairperson, 410-706-7773, Fax: 410-706-0349. *Application contact:* Keith T. Brooks, Assistant Dean, 410-706-7131, Fax: 410-706-3473, E-mail: kbrooks@umaryland.edu.

University of Michigan, School of Dentistry and Rackham Graduate School, Graduate Programs in Dentistry, Dental Hygiene Program, Ann Arbor, MI 48109-1078. Offers MS. *Students:* 10 full-time (all women). 2 applicants, 100% accepted, 2 enrolled. In 2013, 1 master's awarded. *Degree requirements:* For master's, thesis. *Entrance requirements:* For master's, bachelor's degree in dental hygiene. Additional exam requirements/recommendations for international students: Required—TOEFL (minimum score 84 iBT). *Application deadline:* Applications are processed on a rolling basis. Application fee: $75 ($90 for international students). Electronic applications accepted. Tuition and fees vary according to course level, course load, degree level, program and student level. *Unit head:* Karen Ridley, Director, 734-763-1068, E-mail: kjr@umich.edu. *Application contact:* Patricia Katcher, Associate Admissions Director, 734-763-3316, Fax: 734-764-1922, E-mail: graddentinquiry@umich.edu.
Website: http://www.dent.umich.edu/dentalhygiene/education/MShome

University of Missouri–Kansas City, School of Dentistry, Kansas City, MO 64110-2499. Offers advanced education in dentistry (Graduate Dental Certificate); dental hygiene education (MS); dentistry (DDS); endodontics (Graduate Dental Certificate); oral and maxillofacial surgery (Graduate Dental Certificate); oral biology (MS, PhD); orthodontics and dentofacial orthopedics (Graduate Dental Certificate); periodontics (Graduate Dental Certificate). PhD (interdisciplinary) offered through the School of Graduate Studies. *Accreditation:* ADA (one or more programs are accredited). *Faculty:* 97 full-time (45 women), 61 part-time/adjunct (18 women). *Students:* 425 full-time (178 women), 50 part-time (26 women); includes 87 minority (12 Black or African American, non-Hispanic/Latino; 3 American Indian or Alaska Native, non-Hispanic/Latino; 51 Asian, non-Hispanic/Latino; 15 Hispanic/Latino; 6 Two or more races, non-Hispanic/Latino), 3 international. Average age 27. 807 applicants, 17% accepted, 131 enrolled. In 2013, 10 master's, 106 doctorates, 17 other advanced degrees awarded. *Degree requirements:* For master's, thesis; for doctorate, thesis/dissertation (for some programs). *Entrance requirements:* For master's, DAT, letters of evaluation, personal

interview; for doctorate, DAT (for DDS); for Graduate Dental Certificate, DDS. Additional exam requirements/recommendations for international students: Required—TOEFL (minimum score 550 paper-based; 80 iBT). *Application deadline:* For fall admission, 2/1 for domestic and international students. Application fee: $45 ($50 for international students). *Expenses:* Contact institution. *Financial support:* In 2013–14, 2 research assistantships (averaging $23,800 per year) were awarded; career-related internships or fieldwork, Federal Work-Study, institutionally sponsored loans, and tuition waivers (full and partial) also available. Support available to part-time students. Financial award application deadline: 3/1; financial award applicants required to submit FAFSA. *Faculty research:* Biomaterials, dental use of lasers, effectiveness of periodontal treatments, temporomandibular joint dysfunction. *Unit head:* Dr. Marsha Pyle, Dean, 816-235-2010, E-mail: pylem@umkc.edu. *Application contact:* Richard Bigham, Assistant Dean for Student Programs, 816-235-2082, E-mail: bighamr@umkc.edu.
Website: http://dentistry.umkc.edu/

University of New Mexico, School of Medicine, Program in Dental Hygiene, Albuquerque, NM 87131. Offers MS. Part-time and evening/weekend programs available. Postbaccalaureate distance learning degree programs offered (no on-campus study). *Faculty:* 5 full-time (all women). *Students:* 5 full-time (3 women), 13 part-time (all women); includes 16 minority (1 Black or African American, non-Hispanic/Latino; 2 Asian, non-Hispanic/Latino; 13 Hispanic/Latino). Average age 35. 8 applicants, 63% accepted, 4 enrolled. In 2013, 2 master's awarded. *Application deadline:* For fall admission, 4/15 for domestic and international students; for winter admission, 1/31 priority date for domestic and international students. Application fee: $50. *Financial support:* In 2013–14, 7 students received support. *Unit head:* Prof. Christine N. Nathe, Director, 505-272-8147, Fax: 505-272-5584, E-mail: cnathe@unm.edu. *Application contact:* Prof. Demetra D. Logothetis, Graduate Program Director, 505-272-6687, Fax: 505-272-5584, E-mail: dlogothetis@salud.unm.edu.
Website: http://dentalmedicine.unm.edu/dentalhy/index.html

The University of North Carolina at Chapel Hill, School of Dentistry and Graduate School, Graduate Programs in Dentistry, Chapel Hill, NC 27599. Offers dental hygiene (MS); endodontics (MS); epidemiology (PhD); operative dentistry (MS); oral and maxillofacial pathology (MS); oral and maxillofacial radiology (MS); oral biology (PhD); orthodontics (MS); pediatric dentistry (MS); periodontology (MS); prosthodontics (MS). *Degree requirements:* For master's, thesis; for doctorate, thesis/dissertation. *Entrance requirements:* For master's, GRE General Test (for orthodontics and oral biology only); National Dental Board Part I (Part II if available), dental degree (for all except dental hygiene); for doctorate, GRE General Test. Additional exam requirements/recommendations for international students: Required—TOEFL (minimum score 550 paper-based; 79 iBT). Electronic applications accepted. *Expenses:* Contact institution. *Faculty research:* Clinical research, inflammation, immunology, neuroscience, molecular biology.

Emergency Medical Services

Baylor University, Graduate School, Military Programs, Program in Emergency Medicine, Waco, TX 76798. Offers D Sc PA. *Students:* 16 full-time (1 woman); includes 2 minority (1 Asian, non-Hispanic/Latino; 1 Hispanic/Latino). In 2013, 10 doctorates awarded. *Expenses: Tuition:* Full-time $25,866; part-time $1437 per credit hour. *Required fees:* $2736; $152 per credit hour. Tuition and fees vary according to course load and program. *Unit head:* Maj. Larry Lindsay, Graduate Program Director, 210-916-4542, Fax: 210-221-7306, E-mail: larry.lindsay1@us.army.mil. *Application contact:* Maj. Sue Love, 210-916-4542, Fax: 254-710-3870, E-mail: sue.love@us.army.mil.

Drexel University, College of Nursing and Health Professions, Emergency and Public Safety Services Program, Philadelphia, PA 19104-2875. Offers MS. Part-time and evening/weekend programs available. *Degree requirements:* For master's, comprehensive exam. *Entrance requirements:* For master's, GRE General Test, minimum GPA of 2.75.

San Diego State University, Graduate and Research Affairs, College of Health and Human Services, Graduate School of Public Health, San Diego, CA 92182. Offers environmental health (MPH); epidemiology (MPH, PhD), including biostatistics (MPH); global emergency preparedness and response (MS); global health (PhD); health behavior (PhD); health promotion (MPH); health services administration (MPH); toxicology (MS); MPH/MA; MSW/MPH. *Accreditation:* CAHME (one or more programs are accredited); CEPH (one or more programs are accredited). Part-time programs available. *Degree requirements:* For master's, comprehensive exam (for some programs), thesis (for some programs); for doctorate, thesis/dissertation. *Entrance requirements:* For master's, GMAT (MPH in health services administration), GRE General Test; for doctorate, GRE General Test. Additional exam requirements/recommendations for international students: Required—TOEFL. *Faculty research:* Evaluation of tobacco, AIDS prevalence and prevention, mammography, infant death project, Alzheimer's in elderly Chinese.

Université Laval, Faculty of Medicine, Post-Professional Programs in Medical Studies, Québec, QC G1K 7P4, Canada. Offers anatomy–pathology (DESS); anesthesiology (DESS); cardiology (DESS); care of older people (Diploma); clinical research (DESS); community health (DESS); dermatology (DESS); diagnostic radiology (DESS); emergency medicine (Diploma); family medicine (DESS); general surgery (DESS); geriatrics (DESS); hematology (DESS); internal medicine (DESS); maternal and fetal medicine (Diploma); medical biochemistry (DESS); medical microbiology and infectious diseases (DESS); medical oncology (DESS); nephrology (DESS); neurology (DESS); neurosurgery (DESS); obstetrics and gynecology (DESS); ophthalmology (DESS); orthopedic surgery (DESS); oto-rhino-laryngology (DESS); palliative medicine (Diploma); pediatrics (DESS); plastic surgery (DESS); psychiatry (DESS); pulmonary medicine (DESS); radiology–oncology (DESS); thoracic surgery (DESS); urology (DESS). *Degree requirements:* For other advanced degree, comprehensive exam. *Entrance requirements:* For degree, knowledge of French. Electronic applications accepted.

University of Guelph, Ontario Veterinary College and Graduate Studies, Graduate Programs in Veterinary Sciences, Department of Clinical Studies, Guelph, ON N1G 2W1, Canada. Offers anesthesiology (M Sc, DV Sc); cardiology (DV Sc, Diploma); clinical studies (Diploma); dermatology (M Sc); diagnostic imaging (M Sc, DV Sc); emergency/critical care (M Sc, DV Sc, Diploma); medicine (M Sc, DV Sc); neurology (M Sc, DV Sc); ophthalmology (M Sc, DV Sc); surgery (M Sc, DV Sc). *Degree requirements:* For master's, thesis; for doctorate, comprehensive exam, thesis/dissertation. *Entrance requirements:* Additional exam requirements/recommendations for international students: Required—TOEFL (minimum score 550 paper-based), IELTS (minimum score 6.5). Electronic applications accepted. *Faculty research:* Orthopedics, respirology, oncology, exercise physiology, cardiology.

Occupational Therapy

Alabama State University, College of Health Sciences, Department of Occupational Therapy, Montgomery, AL 36101-0271. Offers MS. *Accreditation:* AOTA. *Faculty:* 5 full-time (all women). *Students:* 56 full-time (47 women), 1 (woman) part-time; includes 18 minority (17 Black or African American, non-Hispanic/Latino; 1 Hispanic/Latino). 41 applicants, 59% accepted, 23 enrolled. In 2013, 16 master's awarded. *Entrance requirements:* For master's, interview. Application fee: $25. Electronic applications accepted. *Expenses:* Tuition, state resident: full-time $7958; part-time $343 per credit hour. Tuition, nonresident: full-time $14,132; part-time $686 per credit hour. *Required fees:* $446 per term. One-time fee: $1784 full-time; $892 part-time. Tuition and fees vary according to course load. *Unit head:* Dr. Susan Denham, Chair, 334-229-5611, E-mail: sdenham@alasu.edu. *Application contact:* Dr. William Person, Dean of Graduate Studies, 334-229-4274, Fax: 334-229-4928, E-mail: wperson@alasu.edu.
Website: http://www.alasu.edu/academics/colleges—departments/health-sciences/occupational-therapy/index.aspx

Alvernia University, Graduate Studies, Program in Occupational Therapy, Reading, PA 19607-1799. Offers MSOT. *Accreditation:* AOTA. Part-time and evening/weekend programs available. *Degree requirements:* For master's, thesis optional. Electronic applications accepted.

American International College, School of Health Sciences, Occupational Therapy Program, Springfield, MA 01109-3189. Offers MSOT. *Accreditation:* AOTA. *Faculty:* 5 full-time (all women), 2 part-time/adjunct (both women). *Students:* 37 full-time (33 women), 23 part-time (14 women); includes 19 minority (8 Black or African American, non-Hispanic/Latino; 7 Asian, non-Hispanic/Latino; 2 Hispanic/Latino; 1 Native Hawaiian or other Pacific Islander, non-Hispanic/Latino; 1 Two or more races, non-Hispanic/Latino), 1 international. Average age 25. 98 applicants, 47% accepted, 22 enrolled. In 2013, 22 master's awarded. *Degree requirements:* For master's, comprehensive exam, thesis (for some programs), clinical observation. *Entrance requirements:* For master's, bachelor's degree with minimum GPA of 2.85. Additional exam requirements/recommendations for international students: Required—TOEFL or IELTS. *Application deadline:* For fall admission, 4/1 priority date for domestic and international students; for spring admission, 12/1 for domestic and international students. Applications are processed on a rolling basis. Application fee: $50. Electronic applications accepted. *Expenses:* Contact institution. *Financial support:* Career-related internships or fieldwork available. Support available to part-time students. Financial award application deadline: 4/1; financial award applicants required to submit FAFSA. *Faculty research:* Occupational therapy education, use of social media in occupational therapy education, interprofessional collaboration in the health sciences. *Unit head:* Dr. Cathy Dow-Royer, Director, 413-205-3262, Fax: 413-654-1430, E-mail: cathy.dowroyer@aic.edu. *Application contact:* Kerry Barnes, Director of Graduate Admissions, 413-205-3703, Fax: 413-205-3051, E-mail: kerry.barnes@aic.edu.
Website: http://www.aic.edu/academics

A.T. Still University, Arizona School of Health Sciences, Mesa, AZ 85206. Offers advanced occupational therapy (MS); advanced physician assistant studies (MS); athletic training (MS); audiology (Au D); health sciences (DHSc); human movement (MS); occupational therapy (MS, DOT); physical therapy (DPT); physician assistant (MS); transitional audiology (Au D); transitional physical therapy (DPT). *Accreditation:* AOTA (one or more programs are accredited); ASHA. Part-time and evening/weekend programs available. Postbaccalaureate distance learning degree programs offered (minimal on-campus study). *Faculty:* 47 full-time (27 women), 279 part-time/adjunct (173 women). *Students:* 531 full-time (354 women), 865 part-time (547 women); includes 315 minority (79 Black or African American, non-Hispanic/Latino; 10 American Indian or Alaska Native, non-Hispanic/Latino; 114 Asian, non-Hispanic/Latino; 83 Hispanic/Latino; 6 Native Hawaiian or other Pacific Islander, non-Hispanic/Latino; 23 Two or more races, non-Hispanic/Latino), 82 international. Average age 36. 3,325 applicants, 14% accepted, 329 enrolled. In 2013, 252 master's, 370 doctorates awarded. *Degree requirements:* For master's, thesis (for some programs); for doctorate, thesis/dissertation (for some programs). *Entrance requirements:* For master's, GRE General Test; for doctorate, GRE, Evaluation of Practicing Audiologists Capabilities (Au D), Physical Therapist Evaluation Tool (DPT), current state licensure, master's degree or equivalent (Au D). Additional exam requirements/recommendations for international students: Required—TOEFL (minimum score 550 paper-based; 80 iBT). *Application deadline:* For fall admission, 8/1 for domestic and international students. Applications are processed on a rolling basis. Application fee: $70. Electronic applications accepted. *Expenses:* Contact institution. *Financial support:* In 2013–14, 151 students received support. Federal Work-Study and scholarships/grants available. Financial award application deadline: 5/1; financial award applicants required to submit FAFSA. *Faculty research:* Pediatric sport-related concussion, adolescent athlete health-related quality of life; geriatric and pediatric well-being, pain management for participation, practice-based research network, BMI and dental caries. *Total annual research expenditures:* $174,826. *Unit head:* Dr. Randy Danielsen, Dean, 480-219-6000, Fax: 480-219-6110,

E-mail: rdanielsen@atsu.edu. *Application contact:* Donna Sparks, Associate Director, Admissions Processing, 660-626-2117, Fax: 660-626-2969, E-mail: admissions@atsu.edu.
Website: http://www.atsu.edu/ashs

Barry University, College of Health Sciences, Program in Occupational Therapy, Miami Shores, FL 33161-6695. Offers MS. *Accreditation:* AOTA. Electronic applications accepted.

Bay Path College, Program in Occupational Therapy, Longmeadow, MA 01106-2292. Offers MOT. *Accreditation:* AOTA. Part-time programs available. *Students:* 217 full-time (185 women), 13 part-time (all women); includes 36 minority (9 Black or African American, non-Hispanic/Latino; 1 American Indian or Alaska Native, non-Hispanic/Latino; 12 Asian, non-Hispanic/Latino; 7 Hispanic/Latino; 7 Two or more races, non-Hispanic/Latino). Average age 26. 270 applicants, 56% accepted, 99 enrolled. In 2013, 63 master's awarded. *Degree requirements:* For master's, 78 credits and 24 weeks of full-time level II fieldwork following completion of all academic courses. *Entrance requirements:* For master's, bachelor's degree with minimum GPA of 3.0; two courses in anatomy and physiology, and one course each in developmental psychology, statistics, and sociology or culture (for occupational therapy). *Application deadline:* For fall admission, 3/1 priority date for domestic students. Applications are processed on a rolling basis. Application fee: $45. Electronic applications accepted. Application fee is waived when completed online. *Expenses:* Contact institution. *Financial support:* In 2013–14, 118 students received support. Scholarships/grants available. Financial award applicants required to submit FAFSA. *Unit head:* Lori Vaughn, Chair, 413-565-1012. *Application contact:* Lisa Adams, Director of Graduate Admissions, 413-565-1317, Fax: 413-565-1250, E-mail: ladams@baypath.edu.
Website: http://graduate.baypath.edu/Graduate-Programs/Programs-On-Campus/MS-Programs/Master-of-Occupational-Therapy

Belmont University, Gordon E. Inman College of Health Sciences and Nursing, Nashville, TN 37212-3757. Offers nursing (MSN, DNP); occupational therapy (MSOT, OTD); physical therapy (DPT). Part-time programs available. Postbaccalaureate distance learning degree programs offered (minimal on-campus study). *Students:* 290 full-time (172 women), 1 part-time (0 women); includes 43 minority (12 Black or African American, non-Hispanic/Latino; 22 Asian, non-Hispanic/Latino; 8 Hispanic/Latino; 1 Two or more races, non-Hispanic/Latino), 3 international. Average age 26. *Degree requirements:* For master's, comprehensive exam, thesis; for doctorate, comprehensive exam. *Entrance requirements:* For master's, GRE, BSN, minimum GPA of 3.0. Additional exam requirements/recommendations for international students: Required—TOEFL (minimum score 550 paper-based). *Application deadline:* Applications are processed on a rolling basis. Application fee: $50. Electronic applications accepted. *Expenses:* Contact institution. *Financial support:* Teaching assistantships with full tuition reimbursements, career-related internships or fieldwork, scholarships/grants, and traineeships available. Financial award application deadline: 3/1; financial award applicants required to submit FAFSA. *Unit head:* Dean, 615-460-6916, Fax: 615-460-6750. *Application contact:* David Mee, Dean of Enrollment Services, 615-460-6785, Fax: 615-460-5434, E-mail: david.mee@belmont.edu.
Website: http://www.belmont.edu/healthsciences/

Boston University, College of Health and Rehabilitation Sciences: Sargent College, Department of Occupational Therapy, Boston, MA 02215. Offers occupational therapy (MSOT, OTD); rehabilitation sciences (PhD). *Accreditation:* AOTA (one or more programs are accredited). Postbaccalaureate distance learning degree programs offered (minimal on-campus study). *Faculty:* 13 full-time (all women), 2 part-time/adjunct (both women). *Students:* 119 full-time (110 women), 10 part-time (9 women); includes 16 minority (8 Asian, non-Hispanic/Latino; 6 Hispanic/Latino; 2 Two or more races, non-Hispanic/Latino), 2 international. Average age 25. 298 applicants, 29% accepted, 29 enrolled. In 2013, 52 master's, 5 doctorates awarded. *Degree requirements:* For master's, thesis optional, full-time internship; for doctorate, comprehensive exam, thesis/dissertation. *Entrance requirements:* For master's, minimum GPA of 3.0; BS in area related to occupational therapy; for doctorate, GRE General Test. Additional exam requirements/recommendations for international students: Required—TOEFL (minimum score 550 paper-based), TWE (minimum score 5). *Application deadline:* For fall admission, 1/15 priority date for domestic and international students. Applications are processed on a rolling basis. Application fee: $125. Electronic applications accepted. *Expenses: Tuition:* Full-time $43,970; part-time $1374 per credit hour. *Required fees:* $60 per semester. Tuition and fees vary according to class time, course level and program. *Financial support:* In 2013–14, 64 students received support, including 60 fellowships (averaging $12,300 per year), 10 teaching assistantships (averaging $4,000 per year); career-related internships or fieldwork, Federal Work-Study, institutionally sponsored loans, scholarships/grants, and tuition waivers (partial) also available. Financial award application deadline: 4/15; financial award applicants required to submit FAFSA. *Faculty research:* Sensory integration, outcomes measurement, impact of Parkinson's disease, families of people with autism. *Total annual research expenditures:* $378,582. *Unit head:* Dr. Wendy J. Coster, Department Chair, 617-353-2727, Fax: 617-353-2926, E-mail: wjcoster@bu.edu. *Application contact:* Sharon Sankey, Director, Student Services, 617-353-2713, Fax: 617-353-7500, E-mail: ssankey@bu.edu.
Website: http://www.bu.edu/sargent/

Brenau University, Sydney O. Smith Graduate School, College of Health and Science, Gainesville, GA 30501. Offers family nurse practitioner (MSN); nurse educator (MSN); nursing management (MSN); occupational therapy (MS); psychology (MS). *Accreditation:* AOTA. Part-time and evening/weekend programs available. *Degree requirements:* For master's, comprehensive exam (for some programs), thesis (for some programs), clinical practicum hours. *Entrance requirements:* For master's, GRE General Test or MAT (for some programs), interview, writing sample, references (for some programs). Additional exam requirements/recommendations for international students: Required—TOEFL (minimum score 500 paper-based; 61 iBT); Recommended—IELTS (minimum score 5). Electronic applications accepted. *Expenses:* Contact institution.

California State University, Dominguez Hills, College of Health, Human Services and Nursing, Program in Occupational Therapy, Carson, CA 90747-0001. Offers MS. *Accreditation:* AOTA. *Faculty:* 4 full-time (3 women), 6 part-time/adjunct (all women). *Students:* 133 full-time (114 women), 2 part-time (0 women); includes 66 minority (3 Black or African American, non-Hispanic/Latino; 36 Asian, non-Hispanic/Latino; 18 Hispanic/Latino; 1 Native Hawaiian or other Pacific Islander, non-Hispanic/Latino; 8 Two or more races, non-Hispanic/Latino), 3 international. Average age 29. In 2013, 69 master's awarded. *Degree requirements:* For master's, comprehensive exam. *Entrance requirements:* For master's, GRE. Additional exam requirements/recommendations for international students: Required—TOEFL, TWE. *Application deadline:* For fall admission, 9/15 priority date for domestic students. Electronic applications accepted. *Expenses:* Tuition, state resident: full-time $6738. Tuition, nonresident: full-time $13,434. *Required fees:* $622. *Faculty research:* Child school functioning, assessment, lifespan occupational development, low vision occupational therapy intervention. *Unit head:* Dr. Terry Peralta-Catipon, Chair, 310-243-2812, E-mail: tperalta@csudh.edu. *Application contact:* Brandy McLelland, Director of Student Information Services and Registrar, 310-243-3645, E-mail: bmclelland@csudh.edu.
Website: http://www4.csudh.edu/ot/

Chatham University, Program in Occupational Therapy, Pittsburgh, PA 15232-2826. Offers MOT, OTD. *Accreditation:* AOTA. *Faculty:* 6 full-time (all women), 5 part-time/adjunct (4 women). *Students:* 124 full-time (116 women), 12 part-time (10 women); includes 14 minority (6 Black or African American, non-Hispanic/Latino; 3 Asian, non-Hispanic/Latino; 4 Hispanic/Latino; 1 Two or more races, non-Hispanic/Latino), 6 international. Average age 32. 321 applicants, 27% accepted, 64 enrolled. In 2013, 67 master's, 35 doctorates awarded. *Entrance requirements:* For master's, recommendation letter, community service, volunteer service. Additional exam requirements/recommendations for international students: Required—TOEFL (minimum score 600 paper-based; 100 iBT), IELTS (minimum score 7), TWE. *Application deadline:* For fall admission, 12/5 priority date for domestic and international students. Applications are processed on a rolling basis. Application fee: $45. Electronic applications accepted. Application fee is waived when completed online. *Expenses:* Contact institution. *Financial support:* Applicants required to submit FAFSA. *Unit head:* Dr. Joyce Salls, Director, 412-365-1177, E-mail: salls@chatham.edu. *Application contact:* Ashlee Bartko, Senior Assistant Director of Graduate Admission, 412-365-1115, Fax: 412-365-1609, E-mail: gradadmissions@chatham.edu.
Website: http://www.chatham.edu/ot

Chicago State University, School of Graduate and Professional Studies, College of Health Sciences, Department of Occupational Therapy, Chicago, IL 60628. Offers MOT. *Accreditation:* AOTA. Part-time programs available. *Entrance requirements:* For master's, bachelor's degree from accredited college or university with minimum GPA of 3.0 in final 60 semester credit hours; two recommendations; human service experience; essay; interview.

Cleveland State University, College of Graduate Studies, College of Sciences and Health Professions, School of Health Sciences, Program in Occupational Therapy, Cleveland, OH 44115. Offers MOT. *Accreditation:* AOTA. *Faculty:* 7 full-time (5 women), 2 part-time/adjunct (both women). *Students:* 85 full-time (69 women), 33 part-time (29 women); includes 10 minority (5 Black or African American, non-Hispanic/Latino; 2 Asian, non-Hispanic/Latino; 2 Hispanic/Latino; 1 Two or more races, non-Hispanic/Latino), 1 international. Average age 29. 163 applicants, 30% accepted, 40 enrolled. In 2013, 32 master's awarded. *Degree requirements:* For master's, fieldwork, capstone research project. *Entrance requirements:* For master's, GRE (if overall GPA less than 3.0). Additional exam requirements/recommendations for international students: Recommended—TOEFL (minimum score 525 paper-based; 14 iBT), IELTS (minimum score 6). *Application deadline:* For fall admission, 1/15 priority date for domestic and international students. Application fee: $55. Electronic applications accepted. *Expenses:* Tuition, state resident: full-time $8335; part-time $521 per credit hour. Tuition, nonresident: full-time $15,670; part-time $979 per credit hour. *Required fees:* $50; $25 per semester. *Financial support:* In 2013–14, 9 students received support, including 9 teaching assistantships (averaging $11,000 per year); unspecified assistantships also available. Financial award application deadline: 3/15; financial award applicants required to submit FAFSA. *Faculty research:* Pediatrics, psychology, daily living, exercise physiology, neuromuscular disorders. *Total annual research expenditures:* $620,000. *Unit head:* Dr. Glenn D. Goodman, Director, 216-687-2493, Fax: 216-687-9316, E-mail: g.goodman@csuohio.edu. *Application contact:* Karen Armstrong, Administrative Assistant, 216-687-3567, Fax: 216-687-9316, E-mail: k.bradley@csuohio.edu.
Website: http://www.csuohio.edu/sciences/dept/healthsciences/graduate/MOT/index.html

College of Saint Mary, Program in Occupational Therapy, Omaha, NE 68106. Offers MOT. *Accreditation:* AOTA.

The College of St. Scholastica, Graduate Studies, Department of Occupational Therapy, Duluth, MN 55811-4199. Offers MA. *Accreditation:* AOTA. Part-time programs available. *Faculty:* 5 full-time (4 women). *Students:* 67 full-time (59 women), 1 international. Average age 24. 67 applicants, 15% accepted, 6 enrolled. In 2013, 32 master's awarded. *Degree requirements:* For master's, thesis. *Entrance requirements:* Additional exam requirements/recommendations for international students: Required—TOEFL (minimum score 550 paper-based; 79 iBT). *Application deadline:* For fall admission, 11/15 for domestic and international students. Applications are processed on a rolling basis. Electronic applications accepted. Tuition and fees vary according to course load, program and student level. *Financial support:* In 2013–14, 32 students received support, including 1 teaching assistantship (averaging $1,192 per year); scholarships/grants also available. Support available to part-time students. Financial award applicants required to submit FAFSA. *Faculty research:* Gerontology, occupational therapy administration, neurorehabilitation, occupational therapy in nontraditional settings, clinical fieldwork issues. *Unit head:* Steven Cope, Director, 218-723-5915, Fax: 218-723-6290, E-mail: scope@css.edu. *Application contact:* Lindsay Lahti, Director of Graduate and Extended Studies Recruitment, 218-733-2240, Fax: 218-733-2275, E-mail: gradstudies@css.edu.
Website: http://www.css.edu/Graduate/Masters-Doctoral-and-Professional-Programs/Areas-of-Study/MS-Occupational-Therapy.html

Colorado State University, Graduate School, College of Health and Human Sciences, Department of Occupational Therapy, Fort Collins, CO 80523-1573. Offers MOT, MS, PhD. *Accreditation:* AOTA. *Faculty:* 10 full-time (7 women). *Students:* 111 full-time (106 women), 7 part-time (6 women); includes 11 minority (1 Black or African American, non-Hispanic/Latino; 1 American Indian or Alaska Native, non-Hispanic/Latino; 3 Asian, non-Hispanic/Latino; 3 Hispanic/Latino; 3 Two or more races, non-Hispanic/Latino), 3 international. Average age 29. 414 applicants, 14% accepted, 53 enrolled. In 2013, 34 master's awarded. *Degree requirements:* For master's, comprehensive exam, thesis optional; for doctorate, comprehensive exam, thesis/dissertation. *Entrance requirements:* For master's, GRE General Test, minimum cumulative undergraduate or master's GPA of 3.0, essay; for doctorate, GRE General Test, minimum cumulative undergraduate or master's GPA of 3.0. Additional exam requirements/recommendations for international students: Required—TOEFL. *Application deadline:* For fall admission, 1/15 priority date for domestic and international students; for spring admission, 10/15 for domestic and international students. Application fee: $50. Electronic applications accepted. *Expenses:* Tuition, state resident: full-time $9075.40; part-time $504 per credit. Tuition, nonresident: full-time $22,248; part-time $1236 per credit. *Required fees:* $1819; $60 per credit. *Financial support:* In 2013–14, 5 students received support, including 2 research assistantships with partial tuition reimbursements available (averaging $6,540 per year), 3 teaching assistantships with partial tuition reimbursements available (averaging $5,329 per year); scholarships/grants and unspecified assistantships also available. Financial award application deadline: 1/1. *Faculty research:* Stroke rehabilitation, environmental influences on participation of children with disabilities, student veterans in higher education, equine assisted activities and therapy, EEG measures of cognitive and sensory processing. *Total annual research expenditures:* $547,060. *Unit head:* Dr. Wendy Wood, Department Head, 970-491-1882, Fax: 970-491-6920, E-mail: wendy.wood@colostate.edu. *Application contact:* Linda McDowell, Graduate Coordinator, 970-491-6243, Fax: 970-491-6290, E-mail: linda.mcdowell@colostate.edu.
Website: http://www.ot.chhs.colostate.edu/

Columbia University, College of Physicians and Surgeons, Programs in Occupational Therapy, New York, NY 10032. Offers movement science (Ed D), including occupational therapy; occupational therapy (professional) (MS); occupational therapy administration or education (post-professional) (MS); MPH/MS. *Accreditation:* AOTA. *Degree requirements:* For master's, project, 6 months of fieldwork, thesis (for post-professional students); for doctorate, comprehensive exam, thesis/dissertation. *Entrance requirements:* For master's, undergraduate course work in anatomy, physiology, statistics, psychology, social sciences, humanities, English composition; NBCOT eligibility; for doctorate, NBCOT certification, MS. Additional exam requirements/ recommendations for international students: Required—TOEFL (minimum score 100 iBT), TWE (minimum score 4). Electronic applications accepted. *Expenses:* Contact institution. *Faculty research:* Community mental health, developmental tasks of late life, infant play, cognition, obesity, motor learning.

Concordia University Wisconsin, Graduate Programs, School of Human Services, Program in Occupational Therapy, Mequon, WI 53097-2402. Offers MOT. *Accreditation:* AOTA. *Degree requirements:* For master's, comprehensive exam, thesis or alternative. *Entrance requirements:* Additional exam requirements/recommendations for international students: Required—TOEFL.

Creighton University, School of Pharmacy and Health Professions, Program in Occupational Therapy, Omaha, NE 68178-0001. Offers OTD. *Accreditation:* AOTA. Postbaccalaureate distance learning degree programs offered (minimal on-campus study). *Entrance requirements:* Additional exam requirements/recommendations for international students: Required—TOEFL. Electronic applications accepted. *Expenses: Tuition:* Full-time $13,608; part-time $756 per credit hour. *Required fees:* $149 per semester. Tuition and fees vary according to course load, campus/location, program, reciprocity agreements and student's religious affiliation. *Faculty research:* Patient safety in health services research, health information technology and health services research, health care services in minority and underserved populations, occupational therapy in school-based programs, educational technology use in the classroom.

Dalhousie University, Faculty of Health Professions, School of Occupational Therapy, Halifax, NS B3H3J5, Canada. Offers occupational therapy (entry to profession) (M Sc); occupational therapy (post-professional) (M Sc). Part-time and evening/weekend programs available. Postbaccalaureate distance learning degree programs offered (no on-campus study). *Degree requirements:* For master's, thesis. *Entrance requirements:* Additional exam requirements/recommendations for international students: Required—TOEFL, IELTS, CANTEST, CAEL, or Michigan English Language Assessment Battery. Electronic applications accepted. *Faculty research:* Gender, health systems, design, geriatrics power and empowerment.

Dominican College, Division of Allied Health, Department of Occupational Therapy, Orangeburg, NY 10962-1210. Offers MS. Students enter program as undergraduates. *Accreditation:* AOTA. Part-time and evening/weekend programs available. *Faculty:* 3 full-time (all women), 12 part-time/adjunct (11 women). *Students:* 84 full-time (69 women), 23 part-time (20 women). In 2013, 27 master's awarded. *Degree requirements:* For master's, 2 clinical affiliations. *Entrance requirements:* For master's, minimum GPA of 3.0, writing sample, 3 letters of recommendation. Additional exam requirements/ recommendations for international students: Required—TOEFL (minimum score 550 paper-based). *Application deadline:* Applications are processed on a rolling basis. Application fee: $50. *Expenses: Tuition:* Part-time $815 per credit. *Required fees:* $180 per semester. *Financial support:* Applicants required to submit FAFSA. *Unit head:* Dr. Sandra Countee, Program Director, 845-848-7900 Ext. 1219, Fax: 845-398-4893, E-mail: sandra.countee@dc.edu. *Application contact:* Director of Admissions, 845-848-7900, Fax: 845-365-3150, E-mail: admissions@dc.edu.
Website: http://www.dc.edu/

Dominican University of California, School of Health and Natural Sciences, Program in Occupational Therapy, San Rafael, CA 94901-2298. Offers MS. *Accreditation:* AOTA. *Faculty:* 4 full-time (all women), 11 part-time/adjunct (10 women). *Students:* 74 full-time (67 women), 24 part-time (20 women); includes 40 minority (3 Black or African American, non-Hispanic/Latino; 2 American Indian or Alaska Native, non-Hispanic/ Latino; 15 Asian, non-Hispanic/Latino; 17 Hispanic/Latino; 1 Native Hawaiian or other Pacific Islander, non-Hispanic/Latino; 2 Two or more races, non-Hispanic/Latino). Average age 28. 264 applicants, 23% accepted, 40 enrolled. *Degree requirements:* For master's, thesis. *Entrance requirements:* For master's, GRE, minimum GPA of 3.0, minimum of 60 hours of volunteer experience. Additional exam requirements/ recommendations for international students: Required—TOEFL (minimum score 550 paper-based; 80 iBT), IELTS (minimum score 6.5). *Application deadline:* For fall admission, 2/1 priority date for domestic students. Applications are processed on a rolling basis. Electronic applications accepted. *Financial support:* Application deadline: 3/2; applicants required to submit FAFSA. *Unit head:* Dr. Ruth Ramsey, Department Chair and Program Director, 415-257-1393, E-mail: rramsey@dominican.edu. *Application contact:* Ryan Purtill, Admissions Counselor, 415-458-3748, Fax: 415-485-3214, E-mail: ryan.purtill@dominican.edu.
Website: http://www.dominican.edu/academics/hns/ot/grad

Duquesne University, John G. Rangos, Sr. School of Health Sciences, Pittsburgh, PA 15282-0001. Offers health management systems (MHMS); occupational therapy (MS, OTD); physical therapy (DPT); physician assistant studies (MPAS); rehabilitation science (MS, PhD); speech-language pathology (MS); MBA/MHMS. *Accreditation:* AOTA (one or more programs are accredited); APTA (one or more programs are accredited); ASHA. Postbaccalaureate distance learning degree programs offered (minimal on-campus study). *Faculty:* 41 full-time (29 women), 32 part-time/adjunct (15 women). *Students:* 232 full-time (174 women), 14 part-time (7 women); includes 12 minority (2 Black or African American, non-Hispanic/Latino; 7 Asian, non-Hispanic/ Latino; 1 Hispanic/Latino; 2 Two or more races, non-Hispanic/Latino), 7 international. Average age 23. 951 applicants, 11% accepted, 35 enrolled. In 2013, 119 master's, 40 doctorates awarded. *Degree requirements:* For doctorate, comprehensive exam (for some programs), thesis/dissertation (for some programs). *Entrance requirements:* For master's, GRE General Test (speech-language pathology), 3 letters of recommendation; minimum GPA of 2.75 (health management systems), 3.0 (speech-language pathology); for doctorate, GRE General Test (for physical therapy and rehabilitation science), 3 letters of recommendation, minimum GPA of 3.0, personal interview. Additional exam requirements/recommendations for international students: Required—TOEFL (minimum score 550 paper-based; 90 iBT). *Application deadline:* For fall admission, 2/1 for domestic and international students; for spring admission, 7/1 for domestic and international students. Applications are processed on a rolling basis. Electronic applications accepted. *Expenses:* Contact institution. *Financial support:* Federal Work-Study available. Financial award applicants required to submit FAFSA. *Faculty research:* Neuronal processing, electrical stimulation on peripheral neuropathy, central nervous system (CNS) stimulatory and inhibitory signals, behavioral genetic methodologies to development disorders of speech, neurogenic communication disorders. *Total annual research expenditures:* $83,650. *Unit head:* Dr. Gregory H. Frazer, Dean, 412-396-5303, Fax: 412-396-5554, E-mail: frazer@duq.edu. *Application contact:* Christopher R. Hilf, Recruiter/Academic Advisor, 412-396-5653, Fax: 412-396-5554, E-mail: hilfc@duq.edu.
Website: http://www.duq.edu/academics/schools/health-sciences

D'Youville College, Occupational Therapy Department, Buffalo, NY 14201-1084. Offers MS. *Accreditation:* AOTA. *Faculty:* 10 full-time (all women), 4 part-time/adjunct (all women). *Students:* 253 full-time (227 women), 19 part-time (18 women); includes 35 minority (8 Black or African American, non-Hispanic/Latino; 2 American Indian or Alaska Native, non-Hispanic/Latino; 11 Asian, non-Hispanic/Latino; 10 Hispanic/Latino; 4 Two or more races, non-Hispanic/Latino), 19 international. Average age 23. 448 applicants, 40% accepted, 76 enrolled. In 2013, 43 master's awarded. *Degree requirements:* For master's, research project or thesis. *Entrance requirements:* For master's, minimum undergraduate GPA of 3.0. Additional exam requirements/recommendations for international students: Required—TOEFL (minimum score 500 paper-based). *Application deadline:* For fall admission, 5/1 priority date for international students; for spring admission, 9/1 priority date for international students. Applications are processed on a rolling basis. Application fee: $25. Electronic applications accepted. *Financial support:* Scholarships/grants, tuition waivers (partial), and unspecified assistantships available. *Faculty research:* Learning styles, range of motion in the elderly, hospice care, culture, health, differences in education and performance of Afro-American children, autistic spectrum disorder and social stories, autistic disorders and listening programs. *Unit head:* Dr. Theresa Vallone, Chair, 716-829-7831, Fax: 716-829-8137. *Application contact:* Mark Pavone, Graduate Admissions Director, 716-829-8400, Fax: 716-829-7900, E-mail: graduateadmissions@dyc.edu.

East Carolina University, Graduate School, School of Allied Health Sciences, Department of Addictions and Rehabilitation Studies, Greenville, NC 27858-4353. Offers military and trauma counseling (Certificate); rehabilitation and career counseling (MS); rehabilitation counseling (Certificate); rehabilitation counseling and administration (PhD); substance abuse and clinical counseling (MS); substance abuse counseling (Certificate); vocational evaluation (Certificate). *Accreditation:* CORE. Part-time and evening/weekend programs available. *Degree requirements:* For master's, comprehensive exam, thesis or alternative, internship. *Entrance requirements:* For master's, GRE General Test or MAT. Additional exam requirements/recommendations for international students: Required—TOEFL. *Application deadline:* For fall admission, 3/1 priority date for domestic students; for spring admission, 10/1 priority date for domestic students. Applications are processed on a rolling basis. Application fee: $50. *Expenses:* Tuition, state resident: full-time $4223. Tuition, nonresident: full-time $16,540. *Required fees:* $2184. *Financial support:* Research assistantships with partial tuition reimbursements, teaching assistantships with partial tuition reimbursements, Federal Work-Study, and scholarships/grants available. Support available to part-time students. Financial award application deadline: 3/1. *Unit head:* Dr. Paul Toriello, Chair, 252-744-6292, E-mail: toriellop@ecu.edu. *Application contact:* Dr. Paul Toriello, Chair, 252-744-6292, E-mail: toriellop@ecu.edu.
Website: http://www.ecu.edu/rehb/

East Carolina University, Graduate School, School of Allied Health Sciences, Department of Occupational Therapy, Greenville, NC 27858-4353. Offers MSOT. *Accreditation:* AOTA. Part-time programs available. Postbaccalaureate distance learning degree programs offered (minimal on-campus study). *Degree requirements:* For master's, comprehensive exam, thesis or research project. *Entrance requirements:* For master's, GRE General Test. Additional exam requirements/recommendations for international students: Required—TOEFL. *Application deadline:* For fall admission, 6/1 for domestic students. Applications are processed on a rolling basis. Application fee: $50. Electronic applications accepted. *Expenses:* Tuition, state resident: full-time $4223. Tuition, nonresident: full-time $16,540. *Required fees:* $2184. *Financial support:* Research assistantships, career-related internships or fieldwork, and Federal Work-Study available. Financial award application deadline: 6/1; financial award applicants required to submit FAFSA. *Faculty research:* Quality of life, assistive technology, environmental contributions, modifications of occupation to health, therapeutic activities. *Unit head:* Dr. Leonard Trujillo, Chair, 252-744-6195, E-mail: trujillol@ecu.edu. *Application contact:* Dean of Graduate School, 252-328-6012, Fax: 252-328-6071, E-mail: gradschool@ecu.edu.
Website: http://www.ecu.edu/ot/

Eastern Kentucky University, The Graduate School, College of Health Sciences, Department of Occupational Therapy, Richmond, KY 40475-3102. Offers MS. *Accreditation:* AOTA. Part-time programs available. *Degree requirements:* For master's, thesis optional. *Entrance requirements:* For master's, GRE General Test, minimum GPA of 3.0. *Faculty research:* Rehabilitation, pediatrics, leadership issues.

Eastern Michigan University, Graduate School, College of Health and Human Services, School of Health Sciences, Program in Occupational Therapy, Ypsilanti, MI 48197. Offers MOT, MS. *Accreditation:* AOTA. Part-time and evening/weekend programs available. Postbaccalaureate distance learning degree programs offered (minimal on-campus study). *Students:* 25 full-time (24 women), 37 part-time (32 women); includes 3 minority (1 Black or African American, non-Hispanic/Latino; 2 Asian, non-Hispanic/Latino). Average age 28. 11 applicants, 73% accepted, 7 enrolled. In 2013, 38 master's awarded. *Entrance requirements:* Additional exam requirements/ recommendations for international students: Required—TOEFL. *Application deadline:* Applications are processed on a rolling basis. Application fee: $35. *Expenses:* Tuition, state resident: full-time $12,300; part-time $466 per credit hour. Tuition, nonresident: full-time $23,159; part-time $918 per credit hour. *Required fees:* $71 per credit hour. $46 per semester. One-time fee: $100. Tuition and fees vary according to course level and degree level. *Financial support:* Fellowships, research assistantships with full tuition reimbursements, teaching assistantships with full tuition reimbursements, career-related internships or fieldwork, Federal Work-Study, institutionally sponsored loans, scholarships/grants, tuition waivers (partial), and unspecified assistantships available. Support available to part-time students. Financial award applicants required to submit FAFSA. *Unit head:* Dr. Colleen Croxall, Director, 734-487-4096, Fax: 734-487-4095, E-mail: ccroxall@emich.edu. *Application contact:* Dr. Amy Lamb, Program Director, 734-487-4096, Fax: 734-487-4095, E-mail: alamb9@emich.edu.

Eastern Washington University, Graduate Studies, College of Science, Health and Engineering, Department of Occupational Therapy, Cheney, WA 99004-2431. Offers MOT. *Accreditation:* AOTA. *Faculty:* 6 full-time (5 women). *Students:* 101 full-time (79 women), 2 part-time (0 women); includes 17 minority (1 Black or African American, non-Hispanic/Latino; 10 Asian, non-Hispanic/Latino; 6 Hispanic/Latino). 12 applicants, 83% accepted, 10 enrolled. In 2013, 31 master's awarded. *Degree requirements:* For master's, comprehensive exam. *Financial support:* Career-related internships or fieldwork, Federal Work-Study, institutionally sponsored loans, scholarships/grants, tuition waivers (partial), and unspecified assistantships available. Support available to part-time students. Financial award applicants required to submit FAFSA. *Unit head:* Dr. Gregory Wintz, Chair, 509-368-6562, Fax: 509-368-6561. *Application contact:* Julie Marr, Associate Dean for Graduate Studies, 509-359-6297, Fax: 509-359-6044, E-mail: gradprograms@ewu.edu.
Website: http://www.ewu.edu/cshe/programs/occupational-therapy.xml

Elizabethtown College, Department of Occupational Therapy, Elizabethtown, PA 17022-2298. Offers MS. *Accreditation:* AOTA.

Florida Agricultural and Mechanical University, Division of Graduate Studies, Research, and Continuing Education, School of Allied Health Sciences, Division of Occupational Therapy, Tallahassee, FL 32307-3200. Offers MOT. *Accreditation:* AOTA.

Occupational Therapy

Florida Gulf Coast University, College of Health Professions, Department of Occupational Therapy, Fort Myers, FL 33965-6565. Offers MS. *Accreditation:* AOTA. *Entrance requirements:* For master's, GRE General Test, MAT, minimum GPA of 3.0. Additional exam requirements/recommendations for international students: Required—TOEFL (minimum score 550 paper-based). Electronic applications accepted.

Florida International University, College of Nursing and Health Sciences, Department of Occupational Therapy, Miami, FL 33199. Offers MSOT. *Accreditation:* AOTA. Part-time programs available. *Degree requirements:* For master's, thesis or alternative. *Entrance requirements:* For master's, minimum undergraduate GPA of 3.0 in upper-level course work, letter of intent, 3 letters of recommendation, resume. Additional exam requirements/recommendations for international students: Required—TOEFL (minimum score 550 paper-based; 80 iBT). Electronic applications accepted. *Expenses:* Contact institution. *Faculty research:* Senior transportation and driving, foster care, adolescent transitions, independent living skills development, family and patient-centered care, aging, quality of life, social justice, cognition.

Gannon University, School of Graduate Studies, Morosky College of Health Professions and Sciences, School of Health Professions, Program in Occupational Therapy, Erie, PA 16541-0001. Offers MS. *Accreditation:* AOTA. *Students:* 48 full-time (43 women), 1 (woman) part-time; includes 1 minority (Black or African American, non-Hispanic/Latino), 1 international. Average age 24. 14 applicants, 7% accepted. In 2013, 37 master's awarded. *Degree requirements:* For master's, thesis, field work. *Entrance requirements:* For master's, letters of recommendation, interview, minimum GPA of 3.0, 40 hours of volunteer experience. Additional exam requirements/recommendations for international students: Required—TOEFL (minimum score 79 iBT). *Application deadline:* For fall admission, 1/15 for domestic students. Application fee: $25. Electronic applications accepted. *Expenses:* Contact institution. *Financial support:* Scholarships/grants and unspecified assistantships available. Financial award application deadline: 7/1; financial award applicants required to submit FAFSA. *Faculty research:* Assistive technology, autism, sexuality in occupational therapy intervention, health and wellness in Parkinson's disease, occupational science. *Unit head:* Dr. David LeVan, Director, 814-871-7730, E-mail: levan005@gannon.edu. *Application contact:* Kara Morgan, Director of Graduate Admissions, 814-871-5831, Fax: 814-871-5827, E-mail: graduate@gannon.edu.

Governors State University, College of Health Professions, Program in Occupational Therapy, University Park, IL 60484. Offers MOT. *Accreditation:* AOTA. *Degree requirements:* For master's, thesis or alternative. *Entrance requirements:* For master's, minimum GPA of 3.0 in field, 2.75 overall.

Grand Valley State University, College of Health Professions, Occupational Therapy Program, Allendale, MI 49401-9403. Offers MS. *Accreditation:* AOTA. *Degree requirements:* For master's, thesis or alternative, fieldwork, project. *Entrance requirements:* For master's, interview, volunteer work, writing sample. Additional exam requirements/recommendations for international students: Required—TOEFL (minimum score 610 paper-based). Electronic applications accepted. *Faculty research:* Teaching/learning methods, continuing professional education, clinical reasoning, geriatrics, performing artists.

Husson University, Master's in Occupational Therapy Program, Bangor, ME 04401-2999. Offers MSOT. *Accreditation:* AOTA. *Faculty:* 5 full-time (all women), 2 part-time/adjunct (0 women). *Students:* 48 full-time (44 women); includes 1 minority (Asian, non-Hispanic/Latino). Average age 23. 47 applicants, 23% accepted, 6 enrolled. In 2013, 37 master's awarded. *Degree requirements:* For master's, research project, paper and presentation. *Entrance requirements:* For master's, GRE, BS with minimum GPA of 3.0. Additional exam requirements/recommendations for international students: Required—TOEFL (minimum score 550 paper-based). *Application deadline:* For fall admission, 5/1 for domestic students. Application fee: $40. Electronic applications accepted. *Expenses:* Contact institution. *Financial support:* Federal Work-Study, scholarships/grants, and unspecified assistantships available. Financial award application deadline: 4/15; financial award applicants required to submit FAFSA. *Unit head:* Dr. Laurie Mouradian, Program Director, 207-404-5630, E-mail: mouradianl@husson.edu. *Application contact:* Kristen Card, Director of Graduate Admissions, 207-404-5660, E-mail: cardk@husson.edu.
Website: http://www.husson.edu/occupational-therapy

Idaho State University, Office of Graduate Studies, Kasiska College of Health Professions, Department of Physical and Occupational Therapy, Program in Occupational Therapy, Pocatello, ID 83209-8045. Offers MOT. *Accreditation:* AOTA. *Degree requirements:* For master's, comprehensive exam, thesis, oral and written exam. *Entrance requirements:* For master's, GRE General Test, minimum GPA of 3.0, 80 hours in 2 practice settings of occupational therapy. Additional exam requirements/recommendations for international students: Required—TOEFL (minimum score 600 paper-based). Electronic applications accepted. *Expenses:* Contact institution. *Faculty research:* Human movement, health care.

Indiana University–Purdue University Indianapolis, School of Health and Rehabilitation Sciences, Indianapolis, IN 46202. Offers health and rehabilitation sciences (PhD); health sciences (MS); nutrition and dietetics (MS); occupational therapy (MS); physical therapy (DPT); physician assistant (MPAS). Part-time and evening/weekend programs available. *Faculty:* 4 full-time (3 women). *Students:* 266 full-time (201 women), 13 part-time (12 women); includes 21 minority (6 Black or African American, non-Hispanic/Latino; 7 Asian, non-Hispanic/Latino; 4 Hispanic/Latino; 1 Native Hawaiian or other Pacific Islander, non-Hispanic/Latino; 3 Two or more races, non-Hispanic/Latino), 11 international. Average age 26. 381 applicants, 23% accepted, 77 enrolled. In 2013, 33 master's, 39 doctorates awarded. *Degree requirements:* For master's, thesis (for some programs). *Entrance requirements:* For master's, GRE General Test, minimum GPA of 3.0 (for MS in health sciences, nutrition and dietetics), 3.2 (for MS in occupational therapy), 3.0 cumulative and prerequisite math/science (for MPAS); for doctorate, GRE, minimum cumulative and prerequisite math/science GPA of 3.2. Additional exam requirements/recommendations for international students: Required—TOEFL (minimum score 550 paper-based; 79 iBT), IELTS (minimum score 6.5), PTE (minimum score 54). *Application deadline:* For fall admission, 10/1 for domestic students; for spring admission, 10/15 for domestic students. Electronic applications accepted. *Expenses:* Contact institution. *Financial support:* Fellowships, research assistantships, Federal Work-Study, institutionally sponsored loans, and scholarships/grants available. Support available to part-time students. Financial award applicants required to submit FAFSA. *Faculty research:* Function and mobility across the lifespan, pediatric nutrition, driving and mobility rehabilitation, neurorehabilitation and biomechanics, rehabilitation and integrative therapy. *Total annual research expenditures:* $1.1 million. *Unit head:* Dr. Augustine Agho, Dean, 317-274-4704, E-mail: aagho@iu.edu. *Application contact:* Kim Crockett, Student Data Coordinator, 317-278-6744, E-mail: kimecroc@iu.edu.
Website: http://shrs.iupui.edu/

Ithaca College, School of Health Sciences and Human Performance, Program in Occupational Therapy, Ithaca, NY 14850. Offers MS. *Accreditation:* AOTA. *Faculty:* 9 full-time (all women). *Students:* 54 full-time (51 women), 3 part-time (2 women); includes 10 minority (1 Asian, non-Hispanic/Latino; 7 Hispanic/Latino; 2 Two or more races, non-Hispanic/Latino). Average age 24. In 2013, 42 master's awarded. *Degree requirements:* For master's, thesis optional, clinical fieldwork. *Entrance requirements:* Additional exam requirements/recommendations for international students: Required—TOEFL (minimum score 550 paper-based; 80 iBT). Tuition and fees vary according to program. *Financial support:* In 2013–14, 41 students received support, including 11 teaching assistantships (averaging $9,084 per year); career-related internships or fieldwork, Federal Work-Study, and scholarships/grants also available. Support available to part-time students. Financial award application deadline: 3/1; financial award applicants required to submit CSS PROFILE or FAFSA. *Faculty research:* Sensory integration intervention, therapeutic listening, motor control intervention for pediatrics and adults, adult neuromuscular facilitation for individuals with neurological impairments, school-aged handwriting assessment, psychosocial community, intervention and assessment, virtual reality and robotic training for children with neurological and or sensory disorders, clinical reasoning, aging and human occupations. *Unit head:* Dr. Melinda Cozzolino, Chair, 607-274-3143, Fax: 607-274-1263, E-mail: gps@ithaca.edu. *Application contact:* Gerard Turbide, Director, Office of Admission, 607-274-3143, Fax: 607-274-1263, E-mail: gps@ithaca.edu.
Website: http://www.ithaca.edu/gps/gradprograms/ot

James Madison University, The Graduate School, College of Health and Behavioral Studies, Department of Health Sciences, Program in Occupational Therapy, Harrisonburg, VA 22807. Offers MOT. *Accreditation:* AOTA. Part-time programs available. *Students:* 63 full-time (56 women), 1 (woman) part-time; includes 11 minority (2 Black or African American, non-Hispanic/Latino; 4 Asian, non-Hispanic/Latino; 4 Hispanic/Latino; 1 Two or more races, non-Hispanic/Latino). Average age 27. In 2013, 22 master's awarded. *Entrance requirements:* For master's, GRE General Test, GRE Subject Test, 3 reference forms, evidence of one instructional experience, documentation of competency in computer technology and information-seeking skills. *Application deadline:* For fall admission, 2/1 priority date for domestic students. Application fee: $55. *Financial support:* Application deadline: 3/1; applicants required to submit FAFSA. *Unit head:* Dr. Jeff Loveland, Director, 540-568-2399, E-mail: lovelajd@jmu.edu. *Application contact:* Lynette M. Bible, Director of Graduate Admissions, 540-568-6395, Fax: 540-568-7860, E-mail: biblelm@jmu.edu.

Jefferson College of Health Sciences, Program in Occupational Therapy, Roanoke, VA 24031-3186. Offers MS. *Accreditation:* AOTA. Part-time programs available. *Entrance requirements:* For master's, GRE. Additional exam requirements/recommendations for international students: Required—TOEFL (minimum score 550 paper-based; 80 iBT). Electronic applications accepted.

Kean University, Nathan Weiss Graduate College, Program in Occupational Therapy, Union, NJ 07083. Offers MS. *Accreditation:* AOTA. Part-time programs available. *Faculty:* 5 full-time (all women). *Students:* 67 full-time (57 women), 27 part-time (22 women); includes 18 minority (1 Black or African American, non-Hispanic/Latino; 5 Asian, non-Hispanic/Latino; 11 Hispanic/Latino; 1 Two or more races, non-Hispanic/Latino), 1 international. Average age 26. 254 applicants, 17% accepted, 34 enrolled. In 2013, 27 master's awarded. *Degree requirements:* For master's, 6 months of field work, final project. *Entrance requirements:* For master's, minimum GPA of 3.0, minimum grade of B in each prerequisite course, official transcripts from all institutions attended, three letters of recommendation (one letter must be from an occupational therapist), documented observation of occupational therapy services in two or more practice settings for a minimum of 40 hours. Additional exam requirements/recommendations for international students: Required—TOEFL (minimum score 550 paper-based; 79 iBT). *Application deadline:* For fall admission, 2/1 for domestic and international students. Applications are processed on a rolling basis. Application fee: $75 ($150 for international students). Electronic applications accepted. *Expenses:* Tuition, state resident: full-time $12,099; part-time $589 per credit. Tuition, nonresident: full-time $16,399; part-time $722 per credit. *Required fees:* $3050; $139 per credit. Part-time tuition and fees vary according to course level, course load, degree level and program. *Financial support:* In 2013–14, 13 research assistantships with full tuition reimbursements (averaging $3,713 per year) were awarded; unspecified assistantships also available. Financial award applicants required to submit FAFSA. *Unit head:* Dr. Laurie Knis-Matthews, Program Coordinator, 908-737-5850, Fax: 908-737-3377, E-mail: ot@kean.edu. *Application contact:* Reenat Hasan, Admissions Counselor, 908-737-5923, Fax: 908-737-5925, E-mail: hasanr@kean.edu.
Website: http://grad.kean.edu/ot

Keuka College, Program in Occupational Therapy, Keuka Park, NY 14478-0098. Offers MS. *Accreditation:* AOTA. *Faculty:* 5 full-time (3 women). *Students:* 29 full-time (27 women). Average age 23. 15 applicants, 100% accepted. In 2013, 21 master's awarded. *Degree requirements:* For master's, thesis or alternative, clinical internships. *Entrance requirements:* For master's, minimum GPA of 3.0, BS in occupational therapy at Keuka College. Additional exam requirements/recommendations for international students: Required—TOEFL (minimum score 550 paper-based). *Application deadline:* For fall admission, 8/15 priority date for domestic students; for winter admission, 12/15 priority date for domestic students; for spring admission, 4/15 priority date for domestic students. Applications are processed on a rolling basis. Application fee: $30. *Expenses:* Contact institution. *Unit head:* Dr. Vicki Smith, Associate Professor and Chair, 315-279-5666, Fax: 315-279-5439, E-mail: vlsmith@mail.keuka.edu. *Application contact:* Mark Petrie, Dean of Enrollment, 315-279-5413, Fax: 315-279-5386, E-mail: admissions@mail.keuka.edu.

Lenoir-Rhyne University, Graduate Programs, School of Occupational Therapy, Hickory, NC 28601. Offers MS. *Accreditation:* AOTA. *Entrance requirements:* For master's, GRE or MAT, minimum GPA of 2.7.

Loma Linda University, School of Allied Health Professions, Department of Occupational Therapy, Loma Linda, CA 92350. Offers MOT, OTD. *Accreditation:* AOTA.

Louisiana State University Health Sciences Center, School of Allied Health Professions, Department of Occupational Therapy, New Orleans, LA 70112-2223. Offers MOT. *Accreditation:* AOTA. *Faculty:* 5 full-time (all women), 1 (woman) part-time/adjunct. *Students:* 60 full-time (50 women); includes 10 minority (5 Black or African American, non-Hispanic/Latino; 1 Asian, non-Hispanic/Latino; 3 Hispanic/Latino; 1 Two or more races, non-Hispanic/Latino). Average age 25. 127 applicants, 24% accepted, 31 enrolled. In 2013, 33 master's awarded. *Entrance requirements:* For master's, GRE (minimum scores: 150 verbal and 141 quantitative), bachelor's degree, 40 hours of observation in occupational therapy. *Application deadline:* For spring admission, 7/1 priority date for domestic students. Application fee: $50. *Financial support:* In 2013–14, 29 students received support. Application deadline: 4/15. *Unit head:* Dr. Rennie U. Jacobs, Interim Head, 504-568-4308, Fax: 504-568-4306, E-mail: rjaco1@lsuhsc.edu. *Application contact:* Yudialys Delgado, Student Affairs Director, 504-568-4253, Fax: 504-568-3185, E-mail: ydelga@lsuhsc.edu.
Website: http://alliedhealth.lsuhsc.edu/ot/

Maryville University of Saint Louis, College of Health Professions, Occupational Therapy Program, St. Louis, MO 63141-7299. Offers MOT. *Accreditation:* AOTA. *Students:* 30 part-time (29 women); includes 1 minority (Hispanic/Latino). Average age 23. In 2013, 27 master's awarded. *Entrance requirements:* For master's, ACT (minimum composite score of 21) or SAT-I (minimum combined score of 990) unless applicant has

completed more than 30 college credits, minimum cumulative GPA of 3.0, resume, interview, writing sample. Additional exam requirements/recommendations for international students: Required—TOEFL (minimum score 550 paper-based). *Application deadline:* Applications are processed on a rolling basis. Application fee: $40 ($60 for international students). Electronic applications accepted. Application fee is waived when completed online. *Expenses:* Contact institution. *Financial support:* Career-related internships or fieldwork, Federal Work-Study, and campus employment available. Financial award application deadline: 3/1; financial award applicants required to submit FAFSA. *Faculty research:* Older driver safety rehabilitation options, adaptive equipment and training remediation, injured workers disability interventions. *Unit head:* Dr. Paula Bohr, Director, 314-529-9682, Fax: 314-529-9191, E-mail: pbohr@maryville.edu. *Application contact:* Crystal Jacobsmeyer, Assistant Director, Graduate Enrollment Advising, 314-529-9654, Fax: 314-529-9927, E-mail: cjacobsmeyer@maryville.edu.
Website: http://www.maryville.edu/hp/occupational-therapy/

McMaster University, Faculty of Health Sciences, Professional Program in Occupational Therapy, Hamilton, ON L8S 4M2, Canada. Offers M Sc. *Degree requirements:* For master's, fieldwork and independent research project. *Entrance requirements:* For master's, minimum B average over last 60 undergraduate units. Additional exam requirements/recommendations for international students: Required—TOEFL (minimum score 600 paper-based).

Medical University of South Carolina, College of Health Professions, Program in Occupational Therapy, Charleston, SC 29425. Offers MSOT. *Accreditation:* AOTA. *Degree requirements:* For master's, thesis or alternative, research project. *Entrance requirements:* For master's, GRE General Test, interview, minimum GPA of 3.0, references. Additional exam requirements/recommendations for international students: Required—TOEFL (minimum score 600 paper-based). Electronic applications accepted. *Faculty research:* Therapeutic interventions for children with cerebral palsy; function, well being, quality of life for adults with chronic conditions and health disparities; driving interventions for adults with head and neck cancer; oral health for adults with tetraplegia; interprofessional education.

Mercy College, School of Health and Natural Sciences, Program in Occupational Therapy, Dobbs Ferry, NY 10522-1189. Offers MS. *Accreditation:* AOTA. Evening/weekend programs available. *Students:* 65 full-time (57 women), 33 part-time (28 women); includes 38 minority (9 Black or African American, non-Hispanic/Latino; 8 Asian, non-Hispanic/Latino; 14 Hispanic/Latino; 5 Native Hawaiian or other Pacific Islander, non-Hispanic/Latino; 2 Two or more races, non-Hispanic/Latino), 3 international. Average age 33. 163 applicants, 25% accepted, 34 enrolled. In 2013, 34 master's awarded. *Degree requirements:* For master's, comprehensive exam (for some programs), thesis, fieldwork. *Entrance requirements:* For master's, essay, 3 letters of recommendation, interview, resume, undergraduate transcripts with minimum GPA of 3.0. Additional exam requirements/recommendations for international students: Required—TOEFL (minimum score 600 paper-based; 100 iBT), IELTS (minimum score 8). *Application deadline:* Applications are processed on a rolling basis. Application fee: $62. Electronic applications accepted. *Expenses:* Contact institution. *Financial support:* Career-related internships or fieldwork, Federal Work-Study, scholarships/grants, and unspecified assistantships available. Support available to part-time students. Financial award applicants required to submit FAFSA. *Unit head:* Dr. Joan Toglia, Dean, School of Health and Natural Sciences, 914-674-7837, E-mail: jtoglia@mercy.edu. *Application contact:* Allison Gurdineer, Senior Director of Admissions, 877-637-2946, Fax: 914-674-7382, E-mail: admissions@mercy.edu.
Website: https://www.mercy.edu/academics/school-of-health-and-natural-sciences/department-of-health-professions/ms-in-occupational-therapy/

MGH Institute of Health Professions, School of Health and Rehabilitation Sciences, Department of Occupational Therapy, Boston, MA 02129. Offers OTD. *Entrance requirements:* For doctorate, GRE, bachelor's degree from regionally-accredited U.S. college or university with minimum undergraduate GPA of 3.0; official transcripts; personal statement; recommendation letters. Additional exam requirements/recommendations for international students: Required—TOEFL (minimum score 80 iBT). *Application deadline:* For summer admission, 12/1 for domestic and international students. Electronic applications accepted. *Expenses: Tuition:* Part-time $1114 per credit. *Required fees:* $620 per term. One-time fee: $475 part-time. *Unit head:* Regina Doherty, Program Director, 617-643-7768, Fax: 617-724-6321, E-mail: rdoherty@mghihp.edu. *Application contact:* Catherine Hamiton, Assistant Director of Admission and Multicultural Recruitment, 617-726-3140, Fax: 617-726-8010, E-mail: admissions@mghihp.edu.
Website: http://www.mghihp.edu/academics/school-of-health-and-rehabilitation-sciences/occupational-therapy/

Midwestern University, Downers Grove Campus, College of Health Sciences, Illinois Campus, Program in Occupational Therapy, Downers Grove, IL 60515-1235. Offers MOT. *Accreditation:* AOTA. *Entrance requirements:* For master's, GRE General Test. *Expenses:* Contact institution.

Midwestern University, Glendale Campus, College of Health Sciences, Arizona Campus, Program in Occupational Therapy, Glendale, AZ 85308. Offers MOT. *Accreditation:* AOTA. *Entrance requirements:* For master's, GRE. *Expenses:* Contact institution.

Milligan College, Program in Occupational Therapy, Milligan College, TN 37682. Offers MSOT. *Accreditation:* AOTA. *Faculty:* 6 full-time (4 women), 5 part-time/adjunct (4 women). *Students:* 92 full-time (82 women). Average age 30. 300 applicants, 13% accepted, 32 enrolled. In 2013, 31 master's awarded. *Degree requirements:* For master's, thesis. *Entrance requirements:* For master's, GRE. Additional exam requirements/recommendations for international students: Required—TOEFL (minimum score 550 paper-based; 80 iBT). *Application deadline:* For spring admission, 1/1 for domestic and international students. Application fee: $30. Electronic applications accepted. *Expenses:* Contact institution. *Financial support:* Career-related internships or fieldwork and institutionally sponsored loans available. Financial award application deadline: 4/15; financial award applicants required to submit FAFSA. *Faculty research:* Handwriting, creativity, leadership in health care and rehabilitation, prevention and rehabilitation of work-related musculoskeletal disorders, parent-child interaction therapy, community-based occupational therapy programs. *Unit head:* Dr. Jeff Snodgrass, Program Director and Associate Professor, 423-975-8010, Fax: 423-975-8019, E-mail: jsnodgrass@milligan.edu. *Application contact:* Kristia Brown, Office Manager and Admissions Representative, 423-975-8010, Fax: 423-975-8019, E-mail: kngarland@milligan.edu.
Website: http://www.milligan.edu/msot/

Misericordia University, College of Health Sciences, Program in Occupational Therapy, Dallas, PA 18612-1098. Offers MSOT, OTD. *Accreditation:* AOTA. *Faculty:* 4 full-time (2 women), 15 part-time/adjunct (13 women). *Students:* 30 full-time (28 women), 67 part-time (62 women); includes 6 minority (2 Asian, non-Hispanic/Latino; 3 Hispanic/Latino; 1 Two or more races, non-Hispanic/Latino), 1 international. Average age 29. In 2013, 44 master's, 5 doctorates awarded. *Entrance requirements:* For master's, minimum undergraduate GPA of 2.8, 2 letters of reference; for doctorate, minimum graduate GPA of 3.0, interview, 3 letters of reference. Additional exam requirements/recommendations for international students: Required—TOEFL. *Application deadline:* Applications are processed on a rolling basis. Application fee: $35. Electronic applications accepted. *Expenses: Tuition:* Full-time $14,450; part-time $680 per credit. Tuition and fees vary according to degree level. *Financial support:* In 2013–14, 35 students received support. Teaching assistantships, career-related internships or fieldwork, and scholarships/grants available. Support available to part-time students. Financial award application deadline: 6/30; financial award applicants required to submit FAFSA. *Unit head:* Dr. Grace Fisher, Chair, 570-674-8015, E-mail: gfisher@misericordia.edu. *Application contact:* Maureen Sheridan, Assistant Director of Admissions, Part-Time Undergraduate and Graduate Programs, 570-674-6451, E-mail: msherida@misericordia.edu.
Website: http://www.misericordia.edu/ot

Mount Mary University, Graduate Division, Program in Occupational Therapy, Milwaukee, WI 53222-4597. Offers MS. *Accreditation:* AOTA. Part-time and evening/weekend programs available. *Faculty:* 7 full-time (all women), 5 part-time/adjunct (4 women). *Students:* 118 full-time (104 women); includes 15 minority (4 Black or African American, non-Hispanic/Latino; 5 Asian, non-Hispanic/Latino; 5 Hispanic/Latino; 1 Two or more races, non-Hispanic/Latino). Average age 28. 72 applicants, 61% accepted, 35 enrolled. In 2013, 43 master's awarded. *Degree requirements:* For master's, comprehensive exam, thesis or alternative, professional development portfolio. *Entrance requirements:* For master's, minimum GPA of 3.0, occupational therapy license, 1 year of work experience. Additional exam requirements/recommendations for international students: Required—TOEFL (minimum score 80 iBT) or IELTS (minimum score 6.5). *Application deadline:* For fall admission, 1/15 priority date for domestic and international students; for spring admission, 3/15 for domestic and international students. Application fee: $45 ($100 for international students). Electronic applications accepted. *Expenses:* Contact institution. *Financial support:* Career-related internships or fieldwork and Federal Work-Study available. Support available to part-time students. Financial award application deadline: 5/1; financial award applicants required to submit FAFSA. *Faculty research:* Clinical reasoning, occupational science, sensory integration. *Unit head:* Dr. Kari Inda, Director, 414-258-4810 Ext. 263, E-mail: indak@mtmary.edu. *Application contact:* Dr. Douglas J. Mickelson, Dean for Graduate Education, 414-256-1252, Fax: 414-256-0167, E-mail: mickelsd@mtmary.edu.
Website: http://www.mtmary.edu/majors-programs/graduate/occupational-therapy/index.html

New England Institute of Technology, Program in Occupational Therapy, East Greenwich, RI 02818. Offers MS. *Accreditation:* AOTA. Part-time and evening/weekend programs available. *Students:* 37 full-time (34 women), 8 part-time (6 women); includes 5 minority (1 Black or African American, non-Hispanic/Latino; 1 American Indian or Alaska Native, non-Hispanic/Latino; 1 Asian, non-Hispanic/Latino; 2 Hispanic/Latino). Average age 34. *Degree requirements:* For master's, fieldwork. *Application deadline:* For fall admission, 10/1 for domestic students. Applications are processed on a rolling basis. Application fee: $25. Electronic applications accepted. *Application contact:* James Jessup, Director of Admissions, 401-467-7744 Ext. 3339, E-mail: jjessup@neit.edu.

New York Institute of Technology, School of Health Professions, Department of Occupational Therapy, Old Westbury, NY 11568-8000. Offers MS. *Accreditation:* AOTA. *Faculty:* 5 full-time (all women), 7 part-time/adjunct (6 women). *Students:* 125 full-time (97 women), 2 part-time (1 woman); includes 36 minority (11 Black or African American, non-Hispanic/Latino; 18 Asian, non-Hispanic/Latino; 6 Hispanic/Latino; 1 Native Hawaiian or other Pacific Islander, non-Hispanic/Latino). Average age 25. 167 applicants, 38% accepted, 45 enrolled. In 2013, 27 master's awarded. *Degree requirements:* For master's, thesis. *Entrance requirements:* For master's, minimum GPA of 2.0 in science or mathematics, 2.5 overall; 100 hours of supervised volunteer work; interview; 2 professional letters of recommendation. Additional exam requirements/recommendations for international students: Required—TOEFL (minimum score 550 paper-based; 79 iBT), IELTS (minimum score 6). *Application deadline:* For fall admission, 7/1 priority date for domestic students, 6/1 for international students; for spring admission, 12/1 priority date for domestic students, 12/1 for international students. Applications are processed on a rolling basis. Application fee: $50. Electronic applications accepted. *Expenses: Tuition:* Full-time $18,900; part-time $1050 per credit. *Financial support:* Research assistantships with partial tuition reimbursements, scholarships/grants, health care benefits, tuition waivers, and unspecified assistantships available. Support available to part-time students. Financial award applicants required to submit FAFSA. *Faculty research:* Health and wellness in aging population, technology in education, caregiver burden in ALS, strategies to increase student learning. *Unit head:* Dr. Gioia Ciani, Department Chairperson, 516-686-3886, E-mail: gciani@nyit.edu. *Application contact:* Alice Dolitsky, Director, Graduate Admissions, 516-686-7520, Fax: 516-686-1116, E-mail: nyitgrad@nyit.edu.
Website: http://www.nyit.edu/occupational_therapy

New York University, Steinhardt School of Culture, Education, and Human Development, Department of Occupational Therapy, New York, NY 10012. Offers advanced occupational therapy (MA); occupational therapy (MS, DPS); research in occupational therapy (PhD). *Accreditation:* AOTA (one or more programs are accredited). Part-time programs available. *Faculty:* 11 full-time (8 women), 12 part-time/adjunct (10 women). *Students:* 176 full-time (162 women), 20 part-time (19 women); includes 67 minority (8 Black or African American, non-Hispanic/Latino; 40 Asian, non-Hispanic/Latino; 14 Hispanic/Latino; 1 Native Hawaiian or other Pacific Islander, non-Hispanic/Latino; 4 Two or more races, non-Hispanic/Latino), 8 international. Average age 33. 575 applicants, 21% accepted, 57 enrolled. In 2013, 54 master's, 1 doctorate awarded. *Degree requirements:* For master's, thesis (for some programs), terminal project; fieldwork; for doctorate, thesis/dissertation, terminal project. *Entrance requirements:* For doctorate, GRE General Test, interview. Additional exam requirements/recommendations for international students: Required—TOEFL (minimum score 100 iBT). *Application deadline:* For fall admission, 12/1 priority date for domestic and international students. Applications are processed on a rolling basis. Application fee: $75. Electronic applications accepted. *Expenses: Tuition:* Full-time $35,856; part-time $1494 per unit. *Required fees:* $1408; $64 per unit. $473 per term. Tuition and fees vary according to course load and program. *Financial support:* Fellowships with full and partial tuition reimbursements, teaching assistantships with full and partial tuition reimbursements, career-related internships or fieldwork, Federal Work-Study, institutionally sponsored loans, scholarships/grants, traineeships, tuition waivers (partial), and unspecified assistantships available. Support available to part-time students. Financial award application deadline: 2/1; financial award applicants required to submit FAFSA. *Faculty research:* Pediatrics, assistive rehabilitation technology, adaptive computer technology for children with disabilities, cognitive bases of adult disablement, upper limb rehabilitation. *Unit head:* Prof. Kristie Patten Koenig, Chairperson, 212-998-5852, Fax: 212-995-4044, E-mail: kpk3@nyu.edu. *Application contact:* 212-998-5030, Fax: 212-995-4328, E-mail: steinhardt.gradadmissions@nyu.edu.
Website: http://steinhardt.nyu.edu/ot

Northeastern State University, College of Science and Health Professions, Department of Health Professions, Program in Occupational Therapy, Tahlequah, OK

74464-2399. Offers MS. *Faculty:* 4 full-time (3 women). *Students:* 1 (woman) part-time. Average age 34. *Application deadline:* For fall admission, 7/1 priority date for domestic and international students. Applications are processed on a rolling basis. Electronic applications accepted. *Expenses:* Tuition, state resident: full-time $3029; part-time $168.25 per credit hour. Tuition, nonresident: full-time $7709; part-time $428.25 per credit hour. *Required fees:* $35.90 per credit hour. *Unit head:* Dr. Judith A. Melvin, Director, 918-444-5232, E-mail: melvin02@nsuok.edu. *Application contact:* Margie Railey, Administrative Assistant, 918-456-5511 Ext. 2093, Fax: 918-458-2061, E-mail: railey@nsouk.edu.
Website: http://academics.nsuok.edu/healthprofessions/DegreePrograms/Graduate/OccupatTherapy.aspx

Nova Southeastern University, College of Health Care Sciences, Fort Lauderdale, FL 33314-7796. Offers audiology (Au D); health science (MH Sc, DHSc, PhD); occupational therapy (MOT, OTD, PhD); physical therapy (DPT, PhD, TDPT); physician assistant (MMS). Postbaccalaureate distance learning degree programs offered (minimal on-campus study). *Faculty:* 117 full-time (68 women), 110 part-time/adjunct (57 women). *Students:* 1,187 full-time (844 women), 509 part-time (340 women); includes 560 minority (184 Black or African American, non-Hispanic/Latino; 2 American Indian or Alaska Native, non-Hispanic/Latino; 120 Asian, non-Hispanic/Latino; 218 Hispanic/Latino; 36 Two or more races, non-Hispanic/Latino), 20 international. Average age 31. 5,996 applicants, 14% accepted, 548 enrolled. In 2013, 374 master's, 132 doctorates awarded. *Degree requirements:* For master's, thesis; for doctorate, comprehensive exam, thesis/dissertation. *Entrance requirements:* For master's and doctorate, GRE General Test. *Application deadline:* Applications are processed on a rolling basis. Application fee: $50. Electronic applications accepted. *Expenses:* Contact institution. *Financial support:* In 2013–14, 10 students received support, including 2 research assistantships (averaging $3,500 per year); institutionally sponsored loans and unspecified assistantships also available. *Unit head:* Dr. Stanley Wilson, Dean, 954-262-1203, E-mail: swilson@nova.edu. *Application contact:* Joey Jankie, Admissions Counselor, 954-262-7249, E-mail: joey@nova.edu.
Website: http://www.nova.edu/chcs/

The Ohio State University, College of Medicine, School of Health and Rehabilitation Sciences, Program in Occupational Therapy, Columbus, OH 43210. Offers MOT, MOT/PhD. *Accreditation:* AOTA. *Faculty:* 9. *Students:* 117 full-time (104 women); includes 2 minority (both Two or more races, non-Hispanic/Latino), 1 international. Average age 25. In 2013, 40 master's awarded. *Degree requirements:* For master's, fieldwork. *Entrance requirements:* For master's, GRE General Test. Additional exam requirements/recommendations for international students: Required—TOEFL (minimum score 550 paper-based; 79 iBT), Michigan English Language Assessment Battery (minimum score 82); Recommended—IELTS (minimum score 7). *Application deadline:* For fall admission, 11/30 for domestic and international students; for winter admission, 12/1 for domestic students, 11/1 for international students; for spring admission, 3/1 for domestic students, 2/1 for international students; for summer admission, 11/1 for domestic and international students. Applications are processed on a rolling basis. Application fee: $60 ($70 for international students). Electronic applications accepted. *Financial support:* Fellowships available. *Unit head:* Dr. Jane D. Case-Smith, Director, 614-292-5824, Fax: 614-292-0210, E-mail: case-smith.1@osu.edu. *Application contact:* 614-292-9444, Fax: 614-292-3895, E-mail: gradadmissions@osu.edu.
Website: http://medicine.osu.edu/hrs/ot

Pacific University, School of Occupational Therapy, Forest Grove, OR 97116-1797. Offers MOT. *Accreditation:* AOTA. *Degree requirements:* For master's, research project, professional project. Electronic applications accepted. *Expenses:* Contact institution. *Faculty research:* Cultural competency development, disability policy, scholarship of teaching and learning, driver rehabilitation and older adult visual perception, neurorehabilitation and motor learning.

Philadelphia University, College of Science, Health and the Liberal Arts, Occupational Therapy Clinical Doctorate Program, Philadelphia, PA 19144. Offers OTD. *Entrance requirements:* For doctorate, proof of occupational therapy certification or eligibility for certification in the U.S.; official transcripts from all colleges and universities attended with minimum GPA of 3.0; statistics; research methods; resume or curriculum vitae; two letters of recommendation; personal statement. Additional exam requirements/recommendations for international students: Required—TOEFL (minimum iBT score 79) or IELTS (minimum score 6.5). Electronic applications accepted.

Philadelphia University, College of Science, Health and the Liberal Arts, Program in Occupational Therapy, Philadelphia, PA 19144. Offers MS. *Accreditation:* AOTA. Evening/weekend programs available. *Degree requirements:* For master's, portfolio. *Entrance requirements:* For master's, GRE or MAT. Additional exam requirements/recommendations for international students: Required—TOEFL (minimum score 550 paper-based; 79 iBT). Electronic applications accepted.

Queen's University at Kingston, School of Graduate Studies, Faculty of Health Sciences, School of Rehabilitation Therapy, Kingston, ON K7L 3N6, Canada. Offers occupational therapy (M Sc OT); physical therapy (M Sc PT); rehabilitation science (M Sc, PhD). Part-time programs available. *Degree requirements:* For master's, thesis; for doctorate, comprehensive exam, thesis/dissertation. *Entrance requirements:* Additional exam requirements/recommendations for international students: Required—TOEFL. *Faculty research:* Disability, community, motor performance, rehabilitation, treatment efficiency.

Quinnipiac University, School of Health Sciences, Program in Occupational Therapy, Hamden, CT 06518-1940. Offers MOT. Students are admitted to the program as undergraduates. *Accreditation:* AOTA. *Faculty:* 11 full-time (10 women), 17 part-time/adjunct (all women). *Students:* 112 full-time (104 women), 6 part-time (5 women); includes 12 minority (1 Black or African American, non-Hispanic/Latino; 5 Asian, non-Hispanic/Latino; 6 Hispanic/Latino). Average age 24. 60 applicants, 100% accepted, 59 enrolled. In 2013, 79 master's awarded. *Entrance requirements:* Additional exam requirements/recommendations for international students: Required—TOEFL (minimum score 575 paper-based; 90 iBT). *Expenses: Tuition:* Part-time $920 per credit. *Required fees:* $37 per credit. *Financial support:* In 2013–14, 45 students received support. Career-related internships or fieldwork, Federal Work-Study, scholarships/grants, and unspecified assistantships available. Support available to part-time students. Financial award application deadline: 6/1; financial award applicants required to submit FAFSA. *Application contact:* Office of Undergraduate Admissions, 800-462-1944, E-mail: admissions@quinnipiac.edu.

Radford University, College of Graduate and Professional Studies, Waldron College of Health and Human Services, Department of Occupational Therapy, Radford, VA 24142. Offers MOT. *Accreditation:* AOTA. Part-time and evening/weekend programs available. *Faculty:* 5 full-time (4 women), 1 (woman) part-time/adjunct. *Students:* 56 full-time (49 women); includes 4 minority (2 Asian, non-Hispanic/Latino; 2 Two or more races, non-Hispanic/Latino). Average age 26. 56 applicants, 39% accepted, 20 enrolled. In 2013, 17 master's awarded. *Degree requirements:* For master's, comprehensive exam. *Entrance requirements:* For master's, GRE, minimum GPA of 3.25, minimum B grade in prerequisite courses, 2 letters of recommendation, professional resume, 40 hours of observation, official transcripts; completion of a college or community course to learn a new occupation. Additional exam requirements/recommendations for international students: Required—TOEFL (minimum score 550 paper-based; 79 iBT). *Application deadline:* For fall admission, 2/15 priority date for domestic students, 12/1 for international students; for spring admission, 7/1 for international students. Applications are processed on a rolling basis. Application fee: $50. Electronic applications accepted. *Expenses:* Contact institution. *Financial support:* In 2013–14, 21 students received support, including 21 research assistantships (averaging $4,500 per year); career-related internships or fieldwork, Federal Work-Study, institutionally sponsored loans, scholarships/grants, and unspecified assistantships also available. Financial award application deadline: 3/1; financial award applicants required to submit FAFSA. *Unit head:* Dr. Douglas Mitchell, Chair, 540-831-2693, Fax: 540-831-6802, E-mail: ot@radford.edu. *Application contact:* Rebecca Conner, Director, Graduate Enrollment, 540-831-6296, Fax: 540-831-6061, E-mail: gradcollege@radford.edu.
Website: http://www.radford.edu/content/wchs/home/occupational-therapy.html

The Richard Stockton College of New Jersey, School of Graduate and Continuing Studies, Program in Occupational Therapy, Galloway, NJ 08205-9441. Offers MSOT. *Accreditation:* AOTA. *Faculty:* 4 full-time (all women), 2 part-time/adjunct (both women). *Students:* 47 full-time (41 women), 21 part-time (16 women); includes 7 minority (1 Black or African American, non-Hispanic/Latino; 3 Hispanic/Latino; 3 Two or more races, non-Hispanic/Latino). Average age 26. 266 applicants, 12% accepted, 26 enrolled. In 2013, 21 master's awarded. *Degree requirements:* For master's, fieldwork, research project. *Entrance requirements:* For master's, minimum GPA of 3.0, 60 hours of work, volunteer or community service. Additional exam requirements/recommendations for international students: Required—TOEFL. *Application deadline:* For fall admission, 11/17 for domestic and international students. Application fee: $50. Electronic applications accepted. *Expenses: Tuition, area resident:* Part-time $559 per credit. Tuition, state resident: part-time $559 per credit. Tuition, nonresident: part-time $861 per credit. *Required fees:* $168.23 per credit. $75 per semester. Tuition and fees vary according to course load and degree level. *Financial support:* In 2013–14, 16 students received support, including 3 fellowships, 32 research assistantships with partial tuition reimbursements available; career-related internships or fieldwork, institutionally sponsored loans, scholarships/grants, and unspecified assistantships also available. Support available to part-time students. Financial award application deadline: 3/1; financial award applicants required to submit FAFSA. *Faculty research:* Home health-based occupational therapy for women with HIV/AIDS. *Unit head:* Dr. Kim Furphy, Program Director, 609-626-3640, E-mail: msot@stockton.edu. *Application contact:* Tara Williams, Assistant Director of Graduate Enrollment Management, 609-626-3640, Fax: 609-626-6050, E-mail: gradschool@stockton.edu.

Rockhurst University, School of Graduate and Professional Studies, Program in Occupational Therapy, Kansas City, MO 64110-2561. Offers MOT. *Accreditation:* AOTA. Part-time programs available. *Faculty:* 6 full-time (all women), 5 part-time/adjunct (3 women). *Students:* 63 full-time (59 women), 2 part-time (both women); includes 6 minority (1 Black or African American, non-Hispanic/Latino; 1 American Indian or Alaska Native, non-Hispanic/Latino; 2 Asian, non-Hispanic/Latino; 1 Hispanic/Latino; 1 Two or more races, non-Hispanic/Latino). Average age 25. 221 applicants, 27% accepted, 40 enrolled. In 2013, 38 master's awarded. *Entrance requirements:* For master's, minimum GPA of 3.0. Additional exam requirements/recommendations for international students: Required—TOEFL (minimum score 550 paper-based; 79 iBT). *Application deadline:* Applications are processed on a rolling basis. Application fee: $25. Electronic applications accepted. Application fee is waived when completed online. Tuition and fees vary according to program. *Financial support:* Career-related internships or fieldwork, institutionally sponsored loans, and unspecified assistantships available. Financial award applicants required to submit FAFSA. *Faculty research:* Problem-based learning, cognitive rehabilitation behavioral state in infants and children, adult neurological defects and prosthetics. *Unit head:* Dr. Kris Vacek, Chair, 816-501-4635, Fax: 816-501-4643, E-mail: kris.vacek@rockhurst.edu. *Application contact:* Cheryl Hooper, Director of Graduate Recruitment and Admission, 816-501-4097, Fax: 816-501-4241, E-mail: cheryl.hooper@rockhurst.edu.
Website: http://www.rockhurst.edu/academic/ot/index.asp

Rocky Mountain University of Health Professions, Program in Occupational Therapy, Provo, UT 84606. Offers OTD. Postbaccalaureate distance learning degree programs offered (minimal on-campus study). *Students:* 78 full-time (63 women); includes 14 minority (2 Black or African American, non-Hispanic/Latino; 5 Asian, non-Hispanic/Latino; 7 Hispanic/Latino). Average age 40. In 2013, 50 doctorates awarded. *Entrance requirements:* For doctorate, bachelor's or master's degree from accredited institution with minimum cumulative GPA of 3.0; current U.S. occupational therapy license; resume/curriculum vitae; two letters of recommendation; official transcripts. *Application deadline:* For fall admission, 8/19 for domestic students. Application fee: $150. Electronic applications accepted. *Unit head:* Dr. Loriann Helgeson, Co-Director, 801-375-5125. *Application contact:* Bryce Greenberg, Director of Admissions, 801-734-6832, Fax: 801-734-6833, E-mail: bgreenberg@rmuohp.edu.
Website: http://rmuohp.edu/academics/post-professional-doctor-of-occupational-therapy/

Rush University, College of Health Sciences, Department of Occupational Therapy, Chicago, IL 60612-3832. Offers MS. *Accreditation:* AOTA. *Degree requirements:* For master's, thesis optional. *Entrance requirements:* For master's, GRE General Test. Electronic applications accepted. *Faculty research:* Intervention and practice strategies in the stroke population and the impact of evidenced based interventions.

Sacred Heart University, Graduate Programs, College of Health Professions, Program in Occupational Therapy, Fairfield, CT 06825-1000. Offers MSOT. *Accreditation:* AOTA. *Faculty:* 4 full-time (all women), 4 part-time/adjunct (all women). *Students:* 89 full-time (78 women), 2 part-time (both women); includes 7 minority (1 Black or African American, non-Hispanic/Latino; 1 Asian, non-Hispanic/Latino; 3 Hispanic/Latino; 2 Two or more races, non-Hispanic/Latino). Average age 26. 316 applicants, 40% accepted, 45 enrolled. In 2013, 38 master's awarded. *Entrance requirements:* For master's, GRE (recommended), minimum overall and prerequisites GPA of 3.2 (science 3.0) with no prerequisite course below a C; statistics and human anatomy and physiology completed in the past 10 years. Additional exam requirements/recommendations for international students: Required—TOEFL (minimum score 570 paper-based; 80 iBT), IELTS (minimum score 6.5), PTE. *Application deadline:* For fall admission, 1/15 priority date for domestic students. Applications are processed on a rolling basis. Application fee: $60. Electronic applications accepted. *Expenses:* Contact institution. *Financial support:* Career-related internships or fieldwork, institutionally sponsored loans, and unspecified assistantships available. Support available to part-time students. Financial award applicants required to submit FAFSA. *Unit head:* Dr. Jody Bortone, Director, 203-396-8023, Fax: 203-365-7508, E-mail: gradstudies@sacredheart.edu. *Application contact:* Kathy Dilks, Executive Director of Graduate Admissions, 203-365-7619, Fax: 203-365-4732, E-mail: dilksk@sacredheart.edu.
Website: http://www.sacredheart.edu/academics/collegeofhealthprofessions/academicprograms/occupationaltherapy/

Sage Graduate School, School of Health Sciences, Program in Occupational Therapy, Troy, NY 12180-4115. Offers MS. *Accreditation:* AOTA. Part-time and evening/weekend programs available. *Faculty:* 7 full-time (all women), 8 part-time/adjunct (all women).

Students: 57 full-time (54 women), 34 part-time (33 women); includes 8 minority (2 Asian, non-Hispanic/Latino; 3 Hispanic/Latino; 1 Native Hawaiian or other Pacific Islander, non-Hispanic/Latino; 2 Two or more races, non-Hispanic/Latino). Average age 27. 158 applicants, 18% accepted, 26 enrolled. In 2013, 30 master's awarded. *Entrance requirements:* For master's, baccalaureate degree, minimum undergraduate GPA of 3.0, completion of program prerequisites with minimum C grade, completion of 20 hours of clinical observation. Additional exam requirements/recommendations for international students: Required—TOEFL (minimum score 550 paper-based). *Application deadline:* For fall admission, 2/1 for domestic students. Applications are processed on a rolling basis. Application fee: $40. *Expenses: Tuition:* Full-time $11,880; part-time $660 per credit hour. *Financial support:* Fellowships, research assistantships, Federal Work-Study, scholarships/grants, and unspecified assistantships available. Support available to part-time students. *Unit head:* Dr. Esther Haskevitz, Dean, School of Health Sciences, 518-244-2296, Fax: 518-244-4571, E-mail: haskve@sage.edu. *Application contact:* Theresa Hand, Chair and Program Director, 518-244-2069, Fax: 518-244-4524, E-mail: handt@sage.edu.

Saginaw Valley State University, Crystal M. Lange College of Nursing and Health Sciences, Program in Occupational Therapy, University Center, MI 48710. Offers MSOT. *Accreditation:* AOTA. Part-time and evening/weekend programs available. *Students:* 108 full-time (84 women), 41 part-time (37 women); includes 5 minority (2 Hispanic/Latino; 3 Two or more races, non-Hispanic/Latino), 4 international. Average age 24. 1 applicant, 100% accepted. In 2013, 39 master's awarded. *Entrance requirements:* For master's, minimum GPA of 3.0. Additional exam requirements/recommendations for international students: Required—TOEFL (minimum score 525 paper-based; 71 iBT). *Application deadline:* For spring admission, 1/16 for domestic and international students. Applications are processed on a rolling basis. Application fee: $30 ($80 for international students). Electronic applications accepted. *Expenses:* Tuition, state resident: full-time $8933; part-time $496.30 per credit hour. Tuition, nonresident: full-time $16,806; part-time $933.65 per credit hour. *Required fees:* $263; $14.60 per credit hour. Tuition and fees vary according to degree level. *Financial support:* Federal Work-Study and scholarships/grants available. Support available to part-time students. *Unit head:* Dr. Ellen Herlache-Pretzer, Graduate Program Coordinator, 989-964-2187, E-mail: echerlac@svsu.edu. *Application contact:* Jenna Briggs, Director, Graduate and International Admissions, 989-964-6096, Fax: 989-964-2788, E-mail: gradadm@svsu.edu.

St. Ambrose University, College of Education and Health Sciences, Program in Occupational Therapy, Davenport, IA 52803-2898. Offers MOT. *Accreditation:* AOTA. *Degree requirements:* For master's, board exams. *Entrance requirements:* For master's, 50 hours of volunteer experience in 2 occupational therapy settings, minimum GPA of 2.7, essay or interview on campus, 3 letters of reference. Additional exam requirements/recommendations for international students: Required—TOEFL. Electronic applications accepted.

St. Catherine University, Graduate Programs, Program in Occupational Therapy, St. Paul, MN 55105. Offers MA, OTD. *Accreditation:* AOTA. Part-time and evening/weekend programs available. *Degree requirements:* For master's, thesis. *Entrance requirements:* For master's, GRE, minimum GPA of 3.0. Additional exam requirements/recommendations for international students: Required—Michigan English Language Assessment Battery or TOEFL.

Saint Francis University, Department of Occupational Therapy, Loretto, PA 15940-0600. Offers MOT. *Accreditation:* AOTA. *Faculty:* 6 full-time (4 women), 2 part-time/adjunct (both women). *Students:* 36 full-time (31 women). Average age 22. 36 applicants, 100% accepted, 36 enrolled. In 2013, 23 master's awarded. *Degree requirements:* For master's, one foreign language, thesis. *Expenses: Tuition:* Full-time $18,848. Tuition and fees vary according to degree level and reciprocity agreements. *Faculty research:* Retention, technology, work injury, distance learning. *Unit head:* Dr. Edward Mihelcic, Chair, 814-472-2760, Fax: 814-472-3950, E-mail: emihelcic@francis.edu. *Application contact:* Dr. Peter Raymond Skoner, Associate Vice President for Academic Affairs, 814-472-3085, Fax: 814-472-3365, E-mail: pskoner@francis.edu.
Website: http://www.francis.edu/ot

Saint Louis University, Graduate Education, Doisy College of Health Sciences, Department of Occupational Science and Occupational Therapy, St. Louis, MO 63103-2097. Offers MOT. *Accreditation:* AOTA. *Degree requirements:* For master's, project. *Entrance requirements:* For master's, minimum GPA of 2.8. Additional exam requirements/recommendations for international students: Required—TOEFL (minimum score 525 paper-based; 55 iBT). Electronic applications accepted. *Faculty research:* Autism spectrum and Asperger's disease, early intervention with children of homeless families, disability awareness program development of developing countries, environmental adaptations and universal design for persons who are disabled and/or aging, physical activity models for persons with dementia.

Salem State University, School of Graduate Studies, Program in Occupational Therapy, Salem, MA 01970-5353. Offers MS. *Accreditation:* AOTA. Part-time and evening/weekend programs available. *Students:* 14 part-time (12 women); includes 2 minority (1 Asian, non-Hispanic/Latino; 1 Hispanic/Latino). In 2013, 8 master's awarded. *Entrance requirements:* For master's, GRE or MAT. Additional exam requirements/recommendations for international students: Required—TOEFL (minimum score 550 paper-based; 80 iBT), IELTS (minimum score 5.5). *Application deadline:* For fall admission, 5/31 for domestic students. Application fee: $50. *Financial support:* Career-related internships or fieldwork, Federal Work-Study, scholarships/grants, and unspecified assistantships available. Support available to part-time students. Financial award application deadline: 5/1; financial award applicants required to submit FAFSA. *Application contact:* Dr. Lee A. Brossoit, Assistant Dean of Graduate Admissions, 978-542-6675, Fax: 978-542-7215, E-mail: lbrossoit@salemstate.edu.
Website: http://www.salemstate.edu/admissions/10886.php

Samuel Merritt University, Department of Occupational Therapy, Oakland, CA 94609-3108. Offers MOT. *Accreditation:* AOTA. *Degree requirements:* For master's, project. *Entrance requirements:* For master's, GRE General Test, minimum GPA of 2.6 in science, 2.8 overall; 40-70 hours of volunteer or professional occupational therapy experience; interview. Additional exam requirements/recommendations for international students: Required—TOEFL. *Expenses:* Contact institution.

San Jose State University, Graduate Studies and Research, College of Applied Sciences and Arts, Department of Occupational Therapy, San Jose, CA 95192-0001. Offers MS. *Accreditation:* AOTA. *Degree requirements:* For master's, thesis or alternative. *Entrance requirements:* For master's, GRE, minimum GPA of 3.0. Electronic applications accepted. *Faculty research:* Generic occupational therapy, psychosocial rehabilitation, physical rehabilitation, organizational development, occupational performance.

Seton Hall University, School of Health and Medical Sciences, Program in Occupational Therapy, South Orange, NJ 07079-2697. Offers MS. *Accreditation:* AOTA. *Entrance requirements:* For master's, health care experience, minimum GPA of 3.0, 50 hours of occupational therapy volunteer work, pre-requisite courses. Additional exam requirements/recommendations for international students: Required—TOEFL. Electronic applications accepted. *Faculty research:* Occupational genesis, occupational technology, pediatric OT, community practice, families of children with special needs; family routines; complementary medicine and wellness.

Shawnee State University, Program in Occupational Therapy, Portsmouth, OH 45662-4344. Offers MOT. *Accreditation:* AOTA.

Shenandoah University, School of Health Professions, Division of Occupational Therapy, Winchester, VA 22601-5195. Offers MS. *Accreditation:* AOTA. *Faculty:* 6 full-time (all women), 4 part-time/adjunct (all women). *Students:* 59 full-time (51 women), 28 part-time (25 women); includes 12 minority (3 Black or African American, non-Hispanic/Latino; 3 Asian, non-Hispanic/Latino; 6 Hispanic/Latino). Average age 30. 239 applicants, 25% accepted, 31 enrolled. In 2013, 22 master's awarded. *Degree requirements:* For master's, comprehensive exam, thesis or alternative, fieldwork. *Entrance requirements:* For master's, GRE (minimum score 480 quantitative), 24 hours of clinical exposure, 2 references, writing sample, bachelor's degree with minimum GPA of 3.0. Additional exam requirements/recommendations for international students: Required—TOEFL (minimum score 550 paper-based; 79 iBT), IELTS (minimum score 6.5), Sakae Institute of Study Abroad (SISA) test (minimum score 15). *Application deadline:* For fall admission, 11/30 for domestic and international students. Application fee: $30. Electronic applications accepted. *Expenses:* Contact institution. *Financial support:* In 2013–14, 11 students received support. Career-related internships or fieldwork and scholarships/grants available. Support available to part-time students. Financial award application deadline: 3/15; financial award applicants required to submit FAFSA. *Faculty research:* Concussion and occupational-based outcomes, development of ecologically valid assessments for soldiers post-concussion to determine return to duty. *Unit head:* Leslie Davidson, Director/Associate Professor, 540-665-5561, Fax: 540-665-5564, E-mail: ldavids2@su.edu. *Application contact:* Andrew Woodall, Executive Director of Recruitment and Admissions, 540-665-4581, Fax: 540-665-4627, E-mail: admit@su.edu.
Website: http://www.occupational-therapy.su.edu/

Sonoma State University, School of Science and Technology, Department of Kinesiology, Rohnert Park, CA 94928. Offers adapted physical education (MA); interdisciplinary (MA); interdisciplinary pre-occupational therapy (MA); lifetime physical activity (MA), including coach education, fitness and wellness; physical education (MA); pre-physical therapy (MA). Part-time programs available. *Faculty:* 5 full-time (3 women). *Students:* 1 full-time (0 women), 11 part-time (3 women); includes 2 minority (1 Hispanic/Latino; 1 Two or more races, non-Hispanic/Latino). Average age 29. *Degree requirements:* For master's, thesis, oral exam. *Entrance requirements:* For master's, minimum GPA of 2.8. Additional exam requirements/recommendations for international students: Required—TOEFL (minimum score 500 paper-based). *Application deadline:* For fall admission, 11/30 for domestic students; for spring admission, 9/1 for domestic students. Applications are processed on a rolling basis. Application fee: $55. *Expenses:* Tuition, state resident: full-time $8500. Tuition, nonresident: full-time $12,964. *Required fees:* $1762. *Financial support:* Career-related internships or fieldwork available. Financial award application deadline: 3/2; financial award applicants required to submit FAFSA. *Unit head:* Dr. Elaine McHugh, Chair, 707-664-2660, E-mail: elaine.mchugh@sonoma.edu. *Application contact:* Dr. Lauren Morimoto, Graduate Coordinator, 707-664-2479, E-mail: morimoto@sonoma.edu.
Website: http://www.sonoma.edu/kinesiology/

Spalding University, Graduate Studies, Kosair College of Health and Natural Sciences, Auerbach School of Occupational Therapy, Louisville, KY 40203-2188. Offers MSOT. *Accreditation:* AOTA. *Faculty:* 9 full-time (6 women), 2 part-time/adjunct (both women). *Students:* 133 full-time (116 women), 28 part-time (24 women); includes 15 minority (8 Black or African American, non-Hispanic/Latino; 3 Asian, non-Hispanic/Latino; 1 Hispanic/Latino; 3 Two or more races, non-Hispanic/Latino). Average age 28. 124 applicants, 42% accepted, 44 enrolled. In 2013, 63 master's awarded. *Entrance requirements:* For master's, interview, letters of recommendation, transcripts, writing sample, 20 observation hours in human service delivery setting. Additional exam requirements/recommendations for international students: Required—TOEFL (minimum score 535 paper-based). *Application deadline:* For spring admission, 6/27 priority date for domestic students. Application fee: $30. *Expenses: Tuition:* Full-time $21,450. *Required fees:* $810. Tuition and fees vary according to course load, degree level, program and student level. *Financial support:* In 2013–14, 9 research assistantships (averaging $3,943 per year) were awarded; unspecified assistantships also available. Financial award applicants required to submit FAFSA. *Faculty research:* High-risk youth, community-dwelling older adults, assistive technology, mother-infant relationships, community accessibility. *Unit head:* Dr. Laura Schluter Strickland, Associate Dean, 502-873-4219, E-mail: lstrickland@spalding.edu. *Application contact:* Arlisa Spaulding, Administrative Office Coordinator, 502-873-7196, E-mail: aspaulding@spalding.edu.
Website: http://spalding.edu/academics/occupational-therapy/

Springfield College, Graduate Programs, Program in Occupational Therapy, Springfield, MA 01109-3797. Offers M Ed, MS, CAGS. *Accreditation:* AOTA (one or more programs are accredited). Part-time programs available. *Faculty:* 6 full-time, 2 part-time/adjunct. *Students:* 77 full-time. Average age 30. 196 applicants, 28% accepted, 23 enrolled. In 2013, 37 master's awarded. *Degree requirements:* For master's, comprehensive exam. *Entrance requirements:* Additional exam requirements/recommendations for international students: Required—TOEFL (minimum score 550 paper-based); Recommended—IELTS (minimum score 6). *Application deadline:* For fall admission, 1/15 for domestic and international students; for winter admission, 11/1 for domestic and international students; for spring admission, 11/1 for domestic and international students. Applications are processed on a rolling basis. Application fee: $50. Electronic applications accepted. *Expenses: Tuition:* Full-time $13,620; part-time $908 per credit. *Financial support:* Fellowships with partial tuition reimbursements, teaching assistantships with partial tuition reimbursements, career-related internships or fieldwork, Federal Work-Study, institutionally sponsored loans, and unspecified assistantships available. Financial award application deadline: 3/1; financial award applicants required to submit FAFSA. *Unit head:* Dr. Katherine Post, Director, 413-748-3785, Fax: 413-748-3796, E-mail: kpost@springfieldcollege.edu. *Application contact:* Evelyn Cohen, Associate Director of Graduate Admissions, 413-748-3479, Fax: 413-748-3694, E-mail: ecohen@springfieldcollege.edu.
Website: http://www.springfieldcollege.edu/academic-programs/occupational-therapy-programs-at-springfield-college/occupational-therapy-programs/graduate-entry/

Stony Brook University, State University of New York, Stony Brook University Medical Center, Health Sciences Center, School of Health Technology and Management, Stony Brook, NY 11794. Offers health care management (Advanced Certificate); health care policy and management (MS); occupational therapy (MS); physical therapy (DPT); physician assistant (MS). *Accreditation:* APTA. Part-time programs available. *Faculty:* 70 full-time (46 women), 51 part-time/adjunct (34 women). *Students:* 349 full-time (225 women), 159 part-time (120 women); includes 140 minority (25 Black or African American, non-Hispanic/Latino; 1 American Indian or Alaska Native, non-Hispanic/Latino; 72 Asian, non-Hispanic/Latino; 34 Hispanic/Latino; 8 Two or more races, non-Hispanic/Latino), 7 international. 2,215 applicants, 11% accepted, 221 enrolled. In 2013, 120 master's, 77 doctorates, 23 other advanced degrees awarded. *Degree requirements:* For master's, thesis. *Entrance requirements:* For master's, GRE General Test, minimum GPA of 3.0, work experience in field, references; for doctorate,

Occupational Therapy

GRE, references. Additional exam requirements/recommendations for international students: Required—TOEFL (minimum score 550 paper-based). *Application deadline:* For fall admission, 1/15 for domestic students; for spring admission, 10/1 for domestic students. Application fee: $100. *Expenses:* Tuition, state resident: full-time $9870; part-time $411 per credit. Tuition, nonresident: full-time $18,350; part-time $765 per credit. *Financial support:* In 2013–14, 1 fellowship was awarded; research assistantships, teaching assistantships, career-related internships or fieldwork, Federal Work-Study, and institutionally sponsored loans also available. Financial award application deadline: 3/15. *Faculty research:* Health promotion and disease prevention. *Total annual research expenditures:* $1.1 million. *Unit head:* Dr. Craig A. Lehmann, Dean, 631-444-2252, Fax: 631-444-7621, E-mail: craig.lehmann@stonybrook.edu. *Application contact:* Dr. Richard W. Johnson, Associate Dean for Graduate Studies, 631-444-3251, Fax: 631-444-7621, E-mail: richard.johnson@stonybrook.edu.
Website: http://healthtechnology.stonybrookmedicine.edu/

Temple University, College of Health Professions and Social Work, Department of Rehabilitation Sciences, Program in Occupational Therapy, Philadelphia, PA 19122. Offers MOT, DOT. *Accreditation:* AOTA. Part-time programs available. Postbaccalaureate distance learning degree programs offered. *Faculty:* 17 full-time (14 women). *Students:* 85 full-time (75 women), 15 part-time (12 women); includes 14 minority (1 Black or African American, non-Hispanic/Latino; 5 Asian, non-Hispanic/Latino; 4 Hispanic/Latino; 4 Two or more races, non-Hispanic/Latino), 2 international. 516 applicants, 23% accepted, 45 enrolled. In 2013, 34 master's, 7 doctorates awarded. *Degree requirements:* For master's, comprehensive exam (for some programs), thesis, capstone, clinical field study. *Entrance requirements:* For master's, GRE General Test or MAT, minimum GPA of 3.0, 3 letters of reference, statement of goals; for doctorate, GRE if GPA less than 3.0, MOT, 2 letters of reference, resume. Additional exam requirements/recommendations for international students: Required—TOEFL (minimum score 550 paper-based; 79 iBT). *Application deadline:* For fall admission, 2/1 for domestic students, 1/1 for international students; for spring admission, 11/1 for domestic students, 10/1 for international students. Applications are processed on a rolling basis. Application fee: $60. Electronic applications accepted. *Expenses:* Contact institution. *Financial support:* Research assistantships, career-related internships or fieldwork, Federal Work-Study, and institutionally sponsored loans available. Financial award application deadline: 1/15. *Faculty research:* Participation, community inclusion, disability issues, leisure/recreation, occupation, quality of life, adaptive equipment and technology. *Unit head:* Dr. Mark Salzer, Chair, 215-204-7879, Fax: 215-707-7656, E-mail: mark.salzer@temple.edu. *Application contact:* Jacquee Lukawski, 215-707-4875, E-mail: jacquee.lukawski@temple.edu.
Website: http://chpsw.temple.edu/rs/home

Tennessee State University, The School of Graduate Studies and Research, College of Health Sciences, Department of Occupational Therapy, Nashville, TN 37209-1561. Offers MOT. *Entrance requirements:* For master's, GRE within the last 5 years, undergraduate degree with minimum GPA of 3.0; 30 hours of observation, volunteer, or work with an occupational therapist; 3 professional and/or academic references.

Texas Tech University Health Sciences Center, School of Allied Health Sciences, Program in Occupational Therapy, Lubbock, TX 79430. Offers MOT. *Accreditation:* AOTA. *Faculty:* 5 full-time (3 women). *Students:* 108 full-time (96 women); includes 20 minority (1 Black or African American, non-Hispanic/Latino; 3 Asian, non-Hispanic/Latino; 14 Hispanic/Latino; 2 Two or more races, non-Hispanic/Latino). Average age 25. 312 applicants, 12% accepted, 37 enrolled. In 2013, 36 master's awarded. *Entrance requirements:* Additional exam requirements/recommendations for international students: Required—TOEFL, IELTS. *Application deadline:* For fall admission, 10/1 priority date for domestic students; for spring admission, 12/15 priority date for domestic students. Applications are processed on a rolling basis. Application fee: $40. Electronic applications accepted. *Financial support:* Application deadline: 9/1; applicants required to submit FAFSA. *Unit head:* Dr. Dawndra Sechrist, Program Director, 806-743-3246, Fax: 806-743-6005, E-mail: dawndra.sechrist@ttuhsc.edu. *Application contact:* Lindsay Johnson, Associate Dean for Admissions and Student Affairs, 806-743-3220, Fax: 806-743-2994, E-mail: lindsay.johnson@ttuhsc.edu.
Website: http://www.ttuhsc.edu/sah/mot/

Texas Woman's University, Graduate School, College of Health Sciences, School of Occupational Therapy, Denton, TX 76201. Offers MA, MOT, PhD. *Accreditation:* AOTA (one or more programs are accredited). Part-time and evening/weekend programs available. Postbaccalaureate distance learning degree programs offered. *Faculty:* 23 full-time (22 women), 7 part-time/adjunct (5 women). *Students:* 337 full-time (316 women), 81 part-time (73 women); includes 121 minority (26 Black or African American, non-Hispanic/Latino; 4 American Indian or Alaska Native, non-Hispanic/Latino; 33 Asian, non-Hispanic/Latino; 58 Hispanic/Latino), 6 international. Average age 30. 683 applicants, 17% accepted, 101 enrolled. In 2013, 116 master's, 1 doctorate awarded. *Degree requirements:* For master's, thesis or alternative; for doctorate, comprehensive exam, thesis/dissertation. *Entrance requirements:* For master's, minimum GPA of 3.0 on prerequisites, interview, recommendation based on 20 hours of observation with one supervising OTR; for doctorate, GRE General Test, essay, interview, 3 letters of reference, certification and master's degree in occupational therapy or related field. Additional exam requirements/recommendations for international students: Required—TOEFL (minimum score 550 paper-based; 79 iBT). *Application deadline:* For fall admission, 9/15 priority date for domestic students, 9/15 for international students. Applications are processed on a rolling basis. Application fee: $50 ($75 for international students). Electronic applications accepted. *Expenses:* Tuition, state resident: full-time $4182; part-time $233.32 per credit hour. Tuition, nonresident: full-time $10,716; part-time $595.32 per credit hour. *Financial support:* In 2013–14, 204 students received support, including 4 research assistantships (averaging $2,968 per year); career-related internships or fieldwork, Federal Work-Study, institutionally sponsored loans, scholarships/grants, traineeships, health care benefits, and unspecified assistantships also available. Support available to part-time students. Financial award application deadline: 3/1; financial award applicants required to submit FAFSA. *Faculty research:* Quality of life/wellness, Alzheimer's disease, hand rehabilitation, psychosocial dysfunction, adaptation/chronic disability, long-term care. *Total annual research expenditures:* $95,953. *Unit head:* Dr. Catherine Candler, Director, 940-898-2801, Fax: 940-898-2806, E-mail: ot@twu.edu. *Application contact:* Dr. Samuel Wheeler, Assistant Director of Admissions, 940-898-3188, Fax: 940-898-3081, E-mail: wheelers@twu.edu.
Website: http://www.twu.edu/occupational-therapy/

Thomas Jefferson University, Jefferson School of Health Professions, Program in Occupational Therapy, Philadelphia, PA 19107. Offers MS, OTD. *Accreditation:* AOTA. Part-time programs available. *Faculty:* 9 full-time (8 women), 3 part-time/adjunct (2 women). *Students:* 111 full-time (104 women), 54 part-time (52 women); includes 18 minority (2 Black or African American, non-Hispanic/Latino; 10 Asian, non-Hispanic/Latino; 6 Hispanic/Latino), 1 international. Average age 30. 678 applicants, 19% accepted, 63 enrolled. In 2013, 64 master's, 8 doctorates awarded. *Degree requirements:* For master's, thesis (for some programs). *Entrance requirements:* For master's, GRE General Test or MAT. Additional exam requirements/recommendations for international students: Required—TOEFL. *Application deadline:* For fall admission, 3/1 for domestic and international students. Applications are processed on a rolling basis. Application fee: $125. Electronic applications accepted. *Expenses:* Contact institution. *Financial support:* In 2013–14, 51 students received support. Fellowships with tuition reimbursements available, research assistantships, Federal Work-Study, institutionally sponsored loans, scholarships/grants, and unspecified assistantships available. Support available to part-time students. Financial award application deadline: 4/1; financial award applicants required to submit FAFSA. *Faculty research:* Functional outcomes in traumatic brain injury, clinical reasoning in therapist/patient interactions, gerontology, sensory integration in pediatrics, effective intervention for homeless. *Total annual research expenditures:* $3.5 million. *Unit head:* Dr. Roseann Schaaf, Chair, Occupational Therapy Department, 215-503-9609, Fax: 215-503-0376, E-mail: roseann.schaaf@jefferson.edu. *Application contact:* Donald Sharples, Director of Graduate Admissions, 215-503-1044, Fax: 215-503-7241, E-mail: jshpadmissions@jefferson.edu.
Website: http://www.jefferson.edu/health_professions/departments/occupational_therapy

Touro College, School of Health Sciences, Bay Shore, NY 11706. Offers occupational therapy (MS); physical therapy (DPT); physicians assistant (MS); speech-language pathology (MS). *Faculty:* 20 full-time, 94 part-time/adjunct. *Students:* 975 full-time (710 women), 160 part-time (114 women); includes 271 minority (58 Black or African American, non-Hispanic/Latino; 1 American Indian or Alaska Native, non-Hispanic/Latino; 132 Asian, non-Hispanic/Latino; 60 Hispanic/Latino; 4 Native Hawaiian or other Pacific Islander, non-Hispanic/Latino; 16 Two or more races, non-Hispanic/Latino), 10 international. *Expenses:* Contact institution. *Financial support:* Fellowships available. *Unit head:* Dr. Louis Primavera, Dean, School of Health Sciences, 516-673-3200, E-mail: louis.primavera@touro.edu. *Application contact:* Brian J. Diele, Associate Director of Central Admissions, 631-665-1600 Ext. 6311, E-mail: brian.diele@touro.edu.

Towson University, Program in Occupational Therapy, Towson, MD 21252-0001. Offers MS. *Accreditation:* AOTA. *Students:* 148 full-time (137 women), 8 part-time (7 women); includes 11 minority (2 Black or African American, non-Hispanic/Latino; 1 American Indian or Alaska Native, non-Hispanic/Latino; 4 Asian, non-Hispanic/Latino; 2 Hispanic/Latino; 2 Two or more races, non-Hispanic/Latino). *Degree requirements:* For master's, thesis optional. *Entrance requirements:* For master's, bachelor's degree with minimum GPA of 3.25; master's degree, or doctorate; 3 letters of recommendation; human service/OT observation hours; personal statement. *Application deadline:* For spring admission, 8/1 for domestic students. Applications are processed on a rolling basis. Application fee: $45. Electronic applications accepted. *Financial support:* Application deadline: 4/1. *Unit head:* Dr. Sonia Lawson, Graduate Program Director, 410-704-2762, E-mail: slawson@towson.edu. *Application contact:* Lynne Murphy, The Graduate School, 410-704-2320, E-mail: lmurphy@towson.edu.
Website: http://grad.towson.edu/program/master/octh-ms/

Tufts University, Graduate School of Arts and Sciences, Department of Occupational Therapy, Medford, MA 02155. Offers MS, OTD. *Accreditation:* AOTA. *Faculty:* 6 full-time, 9 part-time/adjunct. *Students:* 123 full-time (116 women); includes 13 minority (1 Black or African American, non-Hispanic/Latino; 9 Asian, non-Hispanic/Latino; 2 Hispanic/Latino; 1 Two or more races, non-Hispanic/Latino), 4 international. Average age 27. 213 applicants, 36% accepted, 57 enrolled. In 2013, 45 master's, 1 doctorate awarded. *Degree requirements:* For master's, thesis (for some programs); for doctorate, leadership project. *Entrance requirements:* For master's and doctorate, GRE General Test. Additional exam requirements/recommendations for international students: Required—TOEFL (minimum score 550 paper-based; 80 iBT), IELTS (minimum score 6.5). *Application deadline:* For fall admission, 1/15 for domestic and international students; for spring admission, 10/15 for domestic students, 9/15 for international students. Applications are processed on a rolling basis. Application fee: $75. Electronic applications accepted. *Expenses:* Contact institution. *Financial support:* Teaching assistantships with partial tuition reimbursements, Federal Work-Study, scholarships/grants, and tuition waivers (partial) available. Support available to part-time students. Financial award application deadline: 1/15; financial award applicants required to submit FAFSA. *Unit head:* Gary Bedell, Chair, 617-627-5720. *Application contact:* Elizabeth Owen, Staff Assistant, 617-627-5720.
Website: http://ase.tufts.edu/bsot/

Tufts University, Graduate School of Arts and Sciences, Graduate Certificate Programs, Advanced Professional Study in Occupational Therapy Program, Medford, MA 02155. Offers Certificate. Part-time and evening/weekend programs available. Electronic applications accepted. *Expenses:* Contact institution.

Université de Montréal, Faculty of Medicine, Programs in Ergonomics, Montréal, QC H3C 3J7, Canada. Offers occupational therapy (DESS). Program offered jointly with École Polytechnique de Montréal.

University at Buffalo, the State University of New York, Graduate School, School of Public Health and Health Professions, Department of Rehabilitation Science, Program in Occupational Therapy, Buffalo, NY 14260. Offers physical disabilities/developmental disabilities (MS); school-based therapy/early intervention (MS). *Accreditation:* AOTA. *Faculty:* 7 full-time (6 women), 8 part-time/adjunct (all women). *Students:* 87 full-time (71 women), 1 part-time (0 women); includes 13 minority (1 Black or African American, non-Hispanic/Latino; 1 American Indian or Alaska Native, non-Hispanic/Latino; 10 Asian, non-Hispanic/Latino; 1 Native Hawaiian or other Pacific Islander, non-Hispanic/Latino). Average age 25. 54 applicants, 94% accepted, 36 enrolled. In 2013, 44 master's awarded. *Degree requirements:* For master's, project or thesis. *Entrance requirements:* For master's, GRE, BS in occupational therapy. Additional exam requirements/recommendations for international students: Required—TOEFL (minimum score 79 iBT). *Application deadline:* For fall admission, 2/1 priority date for domestic students, 4/1 for international students; for spring admission, 11/1 priority date for domestic students, 9/1 for international students. Application fee: $50. Electronic applications accepted. *Financial support:* In 2013–14, 5 teaching assistantships with full and partial tuition reimbursements (averaging $3,031 per year) were awarded; unspecified assistantships also available. Financial award application deadline: 2/1; financial award applicants required to submit FAFSA. *Faculty research:* Sensory integration, assistive technology, aging and technology, transition for students with emotional/behavioral problems. *Total annual research expenditures:* $391,708. *Unit head:* Dr. Susan Nochajski, Graduate Program Director, 716-829-6942, Fax: 716-829-3217, E-mail: phhpadv@buffalo.edu. *Application contact:* MaryAnn Venezia, Program Coordinator, 716-829-6942, Fax: 716-829-3217, E-mail: venezia3@buffalo.edu.
Website: http://www.sphhp.buffalo.edu/rs/ot/bsms/

The University of Alabama at Birmingham, School of Health Professions, Program in Occupational Therapy, Birmingham, AL 35294. Offers entry-level (MS); low vision rehabilitation (MS); post-professional (MS). *Accreditation:* AOTA. *Entrance requirements:* Additional exam requirements/recommendations for international students: Recommended—TOEFL, IELTS.

University of Alberta, Faculty of Graduate Studies and Research, Department of Occupational Therapy, Edmonton, AB T6G 2E1, Canada. Offers M Sc, PhD. Part-time programs available. *Degree requirements:* For master's, thesis. *Entrance requirements:* For master's, bachelor's degree in occupational therapy, minimum GPA of 6.9 on a 9.0 scale. Additional exam requirements/recommendations for international students:

Required—TOEFL. Electronic applications accepted. *Faculty research:* Work evaluation, pediatrics, geriatrics, program evaluation, community-based rehabilitation.

The University of British Columbia, Faculty of Medicine, Department of Occupational Science and Occupational Therapy, Vancouver, BC V6T 1Z1, Canada. Offers MOT. *Entrance requirements:* Additional exam requirements/recommendations for international students: Required—TOEFL (minimum score 600 paper-based; 100 iBT), IELTS (minimum score 6.5). Electronic applications accepted. *Expenses: Tuition, area resident:* Full-time $8000 Canadian dollars.

University of Central Arkansas, Graduate School, College of Health and Behavioral Sciences, Department of Occupational Therapy, Conway, AR 72035-0001. Offers MS. *Accreditation:* AOTA. *Degree requirements:* For master's, thesis optional, internship. *Entrance requirements:* For master's, GRE General Test, minimum GPA of 2.7. Additional exam requirements/recommendations for international students: Required—TOEFL (minimum score 550 paper-based; 80 iBT). Electronic applications accepted. *Expenses:* Contact institution.

The University of Findlay, Office of Graduate Admissions, Findlay, OH 45840-3653. Offers athletic training (MAT); business (MBA), including health care management, hospitality management, organizational leadership, public management; education (MA Ed), including administration, children's literature, early childhood, human resource development, reading, science, special education, technology; environmental, safety and health management (MSEM); health informatics (MS); occupational therapy (MOT); pharmacy (Pharm D); physical therapy (DPT); physician assistant (MPA); rhetoric and writing (MA); teaching English to speakers of other languages (TESOL) and bilingual education (MA). Part-time and evening/weekend programs available. Postbaccalaureate distance learning degree programs offered (no on-campus study). *Faculty:* 209 full-time (98 women), 69 part-time/adjunct (38 women). *Students:* 551 full-time (332 women), 457 part-time (276 women); includes 77 minority (37 Black or African American, non-Hispanic/Latino; 1 American Indian or Alaska Native, non-Hispanic/Latino; 15 Asian, non-Hispanic/Latino; 23 Hispanic/Latino; 1 Native Hawaiian or other Pacific Islander, non-Hispanic/Latino), 135 international. Average age 28. 637 applicants, 66% accepted, 241 enrolled. In 2013, 267 master's, 91 doctorates awarded. *Degree requirements:* For master's, thesis, cumulative project, capstone project. *Entrance requirements:* For master's, GRE/GMAT, bachelor's degree from accredited institution, minimum undergraduate GPA of 2.5 in last 64 hours of course work; for doctorate, GRE, minimum cumulative GPA of 3.0. Additional exam requirements/recommendations for international students: Required—TOEFL (minimum score 80 iBT). *Application deadline:* Applications are processed on a rolling basis. Application fee: $25. Electronic applications accepted. *Expenses: Required fees:* $146 per semester. Tuition and fees vary according to degree level and program. *Financial support:* In 2013–14, 11 research assistantships with full and partial tuition reimbursements (averaging $4,000 per year), 10 teaching assistantships with full and partial tuition reimbursements (averaging $3,600 per year) were awarded; career-related internships or fieldwork, Federal Work-Study, health care benefits, and unspecified assistantships also available. Financial award application deadline: 4/1; financial award applicants required to submit FAFSA. *Unit head:* Christopher M. Harris, Director of Admissions, 419-434-4347, E-mail: harrisc1@findlay.edu. *Application contact:* Emily Ickes, Graduate Admissions Counselor, 419-434-6933, Fax: 419-434-4898, E-mail: ickese@findlay.edu.
Website: http://www.findlay.edu/admissions/graduate/Pages/default.aspx

University of Florida, Graduate School, College of Public Health and Health Professions, Department of Occupational Therapy, Gainesville, FL 32610. Offers MHS, MOT. *Accreditation:* AOTA. *Faculty:* 2 full-time (both women), 3 part-time/adjunct (1 woman). *Students:* 78 full-time (74 women), 35 part-time (32 women); includes 31 minority (3 Black or African American, non-Hispanic/Latino; 8 Asian, non-Hispanic/Latino; 20 Hispanic/Latino). Average age 26. 138 applicants, 21% accepted, 22 enrolled. In 2013, 43 master's awarded. *Degree requirements:* For master's, clinical rotations. *Entrance requirements:* For master's, GRE General Test, minimum GPA of 3.0. Additional exam requirements/recommendations for international students: Required—TOEFL (minimum score 550 paper-based; 80 iBT), IELTS (minimum score 6). *Application deadline:* For fall admission, 2/15 for domestic and international students; for spring admission, 1/15 for domestic and international students. Application fee: $30. Electronic applications accepted. *Expenses:* Tuition, state resident: full-time $12,640. Tuition, nonresident: full-time $30,000. *Financial support:* Career-related internships or fieldwork, institutionally sponsored loans, scholarships/grants, and unspecified assistantships available. Support available to part-time students. Financial award applicants required to submit FAFSA. *Faculty research:* Rehabilitation intervention outcomes assessment, safe driving and community participation, assessment of driving skills and impact on participation, stroke and upper extremity rehabilitation, effective rehabilitation outcomes, community participation in families and children with muscular dystrophy, assessment of the impact of MD on community participation, assistive technology, AT effectiveness and availability. *Unit head:* William C. Mann, PhD, Professor and Chair, 352-273-6817, Fax: 352-273-6042, E-mail: wmann@phhp.ufl.edu. *Application contact:* Office of Admissions, 352-392-1365, E-mail: webrequests@admissions.ufl.edu.
Website: http://www.phhp.ufl.edu/ot/

University of Illinois at Chicago, Graduate College, College of Applied Health Sciences, Department of Occupational Therapy, Chicago, IL 60607-7128. Offers MS, OTD. *Accreditation:* AOTA. Part-time programs available. *Faculty:* 7 full-time (all women), 10 part-time/adjunct (8 women). *Students:* 84 full-time (77 women), 6 part-time (5 women); includes 24 minority (2 Black or African American, non-Hispanic/Latino; 6 Asian, non-Hispanic/Latino; 13 Hispanic/Latino; 3 Two or more races, non-Hispanic/Latino), 5 international. Average age 27. 553 applicants, 14% accepted, 37 enrolled. In 2013, 38 master's, 8 doctorates awarded. *Degree requirements:* For master's, thesis. *Entrance requirements:* For master's, GRE General Test, minimum GPA of 2.75, previous course work in statistics. Additional exam requirements/recommendations for international students: Required—TOEFL. *Application deadline:* For fall admission, 12/1 priority date for domestic and international students. Application fee: $40 ($50 for international students). Electronic applications accepted. *Expenses:* Tuition, state resident: full-time $11,066; part-time $3689 per term. Tuition, nonresident: full-time $23,064; part-time $7688 per term. *Required fees:* $3004; $1190 per term. Tuition and fees vary according to course level and program. *Financial support:* Fellowships with full tuition reimbursements, research assistantships with full tuition reimbursements, teaching assistantships with full tuition reimbursements, career-related internships or fieldwork, Federal Work-Study, traineeships, tuition waivers (full), and unspecified assistantships available. Financial award application deadline: 3/1; financial award applicants required to submit FAFSA. *Faculty research:* Sensory integration, perception, play, treatment efficacy, instrument development. *Total annual research expenditures:* $376,000. *Unit head:* Dr. Yolanda Suarez-Balcazar, Head, 312-996-3051, Fax: 312-413-0256, E-mail: ysuarez@uic.edu. *Application contact:* Receptionist, 312-413-2550, E-mail: gradcoll@uic.edu.
Website: http://www.ahs.uic.edu/ot/

University of Indianapolis, Graduate Programs, College of Health Sciences, School of Occupational Therapy, Indianapolis, IN 46227-3697. Offers MOT, DHS, OTD. *Accreditation:* AOTA. Part-time and evening/weekend programs available. *Faculty:* 4 full-time (all women), 3 part-time/adjunct (all women). *Students:* 84 full-time (80 women), 88 part-time (77 women); includes 16 minority (6 Black or African American, non-Hispanic/Latino; 5 Asian, non-Hispanic/Latino; 2 Hispanic/Latino; 3 Two or more races, non-Hispanic/Latino), 3 international. Average age 28. In 2013, 60 master's, 2 doctorates awarded. *Degree requirements:* For master's, thesis. *Entrance requirements:* For master's, minimum GPA of 3.0, interview; for doctorate, minimum GPA of 3.3, BA/BS or MA/MS from occupational therapy program, current state license, currently in practice as occupational therapist or have 1000 hours of practice in last 5 years. Additional exam requirements/recommendations for international students: Required—TOEFL (minimum score 550 paper-based; 92 iBT), TWE (minimum score 5). *Application deadline:* For fall admission, 11/1 for domestic students, 2/1 for international students. Application fee: $55. *Expenses:* Contact institution. *Financial support:* Career-related internships or fieldwork, Federal Work-Study, tuition waivers (full and partial), and unspecified assistantships available. Financial award application deadline: 5/1; financial award applicants required to submit FAFSA. *Unit head:* Dr. Stephanie Kelly, Dean, College of Health Sciences, 317-788-3500, Fax: 317-788-3542, E-mail: spkelly@uindy.edu. *Application contact:* Anne Hardwick, Director, Marketing and Admissions, 317-788-3495, Fax: 317-788-3542, E-mail: ahardwick@uindy.edu.
Website: http://ot.uindy.edu/

The University of Kansas, University of Kansas Medical Center, School of Health Professions, Department of Occupational Therapy Education, Kansas City, KS 66160. Offers occupational therapy (MOT, MS, OTD); therapeutic science (PhD). *Accreditation:* AOTA. Part-time programs available. *Faculty:* 16. *Students:* 77 full-time (72 women), 26 part-time (24 women); includes 8 minority (3 Black or African American, non-Hispanic/Latino; 3 Hispanic/Latino; 2 Two or more races, non-Hispanic/Latino), 3 international. Average age 28. 125 applicants, 36% accepted, 45 enrolled. In 2013, 32 master's, 2 doctorates awarded. *Degree requirements:* For doctorate, comprehensive exam, thesis/dissertation, oral defense. *Entrance requirements:* For master's, 40 hours of paid work or volunteer experience working directly with people with special needs, 3 letters of recommendation, personal statement and program statement of interest, 90 hours of elective course work with 40 hours of prerequisite work, minimum GPA of 3.0; for doctorate, 24 hours of master's-level research. Additional exam requirements/recommendations for international students: Required—TOEFL. *Application deadline:* For fall admission, 12/1 for domestic students, 4/1 for international students. Applications are processed on a rolling basis. Application fee: $60. Electronic applications accepted. *Financial support:* Research assistantships with partial tuition reimbursements, teaching assistantships with full and partial tuition reimbursements, traineeships, and unspecified assistantships available. Financial award application deadline: 3/1; financial award applicants required to submit FAFSA. *Faculty research:* Impact of sensory processing in everyday life; improving balance, motor skills, and independence with community nonprofit organizations serving people with special needs; improving self-confidence and self-sufficiency with poverty-based services in community; working with autism population in a community-wide aquatics program; improving quality of life of people living with cancer and chronic illness. *Total annual research expenditures:* $19,000. *Unit head:* Dr. Winifred W. Dunn, Professor/Chair, 913-588-7195, Fax: 913-588-4568, E-mail: wdunn@kumc.edu. *Application contact:* Wendy Hildenbrand, Admissions Representative, 913-588-7174, Fax: 913-588-4568, E-mail: whildenb@kumc.edu.
Website: http://www.kumc.edu/school-of-health-professions/occupational-therapy-education.html

University of Louisiana at Monroe, Graduate School, College of Health and Pharmaceutical Sciences, Department of Occupational Therapy, Monroe, LA 71209-0001. Offers MOT. In 2013, 33 master's awarded. Application fee: $50. *Expenses:* Tuition, state resident: full-time $6607. Tuition, nonresident: full-time $17,179. Full-time tuition and fees vary according to program. *Unit head:* Peggy Meredith, Program Director, 318-342-1617, E-mail: meredith@ulm.edu. *Application contact:* Peggy Meredith, Program Director, 318-342-1617, E-mail: meredith@ulm.edu.
Website: http://www.ulm.edu/ot/

University of Manitoba, Faculty of Graduate Studies, School of Medical Rehabilitation, Winnipeg, MB R3T 2N2, Canada. Offers applied health sciences (PhD); occupational therapy (MOT); physical therapy (MPT); rehabilitation (M Sc).

University of Mary, School of Health Sciences, Program in Occupational Therapy, Bismarck, ND 58504-9652. Offers MSOT. *Accreditation:* AOTA. Part-time programs available. Postbaccalaureate distance learning degree programs offered (minimal on-campus study). *Degree requirements:* For master's, thesis or alternative, practicum. *Entrance requirements:* For master's, ACT or equivalent, minimum GPA of 2.75, 48 hours of volunteer experience. Additional exam requirements/recommendations for international students: Required—TOEFL (minimum score 550 paper-based). Electronic applications accepted. *Expenses:* Contact institution. *Faculty research:* Safe homes for well elderly, occupation and spirituality, professional development in the spiritual domain, case method instruction, ergonomics, assistive technology.

University of Mississippi Medical Center, School of Health Related Professions, Department of Occupational Therapy, Jackson, MS 39216-4505. Offers MOT. *Accreditation:* AOTA.

University of Missouri, School of Health Professions, Program in Occupational Therapy, Columbia, MO 65211. Offers MOT. *Accreditation:* AOTA. *Faculty:* 8 full-time (all women). *Students:* 33 full-time (29 women); includes 1 minority (Hispanic/Latino). Average age 25. 27 applicants, 7% accepted, 2 enrolled. In 2013, 27 master's awarded. *Entrance requirements:* Additional exam requirements/recommendations for international students: Required—TOEFL (minimum score 500 paper-based; 61 iBT). *Application deadline:* For fall admission, 12/31 priority date for domestic and international students; for spring admission, 12/31 for domestic students. Applications are processed on a rolling basis. Application fee: $55 ($75 for international students). Electronic applications accepted. *Faculty research:* Health literacy, disability advocacy, nontraditional students in health professions educational programs, faculty teaching styles vs. student learning style preferences, brain plasticity in health and disease, neurorehabilitation, autism, gender, aging, HIV/AIDS, sub-Saharan Africa, integrating qualitative and quantitative methods. *Unit head:* Dr. Diane L. Smith, Department Chair, 573-882-8403, E-mail: smithdiane@health.missouri.edu. *Application contact:* Leanna Garrison, Department Administrator, 573-884-2113, E-mail: garrisonl@missouri.edu.
Website: http://shp.missouri.edu/ot/degrees.php

University of New England, Westbrook College of Health Professions, Program in Occupational Therapy, Biddeford, ME 04005-9526. Offers MS. *Accreditation:* AOTA. *Faculty:* 9 full-time (8 women), 5 part-time/adjunct (4 women). *Students:* 94 full-time (86 women). Average age 23. 187 applicants, 40% accepted, 45 enrolled. In 2013, 46 master's awarded. *Degree requirements:* For master's, research project, clinical fieldwork. *Entrance requirements:* For master's, minimum undergraduate GPA of 3.0, prerequisite coursework in anatomy and physiology. *Application deadline:* For fall admission, 1/15 for domestic students. Applications are processed on a rolling basis. Electronic applications accepted. *Financial support:* Application deadline: 5/1; applicants required to submit FAFSA. *Unit head:* Dr. Jane Clifford O'Brien, Director, Occupational Therapy Program/Associate Professor, 207-221-4107, E-mail: jobrien@

une.edu. *Application contact:* Dr. Cynthia Forrest, Vice President for Student Affairs, 207-221-4225, Fax: 207-523-1925, E-mail: gradadmissions@une.edu.
Website: http://www.une.edu/wchp/ot

University of New Hampshire, Graduate School, School of Health and Human Services, Department of Occupational Therapy, Durham, NH 03824. Offers MS, Postbaccalaureate Certificate. *Accreditation:* AOTA. Part-time programs available. *Faculty:* 6 full-time (5 women). *Students:* 129 full-time (125 women), 6 part-time (all women); includes 8 minority (2 Black or African American, non-Hispanic/Latino; 3 Asian, non-Hispanic/Latino; 2 Hispanic/Latino; 1 Two or more races, non-Hispanic/Latino). Average age 24. 155 applicants, 45% accepted, 66 enrolled. In 2013, 60 master's, 10 other advanced degrees awarded. *Degree requirements:* For master's, thesis or alternative. *Entrance requirements:* For master's, GRE General Test, current certification as an OTR from the American Occupational Therapy Board or World Federation of Occupational Therapy. Additional exam requirements/recommendations for international students: Required—TOEFL (minimum score 550 paper-based; 80 iBT). *Application deadline:* For fall admission, 4/1 for domestic and international students. Applications are processed on a rolling basis. Application fee: $65. Electronic applications accepted. *Expenses:* Tuition, state resident: full-time $13,500; part-time $750 per credit hour. Tuition, nonresident: full-time $26,200; part-time $1100 per credit hour. *Required fees:* $1741; $435.25 per term. Tuition and fees vary according to course level, course load, campus/location and program. *Financial support:* In 2013–14, 2 students received support. Fellowships, research assistantships, teaching assistantships, career-related internships or fieldwork, Federal Work-Study, and scholarships/grants available. Support available to part-time students. Financial award application deadline: 2/15. *Unit head:* Kerryellen Vroman, Chairperson, 603-862-4932. *Application contact:* Janice Mutschler, Administrative Assistant, 603-862-2110, E-mail: ot.dept@unh.edu.
Website: http://www.chhs.unh.edu/ot/index

University of New Mexico, School of Medicine, Program in Occupational Therapy, Albuquerque, NM 87131-5196. Offers MOT. *Accreditation:* AOTA. Part-time programs available. *Faculty:* 6 full-time (3 women). *Students:* 71 full-time (61 women), 2 part-time (both women); includes 29 minority (1 Asian, non-Hispanic/Latino; 27 Hispanic/Latino; 1 Two or more races, non-Hispanic/Latino). Average age 32. 80 applicants, 30% accepted, 24 enrolled. In 2013, 30 master's awarded. *Degree requirements:* For master's, thesis, clinical fieldwork. *Entrance requirements:* For master's, interview, writing sample, volunteer experience. *Application deadline:* For fall admission, 12/1 priority date for domestic students. Applications are processed on a rolling basis. Application fee: $50. Electronic applications accepted. *Financial support:* In 2013–14, 21 students received support. Research assistantships, Federal Work-Study, institutionally sponsored loans, scholarships/grants, traineeships, and unspecified assistantships available. Financial award application deadline: 3/1; financial award applicants required to submit FAFSA. *Faculty research:* Sensory processing, scleroderma treatment, use of therapy dogs, educational scholarship. *Unit head:* Dr. Betsy VanLeit, Director, 505-272-1753, Fax: 505-272-3583, E-mail: bvanleit@salud.unm.edu. *Application contact:* Janet Werner, Coordinator, 505-272-1753, Fax: 505-272-3583, E-mail: werner@salud.unm.edu.
Website: http://hsc.unm.edu/som/ot/

The University of North Carolina at Chapel Hill, School of Medicine and Graduate School, Graduate Programs in Medicine, Chapel Hill, NC 27599. Offers allied health sciences (MPT, MS, Au D, DPT, PhD), including human movement science (MS, PhD), occupational science (MS, PhD), physical therapy (MPT, MS, DPT), rehabilitation counseling and psychology (MS), speech and hearing sciences (MS, Au D, PhD); biochemistry and biophysics (MS, PhD); bioinformatics and computational biology (PhD); biomedical engineering (MS, PhD); cell and developmental biology (PhD); cell and molecular physiology (PhD); genetics and molecular biology (PhD); microbiology and immunology (MS, PhD), including immunology, microbiology; neurobiology (PhD); pathology and laboratory medicine (PhD), including experimental pathology; pharmacology (PhD); MD/PhD. Postbaccalaureate distance learning degree programs offered. Terminal master's awarded for partial completion of doctoral program. *Degree requirements:* For master's, comprehensive exam; for doctorate, thesis/dissertation. Electronic applications accepted. *Expenses:* Contact institution.

The University of North Carolina at Chapel Hill, School of Medicine and Graduate School, Graduate Programs in Medicine, Department of Allied Health Sciences, Division of Occupational Science and Occupational Therapy, Chapel Hill, NC 27599. Offers occupational science (PhD); occupational therapy (MS). *Accreditation:* AOTA. *Degree requirements:* For master's, comprehensive exam, thesis optional, collaborative research project; for doctorate, thesis/dissertation. *Entrance requirements:* For master's, GRE General Test; for doctorate, GRE, master's degree in occupational therapy, relevant social behavioral sciences or health field. Additional exam requirements/recommendations for international students: Required—TOEFL (minimum score 550 paper-based). Electronic applications accepted. *Faculty research:* Parents and infants in co-occupations, psychosocial dysfunction, predictors of autism, factors influencing the occupation of primates, factors influencing occupations of people with dementia, occupational development of young children.

University of North Dakota, Graduate School and Graduate School, Graduate Programs in Medicine, Department of Occupational Therapy, Grand Forks, ND 58202. Offers MOT. *Accreditation:* AOTA. Part-time programs available. *Entrance requirements:* For master's, letter of reference; volunteer or work experience, preferably from health-related field; interview; minimum GPA of 2.7. Additional exam requirements/recommendations for international students: Required—TOEFL (minimum score 550 paper-based; 79 iBT), IELTS (minimum score 6.5). Electronic applications accepted.

University of Oklahoma Health Sciences Center, Graduate College, College of Allied Health, Department of Occupational Therapy, Oklahoma City, OK 73190. Offers MOT. *Accreditation:* AOTA. *Faculty:* 4 full-time (all women). *Students:* 61 full-time (52 women), 19 part-time (17 women); includes 13 minority (1 Black or African American, non-Hispanic/Latino; 5 American Indian or Alaska Native, non-Hispanic/Latino; 2 Asian, non-Hispanic/Latino; 5 Two or more races, non-Hispanic/Latino), 11 international. Average age 24. 119 applicants, 31% accepted, 29 enrolled. In 2013, 32 master's awarded. *Application deadline:* For fall admission, 6/1 for domestic students; for winter admission, 4/1 for domestic students; for spring admission, 10/1 for domestic students. *Expenses:* Tuition, state resident: full-time $3504; part-time $175.20 per credit hour. Tuition, nonresident: full-time $13,504; part-time $675.20 per credit hour. *Required fees:* $1545; $52.70 per credit hour. $245.25 per semester. Tuition and fees vary according to course load. *Unit head:* Dr. Kevin Rudeen, Dean, 405-271-2288, Fax: 405-271-1190, E-mail: kevin-rudeen@ouhsc.edu. *Application contact:* Susan Tucker, Associate Dean for Finance, 405-271-2288, Fax: 405-271-1190, E-mail: susan-tucker@ouhsc.edu.

University of Pittsburgh, School of Health and Rehabilitation Sciences, Master of Occupational Therapy Program, Pittsburgh, PA 15260. Offers MOT. *Accreditation:* AOTA. *Faculty:* 5 full-time (all women), 2 part-time/adjunct (1 woman). *Students:* 97 full-time (87 women), 6 part-time (all women); includes 9 minority (1 Black or African American, non-Hispanic/Latino; 5 Asian, non-Hispanic/Latino; 3 Hispanic/Latino), 2 international. Average age 27. 640 applicants, 16% accepted, 51 enrolled. In 2013, 49 master's awarded. *Entrance requirements:* For master's, GRE General Test, volunteer experience. Additional exam requirements/recommendations for international students: Required—TOEFL (minimum score 550 paper-based; 80 iBT), IELTS (minimum score 6.5). *Application deadline:* For fall admission, 4/1 for domestic students, 2/1 for international students. Applications are processed on a rolling basis. Application fee: $125. Electronic applications accepted. *Expenses:* Contact institution. *Financial support:* In 2013–14, 1 fellowship (averaging $17,370 per year) was awarded; Federal Work-Study also available. *Faculty research:* Expertise in evidence-based practice, measuring occupational performance, ergonomics, geriatrics, mental health, neurorehabilitation, research. *Total annual research expenditures:* $441,440. *Unit head:* Dr. Joan Rogers, Associate Dean of Graduate Studies, 412-383-6620, Fax: 412-383-6613, E-mail: jcr@pitt.edu. *Application contact:* Joyce Broadwick, Administrator, 412-383-6620, Fax: 412-383-6613, E-mail: otpitt@shrs.pitt.edu.
Website: http://www.shrs.pitt.edu/mot/

University of Pittsburgh, School of Health and Rehabilitation Sciences, Master's Programs in Health and Rehabilitation Sciences, Pittsburgh, PA 15260. Offers health and rehabilitation sciences (MS), including health care supervision and management, health information systems, occupational therapy, physical therapy, rehabilitation counseling, rehabilitation science and technology, sports medicine, wellness and human performance. *Accreditation:* APTA. Part-time and evening/weekend programs available. *Faculty:* 63 full-time (37 women), 4 part-time/adjunct (2 women). *Students:* 117 full-time (70 women), 44 part-time (27 women); includes 18 minority (8 Black or African American, non-Hispanic/Latino; 1 American Indian or Alaska Native, non-Hispanic/Latino; 6 Asian, non-Hispanic/Latino; 3 Hispanic/Latino), 52 international. Average age 30. 368 applicants, 57% accepted, 96 enrolled. In 2013, 90 master's awarded. *Degree requirements:* For master's, comprehensive exam (for some programs), thesis optional. *Entrance requirements:* For master's, minimum GPA of 3.0. Additional exam requirements/recommendations for international students: Required—TOEFL (minimum score 550 paper-based; 80 iBT), IELTS (minimum score 6.5). *Application deadline:* For fall admission, 3/1 for international students; for spring admission, 9/1 for international students. Applications are processed on a rolling basis. Application fee: $50. Electronic applications accepted. *Expenses:* Contact institution. *Financial support:* In 2013–14, 3 fellowships (averaging $20,460 per year) were awarded; Federal Work-Study, institutionally sponsored loans, scholarships/grants, traineeships, and unspecified assistantships available. Financial award applicants required to submit FAFSA. *Faculty research:* Assistive technology, seating and wheeled mobility, cellular neurophysiology, low back syndrome, augmentative communication. *Total annual research expenditures:* $8.1 million. *Unit head:* Dr. Clifford E. Brubaker, Dean, 412-383-6560, Fax: 412-383-6535, E-mail: cliffb@pitt.edu. *Application contact:* Jessica Maguire, Director of Admissions, 412-383-6557, Fax: 412-383-6535, E-mail: maguire@pitt.edu.
Website: http://www.shrs.pitt.edu/

University of Puerto Rico, Medical Sciences Campus, School of Health Professions, Program in Occupational Therapy, San Juan, PR 00936-5067. Offers MS. *Accreditation:* AOTA.

University of Puget Sound, Graduate Studies, School of Occupational Therapy, Tacoma, WA 98416. Offers policy, advocacy, and leadership (MOT); research (MSOT). *Accreditation:* AOTA. *Degree requirements:* For master's, thesis, publishable paper or program development project. *Entrance requirements:* For master's, GRE General Test, minimum baccalaureate GPA of 3.0, three letters of recommendation. Additional exam requirements/recommendations for international students: Required—TOEFL (minimum score 550 paper-based; 90 iBT). Electronic applications accepted. *Expenses:* Contact institution. *Faculty research:* Scope of practice for school-based occupational therapy, family occupational adaptation to autism, clinical decision-making, low vision adaptation, assistive technology.

University of St. Augustine for Health Sciences, Graduate Programs, Division of Occupational Therapy, St. Augustine, FL 32086. Offers MOT; OTD. *Accreditation:* AOTA. *Entrance requirements:* For master's, GRE General Test. *Application deadline:* For fall admission, 12/15 for domestic students; for spring admission, 6/15 for domestic students; for summer admission, 10/1 for domestic students. Applications are processed on a rolling basis. Application fee: $50. Tuition and fees vary according to course level, course load, campus/location and program. *Unit head:* Dr. Karen S. Howell, Director of Occupational Therapy, 904-826-0084 Ext. 222, Fax: 904-826-0085, E-mail: kclayton@usa.edu. *Application contact:* Dian Hartley, Director of Admissions, 904-826-0084 Ext. 207, Fax: 904-826-0085, E-mail: dhartley@usa.edu.
Website: http://www.usa.edu/

The University of Scranton, College of Graduate and Continuing Education, Program in Occupational Therapy, Scranton, PA 18510. Offers MS. *Accreditation:* AOTA. *Faculty:* 6 full-time (5 women). *Students:* 49 full-time (48 women), 1 part-time (0 women); includes 2 minority (1 Hispanic/Latino; 1 Two or more races, non-Hispanic/Latino). Average age 23. 10 applicants, 100% accepted. In 2013, 39 master's awarded. *Degree requirements:* For master's, thesis, capstone experience. *Entrance requirements:* For master's, minimum GPA of 3.0. Additional exam requirements/recommendations for international students: Required—TOEFL (minimum score 500 paper-based), IELTS (minimum score 6). *Application deadline:* Applications are processed on a rolling basis. Application fee: $0. *Financial support:* In 2013–14, 7 students received support, including 7 teaching assistantships with full tuition reimbursements available; career-related internships or fieldwork, Federal Work-Study, and unspecified assistantships also available. Support available to part-time students. Financial award application deadline: 3/1. *Unit head:* Dr. Marlene Joy Morgan, Director, 570-941-5789, Fax: 570-941-4380. *Application contact:* Joseph M. Roback, Director of Admissions, 570-941-4385, Fax: 570-941-5928, E-mail: robackj2@scranton.edu.

University of South Alabama, Graduate School, College of Allied Health Professions, Department of Occupational Therapy, Mobile, AL 36688-0002. Offers MS. *Accreditation:* AOTA. *Faculty:* 5 full-time (all women). *Students:* 75 full-time (64 women); includes 9 minority (3 Black or African American, non-Hispanic/Latino; 2 American Indian or Alaska Native, non-Hispanic/Latino; 1 Asian, non-Hispanic/Latino; 2 Hispanic/Latino; 1 Two or more races, non-Hispanic/Latino). 105 applicants, 37% accepted, 21 enrolled. In 2013, 25 master's awarded. *Degree requirements:* For master's, clinical externship. *Entrance requirements:* For master's, GRE, minimum GPA of 3.0; bachelor's degree or 96 semester hours of prerequisites and electives. Additional exam requirements/recommendations for international students: Required—TOEFL (minimum score 525 paper-based). *Application deadline:* For fall admission, 1/2 for domestic and international students. Application fee: $75. *Expenses:* Tuition, state resident: full-time $8976; part-time $374 per credit hour. Tuition, nonresident: full-time $17,952; part-time $748 per credit hour. *Unit head:* Dr. Majorie Scaffa, Chair, 251-445-9222, Fax: 251-445-9211, E-mail: otdept@usouthal.edu. *Application contact:* Dr. Julio Turrens, Director of Graduate Studies, 251-445-9250.
Website: http://www.southalabama.edu/alliedhealth/ot/

The University of South Dakota, Graduate School, School of Health Sciences, Department of Occupational Therapy, Vermillion, SD 57069-2390. Offers MS. *Accreditation:* AOTA. Part-time programs available. *Degree requirements:* For master's, thesis optional, 6 months of supervised fieldwork. *Entrance requirements:* For master's, courses in human anatomy, human physiology, general psychology, abnormal psychology, lifespan development, statistics. Additional exam requirements/

recommendations for international students: Required—TOEFL (minimum score 550 paper-based). *Expenses:* Contact institution. *Faculty research:* Low vision in youth and adults, agricultural/rural health, childhood obesity, adolescent mental health, elder health and well being.

University of Southern California, Graduate School, Herman Ostrow School of Dentistry, Division of Occupational Science and Occupational Therapy, Graduate Program in Occupational Science, Los Angeles, CA 90089. Offers PhD. *Degree requirements:* For doctorate, thesis/dissertation, qualifying exam. *Entrance requirements:* For doctorate, GRE (minimum combined score of 1100), minimum GPA of 3.0. Additional exam requirements/recommendations for international students: Required—TOEFL (minimum score 600 paper-based; 100 iBT). Electronic applications accepted. *Faculty research:* Health and well-being; health disparities and cultural influences on health and recovery; family life; community re-integration and social participation; engagement, activity and neuroscience; rehabilitation science and ethics; society and social justice; autism and sensory integration; interventions; health disparities in autism diagnosis.

University of Southern California, Graduate School, Herman Ostrow School of Dentistry, Division of Occupational Science and Occupational Therapy, Graduate Programs in Occupational Therapy, Los Angeles, CA 90089. Offers MA, OTD. *Accreditation:* AOTA. Part-time programs available. *Degree requirements:* For master's, comprehensive exam (for some programs), thesis or alternative; for doctorate, residency, portfolio. *Entrance requirements:* For master's and doctorate, GRE (minimum score 1000), minimum cumulative GPA of 3.0. Additional exam requirements/recommendations for international students: Required—TOEFL (minimum score 600 paper-based; 100 iBT). Electronic applications accepted. *Faculty research:* Health and well-being; health disparities and cultural influences on health and recovery; family life; community re-integration and social participation; engagement, activity and neuroscience; rehabilitation science and ethics; society and social justice; autism and sensory integration; interventions; health disparities in autism diagnosis.

University of Southern Indiana, Graduate Studies, College of Nursing and Health Professions, Program in Occupational Therapy, Evansville, IN 47712-3590. Offers MSOT. *Accreditation:* AOTA. Part-time programs available. Postbaccalaureate distance learning degree programs offered (minimal on-campus study). *Faculty:* 7 full-time (6 women). *Students:* 29 full-time (24 women); includes 1 minority (Hispanic/Latino). Average age 24. 5 applicants. In 2013, 27 master's awarded. *Entrance requirements:* Additional exam requirements/recommendations for international students: Required—TOEFL (minimum score 550 paper-based; 79 iBT), IELTS (minimum score 6). *Application deadline:* For fall admission, 2/15 priority date for domestic and international students. Applications are processed on a rolling basis. Application fee: $40. Electronic applications accepted. *Expenses:* Tuition, state resident: full-time $5567; part-time $309 per credit hour. Tuition, nonresident: full-time $10,977; part-time $610 per credit. *Required fees:* $23 per semester. *Financial support:* In 2013–14, 9 students received support. Federal Work-Study, scholarships/grants, tuition waivers (full and partial), and unspecified assistantships available. Financial award application deadline: 3/1; financial award applicants required to submit FAFSA. *Unit head:* Dr. Janet Kilbane, Interim Program Chair, 812-465-1179, E-mail: bjwilliams4@usi.edu. *Application contact:* Dr. Mayola Rowser, Interim Director, Graduate Studies, 812-465-7016, Fax: 812-464-1956, E-mail: mrowser@usi.edu.
Website: http://www.usi.edu/health/occupational-therapy

University of Southern Maine, Lewiston-Auburn College, Program in Occupational Therapy, Lewiston, ME 04240. Offers occupational therapy (MOT); occupational therapy: return to practice (CGS). *Accreditation:* AOTA. *Faculty:* 5 full-time (4 women), 3 part-time/adjunct (all women). *Students:* 41 full-time (36 women), 36 part-time (30 women); includes 2 minority (1 Black or African American, non-Hispanic/Latino; 1 American Indian or Alaska Native, non-Hispanic/Latino). Average age 29. 45 applicants, 71% accepted, 24 enrolled. In 2013, 21 master's awarded. *Degree requirements:* For master's, fieldwork, original research. *Entrance requirements:* For master's, minimum GPA of 3.0, writing sample, interview, reference letters, job shadow observation. *Application deadline:* Applications are processed on a rolling basis. Application fee: $65. Electronic applications accepted. *Expenses:* Tuition, state resident: part-time $380 per credit. Tuition, nonresident: part-time $1026 per credit. Part-time tuition and fees vary according to program. *Financial support:* Fellowships, research assistantships, teaching assistantships, Federal Work-Study, scholarships/grants, tuition waivers (partial), and unspecified assistantships available. Financial award application deadline: 3/1; financial award applicants required to submit FAFSA. *Faculty research:* Multicultural curricula, cultural competence, parents responses to fussy infants, chronic pain, early childhood eating disorders. *Unit head:* Dr. Roxie M. Black, Professor and Program Director, 207-753-6515, Fax: 207-753-6555, E-mail: rblack@usm.maine.edu. *Application contact:* Luisa Scott, 207-753-6523, E-mail: lscott@usm.maine.edu.
Website: http://usm.maine.edu/ot

The University of Tennessee Health Science Center, College of Health Professions, Memphis, TN 38163-0002. Offers audiology (MS, Au D); clinical laboratory science (MSCLS); cytopathology practice (MCP); health informatics and information management (MHIIM); occupational therapy (MOT); physical therapy (DPT, ScDPT); physician assistant (MMS); speech-language pathology (MS). *Accreditation:* AOTA; APTA. Part-time and evening/weekend programs available. Postbaccalaureate distance learning degree programs offered (minimal on-campus study). Terminal master's awarded for partial completion of doctoral program. *Degree requirements:* For master's, comprehensive exam, thesis; for doctorate, comprehensive exam, residency. *Entrance requirements:* For master's, GRE (MOT, MSCLS), minimum GPA of 3.0, 3 letters of reference, national accreditation (MSCLS), GRE if GPA is less than 3.0 (MCP); for doctorate, GRE. Additional exam requirements/recommendations for international students: Required—TOEFL (minimum score 550 paper-based; 80 iBT). *Application deadline:* For fall admission, 1/30 priority date for domestic students; for winter admission, 10/1 priority date for domestic students. Application fee: $50. Electronic applications accepted. *Expenses:* Contact institution. *Financial support:* Teaching assistantships, Federal Work-Study, institutionally sponsored loans, and scholarships/grants available. Support available to part-time students. Financial award application deadline: 2/15; financial award applicants required to submit FAFSA. *Faculty research:* Gait deviation, muscular dystrophy and strength, hemophilia and exercise, pediatric neurology, self-efficacy. *Unit head:* Dr. Noma Anderson, Dean, 901-528-5588, Fax: 901-528-7545, E-mail: nander13@uthsc.edu. *Application contact:* Dr. Noma Anderson, Dean, 901-528-5588, Fax: 901-528-7545, E-mail: nander13@uthsc.edu.
Website: http://www.uthsc.edu/health-professions/

The University of Texas at El Paso, Graduate School, College of Health Sciences, Master of Occupational Therapy (MOT) Program, El Paso, TX 79968-0001. Offers MOT. *Accreditation:* AOTA. *Degree requirements:* For master's, thesis optional. *Entrance requirements:* For master's, GRE, minimum cumulative and prerequisite GPA of 3.0, bachelor's degree, 40 clock hours of supervised observations with an OT. Additional exam requirements/recommendations for international students: Required—TOEFL; Recommended—IELTS. *Faculty research:* Falls prevention, coping of mothers with children with disabilities.

The University of Texas Health Science Center at San Antonio, School of Health Professions, San Antonio, TX 78229-3900. Offers occupational therapy (MOT); physical therapy (DPT); physician assistant studies (MS); toxicology (MS). *Accreditation:* AOTA; APTA; ARC-PA. *Faculty:* 75 full-time (31 women), 49 part-time/adjunct (19 women). *Students:* 353 full-time (258 women), 2 part-time (1 woman); includes 180 minority (15 Black or African American, non-Hispanic/Latino; 29 Asian, non-Hispanic/Latino; 129 Hispanic/Latino; 1 Native Hawaiian or other Pacific Islander, non-Hispanic/Latino; 6 Two or more races, non-Hispanic/Latino), 3 international. Average age 28. 605 applicants, 21% accepted, 125 enrolled. In 2013, 73 master's, 63 doctorates awarded. *Degree requirements:* For master's, comprehensive exam, thesis (for some programs); for doctorate, comprehensive exam. *Entrance requirements:* For master's, GRE (for toxicology), minimum GPA of 3.0 and bachelor's degree in clinical laboratory science or closely-related science discipline (for MS in toxicology); minimum GPA of 3.0, bachelor's degree, PA shadowing, and community service (for MS in physician assistant); for doctorate, GRE, minimum GPA of 3.0, bachelor's degree, PT shadowing, observation hours. Additional exam requirements/recommendations for international students: Required—TOEFL (minimum score 560 paper-based). *Application deadline:* For fall admission, 6/1 for domestic and international students; for spring admission, 10/1 for domestic and international students. Application fee: $60. Electronic applications accepted. *Financial support:* In 2013–14, 219 students received support. Federal Work-Study, scholarships/grants, and stipends, department payments available. Financial award application deadline: 6/30; financial award applicants required to submit FAFSA. *Total annual research expenditures:* $760,563. *Unit head:* Dr. Susan Dollar, Assistant Dean, 210-567-4837, Fax: 210-567-4828, E-mail: dollar@uthscsa.edu. *Application contact:* Dr. David L. Henzi, Assistant Dean for Admissions, 210-567-4818, Fax: 210-567-4828, E-mail: henzi@uthscsa.edu.
Website: http://www.uthscsa.edu/shp/

The University of Texas Medical Branch, School of Health Professions, Department of Occupational Therapy, Galveston, TX 77555. Offers MOT. *Accreditation:* AOTA. *Entrance requirements:* For master's, MAT, 20 volunteer hours, telephone interview, 2 references.

The University of Texas–Pan American, College of Health Sciences and Human Services, Department of Occupational Therapy, Edinburg, TX 78539. Offers MS. *Accreditation:* AOTA. Evening/weekend programs available. *Entrance requirements:* For master's, Health Occupations Aptitude Examination. *Expenses:* Tuition, state resident: full-time $5986; part-time $333 per credit hour. Tuition, nonresident: full-time $12,358; part-time $687 per credit hour. *Required fees:* $782. Tuition and fees vary according to program. *Faculty research:* Parenting of children with disabilities, effects of healing touch on student stress.

The University of Toledo, College of Graduate Studies, College of Health Sciences, Department of Rehabilitation Sciences, Toledo, OH 43606-3390. Offers occupational therapy (OTD); physical therapy (DPT); speech-language pathology (MA). *Faculty:* 30. *Students:* 180 full-time (148 women), 31 part-time (29 women); includes 11 minority (2 Black or African American, non-Hispanic/Latino; 3 Asian, non-Hispanic/Latino; 2 Hispanic/Latino; 4 Two or more races, non-Hispanic/Latino). Average age 25. 230 applicants, 58% accepted, 61 enrolled. In 2013, 25 master's, 43 doctorates awarded. *Degree requirements:* For master's, comprehensive exam, thesis; for doctorate, thesis/dissertation or alternative. *Entrance requirements:* For master's, GRE, minimum cumulative GPA of 2.7 for all previous academic work, letters of recommendation; for doctorate, GRE; minimum cumulative GPA of 3.0 for all previous academic work, letters of recommendation; OTCAS or PTCAS application and UT supplemental application (for OTD and DPT). Additional exam requirements/recommendations for international students: Required—TOEFL (minimum score 550 paper-based; 80 iBT). *Application deadline:* For fall admission, 11/1 for domestic and international students. Application fee: $45 ($75 for international students). Electronic applications accepted. *Financial support:* In 2013–14, 16 teaching assistantships with full and partial tuition reimbursements (averaging $5,002 per year) were awarded; Federal Work-Study, scholarships/grants, tuition waivers (full and partial), unspecified assistantships, and administrative assistantships also available. Financial award applicants required to submit FAFSA. *Unit head:* Dr. Michelle Masterson, Chair, 419-530-6671, Fax: 419-530-4780, E-mail: michelle.masterson@utoledo.edu. *Application contact:* College of Graduate Studies, 419-383-4112, Fax: 419-383-6140, E-mail: grdsch@utnet.utoledo.edu.
Website: http://www.utoledo.edu/eduhshs/

University of Toronto, Faculty of Medicine, Department of Occupational Science and Occupational Therapy, Toronto, ON M5S 1A1, Canada. Offers occupational therapy (M Sc OT). *Entrance requirements:* For master's, bachelor's degree with high academic standing from recognized university with minimum B average in final year, personal statement. Additional exam requirements/recommendations for international students: Required—TOEFL (minimum score 600 paper-based; 100 iBT), TWE (minimum score 5). Electronic applications accepted.

University of Utah, Graduate School, College of Health, Division of Occupational Therapy, Salt Lake City, UT 84108. Offers MOT, OTD. *Accreditation:* AOTA. Part-time and evening/weekend programs available. Postbaccalaureate distance learning degree programs offered (no on-campus study). *Faculty:* 2 full-time (both women), 12 part-time/adjunct (10 women). *Students:* 97 full-time (64 women), 19 part-time (16 women); includes 9 minority (5 Asian, non-Hispanic/Latino; 3 Hispanic/Latino; 1 Native Hawaiian or other Pacific Islander, non-Hispanic/Latino). Average age 30. 130 applicants, 36% accepted, 47 enrolled. In 2013, 31 master's awarded. *Degree requirements:* For master's, thesis or alternative, project; for doctorate, thesis/dissertation or alternative, capstone. *Entrance requirements:* For master's, GRE General Test. Additional exam requirements/recommendations for international students: Required—TOEFL (minimum score 575 paper-based). *Application deadline:* For fall admission, 12/1 for domestic and international students. Application fee: $125. *Expenses:* Contact institution. *Financial support:* In 2013–14, 10 students received support. Career-related internships or fieldwork, Federal Work-Study, institutionally sponsored loans, scholarships/grants, and unspecified assistantships available. Financial award application deadline: 2/15; financial award applicants required to submit FAFSA. *Faculty research:* Community-based practice, occupational science, refugees, resilience, low vision, traumatic brain injury, pediatrics. *Total annual research expenditures:* $13,409. *Unit head:* Dr. Lorie Richards, Chairperson, 801-585-1069, Fax: 801-585-1001, E-mail: lorie.richards@hsc.utah.edu. *Application contact:* Kelly C. Brown, Academic Advisor, 801-585-0555, Fax: 801-585-1001, E-mail: kelly.brown@hsc.utah.edu.
Website: http://www.health.utah.edu/ot/

University of Washington, Graduate School, School of Medicine, Graduate Programs in Medicine, Department of Rehabilitation Medicine, Seattle, WA 98195-6490. Offers occupational therapy (MOT); physical therapy (DPT); prosthetics and orthotics (MPO); rehabilitation science (PhD). *Degree requirements:* For doctorate, comprehensive exam (for some programs), thesis/dissertation (for some programs). *Entrance requirements:* For master's and doctorate, GRE. Additional exam requirements/recommendations for international students: Required—TOEFL. *Faculty research:* Biomechanics, balance, brain injury, spinal cord injury, pain, degenerative diseases.

Occupational Therapy

The University of Western Ontario, Faculty of Graduate Studies, Health Sciences Division, School of Occupational Therapy, London, ON N6A 5B8, Canada. Offers M Sc. Part-time programs available. *Degree requirements:* For master's, thesis. *Entrance requirements:* For master's, Canadian BA in occupational therapy or equivalent, minimum B+ average in last 2 years of 4 year degree. Additional exam requirements/recommendations for international students: Required—TOEFL (minimum score 570 paper-based). *Faculty research:* Human occupation, clumsy children, biomechanics, learning disabilities, ergonomics.

University of Wisconsin–La Crosse, Graduate Studies, College of Science and Health, Department of Health Professions, Program in Occupational Therapy, La Crosse, WI 54601-3742. Offers MS. *Accreditation:* AOTA. *Faculty:* 5 full-time (all women). *Students:* 47 full-time (44 women), 26 part-time (24 women); includes 3 minority (2 Asian, non-Hispanic/Latino; 1 Two or more races, non-Hispanic/Latino). Average age 25. 101 applicants, 33% accepted, 23 enrolled. In 2013, 26 master's awarded. *Degree requirements:* For master's, 6-month clinical internship. *Entrance requirements:* For master's, minimum GPA of 3.0, 20 job shadowing hours. Additional exam requirements/recommendations for international students: Required—TOEFL (minimum score 550 paper-based; 79 iBT). *Application deadline:* For fall admission, 1/4 for domestic students. Electronic applications accepted. *Expenses:* Contact institution. *Financial support:* Federal Work-Study, scholarships/grants, and health care benefits available. Support available to part-time students. Financial award application deadline: 3/15; financial award applicants required to submit FAFSA. *Unit head:* Dr. Peggy Denton, Director, 608-785-8470, E-mail: pdenton@uwlax.edu. *Application contact:* Corey Sjoquist, Director of Admissions, 608-785-8939, E-mail: admissions@uwlax.edu. Website: http://www.uwlax.edu/ot/

University of Wisconsin–Madison, Graduate School, School of Education, Department of Kinesiology, Occupational Therapy Program, Madison, WI 53706-1380. Offers MS, PhD. *Accreditation:* AOTA. *Degree requirements:* For doctorate, thesis/dissertation. Application fee: $56. *Expenses:* Tuition, state resident: full-time $10,728; part-time $790 per credit. Tuition, nonresident: full-time $24,054; part-time $1623 per credit. *Required fees:* $1130; $119 per credit. *Financial support:* Fellowships with full tuition reimbursements, research assistantships with full tuition reimbursements, teaching assistantships with full tuition reimbursements, traineeships, and project assistantships available. *Unit head:* Dr. Dorothy Edwards, Chair, 608-262-2936, E-mail: kines@education.wisc.edu. *Application contact:* Admissions Coordinator. Website: http://kinesiology.education.wisc.edu/ot/about

University of Wisconsin–Milwaukee, Graduate School, College of Health Sciences, Department of Occupational Science and Technology, Milwaukee, WI 53201-0413. Offers ergonomics (Certificate); occupational therapy (MS); therapeutic recreation (Certificate). *Accreditation:* AOTA. *Faculty:* 11 full-time (6 women), 1 (woman) part-time/adjunct. *Students:* 45 full-time (37 women), 4 part-time (3 women); includes 4 minority (2 Asian, non-Hispanic/Latino; 2 Two or more races, non-Hispanic/Latino), 1 international. Average age 27. 54 applicants, 24% accepted, 11 enrolled. In 2013, 33 master's awarded. *Degree requirements:* For master's, thesis or alternative. *Entrance requirements:* Additional exam requirements/recommendations for international students: Required—TOEFL (minimum score 550 paper-based; 79 iBT), IELTS (minimum score 6.5). *Application deadline:* For fall admission, 1/1 priority date for domestic students; for spring admission, 9/1 for domestic students. Applications are processed on a rolling basis. Application fee: $45 ($75 for international students). *Financial support:* Fellowships, research assistantships, teaching assistantships, and unspecified assistantships available. Support available to part-time students. Financial award application deadline: 4/15. *Unit head:* Carol Haertlein Sells, Department Chair, 414-229-6933, E-mail: chaert@uwm.edu. *Application contact:* Roger O. Smith, General Information Contact, 414-229-6697, Fax: 414-229-6697, E-mail: smithro@uwm.edu. Website: http://www4.uwm.edu/chs/academics/occupational_therapy/

Utica College, Program in Occupational Therapy, Utica, NY 13502-4892. Offers MS. *Accreditation:* AOTA. Part-time and evening/weekend programs available. *Faculty:* 7 full-time (all women). *Students:* 82 full-time (67 women), 3 part-time (1 woman); includes 13 minority (6 Black or African American, non-Hispanic/Latino; 4 Asian, non-Hispanic/Latino; 3 Hispanic/Latino), 2 international. Average age 27. In 2013, 57 master's awarded. *Degree requirements:* For master's, thesis. *Entrance requirements:* For master's, physical health exam, CPR certification, 60 hours of volunteer experience, minimum GPA of 3.0. Additional exam requirements/recommendations for international students: Required—TOEFL (minimum score 525 paper-based). *Application deadline:* Applications are processed on a rolling basis. Application fee: $50. Electronic applications accepted. *Expenses:* Contact institution. *Financial support:* Career-related internships or fieldwork, scholarships/grants, tuition waivers (partial), and unspecified assistantships available. Support available to part-time students. Financial award application deadline: 3/15; financial award applicants required to submit FAFSA. *Unit head:* Cora Bruns, Director, 315-792-3125, E-mail: cbruns@utica.edu. *Application contact:* John D. Rowe, Director of Graduate Admissions, 315-792-3824, Fax: 315-792-3003, E-mail: jrowe@utica.edu.

Virginia Commonwealth University, Graduate School, School of Allied Health Professions, Department of Occupational Therapy, Richmond, VA 23284-9005. Offers MS, MSOT, OTD. *Accreditation:* AOTA (one or more programs are accredited). *Degree requirements:* For master's, fieldwork. *Entrance requirements:* For master's, GRE General Test. Additional exam requirements/recommendations for international students: Required—TOEFL (minimum score 600 paper-based; 100 iBT); Recommended—IELTS (minimum score 6.5). Electronic applications accepted. *Faculty research:* Children with complex care needs, instrument development, carpal tunnel syndrome, development of oral-motor feeding programs, school system practice.

Virginia Commonwealth University, Graduate School, School of Allied Health Professions, Doctoral Program in Health Related Sciences, Richmond, VA 23284-9005. Offers clinical laboratory sciences (PhD); gerontology (PhD); health administration (PhD); nurse anesthesia (PhD); occupational therapy (PhD); physical therapy (PhD); radiation sciences (PhD); rehabilitation leadership (PhD). *Entrance requirements:* For doctorate, GRE General Test or MAT, minimum GPA of 3.3 in master's degree. Additional exam requirements/recommendations for international students: Required—TOEFL (minimum score 600 paper-based; 100 iBT); Recommended—IELTS (minimum score 6.5). Electronic applications accepted.

Washington University in St. Louis, School of Medicine, Program in Occupational Therapy, Saint Louis, MO 63108. Offers MSOT, OTD. *Accreditation:* AOTA. Terminal master's awarded for partial completion of doctoral program. *Degree requirements:* For master's, fieldwork experiences; for doctorate, fieldwork and apprenticeship experiences. *Entrance requirements:* For master's and doctorate, GRE General Test, bachelor's degree in another field or enrollment in an affiliated institution. Additional exam requirements/recommendations for international students: Required—TOEFL, TWE (minimum score 5). Electronic applications accepted. *Faculty research:* Brain injury, ergonomics, work performance, care giving, quality of life, rehabilitation.

Wayne State University, Eugene Applebaum College of Pharmacy and Health Sciences, Department of Health Care Sciences, Program in Occupational Therapy, Detroit, MI 48202. Offers MOT. Students begin the program as undergraduates. *Accreditation:* AOTA. Part-time programs available. *Faculty:* 6 full-time (all women), 6 part-time/adjunct (all women). *Students:* 30 full-time (24 women); includes 5 minority (2 Black or African American, non-Hispanic/Latino; 2 Asian, non-Hispanic/Latino; 1 Two or more races, non-Hispanic/Latino), 1 international. Average age 26. In 2013, 30 master's awarded. *Entrance requirements:* For master's, personal resume; 20 contact hours under supervision of an OTR; two professional recommendations; interview, background check. Additional exam requirements/recommendations for international students: Required—TOEFL (minimum score 550 paper-based; 79 iBT), Michigan English Language Assessment Battery (minimum score 85); Recommended—IELTS (minimum score 6.5), TWE (minimum score 5.5). *Application deadline:* For fall admission, 2/28 for domestic and international students. Application fee: $0. Electronic applications accepted. *Expenses:* Contact institution. *Financial support:* In 2013–14, 21 students received support. Teaching assistantships, career-related internships or fieldwork, scholarships/grants, and unspecified assistantships available. Support available to part-time students. Financial award application deadline: 3/31; financial award applicants required to submit FAFSA. *Faculty research:* Technology for neurorehabilitation, body shape and movement analysis, grasp and manipulation, methods of measurement of quality-of-life outcomes of the entire family of a person with chronic illnesses or disabilities, evaluating the efficacy of different types of family support interventions for persons of low socio-economic status, program evaluation for persons with disabilities across the lifespan. *Unit head:* Dr. Doreen Head, Program Director, 313-577-5884, E-mail: doreen.head@wayne.edu. *Application contact:* Dr. Regina N. Parnell, Assistant Professor, 313-577-6794, Fax: 313-577-5822, E-mail: ad9049@wayne.edu. Website: http://www.cphs.wayne.edu/ot/

Western Michigan University, Graduate College, College of Health and Human Services, Department of Occupational Therapy, Kalamazoo, MI 49008. Offers MS. *Accreditation:* AOTA. *Entrance requirements:* For master's, GRE General Test.

Western New Mexico University, Graduate Division, Program in Occupational Therapy, Silver City, NM 88062-0680. Offers MOT. *Accreditation:* AOTA. Part-time programs available. Postbaccalaureate distance learning degree programs offered.

West Virginia University, School of Medicine, Graduate Programs in Human Performance, Division of Occupational Therapy, Morgantown, WV 26506. Offers MOT. Students enter program as undergraduates. *Accreditation:* AOTA. Postbaccalaureate distance learning degree programs offered. *Degree requirements:* For master's, clinical rotation. *Entrance requirements:* For master's, interview, 2 reference forms, minimum GPA of 3.0, 60 hours of volunteer experience with people with disabilities. *Expenses:* Contact institution.

Winston-Salem State University, Department of Occupational Therapy, Winston-Salem, NC 27110-0003. Offers MS. *Accreditation:* AOTA. *Entrance requirements:* For master's, GRE, 3 letters of recommendation (one from a licensed occupational therapist where volunteer or work experiences were performed; the other two from former professors or persons acquainted with academic potential); writing sample. Additional exam requirements/recommendations for international students: Required—TOEFL. Electronic applications accepted. *Faculty research:* Assistive technology, environmental adaptations, comprehensive performance evaluations.

Worcester State University, Graduate Studies, Program in Occupational Therapy, Worcester, MA 01602-2597. Offers MOT. *Accreditation:* AOTA. *Faculty:* 3 full-time (all women). *Students:* 29 full-time (27 women), 30 part-time (27 women); includes 4 minority (1 Black or African American, non-Hispanic/Latino; 3 Two or more races, non-Hispanic/Latino), 1 international. Average age 26. 70 applicants, 44% accepted, 18 enrolled. In 2013, 24 master's awarded. *Degree requirements:* For master's, comprehensive exam (for some programs), thesis optional, fieldwork. *Entrance requirements:* For master's, GRE General Test or MAT, minimum undergraduate GPA of 3.2. Additional exam requirements/recommendations for international students: Required—TOEFL (minimum score 500 paper-based; 61 iBT). *Application deadline:* For fall admission, 3/1 priority date for domestic and international students. Applications are processed on a rolling basis. Application fee: $40. Electronic applications accepted. *Expenses:* Contact institution. *Financial support:* In 2013–14, 5 students received support, including 5 research assistantships with full tuition reimbursements available (averaging $4,800 per year); career-related internships or fieldwork, scholarships/grants, and unspecified assistantships also available. Financial award application deadline: 3/1; financial award applicants required to submit FAFSA. *Unit head:* Dr. Joanne Gallagher, Coordinator, 508-929-8783, Fax: 508-929-8178, E-mail: jgallagher@worcester.edu. *Application contact:* Sara Grady, Assistant Dean of Continuing Education, 508-929-8787, Fax: 508-929-8100, E-mail: sara.grady@worcester.edu.

Xavier University, College of Social Sciences, Health and Education, Occupational Therapy Program, Cincinnati, OH 45207. Offers MOT. *Accreditation:* AOTA. *Faculty:* 6 full-time (all women), 2 part-time/adjunct (both women). *Students:* 37 full-time (34 women), 28 part-time (26 women); includes 4 minority (3 Black or African American, non-Hispanic/Latino; 1 Asian, non-Hispanic/Latino). Average age 24. 40 applicants, 75% accepted, 31 enrolled. In 2013, 28 master's awarded. *Degree requirements:* For master's, one foreign language, group research project. *Entrance requirements:* For master's, GRE (minimum of 33% average across all GRE sections - verbal, quantitative, analytical writing), minimum GPA of 3.0, completion of 40 volunteer hours, completion of all prerequisite courses with no more than 2 grades of C or lower. Additional exam requirements/recommendations for international students: Required—TOEFL or IELTS. *Application deadline:* For winter admission, 6/1 priority date for domestic and international students. Application fee: $35. Electronic applications accepted. *Expenses:* Contact institution. *Financial support:* In 2013–14, 25 students received support. Scholarships/grants and tuition waivers (partial) available. Financial award application deadline: 5/23; financial award applicants required to submit FAFSA. *Faculty research:* Occupation, ethics, pediatric, occupational therapy interventions, pediatric occupational therapy assessment. *Unit head:* Dr. Carol Scheerer, Chair, 513-745-3310, Fax: 513-745-3261, E-mail: scheerer@xavier.edu. *Application contact:* Georganna Miller, Academic Advisor, 513-745-3104, Fax: 513-745-3261, E-mail: millerg@xavier.edu. Website: http://www.xavier.edu/OT/

Perfusion

Long Island University–LIU Post, School of Health Professions and Nursing, Department of Biomedical Sciences, Brookville, NY 11548-1300. Offers cardiovascular perfusion (MS); clinical laboratory management (MS); medical biology (MS), including hematology, immunology, medical biology, medical chemistry, medical microbiology. Part-time and evening/weekend programs available. Postbaccalaureate distance learning degree programs offered. *Degree requirements:* For master's, thesis. *Entrance requirements:* For master's, minimum GPA of 2.75 in major. Electronic applications accepted.

Milwaukee School of Engineering, Department of Electrical Engineering and Computer Science, Program in Perfusion, Milwaukee, WI 53202-3109. Offers MS. Part-time and evening/weekend programs available. *Faculty:* 1 full-time (0 women), 8 part-time/adjunct (3 women). *Students:* 12 full-time (4 women). Average age 33. 46 applicants, 15% accepted, 7 enrolled. In 2013, 4 master's awarded. *Degree requirements:* For master's, comprehensive exam, thesis, exam. *Entrance requirements:* For master's, GRE General Test or GMAT (percentiles must average 50% or better), BS in appropriate discipline (biomedical engineering, biology, biomedical sciences, etc.), 3 letters of recommendation, personal interview, observation of 2 perfusion clinical cases. Additional exam requirements/recommendations for international students: Required—TOEFL (minimum score 79 iBT), IELTS (minimum score 6.5). *Application deadline:* Applications are processed on a rolling basis. Application fee: $0. Electronic applications accepted. Application fee is waived when completed online. *Expenses: Tuition:* Full-time $6939; part-time $771 per credit. *Financial support:* Career-related internships or fieldwork, institutionally sponsored loans, and scholarships/grants available. Financial award application deadline: 3/15; financial award applicants required to submit FAFSA. *Faculty research:* Heart medicine. *Unit head:* Dr. Ronald Gerrits, Director, 414-277-7561, Fax: 414-277-7494, E-mail: gerrits@msoe.edu. *Application contact:* Katie Weinschenk, Graduate Program Associate, 800-321-6763, Fax: 414-277-7208, E-mail: weinschenk@msoe.edu.
Website: http://www.msoe.edu/academics/academic_departments/eecs/msp/

Quinnipiac University, School of Health Sciences, Program in Cardiovascular Perfusion, Hamden, CT 06518-1940. Offers MHS. *Faculty:* 1 full-time (0 women), 3 part-time/adjunct (0 women). *Students:* 14 full-time (10 women); includes 3 minority (2 Black or African American, non-Hispanic/Latino; 1 Asian, non-Hispanic/Latino). 34 applicants, 38% accepted, 9 enrolled. In 2013, 3 master's awarded. *Entrance requirements:* For master's, bachelor's degree in science or health-related discipline from an accredited American or Canadian college or university; 2 years of health care work experience; interview. *Application deadline:* For fall admission, 2/1 priority date for domestic students, 4/30 for international students. Applications are processed on a rolling basis. Application fee: $45. Electronic applications accepted. *Expenses: Tuition:* Part-time $920 per credit. *Required fees:* $37 per credit. *Financial support:* In 2013–14, 5 students received support. Career-related internships or fieldwork, Federal Work-Study, scholarships/grants, and unspecified assistantships available. Support available to part-time students. Financial award application deadline: 6/1; financial award applicants required to submit FAFSA. *Faculty research:* Methods of preventing systemic inflammatory response syndrome (SIRS) during extracorporeal circulation of blood, investigations into the role of P-selectin in causing monocyte-platelet interaction, effect of simulated cardiopulmonary bypass on platelets and other formed elements in the blood. *Unit head:* Dr. Michael Smith, Director, 203-582-3427, E-mail: michael.smith@quinnipiac.edu. *Application contact:* Office of Graduate Admissions, 800-462-1944, Fax: 208-582-3443, E-mail: graduate@quinnipiac.edu.
Website: http://www.quinnipiac.edu/gradperfusion

The University of Arizona, College of Pharmacy, Department of Pharmacology and Toxicology, Graduate Program in Medical Pharmacology, Tucson, AZ 85721. Offers medical pharmacology (PhD); perfusion science (MS). *Faculty:* 11 full-time (3 women). *Students:* 24 full-time (18 women); includes 11 minority (2 Black or African American, non-Hispanic/Latino; 4 Asian, non-Hispanic/Latino; 3 Hispanic/Latino; 2 Two or more races, non-Hispanic/Latino), 3 international. Average age 27. 34 applicants, 18% accepted, 5 enrolled. In 2013, 3 master's, 3 doctorates awarded. *Degree requirements:* For master's, thesis; for doctorate, comprehensive exam, thesis/dissertation. *Entrance requirements:* For master's, GRE General Test, 3 letters of recommendation; for doctorate, GRE General Test, personal statement, 3 letters of recommendation. Additional exam requirements/recommendations for international students: Required—TOEFL (minimum score 550 paper-based; 79 iBT). *Application deadline:* For fall admission, 1/1 for domestic and international students. Applications are processed on a rolling basis. Application fee: $75. Electronic applications accepted. *Expenses:* Tuition, state resident: full-time $11,526. Tuition, nonresident: full-time $27,398. *Financial support:* In 2013–14, 17 research assistantships with full tuition reimbursements (averaging $23,929 per year) were awarded; institutionally sponsored loans and tuition waivers (partial) also available. Financial award applicants required to submit FAFSA. *Faculty research:* Immunopharmacology, pharmacogenetics, pharmacogenomics, clinical pharmacology, ocularpharmacology and neuropharmacology. *Unit head:* Dr. I. Glenn Sipes, Head, 520-626-7123, Fax: 520-626-2204, E-mail: sipes@email.arizona.edu. *Application contact:* Vicki Healey, Coordinator, 520-626-7218, Fax: 520-626-2204, E-mail: stanley@email.arizona.edu.
Website: http://www.pharmacology.arizona.edu/

University of Nebraska Medical Center, School of Allied Health Professions, Program in Clinical Perfusion Education, Omaha, NE 68198-4144. Offers distance education perfusion education (MPS); perfusion science (MPS). *Accreditation:* NAACLS. Postbaccalaureate distance learning degree programs offered. *Degree requirements:* For master's, comprehensive exam, thesis. *Entrance requirements:* For master's, GRE. Electronic applications accepted. *Expenses: Required fees:* $300 per semester. Tuition and fees vary according to program. *Faculty research:* Platelet gel, hemoconcentrators.

Physical Therapy

Alabama State University, College of Health Sciences, Department of Physical Therapy, Montgomery, AL 36101-0271. Offers DPT. *Accreditation:* APTA. *Faculty:* 7 full-time (5 women). *Students:* 67 full-time (38 women), 27 part-time (19 women); includes 50 minority (42 Black or African American, non-Hispanic/Latino; 3 American Indian or Alaska Native, non-Hispanic/Latino; 2 Asian, non-Hispanic/Latino; 2 Hispanic/Latino; 1 Two or more races, non-Hispanic/Latino), 1 international. Average age 29. 153 applicants, 26% accepted, 40 enrolled. In 2013, 31 doctorates awarded. Terminal master's awarded for partial completion of doctoral program. *Entrance requirements:* Additional exam requirements/recommendations for international students: Required—TOEFL (minimum score 500 paper-based). *Application deadline:* For fall admission, 7/15 for domestic students; for spring admission, 12/15 for domestic students. Applications are processed on a rolling basis. Application fee: $10. *Expenses:* Tuition, state resident: full-time $7958; part-time $343 per credit hour. Tuition, nonresident: full-time $14,132; part-time $686 per credit hour. *Required fees:* $446 per term. One-time fee: $1784 full-time; $892 part-time. Tuition and fees vary according to course load. *Financial support:* In 2013–14, 4 research assistantships (averaging $9,450 per year) were awarded. *Unit head:* Dr. Bernadette Williams-York, Chair, 334-229-4707, Fax: 334-229-4964, E-mail: asupt@alasu.edu. *Application contact:* Dr. William Person, Dean of Graduate Studies, 334-229-4274, Fax: 334-229-4928, E-mail: wperson@alasu.edu.
Website: http://www.alasu.edu/academics/colleges—departments/health-sciences/physical-therapy/index.aspx

American International College, School of Health Sciences, Program in Physical Therapy, Springfield, MA 01109-3189. Offers DPT. *Accreditation:* APTA. *Faculty:* 7 full-time (6 women), 7 part-time/adjunct (6 women). *Students:* 80 full-time (48 women), 1 part-time (0 women); includes 9 minority (4 Black or African American, non-Hispanic/Latino; 2 Asian, non-Hispanic/Latino; 1 Hispanic/Latino; 2 Two or more races, non-Hispanic/Latino). Average age 26. 71 applicants, 46% accepted, 16 enrolled. In 2013, 29 doctorates awarded. *Degree requirements:* For doctorate, thesis/dissertation. *Entrance requirements:* For doctorate, minimum GPA of 3.2. Additional exam requirements/recommendations for international students: Required—TOEFL or IELTS. *Application deadline:* For fall admission, 4/1 priority date for domestic and international students; for spring admission, 12/1 priority date for domestic and international students. Application fee: $50. Electronic applications accepted. *Expenses:* Contact institution. *Financial support:* Career-related internships or fieldwork available. Support available to part-time students. Financial award application deadline: 4/1; financial award applicants required to submit FAFSA. *Faculty research:* Ergonomics, orthopedics, teaching simulations. *Unit head:* Dr. Cesarina Thompson, Director, 413-205-3056, Fax: 413-654-1430, E-mail: cesarina.thompson@aic.edu. *Application contact:* Kerry Barnes, Director of Graduate Admissions, 413-205-3703, Fax: 413-205-3051, E-mail: kerry.barnes@aic.edu.
Website: http://www.aic.edu/academics/hs/physical_therapy/dpt

Andrews University, School of Health Professions, Department of Physical Therapy, Postprofessional Physical Therapy Program, Berrien Springs, MI 49104. Offers Dr Sc PT, TDPT. *Accreditation:* APTA. *Students:* 6 full-time (3 women), 48 part-time (25 women); includes 11 minority (1 Black or African American, non-Hispanic/Latino; 1 American Indian or Alaska Native, non-Hispanic/Latino; 6 Asian, non-Hispanic/Latino; 1 Native Hawaiian or other Pacific Islander, non-Hispanic/Latino; 2 Two or more races, non-Hispanic/Latino), 12 international. Average age 41. 9 applicants, 56% accepted, 1 enrolled. *Application deadline:* For fall admission, 12/1 priority date for domestic students. Applications are processed on a rolling basis. Application fee: $40. *Expenses:* Contact institution. *Financial support:* Federal Work-Study, institutionally sponsored loans, and scholarships/grants available. Financial award application deadline: 9/1; financial award applicants required to submit FAFSA. *Faculty research:* Home health patient profile, clinical education, breeding success of marine birds, trends in home health care for physical therapy, patient motivation in acute rehabilitation. *Unit head:* Kathy Berglund, Director of Professional Programs, 269-471-6076, Fax: 269-471-2866, E-mail: berglund@andrews.edu. *Application contact:* Jillian Panigot, Director of Admissions, 800-827-2878, Fax: 269-471-2867, E-mail: pt-info@andrews.edu.
Website: http://www.andrews.edu/PHTH/

Angelo State University, College of Graduate Studies, College of Health and Human Services, Department of Physical Therapy, San Angelo, TX 76909. Offers DPT. *Accreditation:* APTA. *Entrance requirements:* Additional exam requirements/recommendations for international students: Required—TOEFL or IELTS. Electronic applications accepted. *Faculty research:* Women and lipoproteins, international distance education, quadriceps femoris and the vastus medialis obliquus (VMO), ergonomics, children and obesity.

Arcadia University, Graduate Studies, Department of Physical Therapy, Glenside, PA 19038-3295. Offers DPT. *Accreditation:* APTA. *Expenses:* Contact institution.

Arkansas State University, Graduate School, College of Nursing and Health Professions, Department of Physical Therapy, State University, AR 72467. Offers DPT. *Accreditation:* APTA. Part-time programs available. *Faculty:* 8 full-time (4 women). *Students:* 87 full-time (48 women), 6 part-time (all women); includes 10 minority (6 Black or African American, non-Hispanic/Latino; 2 Asian, non-Hispanic/Latino; 1 Hispanic/Latino; 1 Two or more races, non-Hispanic/Latino), 1 international. Average age 25. 454 applicants, 7% accepted, 16 enrolled. In 2013, 30 doctorates awarded. *Degree requirements:* For doctorate, comprehensive exam, thesis/dissertation. *Entrance requirements:* For doctorate, GRE, Allied Health Professions Admissions Test, appropriate bachelor's or master's degree, letters of reference, resume, official transcript, volunteer experience, criminal background check, immunization records, writing sample. Additional exam requirements/recommendations for international students: Required—TOEFL (minimum score 550 paper-based; 79 iBT), IELTS (minimum score 6), PTE (minimum score 56). *Application deadline:* For fall admission, 2/1 for domestic and international students. Applications are processed on a rolling basis. Application fee: $50. Electronic applications accepted. *Expenses:* Contact institution. *Financial support:* In 2013–14, 12 students received support. Fellowships, career-related internships or fieldwork, scholarships/grants, and unspecified assistantships available. Financial award application deadline: 7/1; financial award applicants required to submit FAFSA. *Unit head:* Dr. Shawn Drake, Chair, 870-972-3591, Fax: 870-972-3652, E-mail: sdrake@astate.edu. *Application contact:* Vickey Ring,

Graduate Admissions Coordinator, 870-972-3029, Fax: 870-972-3857, E-mail: vickeyring@astate.edu.
Website: http://www.astate.edu/college/conhp/departments/physical-therapy/

Armstrong State University, School of Graduate Studies, Program in Physical Therapy, Savannah, GA 31419-1997. Offers DPT. *Accreditation:* APTA. *Faculty:* 9 full-time (6 women). *Students:* 62 full-time (42 women), 1 part-time (0 women); includes 6 minority (3 Black or African American, non-Hispanic/Latino; 1 Hispanic/Latino; 2 Two or more races, non-Hispanic/Latino). Average age 25. 546 applicants, 5% accepted, 24 enrolled. In 2013, 21 doctorates awarded. *Degree requirements:* For doctorate, thesis/dissertation, licensure exam. *Entrance requirements:* For doctorate, GRE General Test, course work in general biology, chemistry, physical anatomy, physiology, and statistics; letters of recommendation; bachelor's degree; minimum GPA of 3.0; observation hours. Additional exam requirements/recommendations for international students: Required—TOEFL (minimum score 600 paper-based). *Application deadline:* For fall admission, 10/15 priority date for domestic students; for summer admission, 8/15 priority date for domestic students. Applications are processed on a rolling basis. Application fee: $30. Electronic applications accepted. *Expenses:* Contact institution. *Financial support:* In 2013–14, research assistantships with full tuition reimbursements (averaging $5,000 per year) were awarded; career-related internships or fieldwork, scholarships/grants, and unspecified assistantships also available. Financial award application deadline: 3/5; financial award applicants required to submit FAFSA. *Faculty research:* Therapeutic exercise, effectiveness of therapeutic interventions, injury prevention and prediction, effective teaching and learning in health professions. *Unit head:* Dr. Anne Thompson, Department Head, 912-344-2737, Fax: 912-344-3469, E-mail: anne.thompson@armstrong.edu. *Application contact:* Jill Bell, Director, Graduate Enrollment Services, 912-344-2798, Fax: 912-344-3488, E-mail: graduate@armstrong.edu.
Website: http://www.armstrong.edu/Health_Professions/rehabilitation_sciences/rehab_sci_doctor_physical_therapy

A.T. Still University, Arizona School of Health Sciences, Mesa, AZ 85206. Offers advanced occupational therapy (MS); advanced physician assistant studies (MS); athletic training (MS); audiology (Au D); health sciences (DHSc); human movement (MS); occupational therapy (MS, DOT); physical therapy (DPT); physician assistant (MS); transitional audiology (Au D); transitional physical therapy (DPT). *Accreditation:* AOTA (one or more programs are accredited); ASHA. Part-time and evening/weekend programs available. Postbaccalaureate distance learning degree programs offered (minimal on-campus study). *Faculty:* 47 full-time (27 women), 279 part-time/adjunct (173 women). *Students:* 531 full-time (354 women), 865 part-time (547 women); includes 315 minority (79 Black or African American, non-Hispanic/Latino; 10 American Indian or Alaska Native, non-Hispanic/Latino; 114 Asian, non-Hispanic/Latino; 83 Hispanic/Latino; 6 Native Hawaiian or other Pacific Islander, non-Hispanic/Latino; 23 Two or more races, non-Hispanic/Latino), 82 international. Average age 36. 3,325 applicants, 14% accepted, 329 enrolled. In 2013, 252 master's, 370 doctorates awarded. *Degree requirements:* For master's, thesis (for some programs); for doctorate, thesis/dissertation (for some programs). *Entrance requirements:* For master's, GRE General Test; for doctorate, GRE, Evaluation of Practicing Audiologists Capabilities (Au D), Physical Therapist Evaluation Tool (DPT), current state licensure, master's degree or equivalent (Au D). Additional exam requirements/recommendations for international students: Required—TOEFL (minimum score 550 paper-based; 80 iBT). *Application deadline:* For fall admission, 8/1 for domestic and international students. Applications are processed on a rolling basis. Application fee: $70. Electronic applications accepted. *Expenses:* Contact institution. *Financial support:* In 2013–14, 151 students received support. Federal Work-Study and scholarships/grants available. Financial award application deadline: 5/1; financial award applicants required to submit FAFSA. *Faculty research:* Pediatric sport-related concussion, adolescent athlete health-related quality of life; geriatric and pediatric well-being, pain management for participation, practice-based research network, BMI and dental caries. *Total annual research expenditures:* $174,826. *Unit head:* Dr. Randy Danielsen, Dean, 480-219-6000, Fax: 480-219-6110, E-mail: rdanielsen@atsu.edu. *Application contact:* Donna Sparks, Associate Director, Admissions Processing, 660-626-2117, Fax: 660-626-2969, E-mail: admissions@atsu.edu.
Website: http://www.atsu.edu/ashs

Azusa Pacific University, School of Behavioral and Applied Sciences, Department of Physical Therapy, Azusa, CA 91702-7000. Offers DPT. *Accreditation:* APTA. *Degree requirements:* For doctorate, thesis/dissertation. *Entrance requirements:* For doctorate, GRE General Test. Additional exam requirements/recommendations for international students: Required—TOEFL (minimum score 600 paper-based). Electronic applications accepted. *Expenses:* Contact institution. *Faculty research:* Antioxidants and endothelial function, EEG and pain, imaging ultrasound for MSK, metabolic function in obesity.

Baylor University, Graduate School, Military Programs, Program in Orthopedics, Waco, TX 76798. Offers D Sc. *Students:* 23 full-time (11 women); includes 3 minority (1 Asian, non-Hispanic/Latino; 2 Hispanic/Latino). In 2013, 16 doctorates awarded. *Expenses: Tuition:* Full-time $25,866; part-time $1437 per credit hour. *Required fees:* $2736; $152 per credit hour. Tuition and fees vary according to course load and program. *Unit head:* Maj. Craig Paige, Graduate Program Director, 915-443-4215, Fax: 210-221-7306, E-mail: craig.v.paige@us.army.mil. *Application contact:* Lori McNamara, Administrative Assistant, 254-710-3588, Fax: 254-710-3870.

Baylor University, Graduate School, Military Programs, Program in Physical Therapy, Waco, TX 76798. Offers DPT. Program offered jointly with the U.S. Army. *Accreditation:* APTA. *Students:* 55 full-time (28 women); includes 1 minority (Hispanic/Latino). In 2013, 26 doctorates awarded. *Application deadline:* For fall admission, 2/1 for domestic students. Applications are processed on a rolling basis. Application fee: $25. *Expenses: Tuition:* Full-time $25,866; part-time $1437 per credit hour. *Required fees:* $2736; $152 per credit hour. Tuition and fees vary according to course load and program. *Faculty research:* Effect of electrical stimulation on normal and immobilized muscle, effects of inversion traction. *Unit head:* Col. Josef Moore, Graduate Program Director, 210-221-8410, Fax: 210-221-7585, E-mail: josef.moore@cen.amedd.army.mil. *Application contact:* Cindy Quiroz, Training Technician, 210-221-8410, E-mail: cynthia.quiroz@cen.amedd.army.mil.
Website: http://www.cs.amedd.army.mil/baylorpt/

Bellarmine University, Donna and Allan Lansing School of Nursing and Health Sciences, Louisville, KY 40205. Offers family nurse practitioner (MSN); health science (MHS); nursing administration (MSN); nursing education (MSN); nursing practice (DNP); physical therapy (DPT). *Accreditation:* AACN; APTA. Part-time and evening/weekend programs available. *Faculty:* 21 full-time (19 women), 8 part-time/adjunct (5 women). *Students:* 162 full-time (111 women), 120 part-time (113 women); includes 16 minority (6 Black or African American, non-Hispanic/Latino; 1 American Indian or Alaska Native, non-Hispanic/Latino; 3 Asian, non-Hispanic/Latino; 3 Hispanic/Latino; 3 Two or more races, non-Hispanic/Latino). Average age 29. In 2013, 30 master's, 54 doctorates awarded. *Degree requirements:* For doctorate, comprehensive exam, thesis/dissertation. *Entrance requirements:* For master's, GRE General Test, RN license; for doctorate, GRE General Test, Physical Therapist Centralized Application Service (for DPT). Additional exam requirements/recommendations for international students: Required—TOEFL (minimum score 550 paper-based; 80 iBT). Application fee: $25. Electronic applications accepted. *Expenses:* Contact institution. *Financial support:* Career-related internships or fieldwork and scholarships/grants available. *Faculty research:* Nursing: pain, empathy, leadership styles, control; physical therapy: service-learning; exercise in chronic and pre-operative conditions, athletes; women's health; aging. *Unit head:* Dr. Mark Wiegand, Dean, 800-274-4723 Ext. 8368, E-mail: mwiegand@bellarmine.edu. *Application contact:* Julie Armstrong-Binnix, Health Science Recruiter, 800-274-4723 Ext. 8364, E-mail: julieab@bellarmine.edu.
Website: http://www.bellarmine.edu/lansing

Belmont University, Gordon E. Inman College of Health Sciences and Nursing, Nashville, TN 37212-3757. Offers nursing (MSN, DNP); occupational therapy (MSOT, OTD); physical therapy (DPT). Part-time programs available. Postbaccalaureate distance learning degree programs offered (minimal on-campus study). *Students:* 290 full-time (172 women), 1 part-time (0 women); includes 43 minority (12 Black or African American, non-Hispanic/Latino; 22 Asian, non-Hispanic/Latino; 8 Hispanic/Latino; 1 Two or more races, non-Hispanic/Latino), 3 international. Average age 26. *Degree requirements:* For master's, comprehensive exam, thesis; for doctorate, comprehensive exam. *Entrance requirements:* For master's, GRE, BSN, minimum GPA of 3.0. Additional exam requirements/recommendations for international students: Required—TOEFL (minimum score 550 paper-based). *Application deadline:* Applications are processed on a rolling basis. Application fee: $50. Electronic applications accepted. *Expenses:* Contact institution. *Financial support:* Teaching assistantships with full tuition reimbursements, career-related internships or fieldwork, scholarships/grants, and traineeships available. Financial award application deadline: 3/1; financial award applicants required to submit FAFSA. *Unit head:* Dean, 615-460-6916, Fax: 615-460-6750. *Application contact:* David Mee, Dean of Enrollment Services, 615-460-6785, Fax: 615-460-5434, E-mail: david.mee@belmont.edu.
Website: http://www.belmont.edu/healthsciences/

Boston University, College of Health and Rehabilitation Sciences: Sargent College, Department of Physical Therapy and Athletic Training, Boston, MA 02215. Offers physical therapy (DPT); rehabilitation sciences (PhD). *Accreditation:* APTA (one or more programs are accredited). *Faculty:* 13 full-time (10 women), 26 part-time/adjunct (12 women). *Students:* 139 full-time (100 women), 25 part-time (21 women); includes 29 minority (17 Asian, non-Hispanic/Latino; 7 Hispanic/Latino; 5 Two or more races, non-Hispanic/Latino), 6 international. Average age 27. 836 applicants, 17% accepted, 37 enrolled. In 2013, 72 doctorates awarded. *Degree requirements:* For doctorate, comprehensive exam and thesis (for PhD). *Entrance requirements:* For doctorate, GRE General Test, master's degree (for PhD), bachelor's degree (for DPT). Additional exam requirements/recommendations for international students: Required—TOEFL (minimum score 550 paper-based). *Application deadline:* For fall admission, 1/7 priority date for domestic and international students. Applications are processed on a rolling basis. Application fee: $120. Electronic applications accepted. *Expenses: Tuition:* Full-time $43,970; part-time $1374 per credit hour. *Required fees:* $60 per semester. Tuition and fees vary according to class time, course level and program. *Financial support:* In 2013–14, 120 students received support, including 113 fellowships (averaging $10,000 per year), 6 teaching assistantships (averaging $3,000 per year); career-related internships or fieldwork, Federal Work-Study, institutionally sponsored loans, scholarships/grants, and tuition waivers (partial) also available. Financial award application deadline: 4/15; financial award applicants required to submit FAFSA. *Faculty research:* Gait, balance, motor control, dynamic systems analysis, spinal cord injury. *Total annual research expenditures:* $1.5 million. *Unit head:* Dr. Melanie Matthies, Department Chair, 617-353-2724, E-mail: pt@bu.edu. *Application contact:* Sharon Sankey, Director, Student Services, 617-353-2713, Fax: 617-353-7500, E-mail: ssankey@bu.edu.
Website: http://www.bu.edu/sargent/

Bradley University, Graduate School, College of Education and Health Sciences, Department of Physical Therapy and Health Science, Peoria, IL 61625-0002. Offers physical therapy (DPT). *Accreditation:* APTA. *Entrance requirements:* For doctorate, GRE, 2 letters of recommendation. Additional exam requirements/recommendations for international students: Required—TOEFL (minimum score 600 paper-based; 100 iBT). *Expenses:* Contact institution.

California State University, Fresno, Division of Graduate Studies, College of Health and Human Services, Department of Physical Therapy, Fresno, CA 93740-8027. Offers MPT, DPT. *Accreditation:* APTA. *Degree requirements:* For master's, comprehensive exam. *Entrance requirements:* For master's, GRE General Test, minimum GPA of 3.0. Additional exam requirements/recommendations for international students: Required—TOEFL. Electronic applications accepted. *Faculty research:* Dance, occupational health, ethics.

California State University, Long Beach, Graduate Studies, College of Health and Human Services, Department of Physical Therapy, Long Beach, CA 90840. Offers DPT. *Accreditation:* APTA. *Entrance requirements:* Additional exam requirements/recommendations for international students: Required—TOEFL. Electronic applications accepted.

California State University, Northridge, Graduate Studies, College of Health and Human Development, Department of Physical Therapy, Northridge, CA 91330. Offers MPT. *Accreditation:* APTA. *Entrance requirements:* For master's, GRE General Test or minimum GPA of 3.0. Additional exam requirements/recommendations for international students: Required—TOEFL.

Carroll University, Program in Physical Therapy, Waukesha, WI 53186-5593. Offers MPT, DPT. *Accreditation:* APTA. *Degree requirements:* For master's, thesis (for some programs). *Entrance requirements:* For master's, GRE General Test, recommendations, clinical observation. Additional exam requirements/recommendations for international students: Required—TOEFL. *Expenses:* Contact institution. *Faculty research:* Physical therapy education, geriatrics, neural control of movement, wellness and prevention in apparently healthy individuals with disease and disability.

Central Michigan University, College of Graduate Studies, The Herbert H. and Grace A. Dow College of Health Professions, School of Rehabilitation and Medical Sciences, Mount Pleasant, MI 48859. Offers physical therapy (DPT); physician assistant (MS). *Accreditation:* APTA; ARC-PA. *Degree requirements:* For master's, thesis or alternative; for doctorate, thesis/dissertation or alternative. *Entrance requirements:* For master's and doctorate, GRE. Electronic applications accepted.

Chapman University, Schmid College of Science and Technology, Department of Physical Therapy, Orange, CA 92866. Offers DPT. *Accreditation:* APTA. *Faculty:* 9 full-time (7 women), 8 part-time/adjunct (6 women). *Students:* 105 full-time (68 women), 58 part-time (34 women); includes 62 minority (2 Black or African American, non-Hispanic/Latino; 33 Asian, non-Hispanic/Latino; 14 Hispanic/Latino; 13 Two or more races, non-Hispanic/Latino), 4 international. Average age 27. 1,321 applicants, 15% accepted, 66 enrolled. In 2013, 45 doctorates awarded. *Degree requirements:* For doctorate, 1440 hours of clinical experience. *Entrance requirements:* For doctorate, GRE, minimum undergraduate GPA of 3.0; 40 hours of physical therapy observation (or paid work). Additional exam requirements/recommendations for international students: Required—TOEFL (minimum score 550 paper-based; 80 iBT). *Application deadline:* For fall admission, 11/15 for domestic students. Application fee: $65. Electronic applications accepted. *Expenses:* Contact institution. *Financial support:* Fellowships, Federal Work-Study, and scholarships/grants available. Financial award applicants required to submit FAFSA. *Unit head:* Dr. Jacki Brechter, Chair, 714-744-7649, E-mail: brechter@chapman.edu. *Application contact:* Derek Robinson, Admission Counselor, 714-997-6711, E-mail: drobinso@chapman.edu.

Chatham University, Program in Physical Therapy, Pittsburgh, PA 15232-2826. Offers DPT, TDPT. *Accreditation:* APTA. *Faculty:* 7 full-time (4 women). *Students:* 113 full-time (82 women); includes 9 minority (2 Black or African American, non-Hispanic/Latino; 5 Asian, non-Hispanic/Latino; 2 Hispanic/Latino), 1 international. Average age 25. 559 applicants, 13% accepted, 41 enrolled. In 2013, 50 doctorates awarded. *Entrance requirements:* For doctorate, GRE, community service, interview, minimum GPA of 3.0, writing sample, volunteer/work experience, 3 references. Additional exam requirements/recommendations for international students: Required—TOEFL (minimum score 600 paper-based; 100 iBT), IELTS (minimum score 7), TWE. *Application deadline:* For fall admission, 12/1 priority date for domestic and international students. Application fee: $0. *Expenses:* Contact institution. *Financial support:* Career-related internships or fieldwork available. Financial award applicants required to submit FAFSA. *Faculty research:* Stroke rehabilitation, osteoporosis and fall prevention, physical therapy for children with disabilities, evidence-based practice and decision-making, low back pain in children and adolescents. *Unit head:* Dr. Patricia Downey, Director, 412-365-1199, Fax: 412-365-1505, E-mail: downey@chatham.edu. *Application contact:* Ashlee Bartko, Senior Assistant Director of Graduate Admission, 412-365-2988, Fax: 412-365-1609, E-mail: gradadmissions@chatham.edu.
Website: http://www.chatham.edu/departments/healthmgmt/graduate/pt

Clarke University, Physical Therapy Program, Dubuque, IA 52001-3198. Offers DPT. *Accreditation:* APTA. *Faculty:* 6 full-time (4 women). *Students:* 73 full-time (45 women), 4 part-time (3 women); includes 4 minority (1 Black or African American, non-Hispanic/Latino; 2 Asian, non-Hispanic/Latino; 1 Hispanic/Latino). In 2013, 19 doctorates awarded. *Entrance requirements:* For doctorate, minimum GPA of 3.0, 16-24 hours of clinical experience in 3 different areas. *Application deadline:* For spring admission, 3/31 for domestic students. Application fee: $0. *Expenses: Tuition:* Part-time $660 per credit. *Required fees:* $15 per credit. *Financial support:* In 2013–14, 4 students received support. Career-related internships or fieldwork available. Support available to part-time students. Financial award applicants required to submit FAFSA. *Faculty research:* Qualitative research, occupational health, discontinuous anaerobic studies, low back dysfunction. *Unit head:* Dr. Bill O'Dell, Chair, 319-588-6382, Fax: 319-588-8684. *Application contact:* Kara Shroeder, Information Contact, 563-588-6354, Fax: 563-588-6789, E-mail: graduate@clarke.edu.
Website: http://www.clarke.edu/

Clarkson University, Graduate School, School of Arts and Sciences, Department of Physical Therapy, Potsdam, NY 13699. Offers DPT. *Accreditation:* APTA. *Faculty:* 7 full-time (4 women), 5 part-time/adjunct (3 women). *Students:* 73 full-time (55 women); includes 12 minority (3 Black or African American, non-Hispanic/Latino; 1 American Indian or Alaska Native, non-Hispanic/Latino; 2 Asian, non-Hispanic/Latino; 3 Hispanic/Latino; 3 Two or more races, non-Hispanic/Latino). Average age 24. 46 applicants, 76% accepted, 27 enrolled. In 2013, 20 doctorates awarded. *Entrance requirements:* For doctorate, GRE, Physical Therapy Centralized Application Service (PTCAS) application, including transcripts of all college coursework, two personal essays, and three letters of recommendation. Additional exam requirements/recommendations for international students: Required—TOEFL. *Application deadline:* Applications are processed on a rolling basis. Application fee: $125. Electronic applications accepted. *Expenses: Tuition:* Full-time $15,888; part-time $1324 per credit. *Required fees:* $295 per semester. *Financial support:* In 2013–14, 70 students received support. Scholarships/grants and tuition waivers (partial) available. *Faculty research:* Longitudinal assessment of the risk of falling. *Total annual research expenditures:* $27,804. *Unit head:* Dr. George Fulk, Chair, 315-268-3786, Fax: 315-268-1539, E-mail: gfulk@clarkson.edu. *Application contact:* Jennifer Reed, Graduate Coordinator, School of Arts and Sciences, 315-268-3802, Fax: 315-268-3989, E-mail: sciencegrad@clarkson.edu.
Website: http://www.clarkson.edu/pt/

Cleveland State University, College of Graduate Studies, College of Sciences and Health Professions, School of Health Sciences, Program in Physical Therapy, Cleveland, OH 44115. Offers DPT. *Accreditation:* APTA. *Faculty:* 7 full-time (6 women), 7 part-time/adjunct (5 women). *Students:* 109 full-time (68 women), 2 part-time (1 woman); includes 6 minority (2 Black or African American, non-Hispanic/Latino; 3 Asian, non-Hispanic/Latino; 1 Hispanic/Latino), 1 international. Average age 26. 23 applicants, 13% accepted, 1 enrolled. In 2013, 23 doctorates awarded. *Degree requirements:* For doctorate, comprehensive exam. *Entrance requirements:* For doctorate, GRE (minimum scores: 450 verbal; 550 quantitative; 4.0 analytical writing), minimum overall GPA of 3.0. Additional exam requirements/recommendations for international students: Required—TOEFL (minimum score 525 paper-based; 65 iBT). *Application deadline:* For spring admission, 2/15 priority date for domestic and international students. Electronic applications accepted. Application fee is waived when completed online. *Expenses:* Contact institution. *Financial support:* In 2013–14, 11 teaching assistantships with partial tuition reimbursements (averaging $9,122 per year) were awarded; scholarships/grants also available. Financial award application deadline: 1/1; financial award applicants required to submit FAFSA. *Faculty research:* Biomechanics, exercise physiology, motor control/motor learning, physical dysfunctions, health disparities/urban health, health promotion and fitness. *Unit head:* Dr. Karen Ann O'Loughlin, Director, 216-687-3581, Fax: 216-687-9316, E-mail: k.oloughlin@@csuohio.edu. *Application contact:* Lisa Pistone, Administrative Secretary, 216-687-3566, Fax: 216-687-9316, E-mail: l.pistone@csuohio.edu.

The College of St. Scholastica, Graduate Studies, Department of Physical Therapy, Duluth, MN 55811-4199. Offers DPT. *Accreditation:* APTA. *Faculty:* 9 full-time (7 women), 3 part-time/adjunct (1 woman). *Students:* 107 full-time (73 women), 158 part-time (123 women); includes 23 minority (3 Black or African American, non-Hispanic/Latino; 9 Asian, non-Hispanic/Latino; 5 Hispanic/Latino; 6 Two or more races, non-Hispanic/Latino), 8 international. Average age 36. In 2013, 79 doctorates awarded. *Entrance requirements:* For doctorate, GRE. Additional exam requirements/recommendations for international students: Required—TOEFL (minimum score 550 paper-based; 79 iBT). *Application deadline:* For fall admission, 10/1 for domestic and international students. Applications are processed on a rolling basis. Electronic applications accepted. Tuition and fees vary according to course load, program and student level. *Financial support:* In 2013–14, 81 students received support, including 4 teaching assistantships (averaging $1,042 per year); scholarships/grants also available. Support available to part-time students. Financial award applicants required to submit FAFSA. *Faculty research:* Postural control, reliability and validity of spinal assessment tools, biomechanics of golf swing and low back pain, gait assessment and treatment, ethical issues. *Unit head:* Dr. Denise Wise, Director, 218-723-6523, E-mail: dwise@css.edu. *Application contact:* Lindsay Lahti, Director of Graduate and Extended Studies Recruitment, 218-733-2240, Fax: 218-733-2275, E-mail: gradstudies@css.edu.
Website: http://www.css.edu/Graduate/Masters-Doctoral-and-Professional-Programs/Areas-of-Study/Doctor-of-Physical-Therapy.html

Columbia University, College of Physicians and Surgeons, Program in Physical Therapy, New York, NY 10032. Offers DPT. *Accreditation:* APTA. *Faculty:* 13 full-time (9 women), 15 part-time/adjunct (6 women). *Students:* 175 full-time (141 women); includes 34 minority (2 Black or African American, non-Hispanic/Latino; 20 Asian, non-Hispanic/Latino; 6 Hispanic/Latino; 6 Two or more races, non-Hispanic/Latino). Average age 24. 450 applicants, 24% accepted, 55 enrolled. In 2013, 60 doctorates awarded. *Degree requirements:* For doctorate, fieldwork, capstone project. *Entrance requirements:* For doctorate, GRE General Test, undergraduate course work in biology, chemistry, physics, psychology, statistics and humanities. Additional exam requirements/recommendations for international students: Required—TOEFL. *Application deadline:* For fall admission, 12/1 priority date for domestic and international students. Applications are processed on a rolling basis. Application fee: $0. Electronic applications accepted. *Expenses:* Contact institution. *Financial support:* In 2013–14, 111 students received support. Career-related internships or fieldwork, Federal Work-Study, institutionally sponsored loans, and scholarships/grants available. Financial award application deadline: 4/15; financial award applicants required to submit FAFSA. *Faculty research:* Motor control, motion analysis, back assessment, recovery of function following neurological injury, women's health, disability awareness, pediatrics, orthopedics. *Total annual research expenditures:* $2.5 million. *Unit head:* Dr. Risa Granick, Director, 212-305-6907, Fax: 212-305-4569, E-mail: rg2135@cumc.columbia.edu. *Application contact:* Cynthia Worthington, Admissions Coordinator, 212-305-0470, Fax: 212-305-4569, E-mail: cw75@cumc.columbia.edu.
Website: http://www.columbiaphysicaltherapy.org

Concordia University Wisconsin, Graduate Programs, School of Human Services, Program in Physical Therapy, Mequon, WI 53097-2402. Offers MSPT, DPT. *Accreditation:* APTA. *Degree requirements:* For master's, comprehensive exam, thesis or alternative. *Entrance requirements:* Additional exam requirements/recommendations for international students: Required—TOEFL. *Expenses:* Contact institution.

Creighton University, School of Pharmacy and Health Professions, Program in Physical Therapy, Omaha, NE 68178-0001. Offers DPT. *Accreditation:* APTA. *Entrance requirements:* For doctorate, GRE. Additional exam requirements/recommendations for international students: Required—TOEFL. Electronic applications accepted. *Expenses: Tuition:* Full-time $13,608; part-time $756 per credit hour. *Required fees:* $149 per semester. Tuition and fees vary according to course load, campus/location, program, reciprocity agreements and student's religious affiliation. *Faculty research:* Patient safety in health services research, health information technology and health services research, Parkinson's rigidity and rehabilitation sciences, prion disease transmission, outcomes research in the rehabilitation sciences.

Daemen College, Department of Physical Therapy, Amherst, NY 14226-3592. Offers orthopedic manual physical therapy (Advanced Certificate); physical therapy-direct entry (DPT); transitional (DPT). *Accreditation:* APTA. Part-time programs available. *Degree requirements:* For doctorate, minimum C grade in all coursework; for Advanced Certificate, minimum GPA of 3.0; degree completion in maximum of 3 years. *Entrance requirements:* For doctorate, baccalaureate degree with minimum GPA of 2.8 in science coursework; letter of intent; resume; 2 letters of reference; 120 hours of PT exposure; transcripts; for Advanced Certificate, BS/BA; license to practice physical therapy; current registration; 2 recommendations; letter of intent; 2 years of physical therapy experience. Additional exam requirements/recommendations for international students: Required—TOEFL (minimum score 500 paper-based; 63 iBT), IELTS (minimum score 5.5). Electronic applications accepted. *Faculty research:* Athletic injuries, myofacial pain syndrome, electrical stimulation and tissue healing, lumbar spine dysfunction, temporomandibular joint syndrome.

Dalhousie University, Faculty of Health Professions, School of Physiotherapy, Halifax, NS B3H 3J5, Canada. Offers physiotherapy (entry to profession) (M Sc); physiotherapy (rehabilitation research) (M Sc). *Entrance requirements:* Additional exam requirements/recommendations for international students: Required—TOEFL, IELTS, CANTEST, CAEL, or Michigan English Language Assessment Battery. Electronic applications accepted.

DeSales University, Graduate Division, Division of Healthcare and Natural Sciences, Center Valley, PA 18034-9568. Offers adult clinical nurse specialist (MSN); certified nurse midwives (MSN); certified nurse practitioners (MSN); clinical leadership (DNP); family nurse practitioner (MSN); information systems (MSIS); nurse educator (MSN); nurse practitioner (Post-Master's Certificate); physical therapy (DPT); physician assistant studies (MSPAS); MSN/MBA. Part-time programs available. In 2013, 5 doctorates awarded. *Degree requirements:* For master's, thesis optional. *Entrance requirements:* For master's, GRE General Test, MAT, minimum B average in undergraduate course work, health assessment course or equivalent, course work in statistics. Additional exam requirements/recommendations for international students: Required—TOEFL. *Application deadline:* Applications are processed on a rolling basis. Application fee: $35. Electronic applications accepted. *Expenses: Tuition:* Part-time $790 per credit. *Financial support:* Applicants required to submit FAFSA. *Unit head:* Dr. Mary Liz Doyle-Tadduni, Department Chair, Nursing, 610-282-1100 Ext. 1394, Fax: 610-282-2091, E-mail: carol.mest@desales.edu. *Application contact:* Abagail Wernicki, Director of Graduate Admissions, 610-282-1100 Ext. 1768, Fax: 610-282-2869, E-mail: abagail.wernicki@desales.edu.

Des Moines University, College of Health Sciences, Program in Physical Therapy, Des Moines, IA 50312-4104. Offers DPT. *Accreditation:* APTA. *Entrance requirements:* For doctorate, GRE. Additional exam requirements/recommendations for international students: Required—TOEFL. Electronic applications accepted. *Expenses:* Contact institution.

Dominican College, Division of Allied Health, Department of Physical Therapy, Orangeburg, NY 10962-1210. Offers MS, DPT. *Accreditation:* APTA. Part-time and evening/weekend programs available. *Faculty:* 7 full-time (6 women), 7 part-time/adjunct (5 women). *Students:* 54 full-time (27 women), 168 part-time (78 women). Average age 30. In 2013, 126 doctorates awarded. *Degree requirements:* For master's, 3 clinical affiliations. *Entrance requirements:* For master's, minimum GPA of 3.0. Additional exam requirements/recommendations for international students: Required—TOEFL (minimum score 550 paper-based). *Application deadline:* Applications are processed on a rolling basis. Application fee: $50. *Expenses: Tuition:* Part-time $815 per credit. *Required fees:* $180 per semester. *Financial support:* Applicants required to submit FAFSA. *Unit head:* Dr. Valerie Olson, Program Director, 845-848-6048, Fax: 845-398-4893, E-mail: valerie.olson@dc.edu. *Application contact:* Director of Admissions, 845-848-7900, Fax: 845-365-3150, E-mail: admissions@dc.edu.

Drexel University, College of Nursing and Health Professions, Department of Physical Therapy and Rehabilitation Sciences, Philadelphia, PA 19102. Offers clinical biomechanics and orthopedics (PhD); hand and upper quarter rehabilitation (Certificate); hand therapy (MHS, PPDPT); orthopedics (MHS, PPDPT); pediatric rehabilitation (Certificate); pediatrics (MHS, PPDPT, PhD); physical therapy (DPT). *Accreditation:* APTA. Part-time programs available. Terminal master's awarded for partial completion of doctoral program. *Degree requirements:* For master's, comprehensive exam; for doctorate, thesis/dissertation, qualifying exam. *Entrance requirements:* For master's and doctorate, GRE General Test. Additional exam requirements/recommendations for international students: Required—TOEFL. Electronic applications accepted. *Faculty research:* Cerebral palsy, chronic low back pain, shoulder dysfunction, early intervention/community programs.

Duke University, School of Medicine, Physical Therapy Division, Durham, NC 27708. Offers DPT. *Accreditation:* APTA. *Faculty:* 19 full-time (9 women), 6 part-time/adjunct (5 women). *Students:* 192 full-time (147 women); includes 19 minority (3 Black or African American, non-Hispanic/Latino; 1 American Indian or Alaska Native, non-Hispanic/Latino; 9 Asian, non-Hispanic/Latino; 5 Hispanic/Latino; 1 Native Hawaiian or other Pacific Islander, non-Hispanic/Latino), 4 international. 594 applicants, 19% accepted, 62 enrolled. In 2013, 63 doctorates awarded. *Degree requirements:* For doctorate, comprehensive exam, scholarly project. *Entrance requirements:* For doctorate, GRE, previous course work in anatomy, physiology, biological sciences, chemistry, physics, psychology, and statistics. *Application deadline:* For fall admission, 11/1 priority date for domestic and international students. Applications are processed on a rolling basis. Application fee: $0. Electronic applications accepted. *Expenses:* Contact institution. *Financial support:* In 2013–14, 92 students received support. Fellowships, research assistantships, and teaching assistantships available. Financial award application deadline: 5/1; financial award applicants required to submit FAFSA. *Faculty research:* Geriatrics, visual plasticity, educational outcomes, orthopedics, neurology. *Unit head:* Dr. Michel D. Landry, Chief, 919-613-4520, Fax: 919-684-1846, E-mail: mike.landry@duke.edu. *Application contact:* Mya Shackleford, Admissions Coordinator, 919-668-5206, Fax: 919-684-1846, E-mail: mya.shackleford@duke.edu.
Website: http://dpt.duhs.duke.edu

Duquesne University, John G. Rangos, Sr. School of Health Sciences, Pittsburgh, PA 15282-0001. Offers health management systems (MHMS); occupational therapy (MS, OTD); physical therapy (DPT); physician assistant studies (MPAS); rehabilitation science (MS, PhD); speech-language pathology (MS); MBA/MHMS. *Accreditation:* AOTA (one or more programs are accredited); APTA (one or more programs are accredited); ASHA. Postbaccalaureate distance learning degree programs offered (minimal on-campus study). *Faculty:* 41 full-time (29 women), 32 part-time/adjunct (15 women). *Students:* 232 full-time (174 women), 14 part-time (7 women); includes 12 minority (2 Black or African American, non-Hispanic/Latino; 7 Asian, non-Hispanic/Latino; 1 Hispanic/Latino; 2 Two or more races, non-Hispanic/Latino), 7 international. Average age 23. 951 applicants, 11% accepted, 35 enrolled. In 2013, 119 master's, 40 doctorates awarded. *Degree requirements:* For doctorate, comprehensive exam (for some programs), thesis/dissertation (for some programs). *Entrance requirements:* For master's, GRE General Test (speech-language pathology), 3 letters of recommendation; minimum GPA of 2.75 (health management systems), 3.0 (speech-language pathology); for doctorate, GRE General Test (for physical therapy and rehabilitation science), 3 letters of recommendation, minimum GPA of 3.0, personal interview. Additional exam requirements/recommendations for international students: Required—TOEFL (minimum score 550 paper-based; 90 iBT). *Application deadline:* For fall admission, 2/1 for domestic and international students; for spring admission, 7/1 for domestic and international students. Applications are processed on a rolling basis. Electronic applications accepted. *Expenses:* Contact institution. *Financial support:* Federal Work-Study available. Financial award applicants required to submit FAFSA. *Faculty research:* Neuronal processing, electrical stimulation on peripheral neuropathy, central nervous system (CNS) stimulatory and inhibitory signals, behavioral genetic methodologies to development disorders of speech, neurogenic communication disorders. *Total annual research expenditures:* $83,650. *Unit head:* Dr. Gregory H. Frazer, Dean, 412-396-5303, Fax: 412-396-5554, E-mail: frazer@duq.edu. *Application contact:* Christopher R. Hilf, Recruiter/Academic Advisor, 412-396-5653, Fax: 412-396-5554, E-mail: hilfc@duq.edu.
Website: http://www.duq.edu/academics/schools/health-sciences

D'Youville College, Department of Physical Therapy, Buffalo, NY 14201-1084. Offers advanced orthopedic physical therapy (Certificate); manual physical therapy (Certificate); physical therapy (DPT). *Accreditation:* APTA. Part-time programs available. Postbaccalaureate distance learning degree programs offered (minimal on-campus study). *Students:* 145 full-time (83 women), 16 part-time (13 women); includes 15 minority (5 Black or African American, non-Hispanic/Latino; 5 Asian, non-Hispanic/Latino; 5 Hispanic/Latino), 40 international. Average age 25. 373 applicants, 28% accepted, 57 enrolled. In 2013, 48 doctorates awarded. *Degree requirements:* For doctorate, comprehensive exam, project or thesis. *Entrance requirements:* For doctorate, bachelor's degree, minimum GPA of 3.0. Additional exam requirements/recommendations for international students: Required—TOEFL (minimum score 500 paper-based). *Application deadline:* For fall admission, 5/1 priority date for international students; for spring admission, 9/1 priority date for international students. Applications are processed on a rolling basis. Application fee: $25. Electronic applications accepted. *Financial support:* Federal Work-Study and scholarships/grants available. Financial award application deadline: 3/1; financial award applicants required to submit FAFSA. *Faculty research:* Therapeutic effects of Tai Chi, orthopedics, health promotion in type 2 diabetes, athletic performance in youth and college sports, behavioral determinants in childhood obesity. *Total annual research expenditures:* $4,000. *Unit head:* Dr. Lynn Rivers, Chair, 716-829-7708, Fax: 716-829-8137, E-mail: riversl@dyc.edu. *Application contact:* Mark Pavone, Graduate Admissions Director, 716-829-8400, Fax: 716-829-7900, E-mail: graduateadmissions@dyc.edu.

East Carolina University, Graduate School, School of Allied Health Sciences, Department of Physical Therapy, Greenville, NC 27858-4353. Offers DPT. *Accreditation:* APTA. *Entrance requirements:* Additional exam requirements/recommendations for international students: Required—TOEFL. *Application deadline:* For fall admission, 1/15 for domestic students. Application fee: $50. *Expenses:* Tuition, state resident: full-time $4223. Tuition, nonresident: full-time $16,540. *Required fees:* $2184. *Financial support:* Application deadline: 6/1. *Faculty research:* Diabetes and obesity, diabetic foot, ACL injury. *Unit head:* Dr. Walter L. Jenkins, Chair, 252-744-6234, E-mail: jenkinsw@ecu.edu. *Application contact:* Dean of Graduate School, 252-328-6012, Fax: 252-328-6071, E-mail: gradschool@ecu.edu.

Eastern Washington University, Graduate Studies, College of Science, Health and Engineering, Department of Physical Therapy, Cheney, WA 99004-2431. Offers DPT. *Accreditation:* APTA. *Faculty:* 5 full-time (2 women). *Students:* 123 full-time (69 women), 1 part-time (0 women); includes 15 minority (3 American Indian or Alaska Native, non-Hispanic/Latino; 8 Asian, non-Hispanic/Latino; 4 Hispanic/Latino). Average age 26. 465 applicants, 8% accepted, 38 enrolled. In 2013, 43 doctorates awarded. *Degree requirements:* For doctorate, comprehensive exam, thesis/dissertation or final project. *Entrance requirements:* For doctorate, GRE General Test, minimum GPA of 3.0, 75 hours of experience, 3 letters of recommendation. Application fee: $75. *Financial support:* In 2013–14, 6 teaching assistantships were awarded; career-related internships or fieldwork, Federal Work-Study, institutionally sponsored loans, scholarships/grants, health care benefits, tuition waivers (partial), and unspecified assistantships also available. Support available to part-time students. Financial award application deadline: 2/1; financial award applicants required to submit FAFSA. *Unit head:* Dr. Byron Russell, Chair, 509-368-6608, Fax: 509-623-4321. *Application contact:* Prof. Meryl Gersh, Director of Admissions, 509-623-4302.

East Tennessee State University, School of Graduate Studies, College of Clinical and Rehabilitative Health Sciences, Department of Physical Therapy, Johnson City, TN 37614. Offers DPT. *Accreditation:* APTA. *Faculty:* 9 full-time (5 women), 3 part-time/adjunct (all women). *Students:* 108 full-time (55 women); includes 7 minority (2 Black or African American, non-Hispanic/Latino; 1 Asian, non-Hispanic/Latino; 2 Hispanic/Latino; 2 Two or more races, non-Hispanic/Latino). Average age 26. In 2013, 29 doctorates awarded. *Degree requirements:* For doctorate, comprehensive exam, internship. *Entrance requirements:* For doctorate, GRE General Test, minimum GPA of 3.0. Additional exam requirements/recommendations for international students: Required—TOEFL (minimum score 550 paper-based; 79 iBT). *Application deadline:* For spring admission, 7/1 for domestic and international students. Application fee: $35 ($45 for international students). Electronic applications accepted. *Expenses:* Tuition, state resident: full-time $7900; part-time $395 per credit hour. Tuition, nonresident: full-time $21,960; part-time $1098 per credit hour. *Required fees:* $1345; $84 per credit hour. *Financial support:* In 2013–14, 17 students received support, including 2 research assistantships with full tuition reimbursements available (averaging $6,000 per year); career-related internships or fieldwork, institutionally sponsored loans, scholarships/grants, and unspecified assistantships also available. Financial award application deadline: 7/1; financial award applicants required to submit FAFSA. *Faculty research:* Health and wellness across the lifespan; relationships between scapular kinematics, pain, and function; cognitive training and dual-task ability in older adult; vestibular rehabilitation and dizziness in geriatric patients; assessment tools for patients with TMJ dysfunction; proprioceptive training and gait variability in older adults. *Unit head:* Dr. Mary Jo Davenport, Interim Chair, 423-439-8792, Fax: 423-439-8077, E-mail: davenpom@etsu.edu. *Application contact:* Mary Duncan, Graduate Specialist, 423-439-4302, Fax: 423-439-5624, E-mail: duncanm@etsu.edu.
Website: http://www.etsu.edu/crhs/physther/default.aspx

Elon University, Program in Physical Therapy, Elon, NC 27244-2010. Offers DPT. *Accreditation:* APTA. *Faculty:* 14 full-time (9 women), 6 part-time/adjunct (4 women). *Students:* 153 full-time (102 women); includes 8 minority (1 Black or African American, non-Hispanic/Latino; 2 American Indian or Alaska Native, non-Hispanic/Latino; 1 Asian, non-Hispanic/Latino; 2 Hispanic/Latino; 2 Two or more races, non-Hispanic/Latino). Average age 26. 689 applicants, 17% accepted, 53 enrolled. *Entrance requirements:* For doctorate, GRE General Test. Additional exam requirements/recommendations for international students: Required—TOEFL (minimum score 550 paper-based; 79 iBT). *Application deadline:* For winter admission, 12/1 priority date for domestic students. Applications are processed on a rolling basis. Application fee: $50. Electronic applications accepted. *Expenses:* Contact institution. *Financial support:* In 2013–14, 20 students received support. Federal Work-Study and scholarships/grants available. Financial award application deadline: 10/1; financial award applicants required to submit FAFSA. *Faculty research:* Exercise readiness in female survivors of domestic violence, animal-assisted therapy, locomotor training for multiple sclerosis patients, effect of infant positioning on the attainment of gross motor skills, physical activity levels for methadone maintenance treatment patients. *Unit head:* Dr. Elizabeth A. Rogers, Chair, 336-278-6400, Fax: 336-278-6414, E-mail: rogers@elon.edu. *Application contact:* Art Fadde, Director of Graduate Admissions, 800-334-8448 Ext. 3, Fax: 336-278-7699, E-mail: afadde@elon.edu.
Website: http://www.elon.edu/dpt/

Emory University, School of Medicine, Programs in Allied Health Professions, Doctor of Physical Therapy Program, Atlanta, GA 30322. Offers DPT. *Accreditation:* APTA. *Faculty:* 16 full-time (11 women), 7 part-time/adjunct (4 women). *Students:* 195 full-time (145 women); includes 31 minority (7 Black or African American, non-Hispanic/Latino; 1 American Indian or Alaska Native, non-Hispanic/Latino; 18 Asian, non-Hispanic/Latino; 1 Hispanic/Latino; 4 Two or more races, non-Hispanic/Latino). Average age 22. 618 applicants, 25% accepted, 70 enrolled. In 2013, 62 doctorates awarded. *Entrance requirements:* For doctorate, GRE General Test. Additional exam requirements/recommendations for international students: Recommended—TOEFL. *Application deadline:* For fall admission, 10/1 priority date for domestic and international students. Applications are processed on a rolling basis. Application fee: $65. Electronic applications accepted. *Expenses:* Contact institution. *Financial support:* In 2013–14, 81 students received support. Institutionally sponsored loans and scholarships/grants available. Financial award application deadline: 3/1; financial award applicants required to submit FAFSA. *Faculty research:* Sensorimotor plasticity, biomechanics of walking, qualitative distinctions of moral practice, constraint induced therapy following stroke. *Unit head:* Dr. Zoher F. Kapasi, Director and Associate Professor, 404-712-5683, Fax: 404-712-4130, E-mail: dptadmissions@emory.edu. *Application contact:* Monica George-Komi, Admission Coordinator, 404-712-5657, Fax: 404-712-4130, E-mail: mgeorg2@emory.edu.
Website: http://www.rehabmed.emory.edu/pt/

Florida Agricultural and Mechanical University, Division of Graduate Studies, Research, and Continuing Education, School of Allied Health Sciences, Division of Physical Therapy, Tallahassee, FL 32307-3200. Offers MPT. *Accreditation:* APTA. *Entrance requirements:* For master's, GRE General Test or GMAT, minimum GPA of 3.0. Additional exam requirements/recommendations for international students: Required—TOEFL.

Florida Gulf Coast University, College of Health Professions, Department of Physical Therapy, Fort Myers, FL 33965-6565. Offers MS, DPT. *Accreditation:* APTA. Part-time programs available. Postbaccalaureate distance learning degree programs offered (minimal on-campus study). *Degree requirements:* For master's, thesis or alternative. *Entrance requirements:* For master's, GRE General Test or MAT, minimum GPA of 3.0. Additional exam requirements/recommendations for international students: Required—TOEFL (minimum score 550 paper-based). Electronic applications accepted. *Faculty research:* Physical therapy practice and education.

Florida International University, College of Nursing and Health Sciences, Department of Physical Therapy, Miami, FL 33199. Offers DPT. *Accreditation:* APTA. Part-time programs available. *Degree requirements:* For doctorate, comprehensive exam. *Entrance requirements:* For doctorate, minimum undergraduate GPA of 3.0 in upper-level coursework; letter of intent; resume; at least 40 hours of observation within physical therapy clinic or facility. Additional exam requirements/recommendations for international students: Required—TOEFL (minimum score 550 paper-based; 80 iBT). Electronic applications accepted. *Faculty research:* Isokinetic test results and gait abnormalities after knee arthroscopy.

Franklin Pierce University, Graduate Studies, Rindge, NH 03461-0060. Offers curriculum and instruction (M Ed); emerging network technologies (Graduate Certificate); energy and sustainability studies (MBA); health administration (MBA, Graduate Certificate); human resource management (MBA, Graduate Certificate); information technology (MBA); information technology management (MS); leadership (MBA, DA); nursing (MS); physical therapy (DPT); physician assistant studies (MPAS); special education (M Ed); sports management (MBA). *Accreditation:* APTA. Part-time programs available. Postbaccalaureate distance learning degree programs offered (no on-campus study). *Degree requirements:* For master's, concentrated original research projects; student teaching; fieldwork and/or internship; leadership project; PRAXIS I and II (for M Ed); for doctorate, concentrated original research projects, clinical fieldwork and/or internship, leadership project. *Entrance requirements:* For master's, minimum GPA of 2.5, 3 letters of recommendation; competencies in accounting, economics, statistics, and computer skills through life experience or undergraduate coursework (for MBA); certification/e-portfolio, minimum C grade in all education courses (for M Ed); license to practice as RN (for MS in nursing); for doctorate, GRE, BA/BS, 3 letters of recommendation, personal mission statement, interview, writing sample, minimum cumulative GPA of 2.8, master's degree (for DA); 80 hours of observation/work in PT settings, completion of anatomy, chemistry, physics, and statistics, minimum GPA of 3.0 (for DPT). Additional exam requirements/recommendations for international students: Required—TOEFL (minimum score 550 paper-based; 61 iBT). Electronic applications accepted. *Faculty research:* Evidence-based practice in sports physical therapy, human resource management in economic crisis, leadership in nursing, innovation in sports facility management, differentiated learning and understanding by design.

Gannon University, School of Graduate Studies, Morosky College of Health Professions and Sciences, School of Health Professions, Program in Physical Therapy, Erie, PA 16541-0001. Offers DPT. *Accreditation:* APTA. *Students:* 129 full-time (74 women); includes 6 minority (1 Black or African American, non-Hispanic/Latino; 4 Asian, non-Hispanic/Latino; 1 Hispanic/Latino), 2 international. Average age 23. 206 applicants, 53% accepted, 51 enrolled. In 2013, 42 doctorates awarded. *Degree requirements:* For doctorate, thesis/dissertation or alternative, research project, practicum. *Entrance requirements:* For doctorate, interview, minimum QPA of 3.0. Additional exam requirements/recommendations for international students: Required—TOEFL (minimum score 79 iBT). *Application deadline:* For fall admission, 1/15 for domestic students. Application fee: $50. Electronic applications accepted. *Expenses:* Contact institution. *Financial support:* Federal Work-Study, scholarships/grants, and unspecified assistantships available. Financial award application deadline: 7/1; financial award applicants required to submit FAFSA. *Faculty research:* Ergonomics and cervical dysfunction, thoracic spine mobilization, anterior cruciate ligament injury in adolescent female athletes, ethics in physical therapy, admission requirements of entry-level physical therapy students. *Unit head:* Dr. Kristine Legters, Chair, 814-871-5641, E-mail: legters001@gannon.edu. *Application contact:* Kara Morgan, Director of Graduate Admissions, 814-871-5831, Fax: 814-871-5827, E-mail: graduate@gannon.edu.

George Fox University, Department of Physical Therapy, Newberg, OR 97132-2697. Offers DPT. *Faculty:* 3 full-time (1 woman), 6 part-time/adjunct (3 women). *Students:* 67 full-time (38 women); includes 15 minority (1 Black or African American, non-Hispanic/Latino; 6 Asian, non-Hispanic/Latino; 2 Hispanic/Latino; 2 Native Hawaiian or other Pacific Islander, non-Hispanic/Latino; 4 Two or more races, non-Hispanic/Latino). Average age 25. 156 applicants, 30% accepted, 36 enrolled. *Entrance requirements:* For doctorate, bachelor's degree from regionally-accredited university or college, minimum GPA of 3.0. Additional exam requirements/recommendations for international students: Required—TOEFL, IELTS. *Application deadline:* For fall admission, 12/1 for domestic and international students. Application fee: $40. Electronic applications accepted. *Financial support:* Applicants required to submit FAFSA. *Unit head:* Dr. Tyler Cuddeford, Director/Assistant Professor, 503-554-2452, E-mail: tcuddeford@georgefox.edu. *Application contact:* Cristina Schmitt, Director of Graduate Admissions, 503-554-6097, Fax: 503-554-3110, E-mail: dpt@georgefox.edu.
Website: http://www.georgefox.edu/physical-therapy/index.html

The George Washington University, School of Medicine and Health Sciences, Health Sciences Programs, Program in Physical Therapy, Washington, DC 20052. Offers DPT. *Accreditation:* APTA. *Students:* 109 full-time (82 women), 2 part-time (both women); includes 28 minority (6 Black or African American, non-Hispanic/Latino; 2 American Indian or Alaska Native, non-Hispanic/Latino; 14 Asian, non-Hispanic/Latino; 5 Hispanic/Latino; 1 Native Hawaiian or other Pacific Islander, non-Hispanic/Latino). Average age 27. 629 applicants, 15% accepted, 41 enrolled. In 2013, 33 doctorates awarded. *Entrance requirements:* Additional exam requirements/recommendations for international students: Required—TOEFL (minimum score 550 paper-based). *Application deadline:* For spring admission, 7/31 priority date for domestic students. Applications are processed on a rolling basis. Application fee: $75. *Unit head:* Dr. Joyce Maring, Director, E-mail: maringj@gwu.edu. *Application contact:* Marsha White, Information Contact, 202-994-8184, E-mail: hspmkw@gwumc.edu.

Georgia State University, Byrdine F. Lewis School of Nursing, Division of Physical Therapy, Atlanta, GA 30302-3083. Offers DPT. *Accreditation:* APTA. *Faculty:* 4 full-time (1 woman). *Students:* 100 full-time (55 women), 3 part-time (all women); includes 16 minority (4 Black or African American, non-Hispanic/Latino; 9 Asian, non-Hispanic/Latino; 1 Hispanic/Latino; 2 Native Hawaiian or other Pacific Islander, non-Hispanic/Latino), 4 international. Average age 27. 339 applicants, 13% accepted, 36 enrolled. In 2013, 37 doctorates awarded. *Degree requirements:* For doctorate, comprehensive exam, thesis/dissertation or alternative, clinical education. *Entrance requirements:* For doctorate, GRE, transcripts, documentation of Physical Therapy Experience Form, statement of goals. Additional exam requirements/recommendations for international students: Required—TOEFL (minimum score 550 paper-based; 80 iBT). *Application deadline:* For fall admission, 11/15 for domestic and international students. Application fee: $50. Electronic applications accepted. *Expenses:* Contact institution. *Financial support:* In 2013–14, research assistantships with full tuition reimbursements (averaging $2,000 per year), teaching assistantships with full tuition reimbursements (averaging $2,000 per year) were awarded; scholarships/grants, tuition waivers (partial), and unspecified assistantships also available. Financial award application deadline: 4/1. *Faculty research:* Tissue regeneration, wheelchair propulsion, neurophysiology, function in cerebral palsy, musculoskeletal anatomy and function. *Unit head:* Dr. Andrew Butler, Department Head, 404-413-1415, Fax: 404-413-1230, E-mail: andrewbutler@gsu.edu. *Application contact:* Vanessa Thomas-Meikle, Academic Advisor, 404-413-1000, Fax: 404-413-1001, E-mail: vthomas@gsu.edu.
Website: http://physicaltherapy.gsu.edu/

Governors State University, College of Health Professions, Program in Physical Therapy, University Park, IL 60484. Offers MPT, DPT. *Accreditation:* APTA. *Degree requirements:* For master's, thesis or alternative. *Entrance requirements:* For master's, minimum GPA of 3.0 in field, 2.75 overall.

The Graduate Center, City University of New York, Graduate Studies, Program in Physical Therapy, New York, NY 10016-4039. Offers DPT. Program offered jointly with College of Staten Island of the City University of New York and Hunter College of the City University of New York. *Accreditation:* APTA. *Degree requirements:* For doctorate, exams, publishable research project. *Entrance requirements:* For doctorate, GRE, CPR certification, 100 hours of clinical experience, minimum undergraduate GPA of 3.0. Additional exam requirements/recommendations for international students: Required—TOEFL.

Grand Valley State University, College of Health Professions, Physical Therapy Program, Allendale, MI 49401-9403. Offers DPT. *Accreditation:* APTA. *Entrance requirements:* For doctorate, GRE, minimum GPA of 3.0 in most recent 60 hours and in prerequisites, 50 hours of volunteer work, interview, writing sample. Additional exam requirements/recommendations for international students: Required—TOEFL (minimum score 610 paper-based). Electronic applications accepted. *Faculty research:* Balance deficits, motion analysis, nutritional knowledge of female athletes, trust in athletic performance, spinal functions dysfunction.

Hampton University, Graduate College, Department of Physical Therapy, Hampton, VA 23668. Offers DPT. *Accreditation:* APTA. *Degree requirements:* For doctorate, thesis/dissertation, oral defense, qualifying exam. *Entrance requirements:* For doctorate, GRE General Test, minimum GPA of 3.0 or master's degree in physics or related field.

Harding University, College of Allied Health, Program in Physical Therapy, Searcy, AR 72149-0001. Offers DPT. *Faculty:* 9 full-time (3 women). *Students:* 86 full-time (44 women); includes 5 minority (2 Black or African American, non-Hispanic/Latino; 3 Hispanic/Latino). Average age 25. 62 applicants, 82% accepted, 35 enrolled. *Entrance requirements:* For doctorate, GRE. Additional exam requirements/recommendations for international students: Required—TOEFL (minimum score 550 paper-based). Application fee: $50. *Expenses: Tuition:* Full-time $11,574; part-time $643 per credit hour. *Required fees:* $432; $24 per credit hour. Tuition and fees vary according to course load, degree level and program. *Unit head:* Dr. Michael McGalliard, Chair and Associate Professor, 501-279-5990, E-mail: mmcgalliard@harding.edu. *Application contact:* Dr. Cheri Yecke, Dean of Graduate Programs, 501-279-4335, Fax: 501-279-5192, E-mail: cyecke@harding.edu.
Website: http://www.harding.edu/pt/

Hardin-Simmons University, Graduate School, Holland School of Sciences and Mathematics, Doctoral Program in Physical Therapy, Abilene, TX 79698. Offers physical therapy (DPT). *Accreditation:* APTA. *Faculty:* 8 full-time (4 women), 1 part-time/adjunct (0 women). *Students:* 78 full-time (54 women); includes 10 minority (1 Asian, non-Hispanic/Latino; 9 Hispanic/Latino). Average age 24. 150 applicants, 23% accepted, 28 enrolled. In 2013, 22 doctorates awarded. *Degree requirements:* For doctorate, comprehensive exam, thesis/dissertation or alternative. *Entrance requirements:* For doctorate, GRE, letters of recommendation, interview, writing sample, transcripts from all colleges attended. Additional exam requirements/recommendations for international students: Required—TOEFL (minimum score 550 paper-based; 75 iBT). *Application deadline:* For fall admission, 10/15 priority date for domestic students, 10/1 priority date for international students. Application fee: $50 ($100 for international students). *Expenses:* Contact institution. *Financial support:* In 2013–14, 78 students received support. Scholarships/grants available. Financial award application deadline: 3/1; financial award applicants required to submit FAFSA. *Faculty research:* Gait parameters, health promotion for seniors/disabled populations, sports injuries and recovery, spirituality, vibration platforms, sensory integration, postural stability. *Unit head:* Dr. Janelle K. O'Connell, Department Head/Professor, 325-670-5860, Fax: 325-670-5868, E-mail: ptoffice@hsutx.edu. *Application contact:* Dr. Nancy Kucinski, Dean of Graduate Studies, 325-670-1298, Fax: 325-670-1564, E-mail: gradoff@hsutx.edu.
Website: http://www.hsutx.edu/academics/holland/graduate/physicaltherapy

Humboldt State University, Academic Programs, College of Professional Studies, Department of Kinesiology and Recreation Administration, Arcata, CA 95521-8299. Offers athletic training education (MS); exercise science/wellness management (MS); pre-physical therapy (MS); teaching/coaching (MS). *Degree requirements:* For master's, thesis or alternative. *Entrance requirements:* For master's, GMAT, minimum GPA of 2.5. Additional exam requirements/recommendations for international students: Required—TOEFL. *Faculty research:* Human performance, adapted physical education, physical therapy.

Husson University, Doctorate in Physical Therapy Program, Bangor, ME 04401-2999. Offers DPT. *Accreditation:* APTA. *Faculty:* 9 full-time (5 women), 10 part-time/adjunct (6 women). *Students:* 74 full-time (51 women); includes 4 minority (all Two or more races, non-Hispanic/Latino). Average age 23. 171 applicants, 6% accepted, 7 enrolled. In 2013, 27 doctorates awarded. *Entrance requirements:* For doctorate, GRE (minimum score of 1500), essay, minimum GPA of 3.5. Additional exam requirements/recommendations for international students: Required—TOEFL (minimum score 550 paper-based). *Application deadline:* For fall admission, 4/15 for domestic and international students. Application fee: $40. Electronic applications accepted. *Expenses:* Contact institution. *Financial support:* Federal Work-Study and unspecified assistantships available. Financial award application deadline: 4/15; financial award applicants required to submit FAFSA. *Unit head:* Dr. Suzanne Gordon, Director, 207-941-7797, E-mail: gordons@husson.edu. *Application contact:* Cecile Ferguson, Administrative Assistant, 207-941-7101, E-mail: pt@fc.husson.edu.

Idaho State University, Office of Graduate Studies, Kasiska College of Health Professions, Department of Physical and Occupational Therapy, Program in Physical Therapy, Pocatello, ID 83209-8045. Offers DPT. *Accreditation:* APTA. *Degree requirements:* For doctorate, comprehensive exam, thesis/dissertation, oral and written exam. *Entrance requirements:* For doctorate, GRE General Test, minimum GPA of 3.0, 80 hours in 2 practice settings of physical therapy. Additional exam requirements/recommendations for international students: Required—TOEFL (minimum score 600 paper-based). Electronic applications accepted. *Expenses:* Contact institution. *Faculty research:* Cardiovascular/pulmonary balance, neural plasticity, orthopedics, geriatrics, hypertension.

Indiana University–Purdue University Indianapolis, School of Health and Rehabilitation Sciences, Indianapolis, IN 46202. Offers health and rehabilitation sciences (PhD); health sciences (MS); nutrition and dietetics (MS); occupational therapy (MS); physical therapy (DPT); physician assistant (MPAS). Part-time and evening/weekend programs available. *Faculty:* 4 full-time (3 women). *Students:* 266 full-time (201 women), 13 part-time (12 women); includes 21 minority (6 Black or African American, non-Hispanic/Latino; 7 Asian, non-Hispanic/Latino; 4 Hispanic/Latino; 1 Native Hawaiian or other Pacific Islander, non-Hispanic/Latino; 3 Two or more races, non-Hispanic/Latino), 11 international. Average age 26. 381 applicants, 23% accepted, 77 enrolled. In 2013, 33 master's, 39 doctorates awarded. *Degree requirements:* For master's, thesis (for some programs). *Entrance requirements:* For master's, GRE General Test, minimum GPA of 3.0 (for MS in health sciences, nutrition and dietetics), 3.2 (for MS in occupational therapy), 3.0 cumulative and prerequisite math/science (for MPAS); for doctorate, GRE, minimum cumulative and prerequisite math/science GPA of 3.2. Additional exam requirements/recommendations for international students: Required—TOEFL (minimum score 550 paper-based; 79 iBT), IELTS (minimum score 6.5), PTE (minimum score 54). *Application deadline:* For fall admission, 10/1 for domestic students; for spring admission, 10/15 for domestic students. Electronic applications accepted. *Expenses:* Contact institution. *Financial support:* Fellowships, research assistantships, Federal Work-Study, institutionally sponsored loans, and scholarships/grants available. Support available to part-time students. Financial award applicants required to submit FAFSA. *Faculty research:* Function and mobility across the lifespan, pediatric nutrition, driving and mobility rehabilitation, neurorehabilitation and biomechanics, rehabilitation and integrative therapy. *Total annual research expenditures:* $1.1 million. *Unit head:* Dr. Augustine Agho, Dean, 317-274-4704, E-mail: aagho@iu.edu. *Application contact:* Kim Crockett, Student Data Coordinator, 317-278-6744, E-mail: kimecroc@iu.edu.
Website: http://shrs.iupui.edu/

Ithaca College, School of Health Sciences and Human Performance, Program in Physical Therapy, Ithaca, NY 14850. Offers DPT. *Accreditation:* APTA. *Faculty:* 16 full-time (9 women). *Students:* 167 full-time (121 women), 1 (woman) part-time; includes 21 minority (4 Black or African American, non-Hispanic/Latino; 5 Asian, non-Hispanic/Latino; 8 Hispanic/Latino; 4 Two or more races, non-Hispanic/Latino), 1 international.

Average age 22. In 2013, 63 doctorates awarded. *Degree requirements:* For doctorate, thesis/dissertation optional, clinical internships. *Entrance requirements:* Additional exam requirements/recommendations for international students: Required—TOEFL (minimum score 550 paper-based; 80 iBT). Tuition and fees vary according to program. *Financial support:* In 2013–14, 120 students received support. Career-related internships or fieldwork, Federal Work-Study, and scholarships/grants available. Support available to part-time students. Financial award applicants required to submit CSS PROFILE or FAFSA. *Faculty research:* Mindful practice and failure in clinical education; relationships between patient characteristics, health behaviors and patient reported outcomes; prevention and treatment of knee injuries; use of technology in teaching and clinic; mindfulness and its role in failure within the clinical setting; evaluation and treatment of foot and ankle pathologies; shoulder impingement in individuals with spinal cord injury; cognitive-behavioral pain self-management; performing arts medicine; movement analysis. *Unit head:* Dr. Andrew Robinson, Graduate Chair, 607-274-3143, Fax: 607-274-1263, E-mail: gps@ithaca.edu. *Application contact:* Gerard Turbide, Director, Office of Admission, 607-274-3143, Fax: 607-274-1263, E-mail: gps@ithaca.edu.
Website: http://www.ithaca.edu/gps/gradprograms/pt

Langston University, School of Physical Therapy, Langston, OK 73050. Offers DPT. *Accreditation:* APTA.

Lebanon Valley College, Physical Therapy Department, Annville, PA 17003-1400. Offers DPT. *Accreditation:* APTA. *Faculty:* 9 full-time (4 women). *Students:* 66 full-time (54 women), 4 part-time (3 women); includes 2 minority (1 Asian, non-Hispanic/Latino; 1 Hispanic/Latino), 1 international. Average age 23. 66 applicants, 12% accepted, 7 enrolled. In 2013, 27 doctorates awarded. *Entrance requirements:* For doctorate, GRE. *Application deadline:* For winter admission, 2/1 for domestic students. Application fee: $30. Electronic applications accepted. *Expenses:* Contact institution. *Financial support:* Scholarships/grants available. Financial award application deadline: 5/1; financial award applicants required to submit FAFSA. *Unit head:* Dr. Stan M. Dacko, Chairperson/Associate Professor, 717-867-6843, Fax: 717-867-6849, E-mail: dacko@lvc.edu. *Application contact:* E. J. Smith, Assistant Director of Admission, 866-582-4236, Fax: 717-867-6026, E-mail: ejsmith@lvc.edu.
Website: http://www.lvc.edu/physical-therapy/index.aspx?bhiw-952

Loma Linda University, School of Allied Health Professions, Department of Physical Therapy, Loma Linda, CA 92350. Offers MPT, D Sc, DPT, DPTSc. *Accreditation:* APTA. *Entrance requirements:* Additional exam requirements/recommendations for international students: Required—TOEFL (minimum score 550 paper-based). Electronic applications accepted.

Long Island University–LIU Brooklyn, School of Health Professions, Division of Physical Therapy, Brooklyn, NY 11201-8423. Offers DPT, TDPT. *Accreditation:* APTA. Part-time and evening/weekend programs available. *Entrance requirements:* Additional exam requirements/recommendations for international students: Required—TOEFL (minimum score 500 paper-based). Electronic applications accepted.

Louisiana State University Health Sciences Center, School of Allied Health Professions, Department of Physical Therapy, New Orleans, LA 70112-2223. Offers DPT. *Accreditation:* APTA. *Faculty:* 8 full-time (4 women). *Students:* 103 full-time (69 women); includes 12 minority (5 Black or African American, non-Hispanic/Latino; 2 Asian, non-Hispanic/Latino; 1 Hispanic/Latino; 4 Two or more races, non-Hispanic/Latino). Average age 26. 306 applicants, 11% accepted, 35 enrolled. In 2013, 30 doctorates awarded. *Degree requirements:* For doctorate, thesis/dissertation optional. *Entrance requirements:* For doctorate, GRE General Test (minimum combined score: 296), 60 hours of experience in physical therapy, minimum GPA of 3.0 in math and science, bachelor's degree, reference letter from physical therapist that observed student. *Application deadline:* For fall admission, 11/15 for domestic students; for summer admission, 10/1 for domestic students. Application fee: $140. Electronic applications accepted. *Financial support:* Application deadline: 4/15; applicants required to submit FAFSA. *Faculty research:* Wound healing, spinal cord injury, pain management, geriatrics, muscle physiology, muscle damage, motor control, balance. *Total annual research expenditures:* $101,546. *Unit head:* Dr. Jane M. Eason, Head, 504-568-4288, Fax: 504-568-6552, E-mail: jeason@lsuhsc.edu. *Application contact:* Yudialys Delgado, Student Affairs Director, 504-568-4253, Fax: 504-568-3185, E-mail: ydelga@lsuhsc.edu.
Website: http://alliedhealth.lsuhsc.edu/pt/

Lynchburg College, Graduate Studies, School of Health Sciences and Human Performance, Doctor of Physical Therapy Program, Lynchburg, VA 24501-3199. Offers DPT. *Faculty:* 9 full-time (5 women), 3 part-time/adjunct (1 woman). *Students:* 132 full-time (78 women), 1 (woman) part-time; includes 12 minority (1 Black or African American, non-Hispanic/Latino; 1 American Indian or Alaska Native, non-Hispanic/Latino; 3 Asian, non-Hispanic/Latino; 3 Hispanic/Latino; 1 Native Hawaiian or other Pacific Islander, non-Hispanic/Latino; 3 Two or more races, non-Hispanic/Latino), 1 international. Average age 25. In 2013, 43 doctorates awarded. *Degree requirements:* For doctorate, comprehensive exam. *Entrance requirements:* For doctorate, GRE, graduation from a 4-year program, observation hours, references, bachelor's degree. Additional exam requirements/recommendations for international students: Required—TOEFL. *Application deadline:* For spring admission, 2/1 priority date for domestic and international students. Applications are processed on a rolling basis. Application fee: $135. Electronic applications accepted. *Expenses:* Contact institution. *Financial support:* Scholarships/grants, tuition waivers (partial), and unspecified assistantships available. Financial award application deadline: 7/31; financial award applicants required to submit FAFSA. *Unit head:* Dr. A. Russell Smith, Jr., Associate Professor/Director of DPT Program, 434-544-8880, E-mail: smith.ar@lynchburg.edu. *Application contact:* Savannah G. Cook, Admissions Coordinator, 434-544-8885, Fax: 434-544-8887, E-mail: cook.s@lynchburg.edu.
Website: http://www.lynchburg.edu/doctor-physical-therapy

Marquette University, Graduate School, College of Health Sciences, Program in Physical Therapy, Milwaukee, WI 53201-1881. Offers DPT. *Accreditation:* APTA. *Faculty:* 14 full-time (7 women), 37 part-time/adjunct (25 women). *Students:* 94 full-time (76 women), 2 part-time (0 women); includes 17 minority (2 Black or African American, non-Hispanic/Latino; 6 Asian, non-Hispanic/Latino; 3 Hispanic/Latino; 2 Native Hawaiian or other Pacific Islander, non-Hispanic/Latino; 4 Two or more races, non-Hispanic/Latino), 1 international. Average age 23. *Degree requirements:* For doctorate, clinical rotations. *Entrance requirements:* For doctorate, GRE General Test. Additional exam requirements/recommendations for international students: Required—TOEFL. Application fee: $50. Electronic applications accepted. *Expenses:* Contact institution. *Financial support:* In 2013–14, 2 students received support, including 2 research assistantships with full tuition reimbursements available (averaging $21,750 per year); health care benefits and unspecified assistantships also available. Financial award application deadline: 2/15. *Faculty research:* Urban health issues, mechanisms and management of pain, kinesiologic principles, brain and spinal cord control of human locomotion, mechanisms of motor impairment. *Total annual research expenditures:* $776,347. *Unit head:* Dr. Lawrence Pan, Dean, 414-288-7161, Fax: 414-288-5987, E-mail: lawrence.pan@marquette.edu. *Application contact:* Dr. Lawrence Pan, Dean, 414-288-7161, Fax: 414-288-5987, E-mail: lawrence.pan@marquette.edu.
Website: http://www.marquette.edu/physical-therapy/

Marshall University, Academic Affairs Division, College of Health Professions, School of Physical Therapy, Huntington, WV 25755. Offers DPT. *Students:* 62 part-time (26 women). Average age 25. *Application deadline:* Applications are processed on a rolling basis. *Unit head:* Dr. Penny G. Kroll, Program Director, 800-642-3463, E-mail: kroll@marshall.edu. *Application contact:* Information Contact, 304-746-1900, Fax: 304-746-1902, E-mail: services@marshall.edu.

Marymount University, School of Health Professions, Program in Physical Therapy, Arlington, VA 22207-4299. Offers DPT. *Accreditation:* APTA. *Faculty:* 8 full-time (6 women), 2 part-time/adjunct (both women). *Students:* 106 full-time (75 women); includes 20 minority (4 Black or African American, non-Hispanic/Latino; 9 Asian, non-Hispanic/Latino; 5 Hispanic/Latino; 2 Two or more races, non-Hispanic/Latino), 3 international. Average age 26. 616 applicants, 30% accepted, 39 enrolled. In 2013, 28 doctorates awarded. *Degree requirements:* For doctorate, comprehensive exam, thesis/dissertation. *Entrance requirements:* For doctorate, GRE, 2 letters of recommendation, interview, resume, 40 hours of clinical work experience, essay, minimum GPA of 3.0 from previous university coursework. Additional exam requirements/recommendations for international students: Required—TOEFL (minimum score 600 paper-based; 96 iBT), IELTS (minimum score 6.5). *Application deadline:* For fall admission, 12/2 priority date for domestic students, 12/13 for international students. Application fee: $180. Electronic applications accepted. *Expenses:* Contact institution. *Financial support:* In 2013–14, 13 students received support, including 2 research assistantships with partial tuition reimbursements available, 5 teaching assistantships with partial tuition reimbursements available; career-related internships or fieldwork, Federal Work-Study, scholarships/grants, and unspecified assistantships also available. Financial award applicants required to submit FAFSA. *Unit head:* Dr. Jason Craig, Chair, 703-284-5988, Fax: 703-284-5981, E-mail: jason.craig@marymount.edu. *Application contact:* Francesca Reed, Director, Graduate Admissions, 703-284-5901, Fax: 703-527-3815, E-mail: grad.admissions@marymount.edu.
Website: http://www.marymount.edu/academics/programs/physicalTherapy

Maryville University of Saint Louis, College of Health Professions, Physical Therapy Program, St. Louis, MO 63141-7299. Offers DPT. *Accreditation:* APTA. *Students:* 69 full-time (53 women), 36 part-time (31 women); includes 2 minority (both Asian, non-Hispanic/Latino). Average age 24. In 2013, 33 doctorates awarded. *Degree requirements:* For doctorate, clinical rotations. *Entrance requirements:* For doctorate, minimum cumulative GPA of 3.0, 2 letters of recommendation, interview. Additional exam requirements/recommendations for international students: Required—TOEFL (minimum score 560 paper-based). *Application deadline:* Applications are processed on a rolling basis. Application fee: $40 ($60 for international students). Electronic applications accepted. Application fee is waived when completed online. *Expenses:* *Tuition:* Full-time $23,812; part-time $728 per credit hour. *Required fees:* $395 per year. Tuition and fees vary according to course load, degree level and program. *Financial support:* Career-related internships or fieldwork, Federal Work-Study, and campus employment available. Financial award application deadline: 3/1; financial award applicants required to submit FAFSA. *Faculty research:* Memory and exercise. *Unit head:* Dr. Michelle Unterberg, Director, 314-529-9590, Fax: 314-529-9946, E-mail: munterberg@maryville.edu. *Application contact:* Crystal Jacobsmeyer, Assistant Director, Graduate Enrollment Advising, 314-529-9654, Fax: 314-529-9927, E-mail: cjacobsmeyer@maryville.edu.
Website: http://www.maryville.edu/hp/physical-therapy/

Mayo School of Health Sciences, Program in Physical Therapy, Rochester, MN 55905. Offers DPT. *Accreditation:* APTA. *Faculty:* 5 full-time (0 women), 3 part-time/adjunct (all women). *Students:* 84 full-time (57 women); includes 6 minority (3 Black or African American, non-Hispanic/Latino; 1 American Indian or Alaska Native, non-Hispanic/Latino; 1 Asian, non-Hispanic/Latino; 1 Hispanic/Latino). Average age 25. 629 applicants, 9% accepted, 28 enrolled. In 2013, 28 doctorates awarded. *Degree requirements:* For doctorate, comprehensive exam. *Entrance requirements:* For doctorate, GRE. Additional exam requirements/recommendations for international students: Required—TOEFL. *Application deadline:* For fall admission, 10/15 for domestic and international students. Applications are processed on a rolling basis. Electronic applications accepted. *Expenses:* *Tuition:* Full-time $17,820. *Required fees:* $250. *Financial support:* In 2013–14, 75 students received support. Scholarships/grants available. Financial award applicants required to submit FAFSA. *Faculty research:* Biomechanics, gait analysis, growth factor-mediated plasticity in muscle, musculoskeletal clinical tests and measures, Parkinson's disease, coordination testing. *Unit head:* Dr. John Hollman, Director, 507-284-9547, Fax: 507-284-0656, E-mail: hollman.john@mayo.edu. *Application contact:* Carol Cooper, Administrative Assistant, 507-284-2054, Fax: 507-284-0656, E-mail: cooper.carol@mayo.edu.
Website: http://www.mayo.edu/mshs/careers/physical-therapy/physical-therapy-doctoral-program-minnesota

McMaster University, Faculty of Health Sciences, Professional Program in Physiotherapy, Hamilton, ON L8S 4M2, Canada. Offers M Sc. *Degree requirements:* For master's, clinical placements, independent research project. *Entrance requirements:* For master's, minimum B average over last 60 undergraduate units. Additional exam requirements/recommendations for international students: Required—TOEFL (minimum score 600 paper-based).

Medical University of South Carolina, College of Health Professions, Program in Physical Therapy, Charleston, SC 29425. Offers DPT. *Accreditation:* APTA. Postbaccalaureate distance learning degree programs offered (minimal on-campus study). *Entrance requirements:* For doctorate, GRE, references, minimum GPA of 3.0, volunteer hours. Additional exam requirements/recommendations for international students: Required—TOEFL (minimum score 600 paper-based). Electronic applications accepted. *Faculty research:* Low back pain, spinal cord injury.

Mercer University, Graduate Studies, Cecil B. Day Campus, College of Health Professions, Atlanta, GA 30341. Offers physical therapy (DPT); physician assistant (MM Sc); public health (MPH). *Faculty:* 23 full-time (17 women), 3 part-time/adjunct (2 women). *Students:* 281 full-time (208 women), 3 part-time (1 woman); includes 105 minority (70 Black or African American, non-Hispanic/Latino; 17 Asian, non-Hispanic/Latino; 6 Hispanic/Latino; 12 Two or more races, non-Hispanic/Latino), 3 international. Average age 26. In 2013, 42 master's, 26 doctorates awarded. *Unit head:* Richard V. Swindle, Senior Vice President, 678-547-6397, E-mail: swindle_rv@mercer.edu. *Application contact:* Tracey M. Wofford, Associate Director of Admissions, 678-547-6422, E-mail: wofford_tm@mercer.edu.
Website: http://chp.mercer.edu/

Mercy College, School of Health and Natural Sciences, Program in Physical Therapy, Dobbs Ferry, NY 10522-1189. Offers DPT. *Accreditation:* APTA. Evening/weekend programs available. *Students:* 67 full-time (34 women), 26 part-time (14 women); includes 30 minority (8 Black or African American, non-Hispanic/Latino; 12 Asian, non-Hispanic/Latino; 7 Hispanic/Latino; 1 Native Hawaiian or other Pacific Islander, non-Hispanic/Latino; 2 Two or more races, non-Hispanic/Latino), 2 international. Average

age 33. 315 applicants, 15% accepted, 30 enrolled. In 2013, 24 doctorates awarded. *Entrance requirements:* For doctorate, interview, two letters of recommendations, official college transcripts with minimum GPA of 3.0, two-page typewritten essay on reasons for pursuing career in physical therapy, volunteer/work experience forms demonstrating at least eighty hours of volunteer work or work-related experience. Additional exam requirements/recommendations for international students: Required—TOEFL (minimum score 600 paper-based; 100 iBT), IELTS (minimum score 8). *Application deadline:* Applications are processed on a rolling basis. Application fee: $62. Electronic applications accepted. *Expenses:* Contact institution. *Financial support:* Career-related internships or fieldwork, Federal Work-Study, scholarships/grants, and unspecified assistantships available. Support available to part-time students. Financial award applicants required to submit FAFSA. *Unit head:* Dr. Joan Toglia, Dean, School of Health and Natural Sciences, 914-674-7837, E-mail: jtoglia@mercy.edu. *Application contact:* Allison Gurdineer, Senior Director of Admissions, 877-637-2946, Fax: 914-674-7382, E-mail: admissions@mercy.edu.
Website: https://www.mercy.edu/DPTprogram

MGH Institute of Health Professions, School of Health and Rehabilitation Sciences, Post-Professional Graduate Program in Physical Therapy, Boston, MA 02129. Offers MS, DPT, Certificate. Part-time and evening/weekend programs available. *Faculty:* 14 full-time (11 women), 6 part-time/adjunct (all women). *Students:* 19 full-time (14 women), 82 part-time (61 women); includes 49 minority (1 Black or African American, non-Hispanic/Latino; 48 Asian, non-Hispanic/Latino). Average age 35. 168 applicants, 80% accepted, 109 enrolled. In 2013, 42 master's, 58 doctorates, 5 other advanced degrees awarded. *Degree requirements:* For master's, thesis, clinical preceptorship. *Entrance requirements:* For master's, GRE General Test, graduation from an approved program in physical therapy. Additional exam requirements/recommendations for international students: Required—TOEFL (minimum score 550 paper-based; 80 iBT). *Application deadline:* For fall admission, 3/1 priority date for domestic students, 3/1 for international students; for winter admission, 7/1 priority date for domestic students, 7/1 for international students; for spring admission, 11/1 priority date for domestic students, 11/1 for international students. Applications are processed on a rolling basis. Application fee: $100. Electronic applications accepted. *Expenses: Tuition:* Part-time $1114 per credit. *Required fees:* $620 per term. One-time fee: $475 part-time. *Financial support:* In 2013–14, 4 students received support. Career-related internships or fieldwork, scholarships/grants, and unspecified assistantships available. Support available to part-time students. Financial award application deadline: 4/1; financial award applicants required to submit FAFSA. *Faculty research:* Disability in the elderly; gait, balance and posture; cardiac rehabilitation; relationship of impairment to disability; effect of muscle strengthening in the elderly. *Unit head:* Dr. Leslie G. Portney, Dean, 617-726-3170, Fax: 617-724-6321, E-mail: lportney@mghihp.edu. *Application contact:* Catherine Hamilton, Assistant Director of Admission and Multicultural Recruitment, 617-726-3140, Fax: 617-726-8010, E-mail: admissions@mghihp.edu.
Website: http://www.mghihp.edu/academics/school-of-health-and-rehabilitation-sciences/

MGH Institute of Health Professions, School of Health and Rehabilitation Sciences, Professional Graduate Program in Physical Therapy, Boston, MA 02129. Offers DPT. *Accreditation:* APTA. *Faculty:* 14 full-time (11 women), 6 part-time/adjunct (all women). *Students:* 126 full-time (85 women), 51 part-time (38 women); includes 34 minority (4 Black or African American, non-Hispanic/Latino; 1 American Indian or Alaska Native, non-Hispanic/Latino; 19 Asian, non-Hispanic/Latino; 10 Hispanic/Latino). Average age 26. 609 applicants, 19% accepted, 70 enrolled. In 2013, 95 doctorates awarded. *Degree requirements:* For doctorate, thesis/dissertation or alternative, research project. *Entrance requirements:* For doctorate, GRE General Test, interview, minimum of 10 physical therapy observation hours, bachelor's degree from regionally-accredited college or university. Additional exam requirements/recommendations for international students: Required—TOEFL (minimum score 550 paper-based; 80 iBT). *Application deadline:* For spring admission, 10/15 for domestic students, 11/15 for international students; for summer admission, 11/1 for domestic and international students. Application fee: $0. Electronic applications accepted. *Expenses: Tuition:* Part-time $1114 per credit. *Required fees:* $620 per term. One-time fee: $475 part-time. *Financial support:* In 2013–14, 36 students received support, including 4 research assistantships, 9 teaching assistantships; career-related internships or fieldwork, scholarships/grants, and unspecified assistantships also available. Support available to part-time students. Financial award application deadline: 4/1; financial award applicants required to submit FAFSA. *Faculty research:* Disability in the elderly; gait, balance, and posture; cardiac rehabilitation: relationship of impairment to disability. *Unit head:* Dr. Pamela Levangie, Chair, 617-726-3170, Fax: 617-724-6446, E-mail: plevangie@mghihp.edu. *Application contact:* Catherine Hamilton, Assistant Director of Admission and Multicultural Recruitment, 617-726-3140, Fax: 617-726-8010, E-mail: admissions@mghihp.edu.
Website: http://www.mghihp.edu/academics/school-of-health-and-rehabilitation-sciences/

Midwestern University, Downers Grove Campus, College of Health Sciences, Illinois Campus, Program in Physical Therapy, Downers Grove, IL 60515-1235. Offers DPT. *Accreditation:* APTA. *Entrance requirements:* For doctorate, GRE General Test. *Expenses:* Contact institution.

Midwestern University, Glendale Campus, College of Health Sciences, Arizona Campus, Program in Physical Therapy, Glendale, AZ 85308. Offers DPT. *Accreditation:* APTA. *Entrance requirements:* For doctorate, GRE General Test, bachelor's degree, minimum cumulative GPA of 2.75.

Misericordia University, College of Health Sciences, Program in Physical Therapy, Dallas, PA 18612-1098. Offers DPT. *Accreditation:* APTA. *Faculty:* 9 full-time (6 women), 6 part-time/adjunct (3 women). *Students:* 138 full-time (89 women), 51 part-time (37 women); includes 11 minority (3 Black or African American, non-Hispanic/Latino; 1 American Indian or Alaska Native, non-Hispanic/Latino; 1 Asian, non-Hispanic/Latino; 4 Hispanic/Latino; 2 Two or more races, non-Hispanic/Latino), 1 international. Average age 25. In 2013, 21 doctorates awarded. *Entrance requirements:* For doctorate, GRE General Test, minimum undergraduate GPA of 3.0, volunteer experience. Additional exam requirements/recommendations for international students: Required—TOEFL. *Application deadline:* For fall admission, 12/15 priority date for domestic students. Applications are processed on a rolling basis. Application fee: $35. Electronic applications accepted. *Expenses: Tuition:* Full-time $14,450; part-time $680 per credit. Tuition and fees vary according to degree level. *Financial support:* In 2013–14, 141 students received support. Teaching assistantships, career-related internships or fieldwork, scholarships/grants, and tuition waivers (partial) available. Support available to part-time students. Financial award application deadline: 6/30; financial award applicants required to submit FAFSA. *Faculty research:* Wound care, computer-assisted instruction, instruction in applied physiology, isokinetics, prosthetics. *Unit head:* Dr. Susan Barker, Chair, 570-674-6422, E-mail: sbarker@misericordia.edu. *Application contact:* Kristen Andrews, Assistant Director of Admissions, 570-674-6255, Fax: 570-674-6232, E-mail: kandrews@misericordia.edu.
Website: http://www.misericordia.edu/pt

Missouri State University, Graduate College, College of Health and Human Services, Department of Physical Therapy, Springfield, MO 65897. Offers DPT. *Accreditation:* APTA. *Faculty:* 7 full-time (4 women), 8 part-time/adjunct (2 women). *Students:* 99 full-time (62 women), 3 part-time (all women); includes 3 minority (1 Asian, non-Hispanic/Latino; 1 Hispanic/Latino; 1 Two or more races, non-Hispanic/Latino), 2 international. Average age 26. 48 applicants, 98% accepted, 38 enrolled. In 2013, 33 doctorates awarded. *Degree requirements:* For doctorate, comprehensive exam, thesis/dissertation or alternative. *Entrance requirements:* For doctorate, GRE, minimum GPA of 3.0. Additional exam requirements/recommendations for international students: Required—TOEFL (minimum score 550 paper-based; 79 iBT). *Application deadline:* For fall admission, 12/15 for domestic and international students. Application fee: $35 ($50 for international students). Electronic applications accepted. *Expenses:* Tuition, state resident: full-time $4500; part-time $250 per credit hour. Tuition, nonresident: full-time $9018; part-time $501 per credit hour. *Required fees:* $361 per semester. Tuition and fees vary according to course level, course load and program. *Financial support:* Federal Work-Study, institutionally sponsored loans, and unspecified assistantships available. Financial award application deadline: 3/31; financial award applicants required to submit FAFSA. *Faculty research:* Complex regional pain syndrome (CRPS), posture and the temporomandibular joint, clinical orthopedics, aging of the motor system. *Unit head:* Dr. Jeanne Cook, Head, 417-836-6179, Fax: 417-836-6229, E-mail: physicaltherapy@missouristate.edu. *Application contact:* Misty Stewart, Coordinator of Graduate Recruitment, 417-836-6079, Fax: 417-836-6200, E-mail: mistystewart@missouristate.edu.
Website: http://www.missouristate.edu/physicaltherapy/

Mount St. Joseph University, Physical Therapy Program, Cincinnati, OH 45233-1670. Offers DPT. *Accreditation:* APTA. *Faculty:* 7 full-time (5 women), 9 part-time/adjunct (4 women). *Students:* 72 full-time (47 women), 40 part-time (23 women); includes 1 minority (Two or more races, non-Hispanic/Latino). Average age 24. 207 applicants, 25% accepted, 37 enrolled. In 2013, 24 doctorates awarded. *Degree requirements:* For doctorate, clinical internship; integrative project. *Entrance requirements:* For doctorate, GRE, minimum GPA of 3.0; prerequisite coursework in sciences, humanities, social sciences, and statistics; 80 observation hours; at least 80 hours of clinical observation in 2 different physical therapy settings; PTCAS application. Additional exam requirements/recommendations for international students: Required—TOEFL (minimum score 560 paper-based; 83 iBT). *Application deadline:* For fall admission, 11/1 for domestic students. Application fee: $50. Electronic applications accepted. *Expenses:* Contact institution. *Financial support:* In 2013–14, 1 student received support. Application deadline: 6/1; applicants required to submit FAFSA. *Faculty research:* Utilizing technology in learning, neurobiology, assessment of student learning, critical thinking, effectiveness of distance education methods. *Unit head:* Dr. Rosanne Thomas, Chair, 513-244-4519, Fax: 513-451-2547, E-mail: rosanne_thomas@mail.msj.edu. *Application contact:* Mary Brigham, Assistant Director of Graduate Recruitment, 513-244-4233, Fax: 513-244-4629, E-mail: mary_brigham@mail.msj.edu.
Website: http://www.msj.edu/academics/graduate-programs/doctor-of-physical-therapy1/

Mount St. Mary's College, Graduate Division, Los Angeles, CA 90049-1599. Offers business administration (MBA); counseling psychology (MS); creative writing (MFA); education (MS, Certificate); humanities (MA); nursing (MSN, Certificate); physical therapy (DPT); religious studies (MA); MFA/MA. Part-time and evening/weekend programs available. *Faculty:* 35 full-time (26 women), 112 part-time/adjunct (76 women). *Students:* 416 full-time (324 women), 233 part-time (184 women); includes 376 minority (64 Black or African American, non-Hispanic/Latino; 2 American Indian or Alaska Native, non-Hispanic/Latino; 57 Asian, non-Hispanic/Latino; 229 Hispanic/Latino; 8 Native Hawaiian or other Pacific Islander, non-Hispanic/Latino; 16 Two or more races, non-Hispanic/Latino), 4 international. Average age 33. 1,041 applicants, 22% accepted, 183 enrolled. In 2013, 168 master's, 29 doctorates awarded. *Entrance requirements:* Additional exam requirements/recommendations for international students: Required—TOEFL. *Application deadline:* Applications are processed on a rolling basis. Application fee: $50. Electronic applications accepted. *Expenses: Tuition:* Part-time $798 per unit. *Required fees:* $125 per semester. Tuition and fees vary according to program. *Financial support:* Career-related internships or fieldwork, Federal Work-Study, institutionally sponsored loans, and tuition waivers (full and partial) available. Support available to part-time students. Financial award application deadline: 3/15; financial award applicants required to submit FAFSA. *Unit head:* Dr. Linda Moody, Graduate Dean, 213-477-2800, E-mail: gradprograms@msmc.la.edu. *Application contact:* Natalie Dymchenko, Senior Graduate Admission Counselor, 213-477-2800, E-mail: gradprograms@msmc.la.edu.
Website: http://www.msmc.la.edu/admission/graduate-admission.asp

Nazareth College of Rochester, Graduate Studies, Department of Physical Therapy, Doctoral Program in Physical Therapy, Rochester, NY 14618-3790. Offers DPT. *Accreditation:* APTA. *Entrance requirements:* For doctorate, minimum GPA of 3.0.

Nazareth College of Rochester, Graduate Studies, Department of Physical Therapy, Master's Program in Physical Therapy, Rochester, NY 14618-3790. Offers MS. *Accreditation:* APTA. *Entrance requirements:* For master's, minimum GPA of 3.0.

Neumann University, Program in Physical Therapy, Aston, PA 19014-1298. Offers DPT. *Accreditation:* APTA. Evening/weekend programs available. *Entrance requirements:* Additional exam requirements/recommendations for international students: Required—TOEFL. Electronic applications accepted. *Expenses:* Contact institution.

New York Institute of Technology, School of Health Professions, Department of Physical Therapy, Old Westbury, NY 11568-8000. Offers DPT. *Accreditation:* APTA. *Faculty:* 9 full-time (5 women), 12 part-time/adjunct (6 women). *Students:* 101 full-time (59 women); includes 24 minority (4 Black or African American, non-Hispanic/Latino; 15 Asian, non-Hispanic/Latino; 5 Hispanic/Latino), 2 international. Average age 25. 861 applicants, 11% accepted, 39 enrolled. In 2013, 30 doctorates awarded. *Entrance requirements:* Additional exam requirements/recommendations for international students: Required—TOEFL (minimum score 550 paper-based; 79 iBT), IELTS (minimum score 6). *Application deadline:* For fall admission, 7/1 priority date for domestic students, 6/1 for international students; for spring admission, 12/1 priority date for domestic students, 12/1 for international students. Application fee: $50. *Expenses: Tuition:* Full-time $18,900; part-time $1050 per credit. *Financial support:* Research assistantships with partial tuition reimbursements, scholarships/grants, health care benefits, tuition waivers, and unspecified assistantships available. Support available to part-time students. Financial award applicants required to submit FAFSA. *Faculty research:* Parkinson's disease, spinal cord injury, manual therapy, educational technology, response to exercise, geriatrics, balance. *Unit head:* Dr. Karen Friel, Department Chair, 516-686-7651, Fax: 516-686-7699, E-mail: kfriel@nyit.edu. *Application contact:* Alice Dolitsky, Director, Graduate Admissions, 516-686-7520, Fax: 516-686-1116, E-mail: nyitgrad@nyit.edu.
Website: http://www.nyit.edu/physical_therapy

New York Medical College, School of Health Sciences and Practice, Department of Physical Therapy, Valhalla, NY 10595-1691. Offers DPT. *Accreditation:* APTA. *Faculty:* 6 full-time, 15 part-time/adjunct. *Students:* 38 full-time. Average age 27. 400 applicants, 25% accepted, 38 enrolled. In 2013, 38 doctorates awarded. *Degree requirements:* For doctorate, comprehensive exam, thesis/dissertation, final project. *Entrance*

requirements: For doctorate, GRE, minimum GPA of 3.2. Additional exam requirements/recommendations for international students: Required—TOEFL (minimum score 637 paper-based; 117 iBT), IELTS (minimum score 7). *Application deadline:* For winter admission, 2/3 priority date for domestic and international students. Applications are processed on a rolling basis. Application fee: $75 ($100 for international students). Electronic applications accepted. *Expenses:* Contact institution. *Financial support:* Applicants required to submit FAFSA. *Unit head:* Dr. Michael Majsak, Chair, 914-594-4916, Fax: 914-594-4292, E-mail: michael_majsak@nymc.edu. *Application contact:* Pamela Suett, Director of Recruitment, 914-594-4510, Fax: 914-594-4292, E-mail: shsp_admissions@nymc.edu.
Website: http://www.nymc.edu/pt

New York University, Steinhardt School of Culture, Education, and Human Development, Department of Physical Therapy, New York, NY 10010-5615. Offers orthopedic physical therapy (Advanced Certificate); physical therapy (MA, DPT, PhD), including pathokinesiology (MA). *Accreditation:* APTA (one or more programs are accredited). Part-time programs available. *Faculty:* 10 full-time (5 women), 15 part-time/adjunct (6 women). *Students:* 116 full-time (82 women), 9 part-time (6 women); includes 41 minority (8 Black or African American, non-Hispanic/Latino; 14 Asian, non-Hispanic/Latino; 15 Hispanic/Latino; 2 Native Hawaiian or other Pacific Islander, non-Hispanic/Latino; 2 Two or more races, non-Hispanic/Latino), 15 international. Average age 29. 496 applicants, 19% accepted, 48 enrolled. In 2013, 4 master's, 42 doctorates, 3 other advanced degrees awarded. *Degree requirements:* For master's, thesis (for some programs); for doctorate, thesis/dissertation. *Entrance requirements:* For master's, physical therapy certificate; for doctorate, GRE General Test, interview, physical therapy certificate. Additional exam requirements/recommendations for international students: Required—TOEFL (minimum score 100 iBT). *Application deadline:* For fall admission, 12/1 priority date for domestic and international students; for spring admission, 10/1 for domestic and international students. Applications are processed on a rolling basis. Application fee: $75. Electronic applications accepted. *Expenses: Tuition:* Full-time $35,856; part-time $1494 per unit. *Required fees:* $1408; $64 per unit. $473 per term. Tuition and fees vary according to course load and program. *Financial support:* Fellowships with full and partial tuition reimbursements, research assistantships with full and partial tuition reimbursements, career-related internships or fieldwork, Federal Work-Study, scholarships/grants, tuition waivers (partial), and unspecified assistantships available. Support available to part-time students. Financial award application deadline: 2/1; financial award applicants required to submit FAFSA. *Faculty research:* Motor learning and control, neuromuscular disorders, biomechanics and ergonomics, movement analysis, pathomechanics. *Unit head:* Prof. Mitchell Batavia, Chairperson, 212-998-9400, Fax: 212-995-4190, E-mail: mitchell.batavia@nyu.edu. *Application contact:* 212-998-5030, Fax: 212-995-4328, E-mail: steinhardt.gradadmissions@nyu.edu.
Website: http://steinhardt.nyu.edu/pt

Northeastern University, Bouvé College of Health Sciences, Boston, MA 02115-5096. Offers audiology (Au D); biotechnology (MS); counseling psychology (MS, PhD, CAGS); counseling/school psychology (PhD); exercise physiology (MS), including exercise physiology, public health; health informatics (MS); nursing (MS, PhD, CAGS), including acute care (MS), administration (MS), anesthesia (MS), primary care (MS), psychiatric mental health (MS); pharmaceutical sciences (PhD); pharmaceutics and drug delivery systems (MS); pharmacology (MS); physical therapy (DPT); physician assistant (MS); school psychology (PhD, CAGS); school/counseling psychology (PhD); speech language pathology (MS); urban public health (MPH); MS/MBA. *Accreditation:* ACPE (one or more programs are accredited). Part-time and evening/weekend programs available. *Degree requirements:* For doctorate, thesis/dissertation (for some programs); for CAGS, comprehensive exam.

Northern Arizona University, Graduate College, College of Health and Human Services, Department of Physical Therapy, Flagstaff, AZ 86011. Offers DPT. *Accreditation:* APTA. *Faculty:* 17 full-time (10 women), 6 part-time/adjunct (3 women). *Students:* 193 full-time (110 women); includes 33 minority (1 Black or African American, non-Hispanic/Latino; 2 American Indian or Alaska Native, non-Hispanic/Latino; 6 Asian, non-Hispanic/Latino; 17 Hispanic/Latino; 7 Two or more races, non-Hispanic/Latino). Average age 27. 886 applicants, 10% accepted, 78 enrolled. In 2013, 47 doctorates awarded. *Entrance requirements:* For doctorate, GRE General Test, minimum GPA of 3.0. Additional exam requirements/recommendations for international students: Required—TOEFL (minimum score 550 paper-based; 80 iBT), IELTS (minimum score 7). *Application deadline:* For fall admission, 11/1 priority date for domestic and international students. Applications are processed on a rolling basis. Application fee: $65. Electronic applications accepted. *Expenses:* Contact institution. *Financial support:* Career-related internships or fieldwork, Federal Work-Study, scholarships/grants, health care benefits, tuition waivers (full and partial), and unspecified assistantships available. Financial award applicants required to submit FAFSA. *Unit head:* Dr. Mark Cornwall, Chair, 928-523-1606, Fax: 928-523-0148, E-mail: mark.cornwall@nau.edu. *Application contact:* John Hammond, Program Coordinator, 928-523-4270, Fax: 928-523-9289, E-mail: physical.therapy@nau.edu.
Website: http://nau.edu/chhs/physical-therapy/

Northern Illinois University, Graduate School, College of Health and Human Sciences, School of Allied Health and Communicative Disorders, Program in Physical Therapy, De Kalb, IL 60115-2854. Offers MPT, DPT, TDPT. *Accreditation:* APTA; CEPH. Part-time programs available. *Students:* 109 full-time (62 women), 19 part-time (all women); includes 16 minority (3 Black or African American, non-Hispanic/Latino; 2 Asian, non-Hispanic/Latino; 8 Hispanic/Latino; 3 Two or more races, non-Hispanic/Latino). Average age 26. 193 applicants, 16% accepted, 29 enrolled. In 2013, 2 master's, 42 doctorates awarded. *Degree requirements:* For master's, comprehensive exam, thesis optional, internship, research paper in public health. *Entrance requirements:* For master's, GRE General Test, minimum GPA of 2.75. Additional exam requirements/recommendations for international students: Required—TOEFL (minimum score 550 paper-based). *Application deadline:* For fall admission, 6/1 for domestic students, 5/1 for international students; for spring admission, 11/1 for domestic students, 10/1 for international students. Applications are processed on a rolling basis. Application fee: $40. Electronic applications accepted. *Financial support:* Fellowships with full tuition reimbursements, research assistantships with full tuition reimbursements, teaching assistantships with full tuition reimbursements, career-related internships or fieldwork, Federal Work-Study, scholarships/grants, tuition waivers (full), and unspecified assistantships available. Support available to part-time students. Financial award applicants required to submit FAFSA. *Faculty research:* Stroke rehabilitation, radon exposure prevention, environmental causes of cancer, body image in young girls. *Unit head:* Dr. Mary Jo Blaschak, Chair, 815-753-1486, Fax: 815-753-6169, E-mail: ahcd@niu.edu. *Application contact:* Graduate School Office, 815-753-0395, E-mail: gradsch@niu.edu.
Website: http://www.chhs.niu.edu/physical_therapy/

Northwestern University, Fienberg School of Medicine, Department of Physical Therapy and Human Movement Sciences, Chicago, IL 60611-2814. Offers neuroscience (PhD), including movement and rehabilitation science; physical therapy (DPT); DPT/PhD. *Accreditation:* APTA. *Degree requirements:* For doctorate, synthesis research project. *Entrance requirements:* For doctorate, GRE General Test (for DPT), baccalaureate degree with minimum GPA of 3.0 in required course work (DPT). Additional exam requirements/recommendations for international students: Required—TOEFL. Electronic applications accepted. *Expenses:* Contact institution. *Faculty research:* Motor control, robotics, neuromuscular imaging, student performance (academic/professional), clinical outcomes.

Nova Southeastern University, College of Health Care Sciences, Fort Lauderdale, FL 33314-7796. Offers audiology (Au D); health science (MH Sc, DHSc, PhD); occupational therapy (MOT, OTD, PhD); physical therapy (DPT, PhD, TDPT); physician assistant (MMS). Postbaccalaureate distance learning degree programs offered (minimal on-campus study). *Faculty:* 117 full-time (68 women), 110 part-time/adjunct (57 women). *Students:* 1,187 full-time (844 women), 509 part-time (340 women); includes 560 minority (184 Black or African American, non-Hispanic/Latino; 2 American Indian or Alaska Native, non-Hispanic/Latino; 120 Asian, non-Hispanic/Latino; 218 Hispanic/Latino; 36 Two or more races, non-Hispanic/Latino), 20 international. Average age 31. 5,996 applicants, 14% accepted, 548 enrolled. In 2013, 374 master's, 132 doctorates awarded. *Degree requirements:* For master's, thesis; for doctorate, comprehensive exam, thesis/dissertation. *Entrance requirements:* For master's and doctorate, GRE General Test. *Application deadline:* Applications are processed on a rolling basis. Application fee: $50. Electronic applications accepted. *Expenses:* Contact institution. *Financial support:* In 2013–14, 10 students received support, including 2 research assistantships (averaging $3,500 per year); institutionally sponsored loans and unspecified assistantships also available. *Unit head:* Dr. Stanley Wilson, Dean, 954-262-1203, E-mail: swilson@nova.edu. *Application contact:* Joey Jankie, Admissions Counselor, 954-262-7249, E-mail: joey@nova.edu.
Website: http://www.nova.edu/chcs/

Oakland University, Graduate Study and Lifelong Learning, School of Health Sciences, Program in Physical Therapy, Rochester, MI 48309-4401. Offers neurological rehabilitation (Certificate); orthopedic manual physical therapy (Certificate); orthopedic physical therapy (Certificate); pediatric rehabilitation (Certificate); physical therapy (MSPT, DPT, Dr Sc PT); teaching and learning for rehabilitation professionals (Certificate). *Accreditation:* APTA. *Faculty:* 11 full-time (9 women), 1 part-time/adjunct (0 women). *Students:* 134 full-time (92 women), 36 part-time (22 women); includes 6 minority (1 Black or African American, non-Hispanic/Latino; 3 Asian, non-Hispanic/Latino; 2 Hispanic/Latino), 3 international. Average age 26. 448 applicants, 12% accepted, 47 enrolled. In 2013, 7 master's, 38 doctorates, 22 other advanced degrees awarded. *Degree requirements:* For master's, thesis (for some programs). *Entrance requirements:* For master's, minimum GPA of 3.0; for doctorate, GRE General Test. Additional exam requirements/recommendations for international students: Required—TOEFL (minimum score 550 paper-based). *Application deadline:* For fall admission, 10/15 for domestic and international students. Application fee: $0. *Expenses:* Contact institution. *Financial support:* Federal Work-Study, institutionally sponsored loans, and tuition waivers (full) available. Financial award application deadline: 3/1; financial award applicants required to submit FAFSA. *Unit head:* Dr. Kristine A. Thompson, Program Director, 248-370-4041, E-mail: marcoux@oakland.edu. *Application contact:* Christina J. Grabowski, Associate Director of Graduate Study and Lifelong Learning, 248-370-3167, Fax: 248-370-4114, E-mail: grabowsk@oakland.edu.

The Ohio State University, College of Medicine, School of Health and Rehabilitation Sciences, Program in Physical Therapy, Columbus, OH 43210. Offers DPT. *Accreditation:* APTA. *Faculty:* 16. *Students:* 144 full-time (98 women), 1 part-time (0 women); includes 11 minority (2 Black or African American, non-Hispanic/Latino; 3 Asian, non-Hispanic/Latino; 3 Hispanic/Latino; 3 Two or more races, non-Hispanic/Latino). Average age 24. In 2013, 39 doctorates awarded. *Degree requirements:* For doctorate, thesis/dissertation. *Entrance requirements:* For doctorate, GRE General Test. Additional exam requirements/recommendations for international students: Required—TOEFL (minimum score 550 paper-based; 79 iBT), Michigan English Language Assessment Battery (minimum score 82); Recommended—IELTS (minimum score 7). *Application deadline:* For fall admission, 11/30 for domestic and international students; for winter admission, 12/1 for domestic students, 11/1 for international students; for spring admission, 3/1 for domestic students, 2/1 for international students; for summer admission, 10/1 priority date for domestic and international students. Applications are processed on a rolling basis. Application fee: $60 ($70 for international students). Electronic applications accepted. *Financial support:* Fellowships with tuition reimbursements available. *Unit head:* John Buford, Program Director, 614-292-1520, Fax: 614-292-0210, E-mail: buford.5@osu.edu. *Application contact:* 614-292-9444, Fax: 614-292-3895, E-mail: gradadmissions@osu.edu.
Website: http://medicine.osu.edu/hrs/pt

Ohio University, Graduate College, College of Health Sciences and Professions, School of Rehabilitation and Communication Sciences, Division of Physical Therapy, Athens, OH 45701-2979. Offers DPT. Applications accepted for summer term only. *Accreditation:* APTA. *Entrance requirements:* For doctorate, GRE. Additional exam requirements/recommendations for international students: Required—TOEFL (minimum score 550 paper-based; 80 iBT) or IELTS (minimum score 6.5). Electronic applications accepted. *Faculty research:* Motor control, muscle architecture, postural control, morphonetrics, sensory integration.

Old Dominion University, College of Health Sciences, School of Physical Therapy and Athletic Training, Norfolk, VA 23529. Offers DPT. *Accreditation:* APTA. *Faculty:* 13 full-time (8 women), 5 part-time/adjunct (3 women). *Students:* 127 full-time (85 women), 1 (woman) part-time; includes 26 minority (5 Black or African American, non-Hispanic/Latino; 8 Asian, non-Hispanic/Latino; 7 Hispanic/Latino; 6 Two or more races, non-Hispanic/Latino). Average age 25. 607 applicants, 13% accepted, 45 enrolled. In 2013, 44 doctorates awarded. *Degree requirements:* For doctorate, comprehensive exam, clinical internships. *Entrance requirements:* For doctorate, GRE, 3 letters of recommendation (1 of which is from a physical therapist); 80 hours of volunteer experience. Additional exam requirements/recommendations for international students: Required—TOEFL. *Application deadline:* For fall admission, 11/1 for domestic and international students. Application fee: $50. Electronic applications accepted. *Expenses:* Contact institution. *Financial support:* In 2013–14, 4 students received support, including 1 fellowship (averaging $15,000 per year), 4 teaching assistantships with partial tuition reimbursements available (averaging $7,500 per year); career-related internships or fieldwork, scholarships/grants, and unspecified assistantships also available. Financial award applicants required to submit FAFSA. *Faculty research:* Virtual reality and rehabilitation, rehabilitation for amputees, electromyography, biomechanics, gait and balance. *Total annual research expenditures:* $103,022. *Unit head:* Dr. George Maihafer, Graduate Program Director, 757-683-4519, Fax: 757-683-4410, E-mail: ptgpd@odu.edu. *Application contact:* William Heffelfinger, Director of Graduate Admissions, 757-683-5554, Fax: 757-683-3255, E-mail: gradadmit@odu.edu.
Website: http://hs.odu.edu/physther/

Pacific University, School of Physical Therapy, Forest Grove, OR 97116-1797. Offers entry level (DPT); post-professional (DPT). *Accreditation:* APTA. *Degree requirements:* For doctorate, evidence-based capstone project thesis. *Entrance requirements:* For doctorate, 100 hours of volunteer/observational hours, minimum cumulative GPA of 3.0, prerequisite courses with a C grade or better, minimum GPA of 2.5 in science/statistics.

Additional exam requirements/recommendations for international students: Required—TOEFL (minimum score 600 paper-based). Electronic applications accepted. *Expenses:* Contact institution. *Faculty research:* Balance disorders, geriatrics, orthopedic treatment outcomes, obesity, women's health.

Queen's University at Kingston, School of Graduate Studies, Faculty of Health Sciences, School of Rehabilitation Therapy, Kingston, ON K7L 3N6, Canada. Offers occupational therapy (M Sc OT); physical therapy (M Sc PT); rehabilitation science (M Sc, PhD). Part-time programs available. *Degree requirements:* For master's, thesis; for doctorate, comprehensive exam, thesis/dissertation. *Entrance requirements:* Additional exam requirements/recommendations for international students: Required—TOEFL. *Faculty research:* Disability, community, motor performance, rehabilitation, treatment efficiency.

Quinnipiac University, School of Health Sciences, Program in Physical Therapy, Hamden, CT 06518-1940. Offers DPT. Stuents are accepted into the program as undergraduates. *Accreditation:* APTA. *Faculty:* 18 full-time (14 women), 24 part-time/adjunct (10 women). *Students:* 276 full-time (221 women); includes 25 minority (3 Black or African American, non-Hispanic/Latino; 2 American Indian or Alaska Native, non-Hispanic/Latino; 13 Asian, non-Hispanic/Latino; 6 Hispanic/Latino; 1 Two or more races, non-Hispanic/Latino). 539 applicants, 14% accepted, 63 enrolled. In 2013, 69 doctorates awarded. *Degree requirements:* For doctorate, capstone research project. *Expenses: Tuition:* Part-time $920 per credit. *Required fees:* $37 per credit. *Financial support:* In 2013–14, 208 students received support. Career-related internships or fieldwork, Federal Work-Study, scholarships/grants, and unspecified assistantships available. Support available to part-time students. Financial award application deadline: 6/1; financial award applicants required to submit FAFSA. *Application contact:* Office of Undergraduate Admissions, 800-462-1944, Fax: 203-582-8901, E-mail: admissions@quinnipiac.edu.
Website: http://www.quinnipiac.edu/academics/colleges-schools-and-departments/school-of-health-sciences/departments-and-faculty/department-of-physical-therapy/

Radford University, College of Graduate and Professional Studies, Waldron College of Health and Human Services, Department of Physical Therapy, Roanoke, VA 24013. Offers DPT. *Faculty:* 7 full-time (2 women), 3 part-time/adjunct (all women). *Students:* 58 full-time (37 women); includes 2 minority (1 Black or African American, non-Hispanic/Latino; 1 Asian, non-Hispanic/Latino). Average age 25. 224 applicants, 21% accepted, 26 enrolled. *Degree requirements:* For doctorate, comprehensive exam, capstone research project suitable for publication. *Entrance requirements:* For doctorate, GRE, completed PTCAS application with 3 letters of reference, personal essay, resume, 40 hours of clinical experience, minimum overall GPA of 3.25, 3.0 in math and science prerequisites. Additional exam requirements/recommendations for international students: Required—TOEFL (minimum score 575 paper-based; 88 iBT), IELTS (minimum score 6.5). *Application deadline:* For fall admission, 11/1 priority date for domestic students. Applications are processed on a rolling basis. Application fee: $50. Electronic applications accepted. *Expenses:* Contact institution. *Financial support:* In 2013–14, 8 students received support. Application deadline: 3/1; applicants required to submit FAFSA. *Unit head:* Dr. Edward C. Swanson, Chair, 540-224-6657, Fax: 540-224-6660, E-mail: dpt@radford.edu. *Application contact:* Rebecca Conner, Director, Graduate Enrollment, 540-831-6296, Fax: 540-831-6061, E-mail: gradcollege@radford.edu.
Website: http://www.radford.edu/content/wchs/home/pt.html

The Richard Stockton College of New Jersey, School of Graduate and Continuing Studies, Program in Physical Therapy, Galloway, NJ 08205-9441. Offers DPT. *Accreditation:* APTA. *Faculty:* 9 full-time (6 women), 5 part-time/adjunct (4 women). *Students:* 62 full-time (39 women), 52 part-time (42 women); includes 20 minority (2 Black or African American, non-Hispanic/Latino; 1 American Indian or Alaska Native, non-Hispanic/Latino; 15 Asian, non-Hispanic/Latino; 2 Hispanic/Latino), 1 international. Average age 33. 323 applicants, 24% accepted, 43 enrolled. In 2013, 39 doctorates awarded. *Entrance requirements:* Additional exam requirements/recommendations for international students: Required—TOEFL. *Application deadline:* For fall admission, 10/15 priority date for domestic students, 10/15 for international students. Applications are processed on a rolling basis. Application fee: $50. Electronic applications accepted. *Expenses: Tuition, area resident:* Part-time $559 per credit. Tuition, state resident: part-time $559 per credit. Tuition, nonresident: part-time $861 per credit. *Required fees:* $168.23 per credit. $75 per semester. Tuition and fees vary according to course load and degree level. *Financial support:* In 2013–14, 33 students received support, including 16 fellowships, 56 research assistantships with partial tuition reimbursements available; career-related internships or fieldwork, Federal Work-Study, scholarships/grants, and unspecified assistantships also available. Support available to part-time students. Financial award application deadline: 3/1; financial award applicants required to submit FAFSA. *Faculty research:* Spinal flexibility in the well elderly, use of traditional Chinese medicine concepts in physical therapy, computerized vs. traditional study in human gross anatomy. *Unit head:* Dr. Tom Nolan, Program Director, 609-626-3640, E-mail: gradschool@stockton.edu. *Application contact:* Tara Williams, Assistant Director of Graduate Enrollment Management, 609-626-3640, Fax: 609-626-6050, E-mail: gradschool@stockton.edu.

Rockhurst University, School of Graduate and Professional Studies, Program in Physical Therapy, Kansas City, MO 64110-2561. Offers DPT. *Accreditation:* APTA. *Faculty:* 9 full-time (8 women), 9 part-time/adjunct (6 women). *Students:* 137 full-time (85 women); includes 20 minority (1 Black or African American, non-Hispanic/Latino; 6 Asian, non-Hispanic/Latino; 2 Hispanic/Latino; 11 Two or more races, non-Hispanic/Latino), 2 international. Average age 25. 534 applicants, 21% accepted, 47 enrolled. In 2013, 46 doctorates awarded. *Entrance requirements:* For doctorate, 3 letters of recommendation, interview, minimum GPA of 3.0, physical therapy experience. Additional exam requirements/recommendations for international students: Required—TOEFL (minimum score 550 paper-based; 79 iBT). *Application deadline:* Applications are processed on a rolling basis. Application fee: $25. Electronic applications accepted. Application fee is waived when completed online. Tuition and fees vary according to program. *Financial support:* In 2013–14, 5 research assistantships, 10 teaching assistantships were awarded; career-related internships or fieldwork, institutionally sponsored loans, and unspecified assistantships also available. Financial award application deadline: 4/1; financial award applicants required to submit FAFSA. *Faculty research:* Clinical decision-making, geriatrics, balance in persons with neurological disorders, physical rehabilitation following total joint replacement, clinical education. *Unit head:* Dr. Jean Hiebert, Chair, 816-501-4059, Fax: 816-501-4169, E-mail: jean.hiebert@rockhurst.edu. *Application contact:* Cheryl Hooper, Director of Graduate Admission, 816-501-4097, Fax: 816-501-4241, E-mail: cheryl.hooper@rockhurst.edu.
Website: http://www.rockhurst.edu/academic/pt/index.asp

Rocky Mountain University of Health Professions, Programs in Physical Therapy, Provo, UT 84606. Offers DPT, TDPT. *Students:* 156 full-time (59 women); includes 14 minority (3 Black or African American, non-Hispanic/Latino; 2 Asian, non-Hispanic/Latino; 5 Hispanic/Latino; 1 Native Hawaiian or other Pacific Islander, non-Hispanic/Latino; 3 Two or more races, non-Hispanic/Latino). Average age 31. In 2013, 56 doctorates awarded. *Entrance requirements:* For doctorate, GRE, bachelor's degree; two courses each of general chemistry and general physics with lab (for science majors); one course each in biology, human anatomy (with lab), and physiology (with lab); three semester hours of statistics; six semester hours in the behavioral sciences (life span development preferred); minimum cumulative GPA of 3.0. *Application deadline:* For fall admission, 2/1 priority date for domestic students. Applications are processed on a rolling basis. *Unit head:* Dr. J. Wesley McWhorter, Director, 801-375-5125, E-mail: wmcwhorter@rmuohp.edu. *Application contact:* Bryce Greenberg, Director of Admissions, 801-734-6832, Fax: 801-734-6833, E-mail: bgreenberg@rmuohp.edu.
Website: http://rmuohp.edu/academics/physical-therapy/

Rosalind Franklin University of Medicine and Science, College of Health Professions, Department of Physical Therapy, North Chicago, IL 60064-3095. Offers MS, DPT, TDPT. *Accreditation:* APTA. Postbaccalaureate distance learning degree programs offered (minimal on-campus study). *Degree requirements:* For master's, thesis. *Entrance requirements:* For master's, physical therapy license. Additional exam requirements/recommendations for international students: Required—TOEFL. *Faculty research:* Clinical research, development/analysis of tests, measures, education.

Rutgers, The State University of New Jersey, Camden, Graduate School of Arts and Sciences, Program in Physical Therapy, Stratford, NJ 08084. Offers DPT. Program offered jointly with University of Medicine and Dentistry of New Jersey. *Accreditation:* APTA. *Entrance requirements:* For doctorate, GRE, physical therapy experience, 3 letters of recommendation, statement of personal, professional and academic goals, resume. Additional exam requirements/recommendations for international students: Required—TOEFL, IELTS. Electronic applications accepted. *Faculty research:* Clinical education, migrant workers, biomechanical constraints on motor control, high intensity strength training and the elderly, posture and ergonomics.

Rutgers, The State University of New Jersey, Newark, School of Health Related Professions, Department of Rehabilitation and Movement Sciences, Program in Physical Therapy–Newark, Newark, NJ 07102. Offers DPT. *Accreditation:* APTA. *Entrance requirements:* For doctorate, GRE, chemistry, physics, calculus, psychology, statistics, interview, 3 reference letters. Additional exam requirements/recommendations for international students: Required—TOEFL (minimum score 500 paper-based; 79 iBT). Electronic applications accepted.

Rutgers, The State University of New Jersey, Newark, School of Health Related Professions, Department of Rehabilitation and Movement Sciences, Program in Physical Therapy–Stratford, Newark, NJ 07102. Offers DPT. *Accreditation:* APTA. *Entrance requirements:* For doctorate, GRE, BS, 3 reference letters, interview. Additional exam requirements/recommendations for international students: Required—TOEFL (minimum score 500 paper-based; 79 iBT). Electronic applications accepted.

Sacred Heart University, Graduate Programs, College of Health Professions, Department of Physical Therapy, Fairfield, CT 06825-1000. Offers DPT. *Accreditation:* APTA. *Faculty:* 11 full-time (5 women), 29 part-time/adjunct (21 women). *Students:* 181 full-time (132 women), 4 part-time (1 woman); includes 9 minority (7 Asian, non-Hispanic/Latino; 2 Hispanic/Latino), 1 international. Average age 24. 366 applicants, 50% accepted, 73 enrolled. In 2013, 57 doctorates awarded. *Entrance requirements:* For doctorate, GRE (recommended). Additional exam requirements/recommendations for international students: Required—PTE; Recommended—TOEFL (minimum score 570 paper-based; 80 iBT), IELTS (minimum score 6.5). *Application deadline:* For fall admission, 1/15 priority date for domestic students. Applications are processed on a rolling basis. Application fee: $60. Electronic applications accepted. *Expenses:* Contact institution. *Financial support:* Career-related internships or fieldwork, institutionally sponsored loans, and unspecified assistantships available. Support available to part-time students. Financial award applicants required to submit FAFSA. *Unit head:* Dr. Michael Emery, Director, 203-365-7656, Fax: 203-365-4723, E-mail: emerym@sacredheart.edu. *Application contact:* Kathy Dilks, Executive Director of Graduate Admissions, 203-396-8259, Fax: 203-365-4732, E-mail: gradstudies@sacredheart.edu.
Website: http://www.sacredheart.edu/academics/collegeofhealthprofessions/academicprograms/physicaltherapy/

Sage Graduate School, School of Health Sciences, Program in Physical Therapy, Troy, NY 12180-4115. Offers DPT. *Accreditation:* APTA. *Faculty:* 12 full-time (11 women), 10 part-time/adjunct (9 women). *Students:* 99 full-time (76 women), 2 part-time (1 woman); includes 10 minority (2 Black or African American, non-Hispanic/Latino; 5 Asian, non-Hispanic/Latino; 1 Hispanic/Latino; 2 Two or more races, non-Hispanic/Latino), 1 international. Average age 25. 309 applicants, 95% accepted, 29 enrolled. In 2013, 46 doctorates awarded. *Entrance requirements:* For doctorate, current resume; 2 letters of recommendation; minimum GPA of 3.0 overall and in science prerequisites; completion of 40 hours of physical therapy observation. Additional exam requirements/recommendations for international students: Required—TOEFL (minimum score 550 paper-based). *Application deadline:* Applications are processed on a rolling basis. Application fee: $40. *Expenses: Tuition:* Full-time $11,880; part-time $660 per credit hour. *Financial support:* Federal Work-Study, scholarships/grants, and unspecified assistantships available. Support available to part-time students. Financial award application deadline: 3/1; financial award applicants required to submit FAFSA. *Unit head:* Dr. Esther Haskevitz, Dean, School of Health Sciences, 518-244-2296, Fax: 518-244-4571, E-mail: haskve@sage.edu. *Application contact:* Dr. Patricia Pohl, Professor and Chair, 518-244-2056, Fax: 518-244-4524, E-mail: pohlp@sage.edu.

St. Ambrose University, College of Education and Health Sciences, Department of Physical Therapy, Davenport, IA 52803-2898. Offers DPT. *Accreditation:* APTA. *Degree requirements:* For doctorate, board exams. *Entrance requirements:* For doctorate, GRE, interview. Additional exam requirements/recommendations for international students: Required—TOEFL. *Faculty research:* Human motor control, orthopedic physical therapy, cardiopulmonary physical therapy, kinesiology/biomechanics.

St. Catherine University, Graduate Programs, Program in Physical Therapy, St. Paul, MN 55105. Offers DPT. Offered on the Minneapolis campus only. *Accreditation:* APTA. *Degree requirements:* For doctorate, research project. *Entrance requirements:* For doctorate, GRE, minimum GPA of 3.0, coursework in biology/zoology, anatomy, physiology, chemistry, physics, psychology, statistics, mathematics and medical terminology. Additional exam requirements/recommendations for international students: Required—Michigan English Language Assessment Battery or TOEFL (minimum score 600 paper-based; 100 iBT). *Expenses:* Contact institution.

Saint Francis University, Department of Physical Therapy, Loretto, PA 15940-0600. Offers DPT. *Accreditation:* APTA. *Faculty:* 8 full-time (3 women), 22 part-time/adjunct (14 women). *Students:* 111 full-time (70 women); includes 5 minority (2 Black or African American, non-Hispanic/Latino; 3 Hispanic/Latino). Average age 23. 66 applicants, 23% accepted, 3 enrolled. In 2013, 36 doctorates awarded. *Entrance requirements:* Additional exam requirements/recommendations for international students: Required—TOEFL. *Application deadline:* For winter admission, 1/15 for domestic and international students. Application fee: $30. Electronic applications accepted. *Expenses: Tuition:* Full-time $18,848. Tuition and fees vary according to degree level and reciprocity agreements. *Financial support:* In 2013–14, 8 students received support, including 8 teaching assistantships with partial tuition reimbursements available; unspecified assistantships also available. *Faculty research:* Childhood asthma, athletic performance, energy expenditure, sports injuries, balance and falls, concussion management, physical therapy administration, orthopedic assignment. *Unit head:* Dr. Ivan J. Mulligan, Chair/Associate Professor, 814-472-3123, Fax: 814-472-3140, E-mail: imulligan@francis.edu. *Application contact:* Dr. Peter Raymond Skoner, Associate Provost, 814-472-3085, Fax: 814-472-3365, E-mail: pskoner@francis.edu.

Saint Louis University, Graduate Education, Doisy College of Health Sciences, Department of Physical Therapy, St. Louis, MO 63103-2097. Offers athletic training (MAT); physical therapy (DPT). *Accreditation:* APTA. Part-time programs available. *Entrance requirements:* Additional exam requirements/recommendations for international students: Required—TOEFL (minimum score 525 paper-based; 55 iBT). Electronic applications accepted. *Faculty research:* Patellofemoral pain and associated risk factors; prevalence of disordered eating in physical therapy students; effects of selected interventions for children with cerebral palsy on gait and posture: hippotherapy, ankle strengthening, supported treadmill training, spirituality in physical therapy/patient care, risk factors for exercise-related leg pain in running athletes.

Samuel Merritt University, Department of Physical Therapy, Oakland, CA 94609-3108. Offers DPT. *Accreditation:* APTA. *Entrance requirements:* Additional exam requirements/recommendations for international students: Required—TOEFL. *Expenses:* Contact institution. *Faculty research:* Human movement, motor control, falls prevention in the elderly.

San Diego State University, Graduate and Research Affairs, College of Health and Human Services, School of Exercise and Nutritional Sciences, Program in Physical Therapy, San Diego, CA 92182. Offers DPT.

San Francisco State University, Division of Graduate Studies, College of Health and Social Sciences, Program in Physical Therapy, San Francisco, CA 94132-1722. Offers DPT, Dr Sc PT. Dr Sc PT and DPT offered jointly with University of California, San Francisco. *Accreditation:* APTA. *Financial support:* Career-related internships or fieldwork and institutionally sponsored loans available. *Unit head:* Dr. Linda Wanek, Director, 415-338-2001, E-mail: gppt@sfsu.edu. *Application contact:* Jill Lienau, Academic Office Coordinator, 415-338-2001, E-mail: jlineau@sfsu.edu.
Website: http://www.pt.sfsu.edu/

Seton Hall University, School of Health and Medical Sciences, Program in Physical Therapy, South Orange, NJ 07079-2697. Offers professional physical therapy (DPT). *Accreditation:* APTA. *Degree requirements:* For doctorate, research project. *Entrance requirements:* Additional exam requirements/recommendations for international students: Required—TOEFL. Electronic applications accepted. *Faculty research:* Electrical stimulation, motor learning, backpacks, gait and balance, orthopedic injury, women's health, pediatric obesity.

Shenandoah University, School of Health Professions, Division of Physical Therapy, Winchester, VA 22601-5195. Offers DPT. *Accreditation:* APTA. Postbaccalaureate distance learning degree programs offered (minimal on-campus study). *Faculty:* 10 full-time (7 women), 2 part-time/adjunct (1 woman). *Students:* 120 full-time (92 women), 91 part-time (66 women); includes 37 minority (5 Black or African American, non-Hispanic/Latino; 1 American Indian or Alaska Native, non-Hispanic/Latino; 18 Asian, non-Hispanic/Latino; 12 Hispanic/Latino; 1 Two or more races, non-Hispanic/Latino), 6 international. Average age 31. 716 applicants, 19% accepted, 68 enrolled. In 2013, 94 doctorates awarded. *Degree requirements:* For doctorate, comprehensive exam, evidence-based practice research project. *Entrance requirements:* For doctorate, GRE General Test, minimum GPA of 2.8 in completed coursework and in all prerequisite coursework; 2 letters of recommendation, one from a licensed practicing physical therapist, one from a college professor; 40 documented hours (volunteer or paid) of exposure to PT practice. Additional exam requirements/recommendations for international students: Required—TOEFL (minimum score 550 paper-based; 79 iBT), IELTS (minimum score 6.5), Sakae Institute of Study Abroad (SISA) test (minimum score 15). *Application deadline:* For fall admission, 10/1 for domestic and international students. Application fee: $30. Electronic applications accepted. *Expenses:* Contact institution. *Financial support:* In 2013–14, 12 students received support. Career-related internships or fieldwork and scholarships/grants available. Support available to part-time students. Financial award application deadline: 3/15; financial award applicants required to submit FAFSA. *Faculty research:* Blood pressure, women's health, cross cultural, motion analysis, four-square step test. *Total annual research expenditures:* $4,500. *Unit head:* Dr. Karen Abraham-Justice, Director, 540-665-5520, Fax: 540-545-7387, E-mail: kabraham@su.edu. *Application contact:* Andrew Woodall, Executive Director of Recruitment and Admissions, 540-665-4581, Fax: 540-665-4627, E-mail: admit@su.edu.
Website: http://www.physical-therapy.su.edu

Simmons College, School of Nursing and Health Sciences, Boston, MA 02115. Offers didactic dietetics (Certificate); dietetic internship (Certificate); health professions education (CAGS); nursing (MS); nursing practice (DNP); nutrition and health promotion (MS); physical therapy (DPT); sports nutrition (Certificate). Part-time programs available. Postbaccalaureate distance learning degree programs offered (minimal on-campus study). *Students:* 143 full-time (129 women), 347 part-time (329 women); includes 72 minority (31 Black or African American, non-Hispanic/Latino; 17 Asian, non-Hispanic/Latino; 15 Hispanic/Latino; 9 Two or more races, non-Hispanic/Latino), 4 international. 196 applicants, 56% accepted, 88 enrolled. In 2013, 70 master's, 45 doctorates awarded. *Entrance requirements:* For doctorate, GRE. Additional exam requirements/recommendations for international students: Required—TOEFL (minimum score 570 paper-based; 88 iBT). *Application deadline:* For fall admission, 6/1 for international students. Application fee: $50. Electronic applications accepted. *Financial support:* In 2013–14, 33 students received support, including 24 teaching assistantships (averaging $6,000 per year); scholarships/grants and unspecified assistantships also available. *Unit head:* Dr. Judy Beal, Dean, 617-521-2139. *Application contact:* Carmen Fortin, Assistant Dean/Director of Admission, 617-521-2651, Fax: 617-521-3137, E-mail: gshsadm@simmons.edu.
Website: http://www.simmons.edu/snhs/

Slippery Rock University of Pennsylvania, Graduate Studies (Recruitment), College of Health, Environment, and Science, School of Physical Therapy, Slippery Rock, PA 16057-1383. Offers DPT. *Accreditation:* APTA. *Faculty:* 9 full-time (7 women), 1 (woman) part-time/adjunct. *Students:* 135 full-time (87 women); includes 3 minority (1 Hispanic/Latino; 1 Native Hawaiian or other Pacific Islander, non-Hispanic/Latino; 1 Two or more races, non-Hispanic/Latino), 1 international. Average age 23. 315 applicants, 23% accepted, 35 enrolled. In 2013, 51 doctorates awarded. *Degree requirements:* For doctorate, clinical residency. *Entrance requirements:* For doctorate, GRE General Test, minimum GPA of 3.0, three letters of recommendation, essay, 100 hours of PT experience with a licensed physical therapist, CPR certification. Additional exam requirements/recommendations for international students: Required—TOEFL (minimum score 550 paper-based; 80 iBT). *Application deadline:* For fall admission, 11/1 priority date for domestic and international students. Application fee: $35. Electronic applications accepted. *Expenses:* Contact institution. *Financial support:* Career-related internships or fieldwork, Federal Work-Study, institutionally sponsored loans, scholarships/grants, tuition waivers (partial), and unspecified assistantships available. Financial award application deadline: 5/1; financial award applicants required to submit FAFSA. *Unit head:* Dr. Carol Martin-Elkins, Graduate Coordinator, 724-738-2080, Fax: 724-738-2113, E-mail: carol.martin-elkins@sru.edu. *Application contact:* Brandi Weber-Mortimer, Director of Graduate Admissions, 724-738-2051, Fax: 724-738-2146, E-mail: graduate.admissions@sru.edu.

Sonoma State University, School of Science and Technology, Department of Kinesiology, Rohnert Park, CA 94928. Offers adapted physical education (MA); interdisciplinary (MA); interdisciplinary pre-occupational therapy (MA); lifetime physical activity (MA), including coach education, fitness and wellness; physical education (MA); pre-physical therapy (MA). Part-time programs available. *Faculty:* 5 full-time (3 women). *Students:* 1 full-time (0 women), 11 part-time (3 women); includes 2 minority (1 Hispanic/Latino; 1 Two or more races, non-Hispanic/Latino). Average age 29. *Degree requirements:* For master's, thesis, oral exam. *Entrance requirements:* For master's, minimum GPA of 2.8. Additional exam requirements/recommendations for international students: Required—TOEFL (minimum score 500 paper-based). *Application deadline:* For fall admission, 11/30 for domestic students; for spring admission, 9/1 for domestic students. Applications are processed on a rolling basis. Application fee: $55. *Expenses:* Tuition, state resident: full-time $8500. Tuition, nonresident: full-time $12,964. *Required fees:* $1762. *Financial support:* Career-related internships or fieldwork available. Financial award application deadline: 3/2; financial award applicants required to submit FAFSA. *Unit head:* Dr. Elaine McHugh, Chair, 707-664-2660, E-mail: elaine.mchugh@sonoma.edu. *Application contact:* Dr. Lauren Morimoto, Graduate Coordinator, 707-664-2479, E-mail: morimoto@sonoma.edu.
Website: http://www.sonoma.edu/kinesiology/

Southwest Baptist University, Program in Physical Therapy, Bolivar, MO 65613-2597. Offers DPT. *Accreditation:* APTA. *Degree requirements:* For doctorate, comprehensive exam, 3-4 clinical education experiences. *Entrance requirements:* Additional exam requirements/recommendations for international students: Required—TOEFL (minimum score 550 paper-based). *Expenses:* Contact institution. *Faculty research:* Balance and falls prevention, distance and web based learning, foot and ankle intervention, pediatrics, musculoskeletal management.

Springfield College, Graduate Programs, Program in Physical Therapy, Springfield, MA 01109-3797. Offers DPT. *Accreditation:* APTA. Part-time programs available. *Faculty:* 9 full-time, 4 part-time/adjunct. *Students:* 68 full-time. Average age 30. 56 applicants, 45% accepted, 11 enrolled. In 2013, 32 doctorates awarded. *Degree requirements:* For doctorate, comprehensive exam, thesis/dissertation, research project. *Entrance requirements:* For doctorate, GRE General Test. Additional exam requirements/recommendations for international students: Required—TOEFL (minimum score 550 paper-based); Recommended—IELTS (minimum score 6). *Application deadline:* For fall admission, 12/1 for domestic and international students. Applications are processed on a rolling basis. Application fee: $50. Electronic applications accepted. *Expenses: Tuition:* Full-time $13,620; part-time $908 per credit. *Financial support:* Fellowships with partial tuition reimbursements, teaching assistantships with partial tuition reimbursements, career-related internships or fieldwork, Federal Work-Study, institutionally sponsored loans, and unspecified assistantships available. Financial award application deadline: 3/1; financial award applicants required to submit FAFSA. *Unit head:* Dr. Kathy Pappas, Director, 413-748-3028, Fax: 413-748-3371, E-mail: kpappas@springfieldcollege.edu. *Application contact:* Evelyn Cohen, Associate Director of Graduate Admissions, 413-748-3479, Fax: 413-748-3694, E-mail: ecohen@springfieldcollege.edu.
Website: http://www.springfieldcollege.edu/academic-programs/physical-therapy-program-at-springfield-college/index

State University of New York Upstate Medical University, Department of Physical Therapy, Syracuse, NY 13210-2334. Offers DPT. *Accreditation:* APTA. Part-time and evening/weekend programs available. Postbaccalaureate distance learning degree programs offered (minimal on-campus study). Electronic applications accepted.

Stony Brook University, State University of New York, Stony Brook University Medical Center, Health Sciences Center, School of Health Technology and Management, Stony Brook, NY 11794. Offers health care management (Advanced Certificate); health care policy and management (MS); occupational therapy (MS); physical therapy (DPT); physician assistant (MS). *Accreditation:* APTA. Part-time programs available. *Faculty:* 70 full-time (46 women), 51 part-time/adjunct (34 women). *Students:* 349 full-time (225 women), 159 part-time (120 women); includes 140 minority (25 Black or African American, non-Hispanic/Latino; 1 American Indian or Alaska Native, non-Hispanic/Latino; 72 Asian, non-Hispanic/Latino; 34 Hispanic/Latino; 8 Two or more races, non-Hispanic/Latino), 7 international. 2,215 applicants, 11% accepted, 221 enrolled. In 2013, 120 master's, 77 doctorates, 23 other advanced degrees awarded. *Degree requirements:* For master's, thesis. *Entrance requirements:* For master's, GRE General Test, minimum GPA of 3.0, work experience in field, references; for doctorate, GRE, references. Additional exam requirements/recommendations for international students: Required—TOEFL (minimum score 550 paper-based). *Application deadline:* For fall admission, 1/15 for domestic students; for spring admission, 10/1 for domestic students. Application fee: $100. *Expenses:* Tuition, state resident: full-time $9870; part-time $411 per credit. Tuition, nonresident: full-time $18,350; part-time $765 per credit. *Financial support:* In 2013–14, 1 fellowship was awarded; research assistantships, teaching assistantships, career-related internships or fieldwork, Federal Work-Study, and institutionally sponsored loans also available. Financial award application deadline: 3/15. *Faculty research:* Health promotion and disease prevention. *Total annual research expenditures:* $1.1 million. *Unit head:* Dr. Craig A. Lehmann, Dean, 631-444-2252, Fax: 631-444-7621, E-mail: craig.lehmann@stonybrook.edu. *Application contact:* Dr. Richard W. Johnson, Associate Dean for Graduate Studies, 631-444-3251, Fax: 631-444-7621, E-mail: richard.johnson@stonybrook.edu.
Website: http://healthtechnology.stonybrookmedicine.edu/

Temple University, College of Health Professions and Social Work, Department of Physical Therapy, Philadelphia, PA 19140. Offers DPT, PhD. *Accreditation:* APTA (one or more programs are accredited). Part-time programs available. Postbaccalaureate distance learning degree programs offered. *Faculty:* 14 full-time (8 women). *Students:* 152 full-time (108 women), 86 part-time (61 women); includes 34 minority (5 Black or African American, non-Hispanic/Latino; 1 American Indian or Alaska Native, non-Hispanic/Latino; 14 Asian, non-Hispanic/Latino; 10 Hispanic/Latino; 2 Native Hawaiian or other Pacific Islander, non-Hispanic/Latino; 2 Two or more races, non-Hispanic/Latino), 2 international. 67 applicants, 61% accepted, 37 enrolled. In 2013, 105 doctorates awarded. *Degree requirements:* For doctorate, comprehensive exam, thesis/dissertation. *Entrance requirements:* For doctorate, GRE General Test, essay, interview, clinical experience. Additional exam requirements/recommendations for international students: Required—TOEFL (minimum score 550 paper-based; 79 iBT). *Application deadline:* For fall admission, 3/1 for domestic students, 2/1 for international students; for spring admission, 11/1 for domestic students, 10/1 for international students; for summer admission, 3/1 for domestic students, 2/1 for international students. Applications are processed on a rolling basis. Application fee: $60. Electronic applications accepted. *Expenses:* Contact institution. *Financial support:* In 2013–14, 2 teaching assistantships with full and partial tuition reimbursements (averaging $23,627 per year) were awarded; career-related internships or fieldwork, Federal Work-Study, scholarships/grants, and unspecified assistantships also available. Financial award application deadline: 1/1; financial award applicants required to submit FAFSA. *Faculty research:* Balance

dysfunction, biomechanics, development, qualitative research, developmental neuroscience, health services. *Total annual research expenditures:* $231,410. *Unit head:* Dr. Emily A. Keshner, Chair, 215-707-4815, Fax: 215-707-7500, E-mail: deptpt@temple.edu. *Application contact:* Sarah Carroll, 215-204-4828, E-mail: sarah.carroll@temple.edu.
Website: http://chpsw.temple.edu/pt/home

Tennessee State University, The School of Graduate Studies and Research, College of Health Sciences, Department of Physical Therapy, Nashville, TN 37209-1561. Offers DPT. *Accreditation:* APTA. Part-time programs available. Postbaccalaureate distance learning degree programs offered (minimal on-campus study). *Entrance requirements:* For doctorate, GRE, baccalaureate degree, 2 letters of recommendation, interview, essay. Electronic applications accepted. *Faculty research:* Evidence-based research clinical research case studies/reports qualitative research education assessment total knee anthroplasty; ergonomics; childhood obesity.

Texas State University, Graduate School, College of Health Professions, Doctor of Physical Therapy Program, San Marcos, TX 78666. Offers DPT. *Accreditation:* APTA. *Faculty:* 12 full-time (10 women), 3 part-time/adjunct (0 women). *Students:* 117 full-time (61 women); includes 39 minority (2 Black or African American, non-Hispanic/Latino; 5 Asian, non-Hispanic/Latino; 27 Hispanic/Latino; 5 Two or more races, non-Hispanic/Latino), 1 international. Average age 27. 417 applicants, 17% accepted, 41 enrolled. *Degree requirements:* For doctorate, comprehensive exam. *Entrance requirements:* For doctorate, GRE General Test (minimum combined score of 1000 Verbal and Quantitative), bachelor's degree in physical therapy; minimum GPA of 3.0 on last 60 hours of undergraduate and science courses. Additional exam requirements/recommendations for international students: Required—TOEFL (minimum score 550 paper-based; 78 iBT). *Application deadline:* For summer admission, 10/15 for domestic and international students. Applications are processed on a rolling basis. Application fee: $65 ($115 for international students). Electronic applications accepted. *Expenses:* Tuition, state resident: full-time $6663; part-time $278 per credit hour. Tuition, nonresident: full-time $15,159; part-time $632 per credit hour. *Required fees:* $1872; $54 per credit hour. $306 per term. Tuition and fees vary according to course load. *Financial support:* In 2013–14, 91 students received support, including 10 teaching assistantships (averaging $7,730 per year); research assistantships, career-related internships or fieldwork, Federal Work-Study, institutionally sponsored loans, scholarships/grants, and unspecified assistantships also available. Support available to part-time students. Financial award application deadline: 4/1; financial award applicants required to submit FAFSA. *Faculty research:* Effect of a cultural competence education module on student physical therapists. *Total annual research expenditures:* $2,199. *Unit head:* Dr. Barbara Sanders, Chair/Graduate Advisor, 512-245-8351, Fax: 512-245-8736, E-mail: bs04@txstate.edu. *Application contact:* Dr. Andrea Golato, Dean of Graduate School, 512-245-2581, Fax: 512-245-8365, E-mail: gradcollege@txstate.edu.
Website: http://www.health.txstate.edu/pt/

Texas Tech University Health Sciences Center, School of Allied Health Sciences, Program in Physical Therapy, Lubbock, TX 79430. Offers DPT, Sc D, TDPT. *Accreditation:* APTA. *Faculty:* 19 full-time (5 women). *Students:* 197 full-time (109 women), 102 part-time (45 women); includes 95 minority (5 Black or African American, non-Hispanic/Latino; 6 American Indian or Alaska Native, non-Hispanic/Latino; 29 Asian, non-Hispanic/Latino; 41 Hispanic/Latino; 1 Native Hawaiian or other Pacific Islander, non-Hispanic/Latino; 13 Two or more races, non-Hispanic/Latino), 3 international. Average age 30. 550 applicants, 20% accepted, 111 enrolled. In 2013, 95 doctorates awarded. *Entrance requirements:* For doctorate, GRE. Additional exam requirements/recommendations for international students: Required—TOEFL, IELTS. *Application deadline:* For fall admission, 10/1 priority date for domestic students; for winter admission, 1/15 for domestic students; for spring admission, 1/15 for domestic students. Applications are processed on a rolling basis. Application fee: $40. Electronic applications accepted. *Financial support:* Institutionally sponsored loans and scholarships/grants available. Financial award application deadline: 10/1; financial award applicants required to submit FAFSA. *Unit head:* Dr. Kerry Gilbert, Program Director, 806-743-2958, Fax: 806-743-6005, E-mail: kerry.gilbert@ttuhsc.edu. *Application contact:* Lindsay Johnson, Associate Dean for Admissions and Student Affairs, 806-743-3220, Fax: 806-743-2994, E-mail: lindsay.johnson@ttuhsc.edu.

Texas Woman's University, Graduate School, College of Health Sciences, School of Physical Therapy, Denton, TX 76201. Offers DPT, PhD. *Accreditation:* APTA (one or more programs are accredited). Part-time programs available. *Faculty:* 22 full-time (17 women), 5 part-time/adjunct (4 women). *Students:* 307 full-time (226 women), 72 part-time (57 women); includes 98 minority (14 Black or African American, non-Hispanic/Latino; 4 American Indian or Alaska Native, non-Hispanic/Latino; 38 Asian, non-Hispanic/Latino; 41 Hispanic/Latino; 1 Native Hawaiian or other Pacific Islander, non-Hispanic/Latino), 6 international. Average age 28. 454 applicants, 35% accepted, 109 enrolled. In 2013, 105 doctorates awarded. *Degree requirements:* For doctorate, comprehensive exam, thesis/dissertation. *Entrance requirements:* For doctorate, interview, resume, essay; eligibility for licensure and 2 letters of recommendation (PhD); 3 letters of recommendation on department form (DPT). Additional exam requirements/recommendations for international students: Required—TOEFL (minimum score 550 paper-based; 79 iBT). *Application deadline:* For fall admission, 11/1 priority date for domestic students, 11/1 for international students. Applications are processed on a rolling basis. Application fee: $50 ($75 for international students). Electronic applications accepted. *Expenses:* Tuition, state resident: full-time $4182; part-time $233.32 per credit hour. Tuition, nonresident: full-time $10,716; part-time $595.32 per credit hour. *Financial support:* In 2013–14, 228 students received support, including 4 research assistantships (averaging $10,215 per year); career-related internships or fieldwork, Federal Work-Study, institutionally sponsored loans, scholarships/grants, traineeships, health care benefits, and unspecified assistantships also available. Support available to part-time students. Financial award application deadline: 3/1; financial award applicants required to submit FAFSA. *Faculty research:* Gait training in stroke survivors, physical activity to promote health in youth and adults, exercise training for individuals with amputation, treatment of balance and gait deficits in persons with multiple sclerosis. *Total annual research expenditures:* $187,166. *Unit head:* Dr. Sharon Olson, Director, 713-794-2070, Fax: 713-794-2071, E-mail: pt@twu.edu. *Application contact:* Dr. Samuel Wheeler, Assistant Director of Admissions, 940-898-3188, Fax: 940-898-3081, E-mail: wheelersr@twu.edu.
Website: http://www.twu.edu/physical-therapy/

Thomas Jefferson University, Jefferson School of Health Professions, Program in Physical Therapy, Philadelphia, PA 19107. Offers DPT. *Accreditation:* APTA. *Faculty:* 7 full-time (3 women), 1 (woman) part-time/adjunct. *Students:* 159 full-time (114 women); includes 11 minority (6 Black or African American, non-Hispanic/Latino; 3 Asian, non-Hispanic/Latino; 2 Hispanic/Latino), 1 international. Average age 25. 1,310 applicants, 7% accepted, 60 enrolled. In 2013, 46 doctorates awarded. *Entrance requirements:* Additional exam requirements/recommendations for international students: Required—TOEFL. *Application deadline:* For fall admission, 3/1 priority date for domestic and international students. Applications are processed on a rolling basis. Application fee: $140. Electronic applications accepted. *Expenses:* Contact institution. *Financial support:* In 2013–14, 104 students received support. Federal Work-Study, institutionally sponsored loans, scholarships/grants, and unspecified assistantships available. Support available to part-time students. Financial award application deadline: 4/1; financial award applicants required to submit FAFSA. *Faculty research:* Gait and motion analysis, motor control and learning, single motor unit discharge in human muscle, musculoskeletal injuries, cancer rehabilitation. *Unit head:* Dr. Susan Wainwright, Chair, Department of Physical Therapy, 215-503-8961, Fax: 215-503-3499, E-mail: susan.wainwright@jefferson.edu. *Application contact:* Donald Sharples, Director of Graduate Admissions, 215-503-1044, Fax: 215-503-7241, E-mail: jshpadmissions@jefferson.edu.
Website: http://www.jefferson.edu/health_professions/departments/physical_therapy

Touro College, School of Health Sciences, Bay Shore, NY 11706. Offers occupational therapy (MS); physical therapy (DPT); physicians assistant (MS); speech-language pathology (MS). *Faculty:* 20 full-time, 94 part-time/adjunct. *Students:* 975 full-time (710 women), 160 part-time (114 women); includes 271 minority (58 Black or African American, non-Hispanic/Latino; 1 American Indian or Alaska Native, non-Hispanic/Latino; 132 Asian, non-Hispanic/Latino; 60 Hispanic/Latino; 4 Native Hawaiian or other Pacific Islander, non-Hispanic/Latino; 16 Two or more races, non-Hispanic/Latino), 10 international. *Expenses:* Contact institution. *Financial support:* Fellowships available. *Unit head:* Dr. Louis Primavera, Dean, School of Health Sciences, 516-673-3200, E-mail: louis.primavera@touro.edu. *Application contact:* Brian J. Diele, Associate Director of Central Admissions, 631-665-1600 Ext. 6311, E-mail: brian.diele@touro.edu.

University at Buffalo, the State University of New York, Graduate School, School of Public Health and Health Professions, Department of Rehabilitation Science, Program in Physical Therapy, Buffalo, NY 14214. Offers DPT. *Accreditation:* APTA. *Faculty:* 9 full-time (5 women), 3 part-time/adjunct (1 woman). *Students:* 127 full-time (66 women); includes 14 minority (11 Asian, non-Hispanic/Latino; 3 Hispanic/Latino). Average age 22. 82 applicants, 57% accepted, 42 enrolled. In 2013, 43 doctorates awarded. *Entrance requirements:* For doctorate, GRE. Additional exam requirements/recommendations for international students: Required—TOEFL (minimum score 79 iBT). *Application deadline:* For fall admission, 11/1 for domestic and international students. Application fee: $50. Electronic applications accepted. *Financial support:* Career-related internships or fieldwork and Federal Work-Study available. Financial award application deadline: 2/1; financial award applicants required to submit FAFSA. *Faculty research:* Functional limitations and rehabilitation for individuals with osteoporosis, multiple sclerosis, juvenile arthritis and aging; neuroscience concepts as they relate to rehabilitation in stroke and cerebral palsy; neural mechanisms associated with development, aging and neuromuscular disorders; sleep apnea and episodic hypoxia as it relates to muscles in the upper airway and cardiovascular system, neurobiological changes in ventilator control. *Total annual research expenditures:* $391,708. *Unit head:* Dr. Kirkwood Personious, Program Director, 716-829-6742, Fax: 716-829-3217, E-mail: phhpadv@buffalo.edu. *Application contact:* MaryAnn Venezia, Program Coordinator, 716-829-6742, Fax: 716-829-3217, E-mail: venezia3@buffalo.edu.
Website: http://sphhp.buffalo.edu/rs/dpt/

The University of Alabama at Birmingham, School of Health Professions, Program in Physical Therapy, Birmingham, AL 35294. Offers DPT. *Accreditation:* APTA. *Entrance requirements:* For doctorate, GRE, interview, letters of recommendation, minimum GPA of 3.0 overall, in prerequisite courses, and last 60 hours. *Faculty research:* Geriatrics, exercise physiology, aquatic therapy, industrial rehabilitation, outcome measurement.

University of Alberta, Faculty of Graduate Studies and Research, Department of Physical Therapy, Edmonton, AB T6G 2E1, Canada. Offers M Sc, PhD. Part-time programs available. *Degree requirements:* For master's, thesis. *Entrance requirements:* For master's, bachelor's degree in physical therapy, minimum GPA of 6.5 on a 9.0 scale. Additional exam requirements/recommendations for international students: Required—TOEFL. Electronic applications accepted. *Faculty research:* Spinal disorders, musculoskeletal disorders, ergonomics, sports therapy, motor development, cardiac rehabilitation/therapeutic exercise.

University of California, San Francisco, Graduate Division, Program in Physical Therapy, San Francisco, CA 94143. Offers DPT, DPTSc. Programs offered jointly with San Francisco State University. *Accreditation:* APTA. *Entrance requirements:* For doctorate, GRE General Test, letters of recommendation. *Application deadline:* For fall admission, 10/1 for domestic students. Application fee: $40. *Expenses:* Tuition, state resident: full-time $11,220. Tuition, nonresident: full-time $26,322. *Required fees:* $5204. Full-time tuition and fees vary according to degree level and program. *Financial support:* Institutionally sponsored loans available. Financial award application deadline: 1/10. *Unit head:* Dr. Kimberly Topp, Chair, 415-476-9449, E-mail: toppk@ptrehab.ucsf.edu. *Application contact:* Dr. Kimberly Topp, Chair, 415-476-9449, E-mail: toppk@ptrehab.ucsf.edu.

University of Central Arkansas, Graduate School, College of Health and Behavioral Sciences, Department of Physical Therapy, Conway, AR 72035-0001. Offers DPT, PhD. *Accreditation:* APTA. *Degree requirements:* For doctorate, comprehensive exam, thesis/dissertation. *Entrance requirements:* Additional exam requirements/recommendations for international students: Required—TOEFL (minimum score 550 paper-based; 80 iBT). Electronic applications accepted. *Expenses:* Contact institution.

University of Central Florida, College of Health and Public Affairs, Department of Health Professions, Program in Physical Therapy, Orlando, FL 32816. Offers DPT. *Accreditation:* APTA. *Faculty:* 18 full-time (10 women), 14 part-time/adjunct (9 women). *Students:* 116 full-time (75 women); includes 21 minority (4 Black or African American, non-Hispanic/Latino; 1 American Indian or Alaska Native, non-Hispanic/Latino; 2 Asian, non-Hispanic/Latino; 13 Hispanic/Latino; 1 Two or more races, non-Hispanic/Latino), 2 international. Average age 26. 282 applicants, 22% accepted, 36 enrolled. In 2013, 2 doctorates awarded. Application fee: $30. Electronic applications accepted. *Expenses:* Contact institution. *Financial support:* In 2013–14, 2 students received support, including 1 fellowship (averaging $2,000 per year), 1 teaching assistantship (averaging $7,700 per year); career-related internships or fieldwork, institutionally sponsored loans, scholarships/grants, tuition waivers (partial), and unspecified assistantships also available. *Unit head:* Dr. Patrick Pabian, Interim Director, 407-823-3457, E-mail: patrick.pabian@ucf.edu. *Application contact:* Barbara Rodriguez Lamas, Director, Admissions and Student Services, 407-823-2766, Fax: 407-823-6442, E-mail: gradadmissions@ucf.edu.

University of Colorado Denver, School of Medicine, Program in Physical Therapy, Aurora, CO 80045. Offers DPT. *Accreditation:* APTA. Part-time programs available. *Students:* 181 full-time (142 women); includes 13 minority (1 American Indian or Alaska Native, non-Hispanic/Latino; 3 Asian, non-Hispanic/Latino; 9 Hispanic/Latino). Average age 27. 550 applicants, 13% accepted, 61 enrolled. In 2013, 75 doctorates awarded. *Degree requirements:* For doctorate, thesis/dissertation or alternative, 116 credit hours, 44 weeks of clinical experiences, capstone project at end of year 3. *Entrance requirements:* For doctorate, GRE, minimum GPA of 3.0; prerequisite coursework in anatomy, physiology, chemistry, physics, psychology, English composition or writing, college-level math, statistics, and upper-level science, 45 hours of observation. Additional exam requirements/recommendations for international students: Required—TOEFL (minimum score 550 paper-based). *Application deadline:* For fall admission, 10/1 for domestic students, 8/8 priority date for international students. Application fee:

$120. Electronic applications accepted. *Expenses:* Contact institution. *Financial support:* In 2013–14, 128 students received support. Fellowships, research assistantships, teaching assistantships, Federal Work-Study, institutionally sponsored loans, scholarships/grants, traineeships, and unspecified assistantships available. Financial award application deadline: 3/15; financial award applicants required to submit FAFSA. *Faculty research:* Interventions for early and mid-stages of Parkinson's disease, physical therapy for individuals with recurrent lower back pain. *Unit head:* Margaret Schenkman, Program Director, 303-724-9375, E-mail: margaret.schenkman@ucdenver.edu. *Application contact:* Betti Krapfl, Admissions Advisor, 303-724-9135, E-mail: betti.krapfl@ucdenver.edu.
Website: http://www.ucdenver.edu/academics/colleges/medicalschool/education/degree_programs/pt/Pages/PT.aspx

University of Connecticut, Graduate School, Neag School of Education, Department of Physical Therapy, Storrs, CT 06269. Offers DPT. *Accreditation:* APTA. *Entrance requirements:* Additional exam requirements/recommendations for international students: Required—TOEFL (minimum score 550 paper-based). Electronic applications accepted.

University of Dayton, Department of Health and Sport Science, Dayton, OH 45469-1300. Offers exercise science (MS Ed); physical therapy (DPT). Part-time programs available. *Faculty:* 17 full-time (8 women). *Students:* 119 full-time (76 women), 6 part-time (5 women); includes 4 minority (2 Black or African American, non-Hispanic/Latino; 2 Asian, non-Hispanic/Latino), 7 international. Average age 25. 150 applicants, 45% accepted, 38 enrolled. In 2013, 3 master's, 33 doctorates awarded. *Degree requirements:* For master's, thesis; for doctorate, thesis/dissertation or alternative, research project. *Entrance requirements:* For master's, GRE General Test, MAT, minimum GPA of 2.75; for doctorate, GRE General Test, bachelor's degree from accredited college or university; minimum GPA of 3.0, across all schools attended; 80 observation hours; science prerequisites of human anatomy/physiology, general biology, general chemistry, general physics, and exercise physiology. Additional exam requirements/recommendations for international students: Required—TOEFL (minimum score 550 paper-based; 80 iBT). *Application deadline:* For fall admission, 2/15 priority date for domestic students, 5/1 priority date for international students; for winter admission, 7/1 for international students; for spring admission, 11/1 priority date for international students. Applications are processed on a rolling basis. Application fee: $0 ($50 for international students). Electronic applications accepted. *Expenses: Tuition:* Full-time $10,296; part-time $858 per credit hour. *Required fees:* $50; $25. *Financial support:* In 2013–14, 1 research assistantship with full tuition reimbursement (averaging $8,720 per year), 10 teaching assistantships with full tuition reimbursements (averaging $8,720 per year) were awarded; career-related internships or fieldwork, institutionally sponsored loans, health care benefits, and unspecified assistantships also available. Financial award application deadline: 3/1; financial award applicants required to submit FAFSA. *Faculty research:* Energy expenditure, strength, training, teaching nutrition and calcium intake for children and families in Head Start; motion analysis of human gait, pediatric physical therapy, arm function of breast cancer survivors, predicting injury in athletes, neurological rehab in persons with multiple sclerosis. *Unit head:* Dr. Lloyd Laubach, Chair, 937-229-4240, Fax: 937-229-4244, E-mail: llaubach1@udayton.edu. *Application contact:* Laura Greger, Administrative Assistant, 937-229-4225, E-mail: lgreger1@udayton.edu.

University of Delaware, College of Health Sciences, Department of Physical Therapy, Newark, DE 19716. Offers DPT. *Accreditation:* APTA. *Entrance requirements:* For doctorate, GRE, 100 hours clinical experience, 3 letters of recommendation. Additional exam requirements/recommendations for international students: Required—TOEFL (minimum score 550 paper-based). Electronic applications accepted. *Faculty research:* Movement sciences, applied physiology, physical rehabilitation.

University of Evansville, College of Education and Health Sciences, Department of Physical Therapy, Evansville, IN 47722. Offers DPT. *Accreditation:* APTA. *Degree requirements:* For doctorate, 30 weeks of full-time clinical internships (20 credit hours). *Entrance requirements:* For doctorate, bachelor's degree, science and math prerequisite courses, minimum GPA of 2.75, interview, recommendations. Additional exam requirements/recommendations for international students: Required—TOEFL (minimum score 88 iBT), IELTS (minimum score 6.5). *Expenses:* Contact institution.

The University of Findlay, Office of Graduate Admissions, Findlay, OH 45840-3653. Offers athletic training (MAT); business (MBA), including health care management, hospitality management, organizational leadership, public management; education (MA Ed), including administration, children's literature, early childhood, human resource development, reading, science, special education, technology; environmental, safety and health management (MSEM); health informatics (MS); occupational therapy (MOT); pharmacy (Pharm D); physical therapy (DPT); physician assistant (MPA); rhetoric and writing (MA); teaching English to speakers of other languages (TESOL) and bilingual education (MA). Part-time and evening/weekend programs available. Postbaccalaureate distance learning degree programs offered (no on-campus study). *Faculty:* 209 full-time (98 women), 69 part-time/adjunct (38 women). *Students:* 551 full-time (332 women), 457 part-time (276 women); includes 77 minority (37 Black or African American, non-Hispanic/Latino; 1 American Indian or Alaska Native, non-Hispanic/Latino; 15 Asian, non-Hispanic/Latino; 23 Hispanic/Latino; 1 Native Hawaiian or other Pacific Islander, non-Hispanic/Latino), 135 international. Average age 28. 637 applicants, 66% accepted, 241 enrolled. In 2013, 267 master's, 91 doctorates awarded. *Degree requirements:* For master's, thesis, cumulative project, capstone project. *Entrance requirements:* For master's, GRE/GMAT, bachelor's degree from accredited institution, minimum undergraduate GPA of 2.5 in last 64 hours of course work; for doctorate, GRE, minimum cumulative GPA of 3.0. Additional exam requirements/recommendations for international students: Required—TOEFL (minimum score 80 iBT). *Application deadline:* Applications are processed on a rolling basis. Application fee: $25. Electronic applications accepted. *Expenses: Required fees:* $146 per semester. Tuition and fees vary according to degree level and program. *Financial support:* In 2013–14, 11 research assistantships with full and partial tuition reimbursements (averaging $4,000 per year), 10 teaching assistantships with full and partial tuition reimbursements (averaging $3,600 per year) were awarded; career-related internships or fieldwork, Federal Work-Study, health care benefits, and unspecified assistantships also available. Financial award application deadline: 4/1; financial award applicants required to submit FAFSA. *Unit head:* Christopher M. Harris, Director of Admissions, 419-434-4347, E-mail: harrisc1@findlay.edu. *Application contact:* Emily Ickes, Graduate Admissions Counselor, 419-434-6933, Fax: 419-434-4898, E-mail: ickese@findlay.edu.
Website: http://www.findlay.edu/admissions/graduate/Pages/default.aspx

University of Florida, Graduate School, College of Public Health and Health Professions, Department of Physical Therapy, Gainesville, FL 32611. Offers DPT, DPT/MPH. *Accreditation:* APTA (one or more programs are accredited). *Entrance requirements:* For doctorate, GRE General Test, minimum GPA of 3.0. Additional exam requirements/recommendations for international students: Required—TOEFL (minimum score 515 paper-based; 80 iBT), IELTS (minimum score 6). *Application deadline:* For fall admission, 11/1 for domestic students; for spring admission, 11/1 for domestic students. Applications are processed on a rolling basis. Application fee: $30. Electronic applications accepted. *Expenses:* Tuition, state resident: full-time $12,640. Tuition, nonresident: full-time $30,000. *Financial support:* Career-related internships or fieldwork available. Financial award applicants required to submit FAFSA. *Faculty research:* Exercise physiology, motor control, rehabilitation, geriatrics. *Unit head:* Krista Vandenborne, PhD, Department Chair and Associate Dean for Research and Planning, 352-273-6085, Fax: 352-273-6109, E-mail: kvandenb@phhp.ufl.edu. *Application contact:* Steven Z. George, PhD, Associate Professor/Assistant Department Chair, 352-273-6432, Fax: 352-273-6109, E-mail: szgeorge@phhp.ufl.edu.
Website: http://pt.phhp.ufl.edu/

University of Hartford, College of Education, Nursing, and Health Professions, Program in Physical Therapy, West Hartford, CT 06117-1599. Offers MSPT, DPT. *Accreditation:* APTA. *Entrance requirements:* For master's, GRE, 3 letters of recommendation. Additional exam requirements/recommendations for international students: Required—TOEFL (minimum score 550 paper-based).

University of Illinois at Chicago, Graduate College, College of Applied Health Sciences, Department of Physical Therapy, Chicago, IL 60607-7128. Offers physical therapy (DPT); rehabilitation science (MS). *Accreditation:* APTA. *Faculty:* 12 full-time (7 women), 6 part-time/adjunct (2 women). *Students:* 171 full-time (117 women), 3 part-time (1 woman); includes 32 minority (4 Black or African American, non-Hispanic/Latino; 1 American Indian or Alaska Native, non-Hispanic/Latino; 14 Asian, non-Hispanic/Latino; 8 Hispanic/Latino; 1 Native Hawaiian or other Pacific Islander, non-Hispanic/Latino; 4 Two or more races, non-Hispanic/Latino), 14 international. Average age 26. 1,081 applicants, 15% accepted, 51 enrolled. In 2013, 6 master's, 46 doctorates awarded. *Degree requirements:* For master's, thesis. *Entrance requirements:* For master's, GRE General Test, minimum GPA of 2.75. Additional exam requirements/recommendations for international students: Required—TOEFL. *Application deadline:* For fall admission, 2/15 for domestic and international students. Electronic applications accepted. *Expenses:* Tuition, state resident: full-time $11,066; part-time $3689 per term. Tuition, nonresident: full-time $23,064; part-time $7688 per term. *Required fees:* $3004; $1190 per term. Tuition and fees vary according to course level and program. *Financial support:* Fellowships with full tuition reimbursements, research assistantships with full tuition reimbursements, teaching assistantships with full tuition reimbursements, Federal Work-Study, tuition waivers (full), and tuition service fee waivers available. Financial award applicants required to submit FAFSA. *Total annual research expenditures:* $1.1 million. *Unit head:* Prof. Ross Anthony Arena, Department Head, 312-996-3338, E-mail: raarena@uic.edu. *Application contact:* Alexander Aruin, Receptionist, 312-355-0904, E-mail: aaruin@uic.edu.
Website: http://www.ahs.uic.edu/pt/

University of Indianapolis, Graduate Programs, College of Health Sciences, Krannert School of Physical Therapy, Indianapolis, IN 46227-3697. Offers MHS, DHS, DPT. *Accreditation:* APTA (one or more programs are accredited). Part-time and evening/weekend programs available. *Faculty:* 9 full-time (4 women), 5 part-time/adjunct (4 women). *Students:* 126 full-time (91 women), 72 part-time (58 women); includes 9 minority (4 Black or African American, non-Hispanic/Latino; 4 Asian, non-Hispanic/Latino; 1 Hispanic/Latino), 41 international. Average age 27. In 2013, 22 master's, 47 doctorates awarded. *Entrance requirements:* For doctorate, GRE General Test (for DPT), minimum GPA of 3.0 (for DPT), 3 letters of recommendation. Additional exam requirements/recommendations for international students: Required—TOEFL (minimum score 100 iBT), TWE (minimum score 5). *Application deadline:* For fall admission, 10/10 for domestic students. Application fee: $50. Electronic applications accepted. *Expenses:* Contact institution. *Financial support:* Teaching assistantships, career-related internships or fieldwork, Federal Work-Study, scholarships/grants, tuition waivers (full and partial), and unspecified assistantships available. Support available to part-time students. Financial award application deadline: 5/1; financial award applicants required to submit FAFSA. *Faculty research:* Patella positioning, reaction time, allocation of physical therapy resources. *Unit head:* Dr. Stephanie Kelly, Dean, College of Health Sciences, 317-788-3500, Fax: 317-788-3542, E-mail: huerm@uindy.edu. *Application contact:* Anne Hardwick, Director, Marketing and Admissions, 317-788-3495, Fax: 317-788-3542, E-mail: ahardwick@uindy.edu.
Website: http://pt.uindy.edu/

The University of Iowa, Roy J. and Lucille A. Carver College of Medicine and Graduate College, Biosciences Program, Iowa City, IA 52242-1316. Offers anatomy and cell biology (PhD); biochemistry (PhD); biology (PhD); biomedical engineering (PhD); chemistry (PhD); free radical and radiation biology (PhD); genetics (PhD); human toxicology (PhD); immunology (PhD); microbiology (PhD); molecular and cellular biology (PhD); molecular physiology and biophysics (PhD); neuroscience (PhD); pharmacology (PhD); physical therapy and rehabilitation science (PhD); rehabilitation science (PhD); speech and hearing (PhD). *Faculty:* 332 full-time. *Students:* 8 full-time (3 women); includes 2 minority (1 Black or African American, non-Hispanic/Latino; 1 Asian, non-Hispanic/Latino), 1 international. 200 applicants. *Degree requirements:* For doctorate, thesis/dissertation. *Entrance requirements:* For doctorate, GRE General Test, minimum GPA of 3.0. Additional exam requirements/recommendations for international students: Required—TOEFL (minimum score 600 paper-based; 100 iBT). *Application deadline:* For fall admission, 1/1 priority date for domestic and international students. Applications are processed on a rolling basis. Application fee: $60 ($100 for international students). Electronic applications accepted. *Expenses:* Contact institution. *Financial support:* In 2013–14, 8 students received support, including 8 research assistantships with full tuition reimbursements available (averaging $26,000 per year); fellowships, teaching assistantships, health care benefits, and unspecified assistantships also available. *Unit head:* Dr. Douglas Spitz, Director, 319-335-8001, E-mail: douglas-spitz@uiowa.edu. *Application contact:* Jodi Graff, Director, Admissions and First-Year Experience, 319-335-8306, E-mail: biosciences-admissions@uiowa.edu.
Website: http://www.medicine.uiowa.edu/biosciences/

The University of Iowa, Roy J. and Lucille A. Carver College of Medicine and Graduate College, Graduate Programs in Medicine, Graduate Program in Physical Therapy and Rehabilitation Science, Iowa City, IA 52242-1316. Offers physical therapy (DPT). *Accreditation:* APTA. *Faculty:* 7 full-time (3 women), 66 part-time/adjunct (39 women). *Students:* 115 full-time (64 women), 4 part-time (1 woman); includes 3 minority (1 Black or African American, non-Hispanic/Latino; 1 Asian, non-Hispanic/Latino; 1 Native Hawaiian or other Pacific Islander, non-Hispanic/Latino), 1 international. Average age 24. 455 applicants, 9% accepted, 40 enrolled. In 2013, 4 doctorates awarded. *Degree requirements:* For doctorate, thesis/dissertation (for some programs). *Entrance requirements:* For doctorate, GRE. Additional exam requirements/recommendations for international students: Required—TOEFL. *Application deadline:* For fall admission, 11/1 priority date for domestic students, 5/15 for international students; for winter admission, 10/15 for international students; for spring admission, 3/15 for international students. Application fee: $60 ($85 for international students). Electronic applications accepted. *Expenses:* Contact institution. *Financial support:* In 2013–14, 94 students received support, including 1 fellowship with partial tuition reimbursement available (averaging $9,000 per year), 2 research assistantships with partial tuition reimbursements available (averaging $10,802 per year), 6 teaching assistantships with partial tuition reimbursements available (averaging $10,802 per year); Federal Work-Study, institutionally sponsored loans, scholarships/grants, health care benefits, and unspecified assistantships also available. Support available to part-time students.

Financial award application deadline: 6/30; financial award applicants required to submit FAFSA. *Faculty research:* Muscle fatigue, motor control, pain mechanisms, body composition, sports medicine, occupational safety, neuromuscular physiology, neural control of movement. *Total annual research expenditures:* $1.4 million. *Unit head:* Dr. Richard K. Shields, Chair and Department Executive Officer, 319-335-9791, Fax: 319-335-9707, E-mail: physical-therapy@uiowa.edu. *Application contact:* Carol Leigh, Project Assistant, 319-335-9792, Fax: 319-335-9707, E-mail: carol-leigh@uiowa.edu. Website: http://www.medicine.uiowa.edu/pt/

University of Jamestown, Program in Physical Therapy, Jamestown, ND 58405. Offers DPT. *Entrance requirements:* For doctorate, bachelor's degree. *Expenses: Tuition:* Full-time $24,600; part-time $425 per credit. *Required fees:* $180. Tuition and fees vary according to degree level.

The University of Kansas, University of Kansas Medical Center, School of Health Professions, Department of Physical Therapy and Rehabilitation Science, Kansas City, KS 66160. Offers physical therapy (DPT); rehabilitation science (PhD). *Accreditation:* APTA. *Faculty:* 19. *Students:* 134 full-time (85 women), 16 part-time (12 women); includes 11 minority (4 Black or African American, non-Hispanic/Latino; 2 Asian, non-Hispanic/Latino; 4 Hispanic/Latino; 1 Two or more races, non-Hispanic/Latino), 15 international. Average age 27. 327 applicants, 23% accepted, 48 enrolled. In 2013, 46 doctorates awarded. *Degree requirements:* For doctorate, comprehensive exam, research project with paper. *Entrance requirements:* For doctorate, GRE General Test, minimum GPA of 3.0. Additional exam requirements/recommendations for international students: Required—TOEFL. *Application deadline:* For fall admission, 11/1 for domestic students. Applications are processed on a rolling basis. Application fee: $60. Electronic applications accepted. *Expenses:* Contact institution. *Financial support:* Research assistantships with tuition reimbursements, teaching assistantships with full and partial tuition reimbursements, career-related internships or fieldwork, Federal Work-Study, institutionally sponsored loans, scholarships/grants, traineeships, and unspecified assistantships available. Financial award application deadline: 3/1; financial award applicants required to submit FAFSA. *Faculty research:* Stroke rehabilitation and the effects on balance and coordination; deep brain stimulation and Parkinson's Disease; peripheral neuropathies, pain and the effects of exercise; islet transplants for Type 1 diabetes; cardiac disease associated with diabetes. *Total annual research expenditures:* $696,000. *Unit head:* Dr. Lisa Stehno-Bittel, Chair, 913-588-6733, Fax: 913-588-4568, E-mail: lbittel@kumc.edu. *Application contact:* Robert Bagley, Admission Coordinator, 913-588-6799, Fax: 913-588-4568, E-mail: rbagley@kumc.edu.
Website: http://www.kumc.edu/school-of-health-professions/physical-therapy-and-rehabilitation-science.html

University of Kentucky, Graduate School, College of Health Sciences, Program in Physical Therapy, Lexington, KY 40506-0032. Offers DPT. *Accreditation:* APTA. *Degree requirements:* For doctorate, comprehensive exam, thesis/dissertation optional. *Entrance requirements:* For doctorate, GRE General Test, minimum undergraduate GPA of 2.75, U.S. physical therapist license. Additional exam requirements/recommendations for international students: Required—TOEFL (minimum score 550 paper-based). Electronic applications accepted. *Faculty research:* Orthopedics, biomechanics, electrophysiological stimulation, neural plasticity, brain damage and mechanism.

University of Manitoba, Faculty of Graduate Studies, School of Medical Rehabilitation, Winnipeg, MB R3T 2N2, Canada. Offers applied health sciences (PhD); occupational therapy (MOT); physical therapy (MPT); rehabilitation (M Sc).

University of Mary, School of Health Sciences, Program in Physical Therapy, Bismarck, ND 58504-9652. Offers DPT. *Accreditation:* APTA. *Degree requirements:* For doctorate, comprehensive exam, professional paper. *Entrance requirements:* For doctorate, minimum GPA of 3.0 in core requirements, 40 hours of paid/volunteer experience, interview. Additional exam requirements/recommendations for international students: Required—TOEFL (minimum score 500 paper-based; 71 iBT). Electronic applications accepted. *Expenses:* Contact institution. *Faculty research:* Proprioception, falls and elderly, clinical biomechanics, admission predictors, electromyography and muscle performance, wellness.

University of Maryland, Baltimore, School of Medicine, Department of Physical Therapy and Rehabilitation Science, Baltimore, MD 21201. Offers physical rehabilitation science (PhD); physical therapy and rehabilitation science (DPT). *Accreditation:* APTA. *Students:* 170 full-time (120 women), 3 part-time (2 women); includes 27 minority (8 Black or African American, non-Hispanic/Latino; 10 Asian, non-Hispanic/Latino; 6 Hispanic/Latino; 3 Two or more races, non-Hispanic/Latino), 1 international. Average age 24. 545 applicants, 20% accepted, 55 enrolled. In 2013, 59 doctorates awarded. *Entrance requirements:* For doctorate, GRE General Test, BS, science coursework. Additional exam requirements/recommendations for international students: Required—TOEFL (minimum score 80 iBT). Electronic applications accepted. *Expenses:* Contact institution. *Financial support:* Career-related internships or fieldwork, Federal Work-Study, scholarships/grants, traineeships, health care benefits, and unspecified assistantships available. Financial award application deadline: 3/1; financial award applicants required to submit FAFSA. *Unit head:* Dr. Mary Rodgers, Chair, 410-706-5216, Fax: 410-706-4903, E-mail: mrodgers@som.umaryland.edu. *Application contact:* Terry Heron, Program Coordinator, 410-706-5215, Fax: 410-706-6387, E-mail: theron@som.umaryland.edu.
Website: http://pt.umaryland.edu/pros.asp

University of Maryland Eastern Shore, Graduate Programs, Department of Physical Therapy, Princess Anne, MD 21853-1299. Offers DPT. *Accreditation:* APTA. *Degree requirements:* For doctorate, thesis/dissertation, clinical practicum, research project. *Entrance requirements:* For doctorate, minimum GPA of 3.0, course work in science and mathematics, interview, knowledge of the physical therapy field. Additional exam requirements/recommendations for international students: Required—TOEFL (minimum score 80 iBT). Electronic applications accepted. *Faculty research:* Allied health projects.

University of Massachusetts Lowell, College of Health Sciences, Department of Physical Therapy, Lowell, MA 01854-2881. Offers DPT. *Accreditation:* APTA. *Entrance requirements:* For doctorate, GRE General Test, minimum GPA of 3.0, 3 letters of recommendation. Additional exam requirements/recommendations for international students: Required—TOEFL (minimum score 560 paper-based). *Faculty research:* Orthopedics, pediatrics, electrophysiology, cardiopulmonary, neurology.

University of Miami, Graduate School, Miller School of Medicine, Graduate Programs in Medicine, Department of Physical Therapy, Coral Gables, FL 33124. Offers DPT, PhD. *Accreditation:* APTA (one or more programs are accredited). *Degree requirements:* For doctorate, comprehensive exam, thesis/dissertation. *Entrance requirements:* For doctorate, GRE General Test. Additional exam requirements/recommendations for international students: Required—TOEFL. Electronic applications accepted. *Expenses:* Contact institution. *Faculty research:* Central pattern generators in SCI balance and vestibular function in children, amputee rehabilitation.

University of Michigan–Flint, School of Health Professions and Studies, Program in Physical Therapy, Flint, MI 48502-1950. Offers DPT, PhD. *Accreditation:* APTA. Part-time programs available. Postbaccalaureate distance learning degree programs offered. *Faculty:* 12 full-time (9 women), 3 part-time/adjunct (all women). *Students:* 189 full-time (122 women), 53 part-time (37 women); includes 23 minority (4 Black or African American, non-Hispanic/Latino; 10 Asian, non-Hispanic/Latino; 7 Hispanic/Latino; 2 Two or more races, non-Hispanic/Latino), 26 international. Average age 33. 333 applicants, 26% accepted, 85 enrolled. In 2013, 52 doctorates awarded. *Degree requirements:* For doctorate, comprehensive exam, thesis/dissertation or alternative. *Entrance requirements:* For doctorate, GRE (minimum Verbal score between 340-480; Quantitative 370-710), minimum GPA of 3.16. Additional exam requirements/recommendations for international students: Required—TOEFL (minimum score 560 paper-based; 84 iBT), IELTS (minimum score 6.5). *Application deadline:* For fall admission, 12/1 priority date for domestic students, 9/1 priority date for international students; for winter admission, 11/15 for domestic students, 9/1 for international students; for spring admission, 3/15 for domestic students, 1/1 for international students. Application fee: $55. Electronic applications accepted. *Expenses:* Contact institution. *Financial support:* Career-related internships or fieldwork, Federal Work-Study, scholarships/grants, and unspecified assistantships available. Support available to part-time students. Financial award application deadline: 3/1; financial award applicants required to submit FAFSA. *Faculty research:* Cumulative trauma disorders, oncology rehabilitation, neurological rehabilitation, musculoskeletal rehabilitation, cardiopulmonary rehabilitation. *Unit head:* Dr. Amy Yorke, Admissions Chair, 810-762-3373, E-mail: amyorke@umflint.edu. *Application contact:* Crystal Quaderer, Administrative Assistant, 810-762-3373, Fax: 810-766-6668, E-mail: quaderer@umflint.edu.
Website: http://www.umflint.edu/graduateprograms/physical-therapy-entry-level-dpt

University of Minnesota, Twin Cities Campus, Medical School, Minneapolis, MN 55455-0213. Offers MA, MS, DPT, MD, PhD, JD/MD, MD/MBA, MD/MHI, MD/MPH, MD/MS, MD/PhD. Part-time and evening/weekend programs available. *Expenses:* Contact institution.

University of Mississippi Medical Center, School of Health Related Professions, Department of Physical Therapy, Jackson, MS 39216-4505. Offers MPT. *Accreditation:* APTA. *Faculty research:* Pain, acupressure, seating, patient satisfaction, physical therapy educational issues.

University of Missouri, School of Health Professions, Program in Physical Therapy, Columbia, MO 65211. Offers MPT, DPT. *Accreditation:* APTA. *Faculty:* 8 full-time (6 women), 1 (woman) part-time/adjunct. *Students:* 121 full-time (82 women), 1 (woman) part-time; includes 6 minority (2 Black or African American, non-Hispanic/Latino; 1 Asian, non-Hispanic/Latino; 3 Two or more races, non-Hispanic/Latino). Average age 24. 230 applicants, 22% accepted, 44 enrolled. In 2013, 45 doctorates awarded. *Entrance requirements:* For master's, GRE General Test, minimum GPA of 3.0. Additional exam requirements/recommendations for international students: Required—TOEFL (minimum score 600 paper-based; 100 iBT). *Application deadline:* For spring admission, 1/10 priority date for domestic and international students. Applications are processed on a rolling basis. Application fee: $55 ($75 for international students). Electronic applications accepted. *Financial support:* Research assistantships, teaching assistantships, and institutionally sponsored loans available. *Faculty research:* Fall prevention, early identification of motor impairments in high risk infants, the impact of treadmill training on gait in children with motor impairments, the clinical use of motion analysis to assess functional changes in movement in the pediatric population, injuries common in endurance athletes, patellofemoral dysfunction, manual therapy for the treatment of spinal disorders, estrogen action in skeletal muscle, biopsychosocial factors, exercise in an older adult population. *Unit head:* Dr. Kyle Gibson, Department Chair, 573-882-7103, E-mail: gibsonk@health.missouri.edu. *Application contact:* Beverly Denbigh, Office Support Staff III, 573-882-7103, E-mail: denbighb@missouri.edu.
Website: http://shp.missouri.edu/pt/index.php

The University of Montana, Graduate School, College of Health Professions and Biomedical Sciences, School of Physical Therapy and Rehabilitation Science, Missoula, MT 59812-0002. Offers physical therapy (DPT). *Accreditation:* APTA. *Degree requirements:* For doctorate, professional paper. *Entrance requirements:* For doctorate, GRE General Test. Additional exam requirements/recommendations for international students: Required—TOEFL. *Application deadline:* For winter admission, 1/15 priority date for domestic and international students. Application fee: $120. Electronic applications accepted. *Expenses:* Contact institution. *Financial support:* Career-related internships or fieldwork, Federal Work-Study, institutionally sponsored loans, and scholarships/grants available. Financial award application deadline: 2/15; financial award applicants required to submit FAFSA. *Faculty research:* Muscle stiffness, fitness with a disability, psychosocial aspects of disability, clinical learning, motion analysis. *Unit head:* Reed Humphrey, Chair, 406-243-2417, E-mail: reed.humphrey@umontana.edu. *Application contact:* Kathy Frantzreb, Administrative Associate, 406-243-4027, Fax: 406-243-2795, E-mail: physical.therapy@umontana.edu.
Website: http://www.health.umt.edu/schools/pt/

University of Nebraska Medical Center, School of Allied Health Professions, Division of Physical Therapy Education, Omaha, NE 68198. Offers DPT. *Accreditation:* APTA. *Expenses: Required fees:* $300 per semester. Tuition and fees vary according to program.

University of Nevada, Las Vegas, Graduate College, School of Allied Health Sciences, Department of Physical Therapy, Las Vegas, NV 89154-3029. Offers DPT. *Accreditation:* APTA. *Faculty:* 6 full-time (2 women), 3 part-time/adjunct (all women). *Students:* 91 full-time (52 women); includes 20 minority (7 Asian, non-Hispanic/Latino; 4 Hispanic/Latino; 9 Two or more races, non-Hispanic/Latino). Average age 28. In 2013, 28 doctorates awarded. *Entrance requirements:* Additional exam requirements/recommendations for international students: Required—TOEFL (minimum score 550 paper-based; 80 iBT), IELTS (minimum score 7). *Application deadline:* For fall admission, 5/1 for international students; for spring admission, 10/1 for international students; for summer admission, 12/1 priority date for domestic students. Application fee: $60 ($95 for international students). Electronic applications accepted. *Expenses:* Tuition, state resident: full-time $4752; part-time $264 per credit. Tuition, nonresident: full-time $18,662; part-time $554.50 per credit. *International tuition:* $18,952 full-time. *Required fees:* $532; $12 per credit. $266 per semester. One-time fee: $35. Tuition and fees vary according to course load and program. *Financial support:* In 2013–14, 9 students received support, including 6 research assistantships with partial tuition reimbursements available (averaging $13,000 per year), 3 teaching assistantships with partial tuition reimbursements available (averaging $13,000 per year); institutionally sponsored loans, scholarships/grants, health care benefits, and unspecified assistantships also available. Financial award application deadline: 3/1. *Faculty research:* Spinal manipulation, balance assessment and impairment, falls and fall avoidance behavior, wound care and acute care delivery services, pediatric physical therapy, pain reduction and pain science education. *Total annual research expenditures:* $1,556. *Unit head:* Dr. Merrill Landers, Chair/Associate Professor, 702-895-1377, Fax: 702-895-4883, E-mail: merrill.landers@unlv.edu. *Application contact:* Graduate College Admissions Evaluator, 702-895-3320, Fax: 702-895-4180, E-mail: gradcollege@unlv.edu.
Website: http://pt.unlv.edu/

Physical Therapy

University of New England, Westbrook College of Health Professions, Program in Physical Therapy, Biddeford, ME 04005-9526. Offers physical therapy (DPT); post professional physical therapy (DPT). *Accreditation:* APTA. Postbaccalaureate distance learning degree programs offered (no on-campus study). *Faculty:* 11 full-time (7 women), 5 part-time/adjunct (4 women). *Students:* 197 full-time (128 women); includes 21 minority (1 Black or African American, non-Hispanic/Latino; 9 Asian, non-Hispanic/Latino; 6 Hispanic/Latino; 2 Native Hawaiian or other Pacific Islander, non-Hispanic/Latino; 3 Two or more races, non-Hispanic/Latino), 1 international. Average age 27. 975 applicants, 14% accepted, 67 enrolled. In 2013, 51 doctorates awarded. *Degree requirements:* For doctorate, clinical rotations. *Entrance requirements:* For doctorate, GRE. *Application deadline:* For fall admission, 1/15 for domestic students. Applications are processed on a rolling basis. Electronic applications accepted. *Financial support:* Scholarships/grants available. Financial award application deadline: 5/1; financial award applicants required to submit FAFSA. *Unit head:* Dr. Michael Sheldon, Program Director/Associate Professor, 207-221-4591, Fax: 207-523-1910, E-mail: msheldon@une.edu. *Application contact:* Dr. Cynthia Forrest, Vice President for Student Affairs, 207-221-4225, Fax: 207-523-1925, E-mail: gradadmissions@une.edu.
Website: http://www.une.edu/wchp/pt

University of New Mexico, School of Medicine, Division of Physical Therapy, Albuquerque, NM 87131. Offers DPT. *Accreditation:* APTA. *Faculty:* 6 full-time (3 women). *Students:* 88 full-time (62 women); includes 29 minority (1 Black or African American, non-Hispanic/Latino; 1 American Indian or Alaska Native, non-Hispanic/Latino; 2 Asian, non-Hispanic/Latino; 25 Hispanic/Latino). Average age 29. 31 applicants, 100% accepted, 30 enrolled. In 2013, 1 doctorate awarded. *Degree requirements:* For doctorate, comprehensive exam, thesis/dissertation or alternative. *Entrance requirements:* For doctorate, GRE General Test, GRE Writing Assessment Test, interview, minimum GPA of 3.0. *Application deadline:* For fall admission, 12/15 priority date for domestic students. Applications are processed on a rolling basis. Application fee: $50. *Financial support:* In 2013–14, 3 students received support, including 1 fellowship (averaging $2,000 per year); Federal Work-Study, institutionally sponsored loans, and scholarships/grants also available. Financial award application deadline: 3/1; financial award applicants required to submit FAFSA. *Faculty research:* Gait analysis, motion analysis, balance, articular cartilage, quality of life. *Total annual research expenditures:* $7,800. *Unit head:* Dr. Susan A. Queen, Director, 505-272-5756, Fax: 505-272-8079, E-mail: squeen@salud.unm.edu. *Application contact:* Rosalia Loya Vejar, Administrative Assistant, 505-272-6956, Fax: 505-272-8079, E-mail: rloyavejar@salud.unm.edu.
Website: http://hsc.unm.edu/som/physther/

The University of North Carolina at Chapel Hill, School of Medicine and Graduate School, Graduate Programs in Medicine, Chapel Hill, NC 27599. Offers allied health sciences (MPT, MS, Au D, DPT, PhD), including human movement science (MS, PhD), occupational science (MS, PhD), physical therapy (MPT, MS, DPT), rehabilitation counseling and psychology (MS), speech and hearing sciences (MS, Au D, PhD); biochemistry and biophysics (MS, PhD); bioinformatics and computational biology (PhD); biomedical engineering (MS, PhD); cell and developmental biology (PhD); cell and molecular physiology (PhD); genetics and molecular biology (PhD); microbiology and immunology (MS, PhD), including immunology, microbiology; neurobiology (PhD); pathology and laboratory medicine (PhD), including experimental pathology; pharmacology (PhD); MD/PhD. Postbaccalaureate distance learning degree programs offered. Terminal master's awarded for partial completion of doctoral program. *Degree requirements:* For master's, comprehensive exam; for doctorate, thesis/dissertation. Electronic applications accepted. *Expenses:* Contact institution.

The University of North Carolina at Chapel Hill, School of Medicine and Graduate School, Graduate Programs in Medicine, Department of Allied Health Sciences, Program in Physical Therapy, Chapel Hill, NC 27599. Offers physical therapy - off campus (DPT); physical therapy - on campus (DPT). *Accreditation:* APTA. Part-time and evening/weekend programs available. Postbaccalaureate distance learning degree programs offered (no on-campus study). *Degree requirements:* For doctorate, thesis/dissertation or alternative. *Entrance requirements:* For doctorate, physical therapy license. Additional exam requirements/recommendations for international students: Required—TOEFL (minimum score 550 paper-based). Electronic applications accepted. *Faculty research:* Traumatic brain injury, quality of life after heart and/or lung transplant, cultural diversity, life care planning, rehabilitation education and supervision.

University of North Dakota, Graduate School and Graduate School, Graduate Programs in Medicine, Department of Physical Therapy, Grand Forks, ND 58202. Offers MPT, DPT. *Accreditation:* APTA. *Degree requirements:* For master's, comprehensive exam, thesis or alternative. *Entrance requirements:* For master's and doctorate, minimum GPA of 3.0, pre-physical therapy program. Additional exam requirements/recommendations for international students: Required—TOEFL (minimum score 550 paper-based; 79 iBT), IELTS (minimum score 6.5). *Faculty research:* Practice-based program.

University of North Florida, Brooks College of Health, Department of Clinical and Applied Movement Sciences, Jacksonville, FL 32224. Offers exercise science and chronic disease (MSH); physical therapy (DPT). *Accreditation:* APTA. Part-time and evening/weekend programs available. *Faculty:* 14 full-time (8 women), 2 part-time/adjunct (0 women). *Students:* 86 full-time (50 women), 2 part-time (both women); includes 22 minority (3 Black or African American, non-Hispanic/Latino; 3 Asian, non-Hispanic/Latino; 11 Hispanic/Latino; 5 Two or more races, non-Hispanic/Latino). Average age 25. 464 applicants, 9% accepted, 30 enrolled. In 2013, 28 doctorates awarded. *Degree requirements:* For master's, internship. *Entrance requirements:* For master's, GRE General Test, minimum GPA of 3.0 in last 60 hours, volunteer/observation experience. Additional exam requirements/recommendations for international students: Required—TOEFL (minimum score 500 paper-based). *Application deadline:* For fall admission, 2/15 for domestic students, 1/15 for international students. Application fee: $30. Electronic applications accepted. *Expenses:* Tuition, state resident: full-time $9794; part-time $408.10 per credit hour. Tuition, nonresident: full-time $22,383; part-time $932.61 per credit hour. *Required fees:* $2020; $84.20 per credit hour. Tuition and fees vary according to course load and program. *Financial support:* In 2013–14, 29 students received support. Teaching assistantships, career-related internships or fieldwork, Federal Work-Study, scholarships/grants, and tuition waivers (partial) available. Support available to part-time students. Financial award application deadline: 4/1; financial award applicants required to submit FAFSA. *Faculty research:* Clinical outcomes related to orthopedic physical therapy interventions, instructional multimedia in physical therapy education, effect of functional electrical stimulation orthostatic hypotension in acute complete spinal cord injury individuals. *Total annual research expenditures:* $123,734. *Unit head:* Dr. Joel Beam, Chair, 904-620-1424, E-mail: jbeam@unf.edu. *Application contact:* Beth Dibble, Program Director, 904-620-2418, E-mail: ptadmissions@unf.edu.
Website: http://www.unf.edu/brooks/movement_science/

University of North Georgia, Department of Physical Therapy, Dahlonega, GA 30597. Offers DPT. *Accreditation:* APTA. *Entrance requirements:* For doctorate, GRE, interview, recommendations, physical therapy observations hours, minimum GPA of 2.8. Additional exam requirements/recommendations for international students: Required—TOEFL (minimum score 550 paper-based; 79 iBT), IELTS (minimum score 6.5). Electronic applications accepted. *Faculty research:* Ergonomics, spinal mobility measurements, electrophysiology, orthopedic physical therapy.

University of Oklahoma Health Sciences Center, Graduate College, College of Allied Health, Department of Physical Therapy, Oklahoma City, OK 73190. Offers MPT. *Accreditation:* APTA. *Faculty:* 6 full-time (3 women). *Students:* 182 full-time (125 women), 2 part-time (1 woman); includes 45 minority (7 Black or African American, non-Hispanic/Latino; 8 American Indian or Alaska Native, non-Hispanic/Latino; 6 Asian, non-Hispanic/Latino; 14 Hispanic/Latino; 10 Two or more races, non-Hispanic/Latino). Average age 25. 286 applicants, 29% accepted, 62 enrolled. *Expenses:* Tuition, state resident: full-time $3504; part-time $175.20 per credit hour. Tuition, nonresident: full-time $13,504; part-time $675.20 per credit hour. *Required fees:* $1545; $52.70 per credit hour. $245.25 per semester. Tuition and fees vary according to course load. *Unit head:* Dr. Kevin Rudeen, Dean, 405-271-2288, Fax: 405-271-1190, E-mail: carole-sullivan@ouhsc.edu. *Application contact:* Jenielle Greenlee, Associate Dean for Finance, 405-271-2288, Fax: 405-271-1190, E-mail: jenielle-greenlee@ouhse.edu.

University of Pittsburgh, School of Health and Rehabilitation Sciences, Doctor of Physical Therapy Program, Pittsburgh, PA 15260. Offers DPT. *Accreditation:* APTA. *Faculty:* 12 full-time (7 women), 3 part-time/adjunct (1 woman). *Students:* 167 full-time (116 women); includes 5 minority (2 Black or African American, non-Hispanic/Latino; 1 Asian, non-Hispanic/Latino; 2 Hispanic/Latino), 1 international. Average age 26. 857 applicants, 14% accepted, 55 enrolled. In 2013, 51 doctorates awarded. *Degree requirements:* For doctorate, clinical practice. *Entrance requirements:* For doctorate, GRE, volunteer work in physical therapy. Additional exam requirements/recommendations for international students: Required—TOEFL (minimum score 550 paper-based; 80 iBT), IELTS (minimum score 6.5). *Application deadline:* For fall admission, 12/17 for domestic and international students. Applications are processed on a rolling basis. Application fee: $130. Electronic applications accepted. *Expenses:* Contact institution. *Financial support:* Federal Work-Study, scholarships/grants, and traineeships available. Support available to part-time students. Financial award applicants required to submit FAFSA. *Faculty research:* Biomechanics, neuromuscular system, sports medicine, movement analysis, validity/outcomes of clinical procedures. *Total annual research expenditures:* $1.1 million. *Unit head:* Dr. Anthony Delitto, Chairman, 412-383-6630, Fax: 412-383-6629, E-mail: delitto@pitt.edu. *Application contact:* Corinne Grubb, Administrator, PT Student Services, 412-383-8169, Fax: 412-648-5970, E-mail: cgrubb@pitt.edu.
Website: http://www.shrs.pitt.edu/dpt/

University of Pittsburgh, School of Health and Rehabilitation Sciences, Master's Programs in Health and Rehabilitation Sciences, Pittsburgh, PA 15260. Offers health and rehabilitation sciences (MS), including health care supervision and management, health information systems, occupational therapy, physical therapy, rehabilitation counseling, rehabilitation science and technology, sports medicine, wellness and human performance. *Accreditation:* APTA. Part-time and evening/weekend programs available. *Faculty:* 63 full-time (37 women), 4 part-time/adjunct (2 women). *Students:* 117 full-time (70 women), 44 part-time (27 women); includes 18 minority (8 Black or African American, non-Hispanic/Latino; 1 American Indian or Alaska Native, non-Hispanic/Latino; 6 Asian, non-Hispanic/Latino; 3 Hispanic/Latino), 52 international. Average age 30. 368 applicants, 57% accepted, 96 enrolled. In 2013, 90 master's awarded. *Degree requirements:* For master's, comprehensive exam (for some programs), thesis optional. *Entrance requirements:* For master's, minimum GPA of 3.0. Additional exam requirements/recommendations for international students: Required—TOEFL (minimum score 550 paper-based; 80 iBT), IELTS (minimum score 6.5). *Application deadline:* For fall admission, 3/1 for international students; for spring admission, 9/1 for international students. Applications are processed on a rolling basis. Application fee: $50. Electronic applications accepted. *Expenses:* Contact institution. *Financial support:* In 2013–14, 3 fellowships (averaging $20,460 per year) were awarded; Federal Work-Study, institutionally sponsored loans, scholarships/grants, traineeships, and unspecified assistantships also available. Financial award applicants required to submit FAFSA. *Faculty research:* Assistive technology, seating and wheeled mobility, cellular neurophysiology, low back syndrome, augmentative communication. *Total annual research expenditures:* $8.1 million. *Unit head:* Dr. Clifford E. Brubaker, Dean, 412-383-6560, Fax: 412-383-6535, E-mail: cliffb@pitt.edu. *Application contact:* Jessica Maguire, Director of Admissions, 412-383-6557, Fax: 412-383-6535, E-mail: maguire@pitt.edu.
Website: http://www.shrs.pitt.edu/

University of Puerto Rico, Medical Sciences Campus, School of Health Professions, Program in Physical Therapy, San Juan, PR 00936-5067. Offers MS. *Accreditation:* APTA. Part-time and evening/weekend programs available. *Degree requirements:* For master's, one foreign language, thesis. *Entrance requirements:* For master's, EXADEP, minimum GPA of 2.8, interview, first aid training and CPR certification.

University of Puget Sound, Graduate Studies, School of Physical Therapy, Tacoma, WA 98416. Offers DPT. *Accreditation:* APTA. *Degree requirements:* For doctorate, comprehensive exam, thesis/dissertation or alternative, successful completion of 36 weeks of full-time internships and a research project. *Entrance requirements:* For doctorate, GRE General Test, minimum baccalaureate GPA of 3.0, observation hours (at least 100 recommended), three letters of recommendation. Additional exam requirements/recommendations for international students: Required—TOEFL (minimum score 550 paper-based; 90 iBT). Electronic applications accepted. *Expenses:* Contact institution. *Faculty research:* Manual therapy, assessment of chronic pain, movement assessment of children, pediatric gait, seating interventions, electro-physical agents, injury prevention.

University of Rhode Island, Graduate School, College of Human Science and Services, Physical Therapy Department, Kingston, RI 02881. Offers DPT. *Accreditation:* APTA. Part-time programs available. *Faculty:* 8 full-time (5 women). *Students:* 63 full-time (49 women), 29 part-time (16 women); includes 1 minority (Asian, non-Hispanic/Latino), 2 international. In 2013, 26 doctorates awarded. *Degree requirements:* For doctorate, comprehensive exam. *Entrance requirements:* For doctorate, GRE, 2 letters of recommendation (one must be a physical therapist). Additional exam requirements/recommendations for international students: Required—TOEFL (minimum score 550 paper-based). *Application deadline:* For fall admission, 12/15 for domestic and international students; for summer admission, 11/1 for domestic and international students. Application fee: $65. Electronic applications accepted. *Expenses:* Tuition, state resident: full-time $11,532; part-time $641 per credit. Tuition, nonresident: full-time $23,606; part-time $1311 per credit. *Required fees:* $1388; $36 per credit. $35 per semester. One-time fee: $130. *Financial support:* In 2013–14, 2 teaching assistantships with full and partial tuition reimbursements (averaging $5,093 per year) were awarded. Financial award application deadline: 11/1; financial award applicants required to submit FAFSA. *Total annual research expenditures:* $180,819. *Unit head:* Dr. Jeff Konin, Chair, 401-574-5627, E-mail: jkonin@mail.uri.edu. *Application contact:* Graduate Admissions, 401-874-2872, E-mail: gradadm@etal.uri.edu.
Website: http://www.uri.edu/hss/pt/

University of St. Augustine for Health Sciences, Graduate Programs, Division of Physical Therapy, St. Augustine, FL 32086. Offers DPT, TDPT, Certificate. *Accreditation:* APTA. *Entrance requirements:* Additional exam requirements/

recommendations for international students: Required—TOEFL. *Application deadline:* Applications are processed on a rolling basis. Application fee: $50. Tuition and fees vary according to course level, course load, campus/location and program. *Unit head:* Dr. Catherine K. Patla, Director of Clinical Fellowship, 904-826-0084 Ext. 254, Fax: 904-826-0085, E-mail: cpatla@usa.edu. *Application contact:* Dian Hartley, Director of Admissions, 904-826-0084 Ext. 207, Fax: 904-826-0085, E-mail: dhartley@usa.edu.
Website: http://www.usa.edu/

University of Saint Mary, Graduate Programs, Program in Physical Therapy, Leavenworth, KS 66048-5082. Offers DPT. *Students:* 78 full-time (50 women); includes 6 minority (2 Black or African American, non-Hispanic/Latino; 1 Asian, non-Hispanic/Latino; 3 Hispanic/Latino). *Expenses: Tuition:* Part-time $550 per credit hour. *Application contact:* Christi Sumpter, Department Secretary, 913-758-4398, Fax: 913-345-2802, E-mail: dpt@stmary.edu.
Website: http://www.stmary.edu/DPT

The University of Scranton, College of Graduate and Continuing Education, Department of Physical Therapy, Scranton, PA 18510. Offers DPT. *Accreditation:* APTA. Part-time programs available. Postbaccalaureate distance learning degree programs offered (no on-campus study). *Faculty:* 7 full-time (3 women). *Students:* 111 full-time (68 women), 12 part-time (8 women); includes 9 minority (1 Black or African American, non-Hispanic/Latino; 2 Asian, non-Hispanic/Latino; 4 Hispanic/Latino; 1 Native Hawaiian or other Pacific Islander, non-Hispanic/Latino; 1 Two or more races, non-Hispanic/Latino). Average age 25. 710 applicants, 8% accepted. In 2013, 65 doctorates awarded. *Entrance requirements:* For doctorate, physical therapist license. Additional exam requirements/recommendations for international students: Required—TOEFL (minimum score 500 paper-based), IELTS (minimum score 5.5). *Application deadline:* Applications are processed on a rolling basis. Application fee: $0. *Financial support:* In 2013–14, 14 students received support, including 14 teaching assistantships (averaging $4,400 per year); career-related internships or fieldwork, Federal Work-Study, and unspecified assistantships also available. Support available to part-time students. Financial award application deadline: 3/1. *Unit head:* Dr. John P. Sanko, Chair, 570-941-7934, Fax: 570-941-7940, E-mail: sankoi1@scranton.edu. *Application contact:* Joseph M. Roback, Director of Admissions, 570-941-4385, Fax: 570-941-5928, E-mail: robackj2@scranton.edu.

University of South Alabama, Graduate School, College of Allied Health Professions, Department of Physical Therapy, Mobile, AL 36688-0002. Offers DPT. *Accreditation:* APTA. *Faculty:* 7 full-time (5 women), 1 part-time/adjunct (0 women). *Students:* 105 full-time (61 women); includes 3 minority (1 Black or African American, non-Hispanic/Latino; 1 Asian, non-Hispanic/Latino; 1 Hispanic/Latino), 1 international. 302 applicants, 32% accepted, 34 enrolled. In 2013, 33 doctorates awarded. *Entrance requirements:* For doctorate, GRE, minimum GPA of 3.0. Additional exam requirements/recommendations for international students: Required—TOEFL (minimum score 600 paper-based). *Application deadline:* For fall admission, 12/15 priority date for domestic students. Applications are processed on a rolling basis. Application fee: $75. *Expenses:* Tuition, state resident: full-time $8976; part-time $374 per credit hour. Tuition, nonresident: full-time $17,952; part-time $748 per credit hour. *Financial support:* Application deadline: 4/1. *Unit head:* Dr. Dennis Fell, Chair, 251-445-9330, E-mail: ptdept@jaguar1.usouthal.edu. *Application contact:* Dr. Julio Turrens, Director of Graduate Studies, 251-445-9250.
Website: http://www.southalabama.edu/alliedhealth/pt/

The University of South Dakota, Graduate School, School of Health Sciences, Department of Physical Therapy, Vermillion, SD 57069-2390. Offers DPT. *Accreditation:* APTA. *Entrance requirements:* For doctorate, GRE General Test. Additional exam requirements/recommendations for international students: Required—TOEFL. *Expenses:* Contact institution. *Faculty research:* Physical therapy, knee rehabilitation, pediatric intervention, wound care, motion analysis.

University of Southern California, Graduate School, Herman Ostrow School of Dentistry, Division of Biokinesiology and Physical Therapy, Los Angeles, CA 90089. Offers biokinesiology (MS, PhD); physical therapy (DPT). *Accreditation:* APTA (one or more programs are accredited). *Degree requirements:* For master's, comprehensive exam; for doctorate, thesis/dissertation. *Entrance requirements:* For master's and doctorate, GRE (minimum combined score 1200, verbal 600, quantitative 600). Additional exam requirements/recommendations for international students: Required—TOEFL. Electronic applications accepted. *Expenses:* Contact institution. *Faculty research:* Exercise and aging biomechanics, musculoskeletal biomechanics, exercise and hormones related to muscle wasting, computational neurorehabilitation, motor behavior and neurorehabilitation, motor development, infant motor performance.

University of South Florida, Morsani College of Medicine, School of Physical Therapy, Tampa, FL 33620-9951. Offers DPT. *Accreditation:* APTA. *Faculty:* 2 full-time (both women). *Students:* 117 full-time (88 women), 224 part-time (152 women); includes 103 minority (20 Black or African American, non-Hispanic/Latino; 1 American Indian or Alaska Native, non-Hispanic/Latino; 57 Asian, non-Hispanic/Latino; 25 Hispanic/Latino). Average age 34. 1,011 applicants, 17% accepted, 162 enrolled. In 2013, 42 doctorates awarded. *Entrance requirements:* For doctorate, GRE General Test, bachelor's degree from regionally-accredited university with minimum GPA of 3.0 in all upper-division coursework; interview; at least 20 hours of documented volunteer or work experience in hospital outpatient/inpatient physical therapy settings; written personal statement of values and purpose for attending. Additional exam requirements/recommendations for international students: Required—TOEFL (minimum score 600 paper-based). *Application deadline:* For fall admission, 9/1 for domestic students, 2/1 for international students. Application fee: $30. *Faculty research:* Veteran's reintegration and resilience, prosthetics and orthotics (microprocessor prosthetic knee), neuromusculoskeletal disorders (occupational ergonomics, fall risk and prevention, exercise adherence and compliance, and orthotic and prosthetic wear and use), human movement and function. *Total annual research expenditures:* $1.7 million. *Unit head:* Dr. William S. Quillen, Director, 813-974-9863, Fax: 813-974-8915, E-mail: wquillen@health.usf.edu. *Application contact:* Dr. Gina Maria Musolino, Associate Professor and Coordinator for Clinical Education, 813-974-2254, Fax: 813-974-8915, E-mail: gmusolin@health.usf.edu.
Website: http://health.usf.edu/medicine/dpt/index.htm

The University of Tennessee at Chattanooga, Graduate School, College of Health, Education and Professional Studies, Program in Physical Therapy, Chattanooga, TN 37403. Offers DPT. *Accreditation:* APTA. *Faculty:* 8 full-time (5 women), 5 part-time/adjunct (3 women). *Students:* 92 full-time (66 women), 12 part-time (9 women); includes 8 minority (1 Black or African American, non-Hispanic/Latino; 4 Asian, non-Hispanic/Latino; 2 Hispanic/Latino; 1 Two or more races, non-Hispanic/Latino). Average age 27. 180 applicants, 21% accepted, 37 enrolled. In 2013, 48 doctorates awarded. *Degree requirements:* For doctorate, qualifying exams, internship. *Entrance requirements:* For doctorate, interview, minimum GPA of 3.0 in science and overall. Additional exam requirements/recommendations for international students: Required—TOEFL (minimum score 550 paper-based; 79 iBT); Recommended—IELTS (minimum score 6). *Application deadline:* For fall admission, 6/13 priority date for domestic students, 6/1 for international students; for spring admission, 10/15 priority date for domestic students, 10/1 for international students. Applications are processed on a rolling basis. Application fee: $30 ($35 for international students). Electronic applications accepted. *Financial support:* In 2013–14, 9 research assistantships with tuition reimbursements (averaging $3,430 per year), 1 teaching assistantship with tuition reimbursement (averaging $3,430 per year) were awarded; career-related internships or fieldwork, scholarships/grants, and unspecified assistantships also available. Support available to part-time students. *Faculty research:* Diabetes and wound management, disabilities, animal physical therapy and rehabilitation, orthopedics. *Total annual research expenditures:* $3,270. *Unit head:* Dr. Debbie Ingram, Interim Department Head, 423-425-4767, Fax: 423-425-2215, E-mail: debbie-ingram@utc.edu. *Application contact:* Dr. J. Randy Walker, Dean of Graduate Studies, 423-425-4478, Fax: 423-425-5223, E-mail: randy-walker@utc.edu.
Website: http://www.utc.edu/Academic/PhysicalTherapy/

The University of Tennessee Health Science Center, College of Health Professions, Memphis, TN 38163-0002. Offers audiology (MS, Au D); clinical laboratory science (MSCLS); cytopathology practice (MCP); health informatics and information management (MHIIM); occupational therapy (MOT); physical therapy (DPT, ScDPT); physician assistant (MMS); speech-language pathology (MS). *Accreditation:* AOTA; APTA. Part-time and evening/weekend programs available. Postbaccalaureate distance learning degree programs offered (minimal on-campus study). Terminal master's awarded for partial completion of doctoral program. *Degree requirements:* For master's, comprehensive exam, thesis; for doctorate, comprehensive exam, residency. *Entrance requirements:* For master's, GRE (MOT, MSCLS), minimum GPA of 3.0, 3 letters of reference, national accreditation (MSCLS), GRE if GPA is less than 3.0 (MCP); for doctorate, GRE. Additional exam requirements/recommendations for international students: Required—TOEFL (minimum score 550 paper-based; 80 iBT). *Application deadline:* For fall admission, 1/30 priority date for domestic students; for winter admission, 10/1 priority date for domestic students. Application fee: $50. Electronic applications accepted. *Expenses:* Contact institution. *Financial support:* Teaching assistantships, Federal Work-Study, institutionally sponsored loans, and scholarships/grants available. Support available to part-time students. Financial award application deadline: 2/15; financial award applicants required to submit FAFSA. *Faculty research:* Gait deviation, muscular dystrophy and strength, hemophilia and exercise, pediatric neurology, self-efficacy. *Unit head:* Dr. Noma Anderson, Dean, 901-528-5588, Fax: 901-528-7545, E-mail: nander13@uthsc.edu. *Application contact:* Dr. Noma Anderson, Dean, 901-528-5588, Fax: 901-528-7545, E-mail: nander13@uthsc.edu.
Website: http://www.uthsc.edu/health-professions/

The University of Texas at El Paso, Graduate School, College of Health Sciences, Program in Physical Therapy, El Paso, TX 79968-0001. Offers DPT. *Accreditation:* APTA. *Entrance requirements:* For doctorate, GRE General Test. Additional exam requirements/recommendations for international students: Required—TOEFL. Electronic applications accepted.

The University of Texas Health Science Center at San Antonio, School of Health Professions, San Antonio, TX 78229-3900. Offers occupational therapy (MOT); physical therapy (DPT); physician assistant studies (MS); toxicology (MS). *Accreditation:* AOTA; APTA; ARC-PA. *Faculty:* 75 full-time (31 women), 49 part-time/adjunct (19 women). *Students:* 353 full-time (258 women), 2 part-time (1 woman); includes 180 minority (15 Black or African American, non-Hispanic/Latino; 29 Asian, non-Hispanic/Latino; 129 Hispanic/Latino; 1 Native Hawaiian or other Pacific Islander, non-Hispanic/Latino; 6 Two or more races, non-Hispanic/Latino), 3 international. Average age 28. 605 applicants, 21% accepted, 125 enrolled. In 2013, 73 master's, 63 doctorates awarded. *Degree requirements:* For master's, comprehensive exam, thesis (for some programs); for doctorate, comprehensive exam. *Entrance requirements:* For master's, GRE (for toxicology), minimum GPA of 3.0 and bachelor's degree in clinical laboratory science or closely-related science discipline (for MS in toxicology); minimum GPA of 3.0, bachelor's degree, PA shadowing, and community service (for MS in physician assistant); for doctorate, GRE, minimum GPA of 3.0, bachelor's degree, PT shadowing, observation hours. Additional exam requirements/recommendations for international students: Required—TOEFL (minimum score 560 paper-based). *Application deadline:* For fall admission, 6/1 for domestic and international students; for spring admission, 10/1 for domestic and international students. Application fee: $60. Electronic applications accepted. *Financial support:* In 2013–14, 219 students received support. Federal Work-Study, scholarships/grants, and stipends, department payments available. Financial award application deadline: 6/30; financial award applicants required to submit FAFSA. *Total annual research expenditures:* $760,563. *Unit head:* Dr. Susan Dollar, Assistant Dean, 210-567-4837, Fax: 210-567-4828, E-mail: dollar@uthscsa.edu. *Application contact:* Dr. David L. Henzi, Assistant Dean for Admissions, 210-567-4818, Fax: 210-567-4828, E-mail: henzi@uthscsa.edu.
Website: http://www.uthscsa.edu/shp/

The University of Texas Medical Branch, School of Health Professions, Department of Physical Therapy, Galveston, TX 77555. Offers MPT, DPT. *Accreditation:* APTA. *Degree requirements:* For master's, thesis or alternative. *Entrance requirements:* For master's and doctorate, GRE, documentation of 40 hours' experience. Electronic applications accepted.

The University of Texas Southwestern Medical Center, Southwestern School of Health Professions, Physical Therapy Program, Dallas, TX 75390. Offers DPT. *Accreditation:* APTA. *Faculty:* 85 full-time (58 women). *Students:* 109 full-time (88 women); includes 17 minority (3 Black or African American, non-Hispanic/Latino; 1 American Indian or Alaska Native, non-Hispanic/Latino; 7 Asian, non-Hispanic/Latino; 4 Hispanic/Latino; 2 Two or more races, non-Hispanic/Latino), 3 international. Average age 25. 416 applicants, 15% accepted, 43 enrolled. In 2013, 35 doctorates awarded. *Entrance requirements:* For doctorate, GRE, minimum GPA of 3.0. Additional exam requirements/recommendations for international students: Required—TOEFL (minimum score 600 paper-based). *Application deadline:* For spring admission, 9/1 priority date for domestic students. Application fee: $10. Electronic applications accepted. *Financial support:* Application deadline: 3/1; applicants required to submit FAFSA. *Unit head:* Dr. Patricia Winchester, Chair, 214-648-1551, Fax: 214-648-1511, E-mail: patricia.winchester@utsouthwestern.edu. *Application contact:* Billy Crawford, Education Coordinator, 214-648-1566, Fax: 214-648-1511, E-mail: billy.crawford@utsouthwestern.edu.
Website: http://www8.utsouthwestern.edu/utsw/cda/dept28445/files/51683.html

University of the Pacific, Thomas J. Long School of Pharmacy and Health Sciences, Department of Physical Therapy, Stockton, CA 95211-0197. Offers MS, DPT. *Accreditation:* APTA. *Faculty:* 10 full-time (7 women), 9 part-time/adjunct (7 women). *Students:* 69 full-time (39 women), 2 part-time (both women); includes 25 minority (14 Asian, non-Hispanic/Latino; 8 Hispanic/Latino; 3 Two or more races, non-Hispanic/Latino). Average age 25. 550 applicants, 13% accepted, 35 enrolled. In 2013, 36 doctorates awarded. *Entrance requirements:* For master's, GRE General Test, minimum GPA of 3.0. Additional exam requirements/recommendations for international students: Required—TOEFL (minimum score 475 paper-based). *Application deadline:* For fall admission, 1/4 for domestic students. Application fee: $75. *Financial support:* Federal Work-Study available. Financial award application deadline: 3/1; financial award applicants required to submit FAFSA. *Unit head:* Dr. Cathy Peterson, Chair, 209-946-2947, Fax: 209-946-2410. *Application contact:* Ron Espejo, Recruitment Specialist, 209-946-3957, Fax: 209-946-3147, E-mail: respejo@pacific.edu.

Physical Therapy

The University of Toledo, College of Graduate Studies, College of Health Sciences, Department of Rehabilitation Sciences, Toledo, OH 43606-3390. Offers occupational therapy (OTD); physical therapy (DPT); speech-language pathology (MA). *Faculty:* 30. *Students:* 180 full-time (148 women), 31 part-time (29 women); includes 11 minority (2 Black or African American, non-Hispanic/Latino; 3 Asian, non-Hispanic/Latino; 2 Hispanic/Latino; 4 Two or more races, non-Hispanic/Latino). Average age 25. 230 applicants, 58% accepted, 61 enrolled. In 2013, 25 master's, 43 doctorates awarded. *Degree requirements:* For master's, comprehensive exam, thesis; for doctorate, thesis/dissertation or alternative. *Entrance requirements:* For master's, GRE, minimum cumulative GPA of 2.7 for all previous academic work, letters of recommendation; for doctorate, GRE, minimum cumulative GPA of 3.0 for all previous academic work, letters of recommendation; OTCAS or PTCAS application and UT supplemental application (for OTD and DPT). Additional exam requirements/recommendations for international students: Required—TOEFL (minimum score 550 paper-based; 80 iBT). *Application deadline:* For fall admission, 11/1 for domestic and international students. Application fee: $45 ($75 for international students). Electronic applications accepted. *Financial support:* In 2013–14, 16 teaching assistantships with full and partial tuition reimbursements (averaging $5,002 per year) were awarded; Federal Work-Study, scholarships/grants, tuition waivers (full and partial), unspecified assistantships, and administrative assistantships also available. Financial award applicants required to submit FAFSA. *Unit head:* Dr. Michelle Masterson, Chair, 419-530-6671, Fax: 419-530-4780, E-mail: michelle.masterson@utoledo.edu. *Application contact:* College of Graduate Studies, 419-383-4112, Fax: 419-383-6140, E-mail: grdsch@utnet.utoledo.edu.
Website: http://www.utoledo.edu/eduhshs/

The University of Toledo, College of Graduate Studies, College of Medicine and Life Sciences, Department of Orthopedic Surgery, Toledo, OH 43606-3390. Offers MSBS. *Faculty:* 8. *Students:* 4 applicants. In 2013, 1 master's awarded. *Degree requirements:* For master's, thesis or alternative. *Entrance requirements:* For master's, GRE, minimum undergraduate GPA of 3.0, three letters of recommendation, statement of purpose, transcripts from all prior institutions attended, resume. Additional exam requirements/recommendations for international students: Required—TOEFL (minimum score 550 paper-based; 80 iBT). *Application deadline:* For fall admission, 1/15 priority date for domestic and international students. Application fee: $45 ($75 for international students). Electronic applications accepted. *Financial support:* In 2013–14, 1 research assistantship with full and partial tuition reimbursement (averaging $10,000 per year) was awarded; institutionally sponsored loans and tuition waivers (full and partial) also available. *Unit head:* Dr. Martin Skie, Chair, 419-383-3761, E-mail: nabil.ebraheim@utoledo.edu. *Application contact:* Admissions Analyst, 419-383-4112, Fax: 419-383-6140.
Website: http://www.utoledo.edu/med/grad/

University of Toronto, Faculty of Medicine, Department of Physical Therapy, Toronto, ON M5S 1A1, Canada. Offers M Sc PT. *Accreditation:* APTA. *Entrance requirements:* For master's, minimum B average in final year, 2 references. Additional exam requirements/recommendations for international students: Required—TOEFL (minimum score 600 paper-based; 100 iBT), TWE (minimum score 5). Electronic applications accepted.

University of Utah, Graduate School, College of Health, Department of Physical Therapy, Salt Lake City, UT 84112-1290. Offers physical therapy (DPT); rehabilitation science (PhD). *Accreditation:* APTA. *Faculty:* 7 full-time (1 woman), 15 part-time/adjunct (8 women). *Students:* 151 full-time (84 women), 3 part-time (1 woman); includes 10 minority (1 American Indian or Alaska Native, non-Hispanic/Latino; 2 Asian, non-Hispanic/Latino; 3 Hispanic/Latino; 3 Native Hawaiian or other Pacific Islander, non-Hispanic/Latino; 1 Two or more races, non-Hispanic/Latino), 4 international. Average age 28. 340 applicants, 14% accepted, 48 enrolled. In 2013, 48 doctorates awarded. *Degree requirements:* For doctorate, thesis/dissertation, clinical project. *Entrance requirements:* For doctorate, GRE, minimum GPA of 3.0, volunteer work, bachelor's degree. Additional exam requirements/recommendations for international students: Required—TOEFL (minimum score 90 iBT); Recommended—IELTS (minimum score 7). *Application deadline:* For fall admission, 10/1 priority date for domestic students, 10/1 for international students. Application fee: $55 ($65 for international students). Electronic applications accepted. *Expenses:* Contact institution. *Financial support:* Research assistantships with full tuition reimbursements, teaching assistantships with full tuition reimbursements, Federal Work-Study, scholarships/grants, tuition waivers (partial), and unspecified assistantships available. Financial award application deadline: 10/1; financial award applicants required to submit FAFSA. *Faculty research:* Rehabilitation and Parkinson's Disease, motor control and musculoskeletal dysfunction, burns/wound care, rehabilitation and multiple sclerosis, cancer. *Total annual research expenditures:* $983,166. *Unit head:* Dr. R. Scott Ward, Chair, 801-581-4895, E-mail: scott.ward@hsc.utah.edu. *Application contact:* Dee-Dee Darby-Duffin, Academic Advisor, 801-581-5146, E-mail: darbyduffinfamily@gmail.com.
Website: http://www.health.utah.edu/pt

University of Vermont, Graduate College, College of Nursing and Health Sciences, Program in Physical Therapy, Burlington, VT 05405. Offers DPT. *Accreditation:* APTA. *Students:* 91 (66 women); includes 6 minority (2 Black or African American, non-Hispanic/Latino; 4 Hispanic/Latino), 1 international. 398 applicants, 22% accepted, 1 enrolled. In 2013, 38 doctorates awarded. *Entrance requirements:* For doctorate, GRE General Test. Additional exam requirements/recommendations for international students: Required—TOEFL (minimum score 550 paper-based; 80 iBT). *Application deadline:* For fall admission, 12/15 for domestic and international students. Applications are processed on a rolling basis. Application fee: $65. Electronic applications accepted. *Financial support:* Fellowships, research assistantships, teaching assistantships, and Federal Work-Study available. Financial award application deadline: 3/1. *Unit head:* Dr. Patricia Prelock, Dean, 802-656-3858. *Application contact:* Dr. Diane Jette, Coordinator, 802-656-3858.

University of Washington, Graduate School, School of Medicine, Graduate Programs in Medicine, Department of Rehabilitation Medicine, Seattle, WA 98195-6490. Offers occupational therapy (MOT); physical therapy (DPT); prosthetics and orthotics (MPO); rehabilitation science (PhD). *Degree requirements:* For doctorate, comprehensive exam (for some programs), thesis/dissertation (for some programs). *Entrance requirements:* For master's and doctorate, GRE. Additional exam requirements/recommendations for international students: Required—TOEFL. *Faculty research:* Biomechanics, balance, brain injury, spinal cord injury, pain, degenerative diseases.

The University of Western Ontario, Faculty of Graduate Studies, Biosciences Division, School of Physical Therapy, London, ON N6A 5B8, Canada. Offers manipulative therapy (CAS); physical therapy (MPT); wound healing (CAS). *Accreditation:* APTA. Part-time programs available. *Degree requirements:* For master's, thesis. *Entrance requirements:* For master's, B Sc in physical therapy. Additional exam requirements/recommendations for international students: Required—TOEFL. *Faculty research:* Muscle strength, wound healing, motor control, respiratory physiology, exercise physiology.

University of Wisconsin–La Crosse, Graduate Studies, College of Science and Health, Department of Health Professions, Program in Physical Therapy, La Crosse, WI 54601-3742. Offers DPT. *Accreditation:* APTA. *Faculty:* 8 full-time (2 women), 2 part-time/adjunct (both women). *Students:* 88 full-time (48 women), 45 part-time (30 women); includes 3 minority (2 Hispanic/Latino; 1 Two or more races, non-Hispanic/Latino). Average age 24. 564 applicants, 13% accepted, 45 enrolled. In 2013, 44 doctorates awarded. *Entrance requirements:* Additional exam requirements/recommendations for international students: Required—TOEFL (minimum score 550 paper-based; 79 iBT). Electronic applications accepted. *Expenses:* Contact institution. *Financial support:* Federal Work-Study, scholarships/grants, and health care benefits available. Support available to part-time students. Financial award application deadline: 11/1; financial award applicants required to submit FAFSA. *Unit head:* Dr. Michele Thorman, Director, 608-785-8466, E-mail: thorman.mich@uwlax.edu. *Application contact:* Corey Sjoquist, Director of Admissions, 608-785-8939, E-mail: admissions@uwlax.edu.
Website: http://www.uwlax.edu/pt/

University of Wisconsin–Milwaukee, Graduate School, College of Health Sciences, Doctor of Physical Therapy Program, Milwaukee, WI 53201-0413. Offers DPT. *Accreditation:* APTA. *Students:* 69 full-time (45 women), 1 (woman) part-time; includes 6 minority (4 Asian, non-Hispanic/Latino; 2 Two or more races, non-Hispanic/Latino). Average age 26. 3 applicants. *Degree requirements:* For doctorate, thesis/dissertation optional. *Entrance requirements:* For doctorate, GRE General Test, minimum GPA of 3.0. Additional exam requirements/recommendations for international students: Required—TOEFL (minimum score 550 paper-based; 79 iBT), IELTS (minimum score 6.5). *Financial support:* In 2013–14, 1 teaching assistantship was awarded; fellowships, research assistantships, and project assistantships also available. *Unit head:* Kristian O'Connor, Department Chair, 414-229-2680, E-mail: krisocon@uwm.edu. *Application contact:* General Information Contact, 414-229-4982, Fax: 414-229-6967, E-mail: gradschool@uwm.edu.

Utica College, Department of Physical Therapy, Utica, NY 13502-4892. Offers DPT, TDPT. *Accreditation:* APTA. Part-time and evening/weekend programs available. Postbaccalaureate distance learning degree programs offered (minimal on-campus study). *Faculty:* 10 full-time (4 women). *Students:* 81 full-time (44 women), 319 part-time (210 women); includes 211 minority (21 Black or African American, non-Hispanic/Latino; 180 Asian, non-Hispanic/Latino; 7 Hispanic/Latino; 3 Two or more races, non-Hispanic/Latino), 3 international. Average age 36. In 2013, 241 doctorates awarded. *Degree requirements:* For doctorate, comprehensive exam, thesis/dissertation (for some programs). *Entrance requirements:* For doctorate, GRE, MCAT, DAT or OPT, BS, minimum GPA of 3.0. Additional exam requirements/recommendations for international students: Required—TOEFL (minimum score 525 paper-based). *Application deadline:* Applications are processed on a rolling basis. Application fee: $50. Electronic applications accepted. *Expenses:* Contact institution. *Financial support:* Career-related internships or fieldwork, scholarships/grants, tuition waivers (partial), and unspecified assistantships available. Support available to part-time students. Financial award application deadline: 3/15; financial award applicants required to submit FAFSA. *Faculty research:* Forensic paleopathology, biomechanical analysis of movement, neuronal plasticity, somatosensory mechanotransduction. *Unit head:* Dr. Shauna Malta, Director, 315-792-3313, E-mail: smalta@utica.edu. *Application contact:* John D. Rowe, Director of Graduate Admissions, 315-792-3824, Fax: 315-792-3003, E-mail: jrowe@utica.edu.

Virginia Commonwealth University, Graduate School, School of Allied Health Professions, Department of Physical Therapy, Richmond, VA 23284-9005. Offers advanced physical therapy (DPT); entry-level physical therapy (DPT); health related sciences (PhD); physiology/physical therapy (PhD). *Accreditation:* APTA (one or more programs are accredited). *Degree requirements:* For doctorate, thesis/dissertation. *Entrance requirements:* For doctorate, GRE General Test, Physical Therapist Centralized Application Service (PTCAS). Additional exam requirements/recommendations for international students: Required—TOEFL (minimum score 600 paper-based; 100 iBT). Electronic applications accepted. *Faculty research:* Eye movement, bilabyrinthectomy on ferret muscle fiber typing, neck disability index, cost-effective care, training effect on muscle.

Virginia Commonwealth University, Medical College of Virginia-Professional Programs, School of Medicine, School of Medicine Graduate Programs, Department of Physiology and Biophysics, Richmond, VA 23284-9005. Offers physical therapy (PhD); physiology (MS, PhD); MD/PhD. Terminal master's awarded for partial completion of doctoral program. *Degree requirements:* For master's, thesis; for doctorate, thesis/dissertation, comprehensive oral and written exams. *Entrance requirements:* For master's, GRE General Test, MCAT, or DAT; for doctorate, GRE, MCAT or DAT. Additional exam requirements/recommendations for international students: Required—TOEFL (minimum score 600 paper-based; 100 iBT). Electronic applications accepted.

Walsh University, Graduate Studies, Program in Physical Therapy, North Canton, OH 44720-3396. Offers DPT. *Accreditation:* APTA. *Faculty:* 7 full-time (5 women), 10 part-time/adjunct (5 women). *Students:* 92 full-time (66 women); includes 1 minority (Black or African American, non-Hispanic/Latino). Average age 24. 149 applicants, 40% accepted, 32 enrolled. In 2013, 29 doctorates awarded. *Degree requirements:* For doctorate, comprehensive exam, research project, 3 clinical placements. *Entrance requirements:* For doctorate, GRE General Test (minimum scores: verbal 150; quantitative 150, or combined score of 291), previous coursework in anatomy, human physiology, exercise physiology, chemistry, statistics, psychology, biology, and physics; minimum GPA of 3.0. Additional exam requirements/recommendations for international students: Required—TOEFL (minimum score 500 paper-based; 61 iBT). *Application deadline:* For fall admission, 7/15 priority date for domestic students. Applications are processed on a rolling basis. Application fee: $0. Electronic applications accepted. *Expenses:* Contact institution. *Financial support:* In 2013–14, 8 students received support, including 18 fellowships (averaging $1,000 per year), 5 research assistantships with partial tuition reimbursements available (averaging $12,545 per year), 3 teaching assistantships (averaging $2,163 per year); unspecified assistantships also available. Support available to part-time students. Financial award application deadline: 12/31; financial award applicants required to submit FAFSA. *Faculty research:* Interventions, diagnosis, adherence, advancing and improving learning with information technology, consumer-driven healthcare, service provider training and customer satisfaction. *Total annual research expenditures:* $600. *Unit head:* Dr. Chad Cook, Chair, 330-490-7370, Fax: 330-490-7371, E-mail: ccook@walsh.edu. *Application contact:* Audra Dice, Graduate Admissions Counselor, 330-490-7181, Fax: 330-244-4680, E-mail: adice@walsh.edu.

Washington University in St. Louis, School of Medicine, Program in Physical Therapy, Saint Louis, MO 63108. Offers DPT, PPDPT. *Accreditation:* APTA (one or more programs are accredited). Part-time and evening/weekend programs available. Postbaccalaureate distance learning degree programs offered (minimal on-campus study). *Degree requirements:* For doctorate, thesis/dissertation (for some programs). *Entrance requirements:* For doctorate, GRE. Additional exam requirements/recommendations for international students: Required—TOEFL (minimum score 600 paper-based; 100 iBT), TWE (minimum score 5). Electronic applications accepted. *Expenses:* Contact institution. *Faculty research:* Movement and movement dysfunction.

Wayne State University, Eugene Applebaum College of Pharmacy and Health Sciences, Department of Health Care Sciences, Program in Physical Therapy, Detroit, MI 48202. Offers DPT. *Accreditation:* APTA. Part-time programs available. *Faculty:* 10

full-time (5 women), 18 part-time/adjunct (15 women). *Students:* 137 full-time (87 women), 13 part-time (7 women); includes 29 minority (6 Black or African American, non-Hispanic/Latino; 1 American Indian or Alaska Native, non-Hispanic/Latino; 14 Asian, non-Hispanic/Latino; 4 Hispanic/Latino; 1 Native Hawaiian or other Pacific Islander, non-Hispanic/Latino; 3 Two or more races, non-Hispanic/Latino), 8 international. Average age 27. 208 applicants, 18% accepted, 36 enrolled. In 2013, 41 doctorates awarded. *Entrance requirements:* For doctorate, interview; minimum of 90 undergraduate credit hours with minimum GPA of 3.0 (calculated by PTCAS) and no less than a C in prerequisite courses; PTCAS application; essay. Additional exam requirements/recommendations for international students: Required—TOEFL (minimum score 550 paper-based; 79 iBT), Michigan English Language Assessment Battery (minimum score 85); Recommended—IELTS (minimum score 6.5), TWE (minimum score 5.5). *Application deadline:* For fall admission, 10/15 for domestic and international students. Applications are processed on a rolling basis. Application fee: $0. Electronic applications accepted. *Expenses:* Contact institution. *Financial support:* In 2013–14, 49 students received support. Scholarships/grants available. Financial award application deadline: 3/31; financial award applicants required to submit FAFSA. *Faculty research:* Muscle dysfunction, response to immobility and exercise. *Unit head:* Dr. Sara Maher, Associate Professor/Clinical and Program Director, 313-577-5630. *Application contact:* Dr. Vicky Pardo, Assistant Professor of Physical Therapy/Chair of Admissions Committee, 313-577-9166, Fax: 313-577-8685.
Website: http://pt.cphs.wayne.edu/

Western Carolina University, Graduate School, College of Health and Human Sciences, Department of Physical Therapy, Cullowhee, NC 28723. Offers MPT, DPT. *Accreditation:* APTA. *Degree requirements:* For master's, comprehensive exam. *Entrance requirements:* For master's, GRE General Test, appropriate undergraduate degree with minimum GPA of 3.0, 3 letters of recommendation. Additional exam requirements/recommendations for international students: Required—TOEFL (minimum score 550 paper-based; 79 iBT). *Faculty research:* Bone density, disability in older adults, neuroanatomy, intervention of musculoskeletal conditions.

Western Kentucky University, Graduate Studies, College of Health and Human Services, Department of Allied Health, Bowling Green, KY 42101. Offers physical therapy (DPT).

Western University of Health Sciences, College of Allied Health Professions, Program in Physical Therapy, Pomona, CA 91766-1854. Offers DPT. *Accreditation:* APTA. *Faculty:* 10 full-time (7 women), 2 part-time/adjunct (both women). *Students:* 157 full-time (90 women), 23 part-time (12 women); includes 81 minority (4 Black or African American, non-Hispanic/Latino; 50 Asian, non-Hispanic/Latino; 22 Hispanic/Latino; 5 Two or more races, non-Hispanic/Latino), 2 international. Average age 29. 877 applicants, 14% accepted, 54 enrolled. In 2013, 60 doctorates awarded. *Degree requirements:* For doctorate, comprehensive exam (for some programs). *Entrance requirements:* For doctorate, GRE, bachelor's degree, letters of recommendation, minimum GPA of 2.8, volunteer or paid work experience. *Application deadline:* For fall admission, 11/1 priority date for domestic students, 11/1 for international students. Application fee: $60. Electronic applications accepted. *Expenses:* Contact institution. *Financial support:* Institutionally sponsored loans, scholarships/grants, and veterans educational benefits available. Financial award application deadline: 3/2; financial award applicants required to submit FAFSA. *Unit head:* Dr. Dee Schilling, Chair, 909-469-3526, Fax: 909-469-5692, E-mail: dschilling@westernu.edu. *Application contact:* Karen Hutton-Lopez, Director of Admissions, 909-469-5335, Fax: 909-469-5570, E-mail: admissions@westernu.edu.
Website: http://www.westernu.edu/allied-health/allied-health-dpt/

West Virginia University, School of Medicine, Graduate Programs in Human Performance, Division of Physical Therapy, Morgantown, WV 26506. Offers DPT. *Accreditation:* APTA. Evening/weekend programs available. Postbaccalaureate distance learning degree programs offered (minimal on-campus study). *Entrance requirements:* For doctorate, GRE, minimum cumulative GPA and prerequisite science GPA of 3.0; volunteer/work experience in physical therapy; letters of recommendation. *Expenses:* Contact institution.

Wheeling Jesuit University, Department of Physical Therapy, Wheeling, WV 26003-6295. Offers DPT. *Accreditation:* APTA. *Degree requirements:* For doctorate, comprehensive exam, thesis/dissertation. *Entrance requirements:* For doctorate, GRE, minimum GPA of 3.0. Additional exam requirements/recommendations for international students: Required—TOEFL (minimum score 650 paper-based). Electronic applications accepted. Application fee is waived when completed online. *Expenses:* Contact institution. *Faculty research:* Service-learning, clinical prediction rules, ergonomics, public health, pediatrics.

Wichita State University, Graduate School, College of Health Professions, Department of Physical Therapy, Wichita, KS 67260. Offers DPT. *Accreditation:* APTA. *Unit head:* Dr. Robert C. Manske, Chair, 316-978-3604, Fax: 316-978-3025, E-mail: robert.manske@wichita.edu. *Application contact:* Jordan Oleson, Admissions Coordinator, 316-978-3095, Fax: 316-978-3253, E-mail: jordan.oleson@wichita.edu.
Website: http://www.wichita.edu/

Widener University, School of Human Service Professions, Institute for Physical Therapy Education, Chester, PA 19013-5792. Offers MS, DPT. *Accreditation:* APTA. *Faculty:* 8 full-time (5 women), 1 (woman) part-time/adjunct. *Students:* 218 full-time (172 women), 21 part-time (12 women); includes 10 minority (3 Black or African American, non-Hispanic/Latino; 1 American Indian or Alaska Native, non-Hispanic/Latino; 5 Asian, non-Hispanic/Latino; 1 Hispanic/Latino). 82 applicants, 93% accepted. In 2013, 53 doctorates awarded. *Degree requirements:* For master's, thesis. *Entrance requirements:* For master's, GRE. *Application deadline:* For fall admission, 1/30 for domestic students. Applications are processed on a rolling basis. Application fee: $40. *Expenses:* Contact institution. *Financial support:* Teaching assistantships, Federal Work-Study, institutionally sponsored loans, and scholarships/grants available. Financial award application deadline: 5/1; financial award applicants required to submit FAFSA. *Faculty research:* Social support, aquatics, children and adults with movement dysfunction, physical therapy modalities. *Unit head:* Dr. Robin L. Dole, Associate Dean and Director, 610-499-1159, Fax: 610-499-1231, E-mail: robin.l.dole@widener.edu. *Application contact:* 610-499-4372, E-mail: gradmc@mail.widener.edu.

Winston-Salem State University, Department of Physical Therapy, Winston-Salem, NC 27110-0003. Offers MPT. *Accreditation:* APTA. *Entrance requirements:* For master's, GRE, 3 letters of recommendation. Electronic applications accepted. *Faculty research:* Tissue healing; neuroimaging with functional recovery; visual, proprioceptive and vestibular sensor inputs roles.

Youngstown State University, Graduate School, Bitonte College of Health and Human Services, Department of Physical Therapy, Youngstown, OH 44555-0001. Offers DPT. *Accreditation:* APTA. *Entrance requirements:* Additional exam requirements/recommendations for international students: Required—TOEFL.

Physician Assistant Studies

Albany Medical College, Center for Physician Assistant Studies, Albany, NY 12208-3479. Offers MS. *Accreditation:* ARC-PA. *Degree requirements:* For master's, comprehensive exam, clinical portfolio. *Entrance requirements:* For master's, GRE. Additional exam requirements/recommendations for international students: Required—TOEFL. Electronic applications accepted. *Expenses:* Contact institution. *Faculty research:* Genetics, education, informatics.

Alderson Broaddus University, Program in Physician Assistant Studies, Philippi, WV 26416. Offers MPAS. *Degree requirements:* For master's, comprehensive exam, thesis. *Entrance requirements:* For master's, minimum 60 semester hours plus specific science. Electronic applications accepted.

Arcadia University, Graduate Studies, Department of Medical Science and Community Health, Glenside, PA 19038-3295. Offers health education (MA, MSHE); physician assistant (MM Sc); MM Sc/MAHE; MM Sc/MSPH. *Entrance requirements:* For master's, GRE General Test or MCAT. Additional exam requirements/recommendations for international students: Required—TOEFL. *Expenses:* Contact institution.

A.T. Still University, Arizona School of Health Sciences, Mesa, AZ 85206. Offers advanced occupational therapy (MS); advanced physician assistant studies (MS); athletic training (MS); audiology (Au D); health sciences (DHSc); human movement (MS); occupational therapy (MS, DOT); physical therapy (DPT); physician assistant (MS); transitional audiology (Au D); transitional physical therapy (DPT). *Accreditation:* AOTA (one or more programs are accredited); ASHA. Part-time and evening/weekend programs available. Postbaccalaureate distance learning degree programs offered (minimal on-campus study). *Faculty:* 47 full-time (27 women), 279 part-time/adjunct (173 women). *Students:* 531 full-time (354 women), 865 part-time (547 women); includes 315 minority (79 Black or African American, non-Hispanic/Latino; 10 American Indian or Alaska Native, non-Hispanic/Latino; 114 Asian, non-Hispanic/Latino; 83 Hispanic/Latino; 6 Native Hawaiian or other Pacific Islander, non-Hispanic/Latino; 23 Two or more races, non-Hispanic/Latino), 82 international. Average age 36. 3,325 applicants, 14% accepted, 329 enrolled. In 2013, 252 master's, 370 doctorates awarded. *Degree requirements:* For master's, thesis (for some programs); for doctorate, thesis/dissertation (for some programs). *Entrance requirements:* For master's, GRE General Test; for doctorate, GRE, Evaluation of Practicing Audiologists Capabilities (Au D), Physical Therapist Evaluation Tool (DPT), current state licensure, master's degree or equivalent (Au D). Additional exam requirements/recommendations for international students: Required—TOEFL (minimum score 550 paper-based; 80 iBT). *Application deadline:* For fall admission, 8/1 for domestic and international students. Applications are processed on a rolling basis. Application fee: $70. Electronic applications accepted. *Expenses:* Contact institution. *Financial support:* In 2013–14, 151 students received support. Federal Work-Study and scholarships/grants available. Financial award application deadline: 5/1; financial award applicants required to submit FAFSA. *Faculty research:* Pediatric sport-related concussion, adolescent athlete health-related quality of life; geriatric and pediatric well-being, pain management for participation, practice-based research network, BMI and dental caries. *Total annual research expenditures:* $174,826. *Unit head:* Dr. Randy Danielsen, Dean, 480-219-6000, Fax: 480-219-6110, E-mail: rdanielsen@atsu.edu. *Application contact:* Donna Sparks, Associate Director, Admissions Processing, 660-626-2117, Fax: 660-626-2969, E-mail: admissions@atsu.edu.
Website: http://www.atsu.edu/ashs

Augsburg College, Program in Physicians Assistant Studies, Minneapolis, MN 55454-1351. Offers MS. *Accreditation:* ARC-PA.

Baldwin Wallace University, Graduate Programs, Physician Assistant Program, Berea, OH 44017-2088. Offers MMS. *Faculty:* 5 full-time (2 women), 3 part-time/adjunct (1 woman). *Students:* 19 full-time (15 women); includes 1 minority (Two or more races, non-Hispanic/Latino). Average age 24. 450 applicants, 9% accepted, 25 enrolled. *Degree requirements:* For master's, comprehensive exam (for some programs), thesis or alternative, capstone project. *Entrance requirements:* For master's, GRE, 3 letters of recommendation, personal statement, 40 hours of shadowing. Additional exam requirements/recommendations for international students: Required—TOEFL. *Application deadline:* For spring admission, 1/31 for domestic students. *Expenses:* Contact institution. *Unit head:* Jared R. Pennington, Department Chair, 440-826-2221, E-mail: jpenning@bw.edu. *Application contact:* Jared R. Pennington, Program Director and Department Chair, 440-826-2221, E-mail: jpenning@bw.edu.
Website: http://www.bw.edu/PA

Barry University, Physician Assistant Program, Miami Shores, FL 33161-6695. Offers MCMS. *Accreditation:* ARC-PA. *Entrance requirements:* For master's, GRE General Test. Electronic applications accepted.

Baylor College of Medicine, School of Allied Health Sciences, Physician Assistant Program, Houston, TX 77030-3498. Offers MS. *Accreditation:* ARC-PA. *Degree requirements:* For master's, comprehensive exam, thesis. *Entrance requirements:* For master's, GRE General Test, bachelor's degree; minimum GPA of 3.0; prerequisite courses in general chemistry, organic chemistry, microbiology, general psychology, human anatomy, human physiology, statistics, and expository writing. Additional exam requirements/recommendations for international students: Required—TOEFL. Electronic applications accepted. *Expenses:* Contact institution. *Faculty research:* Cultural competency attainment, health behavioral counseling skills mastery, readiness for inter-professional learning, probability error in differential diagnosis, shared decision-making.

Bay Path College, Program in Physician Assistant Studies, Longmeadow, MA 01106-2292. Offers MS. *Students:* 48 full-time (27 women); includes 12 minority (2 Black or African American, non-Hispanic/Latino; 4 Asian, non-Hispanic/Latino; 6 Hispanic/Latino). Average age 29. 31 applicants, 84% accepted, 24 enrolled. *Degree requirements:* For master's, 116 credits with minimum cumulative GPA of 3.0 and no grade below a B. *Entrance requirements:* For master's, minimum of 500 hours of patient contact hours; minimum of 24 hours of documented PA shadowing; all prerequisite courses completed with minimum C grade and cumulative GPA of 3.0. Additional exam

requirements/recommendations for international students: Required—TOEFL. *Application deadline:* For fall admission, 10/1 for domestic students. Application fee: $45. *Unit head:* Dr. Jennifer Hixon, Director, 413-565-1206. *Application contact:* Lisa Adams, Director of Graduate Admissions, 413-565-1317, Fax: 413-565-1250, E-mail: ladams@baypath.edu.
Website: http://graduate.baypath.edu/Graduate-Programs/Programs-On-Campus/MS-Programs/Physician-Assistant-Studies

Bethel University, Graduate Programs, McKenzie, TN 38201. Offers administration and supervision (MA Ed); business administration (MBA); conflict resolution (MA); physician assistant studies (MS). Part-time and evening/weekend programs available. *Degree requirements:* For master's, thesis (for some programs). *Entrance requirements:* For master's, GRE General Test or MAT, minimum undergraduate GPA of 2.5.

Bethel University, Graduate School, St. Paul, MN 55112-6999. Offers autism spectrum disorders (Certificate); business administration (MBA); communication (MA); counseling psychology (MA); educational leadership (Ed D); gerontology (MA); international baccalaureate education (Certificate); K-12 education (MA); literacy education (MA, Certificate); nurse educator (Certificate); nurse leader (Certificate); nurse-midwifery (MS); nursing (MS); physician assistant (MS); postsecondary teaching (Certificate); special education (MA); strategic leadership (MA); teaching (MA). Part-time and evening/weekend programs available. Postbaccalaureate distance learning degree programs offered (no on-campus study). *Faculty:* 13 full-time (7 women), 89 part-time/adjunct (43 women). *Students:* 692 full-time (457 women), 573 part-time (371 women); includes 170 minority (86 Black or African American, non-Hispanic/Latino; 1 American Indian or Alaska Native, non-Hispanic/Latino; 49 Asian, non-Hispanic/Latino; 20 Hispanic/Latino; 1 Native Hawaiian or other Pacific Islander, non-Hispanic/Latino; 13 Two or more races, non-Hispanic/Latino), 21 international. Average age 37. In 2013, 166 master's, 9 doctorates, 11 other advanced degrees awarded. *Degree requirements:* For master's, comprehensive exam (for some programs), thesis (for some programs); for doctorate, comprehensive exam, thesis/dissertation. *Entrance requirements:* Additional exam requirements/recommendations for international students: Required—TOEFL (minimum score 550 paper-based; 80 iBT). *Application deadline:* Applications are processed on a rolling basis. Electronic applications accepted. Tuition and fees vary according to course load, degree level and program. *Financial support:* Teaching assistantships, career-related internships or fieldwork, and scholarships/grants available. Support available to part-time students. Financial award applicants required to submit FAFSA. *Unit head:* Dick Crombie, Vice-President/Dean, 651-635-8000, Fax: 651-635-8004, E-mail: gs@bethel.edu. *Application contact:* Director of Admissions, 651-635-8000, Fax: 651-635-8004, E-mail: gs@bethel.edu.
Website: http://gs.bethel.edu/

Boston University, School of Medicine, Division of Graduate Medical Sciences, Physician Assistant Program, Boston, MA 02215. Offers MS. *Students:* 24. *Entrance requirements:* For master's, GRE, three letters of recommendation. Additional exam requirements/recommendations for international students: Required—TOEFL (minimum score 550 paper-based; 80 iBT). *Application deadline:* For spring admission, 10/1 for domestic students. Electronic applications accepted. *Expenses: Tuition:* Full-time $43,970; part-time $1374 per credit hour. *Required fees:* $60 per semester. Tuition and fees vary according to class time, course level and program. *Unit head:* Madeline Brisotti, Administrative Coordinator, 617-638-5744, E-mail: paoffice@bu.edu. *Application contact:* GMS Admissions Office, 617-638-5255, Fax: 617-638-5740, E-mail: natashah@bu.edu.
Website: http://www.bu.edu/paprogram/

Butler University, College of Pharmacy and Health Sciences, Indianapolis, IN 46208-3485. Offers pharmaceutical science (MS, Pharm D); physician assistance studies (MS). *Accreditation:* ACPE (one or more programs are accredited). Part-time and evening/weekend programs available. *Faculty:* 6 full-time (2 women). *Students:* 296 full-time (196 women), 12 part-time (7 women); includes 24 minority (7 Black or African American, non-Hispanic/Latino; 1 American Indian or Alaska Native, non-Hispanic/Latino; 10 Asian, non-Hispanic/Latino; 4 Hispanic/Latino; 2 Two or more races, non-Hispanic/Latino), 11 international. Average age 24. 52 applicants, 6% accepted, 2 enrolled. In 2013, 50 master's awarded. *Degree requirements:* For master's, research paper or thesis. *Application deadline:* For fall admission, 8/1 priority date for domestic students; for spring admission, 12/15 for domestic students. Applications are processed on a rolling basis. Application fee: $35. Electronic applications accepted. *Expenses:* Contact institution. *Financial support:* Applicants required to submit FAFSA. *Unit head:* Dr. Mary Andritz, Dean, 317-940-8056, E-mail: mandritz@butler.edu. *Application contact:* Diane Dubord, Graduate Student Services Specialist, 317-940-8107, E-mail: ddubord@butler.edu.
Website: http://www.butler.edu/academics/graduate-cophs/

Carroll University, Program in Physician Assistant Studies, Waukesha, WI 53186-5593. Offers MS. *Entrance requirements:* For master's, GRE, three letters of reference, personal essay, documentation of college or community service activities, transcripts. Additional exam requirements/recommendations for international students: Required—TOEFL.

Central Michigan University, College of Graduate Studies, The Herbert H. and Grace A. Dow College of Health Professions, School of Rehabilitation and Medical Sciences, Mount Pleasant, MI 48859. Offers physical therapy (DPT); physician assistant (MS). *Accreditation:* APTA; ARC-PA. *Degree requirements:* For master's, thesis or alternative; for doctorate, thesis/dissertation or alternative. *Entrance requirements:* For master's and doctorate, GRE. Electronic applications accepted.

Chapman University, Schmid College of Science and Technology, Physician Assistant Studies Program, Orange, CA 92866. Offers MMS. Tuition and fees vary according to program. *Unit head:* Michael Estrada, Director, E-mail: paprogram@chapman.edu. *Application contact:* Saundra Hoover, Director of Graduate Admissions, 714-997-6786, Fax: 714-997-6713, E-mail: shoover@chapman.edu.
Website: http://www.chapman.edu/scst/crean-school-health/academic-programs/physician-assistant/index.aspx

Chatham University, Program in Physician Assistant Studies, Pittsburgh, PA 15232-2826. Offers MPAS. *Accreditation:* ARC-PA. *Faculty:* 10 full-time (6 women), 8 part-time/adjunct (7 women). *Students:* 150 full-time (118 women), 1 (woman) part-time; includes 19 minority (9 Black or African American, non-Hispanic/Latino; 4 Asian, non-Hispanic/Latino; 5 Hispanic/Latino; 1 Two or more races, non-Hispanic/Latino), 11 international. Average age 27. 1,003 applicants, 15% accepted, 77 enrolled. In 2013, 65 master's awarded. *Degree requirements:* For master's, thesis, clinical experience, research project. *Entrance requirements:* For master's, community service, minimum GPA of 3.0, health science work or shadowing, volunteer work experience, PA shadowing form, 3 references. Additional exam requirements/recommendations for international students: Required—TOEFL (minimum score 600 paper-based; 100 iBT), IELTS (minimum score 7), TWE. *Application deadline:* For fall admission, 10/1 priority date for domestic and international students. Application fee: $0. Electronic applications accepted. *Expenses:* Contact institution. *Financial support:* Career-related internships or fieldwork available. Financial award applicants required to submit FAFSA. *Faculty research:* Complementary and alternative medicine, education methods, physician assistant practice. *Unit head:* Carl Garrubba, Director, 412-365-1425, Fax: 412-365-1213, E-mail: cgarrubba@chatham.edu. *Application contact:* Maureen Stokan, Assistant Director of Graduate Admission, 412-365-2988, Fax: 412-365-1609, E-mail: gradadmissions@chatham.edu.
Website: http://www.chatham.edu/departments/healthmgmt/graduate/pa

Christian Brothers University, School of Sciences, Memphis, TN 38104-5581. Offers physician assistant studies (MS).

Clarkson University, Graduate School, School of Arts and Sciences, Department of Physician Assistant Studies, Potsdam, NY 13699. Offers MS. *Faculty:* 6 full-time (3 women), 2 part-time/adjunct (1 woman). *Students:* 36 full-time (26 women); includes 4 minority (3 Asian, non-Hispanic/Latino; 1 Hispanic/Latino). Average age 27. 26 applicants, 81% accepted, 20 enrolled. *Entrance requirements:* Additional exam requirements/recommendations for international students: Required—TOEFL. *Application deadline:* Applications are processed on a rolling basis. Application fee: $185. Electronic applications accepted. *Expenses: Tuition:* Full-time $15,888; part-time $1324 per credit. *Required fees:* $295 per semester. *Financial support:* Scholarships/grants and tuition waivers (partial) available. *Unit head:* Dr. Michael Whitehead, Chair, 315-268-7942, Fax: 315-268-7944, E-mail: mwhitehe@clarkson.edu. *Application contact:* Jennifer Reed, Graduate Coordinator, School of Arts and Sciences, 315-268-3802, Fax: 315-268-3989, E-mail: sciencegrad@clarkson.edu.
Website: http://www.clarkson.edu/pa/

Cleveland State University, College of Graduate Studies, College of Sciences and Health Professions, School of Health Sciences, Cleveland, OH 44115. Offers health sciences (MS); occupational therapy (MOT); physical therapy (DPT); physician's assistant (MS); speech pathology and audiology (MA). Part-time programs available. Postbaccalaureate distance learning degree programs offered (no on-campus study). *Faculty:* 22 full-time (15 women), 7 part-time/adjunct (6 women). *Students:* 261 full-time (188 women), 111 part-time (87 women); includes 39 minority (20 Black or African American, non-Hispanic/Latino; 12 Asian, non-Hispanic/Latino; 4 Hispanic/Latino; 3 Two or more races, non-Hispanic/Latino), 6 international. Average age 28. 527 applicants, 35% accepted, 90 enrolled. In 2013, 82 master's, 23 doctorates awarded. *Degree requirements:* For master's, comprehensive exam (for some programs), thesis optional, clinical/fieldwork education. *Entrance requirements:* For master's, GRE, minimum cumulative GPA of 3.0; for doctorate, GRE, BA, minimum cumulative GPA of 3.0. Additional exam requirements/recommendations for international students: Required—TOEFL (minimum score 523 paper-based), IELTS (minimum score 6). *Application deadline:* For fall admission, 7/1 for domestic and international students; for spring admission, 3/15 for domestic and international students. Application fee: $55. *Expenses:* Tuition, state resident: full-time $8335; part-time $521 per credit hour. Tuition, nonresident: full-time $15,670; part-time $979 per credit hour. *Required fees:* $50; $25 per semester. *Financial support:* In 2013–14, 22 students received support, including 2 research assistantships, 20 teaching assistantships. Financial award applicants required to submit FAFSA. *Faculty research:* Psychosocial needs of children, use of technology with disabilities, effects of stroke on gait, communication variables with accentedness, grasp patterns of possums. *Unit head:* Dr. John J. Bazyk, Director of School of Health Sciences, 216-687-2379, Fax: 216-687-9316, E-mail: j.bazyk@csuohio.edu. *Application contact:* Karen Armstrong, Administrative Secretary, 216-687-3567, Fax: 216-687-9316, E-mail: k.bradley@csuohio.edu.
Website: http://www.csuohio.edu/sciences/dept/healthsciences/

Daemen College, Physician Assistant Department, Amherst, NY 14226-3592. Offers MS. *Accreditation:* ARC-PA. *Degree requirements:* For master's, 30 credits (40 weeks) in clinical clerk-ships; 2 research courses; 3 final year seminars. *Entrance requirements:* For master's, minimum GPA of 3.0 overall and in math and science prerequisites; 120 hours of direct patient contact; admission to professional phase. Additional exam requirements/recommendations for international students: Required—TOEFL (minimum score 500 paper-based; 63 iBT), IELTS (minimum score 5.5). Electronic applications accepted.

DeSales University, Graduate Division, Division of Healthcare and Natural Sciences, Program in Physician Assistant Studies, Center Valley, PA 18034-9568. Offers MSPAS. *Accreditation:* ARC-PA. *Faculty:* 10 full-time (7 women). *Students:* 70 full-time. 1,159 applicants, 5% accepted, 26 enrolled. In 2013, 40 master's awarded. *Degree requirements:* For master's, comprehensive exam. *Entrance requirements:* For master's, GRE General Test. Additional exam requirements/recommendations for international students: Required—TOEFL (minimum score 610 paper-based; 102 iBT). *Application deadline:* For fall admission, 1/15 for domestic and international students. Electronic applications accepted. *Expenses: Tuition:* Part-time $790 per credit. *Financial support:* Applicants required to submit FAFSA. *Unit head:* Dr. Wayne Stuart, Director, 610-282-1100 Ext. 1344, Fax: 610-282-1893, E-mail: wayne.stuart@desales.edu. *Application contact:* Anne Lobley, Program Assistant, 610-282-1100 Ext. 2780, E-mail: anne.lobley@desales.edu.

Des Moines University, College of Health Sciences, Physician Assistant Program, Des Moines, IA 50312-4104. Offers MS. *Accreditation:* ARC-PA. *Degree requirements:* For master's, research project. *Entrance requirements:* For master's, GRE, interview, minimum GPA of 2.8, related work experience. Additional exam requirements/recommendations for international students: Recommended—TOEFL. Electronic applications accepted. *Expenses:* Contact institution.

Drexel University, College of Nursing and Health Professions, Physician Assistant Department, Philadelphia, PA 19104-2875. Offers MHS. *Accreditation:* ARC-PA. Electronic applications accepted.

Duke University, School of Medicine, Physician Assistant Program, Durham, NC 27701. Offers MHS. *Accreditation:* ARC-PA. *Faculty:* 18 full-time (15 women), 5 part-time/adjunct (4 women). *Students:* 172 full-time (134 women); includes 43 minority (11 Black or African American, non-Hispanic/Latino; 14 Asian, non-Hispanic/Latino; 17 Hispanic/Latino; 1 Native Hawaiian or other Pacific Islander, non-Hispanic/Latino). Average age 28. 1,020 applicants, 11% accepted, 88 enrolled. In 2013, 79 master's awarded. *Entrance requirements:* For master's, GRE, minimum of 5 courses in biological sciences with courses in anatomy, physiology and microbiology, 8 undergraduate hours in chemistry and statistics, patient care experience. *Application deadline:* For fall admission, 10/1 for domestic students. Application fee: $50. Electronic applications accepted. *Expenses:* Contact institution. *Financial support:* In 2013–14, 72 students received support. Fellowships, research assistantships, teaching assistantships, institutionally sponsored loans, and scholarships/grants available. Financial award application deadline: 5/1; financial award applicants required to submit FAFSA. *Unit head:* Karen J. Hills, Program Director/Associate Professor, 919-681-3161, Fax: 919-681-9666, E-mail: karen.hills@duke.edu. *Application contact:* Wendy Z. Elwell, Program Coordinator, 919-668-4710, Fax: 919-681-9666, E-mail: wendy.elwell@duke.edu.
Website: http://paprogram.mc.duke.edu/

Duquesne University, John G. Rangos, Sr. School of Health Sciences, Pittsburgh, PA 15282-0001. Offers health management systems (MHMS); occupational therapy (MS, OTD); physical therapy (DPT); physician assistant studies (MPAS); rehabilitation science (MS, PhD); speech-language pathology (MS); MBA/MHMS. *Accreditation:*

AOTA (one or more programs are accredited); APTA (one or more programs are accredited); ASHA. Postbaccalaureate distance learning degree programs offered (minimal on-campus study). *Faculty:* 41 full-time (29 women), 32 part-time/adjunct (15 women). *Students:* 232 full-time (174 women), 14 part-time (7 women); includes 12 minority (2 Black or African American, non-Hispanic/Latino; 7 Asian, non-Hispanic/Latino; 1 Hispanic/Latino; 2 Two or more races, non-Hispanic/Latino), 7 international. Average age 23. 951 applicants, 11% accepted, 35 enrolled. In 2013, 119 master's, 40 doctorates awarded. *Degree requirements:* For doctorate, comprehensive exam (for some programs), thesis/dissertation (for some programs). *Entrance requirements:* For master's, GRE General Test (speech-language pathology), 3 letters of recommendation; minimum GPA of 2.75 (health management systems), 3.0 (speech-language pathology); for doctorate, GRE General Test (for physical therapy and rehabilitation science), 3 letters of recommendation, minimum GPA of 3.0, personal interview. Additional exam requirements/recommendations for international students: Required—TOEFL (minimum score 550 paper-based; 90 iBT). *Application deadline:* For fall admission, 2/1 for domestic and international students; for spring admission, 7/1 for domestic and international students. Applications are processed on a rolling basis. Electronic applications accepted. *Expenses:* Contact institution. *Financial support:* Federal Work-Study available. Financial award applicants required to submit FAFSA. *Faculty research:* Neuronal processing, electrical stimulation on peripheral neuropathy, central nervous system (CNS) stimulatory and inhibitory signals, behavioral genetic methodologies to development disorders of speech, neurogenic communication disorders. *Total annual research expenditures:* $83,650. *Unit head:* Dr. Gregory H. Frazer, Dean, 412-396-5303, Fax: 412-396-5554, E-mail: frazer@duq.edu. *Application contact:* Christopher R. Hilf, Recruiter/Academic Advisor, 412-396-5653, Fax: 412-396-5554, E-mail: hilfc@duq.edu.
Website: http://www.duq.edu/academics/schools/health-sciences

D'Youville College, Physician Assistant Department, Buffalo, NY 14201-1084. Offers MS. *Accreditation:* ARC-PA. *Students:* 160 full-time (106 women), 8 part-time (3 women); includes 13 minority (3 Black or African American, non-Hispanic/Latino; 4 Asian, non-Hispanic/Latino; 3 Hispanic/Latino; 3 Two or more races, non-Hispanic/Latino), 6 international. Average age 26. 275 applicants, 24% accepted, 38 enrolled. In 2013, 39 master's awarded. *Entrance requirements:* For master's, BS, patient contact, 3 letters of recommendation. Additional exam requirements/recommendations for international students: Required—TOEFL (minimum score 500 paper-based). *Application deadline:* For fall admission, 5/1 priority date for international students; for spring admission, 9/1 priority date for international students. Applications are processed on a rolling basis. Application fee: $25. Electronic applications accepted. *Unit head:* Dr. Maureen F. Finney, Chair, 716-829-7730, E-mail: finneym@dyc.edu. *Application contact:* Dr. Stephen Smith, Admissions Director, 716-829-7600, Fax: 716-829-7900, E-mail: admissions@dyc.edu.

East Carolina University, Graduate School, School of Allied Health Sciences, Department of Physician Assistant Studies, Greenville, NC 27858-4353. Offers MS. *Accreditation:* ARC-PA. Application fee: $50. *Expenses:* Tuition, state resident: full-time $4223. Tuition, nonresident: full-time $16,540. *Required fees:* $2184. *Unit head:* Dr. Alan Gindoff, Chair, 252-744-6271, E-mail: gindoffa@ecu.edu. *Application contact:* Dean of Graduate School, 252-328-6012, Fax: 252-328-6071, E-mail: gradschool@ecu.edu.

Eastern Virginia Medical School, Master of Physician Assistant Program, Norfolk, VA 23501-1980. Offers MPA. *Accreditation:* ARC-PA. *Faculty:* 11 full-time (7 women), 2 part-time/adjunct (1 woman). *Students:* 146 full-time (107 women); includes 47 minority (12 Black or African American, non-Hispanic/Latino; 29 Asian, non-Hispanic/Latino; 1 Native Hawaiian or other Pacific Islander, non-Hispanic/Latino; 5 Two or more races, non-Hispanic/Latino). 1,225 applicants, 0% accepted, 85 enrolled. In 2013, 55 master's awarded. *Entrance requirements:* Additional exam requirements/recommendations for international students: Required—TOEFL. *Application deadline:* For spring admission, 3/1 for domestic students. Applications are processed on a rolling basis. Application fee: $60. Electronic applications accepted. *Expenses:* Contact institution. *Financial support:* Applicants required to submit FAFSA. *Unit head:* Dr. Thomas Parish, Director, 757-446-7126, Fax: 757-446-7403, E-mail: parishtg@evms.edu. *Application contact:* Rose Mwayungu, Admissions and Enrollment Manager, 757-446-7153, Fax: 757-446-8915, E-mail: mwayunra@evms.edu.
Website: http://www.evms.edu/education/masters_programs/physician_assistant_program/

Elon University, Program in Physician Assistant Studies, Elon, NC 27244-2010. Offers MS. *Faculty:* 8 full-time (7 women), 6 part-time/adjunct (4 women). *Students:* 37 full-time (33 women); includes 7 minority (1 Black or African American, non-Hispanic/Latino; 1 American Indian or Alaska Native, non-Hispanic/Latino; 2 Asian, non-Hispanic/Latino; 2 Hispanic/Latino; 1 Two or more races, non-Hispanic/Latino). Average age 26. 200 applicants, 24% accepted, 36 enrolled. *Entrance requirements:* Additional exam requirements/recommendations for international students: Required—TOEFL. *Application deadline:* For fall admission, 11/1 for domestic students. Applications are processed on a rolling basis. Application fee: $50. Electronic applications accepted. *Financial support:* Federal Work-Study and scholarships/grants available. Financial award application deadline: 10/1; financial award applicants required to submit FAFSA. *Unit head:* Dr. Elizabeth A. Rogers, 336-278-6400, E-mail: rogers@elon.edu. *Application contact:* Art Fadde, Director of Graduate Admissions, 800-334-8448 Ext. 3, Fax: 336-278-7699, E-mail: afadde@elon.edu.
Website: http://www.elon.edu/e-web/academics/pa/

Emory University, School of Medicine, Programs in Allied Health Professions, Physician Assistant Program, Atlanta, GA 30322. Offers MM Sc. *Accreditation:* ARC-PA. *Faculty:* 8 full-time (7 women), 6 part-time/adjunct (4 women). *Students:* 165 full-time (116 women); includes 38 minority (14 Black or African American, non-Hispanic/Latino; 8 Asian, non-Hispanic/Latino; 12 Hispanic/Latino; 4 Two or more races, non-Hispanic/Latino). Average age 29. 1,280 applicants, 5% accepted, 56 enrolled. In 2013, 49 master's awarded. *Entrance requirements:* For master's, GRE General Test. Additional exam requirements/recommendations for international students: Required—TOEFL (minimum score 69 iBT). *Application deadline:* For fall admission, 10/1 for domestic and international students. Applications are processed on a rolling basis. Application fee: $60. Electronic applications accepted. *Expenses:* Contact institution. *Financial support:* In 2013–14, 59 students received support. Institutionally sponsored loans and scholarships/grants available. Financial award application deadline: 3/1; financial award applicants required to submit FAFSA. *Faculty research:* Cultural competency in medical education, farm worker health, technology in medicine, physician assistants in primary care, interprofessional education. *Unit head:* Dr. Douglas Ander, Director, 404-727-7825, Fax: 404-727-7836, E-mail: dander@emory.edu. *Application contact:* Kaye Johnson, Assistant Director of Admissions, 404-727-7857, Fax: 404-727-7836, E-mail: ljohn07@emory.edu.
Website: http://med.emory.edu/pa/

Franklin Pierce University, Graduate Studies, Rindge, NH 03461-0060. Offers curriculum and instruction (M Ed); emerging network technologies (Graduate Certificate); energy and sustainability studies (MBA); health administration (MBA, Graduate Certificate); human resource management (MBA, Graduate Certificate); information technology (MBA); information technology management (MS); leadership (MBA, DA); nursing (MS); physical therapy (DPT); physician assistant studies (MPAS); special education (M Ed); sports management (MBA). *Accreditation:* APTA. Part-time programs available. Postbaccalaureate distance learning degree programs offered (no on-campus study). *Degree requirements:* For master's, concentrated original research projects; student teaching; fieldwork and/or internship; leadership project; PRAXIS I and II (for M Ed); for doctorate, concentrated original research projects, clinical fieldwork and/or internship, leadership project. *Entrance requirements:* For master's, minimum GPA of 2.5, 3 letters of recommendation; competencies in accounting, economics, statistics, and computer skills through life experience or undergraduate coursework (for MBA); certification/e-portfolio, minimum C grade in all education courses (for M Ed); license to practice as RN (for MS in nursing); for doctorate, GRE, BA/BS, 3 letters of recommendation, personal mission statement, interview, writing sample, minimum cumulative GPA of 2.8, master's degree (for DA); 80 hours of observation/work in PT settings, completion of anatomy, chemistry, physics, and statistics, minimum GPA of 3.0 (for DPT). Additional exam requirements/recommendations for international students: Required—TOEFL (minimum score 550 paper-based; 61 iBT). Electronic applications accepted. *Faculty research:* Evidence-based practice in sports physical therapy, human resource management in economic crisis, leadership in nursing, innovation in sports facility management, differentiated learning and understanding by design.

Gannon University, School of Graduate Studies, Morosky College of Health Professions and Sciences, School of Health Professions, Program in Physician Assistant Science, Erie, PA 16541-0001. Offers MPAS. *Accreditation:* ARC-PA. *Students:* 47 full-time (44 women); includes 1 minority (Asian, non-Hispanic/Latino). Average age 22. In 2013, 46 master's awarded. *Degree requirements:* For master's, thesis or alternative, research project, practicum. *Entrance requirements:* For master's, interview, minimum QPA of 3.0, 30 hours of volunteer or paid medical experience or 30 hours shadowing a Physician Assistant. Additional exam requirements/recommendations for international students: Required—TOEFL (minimum score 79 iBT). *Application deadline:* For fall admission, 1/15 for domestic students. Application fee: $25. Electronic applications accepted. *Expenses:* Contact institution. *Financial support:* Scholarships/grants available. Financial award application deadline: 7/1; financial award applicants required to submit FAFSA. *Faculty research:* Cardiology, assessment and evaluation, cervical cancer screening and prevention, simulation. *Unit head:* Michele Roth-Kauffman, Chair, 814-871-5643, E-mail: rothkauf001@gannon.edu. *Application contact:* Kara Morgan, Director of Graduate Admissions, 814-871-5831, Fax: 814-871-5827, E-mail: graduate@gannon.edu.

The George Washington University, School of Medicine and Health Sciences, Health Sciences Programs, Physician Assistant Program, Washington, DC 20052. Offers MSHS, MSHS/MPH. *Accreditation:* ARC-PA. *Students:* 141 full-time (115 women), 1 (woman) part-time; includes 29 minority (2 Black or African American, non-Hispanic/Latino; 1 American Indian or Alaska Native, non-Hispanic/Latino; 14 Asian, non-Hispanic/Latino; 11 Hispanic/Latino; 1 Native Hawaiian or other Pacific Islander, non-Hispanic/Latino), 2 international. Average age 28. 883 applicants, 12% accepted, 61 enrolled. In 2013, 62 master's awarded. *Entrance requirements:* For master's, GRE General Test, BA/BS with clinical experience. *Application deadline:* For fall admission, 10/15 for domestic students. Applications are processed on a rolling basis. Application fee: $75. Electronic applications accepted. *Unit head:* Lisa L. Alexander, Director, E-mail: lmapa@gwu.edu. *Application contact:* Jamie Lewis, Executive Assistant, 202-994-6661, E-mail: npajsl@gwumc.edu.

Grand Valley State University, College of Health Professions, Physician Assistant Studies Program, Allendale, MI 49401-9403. Offers MPAS. *Accreditation:* ARC-PA. *Degree requirements:* For master's, thesis, clinical rotations, project. *Entrance requirements:* For master's, interview, 250 hours of health care experience. Additional exam requirements/recommendations for international students: Required—TOEFL (minimum score 610 paper-based). Electronic applications accepted. *Faculty research:* Women's health, pain management, PA practice issues, hematology/hemostasis, patient education.

Harding University, College of Allied Health, Program in Physician Assistant, Searcy, AR 72149-0001. Offers MS. *Faculty:* 6 full-time (3 women), 2 part-time/adjunct (1 woman). *Students:* 107 full-time (77 women); includes 6 minority (1 Black or African American, non-Hispanic/Latino; 1 Asian, non-Hispanic/Latino; 3 Hispanic/Latino; 1 Two or more races, non-Hispanic/Latino). Average age 28. 631 applicants, 6% accepted, 36 enrolled. In 2013, 31 master's awarded. *Entrance requirements:* For master's, GRE. *Application deadline:* For fall admission, 11/1 for domestic and international students. Application fee: $25. *Expenses: Tuition:* Full-time $11,574; part-time $643 per credit hour. *Required fees:* $432; $24 per credit hour. Tuition and fees vary according to course load, degree level and program. *Unit head:* Dr. Mike Murphy, Professor/Program Director, 501-279-5642, E-mail: mmurphy1@harding.edu. *Application contact:* Dr. Cheri Yecke, Dean of Graduate Programs, 501-279-4335, Fax: 501-279-5192, E-mail: cyecke@harding.edu.
Website: http://www.harding.edu/paprogram/

Hofstra University, School of Health Sciences and Human Services, Program in Physician Assistant, Hempstead, NY 11549. Offers MS.

Idaho State University, Office of Graduate Studies, Kasiska College of Health Professions, Program in Physician Assistant Studies, Pocatello, ID 83209-8253. Offers MPAS. *Accreditation:* ARC-PA. *Degree requirements:* For master's, comprehensive exam, thesis (for some programs), portfolio, clinical year, oral case presentation. *Entrance requirements:* For master's, GRE General Test, minimum GPA of 3.0, letters of reference. Additional exam requirements/recommendations for international students: Required—TOEFL (minimum score 500 paper-based). Electronic applications accepted. *Expenses:* Contact institution.

James Madison University, The Graduate School, College of Health and Behavioral Studies, Department of Health Sciences, Program in Physician Assistant Studies, Harrisonburg, VA 22807. Offers MPAS. *Accreditation:* ARC-PA. Part-time programs available. *Students:* 75 full-time (54 women), 2 part-time (both women); includes 10 minority (1 Black or African American, non-Hispanic/Latino; 4 Asian, non-Hispanic/Latino; 3 Hispanic/Latino; 2 Two or more races, non-Hispanic/Latino), 1 international. Average age 27. In 2013, 23 master's awarded. *Entrance requirements:* For master's, GRE General Test. *Application deadline:* For fall admission, 1/15 priority date for domestic students. Application fee: $55. *Financial support:* Application deadline: 3/1; applicants required to submit FAFSA. *Unit head:* James Hammond, Director, 540-568-2395, E-mail: hammonjb@jmu.edu. *Application contact:* Lynette M. Bible, Director of Graduate Admissions, 540-568-6395, Fax: 540-568-7860, E-mail: biblelm@jmu.edu.

Jefferson College of Health Sciences, Program in Physician Assistant, Roanoke, VA 24031-3186. Offers MS. *Accreditation:* ARC-PA. *Degree requirements:* For master's, rotations. *Entrance requirements:* For master's, GRE. Additional exam requirements/recommendations for international students: Required—TOEFL (minimum score 550 paper-based; 80 iBT). Electronic applications accepted. *Faculty research:* Community health, chronic disease management, geriatrics, rheumatology, medically underserved populations.

Physician Assistant Studies

Johnson & Wales University, Master of Science Program in Physician Assistant Studies, Providence, RI 02903-3703. Offers MS.

Keiser University, MS in Physician Assistant Program, Ft. Lauderdale, FL 33309. Offers MS.

Kettering College, Program in Physician Assistant Studies, Kettering, OH 45429-1299. Offers MPAS.

King's College, Program in Physician Assistant Studies, Wilkes-Barre, PA 18711-0801. Offers MSPAS. *Accreditation:* ARC-PA. *Degree requirements:* For master's, thesis. *Entrance requirements:* Additional exam requirements/recommendations for international students: Required—TOEFL (minimum score 600 paper-based). Electronic applications accepted.

Le Moyne College, Department of Physician Assistant Studies, Syracuse, NY 13214. Offers MS. *Accreditation:* ARC-PA. *Faculty:* 8 full-time (5 women), 9 part-time/adjunct (6 women). *Students:* 92 full-time (64 women), 3 part-time (all women); includes 14 minority (3 Black or African American, non-Hispanic/Latino; 1 American Indian or Alaska Native, non-Hispanic/Latino; 7 Asian, non-Hispanic/Latino; 3 Hispanic/Latino). Average age 26. 730 applicants, 10% accepted, 54 enrolled. In 2013, 38 master's awarded. *Degree requirements:* For master's, project. *Entrance requirements:* For master's, minimum GPA of 3.0, patient contact, interview, 3 letters of recommendation. Additional exam requirements/recommendations for international students: Required—TOEFL (minimum score 550 paper-based; 79 iBT). *Application deadline:* For fall admission, 10/1 priority date for domestic and international students. Electronic applications accepted. *Expenses:* Contact institution. *Financial support:* In 2013–14, 7 students received support. Career-related internships or fieldwork, scholarships/grants, health care benefits, and U.S. Department of Health and Human Services Affordable Care Act Expansion of PA Training Program (EPAT) available. Financial award applicants required to submit FAFSA. *Faculty research:* Cultural competence, educational outcomes, preventive medicine, health literacy. *Unit head:* Mary E. Springston, Clinical Assistant Professor and Director of Department of Physician Assistant Studies, 315-445-4163, Fax: 315-445-4602, E-mail: springme@lemoyne.edu. *Application contact:* Kristen P. Trapasso, Senior Director of Enrollment Management, 315-445-4265, Fax: 315-445-6092, E-mail: trapaskp@lemoyne.edu.
Website: http://www.lemoyne.edu/pa

Lock Haven University of Pennsylvania, College of Natural, Behavioral and Health Sciences, Lock Haven, PA 17745-2390. Offers physician assistant (MHS). Program also offered at the Clearfield, Coudersport, and Harrisburg campuses. *Accreditation:* ARC-PA. *Entrance requirements:* For master's, minimum undergraduate GPA of 3.0. Additional exam requirements/recommendations for international students: Required—TOEFL. *Application deadline:* Applications are processed on a rolling basis. Application fee: $25. Electronic applications accepted. *Expenses: Tuition, area resident:* Part-time $442 per credit hour. Tuition, state resident: part-time $442 per credit hour. Tuition, nonresident: part-time $663 per credit hour. *Required fees:* $208.45 per credit hour. Tuition and fees vary according to program. *Financial support:* Unspecified assistantships available. Financial award application deadline: 8/1. *Unit head:* Dr. Scott Carnicom, Dean, 570-484-2204, E-mail: carnicom@lhup.edu. *Application contact:* Cherie Dolan, Secretary, 570-484-2204, Fax: 570-484-2734, E-mail: cdolan1@lhup.edu.
Website: http://www.lhup.edu/colleges/natural_behavioral_health/

Loma Linda University, School of Allied Health Professions, Department of Physician Assistant, Loma Linda, CA 92350. Offers MS. *Accreditation:* ARC-PA. *Entrance requirements:* For master's, minimum GPA of 3.0. Additional exam requirements/recommendations for international students: Required—TOEFL (minimum score 550 paper-based).

Marietta College, Program in Physician Assistant Studies, Marietta, OH 45750-4000. Offers MS. *Accreditation:* ARC-PA. *Degree requirements:* For master's, capstone project. *Entrance requirements:* For master's, MCAT and/or GRE, official transcripts.

Marquette University, Graduate School, College of Health Sciences, Department of Physician Assistant Studies, Milwaukee, WI 53201-1881. Offers MPAS. Students enter the program as undergraduates. *Accreditation:* ARC-PA. *Faculty:* 8 full-time (4 women), 4 part-time/adjunct (3 women). *Students:* 107 full-time (83 women), 4 part-time (3 women); includes 11 minority (1 Black or African American, non-Hispanic/Latino; 6 Asian, non-Hispanic/Latino; 3 Hispanic/Latino; 1 Two or more races, non-Hispanic/Latino), 2 international. Average age 25. 966 applicants, 17% accepted, 56 enrolled. In 2013, 47 master's awarded. *Degree requirements:* For master's, clinical clerkship experience, capstone project. *Entrance requirements:* For master's, GRE General Test, three letters of recommendation, minimum GPA of 3.0, official transcripts from all current and previous institutions except Marquette. Additional exam requirements/recommendations for international students: Required—TOEFL (minimum score 530 paper-based). *Application deadline:* For fall admission, 10/1 for domestic students. Application fee: $50. Electronic applications accepted. *Expenses:* Contact institution. *Financial support:* Application deadline: 2/15. *Unit head:* MaryJo Wiemiller, Chair, 414-288-7180, Fax: 414-288-7951, E-mail: maryjo.wiemiller@marquette.edu. *Application contact:* MaryJo Wiemiller, Chair, 414-288-7180, Fax: 414-288-7951, E-mail: maryjo.wiemiller@marquette.edu.
Website: http://www.marquette.edu/chs/pa/index.shtml

Marywood University, Academic Affairs, College of Health and Human Services, Department of Physician Assistant Studies, Clinical Physician Assistant Track, Scranton, PA 18509-1598. Offers emergency medicine (MS); general surgery (MS); hospitalist (MS); orthopedics and sports medicine (MS); pediatrics (MS). *Entrance requirements:* Additional exam requirements/recommendations for international students: Required—TOEFL (minimum score 550 paper-based; 79 iBT). Application fee: $35. Electronic applications accepted. *Expenses: Tuition:* Part-time $775 per credit. Tuition and fees vary according to degree level. *Financial support:* Career-related internships or fieldwork, scholarships/grants, and unspecified assistantships available. Support available to part-time students. Financial award application deadline: 6/30; financial award applicants required to submit FAFSA. *Unit head:* Dr. Lori E. Swanchak, Director, 570-961-4711, E-mail: swanchak@marywood.edu. *Application contact:* Tammy Manka, Assistant Director of Graduate Admissions, 570-348-6211 Ext. 2322, E-mail: tmanka@marywood.edu.
Website: http://www.marywood.edu/academics/gradcatalog/

Marywood University, Academic Affairs, College of Health and Human Services, Department of Physician Assistant Studies, Physician Assistant Studies Program, Scranton, PA 18509-1598. Offers MS. *Accreditation:* ARC-PA. Part-time and evening/weekend programs available. *Entrance requirements:* Additional exam requirements/recommendations for international students: Required—TOEFL (minimum score 550 paper-based; 79 iBT). Application fee: $35. Electronic applications accepted. *Expenses:* Contact institution. *Financial support:* Career-related internships or fieldwork, scholarships/grants, and unspecified assistantships available. Support available to part-time students. Financial award application deadline: 6/30; financial award applicants required to submit FAFSA. *Unit head:* Dr. Lori E. Swanchak, Director, 570-961-4711, E-mail: swanchak@marywood.edu. *Application contact:* Tammy Manka, Assistant Director of Graduate Admissions, 570-348-6211 Ext. 2322, E-mail: tmanka@marywood.edu.
Website: http://www.marywood.edu/academics/gradcatalog/

MCPHS University, Graduate Studies, Programs in Physician Assistant Studies, Accelerated Program in Physician Assistant Studies (Manchester/Worcester), Boston, MA 02115-5896. Offers MPAS. *Accreditation:* ARC-PA. *Entrance requirements:* Additional exam requirements/recommendations for international students: Required—TOEFL (minimum score 550 paper-based; 79 iBT). Electronic applications accepted.

MCPHS University, Graduate Studies, Programs in Physician Assistant Studies, Program in Physician Assistant Studies (Boston), Boston, MA 02115-5896. Offers MPAS. *Entrance requirements:* Additional exam requirements/recommendations for international students: Required—TOEFL (minimum score 550 paper-based; 79 iBT).

Medical University of South Carolina, College of Health Professions, Physician Assistant Studies Program, Charleston, SC 29425. Offers MS. *Accreditation:* ARC-PA. *Degree requirements:* For master's, clinical clerkship, research project. *Entrance requirements:* For master's, GRE General Test, interview, minimum GPA of 3.0, 3 references. Additional exam requirements/recommendations for international students: Required—TOEFL (minimum score 600 paper-based). Electronic applications accepted. *Faculty research:* Oral health, pediatric emergency medicine, simulation technology in education, health manpower needs, cultural competency.

Mercer University, Graduate Studies, Cecil B. Day Campus, College of Health Professions, Atlanta, GA 30341. Offers physical therapy (DPT); physician assistant (MM Sc); public health (MPH). *Faculty:* 23 full-time (17 women), 3 part-time/adjunct (2 women). *Students:* 281 full-time (208 women), 3 part-time (1 woman); includes 105 minority (70 Black or African American, non-Hispanic/Latino; 17 Asian, non-Hispanic/Latino; 6 Hispanic/Latino; 12 Two or more races, non-Hispanic/Latino), 3 international. Average age 26. In 2013, 42 master's, 26 doctorates awarded. *Unit head:* Richard V. Swindle, Senior Vice President, 678-547-6397, E-mail: swindle_rv@mercer.edu. *Application contact:* Tracey M. Wofford, Associate Director of Admissions, 678-547-6422, E-mail: wofford_tm@mercer.edu.
Website: http://chp.mercer.edu/

Mercy College, School of Health and Natural Sciences, Program in Physician Assistant Studies, Dobbs Ferry, NY 10522-1189. Offers MS. *Accreditation:* ARC-PA. Evening/weekend programs available. *Students:* 121 full-time (84 women), 4 part-time (3 women); includes 47 minority (5 Black or African American, non-Hispanic/Latino; 1 American Indian or Alaska Native, non-Hispanic/Latino; 31 Asian, non-Hispanic/Latino; 10 Hispanic/Latino), 1 international. Average age 33. In 2013, 35 master's awarded. *Entrance requirements:* For master's, essay, interview, two letters of reference, undergraduate transcripts with minimum GPA of 3.0. Additional exam requirements/recommendations for international students: Required—TOEFL (minimum score 600 paper-based; 100 iBT), IELTS (minimum score 8). *Application deadline:* Applications are processed on a rolling basis. Application fee: $62. Electronic applications accepted. *Expenses:* Contact institution. *Financial support:* Career-related internships or fieldwork, Federal Work-Study, scholarships/grants, and unspecified assistantships available. Support available to part-time students. Financial award applicants required to submit FAFSA. *Unit head:* Dr. Joan Toglia, Dean, School of Health and Natural Sciences, 914-674-7837, E-mail: jtoglia@mercy.edu. *Application contact:* Allison Gurdineer, Senior Director of Admissions, 877-637-2946, Fax: 914-674-7382, E-mail: admissions@mercy.edu.
Website: https://www.mercy.edu/academics/school-of-health-and-natural-sciences/department-of-health-professions/ms-in-physician-assistant-studies/

Methodist University, School of Graduate Studies, Program in Physician Assistant Studies, Fayetteville, NC 28311-1498. Offers MMS. *Accreditation:* ARC-PA. *Degree requirements:* For master's, comprehensive exam. *Entrance requirements:* For master's, GRE, bachelor's degree from four-year, regionally-accredited college or university; minimum of 500 hours' clinical experience with direct patient contact; minimum GPA of 3.0 on all college level work attempted, 3.2 on medical core prerequisites (recommended). Additional exam requirements/recommendations for international students: Required—TOEFL (minimum score 500 paper-based; 60 iBT).

Midwestern University, Downers Grove Campus, College of Health Sciences, Illinois Campus, Program in Physician Assistant Studies, Downers Grove, IL 60515-1235. Offers MMS. *Accreditation:* ARC-PA. *Entrance requirements:* For master's, GRE General Test. *Expenses:* Contact institution.

Midwestern University, Glendale Campus, College of Health Sciences, Arizona Campus, Program in Physician Assistant Studies, Glendale, AZ 85308. Offers MMS. *Accreditation:* ARC-PA. *Entrance requirements:* For master's, GRE. *Expenses:* Contact institution.

Missouri State University, Graduate College, College of Health and Human Services, Department of Physician Assistant Studies, Springfield, MO 65897. Offers MS. *Accreditation:* ARC-PA. *Faculty:* 6 full-time (4 women), 50 part-time/adjunct (11 women). *Students:* 54 full-time (37 women); includes 3 minority (1 Black or African American, non-Hispanic/Latino; 1 Asian, non-Hispanic/Latino; 1 Native Hawaiian or other Pacific Islander, non-Hispanic/Latino), 2 international. Average age 28. In 2013, 27 master's awarded. *Degree requirements:* For master's, comprehensive exam, thesis or alternative. *Entrance requirements:* For master's, GRE General Test, minimum GPA of 3.0. Additional exam requirements/recommendations for international students: Required—TOEFL (minimum score 550 paper-based; 79 iBT). *Application deadline:* For spring admission, 8/1 for domestic and international students. Application fee: $35 ($50 for international students). *Expenses:* Tuition, state resident: full-time $4500; part-time $250 per credit hour. Tuition, nonresident: full-time $9018; part-time $501 per credit hour. *Required fees:* $361 per semester. Tuition and fees vary according to course level, course load and program. *Financial support:* Application deadline: 3/31; applicants required to submit FAFSA. *Unit head:* Dr. Steven Dodge, Head, 417-836-6151, Fax: 417-836-6406, E-mail: physicianasststudies@missouristate.edu. *Application contact:* Misty Stewart, Coordinator of Graduate Recruitment, 417-836-6079, Fax: 417-836-6200, E-mail: mistystewart@missouristate.edu.
Website: http://www.missouristate.edu/pas/

Monmouth University, The Graduate School, The Marjorie K. Unterberg School of Nursing and Health Studies, West Long Branch, NJ 07764-1898. Offers adult and gerontological nurse practitioner (MSN); adult-gerontological nurse practitioner (Post-Master's Certificate); family nurse practitioner (MSN, Post-Master's Certificate); family psychiatric and mental health advanced practice nursing (MSN); forensic nursing (MSN, Certificate); nursing (MSN); nursing administration (MSN, Post-Master's Certificate); nursing education (MSN, Post-Master's Certificate); nursing practice (DNP); physician assistant (MS); psychiatric-mental health nurse practitioner (Post-Master's Certificate); school nursing (MSN, Certificate). *Accreditation:* AACN. Part-time and evening/weekend programs available. *Faculty:* 14 full-time (all women), 4 part-time/adjunct (3 women). *Students:* 19 full-time (18 women), 269 part-time (252 women); includes 106 minority (35 Black or African American, non-Hispanic/Latino; 2 American Indian or Alaska Native, non-Hispanic/Latino; 51 Asian, non-Hispanic/Latino; 12 Hispanic/Latino; 3 Native Hawaiian or other Pacific Islander, non-Hispanic/Latino; 3 Two or more races, non-Hispanic/Latino), 2 international. Average age 39. 135 applicants, 98% accepted, 96

enrolled. In 2013, 54 master's, 7 doctorates awarded. *Degree requirements:* For master's, practicum (for some tracks). *Entrance requirements:* For master's, GRE General Test, BSN with minimum GPA of 2.75, current RN license, proof of liability and malpractice policy, personal statement, two letters of recommendation, college course work in health assessment, resume; minimum GPA of 3.0, minimum C grade in prerequisite courses, minimum 200 hours' clinical experience, 3 letters of recommendation, and interview (for MS); for doctorate, accredited master's nursing program degree with minimum GPA of 3.2, active RN license, national certification as Nurse Practitioner or Nurse Administrator, working knowledge of statistics, statement of goals and vision for change, 2 letters of recommendation, resume, interview. Additional exam requirements/recommendations for international students: Required—TOEFL (minimum score 550 paper-based; 79 iBT), IELTS (minimum score 6) or Michigan English Language Assessment Battery (minimum score 77). *Application deadline:* For fall admission, 7/15 priority date for domestic students, 6/1 for international students; for spring admission, 11/15 priority date for domestic students, 11/1 for international students; for summer admission, 2/1 for domestic students. Applications are processed on a rolling basis. Application fee: $50. Electronic applications accepted. *Expenses: Tuition:* Part-time $1004 per credit hour. *Required fees:* $157 per semester. *Financial support:* In 2013–14, 163 students received support, including 113 fellowships (averaging $3,093 per year), 27 research assistantships (averaging $6,273 per year); career-related internships or fieldwork, scholarships/grants, and unspecified assistantships also available. Support available to part-time students. Financial award applicants required to submit FAFSA. *Faculty research:* Relationship of undergraduate GPA and GRE to succeeding in a graduate nursing program. *Unit head:* Dr. Janet Mahoney, Dean, 732-571-3443, Fax: 732-263-5131, E-mail: jmahoney@monmouth.edu. *Application contact:* Lauren Vento-Cifelli, Associate Vice President of Undergraduate and Graduate Admission, 732-571-3452, Fax: 732-263-5123, E-mail: gradadm@monmouth.edu.
Website: http://www.monmouth.edu/school-of-nursing-health/graduate-nursing-programs.aspx

New York Institute of Technology, School of Health Professions, Department of Physician Assistant Studies, Old Westbury, NY 11568-8000. Offers MS. *Accreditation:* ARC-PA. *Faculty:* 6 full-time (4 women), 7 part-time/adjunct (3 women). *Students:* 162 full-time (123 women), 2 part-time (both women); includes 41 minority (4 Black or African American, non-Hispanic/Latino; 24 Asian, non-Hispanic/Latino; 9 Hispanic/Latino; 4 Two or more races, non-Hispanic/Latino), 1 international. Average age 25. 1,350 applicants, 8% accepted, 54 enrolled. In 2013, 51 master's awarded. *Degree requirements:* For master's, thesis. *Entrance requirements:* For master's, minimum GPA of 3.0, interview, 100 hours of volunteer work, 2 letters of recommendation. Additional exam requirements/recommendations for international students: Required—TOEFL (minimum score 550 paper-based; 79 iBT), IELTS (minimum score 6). *Application deadline:* For fall admission, 7/1 priority date for domestic students, 6/1 for international students; for spring admission, 12/1 priority date for domestic students, 12/1 for international students. Applications are processed on a rolling basis. Application fee: $50. Electronic applications accepted. *Expenses: Tuition:* Full-time $18,900; part-time $1050 per credit. *Financial support:* Research assistantships with partial tuition reimbursements, scholarships/grants, health care benefits, tuition waivers, and unspecified assistantships available. Support available to part-time students. Financial award applicants required to submit FAFSA. *Faculty research:* Healthcare workforce issues, point-of-care ultrasound, cultural competency, palliative care, diet and disease prevention. *Unit head:* Dr. Lawrence Herman, Department Chair, 516-686-3881, Fax: 516-686-3795, E-mail: lherman@nyit.edu. *Application contact:* Alice Dolitsky, Director, Graduate Admissions, 516-686-7520, Fax: 516-686-1116, E-mail: nyitgrad@nyit.edu.
Website: http://www.nyit.edu/physician_assistant_studies

Northeastern University, Bouvé College of Health Sciences, Boston, MA 02115-5096. Offers audiology (Au D); biotechnology (MS); counseling psychology (MS, PhD, CAGS); counseling/school psychology (PhD); exercise physiology (MS), including exercise physiology, public health; health informatics (MS); nursing (MS, PhD, CAGS), including acute care (MS), administration (MS), anesthesia (MS), primary care (MS), psychiatric mental health (MS); pharmaceutical sciences (PhD); pharmaceutics and drug delivery systems (MS); pharmacology (MS); physical therapy (DPT); physician assistant (MS); school psychology (PhD, CAGS); school/counseling psychology (PhD); speech language pathology (MS); urban public health (MPH); MS/MBA. *Accreditation:* ACPE (one or more programs are accredited). Part-time and evening/weekend programs available. *Degree requirements:* For doctorate, thesis/dissertation (for some programs); for CAGS, comprehensive exam.

Northern Arizona University, Graduate College, College of Health and Human Services, Physician Assistant Program, Phoenix, AZ 86011. Offers MPAS. *Faculty:* 6 full-time (4 women), 3 part-time/adjunct (all women). *Students:* 49 full-time (29 women); includes 15 minority (1 American Indian or Alaska Native, non-Hispanic/Latino; 3 Asian, non-Hispanic/Latino; 10 Hispanic/Latino; 1 Two or more races, non-Hispanic/Latino). Average age 29. 374 applicants, 7% accepted, 25 enrolled. *Unit head:* Dr. Kay Look, Chair, 602-827-2450, E-mail: paprog@nau.edu. *Application contact:* April Sandoval, Coordinator, 928-523-4348, Fax: 928-523-8950, E-mail: april.sandoval@nau.edu.

Nova Southeastern University, College of Health Care Sciences, Fort Lauderdale, FL 33314-7796. Offers audiology (Au D); health science (MH Sc, DHSc, PhD); occupational therapy (MOT, OTD, PhD); physical therapy (DPT, PhD, TDPT); physician assistant (MMS). Postbaccalaureate distance learning degree programs offered (minimal on-campus study). *Faculty:* 117 full-time (68 women), 110 part-time/adjunct (57 women). *Students:* 1,187 full-time (844 women), 509 part-time (340 women); includes 560 minority (184 Black or African American, non-Hispanic/Latino; 2 American Indian or Alaska Native, non-Hispanic/Latino; 120 Asian, non-Hispanic/Latino; 218 Hispanic/Latino; 36 Two or more races, non-Hispanic/Latino), 20 international. Average age 31. 5,996 applicants, 14% accepted, 548 enrolled. In 2013, 374 master's, 132 doctorates awarded. *Degree requirements:* For master's, thesis; for doctorate, comprehensive exam, thesis/dissertation. *Entrance requirements:* For master's and doctorate, GRE General Test. *Application deadline:* Applications are processed on a rolling basis. Application fee: $50. Electronic applications accepted. *Expenses:* Contact institution. *Financial support:* In 2013–14, 10 students received support, including 2 research assistantships (averaging $3,500 per year); institutionally sponsored loans and unspecified assistantships also available. *Unit head:* Dr. Stanley Wilson, Dean, 954-262-1203, E-mail: swilson@nova.edu. *Application contact:* Joey Jankie, Admissions Counselor, 954-262-7249, E-mail: joey@nova.edu.
Website: http://www.nova.edu/chcs/

Ohio Dominican University, Graduate Programs, Division of Math, Computer and Natural Science, Columbus, OH 43219-2099. Offers physician assistant studies (MS). Part-time and evening/weekend programs available. *Degree requirements:* For master's, thesis. *Entrance requirements:* For master's, minimum undergraduate GPA of 3.0, 3 letters of recommendation, interview. Additional exam requirements/recommendations for international students: Required—TOEFL (minimum score 550 paper-based), IELTS (minimum score 6.5).

Oregon Health & Science University, School of Medicine, Graduate Programs in Medicine, Division of Physician Assistant Education, Portland, OR 97239-3098. Offers MPAS. *Accreditation:* ARC-PA. *Faculty:* 6 full-time (4 women), 9 part-time/adjunct (6 women). *Students:* 74 full-time (51 women), 4 part-time (3 women); includes 23 minority (2 Black or African American, non-Hispanic/Latino; 8 Asian, non-Hispanic/Latino; 6 Hispanic/Latino; 1 Native Hawaiian or other Pacific Islander, non-Hispanic/Latino; 6 Two or more races, non-Hispanic/Latino). Average age 28. 1,044 applicants, 4% accepted, 38 enrolled. In 2013, 38 master's awarded. *Application deadline:* For fall admission, 10/1 for domestic students. *Unit head:* Ted Ruback, Program Director/Division Head, 503-494-1408, E-mail: ruback@ohsu.edu. *Application contact:* Colleen Schierholtz, Director of Admissions, 503-494-1408, E-mail: schierhc@ohsu.edu.
Website: http://www.ohsu.edu/xd/education/schools/school-of-medicine/academic-programs/physician-assistant/index.cfm

Our Lady of the Lake College, School of Arts, Sciences and Health Professions, Baton Rouge, LA 70808. Offers health administration (MHA); physician assistant studies (MMS).

Pace University, College of Health Professions, Program in Physician Assistant Studies, New York, NY 10038. Offers MS. *Accreditation:* ARC-PA. *Faculty:* 7 full-time (all women), 5 part-time/adjunct (3 women). *Students:* 83 full-time (74 women), 102 part-time (75 women); includes 59 minority (4 Black or African American, non-Hispanic/Latino; 7 American Indian or Alaska Native, non-Hispanic/Latino; 27 Asian, non-Hispanic/Latino; 4 Hispanic/Latino; 17 Two or more races, non-Hispanic/Latino), 2 international. Average age 28. 1,446 applicants, 9% accepted, 80 enrolled. In 2013, 71 master's awarded. *Entrance requirements:* For master's, 200 hours' volunteer or job related health care experience, 3 references from professionals (1 must be a health care professional). Additional exam requirements/recommendations for international students: Required—TOEFL. *Application deadline:* For spring admission, 11/1 priority date for domestic students, 11/1 for international students. Application fee: $70. *Expenses: Tuition:* Part-time $1075 per credit. *Required fees:* $192 per semester. Tuition and fees vary according to course load, degree level and program. *Unit head:* Kathleen T. Roche, Program Director, 212-618-6050, E-mail: paprogram@pace.edu. *Application contact:* Susan Ford-Goldschein, Director of Graduate Admissions, 212-346-1660, Fax: 212-346-1585, E-mail: gradnyc@pace.edu.
Website: http://www.pace.edu/physician-assistant/

Pacific University, School of Physician Assistant Studies, Forest Grove, OR 97116-1797. Offers MHS, MS. *Accreditation:* ARC-PA. *Degree requirements:* For master's, comprehensive exam, thesis, clinical project. *Entrance requirements:* For master's, minimum of 1000 hours of direct clinical patient care, prerequisite coursework in science with minimum C average. Additional exam requirements/recommendations for international students: Required—TOEFL (minimum score 600 paper-based). *Expenses:* Contact institution. *Faculty research:* Public health, evidenced based medicine.

Philadelphia College of Osteopathic Medicine, Graduate and Professional Programs, Physician Assistant Studies Program, Philadelphia, PA 19131. Offers health sciences (MS). *Accreditation:* ARC-PA. *Faculty:* 9 full-time (6 women), 34 part-time/adjunct (11 women). *Students:* 111 full-time (90 women); includes 26 minority (7 Black or African American, non-Hispanic/Latino; 1 Asian, non-Hispanic/Latino; 3 Hispanic/Latino; 15 Two or more races, non-Hispanic/Latino). Average age 25. 2,341 applicants, 4% accepted, 57 enrolled. In 2013, 55 master's awarded. *Degree requirements:* For master's, thesis. *Entrance requirements:* For master's, minimum GPA of 3.0; 200 hours of patient contact. Additional exam requirements/recommendations for international students: Required—TOEFL (minimum score 79 iBT). *Application deadline:* For fall admission, 12/1 for domestic students. Applications are processed on a rolling basis. Application fee: $50. Electronic applications accepted. *Financial support:* In 2013–14, 80 students received support. Federal Work-Study, institutionally sponsored loans, and scholarships/grants available. Financial award application deadline: 3/15; financial award applicants required to submit FAFSA. *Application contact:* Office of Admissions, 215-871-6700, E-mail: admissions@pcom.edu.
Website: http://www.pcom.edu

See Display on next page and Close-Up on page 557.

Philadelphia University, College of Science, Health and the Liberal Arts, Program in Physician Assistant Studies, Philadelphia, PA 19144. Offers MS. *Accreditation:* ARC-PA. *Entrance requirements:* For master's, MCAT, GRE, or MAT. Additional exam requirements/recommendations for international students: Required—TOEFL (minimum score 550 paper-based; 79 iBT), IELTS (minimum score 6.5).

Quinnipiac University, School of Health Sciences, Program for Pathologists' Assistant, Hamden, CT 06518-1940. Offers MHS. *Accreditation:* NAACLS. *Faculty:* 1 full-time (0 women), 4 part-time/adjunct (3 women). *Students:* 39 full-time (27 women); includes 9 minority (4 Black or African American, non-Hispanic/Latino; 2 Asian, non-Hispanic/Latino; 3 Hispanic/Latino). 150 applicants, 18% accepted, 22 enrolled. In 2013, 18 master's awarded. *Degree requirements:* For master's, residency. *Entrance requirements:* For master's, interview, coursework in biological and health sciences, minimum GPA of 2.8. *Application deadline:* For fall admission, 11/1 for domestic students; for summer admission, 10/1 for domestic students. Applications are processed on a rolling basis. Application fee: $45. Electronic applications accepted. *Expenses: Tuition:* Part-time $920 per credit. *Required fees:* $37 per credit. *Financial support:* In 2013–14, 8 students received support. Career-related internships or fieldwork, scholarships/grants, and unspecified assistantships available. Support available to part-time students. Financial award application deadline: 6/1; financial award applicants required to submit FAFSA. *Faculty research:* ACL injury mechanism and running injuries and performance; transcriptional activators upstream stimulatory factor (USF); identification of novel antimicrobials; vaccines, fomites and opportunistic pathogens; molecular biology of the Lyme Disease agent, Borrelia burgdorferi; molecular and microscopic techniques in host-pathogen interactions; non-invasive vascular biology, external pneumatic compression, sports performance. *Unit head:* Dr. Kenneth Kaloustian, Director, E-mail: kenneth.kaloustian@quinnipiac.edu. *Application contact:* Office of Graduate Admissions, 800-462-1944, Fax: 203-582-3443, E-mail: paadmissions@quinnipiac.edu.
Website: http://www.quinnipiac.edu/gradpathologists

Quinnipiac University, School of Health Sciences, Program for Physician Assistant, Hamden, CT 06518-1940. Offers MHS. *Accreditation:* ARC-PA. *Faculty:* 12 full-time (8 women), 21 part-time/adjunct (8 women). *Students:* 124 full-time (80 women), 6 part-time (5 women); includes 15 minority (2 Black or African American, non-Hispanic/Latino; 9 Asian, non-Hispanic/Latino; 4 Hispanic/Latino). 1,135 applicants, 9% accepted, 71 enrolled. In 2013, 50 master's awarded. *Degree requirements:* For master's, comprehensive exam. *Entrance requirements:* For master's, minimum GPA of 3.0; course work in biological, physical, and behavioral sciences; interviews; 2000 hours of direct patient care experience. *Application deadline:* For fall admission, 9/1 for domestic students; for summer admission, 9/1 for domestic students. *Expenses: Tuition:* Part-time $920 per credit. *Required fees:* $37 per credit. *Financial support:* In 2013–14, 90 students received support. Career-related internships or fieldwork, scholarships/grants, and unspecified assistantships available. Support available to part-time students. Financial award application deadline: 6/1; financial award applicants required to submit

FAFSA. *Unit head:* Cynthia Lord, Director. *Application contact:* Office of Graduate Admissions, 800-462-1944, Fax: 203-582-3443, E-mail: paadmissions@quinnipiac.edu. Website: http://www.quinnipiac.edu/gradphysicianasst

Rocky Mountain College, Program in Physician Assistant Studies, Billings, MT 59102-1796. Offers MPAS. *Accreditation:* ARC-PA. *Entrance requirements:* For master's, GRE. Additional exam requirements/recommendations for international students: Required—TOEFL (minimum score 570 paper-based; 88 iBT), IELTS (minimum score 6.5). Electronic applications accepted. *Expenses:* Contact institution.

Rosalind Franklin University of Medicine and Science, College of Health Professions, Physician Assistant Department, North Chicago, IL 60064-3095. Offers MS. *Accreditation:* ARC-PA. *Degree requirements:* For master's, thesis. *Entrance requirements:* For master's, GRE, writing sample. Additional exam requirements/recommendations for international students: Required—TOEFL. Electronic applications accepted. *Faculty research:* Ortho-spine, diabetes education, cultural competency, interprofessional medical education.

Rush University, College of Health Sciences, Physician Assistant Studies Program, Chicago, IL 60612-3832. Offers MS. *Entrance requirements:* Additional exam requirements/recommendations for international students: Required—TOEFL (minimum score 570 paper-based; 88 iBT).

Rutgers, The State University of New Jersey, Newark, School of Health Related Professions, Department of Primary Care, Physician Assistant Program, Newark, NJ 07102. Offers MS. *Accreditation:* ARC-PA. *Degree requirements:* For master's, internship. *Entrance requirements:* For master's, GRE, interview, minimum GPA of 3.0, BS, 3 reference letters. Additional exam requirements/recommendations for international students: Required—TOEFL. Electronic applications accepted.

St. Catherine University, Graduate Programs, Program in Physician Assistant Studies, St. Paul, MN 55105. Offers MPAS. *Entrance requirements:* For master's, GRE, personal essay, CASPA verification.

Saint Francis University, Department of Physician Assistant Sciences, Loretto, PA 15940-0600. Offers health science (MHS); medical science (MMS); physician assistant sciences (MPAS). *Accreditation:* ARC-PA. *Faculty:* 8 full-time (7 women), 3 part-time/adjunct (0 women). *Students:* 109 full-time (91 women); includes 2 minority (both Hispanic/Latino). Average age 22. In 2013, 55 master's awarded. *Degree requirements:* For master's, capstone, summative evaluation. *Entrance requirements:* For master's, interview. Additional exam requirements/recommendations for international students: Required—TOEFL (minimum score 550 paper-based; 70 iBT). *Application deadline:* For fall admission, 10/1 for domestic and international students. Applications are processed on a rolling basis. Application fee: $175. Electronic applications accepted. *Expenses: Tuition:* Full-time $18,848. Tuition and fees vary according to degree level and reciprocity agreements. *Financial support:* Applicants required to submit FAFSA. *Unit head:* Donna L. Yeisley, Director, 814-472-3131, Fax: 814-472-3137, E-mail: dyeisley@francis.edu. *Application contact:* Marie S. Link, Director of Research and MPAS Admission, 814-472-3138, Fax: 814-472-3137, E-mail: mlink@francis.edu. Website: http://francis.edu/physician-assistant-science/

Saint Louis University, Graduate Education, Doisy College of Health Sciences, Department of Physician Assistant Education, St. Louis, MO 63103-2097. Offers MMS. *Accreditation:* ARC-PA. *Entrance requirements:* Additional exam requirements/recommendations for international students: Required—TOEFL (minimum score 86 iBT). Electronic applications accepted.

Salus University, College of Health Sciences, Elkins Park, PA 19027-1598. Offers physician assistant (MMS); public health (MPH). *Accreditation:* ARC-PA. *Entrance requirements:* For master's, GRE (recommended). Additional exam requirements/recommendations for international students: Required—TOEFL. Electronic applications accepted.

Samuel Merritt University, Department of Physician Assistant Studies, Oakland, CA 94609-3108. Offers MPA. *Accreditation:* ARC-PA. *Entrance requirements:* For master's, health care experience, minimum GPA of 3.0, previous course work in statistics.

Seton Hall University, School of Health and Medical Sciences, Physician Assistant Program, South Orange, NJ 07079-2697. Offers MS. *Accreditation:* ARC-PA. *Entrance requirements:* For master's, GRE, health care experience, interview, minimum GPA of 3.0. Additional exam requirements/recommendations for international students: Required—TOEFL. Electronic applications accepted.

Seton Hill University, Program in Physician Assistant, Greensburg, PA 15601. Offers MS. *Accreditation:* ARC-PA. *Faculty:* 7 full-time (4 women), 22 part-time/adjunct (13 women). *Students:* 61 full-time (45 women); includes 5 minority (all Asian, non-Hispanic/Latino). Average age 25. 718 applicants, 6% accepted, 23 enrolled. In 2013, 36 master's awarded. *Entrance requirements:* For master's, minimum GPA of 3.2 overall undergraduate and prerequisite courses, transcripts, 3 letters of recommendation, personal statement. Additional exam requirements/recommendations for international students: Required—TOEFL (minimum score 650 paper-based; 114 iBT), IELTS (minimum score 7). *Application deadline:* For spring admission, 1/15 priority date for domestic students. Electronic applications accepted. *Expenses: Tuition:* Full-time $14,220; part-time $790 per credit. *Required fees:* $700; $34 per credit. $50 per semester. *Faculty research:* Use of mobile technology in education, role of HCG in weight loss, cadaver use in human gross anatomy education. *Unit head:* Dr. James France, Director, 724-838-2455, E-mail: france@setonhill.edu. *Application contact:* Laurel Komarny, Program Counselor, 724-552-4355, E-mail: komarny@setonhill.edu. Website: http://www.setonhill.edu/academics/gradaute_programs/physician_assistant

Shenandoah University, School of Health Professions, Division of Physician Assistant Studies, Winchester, VA 22601-5195. Offers MS. *Accreditation:* ARC-PA. *Faculty:* 6 full-time (all women), 5 part-time/adjunct (3 women). *Students:* 117 full-time (96 women), 1 (woman) part-time; includes 10 minority (2 Black or African American, non-Hispanic/Latino; 1 American Indian or Alaska Native, non-Hispanic/Latino; 4 Asian, non-Hispanic/Latino; 3 Hispanic/Latino), 1 international. Average age 27. 792 applicants, 9% accepted, 38 enrolled. In 2013, 32 master's awarded. *Degree requirements:* For master's, project, minimum C grade in each course, minimum GPA of 3.0. *Entrance requirements:* For master's, GRE General Test, bachelor's degree with minimum GPA of 3.0, 3 letters of reference, interview. Additional exam requirements/recommendations for international students: Required—TOEFL (minimum score 550 paper-based; 79 iBT), IELTS (minimum score 6.5), Sakae Institute of Study Abroad (SISA) test (minimum score 15). *Application deadline:* For fall admission, 1/15 for domestic students; for summer admission, 1/15 for domestic and international students. Application fee: $30. Electronic applications accepted. *Expenses:* Contact institution. *Financial support:* In 2013–14, 8 students received support. Career-related internships or fieldwork and scholarships/grants available. Support available to part-time students. Financial award application deadline: 3/15; financial award applicants required to submit FAFSA. *Unit head:* Rachel A. Carlson, Director and Associate Professor, 540-542-6208, Fax: 540-542-6210, E-mail: rcarlso2@su.edu. *Application contact:* Andrew Woodall, Executive Director of Recruitment and Admissions, 540-665-4581, Fax: 540-665-4627, E-mail: admit@su.edu.
Website: http://www.physician-assistant.su.edu

South College, Program in Physician Assistant Studies, Knoxville, TN 37917. Offers MHS. *Accreditation:* ARC-PA.

Southern Illinois University Carbondale, Graduate School, Graduate Program in Medicine, Program in Physician Assistant Studies, Carbondale, IL 62901-4701. Offers MSPA. *Accreditation:* ARC-PA. *Faculty:* 12 full-time (8 women). *Students:* 65 full-time (49 women), 1 (woman) part-time; includes 2 minority (1 Black or African American, non-Hispanic/Latino; 1 Asian, non-Hispanic/Latino). 30 applicants. In 2013, 27 master's awarded. *Entrance requirements:* For master's, GRE, MAT, or MCAT. Additional exam requirements/recommendations for international students: Required—TOEFL. Application fee: $50. *Unit head:* Don Diemer, Head, 618-453-8850, E-mail: ddiemer@siumed.edu.

South University, Graduate Programs, College of Health Professions, Program in Physician Assistant Studies, Savannah, GA 31406. Offers MS. *Accreditation:* ARC-PA.

Springfield College, Graduate Programs, Program in Physician Assistant, Springfield, MA 01109-3797. Offers MS. *Accreditation:* ARC-PA. Part-time programs available. *Faculty:* 5 full-time, 2 part-time/adjunct. *Students:* 40 full-time. 1 applicant, 100% accepted, 1 enrolled. In 2013, 30 master's awarded. *Degree requirements:* For master's, comprehensive exam. *Entrance requirements:* Additional exam requirements/recommendations for international students: Required—TOEFL (minimum score 550 paper-based); Recommended—IELTS (minimum score 6). *Application deadline:* For spring admission, 6/15 for domestic and international students. Applications are processed on a rolling basis. Application fee: $50. Electronic applications accepted. *Expenses: Tuition:* Full-time $13,620; part-time $908 per credit. *Financial support:* Fellowships with partial tuition reimbursements, teaching assistantships with partial tuition reimbursements, career-related internships or fieldwork, Federal Work-Study, institutionally sponsored loans, and unspecified assistantships available. Financial award application deadline: 3/1; financial award applicants required to submit FAFSA. *Unit head:* Charles Milch, Director, 413-748-3554, Fax: 413-748-3595, E-mail: cmilch@springfieldcollege.edu. *Application contact:* Evelyn Cohen, Associate Director of Graduate Admissions, 413-748-3479, Fax: 413-748-3694, E-mail: ecohen@springfieldcollege.edu.

Stony Brook University, State University of New York, Stony Brook University Medical Center, Health Sciences Center, School of Health Technology and Management, Stony Brook, NY 11794. Offers health care management (Advanced Certificate); health care policy and management (MS); occupational therapy (MS); physical therapy (DPT); physician assistant (MS). *Accreditation:* APTA. Part-time programs available. *Faculty:* 70 full-time (46 women), 51 part-time/adjunct (34 women). *Students:* 349 full-time (225 women), 159 part-time (120 women); includes 140 minority (25 Black or African American, non-Hispanic/Latino; 1 American Indian or Alaska Native, non-Hispanic/Latino; 72 Asian, non-Hispanic/Latino; 34 Hispanic/Latino; 8 Two or more races, non-Hispanic/Latino), 7 international. 2,215 applicants, 11% accepted, 221 enrolled. In 2013, 120 master's, 77 doctorates, 23 other advanced degrees awarded. *Degree requirements:* For master's, thesis. *Entrance requirements:* For master's, GRE General Test, minimum GPA of 3.0, work experience in field, references; for doctorate, GRE, references. Additional exam requirements/recommendations for international students: Required—TOEFL (minimum score 550 paper-based). *Application deadline:* For fall admission, 1/15 for domestic students; for spring admission, 10/1 for domestic students. Application fee: $100. *Expenses:* Tuition, state resident: full-time $9870; part-time $411 per credit. Tuition, nonresident: full-time $18,350; part-time $765 per credit. *Financial support:* In 2013–14, 1 fellowship was awarded; research assistantships, teaching assistantships, career-related internships or fieldwork, Federal Work-Study, and institutionally sponsored loans also available. Financial award application deadline: 3/15. *Faculty research:* Health promotion and disease prevention. *Total annual research expenditures:* $1.1 million. *Unit head:* Dr. Craig A. Lehmann, Dean, 631-444-2252, Fax: 631-444-7621, E-mail: craig.lehmann@stonybrook.edu. *Application contact:* Dr. Richard W. Johnson, Associate Dean for Graduate Studies, 631-444-3251, Fax: 631-444-7621, E-mail: richard.johnson@stonybrook.edu.
Website: http://healthtechnology.stonybrookmedicine.edu/

Texas Tech University Health Sciences Center, School of Allied Health Sciences, Program in Physician Assistant Studies, Midland, TX 79705. Offers MPAS. *Accreditation:* ARC-PA. *Faculty:* 8 full-time (3 women). *Students:* 110 full-time (82 women), 4 part-time (3 women); includes 34 minority (1 Black or African American, non-Hispanic/Latino; 1 American Indian or Alaska Native, non-Hispanic/Latino; 20 Asian, non-Hispanic/Latino; 5 Hispanic/Latino; 7 Two or more races, non-Hispanic/Latino), 1 international. Average age 27. 1,171 applicants, 5% accepted, 60 enrolled. In 2013, 57 master's awarded. *Entrance requirements:* For master's, GRE. Additional exam requirements/recommendations for international students: Required—TOEFL, IELTS. *Application deadline:* For fall admission, 12/1 for domestic students. Applications are processed on a rolling basis. Application fee: $40. Electronic applications accepted. *Financial support:* Institutionally sponsored loans and scholarships/grants available. Financial award applicants required to submit FAFSA. *Unit head:* Christina Robohm, Program Director, 432-620-9905, Fax: 432-620-8605, E-mail: christina.robohm@ttuhsc.edu. *Application contact:* Lindsay Johnson, Associate Dean for Admissions and Student Affairs, 806-743-3220, Fax: 806-743-2994, E-mail: lindsay.johnson@ttuhsc.edu.
Website: http://www.ttuhsc.edu/sah/mpa/

Touro College, School of Health Sciences, Bay Shore, NY 11706. Offers occupational therapy (MS); physical therapy (DPT); physicians assistant (MS); speech-language pathology (MS). *Faculty:* 20 full-time, 94 part-time/adjunct. *Students:* 975 full-time (710 women), 160 part-time (114 women); includes 271 minority (58 Black or African American, non-Hispanic/Latino; 1 American Indian or Alaska Native, non-Hispanic/Latino; 132 Asian, non-Hispanic/Latino; 60 Hispanic/Latino; 4 Native Hawaiian or other Pacific Islander, non-Hispanic/Latino; 16 Two or more races, non-Hispanic/Latino), 10 international. *Expenses:* Contact institution. *Financial support:* Fellowships available. *Unit head:* Dr. Louis Primavera, Dean, School of Health Sciences, 516-673-3200, E-mail: louis.primavera@touro.edu. *Application contact:* Brian J. Diele, Associate Director of Central Admissions, 631-665-1600 Ext. 6311, E-mail: brian.diele@touro.edu.

Towson University, Program in Physician Assistant Studies, Towson, MD 21252-0001. Offers MS. *Accreditation:* ARC-PA. *Students:* 68 full-time (49 women); includes 19 minority (5 Black or African American, non-Hispanic/Latino; 1 American Indian or Alaska Native, non-Hispanic/Latino; 11 Asian, non-Hispanic/Latino; 1 Hispanic/Latino; 1 Two or more races, non-Hispanic/Latino), 1 international. *Entrance requirements:* For master's, bachelor's degree with minimum GPA of 3.0, completion of prerequisite math and science courses, minimum of 800 hours of patient contact experience or medical/health related experience. Additional exam requirements/recommendations for international students: Required—TOEFL (minimum score 550 paper-based; 80 iBT). *Application deadline:* Applications are processed on a rolling basis. Application fee: $45. Electronic applications accepted. *Expenses:* Contact institution. *Financial support:* Application deadline: 4/1. *Unit head:* Dr. Marcie Weinstein, Graduate Program Director, 410-704-4049, E-mail: mweinstein@towson.edu. *Application contact:* Alicia Arkell-Kleis, Information Contact, 410-704-6004, E-mail: grads@towson.edu.
Website: http://grad.towson.edu/program/master/past-ms/

Trevecca Nazarene University, Graduate Physician Assistant Program, Nashville, TN 37210-2877. Offers MS. *Accreditation:* ARC-PA. *Faculty:* 6 full-time (all women), 5 part-time/adjunct (all women). *Students:* 92 full-time (68 women); includes 3 minority (1 Black or African American, non-Hispanic/Latino; 2 Hispanic/Latino). Average age 26. In 2013, 42 master's awarded. *Degree requirements:* For master's, comprehensive exam, successful completion of 10 clinical skills rotations, professional assessment, OSCE exam. *Entrance requirements:* For master's, GRE (minimum score: 300 combined verbal and quatitative), minimum GPA of 3.25, 3 letters of recommendation (physician or physician assistant familiar with applicant abilities/potential, college professor, employer), clinical preference (highly recommended), prerequisites in human anatomy and physiology, general chemistry, microbiology with lab, general psychology, and developmental psychology. Additional exam requirements/recommendations for international students: Required—TOEFL (minimum score 550 paper-based). *Application deadline:* For fall admission, 11/1 for domestic students. Application fee: $45. *Expenses:* Contact institution. *Financial support:* Applicants required to submit FAFSA. *Unit head:* Dr. Randall Morton, Director, 615-248-1504, E-mail: admissions_pa@trevecca.edu. *Application contact:* 615-248-1225, E-mail: admissions_pa@trevecca.edu.

Tufts University, School of Medicine, Public Health and Professional Degree Programs, Boston, MA 02111. Offers biomedical sciences (MS); development and regulation of medicines and devices (MS); health communication (MS); pain research, education and policy (MS); physician assistant (MS); public health (MPH, Dr PH). MS programs offered jointly with Emerson College. *Accreditation:* CEPH (one or more programs are accredited). Part-time and evening/weekend programs available. *Faculty:* 77 full-time (26 women), 44 part-time/adjunct (22 women). *Students:* 324 full-time (189 women), 80 part-time (61 women); includes 137 minority (13 Black or African American, non-Hispanic/Latino; 87 Asian, non-Hispanic/Latino; 17 Hispanic/Latino; 20 Two or more races, non-Hispanic/Latino), 24 international. Average age 27. 1,267 applicants, 52% accepted, 245 enrolled. In 2013, 171 master's awarded. *Degree requirements:* For master's, thesis (for some programs); for doctorate, thesis/dissertation. *Entrance requirements:* For master's, GRE General Test, MCAT, GMAT. Additional exam requirements/recommendations for international students: Required—TOEFL (minimum score 96 iBT). *Application deadline:* For fall admission, 1/15 priority date for domestic students, 1/15 for international students; for spring admission, 10/25 priority date for domestic students, 10/25 for international students. Applications are processed on a rolling basis. Application fee: $70. Electronic applications accepted. *Expenses:* Contact institution. *Financial support:* In 2013–14, 17 students received support, including 1 fellowship (averaging $3,000 per year), 21 research assistantships (averaging $500 per year), 35 teaching assistantships (averaging $2,000 per year); Federal Work-Study and scholarships/grants also available. Support available to part-time students. Financial award application deadline: 2/4; financial award applicants required to submit FAFSA. *Faculty research:* Environmental and occupational health, nutrition, epidemiology, health communication, health services management and policy, biostatics, protein interaction, mRNA processing, vascular pathology. *Unit head:* Dr. Aviva Must, Dean, 617-636-0935, Fax: 617-636-0898, E-mail: aviva.must@tufts.edu. *Application contact:* Emily Keily, Director of Admissions, 617-636-0935, Fax: 617-636-0898, E-mail: med-phpd@tufts.edu.
Website: http://publichealth.tufts.edu

Union College, Physician Assistant Program, Lincoln, NE 68506-4300. Offers MPAS. *Accreditation:* ARC-PA. *Entrance requirements:* Additional exam requirements/recommendations for international students: Required—TOEFL (minimum score 600 paper-based; 100 iBT). Electronic applications accepted. *Faculty research:* Servant leadership, cultural competency.

The University of Alabama at Birmingham, School of Health Professions, Program in Physician Assistant Studies, Birmingham, AL 35294. Offers MSPAS. *Accreditation:* ARC-PA. *Entrance requirements:* For master's, GRE, three evaluations. Additional exam requirements/recommendations for international students: Required—TOEFL.

University of Arkansas for Medical Sciences, College of Health Professions, Little Rock, AR 72205-7199. Offers audiology (Au D); communication sciences and disorders (MS, PhD); genetic counseling (MS); nuclear medicine advanced associate (MIS); physician assistant studies (MPAS); radiologist assistant (MIS). PhD offered through consortium with University of Arkansas at Little Rock and University of Central Arkansas. Part-time programs available. Postbaccalaureate distance learning degree programs offered (minimal on-campus study). *Faculty:* 54 full-time (34 women), 16 part-time/adjunct (11 women). *Students:* 55 full-time (43 women), 32 part-time (24 women); includes 9 minority (3 Black or African American, non-Hispanic/Latino; 1 American Indian or Alaska Native, non-Hispanic/Latino; 1 Asian, non-Hispanic/Latino; 3 Hispanic/Latino; 1 Two or more races, non-Hispanic/Latino). In 2013, 10 master's, 8 doctorates awarded. *Degree requirements:* For master's, thesis (for some programs); for doctorate, comprehensive exam (for some programs), thesis/dissertation (for some programs). *Entrance requirements:* For master's, GRE. Additional exam requirements/recommendations for international students: Required—TOEFL (minimum score 550 paper-based; 79 iBT). Application fee: $40. Electronic applications accepted. *Expenses:* Contact institution. *Financial support:* Unspecified assistantships available. Financial award application deadline: 6/15; financial award applicants required to submit FAFSA. *Faculty research:* Auditory-based intervention, soy diet, nutrition and cancer. *Unit head:* Dr. Douglas L. Murphy, Dean, 501-686-5730. *Application contact:* Phyllis Fields, Assistant Dean, Student Affairs, 501-686-5730, E-mail: pafields@uams.edu.
Website: http://healthprofessions.uams.edu/

University of Bridgeport, Physician Assistant Institute, Bridgeport, CT 06604. Offers MS. *Faculty:* 4 full-time (2 women), 6 part-time/adjunct (3 women). *Students:* 74 full-time (47 women); includes 16 minority (2 Black or African American, non-Hispanic/Latino; 7 Asian, non-Hispanic/Latino; 5 Hispanic/Latino; 2 Two or more races, non-Hispanic/Latino). Average age 29. 104 applicants, 52% accepted, 40 enrolled. In 2013, 19 master's awarded. *Degree requirements:* For master's, thesis. *Entrance requirements:* Additional exam requirements/recommendations for international students: Recommended—TOEFL (minimum score 550 paper-based; 80 iBT), IELTS (minimum score 6.5). *Application deadline:* For fall admission, 8/1 for domestic and international students; for spring admission, 12/1 priority date for domestic and international students. Applications are processed on a rolling basis. Application fee: $50. *Expenses: Tuition:* Part-time $755 per credit. *Required fees:* $200 per semester. Tuition and fees vary according to program. *Unit head:* Dr. Daniel Cervonka, Director, 203-576-2399, Fax: 203-576-2402, E-mail: cervonka@bridgeport.edu. *Application contact:* Leanne Proctor, Director of Health Science Admissions, 203-576-4552, Fax: 203-576-4941, E-mail: admit@bridgeport.edu.

University of Charleston, Physician Assistant Program, Charleston, WV 25304-1099. Offers MPAS. *Students:* 63 full-time (38 women); includes 7 minority (2 Black or African American, non-Hispanic/Latino; 1 Asian, non-Hispanic/Latino; 3 Hispanic/Latino; 1 Native Hawaiian or other Pacific Islander, non-Hispanic/Latino). Average age 27. *Degree requirements:* For master's, clinical rotations. *Entrance requirements:* For master's, GRE, personal narrative, work and health care experience history, social engagement history, two references, transcripts. *Application deadline:* Applications are processed on a rolling basis. Electronic applications accepted. *Financial support:*

Physician Assistant Studies

Career-related internships or fieldwork available. *Unit head:* Jennifer Pack, Program Director, 304-357-4790, E-mail: jenniferpack@ucwv.edu. *Application contact:* Pam Carden, Admissions Coordinator, 304-357-4968, Fax: 304-357-4832, E-mail: pamcarden@ucwv.edu.
Website: http://www.ucwv.edu/PA/

University of Colorado Denver, School of Medicine, Physician Assistant Program, Aurora, CO 80045. Offers child health associate (MPAS), including global health, leadership, education, advocacy, development, and scholarship, rural health, urban/underserved populations. *Accreditation:* ARC-PA. *Students:* 132 full-time (107 women); includes 15 minority (1 American Indian or Alaska Native, non-Hispanic/Latino; 6 Asian, non-Hispanic/Latino; 8 Hispanic/Latino). Average age 27. 1,313 applicants, 3% accepted, 44 enrolled. In 2013, 43 master's awarded. *Degree requirements:* For master's, comprehensive exam, successful completion of all coursework and rotations. *Entrance requirements:* For master's, GRE General Test, minimum GPA of 2.8, 3 letters of recommendation, prerequisite courses in chemistry, biology, general genetics, psychology and statistics, interviews. Additional exam requirements/recommendations for international students: Required—TOEFL (minimum score 550 paper-based; 80 iBT). *Application deadline:* For fall admission, 9/1 for domestic students, 8/15 for international students. Application fee: $170. Electronic applications accepted. *Expenses:* Contact institution. *Financial support:* In 2013–14, 85 students received support. Fellowships, research assistantships, teaching assistantships, career-related internships or fieldwork, Federal Work-Study, institutionally sponsored loans, scholarships/grants, traineeships, and unspecified assistantships available. Financial award application deadline: 3/15; financial award applicants required to submit FAFSA. *Faculty research:* Clinical genetics and genetic counseling, evidence-based medicine, pediatric allergy and asthma, childhood diabetes, standardized patient assessment. *Unit head:* Jonathan Bowser, Program Director, 303-724-1349, E-mail: jonathan.bowser@ucdenver.edu. *Application contact:* Kay Denler, Director of Admissions, 303-724-7963, E-mail: kay.denler@ucdenver.edu.
Website: http://www.ucdenver.edu/academics/colleges/medicalschool/education/degree_programs/PAProgram/Pages/Home.aspx

University of Detroit Mercy, College of Health Professions, Physician Assistant Program, Detroit, MI 48221. Offers MS. *Accreditation:* ARC-PA. *Degree requirements:* For master's, thesis or alternative. *Entrance requirements:* For master's, GRE General Test, minimum GPA of 3.0. *Expenses:* Contact institution. *Faculty research:* Substance abuse prevention, international health care, public health.

The University of Findlay, Office of Graduate Admissions, Findlay, OH 45840-3653. Offers athletic training (MAT); business (MBA), including health care management, hospitality management, organizational leadership, public management; education (MA Ed), including administration, children's literature, early childhood, human resource development, reading, science, special education, technology; environmental, safety and health management (MSEM); health informatics (MS); occupational therapy (MOT); pharmacy (Pharm D); physical therapy (DPT); physician assistant (MPA); rhetoric and writing (MA); teaching English to speakers of other languages (TESOL) and bilingual education (MA). Part-time and evening/weekend programs available. Postbaccalaureate distance learning degree programs offered (no on-campus study). *Faculty:* 209 full-time (98 women), 69 part-time/adjunct (38 women). *Students:* 551 full-time (332 women), 457 part-time (276 women); includes 77 minority (37 Black or African American, non-Hispanic/Latino; 1 American Indian or Alaska Native, non-Hispanic/Latino; 15 Asian, non-Hispanic/Latino; 23 Hispanic/Latino; 1 Native Hawaiian or other Pacific Islander, non-Hispanic/Latino), 135 international. Average age 28. 637 applicants, 66% accepted, 241 enrolled. In 2013, 267 master's, 91 doctorates awarded. *Degree requirements:* For master's, thesis, cumulative project, capstone project. *Entrance requirements:* For master's, GRE/GMAT, bachelor's degree from accredited institution, minimum undergraduate GPA of 2.5 in last 64 hours of course work; for doctorate, GRE, minimum cumulative GPA of 3.0. Additional exam requirements/recommendations for international students: Required—TOEFL (minimum score 80 iBT). *Application deadline:* Applications are processed on a rolling basis. Application fee: $25. Electronic applications accepted. *Expenses: Required fees:* $146 per semester. Tuition and fees vary according to degree level and program. *Financial support:* In 2013–14, 11 research assistantships with full and partial tuition reimbursements (averaging $4,000 per year), 10 teaching assistantships with full and partial tuition reimbursements (averaging $3,600 per year) were awarded; career-related internships or fieldwork, Federal Work-Study, health care benefits, and unspecified assistantships also available. Financial award application deadline: 4/1; financial award applicants required to submit FAFSA. *Unit head:* Christopher M. Harris, Director of Admissions, 419-434-4347, E-mail: harrisc1@findlay.edu. *Application contact:* Emily Ickes, Graduate Admissions Counselor, 419-434-6933, Fax: 419-434-4898, E-mail: ickese@findlay.edu.
Website: http://www.findlay.edu/admissions/graduate/Pages/default.aspx

University of Florida, College of Medicine, Program in Physician Assistant, Gainesville, FL 32611. Offers MPAS. *Accreditation:* ARC-PA. *Entrance requirements:* For master's, GRE General Test, interview. Electronic applications accepted. *Expenses:* Tuition, state resident: full-time $12,640. Tuition, nonresident: full-time $30,000.

The University of Iowa, Roy J. and Lucille A. Carver College of Medicine and Graduate College, Graduate Programs in Medicine, Department of Physician Assistant Studies and Services, Iowa City, IA 52242-1316. Offers MPAS. *Accreditation:* ARC-PA. *Faculty:* 3 full-time (2 women), 2 part-time/adjunct (1 woman). *Students:* 48 full-time (30 women); includes 11 minority (2 Black or African American, non-Hispanic/Latino; 7 Asian, non-Hispanic/Latino; 2 Hispanic/Latino). Average age 28. 667 applicants, 4% accepted, 25 enrolled. In 2013, 25 master's awarded. *Degree requirements:* For master's, comprehensive exam, comprehensive clinical exam, clinical presentation. *Entrance requirements:* For master's, GRE General Test or MCAT, health care/research experience. Additional exam requirements/recommendations for international students: Required—TOEFL (minimum score 93 iBT). *Application deadline:* For spring admission, 11/1 for domestic students. Applications are processed on a rolling basis. Application fee: $60. Electronic applications accepted. *Financial support:* In 2013–14, 40 students received support. Institutionally sponsored loans and scholarships/grants available. Financial award application deadline: 3/1; financial award applicants required to submit FAFSA. *Unit head:* Dr. David P. Asprey, Chair and Department Executive Officer, 319-335-8922, Fax: 319-335-8923, E-mail: david-asprey@uiowa.edu. *Application contact:* Kaila A. Fairchild, Secretary, 319-335-8922, Fax: 319-335-8923, E-mail: kaila-fairchild@uiowa.edu.
Website: http://www.medicine.uiowa.edu/pa/

University of Kentucky, Graduate School, College of Health Sciences, Program in Physician Assistant Studies, Lexington, KY 40506-0032. Offers MSPAS. *Accreditation:* ARC-PA. *Degree requirements:* For master's, comprehensive exam. *Entrance requirements:* For master's, GRE General Test, minimum undergraduate GPA of 2.75. Additional exam requirements/recommendations for international students: Required—TOEFL (minimum score 550 paper-based). Electronic applications accepted.

University of Missouri–Kansas City, School of Medicine, Kansas City, MO 64110-2499. Offers anesthesia (MS); bioinformatics (MS); health professions education (MS); medicine (MD); physician assistant (MMS); MD/PhD. *Accreditation:* LCME/AMA. *Faculty:* 49 full-time (20 women), 13 part-time/adjunct (6 women). *Students:* 462 full-time (241 women), 16 part-time (8 women); includes 253 minority (33 Black or African American, non-Hispanic/Latino; 2 American Indian or Alaska Native, non-Hispanic/Latino; 196 Asian, non-Hispanic/Latino; 14 Hispanic/Latino; 1 Native Hawaiian or other Pacific Islander, non-Hispanic/Latino; 7 Two or more races, non-Hispanic/Latino), 3 international. Average age 24. 1,070 applicants, 11% accepted, 94 enrolled. In 2013, 12 master's, 88 doctorates awarded. *Degree requirements:* For doctorate, one foreign language, United States Medical Licensing Exam Step 1 and 2. *Entrance requirements:* For doctorate, interview. *Application deadline:* For fall admission, 11/15 for domestic and international students. Application fee: $50. *Expenses:* Contact institution. *Financial support:* In 2013–14, 4 fellowships (averaging $38,964 per year), 4 research assistantships (averaging $17,373 per year) were awarded; career-related internships or fieldwork, Federal Work-Study, institutionally sponsored loans, scholarships/grants, and tuition waivers (partial) also available. Financial award application deadline: 3/1; financial award applicants required to submit FAFSA. *Faculty research:* Cardiovascular disease, women's and children's health, trauma and infectious diseases, neurological, metabolic disease. *Unit head:* Dr. Betty Drees, Dean, 816-235-1808, E-mail: dreesb@umkc.edu. *Application contact:* Janine Kluckhohn, Admissions Coordinator, 816-235-1870, Fax: 816-235-6579, E-mail: kluckhohnj@umkc.edu.
Website: http://www.med.umkc.edu/

University of Mount Union, Program in Physician Assistant Studies, Alliance, OH 44601-3993. Offers MS. *Faculty:* 4 full-time (all women), 2 part-time/adjunct (1 woman). *Students:* 62 full-time (43 women); includes 3 minority (2 Asian, non-Hispanic/Latino; 1 Two or more races, non-Hispanic/Latino), 1 international. Average age 25. 250 applicants, 20% accepted, 32 enrolled. In 2013, 31 master's awarded. *Entrance requirements:* For master's, interview. *Application deadline:* Applications are processed on a rolling basis. Application fee: $500. Electronic applications accepted. *Expenses: Tuition:* Full-time $26,280; part-time $520 per credit hour. *Required fees:* $485; $80 per semester. Tuition and fees vary according to program. *Financial support:* Applicants required to submit FAFSA. *Unit head:* Sharon Luke, Director, 800-992-6682. *Application contact:* Jessie Canavan, Director of Admissions, 330-823-2579, E-mail: canavajl@mountunion.edu.
Website: http://www.mountunion.edu/pa

University of Nebraska Medical Center, School of Allied Health Professions, Division of Physician Assistant Education, Omaha, NE 68198-4300. Offers MPAS. *Accreditation:* ARC-PA. *Degree requirements:* For master's, comprehensive exam, research paper. *Entrance requirements:* For master's, GRE General Test, 16 undergraduate hours of course work in both biology and chemistry, 3 in math, 6 in English, 9 in psychology; minimum GPA of 3.0. Additional exam requirements/recommendations for international students: Required—TOEFL (minimum score 600 paper-based; 100 iBT). Electronic applications accepted. *Expenses: Required fees:* $300 per semester. Tuition and fees vary according to program. *Faculty research:* Substance abuse, mental health, women's health, geriatrics.

University of New England, Westbrook College of Health Professions, Program in Physician Assistant, Biddeford, ME 04005-9526. Offers MS. *Accreditation:* ARC-PA. *Faculty:* 6 full-time, 1 part-time/adjunct. *Students:* 98 full-time (69 women); includes 12 minority (1 Black or African American, non-Hispanic/Latino; 1 American Indian or Alaska Native, non-Hispanic/Latino; 4 Asian, non-Hispanic/Latino; 4 Hispanic/Latino; 2 Two or more races, non-Hispanic/Latino). Average age 27. 1,358 applicants, 5% accepted, 43 enrolled. In 2013, 46 master's awarded. *Degree requirements:* For master's, clinical rotations. *Entrance requirements:* For master's, minimum undergraduate GPA of 3.0, prerequisite courses in anatomy and physiology. *Application deadline:* For fall admission, 10/1 for domestic students. Applications are processed on a rolling basis. Electronic applications accepted. *Financial support:* Scholarships/grants available. Financial award application deadline: 5/1; financial award applicants required to submit FAFSA. *Unit head:* Thomas White, Program Director, Physician Assistant Program/Associate Professor, 207-221-4524, E-mail: twhite4@une.edu. *Application contact:* Dr. Cynthia Forrest, Vice President for Student Affairs, 207-221-4225, Fax: 207-523-1925, E-mail: gradadmissions@une.edu.
Website: http://www.une.edu/wchp/pa/program

University of New Mexico, School of Medicine, Program in Physician Assistant Studies, Albuquerque, NM 87131. Offers MS. *Accreditation:* ARC-PA. *Faculty:* 5 full-time (3 women), 3 part-time/adjunct (2 women). *Students:* 34 full-time (23 women), 2 part-time (both women); includes 16 minority (2 Asian, non-Hispanic/Latino; 12 Hispanic/Latino; 2 Two or more races, non-Hispanic/Latino). Average age 31. 4 applicants, 25% accepted. In 2013, 14 master's awarded. *Degree requirements:* For master's, comprehensive exam. *Entrance requirements:* For master's, GRE. Additional exam requirements/recommendations for international students: Recommended—TOEFL. *Application deadline:* For fall admission, 8/1 for domestic and international students; for winter admission, 8/1 for domestic and international students; for spring admission, 8/8 for domestic students, 8/1 for international students. Applications are processed on a rolling basis. Application fee: $50. Electronic applications accepted. *Financial support:* In 2013–14, 6 students received support. Application deadline: 6/30; applicants required to submit FAFSA. *Unit head:* Dr. Nikki Katalanos, Program Director, 505-272-9864, E-mail: paprogram@salud.unm.edu. *Application contact:* Marlys Harrison, Program Manager, 505-272-9864, E-mail: mharrison@salud.unm.edu.
Website: http://fcm.unm.edu/physician_assistant_program/index.html

University of North Dakota, Graduate School and Graduate School, Graduate Programs in Medicine, Physician Assistant Program, Grand Forks, ND 58202. Offers MPAS. *Accreditation:* ARC-PA. *Entrance requirements:* For master's, current RN licensure, minimum of 4 years of clinical experience, current ACLS certification, interview, letters of recommendation. Additional exam requirements/recommendations for international students: Required—TOEFL (minimum score 550 paper-based; 79 iBT), IELTS (minimum score 6.5).

University of North Texas Health Science Center at Fort Worth, Texas College of Osteopathic Medicine, School of Health Professions, Fort Worth, TX 76107-2699. Offers MPAS. *Accreditation:* ARC-PA. *Degree requirements:* For master's, thesis or alternative, research paper. *Entrance requirements:* For master's, minimum GPA of 2.85. *Faculty research:* Impact of mid-level providers on medical treatment, curriculum development, pain in geriatric patients, biopsychosocial risk factors.

University of Pittsburgh, School of Health and Rehabilitation Sciences, Physician Assistant Studies Program, Pittsburgh, PA 15260. Offers MS. *Faculty:* 5 full-time (3 women), 2 part-time/adjunct (0 women). *Students:* 79 full-time (63 women); includes 4 minority (1 Black or African American, non-Hispanic/Latino; 1 Asian, non-Hispanic/Latino; 2 Hispanic/Latino), 2 international. Average age 26. 658 applicants, 8% accepted, 41 enrolled. In 2013, 31 master's awarded. *Entrance requirements:* For master's, GRE. Additional exam requirements/recommendations for international students: Required—TOEFL (minimum score 550 paper-based; 80 iBT), IELTS (minimum score 6.5). *Application deadline:* For spring admission, 11/1 for domestic students, 10/1 for international students. Application fee: $135. *Expenses:* Contact institution. *Unit head:* Dr. Deborah A. Opacic, Program Director, 412-647-4646, E-mail: dopacic@pitt.edu. *Application contact:* Marsha LaCovey, Program Administrator, 412-624-6719, Fax: 412-624-7934, E-mail: mlacovey@pitt.edu.
Website: http://www.shrs.pitt.edu/pa/

University of St. Francis, College of Arts and Sciences, Joliet, IL 60435-6169. Offers advanced generalist forensic social work (Post-Master's Certificate); physician assistant practice (MS); social work (MSW). *Faculty:* 7 full-time (5 women), 1 (woman) part-time/adjunct. *Students:* 106 full-time (86 women), 22 part-time (20 women); includes 59 minority (21 Black or African American, non-Hispanic/Latino; 7 Asian, non-Hispanic/Latino; 26 Hispanic/Latino; 5 Two or more races, non-Hispanic/Latino). Average age 30. 88 applicants, 42% accepted, 28 enrolled. In 2013, 54 master's, 3 other advanced degrees awarded. *Entrance requirements:* Additional exam requirements/recommendations for international students: Required—TOEFL (minimum score 550 paper-based; 79 iBT). *Application deadline:* Applications are processed on a rolling basis. Application fee: $30. Electronic applications accepted. Application fee is waived when completed online. *Expenses:* Contact institution. *Financial support:* In 2013–14, 11 students received support. Scholarships/grants, tuition waivers (partial), and unspecified assistantships available. Support available to part-time students. Financial award applicants required to submit FAFSA. *Unit head:* Dr. Robert Kase, Dean, 815-740-3367, Fax: 815-740-6366. *Application contact:* Sandra Sloka, Director of Admissions for Graduate and Degree Completion Programs, 800-735-7500, Fax: 815-740-3431, E-mail: ssloka@stfrancis.edu.
Website: http://www.stfrancis.edu/academics/cas

University of Saint Francis, Graduate School, Department of Physician Assistant Studies, Fort Wayne, IN 46808-3994. Offers MS. *Accreditation:* ARC-PA. *Faculty:* 5. *Students:* 49 full-time (31 women); includes 4 minority (1 Asian, non-Hispanic/Latino; 2 Hispanic/Latino; 1 Two or more races, non-Hispanic/Latino), 1 international. Average age 27. In 2013, 23 master's awarded. *Degree requirements:* For master's, comprehensive exam. *Entrance requirements:* For master's, GRE, previous courses in biology, chemistry, and psychology, previous direct patient care. Additional exam requirements/recommendations for international students: Required—TOEFL, IELTS. *Application deadline:* For summer admission, 12/1 for domestic students. Application fee: $20. Application fee is waived when completed online. *Financial support:* Scholarships/grants available. Financial award application deadline: 3/10; financial award applicants required to submit FAFSA. *Unit head:* Dr. Dawn LaBarbera, Chair of the Department of Physician Assistant Studies, 260-399-7700 Ext. 8559, E-mail: dlabarbera@sf.edu. *Application contact:* James Cashdollar, Admissions Counselor, 260-399-7700 Ext. 6302, E-mail: jcashdollar@sf.edu.
Website: http://www.sf.edu/sf/physician-assistant

University of South Alabama, Graduate School, College of Allied Health Professions, Department of Physician Assistant Studies, Mobile, AL 36688-0002. Offers MHS. *Accreditation:* ARC-PA. *Faculty:* 6 full-time (4 women). *Students:* 79 full-time (58 women); includes 11 minority (2 Black or African American, non-Hispanic/Latino; 1 Asian, non-Hispanic/Latino; 4 Hispanic/Latino; 1 Native Hawaiian or other Pacific Islander, non-Hispanic/Latino; 3 Two or more races, non-Hispanic/Latino), 1 international. In 2013, 39 master's awarded. *Degree requirements:* For master's, thesis optional, externship; 121 hours consisting of 73 credit hours of didactic course work and 48 hours of clinical work. *Entrance requirements:* For master's, GRE General Test, minimum GPA of 3.0. *Application deadline:* For fall admission, 11/1 priority date for domestic students. Applications are processed on a rolling basis. Application fee: $110. *Expenses:* Tuition, state resident: full-time $8976; part-time $374 per credit hour. Tuition, nonresident: full-time $17,952; part-time $748 per credit hour. *Financial support:* Application deadline: 4/1. *Unit head:* Dr. Zarrintaj Alibadi, Chair, 251-445-9334. *Application contact:* Dr. Julio Turrens, Director of Graduate Studies, 251-445-9250.
Website: http://www.southalabama.edu/alliedhealth/pa/

The University of South Dakota, Graduate School, School of Health Sciences, Department of Physician Assistant Studies, Vermillion, SD 57069-2390. Offers MS. *Accreditation:* ARC-PA. *Entrance requirements:* Additional exam requirements/recommendations for international students: Required—TOEFL (minimum score 550 paper-based). Electronic applications accepted. *Expenses:* Contact institution. *Faculty research:* Neuroscience, teaching techniques in physician assistant education.

University of Southern California, Keck School of Medicine and Graduate School, Graduate Programs in Medicine, Primary Care Physician Assistant Program, Alhambra, CA 91803. Offers MPAP. *Accreditation:* ARC-PA. *Faculty:* 9 full-time (5 women), 7 part-time/adjunct (5 women). *Students:* 162 full-time (125 women); includes 87 minority (9 Black or African American, non-Hispanic/Latino; 2 American Indian or Alaska Native, non-Hispanic/Latino; 38 Asian, non-Hispanic/Latino; 23 Hispanic/Latino; 3 Native Hawaiian or other Pacific Islander, non-Hispanic/Latino; 12 Two or more races, non-Hispanic/Latino). Average age 24. 957 applicants, 8% accepted, 60 enrolled. In 2013, 50 master's awarded. *Degree requirements:* For master's, comprehensive exam, clinical training. *Entrance requirements:* For master's, GRE or MCAT, bachelor's degree; minimum cumulative GPA of 3.0, cumulative science 2.75. Additional exam requirements/recommendations for international students: Required—TOEFL (minimum score 600 paper-based; 100 iBT). *Application deadline:* For fall admission, 11/1 for domestic and international students. Applications are processed on a rolling basis. Application fee: $85. Electronic applications accepted. *Financial support:* Institutionally sponsored loans and scholarships/grants available. Financial award application deadline: 5/4; financial award applicants required to submit FAFSA. *Unit head:* Dr. Kevin C. Lohenry, Program Director, 626-457-4262, Fax: 626-457-4245, E-mail: lohenry@med.usc.edu. *Application contact:* Dr. John Mabee, Chair, Physician Assistant Admissions Committee, 626-457-4251, Fax: 626-457-4245, E-mail: mabee@med.usc.edu.
Website: http://www.usc.edu/schools/medicine/pa/

The University of Tennessee Health Science Center, College of Health Professions, Memphis, TN 38163-0002. Offers audiology (MS, Au D); clinical laboratory science (MSCLS); cytopathology practice (MCP); health informatics and information management (MHIIM); occupational therapy (MOT); physical therapy (DPT, ScDPT); physician assistant (MMS); speech-language pathology (MS). *Accreditation:* AOTA; APTA. Part-time and evening/weekend programs available. Postbaccalaureate distance learning degree programs offered (minimal on-campus study). Terminal master's awarded for partial completion of doctoral program. *Degree requirements:* For master's, comprehensive exam, thesis; for doctorate, comprehensive exam, residency. *Entrance requirements:* For master's, GRE (MOT, MSCLS), minimum GPA of 3.0, 3 letters of reference, national accreditation (MSCLS), GRE if GPA is less than 3.0 (MCP); for doctorate, GRE. Additional exam requirements/recommendations for international students: Required—TOEFL (minimum score 550 paper-based; 80 iBT). *Application deadline:* For fall admission, 1/30 priority date for domestic students; for winter admission, 10/1 priority date for domestic students. Application fee: $50. Electronic applications accepted. *Expenses:* Contact institution. *Financial support:* Teaching assistantships, Federal Work-Study, institutionally sponsored loans, and scholarships/grants available. Support available to part-time students. Financial award application deadline: 2/15; financial award applicants required to submit FAFSA. *Faculty research:* Gait deviation, muscular dystrophy and strength, hemophilia and exercise, pediatric neurology, self-efficacy. *Unit head:* Dr. Noma Anderson, Dean, 901-528-5588, Fax: 901-528-7545, E-mail: nander13@uthsc.edu. *Application contact:* Dr. Noma Anderson, Dean, 901-528-5588, Fax: 901-528-7545, E-mail: nander13@uthsc.edu.
Website: http://www.uthsc.edu/health-professions/

The University of Texas Health Science Center at San Antonio, School of Health Professions, San Antonio, TX 78229-3900. Offers occupational therapy (MOT); physical therapy (DPT); physician assistant studies (MS); toxicology (MS). *Accreditation:* AOTA; APTA; ARC-PA. *Faculty:* 85 full-time (31 women), 49 part-time/adjunct (19 women). *Students:* 353 full-time (258 women), 2 part-time (1 woman); includes 180 minority (15 Black or African American, non-Hispanic/Latino; 29 Asian, non-Hispanic/Latino; 129 Hispanic/Latino; 1 Native Hawaiian or other Pacific Islander, non-Hispanic/Latino; 6 Two or more races, non-Hispanic/Latino), 3 international. Average age 28. 605 applicants, 21% accepted, 125 enrolled. In 2013, 73 master's, 63 doctorates awarded. *Degree requirements:* For master's, comprehensive exam, thesis (for some programs); for doctorate, comprehensive exam. *Entrance requirements:* For master's, GRE (for toxicology), minimum GPA of 3.0 and bachelor's degree in clinical laboratory science or closely-related science discipline (for MS in toxicology); minimum GPA of 3.0, bachelor's degree, PA shadowing, and community service (for MS in physician assistant); for doctorate, GRE, minimum GPA of 3.0, bachelor's degree, PT shadowing, observation hours. Additional exam requirements/recommendations for international students: Required—TOEFL (minimum score 560 paper-based). *Application deadline:* For fall admission, 6/1 for domestic and international students; for spring admission, 10/1 for domestic and international students. Application fee: $60. Electronic applications accepted. *Financial support:* In 2013–14, 219 students received support. Federal Work-Study, scholarships/grants, and stipends, department payments available. Financial award application deadline: 6/30; financial award applicants required to submit FAFSA. *Total annual research expenditures:* $760,563. *Unit head:* Dr. Susan Dollar, Assistant Dean, 210-567-4837, Fax: 210-567-4828, E-mail: dollar@uthscsa.edu. *Application contact:* Dr. David L. Henzi, Assistant Dean for Admissions, 210-567-4818, Fax: 210-567-4828, E-mail: henzi@uthscsa.edu.
Website: http://www.uthscsa.edu/shp/

The University of Texas Medical Branch, School of Health Professions, Department of Physician Assistant Studies, Galveston, TX 77555. Offers MPAS. *Accreditation:* ARC-PA. *Entrance requirements:* For master's, GRE, interview. Electronic applications accepted.

The University of Texas Southwestern Medical Center, Southwestern School of Health Professions, Physician Assistant Studies Program, Dallas, TX 75390. Offers MPAS. *Accreditation:* ARC-PA. *Faculty:* 85 full-time (58 women). *Students:* 117 full-time (97 women); includes 29 minority (8 Black or African American, non-Hispanic/Latino; 4 Asian, non-Hispanic/Latino; 16 Hispanic/Latino; 1 Two or more races, non-Hispanic/Latino), 1 international. Average age 27. 888 applicants, 5% accepted, 36 enrolled. In 2013, 36 master's awarded. *Entrance requirements:* For master's, GRE, minimum GPA of 3.0. *Application deadline:* For spring admission, 10/1 for domestic students. Electronic applications accepted. *Financial support:* Application deadline: 3/1; applicants required to submit FAFSA. *Unit head:* Dr. Eugene Jones, Chair, 214-648-1701, Fax: 214-648-1003, E-mail: pa.sahss@utsouthwestern.edu. *Application contact:* Isela Perez, Education Coordinator, 214-648-1701, Fax: 214-648-1003, E-mail: isela.perez@utsouthwestern.edu.
Website: http://www8.utsouthwestern.edu/utsw/cda/dept48945/files/54102.html

University of the Cumberlands, Program in Physician Assistant Studies, Williamsburg, KY 40769-1372. Offers MPAS. *Accreditation:* ARC-PA. *Entrance requirements:* Additional exam requirements/recommendations for international students: Required—TOEFL. Electronic applications accepted.

The University of Toledo, College of Graduate Studies, College of Medicine and Life Sciences, Department of Physician Assistant Studies, Toledo, OH 43606-3390. Offers MSBS. *Accreditation:* ARC-PA. *Faculty:* 8. *Students:* 89 full-time (56 women), 42 part-time (28 women); includes 25 minority (17 Black or African American, non-Hispanic/Latino; 3 Asian, non-Hispanic/Latino; 4 Hispanic/Latino; 1 Two or more races, non-Hispanic/Latino). Average age 28. 792 applicants, 6% accepted, 44 enrolled. In 2013, 32 master's awarded. *Degree requirements:* For master's, thesis or alternative, scholarly project. *Entrance requirements:* For master's, GRE, interview, minimum undergraduate GPA of 3.0, writing sample, transcripts. Additional exam requirements/recommendations for international students: Required—TOEFL (minimum score 550 paper-based; 80 iBT). *Application deadline:* For fall admission, 10/1 for domestic and international students. Application fee: $45 ($75 for international students). Electronic applications accepted. *Expenses:* Contact institution. *Financial support:* Federal Work-Study, institutionally sponsored loans, scholarships/grants, and tuition waivers (partial) available. *Unit head:* Dr. Patricia Hogue, Director, 419-383-4807, E-mail: patricia.hogue@utoledo.edu. *Application contact:* Kristi Hayes, Secretary, 419-383-5408, E-mail: kristi.hayes@utoledo.edu.
Website: http://www.utoledo.edu/med/grad/pa/index.html

University of Utah, School of Medicine and Graduate School, Graduate Programs in Medicine, Department of Family and Preventive Medicine, Utah Physician Assistant Program, Salt Lake City, UT 84112-1107. Offers MPAS. *Accreditation:* ARC-PA. *Degree requirements:* For master's, comprehensive exam, thesis or alternative. *Entrance requirements:* Additional exam requirements/recommendations for international students: Required—TOEFL (minimum score 550 paper-based). Electronic applications accepted. *Expenses:* Contact institution. *Faculty research:* Physical assistant education, evidence–based medicine, technology and education, international medicine education.

University of Wisconsin–La Crosse, Graduate Studies, College of Science and Health, Department of Health Professions, Program in Physician Assistant Studies, La Crosse, WI 54601-3742. Offers MS. *Accreditation:* ARC-PA. *Faculty:* 2 full-time (both women), 3 part-time/adjunct (2 women). *Students:* 35 full-time (30 women), 1 (woman) part-time; includes 2 minority (both Asian, non-Hispanic/Latino). Average age 26. 374 applicants, 7% accepted, 19 enrolled. In 2013, 20 master's awarded. *Degree requirements:* For master's, comprehensive exam. *Entrance requirements:* For master's, GRE. Additional exam requirements/recommendations for international students: Required—TOEFL (minimum score 550 paper-based; 79 iBT). Electronic applications accepted. *Expenses:* Contact institution. *Financial support:* Federal Work-Study and scholarships/grants available. Support available to part-time students. *Unit head:* Dr. Edward J. Malone, III, Director, 608-785-8470, E-mail: malone.edwa@uwlax.edu. *Application contact:* Corey Sjoquist, Director of Admissions, 608-785-8939, E-mail: admissions@uwlax.edu.
Website: http://www.uwlax.edu/pastudies/

Wagner College, Division of Graduate Studies, Program in Advanced Physician Assistant Studies, Staten Island, NY 10301-4495. Offers MS. *Accreditation:* ARC-PA. Part-time programs available. *Faculty:* 1 (woman) full-time, 3 part-time/adjunct (2 women). *Students:* 27 full-time (23 women); includes 5 minority (4 Asian, non-Hispanic/Latino; 1 Native Hawaiian or other Pacific Islander, non-Hispanic/Latino). Average age 22. 24 applicants, 100% accepted, 24 enrolled. In 2013, 15 master's awarded. *Degree requirements:* For master's, thesis. *Entrance requirements:* For master's, minimum GPA of 3.0; bachelor's degree in one of the biological sciences, chemistry or physician assistant studies; physician assistant certification. Additional exam requirements/recommendations for international students: Required—TOEFL (minimum score 550 paper-based; 79 iBT). *Application deadline:* For fall admission, 5/1 priority date for domestic and international students; for spring admission, 11/1 for domestic and international students. Applications are processed on a rolling basis. Application fee:

$50. *Expenses: Tuition:* Full-time $17,496; part-time $972 per credit. Tuition and fees vary according to course load. *Financial support:* In 2013–14, 27 students received support. Career-related internships or fieldwork, Federal Work-Study, unspecified assistantships, and alumni fellowship grants available. Financial award applicants required to submit FAFSA. *Unit head:* Nora Lowy, Director, 718-390-4610, Fax: 718-420-4004, E-mail: nora.lowy@wagner.edu. *Application contact:* Patricia Clancy, Administrative Assistant, 718-420-4464, Fax: 718-390-3105, E-mail: patricia.clancy@wagner.edu.

Wayne State University, Eugene Applebaum College of Pharmacy and Health Sciences, Department of Health Care Sciences, Program in Physician Assistant Studies, Detroit, MI 48202. Offers MS. *Accreditation:* ARC-PA. *Faculty:* 3 full-time (2 women), 5 part-time/adjunct (3 women). *Students:* 92 full-time (76 women); includes 6 minority (5 Asian, non-Hispanic/Latino; 1 Hispanic/Latino), 1 international. Average age 27. In 2013, 43 master's awarded. *Entrance requirements:* For master's, GRE General Test, course work in science, 500 hours of work experience in health services, recommendations, interview, bachelor's degree from accredited institution before start of PA program with minimum GPA of 3.0 overall and in prerequisites, CASPA application. Additional exam requirements/recommendations for international students: Required—TOEFL (minimum score 550 paper-based; 79 iBT), TWE (minimum score 5.5), Michigan English Language Assessment Battery (minimum score 85); Recommended—IELTS (minimum score 6.5). *Application deadline:* For fall and spring admission, 9/1 for domestic and international students. Application fee: $0. Electronic applications accepted. *Expenses:* Contact institution. *Financial support:* Scholarships/grants available. Financial award application deadline: 3/31; financial award applicants required to submit FAFSA. *Faculty research:* Professionalism in physician assistant programs, interprofessional education, including advancements in neurological surgery, vestibular dysfunction, special needs populations. *Unit head:* Stephanie Gilkey, Program Director, 313-577-9666, E-mail: sgilkey@wayne.edu. *Application contact:* Heather Sandlin, Academic Services Officer II, 313-577-5523, Fax: 313-577-6367, E-mail: hsandlin@wayne.edu.
Website: http://www.pa.cphs.wayne.edu/

Weill Cornell Medical College, Weill Cornell Graduate School of Medical Sciences, Physician Assistant Program, New York, NY 10022. Offers health sciences (MS), including surgery. *Accreditation:* ARC-PA. *Degree requirements:* For master's, thesis. *Entrance requirements:* For master's, GRE. Additional exam requirements/recommendations for international students: Required—TOEFL. Electronic applications accepted.

Western Michigan University, Graduate College, College of Health and Human Services, Department of Physician Assistant, Kalamazoo, MI 49008. Offers MS. *Accreditation:* ARC-PA. Part-time programs available.

Western University of Health Sciences, College of Allied Health Professions, Program in Physician Assistant Studies, Pomona, CA 91766-1854. Offers MS. *Accreditation:* ARC-PA. *Faculty:* 9 full-time (6 women), 3 part-time/adjunct (2 women). *Students:* 191 full-time (144 women); includes 80 minority (2 Black or African American, non-Hispanic/Latino; 40 Asian, non-Hispanic/Latino; 24 Hispanic/Latino; 14 Two or more races, non-Hispanic/Latino). Average age 27. 1,609 applicants, 8% accepted, 95 enrolled. In 2013, 94 master's awarded. *Degree requirements:* For master's, comprehensive exam, thesis. *Entrance requirements:* For master's, minimum GPA of 2.7, letters of recommendation, interview. *Application deadline:* For fall admission, 11/1 for domestic students; for spring admission, 3/1 for domestic students. Application fee: $50. Electronic applications accepted. *Expenses:* Contact institution. *Financial support:* Institutionally sponsored loans, scholarships/grants, and veterans educational benefits available. Financial award applicants required to submit FAFSA. *Unit head:* Roy Guizado, Chair, 909-469-5445, Fax: 909-469-5407, E-mail: roygpac@westernu.edu. *Application contact:* Karen Hutton-Lopez, Director of Admissions, 909-469-5335, Fax: 909-469-5570, E-mail: admissions@westernu.edu.
Website: http://www.westernu.edu/allied-health/allied-health-mspas/

Wichita State University, Graduate School, College of Health Professions, Department of Physician Assistant, Wichita, KS 67260. Offers MPA. *Accreditation:* ARC-PA. *Unit head:* Dr. Dan Bequillard, Chair, 316-978-3011, Fax: 316-978-3669, E-mail: daniel.bequillard. *Application contact:* Jordan Oleson, Admissions Coordinator, 316-978-3095, Fax: 316-978-3253, E-mail: jordan.oleson@wichita.edu.
Website: http://www.wichita.edu/pa

Yale University, School of Medicine, Physician Associate Program, New Haven, CT 06510. Offers MM Sc, MM Sc/MPH. *Accreditation:* ARC-PA. *Degree requirements:* For master's, thesis. *Entrance requirements:* For master's, GRE General Test, course work in science. Additional exam requirements/recommendations for international students: Required—TOEFL. Electronic applications accepted. *Expenses:* Contact institution. *Faculty research:* Correlation of GRE scores and program performance, relationship of PA programs and pharmaceutical companies, career patterns in physician assistants, PA utilization and satisfaction with care, factors influencing PAs in their decision to pursue postgraduate residencies.

Rehabilitation Sciences

Alabama State University, College of Health Sciences, Department of Prosthetics and Orthotics, Montgomery, AL 36101-0271. Offers MS. *Faculty:* 1 full-time (0 women). *Students:* 11 full-time (2 women); includes 5 minority (2 Black or African American, non-Hispanic/Latino; 1 American Indian or Alaska Native, non-Hispanic/Latino; 1 Asian, non-Hispanic/Latino; 1 Hispanic/Latino). 15 applicants, 47% accepted, 7 enrolled. Application fee: $25. *Expenses:* Tuition, state resident: full-time $7958; part-time $343 per credit hour. Tuition, nonresident: full-time $14,132; part-time $686 per credit hour. *Required fees:* $446 per term. One-time fee: $1784 full-time; $892 part-time. Tuition and fees vary according to course load. *Unit head:* Dr. J. Chad Duncan, Chair, 334-229-5888, E-mail: jduncan@alasu.edu. *Application contact:* Dr. William Person, Dean of Graduate Studies, 334-229-4274, Fax: 334-229-4928, E-mail: wperson@alasu.edu.
Website: http://www.alasu.edu/academics/colleges—departments/health-sciences/prosthetics-orthotics/index.aspx

Appalachian State University, Cratis D. Williams Graduate School, Department of Health, Leisure, and Exercise Science, Boone, NC 28608. Offers exercise science (MS), including clinical exercise physiology, research, strength and conditioning. *Degree requirements:* For master's, comprehensive exam, thesis optional. *Entrance requirements:* For master's, GRE General Test, 3 letters of recommendation. Additional exam requirements/recommendations for international students: Required—TOEFL (minimum score 570 paper-based; 79 iBT), IELTS (minimum score 6.5). Electronic applications accepted. *Faculty research:* Exercise immunology, biomechanics, exercise and chronic disease, muscle damage, strength and conditioning.

Boston University, College of Health and Rehabilitation Sciences: Sargent College, Department of Occupational Therapy, Boston, MA 02215. Offers occupational therapy (MSOT, OTD); rehabilitation sciences (PhD). *Accreditation:* AOTA (one or more programs are accredited). Postbaccalaureate distance learning degree programs offered (minimal on-campus study). *Faculty:* 13 full-time (all women), 2 part-time/adjunct (both women). *Students:* 119 full-time (110 women), 10 part-time (9 women); includes 16 minority (8 Asian, non-Hispanic/Latino; 6 Hispanic/Latino; 2 Two or more races, non-Hispanic/Latino), 2 international. Average age 25. 298 applicants, 29% accepted, 29 enrolled. In 2013, 52 master's, 5 doctorates awarded. *Degree requirements:* For master's, thesis optional, full-time internship; for doctorate, comprehensive exam, thesis/dissertation. *Entrance requirements:* For master's, minimum GPA of 3.0; BS in area related to occupational therapy; for doctorate, GRE General Test. Additional exam requirements/recommendations for international students: Required—TOEFL (minimum score 550 paper-based), TWE (minimum score 5). *Application deadline:* For fall admission, 1/15 priority date for domestic and international students. Applications are processed on a rolling basis. Application fee: $125. Electronic applications accepted. *Expenses: Tuition:* Full-time $43,970; part-time $1374 per credit hour. *Required fees:* $60 per semester. Tuition and fees vary according to class time, course level and program. *Financial support:* In 2013–14, 64 students received support, including 60 fellowships (averaging $12,300 per year), 10 teaching assistantships (averaging $4,000 per year); career-related internships or fieldwork, Federal Work-Study, institutionally sponsored loans, scholarships/grants, and tuition waivers (partial) also available. Financial award application deadline: 4/15; financial award applicants required to submit FAFSA. *Faculty research:* Sensory integration, outcomes measurement, impact of Parkinson's disease, families of people with autism. *Total annual research expenditures:* $378,582. *Unit head:* Dr. Wendy J. Coster, Department Chair, 617-353-2727, Fax: 617-353-2926, E-mail: wjcoster@bu.edu. *Application contact:* Sharon Sankey, Director, Student Services, 617-353-2713, Fax: 617-353-7500, E-mail: ssankey@bu.edu.
Website: http://www.bu.edu/sargent/

Boston University, College of Health and Rehabilitation Sciences: Sargent College, Department of Physical Therapy and Athletic Training, Boston, MA 02215. Offers physical therapy (DPT); rehabilitation sciences (PhD). *Accreditation:* APTA (one or more programs are accredited). *Faculty:* 13 full-time (10 women), 26 part-time/adjunct (12 women). *Students:* 139 full-time (100 women), 25 part-time (21 women); includes 29 minority (17 Asian, non-Hispanic/Latino; 7 Hispanic/Latino; 5 Two or more races, non-Hispanic/Latino), 6 international. Average age 27. 836 applicants, 17% accepted, 37 enrolled. In 2013, 72 doctorates awarded. *Degree requirements:* For doctorate, comprehensive exam and thesis (for PhD). *Entrance requirements:* For doctorate, GRE General Test, master's degree (for PhD), bachelor's degree (for DPT). Additional exam requirements/recommendations for international students: Required—TOEFL (minimum score 550 paper-based). *Application deadline:* For fall admission, 1/7 priority date for domestic and international students. Applications are processed on a rolling basis. Application fee: $120. Electronic applications accepted. *Expenses: Tuition:* Full-time $43,970; part-time $1374 per credit hour. *Required fees:* $60 per semester. Tuition and fees vary according to class time, course level and program. *Financial support:* In 2013–14, 120 students received support, including 113 fellowships (averaging $10,000 per year), 6 teaching assistantships (averaging $3,000 per year); career-related internships or fieldwork, Federal Work-Study, institutionally sponsored loans, scholarships/grants, and tuition waivers (partial) also available. Financial award application deadline: 4/15; financial award applicants required to submit FAFSA. *Faculty research:* Gait, balance, motor control, dynamic systems analysis, spinal cord injury. *Total annual research expenditures:* $1.5 million. *Unit head:* Dr. Melanie Matthies, Department Chair, 617-353-2724, E-mail: pt@bu.edu. *Application contact:* Sharon Sankey, Director, Student Services, 617-353-2713, Fax: 617-353-7500, E-mail: ssankey@bu.edu.
Website: http://www.bu.edu/sargent/

California University of Pennsylvania, School of Graduate Studies and Research, College of Education and Human Services, Program in Exercise Science and Health Promotion, California, PA 15419-1394. Offers performance enhancement and injury prevention (MS); rehabilitation science (MS); sport psychology (MS); wellness and fitness (MS). Part-time and evening/weekend programs available. Postbaccalaureate distance learning degree programs offered (no on-campus study). *Degree requirements:* For master's, comprehensive exam, thesis optional. *Entrance requirements:* For master's, minimum QPA of 3.0. Additional exam requirements/recommendations for international students: Required—TOEFL (minimum score 550 paper-based; 80 iBT). Electronic applications accepted. *Expenses:* Contact institution. *Faculty research:* Reducing obesity in children, sport performance, creating unique biomechanical assessment techniques, Web-based training for fitness professionals, Webcams.

Central Michigan University, College of Graduate Studies, The Herbert H. and Grace A. Dow College of Health Professions, School of Rehabilitation and Medical Sciences, Mount Pleasant, MI 48859. Offers physical therapy (DPT); physician assistant (MS). *Accreditation:* APTA; ARC-PA. *Degree requirements:* For master's, thesis or alternative; for doctorate, thesis/dissertation or alternative. *Entrance requirements:* For master's and doctorate, GRE. Electronic applications accepted.

Clarion University of Pennsylvania, Office of Transfer, Adult and Graduate Admissions, On-Campus Master's Programs, Clarion, PA 16214. Offers rehabilitative sciences (MS); special education (MS); speech language pathology (MS). *Accreditation:* ASHA. Part-time programs available. Postbaccalaureate distance learning degree programs offered (no on-campus study). *Faculty:* 23 full-time (16 women). *Students:* 113 full-time (97 women), 42 part-time (33 women); includes 4 minority (2 Black or African American, non-Hispanic/Latino; 1 American Indian or Alaska Native, non-Hispanic/Latino; 1 Hispanic/Latino). Average age 24. 297 applicants, 18% accepted, 44 enrolled. In 2013, 68 master's awarded. *Degree requirements:* For master's, comprehensive exam (for some programs), thesis or alternative. *Entrance requirements:* For master's, GRE, minimum QPA of 3.0. Additional exam requirements/recommendations for international students: Required—TOEFL (minimum score 600 paper-based; 89 iBT), IELTS (minimum score 7.5). *Application deadline:* For fall admission, 1/31 for domestic and international students. Applications are processed on a rolling basis. Application fee: $40. Electronic applications accepted. *Expenses:* Tuition, state resident: part-time $442 per credit. Tuition, nonresident: part-time $451 per credit. *Required fees:* $142.40

per semester. One-time fee: $150 part-time. *Financial support:* In 2013–14, 21 research assistantships with full and partial tuition reimbursements (averaging $9,240 per year) were awarded; career-related internships or fieldwork also available. Support available to part-time students. Financial award application deadline: 3/1. *Unit head:* Dr. Colleen McAleer, Chair, 814-393-2581, Fax: 814-393-2206, E-mail: cmcaleer@clarion.edu. *Application contact:* Michelle Ritzler, Assistant Director, Graduate Programs, 814-393-2337, Fax: 814-393-2722, E-mail: gradstudies@clarion.edu.
Website: http://www.clarion.edu/991/

Concordia University Wisconsin, Graduate Programs, School of Human Services, Program in Rehabilitation Science, Mequon, WI 53097-2402. Offers MSRS.

Duquesne University, John G. Rangos, Sr. School of Health Sciences, Pittsburgh, PA 15282-0001. Offers health management systems (MHMS); occupational therapy (MS, OTD); physical therapy (DPT); physician assistant studies (MPAS); rehabilitation science (MS, PhD); speech-language pathology (MS); MBA/MHMS. *Accreditation:* AOTA (one or more programs are accredited); APTA (one or more programs are accredited); ASHA. Postbaccalaureate distance learning degree programs offered (minimal on-campus study). *Faculty:* 41 full-time (29 women), 32 part-time/adjunct (15 women). *Students:* 232 full-time (174 women), 14 part-time (7 women); includes 12 minority (2 Black or African American, non-Hispanic/Latino; 7 Asian, non-Hispanic/Latino; 1 Hispanic/Latino; 2 Two or more races, non-Hispanic/Latino), 7 international. Average age 23. 951 applicants, 11% accepted, 35 enrolled. In 2013, 119 master's, 40 doctorates awarded. *Degree requirements:* For doctorate, comprehensive exam (for some programs), thesis/dissertation (for some programs). *Entrance requirements:* For master's, GRE General Test (speech-language pathology), 3 letters of recommendation; minimum GPA of 2.75 (health management systems), 3.0 (speech-language pathology); for doctorate, GRE General Test (for physical therapy and rehabilitation science), 3 letters of recommendation, minimum GPA of 3.0, personal interview. Additional exam requirements/recommendations for international students: Required—TOEFL (minimum score 550 paper-based; 90 iBT). *Application deadline:* For fall admission, 2/1 for domestic and international students; for spring admission, 7/1 for domestic and international students. Applications are processed on a rolling basis. Electronic applications accepted. *Expenses:* Contact institution. *Financial support:* Federal Work-Study available. Financial award applicants required to submit FAFSA. *Faculty research:* Neuronal processing, electrical stimulation on peripheral neuropathy, central nervous system (CNS) stimulatory and inhibitory signals, behavioral genetic methodologies to development disorders of speech, neurogenic communication disorders. *Total annual research expenditures:* $83,650. *Unit head:* Dr. Gregory H. Frazer, Dean, 412-396-5303, Fax: 412-396-5554, E-mail: frazer@duq.edu. *Application contact:* Christopher R. Hilf, Recruiter/Academic Advisor, 412-396-5653, Fax: 412-396-5554, E-mail: hilfc@duq.edu.
Website: http://www.duq.edu/academics/schools/health-sciences

East Carolina University, Graduate School, School of Allied Health Sciences, Department of Addictions and Rehabilitation Studies, Greenville, NC 27858-4353. Offers military and trauma counseling (Certificate); rehabilitation and career counseling (MS); rehabilitation counseling (Certificate); rehabilitation counseling and administration (PhD); substance abuse and clinical counseling (MS); substance abuse counseling (Certificate); vocational evaluation (Certificate). *Accreditation:* CORE. Part-time and evening/weekend programs available. *Degree requirements:* For master's, comprehensive exam, thesis or alternative, internship. *Entrance requirements:* For master's, GRE General Test or MAT. Additional exam requirements/recommendations for international students: Required—TOEFL. *Application deadline:* For fall admission, 3/1 priority date for domestic students; for spring admission, 10/1 priority date for domestic students. Applications are processed on a rolling basis. Application fee: $50. *Expenses:* Tuition, state resident: full-time $4223. Tuition, nonresident: full-time $16,540. *Required fees:* $2184. *Financial support:* Research assistantships with partial tuition reimbursements, teaching assistantships with partial tuition reimbursements, Federal Work-Study, and scholarships/grants available. Support available to part-time students. Financial award application deadline: 3/1. *Unit head:* Dr. Paul Toriello, Chair, 252-744-6292, E-mail: toriellop@ecu.edu. *Application contact:* Dr. Paul Toriello, Chair, 252-744-6292, E-mail: toriellop@ecu.edu.
Website: http://www.ecu.edu/rehb/

East Stroudsburg University of Pennsylvania, Graduate College, College of Health Sciences, Department of Exercise Science, East Stroudsburg, PA 18301-2999. Offers cardiac rehabilitation and exercise science (MS). Part-time and evening/weekend programs available. Postbaccalaureate distance learning degree programs offered. *Faculty:* 7 full-time (2 women). *Students:* 48 full-time (28 women), 2 part-time (1 woman); includes 11 minority (6 Black or African American, non-Hispanic/Latino; 3 Hispanic/Latino; 2 Two or more races, non-Hispanic/Latino), 1 international. Average age 23. 114 applicants, 75% accepted, 54 enrolled. In 2013, 38 master's awarded. *Degree requirements:* For master's, comprehensive exam, thesis or alternative, computer literacy. *Entrance requirements:* Additional exam requirements/recommendations for international students: Required—TOEFL (minimum score 560 paper-based; 83 iBT) or IELTS. *Application deadline:* For fall admission, 3/1 priority date for domestic and international students; for spring admission, 11/30 for domestic students, 10/31 for international students. Applications are processed on a rolling basis. Application fee: $50. Electronic applications accepted. *Expenses:* Tuition, state resident: full-time $7956; part-time $442 per credit. Tuition, nonresident: full-time $11,934; part-time $663 per credit. *Required fees:* $2129; $118 per credit. *Financial support:* Research assistantships with full and partial tuition reimbursements, Federal Work-Study, and institutionally sponsored loans available. Financial award application deadline: 3/1. *Unit head:* Dr. Shala Davis, Graduate Coordinator, 570-422-3302, Fax: 570-422-3616, E-mail: sdavis@po-box.esu.edu. *Application contact:* Kevin Quintero, Graduate Admissions Coordinator, 570-422-3536, Fax: 570-422-2711, E-mail: kquintero@esu.edu.

George Mason University, College of Health and Human Services, Department of Rehabilitation Science, Fairfax, VA 22030. Offers PhD, Certificate. *Faculty:* 6 full-time (2 women), 3 part-time/adjunct (0 women). *Students:* 12 full-time (8 women), 1 (woman) part-time; includes 2 minority (both Asian, non-Hispanic/Latino), 1 international. Average age 32. 23 applicants, 61% accepted, 8 enrolled. *Degree requirements:* For doctorate, comprehensive exam, thesis/dissertation. *Entrance requirements:* For doctorate, GRE, 2 official college transcripts, expanded goals statement, 3 letters of recommendation, resume. Additional exam requirements/recommendations for international students: Required—TOEFL (minimum score 570 paper-based; 88 iBT), IELTS (minimum score 6.5), PTE. *Application deadline:* For fall admission, 2/1 for domestic students. Application fee: $65 ($80 for international students). *Expenses:* Contact institution. *Financial support:* In 2013–14, 10 students received support, including 10 research assistantships (averaging $22,970 per year); teaching assistantships, career-related internships or fieldwork, Federal Work-Study, scholarships/grants, unspecified assistantships, and health care benefits (for full-time research or teaching assistantship recipients) also available. Support available to part-time students. Financial award applicants required to submit FAFSA. *Faculty research:* Physiological determinants of functional loss; biobehavioral factors that contribute to functional disablement; cardiorespiratory function and performance; human motion, function, and performance. *Total annual research expenditures:* $56,181. *Unit head:* Andrew Guccione, Professor/Founding Chair, 703-993-4650, Fax: 703-993-2695, E-mail: aguccion@gmu.edu. *Application contact:* Brett Say, Program Coordinator, 703-993-1950, Fax: 703-993-2695, E-mail: bsay@gmu.edu.
Website: http://chhs.gmu.edu/rehabscience/

Indiana University–Purdue University Indianapolis, School of Health and Rehabilitation Sciences, Indianapolis, IN 46202. Offers health and rehabilitation sciences (PhD); health sciences (MS); nutrition and dietetics (MS); occupational therapy (MS); physical therapy (DPT); physician assistant (MPAS). Part-time and evening/weekend programs available. *Faculty:* 4 full-time (3 women). *Students:* 266 full-time (201 women), 13 part-time (12 women); includes 21 minority (6 Black or African American, non-Hispanic/Latino; 7 Asian, non-Hispanic/Latino; 4 Hispanic/Latino; 1 Native Hawaiian or other Pacific Islander, non-Hispanic/Latino; 3 Two or more races, non-Hispanic/Latino), 11 international. Average age 26. 381 applicants, 23% accepted, 77 enrolled. In 2013, 33 master's, 39 doctorates awarded. *Degree requirements:* For master's, thesis (for some programs). *Entrance requirements:* For master's, GRE General Test, minimum GPA of 3.0 (for MS in health sciences, nutrition and dietetics), 3.2 (for MS in occupational therapy), 3.0 cumulative and prerequisite math/science (for MPAS); for doctorate, GRE, minimum cumulative and prerequisite math/science GPA of 3.2. Additional exam requirements/recommendations for international students: Required—TOEFL (minimum score 550 paper-based; 79 iBT), IELTS (minimum score 6.5), PTE (minimum score 54). *Application deadline:* For fall admission, 10/1 for domestic students; for spring admission, 10/15 for domestic students. Electronic applications accepted. *Expenses:* Contact institution. *Financial support:* Fellowships, research assistantships, Federal Work-Study, institutionally sponsored loans, and scholarships/grants available. Support available to part-time students. Financial award applicants required to submit FAFSA. *Faculty research:* Function and mobility across the lifespan, pediatric nutrition, driving and mobility rehabilitation, neurorehabilitation and biomechanics, rehabilitation and integrative therapy. *Total annual research expenditures:* $1.1 million. *Unit head:* Dr. Augustine Agho, Dean, 317-274-4704, E-mail: aagho@iu.edu. *Application contact:* Kim Crockett, Student Data Coordinator, 317-278-6744, E-mail: kimecroc@iu.edu.
Website: http://shrs.iupui.edu/

Logan University, College of Health Sciences, Chesterfield, MO 63017. Offers nutrition and human performance (MS); sports science and rehabilitation (MS). Part-time programs available. Postbaccalaureate distance learning degree programs offered (no on-campus study). *Faculty:* 10 full-time (3 women), 15 part-time/adjunct (8 women). *Students:* 19 full-time (9 women), 63 part-time (31 women); includes 12 minority (2 Black or African American, non-Hispanic/Latino; 5 Asian, non-Hispanic/Latino; 3 Hispanic/Latino; 2 Two or more races, non-Hispanic/Latino), 1 international. Average age 32. In 2013, 82 master's awarded. *Degree requirements:* For master's, comprehensive exam. *Entrance requirements:* For master's, GRE or National Board of Chiropractic Examiners test, minimum GPA of 2.5; specific undergraduate coursework based on program of interest. Additional exam requirements/recommendations for international students: Required—TOEFL (minimum score 79 iBT). *Application deadline:* For fall admission, 7/15 priority date for domestic and international students; for winter admission, 11/15 priority date for domestic and international students; for spring admission, 3/15 priority date for domestic students, 3/15 for international students. Applications are processed on a rolling basis. Application fee: $50. Electronic applications accepted. *Expenses:* Contact institution. *Financial support:* Federal Work-Study and scholarships/grants available. Support available to part-time students. Financial award applicants required to submit FAFSA. *Faculty research:* Ankle injury prevention in high school athletes, low back pain in college football players, short arc banding and low back pain, the effects of enzymes on inflammatory blood markers, gait analysis in high school and college athletes. *Unit head:* Dr. Sherri Cole, Vice President, Academic Affairs, 636-227-2100 Ext. 2702, Fax: 636-207-2431, E-mail: sherri.cole@logan.edu. *Application contact:* Stacey Till, Director of Admissions, 636-227-2100 Ext. 1749, Fax: 636-207-2425, E-mail: admissions@logan.edu.
Website: http://www.logan.edu

Marquette University, Graduate School, College of Health Sciences, Clinical and Translational Rehabilitation Science Program, Milwaukee, WI 53201-1881. Offers MS, PhD. *Students:* 4 full-time (2 women), 10 part-time (6 women); includes 2 minority (1 Black or African American, non-Hispanic/Latino; 1 Hispanic/Latino). Average age 29. 20 applicants, 60% accepted. In 2013, 1 master's awarded. *Entrance requirements:* For master's and doctorate, GRE, official transcripts, curriculum vitae, personal statement, three letters of recommendation, interview. Additional exam requirements/recommendations for international students: Required—TOEFL (minimum score 90 iBT). *Application deadline:* For fall admission, 8/1 for domestic students, 6/1 for international students; for spring admission, 12/15 for domestic students, 10/15 for international students. Applications are processed on a rolling basis. Application fee: $50. *Financial support:* Research assistantships available. Financial award application deadline: 2/15. *Unit head:* Dr. Lawrence Pan, Professor/Chair, 414-288-7161. *Application contact:* Dr. Paula Papanek, Associate Professor/Director of Exercise Science, 414-288-5069.

McGill University, Faculty of Graduate and Postdoctoral Studies, Faculty of Medicine, School of Physical and Occupational Therapy, Montréal, QC H3A 2T5, Canada. Offers assessing driving capability (PGC); rehabilitation science (M Sc, PhD).

McMaster University, Faculty of Health Sciences and School of Graduate Studies, Program in Rehabilitation Science (course-based), Hamilton, ON L8S 4M2, Canada. Offers M Sc. Part-time programs available. *Degree requirements:* For master's, online courses and scholarly paper. *Entrance requirements:* For master's, minimum B+ average in final year of a 4-year undergraduate health professional program or other relevant program. Additional exam requirements/recommendations for international students: Required—TOEFL (minimum score 600 paper-based).

McMaster University, Faculty of Health Sciences and School of Graduate Studies, Program in Rehabilitation Science (Thesis Option), Hamilton, ON L8S 4M2, Canada. Offers M Sc, PhD. Part-time programs available. *Degree requirements:* For master's, thesis. *Entrance requirements:* For master's, minimum B+ average in final year of a 4-year undergraduate health professional program or other relevant program. Additional exam requirements/recommendations for international students: Required—TOEFL (minimum score 600 paper-based).

Medical University of South Carolina, College of Health Professions, PhD Program in Health and Rehabilitation Science, Charleston, SC 29425. Offers PhD. *Degree requirements:* For doctorate, comprehensive exam, thesis/dissertation. *Entrance requirements:* Additional exam requirements/recommendations for international students: Required—TOEFL (minimum score 600 paper-based). Electronic applications accepted. *Faculty research:* Spinal cord injury, geriatrics, health economics, health psychology, behavioral medicine.

Northwestern University, Feinberg School of Medicine, Department of Physical Therapy and Human Movement Sciences, Chicago, IL 60611-2814. Offers neuroscience (PhD), including movement and rehabilitation science; physical therapy (DPT); DPT/PhD. *Accreditation:* APTA. *Degree requirements:* For doctorate, synthesis research project. *Entrance requirements:* For doctorate, GRE General Test (for DPT), baccalaureate degree with minimum GPA of 3.0 in required course work (DPT). Additional exam requirements/recommendations for international students: Required—TOEFL. Electronic applications accepted. *Expenses:* Contact institution. *Faculty research:* Motor control, robotics, neuromuscular imaging, student performance (academic/professional), clinical outcomes.

The Ohio State University, College of Medicine, School of Health and Rehabilitation Sciences, Columbus, OH 43210. Offers allied health (MS); anatomy (MS, PhD); health and rehabilitation sciences (PhD); occupational therapy (MOT); physical therapy (DPT); MOT/PhD. *Accreditation:* AOTA; APTA. Part-time programs available. *Faculty:* 42. *Students:* 325 full-time (247 women), 19 part-time (15 women); includes 23 minority (2 Black or African American, non-Hispanic/Latino; 1 American Indian or Alaska Native, non-Hispanic/Latino; 6 Asian, non-Hispanic/Latino; 4 Hispanic/Latino; 10 Two or more races, non-Hispanic/Latino), 7 international. Average age 25. In 2013, 74 master's, 85 doctorates awarded. *Degree requirements:* For master's, thesis or alternative; for doctorate, thesis/dissertation. *Entrance requirements:* For master's and doctorate, GRE. *Application deadline:* For fall admission, 8/15 for domestic students, 7/1 for international students; for winter admission, 12/1 for domestic students, 11/1 for international students; for spring admission, 3/1 for domestic students, 2/1 for international students. Applications are processed on a rolling basis. Application fee: $60 ($70 for international students). Electronic applications accepted. *Financial support:* In 2013–14, 14 students received support. Fellowships with tuition reimbursements available, research assistantships with full tuition reimbursements available, teaching assistantships with full tuition reimbursements available, traineeships, and administrative assistantships available. Financial award application deadline: 3/1. *Faculty research:* Geriatrics, quality assurance, nutrition, interdisciplinary health care. *Total annual research expenditures:* $596,453. *Unit head:* Deborah S. Larsen, Director, 614-292-5645, Fax: 614-292-0210, E-mail: larsen.64@osu.edu. *Application contact:* 614-292-9444, Fax: 614-292-3895, E-mail: gradadmissions@osu.edu.
Website: http://medicine.osu.edu/hrs

Queen's University at Kingston, School of Graduate Studies, Faculty of Health Sciences, School of Rehabilitation Therapy, Kingston, ON K7L 3N6, Canada. Offers occupational therapy (M Sc OT); physical therapy (M Sc PT); rehabilitation science (M Sc, PhD). Part-time programs available. *Degree requirements:* For master's, thesis; for doctorate, comprehensive exam, thesis/dissertation. *Entrance requirements:* Additional exam requirements/recommendations for international students: Required—TOEFL. *Faculty research:* Disability, community, motor performance, rehabilitation, treatment efficiency.

Salus University, College of Education and Rehabilitation, Elkins Park, PA 19027-1598. Offers education of children and youth with visual and multiple impairments (M Ed, Certificate); low vision rehabilitation (MS, Certificate); orientation and mobility therapy (MS, Certificate); vision rehabilitation therapy (MS, Certificate); OD/MS. Part-time programs available. Postbaccalaureate distance learning degree programs offered. *Entrance requirements:* For master's, GRE or MAT, letters of reference (3), interviews (2). Additional exam requirements/recommendations for international students: Required—TOEFL, TWE. *Expenses:* Contact institution. *Faculty research:* Knowledge utilization, technology transfer.

Texas Tech University Health Sciences Center, School of Allied Health Sciences, Program in Rehabilitation Sciences, Lubbock, TX 79430. Offers PhD. Part-time programs available. *Faculty:* 7 full-time (2 women). *Students:* 4 full-time (1 woman), 5 part-time (2 women); includes 3 minority (1 Black or African American, non-Hispanic/Latino; 2 Asian, non-Hispanic/Latino). Average age 32. 6 applicants, 33% accepted, 2 enrolled. In 2013, 1 doctorate awarded. *Entrance requirements:* For doctorate, GRE. Additional exam requirements/recommendations for international students: Required—TOEFL, IELTS. *Application deadline:* For fall admission, 3/15 for domestic students; for spring admission, 10/15 for domestic students; for summer admission, 2/1 for domestic students. Applications are processed on a rolling basis. Application fee: $40. Electronic applications accepted. *Financial support:* Application deadline: 9/1; applicants required to submit FAFSA. *Unit head:* Dr. Roger James, Program Director, 806-743-4524, Fax: 806-743-6005, E-mail: roger.james@ttuhsc.edu. *Application contact:* Lindsay Johnson, Associate Dean for Admissions and Student Affairs, 806-743-3220, Fax: 806-743-2994, E-mail: lindsay.johnson@ttuhsc.edu.
Website: http://www.ttuhsc.edu/sah/phdrs/

Université de Montréal, Faculty of Medicine, Program in Mobility and Posture, Montréal, QC H3C 3J7, Canada. Offers DESS.

University at Buffalo, the State University of New York, Graduate School, School of Public Health and Health Professions, Department of Rehabilitation Science, Buffalo, NY 14214. Offers assistive and rehabilitation technology (Certificate); occupational therapy (MS), including physical disabilities/developmental disabilities, school-based therapy/early intervention; physical therapy (DPT); rehabilitation science (PhD). *Faculty:* 7 full-time (4 women), 4 part-time/adjunct (2 women). *Students:* 2 full-time (1 woman), 1 (woman) part-time, 1 international. Average age 28. 5 applicants, 60% accepted, 2 enrolled. *Degree requirements:* For doctorate, comprehensive exam, thesis/dissertation. *Entrance requirements:* For doctorate, GRE General Test. Additional exam requirements/recommendations for international students: Required—TOEFL (minimum score 550 paper-based; 79 iBT). *Application deadline:* For fall admission, 2/1 for domestic students. Applications are processed on a rolling basis. Application fee: $50. Electronic applications accepted. *Financial support:* In 2013–14, 1 fellowship (averaging $4,000 per year), 1 teaching assistantship with full and partial tuition reimbursement (averaging $11,000 per year) were awarded; scholarships/grants and unspecified assistantships also available. *Faculty research:* Occupational therapy, physical therapy, exercise physiology. *Total annual research expenditures:* $392,087. *Unit head:* Dr. Robert Burkard, Chair, 716-829-6720, Fax: 716-829-2317, E-mail: phhpadv@buffalo.edu. *Application contact:* Debbie McDuffie, Assistant to the Chair, 716-829-6729, Fax: 716-829-3217, E-mail: dlm1@buffalo.edu.
Website: http://sphhp.buffalo.edu/rehabilitation-science.html

The University of Alabama at Birmingham, School of Health Professions, Program in Rehabilitation Science, Birmingham, AL 35294. Offers PhD. Program offered jointly by Departments of Occupational Therapy and Physical Therapy. *Entrance requirements:* For doctorate, GRE, evaluation references, minimum GPA of 3.0, interview. Additional exam requirements/recommendations for international students: Required—TOEFL.

University of Alberta, Faculty of Graduate Studies and Research, Faculty of Rehabilitation Medicine, Edmonton, AB T6G 2E1, Canada. Offers PhD. *Degree requirements:* For doctorate, thesis/dissertation. *Entrance requirements:* For doctorate, GRE, minimum GPA of 7.0 on a 9.0 scale. Additional exam requirements/recommendations for international students: Required—TOEFL. Electronic applications accepted. *Faculty research:* Musculoskeletal disorders, neuromotor control, exercise physiology, motor speech disorders, assistive technologies, cardiac rehabilitation/therapeutic exercise.

The University of British Columbia, Faculty of Medicine, School of Rehabilitation Sciences, Vancouver, BC V6T 1Z1, Canada. Offers M Sc, MOT, MPT, MRSc, PhD. *Degree requirements:* For master's, thesis; for doctorate, comprehensive exam, thesis/dissertation. *Entrance requirements:* For master's, minimum B+ average; for doctorate, minimum B+ average, master's degree. Additional exam requirements/recommendations for international students: Required—TOEFL (minimum score 600 paper-based). Electronic applications accepted. *Expenses: Tuition, area resident:* Full-time $8000 Canadian dollars. *Faculty research:* Disability, rehabilitation and society, exercise science and rehabilitation, neurorehabilitation and motor control.

University of Cincinnati, Graduate School, College of Allied Health Sciences, Department of Rehabilitation Sciences, Cincinnati, OH 45221. Offers DPT. *Accreditation:* APTA. *Entrance requirements:* For doctorate, GRE General Test, bachelor's degree with minimum GPA of 3.0, 50 hours volunteer/work in physical therapy setting. Additional exam requirements/recommendations for international students: Required—TOEFL. Electronic applications accepted. *Faculty research:* Biomechanics, sports-related injuries, motor learning, stroke rehabilitation.

University of Colorado Denver, School of Medicine, Program in Rehabilitation Science, Aurora, CO 80045. Offers PhD. *Students:* 7 full-time (4 women). Average age 33. 6 applicants, 50% accepted, 3 enrolled. *Degree requirements:* For doctorate, comprehensive exam, 60 credit hours (30 of core coursework and 30 of thesis). *Entrance requirements:* For doctorate, GRE, bachelor's degree with minimum GPA of 3.0, research experience (preferred), three letters of recommendation, interviews. Additional exam requirements/recommendations for international students: Required—TOEFL (minimum score 570 paper-based; 89 iBT). *Application deadline:* For fall admission, 1/1 for domestic students, 12/1 for international students. Application fee: $50 ($75 for international students). Electronic applications accepted. *Financial support:* In 2013–14, 6 students received support. Fellowships, research assistantships, teaching assistantships, Federal Work-Study, institutionally sponsored loans, scholarships/grants, traineeships, and unspecified assistantships available. Financial award application deadline: 4/1; financial award applicants required to submit FAFSA. *Unit head:* Dr. Katrina Maluf, Director of Physical Therapy Program, 303-724-9139, E-mail: katrina.maluf@ucdenver.edu. *Application contact:* Vonelle Kelly, Program Administrator, 303-724-3102, E-mail: vonelle.kelly@ucdenver.edu.
Website: http://www.ucdenver.edu/academics/colleges/medicalschool/education/degree_programs/pt/EducationPrograms/PhD/Pages/Overview.aspx

University of Florida, Graduate School, College of Public Health and Health Professions, Program in Rehabilitation Science, Gainesville, FL 32610. Offers clinical and translational science (PhD); rehabilitation science (PhD); PhD/MPH. *Faculty:* 10 full-time (6 women). *Students:* 27 full-time (13 women), 6 part-time (4 women); includes 6 minority (2 Black or African American, non-Hispanic/Latino; 2 Asian, non-Hispanic/Latino; 2 Hispanic/Latino), 17 international. Average age 33. 18 applicants, 39% accepted, 7 enrolled. In 2013, 6 doctorates awarded. *Degree requirements:* For doctorate, comprehensive exam, thesis/dissertation. *Entrance requirements:* For doctorate, GRE General Test, minimum GPA of 3.0. Additional exam requirements/recommendations for international students: Required—TOEFL (minimum score 550 paper-based; 80 iBT), IELTS (minimum score 6). *Application deadline:* For fall admission, 3/15 for domestic and international students; for spring admission, 7/15 for domestic and international students. Applications are processed on a rolling basis. Application fee: $30. Electronic applications accepted. *Expenses:* Tuition, state resident: full-time $12,640. Tuition, nonresident: full-time $30,000. *Financial support:* In 2013–14, 24 students received support, including 3 fellowships (averaging $18,695 per year), 18 research assistantships (averaging $19,795 per year), 5 teaching assistantships (averaging $17,555 per year). Financial award application deadline: 4/1; financial award applicants required to submit FAFSA. *Faculty research:* Movement science, applied neuroscience, community mobility, rehabilitation outcomes, assistive technology/environmental interventions. *Unit head:* David Fuller, PhD, Professor and Program Director, 352-273-6634, Fax: 352-273-6109, E-mail: ddf@phhp.ufl.edu. *Application contact:* Amy Ladendorf, Rehabilitation Science Program Admissions, 352-273-6507, E-mail: gradinfo@ufl.edu.
Website: http://rehabsci.phhp.ufl.edu/

University of Illinois at Chicago, Graduate College, College of Applied Health Sciences, Department of Physical Therapy, Chicago, IL 60607-7128. Offers physical therapy (DPT); rehabilitation science (MS). *Accreditation:* APTA. *Faculty:* 12 full-time (7 women), 6 part-time/adjunct (2 women). *Students:* 171 full-time (117 women), 3 part-time (1 woman); includes 32 minority (4 Black or African American, non-Hispanic/Latino; 1 American Indian or Alaska Native, non-Hispanic/Latino; 14 Asian, non-Hispanic/Latino; 8 Hispanic/Latino; 1 Native Hawaiian or other Pacific Islander, non-Hispanic/Latino; 4 Two or more races, non-Hispanic/Latino), 14 international. Average age 26. 1,081 applicants, 15% accepted, 51 enrolled. In 2013, 6 master's, 46 doctorates awarded. *Degree requirements:* For master's, thesis. *Entrance requirements:* For master's, GRE General Test, minimum GPA of 2.75. Additional exam requirements/recommendations for international students: Required—TOEFL. *Application deadline:* For fall admission, 2/15 for domestic and international students. Electronic applications accepted. *Expenses:* Tuition, state resident: full-time $11,066; part-time $3689 per term. Tuition, nonresident: full-time $23,064; part-time $7688 per term. *Required fees:* $3004; $1190 per term. Tuition and fees vary according to course level and program. *Financial support:* Fellowships with full tuition reimbursements, research assistantships with full tuition reimbursements, teaching assistantships with full tuition reimbursements, Federal Work-Study, tuition waivers (full), and tuition service fee waivers available. Financial award applicants required to submit FAFSA. *Total annual research expenditures:* $1.1 million. *Unit head:* Prof. Ross Anthony Arena, Department Head, 312-996-3338, E-mail: raarena@uic.edu. *Application contact:* Alexander Aruin, Receptionist, 312-355-0904, E-mail: aaruin@uic.edu.
Website: http://www.ahs.uic.edu/pt/

University of Illinois at Urbana–Champaign, Graduate College, College of Applied Health Sciences, Department of Kinesiology and Community Health, Champaign, IL 61820. Offers community health (MS, MSPH, PhD); kinesiology (MS, PhD); public health (MPH); rehabilitation (MS); PhD/MPH. *Students:* 138 (83 women). Application fee: $75 ($90 for international students). *Unit head:* Wojciech Chodzko-Zajko, Head, 217-244-0823, Fax: 217-244-7322, E-mail: wojtek@illinois.edu. *Application contact:* Julie Jenkins, Office Administrator, 217-333-1083, Fax: 217-244-7322, E-mail: jjenkns@illinois.edu.
Website: http://www.kch.illinois.edu/

The University of Iowa, Roy J. and Lucille A. Carver College of Medicine and Graduate College, Biosciences Program, Iowa City, IA 52242-1316. Offers anatomy and cell biology (PhD); biochemistry (PhD); biology (PhD); biomedical engineering (PhD); chemistry (PhD); free radical and radiation biology (PhD); genetics (PhD); human toxicology (PhD); immunology (PhD); microbiology (PhD); molecular and cellular biology (PhD); molecular physiology and biophysics (PhD); neuroscience (PhD); pharmacology (PhD); physical therapy and rehabilitation science (PhD); rehabilitation science (PhD); speech and hearing (PhD). *Faculty:* 332 full-time. *Students:* 8 full-time (3 women); includes 2 minority (1 Black or African American, non-Hispanic/Latino; 1 Asian, non-Hispanic/Latino), 1 international. 200 applicants. *Degree requirements:* For doctorate, thesis/dissertation. *Entrance requirements:* For doctorate, GRE General Test, minimum GPA of 3.0. Additional exam requirements/recommendations for international students: Required—TOEFL (minimum score 600 paper-based; 100 iBT). *Application deadline:*

For fall admission, 1/1 priority date for domestic and international students. Applications are processed on a rolling basis. Application fee: $60 ($100 for international students). Electronic applications accepted. *Expenses:* Contact institution. *Financial support:* In 2013–14, 8 students received support, including 8 research assistantships with full tuition reimbursements available (averaging $26,000 per year); fellowships, teaching assistantships, health care benefits, and unspecified assistantships also available. *Unit head:* Dr. Douglas Spitz, Director, 319-335-8001, E-mail: douglas-spitz@uiowa.edu. *Application contact:* Jodi Graff, Director, Admissions and First-Year Experience, 319-335-8306, E-mail: biosciences-admissions@uiowa.edu.
Website: http://www.medicine.uiowa.edu/biosciences/

The University of Kansas, University of Kansas Medical Center, School of Health Professions, Department of Occupational Therapy Education, Kansas City, KS 66160. Offers occupational therapy (MOT, MS, OTD); therapeutic science (PhD). *Accreditation:* AOTA. Part-time programs available. *Faculty:* 16. *Students:* 77 full-time (72 women), 26 part-time (24 women); includes 8 minority (3 Black or African American, non-Hispanic/Latino; 3 Hispanic/Latino; 2 Two or more races, non-Hispanic/Latino), 3 international. Average age 28. 125 applicants, 36% accepted, 45 enrolled. In 2013, 32 master's, 2 doctorates awarded. *Degree requirements:* For doctorate, comprehensive exam, thesis/dissertation, oral defense. *Entrance requirements:* For master's, 40 hours of paid work or volunteer experience working directly with people with special needs, 3 letters of recommendation, personal statement and program statement of interest, 90 hours of elective course work with 40 hours of prerequisite work, minimum GPA of 3.0; for doctorate, 24 hours of master's-level research. Additional exam requirements/recommendations for international students: Required—TOEFL. *Application deadline:* For fall admission, 12/1 for domestic students, 4/1 for international students. Applications are processed on a rolling basis. Application fee: $60. Electronic applications accepted. *Financial support:* Research assistantships with partial tuition reimbursements, teaching assistantships with full and partial tuition reimbursements, traineeships, and unspecified assistantships available. Financial award application deadline: 3/1; financial award applicants required to submit FAFSA. *Faculty research:* Impact of sensory processing in everyday life; improving balance, motor skills, and independence with community nonprofit organizations serving people with special needs; improving self-confidence and self-sufficiency with poverty-based services in community; working with autism population in a community-wide aquatics program; improving quality of life of people living with cancer and chronic illness. *Total annual research expenditures:* $19,000. *Unit head:* Dr. Winifred W. Dunn, Professor/Chair, 913-588-7195, Fax: 913-588-4568, E-mail: wdunn@kumc.edu. *Application contact:* Wendy Hildenbrand, Admissions Representative, 913-588-7174, Fax: 913-588-4568, E-mail: whildenb@kumc.edu.
Website: http://www.kumc.edu/school-of-health-professions/occupational-therapy-education.html

The University of Kansas, University of Kansas Medical Center, School of Health Professions, Department of Physical Therapy and Rehabilitation Science, Kansas City, KS 66160. Offers physical therapy (DPT); rehabilitation science (PhD). *Accreditation:* APTA. *Faculty:* 19. *Students:* 134 full-time (85 women), 16 part-time (12 women); includes 11 minority (4 Black or African American, non-Hispanic/Latino; 2 Asian, non-Hispanic/Latino; 4 Hispanic/Latino; 1 Two or more races, non-Hispanic/Latino), 15 international. Average age 27. 327 applicants, 23% accepted, 48 enrolled. In 2013, 46 doctorates awarded. *Degree requirements:* For doctorate, comprehensive exam, research project with paper. *Entrance requirements:* For doctorate, GRE General Test, minimum GPA of 3.0. Additional exam requirements/recommendations for international students: Required—TOEFL. *Application deadline:* For fall admission, 11/1 for domestic students. Applications are processed on a rolling basis. Application fee: $60. Electronic applications accepted. *Expenses:* Contact institution. *Financial support:* Research assistantships with tuition reimbursements, teaching assistantships with full and partial tuition reimbursements, career-related internships or fieldwork, Federal Work-Study, institutionally sponsored loans, scholarships/grants, traineeships, and unspecified assistantships available. Financial award application deadline: 3/1; financial award applicants required to submit FAFSA. *Faculty research:* Stroke rehabilitation and the effects on balance and coordination; deep brain stimulation and Parkinson's Disease; peripheral neuropathies, pain and the effects of exercise; islet transplants for Type 1 diabetes; cardiac disease associated with diabetes. *Total annual research expenditures:* $696,000. *Unit head:* Dr. Lisa Stehno-Bittel, Chair, 913-588-6733, Fax: 913-588-4568, E-mail: lbittel@kumc.edu. *Application contact:* Robert Bagley, Admission Coordinator, 913-588-6799, Fax: 913-588-4568, E-mail: rbagley@kumc.edu.
Website: http://www.kumc.edu/school-of-health-professions/physical-therapy-and-rehabilitation-science.html

University of Kentucky, Graduate School, College of Health Sciences, Program in Rehabilitation Sciences, Lexington, KY 40506-0032. Offers PhD. *Degree requirements:* For doctorate, comprehensive exam, thesis/dissertation. *Entrance requirements:* For doctorate, GRE General Test, minimum undergraduate GPA of 2.75. Additional exam requirements/recommendations for international students: Required—TOEFL (minimum score 550 paper-based). Electronic applications accepted.

University of Manitoba, Faculty of Graduate Studies, School of Medical Rehabilitation, Winnipeg, MB R3T 2N2, Canada. Offers applied health sciences (PhD); occupational therapy (MOT); physical therapy (MPT); rehabilitation (M Sc).

University of Manitoba, Faculty of Medicine and Faculty of Graduate Studies, Graduate Programs in Medicine, Department of Medical Rehabilitation, Winnipeg, MB R3T 2N2, Canada. Offers rehabilitation (M Sc). Part-time programs available. *Faculty research:* Understanding of human dynamics, motor control and neurological dysfunction, exercise physiology, functional motion of the upper extremity and effects of musculoskeletal disorders.

University of Maryland, Baltimore, Graduate School, Graduate Program in Life Sciences, Program in Physical Rehabilitation Science, Baltimore, MD 21201. Offers PhD. *Students:* 6 full-time (3 women), 1 part-time (0 women); includes 1 minority (Black or African American, non-Hispanic/Latino), 3 international. Average age 27. 15 applicants, 7% accepted, 1 enrolled. In 2013, 1 doctorate awarded. *Degree requirements:* For doctorate, comprehensive exam, thesis/dissertation. *Entrance requirements:* For doctorate, GRE. Additional exam requirements/recommendations for international students: Required—TOEFL (minimum score 550 paper-based; 80 iBT); Recommended—IELTS (minimum score 7). *Application deadline:* For fall admission, 7/15 for domestic students, 1/15 for international students. Application fee: $75. Electronic applications accepted. *Financial support:* In 2013–14, research assistantships with partial tuition reimbursements (averaging $25,000 per year) were awarded; health care benefits and unspecified assistantships also available. Financial award application deadline: 3/1; financial award applicants required to submit FAFSA. *Faculty research:* Applied physiology, biomechanics, epidemiology of disability, neuromotor control. *Unit head:* Dr. Larry Forester, Program Director, 410-706-5212, Fax: 410-706-4903, E-mail: lforrester@som.umaryland.edu. *Application contact:* Terry Heron, Academic Coordinator, 410-706-7721, E-mail: theron@som.umaryland.edu.
Website: http://rehabscience.umaryland.edu

University of Maryland, Baltimore, School of Medicine, Department of Physical Therapy and Rehabilitation Science, Baltimore, MD 21201. Offers physical rehabilitation science (PhD); physical therapy and rehabilitation science (DPT). *Accreditation:* APTA. *Students:* 170 full-time (120 women), 3 part-time (2 women); includes 27 minority (8 Black or African American, non-Hispanic/Latino; 10 Asian, non-Hispanic/Latino; 6 Hispanic/Latino; 3 Two or more races, non-Hispanic/Latino), 1 international. Average age 24. 545 applicants, 20% accepted, 55 enrolled. In 2013, 59 doctorates awarded. *Entrance requirements:* For doctorate, GRE General Test, BS, science coursework. Additional exam requirements/recommendations for international students: Required—TOEFL (minimum score 80 iBT). Electronic applications accepted. *Expenses:* Contact institution. *Financial support:* Career-related internships or fieldwork, Federal Work-Study, scholarships/grants, traineeships, health care benefits, and unspecified assistantships available. Financial award application deadline: 3/1; financial award applicants required to submit FAFSA. *Unit head:* Dr. Mary Rodgers, Chair, 410-706-5216, Fax: 410-706-4903, E-mail: mrodgers@som.umaryland.edu. *Application contact:* Terry Heron, Program Coordinator, 410-706-5215, Fax: 410-706-6387, E-mail: theron@som.umaryland.edu.
Website: http://pt.umaryland.edu/pros.asp

University of Maryland Eastern Shore, Graduate Programs, Department of Rehabilitation Services, Princess Anne, MD 21853-1299. Offers rehabilitation counseling (MS). *Accreditation:* CORE. Part-time and evening/weekend programs available. *Degree requirements:* For master's, internship. *Entrance requirements:* For master's, interview. Additional exam requirements/recommendations for international students: Required—TOEFL (minimum score 80 iBT). Electronic applications accepted. *Faculty research:* Long-term rehabilitation training.

University of Oklahoma Health Sciences Center, Graduate College, College of Allied Health, Department of Rehabilitation Sciences, Oklahoma City, OK 73190. Offers MS. *Faculty:* 7 full-time (all women). *Students:* 2 full-time (both women), 18 part-time (16 women). Average age 45. 7 applicants, 71% accepted, 2 enrolled. *Degree requirements:* For master's, comprehensive exam, thesis optional. *Entrance requirements:* For master's, GRE General Test, 2 years of clinical experience, 3 letters of reference. Additional exam requirements/recommendations for international students: Required—TOEFL (minimum score 550 paper-based). *Application deadline:* For fall admission, 7/1 for domestic students; for winter admission, 5/1 for domestic students; for spring admission, 12/1 for domestic students. Application fee: $50. *Expenses:* Tuition, state resident: full-time $3504; part-time $175.20 per credit hour. Tuition, nonresident: full-time $13,504; part-time $675.20 per credit hour. *Required fees:* $1545; $52.70 per credit hour. $245.25 per semester. Tuition and fees vary according to course load. *Financial support:* In 2013–14, 2 research assistantships (averaging $8,000 per year) were awarded. *Unit head:* Martha Ferretti, Chair, 405-271-2131, E-mail: martha-ferretti@ouhsc.edu. *Application contact:* Dr. Carol Dionne, Graduate Liaison, 405-271-2131, E-mail: carol-dionne@ouhsc.edu.

University of Ottawa, Faculty of Graduate and Postdoctoral Studies, Faculty of Health Sciences, School of Rehabilitation Sciences, Ottawa, ON K1N 6N5, Canada. Offers audiology (M Sc); orthophony (M Sc). Part-time and evening/weekend programs available. *Entrance requirements:* For master's, honors degree or equivalent, minimum B average. Electronic applications accepted.

University of Pittsburgh, School of Health and Rehabilitation Sciences, Master's Programs in Health and Rehabilitation Sciences, Pittsburgh, PA 15260. Offers health and rehabilitation sciences (MS), including health care supervision and management, health information systems, occupational therapy, physical therapy, rehabilitation counseling, rehabilitation science and technology, sports medicine, wellness and human performance. *Accreditation:* APTA. Part-time and evening/weekend programs available. *Faculty:* 63 full-time (37 women), 4 part-time/adjunct (2 women). *Students:* 117 full-time (70 women), 44 part-time (27 women); includes 18 minority (8 Black or African American, non-Hispanic/Latino; 1 American Indian or Alaska Native, non-Hispanic/Latino; 6 Asian, non-Hispanic/Latino; 3 Hispanic/Latino), 52 international. Average age 30. 368 applicants, 57% accepted, 96 enrolled. In 2013, 90 master's awarded. *Degree requirements:* For master's, comprehensive exam (for some programs), thesis optional. *Entrance requirements:* For master's, minimum GPA of 3.0. Additional exam requirements/recommendations for international students: Required—TOEFL (minimum score 550 paper-based; 80 iBT), IELTS (minimum score 6.5). *Application deadline:* For fall admission, 3/1 for international students; for spring admission, 9/1 for international students. Applications are processed on a rolling basis. Application fee: $50. Electronic applications accepted. *Expenses:* Contact institution. *Financial support:* In 2013–14, 3 fellowships (averaging $20,460 per year) were awarded; Federal Work-Study, institutionally sponsored loans, scholarships/grants, traineeships, and unspecified assistantships also available. Financial award applicants required to submit FAFSA. *Faculty research:* Assistive technology, seating and wheeled mobility, cellular neurophysiology, low back syndrome, augmentative communication. *Total annual research expenditures:* $8.1 million. *Unit head:* Dr. Clifford E. Brubaker, Dean, 412-383-6560, Fax: 412-383-6535, E-mail: cliffb@pitt.edu. *Application contact:* Jessica Maguire, Director of Admissions, 412-383-6557, Fax: 412-383-6535, E-mail: maguire@pitt.edu.
Website: http://www.shrs.pitt.edu/

University of Pittsburgh, School of Health and Rehabilitation Sciences, PhD Program in Rehabilitation Science, Pittsburgh, PA 15260. Offers PhD. Part-time programs available. *Faculty:* 33 full-time (18 women). *Students:* 71 full-time (35 women), 10 part-time (5 women); includes 8 minority (4 Black or African American, non-Hispanic/Latino; 2 Asian, non-Hispanic/Latino; 2 Hispanic/Latino), 40 international. Average age 34. 42 applicants, 43% accepted, 13 enrolled. In 2013, 15 doctorates awarded. *Degree requirements:* For doctorate, comprehensive exam, thesis/dissertation. *Entrance requirements:* For doctorate, GRE General Test. Additional exam requirements/recommendations for international students: Required—TOEFL (minimum score 550 paper-based; 80 iBT), IELTS (minimum score 6.5). *Application deadline:* For fall admission, 3/1 for international students; for spring admission, 9/1 for international students. Applications are processed on a rolling basis. Application fee: $50. Electronic applications accepted. *Expenses:* Tuition, state resident: full-time $19,964; part-time $807 per credit. Tuition, nonresident: full-time $32,686; part-time $1337 per credit. *Required fees:* $740; $200. Tuition and fees vary according to program. *Financial support:* In 2013–14, 39 research assistantships with full and partial tuition reimbursements (averaging $19,504 per year), 3 teaching assistantships with full tuition reimbursements (averaging $23,860 per year) were awarded; Federal Work-Study, scholarships/grants, and traineeships also available. Support available to part-time students. *Faculty research:* Measurement and study of motion, balance disorders, human performance, neuropsychological parameters, telerehabilitation, wheelchair performance and design, injury prevention and treatment, nutrition, data mining. *Total annual research expenditures:* $9.2 million. *Unit head:* Dr. Joan Rogers, Associate Dean of Graduate Studies, 412-383-6620, Fax: 412-383-6613, E-mail: jcr@pitt.edu. *Application contact:* Jessica Maguire, Director of Admissions, 412-383-6557, Fax: 412-383-6535, E-mail: maguire@pitt.edu.
Website: http://www.shrs.pitt.edu/PHDRS/

University of Pittsburgh, School of Health and Rehabilitation Sciences, Prosthetics and Orthotics Program, Pittsburgh, PA 15260. Offers MS. Part-time programs available. *Faculty:* 5 full-time (2 women), 6 part-time/adjunct (2 women). *Students:* 40 full-time (24 women); includes 3 minority (1 Asian, non-Hispanic/Latino; 2 Hispanic/Latino). Average

age 26. 110 applicants, 43% accepted, 20 enrolled. In 2013, 20 master's awarded. *Entrance requirements:* For master's, GRE. Additional exam requirements/recommendations for international students: Required—TOEFL (minimum score 550 paper-based; 80 iBT), IELTS (minimum score 6.5). *Application deadline:* For fall admission, 1/15 for domestic and international students. Applications are processed on a rolling basis. Application fee: $135. Electronic applications accepted. *Expenses:* Contact institution. *Unit head:* Dr. David Brienza, Associate Dean of Strategic Initiatives and Planning, 412-624-6383, E-mail: dbrienza@pitt.edu. *Application contact:* Jessica Maguire, Director of Admissions, 412-383-6557, Fax: 412-383-6535, E-mail: maguire@pitt.edu.
Website: http://www.shrs.pitt.edu/po/

University of South Carolina, School of Medicine and The Graduate School, Graduate Programs in Medicine, Program in Rehabilitation Counseling, Columbia, SC 29208. Offers psychiatric rehabilitation (Certificate); rehabilitation counseling (MRC). *Accreditation:* CORE. Part-time and evening/weekend programs available. *Degree requirements:* For master's, comprehensive exam, internship, practicum. *Entrance requirements:* For master's and Certificate, GRE General Test or GMAT. Electronic applications accepted. *Expenses:* Contact institution. *Faculty research:* Quality of life, alcohol dependency, technology for disabled, psychiatric rehabilitation, women with disabilities.

The University of Texas Medical Branch, Graduate School of Biomedical Sciences, Department of Preventive Medicine and Community Health, Galveston, TX 77555. Offers population health sciences (MS, PhD); public health (MPH); rehabilitation sciences (PhD). *Accreditation:* CEPH. *Degree requirements:* For master's, thesis; for doctorate, thesis/dissertation. *Entrance requirements:* For master's, GRE General Test or MAT; for doctorate, GRE General Test. Additional exam requirements/recommendations for international students: Required—TOEFL (minimum score 550 paper-based). Electronic applications accepted.

University of Toronto, Faculty of Medicine, Department of Rehabilitation Science, Toronto, ON M5S 1A1, Canada. Offers M Sc, PhD. *Degree requirements:* For master's, thesis. *Entrance requirements:* For master's, B Sc or equivalent; specialization in occupational therapy, physical therapy, or a related field; minimum B+ average in final 2 years. Additional exam requirements/recommendations for international students: Required—TOEFL (minimum score 580 paper-based; 93 iBT), TWE (minimum score 5). Electronic applications accepted.

University of Utah, Graduate School, College of Health, Department of Physical Therapy, Salt Lake City, UT 84112-1290. Offers physical therapy (DPT); rehabilitation science (PhD). *Accreditation:* APTA. *Faculty:* 7 full-time (1 woman), 15 part-time/adjunct (8 women). *Students:* 151 full-time (84 women), 3 part-time (1 woman); includes 10 minority (1 American Indian or Alaska Native, non-Hispanic/Latino; 2 Asian, non-Hispanic/Latino; 3 Hispanic/Latino; 3 Native Hawaiian or other Pacific Islander, non-Hispanic/Latino; 1 Two or more races, non-Hispanic/Latino), 4 international. Average age 28. 340 applicants, 14% accepted, 48 enrolled. In 2013, 48 doctorates awarded. *Degree requirements:* For doctorate, thesis/dissertation, clinical project. *Entrance requirements:* For doctorate, GRE, minimum GPA of 3.0, volunteer work, bachelor's degree. Additional exam requirements/recommendations for international students: Required—TOEFL (minimum score 90 iBT); Recommended—IELTS (minimum score 7). *Application deadline:* For fall admission, 10/1 priority date for domestic students, 10/1 for international students. Application fee: $55 ($65 for international students). Electronic applications accepted. *Expenses:* Contact institution. *Financial support:* Research assistantships with full tuition reimbursements, teaching assistantships with full tuition reimbursements, Federal Work-Study, scholarships/grants, tuition waivers (partial), and unspecified assistantships available. Financial award application deadline: 10/1; financial award applicants required to submit FAFSA. *Faculty research:* Rehabilitation and Parkinson's Disease, motor control and musculoskeletal dysfunction, burns/wound care, rehabilitation and multiple sclerosis, cancer. *Total annual research expenditures:* $983,166. *Unit head:* Dr. R. Scott Ward, Chair, 801-581-4895, E-mail: scott.ward@hsc.utah.edu. *Application contact:* Dee-Dee Darby-Duffin, Academic Advisor, 801-581-5146, E-mail: darbyduffinfamily@gmail.com.
Website: http://www.health.utah.edu/pt

University of Washington, Graduate School, School of Medicine, Graduate Programs in Medicine, Department of Rehabilitation Medicine, Seattle, WA 98195-6490. Offers occupational therapy (MOT); physical therapy (DPT); prosthetics and orthotics (MPO); rehabilitation science (PhD). *Degree requirements:* For doctorate, comprehensive exam (for some programs), thesis/dissertation (for some programs). *Entrance requirements:* For master's and doctorate, GRE. Additional exam requirements/recommendations for international students: Required—TOEFL. *Faculty research:* Biomechanics, balance, brain injury, spinal cord injury, pain, degenerative diseases.

University of Wisconsin–La Crosse, Graduate Studies, College of Science and Health, Department of Exercise and Sport Science, Program in Clinical Exercise Physiology, La Crosse, WI 54601-3742. Offers MS. *Students:* 15 full-time (9 women); includes 2 minority (1 Asian, non-Hispanic/Latino; 1 Two or more races, non-Hispanic/Latino). Average age 23. 42 applicants, 45% accepted, 15 enrolled. In 2013, 17 master's awarded. *Degree requirements:* For master's, thesis optional. *Entrance requirements:* Additional exam requirements/recommendations for international students: Required—TOEFL (minimum score 550 paper-based; 79 iBT). *Application deadline:* For fall admission, 2/1 priority date for domestic and international students. Electronic applications accepted. *Financial support:* Federal Work-Study, scholarships/grants, health care benefits, and tuition waivers (partial) available. Support available to part-time students. Financial award application deadline: 3/15; financial award applicants required to submit FAFSA. *Unit head:* Dr. John Porcari, Director, 608-785-8684, Fax: 608-785-8686, E-mail: porcari.john@uwlax.edu. *Application contact:* Corey Sjoquist, Director of Admissions, 608-785-8939, E-mail: admissions@uwlax.edu.
Website: http://www.uwlax.edu/sah/ess/cep/

Virginia Commonwealth University, Graduate School, School of Education, Department of Health and Human Performance, Program in Rehabilitation and Movement Science, Richmond, VA 23284-9005. Offers PhD. *Entrance requirements:* Additional exam requirements/recommendations for international students: Required—TOEFL (minimum score 600 paper-based; 100 iBT). Electronic applications accepted.

Washington University in St. Louis, School of Medicine, Program in Rehabilitation and Participation Science, St. Louis, MO 63130-4899. Offers PhD.

Western Michigan University, Graduate College, College of Health and Human Services, Department of Blindness and Low Vision Studies, Kalamazoo, MI 49008. Offers orientation and mobility (MA); orientation and mobility of children (MA); vision rehabilitation teaching (MA). *Accreditation:* CORE.

PHILADELPHIA COLLEGE OF OSTEOPATHIC MEDICINE

Physician Assistant Program

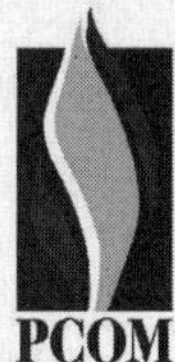

Program of Study

The Physician Assistant (PA) Studies program is a twenty-six-month program that leads to a Master of Science degree in health sciences. Students are prepared for clinical practice, using a variety of learning strategies: formal lectures, practical laboratory classes, and clinical education. Students develop patient communication skills and advanced clinical problem-solving skills in addition to acquiring technical proficiency in areas related to professional practice. The program is highly intensive. Most of the program is provided by experienced physician assistants with clinical backgrounds in multiple specialties.

In addition to admission through the standard application process, there are also two 5-year cooperative programs with Philadelphia College of Osteopathic Medicine (PCOM) and either University of the Sciences in Philadelphia (USP) or Brenau University in Gainesville, Georgia. The programs consist of two distinct phases: the preprofessional phase and the professional phase. After successful completion of the fourth year, students earn a B.S. in health science from USP or Brenau and an M.S. from PCOM after completion of the fifth year. The B.S. degree does not qualify the student as a PA. Students must complete the entire professional phase of the program (years four and five) and obtain an M.S. from PCOM to become eligible to be certified as a PA. PCOM has the ultimate responsibility for granting the M.S. degree. PCOM has a third cooperative program with Thomas University in Thomasville, Georgia where students may apply to the PA Studies program in their fourth year of study. Applicants from institutions without cooperative agreements are certainly admitted into each entering class as affiliation agreement students are not provided preferential admission

The Physician Assistant Studies program at PCOM provides students with the ability to positively affect the lives of their patients, their families, their employers, and their communities. Students become lifelong learners, developing a baseline of analytic and critical thinking skills that prepare them for the challenges of caring for the entire patient, young or old, from the emergency room to the operating room.

Research Facilities

PCOM's library features both a well-developed collection of medical journals and texts and new capabilities for access to online medical references and Internet searching in a facility that provides individual student stations, Internet terminals, advanced audiovisual resources, and a large student computer lab.

Financial Aid

The Financial Aid Office at PCOM offers financial assistance to students through the Federal Direct Loan program, institutional grants, and various alternative private loan programs.

Cost of Study

In 2014–15, the tuition for PCOM's Physician Assistant Studies program is $70,773.

Living and Housing Costs

Students live off campus within the Philadelphia metropolitan and suburban areas, as there is no on-campus housing. Room and board costs vary by each student's individual preferences.

Student Group

Admission to the PA Studies program is competitive and selective. The Faculty Committee on Admissions looks for academically and socially well-rounded individuals who are committed to caring for patients. The class of 2016 totals 57 students, 41 women and 16 men, ranging in age from 21 to 33. Twenty-three percent of the class self-identified as minority. Fifteen were residents of Pennsylvania. The average GPA of the entering class was 3.62.

Location

Philadelphia College of Osteopathic Medicine is one of the largest of twenty-nine osteopathic colleges in the United States, with campuses in both Philadelphia and suburban Atlanta. The PA Studies program is offered only on the Philadelphia campus, which is located in a suburban setting on City Avenue, minutes away from Fairmount Park, Philadelphia's historic district, art museums, theaters, restaurants, and professional sports complexes. PCOM's facilities include two large lecture halls, small classrooms, labs for teaching, clinical skills, robotic simulation, and research, a state-of-the-art library, and scenic landscaping, all in a suburban setting.

The College

PCOM, chartered in 1899, enrolls approximately 2,580 students in its various programs across both campuses, and is committed to educating community-responsive, primary-care–oriented physicians and physician assistants to practice medicine in the twenty-first century. Supported by the latest in medical and educational technology, PCOM emphasizes treating the whole person, not merely the symptoms. Students have a committed, professional, humanistic faculty who are leaders in the osteopathic and physician assistant national health-care community. The PA Studies program provides a thorough foundation in health-care delivery that focuses on comprehensive, humanistic health care.

Applying

Selection for the Physician Assistant Studies program is very competitive. Applicants must complete a baccalaureate degree at a regionally accredited college or university in the United States, Canada, or the United Kingdom with a minimum science and cumulative GPA of 3.0 (on a 4.0 scale), document in their CASPA application 200 hours of experience in volunteer or employment in or related to the health-care industry, and fulfill the following course requirements: five semesters of biology, three semesters of chemistry, one semester of physics or another health related science, two semesters of mathematics, and three semesters of social science courses. All requirements must have been completed within the last ten years, unless the applicant has completed an advanced degree or has extensive experience in the field of patient care. Applications are not accepted from graduates of medical schools. Selected applicants are invited to interview on campus. Application and deadline information is available online at http://www.caspaonline.org and http://admissions.pcom.edu/app-process/physician-assistant-studies-ms/.

Correspondence and Information

Philadelphia College of Osteopathic Medicine
4170 City Avenue
Philadelphia, Pennsylvania 19131
Phone: 215-871-6700
800-999-6998 (toll-free)
Fax: 215-871-6719
E-mail: PAAdmissions@pcom.edu
Website: http://admissions.pcom.edu

THE FACULTY AND THEIR RESEARCH

Full-Time Faculty

Gregory McDonald, D.O., Philadelphia College of Osteopathic Medicine. Medical Director, Department of Physician Assistant Studies. Pathology.

John Cavenagh, Ph.D., Union (Ohio); PA-C. Professor, Chairman, Department of Physician Assistant Studies. Emergency medicine.

Jill Cunningham, M.H.S., Drexel; PA-C. Assistant Professor, Department of Physician Assistant Studies. Internal medicine.

Marilyn DeFeliciantonio, M.S.L.S., Villanova; PA-C. Assistant Professor, Department of Physician Assistant Studies. Hematology and oncology.

Sean Guinane, M.S., Philadelphia College of Osteopathic Medicine; PA-C. Assistant Professor, Department of Physician Assistant Studies. Family medicine.

Paul Krajewski, M.S., Philadelphia College of Osteopathic Medicine; PA-C. Associate Professor, Department of Physician Assistant Studies. Orthopedic surgery, emergency medicine.

Laura Levy, M.M.S., Saint Francis (Pennsylvania); PA-C. Associate Professor, Assistant Program Director, Department of Physician Assistant Studies. Family medicine, women's health.

Nancy E. McLaughlin, M.H.A., D.H.Sc., Nova Southeastern; PA-C. Assistant Professor, Assistant Program Director, and Georgia Campus Site Director, Department of Physician Assistant Studies. Surgical medicine.

Christine Mount, M.S., University of Medicine and Dentistry of New Jersey; PA-C. Assistant Professor, Department of Physician Assistant Studies. Neurology, emergency medicine, trauma.

Jennifer Windstein, M.S., Wagner; PA-C. Assistant Professor, Department of Physician Assistant Studies. Family practice.

Adjunct Faculty

Patrick Auth, Ph.D., Drexel; PA-C. Emergency medicine, orthopedics.

Matt Baker, D.H.Sc., Nova Southeastern; PA-C. Geriatrics and gerontology.

Robert Cuzzolino, Ed.D., Temple. Academic policy.

Jeff Gutting, M.S., Philadelphia College of Osteopathic Medicine; PA-C. Cardiology.

Michael Kirifides, Ph.D., Maryland. Human physiology.

Brian Levine, M.D., Vermont. Emergency medicine.

Burton Mark, D.O., Kirksville College of Osteopathic Medicine. Psychiatry.

Amanda Murphy, M.S., Philadelphia College of Osteopathic Medicine; PA-C. Dermatology.

Joseph Norris, M.S., D.C., Philadelphia College of Osteopathic Medicine; PA-C. Family medicine.

Richard Pascucci, D.O., Philadelphia College of Osteopathic Medicine; FACOI. Rheumatology.

Margaret Reinhart, M.M.A.; M.T., Penn State; ASCP. Laboratory diagnostics.

Gretchen Reynolds, M.S., Philadelphia College of Osteopathic Medicine; PA-C. Occupational health.

Lauren Tavani, M.S., Philadelphia College of Osteopathic Medicine; PA-C. Critical care.

Rosemary Vickers, D.O., Philadelphia College of Osteopathic Medicine. Pediatrics.

Tracy Offerdahl, Pharm.D., Temple. Pharmacology.

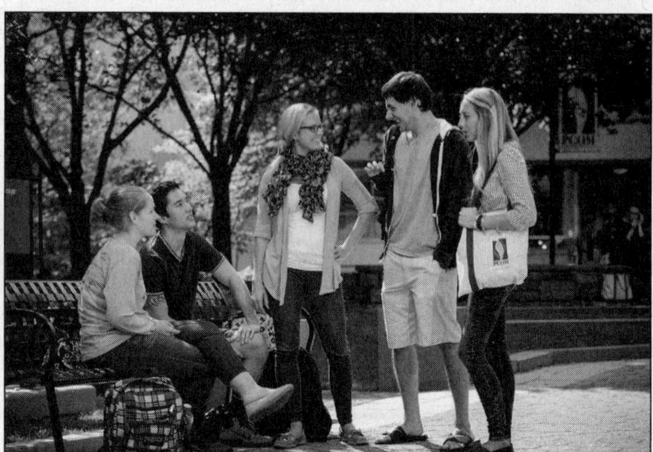

PCOM provides a collaborative learning environment for students.

Section 21
Health Sciences

This section contains a directory of institutions offering graduate work in health sciences. Additional information about programs listed in the directory may be obtained by writing directly to the dean of a graduate school or chair of a department at the address given in the directory.

For programs offering related work, see also in this book *Biological and Biomedical Sciences, Biophysics (Radiation Biology), Dentistry and Dental Sciences, Health Services, Medicine, Nursing,* and *Public Health.* In the other guides in this series:

Graduate Programs in the Physical Sciences, Mathematics, Agricultural Sciences, the Environment & Natural Resources

See *Physics*

Graduate Programs in Engineering & Applied Sciences

See *Agricultural Engineering and Bioengineering (Bioengineering), Biomedical Engineering and Biotechnology,* and *Energy and Power Engineering (Nuclear Engineering)*

CONTENTS

Program Directories

Health Physics/Radiological Health

East Carolina University, Graduate School, Thomas Harriot College of Arts and Sciences, Department of Physics, Greenville, NC 27858-4353. Offers applied physics (MS); biomedical physics (PhD); health physics (MS); medical physics (MS). Part-time programs available. *Degree requirements:* For master's, one foreign language, comprehensive exam. *Entrance requirements:* For master's, GRE General Test. Additional exam requirements/recommendations for international students: Required—TOEFL. *Application deadline:* Applications are processed on a rolling basis. Application fee: $50. *Expenses:* Tuition, state resident: full-time $4223. Tuition, nonresident: full-time $16,540. *Required fees:* $2184. *Financial support:* Research assistantships with partial tuition reimbursements, teaching assistantships with partial tuition reimbursements, and Federal Work-Study available. Support available to part-time students. Financial award application deadline: 6/1. *Unit head:* Dr. John Sutherland, Chair, 252-328-6739, E-mail: sutherlandj@ecu.edu. *Application contact:* Dean of Graduate School, 252-328-6012, Fax: 252-328-6071, E-mail: gradschool@ecu.edu.
Website: http://www.ecu.edu/cs-cas/physics/Graduate-Program.cfm#

Georgia Institute of Technology, Graduate Studies and Research, College of Engineering, George W. Woodruff School of Mechanical Engineering, Nuclear and Radiological Engineering and Medical Physics Programs, Atlanta, GA 30332-0001. Offers medical physics (MS); nuclear and radiological engineering (MSNE, PhD). Part-time programs available. Postbaccalaureate distance learning degree programs offered (no on-campus study). Terminal master's awarded for partial completion of doctoral program. *Degree requirements:* For master's, thesis optional; for doctorate, comprehensive exam, thesis/dissertation. *Entrance requirements:* For master's and doctorate, GRE General Test, minimum GPA of 3.0. Additional exam requirements/recommendations for international students: Required—TOEFL (minimum score 580 paper-based). *Faculty research:* Reactor physics, nuclear materials, plasma physics, radiation detection, radiological assessment.

Idaho State University, Office of Graduate Studies, College of Science and Engineering, Department of Physics, Pocatello, ID 83209-8106. Offers applied physics (PhD); health physics (MS); physics (MNS). Part-time programs available. *Degree requirements:* For master's, comprehensive exam, thesis (for some programs), oral exam (for some programs); for doctorate, comprehensive exam, thesis/dissertation (for some programs), oral exam, written qualifying exam in physics or health physics after 1st year. *Entrance requirements:* For master's, GRE General Test, 3 letters of recommendation, BS or BA in physics, teaching certificate (MNS); for doctorate, GRE General Test (minimum 50th percentile), 3 letters of recommendation, statement of career goals. Additional exam requirements/recommendations for international students: Required—TOEFL (minimum score 550 paper-based; 80 iBT). Electronic applications accepted. *Faculty research:* Ion beam applications, low-energy nuclear physics, relativity and cosmology, observational astronomy.

Illinois Institute of Technology, Graduate College, College of Science and Letters, Department of Physics, Chicago, IL 60616. Offers applied physics (MS); health physics (MHP); physics (MS, PhD). Part-time and evening/weekend programs available. Postbaccalaureate distance learning degree programs offered (minimal on-campus study). Terminal master's awarded for partial completion of doctoral program. *Degree requirements:* For master's, comprehensive exam (for some programs), thesis (for some programs); for doctorate, comprehensive exam, thesis/dissertation. *Entrance requirements:* For master's, GRE General Test (minimum score 1000 Quantitative and Verbal, 2.5 Analytical Writing), minimum undergraduate GPA of 3.0; for doctorate, GRE General Test (minimum score 1100 Quantitative and Verbal, 3.0 Analytical Writing), minimum undergraduate GPA of 3.0. Additional exam requirements/recommendations for international students: Required—TOEFL (minimum score 523 paper-based; 70 iBT); Recommended—IELTS (minimum score 5.5). Electronic applications accepted. *Faculty research:* Elementary particle physics, accelerator and plasma physics, condensed-matter physics, biological physics, x-ray optics, x-ray imaging, quantum theory.

McMaster University, School of Graduate Studies, Faculty of Science, Department of Medical Physics and Applied Radiation Sciences, Hamilton, ON L8S 4M2, Canada. Offers health and radiation physics (M Sc); medical physics (M Sc, PhD). Part-time programs available. *Degree requirements:* For master's, thesis or alternative. *Entrance requirements:* For master's, minimum B+ average. Additional exam requirements/recommendations for international students: Required—TOEFL (minimum score 550 paper-based). *Faculty research:* Imaging, toxicology, dosimetry, body composition, medical lasers.

Midwestern State University, Graduate School, Robert D. and Carol Gunn College of Health Sciences and Human Services, Program in Radiologic Sciences, Wichita Falls, TX 76308. Offers radiologic administration (MSR); radiologic education (MSR); radiologic sciences (MSR); radiologist assistant (MSR). Part-time and evening/weekend programs available. Postbaccalaureate distance learning degree programs offered (minimal on-campus study). *Degree requirements:* For master's, comprehensive exam, thesis optional. *Entrance requirements:* For master's, GRE General Test, MAT or GMAT, credentials in one of the medical imaging modalities or radiation therapy; 1 year of experience; 3 letters of recommendation from past and/or present educators and employers. Additional exam requirements/recommendations for international students: Required—TOEFL (minimum score 550 paper-based). *Application deadline:* For fall admission, 7/1 priority date for domestic students, 4/1 for international students; for spring admission, 11/1 priority date for domestic students, 8/1 for international students. Applications are processed on a rolling basis. Application fee: $35 ($50 for international students). Electronic applications accepted. *Expenses:* Tuition, state resident: full-time $3627; part-time $201.50 per credit hour. Tuition, nonresident: full-time $10,899; part-time $605.50 per credit hour. *Required fees:* $1357. *Financial support:* Career-related internships or fieldwork, Federal Work-Study, institutionally sponsored loans, scholarships/grants, tuition waivers (partial), and unspecified assistantships available. Support available to part-time students. Financial award application deadline: 3/1; financial award applicants required to submit FAFSA. *Faculty research:* Bone densitometry, radiologic dose trends, teaching of radiologic science, radiographic positioning landmarks. *Unit head:* Dr. Jeffery Killion, Chair/Graduate Coordinator, 940-397-4679, Fax: 940-397-4513, E-mail: jeff.killion@mwsu.edu. *Application contact:* Dr. Jeffery Killion, Chair/Graduate Coordinator, 940-397-4679, Fax: 940-397-4513, E-mail: jeff.killion@mwsu.edu.
Website: http://www.mwsu.edu/academics/hs2/radsci/index

New York Chiropractic College, Program in Diagnostic Imaging, Seneca Falls, NY 13148-0800. Offers MS. *Degree requirements:* For master's, thesis. *Entrance requirements:* For master's, DC, minimum GPA of 3.0. *Application deadline:* Applications are processed on a rolling basis. Application fee: $0. *Financial support:* Fellowships with full tuition reimbursements available. Financial award applicants required to submit FAFSA. *Faculty research:* Ultrasound, MRI and back pain, educational theory. *Unit head:* Dr. Chad D. Warshel, Director, 315-568-3297, E-mail: cwarshel@nycc.edu. *Application contact:* Dr. Chad D. Warshel, Director, 315-568-3297, E-mail: cwarshel@nycc.edu.
Website: http://www.nycc.edu/AcademicPrograms_MSDIprogram.htm

Northwestern State University of Louisiana, Graduate Studies and Research, College of Nursing and Allied Health, Department of Radiologic Sciences, Natchitoches, LA 71497. Offers MS. *Degree requirements:* For master's, comprehensive exam, thesis (for some programs). *Entrance requirements:* Additional exam requirements/recommendations for international students: Required—TOEFL. Electronic applications accepted.

Oregon State University, College of Engineering, Program in Radiation Health Physics, Corvallis, OR 97331. Offers MHP, MS, PhD. Part-time programs available. Postbaccalaureate distance learning degree programs offered (no on-campus study). *Faculty:* 11 full-time (3 women), 2 part-time/adjunct (both women). *Students:* 13 full-time (5 women), 44 part-time (17 women); includes 4 minority (3 Asian, non-Hispanic/Latino; 1 Hispanic/Latino), 8 international. Average age 34. 53 applicants, 43% accepted, 17 enrolled. In 2013, 15 master's, 3 doctorates awarded. *Degree requirements:* For master's, thesis. *Entrance requirements:* For master's and doctorate, GRE. Additional exam requirements/recommendations for international students: Required—TOEFL (minimum score 80 iBT), IELTS (minimum score 6.5). *Application deadline:* For fall admission, 8/1 for domestic students. Applications are processed on a rolling basis. Application fee: $60. *Expenses:* Contact institution. *Financial support:* Fellowships, research assistantships, teaching assistantships, and institutionally sponsored loans available. Support available to part-time students. Financial award application deadline: 2/1. *Faculty research:* Radioactive material transport, research reactor health physics, radiation instrumentation, radiation shielding, environmental monitoring. *Unit head:* Dr. Kathryn Higley, Department Head/Professor, 541-737-7063, E-mail: kathryn.higley@oregonstate.edu. *Application contact:* Heidi Braly, Graduate Student Liaison, 541-737-7062, E-mail: heidi.braly@oregonstate.edu.
Website: http://ne.oregonstate.edu/content/health-physics-program

Purdue University, Graduate School, College of Health and Human Sciences, School of Health Sciences, West Lafayette, IN 47907. Offers health physics (MS, PhD); medical physics (MS, PhD); occupational and environmental health science (MS, PhD), including aerosol deposition and lung disease, ergonomics, exposure and risk assessment, indoor air quality and bioaerosols (PhD), liver/lung toxicology; radiation biology (PhD); toxicology (PhD); MS/PhD. Part-time programs available. *Faculty:* 11 full-time (5 women), 28 part-time/adjunct (5 women). *Students:* 28 full-time (8 women), 10 part-time (3 women); includes 6 minority (1 Black or African American, non-Hispanic/Latino; 3 Asian, non-Hispanic/Latino; 1 Hispanic/Latino; 1 Two or more races, non-Hispanic/Latino), 10 international. Average age 28. 77 applicants, 42% accepted, 13 enrolled. In 2013, 6 master's, 6 doctorates awarded. *Degree requirements:* For master's, thesis optional; for doctorate, one foreign language, thesis/dissertation. *Entrance requirements:* For master's and doctorate, GRE General Test, minimum undergraduate GPA of 3.0 or equivalent. Additional exam requirements/recommendations for international students: Required—TOEFL (minimum score 550 paper-based; 77 iBT); Recommended—TWE. *Application deadline:* For fall admission, 5/15 for domestic and international students; for spring admission, 10/15 for domestic and international students. Applications are processed on a rolling basis. Application fee: $60 ($75 for international students). Electronic applications accepted. *Financial support:* In 2013–14, fellowships with tuition reimbursements (averaging $14,400 per year), research assistantships with tuition reimbursements (averaging $12,000 per year), teaching assistantships with tuition reimbursements (averaging $12,000 per year) were awarded; career-related internships or fieldwork and traineeships also available. Support available to part-time students. Financial award applicants required to submit FAFSA. *Faculty research:* Environmental toxicology, industrial hygiene, radiation dosimetry. *Unit head:* Dr. Wei Zheng, Head, 765-494-1419, E-mail: wz18@purdue.edu. *Application contact:* Jennifer S. Franklin, Graduate Contact, 765-494-0248, E-mail: jfranklin@purdue.edu.
Website: http://www.healthsciences.purdue.edu/

Quinnipiac University, School of Health Sciences, Program for Radiologist Assistant, Hamden, CT 06518-1940. Offers MHS. *Faculty:* 2 full-time (1 woman), 3 part-time/adjunct (1 woman). *Students:* 5 full-time (3 women), 3 part-time (1 woman); includes 1 minority (Asian, non-Hispanic/Latino). 7 applicants, 71% accepted, 5 enrolled. In 2013, 5 master's awarded. *Entrance requirements:* For master's, proof of certification from American Registry of Radiologic Technologists; 2000 hours of direct patient care; CPR certification. Additional exam requirements/recommendations for international students: Required—TOEFL (minimum score 575 paper-based; 90 iBT), IELTS (minimum score 6.5). *Application deadline:* For fall admission, 4/30 priority date for domestic and international students; for summer admission, 4/30 for domestic students. Applications are processed on a rolling basis. Application fee: $45. Electronic applications accepted. *Expenses: Tuition:* Part-time $920 per credit. *Required fees:* $37 per credit. *Financial support:* In 2013–14, 4 students received support. Career-related internships or fieldwork, Federal Work-Study, scholarships/grants, and unspecified assistantships available. Support available to part-time students. Financial award application deadline: 6/1; financial award applicants required to submit FAFSA. *Faculty research:* Curriculum development, assessment of student learning, radiation safety. *Unit head:* John Candler, Director, E-mail: john.candler@quinnipiac.edu. *Application contact:* Office of Graduate Admissions, 800-462-1944, Fax: 203-582-3443, E-mail: graduate@quinnipiac.edu.
Website: http://www.quinnipiac.edu/gradradiologistasst

Rutgers, The State University of New Jersey, Newark, School of Health Related Professions, Department of Medical Imaging Sciences, Newark, NJ 07102. Offers radiologist assistant (MS). Part-time and evening/weekend programs available. *Entrance requirements:* For master's, BS with minimum GPA of 3.0, RT license, coursework in intro to pathopsychology, interview, all transcripts, personal statement, BCLS certification. Additional exam requirements/recommendations for international students: Required—TOEFL (minimum score 500 paper-based; 79 iBT). Electronic applications accepted.

San Diego State University, Graduate and Research Affairs, College of Sciences, Department of Physics, Program in Radiological Physics, San Diego, CA 92182. Offers MS. Part-time programs available. *Degree requirements:* For master's, thesis optional, oral or written exam. *Entrance requirements:* For master's, GRE General Test, GRE Subject Test (physics), 2 letters of recommendation. Additional exam requirements/recommendations for international students: Required—TOEFL. Electronic applications accepted. *Faculty research:* Computational radiological physics, medical physics.

Texas A&M University, College of Engineering, Department of Nuclear Engineering, College Station, TX 77843. Offers health physics (MS); nuclear engineering (M Engr, MS, PhD). *Faculty:* 18. *Students:* 125 full-time (16 women), 21 part-time (6 women);

includes 25 minority (3 Black or African American, non-Hispanic/Latino; 1 American Indian or Alaska Native, non-Hispanic/Latino; 4 Asian, non-Hispanic/Latino; 16 Hispanic/Latino; 1 Two or more races, non-Hispanic/Latino), 30 international. Average age 27. 138 applicants, 44% accepted, 40 enrolled. In 2013, 32 master's, 19 doctorates awarded. *Degree requirements:* For master's, thesis or alternative; for doctorate, thesis/dissertation, departmental qualifying exams. *Entrance requirements:* For master's and doctorate, GRE General Test, 3 letters of recommendation. Additional exam requirements/recommendations for international students: Required—TOEFL. *Application deadline:* For fall admission, 3/1 for domestic and international students; for spring admission, 8/1 for domestic and international students. Applications are processed on a rolling basis. Application fee: $50 ($75 for international students). Electronic applications accepted. *Expenses:* Tuition, state resident: full-time $4078; part-time $226.55 per credit hour. Tuition, nonresident: full-time $10,450; part-time $580.55 per credit hour. *Required fees:* $2328; $278.50 per credit hour. $642.45 per semester. *Financial support:* Fellowships, research assistantships, career-related internships or fieldwork, scholarships/grants, and unspecified assistantships available. Financial award application deadline: 4/1; financial award applicants required to submit FAFSA. *Faculty research:* Accelerators, aerosols, computational transport, fission, fusion. *Unit head:* Dr. Yassin A. Hassan, Head, 979-845-7090, E-mail: y-hassan@tamu.edu. *Application contact:* Dr. Karen Vierow, Graduate Program Coordinator, 979-458-0600, E-mail: vierow@tamu.edu.
Website: https://engineering.tamu.edu/nuclear

Thomas Jefferson University, Jefferson School of Health Professions, Department of Radiologic Sciences, Philadelphia, PA 19107. Offers radiologic and imaging sciences (MS). *Students:* 19 full-time (14 women), 6 part-time (4 women); includes 3 minority (1 Black or African American, non-Hispanic/Latino; 2 Asian, non-Hispanic/Latino), 7 international. Average age 32. 29 applicants, 55% accepted, 13 enrolled. In 2013, 14 master's awarded. *Entrance requirements:* Additional exam requirements/recommendations for international students: Required—TOEFL. *Application deadline:* For fall admission, 7/15 for domestic students. Applications are processed on a rolling basis. Application fee: $95. Electronic applications accepted. *Financial support:* In 2013–14, 2 students received support. Scholarships/grants available. Financial award application deadline: 4/1; financial award applicants required to submit FAFSA. *Unit head:* Frances H. Gilman, Chair, 215-503-1865, E-mail: frances.gilman@jefferson.edu. *Application contact:* Tammi Wrice, Assistant Director of Admission, 215-503-1043, Fax: 215-503-7241, E-mail: jshpadmissions@jefferson.edu.
Website: http://www.jefferson.edu/health_professions/departments/radiologic_sciences/

Université Laval, Faculty of Medicine, Post-Professional Programs in Medical Studies, Québec, QC G1K 7P4, Canada. Offers anatomy–pathology (DESS); anesthesiology (DESS); cardiology (DESS); care of older people (Diploma); clinical research (DESS); community health (DESS); dermatology (DESS); diagnostic radiology (DESS); emergency medicine (Diploma); family medicine (DESS); general surgery (DESS); geriatrics (DESS); hematology (DESS); internal medicine (DESS); maternal and fetal medicine (Diploma); medical biochemistry (DESS); medical microbiology and infectious diseases (DESS); medical oncology (DESS); nephrology (DESS); neurology (DESS); neurosurgery (DESS); obstetrics and gynecology (DESS); ophthalmology (DESS); orthopedic surgery (DESS); oto-rhino-laryngology (DESS); palliative medicine (Diploma); pediatrics (DESS); plastic surgery (DESS); psychiatry (DESS); pulmonary medicine (DESS); radiology–oncology (DESS); thoracic surgery (DESS); urology (DESS). *Degree requirements:* For other advanced degree, comprehensive exam. *Entrance requirements:* For degree, knowledge of French. Electronic applications accepted.

University of Alberta, Faculty of Medicine and Dentistry and Faculty of Graduate Studies and Research, Graduate Programs in Medicine, Department of Radiology and Diagnostic Imaging, Edmonton, AB T6G 2E1, Canada. Offers medical sciences (PhD); radiology and diagnostic imaging (M Sc). Terminal master's awarded for partial completion of doctoral program. *Degree requirements:* For master's, thesis; for doctorate, thesis/dissertation. *Entrance requirements:* For master's, minimum GPA of 6.5 on a 9.0 scale; for doctorate, M Sc. *Faculty research:* Spectroscopic attenuation correction, nuclear medicine technology, monoclonal antibody labeling, bone mineral analysis using ultrasound.

University of Arkansas for Medical Sciences, College of Health Professions, Little Rock, AR 72205-7199. Offers audiology (Au D); communication sciences and disorders (MS, PhD); genetic counseling (MS); nuclear medicine advanced associate (MIS); physician assistant studies (MPAS); radiologist assistant (MIS). PhD offered through consortium with University of Arkansas at Little Rock and University of Central Arkansas. Part-time programs available. Postbaccalaureate distance learning degree programs offered (minimal on-campus study). *Faculty:* 54 full-time (34 women), 16 part-time/adjunct (11 women). *Students:* 55 full-time (43 women), 32 part-time (24 women); includes 9 minority (3 Black or African American, non-Hispanic/Latino; 1 American Indian or Alaska Native, non-Hispanic/Latino; 1 Asian, non-Hispanic/Latino; 3 Hispanic/Latino; 1 Two or more races, non-Hispanic/Latino). In 2013, 10 master's, 8 doctorates awarded. *Degree requirements:* For master's, thesis (for some programs); for doctorate, comprehensive exam (for some programs), thesis/dissertation (for some programs). *Entrance requirements:* For master's, GRE. Additional exam requirements/recommendations for international students: Required—TOEFL (minimum score 550 paper-based; 79 iBT). Application fee: $40. Electronic applications accepted. *Expenses:* Contact institution. *Financial support:* Unspecified assistantships available. Financial award application deadline: 6/15; financial award applicants required to submit FAFSA. *Faculty research:* Auditory-based intervention, soy diet, nutrition and cancer. *Unit head:* Dr. Douglas L. Murphy, Dean, 501-686-5730. *Application contact:* Phyllis Fields, Assistant Dean, Student Affairs, 501-686-5730, E-mail: pafields@uams.edu.
Website: http://healthprofessions.uams.edu/

University of California, San Diego, Office of Graduate Studies, Program in Structural Health Monitoring, La Jolla, CA 92093. Offers MAS. *Entrance requirements:* For master's, 3 letters of recommendation; statement of purpose; bachelor's degree in engineering, science, phsyics, or mathematics from accredited institution; minimum undergraduate GPA of 3.0 in final two years of study; two years of relevant work experience; curriculum vitae/resume. Additional exam requirements/recommendations for international students: Required—TOEFL or IELTS. *Expenses:* Tuition, state resident: full-time $11,220; part-time $1870 per quarter. Tuition, nonresident: full-time $26,322; part-time $4387 per quarter. *Required fees:* $519.50 per quarter. Part-time tuition and fees vary according to course load and program.

University of Cincinnati, Graduate School, College of Engineering and Applied Science, Department of Mechanical, Industrial and Nuclear Engineering, Program in Health Physics, Cincinnati, OH 45221. Offers MS. *Degree requirements:* For master's, thesis or alternative. *Entrance requirements:* For master's, GRE General Test. Additional exam requirements/recommendations for international students: Required—TOEFL (minimum score 575 paper-based). Electronic applications accepted.

University of Cincinnati, Graduate School, College of Medicine, Graduate Programs in Biomedical Sciences, Department of Radiological Sciences, Cincinnati, OH 45267. Offers medical physics (MS). Part-time programs available. *Degree requirements:* For master's, comprehensive exam, project. *Entrance requirements:* For master's, GRE General Test. Additional exam requirements/recommendations for international students: Required—TOEFL (minimum score 575 paper-based). Electronic applications accepted. *Faculty research:* Radiation oncology, radiologic imaging, dosimetry, radiation biology, radiation therapy.

University of Kentucky, Graduate School, Graduate School Programs from the College of Medicine, Program in Radiation Sciences, Lexington, KY 40506-0032. Offers radiological medical physics (MSRMP). Part-time programs available. *Degree requirements:* For master's, comprehensive exam, thesis. *Entrance requirements:* For master's, GRE General Test, minimum undergraduate GPA of 2.75. Additional exam requirements/recommendations for international students: Required—TOEFL (minimum score 550 paper-based). Electronic applications accepted. *Faculty research:* Dosimetry, manpower studies, diagnostic imaging physics, shielding.

University of Massachusetts Lowell, College of Sciences, Department of Physics and Applied Physics, Program in Radiological Science and Protection, Lowell, MA 01854-2881. Offers MS. *Degree requirements:* For master's, one foreign language, thesis. *Entrance requirements:* For master's, GRE General Test, 3 letters of reference. Additional exam requirements/recommendations for international students: Required—TOEFL. Electronic applications accepted.

University of Michigan, College of Engineering, Department of Nuclear Engineering and Radiological Sciences, Ann Arbor, MI 48109. Offers nuclear engineering (Nuc E); nuclear engineering and radiological sciences (MSE, PhD); nuclear science (MS, PhD). *Students:* 114 full-time (14 women). 158 applicants, 49% accepted, 33 enrolled. In 2013, 29 master's, 11 doctorates awarded. Terminal master's awarded for partial completion of doctoral program. *Degree requirements:* For master's, thesis optional; for doctorate, thesis/dissertation, oral defense of dissertation, preliminary exams. *Entrance requirements:* For master's and doctorate, GRE General Test. Additional exam requirements/recommendations for international students: Required—TOEFL (minimum score 560 paper-based). *Application deadline:* Applications are processed on a rolling basis. Electronic applications accepted. Tuition and fees vary according to course level, course load, degree level, program and student level. *Financial support:* Fellowships, research assistantships, teaching assistantships, career-related internships or fieldwork, institutionally sponsored loans, scholarships/grants, traineeships, health care benefits, and unspecified assistantships available. *Faculty research:* Radiation safety, environmental sciences, medical physics, fission systems and radiation transport, materials, plasmas and fusion, radiation measurements and imaging. *Total annual research expenditures:* $14.8 million. *Unit head:* Dr. Ronald Gilgenbach, Chair, 734-936-0122, Fax: 734-763-4540, E-mail: rongilg@umich.edu. *Application contact:* Peggy Jo Gramer, Graduate Program Coordinator, 734-615-8810, Fax: 734-763-4540, E-mail: pjgramer@umich.edu.
Website: http://www.ners.engin.umich.edu/

University of Missouri, School of Health Professions, Department of Clinical and Diagnostic Sciences, Columbia, MO 65211. Offers diagnostic medical ultrasound (MHS). *Faculty:* 12 full-time (9 women), 2 part-time/adjunct (1 woman). *Students:* 20 full-time (14 women), 1 (woman) part-time; includes 4 minority (2 Hispanic/Latino; 2 Two or more races, non-Hispanic/Latino). Average age 25. 9 applicants, 89% accepted, 8 enrolled. In 2013, 6 master's awarded. *Entrance requirements:* Additional exam requirements/recommendations for international students: Required—TOEFL (minimum score 500 paper-based; 61 iBT). *Application deadline:* For fall admission, 12/1 priority date for domestic and international students; for winter admission, 10/15 for domestic students. Applications are processed on a rolling basis. Application fee: $55 ($75 for international students). Electronic applications accepted. *Faculty research:* Nuclear medicine, radiology, respiratory therapy, diagnostic medical ultrasound, clinical laboratory science. *Unit head:* Dr. Glen Heggie, Department Chair, 573-884-7843, E-mail: heggieg@missouri.edu. *Application contact:* Ruth Crozier, Director, Student Affairs, 573-882-8011, E-mail: crozierr@health.missouri.edu.
Website: http://shp.missouri.edu/cds/index.php

University of Nevada, Las Vegas, Graduate College, School of Allied Health Sciences, Department of Health Physics, Las Vegas, NV 89154-3037. Offers MS. *Accreditation:* ABET. Part-time programs available. *Faculty:* 4 full-time (0 women). *Students:* 8 full-time (2 women), 3 part-time (1 woman); includes 5 minority (1 Black or African American, non-Hispanic/Latino; 2 Asian, non-Hispanic/Latino; 2 Two or more races, non-Hispanic/Latino), 1 international. Average age 33. 19 applicants, 63% accepted, 3 enrolled. In 2013, 2 master's awarded. *Degree requirements:* For master's, thesis optional, professional paper, oral exam. *Entrance requirements:* Additional exam requirements/recommendations for international students: Required—TOEFL (minimum score 550 paper-based; 80 iBT), IELTS (minimum score 7). *Application deadline:* For fall admission, 6/15 for domestic students, 5/1 for international students; for spring admission, 11/15 for domestic students, 10/1 for international students. Application fee: $60 ($95 for international students). Electronic applications accepted. *Expenses:* Tuition, state resident: full-time $4752; part-time $264 per credit. Tuition, nonresident: full-time $18,662; part-time $554.50 per credit. *International tuition:* $18,952 full-time. *Required fees:* $532; $12 per credit. $266 per semester. One-time fee: $35. Tuition and fees vary according to course load and program. *Financial support:* In 2013–14, 9 students received support, including 2 research assistantships with partial tuition reimbursements available (averaging $7,250 per year), 7 teaching assistantships with partial tuition reimbursements available (averaging $8,262 per year); institutionally sponsored loans, scholarships/grants, health care benefits, and unspecified assistantships also available. Financial award application deadline: 3/1. *Faculty research:* Fate and transport of radionuclides in the environment, radioanalytical methods and applications, biomedical optics and laser biophysics, microdosimetry and cancer initiation processes, medical imaging. *Total annual research expenditures:* $575,598. *Unit head:* Dr. Steen Madsen, Chair/Associate Professor, 702-895-1805, Fax: 702-895-4819, E-mail: steen.madsen@unlv.edu. *Application contact:* Graduate College Admissions Evaluator, 702-895-3320, Fax: 702-895-4180, E-mail: gradcollege@unlv.edu.
Website: http://healthphysics.unlv.edu/

University of Oklahoma Health Sciences Center, College of Medicine and Graduate College, Graduate Programs in Medicine, Department of Radiological Sciences, Oklahoma City, OK 73190. Offers medical radiation physics (MS, PhD), including diagnostic radiology, nuclear medicine, radiation therapy, ultrasound. Part-time programs available. *Faculty:* 11 full-time (2 women). *Students:* 1 full-time (0 women), 10 part-time (1 woman); includes 2 minority (1 Asian, non-Hispanic/Latino; 1 Two or more races, non-Hispanic/Latino). Average age 27. 28 applicants, 18% accepted, 5 enrolled. In 2013, 2 master's, 1 doctorate awarded. Terminal master's awarded for partial completion of doctoral program. *Degree requirements:* For master's, thesis; for doctorate, thesis/dissertation. *Entrance requirements:* For master's, GRE General Test; for doctorate, GRE General Test, 3 letters of recommendation. Additional exam requirements/recommendations for international students: Required—TOEFL. *Application deadline:* For fall admission, 4/1 priority date for domestic students; for spring admission, 10/1 for domestic students. Applications are processed on a rolling basis. Application fee: $50. *Expenses:* Tuition, state resident: full-time $3504; part-time $175.20 per credit hour. Tuition, nonresident: full-time $13,504; part-time $675.20 per credit hour. *Required fees:* $1545; $52.70 per credit hour. $245.25 per semester. Tuition and fees vary according to course load. *Financial support:* In 2013–14, 2 research assistantships (averaging $17,000 per year) were awarded; fellowships, career-related internships or fieldwork, and institutionally sponsored loans also available. Support available to part-time students. Financial award application deadline: 7/1. *Faculty research:* Monte Carlo applications in radiation therapy, observer-performed studies in diagnostic radiology, error analysis in gated cardiac nuclear medicine studies, nuclear medicine absorbed fraction determinations. *Unit head:* Dr. Susan Edwards, Chair, 405-271-5132, E-mail: susan-edwards@ouhsc.edu. *Application contact:* Dr. Jagadeesh Sonnad, Graduate Liaison, 405-270-8001, E-mail: jagadeesh-sonnad@ouhsc.edu.

University of Toronto, Faculty of Medicine, Institute of Medical Science, Toronto, ON M5S 1A1, Canada. Offers bioethics (MH Sc); biomedical communications (M Sc BMC); medical radiation science (MH Sc); medical science (M Sc, PhD). *Degree requirements:* For master's, thesis; for doctorate, thesis/dissertation, thesis defense. *Entrance requirements:* For master's, minimum GPA of 3.7 in 3 of 4 years (M Sc), interview; for doctorate, M Sc or equivalent, defended thesis, minimum A- average, interview. Additional exam requirements/recommendations for international students: Required—TOEFL (minimum score 600 paper-based; 93 iBT), TWE (minimum score 5). Electronic applications accepted.

Vanderbilt University, Graduate School, Department of Physics and Astronomy, Nashville, TN 37240-1001. Offers astronomy (MS); health physics (MA); physics (MAT, MS, PhD). *Faculty:* 31 full-time (4 women). *Students:* 77 full-time (19 women); includes 14 minority (5 Black or African American, non-Hispanic/Latino; 1 Asian, non-Hispanic/Latino; 6 Hispanic/Latino; 2 Two or more races, non-Hispanic/Latino), 23 international. Average age 27. 193 applicants, 16% accepted, 11 enrolled. In 2013, 7 master's, 11 doctorates awarded. *Degree requirements:* For master's, thesis; for doctorate, comprehensive exam, thesis/dissertation, final and qualifying exams. *Entrance requirements:* For master's, GRE General Test; for doctorate, GRE General Test, GRE Subject Test. Additional exam requirements/recommendations for international students: Required—TOEFL (minimum score 570 paper-based; 88 iBT). *Application deadline:* For fall admission, 1/15 for domestic and international students. Electronic applications accepted. *Financial support:* Fellowships with full and partial tuition reimbursements, research assistantships with full tuition reimbursements, teaching assistantships with full tuition reimbursements, career-related internships or fieldwork, Federal Work-Study, and institutionally sponsored loans available. Financial award application deadline: 1/15; financial award applicants required to submit CSS PROFILE or FAFSA. *Faculty research:* Experimental and theoretical physics, free electron laser, living-state physics, heavy-ion physics, nuclear structure. *Unit head:* Dr. Julia Velkovska, Director of Graduate Studies, 615-322-0656, Fax: 615-343-7263, E-mail: julia.velkovska@vanderbilt.edu. *Application contact:* Donald Pickert, Administrative Assistant, 615-343-1026, Fax: 615-343-7263, E-mail: donald.pickert@vanderbilt.edu.
Website: http://www.vanderbilt.edu/physics/

Virginia Commonwealth University, Graduate School, School of Allied Health Professions, Doctoral Program in Health Related Sciences, Richmond, VA 23284-9005. Offers clinical laboratory sciences (PhD); gerontology (PhD); health administration (PhD); nurse anesthesia (PhD); occupational therapy (PhD); physical therapy (PhD); radiation sciences (PhD); rehabilitation leadership (PhD). *Entrance requirements:* For doctorate, GRE General Test or MAT, minimum GPA of 3.3 in master's degree. Additional exam requirements/recommendations for international students: Required—TOEFL (minimum score 600 paper-based; 100 iBT); Recommended—IELTS (minimum score 6.5). Electronic applications accepted.

Wayne State University, Eugene Applebaum College of Pharmacy and Health Sciences, Department of Health Care Sciences, Program in Radiologist Assistant Studies, Detroit, MI 48202. Offers MS. *Faculty:* 1 (woman) full-time, 1 (woman) part-time/adjunct. *Entrance requirements:* For master's, BS from accredited institution with minimum GPA of 3.0, graduation from radiologic technology program accredited by JRCERT, employment as radiologic technologist for at least 3 years, proof of American Registry of Radiologic Technologist registration, proof of Basic Life support certification, three letters of recommendation, personal statement. Additional exam requirements/recommendations for international students: Required—TOEFL (minimum score 550 paper-based; 79 iBT), Michigan English Language Assessment Battery (minimum score 85); Recommended—IELTS (minimum score 6.5), TWE (minimum score 5.5). *Application deadline:* For fall admission, 11/30 for domestic and international students. Application fee: $0. Electronic applications accepted. *Expenses:* Contact institution. *Financial support:* Scholarships/grants available. Financial award application deadline: 3/31; financial award applicants required to submit FAFSA. *Unit head:* Kathleen Kath, Director, 313-916-1348, E-mail: kathykath@wayne.edu. *Application contact:* 313-577-1716, E-mail: cphsinfo@wayne.edu.
Website: http://www.cphs.wayne.edu/program/ra-ms.php

Wayne State University, School of Medicine, Graduate Programs in Medicine, Department of Radiation Oncology, Detroit, MI 48202. Offers medical physics (PhD); radiological physics (MS). Part-time and evening/weekend programs available. *Students:* 25 full-time (3 women), 12 part-time (3 women); includes 10 minority (6 Asian, non-Hispanic/Latino; 2 Hispanic/Latino; 2 Two or more races, non-Hispanic/Latino), 10 international. Average age 30. 85 applicants, 27% accepted, 14 enrolled. In 2013, 12 master's, 1 doctorate awarded. Terminal master's awarded for partial completion of doctoral program. *Degree requirements:* For master's, thesis, essay, exit exam; for doctorate, thesis/dissertation, qualifying exam. *Entrance requirements:* For master's and doctorate, GRE General Test, BS in physics or related area, admission to the Graduate School. Additional exam requirements/recommendations for international students: Required—TOEFL (minimum score 550 paper-based); Recommended—TWE (minimum score 6). *Application deadline:* For fall admission, 1/15 for domestic students, 6/1 for international students; for winter admission, 10/1 for international students; for spring admission, 2/1 for international students. Application fee: $0. Electronic applications accepted. *Expenses:* Contact institution. *Financial support:* In 2013–14, 5 students received support, including 5 research assistantships (averaging $17,373 per year); fellowships, teaching assistantships, scholarships/grants, health care benefits, and unspecified assistantships also available. Financial award application deadline: 3/31; financial award applicants required to submit FAFSA. *Unit head:* Harold E. Kim, MD, Associate Professor and Interim Chair, 313-745-1538, E-mail: kimh@wayne.edu. *Application contact:* Dr. Jay Burmeister, Director, 313-745-2483, E-mail: burmeist@wayne.edu.
Website: http://radiationoncology.med.wayne.edu/

Wayne State University, School of Medicine, Graduate Programs in Medicine, Department of Radiology, Detroit, MI 48202. Offers medical physics (PhD); radiological physics (MS). Part-time and evening/weekend programs available. *Faculty:* 13 full-time (3 women), 1 part-time/adjunct (0 women). *Students:* 23 full-time (3 women), 13 part-time (3 women); includes 9 minority (7 Asian, non-Hispanic/Latino; 2 Two or more races, non-Hispanic/Latino), 6 international. Average age 30. 100 applicants, 27% accepted, 12 enrolled. In 2013, 9 master's awarded. *Degree requirements:* For master's, essay, exam; for doctorate, thesis/dissertation. *Entrance requirements:* For master's, GRE General Test, BS in physics or related area (preferred); for doctorate, GRE, BS in physics or related area (preferred). Additional exam requirements/recommendations for international students: Required—TOEFL (minimum score 600 paper-based; 100 iBT); Recommended—TWE (minimum score 6). *Application deadline:* For fall admission, 1/15 for domestic and international students; for winter admission, 10/1 for domestic students, 9/1 for international students; for spring admission, 2/1 for domestic students, 1/1 for international students. Application fee: $50. Electronic applications accepted. *Expenses:* Contact institution. *Financial support:* In 2013–14, 8 students received support. Fellowships with tuition reimbursements available, research assistantships with tuition reimbursements available, teaching assistantships with tuition reimbursements available, scholarships/grants, and unspecified assistantships available. Financial award application deadline: 3/1. *Faculty research:* Medical physics of radiation therapy, biological basis of radiotherapy, improvements in clinical protocols for radiation therapy, basic physics and biology of radiation action. *Unit head:* Dr. Andre Konski, Professor and Chair of Radiation Oncology, 313-577-9620, E-mail: ec1595@wayne.edu. *Application contact:* Dr. Jay Burmeister, Professor and Chair of Physics, Karmanos Cancer Center, 313-576-9617, E-mail: burmeist@karmanos.org.
Website: http://radiationoncology.med.wayne.edu/medphys/graduate-program/

Weber State University, College of Health Professions, Department of Radiologic Sciences, Ogden, UT 84408-1001. Offers MSRS. *Faculty:* 5 full-time (3 women). *Students:* 31 full-time (17 women), 1 (woman) part-time; includes 5 minority (1 Asian, non-Hispanic/Latino; 3 Hispanic/Latino; 1 Native Hawaiian or other Pacific Islander, non-Hispanic/Latino). Average age 36. 26 applicants, 92% accepted, 23 enrolled. In 2013, 19 master's awarded. *Entrance requirements:* Additional exam requirements/recommendations for international students: Required—TOEFL (minimum score 550 paper-based). *Application deadline:* For fall admission, 5/1 priority date for domestic and international students. Application fee: $60 ($90 for international students). *Expenses:* Tuition, state resident: full-time $7118; part-time $253 per credit hour. Tuition, nonresident: full-time $12,480; part-time $634 per credit hour. *Required fees:* $34.33; $34.33 per credit hour. $257 per semester. Full-time tuition and fees vary according to course load. *Financial support:* In 2013–14, 13 students received support. Application deadline: 4/1; applicants required to submit FAFSA. *Unit head:* Dr. Robert Walker, Program Director, 801-626-7224, Fax: 801-626-7683, E-mail: sconrey@weber.edu. *Application contact:* Lonnie Lujan, Graduate Enrollment Director, 801-626-6088, Fax: 801-626-7966, E-mail: lonnielujan@weber.edu.
Website: http://www.weber.edu/msrs

Medical Imaging

Boston University, School of Medicine, Division of Graduate Medical Sciences, Program in Bioimaging, Boston, MA 02215. Offers MA. *Degree requirements:* For master's, thesis. *Expenses: Tuition:* Full-time $43,970; part-time $1374 per credit hour. *Required fees:* $60 per semester. Tuition and fees vary according to class time, course level and program. *Financial support:* Applicants required to submit FAFSA. *Unit head:* Dr. Mark Moss, Chair, 617-638-4200, E-mail: markmoss@bu.edu. *Application contact:* Patricia Jones, Program Manager and Admissions Director, 617-414-2315, E-mail: psterlin@bu.edu.
Website: http://www.bumc.bu.edu/mbi/

Cleveland State University, College of Graduate Studies, College of Sciences and Health Professions, Department of Physics, Cleveland, OH 44115. Offers applied optics (MS); condensed matter physics (MS); medical physics (MS); optics and materials (MS); optics and medical imaging (MS). Part-time and evening/weekend programs available. *Faculty:* 4 full-time (0 women), 1 part-time/adjunct (0 women). *Students:* 6 full-time (0 women), 14 part-time (3 women); includes 3 minority (1 Black or African American, non-Hispanic/Latino; 2 Asian, non-Hispanic/Latino), 4 international. Average age 32. 48 applicants, 35% accepted. In 2013, 7 master's awarded. *Entrance requirements:* For master's, undergraduate degree in engineering, physics, chemistry or mathematics. Additional exam requirements/recommendations for international students: Required—TOEFL (minimum score 525 paper-based). *Application deadline:* For fall admission, 7/15 priority date for domestic and international students. Applications are processed on a rolling basis. Application fee: $30. Electronic applications accepted. *Expenses:* Tuition, state resident: full-time $8335; part-time $521 per credit hour. Tuition, nonresident: full-time $15,670; part-time $979 per credit hour. *Required fees:* $50; $25 per semester. *Financial support:* In 2013–14, 1 research assistantship with full and partial tuition reimbursement (averaging $5,666 per year) was awarded; fellowships with tuition reimbursements, teaching assistantships, and tuition waivers (full) also available. *Faculty research:* Statistical physics, experimental solid-state physics, theoretical optics, experimental biological physics (macromolecular crystallography), experimental optics. *Total annual research expenditures:* $350,000. *Unit head:* Dr. Miron Kaufman, Chairperson, 216-687-2436, Fax: 216-523-7268, E-mail: m.kaufman@csuohio.edu. *Application contact:* Dr. James A. Lock, Director, 216-687-2420, Fax: 216-523-7268, E-mail: j.lock@csuohio.edu.
Website: http://www.csuohio.edu/sciences/dept/physics/index.html

The College of William and Mary, Faculty of Arts and Sciences, Department of Applied Science, Williamsburg, VA 23187-8795. Offers accelerator science (PhD); applied mathematics (PhD); applied mechanics (PhD); applied robotics (PhD); applied science (MS); atmospheric and environmental science (PhD); computational neuroscience (PhD); interface, thin film and surface science (PhD); lasers and optics (PhD); magnetic resonance (PhD); materials science and engineering (PhD); mathematical and computational biology (PhD); medical imaging (PhD); nanotechnology (PhD); neuroscience (PhD); non-destructive evaluation (PhD); polymer chemistry (PhD); remote sensing (PhD). *Faculty:* 11 full-time (2 women). *Students:* 27 full-time (8 women), 4 part-time (2 women); includes 4 minority (2 Black or African American, non-Hispanic/Latino; 2 Asian, non-Hispanic/Latino), 14 international. Average age 28. 40 applicants, 45% accepted, 3 enrolled. In 2013, 4 master's, 8 doctorates awarded. *Median time to degree:* Of those who began their doctoral program in fall 2005, 95% received their degree in 8 years or less. *Degree requirements:* For master's, comprehensive exam, thesis; for doctorate, comprehensive exam, thesis/dissertation, 4 core courses. *Entrance requirements:* For master's and doctorate, GRE General Test,

GRE Subject Test. Additional exam requirements/recommendations for international students: Required—TOEFL, TWE. *Application deadline:* For fall admission, 2/3 priority date for domestic students, 2/3 for international students; for spring admission, 10/15 priority date for domestic students, 10/14 for international students. Applications are processed on a rolling basis. Application fee: $45. Electronic applications accepted. *Expenses:* Tuition, state resident: full-time $7120; part-time $405 per credit hour. Tuition, nonresident: full-time $21,639; part-time $1050 per credit hour. *Required fees:* $4764. *Financial support:* Fellowships, research assistantships, teaching assistantships, Federal Work-Study, health care benefits, tuition waivers (full), and unspecified assistantships available. Financial award application deadline: 4/15; financial award applicants required to submit FAFSA. *Faculty research:* Computational biology, non-destructive evaluation, neurophysiology, lasers and optics. *Total annual research expenditures:* $2.3 million. *Unit head:* Dr. Christopher Del Negro, Chair, 757-221-7808, Fax: 757-221-2050, E-mail: cadeln@wm.edu. *Application contact:* Rosario Fox, Graduate Program Coordinator, 757-221-2563, Fax: 757-221-2050, E-mail: rxfoxx@wm.edu.
Website: http://www.wm.edu/as/appliedscience

Illinois Institute of Technology, Graduate College, Armour College of Engineering, Department of Electrical and Computer Engineering, Chicago, IL 60616. Offers biomedical imaging and signals (MBMI); computer engineering (MS, PhD); electrical and computer engineering (MECE); electrical engineering (MS, PhD); electricity markets (MEM); network engineering (MNE); power engineering (MPE); telecommunications and software engineering (MTSE); VLSI and microelectronics (MVM). Part-time and evening/weekend programs available. Postbaccalaureate distance learning degree programs offered (minimal on-campus study). Terminal master's awarded for partial completion of doctoral program. *Degree requirements:* For master's, comprehensive exam (for some programs), thesis (for some programs); for doctorate, comprehensive exam, thesis/dissertation. *Entrance requirements:* For master's and doctorate, GRE General Test (minimum score 1100 Quantitative and Verbal, 3.5 Analytical Writing), minimum undergraduate GPA of 3.0. Additional exam requirements/recommendations for international students: Required—TOEFL (minimum score 550 paper-based; 80 iBT); Recommended—IELTS (minimum score 5.5). Electronic applications accepted. *Faculty research:* Communication systems, wireless networks, computer systems, computer networks, wireless security, cloud computing and micro-electronics; electromagnetics and electronics; power and control systems; signal and image processing.

Medical College of Wisconsin, Graduate School of Biomedical Sciences, Program in Functional Imaging, Milwaukee, WI 53226-0509. Offers PhD.

Medical University of South Carolina, College of Graduate Studies, Program in Molecular and Cellular Biology and Pathobiology, Charleston, SC 29425. Offers cancer biology (PhD); cardiovascular biology (PhD); cardiovascular imaging (PhD); cell regulation (PhD); craniofacial biology (PhD); genetics and development (PhD); marine biomedicine (PhD); DMD/PhD; MD/PhD. *Degree requirements:* For doctorate, thesis/dissertation, oral and written exams. *Entrance requirements:* For doctorate, GRE General Test, interview, minimum GPA of 3.0. Additional exam requirements/recommendations for international students: Required—TOEFL (minimum score 600 paper-based; 100 iBT). Electronic applications accepted.

National University of Health Sciences, Lincoln College of Postprofessional, Graduate and Continuing Education, Lombard, IL 60148-4583. Offers advanced clinical practice (MS); diagnostic imaging (MS). Evening/weekend programs available. *Degree requirements:* For master's, comprehensive exam, thesis, capstone. *Entrance requirements:* Additional exam requirements/recommendations for international students: Required—TOEFL. Electronic applications accepted.

New York University, School of Medicine and Graduate School of Arts and Science, Sackler Institute of Graduate Biomedical Sciences, Program in Biomedical Imaging, New York, NY 10012-1019. Offers PhD. *Faculty:* 18 full-time (3 women). *Students:* 11 full-time (8 women); includes 5 minority (4 Asian, non-Hispanic/Latino; 1 Hispanic/Latino), 3 international. Average age 28. In 2013, 4 doctorates awarded. *Expenses: Tuition:* Full-time $35,856; part-time $1494 per unit. *Required fees:* $1408; $64 per unit. $473 per term. Tuition and fees vary according to course load and program. *Faculty research:* In vivo microimaging of transgenic mice, radio frequency (RF) coil design, magnetic resonance spectroscopic imaging. *Unit head:* Dr. Joel D. Oppenheim, Senior Associate Dean for Graduate Studies, 212-263-8001, Fax: 212-263-7600. *Application contact:* Michael Escosia, Admissions Associate, 212-263-5648, Fax: 212-263-7600, E-mail: sackler-info@med.nyu.edu.

Rutgers, The State University of New Jersey, Newark, School of Health Related Professions, Department of Medical Imaging Sciences, Newark, NJ 07102. Offers radiologist assistant (MS). Part-time and evening/weekend programs available. *Entrance requirements:* For master's, BS with minimum GPA of 3.0, RT license, coursework in intro to pathopsychology, interview, all transcripts, personal statement, BCLS certification. Additional exam requirements/recommendations for international students: Required—TOEFL (minimum score 500 paper-based; 79 iBT). Electronic applications accepted.

University of Cincinnati, Graduate School, College of Engineering and Applied Science, Department of Biomedical Engineering, Cincinnati, OH 45221. Offers bioinformatics (PhD); biomechanics (PhD); medical imaging (PhD); tissue engineering (PhD). Part-time programs available. *Degree requirements:* For doctorate, one foreign language, thesis/dissertation. *Entrance requirements:* For doctorate, GRE General Test. Additional exam requirements/recommendations for international students: Required—TOEFL (minimum score 600 paper-based).

University of Guelph, Ontario Veterinary College and Graduate Studies, Graduate Programs in Veterinary Sciences, Department of Clinical Studies, Guelph, ON N1G 2W1, Canada. Offers anesthesiology (M Sc, DV Sc); cardiology (DV Sc, Diploma); clinical studies (Diploma); dermatology (M Sc); diagnostic imaging (M Sc, DV Sc); emergency/critical care (M Sc, DV Sc, Diploma); medicine (M Sc, DV Sc); neurology (M Sc, DV Sc); ophthalmology (M Sc, DV Sc); surgery (M Sc, DV Sc). *Degree requirements:* For master's, thesis; for doctorate, comprehensive exam, thesis/dissertation. *Entrance requirements:* Additional exam requirements/recommendations for international students: Required—TOEFL (minimum score 550 paper-based), IELTS (minimum score 6.5). Electronic applications accepted. *Faculty research:* Orthopedics, respirology, oncology, exercise physiology, cardiology.

University of Southern California, Graduate School, Viterbi School of Engineering, Department of Biomedical Engineering, Los Angeles, CA 90089. Offers biomedical engineering (PhD); medical device and diagnostic engineering (MS); medical imaging and imaging informatics (MS). Postbaccalaureate distance learning degree programs offered (minimal on-campus study). Terminal master's awarded for partial completion of doctoral program. *Degree requirements:* For master's, thesis optional; for doctorate, thesis/dissertation. *Entrance requirements:* For master's and doctorate, GRE General Test. Additional exam requirements/recommendations for international students: Recommended—TOEFL. Electronic applications accepted. *Faculty research:* Medical ultrasound, BioMEMS, neural prosthetics, computational bioengineering, bioengineering of vision, medical devices.

Medical Physics

Cleveland State University, College of Graduate Studies, College of Sciences and Health Professions, Department of Physics, Cleveland, OH 44115. Offers applied optics (MS); condensed matter physics (MS); medical physics (MS); optics and materials (MS); optics and medical imaging (MS). Part-time and evening/weekend programs available. *Faculty:* 4 full-time (0 women), 1 part-time/adjunct (0 women). *Students:* 6 full-time (0 women), 14 part-time (3 women); includes 3 minority (1 Black or African American, non-Hispanic/Latino; 2 Asian, non-Hispanic/Latino), 4 international. Average age 32. 48 applicants, 35% accepted. In 2013, 7 master's awarded. *Entrance requirements:* For master's, undergraduate degree in engineering, physics, chemistry or mathematics. Additional exam requirements/recommendations for international students: Required—TOEFL (minimum score 525 paper-based). *Application deadline:* For fall admission, 7/15 priority date for domestic and international students. Applications are processed on a rolling basis. Application fee: $30. Electronic applications accepted. *Expenses:* Tuition, state resident: full-time $8335; part-time $521 per credit hour. Tuition, nonresident: full-time $15,670; part-time $979 per credit hour. *Required fees:* $50; $25 per semester. *Financial support:* In 2013–14, 1 research assistantship with full and partial tuition reimbursement (averaging $5,666 per year) was awarded; fellowships with tuition reimbursements, teaching assistantships, and tuition waivers (full) also available. *Faculty research:* Statistical physics, experimental solid-state physics, theoretical optics, experimental biological physics (macromolecular crystallography), experimental optics. *Total annual research expenditures:* $350,000. *Unit head:* Dr. Miron Kaufman, Chairperson, 216-687-2436, Fax: 216-523-7268, E-mail: m.kaufman@csuohio.edu. *Application contact:* Dr. James A. Lock, Director, 216-687-2420, Fax: 216-523-7268, E-mail: j.lock@csuohio.edu.
Website: http://www.csuohio.edu/sciences/dept/physics/index.html

The College of William and Mary, Faculty of Arts and Sciences, Department of Applied Science, Williamsburg, VA 23187-8795. Offers accelerator science (PhD); applied mathematics (PhD); applied mechanics (PhD); applied robotics (PhD); applied science (MS); atmospheric and environmental science (PhD); computational neuroscience (PhD); interface, thin film and surface science (PhD); lasers and optics (PhD); magnetic resonance (PhD); materials science and engineering (PhD); mathematical and computational biology (PhD); medical imaging (PhD); nanotechnology (PhD); neuroscience (PhD); non-destructive evaluation (PhD); polymer chemistry (PhD); remote sensing (PhD). *Faculty:* 11 full-time (2 women). *Students:* 27 full-time (8 women), 4 part-time (2 women); includes 4 minority (2 Black or African American, non-Hispanic/Latino; 2 Asian, non-Hispanic/Latino), 14 international. Average age 28. 40 applicants, 45% accepted, 3 enrolled. In 2013, 4 master's, 8 doctorates awarded. *Median time to degree:* Of those who began their doctoral program in fall 2005, 95% received their degree in 8 years or less. *Degree requirements:* For master's, comprehensive exam, thesis; for doctorate, comprehensive exam, thesis/dissertation, 4 core courses. *Entrance requirements:* For master's and doctorate, GRE General Test, GRE Subject Test. Additional exam requirements/recommendations for international students: Required—TOEFL, TWE. *Application deadline:* For fall admission, 2/3 priority date for domestic students, 2/3 for international students; for spring admission, 10/15 priority date for domestic students, 10/14 for international students. Applications are processed on a rolling basis. Application fee: $45. Electronic applications accepted. *Expenses:* Tuition, state resident: full-time $7120; part-time $405 per credit hour. Tuition, nonresident: full-time $21,639; part-time $1050 per credit hour. *Required fees:* $4764. *Financial support:* Fellowships, research assistantships, teaching assistantships, Federal Work-Study, health care benefits, tuition waivers (full), and unspecified assistantships available. Financial award application deadline: 4/15; financial award applicants required to submit FAFSA. *Faculty research:* Computational biology, non-destructive evaluation, neurophysiology, lasers and optics. *Total annual research expenditures:* $2.3 million. *Unit head:* Dr. Christopher Del Negro, Chair, 757-221-7808, Fax: 757-221-2050, E-mail: cadeln@wm.edu. *Application contact:* Rosario Fox, Graduate Program Coordinator, 757-221-2563, Fax: 757-221-2050, E-mail: rxfoxx@wm.edu.
Website: http://www.wm.edu/as/appliedscience

Columbia University, Fu Foundation School of Engineering and Applied Science, Department of Applied Physics and Applied Mathematics, New York, NY 10027. Offers applied physics (Eng Sc D); applied physics and applied mathematics (MS, PhD, Engr); materials science and engineering (MS, Eng Sc D, PhD); medical physics (MS). Part-time programs available. Postbaccalaureate distance learning degree programs offered (no on-campus study). *Faculty:* 36 full-time (4 women), 31 part-time/adjunct (5 women). *Students:* 117 full-time (25 women), 23 part-time (7 women); includes 20 minority (18 Asian, non-Hispanic/Latino; 1 Hispanic/Latino; 1 Two or more races, non-Hispanic/Latino), 72 international. Average age 28. 456 applicants, 27% accepted, 53 enrolled. In 2013, 42 master's, 10 doctorates awarded. Terminal master's awarded for partial completion of doctoral program. *Degree requirements:* For master's, comprehensive exam; for doctorate, thesis/dissertation, qualifying exam. *Entrance requirements:* For master's, GRE General Test, GRE Subject Test (strongly recommended); for doctorate, GRE General Test, GRE Subject Test (applied physics); for Engr, GRE General Test. Additional exam requirements/recommendations for international students: Required—TOEFL, IELTS, PTE. *Application deadline:* For fall admission, 12/15 priority date for domestic and international students; for spring admission, 10/1 priority date for domestic and international students. Application fee: $85. Electronic applications accepted. *Financial support:* In 2013–14, 73 students received support, including 2 fellowships with full tuition reimbursements available (averaging $31,140 per year), 55 research assistantships with full tuition reimbursements available (averaging $31,133 per year), 16 teaching assistantships with full tuition reimbursements available (averaging $31,133 per year); health care benefits also available. Financial award application deadline: 12/15; financial award applicants required to submit FAFSA. *Faculty research:* Plasma physics and fusion energy; optical and laser physics; atmospheric, oceanic and earth physics; applied mathematics; solid state science and processing of materials, their

properties, and their structure; medical physics. *Unit head:* Dr. I. Cevdet Noyan, Professor and Chair, Applied Physics and Applied Mathematics, 212-854-4457, E-mail: seasinfo.apam@columbia.edu. *Application contact:* Montserrat Fernandez-Pinkley, Student Services Coordinator, 212-854-4457, Fax: 212-854-8257, E-mail: mf2157@columbia.edu.
Website: http://www.apam.columbia.edu/

Duke University, Graduate School, Medical Physics Graduate Program, Durham, NC 27705. Offers MS, PhD. *Faculty:* 51. *Students:* 59 full-time (18 women); includes 8 minority (3 Black or African American, non-Hispanic/Latino; 5 Asian, non-Hispanic/Latino), 20 international. 129 applicants, 34% accepted, 24 enrolled. In 2013, 15 master's, 4 doctorates awarded. *Entrance requirements:* For master's and doctorate, GRE General Test. Additional exam requirements/recommendations for international students: Required—TOEFL (minimum score 577 paper-based; 90 iBT) or IELTS (minimum score 7). *Application deadline:* For fall admission, 12/8 priority date for domestic and international students. Application fee: $80. Electronic applications accepted. *Financial support:* Fellowships, research assistantships, and teaching assistantships available. Financial award application deadline: 12/15. *Unit head:* Timothy Turkington, Director, 919-684-1400, Fax: 919-684-1490, E-mail: olga.baranova@duke.edu. *Application contact:* Elizabeth Hutton, Director of Admissions, 919-684-3913, Fax: 919-684-2277, E-mail: grad-admissions@duke.edu.
Website: http://www.medicalphysics.duke.edu/

East Carolina University, Graduate School, Thomas Harriot College of Arts and Sciences, Department of Physics, Greenville, NC 27858-4353. Offers applied physics (MS); biomedical physics (PhD); health physics (MS); medical physics (MS). Part-time programs available. *Degree requirements:* For master's, one foreign language, comprehensive exam. *Entrance requirements:* For master's, GRE General Test. Additional exam requirements/recommendations for international students: Required—TOEFL. *Application deadline:* Applications are processed on a rolling basis. Application fee: $50. *Expenses:* Tuition, state resident: full-time $4223. Tuition, nonresident: full-time $16,540. *Required fees:* $2184. *Financial support:* Research assistantships with partial tuition reimbursements, teaching assistantships with partial tuition reimbursements, and Federal Work-Study available. Support available to part-time students. Financial award application deadline: 6/1. *Unit head:* Dr. John Sutherland, Chair, 252-328-6739, E-mail: sutherlandj@ecu.edu. *Application contact:* Dean of Graduate School, 252-328-6012, Fax: 252-328-6071, E-mail: gradschool@ecu.edu.
Website: http://www.ecu.edu/cs-cas/physics/Graduate-Program.cfm#

Florida Atlantic University, Charles E. Schmidt College of Science, Department of Physics, Boca Raton, FL 33431-0991. Offers medical physics (MSMP); physics (MS, MST, PhD). Part-time programs available. *Faculty:* 5 full-time (1 woman), 3 part-time/adjunct (1 woman). *Students:* 21 full-time (4 women), 14 part-time (5 women); includes 5 minority (3 Black or African American, non-Hispanic/Latino; 1 Hispanic/Latino; 1 Two or more races, non-Hispanic/Latino), 18 international. Average age 31. 30 applicants, 33% accepted, 6 enrolled. In 2013, 8 master's awarded. *Degree requirements:* For master's, thesis; for doctorate, thesis/dissertation. *Entrance requirements:* For master's, GRE General Test, minimum GPA of 3.0; for doctorate, GRE General Test. Additional exam requirements/recommendations for international students: Required—TOEFL (minimum score 500 paper-based; 61 iBT), IELTS (minimum score 6). *Application deadline:* For fall admission, 7/1 for domestic students, 2/15 for international students; for spring admission, 11/1 for domestic students, 7/15 for international students. Applications are processed on a rolling basis. Application fee: $30. *Expenses:* Tuition, state resident: full-time $6660; part-time $370 per credit hour. Tuition, nonresident: full-time $18,450; part-time $1025 per credit hour. Tuition and fees vary according to course load. *Financial support:* Fellowships, research assistantships with tuition reimbursements, teaching assistantships with tuition reimbursements, Federal Work-Study, and unspecified assistantships available. *Faculty research:* Astrophysics, spectroscopy, mathematical physics, theory of metals, superconductivity. *Unit head:* Dr. Warner A. Miller, Chair, 561-297-3382, Fax: 561-297-2662, E-mail: wam@physics.fau.edu. *Application contact:* Dr. Wolfgang Tichy, Graduate Programs, 561-297-3353, Fax: 561-297-2662.
Website: http://physics.fau.edu/

Georgia Institute of Technology, Graduate Studies and Research, College of Engineering, George W. Woodruff School of Mechanical Engineering, Nuclear and Radiological Engineering and Medical Physics Programs, Atlanta, GA 30332-0001. Offers medical physics (MS); nuclear and radiological engineering (MSNE, PhD). Part-time programs available. Postbaccalaureate distance learning degree programs offered (no on-campus study). Terminal master's awarded for partial completion of doctoral program. *Degree requirements:* For master's, thesis optional; for doctorate, comprehensive exam, thesis/dissertation. *Entrance requirements:* For master's and doctorate, GRE General Test, minimum GPA of 3.0. Additional exam requirements/recommendations for international students: Required—TOEFL (minimum score 580 paper-based). *Faculty research:* Reactor physics, nuclear materials, plasma physics, radiation detection, radiological assessment.

Hampton University, Graduate College, Department of Physics, Hampton, VA 23668. Offers atmospheric physics (MS, PhD); medical physics (MS, PhD); nuclear physics (MS, PhD); optical physics (MS, PhD). Part-time and evening/weekend programs available. Terminal master's awarded for partial completion of doctoral program. *Degree requirements:* For master's, thesis optional; for doctorate, thesis/dissertation, oral defense, qualifying exam. *Entrance requirements:* For master's, GRE General Test; for doctorate, GRE General Test, minimum GPA of 3.0 or master's degree in physics or related field. *Faculty research:* Laser optics, remote sensing.

Harvard University, Graduate School of Arts and Sciences, Department of Physics, Cambridge, MA 02138. Offers experimental physics (PhD); medical engineering/medical physics (PhD), including applied physics, engineering sciences, physics; theoretical physics (PhD). *Degree requirements:* For doctorate, thesis/dissertation, final exams, laboratory experience. *Entrance requirements:* For doctorate, GRE General Test, GRE Subject Test. Additional exam requirements/recommendations for international students: Required—TOEFL. *Expenses: Tuition:* Full-time $38,888. *Required fees:* $958. Tuition and fees vary according to campus/location, program and student level. *Faculty research:* Particle physics, condensed matter physics, atomic physics.

Hofstra University, College of Liberal Arts and Sciences, Programs in Physics, Hempstead, NY 11549. Offers medical physics (MA).

Indiana University Bloomington, University Graduate School, College of Arts and Sciences, Department of Physics, Bloomington, IN 47405. Offers medical physics (MS); physics (MAT, MS, PhD). Part-time programs available. Postbaccalaureate distance learning degree programs offered (no on-campus study). *Faculty:* 35 full-time (4 women), 11 part-time/adjunct (1 woman). *Students:* 105 full-time (19 women), 1 part-time (0 women); includes 9 minority (5 Asian, non-Hispanic/Latino; 4 Hispanic/Latino), 48 international. Average age 27. 186 applicants, 37% accepted, 19 enrolled. In 2013, 10 master's, 8 doctorates awarded. Terminal master's awarded for partial completion of doctoral program. *Degree requirements:* For master's, comprehensive exam (for some programs), thesis (for some programs), qualifying exam; for doctorate, comprehensive exam, thesis/dissertation, qualifying exam. *Entrance requirements:* For master's and doctorate, GRE General Test, GRE Subject Test (physics), minimum GPA of 3.0. Additional exam requirements/recommendations for international students: Required—TOEFL (minimum score 550 paper-based; 80 iBT) or IELTS (minimum score 6.5). *Application deadline:* For fall admission, 1/15 priority date for domestic students, 12/1 priority date for international students; for spring admission, 10/1 priority date for domestic students, 9/1 priority date for international students. Applications are processed on a rolling basis. Application fee: $55 ($65 for international students). Electronic applications accepted. *Financial support:* In 2013–14, 14 students received support, including 3 fellowships with full and partial tuition reimbursements available (averaging $21,500 per year), 56 research assistantships with partial tuition reimbursements available (averaging $16,800 per year), 33 teaching assistantships with partial tuition reimbursements available (averaging $16,659 per year); health care benefits also available. Financial award application deadline: 4/15. *Faculty research:* Accelerator physics, astrophysics and cosmology, biophysics (biocomplexity, neural networks, visual systems, chemical signaling), condensed matter physics (neutron scattering, complex fluids, quantum computing), particle physics (collider physics, hybrid mesons, lattice gauge, symmetries, collider phenomenology), neutrino physics, nuclear physics (proton and neutron physics, neutrinos, symmetries, nuclear astrophysics, hadron structure). *Total annual research expenditures:* $13.2 million. *Unit head:* Prof. Rob de Ruyter, Department Chair, 812-855-1247, Fax: 812-855-5533, E-mail: iubphys@indiana.edu. *Application contact:* June Dizer, Director of Academic Support, 812-856-7059, Fax: 812-855-5533, E-mail: gradphys@indiana.edu.
Website: http://physics.indiana.edu/

Louisiana State University and Agricultural & Mechanical College, Graduate School, College of Science, Department of Physics and Astronomy, Baton Rouge, LA 70803. Offers astronomy (PhD); astrophysics (PhD); medical physics (MS); physics (MS, PhD). *Faculty:* 46 full-time (5 women), 1 part-time/adjunct (0 women). *Students:* 101 full-time (22 women), 6 part-time (3 women); includes 7 minority (2 Black or African American, non-Hispanic/Latino; 1 Asian, non-Hispanic/Latino; 4 Hispanic/Latino), 44 international. Average age 26. 153 applicants, 22% accepted, 20 enrolled. In 2013, 15 master's, 9 doctorates awarded. Terminal master's awarded for partial completion of doctoral program. *Degree requirements:* For master's, thesis or alternative; for doctorate, thesis/dissertation. *Entrance requirements:* For master's and doctorate, GRE General Test, minimum GPA of 3.0. Additional exam requirements/recommendations for international students: Required—TOEFL (minimum score 550 paper-based; 79 iBT), IELTS (minimum score 6.5), or PTE (minimum score 59). *Application deadline:* For fall admission, 1/25 priority date for domestic students, 5/15 for international students; for spring admission, 10/15 for international students. Applications are processed on a rolling basis. Application fee: $50 ($70 for international students). Electronic applications accepted. *Financial support:* In 2013–14, 105 students received support, including 10 fellowships with full tuition reimbursements available (averaging $40,065 per year), 53 research assistantships with full and partial tuition reimbursements available (averaging $23,273 per year), 34 teaching assistantships with full and partial tuition reimbursements available (averaging $20,018 per year); Federal Work-Study, institutionally sponsored loans, health care benefits, tuition waivers (full and partial), and unspecified assistantships also available. Financial award application deadline: 3/15; financial award applicants required to submit FAFSA. *Faculty research:* Experimentation and numerical relativity, condensed matter astrophysics, quantum computing, medical physics. *Total annual research expenditures:* $7.7 million. *Unit head:* Dr. Michael Cherry, Chair, 225-578-2262, Fax: 225-578-5855, E-mail: cherry@phys.lsu.edu. *Application contact:* Arnell Dangerfield, Administrative Coordinator, 225-578-1193, Fax: 225-578-5855, E-mail: adanger@lsu.edu.
Website: http://www.phys.lsu.edu/

Massachusetts Institute of Technology, School of Engineering, Harvard-MIT Health Sciences and Technology Program, Cambridge, MA 02139-4307. Offers health sciences and technology (SM, PhD, Sc D), including bioastronautics (PhD, Sc D), bioinformatics and integrative genomics (PhD, Sc D), medical engineering and medical physics (PhD, Sc D), speech and hearing bioscience and technology (PhD, Sc D). *Students:* 281 full-time (115 women), 10 part-time (0 women); includes 84 minority (1 Black or African American, non-Hispanic/Latino; 1 American Indian or Alaska Native, non-Hispanic/Latino; 68 Asian, non-Hispanic/Latino; 11 Hispanic/Latino; 3 Two or more races, non-Hispanic/Latino), 48 international. Average age 26. 180 applicants, 17% accepted, 18 enrolled. In 2013, 7 master's, 20 doctorates awarded. Terminal master's awarded for partial completion of doctoral program. *Degree requirements:* For master's, thesis; for doctorate, comprehensive exam, thesis/dissertation. *Entrance requirements:* For doctorate, GRE General Test (for medical engineering and medical physics). Additional exam requirements/recommendations for international students: Required—TOEFL (minimum score 600 paper-based; 100 iBT), IELTS (minimum score 7). *Application deadline:* For fall admission, 12/15 for domestic and international students. Application fee: $75. Electronic applications accepted. *Expenses: Tuition:* Full-time $43,210; part-time $670 per credit hour. *Required fees:* $288. *Financial support:* In 2013–14, 144 students received support, including 66 fellowships (averaging $35,700 per year), 49 research assistantships (averaging $31,300 per year), 1 teaching assistantship (averaging $33,300 per year); Federal Work-Study, institutionally sponsored loans, scholarships/grants, traineeships, health care benefits, and unspecified assistantships also available. Financial award application deadline: 12/15. *Faculty research:* Signal processing, biomedical imaging, drug delivery, medical devices, medical diagnostics, regenerative biomedical technologies. *Unit head:* Emery N. Brown, Director, 617-452-4091. *Application contact:* Emery N. Brown, Director, 617-452-4091.
Website: http://hst.mit.edu/

McGill University, Faculty of Graduate and Postdoctoral Studies, Faculty of Medicine, Medical Physics Unit, Montréal, QC H3A 2T5, Canada. Offers M Sc, PhD. *Entrance requirements:* Additional exam requirements/recommendations for international students: Required—TOEFL.

McMaster University, School of Graduate Studies, Faculty of Science, Department of Medical Physics and Applied Radiation Sciences, Hamilton, ON L8S 4M2, Canada. Offers health and radiation physics (M Sc); medical physics (M Sc, PhD). Part-time programs available. *Degree requirements:* For master's, thesis or alternative. *Entrance requirements:* For master's, minimum B+ average. Additional exam requirements/recommendations for international students: Required—TOEFL (minimum score 550 paper-based). *Faculty research:* Imaging, toxicology, dosimetry, body composition, medical lasers.

Oakland University, Graduate Study and Lifelong Learning, College of Arts and Sciences, Department of Physics, Rochester, MI 48309-4401. Offers medical physics (PhD); physics (MS). *Faculty:* 6 full-time (0 women), 2 part-time/adjunct (0 women). *Students:* 16 full-time (6 women), 4 part-time (1 woman); includes 4 minority (2 Black or African American, non-Hispanic/Latino; 2 Asian, non-Hispanic/Latino), 9 international. Average age 32. 27 applicants, 19% accepted, 5 enrolled. In 2013, 2 master's, 2 doctorates awarded. *Degree requirements:* For doctorate, thesis/dissertation. *Entrance requirements:* For master's, minimum GPA of 3.0; for doctorate, GRE Subject Test, GRE General Test, minimum GPA of 3.0. Additional exam requirements/recommendations for international students: Required—TOEFL (minimum score 550 paper-based). *Application deadline:* For fall admission, 7/15 priority date for domestic students, 5/1 priority date for international students; for winter admission, 12/1 priority date for domestic students, 9/1 priority date for international students; for spring admission, 3/15 priority date for domestic students. Applications are processed on a rolling basis. Application fee: $0. Electronic applications accepted. *Expenses:* Contact institution. *Financial support:* Fellowships, career-related internships or fieldwork, Federal Work-Study, institutionally sponsored loans, and tuition waivers (full) available. Financial award application deadline: 3/1; financial award applicants required to submit FAFSA. *Faculty research:* Self-assembled multiferroic nanostructures and studies on magnetoelectric interactions. *Total annual research expenditures:* $1.4 million. *Unit head:* Dr. Andrei N. Slavin, Chair, 248-370-3416, Fax: 248-370-3401, E-mail: slavin@oakland.edu. *Application contact:* Christina J. Grabowski, Associate Director of Graduate Study and Lifelong Learning, 248-370-3167, Fax: 248-370-4114, E-mail: grabowsk@oakland.edu.

Oregon State University, College of Engineering, Program in Medical Physics, Corvallis, OR 97331. Offers MMP, MS, PhD. *Faculty:* 11 full-time (3 women), 2 part-time/adjunct (0 women). *Students:* 9 full-time (3 women), 3 part-time (1 woman); includes 1 minority (Asian, non-Hispanic/Latino). Average age 30. 76 applicants, 17% accepted, 5 enrolled. In 2013, 1 master's awarded. *Entrance requirements:* For master's and doctorate, GRE. Additional exam requirements/recommendations for international students: Required—TOEFL (minimum score 80 iBT), IELTS (minimum score 6.5). *Application deadline:* For fall admission, 8/1 for domestic students. Application fee: $60. *Expenses:* Contact institution. *Unit head:* Dr. Krystina M. Tack, Director, 541-737-2343, E-mail: krystina.tack@oregonstate.edu. *Application contact:* Heidi Braly, Graduate Student Liaison, 541-737-7062, E-mail: heidi.braly@oregonstate.edu.
Website: http://ne.oregonstate.edu/content/medical-physics-program

Purdue University, Graduate School, College of Health and Human Sciences, School of Health Sciences, West Lafayette, IN 47907. Offers health physics (MS, PhD); medical physics (MS, PhD); occupational and environmental health science (MS, PhD), including aerosol deposition and lung disease, ergonomics, exposure and risk assessment, indoor air quality and bioaerosols (PhD), liver/lung toxicology; radiation biology (PhD); toxicology (PhD); MS/PhD. Part-time programs available. *Faculty:* 11 full-time (5 women), 28 part-time/adjunct (5 women). *Students:* 28 full-time (8 women), 10 part-time (3 women); includes 6 minority (1 Black or African American, non-Hispanic/Latino; 3 Asian, non-Hispanic/Latino; 1 Hispanic/Latino; 1 Two or more races, non-Hispanic/Latino), 10 international. Average age 28. 77 applicants, 42% accepted, 13 enrolled. In 2013, 6 master's, 6 doctorates awarded. *Degree requirements:* For master's, thesis optional; for doctorate, one foreign language, thesis/dissertation. *Entrance requirements:* For master's and doctorate, GRE General Test, minimum undergraduate GPA of 3.0 or equivalent. Additional exam requirements/recommendations for international students: Required—TOEFL (minimum score 550 paper-based; 77 iBT); Recommended—TWE. *Application deadline:* For fall admission, 5/15 for domestic and international students; for spring admission, 10/15 for domestic and international students. Applications are processed on a rolling basis. Application fee: $60 ($75 for international students). Electronic applications accepted. *Financial support:* In 2013–14, fellowships with tuition reimbursements (averaging $14,400 per year), research assistantships with tuition reimbursements (averaging $12,000 per year), teaching assistantships with tuition reimbursements (averaging $12,000 per year) were awarded; career-related internships or fieldwork and traineeships also available. Support available to part-time students. Financial award applicants required to submit FAFSA. *Faculty research:* Environmental toxicology, industrial hygiene, radiation dosimetry. *Unit head:* Dr. Wei Zheng, Head, 765-494-1419, E-mail: wz18@purdue.edu. *Application contact:* Jennifer S. Franklin, Graduate Contact, 765-494-0248, E-mail: jfranklin@purdue.edu.
Website: http://www.healthsciences.purdue.edu/

Rosalind Franklin University of Medicine and Science, College of Health Professions, Department of Medical Radiation Physics, North Chicago, IL 60064-3095. Offers MS. Terminal master's awarded for partial completion of doctoral program. *Entrance requirements:* For master's, GRE General Test. Additional exam requirements/recommendations for international students: Required—TOEFL. *Expenses:* Contact institution.

Rush University, Graduate College, Division of Medical Physics, Chicago, IL 60612-3832. Offers MS, PhD. Terminal master's awarded for partial completion of doctoral program. *Degree requirements:* For master's, thesis, qualifying exam; for doctorate, thesis/dissertation, preliminary and qualifying exams. *Entrance requirements:* For master's, GRE General Test, BS in physics or physical science; for doctorate, GRE General Test, GRE Subject Test. Additional exam requirements/recommendations for international students: Required—TOEFL. Electronic applications accepted. *Faculty research:* Radiation therapy treatment planning, dosimetry, diagnostic radiology and nuclear imaging.

Southern Illinois University Carbondale, Graduate School, College of Applied Science, Program in Medical Dosimetry, Carbondale, IL 62901-4701. Offers MS. *Faculty:* 32 full-time (22 women). *Students:* 18 full-time (9 women), 18 part-time (11 women); includes 5 minority (2 Black or African American, non-Hispanic/Latino; 3 Asian, non-Hispanic/Latino), 2 international. Average age 25. 53 applicants, 40% accepted, 21 enrolled. In 2013, 18 master's awarded. *Entrance requirements:* Additional exam requirements/recommendations for international students: Required—TOEFL. *Application deadline:* For fall admission, 2/1 for domestic and international students. Application fee: $50. *Unit head:* Prof. Scott Collins, Coordinator, 618-453-8800, E-mail: kscollin@siu.edu. *Application contact:* Donna Colwell, Office Support Specialist, 618-453-8869, E-mail: dcolwell@siu.edu.

Stony Brook University, State University of New York, Graduate School, College of Engineering and Applied Sciences, Department of Biomedical Engineering, Program in Medical Physics, Stony Brook, NY 11794. Offers MS, PhD. *Entrance requirements:* For doctorate, GRE. *Expenses:* Tuition, state resident: full-time $9870; part-time $411 per credit. Tuition, nonresident: full-time $18,350; part-time $765 per credit. *Financial support:* Fellowships available. *Unit head:* Dr. Terry Button, Director, 631-444-3841, E-mail: terry.button@sunysb.edu. *Application contact:* Anne Dusatko, Assistant to Chair/Graduate Program Coordinator, 631-632-8375, Fax: 631-632-8577, E-mail: ann.dusatko@sunysb.edu.
Website: http://bme.sunysb.edu/grad/medicalphysics.html

University of Alberta, Faculty of Graduate Studies and Research, Department of Physics, Edmonton, AB T6G 2E1, Canada. Offers astrophysics (M Sc, PhD); condensed matter (M Sc, PhD); geophysics (M Sc, PhD); medical physics (M Sc, PhD); subatomic physics (M Sc, PhD). *Degree requirements:* For master's, thesis; for doctorate, thesis/dissertation. *Entrance requirements:* For master's and doctorate, minimum GPA of 7.0 on a 9.0 scale. Additional exam requirements/recommendations for international students: Required—TOEFL. *Faculty research:* Cosmology, astroparticle physics, high-intermediate energy, magnetism, superconductivity.

The University of Arizona, College of Science, Department of Physics, Medical Physics Program, Tucson, AZ 85721. Offers PSM. Part-time programs available. *Students:* 8 full-time (0 women), 1 part-time (0 women); includes 4 minority (1 Black or African American, non-Hispanic/Latino; 2 Asian, non-Hispanic/Latino; 1 Hispanic/Latino), 2 international. Average age 28. 34 applicants, 18% accepted, 5 enrolled. In 2013, 2 master's awarded. *Degree requirements:* For master's, thesis or alternative, internship, colloquium, business courses. *Entrance requirements:* Additional exam requirements/recommendations for international students: Required—TOEFL (minimum score 550 paper-based; 79 iBT). Application fee: $75. Electronic applications accepted. *Expenses:* Tuition, state resident: full-time $11,526. Tuition, nonresident: full-time $27,398. *Financial support:* Career-related internships or fieldwork, Federal Work-Study, and scholarships/grants available. *Faculty research:* Nanotechnology, optics, medical imaging, high energy physics, biophysics. *Unit head:* Dr. Michael Shupe, Department Head, 520-621-2679, E-mail: shupe@physics.arizona.edu. *Application contact:* Lisa Shapouri, Graduate Coordinator, 520-621-2290, Fax: 520-621-4721, E-mail: lisas@physics.arizona.edu.
Website: http://www.physics.arizona.edu/

University of California, Los Angeles, David Geffen School of Medicine and Graduate Division, Graduate Programs in Medicine, Program in Biomedical Physics, Los Angeles, CA 90095. Offers MS, PhD. Terminal master's awarded for partial completion of doctoral program. *Degree requirements:* For master's, comprehensive exam or thesis; for doctorate, thesis/dissertation, oral and written qualifying exams. *Entrance requirements:* For master's and doctorate, GRE General Test. Additional exam requirements/recommendations for international students: Required—TOEFL. Electronic applications accepted.

University of Chicago, Division of Biological Sciences, Committee on Medical Physics, Chicago, IL 60637-1513. Offers PhD. *Degree requirements:* For doctorate, thesis/dissertation, ethics class, 2 teaching assistantships. *Entrance requirements:* For doctorate, GRE General Test, GRE Subject Test. Additional exam requirements/recommendations for international students: Required—TOEFL (minimum score 600 paper-based; 104 iBT), IELTS (minimum score 7). Electronic applications accepted.

University of Cincinnati, Graduate School, College of Medicine, Graduate Programs in Biomedical Sciences, Department of Radiological Sciences, Cincinnati, OH 45267. Offers medical physics (MS). Part-time programs available. *Degree requirements:* For master's, comprehensive exam, project. *Entrance requirements:* For master's, GRE General Test. Additional exam requirements/recommendations for international students: Required—TOEFL (minimum score 575 paper-based). Electronic applications accepted. *Faculty research:* Radiation oncology, radiologic imaging, dosimetry, radiation biology, radiation therapy.

University of Colorado Boulder, Graduate School, College of Arts and Sciences, Department of Physics, Boulder, CO 80309. Offers chemical physics (PhD); geophysics (PhD); liquid crystal science and technology (PhD); mathematical physics (PhD); medical physics (PhD); optical sciences and engineering (PhD); physics (MS, PhD). *Faculty:* 50 full-time (7 women). *Students:* 139 full-time (26 women), 84 part-time (16 women); includes 10 minority (5 Asian, non-Hispanic/Latino; 5 Hispanic/Latino), 68 international. Average age 26. 609 applicants, 22% accepted, 32 enrolled. In 2013, 35 master's, 19 doctorates awarded. Terminal master's awarded for partial completion of doctoral program. *Degree requirements:* For master's, comprehensive exam, thesis or alternative; for doctorate, comprehensive exam, thesis/dissertation. *Entrance requirements:* For master's and doctorate, GRE General Test, GRE Subject Test, minimum undergraduate GPA of 3.0. Additional exam requirements/recommendations for international students: Required—TOEFL. *Application deadline:* For fall admission, 12/15 for domestic and international students. Applications are processed on a rolling basis. Application fee: $50 ($60 for international students). Electronic applications accepted. *Financial support:* In 2013–14, 522 students received support, including 45 fellowships (averaging $17,404 per year), 150 research assistantships with full and partial tuition reimbursements available (averaging $32,230 per year), 52 teaching assistantships with full and partial tuition reimbursements available (averaging $26,294 per year); institutionally sponsored loans, scholarships/grants, health care benefits, and unspecified assistantships also available. Financial award application deadline: 1/15; financial award applicants required to submit FAFSA. *Faculty research:* Physics, theoretical physics, high energy physics, experimental physics, elementary particle physics. *Total annual research expenditures:* $26.3 million.
Website: http://physics.colorado.edu/

University of Florida, Graduate School, College of Engineering, Department of Biomedical Engineering, Gainesville, FL 32611. Offers biomedical engineering (ME, MS, PhD, Certificate); clinical and translational science (PhD); medical physics (MS, PhD); MD/PhD. *Faculty:* 26 full-time (5 women), 25 part-time/adjunct (6 women). *Students:* 119 full-time (48 women), 15 part-time (6 women); includes 24 minority (1 Black or African American, non-Hispanic/Latino; 8 Asian, non-Hispanic/Latino; 15 Hispanic/Latino), 49 international. Average age 27. 227 applicants, 26% accepted, 26 enrolled. In 2013, 31 master's, 18 doctorates awarded. Terminal master's awarded for partial completion of doctoral program. *Degree requirements:* For master's, comprehensive exam (for some programs), thesis (for some programs); for doctorate, comprehensive exam (for some programs), thesis/dissertation (for some programs). *Entrance requirements:* For master's and doctorate, minimum GPA of 3.0. Additional exam requirements/recommendations for international students: Required—TOEFL (minimum score 550 paper-based; 80 iBT), IELTS (minimum score 6). *Application deadline:* For fall admission, 12/15 priority date for domestic students, 12/15 for international students; for spring admission, 7/31 for domestic and international students. Applications are processed on a rolling basis. Application fee: $30. Electronic applications accepted. *Expenses:* Tuition, state resident: full-time $12,640. Tuition, nonresident: full-time $30,000. *Financial support:* In 2013–14, 65 students received support, including 2 fellowships with full tuition reimbursements available (averaging $31,000 per year), 66 research assistantships with full tuition reimbursements available (averaging $21,340 per year), 1 teaching assistantship (averaging $2,610 per year). Financial award application deadline: 12/31; financial award applicants required to submit FAFSA. *Faculty research:* Neural engineering, tissue engineering, biomedical imaging. *Unit head:* Christine E. Schmidt, PhD, Chair, 352-273-9222, Fax: 352-392-9791, E-mail: schmidt@bme.ufl.edu. *Application contact:* Hans Van Oostrom, PhD, Associate Professor/Associate Chair/Graduate Coordinator, 352-273-9315, Fax: 352-392-9221, E-mail: oostrom@ufl.edu.
Website: http://www.bme.ufl.edu/

University of Kentucky, Graduate School, Graduate School Programs from the College of Medicine, Program in Radiation Sciences, Lexington, KY 40506-0032. Offers radiological medical physics (MSRMP). Part-time programs available. *Degree requirements:* For master's, comprehensive exam, thesis. *Entrance requirements:* For master's, GRE General Test, minimum undergraduate GPA of 2.75. Additional exam requirements/recommendations for international students: Required—TOEFL (minimum score 550 paper-based). Electronic applications accepted. *Faculty research:* Dosimetry, manpower studies, diagnostic imaging physics, shielding.

University of Minnesota, Twin Cities Campus, Graduate School, Program in Biophysical Sciences and Medical Physics, Minneapolis, MN 55455-0213. Offers MS, PhD. Part-time programs available. *Degree requirements:* For master's, thesis optional, research paper, oral exam; for doctorate, thesis/dissertation, oral/written preliminary exam, oral final exam. *Faculty research:* Theoretical biophysics, radiological physics, cellular and molecular biophysics.

Medical Physics

University of Missouri, Graduate School, Nuclear Engineering Program, Columbia, MO 65211. Offers environmental and regulatory compliance (MS, PhD); materials (PhD); medical physics (MS); nuclear engineering (Certificate); nuclear safeguards science and technology (Certificate); thermal hydraulics (MS, PhD). *Faculty:* 5 full-time (0 women). *Students:* 43 full-time (8 women), 7 part-time (3 women); includes 4 minority (2 Asian, non-Hispanic/Latino; 2 Hispanic/Latino), 14 international. Average age 29. 42 applicants, 17% accepted, 5 enrolled. In 2013, 15 master's, 11 doctorates, 6 other advanced degrees awarded. *Degree requirements:* For master's, research project; for doctorate, thesis/dissertation. *Entrance requirements:* For master's and doctorate, GRE General Test. Additional exam requirements/recommendations for international students: Required—TOEFL (minimum score 500 paper-based; 61 iBT). *Application deadline:* For fall admission, 3/1 priority date for domestic and international students; for winter admission, 10/1 priority date for domestic students, 9/1 priority date for international students. Application fee: $55 ($75 for international students). Electronic applications accepted. *Financial support:* Fellowships with full and partial tuition reimbursements, research assistantships with full and partial tuition reimbursements, teaching assistantships with full and partial tuition reimbursements, institutionally sponsored loans, scholarships/grants, health care benefits, and unspecified assistantships available. Support available to part-time students. *Faculty research:* Nuclear materials management, aerosol mechanics, reactor safety analysis, nuclear energy conversion, reactor physics, reactor design, nondestructive testing and measurement, radiative heat transfer, neutron spectrometry, neutron and gamma ray transport, neutron activation analysis, nuclear waste management, nuclear plasma research, health physics, magnetic resonance imaging, radiation therapy and alternative and renewable energy concepts. *Unit head:* Dr. John M. Gahl, Director, 573-882-5345, E-mail: gahlj@missouri.edu.
Website: http://engineering.missouri.edu/nuclear/

University of Oklahoma Health Sciences Center, College of Medicine and Graduate College, Graduate Programs in Medicine, Department of Radiological Sciences, Oklahoma City, OK 73190. Offers medical radiation physics (MS, PhD), including diagnostic radiology, nuclear medicine, radiation therapy, ultrasound. Part-time programs available. *Faculty:* 11 full-time (2 women). *Students:* 1 full-time (0 women), 10 part-time (1 woman); includes 2 minority (1 Asian, non-Hispanic/Latino; 1 Two or more races, non-Hispanic/Latino). Average age 27. 28 applicants, 18% accepted, 5 enrolled. In 2013, 2 master's, 1 doctorate awarded. Terminal master's awarded for partial completion of doctoral program. *Degree requirements:* For master's, thesis; for doctorate, thesis/dissertation. *Entrance requirements:* For master's, GRE General Test; for doctorate, GRE General Test, 3 letters of recommendation. Additional exam requirements/recommendations for international students: Required—TOEFL. *Application deadline:* For fall admission, 4/1 priority date for domestic students; for spring admission, 10/1 for domestic students. Applications are processed on a rolling basis. Application fee: $50. *Expenses:* Tuition, state resident: full-time $3504; part-time $175.20 per credit hour. Tuition, nonresident: full-time $13,504; part-time $675.20 per credit hour. *Required fees:* $1545; $52.70 per credit hour. $245.25 per semester. Tuition and fees vary according to course load. *Financial support:* In 2013–14, 2 research assistantships (averaging $17,000 per year) were awarded; fellowships, career-related internships or fieldwork, and institutionally sponsored loans also available. Support available to part-time students. Financial award application deadline: 7/1. *Faculty research:* Monte Carlo applications in radiation therapy, observer-performed studies in diagnostic radiology, error analysis in gated cardiac nuclear medicine studies, nuclear medicine absorbed fraction determinations. *Unit head:* Dr. Susan Edwards, Chair, 405-271-5132, E-mail: susan-edwards@ouhsc.edu. *Application contact:* Dr. Jagadeesh Sonnad, Graduate Liaison, 405-270-8001, E-mail: jagadeesh-sonnad@ouhsc.edu.

University of Pennsylvania, School of Arts and Sciences, College of Liberal and Professional Studies, Philadelphia, PA 19104. Offers applied geosciences (MSAG); applied positive psychology (MAP); chemical sciences (MCS); environmental studies (MES); individualized study (MLA); liberal arts (M Phil); medical physics (MMP); organization dynamics (M Phil). *Students:* 167 full-time (98 women), 310 part-time (165 women); includes 84 minority (29 Black or African American, non-Hispanic/Latino; 1 American Indian or Alaska Native, non-Hispanic/Latino; 25 Asian, non-Hispanic/Latino; 18 Hispanic/Latino; 11 Two or more races, non-Hispanic/Latino), 61 international. 718 applicants, 49% accepted, 281 enrolled. In 2013, 173 master's awarded. *Application deadline:* For fall admission, 12/1 priority date for domestic students. Application fee: $70. Electronic applications accepted. *Unit head:* Nora Lewis, Vice Dean, Professional and Liberal Education, 215-898-7326, E-mail: nlewis@sas.upenn.edu. *Application contact:* 215-898-7326, E-mail: lps@sas.upenn.edu.
Website: http://www.sas.upenn.edu/lps/graduate

University of Pennsylvania, School of Arts and Sciences, Graduate Group in Physics and Astronomy, Philadelphia, PA 19104. Offers medical physics (MS); physics (PhD). Part-time programs available. *Faculty:* 41 full-time (6 women), 11 part-time/adjunct (0 women). *Students:* 102 full-time (23 women), 2 part-time (0 women); includes 15 minority (1 Black or African American, non-Hispanic/Latino; 9 Asian, non-Hispanic/Latino; 3 Hispanic/Latino; 2 Two or more races, non-Hispanic/Latino), 18 international. 427 applicants, 14% accepted, 24 enrolled. In 2013, 11 master's, 15 doctorates awarded. *Degree requirements:* For doctorate, thesis/dissertation, oral, preliminary, and final exams. *Entrance requirements:* For doctorate, GRE General Test, GRE Subject Test (recommended). Additional exam requirements/recommendations for international students: Required—TOEFL. *Application deadline:* For fall admission, 12/1 priority date for domestic students. Application fee: $70. Electronic applications accepted. *Financial support:* Fellowships, research assistantships, teaching assistantships, institutionally sponsored loans, scholarships/grants, traineeships, health care benefits, and unspecified assistantships available. Financial award application deadline: 12/15. *Faculty research:* Astrophysics, condensed matter experiment, condensed matter theory, particle experiment, particle theory. *Total annual research expenditures:* $7.3 million. *Unit head:* Dr. Ralph M. Rosen, Associate Dean for Graduate Studies, 215-898-7156, Fax: 215-573-8068, E-mail: grad-dean@sas.upenn.edu. *Application contact:* Arts and Sciences Graduate Admissions, 215-573-5816, Fax: 215-573-8068, E-mail: gdasadmis@sas.upenn.edu.
Website: http://www.sas.upenn.edu/graduate-division

University of South Florida, College of Arts and Sciences, Department of Physics, Tampa, FL 33620-9951. Offers applied physics (MS, PhD); atmospheric physics (MS); atomic and molecular physics (MS); laser physics (MS); materials physics (MS); materials science and engineering (MSMSE); medical physics (MS); optical physics (MS); semiconductor physics (MS); solid state physics (MS). Part-time programs available. *Faculty:* 26 full-time (3 women). *Students:* 77 full-time (17 women), 4 part-time (1 woman); includes 11 minority (3 Black or African American, non-Hispanic/Latino; 1 Asian, non-Hispanic/Latino; 7 Hispanic/Latino), 38 international. Average age 30. 88 applicants, 24% accepted, 13 enrolled. In 2013, 13 master's, 9 doctorates awarded. *Degree requirements:* For master's, comprehensive exam, thesis optional; for doctorate, comprehensive exam, thesis/dissertation. *Entrance requirements:* For master's and doctorate, GRE General Test; GRE Subject Test in physics (recommended), minimum GPA of 3.0, three letters of recommendation, statement of purpose. Additional exam requirements/recommendations for international students: Required—TOEFL (minimum score 550 paper-based; 79 iBT) or IELTS (minimum score 6.5). *Application deadline:* For fall admission, 2/15 priority date for domestic students, 1/2 for international students; for spring admission, 9/1 for domestic students, 7/1 for international students. Applications are processed on a rolling basis. Application fee: $30. Electronic applications accepted. *Financial support:* In 2013–14, 70 students received support, including 27 research assistantships with tuition reimbursements available (averaging $15,272 per year), 43 teaching assistantships with tuition reimbursements available (averaging $16,267 per year); unspecified assistantships also available. *Faculty research:* The molecular organization of collagen, lipid rafts in biological membranes, the formation of Alzheimer plaques, the role of cellular ion pumps in wound healing, carbon nanotubes as biological detectors, optical imaging of neuronal activity, three-dimensional imaging of intact tissues, motility of cancer cells, the optical detection of pathogens in water. *Total annual research expenditures:* $4 million. *Unit head:* Dr. Pritish Mukherjee, Professor and Chairperson, 813-974-3293, Fax: 813-974-5813, E-mail: pritish@usf.edu. *Application contact:* Dr. Dale Johnson, Professor and Graduate Program Director, 813-974-5125, Fax: 813-974-5813, E-mail: dalejohnson@usf.edu.
Website: http://physics.usf.edu/

The University of Texas Health Science Center at Houston, Graduate School of Biomedical Sciences, Program in Medical Physics, Houston, TX 77225-0036. Offers MS, PhD, MD/PhD. *Degree requirements:* For master's, thesis; for doctorate, thesis/dissertation. *Entrance requirements:* For master's and doctorate, GRE General Test. Additional exam requirements/recommendations for international students: Required—TOEFL. Electronic applications accepted. *Expenses:* Tuition, state resident: full-time $3474; part-time $193 per credit hour. Tuition, nonresident: full-time $13,644; part-time $758 per credit hour. *Required fees:* $226.30; $87 per credit hour. *Faculty research:* Medical physics, radiation oncology physics, diagnostic imaging physics, medical nuclear physics, image-guided therapy.

The University of Texas Health Science Center at San Antonio, Graduate School of Biomedical Sciences, Radiological Sciences Graduate Program, San Antonio, TX 78229-3900. Offers MS, PhD. *Faculty:* 52 full-time (12 women), 32 part-time/adjunct (8 women). *Students:* 14 full-time (5 women), 4 part-time (1 woman); includes 6 minority (2 Asian, non-Hispanic/Latino; 3 Hispanic/Latino; 1 Two or more races, non-Hispanic/Latino), 4 international. Average age 31. 69 applicants, 16% accepted, 6 enrolled. In 2013, 3 master's, 3 doctorates awarded. *Degree requirements:* For master's, thesis; for doctorate, comprehensive exam, thesis/dissertation. *Entrance requirements:* For master's and doctorate, GRE General Test. Additional exam requirements/recommendations for international students: Required—TOEFL (minimum score 550 paper-based; 68 iBT). *Application deadline:* For fall admission, 3/1 priority date for domestic and international students; for spring admission, 10/1 for domestic and international students. Applications are processed on a rolling basis. Application fee: $0. Electronic applications accepted. *Financial support:* In 2013–14, 5 students received support, including 37 teaching assistantships (averaging $24,783 per year); scholarships/grants, health care benefits, and NIH training grants also available. Financial award application deadline: 6/30; financial award applicants required to submit FAFSA. *Faculty research:* Positron emission tomography, functional magnetic resonance imaging, transcranial magnetic stimulation, neuroinformatics through network analysis, statistical parametric imaging, stroke, retinal imaging, primate aging studies, cerebral blood flow and metabolism, attention deficit hyperactivity disorder, depression and schizophrenia, motor speech disorders, motor skills disorders, Parkinson's disease, post-traumatic stress disorders. *Unit head:* Dr. Geoffrey D. Clarke, Program Director, 210-567-5552, Fax: 210-567-5541, E-mail: clarkeg@uthscsa.edu. *Application contact:* Dr. Beth Goins, Applicant Advisor/Graduate Advisor/Committee on Graduate Studies Chair, 210-567-5544, E-mail: goins@uthscsa.edu.
Website: http://radsci.uthscsa.edu

The University of Toledo, College of Graduate Studies, College of Medicine and Life Sciences, Program in Medical Physics, Toledo, OH 43606-3390. Offers MSBS. *Faculty:* 8. *Students:* 17 full-time (7 women), 1 (woman) part-time; includes 1 minority (Two or more races, non-Hispanic/Latino), 8 international. Average age 27. 26 applicants, 58% accepted, 6 enrolled. In 2013, 9 master's awarded. *Degree requirements:* For master's, thesis. *Entrance requirements:* For master's, GRE, minimum undergraduate GPA of 3.0, three letters of recommendation, statement of purpose, transcripts from all prior institutions attended, resume. Additional exam requirements/recommendations for international students: Required—TOEFL (minimum score 550 paper-based; 80 iBT). *Application deadline:* For fall admission, 3/31 priority date for domestic and international students. Applications are processed on a rolling basis. Application fee: $45 ($75 for international students). Electronic applications accepted. *Financial support:* In 2013–14, 4 research assistantships with full tuition reimbursements (averaging $10,000 per year) were awarded; Federal Work-Study, institutionally sponsored loans, scholarships/grants, tuition waivers (full), and unspecified assistantships also available. *Unit head:* Dr. E. Ishmael Parsai, Director, 419-383-4541, E-mail: e.parsai@utoledo.edu. *Application contact:* Dianne Adams, Department Secretary, 419-383-5109, E-mail: dianne.adams@utoledo.edu.
Website: http://www.utoledo.edu/med/grad/

The University of Toledo, College of Graduate Studies, College of Natural Sciences and Mathematics, Department of Physics and Astronomy, Toledo, OH 43606-3390. Offers photovoltaics (PSM); physics (MS, PhD), including astrophysics (PhD), materials science, medical physics (PhD); MS/PhD. *Faculty:* 36. *Students:* 52 full-time (12 women), 11 part-time (1 woman); includes 2 minority (1 Asian, non-Hispanic/Latino; 1 Hispanic/Latino), 28 international. Average age 29. 73 applicants, 19% accepted, 10 enrolled. In 2013, 7 master's, 5 doctorates awarded. *Degree requirements:* For master's, thesis; for doctorate, thesis/dissertation, departmental qualifying exam. *Entrance requirements:* For master's and doctorate, GRE General Test, GRE Subject Test, minimum cumulative point-hour ratio of 2.7 for all previous academic work, three letters of recommendation, statement of purpose, transcripts from all prior institutions attended. Additional exam requirements/recommendations for international students: Required—TOEFL (minimum score 550 paper-based; 80 iBT). *Application deadline:* For fall admission, 1/15 priority date for domestic and international students. Applications are processed on a rolling basis. Application fee: $45 ($75 for international students). Electronic applications accepted. *Financial support:* In 2013–14, 9 research assistantships with full and partial tuition reimbursements (averaging $12,500 per year), 25 teaching assistantships with full and partial tuition reimbursements (averaging $14,550 per year) were awarded; Federal Work-Study, institutionally sponsored loans, scholarships/grants, tuition waivers (full), and unspecified assistantships also available. Support available to part-time students. *Faculty research:* Atomic physics, solid-state physics, materials science, astrophysics. *Unit head:* Dr. Lawrence Anderson-Huang, Chair, 419-530-7257, E-mail: lawrence.anderson@utoledo.edu. *Application contact:* Graduate School Office, 419-530-4723, Fax: 419-537-4724, E-mail: grdsch@utnet.utoledo.edu.
Website: http://www.utoledo.edu/nsm/

University of Utah, Graduate School, College of Science, Department of Physics and Astronomy, Salt Lake City, UT 84112. Offers chemical physics (PhD); medical physics (MS, PhD); physics (MA, MS, PhD); physics teaching (PhD). Part-time programs available. *Faculty:* 32 full-time (4 women), 15 part-time/adjunct (0 women). *Students:* 76 full-time (23 women), 20 part-time (3 women); includes 6 minority (4 Asian, non-

Hispanic/Latino; 2 Hispanic/Latino), 48 international. Average age 29. 141 applicants, 30% accepted, 17 enrolled. In 2013, 9 master's, 13 doctorates awarded. Terminal master's awarded for partial completion of doctoral program. *Degree requirements:* For master's, comprehensive exam (for some programs), thesis or alternative, teaching experience, departmental exam; for doctorate, comprehensive exam, thesis/dissertation, departmental qualifying exam. *Entrance requirements:* For master's and doctorate, GRE General Test, GRE Subject Test, minimum GPA of 3.0. Additional exam requirements/recommendations for international students: Required—TOEFL (minimum score 550 paper-based; 80 iBT). *Application deadline:* For fall admission, 4/1 priority date for domestic and international students. Applications are processed on a rolling basis. Application fee: $55 ($65 for international students). Electronic applications accepted. *Expenses:* Tuition, state resident: full-time $5259. Tuition, nonresident: full-time $18,569. *Required fees:* $841. Tuition and fees vary according to course load. *Financial support:* In 2013–14, 41 research assistantships with full tuition reimbursements (averaging $23,500 per year), 31 teaching assistantships with full tuition reimbursements (averaging $20,641 per year) were awarded; Federal Work-Study, institutionally sponsored loans, and scholarships/grants also available. Financial award application deadline: 2/15; financial award applicants required to submit FAFSA. *Faculty research:* High-energy, cosmic-ray, astrophysics, medical physics, condensed matter, relativity applied physics, biophysics, astronomy. *Total annual research expenditures:* $6.8 million. *Unit head:* Dr. Carleton DeTar, Chair, 801-581-3538, Fax: 801-581-4801, E-mail: detar@physics.utah.edu. *Application contact:* Jackie Hadley, Graduate Secretary, 801-581-6861, Fax: 801-581-4801, E-mail: jackie@physics.utah.edu.
Website: http://www.physics.utah.edu/

University of Victoria, Faculty of Graduate Studies, Faculty of Science, Department of Physics and Astronomy, Victoria, BC V8W 2Y2, Canada. Offers astronomy and astrophysics (M Sc, PhD); condensed matter physics (M Sc, PhD); experimental particle physics (M Sc, PhD); medical physics (M Sc, PhD); ocean physics (M Sc, PhD); theoretical physics (M Sc, PhD). *Degree requirements:* For master's, thesis; for doctorate, comprehensive exam, thesis/dissertation, candidacy exam. *Entrance requirements:* For master's and doctorate, GRE. Additional exam requirements/recommendations for international students: Required—TOEFL (minimum score 575 paper-based), IELTS (minimum score 7). Electronic applications accepted. *Faculty research:* Old stellar populations; observational cosmology and large scale structure; cp violation; atlas.

University of Wisconsin–Madison, School of Medicine and Public Health and Graduate School, Graduate Programs in Medicine, Department of Medical Physics, Madison, WI 53705-2275. Offers health physics (MS); medical physics (MS, PhD). Part-time programs available. *Faculty:* 41 full-time (3 women), 6 part-time/adjunct (0 women). *Students:* 104 full-time (25 women), 2 part-time (0 women); includes 26 minority (2 Black or African American, non-Hispanic/Latino; 3 American Indian or Alaska Native, non-Hispanic/Latino; 7 Asian, non-Hispanic/Latino; 13 Hispanic/Latino; 1 Native Hawaiian or other Pacific Islander, non-Hispanic/Latino), 23 international. Average age 26. 97 applicants, 35% accepted, 17 enrolled. Terminal master's awarded for partial completion of doctoral program. *Degree requirements:* For master's, comprehensive exam; for doctorate, comprehensive exam, thesis/dissertation. *Entrance requirements:* For master's and doctorate, GRE General Test, GRE Subject Test (physics), minimum GPA of 3.0. Additional exam requirements/recommendations for international students: Required—TOEFL. *Application deadline:* For fall admission, 12/1 priority date for domestic students, 11/15 for international students. Application fee: $56. Electronic applications accepted. *Expenses:* Tuition, state resident: full-time $10,728; part-time $790 per credit. Tuition, nonresident: full-time $24,054; part-time $1623 per credit. *Required fees:* $1130; $119 per credit. *Financial support:* In 2013–14, 106 students received support, including 13 fellowships with full tuition reimbursements available (averaging $23,346 per year), 90 research assistantships with full tuition reimbursements available (averaging $23,346 per year), 5 teaching assistantships with full tuition reimbursements available (averaging $18,971 per year); traineeships, health care benefits, and unspecified assistantships also available. Financial award application deadline: 11/15. *Faculty research:* Biomagnetism: imaging and physiology, medical imaging processing, radiation therapy and radiation physics. *Total annual research expenditures:* $3.7 million. *Unit head:* Dr. Edward F. Jackson, Chair, 608-262-2171, Fax: 608-262-2413, E-mail: efjackson@wisc.edu. *Application contact:* Debra A. Torgerson, Graduate Coordinator, 608-265-6504, Fax: 608-262-2413, E-mail: datorger@wisc.edu.
Website: http://www.medphysics.wisc.edu/

Vanderbilt University, School of Medicine, Program in Medical Physics, Nashville, TN 37240-1001. Offers MS. Part-time programs available. *Degree requirements:* For master's, comprehensive exam, thesis optional. *Entrance requirements:* For master's, GRE General Test, physics major, physics minor or physics minor equivalent; minimum undergraduate GPA of 3.0. Additional exam requirements/recommendations for international students: Required—TOEFL (minimum score 600 paper-based). Electronic applications accepted. *Faculty research:* MRI imaging, PET imaging, nuclear medicine dosimetry, Monte Carlo dosimetry.

Virginia Commonwealth University, Graduate School, College of Humanities and Sciences, Department of Physics, Programs in Medical Physics, Richmond, VA 23284-9005. Offers MS, PhD. *Entrance requirements:* For master's and doctorate, GRE General Test. Additional exam requirements/recommendations for international students: Required—TOEFL (minimum score 600 paper-based; 100 iBT); Recommended—IELTS (minimum score 6.5). Electronic applications accepted. *Faculty research:* Functional imaging using PET and NMR, computed tomography (CT) image artifact removal and deformation, intensity-modulated radiation therapy, radiation therapy dose calculations, 4D radiation therapy, brachytherapy dose calculations.

Wayne State University, School of Medicine, Graduate Programs in Medicine, Department of Radiation Oncology, Detroit, MI 48202. Offers medical physics (PhD); radiological physics (MS). Part-time and evening/weekend programs available. *Students:* 25 full-time (3 women), 12 part-time (3 women); includes 10 minority (6 Asian, non-Hispanic/Latino; 2 Hispanic/Latino; 2 Two or more races, non-Hispanic/Latino), 10 international. Average age 30. 85 applicants, 27% accepted, 14 enrolled. In 2013, 12 master's, 1 doctorate awarded. Terminal master's awarded for partial completion of doctoral program. *Degree requirements:* For master's, thesis, essay, exit exam; for doctorate, thesis/dissertation, qualifying exam. *Entrance requirements:* For master's and doctorate, GRE General Test, BS in physics or related area, admission to the Graduate School. Additional exam requirements/recommendations for international students: Required—TOEFL (minimum score 550 paper-based); Recommended—TWE (minimum score 6). *Application deadline:* For fall admission, 1/15 for domestic students, 6/1 for international students; for winter admission, 10/1 for international students; for spring admission, 2/1 for international students. Application fee: $0. Electronic applications accepted. *Expenses:* Contact institution. *Financial support:* In 2013–14, 5 students received support, including 5 research assistantships (averaging $17,373 per year); fellowships, teaching assistantships, scholarships/grants, health care benefits, and unspecified assistantships also available. Financial award application deadline: 3/31; financial award applicants required to submit FAFSA. *Unit head:* Harold E. Kim, MD, Associate Professor and Interim Chair, 313-745-1538, E-mail: kimh@wayne.edu. *Application contact:* Dr. Jay Burmeister, Director, 313-745-2483, E-mail: burmeist@wayne.edu.
Website: http://radiationoncology.med.wayne.edu/

Wayne State University, School of Medicine, Graduate Programs in Medicine, Department of Radiology, Detroit, MI 48202. Offers medical physics (PhD); radiological physics (MS). Part-time and evening/weekend programs available. *Faculty:* 13 full-time (3 women), 1 part-time/adjunct (0 women). *Students:* 23 full-time (3 women), 13 part-time (3 women); includes 9 minority (7 Asian, non-Hispanic/Latino; 2 Two or more races, non-Hispanic/Latino), 6 international. Average age 30. 100 applicants, 27% accepted, 12 enrolled. In 2013, 9 master's awarded. *Degree requirements:* For master's, essay, exam; for doctorate, thesis/dissertation. *Entrance requirements:* For master's, GRE General Test, BS in physics or related area (preferred); for doctorate, GRE, BS in physics or related area (preferred). Additional exam requirements/recommendations for international students: Required—TOEFL (minimum score 600 paper-based; 100 iBT); Recommended—TWE (minimum score 6). *Application deadline:* For fall admission, 1/15 for domestic and international students; for winter admission, 10/1 for domestic students, 9/1 for international students; for spring admission, 2/1 for domestic students, 1/1 for international students. Application fee: $50. Electronic applications accepted. *Expenses:* Contact institution. *Financial support:* In 2013–14, 8 students received support. Fellowships with tuition reimbursements available, research assistantships with tuition reimbursements available, teaching assistantships with tuition reimbursements available, scholarships/grants, and unspecified assistantships available. Financial award application deadline: 3/1. *Faculty research:* Medical physics of radiation therapy, biological basis of radiotherapy, improvements in clinical protocols for radiation therapy, basic physics and biology of radiation action. *Unit head:* Dr. Andre Konski, Professor and Chair of Radiation Oncology, 313-577-9620, E-mail: ec1595@wayne.edu. *Application contact:* Dr. Jay Burmeister, Professor and Chair of Physics, Karmanos Cancer Center, 313-576-9617, E-mail: burmeist@karmanos.org.
Website: http://radiationoncology.med.wayne.edu/medphys/graduate-program/

Wright State University, School of Graduate Studies, College of Science and Mathematics, Department of Physics, Program in Physics, Dayton, OH 45435. Offers geophysics (MS); medical physics (MS). Part-time and evening/weekend programs available. *Degree requirements:* For master's, thesis. *Entrance requirements:* Additional exam requirements/recommendations for international students: Required—TOEFL. *Faculty research:* Solid-state physics, optics, geophysics.

Section 22
Health Services

This section contains a directory of institutions offering graduate work in health services. Additional information about programs listed in the directory may be obtained by writing directly to the dean of a graduate school or chair of a department at the address given in the directory.

For programs offering related work, see also in this book *Allied Health, Nursing,* and *Public Health.* In another book in this series:

Graduate Programs in Business, Education, Information Studies, Law & Social Work

See *Business Administration and Management*

CONTENTS

Program Directories

Health Services Management and Hospital Administration

Alaska Pacific University, Graduate Programs, Business Administration Department, Program in Business Administration, Anchorage, AK 99508-4672. Offers business administration (MBA); health services administration (MBA). Part-time and evening/weekend programs available. *Degree requirements:* For master's, capstone course. *Entrance requirements:* For master's, GMAT or GRE General Test, minimum GPA of 3.0.

Albany State University, College of Arts and Humanities, Albany, GA 31705-2717. Offers English education (M Ed); public administration (MPA), including community and economic development administration, criminal justice administration, general administration, health administration and policy, human resources management, public policy, water resources management; social work (MSW). Part-time programs available. *Degree requirements:* For master's, comprehensive exam, professional portfolio (for MPA), internship, capstone report. *Entrance requirements:* For master's, GRE, MAT, minimum GPA of 3.0, official transcript, pre-medical record/certificate of immunization, letters of reference. Electronic applications accepted. *Faculty research:* HIV prevention for minority students.

Albany State University, College of Business, Albany, GA 31705-2717. Offers accounting (MBA); general (MBA); healthcare (MBA). *Accreditation:* ACBSP. Part-time and evening/weekend programs available. *Degree requirements:* For master's, comprehensive exam, internship, 3 hours of physical education. *Entrance requirements:* For master's, GMAT (minimum score of 450)/GRE (minimum score of 800) for those without earned master's degree or higher, minimum undergraduate GPA of 2.5, 2 letters of reference, official transcript, pre-entrance medical record and certificate of immunization. Electronic applications accepted. *Faculty research:* Diversity issues, ancestry, understanding finance through use of technology.

American InterContinental University Online, Program in Business Administration, Schaumburg, IL 60173. Offers accounting and finance (MBA); finance (MBA); healthcare management (MBA); human resource management (MBA); international business (MBA); management (MBA); marketing (MBA); operations management (MBA); organizational psychology and development (MBA); project management (MBA). *Accreditation:* ACBSP. Evening/weekend programs available. Postbaccalaureate distance learning degree programs offered (no on-campus study). *Entrance requirements:* Additional exam requirements/recommendations for international students: Required—TOEFL (minimum score 550 paper-based). Electronic applications accepted.

American Public University System, AMU/APU Graduate Programs, Charles Town, WV 25414. Offers accounting (MBA, MS); criminal justice (MA), including business administration, emergency and disaster management, general (MA, MS); educational leadership (M Ed); emergency and disaster management (MA); entrepreneurship (MBA); environmental policy and management (MS), including environmental planning, environmental sustainability, fish and wildlife management, general (MA, MS), global environmental management; finance (MBA); general (MBA); global business management (MBA); history (MA), including American history, ancient and classical history, European history, global history, public history; homeland security (MA), including business administration, counter-terrorism studies, criminal justice, cyber, emergency management and public health, intelligence studies, transportation security; homeland security resource allocation (MBA); humanities (MA); information technology (MS), including digital forensics, enterprise software development, information assurance and security, IT project management; information technology management (MBA); intelligence studies (MA), including criminal intelligence, cyber, general (MA, MS), homeland security, intelligence analysis, intelligence collection, intelligence management, intelligence operations, terrorism studies; international relations and conflict resolution (MA), including comparative and security issues, conflict resolution, international and transnational security issues, peacekeeping; legal studies (MA); management (MA), including defense management, general (MA, MS), human resource management, organizational leadership, public administration; marketing (MBA); military history (MA), including American military history, American Revolution, civil war, war since 1945, World War II; military studies (MA), including joint warfare, strategic leadership; national security studies (MA), including general (MA, MS), homeland security, regional security studies, security and intelligence analysis, terrorism studies; nonprofit management (MBA); political science (MA), including American politics and government, comparative government and development, general (MA, MS), international relations, public policy; psychology (MA); public administration (MPA), including disaster management, environmental policy, health policy, human resources, national security, organizational management, security management; public health (MPH); reverse logistics management (MA); school counseling (M Ed); security management (MA); space studies (MS), including aerospace science, general (MA, MS), planetary science; sports and health sciences (MS); teaching (M Ed), including curriculum and instruction for elementary teachers, elementary reading, English language learners, instructional leadership, online learning, special education; transportation and logistics management (MA), including general (MA, MS), maritime engineering management, reverse logistics management. Programs offered via distance learning only. Part-time and evening/weekend programs available. Postbaccalaureate distance learning degree programs offered (no on-campus study). *Faculty:* 432 full-time (242 women), 1,722 part-time/adjunct (829 women). *Students:* 511 full-time (241 women), 10,947 part-time (4,294 women); includes 3,760 minority (2,058 Black or African American, non-Hispanic/Latino; 88 American Indian or Alaska Native, non-Hispanic/Latino; 293 Asian, non-Hispanic/Latino; 876 Hispanic/Latino; 91 Native Hawaiian or other Pacific Islander, non-Hispanic/Latino; 354 Two or more races, non-Hispanic/Latino), 134 international. Average age 36. In 2013, 3,323 master's awarded. *Degree requirements:* For master's, comprehensive exam or practicum. *Entrance requirements:* For master's, official transcript showing earned bachelor's degree from institution accredited by recognized accrediting body. Additional exam requirements/recommendations for international students: Required—TOEFL (minimum score 550 paper-based), IELTS (minimum score 6.5). *Application deadline:* Applications are processed on a rolling basis. Application fee: $0. Electronic applications accepted. *Expenses: Tuition:* Part-time $325 per semester hour. *Financial support:* Applicants required to submit FAFSA. *Faculty research:* Military history, criminal justice, management performance, national security. *Unit head:* Dr. Karan Powell, Executive Vice President and Provost, 877-468-6268, Fax: 304-724-3780. *Application contact:* Terry Grant, Vice President of Enrollment Management, 877-468-6268, Fax: 304-724-3780, E-mail: info@apus.edu.
Website: http://www.apus.edu

American Sentinel University, Graduate Programs, Aurora, CO 80014. Offers business administration (MBA); business intelligence (MS); computer science (MSCS); health information management (MS); healthcare (MBA); information systems (MSIS); nursing (MSN). Part-time and evening/weekend programs available. Postbaccalaureate distance learning degree programs offered (no on-campus study). *Entrance requirements:* Additional exam requirements/recommendations for international students: Required—TOEFL (minimum score 600 paper-based). Electronic applications accepted.

American University of Beirut, Graduate Programs, Faculty of Health Sciences, Beirut, Lebanon. Offers environmental sciences (MS), including environmental health; epidemiology (MS); epidemiology and biostatistics (MPH); health management and policy (MPH); health promotion and community health (MPH); population health (MS). Part-time programs available. *Faculty:* 26 full-time (18 women), 7 part-time/adjunct (4 women). *Students:* 42 full-time (37 women), 103 part-time (84 women). Average age 25. 132 applicants, 65% accepted, 48 enrolled. In 2013, 52 master's awarded. *Degree requirements:* For master's, one foreign language, comprehensive exam, thesis (for some programs). *Entrance requirements:* For master's, 2 letters of recommendation, personal statement, transcripts. Additional exam requirements/recommendations for international students: Required—TOEFL (minimum score 583 paper-based; 97 iBT), IELTS (minimum score 7). *Application deadline:* For fall admission, 2/7 priority date for domestic and international students; for spring admission, 11/1 for domestic and international students. Application fee: $50. Electronic applications accepted. *Expenses: Tuition:* Full-time $14,724; part-time $818 per credit. *Required fees:* $692. Tuition and fees vary according to course load and program. *Financial support:* In 2013–14, 56 students received support. Scholarships/grants, health care benefits, and unspecified assistantships available. Financial award application deadline: 4/1. *Faculty research:* Tobacco control; health of the elderly; youth health; mental health; women's health; reproductive and sexual health, including HIV/AIDS; water quality; health systems; quality in health care delivery; health human resources; health policy; occupational and environmental health; social inequality; social determinants of health; non-communicable diseases. *Total annual research expenditures:* $1 million. *Unit head:* Iman Adel Nuwayhid, Dean, 961-1759683, Fax: 961-1744470, E-mail: nuwayhid@aub.edu.lb. *Application contact:* Mitra Tauk, Administrative Coordinator, 961-1-350000 Ext. 4687, Fax: 96-1-1744470, E-mail: mt12@aub.edu.lb.

Aquinas College, School of Management, Grand Rapids, MI 49506-1799. Offers health care administration (MM); marketing management (MM); organizational leadership (MM); sustainable business (MM, MSB). Part-time and evening/weekend programs available. *Students:* 13 full-time (10 women), 56 part-time (38 women); includes 10 minority (4 Black or African American, non-Hispanic/Latino; 1 American Indian or Alaska Native, non-Hispanic/Latino; 4 Hispanic/Latino; 1 Two or more races, non-Hispanic/Latino), 1 international. Average age 33. In 2013, 18 master's awarded. *Entrance requirements:* For master's, GMAT, minimum undergraduate GPA of 2.75, 2 years of work experience. Additional exam requirements/recommendations for international students: Required—TOEFL (minimum score 550 paper-based). *Application deadline:* Applications are processed on a rolling basis. Application fee: $0. *Expenses:* Contact institution. *Financial support:* Scholarships/grants available. Support available to part-time students. Financial award application deadline: 3/15; financial award applicants required to submit FAFSA. *Unit head:* Brian DiVita, Director, 616-632-2922, Fax: 616-732-4489. *Application contact:* Lynn Atkins-Rykert, Administrative Assistant, 616-632-2924, Fax: 616-732-4489, E-mail: atkinlyn@aquinas.edu.

Aquinas Institute of Theology, Graduate and Professional Programs, St. Louis, MO 63108. Offers biblical studies (Certificate); church music (MM); health care mission (MAHCM); ministry (M Div); pastoral care (Certificate); pastoral ministry (MAPM); pastoral studies (MAPS); preaching (D Min); spiritual direction (Certificate); theology (M Div, MA); Thomistic studies (Certificate); M Div/MA; MA/PhD; MAPS/MSW. *Accreditation:* ATS (one or more programs are accredited). Part-time and evening/weekend programs available. Postbaccalaureate distance learning degree programs offered (minimal on-campus study). *Degree requirements:* For master's, variable foreign language requirement, comprehensive exam (for some programs); for doctorate, thesis/dissertation. *Entrance requirements:* For master's and Certificate, MAT; for doctorate, 3 years of ministerial experience, 6 hours of graduate course work in homiletics, M Div or the equivalent, minimum GPA of 3.0. Additional exam requirements/recommendations for international students: Required—TOEFL. *Faculty research:* Theology of preaching, hermeneutics, lay ecclesial ministry, pastoral and practical theology.

Argosy University, Atlanta, College of Business, Atlanta, GA 30328. Offers accounting (DBA); corporate compliance (MBA); customized professional concentration (MBA, DBA); finance (MBA); healthcare administration (MBA); information systems (DBA); information systems management (MBA); international business (MBA, DBA); management (MBA, MSM, DBA); marketing (MBA, DBA).

Argosy University, Chicago, College of Business, Chicago, IL 60601. Offers accounting (DBA); customized professional concentration (MBA, DBA); finance (MBA); fraud examination (MBA); global business sustainability (DBA); healthcare administration (MBA); information systems (DBA); information systems management (MBA); international business (MBA, DBA); management (MBA, MSM, DBA); marketing (MBA, DBA); organizational leadership (Ed D); public administration (MBA); sustainable management (MBA). Postbaccalaureate distance learning degree programs offered (minimal on-campus study).

Argosy University, Dallas, College of Business, Farmers Branch, TX 75244. Offers accounting (DBA, AGC); corporate compliance (MBA, Graduate Certificate); customized professional concentration (MBA); finance (MBA, Graduate Certificate); fraud examination (MBA, Graduate Certificate); global business sustainability (DBA, AGC); healthcare administration (Graduate Certificate); healthcare management (MBA); information systems (MBA, DBA, AGC); information systems management (Graduate Certificate); international business (MBA, DBA, AGC, Graduate Certificate); management (MBA, DBA, AGC, Graduate Certificate); marketing (MBA, DBA, AGC, Graduate Certificate); public administration (MBA, Graduate Certificate); sustainable management (MBA, Graduate Certificate).

Argosy University, Denver, College of Business, Denver, CO 80231. Offers accounting (DBA); corporate compliance (MBA); customized professional concentration (MBA, DBA); finance (MBA); fraud examination (MBA); global business sustainability (DBA); healthcare administration (MBA); information systems (DBA); information systems management (MBA); international business (MBA, DBA); management (MBA, MSM, DBA); marketing (MBA, DBA); organizational leadership (Ed D); public administration (MBA); sustainable management (MBA).

Argosy University, Hawai`i, College of Business, Honolulu, HI 96813. Offers accounting (DBA); corporate compliance (MBA); customized professional concentration (MBA, DBA); finance (MBA, Certificate); fraud examination (MBA); global business sustainability (DBA); healthcare administration (MBA, Certificate); information systems (DBA); information systems management (MBA, Certificate); international business (MBA, DBA, Certificate); management (MBA, MSM, DBA); marketing (MBA, DBA, Certificate); organizational leadership (Ed D); public administration (MBA); sustainable management (MBA).

Argosy University, Inland Empire, College of Business, Ontario, CA 91761. Offers accounting (DBA); corporate compliance (MBA); customized professional concentration (MBA, DBA); finance (MBA); fraud examination (MBA); global business sustainability (DBA); healthcare administration (MBA); information systems (DBA); information systems management (MBA); international business (MBA, DBA); management (MBA, MSM, DBA); marketing (MBA, DBA); organizational leadership (Ed D); public administration (MBA); sustainable management (MBA).

Argosy University, Los Angeles, College of Business, Santa Monica, CA 90045. Offers accounting (DBA); corporate compliance (MBA); customized professional concentration (MBA, DBA); finance (MBA); fraud examination (MBA); global business sustainability (DBA); healthcare administration (MBA); information systems (DBA); information systems management (MBA); international business (MBA, DBA); management (MBA, MSM, DBA); marketing (MBA, DBA); organizational leadership (Ed D); public administration (MBA); sustainable management (MBA).

Argosy University, Nashville, College of Business, Nashville, TN 37214. Offers accounting (DBA); customized professional concentration (MBA, DBA); finance (MBA); healthcare administration (MBA); information systems (MBA, DBA); international business (MBA, DBA); management (MBA, MSM, DBA); marketing (MBA, DBA).

Argosy University, Orange County, College of Business, Orange, CA 92868. Offers accounting (DBA, Adv C); corporate compliance (MBA); customized professional concentration (MBA, DBA); finance (MBA, Certificate); fraud examination (MBA); global business sustainability (DBA); healthcare administration (MBA, Certificate); information systems (DBA, Adv C, Certificate); information systems management (MBA); international business (MBA, DBA, Adv C, Certificate); management (MBA, MSM, DBA, Adv C); marketing (MBA, DBA, Adv C, Certificate); organizational leadership (Ed D); public administration (MBA, Certificate); sustainable management (MBA).

Argosy University, Phoenix, College of Business, Phoenix, AZ 85021. Offers accounting (DBA); corporate compliance (MBA); customized professional concentration (MBA, DBA); finance (MBA); fraud examination (MBA); global business sustainability (DBA); healthcare administration (MBA); information systems (DBA); information systems management (MBA); international business (MBA, DBA); management (MBA, DBA); marketing (MBA, DBA); public administration (MBA); sustainable management (MBA).

Argosy University, Salt Lake City, College of Business, Draper, UT 84020. Offers accounting (DBA); corporate compliance (MBA); customized professional concentration (MBA, DBA); finance (MBA); fraud examination (MBA); global business sustainability (DBA); healthcare administration (MBA); information systems (DBA); information systems management (MBA); international business (MBA, DBA); management (MBA, DBA); marketing (MBA, DBA); public administration (MBA); sustainable management (MBA).

Argosy University, San Francisco Bay Area, College of Business, Alameda, CA 94501. Offers accounting (DBA); corporate compliance (MBA); customized professional concentration (MBA, DBA); finance (MBA); fraud examination (MBA); global business sustainability (DBA); healthcare administration (MBA); information systems (DBA); information systems management (MBA); international business (MBA, DBA); management (MBA, MSM, DBA); marketing (MBA, DBA); organizational leadership (Ed D); public administration (MBA); sustainable management (MBA).

Argosy University, Sarasota, College of Business, Sarasota, FL 34235. Offers accounting (DBA, Adv C); corporate compliance (MBA, DBA, Certificate); customized professional concentration (MBA, DBA); finance (MBA, Certificate); fraud examination (MBA, Certificate); global business sustainability (DBA, Adv C); healthcare administration (MBA, Certificate); information systems (DBA, Adv C, Certificate); information systems management (MBA); international business (MBA, DBA, Adv C, Certificate); management (MBA, MSM, DBA, Adv C, Certificate); marketing (MBA, DBA, Adv C, Certificate); organizational leadership (Ed D); public administration (MBA, Certificate); sustainable management (MBA, Certificate).

Argosy University, Schaumburg, College of Business, Schaumburg, IL 60173-5403. Offers accounting (DBA, Adv C); customized professional concentration (MBA, DBA); finance (MBA, Certificate); fraud examination (MBA); global business sustainability (DBA); healthcare administration (MBA, Certificate); information systems (DBA, Adv C, Certificate); information systems management (MBA); international business (MBA, DBA, Adv C, Certificate); management (MBA, MSM, DBA, Adv C, Certificate); marketing (MBA, DBA, Adv C, Certificate); organizational leadership (Ed D); public administration (MBA); sustainable management (MBA).

Argosy University, Seattle, College of Business, Seattle, WA 98121. Offers accounting (DBA); corporate compliance (MBA); customized professional concentration (MBA, DBA); finance (MBA); fraud examination (MBA); global business sustainability (DBA); healthcare administration (MBA); information systems (DBA); information systems management (MBA); international business (MBA, DBA); management (MBA, MSM, DBA); marketing (MBA, DBA); organizational leadership (Ed D); public administration (MBA); sustainable management (MBA).

Argosy University, Tampa, College of Business, Tampa, FL 33607. Offers accounting (DBA); corporate compliance (MBA); customized professional concentration (MBA, DBA); finance (MBA); fraud examination (MBA); global business sustainability (DBA); healthcare administration (MBA); information systems (DBA); information systems management (MBA); international business (MBA, DBA); management (MBA, MSM, DBA); marketing (MBA, DBA); organizational leadership (Ed D); public administration (MBA); sustainable management (MBA).

Argosy University, Twin Cities, College of Business, Eagan, MN 55121. Offers accounting (DBA); customized professional concentration (MBA, DBA); finance (MBA); fraud examination (MBA); global business sustainability (DBA); healthcare administration (MBA); information systems (DBA); information systems management (MBA); international business (MBA, DBA); management (MBA, MSM, DBA); marketing (MBA, DBA); organizational leadership (Ed D); public administration (MBA); sustainable management (MBA).

Argosy University, Twin Cities, College of Health Sciences, Eagan, MN 55121. Offers health services management (MS); public health (MPH).

Argosy University, Washington DC, College of Business, Arlington, VA 22209. Offers accounting (DBA); customized professional concentration (MBA, DBA); finance (MBA); fraud examination (MBA); global business sustainability (DBA); healthcare administration (MBA); information systems (DBA); information systems management (MBA); international business (MBA, DBA, Certificate); management (MBA, MSM, DBA); marketing (MBA, DBA, Certificate); organizational leadership (Ed D); public administration (MBA); sustainable management (MBA).

Arkansas State University, Graduate School, College of Nursing and Health Professions, School of Nursing, State University, AR 72467. Offers aging studies (Certificate); health care management (Certificate); health communications (Certificate); health sciences (MS); health sciences education (Certificate); nurse anesthesia (MSN); nursing (MSN); nursing practice (DNP). *Accreditation:* AANA/CANAEP (one or more programs are accredited). Part-time programs available. *Faculty:* 16 full-time (14 women). *Students:* 96 full-time (34 women), 120 part-time (108 women); includes 38 minority (26 Black or African American, non-Hispanic/Latino; 3 American Indian or Alaska Native, non-Hispanic/Latino; 2 Asian, non-Hispanic/Latino; 4 Hispanic/Latino; 3 Two or more races, non-Hispanic/Latino). Average age 33. 153 applicants, 32% accepted, 44 enrolled. In 2013, 103 master's awarded. *Degree requirements:* For master's, comprehensive exam, thesis or alternative; for doctorate, comprehensive exam, thesis/dissertation. *Entrance requirements:* For master's, GRE General Test or MAT, appropriate bachelor's degree, current Arkansas nursing license, CPR certification, physical examination, professional liability insurance, critical care experience, ACLS Certification, PALS Certification, interview, immunization records, personal goal statement, health assessment; for doctorate, GRE or MAT, appropriate master's degree, current Arkansas nursing license, CPR certification, physical examination, professional liability insurance, critical care experience, ACLS Certification, PALS Certification, interview, immunization records, personal goal statement, health assessment, TB skin test, NCLEX-RN Exam, background check. Additional exam requirements/recommendations for international students: Required—TOEFL (minimum score 550 paper-based; 79 iBT), IELTS (minimum score 6), PTE (minimum score 56). *Application deadline:* Applications are processed on a rolling basis. Electronic applications accepted. *Expenses:* Contact institution. *Financial support:* In 2013–14, 9 students received support. Fellowships, career-related internships or fieldwork, scholarships/grants, and unspecified assistantships available. Financial award application deadline: 7/1; financial award applicants required to submit FAFSA. *Unit head:* Dr. Marilyn Duran, Chair, 870-972-3074, Fax: 870-972-2954, E-mail: mduran@astate.edu. *Application contact:* Vickey Ring, Graduate Admissions Coordinator, 870-972-3029, Fax: 870-972-3857, E-mail: vickeyring@astate.edu.
Website: http://www.astate.edu/college/conhp/departments/nursing/

Armstrong State University, School of Graduate Studies, Program in Health Services Administration, Savannah, GA 31419-1997. Offers clinical informatics (Certificate); health services administration (MHSA). *Accreditation:* CAHME; CEPH. Part-time and evening/weekend programs available. *Faculty:* 4 full-time (2 women), 1 (woman) part-time/adjunct. *Students:* 21 full-time (15 women), 12 part-time (11 women); includes 7 minority (4 Black or African American, non-Hispanic/Latino; 2 Asian, non-Hispanic/Latino; 1 Hispanic/Latino), 2 international. Average age 30. 28 applicants, 61% accepted, 13 enrolled. In 2013, 18 master's awarded. *Degree requirements:* For master's, comprehensive exam, thesis optional, capstone project and internship, administration practicum, or research practicum. *Entrance requirements:* For master's, GMAT or GRE General Test, MAT, minimum GPA of 2.8, letter of intent, letters of recommendation. Additional exam requirements/recommendations for international students: Required—TOEFL (minimum score 523 paper-based). *Application deadline:* For fall admission, 6/1 priority date for domestic students, 5/1 priority date for international students; for spring admission, 11/15 priority date for domestic students, 9/15 priority date for international students; for summer admission, 4/15 for domestic students, 9/15 for international students. Applications are processed on a rolling basis. Application fee: $30. Electronic applications accepted. *Expenses:* Contact institution. *Financial support:* In 2013–14, research assistantships with full tuition reimbursements (averaging $5,000 per year) were awarded; career-related internships or fieldwork, Federal Work-Study, scholarships/grants, tuition waivers (full), and unspecified assistantships also available. Support available to part-time students. Financial award applicants required to submit FAFSA. *Faculty research:* Health administration, community health, health education. *Unit head:* Dr. Sandy Streater, Department Head, Health Sciences, 912-344-2548, Fax: 912-344-3490, E-mail: sandy.streater@armstrong.edu. *Application contact:* Jill Bell, Director, Graduate Enrollment Services, 912-344-2798, Fax: 912-344-3488, E-mail: graduate@armstrong.edu.
Website: http://www.armstrong.edu/Health_Professions/Health_Sciences/healthsciences_master_of_health_services_administration

Ashworth College, Graduate Programs, Norcross, GA 30092. Offers business administration (MBA); criminal justice (MS); health care administration (MBA, MS); human resource management (MBA, MS); international business (MBA); management (MS); marketing (MBA, MS).

A.T. Still University, School of Health Management, Kirksville, MO 63501. Offers dental public health (MPH); health administration (MHA, DHA); health education (DH Ed); public health (MPH). Part-time and evening/weekend programs available. Postbaccalaureate distance learning degree programs offered (no on-campus study). *Faculty:* 20 full-time (10 women), 49 part-time/adjunct (27 women). *Students:* 164 full-time (123 women), 256 part-time (144 women); includes 143 minority (61 Black or African American, non-Hispanic/Latino; 4 American Indian or Alaska Native, non-Hispanic/Latino; 46 Asian, non-Hispanic/Latino; 25 Hispanic/Latino; 3 Native Hawaiian or other Pacific Islander, non-Hispanic/Latino; 4 Two or more races, non-Hispanic/Latino), 12 international. Average age 34. 154 applicants, 93% accepted, 114 enrolled. In 2013, 132 master's, 13 doctorates awarded. *Degree requirements:* For master's, thesis, integrated terminal project, practicum; for doctorate, thesis/dissertation. *Entrance requirements:* For master's, minimum GPA of 3.0, bachelor's degree or equivalent, background check, essay, three references; for doctorate, minimum GPA of 3.0, master's or terminal degree, background check, essay, three references. Additional exam requirements/recommendations for international students: Required—TOEFL (minimum score 550 paper-based; 80 iBT). *Application deadline:* For fall admission, 5/31 for domestic and international students; for winter admission, 8/2 for domestic and international students; for spring admission, 11/8 for domestic and international students; for summer admission, 1/24 for domestic and international students. Application fee: $70. Electronic applications accepted. *Expenses:* Contact institution. *Financial support:* Scholarships/grants available. Financial award application deadline: 5/1; financial award applicants required to submit FAFSA. *Faculty research:* Public health: influence of availability of comprehensive wellness resources online, student wellness, oral health care needs assessment of community, oral health knowledge and behaviors of Medicaid-eligible pregnant women and mothers of young children in relations to early childhood caries and tooth decay, alcohol use and alcohol related problems among college students. *Unit head:* Dr. Donald Altman, Interim Dean, 660-626-2820, Fax: 660-626-2826, E-mail: daltman@atsu.edu. *Application contact:* Sarah

Spencer, Associate Director, Admissions, 660-626-2820 Ext. 2669, Fax: 660-626-2826, E-mail: sspencer@atsu.edu.
Website: http://www.atsu.edu/shm

Auburn University at Montgomery, School of Sciences, Department of Public Administration and Political Science, Montgomery, AL 36124-4023. Offers international relations (MIR); nonprofit management and leadership (Certificate); political science (MPS); public administration (MPA); public administration and public policy (PhD); public health care administration and policy (Certificate). PhD offered jointly with Auburn University. *Accreditation:* NASPAA (one or more programs are accredited). Part-time and evening/weekend programs available. *Faculty:* 3 full-time (1 woman), 1 part-time/adjunct (0 women). *Students:* 11 full-time (7 women), 66 part-time (44 women); includes 31 minority (29 Black or African American, non-Hispanic/Latino; 2 Hispanic/Latino), 1 international. Average age 37. In 2013, 24 master's awarded. *Degree requirements:* For master's, comprehensive exam; for doctorate, thesis/dissertation. *Entrance requirements:* For master's, GRE General Test or MAT; for doctorate, GRE General Test. *Application deadline:* Applications are processed on a rolling basis. Electronic applications accepted. *Expenses:* Tuition, state resident: full-time $5994; part-time $333 per credit hour. Tuition, nonresident: full-time $17,982; part-time $999 per credit hour. *Financial support:* Research assistantships, career-related internships or fieldwork, and scholarships/grants available. Support available to part-time students. Financial award application deadline: 3/1; financial award applicants required to submit FAFSA. *Unit head:* Dr. Andrew Cortell, Department Head, 334-244-3622, E-mail: acortell@aum.edu. *Application contact:* Dr. William Ellis, Graduate Coordinator, 334-244-3177, Fax: 334-244-3992, E-mail: wellis3@aum.edu.
Website: http://sciences.aum.edu/departments/political-science-and-public-administration

Avila University, School of Business, Kansas City, MO 64145-1698. Offers accounting (MBA); finance (MBA); health care administration (MBA); international business (MBA); management (MBA); management information systems (MBA); marketing (MBA). Part-time and evening/weekend programs available. *Faculty:* 9 full-time (4 women), 12 part-time/adjunct (3 women). *Students:* 66 full-time (32 women), 46 part-time (27 women); includes 34 minority (22 Black or African American, non-Hispanic/Latino; 1 American Indian or Alaska Native, non-Hispanic/Latino; 4 Asian, non-Hispanic/Latino; 7 Hispanic/Latino), 27 international. Average age 32. 30 applicants, 80% accepted, 24 enrolled. In 2013, 61 master's awarded. *Degree requirements:* For master's, comprehensive exam, capstone course. *Entrance requirements:* For master's, GMAT (minimum score 420), minimum GPA of 3.0, interview. Additional exam requirements/recommendations for international students: Required—TOEFL (minimum score 550 paper-based). *Application deadline:* For fall admission, 7/30 priority date for domestic and international students; for winter admission, 11/30 priority date for domestic and international students; for spring admission, 2/28 priority date for domestic and international students; for summer admission, 6/1 priority date for domestic and international students. Applications are processed on a rolling basis. Application fee: $0. Electronic applications accepted. *Expenses:* Contact institution. *Financial support:* In 2013–14, 11 students received support. Career-related internships or fieldwork and scholarships/grants available. Support available to part-time students. Financial award applicants required to submit FAFSA. *Faculty research:* Leadership characteristics, financial hedging, group dynamics. *Unit head:* Dr. Richard Woodall, Dean, 816-501-3720, Fax: 816-501-2463, E-mail: richard.woodall@avila.edu. *Application contact:* Sarah Belanus, MBA Admissions Director, 816-501-3601, Fax: 816-501-2463, E-mail: sarah.belanus@avila.edu.
Website: http://www.avila.edu/mba

Baker College Center for Graduate Studies - Online, Graduate Programs, Flint, MI 48507-9843. Offers accounting (MBA); business administration (DBA); finance (MBA); general business (MBA); health care management (MBA); human resources management (MBA); information management (MBA); leadership studies (MBA); management information systems (MSIS); marketing (MBA). Part-time and evening/weekend programs available. Postbaccalaureate distance learning degree programs offered. *Degree requirements:* For master's, portfolio. *Entrance requirements:* For master's, 3 years of work experience, minimum undergraduate GPA of 2.5, writing sample, 3 letters of recommendation; for doctorate, MBA or acceptable related master's degree from accredited association, 5 years work experience, minimum graduate GPA of 3.25, writing sample, 3 professional references. Additional exam requirements/recommendations for international students: Required—TOEFL (minimum score 550 paper-based). Electronic applications accepted.

Baldwin Wallace University, Graduate Programs, Division of Business, Program in Health Care Management, Berea, OH 44017-2088. Offers MBA. Part-time and evening/weekend programs available. *Students:* 44 full-time (22 women), 14 part-time (10 women); includes 9 minority (3 Black or African American, non-Hispanic/Latino; 4 Asian, non-Hispanic/Latino; 2 Hispanic/Latino). Average age 39. 21 applicants, 76% accepted, 12 enrolled. In 2013, 28 master's awarded. *Degree requirements:* For master's, minimum overall GPA of 3.0, completion of all required courses. *Entrance requirements:* For master's, GMAT, interview, work experience, bachelor's degree in any field. Additional exam requirements/recommendations for international students: Required—TOEFL (minimum score 523 paper-based; 70 iBT). *Application deadline:* For fall admission, 7/25 priority date for domestic students, 4/30 priority date for international students; for spring admission, 12/10 priority date for domestic students, 9/30 priority date for international students. Applications are processed on a rolling basis. Application fee: $25. Electronic applications accepted. Application fee is waived when completed online. *Expenses:* Contact institution. *Financial support:* Application deadline: 5/1; applicants required to submit FAFSA. *Unit head:* Tom Campanella, Director, 440-826-3818, Fax: 440-826-3868, E-mail: tcampane@bw.edu. *Application contact:* Laura Spencer, Graduate Application Specialist, 440-826-2191, Fax: 440-826-3868, E-mail: lspencer@bw.edu.
Website: http://www.bw.edu/academics/bus/programs/hcmba/

Barry University, Andreas School of Business, Graduate Certificate Programs, Miami Shores, FL 33161-6695. Offers finance (Certificate); health services administration (Certificate); international business (Certificate); management (Certificate); management information systems (Certificate); marketing (Certificate).

Barry University, College of Health Sciences, Graduate Certificate Programs, Miami Shores, FL 33161-6695. Offers health care leadership (Certificate); health care planning and informatics (Certificate); histotechnology (Certificate); long term care management (Certificate); medical group practice management (Certificate); quality improvement and outcomes management (Certificate).

Barry University, College of Health Sciences, Program in Health Services Administration, Miami Shores, FL 33161-6695. Offers MS. Part-time and evening/weekend programs available. *Degree requirements:* For master's, comprehensive exam. *Entrance requirements:* For master's, GMAT or GRE General Test, 2 years of experience in the health field, minimum GPA of 3.0, 1 semester of course work in computer applications or the equivalent (business). Electronic applications accepted.

Baruch College of the City University of New York, School of Public Affairs, Program in Public Administration, New York, NY 10010-5585. Offers general public administration (MPA); health care policy (MPA); nonprofit administration (MPA); policy analysis and evaluation (MPA); public management (MPA); MS/MPA. *Accreditation:* NASPAA. Part-time and evening/weekend programs available. *Degree requirements:* For master's, thesis, capstone. *Entrance requirements:* For master's, GRE General Test. Additional exam requirements/recommendations for international students: Required—TOEFL. Electronic applications accepted. *Expenses:* Contact institution. *Faculty research:* Urbanization, population and poverty in the developing world, housing and community development, labor unions and housing, government-nongovernment relations, immigration policy, social network analysis, cross-sectoral governance, comparative healthcare systems, program evaluation, social welfare policy, health outcomes, educational policy and leadership, transnationalism, infant health, welfare reform, racial/ethnic disparities in health, urban politics, homelessness, race and ethnic relations.

Baruch College of the City University of New York, Zicklin School of Business, Zicklin Executive Programs, Baruch/Mt. Sinai Program in Health Care Administration, New York, NY 10010-5585. Offers MBA. *Accreditation:* CAHME. Part-time and evening/weekend programs available. *Entrance requirements:* For master's, GMAT, personal interview, work experience in health care. Additional exam requirements/recommendations for international students: Required—TOEFL. Electronic applications accepted. *Expenses:* Contact institution. *Faculty research:* Economics of reproductive health, multivariate point estimation.

Baylor University, Graduate School, Military Programs, Program in Health Care Administration, Waco, TX 76798. Offers MHA. Program offered jointly with the U.S. Army. *Accreditation:* CAHME. *Students:* 108 full-time (27 women); includes 7 minority (1 Asian, non-Hispanic/Latino; 4 Hispanic/Latino; 1 Native Hawaiian or other Pacific Islander, non-Hispanic/Latino; 1 Two or more races, non-Hispanic/Latino). In 2013, 54 master's awarded. *Entrance requirements:* For master's, GRE General Test. *Application deadline:* For fall admission, 6/15 for domestic students. Applications are processed on a rolling basis. Application fee: $25. *Expenses:* *Tuition:* Full-time $25,866; part-time $1437 per credit hour. *Required fees:* $2736; $152 per credit hour. Tuition and fees vary according to course load and program. *Faculty research:* Data quality, public health policy, organizational behavior, AIDS. *Unit head:* Lt. Cdr. Lee Bewley, Graduate Program Director, 210-221-8857 Ext. 6443, E-mail: lee.bewley@us.army.mil. *Application contact:* Rene Pryor, Program Administrator, 210-221-6443, Fax: 210-221-6010, E-mail: rene.pryor@cen.amedd.army.mil.
Website: http://www.cs.amedd.army.mil/baylorhca/

Belhaven University, School of Business, Jackson, MS 39202-1789. Offers business administration (MBA); health administration (MBA); human resources (MBA, MSL); leadership (MBA); public administration (MPA); sports administration (MBA). MBA program also offered in Houston, TX, Memphis, TN and Orlando, FL. Part-time and evening/weekend programs available. Postbaccalaureate distance learning degree programs offered. *Faculty:* 21 full-time (4 women), 34 part-time/adjunct (12 women). *Students:* 166 full-time (112 women), 688 part-time (460 women); includes 576 minority (540 Black or African American, non-Hispanic/Latino; 2 American Indian or Alaska Native, non-Hispanic/Latino; 2 Asian, non-Hispanic/Latino; 26 Hispanic/Latino; 6 Two or more races, non-Hispanic/Latino). Average age 36. 325 applicants, 72% accepted, 185 enrolled. In 2013, 189 master's awarded. *Degree requirements:* For master's, comprehensive exam (for some programs), thesis (for some programs). *Entrance requirements:* For master's, GMAT, GRE General Test or MAT, minimum GPA of 2.8. *Application deadline:* Applications are processed on a rolling basis. Application fee: $25. Electronic applications accepted. *Financial support:* Applicants required to submit FAFSA. *Unit head:* Dr. Ralph Mason, Dean, 601-968-8949, Fax: 601-968-8951, E-mail: cmason@belhaven.edu. *Application contact:* Dr. Audrey Kelleher, Vice President of Adult and Graduate Marketing and Development, 407-804-1424, Fax: 407-620-5210, E-mail: akelleher@belhaven.edu.
Website: http://www.belhaven.edu/campuses/index.htm

Bellevue University, Graduate School, College of Arts and Sciences, Bellevue, NE 68005-3098. Offers clinical counseling (MS); healthcare administration (MHA); human services (MA); international security and intelligence studies (MS); managerial communication (MA). Postbaccalaureate distance learning degree programs offered.

Belmont University, Jack C. Massey Graduate School of Business, Nashville, TN 37212. Offers accelerated (MBA); accounting (M Acc); healthcare (MBA); professional (MBA). *Accreditation:* AACSB. Part-time and evening/weekend programs available. *Faculty:* 46 full-time (16 women), 27 part-time/adjunct (11 women). *Students:* 162 full-time (61 women), 50 part-time (25 women); includes 30 minority (14 Black or African American, non-Hispanic/Latino; 1 American Indian or Alaska Native, non-Hispanic/Latino; 7 Asian, non-Hispanic/Latino; 5 Hispanic/Latino; 3 Two or more races, non-Hispanic/Latino), 5 international. Average age 28. 148 applicants, 64% accepted, 77 enrolled. In 2013, 136 master's awarded. *Entrance requirements:* For master's, GMAT, 2 years of work experience (MBA). Additional exam requirements/recommendations for international students: Required—TOEFL (minimum score 550 paper-based). *Application deadline:* For fall admission, 7/1 for domestic and international students; for spring admission, 11/1 for domestic and international students. Applications are processed on a rolling basis. Application fee: $50. Electronic applications accepted. *Expenses:* Contact institution. *Financial support:* Scholarships/grants, tuition waivers (partial), and unspecified assistantships available. Financial award application deadline: 7/1; financial award applicants required to submit FAFSA. *Faculty research:* Music business, strategy, ethics, finance, accounting systems. *Unit head:* Dr. Patrick Raines, Dean, 615-460-6480, Fax: 615-460-6455, E-mail: pat.raines@belmont.edu. *Application contact:* Tonya Hollin, Admissions Assistant, 615-460-6480, Fax: 615-460-6353, E-mail: masseyadmissions@belmont.edu.
Website: http://www.belmont.edu/business/masseyschool/

Benedictine University, Graduate Programs, Program in Business Administration, Lisle, IL 60532-0900. Offers accounting (MBA); entrepreneurship and managing innovation (MBA); financial management (MBA); health administration (MBA); human resource management (MBA); information systems security (MBA); international business (MBA); management consulting (MBA); management information systems (MBA); marketing management (MBA); operations management and logistics (MBA); organizational leadership (MBA). Part-time and evening/weekend programs available. Postbaccalaureate distance learning degree programs offered (minimal on-campus study). *Faculty:* 4 full-time (2 women), 24 part-time/adjunct (3 women). *Students:* 144 full-time (83 women), 599 part-time (328 women); includes 189 minority (115 Black or African American, non-Hispanic/Latino; 5 American Indian or Alaska Native, non-Hispanic/Latino; 43 Asian, non-Hispanic/Latino; 24 Hispanic/Latino; 2 Native Hawaiian or other Pacific Islander, non-Hispanic/Latino), 14 international. Average age 34. 211 applicants, 89% accepted, 155 enrolled. In 2013, 376 master's awarded. *Entrance requirements:* For master's, GMAT. Additional exam requirements/recommendations for international students: Required—TOEFL (minimum score 550 paper-based). *Application deadline:* For fall admission, 9/1 for domestic students; for winter admission, 12/1 for domestic students; for spring admission, 2/15 for domestic students. Applications are processed on a rolling basis. Application fee: $40. Electronic applications accepted. *Expenses:* *Tuition:* Part-time $590 per credit hour. *Financial support:* Career-related internships or fieldwork and health care benefits available.

Support available to part-time students. *Faculty research:* Strategic leadership in professional organizations, sociology of professions, organizational change, social identity theory, applications to change management. *Unit head:* Dr. Sharon Borowicz, Director, 630-829-6219, E-mail: sborowicz@ben.edu. *Application contact:* Kari Gibbons, Director, Admissions, 630-829-6200, Fax: 630-829-6584, E-mail: kgibbons@ben.edu.

Benedictine University, Graduate Programs, Program in Public Health, Lisle, IL 60532-0900. Offers administration of health care institutions (MPH); dietetics (MPH); disaster management (MPH); health education (MPH); health information systems (MPH); MBA/MPH; MPH/MS. Part-time and evening/weekend programs available. Postbaccalaureate distance learning degree programs offered. *Students:* 78 full-time (62 women), 340 part-time (254 women); includes 159 minority (97 Black or African American, non-Hispanic/Latino; 3 American Indian or Alaska Native, non-Hispanic/Latino; 47 Asian, non-Hispanic/Latino; 11 Hispanic/Latino; 1 Native Hawaiian or other Pacific Islander, non-Hispanic/Latino), 14 international. Average age 33. 195 applicants, 86% accepted, 143 enrolled. In 2013, 207 master's awarded. *Entrance requirements:* For master's, MAT, GRE, or GMAT. Additional exam requirements/recommendations for international students: Required—TOEFL (minimum score 550 paper-based). *Application deadline:* For fall admission, 9/1 for domestic students; for winter admission, 12/1 for domestic students; for spring admission, 2/15 for domestic students. Application fee: $40. *Expenses: Tuition:* Part-time $590 per credit hour. *Financial support:* Career-related internships or fieldwork and health care benefits available. Support available to part-time students. *Unit head:* Dr. Georgeen Polyak, Director, 630-829-6217, E-mail: gpolyak@ben.edu. *Application contact:* Kari Gibbons, Associate Vice President, Enrollment Center, 630-829-6200, Fax: 630-829-6584, E-mail: kgibbons@ben.edu.

Benedictine University at Springfield, Program in Business Administration, Springfield, IL 62702. Offers health administration (MBA); organizational leadership (MBA). Part-time and evening/weekend programs available. *Entrance requirements:* For master's, GMAT.

Binghamton University, State University of New York, Graduate School, School of Management, Program in Business Administration, Vestal, NY 13850. Offers business administration (MBA); corporate executive (MBA); executive business administration (MBA); health care professional executive (MBA); management (PhD); professional business administration (MBA). Executive and Professional MBA programs offered in Manhattan. *Accreditation:* AACSB. *Students:* 131 full-time (48 women), 16 part-time (8 women); includes 31 minority (7 Black or African American, non-Hispanic/Latino; 13 Asian, non-Hispanic/Latino; 8 Hispanic/Latino; 3 Native Hawaiian or other Pacific Islander, non-Hispanic/Latino), 57 international. Average age 27. 324 applicants, 49% accepted, 102 enrolled. In 2013, 85 master's, 1 doctorate awarded. *Degree requirements:* For doctorate, thesis/dissertation. *Entrance requirements:* For master's and doctorate, GMAT. Additional exam requirements/recommendations for international students: Required—TOEFL (minimum score 550 paper-based; 80 iBT). *Application deadline:* For fall admission, 3/1 priority date for domestic and international students; for spring admission, 10/15 priority date for domestic and international students. Applications are processed on a rolling basis. Application fee: $75. Electronic applications accepted. *Financial support:* In 2013–14, 37 students received support, including 9 teaching assistantships with full tuition reimbursements available (averaging $17,000 per year); career-related internships or fieldwork, Federal Work-Study, institutionally sponsored loans, scholarships/grants, health care benefits, tuition waivers (full and partial), and unspecified assistantships also available. Financial award application deadline: 2/15; financial award applicants required to submit FAFSA. *Unit head:* Dr. Upinder Dhillon, Dean, 607-777-2314, E-mail: dhillon@binghamton.edu. *Application contact:* Kishan Zuber, Recruiting and Admissions Coordinator, 607-777-2151, Fax: 607-777-2501, E-mail: kzuber@binghamton.edu.

Binghamton University, State University of New York, Graduate School, Thomas J. Watson School of Engineering and Applied Science, Department of Systems Science and Industrial Engineering, Vestal, NY 13850. Offers executive health systems (MS); industrial and systems engineering (M Eng); systems science and industrial engineering (MS, PhD). MS in executive health systems also offered in Manhattan. Part-time and evening/weekend programs available. *Faculty:* 14 full-time (3 women), 5 part-time/adjunct (0 women). *Students:* 120 full-time (48 women), 84 part-time (23 women); includes 28 minority (6 Black or African American, non-Hispanic/Latino; 10 Asian, non-Hispanic/Latino; 8 Hispanic/Latino; 4 Native Hawaiian or other Pacific Islander, non-Hispanic/Latino), 101 international. Average age 28. 241 applicants, 78% accepted, 52 enrolled. In 2013, 32 master's, 11 doctorates awarded. Terminal master's awarded for partial completion of doctoral program. *Degree requirements:* For master's, thesis or alternative; for doctorate, thesis/dissertation. *Entrance requirements:* For master's and doctorate, GRE General Test, GRE Subject Test. Additional exam requirements/recommendations for international students: Required—TOEFL. *Application deadline:* For fall admission, 4/15 priority date for domestic students, 1/15 priority date for international students; for spring admission, 11/1 for domestic students, 10/1 priority date for international students. Applications are processed on a rolling basis. Application fee: $75. Electronic applications accepted. *Financial support:* In 2013–14, 75 students received support, including 42 research assistantships with full tuition reimbursements available (averaging $16,500 per year), 15 teaching assistantships with full tuition reimbursements available (averaging $16,500 per year); career-related internships or fieldwork, Federal Work-Study, institutionally sponsored loans, scholarships/grants, health care benefits, tuition waivers (full and partial), and unspecified assistantships also available. Financial award application deadline: 2/15; financial award applicants required to submit FAFSA. *Faculty research:* Problem restructuring, protein modeling. *Unit head:* Ellen Tilden, Coordinator of Graduate Studies, 607-777-2873, E-mail: etilden@binghamton.edu. *Application contact:* Kishan Zuber, Recruiting and Admissions Coordinator, 607-777-2151, Fax: 607-777-2501, E-mail: kzuber@binghamton.edu.
Website: http://www.ssie.binghamton.edu

Boise State University, College of Health Sciences, Department of Community and Environmental Health, Boise, ID 83725-0399. Offers environmental health (MHS); evaluation and research (MHS); health policy (MHS); health promotion (MHS); health services leadership (MHS).

Boston University, School of Medicine, Division of Graduate Medical Sciences, Program in Healthcare Emergency Management, Boston, MA 02215. Offers MS. *Expenses: Tuition:* Full-time $43,970; part-time $1374 per credit hour. *Required fees:* $60 per semester. Tuition and fees vary according to class time, course level and program. *Financial support:* Applicants required to submit FAFSA. *Unit head:* Dr. Kevin Thomas, Director, 617-414-2316, Fax: 617-414-2332, E-mail: kipthoma@bu.edu. *Application contact:* Patricia Jones, Program Manager and Admissions Director, 617-414-2315, E-mail: psterlin@bu.edu.
Website: http://www.bumc.bu.edu/bmcm/

Boston University, School of Medicine, Division of Graduate Medical Sciences, Program in Medical Sciences, Boston, MA 02215. Offers MA, MA/MA, MBA/MA, MPH/MA. Part-time programs available. *Degree requirements:* For master's, thesis. *Entrance requirements:* For master's, MCAT or GRE. *Application deadline:* Applications are processed on a rolling basis. Application fee: $75. Electronic applications accepted. *Expenses: Tuition:* Full-time $43,970; part-time $1374 per credit hour. *Required fees:* $60 per semester. Tuition and fees vary according to class time, course level and program. *Financial support:* Federal Work-Study available. Financial award applicants required to submit FAFSA. *Unit head:* Dr. Gwynneth D. Offner, Director, 617-638-8221, E-mail: goffner@bu.edu. *Application contact:* GMS Admissions Office, 617-638-5255.
Website: http://www.bumc.bu.edu/gms/academics/masters-in-medical-sciences/

Boston University, School of Public Health, Health Policy and Management Department, Boston, MA 02215. Offers health policy and management (MPH); health services research (MS, PhD). *Accreditation:* CAHME. Part-time and evening/weekend programs available. *Faculty:* 37 full-time, 31 part-time/adjunct. *Students:* 115 full-time (78 women), 88 part-time (62 women); includes 45 minority (7 Black or African American, non-Hispanic/Latino; 22 Asian, non-Hispanic/Latino; 12 Hispanic/Latino; 4 Two or more races, non-Hispanic/Latino), 38 international. Average age 28. 507 applicants, 44% accepted, 77 enrolled. In 2013, 187 master's, 2 doctorates awarded. *Degree requirements:* For master's, comprehensive exam (for some programs), thesis (for some programs); for doctorate, comprehensive exam, thesis/dissertation. *Entrance requirements:* For master's, GRE, MCAT, LSAT, GMAT, or DAT; for doctorate, GRE, MCAT, GMAT, LSAT. Additional exam requirements/recommendations for international students: Required—TOEFL (minimum score 600 paper-based; 100 iBT) or IELTS (minimum score 6). *Application deadline:* For fall admission, 2/1 priority date for domestic and international students; for spring admission, 10/15 priority date for domestic and international students. Applications are processed on a rolling basis. Application fee: $115. Electronic applications accepted. *Expenses: Tuition:* Full-time $43,970; part-time $1374 per credit hour. *Required fees:* $60 per semester. Tuition and fees vary according to class time, course level and program. *Financial support:* Career-related internships or fieldwork, Federal Work-Study, institutionally sponsored loans, scholarships/grants, and tuition waivers (partial) available. Support available to part-time students. Financial award application deadline: 3/1; financial award applicants required to submit FAFSA. *Unit head:* Dr. Alan Jette, Acting Chair, 617-638-5042. *Application contact:* LePhan Quan, Associate Director of Admissions, 617-638-4640, Fax: 617-638-5299, E-mail: asksph@bu.edu.
Website: http://sph.bu.edu/hpm

Brandeis University, The Heller School for Social Policy and Management, Program in Nonprofit Management, Waltham, MA 02454-9110. Offers child, youth, and family management (MBA); health care management (MBA); social impact management (MBA); social policy and management (MBA); sustainable development (MBA); MBA/MA; MBA/MD. MBA/MD program offered in conjunction with Tufts University School of Medicine. *Accreditation:* AACSB. Part-time programs available. *Degree requirements:* For master's, team consulting project. *Entrance requirements:* For master's, GMAT (preferred) or GRE, 2 letters of recommendation, problem statement analysis, 3-5 years of professional experience. Additional exam requirements/recommendations for international students: Required—TOEFL (minimum score 600 paper-based; 100 iBT). Electronic applications accepted. *Expenses:* Contact institution. *Faculty research:* Health care; children and families; elder and disabled services; social impact management; organizations in the non-profit, for-profit, or public sector.

Brandman University, School of Nursing and Health Professions, Irvine, CA 92618. Offers health administration (MHA); health risk and crisis communication (MS).

Brenau University, Sydney O. Smith Graduate School, School of Business and Mass Communication, Gainesville, GA 30501. Offers accounting (MBA); business administration (MBA); healthcare management (MBA); organizational leadership (MS); project management (MBA). *Accreditation:* ACBSP. Part-time and evening/weekend programs available. Postbaccalaureate distance learning degree programs offered (no on-campus study). *Degree requirements:* For master's, comprehensive exam (for some programs). *Entrance requirements:* For master's, resume, minimum undergraduate GPA of 2.5. Additional exam requirements/recommendations for international students: Required—TOEFL (minimum score 500 paper-based; 61 iBT); Recommended—IELTS (minimum score 5). Electronic applications accepted. *Expenses:* Contact institution.

Broadview University–West Jordan, Graduate Programs, West Jordan, UT 84088. Offers business administration (MBA); health care management (MSM); information technology (MSM); managerial leadership (MSM).

Brooklyn College of the City University of New York, School of Natural and Behavioral Sciences, Department of Health and Nutrition Sciences, Program in Public Health, Brooklyn, NY 11210-2889. Offers general public health (MPH); health care policy and administration (MPH). *Accreditation:* CEPH. *Degree requirements:* For master's, thesis or alternative, 46 credits. *Entrance requirements:* For master's, GRE, 2 letters of recommendation, essay, interview. *Application deadline:* For fall admission, 3/1 priority date for domestic students, 2/1 priority date for international students; for spring admission, 11/1 priority date for domestic students, 10/1 priority date for international students. Applications are processed on a rolling basis. Application fee: $125. Electronic applications accepted. *Expenses: Tuition, area resident:* Full-time $4585; part-time $385 per credit. Tuition, state resident: full-time $4585; part-time $385 per credit. Tuition, nonresident: part-time $710 per credit. *Required fees:* $430; $153 per semester. Tuition and fees vary according to course load. *Financial support:* Application deadline: 5/1. *Unit head:* Jean Grassman, Graduate Deputy Chairperson, 718-951-5026, Fax: 718-951-4670. *Application contact:* Jean Grassman, Graduate Deputy Chairperson, 718-951-5026, Fax: 718-951-4670.

California Baptist University, Program in Business Administration, Riverside, CA 92504-3206. Offers accounting (MBA); construction management (MBA); healthcare management (MBA); management (MBA). *Accreditation:* ACBSP. Part-time and evening/weekend programs available. Postbaccalaureate distance learning degree programs offered (minimal on-campus study). *Faculty:* 14 full-time (5 women), 4 part-time/adjunct (1 woman). *Students:* 49 full-time (20 women), 53 part-time (20 women); includes 43 minority (8 Black or African American, non-Hispanic/Latino; 2 American Indian or Alaska Native, non-Hispanic/Latino; 4 Asian, non-Hispanic/Latino; 28 Hispanic/Latino; 1 Two or more races, non-Hispanic/Latino), 6 international. Average age 28. 119 applicants, 60% accepted, 43 enrolled. In 2013, 46 master's awarded. *Degree requirements:* For master's, interdisciplinary capstone project. *Entrance requirements:* For master's, GMAT, minimum GPA of 2.5; two recommendations; comprehensive essay; resume; interview; 4 prerequisite courses. Additional exam requirements/recommendations for international students: Required—TOEFL (minimum score 80 iBT). *Application deadline:* For fall admission, 8/1 priority date for domestic students, 7/1 for international students; for spring admission, 12/1 priority date for domestic students, 11/1 for international students. Applications are processed on a rolling basis. Application fee: $45. Electronic applications accepted. *Expenses:* Contact institution. *Financial support:* Institutionally sponsored loans available. Financial award applicants required to submit CSS PROFILE or FAFSA. *Faculty research:* Econometrics, Biblical financial principles, strategic management and corporate performance, shared leadership models, international culture and economics. *Unit head:* Dr. Franco Gandolfi, Dean, School of Business, 951-343-4968, Fax: 951-343-4361, E-mail: fgandolfi@calbaptist.edu. *Application contact:* Dr. Keanon Alderson, Director, Business Administration Program, 951-343-4768, E-mail: kalderson@calbaptist.edu.
Website: http://www.calbaptist.edu/mba/about/

California Baptist University, Program in Nursing, Riverside, CA 92504-3206. Offers clinical nurse specialist (MSN); family nurse practitioner (MSN); healthcare systems

management (MSN); nursing (MSN); teaching-learning (MSN). Part-time programs available. *Faculty:* 15 full-time (all women), 7 part-time/adjunct (all women). *Students:* 49 full-time (41 women), 69 part-time (55 women); includes 61 minority (18 Black or African American, non-Hispanic/Latino; 1 American Indian or Alaska Native, non-Hispanic/Latino; 17 Asian, non-Hispanic/Latino; 22 Hispanic/Latino; 3 Two or more races, non-Hispanic/Latino). Average age 33. 48 applicants, 65% accepted, 20 enrolled. In 2013, 9 master's awarded. *Degree requirements:* For master's, comprehensive exam (for some programs), thesis or alternative, comprehensive exam or directed project thesis; capstone practicum. *Entrance requirements:* For master's, GRE or California Critical Thinking Skills Test; Test of Essential Academic Skills (TEAS), minimum undergraduate GPA of 3.25; Microsoft Office competency; health clearance; health insurance; CPR certification; vehicle insurance; random drug testing; background check clearance; passport photo; three recommendations; comprehensive essay; interview. Additional exam requirements/recommendations for international students: Required—TOEFL (minimum score 80 iBT). *Application deadline:* For fall admission, 8/1 priority date for domestic students, 7/1 for international students; for spring admission, 12/1 priority date for domestic students, 11/1 for international students. Applications are processed on a rolling basis. Application fee: $45. Electronic applications accepted. *Expenses: Tuition:* Full-time $10,080; part-time $560 per unit. *Required fees:* $175 per semester. One-time fee: $45. Tuition and fees vary according to course load and program. *Financial support:* Institutionally sponsored loans available. Financial award applicants required to submit CSS PROFILE or FAFSA. *Faculty research:* Qualitative research using Parse methodology, gerontology, disaster preparedness, medical-surgical nursing, maternal-child nursing. *Unit head:* Dr. Geneva Oaks, Dean, School of Nursing, 951-343-4702, E-mail: goaks@calbaptist.edu. *Application contact:* Dr. Rebecca Meyer, Director, Graduate Program in Nursing, 951-343-4952, Fax: 951-343-5095, E-mail: rmeyer@calbaptist.edu.
Website: http://www.calbaptist.edu/explore-cbu/schools-colleges/school-nursing/master-science-nursing/

California Baptist University, Program in Public Health, Riverside, CA 92504-3206. Offers food, nutrition and health (MPH); health policy and administration (MPH); physical activity (MPH). Part-time and evening/weekend programs available. *Degree requirements:* For master's, capstone project; practicum. *Entrance requirements:* For master's, minimum undergraduate GPA of 2.75, bachelor's degree transcripts, three recommendations, 500-word essay, resume, interview. Additional exam requirements/recommendations for international students: Required—TOEFL (minimum score 80 iBT). *Application deadline:* For fall admission, 8/1 priority date for domestic students, 7/1 for international students; for spring admission, 12/1 priority date for domestic students, 11/1 for international students. Applications are processed on a rolling basis. Application fee: $45. Electronic applications accepted. *Expenses:* Contact institution. *Financial support:* Applicants required to submit CSS PROFILE or FAFSA. *Unit head:* Dr. Chuck Sands, Dean, College of Allied Health, 951-343-4619, E-mail: csands@calbaptist.edu. *Application contact:* Dr. Wayne Fletcher, Chair, Department of Health Sciences, 951-552-8724, E-mail: wfletcher@calbaptist.edu.
Website: http://www.calbaptist.edu/explore-cbu/schools-colleges/college-allied-health/health-sciences/master-public-health/

California Coast University, School of Administration and Management, Santa Ana, CA 92701. Offers business marketing (MBA); health care management (MBA); human resource management (MBA); management (MBA, MS). Postbaccalaureate distance learning degree programs offered (no on-campus study). Electronic applications accepted.

California Intercontinental University, School of Healthcare, Diamond Bar, CA 91765. Offers healthcare management and leadership (MBA, DBA).

California State University, Bakersfield, Division of Graduate Studies, School of Business and Public Administration, Administration–Health Care Management Program, Bakersfield, CA 93311. Offers MSA. *Entrance requirements:* For master's, official transcripts, two letters of recommendation, personal statement. Additional exam requirements/recommendations for international students: Required—TOEFL (minimum score 550 paper-based; 79 iBT), IELTS (minimum score 7). *Application deadline:* Applications are processed on a rolling basis. Application fee: $55. Electronic applications accepted. *Unit head:* Dr. B.J. Moore, Coordinator, 661-654-3026, E-mail: bjmoore@csub.edu. *Application contact:* Debbie Blowers, Assistant Director of Admissions, 661-664-3381, E-mail: dblowers@csub.edu.

California State University, Chico, Office of Graduate Studies, College of Behavioral and Social Sciences, Department of Political Science, Program in Public Administration, Chico, CA 95929-0722. Offers health administration (MPA); local government management (MPA). *Accreditation:* NASPAA. Part-time programs available. *Degree requirements:* For master's, thesis or culminating practicum. *Entrance requirements:* For master's, 2 letters of recommendation. Additional exam requirements/recommendations for international students: Required—TOEFL (minimum score 550 paper-based; 80 iBT), IELTS (minimum score 6.5). Electronic applications accepted.

California State University, East Bay, Office of Academic Programs and Graduate Studies, College of Letters, Arts, and Social Sciences, Department of Public Affairs and Administration, Program in Health Care Administration, Hayward, CA 94542-3000. Offers management and change in health care (MS). Part-time and evening/weekend programs available. Postbaccalaureate distance learning degree programs offered (no on-campus study). *Degree requirements:* For master's, thesis or alternative, final project. *Entrance requirements:* For master's, minimum undergraduate cumulative GPA of 2.5, statement of purpose, two letters of academic and/or professional recommendation, professional resume/curriculum vitae, all undergraduate/graduate transcripts. Additional exam requirements/recommendations for international students: Required—TOEFL (minimum score 550 paper-based). Electronic applications accepted.

California State University, East Bay, Office of Academic Programs and Graduate Studies, College of Letters, Arts, and Social Sciences, Department of Public Affairs and Administration, Program in Public Administration, Hayward, CA 94542-3000. Offers health care administration (MPA); management of human resources and change (MPA); public management and policy analysis (MPA). Part-time and evening/weekend programs available. *Degree requirements:* For master's, comprehensive exam (for some programs), comprehensive exam or thesis. *Entrance requirements:* For master's, minimum GPA of 2.5; statement of purpose; 2 letters of recommendation; professional resume/curriculum vitae. Additional exam requirements/recommendations for international students: Required—TOEFL (minimum score 550 paper-based; 79 iBT). Electronic applications accepted.

California State University, Fresno, Division of Graduate Studies, College of Health and Human Services, Department of Public Health, Fresno, CA 93740-8027. Offers health policy and management (MPH); health promotion (MPH). *Accreditation:* CEPH. Part-time and evening/weekend programs available. *Degree requirements:* For master's, thesis or alternative. *Entrance requirements:* For master's, GRE General Test, minimum GPA of 2.5. Additional exam requirements/recommendations for international students: Required—TOEFL. Electronic applications accepted. *Faculty research:* Foster parent training, geriatrics, tobacco control.

California State University, Long Beach, Graduate Studies, College of Health and Human Services, Program in Health Care Administration, Long Beach, CA 90840. Offers MS. *Accreditation:* CAHME. Part-time programs available. *Degree requirements:* For master's, comprehensive exam or thesis. *Entrance requirements:* For master's, minimum GPA of 3.0. Electronic applications accepted. *Faculty research:* Long-term care, Immigration Reform Act and health care, physician reimbursement.

California State University, Los Angeles, Graduate Studies, College of Business and Economics, Department of Management, Los Angeles, CA 90032-8530. Offers health care management (MS); management (MBA, MS). *Accreditation:* AACSB. Part-time and evening/weekend programs available. *Faculty:* 1 full-time (0 women), 4 part-time/adjunct (0 women). *Students:* 10 full-time (6 women), 41 part-time (29 women); includes 26 minority (2 Black or African American, non-Hispanic/Latino; 10 Asian, non-Hispanic/Latino; 14 Hispanic/Latino), 11 international. Average age 35. 55 applicants, 55% accepted, 20 enrolled. In 2013, 33 master's awarded. *Entrance requirements:* For master's, GMAT, minimum GPA of 2.5 during previous 2 years of course work. Additional exam requirements/recommendations for international students: Required—TOEFL (minimum score 550 paper-based). *Application deadline:* For fall admission, 5/1 for domestic and international students. Applications are processed on a rolling basis. Application fee: $55. Electronic applications accepted. *Financial support:* Application deadline: 3/1. *Unit head:* Dr. Angela Young, Chair, 323-343-2890, Fax: 323-343-6461, E-mail: ayoung3@calstatela.edu. *Application contact:* Dr. Larry Fritz, Dean of Graduate Studies, 323-343-3827, Fax: 323-343-5653, E-mail: lfritz@calstatela.edu.
Website: http://cbe.calstatela.edu/mgmt/

California State University, Northridge, Graduate Studies, College of Health and Human Development, Department of Health Sciences, Northridge, CA 91330. Offers health administration (MS); public health (MPH). *Accreditation:* CEPH. *Entrance requirements:* For master's, GRE General Test or minimum GPA of 3.0. Additional exam requirements/recommendations for international students: Required—TOEFL. *Faculty research:* Labor market needs assessment, health education products, dental hygiene, independent practice prototype.

California State University, Northridge, Graduate Studies, The Tseng College of Extended Learning, Program in Health Administration, Northridge, CA 91330. Offers MPA. Offered in collaboration with the College of Health and Human Development. Postbaccalaureate distance learning degree programs offered (no on-campus study). *Degree requirements:* For master's, comprehensive exam. *Entrance requirements:* For master's, bachelor's degree from accredited college or university, minimum cumulative GPA of 2.5, at least two years of work experience. Additional exam requirements/recommendations for international students: Required—TOEFL (minimum score of 85 iBT or 563 paper-based) or IELTS (minimum score of 7). Electronic applications accepted.

California State University, San Bernardino, Graduate Studies, College of Natural Sciences, Program in Health Services Administration, San Bernardino, CA 92407-2397. Offers MS. *Students:* 7 full-time (4 women), 4 part-time (3 women); includes 7 minority (2 Asian, non-Hispanic/Latino; 3 Hispanic/Latino; 2 Two or more races, non-Hispanic/Latino), 2 international. Average age 26. 15 applicants, 47% accepted, 4 enrolled. *Degree requirements:* For master's, thesis or alternative. *Entrance requirements:* For master's, GRE, writing exam, minimum GPA of 3.0. *Application deadline:* For fall admission, 8/31 priority date for domestic students. Application fee: $55. *Financial support:* Fellowships, research assistantships, and teaching assistantships available. *Faculty research:* Smoking and health, oral hygiene, menopause, health services research. *Unit head:* Dr. Marsha Greer, Assistant Dean, 909-537-5339, Fax: 909-537-7037, E-mail: mgreer@csusb.edu. *Application contact:* Dr. Jeffrey Thompson, Dean of Graduate Studies, 909-537-5058, E-mail: jthompso@csusb.edu.

Cambridge College, School of Management, Cambridge, MA 02138-5304. Offers business negotiation and conflict resolution (M Mgt); general business (M Mgt); health care informatics (M Mgt); health care management (M Mgt); leadership in human and organizational dynamics (M Mgt); non-profit and public organization management (M Mgt); small business development (M Mgt); technology management (M Mgt). Part-time and evening/weekend programs available. *Degree requirements:* For master's, thesis, seminars. *Entrance requirements:* For master's, resume, 2 professional references. Additional exam requirements/recommendations for international students: Required—TOEFL (minimum score 550 paper-based; 79 iBT), Michigan English Language Assessment Battery (minimum score 85); Recommended—IELTS (minimum score 6). Electronic applications accepted. *Expenses:* Contact institution. *Faculty research:* Negotiation, mediation and conflict resolution; leadership; management of diverse organizations; case studies and simulation methodologies for management education, digital as a second language: social networking for digital immigrants, non-profit and public management.

Capella University, School of Business and Technology, Master's Programs in Business, Minneapolis, MN 55402. Offers accounting (MBA); business analysis (MS); business intelligence (MBA); entrepreneurship (MBA); finance (MBA); general business administration (MBA); general human resource management (MS); general leadership (MS); health care management (MBA); human resource management (MBA); marketing (MBA); project management (MBA, MS).

Capella University, School of Public Service Leadership, Doctoral Programs in Healthcare, Minneapolis, MN 55402. Offers criminal justice (PhD); emergency management (PhD); epidemiology (Dr PH); general health administration (DHA); general public administration (DPA); health advocacy and leadership (Dr PH); health care administration (PhD); health care leadership (DHA); health policy advocacy (DHA); multidisciplinary human services (PhD); nonprofit management and leadership (PhD); public safety leadership (PhD); social and community services (PhD).

Capella University, School of Public Service Leadership, Master's Programs in Healthcare, Minneapolis, MN 55402. Offers criminal justice (MS); emergency management (MS); general public health (MPH); gerontology (MS); health administration (MHA); health care operations (MHA); health management policy (MPH); health policy (MHA); homeland security (MS); multidisciplinary human sevrices (MS); public administration (MPA); public safety leadership (MS); social and community services (MS); social behavioral sciences (MPH); MS/MPA.

Carlow University, School of Management, MBA Program, Pittsburgh, PA 15213-3165. Offers business administration (MBA); global business (MBA); healthcare management (MBA); project management (MBA). Part-time and evening/weekend programs available. Postbaccalaureate distance learning degree programs offered (no on-campus study). *Students:* 121 full-time (96 women), 26 part-time (17 women); includes 30 minority (22 Black or African American, non-Hispanic/Latino; 3 Asian, non-Hispanic/Latino; 3 Hispanic/Latino; 2 Two or more races, non-Hispanic/Latino), 5 international. Average age 32. 53 applicants, 96% accepted, 38 enrolled. In 2013, 41 master's awarded. *Entrance requirements:* For master's, minimum undergraduate GPA of 3.0; essay; resume; transcripts; two recommendations. Additional exam requirements/recommendations for international students: Required—TOEFL (minimum score 550 paper-based). *Application deadline:* Applications are processed on a rolling basis. Application fee: $20. Electronic applications accepted. Application fee is waived when completed online. *Expenses: Tuition:* Full-time $9523; part-time $744 per credit. Tuition

and fees vary according to course load, degree level and program. *Unit head:* Dr. Enrique Mu, Chair, MBA Program, 412-578-8729, E-mail: emu@carlow.edu. *Application contact:* Jo Danhires, Administrative Assistant, Admissions, 412-578-6088, Fax: 412-578-6321, E-mail: gradstudies@carlow.edu.
Website: http://gradstudies.carlow.edu/management/mba.html

Carnegie Mellon University, H. John Heinz III College, School of Public Policy and Management, Master of Science Program in Health Care Policy and Management, Pittsburgh, PA 15213-3891. Offers MSHCPM. Part-time and evening/weekend programs available. *Degree requirements:* For master's, internship. *Entrance requirements:* For master's, GRE or GMAT, college-level course in advanced algebra/pre-calculus; college-level courses in economics and statistics (recommended). Additional exam requirements/recommendations for international students: Required—TOEFL or IELTS. *Application deadline:* For fall admission, 1/10 for domestic students. Applications are processed on a rolling basis. Application fee: $0. Electronic applications accepted. *Financial support:* Scholarships/grants available. *Unit head:* James F. Jordan, Senior Director, 412-268-9952, E-mail: jfjordan@andrew.cmu.edu. *Application contact:* Gerrie Halloran, Program Coordinator, 412-268-5301, E-mail: gh1m@andrew.cmu.edu.
Website: http://www.heinz.cmu.edu/school-of-public-policy-management/healthcare-policy-management-hcpm/

Carnegie Mellon University, H. John Heinz III College, School of Public Policy and Management, Programs in Medical Management, Pittsburgh, PA 15213-3891. Offers MMM. *Application deadline:* For fall admission, 1/10 for domestic students. *Unit head:* James F. Jordan, Senior Director, 412-268-9952, E-mail: jfjordan@andrew.cmu.edu. *Application contact:* Barbara L. Pacella, Executive Programs Specialist, 412-268-4656, E-mail: bpacella@andrew.cmu.edu.
Website: http://info.heinz.cmu.edu/

Central Michigan University, Central Michigan University Global Campus, Program in Administration, Mount Pleasant, MI 48859. Offers acquisitions administration (MSA, Certificate); engineering management administration (MSA, Certificate); general administration (MSA, Certificate); health services administration (MSA, Certificate); human resources administration (MSA, Certificate); information resource management (MSA); information resource management administration (Certificate); international administration (MSA, Certificate); leadership (MSA, Certificate); philanthropy and fundraising administration (MSA, Certificate); public administration (MSA, Certificate); recreation and park administration (MSA); research administration (MSA, Certificate). Part-time and evening/weekend programs available. Postbaccalaureate distance learning degree programs offered (no on-campus study). *Students:* Average age 38. *Entrance requirements:* For master's, minimum GPA of 2.7 in major. *Application deadline:* Applications are processed on a rolling basis. Application fee: $50. Electronic applications accepted. *Financial support:* Scholarships/grants available. Support available to part-time students. Financial award applicants required to submit FAFSA. *Unit head:* Dr. Patricia Chase, Director, 989-774-1845, E-mail: chase1pb@cmich.edu. *Application contact:* 877-268-4636, E-mail: cmuglobal@cmich.edu.

Central Michigan University, Central Michigan University Global Campus, Program in Health Administration, Mount Pleasant, MI 48859. Offers health administration (DHA); international health (Certificate); nutrition and dietetics (MS). Part-time and evening/weekend programs available. Postbaccalaureate distance learning degree programs offered (minimal on-campus study). Electronic applications accepted. *Financial support:* Scholarships/grants available. Support available to part-time students. Financial award applicants required to submit FAFSA. *Unit head:* Dr. Steven D. Berkshire, Director, 989-774-1640, E-mail: berks1sd@cmich.edu. *Application contact:* Off-Campus Programs Call Center, 877-268-4636, E-mail: cmuoffcampus@cmich.edu.

Central Michigan University, College of Graduate Studies, The Herbert H. and Grace A. Dow College of Health Professions, School of Health Sciences, Mount Pleasant, MI 48859. Offers exercise science (MA); health administration (DHA). Part-time and evening/weekend programs available. Postbaccalaureate distance learning degree programs offered (no on-campus study). *Degree requirements:* For doctorate, comprehensive exam, thesis/dissertation. *Entrance requirements:* For doctorate, accredited master's or doctoral degree, 5 years of related work experience. Electronic applications accepted. *Faculty research:* Exercise science.

Central Michigan University, College of Graduate Studies, Interdisciplinary Administration Programs, Mount Pleasant, MI 48859. Offers acquisitions administration (MSA, Graduate Certificate); general administration (MSA, Graduate Certificate); health services administration (MSA, Graduate Certificate); human resource administration (Graduate Certificate); human resources administration (MSA); information resource management (MSA, Graduate Certificate); international administration (MSA, Graduate Certificate); leadership (MSA, Graduate Certificate); public administration (MSA, Graduate Certificate); research administration (Graduate Certificate); sport administration (MSA). *Accreditation:* AACSB. Part-time and evening/weekend programs available. Postbaccalaureate distance learning degree programs offered (no on-campus study). *Degree requirements:* For master's, thesis or alternative. *Entrance requirements:* For master's, bachelor's degree with minimum GPA of 2.7. Electronic applications accepted. *Faculty research:* Interdisciplinary studies in acquisitions administration, health services administration, sport administration, recreation and park administration, and international administration.

Champlain College, Graduate Studies, Burlington, VT 05402-0670. Offers business (MBA); digital forensic management (MS); digital forensic science (MS); early childhood education (M Ed); emergent media (MFA, MS); health care administration (MS); law (MS); managing innovation and information technology (MS); mediation and applied conflict studies (MS). MS in emergent media program held in Shanghai. Part-time programs available. Postbaccalaureate distance learning degree programs offered (no on-campus study). *Faculty:* 13 full-time (2 women), 34 part-time/adjunct (14 women). *Students:* 303 full-time (191 women), 104 part-time (58 women); includes 38 minority (21 Black or African American, non-Hispanic/Latino; 8 Asian, non-Hispanic/Latino; 7 Hispanic/Latino; 2 Two or more races, non-Hispanic/Latino), 4 international. Average age 37. In 2013, 169 master's awarded. *Degree requirements:* For master's, capstone project. *Entrance requirements:* Additional exam requirements/recommendations for international students: Required—TOEFL (minimum score 550 paper-based; 80 iBT). *Application deadline:* For fall admission, 8/1 priority date for domestic and international students; for spring admission, 1/1 priority date for domestic and international students. Applications are processed on a rolling basis. Electronic applications accepted. *Expenses: Tuition:* Full-time $18,456; part-time $769 per credit. Tuition and fees vary according to program. *Financial support:* Applicants required to submit FAFSA. *Unit head:* Dr. Donald Haggerty, Associate Provost of Graduate Studies, 802-865-6496, Fax: 802-865-6447, E-mail: haggerty@champlain.edu. *Application contact:* Matt Manz, Assistant Director, Graduate Admission, 800-383-6603, E-mail: mmanz@champlain.edu.
Website: http://www.champlain.edu/academics/graduate-studies

Clayton State University, School of Graduate Studies, College of Business, Program in Health Administration, Morrow, GA 30260-0285. Offers MHA. Part-time and evening/weekend programs available. *Degree requirements:* For master's, comprehensive exam, thesis. *Entrance requirements:* For master's, GRE/GMAT, 2 official copies of transcripts, 3 letters of recommendation, statement of purpose. Additional exam requirements/recommendations for international students: Required—TOEFL (minimum score 550 paper-based; 80 iBT). Electronic applications accepted. *Expenses:* Contact institution.

Cleary University, Online Program in Business Administration, Ann Arbor, MI 48105-2659. Offers accounting (MBA); financial planning (MBA); financial planning (Graduate Certificate); green business strategy (MBA, Graduate Certificate); health care leadership (MBA); management (MBA); nonprofit management (MBA, Graduate Certificate); organizational leadership (MBA). Part-time and evening/weekend programs available. Postbaccalaureate distance learning degree programs offered (no on-campus study). *Degree requirements:* For master's, thesis. *Entrance requirements:* For master's, bachelor's degree; minimum GPA of 2.5; professional resume indicating minimum of 2 years of management or related experience; undergraduate degree from accredited college or university with at least 18 quarter hours (or 12 semester hours) of accounting study (for MBA in accounting). Additional exam requirements/recommendations for international students: Required—TOEFL (minimum score 550 paper-based; 79 iBT), Michigan English Language Assessment Battery (minimum score 75). Electronic applications accepted.

Cleveland State University, College of Graduate Studies, Maxine Goodman Levin College of Urban Affairs, Program in Public Administration, Cleveland, OH 44115. Offers city management (MPA); economic development (MPA); healthcare administration (MPA); local and urban management (Certificate); non-profit management (MPA, Certificate); public financial management (MPA); public management (MPA); urban economic development (Certificate); JD/MPA. *Accreditation:* NASPAA. Part-time and evening/weekend programs available. *Faculty:* 21 full-time (10 women), 11 part-time/adjunct (3 women). *Students:* 16 full-time (11 women), 64 part-time (40 women); includes 23 minority (19 Black or African American, non-Hispanic/Latino; 3 Hispanic/Latino; 1 Two or more races, non-Hispanic/Latino), 3 international. Average age 36. 67 applicants, 51% accepted, 13 enrolled. In 2013, 56 master's awarded. *Degree requirements:* For master's, thesis or alternative, capstone course. *Entrance requirements:* For master's, GRE General Test (minimum scores in 40th percentile verbal and quantitative, 4.0 writing), minimum GPA of 3.0. Additional exam requirements/recommendations for international students: Required—TOEFL (minimum score 525 paper-based; 65 iBT), IELTS or ITEP. *Application deadline:* For fall admission, 7/15 priority date for domestic students, 5/15 for international students; for spring admission, 11/1 for international students. Applications are processed on a rolling basis. Application fee: $30. Electronic applications accepted. *Expenses:* Tuition, state resident: full-time $8335; part-time $521 per credit hour. Tuition, nonresident: full-time $15,670; part-time $979 per credit hour. *Required fees:* $50; $25 per semester. *Financial support:* In 2013–14, 16 students received support, including 12 research assistantships with full and partial tuition reimbursements available (averaging $4,800 per year), 4 teaching assistantships with full and partial tuition reimbursements available (averaging $3,300 per year); career-related internships or fieldwork, scholarships/grants, traineeships, and unspecified assistantships also available. Support available to part-time students. Financial award application deadline: 3/1; financial award applicants required to submit FAFSA. *Faculty research:* City management, nonprofit management, health care administration, public management, economic development. *Unit head:* Dr. Nicholas Zingale, Director, 216-802-3398, Fax: 216-687-9342, E-mail: n.zingale@csuohio.edu. *Application contact:* David Arrighi, Graduate Academic Advisor, 216-523-7522, Fax: 216-687-5398, E-mail: urbanprograms@csuohio.edu.
Website: http://urban.csuohio.edu/academics/graduate/mpa/

Cleveland State University, College of Graduate Studies, Monte Ahuja College of Business, MBA Programs, Cleveland, OH 44115. Offers business administration (AMBA, MBA); executive business administration (EMBA); health care administration (MBA); JD/MBA; MSN/MBA. Programs also offered at Progressive Insurance Corporation, The Cleveland Clinic, and MetroHealth Medical Center. *Accreditation:* AACSB. Part-time and evening/weekend programs available. Postbaccalaureate distance learning degree programs offered (no on-campus study). *Faculty:* 33 full-time (9 women), 16 part-time/adjunct (2 women). *Students:* 258 full-time (116 women), 467 part-time (198 women); includes 130 minority (69 Black or African American, non-Hispanic/Latino; 3 American Indian or Alaska Native, non-Hispanic/Latino; 25 Asian, non-Hispanic/Latino; 23 Hispanic/Latino; 10 Two or more races, non-Hispanic/Latino), 98 international. Average age 30. 674 applicants, 48% accepted, 139 enrolled. In 2013, 325 master's awarded. *Degree requirements:* For master's, variable foreign language requirement, comprehensive exam (for some programs), thesis (for some programs). *Entrance requirements:* For master's, GMAT or GRE, minimum cumulative GPA of 2.75 from bachelor's degree; resume, statement of purpose and two letters of reference (for health care administration MBA). Additional exam requirements/recommendations for international students: Required—TOEFL (minimum score 550 paper-based; 78 iBT). *Application deadline:* For fall admission, 7/15 priority date for domestic students, 5/15 for international students; for spring admission, 12/15 priority date for domestic students, 11/1 for international students. Applications are processed on a rolling basis. Application fee: $30. *Expenses:* Tuition, state resident: full-time $8335; part-time $521 per credit hour. Tuition, nonresident: full-time $15,670; part-time $979 per credit hour. *Required fees:* $50; $25 per semester. *Financial support:* In 2013–14, 594 students received support, including 45 research assistantships with full and partial tuition reimbursements available (averaging $6,960 per year), 1 teaching assistantship with full and partial tuition reimbursement available (averaging $7,800 per year); tuition waivers (full) and unspecified assistantships also available. Financial award application deadline: 5/15; financial award applicants required to submit FAFSA. *Faculty research:* Accounting and finance, management and organizational behavior, marketing, computer information systems, international business. *Total annual research expenditures:* $70,000. *Unit head:* Ronald John Mickler, Jr., Acting Assistant Director, Graduate Programs, 216-687-3730, Fax: 216-687-5311, E-mail: cbacsu@csuohio.edu. *Application contact:* Kenneth Dippong, Director, Student Services, 216-523-7545, Fax: 216-687-9354, E-mail: k.dippong@csuohio.edu.
Website: http://www.csuohio.edu/cba/

The College at Brockport, State University of New York, School of Education and Human Services, Department of Public Administration, Brockport, NY 14420-2997. Offers arts administration (AGC); nonprofit management (AGC); public administration (MPA), including general public administration, health care management, nonprofit management. *Accreditation:* NASPAA. Part-time and evening/weekend programs available. *Faculty:* 5 full-time (2 women), 1 part-time/adjunct (0 women). *Students:* 24 full-time (16 women), 50 part-time (36 women); includes 11 minority (all Black or African American, non-Hispanic/Latino), 2 international. 38 applicants, 87% accepted, 19 enrolled. In 2013, 32 master's, 7 other advanced degrees awarded. *Degree requirements:* For master's, thesis or alternative. *Entrance requirements:* For master's, GRE or minimum GPA of 3.0, letters of recommendation, statement of objectives, current resume. Additional exam requirements/recommendations for international students: Required—TOEFL (minimum score 550 paper-based; 79 iBT), IELTS (minimum score 6.5). *Application deadline:* For fall admission, 8/15 priority date for domestic and international students; for spring admission, 1/15 priority date for domestic and international students. Application fee: $50. Electronic applications accepted.

Expenses: Tuition, state resident: full-time $9870. Tuition, nonresident: full-time $18,350. *Required fees:* $1848. *Financial support:* In 2013–14, 1 fellowship with full tuition reimbursement (averaging $7,500 per year), 1 teaching assistantship with full tuition reimbursement (averaging $6,000 per year) were awarded; Federal Work-Study, scholarships/grants, and unspecified assistantships also available. Support available to part-time students. Financial award application deadline: 3/15; financial award applicants required to submit FAFSA. *Faculty research:* E-government, performance management, nonprofits and policy implementation, Medicaid and disabilities. *Unit head:* Dr. Celia Watt, Graduate Director, 585-395-5538, Fax: 585-395-2172, E-mail: cwatt@brockport.edu. *Application contact:* Danielle A. Welch, Graduate Admissions Counselor, 585-395-2525, Fax: 585-395-2515.
Website: http://www.brockport.edu/pubadmin

College of Saint Elizabeth, Department of Health Care Management, Morristown, NJ 07960-6989. Offers MS. Part-time programs available. *Faculty:* 3 full-time (2 women), 5 part-time/adjunct (4 women). *Students:* 3 full-time (2 women), 93 part-time (75 women); includes 28 minority (9 Black or African American, non-Hispanic/Latino; 9 Asian, non-Hispanic/Latino; 10 Hispanic/Latino), 4 international. Average age 44. In 2013, 30 master's awarded. *Degree requirements:* For master's, thesis optional, culminating experience. *Entrance requirements:* For master's, minimum cumulative undergraduate GPA of 3.0, personal statement, resume, two letters of professional recommendation. Additional exam requirements/recommendations for international students: Required—TOEFL. *Application deadline:* Applications are processed on a rolling basis. Application fee: $35. Electronic applications accepted. *Expenses: Tuition:* Full-time $19,152; part-time $1064 per credit. *Financial support:* Career-related internships or fieldwork, tuition waivers (partial), and unspecified assistantships available. Support available to part-time students. Financial award application deadline: 3/15; financial award applicants required to submit FAFSA. *Faculty research:* Consumer protection in health care. *Unit head:* Dr. David B. Tataw, Associate Professor, Health Care Management, 973-290-4271, Fax: 973-290-4167, E-mail: dtataw@cse.edu. *Application contact:* Deborah S. Cobo, Associate Director for Graduate Admissions, 973-290-4194, Fax: 973-290-4710, E-mail: dscobo@cse.edu.
Website: http://www.cse.edu/academics/academic-programs/health-wellness/health-care-management/

Columbia Southern University, MBA Program, Orange Beach, AL 36561. Offers finance (MBA); health care management (MBA); human resource management (MBA); marketing (MBA); project management (MBA); public administration (MBA). Part-time and evening/weekend programs available. Postbaccalaureate distance learning degree programs offered (no on-campus study). *Entrance requirements:* For master's, bachelor's degree from accredited/approved institution. Additional exam requirements/recommendations for international students: Required—TOEFL. Electronic applications accepted.

Columbia University, Columbia University Mailman School of Public Health, Department of Health Policy and Management, New York, NY 10032. Offers Exec MPH, MPH. *Accreditation:* CAHME. Evening/weekend programs available. *Students:* 208 full-time (150 women), 132 part-time (82 women); includes 126 minority (26 Black or African American, non-Hispanic/Latino; 1 American Indian or Alaska Native, non-Hispanic/Latino; 63 Asian, non-Hispanic/Latino; 30 Hispanic/Latino; 1 Native Hawaiian or other Pacific Islander, non-Hispanic/Latino; 5 Two or more races, non-Hispanic/Latino), 35 international. Average age 29. 704 applicants, 61% accepted, 169 enrolled. In 2013, 159 master's awarded. *Degree requirements:* For master's, thesis optional. *Entrance requirements:* For master's, GRE General Test. Additional exam requirements/recommendations for international students: Required—TOEFL (minimum score 600 paper-based; 100 iBT). *Application deadline:* For fall admission, 12/1 priority date for domestic and international students. Application fee: $120. Electronic applications accepted. *Financial support:* Research assistantships, teaching assistantships, career-related internships or fieldwork, and Federal Work-Study available. Support available to part-time students. Financial award application deadline: 2/1; financial award applicants required to submit FAFSA. *Faculty research:* Health care reform, health care disparities, state and national and cross-national health policy, health care quality, organization structure and performance. *Unit head:* Dr. Michael Sparer, Chairperson, 212-305-3924. *Application contact:* Dr. Joseph Korevec, Director of Admissions and Financial Aid, 212-305-8698, Fax: 212-342-1861, E-mail: ph-admit@columbia.edu.
Website: http://mailman.hs.columbia.edu/hpm/index.html

Concordia University, St. Paul, College of Business and Organizational Leadership, St. Paul, MN 55104-5494. Offers business and organizational leadership (MBA); criminal justice leadership (MA); forensic mental health (MA); health care management (MBA); human resource management (MA); leadership and management (MA). *Accreditation:* ACBSP. Evening/weekend programs available. Postbaccalaureate distance learning degree programs offered (minimal on-campus study). *Faculty:* 10 full-time (3 women), 20 part-time/adjunct (9 women). *Students:* 336 full-time (222 women), 84 part-time (44 women); includes 82 minority (46 Black or African American, non-Hispanic/Latino; 1 American Indian or Alaska Native, non-Hispanic/Latino; 17 Asian, non-Hispanic/Latino; 9 Hispanic/Latino; 1 Native Hawaiian or other Pacific Islander, non-Hispanic/Latino; 8 Two or more races, non-Hispanic/Latino), 1 international. Average age 34. 405 applicants, 50% accepted, 187 enrolled. In 2013, 253 master's awarded. *Degree requirements:* For master's, thesis (for some programs). *Entrance requirements:* For master's, official transcripts from regionally-accredited institution stating the conferral of a bachelor's degree with minimum cumulative GPA of 3.0; personal statement; professional resume. Additional exam requirements/recommendations for international students: Recommended—TOEFL (minimum score 547 paper-based; 78 iBT), IELTS (minimum score 6). *Application deadline:* For fall admission, 8/1 for domestic and international students; for spring admission, 12/1 for domestic and international students; for summer admission, 5/1 for domestic and international students. Applications are processed on a rolling basis. Application fee: $50. Electronic applications accepted. *Expenses: Tuition:* Full-time $6200; part-time $425 per credit. Tuition and fees vary according to degree level and program. *Financial support:* Applicants required to submit FAFSA. *Unit head:* Lonn Maly, Dean, 651-641-8203, Fax: 651-641-8807, E-mail: maly@csp.edu. *Application contact:* Kimberly Craig, Director of Graduate and Cohort Admission, 651-603-6223, Fax: 651-603-6320, E-mail: craig@csp.edu.

Concordia University Wisconsin, Graduate Programs, School of Business and Legal Studies, MBA Program, Mequon, WI 53097-2402. Offers finance (MBA); health care administration (MBA); human resource management (MBA); international business (MBA); international business-bilingual English/Chinese (MBA); management (MBA); management information systems (MBA); managerial communications (MBA); marketing (MBA); public administration (MBA); risk management (MBA). Postbaccalaureate distance learning degree programs offered (minimal on-campus study). *Degree requirements:* For master's, comprehensive exam, thesis or alternative. *Entrance requirements:* Additional exam requirements/recommendations for international students: Required—TOEFL. *Expenses:* Contact institution.

Copenhagen Business School, Graduate Programs, Copenhagen, Denmark. Offers business administration (Exec MBA, MBA, PhD); business administration and information systems (M Sc); business, language and culture (M Sc); economics and business administration (M Sc); health management (MHM); international business and politics (M Sc); public administration (MPA); shipping and logistics (Exec MBA); technology, market and organization (MBA).

Cornell University, Graduate School, Graduate Fields of Human Ecology, Field of Policy Analysis and Management, Ithaca, NY 14853-0001. Offers consumer policy (PhD); family and social welfare policy (PhD); health administration (MHA); health management and policy (PhD); public policy (PhD). *Faculty:* 33 full-time (12 women). *Students:* 66 full-time (39 women); includes 19 minority (2 Black or African American, non-Hispanic/Latino; 8 Asian, non-Hispanic/Latino; 5 Hispanic/Latino; 4 Two or more races, non-Hispanic/Latino), 9 international. Average age 25. 175 applicants, 30% accepted, 36 enrolled. In 2013, 26 master's, 2 doctorates awarded. *Degree requirements:* For master's, thesis; for doctorate, thesis/dissertation. *Entrance requirements:* For master's, GRE General Test or GMAT, 2 letters of recommendation; for doctorate, GRE General Test, 2 letters of recommendation. Additional exam requirements/recommendations for international students: Required—TOEFL (minimum score 550 paper-based; 77 iBT). *Application deadline:* For fall admission, 1/15 for domestic students. Application fee: $95. Electronic applications accepted. *Financial support:* In 2013–14, 16 students received support, including 3 fellowships with full and partial tuition reimbursements available, 2 research assistantships with full and partial tuition reimbursements available, 11 teaching assistantships with full and partial tuition reimbursements available; institutionally sponsored loans, scholarships/grants, health care benefits, tuition waivers (full and partial), and unspecified assistantships also available. Financial award applicants required to submit FAFSA. *Faculty research:* Health policy, family policy, social welfare policy, program evaluation, consumer policy. *Unit head:* Director of Graduate Studies, 607-255-7772. *Application contact:* Graduate Field Assistant, 607-255-7772, Fax: 607-255-4071, E-mail: pam_phd@cornell.edu.
Website: http://www.gradschool.cornell.edu/fields.php?id-69&a-2

Daemen College, Program in Executive Leadership and Change, Amherst, NY 14226-3592. Offers business (MS); health professions (MS); not-for-profit organizations (MS). Part-time and evening/weekend programs available. *Degree requirements:* For master's, thesis, cohort learning sequence (2 years for weekend cohort; 3 years for weeknight cohort). *Entrance requirements:* For master's, 2 letters of recommendation, interview, goal statement, official transcripts, resume. Additional exam requirements/recommendations for international students: Required—TOEFL (minimum score 500 paper-based; 63 iBT), IELTS (minimum score 5.5). Electronic applications accepted.

Dalhousie University, Faculty of Health Professions, School of Health Administration, Halifax, NS B3H 1R2, Canada. Offers MAHSR, MHA, MPH, PhD, LL B/MHA, MBA/MHA, MHA/MN. *Accreditation:* CAHME. Part-time programs available. Postbaccalaureate distance learning degree programs offered (minimal on-campus study). *Entrance requirements:* For master's, GMAT. Additional exam requirements/recommendations for international students: Required—TOEFL, IELTS, CANTEST, CAEL, or Michigan English Language Assessment Battery. Electronic applications accepted. *Expenses:* Contact institution. *Faculty research:* Hospital, nursing, long-term, public, and community health administration; government administration in health areas.

Dallas Baptist University, College of Business, Business Administration Program, Dallas, TX 75211-9299. Offers accounting (MBA); business communication (MBA); conflict resolution management (MBA); entrepreneurship (MBA); finance (MBA); health care management (MBA); international business (MBA); leading the non-profit organization (MBA); management (MBA); management information systems (MBA); marketing (MBA); project management (MBA); technology and engineering (MBA). *Accreditation:* ACBSP. Part-time and evening/weekend programs available. *Entrance requirements:* For master's, GMAT, minimum GPA of 3.0. Additional exam requirements/recommendations for international students: Required—TOEFL, IELTS. *Application deadline:* Applications are processed on a rolling basis. Application fee: $25. Electronic applications accepted. *Expenses: Tuition:* Full-time $13,410; part-time $745 per credit hour. *Required fees:* $300; $150 per semester. Tuition and fees vary according to degree level. *Financial support:* Federal Work-Study, institutionally sponsored loans, scholarships/grants, and tuition waivers (full and partial) available. Support available to part-time students. Financial award applicants required to submit FAFSA. *Faculty research:* Sports management, services marketing, retailing, strategic management, financial planning/investments. *Unit head:* Dr. Sandra S. Reid, Chair, 214-333-5280, Fax: 214-333-5293, E-mail: graduate@dbu.edu. *Application contact:* Kit P. Montgomery, Director of Graduate Programs, 214-333-5242, Fax: 214-333-5579, E-mail: graduate@dbu.edu.
Website: http://www3.dbu.edu/graduate/mba.asp

Dallas Baptist University, College of Business, Management Program, Dallas, TX 75211-9299. Offers conflict resolution management (MA); general management (MA); health care management (MA); human resource management (MA); organizational management (MA); performance management (MA); professional sales and management optimization (MA). Part-time and evening/weekend programs available. *Entrance requirements:* For master's, GRE General Test, minimum GPA of 3.0. Additional exam requirements/recommendations for international students: Required—TOEFL, IELTS. *Application deadline:* Applications are processed on a rolling basis. Application fee: $25. Electronic applications accepted. *Expenses: Tuition:* Full-time $13,410; part-time $745 per credit hour. *Required fees:* $300; $150 per semester. Tuition and fees vary according to degree level. *Financial support:* Federal Work-Study, institutionally sponsored loans, scholarships/grants, and tuition waivers (full and partial) available. Support available to part-time students. Financial award applicants required to submit FAFSA. *Faculty research:* Organizational behavior, conflict personalities. *Unit head:* Joanne Hix, Director, 214-333-5280, Fax: 214-333-5293, E-mail: graduate@dbu.edu. *Application contact:* Kit P. Montgomery, Director of Graduate Programs, 214-333-5242, Fax: 214-333-5579, E-mail: graduate@dbu.edu.
Website: http://www3.dbu.edu/graduate/maom.asp

Dartmouth College, The Dartmouth Institute, Program in Health Policy and Clinical Practice, Hanover, NH 03755. Offers evaluative clinical sciences (MS, PhD). Part-time programs available. *Degree requirements:* For master's, research project or practicum; for doctorate, thesis/dissertation. *Entrance requirements:* For master's and doctorate, GRE or MCAT, 3 letters of recommendation. Additional exam requirements/recommendations for international students: Required—TOEFL. *Faculty research:* Prevention and treatment of cardiovascular diseases, health care cost containment, variation of delivery of care, health care improvement, decision evaluation.

Davenport University, Sneden Graduate School, Grand Rapids, MI 49512. Offers accounting (MBA); business administration (EMBA); finance (MBA); health care management (MBA); human resources (MBA); information assurance (MS); public health (MPH); strategic management (MBA). Evening/weekend programs available. *Entrance requirements:* For master's, GMAT, minimum undergraduate GPA of 2.75. Additional exam requirements/recommendations for international students: Required—TOEFL. Electronic applications accepted. *Faculty research:* Leadership, management, marketing, organizational culture.

Defiance College, Program in Business Administration, Defiance, OH 43512-1610. Offers criminal justice (MBA); health care (MBA); leadership (MBA); sport management (MBA). Part-time and evening/weekend programs available. *Degree requirements:* For master's, thesis. *Entrance requirements:* For master's, minimum GPA of 2.5. Additional exam requirements/recommendations for international students: Recommended—TOEFL.

Delta State University, Graduate Programs, School of Nursing, Cleveland, MS 38733. Offers family nurse practitioner (MSN); nurse administrator (MSN); nurse educator (MSN). *Accreditation:* AACN. Part-time programs available. *Faculty:* 5 full-time (all women), 1 (woman) part-time/adjunct. *Students:* 35 full-time (31 women), 8 part-time (7 women); includes 10 minority (all Black or African American, non-Hispanic/Latino). Average age 41. 23 applicants, 100% accepted, 19 enrolled. In 2013, 13 master's awarded. *Degree requirements:* For master's, thesis optional. *Entrance requirements:* For master's, GRE General Test. *Application deadline:* For fall admission, 8/1 priority date for domestic students; for spring admission, 12/1 priority date for domestic students. Applications are processed on a rolling basis. Application fee: $0. Electronic applications accepted. *Expenses:* Tuition, state resident: full-time $3006; part-time $334 per credit hour. Tuition, nonresident: full-time $3006; part-time $334 per credit hour. *Financial support:* Research assistantships, career-related internships or fieldwork, Federal Work-Study, and institutionally sponsored loans available. Financial award application deadline: 6/1. *Unit head:* Dr. Lizabeth Carlson, Dean, 662-846-4268, Fax: 662-846-4267, E-mail: lcarlson@deltastate.edu. *Application contact:* Dr. Albert Nylander, Dean of Graduate Studies, 662-846-4875, Fax: 662-846-4313, E-mail: grad-info@deltastate.edu.
Website: http://www.deltastate.edu/pages/252.asp

DePaul University, Charles H. Kellstadt Graduate School of Business, Chicago, IL 60604. Offers accountancy (M Acc, MS, MSA); applied economics (MBA); banking (MBA); behavioral finance (MBA); brand and product management (MBA); business development (MBA); business information technology (MS); business strategy and decision-making (MBA); computational finance (MS); consumer insights (MBA); corporate finance (MBA); economic policy analysis (MS); entrepreneurship (MBA, MS); finance (MBA, MS); financial analysis (MBA); general business (MBA); health sector management (MBA); hospitality leadership (MBA); hospitality leadership and operational performance (MS); human resource management (MBA); human resources (MS); investment management (MBA); leadership and change management (MBA); management accounting (MBA); marketing (MBA, MS); marketing analysis (MS); marketing strategy and planning (MBA); operations management (MBA); organizational diversity (MBA); real estate (MS); real estate finance and investment (MBA); revenue management (MBA); sports management (MBA); strategic global marketing (MBA); strategy, execution and valuation (MBA); sustainable management (MBA, MS); taxation (MS); wealth management (MS); JD/MBA. *Accreditation:* AACSB. Part-time and evening/weekend programs available. Postbaccalaureate distance learning degree programs offered (no on-campus study). *Faculty:* 81 full-time (20 women), 45 part-time/adjunct (8 women). *Students:* 1,238 full-time (605 women), 617 part-time (223 women); includes 295 minority (71 Black or African American, non-Hispanic/Latino; 129 Asian, non-Hispanic/Latino; 74 Hispanic/Latino; 4 Native Hawaiian or other Pacific Islander, non-Hispanic/Latino; 17 Two or more races, non-Hispanic/Latino), 462 international. Average age 29. In 2013, 911 master's awarded. *Entrance requirements:* For master's, GMAT, 2 letters of recommendation, resume, essay, official transcripts. Additional exam requirements/recommendations for international students: Required—TOEFL (minimum score 550 paper-based; 80 iBT). *Application deadline:* For fall admission, 7/1 for domestic students, 6/1 for international students; for winter admission, 10/1 for domestic students, 9/1 for international students; for spring admission, 2/1 for domestic students, 1/1 for international students. Applications are processed on a rolling basis. Application fee: $60. Electronic applications accepted. *Expenses:* Contact institution. *Financial support:* Application deadline: 4/1; applicants required to submit FAFSA. *Unit head:* Robert T. Ryan, Assistant Dean and Director, 312-362-8810, Fax: 312-362-6677, E-mail: rryan1@depaul.edu. *Application contact:* James Parker, Director of Recruitment and Admission, 312-362-8810, Fax: 312-362-6677, E-mail: kgsb@depaul.edu.
Website: http://kellstadt.depaul.edu

DeSales University, Graduate Division, Division of Business, Center Valley, PA 18034-9568. Offers accounting (MBA); computer information systems (MBA); finance (MBA); health care systems management (MBA); human resources management (MBA); management (MBA); marketing (MBA); project management (MBA); self-design (MBA). *Accreditation:* ACBSP. Part-time and evening/weekend programs available. Postbaccalaureate distance learning degree programs offered (no on-campus study). *Students:* 444 part-time. Average age 37. In 2013, 1 master's awarded. *Entrance requirements:* For master's, GMAT, minimum GPA of 3.0, 2 years of work experience. Additional exam requirements/recommendations for international students: Required—TOEFL. *Application deadline:* Applications are processed on a rolling basis. Application fee: $50. Electronic applications accepted. *Expenses: Tuition:* Part-time $790 per credit. *Financial support:* Applicants required to submit FAFSA. *Faculty research:* Quality improvement, executive development, productivity, cross-cultural managerial differences, leadership. *Unit head:* Dr. David Gilfoil, Director, 610-282-1100 Ext. 1828, Fax: 610-282-2869, E-mail: david.gilfoil@desales.edu. *Application contact:* Abigail Wernicki, Director of Graduate Admissions, 610-282-1100 Ext. 1768, E-mail: gradadmissions@desales.edu.

Des Moines University, College of Health Sciences, Program in Healthcare Administration, Des Moines, IA 50312-4104. Offers MHA. Part-time and evening/weekend programs available. *Entrance requirements:* For master's, minimum GPA of 3.0. Additional exam requirements/recommendations for international students: Required—TOEFL (minimum score 600 paper-based). Electronic applications accepted. *Expenses:* Contact institution. *Faculty research:* Quality improvement, rural sociology, women's health, health promotion, patient education.

Dowling College, School of Business, Oakdale, NY 11769. Offers aviation management (MBA, Certificate); corporate finance (MBA, Certificate); health care management (MBA); human resource management (Certificate); information systems management (MBA); management and leadership (MBA); marketing (Certificate); project management (Certificate); public management (MBA); school district business leader (MBA); sport, event and entertainment management (Certificate); JD/MBA. Part-time and evening/weekend programs available. Postbaccalaureate distance learning degree programs offered (minimal on-campus study). *Faculty:* 7 full-time (2 women), 43 part-time/adjunct (7 women). *Students:* 183 full-time (79 women), 299 part-time (142 women); includes 137 minority (84 Black or African American, non-Hispanic/Latino; 14 Asian, non-Hispanic/Latino; 20 Hispanic/Latino; 19 Native Hawaiian or other Pacific Islander, non-Hispanic/Latino). Average age 32. 360 applicants, 58% accepted, 127 enrolled. In 2013, 235 master's, 15 other advanced degrees awarded. *Degree requirements:* For master's, comprehensive exam, thesis optional. *Entrance requirements:* For master's, minimum GPA of 2.8, 2 letters of recommendation, courses or seminar in accounting and finance, resume. Additional exam requirements/recommendations for international students: Required—TOEFL (minimum score 550 paper-based). *Application deadline:* For fall admission, 9/1 priority date for domestic students; for winter admission, 1/1 priority date for domestic students; for spring admission, 2/1 priority date for domestic students. Applications are processed on a rolling basis. Application fee: $50. Electronic applications accepted. *Expenses: Tuition:* Full-time $22,731; part-time $1029 per credit. *Required fees:* $956; $956. *Financial support:* Career-related internships or fieldwork and Federal Work-Study available. Support available to part-time students. Financial award application deadline: 6/30; financial award applicants required to submit FAFSA. *Faculty research:* International finance, computer applications, labor relations, executive development. *Unit head:* Dr. Elana Zolfo, Dean, 631-244-3266, Fax: 631-244-1018, E-mail: zolfoe@dowling.edu. *Application contact:* Mary Boullianne, Dean of Admissions, 631-244-3274, Fax: 631-244-1059, E-mail: boulliam@dowling.edu.

Duke University, The Fuqua School of Business, Cross Continent Executive MBA Program, Durham, NC 27708-0586. Offers business administration (MBA); energy and the environment (MBA); entrepreneurship and innovation (MBA); finance (MBA); health sector management (Certificate); marketing (MBA); strategy (MBA). *Faculty:* 91 full-time (15 women), 53 part-time/adjunct (9 women). *Students:* 121 full-time (34 women); includes 23 minority (3 Black or African American, non-Hispanic/Latino; 15 Asian, non-Hispanic/Latino; 4 Hispanic/Latino; 1 Native Hawaiian or other Pacific Islander, non-Hispanic/Latino), 31 international. Average age 30. In 2013, 147 master's awarded. *Degree requirements:* For master's, one foreign language. *Entrance requirements:* For master's, GMAT or GRE, transcripts, essays, resume, recommendation letters, interview. Additional exam requirements/recommendations for international students: Required—TOEFL, IELTS, PTE. *Application deadline:* For fall admission, 10/16 for domestic students, 10/6 for international students; for winter admission, 2/12 for domestic and international students; for spring admission, 5/6 for domestic and international students; for summer admission, 6/4 for domestic students. Application fee: $225. Electronic applications accepted. *Financial support:* In 2013–14, 16 students received support. Institutionally sponsored loans and scholarships/grants available. Financial award applicants required to submit FAFSA. *Unit head:* John Gallagher, Associate Dean for Executive MBA Programs, 919-660-7641, E-mail: johng@duke.edu. *Application contact:* Liz Riley Hargrove, Associate Dean for Admissions, 919-660-1956, Fax: 919-681-8026, E-mail: admissions-info@fuqua.duke.edu.
Website: http://www.fuqua.duke.edu/programs/duke_mba/cross_continent/

Duke University, The Fuqua School of Business, Daytime MBA Program, Durham, NC 27708-0586. Offers academic excellence in finance (Certificate); business administration (MBA); decision sciences (MBA); energy and environment (MBA); energy finance (MBA); entrepreneurship and innovation (MBA); finance (MBA); financial analysis (MBA); health sector management (Certificate); leadership and ethics (MBA); management (MBA); marketing (MBA); operations management (MBA); social entrepreneurship (MBA); strategy (MBA). *Faculty:* 91 full-time (15 women), 53 part-time/adjunct (9 women). *Students:* 862 full-time (283 women); includes 179 minority (34 Black or African American, non-Hispanic/Latino; 1 American Indian or Alaska Native, non-Hispanic/Latino; 92 Asian, non-Hispanic/Latino; 42 Hispanic/Latino; 2 Native Hawaiian or other Pacific Islander, non-Hispanic/Latino; 8 Two or more races, non-Hispanic/Latino), 342 international. Average age 29. In 2013, 437 master's awarded. *Entrance requirements:* For master's, GMAT or GRE, transcripts, essays, resume, recommendation letters, interview. Additional exam requirements/recommendations for international students: Required—TOEFL, IELTS, PTE. *Application deadline:* For fall admission, 9/18 for domestic and international students; for winter admission, 10/21 for domestic and international students; for spring admission, 1/6 for domestic and international students; for summer admission, 3/20 for domestic and international students. Application fee: $225. Electronic applications accepted. *Financial support:* In 2013–14, 331 students received support. Institutionally sponsored loans and scholarships/grants available. Financial award applicants required to submit FAFSA. *Unit head:* Russ Morgan, Associate Dean for the Daytime MBA Program, 919-660-2931, Fax: 919-684-8742, E-mail: ruskin.morgan@duke.edu. *Application contact:* Liz Riley Hargrove, Associate Dean of Admissions, 919-660-7705, Fax: 919-681-8026, E-mail: liz.riley@duke.edu.
Website: http://www.fuqua.duke.edu/daytime-mba/

Duke University, The Fuqua School of Business, Global Executive MBA Program, Durham, NC 27708-0586. Offers business administration (MBA); energy and the environment (MBA); entrepreneurship and innovation (MBA); finance (MBA); health sector management (Certificate); marketing (MBA); strategy (MBA). *Faculty:* 91 full-time (15 women), 53 part-time/adjunct (9 women). *Students:* 49 full-time (7 women); includes 7 minority (1 Black or African American, non-Hispanic/Latino; 3 Asian, non-Hispanic/Latino; 3 Hispanic/Latino), 17 international. Average age 39. In 2013, 51 master's awarded. *Entrance requirements:* For master's, transcripts, essays, resume, recommendation letters, interview. Additional exam requirements/recommendations for international students: Required—TOEFL, IELTS, PTE. *Application deadline:* For fall admission, 9/4 for domestic and international students; for winter admission, 10/16 for domestic and international students; for spring admission, 12/5 for domestic and international students; for summer admission, 1/13 for domestic and international students. Application fee: $225. *Financial support:* In 2013–14, 8 students received support. Institutionally sponsored loans and scholarships/grants available. Financial award applicants required to submit FAFSA. *Unit head:* John Gallagher, Associate Dean for Executive MBA Programs, 919-660-7728, E-mail: johng@duke.edu. *Application contact:* Liz Riley Hargrove, Director of EMBA Admissions, 919-660-7705, Fax: 919-681-8026, E-mail: admissions-info@fuqua.duke.edu.
Website: http://www.fuqua.duke.edu/programs/duke_mba/global-executive/

Duke University, The Fuqua School of Business, Weekend Executive MBA Program, Durham, NC 27708-0586. Offers business administration (MBA); energy and environment (MBA); entrepreneurship and innovation (MBA); finance (MBA); health sector management (Certificate); marketing (MBA); strategy (MBA). *Faculty:* 91 full-time (15 women), 53 part-time/adjunct (9 women). *Students:* 93 full-time (14 women); includes 33 minority (5 Black or African American, non-Hispanic/Latino; 24 Asian, non-Hispanic/Latino; 3 Hispanic/Latino; 1 Two or more races, non-Hispanic/Latino), 15 international. Average age 36. In 2013, 103 master's awarded. *Degree requirements:* For master's, one foreign language. *Entrance requirements:* For master's, GMAT (preferred) or GRE, transcripts, essays, resume, recommendation letters, interview. Additional exam requirements/recommendations for international students: Required—TOEFL, IELTS, PTE. *Application deadline:* For fall admission, 9/4 for domestic and international students; for winter admission, 10/16 for domestic and international students; for spring admission, 2/12 for domestic and international students; for summer admission, 4/2 for domestic and international students. Application fee: $225. Electronic applications accepted. *Financial support:* In 2013–14, 14 students received support. Institutionally sponsored loans and scholarships/grants available. Financial award applicants required to submit FAFSA. *Unit head:* John Gallagher, Associate Dean for Executive MBA Programs, 919-660-7728, E-mail: johng@duke.edu. *Application contact:* Liz Riley Hargrove, Director of EMBA Admissions, 919-660-7705, Fax: 919-681-8026, E-mail: admissions-info@fuqua.duke.edu.
Website: http://www.fuqua.duke.edu/programs/duke_mba/weekend_executive/

Duquesne University, John G. Rangos, Sr. School of Health Sciences, Pittsburgh, PA 15282-0001. Offers health management systems (MHMS); occupational therapy (MS, OTD); physical therapy (DPT); physician assistant studies (MPAS); rehabilitation science (MS, PhD); speech-language pathology (MS); MBA/MHMS. *Accreditation:* AOTA (one or more programs are accredited); APTA (one or more programs are accredited); ASHA. Postbaccalaureate distance learning degree programs offered

(minimal on-campus study). *Faculty:* 41 full-time (29 women), 32 part-time/adjunct (15 women). *Students:* 232 full-time (174 women), 14 part-time (7 women); includes 12 minority (2 Black or African American, non-Hispanic/Latino; 7 Asian, non-Hispanic/Latino; 1 Hispanic/Latino; 2 Two or more races, non-Hispanic/Latino), 7 international. Average age 23. 951 applicants, 11% accepted, 35 enrolled. In 2013, 119 master's, 40 doctorates awarded. *Degree requirements:* For doctorate, comprehensive exam (for some programs), thesis/dissertation (for some programs). *Entrance requirements:* For master's, GRE General Test (speech-language pathology), 3 letters of recommendation; minimum GPA of 2.75 (health management systems), 3.0 (speech-language pathology); for doctorate, GRE General Test (for physical therapy and rehabilitation science), 3 letters of recommendation, minimum GPA of 3.0, personal interview. Additional exam requirements/recommendations for international students: Required—TOEFL (minimum score 550 paper-based; 90 iBT). *Application deadline:* For fall admission, 2/1 for domestic and international students; for spring admission, 7/1 for domestic and international students. Applications are processed on a rolling basis. Electronic applications accepted. *Expenses:* Contact institution. *Financial support:* Federal Work-Study available. Financial award applicants required to submit FAFSA. *Faculty research:* Neuronal processing, electrical stimulation on peripheral neuropathy, central nervous system (CNS) stimulatory and inhibitory signals, behavioral genetic methodologies to development disorders of speech, neurogenic communication disorders. *Total annual research expenditures:* $83,650. *Unit head:* Dr. Gregory H. Frazer, Dean, 412-396-5303, Fax: 412-396-5554, E-mail: frazer@duq.edu. *Application contact:* Christopher R. Hilf, Recruiter/Academic Advisor, 412-396-5653, Fax: 412-396-5554, E-mail: hilfc@duq.edu.
Website: http://www.duq.edu/academics/schools/health-sciences

Duquesne University, School of Leadership and Professional Advancement, Pittsburgh, PA 15282-0001. Offers leadership (MS), including business ethics, community leadership, global leadership, health care, information technology, leadership, liberal studies, professional administration, sports leadership. Part-time and evening/weekend programs available. Postbaccalaureate distance learning degree programs offered (no on-campus study). *Faculty:* 15 full-time (7 women), 64 part-time/adjunct (26 women). *Students:* 213 full-time (106 women), 170 part-time (86 women); includes 89 minority (59 Black or African American, non-Hispanic/Latino; 2 American Indian or Alaska Native, non-Hispanic/Latino; 7 Asian, non-Hispanic/Latino; 9 Hispanic/Latino; 1 Native Hawaiian or other Pacific Islander, non-Hispanic/Latino; 11 Two or more races, non-Hispanic/Latino), 9 international. Average age 36. 204 applicants, 56% accepted, 103 enrolled. In 2013, 140 master's awarded. *Degree requirements:* For master's, capstone course. *Entrance requirements:* For master's, professional work experience, 500-word essay, resume, interview. Additional exam requirements/recommendations for international students: Required—TOEFL (minimum score 80 iBT). *Application deadline:* Applications are processed on a rolling basis. Application fee: $0. Electronic applications accepted. Application fee is waived when completed online. *Expenses: Tuition:* Full-time $18,162; part-time $1009 per credit. *Required fees:* $1728; $96 per credit. Tuition and fees vary according to program. *Financial support:* Scholarships/grants available. Financial award applicants required to submit FAFSA. *Unit head:* Dr. Dorothy Bassett, Dean, 412-396-2141, Fax: 412-396-4711, E-mail: bassettd@duq.edu. *Application contact:* Marianne Leister, Director of Student Services, 412-396-4933, Fax: 412-396-5072, E-mail: leister@duq.edu.
Website: http://www.duq.edu/academics/schools/leadership-and-professional-advancement

D'Youville College, Department of Health Services Administration, Buffalo, NY 14201-1084. Offers clinical research associate (Certificate); health administration (Ed D); health policy and health education (Ed D); health services administration (MS, Certificate); long term care administration (Certificate). Part-time and evening/weekend programs available. *Students:* 38 full-time (25 women), 80 part-time (60 women); includes 28 minority (24 Black or African American, non-Hispanic/Latino; 2 American Indian or Alaska Native, non-Hispanic/Latino; 1 Hispanic/Latino; 1 Two or more races, non-Hispanic/Latino), 20 international. Average age 38. 81 applicants, 54% accepted, 25 enrolled. In 2013, 5 master's, 2 doctorates, 2 other advanced degrees awarded. *Degree requirements:* For master's, project or thesis. *Entrance requirements:* For master's, minimum GPA of 3.0 in major. Additional exam requirements/recommendations for international students: Required—TOEFL (minimum score 500 paper-based). *Application deadline:* For fall admission, 5/1 priority date for international students; for spring admission, 9/1 priority date for international students. Applications are processed on a rolling basis. Application fee: $25. Electronic applications accepted. *Financial support:* Career-related internships or fieldwork, Federal Work-Study, and scholarships/grants available. Support available to part-time students. Financial award application deadline: 3/1; financial award applicants required to submit FAFSA. *Faculty research:* Outcomes research in rehabilitation medicine, cost/benefit analysis of prospective payment systems. *Unit head:* Dr. Lisa Rafalson, Chair, 716-829-8489, Fax: 716-829-8184. *Application contact:* Linda Fisher, Graduate Admissions Director, 716-829-8400, Fax: 716-829-7900, E-mail: graduateadmissions@dyc.edu.

Eastern Kentucky University, The Graduate School, College of Arts and Sciences, Department of Government, Program in General Public Administration, Richmond, KY 40475-3102. Offers community development (MPA); community health administration (MPA); general public administration (MPA). *Accreditation:* NASPAA. Part-time and evening/weekend programs available. *Entrance requirements:* For master's, GRE General Test, minimum GPA of 2.5.

Eastern Mennonite University, Program in Business Administration, Harrisonburg, VA 22802-2462. Offers business administration (MBA); health services administration (MBA); non-profit management (MBA). Part-time and evening/weekend programs available. *Degree requirements:* For master's, final capstone course. *Entrance requirements:* For master's, GMAT, minimum GPA of 2.5, 2 years of work experience, 2 letters of reference. Additional exam requirements/recommendations for international students: Required—TOEFL (minimum score 500 paper-based). Electronic applications accepted. *Expenses:* Contact institution. *Faculty research:* Information security, Anabaptist/Mennonite experiences and perspectives, limits of multi-cultural education, international development performance criteria.

Eastern Michigan University, Graduate School, College of Arts and Sciences, Department of Political Science, Programs in Public Administration, Ypsilanti, MI 48197. Offers local government management (Graduate Certificate); management of public healthcare services (Graduate Certificate); public administration (MPA, Graduate Certificate); public budget management (Graduate Certificate); public land planning (Graduate Certificate); public management (Graduate Certificate); public personnel management (Graduate Certificate); public policy analysis (Graduate Certificate). *Accreditation:* NASPAA. *Students:* 8 full-time (5 women), 59 part-time (30 women); includes 14 minority (10 Black or African American, non-Hispanic/Latino; 2 Asian, non-Hispanic/Latino; 2 Hispanic/Latino), 1 international. Average age 36. 43 applicants, 63% accepted, 13 enrolled. In 2013, 25 master's, 6 other advanced degrees awarded. Application fee: $35. *Expenses:* Tuition, state resident: full-time $12,300; part-time $466 per credit hour. Tuition, nonresident: full-time $23,159; part-time $918 per credit hour. *Required fees:* $71 per credit hour. $46 per semester. One-time fee: $100. Tuition and fees vary according to course level and degree level. *Unit head:* Dr. Arnold Fleischmann, Department Head, 734-487-3113, Fax: 734-487-3340, E-mail: afleisch@emich.edu. *Application contact:* Dr. Gregory Plagens, Program Director, 734-487-2522, Fax: 734-487-3340, E-mail: gregory.plagens@emich.edu.

Eastern Michigan University, Graduate School, College of Health and Human Services, Interdisciplinary Program in Health and Human Services, Ypsilanti, MI 48197. Offers community building (Graduate Certificate). Part-time and evening/weekend programs available. *Students:* 1 part-time (0 women), all international. Average age 25. 7 applicants, 14% accepted, 1 enrolled. In 2013, 4 Graduate Certificates awarded. *Entrance requirements:* Additional exam requirements/recommendations for international students: Required—TOEFL. Application fee: $35. *Expenses:* Tuition, state resident: full-time $12,300; part-time $466 per credit hour. Tuition, nonresident: full-time $23,159; part-time $918 per credit hour. *Required fees:* $71 per credit hour. $46 per semester. One-time fee: $100. Tuition and fees vary according to course level and degree level. *Unit head:* Dr. Marcia Bombyk, Program Coordinator, 734-487-4173, Fax: 734-487-8536, E-mail: marcia.bombyk@emich.edu. *Application contact:* Graduate Admissions, 734-487-2400, Fax: 734-487-6559, E-mail: graduate.admissions@emich.edu.

Eastern Michigan University, Graduate School, College of Health and Human Services, School of Health Sciences, Programs in Health Administration, Ypsilanti, MI 48197. Offers MHA, MS, Graduate Certificate. *Students:* 19 full-time (14 women), 75 part-time (58 women); includes 24 minority (13 Black or African American, non-Hispanic/Latino; 1 American Indian or Alaska Native, non-Hispanic/Latino; 4 Asian, non-Hispanic/Latino; 4 Hispanic/Latino; 2 Two or more races, non-Hispanic/Latino), 9 international. Average age 34. 76 applicants, 74% accepted, 25 enrolled. In 2013, 24 master's, 1 other advanced degree awarded. Application fee: $35. *Expenses:* Tuition, state resident: full-time $12,300; part-time $466 per credit hour. Tuition, nonresident: full-time $23,159; part-time $918 per credit hour. *Required fees:* $71 per credit hour. $46 per semester. One-time fee: $100. Tuition and fees vary according to course level and degree level. *Unit head:* Dr. Colleen Croxall, Director, 734-487-4096, Fax: 734-487-4095, E-mail: ccroxall@emich.edu. *Application contact:* Dr. Pamela Walsh, Program Director, 734-487-2072, Fax: 734-487-4095, E-mail: pwalsh@emich.edu.

Eastern Michigan University, Graduate School, College of Health and Human Services, School of Nursing, Ypsilanti, MI 48197. Offers nursing (MSN); quality improvement in health care systems (Graduate Certificate); teaching in health care systems (MSN, Graduate Certificate). *Accreditation:* AACN. Part-time and evening/weekend programs available. Postbaccalaureate distance learning degree programs offered (minimal on-campus study). *Faculty:* 23 full-time (21 women). *Students:* 3 full-time (all women), 32 part-time (26 women); includes 11 minority (6 Black or African American, non-Hispanic/Latino; 3 Asian, non-Hispanic/Latino; 2 Hispanic/Latino), 1 international. Average age 47. 31 applicants, 55% accepted, 10 enrolled. In 2013, 8 master's, 2 other advanced degrees awarded. *Degree requirements:* For master's, thesis optional. *Entrance requirements:* For master's, GRE General Test, Michigan RN license. Additional exam requirements/recommendations for international students: Required—TOEFL. *Application deadline:* Applications are processed on a rolling basis. Application fee: $35. *Expenses:* Tuition, state resident: full-time $12,300; part-time $466 per credit hour. Tuition, nonresident: full-time $23,159; part-time $918 per credit hour. *Required fees:* $71 per credit hour. $46 per semester. One-time fee: $100. Tuition and fees vary according to course level and degree level. *Financial support:* Fellowships, research assistantships with full tuition reimbursements, teaching assistantships with full tuition reimbursements, career-related internships or fieldwork, Federal Work-Study, institutionally sponsored loans, scholarships/grants, tuition waivers (partial), and unspecified assistantships available. Support available to part-time students. Financial award applicants required to submit FAFSA. *Unit head:* Dr. Michael Williams, Interim Director, 734-487-2310, Fax: 734-487-6946, E-mail: mwilliams@emich.edu. *Application contact:* Roberta Towns, Coordinator, School of Nursing, 734-487-2340, Fax: 734-487-6946, E-mail: rtowne1@emich.edu.
Website: http://www.emich.edu/nursing

Eastern University, School of Management Studies, St. Davids, PA 19087-3696. Offers health administration (MBA); health services management (MS); management (MBA). Part-time and evening/weekend programs available. Postbaccalaureate distance learning degree programs offered (no on-campus study). *Faculty:* 7 full-time (5 women), 40 part-time/adjunct (13 women). *Students:* 185 full-time (125 women), 66 part-time (44 women); includes 122 minority (100 Black or African American, non-Hispanic/Latino; 8 Asian, non-Hispanic/Latino; 13 Hispanic/Latino; 1 Two or more races, non-Hispanic/Latino), 38 international. Average age 35. 72 applicants, 99% accepted, 55 enrolled. In 2013, 96 master's awarded. *Entrance requirements:* Additional exam requirements/recommendations for international students: Required—TOEFL (minimum score 550 paper-based; 79 iBT). *Application deadline:* For fall admission, 8/16 for domestic students; for spring admission, 3/14 for domestic students. Applications are processed on a rolling basis. Application fee: $35. Application fee is waived when completed online. *Expenses: Tuition:* Full-time $15,600; part-time $650 per credit. *Required fees:* $27.50 per semester. One-time fee: $50. Tuition and fees vary according to course load, degree level and program. *Financial support:* In 2013–14, 34 students received support. Scholarships/grants available. Financial award applicants required to submit FAFSA. *Unit head:* Dr. Pat Bleil, Chair, 610-341-1468. *Application contact:* Nicholas Snyder, Enrollment Counselor, 610-225-5557, Fax: 610-341-1468, E-mail: nsnyder@eastern.edu.
Website: http://www.eastern.edu/academics/programs/school-management-studies

East Tennessee State University, School of Graduate Studies, College of Business and Technology, Department of Management and Marketing, Johnson City, TN 37614. Offers business administration (MBA, Postbaccalaureate Certificate); health care management (Postbaccalaureate Certificate). Part-time and evening/weekend programs available. *Faculty:* 33 full-time (5 women), 2 part-time/adjunct (1 woman). *Students:* 85 full-time (25 women), 23 part-time (12 women); includes 10 minority (2 Black or African American, non-Hispanic/Latino; 1 Asian, non-Hispanic/Latino; 5 Hispanic/Latino; 2 Two or more races, non-Hispanic/Latino), 10 international. Average age 29. 135 applicants, 54% accepted, 63 enrolled. In 2013, 54 master's, 6 other advanced degrees awarded. *Degree requirements:* For master's, comprehensive exam, capstone, strategic experience. *Entrance requirements:* For master's, GMAT, minimum GPA of 2.5. Additional exam requirements/recommendations for international students: Required—TOEFL (minimum score 550 paper-based; 79 iBT). *Application deadline:* For fall admission, 6/1 for domestic students, 4/30 for international students; for spring admission, 11/1 for domestic students, 9/30 for international students. Application fee: $35 ($45 for international students). Electronic applications accepted. *Expenses:* Tuition, state resident: full-time $7900; part-time $395 per credit hour. Tuition, nonresident: full-time $21,960; part-time $1098 per credit hour. *Required fees:* $1345; $84 per credit hour. *Financial support:* In 2013–14, 40 students received support, including 19 research assistantships with full tuition reimbursements available (averaging $6,000 per year), 2 teaching assistantships with full tuition reimbursements available (averaging $6,000 per year); career-related internships or fieldwork, institutionally sponsored loans, scholarships/grants, and unspecified assistantships also available. Financial award application deadline: 7/1; financial award applicants required to submit FAFSA. *Faculty research:* Sustainability, healthcare effectiveness, consumer behavior, merchandizing trends, organizational management issues. *Unit head:* Dr. Phillip E. Miller, Chair, 423-439-4422, Fax: 423-439-5661, E-mail: millerpe@etsu.edu. *Application contact:* Cindy Hill, Graduate Specialist, 423-439-6590, Fax: 423-439-5624, E-mail: hillcc@etsu.edu.

Emory University, Rollins School of Public Health, Department of Health Policy and Management, Atlanta, GA 30322-1100. Offers health policy (MPH); health policy research (MSPH); health services management (MPH); health services research and health policy (PhD). Part-time programs available. *Degree requirements:* For master's, thesis (for some programs), practicum, capstone course. *Entrance requirements:* For master's, GRE General Test. Additional exam requirements/recommendations for international students: Required—TOEFL (minimum score 550 paper-based; 80 iBT). Electronic applications accepted. *Faculty research:* U.S. health policy and financing, healthcare organization and financing.

Excelsior College, School of Business and Technology, Albany, NY 12203-5159. Offers business administration (MBA); cybersecurity (MS); cybersecurity management (MBA, Graduate Certificate); health care management (MBA); human performance technology (MBA); information security (MBA); leadership (MBA); social media management (MBA); technology management (MBA). Part-time and evening/weekend programs available. Postbaccalaureate distance learning degree programs offered (no on-campus study). *Faculty:* 36 part-time/adjunct (15 women). *Students:* 1,040 part-time (332 women); includes 411 minority (234 Black or African American, non-Hispanic/Latino; 3 American Indian or Alaska Native, non-Hispanic/Latino; 42 Asian, non-Hispanic/Latino; 104 Hispanic/Latino; 3 Native Hawaiian or other Pacific Islander, non-Hispanic/Latino; 25 Two or more races, non-Hispanic/Latino). Average age 41. In 2013, 75 master's awarded. *Application deadline:* Applications are processed on a rolling basis. Application fee: $100. *Expenses: Tuition:* Part-time $565 per credit. *Unit head:* Dr. Murray Block, Interim Dean, 888-647-2388. *Application contact:* Admissions, 888-647-2388 Ext. 133, Fax: 518-464-8777, E-mail: admissions@excelsior.edu.

Fairleigh Dickinson University, College at Florham, Silberman College of Business, Executive MBA Programs, Executive MBA Program for Health Care and Life Sciences Professionals, Madison, NJ 07940-1099. Offers EMBA.

Fairleigh Dickinson University, Metropolitan Campus, Silberman College of Business, Program in Healthcare and Life Sciences, Teaneck, NJ 07666-1914. Offers EMBA.

Felician College, Program in Health Care Administration, Lodi, NJ 07644-2117. Offers MSHA. *Students:* 15 part-time (13 women); includes 8 minority (3 Black or African American, non-Hispanic/Latino; 1 Asian, non-Hispanic/Latino; 4 Hispanic/Latino). *Expenses: Tuition:* Part-time $945 per credit. *Required fees:* $317.50 per semester. *Application contact:* Nicole Vitale, Assistant Director of Graduate Admissions, 201-559-6077, Fax: 201-559-6138, E-mail: graduate@felician.edu.

Florida Atlantic University, College of Business, Department of Management, Boca Raton, FL 33431-0991. Offers business administration (Exec MBA, MBA); entrepreneurship (MBA); health administration (MBA, MHA, MS); international business (MBA); management (PhD); sports management (MBA). *Faculty:* 22 full-time (10 women), 11 part-time/adjunct (6 women). *Students:* 267 full-time (120 women), 397 part-time (194 women); includes 279 minority (92 Black or African American, non-Hispanic/Latino; 31 Asian, non-Hispanic/Latino; 147 Hispanic/Latino; 9 Two or more races, non-Hispanic/Latino), 37 international. Average age 32. 551 applicants, 50% accepted, 216 enrolled. In 2013, 255 master's, 7 doctorates awarded. *Entrance requirements:* For master's, GMAT or GRE General Test, minimum GPA of 3.0 in last 60 hours of course work. Additional exam requirements/recommendations for international students: Required—TOEFL (minimum score 600 paper-based; 61 iBT), IELTS (minimum score 6). *Application deadline:* For fall admission, 7/25 for domestic students, 2/15 for international students; for spring admission, 12/10 for domestic students, 7/15 for international students. Applications are processed on a rolling basis. Application fee: $30. Electronic applications accepted. *Expenses:* Tuition, state resident: full-time $6660; part-time $370 per credit hour. Tuition, nonresident: full-time $18,450; part-time $1025 per credit hour. Tuition and fees vary according to course load. *Financial support:* Research assistantships with full tuition reimbursements, career-related internships or fieldwork, tuition waivers (partial), and unspecified assistantships available. *Faculty research:* Sports administration, healthcare, policy, finance, real estate, senior living. *Unit head:* Dr. Peggy Golden, Chair, 561-297-2675, E-mail: golden@fau.edu. *Application contact:* Dr. Marcy Krugel, Graduate Adviser, 561-297-3633, Fax: 561-297-1315, E-mail: krugel@fau.edu.
Website: http://business.fau.edu/departments/management/index.aspx

Florida Institute of Technology, Graduate Programs, Nathan M. Bisk College of Business, Online Programs, Melbourne, FL 32901-6975. Offers accounting (MBA); accounting and finance (MBA); business administration (MBA); finance (MBA); healthcare management (MBA); information assurance and cybersecurity (MS); information technology (MS); information technology cybersecurity (MS); information technology management (MBA); international business (MBA); Internet marketing (MBA); management (MBA); marketing (MBA); project management (MBA); supply chain management (MS). Part-time and evening/weekend programs available. Postbaccalaureate distance learning degree programs offered (no on-campus study). *Faculty:* 3 full-time (1 woman), 41 part-time/adjunct (13 women). *Students:* 6 full-time (1 woman), 1,121 part-time (530 women); includes 424 minority (276 Black or African American, non-Hispanic/Latino; 10 American Indian or Alaska Native, non-Hispanic/Latino; 45 Asian, non-Hispanic/Latino; 88 Hispanic/Latino; 5 Native Hawaiian or other Pacific Islander, non-Hispanic/Latino), 32 international. Average age 36. 348 applicants, 42% accepted, 146 enrolled. In 2013, 475 master's awarded. *Entrance requirements:* For master's, GMAT or resume showing 8 years of supervised experience, 2 letters of recommendation, resume, competency in math past college algebra. Additional exam requirements/recommendations for international students: Required—TOEFL (minimum score 550 paper-based; 79 iBT). *Application deadline:* For fall admission, 4/1 for international students; for spring admission, 9/30 for international students. Applications are processed on a rolling basis. Electronic applications accepted. *Expenses:* Contact institution. *Financial support:* Available to part-time students. Application deadline: 3/1; applicants required to submit FAFSA. *Unit head:* Brian Ehrlich, Associate Vice President/Director of Online Learning, 321-674-8202, E-mail: behrlich@fit.edu. *Application contact:* Carolyn Farrior, Director of Graduate Admissions, Online Learning and Off-Campus Programs, 321-674-7118.
Website: http://online.fit.edu

Florida International University, Robert Stempel College of Public Health and Social Work, Department of Health Policy and Management, Miami, FL 33199. Offers MPH. *Accreditation:* CAHME. Part-time and evening/weekend programs available. *Entrance requirements:* For master's, GRE General Test, minimum GPA of 3.0. Additional exam requirements/recommendations for international students: Required—TOEFL (minimum score 550 paper-based; 80 iBT). Electronic applications accepted.

Florida International University, Robert Stempel College of Public Health and Social Work, Programs in Public Health, Miami, FL 33199. Offers biostatistics (MPH); environmental and occupational health (MPH, PhD); epidemiology (MPH, PhD); health policy and management (MPH); health promotion and disease prevention (PhD); health promotion and diseases prevention (MPH). Ph D program has fall admissions only; MPH offered jointly with University of Miami. *Accreditation:* CEPH. Part-time and evening/weekend programs available. Postbaccalaureate distance learning degree programs offered (no on-campus study). *Degree requirements:* For master's, thesis optional; for doctorate, comprehensive exam, thesis/dissertation. *Entrance requirements:* For master's, minimum GPA of 3.0, letters of recommendation; for doctorate, GRE, resume, minimum GPA of 3.0, letters of recommendation, letter of intent. Additional exam requirements/recommendations for international students: Required—TOEFL (minimum score 550 paper-based; 80 iBT). Electronic applications accepted. *Expenses:* Contact institution. *Faculty research:* Drugs/AIDS intervention among migrant workers, provision of services for active/recovering drug users with HIV.

Florida State University, The Graduate School, College of Nursing, Tallahassee, FL 32312. Offers family nurse practitioner (DNP); health systems leadership (DNP); nurse educator (MSN, Certificate); nurse leader (MSN); nursing leadership (Certificate, Post-Graduate Certificate). *Accreditation:* AACN. Part-time programs available. Postbaccalaureate distance learning degree programs offered (minimal on-campus study). *Faculty:* 13 full-time (12 women). *Students:* 53 full-time (49 women), 26 part-time (all women); includes 16 minority (4 Black or African American, non-Hispanic/Latino; 1 Asian, non-Hispanic/Latino; 9 Hispanic/Latino; 2 Two or more races, non-Hispanic/Latino). Average age 38. 56 applicants, 61% accepted, 25 enrolled. In 2013, 5 master's, 18 doctorates awarded. *Degree requirements:* For master's, thesis optional. *Entrance requirements:* For master's, GRE General Test, MAT, minimum GPA of 3.0, BSN, Florida RN license; for doctorate, GRE General Test, MAT, minimum GPA of 3.0, BSN or MSN, Florida RN license. Additional exam requirements/recommendations for international students: Required—TOEFL (minimum score 550 paper-based). *Application deadline:* For fall admission, 7/1 for domestic and international students. Application fee: $30. Electronic applications accepted. *Expenses:* Tuition, state resident: part-time $403.51 per credit hour. Tuition, nonresident: part-time $1004.85 per credit hour. *Required fees:* $75.81 per credit hour. One-time fee: $20 part-time. Tuition and fees vary according to course load, campus/location and student level. *Financial support:* In 2013–14, 75 students received support, including fellowships with partial tuition reimbursements available (averaging $6,300 per year), research assistantships with partial tuition reimbursements available (averaging $3,000 per year), 3 teaching assistantships with partial tuition reimbursements available (averaging $3,000 per year); career-related internships or fieldwork, Federal Work-Study, institutionally sponsored loans, scholarships/grants, traineeships, and tuition waivers (partial) also available. Financial award application deadline: 4/15; financial award applicants required to submit FAFSA. *Faculty research:* Distance learning, gerontology, health promotion, educational strategies, rehabilitation of brain injured patients. *Unit head:* Dr. Judith McFetridge-Durdle, Dean, 850-644-6846, Fax: 850-644-7660, E-mail: jdurdle@nursing.fsu.edu. *Application contact:* Carlos G. Urrutia, Director of Student Services, 850-644-5638, Fax: 850-645-7249, E-mail: currutia@fsu.edu.
Website: http://nursing.fsu.edu/

Framingham State University, Continuing Education, Program in Health Care Administration, Framingham, MA 01701-9101. Offers MA. Part-time and evening/weekend programs available.

Francis Marion University, Graduate Programs, School of Business, Florence, SC 29502-0547. Offers business (MBA); health management (MBA). *Accreditation:* AACSB. Part-time and evening/weekend programs available. *Faculty:* 23 full-time (9 women). *Students:* 3 full-time (0 women), 26 part-time (13 women); includes 8 minority (5 Black or African American, non-Hispanic/Latino; 2 Asian, non-Hispanic/Latino; 1 Hispanic/Latino), 1 international. Average age 30. 18 applicants, 44% accepted, 7 enrolled. In 2013, 12 master's awarded. *Degree requirements:* For master's, comprehensive exam. *Entrance requirements:* For master's, GMAT. *Application deadline:* For fall admission, 3/15 for domestic students; for spring admission, 10/15 for domestic students. Applications are processed on a rolling basis. Application fee: $33. *Expenses:* Tuition, state resident: full-time $9184; part-time $459.20 per credit hour. Tuition, nonresident: full-time $18,368; part-time $918.40 per credit hour. *Required fees:* $13.50 per credit hour. $92 per semester. Tuition and fees vary according to program. *Financial support:* Available to part-time students. Application deadline: 3/1; applicants required to submit FAFSA. *Faculty research:* Ethics, directions of MBA, international business, regional economics, environmental issues. *Unit head:* Dr. M. Barry O'Brien, Dean, 843-661-1419, Fax: 843-661-1432, E-mail: mbobrien@fmarion.edu. *Application contact:* Rannie Gamble, Administrative Manager, 843-661-1286, Fax: 843-661-4688, E-mail: rgamble@fmarion.edu.
Website: http://www.fmarion.edu/academics/schoolofbusiness

Franklin Pierce University, Graduate Studies, Rindge, NH 03461-0060. Offers curriculum and instruction (M Ed); emerging network technologies (Graduate Certificate); energy and sustainability studies (MBA); health administration (MBA, Graduate Certificate); human resource management (MBA, Graduate Certificate); information technology (MBA); information technology management (MS); leadership (MBA, DA); nursing (MS); physical therapy (DPT); physician assistant studies (MPAS); special education (M Ed); sports management (MBA). *Accreditation:* APTA. Part-time programs available. Postbaccalaureate distance learning degree programs offered (no on-campus study). *Degree requirements:* For master's, concentrated original research projects; student teaching; fieldwork and/or internship; leadership project; PRAXIS I and II (for M Ed); for doctorate, concentrated original research projects, clinical fieldwork and/or internship, leadership project. *Entrance requirements:* For master's, minimum GPA of 2.5, 3 letters of recommendation; competencies in accounting, economics, statistics, and computer skills through life experience or undergraduate coursework (for MBA); certification/e-portfolio, minimum C grade in all education courses (for M Ed); license to practice as RN (for MS in nursing); for doctorate, GRE, BA/BS, 3 letters of recommendation, personal mission statement, interview, writing sample, minimum cumulative GPA of 2.8, master's degree (for DA); 80 hours of observation/work in PT settings, completion of anatomy, chemistry, physics, and statistics, minimum GPA of 3.0 (for DPT). Additional exam requirements/recommendations for international students: Required—TOEFL (minimum score 550 paper-based; 61 iBT). Electronic applications accepted. *Faculty research:* Evidence-based practice in sports physical therapy, human resource management in economic crisis, leadership in nursing, innovation in sports facility management, differentiated learning and understanding by design.

Friends University, Graduate School, Wichita, KS 67213. Offers business law (MBL); Christian ministry (MACM); family therapy (MSFT); global (MBA), including accounting, business law, change management, health care leadership, management information systems, supply chain management and logistics; health care leadership (MHCL); management information systems (MMIS); operations management (MSOM); professional (MBA), including accounting, business law, change management, health care leadership, management information systems, supply chain management and logistics; teaching (MAT). Part-time and evening/weekend programs available. Postbaccalaureate distance learning degree programs offered (no on-campus study). *Faculty:* 18 full-time (8 women), 62 part-time/adjunct (28 women). *Students:* 161 full-time (111 women), 408 part-time (258 women); includes 157 minority (68 Black or African American, non-Hispanic/Latino; 7 American Indian or Alaska Native, non-Hispanic/Latino; 28 Asian, non-Hispanic/Latino; 18 Hispanic/Latino; 1 Native Hawaiian or other

Pacific Islander, non-Hispanic/Latino; 35 Two or more races, non-Hispanic/Latino). Average age 36. 371 applicants, 90% accepted, 178 enrolled. In 2013, 432 master's awarded. *Degree requirements:* For master's, research project. *Entrance requirements:* For master's, bachelor's degree from accredited institution, official transcripts, interview with program director, letter(s) of recommendation. Additional exam requirements/recommendations for international students: Required—TOEFL (minimum score 560 paper-based). *Application deadline:* Applications are processed on a rolling basis. Application fee: $35 ($50 for international students). Electronic applications accepted. *Expenses: Tuition:* Part-time $631 per credit hour. Tuition and fees vary according to program. *Financial support:* In 2013–14, 30 students received support. Applicants required to submit FAFSA. *Unit head:* Dr. David Hofmeister, Dean of the Graduate School, 800-794-6945 Ext. 5858, Fax: 316-295-5040, E-mail: david_hofmeister@friends.edu. *Application contact:* Rachel Steiner, Manager, Graduate Recruiting Services, 800-794-6945, Fax: 316-295-5872, E-mail: rachel_steiner@friends.edu.
Website: http://www.friends.edu/

George Mason University, College of Health and Human Services, Department of Health Administration and Policy, Fairfax, VA 22030. Offers health and medical policy (MS); health informatics (MS); health informatics and data analytics (Certificate); health policy (Certificate); health systems management (MHA); physician practice management (Certificate); public health leadership and management (Certificate); quality improvement and outcomes management in health care systems (Certificate); senior housing administration (Certificate). *Accreditation:* CAHME. *Faculty:* 17 full-time (5 women), 17 part-time/adjunct (7 women). *Students:* 78 full-time (55 women), 105 part-time (74 women); includes 85 minority (37 Black or African American, non-Hispanic/Latino; 33 Asian, non-Hispanic/Latino; 12 Hispanic/Latino; 1 Native Hawaiian or other Pacific Islander, non-Hispanic/Latino; 2 Two or more races, non-Hispanic/Latino), 21 international. Average age 33. 140 applicants, 66% accepted, 58 enrolled. In 2013, 45 master's, 4 other advanced degrees awarded. *Degree requirements:* For master's, comprehensive exam, internship. *Entrance requirements:* For master's, GRE recommended if undergraduate GPA is below 3.0 (for senior housing administration MS only), 2 official transcripts; expanded goals statement; 3 letters of recommendation; resume; 1 year of work experience (for MHA in health systems management); for Certificate, 2 official transcripts; expanded goals statement; 3 letters of recommendation; resume. Additional exam requirements/recommendations for international students: Required—TOEFL (minimum score 570 paper-based; 88 iBT), IELTS (minimum score 6.5), PTE. *Application deadline:* For fall admission, 4/1 priority date for domestic students; for spring admission, 11/1 priority date for domestic students. Applications are processed on a rolling basis. Application fee: $65 ($80 for international students). Electronic applications accepted. *Expenses:* Contact institution. *Financial support:* In 2013–14, 3 students received support, including 3 research assistantships with full and partial tuition reimbursements available (averaging $16,333 per year); career-related internships or fieldwork, Federal Work-Study, scholarships/grants, unspecified assistantships, and health care benefits (for full-time research or teaching assistantship recipients) also available. Support available to part-time students. Financial award application deadline: 3/1; financial award applicants required to submit FAFSA. *Faculty research:* Universal health care, publications, relationships between malpractice pressure and rates of Cesarean section and VBAC, seniors and Wii gaming, relationships between changes in physician's incomes and practice settings and their care to Medicaid and charity patients. *Total annual research expenditures:* $306,284. *Unit head:* Dr. P. J. Maddox, Chair, 703-993-1982, Fax: 703-993-1953, E-mail: pmaddox@gmu.edu. *Application contact:* Valerie Bartush, Office Manager, 703-993-1929, Fax: 703-993-1953, E-mail: vbartush@gmu.edu.
Website: http://chhs.gmu.edu/hap/index

George Mason University, School of Policy, Government, and International Affairs, Program in Health and Medical Policy, Fairfax, VA 22030. Offers MS. *Faculty:* 6 full-time (1 woman), 4 part-time/adjunct (1 woman). *Students:* 18 full-time (14 women), 16 part-time (12 women); includes 11 minority (4 Black or African American, non-Hispanic/Latino; 3 Asian, non-Hispanic/Latino; 3 Hispanic/Latino; 1 Two or more races, non-Hispanic/Latino), 2 international. Average age 28. 13 applicants, 77% accepted, 7 enrolled. *Entrance requirements:* For master's, minimum undergraduate GPA of 3.0, expanded goals statement, resume, 2 official college transcripts, 2 letters of recommendation. Additional exam requirements/recommendations for international students: Required—TOEFL (minimum score 575 paper-based; 88 iBT), IELTS (minimum score 6.5), PTE. *Application deadline:* For fall admission, 6/1 for domestic students, 2/1 for international students; for spring admission, 12/1 for domestic students, 11/1 for international students. Application fee: $65 ($80 for international students). *Expenses:* Contact institution. *Financial support:* Career-related internships or fieldwork, Federal Work-Study, scholarships/grants, unspecified assistantships, and health care benefits (for full-time research or teaching assistantship recipients) available. Financial award application deadline: 3/1; financial award applicants required to submit FAFSA. *Faculty research:* Global and regional health policy research. *Unit head:* Dr. Salim Habayeb, Director, Health and Medical Policy, 703-993-4865, Fax: 703-993-2284, E-mail: shabayeb@gmu.edu. *Application contact:* Travis Major, Director of Graduate Admissions, School of Public Policy, 703-993-1383, E-mail: tmajor@gmu.edu.
Website: http://policy.gmu.edu/academic-professional-programs/masters-programs/health-and-medical-policy/

The George Washington University, College of Professional Studies, Program in Healthcare Corporate Compliance, Washington, DC 20052. Offers Graduate Certificate. Program offered with Milken Institute School of Public Health in partnership with the law firm of Feldesman Tucker Leifer Fidel LLP. Postbaccalaureate distance learning degree programs offered (minimal on-campus study). *Students:* 34 part-time (24 women); includes 9 minority (7 Black or African American, non-Hispanic/Latino; 1 American Indian or Alaska Native, non-Hispanic/Latino; 1 Asian, non-Hispanic/Latino). Average age 47. 35 applicants, 94% accepted, 17 enrolled. In 2013, 30 degrees awarded. *Application deadline:* For fall admission, 8/31 for domestic students. *Unit head:* Phyllis C. Borzi, Director, 202-530-2312, E-mail: borziph@gwu.edu. *Application contact:* Kristin Williams, Assistant Vice President for Graduate and Special Enrollment Management, 202-994-0467, Fax: 202-994-0371, E-mail: ksw@gwu.edu.
Website: http://cps.gwu.edu/hcc.html

The George Washington University, School of Medicine and Health Sciences, Health Sciences Programs, Washington, DC 20052. Offers clinical practice management (MSHS); clinical research administration (MSHS); emergency services management (MSHS); end-of-life care (MSHS); immunohematology (MSHS); physical therapy (DPT); physician assistant (MSHS); MSHS/MPH. Postbaccalaureate distance learning degree programs offered (no on-campus study). *Students:* 264 full-time (205 women), 216 part-time (162 women); includes 140 minority (54 Black or African American, non-Hispanic/Latino; 4 American Indian or Alaska Native, non-Hispanic/Latino; 48 Asian, non-Hispanic/Latino; 31 Hispanic/Latino; 3 Native Hawaiian or other Pacific Islander, non-Hispanic/Latino), 12 international. Average age 32. 1,581 applicants, 17% accepted. In 2013, 143 master's, 33 doctorates awarded. *Entrance requirements:* Additional exam requirements/recommendations for international students: Required—TOEFL (minimum score 550 paper-based). *Application deadline:* Applications are processed on a rolling basis. Application fee: $75. *Expenses:* Contact institution. *Unit head:* Jean E. Johnson, Senior Associate Dean, 202-994-3725, E-mail: jejohns@gwu.edu. *Application contact:* Joke Ogundiran, Director of Admission, 202-994-1668, Fax: 202-994-0870, E-mail: jokeogun@gwu.edu.

The George Washington University, School of Public Health and Health Services, Department of Health Policy, Washington, DC 20052. Offers MPH, MS. *Faculty:* 31 full-time (21 women). *Students:* 109 full-time (76 women), 136 part-time (100 women); includes 79 minority (40 Black or African American, non-Hispanic/Latino; 30 Asian, non-Hispanic/Latino; 7 Hispanic/Latino; 2 Two or more races, non-Hispanic/Latino), 9 international. Average age 29. 317 applicants, 86% accepted, 73 enrolled. In 2013, 88 master's awarded. *Degree requirements:* For master's, case study or special project. *Entrance requirements:* For master's, GMAT, GRE General Test, or MCAT. Additional exam requirements/recommendations for international students: Required—TOEFL. *Application deadline:* For fall admission, 4/15 priority date for domestic students, 4/15 for international students; for spring admission, 11/1 for domestic and international students. Applications are processed on a rolling basis. Application fee: $75. *Financial support:* In 2013–14, 10 students received support. Tuition waivers available. Financial award application deadline: 2/15. *Unit head:* Paula Lantz, Chair, 202-994-6568, Fax: 202-296-0025, E-mail: plantz@gwu.edu. *Application contact:* Jane Smith, Director of Admissions, 202-994-0248, Fax: 202-994-1860, E-mail: sphhsinfo@gwumc.edu.

The George Washington University, School of Public Health and Health Services, Department of Health Services Management and Leadership, Washington, DC 20052. Offers health management and leadership (MHSA); health policy (MHSA); health services administration (Specialist); public health management (MPH). *Accreditation:* CAHME (one or more programs are accredited). *Faculty:* 7 full-time (3 women). *Degree requirements:* For master's, internship or residency. *Entrance requirements:* For master's, GMAT or GRE; for Specialist, GMAT or GRE, master's degree in related field. Additional exam requirements/recommendations for international students: Required—TOEFL. *Application deadline:* For fall admission, 5/15 priority date for domestic students; for winter admission, 11/15 for domestic students; for spring admission, 4/1 for domestic students. Applications are processed on a rolling basis. Application fee: $75. *Financial support:* Career-related internships or fieldwork, Federal Work-Study, and institutionally sponsored loans available. Financial award application deadline: 6/1. *Faculty research:* Hospital administration, ambulatory health care, social gerontology, health care financing, health care ethics. *Unit head:* Dr. Robert Burke, Chair, 202-994-5560, Fax: 202-416-0075, E-mail: bobburke@gwu.edu. *Application contact:* Jane Smith, Director of Admissions, 202-994-0248, Fax: 202-994-1860, E-mail: sphhsinfo@gwumc.edu.
Website: http://publichealth.gwu.edu/departments/health-services-management-and-leadership

Georgia Institute of Technology, Graduate Studies and Research, College of Engineering, School of Industrial and Systems Engineering, Program in Health Systems, Atlanta, GA 30332-0001. Offers MSHS. *Entrance requirements:* For master's, GRE General Test, minimum GPA of 3.0. Additional exam requirements/recommendations for international students: Required—TOEFL. Electronic applications accepted. *Faculty research:* Emergency medical services, health development planning, health services evaluations.

Georgia Southern University, Jack N. Averitt College of Graduate Studies, Jiann-Ping Hsu College of Public Health, Program in Healthcare Administration, Statesboro, GA 30460. Offers MHA. Part-time and evening/weekend programs available. *Students:* 31 full-time (20 women), 6 part-time (3 women); includes 19 minority (14 Black or African American, non-Hispanic/Latino; 4 Asian, non-Hispanic/Latino; 1 Two or more races, non-Hispanic/Latino), 1 international. Average age 27. 25 applicants, 92% accepted, 15 enrolled. In 2013, 5 master's awarded. *Degree requirements:* For master's, practicum. *Entrance requirements:* For master's, GRE, GMAT, personal statement, minimum cumulative undergraduate GPA of 2.75, resume, 3 letters of recommendation. Additional exam requirements/recommendations for international students: Required—TOEFL (minimum score 550 paper-based; 80 iBT), IELTS (minimum score 6). *Application deadline:* For fall admission, 3/1 priority date for domestic and international students; for spring admission, 10/1 priority date for domestic students, 10/1 for international students. Applications are processed on a rolling basis. Electronic applications accepted. *Expenses:* Contact institution. *Financial support:* In 2013–14, 9 students received support, including research assistantships with partial tuition reimbursements available (averaging $7,200 per year); Federal Work-Study, scholarships/grants, tuition waivers, and unspecified assistantships also available. Financial award application deadline: 4/15; financial award applicants required to submit FAFSA. *Faculty research:* Health disparity elimination, cost effectiveness analysis, epidemiology of rural public health, health care system assessment, rural health care, health policy and healthcare financing. *Total annual research expenditures:* $57,935. *Unit head:* Dr. James Stephens, Program Director, 912-478-5958, Fax: 912-478-0171, E-mail: jstephens@georgiasouthern.edu. *Application contact:* Amanda Gilliland, Coordinator for Graduate Student Recruitment, 912-478-5384, Fax: 912-478-0740, E-mail: gradadmissions@georgiasouthern.edu.

Georgia Southern University, Jack N. Averitt College of Graduate Studies, Jiann-Ping Hsu College of Public Health, Program in Public Health, Statesboro, GA 30460. Offers biostatistics (MPH, Dr PH); community health behavior and education (Dr PH); community health education (MPH); environmental health sciences (MPH); epidemiology (MPH); health policy and management (MPH, Dr PH). *Accreditation:* CEPH. Part-time programs available. *Students:* 130 full-time (96 women), 50 part-time (39 women); includes 95 minority (80 Black or African American, non-Hispanic/Latino; 5 Asian, non-Hispanic/Latino; 4 Hispanic/Latino; 1 Native Hawaiian or other Pacific Islander, non-Hispanic/Latino; 5 Two or more races, non-Hispanic/Latino), 32 international. Average age 30. 213 applicants, 68% accepted, 61 enrolled. In 2013, 29 master's, 9 doctorates awarded. *Degree requirements:* For master's, thesis optional, practicum; for doctorate, comprehensive exam, thesis/dissertation, practicum. *Entrance requirements:* For master's, GRE General Test, minimum GPA of 2.75, resume, 3 letters of reference; for doctorate, GRE, GMAT, MCAT, LSAT, 3 letters of reference, statement of purpose, resume or curriculum vitae. Additional exam requirements/recommendations for international students: Required—TOEFL (minimum score 550 paper-based; 80 iBT), IELTS (minimum score 6). *Application deadline:* For fall admission, 3/1 priority date for domestic and international students; for spring admission, 10/1 priority date for domestic students, 10/1 for international students. Applications are processed on a rolling basis. Application fee: $50. Electronic applications accepted. *Expenses:* Contact institution. *Financial support:* In 2013–14, 54 students received support, including research assistantships with partial tuition reimbursements available (averaging $7,200 per year), teaching assistantships with partial tuition reimbursements available (averaging $7,200 per year); career-related internships or fieldwork, Federal Work-Study, scholarships/grants, tuition waivers (partial), and unspecified assistantships also available. Support available to part-time students. Financial award application deadline: 4/15; financial award applicants required to submit FAFSA. *Faculty research:* Rural public health best practices, health disparity elimination, community initiatives to enhance public health, cost effectiveness analysis, epidemiology of rural public health, environmental health issues, health care system assessment, rural health care, health policy and healthcare financing, survival analysis, nonparametric statistics and resampling methods, micro-arrays and genomics, data

imputation techniques and clinical trial methodology. *Total annual research expenditures:* $281,707. *Unit head:* Sarah Peterson, Student Services Coordinator, 912-478-2413, Fax: 912-478-5811, E-mail: speterson@georgiasouthern.edu. *Application contact:* Amanda Gilliland, Coordinator for Graduate Student Recruitment, 912-478-5384, Fax: 912-478-0740, E-mail: gradadmissions@georgiasouthern.edu.
Website: http://chhs.georgiasouthern.edu/health/

Georgia State University, Andrew Young School of Policy Studies, Department of Public Management and Policy, Atlanta, GA 30303. Offers criminal justice (MPA); disaster management (Certificate); disaster policy (MPA); environmental policy (PhD); health policy (PhD); management and finance (MPA); nonprofit management (MPA, Certificate); nonprofit policy (MPA); planning and economic development (MPP, Certificate); policy analysis and evaluation (MPA), including planning and economic development; public and nonprofit management (PhD); public finance and budgeting (PhD), including science and technology policy, urban and regional economic development; public finance policy (MPA), including social policy; public health (MPA). *Accreditation:* NASPAA (one or more programs are accredited). Part-time programs available. *Faculty:* 17 full-time (8 women), 3 part-time/adjunct (0 women). *Students:* 139 full-time (76 women), 95 part-time (59 women); includes 98 minority (69 Black or African American, non-Hispanic/Latino; 9 Asian, non-Hispanic/Latino; 11 Hispanic/Latino; 9 Two or more races, non-Hispanic/Latino), 19 international. Average age 29. 310 applicants, 55% accepted, 68 enrolled. In 2013, 68 master's, 9 other advanced degrees awarded. Terminal master's awarded for partial completion of doctoral program. *Degree requirements:* For master's, thesis optional; for doctorate, comprehensive exam, thesis/dissertation. *Entrance requirements:* For master's and doctorate, GRE. Additional exam requirements/recommendations for international students: Required—TOEFL (minimum score 603 paper-based; 100 iBT) or IELTS (minimum score 7). *Application deadline:* For fall admission, 2/15 for domestic and international students; for spring admission, 10/1 for domestic and international students. Application fee: $50. Electronic applications accepted. *Expenses: Tuition, area resident:* Full-time $4176; part-time $348 per credit hour. Tuition, state resident: full-time $14,544; part-time $1212 per credit hour. Tuition, nonresident: full-time $14,544; part-time $1212 per credit hour. Tuition and fees vary according to course load and program. *Financial support:* In 2013–14, fellowships (averaging $8,194 per year), research assistantships (averaging $8,068 per year), teaching assistantships (averaging $3,600 per year) were awarded; institutionally sponsored loans, scholarships/grants, health care benefits, and unspecified assistantships also available. Financial award application deadline: 2/1. *Faculty research:* Public budgeting and finance, public management, nonprofit management, performance measurement and management, urban development. *Unit head:* Dr. Gregory Burr Lewis, Chair and Professor, 404-413-0114, Fax: 404-413-0104, E-mail: glewis@gsu.edu. *Application contact:* Charisma Parker, Admissions Coordinator, 404-413-0030, Fax: 404-413-0023, E-mail: cparker28@gsu.edu.
Website: http://aysps.gsu.edu/pmap/

Georgia State University, J. Mack Robinson College of Business, Institute of Health Administration, Atlanta, GA 30302-3083. Offers health administration (MBA, MSHA); health informatics (MBA, MSCIS); MBA/MHA; PMBA/MHA. *Accreditation:* CAHME. Part-time and evening/weekend programs available. *Faculty:* 4 full-time (1 woman). *Students:* 39 full-time (20 women), 17 part-time (8 women); includes 18 minority (10 Black or African American, non-Hispanic/Latino; 8 Asian, non-Hispanic/Latino), 2 international. Average age 30. 68 applicants, 32% accepted, 16 enrolled. In 2013, 64 master's awarded. *Entrance requirements:* For master's, GRE or GMAT, transcripts from all institutions attended, resume, essays. Additional exam requirements/recommendations for international students: Required—TOEFL (minimum score 610 paper-based; 101 iBT), IELTS (minimum score 7). *Application deadline:* For fall admission, 5/1 priority date for domestic students, 2/1 priority date for international students; for spring admission, 9/15 priority date for domestic students, 4/1 priority date for international students. Applications are processed on a rolling basis. Application fee: $50. Electronic applications accepted. *Expenses: Tuition, area resident:* Full-time $4176; part-time $348 per credit hour. Tuition, state resident: full-time $14,544; part-time $1212 per credit hour. Tuition, nonresident: full-time $14,544; part-time $1212 per credit hour. Tuition and fees vary according to course load and program. *Financial support:* Research assistantships, teaching assistantships, scholarships/grants, tuition waivers, and unspecified assistantships available. *Faculty research:* Health information technology, health insurance exchanges, health policy and economic impact, healthcare quality, healthcare transformation. *Unit head:* Dr. Andrew T. Sumner, Chair in Health Administration/Director of the Institute of Health, 404-413-7630, Fax: 404-413-7631. *Application contact:* Toby McChesney, Assistant Dean for Graduate Recruiting and Student Services, 404-413-7167, Fax: 404-413-7162, E-mail: rcbgradadmissions@gsu.edu.
Website: http://www.hagsu.org/

Globe University–Woodbury, Minnesota School of Business, Woodbury, MN 55125. Offers business administration (MBA); health care management (MSM); information technology (MSM); managerial leadership (MSM).

Goldey-Beacom College, Graduate Program, Wilmington, DE 19808-1999. Offers business administration (MBA); finance (MS); financial management (MBA); health care management (MBA); human resource management (MBA); information technology (MBA); international business management (MBA); major finance (MBA); major taxation (MBA); management (MM); marketing management (MBA); taxation (MBA, MS). *Accreditation:* ACBSP. Part-time and evening/weekend programs available. *Entrance requirements:* For master's, GMAT, MAT, GRE, minimum GPA of 3.0. Additional exam requirements/recommendations for international students: Required—TOEFL (minimum score 65 iBT); Recommended—IELTS (minimum score 6). Electronic applications accepted.

Goldfarb School of Nursing at Barnes-Jewish College, Graduate Programs, St. Louis, MO 63110. Offers adult acute care nurse practitioner (MSN); adult nurse practitioner (MSN); nurse anesthesia (MSN); nurse educator (MSN); nurse executive (MSN); DNP/PhD. *Accreditation:* AACN; AANA/CANAEP. Part-time and evening/weekend programs available. Postbaccalaureate distance learning degree programs offered (minimal on-campus study). *Faculty:* 42 full-time (39 women), 6 part-time/adjunct (all women). *Students:* 81 full-time (67 women), 85 part-time (77 women); includes 28 minority (18 Black or African American, non-Hispanic/Latino; 2 Asian, non-Hispanic/Latino; 3 Hispanic/Latino; 3 Native Hawaiian or other Pacific Islander, non-Hispanic/Latino; 2 Two or more races, non-Hispanic/Latino). *Degree requirements:* For master's, thesis or alternative. *Entrance requirements:* For master's, 2 references, personal statement, curriculum vitae or resume. Additional exam requirements/recommendations for international students: Required—TOEFL (minimum score 575 paper-based; 85 iBT). *Application deadline:* For fall admission, 2/1 priority date for international students; for spring admission, 10/1 priority date for international students. Applications are processed on a rolling basis. Application fee: $50. *Expenses: Tuition:* Full-time $12,960; part-time $720 per credit hour. *Required fees:* $295; $720 per credit hour. Tuition and fees vary according to course load. *Financial support:* Fellowships, research assistantships, Federal Work-Study, institutionally sponsored loans, and scholarships/grants available. Support available to part-time students. Financial award applicants required to submit FAFSA. *Faculty research:* HIV stigma, HIV symptom management, palliative care with children and their families, heart disease prevention in Hispanic women, depression in the well elderly, alternative therapies in pre-term infants. *Unit head:* Dr. Michael Bleich, Dean, 314-362-0956, Fax: 314-362-0984, E-mail: mbleich@bjc.org. *Application contact:* Margaret Anne O'Connor, Program Officer, 314-454-7557, Fax: 314-362-0984, E-mail: maoconnor@bjc.org.

Governors State University, College of Health Professions, Program in Health Administration, University Park, IL 60484. Offers MHA. *Accreditation:* CAHME. *Degree requirements:* For master's, comprehensive exam, field experience or internship. *Entrance requirements:* For master's, minimum GPA of 3.0 in last 60 hours of undergraduate course work or 9 hours of graduate course work.

Grambling State University, School of Graduate Studies and Research, College of Arts and Sciences, Department of Political Science and Public Administration, Grambling, LA 71270. Offers health services administration (MPA); human resource management (MPA); public management (MPA); state and local government (MPA). *Accreditation:* NASPAA. Part-time programs available. *Faculty:* 5 full-time (1 woman). *Students:* 47 full-time (33 women), 28 part-time (23 women); includes 62 minority (61 Black or African American, non-Hispanic/Latino; 1 Asian, non-Hispanic/Latino), 13 international. Average age 29. In 2013, 11 master's awarded. *Degree requirements:* For master's, comprehensive exam (for some programs), thesis optional. *Entrance requirements:* For master's, GRE, minimum GPA of 2.75 on last degree. Additional exam requirements/recommendations for international students: Required—TOEFL (minimum score 500 paper-based; 62 iBT). *Application deadline:* For fall admission, 7/1 for domestic and international students; for spring admission, 12/1 for domestic and international students; for summer admission, 5/1 for domestic and international students. Applications are processed on a rolling basis. Application fee: $20 ($30 for international students). Electronic applications accepted. *Financial support:* Research assistantships, health care benefits, tuition waivers (full), and unspecified assistantships available. Financial award application deadline: 5/31. *Unit head:* Dr. Rose M. Harris, Department Head, 318-274-2310, Fax: 318-274-3427, E-mail: harrisr@gram.edu. *Application contact:* Katina S. Crowe-Fields, Special Assistant to Associate Vice President/Dean, 318-274-2158, Fax: 318-274-7373, E-mail: croweks@gram.edu.
Website: http://www.gram.edu/academics/majors/arts%20and%20sciences/departments/poli-science/mpa/

Grand Canyon University, College of Business, Phoenix, AZ 85017-1097. Offers accounting (MBA); corporate business administration (MBA); disaster preparedness and crisis management (MBA); executive fire service leadership (MS); finance (MBA); general management (MBA); government and policy (MPA); health care management (MPA); health systems management (MBA); human resource management (MBA); innovation (MBA); leadership (MBA, MS); management of information system (MBA); marketing (MBA); project-based (MBA); six sigma (MBA); strategic human resource management (MBA). *Accreditation:* ACBSP. Part-time and evening/weekend programs available. Postbaccalaureate distance learning degree programs offered (no on-campus study). *Entrance requirements:* For master's, equivalent of two years full-time professional work experience. Additional exam requirements/recommendations for international students: Required—TOEFL (minimum score 575 paper-based; 90 iBT), IELTS (minimum score 7). Electronic applications accepted.

Grand Canyon University, College of Nursing, Phoenix, AZ 85017-1097. Offers acute care nurse practitioner (MS, PMC); clinical nurse specialist (PMC), including clinical nurse specialist, education; family nurse practitioner (MS); leadership in health care systems (MS); nurse education (MS). *Accreditation:* AACN. Part-time and evening/weekend programs available. Postbaccalaureate distance learning degree programs offered (no on-campus study). *Degree requirements:* For master's and PMC, comprehensive exam (for some programs). *Entrance requirements:* For master's, minimum cumulative and science course undergraduate GPA of 3.0. Additional exam requirements/recommendations for international students: Required—TOEFL (minimum score 575 paper-based; 90 iBT), IELTS (minimum score 7).

Grand Canyon University, College of Nursing and Health Sciences, Phoenix, AZ 85017-1097. Offers addiction counseling (MS); health care administration (MS); health care informatics (MS); marriage and family therapy (MS); professional counseling (MS); public health (MS). Part-time and evening/weekend programs available. Postbaccalaureate distance learning degree programs offered (no on-campus study). *Entrance requirements:* For master's, undergraduate degree with minimum GPA of 2.8. Additional exam requirements/recommendations for international students: Required—TOEFL (minimum score 575 paper-based; 90 iBT), IELTS (minimum score 7).

Grand Valley State University, College of Community and Public Service, School of Public and Nonprofit Administration, Program in Health Administration, Allendale, MI 49401-9403. Offers MHA. Part-time and evening/weekend programs available. *Entrance requirements:* Additional exam requirements/recommendations for international students: Required—TOEFL. Electronic applications accepted. *Faculty research:* Long-term care and aging, Medicare and Medicaid finance and administration, health economics.

Grand Valley State University, Kirkhof College of Nursing, Allendale, MI 49401-9403. Offers advanced practice (MSN); case management (MSN); nursing administration (MSN); nursing education (MSN); nursing practice (DNP); MSN/MBA. *Accreditation:* AACN. Part-time programs available. *Degree requirements:* For master's, thesis optional. *Entrance requirements:* For master's, GRE, minimum GPA of 3.0 in upper-division course work, course work in statistics, Michigan RN license. Additional exam requirements/recommendations for international students: Required—TOEFL. Electronic applications accepted. *Faculty research:* Multigenerational health promotion, chronic disease prevention, end-of-life issues, nursing workload, family caregiver health.

Grantham University, College of Nursing and Allied Health, Lenexa, KS 66219. Offers case management (MSN); health systems management (MS); healthcare administration (MHA); nursing education (MSN); nursing informatics (MSN); nursing management and organizational leadership (MSN). Part-time and evening/weekend programs available. Postbaccalaureate distance learning degree programs offered (no on-campus study). *Faculty:* 1 (woman) full-time, 11 part-time/adjunct (5 women). *Students:* 64 full-time (43 women), 166 part-time (123 women); includes 116 minority (94 Black or African American, non-Hispanic/Latino; 4 Asian, non-Hispanic/Latino; 9 Hispanic/Latino; 1 Native Hawaiian or other Pacific Islander, non-Hispanic/Latino; 8 Two or more races, non-Hispanic/Latino). Average age 40. 230 applicants, 100% accepted, 230 enrolled. In 2013, 61 master's awarded. *Degree requirements:* For master's, thesis, major applied research paper and practicum (MSN). *Entrance requirements:* For master's, bachelor's degree from accredited degree-granting institution with minimum GPA of 2.5, BSN from an accredited nursing program, valid RN license. Additional exam requirements/recommendations for international students: Required—TOEFL (minimum score 530 paper-based; 71 iBT). *Application deadline:* Applications are processed on a rolling basis. Application fee: $30. Electronic applications accepted. *Expenses: Tuition:* Full-time $3900; part-time $325 per credit hour. *Required fees:* $35 per term. One-time fee: $100. *Financial support:* In 2013–14, 230 students received support. Scholarships/grants available. *Faculty research:* Pharmacy licensure, vaccination certification. *Unit head:* Dr. Susan Fairchild, Dean, School of Nursing, 800-955-2527, E-mail:

admissions@grantham.edu. *Application contact:* Jared Parlette, Vice President of Admissions, 800-955-2527, E-mail: admissions@grantham.edu.
Website: http://www.grantham.edu/colleges-and-schools/college-of-nursing-and-allied-health/

Hampton University, Hampton U Online, Hampton, VA 23668. Offers business administration (PhD); educational management (PhD); health administration (MHA); nursing (MSN, PhD).

Harding University, Paul R. Carter College of Business Administration, Searcy, AR 72149-0001. Offers health care management (MBA); information technology management (MBA); international business (MBA); leadership and organizational management (MBA). *Accreditation:* ACBSP. Part-time and evening/weekend programs available. Postbaccalaureate distance learning degree programs offered (no on-campus study). *Faculty:* 25 part-time/adjunct (5 women). *Students:* 55 full-time (36 women), 115 part-time (50 women); includes 22 minority (17 Black or African American, non-Hispanic/Latino; 2 American Indian or Alaska Native, non-Hispanic/Latino; 3 Asian, non-Hispanic/Latino), 27 international. Average age 34. 48 applicants, 100% accepted, 48 enrolled. In 2013, 88 master's awarded. *Degree requirements:* For master's, portfolio. *Entrance requirements:* For master's, GMAT (minimum score of 500) or GRE (minimum score of 300), minimum GPA of 3.0, 2 letters of recommendation, resume, 3 essays, all official transcripts. Additional exam requirements/recommendations for international students: Required—TOEFL (minimum score 550 paper-based; 79 iBT). *Application deadline:* For fall admission, 8/1 priority date for domestic and international students; for spring admission, 12/1 priority date for domestic and international students. Applications are processed on a rolling basis. Application fee: $40. *Expenses: Tuition:* Full-time $11,574; part-time $643 per credit hour. *Required fees:* $432; $24 per credit hour. Tuition and fees vary according to course load, degree level and program. *Financial support:* Unspecified assistantships available. Financial award application deadline: 7/30; financial award applicants required to submit FAFSA. *Unit head:* Glen Metheny, Director of Graduate Studies, 501-279-5851, Fax: 501-279-4805, E-mail: gmetheny@harding.edu. *Application contact:* Melanie Kiihnl, Recruiting Manager/Director of Marketing, 501-279-4523, Fax: 501-279-4805, E-mail: mba@harding.edu.
Website: http://www.harding.edu/mba

Harrisburg University of Science and Technology, Program in Information Systems Engineering and Management, Harrisburg, PA 17101. Offers digital government (MS); digital health (MS); entrepreneurship (MS). Part-time programs available. *Degree requirements:* For master's, comprehensive exam, thesis optional. *Entrance requirements:* For master's, baccalaureate degree. Additional exam requirements/recommendations for international students: Required—TOEFL (minimum score 520 paper-based; 80 iBT). Electronic applications accepted.

Harvard University, Graduate School of Arts and Sciences, Committee on Higher Degrees in Health Policy, Cambridge, MA 02138. Offers PhD. *Degree requirements:* For doctorate, thesis/dissertation. *Entrance requirements:* For doctorate, GMAT, GRE General Test, or MCAT. Additional exam requirements/recommendations for international students: Required—TOEFL. *Expenses: Tuition:* Full-time $38,888. *Required fees:* $958. Tuition and fees vary according to campus/location, program and student level.

Harvard University, Harvard Business School, Doctoral Programs in Management, Boston, MA 02163. Offers accounting and management (DBA); business economics (PhD); health policy management (PhD); management (DBA); marketing (DBA); organizational behavior (PhD); science, technology and management (PhD); strategy (DBA); technology and operations management (DBA). *Degree requirements:* For doctorate, comprehensive exam (for some programs), thesis/dissertation. *Entrance requirements:* For doctorate, GRE General Test or GMAT. Additional exam requirements/recommendations for international students: Required—TOEFL. *Expenses: Tuition:* Full-time $38,888. *Required fees:* $958. Tuition and fees vary according to campus/location, program and student level.

Harvard University, Harvard School of Public Health, Department of Health Policy and Management, Boston, MA 02115-6096. Offers health policy (PhD); health policy and management (SM, SD). Part-time programs available. *Faculty:* 26 full-time (11 women), 43 part-time/adjunct (11 women). *Students:* 111 full-time, 62 part-time; includes 48 minority (6 Black or African American, non-Hispanic/Latino; 30 Asian, non-Hispanic/Latino; 7 Hispanic/Latino; 5 Two or more races, non-Hispanic/Latino), 23 international. Average age 31. 382 applicants, 20% accepted, 63 enrolled. In 2013, 26 master's, 1 doctorate awarded. *Degree requirements:* For doctorate, thesis/dissertation, qualifying exam. *Entrance requirements:* For master's, GRE, GMAT, MCAT; for doctorate, GRE. Additional exam requirements/recommendations for international students: Required—TOEFL (minimum score 600 paper-based; 100 iBT); Recommended—IELTS (minimum score 7). *Application deadline:* For fall admission, 12/15 for domestic and international students. Application fee: $120. *Expenses: Tuition:* Full-time $38,888. *Required fees:* $958. Tuition and fees vary according to campus/location, program and student level. *Financial support:* Fellowships, research assistantships, teaching assistantships, Federal Work-Study, scholarships/grants, traineeships, and unspecified assistantships available. Support available to part-time students. Financial award application deadline: 2/17; financial award applicants required to submit FAFSA. *Faculty research:* Environmental science and risk management. *Unit head:* Dr. Arnold Epstein, Chair, 617-432-3895, Fax: 617-432-4494, E-mail: aepstein@hsph.harvard.edu. *Application contact:* Vincent W. James, Director of Admissions, 617-432-1031, Fax: 617-432-7080, E-mail: admissions@hsph.harvard.edu.
Website: http://www.hsph.harvard.edu/departments/health-policy-and-management/

Hawai`i Pacific University, College of Business Administration, Honolulu, HI 96813. Offers accounting/CPA (MBA); e-business (MBA); economics (MBA); finance (MBA); healthcare management (MBA); human resource management (MA, MBA); information systems (MBA, MSIS); international business (MBA); management (MBA); marketing (MBA); organizational change (MA, MBA); travel industry management (MBA). Part-time and evening/weekend programs available. *Faculty:* 22 full-time (9 women), 6 part-time/adjunct (0 women). *Students:* 232 full-time (100 women), 174 part-time (84 women); includes 241 minority (18 Black or African American, non-Hispanic/Latino; 112 Asian, non-Hispanic/Latino; 33 Hispanic/Latino; 11 Native Hawaiian or other Pacific Islander, non-Hispanic/Latino; 67 Two or more races, non-Hispanic/Latino). Average age 31. 240 applicants, 81% accepted, 102 enrolled. In 2013, 206 master's awarded. *Degree requirements:* For master's, thesis. *Entrance requirements:* For master's, GMAT. Additional exam requirements/recommendations for international students: Recommended—TOEFL (minimum score 550 paper-based; 80 iBT), TWE (minimum score 5). *Application deadline:* For fall admission, 2/15 priority date for domestic students; for spring admission, 10/15 priority date for domestic students. Applications are processed on a rolling basis. Application fee: $50. Electronic applications accepted. *Financial support:* In 2013–14, 90 students received support. Research assistantships, career-related internships or fieldwork, Federal Work-Study, scholarships/grants, tuition waivers, and unspecified assistantships available. Financial award application deadline: 3/1; financial award applicants required to submit FAFSA. *Faculty research:* Statistical control process as used by management, studies in comparative cross-cultural management styles, not-for-profit management. *Unit head:* Dr. Deborah Crown, Dean, 808-544-0275, Fax: 808-544-0283, E-mail: dcrown@hpu.edu. *Application contact:* Rumi Yoshida, Associate Director of Graduate Admissions, 808-543-8034, Fax: 808-544-0280, E-mail: grad@hpu.edu.
Website: http://www.hpu.edu/CBA/Graduate/index.html

Herzing University Online, Program in Business Administration, Milwaukee, WI 53203. Offers accounting (MBA); business administration (MBA); business management (MBA); healthcare management (MBA); human resources (MBA); marketing (MBA); project management (MBA); technology management (MBA). Postbaccalaureate distance learning degree programs offered (no on-campus study).

Hofstra University, Frank G. Zarb School of Business, Programs in Management and General Business, Hempstead, NY 11549. Offers business administration (MBA), including health services management, management, sports and entertainment management; general management (Advanced Certificate); human resource management (MS, Advanced Certificate).

Hofstra University, School of Health Sciences and Human Services, Programs in Health, Hempstead, NY 11549. Offers community health (MS); health administration (MHA); public health (MPH).

Holy Family University, Division of Extended Learning, Bensalem, PA 19020. Offers business administration (MBA); finance (MBA); health care administration (MBA); human resources management (MBA). *Accreditation:* ACBSP. Part-time and evening/weekend programs available. *Faculty:* 13 part-time/adjunct (3 women). *Students:* 116 part-time (59 women); includes 4 minority (2 Black or African American, non-Hispanic/Latino; 1 Asian, non-Hispanic/Latino; 1 Hispanic/Latino). Average age 34. 25 applicants, 96% accepted, 6 enrolled. In 2013, 52 master's awarded. *Entrance requirements:* For master's, minimum GPA of 3.0, interview, essay/professional statement, 2 recommendations, current resume, official transcripts of college or university work. Additional exam requirements/recommendations for international students: Required—TOEFL (minimum score 550 paper-based; 79 iBT). *Application deadline:* For fall admission, 7/1 priority date for domestic and international students; for spring admission, 11/1 priority date for domestic and international students; for summer admission, 4/1 priority date for domestic and international students. Applications are processed on a rolling basis. Application fee: $50. Electronic applications accepted. *Expenses: Tuition:* Full-time $12,060. *Required fees:* $250. Tuition and fees vary according to degree level. *Financial support:* In 2013–14, 3 students received support. Available to part-time students. Applicants required to submit FAFSA. *Unit head:* Chris Quinn, Director of Academic Services, 267-341-5006, Fax: 215-633-0558, E-mail: cquinn1@holyfamily.edu. *Application contact:* Don Reinmold, Director of Admissions, 267-341-5001 Ext. 3230, Fax: 215-633-0558, E-mail: dreinmold@holyfamily.edu.

Hunter College of the City University of New York, Graduate School, Schools of the Health Professions, School of Health Sciences, Programs in Urban Public Health, Program in Health Policy Management, New York, NY 10065-5085. Offers MPH. Part-time and evening/weekend programs available. *Faculty:* 14 full-time (11 women), 6 part-time/adjunct (2 women). *Students:* 4 full-time (all women), 59 part-time (47 women); includes 17 minority (8 Black or African American, non-Hispanic/Latino; 4 Asian, non-Hispanic/Latino; 5 Hispanic/Latino). Average age 31. 105 applicants, 50% accepted, 22 enrolled. In 2013, 20 master's awarded. *Degree requirements:* For master's, comprehensive exam, thesis optional, internship. *Entrance requirements:* For master's, GRE General Test, previous course work in calculus and statistics. Additional exam requirements/recommendations for international students: Required—TOEFL. *Application deadline:* For fall admission, 4/1 for domestic students; for spring admission, 11/1 for domestic students. Application fee: $125. *Financial support:* In 2013–14, 6 fellowships were awarded; career-related internships or fieldwork, Federal Work-Study, institutionally sponsored loans, and tuition waivers (partial) also available. Support available to part-time students. *Unit head:* Prof. Barbara Berney, Program Director, 212-396-7756, Fax: 212-481-5260, E-mail: bberney@hunter.cuny.edu. *Application contact:* Milena Solo, Director for Graduate Admissions, 212-772-4280, E-mail: milena.solo@hunter.cuny.edu.
Website: http://www.cuny.edu/site/sph/hunter-college/a-programs/graduate/hpm-mph.html

Husson University, Master of Business Administration Program, Bangor, ME 04401-2999. Offers general business administration (MBA); healthcare management (MBA); hospitality and tourism management (MBA); non-profit management (MBA). Part-time and evening/weekend programs available. *Faculty:* 7 full-time (4 women), 16 part-time/adjunct (3 women). *Students:* 91 full-time (55 women), 87 part-time (47 women); includes 21 minority (7 Black or African American, non-Hispanic/Latino; 11 Asian, non-Hispanic/Latino; 3 Two or more races, non-Hispanic/Latino), 4 international. 112 applicants, 88% accepted, 86 enrolled. In 2013, 163 master's awarded. *Degree requirements:* For master's, comprehensive exam (for some programs), thesis optional. *Entrance requirements:* For master's, GMAT or GRE, minimum GPA of 3.0. Additional exam requirements/recommendations for international students: Required—TOEFL (minimum score 550 paper-based). *Application deadline:* Applications are processed on a rolling basis. Application fee: $40. Electronic applications accepted. *Expenses:* Contact institution. *Financial support:* In 2013–14, 6 students received support. Career-related internships or fieldwork, Federal Work-Study, scholarships/grants, and unspecified assistantships available. Financial award application deadline: 4/15; financial award applicants required to submit FAFSA. *Unit head:* Prof. Stephanie Shayne, Director, Graduate and Online Programs, 207-404-5632, Fax: 207-992-4987, E-mail: shaynes@husson.edu. *Application contact:* Kristen Card, Director of Graduate Admissions, 207-404-5660, Fax: 207-941-7935, E-mail: cardk@husson.edu.
Website: http://www.husson.edu/mba

Independence University, Program in Business Administration in Health Care, Salt Lake City, UT 84107. Offers health care administration (MBA). Part-time and evening/weekend programs available. Postbaccalaureate distance learning degree programs offered (no on-campus study). *Degree requirements:* For master's, fieldwork/internship.

Independence University, Program in Health Care Administration, Salt Lake City, UT 84107. Offers MSHCA. Part-time and evening/weekend programs available. Postbaccalaureate distance learning degree programs offered (no on-campus study). *Degree requirements:* For master's, fieldwork, internship. *Entrance requirements:* For master's, previous course work in psychology.

Independence University, Program in Health Services, Salt Lake City, UT 84107. Offers community health (MSHS); wellness promotion (MSHS). Part-time and evening/weekend programs available. Postbaccalaureate distance learning degree programs offered (no on-campus study). *Degree requirements:* For master's, fieldwork, internship, final project (wellness promotion). *Entrance requirements:* For master's, previous course work in psychology.

Indiana Tech, Program in Business Administration, Fort Wayne, IN 46803-1297. Offers accounting (MBA); health care administration (MBA); human resources (MBA); management (MBA); marketing (MBA). Part-time and evening/weekend programs available. Postbaccalaureate distance learning degree programs offered (no on-campus study). *Students:* 160 full-time (94 women), 97 part-time (53 women); includes 69 minority (58 Black or African American, non-Hispanic/Latino; 1 Asian, non-Hispanic/Latino; 8 Hispanic/Latino; 2 Two or more races, non-Hispanic/Latino), 11 international. Average age 36. *Entrance requirements:* For master's, GMAT, bachelor's degree from

regionally-accredited university; minimum undergraduate GPA of 2.5; 2 years of significant work experience; 3 letters of recommendation. *Application deadline:* Applications are processed on a rolling basis. Application fee: $25. Electronic applications accepted. *Expenses: Tuition:* Full-time $8910; part-time $495 per credit. Tuition and fees vary according to course load, degree level and program. *Financial support:* Applicants required to submit FAFSA. *Unit head:* Dr. Andrew I. Nwanne, Associate Dean of Business/Academic Coordinator, 260-422-5561 Ext. 2214, E-mail: ainwanne@indianatech.edu.
Website: http://www.indianatech.edu/

Indiana University Bloomington, School of Public Health, Department of Applied Health Science, Bloomington, IN 47405. Offers behavioral, social, and community health (MPH); family health (MPH); health behavior (PhD); nutrition science (MS); professional health education (MPH); public health administration (MPH); safety management (MS); school and college health education (MS). *Accreditation:* CEPH (one or more programs are accredited). *Faculty:* 30 full-time (19 women). *Students:* 144 full-time (104 women), 26 part-time (16 women); includes 46 minority (23 Black or African American, non-Hispanic/Latino; 1 American Indian or Alaska Native, non-Hispanic/Latino; 8 Asian, non-Hispanic/Latino; 10 Hispanic/Latino; 4 Two or more races, non-Hispanic/Latino), 32 international. Average age 30. 129 applicants, 71% accepted, 58 enrolled. In 2013, 53 master's, 6 doctorates awarded. *Degree requirements:* For master's, thesis optional; for doctorate, comprehensive exam, thesis/dissertation. *Entrance requirements:* For master's, GRE (for MS in nutrition science), 3 recommendations; for doctorate, GRE, 3 recommendations. Additional exam requirements/recommendations for international students: Required—TOEFL (minimum score 550 paper-based; 80 iBT). *Application deadline:* For fall admission, 2/1 priority date for domestic students, 12/1 priority date for international students; for spring admission, 11/15 priority date for domestic students, 9/1 priority date for international students. Application fee: $55 ($65 for international students). Electronic applications accepted. *Financial support:* Fellowships, research assistantships with full and partial tuition reimbursements, teaching assistantships with full and partial tuition reimbursements, career-related internships or fieldwork, Federal Work-Study, institutionally sponsored loans, scholarships/grants, health care benefits, tuition waivers (partial), unspecified assistantships, and fee remissions available. Financial award application deadline: 3/1; financial award applicants required to submit FAFSA. *Faculty research:* Cancer education, HIV/AIDS and drug education, public health, parent-child interactions, safety education, obesity, public health policy, public health administration, school health, health education, human development, nutrition, human sexuality, chronic disease, early childhood health. *Total annual research expenditures:* $1.4 million. *Unit head:* Dr. David K. Lohrmann, Chair, 812-856-5101, Fax: 812-855-3936, E-mail: dlohrman@indiana.edu. *Application contact:* Dr. Susan Middlestadt, Associate Professor and Graduate Coordinator, 812-856-5768, Fax: 812-855-3936, E-mail: semiddle@indiana.edu.
Website: http://www.publichealth.indiana.edu/departments/applied-health-science/index.shtml

Indiana University Northwest, School of Public and Environmental Affairs, Gary, IN 46408-1197. Offers criminal justice (MPA); environmental affairs (Graduate Certificate); health services (MPA); human services (MPA); nonprofit management (Certificate); public management (MPA). *Accreditation:* NASPAA (one or more programs are accredited). Part-time programs available. *Faculty:* 5 full-time (3 women). *Students:* 17 full-time (13 women), 73 part-time (49 women); includes 62 minority (48 Black or African American, non-Hispanic/Latino; 2 Asian, non-Hispanic/Latino; 12 Hispanic/Latino). Average age 38. 25 applicants, 92% accepted, 21 enrolled. In 2013, 27 master's, 26 other advanced degrees awarded. *Entrance requirements:* For master's, GRE General Test or GMAT, letters of recommendation. *Application deadline:* For fall admission, 8/15 priority date for domestic students. Applications are processed on a rolling basis. *Financial support:* Career-related internships or fieldwork, Federal Work-Study, and tuition waivers (partial) available. Support available to part-time students. Financial award application deadline: 3/1. *Faculty research:* Employment in income security policies, evidence in criminal justice, equal employment law, social welfare policy and welfare reform, public finance in developing countries. *Unit head:* Dr. Barbara Peat, Department Chair, 219-981-5645. *Application contact:* Tierra Jackson, Senior Secretary, 219-981-5616, E-mail: jacksoti@iun.edu.
Website: http://www.iun.edu/spea/index.htm

Indiana University of Pennsylvania, School of Graduate Studies and Research, College of Health and Human Services, Department of Employment and Labor Relations, Program in Health Services Administration, Indiana, PA 15705-1087. Offers MS. Program offered at Northpointe Campus near Pittsburgh, PA. Part-time and evening/weekend programs available. *Faculty:* 4 full-time (1 woman). *Students:* 13 full-time (11 women); includes 1 minority (Black or African American, non-Hispanic/Latino). Average age 33. 16 applicants, 56% accepted, 8 enrolled. *Degree requirements:* For master's, thesis optional. *Application deadline:* Applications are processed on a rolling basis. Application fee: $50. Electronic applications accepted. *Expenses:* Tuition, state resident: full-time $3978; part-time $442 per credit. Tuition, nonresident: full-time $5967; part-time $663 per credit. *Required fees:* $2080; $115.55 per credit. $93 per semester. Tuition and fees vary according to degree level and program. *Financial support:* In 2013–14, 2 research assistantships with full and partial tuition reimbursements (averaging $1,000 per year) were awarded; career-related internships or fieldwork, Federal Work-Study, scholarships/grants, and unspecified assistantships also available. Financial award application deadline: 4/15; financial award applicants required to submit FAFSA. *Unit head:* Dr. Michael Korns, Coordinator, 724-357-4424, E-mail: mkorns@iup.edu.
Website: http://www.iup.edu/page.aspx?id=129652

Indiana University of Pennsylvania, School of Graduate Studies and Research, College of Health and Human Services, Department of Nursing and Allied Health, Indiana, PA 15705-1087. Offers health service administration (MS); nursing (MS, PhD); nursing administration (MS); nursing education (MS). Part-time and evening/weekend programs available. *Faculty:* 7 full-time (6 women). *Students:* 1 (woman) full-time, 84 part-time (76 women); includes 2 minority (1 Black or African American, non-Hispanic/Latino; 1 Hispanic/Latino). Average age 40. 68 applicants, 63% accepted, 36 enrolled. In 2013, 21 master's, 2 doctorates awarded. *Degree requirements:* For master's, thesis optional; for doctorate, comprehensive exam, thesis/dissertation. *Entrance requirements:* For master's, 2 letters of recommendation; for doctorate, GRE, 2 letters of recommendation, current nursing license, current curriculum vitae. Additional exam requirements/recommendations for international students: Required—TOEFL (minimum score 540 paper-based). *Application deadline:* Applications are processed on a rolling basis. Application fee: $50. Electronic applications accepted. *Expenses:* Tuition, state resident: full-time $3978; part-time $442 per credit. Tuition, nonresident: full-time $5967; part-time $663 per credit. *Required fees:* $2080; $115.55 per credit. $93 per semester. Tuition and fees vary according to degree level and program. *Financial support:* In 2013–14, 7 fellowships with partial tuition reimbursements (averaging $720 per year), 7 research assistantships with full and partial tuition reimbursements (averaging $1,862 per year), 1 teaching assistantship with partial tuition reimbursement (averaging $22,848 per year) were awarded; career-related internships or fieldwork, Federal Work-Study, scholarships/grants, and unspecified assistantships also available. Support available to part-time students. Financial award application deadline: 4/15; financial award applicants required to submit FAFSA. *Unit head:* Dr. Elizabeth Palmer, Chairperson, 724-357-2558, E-mail: lpalmer@iup.edu. *Application contact:* Dr. Kristy S. Chunta, Assistant Chairperson and Graduate Coordinator, 724-357-2408, E-mail: kchunta@iup.edu.
Website: http://www.iup.edu/rn-alliedhealth

Indiana University–Purdue University Indianapolis, School of Public Health, Indianapolis, IN 46202-2896. Offers biostatistics (MPH); environmental health science (MPH); epidemiology (MPH, PhD); health administration (MHA); health policy and management (MPH, PhD); social and behavioral sciences (MPH). *Accreditation:* CEPH. *Students:* 121 full-time (87 women), 161 part-time (111 women); includes 66 minority (32 Black or African American, non-Hispanic/Latino; 19 Asian, non-Hispanic/Latino; 13 Hispanic/Latino; 1 Native Hawaiian or other Pacific Islander, non-Hispanic/Latino; 1 Two or more races, non-Hispanic/Latino), 10 international. Average age 30. 185 applicants, 70% accepted, 95 enrolled. In 2013, 25 master's awarded. Application fee: $55 ($65 for international students). *Expenses:* Contact institution. *Financial support:* In 2013–14, 1 fellowship (averaging $17,650 per year), 4 research assistantships (averaging $22,000 per year), 8 teaching assistantships (averaging $24,000 per year) were awarded. *Unit head:* Dr. Paul Halverson, Dean, 317-274-4242. *Application contact:* Shawne Mathis, Student Services Coordinator, 317-278-0337, E-mail: snmathis@iupui.edu.
Website: http://www.pbhealth.iupui.edu/

Indiana Wesleyan University, College of Adult and Professional Studies, Graduate Studies in Business, Marion, IN 46953. Offers accounting (MBA, Graduate Certificate); applied management (MBA); business administration (MBA); health care (MBA, Graduate Certificate); human resources (MBA, Graduate Certificate); management (MS); organizational leadership (MA). Part-time and evening/weekend programs available. Postbaccalaureate distance learning degree programs offered (no on-campus study). *Degree requirements:* For master's, applied business or management project. *Entrance requirements:* For master's, minimum GPA of 2.5, 2 years of related work experience. Additional exam requirements/recommendations for international students: Required—TOEFL (minimum score 550 paper-based). Electronic applications accepted. *Expenses: Tuition:* Full-time $8712; part-time $484 per credit hour. *Required fees:* $1673; $105 per credit hour. Tuition and fees vary according to course load, degree level, campus/location and program.

Institute of Public Administration, Programs in Public Administration, Dublin, Ireland. Offers healthcare management (MA); local government management (MA); public management (MA, Diploma).

Iona College, Hagan School of Business, Department of Management, Business Administration and Health Care Management, New Rochelle, NY 10801-1890. Offers business administration (MBA); health care management (MBA, AC); human resource management (MBA, PMC); long term care services management (AC); management (MBA, PMC). Part-time and evening/weekend programs available. *Faculty:* 7 full-time (1 woman), 4 part-time/adjunct (1 woman). *Students:* 31 full-time (20 women), 78 part-time (46 women); includes 20 minority (6 Black or African American, non-Hispanic/Latino; 1 Asian, non-Hispanic/Latino; 13 Hispanic/Latino), 7 international. Average age 30. 28 applicants, 96% accepted, 24 enrolled. In 2013, 62 master's, 60 other advanced degrees awarded. *Entrance requirements:* For master's, GMAT, 2 letters of recommendation, minimum GPA of 3.0; for other advanced degree, GMAT, minimum GPA of 3.0. Additional exam requirements/recommendations for international students: Required—TOEFL (minimum score 550 paper-based; 80 iBT), IELTS (minimum score 6.5). *Application deadline:* For fall admission, 8/15 priority date for domestic students, 8/1 priority date for international students; for winter admission, 11/15 priority date for domestic students, 11/1 priority date for international students; for spring admission, 2/15 priority date for domestic students, 2/1 priority date for international students; for summer admission, 5/15 priority date for domestic students, 5/1 priority date for international students. Applications are processed on a rolling basis. Application fee: $50. Electronic applications accepted. *Expenses:* Contact institution. *Financial support:* In 2013–14, 39 students received support. Scholarships/grants, tuition waivers (partial), and unspecified assistantships available. Support available to part-time students. Financial award application deadline: 4/15; financial award applicants required to submit FAFSA. *Faculty research:* Information systems, strategic management, corporate values and ethics. *Unit head:* Prof. Hugh McCabe, Acting Chair, 914-633-2631, E-mail: hmccabe@iona.edu. *Application contact:* Cameron Hudson, Director of MBA Admissions, 914-633-2288, Fax: 914-637-2708, E-mail: chudson@iona.edu.
Website: http://www.iona.edu/Academics/Hagan-School-of-Business/Departments/Management-Business-Administration-Health-Car/Graduate-Programs.aspx

John Hancock University, MBA Program, Oakbrook Terrace, IL 60181. Offers e-commerce (MBA); finance (MBA); general business (MBA); global management (MBA); health care administration (MBA); leadership (MBA); management of information systems (MBA); marketing (MBA); professional accounting (MBA); project management (MBA); public accounting (MBA); risk management (MBA).

Johns Hopkins University, Bloomberg School of Public Health, Department of Health Policy and Management, Baltimore, MD 21205-1996. Offers bioethics and policy (PhD); health and public policy (PhD); health care management and leadership (Dr PH); health economics (MHS); health economics and policy (PhD); health finance and management (MHA); health policy (MSPH); health services research and policy (PhD); public policy (MPP). *Accreditation:* CAHME (one or more programs are accredited). Part-time programs available. *Faculty:* 60 full-time (32 women), 178 part-time/adjunct (66 women). *Students:* 204 full-time (152 women), 107 part-time (56 women); includes 81 minority (12 Black or African American, non-Hispanic/Latino; 1 American Indian or Alaska Native, non-Hispanic/Latino; 45 Asian, non-Hispanic/Latino; 14 Hispanic/Latino; 1 Native Hawaiian or other Pacific Islander, non-Hispanic/Latino; 8 Two or more races, non-Hispanic/Latino), 92 international. Average age 31. 550 applicants, 42% accepted, 113 enrolled. In 2013, 55 master's, 34 doctorates awarded. *Degree requirements:* For master's, thesis (for some programs), internship (for some programs); for doctorate, comprehensive exam, thesis/dissertation, 1-year full-time residency (for some programs), oral and written exams. *Entrance requirements:* For master's, GRE General Test or GMAT, 3 letters of recommendation, curriculum vitae/resume; for doctorate, GRE General Test or GMAT, 3 letters of recommendation, curriculum vitae, transcripts. Additional exam requirements/recommendations for international students: Recommended—TOEFL (minimum score 600 paper-based; 100 iBT), IELTS. *Application deadline:* For fall admission, 12/1 for domestic and international students. Applications are processed on a rolling basis. Application fee: $45. Electronic applications accepted. *Financial support:* Fellowships, research assistantships, teaching assistantships, career-related internships or fieldwork, Federal Work-Study, institutionally sponsored loans, scholarships/grants, traineeships, and stipends available. Support available to part-time students. Financial award application deadline: 3/15; financial award applicants required to submit FAFSA. *Faculty research:* Quality of care and health outcomes, health care finance and technology, health disparities and vulnerable populations, injury prevention, health policy and health care policy. *Total annual research expenditures:* $14.2 million. *Unit head:* Dr. Ellen J. MacKenzie, Chairman, 410-955-3625, E-mail: emackenz@jhsph.edu. *Application contact:* Mary Sewell, Coordinator, 410-955-2489, Fax: 410-614-9152, E-mail: msewell@jhsph.edu.
Website: http://www.jhsph.edu/hpm/

Health Services Management and Hospital Administration

Johns Hopkins University, Bloomberg School of Public Health, Department of International Health, Baltimore, MD 21205. Offers global disease epidemiology and control (MHS, PhD); health systems (MHS, PhD); human nutrition (MHS, PhD); international health (MSPH, Dr PH); registered dietician (MSPH); social and behavioral interventions (MHS, PhD). *Faculty:* 137 full-time (82 women), 185 part-time/adjunct (63 women). *Students:* 284 full-time (212 women), 4 part-time (3 women); includes 70 minority (11 Black or African American, non-Hispanic/Latino; 1 American Indian or Alaska Native, non-Hispanic/Latino; 41 Asian, non-Hispanic/Latino; 6 Hispanic/Latino; 11 Two or more races, non-Hispanic/Latino), 73 international. Average age 28. 515 applicants, 44% accepted, 104 enrolled. In 2013, 78 master's, 24 doctorates awarded. *Degree requirements:* For master's, comprehensive exam, thesis (for some programs), 1-year full-time residency, 4-9 month internship; for doctorate, comprehensive exam, thesis/dissertation or alternative, 1.5 years' full-time residency, oral and written exams. *Entrance requirements:* For master's, GRE General Test or MCAT, 3 letters of recommendation, resume; for doctorate, GRE General Test or MCAT, 3 letters of recommendation, resume, transcripts. Additional exam requirements/recommendations for international students: Required—TOEFL (minimum score 600 paper-based; 100 iBT); Recommended—IELTS (minimum score 7). *Application deadline:* For fall admission, 1/2 priority date for domestic and international students. Applications are processed on a rolling basis. Application fee: $45. Electronic applications accepted. *Financial support:* Fellowships, Federal Work-Study, institutionally sponsored loans, scholarships/grants, traineeships, and stipends available. Financial award application deadline: 1/2. *Faculty research:* Nutrition, infectious diseases, health systems, health economics, humanitarian emergencies. *Total annual research expenditures:* $72 million. *Unit head:* Dr. David Peters, Chair, 410-955-3928, Fax: 410-955-7159, E-mail: dpeters@jhsph.edu. *Application contact:* Cristina G. Salazar, Academic Program Manager, 410-955-3734, Fax: 410-955-7159, E-mail: csalazar@jhsph.edu.
Website: http://www.jhsph.edu/dept/IH/

Johns Hopkins University, Carey Business School, Health Care Management Programs, Baltimore, MD 21218-2699. Offers business of health care (Certificate); health care management (MS). Part-time and evening/weekend programs available. *Faculty:* 29 full-time (6 women), 135 part-time/adjunct (29 women). *Students:* 2 full-time (both women), 8 part-time (6 women); includes 4 minority (1 Black or African American, non-Hispanic/Latino; 1 Asian, non-Hispanic/Latino; 1 Hispanic/Latino; 1 Two or more races, non-Hispanic/Latino), 1 international. Average age 37. 13 applicants, 92% accepted, 9 enrolled. *Entrance requirements:* For master's, GMAT or GRE, minimum GPA of 3.0, resume, work experience, two letters of recommendation; for Certificate, minimum GPA of 3.0, resume, work experience, two letters of recommendation. Additional exam requirements/recommendations for international students: Required—TOEFL (minimum score 600 paper-based; 100 iBT). *Application deadline:* For fall admission, 4/1 for international students; for spring admission, 9/15 for international students. Applications are processed on a rolling basis. Application fee: $100. Electronic applications accepted. *Financial support:* Scholarships/grants available. Support available to part-time students. Financial award application deadline: 4/15; financial award applicants required to submit FAFSA. *Unit head:* Dr. Dipankar Chakravarti, Vice Dean of Programs, 410-234-9311, E-mail: dipankar.chakravarti@jhu.edu. *Application contact:* Robin Greenberg, Admissions Coordinator, 410-234-9227, Fax: 443-529-1554, E-mail: carey.admissions@jhu.edu.
Website: http://carey.jhu.edu/academics/master-of-science/ms-in-healthcare-management/

Jones International University, School of Business, Centennial, CO 80112. Offers accounting (MBA); business communication (MABC); entrepreneurship (MABC, MBA); finance (MBA); global enterprise management (MBA); health care management (MBA); information security management (MBA); information technology management (MBA); leadership and influence (MABC); leading the customer-driven organization (MABC); negotiation and conflict management (MBA); project management (MABC, MBA). Program only offered online. Part-time and evening/weekend programs available. Postbaccalaureate distance learning degree programs offered (no on-campus study). *Degree requirements:* For master's, capstone project. *Entrance requirements:* For master's, minimum cumulative GPA of 2.5. Additional exam requirements/recommendations for international students: Recommended—TOEFL (minimum score 550 paper-based). Electronic applications accepted.

Kaplan University, Davenport Campus, School of Business, Davenport, IA 52807-2095. Offers business administration (MBA); change leadership (MS); entrepreneurship (MBA); finance (MBA); health care management (MBA, MS); human resource (MBA); international business (MBA); management (MS); marketing (MBA); project management (MBA, MS); supply chain management and logistics (MBA, MS). *Accreditation:* ACBSP. Part-time and evening/weekend programs available. Postbaccalaureate distance learning degree programs offered (no on-campus study). *Entrance requirements:* Additional exam requirements/recommendations for international students: Required—TOEFL (minimum score 550 paper-based; 80 iBT). Electronic applications accepted.

Kaplan University, Davenport Campus, School of Legal Studies, Davenport, IA 52807-2095. Offers health care delivery (MS); pathway to paralegal (Postbaccalaureate Certificate); state and local government (MS). Part-time and evening/weekend programs available. Postbaccalaureate distance learning degree programs offered (no on-campus study). *Entrance requirements:* Additional exam requirements/recommendations for international students: Required—TOEFL (minimum score 550 paper-based; 80 iBT).

Kean University, College of Business and Public Management, Program in Public Administration, Union, NJ 07083. Offers environmental management (MPA); health services administration (MPA); non-profit management (MPA); public administration (MPA). *Accreditation:* NASPAA. Part-time programs available. *Faculty:* 13 full-time (4 women). *Students:* 64 full-time (38 women), 81 part-time (47 women); includes 100 minority (69 Black or African American, non-Hispanic/Latino; 7 Asian, non-Hispanic/Latino; 22 Hispanic/Latino; 2 Two or more races, non-Hispanic/Latino), 3 international. Average age 32. 76 applicants, 82% accepted, 40 enrolled. In 2013, 48 master's awarded. *Degree requirements:* For master's, thesis, internship, research seminar. *Entrance requirements:* For master's, minimum cumulative GPA of 3.0, official transcripts from all institutions attended, two letters of recommendation, personal statement, writing sample, professional resume/curriculum vitae. Additional exam requirements/recommendations for international students: Required—TOEFL (minimum score 550 paper-based; 79 iBT). *Application deadline:* For fall admission, 6/1 for domestic and international students; for spring admission, 12/1 for domestic and international students. Applications are processed on a rolling basis. Application fee: $75 ($150 for international students). Electronic applications accepted. *Expenses:* Tuition, state resident: full-time $12,099; part-time $589 per credit. Tuition, nonresident: full-time $16,399; part-time $722 per credit. *Required fees:* $3050; $139 per credit. Part-time tuition and fees vary according to course level, course load, degree level and program. *Financial support:* In 2013–14, 17 research assistantships with full tuition reimbursements (averaging $3,713 per year) were awarded; unspecified assistantships also available. Financial award applicants required to submit FAFSA. *Unit head:* Dr. Patricia Moore, Program Coordinator, 908-737-4314, E-mail: pmoore@kean.edu. *Application contact:* Reenat Hasan, Admissions Counselor, 908-737-5923, Fax: 908-737-5925, E-mail: hasanr@kean.edu.
Website: http://grad.kean.edu/masters-programs/public-administration

Keiser University, Master of Business Administration Program, Ft. Lauderdale, FL 33309. Offers accounting (MBA); health services management (MBA); information security management (MBA); international business (MBA); leadership for managers (MBA); marketing (MBA). All concentrations except information security management also offered in Mandarin; leadership for managers and international business also offered in Spanish. Part-time programs available. Postbaccalaureate distance learning degree programs offered (minimal on-campus study).

Kennesaw State University, College of Health and Human Services, Program in Advanced Care Management and Leadership, Kennesaw, GA 30144-5591. Offers MSN. Part-time and evening/weekend programs available. Postbaccalaureate distance learning degree programs offered (minimal on-campus study). *Students:* 12 full-time (10 women), 3 part-time (all women); includes 3 minority (all Black or African American, non-Hispanic/Latino). Average age 40. 9 applicants, 89% accepted, 7 enrolled. In 2013, 6 master's awarded. *Entrance requirements:* For master's, GRE General Test, minimum GPA of 3.0, RN license. Additional exam requirements/recommendations for international students: Required—TOEFL (minimum score 550 paper-based; 80 iBT), IELTS (minimum score 6). *Application deadline:* For fall admission, 6/1 for domestic and international students. Application fee: $60. Electronic applications accepted. *Expenses:* Tuition, state resident: full-time $4806; part-time $267 per semester hour. Tuition, nonresident: full-time $17,298; part-time $961 per semester hour. *Required fees:* $1834; $784.50 per semester. *Financial support:* In 2013–14, 2 research assistantships with tuition reimbursements (averaging $8,000 per year) were awarded; unspecified assistantships also available. Financial award application deadline: 4/1; financial award applicants required to submit FAFSA. *Unit head:* Dr. Marilyn King, Director, 770-423-6172, Fax: 770-423-6870, E-mail: mking71@kennesaw.edu. *Application contact:* Jerryl Morris, Admissions Counselor, 678-797-2030, Fax: 770-423-6885, E-mail: ksugrad@kennesaw.edu.

King's College, Program in Health Care Administration, Wilkes-Barre, PA 18711-0801. Offers MS. *Accreditation:* AACSB. Part-time programs available. *Entrance requirements:* Additional exam requirements/recommendations for international students: Required—TOEFL (minimum score 600 paper-based).

Lake Erie College, School of Business, Painesville, OH 44077-3389. Offers general management (MBA); health care administration (MBA). Part-time and evening/weekend programs available. *Faculty:* 8 full-time (3 women), 2 part-time/adjunct (0 women). *Students:* 23 full-time (12 women), 135 part-time (56 women); includes 19 minority (12 Black or African American, non-Hispanic/Latino; 5 Asian, non-Hispanic/Latino; 1 Hispanic/Latino; 1 Two or more races, non-Hispanic/Latino), 3 international. Average age 34. 100 applicants, 77% accepted, 65 enrolled. In 2013, 53 master's awarded. *Entrance requirements:* For master's, GMAT or minimum GPA of 3.0, resume, references. Additional exam requirements/recommendations for international students: Required—TOEFL (minimum score 550 paper-based). *Application deadline:* For fall admission, 8/1 priority date for domestic students, 6/1 for international students; for spring admission, 12/15 for domestic students, 10/1 for international students. Applications are processed on a rolling basis. Application fee: $30. Electronic applications accepted. Application fee is waived when completed online. Tuition and fees vary according to course load and program. *Financial support:* Career-related internships or fieldwork, tuition waivers (full and partial), and unspecified assistantships available. Financial award applicants required to submit FAFSA. *Unit head:* Prof. Robert Trebar, Dean of the School of Business, 440-375-7115, Fax: 440-375-7005, E-mail: rtrebar@lec.edu. *Application contact:* Milena Velez, Senior Admissions Counselor, 800-533-4996, Fax: 440-375-7000, E-mail: admissions@lec.edu.
Website: http://www.lec.edu/parkermba

Lake Forest Graduate School of Management, The Leadership MBA Program, Lake Forest, IL 60045. Offers finance (MBA); global business (MBA); healthcare management (MBA); management (MBA); marketing (MBA); organizational behavior (MBA). Part-time and evening/weekend programs available. *Entrance requirements:* For master's, 4 years of work experience in field, interview, 2 letters of recommendation. Electronic applications accepted.

Lakeland College, Graduate Studies Division, Program in Business Administration, Sheboygan, WI 53082-0359. Offers accounting (MBA); finance (MBA); healthcare management (MBA); project management (MBA). *Entrance requirements:* For master's, GMAT. *Expenses:* Contact institution.

Lamar University, College of Graduate Studies, College of Business, Beaumont, TX 77710. Offers accounting (MBA); experiential business and entrepreneurship (MBA); financial management (MBA); healthcare administration (MBA); information systems (MBA); management (MBA). *Accreditation:* AACSB. Part-time and evening/weekend programs available. *Degree requirements:* For master's, comprehensive exam (for some programs), thesis optional. *Entrance requirements:* For master's, GMAT. Additional exam requirements/recommendations for international students: Required—TOEFL (minimum score 525 paper-based). *Faculty research:* Marketing, finance, quantitative methods, management information systems, legal, environmental.

Lasell College, Graduate and Professional Studies in Management, Newton, MA 02466-2709. Offers business administration (PMBA); elder care management (MSM, Graduate Certificate); elder care marketing (MSM); human resource management (Graduate Certificate); human resources management (MSM); integrated marketing communication (Graduate Certificate); management (MSM, Graduate Certificate); marketing (MSM, Graduate Certificate); non-profit management (MSM, Graduate Certificate); project management (MSM, Graduate Certificate); public relations (Graduate Certificate). Part-time and evening/weekend programs available. Postbaccalaureate distance learning degree programs offered (no on-campus study). *Faculty:* 3 full-time (1 woman), 16 part-time/adjunct (9 women). *Students:* 46 full-time (33 women), 105 part-time (73 women); includes 35 minority (24 Black or African American, non-Hispanic/Latino; 1 American Indian or Alaska Native, non-Hispanic/Latino; 3 Asian, non-Hispanic/Latino; 7 Hispanic/Latino), 22 international. Average age 32. 88 applicants, 55% accepted, 29 enrolled. In 2013, 61 master's awarded. *Entrance requirements:* For master's and Graduate Certificate, bachelor's degree from an accredited institution. Additional exam requirements/recommendations for international students: Required—TOEFL (minimum score 550 paper-based; 79 iBT). *Application deadline:* For fall admission, 8/31 priority date for domestic students, 6/30 priority date for international students; for spring admission, 12/31 priority date for domestic students, 10/31 priority date for international students. Applications are processed on a rolling basis. Electronic applications accepted. *Expenses: Tuition:* Part-time $575 per credit. *Required fees:* $80 per semester. *Financial support:* Available to part-time students. Application deadline: 8/31; applicants required to submit FAFSA. *Unit head:* Dr. Joan Dolamore, Dean of Graduate and Professional Studies, 617-243-2485, Fax: 617-243-2450, E-mail: gradinfo@lasell.edu. *Application contact:* Adrienne Franciosi, Director of Graduate Admission, 617-243-2214, Fax: 617-243-2450, E-mail: gradinfo@lasell.edu.
Website: http://www.lasell.edu/Academics/Graduate-and-Professional-Studies/MS-in-Management.html

Lebanon Valley College, Program in Business Administration, Annville, PA 17003-1400. Offers business administration (MBA); healthcare management (MBA); school leadership (MBA). *Accreditation:* ACBSP. Part-time and evening/weekend programs available. *Faculty:* 3 full-time (0 women), 16 part-time/adjunct (2 women). *Students:* 14 full-time (6 women), 156 part-time (82 women); includes 12 minority (4 Black or African American, non-Hispanic/Latino; 1 American Indian or Alaska Native, non-Hispanic/Latino; 4 Asian, non-Hispanic/Latino; 3 Hispanic/Latino). Average age 38. In 2013, 48 master's awarded. *Entrance requirements:* For master's, 3 years of work experience. *Application deadline:* Applications are processed on a rolling basis. Application fee: $30. Electronic applications accepted. *Expenses:* Contact institution. *Financial support:* Application deadline: 5/1; applicants required to submit FAFSA. *Unit head:* Brenda Adams, Director of the MBA Program, 717-867-6335, Fax: 717-867-6018, E-mail: badams@lvc.edu. *Application contact:* Susan Greenawalt, Graduate Studies and Continuing Education Assistant/Records Coordinator, 717-867-6213, Fax: 717-867-6018, E-mail: greenawa@lvc.edu.
Website: http://www.lvc.edu/mba

Lehigh University, P.C. Rossin College of Engineering and Applied Science, Department of Industrial and Systems Engineering, Program in Healthcare Systems Engineering, Bethlehem, PA 18015. Offers M Eng. Part-time programs available. Postbaccalaureate distance learning degree programs offered (no on-campus study). *Faculty:* 3 part-time/adjunct (1 woman). *Students:* 24 full-time (15 women), 20 part-time (6 women); includes 5 minority (3 Black or African American, non-Hispanic/Latino; 2 Asian, non-Hispanic/Latino), 18 international. Average age 29. 35 applicants, 97% accepted, 12 enrolled. In 2013, 12 master's awarded. *Degree requirements:* For master's, 30 credits. *Entrance requirements:* For master's, GRE (minimum scores in the 75th percentile). Additional exam requirements/recommendations for international students: Required—TOEFL. *Application deadline:* For fall admission, 7/15 for domestic and international students; for spring admission, 12/1 for domestic and international students. Applications are processed on a rolling basis. Application fee: $75. Electronic applications accepted. *Financial support:* In 2013–14, 10 students received support. Application deadline: 1/15. *Faculty research:* Project management, engineering economics, statistics and stochastic processes, operations research, simulation and optimization and IT. *Unit head:* Prof. Hisham Nabaa, Professor of Practice, 610-758-3865, Fax: 610-758-6766, E-mail: hia206@lehigh.edu. *Application contact:* Linda Wismer, Coordinator, 610-758-5867, Fax: 610-758-6766, E-mail: liw511@lehigh.edu.
Website: http://www.lehigh.edu/ise/hse.html

LeTourneau University, Graduate Programs, Longview, TX 75607-7001. Offers business administration (MBA); counseling (MA); education (M Ed); engineering (MS); health care administration (MS); marriage and family therapy (MA); psychology (MA); strategic leadership (MSL). Part-time programs available. Postbaccalaureate distance learning degree programs offered (no on-campus study). *Faculty:* 15 full-time (7 women), 54 part-time/adjunct (23 women). *Students:* 58 full-time (45 women), 365 part-time (287 women); includes 106 minority (51 Black or African American, non-Hispanic/Latino; 3 American Indian or Alaska Native, non-Hispanic/Latino; 1 Asian, non-Hispanic/Latino; 45 Hispanic/Latino; 6 Two or more races, non-Hispanic/Latino), 4 international. Average age 38. 263 applicants, 68% accepted, 116 enrolled. In 2013, 112 master's awarded. *Degree requirements:* For master's, thesis (for some programs). *Entrance requirements:* For master's, GRE (for engineering programs), minimum GPA of 2.8 (3.0 for counseling and engineering programs). Additional exam requirements/recommendations for international students: Required—TOEFL. *Application deadline:* For fall admission, 8/22 for domestic students, 8/29 for international students; for winter admission, 10/10 for domestic students; for spring admission, 1/2 for domestic students, 1/10 for international students; for summer admission, 5/1 for domestic and international students. Applications are processed on a rolling basis. Electronic applications accepted. Application fee is waived when completed online. *Financial support:* In 2013–14, 11 students received support, including 13 research assistantships (averaging $9,122 per year); institutionally sponsored loans and unspecified assistantships also available. Financial award applicants required to submit FAFSA. *Unit head:* Dr. Robert Hudson, Vice President and Dean of the Graduate School, 903-233-1110, E-mail: roberthudson@letu.edu. *Application contact:* Chris Fontaine, Assistant Vice President for Global Campus Admissions, 903-233-4312, E-mail: chrisfontaine@letu.edu.
Website: http://www.adults.letu.edu/

Lewis University, College of Business, Graduate School of Management, Program in Business Administration, Romeoville, IL 60446. Offers accounting (MBA); custom elective option (MBA); e-business (MBA); finance (MBA); healthcare management (MBA); human resources management (MBA); international business (MBA); management information systems (MBA); marketing (MBA); project management (MBA); technology and operations management (MBA). Part-time and evening/weekend programs available. *Students:* 115 full-time (55 women), 227 part-time (129 women); includes 128 minority (74 Black or African American, non-Hispanic/Latino; 1 American Indian or Alaska Native, non-Hispanic/Latino; 9 Asian, non-Hispanic/Latino; 40 Hispanic/Latino; 4 Two or more races, non-Hispanic/Latino), 10 international. Average age 31. In 2013, 99 master's awarded. *Entrance requirements:* For master's, interview, bachelor's degree, resume, 2 recommendations. Additional exam requirements/recommendations for international students: Required—TOEFL (minimum score 550 paper-based). *Application deadline:* For fall admission, 8/15 priority date for domestic students, 5/1 priority date for international students; for spring admission, 11/15 priority date for international students. Applications are processed on a rolling basis. Application fee: $40. Electronic applications accepted. *Financial support:* Career-related internships or fieldwork, Federal Work-Study, scholarships/grants, and unspecified assistantships available. Financial award application deadline: 5/1; financial award applicants required to submit FAFSA. *Unit head:* Dr. Maureen Culleeney, Academic Program Director, 815-838-0500 Ext. 5631, E-mail: culleema@lewisu.edu. *Application contact:* Michele Ryan, Director of Admission, 815-838-0500 Ext. 5384, E-mail: gsm@lewisu.edu.

Liberty University, School of Business, Lynchburg, VA 24515. Offers accounting (MBA, MS, DBA); business administration (MBA); criminal justice (MBA); cyber security (MS); executive leadership (MA); healthcare (MBA); human resources (DBA); information systems (MS), including information assurance, technology management; international business (MBA, DBA); leadership (MBA, DBA); management and leadership (MA); marketing (MBA, MS, DBA), including digital marketing and advertising (MS), project management (MS), public relations (MS), sports marketing and media (MS); project management (MBA, DBA); public administration (MBA); public relations (MBA). Part-time programs available. Postbaccalaureate distance learning degree programs offered (minimal on-campus study). *Students:* 1,342 full-time (749 women), 3,704 part-time (1,820 women); includes 1,657 minority (1,221 Black or African American, non-Hispanic/Latino; 11 American Indian or Alaska Native, non-Hispanic/Latino; 74 Asian, non-Hispanic/Latino; 209 Hispanic/Latino; 13 Native Hawaiian or other Pacific Islander, non-Hispanic/Latino; 129 Two or more races, non-Hispanic/Latino), 40 international. Average age 35. 5,899 applicants, 48% accepted, 1716 enrolled. In 2013, 1,535 master's awarded. *Entrance requirements:* For master's, minimum undergraduate GPA of 3.0, 15 hours of upper-level business courses. Additional exam requirements/recommendations for international students: Required—TOEFL (minimum score 600 paper-based; 100 iBT). *Application deadline:* Applications are processed on a rolling basis. Application fee: $50. Electronic applications accepted. *Expenses:* Contact institution. *Unit head:* Dr. Scott Hicks, Dean, 434-592-4808, Fax: 434-582-2366, E-mail: smhicks@liberty.edu. *Application contact:* Jay Bridge, Director of Graduate Admissions, 800-424-9595, Fax: 800-628-7977, E-mail: gradadmissions@liberty.edu.
Website: http://www.liberty.edu/academics/business/index.cfm?PID-149

Lindenwood University, Graduate Programs, College of Individualized Education, St. Charles, MO 63301-1695. Offers administration (MSA); business administration (MBA); communications (MA); criminal justice and administration (MS); gerontology (MA); healthcare administration (MS); human resource management (MS); information technology (MBA, Certificate); managing information technology (MS); writing (MFA). Part-time and evening/weekend programs available. *Faculty:* 20 full-time (7 women), 96 part-time/adjunct (36 women). *Students:* 928 full-time (587 women), 85 part-time (53 women); includes 394 minority (336 Black or African American, non-Hispanic/Latino; 2 American Indian or Alaska Native, non-Hispanic/Latino; 7 Asian, non-Hispanic/Latino; 24 Hispanic/Latino; 2 Native Hawaiian or other Pacific Islander, non-Hispanic/Latino; 23 Two or more races, non-Hispanic/Latino), 33 international. Average age 34. 569 applicants, 62% accepted, 331 enrolled. In 2013, 487 master's awarded. *Degree requirements:* For master's, thesis (for some programs). *Entrance requirements:* For master's, interview, minimum GPA of 3.0. Additional exam requirements/recommendations for international students: Required—TOEFL (minimum score 550 paper-based; 80 iBT). *Application deadline:* For fall admission, 10/5 priority date for domestic and international students; for winter admission, 1/6 priority date for domestic and international students; for spring admission, 4/7 priority date for domestic and international students. Applications are processed on a rolling basis. Application fee: $30 ($100 for international students). Electronic applications accepted. *Expenses: Tuition:* Full-time $14,800; part-time $428 per credit hour. *Required fees:* $350. Tuition and fees vary according to course level and course load. *Financial support:* In 2013–14, 654 students received support. Career-related internships or fieldwork, institutionally sponsored loans, scholarships/grants, tuition waivers (partial), and unspecified assistantships available. Financial award application deadline: 6/30; financial award applicants required to submit FAFSA. *Unit head:* Dan Kemper, Dean, 636-949-4501, Fax: 636-949-4505, E-mail: dkemper@lindenwood.edu. *Application contact:* Brett Barger, Dean of Evening Admissions and Extension Campuses, 636-949-4934, Fax: 636-949-4109, E-mail: adultadmissions@lindenwood.edu.

Lindenwood University–Belleville, Graduate Programs, Belleville, IL 62226. Offers business administration (MBA); communications (MA), including digital and multimedia, media management, promotions, training and development; counseling (MA); criminal justice administration (MS); education (MA); healthcare administration (MS); human resource management (MS); school administration (MA); teaching (MAT).

Lipscomb University, College of Business, Nashville, TN 37204-3951. Offers accountancy (M Acc); accounting (MBA); conflict management (MBA); financial services (MBA); health care informatics (MBA); healthcare management (MBA); human resources (MHR); information security (MBA); leadership (MBA); nonprofit management (MBA); professional accountancy (Certificate); sports management (MBA); strategic human resources (MBA); sustainability (MBA); MBA/MS. *Accreditation:* ACBSP. Part-time and evening/weekend programs available. *Faculty:* 12 full-time (1 woman), 12 part-time/adjunct (2 women). *Students:* 90 full-time (44 women), 104 part-time (51 women); includes 28 minority (24 Black or African American, non-Hispanic/Latino; 3 Hispanic/Latino; 1 Two or more races, non-Hispanic/Latino), 6 international. Average age 33. 145 applicants, 79% accepted, 69 enrolled. In 2013, 98 master's, 1 other advanced degree awarded. *Entrance requirements:* For master's, GMAT, transcripts, interview, 2 references, resume. Additional exam requirements/recommendations for international students: Required—TOEFL (minimum score 570 paper-based). *Application deadline:* For fall admission, 6/15 for domestic students, 2/1 for international students; for winter admission, 6/1 for international students; for spring admission, 11/15 for domestic students. Applications are processed on a rolling basis. Application fee: $50 ($75 for international students). Electronic applications accepted. *Expenses:* Contact institution. *Financial support:* Career-related internships or fieldwork, scholarships/grants, tuition waivers (partial), and unspecified assistantships available. Support available to part-time students. Financial award application deadline: 7/1; financial award applicants required to submit FAFSA. *Faculty research:* Impact of spirituality on organization commitment, women in corporate leadership, psychological empowerment, training. *Unit head:* Joe Ivey, Associate Dean of Graduate Business Programs, 615-966-6229, Fax: 615-966-1818, E-mail: joe.ivey@lipscomb.edu. *Application contact:* Lisa Shacklett, Assistant Dean of Enrollment and Marketing, 615-966-5968, E-mail: lisa.shacklett@lipscomb.edu.
Website: http://www.lipscomb.edu/business/Graduate-Programs

Loma Linda University, School of Public Health, Programs in Health Administration, Loma Linda, CA 92350. Offers MBA, MHA, MPH. *Entrance requirements:* For master's, GMAT (MHA). Additional exam requirements/recommendations for international students: Required—Michigan Test of English Language Proficiency or TOEFL.

Long Island University–Hudson at Rockland, Graduate School, Master of Business Administration Program, Orangeburg, NY 10962. Offers business administration (Post Master's Certificate); entrepreneurship (MBA); finance (MBA); healthcare sector management (MBA); management (MBA). Part-time and evening/weekend programs available. *Entrance requirements:* For master's, GMAT, college transcripts, two letters of recommendation, personal statement, resume.

Long Island University–Hudson at Rockland, Graduate School, Programs in Health and Public Administration, Orangeburg, NY 10962. Offers gerontology (Advanced Certificate); health administration (MPA); public administration (MPA). Part-time and evening/weekend programs available. *Degree requirements:* For master's, thesis. *Entrance requirements:* For master's, college transcripts, letters of recommendation, personal statement, resume.

Long Island University–LIU Brooklyn, School of Health Professions, Department of Community Health, Brooklyn, NY 11201-8423. Offers community mental health (MS); family health (MS); health management (MS). Part-time and evening/weekend programs available. *Entrance requirements:* For master's, 2 letters of recommendation. Additional exam requirements/recommendations for international students: Required—TOEFL (minimum score 500 paper-based). Electronic applications accepted.

Long Island University–LIU Post, College of Management, Department of Health Care and Public Administration, Brookville, NY 11548-1300. Offers gerontology (Certificate); health care administration (MPA); health care administration/gerontology (MPA); nonprofit management (MPA, Certificate); public administration (MPA). *Accreditation:* NASPAA (one or more programs are accredited). Part-time and evening/weekend programs available. *Degree requirements:* For master's, thesis. *Entrance requirements:* For master's, GMAT, minimum GPA of 2.5; for Certificate, minimum GPA of 2.5. Electronic applications accepted. *Faculty research:* Critical issues in sexuality, social work in religious communities, gerontological social work.

Louisiana State University Health Sciences Center, School of Public Health, New Orleans, LA 70112. Offers behavioral and community health sciences (MPH); biostatistics (MPH, MS, PhD); community health sciences (PhD); environmental and occupational health sciences (MPH); epidemiology (MPH, PhD); health policy and systems management (MPH). *Accreditation:* CEPH. Part-time programs available. *Entrance requirements:* For master's, GRE General Test.

Health Services Management and Hospital Administration

Louisiana State University in Shreveport, College of Business, Education, and Human Development, Program in Health Administration, Shreveport, LA 71115-2399. Offers MHA. Part-time and evening/weekend programs available. Postbaccalaureate distance learning degree programs offered (no on-campus study). *Students:* 9 full-time (6 women), 20 part-time (11 women); includes 6 minority (4 Black or African American, non-Hispanic/Latino; 1 Asian, non-Hispanic/Latino; 1 Hispanic/Latino). Average age 31. 30 applicants, 80% accepted, 8 enrolled. In 2013, 8 master's awarded. *Entrance requirements:* For master's, GRE or GMAT, minimum GPA of 3.0, recommendations. Additional exam requirements/recommendations for international students: Required—TOEFL (minimum score 550 paper-based; 80 iBT). *Application deadline:* For fall admission, 6/30 for domestic and international students; for spring admission, 11/30 for domestic and international students. Applications are processed on a rolling basis. Application fee: $10 ($20 for international students). *Expenses: Tuition, area resident:* Part-time $182 per credit hour. *Required fees:* $51. *Financial support:* In 2013–14, 3 students received support. *Faculty research:* Healthcare marketing, law and ethics, leadership. *Unit head:* Dr. John Fortenberry, Program Director, 318-212-0240, E-mail: john.fortenberry@lsus.edu. *Application contact:* Christianne Wojcik, Secretary, Graduate Studies, 318-797-5247, Fax: 318-798-4120, E-mail: christianne.wojcik@lsus.edu.

Loyola University Chicago, Graduate School, Marcella Niehoff School of Nursing, Nursing Administration Program, Chicago, IL 60660. Offers MSN. Part-time and evening/weekend programs available. Postbaccalaureate distance learning degree programs offered (minimal on-campus study). *Faculty:* 45 full-time (44 women). *Students:* 1 (woman) full-time, 35 part-time (31 women); includes 13 minority (3 Black or African American, non-Hispanic/Latino; 6 Asian, non-Hispanic/Latino; 2 Hispanic/Latino; 2 Native Hawaiian or other Pacific Islander, non-Hispanic/Latino). Average age 38. 16 applicants, 56% accepted, 6 enrolled. In 2013, 10 master's awarded. *Degree requirements:* For master's, comprehensive exam or oral thesis defense. *Entrance requirements:* For master's, BSN, minimum nursing GPA of 3.0, IL nursing license, 1000 hours of experience before starting clinical. *Application deadline:* Applications are processed on a rolling basis. Application fee: $50. Electronic applications accepted. *Expenses: Tuition:* Full-time $16,740; part-time $930 per credit. *Required fees:* $135 per semester. *Financial support:* Traineeships available. Financial award application deadline: 3/1. *Faculty research:* Patient classification systems, career/job mobility. *Unit head:* Dr. Marijo Letizia, Associate Dean, 708-216-9325, Fax: 708-216-9555, E-mail: mletizi@luc.edu. *Application contact:* Amy Weatherford, Enrollment Advisor, School of Nursing, 708-216-3751, Fax: 708-216-9555, E-mail: aweatherford@luc.edu.
Website: http://www.luc.edu/nursing/

Loyola University Chicago, Graduate School, Program in Bioethics and Health Policy, Chicago, IL 60660. Offers D Be, Certificate, MD/MA. Postbaccalaureate distance learning degree programs offered (no on-campus study). *Students:* 13 full-time (9 women), 94 part-time (56 women); includes 13 minority (7 Black or African American, non-Hispanic/Latino; 4 Asian, non-Hispanic/Latino; 2 Hispanic/Latino), 1 international. Average age 47. 55 applicants, 67% accepted, 31 enrolled. In 2013, 8 doctorates, 4 Certificates awarded. *Expenses: Tuition:* Full-time $16,740; part-time $930 per credit. *Required fees:* $135 per semester. *Financial support:* Scholarships/grants available. *Unit head:* Dr. Samuel Attoh, Dean, 773-508-8948, Fax: 773-508-2460, E-mail: sattoh@luc.edu. *Application contact:* Ron Martin, Assistant Director of Enrollment Management, 312-915-8950, Fax: 312-915-8905, E-mail: gradapp@luc.edu.

Loyola University Chicago, Institute of Pastoral Studies, Master of Arts in Pastoral Studies Program, Chicago, IL 60660. Offers healthcare (MA); religious education (MA); youth ministry (MA). *Accreditation:* ACIPE. Part-time programs available. Postbaccalaureate distance learning degree programs offered (no on-campus study). *Faculty:* 11 full-time (5 women). *Students:* 9 full-time (6 women), 73 part-time (54 women); includes 15 minority (6 Black or African American, non-Hispanic/Latino; 2 Asian, non-Hispanic/Latino; 7 Hispanic/Latino), 4 international. Average age 46. 30 applicants, 90% accepted, 17 enrolled. In 2013, 14 master's awarded. *Entrance requirements:* Additional exam requirements/recommendations for international students: Required—TOEFL. *Application deadline:* For fall admission, 8/1 priority date for domestic students; for spring admission, 12/1 for domestic students. Applications are processed on a rolling basis. Application fee: $50. Electronic applications accepted. *Expenses: Tuition:* Full-time $16,740; part-time $930 per credit. *Required fees:* $135 per semester. *Financial support:* Career-related internships or fieldwork, Federal Work-Study, institutionally sponsored loans, and scholarships/grants available. Support available to part-time students. Financial award application deadline: 3/1. *Faculty research:* Karl Rahner, Daniel Berrigan. *Unit head:* Dr. Heidi Russell, Director, 312-915-7476, Fax: 312-915-7410, E-mail: hrussell@luc.edu. *Application contact:* Rachel D. Gibbons, Assistant Director, 312-915-7450, Fax: 312-915-7410, E-mail: rgibbon@luc.edu.
Website: http://www.luc.edu/ips/academics/maps/index.shtml

Loyola University Chicago, Quinlan School of Business, MBA Programs, Chicago, IL 60610. Offers accounting (MBA); business ethics (MBA); derivative markets (MBA); economics (MBA); entrepreneurship (MBA); executive business administration (MBA); finance (MBA); healthcare management (MBA); human resources management (MBA); information systems management (MBA); intercontinental (MBA); international business (MBA); marketing (MBA); operations management (MBA); risk management (MBA); JD/MBA. Part-time and evening/weekend programs available. *Faculty:* 76 full-time (20 women), 10 part-time/adjunct (4 women). *Students:* 73 full-time (34 women), 294 part-time (129 women); includes 60 minority (18 Black or African American, non-Hispanic/Latino; 28 Asian, non-Hispanic/Latino; 14 Hispanic/Latino), 19 international. Average age 31. 529 applicants, 51% accepted, 153 enrolled. In 2013, 229 master's awarded. *Entrance requirements:* For master's, GMAT or GRE, official transcripts, two letters of recommendation, statement of purpose, resume. Additional exam requirements/recommendations for international students: Required—TOEFL (minimum score 90 iBT) or IELTS (minimum score 6.5). *Application deadline:* For fall admission, 7/15 for domestic and international students; for winter admission, 10/1 for domestic and international students; for spring admission, 1/15 for domestic and international students; for summer admission, 4/1 for domestic and international students. Applications are processed on a rolling basis. Application fee: $50. Electronic applications accepted. Application fee is waived when completed online. *Expenses: Tuition:* Full-time $16,740; part-time $930 per credit. *Required fees:* $135 per semester. *Financial support:* Scholarships/grants and unspecified assistantships available. *Faculty research:* Social enterprise and responsibility, emerging markets, supply chain management, risk management. *Unit head:* Jennifer Huntley, Assistant Dean for Graduate Programs, 312-915-6124, Fax: 312-915-7207, E-mail: jhuntle@luc.edu. *Application contact:* Jessica Gagle, Enrollment Advisor, Quinlan School of Business Graduate Programs, 312-915-8908, Fax: 312-915-7207, E-mail: jgagle@luc.edu.

Loyola University New Orleans, College of Social Sciences, School of Nursing, New Orleans, LA 70118-6195. Offers health care systems management (MSN); nursing (MSN, DNP). Part-time and evening/weekend programs available. Postbaccalaureate distance learning degree programs offered. *Faculty:* 16 full-time (15 women), 9 part-time/adjunct (7 women). *Students:* 432 full-time (388 women), 108 part-time (102 women); includes 160 minority (113 Black or African American, non-Hispanic/Latino; 2 American Indian or Alaska Native, non-Hispanic/Latino; 13 Asian, non-Hispanic/Latino; 29 Hispanic/Latino; 2 Native Hawaiian or other Pacific Islander, non-Hispanic/Latino; 1 Two or more races, non-Hispanic/Latino). Average age 42. 285 applicants, 83% accepted, 200 enrolled. In 2013, 185 master's, 15 doctorates awarded. *Degree requirements:* For doctorate, capstone project. *Entrance requirements:* For master's, BSN, Louisiana nursing license, 1 year of work experience in clinical nursing, minimum undergraduate GPA of 2.8, interview, resume. Additional exam requirements/recommendations for international students: Required—TOEFL (minimum score 550 paper-based). *Application deadline:* For fall admission, 8/1 priority date for domestic and international students; for winter admission, 12/15 priority date for domestic and international students; for spring admission, 5/15 priority date for domestic and international students. Applications are processed on a rolling basis. Application fee: $20. Electronic applications accepted. *Expenses: Tuition:* Part-time $818 per hour. Part-time tuition and fees vary according to program. *Financial support:* Traineeships and Incumbent Workers Training Program grants available. Financial award application deadline: 5/1; financial award applicants required to submit FAFSA. *Faculty research:* Increasing compliance with treatment, patient satisfaction with care provided by nurse practitioners. *Unit head:* Dr. Mary D. Oriol, Interim Director, 800-488-6257, Fax: 504-865-3254, E-mail: nursing@loyno.edu. *Application contact:* Deborah Smith, Assistant to the Director, 504-865-2823, Fax: 504-865-3254, E-mail: dhsmith@loyno.edu.
Website: http://css.loyno.edu/nursing

Madonna University, Program in Health Services, Livonia, MI 48150-1173. Offers MSHS. Part-time programs available. *Degree requirements:* For master's, thesis or alternative. *Entrance requirements:* For master's, GRE General Test or minimum GPA of 3.25. Additional exam requirements/recommendations for international students: Required—TOEFL, TWE. Electronic applications accepted.

Marlboro College, Graduate and Professional Studies, Program in Healthcare Administration, Brattleboro, VT 05301. Offers MSM. Part-time and evening/weekend programs available. Postbaccalaureate distance learning degree programs offered (minimal on-campus study). *Faculty:* 8 part-time/adjunct (3 women). *Students:* 14 part-time (12 women); includes 1 minority (Black or African American, non-Hispanic/Latino). Average age 40. 8 applicants, 88% accepted, 6 enrolled. In 2013, 4 master's awarded. *Degree requirements:* For master's, 36 credits including capstone project. *Entrance requirements:* For master's, letter of intent, 2 letters of recommendation, transcripts. *Application deadline:* For fall admission, 7/1 priority date for domestic students. Applications are processed on a rolling basis. Application fee: $0. Electronic applications accepted. *Expenses: Tuition:* Part-time $685 per credit. Tuition and fees vary according to course load and program. *Financial support:* Applicants required to submit FAFSA. *Unit head:* Ariane Krumholz, Degree Chair, 888-251-5665 Ext. 209, E-mail: akrumholz@gradschool.marlboro.edu. *Application contact:* Matthew Livingston, Director of Graduate Admissions, 802-258-9209, Fax: 802-258-9201, E-mail: mlivingston@marlboro.edu.
Website: https://www.marlboro.edu/academics/graduate/hca

Marquette University, Graduate School, College of Professional Studies, Milwaukee, WI 53201-1881. Offers criminal justice administration (MLS, Certificate); dispute resolution (MDR, MLS); health care administration (MLS); leadership studies (Certificate); non-profit sector administration (MLS); public service (MAPS, MLS); sports leadership (MLS). Part-time and evening/weekend programs available. Postbaccalaureate distance learning degree programs offered (no on-campus study). *Faculty:* 3 full-time (2 women), 25 part-time/adjunct (11 women). *Students:* 29 full-time (14 women), 109 part-time (61 women); includes 28 minority (17 Black or African American, non-Hispanic/Latino; 2 American Indian or Alaska Native, non-Hispanic/Latino; 2 Asian, non-Hispanic/Latino; 5 Hispanic/Latino; 2 Two or more races, non-Hispanic/Latino), 1 international. Average age 36. 81 applicants, 81% accepted, 36 enrolled. In 2013, 42 master's, 18 Certificates awarded. *Degree requirements:* For master's, comprehensive exam (for some programs). *Entrance requirements:* For master's, GRE General Test (preferred), GMAT, or LSAT, official transcripts from all current and previous colleges/universities except Marquette, three letters of recommendation, statement of purpose. Additional exam requirements/recommendations for international students: Required—TOEFL. *Application deadline:* Applications are processed on a rolling basis. Electronic applications accepted. *Financial support:* In 2013–14, 9 students received support, including 8 fellowships with full tuition reimbursements available (averaging $16,247 per year). Financial award application deadline: 2/15. *Unit head:* Dr. Robert Deahl, Dean/Assistant Professor, 414-288-3156. *Application contact:* Eva Soeka, Director and Associate Professor, 414-288-5535.
Website: http://www.marquette.edu/cps/

Marshall University, Academic Affairs Division, College of Business, Program in Health Care Administration, Huntington, WV 25755. Offers MS. Part-time and evening/weekend programs available. *Students:* 41 full-time (18 women), 17 part-time (10 women); includes 5 minority (2 Black or African American, non-Hispanic/Latino; 2 Asian, non-Hispanic/Latino; 1 Two or more races, non-Hispanic/Latino), 1 international. Average age 30. In 2013, 33 master's awarded. *Degree requirements:* For master's, comprehensive assessment. *Entrance requirements:* For master's, GMAT or GRE General Test. *Application deadline:* Applications are processed on a rolling basis. Application fee: $40. *Financial support:* Career-related internships or fieldwork and tuition waivers (full) available. Support available to part-time students. Financial award applicants required to submit FAFSA. *Unit head:* Dr. Margie McInerney, Associate Dean, 304-696-2575, E-mail: mcinerney@marshall.edu. *Application contact:* Wesley Spradlin, Academic Advisor, 304-746-8964, Fax: 304-746-1902, E-mail: spradlin2@marshall.edu.

Marylhurst University, Department of Business Administration, Marylhurst, OR 97036-0261. Offers finance (MBA); general management (MBA); government policy and administration (MBA); green development (MBA); health care management (MBA); marketing (MBA); natural and organic resources (MBA); nonprofit management (MBA); organizational behavior (MBA); real estate (MBA); renewable energy (MBA); sustainable business (MBA). Part-time and evening/weekend programs available. Postbaccalaureate distance learning degree programs offered (no on-campus study). *Degree requirements:* For master's, comprehensive exam, capstone course. *Entrance requirements:* For master's, GMAT (if GPA less than 3.0 and fewer than 5 years of work experience), interview, resume, 2 letters of recommendation. Additional exam requirements/recommendations for international students: Recommended—TOEFL (minimum score 550 paper-based; 80 iBT). Electronic applications accepted.

Marymount University, School of Business Administration, Program in Health Care Management, Arlington, VA 22207-4299. Offers MS. *Accreditation:* CAHME. Part-time and evening/weekend programs available. *Faculty:* 5 full-time (3 women), 2 part-time/adjunct (0 women). *Students:* 16 full-time (10 women), 22 part-time (17 women); includes 24 minority (12 Black or African American, non-Hispanic/Latino; 8 Asian, non-Hispanic/Latino; 4 Hispanic/Latino), 1 international. Average age 31. 12 applicants, 83% accepted, 5 enrolled. In 2013, 26 master's awarded. *Degree requirements:* For master's, thesis or alternative. *Entrance requirements:* For master's, GMAT or GRE General Test, resume. Additional exam requirements/recommendations for international students: Required—TOEFL (minimum score 600 paper-based; 96 iBT), IELTS (minimum score 6.5). *Application deadline:* For fall admission, 7/15 priority date for domestic students, 7/1 for international students; for spring admission, 11/15 priority date for domestic

students, 11/15 for international students. Applications are processed on a rolling basis. Application fee: $40. Electronic applications accepted. *Expenses: Tuition:* Part-time $850 per credit. *Required fees:* $10 per credit. One-time fee: $200 part-time. Tuition and fees vary according to program. *Financial support:* In 2013–14, 2 students received support. Research assistantships with full and partial tuition reimbursements available, career-related internships or fieldwork, Federal Work-Study, scholarships/grants, and unspecified assistantships available. Support available to part-time students. Financial award applicants required to submit FAFSA. *Unit head:* Dr. Alyson Eisenhardt, Interim Director, 703-284-4984, Fax: 703-527-3830, E-mail: alyson.eisenhardt@marymount.edu. *Application contact:* Francesca Reed, Director, Graduate Admissions, 703-284-5901, Fax: 703-527-3815, E-mail: grad.admissions@marymount.edu.
Website: http://www.marymount.edu/academics/programs/healthcareMgt

Marywood University, Academic Affairs, College of Health and Human Services, School of Social Work and Administrative Studies, Program in Health Services Administration, Scranton, PA 18509-1598. Offers MHSA. *Entrance requirements:* Additional exam requirements/recommendations for international students: Required—TOEFL (minimum score 550 paper-based; 79 iBT). *Application deadline:* For fall admission, 4/1 priority date for domestic students, 3/31 priority date for international students; for spring admission, 11/1 priority date for domestic students, 8/31 priority date for international students. Applications are processed on a rolling basis. Application fee: $35. Electronic applications accepted. *Expenses: Tuition:* Part-time $775 per credit. Tuition and fees vary according to degree level. *Financial support:* Career-related internships or fieldwork, scholarships/grants, and unspecified assistantships available. Support available to part-time students. Financial award application deadline: 6/30; financial award applicants required to submit FAFSA. *Unit head:* Dr. Lloyd L. Lyter, Director, School of Social Work and Administrative Studies, 570-348-6282 Ext. 2388, E-mail: lyter@marywood.edu. *Application contact:* Tammy Manka, Assistant Director of Graduate Admissions, 570-348-6211 Ext. 2322, E-mail: tmanka@marywood.edu.
Website: http://www.marywood.edu/academics/gradcatalog/

McGill University, Faculty of Graduate and Postdoctoral Studies, Faculty of Medicine, Department of Epidemiology and Biostatistics, Montréal, QC H3A 2T5, Canada. Offers community health (M Sc); environmental health (M Sc); epidemiology and biostatistics (M Sc, PhD, Diploma); health care evaluation (M Sc); medical statistics (M Sc). *Accreditation:* CEPH (one or more programs are accredited).

MCPHS University, Graduate Studies, Program in Drug Regulatory Affairs and Health Policy, Boston, MA 02115-5896. Offers MS. Part-time and evening/weekend programs available. *Degree requirements:* For master's, thesis, oral defense of thesis. *Entrance requirements:* For master's, GRE General Test, minimum GPA of 3.0. Additional exam requirements/recommendations for international students: Required—TOEFL (minimum score 550 paper-based; 79 iBT). Electronic applications accepted. *Faculty research:* Epidemiology, drug policy, drug regulation, ethics.

Medical University of South Carolina, College of Health Professions, Doctoral Program in Health Administration, Charleston, SC 29425. Offers DHA. *Degree requirements:* For doctorate, comprehensive exam, thesis/dissertation. *Entrance requirements:* For doctorate, experience in health care, interview, master's degree in relevant field, resume, 3 references. Additional exam requirements/recommendations for international students: Required—TOEFL (minimum score 600 paper-based). *Faculty research:* HIV outcomes, health outcomes and statistics, inter-professional education.

Medical University of South Carolina, College of Health Professions, Program in Health Administration-Executive, Charleston, SC 29425. Offers MHA. Part-time programs available. Postbaccalaureate distance learning degree programs offered (no on-campus study). *Degree requirements:* For master's, 20 hours of community service. *Entrance requirements:* For master's, GRE General Test or GMAT, minimum GPA of 3.0. Additional exam requirements/recommendations for international students: Required—TOEFL (minimum score 600 paper-based). Electronic applications accepted. *Faculty research:* Electronic health records; telemedicine; fraud prediction and prevention; decision modeling; continuous quality improvement; empathy, caring, patient-centered health care and health outcomes; heath policy.

Medical University of South Carolina, College of Health Professions, Program in Health Administration-Global, Charleston, SC 29425. Offers MHA. *Entrance requirements:* Additional exam requirements/recommendations for international students: Required—TOEFL.

Medical University of South Carolina, College of Health Professions, Program in Health Administration-Residential, Charleston, SC 29425. Offers MHA. *Accreditation:* CAHME. Part-time programs available. Postbaccalaureate distance learning degree programs offered (minimal on-campus study). *Degree requirements:* For master's, 20 hours of community service, internship or field project. *Entrance requirements:* For master's, GRE General Test, GMAT, minimum GPA of 3.0, 3 references, interview. Additional exam requirements/recommendations for international students: Required—TOEFL (minimum score 550 paper-based). *Faculty research:* Electronic health records; telemedicine; fraud prediction and prevention; decision modeling; continuous quality improvement; empathy, caring, patient-centered health care; health policy; health outcomes.

Meharry Medical College, School of Graduate Studies, Division of Community Health Sciences, Nashville, TN 37208-9989. Offers occupational medicine (MSPH); public health administration (MSPH). *Accreditation:* CEPH. Part-time and evening/weekend programs available. *Degree requirements:* For master's, thesis, externship. *Entrance requirements:* For master's, GRE General Test, GMAT. *Expenses:* Contact institution. *Faculty research:* Policy and management, health care financing, health education and promotion.

Mercy College, School of Social and Behavioral Sciences, Program in Health Services Management, Dobbs Ferry, NY 10522-1189. Offers MPA, MS. Part-time and evening/weekend programs available. Postbaccalaureate distance learning degree programs offered (no on-campus study). *Students:* 52 full-time (46 women), 19 part-time (16 women); includes 55 minority (32 Black or African American, non-Hispanic/Latino; 4 Asian, non-Hispanic/Latino; 17 Hispanic/Latino; 1 Native Hawaiian or other Pacific Islander, non-Hispanic/Latino; 1 Two or more races, non-Hispanic/Latino). Average age 34. 86 applicants, 38% accepted, 17 enrolled. In 2013, 25 master's awarded. *Entrance requirements:* For master's, interview, resume, undergraduate transcript. Additional exam requirements/recommendations for international students: Required—TOEFL (minimum score 600 paper-based; 100 iBT), IELTS (minimum score 8). *Application deadline:* For fall admission, 8/1 for international students. Applications are processed on a rolling basis. Application fee: $40. Electronic applications accepted. *Expenses: Tuition:* Full-time $19,344; part-time $806 per credit. *Required fees:* $580; $806 per credit. $145 per term. Tuition and fees vary according to course load, degree level and program. *Financial support:* Career-related internships or fieldwork, Federal Work-Study, scholarships/grants, and unspecified assistantships available. Support available to part-time students. Financial award applicants required to submit FAFSA. *Unit head:* Dr. Mary Knopp Kelly, Interim Dean, School of Social and Behavioral Sciences, 914-674-7809, E-mail: mkkelly@mercy.edu. *Application contact:* Allison Gurdineer, Senior Director of Admissions, 877-637-2946, Fax: 914-674-7382, E-mail: admissions@mercy.edu.
Website: https://www.mercy.edu/academics/school-of-social-and-behavioral-sciences/department-of-social-sciences/

Middle Tennessee State University, College of Graduate Studies, College of Basic and Applied Sciences, Program in Health Care Management, Murfreesboro, TN 37132. Offers Graduate Certificate. *Students:* 3 part-time (2 women). 13 applicants, 46% accepted. In 2013, 4 Graduate Certificates awarded. *Entrance requirements:* Additional exam requirements/recommendations for international students: Required—TOEFL (minimum score 525 paper-based; 71 iBT) or IELTS (minimum score 6). *Financial support:* Application deadline: 5/1. *Unit head:* Dr. Robert W. Fischer, Jr., Dean, 615-898-2613, Fax: 615-898-2615, E-mail: bud.fischer@mtsu.edu. *Application contact:* Dr. Michael D. Allen, Vice Provost for Research/Dean, 615-898-2840, Fax: 615-904-8020, E-mail: michael.allen@mtsu.edu.

Midwestern State University, Graduate School, Robert D. and Carol Gunn College of Health Sciences and Human Services, Department of Criminal Justice and Health Services Administration, Wichita Falls, TX 76308. Offers criminal justice (MA); health information management (MHA); medical practice management (MHA); public and community sector health care management (MHA); rural and urban hospital management (MHA). Part-time and evening/weekend programs available. *Degree requirements:* For master's, comprehensive exam, thesis. *Entrance requirements:* For master's, GRE. Additional exam requirements/recommendations for international students: Required—TOEFL (minimum score 550 paper-based). *Application deadline:* For fall admission, 7/1 priority date for domestic students, 4/1 for international students; for spring admission, 11/1 priority date for domestic students, 8/1 for international students. Applications are processed on a rolling basis. Application fee: $35 ($50 for international students). Electronic applications accepted. *Expenses:* Tuition, state resident: full-time $3627; part-time $201.50 per credit hour. Tuition, nonresident: full-time $10,899; part-time $605.50 per credit hour. *Required fees:* $1357. *Financial support:* Teaching assistantships with partial tuition reimbursements, career-related internships or fieldwork, Federal Work-Study, institutionally sponsored loans, scholarships/grants, tuition waivers (partial), and unspecified assistantships available. Support available to part-time students. Financial award application deadline: 3/1; financial award applicants required to submit FAFSA. *Faculty research:* Universal service policy, telehealth, bullying, healthcare financial management, public health ethics. *Unit head:* Dr. Nathan R. Moran, Chair, 940-397-4752, Fax: 940-397-6291, E-mail: nathan.moran@mwsu.edu.
Website: http://www.mwsu.edu/academics/hs2/health-admin/

Milwaukee School of Engineering, Program in Health Care Systems Management, Milwaukee, WI 53202-3109. Offers MSN. *Expenses: Tuition:* Full-time $6939; part-time $771 per credit.

Mississippi College, Graduate School, Program in Health Services Administration, Clinton, MS 39058. Offers MHSA. Part-time programs available. *Degree requirements:* For master's, comprehensive exam. *Entrance requirements:* For master's, GRE General Test, minimum GPA of 2.5. Additional exam requirements/recommendations for international students: Recommended—TOEFL, IELTS. Electronic applications accepted.

Missouri State University, Graduate College, College of Business Administration, Department of Management, Springfield, MO 65897. Offers health administration (MHA). Part-time and evening/weekend programs available. *Faculty:* 11 full-time (3 women). *Students:* 48 full-time (18 women), 60 part-time (37 women); includes 19 minority (4 Black or African American, non-Hispanic/Latino; 3 Asian, non-Hispanic/Latino; 12 Two or more races, non-Hispanic/Latino), 8 international. Average age 31. 61 applicants, 93% accepted, 34 enrolled. In 2013, 14 master's awarded. *Degree requirements:* For master's, thesis optional. *Entrance requirements:* For master's, GMAT or GRE, minimum GPA of 2.75. Additional exam requirements/recommendations for international students: Required—TOEFL (minimum score 550 paper-based; 79 iBT), IELTS (minimum score 6). *Application deadline:* For fall admission, 7/20 priority date for domestic students, 5/1 for international students; for spring admission, 12/20 priority date for domestic students, 9/1 for international students. Applications are processed on a rolling basis. Application fee: $35 ($50 for international students). Electronic applications accepted. *Expenses:* Tuition, state resident: full-time $4500; part-time $250 per credit hour. Tuition, nonresident: full-time $9018; part-time $501 per credit hour. *Required fees:* $361 per semester. Tuition and fees vary according to course level, course load and program. *Financial support:* Career-related internships or fieldwork, institutionally sponsored loans, scholarships/grants, tuition waivers, and unspecified assistantships available. Support available to part-time students. Financial award application deadline: 3/31; financial award applicants required to submit FAFSA. *Faculty research:* Health care management, human resource management, strategic management. *Unit head:* Dr. William Donoher, Department Head, 417-836-5415, E-mail: management@missouristate.edu. *Application contact:* Misty Stewart, Coordinator of Graduate Admissions and Recruitment, 417-836-6079, E-mail: mistystewart@missouristate.edu.
Website: http://mgt.missouristate.edu/

Molloy College, Graduate Business Program, Rockville Centre, NY 11571-5002. Offers accounting (MBA); accounting and finance (MBA); accounting and management (MBA); finance (MBA); finance and management (MBA); finance and personal financial planning (MBA); healthcare administration (MBA); management (MBA); management and personal financial planning (MBA); marketing (MBA); personal financial planning (MBA). Part-time programs available. *Faculty:* 8 full-time (3 women), 7 part-time/adjunct (1 woman). *Students:* 41 full-time (19 women), 104 part-time (36 women); includes 45 minority (21 Black or African American, non-Hispanic/Latino; 8 Asian, non-Hispanic/Latino; 14 Hispanic/Latino; 1 Native Hawaiian or other Pacific Islander, non-Hispanic/Latino; 1 Two or more races, non-Hispanic/Latino), 4 international. Average age 29. 48 applicants, 71% accepted, 27 enrolled. In 2013, 33 master's awarded. *Application deadline:* Applications are processed on a rolling basis. Application fee: $60. *Expenses: Tuition:* Full-time $16,920; part-time $940 per credit. *Required fees:* $880. *Faculty research:* Leadership, marketing, accounting, finance, international. *Unit head:* Dr. Daniel Cillis, Associate Dean and Director, MBA Program, 516-323-3080, E-mail: dcillis@molloy.edu. *Application contact:* Alina Haitz, Assistant Director of Graduate Admissions, 516-323-4008, E-mail: ahaitz@molloy.edu.

Montana State University Billings, College of Allied Health Professions, Department of Health Administration, Billings, MT 59101-0298. Offers MHA. Postbaccalaureate distance learning degree programs offered (minimal on-campus study). *Degree requirements:* For master's, thesis or professional paper and/or field experience. *Entrance requirements:* For master's, GRE General Test or GMAT, minimum undergraduate GPA of 3.0, graduate 3.25; 3 years' clinical or administrative experience in health care delivery or 5 years' experience in business or industry management. *Application deadline:* For fall admission, 4/20 for domestic students. Applications are processed on a rolling basis. Application fee: $40. *Expenses:* Tuition, state resident: full-time $2653.75; part-time $1718 per semester. Tuition, nonresident: full-time $7015; part-time $4640 per semester. *Required fees:* $2445; $444 per credit. *Financial support:* Career-related internships or fieldwork, Federal Work-Study, institutionally sponsored loans, scholarships/grants, tuition waivers (partial), and unspecified assistantships available. Support available to part-time students. Financial award application deadline: 5/1; financial award applicants required to submit FAFSA. *Unit head:* Deborah Peters, Program Director, 406-896-5832. *Application contact:* David M. Sullivan, Graduate Studies Counselor, 406-657-2053, Fax: 406-657-2299, E-mail: dsullivan@msubillings.edu.

Moravian College, Moravian College Comenius Center, Business and Management Programs, Bethlehem, PA 18018-6650. Offers accounting (MBA); business analytics (MBA); general management (MBA); health administration (MHA); healthcare management (MBA); human resource management (MBA); leadership (MSHRM); learning and performance management (MSHRM); supply chain management (MBA). Part-time and evening/weekend programs available. *Entrance requirements:* For master's, GMAT. Additional exam requirements/recommendations for international students: Required—TOEFL (minimum score 550 paper-based; 90 iBT). Application fee is waived when completed online. *Expenses:* Contact institution. *Faculty research:* Leadership, change management, human resources.

Morehouse School of Medicine, Master of Public Health Program, Atlanta, GA 30310-1495. Offers epidemiology (MPH); health administration, management and policy (MPH); health education/health promotion (MPH); international health (MPH). *Accreditation:* CEPH. Part-time programs available. *Students:* 37 full-time (27 women), 5 part-time (3 women); includes 33 minority (32 Black or African American, non-Hispanic/Latino; 1 American Indian or Alaska Native, non-Hispanic/Latino). Average age 28. In 2013, 13 master's awarded. *Degree requirements:* For master's, thesis, practicum, public health leadership seminar. *Entrance requirements:* For master's, GRE General Test, writing test, public health or human service experience. Additional exam requirements/recommendations for international students: Required—TOEFL (minimum score 550 paper-based). *Application deadline:* For fall admission, 3/1 for domestic and international students. Application fee: $50. Electronic applications accepted. *Expenses:* Contact institution. *Financial support:* Fellowships, research assistantships with partial tuition reimbursements, teaching assistantships, career-related internships or fieldwork, Federal Work-Study, institutionally sponsored loans, scholarships/grants, and unspecified assistantships available. Support available to part-time students. Financial award application deadline: 5/1; financial award applicants required to submit FAFSA. *Faculty research:* Women's and adolescent health, violence prevention, cancer epidemiology/disparities, substance abuse prevention. *Unit head:* Dr. Stephanie Miles-Richardson, Interim Director, 404-752-1944, Fax: 404-752-1051, E-mail: smiles-richardson@msm.edu. *Application contact:* Brandon Hunter, Director of Admissions, 404-752-1650, Fax: 404-752-1512, E-mail: mphadmissions@msm.edu.
Website: http://www.msm.edu/educationTraining/degreePrograms/mph.aspx

Mount St. Mary's University, Program in Health Administration, Emmitsburg, MD 21727-7799. Offers MHA. Part-time and evening/weekend programs available. *Faculty:* 7 part-time/adjunct (2 women). *Students:* 1 (woman) full-time, 60 part-time (44 women); includes 21 minority (8 Black or African American, non-Hispanic/Latino; 2 American Indian or Alaska Native, non-Hispanic/Latino; 8 Asian, non-Hispanic/Latino; 2 Hispanic/Latino; 1 Two or more races, non-Hispanic/Latino), 1 international. Average age 36. 26 applicants, 58% accepted, 11 enrolled. *Degree requirements:* For master's, health care field practicum. *Entrance requirements:* For master's, undergraduate degree, minimum cumulative undergraduate GPA of 2.75. Additional exam requirements/recommendations for international students: Required—TOEFL (minimum score 550 paper-based). Application fee: $35. *Expenses: Tuition:* Full-time $9846; part-time $547 per credit hour. Tuition and fees vary according to program. *Financial support:* In 2013–14, 3 students received support. *Unit head:* Dr. Edward A. Dolan, Director, 301-447-6122. *Application contact:* Deb Powell, Director of Graduate and Adult Business Programs, 301-447-5326, Fax: 301-447-5335, E-mail: dpowell@msmary.edu.
Website: http://www.msmary.edu/School_of_business/Graduate_Programs/mha/

National University, Academic Affairs, School of Health and Human Services, La Jolla, CA 92037-1011. Offers clinical affairs (MS); clinical informatics (Certificate); clinical regulatory affairs (MS); health and life science analytics (MS); health coaching (Certificate); health informatics (MS); healthcare administration (MHA); nurse anesthesia (MS); nursing (MS), including forensic nursing, nursing administration, nursing informatics; nursing administration (Certificate); nursing informatics (Certificate); nursing practice (DNP); public health (MPH), including health promotion, healthcare administration, mental health. Part-time and evening/weekend programs available. Postbaccalaureate distance learning degree programs offered (no on-campus study). *Faculty:* 20 full-time (12 women), 27 part-time/adjunct (16 women). *Students:* 229 full-time (176 women), 89 part-time (52 women); includes 215 minority (58 Black or African American, non-Hispanic/Latino; 1 American Indian or Alaska Native, non-Hispanic/Latino; 68 Asian, non-Hispanic/Latino; 63 Hispanic/Latino; 8 Native Hawaiian or other Pacific Islander, non-Hispanic/Latino; 17 Two or more races, non-Hispanic/Latino), 18 international. Average age 33. 118 applicants, 100% accepted, 92 enrolled. In 2013, 29 master's awarded. *Degree requirements:* For master's, thesis (for some programs). *Entrance requirements:* For master's, interview, minimum GPA of 2.5. Additional exam requirements/recommendations for international students: Required—TOEFL (minimum score 550 paper-based; 79 iBT), IELTS (minimum score 6). *Application deadline:* Applications are processed on a rolling basis. Application fee: $60 ($65 for international students). Electronic applications accepted. *Expenses: Tuition:* Full-time $13,824; part-time $1728 per course. One-time fee: $160. *Financial support:* Career-related internships or fieldwork, institutionally sponsored loans, scholarships/grants, and tuition waivers (partial) available. Support available to part-time students. Financial award application deadline: 6/30; financial award applicants required to submit FAFSA. *Faculty research:* Nursing education, obesity prevention, workforce diversity. *Unit head:* School of Health and Human Services, 800-628-8648, E-mail: shhs@nu.edu. *Application contact:* Louis Cruz, Interim Vice President for Enrollment Services, 800-628-8648, E-mail: advisor@nu.edu.
Website: http://www.nu.edu/OurPrograms/SchoolOfHealthAndHumanServices.html

National University of Health Sciences, Lincoln College of Postprofessional, Graduate and Continuing Education, Lombard, IL 60148-4583. Offers advanced clinical practice (MS); diagnostic imaging (MS). Evening/weekend programs available. *Degree requirements:* For master's, comprehensive exam, thesis, capstone. *Entrance requirements:* Additional exam requirements/recommendations for international students: Required—TOEFL. Electronic applications accepted.

Nebraska Methodist College, Program in Healthcare Operations Management, Omaha, NE 68114. Offers MS. Part-time and evening/weekend programs available. Postbaccalaureate distance learning degree programs offered (no on-campus study). *Faculty:* 3 full-time (2 women), 16 part-time/adjunct (9 women). *Students:* 16 full-time (10 women), 25 part-time (18 women); includes 6 minority (2 Black or African American, non-Hispanic/Latino; 2 Asian, non-Hispanic/Latino; 1 Hispanic/Latino; 1 Two or more races, non-Hispanic/Latino). Average age 38. 46 applicants, 35% accepted, 16 enrolled. *Degree requirements:* For master's, thesis or alternative, capstone. *Entrance requirements:* Additional exam requirements/recommendations for international students: Required—TOEFL (minimum score 550 paper-based; 80 iBT). *Application deadline:* Applications are processed on a rolling basis. Application fee: $25. *Expenses: Tuition:* Full-time $12,258; part-time $681 per credit hour. *Required fees:* $450; $450 per year. *Financial support:* Scholarships/grants available. Financial award applicants required to submit FAFSA. *Unit head:* Ann Greiman, Academic Program Director, 402-354-7138, E-mail: ann.greiman@methodistcollege.edu. *Application contact:* Laurel Zentner, Recruitment and Admissions Coordinator, 402-354-7170, Fax: 402-354-7020, E-mail: admissions@methodistcollege.edu.
Website: http://www.methodistcollege.edu/healthcare-operations-management

New Charter University, College of Business, San Francisco, CA 94105. Offers finance (MBA); health care management (MBA); management (MBA). Part-time and evening/weekend programs available. Postbaccalaureate distance learning degree programs offered (no on-campus study). *Entrance requirements:* For master's, course work in calculus, statistics, macroeconomics. Additional exam requirements/recommendations for international students: Required—TOEFL (minimum score 550 paper-based). Electronic applications accepted.

New England College, Program in Management, Henniker, NH 03242-3293. Offers accounting (MSA); healthcare administration (MS); international relations (MA); marketing management (MS); nonprofit leadership (MS); project management (MS); strategic leadership (MS). Part-time and evening/weekend programs available. *Degree requirements:* For master's, independent research project. Electronic applications accepted.

New Jersey City University, Graduate Studies and Continuing Education, College of Professional Studies, Department of Health Sciences, Jersey City, NJ 07305-1597. Offers community health education (MS); health administration (MS); school health education (MS). Part-time and evening/weekend programs available. *Faculty:* 5 full-time (all women), 7 part-time/adjunct (2 women). *Students:* 10 full-time (7 women), 58 part-time (50 women); includes 32 minority (15 Black or African American, non-Hispanic/Latino; 7 Asian, non-Hispanic/Latino; 10 Hispanic/Latino), 2 international. Average age 40. In 2013, 18 master's awarded. *Degree requirements:* For master's, thesis or alternative, internship. *Entrance requirements:* Additional exam requirements/recommendations for international students: Required—TOEFL (minimum score 61 iBT). *Application deadline:* For fall admission, 8/1 priority date for domestic students; for spring admission, 12/1 for domestic students. Applications are processed on a rolling basis. Application fee: $0. *Expenses: Tuition, area resident:* Part-time $527.90 per credit. Tuition, nonresident: part-time $947.75 per credit. *Financial support:* Career-related internships or fieldwork and unspecified assistantships available. *Unit head:* Dr. Lilliam Rosado, Chairperson, 201-200-3431, E-mail: lrosado@njcu.edu. *Application contact:* Dr. William Bajor, Dean of Graduate Studies, 201-200-3409, Fax: 201-200-3411, E-mail: wbajor@njcu.edu.

New Jersey Institute of Technology, Newark College of Engineering, Newark, NJ 07102. Offers biomedical engineering (MS, PhD); chemical engineering (MS, PhD); computer engineering (MS, PhD); electrical engineering (MS, PhD); engineering management (MS); healthcare systems management (MS); industrial engineering (MS, PhD); Internet engineering (MS); manufacturing engineering (MS); mechanical engineering (MS, PhD); occupational safety and health engineering (MS); pharmaceutical bioprocessing (MS); pharmaceutical engineering (MS); pharmaceutical systems management (MS); power and energy systems (MS); telecommunications (MS); transportation (MS, PhD). Part-time and evening/weekend programs available. *Faculty:* 133 full-time (18 women), 101 part-time/adjunct (14 women). *Students:* 823 full-time (222 women), 535 part-time (130 women); includes 361 minority (92 Black or African American, non-Hispanic/Latino; 4 American Indian or Alaska Native, non-Hispanic/Latino; 142 Asian, non-Hispanic/Latino; 123 Hispanic/Latino), 605 international. Average age 29. 2,800 applicants, 68% accepted, 523 enrolled. In 2013, 471 master's, 32 doctorates awarded. Terminal master's awarded for partial completion of doctoral program. *Degree requirements:* For master's, thesis optional; for doctorate, thesis/dissertation. *Entrance requirements:* For master's, GRE General Test; for doctorate, GRE General Test, minimum graduate GPA of 3.5. Additional exam requirements/recommendations for international students: Required—TOEFL (minimum score 550 paper-based; 79 iBT). *Application deadline:* For fall admission, 6/1 priority date for domestic students, 5/1 priority date for international students; for spring admission, 11/15 priority date for domestic and international students. Applications are processed on a rolling basis. Application fee: $65. Electronic applications accepted. *Expenses:* Tuition, state resident: full-time $17,384; part-time $945 per credit. Tuition, nonresident: full-time $25,404; part-time $1341 per credit. *Required fees:* $2396; $118 per credit. *Financial support:* Fellowships with full and partial tuition reimbursements, research assistantships with full and partial tuition reimbursements, and teaching assistantships with full and partial tuition reimbursements available. Financial award application deadline: 1/15. *Total annual research expenditures:* $16 million. *Unit head:* Dr. Basil Baltzis, Dean, 973-596-3000, E-mail: sunil.saigal@njit.edu. *Application contact:* Stephen Eck, Director of Admissions, 973-596-3300, Fax: 973-596-3461, E-mail: admissions@njit.edu.
Website: http://engineering.njit.edu/

New Mexico State University, Graduate School, College of Health and Social Services, Department of Public Health Sciences, Las Cruces, NM 88003-8001. Offers community health education (MPH); health management, administration and policy (MPH). Part-time programs available. Postbaccalaureate distance learning degree programs offered (minimal on-campus study). *Faculty:* 11 full-time (6 women), 2 part-time/adjunct (1 woman). *Students:* 32 full-time (30 women), 28 part-time (21 women); includes 24 minority (3 Black or African American, non-Hispanic/Latino; 4 American Indian or Alaska Native, non-Hispanic/Latino; 2 Asian, non-Hispanic/Latino; 14 Hispanic/Latino; 1 Two or more races, non-Hispanic/Latino), 1 international. Average age 34. 37 applicants, 68% accepted, 18 enrolled. In 2013, 25 master's awarded. *Degree requirements:* For master's, thesis optional. *Entrance requirements:* For master's, GRE. Additional exam requirements/recommendations for international students: Required—TOEFL (minimum score 550 paper-based; 79 iBT), IELTS (minimum score 6.5). *Application deadline:* For fall admission, 2/15 for domestic and international students. Application fee: $40 ($50 for international students). Electronic applications accepted. *Expenses:* Tuition, state resident: full-time $5398; part-time $224.90 per credit. Tuition, nonresident: full-time $18,821; part-time $784.20 per credit. *Required fees:* $1310; $54.60 per credit. *Financial support:* In 2013–14, 19 students received support, including 8 teaching assistantships (averaging $8,131 per year); career-related internships or fieldwork, Federal Work-Study, health care benefits, and unspecified assistantships also available. Financial award application deadline: 4/1. *Faculty research:* Community health education, health issues of U.S.-Mexico border, health policy and management, victims of violence, environmental and occupational health issues. *Total annual research expenditures:* $79,183. *Unit head:* Dr. Mark J. Kittleson, Head, 575-646-4300, Fax: 575-646-4343, E-mail: kittle@nmsu.edu. *Application contact:* Dr. James Robinson, III, Graduate Coordinator, 575-646-7431, E-mail: jrobin3@nmsu.edu.
Website: http://publichealth.nmsu.edu

New York Medical College, School of Health Sciences and Practice, Department of Health Policy and Management, Valhalla, NY 10595-1691. Offers emergency preparedness (Graduate Certificate); global health (Graduate Certificate); health policy and management (MPH, Dr PH). Part-time and evening/weekend programs available. *Faculty:* 6 full-time, 23 part-time/adjunct. *Students:* 55 full-time, 98 part-time. Average

age 32. 125 applicants, 62% accepted, 59 enrolled. In 2013, 95 master's, 5 doctorates awarded. *Degree requirements:* For master's, comprehensive exam, thesis; for doctorate, comprehensive exam, thesis/dissertation. *Entrance requirements:* For master's, minimum GPA of 3.0, some work experience; for doctorate, GRE, minimum graduate GPA of 3.5. Additional exam requirements/recommendations for international students: Required—TOEFL (minimum score 600 paper-based; 100 iBT), IELTS (minimum score 7). *Application deadline:* For fall admission, 8/1 priority date for domestic students, 5/15 for international students; for spring admission, 12/1 priority date for domestic students, 10/15 for international students; for summer admission, 5/1 for domestic students, 4/1 for international students. Applications are processed on a rolling basis. Application fee: $50 ($100 for international students). Electronic applications accepted. *Expenses: Tuition:* Full-time $49,170; part-time $910 per credit. Tuition and fees vary according to program. *Financial support:* Research assistantships, teaching assistantships, career-related internships or fieldwork, Federal Work-Study, institutionally sponsored loans, health care benefits, and tuition reimbursements available. Support available to part-time students. Financial award applicants required to submit FAFSA. *Unit head:* Annette Choolfaian, Chair, 914-594-4250, Fax: 914-594-4292, E-mail: annette_choolfaian@nymc.edu. *Application contact:* Pamela Suett, Director of Recruitment, 914-594-4510, Fax: 914-594-4292, E-mail: shsp_admissions@nymc.edu.
Website: http://www.nymc.edu/shsp

New York University, Robert F. Wagner Graduate School of Public Service, Program in Health Policy and Management, New York, NY 10012. Offers health finance (MPA); health policy analysis (MPA); health policy and management (Advanced Certificate); health services management (MPA); international health (MPA); MBA/MPA; MD/MPA; MPA/MPH. *Accreditation:* CAHME (one or more programs are accredited). Part-time programs available. *Faculty:* 9 full-time (5 women), 10 part-time/adjunct (4 women). *Students:* 82 full-time (62 women), 89 part-time (65 women); includes 64 minority (15 Black or African American, non-Hispanic/Latino; 1 American Indian or Alaska Native, non-Hispanic/Latino; 32 Asian, non-Hispanic/Latino; 9 Hispanic/Latino; 7 Two or more races, non-Hispanic/Latino), 20 international. Average age 29. 227 applicants, 60% accepted, 63 enrolled. In 2013, 67 master's awarded. *Degree requirements:* For master's, thesis or alternative, capstone end event. *Entrance requirements:* Additional exam requirements/recommendations for international students: Required—TOEFL (minimum score 100 iBT), IELTS (minimum score 7.5), TWE. *Application deadline:* For fall admission, 1/6 for domestic students, 1/5 for international students; for spring admission, 10/1 for domestic and international students. Application fee: $85. Electronic applications accepted. *Expenses:* Contact institution. *Financial support:* In 2013–14, 30 students received support, including 28 fellowships with partial tuition reimbursements available (averaging $12,410 per year), 2 research assistantships with full tuition reimbursements available (averaging $56,524 per year); career-related internships or fieldwork, Federal Work-Study, scholarships/grants, health care benefits, and unspecified assistantships also available. Support available to part-time students. Financial award application deadline: 1/5; financial award applicants required to submit FAFSA. *Unit head:* Prof. John Billings, Director, 212-998-7455, Fax: 212-995-4162. *Application contact:* Janet Barzilay, Admissions Officer, 212-998-7414, Fax: 212-995-4611, E-mail: wagner.admissions@nyu.edu.
Website: http://www.nyu.edu/wagner/

Northeast Ohio Medical University, College of Graduate Studies, Rootstown, OH 44272-0095. Offers bioethics (Certificate); health-system pharmacy administration (MS); integrated pharmaceutical medicine (MS, PhD); public health (MS). *Faculty:* 80 part-time/adjunct (26 women). *Students:* 38 full-time (21 women); includes 4 minority (3 Asian, non-Hispanic/Latino; 1 Hispanic/Latino). Average age 28. 45 applicants, 84% accepted, 38 enrolled. In 2013, 9 master's, 1 doctorate awarded. *Application deadline:* For fall admission, 9/1 priority date for domestic students; for winter admission, 1/5 priority date for domestic students. Applications are processed on a rolling basis. Application fee: $45. Electronic applications accepted. Full-time tuition and fees vary according to program. Part-time tuition and fees vary according to degree level. *Unit head:* Dr. Walter E. Horton, Jr., Dean of the College of Graduate Studies. *Application contact:* Luke Gloeckner, Associate Director for Enrollment Services and Registration, 330-325-6274, E-mail: lgloeckner@gmail.com.
Website: http://www.neomed.edu/academics/graduatestudies

Northern Arizona University, Graduate College, College of Health and Human Services, Program in Interdisciplinary Health Policy, Flagstaff, AZ 86011. Offers Certificate. Part-time programs available. *Entrance requirements:* For degree, bachelor's degree from regionally-accredited university. Additional exam requirements/recommendations for international students: Required—TOEFL (minimum score 550 paper-based; 80 iBT), IELTS (minimum score 7). *Application deadline:* For fall admission, 3/1 priority date for international students; for spring admission, 9/15 priority date for international students. Applications are processed on a rolling basis. Application fee: $65. Electronic applications accepted. *Financial support:* Applicants required to submit FAFSA. *Unit head:* Paul V. Dutton, Executive Director, Interdisciplinary Health Policy Institute, 928-523-8830, Fax: 928-523-1277, E-mail: paul.dutton@nau.edu.
Website: http://nau.edu/CHHS/IHPI/

Northern Michigan University, College of Graduate Studies, College of Health Sciences and Professional Studies, School of Education, Leadership and Public Service, Program in Public Administration, Marquette, MI 49855-5301. Offers criminal justice administration (MPA); healthcare administration (MPA); human resource administration (MPA); public management (MPA); state and local government (MPA). Part-time and evening/weekend programs available. Postbaccalaureate distance learning degree programs offered (no on-campus study). *Faculty:* 1 (woman) full-time, 4 part-time/adjunct (1 woman). *Students:* 18 full-time (14 women), 12 part-time (4 women). In 2013, 11 master's awarded. *Degree requirements:* For master's, thesis or alternative. *Entrance requirements:* For master's, minimum GPA of 3.0, resume, personal interview. Additional exam requirements/recommendations for international students: Required—TOEFL (minimum score 550 paper-based; 70 iBT), IELTS (minimum score 6.5). *Application deadline:* For fall admission, 7/1 for domestic students; for winter admission, 11/15 for domestic students; for spring admission, 3/17 for domestic students. Applications are processed on a rolling basis. Application fee: $50. Electronic applications accepted. *Expenses:* Tuition, state resident: part-time $427 per credit. Tuition, nonresident: part-time $614.50 per credit. *Required fees:* $325 per semester. Tuition and fees vary according to course load and program. *Financial support:* Fellowships, research assistantships with full and partial tuition reimbursements, teaching assistantships with full and partial tuition reimbursements, career-related internships or fieldwork, Federal Work-Study, institutionally sponsored loans, tuition waivers (full and partial), and unspecified assistantships available. Support available to part-time students. Financial award application deadline: 3/1; financial award applicants required to submit FAFSA. *Unit head:* Dr. Joseph Lubig, Department Head, 906-227-1880, E-mail: jlubig@nmu.edu. *Application contact:* Dr. Jennifer James-Mesloh, MPA Program Coordinator/Assistant Professor, 906-227-1858, Fax: 906-227-2315, E-mail: jjamesme@nmu.edu.
Website: http://www.nmu.edu/education/MPA-online

Northwestern University, Fienberg School of Medicine and Interdepartmental Programs, Integrated Graduate Programs in the Life Sciences, Chicago, IL 60611. Offers biostatistics (PhD); epidemiology (PhD); health and biomedical informatics (PhD); health services and outcomes research (PhD); healthcare quality and patient safety (PhD); translational outcomes in science (PhD). *Degree requirements:* For doctorate, comprehensive exam, thesis/dissertation, written and oral qualifying exams. *Entrance requirements:* For doctorate, GRE General Test. Additional exam requirements/recommendations for international students: Required—TOEFL (minimum score 600 paper-based). Electronic applications accepted.

Northwestern University, The Graduate School, Kellogg School of Management, Management Programs, Evanston, IL 60208. Offers accounting information and management (MBA, PhD); analytical finance (MBA); business administration (MBA); decision sciences (MBA); entrepreneurship and innovation (MBA); finance (MBA, PhD); health enterprise management (MBA); human resources management (MBA); international business (MBA); management and organizations (MBA, PhD); management and organizations and sociology (PhD); management and strategy (MBA); management studies (MS); managerial analytics (MBA); managerial economics (MBA); managerial economics and strategy (PhD); marketing (MBA, PhD); marketing management (MBA); media management (MBA); operations management (MBA, PhD); real estate (MBA); social enterprise at Kellogg (MBA); JD/MBA. Part-time and evening/weekend programs available. Terminal master's awarded for partial completion of doctoral program. *Degree requirements:* For doctorate, thesis/dissertation, 2 years of coursework, qualifying (field) exam and candidacy, summer research papers and presentations to faculty, proposal defense, final exam/defense. *Entrance requirements:* For master's, GMAT, GRE, interview, 2 letters of recommendation, college transcripts, resume, essays, Kellogg honor code; for doctorate, GMAT, GRE, statement of purpose, transcripts, 2 letters of recommendation, resume, interview. Additional exam requirements/recommendations for international students: Required—TOEFL, IELTS. Electronic applications accepted. *Expenses:* Contact institution. *Faculty research:* Business cycles and international finance, health policy, networks, non-market strategy, consumer psychology.

Northwestern University, School of Professional Studies, Program in Public Policy and Administration, Evanston, IL 60208. Offers global policy (MA); health services policy (MA); public administration (MA); public policy (MA). Postbaccalaureate distance learning degree programs offered.

Northwest Nazarene University, Graduate Studies, Program in Business Administration, Nampa, ID 83686-5897. Offers business administration (MBA); healthcare (MBA). *Accreditation:* ACBSP. Part-time and evening/weekend programs available. Postbaccalaureate distance learning degree programs offered (no on-campus study). *Faculty:* 12 full-time (4 women), 14 part-time/adjunct (2 women). *Students:* 103 full-time (31 women), 36 part-time (14 women); includes 17 minority (1 Black or African American, non-Hispanic/Latino; 1 American Indian or Alaska Native, non-Hispanic/Latino; 2 Asian, non-Hispanic/Latino; 9 Hispanic/Latino; 4 Two or more races, non-Hispanic/Latino), 5 international. Average age 34. 26 applicants, 62% accepted, 11 enrolled. In 2013, 41 master's awarded. *Degree requirements:* For master's, comprehensive exam, thesis or alternative. *Entrance requirements:* For master's, minimum GPA of 3.0. *Application deadline:* Applications are processed on a rolling basis. Application fee: $50. Electronic applications accepted. *Expenses:* Contact institution. *Unit head:* Dr. Brenda Johnson, Director, 208-467-8415, Fax: 208-467-8440, E-mail: mba@nnu.edu. *Application contact:* Wendy Rhodes, MBA Program Coordinator, 208-467-8123, Fax: 208-467-8440, E-mail: nnu-mba@nnu.edu.
Website: http://nnu.edu/mba

The Ohio State University, College of Public Health, Columbus, OH 43210. Offers MHA, MPH, MS, PhD, JD/MHA, MHA/MBA, MHA/MD, MHA/MPA, MHA/MS, MPH/JD, MPH/MD, OD/MPH. *Accreditation:* CAHME; CEPH. Part-time programs available. *Faculty:* 40. *Students:* 244 full-time (180 women), 59 part-time (40 women); includes 56 minority (24 Black or African American, non-Hispanic/Latino; 1 American Indian or Alaska Native, non-Hispanic/Latino; 19 Asian, non-Hispanic/Latino; 8 Hispanic/Latino; 4 Two or more races, non-Hispanic/Latino), 20 international. Average age 29. In 2013, 106 master's, 7 doctorates awarded. Terminal master's awarded for partial completion of doctoral program. *Degree requirements:* For master's, thesis optional, practicum. *Entrance requirements:* For master's and doctorate, GRE. Additional exam requirements/recommendations for international students: Required—TOEFL (minimum score 600 paper-based; 100 iBT); Recommended—IELTS (minimum score 8). *Application deadline:* For fall admission, 11/15 for domestic and international students. Applications are processed on a rolling basis. Application fee: $60 ($70 for international students). Electronic applications accepted. *Financial support:* Fellowships with tuition reimbursements and research assistantships with tuition reimbursements available. *Unit head:* Dr. William J. Martin, II, Dean, 614-292-8350, E-mail: martin.3047@osu.edu. *Application contact:* 614-292-8350, Fax: 614-247-1846, E-mail: cph@cph.osu.edu.
Website: http://cph.osu.edu/

Ohio University, Graduate College, College of Business, Program in Business Administration, Athens, OH 45701-2979. Offers executive management (MBA); finance (MBA); healthcare (MBA). *Accreditation:* AACSB. Part-time and evening/weekend programs available. Postbaccalaureate distance learning degree programs offered (minimal on-campus study). *Entrance requirements:* For master's, minimum GPA of 3.0. Additional exam requirements/recommendations for international students: Required—TOEFL (minimum score 600 paper-based). Electronic applications accepted. *Expenses:* Contact institution.

Ohio University, Graduate College, College of Health Sciences and Professions, Department of Social and Public Health, Athens, OH 45701-2979. Offers early child development and family life (MS); family studies (MS); health administration (MHA); public health (MPH); social work (MSW). *Accreditation:* CEPH. Part-time and evening/weekend programs available. Postbaccalaureate distance learning degree programs offered (no on-campus study). *Degree requirements:* For master's, capstone (MPH). *Entrance requirements:* For master's, GMAT, GRE General Test, previous course work in accounting, management, and statistics, previous public health background (MHA, MPH). Additional exam requirements/recommendations for international students: Required—TOEFL (minimum score 550 paper-based; 80 iBT) or IELTS (minimum score 6.5). Electronic applications accepted. *Expenses:* Contact institution. *Faculty research:* Health care management, health policy, managed care, health behavior, disease prevention.

Oklahoma Christian University, Graduate School of Business, Oklahoma City, OK 73136-1100. Offers accounting (MBA); electronic business (MBA); financial services (MBA); health services management (MBA); human resources (MBA); international business (MBA); leadership and organizational development (MBA); marketing (MBA); project management (MBA). Postbaccalaureate distance learning degree programs offered (no on-campus study). *Entrance requirements:* For master's, bachelor's degree. Electronic applications accepted.

Oklahoma City University, Kramer School of Nursing, Oklahoma City, OK 73106-1402. Offers health care systems leadership and administration (MSN); nursing (PhD); nursing education (MSN); nursing practice (DNP). Part-time and evening/weekend

programs available. *Faculty:* 14 full-time (12 women), 5 part-time/adjunct (3 women). *Students:* 78 full-time (51 women), 116 part-time (101 women); includes 43 minority (10 Black or African American, non-Hispanic/Latino; 16 American Indian or Alaska Native, non-Hispanic/Latino; 9 Asian, non-Hispanic/Latino; 3 Hispanic/Latino; 5 Two or more races, non-Hispanic/Latino), 55 international. Average age 36. 97 applicants, 69% accepted, 37 enrolled. In 2013, 14 master's, 8 doctorates awarded. *Degree requirements:* For master's, thesis, minimum GPA of 3.0; for doctorate, comprehensive exam, thesis/dissertation, minimum GPA of 3.0. *Entrance requirements:* For master's, registered nurse licensure, minimum undergraduate GPA of 3.0, BSN from nationally-accredited nursing program, completion of courses in health assessment and statistics; for doctorate, GRE, approved scholarly paper, or published article/paper in a refereed journal, current RN licensure, bachelor's and master's degrees from accredited programs (at least one of which must be in nursing), minimum graduate GPA of 3.5, personal essay. Additional exam requirements/recommendations for international students: Required—TOEFL (minimum score 550 paper-based; 80 iBT), IELTS (minimum score 6). *Application deadline:* Applications are processed on a rolling basis. Application fee: $50. Electronic applications accepted. *Expenses: Tuition:* Full-time $16,848; part-time $936 per credit hour. Tuition and fees vary according to course load, degree level and program. *Financial support:* Federal Work-Study, institutionally sponsored loans, scholarships/grants, and tuition waivers available. Support available to part-time students. Financial award applicants required to submit FAFSA. *Unit head:* Dr. Lois Salmeron, Dean, Kramer School of Nursing, 405-208-5900, Fax: 405-208-5914, E-mail: lsalmeron@okcu.edu. *Application contact:* Heidi Puckett, Director of Graduate Admissions, 800-633-7242, Fax: 405-208-5916, E-mail: gadmissions@okcu.edu.
Website: http://www.okcu.edu/nursing/

Oklahoma State University Center for Health Sciences, Program in Health Care Administration, Tulsa, OK 74107-1898. Offers MS. *Degree requirements:* For master's, thesis or alternative. *Entrance requirements:* For master's, official transcripts, health care experience. *Application deadline:* For fall admission, 7/1 for domestic students; for spring admission, 12/1 for domestic students. Application fee: $50 ($75 for international students). *Expenses:* Tuition, state resident: full-time $22,127; part-time $178 per credit hour. Tuition, nonresident: full-time $43,572; part-time $728 per credit hour. *Required fees:* $910.79; $200 per semester. *Unit head:* Dr. James D. Hess, Director, 918-561-1105, Fax: 918-561-1416, E-mail: jim.hess@okstate.edu. *Application contact:* Patrick Anderson, Coordinator of Graduate Admissions, 918-561-1228, Fax: 918-561-8243, E-mail: patrick.anderson@okstate.edu.
Website: http://www.healthsciences.okstate.edu/hca/index.cfm

Old Dominion University, College of Business and Public Administration, MBA Program, Norfolk, VA 23529. Offers business and economic forecasting (MBA); financial analysis and valuation (MBA); health sciences administration (MBA); information technology and enterprise integration (MBA); international business (MBA); maritime and port management (MBA); public administration (MBA). *Accreditation:* AACSB. Part-time and evening/weekend programs available. Postbaccalaureate distance learning degree programs offered (no on-campus study). *Faculty:* 83 full-time (19 women), 5 part-time/adjunct (2 women). *Students:* 42 full-time (20 women), 103 part-time (42 women); includes 18 minority (8 Black or African American, non-Hispanic/Latino; 4 Asian, non-Hispanic/Latino; 1 Hispanic/Latino; 1 Native Hawaiian or other Pacific Islander, non-Hispanic/Latino; 4 Two or more races, non-Hispanic/Latino), 16 international. Average age 30. 161 applicants, 71% accepted, 75 enrolled. In 2013, 61 master's awarded. *Entrance requirements:* For master's, GMAT, GRE, letter of reference, resume, essay. Additional exam requirements/recommendations for international students: Required—TOEFL (minimum score 550 paper-based; 80 iBT). *Application deadline:* For fall admission, 6/1 priority date for domestic students, 4/15 priority date for international students; for spring admission, 11/1 priority date for domestic students, 10/1 priority date for international students. Applications are processed on a rolling basis. Application fee: $50. Electronic applications accepted. *Expenses:* Tuition, state resident: full-time $9888; part-time $412 per credit. Tuition, nonresident: full-time $25,152; part-time $1048 per credit. *Required fees:* $59 per semester. One-time fee: $50. *Financial support:* In 2013–14, 47 students received support, including 94 research assistantships with partial tuition reimbursements available (averaging $8,900 per year); career-related internships or fieldwork, scholarships/grants, and unspecified assistantships also available. Support available to part-time students. Financial award application deadline: 2/15; financial award applicants required to submit FAFSA. *Faculty research:* International business, buyer behavior, financial markets, strategy, operations research, maritime and transportation economics. *Unit head:* Dr. Kiran Karaude, Graduate Program Director, 757-683-3585, Fax: 757-683-5750, E-mail: mbainfo@odu.edu. *Application contact:* Sandi Phillips, MBA Program Assistant, 757-683-3585, Fax: 757-683-5750, E-mail: mbainfo@odu.edu.
Website: http://www.odu.edu/mba/

Oregon Health & Science University, School of Medicine, Graduate Programs in Medicine, Division of Management, Portland, OR 97239-3098. Offers healthcare management (MBA, MS). Part-time programs available. *Faculty:* 5 full-time (2 women), 27 part-time/adjunct (7 women). *Students:* 160 part-time (103 women); includes 32 minority (3 Black or African American, non-Hispanic/Latino; 18 Asian, non-Hispanic/Latino; 7 Hispanic/Latino; 4 Two or more races, non-Hispanic/Latino), 2 international. Average age 38. 88 applicants, 80% accepted, 70 enrolled. In 2013, 39 master's awarded. *Degree requirements:* For master's, thesis optional. *Entrance requirements:* For master's, GRE General Test (minimum scores: 153 Verbal/148 Quantitative/4.5 Analytical) or GMAT. Additional exam requirements/recommendations for international students: Required—TOEFL (minimum score 625 paper-based). *Application deadline:* For fall admission, 7/15 for domestic and international students; for winter admission, 10/15 for domestic and international students; for spring admission, 1/15 for domestic and international students. Applications are processed on a rolling basis. Application fee: $70. Electronic applications accepted. *Financial support:* Health care benefits available. *Faculty research:* Enhancing quality and reducing cost for healthcare by improving patient activation, identifying factors in hospital readmissions using system dynamics modeling, human and organizational dimensions of creating healthy communities. *Unit head:* Jim Huntzicker, Division Head, 503-346-0368, E-mail: hcmanagement@ohsu.edu. *Application contact:* Jessica Walter, Program Coordinator, 503-346-0369, E-mail: hcmanagement@ohsu.edu.

Oregon State University, College of Public Health and Human Sciences, Program in Public Health, Corvallis, OR 97331. Offers biostatistics (MPH); environmental and occupational health and safety (MPH, PhD); epidemiology (MPH); health management and policy (MPH); health policy (PhD); health promotion and health behavior (MPH, PhD); international health (MPH). *Accreditation:* CEPH. Part-time programs available. *Faculty:* 29 full-time (16 women), 4 part-time/adjunct (3 women). *Students:* 137 full-time (102 women), 29 part-time (18 women); includes 37 minority (4 Black or African American, non-Hispanic/Latino; 7 Asian, non-Hispanic/Latino; 17 Hispanic/Latino; 9 Two or more races, non-Hispanic/Latino), 15 international. Average age 32. 163 applicants, 58% accepted, 48 enrolled. In 2013, 39 master's, 3 doctorates awarded. Terminal master's awarded for partial completion of doctoral program. *Degree requirements:* For doctorate, one foreign language, thesis/dissertation. *Entrance requirements:* For master's and doctorate, GRE, minimum GPA of 3.0 in last 90 hours. Additional exam requirements/recommendations for international students: Required—TOEFL (minimum score 80 iBT), IELTS (minimum score 6.5). *Application deadline:* For fall admission, 12/1 for domestic students. Applications are processed on a rolling basis. Application fee: $60. *Expenses:* Contact institution. *Financial support:* Fellowships, research assistantships, teaching assistantships, career-related internships or fieldwork, Federal Work-Study, and institutionally sponsored loans available. Support available to part-time students. Financial award application deadline: 2/1. *Faculty research:* Traffic safety, health safety, injury control, health promotion. *Unit head:* Dr. Sheryl Thorburn, Professor/Co-Director, 541-737-9493. *Application contact:* Eileen Kaspar, Public Health Graduate Programs Manager, 541-737-3825, E-mail: eileen.kaspar@oregonstate.edu.

Our Lady of the Lake College, School of Arts, Sciences and Health Professions, Baton Rouge, LA 70808. Offers health administration (MHA); physician assistant studies (MMS).

Our Lady of the Lake University of San Antonio, School of Business and Leadership, Program in Healthcare Management, San Antonio, TX 78207-4689. Offers MBA. Part-time and evening/weekend programs available. Postbaccalaureate distance learning degree programs offered (no on-campus study). *Faculty:* 3 full-time (0 women), 1 (woman) part-time/adjunct. *Students:* 81 full-time (54 women), 7 part-time (5 women); includes 59 minority (14 Black or African American, non-Hispanic/Latino; 4 Asian, non-Hispanic/Latino; 41 Hispanic/Latino), 1 international. Average age 35. 54 applicants, 96% accepted, 33 enrolled. In 2013, 20 master's awarded. *Entrance requirements:* For master's, GMAT, GRE General Test, or MAT. Additional exam requirements/recommendations for international students: Required—TOEFL. *Application deadline:* Applications are processed on a rolling basis. Application fee: $25 ($50 for international students). Electronic applications accepted. *Expenses: Tuition:* Full-time $9120; part-time $760 per credit. *Required fees:* $698; $334 per trimester. Tuition and fees vary according to course load, degree level, campus/location and program. *Financial support:* Fellowships, career-related internships or fieldwork, Federal Work-Study, institutionally sponsored loans, scholarships/grants, and tuition waivers (partial) available. Support available to part-time students. Financial award application deadline: 4/15. *Faculty research:* Decision-making, problem-solving, administration, leadership, management. *Unit head:* Dr. Kathryn Winney Bisking, Chair of the Business Department, 210-434-6711 Ext. 2297, Fax: 210-434-0821, E-mail: kmwinney@lake.ollusa.edu. *Application contact:* Graduate Admission, 210-431-3961, Fax: 210-431-4013, E-mail: gradadm@ollusa.edu.
Website: http://www.ollusa.edu/s/1190/ollu-3-column-noads.aspx?sid=1190&gid=1&pgid=6459

Pace University, Dyson College of Arts and Sciences, Department of Public Administration, New York, NY 10038. Offers environmental management (MPA); government management (MPA); health care administration (MPA); management for public safety and homeland security (MA); nonprofit management (MPA); JD/MPA. Offered at White Plains, NY location only. Part-time and evening/weekend programs available. *Faculty:* 5 full-time (2 women), 5 part-time/adjunct (1 woman). *Students:* 78 full-time (60 women), 68 part-time (37 women); includes 82 minority (49 Black or African American, non-Hispanic/Latino; 1 American Indian or Alaska Native, non-Hispanic/Latino; 5 Asian, non-Hispanic/Latino; 22 Hispanic/Latino; 5 Two or more races, non-Hispanic/Latino), 31 international. Average age 29. 101 applicants, 86% accepted, 51 enrolled. In 2013, 43 master's awarded. *Degree requirements:* For master's, capstone project. *Entrance requirements:* For master's, GRE General Test. Additional exam requirements/recommendations for international students: Required—TOEFL. *Application deadline:* For fall admission, 8/1 priority date for domestic students, 6/1 for international students; for spring admission, 12/1 priority date for domestic students, 10/1 for international students. Applications are processed on a rolling basis. Application fee: $70. Electronic applications accepted. *Expenses: Tuition:* Part-time $1075 per credit. *Required fees:* $192 per semester. Tuition and fees vary according to course load, degree level and program. *Financial support:* Research assistantships, career-related internships or fieldwork, Federal Work-Study, and tuition waivers (partial) available. Support available to part-time students. Financial award applicants required to submit FAFSA. *Unit head:* Dr. Farrokh Hormozi, Chairperson, 914-422-4285, E-mail: fhormozi@pace.edu. *Application contact:* Susan Ford-Goldschein, Director of Admissions, 914-422-4283, Fax: 914-422-4287, E-mail: gradwp@pace.edu.
Website: http://www.pace.edu/dyson/academic-departments-and-programs/public-admin

Pacific University, Healthcare Administration Program, Forest Grove, OR 97116-1797. Offers MHA.

Park University, School of Graduate and Professional Studies, Kansas City, MO 54105. Offers adult education (M Ed); business and government leadership (Graduate Certificate); business, government, and global society (MPA); communication and leadership (MA); creative and life writing (Graduate Certificate); disaster and emergency management (MPA, Graduate Certificate); educational leadership (M Ed); finance (MBA, Graduate Certificate); general business (MBA); global business (Graduate Certificate); healthcare administration (MHA); healthcare services management and leadership (Graduate Certificate); international business (MBA); language and literacy (M Ed), including English for speakers of other languages, special reading teacher/literacy coach; leadership of international healthcare organizations (Graduate Certificate); management information systems (MBA, Graduate Certificate); music performance (ADP, Graduate Certificate), including cello (MM, ADP), piano (MM, ADP), viola (MM, ADP), violin (MM, ADP); nonprofit and community services management (MPA); nonprofit leadership (Graduate Certificate); performance (MM), including cello (MM, ADP), piano (MM, ADP), viola (MM, ADP), violin (MM, ADP); public management (MPA); social work (MSW); teacher leadership (M Ed), including curriculum and assessment, instructional leader. Part-time and evening/weekend programs available. Postbaccalaureate distance learning degree programs offered (no on-campus study). *Students:* 862 full-time (482 women); includes 55 minority (30 Black or African American, non-Hispanic/Latino; 2 American Indian or Alaska Native, non-Hispanic/Latino; 4 Asian, non-Hispanic/Latino; 14 Hispanic/Latino; 5 Two or more races, non-Hispanic/Latino), 141 international. Average age 34. 497 applicants, 62% accepted, 119 enrolled. In 2013, 281 master's, 14 other advanced degrees awarded. *Degree requirements:* For master's, comprehensive exam (for some programs), thesis (for some programs), internship (for some programs); exam (for some programs). *Entrance requirements:* For master's, GRE or GMAT (for some programs), teacher certification (for some M Ed programs), letters of recommendation, essay, resume (for some programs). Additional exam requirements/recommendations for international students: Required—TOEFL (minimum score 550 paper-based; 79 iBT), IELTS (minimum score 6). *Application deadline:* For fall admission, 8/1 priority date for domestic students, 7/15 priority date for international students; for spring admission, 1/1 priority date for domestic students, 11/1 priority date for international students. Applications are processed on a rolling basis. Application fee: $50 ($100 for international students). Electronic applications accepted. *Financial support:* In 2013–14, 2 research assistantships with full tuition reimbursements (averaging $15,760 per year) were awarded. Financial award applicants required to submit FAFSA. *Unit head:* Dr. Laurie Dipadova-Stocks, Dean of Graduate and Professional Studies, 816-559-5624, Fax: 816-472-1173, E-mail: ldipadovastocks@park.edu. *Application contact:* Judith Appollis, Director of Graduate

Admissions and Internationalization, School of Graduate and Professional Studies, 816-559-5627, Fax: 816-472-1173, E-mail: gradschool@park.edu.
Website: http://www.park.edu/grad

Penn State Harrisburg, Graduate School, School of Public Affairs, Middletown, PA 17057-4898. Offers criminal justice (MA); health administration (MHA); public administration (MPA, PhD). *Accreditation:* NASPAA. *Unit head:* Dr. Mukund S. Kulkarni, Chancellor, 717-948-6105, Fax: 717-948-6452, E-mail: msk5@psu.edu. *Application contact:* Robert W. Coffman, Jr., Director of Enrollment Management, Admissions, 717-948-6250, Fax: 717-948-6325, E-mail: ric1@psu.edu.
Website: http://harrisburg.psu.edu/public-affairs

Penn State University Park, Graduate School, College of Health and Human Development, Department of Health Policy and Administration, University Park, PA 16802. Offers MHA, MS, PhD. *Accreditation:* CAHME. *Unit head:* Dr. Ann C. Crouter, Dean, 814-865-1420, Fax: 814-865-3282, E-mail: ac1@psu.edu. *Application contact:* Cynthia E. Nicosia, Director, Graduate Enrollment Services, 814-865-1834, Fax: 814-863-4627, E-mail: cey1@psu.edu.
Website: http://www.hhdev.psu.edu/hpa

Pfeiffer University, Program in Health Administration, Misenheimer, NC 28109-0960. Offers MHA, MBA/MHA.

Point Loma Nazarene University, Fermanian School of Business, San Diego, CA 92106-2899. Offers general business (MBA); healthcare (MBA); not-for-profit management (MBA); organizational leadership (MBA); sustainability (MBA). *Accreditation:* ACBSP. Part-time and evening/weekend programs available. *Students:* 37 full-time (12 women), 70 part-time (35 women); includes 33 minority (3 Black or African American, non-Hispanic/Latino; 9 Asian, non-Hispanic/Latino; 14 Hispanic/Latino; 1 Native Hawaiian or other Pacific Islander, non-Hispanic/Latino; 6 Two or more races, non-Hispanic/Latino), 1 international. Average age 29. 51 applicants, 65% accepted, 28 enrolled. In 2013, 59 master's awarded. *Entrance requirements:* For master's, GMAT, letters of recommendation, essay, interview. Additional exam requirements/recommendations for international students: Required—TOEFL. *Application deadline:* For fall admission, 8/4 priority date for domestic students; for spring admission, 12/8 priority date for domestic students; for summer admission, 4/13 priority date for domestic students. Applications are processed on a rolling basis. Application fee: $50. Electronic applications accepted. *Expenses: Tuition:* Full-time $6900; part-time $567 per credit hour. *Financial support:* Applicants required to submit FAFSA. *Unit head:* Dr. Ken Armstrong, Interim Dean, 619-849-2290, E-mail: kenarmstrong@pointloma.edu. *Application contact:* Laura Leinweber, Director of Graduate Admission, 866-692-4723, E-mail: lauraleinweber@pointloma.edu.
Website: http://www.pointloma.edu/discover/graduate-school-san-diego/san-diego-graduate-programs-masters-degree-san-diego/mba

Portland State University, Graduate Studies, College of Urban and Public Affairs, School of Community Health, Program in Health Studies, Portland, OR 97207-0751. Offers health administration (MPA, MPH). Part-time and evening/weekend programs available. *Students:* 39 full-time (33 women), 28 part-time (27 women); includes 13 minority (2 Black or African American, non-Hispanic/Latino; 1 American Indian or Alaska Native, non-Hispanic/Latino; 2 Asian, non-Hispanic/Latino; 4 Hispanic/Latino; 4 Two or more races, non-Hispanic/Latino), 3 international. Average age 30. 127 applicants, 40% accepted, 45 enrolled. *Degree requirements:* For master's, internship (MPA), practicum (MPH). *Entrance requirements:* For master's, minimum GPA of 3.0 in upper-division course work or 2.75 overall, resume, 3 recommendation forms. Additional exam requirements/recommendations for international students: Required—TOEFL (minimum score 550 paper-based). *Application deadline:* For fall admission, 2/1 for domestic and international students. Application fee: $50. *Expenses:* Tuition, state resident: full-time $9207; part-time $341 per credit. Tuition, nonresident: full-time $14,391; part-time $533 per credit. *Required fees:* $1263; $22 per credit. $98 per quarter. One-time fee: $150. Tuition and fees vary according to program. *Financial support:* In 2013–14, 6 research assistantships with full and partial tuition reimbursements (averaging $6,114 per year), 1 teaching assistantship with full tuition reimbursement (averaging $3,186 per year) were awarded; career-related internships or fieldwork, Federal Work-Study, and institutionally sponsored loans also available. Support available to part-time students. Financial award application deadline: 3/1; financial award applicants required to submit FAFSA. *Total annual research expenditures:* $501,625. *Unit head:* Dr. Carlos J. Crespo, Director, 503-725-5120, Fax: 503-725-5100, E-mail: ccrespo@pdx.edu. *Application contact:* Elizabeth Bull, Assistant to the Director, 503-725-4592, Fax: 503-725-5100, E-mail: bulle@pdx.edu.

Post University, Program in Business Administration, Waterbury, CT 06723-2540. Offers accounting (MSA); business administration (MBA); corporate innovation (MBA); entrepreneurship (MBA); finance (MBA); healthcare (MBA); leadership (MBA); marketing (MBA); project management (MBA). *Accreditation:* ACBSP. Postbaccalaureate distance learning degree programs offered.

Queen's University at Kingston, School of Graduate Studies, Faculty of Health Sciences, Department of Community Health and Epidemiology, Kingston, ON K7L 3N6, Canada. Offers epidemiology (PhD); epidemiology and population health (M Sc); health services (M Sc); policy research and clinical epidemiology (M Sc); public health (MPH). Part-time programs available. *Degree requirements:* For master's, thesis. *Entrance requirements:* For master's, GRE General Test (strongly recommended). Additional exam requirements/recommendations for international students: Required—TOEFL (minimum score 600 paper-based). *Faculty research:* Cancer epidemiology, clinical trials, biostatistics health services research, health policy.

Regis College, School of Nursing, Science and Health Professions, Weston, MA 02493. Offers applied behavior analysis (MS); biomedical sciences (MS); health administration (MS); nurse practitioner (Certificate); nursing (MS, DNP); nursing education (Certificate). Part-time and evening/weekend programs available. *Degree requirements:* For master's, thesis. *Entrance requirements:* For master's, GRE General Test or MAT, minimum GPA of 3.0; for doctorate, MAT or GRE if GPA from master's lower than 3.5. Additional exam requirements/recommendations for international students: Required—TOEFL (minimum score 550 paper-based). Electronic applications accepted. *Faculty research:* Health policy, education, aging, job satisfaction, psychiatric nursing, critical thinking.

Regis University, College for Professional Studies, School of Management, MBA Program, Denver, CO 80221-1099. Offers finance and accounting (MBA); general business (MBA); health industry leadership (MBA); marketing (MBA); operations management (MBA); organizational performance management (MBA); strategic management (MBA). Part-time and evening/weekend programs available. Postbaccalaureate distance learning degree programs offered (no on-campus study). *Faculty:* 10 full-time (3 women), 74 part-time/adjunct (17 women). *Students:* 386 full-time (183 women), 269 part-time (134 women); includes 190 minority (38 Black or African American, non-Hispanic/Latino; 2 American Indian or Alaska Native, non-Hispanic/Latino; 30 Asian, non-Hispanic/Latino; 109 Hispanic/Latino; 1 Native Hawaiian or other Pacific Islander, non-Hispanic/Latino; 10 Two or more races, non-Hispanic/Latino), 11 international. Average age 42. 152 applicants, 91% accepted, 112 enrolled. In 2013, 318 master's awarded. *Degree requirements:* For master's, thesis (for some programs), final research project. *Entrance requirements:* For master's, official transcript reflecting baccalaureate degree awarded from regionally-accredited college or university, work experience, resume, letters of recommendation. Additional exam requirements/recommendations for international students: Required—TOEFL (minimum score 550 paper-based; 82 iBT). *Application deadline:* Applications are processed on a rolling basis. Application fee: $75. Electronic applications accepted. *Expenses:* Contact institution. *Financial support:* In 2013–14, 22 students received support. Federal Work-Study and scholarships/grants available. Financial award application deadline: 4/15; financial award applicants required to submit FAFSA. *Unit head:* Dr. Anthony Vrba, Interim Dean, 303-964-5384, Fax: 303-964-5538, E-mail: avrba@regis.edu. *Application contact:* Sarah Engel, Director of Admissions, 303-458-4900, Fax: 303-964-5534, E-mail: regisadm@regis.edu.
Website: http://www.regis.edu/CPS/Academics/Degrees-and-Programs/Graduate-Programs/MBA-College-for-Professional-Studies.aspx

Regis University, Rueckert-Hartman College for Health Professions, Division of Health Services Administration, Denver, CO 80221-1099. Offers health care informatics and information management (MS); health information management (Postbaccalaureate Certificate); health services administration (MS). Part-time and evening/weekend programs available. Postbaccalaureate distance learning degree programs offered (no on-campus study). *Faculty:* 6 full-time (all women), 19 part-time/adjunct (12 women). *Students:* 43 full-time (38 women), 14 part-time (10 women); includes 15 minority (4 Black or African American, non-Hispanic/Latino; 4 Asian, non-Hispanic/Latino; 5 Hispanic/Latino; 2 Two or more races, non-Hispanic/Latino). Average age 39. 80 applicants, 75% accepted, 40 enrolled. In 2013, 19 master's awarded. *Degree requirements:* For master's, thesis, final research project. *Entrance requirements:* For master's, official transcript reflecting baccalaureate degree awarded from regionally-accredited college or university with minimum cumulative GPA of 3.0 or GRE/GMAT; letters of recommendation; essay; resume; interview. Additional exam requirements/recommendations for international students: Required—TOEFL (minimum score 550 paper-based; 82 iBT). *Application deadline:* Applications are processed on a rolling basis. Application fee: $75. Electronic applications accepted. *Expenses:* Contact institution. *Financial support:* In 2013–14, 4 students received support. Federal Work-Study and scholarships/grants available. Financial award application deadline: 4/15; financial award applicants required to submit FAFSA. *Unit head:* Dr. Sheila Carlon, Director, 303-458-4108, Fax: 303-964-5430, E-mail: scarlon@regis.edu. *Application contact:* Sarah Engel, Director of Admissions, 303-458-4900, Fax: 303-964-5534, E-mail: regisadm@regis.edu.
Website: http://www.regis.edu/RHCHP/Schools/Division-of-Health-Services-Administration.aspx

Rice University, Graduate Programs, Wiess School–Professional Science Master's Programs, Professional Master's Program in Bioscience Research and Health Policy, Houston, TX 77251-1892. Offers MS.

Robert Morris University Illinois, Morris Graduate School of Management, Chicago, IL 60605. Offers accounting (MBA); accounting/finance (MBA); business analytics (MIS); design and media (MM); educational technology (MM); health care administration (MM); higher education administration (MM); human resource management (MBA); information security (MIS); information systems (MIS); law enforcement administration (MM); management (MBA); management/finance (MBA); management/human resource management (MBA); mobile computing (MIS); sports administration (MM). Part-time and evening/weekend programs available. *Faculty:* 12 full-time (5 women), 18 part-time/adjunct (4 women). *Students:* 240 full-time (128 women), 195 part-time (127 women); includes 242 minority (147 Black or African American, non-Hispanic/Latino; 2 American Indian or Alaska Native, non-Hispanic/Latino; 24 Asian, non-Hispanic/Latino; 63 Hispanic/Latino; 1 Native Hawaiian or other Pacific Islander, non-Hispanic/Latino; 5 Two or more races, non-Hispanic/Latino), 26 international. Average age 33. 210 applicants, 63% accepted, 116 enrolled. In 2013, 278 master's awarded. *Entrance requirements:* For master's, official transcripts, two letters of recommendation. Additional exam requirements/recommendations for international students: Required—TOEFL (minimum score 550 paper-based). *Application deadline:* Applications are processed on a rolling basis. Application fee: $20 ($100 for international students). Electronic applications accepted. *Expenses: Tuition:* Full-time $14,400; part-time $2400 per course. *Financial support:* In 2013–14, 488 students received support. Federal Work-Study and scholarships/grants available. Support available to part-time students. Financial award applicants required to submit FAFSA. *Unit head:* Kayed Akkawi, Dean for Morris Graduate School of Management, 312-935-6050, Fax: 312-935-6020, E-mail: kakkawi@robertmorris.edu. *Application contact:* Fernando Villeda, Dean of Graduate Enrollment, 312-935-6050, Fax: 312-935-6020, E-mail: fvilleda@robertmorris.edu.

Roberts Wesleyan College, Health Administration Programs, Rochester, NY 14624-1997. Offers health administration (MS); healthcare informatics administration (MS). Evening/weekend programs available. Postbaccalaureate distance learning degree programs offered (no on-campus study). *Faculty:* 2 full-time (0 women), 4 part-time/adjunct (all women). *Students:* 73 full-time (60 women). Average age 34. In 2013, 23 degrees awarded. *Degree requirements:* For master's, thesis or alternative. *Entrance requirements:* For master's, minimum GPA of 3.0, verifiable work experience or recommendation. *Application deadline:* Applications are processed on a rolling basis. Application fee: $35. *Expenses: Tuition:* Full-time $12,816; part-time $712 per credit hour. One-time fee: $300. Tuition and fees vary according to course load and program. *Financial support:* Applicants required to submit FAFSA. *Unit head:* Joe McCarthy, Chair, 585-594-6990, Fax: 585-594-6940, E-mail: mccarthyj@roberts.edu. *Application contact:* Cheryl Johnson, Program Coordinator, 585-594-6452, Fax: 585-594-6940, E-mail: johnson_cheryl@roberts.edu.
Website: http://www.roberts.edu/health-administration-programs.aspx

Rochester Institute of Technology, Graduate Enrollment Services, College of Health Sciences and Technology, Program in Health Systems Administration, Rochester, NY 14623-5603. Offers elements of health care leadership (AC); health information resources (AC); health systems administration (MS); health systems administration executive leader (MS); health systems-finance (AC). Part-time and evening/weekend programs available. Postbaccalaureate distance learning degree programs offered (no on-campus study). *Students:* 5 full-time (3 women), 16 part-time (8 women); includes 5 minority (2 Black or African American, non-Hispanic/Latino; 3 Asian, non-Hispanic/Latino), 4 international. Average age 40. 44 applicants, 39% accepted, 11 enrolled. In 2013, 15 master's awarded. *Degree requirements:* For master's, thesis. *Entrance requirements:* For master's, minimum GPA of 3.0; related professional work experience; for AC, minimum GPA of 3.0. Additional exam requirements/recommendations for international students: Required—TOEFL (minimum score 550 paper-based; 79 iBT) or IELTS (minimum score 6.5). *Application deadline:* For fall admission, 2/15 priority date for domestic and international students; for winter admission, 11/1 for domestic students; for spring admission, 2/1 priority date for domestic students. Applications are processed on a rolling basis. Application fee: $60. Electronic applications accepted. *Expenses: Tuition:* Full-time $37,236; part-time $1552 per credit hour. *Required fees:* $250. *Financial support:* Research assistantships with partial tuition reimbursements, teaching assistantships with partial tuition reimbursements, career-related internships or fieldwork, scholarships/grants, and unspecified assistantships available. Support available to part-time students. Financial award applicants required to submit FAFSA. *Unit head:* Dr. Linda Underhill, Program Director, 585-475-7359, E-mail: lmuism@rit.edu. *Application contact:* Diane Ellison, Assistant Vice President, Graduate Enrollment Services, 585-475-2229, Fax: 585-475-7164, E-mail: gradinfo@rit.edu.

Roger Williams University, School of Justice Studies, Program in Public Administration, Bristol, RI 02809. Offers health care administration (MPA); public management (MPA). Part-time and evening/weekend programs available. Postbaccalaureate distance learning degree programs offered (minimal on-campus study). *Faculty:* 2 full-time (1 woman), 1 part-time/adjunct (0 women). *Students:* 3 full-time (2 women), 46 part-time (28 women); includes 8 minority (7 Black or African American, non-Hispanic/Latino; 1 Two or more races, non-Hispanic/Latino), 6 international. Average age 34. 39 applicants, 82% accepted, 15 enrolled. In 2013, 16 master's awarded. *Degree requirements:* For master's, internship/research project. *Entrance requirements:* For master's, 2 letters of recommendation, curriculum vitae/resume. Additional exam requirements/recommendations for international students: Recommended—TOEFL (minimum score 85 iBT), IELTS. *Application deadline:* Applications are processed on a rolling basis. Application fee: $50. Electronic applications accepted. *Expenses:* Contact institution. *Financial support:* In 2013–14, 12 students received support. Application deadline: 6/15; applicants required to submit FAFSA. *Unit head:* Dr. Michael Hall, Head, 401-254-5746, E-mail: mhall@rwu.edu. *Application contact:* Jamie Grenon, Director of Graduate Admissions, 401-254-6000, Fax: 401-254-3557, E-mail: gradadmit@rwu.edu.

Rosalind Franklin University of Medicine and Science, College of Health Professions, Department of Interprofessional Healthcare Studies, Healthcare Administration and Management Program, North Chicago, IL 60064-3095. Offers MS, Certificate. Part-time and evening/weekend programs available. Postbaccalaureate distance learning degree programs offered (no on-campus study). *Degree requirements:* For master's, capstone portfolio. *Entrance requirements:* For master's, minimum GPA of 2.75, BS/BA from accredited college or university. Additional exam requirements/recommendations for international students: Required—TOEFL.

Royal Roads University, Graduate Studies, Applied Leadership and Management Program, Victoria, BC V9B 5Y2, Canada. Offers executive coaching (Graduate Certificate); health systems leadership (Graduate Certificate); project management (Graduate Certificate); public relations management (Graduate Certificate); strategic human resources management (Graduate Certificate).

Rush University, College of Health Sciences, Department of Health Systems Management, Chicago, IL 60612-3832. Offers MS, DHSc. *Accreditation:* CAHME. Part-time and evening/weekend programs available. *Degree requirements:* For master's, thesis; for doctorate, thesis/dissertation. *Entrance requirements:* For master's, GMAT or GRE General Test, previous undergraduate course work in accounting and statistics; for doctorate, GRE General Test, master's degree preferably in a health discipline. Additional exam requirements/recommendations for international students: Required—TOEFL. Electronic applications accepted. *Faculty research:* Organizational performance, occupational health, quality of care indicators, leadership development, entrepreneurship, health insurance and disability, managed care.

Rutgers, The State University of New Jersey, Camden, School of Public Health, Stratford, NJ 08084. Offers general public health (Certificate); health systems and policy (MPH); DO/MPH. *Accreditation:* CEPH. Part-time and evening/weekend programs available. *Degree requirements:* For master's, thesis, internship. *Entrance requirements:* For master's, GRE General Test. Additional exam requirements/recommendations for international students: Required—TOEFL. Electronic applications accepted.

Rutgers, The State University of New Jersey, Newark, Graduate School, Program in Public Administration, Newark, NJ 07102. Offers health care administration (MPA); human resources administration (MPA); public administration (PhD); public management (MPA); public policy analysis (MPA); urban systems and issues (MPA). *Accreditation:* NASPAA (one or more programs are accredited). Part-time and evening/weekend programs available. *Degree requirements:* For master's, comprehensive exam, thesis or alternative; for doctorate, thesis/dissertation. *Entrance requirements:* For master's, GRE, minimum undergraduate B average; for doctorate, GRE, MPA, minimum B average. Electronic applications accepted. *Faculty research:* Government finance, municipal and state government, public productivity.

Rutgers, The State University of New Jersey, Newark, School of Health Related Professions, Department of Interdisciplinary Studies, Program in Health Care Management, Newark, NJ 07102. Offers MS. Part-time and evening/weekend programs available. Postbaccalaureate distance learning degree programs offered (no on-campus study). *Entrance requirements:* For master's, minimum GPA of 3.0, bachelor's degree, statement of career goals, curriculum vitae, transcript of highest degree. Additional exam requirements/recommendations for international students: Required—TOEFL (minimum score 500 paper-based; 79 iBT). Electronic applications accepted.

Rutgers, The State University of New Jersey, Newark, School of Public Health, Newark, NJ 07107-1709. Offers clinical epidemiology (Certificate); dental public health (MPH); general public health (Certificate); public policy and oral health services administration (Certificate); quantitative methods (MPH); urban health (MPH); DMD/MPH; MD/MPH; MS/MPH. *Accreditation:* CEPH. Part-time and evening/weekend programs available. *Degree requirements:* For master's, thesis, internship. *Entrance requirements:* For master's, GRE General Test. Additional exam requirements/recommendations for international students: Required—TOEFL. Electronic applications accepted.

Rutgers, The State University of New Jersey, New Brunswick, School of Public Health, Piscataway, NJ 08854. Offers biostatistics (MPH, MS, Dr PH, PhD); clinical epidemiology (Certificate); environmental and occupational health (MPH, Dr PH, PhD, Certificate); epidemiology (MPH, Dr PH, PhD); general public health (Certificate); health education and behavioral science (MPH, Dr PH, PhD); health systems and policy (MPH, PhD); public health preparedness (Certificate); DO/MPH; JD/MPH; MD/MPH; MPH/MBA; MPH/MSPA; MS/MPH; Psy D/MPH. *Accreditation:* CEPH. Part-time and evening/weekend programs available. *Degree requirements:* For master's, thesis, internship; for doctorate, comprehensive exam, thesis/dissertation. *Entrance requirements:* For master's, GRE General Test; for doctorate, GRE General Test, MPH (Dr PH); MA, MPH, or MS (PhD). Additional exam requirements/recommendations for international students: Required—TOEFL. Electronic applications accepted.

Sacred Heart University, Graduate Programs, College of Health Professions, Department of Nursing, Fairfield, CT 06825-1000. Offers clinical nurse leader (MSN); clinical practice in health care (DNP); family nurse practitioner (MSN); leadership in health care (DNP); nursing (DN Sc); nursing educator (MSN); patient care services administration (MSN). *Accreditation:* AACN. Part-time and evening/weekend programs available. Postbaccalaureate distance learning degree programs offered (no on-campus study). *Faculty:* 7 full-time (all women), 5 part-time/adjunct (all women). *Students:* 34 full-time (32 women), 645 part-time (595 women); includes 117 minority (50 Black or African American, non-Hispanic/Latino; 1 American Indian or Alaska Native, non-Hispanic/Latino; 26 Asian, non-Hispanic/Latino; 29 Hispanic/Latino; 1 Native Hawaiian or other Pacific Islander, non-Hispanic/Latino; 10 Two or more races, non-Hispanic/Latino). Average age 39. 110 applicants, 58% accepted, 46 enrolled. In 2013, 67 master's, 11 doctorates awarded. *Entrance requirements:* For master's, minimum GPA of 3.0, BSN or RN plus BS (for MSN); for doctorate, minimum GPA of 3.0, MSN or BSN plus MS (for DNP). Additional exam requirements/recommendations for international students: Required—PTE; Recommended—TOEFL (minimum score 570 paper-based; 80 iBT), IELTS (minimum score 6.5). *Application deadline:* Applications are processed on a rolling basis. Application fee: $60. Electronic applications accepted. *Expenses:* Contact institution. *Financial support:* Career-related internships or fieldwork and institutionally sponsored loans available. Support available to part-time students. Financial award applicants required to submit FAFSA. *Unit head:* Dr. Sue DeNisco, Chair, 203-365-7661, Fax: 203-365-7662, E-mail: deniscos@sacredheart.edu. *Application contact:* Kathy Dilks, Executive Director of Graduate Admissions, 203-365-4716, Fax: 203-365-4732, E-mail: gradstudies@sacredheart.edu.
Website: http://www.sacredheart.edu/graduate/nursing/

Sage Graduate School, School of Health Sciences, Department of Nursing, Troy, NY 12180-4115. Offers adult geriatric advanced nursing (MS); adult gerontology nurse practitioner (MS); adult health (MS); adult nurse practitioner (MS, Post Master's Certificate); clinical nurse leader/specialist (Post Master's Certificate); community health (MS); counseling for nursing (Postbaccalaureate Certificate); education and leadership (DNS); family nurse practitioner (MS, Post Master's Certificate); gerontological nurse practitioner (Post Master's Certificate); nurse administrator/executive (Post Master's Certificate); nurse education (Post Master's Certificate); nursing (Post Master's Certificate); psychiatric mental health nurse clinical nurse specialist (MS); psychiatric mental health nurse practitioner (MS, Post Master's Certificate), including psychiatric mental health. *Accreditation:* AACN. Part-time and evening/weekend programs available. *Faculty:* 5 full-time (all women), 10 part-time/adjunct (all women). *Students:* 32 full-time (30 women), 174 part-time (161 women); includes 28 minority (12 Black or African American, non-Hispanic/Latino; 2 American Indian or Alaska Native, non-Hispanic/Latino; 8 Asian, non-Hispanic/Latino; 4 Hispanic/Latino; 2 Two or more races, non-Hispanic/Latino), 3 international. Average age 40. 171 applicants, 43% accepted, 35 enrolled. In 2013, 53 master's, 5 doctorates, 11 other advanced degrees awarded. *Degree requirements:* For master's, thesis or alternative. *Entrance requirements:* For master's, BS in nursing, minimum GPA of 2.75, resume, 2 letters of recommendation. Additional exam requirements/recommendations for international students: Required—TOEFL (minimum score 550 paper-based). *Application deadline:* Applications are processed on a rolling basis. Application fee: $40. *Expenses: Tuition:* Full-time $11,880; part-time $660 per credit hour. *Financial support:* Fellowships, research assistantships, Federal Work-Study, scholarships/grants, and unspecified assistantships available. Support available to part-time students. Financial award application deadline: 3/1; financial award applicants required to submit FAFSA. *Unit head:* Dr. Esther Haskevitz, Dean, School of Health Sciences, 518-244-2296, Fax: 518-244-4571, E-mail: haskve@sage.edu. *Application contact:* Dr. Glenda Kelman, Director, 518-244-2001, Fax: 518-244-2009, E-mail: kelmag@sage.edu.

Sage Graduate School, School of Management, Program in Health Services Administration, Troy, NY 12180-4115. Offers dietetic internship (Certificate); gerontology (MS). Part-time and evening/weekend programs available. *Faculty:* 2 full-time (both women), 28 part-time/adjunct (21 women). *Students:* 3 full-time (all women), 38 part-time (27 women); includes 6 minority (3 Black or African American, non-Hispanic/Latino; 3 Asian, non-Hispanic/Latino). Average age 33. 46 applicants, 41% accepted, 13 enrolled. In 2013, 8 master's awarded. *Entrance requirements:* For master's, minimum GPA of 2.75, resume, 2 letters of recommendation. Additional exam requirements/recommendations for international students: Required—TOEFL (minimum score 550 paper-based). Application fee: $40. *Expenses: Tuition:* Full-time $11,880; part-time $660 per credit hour. *Financial support:* Fellowships, research assistantships, Federal Work-Study, scholarships/grants, and unspecified assistantships available. Support available to part-time students. Financial award application deadline: 3/1; financial award applicants required to submit FAFSA. *Unit head:* Dr. Kimberly Fredricks, Associate Dean, School of Management, 518-292-1700, Fax: 518-292-1964, E-mail: fredek1@sage.edu. *Application contact:* Wendy D. Diefendorf, Director of Graduate and Adult Admission, 518-244-2443, Fax: 518-244-6880, E-mail: diefew@sage.edu.

Saginaw Valley State University, Crystal M. Lange College of Nursing and Health Sciences, Program in Health Leadership, University Center, MI 48710. Offers MS. Part-time and evening/weekend programs available. *Students:* 18 full-time (14 women), 20 part-time (15 women); includes 6 minority (3 Black or African American, non-Hispanic/Latino; 2 Asian, non-Hispanic/Latino; 1 Hispanic/Latino), 2 international. Average age 30. 22 applicants, 95% accepted, 14 enrolled. In 2013, 11 master's awarded. *Entrance requirements:* For master's, minimum GPA of 3.0. Additional exam requirements/recommendations for international students: Required—TOEFL (minimum score 580 paper-based; 92 iBT). *Application deadline:* For fall admission, 7/15 for international students; for winter admission, 11/15 for international students; for spring admission, 4/15 for international students. Applications are processed on a rolling basis. Application fee: $30 ($80 for international students). Electronic applications accepted. *Expenses:* Tuition, state resident: full-time $8933; part-time $496.30 per credit hour. Tuition, nonresident: full-time $16,806; part-time $933.65 per credit hour. *Required fees:* $263; $14.60 per credit hour. Tuition and fees vary according to degree level. *Financial support:* Federal Work-Study and scholarships/grants available. Support available to part-time students. *Unit head:* Dr. Marilyn Skrocki, Program Coordinator, 989-964-7394, E-mail: mskrocki@svsu.edu. *Application contact:* Jenna Briggs, Director, Graduate and International Admissions, 989-964-6096, Fax: 989-964-2788, E-mail: gradadm@svsu.edu.

St. Ambrose University, College of Business, Program in Business Administration, Davenport, IA 52803-2898. Offers business administration (DBA); health care (MBA); human resources (MBA). *Accreditation:* ACBSP. Part-time and evening/weekend programs available. *Degree requirements:* For master's, comprehensive exam (for some programs), thesis or alternative, capstone seminar; for doctorate, comprehensive exam, thesis/dissertation, oral and written exams. *Entrance requirements:* For master's, GMAT; for doctorate, GMAT, master's degree. Additional exam requirements/recommendations for international students: Required—TOEFL. Electronic applications accepted. *Expenses:* Contact institution.

St. Joseph's College, Long Island Campus, Program in Management, Patchogue, NY 11772-2399. Offers health care (AC); health care management (MS); human resource management (AC); human resources management (MS); organizational management (MS).

St. Joseph's College, New York, Graduate Programs, Program in Health Care Management, Brooklyn, NY 11205-3688. Offers MBA.

Saint Joseph's College of Maine, Master of Health Administration Program, Standish, ME 04084. Offers MHA. Degree program is external; available only by correspondence and online. Part-time programs available. Postbaccalaureate distance learning degree programs offered (minimal on-campus study). *Entrance requirements:* For master's, two years of experience in health care. Electronic applications accepted. *Faculty research:* Health care organization, policy, and management; long-term care.

Saint Joseph's University, College of Arts and Sciences, Department of Health Services, Philadelphia, PA 19131-1395. Offers health administration (MS, Post-Master's

Certificate); health care ethics (Post-Master's Certificate); health education (MS, Post-Master's Certificate); health informatics (Post-Master's Certificate); healthcare ethics (MS); long-term care administration (MS); nurse anesthesia (MS); school nurse certification (MS). Part-time and evening/weekend programs available. *Faculty:* 5 full-time (1 woman), 16 part-time/adjunct (6 women). *Students:* 46 full-time (25 women), 431 part-time (315 women); includes 168 minority (120 Black or African American, non-Hispanic/Latino; 29 Asian, non-Hispanic/Latino; 15 Hispanic/Latino; 2 Native Hawaiian or other Pacific Islander, non-Hispanic/Latino; 2 Two or more races, non-Hispanic/Latino), 14 international. Average age 34. 234 applicants, 74% accepted, 135 enrolled. In 2013, 83 master's awarded. *Entrance requirements:* For master's, GRE (if GPA less than 3.0), 2 letters of recommendation, resume, personal statement, official transcripts. Additional exam requirements/recommendations for international students: Required—TOEFL (minimum score 550 paper-based; 80 iBT), IELTS (minimum score 6.5). *Application deadline:* For fall admission, 7/15 priority date for domestic students, 4/15 for international students; for winter admission, 1/15 for international students; for spring admission, 11/15 priority date for domestic students, 10/15 for international students. Applications are processed on a rolling basis. Application fee: $35. Electronic applications accepted. *Expenses: Tuition:* Part-time $786 per credit hour. Tuition and fees vary according to degree level and program. *Financial support:* Career-related internships or fieldwork and unspecified assistantships available. Financial award applicants required to submit FAFSA. *Unit head:* Nakia Henderson, Director, 610-660-3131, E-mail: gradstudies@sju.edu. *Application contact:* Elisabeth Woodward, Director of Marketing and Admissions, Graduate Arts and Sciences, 610-660-3131, Fax: 610-660-3230, E-mail: gradstudies@sju.edu.
Website: http://sju.edu/majors-programs/graduate-arts-sciences/masters/health-administration-ms

Saint Joseph's University, Erivan K. Haub School of Business, Professional MBA Program, Philadelphia, PA 19131-1395. Offers accounting (MBA, Postbaccalaureate Certificate); business intelligence (MBA); finance (MBA); general business (MBA); health and medical services administration (MBA); international business (MBA); international marketing (MBA); managing human capital (MBA); marketing (MBA); DO/MBA. DO/MBA offered jointly with Philadelphia College of Osteopathic Medicine. Part-time and evening/weekend programs available. *Students:* 81 full-time (37 women), 478 part-time (195 women); includes 85 minority (35 Black or African American, non-Hispanic/Latino; 1 American Indian or Alaska Native, non-Hispanic/Latino; 23 Asian, non-Hispanic/Latino; 13 Hispanic/Latino; 1 Native Hawaiian or other Pacific Islander, non-Hispanic/Latino; 12 Two or more races, non-Hispanic/Latino), 44 international. Average age 30. In 2013, 195 master's awarded. *Degree requirements:* For master's and Postbaccalaureate Certificate, minimum GPA of 3.0. *Entrance requirements:* For master's, GMAT or GRE, 2 letters of recommendation, resume, personal statement, official undergraduate and graduate transcripts; for Postbaccalaureate Certificate, official master's-level transcripts. Additional exam requirements/recommendations for international students: Required—TOEFL (minimum score 550 paper-based, 80 iBT), IELTS (minimum score 6.5), or PTE (minimum score 60). *Application deadline:* For fall admission, 7/15 priority date for domestic students, 5/15 priority date for international students; for spring admission, 11/15 priority date for domestic students, 10/15 priority date for international students; for summer admission, 4/15 priority date for domestic students, 2/15 priority date for international students. Applications are processed on a rolling basis. Application fee: $35. Electronic applications accepted. *Expenses: Tuition:* Part-time $786 per credit hour. Tuition and fees vary according to degree level and program. *Financial support:* In 2013–14, 2 research assistantships with partial tuition reimbursements (averaging $4,000 per year) were awarded; scholarships/grants and unspecified assistantships also available. Support available to part-time students. Financial award application deadline: 5/1; financial award applicants required to submit FAFSA. *Unit head:* Christine Hartmann, Director, MBA Program, 610-660-1659, Fax: 610-660-1599, E-mail: chartman@sju.edu. *Application contact:* Jeannine Lajeunesse, Assistant Director, MBA Program, 610-660-1695, Fax: 610-660-1599, E-mail: jlajeune@sju.edu.
Website: http://www.sju.edu/haubmba

Saint Leo University, Graduate Business Studies, Saint Leo, FL 33574-6665. Offers accounting (M Acc, MBA); business (MBA); health care management (MBA); human resource management (MBA); information security management (MBA); marketing (MBA); marketing research and social media analytics (MBA); project management (MBA); sport business (MBA). Part-time and evening/weekend programs available. Postbaccalaureate distance learning degree programs offered (no on-campus study). *Faculty:* 48 full-time (12 women), 61 part-time/adjunct (21 women). *Students:* 1,855 full-time (1,020 women); includes 810 minority (587 Black or African American, non-Hispanic/Latino; 7 American Indian or Alaska Native, non-Hispanic/Latino; 36 Asian, non-Hispanic/Latino; 161 Hispanic/Latino; 3 Native Hawaiian or other Pacific Islander, non-Hispanic/Latino; 16 Two or more races, non-Hispanic/Latino), 33 international. Average age 38. In 2013, 905 master's awarded. *Entrance requirements:* For master's, GMAT (minimum score 500 if applicant has less than 3.0 in the last two years of undergraduate study), bachelor's degree with minimum GPA of 3.0 in the last 60 hours of coursework from regionally-accredited college or university; 2 years of professional work experience; resume; 2 letters of recommendation. Additional exam requirements/recommendations for international students: Required—TOEFL (minimum score 550 paper-based; 80 iBT). *Application deadline:* For fall admission, 7/1 priority date for domestic and international students; for spring admission, 11/12 priority date for domestic students, 11/1 for international students. Applications are processed on a rolling basis. Application fee: $80. Electronic applications accepted. *Expenses: Tuition:* Full-time $12,114; part-time $673 per semester hour. Tuition and fees vary according to degree level, campus/location and program. *Financial support:* In 2013–14, 116 students received support. Career-related internships or fieldwork, Federal Work-Study, scholarships/grants, and health care benefits available. Financial award application deadline: 3/1; financial award applicants required to submit FAFSA. *Unit head:* Dr. Lorrie McGovern, Assistant Dean, Graduate Studies in Business, 352-588-7390, Fax: 352-588-8585, E-mail: mbaslu@saintleo.edu. *Application contact:* Joshua Stagner, Director of Graduate Admission, 800-707-8846, Fax: 352-588-7873, E-mail: grad.admissions@saintleo.edu.
Website: http://www.saintleo.edu/academics/graduate.aspx

Saint Louis University, Graduate Education, School of Public Health and Graduate Education, Department of Health Management and Policy, St. Louis, MO 63103-2097. Offers health administration (MHA); health policy (MPH); public health studies (PhD). *Accreditation:* CAHME. Part-time programs available. *Degree requirements:* For master's, comprehensive exam, internship. *Entrance requirements:* For master's, GMAT or GRE General Test, LSAT, MCAT, letters of recommendation, resume. Additional exam requirements/recommendations for international students: Required—TOEFL (minimum score 525 paper-based). *Faculty research:* Management of HIV/AIDS, rural health services, prevention of asthma, genetics and health services use, health insurance and access to care.

Saint Mary's University of Minnesota, Schools of Graduate and Professional Programs, Graduate School of Health and Human Services, Health and Human Services Administration Program, Winona, MN 55987-1399. Offers MA. *Unit head:* Laurel Anderson, Director, 612-728-5549, E-mail: lqander@smumn.edu. *Application contact:* Russell Kreager, Director of Admissions for Graduate and Professional Programs, 612-728-5207, Fax: 612-728-5121, E-mail: rkreager@smumn.edu.
Website: http://www.smumn.edu/graduate-home/areas-of-study/graduate-school-of-health-human-services/ma-in-health-human-services-administration

Saint Peter's University, Graduate Business Programs, MBA Program, Jersey City, NJ 07306-5997. Offers finance (MBA); health care administration (MBA); human resource management (MBA); international business (MBA); management (MBA); management information systems (MBA); marketing (MBA); risk management (MBA); MBA/MS. Part-time and evening/weekend programs available. *Entrance requirements:* Additional exam requirements/recommendations for international students: Required—TOEFL. Electronic applications accepted. *Faculty research:* Finance, health care management, human resource management, international business, management, management information systems, marketing, risk management.

St. Thomas University, School of Business, Department of Management, Miami Gardens, FL 33054-6459. Offers accounting (MBA); general management (MSM, Certificate); health management (MBA, MSM, Certificate); human resource management (MBA, MSM, Certificate); international business (MBA, MIB, MSM, Certificate); justice administration (MSM, Certificate); management accounting (MSM, Certificate); public management (MSM, Certificate); sports administration (MS). Part-time and evening/weekend programs available. *Degree requirements:* For master's, comprehensive exam. *Entrance requirements:* For master's, interview, minimum GPA of 3.0 or GMAT. Additional exam requirements/recommendations for international students: Required—TOEFL (minimum score 550 paper-based; 79 iBT). Electronic applications accepted.

Saint Xavier University, Graduate Studies, Graham School of Management, Chicago, IL 60655-3105. Offers employee health benefits (Certificate); finance (MBA); financial fraud examination and management (MBA, Certificate); financial planning (MBA, Certificate); generalist/individualized (MBA); health administration (MBA); managed care (Certificate); management (MBA); marketing (MBA); project management (MBA, Certificate); MBA/MS. *Accreditation:* ACBSP. Part-time and evening/weekend programs available. *Entrance requirements:* For master's, GMAT, minimum GPA of 3.0, 2 years of work experience. Electronic applications accepted. *Expenses:* Contact institution.

Salve Regina University, Program in Business Administration, Newport, RI 02840-4192. Offers cybersecurity issues in business (MBA); entrepreneurial enterprise (MBA); health care administration and management (MBA); social ventures (MBA). Part-time and evening/weekend programs available. Postbaccalaureate distance learning degree programs offered (no on-campus study). *Faculty:* 3 full-time (2 women), 12 part-time/adjunct (5 women). *Students:* 32 full-time (15 women), 67 part-time (31 women); includes 8 minority (4 Black or African American, non-Hispanic/Latino; 1 American Indian or Alaska Native, non-Hispanic/Latino; 2 Hispanic/Latino; 1 Two or more races, non-Hispanic/Latino), 2 international. Average age 29. 49 applicants, 82% accepted, 20 enrolled. In 2013, 68 master's awarded. *Entrance requirements:* For master's, GMAT, GRE General Test, or MAT, 6 undergraduate credits each in accounting, economics, quantitative analysis and calculus or statistics. Additional exam requirements/recommendations for international students: Required—TOEFL (minimum score 600 paper-based; 100 iBT) or IELTS. *Application deadline:* For fall admission, 3/15 priority date for domestic and international students; for spring admission, 9/15 priority date for domestic and international students. Applications are processed on a rolling basis. Application fee: $60. Electronic applications accepted. *Expenses: Tuition:* Full-time $8280; part-time $460 per credit. *Required fees:* $40 per term. Tuition and fees vary according to course level, course load, degree level and program. *Financial support:* Career-related internships or fieldwork and Federal Work-Study available. Support available to part-time students. Financial award application deadline: 3/1; financial award applicants required to submit FAFSA. *Unit head:* Dr. Arlene Nicholas, Director, 401-341-3280, E-mail: arlene.nicholas@salve.edu. *Application contact:* Kelly Alverson, Director of Graduate Admissions, 401-341-2153, Fax: 401-341-2973, E-mail: kelly.alverson@salve.edu.
Website: http://salve.edu/graduate-studies/business-administration-and-management

Salve Regina University, Program in Healthcare Administration and Management, Newport, RI 02840-4192. Offers MS, Certificate. Part-time and evening/weekend programs available. Postbaccalaureate distance learning degree programs offered (no on-campus study). *Faculty:* 1 full-time (0 women), 4 part-time/adjunct (0 women). *Students:* 3 full-time (1 woman), 54 part-time (44 women); includes 8 minority (1 Black or African American, non-Hispanic/Latino; 4 Asian, non-Hispanic/Latino; 3 Hispanic/Latino). Average age 41. 5 applicants, 100% accepted, 4 enrolled. In 2013, 24 master's awarded. *Degree requirements:* For master's, internship. *Entrance requirements:* For master's, GMAT, GRE General Test, or MAT, health care work experience or 250 internship hours. Additional exam requirements/recommendations for international students: Required—TOEFL (minimum score 600 paper-based; 100 iBT) or IELTS. *Application deadline:* For fall admission, 3/15 priority date for domestic and international students; for spring admission, 9/15 priority date for domestic and international students. Applications are processed on a rolling basis. Application fee: $60. Electronic applications accepted. *Expenses: Tuition:* Full-time $8280; part-time $460 per credit. *Required fees:* $40 per term. Tuition and fees vary according to course level, course load, degree level and program. *Financial support:* Career-related internships or fieldwork and Federal Work-Study available. Support available to part-time students. Financial award application deadline: 3/1; financial award applicants required to submit FAFSA. *Unit head:* Mark Hough, Director, 401-341-3123, E-mail: mark.hough@salve.edu. *Application contact:* Kelly Alverson, Director of Graduate Admissions, 401-341-2153, Fax: 401-341-2973, E-mail: kelly.alverson@salve.edu.
Website: http://www.salve.edu/graduate-studies/health-care-administration-and-management

San Diego State University, Graduate and Research Affairs, College of Health and Human Services, Graduate School of Public Health, San Diego, CA 92182. Offers environmental health (MPH); epidemiology (MPH, PhD), including biostatistics (MPH); global emergency preparedness and response (MS); global health (PhD); health behavior (PhD); health promotion (MPH); health services administration (MPH); toxicology (MS); MPH/MA; MSW/MPH. *Accreditation:* CAHME (one or more programs are accredited); CEPH (one or more programs are accredited). Part-time programs available. *Degree requirements:* For master's, comprehensive exam (for some programs), thesis (for some programs); for doctorate, thesis/dissertation. *Entrance requirements:* For master's, GMAT (MPH in health services administration), GRE General Test; for doctorate, GRE General Test. Additional exam requirements/recommendations for international students: Required—TOEFL. *Faculty research:* Evaluation of tobacco, AIDS prevalence and prevention, mammography, infant death project, Alzheimer's in elderly Chinese.

Seton Hall University, College of Arts and Sciences, Department of Political Science and Public Affairs, South Orange, NJ 07079-2697. Offers healthcare administration (MHA, Graduate Certificate); nonprofit organization management (Graduate Certificate); public administration (MPA), including health policy and management, nonprofit organization management, public service: leadership, governance, and policy. *Accreditation:* NASPAA. Part-time and evening/weekend programs available. Postbaccalaureate distance learning degree programs offered (minimal on-campus study). *Degree requirements:* For master's, thesis or alternative, internship or practicum. *Entrance requirements:* Additional exam requirements/recommendations for international students: Required—TOEFL. Electronic applications accepted.

Seton Hall University, College of Nursing, South Orange, NJ 07079-2697. Offers advanced practice in primary health care (MSN, DNP), including adult/gerontological nurse practitioner, pediatric nurse practitioner; entry into practice (MSN); health systems administration (MSN, DNP); nursing (PhD); nursing case management (MSN); nursing education (MA); school nurse (MSN); MSN/MA. *Accreditation:* AACN. Part-time programs available. Postbaccalaureate distance learning degree programs offered (minimal on-campus study). *Degree requirements:* For master's, research project; for doctorate, dissertation or scholarly project. *Entrance requirements:* For doctorate, GRE (waived for students with GPA of 3.5 or higher). Additional exam requirements/recommendations for international students: Required—TOEFL. Electronic applications accepted. *Faculty research:* Parent/child, adult, and gerontological nursing; breast cancer; families of children with HIV; parish nursing.

Siena Heights University, Graduate College, Adrian, MI 49221-1796. Offers clinical mental health counseling (MA); educational leadership (Specialist); leadership (MA), including health care leadership, organizational leadership; teacher education (MA), including early childhood education, early childhood education: Montessori, education leadership: principal, elementary education: reading K-12, leadership: higher education, secondary education: reading K-12, special education: cognitive impairment, special education: learning disabilities. Part-time and evening/weekend programs available. *Faculty:* 37. *Students:* 9 full-time (7 women), 251 part-time (179 women). In 2013, 32 master's awarded. *Degree requirements:* For master's, thesis, presentation. *Entrance requirements:* For master's, minimum GPA of 3.0, current resume, essay, all post-secondary transcripts, 3 letters of reference, conviction disclosure form; copy of teaching certificate (for some education programs); for Specialist, master's degree, minimum GPA of 3.0, current resume, essay, all post-secondary transcripts, 3 letters of reference, conviction disclosure form; copy of teaching certificate (for some education programs). *Application deadline:* Applications are processed on a rolling basis. Application fee: $50. *Expenses: Tuition:* Part-time $535 per semester hour. *Required fees:* $130 per semester. *Financial support:* Career-related internships or fieldwork, Federal Work-Study, and resident assistantships available. Financial award application deadline: 9/1; financial award applicants required to submit FAFSA. *Unit head:* Dr. Linda S. Pettit, Dean, Graduate College, 517-264-7661, Fax: 517-264-7714, E-mail: lpettit@sienahts.edu.
Website: http://www.sienaheights.edu

Simmons College, School of Management, Boston, MA 02115. Offers business administration (MBA); business and financial analytics (MBA); corporate social responsibility and sustainability (MBA); entrepreneurship (MBA); healthcare management (MBA); management (MS), including communications management, non-profit management; marketing (MBA); nonprofit management (MBA); organizational leadership (MBA); MBA/MSW; MS/MA. *Accreditation:* AACSB. Part-time and evening/weekend programs available. *Students:* 34 full-time (33 women), 233 part-time (214 women); includes 67 minority (41 Black or African American, non-Hispanic/Latino; 1 American Indian or Alaska Native, non-Hispanic/Latino; 9 Asian, non-Hispanic/Latino; 10 Hispanic/Latino; 2 Native Hawaiian or other Pacific Islander, non-Hispanic/Latino; 4 Two or more races, non-Hispanic/Latino), 7 international. In 2013, 133 master's awarded. *Entrance requirements:* For master's, GMAT or GRE. Additional exam requirements/recommendations for international students: Required—TOEFL. *Application deadline:* Applications are processed on a rolling basis. Application fee: $75. Electronic applications accepted. *Financial support:* Scholarships/grants and unspecified assistantships available. Financial award applicants required to submit FAFSA. *Faculty research:* Gender and organizations, leadership, health care management. *Unit head:* Cathy Minehan, Dean, 617-521-2846. *Application contact:* Melissa Terrio, Director of Graduate Admissions, 617-521-3840, Fax: 617-521-3880, E-mail: somadm@simmons.edu.
Website: http://www.simmons.edu/som

Southeast Missouri State University, School of Graduate Studies, Harrison College of Business, Cape Girardeau, MO 63701-4799. Offers accounting (MBA); entrepreneurship (MBA); environmental management (MBA); financial management (MBA); general management (MBA); health administration (MBA); industrial management (MBA); international business (MBA); organizational management (MS); sport management (MBA). *Accreditation:* AACSB. Part-time and evening/weekend programs available. Postbaccalaureate distance learning degree programs offered (no on-campus study). *Faculty:* 27 full-time (7 women), 1 (woman) part-time/adjunct. *Students:* 59 full-time (27 women), 83 part-time (28 women); includes 10 minority (5 Black or African American, non-Hispanic/Latino; 3 Asian, non-Hispanic/Latino; 1 Hispanic/Latino; 1 Two or more races, non-Hispanic/Latino), 40 international. Average age 28. 77 applicants, 79% accepted, 48 enrolled. In 2013, 50 master's awarded. *Degree requirements:* For master's, variable foreign language requirement, comprehensive exam (for some programs), thesis or alternative, applied research project. *Entrance requirements:* For master's, GMAT or GRE, minimum undergraduate GPA of 2.5, C or better in prerequisite courses. Additional exam requirements/recommendations for international students: Required—TOEFL (minimum score 550 paper-based; 79 iBT), IELTS (minimum score 6), PTE (minimum score 53). *Application deadline:* For fall admission, 8/1 for domestic students, 6/1 for international students; for spring admission, 11/21 for domestic students, 10/1 for international students; for summer admission, 5/15 for domestic students. Applications are processed on a rolling basis. Application fee: $30 ($40 for international students). Electronic applications accepted. *Expenses:* Tuition, state resident: full-time $5139; part-time $285.50 per credit hour. Tuition, nonresident: full-time $9099; part-time $505.50 per credit hour. *Financial support:* In 2013–14, 52 students received support, including 12 teaching assistantships with full tuition reimbursements available (averaging $8,144 per year); career-related internships or fieldwork, Federal Work-Study, scholarships/grants, traineeships, tuition waivers (full), and unspecified assistantships also available. Financial award application deadline: 6/30; financial award applicants required to submit FAFSA. *Faculty research:* Ethics, corporate finance, generational difference, leadership, organizational justice. *Unit head:* Dr. Kenneth A. Heischmidt, Director, Graduate Business Studies, 573-651-2912, Fax: 573-651-5032, E-mail: kheischmidt@semo.edu. *Application contact:* Gail Amick, Admissions Specialist, 573-651-2590, Fax: 573-651-5936, E-mail: gamick@semo.edu.
Website: http://www.semo.edu/mba

Southern Adventist University, School of Business and Management, Collegedale, TN 37315-0370. Offers accounting (MBA); church administration (MSA); church and nonprofit leadership (MBA); financial management (MFM); healthcare administration (MBA); management (MBA); marketing management (MBA); outdoor education (MSA). Part-time and evening/weekend programs available. Postbaccalaureate distance learning degree programs offered (no on-campus study). *Entrance requirements:* For master's, GMAT. Additional exam requirements/recommendations for international students: Required—TOEFL (minimum score 600 paper-based; 100 iBT). Electronic applications accepted.

Southern Illinois University Carbondale, School of Law, Program in Legal Studies, Carbondale, IL 62901-4701. Offers general law (MLS); health law and policy (MLS). *Students:* 5 full-time (2 women), 7 part-time (4 women), 1 international. 10 applicants, 70% accepted, 7 enrolled. In 2013, 6 master's awarded. Application fee: $50. *Unit head:* Lisa David, Admissions Coordinator, 618-453-8767, E-mail: ldavid@law.siu.edu.

Southern Nazarene University, College of Professional and Graduate Studies, School of Business, Bethany, OK 73008. Offers business administration (MBA); health care management (MBA); management (MS Mgt). *Accreditation:* ACBSP. Part-time and evening/weekend programs available. Postbaccalaureate distance learning degree programs offered (minimal on-campus study). *Degree requirements:* For master's, thesis optional. *Entrance requirements:* For master's, resume. Additional exam requirements/recommendations for international students: Required—TOEFL (minimum score 550 paper-based; 80 iBT), IELTS (minimum score 7). *Application deadline:* For fall admission, 8/1 priority date for domestic students. Applications are processed on a rolling basis. Application fee: $0. Electronic applications accepted. *Unit head:* Dr. Randall Spindle, Chair, 405-491-6358, E-mail: rspindle@snu.edu. *Application contact:* Casey Cole, GSM Enrollment Coordinator, 405-491-6628, E-mail: cacole@snu.edu.
Website: http://snu.edu/school-of-business

Southern New Hampshire University, School of Business, Manchester, NH 03106-1045. Offers accounting (MBA, MS, Graduate Certificate); accounting finance (MS); accounting/auditing (MS); accounting/forensic accounting (MS); accounting/taxation (MS); athletic administration (MBA, Graduate Certificate); business administration (IMBA, MBA, Certificate, Graduate Certificate), including accounting (Certificate), business administration (MBA), business information systems (Graduate Certificate), human resource management (Certificate); corporate social responsibility (MBA); entrepreneurship (MBA); finance (MBA, MS, Graduate Certificate); finance/corporate finance (MS); finance/investments and securities (MS); forensic accounting (MBA); healthcare informatics (MBA); healthcare management (MBA); human resource management (Graduate Certificate); information technology (MS, Graduate Certificate); information technology management (MBA); international business (Graduate Certificate); international business and information technology (Graduate Certificate); international finance (Graduate Certificate); international sport management (Graduate Certificate); justice studies (MBA); leadership of nonprofit organizations (Graduate Certificate); marketing (MBA, MS, Graduate Certificate); operations and project management (MS); operations and supply chain management (MBA, Graduate Certificate); organizational leadership (MS); project management (MBA, Graduate Certificate); Six Sigma (MBA); Six Sigma quality (Graduate Certificate); social media marketing (MBA); sport management (MBA, MS, Graduate Certificate); sustainability and environmental compliance (MBA); workplace conflict management (MBA); MBA/Certificate. *Accreditation:* ACBSP. Part-time and evening/weekend programs available. Postbaccalaureate distance learning degree programs offered (no on-campus study). Terminal master's awarded for partial completion of doctoral program. *Degree requirements:* For master's, one foreign language, comprehensive exam (for some programs), thesis or alternative. *Entrance requirements:* For master's, minimum GPA of 2.5. Additional exam requirements/recommendations for international students: Required—TOEFL (minimum score 500 paper-based). Electronic applications accepted.

South University, Graduate Programs, College of Business, Program in Healthcare Administration, Savannah, GA 31406. Offers MBA.

South University, Program in Business Administration, Royal Palm Beach, FL 33411. Offers business administration (MBA); healthcare administration (MBA).

South University, Program in Healthcare Administration, Columbia, SC 29203. Offers MBA.

South University, Program in Healthcare Administration, Montgomery, AL 36116-1120. Offers MBA.

South University, Program in Healthcare Administration, Tampa, FL 33614. Offers MBA.

Southwest Baptist University, Program in Business, Bolivar, MO 65613-2597. Offers business administration (MBA); health administration (MBA). *Accreditation:* ACBSP. Part-time programs available. Postbaccalaureate distance learning degree programs offered (no on-campus study). *Degree requirements:* For master's, comprehensive exam. *Entrance requirements:* For master's, interviews, minimum GPA of 2.75. Additional exam requirements/recommendations for international students: Required—TOEFL (minimum score 550 paper-based).

Stony Brook University, State University of New York, Graduate School, College of Business, Program in Business Administration, Stony Brook, NY 11794. Offers finance (MBA, Certificate); health care management (MBA, Certificate); human resource management (Certificate); human resources (MBA); information systems management (MBA, Certificate); management (MBA); marketing (MBA). *Faculty:* 32 full-time (7 women), 29 part-time/adjunct (8 women). *Students:* 189 full-time (102 women), 111 part-time (40 women); includes 50 minority (10 Black or African American, non-Hispanic/Latino; 1 American Indian or Alaska Native, non-Hispanic/Latino; 25 Asian, non-Hispanic/Latino; 14 Hispanic/Latino), 114 international. 255 applicants, 53% accepted, 70 enrolled. In 2013, 157 master's, 1 other advanced degree awarded. *Entrance requirements:* For master's, GMAT, 3 letters of recommendation from current or former employers or professors, transcripts, personal statement, resume. Additional exam requirements/recommendations for international students: Required—TOEFL (minimum score 550 paper-based; 90 iBT), IELTS (minimum score 6.5). *Application deadline:* For fall admission, 6/1 for domestic students, 3/15 for international students; for spring admission, 12/1 for domestic students, 11/1 for international students. Application fee: $100. *Expenses:* Tuition, state resident: full-time $9870; part-time $411 per credit. Tuition, nonresident: full-time $18,350; part-time $765 per credit. *Financial support:* Teaching assistantships available. *Total annual research expenditures:* $53,718. *Unit head:* Dr. Manuel London, Dean and Director, Center for Human Resource Management, 631-632-7159, Fax: 631-632-8181, E-mail: manuel.london@stonybrook.edu. *Application contact:* Dr. Dmytro Holod, Interim Associate Dean/Graduate Program Director, 631-632-7183, Fax: 631-632-8181, E-mail: dmytro.holod@stonybrook.edu.

Stony Brook University, State University of New York, Stony Brook University Medical Center, Health Sciences Center, School of Health Technology and Management, Stony Brook, NY 11794. Offers health care management (Advanced Certificate); health care policy and management (MS); occupational therapy (MS); physical therapy (DPT); physician assistant (MS). *Accreditation:* APTA. Part-time programs available. *Faculty:* 70 full-time (46 women), 51 part-time/adjunct (34 women). *Students:* 349 full-time (225 women), 159 part-time (120 women); includes 140 minority (25 Black or African American, non-Hispanic/Latino; 1 American Indian or Alaska Native, non-Hispanic/Latino; 72 Asian, non-Hispanic/Latino; 34 Hispanic/Latino; 8 Two or more races, non-Hispanic/Latino), 7 international. 2,215 applicants, 11% accepted, 221 enrolled. In 2013, 120 master's, 77 doctorates, 23 other advanced degrees awarded. *Degree requirements:* For master's, thesis. *Entrance requirements:* For master's, GRE General Test, minimum GPA of 3.0, work experience in field, references; for doctorate, GRE, references. Additional exam requirements/recommendations for international students: Required—TOEFL (minimum score 550 paper-based). *Application deadline:*

For fall admission, 1/15 for domestic students; for spring admission, 10/1 for domestic students. Application fee: $100. *Expenses:* Tuition, state resident: full-time $9870; part-time $411 per credit. Tuition, nonresident: full-time $18,350; part-time $765 per credit. *Financial support:* In 2013–14, 1 fellowship was awarded; research assistantships, teaching assistantships, career-related internships or fieldwork, Federal Work-Study, and institutionally sponsored loans also available. Financial award application deadline: 3/15. *Faculty research:* Health promotion and disease prevention. *Total annual research expenditures:* $1.1 million. *Unit head:* Dr. Craig A. Lehmann, Dean, 631-444-2252, Fax: 631-444-7621, E-mail: craig.lehmann@stonybrook.edu. *Application contact:* Dr. Richard W. Johnson, Associate Dean for Graduate Studies, 631-444-3251, Fax: 631-444-7621, E-mail: richard.johnson@stonybrook.edu.
Website: http://healthtechnology.stonybrookmedicine.edu/

Stony Brook University, State University of New York, Stony Brook University Medical Center, Health Sciences Center, School of Nursing, Program in Nursing Practice, Stony Brook, NY 11794. Offers DNP. Postbaccalaureate distance learning degree programs offered. *Students:* 54 part-time (52 women); includes 25 minority (10 Black or African American, non-Hispanic/Latino; 1 American Indian or Alaska Native, non-Hispanic/Latino; 6 Asian, non-Hispanic/Latino; 7 Hispanic/Latino; 1 Two or more races, non-Hispanic/Latino). In 2013, 1 doctorate awarded. *Degree requirements:* For doctorate, project. *Entrance requirements:* For doctorate, minimum GPA of 3.0. Additional exam requirements/recommendations for international students: Required—TOEFL. *Application deadline:* For fall admission, 1/15 for domestic students, 12/1 for international students. Application fee: $100. *Expenses:* Tuition, state resident: full-time $9870; part-time $411 per credit. Tuition, nonresident: full-time $18,350; part-time $765 per credit. *Unit head:* Dr. Lee Anne Xippolitos, Dean, 631-444-3200, Fax: 631-444-6628. *Application contact:* Dr. Kathleen Shurpin, Professor/Director, 631-444-3267, Fax: 631-444-3136, E-mail: kathleen.shurpin@stonybrook.edu.
Website: http://www.nursing.stonybrookmedicine.edu/

Strayer University, Graduate Studies, Washington, DC 20005-2603. Offers accounting (MS); acquisition (MBA); business administration (MBA); communications technology (MS); educational management (M Ed); finance (MBA); health services administration (MHSA); hospitality and tourism management (MBA); human resource management (MBA); information systems (MS), including computer security management, decision support system management, enterprise resource management, network management, software engineering management, systems development management; management (MBA); management information systems (MS); marketing (MBA); professional accounting (MS), including accounting information systems, controllership, taxation; public administration (MPA); supply chain management (MBA); technology in education (M Ed). Programs also offered at campus locations in Birmingham, AL; Chamblee, GA; Cobb County, GA; Morrow, GA; White Marsh, MD; Charleston, SC; Columbia, SC; Greensboro, NC; Greenville, SC; Lexington, KY; Louisville, KY; Nashville, TN; North Raleigh, NC; Washington, DC. Part-time and evening/weekend programs available. Postbaccalaureate distance learning degree programs offered (minimal on-campus study). *Degree requirements:* For master's, thesis. *Entrance requirements:* For master's, GMAT, GRE General Test, bachelor's degree from an accredited college or university, minimum undergraduate GPA of 2.75. Electronic applications accepted.

Suffolk University, Sawyer Business School, Master of Business Administration Program, Boston, MA 02108-2770. Offers accounting (MBA); business administration (APC); entrepreneurship (MBA); executive business administration (EMBA); finance (MBA); global business administration (GMBA); health administration (MBA); international business (MBA); marketing (MBA); nonprofit management (MBA); organizational behavior (MBA); strategic management (MBA); supply chain management (MBA); taxation (MBA); JD/MBA; MBA/GDPA; MBA/MHA; MBA/MSA; MBA/MSF; MBA/MST. *Accreditation:* AACSB. Part-time and evening/weekend programs available. Postbaccalaureate distance learning degree programs offered (no on-campus study). *Faculty:* 29 full-time (9 women), 12 part-time/adjunct (2 women). *Students:* 106 full-time (44 women), 334 part-time (184 women); includes 57 minority (20 Black or African American, non-Hispanic/Latino; 1 American Indian or Alaska Native, non-Hispanic/Latino; 18 Asian, non-Hispanic/Latino; 14 Hispanic/Latino; 4 Two or more races, non-Hispanic/Latino), 61 international. Average age 30. 448 applicants, 61% accepted, 135 enrolled. In 2013, 217 master's awarded. *Entrance requirements:* For master's, GMAT, minimum undergraduate GPA of 2.75 (MBA), 5 years of managerial experience (EMBA). Additional exam requirements/recommendations for international students: Required—TOEFL (minimum score 550 paper-based; 80 iBT). *Application deadline:* For fall admission, 6/15 priority date for domestic students, 6/15 for international students; for spring admission, 11/1 priority date for domestic students, 11/1 for international students. Applications are processed on a rolling basis. Application fee: $50. Electronic applications accepted. *Expenses: Tuition:* Full-time $38,374; part-time $1279 per credit. *Required fees:* $40; $20 per semester. Tuition and fees vary according to program. *Financial support:* In 2013–14, 107 students received support, including 91 fellowships with full and partial tuition reimbursements available (averaging $12,428 per year); career-related internships or fieldwork, Federal Work-Study, and institutionally sponsored loans also available. Support available to part-time students. Financial award application deadline: 4/1; financial award applicants required to submit FAFSA. *Faculty research:* Foreign investments; career strategies and boundaryless careers; corporate ethics codes; interest rates, inflation, and growth options; innovation and product development performance. *Unit head:* Heather Hewitt, Assistant Dean of Graduate Programs/Director of MBA Programs, 617-573-8306, E-mail: hhewitt@suffolk.edu. *Application contact:* Cory Meyers, Director of Graduate Admissions, 617-573-8302, Fax: 617-305-1733, E-mail: grad.admission@suffolk.edu.
Website: http://www.suffolk.edu/mba

Suffolk University, Sawyer Business School, Program in Health Administration, Boston, MA 02108-2770. Offers MBAH, MHA. Part-time and evening/weekend programs available. *Faculty:* 4 full-time (1 woman), 3 part-time/adjunct (all women). *Students:* 23 full-time (14 women), 68 part-time (49 women); includes 17 minority (9 Black or African American, non-Hispanic/Latino; 4 Asian, non-Hispanic/Latino; 4 Hispanic/Latino), 9 international. Average age 29. 55 applicants, 80% accepted, 26 enrolled. In 2013, 30 master's awarded. *Entrance requirements:* Additional exam requirements/recommendations for international students: Required—TOEFL (minimum score 550 paper-based; 80 iBT). *Application deadline:* For fall admission, 6/15 priority date for domestic students, 6/15 for international students; for spring admission, 11/1 priority date for domestic students, 11/1 for international students. Applications are processed on a rolling basis. Application fee: $50. Electronic applications accepted. *Expenses:* Contact institution. *Financial support:* In 2013–14, 31 students received support, including 30 fellowships (averaging $9,744 per year); career-related internships or fieldwork, Federal Work-Study, and institutionally sponsored loans also available. Support available to part-time students. Financial award application deadline: 4/1; financial award applicants required to submit FAFSA. *Faculty research:* Mental health, federal policy, health care. *Unit head:* Richard Gregg, Director of Programs in Healthcare Administration/Chair of Healthcare Department, 617-994-4246, E-mail: rgregg@suffolk.edu. *Application contact:* Cory Meyers, Director of Graduate Admissions, 617-573-8302, Fax: 617-305-1733, E-mail: grad.admission@suffolk.edu.
Website: http://www.suffolk.edu/business/graduate/11532.php

Syracuse University, Maxwell School of Citizenship and Public Affairs, Program in Health Services Management and Policy, Syracuse, NY 13244. Offers CAS. Part-time programs available. *Students:* 24 applicants, 100% accepted. In 2013, 17 CASs awarded. *Entrance requirements:* For degree, 7 years of mid-career experience. Additional exam requirements/recommendations for international students: Required—TOEFL (minimum score 100 iBT). *Application deadline:* For fall admission, 2/1 for domestic students, 2/1 priority date for international students; for spring admission, 8/15 priority date for domestic and international students. Applications are processed on a rolling basis. Application fee: $75. Electronic applications accepted. *Financial support:* Application deadline: 1/1. *Unit head:* Dr. Thomas H. Dennison, Head, 315-443-9215, Fax: 315-443-9721, E-mail: thdennis@syr.edu. *Application contact:* Tammy Salisbury, Graduate Coordinator, 315-443-3192, Fax: 315-443-3423, E-mail: mtsalisb@maxwell.syr.edu.
Website: http://www.maxwell.syr.edu/

Temple University, College of Health Professions and Social Work, Department of Public Health, Philadelphia, PA 19122. Offers clinical research and translational medicine (MS); environmental health (MPH); epidemiology (MS); epidemiology and biostatistics (MPH); health policy (PhD); health policy and management (MPH); school health education (Ed M); social and behavioral sciences (MPH, PhD). *Accreditation:* CEPH (one or more programs are accredited). Part-time and evening/weekend programs available. *Faculty:* 27 full-time (18 women). *Students:* 47 full-time (30 women), 45 part-time (37 women); includes 27 minority (9 Black or African American, non-Hispanic/Latino; 10 Asian, non-Hispanic/Latino; 7 Hispanic/Latino; 1 Two or more races, non-Hispanic/Latino), 9 international. 188 applicants, 45% accepted, 29 enrolled. In 2013, 29 master's, 3 doctorates awarded. Terminal master's awarded for partial completion of doctoral program. *Degree requirements:* For master's, thesis (for some programs), capstone project; for doctorate, comprehensive exam, thesis/dissertation. *Entrance requirements:* For master's, GRE General Test (for MS only); DAT, GMAT, MCAT, OAT, PCAT (alternates for MPH, Ed M), minimum undergraduate GPA of 3.0, letters of reference, statement of goals, writing sample, resume, interview (only for MS); for doctorate, GRE General Test, minimum undergraduate GPA of 3.0, 3 letters of reference, statement of goals, writing sample, resume. Additional exam requirements/recommendations for international students: Required—TOEFL (minimum score 550 paper-based; 79 iBT). *Application deadline:* For fall admission, 3/1 for domestic students, 2/1 for international students; for spring admission, 10/15 for domestic students, 8/1 for international students. Applications are processed on a rolling basis. Application fee: $60. Electronic applications accepted. *Financial support:* In 2013–14, 1 fellowship with tuition reimbursement, 4 research assistantships with tuition reimbursements, 8 teaching assistantships with tuition reimbursements were awarded; career-related internships or fieldwork, Federal Work-Study, scholarships/grants, tuition waivers (partial), and unspecified assistantships also available. Financial award application deadline: 1/15. *Faculty research:* Smoking cessation, obesity prevention, tobacco policy, community engagement, health communication. *Total annual research expenditures:* $3.9 million. *Unit head:* Dr. Alice J. Hausman, Chair, 215-204-5112, Fax: 215-204-1854, E-mail: hausman@temple.edu. *Application contact:* Joyce Hankins, 215-204-7213, E-mail: joyce.hankins@temple.edu.
Website: http://chpsw.temple.edu/publichealth/home

Temple University, Fox School of Business, MBA Programs, Philadelphia, PA 19122-6096. Offers accounting (MBA); business management (MBA); financial management (MBA); healthcare and life sciences innovation (MBA); human resource management (MBA); international business (IMBA); IT management (MBA); marketing management (MBA); pharmaceutical management (MBA); strategic management (EMBA, MBA). EMBA offered in Philadelphia, PA and Tokyo, Japan. *Accreditation:* AACSB. Part-time and evening/weekend programs available. Postbaccalaureate distance learning degree programs offered (minimal on-campus study). *Entrance requirements:* For master's, GMAT, minimum undergraduate GPA of 3.0. Additional exam requirements/recommendations for international students: Required—TOEFL (minimum score 600 paper-based; 100 iBT), IELTS (minimum score 7.5).

Texas A&M Health Science Center, School of Rural Public Health, College Station, TX 77840. Offers environmental/occupational health (MPH); epidemiology/biostatistics (MPH); health policy/management (MPH); social and behavioral health (MPH). *Accreditation:* CEPH. Part-time programs available. Postbaccalaureate distance learning degree programs offered (no on-campus study). *Degree requirements:* For master's, thesis optional. *Entrance requirements:* For master's, GRE General Test, minimum undergraduate GPA of 3.0. Electronic applications accepted. *Faculty research:* Tobacco cessation, youth health risk.

Texas A&M University–Corpus Christi, Graduate Studies and Research, College of Business, Corpus Christi, TX 78412-5503. Offers accounting (M Acc); health care administration (MBA); international business (MBA). *Accreditation:* AACSB. Part-time and evening/weekend programs available. *Degree requirements:* For master's, comprehensive exam, thesis (for some programs). *Entrance requirements:* For master's, GMAT. Additional exam requirements/recommendations for international students: Required—TOEFL. Electronic applications accepted.

Texas A&M University–Corpus Christi, Graduate Studies and Research, College of Nursing and Health Sciences, Corpus Christi, TX 78412-5503. Offers clinical nurse specialist (MSN); family nurse practitioner (MSN); health care administration (MSN); leadership in nursing systems (MSN). *Accreditation:* AACN. Part-time and evening/weekend programs available. *Degree requirements:* For master's, comprehensive exam, thesis (for some programs). *Entrance requirements:* For master's, GRE General Test. Additional exam requirements/recommendations for international students: Required—TOEFL. Electronic applications accepted.

Texas A&M University–San Antonio, School of Business, San Antonio, TX 78224. Offers business administration (MBA); enterprise resource planning systems (MBA); finance (MBA); healthcare management (MBA); human resources management (MBA); information assurance and security (MBA); international business (MBA); professional accounting (MPA); project management (MBA); supply chain management (MBA). Part-time and evening/weekend programs available. *Entrance requirements:* For master's, GMAT. Additional exam requirements/recommendations for international students: Required—TOEFL (minimum score 550 paper-based; 80 iBT), IELTS (minimum score 6). Electronic applications accepted.

Texas Southern University, College of Pharmacy and Health Sciences, Department of Health Sciences, Houston, TX 77004-4584. Offers health care administration (MS). Postbaccalaureate distance learning degree programs offered. *Faculty:* 2 full-time (both women), 3 part-time/adjunct (1 woman). *Students:* 28 full-time (21 women), 2 part-time (both women); includes 28 minority (26 Black or African American, non-Hispanic/Latino; 2 Asian, non-Hispanic/Latino), 2 international. Average age 30. 46 applicants, 39% accepted, 10 enrolled. In 2013, 4 master's awarded. *Entrance requirements:* For master's, PCAT. *Application deadline:* For fall admission, 2/15 for domestic and international students. Applications are processed on a rolling basis. Application fee: $50 ($75 for international students). Electronic applications accepted. *Financial support:* In 2013–14, 1 teaching assistantship (averaging $1,600 per year) was awarded; fellowships, research assistantships, scholarships/grants, and tuition waivers (partial) also available. Financial award application deadline: 5/1; financial award applicants

required to submit FAFSA. *Unit head:* Dr. Renard Thomas, Interim Chair, 713-313-4463, E-mail: thomas_rl@tsu.edu. *Application contact:* Dr. Gregory Maddox, Dean of the Graduate School, 713-313-7011, E-mail: maddox_gh@tsu.edu.
Website: http://www.tsu.edu/academics/colleges__schools/College_of_Pharmacy_and_Health_Sciences/

Texas State University, Graduate School, College of Health Professions, School of Health Administration, Program in Healthcare Administration, San Marcos, TX 78666. Offers MHA. Part-time and evening/weekend programs available. *Faculty:* 10 full-time (4 women), 1 part-time/adjunct (0 women). *Students:* 37 full-time (21 women), 17 part-time (12 women); includes 25 minority (6 Black or African American, non-Hispanic/Latino; 5 Asian, non-Hispanic/Latino; 12 Hispanic/Latino; 2 Two or more races, non-Hispanic/Latino), 2 international. Average age 28. 65 applicants, 85% accepted, 20 enrolled. In 2013, 35 master's awarded. *Degree requirements:* For master's, comprehensive exam, thesis optional, committee review. *Entrance requirements:* For master's, GRE General Test, 3 letters of reference; resume; interview. Additional exam requirements/recommendations for international students: Required—TOEFL (minimum score 550 paper-based; 78 iBT). *Application deadline:* For fall admission, 6/1 priority date for domestic students, 6/1 for international students; for spring admission, 10/1 priority date for domestic students, 10/1 for international students. Applications are processed on a rolling basis. Application fee: $40 ($90 for international students). Electronic applications accepted. *Expenses:* Tuition, state resident: full-time $6663; part-time $278 per credit hour. Tuition, nonresident: full-time $15,159; part-time $632 per credit hour. *Required fees:* $1872; $54 per credit hour. $306 per term. Tuition and fees vary according to course load. *Financial support:* In 2013–14, 33 students received support, including 2 research assistantships (averaging $10,950 per year), 4 teaching assistantships (averaging $11,352 per year); career-related internships or fieldwork, Federal Work-Study, institutionally sponsored loans, scholarships/grants, and unspecified assistantships also available. Support available to part-time students. Financial award application deadline: 4/1; financial award applicants required to submit FAFSA. *Unit head:* Dr. Matthew Brooks, Graduate Programs Director, 512-245-2238, E-mail: sohagradadvisor@txstate.edu. *Application contact:* Dr. Andrea Golato, Dean of Graduate School, 512-245-2581, Fax: 512-245-8365, E-mail: gradcollege@txstate.edu.
Website: http://www.health.txstate.edu/ha/degs-progs/mha.html

Texas State University, Graduate School, College of Health Professions, School of Health Administration, Program in Healthcare Human Resources, San Marcos, TX 78666. Offers MS. *Accreditation:* CAHME. Part-time and evening/weekend programs available. *Faculty:* 10 full-time (4 women), 1 part-time/adjunct (0 women). *Students:* 2 part-time (both women); includes 1 minority (Hispanic/Latino). Average age 44. 4 applicants. In 2013, 6 master's awarded. *Degree requirements:* For master's, comprehensive exam, thesis optional, committee review. *Entrance requirements:* For master's, GRE General Test, department interview; 3 letters of reference; resume. Additional exam requirements/recommendations for international students: Required—TOEFL (minimum score 550 paper-based; 78 iBT). *Application deadline:* For fall admission, 6/15 priority date for domestic students, 6/1 for international students; for spring admission, 10/15 priority date for domestic students, 10/1 for international students. Applications are processed on a rolling basis. Application fee: $40 ($90 for international students). Electronic applications accepted. *Expenses:* Tuition, state resident: full-time $6663; part-time $278 per credit hour. Tuition, nonresident: full-time $15,159; part-time $632 per credit hour. *Required fees:* $1872; $54 per credit hour. $306 per term. Tuition and fees vary according to course load. *Financial support:* Research assistantships, teaching assistantships, career-related internships or fieldwork, Federal Work-Study, institutionally sponsored loans, scholarships/grants, and unspecified assistantships available. Support available to part-time students. Financial award application deadline: 4/1; financial award applicants required to submit FAFSA. *Total annual research expenditures:* $35,381. *Unit head:* Dr. Michael Nowicki, Program Advisor, 512-245-3556, Fax: 512-245-8712, E-mail: mn03@txstate.edu. *Application contact:* Dr. J. Michael Willoughby, Dean of Graduate School, 512-245-2581, Fax: 512-245-8365, E-mail: gradcollege@txstate.edu.
Website: http://www.health.txstate.edu/hsr

Texas Tech University, Graduate School, Rawls College of Business Administration, Area of Information Systems and Quantitative Sciences, Lubbock, TX 79409. Offers business statistics (MS, PhD); healthcare management (MS); management information systems (MS, PhD); production and operations management (PhD). Part-time programs available. *Faculty:* 13 full-time (0 women). *Students:* 107 full-time (24 women); includes 3 minority (1 Black or African American, non-Hispanic/Latino; 1 American Indian or Alaska Native, non-Hispanic/Latino; 1 Asian, non-Hispanic/Latino), 79 international. Average age 27. 125 applicants, 55% accepted, 40 enrolled. In 2013, 17 master's, 5 doctorates awarded. Terminal master's awarded for partial completion of doctoral program. *Degree requirements:* For master's, comprehensive exam or capstone course; for doctorate, thesis/dissertation, qualifying exams. *Entrance requirements:* For master's and doctorate, GMAT, holistic profile of academic credentials. Additional exam requirements/recommendations for international students: Required—TOEFL (minimum score 550 paper-based; 79 iBT). *Application deadline:* For fall admission, 7/1 priority date for domestic students, 1/15 for international students; for spring admission, 11/1 priority date for domestic students, 6/15 priority date for international students. Applications are processed on a rolling basis. Application fee: $60. Electronic applications accepted. *Expenses:* Tuition, state resident: full-time $6062; part-time $252.57 per credit hour. Tuition, nonresident: full-time $14,558; part-time $606.57 per credit hour. *Required fees:* $2655; $35 per credit hour. $907.50 per semester. Tuition and fees vary according to course load. *Financial support:* In 2013–14, 5 research assistantships (averaging $16,160 per year), 5 teaching assistantships (averaging $18,000 per year) were awarded; Federal Work-Study, scholarships/grants, and unspecified assistantships also available. Financial award applicants required to submit FAFSA. *Faculty research:* Database management systems, systems management and engineering, expert systems and adaptive knowledge-based sciences, statistical analysis and design. *Unit head:* Dr. Glenn Browne, Area Coordinator, 806-834-0969, Fax: 806-742-3193, E-mail: glenn.browne@ttu.edu. *Application contact:* Terri Boston, Applications Manager, Graduate and Professional Programs, 806-742-3184, Fax: 806-742-3958, E-mail: rawlsgrad@ttu.edu.
Website: http://is.ba.ttu.edu

Texas Tech University, Graduate School, Rawls College of Business Administration, Programs in Business Administration, Lubbock, TX 79409. Offers business administration (IMBA); general business (MBA); health organization management (MBA); STEM (MBA); JD/MBA; MBA/M Arch; MBA/MD; MBA/MS; MBA/Pharm D. Part-time and evening/weekend programs available. *Faculty:* 56 full-time (9 women), 1 part-time/adjunct (0 women). *Students:* 97 full-time (63 women), 296 part-time (88 women); includes 73 minority (21 Black or African American, non-Hispanic/Latino; 3 American Indian or Alaska Native, non-Hispanic/Latino; 30 Asian, non-Hispanic/Latino; 19 Hispanic/Latino), 19 international. Average age 31. 155 applicants, 79% accepted, 116 enrolled. In 2013, 225 master's awarded. *Degree requirements:* For master's, capstone course. *Entrance requirements:* For master's, GMAT, holistic review of academic credentials. Additional exam requirements/recommendations for international students: Required—TOEFL (minimum score 550 paper-based; 79 iBT). *Application deadline:* For fall admission, 6/1 priority date for domestic students, 1/15 for international students; for spring admission, 11/1 priority date for domestic students, 6/15 for international students; for summer admission, 4/15 for domestic students. Applications are processed on a rolling basis. Application fee: $60. Electronic applications accepted. *Expenses:* Tuition, state resident: full-time $6062; part-time $252.57 per credit hour. Tuition, nonresident: full-time $14,558; part-time $606.57 per credit hour. *Required fees:* $2655; $35 per credit hour. $907.50 per semester. Tuition and fees vary according to course load. *Financial support:* Research assistantships, teaching assistantships, Federal Work-Study, scholarships/grants, and unspecified assistantships available. Support available to part-time students. Financial award applicants required to submit FAFSA. *Unit head:* Dr. William J. Pasewark, Associate Dean, 806-742-3184, Fax: 806-742-3958, E-mail: w.pasewark@ttu.edu. *Application contact:* Terri Boston, Application Manager, 806-742-3184, Fax: 806-742-3958, E-mail: rawlsgrad@ttu.edu.
Website: http://mba.ba.ttu.edu/

Texas Tech University Health Sciences Center, School of Allied Health Sciences, Program in Clinical Practice Management, Lubbock, TX 79430. Offers MS. *Accreditation:* CORE. Part-time programs available. Postbaccalaureate distance learning degree programs offered (no on-campus study). *Faculty:* 6 full-time (2 women). *Students:* 29 full-time (20 women), 140 part-time (95 women); includes 82 minority (28 Black or African American, non-Hispanic/Latino; 1 American Indian or Alaska Native, non-Hispanic/Latino; 15 Asian, non-Hispanic/Latino; 28 Hispanic/Latino; 1 Native Hawaiian or other Pacific Islander, non-Hispanic/Latino; 9 Two or more races, non-Hispanic/Latino), 2 international. Average age 35. 154 applicants, 70% accepted, 108 enrolled. In 2013, 60 master's awarded. *Entrance requirements:* Additional exam requirements/recommendations for international students: Required—TOEFL, IELTS. *Application deadline:* For fall admission, 8/1 for domestic students; for spring admission, 12/1 for domestic students; for summer admission, 5/1 for domestic students. Applications are processed on a rolling basis. Application fee: $40. Electronic applications accepted. *Financial support:* Institutionally sponsored loans available. *Unit head:* Dr. Nick Coppola, Program Director, 806-743-2260, Fax: 806-743-3244, E-mail: nick.coppola@ttuhsc.edu. *Application contact:* Lindsay Johnson, Associate Dean for Admissions and Student Affairs, 806-743-3220, Fax: 806-743-2994, E-mail: lindsay.johnson@ttuhsc.edu.
Website: http://www.ttuhsc.edu/sah/mscpm

Texas Wesleyan University, Graduate Programs, Graduate Business Programs, Fort Worth, TX 76105-1536. Offers business administration (MBA); health services administration (MS); management (MiM). *Accreditation:* ACBSP. Part-time and evening/weekend programs available. *Degree requirements:* For master's, capstone course. *Entrance requirements:* For master's, GMAT, 3 letters of recommendation. *Expenses:* Contact institution.

Texas Woman's University, Graduate School, College of Arts and Sciences, School of Management, Denton, TX 76201. Offers business administration (MBA); health systems management (MHSM). *Accreditation:* ACBSP. Part-time programs available. *Faculty:* 12 full-time (5 women), 2 part-time/adjunct (0 women). *Students:* 660 full-time (556 women), 474 part-time (379 women); includes 758 minority (461 Black or African American, non-Hispanic/Latino; 14 American Indian or Alaska Native, non-Hispanic/Latino; 139 Asian, non-Hispanic/Latino; 142 Hispanic/Latino; 2 Native Hawaiian or other Pacific Islander, non-Hispanic/Latino), 30 international. Average age 34. 429 applicants, 77% accepted, 259 enrolled. In 2013, 600 master's awarded. *Degree requirements:* For master's, thesis optional. *Entrance requirements:* For master's, 2 letters of reference, resume, 5 years of relevant experience (EMBA only). Additional exam requirements/recommendations for international students: Required—TOEFL (minimum score 550 paper-based; 79 iBT). *Application deadline:* For fall admission, 8/1 priority date for domestic students, 3/1 for international students; for spring admission, 12/1 priority date for domestic students, 7/1 for international students. Applications are processed on a rolling basis. Application fee: $50 ($75 for international students). Electronic applications accepted. *Expenses:* Tuition, state resident: full-time $4182; part-time $233.32 per credit hour. Tuition, nonresident: full-time $10,716; part-time $595.32 per credit hour. *Financial support:* In 2013–14, 254 students received support, including 15 research assistantships (averaging $11,520 per year); career-related internships or fieldwork, Federal Work-Study, institutionally sponsored loans, scholarships/grants, traineeships, health care benefits, and unspecified assistantships also available. Support available to part-time students. Financial award application deadline: 3/1; financial award applicants required to submit FAFSA. *Faculty research:* Tax research, privacy issues in Web-based marketing, multitasking, leadership, women in management, global comparative studies, corporate sustainability and responsibility. *Unit head:* Ron Hovis, Interim Director, 940-898-2121, Fax: 940-898-2120, E-mail: rhovis@twu.edu. *Application contact:* Dr. Samuel Wheeler, Assistant Director of Admissions, 940-898-3188, Fax: 940-898-3081, E-mail: wheelersr@twu.edu.
Website: http://www.twu.edu/som/

Texas Woman's University, Graduate School, College of Health Sciences, Program in Health Care Administration, Houston, TX 77030. Offers MHA. Program offered at Texas Medical Center in Houston. *Accreditation:* CAHME. Part-time and evening/weekend programs available. *Faculty:* 4 full-time (1 woman), 3 part-time/adjunct (1 woman). *Students:* 70 full-time (61 women), 40 part-time (27 women); includes 64 minority (33 Black or African American, non-Hispanic/Latino; 21 Asian, non-Hispanic/Latino; 10 Hispanic/Latino), 5 international. Average age 29. 58 applicants, 67% accepted, 20 enrolled. In 2013, 31 master's awarded. *Degree requirements:* For master's, comprehensive exam, thesis or alternative. *Entrance requirements:* For master's, GMAT (preferred minimum score 450) or GRE General Test (preferred minimum scores 150 [450 old version] Verbal, 141 [450 old version] Quantitative), interview, resume, 3 letters of reference, essay. Additional exam requirements/recommendations for international students: Required—TOEFL (minimum score 550 paper-based; 79 iBT). *Application deadline:* For fall admission, 5/30 priority date for domestic students, 3/1 for international students; for spring admission, 9/30 priority date for domestic students, 7/1 for international students. Applications are processed on a rolling basis. Application fee: $50 ($75 for international students). Electronic applications accepted. *Expenses:* Tuition, state resident: full-time $4182; part-time $233.32 per credit hour. Tuition, nonresident: full-time $10,716; part-time $595.32 per credit hour. *Financial support:* In 2013–14, 30 students received support, including 1 research assistantship (averaging $11,520 per year); career-related internships or fieldwork, Federal Work-Study, institutionally sponsored loans, scholarships/grants, traineeships, health care benefits, and unspecified assistantships also available. Support available to part-time students. Financial award application deadline: 3/1; financial award applicants required to submit FAFSA. *Faculty research:* Organizational culture, medical errors, ethical analysis in health care, leadership and professional development, strategic management, recruitment and retention issues, elderly health care. *Unit head:* Dr. Gerald Goodman, Program Director, 713-794-2061, Fax: 713-794-2350, E-mail: healthcareadministration@twu.edu. *Application contact:* Dr. Samuel Wheeler, Assistant Director of Admissions, 940-898-3188, Fax: 940-898-3081, E-mail: wheelersr@twu.edu.
Website: http://www.twu.edu/health-care-administration/

Texas Woman's University, Graduate School, College of Nursing, Denton, TX 76201. Offers acute care nurse practitioner (MS); adult health clinical nurse specialist (MS); adult health nurse practitioner (MS); child health clinical nurse specialist (MS); clinical

nurse leader (MS); family nurse practitioner (MS); health systems management (MS); nursing education (MS); nursing practice (DNP); nursing science (PhD); pediatric nurse practitioner (MS); women's health clinical nurse specialist (MS); women's health nurse practitioner (MS). *Accreditation:* AACN. Part-time programs available. Postbaccalaureate distance learning degree programs offered. *Faculty:* 60 full-time (59 women), 46 part-time/adjunct (39 women). *Students:* 54 full-time (49 women), 910 part-time (848 women); includes 489 minority (221 Black or African American, non-Hispanic/ Latino; 11 American Indian or Alaska Native, non-Hispanic/Latino; 184 Asian, non-Hispanic/Latino; 70 Hispanic/Latino; 3 Native Hawaiian or other Pacific Islander, non-Hispanic/Latino), 16 international. Average age 38. 430 applicants, 65% accepted, 193 enrolled. In 2013, 258 master's, 22 doctorates awarded. *Degree requirements:* For master's, comprehensive exam, thesis or alternative; for doctorate, comprehensive exam, thesis/dissertation. *Entrance requirements:* For master's, GRE or MAT, minimum GPA of 3.0 on last 60 hours in undergraduate nursing degree and overall, RN license, BS in nursing, basic statistics course; for doctorate, GRE (preferred minimum score 153 [500 old version] Verbal, 144 [500 old version] Quantitative, 4 Analytical), MS in nursing, minimum preferred GPA of 3.5, RN license, statistics, 2 letters of reference, curriculum vitae, graduate nursing-theory course, graduate research course, statement of professional goals and research interests. Additional exam requirements/ recommendations for international students: Required—TOEFL (minimum score 550 paper-based; 79 iBT). *Application deadline:* For fall admission, 5/1 priority date for domestic students, 3/1 for international students; for spring admission, 9/15 priority date for domestic students, 7/1 for international students. Applications are processed on a rolling basis. Application fee: $50 ($75 for international students). Electronic applications accepted. *Expenses:* Tuition, state resident: full-time $4182; part-time $233.32 per credit hour. Tuition, nonresident: full-time $10,716; part-time $595.32 per credit hour. *Financial support:* In 2013–14, 149 students received support, including 10 research assistantships (averaging $5,600 per year), 1 teaching assistantship (averaging $5,600 per year); career-related internships or fieldwork, Federal Work-Study, institutionally sponsored loans, scholarships/grants, traineeships, health care benefits, and unspecified assistantships also available. Support available to part-time students. Financial award application deadline: 3/1; financial award applicants required to submit FAFSA. *Faculty research:* Screening, prevention, and treatment for intimate partner violence; needs of adolescents during childbirth intervention; a network analysis decision tool for nurse managers (social network analysis); support for adolescents with implantable cardioverter defibrillators; informatics: nurse staffing, safety, quality, and financial data as they relate to patient care outcomes; prevention and treatment of obesity; improving infant outcomes related to premature birth. *Total annual research expenditures:* $1.7 million. *Unit head:* Dr. Gayle Roux, Interim Dean and Associate Dean for Research and Clinical Scholarship, 940-898-2401, Fax: 940-898-2437, E-mail: nursing@twu.edu. *Application contact:* Dr. Samuel Wheeler, Assistant Director of Admissions, 940-898-3188, Fax: 940-898-3081, E-mail: wheelersr@twu.edu.
Website: http://www.twu.edu/nursing/

Thomas Jefferson University, Jefferson School of Population Health, Program in Healthcare Quality and Safety, Philadelphia, PA 19107. Offers MS, PhD, Certificate. Part-time and evening/weekend programs available. Postbaccalaureate distance learning degree programs offered (no on-campus study). *Entrance requirements:* For master's, GRE or other graduate examination, 2 letters of recommendation, interview, curriculum vitae; for doctorate, GRE (within the last 5 years), 3 letters of recommendation, interview, curriculum vitae. Additional exam requirements/ recommendations for international students: Required—TOEFL.

Thomas Jefferson University, Jefferson School of Population Health, Program in Health Policy, Philadelphia, PA 19107. Offers MS, PhD, Certificate. Part-time and evening/weekend programs available. Postbaccalaureate distance learning degree programs offered. *Entrance requirements:* For master's, GRE or other graduate exam, two letters of recommendation, curriculum vitae/resume, interview; for doctorate, GRE (within the last 5 years), three letters of recommendation, curriculum vitae/resume, interview. Additional exam requirements/recommendations for international students: Required—TOEFL. Electronic applications accepted.

Tiffin University, Program in Business Administration, Tiffin, OH 44883-2161. Offers finance (MBA); general management (MBA); healthcare administration (MBA); human resource management (MBA); international business (MBA); leadership (MBA); marketing (MBA); sports management (MBA). *Accreditation:* ACBSP. Part-time and evening/weekend programs available. Postbaccalaureate distance learning degree programs offered (no on-campus study). *Entrance requirements:* For master's, minimum undergraduate GPA of 2.5, work experience. Additional exam requirements/ recommendations for international students: Required—TOEFL (minimum score 550 paper-based; 79 iBT). *Application deadline:* For fall admission, 8/15 for domestic students, 8/1 for international students; for spring admission, 1/9 for domestic students, 12/1 for international students. Applications are processed on a rolling basis. Application fee: $50. Electronic applications accepted. *Financial support:* Available to part-time students. Application deadline: 7/31; applicants required to submit FAFSA. *Faculty research:* Small business, executive development operations, research and statistical analysis, market research, management information systems. *Unit head:* Dr. Bonnie Tiell, Dean of Graduate Studies, 419-448-3261, Fax: 419-443-5002, E-mail: btiell@ tiffin.edu. *Application contact:* Nikki Hintze, Director of Graduate and Distance Education Academic Advising, 800-968-6446 Ext. 3596, Fax: 419-443-5002, E-mail: hintzenm@ tiffin.edu.
Website: http://www.tiffin.edu/graduateprograms/

Towson University, Program in Clinician-Administrator Transition, Towson, MD 21252-0001. Offers Postbaccalaureate Certificate. *Students:* 14 full-time (all women), 9 part-time (all women); includes 3 minority (all Black or African American, non-Hispanic/ Latino). *Entrance requirements:* For degree, minimum GPA of 3.0; bachelor's or master's degree in a clinical field; licensure, licensure eligibility, or certificate in a clinical field. *Application deadline:* Applications are processed on a rolling basis. Application fee: $45. Electronic applications accepted. *Financial support:* Application deadline: 4/1. *Unit head:* Dr. Marcie Weinstein, Graduate Program Director, 410-704-4049, E-mail: mweinstein@towson.edu. *Application contact:* Alicia Arkell-Kleis, Information Contact, 410-704-6004, E-mail: grads@towson.edu.
Website: http://grad.towson.edu/program/certificate/catp-pbc/

Trevecca Nazarene University, Graduate Business Programs, Nashville, TN 37210-2877. Offers business administration (MBA); healthcare administration (Certificate); information technology (MBA, MS, Certificate); management (MSM); management and leadership (Certificate); project management (Certificate). Evening/weekend programs available. Postbaccalaureate distance learning degree programs offered. *Faculty:* 7 full-time (0 women), 3 part-time/adjunct (0 women). *Students:* 101 full-time (55 women), 21 part-time (8 women); includes 30 minority (27 Black or African American, non-Hispanic/ Latino; 2 Asian, non-Hispanic/Latino; 1 Hispanic/Latino), 3 international. Average age 36. In 2013, 33 master's awarded. *Entrance requirements:* For master's, minimum GPA of 2.75, resume, official transcript from regionally-accredited institution, minimum math grade of C, minimum English composition grade of C; undergraduate computing degree (for MS). Additional exam requirements/recommendations for international students: Required—TOEFL (minimum score 550 paper-based; 80 iBT). *Application deadline:* Applications are processed on a rolling basis. Application fee: $25. *Expenses:* Contact institution. *Financial support:* Applicants required to submit FAFSA. *Unit head:* Dr. Rick Mann, Director of Graduate and Professional Programs for School of Business, 615-248-1529, E-mail: management@trevecca.edu. *Application contact:* 615-248-1529, E-mail: cll@trevecca.edu.

Trident University International, College of Health Sciences, Cypress, CA 90630. Offers MS, PhD, Certificate. Part-time and evening/weekend programs available. Postbaccalaureate distance learning degree programs offered (no on-campus study). *Degree requirements:* For doctorate, comprehensive exam, thesis/dissertation. *Entrance requirements:* For master's, minimum GPA of 2.5 (students with GPA 3.0 or greater may transfer up to 30% of graduate level credits); for doctorate, minimum GPA of 3.4. Additional exam requirements/recommendations for international students: Required—TOEFL. Electronic applications accepted.

Trinity University, Department of Health Care Administration, San Antonio, TX 78212-7200. Offers MS. *Accreditation:* CAHME. Part-time programs available. Postbaccalaureate distance learning degree programs offered (minimal on-campus study). *Degree requirements:* For master's, research projects. *Entrance requirements:* For master's, GMAT, GRE General Test, previous course work in accounting, economics, and statistics.

Trinity Western University, School of Graduate Studies, Program in Leadership, Langley, BC V2Y 1Y1, Canada. Offers business (MA, Certificate); Christian ministry (MA); education (MA, Certificate); healthcare (MA, Certificate); non-profit (MA, Certificate). Postbaccalaureate distance learning degree programs offered (minimal on-campus study). *Degree requirements:* For master's, major project. *Entrance requirements:* For master's, minimum GPA of 2.7. Additional exam requirements/ recommendations for international students: Required—TOEFL (minimum score 620 paper-based; 105 iBT). Electronic applications accepted. *Expenses:* Contact institution. *Faculty research:* Servant leadership.

Troy University, Graduate School, College of Arts and Sciences, Program in Public Administration, Troy, AL 36082. Offers education (MPA); environmental management (MPA); government contracting (MPA); health care administration (MPA); justice administration (MPA); national security affairs (MPA); nonprofit management (MPA); public human resources management (MPA); public management (MPA). *Accreditation:* NASPAA. Part-time and evening/weekend programs available. Postbaccalaureate distance learning degree programs offered (no on-campus study). *Faculty:* 15 full-time (9 women), 7 part-time/adjunct (4 women). *Students:* 95 full-time (62 women), 307 part-time (204 women); includes 231 minority (195 Black or African American, non-Hispanic/ Latino; 3 American Indian or Alaska Native, non-Hispanic/Latino; 5 Asian, non-Hispanic/ Latino; 15 Hispanic/Latino; 13 Two or more races, non-Hispanic/Latino). Average age 32. 172 applicants, 87% accepted, 107 enrolled. In 2013, 159 master's awarded. *Degree requirements:* For master's, capstone course with minimum B grade, minimum GPA of 3.0, admission to candidacy. *Entrance requirements:* For master's, GRE (minimum score of 850 on old exam or 294 on new exam), MAT (minimum score of 400) or GMAT (minimum score of 490), bachelor's degree; minimum undergraduate GPA of 2.5 or 3.0 on last 30 semester hours, letter of recommendation; essay. Additional exam requirements/recommendations for international students: Required—TOEFL (minimum score 523 paper-based; 70 iBT), IELTS (minimum score 6). *Application deadline:* Applications are processed on a rolling basis. Application fee: $50. Electronic applications accepted. *Expenses:* Tuition, state resident: full-time $6084; part-time $338 per credit hour. Tuition, nonresident: full-time $12,168; part-time $676 per credit hour. *Required fees:* $630; $35 per credit hour. $50 per semester. *Financial support:* Available to part-time students. Applicants required to submit FAFSA. *Unit head:* Dr. Sam Shelton, Chairman, 334-670-3754, Fax: 334-670-5647, E-mail: ssheltonl@ troy.edu. *Application contact:* Brenda K. Campbell, Director of Graduate Admissions, 334-670-3178, Fax: 334-670-3733, E-mail: bcamp@troy.edu.

Troy University, Graduate School, College of Business, Program in Business Administration, Troy, AL 36082. Offers accounting (EMBA, MBA); criminal justice (EMBA); finance (MBA); general management (EMBA, MBA); healthcare management (EMBA); information systems (EMBA, MBA); international economic development (MBA). *Accreditation:* ACBSP. Part-time and evening/weekend programs available. *Faculty:* 56 full-time (20 women), 3 part-time/adjunct (0 women). *Students:* 142 full-time (89 women), 310 part-time (192 women); includes 265 minority (185 Black or African American, non-Hispanic/Latino; 3 American Indian or Alaska Native, non-Hispanic/ Latino; 62 Asian, non-Hispanic/Latino; 8 Hispanic/Latino; 1 Native Hawaiian or other Pacific Islander, non-Hispanic/Latino; 6 Two or more races, non-Hispanic/Latino). Average age 29. 472 applicants, 68% accepted, 51 enrolled. In 2013, 293 master's awarded. *Degree requirements:* For master's, minimum GPA of 3.0, capstone course, research course. *Entrance requirements:* For master's, GMAT (minimum score 500) or GRE General Test (minimum score 900 on old exam or 294 on new exam), bachelor's degree; minimum undergraduate GPA of 2.5 or 3.0 on last 30 semester hours, letter of recommendation. Additional exam requirements/recommendations for international students: Required—TOEFL (minimum score 523 paper-based; 70 iBT), IELTS (minimum score 6). *Application deadline:* Applications are processed on a rolling basis. Application fee: $50. *Expenses:* Tuition, state resident: full-time $6084; part-time $338 per credit hour. Tuition, nonresident: full-time $12,168; part-time $676 per credit hour. *Required fees:* $630; $35 per credit hour. $50 per semester. *Unit head:* Dr. Bob Wheatley, Director, Graduate Business Programs, 334-670-3194, Fax: 334-670-3599, E-mail: rwheat@troy.edu. *Application contact:* Brenda K. Campbell, Director of Graduate Admissions, 334-670-3178, Fax: 334-670-3733, E-mail: bcamp@troy.edu.

Troy University, Graduate School, College of Business, Program in Management, Troy, AL 36082. Offers applied management (MSM); healthcare management (MSM); human resources management (MSM); information systems (MSM); international hospitality management (MSM); international management (MSM); leadership and organizational effectiveness (MSM); public management (MS, MSM). *Accreditation:* ACBSP. Part-time and evening/weekend programs available. *Faculty:* 15 full-time (8 women), 3 part-time/adjunct (0 women). *Students:* 18 full-time (14 women), 148 part-time (86 women); includes 95 minority (75 Black or African American, non-Hispanic/ Latino; 1 American Indian or Alaska Native, non-Hispanic/Latino; 4 Asian, non-Hispanic/ Latino; 8 Hispanic/Latino; 7 Two or more races, non-Hispanic/Latino). Average age 35. 124 applicants, 79% accepted, 30 enrolled. In 2013, 75 master's awarded. *Degree requirements:* For master's, Graduate Educational Testing Service Major Field Test, capstone exam, minimum GPA of 3.0. *Entrance requirements:* For master's, GRE (minimum score of 900 on old exam or 294 on new exam) or GMAT (minimum score of 500), bachelor's degree; minimum undergraduate GPA of 2.5 or 3.0 on last 30 semester hours, letter of recommendation. Additional exam requirements/recommendations for international students: Required—TOEFL (minimum score 523 paper-based; 70 iBT), IELTS (minimum score 6). *Application deadline:* Applications are processed on a rolling basis. Application fee: $50. Electronic applications accepted. *Expenses:* Contact institution. *Unit head:* Dr. Bob Wheatley, Director, Graduate Business Programs, 334-670-3143, Fax: 334-670-3599, E-mail: rwheat@troy.edu. *Application contact:* Brenda K. Campbell, Director of Graduate Admissions, 334-670-3178, Fax: 334-670-3733, E-mail: bcamp@troy.edu.

Health Services Management and Hospital Administration

Tulane University, School of Public Health and Tropical Medicine, Department of Health Systems Management, New Orleans, LA 70118-5669. Offers MHA, MMM, MPH, PhD, Sc D, JD/MHA, MD/MPH. *Accreditation:* CAHME (one or more programs are accredited). *Degree requirements:* For doctorate, comprehensive exam, thesis/dissertation. *Entrance requirements:* For master's, GMAT, GRE General Test; for doctorate, GRE General Test. Additional exam requirements/recommendations for international students: Required—TOEFL. Electronic applications accepted. *Faculty research:* Health policy, organizational governance, international health administration.

Uniformed Services University of the Health Sciences, School of Medicine, Graduate Programs in the Biomedical Sciences and Public Health, Bethesda, MD 20814. Offers emerging infectious diseases (PhD); medical and clinical psychology (PhD), including clinical psychology, medical psychology; molecular and cell biology (MS, PhD); neuroscience (PhD); preventive medicine and biometrics (MPH, MS, MSPH, MTMH, Dr PH, PhD), including environmental health sciences (PhD), healthcare administration and policy (MS), medical zoology (PhD), public health (MPH, MSPH, Dr PH), tropical medicine and hygiene (MTMH). *Faculty:* 372 full-time (119 women), 4,044 part-time/adjunct (908 women). *Students:* 240 full-time (133 women); includes 40 minority (15 Black or African American, non-Hispanic/Latino; 13 Asian, non-Hispanic/Latino; 12 Hispanic/Latino), 30 international. Average age 25. 598 applicants, 17% accepted, 77 enrolled. In 2013, 19 master's, 50 doctorates awarded. Terminal master's awarded for partial completion of doctoral program. *Degree requirements:* For master's, comprehensive exam, thesis or alternative; for doctorate, comprehensive exam, thesis/dissertation, qualifying exam. *Entrance requirements:* For master's, GRE General Test; for doctorate, GRE General Test, minimum GPA of 3.0. Additional exam requirements/recommendations for international students: Required—TOEFL. *Application deadline:* For fall admission, 1/1 priority date for domestic and international students. Applications are processed on a rolling basis. Application fee: $0. Electronic applications accepted. *Financial support:* In 2013–14, fellowships with full tuition reimbursements (averaging $27,000 per year), research assistantships with full tuition reimbursements (averaging $27,000 per year) were awarded; career-related internships or fieldwork, scholarships/grants, health care benefits, and tuition waivers (full) also available. *Unit head:* Dr. Eleanor S. Metcalf, Associate Dean, 301-295-1104, E-mail: emetcalf@usuhs.edu. *Application contact:* Tina Finley, Administrative Officer, 301-295-3642, Fax: 301-295-6772, E-mail: netina.finley@usuhs.edu.
Website: http://www.usuhs.mil/graded

Uniformed Services University of the Health Sciences, School of Medicine, Graduate Programs in the Biomedical Sciences and Public Health, Department of Preventive Medicine and Biometrics, Program in Healthcare Administration and Policy, Bethesda, MD 20814-4799. Offers MS. *Unit head:* Dr. David Cruess, Director, 301-295-9769, E-mail: david.cruess@usuhs.edu. *Application contact:* Elena Marina Sherman, Program Administrative Specialist, 301-295-3913, Fax: 301-295-6772, E-mail: elena.sherman@usuhs.edu.

Union Graduate College, Center for Bioethics and Clinical Leadership, Schenectady, NY 12308-3107. Offers bioethics (MS); clinical ethics (AC); clinical leadership in health management (MS); health, policy and law (AC); research ethics (AC). Part-time and evening/weekend programs available. Postbaccalaureate distance learning degree programs offered (minimal on-campus study). *Faculty:* 2 full-time (0 women), 9 part-time/adjunct (7 women). *Students:* 2 full-time (both women), 59 part-time (39 women); includes 17 minority (3 Black or African American, non-Hispanic/Latino; 8 Asian, non-Hispanic/Latino; 2 Hispanic/Latino; 4 Two or more races, non-Hispanic/Latino), 4 international. Average age 36. In 2013, 19 master's, 3 other advanced degrees awarded. *Entrance requirements:* For master's, letters of recommendation. Additional exam requirements/recommendations for international students: Required—TOEFL (minimum score 550 paper-based). *Application deadline:* Applications are processed on a rolling basis. Electronic applications accepted. *Expenses:* Contact institution. *Financial support:* Federal Work-Study, scholarships/grants, health care benefits, and tuition waivers (partial) available. Support available to part-time students. Financial award applicants required to submit FAFSA. *Faculty research:* Bioethics education, clinical ethics consultation, research ethics, history of biomedical ethics, international bioethics/research ethics. *Unit head:* Dr. Sean Philpott, Director, 518-631-9860, Fax: 518-631-9903, E-mail: philpotts@uniongraduatecollege.edu. *Application contact:* Ann Nolte, Assistant Director, 518-631-9860, Fax: 518-631-9903, E-mail: noltea@uniongraduatecollege.edu.

Union Graduate College, School of Management, Schenectady, NY 12308-3107. Offers business administration (MBA); general management (Certificate); health systems administration (MBA, Certificate); human resources (Certificate). *Accreditation:* AACSB. Part-time and evening/weekend programs available. Postbaccalaureate distance learning degree programs offered (minimal on-campus study). *Faculty:* 16 full-time (3 women), 9 part-time/adjunct (4 women). *Students:* 77 full-time (31 women), 70 part-time (31 women); includes 23 minority (2 Black or African American, non-Hispanic/Latino; 19 Asian, non-Hispanic/Latino; 2 Two or more races, non-Hispanic/Latino), 5 international. Average age 27. In 2013, 94 master's, 11 other advanced degrees awarded. *Degree requirements:* For master's, internship, capstone course. *Entrance requirements:* For master's, GMAT, GRE, minimum GPA of 3.0, 3 letters of recommendation. Additional exam requirements/recommendations for international students: Required—TOEFL (minimum score 550 paper-based). *Application deadline:* Applications are processed on a rolling basis. Application fee: $60. *Financial support:* Research assistantships, career-related internships or fieldwork, Federal Work-Study, scholarships/grants, health care benefits, and tuition waivers (partial) available. Support available to part-time students. Financial award applicants required to submit FAFSA. *Unit head:* Bela Musits, Dean, 518-631-9890, Fax: 518-631-9902, E-mail: musitsb@uniongraduatecollege.edu. *Application contact:* Diane Trzaskos, Admissions Coordinator, 518-631-9837, Fax: 518-631-9901, E-mail: trzaskod@uniongraduatecollege.edu.
Website: http://www.uniongraduatecollege.edu

Universidad de Ciencias Medicas, Graduate Programs, San Jose, Costa Rica. Offers dermatology (SP); family health (MS); health service center administration (MHA); human anatomy (MS); medical and surgery (MD); occupational medicine (MS); pharmacy (Pharm D). Part-time programs available. *Degree requirements:* For master's, thesis; for doctorate and SP, comprehensive exam. *Entrance requirements:* For master's, MD or bachelor's degree; for doctorate, admissions test; for SP, admissions test, MD.

Universidad de Iberoamerica, Graduate School, San Jose, Costa Rica. Offers clinical neuropsychology (PhD); clinical psychology (M Psych); educational psychology (M Psych); forensic psychology (M Psych); hospital management (MHA); intensive care nursing (MN); medicine (MD).

Université de Montréal, Faculty of Medicine, Department of Health Administration, Montréal, QC H3C 3J7, Canada. Offers M Sc, DESS. *Accreditation:* CAHME. *Degree requirements:* For master's, thesis. *Entrance requirements:* For master's, proficiency in French. Electronic applications accepted.

University at Albany, State University of New York, School of Public Health, Department of Health Policy, Management, and Behavior, Albany, NY 12222-0001. Offers MS. *Degree requirements:* For master's, thesis. *Entrance requirements:* For master's, GRE General Test. Additional exam requirements/recommendations for international students: Required—TOEFL (minimum score 550 paper-based). Electronic applications accepted.

University at Buffalo, the State University of New York, Graduate School, School of Nursing, Buffalo, NY 14214. Offers adult gerontology nurse practitioner (DNP); family nurse practitioner (DNP); health care systems and leadership (MS); nurse anesthetist (DNP); nursing (PhD); nursing education (Certificate); psychiatric/mental health nurse practitioner (DNP). *Accreditation:* AACN; AANA/CANAEP (one or more programs are accredited). Part-time programs available. Postbaccalaureate distance learning degree programs offered (no on-campus study). *Faculty:* 24 full-time (21 women), 2 part-time/adjunct (1 woman). *Students:* 80 full-time (60 women), 97 part-time (84 women); includes 35 minority (20 Black or African American, non-Hispanic/Latino; 2 American Indian or Alaska Native, non-Hispanic/Latino; 9 Asian, non-Hispanic/Latino; 1 Hispanic/Latino; 3 Native Hawaiian or other Pacific Islander, non-Hispanic/Latino). 118 applicants, 67% accepted, 58 enrolled. In 2013, 41 master's, 15 doctorates awarded. *Degree requirements:* For master's, thesis optional; for doctorate, comprehensive exam (for some programs), capstone (for DNP), dissertation (for PhD). *Entrance requirements:* For doctorate, GRE or MAT, minimum GPA of 3.0 (3.25 for PhD), RN license, BS or MS in nursing, 3 references, writing sample; for Certificate, interview, minimum GPA of 3.0 or GRE General Test, RN license, MS in nursing. Additional exam requirements/recommendations for international students: Required—TOEFL (minimum score 550 paper-based; 79 iBT), IELTS (minimum score 6.5). *Application deadline:* For fall admission, 7/1 for domestic students, 4/1 for international students; for spring admission, 12/1 for domestic students, 10/1 for international students; for summer admission, 4/1 for domestic students. Application fee: $75. Electronic applications accepted. *Financial support:* In 2013–14, 80 students received support, including 2 fellowships with full and partial tuition reimbursements available (averaging $17,000 per year), 7 research assistantships with full and partial tuition reimbursements available (averaging $10,600 per year), 7 teaching assistantships with full and partial tuition reimbursements available (averaging $10,600 per year); scholarships/grants, traineeships, health care benefits, and unspecified assistantships also available. Financial award application deadline: 3/15; financial award applicants required to submit FAFSA. *Faculty research:* Oncology, palliative care, gerontology, addictions, mental health, community wellness, sleep, workforce, care of underserved populations, quality and safety, person-centered care, adolescent health. *Total annual research expenditures:* $1.1 million. *Unit head:* Dr. Marsha L. Lewis, Dean and Professor, 716-829-2533, Fax: 716-829-2566, E-mail: ubnursingdean@buffalo.edu. *Application contact:* Dr. David J. Lang, Director of Student Affairs, 716-829-2537, Fax: 716-829-2067, E-mail: nursing@buffalo.edu.
Website: http://nursing.buffalo.edu/

The University of Akron, Graduate School, College of Business Administration, Department of Management, Program in Healthcare Management, Akron, OH 44325. Offers MBA. *Students:* 19 full-time (9 women), 47 part-time (17 women); includes 1 minority (Black or African American, non-Hispanic/Latino), 5 international. Average age 32. 19 applicants, 74% accepted, 7 enrolled. In 2013, 4 master's awarded. *Entrance requirements:* For master's, GMAT, minimum GPA of 2.75, two letters of recommendation, statement of purpose, resume. Additional exam requirements/recommendations for international students: Required—TOEFL (minimum score 550 paper-based; 79 iBT). *Application deadline:* For fall admission, 7/15 for domestic and international students; for spring admission, 11/15 for domestic and international students. Application fee: $40 ($60 for international students). Electronic applications accepted. *Expenses:* Tuition, state resident: full-time $7430; part-time $412.80 per credit hour. Tuition, nonresident: full-time $12,722; part-time $706.80 per credit hour. *Required fees:* $53 per credit hour. $12 per semester. Tuition and fees vary according to course load and program. *Unit head:* Dr. Steve Ash, Interim Chair, 330-972-6429, E-mail: ash@uakron.edu. *Application contact:* Dr. William Hauser, Director of Graduate Business Programs, 330-972-7043, Fax: 330-972-6588, E-mail: whauser@uakron.edu.

The University of Alabama at Birmingham, School of Business, Program in Business Administration, Birmingham, AL 35294-4460. Offers business administration (MBA), including finance, health care management, information technology management, marketing. Part-time and evening/weekend programs available. *Students:* 59 full-time (25 women), 249 part-time (93 women); includes 74 minority (53 Black or African American, non-Hispanic/Latino; 13 Asian, non-Hispanic/Latino; 7 Hispanic/Latino; 1 Two or more races, non-Hispanic/Latino), 16 international. Average age 32. In 2013, 128 master's awarded. *Entrance requirements:* For master's, GMAT. Additional exam requirements/recommendations for international students: Required—TOEFL. *Application deadline:* For fall admission, 7/1 for domestic and international students; for spring admission, 11/1 for domestic and international students; for summer admission, 4/1 for domestic and international students. Application fee: $60 ($75 for international students). *Unit head:* Dr. Ken Miller, Executive Director, MBA Programs, 205-934-8855, E-mail: klmiller@uab.edu. *Application contact:* Christy Manning, Coordinator of Graduate Programs in Business, 205-934-8817, E-mail: cmanning@uab.edu.
Website: http://www.uab.edu/business/degrees-certificates/MBA

The University of Alabama at Birmingham, School of Health Professions, Program in Administration/Health Services, Birmingham, AL 35294. Offers D Sc, PhD. *Degree requirements:* For doctorate, thesis/dissertation. *Entrance requirements:* For doctorate, GMAT or GRE General Test. *Faculty research:* Healthcare strategic management, marketing, and organization studies.

The University of Alabama at Birmingham, School of Health Professions, Program in Health Administration, Birmingham, AL 35294. Offers MSHA. *Accreditation:* CAHME. *Degree requirements:* For master's, administrative residency. *Entrance requirements:* For master's, GMAT or GRE General Test, minimum GPA of 3.0 in final 60 hours of undergraduate course work; 5 years of experience in health care organizations, either as managers or as clinical professionals (for executive program). Additional exam requirements/recommendations for international students: Required—TOEFL, TWE. Electronic applications accepted.

The University of Alabama at Birmingham, School of Public Health, Program in Public Health, Birmingham, AL 35294. Offers accelerated industrial hygiene (MPH); applied epidemiology (MSPH); biostatistics (MPH); clinical and translational science (MSPH); environmental health (MPH); environmental health and toxicology (MSPH); epidemiology (MPH); general theory and practice (MPH); health behavior (MPH); health care organization (MPH); health policy quantitative policy analysis (MPH); industrial hygiene (MPH, MSPH); maternal and child health policy (Dr PH); maternal and child health policy and leadership (MPH); occupational health and safety (MPH); outcomes research (MSPH, Dr PH); pharmacoepidemiology and comparative effectiveness research (MSPH); public health (PhD); public health management (Dr PH); public health preparedness management (MPH). *Accreditation:* CEPH. *Entrance requirements:* For master's and doctorate, GRE, evaluations. Additional exam requirements/recommendations for international students: Recommended—TOEFL (minimum score 550 paper-based; 79 iBT), IELTS (minimum score 6.5).

The University of Alabama in Huntsville, School of Graduate Studies, College of Nursing, Huntsville, AL 35899. Offers family nurse practitioner (Certificate); nursing

(MSN, DNP), including acute care nurse practitioner (MSN), adult clinical nurse specialist (MSN), clinical nurse leader (MSN), family nurse practitioner (MSN), leadership in health care systems (MSN); nursing education (Certificate). DNP offered jointly with The University of Alabama at Birmingham. *Accreditation:* AACN. Part-time and evening/weekend programs available. Postbaccalaureate distance learning degree programs offered (minimal on-campus study). *Faculty:* 16 full-time (15 women), 4 part-time/adjunct (all women). *Students:* 67 full-time (63 women), 235 part-time (192 women); includes 40 minority (27 Black or African American, non-Hispanic/Latino; 5 American Indian or Alaska Native, non-Hispanic/Latino; 4 Asian, non-Hispanic/Latino; 3 Hispanic/Latino; 1 Two or more races, non-Hispanic/Latino), 10 international. Average age 36. 265 applicants, 59% accepted, 128 enrolled. In 2013, 75 master's, 10 doctorates, 5 other advanced degrees awarded. *Degree requirements:* For master's, comprehensive exam, thesis or alternative, oral and written exams. *Entrance requirements:* For master's, MAT or GRE, Alabama RN license, BSN, minimum GPA of 3.0; for doctorate, master's degree in nursing in an advanced practice area; for Certificate, MAT or GRE, minimum GPA of 3.0. Additional exam requirements/recommendations for international students: Required—TOEFL (minimum score 500 paper-based; 80 iBT), IELTS (minimum score 6.5). *Application deadline:* For fall admission, 7/15 for domestic students, 4/1 for international students; for spring admission, 11/30 for domestic students, 9/1 for international students. Applications are processed on a rolling basis. Application fee: $50. Electronic applications accepted. *Expenses:* Tuition, state resident: full-time $8912; part-time $540 per credit hour. Tuition, nonresident: full-time $20,774; part-time $1252 per credit hour. *Required fees:* $148 per semester. One-time fee: $150. *Financial support:* In 2013–14, 19 students received support, including 19 teaching assistantships with full tuition reimbursements available (averaging $7,876 per year); career-related internships or fieldwork, Federal Work-Study, institutionally sponsored loans, scholarships/grants, traineeships, health care benefits, and unspecified assistantships also available. Support available to part-time students. Financial award application deadline: 4/1; financial award applicants required to submit FAFSA. *Faculty research:* Health care informatics, chronic illness management, maternal and child health, genetics/genomics, technology and health care. *Total annual research expenditures:* $557,830. *Unit head:* Dr. Fay Raines, Dean, 256-824-6345, Fax: 256-824-6026, E-mail: rainesc@uah.edu. *Application contact:* Charles Davis, Director of Graduate Nursing Admissions and Advising, 256-824-2433, Fax: 256-824-6026, E-mail: charles.davis@uah.edu.
Website: http://www.uah.edu/nursing/welcome

University of Alberta, School of Public Health, Department of Public Health Sciences, Edmonton, AB T6G 2E1, Canada. Offers clinical epidemiology (M Sc, MPH); environmental and occupational health (MPH); environmental health sciences (M Sc); epidemiology (M Sc); global health (M Sc, MPH); health policy and management (MPH); health policy research (M Sc); health technology assessment (MPH); occupational health (M Sc); population health (M Sc); public health leadership (MPH); public health sciences (PhD); quantitative methods (MPH). *Accreditation:* CEPH (one or more programs are accredited). Terminal master's awarded for partial completion of doctoral program. *Degree requirements:* For master's, thesis (for some programs); for doctorate, thesis/dissertation. *Entrance requirements:* For master's, GMAT or GRE General Test. Additional exam requirements/recommendations for international students: Required—TOEFL (minimum score 550 paper-based) or IELTS (minimum score 6). Electronic applications accepted. *Faculty research:* Biostatistics, health promotion and socio-behavioral health science.

University of Arkansas for Medical Sciences, College of Public Health, Little Rock, AR 72205-7199. Offers biostatistics (MPH); environmental and occupational health (MPH, Certificate); epidemiology (MPH, PhD); health behavior and health education (MPH); health policy and management (MPH); health promotion and prevention research (PhD); health services administration (MHSA); health systems research (PhD); public health (Certificate); public health leadership (Dr PH). Part-time programs available. *Faculty:* 37 full-time (19 women), 9 part-time/adjunct (5 women). *Students:* 56 full-time (35 women), 85 part-time (58 women); includes 54 minority (38 Black or African American, non-Hispanic/Latino; 1 American Indian or Alaska Native, non-Hispanic/Latino; 8 Asian, non-Hispanic/Latino; 3 Hispanic/Latino; 1 Native Hawaiian or other Pacific Islander, non-Hispanic/Latino; 3 Two or more races, non-Hispanic/Latino), 5 international. Average age 30. 70 applicants, 91% accepted, 33 enrolled. In 2013, 2 master's, 1 doctorate, 2 other advanced degrees awarded. *Degree requirements:* For master's, preceptorship, culminating experience, internship; for doctorate, comprehensive exam, capstone. *Entrance requirements:* For master's, GRE, GMAT, LSAT, PCAT, MCAT, DAT; for doctorate, GRE. Additional exam requirements/recommendations for international students: Required—TOEFL (minimum score 80 iBT), IELTS. *Application deadline:* For fall admission, 3/1 for domestic students, 2/1 for international students; for spring admission, 8/1 for domestic and international students; for summer admission, 2/1 for domestic and international students. Application fee: $25 ($50 for international students). Electronic applications accepted. *Expenses:* Contact institution. *Financial support:* In 2013–14, 8 research assistantships with full tuition reimbursements (averaging $13,000 per year) were awarded; scholarships/grants and tuition waivers (full and partial) also available. *Faculty research:* Health systems, tobacco prevention control, obesity prevention, environmental and occupational exposure, cancer prevention. *Unit head:* Dr. James M. Raczynski, Dean, 501-526-6600, E-mail: raczynskijameson@uams.edu. *Application contact:* Angie Choi, Director of Admission, 501-526-4620, Fax: 501-526-6750, E-mail: anchoi@uams.edu.
Website: http://publichealth.uams.edu/

University of Baltimore, Graduate School, The Yale Gordon College of Liberal Arts, Program in Health Systems Management, Baltimore, MD 21201-5779. Offers MS. Part-time and evening/weekend programs available. *Entrance requirements:* For master's, minimum undergraduate GPA of 3.0. Additional exam requirements/recommendations for international students: Required—TOEFL (minimum score 550 paper-based).

The University of British Columbia, Faculty of Medicine, School of Population and Public Health, Vancouver, BC V6T 1Z3, Canada. Offers health administration (MHA); health care and epidemiology (MH Sc, PhD); public health (MPH). *Accreditation:* CEPH (one or more programs are accredited). Postbaccalaureate distance learning degree programs offered (minimal on-campus study). *Degree requirements:* For master's, thesis (for some programs), major paper (MH Sc), research project (MHA); for doctorate, thesis/dissertation. *Entrance requirements:* For master's, GRE General Test or GMAT, PCAT, MCAT (MHA), MD or equivalent (for MH Sc); 4-year undergraduate degree from accredited university with minimum B+ overall academic average and in math or statistics course at undergraduate level (for MPH); 4-year undergraduate degree from accredited university with minimum B+ overall academic average plus work experience (for MHA); for doctorate, master's degree from accredited university with minimum B+ overall academic average and in math or statistics course at undergraduate level. Additional exam requirements/recommendations for international students: Required—TOEFL. Electronic applications accepted. *Expenses: Tuition, area resident:* Full-time $8000 Canadian dollars. *Faculty research:* Population and public health, clinical epidemiology, epidemiology and biostatistics, global health and vulnerable populations, health care services and systems, occupational and environmental health, public health emerging threats and rapid response, social and life course determinants of health, health administration.

University of California, Berkeley, Graduate Division, School of Public Health, Group in Health Services and Policy Analysis, Berkeley, CA 94720-1500. Offers PhD. *Degree requirements:* For doctorate, thesis/dissertation, qualifying exam. *Entrance requirements:* For doctorate, GRE General Test, minimum GPA of 3.0, 3 letters of recommendation.

University of California, Irvine, The Paul Merage School of Business, Health Care Executive MBA Program, Irvine, CA 92697. Offers MBA. *Students:* 25 full-time (10 women), 24 part-time (9 women); includes 19 minority (3 American Indian or Alaska Native, non-Hispanic/Latino; 16 Asian, non-Hispanic/Latino), 5 international. Average age 40. 60 applicants, 75% accepted, 24 enrolled. In 2013, 32 master's awarded. Application fee: $80 ($100 for international students). *Unit head:* Anthony Hansford, Senior Assistant Dean, 949-824-3801, E-mail: hansfora@uci.edu. *Application contact:* Sofia Trinidad Dang, Associate Director, Student Affairs, 949-824-5374, Fax: 949-824-0522, E-mail: sofia.dang@uci.edu.
Website: http://merage.uci.edu/HealthCareExecutiveMBA/Default.aspx

University of California, Los Angeles, Graduate Division, School of Public Health, Department of Health Services, Los Angeles, CA 90095. Offers MPH, MS, Dr PH, PhD, JD/MPH, MBA/MPH, MD/MPH. *Degree requirements:* For master's, comprehensive exam or thesis; for doctorate, thesis/dissertation, oral and written qualifying exams. *Entrance requirements:* For master's, GRE General Test, minimum GPA of 3.0; for doctorate, GRE General Test, minimum undergraduate GPA of 3.0. Electronic applications accepted.

University of California, San Diego, Office of Graduate Studies, Program in Health Policy and Law, La Jolla, CA 92093. Offers MAS. Program offered jointly with School of Medicine and California Western School of Law. Part-time programs available. *Students:* 36 part-time (26 women); includes 14 minority (2 Black or African American, non-Hispanic/Latino; 6 Asian, non-Hispanic/Latino; 6 Hispanic/Latino). 26 applicants, 77% accepted, 15 enrolled. In 2013, 12 master's awarded. *Entrance requirements:* For master's, appropriate medical, healthcare, legal or related degree; minimum GPA of 3.0 in final two years of study; minimum 3 years of relevant work experience or equivalent. Additional exam requirements/recommendations for international students: Required—TOEFL, IELTS. *Application deadline:* For fall admission, 4/7 for domestic students. Applications are processed on a rolling basis. Application fee: $80 ($100 for international students). Electronic applications accepted. *Expenses:* Tuition, state resident: full-time $11,220; part-time $1870 per quarter. Tuition, nonresident: full-time $26,322; part-time $4387 per quarter. *Required fees:* $519.50 per quarter. Part-time tuition and fees vary according to course load and program. *Financial support:* Scholarships/grants available. *Unit head:* Gerard Manecke, Program Co-Director, 619-543-3164, E-mail: gmanecke@ucsd.edu. *Application contact:* Jenna Lucius, Program Coordinator, 858-534-9162, E-mail: healthlaw@ucsd.edu.
Website: http://hlaw.ucsd.edu/

University of California, San Diego, School of Medicine, Program in the Leadership of Healthcare Organizations, La Jolla, CA 92093. Offers MAS. Part-time programs available. *Students:* 27 part-time (19 women); includes 10 minority (2 Black or African American, non-Hispanic/Latino; 7 Asian, non-Hispanic/Latino; 1 Hispanic/Latino), 5 international. 14 applicants, 57% accepted, 6 enrolled. In 2013, 8 master's awarded. *Entrance requirements:* For master's, minimum GPA of 3.0; minimum 5 years of professional work in health care or a related field (internship counts). Additional exam requirements/recommendations for international students: Required—TOEFL, IELTS. *Application deadline:* For fall admission, 7/1 for domestic students; for winter admission, 10/14 for domestic students; for spring admission, 1/8 for domestic students. Applications are processed on a rolling basis. Application fee: $80 ($100 for international students). Electronic applications accepted. *Expenses:* Tuition, state resident: full-time $11,220; part-time $1870 per quarter. Tuition, nonresident: full-time $26,322; part-time $4387 per quarter. *Required fees:* $519.50 per quarter. Part-time tuition and fees vary according to course load and program. *Financial support:* Scholarships/grants available. Financial award applicants required to submit FAFSA. *Unit head:* Todd Gilmer, Program Director, 858-534-7596, E-mail: tgilmer@ucsd.edu. *Application contact:* Jenna Lucius, Information Contact, 858-534-9162, E-mail: lhco@ucsd.edu.
Website: http://lhco.ucsd.edu/

University of Central Florida, College of Health and Public Affairs, Department of Health Management and Informatics, Orlando, FL 32816. Offers health care informatics (MS, Certificate); health sciences (MS). *Accreditation:* CAHME. Part-time and evening/weekend programs available. *Faculty:* 19 full-time (12 women), 23 part-time/adjunct (9 women). *Students:* 166 full-time (109 women), 222 part-time (152 women); includes 183 minority (85 Black or African American, non-Hispanic/Latino; 1 American Indian or Alaska Native, non-Hispanic/Latino; 41 Asian, non-Hispanic/Latino; 45 Hispanic/Latino; 2 Native Hawaiian or other Pacific Islander, non-Hispanic/Latino; 9 Two or more races, non-Hispanic/Latino), 8 international. Average age 30. 262 applicants, 77% accepted, 136 enrolled. In 2013, 120 master's awarded. *Degree requirements:* For master's, comprehensive exam, thesis or alternative, research report. *Entrance requirements:* For master's, GRE General Test. Additional exam requirements/recommendations for international students: Required—TOEFL. *Application deadline:* For fall admission, 7/15 for domestic students; for spring admission, 10/1 for domestic students. Application fee: $30. Electronic applications accepted. *Financial support:* Career-related internships or fieldwork, Federal Work-Study, institutionally sponsored loans, and unspecified assistantships available. Financial award application deadline: 3/1; financial award applicants required to submit FAFSA. *Unit head:* Dr. Reid Oetjen, Interim Chair, 407-823-5668, E-mail: reid.oetjen@ucf.edu. *Application contact:* Barbara Rodriguez Lamas, Director, Admissions and Student Services, 407-823-2766, Fax: 407-823-6442, E-mail: gradadmissions@ucf.edu.
Website: http://www.cohpa.ucf.edu/hmi/

University of Chicago, Booth School of Business, Full-Time MBA Program, Chicago, IL 60637. Offers accounting (MBA); analytic finance (MBA); analytic management (MBA); econometrics and statistics (MBA); economics (MBA); entrepreneurship (MBA); finance (MBA); general management (MBA); health administration and policy (Certificate); human resource management (MBA); international business (MBA); managerial and organizational behavior (MBA); marketing management (MBA); operations management (MBA); strategic management (MBA); MBA/AM; MBA/JD; MBA/MA; MBA/MD; MBA/MPP. *Accreditation:* AACSB. Part-time and evening/weekend programs available. Terminal master's awarded for partial completion of doctoral program. *Entrance requirements:* For master's, GMAT, 2 letters of recommendation, 3 essays, resume, interview. Additional exam requirements/recommendations for international students: Required—TOEFL (minimum score 600 paper-based; 104 iBT), IELTS. Electronic applications accepted. *Expenses:* Contact institution. *Faculty research:* Finance, marketing, economics, entrepreneurship, strategy, management.

University of Colorado Denver, Business School, Master of Business Administration Program, Denver, CO 80217. Offers bioinnovation and entrepreneurship (MBA); business intelligence (MBA); business strategy (MBA); business to business marketing (MBA); business to consumer marketing (MBA); change management (MBA); corporate financial management (MBA); enterprise technology management (MBA); entrepreneurship (MBA); health administration (MBA), including financial management, health administration, health information technologies, international health management

and policy; human resources management (MBA); international business (MBA); investment management (MBA); managing for sustainability (MBA); sports and entertainment management (MBA). *Accreditation:* AACSB. Part-time and evening/weekend programs available. Postbaccalaureate distance learning degree programs offered (no on-campus study). *Students:* 611 full-time (246 women), 144 part-time (58 women); includes 102 minority (14 Black or African American, non-Hispanic/Latino; 2 American Indian or Alaska Native, non-Hispanic/Latino; 38 Asian, non-Hispanic/Latino; 42 Hispanic/Latino; 6 Two or more races, non-Hispanic/Latino), 26 international. Average age 32. 330 applicants, 64% accepted, 125 enrolled. In 2013, 398 master's awarded. *Degree requirements:* For master's, 48 semester hours, including 30 of core courses, 3 in international business, and 15 in electives from over 50 other graduate business courses. *Entrance requirements:* For master's, GMAT, resume, official transcripts, essay, two letters of recommendation, financial statements (for international applicants). Additional exam requirements/recommendations for international students: Required—TOEFL (minimum score 560 paper-based; 83 iBT); Recommended—IELTS (minimum score 6.5). *Application deadline:* For fall admission, 4/15 priority date for domestic students, 3/15 priority date for international students; for spring admission, 10/15 priority date for domestic students, 9/15 priority date for international students. Applications are processed on a rolling basis. Application fee: $50 ($75 for international students). Electronic applications accepted. *Expenses:* Contact institution. *Financial support:* In 2013–14, 62 students received support. Fellowships, research assistantships, teaching assistantships, Federal Work-Study, institutionally sponsored loans, scholarships/grants, traineeships, and unspecified assistantships available. Financial award application deadline: 4/1; financial award applicants required to submit FAFSA. *Faculty research:* Marketing, management, entrepreneurship, finance, health administration. *Unit head:* Elizabeth Cooperman, Professor of Finance and Managing for Sustainability/MBA Program Director, 303-315-8422, E-mail: elizabeth.cooperman@ucdenver.edu. *Application contact:* Shelly Townley, Admissions Director, Graduate Programs, 303-315-8202, E-mail: shelly.townley@ucdenver.edu.
Website: http://www.ucdenver.edu/academics/colleges/business/degrees/mba/Pages/MBA.aspx

University of Colorado Denver, Business School, Program in Health Administration, Denver, CO 80217. Offers MS. *Accreditation:* CAHME. Part-time and evening/weekend programs available. *Students:* 3 full-time (1 woman), 2 part-time (1 woman), 1 international. Average age 33. 7 applicants, 29% accepted. In 2013, 3 master's awarded. *Degree requirements:* For master's, 30 credit hours. *Entrance requirements:* For master's, GMAT, resume, essay, two letters of reference, financial statements (for international applicants). Additional exam requirements/recommendations for international students: Required—TOEFL (minimum score 537 paper-based; 75 iBT); Recommended—IELTS (minimum score 6.5). *Application deadline:* For fall admission, 4/15 for domestic students, 3/15 for international students; for spring admission, 10/15 for domestic students, 9/15 for international students. Applications are processed on a rolling basis. Application fee: $50 ($75 for international students). Electronic applications accepted. *Expenses:* Contact institution. *Financial support:* In 2013–14, 1 student received support. Fellowships, research assistantships, teaching assistantships, Federal Work-Study, institutionally sponsored loans, scholarships/grants, and traineeships available. Financial award application deadline: 4/1; financial award applicants required to submit FAFSA. *Faculty research:* Cost containment, financial management, governance, rural health-care delivery systems. *Unit head:* Dr. Errol Biggs, Director, 303-315-8851, E-mail: errol.biggs@ucdenver.edu. *Application contact:* Shelly Townley, Admissions Director, Graduate Programs, 303-315-8202, E-mail: shelly.townley@ucdenver.edu.
Website: http://www.ucdenver.edu/academics/colleges/business/degrees/ms/health-admin/Pages/Health-Administration.aspx

University of Colorado Denver, Business School, Program in Information Systems, Denver, CO 80217. Offers accounting and information systems audit and control (MS); business intelligence systems (MS); ehealth and healthcare service entrepreneurship (MS); enterprise risk management (MS); enterprise technology management (MS); geographic information systems (MS); health information technology (MS); technology innovation and entrepreneurship (MS); Web and mobile computing (MS). Part-time and evening/weekend programs available. Postbaccalaureate distance learning degree programs offered (no on-campus study). *Students:* 55 full-time (14 women), 23 part-time (8 women); includes 10 minority (2 Black or African American, non-Hispanic/Latino; 7 Asian, non-Hispanic/Latino; 1 Hispanic/Latino), 15 international. Average age 33. 54 applicants, 78% accepted, 14 enrolled. In 2013, 27 master's awarded. *Degree requirements:* For master's, 30 credit hours. *Entrance requirements:* For master's, GMAT, resume, essay, two letters of recommendation, financial statements (for international applicants). Additional exam requirements/recommendations for international students: Required—TOEFL (minimum score 537 paper-based; 75 iBT); Recommended—IELTS (minimum score 6.5). *Application deadline:* For fall admission, 4/15 for domestic students, 3/15 for international students; for spring admission, 10/15 for domestic students, 9/15 for international students. Applications are processed on a rolling basis. Application fee: $50 ($75 for international students). Electronic applications accepted. *Expenses:* Contact institution. *Financial support:* In 2013–14, 18 students received support. Fellowships, research assistantships, teaching assistantships, Federal Work-Study, institutionally sponsored loans, scholarships/grants, and traineeships available. Financial award application deadline: 4/1; financial award applicants required to submit FAFSA. *Faculty research:* Human-computer interaction, expert systems, database management, electronic commerce, object-oriented software development. *Unit head:* Dr. Jahangir Karimi, Director of Information Systems Programs, 303-315-8430, E-mail: jahangir.karimi@ucdenver.edu. *Application contact:* Shelly Townley, Admissions Director, Graduate Programs, 303-315-8202, E-mail: shelly.townley@ucdenver.edu.
Website: http://www.ucdenver.edu/academics/colleges/business/degrees/ms/IS/Pages/Information-Systems.aspx

University of Colorado Denver, Colorado School of Public Health, Program in Public Health, Aurora, CO 80045. Offers community and behavioral health (MPH, Dr PH); environmental and occupational health (MPH); epidemiology (MPH); health systems, management and policy (MPH). *Accreditation:* CEPH. Part-time and evening/weekend programs available. *Faculty:* 14 full-time (13 women). *Students:* 295 full-time (247 women), 49 part-time (39 women); includes 77 minority (17 Black or African American, non-Hispanic/Latino; 3 American Indian or Alaska Native, non-Hispanic/Latino; 16 Asian, non-Hispanic/Latino; 31 Hispanic/Latino; 10 Two or more races, non-Hispanic/Latino), 5 international. Average age 30. 657 applicants, 71% accepted, 132 enrolled. In 2013, 106 master's awarded. *Degree requirements:* For master's, thesis or alternative, 42 credit hours; for doctorate, comprehensive exam, thesis/dissertation, 67 credit hours. *Entrance requirements:* For master's, GRE, MCAT, DAT, LSAT, PCAT, GMAT or master's degree from accredited institution, baccalaureate degree or equivalent; minimum GPA of 3.0; transcripts; references; resume; essay; for doctorate, GRE, MCAT, DAT, LSAT, PCAT or GMAT, MPH or master's or higher degree in related field or equivalent; 2 years of previous work experience in public health; essay; resume. Additional exam requirements/recommendations for international students: Required—TOEFL (minimum score 550 paper-based; 80 iBT). *Application deadline:* For fall admission, 12/15 priority date for domestic students, 12/1 priority date for international students. Application fee: $65. Electronic applications accepted. *Expenses:* Contact institution. *Financial support:* In 2013–14, 125 students received support. Fellowships, research assistantships, teaching assistantships, Federal Work-Study, institutionally sponsored loans, scholarships/grants, traineeships, and unspecified assistantships available. Financial award application deadline: 3/15; financial award applicants required to submit FAFSA. *Faculty research:* Cancer prevention by nutrition, cancer survivorship outcomes, social and cultural factors related to health. *Unit head:* Dr. Lori Crane, Chair, 303-724-4385, E-mail: lori.crane@ucdenver.edu. *Application contact:* Carla Denerstein, Departmental Assistant, 303-724-4446, E-mail: carla.denerstein@ucdenver.edu.
Website: http://www.ucdenver.edu/academics/colleges/PublicHealth/departments/CommunityBehavioralHealth/Pages/CommunityBehavioralHealth.aspx

University of Connecticut, Graduate School, School of Business, Storrs, CT 06269. Offers accounting (MS, PhD); business administration (Exec MBA, MBA, PhD); finance (PhD); health care management and insurance studies (MBA); management (PhD); management consulting (MBA); marketing (PhD); marketing intelligence (MBA); MA/MBA; MBA/MSW. *Accreditation:* AACSB. *Degree requirements:* For master's, comprehensive exam; for doctorate, thesis/dissertation. *Entrance requirements:* For master's and doctorate, GMAT. Additional exam requirements/recommendations for international students: Required—TOEFL (minimum score 550 paper-based). Electronic applications accepted.

University of Dallas, Graduate School of Management, Irving, TX 75062-4736. Offers accounting (MBA, MM, MS); business management (MBA, MM); corporate finance (MBA, MM); financial services (MBA); global business (MBA, MM); health services management (MBA, MM); human resource management (MBA, MM); information assurance (MBA, MM, MS); information technology (MBA, MM, MS); information technology service management (MBA, MM, MS); marketing management (MBA, MM); organization development (MBA, MM); project management (MBA, MM); sports and entertainment management (MBA, MM); strategic leadership (MBA, MM); supply chain management (MBA); supply chain management and market logistics (MM). *Accreditation:* ACBSP. Part-time and evening/weekend programs available. Postbaccalaureate distance learning degree programs offered (no on-campus study). *Entrance requirements:* Additional exam requirements/recommendations for international students: Required—TOEFL. Electronic applications accepted. *Expenses:* Contact institution.

University of Denver, University College, Denver, CO 80208. Offers arts and culture (MLS, Certificate), including art, literature, and culture, arts development and program management (Certificate), creative writing; environmental policy and management (MAS, Certificate), including energy and sustainability (Certificate), environmental assessment of nuclear power (Certificate), environmental health and safety (Certificate), environmental management, natural resource management (Certificate); geographic information systems (MAS, Certificate); global affairs (MLS, Certificate), including translation studies, world history and culture; healthcare leadership (MPH, Certificate), including healthcare policy, law, and ethics, medical and healthcare information technologies, strategic management of healthcare; information and communications technology (MCIS, Certificate), including database design and administration (Certificate), geographic information systems (MCIS), information security systems security (Certificate), information systems security (MCIS), project management (MCIS, MPS, Certificate), software design and administration (Certificate), software design and programming (MCIS), technology management, telecommunications technology (MCIS), Web design and development; leadership and organizations (MPS, Certificate), including human capital in organizations, philanthropic leadership, project management (MCIS, MPS, Certificate), strategic innovation and change; organizational and professional communication (MPS, Certificate), including alternative dispute resolution, organizational communication, organizational development and training, public relations and marketing; security management (MAS, Certificate), including emergency planning and response, information security (MAS), organizational security; strategic human resource management (MPS, Certificate), including global human resources (MPS), human resource management and development (MPS). Part-time and evening/weekend programs available. Postbaccalaureate distance learning degree programs offered (no on-campus study). *Faculty:* 139 part-time/adjunct (61 women). *Students:* 49 full-time (16 women), 1,297 part-time (732 women); includes 272 minority (92 Black or African American, non-Hispanic/Latino; 5 American Indian or Alaska Native, non-Hispanic/Latino; 30 Asian, non-Hispanic/Latino; 114 Hispanic/Latino; 3 Native Hawaiian or other Pacific Islander, non-Hispanic/Latino; 28 Two or more races, non-Hispanic/Latino), 92 international. Average age 35. 542 applicants, 95% accepted, 362 enrolled. In 2013, 374 master's, 128 other advanced degrees awarded. *Degree requirements:* For master's, capstone project. *Entrance requirements:* For master's, transcripts, two letters of recommendation, personal statement, resume. Additional exam requirements/recommendations for international students: Required—TOEFL (minimum score 550 paper-based; 80 iBT). *Application deadline:* For fall admission, 7/18 priority date for domestic students, 5/2 priority date for international students; for winter admission, 10/24 priority date for domestic students, 9/19 priority date for international students; for spring admission, 2/1 for domestic students, 12/14 for international students; for summer admission, 4/18 priority date for domestic students, 3/7 priority date for international students. Applications are processed on a rolling basis. Application fee: $75. Electronic applications accepted. *Expenses:* Contact institution. *Financial support:* In 2013–14, 28 students received support. Applicants required to submit FAFSA. *Unit head:* Dr. Michael McGuire, Interim Dean, 303-871-3518, E-mail: mmcguire@du.edu. *Application contact:* Information Contact, 303-871-2291, E-mail: ucoladm@du.edu.
Website: http://www.universitycollege.du.edu/

University of Detroit Mercy, College of Health Professions, Program in Health Services Administration, Detroit, MI 48221. Offers MHSA. *Degree requirements:* For master's, thesis. *Entrance requirements:* For master's, GRE General Test, minimum GPA of 3.0. *Faculty research:* Health systems issues, organizational theory.

University of Detroit Mercy, College of Health Professions, Program in Health Systems Management, Detroit, MI 48221. Offers MSN.

University of Evansville, College of Education and Health Sciences, Department of Nursing and Health Sciences, Evansville, IN 47722. Offers health services administration (MS). Part-time and evening/weekend programs available. *Entrance requirements:* For master's, GRE or GMAT, 2 letters of reference, interview, resume. Additional exam requirements/recommendations for international students: Required—TOEFL (minimum score 71 iBT), IELTS (minimum score 6.5). *Expenses:* Contact institution.

The University of Findlay, Office of Graduate Admissions, Findlay, OH 45840-3653. Offers athletic training (MAT); business (MBA), including health care management, hospitality management, organizational leadership, public management; education (MA Ed), including administration, children's literature, early childhood, human resource development, reading, science, special education, technology; environmental, safety and health management (MSEM); health informatics (MS); occupational therapy (MOT); pharmacy (Pharm D); physical therapy (DPT); physician assistant (MPA); rhetoric and writing (MA); teaching English to speakers of other languages (TESOL) and bilingual education (MA). Part-time and evening/weekend programs available. Postbaccalaureate distance learning degree programs offered (no on-campus study). *Faculty:* 209 full-time

(98 women), 69 part-time/adjunct (38 women). *Students:* 551 full-time (332 women), 457 part-time (276 women); includes 77 minority (37 Black or African American, non-Hispanic/Latino; 1 American Indian or Alaska Native, non-Hispanic/Latino; 15 Asian, non-Hispanic/Latino; 23 Hispanic/Latino; 1 Native Hawaiian or other Pacific Islander, non-Hispanic/Latino), 135 international. Average age 28. 637 applicants, 66% accepted, 241 enrolled. In 2013, 267 master's, 91 doctorates awarded. *Degree requirements:* For master's, thesis, cumulative project, capstone project. *Entrance requirements:* For master's, GRE/GMAT, bachelor's degree from accredited institution, minimum undergraduate GPA of 2.5 in last 64 hours of course work; for doctorate, GRE, minimum cumulative GPA of 3.0. Additional exam requirements/recommendations for international students: Required—TOEFL (minimum score 80 iBT). *Application deadline:* Applications are processed on a rolling basis. Application fee: $25. Electronic applications accepted. *Expenses: Required fees:* $146 per semester. Tuition and fees vary according to degree level and program. *Financial support:* In 2013–14, 11 research assistantships with full and partial tuition reimbursements (averaging $4,000 per year), 10 teaching assistantships with full and partial tuition reimbursements (averaging $3,600 per year) were awarded; career-related internships or fieldwork, Federal Work-Study, health care benefits, and unspecified assistantships also available. Financial award application deadline: 4/1; financial award applicants required to submit FAFSA. *Unit head:* Christopher M. Harris, Director of Admissions, 419-434-4347, E-mail: harrisc1@findlay.edu. *Application contact:* Emily Ickes, Graduate Admissions Counselor, 419-434-6933, Fax: 419-434-4898, E-mail: ickese@findlay.edu.
Website: http://www.findlay.edu/admissions/graduate/Pages/default.aspx

University of Florida, Graduate School, College of Pharmacy and Graduate School, Graduate Programs in Pharmacy, Department of Pharmaceutical Outcomes and Policy, Gainesville, FL 32610. Offers medication therapy management (MSP); pharmaceutical outcomes and policy (MSP, PhD). Part-time programs available. Postbaccalaureate distance learning degree programs offered (minimal on-campus study). *Faculty:* 9 full-time (4 women), 5 part-time/adjunct (3 women). *Students:* 33 full-time (20 women), 142 part-time (88 women); includes 54 minority (26 Black or African American, non-Hispanic/Latino; 1 American Indian or Alaska Native, non-Hispanic/Latino; 19 Asian, non-Hispanic/Latino; 8 Hispanic/Latino), 20 international. Average age 39. 112 applicants, 53% accepted, 51 enrolled. In 2013, 78 master's, 4 doctorates awarded. *Degree requirements:* For doctorate, thesis/dissertation. *Entrance requirements:* For master's, GRE General Test, minimum GPA of 3.0; for doctorate, GRE General Test, minimum GPA of 3.0. Additional exam requirements/recommendations for international students: Required—TOEFL (minimum score 550 paper-based; 80 iBT), IELTS (minimum score 6). *Application deadline:* For fall admission, 1/15 priority date for domestic students. Applications are processed on a rolling basis. Application fee: $30. Electronic applications accepted. *Expenses:* Tuition, state resident: full-time $12,640. Tuition, nonresident: full-time $30,000. *Financial support:* In 2013–14, 18 students received support, including 2 fellowships (averaging $32,625 per year), 1 research assistantship (averaging $16,122 per year), 17 teaching assistantships (averaging $21,910 per year); tuition waivers (full) also available. Financial award applicants required to submit FAFSA. *Faculty research:* Pharmaceutical care, drug use systems, drug-related morbidity. *Unit head:* Richard Segal, PhD, Chair, 352-273-6265, Fax: 352-273-6270, E-mail: segal@cop.health.ufl.edu. *Application contact:* Almut Winterstein, PhD, Professor and Graduate Program Director, 352-273-6258, Fax: 352-273-6270, E-mail: almut@cop.ufl.edu.
Website: http://www.cop.ufl.edu/education/graduate-programs/pharmaceutical-outcomes-and-policy/

University of Florida, Graduate School, College of Public Health and Health Professions, Department of Health Services Research, Management and Policy, Gainesville, FL 32610. Offers health administration (MHA); health services research (PhD). *Accreditation:* CAHME. Part-time programs available. *Faculty:* 5 full-time (2 women), 3 part-time/adjunct (0 women). *Students:* 52 full-time (28 women), 5 part-time (1 woman); includes 15 minority (2 Black or African American, non-Hispanic/Latino; 5 Asian, non-Hispanic/Latino; 8 Hispanic/Latino), 5 international. Average age 29. 108 applicants, 29% accepted, 20 enrolled. In 2013, 22 master's, 6 doctorates awarded. *Degree requirements:* For master's, internship. *Entrance requirements:* For master's and doctorate, GRE General Test, minimum GPA of 3.0. Additional exam requirements/recommendations for international students: Required—TOEFL (minimum score 550 paper-based; 80 iBT), IELTS (minimum score 6). *Application deadline:* For fall admission, 2/1 for domestic students. Applications are processed on a rolling basis. Application fee: $30. Electronic applications accepted. *Expenses:* Tuition, state resident: full-time $12,640. Tuition, nonresident: full-time $30,000. *Financial support:* In 2013–14, 11 students received support, including 7 research assistantships (averaging $16,210 per year), 5 teaching assistantships (averaging $10,045 per year); career-related internships or fieldwork and unspecified assistantships also available. Financial award applicants required to submit FAFSA. *Faculty research:* Hospital profitability, indigent care, rural health care systems, AIDS education, managed care, outcomes. *Unit head:* Dr. Arch G. Mainous, III, Department Chair/Professor, 352-273-6073, Fax: 352-273-6075, E-mail: arch.mainous@phhp.ufl.edu. *Application contact:* Barbara Ross, Student Services Coordinator, 352-273-6074, Fax: 352-273-6075, E-mail: bross@phhp.ufl.edu.
Website: http://www.phhp.ufl.edu/hsrmp/

University of Georgia, College of Public Health, Department of Health Policy and Management, Athens, GA 30602. Offers MPH.

University of Houston–Clear Lake, School of Business, Program in Healthcare Administration, Houston, TX 77058-1002. Offers MHA, MHA/MBA. *Degree requirements:* For master's, thesis optional. *Entrance requirements:* For master's, GMAT. Additional exam requirements/recommendations for international students: Required—TOEFL (minimum score 550 paper-based).

University of Illinois at Chicago, Graduate College, School of Public Health, Division of Health Policy and Administration, Chicago, IL 60607-7128. Offers clinical translational science (MS); health policy (PhD); health policy and administration (Dr PH); health services research (PhD); healthcare (MHA); public health policy management (MPH). Part-time programs available. *Faculty:* 16 full-time (8 women), 17 part-time/adjunct (4 women). *Students:* 114 full-time (77 women), 105 part-time (66 women); includes 106 minority (38 Black or African American, non-Hispanic/Latino; 36 Asian, non-Hispanic/Latino; 23 Hispanic/Latino; 1 Native Hawaiian or other Pacific Islander, non-Hispanic/Latino; 8 Two or more races, non-Hispanic/Latino), 18 international. Average age 31. 480 applicants, 56% accepted, 94 enrolled. In 2013, 97 master's, 3 doctorates awarded. Terminal master's awarded for partial completion of doctoral program. *Degree requirements:* For master's, thesis, field practicum; for doctorate, thesis/dissertation, independent research, internship. *Entrance requirements:* For master's and doctorate, GRE General Test, minimum GPA of 2.75. Additional exam requirements/recommendations for international students: Required—TOEFL. *Application deadline:* For fall admission, 2/1 for domestic students, 1/1 priority date for international students. Application fee: $40 ($50 for international students). Electronic applications accepted. *Expenses:* Tuition, state resident: full-time $11,066; part-time $3689 per term. Tuition, nonresident: full-time $23,064; part-time $7688 per term. *Required fees:* $3004; $1190 per term. Tuition and fees vary according to course level and program. *Financial support:* In 2013–14, 4 fellowships with full tuition reimbursements were awarded; research assistantships with full tuition reimbursements, teaching assistantships with full tuition reimbursements, career-related internships or fieldwork, Federal Work-Study, institutionally sponsored loans, scholarships/grants, traineeships, and unspecified assistantships also available. Support available to part-time students. Financial award application deadline: 3/1; financial award applicants required to submit FAFSA. *Faculty research:* Cancer screening in underserved populations, practices and devices used to reduce firefighter injury, the relationship between communal housing and substance abuse recovery. *Total annual research expenditures:* $1.7 million. *Unit head:* Prof. Jack Zwanziger, Director, 312-996-1062, Fax: 312-996-5356, E-mail: jzwanzig@uic.edu. *Application contact:* Aimee Wiebel, Academic Coordinator, 312-996-7816, Fax: 312-996-5356, E-mail: aimee@uic.edu.
Website: http://publichealth.uic.edu/departments/healthpolicyandadministration/

University of Illinois at Urbana–Champaign, Graduate College, School of Social Work, Champaign, IL 61820. Offers advocacy, leadership, and social change (MSW); children, youth and family services (MSW); health care (MSW); mental health (MSW); school social work (MSW); social work (PhD). *Accreditation:* CSWE (one or more programs are accredited). *Students:* 259 (225 women). *Entrance requirements:* For master's and doctorate, minimum GPA of 3.0. Application fee: $75 ($90 for international students). *Unit head:* Wynne S. Korr, Dean, 217-333-2260, Fax: 217-244-5220, E-mail: wkorr@illinois.edu. *Application contact:* Cheryl M. Street, Admissions and Records Officer, 217-333-2261, Fax: 217-244-5220, E-mail: street@illinois.edu.
Website: http://socialwork.illinois.edu/

The University of Iowa, Graduate College, College of Public Health, Department of Health Management and Policy, Iowa City, IA 52242-1316. Offers MHA, PhD, JD/MHA, MBA/MHA, MHA/MA, MHA/MS. *Accreditation:* CAHME (one or more programs are accredited). *Degree requirements:* For doctorate, comprehensive exam, thesis/dissertation. *Entrance requirements:* For master's, GRE General Test or equivalent, minimum GPA of 3.0; for doctorate, GRE General Test, minimum GPA of 3.0. Additional exam requirements/recommendations for international students: Required—TOEFL (minimum score 550 paper-based; 81 iBT). Electronic applications accepted. *Expenses:* Contact institution.

The University of Kansas, University of Kansas Medical Center, School of Medicine, Department of Health Policy and Management, Kansas City, KS 66160. Offers health policy and management (PhD); health services administration (MHSA); JD/MHSA; MD/MHSA; MHSA/MS. *Accreditation:* CAHME. Part-time programs available. *Faculty:* 12. *Students:* 31 full-time (14 women), 31 part-time (21 women); includes 11 minority (2 Black or African American, non-Hispanic/Latino; 6 Asian, non-Hispanic/Latino; 2 Hispanic/Latino; 1 Two or more races, non-Hispanic/Latino). Average age 32. 57 applicants, 40% accepted, 19 enrolled. In 2013, 18 master's awarded. *Degree requirements:* For master's, internship or research practicum; for doctorate, comprehensive exam, thesis/dissertation. *Entrance requirements:* For master's, college-level statistics; for doctorate, GRE, course work in health delivery system, healthcare finance, health behavior/organizations, healthcare economics, healthcare management, health policy, and graduate statistics. Additional exam requirements/recommendations for international students: Required—TOEFL. *Application deadline:* For fall admission, 3/1 for domestic and international students. Applications are processed on a rolling basis. Application fee: $60. Electronic applications accepted. *Financial support:* Research assistantships with full tuition reimbursements, teaching assistantships with full tuition reimbursements, career-related internships or fieldwork, and departmental scholarships available. Financial award application deadline: 3/1; financial award applicants required to submit FAFSA. *Faculty research:* Economic analysis of long-term care facilities, healthcare workforce supply and demand, tele-medicine, impacts of Affordable Care Act and Medicaid reforms, gender issues in health roles and functions. *Total annual research expenditures:* $23,000. *Unit head:* Dr. Glendon G. Cox, Chair, 913-588-0357, Fax: 913-588-8236, E-mail: gcox@kumc.edu. *Application contact:* Deborah S. Lewis, Student Support Manager, 913-588-3763, Fax: 913-588-8236, E-mail: dlewis4@kumc.edu.
Website: http://www.kumc.edu/school-of-medicine/hpm.html

University of Kentucky, Graduate School, Program in Health Administration, Lexington, KY 40506-0032. Offers MHA. *Accreditation:* CAHME. *Degree requirements:* For master's, comprehensive exam. *Entrance requirements:* For master's, GRE General Test, minimum undergraduate GPA of 2.75. Additional exam requirements/recommendations for international students: Required—TOEFL (minimum score 550 paper-based). Electronic applications accepted. *Faculty research:* Health economy, health finance, health policy.

University of La Verne, College of Business and Public Management, Graduate Programs in Business Administration, La Verne, CA 91750-4443. Offers accounting (MBA); executive management (MBA-EP); finance (MBA, MBA-EP); health services management (MBA); information technology (MBA, MBA-EP); international business (MBA, MBA-EP); leadership (MBA-EP); managed care (MBA); management (MBA, MBA-EP); marketing (MBA, MBA-EP). Part-time and evening/weekend programs available. *Faculty:* 22 full-time (9 women), 37 part-time/adjunct (10 women). *Students:* 793 full-time (356 women), 164 part-time (80 women); includes 153 minority (17 Black or African American, non-Hispanic/Latino; 21 Asian, non-Hispanic/Latino; 110 Hispanic/Latino; 5 Two or more races, non-Hispanic/Latino), 691 international. Average age 27. In 2013, 514 master's awarded. *Entrance requirements:* For master's, GMAT, MAT, or GRE, minimum undergraduate GPA of 3.0, 2 letters of recommendation, resume, statement of purpose. Additional exam requirements/recommendations for international students: Required—TOEFL (minimum score 550 paper-based; 85 iBT). *Application deadline:* Applications are processed on a rolling basis. Application fee: $50. *Expenses:* Contact institution. *Financial support:* Career-related internships or fieldwork, institutionally sponsored loans, and scholarships/grants available. Financial award application deadline: 3/2; financial award applicants required to submit FAFSA. *Unit head:* Dr. Abe Helou, Chairperson, 909-593-3511 Ext. 4211, Fax: 909-392-2704, E-mail: ihelou@laverne.edu. *Application contact:* Rina Lazarian-Chehab, Senior Associate Director of Graduate Admissions, 909-593-3511 Ext. 4317, Fax: 909-392-2704, E-mail: rlazarian@laverne.edu.

University of La Verne, College of Business and Public Management, Program in Gerontology, La Verne, CA 91750-4443. Offers business administration (MS); gerontology (MS, Certificate); gerontology administration (MS); health services management (MS). Part-time programs available. *Faculty:* 1 (woman) full-time, 3 part-time/adjunct (2 women). *Students:* 15 full-time (all women), 16 part-time (12 women); includes 18 minority (5 Black or African American, non-Hispanic/Latino; 13 Hispanic/Latino), 3 international. Average age 40. In 2013, 10 master's awarded. *Entrance requirements:* For master's, minimum GPA of 2.5, 2 recommendations, personal statement. Additional exam requirements/recommendations for international students: Required—TOEFL (minimum score 550 paper-based). *Application deadline:* Applications are processed on a rolling basis. Application fee: $50. *Expenses:* Contact institution. *Financial support:* Institutionally sponsored loans available. Financial award application deadline: 3/2; financial award applicants required to submit FAFSA. *Unit head:* Dr. Kathy Duncan, Program Director, 909-593-3511 Ext. 4796, E-mail: tford@

laverne.edu. *Application contact:* Barbara Cox, Program and Admissions Specialist, 909-593-3511 Ext. 4004, Fax: 909-392-2761, E-mail: bcox@laverne.edu.
Website: http://www.laverne.edu/business-and-public-administration/healthadmin-gerontology/

University of La Verne, College of Business and Public Management, Program in Health Administration, La Verne, CA 91750-4443. Offers financial management (MHA); health information systems (MHA); human resource management (MHA); managed care (MHA); management and leadership (MHA); marketing and business development (MHA). Part-time programs available. *Faculty:* 3 full-time (1 woman), 5 part-time/adjunct (1 woman). *Students:* 43 full-time (31 women), 35 part-time (20 women); includes 29 minority (9 Black or African American, non-Hispanic/Latino; 9 Asian, non-Hispanic/Latino; 11 Hispanic/Latino), 13 international. Average age 31. In 2013, 31 master's awarded. *Entrance requirements:* For master's, minimum undergraduate GPA of 2.5, 3 letters of reference, curriculum vitae or resume, writing sample. Additional exam requirements/recommendations for international students: Required—TOEFL (minimum score 550 paper-based). *Application deadline:* Applications are processed on a rolling basis. Application fee: $50. *Expenses:* Contact institution. *Financial support:* Application deadline: 3/2; applicants required to submit FAFSA. *Unit head:* Dr. Kathy Duncan, Program Chairperson, 909-593-3511 Ext. 4415, E-mail: kduncan2@laverne.edu. *Application contact:* Barbara Cox, Program and Admissions Specialist, 909-593-3511 Ext. 4004, Fax: 909-392-2761, E-mail: bcox@laverne.edu.
Website: http://www.laverne.edu/business-and-public-administration/healthadmin-gerontology/

University of La Verne, Regional and Online Campuses, Graduate Programs, Central Coast/Vandenberg Air Force Base Campuses, La Verne, CA 91750-4443. Offers business administration for experienced professionals (MBA), including health services management, information technology; education (special emphasis) (M Ed); educational counseling (MS); educational leadership (M Ed); multiple subject (elementary) (Credential); preliminary administrative services (Credential); pupil personnel services (Credential); single subject (secondary) (Credential). Part-time programs available. *Faculty:* 11 part-time/adjunct (2 women). *Students:* 17 full-time (7 women), 34 part-time (22 women); includes 15 minority (1 Black or African American, non-Hispanic/Latino; 1 American Indian or Alaska Native, non-Hispanic/Latino; 1 Asian, non-Hispanic/Latino; 10 Hispanic/Latino; 2 Two or more races, non-Hispanic/Latino). Average age 38. In 2013, 25 master's awarded. *Application deadline:* Applications are processed on a rolling basis. Application fee: $50. *Expenses:* Contact institution. *Financial support:* Institutionally sponsored loans available. Financial award application deadline: 3/2; financial award applicants required to submit FAFSA. *Unit head:* Kitt Vincent, Director, Central Coast Campus, 805-788-6202, Fax: 805-788-6201, E-mail: kvincent@laverne.edu. *Application contact:* Gene Teal, Admissions, 805-788-6205, Fax: 805-788-6201, E-mail: eteal@laverne.edu.
Website: http://www.laverne.edu/locations

University of La Verne, Regional and Online Campuses, Graduate Programs, Inland Empire Campus, Ontario, CA 91761. Offers business administration (MBA, MBA-EP), including accounting (MBA), finance (MBA), health services management (MBA-EP), information technology (MBA-EP), international business (MBA), managed care (MBA), management and leadership (MBA-EP), marketing (MBA-EP), supply chain management (MBA); leadership and management (MS), including human resource management, nonprofit management, organizational development. Part-time and evening/weekend programs available. *Faculty:* 1 full-time (0 women), 14 part-time/adjunct (6 women). *Students:* 26 full-time (15 women), 106 part-time (65 women); includes 92 minority (15 Black or African American, non-Hispanic/Latino; 29 Asian, non-Hispanic/Latino; 43 Hispanic/Latino; 1 Native Hawaiian or other Pacific Islander, non-Hispanic/Latino; 4 Two or more races, non-Hispanic/Latino). Average age 37. In 2013, 49 master's awarded. *Application deadline:* Applications are processed on a rolling basis. Application fee: $50. *Expenses:* Contact institution. *Financial support:* Institutionally sponsored loans available. Financial award application deadline: 3/2; financial award applicants required to submit FAFSA. *Unit head:* Allen Stout, Campus Director, Inland Empire Regional Campus in Ontario, 909-937-6987, E-mail: astout@laverne.edu. *Application contact:* Karen Schumann, Senior Associate Director of Admissions, Inland Empire Regional Campus in Ontario, 909-937-6991, E-mail: kschumann@laverne.edu.
Website: http://laverne.edu/locations/inland-empire/

University of La Verne, Regional and Online Campuses, Graduate Programs, Kern County Campus, Bakersfield, CA 93301. Offers business administration for experienced professionals (MBA-EP); education (special emphasis) (M Ed); educational counseling (MS); educational leadership (M Ed); health administration (MHA); leadership and management (MS); mild/moderate education specialist preliminary (Credential); multiple subject (elementary) (Credential); organizational leadership (Ed D); preliminary administrative services (Credential); single subject (secondary) (Credential); special education studies (MS). Part-time and evening/weekend programs available. *Faculty:* 2 part-time/adjunct (1 woman). *Students:* 1 (woman) full-time, 5 part-time (3 women); includes 4 minority (3 Hispanic/Latino; 1 Two or more races, non-Hispanic/Latino). Average age 36. In 2013, 4 master's awarded. *Application deadline:* Applications are processed on a rolling basis. Application fee: $50. *Expenses:* Contact institution. *Financial support:* Institutionally sponsored loans available. Financial award application deadline: 3/2; financial award applicants required to submit FAFSA. *Unit head:* Nora Dominguez, Regional Campus Director, 661-861-6802, E-mail: ndominguez@laverne.edu. *Application contact:* Regina Benavides, Associate Director of Admissions, 661-861-6807, E-mail: rbenavides@laverne.edu.
Website: http://laverne.edu/locations/bakersfield/

University of La Verne, Regional and Online Campuses, Graduate Programs, Orange County Campus, Irvine, CA 92606. Offers business administration for experienced professionals (MBA); educational counseling (MS); educational leadership (M Ed); health administration (MHA); leadership and management (MS); preliminary administrative services (Credential); pupil personnel services (Credential). Part-time programs available. *Faculty:* 3 full-time (all women), 12 part-time/adjunct (3 women). *Students:* 38 full-time (21 women), 78 part-time (36 women); includes 69 minority (7 Black or African American, non-Hispanic/Latino; 1 American Indian or Alaska Native, non-Hispanic/Latino; 19 Asian, non-Hispanic/Latino; 40 Hispanic/Latino; 1 Native Hawaiian or other Pacific Islander, non-Hispanic/Latino; 1 Two or more races, non-Hispanic/Latino). Average age 37. In 2013, 30 master's awarded. *Application deadline:* Applications are processed on a rolling basis. Application fee: $50. *Expenses:* Contact institution. *Financial support:* Institutionally sponsored loans available. Financial award application deadline: 3/2; financial award applicants required to submit FAFSA. *Unit head:* Pam Bergovoy, Director, Center for Educators, 909-448-4953, E-mail: pbergovoy@laverne.edu. *Application contact:* Alison Rodriguez-Balles, Associate Director of Admissions, 714-505-6943, E-mail: arodriguez2@laverne.edu.
Website: http://laverne.edu/locations/irvine/

University of Louisville, Graduate School, College of Business, MBA Programs, Louisville, KY 40292-0001. Offers entrepreneurship (MBA); global business (MBA); health sector management (MBA). *Accreditation:* AACSB. Part-time and evening/weekend programs available. *Students:* 202 full-time (65 women), 42 part-time (15 women); includes 21 minority (9 Black or African American, non-Hispanic/Latino; 1 American Indian or Alaska Native, non-Hispanic/Latino; 7 Asian, non-Hispanic/Latino; 3 Hispanic/Latino; 1 Two or more races, non-Hispanic/Latino), 38 international. Average age 29. 314 applicants, 42% accepted, 116 enrolled. In 2013, 61 master's awarded. *Degree requirements:* For master's, international learning experience. *Entrance requirements:* For master's, GMAT, 2 letters of reference, personal interview, resume, personal statement, college transcript(s). Additional exam requirements/recommendations for international students: Required—TOEFL (minimum score 83 iBT). *Application deadline:* For fall admission, 7/1 for domestic students; for spring admission, 12/1 for domestic students. Applications are processed on a rolling basis. Application fee: $60. *Expenses:* Tuition, state resident: full-time $10,788; part-time $599 per credit hour. Tuition, nonresident: full-time $22,446; part-time $1247 per credit hour. *Required fees:* $196. Tuition and fees vary according to program and reciprocity agreements. *Financial support:* Fellowships with full tuition reimbursements, research assistantships with full tuition reimbursements, health care benefits, and unspecified assistantships available. Financial award application deadline: 3/31; financial award applicants required to submit FAFSA. *Faculty research:* Entrepreneurship, venture capital, retailing/franchising, corporate governance and leadership, supply chain management. *Unit head:* Dr. Carolyn M. Callahan, Dean, 502-852-6440, Fax: 502-852-7557, E-mail: cmcall04@louisville.edu. *Application contact:* Susan E. Hildebrand, Program Director, 502-852-7257, Fax: 502-852-4901, E-mail: s.hildebrand@louisville.edu.
Website: http://business.louisville.edu/mba

University of Louisville, Graduate School, School of Public Health and Information Sciences, Department of Health Management and Systems Sciences, Louisville, KY 40202. Offers public health sciences - health management (PhD). Part-time programs available. *Degree requirements:* For doctorate, comprehensive exam, thesis/dissertation. *Entrance requirements:* For doctorate, GRE General Test. Additional exam requirements/recommendations for international students: Required—TOEFL (minimum score 600 paper-based; 100 iBT). *Application deadline:* For fall admission, 5/1 for domestic and international students. Application fee: $60. Electronic applications accepted. *Expenses:* Tuition, state resident: full-time $10,788; part-time $599 per credit hour. Tuition, nonresident: full-time $22,446; part-time $1247 per credit hour. *Required fees:* $196. Tuition and fees vary according to program and reciprocity agreements. *Financial support:* Research assistantships with full tuition reimbursements, scholarships/grants, health care benefits, and unspecified assistantships available. Financial award applicants required to submit FAFSA. *Faculty research:* Program evaluation, breast cancer, electronic medical records, children's environmental health, lung injury. *Unit head:* Dr. Robert Esterhay, Department Chair, 502-852-6135, Fax: 502-852-3294, E-mail: robert.esterhay@louisville.edu.
Website: http://louisville.edu/sphis/departments/health-management-systems-science

University of Management and Technology, Program in Health Administration, Arlington, VA 22209. Offers MHA.

University of Mary, Gary Tharaldson School of Business, Bismarck, ND 58504-9652. Offers accountancy (MBA); business administration (MBA); health care (MBA); human resource management (MBA); management (MBA); project management (MPM); strategic leadership (MSSL). Part-time and evening/weekend programs available. *Degree requirements:* For master's, strategic planning seminar. *Entrance requirements:* For master's, minimum GPA of 2.5. Additional exam requirements/recommendations for international students: Required—TOEFL (minimum score 500 paper-based; 71 iBT).

University of Maryland, Baltimore County, Graduate School, College of Arts, Humanities and Social Sciences, Department of Emergency Health Services, Baltimore, MD 21250. Offers administration, planning, and policy (MS); education (MS); emergency health services (MS); emergency management (Postbaccalaureate Certificate); preventive medicine and epidemiology (MS). Part-time and evening/weekend programs available. Postbaccalaureate distance learning degree programs offered (no on-campus study). *Faculty:* 1 full-time (0 women), 9 part-time/adjunct (1 woman). *Students:* 20 full-time (8 women), 21 part-time (10 women); includes 2 minority (both Black or African American, non-Hispanic/Latino), 6 international. Average age 32. 13 applicants, 85% accepted, 10 enrolled. In 2013, 13 master's awarded. *Degree requirements:* For master's, comprehensive exam, thesis (for some programs), capstone project. *Entrance requirements:* For master's, GRE General Test, minimum GPA of 3.0. Additional exam requirements/recommendations for international students: Required—TOEFL (minimum score 85 iBT). *Application deadline:* For fall admission, 7/1 for domestic students, 4/1 for international students; for spring admission, 10/15 for domestic students, 9/1 for international students. Applications are processed on a rolling basis. Application fee: $50. Electronic applications accepted. One-time fee: $200 full-time. *Financial support:* In 2013–14, 2 students received support, including 1 fellowship with tuition reimbursement available (averaging $70,000 per year), 1 research assistantship with tuition reimbursement available (averaging $21,000 per year); career-related internships or fieldwork, Federal Work-Study, scholarships/grants, health care benefits, and unspecified assistantships also available. Financial award application deadline: 5/30; financial award applicants required to submit FAFSA. *Faculty research:* EMS management, disaster health services, emergency management. *Total annual research expenditures:* $50,000. *Unit head:* Dr. Bruce Walz, Chairman, 410-455-3223. *Application contact:* Dr. Rick Bissell, Program Director, 410-455-3776, Fax: 410-455-3045, E-mail: bissell@umbc.edu.
Website: http://ehs.umbc.edu/

University of Maryland, Baltimore County, Graduate School, College of Arts, Humanities and Social Sciences, Department of Public Policy, Program in Public Policy, Baltimore, MD 21250. Offers economics (PhD); educational policy (MPP, PhD); evaluation and analytical methods (MPP, PhD); health policy (MPP, PhD); policy history (PhD); public management (MPP, PhD); urban policy (MPP, PhD). Part-time and evening/weekend programs available. *Faculty:* 10 full-time (2 women). *Students:* 60 full-time (35 women), 76 part-time (41 women); includes 29 minority (15 Black or African American, non-Hispanic/Latino; 8 Asian, non-Hispanic/Latino; 3 Hispanic/Latino; 1 Native Hawaiian or other Pacific Islander, non-Hispanic/Latino; 2 Two or more races, non-Hispanic/Latino), 13 international. Average age 36. 91 applicants, 55% accepted, 22 enrolled. In 2013, 11 master's, 8 doctorates awarded. Terminal master's awarded for partial completion of doctoral program. *Degree requirements:* For master's, thesis optional, public analysis paper, internship for pre-service students; for doctorate, comprehensive exam, thesis/dissertation, comprehensive and field qualifying exams. *Entrance requirements:* For master's and doctorate, GRE General Test, 3 academic letters of reference, transcripts, resume, research paper. Additional exam requirements/recommendations for international students: Required—TOEFL (minimum score 550 paper-based; 80 iBT). *Application deadline:* For fall admission, 1/15 priority date for domestic students, 1/1 priority date for international students; for spring admission, 11/1 priority date for domestic students, 5/1 priority date for international students. Applications are processed on a rolling basis. Application fee: $50. Electronic applications accepted. One-time fee: $200 full-time. *Financial support:* In 2013–14, 26 students received support, including 4 fellowships with full tuition reimbursements available (averaging $12,000 per year), 23 research assistantships with full tuition reimbursements available (averaging $20,000 per year), 1 teaching assistantship with

full tuition reimbursement available (averaging $20,000 per year); career-related internships or fieldwork, Federal Work-Study, scholarships/grants, health care benefits, and unspecified assistantships also available. Support available to part-time students. Financial award application deadline: 1/15; financial award applicants required to submit FAFSA. *Faculty research:* Health policy, education policy, urban policy, public management, evaluation and analytical methods. *Unit head:* Dr. Donald F. Norris, Chair, 410-455-1455, E-mail: norris@umbc.edu. *Application contact:* Sally F. Helms, Administrator of Academic Affairs, 410-455-3202, Fax: 410-455-1172, E-mail: gradposi@umbc.edu.
Website: http://www.umbc.edu/pubpol

University of Maryland, Baltimore County, Graduate School, Erickson School of Aging Studies, Baltimore, MD 21228. Offers management of aging services (MA). *Faculty:* 3 full-time (0 women), 4 part-time/adjunct (0 women). *Students:* 13 full-time (7 women); includes 4 minority (1 Black or African American, non-Hispanic/Latino; 2 Asian, non-Hispanic/Latino; 1 Hispanic/Latino). Average age 38. 24 applicants, 75% accepted, 13 enrolled. In 2013, 11 master's awarded. *Degree requirements:* For master's, thesis or alternative. *Entrance requirements:* For master's, essays. *Application deadline:* Applications are processed on a rolling basis. Application fee: $50. Electronic applications accepted. *Expenses:* Contact institution. *Financial support:* In 2013–14, 8 students received support, including 1 teaching assistantship with tuition reimbursement available (averaging $21,600 per year). Financial award applicants required to submit FAFSA. *Faculty research:* Policy implications of entitlement programs, demographic impact of aging population, person-centered care for dementia, changing culture in long-term care. *Unit head:* Dr. Joseph Gribbin, Graduate Program Director, 443-543-5603, E-mail: gribbin@umbc.edu. *Application contact:* Michelle Howell, Administrative Assistant, 443-543-5607, E-mail: mhowell@umbc.edu.
Website: http://www.umbc.edu/erickson/

University of Maryland, College Park, Academic Affairs, School of Public Health, Department of Health Services Administration, College Park, MD 20742. Offers MHA, PhD. *Faculty:* 14 full-time (8 women), 12 part-time/adjunct (8 women). *Students:* 43 full-time (35 women), 25 part-time (20 women); includes 36 minority (21 Black or African American, non-Hispanic/Latino; 12 Asian, non-Hispanic/Latino; 3 Hispanic/Latino), 2 international. 144 applicants, 48% accepted, 43 enrolled. In 2013, 6 master's, 2 doctorates awarded. *Application deadline:* For fall admission, 1/15 for domestic and international students; for spring admission, 6/1 for international students. Application fee: $75. *Expenses:* Tuition, state resident: full-time $10,314; part-time $573 per credit hour. Tuition, nonresident: full-time $22,248; part-time $1236 per credit. *Required fees:* $1446; $403.15 per semester. Tuition and fees vary according to program. *Financial support:* In 2013–14, 3 fellowships with full and partial tuition reimbursements (averaging $13,333 per year), 7 teaching assistantships (averaging $15,455 per year) were awarded. *Total annual research expenditures:* $1.3 million. *Unit head:* Dr. Laura Wilson, Chair, 301-405-2469, E-mail: lwilson@umd.edu. *Application contact:* Dr. Charles A. Caramello, Dean of Graduate School, 301-405-0358, Fax: 301-314-9305, E-mail: ccaramel@umd.edu.

University of Maryland University College, Graduate School of Management and Technology, Program in Health Care Administration, Adelphi, MD 20783. Offers MS, Certificate. Part-time and evening/weekend programs available. Postbaccalaureate distance learning degree programs offered (no on-campus study). *Students:* 18 full-time (15 women), 504 part-time (390 women); includes 321 minority (241 Black or African American, non-Hispanic/Latino; 36 Asian, non-Hispanic/Latino; 27 Hispanic/Latino; 2 Native Hawaiian or other Pacific Islander, non-Hispanic/Latino; 15 Two or more races, non-Hispanic/Latino), 16 international. Average age 36. 183 applicants, 100% accepted, 107 enrolled. In 2013, 130 master's awarded. *Degree requirements:* For master's, thesis or alternative. *Application deadline:* Applications are processed on a rolling basis. Application fee: $50. Electronic applications accepted. *Financial support:* Federal Work-Study and scholarships/grants available. Support available to part-time students. Financial award application deadline: 6/1; financial award applicants required to submit FAFSA. *Unit head:* Dr. Diane Bartoo, Head, 240-684-2400, Fax: 240-684-2401, E-mail: diane.bartoo@umuc.edu. *Application contact:* Coordinator, Graduate Admissions, 800-888-8682, Fax: 240-684-2151, E-mail: newgrad@umuc.edu.
Website: http://www.umuc.edu/grad/hcad/hcad_home.shtml

University of Massachusetts Amherst, Graduate School, Isenberg School of Management, Program in Management, Amherst, MA 01003. Offers accounting (PhD); business administration (MBA); entrepreneurship (MBA); finance (MBA, PhD); healthcare administration (MBA); hospitality and tourism management (PhD); management science (PhD); marketing (MBA, PhD); organization studies (PhD); sport management (PhD); strategic management (PhD); MBA/MS. *Accreditation:* AACSB. Part-time and evening/weekend programs available. Postbaccalaureate distance learning degree programs offered. *Faculty:* 68 full-time (14 women). *Students:* 140 full-time (59 women), 1,127 part-time (319 women); includes 229 minority (24 Black or African American, non-Hispanic/Latino; 2 American Indian or Alaska Native, non-Hispanic/Latino; 135 Asian, non-Hispanic/Latino; 51 Hispanic/Latino; 6 Native Hawaiian or other Pacific Islander, non-Hispanic/Latino; 11 Two or more races, non-Hispanic/Latino), 131 international. Average age 36. 828 applicants, 56% accepted, 351 enrolled. In 2013, 361 master's, 12 doctorates awarded. Terminal master's awarded for partial completion of doctoral program. *Degree requirements:* For doctorate, comprehensive exam, thesis/dissertation. *Entrance requirements:* For master's and doctorate, GMAT or GRE General Test. Additional exam requirements/recommendations for international students: Required—TOEFL (minimum score 550 paper-based; 80 iBT), IELTS (minimum score 6.5). *Application deadline:* For fall admission, 1/20 for domestic and international students. Applications are processed on a rolling basis. Application fee: $75. Electronic applications accepted. *Financial support:* Fellowships with full and partial tuition reimbursements, research assistantships with full and partial tuition reimbursements, teaching assistantships with full and partial tuition reimbursements, career-related internships or fieldwork, Federal Work-Study, scholarships/grants, traineeships, health care benefits, tuition waivers (full and partial), and unspecified assistantships available. Support available to part-time students. Financial award application deadline: 1/20; financial award applicants required to submit FAFSA. *Unit head:* Dr. John Wells, Chair, 413-545-7609, Fax: 413-577-2234. *Application contact:* Lindsay DeSantis, Supervisor of Admissions, 413-545-0722, Fax: 413-577-0010, E-mail: gradadm@grad.umass.edu.
Website: http://www.isenberg.umass.edu/

University of Massachusetts Amherst, Graduate School, School of Public Health and Health Sciences, Department of Public Health, Amherst, MA 01003. Offers biostatistics (MPH, MS, PhD); community health education (MPH, MS, PhD); environmental health sciences (MPH, MS, PhD); epidemiology (MPH, MS, PhD); health policy and management (MPH, MS, PhD); nutrition (MPH, PhD); public health practice (MPH); MPH/MPPA. *Accreditation:* CEPH (one or more programs are accredited). Part-time and evening/weekend programs available. Postbaccalaureate distance learning degree programs offered (no on-campus study). *Faculty:* 53 full-time (29 women). *Students:* 117 full-time (83 women), 271 part-time (213 women); includes 89 minority (34 Black or African American, non-Hispanic/Latino; 23 Asian, non-Hispanic/Latino; 25 Hispanic/Latino; 7 Two or more races, non-Hispanic/Latino), 45 international. Average age 36. 359 applicants, 69% accepted, 94 enrolled. In 2013, 120 master's, 1 doctorate awarded. Terminal master's awarded for partial completion of doctoral program. *Degree requirements:* For master's, thesis (for some programs); for doctorate, comprehensive exam, thesis/dissertation. *Entrance requirements:* For master's and doctorate, GRE General Test. Additional exam requirements/recommendations for international students: Required—TOEFL (minimum score 550 paper-based; 80 iBT), IELTS (minimum score 6.5). *Application deadline:* For fall admission, 2/1 for domestic and international students. Applications are processed on a rolling basis. Application fee: $75. Electronic applications accepted. *Financial support:* Fellowships with full and partial tuition reimbursements, research assistantships with full and partial tuition reimbursements, teaching assistantships with full and partial tuition reimbursements, career-related internships or fieldwork, Federal Work-Study, scholarships/grants, traineeships, health care benefits, tuition waivers (full and partial), and unspecified assistantships available. Support available to part-time students. Financial award application deadline: 2/1; financial award applicants required to submit FAFSA. *Unit head:* Dr. Paula Stamps, Graduate Program Director, 413-545-2861, Fax: 413-545-1645. *Application contact:* Lindsay DeSantis, Supervisor of Admissions, 413-545-0722, Fax: 413-577-0010, E-mail: gradadm@grad.umass.edu.
Website: http://www.umass.edu/sphhs/public_health/

University of Massachusetts Boston, Office of Graduate Studies, John W. McCormack Graduate School of Policy and Global Studies, Program in Gerontology, Boston, MA 02125-3393. Offers gerontology (MS, PhD, Certificate); gerontology research (MA); management in aging services (MA). Part-time programs available. *Degree requirements:* For doctorate, comprehensive exam, thesis/dissertation. *Entrance requirements:* For doctorate, GRE General Test, minimum GPA of 3.0. *Faculty research:* Aging with a chronic disability, pension policy and social security system, elderly minorities, health services research, living arrangements.

University of Massachusetts Lowell, College of Health Sciences, Department of Community Health and Sustainability, Lowell, MA 01854-2881. Offers health management and policy (MS, Graduate Certificate). Part-time programs available. *Degree requirements:* For master's, thesis optional. *Entrance requirements:* For master's, GRE General Test. *Faculty research:* Alzheimer's disease, total quality management systems, information systems, market analysis.

University of Memphis, Graduate School, School of Public Health, Memphis, TN 38152. Offers biostatistics (MPH); environmental health (MPH); epidemiology (MPH); health systems management (MPH); public health (MHA); social and behavioral sciences (MPH). Part-time and evening/weekend programs available. Postbaccalaureate distance learning degree programs offered. *Faculty:* 14 full-time (2 women), 5 part-time/adjunct (1 woman). *Students:* 64 full-time (42 women), 36 part-time (24 women); includes 34 minority (21 Black or African American, non-Hispanic/Latino; 6 Asian, non-Hispanic/Latino; 5 Hispanic/Latino; 2 Two or more races, non-Hispanic/Latino), 15 international. Average age 32. 102 applicants, 51% accepted, 24 enrolled. In 2013, 17 master's awarded. *Degree requirements:* For master's, comprehensive exam, thesis. *Entrance requirements:* For master's, GRE, letters of recommendation. Additional exam requirements/recommendations for international students: Required—TOEFL. *Application deadline:* For fall admission, 4/1 for domestic students; for spring admission, 11/1 for domestic students. Application fee: $35 ($60 for international students). Electronic applications accepted. *Financial support:* In 2013–14, 46 students received support. Research assistantships with full tuition reimbursements available, Federal Work-Study, scholarships/grants, and unspecified assistantships available. Financial award application deadline: 2/15; financial award applicants required to submit FAFSA. *Faculty research:* Health and medical savings accounts, adoption rates, health informatics, Telehealth technologies, biostatistics, environmental health, epidemiology, health systems management, social and behavioral sciences. *Unit head:* Dr. Lisa M. Klesges, Director, 901-678-4637, E-mail: lmklsges@memphis.edu. *Application contact:* Dr. Karen Weddle-West, Information Contact, 901-678-2531, Fax: 901-678-5023, E-mail: gradsch@memphis.edu.
Website: http://www.memphis.edu/sph/

University of Michigan, School of Public Health, Department of Health Management and Policy, Ann Arbor, MI 48109. Offers health management and policy (MHSA, MPH, MS); health services organization and policy (PhD); JD/MHSA; MD/MPH; MHSA/MBA; MHSA/MNA; MHSA/MPP; MHSA/MSIOE; MPH/JD; MPH/MBA; MPH/MPP. PhD and MS offered through the Horace H. Rackham School of Graduate Studies. *Accreditation:* CAHME (one or more programs are accredited). *Degree requirements:* For doctorate, thesis/dissertation, oral defense of dissertation, preliminary exam. *Entrance requirements:* For master's, GMAT, GRE General Test; for doctorate, GRE General Test. Additional exam requirements/recommendations for international students: Required—TOEFL (minimum score 600 paper-based; 100 iBT). Electronic applications accepted. Tuition and fees vary according to course level, course load, degree level, program and student level. *Faculty research:* Health insurance, long-term care and aging, tobacco policy, health information technology, understanding organization.

University of Michigan–Flint, Graduate Programs, Program in Public Administration, Flint, MI 48502-1950. Offers administration of non-profit agencies (MPA); criminal justice administration (MPA); educational administration (MPA); healthcare administration (MPA). Part-time programs available. *Faculty:* 6 full-time (2 women), 12 part-time/adjunct (4 women). *Students:* 16 full-time (6 women), 112 part-time (74 women); includes 34 minority (24 Black or African American, non-Hispanic/Latino; 1 American Indian or Alaska Native, non-Hispanic/Latino; 1 Asian, non-Hispanic/Latino; 5 Hispanic/Latino; 3 Two or more races, non-Hispanic/Latino), 4 international. Average age 33. 75 applicants, 65% accepted, 44 enrolled. In 2013, 59 master's awarded. *Degree requirements:* For master's, thesis or alternative, internship. *Entrance requirements:* For master's, minimum GPA of 3.0, 1 course each in American government, microeconomics and statistics. Additional exam requirements/recommendations for international students: Required—TOEFL (minimum score 560 paper-based; 84 iBT), IELTS (minimum score 6.5). *Application deadline:* For fall admission, 8/1 for domestic students, 5/1 for international students; for winter admission, 11/15 for domestic students, 9/1 for international students; for spring admission, 3/15 for domestic students, 1/1 for international students; for summer admission, 5/15 for domestic students. Applications are processed on a rolling basis. Application fee: $55. Electronic applications accepted. *Expenses:* Contact institution. *Financial support:* Career-related internships or fieldwork, Federal Work-Study, and scholarships/grants available. Support available to part-time students. Financial award application deadline: 3/1; financial award applicants required to submit FAFSA. *Unit head:* Dr. Kathryn Schellenberg, Director, 810-762-3340, E-mail: kathsch@umflint.edu. *Application contact:* Bradley T. Maki, Director of Graduate Admissions, 810-762-3171, Fax: 810-766-6789, E-mail: bmaki@umflint.edu.
Website: http://www.umflint.edu/graduateprograms/public-administration-mpa

University of Michigan–Flint, School of Health Professions and Studies, Flint, MI 48502-1950. Offers anesthesia (MS, DrAP); health education (MS); nursing (MSN, DNP, Certificate), including family nurse practitioner (MSN), nursing (Certificate), nursing practice (DNP); physical therapy (DPT, PhD), including entry-level (DPT), physical therapy (PhD), transitional (DPT); public health (MPH), including health administration, health education. Part-time programs available. *Faculty:* 30 full-time (25 women), 23

part-time/adjunct (17 women). *Students:* 338 full-time (243 women), 204 part-time (155 women); includes 86 minority (37 Black or African American, non-Hispanic/Latino; 3 American Indian or Alaska Native, non-Hispanic/Latino; 21 Asian, non-Hispanic/Latino; 13 Hispanic/Latino; 1 Native Hawaiian or other Pacific Islander, non-Hispanic/Latino; 11 Two or more races, non-Hispanic/Latino), 34 international. Average age 33. 711 applicants, 30% accepted, 198 enrolled. In 2013, 40 master's, 73 doctorates awarded. *Entrance requirements:* Additional exam requirements/recommendations for international students: Required—TOEFL (minimum score 560 paper-based; 84 iBT), IELTS (minimum score 6.5). *Application deadline:* For fall admission, 8/1 priority date for domestic students, 5/1 priority date for international students; for winter admission, 11/15 priority date for domestic students, 9/1 priority date for international students; for spring admission, 3/15 priority date for domestic students, 1/1 priority date for international students. Application fee: $55. Electronic applications accepted. *Expenses:* Contact institution. *Financial support:* Career-related internships or fieldwork, Federal Work-Study, scholarships/grants, and traineeships available. Support available to part-time students. Financial award application deadline: 3/1; financial award applicants required to submit FAFSA. *Faculty research:* Male colorectal cancer, Flint health careers, auditory stimulation, nurse preparation training, healthy aging and physical therapy. *Unit head:* Dr. David Gordon, Dean, 810-237-6503, Fax: 810-237-6532, E-mail: dgordon@umflint.edu. *Application contact:* Brad T. Maki, Executive Secretary, 810-762-3171, Fax: 810-766-6789, E-mail: bmaki@umflint.edu.
Website: http://www.umflint.edu/shps/

University of Michigan–Flint, School of Management, Flint, MI 48502-1950. Offers accounting (MBA, MSA); business (Graduate Certificate); computer information systems (MBA); finance (MBA); health care management (MBA); international business (MBA); lean manufacturing (MBA); marketing (MBA); organizational leadership (MBA). *Accreditation:* AACSB. Part-time and evening/weekend programs available. Postbaccalaureate distance learning degree programs offered (minimal on-campus study). *Faculty:* 13 full-time (3 women), 4 part-time/adjunct (0 women). *Students:* 19 full-time (6 women), 234 part-time (72 women); includes 50 minority (21 Black or African American, non-Hispanic/Latino; 5 American Indian or Alaska Native, non-Hispanic/Latino; 12 Asian, non-Hispanic/Latino; 5 Hispanic/Latino; 7 Two or more races, non-Hispanic/Latino), 30 international. Average age 32. 195 applicants, 56% accepted, 88 enrolled. In 2013, 73 master's awarded. *Degree requirements:* For master's, thesis or alternative. *Entrance requirements:* For master's, GMAT or GRE, minimum GPA of 3.0. Additional exam requirements/recommendations for international students: Required—TOEFL (minimum score 560 paper-based; 84 iBT), IELTS (minimum score 6.5). *Application deadline:* For fall admission, 8/1 for domestic students, 5/1 for international students; for winter admission, 11/1 for domestic students, 9/1 for international students; for spring admission, 2/15 for domestic students, 1/15 for international students. Applications are processed on a rolling basis. Application fee: $55. Electronic applications accepted. *Financial support:* Federal Work-Study, scholarships/grants, and unspecified assistantships available. Support available to part-time students. Financial award application deadline: 3/1; financial award applicants required to submit FAFSA. *Unit head:* Dr. Scott Johnson, Dean, School of Management, 810-762-3164, Fax: 810-237-6685, E-mail: scotjohn@umflint.edu. *Application contact:* Jeremiah Cook, Marketing Communications Specialist, 810-424-5583, Fax: 810-766-6789, E-mail: jecook@umflint.edu.
Website: http://www.umflint.edu/som/

University of Minnesota, Twin Cities Campus, Carlson School of Management, Carlson Full-Time MBA Program, Minneapolis, MN 55455. Offers finance (MBA); information technology (MBA); management (MBA); marketing (MBA); medical industry orientation (MBA); supply chain and operations (MBA); JD/MBA; MBA/MPP; MD/MBA; MHA/MBA; Pharm D/MBA. *Accreditation:* AACSB. *Faculty:* 137 full-time (42 women), 16 part-time/adjunct (5 women). *Students:* 222 full-time (62 women); includes 30 minority (2 Black or African American, non-Hispanic/Latino; 17 Asian, non-Hispanic/Latino; 5 Hispanic/Latino; 6 Two or more races, non-Hispanic/Latino), 60 international. Average age 28. 565 applicants, 44% accepted, 113 enrolled. In 2013, 96 master's awarded. *Entrance requirements:* For master's, GMAT or GRE. Additional exam requirements/recommendations for international students: Required—TOEFL (minimum score 580 paper-based; 84 iBT), IELTS (minimum score 7), PTE. *Application deadline:* For fall admission, 4/1 for domestic students, 2/1 for international students. Application fee: $60 ($90 for international students). Electronic applications accepted. *Expenses:* Contact institution. *Financial support:* In 2013–14, 133 students received support, including 133 fellowships with full and partial tuition reimbursements available (averaging $29,445 per year); research assistantships with partial tuition reimbursements available, teaching assistantships with partial tuition reimbursements available, career-related internships or fieldwork, Federal Work-Study, institutionally sponsored loans, scholarships/grants, health care benefits, and unspecified assistantships also available. Financial award application deadline: 4/1; financial award applicants required to submit FAFSA. *Faculty research:* Finance and accounting: financial reporting, asset pricing models and corporate finance; information and decision sciences: on-line auctions, information transparency and recommender systems; marketing: psychological influences on consumer behavior, brand equity, pricing and marketing channels; operations: lean manufacturing, quality management and global supply chains; strategic management and organization: global strategy, networks, entrepreneurship and innovation, sustainability. *Unit head:* Philip J. Miller, Assistant Dean, MBA Programs and Graduate Business Career Center, 612-625-5555, Fax: 612-625-1012, E-mail: mba@umn.edu. *Application contact:* Linh Gilles, Director of Admissions and Recruiting, 612-625-5555, Fax: 612-625-1012, E-mail: ftmba@umn.edu.
Website: http://www.csom.umn.edu/MBA/full-time/

University of Minnesota, Twin Cities Campus, Carlson School of Management, Carlson Part-Time MBA Program, Minneapolis, MN 55455. Offers finance (MBA); information technology (MBA); management (MBA); marketing (MBA); medical industry orientation (MBA); supply chain and operations (MBA). Part-time and evening/weekend programs available. *Faculty:* 137 full-time (42 women), 15 part-time/adjunct (3 women). *Students:* 1,207 part-time (393 women); includes 108 minority (21 Black or African American, non-Hispanic/Latino; 4 American Indian or Alaska Native, non-Hispanic/Latino; 72 Asian, non-Hispanic/Latino; 5 Hispanic/Latino; 1 Native Hawaiian or other Pacific Islander, non-Hispanic/Latino; 5 Two or more races, non-Hispanic/Latino), 66 international. Average age 28. 291 applicants, 86% accepted, 205 enrolled. In 2013, 372 master's awarded. *Entrance requirements:* For master's, GMAT or GRE. Additional exam requirements/recommendations for international students: Required—TOEFL (minimum score 580 paper-based; 84 iBT), IELTS (minimum score 7), PTE. *Application deadline:* For fall admission, 5/1 priority date for domestic and international students; for spring admission, 10/1 priority date for domestic and international students. Applications are processed on a rolling basis. Application fee: $60 ($90 for international students). Electronic applications accepted. *Expenses:* Contact institution. *Financial support:* Applicants required to submit FAFSA. *Faculty research:* Finance and accounting: financial reporting, asset pricing models and corporate finance; information and decision sciences: on-line auctions, information transparency and recommender systems; marketing: psychological influences on consumer behavior, brand equity, pricing and marketing channels; operations: lean manufacturing, quality management and global supply chains; strategic management and organization: global strategy, networks, entrepreneurship and innovation, sustainability. *Unit head:* Philip J. Miller, Assistant Dean, MBA Programs and Graduate Business Career Center, 612-624-2039, Fax: 612-625-1012, E-mail: mba@umn.edu. *Application contact:* Linh Gilles, Director of Admissions and Recruiting, 612-625-5555, Fax: 612-625-1012, E-mail: ptmba@umn.edu.
Website: http://www.carlsonschool.umn.edu/ptmba

University of Minnesota, Twin Cities Campus, Graduate School, Program in Health Informatics, Minneapolis, MN 55455-0213. Offers MHI, MS, PhD, MD/MHI. Part-time programs available. *Degree requirements:* For master's, thesis or alternative; for doctorate, thesis/dissertation. *Entrance requirements:* For master's and doctorate, GRE General Test, previous course work in life sciences, programming, calculus. Additional exam requirements/recommendations for international students: Required—TOEFL (minimum score 550 paper-based). Electronic applications accepted. *Faculty research:* Medical decision making, physiological control systems, population studies, clinical information systems, telemedicine.

University of Minnesota, Twin Cities Campus, School of Public Health, Major in Health Services Research, Policy, and Administration, Minneapolis, MN 55455-0213. Offers MS, PhD, JD/MS, JD/PhD, MD/PhD, MPP/MS. Part-time programs available. Terminal master's awarded for partial completion of doctoral program. *Degree requirements:* For master's, thesis, internship, final oral exam; for doctorate, thesis/dissertation, teaching experience, written preliminary exam, final oral exam, dissertation. *Entrance requirements:* For master's, GRE General Test, course work in mathematics; for doctorate, GRE General Test, prerequisite courses in calculus and statistics. Additional exam requirements/recommendations for international students: Required—TOEFL (minimum score 600 paper-based; 100 iBT). *Faculty research:* Outcomes, economics and statistics, sociology, health care management.

University of Minnesota, Twin Cities Campus, School of Public Health, Major in Public Health Administration and Policy, Minneapolis, MN 55455-0213. Offers MPH, MPH/JD, MPH/MSN. Part-time programs available. *Degree requirements:* For master's, thesis, field experience. *Entrance requirements:* For master's, GRE General Test. Additional exam requirements/recommendations for international students: Required—TOEFL. Electronic applications accepted. *Faculty research:* Community health service organizations, nursing services, dental services, the elderly, insurance coverage.

University of Minnesota, Twin Cities Campus, School of Public Health, Program in Healthcare Administration, Minneapolis, MN 55455-0213. Offers MHA. *Accreditation:* AACSB; CAHME. Part-time and evening/weekend programs available. Postbaccalaureate distance learning degree programs offered (minimal on-campus study). *Degree requirements:* For master's, thesis, project. *Entrance requirements:* For master's, GMAT or GRE General Test, minimum GPA of 3.0. Additional exam requirements/recommendations for international students: Required—TOEFL (minimum score 600 paper-based; 100 iBT). Electronic applications accepted. *Expenses:* Contact institution. *Faculty research:* Managed care, physician payment, structure and performance of healthcare systems, long-term care.

University of Missouri, Graduate School, Department of Health Management and Informatics, Columbia, MO 65211. Offers health administration (MHA); health ethics (Graduate Certificate); health informatics (MS, Graduate Certificate). *Accreditation:* CAHME. Part-time programs available. *Faculty:* 18 full-time (5 women), 2 part-time/adjunct (0 women). *Students:* 100 full-time (47 women), 35 part-time (24 women); includes 26 minority (10 Black or African American, non-Hispanic/Latino; 9 Asian, non-Hispanic/Latino; 3 Hispanic/Latino; 4 Two or more races, non-Hispanic/Latino), 17 international. Average age 30. 61 applicants, 56% accepted, 31 enrolled. In 2013, 53 master's, 10 other advanced degrees awarded. *Entrance requirements:* For master's, GRE General Test or GMAT, minimum GPA of 3.0. Additional exam requirements/recommendations for international students: Required—TOEFL (minimum score 500 paper-based; 61 iBT). *Application deadline:* Applications are processed on a rolling basis. Application fee: $55 ($75 for international students). Electronic applications accepted. *Financial support:* Fellowships, research assistantships, teaching assistantships, institutionally sponsored loans, scholarships/grants, traineeships, health care benefits, and unspecified assistantships available. Support available to part-time students. *Faculty research:* Application of informatics tools to day-to-day clinical operations, consumer health informatics, decision support, health literacy and numeracy, information interventions for persons with chronic illnesses, use of simulation in the education of health care professionals, statistical bioinformatics, classification, dimension reduction, ethics and end of life care, telehealth and tele-ethics, research ethics, health literacy, clinical informatics, human factors. *Unit head:* Dr. Suzanne Boren, Director of Graduate Studies, 573-882-1492, E-mail: borens@missouri.edu. *Application contact:* Veronica Kramer, Coordinator of Student Recruitment and Admissions, 573-884-0698, E-mail: kramerv@missouri.edu.
Website: http://www.hmi.missouri.edu/

University of Missouri, Graduate School, Master of Public Health Program, Columbia, MO 65211. Offers global public health (Graduate Certificate); health promotion and policy (MPH); public health (Graduate Certificate); veterinary public health (MPH); DVM/MPH; MPH/MA; MPH/MPA. *Accreditation:* CEPH. *Students:* 88 full-time (67 women), 104 part-time (83 women); includes 43 minority (19 Black or African American, non-Hispanic/Latino; 9 Asian, non-Hispanic/Latino; 10 Hispanic/Latino; 5 Two or more races, non-Hispanic/Latino), 16 international. Average age 30. 133 applicants, 84% accepted, 79 enrolled. In 2013, 40 master's, 49 other advanced degrees awarded. *Entrance requirements:* Additional exam requirements/recommendations for international students: Required—TOEFL (minimum score 550 paper-based; 80 iBT). *Application deadline:* For fall admission, 6/30 priority date for domestic and international students. Applications are processed on a rolling basis. Application fee: $55 ($75 for international students). Electronic applications accepted. *Financial support:* Fellowships with tuition reimbursements, research assistantships with tuition reimbursements, teaching assistantships with tuition reimbursements, scholarships/grants, traineeships, health care benefits, and unspecified assistantships available. Support available to part-time students. *Faculty research:* Health professions, health care equality, global health, communicable diseases, public health; zoonosis and infectious diseases, medical education, inquiry-based learning, social determinants of health, violence against women, health disparities, breast cancer screening, epigenetic, nursing, environmental health, cancer and chronic diseases, environmental exposures with metals, geographical information systems, substance use disorders/addictions, mental health. *Unit head:* Lise Saffran, Interim Director, 573-884-6835, E-mail: saffranl@health.missouri.edu. *Application contact:* Sandra Gummersheimer, Academic Advisor, 573-884-6836, E-mail: gummersheimers@health.missouri.edu.
Website: http://publichealth.missouri.edu/

University of Missouri, School of Medicine and Graduate School, Graduate Programs in Medicine, Columbia, MO 65211. Offers family and community medicine (MS); health administration (MS); medical pharmacology and physiology (MS, PhD); molecular microbiology and immunology (MS, PhD); pathology and anatomical sciences (MS). Part-time programs available. *Faculty:* 71 full-time (16 women), 12 part-time/adjunct (4 women). *Students:* 55 full-time (30 women), 3 part-time (all women); includes 6 minority (4 Black or African American, non-Hispanic/Latino; 1 American Indian or Alaska Native, non-Hispanic/Latino; 1 Hispanic/Latino), 25 international. Average age 28. 73

applicants, 16% accepted, 11 enrolled. In 2013, 1 master's, 13 doctorates awarded. *Degree requirements:* For doctorate, thesis/dissertation. *Entrance requirements:* For master's and doctorate, GRE General Test, minimum GPA of 3.0. Additional exam requirements/recommendations for international students: Required—TOEFL. *Application deadline:* Applications are processed on a rolling basis. Application fee: $55 ($75 for international students). *Expenses:* Contact institution. *Financial support:* Fellowships, research assistantships, teaching assistantships, career-related internships or fieldwork, and institutionally sponsored loans available. *Faculty research:* HIV enzymes, calcium and heart function, gene study and Muscular Dystrophy, military medical training using simulation technology, clinical and translational science. *Unit head:* William M. Crist, Dean Emeritus, 573-884-8733, E-mail: cristwm@missouri.edu. *Application contact:* Charles Rudkin, Graduate Programs Assistant, 573-882-4637, E-mail: rudkinc@health.missouri.edu.
Website: http://som.missouri.edu/departments.shtml

University of Missouri–St. Louis, College of Arts and Sciences, School of Social Work, St. Louis, MO 63121. Offers gerontology (MS, Certificate); long term care administration (Certificate); social work (MSW). *Accreditation:* CSWE. *Faculty:* 10 full-time (8 women), 9 part-time/adjunct (6 women). *Students:* 73 full-time (65 women), 75 part-time (66 women); includes 27 minority (24 Black or African American, non-Hispanic/Latino; 1 Asian, non-Hispanic/Latino; 1 Hispanic/Latino; 1 Two or more races, non-Hispanic/Latino), 1 international. Average age 32. 155 applicants, 51% accepted, 50 enrolled. In 2013, 53 master's awarded. *Entrance requirements:* For master's, 3 letters of recommendation. Additional exam requirements/recommendations for international students: Required—TOEFL (minimum score 550 paper-based; 79 iBT), IELTS (minimum score 6.5). *Application deadline:* For fall admission, 2/15 for domestic and international students. Application fee: $50 ($40 for international students). Electronic applications accepted. *Expenses:* Tuition, state resident: full-time $7364; part-time $409.10 per credit hour. Tuition, nonresident: full-time $19,162; part-time $1008.50 per credit hour. *Financial support:* In 2013–14, 3 research assistantships with full and partial tuition reimbursements (averaging $6,750 per year), 7 teaching assistantships with full and partial tuition reimbursements (averaging $5,440 per year) were awarded. Financial award applicants required to submit FAFSA. *Faculty research:* Family violence, child abuse/neglect, immigration, community economic development. *Unit head:* Dr. Margaret Sherraden, Graduate Program Director, 314-516-6364, Fax: 314-516-5816, E-mail: socialwork@umsl.edu. *Application contact:* 314-516-5458, Fax: 314-516-6996, E-mail: gradadm@umsl.edu.
Website: http://www.umsl.edu/~socialwk/

University of Nevada, Las Vegas, Graduate College, School of Community Health Sciences, Department of Health Care Administration, Las Vegas, NV 89154-3023. Offers MHA. *Faculty:* 4 full-time (0 women), 4 part-time/adjunct (3 women). *Students:* 28 full-time (18 women), 28 part-time (15 women); includes 19 minority (10 Black or African American, non-Hispanic/Latino; 8 Asian, non-Hispanic/Latino; 1 Hispanic/Latino), 5 international. Average age 35. 30 applicants, 80% accepted, 13 enrolled. In 2013, 21 master's awarded. *Entrance requirements:* Additional exam requirements/recommendations for international students: Required—TOEFL (minimum score 550 paper-based; 80 iBT), IELTS (minimum score 7). *Application deadline:* For fall admission, 4/1 for domestic students, 5/1 for international students; for spring admission, 11/1 for domestic students, 10/1 for international students. Application fee: $60 ($95 for international students). Electronic applications accepted. *Expenses:* Tuition, state resident: full-time $4752; part-time $264 per credit. Tuition, nonresident: full-time $18,662; part-time $554.50 per credit. *International tuition:* $18,952 full-time. *Required fees:* $532; $12 per credit. $266 per semester. One-time fee: $35. Tuition and fees vary according to course load and program. *Financial support:* In 2013–14, 3 students received support, including 3 research assistantships with partial tuition reimbursements available (averaging $8,333 per year); institutionally sponsored loans, scholarships/grants, health care benefits, and unspecified assistantships also available. Financial award application deadline: 3/1. *Faculty research:* Effects of the EHR on healthcare outcome, quality and financial performance; patient satisfactions on hospital services; mediation errors, medical home performance, ER use among patients with mental illness. *Total annual research expenditures:* $107,458. *Unit head:* Dr. James Busser, Chair/Associate Professor, 702-895-1052, E-mail: james.busser@unlv.edu. *Application contact:* Graduate College Admissions Evaluator, 702-895-3320, Fax: 702-895-4180, E-mail: gradcollege@unlv.edu.
Website: http://hca.unlv.edu

University of New Haven, Graduate School, College of Business, Program in Health Care Administration, West Haven, CT 06516-1916. Offers health care administration (MS); health care management (Certificate); health care marketing (MS); health policy and finance (MS); human resource management in health care (MS); long-term care (MS); long-term health care (Certificate); managed care (MS); medical group management (MS). Part-time and evening/weekend programs available. *Students:* 49 full-time (33 women), 50 part-time (37 women); includes 26 minority (15 Black or African American, non-Hispanic/Latino; 3 Asian, non-Hispanic/Latino; 7 Hispanic/Latino; 1 Two or more races, non-Hispanic/Latino), 33 international. 114 applicants, 82% accepted, 53 enrolled. In 2013, 65 master's, 2 other advanced degrees awarded. *Degree requirements:* For master's, thesis or alternative. *Entrance requirements:* Additional exam requirements/recommendations for international students: Required—TOEFL (minimum score 80 iBT), IELTS, PTE (minimum score 53). *Application deadline:* For fall admission, 5/31 for international students; for winter admission, 10/15 for international students; for spring admission, 1/15 for international students. Applications are processed on a rolling basis. Application fee: $75. Electronic applications accepted. Application fee is waived when completed online. *Expenses: Tuition:* Full-time $21,600; part-time $800 per credit hour. *Required fees:* $45 per trimester. *Financial support:* Research assistantships with partial tuition reimbursements, teaching assistantships with partial tuition reimbursements, career-related internships or fieldwork, Federal Work-Study, scholarships/grants, and unspecified assistantships available. Support available to part-time students. Financial award applicants required to submit FAFSA. *Unit head:* Cynthia Conrad, Chair, 203-932-7486, E-mail: cconrad@newhaven.edu. *Application contact:* Eloise Gormley, Director of Graduate Admissions, 203-932-7440, E-mail: gradinfo@newhaven.edu.
Website: http://www.newhaven.edu/6848/

University of New Haven, Graduate School, College of Business, Program in Public Administration, West Haven, CT 06516-1916. Offers city management (MPA); community-clinical services (MPA); health care management (MPA); long-term health care (MPA); personnel and labor relations (MPA); public administration (MPA, Certificate); public management (Certificate); MBA/MPA. Part-time and evening/weekend programs available. *Students:* 39 full-time (21 women), 20 part-time (9 women); includes 16 minority (12 Black or African American, non-Hispanic/Latino; 2 Asian, non-Hispanic/Latino; 1 Hispanic/Latino; 1 Native Hawaiian or other Pacific Islander, non-Hispanic/Latino), 11 international. 44 applicants, 84% accepted, 13 enrolled. In 2013, 15 master's, 12 other advanced degrees awarded. *Degree requirements:* For master's, thesis or alternative. *Entrance requirements:* Additional exam requirements/recommendations for international students: Required—TOEFL (minimum score 80 iBT), IELTS, PTE (minimum score 53). *Application deadline:* For fall admission, 5/31 for international students; for winter admission, 10/15 for international students; for spring admission, 1/15 for international students. Applications are processed on a rolling basis. Application fee: $75. Electronic applications accepted. Application fee is waived when completed online. *Expenses:* Contact institution. *Financial support:* Research assistantships with partial tuition reimbursements, teaching assistantships with partial tuition reimbursements, career-related internships or fieldwork, Federal Work-Study, scholarships/grants, and unspecified assistantships available. Support available to part-time students. Financial award application deadline: 5/1; financial award applicants required to submit FAFSA. *Unit head:* Cynthia Conrad, Chair, 203-932-7486, E-mail: cconrad@newhaven.edu. *Application contact:* Eloise Gormley, Director of Graduate Admissions, 203-932-7440, E-mail: gradinfo@newhaven.edu.
Website: http://www.newhaven.edu/6854/

University of New Mexico, Graduate School, School of Public Administration, Program in Health Administration, Albuquerque, NM 87131-2039. Offers MHA. *Students:* 5 full-time (4 women), 14 part-time (11 women); includes 9 minority (1 Black or African American, non-Hispanic/Latino; 1 American Indian or Alaska Native, non-Hispanic/Latino; 1 Asian, non-Hispanic/Latino; 5 Hispanic/Latino; 1 Two or more races, non-Hispanic/Latino). 22 applicants, 82% accepted, 18 enrolled. *Entrance requirements:* For master's, baccalaureate degree from accredited college or university with minimum undergraduate GPA of 3.0 for last 60 hours or overall major; letter of intent; three letters of recommendation; resume; official transcripts. *Application deadline:* For fall admission, 4/1 for domestic students, 3/1 for international students. Application fee: $50. Electronic applications accepted. *Unit head:* Dr. Uday Desai, Director, 505-277-1092, Fax: 505-277-2529, E-mail: ucdesai@unm.edu. *Application contact:* Gene V. Henley, Associate Director and Graduate Academic Advisor, 505-277-9196, Fax: 505-277-2529, E-mail: spadvise@unm.edu.
Website: http://spa.unm.edu//mha-graduate-program/

University of New Mexico, School of Medicine, Program in Public Health, Albuquerque, NM 87131-5196. Offers community health (MPH); epidemiology (MPH); health systems, services and policy (MPH). *Accreditation:* CEPH. Part-time programs available. Postbaccalaureate distance learning degree programs offered. *Faculty:* 11 full-time (7 women), 4 part-time/adjunct (3 women). *Students:* 17 full-time (15 women), 16 part-time (12 women); includes 16 minority (3 Black or African American, non-Hispanic/Latino; 2 American Indian or Alaska Native, non-Hispanic/Latino; 1 Asian, non-Hispanic/Latino; 9 Hispanic/Latino; 1 Two or more races, non-Hispanic/Latino), 1 international. Average age 36. 46 applicants, 59% accepted, 17 enrolled. In 2013, 15 master's awarded. *Degree requirements:* For master's, thesis. *Entrance requirements:* For master's, GRE, MCAT, 2 years of experience in health field. Additional exam requirements/recommendations for international students: Required—TOEFL. *Application deadline:* For fall admission, 2/1 for domestic students. Application fee: $50. *Financial support:* Fellowships, research assistantships with tuition reimbursements, and Federal Work-Study available. Financial award application deadline: 12/15; financial award applicants required to submit FAFSA. *Faculty research:* Epidemiology, rural health, environmental health, Native American health issues. *Total annual research expenditures:* $1 million. *Unit head:* Dr. Kristine Tollestrup, Director, 505-272-4173, Fax: 505-272-4494, E-mail: ktollestrup@salud.unm.edu. *Application contact:* Gayle Garcia, Education Coordinator, 505-272-3982, Fax: 505-272-4494, E-mail: garciag@salud.unm.edu.
Website: http://fcm.unm.edu/

University of New Orleans, Graduate School, College of Business Administration, Program in Health Care Management, New Orleans, LA 70148. Offers MS. *Degree requirements:* For master's, thesis optional. *Entrance requirements:* For master's, GRE or GMAT. Additional exam requirements/recommendations for international students: Required—TOEFL (minimum score 550 paper-based; 79 iBT). Electronic applications accepted.

University of North Alabama, College of Business, Florence, AL 35632-0001. Offers accounting (MBA); enterprise resource planning systems (MBA); finance (MBA); health care management (MBA); information systems (MBA); professional (MBA); project management (MBA). *Accreditation:* ACBSP. Part-time and evening/weekend programs available. *Faculty:* 20 full-time (2 women). *Students:* 118 full-time (50 women), 273 part-time (130 women); includes 115 minority (37 Black or African American, non-Hispanic/Latino; 4 American Indian or Alaska Native, non-Hispanic/Latino; 68 Asian, non-Hispanic/Latino; 4 Hispanic/Latino; 2 Two or more races, non-Hispanic/Latino), 36 international. Average age 34. 296 applicants, 82% accepted, 149 enrolled. In 2013, 179 master's awarded. *Entrance requirements:* For master's, GMAT, GRE, minimum GPA of 2.75 in last 60 hours, 2.5 overall on a 3.0 scale; 27 hours of course work in business and economics. Additional exam requirements/recommendations for international students: Required—TOEFL (minimum score 500 paper-based; 79 iBT), IELTS (minimum score 6). *Application deadline:* For fall admission, 7/1 priority date for domestic students, 7/1 for international students; for spring admission, 12/1 for domestic and international students. Applications are processed on a rolling basis. Application fee: $25 ($50 for international students). Electronic applications accepted. *Expenses:* Tuition, state resident: full-time $4968; part-time $3312 per year. Tuition, nonresident: full-time $9936; part-time $6624 per year. *Required fees:* $970; $60.33 per credit. $362 per semester. *Financial support:* Federal Work-Study available. Support available to part-time students. Financial award application deadline: 4/1; financial award applicants required to submit FAFSA. *Unit head:* Dr. Kerry Gatlin, Dean, 256-765-4261, Fax: 256-765-4170, E-mail: kpgatlin@una.edu. *Application contact:* Russ Darracott, Graduate Admissions Counselor, 256-765-4447, E-mail: erdarracott@una.edu.
Website: http://www.una.edu/business/

The University of North Carolina at Chapel Hill, Graduate School, Gillings School of Global Public Health, Department of Health Policy and Management, Chapel Hill, NC 27599-7411. Offers MHA, MPH, MSPH, Dr PH, PhD, DDS/MPH, JD/MPH, MBA/MHA, MBA/MSPH, MD/MPH, MHA/MBA, MHA/MCRP, MHA/MSIS, MHA/MSLS, MSPH/MCRP, MSPH/MSIS, MSPH/MSLS. *Accreditation:* CAHME (one or more programs are accredited). Part-time programs available. Postbaccalaureate distance learning degree programs offered (minimal on-campus study). *Degree requirements:* For master's, comprehensive exam, capstone course or paper; for doctorate, comprehensive exam, thesis/dissertation. *Entrance requirements:* For master's and doctorate, GRE General Test, minimum GPA of 3.0 (recommended). Additional exam requirements/recommendations for international students: Required—TOEFL, IELTS. Electronic applications accepted. *Faculty research:* Organizational behavior; human resource management in healthcare; health services finance; mental health economics, service, and research; strategic planning and marketing.

The University of North Carolina at Charlotte, The Graduate School, College of Health and Human Services, Department of Health Behavior and Administration, Charlotte, NC 28223-0001. Offers community health (Certificate); health administration (MHA); health services research (PhD); public health (MSPH). *Accreditation:* CAHME. Part-time programs available. *Degree requirements:* For master's, thesis or comprehensive exam; for doctorate, thesis/dissertation. *Entrance requirements:* For master's, GRE or MAT (public health), GRE or GMAT (health administration), minimum GPA of 3.0 during previous 2 years, 2.75 overall. Additional exam requirements/recommendations for international students: Required—TOEFL (minimum score 557

paper-based; 83 iBT). *Application deadline:* For fall admission, 7/1 for domestic students, 5/1 for international students; for spring admission, 11/1 for domestic students, 10/1 for international students. Applications are processed on a rolling basis. Application fee: $65 ($75 for international students). Electronic applications accepted. *Expenses:* Tuition, state resident: full-time $3522. Tuition, nonresident: full-time $16,051. *Required fees:* $2585. Tuition and fees vary according to course load and program. *Financial support:* Research assistantships, teaching assistantships, career-related internships or fieldwork, Federal Work-Study, institutionally sponsored loans, scholarships/grants, and unspecified assistantships available. Support available to part-time students. Financial award application deadline: 4/1; financial award applicants required to submit FAFSA. *Faculty research:* Pediatric asthma self-management, reproductive epidemiology, social aspects of injury prevention, chronic illness self-care, competency-based professional education, cognitive health, aging and dementia, infant health outcomes, policing and suicide, data mining for health executive decision support, segmentation analyses in identifying patient satisfaction problems in the primary care setting, enhancing community capacity through data sharing. *Unit head:* Dr. Gary S. Silverman, Chair, 704-687-7191, Fax: 704-687-6122, E-mail: arharver@uncc.edu. *Application contact:* Kathy B. Giddings, Director of Graduate Admissions, 704-687-5503, Fax: 704-687-1668, E-mail: gradadm@uncc.edu.
Website: http://publichealth.uncc.edu/degrees-and-programs/phs-graduate-programs

The University of North Carolina at Charlotte, The Graduate School, College of Health and Human Services, School of Nursing, Charlotte, NC 28223-0001. Offers administration (Post-Master's Certificate); advanced clinical (MSN, Post-Master's Certificate); anesthesia (MSN, Post-Master's Certificate); community health (MSN); family nurse practitioner (MSN, Post-Master's Certificate); health administration (MSN); mental health (MSN); nurse educator (MSN, Post-Master's Certificate); nursing (DNP); systems population (MSN). *Accreditation:* AACN. Part-time programs available. *Faculty:* 17 full-time (16 women), 6 part-time/adjunct (5 women). *Students:* 96 full-time (80 women), 124 part-time (119 women); includes 45 minority (30 Black or African American, non-Hispanic/Latino; 1 American Indian or Alaska Native, non-Hispanic/Latino; 8 Asian, non-Hispanic/Latino; 4 Hispanic/Latino; 2 Two or more races, non-Hispanic/Latino), 1 international. Average age 34. 216 applicants, 38% accepted, 72 enrolled. In 2013, 70 master's, 8 other advanced degrees awarded. Terminal master's awarded for partial completion of doctoral program. *Degree requirements:* For master's, thesis or alternative, practicum; for doctorate, thesis/dissertation or alternative, residency. *Entrance requirements:* For master's, GRE General Test, minimum GPA of 3.0 in undergraduate major; for doctorate, GRE, MAT, or GMAT, minimum GPA of 3.5. Additional exam requirements/recommendations for international students: Required—TOEFL (minimum score 570 paper-based; 83 iBT). *Application deadline:* For fall admission, 5/1 priority date for domestic students, 5/1 for international students; for spring admission, 10/1 priority date for domestic students, 10/1 for international students. Application fee: $75. Electronic applications accepted. *Expenses:* Tuition, state resident: full-time $3522. Tuition, nonresident: full-time $16,051. *Required fees:* $2585. Tuition and fees vary according to course load and program. *Financial support:* In 2013–14, 5 students received support, including 5 teaching assistantships (averaging $4,785 per year); research assistantships, career-related internships or fieldwork, institutionally sponsored loans, scholarships/grants, traineeships, and unspecified assistantships also available. Support available to part-time students. Financial award application deadline: 4/1; financial award applicants required to submit FAFSA. *Faculty research:* Improving care outcomes for the elderly; vulnerable populations; symptom management; self management/health promotion strategies of older adults; migration and maternal child health; health disparities, health literacy, and access to healthcare in Latino adults with diabetes; psychiatric nursing. *Total annual research expenditures:* $572,410. *Unit head:* Dr. Dee Baldwin, Associate Dean, 704-687-7952, Fax: 704-687-6017, E-mail: dbaldwi5@uncc.edu. *Application contact:* Kathy B. Giddings, Director of Graduate Admissions, 704-687-5503, Fax: 704-687-1668, E-mail: gradadm@uncc.edu.
Website: http://nursing.uncc.edu/

University of North Florida, Brooks College of Health, Department of Public Health, Jacksonville, FL 32224. Offers aging services (Certificate); community health (MPH); geriatric management (MSH); health administration (MHA); rehabilitation counseling (MS). *Accreditation:* CEPH. Part-time and evening/weekend programs available. *Faculty:* 16 full-time (9 women), 4 part-time/adjunct (3 women). *Students:* 119 full-time (79 women), 59 part-time (34 women); includes 52 minority (20 Black or African American, non-Hispanic/Latino; 2 American Indian or Alaska Native, non-Hispanic/Latino; 9 Asian, non-Hispanic/Latino; 18 Hispanic/Latino; 3 Two or more races, non-Hispanic/Latino), 6 international. Average age 30. 271 applicants, 40% accepted, 72 enrolled. In 2013, 57 master's awarded. *Degree requirements:* For master's, thesis optional. *Entrance requirements:* For master's, GRE General Test (MSH, MS, MPH); GMAT or GRE General Test (MHA), minimum GPA of 3.0 in last 60 hours. Additional exam requirements/recommendations for international students: Required—TOEFL (minimum score 500 paper-based). *Application deadline:* For fall admission, 7/1 for domestic students, 5/1 for international students; for spring admission, 11/1 for domestic students, 10/1 for international students. Application fee: $30. Electronic applications accepted. *Expenses:* Tuition, state resident: full-time $9794; part-time $408.10 per credit hour. Tuition, nonresident: full-time $22,383; part-time $932.61 per credit hour. *Required fees:* $2020; $84.20 per credit hour. Tuition and fees vary according to course load and program. *Financial support:* In 2013–14, 38 students received support, including 2 teaching assistantships (averaging $1,500 per year); research assistantships, career-related internships or fieldwork, Federal Work-Study, scholarships/grants, and tuition waivers (partial) also available. Support available to part-time students. Financial award application deadline: 4/1; financial award applicants required to submit FAFSA. *Faculty research:* Dietary supplements; alcohol, tobacco, and other drug use prevention; turnover among health professionals; aging; psychosocial aspects of disabilities. *Total annual research expenditures:* $21,747. *Unit head:* Dr. Jeffrey Harrison, Chair, 904-620-1440, Fax: 904-620-2848, E-mail: jeffrey.harrison@unf.edu. *Application contact:* Dr. Heather Kenney, Director of Advising, 904-620-2810, Fax: 904-620-1030, E-mail: heather.kenney@unf.edu.
Website: http://www.unf.edu/brooks/public_health/

University of North Texas, Robert B. Toulouse School of Graduate Studies, Denton, TN 76203-5017. Offers accounting (MS, PhD); applied anthropology (MA, MS); applied behavior analysis (Certificate); applied technology and performance improvement (M Ed, MS, PhD); art education (MA, PhD); art history (MA); art museum education (Certificate); arts leadership (Certificate); audiology (Au D); behavior analysis (MS); biochemistry and molecular biology (MS, PhD); biology (MA, MS, PhD); business (PhD); business computer information systems (PhD); chemistry (MS, PhD); clinical psychology (PhD); communication studies (MA, MS); computer engineering (MS); computer science (MS); computer science and engineering (PhD); counseling (M Ed, MS, PhD), including clinical mental health counseling (MS), college and university counseling (M Ed, MS), elementary school counseling (M Ed, MS), secondary school counseling (M Ed, MS); counseling psychology (PhD); creative writing (MA); criminal justice (MS); curriculum and instruction (M Ed, PhD), including curriculum studies (PhD), early childhood studies (PhD), language and literacy studies (PhD); decision sciences (MBA); design (MA, MFA), including fashion design (MFA), innovation studies, interior design (MFA); early childhood studies (MS); economics (MS); educational leadership (M Ed, Ed D, PhD); educational psychology (MS), including family studies, gifted and talented (MS, PhD), human development, learning and cognition, research, measurement and evaluation; educational research (PhD), including gifted and talented (MS, PhD), human development and family studies, psychological aspects of sports and exercise, research, measurement and statistics; electrical engineering (MS); emergency management (MPA); engineering systems (MS); English (MA, PhD); environmental science (MS, PhD); experimental psychology (PhD); finance (MBA, MS, PhD); financial management (MPA); French (MA); health psychology and behavioral medicine (PhD); health services management (MBA); higher education (M Ed, Ed D, PhD); history (MA, MS, PhD), including European history (PhD), military history (PhD), United States history (PhD); hospitality management (MS); human resources management (MPA); information science (MS, PhD); information technologies (MBA); information technology and decision sciences (MS); interdisciplinary studies (MA, MS); international sustainable tourism (MS); jazz studies (MM); journalism (MA, MJ, Graduate Certificate), including interactive and virtual digital communication (Graduate Certificate), narrative journalism (Graduate Certificate), public relations (Graduate Certificate); kinesiology (MS); learning technologies (MS, PhD); library science (MS); local government management (MPA); logistics and supply chain management (MBA, PhD); long-term care, senior housing, and aging services (MA, MS); management science (PhD); marketing (MBA, PhD); materials science and engineering (MS, PhD); mathematics (MA, PhD); merchandising (MS); music (MA, MM Ed, PhD), including ethnomusicology (MA), music education (MM Ed, PhD), music theory (MA, PhD), musicology (MA, PhD), performance (MA); nonprofit management (MPA); operations and supply chain management (MBA); performance (MM, DMA); philosophy (MA, PhD); physics (MS, PhD); political science (MA, MS, PhD); public administration and management (PhD), including emergency management, nonprofit management, public financial management, urban management; radio, television and film (MA, MFA); recreation, event and sport management (MS); rehabilitation counseling (MS, Certificate); sociology (MA, MS, PhD); Spanish (MA); special education (M Ed, PhD), including autism intervention (PhD), emotional/behavioral disorders (PhD), mild/moderate disabilities (PhD); speech-language pathology (MA, MS); strategic management (MBA); studio art (MFA); taxation (MS); teaching (M Ed); MBA/MS; MS/MPH; MSES/MBA. Part-time and evening/weekend programs available. Postbaccalaureate distance learning degree programs offered. *Faculty:* 661 full-time (213 women), 240 part-time/adjunct (144 women). *Students:* 3,106 full-time (1,620 women), 3,543 part-time (2,221 women); includes 1,740 minority (533 Black or African American, non-Hispanic/Latino; 15 American Indian or Alaska Native, non-Hispanic/Latino; 286 Asian, non-Hispanic/Latino; 746 Hispanic/Latino; 3 Native Hawaiian or other Pacific Islander, non-Hispanic/Latino; 157 Two or more races, non-Hispanic/Latino), 1,145 international. Average age 32. 6,289 applicants, 43% accepted, 1751 enrolled. In 2013, 1,778 master's, 239 doctorates, 10 other advanced degrees awarded. Terminal master's awarded for partial completion of doctoral program. *Degree requirements:* For master's, variable foreign language requirement, comprehensive exam (for some programs), thesis (for some programs); for doctorate, variable foreign language requirement, comprehensive exam (for some programs), thesis/dissertation; for other advanced degree, variable foreign language requirement, comprehensive exam (for some programs). *Entrance requirements:* For master's and doctorate, GRE, GMAT. Additional exam requirements/recommendations for international students: Required—TOEFL (minimum score 550 paper-based; 79 iBT). *Application deadline:* For fall admission, 7/15 for domestic students, 3/15 for international students; for spring admission, 11/15 for domestic students, 9/15 for international students; for summer admission, 5/1 for domestic students. Applications are processed on a rolling basis. Application fee: $60. Electronic applications accepted. *Financial support:* Fellowships with partial tuition reimbursements, research assistantships with partial tuition reimbursements, teaching assistantships, career-related internships or fieldwork, Federal Work-Study, institutionally sponsored loans, scholarships/grants, health care benefits, and library assistantships available. Support available to part-time students. Financial award applicants required to submit FAFSA. *Unit head:* Mark Wardell, Dean, 940-565-2383, E-mail: mark.wardell@unt.edu. *Application contact:* Toulouse School of Graduate Studies, 940-565-2383, Fax: 940-565-2141, E-mail: gradsch@unt.edu.
Website: http://tsgs.unt.edu/

University of North Texas Health Science Center at Fort Worth, School of Public Health, Fort Worth, TX 76107-2699. Offers biostatistics (MPH); community health (MPH); disease control and prevention (Dr PH); environmental and occupational health sciences (MPH); epidemiology (MPH); health administration (MHA); health policy and management (MPH, Dr PH); DO/MPH; MS/MPH; MSN/MPH. MPH offered jointly with University of North Texas; DO/MPH with Texas College of Osteopathic Medicine. *Accreditation:* CEPH. Part-time and evening/weekend programs available. *Degree requirements:* For master's, thesis or alternative, supervised internship; for doctorate, thesis/dissertation, supervised internship. *Entrance requirements:* For master's, GRE General Test. Additional exam requirements/recommendations for international students: Required—TOEFL. Electronic applications accepted.

University of Oklahoma, College of Liberal Studies, Norman, OK 73019. Offers administrative leadership (MA Ed, Graduate Certificate); criminal justice (MS); liberal studies (MA, MA Ed), including human and health services administration (MA Ed), integrated studies (MA), museum studies (MA Ed); prevention science (MPS). Part-time and evening/weekend programs available. Postbaccalaureate distance learning degree programs offered (no on-campus study). *Faculty:* 16 full-time (11 women), 2 part-time/adjunct (0 women). *Students:* 33 full-time (13 women), 562 part-time (262 women); includes 147 minority (57 Black or African American, non-Hispanic/Latino; 27 American Indian or Alaska Native, non-Hispanic/Latino; 7 Asian, non-Hispanic/Latino; 29 Hispanic/Latino; 2 Native Hawaiian or other Pacific Islander, non-Hispanic/Latino; 25 Two or more races, non-Hispanic/Latino), 2 international. Average age 36. 203 applicants, 94% accepted, 122 enrolled. In 2013, 161 master's, 27 other advanced degrees awarded. Terminal master's awarded for partial completion of doctoral program. *Degree requirements:* For master's, comprehensive exam (for some programs), thesis optional, practicum (for museum studies only); for Graduate Certificate, comprehensive exam (for some programs), thesis optional. *Entrance requirements:* For master's and Graduate Certificate, minimum cumulative GPA of 3.0 in previous undergraduate/graduate coursework. Additional exam requirements/recommendations for international students: Required—TOEFL (minimum score 79 iBT). *Application deadline:* For fall admission, 7/1 for domestic students, 1/1 for international students; for winter admission, 12/1 for domestic and international students; for spring admission, 5/1 for domestic and international students. Application fee: $50 ($100 for international students). Electronic applications accepted. *Expenses:* Tuition, state resident: full-time $4205; part-time $175.20 per credit hour. Tuition, nonresident: full-time $16,205; part-time $675.20 per credit hour. *Required fees:* $2745; $103.85 per credit hour. $126.50 per semester. *Financial support:* In 2013–14, 109 students received support. Career-related internships or fieldwork, Federal Work-Study, institutionally sponsored loans, scholarships/grants, health care benefits, and tuition waivers (partial) available. Support available to part-time students. Financial award application deadline: 6/1; financial award applicants required to submit FAFSA. *Faculty research:* Race, crime, and class inequality; human trafficking; textual analysis and early Christianity; drug policy implementation; professionalism in police practice; service-learning; Chinese cultural

studies. *Total annual research expenditures:* $31,745. *Unit head:* Dr. James Pappas, Dean/Vice President of OU Outreach, 405-325-6361, Fax: 405-325-7132, E-mail: jpappas@ou.edu. *Application contact:* Missy Heinze, Recruitment Coordinator, 800-522-0559, Fax: 405-325-7132, E-mail: mheinze@ou.edu.
Website: http://www.ou.edu/cls/

University of Oklahoma Health Sciences Center, Graduate College, College of Public Health, Department of Health Administration and Policy, Oklahoma City, OK 73190. Offers MHA, MPH, MS, Dr PH, PhD, JD/MPH, MBA/MPH. MBA/MPH offered jointly with Oklahoma State University; JD/MPH with University of Oklahoma. *Accreditation:* CAHME. Part-time programs available. *Faculty:* 9 full-time (5 women), 5 part-time/adjunct (3 women). *Students:* 27 full-time (15 women), 13 part-time (7 women); includes 16 minority (3 Black or African American, non-Hispanic/Latino; 2 American Indian or Alaska Native, non-Hispanic/Latino; 6 Asian, non-Hispanic/Latino; 2 Hispanic/Latino; 3 Two or more races, non-Hispanic/Latino), 2 international. Average age 29. 32 applicants, 69% accepted, 10 enrolled. In 2013, 21 master's awarded. *Degree requirements:* For master's, comprehensive exam, thesis (for some programs); for doctorate, 2 foreign languages, comprehensive exam, thesis/dissertation. *Entrance requirements:* For master's, 3 letters of recommendation, resume; for doctorate, GRE General Test, letters of recommendation. Additional exam requirements/recommendations for international students: Required—TOEFL (minimum score 570 paper-based). *Application deadline:* For fall admission, 7/1 for domestic students; for winter admission, 4/1 for domestic students; for spring admission, 12/1 for domestic students. Applications are processed on a rolling basis. Application fee: $50. *Expenses:* Tuition, state resident: full-time $3504; part-time $175.20 per credit hour. Tuition, nonresident: full-time $13,504; part-time $675.20 per credit hour. *Required fees:* $1545; $52.70 per credit hour. $245.25 per semester. Tuition and fees vary according to course load. *Financial support:* In 2013–14, 3 research assistantships (averaging $13,000 per year) were awarded; fellowships, career-related internships or fieldwork, institutionally sponsored loans, traineeships, and tuition waivers (partial) also available. Support available to part-time students. Financial award application deadline: 5/1. *Faculty research:* Public health administration, health institutions management, public policy and the aged, injury control. *Unit head:* Dr. Steven Mattachione, JD, Chair, 405-271-2114, E-mail: steven-mattachione@ouhsc.edu. *Application contact:* Robin Howell, Information Contact, 405-271-2308, E-mail: robin-howell@ouhsc.edu.

University of Ottawa, Faculty of Graduate and Postdoctoral Studies, Telfer School of Management, Health Administration Program, Ottawa, ON K1N 6N5, Canada. Offers MHA. Part-time programs available. *Degree requirements:* For master's, thesis optional, residency. *Entrance requirements:* For master's, GMAT, bachelor's degree or equivalent, minimum B average. Additional exam requirements/recommendations for international students: Recommended—TOEFL. Electronic applications accepted.

University of Pennsylvania, Wharton School, Health Care Management Department, Philadelphia, PA 19104. Offers MBA, PhD. *Degree requirements:* For doctorate, comprehensive exam, thesis/dissertation. *Entrance requirements:* For master's, GMAT; for doctorate, GMAT or GRE. Electronic applications accepted. *Faculty research:* Health economics, health policy, health care management, health insurance and financing.

University of Phoenix–Atlanta Campus, College of Nursing, Sandy Springs, GA 30350-4153. Offers health administration (MHA); nursing (MSN); nursing/health care education (MSN); MSN/MBA; MSN/MHA. Evening/weekend programs available. Postbaccalaureate distance learning degree programs offered. *Degree requirements:* For master's, thesis (for some programs). *Entrance requirements:* For master's, minimum undergraduate GPA of 2.5, 3 years of work experience. Additional exam requirements/recommendations for international students: Required—TOEFL (minimum score 550 paper-based; 79 iBT). Electronic applications accepted.

University of Phoenix–Augusta Campus, College of Nursing, Augusta, GA 30909-4583. Offers health administration (MHA); nursing (MSN); nursing/health care education (MSN); MSN/MBA; MSN/MHA. Postbaccalaureate distance learning degree programs offered.

University of Phoenix–Austin Campus, College of Nursing, Austin, TX 78759. Offers health administration (MHA). Postbaccalaureate distance learning degree programs offered.

University of Phoenix–Bay Area Campus, School of Business, San Jose, CA 95134-1805. Offers accountancy (MS); accounting (MBA); business administration (MBA, DBA); energy management (MBA); global management (MBA); health care management (MBA); human resource management (MBA); human resources management (MM); management (MM); marketing (MBA); organizational leadership (DM); project management (MBA); public administration (MPA); technology management (MBA). Evening/weekend programs available. Postbaccalaureate distance learning degree programs offered (no on-campus study). *Degree requirements:* For master's, thesis (for some programs). *Entrance requirements:* For master's, minimum undergraduate GPA of 3.0, 3 years of work experience. Additional exam requirements/recommendations for international students: Required—TOEFL (minimum score 550 paper-based; 79 iBT). Electronic applications accepted.

University of Phoenix–Birmingham Campus, College of Health and Human Services, Birmingham, AL 35242. Offers education (MHA); gerontology (MHA); health administration (MHA); health care management (MBA); informatics (MHA); nursing (MSN); nursing/health care education (MSN); MSN/MBA; MSN/MHA.

University of Phoenix–Central Valley Campus, College of Nursing, Fresno, CA 93720-1562. Offers education (MHA); gerontology (MHA); health administration (MHA); nursing (MSN); MSN/MBA.

University of Phoenix–Charlotte Campus, College of Nursing, Charlotte, NC 28273-3409. Offers education (MHA); gerontology (MHA); health administration (MHA); informatics (MHA, MSN); nursing (MSN); nursing/health care education (MSN). Evening/weekend programs available. *Degree requirements:* For master's, thesis (for some programs). *Entrance requirements:* For master's, minimum undergraduate GPA of 2.5, 3 years work experience. Additional exam requirements/recommendations for international students: Required—TOEFL (minimum score 550 paper-based; 79 iBT). Electronic applications accepted.

University of Phoenix–Chattanooga Campus, College of Nursing, Chattanooga, TN 37421-3707. Offers education (MHA); gerontology (MHA); health administration (MHA).

University of Phoenix–Cheyenne Campus, College of Nursing, Cheyenne, WY 82009. Offers health administration (MHA); nursing (MSN); nursing/health care education (MSN); MSN/MBA; MSN/MHA. Postbaccalaureate distance learning degree programs offered.

University of Phoenix–Denver Campus, College of Nursing, Lone Tree, CO 80124-5453. Offers health administration (MHA); nursing (MSN); MSN/MBA; MSN/MHA. Evening/weekend programs available. Postbaccalaureate distance learning degree programs offered. *Degree requirements:* For master's, thesis (for some programs). *Entrance requirements:* For master's, minimum undergraduate GPA of 2.5, 3 years work experience, RN license. Additional exam requirements/recommendations for international students: Required—TOEFL (minimum score 550 paper-based; 79 iBT). Electronic applications accepted.

University of Phoenix–Des Moines Campus, College of Nursing, Des Moines, IA 50309. Offers education (MHA); gerontology (MHA); health administration (MHA, DHA); informatics (MHA, MSN); nursing (MSN, PhD); nursing/health care education (MSN).

University of Phoenix–Hawaii Campus, College of Nursing, Honolulu, HI 96813-4317. Offers education (MHA); family nurse practitioner (MSN); gerontology (MHA); health administration (MHA); nursing (MSN); nursing/health care education (MSN); MSN/MBA. Evening/weekend programs available. *Degree requirements:* For master's, thesis (for some programs). *Entrance requirements:* For master's, minimum undergraduate GPA of 2.5, 3 years of work experience, RN license. Additional exam requirements/recommendations for international students: Required—TOEFL (minimum score 550 paper-based; 79 iBT). Electronic applications accepted.

University of Phoenix–Houston Campus, College of Nursing, Houston, TX 77079-2004. Offers health administration (MHA). Postbaccalaureate distance learning degree programs offered. *Degree requirements:* For master's, thesis (for some programs). *Entrance requirements:* For master's, minimum undergraduate GPA of 2.5, 3 years of work experience. Additional exam requirements/recommendations for international students: Required—TOEFL (minimum score 550 paper-based; 79 iBT). Electronic applications accepted.

University of Phoenix–Indianapolis Campus, College of Nursing, Indianapolis, IN 46250-932. Offers health administration (MHA); nursing (MSN); nursing/health care education (MSN); MSN/MBA; MSN/MHA. Evening/weekend programs available. Postbaccalaureate distance learning degree programs offered. *Degree requirements:* For master's, thesis. *Entrance requirements:* For master's, 3 years work experience, minimum undergraduate GPA of 2.5. Additional exam requirements/recommendations for international students: Required—TOEFL (minimum score 500 paper-based). Electronic applications accepted.

University of Phoenix–Memphis Campus, College of Nursing, Cordova, TN 38018. Offers health administration (MHA, DHA).

University of Phoenix–Milwaukee Campus, School of Business, Milwaukee, WI 53224. Offers accounting (MBA); business administration (MBA); energy management (MBA); global management (MBA); health care management (MBA); human resource management (MBA); management (MM); marketing (MBA); project management (MBA); technology management (MBA). Evening/weekend programs available. Postbaccalaureate distance learning degree programs offered. *Entrance requirements:* Additional exam requirements/recommendations for international students: Required—TOEFL, TOEIC (Test of English as an International Communication), Berlitz Online English Proficiency Exam, PTE, or IELTS. Electronic applications accepted. *Expenses:* Contact institution.

University of Phoenix–Nashville Campus, College of Nursing, Nashville, TN 37214-5048. Offers health administration (MHA). Evening/weekend programs available. *Degree requirements:* For master's, thesis (for some programs). *Entrance requirements:* For master's, minimum undergraduate GPA of 2.5, 3 years of work experience. Additional exam requirements/recommendations for international students: Required—TOEFL (minimum score 550 paper-based). Electronic applications accepted.

University of Phoenix–New Mexico Campus, College of Nursing, Albuquerque, NM 87113-1570. Offers health administration (MHA); health care education (MSN); nursing (MSN); MSN/MBA. Evening/weekend programs available. *Degree requirements:* For master's, thesis (for some programs). *Entrance requirements:* For master's, minimum undergraduate GPA of 2.5, 3 years of work experience, RN license. Additional exam requirements/recommendations for international students: Required—TOEFL (minimum score 550 paper-based; 79 iBT). Electronic applications accepted.

University of Phoenix–North Florida Campus, College of Nursing, Jacksonville, FL 32216-0959. Offers health administration (MHA); health care education (MSN); nursing (MSN); MSN/MBA; MSN/MHA. Evening/weekend programs available. *Degree requirements:* For master's, thesis (for some programs). *Entrance requirements:* For master's, minimum undergraduate GPA of 2.5, 3 years work experience, RN license. Additional exam requirements/recommendations for international students: Required—TOEFL (minimum score 550 paper-based; 79 iBT). Electronic applications accepted.

University of Phoenix–Northwest Arkansas Campus, College of Nursing, Rogers, AR 72756-9615. Offers health administration (MHA); health care education (MSN); nursing (MSN); MSN/MBA.

University of Phoenix–Omaha Campus, College of Nursing, Omaha, NE 68154-5240. Offers health administration (MHA).

University of Phoenix–Online Campus, School of Advanced Studies, Phoenix, AZ 85034-7209. Offers business administration (DBA); education (Ed S); educational leadership (Ed D), including curriculum and instruction, education technology, educational leadership; health administration (DHA); higher education administration (PhD); industrial/organizational psychology (PhD); nursing (PhD); organizational leadership (DM), including information systems and technology, organizational leadership. Evening/weekend programs available. Postbaccalaureate distance learning degree programs offered. *Degree requirements:* For doctorate, thesis/dissertation. *Entrance requirements:* Additional exam requirements/recommendations for international students: Required—TOEFL, TOEIC (Test of English as an International Communication), Berlitz Online English Proficiency Exam, PTE, or IELTS. Electronic applications accepted. *Expenses:* Contact institution.

University of Phoenix–Online Campus, School of Business, Phoenix, AZ 85034-7209. Offers accountancy (MS); accounting (MBA, Certificate); business administration (MBA); energy management (MBA); global management (MBA); health care management (MBA); human resource management (MBA, Certificate); human resources management (MM); management (MM); marketing (MBA, Certificate); project management (MBA, Certificate); public administration (MBA, MM); technology management (MBA). Evening/weekend programs available. Postbaccalaureate distance learning degree programs offered. *Entrance requirements:* Additional exam requirements/recommendations for international students: Required—TOEFL, TOEIC (Test of English as an International Communication), Berlitz Online English Proficiency Exam, PTE, or IELTS. Electronic applications accepted. *Expenses:* Contact institution.

University of Phoenix–Oregon Campus, College of Nursing, Tigard, OR 97223. Offers health administration (MHA); nursing (MSN); MSN/MBA. Evening/weekend programs available. *Degree requirements:* For master's, thesis (for some programs). *Entrance requirements:* For master's, minimum undergraduate GPA of 2.5, 3 years of work experience, current RN license (nursing). Additional exam requirements/recommendations for international students: Required—TOEFL (minimum score 550 paper-based; 79 iBT). Electronic applications accepted.

University of Phoenix–Phoenix Campus, School of Business, Tempe, AZ 85282-2371. Offers accounting (MBA, MS, Certificate); business administration (MBA); energy management (MBA); global management (MBA); health care management (MBA); human resource management (MBA, Certificate); management (MM); marketing (MBA); project management (MBA); technology management (MBA). Evening/weekend programs available. Postbaccalaureate distance learning degree programs offered. *Entrance requirements:* Additional exam requirements/recommendations for international students: Required—TOEFL, TOEIC (Test of English as an International Communication), Berlitz Online English Proficiency Exam, PTE, or IELTS. Electronic applications accepted. *Expenses:* Contact institution.

University of Phoenix–Pittsburgh Campus, College of Nursing, Pittsburgh, PA 15276. Offers health administration (MHA); health care education (MSN); nursing (MSN); MSN/MBA; MSN/MHA. Evening/weekend programs available. *Degree requirements:* For master's, thesis (for some programs). *Entrance requirements:* For master's, minimum undergraduate GPA of 2.5, 3 years work experience, current RN license (nursing). Additional exam requirements/recommendations for international students: Required—TOEFL (minimum score 550 paper-based; 79 iBT). Electronic applications accepted.

University of Phoenix–Richmond-Virginia Beach Campus, College of Nursing, Glen Allen, VA 23060. Offers health administration (MHA); health care education (MSN); nursing (MSN); MSN/MBA; MSN/MHA. Evening/weekend programs available. *Degree requirements:* For master's, thesis (for some programs). *Entrance requirements:* For master's, minimum undergraduate GPA of 2.5, 3 years work experience, current RN license for nursing programs. Additional exam requirements/recommendations for international students: Required—TOEFL (minimum score 500 paper-based; 79 iBT). Electronic applications accepted.

University of Phoenix–Sacramento Valley Campus, College of Nursing, Sacramento, CA 95833-3632. Offers family nurse practitioner (MSN); health administration (MHA); health care education (MSN); nursing (MSN); MSN/MBA. Evening/weekend programs available. *Degree requirements:* For master's, thesis (for some programs). *Entrance requirements:* For master's, RN license, minimum undergraduate GPA of 2.5, 3 years work experience. Additional exam requirements/recommendations for international students: Required—TOEFL (minimum score 550 paper-based; 79 iBT). Electronic applications accepted.

University of Phoenix–San Antonio Campus, College of Nursing, San Antonio, TX 78230. Offers health administration (MHA).

University of Phoenix–Savannah Campus, College of Nursing, Savannah, GA 31405-7400. Offers health administration (MHA); nursing (MSN); nursing/health care education (MSN); MSN/MBA; MSN/MHA.

University of Phoenix–Southern California Campus, School of Business, Costa Mesa, CA 92626. Offers accounting (MBA); business administration (MBA); energy management (MBA); global management (MBA); health care management (MBA); human resource management (MBA); management (MM); marketing (MBA); project management (MBA); technology management (MBA). Evening/weekend programs available. Postbaccalaureate distance learning degree programs offered. *Entrance requirements:* Additional exam requirements/recommendations for international students: Required—TOEFL, TOEIC (Test of English as an International Communication), Berlitz Online English Proficiency Exam, PTE, or IELTS. Electronic applications accepted. *Expenses:* Contact institution.

University of Phoenix–Southern Colorado Campus, College of Nursing, Colorado Springs, CO 80903. Offers education (MHA); gerontology (MHA); health administration (MHA); nursing (MSN); MSN/MBA. Evening/weekend programs available. *Degree requirements:* For master's, thesis (for some programs). *Entrance requirements:* For master's, minimum undergraduate GPA of 2.5, 3 years of work experience, RN license. Additional exam requirements/recommendations for international students: Required—TOEFL (minimum score 550 paper-based; 79 iBT). Electronic applications accepted.

University of Phoenix–South Florida Campus, College of Nursing, Miramar, FL 33030. Offers health administration (MHA); health care education (MSN); nursing (MSN); MSN/MBA; MSN/MHA. Evening/weekend programs available. *Degree requirements:* For master's, thesis (for some programs). *Entrance requirements:* For master's, minimum undergraduate GPA of 2.5, 3 years work experience, RN license. Additional exam requirements/recommendations for international students: Required—TOEFL (minimum score 550 paper-based; 79 iBT). Electronic applications accepted.

University of Phoenix–Springfield Campus, College of Nursing, Springfield, MO 65804-7211. Offers health administration (MHA); nursing (MSN); MSN/MBA; MSN/MHA.

University of Phoenix–Washington D.C. Campus, College of Nursing, Washington, DC 20001. Offers education (MHA); gerontology (MHA); health administration (MHA, DHA); informatics (MHA, MSN); nursing (MSN, PhD); nursing/health care education (MSN); MSN/MBA; MSN/MHA.

University of Phoenix–West Florida Campus, College of Nursing, Temple Terrace, FL 33637. Offers health administration (MHA); health care education (MSN); nursing (MSN); MSN/MBA; MSN/MHA. Evening/weekend programs available. Postbaccalaureate distance learning degree programs offered. *Degree requirements:* For master's, thesis (for some programs). *Entrance requirements:* For master's, minimum undergraduate GPA of 2.5, RN license, 3 years work experience. Additional exam requirements/recommendations for international students: Required—TOEFL (minimum score 550 paper-based; 79 iBT). Electronic applications accepted.

University of Pittsburgh, Graduate School of Public Health, Department of Behavioral and Community Health Science, Pittsburgh, PA 15260. Offers behavioral and community health sciences (MPH, Dr PH); community-based participatory research and practice (Certificate); health equity (Certificate); lesbian, gay, bisexual and transgender health and wellness (Certificate); program evaluation (Certificate); MID/MPH; MPH/MPA; MPH/MSW; MPH/PhD. *Accreditation:* CAHME (one or more programs are accredited). Part-time programs available. *Faculty:* 14 full-time (7 women), 18 part-time/adjunct (6 women). *Students:* 61 full-time (47 women), 47 part-time (37 women); includes 27 minority (10 Black or African American, non-Hispanic/Latino; 9 Asian, non-Hispanic/Latino; 8 Hispanic/Latino), 5 international. Average age 29. 296 applicants, 58% accepted, 34 enrolled. In 2013, 34 master's, 6 doctorates awarded. *Degree requirements:* For master's, thesis; for doctorate, comprehensive exam, thesis/dissertation, preliminary exams. *Entrance requirements:* For master's and Certificate, GRE; for doctorate, GRE, master's degree in public health or related field. Additional exam requirements/recommendations for international students: Required—TOEFL (minimum score 550 paper-based; 80 iBT) or IELTS (minimum score 6.5). *Application deadline:* For fall admission, 1/15 for domestic and international students; for winter admission, 9/1 for international students; for spring admission, 10/15 for domestic students, 8/1 for international students; for summer admission, 12/1 for international students. Applications are processed on a rolling basis. Application fee: $120. Electronic applications accepted. *Expenses:* Tuition, state resident: full-time $19,964; part-time $807 per credit. Tuition, nonresident: full-time $32,686; part-time $1337 per credit. *Required fees:* $740; $200. Tuition and fees vary according to program. *Financial support:* In 2013–14, 11 students received support, including 2 fellowships with partial tuition reimbursements available (averaging $225 per year), 6 research assistantships with full and partial tuition reimbursements available (averaging $25,843 per year), 4 teaching assistantships with full and partial tuition reimbursements available (averaging $16,970 per year); unspecified assistantships also available. Financial award applicants required to submit FAFSA. *Faculty research:* Community-based participatory research, health equity, evaluation science, LGBT health, aging. *Total annual research expenditures:* $2.8 million. *Unit head:* Dr. Steven Albert, Chairman, 412-624-3102, Fax: 412-648-5975, E-mail: smalbert@pitt.edu. *Application contact:* Natalie C. Arnold, Recruitment and Academic Affairs Administrator, 412-624-3107, Fax: 412-624-5510, E-mail: narnold@pitt.edu.
Website: http://www.bchs.pitt.edu/

University of Pittsburgh, Graduate School of Public Health, Department of Health Policy and Management, Pittsburgh, PA 15260. Offers health administration (MHA); public health (MPH); JD/MPH. *Accreditation:* CAHME. Part-time programs available. *Faculty:* 17 full-time (7 women), 29 part-time/adjunct (9 women). *Students:* 52 full-time (35 women), 23 part-time (14 women); includes 18 minority (7 Black or African American, non-Hispanic/Latino; 7 Asian, non-Hispanic/Latino; 1 Hispanic/Latino; 3 Two or more races, non-Hispanic/Latino), 12 international. Average age 27. 252 applicants, 50% accepted, 36 enrolled. In 2013, 37 master's awarded. *Degree requirements:* For master's, comprehensive exam (for some programs), thesis, essay. *Entrance requirements:* For master's, GRE, 3 credits each of course work in mathematics and biology, 6 in social science; bachelor's degree; recommendations; professional statement; transcripts. Additional exam requirements/recommendations for international students: Required—TOEFL (minimum score 550 paper-based; 80 iBT) or IELTS (minimum score 6.5). *Application deadline:* For fall admission, 3/15 for domestic students, 1/15 for international students; for winter admission, 11/1 for domestic students, 8/1 for international students; for spring admission, 10/1 for domestic students, 8/1 for international students; for summer admission, 12/1 for international students. Applications are processed on a rolling basis. Application fee: $120. Electronic applications accepted. *Expenses:* Tuition, state resident: full-time $19,964; part-time $807 per credit. Tuition, nonresident: full-time $32,686; part-time $1337 per credit. *Required fees:* $740; $200. Tuition and fees vary according to program. *Financial support:* In 2013–14, 15 students received support, including 1 fellowship with partial tuition reimbursement available (averaging $100 per year), 11 research assistantships with full and partial tuition reimbursements available (averaging $17,280 per year), 5 teaching assistantships with full and partial tuition reimbursements available (averaging $15,353 per year); career-related internships or fieldwork, scholarships/grants, health care benefits, and unspecified assistantships also available. Support available to part-time students. Financial award applicants required to submit FAFSA. *Faculty research:* Cost effectiveness analysis, mathematical modeling and decision science, long-term care and nursing home quality health policy and pharmaceutical policy, organization theory, health economics. *Total annual research expenditures:* $2.1 million. *Unit head:* Dr. Mark S. Roberts, Professor/Chair, 412-383-7049, Fax: 412-624-3146, E-mail: mroberts@pitt.edu. *Application contact:* Donna Schultz, Program Coordinator, 412-624-3123, Fax: 412-624-3146, E-mail: dschultz@pitt.edu.
Website: http://www.hpm.pitt.edu/

University of Pittsburgh, School of Health and Rehabilitation Sciences, Master's Programs in Health and Rehabilitation Sciences, Pittsburgh, PA 15260. Offers health and rehabilitation sciences (MS), including health care supervision and management, health information systems, occupational therapy, physical therapy, rehabilitation counseling, rehabilitation science and technology, sports medicine, wellness and human performance. *Accreditation:* APTA. Part-time and evening/weekend programs available. *Faculty:* 63 full-time (37 women), 4 part-time/adjunct (2 women). *Students:* 117 full-time (70 women), 44 part-time (27 women); includes 18 minority (8 Black or African American, non-Hispanic/Latino; 1 American Indian or Alaska Native, non-Hispanic/Latino; 6 Asian, non-Hispanic/Latino; 3 Hispanic/Latino), 52 international. Average age 30. 368 applicants, 57% accepted, 96 enrolled. In 2013, 90 master's awarded. *Degree requirements:* For master's, comprehensive exam (for some programs), thesis optional. *Entrance requirements:* For master's, minimum GPA of 3.0. Additional exam requirements/recommendations for international students: Required—TOEFL (minimum score 550 paper-based; 80 iBT), IELTS (minimum score 6.5). *Application deadline:* For fall admission, 3/1 for international students; for spring admission, 9/1 for international students. Applications are processed on a rolling basis. Application fee: $50. Electronic applications accepted. *Expenses:* Contact institution. *Financial support:* In 2013–14, 3 fellowships (averaging $20,460 per year) were awarded; Federal Work-Study, institutionally sponsored loans, scholarships/grants, traineeships, and unspecified assistantships also available. Financial award applicants required to submit FAFSA. *Faculty research:* Assistive technology, seating and wheeled mobility, cellular neurophysiology, low back syndrome, augmentative communication. *Total annual research expenditures:* $8.1 million. *Unit head:* Dr. Clifford E. Brubaker, Dean, 412-383-6560, Fax: 412-383-6535, E-mail: cliffb@pitt.edu. *Application contact:* Jessica Maguire, Director of Admissions, 412-383-6557, Fax: 412-383-6535, E-mail: maguire@pitt.edu.
Website: http://www.shrs.pitt.edu/

University of Portland, Dr. Robert B. Pamplin, Jr. School of Business, Portland, OR 97203-5798. Offers entrepreneurship (MBA); finance (MBA, MS); health care management (MBA); marketing (MBA); nonprofit management (EMBA); operations and technology management (MBA, MS); sustainability (MBA). *Accreditation:* AACSB. Part-time and evening/weekend programs available. *Faculty:* 26 full-time (5 women), 8 part-time/adjunct (1 woman). *Students:* 37 full-time (11 women), 93 part-time (44 women); includes 15 minority (1 Black or African American, non-Hispanic/Latino; 7 Asian, non-Hispanic/Latino; 5 Hispanic/Latino; 2 Two or more races, non-Hispanic/Latino), 21 international. Average age 32. In 2013, 68 master's awarded. *Entrance requirements:* For master's, GMAT, minimum GPA of 3.0, resume, 2 letters of recommendation. Additional exam requirements/recommendations for international students: Required—TOEFL (minimum score 570 paper-based; 89 iBT), IELTS (minimum score 7). *Application deadline:* For fall admission, 7/15 priority date for domestic and international students; for spring admission, 12/15 priority date for domestic and international students. Applications are processed on a rolling basis. Application fee: $50. *Expenses:* Contact institution. *Financial support:* Federal Work-Study, scholarships/grants, and tuition waivers (partial) available. Support available to part-time students. Financial award application deadline: 3/1; financial award applicants required to submit FAFSA. *Unit head:* Melissa McCarthy, Director, 503-943-7224, E-mail: mba-up@up.edu.
Website: http://business.up.edu/mba/default.aspx?cid-1179&pid-6450

University of Puerto Rico, Medical Sciences Campus, Graduate School of Public Health, Department of Health Services Administration, Program in Health Services Administration, San Juan, PR 00936-5067. Offers MHSA. *Accreditation:* CAHME. Part-time programs available. *Degree requirements:* For master's, thesis. *Entrance requirements:* For master's, GRE, previous course work in accounting, statistics, economics, algebra, and managerial finance.

University of Regina, Faculty of Graduate Studies and Research, Johnson-Shoyama Graduate School of Public Policy, Regina, SK S4S 0A2, Canada. Offers economic analysis for public policy (Master's Certificate); health administration (MHA); health systems management (Master's Certificate); health systems research (MPP); public management (MPA, Master's Certificate); public policy (MPA, MPP, PhD); public policy analysis (Master's Certificate). Part-time programs available. *Faculty:* 8 full-time (4 women), 16 part-time/adjunct (5 women). *Students:* 51 full-time (32 women), 75 part-time (44 women). 175 applicants, 61% accepted. In 2013, 41 master's, 10 other advanced degrees awarded. *Degree requirements:* For master's, thesis (for some programs); for doctorate, thesis/dissertation. *Entrance requirements:* For doctorate, master's degree, intended research program in an area of public policy. Additional exam

requirements/recommendations for international students: Required—TOEFL (minimum score 580 paper-based; 80 iBT), IELTS (minimum score 6.5). *Application deadline:* For fall admission, 2/1 for domestic and international students. Application fee: $100. Electronic applications accepted. *Expenses:* Contact institution. *Financial support:* In 2013–14, 15 fellowships (averaging $6,133 per year), 1 research assistantship (averaging $5,500 per year), 14 teaching assistantships (averaging $2,356 per year) were awarded; scholarships/grants also available. Financial award application deadline: 6/15. *Faculty research:* Governance and administration, public finance, public policy analysis, non-governmental organizations and alternative service delivery, micro-economics for policy analysis. *Unit head:* Dr. Michael Atkinson, Executive Director, 306-996-1984, Fax: 306-585-5461, E-mail: michael.atkinson@usask.ca. *Application contact:* Sarina Wowchuk, Program Advisor and Administrative Manager, 306-585-5462, Fax: 306-585-5461, E-mail: sarina.wowchuk@uregina.ca.
Website: http://www.schoolofpublicpolicy.sk.ca/

University of Rochester, School of Nursing, Rochester, NY 14642. Offers acute care nurse practitioner (MS); adult nurse practitioner (MS); adult/geriatric nurse practitioner (MS); clinical nurse leader (MS); clinical research coordinator (MS); family nurse practitioner (MS); family psychiatric mental health nurse practitioner (MS); health care organization management and leadership (MS); health practice research (PhD); nursing (DNP); pediatric nurse practitioner (MS); pediatric nurse practitioner/neonatal nurse practitioner (MS). *Accreditation:* AACN. Part-time programs available. Postbaccalaureate distance learning degree programs offered (minimal on-campus study). *Faculty:* 60 full-time (52 women), 61 part-time/adjunct (47 women). *Students:* 33 full-time (29 women), 213 part-time (195 women); includes 32 minority (8 Black or African American, non-Hispanic/Latino; 10 Asian, non-Hispanic/Latino; 8 Hispanic/Latino; 6 Two or more races, non-Hispanic/Latino), 4 international. Average age 34. 41 applicants, 54% accepted, 16 enrolled. In 2013, 58 master's, 11 doctorates awarded. Terminal master's awarded for partial completion of doctoral program. *Degree requirements:* For master's, comprehensive exam (for some programs); for doctorate, thesis/dissertation. *Entrance requirements:* For master's, BS in nursing, minimum GPA of 3.0, course work in statistics; for doctorate, GRE General Test, MS in nursing, minimum GPA of 3.5. Additional exam requirements/recommendations for international students: Required—TOEFL (minimum score 560 paper-based; 88 iBT) or IELTS (minimum score 6.5) recommended. *Application deadline:* For fall admission, 4/1 for domestic and international students; for spring admission, 9/1 for domestic and international students; for summer admission, 1/2 for domestic and international students. Application fee: $50. Electronic applications accepted. *Expenses: Tuition:* Full-time $44,580; part-time $1394 per credit hour. *Required fees:* $492. *Financial support:* In 2013–14, 41 students received support, including 2 fellowships with full and partial tuition reimbursements available (averaging $30,200 per year); scholarships/grants, traineeships, health care benefits, tuition waivers (partial), and unspecified assistantships also available. Support available to part-time students. Financial award application deadline: 6/30. *Faculty research:* Symptom assessment and self-management, illness prevention, nursing intervention research with vulnerable populations, palliative care, aging. *Total annual research expenditures:* $3.5 million. *Unit head:* Dr. Kathy H. Rideout, Dean, 585-273-8902, Fax: 585-273-1268, E-mail: kathy_rideout@urmc.rochester.edu. *Application contact:* Elaine Andolina, Director of Admissions, 585-275-2375, Fax: 585-756-8299, E-mail: elaine_andolina@urmc.rochester.edu.
Website: http://www.son.rochester.edu

University of Rochester, Simon Business School, Full-Time Master's Program in Business Administration, Rochester, NY 14627. Offers accounting and information systems (MBA); business environment and public policy (MBA); business systems consulting (MBA); competitive and organizational strategy - pricing (MBA); computers and information systems (MBA); corporate accounting (MBA); electronic commerce (MBA); entrepreneurship (MBA); finance (MBA); health sciences management (MBA); international management (MBA); marketing - brand management and pricing (MBA); operations management - manufacturing (MBA); operations management - services (MBA); public accounting (MBA). *Accreditation:* AACSB. Part-time and evening/weekend programs available. *Faculty:* 60 full-time (11 women), 23 part-time/adjunct (3 women). *Students:* 282 full-time (74 women); includes 55 minority (29 Black or African American, non-Hispanic/Latino; 1 American Indian or Alaska Native, non-Hispanic/Latino; 11 Asian, non-Hispanic/Latino; 12 Hispanic/Latino; 2 Two or more races, non-Hispanic/Latino), 144 international. 673 applicants, 33% accepted, 65 enrolled. In 2013, 176 master's awarded. *Entrance requirements:* For master's, GMAT/GRE, previous course work in calculus. Additional exam requirements/recommendations for international students: Required—TOEFL. *Application deadline:* For fall admission, 10/15 for domestic and international students; for winter admission, 1/5 for domestic and international students; for spring admission, 3/15 for domestic and international students; for summer admission, 5/15 for domestic students. Applications are processed on a rolling basis. Application fee: $150. Electronic applications accepted. *Expenses: Tuition:* Full-time $44,580; part-time $1394 per credit hour. *Required fees:* $492. *Financial support:* In 2013–14, 72 students received support. Fellowships, research assistantships, teaching assistantships, institutionally sponsored loans, scholarships/grants, and tuition waivers (partial) available. Financial award application deadline: 3/1; financial award applicants required to submit CSS PROFILE or FAFSA. *Unit head:* Mark Zupan, Dean, 585-275-3316. *Application contact:* Rebekah S. Lewin, Assistant Dean of Admissions and Student Engagement, 585-275-3533, E-mail: admissions@simon.rochester.edu.

University of Rochester, Simon Business School, Part-Time MBA Program, Rochester, NY 14627. Offers accounting and information systems (MBA); business environment and public policy (MBA); business systems consulting (MBA); competitive and organizational strategy (MBA); computers and information systems (MBA); corporate accounting (MBA); electronic commerce (MBA); entrepreneurship (MBA); finance (MBA); health sciences management (MBA); international management (MBA); manufacturing management (MBA); marketing (MBA); operations management - services (MBA); public accounting (MBA). Part-time and evening/weekend programs available. *Faculty:* 59 full-time (10 women), 23 part-time/adjunct (3 women). *Students:* 270 part-time (75 women); includes 38 minority (5 Black or African American, non-Hispanic/Latino; 1 American Indian or Alaska Native, non-Hispanic/Latino; 24 Asian, non-Hispanic/Latino; 5 Hispanic/Latino; 3 Two or more races, non-Hispanic/Latino). Average age 32. 56 applicants, 98% accepted, 51 enrolled. In 2013, 77 master's awarded. *Entrance requirements:* For master's, GRE or GMAT, resume, recommendation letters, essays, transcipts. *Application deadline:* For fall admission, 8/15 for domestic students; for winter admission, 11/15 for domestic students; for spring admission, 2/15 for domestic students; for summer admission, 5/15 for domestic students. Applications are processed on a rolling basis. Application fee: $150. Electronic applications accepted. *Expenses: Tuition:* Full-time $44,580; part-time $1394 per credit hour. *Required fees:* $492. *Financial support:* Scholarships/grants and tuition waivers available. Financial award applicants required to submit CSS PROFILE. *Unit head:* Mark Zupan, Dean, 585-275-3316, E-mail: mark.zupan@simon.rochester.edu. *Application contact:* Jennifer Mossotti, Associate Director of Part-Time Programs, 585-275-3803, E-mail: jennifer.mossotti@simon.rochester.edu.
Website: http://www.simon.rochester.edu/programs/part-time-mba-programs/index.aspx

University of St. Francis, College of Business and Health Administration, School of Health Administration, Joliet, IL 60435-6169. Offers MS. Part-time and evening/weekend programs available. Postbaccalaureate distance learning degree programs offered (no on-campus study). *Faculty:* 2 full-time (0 women), 8 part-time/adjunct (3 women). *Students:* 72 full-time (64 women), 201 part-time (160 women); includes 66 minority (31 Black or African American, non-Hispanic/Latino; 1 American Indian or Alaska Native, non-Hispanic/Latino; 8 Asian, non-Hispanic/Latino; 18 Hispanic/Latino; 1 Native Hawaiian or other Pacific Islander, non-Hispanic/Latino; 7 Two or more races, non-Hispanic/Latino), 4 international. Average age 43. 137 applicants, 50% accepted, 49 enrolled. In 2013, 145 master's awarded. *Degree requirements:* For master's, comprehensive exam. *Entrance requirements:* For master's, minimum GPA of 2.75, 2 letters recommendation, personal essay, computer proficiency. Additional exam requirements/recommendations for international students: Required—TOEFL (minimum score 550 paper-based; 79 iBT), IELTS (minimum score 6.5). *Application deadline:* Applications are processed on a rolling basis. Application fee: $30. Electronic applications accepted. Application fee is waived when completed online. *Expenses: Tuition:* Part-time $710 per credit hour. *Required fees:* $125 per semester. Part-time tuition and fees vary according to degree level and program. *Financial support:* In 2013–14, 67 students received support. Tuition waivers (partial) and unspecified assistantships available. Support available to part-time students. Financial award applicants required to submit FAFSA. *Unit head:* Dr. Christopher Clott, Dean, 815-740-3395, Fax: 815-740-3537, E-mail: cclott@stfrancis.edu. *Application contact:* Sandra Sloka, Director of Admissions for Graduate and Degree Completion Programs, 800-735-7500, Fax: 815-740-3431, E-mail: ssloka@stfrancis.edu.
Website: http://www.stfrancis.edu/academics/college-of-business-health-administration/

University of Saint Francis, Graduate School, Keith Busse School of Business and Entrepreneurial Leadership, Fort Wayne, IN 46808-3994. Offers business administration (MBA); environmental health (MEH); healthcare administration (MHA); sustainability (MBA). *Accreditation:* ACBSP. Part-time and evening/weekend programs available. Postbaccalaureate distance learning degree programs offered (no on-campus study). *Faculty:* 8. *Students:* 74 full-time (38 women), 69 part-time (35 women); includes 22 minority (12 Black or African American, non-Hispanic/Latino; 2 Asian, non-Hispanic/Latino; 7 Hispanic/Latino; 1 Two or more races, non-Hispanic/Latino), 3 international. Average age 34. 73 applicants, 97% accepted, 71 enrolled. In 2013, 12 master's awarded. *Entrance requirements:* For master's, minimum undergraduate GPA of 2.75. *Application deadline:* For fall admission, 7/1 priority date for domestic students; for spring admission, 11/1 priority date for domestic students. Applications are processed on a rolling basis. Application fee: $20. Application fee is waived when completed online. *Financial support:* Federal Work-Study, scholarships/grants, and unspecified assistantships available. Support available to part-time students. Financial award application deadline: 3/10; financial award applicants required to submit FAFSA. *Unit head:* Dr. Karen Palumbo, Professor/Graduate Program Director, 260-399-7700 Ext. 8312, Fax: 260-399-8174, E-mail: kpalumbo@sf.edu. *Application contact:* James Cashdollar, Admissions Counselor, 260-399-7700 Ext. 6302, Fax: 260-399-8152, E-mail: jcashdollar@sf.edu.
Website: http://www.sf.edu/sf/graduate/business

University of Saint Mary, Graduate Programs, Program in Business Administration, Leavenworth, KS 66048-5082. Offers enterprise risk management (MBA); finance (MBA); general management (MBA); health care management (MBA); human resource management (MBA); marketing and advertising management (MBA). Part-time and evening/weekend programs available. Postbaccalaureate distance learning degree programs offered (no on-campus study). *Students:* 151 full-time (87 women), 61 part-time (39 women); includes 60 minority (38 Black or African American, non-Hispanic/Latino; 1 American Indian or Alaska Native, non-Hispanic/Latino; 10 Asian, non-Hispanic/Latino; 11 Hispanic/Latino). *Degree requirements:* For master's, thesis. *Entrance requirements:* For master's, minimum undergraduate GPA of 2.75, official transcripts, two letters of recommendation. *Application deadline:* Applications are processed on a rolling basis. Application fee: $25. *Expenses: Tuition:* Part-time $550 per credit hour. *Unit head:* Rick Gunter, Director, 913-319-3007. *Application contact:* Patrick Smith, Coordinator of Business Programs, 913-319-3007, E-mail: smithp@stmary.edu.

University of St. Thomas, Graduate Studies, Opus College of Business, Health Care UST MBA Program, Minneapolis, MN 55403. Offers MBA. *Accreditation:* CAHME. Postbaccalaureate distance learning degree programs offered (minimal on-campus study). *Students:* 145 part-time (62 women); includes 16 minority (2 Black or African American, non-Hispanic/Latino; 8 Asian, non-Hispanic/Latino; 5 Hispanic/Latino; 1 Two or more races, non-Hispanic/Latino). Average age 40. 63 applicants, 98% accepted, 62 enrolled. In 2013, 52 master's awarded. *Entrance requirements:* For master's, minimum 5 years of work experience in related field, letters of recommendation, essays, interview. Additional exam requirements/recommendations for international students: Required—TOEFL (minimum score 80 iBT), IELTS, or Michigan English Language Assessment Battery. *Application deadline:* For fall admission, 2/1 for domestic students; for winter admission, 5/1 for domestic students; for spring admission, 6/1 for domestic students. Applications are processed on a rolling basis. Application fee: $75. Electronic applications accepted. *Expenses:* Contact institution. *Financial support:* Scholarships/grants available. *Unit head:* Kathryn DiAna, Program Director, 651-962-4135, Fax: 651-962-8810, E-mail: medmba@stthomas.edu. *Application contact:* Kathryn DiAna, Program Director, 651-962-4135, Fax: 651-962-8810, E-mail: medmba@stthomas.edu.
Website: http://www.stthomas.edu/healthcaremba

University of San Francisco, School of Management, Master of Public Administration Program, Concentration in Health Services Administration, San Francisco, CA 94117-1080. Offers MPA. Part-time and evening/weekend programs available. *Faculty:* 4 full-time (1 woman), 3 part-time/adjunct (1 woman). *Students:* 40 full-time (33 women), 1 (woman) part-time; includes 31 minority (6 Black or African American, non-Hispanic/Latino; 15 Asian, non-Hispanic/Latino; 9 Hispanic/Latino; 1 Two or more races, non-Hispanic/Latino). Average age 34. 12 applicants, 83% accepted, 9 enrolled. In 2013, 12 master's awarded. *Degree requirements:* For master's, thesis optional. *Entrance requirements:* For master's, minimum GPA of 3.0. Application fee: $55 ($65 for international students). *Expenses: Tuition:* Full-time $21,150; part-time $1175 per unit. Tuition and fees vary according to course load, campus/location and program. *Financial support:* In 2013–14, 1 student received support. Application deadline: 3/2; applicants required to submit FAFSA. *Unit head:* Dr. Maurice Penner, Professor, 415-422-2144. *Application contact:* 415-422-6000, E-mail: graduate@usfca.edu.

University of Saskatchewan, College of Graduate Studies and Research, Edwards School of Business, Program in Business Administration, Saskatoon, SK S7N 5A2, Canada. Offers agribusiness management (MBA); biotechnology management (MBA); health services management (MBA); indigenous management (MBA); international business management (MBA). *Expenses: Tuition, area resident:* Full-time $3585 Canadian dollars; part-time $585 Canadian dollars per course. Tuition, nonresident: part-time $877 Canadian dollars per course. *International tuition:* $5377 Canadian dollars full-time. *Required fees:* $889.51 Canadian dollars.

The University of Scranton, College of Graduate and Continuing Education, Department of Health Administration and Human Resources, Program in Health Administration, Scranton, PA 18510. Offers MHA. *Accreditation:* CAHME. Part-time and evening/weekend programs available. *Students:* 70 full-time (29 women), 4 part-time (3 women); includes 17 minority (5 Black or African American, non-Hispanic/Latino; 7 Asian, non-Hispanic/Latino; 5 Hispanic/Latino), 6 international. Average age 27. 79 applicants, 89% accepted. In 2013, 24 master's awarded. *Degree requirements:* For master's, capstone experience. *Entrance requirements:* For master's, minimum GPA of 3.0. Additional exam requirements/recommendations for international students: Required—TOEFL (minimum score 550 paper-based), IELTS (minimum score 6). *Application deadline:* For fall admission, 4/15 priority date for domestic students. Applications are processed on a rolling basis. Application fee: $0. *Financial support:* Fellowships, teaching assistantships, career-related internships or fieldwork, and unspecified assistantships available. Financial award application deadline: 3/1. *Unit head:* Steven J. Szydlowski, Director, 570-941-4367, Fax: 570-941-4201, E-mail: sjs14@scranton.edu. *Application contact:* Joseph M. Roback, Director of Admissions, 570-941-4385, Fax: 570-941-5928, E-mail: robackj2@scranton.edu.

The University of Scranton, College of Graduate and Continuing Education, Program in Business Administration, Scranton, PA 18510. Offers accounting (MBA); finance (MBA); general business administration (MBA); health care management (MBA); international business (MBA); management information systems (MBA); marketing (MBA); operations management (MBA). *Accreditation:* AACSB. Part-time and evening/weekend programs available. Postbaccalaureate distance learning degree programs offered (no on-campus study). *Faculty:* 34 full-time (8 women). *Students:* 316 full-time (134 women), 241 part-time (94 women); includes 104 minority (43 Black or African American, non-Hispanic/Latino; 3 American Indian or Alaska Native, non-Hispanic/Latino; 29 Asian, non-Hispanic/Latino; 27 Hispanic/Latino; 2 Two or more races, non-Hispanic/Latino), 47 international. Average age 34. 249 applicants, 85% accepted. In 2013, 200 master's awarded. *Degree requirements:* For master's, capstone experience. *Entrance requirements:* For master's, GMAT, minimum GPA of 3.0. Additional exam requirements/recommendations for international students: Required—TOEFL (minimum score 500 paper-based), IELTS (minimum score 6). *Application deadline:* Applications are processed on a rolling basis. Application fee: $0. *Financial support:* In 2013–14, 13 students received support, including 13 teaching assistantships with full and partial tuition reimbursements available (averaging $8,800 per year); fellowships, career-related internships or fieldwork, Federal Work-Study, and unspecified assistantships also available. Support available to part-time students. Financial award application deadline: 3/1. *Faculty research:* Financial markets, strategic impact of total quality management, internal accounting controls, consumer preference, information systems and the Internet. *Unit head:* Dr. Murli Rajan, Director, 570-941-4043, Fax: 570-941-4342. *Application contact:* Joseph M. Roback, Director of Admissions, 570-941-4385, Fax: 570-941-5928, E-mail: robackj2@scranton.edu.
Website: http://www.scranton.edu/academics/cgce/busad.shtml

University of Sioux Falls, Vucurevich School of Business, Sioux Falls, SD 57105-1699. Offers entrepreneurial leadership (MBA); general management (MBA); health care management (MBA); marketing (MBA). Part-time and evening/weekend programs available. *Degree requirements:* For master's, project. *Entrance requirements:* For master's, minimum GPA of 3.0. Additional exam requirements/recommendations for international students: Required—TOEFL. *Expenses:* Contact institution.

University of South Africa, College of Human Sciences, Pretoria, South Africa. Offers adult education (M Ed); African languages (MA, PhD); African politics (MA, PhD); Afrikaans (MA, PhD); ancient history (MA, PhD); ancient Near Eastern studies (MA, PhD); anthropology (MA, PhD); applied linguistics (MA); Arabic (MA, PhD); archaeology (MA); art history (MA); Biblical archaeology (MA); Biblical studies (M Th, D Th, PhD); Christian spirituality (M Th, D Th); church history (M Th, D Th); classical studies (MA, PhD); clinical psychology (MA); communication (MA, PhD); comparative education (M Ed, Ed D); consulting psychology (D Admin, D Com, PhD); curriculum studies (M Ed, Ed D); development studies (M Admin, MA, D Admin, PhD); didactics (M Ed, Ed D); education (M Tech); education management (M Ed, Ed D); educational psychology (M Ed); English (MA); environmental education (M Ed); French (MA, PhD); German (MA, PhD); Greek (MA); guidance and counseling (M Ed); health studies (MA, PhD), including health sciences education (MA), health services management (MA), medical and surgical nursing science (critical care general) (MA), midwifery and neonatal nursing science (MA), trauma and emergency care (MA); history (MA, PhD); history of education (Ed D); inclusive education (M Ed, Ed D); information and communications technology policy and regulation (MA); information science (MA, MIS, PhD); international politics (MA, PhD); Islamic studies (MA, PhD); Italian (MA, PhD); Judaica (MA, PhD); linguistics (MA, PhD); mathematical education (M Ed); mathematics education (MA); missiology (M Th, D Th); modern Hebrew (MA, PhD); musicology (MA, MMus, D Mus, PhD); natural science education (M Ed); New Testament (M Th, D Th); Old Testament (D Th); pastoral therapy (M Th, D Th); philosophy (MA); philosophy of education (M Ed, Ed D); politics (MA, PhD); Portuguese (MA, PhD); practical theology (M Th, D Th); psychology (MA, MS, PhD); psychology of education (M Ed, Ed D); public health (MA); religious studies (MA, D Th, PhD); Romance languages (MA); Russian (MA, PhD); Semitic languages (MA, PhD); social behavior studies in HIV/AIDS (MA); social science (mental health) (MA); social science in development studies (MA); social science in psychology (MA); social science in social work (MA); social science in sociology (MA); social work (MSW, DSW, PhD); socio-education (M Ed, Ed D); sociolinguistics (MA); sociology (MA, PhD); Spanish (MA, PhD); systematic theology (M Th, D Th); TESOL (teaching English to speakers of other languages) (MA); theological ethics (M Th, D Th); theory of literature (MA, PhD); urban ministries (D Th); urban ministry (M Th).

University of South Carolina, The Graduate School, Arnold School of Public Health, Department of Health Services Policy and Management, Columbia, SC 29208. Offers MHA, MPH, Dr PH, PhD, JD/MHA, MPH/MSN, MSW/MPH. *Accreditation:* CAHME (one or more programs are accredited). Part-time and evening/weekend programs available. *Degree requirements:* For master's, comprehensive exam, thesis or alternative, internship (MHA); for doctorate, comprehensive exam, thesis/dissertation. *Entrance requirements:* For master's, GMAT (MHA), GRE General Test (MPH); for doctorate, GRE General Test. Additional exam requirements/recommendations for international students: Required—TOEFL (minimum score 570 paper-based). Electronic applications accepted. *Faculty research:* Health systems management, evaluation, and planning; forecast applications in health care; Medicaid process to health care services.

The University of South Dakota, Graduate School, College of Arts and Sciences, Program in Administrative Studies, Vermillion, SD 57069-2390. Offers alcohol and drug studies (MSA); criminal justice (MSA); health services administration (MSA); human resource management (MSA); interdisciplinary (MSA); long term care administration (MSA); organizational leadership (MSA). Part-time and evening/weekend programs available. Postbaccalaureate distance learning degree programs offered (no on-campus study). *Degree requirements:* For master's, thesis or alternative. *Entrance requirements:* For master's, 3 years of work or experience, minimum GPA of 2.7, resume. Additional exam requirements/recommendations for international students: Required—TOEFL (minimum score 550 paper-based; 79 iBT). Electronic applications accepted.

The University of South Dakota, Graduate School, School of Business, Department of Business Administration, Vermillion, SD 57069-2390. Offers business administration (MBA); health services administration (MBA); JD/MBA. *Accreditation:* AACSB. Part-time and evening/weekend programs available. Postbaccalaureate distance learning degree programs offered (no on-campus study). *Degree requirements:* For master's, thesis or alternative. *Entrance requirements:* For master's, GMAT, minimum GPA of 2.7, resume. Additional exam requirements/recommendations for international students: Required—TOEFL (minimum score 550 paper-based; 79 iBT). Electronic applications accepted. *Expenses:* Contact institution.

University of Southern California, Graduate School, School of Policy, Planning, and Development, Executive Master of Health Administration Program, Los Angeles, CA 90089. Offers EMHA. Part-time and evening/weekend programs available. Postbaccalaureate distance learning degree programs offered (minimal on-campus study). *Entrance requirements:* Additional exam requirements/recommendations for international students: Required—TOEFL (minimum score 600 paper-based; 100 iBT). Electronic applications accepted. *Expenses:* Contact institution. *Faculty research:* Health management and policy, health care systems, health care economics and financing, health care access, community health, healthy communities.

University of Southern California, Graduate School, School of Policy, Planning, and Development, Master of Health Administration Program, Los Angeles, CA 90089. Offers ambulatory care (Graduate Certificate); health administration (MHA); long-term care (Graduate Certificate); MHA/MS. *Accreditation:* CAHME. Part-time programs available. *Degree requirements:* For master's, residency placement. *Entrance requirements:* For master's, GRE, GMAT. Additional exam requirements/recommendations for international students: Required—TOEFL (minimum score 600 paper-based; 100 iBT). Electronic applications accepted. *Faculty research:* Health administration, health management and policy, health care economics and financing, health care access, community health, healthy communities.

University of Southern Indiana, Graduate Studies, College of Nursing and Health Professions, Program in Health Administration, Evansville, IN 47712-3590. Offers MHA. Part-time programs available. Postbaccalaureate distance learning degree programs offered (minimal on-campus study). *Faculty:* 1 full-time (0 women), 1 part-time/adjunct (0 women). *Students:* 1 (woman) full-time, 37 part-time (29 women); includes 1 minority (Hispanic/Latino). Average age 34. 28 applicants, 57% accepted, 16 enrolled. In 2013, 15 master's awarded. *Entrance requirements:* For master's, GRE and one focused essay or three focused essays, minimum GPA of 3.0, curriculum vitae, letter of intent, three professional references. Additional exam requirements/recommendations for international students: Required—TOEFL (minimum score 550 paper-based; 79 iBT), IELTS (minimum score 6). *Application deadline:* For fall admission, 6/1 for domestic students, 1/1 priority date for international students. Applications are processed on a rolling basis. Application fee: $40. Electronic applications accepted. *Expenses:* Tuition, state resident: full-time $5567; part-time $309 per credit hour. Tuition, nonresident: full-time $10,977; part-time $610 per credit. *Required fees:* $23 per semester. *Financial support:* In 2013–14, 9 students received support. Federal Work-Study, scholarships/grants, tuition waivers (full and partial), and unspecified assistantships available. Financial award application deadline: 3/1; financial award applicants required to submit FAFSA. *Unit head:* Dr. Kevin Valadares, Program Chair, 812-461-5277, E-mail: kvaladar@usi.edu. *Application contact:* Dr. Mayola Rowser, Interim Director, Graduate Studies, 812-465-7016, Fax: 812-464-1956, E-mail: mrowser@usi.edu.
Website: http://www.usi.edu/health/master-of-health-administration

University of Southern Maine, College of Management and Human Service, School of Business, Portland, ME 04104-9300. Offers accounting (MBA); business administration (MBA); finance (MBA); health management and policy (MBA); sustainability (MBA); JD/MBA; MBA/MSA; MBA/MSN; MS/MBA. *Accreditation:* AACSB. Part-time and evening/weekend programs available. *Faculty:* 10 part-time/adjunct (2 women). *Students:* 89 part-time (37 women); includes 4 minority (3 American Indian or Alaska Native, non-Hispanic/Latino; 1 Asian, non-Hispanic/Latino), 2 international. Average age 31. 36 applicants, 56% accepted, 16 enrolled. In 2013, 34 master's awarded. *Entrance requirements:* For master's, GMAT or GRE, minimum AACSB index of 1100. Additional exam requirements/recommendations for international students: Required—TOEFL (minimum score 550 paper-based; 79 iBT). *Application deadline:* For fall admission, 8/1 priority date for domestic students, 5/1 priority date for international students; for spring admission, 12/1 priority date for domestic students, 9/1 priority date for international students. Applications are processed on a rolling basis. Application fee: $65. Electronic applications accepted. *Expenses:* Tuition, state resident: part-time $380 per credit. Tuition, nonresident: part-time $1026 per credit. Part-time tuition and fees vary according to program. *Financial support:* In 2013–14, 3 research assistantships with partial tuition reimbursements (averaging $9,000 per year), 3 teaching assistantships with partial tuition reimbursements (averaging $9,000 per year) were awarded; career-related internships or fieldwork, Federal Work-Study, scholarships/grants, tuition waivers (full and partial), and unspecified assistantships also available. Support available to part-time students. Financial award application deadline: 2/15; financial award applicants required to submit FAFSA. *Faculty research:* Economic development, management information systems, real options, system dynamics, simulation. *Unit head:* Joseph W. McDonnell, Dean, 207-228-8002, Fax: 207-780-4060, E-mail: jmcdonnell@usm.maine.edu. *Application contact:* Alice B. Cash, Assistant Director for Student Affairs, 207-780-4184, Fax: 207-780-4662, E-mail: acash@usm.maine.edu.
Website: http://www.usm.maine.edu/sb

University of Southern Mississippi, Graduate School, College of Health, Department of Community Health Sciences, Hattiesburg, MS 39406-0001. Offers epidemiology and biostatistics (MPH); health education (MPH); health policy/administration (MPH); occupational/environmental health (MPH); public health nutrition (MPH). *Accreditation:* CEPH. Part-time and evening/weekend programs available. *Faculty:* 8 full-time (4 women), 1 part-time/adjunct (0 women). *Students:* 92 full-time (60 women), 9 part-time (4 women); includes 38 minority (29 Black or African American, non-Hispanic/Latino; 1 American Indian or Alaska Native, non-Hispanic/Latino; 2 Asian, non-Hispanic/Latino; 6 Two or more races, non-Hispanic/Latino), 13 international. Average age 34. 71 applicants, 93% accepted, 45 enrolled. *Degree requirements:* For master's, comprehensive exam, thesis (for some programs). *Entrance requirements:* For master's, GRE General Test, minimum GPA of 2.75 in last 60 hours. Additional exam requirements/recommendations for international students: Required—TOEFL, IELTS. *Application deadline:* For fall admission, 3/1 priority date for domestic and international students; for spring admission, 1/10 priority date for domestic and international students. Applications are processed on a rolling basis. Application fee: $50. Electronic applications accepted. *Financial support:* In 2013–14, 5 research assistantships with full tuition reimbursements (averaging $7,000 per year), 1 teaching assistantship with full tuition reimbursement (averaging $8,263 per year) were awarded; career-related internships or fieldwork, Federal Work-Study, institutionally sponsored loans, scholarships/grants, health care benefits, and unspecified assistantships also available. Financial award application deadline: 3/15; financial award applicants required to submit FAFSA. *Faculty research:* Rural health care delivery, school health, nutrition of pregnant teens, risk factor reduction, sexually transmitted diseases. *Unit head:* Dr. Ray Newman, Interim Chair, 601-266-5437, Fax: 601-266-5043. *Application contact:* Shonna Breland, Manager of Graduate Admissions, 601-266-6563, Fax: 601-266-5138.
Website: http://www.usm.edu/chs

University of South Florida, College of Public Health, Department of Health Policy and Management, Tampa, FL 33620-9951. Offers MHA, MPH, MSPH, PhD. *Accreditation:*

CAHME. Part-time and evening/weekend programs available. *Degree requirements:* For master's, comprehensive exam, thesis (for some programs); for doctorate, comprehensive exam, thesis/dissertation. *Entrance requirements:* For master's, GRE General Test or GMAT, minimum GPA of 3.0 in upper-level course work, 3 professional letters of recommendation, resume/curriculum vitae; for doctorate, GRE General Test, minimum GPA of 3.0 in upper-level course work, goal statement letter, three professional letters of recommendation, resume/curriculum vitae, writing sample. Additional exam requirements/recommendations for international students: Required—TOEFL (minimum score 550 paper-based; 79 iBT). Electronic applications accepted. *Faculty research:* Tracking community health, inpatient care, discharge policies, stroke education, leadership practices.

University of South Florida, Innovative Education Graduate Certificate Programs, Tampa, FL 33620-9951. *Unit head:* Kathy Barnes, Interdisciplinary Programs Coordinator, 813-974-8031, Fax: 813-974-7061, E-mail: barnesk@usf.edu. *Application contact:* Karen Tylinski, Metro Initiatives, 813-974-9943, Fax: 813-974-7061, E-mail: ktylinsk@usf.edu.
Website: http://www.usf.edu/innovative-education/

The University of Tennessee, Graduate School, College of Education, Health and Human Sciences, Program in Public Health, Knoxville, TN 37996. Offers community health education (MPH); gerontology (MPH); health planning/administration (MPH); MS/MPH. *Accreditation:* CEPH. *Degree requirements:* For master's, thesis optional. *Entrance requirements:* For master's, minimum GPA of 2.7. Additional exam requirements/recommendations for international students: Required—TOEFL. Electronic applications accepted. *Expenses:* Tuition, state resident: full-time $9540; part-time $531 per credit hour. Tuition, nonresident: full-time $27,728; part-time $1542 per credit hour. *Required fees:* $1404; $67 per credit hour.

The University of Texas at Arlington, Graduate School, College of Business, Program in Health Care Administration, Arlington, TX 76019. Offers MS. Part-time and evening/weekend programs available. *Degree requirements:* For master's, one foreign language, thesis optional. *Entrance requirements:* For master's, GRE General Test or GMAT, minimum GPA of 3.0, official undergraduate and graduate transcripts, current professional resume, personal statement, three letters of recommendation. Additional exam requirements/recommendations for international students: Required—TOEFL (minimum score 550 paper-based; 79 iBT).

The University of Texas at Dallas, Naveen Jindal School of Management, Program in Business Administration, Richardson, TX 75080. Offers business administration (MBA, PMBA); executive business administration (EMBA); global leadership (EMBA); healthcare management for physicians (EMBA); product lifecycle and supply chain management (EMBA); project management (EMBA); real estate (MBA). *Accreditation:* AACSB. Part-time and evening/weekend programs available. Postbaccalaureate distance learning degree programs offered (no on-campus study). *Faculty:* 100 full-time (21 women), 52 part-time/adjunct (18 women). *Students:* 421 full-time (196 women), 630 part-time (398 women); includes 295 minority (45 Black or African American, non-Hispanic/Latino; 4 American Indian or Alaska Native, non-Hispanic/Latino; 151 Asian, non-Hispanic/Latino; 76 Hispanic/Latino; 19 Two or more races, non-Hispanic/Latino), 275 international. Average age 31. 940 applicants, 44% accepted, 375 enrolled. In 2013, 384 master's awarded. *Degree requirements:* For master's, thesis optional. *Entrance requirements:* For master's, GMAT, 10 years of business experience (EMBA), minimum GPA of 3.0. Additional exam requirements/recommendations for international students: Required—TOEFL (minimum score 550 paper-based). *Application deadline:* For fall admission, 7/15 for domestic students, 5/1 priority date for international students; for spring admission, 11/15 for domestic students, 9/1 priority date for international students. Applications are processed on a rolling basis. Application fee: $50 ($100 for international students). Electronic applications accepted. *Expenses:* Contact institution. *Financial support:* In 2013–14, 336 students received support. Research assistantships with partial tuition reimbursements available, teaching assistantships with partial tuition reimbursements available, career-related internships or fieldwork, Federal Work-Study, institutionally sponsored loans, scholarships/grants, and unspecified assistantships available. Support available to part-time students. Financial award application deadline: 4/30; financial award applicants required to submit FAFSA. *Faculty research:* Production scheduling, trade and finance, organizational decision-making, life/work planning. *Unit head:* Lisa Shatz, Assistant Dean, MBA Programs, 972-883-6191, E-mail: lisa.shatz@utdallas.edu. *Application contact:* Anna Walls, Enrollment Services Advisor, MBA Programs, 972-883-5951, E-mail: anna.walls@utdallas.edu.
Website: http://jindal.utdallas.edu/academic-programs/mba-programs/

The University of Texas at Dallas, Naveen Jindal School of Management, Program in Organizations, Strategy and International Management, Richardson, TX 75080. Offers healthcare management (MS); international management studies (MS, PhD); management and administrative sciences (MS); project management (MS). Part-time and evening/weekend programs available. *Faculty:* 13 full-time (4 women), 8 part-time/adjunct (4 women). *Students:* 101 full-time (59 women), 198 part-time (119 women); includes 88 minority (27 Black or African American, non-Hispanic/Latino; 38 Asian, non-Hispanic/Latino; 19 Hispanic/Latino; 1 Native Hawaiian or other Pacific Islander, non-Hispanic/Latino; 3 Two or more races, non-Hispanic/Latino), 72 international. Average age 35. 282 applicants, 53% accepted, 139 enrolled. In 2013, 131 master's, 5 doctorates awarded. *Degree requirements:* For doctorate, thesis/dissertation. *Entrance requirements:* For master's and doctorate, GMAT. Additional exam requirements/recommendations for international students: Required—TOEFL (minimum score 550 paper-based). *Application deadline:* For fall admission, 7/15 for domestic students, 5/1 priority date for international students; for spring admission, 11/15 for domestic students, 9/1 priority date for international students. Applications are processed on a rolling basis. Application fee: $50 ($100 for international students). Electronic applications accepted. *Expenses:* Tuition, state resident: full-time $11,940; part-time $663.33 per credit hour. Tuition, nonresident: full-time $21,606; part-time $1200.33 per credit hour. *Financial support:* In 2013–14, 58 students received support. Research assistantships with partial tuition reimbursements available, teaching assistantships with partial tuition reimbursements available, Federal Work-Study, institutionally sponsored loans, scholarships/grants, and unspecified assistantships available. Support available to part-time students. Financial award application deadline: 4/30; financial award applicants required to submit FAFSA. *Faculty research:* International accounting, international trade and finance, economic development, international economics. *Unit head:* Dr. Mike Peng, Area Coordinator, 972-883-2714, Fax: 972-883-5977, E-mail: mikepeng@utdallas.edu. *Application contact:* Dr. Habte Woldu, Director, International Management Studies, 972-883-6357, Fax: 972-883-5977, E-mail: wolduh@utdallas.edu.
Website: http://jindal.utdallas.edu/academic-areas/organizations-strategy-and-international-management/

The University of Texas at El Paso, Graduate School, School of Nursing, El Paso, TX 79968-0001. Offers family nurse practitioner (MSN); health care leadership and management (Certificate); interdisciplinary health sciences (PhD); nursing (DNP); nursing education (MSN, Certificate); nursing systems management (MSN). *Accreditation:* AACN. Postbaccalaureate distance learning degree programs offered (minimal on-campus study). *Degree requirements:* For master's, thesis optional; for doctorate, thesis/dissertation. *Entrance requirements:* For master's, minimum GPA of 3.0, resume; for doctorate, GRE, letters of reference, relevant personal/professional experience; master's degree in nursing (for DNP); for Certificate, bachelor's degree in nursing. Additional exam requirements/recommendations for international students: Required—TOEFL; Recommended—IELTS. Electronic applications accepted.

The University of Texas at Tyler, College of Business and Technology, School of Business Administration, Tyler, TX 75799-0001. Offers business administration (MBA); general management (MBA); health care (MBA). Part-time programs available. Postbaccalaureate distance learning degree programs offered (no on-campus study). *Entrance requirements:* Additional exam requirements/recommendations for international students: Required—TOEFL (minimum score 550 paper-based). *Faculty research:* General business, inventory control, institutional markets, service marketing, product distribution, accounting fraud, financial reporting and recognition.

University of the Incarnate Word, School of Graduate Studies and Research, H-E-B School of Business and Administration, Program in Health Administration, San Antonio, TX 78209-6397. Offers MHA. *Faculty:* 2 full-time (1 woman), 1 (woman) part-time/adjunct. *Students:* 32 full-time (23 women), 1 (woman) part-time; includes 23 minority (1 Black or African American, non-Hispanic/Latino; 1 American Indian or Alaska Native, non-Hispanic/Latino; 3 Asian, non-Hispanic/Latino; 18 Hispanic/Latino), 1 international. Average age 28. 58 applicants, 50% accepted, 21 enrolled. In 2013, 19 master's awarded. *Entrance requirements:* For master's, GRE or GMAT if applicant has GPA of at least 2.5 but less than 3.0, baccalaureate degree with minimum GPA of 3.5, official transcripts of all undergraduate work, letter of intent, interview and evaluation by MHA admissions committee. Additional exam requirements/recommendations for international students: Required—TOEFL (minimum score 560 paper-based; 83 iBT). *Expenses: Tuition:* Part-time $815 per credit hour. *Required fees:* $86 per credit hour. One-time fee: $40 part-time. Tuition and fees vary according to degree level and program. *Unit head:* Dr. Daniel G. Dominguez, Director, 210-829-3180, E-mail: domingue@uiwtx.edu. *Application contact:* Andrea Cyterski-Acosta, Dean of Enrollment, 210-829-6005, Fax: 210-829-3921, E-mail: admis@uiwtx.edu.
Website: http://www.uiw.edu/mha/

University of the Incarnate Word, School of Graduate Studies and Research, H-E-B School of Business and Administration, Programs in Administration, San Antonio, TX 78209-6397. Offers adult education (MAA); communication arts (MAA); healthcare administration (MAA); instructional technology (MAA); nutrition (MAA); organizational development (MAA); sports management (MAA). Part-time and evening/weekend programs available. Postbaccalaureate distance learning degree programs offered (no on-campus study). *Faculty:* 20 full-time (10 women), 14 part-time/adjunct (6 women). *Students:* 31 full-time (22 women), 54 part-time (36 women); includes 61 minority (14 Black or African American, non-Hispanic/Latino; 1 Asian, non-Hispanic/Latino; 46 Hispanic/Latino), 6 international. Average age 31. 63 applicants, 68% accepted, 21 enrolled. In 2013, 35 master's awarded. *Degree requirements:* For master's, capstone. *Entrance requirements:* For master's, GRE, GMAT, undergraduate degree, minimum GPA of 2.5. Additional exam requirements/recommendations for international students: Required—TOEFL (minimum score 560 paper-based; 83 iBT). *Application deadline:* Applications are processed on a rolling basis. Application fee: $20. Electronic applications accepted. *Expenses: Tuition:* Part-time $815 per credit hour. *Required fees:* $86 per credit hour. One-time fee: $40 part-time. Tuition and fees vary according to degree level and program. *Financial support:* Federal Work-Study and scholarships/grants available. Financial award applicants required to submit FAFSA. *Unit head:* Dr. Mark Teachout, MAA Programs Director, 210-829-3177, Fax: 210-805-3564, E-mail: teachout@uiwtx.edu. *Application contact:* Andrea Cyterski-Acosta, Dean of Enrollment, 210-829-6005, Fax: 210-829-3921, E-mail: admis@uiwtx.edu.
Website: http://www.uiw.edu/maa/

University of the Sciences, College of Graduate Studies, Mayes College of Healthcare Business and Policy, Program in Public Health, Philadelphia, PA 19104-4495. Offers MPH. Part-time and evening/weekend programs available. Postbaccalaureate distance learning degree programs offered (no on-campus study). *Students:* 47. In 2013, 10 master's awarded. *Entrance requirements:* Additional exam requirements/recommendations for international students: Required—TOEFL, TWE. *Expenses: Tuition:* Part-time $1447 per credit. Tuition and fees vary according to campus/location and program. *Unit head:* Dr. Glenn Beamer, Graduate Program Director, 267-295-3178, E-mail: g.beamer@usp.edu. *Application contact:* Joyce D'Angelo, Administrative Assistant, 215-596-8937, E-mail: j.dangel@usp.edu.

University of the Sciences, College of Graduate Studies, Program in Health Policy and Public Health, Philadelphia, PA 19104-4495. Offers health policy (MPH, MS, PhD); public health (MPH). Part-time and evening/weekend programs available. Postbaccalaureate distance learning degree programs offered (no on-campus study). *Faculty:* 11 full-time (5 women), 4 part-time/adjunct (2 women). *Students:* 18 full-time (10 women), 55 part-time (32 women); includes 13 minority (5 Black or African American, non-Hispanic/Latino; 6 Asian, non-Hispanic/Latino; 2 Hispanic/Latino), 6 international. Average age 40. 54 applicants, 61% accepted, 17 enrolled. In 2013, 12 master's, 1 doctorate awarded. *Degree requirements:* For doctorate, comprehensive exam, thesis/dissertation. *Entrance requirements:* For master's and doctorate, GRE General Test. Additional exam requirements/recommendations for international students: Required—TOEFL, TWE. *Application deadline:* For fall admission, 6/1 for domestic students, 5/1 for international students; for winter admission, 12/1 for domestic students, 10/1 for international students; for spring admission, 3/1 for international students. Applications are processed on a rolling basis. Application fee: $50. *Expenses:* Contact institution. *Financial support:* Tuition waivers (partial) and unspecified assistantships available. Support available to part-time students. Financial award application deadline: 5/1. *Faculty research:* Managed care, pharmacoeconomics, health law and regulation, rehabilitation, genetic technologies. *Unit head:* Dr. Shenaz Tejani-Butt, Associate Dean, Graduate Studies, E-mail: graduate@usciences.edu. *Application contact:* Christopher Miciek, Associate Director, Graduate Admissions, 215-596-8597, E-mail: c.miciek@usciences.edu.

The University of Toledo, College of Graduate Studies, College of Languages, Literature and Social Sciences, Department of Political Science and Public Administration, Toledo, OH 43606-3390. Offers health care policy and administration (Certificate); management of non-profit organizations (Certificate); municipal administration (Certificate); political science (MA); public administration (MPA); JD/MPA. Part-time programs available. *Faculty:* 8. *Students:* 15 full-time (11 women), 18 part-time (12 women); includes 7 minority (4 Black or African American, non-Hispanic/Latino; 1 Asian, non-Hispanic/Latino; 2 Hispanic/Latino), 2 international. Average age 31. 27 applicants, 89% accepted, 19 enrolled. In 2013, 13 master's, 9 other advanced degrees awarded. *Degree requirements:* For master's, comprehensive exam (for some programs), thesis. *Entrance requirements:* For master's, GRE General Test, minimum cumulative point-hour ratio of 2.7 (3.0 for MPA) for all previous academic work, three letters of recommendation, statement of purpose, transcripts from all prior institutions attended; for Certificate, minimum cumulative point-hour ratio of 2.7 for all previous academic work, three letters of recommendation, statement of purpose, transcripts from all prior institutions attended. Additional exam requirements/recommendations for international students: Required—TOEFL (minimum score 550 paper-based; 80 iBT). *Application deadline:* For fall admission, 1/15 priority date for domestic and international

students. Applications are processed on a rolling basis. Application fee: $45 ($75 for international students). Electronic applications accepted. *Financial support:* In 2013–14, 11 teaching assistantships with full and partial tuition reimbursements (averaging $6,682 per year) were awarded; career-related internships or fieldwork, Federal Work-Study, institutionally sponsored loans, scholarships/grants, tuition waivers (full), unspecified assistantships, and administrative assistantships also available. Support available to part-time students. *Faculty research:* Economic development, health care, Third World, criminal justice, Eastern Europe. *Unit head:* Dr. Sam Nelson, Chair, 419-530-4974, E-mail: sam.nelson@utoledo.edu. *Application contact:* Graduate School Office, 419-530-4723, Fax: 419-530-4724, E-mail: grdsch@utnet.utoledo.edu.
Website: http://www.utoledo.edu/llss/

The University of Toledo, College of Graduate Studies, College of Medicine and Life Sciences, Department of Public Health and Preventative Medicine, Toledo, OH 43606-3390. Offers biostatistics and epidemiology (Certificate); contemporary gerontological practice (Certificate); environmental and occupational health and safety (MPH); epidemiology (Certificate); global public health (Certificate); health promotion and education (MPH); industrial hygiene (MSOH); medical and health science teaching and learning (Certificate); occupational health (Certificate); public health administration (MPH); public health and emergency response (Certificate); public health epidemiology (MPH); public health nutrition (MPH); MD/MPH. Part-time and evening/weekend programs available. *Faculty:* 9. *Students:* 69 full-time (50 women), 88 part-time (66 women); includes 50 minority (35 Black or African American, non-Hispanic/Latino; 10 Asian, non-Hispanic/Latino; 4 Hispanic/Latino; 1 Two or more races, non-Hispanic/Latino), 6 international. Average age 30. 92 applicants, 80% accepted, 52 enrolled. In 2013, 59 master's, 15 other advanced degrees awarded. *Degree requirements:* For master's, thesis or alternative. *Entrance requirements:* For master's, GRE, minimum undergraduate GPA of 3.0, three letters of recommendation, statement of purpose, transcripts from all prior institutions attended, resume; for Certificate, minimum undergraduate GPA of 3.0, three letters of recommendation, statement of purpose, transcripts from all prior institutions attended, resume. Additional exam requirements/recommendations for international students: Required—TOEFL (minimum score 550 paper-based; 80 iBT), IELTS (minimum score 6.5). *Application deadline:* For fall admission, 6/15 for domestic students, 3/15 priority date for international students; for spring admission, 10/15 for domestic students, 6/15 for international students; for summer admission, 3/15 for domestic students, 10/15 for international students. Applications are processed on a rolling basis. Application fee: $45 ($75 for international students). Electronic applications accepted. *Financial support:* In 2013–14, 4 research assistantships with full tuition reimbursements (averaging $10,000 per year) were awarded; Federal Work-Study, institutionally sponsored loans, scholarships/grants, tuition waivers (full and partial), and unspecified assistantships also available. *Unit head:* Dr. Sheryl A. Milz, Chair, 419-383-3976, Fax: 419-383-6140, E-mail: sheryl.milz@utoledo.edu. *Application contact:* Admissions Analyst, 419-383-4112, Fax: 419-383-6140.
Website: http://nocphmph.org/

University of Toronto, Faculty of Medicine, Program in Health Administration, Toronto, ON M5S 1A1, Canada. Offers MHS. *Entrance requirements:* For master's, minimum B+ average on each of the last two years of a four-year undergraduate program, minimum of three years relevant clinical or management experience. Additional exam requirements/recommendations for international students: Required—TOEFL (minimum score 580 paper-based; 93 iBT), TWE (minimum score 5). Electronic applications accepted.

University of Toronto, Faculty of Medicine, Program in Health Policy, Management and Evaluation, Toronto, ON M5S 1A1, Canada. Offers M Sc, PhD. *Entrance requirements:* For master's, 4-year undergraduate degree with minimum B+ standing in last two years of study, 2 reference letters, statement of intent; for doctorate, master's degree with minimum B+ average, 2 reference letters, statement of intent. Additional exam requirements/recommendations for international students: Required—TOEFL (minimum score 580 paper-based; 93 iBT), TWE (minimum score 5). Electronic applications accepted.

University of Utah, Graduate School, College of Pharmacy, Department of Pharmacotherapy, Salt Lake City, UT 84112. Offers health system pharmacy administration (MS); outcomes research and health policy (PhD). *Faculty:* 5 full-time (3 women), 28 part-time/adjunct (17 women). *Students:* 7 full-time (4 women), 5 international. Average age 27. 26 applicants, 19% accepted, 2 enrolled. In 2013, 4 master's awarded. Terminal master's awarded for partial completion of doctoral program. *Degree requirements:* For master's, comprehensive exam, thesis or alternative, project; for doctorate, comprehensive exam, thesis/dissertation. *Entrance requirements:* For doctorate, GRE. Additional exam requirements/recommendations for international students: Required—TOEFL (minimum score 550 paper-based; 80 iBT). *Application deadline:* For fall admission, 1/10 for domestic students, 12/15 for international students. Application fee: $55 ($65 for international students). *Expenses:* Tuition, state resident: full-time $5259. Tuition, nonresident: full-time $18,569. *Required fees:* $841. Tuition and fees vary according to course load. *Financial support:* In 2013–14, 7 students received support, including 5 research assistantships with full tuition reimbursements available (averaging $21,400 per year); health care benefits and unspecified assistantships also available. Financial award application deadline: 12/15. *Faculty research:* Outcomes in pharmacy, pharmacotherapy. *Total annual research expenditures:* $131,217. *Unit head:* Dr. Diana I. Brixner, Department Chair and Professor, 801-581-6731. *Application contact:* Sara Ray, Academic Program Manager, 801-581-5984, Fax: 801-585-6160, E-mail: sara.ray@pharm.utah.edu.
Website: http://www.pharmacy.utah.edu/pharmacotherapy/

University of Utah, Graduate School, David Eccles School of Business, Master in Healthcare Administration Program, Salt Lake City, UT 84112. Offers MHA, MBA/MHA, MHA/MPA, MPH/MHA, PMBA/MHA. Part-time programs available. *Students:* 36 full-time (5 women), 4 part-time (1 woman); includes 4 minority (3 Asian, non-Hispanic/Latino; 1 Hispanic/Latino). Average age 29. 40 applicants, 70% accepted, 14 enrolled. In 2013, 13 master's awarded. *Degree requirements:* For master's, administrative internship. *Entrance requirements:* For master's, GMAT, GRE, statistics course with minimum B grade; minimum undergraduate GPA of 3.0. Additional exam requirements/recommendations for international students: Required—TOEFL (minimum score 600 paper-based; 100 iBT), IELTS (minimum score 7). *Application deadline:* For fall admission, 2/15 priority date for domestic and international students. Applications are processed on a rolling basis. Application fee: $55 ($65 for international students). Electronic applications accepted. *Expenses:* Contact institution. *Financial support:* In 2013–14, 9 students received support, including 9 fellowships with partial tuition reimbursements available (averaging $7,500 per year); scholarships/grants and unspecified assistantships also available. Financial award application deadline: 2/15; financial award applicants required to submit FAFSA. *Faculty research:* Healthcare leadership, problem-solving, primary care delivery redesign, patient engagement, patient-reported outcomes. *Unit head:* Dr. Debra Scammon, Professor, 801-581-4754, Fax: 801-581-3666, E-mail: debra.scammon@business.utah.edu. *Application contact:* Paige Williams, Director of Graduate Admissions, 801-581-7785, Fax: 801-587-3666, E-mail: mastersinfo@business.utah.edu.

University of Virginia, School of Medicine, Department of Public Health Sciences, Charlottesville, VA 22903. Offers clinical research (MS), including clinical investigation and patient-oriented research, informatics in medicine; public health (MPH); MPP/MPH. Part-time programs available. *Faculty:* 36 full-time (17 women), 4 part-time/adjunct (2 women). *Students:* 40 full-time (31 women), 9 part-time (6 women); includes 14 minority (4 Black or African American, non-Hispanic/Latino; 7 Asian, non-Hispanic/Latino; 3 Hispanic/Latino). Average age 27. 106 applicants, 59% accepted, 29 enrolled. In 2013, 38 master's awarded. *Entrance requirements:* For master's, GRE General Test or MCAT. Additional exam requirements/recommendations for international students: Required—TOEFL. *Application deadline:* Applications are processed on a rolling basis. Application fee: $60. Electronic applications accepted. *Expenses:* Tuition, state resident: part-time $334 per credit hour. Tuition, nonresident: part-time $1224 per credit hour. *Financial support:* Career-related internships or fieldwork available. Financial award applicants required to submit FAFSA. *Unit head:* Dr. Ruth Gaare Bernheim, Chair, 434-924-8430, Fax: 434-924-8437, E-mail: rg3r@virginia.edu. *Application contact:* Tracey L. Brookman, Academic Programs Administrator, 434-924-8430, Fax: 434-924-8437, E-mail: phsdegrees@virginia.edu.
Website: http://www.medicine.virginia.edu/clinical/departments/phs

University of Washington, Graduate School, School of Public Health, Department of Health Services, Programs in Health Services Administration, Seattle, WA 98195. Offers EMHA, MHA, JD/MHA, MHA/MBA, MHA/MD, MHA/MPA. *Accreditation:* CAHME. Part-time programs available. *Students:* 55 full-time (29 women), 70 part-time (41 women); includes 31 minority (5 Black or African American, non-Hispanic/Latino; 2 American Indian or Alaska Native, non-Hispanic/Latino; 23 Asian, non-Hispanic/Latino; 1 Native Hawaiian or other Pacific Islander, non-Hispanic/Latino), 3 international. Average age 34. 198 applicants, 54% accepted, 51 enrolled. In 2013, 60 master's awarded. *Degree requirements:* For master's, capstone project. *Entrance requirements:* For master's, GRE General Test or GMAT (for MHA), minimum GPA of 3.0. Additional exam requirements/recommendations for international students: Required—TOEFL (minimum score 580 paper-based; 92 iBT), IELTS (minimum score 7). *Application deadline:* For fall admission, 12/1 for domestic students, 11/1 for international students. Application fee: $85. Electronic applications accepted. *Financial support:* In 2013–14, 8 students received support. Federal Work-Study, scholarships/grants, tuition waivers (partial), and unspecified assistantships available. Financial award applicants required to submit FAFSA. *Faculty research:* Health economics, health information management, research design in health services, health policy, clinical effectiveness. *Unit head:* Dr. Chirstopher Johnson, Director, 206-543-8778, Fax: 206-543-3964, E-mail: chrisj26@uw.edu. *Application contact:* Jennifer Gill, Program Coordinator, 206-685-8878, E-mail: mhap@uw.edu.
Website: http://depts.washington.edu/mhap

The University of Western Ontario, Richard Ivey School of Business, London, ON N6A 3K7, Canada. Offers business (EMBA, PhD); corporate strategy and leadership elective (MBA); entrepreneurship elective (MBA); finance elective (MBA); health sector stream (MBA); international management elective (MBA); marketing elective (MBA); JD/MBA. *Degree requirements:* For master's, thesis (for some programs); for doctorate, thesis/dissertation. *Entrance requirements:* For master's, GMAT, 2 years of full-time work experience, interview. Additional exam requirements/recommendations for international students: Required—TOEFL (minimum score 100 iBT) or IELTS (minimum score 6). Electronic applications accepted. *Faculty research:* Strategy, organizational behavior, international business, finance, operations management.

University of West Georgia, Tanner Health System School of Nursing, Carrollton, GA 30118. Offers health systems leadership (Post-Master's Certificate); nursing (MSN); nursing education (Ed D, Post-Master's Certificate). *Accreditation:* AACN. Part-time programs available. Postbaccalaureate distance learning degree programs offered (no on-campus study). *Faculty:* 11 full-time (10 women), 1 (woman) part-time/adjunct. *Students:* 70 full-time (67 women), 52 part-time (48 women); includes 35 minority (31 Black or African American, non-Hispanic/Latino; 4 Hispanic/Latino). Average age 42. 96 applicants, 83% accepted, 56 enrolled. In 2013, 23 master's awarded. *Degree requirements:* For master's, comprehensive exam, thesis optional; for doctorate, comprehensive exam, thesis/dissertation. *Entrance requirements:* For master's, BSN, RN license, minimum GPA of 3.0 for upper-division nursing courses, two letters of recommendation, resume, official transcript, undergraduate statistics course with minimum C grade; for doctorate, GRE, MSN, minimum GPA of 3.0 in graduate nursing program, three letters of recommendation, 5-page sample of academic writing, RN license, resume or curriculum vitae, official transcripts; for Post-Master's Certificate, MSN, official transcripts, curriculum vitae/resume, two letters of recommendation. Additional exam requirements/recommendations for international students: Required—TOEFL (minimum score 523 paper-based; 69 iBT); Recommended—IELTS (minimum score 6.5). *Application deadline:* For fall admission, 6/1 for domestic and international students. Applications are processed on a rolling basis. Application fee: $40. Electronic applications accepted. *Expenses:* Contact institution. *Financial support:* In 2013–14, 8 students received support, including 1 research assistantship with full tuition reimbursement available (averaging $6,000 per year); scholarships/grants and unspecified assistantships also available. Financial award application deadline: 4/1; financial award applicants required to submit FAFSA. *Faculty research:* Caring in nursing education, pain assessment in older adults, pain outcomes. *Unit head:* Dr. Kathryn Mary Grams, Dean, 678-839-5642, Fax: 678-839-6553, E-mail: kgrams@westga.edu. *Application contact:* Embry Ice, Graduate Studies Associate, 678-839-5115, Fax: 678-839-6553, E-mail: eice@westga.edu.
Website: http://nursing.westga.edu

University of Wisconsin–Oshkosh, Graduate Studies, College of Letters and Science, Department of Public Administration, Oshkosh, WI 54901. Offers general agency (MPA); health care (MPA). Part-time and evening/weekend programs available. *Degree requirements:* For master's, thesis or alternative. *Entrance requirements:* For master's, public service-related experience, resume, sample of written work. Additional exam requirements/recommendations for international students: Required—TOEFL (minimum score 550 paper-based; 79 iBT). Electronic applications accepted. *Faculty research:* Drug policy, local government state revenues and expenditures, health care regulation.

Utica College, Program in Health Care Administration, Utica, NY 13502-4892. Offers MS. Part-time and evening/weekend programs available. Postbaccalaureate distance learning degree programs offered (no on-campus study). *Students:* 17 full-time (14 women), 137 part-time (102 women); includes 33 minority (16 Black or African American, non-Hispanic/Latino; 6 Asian, non-Hispanic/Latino; 9 Hispanic/Latino; 2 Two or more races, non-Hispanic/Latino). Average age 33. In 2013, 39 master's awarded. *Degree requirements:* For master's, capstone (internship or research/program development project). *Entrance requirements:* For master's, BS, minimum GPA of 3.0, 2 recommendation letters, personal essay. Additional exam requirements/recommendations for international students: Required—TOEFL (minimum score 525 paper-based). *Application deadline:* Applications are processed on a rolling basis. Electronic applications accepted. *Financial support:* Application deadline: 3/15; applicants required to submit FAFSA. *Unit head:* Dr. Dana Hart, Head, 315-792-3375, E-mail: dhart@utica.edu. *Application contact:* John D. Rowe, Director of Graduate Admissions, 315-792-3824, Fax: 315-792-3003, E-mail: jrowe@utica.edu.

Valdosta State University, Program in Business Administration, Valdosta, GA 31698. Offers business administration (MBA); healthcare administration (MBA). Program is also a member of the Georgia WebMBA. *Accreditation:* AACSB. Part-time and evening/weekend programs available. Postbaccalaureate distance learning degree programs offered (no on-campus study). *Faculty:* 8 full-time (1 woman). *Students:* 13 full-time (3 women), 59 part-time (34 women); includes 22 minority (19 Black or African American, non-Hispanic/Latino; 1 Hispanic/Latino; 2 Two or more races, non-Hispanic/Latino), 5 international. Average age 25. 38 applicants, 82% accepted, 29 enrolled. In 2013, 39 master's awarded. *Degree requirements:* For master's, comprehensive written and/or oral exams. *Entrance requirements:* For master's, GMAT or GRE, minimum GPA of 2.75. Additional exam requirements/recommendations for international students: Required—TOEFL (minimum score 523 paper-based). *Application deadline:* For fall admission, 7/1 for domestic and international students; for spring admission, 11/1 for domestic students. Applications are processed on a rolling basis. Application fee: $35. Electronic applications accepted. *Expenses:* Tuition, state resident: full-time $4140; part-time $230 per credit hour. Tuition, nonresident: full-time $14,904; part-time $828 per credit hour. *Required fees:* $995 per semester. Tuition and fees vary according to course load. *Financial support:* In 2013–14, 5 students received support, including 5 research assistantships with full tuition reimbursements available (averaging $3,652 per year); institutionally sponsored loans and scholarships/grants also available. Support available to part-time students. Financial award application deadline: 7/1; financial award applicants required to submit FAFSA. *Unit head:* Dr. Mel Schnake, Director, 229-245-2233, Fax: 229-245-2795, E-mail: mschnake@valdosta.edu. *Application contact:* Jessica Powers, Coordinator of Graduate Admissions, 229-333-5694, Fax: 229-245-3853, E-mail: jldevane@valdosta.edu.
Website: http://www.valdosta.edu/academics/graduate-school/our-programs/business-administration.php

Valparaiso University, Graduate School, Program in Health Administration, Valparaiso, IN 46383. Offers MHA. Part-time and evening/weekend programs available. *Students:* 8 full-time (6 women), 11 part-time (7 women); includes 5 minority (1 Black or African American, non-Hispanic/Latino; 1 Asian, non-Hispanic/Latino; 2 Hispanic/Latino; 1 Two or more races, non-Hispanic/Latino), 2 international. Average age 33. *Degree requirements:* For master's, practicum, internship. *Entrance requirements:* For master's, minimum overall GPA of 3.0 or 5 years of work experience in the field; basic course in statistics; official transcripts; two letters of recommendation; essay. Additional exam requirements/recommendations for international students: Required—TOEFL (minimum score 550 paper-based; 80 iBT), IELTS (minimum score 6). *Application deadline:* Applications are processed on a rolling basis. Application fee: $30 ($50 for international students). Electronic applications accepted. *Expenses: Tuition:* Full-time $10,350; part-time $575 per credit hour. *Required fees:* $378; $101 per term. Tuition and fees vary according to course load and program. *Financial support:* Available to part-time students. Applicants required to submit FAFSA. *Unit head:* Dr. Jennifer A. Ziegler, Dean, Graduate School and Continuing Education, 219-464-5313, Fax: 219-464-5381, E-mail: jennifer.ziegler@valpo.edu. *Application contact:* Jessica Choquette, Graduate Admissions Specialist, 219-464-5313, Fax: 219-464-5381, E-mail: jessica.choquette@valpo.edu.
Website: http://www.valpo.edu/grad/healthadministration/index.php

Villanova University, College of Nursing, Villanova, PA 19085-1699. Offers adult nurse practitioner (MSN, Post Master's Certificate); family nurse practitioner (MSN, Post Master's Certificate); health care administration (MSN, Post Master's Certificate); nurse anesthetist (MSN, Post Master's Certificate); nursing (PhD); nursing education (MSN, Post Master's Certificate); nursing practice (DNP); pediatric nurse practitioner (MSN, Post Master's Certificate). *Accreditation:* AACN; AANA/CANAEP. Part-time programs available. Postbaccalaureate distance learning degree programs offered (minimal on-campus study). *Faculty:* 17 full-time (all women), 4 part-time/adjunct (all women). *Students:* 28 full-time (26 women), 191 part-time (161 women); includes 22 minority (2 Black or African American, non-Hispanic/Latino; 6 Asian, non-Hispanic/Latino; 7 Hispanic/Latino; 7 Two or more races, non-Hispanic/Latino), 18 international. Average age 30. 176 applicants, 65% accepted, 82 enrolled. In 2013, 64 master's, 7 doctorates, 5 other advanced degrees awarded. *Degree requirements:* For master's, independent study project; for doctorate, comprehensive exam, thesis/dissertation. *Entrance requirements:* For master's, GRE or MAT, BSN, 1 year of recent nursing experience, physical assessment, course work in statistics; for doctorate, GRE, MSN. Additional exam requirements/recommendations for international students: Required—TOEFL (minimum score 540 paper-based; 83 iBT), IELTS (minimum score 6.5). *Application deadline:* For fall admission, 7/1 priority date for domestic students, 7/1 for international students; for spring admission, 11/1 priority date for domestic students, 11/1 for international students. Applications are processed on a rolling basis. Application fee: $50. Electronic applications accepted. *Expenses:* Contact institution. *Financial support:* In 2013–14, 39 students received support, including 5 teaching assistantships with full tuition reimbursements available (averaging $14,475 per year); institutionally sponsored loans, scholarships/grants, traineeships, tuition waivers (full), and unspecified assistantships also available. Financial award application deadline: 7/1; financial award applicants required to submit FAFSA. *Faculty research:* Genetics, ethics, cognitive development of students, women with disabilities, nursing leadership. *Unit head:* Dr. Marguerite K. Schlag, Assistant Dean/Director, Graduate Programs, 610-519-4907, Fax: 610-519-7650, E-mail: marguerite.schlag@villanova.edu.
Website: http://www.nursing.villanova.edu/

Villanova University, Villanova School of Business, MBA - The Fast Track Program, Villanova, PA 19085. Offers finance (MBA); health care management (MBA); international business (MBA); management information systems (MBA); marketing (MBA); real estate (MBA); strategic management (MBA). *Accreditation:* AACSB. Part-time and evening/weekend programs available. *Faculty:* 101 full-time (33 women), 36 part-time/adjunct (3 women). *Students:* 140 part-time (44 women); includes 22 minority (1 Black or African American, non-Hispanic/Latino; 17 Asian, non-Hispanic/Latino; 3 Hispanic/Latino; 1 Two or more races, non-Hispanic/Latino), 3 international. Average age 29. 127 applicants, 72% accepted, 75 enrolled. In 2013, 61 master's awarded. *Degree requirements:* For master's, minimum GPA of 3.0. *Entrance requirements:* For master's, GMAT or GRE, work experience. Additional exam requirements/recommendations for international students: Required—TOEFL (minimum score 550 paper-based; 90 iBT). *Application deadline:* For fall admission, 6/30 for domestic and international students. Application fee: $50. Electronic applications accepted. *Financial support:* Scholarships/grants available. Financial award application deadline: 6/30; financial award applicants required to submit FAFSA. *Faculty research:* Business analytics; creativity, innovation and entrepreneurship; global leadership; real estate; church management; business ethics. *Unit head:* Zelon Crawford, Director of Graduate Business Programs, 610-519-6283, Fax: 610-519-6273, E-mail: zelon.crawford@villanova.edu. *Application contact:* Meredith L. Lockyer, Manager of Recruiting, 610-519-7016, Fax: 610-519-6273, E-mail: meredith.lockyer@villanova.edu.
Website: http://www1.villanova.edu/villanova/business/graduate/mba/fasttrack.html

Villanova University, Villanova School of Business, MBA - The Flex Track Program, Villanova, PA 19085. Offers finance (MBA); health care management (MBA); international business (MBA); management information systems (MBA); marketing (MBA); real estate (MBA); strategic management (MBA); JD/MBA. *Accreditation:* AACSB. Part-time and evening/weekend programs available. Postbaccalaureate distance learning degree programs offered (minimal on-campus study). *Faculty:* 101 full-time (33 women), 36 part-time/adjunct (3 women). *Students:* 13 full-time (5 women), 413 part-time (127 women); includes 63 minority (13 Black or African American, non-Hispanic/Latino; 1 American Indian or Alaska Native, non-Hispanic/Latino; 29 Asian, non-Hispanic/Latino; 14 Hispanic/Latino; 1 Native Hawaiian or other Pacific Islander, non-Hispanic/Latino; 5 Two or more races, non-Hispanic/Latino), 9 international. Average age 29. 84 applicants, 83% accepted, 66 enrolled. In 2013, 133 master's awarded. *Degree requirements:* For master's, minimum GPA of 3.0. *Entrance requirements:* For master's, GMAT or GRE, work experience. Additional exam requirements/recommendations for international students: Required—TOEFL (minimum score 550 paper-based; 90 iBT). *Application deadline:* For fall admission, 6/30 for domestic and international students; for winter admission, 11/15 for domestic and international students; for spring admission, 11/15 for domestic and international students; for summer admission, 3/31 for domestic and international students. Applications are processed on a rolling basis. Application fee: $50. Electronic applications accepted. *Financial support:* In 2013–14, 13 research assistantships with full tuition reimbursements (averaging $13,100 per year) were awarded; scholarships/grants and unspecified assistantships also available. Financial award application deadline: 6/30; financial award applicants required to submit FAFSA. *Faculty research:* Business analytics; creativity, innovation and entrepreneurship; global leadership; real estate; church management; business ethics. *Unit head:* Zelon Crawford, Director of Graduate Business Programs, 610-610-6283, Fax: 610-519-6273, E-mail: zelon.crawford@villanova.edu. *Application contact:* Meredith L. Lockyer, Manager of Recruiting, 610-519-7016, Fax: 610-519-6273, E-mail: meredith.lockyer@villanova.edu.
Website: http://www1.villanova.edu/villanova/business/graduate/mba/flextrack.html

Virginia College in Birmingham, Program in Business Administration, Birmingham, AL 35209. Offers healthcare (MBA); management (MBA). Part-time and evening/weekend programs available. Postbaccalaureate distance learning degree programs offered (no on-campus study). *Entrance requirements:* For master's, bachelor's degree in related academic area.

Virginia Commonwealth University, Graduate School, School of Allied Health Professions, Department of Health Administration, Doctoral Program in Health Services Organization and Research, Richmond, VA 23284-9005. Offers PhD. *Degree requirements:* For doctorate, thesis/dissertation, residency. *Entrance requirements:* For doctorate, GMAT or GRE General Test, minimum graduate GPA of 3.0. Additional exam requirements/recommendations for international students: Required—TOEFL (minimum score 600 paper-based; 100 iBT). Electronic applications accepted. *Faculty research:* Organizational studies, theory, associated analytical techniques.

Virginia Commonwealth University, Graduate School, School of Allied Health Professions, Department of Health Administration, Master's Program in Health Administration, Richmond, VA 23284-9005. Offers MHA, JD/MHA, MD/MHA. *Accreditation:* CAHME. *Degree requirements:* For master's, residency. *Entrance requirements:* For master's, GMAT or GRE General Test (preferred minimum score of 5.0 on analytical writing), course work in accounting, economics, and statistics; minimum GPA of 3.0. Additional exam requirements/recommendations for international students: Required—TOEFL (minimum score 600 paper-based; 100 iBT). Electronic applications accepted.

Virginia Commonwealth University, Graduate School, School of Allied Health Professions, Department of Health Administration, Professional Online Master of Science in Health Administration Program, Richmond, VA 23284-9005. Offers MSHA. *Accreditation:* CAHME. Postbaccalaureate distance learning degree programs offered (minimal on-campus study). *Degree requirements:* For master's, residency. *Entrance requirements:* For master's, GMAT or GRE General Test. Additional exam requirements/recommendations for international students: Required—TOEFL (minimum score 600 paper-based; 100 iBT). Electronic applications accepted.

Virginia Commonwealth University, Graduate School, School of Allied Health Professions, Doctoral Program in Health Related Sciences, Richmond, VA 23284-9005. Offers clinical laboratory sciences (PhD); gerontology (PhD); health administration (PhD); nurse anesthesia (PhD); occupational therapy (PhD); physical therapy (PhD); radiation sciences (PhD); rehabilitation leadership (PhD). *Entrance requirements:* For doctorate, GRE General Test or MAT, minimum GPA of 3.3 in master's degree. Additional exam requirements/recommendations for international students: Required—TOEFL (minimum score 600 paper-based; 100 iBT); Recommended—IELTS (minimum score 6.5). Electronic applications accepted.

Virginia Commonwealth University, Medical College of Virginia-Professional Programs, School of Medicine, School of Medicine Graduate Programs, Department of Healthcare Policy and Research, Richmond, VA 23284-9005. Offers PhD. *Entrance requirements:* For doctorate, GRE General Test. Additional exam requirements/recommendations for international students: Required—TOEFL (minimum score 600 paper-based; 100 iBT). Electronic applications accepted. *Faculty research:* Evaluation of healthcare services and systems to enhance quality of care and patient safety outcomes; examination of chronic disease (e.g. cancer, HIV/AIDS) policies and practices to improve health outcomes and economic efficiency; impact of uninsurance, public insurance (such as Medicaid) and the safety net on access to care and the health of low-income, underserved, and foreign-born populations; the study of labor supply and healthcare coverage in response to health behaviors and shocks.

Virginia International University, School of Business, Fairfax, VA 22030. Offers accounting (MBA); executive management (Graduate Certificate); global logistics (MBA); health care management (MBA); human resources management (MBA); international business management (MBA); international finance (MBA); marketing management (MBA). Part-time programs available. *Entrance requirements:* For master's and Graduate Certificate, bachelor's degree. Additional exam requirements/recommendations for international students: Required—TOEFL (minimum score 550 paper-based; 80 iBT), IELTS (minimum score 6). Electronic applications accepted.

Viterbo University, Master of Business Administration Program, La Crosse, WI 54601-4797. Offers general business administration (MBA); health care management (MBA); international business (MBA); leadership (MBA); project management (MBA). *Accreditation:* ACBSP. Part-time and evening/weekend programs available. *Faculty:* 3 full-time (2 women), 4 part-time/adjunct (2 women). *Students:* 86 full-time (47 women), 11 part-time (8 women); includes 5 minority (1 Black or African American, non-Hispanic/Latino; 3 Asian, non-Hispanic/Latino; 1 Hispanic/Latino), 11 international. Average age 34. In 2013, 59 master's awarded. *Degree requirements:* For master's, 34 credits. *Entrance requirements:* For master's, BS, transcripts, minimum undergraduate cumulative GPA of 3.0, 2 letters of reference, 3-5 page essay. Additional exam requirements/recommendations for international students: Recommended—TOEFL (minimum score 550 paper-based). Application fee: $50. Electronic applications accepted. *Expenses: Tuition:* Full-time $7140; part-time $444 per credit hour. *Required fees:* $100. *Unit head:* Dr. Barbara Gayle, Dean of Graduate Studies, 608-796-3080, E-mail: bmgayle@viterbo.edu. *Application contact:* Tiffany Morey, MBA Coordinator, 608-796-3379, E-mail: tlmorey@viterbo.edu.

Health Services Management and Hospital Administration

Wagner College, Division of Graduate Studies, Department of Business Administration, Program in Health Care Administration, Staten Island, NY 10301-4495. Offers MBA. *Faculty:* 2 part-time/adjunct (1 woman). *Students:* 5 full-time (3 women), 6 part-time (2 women); includes 2 minority (both Black or African American, non-Hispanic/Latino). Average age 27. 2 applicants, 100% accepted, 2 enrolled. In 2013, 3 master's awarded. *Degree requirements:* For master's, thesis optional. *Entrance requirements:* For master's, GMAT, minimum GPA of 2.6. Additional exam requirements/recommendations for international students: Required—TOEFL (minimum score 550 paper-based; 79 iBT). *Application deadline:* For fall admission, 5/1 priority date for domestic students, 3/1 priority date for international students; for spring admission, 10/1 priority date for domestic and international students. Applications are processed on a rolling basis. Application fee: $50. *Expenses: Tuition:* Full-time $17,496; part-time $972 per credit. Tuition and fees vary according to course load. *Financial support:* In 2013–14, 6 students received support. Unspecified assistantships and alumni fellowship grants available. Financial award applicants required to submit FAFSA. *Unit head:* Dr. John J. Moran, Director, 718-390-3255, Fax: 718-420-3255, E-mail: jmoran@wagner.edu. *Application contact:* Patricia Clancy, Assistant Coordinator of Graduate Studies, 718-420-4464, Fax: 718-390-3105, E-mail: patricia.clancy@wagner.edu.

Walden University, Graduate Programs, School of Health Sciences, Minneapolis, MN 55401. Offers clinical research administration (MS, Graduate Certificate); health education and promotion (MS); health informatics (MS); health services (PhD), including community health, healthcare administration, leadership, public health policy, self-designed; healthcare administration (MHA); public health (MPH, Dr PH, PhD), including community health and education (PhD), epidemiology (PhD). Part-time and evening/weekend programs available. Postbaccalaureate distance learning degree programs offered (minimal on-campus study). *Faculty:* 18 full-time (12 women), 236 part-time/adjunct (120 women). *Students:* 2,563 full-time (1,867 women), 1,775 part-time (1,233 women); includes 2,532 minority (1,963 Black or African American, non-Hispanic/Latino; 29 American Indian or Alaska Native, non-Hispanic/Latino; 212 Asian, non-Hispanic/Latino; 238 Hispanic/Latino; 15 Native Hawaiian or other Pacific Islander, non-Hispanic/Latino; 75 Two or more races, non-Hispanic/Latino), 97 international. Average age 39. 1,191 applicants, 94% accepted, 861 enrolled. In 2013, 723 master's, 121 doctorates, 17 other advanced degrees awarded. *Degree requirements:* For doctorate, thesis/dissertation, residency. *Entrance requirements:* For master's, bachelor's degree or higher; minimum GPA of 2.5; official transcripts; goal statement (for some programs); access to computer and Internet; for doctorate, master's degree or higher; three years of related professional or academic experience (preferred); minimum GPA of 3.0; goal statement and current resume (select programs); official transcripts; access to computer and Internet; for Graduate Certificate, relevant work experience; access to computer and Internet. Additional exam requirements/recommendations for international students: Required—TOEFL (minimum score 550 paper-based; 79 iBT), IELTS (minimum score 6.5), Michigan English Language Assessment Battery (minimum score 82), or PTE. *Application deadline:* Applications are processed on a rolling basis. Application fee: $0. Electronic applications accepted. *Expenses: Tuition:* Full-time $11,813.55; part-time $500 per credit. *Required fees:* $618.76. *Financial support:* Fellowships, Federal Work-Study, scholarships/grants, unspecified assistantships, and family tuition reduction, active duty/veteran tuition reduction, group tuition reduction, interest-free payment plans, employee tuition reduction available. Support available to part-time students. Financial award applicants required to submit FAFSA. *Unit head:* Dr. Jorg Westermann, Associate Dean, 800-925-3368. *Application contact:* Jennifer Hall, Vice President of Enrollment Management, 866-4-WALDEN, E-mail: info@waldenu.edu.
Website: http://www.waldenu.edu/colleges-schools/school-of-health-sciences

Walden University, Graduate Programs, School of Management, Minneapolis, MN 55401. Offers accounting (MBA, MS, DBA), including accounting for the professional (MS), accounting with CPA emphasis (MS), self-designed (MS, PhD); accounting and management (MS), including accountants as strategic managers, self-designed (MS, PhD); advanced project management (Graduate Certificate); applied project management (Graduate Certificate); bridge to business administration (Post-Doctoral Certificate); bridge to management (Post-Doctoral Certificate); business administration (EMBA); business management (Graduate Certificate); communication (MS, Graduate Certificate); corporate finance (MBA); entrepreneurship (DBA); entrepreneurship and small business (MBA); finance (DBA); global supply chain management (DBA); healthcare management (MBA, DBA); human resource management (MBA, MS, Graduate Certificate), including functional human resource management (MS), general program (MS), integrating functional and strategic human resource management (MS), organizational strategy (MS); human resources management (DBA); information systems management (DBA); international business (MBA, DBA); leadership (MBA, MS, DBA), including general program (MS), human resources leadership (MS), leader development (MS), self-designed (MS, PhD); management (MS, PhD), including accounting (PhD), engineering management (PhD), finance (PhD), general program (MS), healthcare management (MS), human resource management (MS), human resources management (PhD), information systems management (PhD), leadership (MS), leadership and organizational change (PhD), marketing (MS), operations research (PhD), project management (MS), self-designed, strategy and operations (MS); marketing (MBA, DBA); project management (MBA, MS, DBA); self-designed (MBA, DBA); social impact management (DBA); technology entrepreneurship (DBA). Part-time and evening/weekend programs available. Postbaccalaureate distance learning degree programs offered (minimal on-campus study). *Faculty:* 24 full-time (9 women), 337 part-time/adjunct (127 women). *Students:* 4,369 full-time (2,379 women), 2,181 part-time (1,304 women); includes 3,669 minority (3,020 Black or African American, non-Hispanic/Latino; 22 American Indian or Alaska Native, non-Hispanic/Latino; 156 Asian, non-Hispanic/Latino; 331 Hispanic/Latino; 11 Native Hawaiian or other Pacific Islander, non-Hispanic/Latino; 129 Two or more races, non-Hispanic/Latino), 107 international. Average age 41. 2,030 applicants, 94% accepted, 1436 enrolled. In 2013, 757 master's, 128 doctorates, 32 other advanced degrees awarded. *Degree requirements:* For master's, residency (for some programs); for doctorate, thesis/dissertation (for some programs), residency. *Entrance requirements:* For master's, bachelor's degree or higher; minimum GPA of 2.5; official transcripts; goal statement (for some programs); access to computer and Internet; for doctorate, master's degree or higher; three years of related professional or academic experience (preferred); minimum GPA of 3.0; goal statement and current resume (select programs); official transcripts; access to computer and Internet; for other advanced degree, relevant work experience; access to computer and Internet. Additional exam requirements/recommendations for international students: Required—TOEFL (minimum score 550 paper-based; 79 iBT), IELTS (minimum score 6.5), Michigan English Language Assessment Battery (minimum score 82), or PTE. *Application deadline:* Applications are processed on a rolling basis. Application fee: $0. Electronic applications accepted. *Expenses: Tuition:* Full-time $11,813.55; part-time $500 per credit. *Required fees:* $618.76. *Financial support:* Fellowships, Federal Work-Study, scholarships/grants, unspecified assistantships, and family tuition reduction, active duty/veteran tuition reduction, group tuition reduction, interest-free payment plans, employee tuition reduction available. Support available to part-time students. Financial award applicants required to submit FAFSA. *Unit head:* Dr. Ward Ulmer, III, Associate Dean, 800-925-3368. *Application contact:* Jennifer Hall, Vice President of Enrollment Management, 866-4-WALDEN, E-mail: info@waldenu.edu.
Website: http://www.waldenu.edu/programs/colleges-schools/management

Walden University, Graduate Programs, School of Nursing, Minneapolis, MN 55401. Offers adult-gerontology acute care nurse practitioner (MSN); adult-gerontology nurse practitioner (MSN); education (MSN); family nurse practitioner (MSN); informatics (MSN); leadership and management (MSN); nursing (DNP, PhD, Post-Master's Certificate), including education (PhD), healthcare administration (PhD), interdisciplinary health (PhD), leadership (PhD), nursing education (Post-Master's Certificate), nursing informatics (Post-Master's Certificate), nursing leadership and management (Post-Master's Certificate), public health policy (PhD). *Accreditation:* AACN. Part-time and evening/weekend programs available. Postbaccalaureate distance learning degree programs offered (no on-campus study). *Faculty:* 22 full-time (19 women), 343 part-time/adjunct (301 women). *Students:* 5,828 full-time (5,240 women), 2,803 part-time (2,578 women); includes 2,920 minority (1,893 Black or African American, non-Hispanic/Latino; 40 American Indian or Alaska Native, non-Hispanic/Latino; 438 Asian, non-Hispanic/Latino; 391 Hispanic/Latino; 35 Native Hawaiian or other Pacific Islander, non-Hispanic/Latino; 123 Two or more races, non-Hispanic/Latino), 147 international. Average age 41. 1,795 applicants, 95% accepted, 1375 enrolled. In 2013, 1,879 master's, 1 doctorate, 36 other advanced degrees awarded. *Degree requirements:* For doctorate, thesis/dissertation (for some programs), residency (for some programs), field experience (for some programs). *Entrance requirements:* For master's, bachelor's degree or equivalent in related field or RN; minimum GPA of 2.5; official transcripts; goal statement (for some programs); access to computer and Internet; for doctorate, master's degree or higher, three years of related professional or academic experience, RN, goal statement (for some programs); access to computer and Internet; for Post-Master's Certificate, relevant work experience; access to computer and Internet. Additional exam requirements/recommendations for international students: Required—TOEFL (minimum score 550 paper-based; 79 iBT), IELTS (minimum score 6.5), Michigan English Language Assessment Battery (minimum score 82), or PTE. *Application deadline:* Applications are processed on a rolling basis. Application fee: $0. Electronic applications accepted. *Expenses: Tuition:* Full-time $11,813.55; part-time $500 per credit. *Required fees:* $618.76. *Financial support:* Fellowships, Federal Work-Study, scholarships/grants, unspecified assistantships, and family tuition reduction, active duty/veteran tuition reduction, group tuition reduction, interest-free payment plans, employee tuition reduction available. Support available to part-time students. Financial award applicants required to submit FAFSA. *Unit head:* Dr. Andrea Lindell, Associate Dean, 800-925-3368. *Application contact:* Jennifer Hall, Vice President of Enrollment Management, 866-4-WALDEN, E-mail: info@waldenu.edu.
Website: http://www.waldenu.edu/programs/colleges-schools/nursing

Walden University, Graduate Programs, School of Public Policy and Administration, Minneapolis, MN 55401. Offers criminal justice (MPA, MPP, MS, Graduate Certificate), including emergency management (MS, PhD), general program (MS, PhD), homeland security and policy coordination (MS, PhD), law and public policy (MS, PhD), policy analysis (MS, PhD), public management and leadership (MS, PhD), self-designed (MS), terrorism, mediation, and peace (MS, PhD); criminal justice leadership and executive management (MS), including emergency management (MS, PhD), general program (MS, PhD), homeland security and policy coordination (MS, PhD), law and public policy (MS, PhD), policy analysis (MS, PhD), public management and leadership (MS, PhD), self-designed, terrorism, mediation, and peace (MS, PhD); emergency management (MPA, MPP, MS), including criminal justice (MS, PhD), general program (MS, PhD), homeland security (MS), public management and leadership (MS, PhD), terrorism and emergency management (MS); general program (MPA, MPP); government management (Graduate Certificate); health policy (MPA, MPP); homeland security (Graduate Certificate); homeland security and policy coordination (MPA, MPP); international nongovernmental organizations (MPA, MPP); law and public policy (MPA, MPP); local government management for sustainable communities (MPA, MPP); nonprofit management (Graduate Certificate); nonprofit management and leadership (MPA, MPP, MS); policy analysis (MPA); public management and leadership (MPA, MPP, Graduate Certificate); public policy (Graduate Certificate); public policy and administration (PhD), including criminal justice (MS, PhD), emergency management (MS, PhD), general program (MS, PhD), health policy, homeland security and policy coordination (MS, PhD), international nongovernmental organizations, law and public policy (MS, PhD), local government management for sustainable communities, nonprofit management and leadership, policy analysis (MS, PhD), public management and leadership (MS, PhD), terrorism, mediation, and peace (MS, PhD); strategic planning and public policy (Graduate Certificate); terrorism, mediation, and peace (MPA, MPP). Part-time and evening/weekend programs available. Postbaccalaureate distance learning degree programs offered (minimal on-campus study). *Faculty:* 10 full-time (4 women), 123 part-time/adjunct (55 women). *Students:* 1,029 full-time (640 women), 1,601 part-time (981 women); includes 1,579 minority (1,326 Black or African American, non-Hispanic/Latino; 18 American Indian or Alaska Native, non-Hispanic/Latino; 39 Asian, non-Hispanic/Latino; 127 Hispanic/Latino; 3 Native Hawaiian or other Pacific Islander, non-Hispanic/Latino; 66 Two or more races, non-Hispanic/Latino), 27 international. Average age 42. 566 applicants, 93% accepted, 412 enrolled. In 2013, 257 master's, 44 doctorates, 18 other advanced degrees awarded. *Degree requirements:* For doctorate, thesis/dissertation, residency. *Entrance requirements:* For master's, bachelor's degree or higher; minimum GPA of 2.5; official transcripts; goal statement (for some programs); access to computer and Internet; for doctorate, master's degree or higher; three years of related professional or academic experience (preferred); minimum GPA of 3.0; goal statement and current resume (select programs); official transcripts; access to computer and Internet; for Graduate Certificate, relevant work experience; access to computer and Internet. Additional exam requirements/recommendations for international students: Required—TOEFL (minimum score 550 paper-based; 79 iBT), IELTS (minimum score 6.5), Michigan English Language Assessment Battery (minimum score 82), or PTE. *Application deadline:* Applications are processed on a rolling basis. Application fee: $0. Electronic applications accepted. *Expenses: Tuition:* Full-time $11,813.55; part-time $500 per credit. *Required fees:* $618.76. *Financial support:* Fellowships, Federal Work-Study, scholarships/grants, unspecified assistantships, and family tuition reduction, active duty/veteran tuition reduction, group tuition reduction, interest-free payment plans, employee tuition reduction available. Support available to part-time students. Financial award applicants required to submit FAFSA. *Unit head:* Dr. Mark Gordon, Associate Dean, 800-925-3368. *Application contact:* Jennifer Hall, Vice President of Enrollment Management, 866-4-WALDEN, E-mail: info@waldenu.edu.
Website: http://www.waldenu.edu/programs/colleges-schools/public-policy-and-administration

Walsh University, Graduate Studies, MBA Program, North Canton, OH 44720-3396. Offers entrepreneurship (MBA); healthcare management (MBA); management (MBA); marketing (MBA). Part-time and evening/weekend programs available. Postbaccalaureate distance learning degree programs offered (no on-campus study). *Faculty:* 5 full-time (1 woman), 16 part-time/adjunct (4 women). *Students:* 29 full-time (15 women), 147 part-time (77 women); includes 6 minority (5 Black or African American, non-Hispanic/Latino; 1 American Indian or Alaska Native, non-Hispanic/Latino), 2 international. Average age 34. 69 applicants, 94% accepted, 31 enrolled. In

2013, 63 master's awarded. *Degree requirements:* For master's, capstone course in strategic management. *Entrance requirements:* For master's, GMAT (minimum score of 490), minimum GPA of 3.0. Additional exam requirements/recommendations for international students: Required—TOEFL (minimum score 500 paper-based; 61 iBT). *Application deadline:* For fall admission, 7/15 priority date for domestic students. Applications are processed on a rolling basis. Application fee: $25. Electronic applications accepted. *Expenses: Tuition:* Full-time $10,890; part-time $605 per credit hour. *Required fees:* $100; $100. *Financial support:* In 2013–14, 91 students received support, including 4 research assistantships with partial tuition reimbursements available (averaging $8,088 per year), 4 teaching assistantships (averaging $6,806 per year); scholarships/grants, tuition waivers (partial), unspecified assistantships, and tuition discounts also available. Support available to part-time students. Financial award application deadline: 12/31; financial award applicants required to submit FAFSA. *Faculty research:* Patient and physician satisfaction, advancing and improving learning with information technology, consumer-driven healthcare, branding and the service industry, service provider training and customer satisfaction, entrepreneurship, business strategy, social media, curriculum redesign, leadership, educational funding. *Total annual research expenditures:* $3,100. *Unit head:* Dr. Michael A. Petrochuk, Director of the MBA Program/Assistant Professor, 330-244-4764, Fax: 330-490-7359, E-mail: mpetrochuk@walsh.edu. *Application contact:* Audra Dice, Graduate and Transfer Admissions Counselor, 330-490-7181, Fax: 330-244-4925, E-mail: adice@walsh.edu.
Website: http://www.walsh.edu/mba-program

Walsh University, Graduate Studies, Program in Healthcare Management, North Canton, OH 44720-3396. Offers Graduate Certificate. *Entrance requirements:* For degree, minimum GPA of 3.0, official transcripts, current resume. Application fee: $25. *Expenses: Tuition:* Full-time $10,890; part-time $605 per credit hour. *Required fees:* $100; $100. *Unit head:* Dr. Michael Petrochuk, Director of the MBA Program, 330-244-4764, Fax: 330-490-7371, E-mail: mpetrochuk@walsh.edu. *Application contact:* Audra Dice, Assistant Director for Graduate and Transfer Admissions, 330-490-7181, Fax: 330-244-4925, E-mail: adice@walsh.edu.
Website: http://www.walsh.edu/certificate-in-healthcare-management

Washington Adventist University, Program in Health Care Administration, Takoma Park, MD 20912. Offers MA. Part-time programs available. *Entrance requirements:* Additional exam requirements/recommendations for international students: Required—TOEFL (minimum score 550 paper-based), IELTS (minimum score 5).

Washington State University Spokane, Graduate Programs, Program in Health Policy and Administration, Spokane, WA 99210. Offers MHPA. *Accreditation:* CAHME. Part-time and evening/weekend programs available. *Degree requirements:* For master's, comprehensive exam (for some programs), thesis (for some programs), oral exam. *Entrance requirements:* For master's, GRE General Test or GMAT, minimum GPA of 3.0, 3 letters of recommendation. Additional exam requirements/recommendations for international students: Required—TOEFL (minimum score 550 paper-based) or IELTS (minimum score 7).

Wayland Baptist University, Graduate Programs, Programs in Business Administration/Management, Plainview, TX 79072-6998. Offers accounting (MBA); general business (MBA); health care administration (MAM, MBA); healthcare administration (MBA); human resource management (MAM, MBA); international management (MBA); management (MBA); management information systems (MBA); organization management (MAM); project management (MBA). Part-time and evening/weekend programs available. Postbaccalaureate distance learning degree programs offered (no on-campus study). *Faculty:* 30 full-time (5 women), 38 part-time/adjunct (9 women). *Students:* 44 full-time (20 women), 702 part-time (315 women); includes 348 minority (149 Black or African American, non-Hispanic/Latino; 4 American Indian or Alaska Native, non-Hispanic/Latino; 23 Asian, non-Hispanic/Latino; 139 Hispanic/Latino; 9 Native Hawaiian or other Pacific Islander, non-Hispanic/Latino; 24 Two or more races, non-Hispanic/Latino), 5 international. Average age 40. 147 applicants, 94% accepted, 73 enrolled. In 2013, 296 master's awarded. *Degree requirements:* For master's, capstone course. *Entrance requirements:* For master's, GMAT, GRE or MAT. Additional exam requirements/recommendations for international students: Required—TOEFL (minimum score 500 paper-based; 61 iBT). *Application deadline:* Applications are processed on a rolling basis. Application fee: $50. Electronic applications accepted. *Expenses: Tuition:* Full-time $8190; part-time $455 per credit hour. *Required fees:* $970; $455 per credit hour. $485 per semester. *Financial support:* Federal Work-Study, institutionally sponsored loans, and scholarships/grants available. Support available to part-time students. Financial award application deadline: 5/1; financial award applicants required to submit FAFSA. *Unit head:* Dr. Otto Schacht, Chairman, 806-291-1020, Fax: 806-291-1957, E-mail: schachto@wbu.edu. *Application contact:* Amanda Stanton, Graduate Studies, 806-291-3423, Fax: 806-291-1950, E-mail: stanton@wbu.edu.

Waynesburg University, Graduate and Professional Studies, Canonsburg, PA 15370. Offers business (MBA), including energy management, finance, health systems, human resources, leadership, market development; counseling (MA), including addictions counseling, clinical mental health; education (M Ed, MAT), including autism (M Ed), curriculum and instruction (M Ed), educational leadership (M Ed), online teaching (M Ed); nursing (MSN), including administration, education, informatics; nursing practice (DNP); special education (M Ed); technology (M Ed); MSN/MBA. *Accreditation:* AACN. Part-time and evening/weekend programs available. *Faculty:* 11 full-time (5 women), 136 part-time/adjunct (80 women). *Students:* 146 full-time (99 women), 419 part-time (268 women). In 2013, 290 master's, 7 doctorates awarded. *Degree requirements:* For doctorate, thesis/dissertation. *Entrance requirements:* Additional exam requirements/recommendations for international students: Required—TOEFL. *Application deadline:* For fall admission, 8/1 priority date for domestic students. Applications are processed on a rolling basis. Electronic applications accepted. *Financial support:* Available to part-time students. Application deadline: 5/1. *Unit head:* David Mariner, Dean, 724-743-4420, Fax: 724-743-4425, E-mail: dmariner@waynesburg.edu. *Application contact:* Dr. Michael Bednarski, Director of Enrollment, 724-743-4420, Fax: 724-743-4425, E-mail: mbednars@waynesburg.edu.
Website: http://www.waynesburg.edu/

Wayne State University, College of Liberal Arts and Sciences, Department of Political Science, Program in Public Administration, Detroit, MI 48202. Offers aging policy and management (MPA); criminal justice policy and management (MPA); economic development policy and management (MPA); health and human services policy and management (MPA); human and fiscal resource management (MPA); information technology management (MPA); nonprofit policy and management (MPA); organizational behavior and management (MPA); public budgeting and financial management (MPA); public policy analysis and program evaluation (MPA); social welfare policy and management (MPA); urban and metropolitan policy and management (MPA). *Accreditation:* NASPAA. Evening/weekend programs available. *Students:* 11 full-time (5 women), 55 part-time (43 women); includes 20 minority (14 Black or African American, non-Hispanic/Latino; 2 Asian, non-Hispanic/Latino; 2 Hispanic/Latino; 2 Two or more races, non-Hispanic/Latino), 1 international. Average age 33. 83 applicants, 34% accepted, 17 enrolled. In 2013, 19 master's awarded. *Degree requirements:* For master's, comprehensive exam. *Entrance requirements:* For master's, GRE General Test, minimum undergraduate upper-division GPA of 3.0 or master's degree. Additional exam requirements/recommendations for international students: Required—TOEFL (minimum score 550 paper-based; 79 iBT), TWE (minimum score 5.5), Michigan English Language Assessment Battery (minimum score 85); Recommended—IELTS (minimum score 6.5). *Application deadline:* For fall admission, 6/1 priority date for domestic students, 5/1 priority date for international students; for winter admission, 10/1 priority date for domestic students, 9/1 priority date for international students; for spring admission, 2/1 priority date for domestic students, 1/1 priority date for international students. Applications are processed on a rolling basis. Application fee: $0. Electronic applications accepted. *Expenses:* Tuition, state resident: part-time $554.15 per credit. Tuition, nonresident: part-time $1200.35 per credit. *Required fees:* $42.15 per credit. $268.30 per semester. Tuition and fees vary according to course load and program. *Financial support:* In 2013–14, 21 students received support. Fellowships, teaching assistantships, scholarships/grants, and unspecified assistantships available. Financial award application deadline: 3/31; financial award applicants required to submit FAFSA. *Faculty research:* Urban politics, urban education, state administration. *Unit head:* Dr. Daniel Geller, Department Chair, 313-577-6328, E-mail: dgeller@wayne.edu. *Application contact:* Dr. Brady Baybeck, Associate Professor/Director, Graduate Program in Public Administration, E-mail: mpa@wayne.edu.
Website: http://clasweb.clas.wayne.edu/mpa

Weber State University, College of Health Professions, Program of Health Administration, Ogden, UT 84408-1001. Offers MHA. *Accreditation:* CAHME. Part-time and evening/weekend programs available. *Faculty:* 5 full-time (2 women). *Students:* 37 full-time (6 women), 13 part-time (6 women); includes 2 minority (both Hispanic/Latino). Average age 32. 44 applicants, 70% accepted, 31 enrolled. In 2013, 23 master's awarded. *Entrance requirements:* For master's, GMAT or GRE. Additional exam requirements/recommendations for international students: Required—TOEFL. *Application deadline:* For fall admission, 7/1 for domestic students. Applications are processed on a rolling basis. Application fee: $60 ($90 for international students). *Expenses:* Tuition, state resident: full-time $7118; part-time $253 per credit hour. Tuition, nonresident: full-time $12,480; part-time $634 per credit hour. *Required fees:* $34.33; $34.33 per credit hour. $257 per semester. Full-time tuition and fees vary according to course load. *Financial support:* In 2013–14, 1 student received support. Application deadline: 4/1; applicants required to submit FAFSA. *Unit head:* Dr. Ken Johnson, Chair, 801-626-6988, Fax: 801-626-7683, E-mail: kjohnson@weber.edu. *Application contact:* Cory Moss, 801-626-7237, Fax: 801-626-6475, E-mail: cmoss@weber.edu.
Website: http://www.weber.edu/MHA/

Webster University, George Herbert Walker School of Business and Technology, Department of Management, St. Louis, MO 63119-3194. Offers business and organizational security management (MA); health administration (MHA); health care management (MA); health services management (MA); human resources development (MA); human resources management (MA); information technology management (MS); management and leadership (MA); marketing (MA); nonprofit leadership (MA); procurement and acquisitions management (MA); public administration (MPA); space systems operations management (MS). Part-time and evening/weekend programs available. Postbaccalaureate distance learning degree programs offered (no on-campus study). *Degree requirements:* For master's, thesis (for some programs). *Entrance requirements:* Additional exam requirements/recommendations for international students: Required—TOEFL. *Expenses: Tuition:* Full-time $11,610; part-time $645 per credit hour. Tuition and fees vary according to campus/location and program.

West Chester University of Pennsylvania, College of Health Sciences, Department of Health, West Chester, PA 19383. Offers community health (MPH); emergency preparedness (Certificate); environmental health (MPH); health care management (MPH, Certificate); integrative health (MPH, Certificate); nutrition (MPH); school health (M Ed). *Accreditation:* CEPH. Part-time and evening/weekend programs available. *Faculty:* 17 full-time (13 women), 3 part-time/adjunct (all women). *Students:* 115 full-time (85 women), 95 part-time (73 women); includes 79 minority (66 Black or African American, non-Hispanic/Latino; 1 American Indian or Alaska Native, non-Hispanic/Latino; 5 Asian, non-Hispanic/Latino; 3 Hispanic/Latino; 4 Two or more races, non-Hispanic/Latino), 15 international. Average age 31. 156 applicants, 83% accepted, 76 enrolled. In 2013, 101 master's, 18 other advanced degrees awarded. *Degree requirements:* For master's, thesis or alternative, minimum GPA of 3.0; research report (for M Ed); major project and practicum (for MPH); for Certificate, minimum GPA of 3.0. *Entrance requirements:* For master's, goal statement, two letters of recommendation, undergraduate Introduction to Statistics course. Additional exam requirements/recommendations for international students: Required—TOEFL (minimum score 550 paper-based; 80 iBT). *Application deadline:* For fall admission, 4/15 priority date for domestic students, 3/15 for international students; for spring admission, 10/15 priority date for domestic students, 9/1 for international students. Applications are processed on a rolling basis. Application fee: $45. Electronic applications accepted. *Expenses:* Tuition, state resident: full-time $7956; part-time $442 per credit. Tuition, nonresident: full-time $11,934; part-time $663 per credit. *Required fees:* $2134.20; $106.24 per credit. Tuition and fees vary according to campus/location and program. *Financial support:* Unspecified assistantships available. Support available to part-time students. Financial award application deadline: 2/15; financial award applicants required to submit FAFSA. *Faculty research:* Healthy school communities, community health issues and evidence-based programs, environment and health, nutrition and health, integrative health. *Unit head:* Dr. Bethann Cinelli, Chair, 610-436-2267, E-mail: bcinelli@wcupa.edu. *Application contact:* Dr. Lynn Carson, Graduate Coordinator, 610-436-2138, E-mail: lcarson@wcupa.edu.
Website: http://www.wcupa.edu/_ACADEMICS/HealthSciences/health/

Western Carolina University, Graduate School, College of Health and Human Sciences, School of Health Sciences, Cullowhee, NC 28723. Offers MHS. Part-time and evening/weekend programs available. *Degree requirements:* For master's, thesis or alternative. *Entrance requirements:* For master's, GRE General Test, appropriate undergraduate degree with minimum GPA of 3.0, 3 letters of recommendation. Additional exam requirements/recommendations for international students: Required—TOEFL (minimum score 550 paper-based; 79 iBT). *Faculty research:* Epidemiology, dietetics, public health, environmental technology, water quality, occupational health.

Western Connecticut State University, Division of Graduate Studies, Ancell School of Business, Program in Health Administration, Danbury, CT 06810-6885. Offers MHA. Part-time programs available. *Degree requirements:* For master's, comprehensive exam, completion of program within 6 years. *Entrance requirements:* For master's, GMAT, GRE, or MAT, minimum GPA of 2.5. Additional exam requirements/recommendations for international students: Recommended—TOEFL (minimum score 550 paper-based; 79 iBT), IELTS (minimum score 6). *Faculty research:* Organizational behavior, human resource management, health delivery systems, health services financial management, managing health services organizations, health services quality management, health policy and strategic management for health services, long-term care administration, health services marketing, health care law.

Western Governors University, College of Health Professions, Salt Lake City, UT 84107. Offers healthcare management (MBA); leadership and management (MSN); nursing education (MSN). Evening/weekend programs available. *Degree requirements:*

For master's, capstone project. *Entrance requirements:* For master's, Readiness Assessment, transcripts. Additional exam requirements/recommendations for international students: Required—TOEFL (minimum score 450 paper-based; 80 iBT). Electronic applications accepted.

Western Illinois University, School of Graduate Studies, College of Education and Human Services, Department of Health Sciences, Macomb, IL 61455-1390. Offers health education (MS); health services administration (Certificate). *Accreditation:* NCATE. Part-time programs available. *Students:* 24 full-time (18 women), 24 part-time (17 women); includes 10 minority (5 Black or African American, non-Hispanic/Latino; 3 Asian, non-Hispanic/Latino; 2 Hispanic/Latino), 7 international. Average age 29. In 2013, 15 master's, 8 other advanced degrees awarded. *Degree requirements:* For master's, comprehensive exam, thesis or alternative. *Entrance requirements:* Additional exam requirements/recommendations for international students: Required—TOEFL (minimum score 550 paper-based; 80 iBT). *Application deadline:* Applications are processed on a rolling basis. Application fee: $30. Electronic applications accepted. *Financial support:* In 2013–14, 11 students received support, including 9 research assistantships with full tuition reimbursements available (averaging $7,544 per year), 2 teaching assistantships with full tuition reimbursements available (averaging $8,688 per year). Financial award applicants required to submit FAFSA. *Unit head:* Dr. Lorette Oden, Interim Chairperson, 309-298-1076. *Application contact:* Dr. Nancy Parsons, Associate Provost and Director of Graduate Studies, 309-298-1806, Fax: 309-298-2345, E-mail: grad-office@wiu.edu.
Website: http://wiu.edu/health

Western Kentucky University, Graduate Studies, College of Health and Human Services, Department of Public Health, Bowling Green, KY 42101. Offers healthcare administration (MHA); public health (MPH). *Accreditation:* CEPH. Part-time and evening/weekend programs available. *Degree requirements:* For master's, comprehensive exam, thesis or alternative. *Entrance requirements:* For master's, GRE General Test, minimum GPA of 2.75. Additional exam requirements/recommendations for international students: Required—TOEFL (minimum score 555 paper-based; 79 iBT). *Faculty research:* Health education training, driver traffic safety, community readiness, occupational injuries, local health departments.

Western Michigan University, Graduate College, College of Arts and Sciences, School of Public Affairs and Administration, Kalamazoo, MI 49008. Offers health care administration (Graduate Certificate); nonprofit leadership and administration (Graduate Certificate); public administration (MPA, PhD). *Accreditation:* NASPAA (one or more programs are accredited). *Degree requirements:* For doctorate, thesis/dissertation, oral exams. *Entrance requirements:* For doctorate, GRE General Test.

Widener University, School of Business Administration, Program in Health and Medical Services Administration, Chester, PA 19013-5792. Offers MBA, MHA, MD/MBA, MD/MHA, Psy D/MBA, Psy D/MHA. *Accreditation:* CAHME (one or more programs are accredited). Part-time and evening/weekend programs available. *Faculty:* 3 full-time (1 woman), 6 part-time/adjunct (1 woman). *Students:* 30 applicants, 80% accepted. In 2013, 1 master's awarded. *Degree requirements:* For master's, clerkship, residency. *Entrance requirements:* For master's, GMAT, interview, minimum GPA of 2.5. *Application deadline:* For fall admission, 8/1 priority date for domestic students; for spring admission, 12/1 for domestic students. Applications are processed on a rolling basis. Application fee: $25 ($300 for international students). Electronic applications accepted. *Expenses: Tuition:* Full-time $30,000; part-time $950 per credit. *Financial support:* Research assistantships, career-related internships or fieldwork, and traineeships available. Support available to part-time students. Financial award application deadline: 5/1. *Faculty research:* Cost containment in health care, reimbursement of hospitals, strategic behavior. *Unit head:* Dr. Caryl Carpenter, Director, 610-499-4109. *Application contact:* Ann Seltzer, Graduate Enrollment Administrator, 610-499-4305, E-mail: apseltzer@widener.edu.
Website: http://www.widener.edu

Widener University, School of Human Service Professions, Institute for Graduate Clinical Psychology, Program in Clinical Psychology and Health and Medical Services Administration, Chester, PA 19013-5792. Offers Psy D/MBA, Psy D/MHA. *Accreditation:* APA (one or more programs are accredited); CAHME. *Faculty:* 15 full-time (6 women), 18 part-time/adjunct (10 women). *Students:* 3 full-time (2 women). Average age 28. *Application deadline:* For fall admission, 12/31 for domestic students. Application fee: $75. Electronic applications accepted. *Expenses: Tuition:* Full-time $30,000; part-time $950 per credit. *Financial support:* Career-related internships or fieldwork, Federal Work-Study, and institutionally sponsored loans available. Financial award application deadline: 5/31. *Faculty research:* Psychosocial competence, family systems, medical care systems and financing. *Unit head:* Dr. Hal Shorey, Director, 610-499-4598, Fax: 610-499-4625.

Wilkes University, College of Graduate and Professional Studies, Jay S. Sidhu School of Business and Leadership, Wilkes-Barre, PA 18766-0002. Offers accounting (MBA); entrepreneurship (MBA); finance (MBA); health care administration (MBA); human resource management (MBA); international business (MBA); marketing (MBA); operations management (MBA); organizational leadership and development (MBA). *Accreditation:* ACBSP. Part-time and evening/weekend programs available. *Students:* 41 full-time (20 women), 119 part-time (48 women); includes 20 minority (5 Black or African American, non-Hispanic/Latino; 3 Asian, non-Hispanic/Latino; 7 Hispanic/Latino; 5 Two or more races, non-Hispanic/Latino), 7 international. Average age 31. In 2013, 55 master's awarded. *Entrance requirements:* For master's, GMAT. Additional exam requirements/recommendations for international students: Required—TOEFL (minimum score 550 paper-based; 79 iBT). *Application deadline:* Applications are processed on a rolling basis. Application fee: $45 ($65 for international students). Electronic applications accepted. *Expenses:* Contact institution. *Financial support:* Federal Work-Study and unspecified assistantships available. Financial award application deadline: 3/1; financial award applicants required to submit FAFSA. *Unit head:* Dr. Jeffrey Alves, Dean, 570-408-4702, Fax: 570-408-7846, E-mail: jeffrey.alves@wilkes.edu. *Application contact:* Joanne Thomas, Interim Director of Graduate Enrollment, 570-408-4234, Fax: 570-408-7846, E-mail: joanne.thomas1@wilkes.edu.
Website: http://www.wilkes.edu/pages/457.asp

William Woods University, Graduate and Adult Studies, Fulton, MO 65251-1098. Offers administration (M Ed, Ed S); athletic/activities administration (M Ed); curriculum and instruction (M Ed, Ed S); educational leadership (Ed D); equestrian education (M Ed); health management (MBA); human resources (MBA); leadership (MBA); marketing, advertising, and public relations (MBA); teaching and technology (M Ed). Part-time and evening/weekend programs available. *Faculty:* 231 part-time/adjunct (87 women). *Students:* 418 full-time (276 women), 716 part-time (433 women); includes 51 minority (34 Black or African American, non-Hispanic/Latino; 4 American Indian or Alaska Native, non-Hispanic/Latino; 5 Asian, non-Hispanic/Latino; 3 Hispanic/Latino; 5 Two or more races, non-Hispanic/Latino), 4 international. Average age 35. In 2013, 507 master's, 8 doctorates, 143 other advanced degrees awarded. *Degree requirements:* For master's, capstone course (MBA), action research (M Ed); for Ed S, field experience. *Entrance requirements:* Additional exam requirements/recommendations for international students: Required—TOEFL (minimum score 550 paper-based). *Application deadline:* Applications are processed on a rolling basis. Application fee: $0. Electronic applications accepted. *Expenses:* Contact institution. *Financial support:* Institutionally sponsored loans available. Financial award applicants required to submit FAFSA. *Unit head:* Dr. Michael Westerfield, Vice President and Dean of the Graduate College, 573-592-4383, Fax: 573-592-1164. *Application contact:* Jessica Brush, Director of Operations, 573-592-4227, Fax: 573-592-1164, E-mail: jessica.brush@williamwoods.ede.
Website: http://www.williamwoods.edu/evening_programs/index.asp

Wilmington University, College of Business, New Castle, DE 19720-6491. Offers accounting (MBA, MS); business administration (MBA, DBA); environmental stewardship (MBA); finance (MBA); health care administration (MBA, MSM); homeland security (MBA, MSM); human resource management (MSM); management information systems (MBA, MSN); marketing (MSM); marketing management (MBA); military leadership (MSM); organizational leadership (MBA, MSM); public administration (MSM). Part-time and evening/weekend programs available. *Entrance requirements:* Additional exam requirements/recommendations for international students: Required—TOEFL (minimum score 500 paper-based). Electronic applications accepted.

Worcester State University, Graduate Studies, Program in Health Care Administration, Worcester, MA 01602-2597. Offers MS. *Faculty:* 1 full-time (0 women), 2 part-time/adjunct (0 women). *Students:* 3 full-time (all women), 14 part-time (12 women); includes 1 minority (Black or African American, non-Hispanic/Latino), 1 international. Average age 37. 27 applicants, 59% accepted, 3 enrolled. In 2013, 9 master's awarded. *Degree requirements:* For master's, comprehensive exam (for some programs), thesis optional. *Entrance requirements:* For master's, MAT, GRE. Additional exam requirements/recommendations for international students: Required—TOEFL (minimum score 500 paper-based; 61 iBT). *Application deadline:* For fall admission, 6/15 for domestic and international students; for spring admission, 4/1 for domestic and international students. Applications are processed on a rolling basis. Application fee: $40. Electronic applications accepted. *Expenses: Tuition, area resident:* Part-time $150 per credit. Tuition, state resident: part-time $150 per credit. Tuition, nonresident: part-time $150 per credit. *Required fees:* $114.50 per credit. *Financial support:* Career-related internships or fieldwork, scholarships/grants, and unspecified assistantships available. Financial award application deadline: 3/1; financial award applicants required to submit FAFSA. *Unit head:* Dr. Robert Holmes, Coordinator, 508-929-8343, Fax: 508-929-8175, E-mail: rholmes3@worcester.edu. *Application contact:* Sara Grady, Assistant Dean of Graduate and Continuing Education, 508-929-8787, Fax: 508-929-8100, E-mail: sara.grady@worcester.edu.

Wright State University, School of Graduate Studies, Raj Soin College of Business, Department of Management, Dayton, OH 45435. Offers flexible business (MBA); health care management (MBA); international business (MBA); management, innovation and change (MBA); project management (MBA); supply chain management (MBA); MBA/MS. *Entrance requirements:* For master's, GMAT, minimum AACSB index of 1000. Additional exam requirements/recommendations for international students: Required—TOEFL.

Xavier University, College of Social Sciences, Health and Education, Program in Health Services Administration, Cincinnati, OH 45207. Offers MHSA, MHSA/MBA. *Accreditation:* CAHME. Part-time programs available. *Faculty:* 7 full-time (2 women), 7 part-time/adjunct (2 women). *Students:* 51 full-time (26 women), 39 part-time (21 women); includes 12 minority (5 Black or African American, non-Hispanic/Latino; 1 American Indian or Alaska Native, non-Hispanic/Latino; 3 Asian, non-Hispanic/Latino; 3 Hispanic/Latino), 1 international. Average age 26. 36 applicants, 100% accepted, 31 enrolled. In 2013, 34 master's awarded. *Degree requirements:* For master's, thesis. *Entrance requirements:* For master's, GMAT or GRE, resume, two letters of recommendation, statement of intent, official transcripts. Additional exam requirements/recommendations for international students: Required—TOEFL (minimum score 550 paper-based; 80 iBT). *Application deadline:* For fall admission, 6/1 priority date for domestic students, 1/1 priority date for international students. Applications are processed on a rolling basis. Application fee: $35. Electronic applications accepted. Application fee is waived when completed online. *Expenses: Tuition:* Part-time $594 per credit hour. *Required fees:* $3 per semester. *Financial support:* In 2013–14, 24 students received support. Scholarships/grants and unspecified assistantships available. Financial award application deadline: 4/30; financial award applicants required to submit FAFSA. *Faculty research:* Success factors of ethics committees in health care, early hospital readmission and quality, health and labor economics, clinical emergency medicine and uncompensated care. *Unit head:* Dr. Nancy Linenkugel, Director/Chair, 513-745-3716, Fax: 513-745-4301, E-mail: linenkugeln@xavier.edu. *Application contact:* Amy Hellkamp, Recruitment/Promotions Coordinator, 513-745-3687, Fax: 513-745-4301, E-mail: hellkampal@xavier.edu.
Website: http://www.xavier.edu/mhsa/

Xavier University, Williams College of Business, Master of Business Administration Program, Cincinnati, OH 45207-3221. Offers business administration (Exec MBA, MBA); business intelligence (MBA); finance (MBA); health industry (MBA); international business (MBA); marketing (MBA); values-based leadership (MBA); MBA/MHSA; MSN/MBA. *Accreditation:* AACSB. Part-time and evening/weekend programs available. *Faculty:* 39 full-time (17 women), 12 part-time/adjunct (2 women). *Students:* 163 full-time (47 women), 483 part-time (162 women); includes 91 minority (28 Black or African American, non-Hispanic/Latino; 3 American Indian or Alaska Native, non-Hispanic/Latino; 42 Asian, non-Hispanic/Latino; 14 Hispanic/Latino; 4 Two or more races, non-Hispanic/Latino), 33 international. Average age 30. 190 applicants, 86% accepted, 110 enrolled. In 2013, 319 master's awarded. *Degree requirements:* For master's, capstone course. *Entrance requirements:* For master's, GMAT or GRE. Additional exam requirements/recommendations for international students: Required—TOEFL (minimum score 550 paper-based; 79 iBT). *Application deadline:* For fall admission, 8/1 priority date for domestic students, 5/1 for international students; for spring admission, 12/1 priority date for domestic students, 9/1 for international students. Applications are processed on a rolling basis. Application fee: $0. Electronic applications accepted. *Expenses:* Contact institution. *Financial support:* In 2013–14, 115 students received support. Scholarships/grants, tuition waivers (partial), and unspecified assistantships available. Financial award application deadline: 3/1; financial award applicants required to submit FAFSA. *Unit head:* Jennifer Bush, Assistant Dean of Graduate Programs, Williams College of Business, 513-745-3527, Fax: 513-745-2929, E-mail: bush@xavier.edu. *Application contact:* Lauren Parcell, MBA Advisor, 513-745-1014, Fax: 513-745-2929, E-mail: parcelll@xavier.edu.
Website: http://www.xavier.edu/williams/mba/

Yale University, School of Medicine, Yale School of Public Health, New Haven, CT 06520. Offers applied biostatistics and epidemiology (APMPH); biostatistics (MPH, MS, PhD), including global health (MPH); chronic disease epidemiology (MPH, PhD), including global health (MPH); environmental health sciences (MPH, PhD), including global health (MPH); epidemiology of microbial diseases (MPH, PhD), including global health (MPH); global health (APMPH); health management (MPH), including global health; health policy (MPH), including global health; health policy and administration (APMPH, PhD); occupational and environmental medicine (APMPH); preventive medicine (APMPH); social and behavioral sciences (APMPH, MPH), including global health (MPH); JD/MPH; M Div/MPH; MBA/MPH; MD/MPH; MEM/MPH; MFS/MPH; MM Sc/MPH; MPH/MA; MSN/MPH. MS and PhD offered through the Graduate School.

Accreditation: CEPH. Part-time programs available. Terminal master's awarded for partial completion of doctoral program. *Degree requirements:* For master's, thesis, summer internship; for doctorate, comprehensive exam, thesis/dissertation, residency. *Entrance requirements:* For master's, GMAT, GRE, or MCAT, two years of undergraduate coursework in math and science; for doctorate, GRE General Test. Additional exam requirements/recommendations for international students: Required—TOEFL (minimum score 100 iBT). Electronic applications accepted. *Expenses:* Contact institution. *Faculty research:* Genetic and emerging infections epidemiology, virology, cost/quality, vector biology, quantitative methods, aging, asthma, cancer.

York College of Pennsylvania, Graham School of Business, York, PA 17405-7199. Offers continuous improvement (MBA); financial management (MBA); health care management (MBA); management (MBA); marketing (MBA); self-designed focus (MBA). *Accreditation:* ACBSP. Part-time and evening/weekend programs available. *Faculty:* 13 full-time (3 women), 2 part-time/adjunct (0 women). *Students:* 6 full-time (all women), 109 part-time (40 women); includes 8 minority (2 Black or African American, non-Hispanic/Latino; 1 Asian, non-Hispanic/Latino; 1 Hispanic/Latino; 4 Two or more races, non-Hispanic/Latino), 3 international. Average age 30. 62 applicants, 63% accepted, 23 enrolled. In 2013, 24 master's awarded. *Entrance requirements:* For master's, GMAT. Additional exam requirements/recommendations for international students: Required—TOEFL (minimum score 530 paper-based; 72 iBT). *Application deadline:* For fall admission, 7/15 priority date for domestic students; for spring admission, 12/15 priority date for domestic students. Applications are processed on a rolling basis. Application fee: $50. Electronic applications accepted. *Expenses: Tuition:* Full-time $12,870; part-time $715 per credit. *Required fees:* $1660; $360 per semester. Tuition and fees vary according to degree level. *Financial support:* In 2013–14, 4 students received support. Scholarships/grants available. Financial award application deadline: 4/15; financial award applicants required to submit FAFSA. *Unit head:* Dr. David Greisler, MBA Director, 717-815-6410, Fax: 717-600-3999, E-mail: dgreisle@ycp.edu. *Application contact:* Brenda Adams, Assistant Director, MBA Program, 717-815-1749, Fax: 717-600-3999, E-mail: badams@ycp.edu.
Website: http://www.ycp.edu/mba

Youngstown State University, Graduate School, Bitonte College of Health and Human Services, Department of Health Professions, Youngstown, OH 44555-0001. Offers health and human services (MHHS); public health (MPH). *Accreditation:* NAACLS. Part-time and evening/weekend programs available. *Degree requirements:* For master's, thesis optional. *Entrance requirements:* For master's, GRE General Test, minimum GPA of 3.0. Additional exam requirements/recommendations for international students: Required—TOEFL. *Faculty research:* Drug prevention, multiskilling in health care, organizational behavior, health care management, health behaviors, research management.

Health Services Research

Albany College of Pharmacy and Health Sciences, School of Pharmacy and Pharmaceutical Sciences, Albany, NY 12208. Offers health outcomes research (MS); pharmaceutical sciences (MS), including pharmaceutics, pharmacology; pharmacy (Pharm D). *Accreditation:* ACPE. *Students:* 527 full-time (308 women), 15 part-time (10 women); includes 138 minority (19 Black or African American, non-Hispanic/Latino; 95 Asian, non-Hispanic/Latino; 13 Hispanic/Latino; 1 Native Hawaiian or other Pacific Islander, non-Hispanic/Latino; 10 Two or more races, non-Hispanic/Latino), 64 international. Average age 24. 1,209 applicants, 15% accepted, 78 enrolled. In 2013, 6 master's, 283 doctorates awarded. *Degree requirements:* For master's, thesis; for doctorate, practice experience. *Entrance requirements:* For master's, GRE, minimum GPA of 3.0; for doctorate, PCAT, minimum GPA of 2.5. Additional exam requirements/recommendations for international students: Required—TOEFL (minimum score 84 iBT). *Application deadline:* For fall admission, 3/1 for domestic and international students. Applications are processed on a rolling basis. Application fee: $75. Electronic applications accepted. *Financial support:* In 2013–14, 20 students received support. Federal Work-Study and scholarships/grants available. Support available to part-time students. Financial award application deadline: 3/1; financial award applicants required to submit FAFSA. *Faculty research:* Therapeutic use of drugs, pharmacokinetics, drug delivery and design. *Unit head:* Dr. Angela Dominelli, Dean, School of Pharmacy and Pharmaceutical Sciences, 518-694-7333. *Application contact:* Ann Bruno, Coordinator, Graduate Programs, 518-694-7130, E-mail: graduate@acphs.edu.
Website: http://www.acphs.edu/academics/schools-departments/school-pharmacy-pharmaceutical-sciences

Boise State University, College of Health Sciences, Department of Community and Environmental Health, Boise, ID 83725-0399. Offers environmental health (MHS); evaluation and research (MHS); health policy (MHS); health promotion (MHS); health services leadership (MHS).

Brown University, Graduate School, Division of Biology and Medicine, School of Public Health, Department of Health Services, Policy and Practice, Providence, RI 02912. Offers PhD.

Case Western Reserve University, School of Medicine and School of Graduate Studies, Graduate Programs in Medicine, Department of Epidemiology and Biostatistics, Program in Health Services Research, Cleveland, OH 44106. Offers MS, PhD. *Degree requirements:* For master's, comprehensive exam, thesis; for doctorate, comprehensive exam, thesis/dissertation. *Entrance requirements:* For master's and doctorate, GRE. Additional exam requirements/recommendations for international students: Required—TOEFL (minimum score 550 paper-based).

Clarkson University, Graduate School, School of Arts and Sciences, Program in Basic Science, Potsdam, NY 13699. Offers MS. *Students:* 2 full-time (1 woman). Average age 27. 1 applicant, 100% accepted, 1 enrolled. In 2013, 1 master's awarded. *Entrance requirements:* For master's, GRE, transcripts of all college coursework, three letters of recommendation; resume and personal statement (recommended). Additional exam requirements/recommendations for international students: Required—TOEFL. *Application deadline:* For fall admission, 1/30 priority date for domestic and international students; for spring admission, 9/1 priority date for domestic and international students. Applications are processed on a rolling basis. Application fee: $25 ($35 for international students). Electronic applications accepted. *Expenses: Tuition:* Full-time $15,888; part-time $1324 per credit. *Required fees:* $295 per semester. *Financial support:* In 2013–14, 2 students received support, including 1 research assistantship with full tuition reimbursement available (averaging $23,329 per year), 1 teaching assistantship with full tuition reimbursement available (averaging $23,329 per year); scholarships/grants, tuition waivers (partial), and unspecified assistantships also available. *Faculty research:* Health science, environmental health. *Unit head:* Dr. Peter Turner, Dean, 315-268-6544, Fax: 315-268-3989, E-mail: pturner@clarkson.edu. *Application contact:* Jennifer Reed, Graduate Coordinator, School of Arts and Sciences, 315-268-3802, Fax: 315-268-3989, E-mail: sciencegrad@clarkson.edu.
Website: http://www.clarkson.edu/artsandsci/grad/admissions/basic_sci.html

Dartmouth College, The Dartmouth Institute, Hanover, NH 03755. Offers MPH, MS, PhD. Part-time programs available. *Degree requirements:* For master's, research project or practicum; for doctorate, thesis/dissertation. *Entrance requirements:* For master's and doctorate, GRE or MCAT, 3 letters of recommendation.

Emory University, Rollins School of Public Health, Department of Health Policy and Management, Atlanta, GA 30322-1100. Offers health policy (MPH); health policy research (MSPH); health services management (MPH); health services research and health policy (PhD). Part-time programs available. *Degree requirements:* For master's, thesis (for some programs), practicum, capstone course. *Entrance requirements:* For master's, GRE General Test. Additional exam requirements/recommendations for international students: Required—TOEFL (minimum score 550 paper-based; 80 iBT). Electronic applications accepted. *Faculty research:* U.S. health policy and financing, healthcare organization and financing.

The George Washington University, School of Medicine and Health Sciences, Health Sciences Programs, Washington, DC 20052. Offers clinical practice management (MSHS); clinical research administration (MSHS); emergency services management (MSHS); end-of-life care (MSHS); immunohematology (MSHS); physical therapy (DPT); physician assistant (MSHS); MSHS/MPH. Postbaccalaureate distance learning degree programs offered (no on-campus study). *Students:* 264 full-time (205 women), 216 part-time (162 women); includes 140 minority (54 Black or African American, non-Hispanic/Latino; 4 American Indian or Alaska Native, non-Hispanic/Latino; 48 Asian, non-Hispanic/Latino; 31 Hispanic/Latino; 3 Native Hawaiian or other Pacific Islander, non-Hispanic/Latino), 12 international. Average age 32. 1,581 applicants, 17% accepted. In 2013, 143 master's, 33 doctorates awarded. *Entrance requirements:* Additional exam requirements/recommendations for international students: Required—TOEFL (minimum score 550 paper-based). *Application deadline:* Applications are processed on a rolling basis. Application fee: $75. *Expenses:* Contact institution. *Unit head:* Jean E. Johnson, Senior Associate Dean, 202-994-3725, E-mail: jejohns@gwu.edu. *Application contact:* Joke Ogundiran, Director of Admission, 202-994-1668, Fax: 202-994-0870, E-mail: jokeogun@gwu.edu.

Johns Hopkins University, Bloomberg School of Public Health, Department of Health Policy and Management, Baltimore, MD 21205-1996. Offers bioethics and policy (PhD); health and public policy (PhD); health care management and leadership (Dr PH); health economics (MHS); health economics and policy (PhD); health finance and management (MHA); health policy (MSPH); health services research and policy (PhD); public policy (MPP). *Accreditation:* CAHME (one or more programs are accredited). Part-time programs available. *Faculty:* 60 full-time (32 women), 178 part-time/adjunct (66 women). *Students:* 204 full-time (152 women), 107 part-time (56 women); includes 81 minority (12 Black or African American, non-Hispanic/Latino; 1 American Indian or Alaska Native, non-Hispanic/Latino; 45 Asian, non-Hispanic/Latino; 14 Hispanic/Latino; 1 Native Hawaiian or other Pacific Islander, non-Hispanic/Latino; 8 Two or more races, non-Hispanic/Latino), 92 international. Average age 31. 550 applicants, 42% accepted, 113 enrolled. In 2013, 55 master's, 34 doctorates awarded. *Degree requirements:* For master's, thesis (for some programs), internship (for some programs); for doctorate, comprehensive exam, thesis/dissertation, 1-year full-time residency (for some programs), oral and written exams. *Entrance requirements:* For master's, GRE General Test or GMAT, 3 letters of recommendation, curriculum vitae/resume; for doctorate, GRE General Test or GMAT, 3 letters of recommendation, curriculum vitae, transcripts. Additional exam requirements/recommendations for international students: Recommended—TOEFL (minimum score 600 paper-based; 100 iBT), IELTS. *Application deadline:* For fall admission, 12/1 for domestic and international students. Applications are processed on a rolling basis. Application fee: $45. Electronic applications accepted. *Financial support:* Fellowships, research assistantships, teaching assistantships, career-related internships or fieldwork, Federal Work-Study, institutionally sponsored loans, scholarships/grants, traineeships, and stipends available. Support available to part-time students. Financial award application deadline: 3/15; financial award applicants required to submit FAFSA. *Faculty research:* Quality of care and health outcomes, health care finance and technology, health disparities and vulnerable populations, injury prevention, health policy and health care policy. *Total annual research expenditures:* $14.2 million. *Unit head:* Dr. Ellen J. MacKenzie, Chairman, 410-955-3625, E-mail: emackenz@jhsph.edu. *Application contact:* Mary Sewell, Coordinator, 410-955-2489, Fax: 410-614-9152, E-mail: msewell@jhsph.edu.
Website: http://www.jhsph.edu/hpm/

Lakehead University, Graduate Studies, Faculty of Social Sciences and Humanities, Department of Sociology, Thunder Bay, ON P7B 5E1, Canada. Offers gerontology (MA); health services and policy research (MA); sociology (MA); women's studies (MA). Part-time and evening/weekend programs available. *Degree requirements:* For master's, research project or thesis. *Entrance requirements:* For master's, minimum B average. Additional exam requirements/recommendations for international students: Required—TOEFL. *Faculty research:* Sociology of medicine, cultural and social change, health human resources, gerontology, women's studies.

McMaster University, Faculty of Health Sciences and School of Graduate Studies, Program in Health Research Methodology (course-based), Hamilton, ON L8S 4M2, Canada. Offers M Sc. Part-time programs available. *Degree requirements:* For master's, research internship, scholarly paper courses. *Entrance requirements:* For master's, 4 year honors degree, minimum B+ average in last year of course work. Additional exam requirements/recommendations for international students: Required—TOEFL (minimum score 580 paper-based).

McMaster University, Faculty of Health Sciences and School of Graduate Studies, Program in Health Research Methodology (thesis), Hamilton, ON L8S 4M2, Canada. Offers M Sc, PhD. Part-time programs available. *Degree requirements:* For master's, thesis; for doctorate, comprehensive exam, thesis/dissertation. *Entrance requirements:* For master's, honors degree, minimum B+ average in last year of undergraduate course work; for doctorate, M Sc, minimum B+ average. Additional exam requirements/recommendations for international students: Required—TOEFL (minimum score 580 paper-based; 92 iBT).

Northwestern University, Fienberg School of Medicine and Interdepartmental Programs, Integrated Graduate Programs in the Life Sciences, Chicago, IL 60611.

Offers biostatistics (PhD); epidemiology (PhD); health and biomedical informatics (PhD); health services and outcomes research (PhD); healthcare quality and patient safety (PhD); translational outcomes in science (PhD). *Degree requirements:* For doctorate, comprehensive exam, thesis/dissertation, written and oral qualifying exams. *Entrance requirements:* For doctorate, GRE General Test. Additional exam requirements/recommendations for international students: Required—TOEFL (minimum score 600 paper-based). Electronic applications accepted.

Old Dominion University, College of Health Sciences, Program in Health Services Research, Norfolk, VA 23529. Offers PhD. Evening/weekend programs available. *Faculty:* 12 full-time (8 women), 10 part-time/adjunct (5 women). *Students:* 15 full-time (12 women), 11 part-time (9 women); includes 7 minority (4 Black or African American, non-Hispanic/Latino; 2 Asian, non-Hispanic/Latino; 1 Hispanic/Latino), 4 international. Average age 36. 16 applicants, 38% accepted, 6 enrolled. In 2013, 3 doctorates awarded. *Degree requirements:* For doctorate, comprehensive exam, thesis/dissertation, oral presentation of dissertation. *Entrance requirements:* For doctorate, GRE, minimum GPA of 3.25, master's degree, degree in health profession or health services, interview. Additional exam requirements/recommendations for international students: Required—TOEFL (minimum score 550 paper-based). *Application deadline:* For fall admission, 7/1 for domestic students, 6/1 for international students. Applications are processed on a rolling basis. Application fee: $50. Electronic applications accepted. *Expenses:* Tuition, state resident: full-time $9888; part-time $412 per credit. Tuition, nonresident: full-time $25,152; part-time $1048 per credit. *Required fees:* $59 per semester. One-time fee: $50. *Financial support:* In 2013–14, 9 students received support, including 5 fellowships with full tuition reimbursements available (averaging $15,000 per year), 5 research assistantships with partial tuition reimbursements available (averaging $10,000 per year); career-related internships or fieldwork, scholarships/grants, and tuition waivers (partial) also available. Financial award application deadline: 7/1; financial award applicants required to submit FAFSA. *Faculty research:* Access to health services, women's health, domestic violence, health policy and planning, economics of obesity, substance abuse, health disparities. *Unit head:* Dr. Deanne Shuman, Graduate Program Director, 757-683-4259, Fax: 757-683-5674, E-mail: dshuman@odu.edu. *Application contact:* William Heffelfinger, Director of Graduate Admissions, 757-683-5554, Fax: 757-683-3255, E-mail: gradadmit@odu.edu.
Website: http://hs.odu.edu/commhealth/academics/phd/

Penn State Hershey Medical Center, College of Medicine, Graduate School Programs in the Biomedical Sciences, Graduate Program in Public Health Sciences, Hershey, PA 17033. Offers MS. Part-time programs available. *Students:* 10 full-time (7 women); includes 1 minority (Asian, non-Hispanic/Latino), 3 international. 26 applicants, 12% accepted, 3 enrolled. In 2013, 9 master's awarded. *Degree requirements:* For master's, thesis or alternative. *Entrance requirements:* Additional exam requirements/recommendations for international students: Required—TOEFL (minimum score 550 paper-based). *Application deadline:* For fall admission, 1/31 priority date for domestic students, 2/1 priority date for international students. Applications are processed on a rolling basis. Application fee: $65. Electronic applications accepted. *Financial support:* Fellowships available. Financial award applicants required to submit FAFSA. *Faculty research:* Clinical trials, statistical methods in genetic epidemiology, genetic factors in nicotine dependence and dementia syndromes, health economics, cancer. *Unit head:* Dr. Douglas Leslie, Chair, 717-531-7178, Fax: 717-531-5779, E-mail: hes-grad-hmc@psu.edu. *Application contact:* Mardi Sawyer, Program Administrator, 717-531-7178, Fax: 717-531-5779, E-mail: hes-grad-hmc@psu.edu.
Website: http://www.pennstatehershey.org/web/phs/programs

Stanford University, School of Medicine, Graduate Programs in Medicine, Department of Health Research and Policy, Stanford, CA 94305-9991. Offers epidemiology (MS); health services research (MS). *Degree requirements:* For master's, thesis. Electronic applications accepted. *Expenses: Tuition:* Full-time $42,690; part-time $949 per credit. *Required fees:* $185. *Faculty research:* Cost and quality of life in cardiovascular disease, technology assessment, physician decision-making.

Texas State University, Graduate School, College of Health Professions, School of Health Administration, Program in Health Services Research, San Marcos, TX 78666. Offers MS. Part-time and evening/weekend programs available. *Faculty:* 10 full-time (6 women), 1 (woman) part-time/adjunct. *Students:* 4 full-time (3 women), 2 part-time (both women); includes 4 minority (1 Asian, non-Hispanic/Latino; 2 Hispanic/Latino; 1 Two or more races, non-Hispanic/Latino), 1 international. Average age 31. 10 applicants, 50% accepted, 2 enrolled. In 2013, 4 master's awarded. *Degree requirements:* For master's, comprehensive exam, thesis optional, committee review. *Entrance requirements:* For master's, GRE General Test, 3 letters of reference, resume, department interview. Additional exam requirements/recommendations for international students: Required—TOEFL (minimum score 550 paper-based; 78 iBT). *Application deadline:* For fall admission, 6/15 priority date for domestic students, 6/1 for international students; for spring admission, 10/15 priority date for domestic students, 10/1 for international students. Applications are processed on a rolling basis. Application fee: $40 ($90 for international students). Electronic applications accepted. *Expenses:* Tuition, state resident: full-time $6663; part-time $278 per credit hour. Tuition, nonresident: full-time $15,159; part-time $632 per credit hour. *Required fees:* $1872; $54 per credit hour. $306 per term. Tuition and fees vary according to course load. *Financial support:* In 2013–14, 2 students received support, including 2 teaching assistantships (averaging $11,640 per year); research assistantships, career-related internships or fieldwork, Federal Work-Study, and institutionally sponsored loans also available. Support available to part-time students. Financial award application deadline: 4/1; financial award applicants required to submit FAFSA. *Unit head:* Dr. Matthew Brooks, Graduate Program Director, 512-245-3556, E-mail: mb96@txstate.edu. *Application contact:* Dr. Andrea Golato, Dean of Graduate School, 512-245-2581, Fax: 512-245-8365, E-mail: gradcollege@txstate.edu.
Website: http://www.health.txstate.edu/hsr

Thomas Jefferson University, Jefferson Graduate School of Biomedical Sciences, Certificate Programs in Clinical Research, Human Clinical Investigation, and Infectious Diseases, Philadelphia, PA 19107. Offers clinical research and trials (Certificate); human clinical investigation (Certificate); infectious disease control (Certificate). *Faculty:* 44 full-time (14 women), 27 part-time/adjunct (11 women). *Students:* 15 part-time (9 women); includes 3 minority (1 Black or African American, non-Hispanic/Latino; 1 Asian, non-Hispanic/Latino; 1 Hispanic/Latino), 1 international. 8 applicants, 100% accepted, 6 enrolled. In 2013, 3 Certificates awarded. *Entrance requirements:* For degree, GRE General Test (recommended). Additional exam requirements/recommendations for international students: Required—TOEFL (minimum score 100 iBT) or IELTS (minimum score 7). *Application deadline:* For fall admission, 8/1 priority date for domestic students, 3/1 priority date for international students; for winter admission, 12/1 priority date for domestic students, 6/1 priority date for international students; for spring admission, 4/1 priority date for domestic students. Applications are processed on a rolling basis. Application fee: $75. Electronic applications accepted. *Financial support:* Federal Work-Study and institutionally sponsored loans available. Support available to part-time students. Financial award application deadline: 5/1; financial award applicants required to submit FAFSA. *Faculty research:* Epidemiology, clinical research, statistics, planning and management, disease control. *Unit head:* Dr. Dennis M. Gross, Associate Dean, 215-503-0156, Fax: 215-503-3433, E-mail: dennis.gross@jefferson.edu. *Application contact:* Marc E. Stearns, Director of Admissions, 215-503-0155, Fax: 215-503-3433, E-mail: jgsbs-info@jefferson.edu.
Website: http://www.jefferson.edu/university/biomedical_sciences/programs/certificates.html

Thomas Jefferson University, Jefferson School of Population Health, Philadelphia, PA 19107. Offers applied health economics and outcomes research (MS, PhD, Certificate); behavioral health science (PhD); health policy (MS, Certificate); healthcare quality and safety (MS, PhD); healthcare quality and safety management (MS); population health (Certificate); public health (MPH, Certificate). Part-time and evening/weekend programs available. Postbaccalaureate distance learning degree programs offered (no on-campus study). Terminal master's awarded for partial completion of doctoral program. *Degree requirements:* For master's, thesis; for doctorate, comprehensive exam, thesis/dissertation. *Entrance requirements:* For master's, GRE or other graduate entrance exam (MCAT, LSAT, DAT, etc.), two letters of recommendation, curriculum vitae, transcripts from all undergraduate and graduate institutions; for doctorate, GRE (taken within the last 5 years), three letters of recommendation, curriculum vitae, transcripts from all undergraduate and graduate institutions. Additional exam requirements/recommendations for international students: Required—TOEFL. Electronic applications accepted. *Faculty research:* Applied health economics and outcomes research, behavioral and health sciences, chronic disease management, health policy, healthcare quality and patient safety, wellness and prevention.

The University of Alabama at Birmingham, School of Public Health, Program in Public Health, Birmingham, AL 35294. Offers accelerated industrial hygiene (MPH); applied epidemiology (MSPH); biostatistics (MPH); clinical and translational science (MSPH); environmental health (MPH); environmental health and toxicology (MSPH); epidemiology (MPH); general theory and practice (MPH); health behavior (MPH); health care organization (MPH); health policy quantitative policy analysis (MPH); industrial hygiene (MPH, MSPH); maternal and child health policy (Dr PH); maternal and child health policy and leadership (MPH); occupational health and safety (MPH); outcomes research (MSPH, Dr PH); pharmacoepidemiology and comparative effectiveness research (MSPH); public health (PhD); public health management (Dr PH); public health preparedness management (MPH). *Accreditation:* CEPH. *Entrance requirements:* For master's and doctorate, GRE, evaluations. Additional exam requirements/recommendations for international students: Recommended—TOEFL (minimum score 550 paper-based; 79 iBT), IELTS (minimum score 6.5).

University of Alberta, School of Public Health, Department of Public Health Sciences, Edmonton, AB T6G 2E1, Canada. Offers clinical epidemiology (M Sc, MPH); environmental and occupational health (MPH); environmental health sciences (M Sc); epidemiology (M Sc); global health (M Sc, MPH); health policy and management (MPH); health policy research (M Sc); health technology assessment (MPH); occupational health (M Sc); population health (M Sc); public health leadership (MPH); public health sciences (PhD); quantitative methods (MPH). *Accreditation:* CEPH (one or more programs are accredited). Terminal master's awarded for partial completion of doctoral program. *Degree requirements:* For master's, thesis (for some programs); for doctorate, thesis/dissertation. *Entrance requirements:* For master's, GMAT or GRE General Test. Additional exam requirements/recommendations for international students: Required—TOEFL (minimum score 550 paper-based) or IELTS (minimum score 6). Electronic applications accepted. *Faculty research:* Biostatistics, health promotion and socio-behavioral health science.

University of Arkansas for Medical Sciences, College of Public Health, Little Rock, AR 72205-7199. Offers biostatistics (MPH); environmental and occupational health (MPH, Certificate); epidemiology (MPH, PhD); health behavior and health education (MPH); health policy and management (MPH); health promotion and prevention research (PhD); health services administration (MHSA); health systems research (PhD); public health (Certificate); public health leadership (Dr PH). Part-time programs available. *Faculty:* 37 full-time (19 women), 9 part-time/adjunct (5 women). *Students:* 56 full-time (35 women), 85 part-time (58 women); includes 54 minority (38 Black or African American, non-Hispanic/Latino; 1 American Indian or Alaska Native, non-Hispanic/Latino; 8 Asian, non-Hispanic/Latino; 3 Hispanic/Latino; 1 Native Hawaiian or other Pacific Islander, non-Hispanic/Latino; 3 Two or more races, non-Hispanic/Latino), 5 international. Average age 30. 70 applicants, 91% accepted, 33 enrolled. In 2013, 2 master's, 1 doctorate, 2 other advanced degrees awarded. *Degree requirements:* For master's, preceptorship, culminating experience, internship; for doctorate, comprehensive exam, capstone. *Entrance requirements:* For master's, GRE, GMAT, LSAT, PCAT, MCAT, DAT; for doctorate, GRE. Additional exam requirements/recommendations for international students: Required—TOEFL (minimum score 80 iBT), IELTS. *Application deadline:* For fall admission, 3/1 for domestic students, 2/1 for international students; for spring admission, 8/1 for domestic and international students; for summer admission, 2/1 for domestic and international students. Application fee: $25 ($50 for international students). Electronic applications accepted. *Expenses:* Contact institution. *Financial support:* In 2013–14, 8 research assistantships with full tuition reimbursements (averaging $13,000 per year) were awarded; scholarships/grants and tuition waivers (full and partial) also available. *Faculty research:* Health systems, tobacco prevention control, obesity prevention, environmental and occupational exposure, cancer prevention. *Unit head:* Dr. James M. Raczynski, Dean, 501-526-6600, E-mail: raczynskijameson@uams.edu. *Application contact:* Angie Choi, Director of Admission, 501-526-4620, Fax: 501-526-6750, E-mail: anchoi@uams.edu.
Website: http://publichealth.uams.edu/

University of Colorado Denver, Colorado School of Public Health, Health Services Research Program, Aurora, CO 80045. Offers PhD. Part-time programs available. *Faculty:* 8 full-time (4 women), 3 part-time/adjunct (2 women). *Students:* 9 full-time (8 women), 8 part-time (6 women); includes 4 minority (1 Black or African American, non-Hispanic/Latino; 2 Asian, non-Hispanic/Latino; 1 Hispanic/Latino), 1 international. Average age 40. 12 applicants, 33% accepted, 4 enrolled. In 2013, 1 doctorate awarded. *Degree requirements:* For doctorate, comprehensive exam, thesis/dissertation, minimum of 65 credit hours including 30 credit hours for thesis research. *Entrance requirements:* For doctorate, GRE, MCAT, or MA, MS or PhD from an accredited school, minimum undergraduate GPA of 3.0. Additional exam requirements/recommendations for international students: Required—TOEFL (minimum score 550 paper-based; 80 iBT). *Application deadline:* For fall admission, 2/1 for domestic students, 1/15 for international students. Application fee: $65. Electronic applications accepted. *Expenses:* Contact institution. *Financial support:* In 2013–14, 4 students received support. Fellowships, research assistantships, teaching assistantships, Federal Work-Study, institutionally sponsored loans, scholarships/grants, traineeships, and unspecified assistantships available. Financial award application deadline: 3/1; financial award applicants required to submit FAFSA. *Faculty research:* Drug safety and risk management, health care financing and cost, health interaction with environmental factors, quality improvement and strategic research, cardiovascular health promotion. *Unit head:* Dr. Adam Atherly, Chair, 303-724-4471, E-mail: adam.atherly@ucdenver.edu. *Application contact:* Mary Baitinger, Departmental Assistant, 303-724-6698, E-mail: mary.baitinger@ucdenver.edu.
Website: http://www.ucdenver.edu/academics/colleges/PublicHealth/departments/HealthSystems/Pages/welcome.aspx

University of Colorado Denver, School of Medicine, Clinical Science Graduate Program, Aurora, CO 80045. Offers clinical investigation (PhD); clinical sciences (MS); health information technology (PhD); health services research (PhD). *Students:* 25 full-time (17 women), 29 part-time (15 women); includes 10 minority (2 Black or African American, non-Hispanic/Latino; 2 Asian, non-Hispanic/Latino; 2 Hispanic/Latino; 1 Native Hawaiian or other Pacific Islander, non-Hispanic/Latino; 3 Two or more races, non-Hispanic/Latino), 1 international. Average age 34. 16 applicants, 81% accepted, 13 enrolled. In 2013, 11 master's, 7 doctorates awarded. *Degree requirements:* For master's, thesis, minimum of 30 credit hours, defense/final exam of thesis or publishable paper; for doctorate, comprehensive exam, thesis/dissertation, at least 30 credit hours of thesis work. *Entrance requirements:* For master's, GRE General Test or MCAT (waived if candidate has earned MS/MA or PhD from accredited U.S. school), minimum undergraduate GPA of 3.0, 3-4 letters of recommendation; for doctorate, GRE General Test or MCAT (waived if candidate has earned MS/MA or PhD from accredited U.S. school), health care graduate, professional degree, or graduate degree related to health sciences; minimum GPA of 3.0, 3-4 letters of recommendation. Additional exam requirements/recommendations for international students: Required—TOEFL (minimum score 550 paper-based; 80 iBT). *Application deadline:* For fall admission, 2/1 for domestic students, 1/15 priority date for international students; for spring admission, 10/1 for domestic students. Application fee: $50 ($75 for international students). Electronic applications accepted. *Expenses:* Contact institution. *Financial support:* In 2013–14, 18 students received support. Fellowships, research assistantships, teaching assistantships, Federal Work-Study, institutionally sponsored loans, scholarships/grants, traineeships, and unspecified assistantships available. Financial award application deadline: 3/15; financial award applicants required to submit FAFSA. *Unit head:* Dr. Ronald Sokol, Program Director, 720-777-6669, E-mail: ronald.sokol@childrenscolorado.org. *Application contact:* Galit Mankin, Program Administrator, 720-848-6249, Fax: 303-848-7381, E-mail: galit.mankin@ucdenver.edu.
Website: http://cctsi.ucdenver.edu/training-and-education/CLSC/Pages/default.aspx

University of Florida, Graduate School, College of Public Health and Health Professions, Department of Health Services Research, Management and Policy, Gainesville, FL 32610. Offers health administration (MHA); health services research (PhD). *Accreditation:* CAHME. Part-time programs available. *Faculty:* 5 full-time (2 women), 3 part-time/adjunct (0 women). *Students:* 52 full-time (28 women), 5 part-time (1 woman); includes 15 minority (2 Black or African American, non-Hispanic/Latino; 5 Asian, non-Hispanic/Latino; 8 Hispanic/Latino), 5 international. Average age 29. 108 applicants, 29% accepted, 20 enrolled. In 2013, 22 master's, 6 doctorates awarded. *Degree requirements:* For master's, internship. *Entrance requirements:* For master's and doctorate, GRE General Test, minimum GPA of 3.0. Additional exam requirements/recommendations for international students: Required—TOEFL (minimum score 550 paper-based; 80 iBT), IELTS (minimum score 6). *Application deadline:* For fall admission, 2/1 for domestic students. Applications are processed on a rolling basis. Application fee: $30. Electronic applications accepted. *Expenses:* Tuition, state resident: full-time $12,640. Tuition, nonresident: full-time $30,000. *Financial support:* In 2013–14, 11 students received support, including 7 research assistantships (averaging $16,210 per year), 5 teaching assistantships (averaging $10,045 per year); career-related internships or fieldwork and unspecified assistantships also available. Financial award applicants required to submit FAFSA. *Faculty research:* Hospital profitability, indigent care, rural health care systems, AIDS education, managed care, outcomes. *Unit head:* Dr. Arch G. Mainous, III, Department Chair/Professor, 352-273-6073, Fax: 352-273-6075, E-mail: arch.mainous@phhp.ufl.edu. *Application contact:* Barbara Ross, Student Services Coordinator, 352-273-6074, Fax: 352-273-6075, E-mail: bross@phhp.ufl.edu.
Website: http://www.phhp.ufl.edu/hsrmp/

University of Illinois at Chicago, Graduate College, School of Public Health, Division of Health Policy and Administration, Chicago, IL 60607-7128. Offers clinical translational science (MS); health policy (PhD); health policy and administration (Dr PH); health services research (PhD); healthcare (MHA); public health policy management (MPH). Part-time programs available. *Faculty:* 16 full-time (8 women), 17 part-time/adjunct (4 women). *Students:* 114 full-time (77 women), 105 part-time (66 women); includes 106 minority (38 Black or African American, non-Hispanic/Latino; 36 Asian, non-Hispanic/Latino; 23 Hispanic/Latino; 1 Native Hawaiian or other Pacific Islander, non-Hispanic/Latino; 8 Two or more races, non-Hispanic/Latino), 18 international. Average age 31. 480 applicants, 56% accepted, 94 enrolled. In 2013, 97 master's, 3 doctorates awarded. Terminal master's awarded for partial completion of doctoral program. *Degree requirements:* For master's, thesis, field practicum; for doctorate, thesis/dissertation, independent research, internship. *Entrance requirements:* For master's and doctorate, GRE General Test, minimum GPA of 2.75. Additional exam requirements/recommendations for international students: Required—TOEFL. *Application deadline:* For fall admission, 2/1 for domestic students, 1/1 priority date for international students. Application fee: $40 ($50 for international students). Electronic applications accepted. *Expenses:* Tuition, state resident: full-time $11,066; part-time $3689 per term. Tuition, nonresident: full-time $23,064; part-time $7688 per term. *Required fees:* $3004; $1190 per term. Tuition and fees vary according to course level and program. *Financial support:* In 2013–14, 4 fellowships with full tuition reimbursements were awarded; research assistantships with full tuition reimbursements, teaching assistantships with full tuition reimbursements, career-related internships or fieldwork, Federal Work-Study, institutionally sponsored loans, scholarships/grants, traineeships, and unspecified assistantships also available. Support available to part-time students. Financial award application deadline: 3/1; financial award applicants required to submit FAFSA. *Faculty research:* Cancer screening in underserved populations, practices and devices used to reduce firefighter injury, the relationship between communal housing and substance abuse recovery. *Total annual research expenditures:* $1.7 million. *Unit head:* Prof. Jack Zwanziger, Director, 312-996-1062, Fax: 312-996-5356, E-mail: jzwanzig@uic.edu. *Application contact:* Aimee Wiebel, Academic Coordinator, 312-996-7816, Fax: 312-996-5356, E-mail: aimee@uic.edu.
Website: http://publichealth.uic.edu/departments/healthpolicyandadministration/

University of La Verne, College of Business and Public Management, Program in Health Administration, La Verne, CA 91750-4443. Offers financial management (MHA); health information systems (MHA); human resource management (MHA); managed care (MHA); management and leadership (MHA); marketing and business development (MHA). Part-time programs available. *Faculty:* 3 full-time (1 woman), 5 part-time/adjunct (1 woman). *Students:* 43 full-time (31 women), 35 part-time (20 women); includes 29 minority (9 Black or African American, non-Hispanic/Latino; 9 Asian, non-Hispanic/Latino; 11 Hispanic/Latino), 13 international. Average age 31. In 2013, 31 master's awarded. *Entrance requirements:* For master's, minimum undergraduate GPA of 2.5, 3 letters of reference, curriculum vitae or resume, writing sample. Additional exam requirements/recommendations for international students: Required—TOEFL (minimum score 550 paper-based). *Application deadline:* Applications are processed on a rolling basis. Application fee: $50. *Expenses:* Contact institution. *Financial support:* Application deadline: 3/2; applicants required to submit FAFSA. *Unit head:* Dr. Kathy Duncan, Program Chairperson, 909-593-3511 Ext. 4415, E-mail: kduncan2@laverne.edu. *Application contact:* Barbara Cox, Program and Admissions Specialist, 909-593-3511 Ext. 4004, Fax: 909-392-2761, E-mail: bcox@laverne.edu.
Website: http://www.laverne.edu/business-and-public-administration/healthadmin-gerontology/

University of Maryland, Baltimore, Graduate School, Graduate Programs in Pharmacy, Department of Pharmaceutical Health Service Research, Baltimore, MD 21201. Offers epidemiology (MS); pharmacy administration (PhD); Pharm D/PhD. *Degree requirements:* For doctorate, comprehensive exam, thesis/dissertation. *Entrance requirements:* For doctorate, GRE General Test. Additional exam requirements/recommendations for international students: Required—TOEFL, IELTS. Electronic applications accepted. *Faculty research:* Pharmacoeconomics, outcomes research, public health policy, drug therapy and aging.

University of Massachusetts Worcester, Graduate School of Biomedical Sciences, Worcester, MA 01655-0115. Offers biochemistry and molecular pharmacology (PhD); bioinformatics and computational biology (PhD); cancer biology (PhD); cell biology (PhD); clinical and population health research (PhD); clinical investigation (MS); immunology and virology (PhD); interdisciplinary biomedical research (PhD); millennium (PhD); molecular genetics and microbiology (PhD); neuroscience (PhD); translational science (PhD); MD/PhD. *Faculty:* 1,388 full-time (521 women), 309 part-time/adjunct (198 women). *Students:* 385 full-time (210 women); includes 53 minority (13 Black or African American, non-Hispanic/Latino; 30 Asian, non-Hispanic/Latino; 10 Hispanic/Latino), 138 international. Average age 28. 491 applicants, 19% accepted, 39 enrolled. In 2013, 5 master's, 50 doctorates awarded. Terminal master's awarded for partial completion of doctoral program. *Median time to degree:* Of those who began their doctoral program in fall 2005, 67% received their degree in 8 years or less. *Degree requirements:* For master's, comprehensive exam, thesis; for doctorate, comprehensive exam, thesis/dissertation. *Entrance requirements:* For master's, MD, PhD, DVM, or PharmD; for doctorate, GRE General Test, bachelor's degree. Additional exam requirements/recommendations for international students: Required—TOEFL (minimum score 100 iBT) or IELTS (minimum score 7.5). *Application deadline:* For fall admission, 12/15 for domestic and international students; for spring admission, 5/15 for domestic students. Application fee: $80. Electronic applications accepted. *Expenses:* Contact institution. *Financial support:* In 2013–14, 431 students received support, including research assistantships with full tuition reimbursements available (averaging $29,500 per year); scholarships/grants, health care benefits, tuition waivers (full), and unspecified assistantships also available. Financial award application deadline: 5/16. *Faculty research:* RNA interference, cell/molecular/developmental biology, bioinformatics, clinical/translational research, infectious disease. *Total annual research expenditures:* $245.9 million. *Unit head:* Dr. Anthony Carruthers, Dean, 508-856-4135, E-mail: anthony.carruthers@umassmed.edu. *Application contact:* Dr. Kendall Knight, Associate Dean and Interim Director of Admissions and Recruitment, 508-856-5628, Fax: 508-856-3659, E-mail: kendall.knight@umassmed.edu.
Website: http://www.umassmed.edu/gsbs/

University of Minnesota, Twin Cities Campus, School of Public Health, Major in Health Services Research, Policy, and Administration, Minneapolis, MN 55455-0213. Offers MS, PhD, JD/MS, JD/PhD, MD/PhD, MPP/MS. Part-time programs available. Terminal master's awarded for partial completion of doctoral program. *Degree requirements:* For master's, thesis, internship, final oral exam; for doctorate, thesis/dissertation, teaching experience, written preliminary exam, final oral exam, dissertation. *Entrance requirements:* For master's, GRE General Test, course work in mathematics; for doctorate, GRE General Test, prerequisite courses in calculus and statistics. Additional exam requirements/recommendations for international students: Required—TOEFL (minimum score 600 paper-based; 100 iBT). *Faculty research:* Outcomes, economics and statistics, sociology, health care management.

University of New Brunswick Fredericton, School of Graduate Studies, Applied Health Services Research Program, Fredericton, NB E3B 5A3, Canada. Offers MAHSR. Part-time programs available. Postbaccalaureate distance learning degree programs offered. *Students:* 5 full-time (all women), 6 part-time (5 women). In 2013, 1 master's awarded. *Degree requirements:* For master's, thesis. *Entrance requirements:* For master's, honours BA, minimum GPA of 3.0. Additional exam requirements/recommendations for international students: Required—TWE (minimum score 4), TOEFL (minimum score 600 paper-based; 100 iBT) or IELTS (minimum score 7). *Application deadline:* For winter admission, 3/31 for domestic and international students. Applications are processed on a rolling basis. Application fee: $50 Canadian dollars. Electronic applications accepted. *Faculty research:* Applied health services research. *Unit head:* Dr. Linda Eyre, Associate Dean of Graduate Studies, 506-447-3044, Fax: 506-453-4817, E-mail: gradidst@unb.ca. *Application contact:* Janet Amirault, Graduate Secretary, 506-458-7558, Fax: 506-453-4817, E-mail: jamiraul@unb.ca.
Website: http://www.artc-hsr.ca

The University of North Carolina at Charlotte, The Graduate School, College of Health and Human Services, Program in Health Services Research, Charlotte, NC 28223-0001. Offers PhD. Part-time programs available. *Students:* 13 full-time (9 women), 12 part-time (7 women); includes 4 minority (all Black or African American, non-Hispanic/Latino), 5 international. Average age 39. 11 applicants, 45% accepted, 4 enrolled. In 2013, 2 doctorates awarded. *Degree requirements:* For doctorate, thesis/dissertation. *Entrance requirements:* For doctorate, GRE, letters of recommendation. Additional exam requirements/recommendations for international students: Required—TOEFL (minimum score 557 paper-based; 83 iBT). *Application deadline:* For fall admission, 2/1 priority date for domestic students, 5/1 priority date for international students; for spring admission, 11/1 for domestic students, 10/1 for international students. Applications are processed on a rolling basis. Application fee: $75. Electronic applications accepted. *Expenses:* Tuition, state resident: full-time $3522. Tuition, nonresident: full-time $16,051. *Required fees:* $2585. Tuition and fees vary according to course load and program. *Financial support:* Research assistantships, teaching assistantships, career-related internships or fieldwork, scholarships/grants, and unspecified assistantships available. Support available to part-time students. Financial award applicants required to submit FAFSA. *Faculty research:* Epidemiology of asthma, mental health services research, healthcare disparities, building research capacity within organizations, health policy and administration, reproductive epidemiology, data warehousing/mining of large scale databases for decision support, program evaluation, health care ethics, informatics and technology, health economics. *Unit head:* Dr. Nancy Fey-Yensan, Dean, 704-687-7917, Fax: 704-687-3180, E-mail: nfeyyens@uncc.edu. *Application contact:* Kathy B. Giddings, Director of Graduate Admissions, 704-687-5503, Fax: 704-687-1668, E-mail: gradadm@uncc.edu.
Website: http://health.uncc.edu/degrees-and-programs/hsr-phd

University of Ottawa, Faculty of Graduate and Postdoctoral Studies, Interdisciplinary Programs, Ottawa, ON K1N 6N5, Canada. Offers e-business (Certificate); e-commerce (Certificate); finance (Certificate); health services and policies research (Diploma); population health (PhD); population health risk assessment and management (Certificate); public management and governance (Certificate); systems science (Certificate).

University of Pennsylvania, Perelman School of Medicine, Program in Health Policy Research, Philadelphia, PA 19104. Offers MS, MD/MS. Part-time programs available.

Faculty: 22 full-time (10 women). *Students:* 46 full-time (32 women); includes 17 minority (7 Black or African American, non-Hispanic/Latino; 10 Asian, non-Hispanic/Latino). Average age 33. 94 applicants, 24% accepted, 21 enrolled. In 2013, 18 master's awarded. *Degree requirements:* For master's, thesis. *Entrance requirements:* Additional exam requirements/recommendations for international students: Recommended—TOEFL. *Application deadline:* For fall admission, 11/30 for domestic and international students. Applications are processed on a rolling basis. Electronic applications accepted. *Financial support:* In 2013–14, 18 fellowships with partial tuition reimbursements were awarded. *Faculty research:* Disparities in health care; cost effectiveness analysis; outcomes research; biological, clinical, behavioral and environmental factors in health care; diffusion of health care innovation; medical ethics; innovation; lay support with peer mentors and community health workers; evaluating medical homes; quality improvement research, health literacy, health numeracy, and medical decision-making. *Unit head:* Dr. Judith A. Long, Director, 215-898-4311. *Application contact:* Elliot M. Adler, Admissions Coordinator, 215-573-2740, Fax: 215-573-2742, E-mail: elliota@mail.med.upenn.edu.
Website: http://www.med.upenn.edu/mshp/

University of Puerto Rico, Medical Sciences Campus, Graduate School of Public Health, Department of Health Services Administration, Program in Evaluative Research of Health Systems, San Juan, PR 00936-5067. Offers MS. Part-time programs available. *Degree requirements:* For master's, thesis. *Entrance requirements:* For master's, GRE, previous course work in algebra and statistics. *Expenses:* Contact institution.

University of Regina, Faculty of Graduate Studies and Research, Johnson-Shoyama Graduate School of Public Policy, Regina, SK S4S 0A2, Canada. Offers economic analysis for public policy (Master's Certificate); health administration (MHA); health systems management (Master's Certificate); health systems research (MPP); public management (MPA, Master's Certificate); public policy (MPA, MPP, PhD); public policy analysis (Master's Certificate). Part-time programs available. *Faculty:* 8 full-time (4 women), 16 part-time/adjunct (5 women). *Students:* 51 full-time (32 women), 75 part-time (44 women). 175 applicants, 61% accepted. In 2013, 41 master's, 10 other advanced degrees awarded. *Degree requirements:* For master's, thesis (for some programs); for doctorate, thesis/dissertation. *Entrance requirements:* For doctorate, master's degree, intended research program in an area of public policy. Additional exam requirements/recommendations for international students: Required—TOEFL (minimum score 580 paper-based; 80 iBT), IELTS (minimum score 6.5). *Application deadline:* For fall admission, 2/1 for domestic and international students. Application fee: $100. Electronic applications accepted. *Expenses:* Contact institution. *Financial support:* In 2013–14, 15 fellowships (averaging $6,133 per year), 1 research assistantship (averaging $5,500 per year), 14 teaching assistantships (averaging $2,356 per year) were awarded; scholarships/grants also available. Financial award application deadline: 6/15. *Faculty research:* Governance and administration, public finance, public policy analysis, non-governmental organizations and alternative service delivery, micro-economics for policy analysis. *Unit head:* Dr. Michael Atkinson, Executive Director, 306-996-1984, Fax: 306-585-5461, E-mail: michael.atkinson@usask.ca. *Application contact:* Sarina Wowchuk, Program Advisor and Administrative Manager, 306-585-5462, Fax: 306-585-5461, E-mail: sarina.wowchuk@uregina.ca.
Website: http://www.schoolofpublicpolicy.sk.ca/

University of Rochester, School of Medicine and Dentistry, Graduate Programs in Medicine and Dentistry, Department of Community and Preventive Medicine, Program in Health Services Research and Policy, Rochester, NY 14627. Offers PhD, MPH/PhD. *Degree requirements:* For doctorate, thesis/dissertation, qualifying exam. *Entrance requirements:* For doctorate, GRE General Test. *Expenses: Tuition:* Full-time $44,580; part-time $1394 per credit hour. *Required fees:* $492.

University of Rochester, School of Nursing, Rochester, NY 14642. Offers acute care nurse practitioner (MS); adult nurse practitioner (MS); adult/geriatric nurse practitioner (MS); clinical nurse leader (MS); clinical research coordinator (MS); family nurse practitioner (MS); family psychiatric mental health nurse practitioner (MS); health care organization management and leadership (MS); health practice research (PhD); nursing (DNP); pediatric nurse practitioner (MS); pediatric nurse practitioner/neonatal nurse practitioner (MS). *Accreditation:* AACN. Part-time programs available. Postbaccalaureate distance learning degree programs offered (minimal on-campus study). *Faculty:* 60 full-time (52 women), 61 part-time/adjunct (47 women). *Students:* 33 full-time (29 women), 213 part-time (195 women); includes 32 minority (8 Black or African American, non-Hispanic/Latino; 10 Asian, non-Hispanic/Latino; 8 Hispanic/Latino; 6 Two or more races, non-Hispanic/Latino), 4 international. Average age 34. 41 applicants, 54% accepted, 16 enrolled. In 2013, 58 master's, 11 doctorates awarded. Terminal master's awarded for partial completion of doctoral program. *Degree requirements:* For master's, comprehensive exam (for some programs); for doctorate, thesis/dissertation. *Entrance requirements:* For master's, BS in nursing, minimum GPA of 3.0, course work in statistics; for doctorate, GRE General Test, MS in nursing, minimum GPA of 3.5. Additional exam requirements/recommendations for international students: Required—TOEFL (minimum score 560 paper-based; 88 iBT) or IELTS (minimum score 6.5) recommended. *Application deadline:* For fall admission, 4/1 for domestic and international students; for spring admission, 9/1 for domestic and international students; for summer admission, 1/2 for domestic and international students. Application fee: $50. Electronic applications accepted. *Expenses: Tuition:* Full-time $44,580; part-time $1394 per credit hour. *Required fees:* $492. *Financial support:* In 2013–14, 41 students received support, including 2 fellowships with full and partial tuition reimbursements available (averaging $30,200 per year); scholarships/grants, traineeships, health care benefits, tuition waivers (partial), and unspecified assistantships also available. Support available to part-time students. Financial award application deadline: 6/30. *Faculty research:* Symptom assessment and self-management, illness prevention, nursing intervention research with vulnerable populations, palliative care, aging. *Total annual research expenditures:* $3.5 million. *Unit head:* Dr. Kathy H. Rideout, Dean, 585-273-8902, Fax: 585-273-1268, E-mail: kathy_rideout@urmc.rochester.edu. *Application contact:* Elaine Andolina, Director of Admissions, 585-275-2375, Fax: 585-756-8299, E-mail: elaine_andolina@urmc.rochester.edu.
Website: http://www.son.rochester.edu

University of Southern California, Keck School of Medicine and Graduate School, Graduate Programs in Medicine, Department of Preventive Medicine, Program in Health Behavior Research, Los Angeles, CA 90032. Offers PhD. *Faculty:* 19 full-time (12 women). *Students:* 27 full-time (14 women); includes 11 minority (2 Black or African American, non-Hispanic/Latino; 7 Asian, non-Hispanic/Latino; 2 Hispanic/Latino), 3 international. Average age 32. 43 applicants, 26% accepted, 7 enrolled. In 2013, 6 doctorates awarded. *Degree requirements:* For doctorate, comprehensive exam, thesis/dissertation. *Entrance requirements:* For doctorate, GRE General Test, minimum GPA of 3.0 (3.5 preferred). Additional exam requirements/recommendations for international students: Required—TOEFL (minimum score 600 paper-based; 100 iBT). *Application deadline:* For fall admission, 12/1 priority date for domestic and international students. Application fee: $85. Electronic applications accepted. *Financial support:* In 2013–14, 27 students received support, including 10 fellowships with full tuition reimbursements available (averaging $33,395 per year), 7 research assistantships with full and partial tuition reimbursements available (averaging $33,395 per year), 8 teaching assistantships with full and partial tuition reimbursements available (averaging $33,395 per year); institutionally sponsored loans, scholarships/grants, traineeships, health care benefits, and unspecified assistantships also available. Financial award application deadline: 5/4; financial award applicants required to submit CSS PROFILE or FAFSA. *Faculty research:* Obesity prevention; etiology and prevention of substance abuse, other addictive behaviors, and chronic diseases; health disparities; translational research. *Unit head:* Dr. Jennifer Unger, Director, 323-442-8234, E-mail: unger@usc.edu. *Application contact:* Marny Barovich, Program Manager, 323-442-8299, E-mail: barovich@hsc.usc.edu.
Website: http://phdhbr.usc.edu

The University of Tennessee Health Science Center, College of Graduate Health Sciences, Memphis, TN 38163-0002. Offers biomedical engineering (MS, PhD); biomedical sciences (PhD); dental sciences (MDS); epidemiology (MS); health outcomes and policy research (PhD); laboratory research and management (MS); nursing science (PhD); pharmaceutical sciences (PhD); pharmacology (MS); speech and hearing science (PhD); DDS/PhD; DNP/PhD; MD/PhD; Pharm D/PhD. *Faculty:* 318 full-time (92 women), 59 part-time/adjunct (16 women). *Students:* 220 full-time (102 women), 22 part-time (13 women); includes 194 minority (22 Black or African American, non-Hispanic/Latino; 161 Asian, non-Hispanic/Latino; 7 Hispanic/Latino; 3 Native Hawaiian or other Pacific Islander, non-Hispanic/Latino; 1 Two or more races, non-Hispanic/Latino), 106 international. Average age 25. 404 applicants, 17% accepted, 64 enrolled. In 2013, 13 master's, 25 doctorates awarded. Terminal master's awarded for partial completion of doctoral program. *Degree requirements:* For master's, comprehensive exam, thesis; for doctorate, comprehensive exam, thesis/dissertation, oral and written preliminary and comprehensive exams. *Entrance requirements:* For master's and doctorate, GRE General Test, minimum GPA of 3.0. Additional exam requirements/recommendations for international students: Required—TOEFL (minimum score 79 iBT); Recommended—IELTS (minimum score 6.5). *Application deadline:* For fall admission, 5/15 priority date for domestic students. Applications are processed on a rolling basis. Application fee: $0. Electronic applications accepted. *Financial support:* In 2013–14, 125 students received support, including 125 research assistantships (averaging $23,000 per year); career-related internships or fieldwork, Federal Work-Study, institutionally sponsored loans, and tuition waivers (full and partial) also available. Support available to part-time students. Financial award application deadline: 2/25; financial award applicants required to submit FAFSA. *Unit head:* Dr. Donald B. Thomason, Dean, 901-448-5538, E-mail: dthomaso@uthsc.edu. *Application contact:* William Carter, Director for Admissions, 901-448-1687, E-mail: wcarte17@uthsc.edu.
Website: http://www.uthsc.edu/grad/

University of Utah, Graduate School, College of Pharmacy, Department of Pharmacotherapy, Salt Lake City, UT 84112. Offers health system pharmacy administration (MS); outcomes research and health policy (PhD). *Faculty:* 5 full-time (3 women), 28 part-time/adjunct (17 women). *Students:* 7 full-time (4 women), 5 international. Average age 27. 26 applicants, 19% accepted, 2 enrolled. In 2013, 4 master's awarded. Terminal master's awarded for partial completion of doctoral program. *Degree requirements:* For master's, comprehensive exam, thesis or alternative, project; for doctorate, comprehensive exam, thesis/dissertation. *Entrance requirements:* For doctorate, GRE. Additional exam requirements/recommendations for international students: Required—TOEFL (minimum score 550 paper-based; 80 iBT). *Application deadline:* For fall admission, 1/10 for domestic students, 12/15 for international students. Application fee: $55 ($65 for international students). *Expenses:* Tuition, state resident: full-time $5259. Tuition, nonresident: full-time $18,569. *Required fees:* $841. Tuition and fees vary according to course load. *Financial support:* In 2013–14, 7 students received support, including 5 research assistantships with full tuition reimbursements available (averaging $21,400 per year); health care benefits and unspecified assistantships also available. Financial award application deadline: 12/15. *Faculty research:* Outcomes in pharmacy, pharmacotherapy. *Total annual research expenditures:* $131,217. *Unit head:* Dr. Diana I. Brixner, Department Chair and Professor, 801-581-6731. *Application contact:* Sara Ray, Academic Program Manager, 801-581-5984, Fax: 801-585-6160, E-mail: sara.ray@pharm.utah.edu.
Website: http://www.pharmacy.utah.edu/pharmacotherapy/

University of Virginia, School of Medicine, Department of Public Health Sciences, Charlottesville, VA 22903. Offers clinical research (MS), including clinical investigation and patient-oriented research, informatics in medicine; public health (MPH); MPP/MPH. Part-time programs available. *Faculty:* 36 full-time (17 women), 4 part-time/adjunct (2 women). *Students:* 40 full-time (31 women), 9 part-time (6 women); includes 14 minority (4 Black or African American, non-Hispanic/Latino; 7 Asian, non-Hispanic/Latino; 3 Hispanic/Latino). Average age 27. 106 applicants, 59% accepted, 29 enrolled. In 2013, 38 master's awarded. *Entrance requirements:* For master's, GRE General Test or MCAT. Additional exam requirements/recommendations for international students: Required—TOEFL. *Application deadline:* Applications are processed on a rolling basis. Application fee: $60. Electronic applications accepted. *Expenses:* Tuition, state resident: part-time $334 per credit hour. Tuition, nonresident: part-time $1224 per credit hour. *Financial support:* Career-related internships or fieldwork available. Financial award applicants required to submit FAFSA. *Unit head:* Dr. Ruth Gaare Bernheim, Chair, 434-924-8430, Fax: 434-924-8437, E-mail: rg3r@virginia.edu. *Application contact:* Tracey L. Brookman, Academic Programs Administrator, 434-924-8430, Fax: 434-924-8437, E-mail: phsdegrees@virginia.edu.
Website: http://www.medicine.virginia.edu/clinical/departments/phs

University of Washington, Graduate School, School of Public Health, Department of Health Services, Seattle, WA 98195. Offers clinical research (MS); community-oriented public health practice (MPH); evaluative sciences and statistics (PhD); health behavior and social determinants of health (PhD); health economics (PhD); health informatics and health information management (MHIHIM); health services (MS, PhD); health services administration (EMHA, MHA); health systems and policy (MPH); health systems research (PhD); maternal and child health (MPH); social and behavioral sciences (MPH); JD/MHA; MHA/MBA; MHA/MD; MHA/MPA; MPH/JD; MPH/MD; MPH/MN; MPH/MPA; MPH/MS; MPH/MSD; MPH/MSW; MPH/PhD. *Faculty:* 63 full-time (30 women), 56 part-time/adjunct (25 women). *Students:* 121 full-time (101 women), 19 part-time (11 women); includes 28 minority (3 Black or African American, non-Hispanic/Latino; 2 American Indian or Alaska Native, non-Hispanic/Latino; 23 Asian, non-Hispanic/Latino), 5 international. Average age 30. 242 applicants, 48% accepted, 36 enrolled. In 2013, 43 master's, 9 doctorates awarded. Terminal master's awarded for partial completion of doctoral program. *Degree requirements:* For master's, thesis (for some programs), practicum (MPH); for doctorate, comprehensive exam, thesis/dissertation. *Entrance requirements:* For master's and doctorate, GRE General Test, minimum GPA of 3.0. Additional exam requirements/recommendations for international students: Required—TOEFL (minimum score 580 paper-based; 92 iBT), IELTS (minimum score 7). *Application deadline:* For fall admission, 1/1 for domestic students, 11/1 for international students. Application fee: 85 Albanian leks. Electronic applications accepted. *Financial support:* In 2013–14, 45 students received support, including 12 fellowships with full and partial tuition reimbursements available (averaging $22,000 per year), 9 research assistantships with full and partial tuition reimbursements available (averaging $18,700 per year), 9 teaching assistantships with full and partial tuition reimbursements available

(averaging $4,575 per year); institutionally sponsored loans, traineeships, and health care benefits also available. Financial award application deadline: 2/28; financial award applicants required to submit FAFSA. *Faculty research:* Public health practice, health promotion and disease prevention, maternal and child health, organizational behavior and culture, health policy. *Unit head:* Dr. Larry Kessler, Chair, 206-543-2930. *Application contact:* Kitty A. Andert, MPH/MS/PhD Programs Manager, 206-616-2926, Fax: 206-543-3964, E-mail: hservmph@u.washington.edu.
Website: http://depts.washington.edu/hserv/

Virginia Commonwealth University, Graduate School, School of Allied Health Professions, Department of Health Administration, Doctoral Program in Health Services Organization and Research, Richmond, VA 23284-9005. Offers PhD. *Degree requirements:* For doctorate, thesis/dissertation, residency. *Entrance requirements:* For doctorate, GMAT or GRE General Test, minimum graduate GPA of 3.0. Additional exam requirements/recommendations for international students: Required—TOEFL (minimum score 600 paper-based; 100 iBT). Electronic applications accepted. *Faculty research:* Organizational studies, theory, associated analytical techniques.

Virginia Commonwealth University, Medical College of Virginia-Professional Programs, School of Medicine, School of Medicine Graduate Programs, Department of Healthcare Policy and Research, Richmond, VA 23284-9005. Offers PhD. *Entrance requirements:* For doctorate, GRE General Test. Additional exam requirements/recommendations for international students: Required—TOEFL (minimum score 600 paper-based; 100 iBT). Electronic applications accepted. *Faculty research:* Evaluation of healthcare services and systems to enhance quality of care and patient safety outcomes; examination of chronic disease (e.g. cancer, HIV/AIDS) policies and practices to improve health outcomes and economic efficiency; impact of uninsurance, public insurance (such as Medicaid) and the safety net on access to care and the health of low-income, underserved, and foreign-born populations; the study of labor supply and healthcare coverage in response to health behaviors and shocks.

Wake Forest University, School of Medicine and Graduate School of Arts and Sciences, Graduate Programs in Medicine, Program in Health Sciences Research, Winston-Salem, NC 27109. Offers MS. *Degree requirements:* For master's, thesis. *Entrance requirements:* For master's, GRE General Test. Additional exam requirements/recommendations for international students: Required—TOEFL. Electronic applications accepted. *Faculty research:* Research methodologies, statistical methods, measurement of health outcomes, health economics.

Washington University in St. Louis, School of Medicine, Program in Applied Health Behavior Research, Saint Louis, MO 63110. Offers health behavior planning and evaluation (Graduate Certificate); health behavior research (MS); health education, program planning and evaluation (MS). Part-time and evening/weekend programs available. *Faculty:* 15 part-time/adjunct (10 women). *Students:* 1 full-time (0 women), 17 part-time (12 women); includes 4 minority (1 Black or African American, non-Hispanic/Latino; 2 Asian, non-Hispanic/Latino; 1 Hispanic/Latino). Average age 40. In 2013, 1 master's, 1 other advanced degree awarded. *Entrance requirements:* For master's and Graduate Certificate, baccalaureate degree in psychology, biology, social work, public health, anthropology or other related field; experience working in the health care field, including health promotion research, social research, or community programs. Additional exam requirements/recommendations for international students: Required—TOEFL. *Application deadline:* Applications are processed on a rolling basis. Application fee: $35. *Financial support:* Applicants required to submit FAFSA. *Faculty research:* Health behavior, health disparities, health education, program management, program evaluation. *Unit head:* Dr. Anjali Deshpande, Program Director, 314-286-0148, E-mail: adeshpan@wustl.edu. *Application contact:* Debbie Pfeiffer, Program Manager, 314-454-8956, Fax: 314-454-8279, E-mail: dpfeiffer@wustl.edu.
Website: http://crtc.wustl.edu/degrees/ahbr.html

Weill Cornell Medical College, Weill Cornell Graduate School of Medical Sciences, Program in Clinical Epidemiology and Health Services Research, New York, NY 10021. Offers MS. *Degree requirements:* For master's, thesis. *Entrance requirements:* For master's, 3 years of work experience, MD or RN certificate. *Faculty research:* Research methodology, biostatistical techniques, data management, decision analysis, health economics.

Section 23
Nursing

This section contains a directory of institutions offering graduate work in nursing, followed by in-depth entries submitted by institutions that chose to prepare detailed program descriptions. Additional information about programs listed in the directory but not augmented by an in-depth entry may be obtained by writing directly to the dean of a graduate school or chair of a department at the address given in the directory.

For programs offering related work, see also in this book *Health Services* and *Public Health.* In another guide in this series:

Graduate Programs in the Humanities, Arts & Social Sciences
See *Family and Consumer Sciences (Gerontology)*

CONTENTS

Program Directories

Displays and Close-Ups

Nursing—General

Abilene Christian University, Graduate School, School of Nursing, Abilene, TX 79699-9100. Offers education and administration (MSN); family nurse practitioner (MSN); nursing (Certificate). *Accreditation:* AACN. Part-time programs available. *Faculty:* 7 part-time/adjunct (all women). *Students:* 1 (woman) part-time. 11 applicants. In 2013, 3 master's awarded. *Degree requirements:* For master's, practicum. *Entrance requirements:* For master's, GRE General Test. Additional exam requirements/recommendations for international students: Required—TOEFL (minimum score 550 paper-based; 90 iBT), IELTS (minimum score 6.5). *Application deadline:* For fall admission, 4/1 priority date for domestic students; for spring admission, 11/1 for domestic students. Applications are processed on a rolling basis. Application fee: $50. Electronic applications accepted. *Expenses: Tuition:* Full-time $17,100; part-time $950 per credit hour. *Financial support:* Application deadline: 4/1; applicants required to submit FAFSA. *Unit head:* Dr. Becky Hammack, Graduate Director, 325-674-2265, Fax: 325-674-6256, E-mail: rsh12a@acu.edu. *Application contact:* Corey Patterson, Director of Graduate Admission and Recruiting, 325-674-6566, Fax: 325-674-6717, E-mail: gradinfo@acu.edu.

Adelphi University, College of Nursing and Public Health, PhD in Nursing Program, Garden City, NY 11530-0701. Offers PhD. *Students:* 6 full-time (5 women), 29 part-time (28 women); includes 15 minority (9 Black or African American, non-Hispanic/Latino; 2 Asian, non-Hispanic/Latino; 3 Hispanic/Latino; 1 Two or more races, non-Hispanic/Latino). Average age 50. In 2013, 3 doctorates awarded. *Expenses: Tuition:* Full-time $32,530; part-time $1010 per credit. *Required fees:* $1150. Tuition and fees vary according to degree level and program. *Unit head:* Patricia Donohue-Porter, Director, 516-877-4532, E-mail: donohue-porter@adelphi.edu. *Application contact:* Christine Murphy, Director of Admissions, 516-877-3050, Fax: 516-877-3039, E-mail: graduateadmissions@adelphi.edu.

See Display below and Close-Up on page 813.

Albany State University, College of Sciences and Health Professions, Albany, GA 31705-2717. Offers criminal justice (MS), including corrections, forensic science, law enforcement, public administration; mathematics education (M Ed); nursing (MSN), including RN to MSN family nurse practitioner, RN to MSN nurse educator; science education (M Ed). Part-time and evening/weekend programs available. Postbaccalaureate distance learning degree programs offered. *Degree requirements:* For master's, comprehensive exam, thesis. *Entrance requirements:* For master's, GRE or MAT, official transcript, letters of recommendations, pre-medical/certificate of immunizations. Electronic applications accepted.

Alcorn State University, School of Graduate Studies, School of Nursing, Natchez, MS 39122-8399. Offers rural nursing (MSN).

Allen College, Program in Nursing, Waterloo, IA 50703. Offers acute care nurse practitioner (MSN, Post-Master's Certificate); adult nurse practitioner (MSN, Post-Master's Certificate); adult psychiatric-mental health nurse practitioner (MSN, Post-Master's Certificate); community public health (MSN, Post-Master's Certificate); family nurse practitioner (MSN, Post-Master's Certificate); gerontological nurse practitioner (MSN, Post-Master's Certificate); health education (MSN); leadership in health care delivery (MSN, Post-Master's Certificate); nursing (DNP). Part-time programs available. Postbaccalaureate distance learning degree programs offered (minimal on-campus study). *Faculty:* 3 full-time (all women), 21 part-time/adjunct (20 women). *Students:* 21 full-time (19 women), 162 part-time (150 women); includes 5 minority (1 Black or African American, non-Hispanic/Latino; 2 Asian, non-Hispanic/Latino; 1 Hispanic/Latino; 1 Two or more races, non-Hispanic/Latino). Average age 34. 213 applicants, 57% accepted, 94 enrolled. In 2013, 41 master's, 4 other advanced degrees awarded. *Degree requirements:* For master's, thesis optional. *Entrance requirements:* For master's, minimum GPA of 3.0 in the last 60 hours of undergraduate coursework; for doctorate, minimum GPA of 3.25 in graduate coursework. Additional exam requirements/recommendations for international students: Recommended—TOEFL (minimum score 580 paper-based; 92 iBT), IELTS (minimum score 6). *Application deadline:* For fall admission, 2/1 priority date for domestic students; for spring admission, 9/1 priority date for domestic students. Applications are processed on a rolling basis. Application fee: $50. Electronic applications accepted. *Expenses: Tuition:* Full-time $14,534; part-time $755 per credit hour. *Required fees:* $935; $75 per credit hour. One-time fee: $275 part-time. Tuition and fees vary according to course load. *Financial support:* In 2013–14, 60 students received support. Institutionally sponsored loans, scholarships/grants, and traineeships available. Support available to part-time students. Financial award application deadline: 8/15; financial award applicants required to submit FAFSA. *Unit head:* Kendra Williams-Perez, Dean, School of Nursing, 319-226-2044, Fax: 319-226-2070, E-mail: kendra.williams-perez@allencollege.edu. *Application contact:* Molly Quinn, Admissions Counselor, 319-226-2001, Fax: 319-226-2010, E-mail: molly.quinn@allencollege.edu.
Website: http://www.allencollege.edu/

Alverno College, School of Nursing, Milwaukee, WI 53234-3922. Offers family nurse practitioner (MSN); mental health nurse practitioner (MSN); nursing education (MSN). *Accreditation:* AACN. Part-time and evening/weekend programs available. *Faculty:* 7 full-time (all women), 8 part-time/adjunct (4 women). *Students:* 82 full-time (79 women), 84 part-time (79 women); includes 48 minority (24 Black or African American, non-Hispanic/Latino; 1 American Indian or Alaska Native, non-Hispanic/Latino; 6 Asian, non-Hispanic/Latino; 11 Hispanic/Latino; 6 Two or more races, non-Hispanic/Latino), 1 international. Average age 36. 59 applicants, 100% accepted, 47 enrolled. In 2013, 33 master's awarded. *Degree requirements:* For master's, 500 clinical hours, capstone. *Entrance requirements:* For master's, BSN, current license. Additional exam requirements/recommendations for international students: Required—TOEFL. *Application deadline:* For fall admission, 7/15 priority date for domestic and international students; for spring admission, 12/15 priority date for domestic and international students. Applications are processed on a rolling basis. Application fee: $0. Electronic applications accepted. Application fee is waived when completed online. *Expenses:* Contact institution. *Financial support:* In 2013–14, 4 students received support. Federal Work-Study and scholarships/grants available. Support available to part-time students. Financial award application deadline: 4/15; financial award applicants required to submit FAFSA. *Faculty research:* Impact of stroke on sexuality, children's asthma management, factors affecting baccalaureate student success. *Unit head:* Dr. Carol Sabel, Associate Dean for MSN Program, 414-382-6309, Fax: 414-382-6354, E-mail: carol.sabel@alverno.edu. *Application contact:* Janet Stikel, Associate Director of Admissions - Adult and Graduate, 414-382-6112, Fax: 414-382-6354, E-mail: janet.stikel@alverno.edu.

American International College, School of Health Sciences, Department of Nursing, Springfield, MA 01109-3189. Offers nursing administration (MSN); nursing education (MSN). *Accreditation:* AACN. Part-time and evening/weekend programs available. Postbaccalaureate distance learning degree programs offered (minimal on-campus study). *Faculty:* 1 (woman) full-time, 1 (woman) part-time/adjunct. *Students:* 12 full-time (all women), 11 part-time (9 women); includes 4 minority (all Black or African American, non-Hispanic/Latino). Average age 39. 17 applicants, 94% accepted, 12 enrolled. In 2013, 10 master's awarded. *Entrance requirements:* For master's, BSN, minimum GPA of 3.0. Additional exam requirements/recommendations for international students: Required—TOEFL or IELTS. *Application deadline:* For fall admission, 7/1 for domestic and international students; for spring admission, 12/1 for domestic and international students. Applications are processed on a rolling basis. Application fee: $50. Electronic applications accepted. *Expenses: Tuition:* Full-time $14,040; part-time $780 per credit. Tuition and fees vary according to course load, degree level and program. *Financial support:* Applicants required to submit FAFSA. *Unit head:* Dr. Ellen Furman, Associate Director of Graduate Nursing, 413-205-3918, Fax: 413-654-1430, E-mail: ellen.furman@aic.edu. *Application contact:* Kerry Barnes, Director of Graduate Admissions, 413-205-3703, Fax: 413-205-3051, E-mail: kerry.barnes@aic.edu.
Website: http://www.aic.edu/academics/hs/nursing

American Sentinel University, Graduate Programs, Aurora, CO 80014. Offers business administration (MBA); business intelligence (MS); computer science (MSCS); health information management (MS); healthcare (MBA); information systems (MSIS); nursing (MSN). Part-time and evening/weekend programs available. Postbaccalaureate distance learning degree programs offered (no on-campus study). *Entrance requirements:* Additional exam requirements/recommendations for international students: Required—TOEFL (minimum score 600 paper-based). Electronic applications accepted.

American University of Beirut, Graduate Programs, Rafic Hariri School of Nursing, Beirut, Lebanon. Offers adult care nursing (MSN); community and public health nursing (MSN); nursing administration (MSN); psychiatry mental health nursing (MSN). *Accreditation:* AACN. Part-time programs available. *Faculty:* 9 full-time (8 women), 12 part-time/adjunct (10 women). *Students:* 4 full-time (3 women), 56 part-time (44 women). Average age 29. 38 applicants, 87% accepted, 26 enrolled. In 2013, 17 master's awarded. *Degree requirements:* For master's, one foreign language, comprehensive exam, thesis optional. *Entrance requirements:* For master's, letter of recommendation. Additional exam requirements/recommendations for international students: Required—TOEFL (minimum score 600 paper-based); Recommended—IELTS. *Application deadline:* For fall admission, 4/1 for domestic and international students; for spring admission, 11/1 for domestic and international students. Applications are processed on a rolling basis. Application fee: $50. Electronic applications accepted. *Expenses: Tuition:* Full-time $14,724; part-time $818 per credit. *Required fees:* $692. Tuition and fees vary according to course load and program. *Financial support:* In 2013–14, 24 teaching assistantships with partial tuition reimbursements were awarded; unspecified assistantships also available. Financial award application deadline: 12/20. *Faculty research:* Pain management and palliative care, stress and post-traumatic stress disorder, health benefits and chronic illness, health promotion and community interventions. *Unit head:* Dr. Huda Huijer Abu-Saad, Director, 961-1374374 Ext. 5952, Fax: 961-1744476, E-mail: hh35@aub.edu.lb. *Application contact:* Dr. Salim Kanaan, Director, Admissions Office, 961-1-350000 Ext. 2594, Fax: 96-1-1750775, E-mail: sk00@aub.edu.lb.
Website: http://staff.aub.edu.lb/~webson

Andrews University, School of Health Professions, Department of Nursing, Berrien Springs, MI 49104. Offers MS. Part-time and evening/weekend programs available. *Faculty:* 10 full-time (all women), 1 (woman) part-time/adjunct. In 2013, 8 master's awarded. *Degree requirements:* For master's, thesis. *Entrance requirements:* For master's, GRE, minimum GPA of 2.5, 1 year of nursing experience, RN license. Additional exam requirements/recommendations for international students: Required—TOEFL (minimum score 550 paper-based). *Application deadline:* Applications are processed on a rolling basis. Application fee: $40. *Financial support:* Institutionally sponsored loans available. *Faculty research:* Theory for nursing, salary equitability. *Unit head:* Dr. Karen A. Allen, Chairperson, 269-471-3364. *Application contact:* Monica Wringer, Supervisor of Graduate Admission, 800-253-2874, Fax: 269-471-6321, E-mail: graduate@andrews.edu.
Website: http://www.andrews.edu/shp/nursing/

Arizona State University at the Tempe campus, College of Nursing and Health Innovation, Phoenix, AZ 85004. Offers advanced nursing practice (DNP); child/family mental health nurse practitioner (Graduate Certificate); clinical research management (MS); community and public health practice (Graduate Certificate); community health (MS); exercise and wellness (MS), including exercise and wellness; family nurse practitioner (Graduate Certificate); healthcare innovation (MHI); international health for healthcare (Graduate Certificate); kinesiology (MS, PhD); nursing (MS, Graduate Certificate); nursing and healthcare innovation (PhD); nutrition (MS); physical activity nutrition and wellness (PhD), including physical activity, nutrition and wellness; public health (MPH); regulatory science and health safety (MS). *Accreditation:* AACN. Postbaccalaureate distance learning degree programs offered (minimal on-campus study). *Degree requirements:* For master's, comprehensive exam (for some programs), thesis (for some programs), interactive Program of Study (iPOS) submitted before completing 50 percent of required credit hours; for doctorate, comprehensive exam, thesis/dissertation, interactive Program of Study (iPOS) submitted before completing 50 percent of required credit hours. *Entrance requirements:* For master's and doctorate, GRE, minimum GPA of 3.0 or equivalent in last 2 years of work leading to bachelor's degree. Additional exam requirements/recommendations for international students: Required—TOEFL (minimum score 80 iBT), TOEFL, IELTS, or PTE. Electronic applications accepted. *Expenses:* Contact institution.

Arkansas State University, Graduate School, College of Nursing and Health Professions, School of Nursing, State University, AR 72467. Offers aging studies (Certificate); health care management (Certificate); health communications (Certificate); health sciences (MS); health sciences education (Certificate); nurse anesthesia (MSN); nursing (MSN); nursing practice (DNP). *Accreditation:* AANA/CANAEP (one or more programs are accredited). Part-time programs available. *Faculty:* 16 full-time (14 women). *Students:* 96 full-time (34 women), 120 part-time (108 women); includes 38 minority (26 Black or African American, non-Hispanic/Latino; 3 American Indian or Alaska Native, non-Hispanic/Latino; 2 Asian, non-Hispanic/Latino; 4 Hispanic/Latino; 3 Two or more races, non-Hispanic/Latino). Average age 33. 153 applicants, 32% accepted, 44 enrolled. In 2013, 103 master's awarded. *Degree requirements:* For master's, comprehensive exam, thesis or alternative; for doctorate, comprehensive exam, thesis/dissertation. *Entrance requirements:* For master's, GRE General Test or MAT, appropriate bachelor's degree, current Arkansas nursing license, CPR certification, physical examination, professional liability insurance, critical care experience, ACLS Certification, PALS Certification, interview, immunization records, personal goal statement, health assessment; for doctorate, GRE or MAT, appropriate master's degree, current Arkansas nursing license, CPR certification, physical examination, professional liability insurance, critical care experience, ACLS Certification, PALS Certification, interview, immunization records, personal goal statement, health assessment, TB skin test, NCLEX-RN Exam, background check. Additional exam requirements/recommendations for international students: Required—TOEFL (minimum score 550 paper-based; 79 iBT), IELTS (minimum score 6), PTE (minimum score 56). *Application deadline:* Applications are processed on a rolling basis. Electronic applications accepted. *Expenses:* Contact institution. *Financial support:* In 2013–14, 9 students received support. Fellowships, career-related internships or fieldwork, scholarships/grants, and unspecified assistantships available. Financial award application deadline: 7/1; financial award applicants required to submit FAFSA. *Unit head:* Dr. Marilyn Duran, Chair, 870-972-3074, Fax: 870-972-2954, E-mail: mduran@astate.edu. *Application contact:* Vickey Ring, Graduate Admissions Coordinator, 870-972-3029, Fax: 870-972-3857, E-mail: vickeyring@astate.edu.
Website: http://www.astate.edu/college/conhp/departments/nursing/

Arkansas Tech University, College of Natural and Health Sciences, Russellville, AR 72801. Offers fisheries and wildlife biology (MS); health informatics (MS); nursing (MSN). Part-time programs available. *Students:* 14 full-time (11 women), 56 part-time (41 women); includes 10 minority (6 Black or African American, non-Hispanic/Latino; 1 American Indian or Alaska Native, non-Hispanic/Latino; 2 Asian, non-Hispanic/Latino; 1 Two or more races, non-Hispanic/Latino), 5 international. Average age 35. In 2013, 22 master's awarded. *Degree requirements:* For master's, thesis (for some programs), project. *Entrance requirements:* For master's, GRE General Test. Additional exam requirements/recommendations for international students: Required—TOEFL (minimum score 550 paper-based; 79 iBT), IELTS (minimum score 6). *Application deadline:* For fall admission, 3/1 priority date for domestic students, 5/1 priority date for international students; for spring admission, 10/1 priority date for domestic and international students. Applications are processed on a rolling basis. Application fee: $25 ($75 for international students). Electronic applications accepted. *Expenses:* Tuition, state resident: full-time $5976; part-time $249 per credit hour. Tuition, nonresident: full-time $11,952; part-time $498 per credit hour. *Required fees:* $411 per semester. Tuition and fees vary according to course load. *Financial support:* In 2013–14, research assistantships with full tuition reimbursements (averaging $4,800 per year), teaching assistantships with full tuition reimbursements (averaging $4,800 per year) were awarded; career-related internships or fieldwork, Federal Work-Study, scholarships/grants, health care benefits, and unspecified assistantships also available. Support available to part-time students. Financial award application deadline: 4/15; financial award applicants required to submit FAFSA. *Unit head:* Dr. Jeff Robertson, Dean, 479-968-0498, E-mail: jrobertson@atu.edu. *Application contact:* Dr. Mary B. Gunter, Dean of Graduate College, 479-968-0398, Fax: 479-964-0542, E-mail: gradcollege@atu.edu.
Website: http://www.atu.edu/nhs/

Armstrong State University, School of Graduate Studies, Program in Nursing, Savannah, GA 31419-1997. Offers adult-gerontological acute care nurse practitioner (MSN); adult-gerontological clinical nurse specialist (MSN); adult-gerontological primary care nurse practitioner (MSN). *Accreditation:* AACN. Part-time and evening/weekend programs available. *Faculty:* 10 full-time (all women), 1 (woman) part-time/adjunct. *Students:* 24 full-time (21 women), 17 part-time (16 women); includes 5 minority (2 Black or African American, non-Hispanic/Latino; 1 Hispanic/Latino; 2 Two or more races, non-Hispanic/Latino). Average age 34. 17 applicants, 65% accepted, 10 enrolled. In 2013, 13 master's awarded. *Degree requirements:* For master's, comprehensive exam, project or thesis. *Entrance requirements:* For master's, GRE General Test or MAT, minimum GPA of 3.0, letter of recommendation, letter of intent. Additional exam requirements/recommendations for international students: Required—TOEFL (minimum score 523 paper-based; 70 iBT). *Application deadline:* For fall admission, 2/28 for domestic and international students; for spring admission, 11/15 for domestic students, 9/15 for international students. Applications are processed on a rolling basis. Application fee: $30. Electronic applications accepted. *Expenses:* Tuition, state resident: part-time $201 per credit hour. Tuition, nonresident: part-time $745 per credit hour. *Required fees:* $310 per semester. Tuition and fees vary according to course load, campus/location and program. *Financial support:* In 2013–14, research assistantships with full tuition reimbursements (averaging $5,000 per year) were awarded; Federal Work-Study, scholarships/grants, and unspecified assistantships also available. Support available to part-time students. Financial award application deadline: 3/1; financial award applicants required to submit FAFSA. *Faculty research:* Midwifery, mental health, nursing simulation, smoking cessation during pregnancy, asthma education, vulnerable populations, geriatrics, disaster nursing, complementary and alternative modalities, nephrology. *Unit head:* Dr. Catherine Gilbert, Department Head, 912-344-3145, E-mail: catherine.gilbert@armstrong.edu. *Application contact:* Jill Bell, Director/Graduate Enrollment Coordinator, 912-344-2798, Fax: 912-344-3488, E-mail: graduate@armstrong.edu.
Website: http://www.armstrong.edu/Health_professions/nursing/nursing_graduate_programs

Athabasca University, Centre for Nursing and Health Studies, Athabasca, AB T9S 3A3, Canada. Offers advanced nursing practice (MN, Advanced Diploma); generalist (MN); health studies-leadership (MHS). Part-time programs available. Postbaccalaureate distance learning degree programs offered. *Degree requirements:* For master's, comprehensive exam (for some programs). *Entrance requirements:* For master's, bachelor's degree in health-related field, 2 years professional health service experience (MHS), bachelor's degree in nursing, 2 years nursing experience (MN), minimum GPA of 3.0 in final 30 credits; for Advanced Diploma, RN license, 2 years health care experience. Electronic applications accepted. *Expenses:* Contact institution.

Auburn University, Graduate School, School of Nursing, Auburn University, AL 36849. Offers nursing educator (MSN); primary care practitioner (MSN). *Accreditation:* AACN. *Faculty:* 17 full-time (15 women). *Students:* 2 full-time (both women), 77 part-time (72 women); includes 12 minority (9 Black or African American, non-Hispanic/Latino; 1 American Indian or Alaska Native, non-Hispanic/Latino; 1 Asian, non-Hispanic/Latino; 1 Hispanic/Latino), 1 international. Average age 31. 87 applicants, 79% accepted, 47 enrolled. In 2013, 29 master's awarded. *Expenses:* Tuition, state resident: full-time $8262; part-time $459 per credit hour. Tuition, nonresident: full-time $24,786; part-time $1377 per credit hour. Tuition and fees vary according to degree level and program. *Unit head:* Dr. Gregg Newschwander, Dean, 334-844-3658, E-mail: gen0002@auburn.edu. *Application contact:* Dr. George Flowers, Dean of the Graduate School, 334-844-4700, E-mail: gradadm@auburn.edu.
Website: http://www.auburn.edu/academic/nursing/

Augsburg College, Program in Transcultural Community Health Nursing, Minneapolis, MN 55454-1351. Offers MA. *Accreditation:* AACN. *Degree requirements:* For master's, thesis or alternative.

Aurora University, College of Professional Studies, Aurora, IL 60506-4892. Offers business (MBA); criminal justice (MS); nursing (MSN); social work (MSW, DSW). Part-time and evening/weekend programs available. *Entrance requirements:* Additional exam requirements/recommendations for international students: Required—TOEFL (minimum score 550 paper-based). Electronic applications accepted.

Austin Peay State University, College of Graduate Studies, College of Behavioral and Health Sciences, School of Nursing, Clarksville, TN 37044. Offers advanced practice (MSN); nursing administration (MSN); nursing education (MSN); nursing informatics

(MSN). Part-time programs available. Postbaccalaureate distance learning degree programs offered. *Faculty:* 9 full-time (all women), 7 part-time/adjunct (all women). *Students:* 47 full-time (43 women), 136 part-time (129 women); includes 30 minority (18 Black or African American, non-Hispanic/Latino; 4 Asian, non-Hispanic/Latino; 4 Hispanic/Latino; 4 Two or more races, non-Hispanic/Latino). Average age 35. 47 applicants, 85% accepted, 37 enrolled. In 2013, 39 master's awarded. *Degree requirements:* For master's, comprehensive exam. *Entrance requirements:* For master's, GRE General Test, minimum GPA of 3.0, RN license eligibility, 3 letters of recommendation. Additional exam requirements/recommendations for international students: Required—TOEFL (minimum score 600 paper-based). *Application deadline:* For fall admission, 8/5 priority date for domestic students. Applications are processed on a rolling basis. Application fee: $25. Electronic applications accepted. *Expenses:* Tuition, state resident: full-time $7500; part-time $375 per credit hour. Tuition, nonresident: full-time $20,800; part-time $1040 per credit hour. *Required fees:* $1284; $64.20 per credit hour. *Financial support:* In 2013–14, research assistantships with full tuition reimbursements (averaging $6,500 per year) were awarded; career-related internships or fieldwork, Federal Work-Study, institutionally sponsored loans, scholarships/grants, and unspecified assistantships also available. Support available to part-time students. *Unit head:* Dr. Patty Orr, Director, 931-221-7710, Fax: 931-221-7595, E-mail: orrp@apsu.edu. *Application contact:* June D. Lee, Graduate Coordinator, 800-859-4723, Fax: 931-221-7641, E-mail: gradadmissions@apsu.edu.
Website: http://www.apsu.edu/nursing

Azusa Pacific University, School of Nursing, Azusa, CA 91702-7000. Offers nursing (MSN); nursing education (PhD). *Accreditation:* AACN. Part-time and evening/weekend programs available. *Degree requirements:* For master's, thesis optional. *Entrance requirements:* For master's, BSN.

Ball State University, Graduate School, College of Applied Science and Technology, School of Nursing, Muncie, IN 47306. Offers MA, MS, DNP. *Accreditation:* AACN. Part-time programs available. *Faculty:* 15 full-time (all women), 6 part-time/adjunct (5 women). *Students:* 6 full-time (4 women), 410 part-time (383 women); includes 38 minority (16 Black or African American, non-Hispanic/Latino; 3 American Indian or Alaska Native, non-Hispanic/Latino; 5 Asian, non-Hispanic/Latino; 11 Hispanic/Latino; 1 Native Hawaiian or other Pacific Islander, non-Hispanic/Latino; 2 Two or more races, non-Hispanic/Latino). Average age 42. 115 applicants, 25% accepted. In 2013, 115 master's, 4 doctorates awarded. *Entrance requirements:* For master's, bachelor's degree in nursing, minimum GPA of 2.8 in upper-level course work, interview, resume. Application fee: $50. *Financial support:* In 2013–14, 7 teaching assistantships with full tuition reimbursements (averaging $11,069 per year) were awarded; research assistantships and career-related internships or fieldwork also available. Financial award application deadline: 3/1. *Unit head:* Dr. Linda Siktberg, Director, 765-285-8718, Fax: 765-285-2169, E-mail: lsiktberg@bsu.edu. *Application contact:* Dr. Robert Morris, Associate Provost for Research and Dean of the Graduate School, 765-285-5723, Fax: 765-285-1328, E-mail: rmorris@bsu.edu.
Website: http://www.bsu.edu/nursing/

Barry University, School of Adult and Continuing Education, Division of Nursing, Miami Shores, FL 33161-6695. Offers MSN, PhD, Certificate, MSN/MBA. Part-time and evening/weekend programs available. *Degree requirements:* For master's, research project or thesis; for doctorate, thesis/dissertation. *Entrance requirements:* For master's, GRE General Test or MAT, BSN, minimum GPA of 3.0, course work in statistics and research, Florida RN license; for doctorate, GRE General Test or MAT, minimum GPA of 3.3, MSN. Electronic applications accepted. *Faculty research:* Adult education, nurse practitioner, stress reduction in pregnancy, prevention of cardiac problems, in children, level of school age children.

Baylor University, Graduate School, Louise Herrington School of Nursing, Dallas, TX 75246. Offers family nurse practitioner (MSN); neonatal nurse practitioner (MSN); nurse-midwifery (DNP). *Accreditation:* AACN. Part-time programs available. Postbaccalaureate distance learning degree programs offered (minimal on-campus study). *Faculty:* 11 full-time (all women), 3 part-time/adjunct (2 women). *Students:* 25 full-time (24 women), 41 part-time (37 women); includes 15 minority (5 Black or African American, non-Hispanic/Latino; 5 Asian, non-Hispanic/Latino; 4 Hispanic/Latino; 1 Two or more races, non-Hispanic/Latino). Average age 35. 47 applicants, 70% accepted, 26 enrolled. In 2013, 25 master's, 5 doctorates awarded. *Degree requirements:* For doctorate, comprehensive exam (for some programs), capstone project. *Entrance requirements:* For master's, GRE General Test or MAT; for doctorate, GRE General Test. Additional exam requirements/recommendations for international students: Required—TOEFL. *Application deadline:* For fall admission, 2/1 for domestic students. Application fee: $50. Electronic applications accepted. *Expenses: Tuition:* Full-time $25,866; part-time $1437 per credit hour. *Required fees:* $2736; $152 per credit hour. Tuition and fees vary according to course load and program. *Financial support:* In 2013–14, 66 students received support, including 1 teaching assistantship (averaging $4,167 per year); Federal Work-Study, scholarships/grants, and unspecified assistantships also available. Support available to part-time students. Financial award application deadline: 6/30; financial award applicants required to submit FAFSA. *Faculty research:* Women and strokes, obesity and pregnancy, educational environmental factors, international undeserved populations, midwifery. *Total annual research expenditures:* $5,000. *Unit head:* Dr. Barbara Camune, Graduate Program Director, 214-367-3754, Fax: 214-820-3375, E-mail: barbara_camune@baylor.edu. *Application contact:* Elaine Lark, Coordinator of Recruitment and Enrollment, 214-818-7839, Fax: 214-820-3835, E-mail: elaine_lark@baylor.edu.
Website: http://www.baylor.edu/nursing/

Bellarmine University, Donna and Allan Lansing School of Nursing and Health Sciences, Louisville, KY 40205. Offers family nurse practitioner (MSN); health science (MHS); nursing administration (MSN); nursing education (MSN); nursing practice (DNP); physical therapy (DPT). *Accreditation:* AACN; APTA. Part-time and evening/weekend programs available. *Faculty:* 21 full-time (19 women), 8 part-time/adjunct (5 women). *Students:* 162 full-time (111 women), 120 part-time (113 women); includes 16 minority (6 Black or African American, non-Hispanic/Latino; 1 American Indian or Alaska Native, non-Hispanic/Latino; 3 Asian, non-Hispanic/Latino; 3 Hispanic/Latino; 3 Two or more races, non-Hispanic/Latino). Average age 29. In 2013, 30 master's, 54 doctorates awarded. *Degree requirements:* For doctorate, comprehensive exam, thesis/dissertation. *Entrance requirements:* For master's, GRE General Test, RN license; for doctorate, GRE General Test, Physical Therapist Centralized Application Service (for DPT). Additional exam requirements/recommendations for international students: Required—TOEFL (minimum score 550 paper-based; 80 iBT). Application fee: $25. Electronic applications accepted. *Expenses:* Contact institution. *Financial support:* Career-related internships or fieldwork and scholarships/grants available. *Faculty research:* Nursing: pain, empathy, leadership styles, control; physical therapy: service-learning; exercise in chronic and pre-operative conditions, athletes; women's health; aging. *Unit head:* Dr. Mark Wiegand, Dean, 800-274-4723 Ext. 8368, E-mail: mwiegand@bellarmine.edu. *Application contact:* Julie Armstrong-Binnix, Health Science Recruiter, 800-274-4723 Ext. 8364, E-mail: julieab@bellarmine.edu.
Website: http://www.bellarmine.edu/lansing

Bellin College, School of Nursing, Green Bay, WI 54305. Offers family nurse practitioner (MSN); nurse educator (MSN). *Accreditation:* AACN. *Faculty:* 1 (woman) full-time, 3 part-time/adjunct (2 women). *Students:* 37 part-time (all women). *Expenses: Tuition:* Part-time $714 per credit. *Required fees:* $100 per year. *Unit head:* Dr. Kimberly Udlis, Graduate Program Director, 920-433-6624, Fax: 920-433-1921, E-mail: kimberly.udlis@bellincollege.edu.

Belmont University, Gordon E. Inman College of Health Sciences and Nursing, Nashville, TN 37212-3757. Offers nursing (MSN, DNP); occupational therapy (MSOT, OTD); physical therapy (DPT). Part-time programs available. Postbaccalaureate distance learning degree programs offered (minimal on-campus study). *Students:* 290 full-time (172 women), 1 part-time (0 women); includes 43 minority (12 Black or African American, non-Hispanic/Latino; 22 Asian, non-Hispanic/Latino; 8 Hispanic/Latino; 1 Two or more races, non-Hispanic/Latino), 3 international. Average age 26. *Degree requirements:* For master's, comprehensive exam, thesis; for doctorate, comprehensive exam. *Entrance requirements:* For master's, GRE, BSN, minimum GPA of 3.0. Additional exam requirements/recommendations for international students: Required—TOEFL (minimum score 550 paper-based). *Application deadline:* Applications are processed on a rolling basis. Application fee: $50. Electronic applications accepted. *Expenses:* Contact institution. *Financial support:* Teaching assistantships with full tuition reimbursements, career-related internships or fieldwork, scholarships/grants, and traineeships available. Financial award application deadline: 3/1; financial award applicants required to submit FAFSA. *Unit head:* Dean, 615-460-6916, Fax: 615-460-6750. *Application contact:* David Mee, Dean of Enrollment Services, 615-460-6785, Fax: 615-460-5434, E-mail: david.mee@belmont.edu.
Website: http://www.belmont.edu/healthsciences/

Benedictine University, Graduate Programs, Program in Nursing, Lisle, IL 60532-0900. Offers MSN. *Accreditation:* AACN. *Students:* 7 full-time (all women), 375 part-time (359 women); includes 76 minority (42 Black or African American, non-Hispanic/Latino; 3 American Indian or Alaska Native, non-Hispanic/Latino; 24 Asian, non-Hispanic/Latino; 6 Hispanic/Latino; 1 Native Hawaiian or other Pacific Islander, non-Hispanic/Latino). 95 applicants, 100% accepted, 84 enrolled. In 2013, 170 master's awarded. *Expenses: Tuition:* Part-time $590 per credit hour. *Unit head:* Elizabeth Ritt, Department Chair, 630-829-1933, E-mail: eritt@ben.edu. *Application contact:* Kari Gibbons, Associate Vice President, Enrollment Center, 630-829-6200, Fax: 630-829-6584, E-mail: kgibbons@ben.edu.

Bethel College, Adult and Graduate Programs, Program in Nursing, Mishawaka, IN 46545-5591. Offers MSN. Part-time and evening/weekend programs available. *Faculty:* 4 part-time/adjunct (all women). *Students:* 22 part-time (21 women); includes 2 minority (1 Black or African American, non-Hispanic/Latino; 1 American Indian or Alaska Native, non-Hispanic/Latino). 12 applicants, 100% accepted, 11 enrolled. In 2013, 7 master's awarded. *Degree requirements:* For master's, thesis. *Entrance requirements:* Additional exam requirements/recommendations for international students: Required—TOEFL (minimum score 540 paper-based). *Application deadline:* For fall admission, 8/15 for domestic students, 5/1 for international students; for spring admission, 10/1 for international students. Application fee: $25. Electronic applications accepted. *Expenses: Required fees:* $75 per semester. Tuition and fees vary according to program. *Financial support:* Career-related internships or fieldwork available. Financial award applicants required to submit FAFSA. *Unit head:* Dr. Deborah Gillum, Dean of Nursing, 574-807-7015, E-mail: gillumd@bethelcollege.edu. *Application contact:* -, Fax: -.

Bethel University, Graduate School, St. Paul, MN 55112-6999. Offers autism spectrum disorders (Certificate); business administration (MBA); communication (MA); counseling psychology (MA); educational leadership (Ed D); gerontology (MA); international baccalaureate education (Certificate); K-12 education (MA); literacy education (MA, Certificate); nurse educator (Certificate); nurse leader (Certificate); nurse-midwifery (MS); nursing (MS); physician assistant (MS); postsecondary teaching (Certificate); special education (MA); strategic leadership (MA); teaching (MA). Part-time and evening/weekend programs available. Postbaccalaureate distance learning degree programs offered (no on-campus study). *Faculty:* 13 full-time (7 women), 89 part-time/adjunct (43 women). *Students:* 692 full-time (457 women), 573 part-time (371 women); includes 170 minority (86 Black or African American, non-Hispanic/Latino; 1 American Indian or Alaska Native, non-Hispanic/Latino; 49 Asian, non-Hispanic/Latino; 20 Hispanic/Latino; 1 Native Hawaiian or other Pacific Islander, non-Hispanic/Latino; 13 Two or more races, non-Hispanic/Latino), 21 international. Average age 37. In 2013, 166 master's, 9 doctorates, 11 other advanced degrees awarded. *Degree requirements:* For master's, comprehensive exam (for some programs), thesis (for some programs); for doctorate, comprehensive exam, thesis/dissertation. *Entrance requirements:* Additional exam requirements/recommendations for international students: Required—TOEFL (minimum score 550 paper-based; 80 iBT). *Application deadline:* Applications are processed on a rolling basis. Electronic applications accepted. Tuition and fees vary according to course load, degree level and program. *Financial support:* Teaching assistantships, career-related internships or fieldwork, and scholarships/grants available. Support available to part-time students. Financial award applicants required to submit FAFSA. *Unit head:* Dick Crombie, Vice-President/Dean, 651-635-8000, Fax: 651-635-8004, E-mail: gs@bethel.edu. *Application contact:* Director of Admissions, 651-635-8000, Fax: 651-635-8004, E-mail: gs@bethel.edu.
Website: http://gs.bethel.edu/

Binghamton University, State University of New York, Graduate School, Decker School of Nursing, Vestal, NY 13902-6000. Offers MS, DNP, PhD, Certificate. *Accreditation:* AACN. Part-time and evening/weekend programs available. *Faculty:* 45 full-time (43 women), 50 part-time/adjunct (44 women). *Students:* 110 full-time (88 women), 122 part-time (110 women); includes 36 minority (7 Black or African American, non-Hispanic/Latino; 3 American Indian or Alaska Native, non-Hispanic/Latino; 15 Asian, non-Hispanic/Latino; 10 Hispanic/Latino; 1 Native Hawaiian or other Pacific Islander, non-Hispanic/Latino), 15 international. Average age 37. 102 applicants, 93% accepted, 65 enrolled. In 2013, 54 master's, 5 doctorates, 18 other advanced degrees awarded. *Degree requirements:* For master's, comprehensive exam, thesis; for doctorate, thesis/dissertation. *Entrance requirements:* For master's, GRE General Test. Additional exam requirements/recommendations for international students: Required—TOEFL. *Application deadline:* For fall admission, 4/15 priority date for domestic students, 1/15 priority date for international students; for spring admission, 11/1 for domestic students, 10/1 priority date for international students. Applications are processed on a rolling basis. Application fee: $75. Electronic applications accepted. *Financial support:* In 2013–14, 55 students received support, including 3 fellowships with partial tuition reimbursements available (averaging $16,500 per year), 2 research assistantships with full tuition reimbursements available (averaging $12,500 per year), 5 teaching assistantships with full tuition reimbursements available (averaging $16,500 per year); career-related internships or fieldwork, Federal Work-Study, institutionally sponsored loans, traineeships, health care benefits, tuition waivers (full and partial), and unspecified assistantships also available. Financial award application deadline: 2/15; financial award applicants required to submit FAFSA. *Unit head:* Dr. Joyce Ferrario, Dean, 607-777-2311, Fax: 607-777-4440, E-mail: jferrari@binghamton.edu. *Application*

contact: Kishan Zuber, Director of Graduate Studies, 607-777-2151, Fax: 607-777-2501, E-mail: kzuber@binghamton.edu.
Website: http://dson.binghamton.edu/

Blessing-Rieman College of Nursing, Program in Nursing, Quincy, IL 62305-7005. Offers MSN. *Accreditation:* AACN. Part-time programs available. *Faculty:* 7 full-time (all women). *Students:* 10 part-time (all women). 17 applicants, 100% accepted, 17 enrolled. *Degree requirements:* For master's, thesis. *Entrance requirements:* For master's, proof of RN license; BSN from CCNE- or NLNAC-accredited program; minimum GPA of 3.0 for last 60 semester hours of undergraduate course work; completion of statistics, nursing research, physical assessment or equivalent with minimum grade of C. Additional exam requirements/recommendations for international students: Required—TOEFL. *Application deadline:* For fall admission, 4/1 for domestic students. Applications are processed on a rolling basis. Application fee: $0. Electronic applications accepted. *Unit head:* Dr. Karen Mayville, Administrative Coordinator for Assessment/Director of the Master's Program, 217-228-5520 Ext. 6968, Fax: 217-223-1781, E-mail: kmayville@brcn.edu. *Application contact:* Heather Mutter, Admissions Counselor, 217-228-5520 Ext. 6964, Fax: 217-223-4661, E-mail: hmutter@brcn.edu.

Bloomsburg University of Pennsylvania, School of Graduate Studies, College of Science and Technology, Department of Nursing, Bloomsburg, PA 17815. Offers adult and family nurse practitioner (MSN); community health (MSN); nurse anesthesia (MSN); nursing (MSN); nursing administration (MSN). *Accreditation:* AACN; AANA/CANAEP. *Faculty:* 5 full-time (all women), 7 part-time/adjunct (all women). *Students:* 62 full-time (52 women), 26 part-time (17 women); includes 8 minority (6 Black or African American, non-Hispanic/Latino; 1 Asian, non-Hispanic/Latino; 1 Hispanic/Latino). Average age 35. 61 applicants, 84% accepted, 14 enrolled. In 2013, 36 master's awarded. *Degree requirements:* For master's, thesis (for some programs), clinical experience. *Entrance requirements:* For master's, minimum QPA of 3.0, personal statement, 2 letters of recommendation, nursing license. Additional exam requirements/recommendations for international students: Required—TOEFL. *Application deadline:* For fall admission, 1/1 for domestic students; for spring admission, 8/1 for domestic students. Applications are processed on a rolling basis. Application fee: $35 ($60 for international students). Electronic applications accepted. *Expenses:* Tuition, state resident: full-time $7956; part-time $442 per credit. Tuition, nonresident: full-time $11,934; part-time $663 per credit. *Required fees:* $95.50 per credit. $55 per semester. Tuition and fees vary according to course load. *Financial support:* Unspecified assistantships available. *Unit head:* Dr. Noreen Chikotas, Coordinator, 570-389-4609, Fax: 570-389-5008, E-mail: nchikota@bloomu.edu. *Application contact:* Jennifer Richard, Administrative Assistant, 570-389-4015, Fax: 570-389-3054, E-mail: jrichard@bloomu.edu.
Website: http://www.bloomu.edu/nursing

Boise State University, College of Health Sciences, School of Nursing, Boise, ID 83725-0399. Offers MN, MSN, Graduate Certificate.

Boston College, William F. Connell School of Nursing, Chestnut Hill, MA 02467-3800. Offers adult-gerontology nursing (MS); community health nursing (MS); family health (MS); forensic nursing (MS); maternal/child health nursing (MS), including pediatric and women's health; nurse anesthesia (MS); nursing (PhD); palliative care (MS), including adult and pediatric; psychiatric-mental health nursing (MS); MBA/MS; MS/MA; MS/PhD. *Accreditation:* AACN; AANA/CANAEP (one or more programs are accredited). Part-time programs available. *Faculty:* 47 full-time (43 women), 42 part-time/adjunct (39 women). *Students:* 199 full-time (180 women), 79 part-time (73 women); includes 44 minority (14 Black or African American, non-Hispanic/Latino; 1 American Indian or Alaska Native, non-Hispanic/Latino; 13 Asian, non-Hispanic/Latino; 12 Hispanic/Latino; 4 Two or more races, non-Hispanic/Latino), 7 international. Average age 31. 502 applicants, 39% accepted, 87 enrolled. In 2013, 105 master's, 8 doctorates awarded. *Degree requirements:* For master's, comprehensive exam, research project; for doctorate, comprehensive exam, thesis/dissertation, computer literacy exam or foreign language. *Entrance requirements:* For master's, bachelor's degree in nursing; for doctorate, GRE General Test, MS in nursing. Additional exam requirements/recommendations for international students: Required—TOEFL (minimum score 600 paper-based; 100 iBT). *Application deadline:* For fall admission, 9/30 for domestic and international students; for winter admission, 1/15 for domestic and international students; for spring admission, 3/15 for domestic and international students. Applications are processed on a rolling basis. Application fee: $40. Electronic applications accepted. *Financial support:* In 2013–14, 174 students received support, including 7 fellowships with full tuition reimbursements available (averaging $20,000 per year), 21 teaching assistantships (averaging $4,800 per year); research assistantships, scholarships/grants, health care benefits, tuition waivers (partial), and unspecified assistantships also available. Support available to part-time students. Financial award application deadline: 3/1; financial award applicants required to submit FAFSA. *Faculty research:* Sexual and reproductive health, health promotion/illness prevention, eating disorders, violence, symptom management. *Total annual research expenditures:* $1.1 million. *Unit head:* Dr. Susan Gennaro, Dean, 617-552-4251, Fax: 617-552-0931, E-mail: susan.gennaro@bc.edu. *Application contact:* MaryBeth Crowley, Graduate Programs Assistant, 617-552-4928, Fax: 617-552-2121, E-mail: csongrad@bc.edu.
Website: http://www.bc.edu/schools/son/

Bowie State University, Graduate Programs, Department of Nursing, Bowie, MD 20715-9465. Offers administration of nursing services (MS); family nurse practitioner (MS); nursing education (MS). Part-time programs available. *Degree requirements:* For master's, comprehensive exam, thesis, research paper. *Entrance requirements:* For master's, minimum GPA of 2.5. Electronic applications accepted. *Expenses:* Tuition, state resident: full-time $8665. Tuition, nonresident: full-time $16,007. *Required fees:* $1927. *Faculty research:* Minority health, women's health, gerontology, leadership management.

Bradley University, Graduate School, College of Education and Health Sciences, Department of Nursing, Peoria, IL 61625-0002. Offers nurse administered anesthesia (MSN); nursing administration (MSN). Part-time and evening/weekend programs available. *Degree requirements:* For master's, comprehensive exam, thesis optional. *Entrance requirements:* For master's, GRE General Test or MAT, interview, Illinois RN license, advanced cardiac life support certification, pediatric advanced life support certification, 3 letters of recommendation. Additional exam requirements/recommendations for international students: Required—TOEFL (minimum score 550 paper-based; 79 iBT). *Expenses: Tuition:* Full-time $14,580; part-time $810 per credit hour. Tuition and fees vary according to course load and program.

Briar Cliff University, Program in Nursing, Sioux City, IA 51104-0100. Offers MSN. *Accreditation:* AACN. Part-time and evening/weekend programs available. *Degree requirements:* For master's, thesis optional. *Entrance requirements:* For master's, minimum undergraduate GPA of 3.0 for last 60 undergraduate credits; current RN license. *Expenses:* Contact institution. *Faculty research:* The process/experience of trying something new (or change), the experience of taking a risk.

Brigham Young University, Graduate Studies, College of Nursing, Provo, UT 84602. Offers family nurse practitioner (MS). *Accreditation:* AACN. *Faculty:* 10 full-time (7 women), 1 part-time/adjunct (0 women). *Students:* 28 full-time (11 women). Average age 34. 44 applicants, 34% accepted, 15 enrolled. In 2013, 15 master's awarded. *Degree requirements:* For master's, thesis. *Entrance requirements:* For master's, GRE, minimum GPA of 3.0 in last 60 hours, interview, BS in nursing, pathophysiology class within undergraduate program, course work in basic statistics. Additional exam requirements/recommendations for international students: Required—TOEFL; Recommended—IELTS. *Application deadline:* For spring admission, 12/1 for domestic students. Applications are processed on a rolling basis. Application fee: $50. Electronic applications accepted. *Expenses: Tuition:* Full-time $6130; part-time $340 per credit hour. Tuition and fees vary according to program and student's religious affiliation. *Financial support:* In 2013–14, 28 students received support, including 2 research assistantships with full and partial tuition reimbursements available (averaging $10,000 per year), 3 teaching assistantships with full and partial tuition reimbursements available (averaging $10,000 per year); institutionally sponsored loans, scholarships/grants, tuition waivers (full), and unspecified assistantships also available. Support available to part-time students. Financial award application deadline: 2/1; financial award applicants required to submit FAFSA. *Faculty research:* Critical care issues, end of life, childhood immunizations, children with diabetes, global health. *Total annual research expenditures:* $1,200. *Unit head:* Dr. Patricia Ravert, Dean, 801-422-1167, Fax: 801-422-0536, E-mail: patricia_ravert@byu.edu. *Application contact:* Lynette Jakins, Graduate Secretary, 801-422-4142, Fax: 801-422-0538, E-mail: lynette-jakins@byu.edu.
Website: http://nursing.byu.edu/

California Baptist University, Program in Nursing, Riverside, CA 92504-3206. Offers clinical nurse specialist (MSN); family nurse practitioner (MSN); healthcare systems management (MSN); nursing (MSN); teaching-learning (MSN). Part-time programs available. *Faculty:* 15 full-time (all women), 7 part-time/adjunct (all women). *Students:* 49 full-time (41 women), 69 part-time (55 women); includes 61 minority (18 Black or African American, non-Hispanic/Latino; 1 American Indian or Alaska Native, non-Hispanic/Latino; 17 Asian, non-Hispanic/Latino; 22 Hispanic/Latino; 3 Two or more races, non-Hispanic/Latino). Average age 33. 48 applicants, 65% accepted, 20 enrolled. In 2013, 9 master's awarded. *Degree requirements:* For master's, comprehensive exam (for some programs), thesis or alternative, comprehensive exam or directed project thesis; capstone practicum. *Entrance requirements:* For master's, GRE or California Critical Thinking Skills Test; Test of Essential Academic Skills (TEAS), minimum undergraduate GPA of 3.25; Microsoft Office competency; health clearance; health insurance; CPR certification; vehicle insurance; random drug testing; background check clearance; passport photo; three recommendations; comprehensive essay; interview. Additional exam requirements/recommendations for international students: Required—TOEFL (minimum score 80 iBT). *Application deadline:* For fall admission, 8/1 priority date for domestic students, 7/1 for international students; for spring admission, 12/1 priority date for domestic students, 11/1 for international students. Applications are processed on a rolling basis. Application fee: $45. Electronic applications accepted. *Expenses: Tuition:* Full-time $10,080; part-time $560 per unit. *Required fees:* $175 per semester. One-time fee: $45. Tuition and fees vary according to course load and program. *Financial support:* Institutionally sponsored loans available. Financial award applicants required to submit CSS PROFILE or FAFSA. *Faculty research:* Qualitative research using Parse methodology, gerontology, disaster preparedness, medical-surgical nursing, maternal-child nursing. *Unit head:* Dr. Geneva Oaks, Dean, School of Nursing, 951-343-4702, E-mail: goaks@calbaptist.edu. *Application contact:* Dr. Rebecca Meyer, Director, Graduate Program in Nursing, 951-343-4952, Fax: 951-343-5095, E-mail: rmeyer@calbaptist.edu.
Website: http://www.calbaptist.edu/explore-cbu/schools-colleges/school-nursing/master-science-nursing/

California State University, Chico, Office of Graduate Studies, College of Natural Sciences, School of Nursing, Chico, CA 95929-0722. Offers MS. *Accreditation:* AACN. Part-time programs available. Postbaccalaureate distance learning degree programs offered. *Degree requirements:* For master's, project or thesis and oral exam. *Entrance requirements:* For master's, GRE, statement of purpose, course work in statistics in the last seven years, BSN, California nursing license. Additional exam requirements/recommendations for international students: Required—TOEFL (minimum score 550 paper-based; 80 iBT), IELTS (minimum score 6.5), PTE (minimum score 59). Electronic applications accepted.

California State University, Dominguez Hills, College of Health, Human Services and Nursing, Program in Nursing, Carson, CA 90747-0001. Offers MSN. *Accreditation:* AACN. Part-time programs available. Postbaccalaureate distance learning degree programs offered. *Faculty:* 11 full-time (10 women), 16 part-time/adjunct (12 women). *Students:* 64 full-time (58 women), 340 part-time (312 women); includes 234 minority (58 Black or African American, non-Hispanic/Latino; 4 American Indian or Alaska Native, non-Hispanic/Latino; 93 Asian, non-Hispanic/Latino; 67 Hispanic/Latino; 12 Two or more races, non-Hispanic/Latino), 2 international. Average age 39. 281 applicants, 83% accepted, 139 enrolled. In 2013, 121 master's awarded. *Degree requirements:* For master's, comprehensive exam. *Entrance requirements:* For master's, minimum GPA of 2.5, 3.0 in prior coursework in statistics, research, pathophysiology and assessment. Additional exam requirements/recommendations for international students: Required—TOEFL. *Application deadline:* For fall admission, 6/1 for domestic students; for spring admission, 11/1 for domestic students. Applications are processed on a rolling basis. Application fee: $55. Electronic applications accepted. *Expenses:* Tuition, state resident: full-time $6738. Tuition, nonresident: full-time $13,434. *Required fees:* $622. *Faculty research:* AIDS/HIV, health promotion, elderly. *Unit head:* Dr. Cynthia Johnson, Director, 310-243-2522, E-mail: cjohnson@csudh.edu. *Application contact:* 310-243-3426.
Website: http://www.csudh.edu/cps/son/

California State University, Fresno, Division of Graduate Studies, College of Health and Human Services, Department of Nursing, Fresno, CA 93740-8027. Offers nursing (MS), including clinical nurse, primary care nurse practitioner, specialist/nurse educator. *Accreditation:* AACN. Part-time and evening/weekend programs available. *Degree requirements:* For master's, thesis or alternative. *Entrance requirements:* For master's, GRE General Test, 1 year of clinical practice, previous course work in statistics, BSN, minimum GPA of 3.0 in nursing. Additional exam requirements/recommendations for international students: Required—TOEFL. Electronic applications accepted. *Faculty research:* Training grant, HIV assessment.

California State University, Fullerton, Graduate Studies, College of Health and Human Development, Department of Nursing, Fullerton, CA 92834-9480. Offers leadership (MSN); nurse anesthesia (MSN); nurse educator (MSN); nursing (DNP); women's health care (MSN). *Accreditation:* AACN; AANA/CANAEP. Part-time programs available. *Students:* 186 full-time (138 women), 134 part-time (120 women); includes 174 minority (15 Black or African American, non-Hispanic/Latino; 3 American Indian or Alaska Native, non-Hispanic/Latino; 92 Asian, non-Hispanic/Latino; 50 Hispanic/Latino; 2 Native Hawaiian or other Pacific Islander, non-Hispanic/Latino; 12 Two or more races, non-Hispanic/Latino), 3 international. Average age 35. 431 applicants, 38% accepted, 131 enrolled. In 2013, 117 master's awarded. Application fee: $55. *Financial support:* Career-related internships or fieldwork, Federal Work-Study, institutionally sponsored loans, scholarships/grants, and traineeships available. Support available to part-time students. Financial award application deadline: 3/1; financial award applicants required

to submit FAFSA. *Unit head:* Dr. Cindy Greenberg, Chair, 657-278-3336. *Application contact:* Admissions/Applications, 657-278-2371.
Website: http://nursing.fullerton.edu/

California State University, Long Beach, Graduate Studies, College of Health and Human Services, School of Nursing, Long Beach, CA 90840. Offers MSN, DNP, MSN/MPH. DNP offered jointly with California State University, Fullerton and California State University, Los Angeles. *Accreditation:* AACN. Part-time programs available. *Degree requirements:* For master's, thesis optional. *Entrance requirements:* For master's, minimum GPA of 3.0. Electronic applications accepted. *Faculty research:* Newborns of drug-dependent mothers, abuse of residents in nursing homes, interventions in care of Alzheimer's patients.

California State University, Los Angeles, Graduate Studies, College of Health and Human Services, School of Nursing, Los Angeles, CA 90032-8530. Offers health science (MA); nursing (MS). *Accreditation:* AACN. Part-time and evening/weekend programs available. *Faculty:* 21 full-time (18 women), 1 (woman) part-time/adjunct. *Students:* 130 full-time (111 women), 61 part-time (52 women); includes 107 minority (11 Black or African American, non-Hispanic/Latino; 65 Asian, non-Hispanic/Latino; 19 Hispanic/Latino; 2 Native Hawaiian or other Pacific Islander, non-Hispanic/Latino; 10 Two or more races, non-Hispanic/Latino), 18 international. Average age 33. 239 applicants, 25% accepted, 50 enrolled. In 2013, 63 master's awarded. *Degree requirements:* For master's, comprehensive exam, project or thesis. *Entrance requirements:* For master's, minimum GPA of 3.0 in nursing, course work in nursing and statistics. Additional exam requirements/recommendations for international students: Required—TOEFL (minimum score 500 paper-based). *Application deadline:* For fall admission, 5/1 for domestic and international students. Applications are processed on a rolling basis. Application fee: $55. *Financial support:* Federal Work-Study available. Support available to part-time students. Financial award application deadline: 3/1. *Faculty research:* Family stress, geripsychiatric nursing, self-care counseling, holistic nursing, adult health. *Unit head:* Dr. Cynthia Hughes, Director, 323-343-4700, Fax: 323-343-6454, E-mail: chughes2@calstatela.edu. *Application contact:* Dr. Larry Fritz, Dean of Graduate Studies, 323-343-3820, Fax: 323-343-5653, E-mail: lfritz@calstatela.edu.
Website: http://web.calstatela.edu/academic/hhs/nursing/

California State University, Sacramento, Office of Graduate Studies, College of Health and Human Services, Division of Nursing, Sacramento, CA 95819. Offers MS. *Accreditation:* AACN. Part-time programs available. *Degree requirements:* For master's, thesis or project; writing proficiency exam. *Entrance requirements:* For master's, GRE, bachelor's degree in nursing, minimum GPA of 3.0. Additional exam requirements/recommendations for international students: Required—TOEFL. *Application deadline:* For fall admission, 3/1 for domestic and international students; for spring admission, 9/30 for international students. Applications are processed on a rolling basis. Application fee: $55. Electronic applications accepted. *Financial support:* Research assistantships, teaching assistantships, career-related internships or fieldwork, and Federal Work-Study available. Support available to part-time students. Financial award application deadline: 3/1; financial award applicants required to submit FAFSA. *Unit head:* Carolyn Goetze, Chair, 916-278-7543, Fax: 916-278-6311, E-mail: cgoetze@csus.edu. *Application contact:* Jose Martinez, Graduate Admissions Supervisor, 916-278-7871, E-mail: martinj@skymail.csus.edu.
Website: http://www.csus.edu/hhs/nrs/programs/graduate.html

California State University, San Bernardino, Graduate Studies, College of Natural Sciences, Department of Nursing, San Bernardino, CA 92407-2397. Offers MS. *Accreditation:* AACN. *Students:* 14 full-time (13 women), 16 part-time (13 women); includes 8 minority (3 Black or African American, non-Hispanic/Latino; 1 Asian, non-Hispanic/Latino; 3 Hispanic/Latino; 1 Two or more races, non-Hispanic/Latino), 1 international. Average age 38. 17 applicants, 47% accepted, 7 enrolled. In 2013, 6 master's awarded. *Degree requirements:* For master's, thesis optional. *Entrance requirements:* For master's, writing exam, BS, minimum GPA of 3.0, California RN license. Application fee: $55. *Unit head:* Dwight P. Sweeney, Interim Chair, 909-537-5385, Fax: 909-537-7089, E-mail: dsweeney@csusb.edu. *Application contact:* Dr. Jeffrey Thompson, Dean of Graduate Studies, 909-537-5058, E-mail: jthompso@csusb.edu.

California State University, Stanislaus, College of Human and Health Sciences, Program in Nursing (MS), Turlock, CA 95382. Offers gerontological nursing (MS); nursing education (MS). *Accreditation:* AACN. Part-time programs available. *Degree requirements:* For master's, comprehensive exam, thesis or alternative. *Entrance requirements:* For master's, GRE or MAT, minimum GPA of 3.0, 3 letters of reference, RN. Additional exam requirements/recommendations for international students: Required—TOEFL (minimum score 550 paper-based). Electronic applications accepted.

Capella University, School of Public Service Leadership, Doctoral Programs in Nursing, Minneapolis, MN 55402. Offers nursing education (PhD); nursing practice (DNP).

Capella University, School of Public Service Leadership, Master's Programs in Nursing, Minneapolis, MN 55402. Offers diabetes nursing (MSN); general nursing (MSN); gerontology nursing (MSN); health information management (MS); nurse educator (MSN); nursing leadership and administration (MSN).

Capital University, School of Nursing, Columbus, OH 43209-2394. Offers administration (MSN); legal studies (MSN); theological studies (MSN); JD/MSN; MBA/MSN; MSN/MTS. *Accreditation:* AACN. Part-time and evening/weekend programs available. *Degree requirements:* For master's, thesis or alternative. *Entrance requirements:* For master's, BSN, current RN license, minimum GPA of 3.0, undergraduate courses in statistics and research. Additional exam requirements/recommendations for international students: Required—TOEFL (minimum score 550 paper-based). *Expenses:* Contact institution. *Faculty research:* Bereavement, wellness/health promotion, emergency cardiac care, critical thinking, complementary and alternative healthcare.

Cardinal Stritch University, College of Nursing, Milwaukee, WI 53217-3985. Offers MSN. Part-time and evening/weekend programs available. *Degree requirements:* For master's, thesis. *Entrance requirements:* For master's, interview; minimum GPA of 3.0; RN license; 3 letters of recommendation; undergraduate coursework in statistics and nursing research; computer literacy; curriculum vitae. Electronic applications accepted. *Expenses:* Contact institution.

Carlow University, School of Nursing, Doctor of Nursing Practice Program, Pittsburgh, PA 15213-3165. Offers DNP. Part-time and evening/weekend programs available. Postbaccalaureate distance learning degree programs offered (minimal on-campus study). *Students:* 31 full-time (29 women), 23 part-time (20 women); includes 7 minority (4 Black or African American, non-Hispanic/Latino; 1 Asian, non-Hispanic/Latino; 1 Hispanic/Latino; 1 Two or more races, non-Hispanic/Latino). Average age 47. 23 applicants, 100% accepted, 14 enrolled. In 2013, 11 doctorates awarded. *Entrance requirements:* For doctorate, master's degree with minimum GPA of 3.0; BSN; current RN license; official transcripts from all undergraduate and graduate institutions; current curriculum vitae; two letters of recommendation; reflective essay. Additional exam requirements/recommendations for international students: Required—TOEFL (minimum score 550 paper-based). *Application deadline:* For fall admission, 4/1 priority date for domestic students. Application fee: $20. Electronic applications accepted. Application fee is waived when completed online. *Expenses: Tuition:* Full-time $9523; part-time $744 per credit. Tuition and fees vary according to course load, degree level and program. *Unit head:* Dr. Peggy Slota, Director, DNP Program, 412-578-6102, Fax: 412-578-6114, E-mail: mmslota@carlow.edu. *Application contact:* Jo Danhires, Administrative Assistant, Admissions, 412-578-6059, Fax: 412-578-6321, E-mail: gradstudies@carlow.edu.
Website: http://www.carlow.edu/Nursing_Doctoral_Offering.aspx

Carson-Newman University, Department of Nursing, Jefferson City, TN 37760. Offers family nurse practitioner (MSN); nurse educator (MSN). *Accreditation:* AACN. *Faculty:* 2 full-time (both women), 10 part-time/adjunct (9 women). *Students:* 4 full-time (2 women), 55 part-time (45 women); includes 2 minority (1 Black or African American, non-Hispanic/Latino; 1 Two or more races, non-Hispanic/Latino), 1 international. Average age 32. In 2013, 20 master's awarded. *Application deadline:* For fall admission, 7/15 priority date for domestic students. Applications are processed on a rolling basis. Application fee: $50. *Expenses: Tuition:* Part-time $390 per credit hour. *Unit head:* Dr. Gregory A. Casalenuovo, Dean, 865-471-3426. *Application contact:* Graduate Admissions and Services Adviser, 865-473-3468, Fax: 865-472-3475.

Case Western Reserve University, Frances Payne Bolton School of Nursing, Doctor of Nursing Practice Program, Cleveland, OH 44106. Offers acute care nurse practitioner (DNP); adult gerontology nurse practitioner (DNP); educational leadership (DNP); family nurse practitioner (DNP); family systems psychiatric mental health nursing (DNP); midwifery/family nursing (DNP); neonatal nurse practitioner (DNP); pediatric nurse practitioner (DNP); practice leadership (DNP); women's health nurse practitioner (DNP). *Accreditation:* AACN. Part-time programs available. Postbaccalaureate distance learning degree programs offered (minimal on-campus study). *Students:* 169 full-time, 9 part-time; includes 10 minority (6 Black or African American, non-Hispanic/Latino; 1 Asian, non-Hispanic/Latino; 2 Hispanic/Latino; 1 Two or more races, non-Hispanic/Latino). 76 applicants, 97% accepted, 59 enrolled. In 2013, 38 doctorates awarded. Terminal master's awarded for partial completion of doctoral program. *Degree requirements:* For doctorate, thesis/dissertation. *Entrance requirements:* For doctorate, GRE General Test or MAT. Additional exam requirements/recommendations for international students: Required—TOEFL (minimum score 577 paper-based; 90 iBT), IELTS (minimum score 7). *Application deadline:* For fall admission, 6/1 priority date for domestic students, 6/1 for international students; for spring admission, 10/1 for domestic and international students. Applications are processed on a rolling basis. Application fee: $75. *Financial support:* In 2013–14, 90 students received support, including 9 fellowships with full tuition reimbursements available (averaging $31,325 per year), 1 research assistantship with partial tuition reimbursement available (averaging $14,472 per year); teaching assistantships, Federal Work-Study, institutionally sponsored loans, scholarships/grants, and tuition waivers (partial) also available. Support available to part-time students. Financial award application deadline: 5/15; financial award applicants required to submit FAFSA. *Faculty research:* Symptom science, family/community care, aging across the lifespan, self-management of health and illness, neuroscience. *Unit head:* Dr. Donna Dowling, Director, 216-368-1869, Fax: 216-368-3542, E-mail: dad10@case.edu. *Application contact:* Donna Hassik, Admissions Coordinator, 216-368-5253, Fax: 216-368-0124, E-mail: dmh7@case.edu.
Website: http://fpb.case.edu/DNP/

Case Western Reserve University, Frances Payne Bolton School of Nursing, Master's Programs in Nursing, Cleveland, OH 44106. Offers nurse anesthesia (MSN); nurse educator (MSN); nurse midwifery (MSN); nurse practitioner (MSN), including acute care cardiovascular nursing, acute care nurse practitioner, acute care/flight nurse, adult gerontology acute care nurse practitioner, adult gerontology nurse practitioner, adult gerontology oncology and palliative care, family nurse practitioner, family systems psychiatric mental health nursing, neonatal nurse practitioner, pediatric nurse practitioner, women's health nurse practitioner; nursing (MN). Part-time programs available. Postbaccalaureate distance learning degree programs offered (minimal on-campus study). *Faculty:* 54 full-time (50 women), 5 part-time/adjunct (3 women). *Students:* 169 (148 women); includes 12 minority (6 Black or African American, non-Hispanic/Latino; 3 Asian, non-Hispanic/Latino; 3 Hispanic/Latino). Average age 35. 70 applicants, 90% accepted, 33 enrolled. In 2013, 119 master's awarded. *Degree requirements:* For master's, thesis optional. *Entrance requirements:* For master's, GRE General Test or MAT. Additional exam requirements/recommendations for international students: Required—TOEFL (minimum score 577 paper-based; 90 iBT), IELTS (minimum score 7). *Application deadline:* For fall admission, 6/1 for domestic and international students; for spring admission, 10/1 for domestic and international students. Applications are processed on a rolling basis. Application fee: $75. *Financial support:* In 2013–14, 25 teaching assistantships with tuition reimbursements (averaging $15,120 per year) were awarded; fellowships, research assistantships, institutionally sponsored loans, traineeships, and tuition waivers (partial) also available. Support available to part-time students. Financial award application deadline: 6/30; financial award applicants required to submit FAFSA. *Faculty research:* Symptom science, family/community care, aging across the lifespan, self-management of health and illness, neuroscience. *Unit head:* Dr. Carol Savrin, Director, 216-368-5304, Fax: 215-368-3542, E-mail: cls18@case.edu. *Application contact:* Donna Hassik, Admissions Coordinator, 216-368-5253, Fax: 216-368-0124, E-mail: dmh7@case.edu.
Website: http://fpb.case.edu/MSN/

Case Western Reserve University, Frances Payne Bolton School of Nursing and Department of Anthropology, Nursing/Anthropology Program, Cleveland, OH 44106. Offers MSN/MA. *Application deadline:* For fall admission, 6/1 for domestic and international students; for spring admission, 10/1 for domestic and international students. Applications are processed on a rolling basis. Application fee: $75. *Financial support:* Fellowships, research assistantships, and teaching assistantships available. Financial award application deadline: 6/30; financial award applicants required to submit FAFSA. *Unit head:* Dr. Carol Savrin, Head, 216-368-6304, E-mail: cls18@case.edu. *Application contact:* Donna Hassik, Admissions Coordinator, 216-368-5253, Fax: 216-368-0124, E-mail: dmh7@case.edu.
Website: http://fpb.case.edu/MSN/

Case Western Reserve University, Frances Payne Bolton School of Nursing, Nursing/Bioethics Program, Cleveland, OH 44106. Offers MSN/MA. *Students:* 1 full-time (0 women). *Application deadline:* For fall admission, 6/1 for domestic and international students; for spring admission, 10/1 for domestic and international students. Applications are processed on a rolling basis. Application fee: $75. *Financial support:* Fellowships, research assistantships, and teaching assistantships available. Financial award application deadline: 6/30; financial award applicants required to submit FAFSA. *Unit head:* Dr. Barbara Daly, Head, 216-368-5994, E-mail: barbara.daly@case.edu. *Application contact:* Donna Hassik, Admissions Coordinator, 216-368-5253, Fax: 216-368-0124, E-mail: dmh7@case.edu.
Website: http://fpb.case.edu/MSN/

Case Western Reserve University, Frances Payne Bolton School of Nursing, PhD in Nursing Program, Cleveland, OH 44106. Offers PhD. Part-time programs available. Postbaccalaureate distance learning degree programs offered (minimal on-campus study). *Faculty:* 34 full-time (32 women), 6 part-time/adjunct (5 women). *Students:* 33

full-time (27 women), 6 part-time (5 women); includes 17 minority (4 Black or African American, non-Hispanic/Latino; 1 American Indian or Alaska Native, non-Hispanic/Latino; 11 Asian, non-Hispanic/Latino; 1 Hispanic/Latino). Average age 40. 21 applicants, 57% accepted, 7 enrolled. In 2013, 55 doctorates awarded. *Degree requirements:* For doctorate, comprehensive exam, thesis/dissertation, 240-hour research practicum. *Entrance requirements:* For doctorate, GRE General Test. Additional exam requirements/recommendations for international students: Required—TOEFL (minimum score 577 paper-based; 90 iBT), IELTS (minimum score 7). *Application deadline:* For fall admission, 6/1 priority date for domestic students, 6/1 for international students; for spring admission, 10/1 for domestic and international students. Applications are processed on a rolling basis. Application fee: $50. Electronic applications accepted. *Financial support:* In 2013–14, 90 students received support, including 9 fellowships with full tuition reimbursements available (averaging $31,325 per year), 1 research assistantship with partial tuition reimbursement available (averaging $14,472 per year); Federal Work-Study, institutionally sponsored loans, and scholarships/grants also available. Support available to part-time students. Financial award application deadline: 5/15; financial award applicants required to submit FAFSA. *Faculty research:* Cardiopulmonary, gerontology, health services, maternal-child, mental health. *Total annual research expenditures:* $5.1 million. *Unit head:* Dr. Jaclene A. Zauszniewski, Associate Dean, 216-368-3612, E-mail: jaz@case.edu. *Application contact:* Donna Hassik, Admissions Coordinator, Graduate Programs, 216-368-5253, Fax: 216-368-0124, E-mail: donna.hassik@case.edu.
Website: http://fpb.cwru.edu/PhD/

The Catholic University of America, School of Nursing, Washington, DC 20064. Offers MSN, DNP, PhD, Certificate. *Accreditation:* AACN. Part-time programs available. *Faculty:* 18 full-time (17 women), 52 part-time/adjunct (43 women). *Students:* 20 full-time (18 women), 99 part-time (89 women); includes 45 minority (28 Black or African American, non-Hispanic/Latino; 8 Asian, non-Hispanic/Latino; 4 Hispanic/Latino; 5 Two or more races, non-Hispanic/Latino), 5 international. Average age 40. 88 applicants, 84% accepted, 43 enrolled. In 2013, 15 master's, 8 doctorates, 1 other advanced degree awarded. *Degree requirements:* For master's, comprehensive exam, thesis optional; for doctorate, comprehensive exam, thesis/dissertation, minimum GPA of 3.0, oral proposal defense. *Entrance requirements:* For master's, GRE General Test, 3 letters of recommendation, BA in nursing, RN registration, official copies of academic transcripts, some post-baccalaureate nursing experience; for doctorate, GRE General Test, BA in nursing, professional portfolio (including statements, resume, copy of RN license, 3 letters of recommendation, narrative description of clinical practice, proposal), copy of research/scholarly paper related to clinical nursing; for Certificate, GRE General Test. Additional exam requirements/recommendations for international students: Required—TOEFL (minimum score 580 paper-based). *Application deadline:* For fall admission, 8/1 priority date for domestic students, 7/15 for international students; for spring admission, 12/1 priority date for domestic students, 10/15 for international students. Applications are processed on a rolling basis. Application fee: $55. Electronic applications accepted. *Expenses: Tuition:* Full-time $38,500; part-time $1490 per credit hour. *Required fees:* $400; $1525 per credit hour. One-time fee: $425. Tuition and fees vary according to program. *Financial support:* Fellowships, research assistantships, teaching assistantships, Federal Work-Study, scholarships/grants, tuition waivers (full and partial), and unspecified assistantships available. Financial award application deadline: 2/1; financial award applicants required to submit FAFSA. *Faculty research:* Community involvement in health care services, primary health care services, pediatrics, chronic illness, cardiovascular disease. *Total annual research expenditures:* $225,949. *Unit head:* Dr. Patricia McMullen, Dean, 202-319-5403, Fax: 202-319-6485, E-mail: mcmullep@cua.edu. *Application contact:* Andrew Woodall, Director of Graduate Admissions, 202-319-5057, Fax: 202-319-6533, E-mail: cua-admissions@cua.edu.
Website: http://nursing.cua.edu/

Cedar Crest College, Program in Nursing, Allentown, PA 18104-6196. Offers nursing administration (MS); nursing education (MS). Part-time programs available. *Faculty:* 6 full-time (all women). *Students:* 34 part-time (31 women); includes 3 minority (1 Asian, non-Hispanic/Latino; 2 Hispanic/Latino). Average age 44. In 2013, 9 master's awarded. *Expenses: Tuition:* Part-time $661 per credit. *Unit head:* Dr. Wendy Robb, Director, 610-606-4666, E-mail: wjrobb@cedarcrest.edu. *Application contact:* Mary Ellen Hickes, Director of School of Adult and Graduate Education, 610-606-4666, E-mail: sage@cedarcrest.edu.
Website: http://sage.cedarcrest.edu/degrees/graduate/nursing-science/

Central Methodist University, College of Graduate and Extended Studies, Fayette, MO 65248-1198. Offers clinical counseling (MS); clinical nurse leader (MSN); education (M Ed); music education (MME); nurse educator (MSN). Part-time and evening/weekend programs available. Postbaccalaureate distance learning degree programs offered (no on-campus study). *Degree requirements:* For master's, thesis. *Entrance requirements:* For master's, GRE General Test, minimum GPA of 2.75. *Application deadline:* Applications are processed on a rolling basis. Application fee: $25. Electronic applications accepted. *Expenses: Tuition:* Part-time $360 per credit hour. Part-time tuition and fees vary according to campus/location and program. *Financial support:* Tuition waivers available. Support available to part-time students. Financial award application deadline: 6/5; financial award applicants required to submit FAFSA. *Unit head:* Dr. Rita Gulstad, Provost, 660-248-6212, Fax: 660-248-6392, E-mail: rgulstad@centralmethodist.edu. *Application contact:* Aimee Sage, Director of Graduate Admissions, 660-248-6651, Fax: 660-248-6392, E-mail: asage@centralmethodist.edu.
Website: http://www.centralmethodist.edu/graduate/

Chatham University, Nursing Programs, Pittsburgh, PA 15232-2826. Offers education/leadership (MSN); nursing (DNP). *Accreditation:* AACN. Postbaccalaureate distance learning degree programs offered (minimal on-campus study). *Faculty:* 9 full-time (8 women), 8 part-time/adjunct (5 women). *Students:* 38 full-time (31 women), 71 part-time (61 women); includes 28 minority (19 Black or African American, non-Hispanic/Latino; 6 Asian, non-Hispanic/Latino; 3 Hispanic/Latino), 1 international. Average age 46. 186 applicants, 47% accepted, 50 enrolled. In 2013, 27 master's, 51 doctorates awarded. *Entrance requirements:* For master's, RN license, BSN, minimum GPA of 3.0; for doctorate, RN license, MSN. Additional exam requirements/recommendations for international students: Required—TOEFL (minimum score 600 paper-based; 100 iBT), IELTS (minimum score 6.5), TWE. *Application deadline:* For fall admission, 5/1 priority date for domestic and international students. Applications are processed on a rolling basis. Application fee: $0. Electronic applications accepted. Application fee is waived when completed online. *Expenses: Tuition:* Full-time $14,886; part-time $827 per credit hour. One-time fee: $396 full-time. *Financial support:* Applicants required to submit FAFSA. *Unit head:* Dr. Diane Hunker, Director, 412-365-1738, E-mail: dhunker@chatham.edu. *Application contact:* David Vey, Admissions Support Specialist, 412-365-1498, Fax: 412-365-1720, E-mail: dvey@chatham.edu.
Website: http://www.chatham.edu/nursing

Chicago State University, School of Graduate and Professional Studies, College of Health Sciences, Department of Nursing, Chicago, IL 60628. Offers MSN.

Clarion University of Pennsylvania, Office of Transfer, Adult and Graduate Admissions, Master of Science in Nursing Program, Clarion, PA 16214. Offers family nurse practitioner (MSN); nurse educator (MSN). Program offered jointly with Slippery Rock University of Pennsylvania. Part-time programs available. Postbaccalaureate distance learning degree programs offered (no on-campus study). *Faculty:* 4 full-time (all women). *Students:* 36 part-time (33 women); includes 2 minority (1 Asian, non-Hispanic/Latino; 1 Two or more races, non-Hispanic/Latino). Average age 39. 64 applicants, 41% accepted, 26 enrolled. In 2013, 21 master's awarded. *Degree requirements:* For master's, comprehensive exam, thesis. *Entrance requirements:* For master's, minimum QPA of 2.75. Additional exam requirements/recommendations for international students: Required—TOEFL (minimum score 550 paper-based; 80 iBT). *Application deadline:* For fall admission, 6/1 for domestic students, 4/15 priority date for international students; for spring admission, 11/1 for domestic students, 9/15 priority date for international students. Application fee: $40. Electronic applications accepted. *Expenses:* Tuition, state resident: part-time $442 per credit. Tuition, nonresident: part-time $451 per credit. *Required fees:* $142.40 per semester. One-time fee: $150 part-time. *Financial support:* In 2013–14, 1 research assistantship with full and partial tuition reimbursement (averaging $9,420 per year) was awarded; career-related internships or fieldwork and unspecified assistantships also available. Financial award application deadline: 3/1. *Unit head:* Dr. Debbie Ciesielka, Graduate Coordinator, 412-578-7277, E-mail: dciesielka@clarion.edu. *Application contact:* Michelle Ritzler, Graduate Programs, 814-393-2337, E-mail: gradstudies@clarion.edu.
Website: http://www.clarion.edu/991/

Clarke University, Department of Nursing and Health, Dubuque, IA 52001-3198. Offers administration of nursing systems (MSN); advanced practice nursing (MSN); education (MSN); family nurse practitioner (MSN, PMC); nursing (DNP). *Accreditation:* AACN. Part-time programs available. *Faculty:* 10 full-time (9 women). *Students:* 42 full-time (41 women), 16 part-time (15 women). In 2013, 13 master's awarded. *Entrance requirements:* For master's, GRE General Test or MAT, BSN, minimum GPA of 3.0. *Application deadline:* For fall admission, 2/15 priority date for domestic students; for spring admission, 12/15 priority date for domestic students. Applications are processed on a rolling basis. Application fee: $25. Electronic applications accepted. *Expenses: Tuition:* Part-time $660 per credit. *Required fees:* $15 per credit. *Financial support:* In 2013–14, 6 students received support. Career-related internships or fieldwork available. Support available to part-time students. Financial award applicants required to submit FAFSA. *Faculty research:* Narrative pedagogy, ethics, end-of-life care, pedagogy, family systems. *Unit head:* Dr. Jan Lee, Chair, 800-224-2736, Fax: 319-584-8684. *Application contact:* Kara Shroeder, Information Contact, 563-588-6635, Fax: 563-588-6789, E-mail: graduate@clarke.edu.
Website: http://www.clarke.edu/

Clarkson College, Master of Science in Nursing Program, Omaha, NE 68131. Offers adult nurse practitioner (MSN, Post-Master's Certificate); family nurse practitioner (MSN, Post-Master's Certificate); nursing education (MSN, Post-Master's Certificate); nursing health care leadership (MSN, Post-Master's Certificate). *Accreditation:* AANA/CANAEP. Part-time and evening/weekend programs available. Postbaccalaureate distance learning degree programs offered (minimal on-campus study). *Degree requirements:* For master's, on-campus skills assessment (family nurse practitioner, adult nurse practitioner), comprehensive exam or thesis. *Entrance requirements:* For master's, minimum GPA of 3.0, 2 references, resume. Additional exam requirements/recommendations for international students: Required—TOEFL (minimum score 600 paper-based; 100 iBT). Electronic applications accepted.

Clayton State University, School of Graduate Studies, College of Health, Program in Nursing, Morrow, GA 30260-0285. Offers MSN. *Accreditation:* AACN. *Degree requirements:* For master's, thesis. *Entrance requirements:* For master's, GRE, 2 official transcripts, 3 letters of recommendation, statement of purpose, on-campus interview. Additional exam requirements/recommendations for international students: Required—TOEFL (minimum score 550 paper-based; 80 iBT). Electronic applications accepted. *Expenses:* Contact institution.

Clemson University, Graduate School, College of Health, Education, and Human Development, School of Nursing, Clemson, SC 29634. Offers healthcare genetics (PhD); nursing (MS). *Accreditation:* AACN. Part-time programs available. *Faculty:* 13 full-time (12 women). *Students:* 75 full-time (67 women), 35 part-time (30 women); includes 12 minority (4 Black or African American, non-Hispanic/Latino; 2 Asian, non-Hispanic/Latino; 2 Hispanic/Latino; 4 Two or more races, non-Hispanic/Latino), 3 international. Average age 31. 43 applicants, 63% accepted, 22 enrolled. In 2013, 38 master's, 2 doctorates awarded. Terminal master's awarded for partial completion of doctoral program. *Degree requirements:* For master's, comprehensive exam, thesis or alternative; for doctorate, comprehensive exam, thesis/dissertation. *Entrance requirements:* For master's, GRE General Test, RN license; for doctorate, GRE General Test. Additional exam requirements/recommendations for international students: Required—TOEFL. *Application deadline:* For fall admission, 4/1 for domestic and international students; for spring admission, 10/1 for domestic and international students. Application fee: $50. Electronic applications accepted. *Expenses:* Contact institution. *Financial support:* In 2013–14, 27 students received support, including 3 fellowships with partial tuition reimbursements available (averaging $7,333 per year), 1 research assistantship with partial tuition reimbursement available (averaging $9,200 per year), 25 teaching assistantships with partial tuition reimbursements available (averaging $9,612 per year); career-related internships or fieldwork, institutionally sponsored loans, scholarships/grants, health care benefits, and unspecified assistantships also available. Financial award applicants required to submit FAFSA. *Faculty research:* Breast cancer, healthcare, genetics, international healthcare, simulation, educational innovation and technology. *Total annual research expenditures:* $381,705. *Unit head:* Dr. Rosanne Harkey Pruitt, Professor/Director, School of Nursing/Associate Dean, College of Health, Education and Human Development, 864-656-7622, Fax: 864-656-5488, E-mail: prosan@clemson.edu. *Application contact:* Dr. Stephanie Clark Davis, Graduate Studies Coordinator, 864-656-2588, Fax: 864-656-5488, E-mail: stephad@clemson.edu.
Website: http://www.clemson.edu/nursing/

Cleveland State University, College of Graduate Studies, School of Nursing, Cleveland, OH 44115. Offers clinical nurse leader (MSN); forensic nursing (MSN); nursing education (MSN); specialized population (MSN); urban education (PhD), including nursing education; MSN/MBA. *Accreditation:* AACN. Part-time programs available. Postbaccalaureate distance learning degree programs offered (no on-campus study). *Faculty:* 6 full-time (all women), 1 (woman) part-time/adjunct. *Students:* 20 full-time (all women), 28 part-time (26 women); includes 12 minority (8 Black or African American, non-Hispanic/Latino; 3 Hispanic/Latino; 1 Two or more races, non-Hispanic/Latino), 1 international. Average age 38. 65 applicants, 62% accepted, 20 enrolled. In 2013, 6 master's awarded. *Degree requirements:* For master's, thesis optional, portfolio, capstone practicum project; for doctorate, comprehensive exam, thesis/dissertation. *Entrance requirements:* For master's, RN license, BSN with minimum cumulative GPA of 3.0, recent (5 years) course work in statistics; for doctorate, GRE, MSN with minimum cumulative GPA of 3.25. Additional exam requirements/recommendations for international students: Required—TOEFL (minimum score 525 paper-based; 65 iBT), IELTS (minimum score 6). *Application deadline:* For fall admission, 3/1 priority date for domestic and international students. Application fee: $55. Electronic applications accepted. *Expenses:* Tuition, state resident: full-time $8335; part-time $521 per credit

hour. Tuition, nonresident: full-time $15,670; part-time $979 per credit hour. *Required fees:* $50; $25 per semester. *Financial support:* In 2013–14, 4 students received support. Tuition waivers (full) and unspecified assistantships available. Financial award application deadline: 3/1; financial award applicants required to submit FAFSA. *Faculty research:* Diabetes management, African-American elders medication compliance, risk in home visiting, suffering, COPD and stress, nursing education, disaster health preparedness. *Total annual research expenditures:* $330,000. *Unit head:* Dr. Vida Lock, Dean, 216-523-7237, Fax: 216-687-3556, E-mail: v.lock@csuohio.edu. *Application contact:* Maureen Mitchell, Assistant Professor and Graduate Program Director, 216-523-7128, Fax: 216-687-3556, E-mail: m.m.mitchell1@csuohio.edu.
Website: http://www.csuohio.edu/nursing/

College of Mount Saint Vincent, School of Professional and Continuing Studies, Department of Nursing, Riverdale, NY 10471-1093. Offers adult nurse practitioner (MSN, PMC); family nurse practitioner (MSN, PMC); nurse educator (PMC); nursing administration (MSN); nursing for the adult and aged (MSN). *Accreditation:* AACN. Part-time programs available. *Entrance requirements:* For master's, BSN, interview, RN license, minimum GPA of 3.0, letters of reference. Additional exam requirements/recommendations for international students: Required—TOEFL. *Expenses:* Contact institution.

The College of New Jersey, Graduate Studies, School of Nursing, Health and Exercise Science, Program in Nursing, Ewing, NJ 08628. Offers MSN, Certificate. *Accreditation:* AACN. Part-time programs available. *Degree requirements:* For master's, comprehensive exam. *Entrance requirements:* For master's, GRE, minimum GPA of 3.0 in field or 2.75 overall. Additional exam requirements/recommendations for international students: Required—TOEFL. Electronic applications accepted.

The College of New Rochelle, Graduate School, Program in Nursing, New Rochelle, NY 10805-2308. Offers acute care nurse practitioner (MS, Certificate); clinical specialist in holistic nursing (MS, Certificate); family nurse practitioner (MS, Certificate); nursing and health care management (MS); nursing education (Certificate). *Accreditation:* AACN. Part-time programs available. *Faculty:* 6 full-time (5 women), 5 part-time/adjunct (4 women). *Students:* 113 part-time (104 women); includes 56 minority (44 Black or African American, non-Hispanic/Latino; 3 Asian, non-Hispanic/Latino; 9 Hispanic/Latino). Average age 40. In 2013, 17 master's awarded. *Entrance requirements:* For master's, GRE General Test or MAT, BSN, malpractice insurance, minimum GPA of 3.0, RN license. *Application deadline:* For fall admission, 8/15 priority date for domestic students; for spring admission, 12/1 priority date for domestic students. Applications are processed on a rolling basis. Application fee: $35. Electronic applications accepted. *Expenses:* Contact institution. *Financial support:* Traineeships available. Support available to part-time students. Financial award application deadline: 8/15. *Unit head:* Dr. Mary McGuinness, Acting Dean, School of Nursing, 914-654-5441, E-mail: mmcguiness@cnr.edu.

College of Saint Elizabeth, Department of Nursing, Morristown, NJ 07960-6989. Offers MSN. Part-time programs available. *Faculty:* 2 full-time (both women), 3 part-time/adjunct (all women). *Students:* 1 full-time (0 women), 37 part-time (34 women); includes 20 minority (7 Black or African American, non-Hispanic/Latino; 5 Asian, non-Hispanic/Latino; 7 Hispanic/Latino; 1 Native Hawaiian or other Pacific Islander, non-Hispanic/Latino). Average age 45. In 2013, 7 master's awarded. *Entrance requirements:* For master's, interview, minimum cumulative GPA of 3.0. Additional exam requirements/recommendations for international students: Required—TOEFL. Application fee: $35. *Expenses: Tuition:* Full-time $19,152; part-time $1064 per credit. *Unit head:* Dr. Dianne DeLong, Nursing Administrator, 973-290-4037, E-mail: ddelong@cse.edu. *Application contact:* Deborah S. Cobo, Associate Director for Graduate Admissions, 973-290-4194, Fax: 973-290-4710, E-mail: dscobo@cse.edu.
Website: http://www.cse.edu/academics/academic-programs/health-wellness/nursing/

College of Saint Mary, Program in Nursing, Omaha, NE 68106. Offers MSN. Part-time programs available. *Entrance requirements:* For master's, bachelor's degree in nursing, Nebraska RN license, essay or scholarly writing, minimum cumulative GPA of 3.0, 2 references. Additional exam requirements/recommendations for international students: Required—TOEFL.

The College of St. Scholastica, Graduate Studies, Department of Nursing, Duluth, MN 55811. Offers MA, PMC. *Accreditation:* AACN. Part-time programs available. Postbaccalaureate distance learning degree programs offered (minimal on-campus study). *Faculty:* 8 full-time (all women), 6 part-time/adjunct (all women). *Students:* 163 full-time (144 women), 20 part-time (18 women); includes 14 minority (6 Black or African American, non-Hispanic/Latino; 1 American Indian or Alaska Native, non-Hispanic/Latino; 3 Asian, non-Hispanic/Latino; 1 Hispanic/Latino; 1 Native Hawaiian or other Pacific Islander, non-Hispanic/Latino; 2 Two or more races, non-Hispanic/Latino), 1 international. Average age 35. In 2013, 46 master's, 7 other advanced degrees awarded. *Degree requirements:* For master's, thesis. *Entrance requirements:* For master's, GRE General Test. Additional exam requirements/recommendations for international students: Required—TOEFL (minimum score 550 paper-based; 79 iBT). *Application deadline:* For fall admission, 12/15 priority date for domestic students, 2/1 for international students. Applications are processed on a rolling basis. Electronic applications accepted. Tuition and fees vary according to course load, program and student level. *Financial support:* In 2013–14, 99 students received support. Scholarships/grants available. Support available to part-time students. Financial award applicants required to submit FAFSA. *Faculty research:* Critical thinking and professional development, social organization of responsibility, rural health HIV/AIDS prevention, Web-based instruction in nursing. *Unit head:* Director. *Application contact:* Lindsay Lahti, Director of Graduate and Extended Studies Recruitment, 218-733-2240, Fax: 218-733-2275, E-mail: gradstudies@css.edu.
Website: http://www.css.edu/Graduate/Masters-Doctoral-and-Professional-Programs/Areas-of-Study/Bachelors-to-DNP.html

College of Staten Island of the City University of New York, Graduate Programs, Department of Nursing, Staten Island, NY 10314-6600. Offers adult health nursing (MS, Post-Master's Certificate); cultural competence (Advanced Certificate); gerontological nursing (MS, Post-Master's Certificate); nursing education (Post-Master's Certificate). *Faculty:* 4 full-time (all women), 5 part-time/adjunct (4 women). *Students:* 74 part-time (66 women). Average age 40. 41 applicants, 59% accepted, 19 enrolled. In 2013, 10 master's, 4 other advanced degrees awarded. *Entrance requirements:* Additional exam requirements/recommendations for international students: Required—TOEFL (minimum score 550 paper-based; 79 iBT). Application fee: $125. *Expenses:* Tuition, state resident: full-time $9240; part-time $385 per credit hour. Tuition, nonresident: full-time $17,040; part-time $710 per credit hour. *Required fees:* $428; $128 per term. *Unit head:* Dr. Mary O'Donnell, Chairperson, 718-982-3812, Fax: 718-982-3813, E-mail: mary.odonnell@csi.cuny.edu. *Application contact:* Sasha Spence, Assistant Director for Graduate Recruitment and Admissions, 718-982-2019, Fax: 718-982-2500, E-mail: sasha.spence@csi.cuny.edu.
Website: http://www.csi.cuny.edu/nursing/graduate.html

Colorado State University–Pueblo, College of Education, Engineering and Professional Studies, Nursing Department, Pueblo, CO 81001-4901. Offers MS. *Degree requirements:* For master's, comprehensive exam or thesis. *Entrance requirements:* Additional exam requirements/recommendations for international students: Required—TOEFL.

Columbia University, School of Nursing, New York, NY 10032. Offers MS, DNP, PhD, Adv C, MBA/MS, MPH/MS. *Accreditation:* AACN. Part-time programs available. *Degree requirements:* For doctorate, thesis/dissertation. *Entrance requirements:* For master's, GRE General Test, bachelor's degree, 1 year of clinical experience (preferred for most, required for some); for doctorate, GRE General Test. Additional exam requirements/recommendations for international students: Required—TOEFL. Electronic applications accepted. *Expenses:* Contact institution. *Faculty research:* HIV/AIDS, health promotion/disease prevention, health policies, advanced practice, urban health.

Columbus State University, Graduate Studies, College of Education and Health Professions, School of Nursing, Columbus, GA 31907-5645. Offers MSN. Program offered in collaboration with Georgia Southwestern University. *Faculty:* 3 full-time (all women). *Students:* 2 full-time (both women), 15 part-time (14 women); includes 6 minority (5 Black or African American, non-Hispanic/Latino; 1 Two or more races, non-Hispanic/Latino). Average age 40. 19 applicants, 89% accepted, 9 enrolled. *Entrance requirements:* For master's, GRE, BSN, minimum undergraduate GPA of 3.0. Additional exam requirements/recommendations for international students: Required—TOEFL (minimum score 550 paper-based; 79 iBT). *Application deadline:* For fall admission, 5/1 for domestic and international students; for spring admission, 11/1 for domestic and international students; for summer admission, 3/1 for domestic and international students. Application fee: $40. *Expenses:* Tuition, state resident: full-time $4572; part-time $382 per credit hour. Tuition, nonresident: full-time $18,292; part-time $1526 per credit hour. *Required fees:* $1800; $196 per credit hour. Tuition and fees vary according to campus/location and program. *Financial support:* In 2013–14, 8 students received support. Applicants required to submit FAFSA. *Unit head:* Cheryl Smith, Interim Director, 706-507-8578, E-mail: smith_cheryl6@columbusstate.edu. *Application contact:* Kristin Williams, Director of International and Graduate Recruitment, 706-507-8848, Fax: 706-568-5091, E-mail: williams_kristin@columbusstate.edu.
Website: http://nursing.columbusstate.edu/

Concordia University Wisconsin, Graduate Programs, School of Human Services, Program in Nursing, Mequon, WI 53097-2402. Offers family nurse practitioner (MSN); geriatric nurse practitioner (MSN); nurse educator (MSN). *Accreditation:* AACN. Postbaccalaureate distance learning degree programs offered (minimal on-campus study). *Degree requirements:* For master's, comprehensive exam, thesis or alternative. *Entrance requirements:* Additional exam requirements/recommendations for international students: Required—TOEFL. *Expenses:* Contact institution.

Coppin State University, Division of Graduate Studies, Helene Fuld School of Nursing, Baltimore, MD 21216-3698. Offers family nurse practitioner (PMC); nursing (MSN). Part-time and evening/weekend programs available. *Degree requirements:* For master's, comprehensive exam, thesis, clinical internship. *Entrance requirements:* For master's, GRE, bachelor's degree in nursing, interview, minimum GPA of 3.0, RN license. Additional exam requirements/recommendations for international students: Required—TOEFL (minimum score 550 paper-based).

Cox College, Programs in Nursing, Springfield, MO 65802. Offers clinical nurse leader (MSN); family nurse practitioner (MSN); nurse educator (MSN). *Accreditation:* AACN. *Entrance requirements:* For master's, RN license, essay, 2 letters of recommendation, official transcripts. Electronic applications accepted.

Creighton University, College of Nursing, Omaha, NE 68178-0001. Offers MSN, DNP. *Accreditation:* AACN. Part-time programs available. Postbaccalaureate distance learning degree programs offered (minimal on-campus study). *Faculty:* 9 full-time (all women), 11 part-time/adjunct (8 women). *Students:* 107 full-time (97 women), 175 part-time (165 women); includes 19 minority (6 Black or African American, non-Hispanic/Latino; 1 American Indian or Alaska Native, non-Hispanic/Latino; 9 Asian, non-Hispanic/Latino; 2 Hispanic/Latino; 1 Native Hawaiian or other Pacific Islander, non-Hispanic/Latino). Average age 33. 108 applicants, 84% accepted, 75 enrolled. In 2013, 42 master's, 21 doctorates awarded. Terminal master's awarded for partial completion of doctoral program. *Degree requirements:* For master's, thesis optional, capstone project; for doctorate, thesis/dissertation, scholarly research project. *Entrance requirements:* For master's, BSN, minimum GPA of 3.0, RN license; for doctorate, BSN or MSN, minimum GPA of 3.0, RN license. Additional exam requirements/recommendations for international students: Required—TOEFL (minimum score 600 paper-based; 100 iBT). *Application deadline:* For fall admission, 6/15 priority date for domestic and international students; for spring admission, 11/15 priority date for domestic and international students; for summer admission, 4/15 for domestic and international students. Applications are processed on a rolling basis. Application fee: $50. Electronic applications accepted. *Expenses: Tuition:* Full-time $13,608; part-time $756 per credit hour. *Required fees:* $149 per semester. Tuition and fees vary according to course load, campus/location, program, reciprocity agreements and student's religious affiliation. *Financial support:* Career-related internships or fieldwork, Federal Work-Study, institutionally sponsored loans, and traineeships available. Financial award applicants required to submit FAFSA. *Faculty research:* Obesity prevention in children, evaluation of simulated clinical experiences, vitamin D3 and calcium for cancer risk education in post menopausal women, online support and education to reduce stress for prenatal patients on bed rest, behavioral counseling to increase physical activity in women. *Unit head:* Dr. Cindy Costanzo, RN, Interim Dean, 402-280-2004, Fax: 402-280-2045. *Application contact:* Shannon R. Cox, Senior Admissions Counselor, 402-280-2067, Fax: 402-280-2045, E-mail: shannoncox@creighton.edu.
Website: http://www.creighton.edu/nursing/

Curry College, Graduate Studies, Program in Nursing, Milton, MA 02186-9984. Offers MSN. *Accreditation:* AACN.

Daemen College, Department of Nursing, Amherst, NY 14226-3592. Offers adult nurse practitioner (MS, Post Master's Certificate); nurse executive leadership (Post Master's Certificate); nursing education (MS, Post Master's Certificate); nursing executive leadership (MS); nursing practice (DNP); palliative care nursing (Post Master's Certificate). Part-time programs available. *Degree requirements:* For master's, thesis or alternative, degree completed in 4 years; minimum GPA of 3.0; for doctorate, degree completed in 5 years; 500 post-master's clinical hours. *Entrance requirements:* For master's, BN, 1 year medical/surgical experience, RN license and state registration, statistics course with minimum C grade, 3 letters of recommendation, minimum GPA of 3.25, interview; for doctorate, MS in advance nursing practice; New York state RN license; goal statement; resume; interview; statistics course with minimum grade of 'C'; for Post Master's Certificate, master's degree in clinical area; RN license and current registration; one year of clinical experience; statistics course with minimum grade of 'C'; 3 letters of recommendation; interview; letter of intent. Additional exam requirements/recommendations for international students: Required—TOEFL (minimum score 500 paper-based; 63 iBT), IELTS (minimum score 5.5). Electronic applications accepted. *Faculty research:* Professional stress, client behavior, drug therapy, treatment modalities and pulmonary cancers, chemical dependency.

Dalhousie University, Faculty of Health Professions, School of Nursing, Halifax, NS B3H 3J5, Canada. Offers MN, PhD, MN/MHSA. Part-time programs available. Postbaccalaureate distance learning degree programs offered (minimal on-campus study). *Degree requirements:* For master's, thesis optional. *Entrance requirements:* For master's, minimum GPA of 3.0; for doctorate, written support of faculty member who has agreed to be thesis supervisor. Additional exam requirements/recommendations for international students: Required—TOEFL, IELTS, CANTEST, CAEL, or Michigan English Language Assessment Battery. Electronic applications accepted. *Faculty research:* Coping, social support, health promotion, aging, feminist studies.

Delaware State University, Graduate Programs, College of Education, Health and Public Policy, Department of Nursing, Dover, DE 19901-2277. Offers MS. *Entrance requirements:* Additional exam requirements/recommendations for international students: Required—TOEFL (minimum score 550 paper-based). Electronic applications accepted.

Delta State University, Graduate Programs, School of Nursing, Cleveland, MS 38733. Offers family nurse practitioner (MSN); nurse administrator (MSN); nurse educator (MSN). *Accreditation:* AACN. Part-time programs available. *Faculty:* 5 full-time (all women), 1 (woman) part-time/adjunct. *Students:* 35 full-time (31 women), 8 part-time (7 women); includes 10 minority (all Black or African American, non-Hispanic/Latino). Average age 41. 23 applicants, 100% accepted, 19 enrolled. In 2013, 13 master's awarded. *Degree requirements:* For master's, thesis optional. *Entrance requirements:* For master's, GRE General Test. *Application deadline:* For fall admission, 8/1 priority date for domestic students; for spring admission, 12/1 priority date for domestic students. Applications are processed on a rolling basis. Application fee: $0. Electronic applications accepted. *Expenses:* Tuition, state resident: full-time $3006; part-time $334 per credit hour. Tuition, nonresident: full-time $3006; part-time $334 per credit hour. *Financial support:* Research assistantships, career-related internships or fieldwork, Federal Work-Study, and institutionally sponsored loans available. Financial award application deadline: 6/1. *Unit head:* Dr. Lizabeth Carlson, Dean, 662-846-4268, Fax: 662-846-4267, E-mail: lcarlson@deltastate.edu. *Application contact:* Dr. Albert Nylander, Dean of Graduate Studies, 662-846-4875, Fax: 662-846-4313, E-mail: grad-info@deltastate.edu.
Website: http://www.deltastate.edu/pages/252.asp

DePaul University, College of Science and Health, Chicago, IL 60614. Offers applied mathematics (MS); applied statistics (MS); biological sciences (MA, MS); chemistry (MS); mathematics education (MA); mathematics for teaching (MS); nursing (MS); nursing practice (DNP); physics (MS); psychology (MS); pure mathematics (MS); science education (MS); MA/PhD. *Faculty:* 66 full-time (40 women), 23 part-time/adjunct (21 women). *Students:* 485 full-time (338 women), 207 part-time (132 women); includes 198 minority (55 Black or African American, non-Hispanic/Latino; 1 American Indian or Alaska Native, non-Hispanic/Latino; 64 Asian, non-Hispanic/Latino; 53 Hispanic/Latino; 2 Native Hawaiian or other Pacific Islander, non-Hispanic/Latino; 23 Two or more races, non-Hispanic/Latino), 48 international. Average age 29. In 2013, 244 master's, 20 doctorates awarded. *Application deadline:* Applications are processed on a rolling basis. Application fee: $40. Electronic applications accepted. Tuition and fees vary according to course level, course load and degree level. *Financial support:* Applicants required to submit FAFSA. *Application contact:* Ann Spittle, Director of Graduate Admission, 773-325-7315, Fax: 312-476-3244, E-mail: graddepaul@depaul.edu.
Website: http://csh.depaul.edu/

DeSales University, Graduate Division, Division of Healthcare and Natural Sciences, Center Valley, PA 18034-9568. Offers adult clinical nurse specialist (MSN); certified nurse midwives (MSN); certified nurse practitioners (MSN); clinical leadership (DNP); family nurse practitioner (MSN); information systems (MSIS); nurse educator (MSN); nurse practitioner (Post-Master's Certificate); physical therapy (DPT); physician assistant studies (MSPAS); MSN/MBA. Part-time programs available. In 2013, 5 doctorates awarded. *Degree requirements:* For master's, thesis optional. *Entrance requirements:* For master's, GRE General Test, MAT, minimum B average in undergraduate course work, health assessment course or equivalent, course work in statistics. Additional exam requirements/recommendations for international students: Required—TOEFL. *Application deadline:* Applications are processed on a rolling basis. Application fee: $35. Electronic applications accepted. *Expenses: Tuition:* Part-time $790 per credit. *Financial support:* Applicants required to submit FAFSA. *Unit head:* Dr. Mary Liz Doyle-Tadduni, Department Chair, Nursing, 610-282-1100 Ext. 1394, Fax: 610-282-2091, E-mail: carol.mest@desales.edu. *Application contact:* Abagail Wernicki, Director of Graduate Admissions, 610-282-1100 Ext. 1768, Fax: 610-282-2869, E-mail: abagail.wernicki@desales.edu.

Drexel University, College of Nursing and Health Professions, Division of Graduate Nursing, Philadelphia, PA 19104-2875. Offers adult acute care (MSN); adult psychiatric/mental health (MSN); advanced practice nursing (MSN); clinical trials research (MSN); family nurse practitioner (MSN); leadership in health systems management (MSN); nursing education (MSN); pediatric primary care (MSN); women's health (MSN). *Accreditation:* AACN. Electronic applications accepted.

Drexel University, College of Nursing and Health Professions, Doctor of Nursing Practice Program, Philadelphia, PA 19104-2875. Offers Dr NP.

Duke University, School of Nursing, Ph D Program in Nursing, Durham, NC 27708-0586. Offers PhD. *Faculty:* 36 full-time (30 women). *Students:* 13 full-time (12 women), 7 part-time (6 women); includes 6 minority (3 Black or African American, non-Hispanic/Latino; 3 Asian, non-Hispanic/Latino), 5 international. Average age 32. 25 applicants, 44% accepted, 8 enrolled. In 2013, 4 doctorates awarded. *Degree requirements:* For doctorate, comprehensive exam, thesis/dissertation. *Entrance requirements:* For doctorate, GRE General Test, resume, personal statement, minimum cumulative undergraduate GPA of 3.0, recommendations, previous work in nursing, research course, graduate level statistics course. Additional exam requirements/recommendations for international students: Recommended—TOEFL (minimum score 550 paper-based; 83 iBT), IELTS (minimum score 7). *Application deadline:* For fall admission, 12/8 priority date for domestic students, 12/1 priority date for international students; for spring admission, 5/1 priority date for domestic and international students. Application fee: $80. Electronic applications accepted. *Financial support:* Institutionally sponsored loans, scholarships/grants, and health care benefits available. *Faculty research:* Nursing management practices, adolescents and families undergoing intense treatments, psychosocial and chronic disease. *Unit head:* Dr. Debra H. Brandon, Director, PhD in Nursing Program, 919-684-3813, Fax: 919-681-8899, E-mail: debra.brandon@duke.edu. *Application contact:* Revonda P. Huppert, Program Coordinator, 919-668-4797, Fax: 919-681-8899, E-mail: revonda.huppert@duke.edu.
Website: http://www.nursing.duke.edu

Duquesne University, School of Nursing, Doctor of Nursing Practice Program, Pittsburgh, PA 15282-0001. Offers DNP. Part-time and evening/weekend programs available. Postbaccalaureate distance learning degree programs offered (minimal on-campus study). *Faculty:* 19 full-time (17 women), 2 part-time/adjunct (both women). *Students:* 56 full-time (55 women), 3 part-time (all women); includes 4 minority (3 Black or African American, non-Hispanic/Latino; 1 Hispanic/Latino). Average age 49. 60 applicants, 53% accepted, 25 enrolled. In 2013, 16 doctorates awarded. *Degree requirements:* For doctorate, thesis/dissertation, capstone project. *Entrance requirements:* For doctorate, current RN license; BSN; MSN with minimum GPA of 3.5; current certifications; phone interview. Additional exam requirements/recommendations for international students: Required—TOEFL (minimum score 600 paper-based; 80 iBT). *Application deadline:* For fall admission, 2/1 for domestic and international students. Application fee: $0. Electronic applications accepted. *Expenses: Tuition:* Full-time $18,162; part-time $1009 per credit. *Required fees:* $1728; $96 per credit. Tuition and fees vary according to program. *Financial support:* In 2013–14, 34 students received support, including 5 research assistantships with partial tuition reimbursements available (averaging $1,285 per year); teaching assistantships with partial tuition reimbursements available, institutionally sponsored loans, scholarships/grants, traineeships, and unspecified assistantships also available. Support available to part-time students. Financial award application deadline: 7/1; financial award applicants required to submit FAFSA. *Faculty research:* Vulnerable populations, social justice, cultural competence, health disparities, wellness within chronic illness. *Unit head:* Dr. Joan Such Lockhart, Professor and Associate Dean of Academic Affairs, 412-396-6540, Fax: 412-396-1821, E-mail: lockhart@duq.edu. *Application contact:* Susan Hardner, Nurse Recruiter, 412-396-4945, Fax: 412-396-6346, E-mail: nursing@duq.edu.
Website: http://www.duq.edu/academics/schools/nursing/graduate-programs/doctor-of-nursing-practice

Duquesne University, School of Nursing, Doctor of Philosophy in Nursing Program, Pittsburgh, PA 15282-0001. Offers PhD. Part-time and evening/weekend programs available. Postbaccalaureate distance learning degree programs offered (minimal on-campus study). *Faculty:* 15 full-time (13 women), 2 part-time/adjunct (1 woman). *Students:* 32 full-time (28 women), 25 part-time (23 women); includes 13 minority (7 Black or African American, non-Hispanic/Latino; 1 Asian, non-Hispanic/Latino; 4 Hispanic/Latino; 1 Two or more races, non-Hispanic/Latino), 1 international. Average age 49. 37 applicants, 35% accepted, 12 enrolled. In 2013, 7 doctorates awarded. *Degree requirements:* For doctorate, thesis/dissertation, preliminary exam. *Entrance requirements:* For doctorate, current RN license; BSN; master's degree with minimum GPA of 3.5; phone interview. Additional exam requirements/recommendations for international students: Required—TOEFL (minimum score 600 paper-based; 80 iBT). *Application deadline:* For fall admission, 1/15 for domestic and international students. Application fee: $0. Electronic applications accepted. *Expenses: Tuition:* Full-time $18,162; part-time $1009 per credit. *Required fees:* $1728; $96 per credit. Tuition and fees vary according to program. *Financial support:* In 2013–14, 33 students received support, including 6 research assistantships with partial tuition reimbursements available (averaging $1,285 per year), teaching assistantships with partial tuition reimbursements available (averaging $1,170 per year); institutionally sponsored loans, scholarships/grants, traineeships, and unspecified assistantships also available. Support available to part-time students. Financial award application deadline: 7/1; financial award applicants required to submit FAFSA. *Faculty research:* Vulnerable populations, social justice, cultural competence, health disparities, wellness within chronic illness. *Total annual research expenditures:* $149,737. *Unit head:* Dr. Joan Such Lockhart, Professor and Associate Dean of Academic Affairs, 412-396-6540, Fax: 412-396-1821, E-mail: lockhart@duq.edu. *Application contact:* Susan Hardner, Nurse Recruiter, 412-396-4945, Fax: 412-396-6346, E-mail: nursing@duq.edu.
Website: http://www.duq.edu/academics/schools/nursing/graduate-programs/phd-in-nursing

Duquesne University, School of Nursing, Master of Science in Nursing Program, Pittsburgh, PA 15282-0001. Offers family (individual across the life span) nurse practitioner (MSN); forensic nursing (MSN); nursing education (MSN). *Accreditation:* AACN. Part-time and evening/weekend programs available. Postbaccalaureate distance learning degree programs offered (minimal on-campus study). *Faculty:* 20 full-time (18 women), 4 part-time/adjunct (all women). *Students:* 73 full-time (67 women), 54 part-time (53 women); includes 23 minority (8 Black or African American, non-Hispanic/Latino; 1 American Indian or Alaska Native, non-Hispanic/Latino; 4 Asian, non-Hispanic/Latino; 5 Hispanic/Latino; 5 Two or more races, non-Hispanic/Latino), 1 international. Average age 35. 206 applicants, 35% accepted, 55 enrolled. In 2013, 28 master's awarded. *Degree requirements:* For master's, culminating paper. *Entrance requirements:* For master's, current RN license; BSN with minimum GPA of 3.0; minimum of 1 year full-time work experience as RN prior to registration in clinical or specialty course. Additional exam requirements/recommendations for international students: Required—TOEFL (minimum score 600 paper-based; 80 iBT). *Application deadline:* For fall admission, 3/1 for domestic and international students. Application fee: $0. Electronic applications accepted. *Expenses: Tuition:* Full-time $18,162; part-time $1009 per credit. *Required fees:* $1728; $96 per credit. Tuition and fees vary according to program. *Financial support:* In 2013–14, 5 students received support, including 3 teaching assistantships with partial tuition reimbursements available (averaging $1,285 per year); research assistantships with partial tuition reimbursements available, scholarships/grants, traineeships, and tuition waivers (partial) also available. Support available to part-time students. Financial award application deadline: 7/1; financial award applicants required to submit FAFSA. *Faculty research:* Vulnerable populations, social justice, cultural competence, health disparities, wellness within chronic illness. *Unit head:* Dr. Joan Such Lockhart, Professor and Associate Dean of Academic Affairs, 412-396-6540, Fax: 412-396-1821, E-mail: lockhart@duq.edu. *Application contact:* Susan Hardner, Nurse Recruiter, 412-396-4945, Fax: 412-396-6346, E-mail: nursing@duq.edu.
Website: http://www.duq.edu/academics/schools/nursing/graduate-programs/master-science-nursing

Duquesne University, School of Nursing, Post Master's Certificate Program, Pittsburgh, PA 15282-0001. Offers family (individual across the life span) nurse practitioner (Post-Master's Certificate); forensic nursing (Post-Master's Certificate). Part-time and evening/weekend programs available. Postbaccalaureate distance learning degree programs offered (minimal on-campus study). *Faculty:* 10 full-time (9 women), 4 part-time/adjunct (all women). *Students:* 11 part-time (all women); includes 2 minority (1 Black or African American, non-Hispanic/Latino; 1 Hispanic/Latino). Average age 41. 19 applicants, 26% accepted, 4 enrolled. In 2013, 1 Post-Master's Certificate awarded. *Entrance requirements:* For degree, current RN license, BSN, MSN. Additional exam requirements/recommendations for international students: Required—TOEFL (minimum score 600 paper-based; 80 iBT). *Application deadline:* For fall admission, 3/1 for domestic and international students. Application fee: $0. *Expenses: Tuition:* Full-time $18,162; part-time $1009 per credit. *Required fees:* $1728; $96 per credit. Tuition and fees vary according to program. *Financial support:* Teaching assistantships with partial tuition reimbursements, scholarships/grants, traineeships, and tuition waivers (partial) available. Support available to part-time students. Financial award application deadline: 7/1; financial award applicants required to submit FAFSA. *Faculty research:* Vulnerable populations, social justice, cultural competence, health disparities, wellness within chronic illness. *Unit head:* Dr. Joan Such Lockhart, Professor and Associate Dean of Academic Affairs, 412-396-6540, Fax: 412-396-1821, E-mail: lockhart@duq.edu. *Application contact:* Susan Hardner, Nurse Recruiter, 412-396-4945, Fax: 412-396-6346, E-mail: nursing@duq.edu.
Website: http://www.duq.edu/academics/schools/nursing/graduate-programs/post-masters-certificates

D'Youville College, School of Nursing, Buffalo, NY 14201-1084. Offers advanced practice nursing (DNP); community health nursing/education (MSN); community health nursing/management (MSN); family nurse practitioner (MSN, Certificate); nursing and

health-related professions education (Certificate). *Accreditation:* AACN. Part-time programs available. *Students:* 51 full-time (45 women), 136 part-time (115 women); includes 25 minority (17 Black or African American, non-Hispanic/Latino; 1 American Indian or Alaska Native, non-Hispanic/Latino; 1 Asian, non-Hispanic/Latino; 6 Hispanic/Latino), 76 international. Average age 35. 261 applicants, 36% accepted, 73 enrolled. In 2013, 51 master's, 3 other advanced degrees awarded. *Degree requirements:* For master's, thesis or alternative, membership on board of community agency, publishable paper. *Entrance requirements:* For master's, BS in nursing, minimum GPA of 3.0, course work in statistics and computers. Additional exam requirements/recommendations for international students: Required—TOEFL (minimum score 500 paper-based). *Application deadline:* For fall admission, 5/1 priority date for international students; for spring admission, 9/1 priority date for international students. Applications are processed on a rolling basis. Application fee: $25. Electronic applications accepted. *Financial support:* Federal Work-Study, scholarships/grants, traineeships, and unspecified assistantships available. Support available to part-time students. Financial award application deadline: 3/1; financial award applicants required to submit FAFSA. *Faculty research:* Nursing curriculum, nursing theory-testing, wellness research, communication and socialization patterns. *Unit head:* Dr. Ann Caughill, Chair, 716-829-7892, Fax: 716-829-8159. *Application contact:* Mark Pavone, Graduate Admissions Director, 716-829-8400, Fax: 716-829-7900, E-mail: graduateadmissions@dyc.edu.
Website: http://www.dyc.edu/academics/nursing/

See Display below and Close-Up on page 815.

East Carolina University, Graduate School, College of Nursing, Greenville, NC 27858-4353. Offers MSN, DNP, PhD, PMC. *Accreditation:* AACN; AANA/CANAEP (one or more programs are accredited); ACNM/ACME (one or more programs are accredited). Part-time programs available. *Degree requirements:* For master's, comprehensive exam, thesis optional. *Entrance requirements:* For master's, GRE General Test or MAT, bachelor's degree in nursing, professional license, minimum B average in nursing. *Application deadline:* For fall admission, 6/1 priority date for domestic students. Applications are processed on a rolling basis. Application fee: $50. *Expenses:* Tuition, state resident: full-time $4223. Tuition, nonresident: full-time $16,540. *Required fees:* $2184. *Financial support:* Research assistantships with partial tuition reimbursements, teaching assistantships with partial tuition reimbursements, and Federal Work-Study available. Support available to part-time students. Financial award application deadline: 6/1. *Unit head:* Dr. Sylvia Brown, Dean, 252-744-6372, E-mail: brownsy@ecu.edu. *Application contact:* Dean of Graduate School, 252-328-6012, Fax: 252-328-6071, E-mail: gradschool@ecu.edu.
Website: http://www.nursing.ecu.edu/home.htm

Eastern Kentucky University, The Graduate School, College of Health Sciences, Department of Nursing, Richmond, KY 40475-3102. Offers rural community health care (MSN); rural health family nurse practitioner (MSN). *Accreditation:* AACN. *Entrance requirements:* For master's, GRE General Test, minimum GPA of 2.75.

Eastern Mennonite University, Program in Nursing, Harrisonburg, VA 22802-2462. Offers leadership and management (MSN); leadership/school nursing (MSN). *Accreditation:* AACN. Part-time programs available. Postbaccalaureate distance learning degree programs offered (minimal on-campus study). *Degree requirements:* For master's, leadership project. *Entrance requirements:* For master's, RN license, one year of full-time work experience as RN, minimum GPA of 3.0. Additional exam requirements/recommendations for international students: Required—TOEFL. *Faculty research:* Community health, international health, effectiveness of the nursing school environment, development of caring ability in nursing students, international nursing students.

Eastern New Mexico University, Graduate School, College of Liberal Arts and Sciences, Department of Health and Human Services, Portales, NM 88130. Offers nursing (MSN); speech pathology and audiology (MS). *Accreditation:* ASHA. Part-time programs available. Postbaccalaureate distance learning degree programs offered (minimal on-campus study). *Degree requirements:* For master's, thesis optional, oral and written comprehensive exam, oral presentation of professional portfolio. *Entrance requirements:* For master's, GRE, three letters of recommendation, resume, two essays. Additional exam requirements/recommendations for international students: Required—TOEFL (minimum score 550 paper-based; 79 iBT), IELTS (minimum score 6). Electronic applications accepted.

Edgewood College, Henry Predolin School of Nursing, Madison, WI 53711. Offers MS, DNP. *Accreditation:* AACN. *Students:* 8 full-time (all women), 56 part-time (55 women); includes 3 minority (1 Asian, non-Hispanic/Latino; 1 Hispanic/Latino; 1 Two or more races, non-Hispanic/Latino), 2 international. Average age 37. In 2013, 15 master's awarded. *Degree requirements:* For master's, practicum, research project; for doctorate, practicum, capstone project. *Entrance requirements:* For master's, minimum GPA of 3.0, 2 letters of reference, current RN license. Additional exam requirements/recommendations for international students: Required—TOEFL. *Application deadline:* For fall admission, 8/15 priority date for domestic students, 5/1 for international students; for spring admission, 1/8 priority date for domestic students, 11/1 for international students. Applications are processed on a rolling basis. Application fee: $30. Electronic applications accepted. *Unit head:* Dr. Margaret Noreuil, Dean, 608-663-2820, Fax: 608-663-3291, E-mail: mnoreuil@edgewood.edu. *Application contact:* Tracy Kantor, Enrollment and Applications Manager, 608-663-3297, Fax: 608-663-3496, E-mail: gps@edgewood.edu.
Website: http://www.edgewood.edu/Academics/School-of-Nursing

Edinboro University of Pennsylvania, Department of Nursing, Edinboro, PA 16444. Offers advanced practice nursing (DNP); family nurse practitioner (MSN); nurse educator (MSN). Part-time and evening/weekend programs available. *Degree requirements:* For master's, thesis, competency exam. *Entrance requirements:* For master's, GRE or MAT, minimum QPA of 2.5. *Application deadline:* Applications are processed on a rolling basis. Application fee: $30. Electronic applications accepted. *Expenses:* Tuition, state resident: part-time $454 per credit hour. Tuition, nonresident: part-time $681 per credit hour. *Required fees:* $143.55 per credit hour. Part-time tuition and fees vary according to campus/location and program. *Financial support:* Research assistantships with full and partial tuition reimbursements, career-related internships or fieldwork, Federal Work-Study, scholarships/grants, and unspecified assistantships available. Support available to part-time students. Financial award application deadline: 2/15; financial award applicants required to submit FAFSA. *Unit head:* Dr. Thomas White, Chairperson, 814-732-2900, E-mail: twhite@edinboro.edu. *Application contact:* Dr. Thomas White, Chairperson, 814-732-2900, E-mail: twhite@edinboro.edu.
Website: http://www.edinboro.edu/departments/nursing/nursing.dot

Elmhurst College, Graduate Programs, Program in Nursing, Elmhurst, IL 60126-3296. Offers MSN. *Accreditation:* AACN. Part-time and evening/weekend programs available. *Faculty:* 5 full-time (all women), 1 (woman) part-time/adjunct. *Students:* 46 part-time (43 women); includes 8 minority (3 Black or African American, non-Hispanic/Latino; 5 Asian, non-Hispanic/Latino), 1 international. Average age 40. 41 applicants, 68% accepted, 19 enrolled. In 2013, 8 master's awarded. *Entrance requirements:* For master's, 3 recommendations, resume, statement of purpose, current RN licensure in Illinois, interview. Additional exam requirements/recommendations for international students: Required—TOEFL (minimum score 550 paper-based; 79 iBT). *Application deadline:* Applications are processed on a rolling basis. Application fee: $0. Electronic applications accepted. *Expenses:* Contact institution. *Financial support:* In 2013–14, 3 students received support. Federal Work-Study and scholarships/grants available. Support available to part-time students. Financial award application deadline: 6/1; financial award applicants required to submit FAFSA. *Application contact:* Timothy J. Panfil, Director of Enrollment Management, School for Professional Studies, 630-617-3300 Ext. 3256, Fax: 630-617-6471, E-mail: panfilt@elmhurst.edu.

Elms College, Division of Nursing, Chicopee, MA 01013-2839. Offers nursing and health services management (MSN); nursing education (MSN). *Accreditation:* AACN. Part-time and evening/weekend programs available. *Entrance requirements:* Additional exam requirements/recommendations for international students: Required—TOEFL.

Emmanuel College, Graduate Studies, Graduate Program in Nursing, Boston, MA 02115. Offers nursing education (MSN); nursing management/administration (MSN). Part-time and evening/weekend programs available. *Faculty:* 4 full-time (all women), 4 part-time/adjunct (all women). *Students:* 51 part-time (47 women); includes 9 minority (6 Black or African American, non-Hispanic/Latino; 1 American Indian or Alaska Native, non-Hispanic/Latino; 1 Asian, non-Hispanic/Latino; 1 Hispanic/Latino). Average age 49. *Degree requirements:* For master's, 36 credits, including 6-credit practicum. *Entrance requirements:* For master's, transcripts from all regionally-accredited institutions attended (showing proof of bachelor's degree completion), proof of RN license, 2 letters of recommendation, essay, resume, interview. Additional exam requirements/recommendations for international students: Required—TOEFL (minimum score 600 paper-based; 106 iBT) or IELTS (minimum score 6.5). *Application deadline:* For fall admission, 4/30 for domestic students. Applications are processed on a rolling basis. Application fee: $0. Electronic applications accepted. *Financial support:* Applicants required to submit FAFSA. *Unit head:* Sandy Robbins, Dean of Enrollment, 617-735-9700, Fax: 617-507-0434, E-mail: graduatestudies@emmanuel.edu. *Application contact:* Enrollment Counselor, 617-735-9700, Fax: 617-507-0434, E-mail: graduatestudies@emmanuel.edu.
Website: http://www.emmanuel.edu/graduate-studies-nursing/academics/nursing.html

Emory University, Laney Graduate School, Program in Nursing, Atlanta, GA 30322-1100. Offers PhD. *Accreditation:* AACN. *Degree requirements:* For doctorate, comprehensive exam, thesis/dissertation. *Entrance requirements:* For doctorate, GRE General Test. Additional exam requirements/recommendations for international students: Required—TOEFL. Electronic applications accepted. *Faculty research:* Symptoms, self management, care-giving, biobehavioral approaches, women's health.

Emory University, Nell Hodgson Woodruff School of Nursing, Atlanta, GA 30322-1100. Offers adult nurse practitioner (MSN); emergency nurse practitioner (MSN); family nurse practitioner (MSN); family nurse-midwife (MSN); health systems leadership (MSN); nurse-midwifery (MSN); pediatric nurse practitioner acute and primary care (MSN); women's health care (Title X) (MSN); women's health nurse practitioner (MSN); MSN/MPH. *Accreditation:* AACN; ACNM/ACME (one or more programs are accredited). Part-time programs available. *Entrance requirements:* For master's, GRE General Test or MAT, minimum GPA of 3.0, BS in nursing from an accredited institution, RN license and additional course work, 3 letters of recommendation. Additional exam requirements/recommendations for international students: Required—TOEFL (minimum score 600 paper-based; 100 iBT). Electronic applications accepted. *Expenses:* Contact institution. *Faculty research:* Older adult falls and injuries, minority health issues, cardiac symptoms and quality of life, bio-ethics and decision-making, menopausal issues.

Endicott College, Van Loan School of Graduate and Professional Studies, Program in Nursing, Beverly, MA 01915-2096. Offers MSN. *Faculty:* 2 full-time (both women), 5 part-time/adjunct (all women). *Students:* 27 full-time (25 women), 8 part-time (7 women); includes 1 minority (Hispanic/Latino). Average age 36. 35 applicants, 83% accepted, 26 enrolled. In 2013, 9 master's awarded. *Entrance requirements:* For master's, MAT or GRE, statement of professional goals, official transcripts of all undergraduate and graduate course work, two letters of recommendation, photocopy of current and unrestricted RN license, basic statistics course, interview. Additional exam requirements/recommendations for international students: Required—TOEFL. *Application deadline:* Applications are processed on a rolling basis. Application fee: $50. Electronic applications accepted. *Financial support:* Applicants required to submit FAFSA. *Unit head:* Mary Findeisen, Program Director, 978-232-2332, E-mail: mfindeis@endicott.edu. *Application contact:* Dr. Mary Huegel, Vice President and Dean of the School of Graduate and Professional Studies, 978-232-2084, Fax: 978-232-3000, E-mail: mhuegel@endicott.edu.
Website: http://www.endicott.edu/GradProf/GPSGrad/MasterofScience/GPSGradMSNursing.aspx

Excelsior College, School of Nursing, Albany, NY 12203-5159. Offers clinical systems management (MS); nursing (MS); nursing education (MS); nursing informatics (MS). Part-time and evening/weekend programs available. Postbaccalaureate distance learning degree programs offered (no on-campus study). *Faculty:* 13 part-time/adjunct (all women). *Students:* 550 part-time (448 women); includes 184 minority (106 Black or African American, non-Hispanic/Latino; 4 American Indian or Alaska Native, non-Hispanic/Latino; 30 Asian, non-Hispanic/Latino; 29 Hispanic/Latino; 5 Native Hawaiian or other Pacific Islander, non-Hispanic/Latino; 10 Two or more races, non-Hispanic/Latino). Average age 46. In 2013, 124 master's awarded. *Entrance requirements:* For master's, RN license. *Application deadline:* Applications are processed on a rolling basis. Application fee: $100. Electronic applications accepted. *Expenses: Tuition:* Part-time $565 per credit. *Financial support:* Scholarships/grants and traineeships available. Support available to part-time students. Financial award application deadline: 8/21. *Faculty research:* Leadership development, test anxiety, use of technology in online learning. *Unit head:* Dr. Barbara Pieper, Associate Dean, Graduate Program in Nursing, 518-464-8500, Fax: 518-464-8777, E-mail: msn@excelsior.edu. *Application contact:* Christine McIlwraith, Graduate Advisor, 518-464-8500, Fax: 518-464-8777, E-mail: nursingmasters@excelsior.edu.

Fairfield University, School of Nursing, Fairfield, CT 06824-5195. Offers advanced practice (DNP); executive (DNP); family nurse practitioner (MSN, DNP); nurse anesthesia (DNP); nursing leadership (MSN); psychiatric nurse practitioner (MSN, DNP). *Accreditation:* AACN; AANA/CANAEP. Part-time programs available. *Faculty:* 22 full-time (all women), 28 part-time/adjunct (23 women). *Students:* 27 full-time (23 women), 157 part-time (136 women); includes 37 minority (15 Black or African American, non-Hispanic/Latino; 10 Asian, non-Hispanic/Latino; 8 Hispanic/Latino; 2 Native Hawaiian or other Pacific Islander, non-Hispanic/Latino; 2 Two or more races, non-Hispanic/Latino), 8 international. Average age 37. 132 applicants, 52% accepted, 59 enrolled. In 2013, 39 master's, 3 doctorates awarded. *Degree requirements:* For master's, capstone project. *Entrance requirements:* For master's, minimum QPA of 3.0, RN license, resume, 2 recommendations; for doctorate, GRE (nurse anesthesia applicants only), MSN (minimum QPA of 3.2) or BSN (minimum QPA of 3.0); critical care nursing experience (for nurse anesthesia DNP candidates). Additional exam requirements/recommendations for international students: Required—TOEFL (minimum score 550 paper-based; 80 iBT) or IELTS (minimum score 6.5). *Application deadline:* For fall admission, 5/15 for international students; for spring admission, 10/15 for international students. Applications are processed on a rolling basis. Application fee: $60. Electronic applications accepted. *Expenses:* Contact institution. *Financial support:* In 2013–14, 4 students received support. Unspecified assistantships available. Financial award applicants required to submit FAFSA. *Faculty research:* Aging and sexual health, psychosocial needs of men with prostate cancer, nurse practitioner education, mentoring, psychiatric and mental health, incarceration of the mentally ill, recovery in schizophrenia, palliative and end of life care, maternal and child health, breastfeeding and lactation consultant, stress and emotional eating, care of veterans and their families, falls prevention and the elderly, health care leadership, interprofessional education, academic partnerships. *Total annual research expenditures:* $775,000. *Unit head:* Dr. Lynn Babington, Dean, 203-254-4000 Ext. 2701, Fax: 203-254-4126, E-mail: lbabington@fairfield.edu. *Application contact:* Marianne Gumpper, Director of Graduate and Continuing Studies Admission, 203-254-4184, Fax: 203-254-4073, E-mail: gradadmis@fairfield.edu.
Website: http://fairfield.edu/son

Fairleigh Dickinson University, Metropolitan Campus, University College: Arts, Sciences, and Professional Studies, Henry P. Becton School of Nursing and Allied Health, Program in Nursing, Teaneck, NJ 07666-1914. Offers MSN, Certificate. *Accreditation:* AACN.

Fairleigh Dickinson University, Metropolitan Campus, University College: Arts, Sciences, and Professional Studies, Henry P. Becton School of Nursing and Allied Health, Program in Nursing Practice, Teaneck, NJ 07666-1914. Offers DNP.

Felician College, Doctor of Nursing Practice Program, Lodi, NJ 07644-2117. Offers advanced practice (DNP); executive leadership (DNP). Postbaccalaureate distance learning degree programs offered (no on-campus study). *Students:* 14 part-time (11 women); includes 10 minority (7 Black or African American, non-Hispanic/Latino; 1 American Indian or Alaska Native, non-Hispanic/Latino; 1 Asian, non-Hispanic/Latino; 1 Native Hawaiian or other Pacific Islander, non-Hispanic/Latino). *Degree requirements:* For doctorate, project, residency. *Expenses: Tuition:* Part-time $945 per credit. *Required fees:* $317.50 per semester. *Application contact:* Nicole Vitale, Assistant Director of Graduate Admissions, 201-559-6077, Fax: 201-559-6138, E-mail: graduate@felician.edu.

Felician College, Program in Nursing, Lodi, NJ 07644-2117. Offers adult-gerontology nurse practitioner (MSN, PMC); executive leadership (MSN, PMC); family nurse practitioner (MSN, PMC); nursing education (MSN, PMC). *Accreditation:* AACN. Part-time and evening/weekend programs available. Postbaccalaureate distance learning degree programs offered (no on-campus study). *Students:* 5 full-time (4 women), 85 part-time (78 women); includes 50 minority (20 Black or African American, non-Hispanic/Latino; 14 Asian, non-Hispanic/Latino; 16 Hispanic/Latino). Average age 42. *Degree requirements:* For master's, scholarly project. *Entrance requirements:* For master's, BS in nursing or equivalent, minimum GPA of 3.0, 2 letters of recommendation, RN license; for PMC, RN license, minimum GPA of 2.75. Additional exam requirements/recommendations for international students: Recommended—TOEFL (minimum score 550 paper-based). *Application deadline:* Applications are processed on a rolling basis. Application fee: $40. *Expenses: Tuition:* Part-time $945 per credit. *Required fees:* $317.50 per semester. *Financial support:* In 2013–14, 10 students received support. Traineeships available. Financial award applicants required to submit FAFSA. *Faculty research:* Anxiety and fear, curriculum innovation, health promotion. *Unit head:* Dr. Muriel Shore, Dean, Division of Health Sciences, 201-559-6030, E-mail: shorem@felician.edu. *Application contact:* Elizabeth Barca, Senior Assistant Director, Graduate Admissions, 201-559-6077, Fax: 201-559-6138, E-mail: graduate@felician.edu.

Ferris State University, College of Health Professions, School of Nursing, Big Rapids, MI 49307. Offers nursing (MSN); nursing administration (MSN); nursing education (MSN); nursing informatics (MSN). Part-time and evening/weekend programs available. Postbaccalaureate distance learning degree programs offered (minimal on-campus study). *Faculty:* 5 full-time (all women), 1 (woman) part-time/adjunct. *Students:* 1 (woman) full-time, 103 part-time (91 women); includes 5 minority (2 Black or African American, non-Hispanic/Latino; 1 American Indian or Alaska Native, non-Hispanic/Latino; 1 Native Hawaiian or other Pacific Islander, non-Hispanic/Latino; 1 Two or more races, non-Hispanic/Latino). Average age 40. 25 applicants, 92% accepted, 21 enrolled. In 2013, 20 master's awarded. *Degree requirements:* For master's, comprehensive exam, practicum, practicum project. *Entrance requirements:* For master's, BS in nursing or related field with registered nurse license, writing sample, letters of reference, 2 years' clinical experience. Additional exam requirements/recommendations for international students: Required—TOEFL (minimum score 550 paper-based; 61 iBT). *Application deadline:* For fall admission, 4/15 priority date for domestic students; for spring admission, 10/15 for domestic students. Applications are processed on a rolling basis. Application fee: $30. Electronic applications accepted. Application fee is waived when completed online. *Financial support:* In 2013–14, 3 students received support. Fellowships, research assistantships, teaching assistantships, career-related internships or fieldwork, and scholarships/grants available. Financial award application deadline: 4/15. *Faculty research:* Nursing education-minority student focus, student attitudes toward aging. *Unit head:* Dr. Susan Owens, Program Coordinator, 231-591-2267, Fax: 231-591-2325, E-mail: owenss3@ferris.edu. *Application contact:* Debby Buck, Off-Campus Program Secretary, 231-591-2270, Fax: 231-591-3788, E-mail: buckd@ferris.edu.
Website: http://www.ferris.edu/htmls/colleges/alliedhe/Nursing/homepage.htm

Florida Agricultural and Mechanical University, Division of Graduate Studies, Research, and Continuing Education, School of Nursing, Tallahassee, FL 32307-3200. Offers MS. *Entrance requirements:* Additional exam requirements/recommendations for international students: Required—TOEFL.

Florida Atlantic University, Christine E. Lynn College of Nursing, Boca Raton, FL 33431-0991. Offers administrative and financial leadership in nursing and health care (Post Master's Certificate); adult/gerontological nurse practitioner (Post Master's Certificate); advanced holistic nursing (MS, Post Master's Certificate); clinical nurse leader (MS, Post Master's Certificate); family nurse practitioner (MS, Post Master's Certificate); nurse educator (MS, Post Master's Certificate); nursing (PhD); nursing administration and financial leadership (MS); nursing practice (DNP). *Accreditation:* AACN. Part-time programs available. *Faculty:* 30 full-time (27 women), 9 part-time/adjunct (8 women). *Students:* 29 full-time (27 women), 523 part-time (492 women); includes 254 minority (157 Black or African American, non-Hispanic/Latino; 2 American Indian or Alaska Native, non-Hispanic/Latino; 19 Asian, non-Hispanic/Latino; 62 Hispanic/Latino; 2 Native Hawaiian or other Pacific Islander, non-Hispanic/Latino; 12 Two or more races, non-Hispanic/Latino), 3 international. Average age 39. 463 applicants, 25% accepted, 111 enrolled. In 2013, 148 master's, 15 doctorates awarded. *Degree requirements:* For master's, thesis or alternative; for doctorate, comprehensive exam, thesis/dissertation. *Entrance requirements:* For master's, GRE General Test or MAT, bachelor's degree in nursing, Florida RN license, minimum GPA of 3.0, resume/curriculum vitae, letter of recommendation; for doctorate, GRE General Test or MAT, curriculum vitae, Florida RN license, minimum GPA of 3.5, master's degree in nursing, three letters of recommendation. *Application deadline:* For fall admission, 6/1 for domestic students, 2/15 for international students; for spring admission, 10/1 for domestic students, 7/15 for international students. Applications are processed on a rolling basis. Application fee: $30. *Expenses:* Tuition, state resident: full-time $6660; part-time $370 per credit hour. Tuition, nonresident: full-time $18,450; part-time $1025 per credit hour. Tuition and fees vary according to course load. *Financial support:* Research assistantships with partial tuition reimbursements, teaching assistantships with partial tuition reimbursements, career-related internships or fieldwork, Federal

Work-Study, institutionally sponsored loans, scholarships/grants, and traineeships available. Support available to part-time students. *Faculty research:* Econometrics of nurse-patient relationship, Alzheimer's disease, community-based programs, falls, self-healing. *Unit head:* Dr. Marlaine Smith, Dean, 561-297-3206, Fax: 561-297-3687, E-mail: msmit230@fau.edu. *Application contact:* Carol Kruse, Graduate Coordinator, 561-297-3261, Fax: 561-297-0088, E-mail: ckruse@fau.edu.
Website: http://nursing.fau.edu/

Florida International University, College of Nursing and Health Sciences, Nursing Program, Miami, FL 33199. Offers MSN, PhD. *Accreditation:* AACN; AANA/CANAEP. Part-time and evening/weekend programs available. *Degree requirements:* For master's, thesis or alternative; for doctorate, comprehensive exam, thesis/dissertation. *Entrance requirements:* For master's, bachelor's degree in nursing, minimum undergraduate GPA of 3.0 in upper-level coursework, letters of recommendation; for doctorate, GRE, letters of recommendation, minimum undergraduate GPA of 3.0 in upper-level coursework, interview. Additional exam requirements/recommendations for international students: Required—TOEFL (minimum score 550 paper-based; 80 iBT). Electronic applications accepted. *Faculty research:* Adult health nursing.

Florida Southern College, Program in Nursing, Lakeland, FL 33801-5698. Offers adult gerontology clinical nurse specialist (MSN); adult gerontology primary care nurse practitioner (MSN); nurse educator (MSN); nursing administration (MSN). *Accreditation:* AACN. Part-time and evening/weekend programs available. *Entrance requirements:* For master's, Florida RN license, 3 letters of recommendation, personal statement, minimum GPA of 3.0, resume. Additional exam requirements/recommendations for international students: Required—TOEFL (minimum score 550 paper-based). *Expenses:* Contact institution. *Faculty research:* End of life care, dementia, health promotion.

Florida State University, The Graduate School, College of Nursing, Tallahassee, FL 32312. Offers family nurse practitioner (DNP); health systems leadership (DNP); nurse educator (MSN, Certificate); nurse leader (MSN); nursing leadership (Certificate, Post-Graduate Certificate). *Accreditation:* AACN. Part-time programs available. Postbaccalaureate distance learning degree programs offered (minimal on-campus study). *Faculty:* 13 full-time (12 women). *Students:* 53 full-time (49 women), 26 part-time (all women); includes 16 minority (4 Black or African American, non-Hispanic/Latino; 1 Asian, non-Hispanic/Latino; 9 Hispanic/Latino; 2 Two or more races, non-Hispanic/Latino). Average age 38. 56 applicants, 61% accepted, 25 enrolled. In 2013, 5 master's, 18 doctorates awarded. *Degree requirements:* For master's, thesis optional. *Entrance requirements:* For master's, GRE General Test, MAT, minimum GPA of 3.0, BSN, Florida RN license; for doctorate, GRE General Test, MAT, minimum GPA of 3.0, BSN or MSN, Florida RN license. Additional exam requirements/recommendations for international students: Required—TOEFL (minimum score 550 paper-based). *Application deadline:* For fall admission, 7/1 for domestic and international students. Application fee: $30. Electronic applications accepted. *Expenses:* Tuition, state resident: part-time $403.51 per credit hour. Tuition, nonresident: part-time $1004.85 per credit hour. *Required fees:* $75.81 per credit hour. One-time fee: $20 part-time. Tuition and fees vary according to course load, campus/location and student level. *Financial support:* In 2013–14, 75 students received support, including fellowships with partial tuition reimbursements available (averaging $6,300 per year), research assistantships with partial tuition reimbursements available (averaging $3,000 per year), 3 teaching assistantships with partial tuition reimbursements available (averaging $3,000 per year); career-related internships or fieldwork, Federal Work-Study, institutionally sponsored loans, scholarships/grants, traineeships, and tuition waivers (partial) also available. Financial award application deadline: 4/15; financial award applicants required to submit FAFSA. *Faculty research:* Distance learning, gerontology, health promotion, educational strategies, rehabilitation of brain injured patients. *Unit head:* Dr. Judith McFetridge-Durdle, Dean, 850-644-6846, Fax: 850-644-7660, E-mail: jdurdle@nursing.fsu.edu. *Application contact:* Carlos G. Urrutia, Director of Student Services, 850-644-5638, Fax: 850-645-7249, E-mail: currutia@fsu.edu.
Website: http://nursing.fsu.edu/

Fort Hays State University, Graduate School, College of Health and Life Sciences, Department of Nursing, Hays, KS 67601-4099. Offers MSN. *Accreditation:* AACN. *Degree requirements:* For master's, comprehensive exam, thesis optional. *Entrance requirements:* For master's, GRE General Test or MAT. Additional exam requirements/recommendations for international students: Required—TOEFL (minimum score 550 paper-based). Electronic applications accepted.

Framingham State University, Continuing Education, Program in Nursing, Framingham, MA 01701-9101. Offers nursing education (MSN); nursing leadership (MSN). *Accreditation:* AACN. *Entrance requirements:* For master's, BSN; minimum cumulative undergraduate GPA of 3.0, 3.25 in nursing courses; coursework in statistics; 2 letters of recommendation; interview. Electronic applications accepted.

Franciscan University of Steubenville, Graduate Programs, Department of Nursing, Steubenville, OH 43952-1763. Offers MSN. Part-time and evening/weekend programs available. *Degree requirements:* For master's, thesis. *Entrance requirements:* For master's, GRE General Test, MAT.

Francis Marion University, Graduate Programs, Department of Nursing, Florence, SC 29502-0547. Offers family nurse practitioner (MSN); nurse educator (MSN). Part-time programs available. *Faculty:* 8 full-time (all women). *Students:* 40 full-time (37 women), 7 part-time (4 women); includes 14 minority (12 Black or African American, non-Hispanic/Latino; 1 Asian, non-Hispanic/Latino; 1 Two or more races, non-Hispanic/Latino). Average age 34. 20 applicants, 80% accepted, 16 enrolled. *Entrance requirements:* For master's, GRE, official transcripts, two letters of recommendation, written statement, current SC nursing license. *Application deadline:* For fall admission, 3/15 for domestic students; for spring admission, 10/15 for domestic students. Applications are processed on a rolling basis. Application fee: $33. Electronic applications accepted. *Expenses:* Tuition, state resident: full-time $9184; part-time $459.20 per credit hour. Tuition, nonresident: full-time $18,368; part-time $918.40 per credit hour. *Required fees:* $13.50 per credit hour. $92 per semester. Tuition and fees vary according to program. *Financial support:* Available to part-time students. Application deadline: 3/1; applicants required to submit FAFSA. *Unit head:* Dr. Ruth Wittmann-Price, Chair, 843-661-4625, E-mail: rwittmannprice@fmarion.edu. *Application contact:* Rannie Gamble, Administrative Manager, 843-661-1286, Fax: 843-661-4688, E-mail: rgamble@fmarion.edu.

Franklin Pierce University, Graduate Studies, Rindge, NH 03461-0060. Offers curriculum and instruction (M Ed); emerging network technologies (Graduate Certificate); energy and sustainability studies (MBA); health administration (MBA, Graduate Certificate); human resource management (MBA, Graduate Certificate); information technology (MBA); information technology management (MS); leadership (MBA, DA); nursing (MS); physical therapy (DPT); physician assistant studies (MPAS); special education (M Ed); sports management (MBA). *Accreditation:* APTA. Part-time programs available. Postbaccalaureate distance learning degree programs offered (no on-campus study). *Degree requirements:* For master's, concentrated original research projects; student teaching; fieldwork and/or internship; leadership project; PRAXIS I and II (for M Ed); for doctorate, concentrated original research projects, clinical fieldwork and/or internship, leadership project. *Entrance requirements:* For master's, minimum GPA of 2.5, 3 letters of recommendation; competencies in accounting, economics, statistics, and computer skills through life experience or undergraduate coursework (for MBA); certification/e-portfolio, minimum C grade in all education courses (for M Ed); license to practice as RN (for MS in nursing); for doctorate, GRE, BA/BS, 3 letters of recommendation, personal mission statement, interview, writing sample, minimum cumulative GPA of 2.8, master's degree (for DA); 80 hours of observation/work in PT settings, completion of anatomy, chemistry, physics, and statistics, minimum GPA of 3.0 (for DPT). Additional exam requirements/recommendations for international students: Required—TOEFL (minimum score 550 paper-based; 61 iBT). Electronic applications accepted. *Faculty research:* Evidence-based practice in sports physical therapy, human resource management in economic crisis, leadership in nursing, innovation in sports facility management, differentiated learning and understanding by design.

Frontier Nursing University, Graduate Programs, Hyden, KY 41749. Offers family nurse practitioner (MSN, DNP, Post Master's Certificate); nurse-midwifery (MSN, DNP, Post Master's Certificate); women's health care nurse practitioner (MSN, DNP, Post Master's Certificate). *Accreditation:* ACNM. *Degree requirements:* For doctorate, capstone project, practicum.

Gannon University, School of Graduate Studies, Morosky College of Health Professions and Sciences, Villa Maria School of Nursing, Program in Nursing Practice, Erie, PA 16541-0001. Offers DNP. Part-time and evening/weekend programs available. *Students:* 5 part-time (4 women). Average age 45. 6 applicants, 100% accepted, 6 enrolled. *Entrance requirements:* For doctorate, MSN, minimum GPA of 3.5 in master's work, resume, evidence of thesis, essay, interview. Additional exam requirements/recommendations for international students: Required—TOEFL (minimum score 79 iBT). *Application deadline:* For fall admission, 1/15 for domestic students. Application fee: $50. Electronic applications accepted. *Expenses:* Contact institution. *Unit head:* Dr. Kathleen Patterson, Director, 814-871-5547, E-mail: patterso018@gannon.edu. *Application contact:* Kara Morgan, Director of Graduate Admissions, 814-871-5831, Fax: 814-871-5827, E-mail: graduate@gannon.edu.

Gardner-Webb University, Graduate School, School of Nursing, Boiling Springs, NC 28017. Offers MSN, DNP, PMC. Part-time programs available. Postbaccalaureate distance learning degree programs offered (no on-campus study). *Faculty:* 8 full-time (7 women), 7 part-time/adjunct (5 women). *Students:* 23 full-time (22 women), 177 part-time (166 women); includes 30 minority (22 Black or African American, non-Hispanic/Latino; 1 American Indian or Alaska Native, non-Hispanic/Latino; 4 Asian, non-Hispanic/Latino; 3 Hispanic/Latino), 1 international. Average age 37. 247 applicants, 44% accepted, 95 enrolled. In 2013, 38 master's awarded. *Entrance requirements:* For master's, GRE or MAT, minimum undergraduate GPA of 2.7; unrestricted licensure to practice as an RN. *Expenses: Tuition:* Full-time $7200; part-time $400 per credit hour. Tuition and fees vary according to course load and program. *Unit head:* Dr. Suzie B. Little, Dean, 704-406-4358, Fax: 704-406-4329, E-mail: gradschool@gardner-webb.edu. *Application contact:* Office of Graduate Admissions, 877-498-4723, Fax: 704-406-3895, E-mail: gradinfo@gardner-webb.edu.

George Mason University, College of Health and Human Services, School of Nursing, Fairfax, VA 22030. Offers nursing (MSN, DNP, PhD); nursing administration (Certificate); nursing education (Certificate). *Faculty:* 33 full-time (32 women), 44 part-time/adjunct (42 women). *Students:* 82 full-time (77 women), 187 part-time (175 women); includes 98 minority (47 Black or African American, non-Hispanic/Latino; 2 American Indian or Alaska Native, non-Hispanic/Latino; 26 Asian, non-Hispanic/Latino; 18 Hispanic/Latino; 1 Native Hawaiian or other Pacific Islander, non-Hispanic/Latino; 4 Two or more races, non-Hispanic/Latino), 9 international. Average age 40. 182 applicants, 55% accepted, 71 enrolled. In 2013, 78 master's, 16 doctorates, 3 other advanced degrees awarded. *Degree requirements:* For master's, comprehensive exam (for some programs), thesis in clinical classes; for doctorate, comprehensive exam (for some programs), thesis/dissertation (for some programs). *Entrance requirements:* For master's, 2 official transcripts; expanded goals statement; resume; BSN from accredited institution; minimum GPA of 3.0 in last 60 credits of undergraduate work; 2 letters of recommendation; completion of undergraduate statistics and graduate-level bivariate statistics; certification in professional CPR; for doctorate, 2 official transcripts; expanded goals statement; resume; 3 recommendation letters; nursing license; at least 1 year of work experience as an RN; interview; writing sample; evidence of graduate-level course in applied statistics; master's in nursing with minimum GPA of 3.5; for Certificate, 2 official transcripts; expanded goals statement; resume; master's degree from accredited institution or currently enrolled with minimum GPA of 3.0. Additional exam requirements/recommendations for international students: Required—TOEFL (minimum score 570 paper-based; 88 iBT), IELTS (minimum score 6.5), PTE. *Application deadline:* For fall admission, 2/1 priority date for domestic students; for spring admission, 11/1 for domestic students. Application fee: $65 ($80 for international students). Electronic applications accepted. *Expenses:* Contact institution. *Financial support:* In 2013–14, 14 students received support, including 11 fellowships (averaging $15,091 per year), 3 research assistantships with full and partial tuition reimbursements available (averaging $36,667 per year); career-related internships or fieldwork, Federal Work-Study, scholarships/grants, unspecified assistantships, and health care benefits (for full-time research or teaching assistantship recipients) also available. Financial award application deadline: 3/1; financial award applicants required to submit FAFSA. *Faculty research:* Research in health care, nursing science. *Total annual research expenditures:* $366,930. *Unit head:* Carol Urban, Acting Director, 703-993-2991, Fax: 703-993-3606, E-mail: curban@gmu.edu. *Application contact:* Janice Lee-Beverly, Program Support, 703-993-1947, Fax: 703-993-1943, E-mail: jleebev1@gmu.edu.
Website: http://chhs.gmu.edu/nursing

Georgetown University, Graduate School of Arts and Sciences, School of Nursing and Health Studies, Washington, DC 20057. Offers acute care nurse practitioner (MS); clinical nurse specialist (MS); family nurse practitioner (MS); nurse anesthesia (MS); nurse-midwifery (MS); nursing (DNP); nursing education (MS). *Accreditation:* AACN; AANA/CANAEP (one or more programs are accredited); ACNM/ACME (one or more programs are accredited). *Degree requirements:* For master's, thesis optional. *Entrance requirements:* For master's, GRE General Test or MAT, bachelor's degree in nursing from NLN-accredited school, minimum undergraduate GPA of 3.0. Additional exam requirements/recommendations for international students: Required—TOEFL. Application fee: $50 ($55 for international students). *Financial support:* Scholarships/grants and traineeships available. Financial award applicants required to submit FAFSA. *Unit head:* Dr. Patricia Ann Cloonan, Dean, 202-687-7318. *Application contact:* Graduate School Admissions Office, 202-687-5568.

The George Washington University, School of Nursing, Washington, DC 20052. Offers adult nurse practitioner (MSN, Post-Master's Certificate); clinical research administration (MSN); family nurse practitioner (MSN, Post-Master's Certificate); health care quality (MSN, Post-Master's Certificate); nursing (DNP); nursing leadership and management (MSN); palliative care nurse practitioner (Post-Master's Certificate). *Accreditation:* AACN. *Faculty:* 37 full-time (all women). *Students:* 36 full-time (33 women), 438 part-time (405 women); includes 114 minority (59 Black or African American, non-Hispanic/Latino; 7 American Indian or Alaska Native, non-Hispanic/Latino; 32 Asian, non-Hispanic/Latino; 15 Hispanic/Latino; 1 Two or more races, non-

Hispanic/Latino), 8 international. Average age 38. 360 applicants, 83% accepted, 178 enrolled. In 2013, 79 master's, 26 doctorates awarded. *Unit head:* Jean E. Johnson, Dean, 202-994-3725, E-mail: sonjej@gwumc.edu. *Application contact:* Kristin Williams, Assistant Vice President for Graduate and Special Enrollment Management, 202-994-0467, Fax: 202-994-0371, E-mail: ksw@gwu.edu.
Website: http://nursing.gwumc.edu/

Georgia College & State University, Graduate School, College of Health Sciences, Graduate Nursing Program, Milledgeville, GA 31061. Offers family nurse practitioner (MSN); nursing practice (DNP). Part-time and evening/weekend programs available. *Students:* 87 part-time (80 women); includes 17 minority (all Black or African American, non-Hispanic/Latino). Average age 35. In 2013, 19 master's awarded. *Degree requirements:* For master's, comprehensive exam, thesis optional; for doctorate, capstone project, complete all required courses within a period of 7 years. *Entrance requirements:* For master's, GRE (taken within last 5 years), bachelor's degree in nursing, RN license, 1 year of clinical experience, minimum GPA of 2.75, statistics course; for doctorate, master's degree in nursing or anesthesia, minimum graduate GPA of 3.2, unencumbered RN licensure, 500 faculty-supervised clinical hours in master's program. Additional exam requirements/recommendations for international students: Recommended—TOEFL (minimum score 550 paper-based; 79 iBT). *Application deadline:* For fall admission, 7/1 priority date for domestic students; for spring admission, 4/1 priority date for domestic students. Applications are processed on a rolling basis. Application fee: $40. Electronic applications accepted. *Financial support:* In 2013–14, 2 research assistantships were awarded; unspecified assistantships also available. Financial award applicants required to submit FAFSA. *Unit head:* Dr. Deborah MacMillan, Assistant Director, Graduate Program, 478-751-1074, Fax: 478-757-1077, E-mail: debby.macmillan@gcsu.edu.

Georgia Regents University, The Graduate School, Doctor of Nursing Practice Program, Augusta, GA 30912. Offers DNP. *Degree requirements:* For doctorate, thesis/dissertation or alternative. *Entrance requirements:* For doctorate, GRE General Test or MAT, master's degree in nursing or related field, current professional nurse licensure. Additional exam requirements/recommendations for international students: Required—TOEFL (minimum score 600 paper-based; 100 iBT). Electronic applications accepted.

Georgia Regents University, The Graduate School, Nursing PhD Program, Augusta, GA 30912. Offers PhD. *Degree requirements:* For doctorate, thesis/dissertation. *Entrance requirements:* For doctorate, GRE General Test, current GA nurse licensure. Additional exam requirements/recommendations for international students: Required—TOEFL (minimum score 550 paper-based; 79 iBT). Electronic applications accepted.

Georgia Southern University, Jack N. Averitt College of Graduate Studies, College of Health and Human Sciences, School of Nursing, Program in Nursing Science, Statesboro, GA 30460. Offers DNP. Part-time programs available. Postbaccalaureate distance learning degree programs offered. *Students:* 7 full-time (all women), 14 part-time (13 women); includes 3 minority (all Black or African American, non-Hispanic/Latino). Average age 46. 8 applicants, 63% accepted, 3 enrolled. In 2013, 6 doctorates awarded. *Entrance requirements:* Additional exam requirements/recommendations for international students: Required—TOEFL (minimum score 550 paper-based; 80 iBT), IELTS (minimum score 6). *Application deadline:* For fall admission, 3/1 priority date for domestic and international students; for spring admission, 10/1 priority date for domestic students, 10/1 for international students. Applications are processed on a rolling basis. Application fee: $50. Electronic applications accepted. *Expenses:* Tuition, state resident: full-time $7068; part-time $270 per semester hour. Tuition, nonresident: full-time $26,446; part-time $1077 per semester hour. *Required fees:* $2092. *Financial support:* In 2013–14, 6 students received support. Career-related internships or fieldwork, Federal Work-Study, scholarships/grants, traineeships, and tuition waivers available. Support available to part-time students. Financial award application deadline: 4/15; financial award applicants required to submit FAFSA. *Faculty research:* Vulnerable populations, breast cancer, diabetes mellitus, advanced practice nursing issues. *Unit head:* Dr. Deborah Allen, Chair, 912-478-5770, Fax: 912-478-0536, E-mail: debbieallen@georgiasouthern.edu. *Application contact:* Amanda Gilliland, Coordinator for Graduate Student Recruitment, 912-478-5384, Fax: 912-478-0740, E-mail: gradadmissions@georgiasouthern.edu.

Georgia State University, Byrdine F. Lewis School of Nursing, Atlanta, GA 30303. Offers adult health clinical nurse specialist/nurse practitioner (MS, Certificate); child health clinical nurse specialist/pediatric nurse practitioner (MS, Certificate); family nurse practitioner (MS, Certificate); family psychiatric mental health nurse practitioner (MS, Certificate); nursing (PhD); nursing leadership in healthcare innovations (MS), including nursing administration, nursing informatics; nutrition (MS); perinatal clinical nurse specialist/women's health nurse practitioner (MS, Certificate); physical therapy (DPT); respiratory therapy (MS). *Accreditation:* AACN. Part-time programs available. Postbaccalaureate distance learning degree programs offered (minimal on-campus study). *Faculty:* 22 full-time (16 women). *Students:* 241 full-time (180 women), 262 part-time (236 women); includes 176 minority (120 Black or African American, non-Hispanic/Latino; 31 Asian, non-Hispanic/Latino; 13 Hispanic/Latino; 3 Native Hawaiian or other Pacific Islander, non-Hispanic/Latino; 9 Two or more races, non-Hispanic/Latino), 19 international. Average age 34. 583 applicants, 34% accepted, 160 enrolled. In 2013, 110 master's, 44 doctorates, 6 other advanced degrees awarded. *Degree requirements:* For doctorate, comprehensive exam, thesis/dissertation. *Entrance requirements:* For doctorate, GRE. Additional exam requirements/recommendations for international students: Required—TOEFL. *Application deadline:* For fall admission, 2/1 priority date for domestic and international students; for spring admission, 9/15 for domestic and international students. Applications are processed on a rolling basis. Application fee: $50. Electronic applications accepted. *Expenses:* Contact institution. *Financial support:* In 2013–14, research assistantships with full and partial tuition reimbursements (averaging $1,666 per year), teaching assistantships with full and partial tuition reimbursements (averaging $1,920 per year) were awarded; scholarships/grants, tuition waivers (full and partial), and unspecified assistantships also available. Support available to part-time students. Financial award application deadline: 8/1; financial award applicants required to submit FAFSA. *Faculty research:* Stroke intervention for caregivers, stroke prevention in African Americans; relationships between psychological distress and health outcomes in parents with a medically ill infant; medically fragile children; nursing expertise and patient outcomes. *Unit head:* Joan S. Cranford, Assistant Dean for Nursing, 404-413-1200, Fax: 404-413-1205, E-mail: jcranford2@gsu.edu. *Application contact:* Tiffany Norman, Senior Administrative Coordinator, 404-413-1190, Fax: 404-413-1205, E-mail: tnorman7@gsu.edu.
Website: http://nursing.gsu.edu/

Goldfarb School of Nursing at Barnes-Jewish College, Graduate Programs, St. Louis, MO 63110. Offers adult acute care nurse practitioner (MSN); adult nurse practitioner (MSN); nurse anesthesia (MSN); nurse educator (MSN); nurse executive (MSN); DNP/PhD. *Accreditation:* AACN; AANA/CANAEP. Part-time and evening/weekend programs available. Postbaccalaureate distance learning degree programs offered (minimal on-campus study). *Faculty:* 42 full-time (39 women), 6 part-time/adjunct (all women). *Students:* 81 full-time (67 women), 85 part-time (77 women); includes 28 minority (18 Black or African American, non-Hispanic/Latino; 2 Asian, non-Hispanic/Latino; 3 Hispanic/Latino; 3 Native Hawaiian or other Pacific Islander, non-Hispanic/Latino; 2 Two or more races, non-Hispanic/Latino). *Degree requirements:* For master's, thesis or alternative. *Entrance requirements:* For master's, 2 references, personal statement, curriculum vitae or resume. Additional exam requirements/recommendations for international students: Required—TOEFL (minimum score 575 paper-based; 85 iBT). *Application deadline:* For fall admission, 2/1 priority date for international students; for spring admission, 10/1 priority date for international students. Applications are processed on a rolling basis. Application fee: $50. *Expenses: Tuition:* Full-time $12,960; part-time $720 per credit hour. *Required fees:* $295; $720 per credit hour. Tuition and fees vary according to course load. *Financial support:* Fellowships, research assistantships, Federal Work-Study, institutionally sponsored loans, and scholarships/grants available. Support available to part-time students. Financial award applicants required to submit FAFSA. *Faculty research:* HIV stigma, HIV symptom management, palliative care with children and their families, heart disease prevention in Hispanic women, depression in the well elderly, alternative therapies in pre-term infants. *Unit head:* Dr. Michael Bleich, Dean, 314-362-0956, Fax: 314-362-0984, E-mail: mbleich@bjc.org. *Application contact:* Margaret Anne O'Connor, Program Officer, 314-454-7557, Fax: 314-362-0984, E-mail: maoconnor@bjc.org.

Gonzaga University, School of Nursing and Human Physiology, Spokane, WA 99258. Offers MSN, DNP. *Accreditation:* AACN. Part-time and evening/weekend programs available. Postbaccalaureate distance learning degree programs offered (minimal on-campus study). *Faculty:* 16 full-time (15 women), 8 part-time/adjunct (7 women). *Students:* 16 full-time (13 women), 577 part-time (510 women); includes 78 minority (8 Black or African American, non-Hispanic/Latino; 10 American Indian or Alaska Native, non-Hispanic/Latino; 22 Asian, non-Hispanic/Latino; 19 Hispanic/Latino; 4 Native Hawaiian or other Pacific Islander, non-Hispanic/Latino; 15 Two or more races, non-Hispanic/Latino), 10 international. Average age 40. 64 applicants, 56% accepted, 27 enrolled. In 2013, 125 master's awarded. *Entrance requirements:* For master's, MAT, minimum B average in undergraduate course work; for doctorate, MAT or GRE within the last 5 years, curriculum vitae, personal statement, three letters of recommendation, official transcripts, copy of current RN license, practicum hours. Additional exam requirements/recommendations for international students: Required—TOEFL. *Application deadline:* For fall admission, 7/20 priority date for domestic students; for spring admission, 11/1 for domestic students. Applications are processed on a rolling basis. Application fee: $50. Electronic applications accepted. *Expenses:* Contact institution. *Financial support:* Application deadline: 2/1; applicants required to submit FAFSA. *Unit head:* Dr. Lin Murphy, RN, Chair, 509-313-6644. *Application contact:* Julie McCulloh, Dean of Admissions, 509-313-6592, Fax: 509-313-5780, E-mail: mcculloh@gu.gonzaga.edu.
Website: http://www.gonzaga.edu/Academics/Colleges-and-Schools/School-of-Nursing-Human-Physiology/

Goshen College, Program in Nursing, Goshen, IN 46526-4794. Offers family nurse practitioner (MSN). *Accreditation:* AACN. Part-time and evening/weekend programs available. *Faculty:* 6 full-time (all women), 2 part-time/adjunct (both women). *Students:* 43 part-time (40 women), 3 international. *Degree requirements:* For master's, comprehensive exam (for some programs). *Entrance requirements:* For master's, minimum GPA of 3.0, curriculum vitae, bachelor's degree in nursing, active RN license, three professional recommendations, essay, one year of clinical nursing experience, statistics course, interview. Additional exam requirements/recommendations for international students: Required—TOEFL (minimum score 600 paper-based; 100 iBT). *Application deadline:* For fall admission, 3/14 for domestic students. Applications are processed on a rolling basis. Application fee: $50. Electronic applications accepted. *Expenses:* Contact institution. *Financial support:* Scholarships/grants available. Financial award applicants required to submit FAFSA. *Unit head:* Dr. Ruth Stoltzfus, RN, Director, 574-535-7973, E-mail: ruthas@goshen.edu. *Application contact:* Nina Mishler, Associate Director of Admissions, 574-535-7527, Fax: 574-535-7609, E-mail: ninajm@goshen.edu.
Website: http://www.goshen.edu/nursing/masters

Governors State University, College of Health Professions, Program in Nursing, University Park, IL 60484. Offers MSN. *Degree requirements:* For master's, comprehensive exam, thesis or alternative, practicum. *Entrance requirements:* For master's, GRE General Test, minimum GPA of 3.0 in upper-division nursing course work, 2.5 overall; BSN verification of AAS or employment as registered nurse; Illinois licensure; BSN from NLN-accredited institution.

Graceland University, School of Nursing, Independence, MO 64050-3434. Offers family nurse practitioner (MSN, PMC); nurse educator (MSN, PMC); organizational leadership (DNP). Part-time programs available. Postbaccalaureate distance learning degree programs offered (minimal on-campus study). *Faculty:* 13 full-time (all women), 9 part-time/adjunct (7 women). *Students:* 215 full-time (197 women), 339 part-time (303 women); includes 95 minority (37 Black or African American, non-Hispanic/Latino; 11 American Indian or Alaska Native, non-Hispanic/Latino; 15 Asian, non-Hispanic/Latino; 18 Hispanic/Latino; 2 Native Hawaiian or other Pacific Islander, non-Hispanic/Latino; 12 Two or more races, non-Hispanic/Latino), 4 international. Average age 44. 84 applicants, 89% accepted, 63 enrolled. In 2013, 71 master's awarded. *Degree requirements:* For master's, comprehensive exam (for some programs), thesis optional, scholarly project; for doctorate, capstone project. *Entrance requirements:* For master's, BSN from nationally-accredited program, RN license, minimum GPA of 3.0; satisfactory criminal background check; for doctorate, MSN from nationally-accredited program, RN license, minimum GPA of 3.2; satisfactory criminal background check. Additional exam requirements/recommendations for international students: Recommended—TOEFL. *Application deadline:* For fall admission, 6/1 priority date for domestic students; for winter admission, 10/1 priority date for domestic students; for spring admission, 3/1 priority date for domestic students. Application fee: $50. Electronic applications accepted. *Expenses:* Contact institution. *Financial support:* Institutionally sponsored loans available. Support available to part-time students. Financial award applicants required to submit FAFSA. *Faculty research:* International nursing, family care-giving, health promotion. *Unit head:* Dr. Claudia D. Horton, Dean, 816-423-4670, Fax: 816-423-4753, E-mail: horton@graceland.edu. *Application contact:* Nick Walker, Program Consultant, 816-423-4717, Fax: 816-833-2990, E-mail: nowalker@graceland.edu.
Website: http://www.graceland.edu/nursing

The Graduate Center, City University of New York, Graduate Studies, Program in Nursing Science, New York, NY 10016-4039. Offers DNS. *Degree requirements:* For doctorate, thesis/dissertation, exams. *Entrance requirements:* For doctorate, GRE, 2 letters of recommendation. Additional exam requirements/recommendations for international students: Required—TOEFL. Electronic applications accepted.

Grambling State University, School of Graduate Studies and Research, College of Professional Studies, School of Nursing, Grambling, LA 71245. Offers family nurse practitioner (PMC); nursing (MSN). Part-time programs available. *Faculty:* 5 full-time (all women), 2 part-time/adjunct (both women). *Students:* 43 full-time (40 women), 23 part-time (20 women); includes 41 minority (39 Black or African American, non-Hispanic/Latino; 1 Asian, non-Hispanic/Latino; 1 Hispanic/Latino), 1 international. Average age 36. In 2013, 33 master's awarded. *Degree requirements:* For master's, comprehensive exam (for some programs), thesis (for some programs). *Entrance requirements:* For master's, GRE, minimum GPA of 3.0 on last degree, interview, 2 years of experience as

RN. Additional exam requirements/recommendations for international students: Required—TOEFL (minimum score 500 paper-based; 62 iBT). *Application deadline:* For fall admission, 7/1 for domestic and international students; for spring admission, 12/1 for domestic and international students; for summer admission, 5/1 for domestic and international students. Applications are processed on a rolling basis. Application fee: $20 ($30 for international students). Electronic applications accepted. *Financial support:* Health care benefits and tuition waivers (full and partial) available. Financial award application deadline: 5/31; financial award applicants required to submit FAFSA. *Unit head:* Dr. Danita R. Potter, Interim Associate Dean, 318-274-2632, E-mail: potterd@gram.edu. *Application contact:* Dr. Rhonda Hensley, MSN Program Director, 318-274-2897, Fax: 318-274-3491, E-mail: hensleyr@gram.edu.
Website: http://www.gram.edu/academics/majors/professional%20studies/departments/nursing/

Grand Canyon University, College of Nursing, Phoenix, AZ 85017-1097. Offers acute care nurse practitioner (MS, PMC); clinical nurse specialist (PMC), including clinical nurse specialist, education; family nurse practitioner (MS); leadership in health care systems (MS); nurse education (MS). *Accreditation:* AACN. Part-time and evening/weekend programs available. Postbaccalaureate distance learning degree programs offered (no on-campus study). *Degree requirements:* For master's and PMC, comprehensive exam (for some programs). *Entrance requirements:* For master's, minimum cumulative and science course undergraduate GPA of 3.0. Additional exam requirements/recommendations for international students: Required—TOEFL (minimum score 575 paper-based; 90 iBT), IELTS (minimum score 7).

Grand Valley State University, Kirkhof College of Nursing, Allendale, MI 49401-9403. Offers advanced practice (MSN); case management (MSN); nursing administration (MSN); nursing education (MSN); nursing practice (DNP); MSN/MBA. *Accreditation:* AACN. Part-time programs available. *Degree requirements:* For master's, thesis optional. *Entrance requirements:* For master's, GRE, minimum GPA of 3.0 in upper-division course work, course work in statistics, Michigan RN license. Additional exam requirements/recommendations for international students: Required—TOEFL. Electronic applications accepted. *Faculty research:* Multigenerational health promotion, chronic disease prevention, end-of-life issues, nursing workload, family caregiver health.

Grand View University, Master of Science in Innovative Leadership Program, Des Moines, IA 50316-1599. Offers business (MS); education (MS); nursing (MS). Part-time and evening/weekend programs available. *Degree requirements:* For master's, completion of all required coursework in common core and selected track with minimum cumulative GPA of 3.0 and no more than two grades of C. *Entrance requirements:* For master's, GRE, GMAT, or essay, minimum undergraduate GPA of 3.0, professional resume, 3 letters of recommendation, interview. Additional exam requirements/recommendations for international students: Required—TOEFL (minimum score 550 paper-based). Electronic applications accepted.

Gwynedd Mercy University, School of Nursing, Gwynedd Valley, PA 19437-0901. Offers clinical nurse specialist (MSN), including gerontology, oncology, pediatrics; nurse practitioner (MSN), including adult health, pediatric health. *Degree requirements:* For master's, thesis optional. *Entrance requirements:* For master's, GRE General Test or MAT, current nursing experience, physical assessment, course work in statistics, BSN from NLNAC-accredited program, 2 letters of recommendation, personal interview. Additional exam requirements/recommendations for international students: Required—TOEFL (minimum score 575 paper-based). Electronic applications accepted. *Expenses:* Contact institution. *Faculty research:* Critical thinking, primary care, domestic violence, multiculturalism, nursing centers.

Hampton University, Graduate College, School of Nursing, Hampton, VA 23668. Offers advanced adult nursing (MS); community health nursing (MS); community mental health/psychiatric nursing (MS); family nursing (MS); gerontological nursing for the nurse practitioner (MS); pediatric nursing (MS); women's health nursing (MS). *Accreditation:* AACN. Part-time and evening/weekend programs available. *Degree requirements:* For master's, thesis optional. *Entrance requirements:* For master's, GRE General Test. *Faculty research:* Curriculum development, physical and mental assessment.

Hampton University, Hampton U Online, Hampton, VA 23668. Offers business administration (PhD); educational management (PhD); health administration (MHA); nursing (MSN, PhD).

Hardin-Simmons University, Graduate School, Patty Hanks Shelton School of Nursing, Abilene, TX 79698-0001. Offers advanced healthcare delivery (MSN); family nurse practitioner (MSN). Programs offered jointly with Abilene Christian University and McMurry University. *Accreditation:* AACN. Part-time programs available. *Faculty:* 6 full-time (all women), 2 part-time/adjunct (both women). *Students:* 4 full-time (all women), 7 part-time (4 women); includes 4 minority (3 Black or African American, non-Hispanic/Latino; 1 Hispanic/Latino), 1 international. Average age 37. 7 applicants, 100% accepted, 6 enrolled. In 2013, 8 master's awarded. *Degree requirements:* For master's, comprehensive exam, thesis or alternative. *Entrance requirements:* For master's, GRE, minimum undergraduate GPA of 3.0 in major, 2.8 overall; interview; upper-level course work in statistics; CPR certification; letters of recommendation. Additional exam requirements/recommendations for international students: Required—TOEFL (minimum score 550 paper-based; 75 iBT). *Application deadline:* For fall admission, 8/15 priority date for domestic students, 4/1 for international students; for spring admission, 1/5 priority date for domestic students, 9/1 for international students. Applications are processed on a rolling basis. Application fee: $50. *Expenses:* Contact institution. *Financial support:* In 2013–14, 1 student received support. Career-related internships or fieldwork and scholarships/grants available. Support available to part-time students. Financial award application deadline: 6/30; financial award applicants required to submit FAFSA. *Faculty research:* Child abuse, alternative medicine, pediatric chronic disease, health promotion. *Unit head:* Dr. Indira Tyler, Interim Director, 325-671-2367, Fax: 325-671-2386, E-mail: atoone@phssn.edu. *Application contact:* Dr. Nancy Kucinski, Dean of Graduate Studies, 325-670-1298, Fax: 325-670-1564, E-mail: gradoff@hsutx.edu.
Website: http://www.phssn.edu/

Hawai`i Pacific University, College of Nursing and Health Sciences, Honolulu, HI 96813. Offers community clinical nurse specialist (MSN); family nurse practitioner (MSN). Part-time and evening/weekend programs available. *Faculty:* 6 full-time (all women), 2 part-time/adjunct (both women). *Students:* 39 full-time (33 women), 16 part-time (11 women); includes 40 minority (2 Black or African American, non-Hispanic/Latino; 22 Asian, non-Hispanic/Latino; 7 Hispanic/Latino; 2 Native Hawaiian or other Pacific Islander, non-Hispanic/Latino; 7 Two or more races, non-Hispanic/Latino). Average age 38. 32 applicants, 75% accepted, 15 enrolled. In 2013, 7 master's awarded. *Degree requirements:* For master's, practicum, professional paper. *Entrance requirements:* For master's, bachelor's degree in nursing, minimum GPA of 3.0. Additional exam requirements/recommendations for international students: Recommended—TOEFL (minimum score 550 paper-based; 80 iBT), TWE (minimum score 5). *Application deadline:* Applications are processed on a rolling basis. Application fee: $50. Electronic applications accepted. *Financial support:* In 2013–14, 11 students received support. Career-related internships or fieldwork, Federal Work-Study, scholarships/grants, traineeships, and tuition waivers available. Financial award application deadline: 3/1; financial award applicants required to submit FAFSA. *Faculty research:* Hawaiian elders, traditional healing and nursing center. *Unit head:* Dr. Lynette Landry, Dean, 808-236-5811, E-mail: llandry@hpu.edu. *Application contact:* Rumi Yoshida, Associate Director of Graduate Admissions, 808-543-8034, Fax: 808-544-0280, E-mail: grad@hpu.edu.
Website: http://www.hpu.edu/CNHS/index.html

Herzing University Online, Program in Nursing, Milwaukee, WI 53203. Offers nursing (MSN); nursing education (MSN); nursing management (MSN). *Accreditation:* AACN. Postbaccalaureate distance learning degree programs offered (no on-campus study).

Holy Family University, Graduate School, School of Nursing, Philadelphia, PA 19114. Offers community health nursing (MSN); nursing administration (MSN); nursing education (MSN). *Accreditation:* AACN. Part-time and evening/weekend programs available. *Faculty:* 7 full-time (all women). *Students:* 42 part-time (39 women); includes 9 minority (4 Black or African American, non-Hispanic/Latino; 4 Asian, non-Hispanic/Latino; 1 Hispanic/Latino). Average age 36. 17 applicants, 82% accepted, 6 enrolled. In 2013, 12 master's awarded. *Degree requirements:* For master's, thesis or alternative, comprehensive portfolio, clinical practicum. *Entrance requirements:* For master's, BSN or RN from appropriately-accredited program, minimum GPA of 3.0, professional references, official transcripts of all college or university work, essay/personal statement, current resume, completion of one undergraduate statistics course with minimum grade of C. Additional exam requirements/recommendations for international students: Required—TOEFL (minimum score 550 paper-based; 79 iBT), IELTS (minimum score 6), or PTE (minimum score 54). *Application deadline:* For fall admission, 7/1 priority date for domestic and international students; for winter admission, 1/1 for domestic students; for spring admission, 11/1 priority date for domestic and international students; for summer admission, 4/1 priority date for domestic and international students. Applications are processed on a rolling basis. Application fee: $25. Electronic applications accepted. *Expenses: Tuition:* Full-time $12,060. *Required fees:* $250. Tuition and fees vary according to degree level. *Financial support:* In 2013–14, 1 student received support. Available to part-time students. Application deadline: 2/15; applicants required to submit FAFSA. *Unit head:* Dr. Ana Maria Catanzaro, Dean, 267-341-3292, Fax: 215-637-6598, E-mail: acatanzaro@holyfamily.edu. *Application contact:* Gidget Matie Montelibano, Associate Director of Graduate Admissions, 267-341-3558, Fax: 215-637-1478, E-mail: gmontelibano@holyfamily.edu.
Website: http://www.holyfamily.edu/choosing-holy-family-u/academics/schools-of-study/school-of-nursing

Holy Names University, Graduate Division, Department of Nursing, Oakland, CA 94619-1699. Offers administration/management (MSN, PMC); clinical faculty (MSN, PMC); community health nursing/case manager (MSN); family nurse practitioner (MSN, PMC); MSN/MA; MSN/MBA. *Accreditation:* AACN. Part-time and evening/weekend programs available. *Faculty:* 3 full-time, 22 part-time/adjunct. *Students:* 31 full-time (26 women), 78 part-time (67 women); includes 66 minority (27 Black or African American, non-Hispanic/Latino; 25 Asian, non-Hispanic/Latino; 13 Hispanic/Latino; 1 Two or more races, non-Hispanic/Latino), 5 international. Average age 38. 97 applicants, 61% accepted, 49 enrolled. In 2013, 66 master's, 3 other advanced degrees awarded. *Entrance requirements:* For master's, bachelor's degree in nursing or related field; California RN license or eligibility; minimum cumulative GPA of 2.8, 3.0 in nursing courses from baccalaureate program; courses in pathophysiology, statistics, and research at the undergraduate level. Additional exam requirements/recommendations for international students: Required—TOEFL (minimum score 500 paper-based; 79 iBT). *Application deadline:* For fall admission, 8/1 priority date for domestic students, 7/15 priority date for international students; for spring admission, 12/1 priority date for domestic and international students; for summer admission, 5/1 priority date for domestic and international students. Applications are processed on a rolling basis. Application fee: $65. Electronic applications accepted. Application fee is waived when completed online. *Expenses: Tuition:* Part-time $866 per unit. *Financial support:* Career-related internships or fieldwork, Federal Work-Study, scholarships/grants, and unspecified assistantships available. Support available to part-time students. Financial award application deadline: 3/2; financial award applicants required to submit FAFSA. *Faculty research:* Women's reproductive health, gerontology, attitudes about aging, schizophrenic families, international health issues. *Unit head:* Dr. Miki Goodwin, Associate Professor/Chair of Nursing, 510-436-1374, E-mail: goodwin@hnu.edu. *Application contact:* Graduate Admission Office, 800-430-1321, E-mail: graduateadmissions@hnu.edu.

Howard University, College of Nursing and Allied Health Sciences, Division of Nursing, Washington, DC 20059-0002. Offers nurse practitioner (Certificate); primary family health nursing (MSN). *Accreditation:* AACN. Part-time programs available. *Degree requirements:* For master's, comprehensive exam, thesis optional. *Entrance requirements:* For master's, RN license, minimum GPA of 3.0, BS in nursing. *Faculty research:* Urinary incontinence, breast cancer prevention, depression in the elderly, adolescent pregnancy.

Hunter College of the City University of New York, Graduate School, Schools of the Health Professions, Hunter-Bellevue School of Nursing, New York, NY 10010. Offers MS, AC, MS/MPH. *Accreditation:* AACN. Part-time programs available. *Faculty:* 18 full-time (15 women), 25 part-time/adjunct (21 women). *Students:* 2 full-time (1 woman), 292 part-time (226 women); includes 151 minority (92 Black or African American, non-Hispanic/Latino; 26 Asian, non-Hispanic/Latino; 33 Hispanic/Latino), 24 international. Average age 34. 323 applicants, 47% accepted, 128 enrolled. In 2013, 115 master's, 4 other advanced degrees awarded. *Degree requirements:* For master's, practicum, portfolio. *Entrance requirements:* For master's, BSN, minimum GPA of 3.0, New York RN license, course work in basic statistics, resume; for AC, MSN, minimum GPA of 3.0. Additional exam requirements/recommendations for international students: Required—TOEFL. *Application deadline:* For fall admission, 4/1 for domestic students; for spring admission, 11/1 for domestic students. Applications are processed on a rolling basis. Application fee: $125. *Financial support:* In 2013–14, 9 students received support. Federal Work-Study, scholarships/grants, traineeships, and tuition waivers (partial) available. Support available to part-time students. Financial award application deadline: 5/1; financial award applicants required to submit FAFSA. *Faculty research:* Aging, high-risk mothers and babies, adolescent health, care of HIV/AIDS clients, critical care nursing. *Unit head:* Dr. Gail McCain, Dean, 212-481-7596, Fax: 212-481-5078, E-mail: gmccain@hunter.cuny.edu. *Application contact:* Milena Solo, Director for Graduate Admissions, 212-772-4288, E-mail: milena.solo@hunter.cuny.edu.
Website: http://www.hunter.cuny.edu/nursing/

Husson University, Graduate Nursing Program, Bangor, ME 04401-2999. Offers advanced practice psychiatric nursing (MSN, PMC); family and community nurse practitioner (MSN, PMC); nursing education (MSN, PMC). *Accreditation:* AACN. Part-time programs available. *Faculty:* 3 full-time (all women), 3 part-time/adjunct (all women). *Students:* 10 full-time (8 women), 15 part-time (14 women); includes 1 minority (Two or more races, non-Hispanic/Latino). 29 applicants, 76% accepted, 21 enrolled. In 2013, 16 master's awarded. *Degree requirements:* For master's, comprehensive exam (for some programs). *Entrance requirements:* For master's, MAT or GRE, BSN. Additional exam requirements/recommendations for international students: Required—TOEFL (minimum score 550 paper-based). *Application deadline:* For fall admission, 6/

30 for domestic students; for spring admission, 10/30 for domestic students. Application fee: $40. *Expenses:* Contact institution. *Financial support:* In 2013–14, 16 students received support. Federal Work-Study, institutionally sponsored loans, traineeships, and unspecified assistantships available. Financial award application deadline: 4/15; financial award applicants required to submit FAFSA. *Unit head:* Prof. Chrystal Adams, Director, Nurse Practitioner Program, 207-941-7080, E-mail: adamsc@husson.edu. *Application contact:* Kristen Card, Director of Graduate Admissions, 207-404-5660, Fax: 207-941-7935, E-mail: cardk@husson.edu.

Idaho State University, Office of Graduate Studies, Kasiska College of Health Professions, Department of Nursing, Pocatello, ID 83209-8101. Offers nursing (MS, Post-Master's Certificate). *Accreditation:* AACN. Part-time programs available. *Degree requirements:* For master's, comprehensive exam, thesis optional, practicum and/or clinical hours; for Post-Master's Certificate, comprehensive exam, thesis optional, practicum. *Entrance requirements:* For master's, GRE General Test, interview, 3 letters of reference, active RN license; for Post-Master's Certificate, GRE General Test, 3 letters of reference, practicum or nursing license, graduate degree. Additional exam requirements/recommendations for international students: Required—TOEFL (minimum score 600 paper-based). Electronic applications accepted. *Faculty research:* Health promotions, health of homeless, exercise and elderly, student stress, midwifery.

Illinois State University, Graduate School, Mennonite College of Nursing, Normal, IL 61790. Offers family nurse practitioner (PMC); nursing (MSN, PhD). *Accreditation:* AACN. *Faculty research:* Expanding the teaching-nursing home culture in the state of Illinois, advanced education nursing traineeship program, collaborative doctoral program-caring for older adults.

Immaculata University, College of Graduate Studies, Division of Nursing, Immaculata, PA 19345. Offers nursing administration (MSN); nursing education (MSN). *Accreditation:* AACN. Part-time and evening/weekend programs available. *Entrance requirements:* For master's, MAT or GRE, BSN, minimum undergraduate GPA of 3.0. Additional exam requirements/recommendations for international students: Required—TOEFL. *Application deadline:* Applications are processed on a rolling basis. Application fee: $50. *Expenses: Tuition:* Part-time $660 per credit. Part-time tuition and fees vary according to degree level and program. *Financial support:* Application deadline: 5/1; applicants required to submit FAFSA. *Unit head:* Dr. Jane Tang, RN, Program Director, 610-647-4400 Ext. 3309, Fax: 610-993-8550, E-mail: jtang@immaculata.edu.
Website: http://www.immaculata.edu/nursing/

Independence University, Program in Nursing, Salt Lake City, UT 84107. Offers community health (MSN); gerontology (MSN); nursing administration (MSN); wellness promotion (MSN).

Indiana State University, College of Graduate and Professional Studies, College of Nursing, Health and Human Services, Department of Nursing, Terre Haute, IN 47809. Offers MS. Part-time programs available. *Degree requirements:* For master's, thesis or alternative. *Entrance requirements:* For master's, BSN, RN license, minimum undergraduate GPA of 3.0. Electronic applications accepted. *Faculty research:* Nursing faculty-student interactions, clinical evaluation, program evaluation, sexual dysfunction, faculty attitudes.

Indiana University East, School of Nursing, Richmond, IN 47374-1289. Offers MSN.

Indiana University Kokomo, School of Nursing, Kokomo, IN 46904-9003. Offers nurse administrator (MSN); nurse educator (MSN). *Students:* 3 full-time (all women), 35 part-time (all women), 1 international. 14 applicants, 93% accepted, 11 enrolled. *Unit head:* Dr. Mary P. Bourke, Assistant Dean of Graduate Programs, 765-455-9326, E-mail: mbourke@iuk.edu. *Application contact:* Admissions Office, 765-455-9326.
Website: http://www.iuk.edu/academics/majors/nursing/graduate-programs/index.shtml

Indiana University of Pennsylvania, School of Graduate Studies and Research, College of Health and Human Services, Department of Nursing and Allied Health, PhD in Nursing Program, Indiana, PA 15705-1087. Offers PhD. Part-time programs available. *Faculty:* 7 full-time (6 women). *Students:* 35 part-time (33 women); includes 1 minority (Hispanic/Latino). Average age 44. 16 applicants, 69% accepted, 11 enrolled. In 2013, 2 doctorates awarded. *Degree requirements:* For doctorate, comprehensive exam, thesis/dissertation. *Entrance requirements:* For doctorate, GRE. Additional exam requirements/recommendations for international students: Required—TOEFL (minimum score 540 paper-based). *Application deadline:* Applications are processed on a rolling basis. Application fee: $50. Electronic applications accepted. *Expenses:* Tuition, state resident: full-time $3978; part-time $442 per credit. Tuition, nonresident: full-time $5967; part-time $663 per credit. *Required fees:* $2080; $115.55 per credit. $93 per semester. Tuition and fees vary according to degree level and program. *Financial support:* In 2013–14, 7 fellowships with full tuition reimbursements (averaging $720 per year), 1 teaching assistantship with partial tuition reimbursement (averaging $22,848 per year) were awarded; research assistantships, career-related internships or fieldwork, Federal Work-Study, scholarships/grants, and unspecified assistantships also available. Financial award application deadline: 4/15; financial award applicants required to submit FAFSA. *Unit head:* Dr. Susan Poorman, Doctoral Coordinator, 724-357-3258, E-mail: susan.poorman@iup.edu.
Website: http://www.iup.edu/grad/nursingphd/default.aspx

Indiana University–Purdue University Fort Wayne, College of Health and Human Services, Department of Nursing, Fort Wayne, IN 46805-1499. Offers adult-gerontology primary care nurse practitioner (MS); nurse executive (MS); nursing administration (Certificate); nursing education (MS); women's health nurse practitioner (MS). Part-time programs available. *Faculty:* 12 full-time (all women). *Students:* 5 full-time (all women), 63 part-time (60 women); includes 3 minority (2 Black or African American, non-Hispanic/Latino; 1 Asian, non-Hispanic/Latino). Average age 35. 34 applicants, 100% accepted, 25 enrolled. In 2013, 10 master's awarded. *Entrance requirements:* For master's, GRE Writing Test (if GPA below 3.0), BS in nursing, eligibility for Indiana RN license, minimum GPA of 3.0, essay, copy of resume, three references, undergraduate course work in research and statistics within last 5 years. Additional exam requirements/recommendations for international students: Required—TOEFL (minimum score 550 paper-based; 79 iBT); Recommended—TWE. *Application deadline:* For fall admission, 5/1 priority date for domestic and international students; for spring admission, 11/15 priority date for domestic students. Applications are processed on a rolling basis. Application fee: $55 ($60 for international students). Electronic applications accepted. *Financial support:* In 2013–14, 3 teaching assistantships with partial tuition reimbursements (averaging $13,322 per year) were awarded; scholarships/grants also available. Support available to part-time students. Financial award application deadline: 3/1; financial award applicants required to submit FAFSA. *Faculty research:* Pain management and substance abuse, high-risk alcohol use on campus, pediatric case management. *Unit head:* Dr. Lee-Ellen Kirkhorn, Chair/Professor, 260-481-6789, Fax: 260-481-5767, E-mail: kirkhorl@ipfw.edu. *Application contact:* Dr. Deborah Poling, Director of Graduate Program, 260-481-6276, Fax: 260-481-5767, E-mail: polingd@ipfw.edu.
Website: http://www.ipfw.edu/nursing/

Indiana University–Purdue University Indianapolis, School of Nursing, Doctor of Nursing Practice Program, Indianapolis, IN 46202-2896. Offers DNP. Part-time programs available. Postbaccalaureate distance learning degree programs offered (minimal on-campus study). *Students:* 4 full-time (all women), 25 part-time (all women); includes 5 minority (2 Black or African American, non-Hispanic/Latino; 1 Asian, non-Hispanic/Latino; 2 Hispanic/Latino), 1 international. Average age 48. 13 applicants, 92% accepted, 11 enrolled. In 2013, 1 doctorate awarded. *Degree requirements:* For doctorate, comprehensive exam, inquiry project: evidence-based practice implementation or intervention. *Entrance requirements:* For doctorate, background check. Additional exam requirements/recommendations for international students: Required—TOEFL, IELTS. *Application deadline:* For spring admission, 3/1 for domestic and international students. Electronic applications accepted. *Financial support:* Teaching assistantships with partial tuition reimbursements and tuition waivers (partial) available. Financial award application deadline: 5/1; financial award applicants required to submit FAFSA. *Unit head:* Dr. Mary Beth Riner, Coordinator, 317-274-4325, E-mail: mriner@iupui.edu. *Application contact:* Deborah Jean Grew, Graduate Advisor for Doctoral Programs, 317-274-2806, Fax: 317-274-2996, E-mail: dgrew@iupui.edu.
Website: http://nursing.iu.edu/graduate/programs/dnp/index.shtml

Indiana University–Purdue University Indianapolis, School of Nursing, Master of Science in Nursing Program, Indianapolis, IN 46202-2896. Offers nursing administration (MSN); nursing education (MSN). *Students:* 31 full-time (27 women), 303 part-time (284 women); includes 54 minority (27 Black or African American, non-Hispanic/Latino; 11 Asian, non-Hispanic/Latino; 8 Hispanic/Latino; 8 Two or more races, non-Hispanic/Latino), 3 international. 200 applicants, 59% accepted, 88 enrolled. In 2013, 120 master's awarded. *Entrance requirements:* For master's, background check, statistics. *Unit head:* Associate Dean for Graduate Programs, 317-274-2806, E-mail: nursing@iupui.edu. *Application contact:* Lisa Thompson, Graduate Advisor, 317-274-2806, E-mail: lisrthom@iu.edu.
Website: http://nursing.iu.edu/graduate/programs/msn/index.shtml

Indiana University–Purdue University Indianapolis, School of Nursing, PhD Program in Nursing Science, Indianapolis, IN 46202-2896. Offers PhD. Part-time programs available. Postbaccalaureate distance learning degree programs offered (minimal on-campus study). *Faculty:* 31 full-time (29 women). *Students:* 51 full-time (47 women); includes 7 minority (4 Black or African American, non-Hispanic/Latino; 1 American Indian or Alaska Native, non-Hispanic/Latino; 1 Asian, non-Hispanic/Latino; 1 Hispanic/Latino), 2 international. Average age 45. 2 applicants. In 2013, 9 doctorates awarded. *Degree requirements:* For doctorate, comprehensive exam, thesis/dissertation. *Entrance requirements:* For doctorate, GRE. Additional exam requirements/recommendations for international students: Required—TOEFL, IELTS. *Application deadline:* For fall admission, 8/15 for domestic and international students; for winter admission, 1/15 for domestic and international students. Electronic applications accepted. *Financial support:* In 2013–14, 14 fellowships with full tuition reimbursements (averaging $15,300 per year), 4 research assistantships with partial tuition reimbursements (averaging $11,000 per year) were awarded; teaching assistantships with partial tuition reimbursements, Federal Work-Study, institutionally sponsored loans, scholarships/grants, traineeships, tuition waivers (partial), and unspecified assistantships also available. Support available to part-time students. Financial award application deadline: 5/1; financial award applicants required to submit FAFSA. *Unit head:* Dr. Patricia Ebright, Associate Dean for Graduate Programs, 317-274-2806, E-mail: prebrigh@iupui.edu. *Application contact:* Deborah Jean Grew, Graduate Advisor for Doctoral Programs, 317-274-2806, Fax: 317-274-2996, E-mail: dgrew@iupui.edu.
Website: http://nursing.iu.edu/graduate/programs/phd/index.shtml

Indiana University South Bend, School of Nursing, South Bend, IN 46634-7111. Offers family nurse practitioner (MSN). Part-time and evening/weekend programs available. *Faculty:* 4 full-time (all women). *Students:* 46 part-time (39 women); includes 9 minority (3 Black or African American, non-Hispanic/Latino; 2 Asian, non-Hispanic/Latino; 2 Hispanic/Latino; 2 Two or more races, non-Hispanic/Latino). Average age 43. 33 applicants, 48% accepted, 15 enrolled. In 2013, 10 master's awarded. *Entrance requirements:* For master's, GRE General Test, minimum GPA of 3.0. *Application deadline:* For fall admission, 4/1 for domestic students. *Financial support:* Teaching assistantships and Federal Work-Study available. Support available to part-time students. Financial award application deadline: 3/1; financial award applicants required to submit FAFSA. *Application contact:* Admissions Counselor, 574-520-4839, Fax: 574-520-4834, E-mail: graduate@iusb.edu.
Website: https://www.iusb.edu/nursing/msn.php

Indiana Wesleyan University, Graduate School, School of Nursing, Marion, IN 46953-4974. Offers nursing administration (MS); nursing education (MS); primary care nursing (MS); MSN/MBA. *Accreditation:* AACN. Part-time programs available. Postbaccalaureate distance learning degree programs offered (minimal on-campus study). *Degree requirements:* For master's, capstone project or thesis. *Entrance requirements:* For master's, writing sample, RN license, 1 year of related experience, graduate statistics course. Additional exam requirements/recommendations for international students: Required—TOEFL. *Expenses:* Contact institution. *Faculty research:* Primary health care with international emphasis, international nursing.

Inter American University of Puerto Rico, Arecibo Campus, Program in Nursing, Arecibo, PR 00614-4050. Offers critical care nursing (MSN); surgical nursing (MSN). *Entrance requirements:* For master's, EXADEP or GRE General Test or MAT, 2 letters of recommendation, bachelor's degree in nursing, minimum GPA of 2.5 in last 60 credits, minimum 1 year nursing experience, nursing license.

Jacksonville State University, College of Graduate Studies and Continuing Education, College of Nursing, Jacksonville, AL 36265-1602. Offers MSN. *Accreditation:* AACN. Part-time and evening/weekend programs available. *Degree requirements:* For master's, comprehensive exam, thesis (for some programs). *Entrance requirements:* For master's, GRE General Test or MAT. Additional exam requirements/recommendations for international students: Required—TOEFL (minimum score 500 paper-based; 61 iBT). Electronic applications accepted.

Jacksonville University, School of Nursing, Jacksonville, FL 32211. Offers MSN, DNP. *Accreditation:* AACN. Part-time programs available. *Degree requirements:* For master's, thesis. *Entrance requirements:* For master's, GRE General Test, BS in nursing from an accredited program, course work in statistics within last 5 years, Florida nursing license. Additional exam requirements/recommendations for international students: Required—TOEFL (minimum score 550 paper-based). *Expenses:* Contact institution.

James Madison University, The Graduate School, College of Health and Behavioral Studies, Department of Nursing, Harrisonburg, VA 22807. Offers MSN. *Accreditation:* AACN. *Faculty:* 10 full-time (all women). *Students:* 8 full-time (7 women), 54 part-time (41 women); includes 3 minority (2 Black or African American, non-Hispanic/Latino; 1 Two or more races, non-Hispanic/Latino), 1 international. Average age 27. In 2013, 12 master's awarded. *Entrance requirements:* For master's, GRE General Test. *Application deadline:* For fall admission, 4/1 priority date for domestic students; for spring admission, 4/1 priority date for domestic students. Application fee: $55. *Financial support:* In 2013–14, 1 student received support. 1 graduate assistantship (averaging $7530) available. Financial award application deadline: 3/1; financial award applicants required to submit FAFSA. *Unit head:* Julie Sanford, Academic Unit Head, 540-568-6314, E-mail: sanforjt@jmu.edu. *Application contact:* Dr. Patty Hale, Graduate Program Coordinator, 540-568-1700.

Nursing—General

Jefferson College of Health Sciences, Program in Nursing, Roanoke, VA 24031-3186. Offers nursing education (MSN); nursing management (MSN). *Accreditation:* AACN. Part-time programs available. *Degree requirements:* For master's, project. *Entrance requirements:* For master's, MAT. Additional exam requirements/recommendations for international students: Required—TOEFL (minimum score 550 paper-based; 80 iBT). Electronic applications accepted. *Faculty research:* Nursing, teaching and learning techniques, cultural competence, spirituality and nursing.

Johns Hopkins University, School of Nursing, Certificate Programs in Nursing, Baltimore, MD 21218-2699. Offers Certificate. *Faculty:* 62 full-time (46 women), 160 part-time/adjunct (all women). *Students:* 14 part-time (all women); includes 3 minority (1 Black or African American, non-Hispanic/Latino; 1 Asian, non-Hispanic/Latino; 1 Two or more races, non-Hispanic/Latino). Average age 39. 52 applicants, 42% accepted, 10 enrolled. In 2013, 1 Certificate awarded. *Application deadline:* Applications are processed on a rolling basis. Application fee: $75. *Unit head:* Dr. Patricia M. Davidson, Dean, 410-955-7544, Fax: 410-955-4890, E-mail: sondeansoffice@jhu.edu. *Application contact:* Nadine Marks, Director of Admissions and Student Services, 410-955-7548, Fax: 410-614-7086, E-mail: nmarks3@jhu.edu.

Johns Hopkins University, School of Nursing, Doctoral Programs in Nursing, Baltimore, MD 21218-2699. Offers DNP, PhD. *Faculty:* 62 full-time (46 women), 160 part-time/adjunct (all women). *Students:* 29 full-time (26 women), 39 part-time (36 women); includes 20 minority (7 Black or African American, non-Hispanic/Latino; 7 Asian, non-Hispanic/Latino; 5 Hispanic/Latino; 1 Two or more races, non-Hispanic/Latino), 9 international. Average age 39. 39 applicants, 33% accepted, 9 enrolled. In 2013, 25 doctorates awarded. *Application deadline:* For fall admission, 1/15 for domestic students. Application fee: $100. *Financial support:* Fellowships, research assistantships, teaching assistantships, and unspecified assistantships available. *Unit head:* Dr. Patricia M. Davidson, Dean, 410-955-7544, Fax: 410-955-4890, E-mail: sondeansoffice@jhu.edu. *Application contact:* Nadine Marks, Director of Admissions and Student Services, 410-955-7548, Fax: 410-614-7086, E-mail: nmarks3@jhu.edu.

Johns Hopkins University, School of Nursing, Master's Programs in Nursing, Baltimore, MD 21218-2699. Offers MSN, MSN/MBA, MSN/MPH. *Faculty:* 62 full-time (46 women), 160 part-time/adjunct (all women). *Students:* 60 full-time (57 women), 212 part-time (198 women); includes 69 minority (17 Black or African American, non-Hispanic/Latino; 34 Asian, non-Hispanic/Latino; 11 Hispanic/Latino; 1 Native Hawaiian or other Pacific Islander, non-Hispanic/Latino; 6 Two or more races, non-Hispanic/Latino), 5 international. Average age 31. 299 applicants, 54% accepted, 91 enrolled. In 2013, 83 master's awarded. Application fee: $75. *Unit head:* Dr. Patricia M. Davidson, Dean, 410-955-7544, Fax: 410-955-4890, E-mail: sondeansoffice@jhu.edu. *Application contact:* Nadine Marks, Director of Admissions and Student Services, 410-955-7548, Fax: 410-614-7086, E-mail: nmarks3@jhu.edu.

Kaplan University, Davenport Campus, School of Nursing, Davenport, IA 52807-2095. Offers nurse administrator (MS); nurse educator (MS). Part-time and evening/weekend programs available. Postbaccalaureate distance learning degree programs offered (no on-campus study). *Entrance requirements:* For master's, RN. Additional exam requirements/recommendations for international students: Required—TOEFL (minimum score 550 paper-based).

Kean University, College of Natural, Applied and Health Sciences, Program in Nursing, Union, NJ 07083. Offers clinical management with transcultural focus (MSN); community health nursing (MSN); school nursing (MSN). Part-time programs available. *Faculty:* 8 full-time (all women). *Students:* 14 full-time (12 women), 121 part-time (117 women); includes 62 minority (43 Black or African American, non-Hispanic/Latino; 11 Asian, non-Hispanic/Latino; 7 Hispanic/Latino; 1 Two or more races, non-Hispanic/Latino), 2 international. Average age 42. 72 applicants, 94% accepted, 49 enrolled. In 2013, 35 master's awarded. *Degree requirements:* For master's, thesis or alternative, clinical field experience. *Entrance requirements:* For master's, minimum GPA of 3.0; BS in nursing; RN license; 2 letters of recommendation; interview. Additional exam requirements/recommendations for international students: Required—TOEFL. *Application deadline:* For fall admission, 6/1 for domestic and international students; for spring admission, 12/1 for domestic and international students. Applications are processed on a rolling basis. Application fee: $75 ($150 for international students). Electronic applications accepted. *Expenses:* Tuition, state resident: full-time $12,099; part-time $589 per credit. Tuition, nonresident: full-time $16,399; part-time $722 per credit. *Required fees:* $3050; $139 per credit. Part-time tuition and fees vary according to course level, course load, degree level and program. *Financial support:* In 2013–14, 2 research assistantships with full tuition reimbursements (averaging $3,713 per year) were awarded; unspecified assistantships also available. Financial award applicants required to submit FAFSA. *Unit head:* Dr. Virginia Fitzsimons, Program Coordinator, 908-527-3396, E-mail: vfitzsim@kean.edu. *Application contact:* Ann-Marie Kay, Assistant Director of Graduate Admissions, 908-737-5922, Fax: 908-737-5925, E-mail: akay@kean.edu.
Website: http://grad.kean.edu/masters-programs/nursing-clinical-management

Keiser University, Master of Science in Nursing Program, Ft. Lauderdale, FL 33309. Offers MSN.

Kennesaw State University, College of Health and Human Services, Doctor of Nursing Science Program, Kennesaw, GA 30144-5591. Offers DNS. Part-time programs available. *Students:* 1 (woman) full-time, 9 part-time (8 women). Average age 49. 4 applicants, 25% accepted. *Degree requirements:* For doctorate, thesis/dissertation. *Entrance requirements:* For doctorate, GRE, master's degree in nursing, RN licensure. Additional exam requirements/recommendations for international students: Required—TOEFL (minimum score 550 paper-based; 80 iBT), IELTS (minimum score 6). *Application deadline:* For fall admission, 3/1 for domestic and international students. Applications are processed on a rolling basis. Application fee: $60. Electronic applications accepted. *Expenses:* Tuition, state resident: full-time $4806; part-time $267 per semester hour. Tuition, nonresident: full-time $17,298; part-time $961 per semester hour. *Required fees:* $1834; $784.50 per semester. *Financial support:* In 2013–14, 2 research assistantships with full tuition reimbursements (averaging $8,000 per year) were awarded. Financial award application deadline: 4/1; financial award applicants required to submit FAFSA. *Unit head:* Dr. Tommie Nelms, Director, 678-797-2088, E-mail: tnelms1@kennesaw.edu. *Application contact:* Jerryl Morris, Admissions Counselor, 678-797-2030, Fax: 770-423-6885, E-mail: ksugrad@kennesaw.edu.

Kennesaw State University, College of Health and Human Services, Program in Primary Care Nurse Practitioner, Kennesaw, GA 30144-5591. Offers MSN. *Accreditation:* AACN. Part-time and evening/weekend programs available. *Students:* 66 full-time (59 women), 1 (woman) part-time; includes 15 minority (8 Black or African American, non-Hispanic/Latino; 4 Asian, non-Hispanic/Latino; 2 Hispanic/Latino; 1 Two or more races, non-Hispanic/Latino). Average age 35. 54 applicants, 61% accepted, 30 enrolled. In 2013, 42 master's awarded. *Entrance requirements:* For master's, GRE General Test, minimum GPA of 2.5, RN license, 3 years of professional experience. Additional exam requirements/recommendations for international students: Required—TOEFL (minimum score 550 paper-based), IELTS (minimum score 6). *Application deadline:* For fall admission, 6/1 for domestic and international students. Application fee: $60. Electronic applications accepted. *Expenses:* Tuition, state resident: full-time $4806; part-time $267 per semester hour. Tuition, nonresident: full-time $17,298; part-time $961 per semester hour. *Required fees:* $1834; $784.50 per semester. *Financial support:* In 2013–14, 2 research assistantships with full tuition reimbursements (averaging $8,000 per year) were awarded; Federal Work-Study and unspecified assistantships also available. Support available to part-time students. Financial award application deadline: 4/1; financial award applicants required to submit FAFSA. *Unit head:* Dr. Marilyn King, Director, 770-423-6172, Fax: 770-423-6627, E-mail: mking71@kennesaw.edu. *Application contact:* Jerryl Morris, Admissions Counselor, 678-797-2030, E-mail: ksugrad@kennesaw.edu.

Kent State University, College of Nursing, Kent, OH 44242-0001. Offers acute care nurse practitioner (MSN); adult nurse practitioner (MSN); clinical nurse specialist (MSN); family nurse practitioner (MSN); geriatric nurse practitioner (MSN); health care management (MSN); nurse educator (MSN); nursing (PhD); nursing practice (DNP); pediatric nurse practitioner (MSN); psychiatric/mental health nurse practitioner (MSN); women's health nurse practitioner (MSN). PhD program offered jointly with The University of Akron. *Accreditation:* AACN. Part-time programs available. *Degree requirements:* For master's, thesis optional; for doctorate, comprehensive exam, thesis/dissertation. *Entrance requirements:* For master's, GRE (if undergraduate GPA less than 3.0), minimum GPA of 2.75; for doctorate, GRE, MSN. Additional exam requirements/recommendations for international students: Required—TOEFL. Electronic applications accepted. *Expenses:* Contact institution. *Faculty research:* Women and violence, methodological specialties, osteoporosis in women, new caregivers and the elderly.

Keuka College, Program in Nursing, Keuka Park, NY 14478-0098. Offers MS. *Accreditation:* AACN. *Faculty:* 2 full-time (both women), 4 part-time/adjunct (all women). *Students:* 20 full-time (18 women), 36 part-time (1 woman); includes 5 minority (4 Black or African American, non-Hispanic/Latino; 1 American Indian or Alaska Native, non-Hispanic/Latino). *Unit head:* Dr. Debra Gates, Chair, 315-279-5115 Ext. 5273, E-mail: dgates@keuka.edu. *Application contact:* Mark Petrie, Director of Admissions, 315-279-5434, Fax: 315-279-5386, E-mail: admissions@mail.keuka.edu.
Website: http://academics.keuka.edu/asap/programs/ms_nursing

Lamar University, College of Graduate Studies, College of Arts and Sciences, Department of Nursing, Beaumont, TX 77710. Offers nursing administration (MSN); nursing education (MSN); MSN/MBA. Part-time and evening/weekend programs available. Postbaccalaureate distance learning degree programs offered. *Degree requirements:* For master's, comprehensive exam, practicum project presentation, evidence-based project. *Entrance requirements:* For master's, GRE General Test, MAT, criminal background check, RN license, NLN-accredited BSN, college course work in graduate statistics in past 5 years, letters of recommendation, minimum undergraduate GPA of 3.0. Additional exam requirements/recommendations for international students: Required—TOEFL. *Faculty research:* Student retention, theory, care giving, online course and research.

La Roche College, School of Graduate Studies and Adult Education, Program in Nursing, Pittsburgh, PA 15237-5898. Offers nursing education (MSN); nursing management (MSN). *Accreditation:* AANA/CANAEP. Part-time and evening/weekend programs available. Postbaccalaureate distance learning degree programs offered (minimal on-campus study). *Faculty:* 3 full-time (all women), 2 part-time/adjunct (1 woman). *Students:* 6 full-time (all women), 7 part-time (all women), 1 international. Average age 43. 6 applicants, 50% accepted, 1 enrolled. In 2013, 7 master's awarded. *Degree requirements:* For master's, thesis optional, internship, practicum. *Entrance requirements:* For master's, GRE General Test, BSN, nursing license, work experience. Additional exam requirements/recommendations for international students: Recommended—TOEFL (minimum score 550 paper-based). *Application deadline:* For fall admission, 8/15 priority date for domestic students, 8/15 for international students; for spring admission, 12/15 priority date for domestic students, 12/15 for international students. Applications are processed on a rolling basis. Application fee: $50. Electronic applications accepted. *Expenses:* Contact institution. *Financial support:* Application deadline: 3/31; applicants required to submit FAFSA. *Faculty research:* Patient education, perception. *Unit head:* Dr. Terri Liberto, Division Chair, 412-847-1813, Fax: 412-536-1175, E-mail: terri.liberto@laroche.edu. *Application contact:* Hope Schiffgens, Director of Graduate Studies and Adult Education, 412-536-1266, Fax: 412-536-1283, E-mail: schombh1@laroche.edu.

La Salle University, School of Nursing and Health Sciences, Program in Nursing, Philadelphia, PA 19141-1199. Offers adult gerontology primary care nurse practitioner (MSN, Certificate); adult health and illness clinical nurse specialist (MSN); adult-gerontology clinical nurse specialist (MSN, Certificate); clinical nurse leader (MSN); family primary care nurse practitioner (MSN, Certificate); gerontology (Certificate); nurse anesthetist (MSN, Certificate); nursing (MSN, Certificate); nursing administration (MSN, Certificate); nursing education (Certificate); nursing practice (DNP); nursing service administration (MSN); public health nursing (MSN, Certificate); school nursing (Certificate); MSN/MBA; MSN/MPH. *Accreditation:* AANA/CANAEP. Part-time programs available. Postbaccalaureate distance learning degree programs offered (minimal on-campus study). *Faculty:* 13 full-time (12 women), 10 part-time/adjunct (8 women). *Students:* 4 full-time (all women), 379 part-time (331 women); includes 119 minority (70 Black or African American, non-Hispanic/Latino; 2 American Indian or Alaska Native, non-Hispanic/Latino; 31 Asian, non-Hispanic/Latino; 12 Hispanic/Latino; 4 Two or more races, non-Hispanic/Latino), 1 international. Average age 37. 133 applicants, 85% accepted, 63 enrolled. In 2013, 72 master's, 3 doctorates, 26 other advanced degrees awarded. *Degree requirements:* For doctorate, minimum of 1,000 hours of post baccalaureate clinical practice supervised by preceptors. *Entrance requirements:* For master's, GRE, MAT, or GMAT (for students with BSN GPA of less than 3.2), baccalaureate degree in nursing from an NLNAC- or CCNE-accredited program or an MSN Bridge program; Pennsylvania RN license; 2 letters of reference; resume; statement of philosophy articulating professional values and future educational goal; 1 year of work experience as a registered nurse; for doctorate, GRE (waived for applicants with MSN cumulative GPA of 3.7 or above), MSN from nationally-accredited program or master's degree, MBA or MHA from nationally-accredited program; resume or curriculum vitae; 2 letters of reference; interview; for Certificate, GRE, MAT, or GMAT (for students with BSN GPA of less than 3.2, baccalaureate degree in nursing from an NLNAC- or CCNE-accredited program or an MSN Bridge program; Pennsylvania RN license; 2 letters of reference; resume; statement of philosophy articulating professional values and future educational goal; 1 year of work experience as a registered nurse. Additional exam requirements/recommendations for international students: Required—TOEFL. *Application deadline:* For fall admission, 8/15 priority date for domestic students, 7/15 for international students; for spring admission, 12/15 priority date for domestic students, 11/15 for international students; for summer admission, 4/15 priority date for domestic students, 3/15 for international students. Applications are processed on a rolling basis. Application fee: $35. Electronic applications accepted. Application fee is waived when completed online. *Expenses:* Contact institution. *Financial support:* In 2013–14, 48 students received support. Teaching assistantships, scholarships/grants, and traineeships available. Support available to part-time students. Financial award application deadline: 8/31; financial award applicants required to submit FAFSA. *Unit head:* Dr. Patricia M. Dillon, Director, 215-951-1322, Fax: 215-951-1896, E-mail:

msnapn@lasalle.edu. *Application contact:* Paul J. Reilly, Assistant Vice President, Enrollment Services, 215-951-1946, Fax: 215-951-1462, E-mail: reilly@lasalle.edu.

Laurentian University, School of Graduate Studies and Research, Programme in Nursing, Sudbury, ON P3E 2C6, Canada. Offers M Sc N.

Lehman College of the City University of New York, School of Natural and Social Sciences, Department of Nursing, Bronx, NY 10468-1589. Offers adult health nursing (MS); nursing of older adults (MS); parent-child nursing (MS); pediatric nurse practitioner (MS). *Accreditation:* AACN. Part-time and evening/weekend programs available. *Entrance requirements:* For master's, bachelor's degree in nursing, New York RN license.

Le Moyne College, Department of Nursing, Syracuse, NY 13214. Offers informatics (MS, CAS); nursing administration (MS, CAS); nursing education (MS, CAS); nursing gerontology (MS, CAS); palliative care (MS, CAS). *Accreditation:* AACN. Part-time and evening/weekend programs available. *Faculty:* 4 full-time (all women), 3 part-time/adjunct (2 women). *Students:* 13 part-time (12 women); includes 2 minority (both Black or African American, non-Hispanic/Latino). Average age 41. 14 applicants, 86% accepted, 5 enrolled. In 2013, 6 master's, 6 other advanced degrees awarded. *Degree requirements:* For master's, scholarly project. *Entrance requirements:* For master's, bachelor's degree, interview, minimum GPA of 3.0, New York RN license, 2 letters of recommendation, writing sample, transcripts. Additional exam requirements/recommendations for international students: Required—TOEFL (minimum score 550 paper-based; 79 iBT). *Application deadline:* For fall admission, 8/1 priority date for domestic and international students; for spring admission, 12/15 priority date for domestic and international students; for summer admission, 5/1 priority date for domestic and international students. Applications are processed on a rolling basis. Application fee: $50. *Expenses:* Contact institution. *Financial support:* In 2013–14, 2 students received support. Career-related internships or fieldwork, scholarships/grants, health care benefits, and unspecified assistantships available. Support available to part-time students. Financial award applicants required to submit FAFSA. *Faculty research:* Inter-profession education, gerontology, utilization of free healthcare services by the insured, health promotion education, innovative undergraduate nursing education models, patient and family education, horizontal violence. *Unit head:* Dr. Susan B. Bastable, Chair and Professor, Department of Nursing, 315-445-5436, Fax: 315-445-6024, E-mail: bastabsb@lemoyne.edu. *Application contact:* Kristen P. Trapasso, Senior Director of Enrollment Management, 315-445-4265, Fax: 315-445-6092, E-mail: trapaskp@lemoyne.edu.
Website: http://www.lemoyne.edu/nursing

Lewis University, College of Nursing and Health Professions, Program in Nursing, Romeoville, IL 60446. Offers adult nurse practitioner (MSN); nursing administration (MSN); nursing education (MSN). *Accreditation:* AACN. Part-time and evening/weekend programs available. Postbaccalaureate distance learning degree programs offered (no on-campus study). *Students:* 23 full-time (22 women), 234 part-time (222 women); includes 72 minority (31 Black or African American, non-Hispanic/Latino; 23 Asian, non-Hispanic/Latino; 15 Hispanic/Latino; 1 Native Hawaiian or other Pacific Islander, non-Hispanic/Latino; 2 Two or more races, non-Hispanic/Latino). Average age 38. *Degree requirements:* For master's, clinical practicum. *Entrance requirements:* For master's, minimum undergraduate GPA of 3.0, degree in nursing, RN license, letter of recommendation, interview, resume or curriculum vitae. Additional exam requirements/recommendations for international students: Required—TOEFL (minimum score 550 paper-based; 80 iBT). *Application deadline:* For fall admission, 5/1 priority date for international students; for spring admission, 11/15 priority date for international students. Applications are processed on a rolling basis. Application fee: $40. Electronic applications accepted. *Financial support:* Federal Work-Study, scholarships/grants, tuition waivers (full and partial), and unspecified assistantships available. Financial award application deadline: 5/1; financial award applicants required to submit FAFSA. *Faculty research:* Cancer prevention, phenomenological methods, public policy analysis. *Total annual research expenditures:* $1,000. *Unit head:* 815-836-5610. *Application contact:* Nancy Wiksten, Adult Admission Counselor, 815-836-5628, Fax: 815-836-5578, E-mail: wikstena@lewisu.edu.
Website: http://www.lewisu.edu/

Lewis University, College of Nursing and Health Professions and College of Business, Program in Nursing/Business, Romeoville, IL 60446. Offers MSN/MBA. Part-time and evening/weekend programs available. *Students:* 7 full-time (6 women), 18 part-time (17 women); includes 9 minority (4 Black or African American, non-Hispanic/Latino; 1 Asian, non-Hispanic/Latino; 3 Hispanic/Latino; 1 Native Hawaiian or other Pacific Islander, non-Hispanic/Latino). Average age 36. *Entrance requirements:* Additional exam requirements/recommendations for international students: Required—TOEFL (minimum score 550 paper-based; 80 iBT). *Application deadline:* For fall admission, 4/2 priority date for domestic students, 5/1 priority date for international students; for spring admission, 11/15 priority date for international students. Applications are processed on a rolling basis. Electronic applications accepted. *Financial support:* Scholarships/grants, tuition waivers (full and partial), and unspecified assistantships available. Financial award application deadline: 5/1; financial award applicants required to submit FAFSA. *Faculty research:* Cancer prevention, phenomenological methods, public policy analysis. *Total annual research expenditures:* $1,000. *Unit head:* Dr. Linda Niedringhaus, Interim Director, 815-838-0500 Ext. 5878, E-mail: niedrili@lewisu.edu. *Application contact:* Nancy Wiksten, Adult Admission Counselor, 815-838-0500 Ext. 5628, Fax: 815-836-5578, E-mail: wikstena@lewisu.edu.

Liberty University, School of Health Sciences, Lynchburg, VA 24515. Offers biomedical sciences (MS); clinical mental health counseling (MA); global health (MPH); health promotion (MPH); human services (MA), including addictions and recovery, business, Christian ministry, criminal justice, crisis response and trauma, executive leadership, health and wellness, life coaching, marriage and family, military resilience; marriage and family therapy (MA); nurse educator (MS); nursing (MSN); nursing administration (MSN); nutrition (MPH); pastoral care and counseling (PhD); professional counseling (MA, PhD). *Students:* 2,830 full-time (2,293 women), 6,275 part-time (5,051 women); includes 1,677 minority (1,178 Black or African American, non-Hispanic/Latino; 19 American Indian or Alaska Native, non-Hispanic/Latino; 36 Asian, non-Hispanic/Latino; 278 Hispanic/Latino; 7 Native Hawaiian or other Pacific Islander, non-Hispanic/Latino; 159 Two or more races, non-Hispanic/Latino), 177 international. Average age 37. 9,147 applicants, 50% accepted, 2939 enrolled. In 2013, 2,618 master's, 11 doctorates awarded. *Degree requirements:* For master's, thesis (for some programs); for doctorate, thesis/dissertation. *Entrance requirements:* For doctorate, MAT or GRE, minimum GPA of 3.25 in master's program, 2-3 recommendations, writing samples (for some programs), letter of intent, professional vitae. Additional exam requirements/recommendations for international students: Required—TOEFL (minimum score 600 paper-based; 100 iBT). Application fee: $50. *Expenses: Tuition:* Full-time $9630; part-time $535 per credit hour. *Required fees:* $175 per term. One-time fee: $50. Tuition and fees vary according to course load, degree level, campus/location and program. *Application contact:* Jay Bridge, Director of Admissions, 800-424-9595, Fax: 800-628-7977, E-mail: gradadmissions@liberty.edu.

Lincoln Memorial University, Caylor School of Nursing, Harrogate, TN 37752-1901. Offers family nurse practitioner (MSN); nurse anesthesia (MSN); psychiatric mental health nurse practitioner (MSN). *Accreditation:* AANA/CANAEP. Part-time programs available. *Entrance requirements:* For master's, GRE.

Loma Linda University, Department of Graduate Nursing, Loma Linda, CA 92350. Offers adult and aging family nursing (MS); growing family nursing (MS); nursing administration (MS). *Accreditation:* AACN; AANA/CANAEP. Part-time programs available. *Degree requirements:* For master's, thesis or alternative. *Entrance requirements:* For master's, GRE General Test, BSN, minimum GPA of 3.0, RN license. Additional exam requirements/recommendations for international students: Required—TOEFL (minimum score 550 paper-based). Electronic applications accepted.

Long Island University–LIU Brooklyn, School of Nursing, Brooklyn, NY 11201-8423. Offers MS, Certificate. *Accreditation:* AACN. *Entrance requirements:* For master's, New York RN license, 2 letters of recommendation. Additional exam requirements/recommendations for international students: Required—TOEFL (minimum score 500 paper-based). Electronic applications accepted.

Long Island University–LIU Post, School of Health Professions and Nursing, Department of Nursing, Brookville, NY 11548-1300. Offers clinical nurse specialist (MS); family nurse practitioner (MS, Certificate). *Accreditation:* AACN. Part-time and evening/weekend programs available. *Degree requirements:* For master's, thesis. *Entrance requirements:* For master's, minimum GPA of 3.0 in major, bachelor's degree in nursing, NYS registered nurse, interview. Electronic applications accepted. *Faculty research:* Lactation/breast cancer, early discharge in maternity.

Louisiana State University Health Sciences Center, School of Nursing, New Orleans, LA 70112-2223. Offers advanced public/community health nursing (MN); clinical nurse specialist (MN); nurse anesthesia (MN); nurse practitioner (MN); nursing (DNS). *Accreditation:* AACN; AANA/CANAEP (one or more programs are accredited). Part-time programs available. *Degree requirements:* For master's, thesis optional; for doctorate, thesis/dissertation. *Entrance requirements:* For master's, GRE General Test, MAT, minimum GPA of 3.0; for doctorate, GRE General Test, minimum GPA of 3.5. Additional exam requirements/recommendations for international students: Required—TOEFL. Electronic applications accepted. *Faculty research:* Advanced clinical practice, nursing education, health, social support, nursing administration.

Loyola University Chicago, Graduate School, Marcella Niehoff School of Nursing, Doctor of Nursing Practice Program, Maywood, IL 60153. Offers infection prevention (DNP); informatics and outcomes (DNP). Evening/weekend programs available. Postbaccalaureate distance learning degree programs offered (minimal on-campus study). *Faculty:* 45 full-time (44 women). *Students:* 4 full-time (all women), 27 part-time (24 women); includes 9 minority (3 Black or African American, non-Hispanic/Latino; 2 Asian, non-Hispanic/Latino; 4 Hispanic/Latino). Average age 46. 26 applicants, 62% accepted, 12 enrolled. In 2013, 8 doctorates awarded. *Degree requirements:* For doctorate, capstone project. *Entrance requirements:* For doctorate, BSN or MSN, minimum GPA of 3.25, Illinois nursing license, 3 letters of recommendation, 1000 hours of experience and certification in area of specialty, curriculum vitae. Additional exam requirements/recommendations for international students: Required—TOEFL. *Expenses: Tuition:* Full-time $16,740; part-time $930 per credit. *Required fees:* $135 per semester. *Unit head:* Dr. Marijo Letizia, Associate Dean, 708-216-9325, Fax: 708-216-9555, E-mail: mletizi@luc.edu. *Application contact:* Amy Weatherford, Enrollment Advisor, School of Nursing, 773-508-3249, Fax: 773-508-3241, E-mail: aweatherford@luc.edu.
Website: http://www.luc.edu/nursing/dnp/

Loyola University Chicago, Graduate School, Marcella Niehoff School of Nursing, PhD Program in Nursing, Maywood, IL 60153. Offers PhD. *Faculty:* 45 full-time (44 women). *Students:* 24 full-time (23 women), 7 part-time (all women); includes 2 minority (both Asian, non-Hispanic/Latino), 1 international. Average age 51. 8 applicants, 50% accepted, 4 enrolled. In 2013, 3 doctorates awarded. *Degree requirements:* For doctorate, comprehensive exam, thesis/dissertation, research internship. *Entrance requirements:* For doctorate, GRE General Test, master's degree in nursing or related field, minimum GPA of 3.0, active nursing license, 3 letters of recommendation. Additional exam requirements/recommendations for international students: Required—TOEFL (minimum score 650 paper-based; 114 iBT) or IELTS. *Application deadline:* For fall admission, 7/1 for domestic and international students. Applications are processed on a rolling basis. Application fee: $0. *Expenses: Tuition:* Full-time $16,740; part-time $930 per credit. *Required fees:* $135 per semester. *Financial support:* In 2013–14, 3 students received support, including 3 research assistantships with full tuition reimbursements available (averaging $18,000 per year). Financial award application deadline: 5/1; financial award applicants required to submit FAFSA. *Faculty research:* Women's health, adolescent health and chronic illness, psychoneuroimmunology, grief and bereavement, nurse staffing and outcomes. *Unit head:* Dr. Barbara Velsor-Friedrich, Director, PhD in Nursing Program, 773-508-2892, Fax: 773-508-3241, E-mail: bvelsor@luc.edu. *Application contact:* Amy Weatherford, Enrollment Advisor, School of Nursing, 773-508-3249, Fax: 773-508-3241, E-mail: aweatherford@luc.edu.

Loyola University Chicago, Graduate School, Marcella Niehoff School of Nursing, Program in Emergency Nurse Practitioner, Chicago, IL 60660. Offers MSN. *Entrance requirements:* For master's, Illinois nursing license, 3 letters of recommendation, minimum nursing GPA of 3.0, 1000 hours of experience before starting clinical. Application fee: $50. *Expenses: Tuition:* Full-time $16,740; part-time $930 per credit. *Required fees:* $135 per semester. *Financial support:* Traineeships available. *Unit head:* Dr. Marijo Letizia, Associate Dean, 708-216-9325, Fax: 708-216-9555, E-mail: mletizi@luc.edu. *Application contact:* Amy Weatherford, Enrollment Advisor, School of Nursing, 773-508-3249, Fax: 773-508-3241, E-mail: aweatherford@luc.edu.
Website: http://luc.edu/media/lucedu/nursing/pdfs/FNP-ER.pdf

Loyola University New Orleans, College of Social Sciences, School of Nursing, New Orleans, LA 70118-6195. Offers health care systems management (MSN); nursing (MSN, DNP). Part-time and evening/weekend programs available. Postbaccalaureate distance learning degree programs offered. *Faculty:* 16 full-time (15 women), 9 part-time/adjunct (7 women). *Students:* 432 full-time (388 women), 108 part-time (102 women); includes 160 minority (113 Black or African American, non-Hispanic/Latino; 2 American Indian or Alaska Native, non-Hispanic/Latino; 13 Asian, non-Hispanic/Latino; 29 Hispanic/Latino; 2 Native Hawaiian or other Pacific Islander, non-Hispanic/Latino; 1 Two or more races, non-Hispanic/Latino). Average age 42. 285 applicants, 83% accepted, 200 enrolled. In 2013, 185 master's, 15 doctorates awarded. *Degree requirements:* For doctorate, capstone project. *Entrance requirements:* For master's, BSN, Louisiana nursing license, 1 year of work experience in clinical nursing, minimum undergraduate GPA of 2.8, interview, resume. Additional exam requirements/recommendations for international students: Required—TOEFL (minimum score 550 paper-based). *Application deadline:* For fall admission, 8/1 priority date for domestic and international students; for winter admission, 12/15 priority date for domestic and international students; for spring admission, 5/15 priority date for domestic and international students. Applications are processed on a rolling basis. Application fee: $20. Electronic applications accepted. *Expenses: Tuition:* Part-time $818 per hour. Part-time tuition and fees vary according to program. *Financial support:* Traineeships and Incumbent Workers Training Program grants available. Financial award application deadline: 5/1; financial award applicants required to submit FAFSA. *Faculty research:*

Increasing compliance with treatment, patient satisfaction with care provided by nurse practitioners. *Unit head:* Dr. Mary D. Oriol, Interim Director, 800-488-6257, Fax: 504-865-3254, E-mail: nursing@loyno.edu. *Application contact:* Deborah Smith, Assistant to the Director, 504-865-2823, Fax: 504-865-3254, E-mail: dhsmith@loyno.edu.
Website: http://css.loyno.edu/nursing

Lynchburg College, Graduate Studies, School of Health Sciences and Human Performance, MS Program in Nursing, Lynchburg, VA 24501-3199. Offers clinical nurse leader (MS); nursing education (MS). *Accreditation:* AACN. Part-time and evening/weekend programs available. Postbaccalaureate distance learning degree programs offered (minimal on-campus study). *Faculty:* 4 full-time (all women), 1 (woman) part-time/adjunct. *Students:* 2 full-time (both women), 16 part-time (14 women); includes 2 minority (1 Black or African American, non-Hispanic/Latino; 1 Hispanic/Latino), 1 international. Average age 40. In 2013, 4 master's awarded. *Degree requirements:* For master's, practicum. *Entrance requirements:* For master's, GRE or 2 years of professional nursing experience, official transcripts, personal essay, 3 letters of recommendation, current unrestricted registered nurse license in Virginia. Additional exam requirements/recommendations for international students: Required—TOEFL (minimum score 550 paper-based; 79 iBT), IELTS (minimum score 6.5). *Application deadline:* For fall admission, 7/31 for domestic students, 6/1 for international students; for spring admission, 11/30 for domestic students, 10/15 for international students. Applications are processed on a rolling basis. Application fee: $30. Electronic applications accepted. Application fee is waived when completed online. *Financial support:* Fellowships, Federal Work-Study, scholarships/grants, health care benefits, and unspecified assistantships available. Support available to part-time students. Financial award application deadline: 7/31; financial award applicants required to submit FAFSA. *Unit head:* Dr. Nancy Overstreet, Associate Professor/Director of MSN Program, 434-544-8340, E-mail: overstreet.n@lynchburg.edu. *Application contact:* Anne Pingstock, Executive Assistant, Graduate Studies, 434-544-8383, E-mail: gradstudies@lynchburg.edu.
Website: http://www.lynchburg.edu/master-science-nursing

Madonna University, Program in Nursing, Livonia, MI 48150-1173. Offers adult health: chronic health conditions (MSN); adult nurse practitioner (MSN); nursing administration (MSN); MSN/MSBA. *Accreditation:* AACN. Part-time programs available. *Degree requirements:* For master's, thesis or alternative. *Entrance requirements:* For master's, GRE General Test, Michigan nursing license. Electronic applications accepted. *Faculty research:* Coping, caring.

Malone University, Graduate Program in Nursing, Canton, OH 44709. Offers family nurse practitioner (MSN). *Accreditation:* AACN. Part-time and evening/weekend programs available. *Faculty:* 10 full-time (all women), 14 part-time/adjunct (13 women). *Students:* 65 part-time (62 women); includes 5 minority (2 Black or African American, non-Hispanic/Latino; 1 American Indian or Alaska Native, non-Hispanic/Latino; 1 Asian, non-Hispanic/Latino; 1 Hispanic/Latino). Average age 34. In 2013, 26 master's awarded. *Degree requirements:* For master's, thesis. *Entrance requirements:* For master's, minimum GPA of 3.0 from BSN program, interview, Ohio RN license. Additional exam requirements/recommendations for international students: Required—TOEFL (minimum score 550 paper-based; 79 iBT). *Application deadline:* Applications are processed on a rolling basis. *Expenses:* Contact institution. *Financial support:* Tuition waivers (partial) available. Support available to part-time students. Financial award application deadline: 6/30. *Faculty research:* Home heath care and geriatrics, community settings, culture, Hispanics, tuberculosis, geriatrics, Neuman Systems Model, nursing education. *Unit head:* Dr. Kathleen M. Flaherty, Director, 330-471-8330, Fax: 330-471-8607, E-mail: kflaherty@malone.edu. *Application contact:* Natalie D. Denholm, Recruiter/Adviser, 330-471-8207, Fax: 330-471-8570, E-mail: ndenholm@malone.edu.
Website: http://www.malone.edu/admissions/graduate/nursing/

Mansfield University of Pennsylvania, Graduate Studies, Program in Nursing, Mansfield, PA 16933. Offers MSN. Part-time and evening/weekend programs available. Postbaccalaureate distance learning degree programs offered. *Degree requirements:* For master's, comprehensive exam, thesis optional. *Entrance requirements:* For master's, minimum GPA of 3.0. Additional exam requirements/recommendations for international students: Required—TOEFL (minimum score 550 paper-based). Electronic applications accepted. *Faculty research:* Women's health, gyniatrics, art therapy, nursing empowerment.

Marian University, School of Nursing and Health Professions, Fond du Lac, WI 54935-4699. Offers adult nurse practitioner (MSN); nurse educator (MSN). *Accreditation:* AACN. Part-time and evening/weekend programs available. *Faculty:* 5 full-time (all women), 10 part-time/adjunct (6 women). *Students:* 21 full-time (18 women), 77 part-time (71 women); includes 9 minority (3 Black or African American, non-Hispanic/Latino; 5 Hispanic/Latino; 1 Native Hawaiian or other Pacific Islander, non-Hispanic/Latino). Average age 37. In 2013, 24 master's awarded. *Degree requirements:* For master's, thesis, 675 clinical practicum hours. *Entrance requirements:* For master's, 3 letters of professional recommendation; undergraduate work in nursing research, statistics, health assessment. Additional exam requirements/recommendations for international students: Required—TOEFL (minimum score 525 paper-based; 70 iBT). *Application deadline:* Applications are processed on a rolling basis. Application fee: $50. Electronic applications accepted. *Expenses:* Contact institution. *Financial support:* In 2013–14, 3 students received support. Institutionally sponsored loans and scholarships/grants available. Support available to part-time students. Financial award application deadline: 3/1; financial award applicants required to submit FAFSA. *Unit head:* Dr. Julie Luetschwager, Dean, 920-923-8094, Fax: 920-923-8770, E-mail: jaluetschwager25@marianuniversity.edu. *Application contact:* Selina Scoles, Admissions Counselor, 920-923-8938, Fax: 920-923-8770, E-mail: sascoles30@marianuniversity.edu.
Website: http://www.marianuniversity.edu/nursing/

Marquette University, Graduate School, College of Nursing, Milwaukee, WI 53201-1881. Offers acute care nurse practitioner (Certificate); adult clinical nurse specialist (Certificate); adult nurse practitioner (Certificate); advanced practice nursing (MSN, DNP), including adult-older adult acute care (DNP), adults (MSN), adults-older adults (DNP), clinical nurse leader (MSN), health care systems leadership (DNP), nurse-midwifery (MSN), older adults (MSN), pediatrics acute care (MSN), pediatrics primary care (MSN), pediatrics-acute care (DNP), pediatrics-primary care (DNP), primary care (DNP), systems leadership and healthcare quality (MSN); family nurse practitioner (Certificate); nurse-midwifery (Certificate); nursing (PhD); pediatric acute care (Certificate); pediatric primary care (Certificate); systems leadership and healthcare quality (Certificate). *Accreditation:* AACN. *Faculty:* 35 full-time (34 women), 59 part-time/adjunct (58 women). *Students:* 105 full-time (96 women), 279 part-time (256 women); includes 28 minority (11 Black or African American, non-Hispanic/Latino; 7 Asian, non-Hispanic/Latino; 8 Hispanic/Latino; 2 Two or more races, non-Hispanic/Latino), 3 international. Average age 30. 322 applicants, 62% accepted, 98 enrolled. In 2013, 66 master's, 4 doctorates, 6 other advanced degrees awarded. Terminal master's awarded for partial completion of doctoral program. *Degree requirements:* For master's, comprehensive exam, thesis or alternative. *Entrance requirements:* For master's, GRE General Test, BSN, Wisconsin RN license, official transcripts from all current and previous colleges/universities except Marquette, three completed recommendation forms, resume, written statement of professional goals; for doctorate, GRE General Test, official transcripts from all current and previous colleges/universities except Marquette, three letters of recommendation, resume, written statement of professional goals, sample of scholarly writing. Additional exam requirements/recommendations for international students: Required—TOEFL (minimum score 530 paper-based). *Application deadline:* For fall admission, 2/15 for domestic and international students. Application fee: $50. Electronic applications accepted. *Financial support:* In 2013–14, 41 students received support, including 1 fellowship with partial tuition reimbursement available (averaging $17,500 per year), 2 research assistantships with full tuition reimbursements available (averaging $13,285 per year), 8 teaching assistantships with full tuition reimbursements available (averaging $13,912 per year); career-related internships or fieldwork, Federal Work-Study, scholarships/grants, health care benefits, tuition waivers (partial), and unspecified assistantships also available. Support available to part-time students. Financial award application deadline: 2/15. *Faculty research:* Psychosocial adjustment to chronic illness, gerontology, reminiscence, health policy: uninsured and access, hospital care delivery systems. *Total annual research expenditures:* $769,051. *Unit head:* Dr. Margaret Callahan, Dean, 414-288-3800, Fax: 414-288-1578. *Application contact:* Dr. Maureen O'Brien, Associate Dean/Clinical Associate Professor, 414-288-3823.
Website: http://www.marquette.edu/nursing/academicprograms-graduate.shtml

Marshall University, Academic Affairs Division, College of Health Professions, Department of Nursing, Huntington, WV 25755. Offers MSN. *Students:* 14 full-time (12 women), 126 part-time (117 women); includes 6 minority (3 Black or African American, non-Hispanic/Latino; 2 Asian, non-Hispanic/Latino; 1 Hispanic/Latino), 1 international. Average age 34. In 2013, 61 master's awarded. *Entrance requirements:* For master's, GRE General Test. Application fee: $40. *Unit head:* Dr. Diana Stotts, Associate Dean, 304-696-2623, E-mail: stotts@marshall.edu. *Application contact:* Information Contact, 304-746-1900, Fax: 304-746-1902, E-mail: services@marshall.edu.

Marymount University, School of Health Professions, Program in Nursing, Arlington, VA 22207-4299. Offers family nurse practitioner (MSN, Certificate); nursing (DNP). *Accreditation:* AACN. Part-time and evening/weekend programs available. *Faculty:* 6 full-time (all women), 2 part-time/adjunct (both women). *Students:* 11 full-time (all women), 58 part-time (54 women); includes 32 minority (17 Black or African American, non-Hispanic/Latino; 2 American Indian or Alaska Native, non-Hispanic/Latino; 5 Asian, non-Hispanic/Latino; 5 Hispanic/Latino; 2 Native Hawaiian or other Pacific Islander, non-Hispanic/Latino; 1 Two or more races, non-Hispanic/Latino), 2 international. Average age 38. 54 applicants, 31% accepted, 11 enrolled. In 2013, 18 master's, 2 doctorates, 1 other advanced degree awarded. *Degree requirements:* For master's, comprehensive exam; for doctorate, thesis/dissertation or alternative. *Entrance requirements:* For master's, 2 letters of recommendation, interview, resume, RN license, personal statement; for doctorate, 2 letters of recommendation, interview, resume, RN license, minimum MSN GPA of 3.5 or BSN 3.3; for Certificate, interview, master's degree in nursing. Additional exam requirements/recommendations for international students: Required—TOEFL (minimum score 600 paper-based; 96 iBT), IELTS (minimum score 6.5). *Application deadline:* For fall admission, 5/1 for domestic students, 7/1 for international students; for spring admission, 11/1 for domestic students, 9/16 for international students. Application fee: $40. Electronic applications accepted. *Expenses: Tuition:* Part-time $850 per credit. *Required fees:* $10 per credit. One-time fee: $200 part-time. Tuition and fees vary according to program. *Financial support:* In 2013–14, 7 students received support, including 2 teaching assistantships with partial tuition reimbursements available; research assistantships with partial tuition reimbursements available, career-related internships or fieldwork, Federal Work-Study, scholarships/grants, and unspecified assistantships also available. Support available to part-time students. Financial award applicants required to submit FAFSA. *Unit head:* Dr. Shelli Wolfe Mayer, Chair, 703-284-6886, Fax: 703-284-3819, E-mail: michelle.wolfe@marymount.edu. *Application contact:* Francesca Reed, Director, Graduate Admissions, 703-284-5901, Fax: 703-527-3815, E-mail: grad.admissions@marymount.edu.

Maryville University of Saint Louis, College of Health Professions, The Catherine McAuley School of Nursing, St. Louis, MO 63141-7299. Offers adult nurse practitioner (MSN); advanced practice nursing (DNP); family nurse practitioner (MSN); geriatric nurse practitioner (MSN); nursing education (MSN). *Accreditation:* AACN. Postbaccalaureate distance learning degree programs offered. *Students:* 30 full-time (28 women), 1,551 part-time (1,416 women); includes 361 minority (181 Black or African American, non-Hispanic/Latino; 16 American Indian or Alaska Native, non-Hispanic/Latino; 59 Asian, non-Hispanic/Latino; 71 Hispanic/Latino; 5 Native Hawaiian or other Pacific Islander, non-Hispanic/Latino; 29 Two or more races, non-Hispanic/Latino), 3 international. Average age 36. In 2013, 37 master's awarded. *Degree requirements:* For master's, practicum. *Entrance requirements:* For master's, BSN, current licensure, minimum GPA of 3.0, 3 letters of recommendation, curriculum vitae. Additional exam requirements/recommendations for international students: Required—TOEFL (minimum score 550 paper-based). *Application deadline:* Applications are processed on a rolling basis. Application fee: $40 ($60 for international students). Electronic applications accepted. Application fee is waived when completed online. *Expenses: Tuition:* Full-time $23,812; part-time $728 per credit hour. *Required fees:* $395 per year. Tuition and fees vary according to course load, degree level and program. *Financial support:* Federal Work-Study and campus employment available. Support available to part-time students. Financial award application deadline: 3/1; financial award applicants required to submit FAFSA. *Unit head:* Dr. Elizabeth Buck, Director, 314-529-9453, Fax: 314-529-9139, E-mail: ebuck@maryville.edu. *Application contact:* Crystal Jacobsmeyer, Assistant Director, Graduate Enrollment Advising, 314-929-9654, Fax: 314-529-9927, E-mail: cjacobsmeyer@maryville.edu.
Website: http://www.maryville.edu/hp/nursing/

McGill University, Faculty of Graduate and Postdoctoral Studies, Faculty of Medicine, School of Nursing, Montréal, QC H3A 2T5, Canada. Offers nurse practitioner (Graduate Diploma); nursing (M Sc A, PhD). PhD offered jointly with Université du Québec à Montréal.

McKendree University, Graduate Programs, Master of Science in Nursing Program, Lebanon, IL 62254-1299. Offers nursing education (MSN); nursing management/administration (MSN). *Accreditation:* AACN. Part-time and evening/weekend programs available. Postbaccalaureate distance learning degree programs offered (no on-campus study). *Degree requirements:* For master's, research project or thesis. *Entrance requirements:* For master's, resume, references, valid Professional Registered Nurse license. Additional exam requirements/recommendations for international students: Required—TOEFL. Electronic applications accepted.

McMaster University, Faculty of Health Sciences and School of Graduate Studies, Program in Nursing (course-based), Hamilton, ON L8S 4M2, Canada. Offers M Sc. *Degree requirements:* For master's, scholarly paper. *Entrance requirements:* For master's, 4 year honors BSCN, minimum B+ average in last 60 units. Additional exam requirements/recommendations for international students: Required—TOEFL (minimum score 580 paper-based; 92 iBT).

McMaster University, Faculty of Health Sciences and School of Graduate Studies, Program in Nursing (thesis), Hamilton, ON L8S 4M2, Canada. Offers M Sc, PhD. *Degree requirements:* For master's, thesis; for doctorate, comprehensive exam, thesis/dissertation. *Entrance requirements:* For master's, honors B Sc N, B+ average in last 60 units; for doctorate, M Sc, minimum B+ average. Additional exam requirements/recommendations for international students: Required—TOEFL (minimum score 580 paper-based; 92 iBT).

McMurry University, Graduate Studies, Abilene, TX 79697. Offers education (MSN); family nurse practitioner (MSN).

McNeese State University, Doré School of Graduate Studies, College of Nursing, Lake Charles, LA 70609. Offers MSN, PMC, Postbaccalaureate Certificate. Program offered jointly with Southeastern Louisiana University and Southern University and Agricultural and Mechanical College. *Accreditation:* AACN. *Degree requirements:* For master's, comprehensive exam. *Entrance requirements:* For master's, GRE, eligibility for unencumbered licensure as RN in Louisiana.

McNeese State University, Doré School of Graduate Studies, College of Nursing, Department of Graduate Nursing, Nursing Program, Lake Charles, LA 70609. Offers family nurse practitioner (MSN); family psychiatric/mental health nurse practitioner (MSN); nurse educator (MSN); nurse executive (MSN). *Degree requirements:* For master's, comprehensive exam. *Entrance requirements:* For master's, GRE, baccalaureate degree in nursing, minimum overall GPA of 2.7 for all undergraduate coursework, eligibility for unencumbered licensure as Registered Nurse in Louisiana or Texas, course in introductory statistics with minimum C grade, physical assessment skills, two letters of professional reference, 500-word essay, current resume.

MCPHS University, Graduate Studies, Program in Nursing, Boston, MA 02115-5896. Offers MS. *Accreditation:* AACN. Part-time programs available. Postbaccalaureate distance learning degree programs offered (minimal on-campus study). *Entrance requirements:* For master's, BSN. Additional exam requirements/recommendations for international students: Required—TOEFL (minimum score 550 paper-based; 79 iBT). Electronic applications accepted.

Medical University of South Carolina, College of Nursing, PhD in Nursing Program, Charleston, SC 29425. Offers PhD. *Accreditation:* AACN. Part-time programs available. Postbaccalaureate distance learning degree programs offered (minimal on-campus study). *Degree requirements:* For doctorate, comprehensive exam, thesis/dissertation, mentored teaching and research seminar. *Entrance requirements:* For doctorate, BSN or MSN from accredited NLNAC or CCNE program, minimum GPA of 3.5, documentation of RN license from state of residence, curriculum vitae, personal statement, 3 references, interview, evidence of computer literacy. Additional exam requirements/recommendations for international students: Required—TOEFL (minimum score 550 paper-based; 80 iBT). Electronic applications accepted. *Faculty research:* Rare diseases, vascular ulcer prevention, health disparities, community engagement, health services.

Medical University of South Carolina, College of Nursing, Post-MSN Doctor of Nursing Practice Program, Charleston, SC 29425. Offers advanced practice nursing (DNP). Part-time programs available. Postbaccalaureate distance learning degree programs offered (minimal on-campus study). *Degree requirements:* For doctorate, final project. *Entrance requirements:* For doctorate, BSN and MSN from nationally-accredited program, minimum cumulative GPA of 3.0 for undergraduate and graduate coursework, active APRN License and specialty certification, 3 confidential references, current curriculum vitae or resume, statement of goals. Additional exam requirements/recommendations for international students: Required—TOEFL (minimum score 550 paper-based; 80 iBT). Electronic applications accepted. *Faculty research:* Women's health cardiovascular, hospital roles, HPV, guidelines implementation, adolescent family obesity.

Memorial University of Newfoundland, School of Graduate Studies, School of Nursing, St. John's, NL A1C 5S7, Canada. Offers MN, PMD. Part-time programs available. *Degree requirements:* For master's, thesis optional; for PMD, clinical placement. *Entrance requirements:* For master's, bachelor's degree in nursing, 1 year experience in nursing practice, practicing license; for PMD, 2 years clinical nursing experience, practicing license (Canada) or proof of registration as a practicing nurse (international), letter from a health care agency guaranteeing clinical placement. Electronic applications accepted. *Faculty research:* Women's health, infant feeding practices, nursing management, care of the elderly, children's health.

Mercer University, Graduate Studies, Cecil B. Day Campus, Georgia Baptist College of Nursing, Macon, GA 31207-0003. Offers adult critical care (MSN); family nurse practitioner (MSN); nurse education (MSN, Certificate); nursing (MSN, PhD); nursing practice (DNP). *Accreditation:* AACN. Part-time programs available. *Faculty:* 12 full-time (all women). *Students:* 44 full-time (all women), 49 part-time (45 women); includes 29 minority (24 Black or African American, non-Hispanic/Latino; 2 Asian, non-Hispanic/Latino; 1 Hispanic/Latino; 2 Two or more races, non-Hispanic/Latino), 3 international. Average age 38. In 2013, 24 master's, 4 doctorates awarded. *Degree requirements:* For master's, thesis or alternative; for doctorate, comprehensive exam, thesis/dissertation. *Entrance requirements:* For master's, MAT or GRE, bachelor's degree from an accredited nursing program, registered GA nursing license (unencumbered); for doctorate, GRE, master's degree from accredited nursing program, RN licensure. Additional exam requirements/recommendations for international students: Required—TOEFL (minimum score 80 iBT). *Application deadline:* For fall admission, 6/1 for domestic students, 4/1 for international students; for winter admission, 11/1 for domestic students, 9/1 for international students; for spring admission, 4/1 for domestic students, 2/1 for international students. Applications are processed on a rolling basis. Application fee: $50. *Expenses:* Contact institution. *Financial support:* Institutionally sponsored loans, scholarships/grants, and traineeships available. Support available to part-time students. Financial award application deadline: 5/1; financial award applicants required to submit FAFSA. *Faculty research:* Osteoporosis, honor system, women and alcoholism, nursing assessment measures. *Unit head:* Dr. Linda Streit, Dean/Professor, 678-547-6793, Fax: 678-547-6796, E-mail: gunby_ss@mercer.edu. *Application contact:* Lynn Vines, Director of Admissions, 678-547-6700, Fax: 678-547-6794, E-mail: vines_ml@mercer.edu.
Website: http://www.mercer.edu/nursing

Mercy College, School of Health and Natural Sciences, Programs in Nursing, Dobbs Ferry, NY 10522-1189. Offers nursing administration (MS); nursing education (MS). *Accreditation:* AACN. Part-time and evening/weekend programs available. Postbaccalaureate distance learning degree programs offered (no on-campus study). *Students:* 4 full-time (3 women), 167 part-time (151 women); includes 105 minority (77 Black or African American, non-Hispanic/Latino; 14 Asian, non-Hispanic/Latino; 14 Hispanic/Latino), 3 international. Average age 33. 82 applicants, 77% accepted, 35 enrolled. In 2013, 33 master's awarded. *Degree requirements:* For master's, comprehensive exam (for some programs), written comprehensive exam or the production of a comprehensive project. *Entrance requirements:* For master's, interview, two letters of reference, skills assessment, bachelor's degree, RN registration in the U.S. Additional exam requirements/recommendations for international students: Required—TOEFL (minimum score 600 paper-based; 100 iBT), IELTS (minimum score 8). *Application deadline:* For fall admission, 8/1 for international students. Applications are processed on a rolling basis. Application fee: $62. Electronic applications accepted. *Expenses: Tuition:* Full-time $19,344; part-time $806 per credit. *Required fees:* $580; $806 per credit. $145 per term. Tuition and fees vary according to course load, degree level and program. *Financial support:* Career-related internships or fieldwork, Federal Work-Study, scholarships/grants, and unspecified assistantships available. Support available to part-time students. Financial award applicants required to submit FAFSA. *Unit head:* Dr. Joan Toglia, Dean, School of Health and Natural Sciences, 914-674-7837, E-mail: jtoglia@mercy.edu. *Application contact:* Allison Gurdineer, Senior Director of Admissions, 877-637-2946, Fax: 914-674-7382, E-mail: admissions@mercy.edu.
Website: https://www.mercy.edu/academics/school-of-health-and-natural-sciences/graduate-programs/

Metropolitan State University, College of Health, Community and Professional Studies, St. Paul, MN 55106-5000. Offers advanced dental therapy (MS); leadership and management (MSN); nurse educator (MSN); nursing (DNP); psychology (MA). *Accreditation:* AACN. Part-time programs available. *Degree requirements:* For master's, thesis or alternative; for doctorate, thesis/dissertation or alternative. *Entrance requirements:* For master's, GRE General Test, minimum GPA of 3.0, RN license, BS/BA; for doctorate, minimum GPA of 3.0; RN license, MSN. Additional exam requirements/recommendations for international students: Required—TOEFL (minimum score 550 paper-based). *Expenses:* Tuition, state resident: full-time $5548. Tuition, nonresident: full-time $10,929. *Faculty research:* Women's health, gerontology.

MGH Institute of Health Professions, School of Nursing, Boston, MA 02129-4557. Offers advanced practice nursing (MSN); gerontological nursing (MSN); nursing (DNP); pediatric nursing (MSN); psychiatric nursing (MSN); teaching and learning for health care education (Certificate); women's health nursing (MSN). *Accreditation:* AACN. *Faculty:* 41 full-time (36 women), 14 part-time/adjunct (13 women). *Students:* 494 full-time (428 women), 85 part-time (77 women); includes 108 minority (32 Black or African American, non-Hispanic/Latino; 2 American Indian or Alaska Native, non-Hispanic/Latino; 38 Asian, non-Hispanic/Latino; 33 Hispanic/Latino; 3 Native Hawaiian or other Pacific Islander, non-Hispanic/Latino). Average age 32. 470 applicants, 52% accepted, 133 enrolled. In 2013, 85 master's, 12 doctorates, 98 other advanced degrees awarded. *Degree requirements:* For master's, thesis or alternative. *Entrance requirements:* For master's, GRE General Test, bachelor's degree from regionally-accredited college or university. Additional exam requirements/recommendations for international students: Required—TOEFL (minimum score 550 paper-based; 80 iBT). *Application deadline:* For fall admission, 12/1 for domestic and international students; for spring admission, 10/1 for domestic and international students. Application fee: $100. Electronic applications accepted. *Expenses: Tuition:* Part-time $1114 per credit. *Required fees:* $620 per term. One-time fee: $475 part-time. *Financial support:* In 2013–14, 75 students received support, including 4 research assistantships (averaging $1,200 per year), 17 teaching assistantships (averaging $1,200 per year); career-related internships or fieldwork, scholarships/grants, traineeships, and unspecified assistantships also available. Support available to part-time students. Financial award application deadline: 4/1; financial award applicants required to submit FAFSA. *Faculty research:* Biobehavioral nursing, HIV/AIDS, gerontological nursing, women's health, vulnerable populations, health systems. *Unit head:* Dr. Laurie Lauzon-Clabo, Dean, 617-643-0605, Fax: 617-726-8022, E-mail: llauzonclabo@mghihp.edu. *Application contact:* Lauren Putnam, Assistant Director of Admission, 617-726-3140, Fax: 617-726-8010, E-mail: admissions@mghihp.edu.
Website: http://www.mghihp.edu/academics/nursing/

Michigan State University, The Graduate School, College of Nursing, East Lansing, MI 48824. Offers MSN, PhD. *Accreditation:* AACN; AANA/CANAEP. Part-time programs available. Postbaccalaureate distance learning degree programs offered (no on-campus study). *Entrance requirements:* Additional exam requirements/recommendations for international students: Required—TOEFL (minimum score 580 paper-based), Michigan State University ELT (minimum score 85), Michigan English Language Assessment Battery (minimum score 83). Electronic applications accepted. *Faculty research:* Hormone replacement therapy, end of life research, human-animal bond, chronic disease, family home care for cancer.

Middle Tennessee State University, College of Graduate Studies, College of Behavioral and Health Sciences, School of Nursing, Murfreesboro, TN 37132. Offers MSN, Graduate Certificate. Part-time and evening/weekend programs available. Postbaccalaureate distance learning degree programs offered. *Faculty:* 12 full-time (all women), 13 part-time/adjunct (10 women). *Students:* 52 full-time (47 women), 196 part-time (177 women); includes 35 minority (22 Black or African American, non-Hispanic/Latino; 2 American Indian or Alaska Native, non-Hispanic/Latino; 4 Asian, non-Hispanic/Latino; 3 Hispanic/Latino; 4 Two or more races, non-Hispanic/Latino). 139 applicants, 89% accepted. In 2013, 32 master's awarded. *Entrance requirements:* Additional exam requirements/recommendations for international students: Required—TOEFL (minimum score 525 paper-based; 71 iBT) or IELTS (minimum score 6). *Application deadline:* For fall admission, 6/1 for domestic and international students. Applications are processed on a rolling basis. Application fee: $25 ($30 for international students). Electronic applications accepted. *Financial support:* In 2013–14, 2 students received support. Tuition waivers available. Support available to part-time students. Financial award application deadline: 5/1. *Unit head:* Dr. Jenny Sauls, Director, 615-898-2446, Fax: 615-898-5441, E-mail: jenny.sauls@mtsu.edu. *Application contact:* Dr. Michael D. Allen, Vice Provost for Research/Dean, 615-898-2840, Fax: 615-904-8020, E-mail: michael.allen@mtsu.edu.

Midwestern State University, Graduate School, Robert D. and Carol Gunn College of Health Sciences and Human Services, Wilson School of Nursing, Wichita Falls, TX 76308. Offers family nurse practitioner (MSN); family psychiatric mental health nurse practitioner (MSN); nurse educator (MSN). *Accreditation:* AACN. Part-time and evening/weekend programs available. *Degree requirements:* For master's, comprehensive exam, thesis optional. *Entrance requirements:* For master's, GRE General Test or MAT. Additional exam requirements/recommendations for international students: Required—TOEFL (minimum score 550 paper-based). *Application deadline:* For fall admission, 7/1 priority date for domestic students, 4/1 for international students; for spring admission, 11/1 priority date for domestic students, 8/1 for international students. Applications are processed on a rolling basis. Application fee: $35 ($50 for international students). Electronic applications accepted. *Expenses:* Tuition, state resident: full-time $3627; part-time $201.50 per credit hour. Tuition, nonresident: full-time $10,899; part-time $605.50 per credit hour. *Required fees:* $1357. *Financial support:* Teaching assistantships with partial tuition reimbursements, career-related internships or fieldwork, Federal Work-Study, institutionally sponsored loans, scholarships/grants, tuition waivers (partial), and unspecified assistantships available. Support available to part-time students. Financial award application deadline: 3/1; financial award applicants required to submit FAFSA. *Faculty research:* Infant feeding, musculoskeletal disorders, diabetes, community health education, water quality reporting. *Unit head:* Robin Lockhart, RN, Interim Chair, 940-397-4614, Fax: 940-397-4513, E-mail: robin.lockhart@mwsu.edu.
Website: http://www.mwsu.edu/academics/hs2/nursing/

Millersville University of Pennsylvania, College of Graduate and Professional Studies, School of Science and Mathematics, Department of Nursing, Millersville, PA 17551-0302. Offers family nurse practitioner (MSN); nursing education (MSN). Part-time and evening/weekend programs available. *Faculty:* 5 full-time (all women), 5 part-time/adjunct (all women). *Students:* 5 full-time (all women), 78 part-time (72 women);

includes 10 minority (8 Black or African American, non-Hispanic/Latino; 2 Hispanic/Latino). Average age 38. 43 applicants, 67% accepted, 24 enrolled. In 2013, 25 master's awarded. *Degree requirements:* For master's, internship, scholarly project. *Entrance requirements:* For master's, 3 letters of recommendation; interview; resume; copy of RN license, goal statement, official transcripts. Additional exam requirements/recommendations for international students: Required—TOEFL (minimum score 550 paper-based, 79 iBT) or IELTS (minimum score 6). *Application deadline:* For fall admission, 1/15 for domestic and international students; for winter admission, 10/1 for domestic and international students; for spring admission, 10/1 for domestic and international students. Application fee: $40. Electronic applications accepted. *Expenses:* Tuition, state resident: full-time $7956; part-time $442 per credit. Tuition, nonresident: full-time $11,934; part-time $663 per credit. *Required fees:* $2196; $122 per credit. Tuition and fees vary according to course load. *Financial support:* In 2013–14, 3 students received support, including 3 research assistantships with full tuition reimbursements available (averaging $2,117 per year); institutionally sponsored loans and unspecified assistantships also available. Support available to part-time students. Financial award application deadline: 3/15; financial award applicants required to submit FAFSA. *Faculty research:* Family nurse practitioner, nurse educator. *Unit head:* Dr. Barbara J. Zimmerman, Chair, 717-872-3376, Fax: 717-871-4877, E-mail: barbara.zimmerman@millersville.edu. *Application contact:* Dr. Victor S. DeSantis, Dean of College of Graduate and Professional Studies/Associate Provost for Civic and Community Engagement, 717-872-3099, Fax: 717-872-3453, E-mail: victor.desantis@millersville.edu.
Website: http://www.millersville.edu/nursing/msn/

Millikin University, School of Nursing, Decatur, IL 62522-2084. Offers clinical nurse leader (MSN); entry into nursing practice: pre-licensure (MSN); nurse anesthesia (DNP); nurse educator (MSN); nursing practice (DNP). *Accreditation:* AACN; AANA/CANAEP. Part-time programs available. *Faculty:* 17 full-time (15 women), 5 part-time/adjunct (4 women). *Students:* 41 full-time (30 women), 26 part-time (19 women); includes 7 minority (2 Black or African American, non-Hispanic/Latino; 1 American Indian or Alaska Native, non-Hispanic/Latino; 1 Asian, non-Hispanic/Latino; 3 Hispanic/Latino). Average age 32. 69 applicants, 51% accepted, 21 enrolled. In 2013, 8 master's awarded. *Degree requirements:* For master's, thesis or alternative, research project. *Entrance requirements:* For master's, GRE, official academic transcript(s), essay, immunizations, statistics course, 3 letters of recommendation, CPR certification, professional liability/malpractice insurance; for doctorate, GRE (if undergraduate cumulative GPA is below 3.0), official academic transcript(s); undergraduate courses: nursing research, health assessment, inorganic and organic chemistry, intro to statistics; graduate-level statistics; 3 written recommendations; Assessment of Critical Care Skills form; written statement; resume or curriculum vita. Additional exam requirements/recommendations for international students: Required—TOEFL (minimum score 550 paper-based; 79 iBT). *Application deadline:* For spring admission, 11/1 for domestic students. Applications are processed on a rolling basis. Application fee: $0. Electronic applications accepted. *Expenses: Tuition:* Full-time $20,300; part-time $700 per credit hour. Tuition and fees vary according to program. *Financial support:* In 2013–14, 13 students received support. Institutionally sponsored loans available. Financial award applicants required to submit FAFSA. *Faculty research:* Congestive heart failure, quality of life, transcultural nursing issues, teaching/learning strategies, maternal - newborn. *Unit head:* Dr. Kathy Booker, Director, 217-424-6348, Fax: 217-420-6731, E-mail: kbooker@millikin.edu. *Application contact:* Marianne Taylor, Administrative Assistant, 800-373-7733 Ext. 5034, Fax: 217-420-6677, E-mail: mgtaylor@millikin.edu.
Website: http://www.millikin.edu/academics/cps/nursing/programs

Minnesota State University Mankato, College of Graduate Studies and Research, College of Allied Health and Nursing, School of Nursing, Mankato, MN 56001. Offers family nursing (MSN), including family nurse practitioner; nursing (DNP). MSN offered jointly with Metropolitan State University; DNP with Metropolitan State University, Minnesota State University Moorhead, Winona State University. *Accreditation:* AACN. *Students:* 54 part-time (51 women). *Degree requirements:* For master's, comprehensive exam, internships, research project or thesis; for doctorate, capstone project. *Entrance requirements:* For master's, GRE General Test or on-campus essay, minimum GPA of 3.0 during previous 2 years, BSN or equivalent references; for doctorate, master's degree in nursing. Additional exam requirements/recommendations for international students: Required—TOEFL. *Application deadline:* For fall admission, 2/15 priority date for domestic students, 2/15 for international students. Applications are processed on a rolling basis. Application fee: $40. Electronic applications accepted. *Financial support:* Research assistantships with full tuition reimbursements and teaching assistantships with full tuition reimbursements available. Financial award application deadline: 3/15; financial award applicants required to submit FAFSA. *Faculty research:* Psychosocial nursing, computers in nursing, family adaptation. *Unit head:* Dr. Sue Ellen Bell, Graduate Coordinator, 507-389-6814. *Application contact:* Collaborative MSN Program Admissions, 507-389-6022.
Website: http://www.mnsu.edu/nursing/

Minnesota State University Moorhead, Graduate Studies, College of Education and Human Services, Moorhead, MN 56563-0002. Offers counseling and student affairs (MS); curriculum and instruction (MS); educational leadership (MS, Ed S); nursing (MS); reading (MS); special education (MS); speech-language pathology (MS). *Accreditation:* NCATE. Part-time and evening/weekend programs available. *Degree requirements:* For master's, comprehensive exam, final oral exam, project or thesis. *Entrance requirements:* Additional exam requirements/recommendations for international students: Required—TOEFL. Electronic applications accepted.

Misericordia University, College of Health Sciences, Department of Nursing, Dallas, PA 18612. Offers MSN. *Accreditation:* AACN. Part-time and evening/weekend programs available. Postbaccalaureate distance learning degree programs offered (minimal on-campus study). *Faculty:* 6 full-time (all women), 1 (woman) part-time/adjunct. *Students:* 41 part-time (39 women); includes 3 minority (1 Black or African American, non-Hispanic/Latino; 1 Asian, non-Hispanic/Latino; 1 Two or more races, non-Hispanic/Latino). Average age 35. In 2013, 25 master's awarded. *Degree requirements:* For master's, thesis optional, practicum. *Entrance requirements:* For master's, interview, minimum GPA of 3.0. Additional exam requirements/recommendations for international students: Required—TOEFL. *Application deadline:* For fall admission, 8/7 priority date for domestic students; for spring admission, 1/3 for domestic students. Applications are processed on a rolling basis. Application fee: $35. Electronic applications accepted. *Expenses:* Contact institution. *Financial support:* In 2013–14, 23 students received support. Teaching assistantships, career-related internships or fieldwork, scholarships/grants, traineeships, tuition waivers (partial), and unspecified assistantships available. Support available to part-time students. Financial award application deadline: 6/30; financial award applicants required to submit FAFSA. *Faculty research:* Quality of life, maternal-child, spirituality, critical thinking, adult health. *Unit head:* Dr. Brenda Hage, Coordinator of Graduate Nursing, 570-674-6760, E-mail: bhage@misericordia.edu. *Application contact:* Maureen Sheridan, Assistant Director of Admissions, Part-Time Undergraduate and Graduate Programs, 570-674-6451, Fax: 570-674-6232, E-mail: msherida@misericordia.edu.
Website: http://www.misericordia.edu/nursing

Mississippi University for Women, Graduate School, College of Nursing and Speech Language Pathology, Columbus, MS 39701-9998. Offers nursing (MSN, PMC); speech-language pathology (MS). *Accreditation:* AACN. Part-time programs available. *Degree requirements:* For master's, comprehensive exam, thesis. *Entrance requirements:* For master's, GRE General Test, bachelor's degree in nursing, previous course work in statistics, proficiency in English.

Missouri Southern State University, Program in Nursing, Joplin, MO 64801-1595. Offers MSN. Program offered jointly with University of Missouri–Kansas City. *Accreditation:* AACN. Part-time programs available. *Entrance requirements:* For master's, minimum cumulative GPA of 3.2 for the last 60 hours of the BSN program, resume, RN licensure, CPR certification, course work in statistics and health assessment. Electronic applications accepted.

Missouri State University, Graduate College, College of Health and Human Services, Department of Nursing, Springfield, MO 65897. Offers nursing (MSN), including family nurse practitioner, nurse educator. *Accreditation:* AACN. *Faculty:* 14 full-time (all women), 12 part-time/adjunct (9 women). *Students:* 18 full-time (17 women), 29 part-time (27 women); includes 5 minority (all Black or African American, non-Hispanic/Latino). Average age 37. 11 applicants, 91% accepted, 6 enrolled. In 2013, 17 master's awarded. *Degree requirements:* For master's, comprehensive exam, thesis or alternative. *Entrance requirements:* For master's, GRE General Test, minimum GPA of 3.0, RN license (for MSN), 1 year of work experience (for MPH). Additional exam requirements/recommendations for international students: Required—TOEFL (minimum score 550 paper-based; 79 iBT). *Application deadline:* For fall admission, 7/20 priority date for domestic students, 5/1 for international students; for spring admission, 12/20 priority date for domestic students, 9/1 for international students. Applications are processed on a rolling basis. Application fee: $35 ($50 for international students). Electronic applications accepted. *Expenses:* Tuition, state resident: full-time $4500; part-time $250 per credit hour. Tuition, nonresident: full-time $9018; part-time $501 per credit hour. *Required fees:* $361 per semester. Tuition and fees vary according to course level, course load and program. *Financial support:* In 2013–14, 2 research assistantships with full tuition reimbursements (averaging $8,324 per year) were awarded; Federal Work-Study, institutionally sponsored loans, scholarships/grants, and unspecified assistantships also available. Financial award application deadline: 3/31; financial award applicants required to submit FAFSA. *Faculty research:* Preconceptual health, women's health, nursing satisfaction, nursing education. *Unit head:* Dr. Kathryn Hope, Head, 417-836-5310, Fax: 417-836-5484, E-mail: nursing@missouristate.edu. *Application contact:* Misty Stewart, Coordinator of Admissions and Recruitment, 417-836-6079, Fax: 417-836-6200, E-mail: mistystewart@missouristate.edu.
Website: http://www.missouristate.edu/nursing/

Missouri Western State University, Program in Health Care Leadership, St. Joseph, MO 64507-2294. Offers MSN. Part-time programs available. *Students:* 13 part-time (all women). Average age 39. 3 applicants, 67% accepted, 2 enrolled. In 2013, 5 master's awarded. *Entrance requirements:* For master's, minimum GPA of 2.75, interview. Additional exam requirements/recommendations for international students: Recommended—TOEFL (minimum score 500 paper-based; 61 iBT), IELTS (minimum score 5.5). *Application deadline:* For fall admission, 7/15 for domestic students, 6/15 for international students; for spring admission, 10/1 for domestic students, 10/15 for international students. Applications are processed on a rolling basis. Application fee: $45 ($50 for international students). Electronic applications accepted. *Expenses:* Tuition, state resident: full-time $6019; part-time $300.96 per credit hour. Tuition, nonresident: full-time $11,194; part-time $559.71 per credit hour. *Required fees:* $542; $99 per credit hour. $176 per semester. Tuition and fees vary according to course load and program. *Financial support:* Scholarships/grants and unspecified assistantships available. Support available to part-time students. *Unit head:* Dr. Carolyn Brose, Coordinator, 816-271-5912, E-mail: brose@missouriwestern.edu. *Application contact:* Dr. Benjamin D. Caldwell, Dean of the Graduate School, 816-271-4394, Fax: 816-271-4525, E-mail: graduate@missouriwestern.edu.
Website: https://www.missouriwestern.edu/nursing/master-of-science-in-nursing/

Molloy College, Division of Nursing, Rockville Centre, NY 11571-5002. Offers adult nurse practitioner (Advanced Certificate); clinical nurse specialist: adult health (Advanced Certificate); family nurse practitioner (Advanced Certificate); nurse practitioner psychiatry (Advanced Certificate); nursing (MS, PhD); nursing administration (Advanced Certificate); nursing administration with informatics (Advanced Certificate); nursing education (Advanced Certificate); nursing informatics (Advanced Certificate); pediatric nurse practitioner (Advanced Certificate). *Accreditation:* AACN. Part-time and evening/weekend programs available. *Faculty:* 30 full-time (29 women), 10 part-time/adjunct (7 women). *Students:* 18 full-time (all women), 538 part-time (495 women); includes 289 minority (159 Black or African American, non-Hispanic/Latino; 1 American Indian or Alaska Native, non-Hispanic/Latino; 80 Asian, non-Hispanic/Latino; 43 Hispanic/Latino; 4 Native Hawaiian or other Pacific Islander, non-Hispanic/Latino; 2 Two or more races, non-Hispanic/Latino), 2 international. Average age 38. 241 applicants, 63% accepted, 122 enrolled. In 2013, 84 master's, 2 other advanced degrees awarded. *Degree requirements:* For master's, thesis optional. *Entrance requirements:* For master's, 3 letters of reference, BS in nursing, minimum undergraduate GPA of 3.0; for Advanced Certificate, 3 letters of reference, master's degree in nursing. *Application deadline:* For fall admission, 9/2 priority date for domestic students; for spring admission, 1/20 priority date for domestic students. Applications are processed on a rolling basis. Application fee: $60. *Expenses: Tuition:* Full-time $16,920; part-time $940 per credit. *Required fees:* $880. *Financial support:* Research assistantships with partial tuition reimbursements, teaching assistantships with partial tuition reimbursements, institutionally sponsored loans, scholarships/grants, and unspecified assistantships available. Support available to part-time students. Financial award application deadline: 4/1; financial award applicants required to submit FAFSA. *Unit head:* Dr. Jeannine Muldoon, Dean of Nursing, 516-323-3651, E-mail: jmuldoon@molloy.edu. *Application contact:* Alina Haitz, Assistant Director of Graduate Admissions, 516-323-4008, E-mail: ahaitz@molloy.edu.
Website: http://www.molloy.edu/academics/nursing-division

Monmouth University, The Graduate School, The Marjorie K. Unterberg School of Nursing and Health Studies, West Long Branch, NJ 07764-1898. Offers adult and gerontological nurse practitioner (MSN); adult-gerontological nurse practitioner (Post-Master's Certificate); family nurse practitioner (MSN, Post-Master's Certificate); family psychiatric and mental health advanced practice nursing (MSN); forensic nursing (MSN, Certificate); nursing (MSN); nursing administration (MSN, Post-Master's Certificate); nursing education (MSN, Post-Master's Certificate); nursing practice (DNP); physician assistant (MS); psychiatric-mental health nurse practitioner (Post-Master's Certificate); school nursing (MSN, Certificate). *Accreditation:* AACN. Part-time and evening/weekend programs available. *Faculty:* 14 full-time (all women), 4 part-time/adjunct (3 women). *Students:* 19 full-time (18 women), 269 part-time (252 women); includes 106 minority (35 Black or African American, non-Hispanic/Latino; 2 American Indian or Alaska Native, non-Hispanic/Latino; 51 Asian, non-Hispanic/Latino; 12 Hispanic/Latino; 3 Native Hawaiian or other Pacific Islander, non-Hispanic/Latino; 3 Two or more races, non-Hispanic/Latino), 2 international. Average age 39. 135 applicants, 98% accepted, 96 enrolled. In 2013, 54 master's, 7 doctorates awarded. *Degree requirements:* For

master's, practicum (for some tracks). *Entrance requirements:* For master's, GRE General Test, BSN with minimum GPA of 2.75, current RN license, proof of liability and malpractice policy, personal statement, two letters of recommendation, college course work in health assessment, resume; minimum GPA of 3.0, minimum C grade in prerequisite courses, minimum 200 hours' clinical experience, 3 letters of recommendation, and interview (for MS); for doctorate, accredited master's nursing program degree with minimum GPA of 3.2, active RN license, national certification as Nurse Practitioner or Nurse Administrator, working knowledge of statistics, statement of goals and vision for change, 2 letters of recommendation, resume, interview. Additional exam requirements/recommendations for international students: Required—TOEFL (minimum score 550 paper-based; 79 iBT), IELTS (minimum score 6) or Michigan English Language Assessment Battery (minimum score 77). *Application deadline:* For fall admission, 7/15 priority date for domestic students, 6/1 for international students; for spring admission, 11/15 priority date for domestic students, 11/1 for international students; for summer admission, 2/1 for domestic students. Applications are processed on a rolling basis. Application fee: $50. Electronic applications accepted. *Expenses: Tuition:* Part-time $1004 per credit hour. *Required fees:* $157 per semester. *Financial support:* In 2013–14, 163 students received support, including 113 fellowships (averaging $3,093 per year), 27 research assistantships (averaging $6,273 per year); career-related internships or fieldwork, scholarships/grants, and unspecified assistantships also available. Support available to part-time students. Financial award applicants required to submit FAFSA. *Faculty research:* Relationship of undergraduate GPA and GRE to succeeding in a graduate nursing program. *Unit head:* Dr. Janet Mahoney, Dean, 732-571-3443, Fax: 732-263-5131, E-mail: jmahoney@monmouth.edu. *Application contact:* Lauren Vento-Cifelli, Associate Vice President of Undergraduate and Graduate Admission, 732-571-3452, Fax: 732-263-5123, E-mail: gradadm@monmouth.edu.
Website: http://www.monmouth.edu/school-of-nursing-health/graduate-nursing-programs.aspx

Moravian College, Moravian College Comenius Center, St. Luke's School of Nursing, Bethlehem, PA 18018-6650. Offers clinical nurse leader (MS); nurse administrator (MS); nurse educator (MS). *Accreditation:* AACN. Part-time and evening/weekend programs available. *Degree requirements:* For master's, comprehensive exam (for some programs), evidence-based practice project. *Entrance requirements:* For master's, GRE or MAT. Additional exam requirements/recommendations for international students: Required—TOEFL (minimum score 550 paper-based; 90 iBT).

Morgan State University, School of Graduate Studies, School of Community Health and Policy, Program in Nursing, Baltimore, MD 21251. Offers MS.

Mount Carmel College of Nursing, Nursing Program, Columbus, OH 43222. Offers adult gerontology acute care nurse practitioner (MS); adult health clinical nurse specialist (MS); family nurse practitioner (MS); nursing administration (MS); nursing education (MS). *Accreditation:* AACN. Part-time programs available. *Faculty:* 8 full-time (7 women), 8 part-time/adjunct (7 women). *Students:* 94 full-time (89 women), 76 part-time (73 women); includes 35 minority (21 Black or African American, non-Hispanic/Latino; 2 American Indian or Alaska Native, non-Hispanic/Latino; 6 Asian, non-Hispanic/Latino; 2 Hispanic/Latino; 1 Native Hawaiian or other Pacific Islander, non-Hispanic/Latino; 3 Two or more races, non-Hispanic/Latino). Average age 38. 123 applicants, 50% accepted, 47 enrolled. In 2013, 41 master's awarded. *Degree requirements:* For master's, professional manuscript. *Entrance requirements:* For master's, letters of recommendation, statement of purpose, current resume, baccalaureate degree in nursing, current Ohio RN license, minimum cumulative GPA of 3.0. Additional exam requirements/recommendations for international students: Required—TOEFL (minimum score 550 paper-based; 80 iBT). *Application deadline:* For fall admission, 6/1 priority date for domestic students; for winter admission, 11/1 for domestic students; for spring admission, 10/1 priority date for domestic students; for summer admission, 3/1 for domestic students. Applications are processed on a rolling basis. Application fee: $30. *Expenses: Tuition:* Full-time $8560; part-time $428 per credit. *Required fees:* $75. *Financial support:* In 2013–14, 9 students received support. Institutionally sponsored loans and scholarships/grants available. Financial award application deadline: 3/15; financial award applicants required to submit FAFSA. *Unit head:* Dr. Angela Phillips-Lowe, Associate Dean, 614-234-5717, Fax: 614-234-2875, E-mail: aphillips-lowe@mccn.edu. *Application contact:* Kathleen Walters, Program Coordinator, 614-234-5408, Fax: 614-234-2875, E-mail: kwalters@mccn.edu.
Website: http://www.mccn.edu/

Mount Marty College, Graduate Studies Division, Yankton, SD 57078-3724. Offers business administration (MBA); nurse anesthesia (MS); nursing (MSN); pastoral ministries (MPM). *Accreditation:* AANA/CANAEP (one or more programs are accredited). *Degree requirements:* For master's, thesis or alternative. *Entrance requirements:* For master's, GRE General Test, minimum GPA of 3.0. Electronic applications accepted. *Faculty research:* Clinical anesthesia, professional characteristics, motivations of applicants.

Mount St. Joseph University, Doctor of Nursing Practice Program, Cincinnati, OH 45233-1670. Offers advanced practice (DNP). Part-time programs available. *Faculty:* 10 full-time (9 women), 23 part-time/adjunct (all women). *Students:* 15 part-time (13 women). Average age 49. 4 applicants, 50% accepted, 2 enrolled. *Entrance requirements:* For doctorate, essay; MSN from regionally-accredited university; minimum graduate GPA of 3.5; professional resume; three professional references; interview; 2 years of clinical nursing experience; active RN license; criminal background check; minimum C grade in an undergraduate statistics course; official documentation of practicum. Additional exam requirements/recommendations for international students: Required—TOEFL (minimum score 560 paper-based; 83 iBT). Application fee: $50. Electronic applications accepted. *Expenses:* Contact institution. *Financial support:* Applicants required to submit FAFSA. *Unit head:* Dr. Nancy Hinzman, Director, 513-244-4325, E-mail: nancy_hinzman@mail.msj.edu. *Application contact:* Mary Brigham, Assistant Director for Graduate Recruitment, 513-244-4233, Fax: 513-244-4629, E-mail: mary_brigham@mail.msj.edu.
Website: http://www.msj.edu/academics/graduate-programs/doctor-of-nursing-practice/

Mount St. Joseph University, MAGELIN Program: Master's Graduate Entry-Level into Nursing, Cincinnati, OH 45233-1670. Offers MSN. *Accreditation:* AACN. *Faculty:* 10 full-time (9 women), 23 part-time/adjunct (all women). *Students:* 95 full-time (77 women), 1 part-time (0 women); includes 16 minority (12 Black or African American, non-Hispanic/Latino; 2 American Indian or Alaska Native, non-Hispanic/Latino; 2 Asian, non-Hispanic/Latino). Average age 29. 129 applicants, 80% accepted, 72 enrolled. In 2013, 55 master's awarded. *Degree requirements:* For master's, evidence-based project, preceptorship. *Entrance requirements:* For master's, GRE (or minimum GPA of 3.0), interview; course work in chemistry, anatomy, physiology, microbiology, psychology, sociology, statistics, life span development, and nutrition; non-nursing bachelor's degree; statement of goals; transcripts; criminal background check. Additional exam requirements/recommendations for international students: Required—TOEFL (minimum score 560 paper-based; 83 iBT). *Application deadline:* Applications are processed on a rolling basis. Application fee: $50. Electronic applications accepted. *Expenses:* Contact institution. *Financial support:* In 2013–14, 6 students received support. Scholarships/grants available. Financial award application deadline: 3/1; financial award applicants required to submit FAFSA. *Faculty research:* Utilizing technology in learning, assessment of student learning, critical thinking, women's health and nursing education. *Unit head:* Mary Kishman, Nursing/Program Director, MAGELIN, 513-244-4726, Fax: 513-451-2547, E-mail: mary_kishman@mail.msj.edu. *Application contact:* Mary Brigham, Assistant Director of Graduate Recruitment, 513-244-4233, Fax: 513-244-4629, E-mail: mary_brigham@mail.msj.edu.
Website: http://www.msj.edu/academics/graduate-programs/magelin-masters-graduate-entry-level-into-nursing/

Mount St. Joseph University, Master of Science in Nursing Program, Cincinnati, OH 45233-1670. Offers administration (MSN); clinical nurse leader (MSN); education (MSN). Part-time programs available. *Faculty:* 10 full-time (9 women), 23 part-time/adjunct (all women). *Students:* 33 part-time (31 women); includes 3 minority (all Black or African American, non-Hispanic/Latino). Average age 45. 24 applicants, 67% accepted, 16 enrolled. *Entrance requirements:* For master's, essay; BSN from regionally-accredited university; minimum undergraduate GPA of 3.25 or GRE; professional resume; three professional references; interview; 2 years of clinical nursing experience; active RN license; criminal background check. Additional exam requirements/recommendations for international students: Required—TOEFL (minimum score 560 paper-based; 83 iBT). Application fee: $50. Electronic applications accepted. *Expenses: Tuition:* Full-time $18,400; part-time $575 per credit hour. *Required fees:* $450; $450 per year. Part-time tuition and fees vary according to course load, degree level and program. *Financial support:* Application deadline: 3/1; applicants required to submit FAFSA. *Unit head:* Dr. Nancy Hinzman, MSN/DNP Director, 513-244-4325, E-mail: nancy_hinzman@mail.msj.edu. *Application contact:* Mary Brigham, Assistant Director for Graduate Recruitment, 513-244-4233, Fax: 513-244-4629, E-mail: mary_brigham@mail.msj.edu.
Website: http://www.msj.edu/academics/graduate-programs/master-of-science-in-nursing/

Mount Saint Mary College, Division of Nursing, Newburgh, NY 12550-3494. Offers adult nurse practitioner (MS, Advanced Certificate), including nursing education (MS), nursing management (MS); clinical nurse specialist-adult health (MS), including nursing education, nursing management; family nurse practitioner (Advanced Certificate). *Accreditation:* AACN. Part-time and evening/weekend programs available. *Faculty:* 4 full-time (all women). *Students:* 79 part-time (72 women); includes 19 minority (12 Black or African American, non-Hispanic/Latino; 1 Asian, non-Hispanic/Latino; 5 Hispanic/Latino; 1 Native Hawaiian or other Pacific Islander, non-Hispanic/Latino). Average age 39. 45 applicants, 47% accepted, 9 enrolled. In 2013, 13 master's, 3 other advanced degrees awarded. *Degree requirements:* For master's, research utilization project. *Entrance requirements:* For master's, BSN, minimum GPA of 3.0, RN license. *Application deadline:* For fall admission, 6/3 priority date for domestic students; for spring admission, 10/31 priority date for domestic students. Applications are processed on a rolling basis. Application fee: $45. Application fee is waived when completed online. *Expenses: Tuition:* Full-time $13,356; part-time $742 per credit. *Required fees:* $70 per semester. *Financial support:* In 2013–14, 8 students received support. Unspecified assistantships available. Financial award application deadline: 4/15; financial award applicants required to submit FAFSA. *Unit head:* Linda Ruta, Graduate Coordinator, 845-569-3512, Fax: 845-562-6762, E-mail: linda.ruta@msmc.edu. *Application contact:* Lisa Gallina, Director of Admissions for Graduate Programs and Adult Degree Completion, 845-569-3166, Fax: 845-569-3450, E-mail: lisa.gallina@msmc.edu.
Website: http://www.msmc.edu/Academics/Graduate_Programs/Master_of_Science_in_Nursing

Mount St. Mary's College, Graduate Division, Los Angeles, CA 90049-1599. Offers business administration (MBA); counseling psychology (MS); creative writing (MFA); education (MS, Certificate); humanities (MA); nursing (MSN, Certificate); physical therapy (DPT); religious studies (MA); MFA/MA. Part-time and evening/weekend programs available. *Faculty:* 35 full-time (26 women), 112 part-time/adjunct (76 women). *Students:* 416 full-time (324 women), 233 part-time (184 women); includes 376 minority (64 Black or African American, non-Hispanic/Latino; 2 American Indian or Alaska Native, non-Hispanic/Latino; 57 Asian, non-Hispanic/Latino; 229 Hispanic/Latino; 8 Native Hawaiian or other Pacific Islander, non-Hispanic/Latino; 16 Two or more races, non-Hispanic/Latino), 4 international. Average age 33. 1,041 applicants, 22% accepted, 183 enrolled. In 2013, 168 master's, 29 doctorates awarded. *Entrance requirements:* Additional exam requirements/recommendations for international students: Required—TOEFL. *Application deadline:* Applications are processed on a rolling basis. Application fee: $50. Electronic applications accepted. *Expenses: Tuition:* Part-time $798 per unit. *Required fees:* $125 per semester. Tuition and fees vary according to program. *Financial support:* Career-related internships or fieldwork, Federal Work-Study, institutionally sponsored loans, and tuition waivers (full and partial) available. Support available to part-time students. Financial award application deadline: 3/15; financial award applicants required to submit FAFSA. *Unit head:* Dr. Linda Moody, Graduate Dean, 213-477-2800, E-mail: gradprograms@msmc.la.edu. *Application contact:* Natalie Dymchenko, Senior Graduate Admission Counselor, 213-477-2800, E-mail: gradprograms@msmc.la.edu.
Website: http://www.msmc.la.edu/admission/graduate-admission.asp

Murray State University, College of Health Sciences and Human Services, Program in Nursing, Murray, KY 42071. Offers clinical nurse specialist (MSN); family nurse practitioner (MSN); nurse anesthesia (MSN). *Accreditation:* AACN; AANA/CANAEP. *Degree requirements:* For master's, research project. *Entrance requirements:* For master's, GRE General Test, BSN, interview, RN licensure. Additional exam requirements/recommendations for international students: Required—TOEFL (minimum score 550 paper-based). *Faculty research:* Fibromyalgis, primary care, rural health.

National University, Academic Affairs, School of Health and Human Services, La Jolla, CA 92037-1011. Offers clinical affairs (MS); clinical informatics (Certificate); clinical regulatory affairs (MS); health and life science analytics (MS); health coaching (Certificate); health informatics (MS); healthcare administration (MHA); nurse anesthesia (MS); nursing (MS), including forensic nursing, nursing administration, nursing informatics; nursing administration (Certificate); nursing informatics (Certificate); nursing practice (DNP); public health (MPH), including health promotion, healthcare administration, mental health. Part-time and evening/weekend programs available. Postbaccalaureate distance learning degree programs offered (no on-campus study). *Faculty:* 20 full-time (12 women), 27 part-time/adjunct (16 women). *Students:* 229 full-time (176 women), 89 part-time (52 women); includes 215 minority (58 Black or African American, non-Hispanic/Latino; 1 American Indian or Alaska Native, non-Hispanic/Latino; 68 Asian, non-Hispanic/Latino; 63 Hispanic/Latino; 8 Native Hawaiian or other Pacific Islander, non-Hispanic/Latino; 17 Two or more races, non-Hispanic/Latino), 18 international. Average age 33. 118 applicants, 100% accepted, 92 enrolled. In 2013, 29 master's awarded. *Degree requirements:* For master's, thesis (for some programs). *Entrance requirements:* For master's, interview, minimum GPA of 2.5. Additional exam requirements/recommendations for international students: Required—TOEFL (minimum score 550 paper-based; 79 iBT), IELTS (minimum score 6). *Application deadline:* Applications are processed on a rolling basis. Application fee: $60 ($65 for international students). Electronic applications accepted. *Expenses: Tuition:* Full-time $13,824; part-time $1728 per course. One-time fee: $160. *Financial support:* Career-related

internships or fieldwork, institutionally sponsored loans, scholarships/grants, and tuition waivers (partial) available. Support available to part-time students. Financial award application deadline: 6/30; financial award applicants required to submit FAFSA. *Faculty research:* Nursing education, obesity prevention, workforce diversity. *Unit head:* School of Health and Human Services, 800-628-8648, E-mail: shhs@nu.edu. *Application contact:* Louis Cruz, Interim Vice President for Enrollment Services, 800-628-8648, E-mail: advisor@nu.edu.
Website: http://www.nu.edu/OurPrograms/SchoolOfHealthAndHumanServices.html

Nazareth College of Rochester, Graduate Studies, Department of Nursing, Rochester, NY 14618-3790. Offers gerontological nurse practitioner (MS). *Accreditation:* AACN. Part-time programs available. *Entrance requirements:* For master's, minimum GPA of 3.0, RN license.

Nebraska Methodist College, Program in Nursing, Omaha, NE 68114. Offers nurse educator (MSN); nurse executive (MSN). *Accreditation:* AACN. Evening/weekend programs available. Postbaccalaureate distance learning degree programs offered (no on-campus study). *Faculty:* 2 full-time (both women), 5 part-time/adjunct (all women). *Students:* 82 full-time (81 women), 39 part-time (36 women); includes 5 minority (4 Black or African American, non-Hispanic/Latino; 1 Asian, non-Hispanic/Latino). Average age 37. 156 applicants, 21% accepted, 28 enrolled. In 2013, 20 master's awarded. *Degree requirements:* For master's, thesis or alternative, Evidence Based Practice (EBP) project. *Entrance requirements:* For master's, interview. Additional exam requirements/recommendations for international students: Required—TOEFL (minimum score 550 paper-based; 80 iBT). *Application deadline:* For spring admission, 11/1 for domestic and international students. Applications are processed on a rolling basis. Application fee: $25. *Expenses: Tuition:* Full-time $12,258; part-time $681 per credit hour. *Required fees:* $450; $450 per year. *Financial support:* Research assistantships with full and partial tuition reimbursements and scholarships/grants available. Financial award applicants required to submit FAFSA. *Faculty research:* Spirituality, student outcomes, service-learning, leadership and administration, women's issues. *Unit head:* Dr. Linda Foley, Director, Graduate Nursing, 402-354-7050, Fax: 402-354-7020, E-mail: linda.foley@methodistcollege.edu. *Application contact:* Laurel Zentner, Recruitment and Admissions Coordinator, 402-354-7170, Fax: 402-354-7020, E-mail: admissions@methodistcollege.edu.
Website: http://www.methodistcollege.edu/nursing-online

Nebraska Wesleyan University, University College, Program in Nursing, Lincoln, NE 68504-2796. Offers MSN. Part-time programs available.

Neumann University, Program in Nursing and Health Sciences, Aston, PA 19014-1298. Offers MS. Part-time programs available. *Entrance requirements:* For master's, GRE or MAT. Additional exam requirements/recommendations for international students: Required—TOEFL. *Expenses:* Contact institution.

New Mexico State University, Graduate School, College of Health and Social Services, School of Nursing, Las Cruces, NM 88003. Offers adult/gerontology nurse practitioner (DNP); family nurse practitioner (DNP); nursing (MSN, PhD); public/community health (DNP). *Accreditation:* AACN. Postbaccalaureate distance learning degree programs offered (minimal on-campus study). *Faculty:* 15 full-time (14 women). *Students:* 42 full-time (33 women), 64 part-time (56 women); includes 50 minority (11 Black or African American, non-Hispanic/Latino; 1 American Indian or Alaska Native, non-Hispanic/Latino; 1 Asian, non-Hispanic/Latino; 36 Hispanic/Latino; 1 Two or more races, non-Hispanic/Latino), 1 international. Average age 42. 50 applicants, 86% accepted, 36 enrolled. In 2013, 12 master's, 6 doctorates awarded. *Degree requirements:* For master's, comprehensive exam, thesis optional, clinical practice; for doctorate, comprehensive exam, thesis/dissertation. *Entrance requirements:* For master's, NCLEX exam, BSN, minimum GPA of 3.0, course work in statistics, 3 letters of reference, writing sample, RN license, CPR certification, proof of liability, immunizations, criminal background check; for doctorate, NCLEX exam, MSN, minimum GPA of 3.0, 3 letters of reference, writing sample, RN license, CPR certification, proof of liability, immunizations, criminal background check, statistics course. Additional exam requirements/recommendations for international students: Required—TOEFL (minimum score 550 paper-based; 79 iBT), IELTS (minimum score 6.5). *Application deadline:* For spring admission, 10/1 priority date for domestic students. Application fee: $40 ($50 for international students). Electronic applications accepted. *Expenses:* Tuition, state resident: full-time $5398; part-time $224.90 per credit. Tuition, nonresident: full-time $18,821; part-time $784.20 per credit. *Required fees:* $1310; $54.60 per credit. *Financial support:* In 2013–14, 31 students received support. Career-related internships or fieldwork, Federal Work-Study, scholarships/grants, traineeships, health care benefits, and unspecified assistantships available. Financial award application deadline: 3/1. *Faculty research:* Public policy, community health, health disparities, self efficacy and self management, psychiatric mental health. *Total annual research expenditures:* $3,424. *Unit head:* Dr. Pamela Schultz, Director, 575-646-3812, Fax: 575-646-2167, E-mail: pschultz@nmsu.edu. *Application contact:* Dr. Kathleen Huttlinger, Associate Director for Graduate Studies, 575-646-4387, Fax: 575-646-2167.
Website: http://schoolofnursing.nmsu.edu

New York University, College of Nursing, Doctor of Nursing Practice Program, New York, NY 10012-1019. Offers advanced practice nursing (DNP), including adult acute care, adult nurse practitioner/holistic nursing, adult nurse practitioner/palliative care nursing, adult primary care, adult primary care/geriatrics, family, geriatrics, mental health nursing, nurse-midwifery, pediatrics. Part-time and evening/weekend programs available. *Faculty:* 3 full-time (all women), 1 part-time/adjunct (0 women). *Students:* 1 (woman) full-time, 33 part-time (30 women); includes 7 minority (3 Black or African American, non-Hispanic/Latino; 3 Asian, non-Hispanic/Latino; 1 Hispanic/Latino). Average age 39. 18 applicants, 100% accepted, 12 enrolled. In 2013, 4 doctorates awarded. *Degree requirements:* For doctorate, thesis/dissertation, capstone. *Entrance requirements:* For doctorate, MAT or GRE (either taken within past 5 years), MS, RN license, interview, Nurse Practitioner Certification. Additional exam requirements/recommendations for international students: Required—TOEFL (minimum score 90 iBT), IELTS (minimum score 7). *Application deadline:* For fall admission, 3/1 for domestic students, 4/1 for international students. Applications are processed on a rolling basis. Application fee: $80. Electronic applications accepted. *Expenses: Tuition:* Full-time $35,856; part-time $1494 per unit. *Required fees:* $1408; $64 per unit. $473 per term. Tuition and fees vary according to course load and program. *Financial support:* Scholarships/grants available. Support available to part-time students. Financial award application deadline: 2/1. *Faculty research:* Geriatrics, HIV, elderly black diabetics, families and illness, oral systemic connection. *Unit head:* Dr. Rona Levin, Director, 212-998-5319, Fax: 212-995-3143, E-mail: rfl2039@nyu.edu. *Application contact:* Elizabeth Ensweiler, Assistant Director, Graduate Student Affairs and Admissions, 212-992-7653, Fax: 212-995-4302, E-mail: ee39@nyu.edu.

New York University, College of Nursing, Doctor of Philosophy in Nursing Program, New York, NY 10012-1019. Offers research and theory development in nursing science (PhD). Part-time programs available. *Faculty:* 4 full-time (all women). *Students:* 6 full-time (all women), 22 part-time (18 women); includes 6 minority (2 Black or African American, non-Hispanic/Latino; 2 Asian, non-Hispanic/Latino; 2 Hispanic/Latino), 4 international. Average age 40. 15 applicants, 73% accepted, 7 enrolled. In 2013, 11 doctorates awarded. *Degree requirements:* For doctorate, thesis/dissertation, candidacy exam. *Entrance requirements:* For doctorate, GRE General Test, interview. Additional exam requirements/recommendations for international students: Required—TOEFL (minimum score 90 iBT), IELTS (minimum score 7). *Application deadline:* For fall admission, 1/15 for domestic and international students. Applications are processed on a rolling basis. Application fee: $80. Electronic applications accepted. *Expenses: Tuition:* Full-time $35,856; part-time $1494 per unit. *Required fees:* $1408; $64 per unit. $473 per term. Tuition and fees vary according to course load and program. *Financial support:* In 2013–14, 18 students received support, including 5 research assistantships (averaging $25,061 per year); scholarships/grants also available. Support available to part-time students. Financial award application deadline: 2/1; financial award applicants required to submit FAFSA. *Faculty research:* Geriatrics, infectious diseases/global public health, chronic disease prevention and management, health systems/education. *Unit head:* Dr. Susan Sullivan-Bolyai, Director, 212-998-5264, Fax: 212-995-4561, E-mail: ssb7@nyu.edu. *Application contact:* Elizabeth Ensweiler, Assistant Director, Graduate Student Affairs and Admissions, 212-992-7653, Fax: 212-995-4302, E-mail: ee39@nyu.edu.

New York University, College of Nursing, Programs in Advanced Practice Nursing, New York, NY 10012-1019. Offers advanced practice nursing: adult acute care (MS, Advanced Certificate); advanced practice nursing: adult nurse practitioner/holistic nurse practitioner (Advanced Certificate); advanced practice nursing: adult nurse practitioner/palliative care nurse practitioner (Advanced Certificate); advanced practice nursing: adult primary care (MS, Advanced Certificate); advanced practice nursing: family (MS, Advanced Certificate); advanced practice nursing: geriatrics (Advanced Certificate); advanced practice nursing: mental health (MS); advanced practice nursing: mental health nursing (Advanced Certificate); advanced practice nursing: pediatrics (MS, Advanced Certificate); nurse midwifery (MS, Advanced Certificate); nursing administration (MS, Advanced Certificate); nursing education (MS, Advanced Certificate); nursing informatics (MS, Advanced Certificate); MS/MPA; MS/MPH. *Accreditation:* AACN; ACNM/ACME. Part-time programs available. *Faculty:* 22 full-time (all women), 54 part-time/adjunct (46 women). *Students:* 36 full-time (31 women), 622 part-time (549 women); includes 239 minority (73 Black or African American, non-Hispanic/Latino; 1 American Indian or Alaska Native, non-Hispanic/Latino; 116 Asian, non-Hispanic/Latino; 36 Hispanic/Latino; 6 Native Hawaiian or other Pacific Islander, non-Hispanic/Latino; 7 Two or more races, non-Hispanic/Latino), 16 international. Average age 37. 395 applicants, 67% accepted, 156 enrolled. In 2013, 186 master's, 8 other advanced degrees awarded. *Degree requirements:* For master's, thesis (for some programs). *Entrance requirements:* For master's, BS in nursing, AS in nursing with another BS/BA, interview, RN license, 1 year of clinical experience (3 for nursing education program); for Advanced Certificate, master's degree. Additional exam requirements/recommendations for international students: Required—TOEFL (minimum score 90 iBT), IELTS (minimum score 7). *Application deadline:* For fall admission, 7/1 for domestic and international students; for spring admission, 12/1 for domestic and international students. Application fee: $80. Electronic applications accepted. *Expenses: Tuition:* Full-time $35,856; part-time $1494 per unit. *Required fees:* $1408; $64 per unit. $473 per term. Tuition and fees vary according to course load and program. *Financial support:* In 2013–14, 182 students received support. Research assistantships, career-related internships or fieldwork, Federal Work-Study, scholarships/grants, traineeships, and unspecified assistantships available. Support available to part-time students. Financial award application deadline: 2/1; financial award applicants required to submit FAFSA. *Faculty research:* Geriatrics, HIV, elderly black diabetics, families and illness, oral systemic connection. *Unit head:* Dr. Judith Haber, Associate Dean, Graduate Programs, 212-998-9020, Fax: 212-995-3143, E-mail: jh33@nyu.edu. *Application contact:* Elizabeth Ensweiler, Assistant Director, Graduate Student Affairs and Admissions, 212-992-7653, Fax: 212-995-4302, E-mail: ee39@nyu.edu.

Nicholls State University, Graduate Studies, College of Nursing and Allied Health, Thibodaux, LA 70310. Offers family nurse practitioner (MSN); family psychiatric/mental health nurse practitioner (MSN); nurse executive (MSN).

North Dakota State University, College of Graduate and Interdisciplinary Studies, College of Pharmacy, Nursing and Allied Sciences, Graduate Nursing Program, Fargo, ND 58108. Offers MS, DNP. *Accreditation:* AACN. Part-time programs available. Postbaccalaureate distance learning degree programs offered (minimal on-campus study). *Faculty:* 9 full-time (8 women), 3 part-time/adjunct (2 women). *Students:* 42 full-time (37 women), 11 part-time (all women); includes 3 minority (1 Black or African American, non-Hispanic/Latino; 1 American Indian or Alaska Native, non-Hispanic/Latino; 1 Two or more races, non-Hispanic/Latino), 2 international. Average age 35. 52 applicants, 44% accepted, 20 enrolled. In 2013, 2 master's, 8 doctorates awarded. *Degree requirements:* For master's, thesis or alternative, oral defense; for doctorate, thesis/dissertation or alternative, oral defense. *Entrance requirements:* For master's, bachelor's degree with nursing major, minimum GPA of 3.0 in nursing courses, RN license; for doctorate, bachelor's or master's degree with a nursing major, minimum GPA of 3.0 in nursing courses, RN license. Additional exam requirements/recommendations for international students: Required—TOEFL, IELTS. *Application deadline:* For fall admission, 5/1 priority date for domestic students; for spring admission, 11/1 priority date for domestic students. Applications are processed on a rolling basis. Application fee: $35. Electronic applications accepted. *Expenses:* Contact institution. *Financial support:* In 2013–14, 1 research assistantship with full tuition reimbursement (averaging $1,600 per year), 6 teaching assistantships with full tuition reimbursements (averaging $4,668 per year) were awarded; traineeships and unspecified assistantships also available. Financial award application deadline: 8/15; financial award applicants required to submit CSS PROFILE or FAFSA. *Faculty research:* Prevention of farmers' hearing loss, breast cancer in Native American women, colon cancer, quality improvement in a wellness center. *Unit head:* Dr. Carla Gross, Department Chair, 701-231-5692, Fax: 701-231-7606, E-mail: carla.gross@ndsu.edu. *Application contact:* Dr. Jonathan Sheng, Assistant Professor, 701-231-6140, Fax: 701-231-8333, E-mail: jonathan.sheng@ndsu.edu.
Website: http://www.ndsu.edu/ndsu/nursing

Northeastern University, Bouvé College of Health Sciences, Boston, MA 02115-5096. Offers audiology (Au D); biotechnology (MS); counseling psychology (MS, PhD, CAGS); counseling/school psychology (PhD); exercise physiology (MS), including exercise physiology, public health; health informatics (MS); nursing (MS, PhD, CAGS), including acute care (MS), administration (MS), anesthesia (MS), primary care (MS), psychiatric mental health (MS); pharmaceutical sciences (PhD); pharmaceutics and drug delivery systems (MS); pharmacology (MS); physical therapy (DPT); physician assistant (MS); school psychology (PhD, CAGS); school/counseling psychology (PhD); speech language pathology (MS); urban public health (MPH); MS/MBA. *Accreditation:* ACPE (one or more programs are accredited). Part-time and evening/weekend programs available. *Degree requirements:* For doctorate, thesis/dissertation (for some programs); for CAGS, comprehensive exam.

Northern Arizona University, Graduate College, College of Health and Human Services, School of Nursing, Flagstaff, AZ 86011. Offers family nurse practitioner (MSN, Certificate); nurse generalist (MSN); nursing practice (DNP). *Accreditation:* AACN. Part-time programs available. *Faculty:* 37 full-time (33 women), 7 part-time/adjunct (all women). *Students:* 30 full-time (22 women), 108 part-time (95 women); includes 32

minority (3 Black or African American, non-Hispanic/Latino; 5 American Indian or Alaska Native, non-Hispanic/Latino; 6 Asian, non-Hispanic/Latino; 15 Hispanic/Latino; 1 Native Hawaiian or other Pacific Islander, non-Hispanic/Latino; 2 Two or more races, non-Hispanic/Latino). Average age 42. 105 applicants, 57% accepted, 46 enrolled. In 2013, 34 master's, 5 other advanced degrees awarded. *Degree requirements:* For master's, thesis (for some programs), project or thesis. *Entrance requirements:* For master's, GRE General Test or minimum GPA of 3.0, undergraduate statistics or health assessment with minimum grade of B in last 5 years or 3 years of RN experience (nursing education). Additional exam requirements/recommendations for international students: Required—TOEFL (minimum score 550 paper-based; 80 iBT), IELTS (minimum score 7). *Application deadline:* For fall admission, 1/15 priority date for domestic and international students. Applications are processed on a rolling basis. Application fee: $65. Electronic applications accepted. *Financial support:* Career-related internships or fieldwork, Federal Work-Study, scholarships/grants, traineeships, health care benefits, tuition waivers, and unspecified assistantships available. Financial award applicants required to submit FAFSA. *Unit head:* Dr. Debera Thomas, Chair, 928-523-2656, Fax: 928-523-7171, E-mail: debera.thomas@nau.edu. *Application contact:* Penny Susan Walior, Student Academic Specialist, 928-523-6717, Fax: 928-523-9155, E-mail: graduatenursing@nau.edu.
Website: http://nau.edu/CHHS/Nursing/Welcome/

Northern Illinois University, Graduate School, College of Health and Human Sciences, School of Nursing and Health Studies, De Kalb, IL 60115-2854. Offers nursing (MS); public health (MPH). *Accreditation:* AACN. Part-time programs available. *Faculty:* 12 full-time (11 women), 1 (woman) part-time/adjunct. *Students:* 39 full-time (34 women), 257 part-time (236 women); includes 64 minority (17 Black or African American, non-Hispanic/Latino; 23 Asian, non-Hispanic/Latino; 21 Hispanic/Latino; 3 Two or more races, non-Hispanic/Latino), 7 international. Average age 35. 148 applicants, 40% accepted, 29 enrolled. In 2013, 75 master's awarded. *Degree requirements:* For master's, thesis optional, internship. *Entrance requirements:* For master's, minimum GPA of 3.0 in last 60 hours, BA in nursing, nursing license. Additional exam requirements/recommendations for international students: Required—TOEFL (minimum score 550 paper-based). *Application deadline:* For fall admission, 6/1 for domestic students, 5/1 for international students; for spring admission, 11/1 for domestic students, 10/1 for international students. Applications are processed on a rolling basis. Application fee: $40. Electronic applications accepted. *Financial support:* In 2013–14, 1 research assistantship with full tuition reimbursement, 23 teaching assistantships with full tuition reimbursements were awarded; fellowships with full tuition reimbursements, career-related internships or fieldwork, Federal Work-Study, scholarships/grants, tuition waivers (full), and unspecified assistantships also available. Support available to part-time students. Financial award applicants required to submit FAFSA. *Faculty research:* Neonatal intensive care, stress and coping, refugee and immigrant issues, older adults, autoimmune disorders. *Unit head:* Dr. Janice Strom, Chair, 815-753-6550, Fax: 815-753-0814, E-mail: jstrom@niu.edu. *Application contact:* Graduate School Office, 815-753-0395, E-mail: gradsch@niu.edu.
Website: http://www.chhs.niu.edu/nursing/

Northern Kentucky University, Office of Graduate Programs, School of Nursing and Health Professions, Online Doctor of Nursing Practice Program, Highland Heights, KY 41099. Offers DNP. Part-time programs available. Postbaccalaureate distance learning degree programs offered. *Faculty:* 2 full-time (both women), 2 part-time/adjunct (1 woman). *Students:* 20 part-time (19 women); includes 1 minority (Hispanic/Latino). Average age 48. 28 applicants, 61% accepted, 15 enrolled. *Degree requirements:* For doctorate, thesis/dissertation. *Entrance requirements:* For doctorate, RN license, master's degree in nursing, minimum GPA of 3.25, course in statistics, course in informatics. Additional exam requirements/recommendations for international students: Required—TOEFL (minimum score 550 paper-based; 79 iBT); Recommended—IELTS (minimum score 6.5). *Application deadline:* For fall admission, 4/1 for domestic students, 6/1 for international students. Application fee: $50. *Expenses:* Contact institution. *Financial support:* In 2013–14, 1 student received support. *Faculty research:* Pathways to nursing degree, lead poisoning in children, predictors for NCLEX success in BSN and ABSN programs, work-life balance and deans of baccalaureate nursing programs, heart failure self management. *Unit head:* Dr. Jayne C. Lancaster, Program Director, 859-572-7966, Fax: 859-572-1934, E-mail: lancasterj1@nku.edu. *Application contact:* Dr. Christian Gamm, Director of Graduate Programs, 859-572-6364, Fax: 859-572-6670, E-mail: gammc1@nku.edu.
Website: http://advancednursing.nku.edu/programs/dnp/index.php

Northern Kentucky University, Office of Graduate Programs, School of Nursing and Health Professions, Program in Nursing, Highland Heights, KY 41099. Offers MSHS, MSN, Certificate, Post-Master's Certificate. Part-time and evening/weekend programs available. Postbaccalaureate distance learning degree programs offered (no on-campus study). *Faculty:* 8 full-time (7 women), 19 part-time/adjunct (18 women). *Students:* 26 full-time (all women), 286 part-time (271 women); includes 26 minority (17 Black or African American, non-Hispanic/Latino; 1 American Indian or Alaska Native, non-Hispanic/Latino; 2 Asian, non-Hispanic/Latino; 3 Hispanic/Latino; 3 Two or more races, non-Hispanic/Latino). Average age 37. 215 applicants, 52% accepted, 100 enrolled. In 2013, 76 master's, 7 other advanced degrees awarded. *Degree requirements:* For master's, comprehensive exam. *Entrance requirements:* For master's, minimum cumulative GPA of 2.75; one year of experience as RN; college courses in statistics, nursing research, physical assessment and nursing theory, proof of current nursing licensure, updated resume. Additional exam requirements/recommendations for international students: Required—TOEFL (minimum score 550 paper-based; 79 iBT); Recommended—IELTS (minimum score 6.5). *Application deadline:* For fall admission, 2/15 for domestic students, 2/1 for international students; for spring admission, 10/1 for domestic students, 10/15 for international students. Application fee: $40. Electronic applications accepted. *Expenses:* Tuition, state resident: full-time $4446; part-time $494 per credit hour. Tuition, nonresident: full-time $6885; part-time $765 per credit hour. *Required fees:* $72 per semester. One-time fee: $125.50. Part-time tuition and fees vary according to course load, degree level, program and reciprocity agreements. *Financial support:* In 2013–14, 65 students received support. Unspecified assistantships available. Financial award applicants required to submit FAFSA. *Faculty research:* Career planning for middle school students, technology skills for workforce, diabetes, factors affecting NCLEX scores. *Unit head:* Dr. Thomas D. Baxter, Program Director, 859-572-7869, Fax: 859-572-1934, E-mail: baxtert4@nku.edu. *Application contact:* Dr. Christian Gamm, Director of Graduate Programs, 859-572-6934, Fax: 859-572-6670, E-mail: griffinp@nku.edu.
Website: http://advancednursing.nku.edu/index.php

Northern Michigan University, College of Graduate Studies, College of Health Sciences and Professional Studies, School of Nursing, Marquette, MI 49855-5301. Offers DNP. *Accreditation:* AACN. Part-time programs available. Postbaccalaureate distance learning degree programs offered (minimal on-campus study). *Faculty:* 18 full-time (all women). *Students:* 17 part-time (14 women). Average age 35. *Entrance requirements:* For doctorate, Michigan RN license; minimum undergraduate GPA of 3.0; 3 letters of recommendation; written personal goal statement. Additional exam requirements/recommendations for international students: Required—TOEFL (minimum score 550 paper-based; 79 iBT), IELTS (minimum score 6.5). *Application deadline:* For fall admission, 4/15 for domestic and international students; for winter admission, 11/15 for domestic students; for spring admission, 3/17 for domestic students. Application fee: $50. Electronic applications accepted. *Expenses:* Tuition, state resident: part-time $427 per credit. Tuition, nonresident: part-time $614.50 per credit. *Required fees:* $325 per semester. Tuition and fees vary according to course load and program. *Financial support:* In 2013–14, 3 students received support, including 3 teaching assistantships with full tuition reimbursements available (averaging $8,898 per year); Federal Work-Study, institutionally sponsored loans, and unspecified assistantships also available. Financial award application deadline: 3/1; financial award applicants required to submit FAFSA. *Faculty research:* Grief experiences in Alzheimer's caregivers, nursing students attitudes towards the elderly, using Facebook as a means of simulation and educational means for pediatric undergraduate nursing students, use of a nurse practitioner student educational intervention to reduce sugar sweetened beverage consumption in rural adolescents. *Unit head:* Dr. Brian Cherry, Assistant Provost of Graduate Education and Research, 906-227-2300, E-mail: graduate@nmu.edu. *Application contact:* Dr. Melissa Romero, Associate Professor and Graduate Program Coordinator, 906-227-2488, Fax: 906-227-1658, E-mail: mromero@nmu.edu.
Website: http://www.nmu.edu/nursing/

North Park University, School of Nursing, Chicago, IL 60625-4895. Offers advanced practice nursing (MS); leadership and management (MS); MBA/MS; MM/MSN; MS/MHR; MS/MNA. *Accreditation:* AACN. Part-time and evening/weekend programs available. *Degree requirements:* For master's, thesis. *Entrance requirements:* For master's, GMAT, MAT. *Faculty research:* Aging, consultation roles, critical thinking skills, family breakdown, science of caring.

Northwestern State University of Louisiana, Graduate Studies and Research, College of Nursing and Allied Health, Shreveport, LA 71101-4653. Offers MS, MSN. *Accreditation:* AACN. Part-time programs available. *Degree requirements:* For master's, comprehensive exam, thesis or alternative. *Entrance requirements:* For master's, GRE General Test, 6 months of clinical nursing experience, BS in nursing, minimum GPA of 3.0. Additional exam requirements/recommendations for international students: Required—TOEFL. Electronic applications accepted.

Norwich University, College of Graduate and Continuing Studies, Master of Science in Nursing Program, Northfield, VT 05663. Offers nursing administration (MSN); nursing education (MSN). *Accreditation:* AACN. Evening/weekend programs available. Postbaccalaureate distance learning degree programs offered (minimal on-campus study). *Faculty:* 9 part-time/adjunct (5 women). *Students:* 82 full-time (78 women); includes 7 minority (4 Black or African American, non-Hispanic/Latino; 3 Asian, non-Hispanic/Latino). Average age 43. 114 applicants, 28% accepted, 31 enrolled. In 2013, 37 master's awarded. *Entrance requirements:* For master's, minimum undergraduate GPA of 2.75. Additional exam requirements/recommendations for international students: Required—TOEFL (minimum score 600 paper-based; 94 iBT). *Application deadline:* For fall admission, 8/1 for domestic and international students; for winter admission, 11/1 for domestic and international students; for spring admission, 2/1 for domestic and international students; for summer admission, 5/1 for domestic and international students. Applications are processed on a rolling basis. Application fee: $50. Electronic applications accepted. *Expenses:* Contact institution. *Financial support:* In 2013–14, 20 students received support. Scholarships/grants available. Financial award applicants required to submit FAFSA. *Unit head:* Dr. Sharon Richie-Melvan, Director, 802-485-2600, E-mail: srichiem@norwich.edu. *Application contact:* Rija Ramahatra, Associate Program Director, 802-485-2892, Fax: 802-485-2533, E-mail: rramahatr@norwich.edu.
Website: http://online.norwich.edu/degree-programs/masters/master-science-nursing/overview

Nova Southeastern University, College of Nursing, Fort Lauderdale, FL 33314-7796. Offers advanced practice registered nurse (APRN) (MSN); nursing (MSN); nursing education (PhD); nursing practice (DNP). *Accreditation:* AACN. Part-time and evening/weekend programs available. Postbaccalaureate distance learning degree programs offered (no on-campus study). *Faculty:* 12 full-time (all women), 25 part-time/adjunct (all women). *Students:* 3 full-time (all women), 374 part-time (336 women); includes 215 minority (114 Black or African American, non-Hispanic/Latino; 23 Asian, non-Hispanic/Latino; 76 Hispanic/Latino; 2 Two or more races, non-Hispanic/Latino), 3 international. Average age 41. In 2013, 34 master's, 3 doctorates awarded. *Degree requirements:* For doctorate, comprehensive exam, thesis/dissertation. *Entrance requirements:* For doctorate, minimum GPA of 3.5, BSN, RN. Additional exam requirements/recommendations for international students: Recommended—TOEFL. *Application deadline:* For fall admission, 3/1 priority date for domestic students, 3/1 for international students; for winter admission, 11/1 for domestic and international students. Applications are processed on a rolling basis. Application fee: $50. Electronic applications accepted. *Faculty research:* Nursing education, curriculum, clinical research, interdisciplinary research. *Unit head:* Dr. Marcella Rutherford, Dean, 954-262-1963, E-mail: rmarcell@nova.edu. *Application contact:* Keatta Jerry, E-mail: keatta@nova.edu.
Website: http://www.nova.edu/nursing/

Oakland University, Graduate Study and Lifelong Learning, School of Nursing, Rochester, MI 48309-4401. Offers MSN, DNP, Certificate. *Accreditation:* AACN. Part-time and evening/weekend programs available. *Faculty:* 22 full-time (all women), 3 part-time/adjunct (2 women). *Students:* 110 full-time (86 women), 149 part-time (137 women); includes 32 minority (18 Black or African American, non-Hispanic/Latino; 8 Asian, non-Hispanic/Latino; 5 Hispanic/Latino; 1 Two or more races, non-Hispanic/Latino), 5 international. Average age 36. 314 applicants, 18% accepted, 51 enrolled. In 2013, 39 master's, 22 doctorates, 3 other advanced degrees awarded. *Entrance requirements:* For master's, GRE General Test, minimum GPA of 3.0. Application fee: $0. Electronic applications accepted. *Financial support:* Federal Work-Study, institutionally sponsored loans, and tuition waivers (full) available. Financial award application deadline: 3/1; financial award applicants required to submit FAFSA. *Total annual research expenditures:* $1.1 million. *Unit head:* Dr. Linda Thompson, Dean, 248-370-4081, Fax: 248-370-4279. *Application contact:* Mary Bray, Graduate Program Coordinator, 248-370-4482.

The Ohio State University, Graduate School, College of Nursing, Columbus, OH 43210. Offers MS, DNP, PhD. *Accreditation:* AACN; ACNM/ACME. Part-time programs available. *Faculty:* 39. *Students:* 379 full-time (308 women), 188 part-time (164 women); includes 74 minority (24 Black or African American, non-Hispanic/Latino; 1 American Indian or Alaska Native, non-Hispanic/Latino; 24 Asian, non-Hispanic/Latino; 14 Hispanic/Latino; 11 Two or more races, non-Hispanic/Latino), 1 international. Average age 33. In 2013, 129 master's, 12 doctorates awarded. *Degree requirements:* For master's, thesis optional; for doctorate, thesis/dissertation. *Entrance requirements:* Additional exam requirements/recommendations for international students: Required—TOEFL (minimum score 600 paper-based; 100 iBT); Recommended—IELTS (minimum score 8). *Application deadline:* For fall admission, 1/7 priority date for domestic students, 11/30 priority date for international students; for winter admission, 12/1 for domestic students, 11/1 for international students; for spring admission, 3/1 for domestic students, 2/1 for international students. Applications are processed on a rolling basis. Application fee: $60 ($70 for international students). Electronic applications accepted. *Financial support:* Fellowships, research assistantships, teaching assistantships, Federal Work-

Study, institutionally sponsored loans, and unspecified assistantships available. Support available to part-time students. *Unit head:* Dr. Bernadette M. Melnyk, Dean, 614-292-4844, Fax: 614-292-4535, E-mail: melnyk.15@osu.edu. *Application contact:* Graduate Admissions, 614-292-9444, E-mail: gradadmissions@osu.edu.
Website: http://nursing.osu.edu/

Ohio University, Graduate College, College of Health Sciences and Professions, School of Nursing, Athens, OH 45701-2979. Offers acute care nurse practitioner (MSN); acute care nurse practitioner and family nurse practitioner (MSN); acute care nurse practitioner and nurse administrator (MSN); acute care nurse practitioner and nurse educator (MSN); family nurse practitioner (MSN); nurse administrator (MSN); nurse administrator and family nurse practitioner (MSN); nurse educator (MSN); nurse educator and family nurse practitioner (MSN); nurse educator and nurse administrator (MSN). *Accreditation:* AACN. *Degree requirements:* For master's, capstone project. *Entrance requirements:* For master's, GRE, bachelor's degree in nursing from an accredited college or university, minimum overall undergraduate GPA of 3.0, official transcripts, statement of goals and objectives, resume, 3 letters of recommendation. Additional exam requirements/recommendations for international students: Required—TOEFL (minimum score 550 paper-based; 80 iBT) or IELTS (minimum score 6.5). Electronic applications accepted.

Oklahoma Baptist University, Program in Nursing, Shawnee, OK 74804. Offers global nursing (MSN); nursing education (MSN). *Accreditation:* AACN.

Oklahoma City University, Kramer School of Nursing, Oklahoma City, OK 73106-1402. Offers health care systems leadership and administration (MSN); nursing (PhD); nursing education (MSN); nursing practice (DNP). Part-time and evening/weekend programs available. *Faculty:* 14 full-time (12 women), 5 part-time/adjunct (3 women). *Students:* 78 full-time (51 women), 116 part-time (101 women); includes 43 minority (10 Black or African American, non-Hispanic/Latino; 16 American Indian or Alaska Native, non-Hispanic/Latino; 9 Asian, non-Hispanic/Latino; 3 Hispanic/Latino; 5 Two or more races, non-Hispanic/Latino), 55 international. Average age 36. 97 applicants, 69% accepted, 37 enrolled. In 2013, 14 master's, 8 doctorates awarded. *Degree requirements:* For master's, thesis, minimum GPA of 3.0; for doctorate, comprehensive exam, thesis/dissertation, minimum GPA of 3.0. *Entrance requirements:* For master's, registered nurse licensure, minimum undergraduate GPA of 3.0, BSN from nationally-accredited nursing program, completion of courses in health assessment and statistics; for doctorate, GRE, approved scholarly paper, or published article/paper in a refereed journal, current RN licensure, bachelor's and master's degrees from accredited programs (at least one of which must be in nursing), minimum graduate GPA of 3.5, personal essay. Additional exam requirements/recommendations for international students: Required—TOEFL (minimum score 550 paper-based; 80 iBT), IELTS (minimum score 6). *Application deadline:* Applications are processed on a rolling basis. Application fee: $50. Electronic applications accepted. *Expenses: Tuition:* Full-time $16,848; part-time $936 per credit hour. Tuition and fees vary according to course load, degree level and program. *Financial support:* Federal Work-Study, institutionally sponsored loans, scholarships/grants, and tuition waivers available. Support available to part-time students. Financial award applicants required to submit FAFSA. *Unit head:* Dr. Lois Salmeron, Dean, Kramer School of Nursing, 405-208-5900, Fax: 405-208-5914, E-mail: lsalmeron@okcu.edu. *Application contact:* Heidi Puckett, Director of Graduate Admissions, 800-633-7242, Fax: 405-208-5916, E-mail: gadmissions@okcu.edu.
Website: http://www.okcu.edu/nursing/

Old Dominion University, College of Health Sciences, School of Nursing, Norfolk, VA 23529. Offers family nurse practitioner (MSN); nurse administrator (MSN); nurse anesthesia (MSN); nurse educator (MSN); nurse midwifery (MSN); nursing practice (DNP); women's health nurse practitioner (MSN). *Accreditation:* AACN; AANA/CANAEP (one or more programs are accredited). Part-time programs available. Postbaccalaureate distance learning degree programs offered (no on-campus study). *Faculty:* 6 full-time (5 women), 17 part-time/adjunct (15 women). *Students:* 111 full-time (100 women), 123 part-time (115 women); includes 45 minority (34 Black or African American, non-Hispanic/Latino; 7 Asian, non-Hispanic/Latino; 2 Hispanic/Latino; 2 Two or more races, non-Hispanic/Latino). Average age 38. 258 applicants, 61% accepted, 117 enrolled. In 2013, 60 master's, 29 doctorates awarded. *Degree requirements:* For master's, comprehensive exam; for doctorate, capstone project. *Entrance requirements:* For master's, GRE or MAT, BSN, minimum GPA of 3.0 in nursing and overall. Additional exam requirements/recommendations for international students: Required—TOEFL. *Application deadline:* For fall admission, 5/1 for domestic students, 4/15 for international students. Applications are processed on a rolling basis. Application fee: $50. Electronic applications accepted. *Expenses:* Tuition, state resident: full-time $9888; part-time $412 per credit. Tuition, nonresident: full-time $25,152; part-time $1048 per credit. *Required fees:* $59 per semester. One-time fee: $50. *Financial support:* In 2013–14, 18 students received support, including 2 research assistantships with partial tuition reimbursements available (averaging $10,000 per year), 1 teaching assistantship (averaging $2,500 per year); career-related internships or fieldwork, scholarships/grants, traineeships, and tuition waivers (partial) also available. Support available to part-time students. Financial award application deadline: 2/15; financial award applicants required to submit FAFSA. *Faculty research:* Health and culture, cardiovascular health, transition of military families, genetics, cultural diversity. *Total annual research expenditures:* $231,117. *Unit head:* Dr. Karen Karlowicz, Chair, 757-683-5262, Fax: 757-683-5253, E-mail: nursgpd@odu.edu. *Application contact:* Sue Parker, Coordinator, Graduate Student Services, 757-683-4298, Fax: 757-683-5253, E-mail: sparker@odu.edu.
Website: http://www.odu.edu/nursing

Oregon Health & Science University, School of Nursing, Portland, OR 97239-3098. Offers MN, MPH, MS, DNP, PhD, Post Master's Certificate. *Accreditation:* AACN; ACNM/ACME (one or more programs are accredited). Part-time programs available. *Degree requirements:* For master's, thesis optional; for doctorate, thesis/dissertation. *Entrance requirements:* For master's, GRE General Test, bachelor's degree in nursing, minimum undergraduate GPA of 3.0, previous course work in statistics; for doctorate, GRE General Test, master's degree in nursing; minimum undergraduate GPA of 3.0, 3.5 graduate; for Post Master's Certificate, master's degree in nursing. Electronic applications accepted. *Expenses:* Contact institution. *Faculty research:* Nursing care of older persons; families in health, illness, and transition; family caregiving; end of life care/decision making; mother-infant interactions; pregnancy outcomes; enteral feeding; psychoactive drugs in long-term care.

Otterbein University, Department of Nursing, Westerville, OH 43081. Offers advanced practice nurse educator (Certificate); clinical nurse leader (MSN); family nurse practitioner (MSN, Certificate); nurse anesthesia (MSN, Certificate); nursing (DNP); nursing service administration (MSN). *Accreditation:* AACN; AANA/CANAEP. Part-time and evening/weekend programs available. Postbaccalaureate distance learning degree programs offered (minimal on-campus study). *Degree requirements:* For master's, comprehensive exam (for some programs), thesis (for some programs). *Entrance requirements:* For master's, 2 reference forms, resume; for Certificate, official transcripts, 2 reference forms, essay, resumé. Additional exam requirements/recommendations for international students: Required—TOEFL (minimum score 550 paper-based; 79 iBT). *Faculty research:* Patient education, women's health, trauma curriculum development, administration.

Our Lady of the Lake College, School of Nursing, Baton Rouge, LA 70808. Offers nurse anesthesia (MS); nursing (MS), including administration, education.

Our Lady of the Lake University of San Antonio, School of Professional Studies, Program in Nursing, San Antonio, TX 78207-4689. Offers nurse administration (MSN); nurse education (MSN). Postbaccalaureate distance learning degree programs offered (no on-campus study). *Faculty:* 1 (woman) full-time, 1 (woman) part-time/adjunct. *Students:* 17 full-time (16 women), 4 part-time (all women); includes 12 minority (3 Black or African American, non-Hispanic/Latino; 1 American Indian or Alaska Native, non-Hispanic/Latino; 8 Hispanic/Latino). Average age 43. 20 applicants, 100% accepted, 15 enrolled. *Degree requirements:* For master's, comprehensive exam. *Entrance requirements:* For master's, GRE General Test or MAT. Additional exam requirements/recommendations for international students: Required—TOEFL. *Application deadline:* For fall admission, 4/1 priority date for domestic and international students; for spring admission, 11/1 priority date for domestic and international students; for summer admission, 2/1 priority date for domestic and international students. Applications are processed on a rolling basis. Application fee: $25 ($50 for international students). Electronic applications accepted. *Expenses: Tuition:* Full-time $9120; part-time $760 per credit. *Required fees:* $698; $334 per trimester. Tuition and fees vary according to course load, degree level, campus/location and program. *Financial support:* Career-related internships or fieldwork, institutionally sponsored loans, scholarships/grants, and tuition waivers (partial) available. Support available to part-time students. Financial award application deadline: 4/15. *Unit head:* Dr. Wanda Sparks, Chair, 210-431-4162, E-mail: wrsparks@lake.ollusa.edu. *Application contact:* Graduate Admission, 210-431-3961, Fax: 210-431-4013, E-mail: gradadm@lake.ollusa.edu.

Pace University, College of Health Professions, Lienhard School of Nursing, New York, NY 10038. Offers family nurse practitioner (MS); nurse practitioner (Advanced Certificate); nursing education (MA); nursing leadership (Advanced Certificate); nursing practice (DNP). *Accreditation:* AACN. Part-time and evening/weekend programs available. Postbaccalaureate distance learning degree programs offered. *Faculty:* 13 full-time (12 women), 36 part-time/adjunct (29 women). *Students:* 3 full-time (2 women), 427 part-time (390 women); includes 202 minority (98 Black or African American, non-Hispanic/Latino; 2 American Indian or Alaska Native, non-Hispanic/Latino; 68 Asian, non-Hispanic/Latino; 28 Hispanic/Latino; 1 Native Hawaiian or other Pacific Islander, non-Hispanic/Latino; 5 Two or more races, non-Hispanic/Latino), 2 international. Average age 35. 274 applicants, 69% accepted, 131 enrolled. In 2013, 120 master's, 15 doctorates, 3 other advanced degrees awarded. *Degree requirements:* For master's, thesis. *Entrance requirements:* For master's, GRE General Test or MAT, RN license, resume, personal statement, 2 letters of recommendation, official transcripts; for doctorate, RN license, resume, personal statement, 2 letters of recommendation, official transcripts, accredited master's degree in nursing, minimum GPA of 3.3, state certification; for Advanced Certificate, RN license, completion of 2nd degree in nursing. Additional exam requirements/recommendations for international students: Required—TOEFL. *Application deadline:* For fall admission, 3/1 priority date for domestic and international students; for spring admission, 10/14 for domestic students, 9/14 for international students. Applications are processed on a rolling basis. Application fee: $70. Electronic applications accepted. *Expenses:* Contact institution. *Financial support:* Research assistantships, career-related internships or fieldwork, Federal Work-Study, and tuition waivers (partial) available. Support available to part-time students. Financial award applicants required to submit FAFSA. *Unit head:* Dr. Harriet Feldman, Dean, College of Health Professions, 914-773-3245, E-mail: hfeldman@pace.edu. *Application contact:* Susan Ford-Goldschein, Director of Graduate Admissions, 914-422-4283, Fax: 914-422-4287, E-mail: gradwp@pace.edu.
Website: http://www.pace.edu/lienhard

Pacific Lutheran University, Graduate Programs and Continuing Education, School of Nursing, Tacoma, WA 98447. Offers MSN. *Accreditation:* AACN. *Faculty:* 5 full-time (4 women), 2 part-time/adjunct (1 woman). *Students:* 54 full-time (47 women), 1 (woman) part-time; includes 5 minority (3 Asian, non-Hispanic/Latino; 1 Hispanic/Latino; 1 Two or more races, non-Hispanic/Latino). Average age 31. 89 applicants, 49% accepted, 28 enrolled. In 2013, 21 master's awarded. *Degree requirements:* For master's, thesis or alternative. *Entrance requirements:* For master's, GRE General Test, minimum undergraduate GPA of 3.0. Additional exam requirements/recommendations for international students: Required—TOEFL (minimum score 550 paper-based; 86 iBT). *Application deadline:* For fall admission, 11/15 priority date for domestic and international students. Applications are processed on a rolling basis. Application fee: $40. Electronic applications accepted. *Expenses: Tuition:* Full-time $18,560; part-time $1160. Tuition and fees vary according to program and student level. *Financial support:* In 2013–14, 3 students received support. Fellowships, Federal Work-Study, and scholarships/grants available. Financial award application deadline: 3/1; financial award applicants required to submit FAFSA. *Unit head:* Dr. Teri Woo, Associate Dean of Graduate Nursing Programs/Associate Professor of Nursing, 253-535-7686, Fax: 253-535-7590, E-mail: gradnurs@plu.edu. *Application contact:* Rachel Christopherson, Director, Graduate Admission, 253-535-8570, Fax: 253-536-5136, E-mail: gradadmission@plu.edu.

Penn State University Park, Graduate School, College of Nursing, University Park, PA 16802. Offers MS, MSN, PhD. Part-time and evening/weekend programs available. Postbaccalaureate distance learning degree programs offered. *Students:* 67 full-time (58 women), 38 part-time (32 women); includes 11 minority (2 Black or African American, non-Hispanic/Latino; 4 Asian, non-Hispanic/Latino; 4 Hispanic/Latino; 1 Two or more races, non-Hispanic/Latino), 4 international. Average age 33. 86 applicants, 47% accepted, 34 enrolled. In 2013, 36 master's, 3 doctorates awarded. *Entrance requirements:* Additional exam requirements/recommendations for international students: Required—TOEFL (minimum score 550 paper-based; 80 iBT). *Application deadline:* Applications are processed on a rolling basis. Application fee: $65. Electronic applications accepted. *Financial support:* Fellowships, research assistantships, teaching assistantships, career-related internships or fieldwork, Federal Work-Study, and unspecified assistantships available. Support available to part-time students. Financial award application deadline: 2/15; financial award applicants required to submit FAFSA. *Unit head:* Dr. Ann C. Crouter, Dean, 814-865-1420, Fax: 814-865-3282, E-mail: ac1@psu.edu. *Application contact:* Cynthia E. Nicosia, Director, Graduate Enrollment Services, 814-865-1834, Fax: 814-863-4627, E-mail: cey1@psu.edu.
Website: http://www.nursing.psu.edu/

Piedmont College, School of Nursing and Health Sciences, Demorest, GA 30535-0010. Offers nursing administration (MSN); nursing education (MSN). *Expenses: Tuition:* Full-time $7992; part-time $444 per credit hour.

Pittsburg State University, Graduate School, College of Arts and Sciences, Department of Nursing, Pittsburg, KS 66762. Offers MSN. *Accreditation:* AACN. *Entrance requirements:* For master's, GRE General Test.

Point Loma Nazarene University, School of Nursing, San Diego, CA 92106-2899. Offers adult/gerontology nursing (MSN); family/individual health (MSN); general nursing (MSN); nursing (Post-MSN Certificate); pediatric nursing (MSN); psychiatric mental health (MSN). *Accreditation:* AACN. Part-time programs available. *Faculty:* 9 full-time (8 women). *Students:* 1 (woman) full-time, 82 part-time (70 women); includes 43 minority (9 Black or African American, non-Hispanic/Latino; 1 American Indian or Alaska Native,

non-Hispanic/Latino; 26 Asian, non-Hispanic/Latino; 3 Hispanic/Latino; 3 Native Hawaiian or other Pacific Islander, non-Hispanic/Latino; 1 Two or more races, non-Hispanic/Latino). Average age 36. 32 applicants, 94% accepted, 24 enrolled. In 2013, 26 master's awarded. *Entrance requirements:* For master's, NCLEX, ADN or BSN in nursing, interview, RN license, essay, letters of recommendation, interview. *Application deadline:* For fall admission, 7/18 priority date for domestic students; for spring admission, 10/26 priority date for domestic students; for summer admission, 3/23 priority date for domestic students. Applications are processed on a rolling basis. Application fee: $50. *Expenses: Tuition:* Full-time $6900; part-time $567 per credit hour. *Financial support:* Applicants required to submit FAFSA. *Unit head:* Dr. Barb Taylor, Dean of the School of Nursing, 619-849-2766, E-mail: bataylor@pointloma.edu. *Application contact:* Laura Leinweber, Director of Graduate Admissions, 866-692-4723, E-mail: lauraleinweber@pointloma.edu.
Website: http://www.pointloma.edu/discover/graduate-school/graduate-programs/master-science-nursing-and-post-msn-certification

Pontifical Catholic University of Puerto Rico, College of Sciences, Department of Nursing, Ponce, PR 00717-0777. Offers medical-surgical nursing (MSN); mental health and psychiatric nursing (MSN). Part-time and evening/weekend programs available. *Degree requirements:* For master's, comprehensive exam (for some programs), thesis, clinical research paper. *Entrance requirements:* For master's, GRE General Test, 2 letters of recommendation, interview, minimum GPA of 2.5. Electronic applications accepted.

Prairie View A&M University, College of Nursing, Houston, TX 77030. Offers family nurse practitioner (MSN); nursing administration (MSN); nursing education (MSN). Part-time programs available. *Faculty:* 9 full-time (8 women), 13 part-time/adjunct (11 women). *Students:* 74 full-time (61 women), 107 part-time (99 women); includes 65 minority (63 Black or African American, non-Hispanic/Latino; 2 Hispanic/Latino), 4 international. Average age 37. 121 applicants, 42% accepted, 45 enrolled. In 2013, 46 master's awarded. *Degree requirements:* For master's, comprehensive exam, thesis. *Entrance requirements:* For master's, MAT or GRE, BS in nursing; 2 years of experience as a registered nurse; 1 course each in statistics, basic health and assessment. *Application deadline:* For fall admission, 7/1 priority date for domestic students, 7/1 for international students; for spring admission, 11/1 priority date for domestic students, 11/1 for international students. Applications are processed on a rolling basis. Application fee: $50. *Expenses:* Tuition, state resident: full-time $3776; part-time $209.77 per credit hour. Tuition, nonresident: full-time $10,183; part-time $565.77 per credit hour. *Required fees:* $2037; $446.50 per credit hour. *Financial support:* In 2013–14, 17 students received support. Career-related internships or fieldwork, Federal Work-Study, institutionally sponsored loans, scholarships/grants, and traineeships available. Support available to part-time students. Financial award application deadline: 4/1; financial award applicants required to submit FAFSA. *Faculty research:* Software development and violence prevention, health promotion and disease prevention. *Total annual research expenditures:* $350,000. *Unit head:* Dr. Betty N. Adams, Dean, 713-797-7009, Fax: 713-797-7013, E-mail: bnadams@pvamu.edu. *Application contact:* Dr. Forest Smith, Director of Student Services and Admissions, 713-797-7031, Fax: 713-797-7012, E-mail: fdsmith@pvamu.edu.
Website: http://www.pvamu.edu/nursing/

Purdue University Calumet, Graduate Studies Office, School of Nursing, Hammond, IN 46323-2094. Offers adult health clinical nurse specialist (MS); critical care clinical nurse specialist (MS); family nurse practitioner (MS); nurse executive (MS). Part-time programs available. Postbaccalaureate distance learning degree programs offered (minimal on-campus study). *Entrance requirements:* For master's, BSN. Additional exam requirements/recommendations for international students: Required—TOEFL. Electronic applications accepted. *Faculty research:* Adult health, cardiovascular and pulmonary nursing.

Queen's University at Kingston, School of Graduate Studies, Faculty of Health Sciences, School of Nursing, Kingston, ON K7L 3N6, Canada. Offers health and chronic illness (M Sc); nurse scientist (PhD); primary health care nurse practitioner (Certificate); women's and children's health (M Sc). *Degree requirements:* For master's, thesis. *Entrance requirements:* For master's, RN license. Additional exam requirements/recommendations for international students: Required—TOEFL. *Faculty research:* Women and children's health, health and chronic illness.

Queens University of Charlotte, Presbyterian School of Nursing, Charlotte, NC 28274-0002. Offers nursing management (MSN). *Accreditation:* AACN. *Degree requirements:* For master's, research project. *Entrance requirements:* For master's, minimum GPA of 3.0. Additional exam requirements/recommendations for international students: Required—TOEFL. Electronic applications accepted. *Expenses:* Contact institution.

Quinnipiac University, School of Nursing, Hamden, CT 06518-1940. Offers MSN, DNP. Part-time programs available. *Faculty:* 14 full-time (13 women), 5 part-time/adjunct (3 women). *Students:* 44 full-time (42 women), 76 part-time (68 women); includes 23 minority (10 Black or African American, non-Hispanic/Latino; 8 Asian, non-Hispanic/Latino; 5 Hispanic/Latino), 2 international. 73 applicants, 81% accepted, 48 enrolled. In 2013, 50 master's, 5 doctorates awarded. *Degree requirements:* For master's, thesis optional, clinical practicum. *Entrance requirements:* For master's, RN license, minimum GPA of 3.0. Additional exam requirements/recommendations for international students: Required—TOEFL (minimum score 575 paper-based; 90 iBT), IELTS (minimum score 6.5). *Application deadline:* For fall admission, 6/1 priority date for domestic students, 4/30 priority date for international students. Applications are processed on a rolling basis. Application fee: $45. Electronic applications accepted. *Expenses: Tuition:* Part-time $920 per credit. *Required fees:* $37 per credit. *Financial support:* In 2013–14, 7 students received support. Career-related internships or fieldwork, Federal Work-Study, scholarships/grants, tuition waivers (partial), and unspecified assistantships available. Support available to part-time students. Financial award application deadline: 6/1; financial award applicants required to submit FAFSA. *Faculty research:* Decreasing social isolation of older adults, high fidelity simulation as a teaching method, teaching end of life care to nursing students, nurses with disabilities and practice roles, improving depression care of older home care patients, determining hip labral tears with new physical examination technique. *Unit head:* Dr. Lynn Price, Program Director, E-mail: lynn.price@quinnipiac.edu. *Application contact:* Office of Graduate Admissions, 800-462-1944, Fax: 203-582-3443, E-mail: graduate@quinnipiac.edu.
Website: http://www.quinnipiac.edu/gradnursing

Radford University, College of Graduate and Professional Studies, Waldron College of Health and Human Services, School of Nursing, Radford, VA 24142. Offers MSN, DNP. *Accreditation:* AACN. Part-time and evening/weekend programs available. Postbaccalaureate distance learning degree programs offered (minimal on-campus study). *Faculty:* 11 full-time (10 women), 2 part-time/adjunct (both women). *Students:* 8 full-time (7 women), 49 part-time (44 women); includes 11 minority (6 Black or African American, non-Hispanic/Latino; 3 Asian, non-Hispanic/Latino; 1 Hispanic/Latino; 1 Two or more races, non-Hispanic/Latino), 1 international. Average age 42. 33 applicants, 94% accepted, 23 enrolled. In 2013, 5 doctorates awarded. *Degree requirements:* For master's, comprehensive exam, thesis optional; for doctorate, thesis/dissertation. *Entrance requirements:* For doctorate, GRE, current license to practice as registered nurse; minimum undergraduate GPA of 3.0, graduate 3.5; 3-5 page essay; professional writing sample; three letters of reference; personal interview; resume or curriculum vitae; official transcripts; 2000 hours of RN clinical experience; certification in BLS or ACLS; BSN; MSN (for some areas). Additional exam requirements/recommendations for international students: Required—TOEFL (minimum score 550 paper-based; 79 iBT). *Application deadline:* For fall admission, 2/15 priority date for domestic students, 12/1 for international students; for spring admission, 7/1 for international students. Applications are processed on a rolling basis. Application fee: $50. Electronic applications accepted. *Expenses:* Contact institution. *Financial support:* In 2013–14, 31 students received support. Career-related internships or fieldwork, Federal Work-Study, institutionally sponsored loans, scholarships/grants, and unspecified assistantships available. Financial award application deadline: 3/1; financial award applicants required to submit FAFSA. *Unit head:* Dr. Anthony R. Ramsey, Director, 540-831-7700, Fax: 540-831-7716, E-mail: nurs-web@radford.edu. *Application contact:* Rebecca Conner, Director, Graduate Enrollment, 540-831-6296, Fax: 540-831-6061, E-mail: gradcollege@radford.edu.
Website: http://www.radford.edu/content/wchs/home/nursing.html

Ramapo College of New Jersey, Master of Science in Nursing Program, Mahwah, NJ 07430. Offers nursing education (MSN). Part-time programs available. *Faculty:* 1 (woman) full-time, 2 part-time/adjunct (1 woman). *Students:* 3 full-time (2 women), 37 part-time (34 women); includes 6 minority (1 Black or African American, non-Hispanic/Latino; 4 Asian, non-Hispanic/Latino; 1 Hispanic/Latino), 2 international. Average age 43. In 2013, 15 master's awarded. *Entrance requirements:* For master's, official transcript; personal statement; 2 letters of recommendation; resume; current licensure as a Registered Nurse, or eligibility for licensure; evidence of one year recent experience as a Registered Nurse prior to entry into clinical practicum courses; evidence of undergraduate statistics course; satisfactory completion of criminal background. Additional exam requirements/recommendations for international students: Required—TOEFL (minimum score 550 paper-based; 90 iBT); Recommended—IELTS (minimum score 6). *Application deadline:* Applications are processed on a rolling basis. Application fee: $60. Electronic applications accepted. *Expenses: Tuition, area resident:* Part-time $582.45 per credit. Tuition, nonresident: part-time $748.70 per credit. *Required fees:* $127.05 per credit. *Financial support:* In 2013–14, 10 students received support, including 10 fellowships with partial tuition reimbursements available (averaging $1,992 per year); traineeships also available. Financial award applicants required to submit FAFSA. *Faculty research:* Learning styles and critical thinking, evidence-based education, outcomes measurement. *Unit head:* Dr. Kathleen M. Burke, Assistant Dean, Master of Science in Nursing Program, 201-684-7737, E-mail: kmburke@ramapo.edu. *Application contact:* Ulysses Simpkins, Program Assistant, 201-684-7749, E-mail: usimpkin@ramapo.edu.
Website: http://www.ramapo.edu/msn/

Regis College, School of Nursing, Science and Health Professions, Weston, MA 02493. Offers applied behavior analysis (MS); biomedical sciences (MS); health administration (MS); nurse practitioner (Certificate); nursing (MS, DNP); nursing education (Certificate). Part-time and evening/weekend programs available. *Degree requirements:* For master's, thesis. *Entrance requirements:* For master's, GRE General Test or MAT, minimum GPA of 3.0; for doctorate, MAT or GRE if GPA from master's lower than 3.5. Additional exam requirements/recommendations for international students: Required—TOEFL (minimum score 550 paper-based). Electronic applications accepted. *Faculty research:* Health policy, education, aging, job satisfaction, psychiatric nursing, critical thinking.

Research College of Nursing, Nursing Program, Kansas City, MO 64132. Offers adult-gerontological nurse practitioner (MSN); clinical nurse leader (MSN); executive practice and healthcare leadership (MSN); family nurse practitioner (MSN); nurse educator (MSN); nursing (MSN). *Accreditation:* AACN. Part-time programs available. Postbaccalaureate distance learning degree programs offered (no on-campus study). *Faculty:* 9 full-time (all women), 5 part-time/adjunct (2 women). *Students:* 19 full-time (18 women), 101 part-time (94 women). *Degree requirements:* For master's, research project. *Entrance requirements:* For master's, 3 letters of recommendation, official transcripts, resume. Additional exam requirements/recommendations for international students: Required—TOEFL (minimum score 550 paper-based), TWE. *Application deadline:* Applications are processed on a rolling basis. Application fee: $50. *Expenses: Tuition:* Part-time $445 per credit hour. *Required fees:* $25 per credit hour. Part-time tuition and fees vary according to course load. *Financial support:* Applicants required to submit FAFSA. *Unit head:* Dr. Nancy O. DeBasio, President and Dean, 816-995-2815, Fax: 816-995-2817, E-mail: nancy.debasio@researchcollege.edu. *Application contact:* Leslie Mendenhall, Director of Transfer and Graduate Recruitment, 816-995-2820, Fax: 816-995-2813, E-mail: leslie.mendenhall@researchcollege.edu.

Resurrection University, Nursing Program, Chicago, IL 60622. Offers MSN. *Accreditation:* AACN. *Entrance requirements:* For master's, letter of recommendation.

Rhode Island College, School of Graduate Studies, School of Nursing, Providence, RI 02908-1991. Offers MSN. *Accreditation:* AACN. Part-time programs available. *Faculty:* 9 full-time (all women), 5 part-time/adjunct (all women). *Students:* 4 full-time (all women), 65 part-time (55 women); includes 4 minority (2 Black or African American, non-Hispanic/Latino; 2 Asian, non-Hispanic/Latino), 2 international. Average age 40. In 2013, 14 master's awarded. *Entrance requirements:* For master's, GRE, undergraduate transcripts; minimum undergraduate GPA of 3.0; 3 letters of recommendation; evidence of current unrestricted Rhode Island RN licensure; professional resume; letter of intent. Additional exam requirements/recommendations for international students: Recommended—TOEFL (minimum score 550 paper-based; 79 iBT). *Application deadline:* For fall admission, 2/15 for domestic students. Applications are processed on a rolling basis. Application fee: $50. *Expenses:* Tuition, state resident: full-time $8928; part-time $372 per credit hour. Tuition, nonresident: full-time $17,376; part-time $724 per credit hour. *Required fees:* $602; $22 per credit. $72 per term. *Financial support:* In 2013–14, 5 teaching assistantships with full tuition reimbursements (averaging $1,800 per year) were awarded; Federal Work-Study, scholarships/grants, health care benefits, and unspecified assistantships also available. Support available to part-time students. Financial award application deadline: 5/15; financial award applicants required to submit FAFSA. *Unit head:* Dr. Jane Williams, Dean, 401-456-8013, Fax: 401-456-9608, E-mail: jwilliams@ric.edu. *Application contact:* Graduate Studies, 401-456-8700.
Website: http://www.ric.edu/nursing/

The Richard Stockton College of New Jersey, School of Graduate and Continuing Studies, Program in Nursing, Galloway, NJ 08205-9441. Offers MSN. *Accreditation:* AACN. Part-time programs available. *Faculty:* 4 full-time (all women), 3 part-time/adjunct (all women). *Students:* 7 full-time (5 women), 34 part-time (32 women); includes 9 minority (1 Black or African American, non-Hispanic/Latino; 3 Asian, non-Hispanic/Latino; 2 Hispanic/Latino; 1 Native Hawaiian or other Pacific Islander, non-Hispanic/Latino; 2 Two or more races, non-Hispanic/Latino), 1 international. Average age 34. 23 applicants, 61% accepted, 12 enrolled. In 2013, 9 master's awarded. *Degree requirements:* For master's, 300 clinical hours. *Entrance requirements:* For master's, CPR certification, minimum GPA of 3.0, RN license. Additional exam requirements/recommendations for international students: Required—TOEFL. *Application deadline:* For fall admission, 5/1 for domestic and international students; for spring admission, 12/1 for domestic students, 11/1 for international students. Applications are processed on a rolling basis. Application fee: $50. Electronic applications accepted. *Expenses: Tuition, area resident:* Part-time $559 per credit. Tuition, state resident: part-time $559 per credit. Tuition, nonresident: part-time $861 per credit. *Required fees:* $168.23 per credit. $75 per semester. Tuition and fees vary according to course load and degree level. *Financial support:* In 2013–14, 4 students received support, including 5 research assistantships with partial tuition reimbursements available; fellowships, career-related internships or fieldwork, Federal Work-Study, scholarships/grants, and unspecified assistantships also available. Support available to part-time students. Financial award application deadline: 3/1; financial award applicants required to submit FAFSA. *Faculty research:* Psychoneuroimmunology, relationship of nutrition and disease, mental health as affected by chronic disease states, home care for elderly relatives. *Unit head:* Dr. Edward Walton, Program Director, 609-626-3640, E-mail: edward.walton@stockton.edu. *Application contact:* Tara Williams, Associate Director of Admissions, 609-626-3640, Fax: 609-626-6050, E-mail: gradschool@stockton.edu.

Rivier University, School of Graduate Studies, Division of Nursing, Nashua, NH 03060. Offers adult psychiatric/mental health practitioner (MS); family nurse practitioner (MS); nursing education (MS). Part-time and evening/weekend programs available. *Entrance requirements:* For master's, GRE, MAT. Electronic applications accepted.

Robert Morris University, Graduate Studies, School of Nursing and Health Sciences, Moon Township, PA 15108. Offers MSN, DNP. *Accreditation:* AACN. Part-time and evening/weekend programs available. *Faculty:* 10 full-time (8 women), 6 part-time/adjunct (all women). *Students:* 174 part-time (151 women); includes 33 minority (20 Black or African American, non-Hispanic/Latino; 2 Asian, non-Hispanic/Latino; 2 Hispanic/Latino; 9 Two or more races, non-Hispanic/Latino). Average age 28. 137 applicants, 60% accepted, 67 enrolled. In 2013, 7 master's, 35 doctorates awarded. *Entrance requirements:* For master's, letters of recommendation. Additional exam requirements/recommendations for international students: Required—TOEFL (minimum score 550 paper-based; 79 iBT). *Application deadline:* For fall admission, 7/1 priority date for domestic and international students; for spring admission, 11/1 priority date for domestic and international students. Applications are processed on a rolling basis. Application fee: $35. Electronic applications accepted. *Expenses:* Contact institution. *Financial support:* Federal Work-Study, institutionally sponsored loans, and unspecified assistantships available. Financial award application deadline: 5/1; financial award applicants required to submit FAFSA. *Unit head:* Dr. Valerie M Howard, Dean, 412-397-6801, Fax: 412-397-3277, E-mail: howardv@rmu.edu. *Application contact:* 412-397-5200, Fax: 412-397-5915, E-mail: graduateadmissions@rmu.edu.
Website: http://www.rmu.edu/web/cms/schools/snhs/

Roberts Wesleyan College, Department of Nursing, Rochester, NY 14624-1997. Offers nursing administration (MSN); nursing education (MSN). *Accreditation:* AACN. Evening/weekend programs available. Postbaccalaureate distance learning degree programs offered (no on-campus study). *Faculty:* 13 full-time (all women), 6 part-time/adjunct (4 women). *Students:* 67 full-time (63 women); includes 10 minority (5 Black or African American, non-Hispanic/Latino; 2 American Indian or Alaska Native, non-Hispanic/Latino; 1 Asian, non-Hispanic/Latino; 2 Hispanic/Latino), 7 international. Average age 39. 53 applicants, 100% accepted, 36 enrolled. In 2013, 2 master's awarded. *Degree requirements:* For master's, thesis. *Entrance requirements:* For master's, minimum GPA of 3.0; BS in nursing; interview; RN license; resume; course work in statistics. Additional exam requirements/recommendations for international students: Required—TOEFL (minimum score 90 iBT), IELTS (minimum score 6.5). *Application deadline:* Applications are processed on a rolling basis. Application fee: $0. *Expenses: Tuition:* Full-time $12,816; part-time $712 per credit hour. One-time fee: $300. Tuition and fees vary according to course load and program. *Financial support:* In 2013–14, 21 students received support. Scholarships/grants available. Financial award applicants required to submit FAFSA. *Unit head:* Dr. Cheryl B. Crotser, Chairperson and Director of Graduate Program, 585-594-6668, E-mail: crotser_cheryl@roberts.edu. *Application contact:* Brenda Mutton, Admissions Coordinator, 585-594-6686, E-mail: mutton_brenda@roberts.edu.
Website: http://www.roberts.edu/gradnursing

Rush University, College of Nursing, Chicago, IL 60612. Offers MSN, DNP, PhD, Post-Graduate Certificate. *Accreditation:* AACN; AANA/CANAEP (one or more programs are accredited). Part-time programs available. Postbaccalaureate distance learning degree programs offered (minimal on-campus study). *Faculty:* 75 full-time (71 women), 52 part-time/adjunct (44 women). *Students:* 279 full-time (234 women), 556 part-time (514 women); includes 173 minority (48 Black or African American, non-Hispanic/Latino; 8 American Indian or Alaska Native, non-Hispanic/Latino; 59 Asian, non-Hispanic/Latino; 47 Hispanic/Latino; 4 Native Hawaiian or other Pacific Islander, non-Hispanic/Latino; 7 Two or more races, non-Hispanic/Latino). Average age 36. 770 applicants, 69% accepted, 461 enrolled. In 2013, 592 master's, 62 doctorates, 41 other advanced degrees awarded. *Degree requirements:* For master's, thesis, capstone project; for doctorate, leadership project (for DNP); dissertation (for PhD). *Entrance requirements:* For master's, GRE General Test (waived if cumulative GPA is 3.25 or greater, nursing GPA is 3.0 or greater, or completed graduate program GPA is 3.5 or greater), interview, 3 letters of recommendation, personal statement, current resume; for doctorate, GRE General Test (for DNP in nurse anesthesia and PhD; waived for DNP if cumulative GPA is 3.25 or greater, nursing GPA is 3.0 or greater, or a completed graduate program GPA is 3.5 or greater), interview, 3 letters of recommendation, personal statement, current resume; for Post-Graduate Certificate, MSN in a clinical discipline, 3 letters of recommendation, personal statement, current resume, interview. Additional exam requirements/recommendations for international students: Required—TOEFL. *Application deadline:* For fall admission, 1/2 for domestic students; for winter admission, 10/15 for domestic students; for spring admission, 8/4 for domestic students; for summer admission, 12/1 for domestic students. Applications are processed on a rolling basis. Application fee: $100. Electronic applications accepted. *Financial support:* In 2013–14, 207 students received support. Fellowships, research assistantships, teaching assistantships, Federal Work-Study, scholarships/grants, traineeships, and health care benefits available. Support available to part-time students. Financial award application deadline: 3/1; financial award applicants required to submit FAFSA. *Faculty research:* Physical activity adherence in African-American women; reduction of health disparities; evidence-based interventions for caregivers; benefit of human milk feedings for low birth weight infants; patient-centered quality assessment of psychiatric inpatient environments. *Total annual research expenditures:* $3.8 million. *Unit head:* Dr. Marquis Foreman, Acting Dean, 312-942-7117, Fax: 312-942-3043, E-mail: marquis_d_foreman@rush.edu. *Application contact:* Jennifer Thorndyke, Admissions Specialist for the College of Nursing, 312-563-7526, E-mail: jennifer_thorndyke@rush.edu.
Website: http://www.rushu.rush.edu/nursing/

Rutgers, The State University of New Jersey, Newark, Rutgers School of Nursing, Newark, NJ 07107-3001. Offers adult health (MSN); adult occupational health (MSN); advanced practice nursing (MSN, Post Master's Certificate); family nurse practitioner (MSN); nurse anesthesia (MSN); nursing (MSN); nursing informatics (MSN); urban health (PhD); women's health practitioner (MSN). *Accreditation:* AANA/CANAEP. Part-time programs available. *Entrance requirements:* For master's, GRE, RN license; basic life support, statistics, and health assessment experience. Additional exam requirements/recommendations for international students: Required—TOEFL. Electronic applications accepted. *Expenses:* Contact institution. *Faculty research:* HIV/AIDS, diabetes education, learned helplessness, nursing science, psychoeducation.

Sacred Heart University, Graduate Programs, College of Health Professions, Department of Nursing, Fairfield, CT 06825-1000. Offers clinical nurse leader (MSN); clinical practice in health care (DNP); family nurse practitioner (MSN); leadership in health care (DNP); nursing (DN Sc); nursing educator (MSN); patient care services administration (MSN). *Accreditation:* AACN. Part-time and evening/weekend programs available. Postbaccalaureate distance learning degree programs offered (no on-campus study). *Faculty:* 7 full-time (all women), 5 part-time/adjunct (all women). *Students:* 34 full-time (32 women), 645 part-time (595 women); includes 117 minority (50 Black or African American, non-Hispanic/Latino; 1 American Indian or Alaska Native, non-Hispanic/Latino; 26 Asian, non-Hispanic/Latino; 29 Hispanic/Latino; 1 Native Hawaiian or other Pacific Islander, non-Hispanic/Latino; 10 Two or more races, non-Hispanic/Latino). Average age 39. 110 applicants, 58% accepted, 46 enrolled. In 2013, 67 master's, 11 doctorates awarded. *Entrance requirements:* For master's, minimum GPA of 3.0, BSN or RN plus BS (for MSN); for doctorate, minimum GPA of 3.0, MSN or BSN plus MS (for DNP). Additional exam requirements/recommendations for international students: Required—PTE; Recommended—TOEFL (minimum score 570 paper-based; 80 iBT), IELTS (minimum score 6.5). *Application deadline:* Applications are processed on a rolling basis. Application fee: $60. Electronic applications accepted. *Expenses:* Contact institution. *Financial support:* Career-related internships or fieldwork and institutionally sponsored loans available. Support available to part-time students. Financial award applicants required to submit FAFSA. *Unit head:* Dr. Sue DeNisco, Chair, 203-365-7661, Fax: 203-365-7662, E-mail: deniscos@sacredheart.edu. *Application contact:* Kathy Dilks, Executive Director of Graduate Admissions, 203-365-4716, Fax: 203-365-4732, E-mail: gradstudies@sacredheart.edu.
Website: http://www.sacredheart.edu/graduate/nursing/

Sage Graduate School, School of Health Sciences, Department of Nursing, Troy, NY 12180-4115. Offers adult geriatric advanced nursing (MS); adult gerontology nurse practitioner (MS); adult health (MS); adult nurse practitioner (MS, Post Master's Certificate); clinical nurse leader/specialist (Post Master's Certificate); community health (MS); counseling for nursing (Postbaccalaureate Certificate); education and leadership (DNS); family nurse practitioner (MS, Post Master's Certificate); gerontological nurse practitioner (Post Master's Certificate); nurse administrator/executive (Post Master's Certificate); nurse education (Post Master's Certificate); nursing (Post Master's Certificate); psychiatric mental health nurse clinical nurse specialist (MS); psychiatric mental health nurse practitioner (MS, Post Master's Certificate), including psychiatric mental health. *Accreditation:* AACN. Part-time and evening/weekend programs available. *Faculty:* 5 full-time (all women), 10 part-time/adjunct (all women). *Students:* 32 full-time (30 women), 174 part-time (161 women); includes 28 minority (12 Black or African American, non-Hispanic/Latino; 2 American Indian or Alaska Native, non-Hispanic/Latino; 8 Asian, non-Hispanic/Latino; 4 Hispanic/Latino; 2 Two or more races, non-Hispanic/Latino), 3 international. Average age 40. 171 applicants, 43% accepted, 35 enrolled. In 2013, 53 master's, 5 doctorates, 11 other advanced degrees awarded. *Degree requirements:* For master's, thesis or alternative. *Entrance requirements:* For master's, BS in nursing, minimum GPA of 2.75, resume, 2 letters of recommendation. Additional exam requirements/recommendations for international students: Required—TOEFL (minimum score 550 paper-based). *Application deadline:* Applications are processed on a rolling basis. Application fee: $40. *Expenses: Tuition:* Full-time $11,880; part-time $660 per credit hour. *Financial support:* Fellowships, research assistantships, Federal Work-Study, scholarships/grants, and unspecified assistantships available. Support available to part-time students. Financial award application deadline: 3/1; financial award applicants required to submit FAFSA. *Unit head:* Dr. Esther Haskevitz, Dean, School of Health Sciences, 518-244-2296, Fax: 518-244-4571, E-mail: haskve@sage.edu. *Application contact:* Dr. Glenda Kelman, Director, 518-244-2001, Fax: 518-244-2009, E-mail: kelmag@sage.edu.

Saginaw Valley State University, Crystal M. Lange College of Nursing and Health Sciences, Program in Clinical Nurse Specialist, University Center, MI 48710. Offers MSN. *Accreditation:* AACN. Part-time and evening/weekend programs available. *Degree requirements:* For master's, thesis optional. *Entrance requirements:* Additional exam requirements/recommendations for international students: Required—TOEFL (minimum score 580 paper-based; 92 iBT). *Application deadline:* For fall admission, 7/15 for international students; for winter admission, 11/15 for international students; for spring admission, 4/15 for international students. Applications are processed on a rolling basis. Application fee: $30 ($80 for international students). Electronic applications accepted. *Expenses:* Tuition, state resident: full-time $8933; part-time $496.30 per credit hour. Tuition, nonresident: full-time $16,806; part-time $933.65 per credit hour. *Required fees:* $263; $14.60 per credit hour. Tuition and fees vary according to degree level. *Financial support:* Federal Work-Study and scholarships/grants available. Support available to part-time students. Financial award application deadline: 4/1; financial award applicants required to submit FAFSA. *Unit head:* Dr. Karen Brown-Fackler, Coordinator, 989-964-7112, Fax: 964-4925, E-mail: kmbrown4@svsu.edu. *Application contact:* Jenna Briggs, Director, Graduate and International Admissions, 989-964-6096, Fax: 989-964-2788, E-mail: gradadm@svsu.edu.

Saginaw Valley State University, Crystal M. Lange College of Nursing and Health Sciences, Program in Nursing, University Center, MI 48710. Offers MSN. *Accreditation:* AACN. Part-time and evening/weekend programs available. *Students:* 10 part-time (8 women). Average age 33. 4 applicants, 100% accepted, 4 enrolled. *Entrance requirements:* For master's, GRE, minimum GPA of 3.0. Additional exam requirements/recommendations for international students: Required—TOEFL (minimum score 580 paper-based; 92 iBT). *Application deadline:* For fall admission, 7/15 for international students; for winter admission, 11/15 for international students; for spring admission, 4/15 for international students. Applications are processed on a rolling basis. Application fee: $30 ($80 for international students). Electronic applications accepted. *Expenses:* Tuition, state resident: full-time $8933; part-time $496.30 per credit hour. Tuition, nonresident: full-time $16,806; part-time $933.65 per credit hour. *Required fees:* $263; $14.60 per credit hour. Tuition and fees vary according to degree level. *Financial support:* Federal Work-Study and scholarships/grants available. Support available to part-time students. *Unit head:* Dr. Karen Brown-Fackler, Coordinator, 989-964-7112, Fax: 989-964-4925, E-mail: kmbrown4@svsu.edu. *Application contact:* Jenna Briggs, Director, Graduate and International Admissions, 989-964-6096, Fax: 989-964-2788, E-mail: gradadm@svsu.edu.

St. Ambrose University, College of Education and Health Sciences, Program in Nursing, Davenport, IA 52803-2898. Offers MSN. *Accreditation:* AACN. Part-time and evening/weekend programs available. *Entrance requirements:* Additional exam requirements/recommendations for international students: Required—TOEFL. Electronic applications accepted.

Saint Anthony College of Nursing, Graduate Program, Rockford, IL 61108-2468. Offers MSN. *Accreditation:* AACN. Part-time programs available.

St. Catherine University, Graduate Programs, Program in Nursing, St. Paul, MN 55105. Offers adult gerontological nurse practitioner (MA); neonatal nurse practitioner (MA); nurse educator (MA); nursing (DNP); nursing: entry-level (MA); pediatric nurse practitioner (MA). Part-time and evening/weekend programs available. *Degree requirements:* For master's, thesis; for doctorate, portfolio, systems change project. *Entrance requirements:* For master's, GRE General Test, bachelor's degree in nursing, current nursing license, 2 years of recent clinical practice; for doctorate, master's degree in nursing, RN license, advanced nursing position. Additional exam requirements/recommendations for international students: Required—TOEFL (minimum score 600 paper-based; 100 iBT).

Saint Francis Medical Center College of Nursing, Graduate Programs, Peoria, IL 61603-3783. Offers adult gerontology (MSN); clinical nurse leader (MSN); family nurse practitioner (MSN); family psychiatric mental health nurse practitioner (MSN); neonatal nurse practitioner (MSN); nurse clinician (Post-Graduate Certificate); nurse educator (MSN, Post-Graduate Certificate); nursing (DNP); nursing management leadership (MSN). Part-time programs available. Postbaccalaureate distance learning degree programs offered (minimal on-campus study). *Faculty:* 4 full-time (all women), 4 part-time/adjunct (all women). *Students:* 13 full-time (12 women), 268 part-time (245 women); includes 17 minority (10 Black or African American, non-Hispanic/Latino; 2 Asian, non-Hispanic/Latino; 5 Hispanic/Latino), 2 international. Average age 37. 115 applicants, 89% accepted, 42 enrolled. In 2013, 17 master's, 2 doctorates awarded. *Degree requirements:* For master's, research experience, portfolio, practicum; for doctorate, practicum hours. *Entrance requirements:* For master's, nursing research, health assessment, graduate course work in statistics, RN license; for doctorate, master's degree in nursing, professional portfolio, graduate statistics, transcripts, RN license. Additional exam requirements/recommendations for international students: Required—TOEFL. *Application deadline:* For fall admission, 6/1 priority date for domestic and international students; for spring admission, 11/15 priority date for domestic and international students. Applications are processed on a rolling basis. Application fee: $50. Electronic applications accepted. *Expenses: Tuition:* Full-time $6336; part-time $528 per semester hour. *Required fees:* $436. *Financial support:* In 2013–14, 8 students received support. Scholarships/grants and tuition waivers (partial) available. Support available to part-time students. Financial award application deadline: 6/15; financial award applicants required to submit FAFSA. *Faculty research:* Outcome and curriculum planning, health promotion, NCLEX-RN results, decision-making program evaluation. *Unit head:* Dr. Patti A. Stockert, President of the College, 309-655-4124, Fax: 309-624-8973, E-mail: patricia.a.stockert@osfhealthcare.org. *Application contact:* Dr. Janice F. Boundy, Dean, 309-655-2230, Fax: 309-624-8973, E-mail: jan.f.boundy@osfhealthcare.org.
Website: http://www.sfmccon.edu/graduate-programs/

St. John Fisher College, Wegmans School of Nursing, Advanced Practice Nursing Program, Rochester, NY 14618-3597. Offers advanced practice nursing (MS); clinical nurse specialist (Certificate); family nurse practitioner (Certificate); nurse educator (Certificate). *Accreditation:* AACN. Part-time and evening/weekend programs available. *Faculty:* 13 full-time (12 women). *Students:* 2 full-time (1 woman), 114 part-time (104 women); includes 15 minority (7 Black or African American, non-Hispanic/Latino; 4 Asian, non-Hispanic/Latino; 4 Hispanic/Latino), 2 international. Average age 33. 61 applicants, 49% accepted, 19 enrolled. In 2013, 23 master's awarded. *Degree requirements:* For master's, clinical practice, project; for Certificate, clinical practice. *Entrance requirements:* For master's, BSN; undergraduate course work in statistics, health assessment, and nursing research; current New York State RN license; 2 letters of recommendation; current resume. Additional exam requirements/recommendations for international students: Required—TOEFL (minimum score 575 paper-based; 80 iBT). *Application deadline:* Applications are processed on a rolling basis. Application fee: $30. Electronic applications accepted. *Expenses: Tuition:* Part-time $795 per credit hour. *Required fees:* $10 per credit hour. Tuition and fees vary according to course load, degree level and program. *Financial support:* In 2013–14, 29 students received support. Scholarships/grants and traineeships available. Financial award applicants required to submit FAFSA. *Faculty research:* Chronic illness, pediatric injury, women's health, public health policy, health care teams. *Unit head:* Dr. Cynthia McCloskey, Graduate Director, 585-385-8471, Fax: 585-385-8466, E-mail: cmccloskey@sjfc.edu. *Application contact:* Jose Perales, Director of Graduate Admissions, 585-385-8067, E-mail: jperales@sjfc.edu.

St. John Fisher College, Wegmans School of Nursing, Doctor of Nursing Practice Program, Rochester, NY 14618-3597. Offers DNP. Part-time and evening/weekend programs available. *Faculty:* 6 full-time (5 women), 2 part-time/adjunct (1 woman). *Students:* 15 full-time (14 women), 8 part-time (6 women); includes 4 minority (1 Black or African American, non-Hispanic/Latino; 2 Asian, non-Hispanic/Latino; 1 Two or more races, non-Hispanic/Latino). Average age 44. 9 applicants, 89% accepted, 7 enrolled. In 2013, 8 doctorates awarded. *Degree requirements:* For doctorate, 1,000 hours of clinical practice, clinical scholarship project. *Entrance requirements:* For doctorate, New York State RN License; New York State Certificate as advanced practice nurse or eligibility and National Professional Certification in advanced practice nurse (APN) specialty; currently practicing as APN; 2 letters of recommendation; writing sample. *Application deadline:* For fall admission, 8/1 for domestic students; for spring admission, 12/1 for domestic students. Applications are processed on a rolling basis. Application fee: $0. Electronic applications accepted. *Expenses:* Contact institution. *Financial support:* In 2013–14, 20 students received support. Scholarships/grants available. Financial award applicants required to submit FAFSA. *Unit head:* Dr. Mary S. Collins, Program Director, 585-385-8397, E-mail: mscollins@sjfc.edu. *Application contact:* Jose Perales, Director of Graduate Admissions, 585-385-8067, E-mail: jperales@sjfc.edu.
Website: http://www.sjfc.edu/academics/nursing/departments/dnp/

St. Joseph's College, Long Island Campus, Program in Nursing, Patchogue, NY 11772-2399. Offers MS.

St. Joseph's College, New York, Graduate Programs, Program in Nursing, Brooklyn, NY 11205-3688. Offers MS.

Saint Joseph's College of Maine, Master of Science in Nursing Program, Standish, ME 04084. Offers administration (MSN); education (MSN); family nurse practitioner (MSN); nursing administration and leadership (Certificate); nursing and health care education (Certificate). *Accreditation:* AACN. Part-time programs available. Postbaccalaureate distance learning degree programs offered (no on-campus study). *Entrance requirements:* For master's, MAT. Electronic applications accepted.

Saint Louis University, Graduate Education, Doisy College of Health Sciences, School of Nursing, St. Louis, MO 63104-1099. Offers MSN, DNP, PhD, Certificate. *Accreditation:* AACN. Part-time programs available. Postbaccalaureate distance learning degree programs offered (minimal on-campus study). *Degree requirements:* For master's, comprehensive exam, thesis optional; for doctorate, comprehensive exam, thesis/dissertation, preliminary exams. *Entrance requirements:* For master's, 3 letters of recommendation, resumé, transcripts; for doctorate, GRE General Test, 3 letters of recommendation, curriculum vitae; for Certificate, 3 letters of recommendation, resumé, transcripts, copy of RN license, personal statement. Additional exam requirements/recommendations for international students: Required—TOEFL (minimum score 525 paper-based). Electronic applications accepted. *Faculty research:* Sensory enhancement to the elderly, fall prevention in elderly, tube feeding placement and gastroenterology, patient outcomes, exercise behavior in the older adult.

Saint Peter's University, School of Nursing, Nursing Program, Jersey City, NJ 07306-5997. Offers adult nurse practitioner (MSN, Certificate); advanced practice (DNP); case management (MSN, DNP). *Accreditation:* AACN. Part-time and evening/weekend programs available. *Entrance requirements:* Additional exam requirements/recommendations for international students: Required—TOEFL. Electronic applications accepted.

Saint Xavier University, Graduate Studies, School of Nursing, Chicago, IL 60655-3105. Offers MSN, Certificate, MBA/MS. *Accreditation:* AACN. Part-time and evening/weekend programs available. *Entrance requirements:* For master's, GRE General Test or MAT, minimum GPA of 3.0, RN license.

Salem State University, School of Graduate Studies, Program in Nursing, Salem, MA 01970-5353. Offers adult-gerontology primary care nursing (MSN); nursing administration (MSN); nursing education (MSN); MBA/MSN. *Accreditation:* AACN. Part-time and evening/weekend programs available. *Students:* 31 full-time (24 women), 79 part-time (70 women); includes 12 minority (4 Black or African American, non-Hispanic/Latino; 4 Asian, non-Hispanic/Latino; 3 Hispanic/Latino; 1 Native Hawaiian or other Pacific Islander, non-Hispanic/Latino), 5 international. 18 applicants, 94% accepted, 16 enrolled. In 2013, 15 master's awarded. *Entrance requirements:* For master's, GRE or MAT. Additional exam requirements/recommendations for international students: Required—TOEFL (minimum score 550 paper-based; 80 iBT) or IELTS (minimum score 5.5). *Application deadline:* For fall admission, 5/1 for domestic students; for spring admission, 10/1 for domestic students. Applications are processed on a rolling basis. Application fee: $50. *Financial support:* Career-related internships or fieldwork, Federal Work-Study, scholarships/grants, and unspecified assistantships available. Support available to part-time students. Financial award application deadline: 5/1; financial award applicants required to submit FAFSA. *Application contact:* Dr. Lee A. Brossoit, Assistant Dean of Graduate Admissions, 978-542-6675, Fax: 978-542-7215, E-mail: lbrossoit@salemstate.edu.
Website: http://www.salemstate.edu/academics/schools/1819.php

Salisbury University, DNP Program, Salisbury, MD 21801-6837. Offers DNP. *Accreditation:* AACN. Part-time programs available. Postbaccalaureate distance learning degree programs offered. *Faculty:* 4 full-time (all women). *Students:* 1 (woman) full-time, 8 part-time (7 women); includes 1 minority (Hispanic/Latino). Average age 36. 5 applicants. Terminal master's awarded for partial completion of doctoral program. *Entrance requirements:* For doctorate, GRE, minimum undergraduate GPA of 3.0, RN license, CPR certification, resume, 3 letters of recommendation, essay, interview. Additional exam requirements/recommendations for international students: Required—TOEFL (minimum score 550 paper-based; 79 iBT), IELTS (minimum score 6.5). *Application deadline:* For fall admission, 4/15 priority date for domestic and international students; for spring admission, 10/15 for domestic students. Applications are processed on a rolling basis. Application fee: $50. Electronic applications accepted. *Expenses:* Tuition, state resident: part-time $342 per credit hour. Tuition, nonresident: part-time $631 per credit hour. *Required fees:* $76 per credit hour. Tuition and fees vary according to program. *Financial support:* In 2013–14, 8 students received support. Career-related internships or fieldwork, institutionally sponsored loans, scholarships/grants, and unspecified assistantships available. Support available to part-time students. Financial award application deadline: 3/1; financial award applicants required to submit FAFSA. *Faculty research:* End of life issues, simulation in education. *Unit head:* Dr. Lisa Seldomridge, Chair of Department of Nursing, 410-543-6413, E-mail: laseldomridge@salisbury.edu. *Application contact:* Carmel Boger, Administrative Assistant for Graduate and Second Degree Nursing Program, 410-543-6420, E-mail: ciboger@salisbury.edu.
Website: http://www.salisbury.edu/nursing/dnp/

Salisbury University, Program in Nursing, Salisbury, MD 21801-6837. Offers health care leadership (MS); nurse educator (MS); nursing (MS). Part-time programs available. Postbaccalaureate distance learning degree programs offered. *Faculty:* 5 full-time (4 women). *Students:* 1 (woman) full-time, 18 part-time (all women); includes 6 minority (all Black or African American, non-Hispanic/Latino). Average age 36. 18 applicants, 28% accepted, 3 enrolled. In 2013, 17 master's awarded. *Entrance requirements:* For master's, GRE, minimum undergraduate GPA of 3.0, 2 letters of recommendation, resume, personal statement, current and active RN license, interview, CPR certification, personal statement. Additional exam requirements/recommendations for international students: Required—TOEFL (minimum score 550 paper-based; 79 iBT), IELTS (minimum score 6.5). *Application deadline:* For fall admission, 4/15 priority date for domestic and international students. Applications are processed on a rolling basis. Application fee: $50. Electronic applications accepted. *Expenses:* Tuition, state resident: part-time $342 per credit hour. Tuition, nonresident: part-time $631 per credit hour. *Required fees:* $76 per credit hour. Tuition and fees vary according to program. *Financial support:* In 2013–14, 7 students received support. Institutionally sponsored loans, scholarships/grants, and unspecified assistantships available. Support available to part-time students. Financial award application deadline: 3/1; financial award applicants required to submit FAFSA. *Faculty research:* Geriatrics, dementia, adolescent health, domestic violence. *Unit head:* Dr. Lisa Seldomridge, Chair of Department of Nursing, 410-543-6413, E-mail: laseldomridge@salisbury.edu. *Application contact:* Carmel Boger, Administrative Assistant for Graduate and Second Degree Nursing Program, 410-543-6420, E-mail: ciboger@salisbury.edu.
Website: http://www.salisbury.edu/Nursing/MS.html

Samford University, Ida V. Moffett School of Nursing, Birmingham, AL 35229. Offers administration (DNP); advanced practice (DNP); family nurse practitioner (MSN); health systems management and leadership (MSN); nurse anesthesia (MSN); nurse educator (MSN). *Accreditation:* AACN; AANA/CANAEP (one or more programs are accredited). Part-time programs available. Postbaccalaureate distance learning degree programs offered (minimal on-campus study). *Faculty:* 16 full-time (all women), 4 part-time/adjunct (2 women). *Students:* 249 full-time (191 women), 25 part-time (17 women); includes 48 minority (23 Black or African American, non-Hispanic/Latino; 1 American Indian or Alaska Native, non-Hispanic/Latino; 13 Asian, non-Hispanic/Latino; 7 Hispanic/Latino; 4 Two or more races, non-Hispanic/Latino), 1 international. Average age 36. 89 applicants, 53% accepted, 45 enrolled. In 2013, 107 master's, 29 doctorates awarded. *Degree requirements:* For master's and doctorate, capstone project with oral presentation. *Entrance requirements:* For master's, MAT; GRE (for nurse anesthesia). Additional exam requirements/recommendations for international students: Required—TOEFL (minimum score 550 paper-based; 80 iBT). *Application deadline:* For fall admission, 6/1 priority date for domestic and international students; for spring admission, 9/1 priority date for domestic and international students. Application fee: $65. Electronic applications accepted. *Expenses:* Contact institution. *Financial support:* In 2013–14, 48 students received support. Institutionally sponsored loans, scholarships/grants, and traineeships available. Financial award application deadline: 3/1; financial award applicants required to submit FAFSA. *Faculty research:* Issues in rural health care, vulnerable populations, genetics and disabilities in pediatrics, geriatrics, parish nursing research, interprofessional education, global health disparities. *Unit head:* Dr. Nena F. Sanders, Dean, 205-726-2629, E-mail: nfsander@samford.edu. *Application contact:* Allyson Maddox, Director of Graduate Student Services, 205-726-2047, Fax: 205-726-4179, E-mail: amaddox@samford.edu.
Website: http://samford.edu/nursing

Nursing—General

Samuel Merritt University, School of Nursing, Oakland, CA 94609-3108. Offers case management (MSN); family nurse practitioner (MSN, Certificate); nurse anesthetist (MSN, Certificate); nursing (MSN, DNP). *Accreditation:* AACN; AANA/CANAEP (one or more programs are accredited). Part-time and evening/weekend programs available. *Degree requirements:* For master's, thesis or alternative. *Entrance requirements:* For master's, minimum GPA of 2.5 in science, 3.0 overall; previous course work in statistics; current RN license. Additional exam requirements/recommendations for international students: Required—TOEFL. *Faculty research:* Gerontology, community health, maternal-child health, sexually transmitted diseases, substance abuse, oncology.

San Diego State University, Graduate and Research Affairs, College of Health and Human Services, School of Nursing, San Diego, CA 92182. Offers MS. *Accreditation:* AACN; ACNM/ACME. Part-time and evening/weekend programs available. *Entrance requirements:* For master's, GRE General Test, previous course work in statistics and physical assessment, 3 letters of recommendation, California RN license. Additional exam requirements/recommendations for international students: Required—TOEFL. Electronic applications accepted. *Faculty research:* Health promotion, nursing systems and leadership, maternal-child nursing, advanced practice nursing, child oral health.

San Francisco State University, Division of Graduate Studies, College of Health and Social Sciences, School of Nursing, San Francisco, CA 94132-1722. Offers adult acute care (MS); clinical nurse specialist (MS); community/public health nursing (MS); family nurse practitioner (MS, Certificate); nursing administration (MS); nursing education (MS); pediatrics (MS); women's health (MS). *Accreditation:* AACN. Part-time programs available. *Application deadline:* Applications are processed on a rolling basis. *Financial support:* Career-related internships or fieldwork available. *Unit head:* Dr. Mary-Ann van Dam, Director, 415-338-1802, E-mail: vandam@sfsu.edu. *Application contact:* Robert Strachan, Admission and Student Services Coordinator, 415-338-1802, E-mail: strachan@sfsu.edu.
Website: http://nursing.sfsu.edu

San Jose State University, Graduate Studies and Research, College of Applied Sciences and Arts, School of Nursing, San Jose, CA 95192-0001. Offers gerontology nurse practitioner (MS); nursing (Certificate); nursing administration (MS); nursing education (MS). *Accreditation:* AACN. Part-time and evening/weekend programs available. *Degree requirements:* For master's, thesis. *Entrance requirements:* For master's, BS in nursing, RN license. Electronic applications accepted. *Faculty research:* Nurse-managed clinics, computers in nursing.

Seattle Pacific University, MS in Nursing Program, Seattle, WA 98119-1997. Offers administration (MSN); adult/gerontology nurse practitioner (MSN); clinical nurse specialist (MSN); family nurse practitioner (MSN, Certificate); informatics (MSN); nurse educator (MSN). *Accreditation:* AACN. Part-time programs available. *Students:* 9 full-time (7 women), 37 part-time (33 women); includes 8 minority (2 Black or African American, non-Hispanic/Latino; 5 Asian, non-Hispanic/Latino; 1 Hispanic/Latino), 1 international. Average age 41. 70 applicants, 30% accepted, 21 enrolled. In 2013, 27 master's awarded. *Degree requirements:* For master's, thesis. *Entrance requirements:* For master's, personal statement, transcripts, undergraduate nursing degree, proof of undergraduate statistics course with minimum GPA of 2.0, 2 recommendations. *Application deadline:* For fall admission, 1/15 priority date for domestic students; for spring admission, 1/15 for domestic students. Applications are processed on a rolling basis. Application fee: $50. Electronic applications accepted. *Expenses:* Contact institution. *Financial support:* Fellowships and scholarships/grants available. Financial award applicants required to submit FAFSA. *Unit head:* Dr. Susan Casey, Associate Dean, 206-281-2649, E-mail: caseys@spu.edu.
Website: http://www.spu.edu/depts/health-sciences/grad/index.asp

Seattle University, College of Nursing, Doctor of Nursing Practice Program, Seattle, WA 98122-1090. Offers DNP. Evening/weekend programs available. *Students:* 6 full-time (all women), 7 part-time (6 women); includes 7 minority (1 Black or African American, non-Hispanic/Latino; 4 Asian, non-Hispanic/Latino; 1 Hispanic/Latino; 1 Two or more races, non-Hispanic/Latino). Average age 42. 15 applicants, 67% accepted, 8 enrolled. *Degree requirements:* For doctorate, capstone project. *Entrance requirements:* For doctorate, letter of intent. *Application deadline:* For fall admission, 11/1 priority date for domestic students. *Unit head:* Patricia Hayles, Coordinator, 206-296-6986, E-mail: haylesp@seattleu.edu. *Application contact:* Janet Shandley, Director of Graduate Admissions, 206-296-5900, Fax: 206-298-5656, E-mail: grad_admissions@seattleu.edu.
Website: https://www.seattleu.edu/nursing/dnp/

Seattle University, College of Nursing, Program in Advanced Practice Nursing Immersion, Seattle, WA 98122-1090. Offers adult/gerontological nurse practitioner (MSN); advanced community public health nursing (MSN); family nurse practitioner (MSN); family psychiatric mental health nurse practitioner (MSN); nurse midwifery (MSN). *Faculty:* 17 full-time (15 women), 9 part-time/adjunct (6 women). *Students:* 109 full-time (94 women), 6 part-time (5 women); includes 25 minority (3 Black or African American, non-Hispanic/Latino; 11 Asian, non-Hispanic/Latino; 2 Hispanic/Latino; 9 Two or more races, non-Hispanic/Latino). Average age 31. In 2013, 48 master's awarded. *Degree requirements:* For master's, thesis or scholarly project. *Entrance requirements:* For master's, GRE, bachelor's degree, minimum GPA of 3.0, professional resume, two recommendations, letter of intent. Additional exam requirements/recommendations for international students: Required—TOEFL (minimum score 92 iBT), IELTS. *Application deadline:* For fall admission, 12/1 for domestic and international students. Application fee: $55. Electronic applications accepted. *Financial support:* In 2013–14, 3 students received support. Scholarships/grants and traineeships available. Financial award applicants required to submit FAFSA. *Unit head:* Dr. Janiece DeSocio, Interim Dean, 206-296-5660, E-mail: desocioj@seattleu.edu. *Application contact:* Janet Shandley, Associate Dean of Graduate Admissions, 206-296-5900, Fax: 206-298-5656, E-mail: grad_admissions@seattleu.edu.
Website: http://www.seattleu.edu/nursing/msn/apni/

Seattle University, College of Nursing, Program in Nursing, Seattle, WA 98122-1090. Offers adult/gerontological nurse practitioner (MSN); advanced community public health (MSN); psychiatric mental health nurse practitioner (MSN). *Students:* 11 full-time (10 women), 4 part-time (all women); includes 2 minority (both Hispanic/Latino). Average age 36. 39 applicants, 36% accepted, 8 enrolled. In 2013, 7 master's awarded. *Degree requirements:* For master's, thesis or scholarly project. *Entrance requirements:* For master's, GRE, bachelor's degree in nursing or associate degree in nursing with baccalaureate in different major, 5-quarter statistics course, minimum cumulative GPA of 3.0, professional resume, two recommendations, letter of intent, copy of current RN license or ability to obtain RN license in WA state. Additional exam requirements/recommendations for international students: Required—TOEFL (minimum score 92 iBT), IELTS. *Application deadline:* For fall admission, 12/1 for domestic and international students. Application fee: $55. Electronic applications accepted. *Financial support:* In 2013–14, 1 student received support, including 2 teaching assistantships; scholarships/grants and traineeships also available. Financial award applicants required to submit FAFSA. *Unit head:* Dr. Azita Emami, Dean, 206-296-5660. *Application contact:* Janet Shandley, Associate Dean of Graduate Admissions, 206-296-5900, Fax: 206-298-5656, E-mail: grad_admissions@seattleu.edu.
Website: https://www.seattleu.edu/nursing/msn/

Seton Hall University, College of Nursing, South Orange, NJ 07079-2697. Offers advanced practice in primary health care (MSN, DNP), including adult/gerontological nurse practitioner, pediatric nurse practitioner; entry into practice (MSN); health systems administration (MSN, DNP); nursing (PhD); nursing case management (MSN); nursing education (MA); school nurse (MSN); MSN/MA. *Accreditation:* AACN. Part-time programs available. Postbaccalaureate distance learning degree programs offered (minimal on-campus study). *Degree requirements:* For master's, research project; for doctorate, dissertation or scholarly project. *Entrance requirements:* For doctorate, GRE (waived for students with GPA of 3.5 or higher). Additional exam requirements/recommendations for international students: Required—TOEFL. Electronic applications accepted. *Faculty research:* Parent/child, adult, and gerontological nursing; breast cancer; families of children with HIV; parish nursing.

Shenandoah University, Eleanor Wade Custer School of Nursing, Winchester, VA 22601-5195. Offers family nurse practitioner (Certificate); health informatics (Certificate); nursing (MSN, DNP); nursing education (Certificate); psychiatric mental health nurse practitioner (Certificate). *Accreditation:* AACN; ACNM/ACME. Part-time programs available. *Faculty:* 14 full-time (all women), 7 part-time/adjunct (6 women). *Students:* 39 full-time (35 women), 76 part-time (74 women); includes 23 minority (13 Black or African American, non-Hispanic/Latino; 2 American Indian or Alaska Native, non-Hispanic/Latino; 4 Asian, non-Hispanic/Latino; 4 Hispanic/Latino), 1 international. Average age 38. 56 applicants, 77% accepted, 32 enrolled. In 2013, 28 master's, 4 doctorates, 11 other advanced degrees awarded. *Degree requirements:* For master's, research project, clinical hours; for doctorate, scholarly project, clinical hours; for Certificate, clinical hours. *Entrance requirements:* For master's, United States RN license; minimum GPA of 3.0; appropriate clinical experience; curriculum vitae; 3 letters of recommendation; for doctorate, MSN, minimum GPA of 3.0, 3 letters of recommendation, essay, interview, BSN; for Certificate, MSN, minimum GPA of 3.0, 2 letters of recommendation, minimum of one year (2,080 hours) clinical nursing experience, interview. Additional exam requirements/recommendations for international students: Required—TOEFL (minimum score 610 paper-based; 83 iBT), IELTS (minimum score 7.5). *Application deadline:* For fall admission, 5/1 priority date for domestic and international students; for spring admission, 11/1 priority date for domestic and international students. Applications are processed on a rolling basis. Application fee: $30. Electronic applications accepted. *Expenses: Tuition:* Full-time $19,176; part-time $799 per credit. *Required fees:* $365 per term. Tuition and fees vary according to course level, course load and program. *Financial support:* In 2013–14, 13 students received support, including 3 teaching assistantships with partial tuition reimbursements available (averaging $4,912 per year); career-related internships or fieldwork, scholarships/grants, and unspecified assistantships also available. Support available to part-time students. Financial award application deadline: 3/15; financial award applicants required to submit FAFSA. *Faculty research:* Moral reasoning in nurses, improving health care access to underserved rural women, screening for depression and anxiety in the obese in a rural free clinic, health care outcomes among patients in a free clinic setting cared for by nurse practitioners, effects of depression on diabetes as evidenced by the relationship between the patient healthcare questionnaire (PHQ-9) scores and the patient's glycohemoglobin (HbA1c), policy development, research on a Virginia Nurses Hall of Fame inductee. *Unit head:* Dr. Kathryn Ganske, Director, 540-678-4374, Fax: 540-665-5519, E-mail: kganske@su.edu. *Application contact:* Andrew Woodall, Executive Director of Recruitment and Admissions, 540-665-4581, Fax: 540-665-4627, E-mail: admit@su.edu.
Website: http://www.nursing.su.edu

Simmons College, School of Nursing and Health Sciences, Boston, MA 02115. Offers didactic dietetics (Certificate); dietetic internship (Certificate); health professions education (CAGS); nursing (MS); nursing practice (DNP); nutrition and health promotion (MS); physical therapy (DPT); sports nutrition (Certificate). Part-time programs available. Postbaccalaureate distance learning degree programs offered (minimal on-campus study). *Students:* 143 full-time (129 women), 347 part-time (329 women); includes 72 minority (31 Black or African American, non-Hispanic/Latino; 17 Asian, non-Hispanic/Latino; 15 Hispanic/Latino; 9 Two or more races, non-Hispanic/Latino), 4 international. 196 applicants, 56% accepted, 88 enrolled. In 2013, 70 master's, 45 doctorates awarded. *Entrance requirements:* For doctorate, GRE. Additional exam requirements/recommendations for international students: Required—TOEFL (minimum score 570 paper-based; 88 iBT). *Application deadline:* For fall admission, 6/1 for international students. Application fee: $50. Electronic applications accepted. *Financial support:* In 2013–14, 33 students received support, including 24 teaching assistantships (averaging $6,000 per year); scholarships/grants and unspecified assistantships also available. *Unit head:* Dr. Judy Beal, Dean, 617-521-2139. *Application contact:* Carmen Fortin, Assistant Dean/Director of Admission, 617-521-2651, Fax: 617-521-3137, E-mail: gshsadm@simmons.edu.
Website: http://www.simmons.edu/snhs/

Sonoma State University, School of Science and Technology, Master's in Nursing Program, Rohnert Park, CA 94928. Offers family nurse practitioner (MSN). Part-time programs available. *Faculty:* 3 full-time (all women), 3 part-time/adjunct (all women). *Students:* 20 full-time (15 women), 111 part-time (91 women); includes 44 minority (6 Black or African American, non-Hispanic/Latino; 3 American Indian or Alaska Native, non-Hispanic/Latino; 22 Asian, non-Hispanic/Latino; 8 Hispanic/Latino; 5 Two or more races, non-Hispanic/Latino), 2 international. Average age 36. 91 applicants, 77% accepted, 21 enrolled. In 2013, 51 master's awarded. *Degree requirements:* For master's, comprehensive exam, thesis or alternative, oral exams. *Entrance requirements:* For master's, GRE General Test, BSN, minimum GPA of 3.0, course work in statistics, physical assessment, RN license. Additional exam requirements/recommendations for international students: Required—TOEFL (minimum score 500 paper-based). *Application deadline:* For fall admission, 11/30 for domestic students. Application fee: $55. *Expenses:* Tuition, state resident: full-time $8500. Tuition, nonresident: full-time $12,964. *Required fees:* $1762. *Financial support:* Traineeships available. Financial award applicants required to submit FAFSA. *Faculty research:* Neonatal ethics. *Unit head:* Dr. Deborah A. Roberts, Chair, 707-664-2465, E-mail: deborah.roberts@sonoma.edu. *Application contact:* Dr. Wendy Smith, Director, 707-664-2276, E-mail: wendy.smith@sonoma.edu.
Website: http://www.sonoma.edu/nursing/

South Dakota State University, Graduate School, College of Nursing, Brookings, SD 57007. Offers MS, PhD. *Accreditation:* AACN. Part-time and evening/weekend programs available. Postbaccalaureate distance learning degree programs offered. *Degree requirements:* For master's, comprehensive exam, thesis (for some programs), oral exam. *Entrance requirements:* For master's, nurse registration; for doctorate, nurse registration, MS. Additional exam requirements/recommendations for international students: Required—TOEFL (minimum score 525 paper-based; 71 iBT). *Expenses:* Contact institution. *Faculty research:* Rural health, aging, health promotion, Native American health, woman's health, underserved populations, quality of life.

Southeastern Louisiana University, College of Nursing and Health Sciences, School of Nursing, Hammond, LA 70402. Offers adult psychiatric/mental health nurse practitioner/clinical nurse specialist (MSN); education (MSN); nurse executive (MSN); nurse practice (DNP); nurse practitioner (MSN). *Accreditation:* AACN. Part-time and

evening/weekend programs available. *Faculty:* 14 full-time (13 women), 5 part-time/adjunct (4 women). *Students:* 21 full-time (19 women), 138 part-time (121 women); includes 27 minority (17 Black or African American, non-Hispanic/Latino; 4 Asian, non-Hispanic/Latino; 5 Hispanic/Latino; 1 Two or more races, non-Hispanic/Latino). Average age 34. 72 applicants, 68% accepted, 19 enrolled. In 2013, 29 master's awarded. *Degree requirements:* For master's, thesis. *Entrance requirements:* For master's, GRE (verbal and quantitative), baccalaureate degree in nursing from accredited undergraduate nursing program; minimum GPA of 2.7; all transcripts from undergraduate school and any work attempted at the graduate level; curriculum vitae; valid Louisiana Registered Nurse license; letters of recommendation; letter of intent/statement of purpose. Additional exam requirements/recommendations for international students: Required—TOEFL (minimum score 500 paper-based; 61 iBT). *Application deadline:* For fall admission, 7/15 priority date for domestic students, 6/1 priority date for international students; for spring admission, 12/1 priority date for domestic students, 10/1 priority date for international students. Applications are processed on a rolling basis. Application fee: $20 ($30 for international students). Electronic applications accepted. *Expenses:* Tuition, state resident: full-time $5047. Tuition, nonresident: full-time $17,066. *Required fees:* $1213. Tuition and fees vary according to degree level. *Financial support:* Federal Work-Study, institutionally sponsored loans, scholarships/grants, traineeships, and unspecified assistantships available. Support available to part-time students. Financial award application deadline: 5/1; financial award applicants required to submit FAFSA. *Faculty research:* Gender issues, LGBT issues, occupational health/safety, accelerated students, caring development. *Total annual research expenditures:* $103,409. *Unit head:* Dr. Lorinda J. Sealey, Graduate Nursing Program Director, 985-549-5045, Fax: 985-549-5087, E-mail: vjohnson@selu.edu. *Application contact:* Sandra Meyers, Graduate Admissions Analyst, 985-549-5620, Fax: 985-549-5632, E-mail: admissions@selu.edu.
Website: http://www.selu.edu/acad_research/depts/nurs

Southeast Missouri State University, School of Graduate Studies, Department of Nursing, Cape Girardeau, MO 63701-4799. Offers MSN. *Accreditation:* AACN. *Faculty:* 6 full-time (all women). *Students:* 21 part-time (20 women). Average age 35. 32 applicants, 38% accepted, 12 enrolled. In 2013, 16 master's awarded. *Degree requirements:* For master's, comprehensive exam. *Entrance requirements:* For master's, minimum GPA of 3.25; current Missouri license as a Registered Professional Nurse; CPR certification; BSN; professional liability insurance; course in health assessment or demonstrated proficiency with minimum B grade; minimum B grade in statistics; statement of academic goals and objectives; current CPR certification. Additional exam requirements/recommendations for international students: Required—TOEFL (minimum score 550 paper-based; 79 iBT), IELTS (minimum score 6), PTE (minimum score 53). *Application deadline:* For fall admission, 4/1 for domestic and international students; for spring admission, 11/21 for domestic students, 10/1 for international students. Applications are processed on a rolling basis. Application fee: $30 ($40 for international students). Electronic applications accepted. *Expenses:* Tuition, state resident: full-time $5139; part-time $285.50 per credit hour. Tuition, nonresident: full-time $9099; part-time $505.50 per credit hour. *Financial support:* In 2013–14, 21 students received support, including 2 teaching assistantships with full tuition reimbursements available (averaging $8,144 per year); career-related internships or fieldwork, Federal Work-Study, scholarships/grants, traineeships, tuition waivers (full), and unspecified assistantships also available. Financial award application deadline: 6/30; financial award applicants required to submit FAFSA. *Faculty research:* Rural health, domestic abuse, substance abuse, use of simulation for nursing education. *Unit head:* Dr. Elaine Jackson, Director of Graduate Studies, 573-651-2871, Fax: 573-651-2141, E-mail: ejackson@semo.edu.
Website: http://www2.semo.edu/nursing/

Southern Adventist University, School of Nursing, Collegedale, TN 37315-0370. Offers acute care nurse practitioner (MSN); adult nurse practitioner (MSN); family nurse practitioner (MSN); nurse educator (MSN); MSN/MSBA. Part-time programs available. *Degree requirements:* For master's, thesis or project. *Entrance requirements:* For master's, RN license. Additional exam requirements/recommendations for international students: Required—TOEFL (minimum score 600 paper-based). Electronic applications accepted. *Faculty research:* Pain management, ethics, corporate wellness, caring spirituality, stress.

Southern Connecticut State University, School of Graduate Studies, School of Health and Human Services, Department of Nursing, New Haven, CT 06515-1355. Offers nursing administration (MSN); nursing education (MSN). *Accreditation:* AACN. Part-time and evening/weekend programs available. *Degree requirements:* For master's, thesis. *Entrance requirements:* For master's, GRE, MAT, interview, minimum QPA of 2.8, RN license, minimum 1 year of professional nursing experience. Electronic applications accepted.

Southern Illinois University Edwardsville, Graduate School, School of Nursing, Edwardsville, IL 62026. Offers MS, DNP, Post-Master's Certificate. *Accreditation:* AACN. Part-time programs available. *Faculty:* 26 full-time (24 women). *Students:* 72 full-time (48 women), 196 part-time (186 women); includes 26 minority (11 Black or African American, non-Hispanic/Latino; 11 Asian, non-Hispanic/Latino; 2 Hispanic/Latino; 2 Two or more races, non-Hispanic/Latino). 101 applicants, 71% accepted. In 2013, 64 master's, 12 doctorates awarded. *Degree requirements:* For master's, comprehensive exam (for some programs), thesis or alternative. *Entrance requirements:* For master's, appropriate bachelor's degree, RN license; for Post-Master's Certificate, minimum graduate nursing GPA of 3.0, completion of graduate-level statistics and epidemiology courses with minimum B grade, current unencumbered RN licensure. Additional exam requirements/recommendations for international students: Required—TOEFL (minimum score 550 paper-based, 79 iBT), IELTS (minimum score 6.5), Michigan Test of English Language Proficiency or PTE. *Application deadline:* For fall admission, 3/1 for domestic and international students; for summer admission, 6/1 for domestic and international students. Application fee: $30. Electronic applications accepted. *Expenses:* Tuition, state resident: full-time $3551. Tuition, nonresident: full-time $8378. *Financial support:* In 2013–14, 2 fellowships with full tuition reimbursements (averaging $8,370 per year), 1 research assistantship with full tuition reimbursement (averaging $9,585 per year), 4 teaching assistantships with full tuition reimbursements (averaging $9,585 per year) were awarded; institutionally sponsored loans, scholarships/grants, and unspecified assistantships also available. Financial award application deadline: 3/1; financial award applicants required to submit FAFSA. *Unit head:* Dr. Anne Perry, Interim Dean, 618-650-3956, Fax: 618-650-3854, E-mail: mamaure@siue.edu. *Application contact:* Dr. Kathy Ketchum, Program Director, 618-650-3936, Fax: 618-650-3854, E-mail: kketchu@siue.edu.
Website: http://www.siue.edu/nursing/graduate

Southern Nazarene University, College of Professional and Graduate Studies, School of Nursing, Bethany, OK 73008. Offers nursing education (MS); nursing leadership (MS). *Accreditation:* AACN. Part-time and evening/weekend programs available. *Degree requirements:* For master's, thesis. *Entrance requirements:* For master's, minimum undergraduate cumulative GPA of 3.0; baccalaureate degree in nursing from nationally-accredited program; current unencumbered registered nurse licensure in Oklahoma or eligibility for same; documentation of basic computer skills; basic statistics course; statement of professional goals; three letters of recommendation. Additional exam requirements/recommendations for international students: Required—TOEFL (minimum score 550 paper-based). *Unit head:* Dr. Katie Sigler, Chair, 405-717-6217, E-mail: ksigler@snu.edu.
Website: http://snu.edu/school-of-nursing

Southern University and Agricultural and Mechanical College, School of Nursing, Baton Rouge, LA 70813. Offers educator/administrator (PhD); family health nursing (MSN); family nurse practitioner (Post Master's Certificate); geriatric nurse practitioner/gerontology (PhD). *Accreditation:* AACN. Part-time programs available. *Degree requirements:* For master's, comprehensive exam, thesis; for doctorate, comprehensive exam, thesis/dissertation. *Entrance requirements:* For master's, GRE General Test, BSN, minimum GPA of 2.7; for doctorate, GRE General Test; for Post Master's Certificate, MSN. Additional exam requirements/recommendations for international students: Required—TOEFL (minimum score 525 paper-based). *Faculty research:* Health promotions, vulnerable populations, (community-based) cardiovascular participating research, health disparities chronic diseases, care of the elderly.

South University, Graduate Programs, College of Nursing, Savannah, GA 31406. Offers nurse educator (MS).

South University, Program in Nursing, Tampa, FL 33614. Offers adult health nurse practitioner (MS); family nurse practitioner (MS); nurse educator (MS).

South University, Program in Nursing, Royal Palm Beach, FL 33411. Offers family nurse practitioner (MS).

South University, Program in Nursing, Montgomery, AL 36116-1120. Offers MSN.

South University, Program in Nursing, Columbia, SC 29203. Offers MSN.

South University, Program in Nursing, Novi, MI 48377. Offers MSN.

South University, Program in Nursing, Glen Allen, VA 23060. Offers MSN.

Spalding University, Graduate Studies, Kosair College of Health and Natural Sciences, School of Nursing, Louisville, KY 40203-2188. Offers adult nurse practitioner (MSN, PMC); family nurse practitioner (MSN, PMC); leadership in nursing and healthcare (MSN, PMC); pediatric nurse practitioner (MSN, PMC). *Accreditation:* AACN. Part-time and evening/weekend programs available. *Faculty:* 6 full-time (all women), 6 part-time/adjunct (5 women). *Students:* 98 full-time (85 women), 13 part-time (all women); includes 23 minority (19 Black or African American, non-Hispanic/Latino; 2 Asian, non-Hispanic/Latino; 1 Hispanic/Latino; 1 Two or more races, non-Hispanic/Latino). Average age 36. 136 applicants, 31% accepted, 39 enrolled. In 2013, 48 master's, 5 other advanced degrees awarded. *Degree requirements:* For master's, comprehensive exam (for some programs), thesis. *Entrance requirements:* For master's, GRE General Test, BSN or bachelor's degree, RN licensure, autobiographical statement, transcripts, letters of recommendation. Additional exam requirements/recommendations for international students: Required—TOEFL (minimum score 535 paper-based). *Application deadline:* For fall admission, 2/1 priority date for domestic students. Application fee: $30. *Expenses: Tuition:* Full-time $21,450. *Required fees:* $810. Tuition and fees vary according to course load, degree level, program and student level. *Financial support:* Career-related internships or fieldwork, scholarships/grants, and traineeships available. Support available to part-time students. Financial award application deadline: 3/30; financial award applicants required to submit FAFSA. *Faculty research:* Nurse educational administration, gerontology, bioterrorism, healthcare ethics, leadership. *Unit head:* Dr. Paula Travis, Chair, 502-873-4298, E-mail: clewis@spalding.edu. *Application contact:* Dr. Pam King, Assistant Professor, 502-873-4292, E-mail: pking@spalding.edu.
Website: http://www.spalding.edu/nursing/

Spring Arbor University, School of Human Services, Spring Arbor, MI 49283-9799. Offers counseling (MAC); family studies (MAFS); nursing (MSN). Part-time and evening/weekend programs available. Postbaccalaureate distance learning degree programs offered (no on-campus study). *Faculty:* 12 full-time (5 women), 113 part-time/adjunct (67 women). *Students:* 225 full-time (185 women), 269 part-time (222 women); includes 166 minority (142 Black or African American, non-Hispanic/Latino; 4 American Indian or Alaska Native, non-Hispanic/Latino; 5 Asian, non-Hispanic/Latino; 13 Hispanic/Latino; 2 Two or more races, non-Hispanic/Latino), 1 international. Average age 40. In 2013, 276 master's awarded. *Entrance requirements:* For master's, bachelor's degree from regionally-accredited college or university, minimum GPA of 3.0 for at least the last two years of the bachelor's degree, at least two recommendations from professional/academic individuals. Additional exam requirements/recommendations for international students: Required—TOEFL (minimum score 600 paper-based). *Application deadline:* Applications are processed on a rolling basis. Application fee: $40. Electronic applications accepted. *Financial support:* Scholarships/grants available. Support available to part-time students. Financial award applicants required to submit FAFSA. *Unit head:* Natalie Gianetti, Dean, 517-750-1200 Ext. 1343, Fax: 517-750-6602, E-mail: gianetti@arbor.edu. *Application contact:* Greg Bentle, Coordinator of Graduate Recruitment, 517-750-6763, Fax: 517-750-6624, E-mail: gbentle@arbor.edu.
Website: http://www.arbor.edu/academics/schools/school-of-human-services/

Spring Hill College, Graduate Programs, Program in Nursing, Mobile, AL 36608-1791. Offers clinical nurse leader (MSN, Post-Master's Certificate). *Accreditation:* AACN. Part-time and evening/weekend programs available. Postbaccalaureate distance learning degree programs offered (no on-campus study). *Faculty:* 2 full-time (both women). *Students:* 20 part-time (17 women); includes 13 minority (10 Black or African American, non-Hispanic/Latino; 3 Asian, non-Hispanic/Latino). Average age 43. In 2013, 9 master's, 2 other advanced degrees awarded. *Degree requirements:* For master's, comprehensive exam, capstone courses, completion of program within 6 calendar years; for Post-Master's Certificate, 460 clinical integration hours. *Entrance requirements:* For master's, RN license in state where practicing nursing; 1 year of clinical nursing experience; work in clinical setting or access to health care facility for clinical integration/research; 3 written references; employer verification; resume; 500-word essay explaining how becoming a CNL will help applicant achieve personal and professional goals; for Post-Master's Certificate, RN license; master's degree in nursing. Additional exam requirements/recommendations for international students: Required—TOEFL (minimum score 550 paper-based; 80 iBT), IELTS (minimum score 6.5), CPE or CAE (minimum score C), Michigan English Language Assessment Battery (minimum score 90). *Application deadline:* For fall admission, 8/1 priority date for domestic and international students; for spring admission, 12/1 priority date for domestic and international students. Applications are processed on a rolling basis. Application fee: $25 ($35 for international students). Electronic applications accepted. *Expenses:* Contact institution. *Financial support:* Applicants required to submit FAFSA. *Unit head:* Dr. Ola H. Fox, Director, 251-380-4486, Fax: 251-460-4495, E-mail: ofox@shc.edu. *Application contact:* Donna B. Tarasavage, Associate Director, Academic Affairs, 251-380-3067, Fax: 251-460-2182, E-mail: dtarasavage@shc.edu.
Website: http://www.shc.edu/page/master-science-nursing

State University of New York Downstate Medical Center, College of Nursing, Graduate Program in Nursing, Brooklyn, NY 11203-2098. Offers clinical nurse specialist (MS, Post Master's Certificate); nurse anesthesia (MS); nurse midwifery (MS, Post Master's Certificate); nurse practitioner (MS, Post Master's Certificate); nursing (MS). *Accreditation:* AACN. Part-time programs available. *Degree requirements:* For master's, thesis optional, clinical research project. *Entrance requirements:* For master's, GRE, BSN; minimum GPA of 3.0; previous undergraduate course work in statistics, health assessment, and nursing research; RN license; for Post Master's Certificate, BSN; minimum GPA of 3.0; RN license; previous undergraduate course work in statistics, health assessment, and nursing research. *Faculty research:* AIDS, continuity of care, case management, self-care.

State University of New York Upstate Medical University, College of Nursing, Syracuse, NY 13210-2334. Offers nurse practitioner (Post Master's Certificate); nursing (MS). *Accreditation:* AACN. Part-time programs available. Postbaccalaureate distance learning degree programs offered (no on-campus study). *Degree requirements:* For master's, thesis or alternative. *Entrance requirements:* For master's, 3 years of work experience. Electronic applications accepted.

Stevenson University, Program in Nursing, Owings Mills, MD 21117. Offers MS. *Faculty:* 3 full-time (all women), 10 part-time/adjunct (9 women). *Students:* 1 (woman) full-time, 138 part-time (135 women); includes 62 minority (48 Black or African American, non-Hispanic/Latino; 14 Asian, non-Hispanic/Latino). 56 applicants, 89% accepted, 42 enrolled. In 2013, 9 master's awarded. *Degree requirements:* For master's, capstone course. *Entrance requirements:* Additional exam requirements/recommendations for international students: Required—TOEFL (minimum score 550 paper-based), IELTS (minimum score 6.5). *Application deadline:* Applications are processed on a rolling basis. Application fee: $0. Electronic applications accepted. *Unit head:* Judith Feustle, PhD, Associate Dean, 443-352-4292, Fax: 443-394-0538, E-mail: jfeustle@stevenson.edu. *Application contact:* Amanda Courter, Enrollment Counselor, 443-352-4243, Fax: 443-394-0538, E-mail: acourter@stevenson.edu.
Website: http://gps.stevenson.edu/graduate-studies/graduate-nursing/

Stony Brook University, State University of New York, Stony Brook University Medical Center, Health Sciences Center, School of Nursing, Stony Brook, NY 11794. Offers MS, DNP, Certificate. *Accreditation:* AACN; ACNM/ACME. Postbaccalaureate distance learning degree programs offered. *Faculty:* 35 full-time (32 women), 29 part-time/adjunct (24 women). *Students:* 29 full-time (28 women), 553 part-time (507 women); includes 187 minority (77 Black or African American, non-Hispanic/Latino; 1 American Indian or Alaska Native, non-Hispanic/Latino; 58 Asian, non-Hispanic/Latino; 38 Hispanic/Latino; 1 Native Hawaiian or other Pacific Islander, non-Hispanic/Latino; 12 Two or more races, non-Hispanic/Latino), 5 international. Average age 30. 537 applicants, 56% accepted, 268 enrolled. In 2013, 140 master's, 1 doctorate, 12 other advanced degrees awarded. *Degree requirements:* For master's, thesis. *Entrance requirements:* For master's, BSN, minimum GPA of 3.0, course work in statistics. *Application deadline:* For fall admission, 1/15 for domestic students. Application fee: $100. *Expenses:* Tuition, state resident: full-time $9870; part-time $411 per credit. Tuition, nonresident: full-time $18,350; part-time $765 per credit. *Financial support:* Fellowships, research assistantships, teaching assistantships, career-related internships or fieldwork, Federal Work-Study, institutionally sponsored loans, and traineeships available. Financial award application deadline: 3/15. *Total annual research expenditures:* $87,846. *Unit head:* Dr. Lee Anne Xippolitos, Dean, 631-444-3200, Fax: 631-444-6628, E-mail: lee.xippolitos@stonybrook.edu. *Application contact:* Karen Allard, Admissions Coordinator, School of Nursing, 631-444-3554, Fax: 631-444-6628, E-mail: karen.allard@stonybrook.edu.
Website: http://www.nursing.stonybrookmedicine.edu/

Tarleton State University, College of Graduate Studies, College of Science and Technology, Department of Nursing, Stephenville, TX 76402. Offers MSN. Part-time and evening/weekend programs available. *Faculty:* 2 full-time (both women). *Students:* 4 full-time (3 women), 8 part-time (all women); includes 1 minority (Black or African American, non-Hispanic/Latino), 1 international. Average age 42. 5 applicants, 80% accepted, 4 enrolled. *Degree requirements:* For master's, comprehensive exam. *Entrance requirements:* For master's, GRE General Test, minimum GPA of 3.0. Additional exam requirements/recommendations for international students: Required—TOEFL (minimum score 550 paper-based; 80 iBT). *Application deadline:* For fall admission, 8/15 priority date for domestic students; for spring admission, 1/7 for domestic students. Applications are processed on a rolling basis. Application fee: $30 ($130 for international students). Electronic applications accepted. *Expenses:* Tuition, state resident: full-time $3312; part-time $184 per credit hour. Tuition, nonresident: full-time $9144; part-time $508 per credit hour. *Required fees:* $1916. Tuition and fees vary according to course load and campus/location. *Financial support:* Career-related internships or fieldwork, Federal Work-Study, and institutionally sponsored loans available. Support available to part-time students. *Unit head:* Dr. Elaine Evans, Head, 254-968-9717, E-mail: eevans@tarleton.edu. *Application contact:* Information Contact, 254-968-9104, Fax: 254-968-9670, E-mail: gradoffice@tarleton.edu.
Website: http://www.tarleton.edu/COSTWEB/nursing/

Temple University, College of Health Professions and Social Work, Department of Nursing, Philadelphia, PA 19140. Offers adult-gerontology primary care (DNP); clinical nurse leader (MSN); family-individual across the lifespan (DNP); nurse educator (MSN); nursing (MSN, DNP). *Accreditation:* AACN. Part-time programs available. *Faculty:* 9 full-time (8 women), 3 part-time/adjunct (all women). *Students:* 6 full-time (5 women), 92 part-time (78 women); includes 51 minority (34 Black or African American, non-Hispanic/Latino; 9 Asian, non-Hispanic/Latino; 8 Hispanic/Latino), 1 international. 48 applicants, 58% accepted, 23 enrolled. In 2013, 12 master's, 9 doctorates awarded. *Degree requirements:* For master's and doctorate, evidence based practice project. *Entrance requirements:* For master's and doctorate, GRE General Test or MAT, 2 letters of reference, RN license, interview, statement of purpose, resume. Additional exam requirements/recommendations for international students: Required—TOEFL (minimum score 550 paper-based; 79 iBT). *Application deadline:* For fall admission, 2/15 priority date for domestic students, 1/15 for international students; for spring admission, 10/15 for domestic students, 9/15 for international students. Applications are processed on a rolling basis. Application fee: $60. Electronic applications accepted. *Financial support:* Federal Work-Study, scholarships/grants, traineeships, and tuition waivers available. Support available to part-time students. Financial award application deadline: 1/15. *Faculty research:* Health promotion, chronic illness, family support systems, primary care, health policy, community health services, evidence-based practice. *Total annual research expenditures:* $741,567. *Unit head:* Dr. Jane Kurz, RN, Chair, 215-707-8327, E-mail: jane.kurz@temple.edu. *Application contact:* Naseem Lodhi, Student Services Coordinator, 215-204-4618, E-mail: tunurse@temple.edu.

Tennessee State University, The School of Graduate Studies and Research, College of Health Sciences, Division of Nursing, Nashville, TN 37209-1561. Offers family nurse practitioner (MSN); holistic nurse practitioner (MSN); nursing education (MSN). *Entrance requirements:* For master's, GRE General Test or MAT, BSN, current RN license, minimum GPA of 3.0.

Tennessee Technological University, Whitson-Hester School of Nursing, Cookeville, TN 38505. Offers family nurse practitioner (MSN); informatics (MSN); nursing administration (MSN); nursing education (MSN). Part-time and evening/weekend programs available. Postbaccalaureate distance learning degree programs offered (no on-campus study). *Students:* 22 full-time (19 women), 101 part-time (94 women); includes 11 minority (5 Black or African American, non-Hispanic/Latino; 2 Asian, non-Hispanic/Latino; 1 Hispanic/Latino; 3 Two or more races, non-Hispanic/Latino). 79 applicants, 65% accepted, 38 enrolled. In 2013, 14 master's awarded. *Degree requirements:* For master's, comprehensive exam, thesis or alternative. *Entrance requirements:* Additional exam requirements/recommendations for international students: Required—TOEFL (minimum score 600 paper-based; 100 iBT), IELTS (minimum score 5.5), PTE, or TOEIC (Test of English as an International Communication). *Application deadline:* For fall admission, 8/1 for domestic students, 5/1 for international students; for spring admission, 12/1 for domestic students, 10/1 for international students. Applications are processed on a rolling basis. Application fee: $35 ($40 for international students). Electronic applications accepted. *Expenses:* Tuition, state resident: full-time $9347; part-time $465 per credit hour. Tuition, nonresident: full-time $23,635; part-time $1152 per credit hour. *Financial support:* Application deadline: 4/1. *Unit head:* Dr. Bedelia Russell, Director, 931-372-3203, Fax: 931-372-6244, E-mail: bhrussell@tntech.edu. *Application contact:* Shelia K. Kendrick, Coordinator of Graduate Studies, 931-372-3808, Fax: 931-372-3497, E-mail: skendrick@tntech.edu.

Texas A&M International University, Office of Graduate Studies and Research, College of Nursing and Health Sciences, Laredo, TX 78041-1900. Offers family nurse practitioner (MSN). *Faculty:* 2 full-time (both women), 2 part-time/adjunct (both women). *Students:* 39 part-time (32 women); includes 37 minority (2 Asian, non-Hispanic/Latino; 35 Hispanic/Latino), 1 international. Average age 36. 43 applicants, 67% accepted, 23 enrolled. In 2013, 15 master's awarded. *Entrance requirements:* Additional exam requirements/recommendations for international students: Required—TOEFL (minimum score 550 paper-based; 79 iBT). *Application deadline:* For fall admission, 4/30 for domestic and international students; for spring admission, 11/30 for domestic students, 10/1 for international students. Applications are processed on a rolling basis. Application fee: $35 ($50 for international students). *Expenses:* Tuition, state resident: full-time $5184. *International tuition:* $11,556 full-time. *Unit head:* Glenda Walker, Dean, 956-326-2574, E-mail: glenda.walker@tamiu.edu. *Application contact:* Suzanne Hansen-Alford, Director of Graduate Recruiting, 956-326-3023, Fax: 956-326-3021, E-mail: enroll@tamiu.edu.
Website: http://www.tamiu.edu/cson/

Texas A&M University–Corpus Christi, Graduate Studies and Research, College of Nursing and Health Sciences, Corpus Christi, TX 78412-5503. Offers clinical nurse specialist (MSN); family nurse practitioner (MSN); health care administration (MSN); leadership in nursing systems (MSN). *Accreditation:* AACN. Part-time and evening/weekend programs available. *Degree requirements:* For master's, comprehensive exam, thesis (for some programs). *Entrance requirements:* For master's, GRE General Test. Additional exam requirements/recommendations for international students: Required—TOEFL. Electronic applications accepted.

Texas Christian University, Harris College of Nursing and Health Sciences, Program in Nursing, Fort Worth, TX 76129-0002. Offers advanced practice registered nurse (DNP); clinical nurse leader (MSN); clinical nurse specialist: adult/gerontology nursing (MSN); clinical nurse specialist: pediatric nursing (MSN); nursing administration (DNP); nursing education (MSN). *Accreditation:* AACN; AANA/CANAEP (one or more programs are accredited). Part-time programs available. Postbaccalaureate distance learning degree programs offered (no on-campus study). *Faculty:* 18 full-time (16 women), 1 (woman) part-time/adjunct. *Students:* 44 full-time (35 women), 46 part-time (42 women); includes 8 minority (3 Black or African American, non-Hispanic/Latino; 2 Asian, non-Hispanic/Latino; 3 Hispanic/Latino), 1 international. Average age 43. 72 applicants, 63% accepted, 36 enrolled. In 2013, 19 master's, 17 doctorates awarded. *Degree requirements:* For master's, professional project; for doctorate, capstone project. *Entrance requirements:* For master's, GRE General Test, 3 letters of reference, essay, resume, two official transcripts from every institution attended; for doctorate, APRN recognition (national certification) or master's and experience in nursing administration; 3 letters of reference; essay; resume; two official transcripts from every institution attended. Additional exam requirements/recommendations for international students: Recommended—TOEFL. *Application deadline:* For fall admission, 4/1 for domestic students; for spring admission, 9/1 for domestic students; for summer admission, 2/1 for domestic students. Applications are processed on a rolling basis. Application fee: $60. Electronic applications accepted. *Expenses: Tuition:* Part-time $1270 per credit hour. Tuition and fees vary according to course load and program. *Financial support:* In 2013–14, 4 teaching assistantships (averaging $2,500 per year) were awarded. Financial award applicants required to submit FAFSA. *Unit head:* Dr. Kathy A. Baker, Director, Division of Nursing Graduate Studies and Scholarship, 817-257-6726, Fax: 817-257-8383, E-mail: kathy.baker@tcu.edu. *Application contact:* Mary Jane Allred, Administrative Program Specialist, 817-257-6726, Fax: 817-257-8383, E-mail: m.allred@tcu.edu.
Website: http://www.nursing.tcu.edu/graduate.asp

Texas Tech University Health Sciences Center, School of Nursing, Lubbock, TX 79430. Offers acute care nurse practitioner (MSN, Certificate); administration (MSN); advanced practice (DNP); education (MSN); executive leadership (DNP); family nurse practitioner (MSN, Certificate); geriatric nurse practitioner (MSN, Certificate); pediatric nurse practitioner (MSN, Certificate). *Accreditation:* AACN. Part-time programs available. Postbaccalaureate distance learning degree programs offered (minimal on-campus study). *Degree requirements:* For master's, thesis optional. *Entrance requirements:* For master's, minimum GPA of 3.0, 3 letters of reference, BSN, RN license; for Certificate, minimum GPA of 3.0, 3 letters of reference, RN license. Additional exam requirements/recommendations for international students: Required—TOEFL (minimum score 550 paper-based). *Faculty research:* Diabetes/obesity, nurse competency, disease management, intervention and measurements, health disparities.

Texas Woman's University, Graduate School, College of Nursing, Denton, TX 76201. Offers acute care nurse practitioner (MS); adult health clinical nurse specialist (MS); adult health nurse practitioner (MS); child health clinical nurse specialist (MS); clinical nurse leader (MS); family nurse practitioner (MS); health systems management (MS); nursing education (MS); nursing practice (DNP); nursing science (PhD); pediatric nurse practitioner (MS); women's health clinical nurse specialist (MS); women's health nurse practitioner (MS). *Accreditation:* AACN. Part-time programs available. Postbaccalaureate distance learning degree programs offered. *Faculty:* 60 full-time (59 women), 46 part-time/adjunct (39 women). *Students:* 54 full-time (49 women), 910 part-time (848 women); includes 489 minority (221 Black or African American, non-Hispanic/Latino; 11 American Indian or Alaska Native, non-Hispanic/Latino; 184 Asian, non-Hispanic/Latino; 70 Hispanic/Latino; 3 Native Hawaiian or other Pacific Islander, non-Hispanic/Latino), 16 international. Average age 38. 430 applicants, 65% accepted, 193 enrolled. In 2013, 258 master's, 22 doctorates awarded. *Degree requirements:* For master's, comprehensive exam, thesis or alternative; for doctorate, comprehensive exam, thesis/dissertation. *Entrance requirements:* For master's, GRE or MAT, minimum GPA of 3.0 on last 60 hours in undergraduate nursing degree and overall, RN license, BS in nursing, basic statistics course; for doctorate, GRE (preferred minimum score 153 [500 old version] Verbal, 144 [500 old version] Quantitative, 4 Analytical), MS in nursing, minimum preferred GPA of 3.5, RN license, statistics, 2 letters of reference, curriculum vitae, graduate nursing-theory course, graduate research course, statement of professional goals and research interests. Additional exam requirements/recommendations for international students: Required—TOEFL (minimum score 550

paper-based; 79 iBT). *Application deadline:* For fall admission, 5/1 priority date for domestic students, 3/1 for international students; for spring admission, 9/15 priority date for domestic students, 7/1 for international students. Applications are processed on a rolling basis. Application fee: $50 ($75 for international students). Electronic applications accepted. *Expenses:* Tuition, state resident: full-time $4182; part-time $233.32 per credit hour. Tuition, nonresident: full-time $10,716; part-time $595.32 per credit hour. *Financial support:* In 2013–14, 149 students received support, including 10 research assistantships (averaging $5,600 per year), 1 teaching assistantship (averaging $5,600 per year); career-related internships or fieldwork, Federal Work-Study, institutionally sponsored loans, scholarships/grants, traineeships, health care benefits, and unspecified assistantships also available. Support available to part-time students. Financial award application deadline: 3/1; financial award applicants required to submit FAFSA. *Faculty research:* Screening, prevention, and treatment for intimate partner violence; needs of adolescents during childbirth intervention; a network analysis decision tool for nurse managers (social network analysis); support for adolescents with implantable cardioverter defibrillators; informatics: nurse staffing, safety, quality, and financial data as they relate to patient care outcomes; prevention and treatment of obesity; improving infant outcomes related to premature birth. *Total annual research expenditures:* $1.7 million. *Unit head:* Dr. Gayle Roux, Interim Dean and Associate Dean for Research and Clinical Scholarship, 940-898-2401, Fax: 940-898-2437, E-mail: nursing@twu.edu. *Application contact:* Dr. Samuel Wheeler, Assistant Director of Admissions, 940-898-3188, Fax: 940-898-3081, E-mail: wheelersr@twu.edu.
Website: http://www.twu.edu/nursing/

Thomas Edison State College, School of Nursing, Program in Nursing, Trenton, NJ 08608-1176. Offers MSN. Part-time programs available. Postbaccalaureate distance learning degree programs offered (no on-campus study). *Degree requirements:* For master's, nursing education seminar, onground practicum, online practicum. *Entrance requirements:* For master's, BSN. Additional exam requirements/recommendations for international students: Required—TOEFL (minimum score 550 paper-based; 79 iBT). Electronic applications accepted.

Thomas Jefferson University, Jefferson School of Nursing, Philadelphia, PA 19107. Offers MS, DNP. *Accreditation:* AACN; AANA/CANAEP. Part-time programs available. Postbaccalaureate distance learning degree programs offered (no on-campus study). *Faculty:* 8 full-time (7 women), 2 part-time/adjunct (both women). *Students:* 49 full-time (38 women), 385 part-time (343 women); includes 107 minority (41 Black or African American, non-Hispanic/Latino; 50 Asian, non-Hispanic/Latino; 16 Hispanic/Latino), 6 international. Average age 33. 384 applicants, 15% accepted, 42 enrolled. In 2013, 112 master's, 12 doctorates awarded. *Entrance requirements:* For master's, GRE or MAT, BSN or equivalent, CPR certification, professional RN license, previous undergraduate course work in statistics and nursing research, minimum GPA of 3.0. Additional exam requirements/recommendations for international students: Required—TOEFL. *Application deadline:* For fall admission, 4/1 priority date for domestic and international students; for spring admission, 9/1 priority date for domestic and international students; for summer admission, 1/2 priority date for domestic and international students. Applications are processed on a rolling basis. Application fee: $25. Electronic applications accepted. *Expenses:* Contact institution. *Financial support:* In 2013–14, 87 students received support. Federal Work-Study, institutionally sponsored loans, and scholarships/grants available. Support available to part-time students. Financial award application deadline: 4/1; financial award applicants required to submit FAFSA. *Faculty research:* Interdisciplinary primary care, women and HIV, health promotion and disease prevention, psychosocial impact of disability, ethical decision-making. *Total annual research expenditures:* $498,070. *Unit head:* Dr. Ksenia Zukowsky, Associate Dean, Graduate Programs, 215-503-9426, E-mail: ksenia.zukowsky@jefferson.edu. *Application contact:* Niki M. Kelley, 215-503-1041, Fax: 215-503-7241, E-mail: niki.kelley@jefferson.edu.
Website: http://www.jefferson.edu/nursing

Thomas University, Department of Nursing, Thomasville, GA 31792-7499. Offers MSN. Part-time programs available. *Entrance requirements:* For master's, resume, 3 academic/professional references. Additional exam requirements/recommendations for international students: Required—TOEFL (minimum score 600 paper-based). Electronic applications accepted.

Towson University, Program in Nursing, Towson, MD 21252-0001. Offers nursing (MS); nursing education (Postbaccalaureate Certificate). *Accreditation:* AACN. Part-time programs available. *Students:* 28 full-time (24 women), 56 part-time (55 women); includes 24 minority (20 Black or African American, non-Hispanic/Latino; 1 American Indian or Alaska Native, non-Hispanic/Latino; 1 Asian, non-Hispanic/Latino; 2 Two or more races, non-Hispanic/Latino), 1 international. *Degree requirements:* For master's, thesis optional. *Entrance requirements:* For master's, minimum GPA of 3.0, copy of current nursing license, bachelor's degree in nursing, current resume or curriculum vitae, completion of an elementary statistics and/or nursing research course, completion of an approved physical assessment course; for Postbaccalaureate Certificate, minimum GPA of 3.0, copy of current nursing license, current resume or curriculum vitae, bachelor's degree, completion of an elementary statistics and/or nursing research course, completion of an approved physical assessment course, personal statement. *Application deadline:* Applications are processed on a rolling basis. Application fee: $45. Electronic applications accepted. *Financial support:* Application deadline: 4/1. *Unit head:* Dr. Kathleen Ogle, Graduate Program Director, 410-704-4389, E-mail: kogle@towson.edu. *Application contact:* Alicia Arkell-Kleis, Information Contact, 410-704-6004, E-mail: grads@towson.edu.

Trinity Western University, School of Graduate Studies, School of Nursing, Langley, BC V2Y 1Y1, Canada. Offers MSN.

Troy University, Graduate School, College of Health and Human Services, Program in Nursing, Troy, AL 36082. Offers adult health (MSN); clinical nurse specialist adult health (DNP); clinical nurse specialist maternal infant (DNP); family nurse practitioner (MSN, DNP, PMC); informatics specialist (MSN); maternal infant (MSN). Part-time and evening/weekend programs available. *Faculty:* 15 full-time (8 women), 3 part-time/adjunct (1 woman). *Students:* 61 full-time (56 women), 228 part-time (193 women); includes 97 minority (77 Black or African American, non-Hispanic/Latino; 4 American Indian or Alaska Native, non-Hispanic/Latino; 2 Asian, non-Hispanic/Latino; 5 Hispanic/Latino; 9 Two or more races, non-Hispanic/Latino). Average age 34. 138 applicants, 80% accepted, 39 enrolled. In 2013, 81 master's, 9 doctorates awarded. *Degree requirements:* For master's, comprehensive exam, minimum GPA of 3.0, candidacy; for doctorate, minimum GPA of 3.0, submission of approved comprehensive e-portfolio, completion of residency synthesis project, minimum of 1000 hours of clinical practice, score of 80% or better on qualifying exam. *Entrance requirements:* For master's, GRE (minimum score of 850 on old exam or 294 on new exam) or GMAT (minimum score of 500), minimum GPA of 3.0, BSN, current RN licensure; 2 letters of reference, undergraduate health assessment course; for doctorate, GRE (minimum score of 850 on old exam or 294 on new exam) or GMAT (minimum score of 500), BSN or MSN, minimum GPA of 3.0, 2 letters of reference, current RN licensure, essay. Additional exam requirements/recommendations for international students: Required—TOEFL (minimum score 523 paper-based; 70 iBT), IELTS (minimum score 6). *Application deadline:* Applications are processed on a rolling basis. Application fee: $50. Electronic applications accepted. *Expenses:* Tuition, state resident: full-time $6084; part-time $338 per credit hour. Tuition, nonresident: full-time $12,168; part-time $676 per credit hour. *Required fees:* $630; $35 per credit hour. $50 per semester. *Financial support:* Available to part-time students. Applicants required to submit FAFSA. *Unit head:* Dr. Diane Weed, Director, School of Nursing, 334-670-5864, Fax: 334-670-3745, E-mail: lweed@troy.edu. *Application contact:* Brenda K. Campbell, Director of Graduate Admissions, 334-670-3178, Fax: 334-670-3733, E-mail: bcamp@troy.edu.

Uniformed Services University of the Health Sciences, Graduate School of Nursing, Bethesda, MD 20814-4799. Offers family nurse practitioner (MSN, DNP); nurse anesthesia (MSN); nursing science (PhD); perioperative clinical nurse specialist (MSN); psychiatric nurse practitioner (MSN, DNP). Program available to military officers only. *Accreditation:* AACN; AANA/CANAEP. *Faculty:* 42 full-time (24 women), 5 part-time/adjunct (4 women). *Students:* 62 full-time (31 women); includes 13 minority (7 Black or African American, non-Hispanic/Latino; 5 Asian, non-Hispanic/Latino; 1 Hispanic/Latino). Average age 34. 100 applicants, 62% accepted, 62 enrolled. In 2013, 57 master's, 1 doctorate awarded. *Degree requirements:* For master's, thesis or alternative; for doctorate, thesis/dissertation or alternative. *Entrance requirements:* For master's, GRE, BSN, clinical experience, minimum GPA of 3.0, previous course work in science; for doctorate, GRE. *Application deadline:* For fall admission, 7/1 for domestic students; for winter admission, 2/15 for domestic students. Application fee: $0. Electronic applications accepted. *Faculty research:* Prenatal care, military health care, military readiness, distance learning. *Unit head:* Dr. Carol A. Romano, Associate Dean for Academic Affairs, 301-295-1180, Fax: 301-295-1707, E-mail: carol.romano@usuhs.edu. *Application contact:* Terry Lynn Malavakis, Recording Secretary for Admissions Committee, 301-295-1055, Fax: 301-295-1707, E-mail: terry.malavakis@usuhs.edu.
Website: http://www.usuhs.mil/gsn/

Union University, School of Nursing, Jackson, TN 38305-3697. Offers executive leadership (DNP); nurse anesthesia (DNP); nurse anesthetist (PMC); nurse practitioner (DNP); nursing education (MSN, PMC). *Accreditation:* AACN; AANA/CANAEP. *Degree requirements:* For master's, thesis or alternative. *Entrance requirements:* For master's, GRE, 3 letters of reference, bachelor's degree in nursing, minimum GPA of 3.0. Additional exam requirements/recommendations for international students: Required—TOEFL (minimum score 560 paper-based). Electronic applications accepted. *Faculty research:* Children's health, occupational rehabilitation, informatics, health promotion.

United States University, School of Nursing, Cypress, CA 90630. Offers administrator (MSN); educator (MSN).

Universidad Metropolitana, School of Health Sciences, Department of Nursing, San Juan, PR 00928-1150. Offers case management (Certificate); nursing (MSN); oncology nursing (Certificate).

Université de Montréal, Faculty of Nursing, Montréal, QC H3C 3J7, Canada. Offers M Sc, PhD, Certificate, DESS. PhD offered jointly with McGill University. Part-time programs available. *Degree requirements:* For master's, one foreign language, thesis optional; for doctorate, thesis/dissertation, general exam; for other advanced degree, one foreign language. *Entrance requirements:* For master's, doctorate, and other advanced degree, proficiency in French. Electronic applications accepted. *Faculty research:* Mental and physical care of chronic patients, care of the hospitalized aged, cancer nursing, home care of caregivers, AIDS patients.

Université du Québec à Rimouski, Graduate Programs, Program in Nursing Studies, Rimouski, QC G5L 3A1, Canada. Offers M Sc, Diploma. Programs offered jointly with Université du Québec à Chicoutimi, Université du Québec à Trois-Rivières, and Université du Québec en Outaouais.

Université du Québec à Trois-Rivières, Graduate Programs, Program in Nursing Sciences, Trois-Rivières, QC G9A 5H7, Canada. Offers M Sc, DESS. Part-time programs available.

Université du Québec en Outaouais, Graduate Programs, Program in Nursing, Gatineau, QC J8X 3X7, Canada. Offers M Sc, DESS, Diploma. Part-time and evening/weekend programs available. *Degree requirements:* For master's, thesis (for some programs). *Entrance requirements:* For master's, appropriate bachelor's degree, proficiency in French.

Université Laval, Faculty of Nursing, Programs in Nursing, Québec, QC G1K 7P4, Canada. Offers M Sc, PhD, DESS, Diploma. *Degree requirements:* For master's, thesis (for some programs). *Entrance requirements:* For master's, French exam, knowledge of English; for other advanced degree, knowledge of French. Electronic applications accepted.

University at Buffalo, the State University of New York, Graduate School, School of Nursing, Buffalo, NY 14214. Offers adult gerontology nurse practitioner (DNP); family nurse practitioner (DNP); health care systems and leadership (MS); nurse anesthetist (DNP); nursing (PhD); nursing education (Certificate); psychiatric/mental health nurse practitioner (DNP). *Accreditation:* AACN; AANA/CANAEP (one or more programs are accredited). Part-time programs available. Postbaccalaureate distance learning degree programs offered (no on-campus study). *Faculty:* 24 full-time (21 women), 2 part-time/adjunct (1 woman). *Students:* 80 full-time (60 women), 97 part-time (84 women); includes 35 minority (20 Black or African American, non-Hispanic/Latino; 2 American Indian or Alaska Native, non-Hispanic/Latino; 9 Asian, non-Hispanic/Latino; 1 Hispanic/Latino; 3 Native Hawaiian or other Pacific Islander, non-Hispanic/Latino). 118 applicants, 67% accepted, 58 enrolled. In 2013, 41 master's, 15 doctorates awarded. *Degree requirements:* For master's, thesis optional; for doctorate, comprehensive exam (for some programs), capstone (for DNP), dissertation (for PhD). *Entrance requirements:* For doctorate, GRE or MAT, minimum GPA of 3.0 (3.25 for PhD), RN license, BS or MS in nursing, 3 references, writing sample; for Certificate, interview, minimum GPA of 3.0 or GRE General Test, RN license, MS in nursing. Additional exam requirements/recommendations for international students: Required—TOEFL (minimum score 550 paper-based; 79 iBT), IELTS (minimum score 6.5). *Application deadline:* For fall admission, 7/1 for domestic students, 4/1 for international students; for spring admission, 12/1 for domestic students, 10/1 for international students; for summer admission, 4/1 for domestic students. Application fee: $75. Electronic applications accepted. *Financial support:* In 2013–14, 80 students received support, including 2 fellowships with full and partial tuition reimbursements available (averaging $17,000 per year), 7 research assistantships with full and partial tuition reimbursements available (averaging $10,600 per year), 7 teaching assistantships with full and partial tuition reimbursements available (averaging $10,600 per year); scholarships/grants, traineeships, health care benefits, and unspecified assistantships also available. Financial award application deadline: 3/15; financial award applicants required to submit FAFSA. *Faculty research:* Oncology, palliative care, gerontology, addictions, mental health, community wellness, sleep, workforce, care of underserved populations, quality and safety, person-centered care, adolescent health. *Total annual research expenditures:* $1.1 million. *Unit head:* Dr. Marsha L. Lewis, Dean and Professor, 716-829-2533, Fax: 716-829-2566, E-mail: ubnursingdean@buffalo.edu. *Application contact:* Dr. David J. Lang, Director of Student Affairs, 716-829-2537, Fax: 716-829-2067, E-mail: nursing@buffalo.edu.
Website: http://nursing.buffalo.edu/

Nursing—General

The University of Akron, Graduate School, College of Health Professions, School of Nursing, Akron, OH 44325-3701. Offers nursing (MSN, PhD); nursing practice (DNP); public health (MPH). PhD offered jointly with Kent State University. *Accreditation:* AACN; AANA/CANAEP (one or more programs are accredited). Part-time programs available. *Faculty:* 16 full-time (all women), 42 part-time/adjunct (39 women). *Students:* 46 full-time (34 women), 362 part-time (300 women); includes 59 minority (35 Black or African American, non-Hispanic/Latino; 5 Asian, non-Hispanic/Latino; 12 Hispanic/Latino; 1 Native Hawaiian or other Pacific Islander, non-Hispanic/Latino; 6 Two or more races, non-Hispanic/Latino), 3 international. Average age 34. 117 applicants, 75% accepted, 59 enrolled. In 2013, 75 master's awarded. *Degree requirements:* For doctorate, one foreign language, thesis/dissertation, qualifying exam. *Entrance requirements:* For master's, current Ohio state license as registered nurse, three letters of reference, 300-word essay, interview with program coordinator; for doctorate, GRE, minimum GPA of 3.0, MSN, nursing license or eligibility for licensure, writing sample, letters of recommendation, interview, resume, personal statement of research interests and career goals. Additional exam requirements/recommendations for international students: Required—TOEFL (minimum score 550 paper-based; 79 iBT). *Application deadline:* For fall admission, 7/15 for domestic and international students. Applications are processed on a rolling basis. Application fee: $40 ($60 for international students). Electronic applications accepted. *Expenses:* Tuition, state resident: full-time $7430; part-time $412.80 per credit hour. Tuition, nonresident: full-time $12,722; part-time $706.80 per credit hour. *Required fees:* $53 per credit hour. $12 per semester. Tuition and fees vary according to course load and program. *Financial support:* In 2013–14, 11 teaching assistantships with full tuition reimbursements were awarded; career-related internships or fieldwork and Federal Work-Study also available. *Faculty research:* Health promotion and chronic disease prevention, mental health and psychosocial resilience, gerontological health, trauma and violence, gut oxygenation during shock and trauma, simulation and the pedagogy of teaching and learning. *Total annual research expenditures:* $596,812. *Unit head:* Dr. Elaine Fisher, Director, 330-972-6125, E-mail: efisher@uakron.edu. *Application contact:* Dr. Marlene Huff, Graduate Director, 330-972-7555, E-mail: mhuff@uakron.edu.
Website: http://www.uakron.edu/nursing/

The University of Alabama, Graduate School, Capstone College of Nursing, Tuscaloosa, AL 35487. Offers MSN, DNP, Ed D, MSN/Ed D. *Accreditation:* AACN. Part-time programs available. Postbaccalaureate distance learning degree programs offered (no on-campus study). *Faculty:* 21 full-time (18 women), 1 (woman) part-time/adjunct. *Students:* 90 full-time (76 women), 281 part-time (248 women); includes 142 minority (101 Black or African American, non-Hispanic/Latino; 1 American Indian or Alaska Native, non-Hispanic/Latino; 8 Asian, non-Hispanic/Latino; 22 Hispanic/Latino; 2 Native Hawaiian or other Pacific Islander, non-Hispanic/Latino; 8 Two or more races, non-Hispanic/Latino). Average age 43. 266 applicants, 54% accepted, 119 enrolled. In 2013, 40 master's, 122 doctorates awarded. *Degree requirements:* For master's, thesis optional; for doctorate, comprehensive exam, thesis/dissertation, scholarly practice project. *Entrance requirements:* For master's, GRE or MAT (if GPA is below 3.0), BSN, RN licensure, minimum GPA of 3.0; for doctorate, GRE or MAT, MSN, RN licensure, minimum GPA of 3.0, references, writing sample, curriculum vitae. Additional exam requirements/recommendations for international students: Required—TOEFL. *Application deadline:* For fall admission, 6/1 priority date for domestic students; for winter admission, 11/1 for domestic students; for spring admission, 4/1 priority date for domestic students. Applications are processed on a rolling basis. Application fee: $50 ($60 for international students). Electronic applications accepted. *Expenses:* Tuition, state resident: full-time $9450. Tuition, nonresident: full-time $23,950. *Financial support:* In 2013–14, 2 fellowships with full tuition reimbursements (averaging $15,000 per year) were awarded; scholarships/grants also available. Financial award application deadline: 7/1; financial award applicants required to submit FAFSA. *Faculty research:* Diabetes education, childhood asthma, HIV/AIDS prevention and care, breast cancer in rural minority women, nursing labor cost, nursing case management, sleep, gerontology, health disparities of rural children. *Total annual research expenditures:* $245,736. *Unit head:* Dr. Suzanne Prevost, Dean, 205-348-1040, Fax: 205-348-5559, E-mail: sprevost@ua.edu. *Application contact:* Dr. Marsha H. Adams, Senior Associate Dean, 205-348-1044, Fax: 205-348-5559, E-mail: madams@ua.edu.
Website: http://nursing.ua.edu/

The University of Alabama at Birmingham, School of Nursing, Birmingham, AL 35294. Offers nurse anesthesia (MSN); nursing (MSN, DNP, PhD). *Accreditation:* AACN. Part-time programs available. Terminal master's awarded for partial completion of doctoral program. *Degree requirements:* For doctorate, thesis/dissertation, research mentorship experience. *Entrance requirements:* For master's, GRE, GMAT, or MAT, BS in nursing, interview; for doctorate, GRE General Test, computer literacy, course work in statistics, interview, minimum GPA of 3.0, MS in nursing, references, writing sample. Additional exam requirements/recommendations for international students: Required—TOEFL. Electronic applications accepted. *Expenses:* Contact institution.

The University of Alabama in Huntsville, School of Graduate Studies, College of Nursing, Huntsville, AL 35899. Offers family nurse practitioner (Certificate); nursing (MSN, DNP), including acute care nurse practitioner (MSN), adult clinical nurse specialist (MSN), clinical nurse leader (MSN), family nurse practitioner (MSN), leadership in health care systems (MSN); nursing education (Certificate). DNP offered jointly with The University of Alabama at Birmingham. *Accreditation:* AACN. Part-time and evening/weekend programs available. Postbaccalaureate distance learning degree programs offered (minimal on-campus study). *Faculty:* 16 full-time (15 women), 4 part-time/adjunct (all women). *Students:* 67 full-time (63 women), 235 part-time (192 women); includes 40 minority (27 Black or African American, non-Hispanic/Latino; 5 American Indian or Alaska Native, non-Hispanic/Latino; 4 Asian, non-Hispanic/Latino; 3 Hispanic/Latino; 1 Two or more races, non-Hispanic/Latino), 10 international. Average age 36. 265 applicants, 59% accepted, 128 enrolled. In 2013, 75 master's, 10 doctorates, 5 other advanced degrees awarded. *Degree requirements:* For master's, comprehensive exam, thesis or alternative, oral and written exams. *Entrance requirements:* For master's, MAT or GRE, Alabama RN license, BSN, minimum GPA of 3.0; for doctorate, master's degree in nursing in an advanced practice area; for Certificate, MAT or GRE, minimum GPA of 3.0. Additional exam requirements/recommendations for international students: Required—TOEFL (minimum score 500 paper-based; 80 iBT), IELTS (minimum score 6.5). *Application deadline:* For fall admission, 7/15 for domestic students, 4/1 for international students; for spring admission, 11/30 for domestic students, 9/1 for international students. Applications are processed on a rolling basis. Application fee: $50. Electronic applications accepted. *Expenses:* Tuition, state resident: full-time $8912; part-time $540 per credit hour. Tuition, nonresident: full-time $20,774; part-time $1252 per credit hour. *Required fees:* $148 per semester. One-time fee: $150. *Financial support:* In 2013–14, 19 students received support, including 19 teaching assistantships with full tuition reimbursements available (averaging $7,876 per year); career-related internships or fieldwork, Federal Work-Study, institutionally sponsored loans, scholarships/grants, traineeships, health care benefits, and unspecified assistantships also available. Support available to part-time students. Financial award application deadline: 4/1; financial award applicants required to submit FAFSA. *Faculty research:* Health care informatics, chronic illness management, maternal and child health, genetics/genomics, technology and health care. *Total annual research expenditures:* $557,830. *Unit head:* Dr. Fay Raines, Dean, 256-824-6345, Fax: 256-824-6026, E-mail: rainesc@uah.edu. *Application contact:* Charles Davis, Director of Graduate Nursing Admissions and Advising, 256-824-2433, Fax: 256-824-6026, E-mail: charles.davis@uah.edu.
Website: http://www.uah.edu/nursing/welcome

University of Alaska Anchorage, College of Health, School of Nursing, Anchorage, AK 99508. Offers MS. Part-time and evening/weekend programs available. *Degree requirements:* For master's, comprehensive exam, individual project. *Entrance requirements:* For master's, GRE or MAT, BS in nursing, interview, minimum GPA of 3.0, RN license, 1 year of part-time or 6 months of full-time clinical experience. Additional exam requirements/recommendations for international students: Required—TOEFL (minimum score 550 paper-based).

University of Alberta, Faculty of Graduate Studies and Research, Faculty of Nursing, Edmonton, AB T6G 2E1, Canada. Offers MN, PhD. Part-time programs available. *Degree requirements:* For master's, thesis optional, clinical practice; for doctorate, thesis/dissertation. *Entrance requirements:* For master's, B Sc N, 1 year of clinical nursing experience in specialty area; for doctorate, MN. Additional exam requirements/recommendations for international students: Required—TOEFL (minimum score 550 paper-based). *Faculty research:* Symptom management, healthy human development, health policy, teaching excellence and information.

The University of Arizona, College of Nursing, Tucson, AZ 85721. Offers health care informatics (Certificate); nurse practitioner (MS, Certificate); nursing (DNP, PhD); rural health (Certificate). *Accreditation:* AACN. Part-time programs available. Postbaccalaureate distance learning degree programs offered (minimal on-campus study). *Faculty:* 20 full-time (18 women). *Students:* 352 full-time (298 women), 202 part-time (169 women); includes 152 minority (36 Black or African American, non-Hispanic/Latino; 2 American Indian or Alaska Native, non-Hispanic/Latino; 29 Asian, non-Hispanic/Latino; 54 Hispanic/Latino; 3 Native Hawaiian or other Pacific Islander, non-Hispanic/Latino; 28 Two or more races, non-Hispanic/Latino). Average age 39. 629 applicants, 59% accepted, 266 enrolled. In 2013, 159 master's, 23 doctorates awarded. Terminal master's awarded for partial completion of doctoral program. *Degree requirements:* For master's, thesis optional; for doctorate, comprehensive exam, thesis/dissertation. *Entrance requirements:* For master's, BSN, eligibility for RN license; for doctorate, BSN; for Certificate, GRE General Test, Arizona RN license, BSN, minimum GPA of 3.0. Additional exam requirements/recommendations for international students: Required—TOEFL (minimum score 550 paper-based; 79 iBT). *Application deadline:* For fall admission, 1/15 for domestic and international students. Applications are processed on a rolling basis. Application fee: $75. Electronic applications accepted. *Expenses:* Contact institution. *Financial support:* In 2013–14, 11 research assistantships with full tuition reimbursements (averaging $18,220 per year), 3 teaching assistantships (averaging $18,327 per year) were awarded; career-related internships or fieldwork, institutionally sponsored loans, scholarships/grants, traineeships, health care benefits, tuition waivers (full), and unspecified assistantships also available. Financial award application deadline: 6/1. *Faculty research:* Vulnerable populations, injury mechanisms and biobehavioral responses, health care systems, informatics, rural health. *Total annual research expenditures:* $4.4 million. *Unit head:* Dr. Joan Shaver, Dean, 520-626-7124, Fax: 520-626-6424, E-mail: cmurdaugh@nursing.arizona.edu. *Application contact:* Oscar Parra, Assistant Dean, Student Affairs, 520-626-6154, Fax: 520-626-2211, E-mail: info@nursing.arizona.edu.
Website: http://www.nursing.arizona.edu/

University of Arkansas, Graduate School, College of Education and Health Professions, Eleanor Mann School of Nursing, Fayetteville, AR 72701-1201. Offers MSN. *Accreditation:* AACN. Postbaccalaureate distance learning degree programs offered. Electronic applications accepted.

University of Arkansas for Medical Sciences, College of Nursing, Little Rock, AR 72205-7199. Offers PhD. *Accreditation:* AACN. Part-time programs available. *Faculty:* 34 full-time (32 women), 6 part-time/adjunct (5 women). *Students:* 28 full-time (25 women), 311 part-time (269 women); includes 48 minority (23 Black or African American, non-Hispanic/Latino; 1 American Indian or Alaska Native, non-Hispanic/Latino; 7 Asian, non-Hispanic/Latino; 9 Hispanic/Latino; 1 Native Hawaiian or other Pacific Islander, non-Hispanic/Latino; 7 Two or more races, non-Hispanic/Latino), 1 international. *Entrance requirements:* For doctorate, GRE. Additional exam requirements/recommendations for international students: Required—TOEFL. *Application deadline:* For fall admission, 1/2 for domestic and international students. Application fee: $0. *Expenses:* Contact institution. *Financial support:* Career-related internships or fieldwork and traineeships available. Support available to part-time students. *Unit head:* Dr. Lorraine Frazier, Dean, 501-686-8493. *Application contact:* Dr. Jean McSweeney, Information Contact, 501-296-1892, E-mail: mcsweeney@uams.edu.
Website: http://www.nursing.uams.edu/

The University of British Columbia, Faculty of Applied Science, Program in Nursing, Vancouver, BC V6T 1Z1, Canada. Offers MSN, PhD. Part-time programs available. *Degree requirements:* For master's, essay or thesis; for doctorate, comprehensive exam, thesis/dissertation. *Entrance requirements:* For master's, GRE, bachelor's degree in nursing; for doctorate, GRE, master's degree in nursing. Additional exam requirements/recommendations for international students: Required—TOEFL. Electronic applications accepted. *Expenses: Tuition, area resident:* Full-time $8000 Canadian dollars. *Faculty research:* Women and children, aging, critical care, cross-cultural.

University of Calgary, Faculty of Graduate Studies, Faculty of Nursing, Calgary, AB T2N 1N4, Canada. Offers MN, PhD, PMD. Part-time programs available. *Faculty:* 34 full-time (30 women). *Students:* 110 full-time (99 women), 29 part-time (24 women); includes 4 minority (all Black or African American, non-Hispanic/Latino). Average age 32. 66 applicants, 74% accepted, 37 enrolled. In 2013, 22 master's, 2 doctorates, 8 other advanced degrees awarded. *Degree requirements:* For master's, comprehensive exam (for some programs), thesis (for some programs); for doctorate, thesis/dissertation; for PMD, comprehensive exam. *Entrance requirements:* For master's and PMD, nursing experience, nursing registration; for doctorate, nursing registration. Additional exam requirements/recommendations for international students: Required—TOEFL (minimum score 600 paper-based), IELTS (minimum score 7), Michigan English Language Assessment Battery. *Application deadline:* For fall admission, 2/1 for domestic and international students; for winter admission, 9/15 for domestic and international students. Application fee: $100 ($130 for international students). Electronic applications accepted. *Expenses:* Contact institution. *Financial support:* In 2013–14, 41 students received support, including 14 teaching assistantships (averaging $4,000 per year); institutionally sponsored loans, scholarships/grants, health care benefits, and unspecified assistantships also available. Support available to part-time students. Financial award application deadline: 3/31. *Faculty research:* Health outcomes across multiple populations and multiple settings including patients and families with chronic health problems, culturally diverse, and vulnerable populations; family health; core processes; professional, educational and health services delivery. *Unit head:* Dr. Shelley Raffin Bouchal, Associate Dean, Graduate Programs, 403-220-6258, Fax: 403-284-4803, E-mail: raffin@ucalgary.ca. *Application contact:* Miwa Shibuya, Graduate

Programs Student Advisor, 403-220-6241, Fax: 403-284-4803, E-mail: mmshibuy@ucalgary.ca.
Website: http://nursing.ucalgary.ca

University of California, Irvine, College of Health Sciences, Program in Nursing Science, Irvine, CA 92697. Offers MSN. *Accreditation:* AACN. *Students:* 14 full-time (12 women), 17 part-time (all women); includes 17 minority (10 Asian, non-Hispanic/Latino; 1 Hispanic/Latino; 6 Two or more races, non-Hispanic/Latino). Average age 32. 76 applicants, 41% accepted, 19 enrolled. In 2013, 17 master's awarded. Application fee: $80 ($100 for international students). *Unit head:* Ellen F. Olshankhsky, Director, 949-824-9734, Fax: 949-824-0470, E-mail: e.olshansky@uci.edu. *Application contact:* Julie Aird, Manager of Student Affairs, 949-824-1514, Fax: 949-824-3650, E-mail: jaird@uci.edu.
Website: http://www.nursing.uci.edu/

University of California, Los Angeles, Graduate Division, School of Nursing, Los Angeles, CA 90095. Offers MSN, PhD, MBA/MSN. *Accreditation:* AACN. *Degree requirements:* For master's, comprehensive exam; for doctorate, thesis/dissertation, oral and written qualifying exams. *Entrance requirements:* For master's, bachelor's degree in nursing; minimum undergraduate GPA of 3.0 (or its equivalent if letter grade system not used); for doctorate, bachelor's degree in nursing; minimum undergraduate GPA of 3.5 (or its equivalent if letter grade system not used); writing sample. Additional exam requirements/recommendations for international students: Required—TOEFL. Electronic applications accepted. *Expenses:* Contact institution.

University of California, San Francisco, Graduate Division, School of Nursing, Program in Nursing, San Francisco, CA 94143. Offers MS, PhD. *Accreditation:* AACN; ACNM/ACME (one or more programs are accredited). *Degree requirements:* For master's, comprehensive exam, thesis or alternative; for doctorate, thesis/dissertation. *Entrance requirements:* For master's and doctorate, GRE General Test. *Application deadline:* For fall admission, 3/1 for domestic students. Application fee: $40. *Expenses:* Contact institution. *Financial support:* Fellowships and Federal Work-Study available. Support available to part-time students. Financial award application deadline: 1/10. *Application contact:* Jeff Kilmer, Assistant Dean, Student Affairs, 415-476-0600, E-mail: jeff.kilmer@nursing.ucsf.edu.

University of Central Arkansas, Graduate School, College of Health and Behavioral Sciences, Department of Nursing, Conway, AR 72035-0001. Offers adult nurse practitioner (PMC); clinical nurse leader (PMC); clinical nurse specialist (MSN); family nurse practitioner (PMC); nurse educator (PMC); nurse practitioner (MSN). *Accreditation:* AACN. Part-time and evening/weekend programs available. Postbaccalaureate distance learning degree programs offered (minimal on-campus study). *Degree requirements:* For master's, comprehensive exam, thesis optional, clinicals. *Entrance requirements:* For master's, GRE General Test, minimum GPA of 2.7. Additional exam requirements/recommendations for international students: Required—TOEFL (minimum score 550 paper-based; 80 iBT). Electronic applications accepted. *Expenses:* Contact institution.

University of Central Florida, College of Nursing, Orlando, FL 32816. Offers adult-gerontology nurse practitioner (Post-Master's Certificate); family nurse practitioner (Post-Master's Certificate); nursing (MSN, PhD); nursing education (Post-Master's Certificate); nursing practice (DNP). *Accreditation:* AACN. Part-time and evening/weekend programs available. *Faculty:* 47 full-time (41 women), 78 part-time/adjunct (75 women). *Students:* 54 full-time (49 women), 264 part-time (239 women); includes 72 minority (35 Black or African American, non-Hispanic/Latino; 7 Asian, non-Hispanic/Latino; 25 Hispanic/Latino; 1 Native Hawaiian or other Pacific Islander, non-Hispanic/Latino; 4 Two or more races, non-Hispanic/Latino), 1 international. Average age 39. 179 applicants, 55% accepted, 71 enrolled. In 2013, 96 master's, 12 doctorates, 3 other advanced degrees awarded. *Degree requirements:* For master's, thesis or alternative. *Entrance requirements:* For master's, GRE General Test, minimum GPA of 3.0 in last 60 hours. Additional exam requirements/recommendations for international students: Required—TOEFL. *Application deadline:* For fall admission, 2/15 for domestic students; for spring admission, 9/15 for domestic students. Application fee: $30. Electronic applications accepted. *Financial support:* In 2013–14, 2 students received support, including 3 teaching assistantships with partial tuition reimbursements available (averaging $6,300 per year); fellowships with partial tuition reimbursements available, research assistantships with partial tuition reimbursements available, career-related internships or fieldwork, Federal Work-Study, institutionally sponsored loans, traineeships, and unspecified assistantships also available. Financial award application deadline: 3/1; financial award applicants required to submit FAFSA. *Unit head:* Dr. Mary Lou Sole, Interim Dean, 407-823-5496, Fax: 407-823-5675, E-mail: mary.sole@ucf.edu. *Application contact:* Barbara Rodriguez Lamas, Director, Admissions and Student Services, 407-823-2766, Fax: 407-823-6442, E-mail: gradadmissions@ucf.edu.
Website: http://nursing.ucf.edu/

University of Central Missouri, The Graduate School, Warrensburg, MO 6409. Offers accountancy (MA); accounting (MBA); applied mathematics (MS); aviation safety (MA); biology (MS); business administration (MBA); career and technical education leadership (MS); college student personnel administration (MS); communication (MA); computer science (MS); counseling (MS); criminal justice (MS); educational leadership (Ed D); educational technology (MS); elementary and early childhood education (MSE); English (MA); environmental studies (MA); finance (MBA); history (MA); human services/educational technology (Ed S); human services/learning resources (Ed S); human services/professional counseling (Ed S); industrial hygiene (MS); industrial management (MS); information systems (MBA); information technology (MS); kinesiology (MS); library science and information services (MS); literacy education (MSE); marketing (MBA); mathematics (MS); music (MA); occupational safety management (MS); psychology (MS); rural family nursing (MS); school administration (MSE); social gerontology (MS); sociology (MA); special education (MSE); speech language pathology (MS); superintendency (Ed S); teaching (MAT); teaching English as a second language (MA); technology (MS); technology management (PhD); theatre (MA). Part-time programs available. *Faculty:* 233. *Students:* 890 full-time (396 women), 1,486 part-time (1,001 women); includes 192 minority (97 Black or African American, non-Hispanic/Latino; 9 American Indian or Alaska Native, non-Hispanic/Latino; 32 Asian, non-Hispanic/Latino; 40 Hispanic/Latino; 3 Native Hawaiian or other Pacific Islander, non-Hispanic/Latino; 11 Two or more races, non-Hispanic/Latino), 539 international. Average age 31. 1,953 applicants, 75% accepted. In 2013, 719 master's, 58 other advanced degrees awarded. *Degree requirements:* For master's and Ed S, comprehensive exam (for some programs), thesis (for some programs). *Entrance requirements:* Additional exam requirements/recommendations for international students: Required—TOEFL (minimum score 550 paper-based; 79 iBT). *Application deadline:* For fall admission, 6/1 for domestic students; for spring admission, 10/1 for domestic and international students. Applications are processed on a rolling basis. Application fee: $30 ($75 for international students). Electronic applications accepted. *Expenses:* Tuition, state resident: full-time $7326; part-time $276.25 per credit hour. Tuition, nonresident: full-time $13,956; part-time $552.50 per credit hour. *Required fees:* $29 per credit hour. *Financial support:* In 2013–14, 118 students received support, including 271 research assistantships with full and partial tuition reimbursements available (averaging $7,500 per year), 109 teaching assistantships with full and partial tuition reimbursements available (averaging $7,500 per year); career-related internships or fieldwork, Federal Work-Study, scholarships/grants, and administrative and laboratory assistantships also available. Support available to part-time students. Financial award application deadline: 3/1; financial award applicants required to submit FAFSA. *Unit head:* Dr. Joseph Vaughn, Assistant Provost for Research/Dean, 660-543-4092, Fax: 660-543-4778, E-mail: vaughn@ucmo.edu. *Application contact:* Brittany Lawrence, Graduate Student Services Coordinator, 660-543-4621, Fax: 660-543-4778, E-mail: gradinfo@ucmo.edu.
Website: http://www.ucmo.edu/graduate/

University of Central Oklahoma, The Jackson College of Graduate Studies, College of Mathematics and Science, Department of Nursing, Edmond, OK 73034-5209. Offers MS. Part-time programs available. *Faculty:* 5 full-time (all women). *Students:* 7 full-time (all women), 15 part-time (13 women); includes 8 minority (3 Black or African American, non-Hispanic/Latino; 1 American Indian or Alaska Native, non-Hispanic/Latino; 1 Asian, non-Hispanic/Latino; 3 Two or more races, non-Hispanic/Latino), 2 international. Average age 37. 22 applicants, 77% accepted, 10 enrolled. In 2013, 18 master's awarded. *Entrance requirements:* For master's, minimum undergraduate GPA of 3.0 in nursing; bachelor's degree in nursing; license as an RN. *Application deadline:* For fall admission, 7/1 for international students; for spring admission, 11/1 for international students. Applications are processed on a rolling basis. Application fee: $50. Electronic applications accepted. *Expenses:* Tuition, state resident: full-time $4137; part-time $206.85 per credit hour. Tuition, nonresident: full-time $10,359; part-time $517.95 per credit hour. *Required fees:* $481. Tuition and fees vary according to course load and program. *Financial support:* In 2013–14, 6 students received support. Application deadline: 3/31; applicants required to submit FAFSA. *Unit head:* Dr. Linda Rider, Chair, 405-974-5176. *Application contact:* Dr. Richard Bernard, Dean, College of Graduate Studies, 405-974-3493, Fax: 405-974-3852, E-mail: gradcoll@uco.edu.

University of Cincinnati, Graduate School, College of Nursing, Cincinnati, OH 45221-0038. Offers clinical nurse specialist (MSN), including adult health, community health, neonatal, nursing administration, occupational health, pediatric health, psychiatric nursing, women's health; nurse anesthesia (MSN); nurse midwifery (MSN); nurse practitioner (MSN), including acute care, ambulatory care, family, family/psychiatric, women's health; nursing (PhD); MBA/MSN. *Accreditation:* AACN; AANA/CANAEP (one or more programs are accredited); ACNM/ACME. Part-time programs available. Postbaccalaureate distance learning degree programs offered (no on-campus study). Terminal master's awarded for partial completion of doctoral program. *Degree requirements:* For master's, thesis or alternative; for doctorate, comprehensive exam, thesis/dissertation. *Entrance requirements:* For master's and doctorate, GRE General Test. Additional exam requirements/recommendations for international students: Required—TOEFL (minimum score 520 paper-based). Electronic applications accepted. *Faculty research:* Substance abuse, injury and violence, symptom management.

University of Colorado Colorado Springs, Beth-El College of Nursing and Health Sciences, Colorado Springs, CO 80933-7150. Offers nursing education (MSN); nursing practice (DNP); primary care nurse practitioner (MSN). *Accreditation:* AACN. Part-time programs available. Postbaccalaureate distance learning degree programs offered (minimal on-campus study). *Faculty:* 5 full-time (all women), 1 part-time/adjunct (0 women). *Students:* 14 full-time (13 women), 160 part-time (149 women); includes 32 minority (2 Black or African American, non-Hispanic/Latino; 2 American Indian or Alaska Native, non-Hispanic/Latino; 5 Asian, non-Hispanic/Latino; 21 Hispanic/Latino; 2 Two or more races, non-Hispanic/Latino). Average age 37. 125 applicants, 38% accepted, 42 enrolled. In 2013, 31 master's, 3 doctorates awarded. *Degree requirements:* For master's, comprehensive exam, thesis optional; for doctorate, capstone project. *Entrance requirements:* For master's, GRE General Test or MAT, BSN, minimum GPA of 3.0, unrestricted RN license; for doctorate, interview; active RN license; MA; minimum GPA of 3.3; National Certification as nurse practitioner or clinical nurse specialist; portfolio. Additional exam requirements/recommendations for international students: Required—TOEFL. *Application deadline:* For fall admission, 6/15 priority date for domestic students, 6/15 for international students; for spring admission, 9/15 for domestic and international students. Application fee: $60 ($75 for international students). Electronic applications accepted. *Expenses:* Contact institution. *Financial support:* In 2013–14, 17 students received support, including 17 fellowships (averaging $2,500 per year); career-related internships or fieldwork, Federal Work-Study, and scholarships/grants also available. Support available to part-time students. Financial award application deadline: 3/1; financial award applicants required to submit FAFSA. *Faculty research:* Women's health, uncertainty, empowerment, family experience in chronic illness. *Total annual research expenditures:* $2,568. *Unit head:* Dr. Amy Silva-Smith, Graduate Department Chairperson, 719-255-4490, Fax: 719-255-4416, E-mail: asilvasm@uccs.edu. *Application contact:* Diane Busch, Director, 719-255-4424, Fax: 719-255-4416, E-mail: dbusch@uccs.edu.
Website: http://www.uccs.edu/~bethel/

University of Colorado Denver, College of Nursing, Aurora, CO 80045. Offers adult clinical nurse specialist (MS); adult nurse practitioner (MS); family nurse practitioner (MS); family psychiatric mental health nurse practitioner (MS); health care informatics (MS); nurse-midwifery (MS); nursing (DNP, PhD); nursing leadership and health care systems (MS); pediatric nurse practitioner (MS); special studies (MS); women's health (MS); MS/PhD. *Accreditation:* ACNM/ACME (one or more programs are accredited). Part-time and evening/weekend programs available. Postbaccalaureate distance learning degree programs offered (minimal on-campus study). *Faculty:* 74 full-time (65 women), 58 part-time/adjunct (56 women). *Students:* 351 full-time (327 women), 138 part-time (125 women); includes 79 minority (12 Black or African American, non-Hispanic/Latino; 9 American Indian or Alaska Native, non-Hispanic/Latino; 13 Asian, non-Hispanic/Latino; 32 Hispanic/Latino; 2 Native Hawaiian or other Pacific Islander, non-Hispanic/Latino; 11 Two or more races, non-Hispanic/Latino), 7 international. Average age 33. 354 applicants, 43% accepted, 109 enrolled. In 2013, 108 master's, 28 doctorates awarded. Terminal master's awarded for partial completion of doctoral program. *Degree requirements:* For master's, thesis optional; for doctorate, comprehensive exam, thesis/dissertation, 42 credits of coursework. *Entrance requirements:* For master's, GRE if cumulative undergraduate GPA is less than 3.0, undergraduate nursing degree from NLNAC- or CCNE-accredited school or university; completion of research and statistics courses with minimum grade of C; copy of current and unencumbered nursing license; for doctorate, GRE, bachelor's and/or master's degrees in nursing from NLN- or CCNE-accredited institution; portfolio; minimum undergraduate GPA of 3.0, graduate 3.5; graduate-level intermediate statistics and master's-level nursing theory courses with minimum B grade; interview. Additional exam requirements/recommendations for international students: Required—TOEFL (minimum score 560 paper-based; 83 iBT). *Application deadline:* For fall admission, 2/15 for domestic students, 1/15 for international students; for spring admission, 7/1 for domestic students, 6/1 for international students. Application fee: $50 ($75 for international students). Electronic applications accepted. *Expenses:* Contact institution. *Financial support:* In 2013–14, 113 students received support. Fellowships, research assistantships, teaching assistantships, Federal Work-Study, institutionally sponsored loans, scholarships/grants, traineeships, and unspecified assistantships available. Support available to part-time students. Financial award application deadline: 4/1; financial award applicants required to submit FAFSA. *Faculty research:* Biological and behavioral phenomena in pregnancy and postpartum; patterns of glycemia during the insulin resistance of pregnancy; obesity, gestational diabetes, and relationship to

neonatal adiposity; men's awareness and knowledge of male breast cancer; cognitive-behavioral therapy for chronic insomnia after breast cancer treatment; massage therapy for the treatment of tension-type headaches. *Total annual research expenditures:* $5.9 million. *Unit head:* Dr. Sarah Thompson, Dean, 303-724-1679, E-mail: sarah.a.thompson@ucdenver.edu. *Application contact:* Judy Campbell, Graduate Programs Coordinator, 303-724-8503, E-mail: judy.campbell@ucdenver.edu.
Website: http://www.ucdenver.edu/academics/colleges/nursing/Pages/default.aspx

University of Connecticut, Graduate School, School of Nursing, Storrs, CT 06269. Offers MS, PhD, Post-Master's Certificate. *Accreditation:* AACN. *Degree requirements:* For master's, comprehensive exam; for doctorate, thesis/dissertation. *Entrance requirements:* Additional exam requirements/recommendations for international students: Required—TOEFL (minimum score 550 paper-based). Electronic applications accepted.

University of Delaware, College of Health Sciences, School of Nursing, Newark, DE 19716. Offers adult nurse practitioner (MSN, PMC); cardiopulmonary clinical nurse specialist (MSN, PMC); cardiopulmonary clinical nurse specialist/adult nurse practitioner (MSN, PMC); family nurse practitioner (MSN, PMC); gerontology clinical nurse specialist (MSN, PMC); gerontology clinical nurse specialist geriatric nurse practitioner (PMC); gerontology clinical nurse specialist/geriatric nurse practitioner (MSN); health services administration (MSN, PMC); nursing of children clinical nurse specialist (MSN, PMC); nursing of children clinical nurse specialist/pediatric nurse practitioner (MSN, PMC); oncology/immune deficiency clinical nurse specialist (MSN, PMC); oncology/immune deficiency clinical nurse specialist/adult nurse practitioner (MSN, PMC); perinatal/women's health clinical nurse specialist (MSN, PMC); perinatal/women's health clinical nurse specialist/women's health nurse practitioner (MSN, PMC); psychiatric nursing clinical nurse specialist (MSN, PMC). *Accreditation:* AACN. Part-time and evening/weekend programs available. Postbaccalaureate distance learning degree programs offered (minimal on-campus study). *Degree requirements:* For master's, thesis optional. *Entrance requirements:* For master's, BSN, interview, RN license. Electronic applications accepted. *Faculty research:* Marriage and chronic illness, health promotion, congestive heart failure patient outcomes, school nursing, diabetes in children, culture, health disparities, cardiovascular, prison nursing, oncology, public policy, child obesity, smoking and teen pregnancy, blood pressure measurements, men's health.

University of Florida, Graduate School, College of Nursing, Gainesville, FL 32611. Offers clinical and translational science (PhD); nursing (MSN); nursing sciences (DNP). *Accreditation:* AACN; ACNM/ACME (one or more programs are accredited). Part-time programs available. *Faculty:* 13 full-time (11 women), 5 part-time/adjunct (3 women). *Students:* 72 full-time (64 women), 55 part-time (49 women); includes 20 minority (5 Black or African American, non-Hispanic/Latino; 4 Asian, non-Hispanic/Latino; 11 Hispanic/Latino), 4 international. Average age 36. 51 applicants, 27% accepted, 13 enrolled. In 2013, 79 master's, 5 doctorates awarded. *Degree requirements:* For master's, thesis optional; for doctorate, thesis/dissertation. *Entrance requirements:* For master's and doctorate, GRE General Test, minimum GPA of 3.0. Additional exam requirements/recommendations for international students: Required—TOEFL (minimum score 550 paper-based; 80 iBT), IELTS (minimum score 6). *Application deadline:* For fall admission, 3/15 priority date for domestic students, 3/15 for international students. Applications are processed on a rolling basis. Application fee: $30. Electronic applications accepted. *Expenses:* Tuition, state resident: full-time $12,640. Tuition, nonresident: full-time $30,000. *Financial support:* In 2013–14, 5 students received support, including 5 fellowships with partial tuition reimbursements available (averaging $24,000 per year); career-related internships or fieldwork and Federal Work-Study also available. Support available to part-time students. Financial award applicants required to submit FAFSA. *Faculty research:* Aging and health: cancer survivorship, interventions to promote healthy aging, and symptom management; women's health, fetal and infant development; biobehavioral interventions: interrelationships among the biological, behavioral, psychological, social and spiritual factors that influence wellness and disease; health policy: influence of local and national policy on physical and psychological health. *Unit head:* Anna M. McDaniel, PhD, Dean, College of Nursing, 352-273-6324, Fax: 352-273-6505, E-mail: annammcdaniel@ufl.edu. *Application contact:* Bridgette Hart-Sams, Coordinator, Student Academic Services, 352-273-6331, Fax: 352-273-6440, E-mail: bhart@ufl.edu.
Website: http://nursing.ufl.edu/

University of Hartford, College of Education, Nursing, and Health Professions, Program in Nursing, West Hartford, CT 06117-1599. Offers community/public health nursing (MSN); nursing education (MSN); nursing management (MSN). *Accreditation:* AACN. Part-time and evening/weekend programs available. *Degree requirements:* For master's, research project. *Entrance requirements:* For master's, BSN, Connecticut RN license. Additional exam requirements/recommendations for international students: Required—TOEFL (minimum score 550 paper-based). Electronic applications accepted. *Expenses:* Contact institution. *Faculty research:* Child development, women in doctoral study, applying feminist theory in teaching methods, near death experience, grandmothers as primary care providers.

University of Hawaii at Hilo, Program in Nursing Practice, Hilo, HI 96720-4091. Offers DNP. *Faculty:* 2 full-time (both women), 5 part-time/adjunct (all women). *Students:* 22 full-time (20 women); includes 14 minority (4 Asian, non-Hispanic/Latino; 2 Hispanic/Latino; 2 Native Hawaiian or other Pacific Islander, non-Hispanic/Latino; 6 Two or more races, non-Hispanic/Latino). Average age 39. 24 applicants, 71% accepted, 13 enrolled. *Entrance requirements:* Additional exam requirements/recommendations for international students: Required—TOEFL, IELTS. *Application deadline:* For fall admission, 2/1 priority date for domestic students. Application fee: $50. Electronic applications accepted. *Expenses:* Tuition, state resident: full-time $4668. Tuition, nonresident: full-time $10,704. Tuition and fees vary according to course load and program. *Financial support:* Application deadline: 3/1; applicants required to submit FAFSA. *Unit head:* Alice Davis, Program Director, 808-932-7067, Fax: 808-932-7066. *Application contact:* UH Hilo Admissions Office, 808-932-7446, Fax: 808-932-7459, E-mail: uhhadm@hawaii.edu.
Website: http://hilo.hawaii.edu/depts/nursing/dnp/

University of Hawaii at Manoa, Graduate Division, School of Nursing and Dental Hygiene, Honolulu, HI 96822. Offers clinical nurse specialist (MS), including adult health, community mental health; nurse practitioner (MS), including adult health, community mental health, family nurse practitioner; nursing (PhD, Graduate Certificate); nursing administration (MS). *Accreditation:* AACN. Part-time programs available. Postbaccalaureate distance learning degree programs offered (minimal on-campus study). *Degree requirements:* For master's, thesis optional; for doctorate, comprehensive exam, thesis/dissertation. *Entrance requirements:* For master's, Hawaii RN license. Additional exam requirements/recommendations for international students: Required—TOEFL (minimum score 580 paper-based; 92 iBT), IELTS (minimum score 5). *Expenses:* Contact institution.

University of Houston–Victoria, School of Nursing, Victoria, TX 77901-4450. Offers family nurse practitioner (MSN); nursing administration (MSN); nursing education (MSN). *Accreditation:* AACN. *Faculty:* 13 full-time (12 women). *Students:* 27 full-time (23 women), 42 part-time (35 women); includes 33 minority (18 Black or African American, non-Hispanic/Latino; 8 Asian, non-Hispanic/Latino; 7 Hispanic/Latino), 7 international. *Entrance requirements:* For master's, GRE or MAT, minimum GPA of 3.0 in last 60 hours of academic course work, valid Texas RN licensure, 2 letters of recommendation. *Application deadline:* For fall admission, 7/15 for domestic students, 6/1 for international students. Applications are processed on a rolling basis. Electronic applications accepted. *Expenses:* Tuition, state resident: full-time $4534; part-time $251 per credit hour. Tuition, nonresident: full-time $10,906; part-time $606 per contact hour. *Required fees:* $68 per semester hour. Tuition and fees vary according to course load. *Financial support:* Federal Work-Study, scholarships/grants, and unspecified assistantships available. Support available to part-time students. Financial award application deadline: 4/15. *Unit head:* Dr. Kathryn Tart, Dean, 361-570-4295, E-mail: neilld@uhv.edu. *Application contact:* Tammy Whatley, Senior Recruitment Coordinator, 361-570-4297, E-mail: whatleyt@uhv.edu.
Website: http://www.uhv.edu/nursing/

University of Illinois at Chicago, Graduate College, College of Nursing, Chicago, IL 60607-7128. Offers MS, DNP, PhD, Certificate, MBA/MS, MPH/MS. *Accreditation:* AACN. Part-time programs available. *Faculty:* 101 full-time (94 women), 84 part-time/adjunct (78 women). *Students:* 416 full-time (381 women), 499 part-time (447 women); includes 227 minority (55 Black or African American, non-Hispanic/Latino; 1 American Indian or Alaska Native, non-Hispanic/Latino; 77 Asian, non-Hispanic/Latino; 76 Hispanic/Latino; 2 Native Hawaiian or other Pacific Islander, non-Hispanic/Latino; 16 Two or more races, non-Hispanic/Latino), 33 international. Average age 33. 576 applicants, 72% accepted, 222 enrolled. In 2013, 188 master's, 30 doctorates, 2 other advanced degrees awarded. *Degree requirements:* For master's, thesis or alternative; for doctorate, thesis/dissertation. *Entrance requirements:* For master's and doctorate, GRE General Test, minimum GPA of 2.75. Additional exam requirements/recommendations for international students: Required—TOEFL. *Application deadline:* For fall admission, 5/15 for domestic students, 2/1 for international students; for spring admission, 10/15 for domestic students. Applications are processed on a rolling basis. Application fee: $40 ($50 for international students). Electronic applications accepted. *Expenses:* Contact institution. *Financial support:* In 2013–14, 3 fellowships with full tuition reimbursements were awarded; research assistantships with full tuition reimbursements, teaching assistantships with full tuition reimbursements, career-related internships or fieldwork, Federal Work-Study, institutionally sponsored loans, scholarships/grants, traineeships, tuition waivers (full and partial), and unspecified assistantships also available. Support available to part-time students. Financial award application deadline: 3/1; financial award applicants required to submit FAFSA. *Total annual research expenditures:* $7.1 million. *Unit head:* Dr. Terri E. Weaver, Dean, 312-996-7808, E-mail: teweaver@uic.edu. *Application contact:* Receptionist, 312-413-2550, E-mail: gradcoll@uic.edu.
Website: http://www.nursing.uic.edu

University of Indianapolis, Graduate Programs, School of Nursing, Indianapolis, IN 46227-3697. Offers advanced practice nursing (DNP); family nurse practitioner (MSN); gerontological nurse practitioner (MSN); neonatal nurse practitioner (MSN); nurse-midwifery (MSN); nursing (MSN); nursing and health systems leadership (MSN); nursing education (MSN); women's health nurse practitioner (MSN); MBA/MSN. *Accreditation:* AACN; ACNM. *Faculty:* 5 full-time (4 women), 1 part-time/adjunct (0 women). *Students:* 15 full-time (14 women), 285 part-time (270 women); includes 42 minority (24 Black or African American, non-Hispanic/Latino; 6 Asian, non-Hispanic/Latino; 3 Hispanic/Latino; 9 Two or more races, non-Hispanic/Latino), 2 international. Average age 35. In 2013, 46 master's awarded. *Entrance requirements:* For master's, minimum GPA of 3.0, interview, letters of recommendation, resume, IN nursing license, 1 year of professional practice; for doctorate, graduate of NLNAC- or CCNE-accredited nursing program; MSN or MA with nursing major and minimum cumulative GPA of 3.25; unencumbered RN license with eligibility for licensure in Indiana; completion of graduate-level statistics course within last 5 years with minimum grade of B; resume; essay; official transcripts from all academic institutions. Additional exam requirements/recommendations for international students: Required—TOEFL (minimum score 550 paper-based). *Application deadline:* For fall admission, 8/1 for domestic students; for winter admission, 12/15 for domestic students; for spring admission, 4/15 for domestic students. Applications are processed on a rolling basis. Application fee: $60. Electronic applications accepted. *Expenses: Tuition:* Full-time $5436; part-time $810 per credit hour. *Financial support:* Federal Work-Study available. *Unit head:* Dr. Anne Thomas, Dean, 317-788-3206, E-mail: athomas@uindy.edu. *Application contact:* Sueann Meagher, Graduate Administrative Assistant, 317-788-8005, Fax: 317-788-3542, E-mail: meaghers@uindy.edu.
Website: http://nursing.uindy.edu/

The University of Iowa, Graduate College, College of Nursing, Iowa City, IA 52242-1316. Offers MSN, DNP, PhD. *Accreditation:* AACN; AANA/CANAEP (one or more programs are accredited). *Degree requirements:* For master's, thesis optional, portfolio, project; for doctorate, comprehensive exam, thesis/dissertation. *Entrance requirements:* For master's, minimum GPA of 3.0; for doctorate, GRE General Test, minimum GPA of 3.0. Additional exam requirements/recommendations for international students: Required—TOEFL (minimum score 550 paper-based; 81 iBT). Electronic applications accepted. *Expenses:* Contact institution.

The University of Kansas, University of Kansas Medical Center, School of Nursing, Kansas City, KS 66160. Offers adult/gerontological clinical nurse specialist (PMC); adult/gerontological nurse practitioner (PMC); clinical research management (PMC); health care informatics (PMC); health professions educator (PMC); nurse midwife (PMC); nursing (MS, DNP, PhD); organizational leadership (PMC); psychiatric/mental health nurse practitioner (PMC); public health nursing (PMC). *Accreditation:* AACN; ACNM/ACME. Part-time programs available. Postbaccalaureate distance learning degree programs offered (minimal on-campus study). *Faculty:* 59. *Students:* 55 full-time (53 women), 323 part-time (303 women); includes 57 minority (23 Black or African American, non-Hispanic/Latino; 14 Asian, non-Hispanic/Latino; 16 Hispanic/Latino; 1 Native Hawaiian or other Pacific Islander, non-Hispanic/Latino; 3 Two or more races, non-Hispanic/Latino), 1 international. Average age 38. 113 applicants, 59% accepted, 61 enrolled. In 2013, 77 master's, 18 doctorates, 11 other advanced degrees awarded. Terminal master's awarded for partial completion of doctoral program. *Degree requirements:* For master's, comprehensive exam, thesis (for some programs), general oral exam; for doctorate, variable foreign language requirement, thesis/dissertation, comprehensive oral exam (for DNP); comprehensive written and oral exam (for PhD). *Entrance requirements:* For master's, bachelor's degree in nursing, minimum GPA of 3.0, 1 year of clinical experience, RN license in KS and MO; for doctorate, GRE General Test, bachelor's degree in nursing, minimum GPA of 3.5, RN license in KS and MO. Additional exam requirements/recommendations for international students: Required—TOEFL. *Application deadline:* For fall admission, 4/1 for domestic and international students; for spring admission, 9/1 for domestic and international students. Application fee: $60. Electronic applications accepted. *Financial support:* Research assistantships with full and partial tuition reimbursements, teaching assistantships with full and partial tuition reimbursements, scholarships/grants, and traineeships available. Financial award application deadline: 3/1; financial award applicants required to submit FAFSA. *Faculty research:* Breastfeeding practices of teen mothers, national database of nursing quality indicators, caregiving of families of patients using technology in the home, simulation in nursing education, diaphragm fatigue. *Total annual research expenditures:* $6.4 million.

Unit head: Dr. Karen L. Miller, Dean, 913-588-1601, Fax: 913-588-1660, E-mail: kmiller@kumc.edu. *Application contact:* Dr. Pamela K. Barnes, Associate Dean, Student Affairs, 913-588-1619, Fax: 913-588-1615, E-mail: pbarnes2@kumc.edu.
Website: http://nursing.kumc.edu

University of Kentucky, Graduate School, College of Nursing, Lexington, KY 40506-0032. Offers DNP, PhD. *Degree requirements:* For doctorate, comprehensive exam, thesis/dissertation. *Entrance requirements:* For doctorate, GRE General Test, minimum undergraduate GPA of 3.0. Additional exam requirements/recommendations for international students: Required—TOEFL (minimum score 550 paper-based). Electronic applications accepted.

University of Lethbridge, School of Graduate Studies, Lethbridge, AB T1K 3M4, Canada. Offers accounting (MScM); addictions counseling (M Sc); agricultural biotechnology (M Sc); agricultural studies (M Sc, MA); anthropology (MA); archaeology (M Sc, MA); art (MA, MFA); biochemistry (M Sc); biological sciences (M Sc); biomolecular science (PhD); biosystems and biodiversity (PhD); Canadian studies (MA); chemistry (M Sc); computer science (M Sc); computer science and geographical information science (M Sc); counseling (MC); counseling psychology (M Ed); dramatic arts (MA); earth, space, and physical science (PhD); economics (MA); education (MA); educational leadership (M Ed); English (MA); environmental science (M Sc); evolution and behavior (PhD); exercise science (M Sc); finance (MScM); French (MA); French/German (MA); French/Spanish (MA); general education (M Ed); general management (MScM); geography (M Sc, MA); German (MA); health sciences (M Sc); human resource management and labour relations (MScM); individualized multidisciplinary (M Sc, MA); information systems (MScM); international management (MScM); kinesiology (M Sc, MA); marketing (MScM); mathematics (M Sc); modern languages (MA); music (M Mus, MA); Native American studies (MA); neuroscience (M Sc, PhD); new media (MA, MFA); nursing (M Sc); philosophy (MA); physics (M Sc); policy and strategy (MScM); political science (MA); psychology (M Sc, MA); religious studies (MA); sociology (MA); theatre and dramatic arts (MFA); theoretical and computational science (PhD); urban and regional studies (MA); women and gender studies (MA). Part-time and evening/weekend programs available. *Degree requirements:* For doctorate, comprehensive exam, thesis/dissertation. *Entrance requirements:* For master's, GMAT (for M Sc in management), bachelor's degree in related field, minimum GPA of 3.0 during previous 20 graded semester courses, 2 years teaching or related experience (M Ed); for doctorate, master's degree, minimum graduate GPA of 3.5. Additional exam requirements/recommendations for international students: Required—TOEFL. Application fee: $60 Canadian dollars. *Financial support:* Fellowships, research assistantships, teaching assistantships, scholarships/grants, health care benefits, and unspecified assistantships available. *Faculty research:* Movement and brain plasticity, gibberellin physiology, photosynthesis, carbon cycling, molecular properties of main-group ring components. *Application contact:* School of Graduate Studies, 403-329-2793, Fax: 403-332-5239, E-mail: sgsinquiries@uleth.ca.
Website: http://www.uleth.ca/graduatestudies/

University of Louisiana at Lafayette, College of Nursing, Lafayette, LA 70504. Offers MSN. Program offered jointly with Southern Louisiana University, McNeese State University, Southern University and Agricultural and Mechanical College. *Accreditation:* AACN. *Degree requirements:* For master's, thesis or alternative. *Entrance requirements:* For master's, GRE General Test, minimum GPA of 2.75. Additional exam requirements/recommendations for international students: Required—TOEFL (minimum score 550 paper-based). Electronic applications accepted.

University of Louisville, Graduate School, School of Nursing, Louisville, KY 40202. Offers adult nurse practitioner (MSN); family nurse practitioner (MSN); health professions education (MSN); neonatal nurse practitioner (MSN); nursing research (PhD); psychiatric mental health nurse practitioner (MSN). *Accreditation:* AACN. Part-time programs available. *Students:* 91 full-time (81 women), 47 part-time (42 women); includes 16 minority (8 Black or African American, non-Hispanic/Latino; 3 Asian, non-Hispanic/Latino; 3 Hispanic/Latino; 2 Two or more races, non-Hispanic/Latino), 6 international. Average age 36. 58 applicants, 74% accepted, 36 enrolled. In 2013, 33 master's, 3 doctorates awarded. Terminal master's awarded for partial completion of doctoral program. *Degree requirements:* For master's, thesis optional; for doctorate, comprehensive exam, thesis/dissertation. *Entrance requirements:* For master's, GRE General Test, bachelor's degree in nursing, minimum GPA of 3.0, RN license; for doctorate, GRE General Test, BSN or MSN with recommended minimum GPA of 3.0. Additional exam requirements/recommendations for international students: Required—TOEFL. *Application deadline:* For fall admission, 4/1 priority date for domestic students, 4/1 for international students. Applications are processed on a rolling basis. Application fee: $60. Electronic applications accepted. *Expenses:* Tuition, state resident: full-time $10,788; part-time $599 per credit hour. Tuition, nonresident: full-time $22,446; part-time $1247 per credit hour. *Required fees:* $196. Tuition and fees vary according to program and reciprocity agreements. *Financial support:* Fellowships with full tuition reimbursements, research assistantships with full tuition reimbursements, teaching assistantships with full tuition reimbursements, institutionally sponsored loans, scholarships/grants, traineeships, health care benefits, and unspecified assistantships available. Support available to part-time students. Financial award application deadline: 4/15; financial award applicants required to submit FAFSA. *Faculty research:* Maternal-child/family stress after pregnancy loss, postpartum depression, access to healthcare (underserved populations), quality of life issues, physical activity (impact on chronic/acute conditions). *Total annual research expenditures:* $718,934. *Unit head:* Dr. Marcia J. Hern, Dean, 502-852-8300, Fax: 502-852-5044, E-mail: m.hern@gwise.louisville.edu. *Application contact:* Dr. Lee Ridner, Interim Associate Dean for Academic Affairs and Director of MSN Programs, 502-852-8518, Fax: 502-852-0704, E-mail: romain01@louisville.edu.
Website: http://www.louisville.edu/nursing/

University of Maine, Graduate School, College of Natural Sciences, Forestry, and Agriculture, School of Nursing, Orono, ME 04469. Offers individualized (MS, CAS); nursing education (CGS); rural health family nurse practitioner (MS, CAS). *Accreditation:* AACN. *Faculty:* 17 full-time (13 women), 7 part-time/adjunct (3 women). *Students:* 10 full-time (8 women), 12 part-time (all women); includes 3 minority (2 American Indian or Alaska Native, non-Hispanic/Latino; 1 Hispanic/Latino), 1 international. Average age 38. 12 applicants, 50% accepted, 5 enrolled. In 2013, 8 master's, 2 other advanced degrees awarded. *Entrance requirements:* For master's, GRE General Test; for other advanced degree, master's degree. Additional exam requirements/recommendations for international students: Required—TOEFL. *Application deadline:* For fall admission, 2/1 for domestic students. Applications are processed on a rolling basis. Application fee: $65. Electronic applications accepted. *Expenses:* Tuition, state resident: full-time $7524. Tuition, nonresident: full-time $23,112. *Required fees:* $1970. *Financial support:* In 2013–14, 4 students received support. Career-related internships or fieldwork, Federal Work-Study, institutionally sponsored loans, and tuition waivers (full and partial) available. Support available to part-time students. Financial award application deadline: 3/1. *Unit head:* Dr. Nancy Fishwick, Director, 207-581-2505, Fax: 207-581-2585. *Application contact:* Scott G. Delcourt, Associate Dean of the Graduate School, 207-581-3291, Fax: 207-581-3232, E-mail: graduate@maine.edu.
Website: http://umaine.edu/nursing/

The University of Manchester, School of Nursing, Midwifery and Social Work, Manchester, United Kingdom. Offers nursing (M Phil, PhD); social work (M Phil, PhD).

University of Manitoba, Faculty of Graduate Studies, Faculty of Nursing, Winnipeg, MB R3T 2N2, Canada. Offers cancer nursing (MN); nursing (MN). *Degree requirements:* For master's, thesis.

University of Mary, School of Health Sciences, Division of Nursing, Bismarck, ND 58504-9652. Offers family nurse practitioner (MSN); nurse administrator (MSN); nursing educator (MSN). *Accreditation:* AACN. Part-time and evening/weekend programs available. Postbaccalaureate distance learning degree programs offered (minimal on-campus study). *Degree requirements:* For master's, comprehensive exam (for some programs), thesis (for some programs), internship (family nurse practitioner), teaching practice. *Entrance requirements:* For master's, minimum GPA of 2.75 in nursing, interview, letters of recommendation, criminal background check, immunizations, statement of professional goals. Additional exam requirements/recommendations for international students: Required—TOEFL (minimum score 500 paper-based; 71 iBT). Electronic applications accepted. *Faculty research:* Gerontology issues, rural nursing, health policy, primary care, women's health.

University of Mary Hardin-Baylor, Graduate Studies in Nursing, Belton, TX 76513. Offers clinical nurse leader (MSN); family nurse practitioner (MSN, Post-Master's Certificate); nurse educator (Post-Master's Certificate); nursing education (MSN). *Accreditation:* AACN. Part-time and evening/weekend programs available. *Faculty:* 6 full-time (all women), 4 part-time/adjunct (3 women). *Students:* 44 full-time (all women), 6 part-time (all women); includes 13 minority (5 Black or African American, non-Hispanic/Latino; 2 Asian, non-Hispanic/Latino; 6 Hispanic/Latino). Average age 33. 57 applicants, 67% accepted, 31 enrolled. In 2013, 17 master's awarded. *Degree requirements:* For master's, practicum. *Entrance requirements:* For master's, full-time RN for 1 year, BSN, minimum GPA of 3.0 in last 60 hours of undergraduate program, two letters of recommendation. Additional exam requirements/recommendations for international students: Required—TOEFL (minimum score 550 paper-based; 80 iBT), IELTS (minimum score 6). *Application deadline:* For fall admission, 4/15 for domestic students, 4/15 priority date for international students; for spring admission, 11/1 for domestic students, 10/15 priority date for international students. Applications are processed on a rolling basis. Application fee: $35 ($135 for international students). Electronic applications accepted. *Expenses: Tuition:* Full-time $14,130; part-time $785 per credit hour. *Required fees:* $1350; $75 per credit hour. $50 per term. *Financial support:* Applicants required to submit FAFSA. *Unit head:* Dr. Carrie Johnson, Associate Professor/Director, Master of Science in Nursing Programs, 254-295-4178, E-mail: cjohnson@umhb.edu. *Application contact:* Melissa Ford, Director of Graduate Admissions, 254-295-4020, Fax: 254-295-5038, E-mail: mford@umhb.edu.
Website: http://graduate.umhb.edu/nursing/

University of Maryland, Baltimore, Graduate School, School of Nursing, Doctoral Program in Nursing, Baltimore, MD 21201. Offers PhD. *Students:* 24 full-time (21 women), 33 part-time (27 women); includes 16 minority (8 Black or African American, non-Hispanic/Latino; 4 Asian, non-Hispanic/Latino; 3 Hispanic/Latino; 1 Two or more races, non-Hispanic/Latino), 14 international. Average age 40. 65 applicants, 49% accepted, 16 enrolled. In 2013, 14 doctorates awarded. *Degree requirements:* For doctorate, thesis/dissertation. *Entrance requirements:* For doctorate, GRE General Test, minimum GPA of 3.0, MS in nursing. Additional exam requirements/recommendations for international students: Required—TOEFL (minimum score 550 paper-based; 80 iBT); Recommended—IELTS (minimum score 7). *Application deadline:* For fall admission, 2/15 for domestic students, 1/15 for international students. Application fee: $75. Electronic applications accepted. *Financial support:* Fellowships, research assistantships, and teaching assistantships available. Financial award application deadline: 2/15; financial award applicants required to submit FAFSA. *Faculty research:* Aging populations, cardiovascular health, health systems outcomes, implementation science, occupational health, pain and symptom science, palliative and end-of-life care. *Unit head:* Dr. Meg Johantgen, Director, 410-706-0520, Fax: 410-706-3769, E-mail: johantgen@son.umaryland.edu. *Application contact:* Janice Anarino, Program Coordinator, 410-706-3147, E-mail: janar001@son.umaryland.edu.
Website: http://nursing.umaryland.edu/

University of Maryland, Baltimore, Graduate School, School of Nursing, Doctor of Nursing Practice Program, Baltimore, MD 21201. Offers DNP. *Students:* 10 full-time (all women), 79 part-time (72 women); includes 23 minority (17 Black or African American, non-Hispanic/Latino; 1 American Indian or Alaska Native, non-Hispanic/Latino; 1 Asian, non-Hispanic/Latino; 3 Hispanic/Latino; 1 Two or more races, non-Hispanic/Latino). Average age 47. 66 applicants, 61% accepted, 31 enrolled. In 2013, 17 doctorates awarded. *Unit head:* Dr. Jane Kapustin, Professor/Director of Master's Program, 410-706-3890. *Application contact:* Keith T. Brooks, Assistant Dean, 410-706-7131, Fax: 410-706-3473, E-mail: kbrooks@umaryland.edu.
Website: http://nursing.umaryland.edu/academic-programs/grad/doctoral-degree/dnp

University of Maryland, Baltimore, Graduate School, School of Nursing, Master's Program in Nursing, Baltimore, MD 21201. Offers community health nursing (MS); gerontological nursing (MS); maternal-child nursing (MS); medical-surgical nursing (MS); nurse-midwifery education (MS); nursing administration (MS); nursing education (MS); nursing health policy (MS); primary care nursing (MS); psychiatric nursing (MS); MS/MBA. MS/MBA offered jointly with University of Baltimore. *Accreditation:* AACN; AANA/CANAEP. Part-time programs available. *Students:* 345 full-time (297 women), 508 part-time (469 women); includes 288 minority (152 Black or African American, non-Hispanic/Latino; 2 American Indian or Alaska Native, non-Hispanic/Latino; 72 Asian, non-Hispanic/Latino; 32 Hispanic/Latino; 1 Native Hawaiian or other Pacific Islander, non-Hispanic/Latino; 29 Two or more races, non-Hispanic/Latino), 13 international. Average age 33. 971 applicants, 34% accepted, 253 enrolled. In 2013, 308 master's awarded. *Degree requirements:* For master's, comprehensive exam (for some programs), thesis or alternative. *Entrance requirements:* For master's, minimum GPA of 2.75, course work in statistics, BS in nursing. Additional exam requirements/recommendations for international students: Required—TOEFL (minimum score 550 paper-based; 80 iBT) or IELTS (minimum score 7). *Application deadline:* For fall admission, 2/1 for domestic students, 1/15 for international students. Application fee: $75. Electronic applications accepted. *Financial support:* Fellowships, research assistantships, teaching assistantships, career-related internships or fieldwork, and traineeships available. Support available to part-time students. Financial award application deadline: 2/15; financial award applicants required to submit FAFSA. *Unit head:* Dr. Jane Kapustin, Assistant Dean, 410-706-6741, Fax: 410-706-4231. *Application contact:* Marjorie Fass, Admissions Director, 410-706-0501, Fax: 410-706-7238.

University of Maryland, Baltimore, Graduate School, School of Nursing, Post Baccalaureate Certificate Program in Nursing, Baltimore, MD 21201. Offers Postbaccalaureate Certificate. *Students:* 6 part-time (all women); includes 1 minority (Black or African American, non-Hispanic/Latino). Average age 50. 53 applicants, 23%

accepted, 3 enrolled. *Entrance requirements:* Additional exam requirements/recommendations for international students: Required—TOEFL (minimum score 550 paper-based; 80 iBT); Recommended—IELTS (minimum score 7). *Application deadline:* For fall admission, 5/1 for domestic students, 1/15 for international students. Application fee: $75. Electronic applications accepted. *Unit head:* Dr. Jane Kapustin, Professor/Director of Master's Program, 410-706-3890. *Application contact:* Marjorie Fass, Admissions Director, 410-706-0501, E-mail: fass@son.umaryland.edu.

University of Massachusetts Amherst, Graduate School, School of Nursing, Amherst, MA 01003. Offers adult gerontology primary care (DNP); clinical nurse leader (MS); family nurse practitioner (DNP); nursing (PhD); public health nurse leader (DNP). *Accreditation:* AACN. Part-time programs available. Postbaccalaureate distance learning degree programs offered (minimal on-campus study). *Faculty:* 16 full-time (15 women). *Students:* 74 full-time (61 women), 161 part-time (149 women); includes 62 minority (31 Black or African American, non-Hispanic/Latino; 9 Asian, non-Hispanic/Latino; 19 Hispanic/Latino; 3 Two or more races, non-Hispanic/Latino), 6 international. Average age 40. 133 applicants, 80% accepted, 68 enrolled. In 2013, 9 master's, 32 doctorates awarded. Terminal master's awarded for partial completion of doctoral program. *Degree requirements:* For master's, thesis optional; for doctorate, comprehensive exam, thesis/dissertation. *Entrance requirements:* Additional exam requirements/recommendations for international students: Required—TOEFL (minimum score 550 paper-based; 80 iBT), IELTS (minimum score 6.5). *Application deadline:* For fall admission, 12/15 for domestic and international students. Applications are processed on a rolling basis. Application fee: $75. Electronic applications accepted. *Financial support:* Fellowships with full and partial tuition reimbursements, research assistantships with full and partial tuition reimbursements, teaching assistantships with full and partial tuition reimbursements, career-related internships or fieldwork, Federal Work-Study, scholarships/grants, traineeships, health care benefits, tuition waivers (full and partial), and unspecified assistantships available. Support available to part-time students. Financial award application deadline: 2/1. *Faculty research:* Health of older adults and their caretakers, mental health of individuals and families, health of children and adolescents, power and decision-making, transcultural health. *Unit head:* Dr. Stephen J. Cavanagh, Dean, 413-545-2703, Fax: 413-577-2550, E-mail: dean@nursing.umass.edu. *Application contact:* Lindsay DeSantis, Supervisor of Admissions, 413-545-0722, Fax: 413-577-0010, E-mail: gradadm@grad.umass.edu.
Website: http://www.umass.edu/nursing/

University of Massachusetts Boston, Office of Graduate Studies, College of Nursing and Health Sciences, Boston, MA 02125-3393. Offers MS, PhD, MS/MBA. *Accreditation:* AACN. Part-time and evening/weekend programs available. *Degree requirements:* For master's, comprehensive exam; for doctorate, comprehensive exam, thesis/dissertation. *Entrance requirements:* For master's, minimum GPA of 2.75; for doctorate, GRE General Test, master's degree, minimum GPA of 3.3. *Faculty research:* Domestic abuse and pregnancy, health policy and home health care, caregiving burdens of families, the chronically ill, health care delivery models and their impact on outcomes, health promotion and disease prevention among the elderly.

University of Massachusetts Dartmouth, Graduate School, College of Nursing, Programs in Nursing, North Dartmouth, MA 02747-2300. Offers adult gerontology primary care nurse practitioner (DNP); adult health clinical nurse specialist (DNP); adult health/adult nurse practitioner (MS); adult health/advanced practice (MS); adult health/nurse educator (MS); adult health/nurse manager (MS); adult nurse practitioner (PMC); community health nurse specialist (DNP); community nursing/advanced practice (MS); community nursing/nurse educator (MS); community nursing/nurse manager (MS); individualized nursing (PMC); nursing (MS, PhD); nursing practice (DNP). Part-time programs available. *Faculty:* 25 full-time (all women), 45 part-time/adjunct (44 women). *Students:* 103 part-time (95 women); includes 10 minority (4 Black or African American, non-Hispanic/Latino; 2 Asian, non-Hispanic/Latino; 4 Hispanic/Latino). Average age 40. 49 applicants, 92% accepted, 33 enrolled. In 2013, 25 master's, 1 doctorate, 2 other advanced degrees awarded. *Degree requirements:* For master's, thesis; for doctorate, comprehensive exam, thesis/dissertation, project (for DNP only). *Entrance requirements:* For master's, statement of purpose (minimum of 300 words), resume, 3 letters of recommendation, official transcripts, copy of RN license; for doctorate, GRE (for PhD), statement of purpose (minimum of 300 words), resume, 3 letters of recommendation, official transcripts, copy of RN license, scholarly writing sample (minimum 10 pages for PhD). Additional exam requirements/recommendations for international students: Required—TOEFL (minimum score 533 paper-based; 72 iBT). *Application deadline:* For fall admission, 2/15 priority date for domestic and international students. Applications are processed on a rolling basis. Application fee: $60. Electronic applications accepted. *Expenses:* Tuition, state resident: full-time $2071; part-time $86.29 per credit. Tuition, nonresident: full-time $8099; part-time $337.46 per credit. Tuition and fees vary according to course load and reciprocity agreements. *Financial support:* In 2013–14, 5 teaching assistantships with full and partial tuition reimbursements (averaging $7,500 per year) were awarded; Federal Work-Study and unspecified assistantships also available. Support available to part-time students. Financial award application deadline: 3/1; financial award applicants required to submit FAFSA. *Faculty research:* Pathophysiology, aging with spinal cord injury, relational ontology, severe mental illness, patient care. *Total annual research expenditures:* $1,000. *Unit head:* Kerry Fater, Graduate Program Director for Nursing Master's Programs, 508-999-8525, Fax: 508-999-9127, E-mail: kfater@umassd.edu. *Application contact:* Steven Briggs, Director of Marketing and Recruitment for Graduate Studies, 508-999-8604, Fax: 508-999-8183, E-mail: graduate@umassd.edu.
Website: http://www.umassd.edu/nursing/graduateprograms

University of Massachusetts Lowell, College of Health Sciences, School of Nursing, Lowell, MA 01854-2881. Offers adult/gerontological nursing (MS); family health nursing (MS); nursing (DNP, PhD); psychiatric and mental health nursing (MS, Graduate Certificate). *Accreditation:* AACN. *Degree requirements:* For master's, thesis optional; for doctorate, thesis/dissertation. *Entrance requirements:* For master's and doctorate, GRE General Test. *Faculty research:* Gerontology, women's health issues, long-term care, alcoholism, health promotion.

University of Massachusetts Worcester, Graduate School of Nursing, Worcester, MA 01655-0115. Offers advanced practice nursing (DNP); family nurse practitioner (MS); gerontological adult acute care nurse practitioner (MS, Post Master's Certificate); gerontological adult primary care nurse practitioner (Post Master's Certificate); gerontological primary care nurse practitioner (MS); leadership (DNP); nurse educator (MS, Post Master's Certificate); nursing (PhD). *Accreditation:* AACN. *Faculty:* 19 full-time (17 women), 40 part-time/adjunct (33 women). *Students:* 153 full-time (129 women), 35 part-time (28 women); includes 30 minority (18 Black or African American, non-Hispanic/Latino; 7 Asian, non-Hispanic/Latino; 5 Hispanic/Latino). Average age 34. 254 applicants, 31% accepted, 57 enrolled. In 2013, 50 master's, 4 doctorates, 2 other advanced degrees awarded. *Degree requirements:* For doctorate, thesis/dissertation (for some programs), comprehensive exam (for PhD); capstone project and manuscript (for DNP). *Entrance requirements:* For master's, GRE General Test, bachelor's degree in nursing, course work in statistics, unrestricted Massachusetts license as registered nurse; for doctorate, GRE General Test, bachelor's or master's degree; for Post Master's Certificate, GRE General Test, MS in nursing. Additional exam requirements/recommendations for international students: Required—TOEFL. *Application deadline:* For fall admission, 12/1 priority date for domestic students. Applications are processed on a rolling basis. Application fee: $60. Electronic applications accepted. *Expenses:* Contact institution. *Financial support:* In 2013–14, 43 students received support. Institutionally sponsored loans, scholarships/grants, traineeships, and tuition waivers available. Support available to part-time students. Financial award application deadline: 5/16; financial award applicants required to submit FAFSA. *Faculty research:* Decision-making of partners and men with prostate cancer, coinfection (HIV and Hepatitis C) and treatment decisions, parent management of children with Type 1 diabetes, health literacy and discharge planning, Ghanaian women and self-care. *Total annual research expenditures:* $1.5 million. *Unit head:* Dr. Paulette Seymour-Route, Dean, 508-856-5801, Fax: 508-856-6552, E-mail: paulette.seymour-route@umassmed.edu. *Application contact:* Diane Brescia, Admissions Coordinator, 508-856-3488, Fax: 508-856-5851, E-mail: diane.brescia@umassmed.edu.
Website: http://www.umassmed.edu/gsn/

University of Memphis, Loewenberg School of Nursing, Memphis, TN 38152. Offers advance practice-family nurse practitioner (MSN); executive nursing leadership (MSN); nursing (Graduate Certificate); nursing administration (MSN); nursing education (MSN); nursing informatics (MSN). *Accreditation:* AACN. Part-time and evening/weekend programs available. Postbaccalaureate distance learning degree programs offered. *Faculty:* 18 full-time (16 women), 5 part-time/adjunct (0 women). *Students:* 23 full-time (21 women), 240 part-time (214 women); includes 112 minority (100 Black or African American, non-Hispanic/Latino; 9 Asian, non-Hispanic/Latino; 1 Hispanic/Latino; 2 Two or more races, non-Hispanic/Latino), 1 international. Average age 35. 176 applicants, 38% accepted, 25 enrolled. In 2013, 47 master's, 2 other advanced degrees awarded. *Degree requirements:* For master's, comprehensive exam, thesis optional, scholarly project; completion of clinical practicum hours. *Entrance requirements:* For master's, NCLEX Exam, interview. Additional exam requirements/recommendations for international students: Required—TOEFL (minimum score 550 paper-based; 79 iBT). *Application deadline:* For fall admission, 2/15 for domestic and international students; for spring admission, 10/1 for domestic and international students. Application fee: $35 ($60 for international students). *Financial support:* In 2013–14, 147 students received support. Federal Work-Study and scholarships/grants available. Financial award application deadline: 2/15; financial award applicants required to submit FAFSA. *Faculty research:* Technology in nursing, nurse retention, cultural competence, health policy, health access. *Total annual research expenditures:* $560,619. *Unit head:* Dr. Robert Koch, Associate Dean, 901-678-3908, Fax: 901-678-4907, E-mail: rakoch@memphis.edu. *Application contact:* Dr. Karen Weddle-West, Information Contact, 901-678-2531, Fax: 901-678-5023, E-mail: gradsch@memphis.edu.
Website: http://www.memphis.edu/nursing

University of Miami, Graduate School, School of Nursing and Health Studies, Coral Gables, FL 33124. Offers acute care (MSN), including acute care nurse practitioner, nurse anesthesia; nursing (PhD); primary care (MSN), including adult nurse practitioner, family nurse practitioner, nurse midwifery, women's health practitioner. *Accreditation:* AACN; AANA/CANAEP; ACNM/ACME (one or more programs are accredited). Part-time programs available. *Degree requirements:* For master's, thesis optional; for doctorate, thesis/dissertation. *Entrance requirements:* For master's, GRE General Test, BSN, minimum GPA of 3.0, Florida RN license; for doctorate, GRE General Test, BSN or MSN, minimum GPA of 3.0. Additional exam requirements/recommendations for international students: Required—TOEFL (minimum score 550 paper-based). Electronic applications accepted. *Faculty research:* Transcultural nursing, exercise and depression in Alzheimer's disease, infectious diseases/HIV–AIDS, postpartum depression, outcomes assessment.

University of Michigan, Rackham Graduate School, School of Nursing, Ann Arbor, MI 48109. Offers acute care pediatric nurse practitioner (MS); adult-gerontology acute care clinical nurse specialist (MS); adult-gerontology acute care nurse practitioner (MS); adult-gerontology primary care nurse practitioner (MS); health systems, nursing leadership, and effectiveness science (MS); nurse midwife (MS); nurse midwife and family nurse practitioner (MS); nurse midwife and primary care pediatric nurse practitioner (MS); nursing (DNP, PhD, Post Master's Certificate); primary care family nurse practitioner (MS); primary care pediatric nurse practitioner (MS). *Accreditation:* AACN; ACNM/ACME (one or more programs are accredited). Part-time programs available. Postbaccalaureate distance learning degree programs offered (minimal on-campus study). Terminal master's awarded for partial completion of doctoral program. *Degree requirements:* For doctorate, thesis/dissertation. *Application deadline:* For fall admission, 2/1 for domestic students; for winter admission, 5/1 for domestic students; for spring admission, 11/1 for domestic students. Applications are processed on a rolling basis. Electronic applications accepted. Tuition and fees vary according to course level, course load, degree level, program and student level. *Financial support:* Fellowships with full and partial tuition reimbursements, research assistantships with full and partial tuition reimbursements, teaching assistantships with full tuition reimbursements, Federal Work-Study, institutionally sponsored loans, scholarships/grants, traineeships, and tuition waivers (partial) available. Support available to part-time students. *Faculty research:* Preparation of clinical nurse researchers, biobehavior, women's health, health promotion, substance abuse, psychobiology of menopause, fertility, obesity, health care systems. *Unit head:* Dr. Kathleen Potempa, Dean, 734-764-7185, Fax: 734-764-7186. *Application contact:* James Diesing, Graduate Recruiting and Admissions Coordinator, 734-615-4739, E-mail: sn-osams@umich.edu.
Website: http://www.nursing.umich.edu/

University of Michigan–Flint, School of Health Professions and Studies, Program in Nursing, Flint, MI 48502-1950. Offers family nurse practitioner (MSN); nursing (Certificate); nursing practice (DNP). *Accreditation:* AACN. Part-time programs available. *Faculty:* 9 full-time (all women), 6 part-time/adjunct (5 women). *Students:* 98 full-time (85 women), 80 part-time (71 women); includes 35 minority (15 Black or African American, non-Hispanic/Latino; 3 American Indian or Alaska Native, non-Hispanic/Latino; 6 Asian, non-Hispanic/Latino; 4 Hispanic/Latino; 1 Native Hawaiian or other Pacific Islander, non-Hispanic/Latino; 6 Two or more races, non-Hispanic/Latino), 3 international. Average age 39. 157 applicants, 38% accepted, 55 enrolled. In 2013, 15 master's, 18 doctorates awarded. *Degree requirements:* For master's, thesis. *Entrance requirements:* For master's, current Michigan RN license, minimum GPA of 3.2, three or more credits in college-level chemistry with minimum C grade, three or more credits in college-level statistics with minimum C grade. Additional exam requirements/recommendations for international students: Required—TOEFL (minimum score 560 paper-based; 84 iBT), IELTS (minimum score 6.5). *Application deadline:* For fall admission, 8/1 priority date for domestic students, 5/1 priority date for international students; for winter admission, 11/15 priority date for domestic students, 9/1 priority date for international students; for spring admission, 3/15 priority date for domestic students, 1/1 priority date for international students. Application fee: $55. Electronic applications accepted. *Expenses:* Contact institution. *Financial support:* Federal Work-Study, scholarships/grants, and unspecified assistantships available. Support available to part-time students. Financial award application deadline: 3/1; financial award applicants required to submit FAFSA. *Faculty research:* Family system stress, self breast exam, family roads evaluation, causal model testing for psychosocial development, basic needs. *Unit head:* Dr. Constance J. Creech, Director, 810-762-3420, Fax: 810-766-

6851, E-mail: ccreech@umflint.edu. *Application contact:* Bradley T. Maki, Director of Graduate Admissions, 810-762-3171, Fax: 810-766-6789, E-mail: bmaki@umflint.edu. Website: http://www.umflint.edu/graduateprograms/nursing.htm

University of Minnesota, Twin Cities Campus, Graduate School, School of Nursing, Minneapolis, MN 55455-0213. Offers MN, MS, DNP, PhD. *Accreditation:* AACN; AANA/CANAEP; ACNM/ACME (one or more programs are accredited). Part-time programs available. Postbaccalaureate distance learning degree programs offered (minimal on-campus study). Terminal master's awarded for partial completion of doctoral program. *Degree requirements:* For master's, final oral exam, project or thesis; for doctorate, thesis/dissertation. *Entrance requirements:* For master's and doctorate, GRE General Test. Additional exam requirements/recommendations for international students: Required—TOEFL (minimum score 586 paper-based). *Expenses:* Contact institution. *Faculty research:* Child and family health promotion, nursing research on elders.

University of Mississippi Medical Center, School of Nursing, Jackson, MS 39216-4505. Offers MSN, DNP, PhD. *Accreditation:* AACN. Part-time and evening/weekend programs available. Postbaccalaureate distance learning degree programs offered (minimal on-campus study). *Degree requirements:* For master's, thesis optional; for doctorate, comprehensive exam, thesis/dissertation, publishable paper. *Entrance requirements:* For master's, GRE, 1 year of clinical experience (acute care nurse practitioner only), RN license; for doctorate, GRE, RN license, professional nursing experience. Additional exam requirements/recommendations for international students: Required—TOEFL (minimum score 550 paper-based; 79 iBT). Electronic applications accepted. *Expenses:* Contact institution. *Faculty research:* Predictive biomarkers for head and neck cancer; cellular events in response to demyelization in diseases; health care disparities (various diseases); childhood obesity; psychosocial adaptations to pregnancy and birth.

University of Missouri, Graduate School, Sinclair School of Nursing, Columbia, MO 65211. Offers adult-gerontology clinical nurse specialist (DNP, Certificate); family nurse practitioner (DNP); family psychiatric and mental health nurse practitioner (DNP); nursing (MS, PhD); nursing leadership and innovations in health care (DNP); pediatric clinical nurse specialist (DNP, Certificate); pediatric nurse practitioner (DNP). *Accreditation:* AACN. Part-time programs available. *Faculty:* 20 full-time (18 women), 6 part-time/adjunct (all women). *Students:* 60 full-time (58 women), 232 part-time (211 women); includes 24 minority (9 Black or African American, non-Hispanic/Latino; 4 American Indian or Alaska Native, non-Hispanic/Latino; 2 Asian, non-Hispanic/Latino; 6 Hispanic/Latino; 3 Two or more races, non-Hispanic/Latino), 4 international. Average age 37. 131 applicants, 62% accepted, 61 enrolled. In 2013, 42 master's, 2 doctorates, 7 other advanced degrees awarded. *Degree requirements:* For master's, thesis optional, oral exam; for doctorate, thesis/dissertation. *Entrance requirements:* For master's, GRE General Test, BSN, minimum GPA of 3.0 during last 60 hours, nursing license. Additional exam requirements/recommendations for international students: Required—TOEFL (minimum score 550 paper-based; 79 iBT). *Application deadline:* For fall admission, 2/1 priority date for domestic and international students. Applications are processed on a rolling basis. Application fee: $55 ($75 for international students). Electronic applications accepted. *Financial support:* Fellowships, research assistantships, teaching assistantships, career-related internships or fieldwork, institutionally sponsored loans, scholarships/grants, traineeships, health care benefits, tuition waivers (full), and unspecified assistantships available. Support available to part-time students. *Faculty research:* Pain, stepfamilies, chemotherapy-related nausea and vomiting, stress management, self-care deficit theory. *Unit head:* Dr. Judith F. Miller, Dean, 573-882-0278, E-mail: millerjud@missouri.edu. *Application contact:* Laura Anderson, Senior Academic Advisor, 573-882-0294, E-mail: andersonla@missouri.edu. Website: http://nursing.missouri.edu/

University of Missouri–Kansas City, School of Nursing and Health Studies, Kansas City, MO 64110-2499. Offers adult clinical nurse specialist (MSN), including adult nurse practitioner, women's health nurse practitioner (MSN, DNP); adult clinical nursing practice (DNP), including adult gerontology nurse practitioner, women's health nurse practitioner (MSN, DNP); clinical nursing practice (DNP), including family nurse practitioner; family nurse practitioner (MSN); neonatal nurse practitioner (MSN); nurse educator (MSN); nurse executive (MSN); nursing (PhD); nursing practice (DNP); pediatric clinical nursing practice (DNP), including pediatric nurse practitioner; pediatric nurse practitioner (MSN). *Accreditation:* AACN. Part-time programs available. Postbaccalaureate distance learning degree programs offered (minimal on-campus study). *Faculty:* 44 full-time (38 women), 55 part-time/adjunct (52 women). *Students:* 44 full-time (33 women), 401 part-time (370 women); includes 59 minority (25 Black or African American, non-Hispanic/Latino; 2 American Indian or Alaska Native, non-Hispanic/Latino; 12 Asian, non-Hispanic/Latino; 15 Hispanic/Latino; 5 Two or more races, non-Hispanic/Latino). Average age 37. 182 applicants, 68% accepted, 124 enrolled. In 2013, 106 master's, 15 doctorates awarded. *Degree requirements:* For master's, thesis or alternative. *Entrance requirements:* For master's, minimum undergraduate GPA of 3.2; for doctorate, GRE, 3 letters of reference. Additional exam requirements/recommendations for international students: Required—TOEFL (minimum score 550 paper-based; 80 iBT). *Application deadline:* For fall admission, 2/1 priority date for domestic and international students; for spring admission, 9/1 priority date for domestic and international students. Application fee: $45 ($50 for international students). *Expenses:* Tuition, state resident: full-time $6073; part-time $337.40 per credit hour. Tuition, nonresident: full-time $15,680; part-time $871.10 per credit hour. *Required fees:* $97.59 per credit hour. Full-time tuition and fees vary according to program. *Financial support:* In 2013–14, 13 teaching assistantships with partial tuition reimbursements (averaging $9,470 per year) were awarded; fellowships, research assistantships, career-related internships or fieldwork, Federal Work-Study, institutionally sponsored loans, and tuition waivers (full and partial) also available. Support available to part-time students. Financial award application deadline: 3/1; financial award applicants required to submit FAFSA. *Faculty research:* Geriatrics/gerontology, children's pain, neonatology, Alzheimer's care, cancer caregivers. *Unit head:* Dr. Ann Cary, Dean, 816-235-1723, Fax: 816-235-1701, E-mail: caryah@umkc.edu. *Application contact:* Judy Jellison, Coordinator for Admissions and Recruitment, 816-235-1740, Fax: 816-235-1701, E-mail: jellisonj@umkc.edu. Website: http://nursing.umkc.edu/

University of Missouri–St. Louis, College of Nursing, St. Louis, MO 63121-4400. Offers adult nurse practitioner (DNP, Post Master's Certificate); clinical nurse specialist (DNP); family mental health nurse practitioner (DNP); family nurse practitioner (MSN, DNP, Post Master's Certificate); neonatal nurse practitioner (MSN); nurse educator (MSN); nurse leader (MSN); nurse practitioner (Post Master's Certificate); nursing (PhD); pediatric clinical nurse specialist (DNP); pediatric nurse practitioner (MSN, DNP, Post Master's Certificate); women's health nurse practitioner (MSN, Post Master's Certificate). *Accreditation:* AACN. Part-time programs available. *Faculty:* 14 full-time (13 women), 14 part-time/adjunct (13 women). *Students:* 227 part-time (217 women); includes 40 minority (35 Black or African American, non-Hispanic/Latino; 1 American Indian or Alaska Native, non-Hispanic/Latino; 1 Asian, non-Hispanic/Latino; 1 Hispanic/Latino; 2 Two or more races, non-Hispanic/Latino). Average age 35. 190 applicants, 51% accepted, 76 enrolled. In 2013, 80 master's, 8 doctorates, 2 other advanced degrees awarded. *Degree requirements:* For doctorate, comprehensive exam, thesis/dissertation; for Post Master's Certificate, thesis. *Entrance requirements:* For master's, 2 recommendation letters; minimum GPA of 3.0; BSN; nursing licensure; statement of purpose; course in differential/inferential statistics; for doctorate, GRE, 2 letters of recommendation, MSN, minimum GPA of 3.2, course in differential/inferential statistics; for Post Master's Certificate, 2 recommendation letters; MSN; advanced practice certificate; minimum GPA of 3.0; essay. Additional exam requirements/recommendations for international students: Recommended—TOEFL (minimum score 550 paper-based; 79 iBT), IELTS (minimum score 6.5). *Application deadline:* For fall admission, 2/15 for domestic and international students. Application fee: $50 ($40 for international students). Electronic applications accepted. *Expenses:* Tuition, state resident: full-time $7364; part-time $409.10 per credit hour. Tuition, nonresident: full-time $19,162; part-time $1008.50 per credit hour. *Financial support:* Application deadline: 4/1; applicants required to submit FAFSA. *Faculty research:* Health promotion and restoration, family disruption, violence, abuse, battered women, health survey methods. *Unit head:* Dr. Nancy Magnuson, Director, 314-516-6066. *Application contact:* 314-516-5458, Fax: 314-516-6996, E-mail: gradadm@umsl.edu. Website: http://www.umsl.edu/divisions/nursing/

University of Mobile, Graduate Programs, Program in Nursing, Mobile, AL 36613. Offers MSN. *Accreditation:* AACN. Part-time and evening/weekend programs available. *Faculty:* 2 full-time (both women), 1 (woman) part-time/adjunct. *Students:* 5 full-time (4 women), 10 part-time (8 women); includes 7 minority (all Black or African American, non-Hispanic/Latino), 2 international. Average age 38. 1 applicant, 100% accepted, 1 enrolled. In 2013, 9 master's awarded. *Degree requirements:* For master's, comprehensive exam, thesis or alternative. *Entrance requirements:* For master's, GRE. Additional exam requirements/recommendations for international students: Required—TOEFL (minimum score 550 paper-based; 80 iBT). *Application deadline:* For fall admission, 8/3 for domestic students; for spring admission, 12/23 for domestic students. Applications are processed on a rolling basis. Application fee: $40 ($50 for international students). *Financial support:* Application deadline: 8/1. *Faculty research:* Nursing management, transcultural nursing, spiritual aspects, educational expectations. *Unit head:* Dr. Jan Wood, Dean, School of Nursing, 251-442-2446, Fax: 251-442-2520, E-mail: jwood@umobile.edu. *Application contact:* Danielle M. Riley, Administrative Assistant to Dean of Graduate Programs, 251-442-2270, Fax: 251-442-2523, E-mail: driley@umobile.edu. Website: http://www.umobile.edu/

University of Nebraska Medical Center, Program in Nursing, Omaha, NE 68198-5330. Offers PhD. *Accreditation:* AACN. Part-time programs available. Postbaccalaureate distance learning degree programs offered. *Degree requirements:* For doctorate, comprehensive exam, thesis/dissertation. *Entrance requirements:* For doctorate, GRE General Test, minimum GPA of 3.2. Additional exam requirements/recommendations for international students: Required—TOEFL (minimum score 550 paper-based). Electronic applications accepted. *Expenses:* Contact institution. *Faculty research:* Health promotion, sleep and fatigue in cancer patients, symptoms management in cardiovascular disease, prevention of osteoporosis in breast cancer survivors, impact of quality end of life care in nursing homes.

University of Nevada, Las Vegas, Graduate College, School of Nursing, Las Vegas, NV 89154-3018. Offers family nurse practitioner (Advanced Certificate); nursing (MS, DNP); nursing education (Advanced Certificate); pediatric nurse practitioner (PhD, Post-Master's Certificate). *Accreditation:* AACN. Part-time programs available. Postbaccalaureate distance learning degree programs offered (minimal on-campus study). *Faculty:* 11 full-time (10 women), 9 part-time/adjunct (6 women). *Students:* 48 full-time (40 women), 74 part-time (65 women); includes 30 minority (5 Black or African American, non-Hispanic/Latino; 10 Asian, non-Hispanic/Latino; 6 Hispanic/Latino; 9 Two or more races, non-Hispanic/Latino), 4 international. Average age 41. 114 applicants, 54% accepted, 48 enrolled. In 2013, 16 master's, 8 doctorates, 1 other advanced degree awarded. *Entrance requirements:* For doctorate, GRE General Test. Additional exam requirements/recommendations for international students: Recommended—TOEFL (minimum score 550 paper-based; 80 iBT), IELTS (minimum score 7). *Application deadline:* For fall admission, 2/1 for domestic students, 5/1 for international students; for spring admission, 10/1 for international students. Application fee: $60 ($95 for international students). Electronic applications accepted. *Expenses:* Tuition, state resident: full-time $4752; part-time $264 per credit. Tuition, nonresident: full-time $18,662; part-time $554.50 per credit. *International tuition:* $18,952 full-time. *Required fees:* $532; $12 per credit. $266 per semester. One-time fee: $35. Tuition and fees vary according to course load and program. *Financial support:* In 2013–14, 5 students received support, including 5 teaching assistantships with partial tuition reimbursements available (averaging $9,500 per year); institutionally sponsored loans, scholarships/grants, health care benefits, and unspecified assistantships also available. Financial award application deadline: 3/1. *Faculty research:* Health promotion issues such as obesity and exercise, dance and cardiovascular disease, informal caregiver stress and risk factors for depression, clinical management of hypertension and chronic obstructive pulmonary disease (COPD), childhood obesity and activity. *Total annual research expenditures:* $896,934. *Unit head:* Dr. Carolyn Yucha, Chair, 702-895-5307, E-mail: carolyn.yucha@unlv.edu. *Application contact:* Graduate College Admissions Evaluator, 702-895-3320, Fax: 702-895-4180, E-mail: gradcollege@unlv.edu. Website: http://nursing.unlv.edu/

University of Nevada, Reno, Graduate School, Division of Health Sciences, Orvis School of Nursing, Reno, NV 89557. Offers MSN, DNP, MPH/MSN. *Accreditation:* AACN. *Degree requirements:* For master's, thesis optional. *Entrance requirements:* For master's, minimum GPA of 3.0 in bachelor's degree from accredited school. Additional exam requirements/recommendations for international students: Required—TOEFL (minimum score 500 paper-based; 61 iBT), IELTS (minimum score 6). Electronic applications accepted. *Faculty research:* Analysis and evaluation of nursing theory, strategies for nursing applications.

University of New Brunswick Fredericton, School of Graduate Studies, Faculty of Nursing, Fredericton, NB E3B 5A3, Canada. Offers nurse educator (MN); nurse practitioner (MN); nursing (thesis/report) (MN). Part-time programs available. Postbaccalaureate distance learning degree programs offered. *Faculty:* 22 full-time (all women). *Students:* 11 full-time (10 women), 22 part-time (all women). In 2013, 8 master's awarded. *Degree requirements:* For master's, comprehensive exam (for some programs), thesis (for some programs). *Entrance requirements:* For master's, undergraduate coursework in statistics and nursing research, minimum GPA of 3.3, registration as a nurse (or eligibility) in New Brunswick. Additional exam requirements/recommendations for international students: Required—TOEFL (minimum score 600 paper-based). *Application deadline:* For winter admission, 1/2 priority date for domestic students. Application fee: $50 Canadian dollars. Electronic applications accepted. *Financial support:* In 2013–14, 7 fellowships, 2 research assistantships were awarded. *Faculty research:* Violence and abuse; healthy child development, chronic illness and addiction; rural populations' access to health care and primary healthcare; teaching and learning in the classroom, clinical lab, and by distance; Aboriginal nursing. *Unit head:* Kathy Wilson, Assistant Dean of Graduate and Advanced RN Studies, 506-458-7640,

Fax: 506-447-3057, E-mail: kewilson@unb.ca. *Application contact:* Francis Perry, Graduate Secretary, 506-451-6844, Fax: 506-447-3057, E-mail: fperry@unb.ca.
Website: http://www.unb.ca/fredericton/nursing/graduate/

University of New Hampshire, Graduate School, School of Health and Human Services, Department of Nursing, Durham, NH 03824. Offers family practitioner (Postbaccalaureate Certificate); nursing (MS, DNP). *Accreditation:* AACN. Part-time programs available. *Faculty:* 11 full-time (9 women). *Students:* 57 full-time (46 women), 53 part-time (49 women); includes 11 minority (3 Black or African American, non-Hispanic/Latino; 1 American Indian or Alaska Native, non-Hispanic/Latino; 5 Asian, non-Hispanic/Latino; 2 Hispanic/Latino). Average age 33. 70 applicants, 47% accepted, 19 enrolled. In 2013, 48 master's, 1 other advanced degree awarded. *Degree requirements:* For master's, thesis or alternative. *Entrance requirements:* For master's, GRE General Test or MAT. Additional exam requirements/recommendations for international students: Required—TOEFL (minimum score 550 paper-based; 80 iBT). *Application deadline:* For fall admission, 4/1 priority date for domestic students, 4/1 for international students; for spring admission, 11/1 for domestic students. Applications are processed on a rolling basis. Application fee: $65. Electronic applications accepted. *Expenses:* Tuition, state resident: full-time $13,500; part-time $750 per credit hour. Tuition, nonresident: full-time $26,200; part-time $1100 per credit hour. *Required fees:* $1741; $435.25 per term. Tuition and fees vary according to course level, course load, campus/location and program. *Financial support:* In 2013–14, 2 students received support, including 2 teaching assistantships; fellowships, research assistantships, Federal Work-Study, scholarships/grants, and tuition waivers (full and partial) also available. Financial award application deadline: 2/15. *Faculty research:* Adult health, nursing administration, family nurse practitioner. *Unit head:* Dr. Gene Harkless, Chairperson, 603-862-2285. *Application contact:* Jane Dufresne, Administrative Assistant, 603-862-2299, E-mail: nursing.department@unh.edu.
Website: http://www.chhs.unh.edu/nursing/graduate-programs

University of New Mexico, Graduate School, Program in Nursing, Albuquerque, NM 87131-0001. Offers MSN, DNP, PhD. *Accreditation:* AACN; ACNM/ACME (one or more programs are accredited). Part-time programs available. Postbaccalaureate distance learning degree programs offered (minimal on-campus study). *Faculty:* 44 full-time (35 women), 3 part-time/adjunct (all women). *Students:* 78 full-time (66 women), 80 part-time (72 women); includes 52 minority (3 Black or African American, non-Hispanic/Latino; 8 American Indian or Alaska Native, non-Hispanic/Latino; 8 Asian, non-Hispanic/Latino; 31 Hispanic/Latino; 2 Two or more races, non-Hispanic/Latino), 1 international. Average age 42. 114 applicants, 65% accepted, 71 enrolled. In 2013, 51 master's, 5 doctorates awarded. *Degree requirements:* For master's, comprehensive exam, thesis optional; for doctorate, comprehensive exam, thesis/dissertation. *Entrance requirements:* For master's, minimum GPA of 3.0, course work in statistics (recommended), interview (for some concentrations), BSN or RN with BA; for doctorate, interview, minimum GPA of 3.0, writing sample, MSN or BSN with MA. Additional exam requirements/recommendations for international students: Required—TOEFL. Application fee: $60. Electronic applications accepted. *Financial support:* In 2013–14, 24 students received support, including 11 fellowships (averaging $24,000 per year), 4 research assistantships with partial tuition reimbursements available (averaging $4,054 per year), 13 teaching assistantships with partial tuition reimbursements available (averaging $4,787 per year); institutionally sponsored loans, scholarships/grants, and unspecified assistantships also available. Support available to part-time students. Financial award application deadline: 3/1; financial award applicants required to submit FAFSA. *Faculty research:* Women's and children's health, pregnancy prevention in teens, vulnerable populations, nursing education, chronic illness, symptom appraisal and management. *Unit head:* Dr. Nancy Ridenour, Dean, 505-272-6284, Fax: 505-272-4343, E-mail: nridenour@salud.unm.edu. *Application contact:* Nissane Capps, Senior Academic Advisor, 505-272-4223, Fax: 505-272-3970, E-mail: ncapps@salud.unm.edu.
Website: http://nursing.unm.edu/

University of North Alabama, College of Nursing and Allied Health, Florence, AL 35632-0001. Offers MSN. *Accreditation:* AACN. Postbaccalaureate distance learning degree programs offered. *Faculty:* 5 full-time (all women). *Students:* 10 full-time (all women), 64 part-time (55 women); includes 12 minority (10 Black or African American, non-Hispanic/Latino; 2 Two or more races, non-Hispanic/Latino). Average age 40. 77 applicants, 69% accepted, 35 enrolled. In 2013, 26 master's awarded. *Entrance requirements:* Additional exam requirements/recommendations for international students: Required—TOEFL (minimum score 550 paper-based; 79 iBT), IELTS (minimum score 6). *Application deadline:* For fall admission, 7/1 for domestic and international students; for spring admission, 12/1 for domestic and international students. Applications are processed on a rolling basis. Application fee: $25 ($50 for international students). Electronic applications accepted. *Expenses:* Tuition, state resident: full-time $4968; part-time $3312 per year. Tuition, nonresident: full-time $9936; part-time $6624 per year. *Required fees:* $970; $60.33 per credit. $362 per semester. *Financial support:* Applicants required to submit FAFSA. *Unit head:* Dr. Birdie Bailey, Dean, 256-765-4984, E-mail: bibailey@una.edu. *Application contact:* Russ Durracott, Graduate Admissions Counselor, 256-465-4447, E-mail: erdarracott@una.edu.
Website: http://www.una.edu/nursing/

The University of North Carolina at Chapel Hill, School of Nursing, Chapel Hill, NC 27599-7460. Offers nursing (MSN, DNP, PhD, PMC), including adult nurse practitioner (MSN, PMC), children's health advanced practice (MSN, PMC), family nurse practitioner (MSN, PMC), health care systems (MSN, PMC), psychiatric/mental health nursing (MSN, PMC). Part-time programs available. *Degree requirements:* For master's, comprehensive exam, thesis; for doctorate, thesis/dissertation, 3 exams. *Entrance requirements:* For master's and doctorate, GRE General Test. Additional exam requirements/recommendations for international students: Required—TOEFL (minimum score 550 paper-based; 79 iBT), IELTS (minimum score 7). Electronic applications accepted. *Faculty research:* Preventing and managing chronic illness, reducing health disparities, Improving healthcare quality and patient outcomes, understanding biobehavioral and genetic bases of health and illness, developing innovative ways to enhance science and its clinical translation.

The University of North Carolina at Charlotte, The Graduate School, College of Health and Human Services, School of Nursing, Charlotte, NC 28223-0001. Offers administration (Post-Master's Certificate); advanced clinical (MSN, Post-Master's Certificate); anesthesia (MSN, Post-Master's Certificate); community health (MSN); family nurse practitioner (MSN, Post-Master's Certificate); health administration (MSN); mental health (MSN); nurse educator (MSN, Post-Master's Certificate); nursing (DNP); systems population (MSN). *Accreditation:* AACN. Part-time programs available. *Faculty:* 17 full-time (16 women), 6 part-time/adjunct (5 women). *Students:* 96 full-time (80 women), 124 part-time (119 women); includes 45 minority (30 Black or African American, non-Hispanic/Latino; 1 American Indian or Alaska Native, non-Hispanic/Latino; 8 Asian, non-Hispanic/Latino; 4 Hispanic/Latino; 2 Two or more races, non-Hispanic/Latino), 1 international. Average age 34. 216 applicants, 38% accepted, 72 enrolled. In 2013, 70 master's, 8 other advanced degrees awarded. Terminal master's awarded for partial completion of doctoral program. *Degree requirements:* For master's, thesis or alternative, practicum; for doctorate, thesis/dissertation or alternative, residency. *Entrance requirements:* For master's, GRE General Test, minimum GPA of 3.0 in undergraduate major; for doctorate, GRE, MAT, or GMAT, minimum GPA of 3.5. Additional exam requirements/recommendations for international students: Required—TOEFL (minimum score 570 paper-based; 83 iBT). *Application deadline:* For fall admission, 5/1 priority date for domestic students, 5/1 for international students; for spring admission, 10/1 priority date for domestic students, 10/1 for international students. Application fee: $75. Electronic applications accepted. *Expenses:* Tuition, state resident: full-time $3522. Tuition, nonresident: full-time $16,051. *Required fees:* $2585. Tuition and fees vary according to course load and program. *Financial support:* In 2013–14, 5 students received support, including 5 teaching assistantships (averaging $4,785 per year); research assistantships, career-related internships or fieldwork, institutionally sponsored loans, scholarships/grants, traineeships, and unspecified assistantships also available. Support available to part-time students. Financial award application deadline: 4/1; financial award applicants required to submit FAFSA. *Faculty research:* Improving care outcomes for the elderly; vulnerable populations; symptom management; self management/health promotion strategies of older adults; migration and maternal child health; health disparities, health literacy, and access to healthcare in Latino adults with diabetes; psychiatric nursing. *Total annual research expenditures:* $572,410. *Unit head:* Dr. Dee Baldwin, Associate Dean, 704-687-7952, Fax: 704-687-6017, E-mail: dbaldwi5@uncc.edu. *Application contact:* Kathy B. Giddings, Director of Graduate Admissions, 704-687-5503, Fax: 704-687-1668, E-mail: gradadm@uncc.edu.
Website: http://nursing.uncc.edu/

The University of North Carolina at Greensboro, Graduate School, School of Nursing, Greensboro, NC 27412-5001. Offers adult clinical nurse specialist (MSN, PMC); adult/gerontological nurse practitioner (MSN, PMC); nurse anesthesia (MSN, PMC); nursing (PhD); nursing administration (MSN); nursing education (MSN); MSN/MBA. *Accreditation:* AACN; AANA/CANAEP. *Degree requirements:* For master's, thesis or alternative. *Entrance requirements:* For master's, GRE General Test or MAT, BSN, clinical experience, liability insurance, RN license; for PMC, liability insurance, MSN, RN license. Additional exam requirements/recommendations for international students: Required—TOEFL. Electronic applications accepted.

The University of North Carolina at Pembroke, Graduate Studies, Department of Nursing, Pembroke, NC 28372-1510. Offers clinical nurse leader (MSN); nurse educator (MSN); rural case manager (MSN). Part-time programs available.

The University of North Carolina Wilmington, School of Nursing, Wilmington, NC 28403-5995. Offers clinical research and product development (MS); family nurse practitioner (MSN). *Faculty:* 10 full-time (9 women), 1 (woman) part-time/adjunct. *Students:* 59 full-time (54 women), 61 part-time (53 women); includes 17 minority (6 Black or African American, non-Hispanic/Latino; 5 American Indian or Alaska Native, non-Hispanic/Latino; 5 Hispanic/Latino; 1 Two or more races, non-Hispanic/Latino). Average age 32. 134 applicants, 44% accepted, 43 enrolled. In 2013, 13 master's awarded. *Degree requirements:* For master's, comprehensive exam, thesis or project. *Entrance requirements:* For master's, GRE General Test, bachelor's degree in nursing. Additional exam requirements/recommendations for international students: Required—TOEFL (minimum score 550 paper-based; 79 iBT), IELTS (minimum score 6.5). *Application deadline:* For fall admission, 3/1 for domestic students. Applications are processed on a rolling basis. Application fee: $60. Electronic applications accepted. *Expenses:* Tuition, state resident: full-time $4163. Tuition, nonresident: full-time $16,098. *Financial support:* In 2013–14, 2 teaching assistantships with full and partial tuition reimbursements (averaging $9,500 per year) were awarded. Financial award application deadline: 3/15. *Unit head:* Dr. Deborah Pollard, Interim Director, 910-962-7410, E-mail: pollardd@uncw.edu. *Application contact:* Dr. Julie Taylor, Graduate Coordinator, 910-962-7927, E-mail: taylorjs@uncw.edu.
Website: http://www.uncw.edu/son/

University of North Dakota, Graduate School, College of Nursing, Department of Nursing, Grand Forks, ND 58202. Offers adult-gerontological nurse practitioner (MSN); advanced public health nurse (MSN); family nurse practitioner (MSN); nurse anesthesia (MSN); nurse educator (MSN); nursing (DNP, PhD); psychiatric and mental health nurse practitioner (MSN).

University of Northern Colorado, Graduate School, College of Natural and Health Sciences, School of Nursing, Greeley, CO 80639. Offers clinical nurse specialist in chronic illness (MS); family nurse practitioner (MS); nursing education (MS, PhD). *Accreditation:* AACN. Postbaccalaureate distance learning degree programs offered. *Degree requirements:* For master's, comprehensive exam, thesis or alternative; for doctorate, comprehensive exam, thesis/dissertation. *Entrance requirements:* For master's and doctorate, GRE General Test, minimum GPA of 3.0 in last 60 hours, BS in nursing, 2 letters of recommendation. Electronic applications accepted.

University of North Florida, Brooks College of Health, School of Nursing, Jacksonville, FL 32224. Offers clinical nurse leader (MSN); clinical nurse specialist (MSN); family nurse practitioner (Certificate); nurse anesthetist (CRNA) (MSN); nursing practice (DNP); primary care nurse practitioner (MSN). *Accreditation:* AACN; AANA/CANAEP. Part-time programs available. *Faculty:* 29 full-time (23 women), 1 part-time/adjunct (0 women). *Students:* 93 full-time (70 women), 74 part-time (61 women); includes 33 minority (11 Black or African American, non-Hispanic/Latino; 1 American Indian or Alaska Native, non-Hispanic/Latino; 6 Asian, non-Hispanic/Latino; 12 Hispanic/Latino; 3 Two or more races, non-Hispanic/Latino), 2 international. Average age 34. 133 applicants, 40% accepted, 32 enrolled. In 2013, 45 master's, 3 doctorates awarded. *Degree requirements:* For master's, thesis optional. *Entrance requirements:* For master's, GRE General Test, minimum GPA of 3.0 in last 60 hours of course work, BSN, clinical experience, resume; for doctorate, GRE, master's degree in nursing specialty from nationally-accredited program; national certification in one of the following APRN roles: CNE, CNM, CNS, CRNA, CNP; minimum graduate GPA of 3.3; three letters of reference which address academic ability and clinical skills; active license as registered nurse or advanced practice registered nurse. Additional exam requirements/recommendations for international students: Required—TOEFL (minimum score 500 paper-based; 61 iBT). *Application deadline:* For fall admission, 3/15 for domestic students, 4/1 for international students. Application fee: $30. Electronic applications accepted. *Expenses:* Tuition, state resident: full-time $9794; part-time $408.10 per credit hour. Tuition, nonresident: full-time $22,383; part-time $932.61 per credit hour. *Required fees:* $2020; $84.20 per credit hour. Tuition and fees vary according to course load and program. *Financial support:* In 2013–14, 26 students received support. Research assistantships available. Financial award application deadline: 4/1; financial award applicants required to submit FAFSA. *Faculty research:* Teen pregnancy, diabetes, ethical decision-making, family caregivers. *Total annual research expenditures:* $66,739. *Unit head:* Dr. Li Loriz, Chair, 904-620-1053, E-mail: lloriz@unf.edu. *Application contact:* Beth Dibble, Assistant Director of Admissions for Nursing and Physical Therapy, 904-620-2684, Fax: 904-620-1832, E-mail: nursingadmissions@unf.edu.
Website: http://www.unf.edu/brooks/nursing

University of Oklahoma Health Sciences Center, Graduate College, College of Nursing, Oklahoma City, OK 73190. Offers MS, MS/MBA. MS/MBA offered jointly with Oklahoma State University and University of Oklahoma. Part-time programs available. *Faculty:* 21 full-time (20 women), 7 part-time/adjunct (all women). *Students:* 81 full-time

(67 women), 164 part-time (152 women); includes 57 minority (19 Black or African American, non-Hispanic/Latino; 17 American Indian or Alaska Native, non-Hispanic/ Latino; 4 Asian, non-Hispanic/Latino; 4 Hispanic/Latino; 13 Two or more races, non-Hispanic/Latino), 2 international. Average age 38. 226 applicants, 37% accepted, 46 enrolled. In 2013, 27 master's awarded. *Degree requirements:* For master's, comprehensive exam, thesis optional. *Entrance requirements:* For master's, 3 letters of recommendation, Oklahoma RN license, statistics course, research methods, computer course or completion of a computer literacy test. *Application deadline:* For fall admission, 6/1 for domestic students; for winter admission, 4/1 for domestic students; for spring admission, 11/1 for domestic students. Applications are processed on a rolling basis. Application fee: $50. *Expenses:* Tuition, state resident: full-time $3504; part-time $175.20 per credit hour. Tuition, nonresident: full-time $13,504; part-time $675.20 per credit hour. *Required fees:* $1545; $52.70 per credit hour. $245.25 per semester. Tuition and fees vary according to course load. *Financial support:* In 2013–14, 6 research assistantships (averaging $6,000 per year) were awarded; teaching assistantships, institutionally sponsored loans, scholarships/grants, and traineeships also available. Support available to part-time students. Financial award application deadline: 8/1. *Faculty research:* Parenting and Native Americans, elderly reminiscence, diabetes in Native Americans. *Unit head:* Dr. Lazelle Benefield, Dean, 405-271-2420, E-mail: lazelle-benefield@ouhsc.edu. *Application contact:* Heath Burge, Information Contact, 405-271-2420, Fax: 405-271-3443, E-mail: heath-burge@ouhsc.edu.

University of Ottawa, Faculty of Graduate and Postdoctoral Studies, Faculty of Health Sciences, School of Nursing, Ottawa, ON K1N 6N5, Canada. Offers nurse practitioner (Certificate); nursing (M Sc, PhD); nursing/primary health care (M Sc). Part-time and evening/weekend programs available. *Degree requirements:* For master's, thesis or alternative. *Entrance requirements:* For master's, honors degree or equivalent, minimum B average. Electronic applications accepted. *Faculty research:* Decision making in nursing, evaluating complete nursing interventions.

University of Pennsylvania, School of Nursing, Philadelphia, PA 19104. Offers MSN, PhD, Certificate, MBA/MSN, MBA/PhD, MSN/PhD. *Accreditation:* AACN; AANA/ CANAEP. Part-time programs available. Postbaccalaureate distance learning degree programs offered. *Faculty:* 57 full-time (51 women), 35 part-time/adjunct (32 women). *Students:* 286 full-time (252 women), 291 part-time (259 women); includes 117 minority (46 Black or African American, non-Hispanic/Latino; 42 Asian, non-Hispanic/Latino; 12 Hispanic/Latino; 17 Two or more races, non-Hispanic/Latino), 21 international. 144 applicants, 49% accepted, 65 enrolled. In 2013, 230 master's, 11 doctorates, 9 other advanced degrees awarded. Terminal master's awarded for partial completion of doctoral program. *Degree requirements:* For doctorate, thesis/dissertation. *Entrance requirements:* For master's, GRE General Test, BSN, minimum GPA of 3.0; for doctorate, GRE General Test, BSN or MSN, minimum GPA of 3.0. Additional exam requirements/recommendations for international students: Required—TOEFL. *Application deadline:* For fall admission, 2/15 priority date for domestic students. Applications are processed on a rolling basis. Application fee: $70. *Expenses:* Contact institution. *Financial support:* In 2013–14, 71 students received support. Fellowships, research assistantships, teaching assistantships, institutionally sponsored loans, scholarships/grants, traineeships, health care benefits, and unspecified assistantships available. Financial award application deadline: 12/15. *Faculty research:* Nursing and patient outcomes research. *Unit head:* Assistant Dean of Admissions and Financial Aid, 866-867-6877, Fax: 215-573-8439, E-mail: admissions@nursing.upenn.edu. *Application contact:* Sylvia V. J. English, Enrollment Management Coordinator, 866-867-6877, Fax: 215-573-8439, E-mail: admissions@nursing.upenn.edu.
Website: http://www.nursing.upenn.edu/

University of Phoenix–Atlanta Campus, College of Nursing, Sandy Springs, GA 30350-4153. Offers health administration (MHA); nursing (MSN); nursing/health care education (MSN); MSN/MBA; MSN/MHA. Evening/weekend programs available. Postbaccalaureate distance learning degree programs offered. *Degree requirements:* For master's, thesis (for some programs). *Entrance requirements:* For master's, minimum undergraduate GPA of 2.5, 3 years of work experience. Additional exam requirements/recommendations for international students: Required—TOEFL (minimum score 550 paper-based; 79 iBT). Electronic applications accepted.

University of Phoenix–Augusta Campus, College of Nursing, Augusta, GA 30909-4583. Offers health administration (MHA); nursing (MSN); nursing/health care education (MSN); MSN/MBA; MSN/MHA. Postbaccalaureate distance learning degree programs offered.

University of Phoenix–Austin Campus, College of Nursing, Austin, TX 78759. Offers health administration (MHA). Postbaccalaureate distance learning degree programs offered.

University of Phoenix–Bay Area Campus, College of Nursing, San Jose, CA 95134-1805. Offers education (MHA); gerontology (MHA); health administration (MHA, DHA); informatics (MHA, MSN); nursing (MSN, PhD); nursing/health care education (MSN); MSN/MBA. Evening/weekend programs available. Postbaccalaureate distance learning degree programs offered (no on-campus study). *Degree requirements:* For master's, thesis (for some programs). *Entrance requirements:* For master's, minimum undergraduate GPA of 2.5, 3 years of work experience, RN license. Additional exam requirements/recommendations for international students: Required—TOEFL (minimum score 550 paper-based; 79 iBT). Electronic applications accepted.

University of Phoenix–Birmingham Campus, College of Health and Human Services, Birmingham, AL 35242. Offers education (MHA); gerontology (MHA); health administration (MHA); health care management (MBA); informatics (MHA); nursing (MSN); nursing/health care education (MSN); MSN/MBA; MSN/MHA.

University of Phoenix–Central Valley Campus, College of Nursing, Fresno, CA 93720-1562. Offers education (MHA); gerontology (MHA); health administration (MHA); nursing (MSN); MSN/MBA.

University of Phoenix–Charlotte Campus, College of Nursing, Charlotte, NC 28273-3409. Offers education (MHA); gerontology (MHA); health administration (MHA); informatics (MHA, MSN); nursing (MSN); nursing/health care education (MSN). Evening/ weekend programs available. *Degree requirements:* For master's, thesis (for some programs). *Entrance requirements:* For master's, minimum undergraduate GPA of 2.5, 3 years work experience. Additional exam requirements/recommendations for international students: Required—TOEFL (minimum score 550 paper-based; 79 iBT). Electronic applications accepted.

University of Phoenix–Chattanooga Campus, College of Nursing, Chattanooga, TN 37421-3707. Offers education (MHA); gerontology (MHA); health administration (MHA).

University of Phoenix–Cheyenne Campus, College of Nursing, Cheyenne, WY 82009. Offers health administration (MHA); nursing (MSN); nursing/health care education (MSN); MSN/MBA; MSN/MHA. Postbaccalaureate distance learning degree programs offered.

University of Phoenix–Cleveland Campus, College of Nursing, Independence, OH 44131-2194. Offers MSN, PhD. Evening/weekend programs available. Postbaccalaureate distance learning degree programs offered. *Degree requirements:* For master's, thesis (for some programs). *Entrance requirements:* For master's, minimum undergraduate GPA of 2.5, 3 years of work experience. Additional exam requirements/recommendations for international students: Required—TOEFL (minimum score 550 paper-based; 79 iBT). Electronic applications accepted.

University of Phoenix–Columbus Georgia Campus, College of Nursing, Columbus, GA 31909. Offers health administration (MHA); nursing (MSN). Postbaccalaureate distance learning degree programs offered. *Degree requirements:* For master's, thesis (for some programs). *Entrance requirements:* For master's, minimum undergraduate GPA of 2.5, 3 years of work experience. Additional exam requirements/ recommendations for international students: Required—TOEFL (minimum score 550 paper-based; 79 iBT). Electronic applications accepted.

University of Phoenix–Columbus Ohio Campus, College of Nursing, Columbus, OH 43240-4032. Offers MSN, PhD. Evening/weekend programs available. Postbaccalaureate distance learning degree programs offered. *Degree requirements:* For master's, thesis (for some programs). *Entrance requirements:* For master's, minimum undergraduate GPA of 2.5, 3 years work experience. Additional exam requirements/recommendations for international students: Required—TOEFL (minimum score 550 paper-based; 79 iBT). Electronic applications accepted.

University of Phoenix–Denver Campus, College of Nursing, Lone Tree, CO 80124-5453. Offers health administration (MHA); nursing (MSN); MSN/MBA; MSN/MHA. Evening/weekend programs available. Postbaccalaureate distance learning degree programs offered. *Degree requirements:* For master's, thesis (for some programs). *Entrance requirements:* For master's, minimum undergraduate GPA of 2.5, 3 years work experience, RN license. Additional exam requirements/recommendations for international students: Required—TOEFL (minimum score 550 paper-based; 79 iBT). Electronic applications accepted.

University of Phoenix–Des Moines Campus, College of Nursing, Des Moines, IA 50309. Offers education (MHA); gerontology (MHA); health administration (MHA, DHA); informatics (MHA, MSN); nursing (MSN, PhD); nursing/health care education (MSN).

University of Phoenix–Hawaii Campus, College of Nursing, Honolulu, HI 96813-4317. Offers education (MHA); family nurse practitioner (MSN); gerontology (MHA); health administration (MHA); nursing (MSN); nursing/health care education (MSN); MSN/MBA. Evening/weekend programs available. *Degree requirements:* For master's, thesis (for some programs). *Entrance requirements:* For master's, minimum undergraduate GPA of 2.5, 3 years of work experience, RN license. Additional exam requirements/ recommendations for international students: Required—TOEFL (minimum score 550 paper-based; 79 iBT). Electronic applications accepted.

University of Phoenix–Houston Campus, College of Nursing, Houston, TX 77079-2004. Offers health administration (MHA). Postbaccalaureate distance learning degree programs offered. *Degree requirements:* For master's, thesis (for some programs). *Entrance requirements:* For master's, minimum undergraduate GPA of 2.5, 3 years of work experience. Additional exam requirements/recommendations for international students: Required—TOEFL (minimum score 550 paper-based; 79 iBT). Electronic applications accepted.

University of Phoenix–Idaho Campus, College of Nursing, Meridian, ID 83642-5114. Offers health administration (MHA); nursing (MSN); nursing/health care education (MSN); MSN/MBA. Evening/weekend programs available. Postbaccalaureate distance learning degree programs offered. *Degree requirements:* For master's, thesis (for some programs). *Entrance requirements:* For master's, minimum undergraduate GPA of 2.5, 3 years of work experience. Additional exam requirements/recommendations for international students: Required—TOEFL (minimum score 550 paper-based). Electronic applications accepted.

University of Phoenix–Indianapolis Campus, College of Nursing, Indianapolis, IN 46250-932. Offers health administration (MHA); nursing (MSN); nursing/health care education (MSN); MSN/MBA; MSN/MHA. Evening/weekend programs available. Postbaccalaureate distance learning degree programs offered. *Degree requirements:* For master's, thesis. *Entrance requirements:* For master's, 3 years work experience, minimum undergraduate GPA of 2.5. Additional exam requirements/recommendations for international students: Required—TOEFL (minimum score 500 paper-based). Electronic applications accepted.

University of Phoenix–Louisiana Campus, College of Nursing, Metairie, LA 70001-2082. Offers health administration (MHA); nursing (MSN); MSN/MBA. Evening/weekend programs available. Postbaccalaureate distance learning degree programs offered (no on-campus study). *Degree requirements:* For master's, thesis (for some programs). *Entrance requirements:* For master's, minimum undergraduate GPA of 2.5, 3 years work experience, RN license. Additional exam requirements/recommendations for international students: Required—TOEFL (minimum score 550 paper-based; 79 iBT). Electronic applications accepted.

University of Phoenix–Memphis Campus, College of Nursing, Cordova, TN 38018. Offers health administration (MHA, DHA).

University of Phoenix–Nashville Campus, College of Nursing, Nashville, TN 37214-5048. Offers health administration (MHA). Evening/weekend programs available. *Degree requirements:* For master's, thesis (for some programs). *Entrance requirements:* For master's, minimum undergraduate GPA of 2.5, 3 years of work experience. Additional exam requirements/recommendations for international students: Required—TOEFL (minimum score 550 paper-based). Electronic applications accepted.

University of Phoenix–New Mexico Campus, College of Nursing, Albuquerque, NM 87113-1570. Offers health administration (MHA); health care education (MSN); nursing (MSN); MSN/MBA. Evening/weekend programs available. *Degree requirements:* For master's, thesis (for some programs). *Entrance requirements:* For master's, minimum undergraduate GPA of 2.5, 3 years of work experience, RN license. Additional exam requirements/recommendations for international students: Required—TOEFL (minimum score 550 paper-based; 79 iBT). Electronic applications accepted.

University of Phoenix–North Florida Campus, College of Nursing, Jacksonville, FL 32216-0959. Offers health administration (MHA); health care education (MSN); nursing (MSN); MSN/MBA; MSN/MHA. Evening/weekend programs available. *Degree requirements:* For master's, thesis (for some programs). *Entrance requirements:* For master's, minimum undergraduate GPA of 2.5, 3 years work experience, RN license. Additional exam requirements/recommendations for international students: Required—TOEFL (minimum score 550 paper-based; 79 iBT). Electronic applications accepted.

University of Phoenix–Northwest Arkansas Campus, College of Nursing, Rogers, AR 72756-9615. Offers health administration (MHA); health care education (MSN); nursing (MSN); MSN/MBA.

University of Phoenix–Oklahoma City Campus, College of Nursing, Oklahoma City, OK 73116-8244. Offers MSN.

University of Phoenix–Omaha Campus, College of Nursing, Omaha, NE 68154-5240. Offers health administration (MHA).

University of Phoenix–Online Campus, College of Health Sciences and Nursing, Phoenix, AZ 85034-7209. Offers family nurse practitioner (Certificate); health care (Certificate); health care education (Certificate); health care informatics (Certificate); informatics (MSN); nursing (MSN); nursing and health care education (MSN); MSN/

MBA; MSN/MHA. *Accreditation:* AACN. Evening/weekend programs available. Postbaccalaureate distance learning degree programs offered. *Entrance requirements:* Additional exam requirements/recommendations for international students: Required—TOEFL, TOEIC (Test of English as an International Communication), Berlitz Online English Proficiency Exam, PTE, or IELTS. Electronic applications accepted. *Expenses:* Contact institution.

University of Phoenix–Online Campus, School of Advanced Studies, Phoenix, AZ 85034-7209. Offers business administration (DBA); education (Ed S); educational leadership (Ed D), including curriculum and instruction, education technology, educational leadership; health administration (DHA); higher education administration (PhD); industrial/organizational psychology (PhD); nursing (PhD); organizational leadership (DM), including information systems and technology, organizational leadership. Evening/weekend programs available. Postbaccalaureate distance learning degree programs offered. *Degree requirements:* For doctorate, thesis/dissertation. *Entrance requirements:* Additional exam requirements/recommendations for international students: Required—TOEFL, TOEIC (Test of English as an International Communication), Berlitz Online English Proficiency Exam, PTE, or IELTS. Electronic applications accepted. *Expenses:* Contact institution.

University of Phoenix–Oregon Campus, College of Nursing, Tigard, OR 97223. Offers health administration (MHA); nursing (MSN); MSN/MBA. Evening/weekend programs available. *Degree requirements:* For master's, thesis (for some programs). *Entrance requirements:* For master's, minimum undergraduate GPA of 2.5, 3 years of work experience, current RN license (nursing). Additional exam requirements/recommendations for international students: Required—TOEFL (minimum score 550 paper-based; 79 iBT). Electronic applications accepted.

University of Phoenix–Phoenix Campus, College of Health Sciences and Nursing, Tempe, AZ 85282-2371. Offers family nurse practitioner (MSN, Certificate); gerontology health care (Certificate); health care education (MSN, Certificate); health care informatics (Certificate); informatics (MSN); nursing (MSN); MSN/MHA. Evening/weekend programs available. Postbaccalaureate distance learning degree programs offered. *Entrance requirements:* Additional exam requirements/recommendations for international students: Required—TOEFL, TOEIC (Test of English as an International Communication), Berlitz Online English Proficiency Exam, PTE, or IELTS. Electronic applications accepted. *Expenses:* Contact institution.

University of Phoenix–Pittsburgh Campus, College of Nursing, Pittsburgh, PA 15276. Offers health administration (MHA); health care education (MSN); nursing (MSN); MSN/MBA; MSN/MHA. Evening/weekend programs available. *Degree requirements:* For master's, thesis (for some programs). *Entrance requirements:* For master's, minimum undergraduate GPA of 2.5, 3 years work experience, current RN license (nursing). Additional exam requirements/recommendations for international students: Required—TOEFL (minimum score 550 paper-based; 79 iBT). Electronic applications accepted.

University of Phoenix–Richmond-Virginia Beach Campus, College of Nursing, Glen Allen, VA 23060. Offers health administration (MHA); health care education (MSN); nursing (MSN); MSN/MBA; MSN/MHA. Evening/weekend programs available. *Degree requirements:* For master's, thesis (for some programs). *Entrance requirements:* For master's, minimum undergraduate GPA of 2.5, 3 years work experience, current RN license for nursing programs. Additional exam requirements/recommendations for international students: Required—TOEFL (minimum score 500 paper-based; 79 iBT). Electronic applications accepted.

University of Phoenix–Sacramento Valley Campus, College of Nursing, Sacramento, CA 95833-3632. Offers family nurse practitioner (MSN); health administration (MHA); health care education (MSN); nursing (MSN); MSN/MBA. Evening/weekend programs available. *Degree requirements:* For master's, thesis (for some programs). *Entrance requirements:* For master's, RN license, minimum undergraduate GPA of 2.5, 3 years work experience. Additional exam requirements/recommendations for international students: Required—TOEFL (minimum score 550 paper-based; 79 iBT). Electronic applications accepted.

University of Phoenix–San Antonio Campus, College of Nursing, San Antonio, TX 78230. Offers health administration (MHA).

University of Phoenix–San Diego Campus, College of Nursing, San Diego, CA 92123. Offers health care education (MSN); nursing (MSN); MSN/MBA. Evening/weekend programs available. *Degree requirements:* For master's, thesis (for some programs). *Entrance requirements:* For master's, minimum undergraduate GPA of 2.5, 3 years work experience, RN license. Additional exam requirements/recommendations for international students: Required—TOEFL (minimum score 550 paper-based; 79 iBT). Electronic applications accepted.

University of Phoenix–Savannah Campus, College of Nursing, Savannah, GA 31405-7400. Offers health administration (MHA); nursing (MSN); nursing/health care education (MSN); MSN/MBA; MSN/MHA.

University of Phoenix–Southern California Campus, College of Health Sciences and Nursing, Costa Mesa, CA 92626. Offers family nurse practitioner (MSN, Certificate); health care (Certificate); informatics (MSN); nursing (MSN); nursing/health care education (MSN, Certificate); MSN/MBA; MSN/MHA. Evening/weekend programs available. Postbaccalaureate distance learning degree programs offered. *Entrance requirements:* Additional exam requirements/recommendations for international students: Required—TOEFL, TOEIC (Test of English as an International Communication), Berlitz Online English Proficiency Exam, PTE, or IELTS. Electronic applications accepted. *Expenses:* Contact institution.

University of Phoenix–Southern Colorado Campus, College of Nursing, Colorado Springs, CO 80903. Offers education (MHA); gerontology (MHA); health administration (MHA); nursing (MSN); MSN/MBA. Evening/weekend programs available. *Degree requirements:* For master's, thesis (for some programs). *Entrance requirements:* For master's, minimum undergraduate GPA of 2.5, 3 years of work experience, RN license. Additional exam requirements/recommendations for international students: Required—TOEFL (minimum score 550 paper-based; 79 iBT). Electronic applications accepted.

University of Phoenix–South Florida Campus, College of Nursing, Miramar, FL 33030. Offers health administration (MHA); health care education (MSN); nursing (MSN); MSN/MBA; MSN/MHA. Evening/weekend programs available. *Degree requirements:* For master's, thesis (for some programs). *Entrance requirements:* For master's, minimum undergraduate GPA of 2.5, 3 years work experience, RN license. Additional exam requirements/recommendations for international students: Required—TOEFL (minimum score 550 paper-based; 79 iBT). Electronic applications accepted.

University of Phoenix–Springfield Campus, College of Nursing, Springfield, MO 65804-7211. Offers health administration (MHA); nursing (MSN); MSN/MBA; MSN/MHA.

University of Phoenix–Tulsa Campus, College of Nursing, Tulsa, OK 74134-1412. Offers MSN.

University of Phoenix–Utah Campus, College of Nursing, Salt Lake City, UT 84123-4617. Offers health care education (MSN); nursing (MSN); MSN/MBA. Evening/weekend programs available. *Degree requirements:* For master's, thesis (for some programs). *Entrance requirements:* For master's, minimum undergraduate GPA of 2.5, 3 years work experience, RN license. Additional exam requirements/recommendations for international students: Required—TOEFL (minimum score 550 paper-based; 79 iBT). Electronic applications accepted.

University of Phoenix–Washington D.C. Campus, College of Nursing, Washington, DC 20001. Offers education (MHA); gerontology (MHA); health administration (MHA, DHA); informatics (MHA, MSN); nursing (MSN, PhD); nursing/health care education (MSN); MSN/MBA; MSN/MHA.

University of Phoenix–West Florida Campus, College of Nursing, Temple Terrace, FL 33637. Offers health administration (MHA); health care education (MSN); nursing (MSN); MSN/MBA; MSN/MHA. Evening/weekend programs available. Postbaccalaureate distance learning degree programs offered. *Degree requirements:* For master's, thesis (for some programs). *Entrance requirements:* For master's, minimum undergraduate GPA of 2.5, RN license, 3 years work experience. Additional exam requirements/recommendations for international students: Required—TOEFL (minimum score 550 paper-based; 79 iBT). Electronic applications accepted.

University of Pittsburgh, School of Nursing, Clinical Nurse Specialist Program, Pittsburgh, PA 15260. Offers adult-gerontology clinical nurse specialist (DNP); psychiatric mental health clinical nurse specialist (DNP). *Accreditation:* AACN. Part-time programs available. *Students:* 4 full-time (all women), 16 part-time (14 women); includes 2 minority (both Black or African American, non-Hispanic/Latino), 1 international. Average age 41. 4 applicants, 75% accepted, 2 enrolled. In 2013, 5 doctorates awarded. *Entrance requirements:* Additional exam requirements/recommendations for international students: Required—TOEFL (minimum score 550 paper-based; 80 iBT). *Application deadline:* For fall admission, 6/1 priority date for domestic and international students. Applications are processed on a rolling basis. Application fee: $50. Electronic applications accepted. *Expenses:* Tuition, state resident: full-time $19,964; part-time $807 per credit. Tuition, nonresident: full-time $32,686; part-time $1337 per credit. *Required fees:* $740; $200. Tuition and fees vary according to program. *Financial support:* In 2013–14, 4 students received support, including 1 fellowship with full tuition reimbursement available (averaging $24,108 per year), 3 teaching assistantships with full and partial tuition reimbursements available (averaging $21,884 per year); scholarships/grants, traineeships, health care benefits, and unspecified assistantships also available. Support available to part-time students. *Unit head:* Dr. Sandra Engberg, Associate Dean for Clinical Education, 412-624-3835, Fax: 412-624-8521, E-mail: sje1@pitt.edu. *Application contact:* Laurie Lapsley, Administrator of Graduate Student Services, 412-624-9670, Fax: 412-624-2409, E-mail: lapsleyl@pitt.edu.

University of Pittsburgh, School of Nursing, Nurse Specialty Role Program, Pittsburgh, PA 15260. Offers clinical nurse leader (MSN); nursing (DNP); nursing administration (MSN); nursing informatics (MSN). *Accreditation:* AACN. Part-time programs available. *Students:* 11 full-time (9 women), 70 part-time (60 women); includes 6 minority (3 Black or African American, non-Hispanic/Latino; 3 Asian, non-Hispanic/Latino), 2 international. Average age 38. 43 applicants, 74% accepted, 26 enrolled. In 2013, 13 master's, 10 doctorates awarded. *Degree requirements:* For master's, comprehensive exam, thesis optional. *Entrance requirements:* For master's, GRE or MAT, BSN, RN license, letters of recommendation, resume, course work in statistics, 1-3 years of nursing experience. Additional exam requirements/recommendations for international students: Required—TOEFL (minimum score 550 paper-based; 80 iBT). *Application deadline:* For fall admission, 6/1 priority date for domestic students, 6/1 for international students; for spring admission, 2/15 priority date for domestic students, 2/15 for international students. Applications are processed on a rolling basis. Application fee: $50. Electronic applications accepted. *Expenses:* Tuition, state resident: full-time $19,964; part-time $807 per credit. Tuition, nonresident: full-time $32,686; part-time $1337 per credit. *Required fees:* $740; $200. Tuition and fees vary according to program. *Unit head:* Dr. Sandra Engberg, Associate Dean for Clinical Education, 412-624-3835, Fax: 412-624-8521, E-mail: sje1@pitt.edu. *Application contact:* Laurie Lapsley, Administrator of Graduate Student Services, 412-624-9670, Fax: 412-624-2409, E-mail: lapsleyl@pitt.edu.
Website: http://www.nursing.pitt.edu/

University of Pittsburgh, School of Nursing, PhD Program in Nursing, Pittsburgh, PA 15261. Offers PhD. Part-time programs available. *Students:* 29 full-time (25 women), 8 part-time (7 women); includes 3 minority (2 Black or African American, non-Hispanic/Latino; 1 Asian, non-Hispanic/Latino), 8 international. Average age 35. 12 applicants, 42% accepted, 5 enrolled. In 2013, 7 doctorates awarded. *Degree requirements:* For doctorate, comprehensive exam, thesis/dissertation. *Entrance requirements:* For doctorate, GRE General Test. Additional exam requirements/recommendations for international students: Required—TOEFL (minimum score 550 paper-based; 79 iBT) or IELTS (minimum score 6.5). *Application deadline:* For fall admission, 6/1 priority date for domestic students, 5/1 priority date for international students. Applications are processed on a rolling basis. Application fee: $50. Electronic applications accepted. *Expenses:* Tuition, state resident: full-time $19,964; part-time $807 per credit. Tuition, nonresident: full-time $32,686; part-time $1337 per credit. *Required fees:* $740; $200. Tuition and fees vary according to program. *Financial support:* In 2013–14, 29 students received support, including 16 fellowships with partial tuition reimbursements available (averaging $10,022 per year), 15 research assistantships with partial tuition reimbursements available (averaging $12,166 per year), 3 teaching assistantships with partial tuition reimbursements available (averaging $13,693 per year); scholarships/grants, traineeships, health care benefits, and unspecified assistantships also available. Support available to part-time students. *Faculty research:* Behavioral management of chronic disorders, patient management in critical care, consumer informatics, genetic applications, technology. *Unit head:* Dr. Judith Erlen, Coordinator, 412-624-1905, Fax: 412-624-2401, E-mail: jae001@pitt.edu. *Application contact:* Laurie Lapsley, Administrator of Graduate Student Services, 412-624-9670, Fax: 412-624-2409, E-mail: lapsleyl@pitt.edu.
Website: http://www.nursing.pitt.edu/

University of Portland, School of Nursing, Portland, OR 97203. Offers clinical nurse leader (MS); nurse educator (MS); nursing (DNP). *Accreditation:* AACN. Part-time and evening/weekend programs available. Postbaccalaureate distance learning degree programs offered (minimal on-campus study). *Faculty:* 16 full-time (15 women), 10 part-time/adjunct (8 women). *Students:* 57 part-time (48 women); includes 4 minority (2 Asian, non-Hispanic/Latino; 1 Hispanic/Latino; 1 Two or more races, non-Hispanic/Latino), 2 international. Average age 36. In 2013, 12 master's, 6 doctorates awarded. *Entrance requirements:* For master's, GRE General Test or MAT, Oregon RN license, BSN, course work in statistics, resume, letters of recommendation, writing sample; for doctorate, GRE General Test or MAT, Oregon RN license, BSN or MSN, 2 letters of recommendation, resume, writing sample, official transcripts. Additional exam requirements/recommendations for international students: Required—TOEFL (minimum score 550 paper-based; 80 iBT), IELTS (minimum score 7). *Application deadline:* For fall admission, 11/2 priority date for domestic and international students; for spring admission, 1/7 priority date for domestic and international students. Applications are processed on a rolling basis. Application fee: $50. *Expenses:* Contact institution. *Financial support:* Fellowships, research assistantships, Federal Work-Study, and scholarships/grants available. Support available to part-time students. Financial award

application deadline: 3/1; financial award applicants required to submit FAFSA. *Unit head:* Dr. Katherine Crabtree, Associate Dean, 503-943-7211, E-mail: nursing@up.edu. *Application contact:* Chris Olinger, Assistant to the Provost and Dean of the Graduate School, 503-943-7107, Fax: 503-943-7315, E-mail: olingerc@up.edu.
Website: http://nursing.up.edu/default.aspx?cid-7047&pid-207

University of Puerto Rico, Medical Sciences Campus, School of Nursing, San Juan, PR 00936-5067. Offers adult and elderly nursing (MSN); child and adolescent nursing (MSN); critical care nursing (MSN); family and community nursing (MSN); family nurse practitioner (MSN); maternity nursing (MSN); mental health and psychiatric nursing (MSN). *Accreditation:* AACN. *Entrance requirements:* For master's, GRE or EXADEP, interview, Puerto Rico RN license or professional license for international students, general and specific point average, article analysis. Electronic applications accepted. *Faculty research:* HIV, health disparities, teen violence, women and violence, neurological disorders.

University of Regina, Faculty of Graduate Studies and Research, Faculty of Nursing, Regina, SK S4S 0A2, Canada. Offers MN. *Faculty:* 10 full-time (7 women). *Students:* 1 (woman) full-time. *Entrance requirements:* For master's, proof of licensure or registration as an RN including registration number in a Canadian province or territory, 2 years of clinical practice within last 5 years, written essay, minimum overall GPA of 75% in all 3rd- and 4th-year nursing courses taken at a Canadian-accredited or provincially-approved baccalaureate nursing education program. Additional exam requirements/recommendations for international students: Required—TOEFL (minimum score 580 paper-based; 80 iBT), IELTS (minimum score 6.5). *Application deadline:* For fall admission, 1/15 for domestic and international students. Application fee: $100. Electronic applications accepted. *Expenses: Tuition, area resident:* Full-time $4338 Canadian dollars. *International tuition:* $7338 Canadian dollars full-time. *Required fees:* $449.25 Canadian dollars. *Financial support:* Fellowships, research assistantships, teaching assistantships, and scholarships/grants available. Financial award application deadline: 6/15. *Unit head:* Dr. Laurie Clune, Associate Dean, Graduate Programs and Research, 306-337-3356, Fax: 306-337-8493, E-mail: laurie.clune@uregina.ca.
Website: http://www.uregina.ca/nursing/

University of Rhode Island, Graduate School, College of Nursing, Kingston, RI 02881. Offers administration (MS); clinical nurse leader (MS); clinical specialist in gerontology (MS); clinical specialist in psychiatric/mental health (MS); family nurse practitioner (MS); gerontological nurse practitioner (MS); nursing (DNP, PhD); nursing education (MS). *Accreditation:* AACN; ACNM/ACME (one or more programs are accredited). Part-time programs available. *Faculty:* 26 full-time (25 women), 3 part-time/adjunct (2 women). *Students:* 46 full-time (42 women), 78 part-time (70 women); includes 11 minority (7 Black or African American, non-Hispanic/Latino; 1 Asian, non-Hispanic/Latino; 3 Hispanic/Latino), 4 international. In 2013, 38 master's, 4 doctorates awarded. *Degree requirements:* For master's, comprehensive exam; for doctorate, comprehensive exam, thesis/dissertation. *Entrance requirements:* For master's, GRE or MAT, 2 letters of recommendation, scholarly papers; for doctorate, GRE, 3 letters of recommendation, scholarly papers. Additional exam requirements/recommendations for international students: Required—TOEFL (minimum score 550 paper-based). *Application deadline:* For fall admission, 2/15 for domestic students, 2/1 for international students; for spring admission, 10/15 for domestic students, 7/15 for international students. Application fee: $65. Electronic applications accepted. *Expenses:* Tuition, state resident: full-time $11,532; part-time $641 per credit. Tuition, nonresident: full-time $23,606; part-time $1311 per credit. *Required fees:* $1388; $36 per credit. $35 per semester. One-time fee: $130. *Financial support:* In 2013–14, 4 teaching assistantships with full and partial tuition reimbursements (averaging $8,383 per year) were awarded. Financial award application deadline: 2/15; financial award applicants required to submit FAFSA. *Faculty research:* Group intervention for grieving women in prison, translating best practice in non-drug interventions for postoperative pain management, further development and testing of the pain assessment inventory, preschool motor and functional performance of two cohorts, neuroactivation of brain motor areas in preterm children. *Total annual research expenditures:* $1.2 million. *Unit head:* Dr. Mary Sullivan, Interim Dean, 401-874-5339, Fax: 401-874-2061, E-mail: mcsullivan@uri.edu. *Application contact:* Graduate Admission, 401-874-2872, E-mail: gradadm@etal.uri.edu.
Website: http://www.uri.edu/nursing/

University of Rochester, School of Nursing, Rochester, NY 14642. Offers acute care nurse practitioner (MS); adult nurse practitioner (MS); adult/geriatric nurse practitioner (MS); clinical nurse leader (MS); clinical research coordinator (MS); family nurse practitioner (MS); family psychiatric mental health nurse practitioner (MS); health care organization management and leadership (MS); health practice research (PhD); nursing (DNP); pediatric nurse practitioner (MS); pediatric nurse practitioner/neonatal nurse practitioner (MS). *Accreditation:* AACN. Part-time programs available. Postbaccalaureate distance learning degree programs offered (minimal on-campus study). *Faculty:* 60 full-time (52 women), 61 part-time/adjunct (47 women). *Students:* 33 full-time (29 women), 213 part-time (195 women); includes 32 minority (8 Black or African American, non-Hispanic/Latino; 10 Asian, non-Hispanic/Latino; 8 Hispanic/Latino; 6 Two or more races, non-Hispanic/Latino), 4 international. Average age 34. 41 applicants, 54% accepted, 16 enrolled. In 2013, 58 master's, 11 doctorates awarded. Terminal master's awarded for partial completion of doctoral program. *Degree requirements:* For master's, comprehensive exam (for some programs); for doctorate, thesis/dissertation. *Entrance requirements:* For master's, BS in nursing, minimum GPA of 3.0, course work in statistics; for doctorate, GRE General Test, MS in nursing, minimum GPA of 3.5. Additional exam requirements/recommendations for international students: Required—TOEFL (minimum score 560 paper-based; 88 iBT) or IELTS (minimum score 6.5) recommended. *Application deadline:* For fall admission, 4/1 for domestic and international students; for spring admission, 9/1 for domestic and international students; for summer admission, 1/2 for domestic and international students. Application fee: $50. Electronic applications accepted. *Expenses: Tuition:* Full-time $44,580; part-time $1394 per credit hour. *Required fees:* $492. *Financial support:* In 2013–14, 41 students received support, including 2 fellowships with full and partial tuition reimbursements available (averaging $30,200 per year); scholarships/grants, traineeships, health care benefits, tuition waivers (partial), and unspecified assistantships also available. Support available to part-time students. Financial award application deadline: 6/30. *Faculty research:* Symptom assessment and self-management, illness prevention, nursing intervention research with vulnerable populations, palliative care, aging. *Total annual research expenditures:* $3.5 million. *Unit head:* Dr. Kathy H. Rideout, Dean, 585-273-8902, Fax: 585-273-1268, E-mail: kathy_rideout@urmc.rochester.edu. *Application contact:* Elaine Andolina, Director of Admissions, 585-275-2375, Fax: 585-756-8299, E-mail: elaine_andolina@urmc.rochester.edu.
Website: http://www.son.rochester.edu

University of Saint Francis, Graduate School, Department of Nursing, Fort Wayne, IN 46808. Offers family nurse practitioner (MSN, Post Master's Certificate). *Accreditation:* AACN. Part-time and evening/weekend programs available. Postbaccalaureate distance learning degree programs offered (minimal on-campus study). *Faculty:* 9. *Students:* 33 full-time (30 women), 69 part-time (65 women); includes 7 minority (3 Black or African American, non-Hispanic/Latino; 3 Hispanic/Latino; 1 Two or more races, non-Hispanic/Latino). Average age 33. 10 applicants, 100% accepted, 10 enrolled. In 2013, 33 master's awarded. *Degree requirements:* For master's, research project. *Entrance requirements:* For master's, GRE (if undergraduate GPA is less than 3.0), minimum undergraduate GPA of 3.2; Indiana RN license; graduate or undergraduate statistics course within the last five years. *Application deadline:* For fall admission, 7/1 priority date for domestic students; for spring admission, 11/1 priority date for domestic students. Applications are processed on a rolling basis. Application fee: $20. Application fee is waived when completed online. *Financial support:* Federal Work-Study, scholarships/grants, and unspecified assistantships available. Support available to part-time students. Financial award application deadline: 3/10; financial award applicants required to submit FAFSA. *Unit head:* Dr. Wendy Clark, Assistant Professor/Director of the MSN Program, 260-399-7700 Ext. 8534, Fax: 260-399-8167, E-mail: wclark@sf.edu. *Application contact:* James Cashdollar, Admissions Counselor, 260-399-7700 Ext. 6302, Fax: 260-399-8152, E-mail: jcashdollar@sf.edu.
Website: http://www.sf.edu/sf/graduate/sohs/nursing

University of St. Francis, Leach College of Nursing, Joliet, IL 60435-6169. Offers family nurse practitioner (MSN, Post-Master's Certificate); family psychology/mental health nurse practitioner (MSN, Post-Master's Certificate); nursing administration (MSN); nursing education (MSN); nursing practice (DNP); teaching in nursing (Certificate). *Accreditation:* AACN. Part-time and evening/weekend programs available. Postbaccalaureate distance learning degree programs offered (no on-campus study). *Faculty:* 11 full-time (all women), 12 part-time/adjunct (11 women). *Students:* 90 full-time (76 women), 332 part-time (305 women); includes 122 minority (43 Black or African American, non-Hispanic/Latino; 1 American Indian or Alaska Native, non-Hispanic/Latino; 19 Asian, non-Hispanic/Latino; 45 Hispanic/Latino; 3 Native Hawaiian or other Pacific Islander, non-Hispanic/Latino; 11 Two or more races, non-Hispanic/Latino), 4 international. Average age 42. 343 applicants, 43% accepted, 111 enrolled. In 2013, 82 master's, 6 doctorates, 17 other advanced degrees awarded. *Entrance requirements:* For master's, minimum undergraduate GPA of 3.0, 2 years of full-time clinical experience, 3 letters recommendation, resume, nursing license, interview; for doctorate, MSN with minimum GPA of 3.0, national certification, interview, computer competency, medical/physical requirements, background check, liability insurance, resume, recommendation, graduate-level statistics course. Additional exam requirements/recommendations for international students: Required—TOEFL (minimum score 550 paper-based; 79 iBT), IELTS (minimum score 6.5). *Application deadline:* Applications are processed on a rolling basis. Application fee: $30. Electronic applications accepted. Application fee is waived when completed online. *Expenses:* Contact institution. *Financial support:* In 2013–14, 109 students received support. Scholarships/grants and tuition waivers (partial) available. Support available to part-time students. Financial award applicants required to submit FAFSA. *Unit head:* Dr. Carol Wilson, Dean, 815-740-3840, Fax: 815-740-4243, E-mail: cwilson@stfrancis.edu. *Application contact:* Sandra Sloka, Director of Admissions for Graduate and Degree Completion Programs, 800-735-7500, Fax: 815-740-3431, E-mail: ssloka@stfrancis.edu.
Website: http://www.stfrancis.edu/academics/college-of-nursing/

University of Saint Joseph, Department of Nursing, West Hartford, CT 06117-2700. Offers family nurse practitioner (MS); family psychiatric/mental health nurse practitioner (MS); nurse educator (MS); nursing practice (DNP). *Accreditation:* AACN. Part-time and evening/weekend programs available. *Degree requirements:* For master's, thesis. *Entrance requirements:* For master's, 2 letters of recommendation. *Application deadline:* Applications are processed on a rolling basis. Application fee: $50. Electronic applications accepted. Application fee is waived when completed online. *Financial support:* Career-related internships or fieldwork and unspecified assistantships available. Support available to part-time students. Financial award applicants required to submit FAFSA. *Unit head:* Dr. Patricia Padula Morgan, RN, Chair, 860-231-5591, E-mail: pmorgan@usj.edu. *Application contact:* Graduate Admissions Office, 860-231-5261, E-mail: graduate@usj.edu.
Website: http://www.usj.edu/academics/schools/school-of-health-natural-sciences/nursing/

University of Saint Mary, Graduate Programs, Program in Nursing, Leavenworth, KS 66048-5082. Offers nurse administrator (MSN); nurse educator (MSN). Part-time programs available. Postbaccalaureate distance learning degree programs offered (no on-campus study). *Students:* 8 full-time (7 women), 4 part-time (all women). *Entrance requirements:* For master's, BSN from CCNE- or NLNAC-accredited baccalaureate nursing program at regionally-accredited institution. *Expenses: Tuition:* Part-time $550 per credit hour. *Unit head:* Dr. Glenna Mahoney, Department Chair, 877-307-4915, Fax: 913-345-2802. *Application contact:* Dr. Joyce Lasseter, Director, 877-307-4915, Fax: 913-345-2802.
Website: http://online.stmary.edu/MSN/master-science-nursing.asp

University of San Diego, Hahn School of Nursing and Health Science, San Diego, CA 92110. Offers adult-gerontology clinical nurse specialist (MSN); adult-gerontology nurse practitioner/family nurse practitioner (MSN); clinical nursing (MSN); executive nurse leader (MSN); family nurse practitioner (MSN); family/lifespan psychiatric-mental health nurse practitioner (MSN); healthcare informatics (MS, MSN); nursing (PhD); nursing practice (DNP); pediatric nurse practitioner/family nurse practitioner (MSN). *Accreditation:* AACN. Part-time and evening/weekend programs available. *Faculty:* 23 full-time (19 women), 48 part-time/adjunct (43 women). *Students:* 204 full-time (170 women), 166 part-time (144 women); includes 133 minority (26 Black or African American, non-Hispanic/Latino; 8 American Indian or Alaska Native, non-Hispanic/Latino; 50 Asian, non-Hispanic/Latino; 42 Hispanic/Latino; 1 Native Hawaiian or other Pacific Islander, non-Hispanic/Latino; 6 Two or more races, non-Hispanic/Latino), 7 international. Average age 36. 483 applicants, 58% accepted, 154 enrolled. In 2013, 91 master's, 33 doctorates awarded. *Degree requirements:* For doctorate, thesis/dissertation (for some programs), residency (DNP). *Entrance requirements:* For master's, GRE General Test (for entry-level nursing), BSN, current California RN licensure (except for entry-level nursing); minimum GPA of 3.0; for doctorate, minimum GPA of 3.5, MSN, current California RN licensure. Additional exam requirements/recommendations for international students: Required—TOEFL (minimum score 580 paper-based; 83 iBT), TWE. *Application deadline:* For fall admission, 3/1 priority date for domestic students, 3/1 for international students; for spring admission, 11/1 priority date for domestic students, 11/1 for international students. Applications are processed on a rolling basis. Application fee: $45. Electronic applications accepted. *Expenses: Tuition:* Full-time $23,580; part-time $1310 per credit. *Required fees:* $350. *Financial support:* In 2013–14, 250 students received support. Scholarships/grants and traineeships available. Support available to part-time students. Financial award application deadline: 4/1; financial award applicants required to submit FAFSA. *Faculty research:* Palliative and end of life care, maternal/child health, childhood obesity, health care disparities, cognitive functioning. *Unit head:* Dr. Sally Hardin, Dean, 619-260-4550, Fax: 619-260-6814. *Application contact:* Monica Mahon, Associate Director of Graduate Admissions, 619-260-4524, Fax: 619-260-4158, E-mail: grads@sandiego.edu.
Website: http://www.sandiego.edu/nursing/

University of San Francisco, School of Nursing and Health Professions, San Francisco, CA 94117-1080. Offers MPH, MSBH, MSN, DNP, Psy D. *Accreditation:* AACN. Part-time programs available. *Faculty:* 23 full-time (20 women), 38 part-time/

adjunct (30 women). *Students:* 473 full-time (393 women), 142 part-time (128 women); includes 311 minority (39 Black or African American, non-Hispanic/Latino; 3 American Indian or Alaska Native, non-Hispanic/Latino; 154 Asian, non-Hispanic/Latino; 76 Hispanic/Latino; 6 Native Hawaiian or other Pacific Islander, non-Hispanic/Latino; 33 Two or more races, non-Hispanic/Latino), 6 international. Average age 35. 622 applicants, 55% accepted, 219 enrolled. In 2013, 106 master's, 39 doctorates awarded. *Entrance requirements:* For master's, minimum GPA of 3.0. *Application deadline:* Applications are processed on a rolling basis. *Expenses: Tuition:* Full-time $21,150; part-time $1175 per unit. Tuition and fees vary according to course load, campus/location and program. *Financial support:* In 2013–14, 57 students received support. Institutionally sponsored loans available. Financial award application deadline: 3/2. *Faculty research:* Direct patient/client care, providers of health care. *Unit head:* Dr. Judith Karshmer, Dean, 415-422-6681, Fax: 415-422-6877, E-mail: nursing@usfca.edu. *Application contact:* Ingrid McVanner, Information Contact, 415-422-2746, Fax: 415-422-2217.
Website: http://www.usfca.edu/nursing/

University of Saskatchewan, College of Graduate Studies and Research, College of Nursing, Saskatoon, SK S7N 5E5, Canada. Offers MN. Part-time programs available. *Entrance requirements:* Additional exam requirements/recommendations for international students: Required—TOEFL. *Expenses: Tuition, area resident:* Full-time $3585 Canadian dollars; part-time $585 Canadian dollars per course. Tuition, Canadian resident: part-time $877 Canadian dollars per course. *International tuition:* $5377 Canadian dollars full-time. *Required fees:* $889.51 Canadian dollars.

The University of Scranton, College of Graduate and Continuing Education, Department of Nursing, Scranton, PA 18510-4595. Offers adult health nursing (MSN); family nurse practitioner (MSN, PMC); nurse anesthesia (MSN, PMC). Applicants accepted in odd-numbered years only. *Accreditation:* AACN; AANA/CANAEP. Part-time and evening/weekend programs available. *Faculty:* 13 full-time (all women), 2 part-time/adjunct (both women). *Students:* 42 full-time (37 women), 28 part-time (16 women); includes 9 minority (4 Black or African American, non-Hispanic/Latino; 3 Hispanic/Latino; 2 Two or more races, non-Hispanic/Latino). Average age 34. 58 applicants, 62% accepted. In 2013, 34 master's awarded. *Degree requirements:* For master's, thesis (for some programs), capstone experience. *Entrance requirements:* For master's, BSN, minimum GPA of 3.0, Pennsylvania RN license. Additional exam requirements/recommendations for international students: Required—TOEFL (minimum score 500 paper-based), IELTS (minimum score 5.5). *Application deadline:* For fall admission, 9/1 for domestic students. Applications are processed on a rolling basis. Application fee: $0. *Financial support:* In 2013–14, 6 students received support, including 6 teaching assistantships with full and partial tuition reimbursements available (averaging $6,600 per year); career-related internships or fieldwork, Federal Work-Study, and unspecified assistantships also available. Support available to part-time students. Financial award application deadline: 3/1. *Faculty research:* Home care, doctoral education, health care of women and children, pain, health promotion and adolescence. *Unit head:* Dr. Patricia Harrington, Chair, 570-941-7673, Fax: 570-941-4201, E-mail: harringtonp1@uofs.edu. *Application contact:* Dr. Mary Jane Hanson, Director, 570-941-4060, Fax: 570-941-4201, E-mail: hansonm2@scranton.edu.
Website: http://www.scranton.edu/academics/pcps/nursing/index.shtml

University of South Alabama, Graduate School, College of Nursing, Mobile, AL 36688. Offers adult health nursing (MSN); community/mental health nursing (MSN); maternal/child nursing (MSN); nursing (DNP). *Accreditation:* AACN. *Faculty:* 50 full-time (46 women), 31 part-time/adjunct (30 women). *Students:* 1,878 full-time (1,680 women), 241 part-time (208 women); includes 523 minority (341 Black or African American, non-Hispanic/Latino; 18 American Indian or Alaska Native, non-Hispanic/Latino; 76 Asian, non-Hispanic/Latino; 54 Hispanic/Latino; 7 Native Hawaiian or other Pacific Islander, non-Hispanic/Latino; 27 Two or more races, non-Hispanic/Latino), 10 international. 1,308 applicants, 64% accepted, 602 enrolled. In 2013, 332 master's, 44 doctorates awarded. *Degree requirements:* For master's, thesis optional. *Entrance requirements:* For master's, BSN, RN licensure, minimum GPA of 3.0, resume documenting clinical experience, background check, drug screening; for doctorate, GRE. *Application deadline:* For fall admission, 7/15 for domestic students; for spring admission, 12/1 for domestic students. Application fee: $35. *Expenses:* Tuition, state resident: full-time $8976; part-time $374 per credit hour. Tuition, nonresident: full-time $17,952; part-time $748 per credit hour. *Unit head:* Dr. Debra Davis, Dean, 251-445-9409, Fax: 251-445-9416. *Application contact:* Dr. Rosemary Rhodes, Director of Graduate Education, 251-445-9409, Fax: 251-445-9416, E-mail: kharriso@usouthal.edu.
Website: http://www.southalabama.edu/nursing

University of South Carolina, The Graduate School, College of Nursing, Program in Advanced Practice Clinical Nursing, Columbia, SC 29208. Offers acute care nurse practitioner (Certificate); advanced practice clinical nursing (MSN). *Accreditation:* AACN. Part-time programs available. Postbaccalaureate distance learning degree programs offered (minimal on-campus study). *Entrance requirements:* For master's, master's degree in nursing, RN license; for Certificate, MSN. Additional exam requirements/recommendations for international students: Required—TOEFL (minimum score 570 paper-based). Electronic applications accepted. *Faculty research:* Systems research, evidence based practice, breast cancer, violence.

University of South Carolina, The Graduate School, College of Nursing, Program in Advanced Practice Nursing in Primary Care, Columbia, SC 29208. Offers MSN, Certificate. *Accreditation:* AACN. *Entrance requirements:* For master's, master's degree in nursing, RN license; for Certificate, MSN. Additional exam requirements/recommendations for international students: Required—TOEFL (minimum score 570 paper-based). Electronic applications accepted. *Faculty research:* Systems research, evidence based practice, breast cancer, violence.

University of Southern Indiana, Graduate Studies, College of Nursing and Health Professions, Program in Nursing, Evansville, IN 47712-3590. Offers MSN, DNP. Part-time programs available. Postbaccalaureate distance learning degree programs offered (minimal on-campus study). *Faculty:* 7 full-time (6 women), 2 part-time/adjunct (both women). *Students:* 17 full-time (14 women), 445 part-time (404 women); includes 34 minority (19 Black or African American, non-Hispanic/Latino; 2 American Indian or Alaska Native, non-Hispanic/Latino; 6 Asian, non-Hispanic/Latino; 3 Hispanic/Latino; 1 Native Hawaiian or other Pacific Islander, non-Hispanic/Latino; 3 Two or more races, non-Hispanic/Latino), 12 international. Average age 37. 633 applicants, 34% accepted, 155 enrolled. In 2013, 107 master's, 18 doctorates awarded. *Entrance requirements:* For master's, BSN from nationally-accredited school; minimum cumulative GPA of 3.0; satisfactory completion of a course in undergraduate statistics (minimum grade C); one year full-time or two thousand hours of clinical practice as an RN (recommended); for doctorate, MSN; minimum cumulative graduate GPA of 3.25; satisfactory completion of a course in research; unencumbered RN license; curriculum vitae; three professional references; letters of intent. Additional exam requirements/recommendations for international students: Required—TOEFL (minimum score 550 paper-based; 79 iBT), IELTS (minimum score 6). *Application deadline:* For fall admission, 2/1 for domestic students, 1/1 priority date for international students. Applications are processed on a rolling basis. Application fee: $40. Electronic applications accepted. *Expenses:* Tuition, state resident: full-time $5567; part-time $309 per credit hour. Tuition, nonresident: full-time $10,977; part-time $610 per credit. *Required fees:* $23 per semester. *Financial support:* In 2013–14, 34 students received support. Federal Work-Study, scholarships/grants, tuition waivers (full and partial), and unspecified assistantships available. Financial award application deadline: 3/1; financial award applicants required to submit FAFSA. *Unit head:* Dr. Mellisa Hall, Chair of the Master of Science in Nursing Program, 812-465-1168, E-mail: mrowser@usi.edu. *Application contact:* Dr. Mayola Rowser, Interim Director, Graduate Studies, 812-465-7016, Fax: 812-464-1956, E-mail: mrowser@usi.edu.
Website: https://www.usi.edu/health/nursing/degrees-and-programs

University of Southern Maine, College of Science, Technology, and Health, School of Nursing, Portland, ME 04104-9300. Offers adult-gerontology primary care nurse practitioner (MS, PMC); clinical nurse leader (MS); education (MS); family nurse practitioner (MS, PMC); family psychiatric/mental health nurse practitioner (MS); management (MS); nursing (DNP); psychiatric-mental health nurse practitioner (PMC); MBA/MSN. *Accreditation:* AACN. Part-time programs available. *Faculty:* 11 full-time (all women), 10 part-time/adjunct (8 women). *Students:* 57 full-time (47 women), 53 part-time (46 women); includes 5 minority (1 American Indian or Alaska Native, non-Hispanic/Latino; 2 Asian, non-Hispanic/Latino; 1 Hispanic/Latino; 1 Two or more races, non-Hispanic/Latino). Average age 36. 140 applicants, 44% accepted, 29 enrolled. In 2013, 33 master's, 11 other advanced degrees awarded. *Degree requirements:* For master's, thesis optional. *Entrance requirements:* For master's, GRE General Test or MAT, minimum GPA of 3.0; for doctorate, GRE. Additional exam requirements/recommendations for international students: Required—TOEFL (minimum score 550 paper-based). *Application deadline:* For fall admission, 4/1 for domestic and international students; for spring admission, 10/1 for domestic and international students. Application fee: $65. Electronic applications accepted. *Expenses:* Tuition, state resident: part-time $380 per credit. Tuition, nonresident: part-time $1026 per credit. Part-time tuition and fees vary according to program. *Financial support:* Research assistantships, teaching assistantships, career-related internships or fieldwork, Federal Work-Study, scholarships/grants, traineeships, tuition waivers (full and partial), and unspecified assistantships available. Support available to part-time students. Financial award application deadline: 2/15; financial award applicants required to submit FAFSA. *Faculty research:* Women's health, nursing history, weight control, community services, substance abuse. *Unit head:* Krista M. Meinersmann, Director of Nursing Program, 207-780-4993, E-mail: kmeinersmann@usm.maine.edu. *Application contact:* Mary Sloan, Assistant Dean of Graduate Studies and Director of Graduate Admissions, 207-780-4812, E-mail: gradstudies@usm.maine.edu.
Website: http://www.usm.maine.edu/nursing/

University of Southern Mississippi, Graduate School, College of Health, School of Nursing, Hattiesburg, MS 39406-0001. Offers family nurse practitioner (MSN); nursing (DNP, PhD); nursing executive (MSN); psychiatric nurse practitioner (MSN). *Accreditation:* AACN. Part-time and evening/weekend programs available. *Faculty:* 17 full-time (16 women), 1 part-time/adjunct (0 women). *Students:* 133 full-time (104 women), 42 part-time (40 women); includes 45 minority (33 Black or African American, non-Hispanic/Latino; 1 American Indian or Alaska Native, non-Hispanic/Latino; 1 Asian, non-Hispanic/Latino; 1 Hispanic/Latino; 9 Two or more races, non-Hispanic/Latino). Average age 37. 118 applicants, 61% accepted, 62 enrolled. In 2013, 45 master's, 9 doctorates awarded. *Degree requirements:* For master's, comprehensive exam, thesis optional; for doctorate, comprehensive exam, thesis/dissertation. *Entrance requirements:* For master's, GRE General Test, minimum GPA of 2.75 during last 60 hours, nursing license, BS in nursing; for doctorate, GRE General Test, master's degree in nursing, minimum GPA of 3.5. Additional exam requirements/recommendations for international students: Required—TOEFL, IELTS. *Application deadline:* For fall admission, 3/15 priority date for domestic students, 5/1 for international students; for spring admission, 1/10 priority date for domestic and international students. Applications are processed on a rolling basis. Application fee: $50. Electronic applications accepted. *Financial support:* In 2013–14, 14 research assistantships with full tuition reimbursements (averaging $12,577 per year), teaching assistantships (averaging $12,000 per year) were awarded; Federal Work-Study, institutionally sponsored loans, scholarships/grants, traineeships, health care benefits, and unspecified assistantships also available. Financial award application deadline: 3/15; financial award applicants required to submit FAFSA. *Faculty research:* Gerontology, caregivers, HIV, bereavement, pain, nursing leadership. *Unit head:* Dr. Katherine Nugent, Director and Associate Dean, 601-266-5500, Fax: 601-266-5927. *Application contact:* Dr. Sandra Bishop, Graduate Coordinator, 601-266-5500, Fax: 601-266-5927.
Website: http://www.usm.edu/graduateschool/table.php

University of South Florida, College of Nursing, Tampa, FL 33612. Offers adult gerontology acute care (DNP, PhD); adult gerontology acute care nursing (MS); adult gerontology primary care (DNP, PhD); adult gerontology primary care nursing (MS); adult gerontology primary care/occupational health nursing (MS); adult gerontology primary care/oncology nursing (MS, PhD); clinical nurse leader (MS); family health (DNP, PhD); family nurse practitioner (MS); nurse anesthesia (MS); nursing education (MS); nursing practice (DNP); nursing science (PhD), including nursing education; occupational health/adult-gerontology (DNP); oncology/adult-gerontology primary care (DNP); pediatric health (DNP, PhD); pediatric nurse practitioner (MS). *Accreditation:* AACN; AANA/CANAEP. Part-time programs available. *Faculty:* 46 full-time (40 women), 15 part-time/adjunct (11 women). *Students:* 177 full-time (150 women), 700 part-time (622 women); includes 272 minority (116 Black or African American, non-Hispanic/Latino; 2 American Indian or Alaska Native, non-Hispanic/Latino; 45 Asian, non-Hispanic/Latino; 93 Hispanic/Latino; 2 Native Hawaiian or other Pacific Islander, non-Hispanic/Latino; 14 Two or more races, non-Hispanic/Latino), 12 international. Average age 35. 656 applicants, 43% accepted, 224 enrolled. In 2013, 224 master's, 14 doctorates awarded. *Degree requirements:* For master's, comprehensive exam, thesis optional; for doctorate, comprehensive exam, thesis/dissertation. *Entrance requirements:* For master's, GRE General Test, bachelor's degree from accredited program with minimum GPA of 3.0 in all upper-division coursework; current license as Registered Nurse; 3 letters of recommendation; personal statement of goals; resume or curriculum vitae; personal interview; for doctorate, GRE General Test (recommended), bachelor's degree in nursing from a CCNA/NLNAC regionally-accredited institution with minimum GPA of 3.0 in all coursework or in all upper-division coursework; current license as Registered Nurse in Florida; undergraduate statistics course with minimum B grade; 3 letters of recommendation; statement of goals; resume; interview. Additional exam requirements/recommendations for international students: Required—TOEFL (minimum score 550 paper-based; 79 iBT). *Application deadline:* For fall admission, 2/15 for domestic students, 1/2 for international students; for spring admission, 10/1 for domestic students, 6/1 for international students. Application fee: $30. Electronic applications accepted. *Financial support:* In 2013–14, 36 students received support, including 7 research assistantships with tuition reimbursements available (averaging $18,935 per year), 29 teaching assistantships with tuition reimbursements available (averaging $30,814 per year); tuition waivers (partial) and unspecified assistantships also available. Financial award application deadline: 2/1; financial award applicants required to submit FAFSA. *Faculty research:* Women's health, palliative and end-of-life care, cardiac rehabilitation, complementary therapies for chronic illness and cancer. *Total annual research expenditures:* $3.4 million. *Unit head:* Dr. Dianne C. Morrison-

Beedy, Dean and Professor, College of Nursing, 813-974-9091, Fax: 813-974-5418, E-mail: dmbeedy@health.usf.edu. *Application contact:* Dr. Connie Visovsky, Associate Professor and Associate Dean of Student Affairs, 813-396-9641, Fax: 813-974-5418, E-mail: cvisovsk@health.usf.edu.
Website: http://health.usf.edu/nursing/index.htm

The University of Tampa, Nursing Programs, Tampa, FL 33606-1490. Offers adult nurse practitioner (MSN); family nurse practitioner (MSN). Part-time programs available. *Faculty:* 15 full-time (all women), 15 part-time/adjunct (14 women). *Students:* 2 full-time (both women), 134 part-time (119 women); includes 37 minority (10 Black or African American, non-Hispanic/Latino; 1 American Indian or Alaska Native, non-Hispanic/Latino; 6 Asian, non-Hispanic/Latino; 19 Hispanic/Latino; 1 Two or more races, non-Hispanic/Latino). Average age 34. 79 applicants, 51% accepted, 28 enrolled. In 2013, 39 master's awarded. *Degree requirements:* For master's, comprehensive exam, oral exam, practicum. *Entrance requirements:* For master's, GRE (minimum score of 1000, 4.0 on Analytical Writing portion), bachelor's degree in nursing, current Florida RN license, minimum GPA of 3.0. Additional exam requirements/recommendations for international students: Required—TOEFL or IELTS. *Application deadline:* Applications are processed on a rolling basis. Application fee: $40. Electronic applications accepted. *Expenses: Tuition:* Full-time $8928; part-time $558 per credit hour. *Required fees:* $80; $80 $40 per term. Tuition and fees vary according to program. *Financial support:* In 2013–14, 9 students received support. Unspecified assistantships available. Financial award applicants required to submit FAFSA. *Faculty research:* Vaccinations and public health, osteoporosis, cultural diversity, ethics, nursing practice. *Unit head:* Dr. Maria Warda, Director/Chair, 813-257-3302, Fax: 813-258-7214, E-mail: mwarda@ut.edu. *Application contact:* Brent Benner, Director of Admissions, 813-257-3642, E-mail: bbenner@ut.edu.

The University of Tennessee, Graduate School, College of Nursing, Knoxville, TN 37996. Offers MSN, PhD. *Accreditation:* AACN; AANA/CANAEP. Part-time programs available. *Degree requirements:* For master's, thesis or alternative; for doctorate, thesis/dissertation. *Entrance requirements:* For master's and doctorate, GRE General Test, minimum GPA of 2.7. Additional exam requirements/recommendations for international students: Required—TOEFL. Electronic applications accepted. *Expenses:* Tuition, state resident: full-time $9540; part-time $531 per credit hour. Tuition, nonresident: full-time $27,728; part-time $1542 per credit hour. *Required fees:* $1404; $67 per credit hour.

The University of Tennessee at Chattanooga, Graduate School, College of Health, Education and Professional Studies, School of Nursing, Chattanooga, TN 37403. Offers administration (MSN); certified nurse anesthetist (Post-Master's Certificate); education (MSN); family nurse practitioner (MSN, Post-Master's Certificate); health care informatics (Post-Master's Certificate); nurse anesthesia (MSN); nurse education (Post-Master's Certificate); nursing (DNP). *Accreditation:* AACN; AANA/CANAEP (one or more programs are accredited). *Faculty:* 9 full-time (7 women), 2 part-time/adjunct (1 woman). *Students:* 72 full-time (39 women), 53 part-time (43 women); includes 11 minority (6 Black or African American, non-Hispanic/Latino; 1 Asian, non-Hispanic/Latino; 3 Hispanic/Latino; 1 Two or more races, non-Hispanic/Latino). Average age 33. 3 applicants, 100% accepted, 1 enrolled. In 2013, 35 master's, 10 doctorates, 2 other advanced degrees awarded. *Degree requirements:* For master's, thesis optional, qualifying exams, professional project; for Post-Master's Certificate, thesis or alternative, practicum, seminar. *Entrance requirements:* For master's, GRE General Test, MAT, BSN, minimum GPA of 3.0, eligibility for Tennessee RN license, 1 year of direct patient care experience; for Post-Master's Certificate, GRE General Test, MAT, MSN, minimum GPA of 3.0, eligibility for Tennessee RN license, one year of direct patient care experience. Additional exam requirements/recommendations for international students: Required—TOEFL (minimum score 550 paper-based; 79 iBT), IELTS (minimum score 6). *Application deadline:* For fall admission, 6/13 priority date for domestic students, 6/1 for international students; for spring admission, 10/15 priority date for domestic students, 10/1 for international students. Applications are processed on a rolling basis. Application fee: $30 ($35 for international students). Electronic applications accepted. *Financial support:* Career-related internships or fieldwork and scholarships/grants available. Support available to part-time students. *Faculty research:* Diabetes in women, health care for elderly, alternative medicine, hypertension, nurse anesthesia. *Total annual research expenditures:* $3.4 million. *Unit head:* Dr. Chris Smith, Interim Director, 423-425-1741, Fax: 423-425-4668, E-mail: chris-smith@utc.edu. *Application contact:* Dr. J. Randy Walker, Interim Dean of Graduate Studies, 423-425-4478, Fax: 423-425-5223, E-mail: randy-walker@utc.edu.
Website: http://www.utc.edu/Academic/Nursing/

The University of Tennessee Health Science Center, College of Graduate Health Sciences, Memphis, TN 38163-0002. Offers biomedical engineering (MS, PhD); biomedical sciences (PhD); dental sciences (MDS); epidemiology (MS); health outcomes and policy research (PhD); laboratory research and management (MS); nursing science (PhD); pharmaceutical sciences (PhD); pharmacology (MS); speech and hearing science (PhD); DDS/PhD; DNP/PhD; MD/PhD; Pharm D/PhD. *Faculty:* 318 full-time (92 women), 59 part-time/adjunct (16 women). *Students:* 220 full-time (102 women), 22 part-time (13 women); includes 194 minority (22 Black or African American, non-Hispanic/Latino; 161 Asian, non-Hispanic/Latino; 7 Hispanic/Latino; 3 Native Hawaiian or other Pacific Islander, non-Hispanic/Latino; 1 Two or more races, non-Hispanic/Latino), 106 international. Average age 25. 404 applicants, 17% accepted, 64 enrolled. In 2013, 13 master's, 25 doctorates awarded. Terminal master's awarded for partial completion of doctoral program. *Degree requirements:* For master's, comprehensive exam, thesis; for doctorate, comprehensive exam, thesis/dissertation, oral and written preliminary and comprehensive exams. *Entrance requirements:* For master's and doctorate, GRE General Test, minimum GPA of 3.0. Additional exam requirements/recommendations for international students: Required—TOEFL (minimum score 79 iBT); Recommended—IELTS (minimum score 6.5). *Application deadline:* For fall admission, 5/15 priority date for domestic students. Applications are processed on a rolling basis. Application fee: $0. Electronic applications accepted. *Financial support:* In 2013–14, 125 students received support, including 125 research assistantships (averaging $23,000 per year); career-related internships or fieldwork, Federal Work-Study, institutionally sponsored loans, and tuition waivers (full and partial) also available. Support available to part-time students. Financial award application deadline: 2/25; financial award applicants required to submit FAFSA. *Unit head:* Dr. Donald B. Thomason, Dean, 901-448-5538, E-mail: dthomaso@uthsc.edu. *Application contact:* William Carter, Director for Admissions, 901-448-1687, E-mail: wcarte17@uthsc.edu.
Website: http://www.uthsc.edu/grad/

The University of Tennessee Health Science Center, College of Nursing, Memphis, TN 38163-0002. Offers advanced practice nursing (DNP); clinical nurse leader (MSN). *Accreditation:* AACN; AANA/CANAEP. Postbaccalaureate distance learning degree programs offered (minimal on-campus study). *Degree requirements:* For master's, thesis; for doctorate, thesis/dissertation. *Entrance requirements:* For master's, GRE General Test, BSN, minimum GPA of 3.0; for doctorate, minimum GPA of 3.0. Additional exam requirements/recommendations for international students: Required—TOEFL. *Application deadline:* For fall admission, 2/1 for domestic students; for winter admission, 9/1 for domestic students. Application fee: $50. Electronic applications accepted. *Expenses:* Contact institution. *Financial support:* Fellowships with partial tuition reimbursements, teaching assistantships, Federal Work-Study, institutionally sponsored loans, scholarships/grants, and traineeships available. Support available to part-time students. Financial award application deadline: 2/28; financial award applicants required to submit FAFSA. *Unit head:* Dr. Wendy Likes, Interim Dean, 901-448-6135, Fax: 901-448-4121, E-mail: wlikes@uthsc.edu. *Application contact:* Dr. Wendy Likes, Interim Dean, 901-448-6135, Fax: 901-448-4121, E-mail: wlikes@uthsc.edu.
Website: http://uthsc.edu/nursing/

The University of Texas at Arlington, Graduate School, College of Nursing, Arlington, TX 76019. Offers nurse practitioner (MSN); nursing administration (MSN); nursing education (MSN); nursing practice (DNP); nursing science (PhD). *Accreditation:* AACN. Part-time and evening/weekend programs available. Postbaccalaureate distance learning degree programs offered (no on-campus study). *Degree requirements:* For master's, practicum course; for doctorate, comprehensive exam (for some programs), thesis/dissertation (for some programs), proposal defense dissertation (for PhD); scholarship project (for DNP). *Entrance requirements:* For master's, GRE General Test if GPA less than 3.0, minimum GPA of 3.0, Texas nursing license, minimum C grade in undergraduate statistics course; for doctorate, GRE General Test (waived for MSN-to-PhD applicants), minimum undergraduate, graduate and statistics GPA of 3.0; Texas RN license; interview; written statement of goals. Additional exam requirements/recommendations for international students: Required—TOEFL (minimum score 550 paper-based), IELTS (minimum score 7). *Faculty research:* Simulation in clinical education and practice, cultural diversity, vulnerable populations, substance abuse.

The University of Texas at Austin, Graduate School, School of Nursing, Austin, TX 78712-1111. Offers adult - gerontology clinical nurse specialist (MSN); child health (MSN), including administration, public health nursing, teaching; family nurse practitioner (MSN); family psychiatric/mental health nurse practitioner (MSN); holistic adult health (MSN), including administration, teaching; maternity (MSN), including administration, public health nursing, teaching; nursing (PhD); nursing administration and healthcare systems management (MSN); pediatric nurse practitioner (MSN); public health nursing (MSN). *Accreditation:* AACN. Part-time programs available. *Degree requirements:* For master's, thesis optional; for doctorate, thesis/dissertation. *Entrance requirements:* For master's and doctorate, GRE General Test. Additional exam requirements/recommendations for international students: Required—TOEFL (minimum score 550 paper-based). Electronic applications accepted. *Faculty research:* Chronic illness management, memory and aging, health promotion, women's health, adolescent health.

The University of Texas at Brownsville, Graduate Studies, College of Nursing, Brownsville, TX 78520-4991. Offers MSN. Part-time and evening/weekend programs available. Postbaccalaureate distance learning degree programs offered (no on-campus study). *Faculty:* 8 full-time (all women). *Students:* 26 full-time (21 women), 24 part-time (17 women); includes 43 minority (7 Black or African American, non-Hispanic/Latino; 6 Asian, non-Hispanic/Latino; 30 Hispanic/Latino), 1 international. 32 applicants, 44% accepted, 11 enrolled. In 2013, 12 master's awarded. *Degree requirements:* For master's, comprehensive exam, thesis optional, capstone course. *Entrance requirements:* Additional exam requirements/recommendations for international students: Required—TOEFL (minimum score 550 paper-based; 77 iBT). *Application deadline:* For fall admission, 7/1 priority date for domestic students, 7/1 for international students; for spring admission, 12/1 priority date for domestic students, 12/1 for international students. Applications are processed on a rolling basis. Application fee: $30. Electronic applications accepted. *Expenses:* Tuition, state resident: full-time $3444; part-time $1148 per semester. Tuition, nonresident: full-time $9816. *Required fees:* $1018; $221 per credit hour. $401 per semester. *Financial support:* In 2013–14, 7 students received support, including 1 research assistantship (averaging $10,000 per year); Federal Work-Study, scholarships/grants, and unspecified assistantships also available. Financial award application deadline: 3/1; financial award applicants required to submit FAFSA. *Unit head:* Dr. Anne Rentfro, Associate Professor, 956-882-5070, Fax: 956-882-5100, E-mail: anne.rentfro@utb.edu. *Application contact:* Mari Montelongo, Graduate Studies Specialist, 956-882-7787, Fax: 956-882-7279, E-mail: mari.montelongo@utb.edu.
Website: http://www.utb.edu/vpaa/nursing/msn/Pages/default.aspx

The University of Texas at El Paso, Graduate School, School of Nursing, El Paso, TX 79968-0001. Offers family nurse practitioner (MSN); health care leadership and management (Certificate); interdisciplinary health sciences (PhD); nursing (DNP); nursing education (MSN, Certificate); nursing systems management (MSN). *Accreditation:* AACN. Postbaccalaureate distance learning degree programs offered (minimal on-campus study). *Degree requirements:* For master's, thesis optional; for doctorate, thesis/dissertation. *Entrance requirements:* For master's, minimum GPA of 3.0, resume; for doctorate, GRE, letters of reference, relevant personal/professional experience; master's degree in nursing (for DNP); for Certificate, bachelor's degree in nursing. Additional exam requirements/recommendations for international students: Required—TOEFL; Recommended—IELTS. Electronic applications accepted.

The University of Texas at Tyler, College of Nursing and Health Sciences, Program in Nursing, Tyler, TX 75799-0001. Offers nurse practitioner (MSN); nursing (PhD); nursing administration (MSN); nursing education (MSN); MSN/MBA. *Accreditation:* AACN. Part-time and evening/weekend programs available. Postbaccalaureate distance learning degree programs offered (no on-campus study). *Degree requirements:* For master's, comprehensive exam (for some programs), thesis (for some programs); for doctorate, thesis/dissertation. *Entrance requirements:* For master's, GRE General Test or MAT, GMAT, minimum undergraduate GPA of 3.0, course work in statistics, RN license, BSN. Additional exam requirements/recommendations for international students: Required—TOEFL. Electronic applications accepted. *Faculty research:* Psychosocial adjustment, aging, support/commitment of caregivers, psychological abuse and violence, hope/hopelessness, professional values, end of life care, suicidology, clinical supervision, workforce retention and issues, global health issues, health promotion.

The University of Texas Health Science Center at Houston, School of Nursing, Houston, TX 77030. Offers MSN, DNP, PhD, MSN/MPH. *Accreditation:* AACN; AANA/CANAEP. Part-time programs available. *Degree requirements:* For master's, thesis, research project, or clinical project; for doctorate, thesis/dissertation. *Entrance requirements:* For master's, GRE or MAT, BSN, Texas RN license, related work experience, interview, writing sample; for doctorate, GRE, interview, Texas RN license, portfolio, master's degree. Additional exam requirements/recommendations for international students: Required—TOEFL (minimum score 550 paper-based; 86 iBT). Electronic applications accepted. *Expenses:* Tuition, state resident: full-time $3474; part-time $193 per credit hour. Tuition, nonresident: full-time $13,644; part-time $758 per credit hour. *Required fees:* $226.30; $87 per credit hour. *Faculty research:* Malnutrition in institutionalized elderly, defining nursing, sensitive outcome measures, substance abuse in mothers during pregnancy, psychoeducational intervention among caregivers of stroke patients.

The University of Texas Health Science Center at San Antonio, School of Nursing, San Antonio, TX 78229. Offers administrative management (MSN); adult-gerontology acute care nurse practitioner (PGC); clinical nurse leader (MSN); executive administrative management (DNP); family nurse practitioner (PGC); nurse practitioner (MSN), including adult-gerontology acute care nurse practitioner, family nurse

practitioner, pediatric nurse practitioner primary care, psychiatric mental health nurse practitioner; nurse practitioner leadership (DNP); nursing (MSN, PhD); nursing education (MSN, PGC); pediatric nurse practitioner primary care (PGC); psychiatric mental health nurse practitioner (PGC); public health nurse leader (DNP). *Accreditation:* AACN. Part-time programs available. *Faculty:* 84 full-time (74 women), 42 part-time/adjunct (40 women). *Students:* 115 full-time (93 women), 140 part-time (123 women); includes 123 minority (24 Black or African American, non-Hispanic/Latino; 20 Asian, non-Hispanic/Latino; 74 Hispanic/Latino; 5 Two or more races, non-Hispanic/Latino), 7 international. Average age 37. 174 applicants, 59% accepted, 83 enrolled. In 2013, 67 master's, 6 doctorates, 5 other advanced degrees awarded. Terminal master's awarded for partial completion of doctoral program. *Degree requirements:* For master's, thesis optional; for doctorate, comprehensive exam, thesis/dissertation, final projects (for DNP). *Entrance requirements:* For master's, minimum GPA of 3.0, references, goal statement, BSN from accredited nursing school, RN licensure in Texas or compact state; for doctorate, GRE, MAT, minimum GPA of 3.0, personal interview, BSN and/or MSN from accredited nursing school, RN licensure in Texas or compact state, statistics course, references, curriculum vitae, goal statement; for PGC, minimum GPA of 3.0; references; goal statement; MSN from accredited nursing school; RN licensure in Texas or compact state; prerequisites in advanced health assessment, advanced pharmacotherapeutics, and advanced pathophysiology. Additional exam requirements/recommendations for international students: Required—TOEFL (minimum score 550 paper-based; 68 iBT), IELTS (minimum score 6.5). *Application deadline:* For fall admission, 1/10 for domestic and international students; for spring admission, 7/1 for domestic students. Application fee: $65. Electronic applications accepted. *Financial support:* In 2013–14, 145 students received support, including 3 fellowships with full tuition reimbursements available (averaging $30,000 per year); institutionally sponsored loans and scholarships/grants also available. Financial award application deadline: 6/30; financial award applicants required to submit FAFSA. *Faculty research:* Pain, organizational structure, aging, quality and safety, health disparity, obesity and nutrition, women's and children's health. *Total annual research expenditures:* $500,265. *Unit head:* Dr. Eileen T. Breslin, Dean, 210-567-5800, Fax: 210-567-5929, E-mail: breslin@uthscsa.edu. *Application contact:* Brandy Finck, Interim Associate Dean for Admissions and Student Services, 210-567-5805, Fax: 210-567-6189, E-mail: finckb@uthscsa.edu.
Website: http://www.nursing.uthscsa.edu/

The University of Texas Medical Branch, Graduate School of Biomedical Sciences, Doctoral Program in Nursing, Galveston, TX 77555. Offers PhD. *Degree requirements:* For doctorate, comprehensive exam, thesis/dissertation. *Entrance requirements:* For doctorate, GRE General Test, minimum GPA of 3.0, BSN and MSN or equivalent advanced degree, 2 writing samples, 3 letters of reference, curriculum vitae or resume. Additional exam requirements/recommendations for international students: Required—TOEFL (minimum score 550 paper-based). Electronic applications accepted.

The University of Texas Medical Branch, School of Nursing, Master's Program in Nursing, Galveston, TX 77555. Offers MSN. Part-time programs available. Postbaccalaureate distance learning degree programs offered. *Entrance requirements:* For master's, GRE General Test or MAT, minimum BSN GPA of 3.0, 3 references, interview, 1 year nursing experience. Additional exam requirements/recommendations for international students: Required—TOEFL (minimum score 550 paper-based).

The University of Texas–Pan American, College of Health Sciences and Human Services, Department of Nursing, Edinburg, TX 78539. Offers adult health nursing (MSN); family nurse practitioner (MSN). *Accreditation:* AACN. Part-time and evening/weekend programs available. *Degree requirements:* For master's, thesis optional. *Entrance requirements:* For master's, Texas RN licensure, undergraduate physical statistic course. Additional exam requirements/recommendations for international students: Required—TOEFL (minimum score 550 paper-based). Electronic applications accepted. *Expenses:* Contact institution. *Faculty research:* Health promotion, adolescent pregnancy, herbal and nontraditional approaches, healing touch stress.

University of the Incarnate Word, School of Graduate Studies and Research, School of Nursing and Health Professions, Program in Nursing, San Antonio, TX 78209-6397. Offers clinical nursing leader (MSN); clinical nursing specialist (MSN); nursing (DNP). *Accreditation:* AACN. Part-time and evening/weekend programs available. *Faculty:* 14 full-time (all women), 1 part-time/adjunct (0 women). *Students:* 12 full-time (8 women), 50 part-time (34 women); includes 54 minority (8 Black or African American, non-Hispanic/Latino; 6 Asian, non-Hispanic/Latino; 39 Hispanic/Latino; 1 Two or more races, non-Hispanic/Latino), 11 international. Average age 41. 44 applicants, 70% accepted, 17 enrolled. In 2013, 14 master's, 2 doctorates awarded. *Degree requirements:* For master's, capstone, clinical hours. *Entrance requirements:* For master's, baccalaureate degree in nursing from CCNE- or NLN-accredited program including courses in statistics and health assessment; minimum undergraduate cumulative GPA of 2.5, 3.0 in upper-division nursing courses; three professional references; license to practice nursing in Texas or recognized state. Additional exam requirements/recommendations for international students: Required—TOEFL (minimum score 560 paper-based; 83 iBT). *Application deadline:* Applications are processed on a rolling basis. Application fee: $20. Electronic applications accepted. *Expenses: Tuition:* Part-time $815 per credit hour. *Required fees:* $86 per credit hour. One-time fee: $40 part-time. Tuition and fees vary according to degree level and program. *Financial support:* Federal Work-Study, scholarships/grants, and traineeships available. Support available to part-time students. Financial award applicants required to submit FAFSA. *Unit head:* Dr. Holly Cassells, Chair, Graduate Programs, 210-829-3977, Fax: 210-829-3174, E-mail: cassells@uiwtx.edu. *Application contact:* Andrea Cyterski-Acosta, Dean of Enrollment, 210-829-6005, Fax: 210-829-3921, E-mail: admis@uiwtx.edu.
Website: http://www.uiw.edu/msn/

The University of Toledo, College of Graduate Studies, College of Nursing, Toledo, OH 43614. Offers MSN, DNP, Certificate. *Accreditation:* AACN. Part-time programs available. Postbaccalaureate distance learning degree programs offered (no on-campus study). *Faculty:* 68. *Students:* 81 full-time (69 women), 229 part-time (202 women); includes 28 minority (12 Black or African American, non-Hispanic/Latino; 1 American Indian or Alaska Native, non-Hispanic/Latino; 3 Asian, non-Hispanic/Latino; 8 Hispanic/Latino; 4 Two or more races, non-Hispanic/Latino), 2 international. Average age 33. 154 applicants, 79% accepted, 93 enrolled. In 2013, 82 master's, 1 doctorate, 10 other advanced degrees awarded. *Degree requirements:* For master's, thesis or scholarly project; for doctorate, thesis/dissertation or alternative, evidence-based project. *Entrance requirements:* For master's, GRE, BS in nursing, minimum undergraduate GPA of 3.0, statement of purpose, two letters of recommendation, transcripts from all prior institutions attended, resume, Nursing CAS application, UT supplemental application; for doctorate, minimum undergraduate GPA of 3.0, statement of purpose, three letters of recommendation, transcripts from all prior institutions attended, resume, Nursing CAS application, UT supplemental application. Additional exam requirements/recommendations for international students: Required—TOEFL (minimum score 550 paper-based; 80 iBT). Application fee: $45 ($75 for international students). Electronic applications accepted. *Expenses:* Contact institution. *Financial support:* In 2013–14, 6 students received support. Research assistantships with full and partial tuition reimbursements available, Federal Work-Study, institutionally sponsored loans, scholarships/grants, traineeships, and tuition waivers (full and partial) available. *Faculty research:* Sexuality issues, prenatal testing, health care of homeless, nursing education, chronic/acute pain, eating disorders, low birth weight infants. *Unit head:* Dr. Timothy Gaspar, Dean, 419-383-5858, E-mail: admitnurse@utoledo.edu. *Application contact:* David Lymanstall, Nursing Advisor, 419-383-5841, E-mail: david.lymanstall@utoledo.edu.
Website: http://www.utoledo.edu/nursing/

University of Toronto, School of Graduate Studies, Lawrence S. Bloomberg Faculty of Nursing, Toronto, ON M5S 1A1, Canada. Offers MN, PhD, MHSc/MN. Part-time programs available. *Degree requirements:* For doctorate, thesis/dissertation, departmental and final oral exam/thesis defense. *Entrance requirements:* For master's, B Sc N or equivalent, minimum B average in next-to-final year, resume, 3 letters of reference; for doctorate, minimum B+ average, master's degree in nursing or a related area, resume, 2 letters of recommendation. Additional exam requirements/recommendations for international students: Required—TOEFL (minimum score 580 paper-based; 93 iBT), TWE (minimum score 5). Electronic applications accepted. *Expenses:* Contact institution.

University of Utah, Graduate School, College of Nursing, Program in Nursing, Salt Lake City, UT 84112. Offers MS, DNP, PhD. Part-time programs available. Postbaccalaureate distance learning degree programs offered (minimal on-campus study). *Students:* 226 full-time (198 women), 74 part-time (60 women); includes 36 minority (6 Black or African American, non-Hispanic/Latino; 8 Asian, non-Hispanic/Latino; 19 Hispanic/Latino; 3 Two or more races, non-Hispanic/Latino), 8 international. Average age 38. 260 applicants, 47% accepted, 98 enrolled. In 2013, 30 master's, 74 doctorates awarded. *Degree requirements:* For master's, thesis or project; for doctorate, comprehensive exam, thesis/dissertation. *Entrance requirements:* For master's, GRE General Test (if cumulative GPA less than 3.2), RN licensure in one of the jurisdictions of the National Council of State Boards of Nursing, goal statement, professional references; for doctorate, GRE General Test, interview, curriculum vitae/resume, goal statement, professional and academic references, writing sample. Additional exam requirements/recommendations for international students: Required—TOEFL (minimum score 500 paper-based; 85 iBT). *Application deadline:* For fall admission, 1/15 for domestic and international students. Application fee: $55 ($65 for international students). Electronic applications accepted. *Expenses:* Contact institution. *Financial support:* In 2013–14, 73 students received support, including 73 fellowships with full and partial tuition reimbursements available (averaging $10,000 per year), 4 research assistantships with full and partial tuition reimbursements available (averaging $13,000 per year), 9 teaching assistantships with partial tuition reimbursements available (averaging $11,555 per year); scholarships/grants, traineeships, health care benefits, and unspecified assistantships also available. Support available to part-time students. Financial award application deadline: 1/15; financial award applicants required to submit FAFSA. *Faculty research:* Symptom management, patient-provider communication, patient safety/informatics, gerontology/geriatric nursing, end-of-life bereavement. *Total annual research expenditures:* $2.2 million. *Unit head:* Patricia Morton, RN, PhD, Dean, 801-581-8262, Fax: 801-581-4642, E-mail: patricia.morton@nurs.utah.edu. *Application contact:* Carrie Radmall, Program Administrator, 801-581-8798, Fax: 801-585-9705, E-mail: carrie.radmall@nurs.utah.edu.
Website: http://www.nursing.utah.edu/

University of Vermont, Graduate College, College of Nursing and Health Sciences, Department of Nursing, Burlington, VT 05405. Offers MS, DNP. *Accreditation:* AACN. *Students:* 84 (72 women); includes 5 minority (1 Black or African American, non-Hispanic/Latino; 1 Asian, non-Hispanic/Latino; 2 Hispanic/Latino; 1 Two or more races, non-Hispanic/Latino). 90 applicants, 52% accepted, 22 enrolled. In 2013, 20 master's awarded. *Entrance requirements:* For master's, GRE General Test. Additional exam requirements/recommendations for international students: Required—TOEFL (minimum score 550 paper-based; 80 iBT). *Application deadline:* For fall admission, 4/3 for domestic and international students. Applications are processed on a rolling basis. Application fee: $65. Electronic applications accepted. *Financial support:* Application deadline: 3/1. *Unit head:* Rosemary Dale, Chair, 802-656-3858. *Application contact:* Prof. Carol Buck-Rolland, Coordinator, 802-656-3858.

University of Victoria, Faculty of Graduate Studies, Faculty of Human and Social Development, School of Nursing, Victoria, BC V8W 2Y2, Canada. Offers advanced nursing practice (advanced practice leadership option) (MN); advanced nursing practice (nurse educator option) (MN); advanced nursing practice (nurse practitioner option) (MN); nursing (PhD). Part-time programs available. Postbaccalaureate distance learning degree programs offered (no on-campus study). *Entrance requirements:* Additional exam requirements/recommendations for international students: Required—TOEFL (minimum score 575 paper-based), IELTS (minimum score 7). Electronic applications accepted.

University of Virginia, School of Nursing, Charlottesville, VA 22903. Offers acute and specialty care (MSN); acute care nurse practitioner (MSN); clinical nurse leadership (MSN); community-public health leadership (MSN); nursing (DNP, PhD); psychiatric mental health counseling (MSN); MSN/MBA. *Accreditation:* AACN. Part-time programs available. *Faculty:* 45 full-time (41 women), 3 part-time/adjunct (all women). *Students:* 177 full-time (155 women), 147 part-time (133 women); includes 53 minority (27 Black or African American, non-Hispanic/Latino; 10 Asian, non-Hispanic/Latino; 11 Hispanic/Latino; 5 Two or more races, non-Hispanic/Latino), 4 international. Average age 36. 236 applicants, 61% accepted, 110 enrolled. In 2013, 94 master's, 14 doctorates awarded. *Degree requirements:* For doctorate, comprehensive exam (for some programs), capstone project (DNP), dissertation (PhD). *Entrance requirements:* For master's, GRE General Test, MAT; for doctorate, GRE General Test. Additional exam requirements/recommendations for international students: Required—TOEFL, IELTS. *Application deadline:* Applications are processed on a rolling basis. Application fee: $60. Electronic applications accepted. *Expenses:* Contact institution. *Financial support:* Fellowships, research assistantships, teaching assistantships, Federal Work-Study, and scholarships/grants available. Financial award applicants required to submit FAFSA. *Unit head:* Dorrie K. Fontaine, Dean, 434-924-0141, Fax: 434-982-1809, E-mail: dkf2u@virginia.edu. *Application contact:* Clay Hysell, Assistant Dean for Admissions and Financial Services, 434-924-0141, Fax: 434-982-1809, E-mail: nur-osa@virginia.edu.
Website: http://www.nursing.virginia.edu/

University of Washington, Graduate School, School of Nursing, Seattle, WA 98195. Offers MN, MS, DNP, PhD, Graduate Certificate, MN/MPH. *Accreditation:* AACN; ACNM/ACME (one or more programs are accredited). Part-time programs available. *Degree requirements:* For master's, thesis (for some programs); for doctorate, thesis/dissertation. *Entrance requirements:* For master's, GRE, minimum GPA of 3.0, resume; for doctorate, GRE, minimum GPA of 3.0. Additional exam requirements/recommendations for international students: Required—TOEFL. *Faculty research:* High risk youth, pain management, women's health, oncology, sleep.

University of Washington, Bothell, Program in Nursing, Bothell, WA 98011-8246. Offers MN. Part-time programs available. *Degree requirements:* For master's, scholarly project. *Entrance requirements:* For master's, BSN (or other bachelor's degree with additional prerequisite work); current license as registered nurse in Washington state; minimum GPA of 3.0 in last 90 college credits, 2.0 in college statistics course. Additional exam requirements/recommendations for international students: Required—TOEFL (minimum score 580 paper-based). Electronic applications accepted. *Expenses:* Contact institution. *Faculty research:* Health of special populations, nursing education, higher education technology, healing through patient's narratives, women's health care issues, end of life issues in nursing.

University of Washington, Tacoma, Graduate Programs, Program in Nursing, Tacoma, WA 98402-3100. Offers communities, populations and health (MN); leadership in healthcare (MN); nurse educator (MN). Part-time programs available. *Degree requirements:* For master's, thesis (for some programs), advance fieldwork. *Entrance requirements:* For master's, Washington State NCLEX exam, minimum GPA of 3.0. Additional exam requirements/recommendations for international students: Required—TOEFL (minimum score 580 paper-based; 70 iBT); Recommended—IELTS (minimum score 7). *Faculty research:* Hospice and palliative care; clinical trial decision-making; minority nurse retention; asthma and public health; injustice, suffering, difference: Linking Them to Us; adolescent health.

The University of Western Ontario, Faculty of Graduate Studies, Health Sciences Division, School of Nursing, London, ON N6A 5B8, Canada. Offers M Sc N, MN NP, PhD. Part-time programs available. *Degree requirements:* For master's, thesis; for doctorate, thesis/dissertation. *Entrance requirements:* Additional exam requirements/recommendations for international students: Required—TOEFL. *Faculty research:* Empowerment, self-efficacy, family health, community health, gerontology.

University of West Florida, College of Arts and Sciences: Sciences, School of Allied Health and Life Sciences, Department of Nursing, Pensacola, FL 32514-5750. Offers MSN. Part-time and evening/weekend programs available. *Entrance requirements:* For master's, GRE or MAT, letter of intent; current curriculum vitae/resume. Additional exam requirements/recommendations for international students: Required—TOEFL (minimum score 550 paper-based).

University of West Georgia, Tanner Health System School of Nursing, Carrollton, GA 30118. Offers health systems leadership (Post-Master's Certificate); nursing (MSN); nursing education (Ed D, Post-Master's Certificate). *Accreditation:* AACN. Part-time programs available. Postbaccalaureate distance learning degree programs offered (no on-campus study). *Faculty:* 11 full-time (10 women), 1 (woman) part-time/adjunct. *Students:* 70 full-time (67 women), 52 part-time (48 women); includes 35 minority (31 Black or African American, non-Hispanic/Latino; 4 Hispanic/Latino). Average age 42. 96 applicants, 83% accepted, 56 enrolled. In 2013, 23 master's awarded. *Degree requirements:* For master's, comprehensive exam, thesis optional; for doctorate, comprehensive exam, thesis/dissertation. *Entrance requirements:* For master's, BSN, RN license, minimum GPA of 3.0 for upper-division nursing courses, two letters of recommendation, resume, official transcript, undergraduate statistics course with minimum C grade; for doctorate, GRE, MSN, minimum GPA of 3.0 in graduate nursing program, three letters of recommendation, 5-page sample of academic writing, RN license, resume or curriculum vitae, official transcripts; for Post-Master's Certificate, MSN, official transcripts, curriculum vitae/resume, two letters of recommendation. Additional exam requirements/recommendations for international students: Required—TOEFL (minimum score 523 paper-based; 69 iBT); Recommended—IELTS (minimum score 6.5). *Application deadline:* For fall admission, 6/1 for domestic and international students. Applications are processed on a rolling basis. Application fee: $40. Electronic applications accepted. *Expenses:* Contact institution. *Financial support:* In 2013–14, 8 students received support, including 1 research assistantship with full tuition reimbursement available (averaging $6,000 per year); scholarships/grants and unspecified assistantships also available. Financial award application deadline: 4/1; financial award applicants required to submit FAFSA. *Faculty research:* Caring in nursing education, pain assessment in older adults, pain outcomes. *Unit head:* Dr. Kathryn Mary Grams, Dean, 678-839-5642, Fax: 678-839-6553, E-mail: kgrams@westga.edu. *Application contact:* Embry Ice, Graduate Studies Associate, 678-839-5115, Fax: 678-839-6553, E-mail: eice@westga.edu.
Website: http://nursing.westga.edu

University of Windsor, Faculty of Graduate Studies, Faculty of Nursing, Windsor, ON N9B 3P4, Canada. Offers M Sc, MN. *Degree requirements:* For master's, thesis or alternative. *Entrance requirements:* For master's, minimum B average, certificate of competence (nurse registration). Additional exam requirements/recommendations for international students: Required—TOEFL (minimum score 560 paper-based). Electronic applications accepted.

University of Wisconsin–Eau Claire, College of Nursing and Health Sciences, Program in Nursing, Eau Claire, WI 54702-4004. Offers adult-gerontological administration (DNP); adult-gerontological clinical nurse specialist (DNP); adult-gerontological education (MSN); adult-gerontological primary care nurse practitioner (DNP); family health administration (DNP); family health in education (MSN); family health nurse practitioner (DNP); nursing (MSN); nursing practice (DNP). Part-time programs available. *Faculty:* 8 full-time (all women), 2 part-time/adjunct (both women). *Students:* 33 full-time (30 women), 40 part-time (36 women); includes 1 minority (Asian, non-Hispanic/Latino). Average age 37. 48 applicants, 85% accepted, 24 enrolled. In 2013, 31 master's, 9 doctorates awarded. Terminal master's awarded for partial completion of doctoral program. *Degree requirements:* For master's, thesis optional, 500-600 hours clinical practicum, oral and written exams. *Entrance requirements:* For master's, Wisconsin RN license, minimum GPA of 3.0, undergraduate statistics, course work in health assessment. Additional exam requirements/recommendations for international students: Required—TOEFL (minimum score 79 iBT). *Application deadline:* For fall admission, 1/15 priority date for domestic and international students. Applications are processed on a rolling basis. Application fee: $86. *Expenses:* Contact institution. *Financial support:* In 2013–14, 10 students received support. Federal Work-Study and unspecified assistantships available. Financial award application deadline: 3/1; financial award applicants required to submit FAFSA. *Unit head:* Dr. Linda Young, Dean, 715-836-4904, Fax: 715-836-5925, E-mail: younglk@uwec.edu. *Application contact:* Dr. Mary Zwygart-Stauffacher, Director, 715-836-5287, E-mail: zwygarmc@uwec.edu.
Website: http://www.uwec.edu/conhs/programs/grad/index.htm

University of Wisconsin–Madison, School of Nursing, Madison, WI 53706-1380. Offers adult/gerontology (DNP); nursing (PhD); pediatrics (DNP); psychiatric mental health (DNP); MS/MPH. *Accreditation:* AACN. Part-time programs available. *Degree requirements:* For doctorate, comprehensive exam, thesis/dissertation. *Entrance requirements:* For doctorate, GRE General Test, 2 samples of scholarly written work, BS in nursing from an accredited program, minimum undergraduate GPA of 3.0 in last 60 credits (for PhD); licensure as professional nurse (for DNP). Additional exam requirements/recommendations for international students: Required—TOEFL (minimum score 600 paper-based; 100 iBT). Electronic applications accepted. *Expenses:* Tuition, state resident: full-time $10,728; part-time $790 per credit. Tuition, nonresident: full-time $24,054; part-time $1623 per credit. *Required fees:* $1130; $119 per credit. *Faculty research:* Nursing informatics to promote self-care and disease management skills among patients and caregivers; quality of care to frail, vulnerable, and chronically ill populations; study of health-related and health-seeking behaviors; eliminating health disparities; pain and symptom management for patients with cancer.

University of Wisconsin–Milwaukee, Graduate School, College of Nursing, Milwaukee, WI 53201. Offers family nursing practitioner (Post Master's Certificate); health professional education (Certificate); nursing (MN, PhD); public health (Certificate). *Accreditation:* AACN. Part-time programs available. *Faculty:* 30 full-time (29 women), 2 part-time/adjunct (both women). *Students:* 157 full-time (142 women), 90 part-time (79 women); includes 32 minority (13 Black or African American, non-Hispanic/Latino; 10 Asian, non-Hispanic/Latino; 1 Hispanic/Latino; 8 Two or more races, non-Hispanic/Latino), 7 international. Average age 38. 160 applicants, 57% accepted, 51 enrolled. In 2013, 42 master's, 8 doctorates awarded. *Degree requirements:* For master's, thesis; for doctorate, thesis/dissertation. *Entrance requirements:* For master's, GRE General Test or MAT, autobiographical sketch; for doctorate, GRE, minimum GPA of 3.2. Additional exam requirements/recommendations for international students: Required—TOEFL (minimum score 550 paper-based; 79 iBT), IELTS (minimum score 6.5). *Application deadline:* For fall admission, 1/1 priority date for domestic students; for spring admission, 9/1 for domestic students. Applications are processed on a rolling basis. Application fee: $56 ($96 for international students). Electronic applications accepted. *Financial support:* In 2013–14, 3 fellowships, 1 research assistantship, 9 teaching assistantships were awarded; career-related internships or fieldwork, Federal Work-Study, health care benefits, unspecified assistantships, and project assistantships also available. Support available to part-time students. Financial award application deadline: 4/15; financial award applicants required to submit FAFSA. *Total annual research expenditures:* $3.2 million. *Unit head:* Dr. Sally Lundeen, Dean, 414-229-4189, E-mail: slundeen@uwm.edu. *Application contact:* Kim Litwack, Representative, 414-229-5098.
Website: http://www.uwm.edu/Dept/Nursing/

University of Wisconsin–Oshkosh, Graduate Studies, College of Nursing, Oshkosh, WI 54901. Offers adult health and illness (MSN); family nurse practitioner (MSN). *Accreditation:* AACN. Part-time programs available. *Degree requirements:* For master's, thesis or alternative, clinical paper. *Entrance requirements:* For master's, RN license, BSN, previous course work in statistics and health assessment, minimum undergraduate GPA of 3.0, letters of recommendation. Additional exam requirements/recommendations for international students: Required—TOEFL (minimum score 550 paper-based; 79 iBT). Electronic applications accepted. *Faculty research:* Adult health and illness, nurse practitioners practice, health care service, advanced practitioner roles, natural alternative complementary healthcare.

University of Wyoming, College of Health Sciences, Fay W. Whitney School of Nursing, Laramie, WY 82071. Offers MS. *Accreditation:* AACN. Part-time programs available. Postbaccalaureate distance learning degree programs offered (no on-campus study). *Degree requirements:* For master's, thesis. *Entrance requirements:* For master's, GRE General Test, BSN from CCNE or NCN-accredited school, minimum GPA of 3.0. Additional exam requirements/recommendations for international students: Required—TOEFL. *Faculty research:* Support systems for the elderly, fetal alcohol syndrome, teen pregnancy, rehabilitation with chronic mental illness, global peace building among women.

Urbana University, College of Nursing and Allied Health, Urbana, OH 43078-2091. Offers nursing (MSN). *Accreditation:* AACN. *Entrance requirements:* For master's, baccalaureate degree in nursing with minimum cumulative undergraduate GPA of 3.0, official transcripts, Ohio RN license, background check, statement of goals and objectives, resume, 3 letters of recommendation, interview.

Ursuline College, School of Graduate Studies, Programs in Nursing, Pepper Pike, OH 44124-4398. Offers care management (MSN); nurse practitioner (MSN); nursing (DNP); nursing education (MSN); palliative care (MSN). *Accreditation:* AACN. Part-time programs available. *Faculty:* 6 full-time (all women), 13 part-time/adjunct (10 women). *Students:* 9 full-time (7 women), 245 part-time (235 women); includes 69 minority (58 Black or African American, non-Hispanic/Latino; 6 Asian, non-Hispanic/Latino; 2 Hispanic/Latino; 3 Two or more races, non-Hispanic/Latino), 1 international. Average age 36. 91 applicants, 79% accepted, 60 enrolled. In 2013, 57 master's, 2 doctorates awarded. *Degree requirements:* For master's, comprehensive exam. *Entrance requirements:* For master's, minimum undergraduate GPA of 3.0, bachelor's degree in nursing, eligibility for or current Ohio RN license. Additional exam requirements/recommendations for international students: Required—TOEFL (minimum score 500 paper-based). *Application deadline:* For fall admission, 8/1 priority date for domestic students. Applications are processed on a rolling basis. Application fee: $25. *Expenses:* *Tuition:* Full-time $16,920; part-time $940 per credit. *Required fees:* $270. *Financial support:* In 2013–14, 9 students received support. Federal Work-Study available. Financial award application deadline: 3/1. *Unit head:* Dr. Janet Baker, Director, 440-864-8172, Fax: 440-684-6053, E-mail: jbaker@ursuline.edu. *Application contact:* Stephanie Pratt, Graduate Admission Coordinator, 440-646-8119, Fax: 440-684-6138, E-mail: graduateadmissions@ursuline.edu.

Utah Valley University, Program in Nursing, Orem, UT 84058-5999. Offers MSN. Part-time programs available. *Faculty:* 8 full-time (7 women). *Students:* 4 full-time (0 women), 4 part-time (all women). Terminal master's awarded for partial completion of doctoral program. *Degree requirements:* For master's, project or thesis. *Entrance requirements:* For master's, GRE, baccalaureate degree in nursing, nurse licensure, undergraduate course in statistics, minimum undergraduate GPA of 3.2 overall or in last 60 semester hours of coursework, 3 letters of recommendation. Additional exam requirements/recommendations for international students: Required—TOEFL (minimum score 83 iBT). *Application deadline:* For fall admission, 4/1 for domestic and international students. Application fee: $45 ($100 for international students). Electronic applications accepted. *Expenses:* Tuition, state resident: full-time $8520; part-time $355 per credit. Tuition, nonresident: full-time $21,232; part-time $885 per credit. *Required fees:* $700; $350 per semester. Tuition and fees vary according to program. *Financial support:* Application deadline: 5/1; applicants required to submit FAFSA. *Unit head:* Dan Fairbanks, Dean of the College of Science and Health, 801-863-6440.
Website: http://www.uvu.edu/csh/nursing/degrees/ms.html

Valparaiso University, Graduate School, College of Nursing and Health Professions, Valparaiso, IN 46383. Offers management (Certificate); nursing education (MSN, Certificate); MSN/MBA. *Accreditation:* AACN. Part-time and evening/weekend programs available. Postbaccalaureate distance learning degree programs offered (minimal on-campus study). *Faculty:* 11 part-time/adjunct (all women). *Students:* 36 full-time (30 women), 55 part-time (51 women); includes 13 minority (8 Black or African American, non-Hispanic/Latino; 5 Hispanic/Latino), 15 international. Average age 37. In 2013, 7 master's awarded. *Entrance requirements:* For master's, minimum GPA of 3.0, undergraduate major in nursing, Indiana registered nursing license, undergraduate courses in research and statistics. Additional exam requirements/recommendations for international students: Required—TOEFL (minimum score 550 paper-based; 80 iBT), IELTS (minimum score 6). *Application deadline:* Applications are processed on a rolling basis. Application fee: $30 ($50 for international students). Electronic applications accepted. *Expenses:* Contact institution. *Financial support:* Available to part-time students. Applicants required to submit FAFSA. *Unit head:* Dr. Janet Brown, Dean, 219-464-5289, Fax: 219-464-5425, E-mail: janet.brown@valpo.edu. *Application contact:*

Nursing—General

Jessica Choquette, Graduate Admissions Specialist, 219-464-5313, Fax: 219-464-5381, E-mail: jessica.choquette@valpo.edu.
Website: http://www.valpo.edu/nursing/

Vanderbilt University, Graduate School, Program in Nursing Science, Nashville, TN 37240-1001. Offers PhD. *Faculty:* 12 full-time (10 women). *Students:* 18 full-time (15 women), 6 part-time (5 women); includes 2 minority (1 Hispanic/Latino; 1 Native Hawaiian or other Pacific Islander, non-Hispanic/Latino). Average age 38. 32 applicants, 31% accepted, 8 enrolled. In 2013, 3 doctorates awarded. *Degree requirements:* For doctorate, comprehensive exam, thesis/dissertation, final and qualifying exams. *Entrance requirements:* For doctorate, GRE General Test. Additional exam requirements/recommendations for international students: Required—TOEFL (minimum score 570 paper-based; 88 iBT). *Application deadline:* For fall admission, 1/15 for domestic and international students. Electronic applications accepted. *Financial support:* Fellowships with full tuition reimbursements, research assistantships with full tuition reimbursements, teaching assistantships with full tuition reimbursements, career-related internships or fieldwork, Federal Work-Study, institutionally sponsored loans, scholarships/grants, health care benefits, and tuition waivers (full and partial) available. Financial award application deadline: 1/15; financial award applicants required to submit CSS PROFILE or FAFSA. *Faculty research:* Adaptation to chronic illness/conditions, health problems related to stress and coping, vulnerable childbearing and child rearing families. *Unit head:* Ann Minnick, Director of Graduate Studies, 615-343-2998, Fax: 615-343-5898, E-mail: ann.minnick@vanderbilt.edu. *Application contact:* Irene McKirgan, Administrative Manager, 615-322-7410, E-mail: irene.mckirgan@vanderbilt.edu.
Website: http://www.nursing.vanderbilt.edu/

Vanderbilt University, Vanderbilt University School of Nursing, Nashville, TN 37240. Offers adult-gerontology acute care nurse practitioner (MSN), including hospitalist, intensivist; adult-gerontology primary care nurse practitioner (MSN); emergency nurse practitioner (MSN); family nurse practitioner (MSN); healthcare leadership (MSN); neonatal nurse practitioner (MSN); nurse midwifery (MSN); nurse midwifery/family nurse practitioner (MSN); nursing informatics (MSN); nursing practice (DNP); nursing science (PhD); pediatric acute care nurse practitioner (MSN); pediatric primary care nurse practitioner (MSN); psychiatric-mental health nurse practitioner (MSN); women's health nurse practitioner (MSN); women's health nurse practitioner/adult gerontology primary care nurse practitioner (MSN); MSN/M Div; MSN/MTS. *Accreditation:* ACNM/ACME (one or more programs are accredited). Part-time programs available. Postbaccalaureate distance learning degree programs offered (minimal on-campus study). *Faculty:* 139 full-time (124 women), 452 part-time/adjunct (319 women). *Students:* 527 full-time (463 women), 369 part-time (333 women); includes 120 minority (46 Black or African American, non-Hispanic/Latino; 8 American Indian or Alaska Native, non-Hispanic/Latino; 26 Asian, non-Hispanic/Latino; 24 Hispanic/Latino; 4 Native Hawaiian or other Pacific Islander, non-Hispanic/Latino; 12 Two or more races, non-Hispanic/Latino), 7 international. Average age 32. 1,257 applicants, 49% accepted, 457 enrolled. In 2013, 364 master's, 43 doctorates awarded. *Degree requirements:* For doctorate, comprehensive exam, thesis/dissertation. *Entrance requirements:* For master's, GRE General Test (within the past 5 years), minimum B average in undergraduate course work, 3 letters of recommendation; for doctorate, GRE General Test, interview, 3 letters of recommendation from doctorally-prepared faculty, MSN, essay. Additional exam requirements/recommendations for international students: Required—TOEFL (minimum score 570 paper-based), IELTS (minimum score 6.5). *Application deadline:* For fall admission, 12/1 priority date for domestic and international students. Applications are processed on a rolling basis. Application fee: $50. Electronic applications accepted. *Expenses:* Contact institution. *Financial support:* In 2013–14, 582 students received support. Scholarships/grants and health care benefits available. Support available to part-time students. Financial award application deadline: 3/15; financial award applicants required to submit FAFSA. *Faculty research:* Lymphedema, palliative care and bereavement, health services research including workforce, safety and quality of care, gerontology, better birth outcomes including nutrition. *Total annual research expenditures:* $2.5 million. *Unit head:* Dr. Linda Norman, Dean, 615-343-8876, Fax: 615-343-7711, E-mail: linda.norman@vanderbilt.edu. *Application contact:* Patricia Peerman, Assistant Dean for Enrollment Management, 615-322-3800, Fax: 615-343-0333, E-mail: vusn-admissions@vanderbilt.edu.
Website: http://www.nursing.vanderbilt.edu

Vanguard University of Southern California, Graduate Program in Nursing, Costa Mesa, CA 92626-9601. Offers MS. Part-time and evening/weekend programs available. *Degree requirements:* For master's, thesis, two 55-hour practicums. *Entrance requirements:* For master's, free and clear RN license in California. *Expenses:* Contact institution.

Villanova University, College of Nursing, Villanova, PA 19085-1699. Offers adult nurse practitioner (MSN, Post Master's Certificate); family nurse practitioner (MSN, Post Master's Certificate); health care administration (MSN, Post Master's Certificate); nurse anesthetist (MSN, Post Master's Certificate); nursing (PhD); nursing education (MSN, Post Master's Certificate); nursing practice (DNP); pediatric nurse practitioner (MSN, Post Master's Certificate). *Accreditation:* AACN; AANA/CANAEP. Part-time programs available. Postbaccalaureate distance learning degree programs offered (minimal on-campus study). *Faculty:* 17 full-time (all women), 4 part-time/adjunct (all women). *Students:* 28 full-time (26 women), 191 part-time (161 women); includes 22 minority (2 Black or African American, non-Hispanic/Latino; 6 Asian, non-Hispanic/Latino; 7 Hispanic/Latino; 7 Two or more races, non-Hispanic/Latino), 18 international. Average age 30. 176 applicants, 65% accepted, 82 enrolled. In 2013, 64 master's, 7 doctorates, 5 other advanced degrees awarded. *Degree requirements:* For master's, independent study project; for doctorate, comprehensive exam, thesis/dissertation. *Entrance requirements:* For master's, GRE or MAT, BSN, 1 year of recent nursing experience, physical assessment, course work in statistics; for doctorate, GRE, MSN. Additional exam requirements/recommendations for international students: Required—TOEFL (minimum score 540 paper-based; 83 iBT), IELTS (minimum score 6.5). *Application deadline:* For fall admission, 7/1 priority date for domestic students, 7/1 for international students; for spring admission, 11/1 priority date for domestic students, 11/1 for international students. Applications are processed on a rolling basis. Application fee: $50. Electronic applications accepted. *Expenses:* Contact institution. *Financial support:* In 2013–14, 39 students received support, including 5 teaching assistantships with full tuition reimbursements available (averaging $14,475 per year); institutionally sponsored loans, scholarships/grants, traineeships, tuition waivers (full), and unspecified assistantships also available. Financial award application deadline: 7/1; financial award applicants required to submit FAFSA. *Faculty research:* Genetics, ethics, cognitive development of students, women with disabilities, nursing leadership. *Unit head:* Dr. Marguerite K. Schlag, Assistant Dean/Director, Graduate Programs, 610-519-4907, Fax: 610-519-7650, E-mail: marguerite.schlag@villanova.edu.
Website: http://www.nursing.villanova.edu/

Virginia Commonwealth University, Graduate School, School of Nursing, Richmond, VA 23284-9005. Offers adult health acute nursing (MS); adult health primary nursing (MS); biobehavioral clinical research (PhD); child health nursing (MS); clinical nurse leader (MS); family health nursing (MS); nurse educator (MS); nurse practitioner (MS); nursing (Certificate); nursing administration (MS), including clinical nurse manager; psychiatric-mental health nursing (MS); women's health nursing (MS). Part-time and evening/weekend programs available. *Degree requirements:* For master's, thesis optional; for doctorate, thesis/dissertation. *Entrance requirements:* For master's, GRE General Test, BSN, minimum GPA of 2.8; for doctorate, GRE General Test. Additional exam requirements/recommendations for international students: Required—TOEFL (minimum score 600 paper-based; 100 iBT). Electronic applications accepted.

Viterbo University, Graduate Program in Nursing, La Crosse, WI 54601-4797. Offers MSN, DNP. *Accreditation:* AACN. Part-time programs available. Postbaccalaureate distance learning degree programs offered (minimal on-campus study). *Faculty:* 5 full-time, 5 part-time/adjunct. *Students:* 43 full-time (38 women), 12 part-time (all women); includes 5 minority (2 Black or African American, non-Hispanic/Latino; 1 American Indian or Alaska Native, non-Hispanic/Latino; 1 Asian, non-Hispanic/Latino; 1 Hispanic/Latino). Average age 35. 29 applicants, 55% accepted, 14 enrolled. *Degree requirements:* For doctorate, project. *Entrance requirements:* For master's and doctorate, GRE General Test or MAT, bachelor's degree in nursing, minimum GPA of 3.0, RN license, one year of practice as an RN prior to beginning classes. *Application deadline:* For spring admission, 1/15 priority date for domestic students. Applications are processed on a rolling basis. Application fee: $50. Electronic applications accepted. *Expenses:* Contact institution. *Financial support:* In 2013–14, 9 students received support. Institutionally sponsored loans and scholarships/grants available. Financial award application deadline: 3/1; financial award applicants required to submit FAFSA. *Unit head:* Dr. Mary E. Stolder, Associate Professor, Graduate Nursing Program, 608-796-3625, Fax: 608-796-3668, E-mail: mestolder@viterbo.edu. *Application contact:* Bobbi Hundt, Graduate Nursing Program Administrative Assistant, 608-796-3671, Fax: 608-796-3668, E-mail: bmhundt@viterbo.edu.
Website: http://www.viterbo.edu/gradnursing

Wagner College, Division of Graduate Studies, Department of Nursing, Program in Nursing, Staten Island, NY 10301-4495. Offers MS. Part-time and evening/weekend programs available. *Faculty:* 6 full-time (all women), 6 part-time/adjunct (5 women). *Students:* 7 full-time (5 women), 80 part-time (69 women); includes 20 minority (7 Black or African American, non-Hispanic/Latino; 9 Asian, non-Hispanic/Latino; 1 Hispanic/Latino; 3 Two or more races, non-Hispanic/Latino). Average age 34. 28 applicants, 96% accepted, 20 enrolled. In 2013, 15 master's awarded. *Degree requirements:* For master's, thesis optional. *Entrance requirements:* For master's, BS in nursing, current clinical experience, minimum GPA of 2.75. *Application deadline:* For fall admission, 5/1 priority date for domestic students; for spring admission, 12/1 for domestic students. Applications are processed on a rolling basis. Application fee: $50. *Expenses: Tuition:* Full-time $17,496; part-time $972 per credit. Tuition and fees vary according to course load. *Financial support:* In 2013–14, 62 students received support. Traineeships, unspecified assistantships, and alumni fellowship grants available. Financial award applicants required to submit FAFSA. *Unit head:* Dr. Paula Tropello, Associate Professor/Chairman, Department of Nursing, 718-390-3452, Fax: 718-420-4009, E-mail: ptropell@wagner.edu. *Application contact:* Patricia Clancy, Administrative Assistant, 718-420-4464, Fax: 718-390-3105, E-mail: patricia.clancy@wagner.edu.

Walden University, Graduate Programs, School of Nursing, Minneapolis, MN 55401. Offers adult-gerontology acute care nurse practitioner (MSN); adult-gerontology nurse practitioner (MSN); education (MSN); family nurse practitioner (MSN); informatics (MSN); leadership and management (MSN); nursing (DNP, PhD, Post-Master's Certificate), including education (PhD), healthcare administration (PhD), interdisciplinary health (PhD), leadership (PhD), nursing education (Post-Master's Certificate), nursing informatics (Post-Master's Certificate), nursing leadership and management (Post-Master's Certificate), public health policy (PhD). *Accreditation:* AACN. Part-time and evening/weekend programs available. Postbaccalaureate distance learning degree programs offered (no on-campus study). *Faculty:* 22 full-time (19 women), 343 part-time/adjunct (301 women). *Students:* 5,828 full-time (5,240 women), 2,803 part-time (2,578 women); includes 2,920 minority (1,893 Black or African American, non-Hispanic/Latino; 40 American Indian or Alaska Native, non-Hispanic/Latino; 438 Asian, non-Hispanic/Latino; 391 Hispanic/Latino; 35 Native Hawaiian or other Pacific Islander, non-Hispanic/Latino; 123 Two or more races, non-Hispanic/Latino), 147 international. Average age 41. 1,795 applicants, 95% accepted, 1375 enrolled. In 2013, 1,879 master's, 1 doctorate, 36 other advanced degrees awarded. *Degree requirements:* For doctorate, thesis/dissertation (for some programs), residency (for some programs), field experience (for some programs). *Entrance requirements:* For master's, bachelor's degree or equivalent in related field or RN; minimum GPA of 2.5; official transcripts; goal statement (for some programs); access to computer and Internet; for doctorate, master's degree or higher, three years of related professional or academic experience, RN, goal statement (for some programs); access to computer and Internet; for Post-Master's Certificate, relevant work experience; access to computer and Internet. Additional exam requirements/recommendations for international students: Required—TOEFL (minimum score 550 paper-based; 79 iBT), IELTS (minimum score 6.5), Michigan English Language Assessment Battery (minimum score 82), or PTE. *Application deadline:* Applications are processed on a rolling basis. Application fee: $0. Electronic applications accepted. *Expenses: Tuition:* Full-time $11,813.55; part-time $500 per credit. *Required fees:* $618.76. *Financial support:* Fellowships, Federal Work-Study, scholarships/grants, unspecified assistantships, and family tuition reduction, active duty/veteran tuition reduction, group tuition reduction, interest-free payment plans, employee tuition reduction available. Support available to part-time students. Financial award applicants required to submit FAFSA. *Unit head:* Dr. Andrea Lindell, Associate Dean, 800-925-3368. *Application contact:* Jennifer Hall, Vice President of Enrollment Management, 866-4-WALDEN, E-mail: info@waldenu.edu.
Website: http://www.waldenu.edu/programs/colleges-schools/nursing

Walsh University, Graduate Studies, School of Nursing, North Canton, OH 44720-3396. Offers academic nurse educator (MSN); clinical nurse leader (MSN); nursing practice (DNP). Part-time and evening/weekend programs available. Postbaccalaureate distance learning degree programs offered (minimal on-campus study). *Faculty:* 6 full-time (all women), 6 part-time/adjunct (5 women). *Students:* 13 full-time (10 women), 29 part-time (all women); includes 2 minority (1 Black or African American, non-Hispanic/Latino; 1 Hispanic/Latino). Average age 39. 27 applicants, 89% accepted, 19 enrolled. *Degree requirements:* For doctorate, scholarly project; residency practicum. *Entrance requirements:* For master's, undergraduate nursing degree, current unencumbered RN license, completion of an undergraduate or graduate statistics course, essay, interview, recommendations; for doctorate, BSN; master's degree; statistics and research courses; essay; interview. Additional exam requirements/recommendations for international students: Required—TOEFL. *Application deadline:* Applications are processed on a rolling basis. Electronic applications accepted. *Expenses: Tuition:* Full-time $10,890; part-time $605 per credit hour. *Required fees:* $100; $100. *Financial support:* In 2013–14, 32 students received support. Research assistantships, tuition waivers (partial), and tuition discounts available. Financial award application deadline: 12/31; financial award applicants required to submit FAFSA. *Faculty research:* Faith community nursing, gerontology, women's health, global nursing education, nursing assessment, grief and reconstitution, health needs of psychiatric patients, psychometric testing. *Unit head:* Dr. Karen Gehrling, Director, Graduate Program in Nursing, 330-244-4649, Fax: 330-490-7371, E-mail: kgehrling@walsh.edu. *Application contact:* Audra Dice, Graduate and

Transfer Admissions Counselor, 330-490-7181, Fax: 330-244-4680, E-mail: adice@walsh.edu.
Website: http://www.walsh.edu/master-of-science-in-nursing

Washburn University, School of Nursing, Topeka, KS 66621. Offers clinical nurse leader (MSN); nursing (DNP). *Accreditation:* AACN. Part-time programs available. *Entrance requirements:* Additional exam requirements/recommendations for international students: Required—TOEFL. *Application deadline:* For fall admission, 3/15 for international students. Application fee: $35. *Expenses:* Tuition, state resident: full-time $5850; part-time $325 per credit hour. Tuition, nonresident: full-time $11,916; part-time $662 per credit hour. *Required fees:* $86; $43 per semester. Tuition and fees vary according to program. *Financial support:* Application deadline: 2/15. *Unit head:* Dr. Monica S. Scheibmeir, Dean, 785-670-1526, E-mail: monica.scheibmeir@washburn.edu. *Application contact:* Mary V. Allen, Director of Student Services, 785-670-1533, E-mail: mary.allen@washburn.edu.
Website: http://www.washburn.edu/sonu

Washington Adventist University, Program in Nursing - Business Leadership, Takoma Park, MD 20912. Offers MSN. Part-time programs available. *Entrance requirements:* Additional exam requirements/recommendations for international students: Required—TOEFL (minimum score 550 paper-based), IELTS (minimum score 5).

Washington State University Spokane, Graduate Programs, College of Nursing, Spokane, WA 99210-1495. Offers advanced population health (MN, DNP); family nurse practitioner (MN, DNP); nursing (PhD); psychiatric/mental health nurse practitioner (DNP); psychiatric/mental health practitioner (MN). *Accreditation:* AACN. *Degree requirements:* For master's, comprehensive exam (for some programs), thesis (for some programs), oral exam, research project. *Entrance requirements:* For master's, minimum GPA of 3.0, Washington state RN license, physical assessment skills, course work in statistics, recommendations, written interview (for nurse practitioner). *Faculty research:* Cardiovascular and Type 2 diabetes in children, evaluation of strategies to increase physical activity in sedentary people.

Washington State University Tri-Cities, Graduate Programs, College of Nursing, Richland, WA 99354. Offers MN, PhD. Part-time programs available. Postbaccalaureate distance learning degree programs offered (minimal on-campus study). *Degree requirements:* For master's, comprehensive exam (for some programs), thesis (for some programs), oral exam, research project. *Entrance requirements:* For master's, current Washington state RN license; minimum cumulative GPA of 2.5, 2.0 in each nursing course. Additional exam requirements/recommendations for international students: Required—TOEFL.

Washington State University Vancouver, Graduate Programs, College of Nursing, Vancouver, WA 98686. Offers MN. *Degree requirements:* For master's, comprehensive exam (for some programs), thesis (for some programs), research project. *Entrance requirements:* For master's, Washington RN license, minimum GPA of 3.0. Additional exam requirements/recommendations for international students: Required—TOEFL. Electronic applications accepted. *Faculty research:* Cultural competence in nursing, prescribing controlled substances by Advanced Registered Nurse Practitioners, decreasing health disparities, workforce diversity.

Wayland Baptist University, Graduate Programs, Program in Multidisciplinary Science, Plainview, TX 79072-6998. Offers multidisciplinary science (MS); nursing (MS). Part-time and evening/weekend programs available. *Faculty:* 29 full-time (16 women), 1 (woman) part-time/adjunct. *Students:* 22 part-time (17 women); includes 8 minority (3 Black or African American, non-Hispanic/Latino; 5 Hispanic/Latino). Average age 41. 3 applicants, 67% accepted, 1 enrolled. *Degree requirements:* For master's, comprehensive exam. *Entrance requirements:* For master's, GRE or MAT. Additional exam requirements/recommendations for international students: Required—TOEFL (minimum score 500 paper-based; 61 iBT). *Application deadline:* Applications are processed on a rolling basis. Application fee: $50. Electronic applications accepted. *Expenses: Tuition:* Full-time $8190; part-time $455 per credit hour. *Required fees:* $970; $455 per credit hour. $485 per semester. *Financial support:* Federal Work-Study, institutionally sponsored loans, and scholarships/grants available. Support available to part-time students. Financial award application deadline: 5/1; financial award applicants required to submit FAFSA. *Unit head:* Dr. Herbert Grover, Chairman, Division of Mathematics and Science, 806-291-1115, Fax: 806-291-1968, E-mail: groverh@wbu.edu. *Application contact:* Amanda Stanton, Coordinator of Graduate Studies, 806-291-3423, Fax: 806-291-1950, E-mail: stanton@wbu.edu.

Waynesburg University, Graduate and Professional Studies, Canonsburg, PA 15370. Offers business (MBA), including energy management, finance, health systems, human resources, leadership, market development; counseling (MA), including addictions counseling, clinical mental health; education (M Ed, MAT), including autism (M Ed), curriculum and instruction (M Ed), educational leadership (M Ed), online teaching (M Ed); nursing (MSN), including administration, education, informatics; nursing practice (DNP); special education (M Ed); technology (M Ed); MSN/MBA. *Accreditation:* AACN. Part-time and evening/weekend programs available. *Faculty:* 11 full-time (5 women), 136 part-time/adjunct (80 women). *Students:* 146 full-time (99 women), 419 part-time (268 women). In 2013, 290 master's, 7 doctorates awarded. *Degree requirements:* For doctorate, thesis/dissertation. *Entrance requirements:* Additional exam requirements/recommendations for international students: Required—TOEFL. *Application deadline:* For fall admission, 8/1 priority date for domestic students. Applications are processed on a rolling basis. Electronic applications accepted. *Financial support:* Available to part-time students. Application deadline: 5/1. *Unit head:* David Mariner, Dean, 724-743-4420, Fax: 724-743-4425, E-mail: dmariner@waynesburg.edu. *Application contact:* Dr. Michael Bednarski, Director of Enrollment, 724-743-4420, Fax: 724-743-4425, E-mail: mbednars@waynesburg.edu.
Website: http://www.waynesburg.edu/

Wayne State University, College of Nursing, Program in Nursing, Detroit, MI 48202. Offers infant mental health (PhD); nursing (PhD). Part-time programs available. *Students:* 22 full-time (21 women), 5 part-time (all women); includes 10 minority (all Black or African American, non-Hispanic/Latino), 3 international. Average age 44. 9 applicants, 56% accepted, 4 enrolled. In 2013, 3 doctorates awarded. *Degree requirements:* For doctorate, thesis/dissertation. *Entrance requirements:* For doctorate, GRE General Test, minimum GPA of 3.3, bachelor's or master's degree in nursing, current RN license, interview, goals statement, curriculum vitae, reference letters from doctorally-prepared individuals (three for PhD applicants, two for DNP). Additional exam requirements/recommendations for international students: Required—TOEFL (minimum score 550 paper-based; 79 iBT); Recommended—TWE (minimum score 6). *Application deadline:* For fall admission, 1/15 for domestic and international students. Application fee: $50. Electronic applications accepted. *Expenses:* Contact institution. *Financial support:* In 2013–14, 11 students received support. Fellowships with tuition reimbursements available, research assistantships with tuition reimbursements available, teaching assistantships with tuition reimbursements available, institutionally sponsored loans, scholarships/grants, and unspecified assistantships available. Support available to part-time students. *Faculty research:* Self-care, transcultural care, adaptation to acute and chronic illness, urban health and health care systems. *Unit head:* Dr. Barbara Redman, Dean, 313-577-4070, Fax: 313-577-4571, E-mail: ae9080@wayne.edu. *Application contact:* Dr. Cynthia Redwine, Assistant Dean for the Office of Student Affairs, 313-577-4082, E-mail: nursinginfo@wayne.edu.
Website: http://www.nursing.wayne.edu/programs/index.php

Wayne State University, College of Nursing, Program in Nursing Practice, Detroit, MI 48202. Offers DNP. *Students:* 38 full-time (35 women), 44 part-time (42 women); includes 28 minority (22 Black or African American, non-Hispanic/Latino; 5 Asian, non-Hispanic/Latino; 1 Two or more races, non-Hispanic/Latino), 3 international. Average age 38. 60 applicants, 58% accepted, 29 enrolled. In 2013, 3 doctorates awarded. *Entrance requirements:* For doctorate, writing sample or GRE, official transcripts, two professional references, curriculum vitae or resume, statement of goals, BSN or MSN, one reference from a doctorally-prepared individual, current Michigan RN license, criminal background check. Additional exam requirements/recommendations for international students: Required—TOEFL (minimum score 550 paper-based; 79 iBT). *Application deadline:* For fall admission, 11/15 for domestic and international students. Application fee: $50. Electronic applications accepted. *Expenses:* Contact institution. *Financial support:* In 2013–14, 47 students received support. Fellowships, research assistantships, teaching assistantships, institutionally sponsored loans, and scholarships/grants available. *Unit head:* Dr. Barbara Redman, Dean, 313-577-4070. *Application contact:* Dr. Cynthia Redwine, Assistant Dean for the Office of Student Affairs, 313-577-4082, Fax: 313-577-6949, E-mail: nursinginfo@wayne.edu.
Website: http://www.nursing.wayne.edu/dnp/index.php

Weber State University, College of Health Professions, School of Nursing, Ogden, UT 84408-1001. Offers MSN. *Faculty:* 5 full-time (all women). *Students:* 43 full-time (37 women), 2 part-time (0 women); includes 4 minority (1 American Indian or Alaska Native, non-Hispanic/Latino; 1 Asian, non-Hispanic/Latino; 2 Hispanic/Latino). Average age 39. 31 applicants, 77% accepted, 24 enrolled. In 2013, 19 master's awarded. *Application deadline:* For fall admission, 3/1 priority date for domestic students. Application fee: $60 ($90 for international students). *Expenses:* Tuition, state resident: full-time $7118; part-time $253 per credit hour. Tuition, nonresident: full-time $12,480; part-time $634 per credit hour. *Required fees:* $34.33; $34.33 per credit hour. $257 per semester. Full-time tuition and fees vary according to course load. *Financial support:* In 2013–14, 4 students received support. Tuition waivers (full and partial) available. Financial award application deadline: 4/1; financial award applicants required to submit FAFSA. *Unit head:* Dr. Melissa Neville, MSN Program Director, 801-626-6204, Fax: 801-626-6397, E-mail: mneville@weber.edu. *Application contact:* Robert Holt, Director of Enrollment, 801-626-6753, Fax: 801-626-6397, E-mail: slove@weber.edu.

Webster University, College of Arts and Sciences, Department of Nursing, St. Louis, MO 63119-3194. Offers MSN. *Degree requirements:* For master's, comprehensive exam. *Entrance requirements:* For master's, 1 year of clinical experience, BSN, interview, minimum C+ average in statistics and physical assessment, minimum GPA of 3.0, RN license. Additional exam requirements/recommendations for international students: Required—TOEFL. *Expenses: Tuition:* Full-time $11,610; part-time $645 per credit hour. Tuition and fees vary according to campus/location and program. *Faculty research:* Health teaching.

Wesley College, Nursing Program, Dover, DE 19901-3875. Offers MSN. Part-time and evening/weekend programs available. *Degree requirements:* For master's, thesis optional, portfolio. *Entrance requirements:* For master's, GRE or MAT. Electronic applications accepted. *Faculty research:* Childhood obesity, organizational behavior, health promotion and wellness.

West Chester University of Pennsylvania, College of Health Sciences, Department of Nursing, West Chester, PA 19383. Offers nursing (DNP); public health nursing (MSN), including administration, education, integrative health. *Accreditation:* AACN. Part-time and evening/weekend programs available. Postbaccalaureate distance learning degree programs offered (minimal on-campus study). *Faculty:* 4 full-time (3 women). *Students:* 12 full-time (11 women), 17 part-time (15 women); includes 9 minority (7 Black or African American, non-Hispanic/Latino; 1 Asian, non-Hispanic/Latino; 1 Hispanic/Latino), 2 international. Average age 42. 11 applicants, 91% accepted, 7 enrolled. In 2013, 17 master's awarded. *Entrance requirements:* For master's, RN license, BSN or RN with bachelor's degree in another discipline, minimum GPA of 2.8, experience as a nurse providing direct clinical care, two letters of recommendation; for doctorate, minimum graduate GPA of 3.0, two letters of reference, interview. Additional exam requirements/recommendations for international students: Required—TOEFL (minimum score 550 paper-based; 80 iBT). *Application deadline:* For fall admission, 4/15 priority date for domestic students, 3/15 for international students; for spring admission, 10/15 priority date for domestic students, 9/1 for international students. Applications are processed on a rolling basis. Application fee: $45. Electronic applications accepted. *Expenses:* Tuition, state resident: full-time $7956; part-time $442 per credit. Tuition, nonresident: full-time $11,934; part-time $663 per credit. *Required fees:* $2134.20; $106.24 per credit. Tuition and fees vary according to campus/location and program. *Financial support:* Unspecified assistantships available. Support available to part-time students. Financial award application deadline: 2/15; financial award applicants required to submit FAFSA. *Unit head:* Dr. Charlotte Mackey, Chair and Graduate Coordinator, 610-436-3474, Fax: 610-436-3083, E-mail: cmackey@wcupa.edu.
Website: http://www.wcupa.edu/_ACADEMICS/HealthSciences/nursing/

Western Carolina University, Graduate School, College of Health and Human Sciences, School of Nursing, Cullowhee, NC 28723. Offers nurse educator (PMC); nursing (MSN). *Accreditation:* AACN; AANA/CANAEP. Part-time and evening/weekend programs available. *Degree requirements:* For master's, comprehensive exam, thesis or alternative. *Entrance requirements:* For master's, GRE General Test, BSN with minimum GPA of 3.0, 3 references, 1 year of clinical experience. Additional exam requirements/recommendations for international students: Required—TOEFL (minimum score 550 paper-based; 79 iBT).

Western Connecticut State University, Division of Graduate Studies, School of Professional Studies, Nursing Department, Danbury, CT 06810-6885. Offers adult nurse practitioner (MSN); clinical nurse specialist (MSN). *Accreditation:* AACN. Part-time programs available. *Degree requirements:* For master's, clinical component, thesis or research project, completion of program in 6 years. *Entrance requirements:* For master's, MAT (if GPA less than 3.0), bachelor's degree in nursing, minimum GPA of 3.0, previous course work in statistics and nursing research, RN license. Additional exam requirements/recommendations for international students: Recommended—TOEFL (minimum score 550 paper-based; 79 iBT), IELTS (minimum score 6). *Expenses:* Contact institution. *Faculty research:* Evaluating effectiveness of Reiki and acupressure on stress reduction.

Western Kentucky University, Graduate Studies, College of Health and Human Services, School of Nursing, Bowling Green, KY 42101. Offers MSN. *Accreditation:* AACN. Part-time and evening/weekend programs available. *Degree requirements:* For master's, comprehensive exam, thesis optional. *Entrance requirements:* For master's, GRE General Test, minimum GPA of 2.75. Additional exam requirements/recommendations for international students: Required—TOEFL (minimum score 555 paper-based; 79 iBT). *Faculty research:* Folic acid, disease and injury prevention, rural mobile health, mental health issues.

Nursing—General

Western Michigan University, Graduate College, College of Health and Human Services, Bronson School of Nursing, Kalamazoo, MI 49008. Offers MSN. *Accreditation:* AACN.

Western University of Health Sciences, College of Graduate Nursing, Doctor of Nursing Practice Program, Pomona, CA 91766-1854. Offers DNP. Postbaccalaureate distance learning degree programs offered (minimal on-campus study). *Faculty:* 5 full-time (4 women), 2 part-time/adjunct (1 woman). *Students:* 31 full-time (28 women), 2 part-time (1 woman); includes 17 minority (1 Black or African American, non-Hispanic/Latino; 10 Asian, non-Hispanic/Latino; 5 Hispanic/Latino; 1 Two or more races, non-Hispanic/Latino). Average age 47. 58 applicants, 47% accepted, 27 enrolled. In 2013, 34 doctorates awarded. *Degree requirements:* For doctorate, thesis/dissertation, project. *Entrance requirements:* For doctorate, MSN or master's degree in related field, or nurse practitioner, minimum GPA of 3.0, 3 letters of recommendation, copies of all applicable licenses and certifications, sample of scholarly writing. Additional exam requirements/recommendations for international students: Required—TOEFL. *Application deadline:* For fall admission, 3/1 for domestic and international students. Application fee: $60. Electronic applications accepted. *Unit head:* Dr. Karen J. Hanford, Dean, 909-469-5523, Fax: 909-469-5521, E-mail: khanford@westernu.edu. *Application contact:* Kathryn Ford, Director of Admissions/International Student Advisor, 909-469-5335, Fax: 909-469-5570, E-mail: admissions@westernu.edu.
Website: http://www.westernu.edu/nursing-dnp

Western University of Health Sciences, College of Graduate Nursing, Master of Science in Nursing Program, Pomona, CA 91766-1854. Offers administrative nurse leader (MSN); ambulatory care (MSN); clinical nurse leader (MSN); family nurse practitioner (MSN); nursing (MSN). *Faculty:* 14 full-time (all women), 11 part-time/adjunct (10 women). *Students:* 255 full-time (218 women), 10 part-time (all women); includes 163 minority (20 Black or African American, non-Hispanic/Latino; 1 American Indian or Alaska Native, non-Hispanic/Latino; 88 Asian, non-Hispanic/Latino; 40 Hispanic/Latino; 1 Native Hawaiian or other Pacific Islander, non-Hispanic/Latino; 13 Two or more races, non-Hispanic/Latino), 2 international. Average age 31. 739 applicants, 23% accepted, 114 enrolled. In 2013, 73 master's awarded. *Degree requirements:* For master's, thesis. *Entrance requirements:* For master's, BSN, minimum GPA of 3.0, 3 letters of recommendation, resume/curriculum vitae. Additional exam requirements/recommendations for international students: Required—TOEFL. *Application deadline:* For fall admission, 10/1 for domestic students. Application fee: $60. Electronic applications accepted. *Unit head:* Dr. Karen J. Hanford, Dean, 909-469-5523, Fax: 909-469-5521, E-mail: khanford@westernu.edu. *Application contact:* Kathryn Ford, Director of Admissions/International Student Advisor, 909-469-5335, Fax: 909-469-5570, E-mail: admissions@westernu.edu.

Westminster College, School of Nursing and Health Sciences, Salt Lake City, UT 84105-3697. Offers family nurse practitioner (MSN); nurse anesthesia (MSNA); nurse education (MSNED); nursing (MSN); public health (MPH). *Accreditation:* AACN; AANA/CANAEP. *Faculty:* 11 full-time (5 women), 7 part-time/adjunct (4 women). *Students:* 119 full-time (75 women), 5 part-time (2 women); includes 21 minority (5 Black or African American, non-Hispanic/Latino; 1 American Indian or Alaska Native, non-Hispanic/Latino; 4 Asian, non-Hispanic/Latino; 7 Hispanic/Latino; 1 Native Hawaiian or other Pacific Islander, non-Hispanic/Latino; 3 Two or more races, non-Hispanic/Latino), 4 international. Average age 32. 246 applicants, 35% accepted, 56 enrolled. In 2013, 49 master's awarded. *Degree requirements:* For master's, clinical practicum, 504 clinical practice hours. *Entrance requirements:* For master's, GRE, resume, Utah RN license in good standing, minimum GPA of 3.0, 3 letters of reference, BSN from accredited nursing program, proof of clear state and federal background check, drug test results, personal interview, current PALS certification, current ACLS certification, document of current immunizations, physical and mental health certificate. Additional exam requirements/recommendations for international students: Required—TOEFL (minimum score 600 paper-based; 100 iBT), IELTS (minimum score 7.5). *Application deadline:* Applications are processed on a rolling basis. Application fee: $50. Electronic applications accepted. *Expenses:* Contact institution. *Financial support:* In 2013–14, 9 students received support. Career-related internships or fieldwork, unspecified assistantships, and tuition reimbursements, tuition remission available. Support available to part-time students. Financial award applicants required to submit FAFSA. *Faculty research:* Collaborative testing in nursing: student outcomes and perspectives, implementing new educational paradigms into pre-licensure nursing curricula. *Unit head:* Dr. Sheryl Steadman, Dean, 801-832-2164, Fax: 801-832-3110, E-mail: ssteadman@westminstercollege.edu. *Application contact:* Dr. John Baworowsky, Vice President of Enrollment Management, 801-832-2200, Fax: 801-832-3101, E-mail: admission@westminstercollege.edu.
Website: http://www.westminstercollege.edu/msn

West Texas A&M University, College of Nursing and Health Sciences, Department of Nursing, Canyon, TX 79016-0001. Offers family nurse practitioner (MSN); nursing (MSN). *Accreditation:* AACN. Part-time programs available. Postbaccalaureate distance learning degree programs offered (minimal on-campus study). *Degree requirements:* For master's, comprehensive exam, thesis optional. *Entrance requirements:* For master's, GRE General Test, bachelor's degree in nursing, minimum GPA of 3.0 in last 60 hours. Additional exam requirements/recommendations for international students: Required—TOEFL (minimum score 550 paper-based). Electronic applications accepted. *Faculty research:* Family-focused nursing, nursing traineeship, professional nursing.

West Virginia University, School of Nursing, Morgantown, WV 26506. Offers nurse practitioner (Certificate); nursing (MSN, DNP, PhD). *Accreditation:* AACN. Part-time programs available. Postbaccalaureate distance learning degree programs offered (minimal on-campus study). *Degree requirements:* For master's, thesis or alternative; for doctorate, comprehensive exam, thesis/dissertation. *Entrance requirements:* For master's, minimum GPA of 3.0, current U.S. RN license, BSN, course work in statistics and physical assessment, GRE General Test; for doctorate, GRE General Test (PhD), minimum graduate GPA of 3.0, minimum grade of B in graduate statistics course work. Additional exam requirements/recommendations for international students: Required—TOEFL. Electronic applications accepted. *Expenses:* Contact institution. *Faculty research:* Rural primary health/health promotion, parent/child/women's health, cardiovascular risk reduction, complementary health modalities, breast cancer detection-care.

West Virginia Wesleyan College, Department of Nursing, Buckhannon, WV 26201. Offers family nurse practitioner (Post Master's Certificate); family nurse practitoner (MS); nurse administrator (MS); nurse educator (MS); nurse-midwifery (MS); nursing administration (Post Master's Certificate); nursing education (Post Master's Certificate); psychiatric mental health nurse practitioner (MS); MSN/MBA.

Wheeling Jesuit University, Department of Nursing, Wheeling, WV 26003-6295. Offers MSN. *Accreditation:* AACN. Part-time and evening/weekend programs available. Postbaccalaureate distance learning degree programs offered (minimal on-campus study). *Degree requirements:* For master's, comprehensive exam (for some programs), thesis (for some programs). *Entrance requirements:* For master's, GRE General Test or MAT, BSN, minimum GPA of 3.0, course work in research and statistics, U.S. nursing license. Additional exam requirements/recommendations for international students: Required—TOEFL (minimum score 600 paper-based; 100 iBT). Electronic applications accepted. Application fee is waived when completed online. *Faculty research:* Obesity in women, underserved populations, spirituality.

Wichita State University, Graduate School, College of Health Professions, School of Nursing, Wichita, KS 67260. Offers nursing (MSN); nursing practice (DNP). *Accreditation:* AACN. Part-time programs available. *Unit head:* Dr. Betty Smith-Campbell, Chairperson, 316-978-3610, Fax: 316-978-3025, E-mail: betty.smith-campbell@wichita.edu. *Application contact:* Jordan Oleson, Admissions Coordinator, 316-978-3095, Fax: 316-978-3253, E-mail: jordan.oleson@wichita.edu.
Website: http://www.wichita.edu/

Widener University, School of Nursing, Chester, PA 19013. Offers MSN, DN Sc, PhD, PMC. *Accreditation:* AACN. Part-time and evening/weekend programs available. *Faculty:* 12 full-time (all women), 4 part-time/adjunct (3 women). *Students:* 13 full-time (11 women), 161 part-time (148 women); includes 41 minority (31 Black or African American, non-Hispanic/Latino; 7 Asian, non-Hispanic/Latino; 2 Hispanic/Latino; 1 Two or more races, non-Hispanic/Latino). Average age 33. 77 applicants, 79% accepted. In 2013, 34 master's, 11 doctorates awarded. *Degree requirements:* For doctorate, thesis/dissertation. *Entrance requirements:* For master's, GRE General Test, BSN, undergraduate course in statistics; for doctorate, GRE General Test, MSN, undergraduate course in statistics. *Application deadline:* For fall admission, 7/1 for domestic students; for winter admission, 3/1 for domestic students; for spring admission, 11/1 for domestic students. Applications are processed on a rolling basis. Application fee: $25 ($300 for international students). Electronic applications accepted. *Expenses:* Contact institution. *Financial support:* Career-related internships or fieldwork, Federal Work-Study, and traineeships available. Support available to part-time students. Financial award application deadline: 4/1. *Faculty research:* Women's health leadership, nursing education, research utilization, program evaluation, health promotion. *Unit head:* Dr. Mary B. Walker, Assistant Dean for Graduate Studies, 610-499-4208, Fax: 610-499-4216, E-mail: mary.b.walker@widener.edu. *Application contact:* Betty A. Boyles, Information Contact, 610-499-4207, Fax: 610-499-4216, E-mail: betty.a.boyles@widener.edu.

Wilkes University, College of Graduate and Professional Studies, Nesbitt College of Pharmacy and Nursing, Department of Nursing, Wilkes-Barre, PA 18766-0002. Offers MSN, DNP. *Accreditation:* AACN. Part-time and evening/weekend programs available. *Students:* 7 full-time (6 women), 132 part-time (114 women); includes 27 minority (15 Black or African American, non-Hispanic/Latino; 3 Asian, non-Hispanic/Latino; 6 Hispanic/Latino; 3 Two or more races, non-Hispanic/Latino). Average age 45. In 2013, 3 master's, 14 doctorates awarded. *Entrance requirements:* Additional exam requirements/recommendations for international students: Required—TOEFL (minimum score 550 paper-based; 79 iBT). *Application deadline:* Applications are processed on a rolling basis. Application fee: $45. Electronic applications accepted. *Financial support:* Federal Work-Study and unspecified assistantships available. Financial award application deadline: 3/1; financial award applicants required to submit FAFSA. *Unit head:* Dr. Mary Ann Merrigan, Chair, 570-408-4070, Fax: 570-408-7807, E-mail: maryann.merrigan@wilkes.edu. *Application contact:* Joanne Thomas, Interim Director of Graduate Enrollment, 570-408-4234, Fax: 570-408-7846, E-mail: joanne.thomas1@wilkes.edu.
Website: http://www.wilkes.edu/pages/391.asp

William Carey University, School of Nursing, Hattiesburg, MS 39401-5499. Offers MSN. *Accreditation:* AACN. Part-time programs available. *Degree requirements:* For master's, thesis or alternative. *Entrance requirements:* For master's, GRE, minimum GPA of 3.0, RN license. Additional exam requirements/recommendations for international students: Required—TOEFL (minimum score 500 paper-based).

William Paterson University of New Jersey, College of Science and Health, Wayne, NJ 07470-8420. Offers biotechnology (MS); communication disorders (MS); exercise and sports studies (MS); general biology (MS); nursing (MSN); nursing practice (DNP). Part-time and evening/weekend programs available. *Faculty:* 29 full-time (10 women), 10 part-time/adjunct (1 woman). *Students:* 67 full-time (56 women), 160 part-time (138 women); includes 76 minority (19 Black or African American, non-Hispanic/Latino; 26 Asian, non-Hispanic/Latino; 29 Hispanic/Latino; 2 Two or more races, non-Hispanic/Latino). Average age 35. 490 applicants, 33% accepted, 83 enrolled. In 2013, 51 master's awarded. *Degree requirements:* For master's, comprehensive exam (for some programs), thesis (for some programs), non-thesis internship/practicum (for some programs). *Entrance requirements:* For master's, GRE/MAT, minimum GPA of 2.75; for doctorate, GRE/MAT, minimum GPA of 3.3. Additional exam requirements/recommendations for international students: Required—TOEFL (minimum score 550 paper-based; 79 iBT), IELTS (minimum score 6). *Application deadline:* For fall admission, 6/1 for domestic students, 5/1 for international students; for spring admission, 11/1 for domestic students, 10/1 for international students. Applications are processed on a rolling basis. Application fee: $50. Electronic applications accepted. *Financial support:* Research assistantships with full tuition reimbursements, career-related internships or fieldwork, and unspecified assistantships available. Support available to part-time students. Financial award application deadline: 4/1; financial award applicants required to submit FAFSA. *Faculty research:* Human biomechanics, autism, nanomaterials, health and environment, red-tide causing algae. *Unit head:* Dr. Kenneth Wolf, Dean, 973-720-2194, E-mail: wolfk@wpunj.edu. *Application contact:* Christina Aiello, Assistant Director, Graduate Admissions, 973-720-2506, Fax: 973-720-2035, E-mail: aielloc@wpunj.edu.
Website: http://www.wpunj.edu/cosh

Wilmington University, College of Health Professions, New Castle, DE 19720-6491. Offers adult nurse practitioner (MSN); family nurse practitioner (MSN); gerontology nurse practitioner (MSN); nursing (MSN); nursing leadership (MSN); nursing practice (DNP). *Accreditation:* AACN. Part-time programs available. *Degree requirements:* For master's, thesis. *Entrance requirements:* For master's, BSN, RN license, interview, 3 letters of recommendation. Additional exam requirements/recommendations for international students: Required—TOEFL (minimum score 500 paper-based). Electronic applications accepted. *Faculty research:* Outcomes assessment, student writing ability.

Winona State University, College of Nursing and Health Sciences, Winona, MN 55987. Offers adult nurse practitioner (MS, Post Master's Certificate); clinical nurse specialist (MS, Post Master's Certificate); family nurse practitioner (MS, Post Master's Certificate); nurse administrator (MS); nurse educator (MS, Post Master's Certificate); nursing (DNP). *Accreditation:* AACN. Part-time programs available. Postbaccalaureate distance learning degree programs offered (no on-campus study). *Degree requirements:* For master's, thesis; for doctorate, capstone. *Entrance requirements:* For master's, GRE (if GPA less than 3.0). Additional exam requirements/recommendations for international students: Required—TOEFL (minimum score 550 paper-based).

Winston-Salem State University, Program in Nursing, Winston-Salem, NC 27110-0003. Offers MSN. *Accreditation:* AACN. Part-time and evening/weekend programs available. Postbaccalaureate distance learning degree programs offered. *Entrance requirements:* For master's, GRE, MAT, resume, NC or state compact license, 3 letters of recommendation. Electronic applications accepted. *Faculty research:* Elimination of health care disparities.

Wright State University, School of Graduate Studies, College of Nursing and Health, Program in Nursing, Dayton, OH 45435. Offers acute care nurse practitioner (MS); administration of nursing and health care systems (MS); adult health (MS); child and adolescent health (MS); community health (MS); family nurse practitioner (MS); nurse practitioner (MS); school nurse (MS); MBA/MS. *Accreditation:* AACN. Part-time and evening/weekend programs available. *Degree requirements:* For master's, thesis or alternative. *Entrance requirements:* For master's, GRE General Test, BSN from NLN-accredited college, Ohio RN license. Additional exam requirements/recommendations for international students: Required—TOEFL. *Faculty research:* Clinical nursing and health, teaching, caring, pain administration, informatics and technology.

Xavier University, College of Social Sciences, Health and Education, School of Nursing, Cincinnati, OH 45207. Offers MSN, MSN/M Ed, MSN/MBA, MSN/MS. *Accreditation:* AACN. Part-time and evening/weekend programs available. *Faculty:* 19 full-time (18 women), 9 part-time/adjunct (all women). *Students:* 76 full-time (63 women), 192 part-time (184 women); includes 46 minority (21 Black or African American, non-Hispanic/Latino; 2 American Indian or Alaska Native, non-Hispanic/Latino; 9 Asian, non-Hispanic/Latino; 13 Hispanic/Latino; 1 Native Hawaiian or other Pacific Islander, non-Hispanic/Latino). Average age 36. 117 applicants, 70% accepted, 100 enrolled. In 2013, 78 master's awarded. *Degree requirements:* For master's, thesis, scholarly project. *Entrance requirements:* For master's, GRE. Additional exam requirements/recommendations for international students: Required—TOEFL (minimum score 550 paper-based; 79 iBT). *Application deadline:* Applications are processed on a rolling basis. Application fee: $35. Electronic applications accepted. *Expenses: Tuition:* Part-time $594 per credit hour. *Required fees:* $3 per semester. *Financial support:* In 2013–14, 69 students received support. Applicants required to submit FAFSA. *Faculty research:* Clinical nurse leader, simulation, employment satisfaction, nontraditional students, holistic nursing. *Unit head:* Dr. Susan M. Schmidt, Director, 513-745-3815, Fax: 513-745-1087, E-mail: schmidt@xavier.edu. *Application contact:* Marilyn Volk Gomez, Director of Nursing Student Services, 513-745-4392, Fax: 513-745-1087, E-mail: gomez@xavier.edu.
Website: http://www.xavier.edu/msn/

Yale University, School of Nursing, West Haven, CT 06516. Offers MSN, DNP, PhD, Post Master's Certificate, MAR/MSN, MSN/M Div, MSN/MPH. *Accreditation:* AACN. Part-time programs available. Postbaccalaureate distance learning degree programs offered (minimal on-campus study). *Faculty:* 54 full-time (51 women), 95 part-time/adjunct (90 women). *Students:* 293 full-time, 58 part-time; includes 75 minority (16 Black or African American, non-Hispanic/Latino; 1 American Indian or Alaska Native, non-Hispanic/Latino; 25 Asian, non-Hispanic/Latino; 17 Hispanic/Latino; 16 Two or more races, non-Hispanic/Latino), 15 international. Average age 29. 557 applicants, 27% accepted, 96 enrolled. In 2013, 108 master's, 7 doctorates, 2 other advanced degrees awarded. Terminal master's awarded for partial completion of doctoral program. *Degree requirements:* For master's, thesis; for doctorate, comprehensive exam, thesis/dissertation. *Entrance requirements:* For master's, GRE General Test, bachelor's degree; for doctorate, GRE General Test, MSN; for Post Master's Certificate, MSN. Additional exam requirements/recommendations for international students: Required—TOEFL or IELTS. *Application deadline:* For fall admission, 11/1 priority date for domestic students, 11/1 for international students. Application fee: $100. Electronic applications accepted. *Expenses:* Contact institution. *Financial support:* In 2013–14, 265 students received support, including 239 fellowships (averaging $5,905 per year), 13 research assistantships with tuition reimbursements available (averaging $28,450 per year); Federal Work-Study, scholarships/grants, traineeships, and health care benefits also available. Support available to part-time students. Financial award application deadline: 2/1; financial award applicants required to submit FAFSA. *Faculty research:* Family-based care, chronic illness, primary care, development, policy. *Total annual research expenditures:* $6.4 million. *Unit head:* Dr. Margaret Grey, Dean, 203-785-2393, Fax: 203-785-6455, E-mail: margaret.grey@yale.edu. *Application contact:* Melissa Pucci, Director of Admissions, 203-737-1793, Fax: 203-737-5409, E-mail: melissa.pucci@yale.edu.
Website: http://nursing.yale.edu/

York College of Pennsylvania, Department of Nursing, York, PA 17405-7199. Offers adult gerontology clinical nurse specialist (MS), including administration, education; adult gerontology nurse practitioner (MS); certified nurse anesthetist (MS); nurse educator (MS); nursing (DNP). *Accreditation:* AACN; AANA/CANAEP. Part-time and evening/weekend programs available. *Faculty:* 10 full-time (all women), 4 part-time/adjunct (1 woman). *Students:* 33 full-time (26 women), 61 part-time (53 women); includes 12 minority (7 Black or African American, non-Hispanic/Latino; 2 American Indian or Alaska Native, non-Hispanic/Latino; 3 Asian, non-Hispanic/Latino), 1 international. Average age 37. 87 applicants, 31% accepted, 24 enrolled. In 2013, 26 master's, 4 doctorates awarded. *Entrance requirements:* For master's, GRE General Test, minimum GPA of 3.0 from CCNE- or NLNAC-accredited institution; for doctorate, master's degree in nursing from a CCNE- or NLNAC-accredited institution; minimum GPA of 3.0. Additional exam requirements/recommendations for international students: Required—TOEFL (minimum score 530 paper-based; 72 iBT). *Application deadline:* For fall admission, 7/15 priority date for domestic students; for spring admission, 11/15 priority date for domestic students. Applications are processed on a rolling basis. Application fee: $50. Electronic applications accepted. *Expenses: Tuition:* Full-time $12,870; part-time $715 per credit. *Required fees:* $1660; $360 per semester. Tuition and fees vary according to degree level. *Financial support:* Federal Work-Study available. *Faculty research:* Student stress response to simulation versus clinical, evidence-based practice in all clinical settings. *Unit head:* Dr. Richard Haas, Graduate Program Director, 717-815-1243, E-mail: rhaas@ycp.edu. *Application contact:* Diane Dube, Administrative Assistant, Graduate Programs in Nursing, 717-815-1462, E-mail: ddube@ycp.edu.
Website: http://www.ycp.edu/academics/academic-departments/nursing/

York University, Faculty of Graduate Studies, Faculty of Health, Program in Nursing, Toronto, ON M3J 1P3, Canada. Offers M Sc N. *Unit head:* Dr. E. Jenson, Graduate Program Director, 416-736-5271. *Application contact:* Dr. S. Walkerley, Program Coordinator, 416-736-5271, E-mail: swalkerl@yorku.ca.
Website: http://www.atkinson.yorku.ca/NURS/graduate/

Youngstown State University, Graduate School, Bitonte College of Health and Human Services, Department of Nursing, Youngstown, OH 44555-0001. Offers MSN. Part-time and evening/weekend programs available. *Degree requirements:* For master's, thesis optional. *Entrance requirements:* For master's, GRE General Test, BSN, CPR certification. Additional exam requirements/recommendations for international students: Required—TOEFL.

Acute Care/Critical Care Nursing

Allen College, Program in Nursing, Waterloo, IA 50703. Offers acute care nurse practitioner (MSN, Post-Master's Certificate); adult nurse practitioner (MSN, Post-Master's Certificate); adult psychiatric-mental health nurse practitioner (MSN, Post-Master's Certificate); community public health (MSN, Post-Master's Certificate); family nurse practitioner (MSN, Post-Master's Certificate); gerontological nurse practitioner (MSN, Post-Master's Certificate); health education (MSN); leadership in health care delivery (MSN, Post-Master's Certificate); nursing (DNP). Part-time programs available. Postbaccalaureate distance learning degree programs offered (minimal on-campus study). *Faculty:* 3 full-time (all women), 21 part-time/adjunct (20 women). *Students:* 21 full-time (19 women), 162 part-time (150 women); includes 5 minority (1 Black or African American, non-Hispanic/Latino; 2 Asian, non-Hispanic/Latino; 1 Hispanic/Latino; 1 Two or more races, non-Hispanic/Latino). Average age 34. 213 applicants, 57% accepted, 94 enrolled. In 2013, 41 master's, 4 other advanced degrees awarded. *Degree requirements:* For master's, thesis optional. *Entrance requirements:* For master's, minimum GPA of 3.0 in the last 60 hours of undergraduate coursework; for doctorate, minimum GPA of 3.25 in graduate coursework. Additional exam requirements/recommendations for international students: Recommended—TOEFL (minimum score 580 paper-based; 92 iBT), IELTS (minimum score 6). *Application deadline:* For fall admission, 2/1 priority date for domestic students; for spring admission, 9/1 priority date for domestic students. Applications are processed on a rolling basis. Application fee: $50. Electronic applications accepted. *Expenses: Tuition:* Full-time $14,534; part-time $755 per credit hour. *Required fees:* $935; $75 per credit hour. One-time fee: $275 part-time. Tuition and fees vary according to course load. *Financial support:* In 2013–14, 60 students received support. Institutionally sponsored loans, scholarships/grants, and traineeships available. Support available to part-time students. Financial award application deadline: 8/15; financial award applicants required to submit FAFSA. *Unit head:* Kendra Williams-Perez, Dean, School of Nursing, 319-226-2044, Fax: 319-226-2070, E-mail: kendra.williams-perez@allencollege.edu. *Application contact:* Molly Quinn, Admissions Counselor, 319-226-2001, Fax: 319-226-2010, E-mail: molly.quinn@allencollege.edu.
Website: http://www.allencollege.edu/

Armstrong State University, School of Graduate Studies, Program in Nursing, Savannah, GA 31419-1997. Offers adult-gerontological acute care nurse practitioner (MSN); adult-gerontological clinical nurse specialist (MSN); adult-gerontological primary care nurse practitioner (MSN). *Accreditation:* AACN. Part-time and evening/weekend programs available. *Faculty:* 10 full-time (all women), 1 (woman) part-time/adjunct. *Students:* 24 full-time (21 women), 17 part-time (16 women); includes 5 minority (2 Black or African American, non-Hispanic/Latino; 1 Hispanic/Latino; 2 Two or more races, non-Hispanic/Latino). Average age 34. 17 applicants, 65% accepted, 10 enrolled. In 2013, 13 master's awarded. *Degree requirements:* For master's, comprehensive exam, project or thesis. *Entrance requirements:* For master's, GRE General Test or MAT, minimum GPA of 3.0, letter of recommendation, letter of intent. Additional exam requirements/recommendations for international students: Required—TOEFL (minimum score 523 paper-based; 70 iBT). *Application deadline:* For fall admission, 2/28 for domestic and international students; for spring admission, 11/15 for domestic students, 9/15 for international students. Applications are processed on a rolling basis. Application fee: $30. Electronic applications accepted. *Expenses:* Tuition, state resident: part-time $201 per credit hour. Tuition, nonresident: part-time $745 per credit hour. *Required fees:* $310 per semester. Tuition and fees vary according to course load, campus/location and program. *Financial support:* In 2013–14, research assistantships with full tuition reimbursements (averaging $5,000 per year) were awarded; Federal Work-Study, scholarships/grants, and unspecified assistantships also available. Support available to part-time students. Financial award application deadline: 3/1; financial award applicants required to submit FAFSA. *Faculty research:* Midwifery, mental health, nursing simulation, smoking cessation during pregnancy, asthma education, vulnerable populations, geriatrics, disaster nursing, complementary and alternative modalities, nephrology. *Unit head:* Dr. Catherine Gilbert, Department Head, 912-344-3145, E-mail: catherine.gilbert@armstrong.edu. *Application contact:* Jill Bell, Director/Graduate Enrollment Coordinator, 912-344-2798, Fax: 912-344-3488, E-mail: graduate@armstrong.edu.
Website: http://www.armstrong.edu/Health_professions/nursing/nursing_graduate_programs

Barry University, School of Adult and Continuing Education, Division of Nursing, Program in Nurse Practitioner, Miami Shores, FL 33161-6695. Offers acute care nurse practitioner (MSN); family nurse practitioner (MSN); nurse practitioner (Certificate). *Accreditation:* AACN. Part-time and evening/weekend programs available. *Degree requirements:* For master's, research project or thesis. *Entrance requirements:* For master's, GRE General Test or MAT, BSN, minimum GPA of 3.0, course work in statistics. Electronic applications accepted. *Faculty research:* Child abuse, health beliefs, teenage pregnancy, cultural and clinical studies across the lifespan.

Case Western Reserve University, Frances Payne Bolton School of Nursing, Doctor of Nursing Practice Program, Cleveland, OH 44106. Offers acute care nurse practitioner (DNP); adult gerontology nurse practitioner (DNP); educational leadership (DNP); family nurse practitioner (DNP); family systems psychiatric mental health nursing (DNP); midwifery/family nursing (DNP); neonatal nurse practitioner (DNP); pediatric nurse practitioner (DNP); practice leadership (DNP); women's health nurse practitioner (DNP). *Accreditation:* AACN. Part-time programs available. Postbaccalaureate distance learning degree programs offered (minimal on-campus study). *Students:* 169 full-time, 9 part-time; includes 10 minority (6 Black or African American, non-Hispanic/Latino; 1 Asian, non-Hispanic/Latino; 2 Hispanic/Latino; 1 Two or more races, non-Hispanic/Latino). 76 applicants, 97% accepted, 59 enrolled. In 2013, 38 doctorates awarded. Terminal master's awarded for partial completion of doctoral program. *Degree requirements:* For doctorate, thesis/dissertation. *Entrance requirements:* For doctorate, GRE General Test or MAT. Additional exam requirements/recommendations for international students: Required—TOEFL (minimum score 577 paper-based; 90 iBT), IELTS (minimum score 7). *Application deadline:* For fall admission, 6/1 priority date for domestic students, 6/1 for international students; for spring admission, 10/1 for domestic and international students. Applications are processed on a rolling basis. Application fee: $75. *Financial support:* In 2013–14, 90 students received support, including 9 fellowships with full tuition reimbursements available (averaging $31,325 per year), 1 research assistantship with partial tuition reimbursement available (averaging $14,472

per year); teaching assistantships, Federal Work-Study, institutionally sponsored loans, scholarships/grants, and tuition waivers (partial) also available. Support available to part-time students. Financial award application deadline: 5/15; financial award applicants required to submit FAFSA. *Faculty research:* Symptom science, family/community care, aging across the lifespan, self-management of health and illness, neuroscience. *Unit head:* Dr. Donna Dowling, Director, 216-368-1869, Fax: 216-368-3542, E-mail: dad10@case.edu. *Application contact:* Donna Hassik, Admissions Coordinator, 216-368-5253, Fax: 216-368-0124, E-mail: dmh7@case.edu.
Website: http://fpb.case.edu/DNP/

Case Western Reserve University, Frances Payne Bolton School of Nursing, Master's Programs in Nursing, Nurse Practitioner Program, Cleveland, OH 44106. Offers acute care cardiovascular nursing (MSN); acute care nurse practitioner (MSN); acute care/flight nurse (MSN); adult gerontology acute care nurse practitioner (MSN); adult gerontology nurse practitioner (MSN); adult gerontology oncology and palliative care (MSN); family nurse practitioner (MSN); family systems psychiatric mental health nursing (MSN); neonatal nurse practitioner (MSN); pediatric nurse practitioner (MSN); women's health nurse practitioner (MSN). Part-time programs available. Postbaccalaureate distance learning degree programs offered (minimal on-campus study). *Faculty:* 54 full-time (50 women), 5 part-time/adjunct (3 women). *Students:* 56 full-time, 145 part-time; includes 9 minority (6 Black or African American, non-Hispanic/Latino; 2 Asian, non-Hispanic/Latino; 1 Hispanic/Latino), 5 international. Average age 35. 70 applicants, 71% accepted, 33 enrolled. In 2013, 79 master's awarded. *Degree requirements:* For master's, thesis optional. *Entrance requirements:* For master's, GRE General Test or MAT. Additional exam requirements/recommendations for international students: Required—TOEFL (minimum score 577 paper-based; 90 iBT), IELTS (minimum score 7). *Application deadline:* For fall admission, 6/1 for domestic students; for spring admission, 10/1 for domestic students. Applications are processed on a rolling basis. Application fee: $75. *Financial support:* In 2013–14, 25 teaching assistantships (averaging $15,120 per year) were awarded; research assistantships, institutionally sponsored loans, and tuition waivers (partial) also available. Support available to part-time students. Financial award application deadline: 6/30; financial award applicants required to submit FAFSA. *Faculty research:* Symptom science, family/community care, aging across the lifespan, self-management of health and illness, neuroscience. *Unit head:* Dr. Carol Savrin, Director, 216-368-5304, Fax: 216-368-3542, E-mail: cls18@case.edu. *Application contact:* Donna Hassik, Admissions Coordinator, 216-368-5253, Fax: 216-368-0124, E-mail: dmh7@case.edu.
Website: http://fpb.cwru.edu/MSN/majors.shtm

The College of New Rochelle, Graduate School, Program in Nursing, New Rochelle, NY 10805-2308. Offers acute care nurse practitioner (MS, Certificate); clinical specialist in holistic nursing (MS, Certificate); family nurse practitioner (MS, Certificate); nursing and health care management (MS); nursing education (Certificate). *Accreditation:* AACN. Part-time programs available. *Faculty:* 6 full-time (5 women), 5 part-time/adjunct (4 women). *Students:* 113 part-time (104 women); includes 56 minority (44 Black or African American, non-Hispanic/Latino; 3 Asian, non-Hispanic/Latino; 9 Hispanic/Latino). Average age 40. In 2013, 17 master's awarded. *Entrance requirements:* For master's, GRE General Test or MAT, BSN, malpractice insurance, minimum GPA of 3.0, RN license. *Application deadline:* For fall admission, 8/15 priority date for domestic students; for spring admission, 12/1 priority date for domestic students. Applications are processed on a rolling basis. Application fee: $35. Electronic applications accepted. *Expenses:* Contact institution. *Financial support:* Traineeships available. Support available to part-time students. Financial award application deadline: 8/15. *Unit head:* Dr. Mary McGuinness, Acting Dean, School of Nursing, 914-654-5441, E-mail: mmcguiness@cnr.edu.

Columbia University, School of Nursing, Program in Adult-Gerontology Acute Care Nurse Practitioner, New York, NY 10032. Offers MS, Adv C. *Accreditation:* AACN. Part-time programs available. *Entrance requirements:* For master's, GRE General Test, NCLEX, 1 year of clinical experience, BSN; for Adv C, MSN. Additional exam requirements/recommendations for international students: Required—TOEFL (minimum score 100 iBT). Electronic applications accepted.

Drexel University, College of Nursing and Health Professions, Division of Graduate Nursing, Philadelphia, PA 19104-2875. Offers adult acute care (MSN); adult psychiatric/mental health (MSN); advanced practice nursing (MSN); clinical trials research (MSN); family nurse practitioner (MSN); leadership in health systems management (MSN); nursing education (MSN); pediatric primary care (MSN); women's health (MSN). *Accreditation:* AACN. Electronic applications accepted.

Duke University, School of Nursing, Durham, NC 27708-0586. Offers acute care pediatric nurse practitioner (MSN); adult-gerontology nurse practitioner - acute care (MSN, Post Master's Certificate); adult-gerontology nurse practitioner - primary care (MSN, Post Master's Certificate), including adult-gerontology nurse practitioner (MSN), cardiology, oncology; family nurse practitioner (MSN); neonatal nurse practitioner (MSN); nurse anesthesia (MSN, DNP); nursing (PhD); nursing and health care leadership (MSN); nursing education (MSN); nursing informatics (MSN, Post Master's Certificate); pediatric nurse practitioner - primary care (MSN). *Accreditation:* AACN; AANA/CANAEP. Part-time and evening/weekend programs available. Postbaccalaureate distance learning degree programs offered (minimal on-campus study). *Faculty:* 74 full-time (64 women), 7 part-time/adjunct (4 women). *Students:* 127 full-time (113 women), 473 part-time (433 women); includes 131 minority (54 Black or African American, non-Hispanic/Latino; 9 American Indian or Alaska Native, non-Hispanic/Latino; 36 Asian, non-Hispanic/Latino; 27 Hispanic/Latino; 5 Native Hawaiian or other Pacific Islander, non-Hispanic/Latino), 14 international. Average age 34. 516 applicants, 50% accepted, 190 enrolled. In 2013, 179 master's, 49 doctorates, 23 other advanced degrees awarded. Terminal master's awarded for partial completion of doctoral program. *Degree requirements:* For master's, thesis optional; for doctorate, capstone project. *Entrance requirements:* For master's, GRE General Test (waived if undergraduate GPA of 3.4 or higher), 1 year of nursing experience (recommended), BSN, minimum GPA of 3.0, previous course work in statistics; for doctorate, GRE General Test (waived if undergraduate GPA of 3.4 or higher), BSN or MSN, minimum GPA of 3.0, portfolio, resume, personal statement, undergraduate statistics course, current licensure as a registered nurse, transcripts from all post-secondary institutions; for Post Master's Certificate, MSN, licensure or eligibility as a professional nurse, transcripts from all post-secondary institutions, previous course work in statistics. Additional exam requirements/recommendations for international students: Recommended—TOEFL (minimum score 550 paper-based; 83 iBT), IELTS (minimum score 7). *Application deadline:* For fall admission, 12/1 for domestic and international students; for spring admission, 5/1 for domestic and international students. Application fee: $50. Electronic applications accepted. *Expenses:* Contact institution. *Financial support:* Career-related internships or fieldwork, institutionally sponsored loans, scholarships/grants, traineeships, and tuition waivers (partial) available. Support available to part-time students. Financial award applicants required to submit FAFSA. *Faculty research:* Cardiovascular disease, caregiver skill training, data mining, prostate cancer, neonatal immune system. *Unit head:* Dr. Catherine L. Gilliss, Dean/Vice Chancellor for Nursing Affairs, 919-684-9444, Fax: 919-684-9414, E-mail: catherine.gilliss@duke.edu. *Application contact:* Ernie Rushing, Lead Admissions Processor/Admissions Officer, 919-668-6274, Fax: 919-668-4693, E-mail: stephen.rushing@dm.duke.edu.
Website: http://www.nursing.duke.edu/

Georgetown University, Graduate School of Arts and Sciences, School of Nursing and Health Studies, Washington, DC 20057. Offers acute care nurse practitioner (MS); clinical nurse specialist (MS); family nurse practitioner (MS); nurse anesthesia (MS); nurse-midwifery (MS); nursing (DNP); nursing education (MS). *Accreditation:* AACN; AANA/CANAEP (one or more programs are accredited); ACNM/ACME (one or more programs are accredited). *Degree requirements:* For master's, thesis optional. *Entrance requirements:* For master's, GRE General Test or MAT, bachelor's degree in nursing from NLN-accredited school, minimum undergraduate GPA of 3.0. Additional exam requirements/recommendations for international students: Required—TOEFL. Application fee: $50 ($55 for international students). *Financial support:* Scholarships/grants and traineeships available. Financial award applicants required to submit FAFSA. *Unit head:* Dr. Patricia Ann Cloonan, Dean, 202-687-7318. *Application contact:* Graduate School Admissions Office, 202-687-5568.

Grand Canyon University, College of Nursing, Phoenix, AZ 85017-1097. Offers acute care nurse practitioner (MS, PMC); clinical nurse specialist (PMC), including clinical nurse specialist, education; family nurse practitioner (MS); leadership in health care systems (MS); nurse education (MS). *Accreditation:* AACN. Part-time and evening/weekend programs available. Postbaccalaureate distance learning degree programs offered (no on-campus study). *Degree requirements:* For master's and PMC, comprehensive exam (for some programs). *Entrance requirements:* For master's, minimum cumulative and science course undergraduate GPA of 3.0. Additional exam requirements/recommendations for international students: Required—TOEFL (minimum score 575 paper-based; 90 iBT), IELTS (minimum score 7).

Indiana University–Purdue University Indianapolis, School of Nursing, Indianapolis, IN 46202-2896. Offers acute care nurse practitioner (MSN); adult health clinical nurse specialist (MSN); adult health nursing (MSN), including adult clinical nurse specialist, adult nurse practitioner (MSN); adult psychiatric/mental health nursing (MSN); child psychiatric/mental health nursing (MSN); community health nursing (MSN); family nurse practitioner (MSN); neonatal nurse practitioner (MSN); nursing (MSN, DNP), including nursing administration (MSN), nursing education (MSN); nursing science (PhD); pediatric clinical nurse specialist (MSN); women's health nurse practitioner (MSN); MSN/MPA; MSN/MPH. Part-time programs available. *Faculty:* 85 full-time (82 women), 60 part-time/adjunct (all women). *Students:* 86 full-time (78 women), 371 part-time (351 women); includes 74 minority (39 Black or African American, non-Hispanic/Latino; 1 American Indian or Alaska Native, non-Hispanic/Latino; 14 Asian, non-Hispanic/Latino; 11 Hispanic/Latino; 9 Two or more races, non-Hispanic/Latino), 6 international. Average age 38. 224 applicants, 61% accepted, 102 enrolled. In 2013, 120 master's, 10 doctorates awarded. Terminal master's awarded for partial completion of doctoral program. *Degree requirements:* For master's, thesis; for doctorate, thesis/dissertation. *Entrance requirements:* For master's, minimum GPA of 3.0, RN license; for doctorate, GRE General Test, minimum GPA of 3.0, MSN, RN license, graduate statistics course with minimum B grade (not older than 3 years). Additional exam requirements/recommendations for international students: Required—TOEFL. *Application deadline:* For fall admission, 2/15 for domestic students; for spring admission, 9/15 for domestic students. Application fee: $55 ($65 for international students). *Financial support:* In 2013–14, 93 students received support. Fellowships with full tuition reimbursements available, research assistantships with full tuition reimbursements available, teaching assistantships with full tuition reimbursements available, Federal Work-Study, institutionally sponsored loans, scholarships/grants, and tuition waivers (full) available. Support available to part-time students. Financial award application deadline: 5/1. *Faculty research:* Clinical science, health systems. *Total annual research expenditures:* $3 million. *Unit head:* Dr. Patricia Ebright, Associate Dean for Graduate Programs, E-mail: nursing@iupui.edu. *Application contact:* Information Contact, 317-274-2806.
Website: http://nursing.iu.edu/

Inter American University of Puerto Rico, Arecibo Campus, Program in Nursing, Arecibo, PR 00614-4050. Offers critical care nursing (MSN); surgical nursing (MSN). *Entrance requirements:* For master's, EXADEP or GRE General Test or MAT, 2 letters of recommendation, bachelor's degree in nursing, minimum GPA of 2.5 in last 60 credits, minimum 1 year nursing experience, nursing license.

Kent State University, College of Nursing, Kent, OH 44242-0001. Offers acute care nurse practitioner (MSN); adult nurse practitioner (MSN); clinical nurse specialist (MSN); family nurse practitioner (MSN); geriatric nurse practitioner (MSN); health care management (MSN); nurse educator (MSN); nursing (PhD); nursing practice (DNP); pediatric nurse practitioner (MSN); psychiatric/mental health nurse practitioner (MSN); women's health nurse practitioner (MSN). PhD program offered jointly with The University of Akron. *Accreditation:* AACN. Part-time programs available. *Degree requirements:* For master's, thesis optional; for doctorate, comprehensive exam, thesis/dissertation. *Entrance requirements:* For master's, GRE (if undergraduate GPA less than 3.0), minimum GPA of 2.75; for doctorate, GRE, MSN. Additional exam requirements/recommendations for international students: Required—TOEFL. Electronic applications accepted. *Expenses:* Contact institution. *Faculty research:* Women and violence, methodological specialties, osteoporosis in women, new caregivers and the elderly.

Loyola University Chicago, Graduate School, Marcella Niehoff School of Nursing, Acute Care Nurse Practitioner Program, Chicago, IL 60660. Offers MSN, Certificate. *Accreditation:* AACN. Part-time programs available. Postbaccalaureate distance learning degree programs offered (minimal on-campus study). *Students:* 12 full-time (9 women), 27 part-time (23 women); includes 6 minority (2 Black or African American, non-Hispanic/Latino; 1 American Indian or Alaska Native, non-Hispanic/Latino; 3 Asian, non-Hispanic/Latino). Average age 33. 21 applicants, 67% accepted, 8 enrolled. In 2013, 11 master's awarded. *Degree requirements:* For master's, comprehensive exam or oral thesis defense. *Entrance requirements:* For master's, Illinois nursing license, BSN, minimum nursing GPA of 3.0, 3 letters of recommendation, 2,000 hours of experience in acute care prior to clinical. *Application deadline:* Applications are processed on a rolling basis. Application fee: $40. Electronic applications accepted. *Expenses: Tuition:* Full-time $16,740; part-time $930 per credit. *Required fees:* $135 per semester. *Financial support:* Traineeships available. Financial award application deadline: 3/1. *Unit head:* Dr. MariJo Letizia, Associate Dean for MSN and DNP Programs, 708-216-9325, Fax: 708-216-9555, E-mail: mletizi@luc.edu. *Application contact:* Amy Weatherford, Enrollment Advisor, 708-216-3751, Fax: 708-216-9555, E-mail: aweatherford@luc.edu.
Website: http://www.luc.edu/nursing/

Marquette University, Graduate School, College of Nursing, Milwaukee, WI 53201-1881. Offers acute care nurse practitioner (Certificate); adult clinical nurse specialist (Certificate); adult nurse practitioner (Certificate); advanced practice nursing (MSN, DNP), including adult-older adult acute care (DNP), adults (MSN), adults-older adults (DNP), clinical nurse leader (MSN), health care systems leadership (DNP), nurse-midwifery (MSN), older adults (MSN), pediatrics acute care (MSN), pediatrics primary care (MSN), pediatrics-acute care (DNP), pediatrics-primary care (DNP), primary care (DNP), systems leadership and healthcare quality (MSN); family nurse practitioner

(Certificate); nurse-midwifery (Certificate); nursing (PhD); pediatric acute care (Certificate); pediatric primary care (Certificate); systems leadership and healthcare quality (Certificate). *Accreditation:* AACN. *Faculty:* 35 full-time (34 women), 59 part-time/adjunct (58 women). *Students:* 105 full-time (96 women), 279 part-time (256 women); includes 28 minority (11 Black or African American, non-Hispanic/Latino; 7 Asian, non-Hispanic/Latino; 8 Hispanic/Latino; 2 Two or more races, non-Hispanic/Latino), 3 international. Average age 30. 322 applicants, 62% accepted, 98 enrolled. In 2013, 66 master's, 4 doctorates, 6 other advanced degrees awarded. Terminal master's awarded for partial completion of doctoral program. *Degree requirements:* For master's, comprehensive exam, thesis or alternative. *Entrance requirements:* For master's, GRE General Test, BSN, Wisconsin RN license, official transcripts from all current and previous colleges/universities except Marquette, three completed recommendation forms, resume, written statement of professional goals; for doctorate, GRE General Test, official transcripts from all current and previous colleges/universities except Marquette, three letters of recommendation, resume, written statement of professional goals, sample of scholarly writing. Additional exam requirements/recommendations for international students: Required—TOEFL (minimum score 530 paper-based). *Application deadline:* For fall admission, 2/15 for domestic and international students. Application fee: $50. Electronic applications accepted. *Financial support:* In 2013–14, 41 students received support, including 1 fellowship with partial tuition reimbursement available (averaging $17,500 per year), 2 research assistantships with full tuition reimbursements available (averaging $13,285 per year), 8 teaching assistantships with full tuition reimbursements available (averaging $13,912 per year); career-related internships or fieldwork, Federal Work-Study, scholarships/grants, health care benefits, tuition waivers (partial), and unspecified assistantships also available. Support available to part-time students. Financial award application deadline: 2/15. *Faculty research:* Psychosocial adjustment to chronic illness, gerontology, reminiscence, health policy: uninsured and access, hospital care delivery systems. *Total annual research expenditures:* $769,051. *Unit head:* Dr. Margaret Callahan, Dean, 414-288-3800, Fax: 414-288-1578. *Application contact:* Dr. Maureen O'Brien, Associate Dean/Clinical Associate Professor, 414-288-3823.
Website: http://www.marquette.edu/nursing/academicprograms-graduate.shtml

Mount Carmel College of Nursing, Nursing Program, Columbus, OH 43222. Offers adult gerontology acute care nurse practitioner (MS); adult health clinical nurse specialist (MS); family nurse practitioner (MS); nursing administration (MS); nursing education (MS). *Accreditation:* AACN. Part-time programs available. *Faculty:* 8 full-time (7 women), 8 part-time/adjunct (7 women). *Students:* 94 full-time (89 women), 76 part-time (73 women); includes 35 minority (21 Black or African American, non-Hispanic/Latino; 2 American Indian or Alaska Native, non-Hispanic/Latino; 6 Asian, non-Hispanic/Latino; 2 Hispanic/Latino; 1 Native Hawaiian or other Pacific Islander, non-Hispanic/Latino; 3 Two or more races, non-Hispanic/Latino). Average age 38. 123 applicants, 50% accepted, 47 enrolled. In 2013, 41 master's awarded. *Degree requirements:* For master's, professional manuscript. *Entrance requirements:* For master's, letters of recommendation, statement of purpose, current resume, baccalaureate degree in nursing, current Ohio RN license, minimum cumulative GPA of 3.0. Additional exam requirements/recommendations for international students: Required—TOEFL (minimum score 550 paper-based; 80 iBT). *Application deadline:* For fall admission, 6/1 priority date for domestic students; for winter admission, 11/1 for domestic students; for spring admission, 10/1 priority date for domestic students; for summer admission, 3/1 for domestic students. Applications are processed on a rolling basis. Application fee: $30. *Expenses: Tuition:* Full-time $8560; part-time $428 per credit. *Required fees:* $75. *Financial support:* In 2013–14, 9 students received support. Institutionally sponsored loans and scholarships/grants available. Financial award application deadline: 3/15; financial award applicants required to submit FAFSA. *Unit head:* Dr. Angela Phillips-Lowe, Associate Dean, 614-234-5717, Fax: 614-234-2875, E-mail: aphillips-lowe@mccn.edu. *Application contact:* Kathleen Walters, Program Coordinator, 614-234-5408, Fax: 614-234-2875, E-mail: kwalters@mccn.edu.
Website: http://www.mccn.edu/

New York University, College of Nursing, Doctor of Nursing Practice Program, New York, NY 10012-1019. Offers advanced practice nursing (DNP), including adult acute care, adult nurse practitioner/holistic nursing, adult nurse practitioner/palliative care nursing, adult primary care, adult primary care/geriatrics, family, geriatrics, mental health nursing, nurse-midwifery, pediatrics. Part-time and evening/weekend programs available. *Faculty:* 3 full-time (all women), 1 part-time/adjunct (0 women). *Students:* 1 (woman) full-time, 33 part-time (30 women); includes 7 minority (3 Black or African American, non-Hispanic/Latino; 3 Asian, non-Hispanic/Latino; 1 Hispanic/Latino). Average age 39. 18 applicants, 100% accepted, 12 enrolled. In 2013, 4 doctorates awarded. *Degree requirements:* For doctorate, thesis/dissertation, capstone. *Entrance requirements:* For doctorate, MAT or GRE (either taken within past 5 years), MS, RN license, interview, Nurse Practitioner Certification. Additional exam requirements/recommendations for international students: Required—TOEFL (minimum score 90 iBT), IELTS (minimum score 7). *Application deadline:* For fall admission, 3/1 for domestic students, 4/1 for international students. Applications are processed on a rolling basis. Application fee: $80. Electronic applications accepted. *Expenses: Tuition:* Full-time $35,856; part-time $1494 per unit. *Required fees:* $1408; $64 per unit. $473 per term. Tuition and fees vary according to course load and program. *Financial support:* Scholarships/grants available. Support available to part-time students. Financial award application deadline: 2/1. *Faculty research:* Geriatrics, HIV, elderly black diabetics, families and illness, oral systemic connection. *Unit head:* Dr. Rona Levin, Director, 212-998-5319, Fax: 212-995-3143, E-mail: rfl2039@nyu.edu. *Application contact:* Elizabeth Ensweiler, Assistant Director, Graduate Student Affairs and Admissions, 212-992-7653, Fax: 212-995-4302, E-mail: ee39@nyu.edu.

New York University, College of Nursing, Programs in Advanced Practice Nursing, New York, NY 10012-1019. Offers advanced practice nursing: adult acute care (MS, Advanced Certificate); advanced practice nursing: adult nurse practitioner/holistic nurse practitioner (Advanced Certificate); advanced practice nursing: adult nurse practitioner/palliative care nurse practitioner (Advanced Certificate); advanced practice nursing: adult primary care (MS, Advanced Certificate); advanced practice nursing: family (MS, Advanced Certificate); advanced practice nursing: geriatrics (Advanced Certificate); advanced practice nursing: mental health (MS); advanced practice nursing: mental health nursing (Advanced Certificate); advanced practice nursing: pediatrics (MS, Advanced Certificate); nurse midwifery (MS, Advanced Certificate); nursing administration (MS, Advanced Certificate); nursing education (MS, Advanced Certificate); nursing informatics (MS, Advanced Certificate); MS/MPA; MS/MPH. *Accreditation:* AACN; ACNM/ACME. Part-time programs available. *Faculty:* 22 full-time (all women), 54 part-time/adjunct (46 women). *Students:* 36 full-time (31 women), 622 part-time (549 women); includes 239 minority (73 Black or African American, non-Hispanic/Latino; 1 American Indian or Alaska Native, non-Hispanic/Latino; 116 Asian, non-Hispanic/Latino; 36 Hispanic/Latino; 6 Native Hawaiian or other Pacific Islander, non-Hispanic/Latino; 7 Two or more races, non-Hispanic/Latino), 16 international. Average age 37. 395 applicants, 67% accepted, 156 enrolled. In 2013, 186 master's, 8 other advanced degrees awarded. *Degree requirements:* For master's, thesis (for some programs). *Entrance requirements:* For master's, BS in nursing, AS in nursing with another BS/BA, interview, RN license, 1 year of clinical experience (3 for nursing education program); for Advanced Certificate, master's degree. Additional exam requirements/recommendations for international students: Required—TOEFL (minimum score 90 iBT), IELTS (minimum score 7). *Application deadline:* For fall admission, 7/1 for domestic and international students; for spring admission, 12/1 for domestic and international students. Application fee: $80. Electronic applications accepted. *Expenses: Tuition:* Full-time $35,856; part-time $1494 per unit. *Required fees:* $1408; $64 per unit. $473 per term. Tuition and fees vary according to course load and program. *Financial support:* In 2013–14, 182 students received support. Research assistantships, career-related internships or fieldwork, Federal Work-Study, scholarships/grants, traineeships, and unspecified assistantships available. Support available to part-time students. Financial award application deadline: 2/1; financial award applicants required to submit FAFSA. *Faculty research:* Geriatrics, HIV, elderly black diabetics, families and illness, oral systemic connection. *Unit head:* Dr. Judith Haber, Associate Dean, Graduate Programs, 212-998-9020, Fax: 212-995-3143, E-mail: jh33@nyu.edu. *Application contact:* Elizabeth Ensweiler, Assistant Director, Graduate Student Affairs and Admissions, 212-992-7653, Fax: 212-995-4302, E-mail: ee39@nyu.edu.

Northeastern University, Bouvé College of Health Sciences, Boston, MA 02115-5096. Offers audiology (Au D); biotechnology (MS); counseling psychology (MS, PhD, CAGS); counseling/school psychology (PhD); exercise physiology (MS), including exercise physiology, public health; health informatics (MS); nursing (MS, PhD, CAGS), including acute care (MS), administration (MS), anesthesia (MS), primary care (MS), psychiatric mental health (MS); pharmaceutical sciences (PhD); pharmaceutics and drug delivery systems (MS); pharmacology (MS); physical therapy (DPT); physician assistant (MS); school psychology (PhD, CAGS); school/counseling psychology (PhD); speech language pathology (MS); urban public health (MPH); MS/MBA. *Accreditation:* ACPE (one or more programs are accredited). Part-time and evening/weekend programs available. *Degree requirements:* For doctorate, thesis/dissertation (for some programs); for CAGS, comprehensive exam.

Ohio University, Graduate College, College of Health Sciences and Professions, School of Nursing, Athens, OH 45701-2979. Offers acute care nurse practitioner (MSN); acute care nurse practitioner and family nurse practitioner (MSN); acute care nurse practitioner and nurse administrator (MSN); acute care nurse practitioner and nurse educator (MSN); family nurse practitioner (MSN); nurse administrator (MSN); nurse administrator and family nurse practitioner (MSN); nurse educator (MSN); nurse educator and family nurse practitioner (MSN); nurse educator and nurse administrator (MSN). *Accreditation:* AACN. *Degree requirements:* For master's, capstone project. *Entrance requirements:* For master's, GRE, bachelor's degree in nursing from an accredited college or university, minimum overall undergraduate GPA of 3.0, official transcripts, statement of goals and objectives, resume, 3 letters of recommendation. Additional exam requirements/recommendations for international students: Required—TOEFL (minimum score 550 paper-based; 80 iBT) or IELTS (minimum score 6.5). Electronic applications accepted.

Purdue University Calumet, Graduate Studies Office, School of Nursing, Hammond, IN 46323-2094. Offers adult health clinical nurse specialist (MS); critical care clinical nurse specialist (MS); family nurse practitioner (MS); nurse executive (MS). Part-time programs available. Postbaccalaureate distance learning degree programs offered (minimal on-campus study). *Entrance requirements:* For master's, BSN. Additional exam requirements/recommendations for international students: Required—TOEFL. Electronic applications accepted. *Faculty research:* Adult health, cardiovascular and pulmonary nursing.

San Francisco State University, Division of Graduate Studies, College of Health and Social Sciences, School of Nursing, San Francisco, CA 94132-1722. Offers adult acute care (MS); clinical nurse specialist (MS); community/public health nursing (MS); family nurse practitioner (MS, Certificate); nursing administration (MS); nursing education (MS); pediatrics (MS); women's health (MS). *Accreditation:* AACN. Part-time programs available. *Application deadline:* Applications are processed on a rolling basis. *Financial support:* Career-related internships or fieldwork available. *Unit head:* Dr. Mary-Ann van Dam, Director, 415-338-1802, E-mail: vandam@sfsu.edu. *Application contact:* Robert Strachan, Admission and Student Services Coordinator, 415-338-1802, E-mail: strachan@sfsu.edu.
Website: http://nursing.sfsu.edu

Southern Adventist University, School of Nursing, Collegedale, TN 37315-0370. Offers acute care nurse practitioner (MSN); adult nurse practitioner (MSN); family nurse practitioner (MSN); nurse educator (MSN); MSN/MSBA. Part-time programs available. *Degree requirements:* For master's, thesis or project. *Entrance requirements:* For master's, RN license. Additional exam requirements/recommendations for international students: Required—TOEFL (minimum score 600 paper-based). Electronic applications accepted. *Faculty research:* Pain management, ethics, corporate wellness, caring spirituality, stress.

Texas Tech University Health Sciences Center, School of Nursing, Lubbock, TX 79430. Offers acute care nurse practitioner (MSN, Certificate); administration (MSN); advanced practice (DNP); education (MSN); executive leadership (DNP); family nurse practitioner (MSN, Certificate); geriatric nurse practitioner (MSN, Certificate); pediatric nurse practitioner (MSN, Certificate). *Accreditation:* AACN. Part-time programs available. Postbaccalaureate distance learning degree programs offered (minimal on-campus study). *Degree requirements:* For master's, thesis optional. *Entrance requirements:* For master's, minimum GPA of 3.0, 3 letters of reference, BSN, RN license; for Certificate, minimum GPA of 3.0, 3 letters of reference, RN license. Additional exam requirements/recommendations for international students: Required—TOEFL (minimum score 550 paper-based). *Faculty research:* Diabetes/obesity, nurse competency, disease management, intervention and measurements, health disparities.

Texas Woman's University, Graduate School, College of Nursing, Denton, TX 76201. Offers acute care nurse practitioner (MS); adult health clinical nurse specialist (MS); adult health nurse practitioner (MS); child health clinical nurse specialist (MS); clinical nurse leader (MS); family nurse practitioner (MS); health systems management (MS); nursing education (MS); nursing practice (DNP); nursing science (PhD); pediatric nurse practitioner (MS); women's health clinical nurse specialist (MS); women's health nurse practitioner (MS). *Accreditation:* AACN. Part-time programs available. Postbaccalaureate distance learning degree programs offered. *Faculty:* 60 full-time (59 women), 46 part-time/adjunct (39 women). *Students:* 54 full-time (49 women), 910 part-time (848 women); includes 489 minority (221 Black or African American, non-Hispanic/Latino; 11 American Indian or Alaska Native, non-Hispanic/Latino; 184 Asian, non-Hispanic/Latino; 70 Hispanic/Latino; 3 Native Hawaiian or other Pacific Islander, non-Hispanic/Latino), 16 international. Average age 38. 430 applicants, 65% accepted, 193 enrolled. In 2013, 258 master's, 22 doctorates awarded. *Degree requirements:* For master's, comprehensive exam, thesis or alternative; for doctorate, comprehensive exam, thesis/dissertation. *Entrance requirements:* For master's, GRE or MAT, minimum GPA of 3.0 on last 60 hours in undergraduate nursing degree and overall, RN license, BS in nursing, basic statistics course; for doctorate, GRE (preferred minimum score 153 [500 old version] Verbal, 144 [500 old version] Quantitative, 4 Analytical), MS in nursing, minimum preferred GPA of 3.5, RN license, statistics, 2 letters of reference, curriculum vitae, graduate nursing-theory course, graduate research course, statement of professional goals and research interests. Additional exam requirements/

recommendations for international students: Required—TOEFL (minimum score 550 paper-based; 79 iBT). *Application deadline:* For fall admission, 5/1 priority date for domestic students, 3/1 for international students; for spring admission, 9/15 priority date for domestic students, 7/1 for international students. Applications are processed on a rolling basis. Application fee: $50 ($75 for international students). Electronic applications accepted. *Expenses:* Tuition, state resident: full-time $4182; part-time $233.32 per credit hour. Tuition, nonresident: full-time $10,716; part-time $595.32 per credit hour. *Financial support:* In 2013–14, 149 students received support, including 10 research assistantships (averaging $5,600 per year), 1 teaching assistantship (averaging $5,600 per year); career-related internships or fieldwork, Federal Work-Study, institutionally sponsored loans, scholarships/grants, traineeships, health care benefits, and unspecified assistantships also available. Support available to part-time students. Financial award application deadline: 3/1; financial award applicants required to submit FAFSA. *Faculty research:* Screening, prevention, and treatment for intimate partner violence; needs of adolescents during childbirth intervention; a network analysis decision tool for nurse managers (social network analysis); support for adolescents with implantable cardioverter defibrillators; informatics: nurse staffing, safety, quality, and financial data as they relate to patient care outcomes; prevention and treatment of obesity; improving infant outcomes related to premature birth. *Total annual research expenditures:* $1.7 million. *Unit head:* Dr. Gayle Roux, Interim Dean and Associate Dean for Research and Clinical Scholarship, 940-898-2401, Fax: 940-898-2437, E-mail: nursing@twu.edu. *Application contact:* Dr. Samuel Wheeler, Assistant Director of Admissions, 940-898-3188, Fax: 940-898-3081, E-mail: wheelersr@twu.edu.
Website: http://www.twu.edu/nursing/

Universidad de Iberoamerica, Graduate School, San Jose, Costa Rica. Offers clinical neuropsychology (PhD); clinical psychology (M Psych); educational psychology (M Psych); forensic psychology (M Psych); hospital management (MHA); intensive care nursing (MN); medicine (MD).

The University of Alabama in Huntsville, School of Graduate Studies, College of Nursing, Huntsville, AL 35899. Offers family nurse practitioner (Certificate); nursing (MSN, DNP), including acute care nurse practitioner (MSN), adult clinical nurse specialist (MSN), clinical nurse leader (MSN), family nurse practitioner (MSN), leadership in health care systems (MSN); nursing education (Certificate). DNP offered jointly with The University of Alabama at Birmingham. *Accreditation:* AACN. Part-time and evening/weekend programs available. Postbaccalaureate distance learning degree programs offered (minimal on-campus study). *Faculty:* 16 full-time (15 women), 4 part-time/adjunct (all women). *Students:* 67 full-time (63 women), 235 part-time (192 women); includes 40 minority (27 Black or African American, non-Hispanic/Latino; 5 American Indian or Alaska Native, non-Hispanic/Latino; 4 Asian, non-Hispanic/Latino; 3 Hispanic/Latino; 1 Two or more races, non-Hispanic/Latino), 10 international. Average age 36. 265 applicants, 59% accepted, 128 enrolled. In 2013, 75 master's, 10 doctorates, 5 other advanced degrees awarded. *Degree requirements:* For master's, comprehensive exam, thesis or alternative, oral and written exams. *Entrance requirements:* For master's, MAT or GRE, Alabama RN license, BSN, minimum GPA of 3.0; for doctorate, master's degree in nursing in an advanced practice area; for Certificate, MAT or GRE, minimum GPA of 3.0. Additional exam requirements/recommendations for international students: Required—TOEFL (minimum score 500 paper-based; 80 iBT), IELTS (minimum score 6.5). *Application deadline:* For fall admission, 7/15 for domestic students, 4/1 for international students; for spring admission, 11/30 for domestic students, 9/1 for international students. Applications are processed on a rolling basis. Application fee: $50. Electronic applications accepted. *Expenses:* Tuition, state resident: full-time $8912; part-time $540 per credit hour. Tuition, nonresident: full-time $20,774; part-time $1252 per credit hour. *Required fees:* $148 per semester. One-time fee: $150. *Financial support:* In 2013–14, 19 students received support, including 19 teaching assistantships with full tuition reimbursements available (averaging $7,876 per year); career-related internships or fieldwork, Federal Work-Study, institutionally sponsored loans, scholarships/grants, traineeships, health care benefits, and unspecified assistantships also available. Support available to part-time students. Financial award application deadline: 4/1; financial award applicants required to submit FAFSA. *Faculty research:* Health care informatics, chronic illness management, maternal and child health, genetics/genomics, technology and health care. *Total annual research expenditures:* $557,830. *Unit head:* Dr. Fay Raines, Dean, 256-824-6345, Fax: 256-824-6026, E-mail: rainesc@uah.edu. *Application contact:* Charles Davis, Director of Graduate Nursing Admissions and Advising, 256-824-2433, Fax: 256-824-6026, E-mail: charles.davis@uah.edu.
Website: http://www.uah.edu/nursing/welcome

University of Cincinnati, Graduate School, College of Nursing, Cincinnati, OH 45221-0038. Offers clinical nurse specialist (MSN), including adult health, community health, neonatal, nursing administration, occupational health, pediatric health, psychiatric nursing, women's health; nurse anesthesia (MSN); nurse midwifery (MSN); nurse practitioner (MSN), including acute care, ambulatory care, family, family/psychiatric, women's health; nursing (PhD); MBA/MSN. *Accreditation:* AACN; AANA/CANAEP (one or more programs are accredited); ACNM/ACME. Part-time programs available. Postbaccalaureate distance learning degree programs offered (no on-campus study). Terminal master's awarded for partial completion of doctoral program. *Degree requirements:* For master's, thesis or alternative; for doctorate, comprehensive exam, thesis/dissertation. *Entrance requirements:* For master's and doctorate, GRE General Test. Additional exam requirements/recommendations for international students: Required—TOEFL (minimum score 520 paper-based). Electronic applications accepted. *Faculty research:* Substance abuse, injury and violence, symptom management.

University of Guelph, Ontario Veterinary College and Graduate Studies, Graduate Programs in Veterinary Sciences, Department of Clinical Studies, Guelph, ON N1G 2W1, Canada. Offers anesthesiology (M Sc, DV Sc); cardiology (DV Sc, Diploma); clinical studies (Diploma); dermatology (M Sc); diagnostic imaging (M Sc, DV Sc); emergency/critical care (M Sc, DV Sc, Diploma); medicine (M Sc, DV Sc); neurology (M Sc, DV Sc); ophthalmology (M Sc, DV Sc); surgery (M Sc, DV Sc). *Degree requirements:* For master's, thesis; for doctorate, comprehensive exam, thesis/dissertation. *Entrance requirements:* Additional exam requirements/recommendations for international students: Required—TOEFL (minimum score 550 paper-based), IELTS (minimum score 6.5). Electronic applications accepted. *Faculty research:* Orthopedics, respirology, oncology, exercise physiology, cardiology.

University of Illinois at Chicago, Graduate College, College of Nursing, Program in Nursing, Chicago, IL 60607-7128. Offers acute care clinical nurse specialist (MS); acute care nurse practitioner (MS); administrative nursing leadership (Certificate); administrative studies in nursing (MS); adult nurse practitioner (MS); adult/geriatric nurse practitioner (MS); advanced community health nurse specialist (MS); family nurse practitioner (MS); geriatric clinical nurse specialist (MS); geriatric nurse practitioner (MS); mental health clinical nurse specialist (MS); mental health nurse practitioner (MS); nurse midwifery (MS); occupational health/advanced community health nurse specialist (MS); occupational health/family nurse practitioner (MS); pediatric clinical nurse specialist (MS); pediatric nurse practitioner (MS); perinatal clinical nurse specialist (MS); school/advanced community health nurse specialist (MS); school/family nurse practitioner (MS); women's health nurse practitioner (MS). *Accreditation:* AACN. Part-time programs available. *Faculty:* 16 full-time (14 women). *Students:* 393 full-time (361 women), 410 part-time (367 women); includes 198 minority (48 Black or African American, non-Hispanic/Latino; 1 American Indian or Alaska Native, non-Hispanic/Latino; 64 Asian, non-Hispanic/Latino; 71 Hispanic/Latino; 2 Native Hawaiian or other Pacific Islander, non-Hispanic/Latino; 12 Two or more races, non-Hispanic/Latino), 29 international. Average age 32. 396 applicants, 62% accepted, 177 enrolled. In 2013, 184 master's awarded. *Degree requirements:* For master's, thesis or alternative. *Entrance requirements:* For master's, GRE General Test, minimum GPA of 2.75. Additional exam requirements/recommendations for international students: Required—TOEFL. *Application deadline:* For fall admission, 5/15 for domestic students, 2/15 for international students; for spring admission, 11/1 for domestic students, 7/15 for international students. Applications are processed on a rolling basis. Application fee: $40 ($50 for international students). Electronic applications accepted. *Expenses:* Tuition, state resident: full-time $11,066; part-time $3689 per term. Tuition, nonresident: full-time $23,064; part-time $7688 per term. *Required fees:* $3004; $1190 per term. Tuition and fees vary according to course level and program. *Financial support:* Fellowships with full tuition reimbursements, research assistantships with full tuition reimbursements, teaching assistantships with full tuition reimbursements, career-related internships or fieldwork, Federal Work-Study, institutionally sponsored loans, scholarships/grants, traineeships, tuition waivers (full and partial), and unspecified assistantships available. Support available to part-time students. Financial award application deadline: 3/1; financial award applicants required to submit FAFSA. *Unit head:* Dr. Terri E. Weaver, Dean, 312-996-7808, E-mail: teweaver@uic.edu. *Application contact:* Receptionist, 312-413-2550, E-mail: gradcoll@uic.edu.

University of Miami, Graduate School, School of Nursing and Health Studies, Coral Gables, FL 33124. Offers acute care (MSN), including acute care nurse practitioner, nurse anesthesia; nursing (PhD); primary care (MSN), including adult nurse practitioner, family nurse practitioner, nurse midwifery, women's health practitioner. *Accreditation:* AACN; AANA/CANAEP; ACNM/ACME (one or more programs are accredited). Part-time programs available. *Degree requirements:* For master's, thesis optional; for doctorate, thesis/dissertation. *Entrance requirements:* For master's, GRE General Test, BSN, minimum GPA of 3.0, Florida RN license; for doctorate, GRE General Test, BSN or MSN, minimum GPA of 3.0. Additional exam requirements/recommendations for international students: Required—TOEFL (minimum score 550 paper-based). Electronic applications accepted. *Faculty research:* Transcultural nursing, exercise and depression in Alzheimer's disease, infectious diseases/HIV–AIDS, postpartum depression, outcomes assessment.

University of Michigan, Rackham Graduate School, School of Nursing, Ann Arbor, MI 48109. Offers acute care pediatric nurse practitioner (MS); adult-gerontology acute care clinical nurse specialist (MS); adult-gerontology acute care nurse practitioner (MS); adult-gerontology primary care nurse practitioner (MS); health systems, nursing leadership, and effectiveness science (MS); nurse midwife (MS); nurse midwife and family nurse practitioner (MS); nurse midwife and primary care pediatric nurse practitioner (MS); nursing (DNP, PhD, Post Master's Certificate); primary care family nurse practitioner (MS); primary care pediatric nurse practitioner (MS). *Accreditation:* AACN; ACNM/ACME (one or more programs are accredited). Part-time programs available. Postbaccalaureate distance learning degree programs offered (minimal on-campus study). Terminal master's awarded for partial completion of doctoral program. *Degree requirements:* For doctorate, thesis/dissertation. *Application deadline:* For fall admission, 2/1 for domestic students; for winter admission, 5/1 for domestic students; for spring admission, 11/1 for domestic students. Applications are processed on a rolling basis. Electronic applications accepted. Tuition and fees vary according to course level, course load, degree level, program and student level. *Financial support:* Fellowships with full and partial tuition reimbursements, research assistantships with full and partial tuition reimbursements, teaching assistantships with full tuition reimbursements, Federal Work-Study, institutionally sponsored loans, scholarships/grants, traineeships, and tuition waivers (partial) available. Support available to part-time students. *Faculty research:* Preparation of clinical nurse researchers, biobehavior, women's health, health promotion, substance abuse, psychobiology of menopause, fertility, obesity, health care systems. *Unit head:* Dr. Kathleen Potempa, Dean, 734-764-7185, Fax: 734-764-7186. *Application contact:* James Diesing, Graduate Recruiting and Admissions Coordinator, 734-615-4739, E-mail: sn-osams@umich.edu.
Website: http://www.nursing.umich.edu/

University of Pennsylvania, School of Nursing, Adult Acute Care Nurse Practitioner Program, Philadelphia, PA 19104. Offers acute care nurse practitioner (MSN). *Accreditation:* AACN. Part-time programs available. *Students:* 59 full-time (55 women), 124 part-time (110 women); includes 32 minority (11 Black or African American, non-Hispanic/Latino; 17 Asian, non-Hispanic/Latino; 1 Hispanic/Latino; 3 Two or more races, non-Hispanic/Latino), 5 international. 50 applicants, 54% accepted, 25 enrolled. In 2013, 69 master's awarded. *Entrance requirements:* For master's, GRE General Test, BSN, minimum GPA of 3.0, previous course work in statistics. *Application deadline:* For fall admission, 2/15 priority date for domestic students. Applications are processed on a rolling basis. Application fee: $70. *Expenses:* Contact institution. *Financial support:* Fellowships, research assistantships, teaching assistantships, Federal Work-Study, and institutionally sponsored loans available. Support available to part-time students. Financial award application deadline: 4/1. *Faculty research:* Post-injury disability, bereavement and attributions in fire survivors, stress in staff nurses. *Unit head:* Assistant Dean of Admissions and Financial Aid, 866-867-6877, Fax: 215-573-8439, E-mail: admissions@nursing.upenn.edu. *Application contact:* Deborah Becker, Program Director, 215-898-0432, E-mail: debecker@nursing.upenn.edu.
Website: http://www.nursing.upenn.edu/

University of Pennsylvania, School of Nursing, Pediatric Acute/Chronic Care Nurse Practitioner Program, Philadelphia, PA 19104. Offers MSN. *Accreditation:* AACN. Part-time programs available. Postbaccalaureate distance learning degree programs offered. *Students:* 17 full-time (16 women), 33 part-time (31 women); includes 8 minority (3 Black or African American, non-Hispanic/Latino; 3 Asian, non-Hispanic/Latino; 1 Hispanic/Latino; 1 Two or more races, non-Hispanic/Latino), 1 international. 16 applicants, 44% accepted, 6 enrolled. In 2013, 18 master's awarded. *Entrance requirements:* For master's, GRE General Test, 1 year of clinical course work, BSN, minimum GPA of 3.0, previous course work in statistics. Additional exam requirements/recommendations for international students: Required—TOEFL. *Application deadline:* For fall admission, 2/15 priority date for domestic students. Applications are processed on a rolling basis. Application fee: $70. *Expenses:* Contact institution. *Financial support:* Research assistantships, teaching assistantships, career-related internships or fieldwork, and institutionally sponsored loans available. Support available to part-time students. Financial award application deadline: 4/1. *Faculty research:* Hispanic health, bereavement, pediatric AIDS, chronically ill children and their families. *Unit head:* Assistant Dean of Admissions and Financial Aid, 866-867-6877, Fax: 215-573-8439, E-mail: admissions@nursing.upenn.edu. *Application contact:* Terri Lipman, Program Director, 215-898-4271, E-mail: lipman@nursing.upenn.edu.
Website: http://www.nursing.upenn.edu/academic_programs/grad/masters/program_detail.asp?prid-16

University of Pennsylvania, School of Nursing, Pediatric Critical Care Nurse Practitioner Program, Philadelphia, PA 19104. Offers MSN. *Accreditation:* AACN. *Students:* 1 (woman) full-time, 8 part-time (7 women); includes 1 minority (Black or African American, non-Hispanic/Latino), 1 international. 3 applicants, 33% accepted, 1 enrolled. In 2013, 9 master's awarded. *Entrance requirements:* For master's, GRE General Test, BSN, minimum GPA of 3.0, previous course work in statistics, 1 year of clinical course work. Additional exam requirements/recommendations for international students: Required—TOEFL. *Application deadline:* For fall admission, 2/15 priority date for domestic students. Applications are processed on a rolling basis. Application fee: $70. *Expenses:* Contact institution. *Financial support:* Application deadline: 4/1. *Unit head:* Assistant Dean of Admissions and Financial Aid, 866-867-6877, Fax: 215-573-8439, E-mail: admissions@nursing.upenn.edu. *Application contact:* Judy Verger, Senior Lecturer, 215-898-4271, E-mail: jtv@nursing.upenn.edu.
Website: http://www.nursing.upenn.edu/peds/

University of Pittsburgh, School of Nursing, Nurse Practitioner Program, Pittsburgh, PA 15261. Offers adult-gerontology acute care nurse practitioner (DNP); adult-gerontology primary care nurse practitioner (DNP); family (individual across the lifespan) nurse practitioner (DNP); neonatal nurse practitioner (MSN, DNP); pediatric primary care nurse practitioner (DNP); psychiatric mental health nurse practitioner (DNP). *Accreditation:* AACN. Part-time programs available. *Students:* 66 full-time (59 women), 84 part-time (75 women); includes 11 minority (5 Black or African American, non-Hispanic/Latino; 2 American Indian or Alaska Native, non-Hispanic/Latino; 3 Asian, non-Hispanic/Latino; 1 Hispanic/Latino), 2 international. Average age 31. 95 applicants, 74% accepted, 57 enrolled. In 2013, 53 master's, 4 doctorates awarded. *Degree requirements:* For master's, comprehensive exam, thesis optional. *Entrance requirements:* For master's, GRE General Test or MAT, BSN, RN license, letters of recommendation, resume, course work in statistics, 1-3 years of nursing experience; for doctorate, GRE General Test, BSN, RN license, minimum GPA of 3.5, 3 letters of recommendation. Additional exam requirements/recommendations for international students: Required—TOEFL (minimum score 550 paper-based; 80 iBT). *Application deadline:* Applications are processed on a rolling basis. Application fee: $50. Electronic applications accepted. *Expenses:* Tuition, state resident: full-time $19,964; part-time $807 per credit. Tuition, nonresident: full-time $32,686; part-time $1337 per credit. *Required fees:* $740; $200. Tuition and fees vary according to program. *Financial support:* In 2013–14, 18 students received support, including 4 fellowships with full and partial tuition reimbursements available (averaging $22,521 per year), 3 research assistantships with full and partial tuition reimbursements available (averaging $21,884 per year), 15 teaching assistantships with full and partial tuition reimbursements available (averaging $13,535 per year); scholarships/grants, traineeships, health care benefits, and unspecified assistantships also available. Support available to part-time students. *Unit head:* Dr. Sandra Engberg, Associate Dean for Clinical Education, 412-624-3835, Fax: 412-624-8521, E-mail: sje1@pitt.edu. *Application contact:* Laurie Lapsley, Administrator of Graduate Student Services, 412-624-9670, Fax: 412-624-2409, E-mail: lapsleyl@pitt.edu.
Website: http://www.nursing.pitt.edu

University of Puerto Rico, Medical Sciences Campus, School of Nursing, San Juan, PR 00936-5067. Offers adult and elderly nursing (MSN); child and adolescent nursing (MSN); critical care nursing (MSN); family and community nursing (MSN); family nurse practitioner (MSN); maternity nursing (MSN); mental health and psychiatric nursing (MSN). *Accreditation:* AACN. *Entrance requirements:* For master's, GRE or EXADEP, interview, Puerto Rico RN license or professional license for international students, general and specific point average, article analysis. Electronic applications accepted. *Faculty research:* HIV, health disparities, teen violence, women and violence, neurological disorders.

University of Rochester, School of Nursing, Rochester, NY 14642. Offers acute care nurse practitioner (MS); adult nurse practitioner (MS); adult/geriatric nurse practitioner (MS); clinical nurse leader (MS); clinical research coordinator (MS); family nurse practitioner (MS); family psychiatric mental health nurse practitioner (MS); health care organization management and leadership (MS); health practice research (PhD); nursing (DNP); pediatric nurse practitioner (MS); pediatric nurse practitioner/neonatal nurse practitioner (MS). *Accreditation:* AACN. Part-time programs available. Postbaccalaureate distance learning degree programs offered (minimal on-campus study). *Faculty:* 60 full-time (52 women), 61 part-time/adjunct (47 women). *Students:* 33 full-time (29 women), 213 part-time (195 women); includes 32 minority (8 Black or African American, non-Hispanic/Latino; 10 Asian, non-Hispanic/Latino; 8 Hispanic/Latino; 6 Two or more races, non-Hispanic/Latino), 4 international. Average age 34. 41 applicants, 54% accepted, 16 enrolled. In 2013, 58 master's, 11 doctorates awarded. Terminal master's awarded for partial completion of doctoral program. *Degree requirements:* For master's, comprehensive exam (for some programs); for doctorate, thesis/dissertation. *Entrance requirements:* For master's, BS in nursing, minimum GPA of 3.0, course work in statistics; for doctorate, GRE General Test, MS in nursing, minimum GPA of 3.5. Additional exam requirements/recommendations for international students: Required—TOEFL (minimum score 560 paper-based; 88 iBT) or IELTS (minimum score 6.5) recommended. *Application deadline:* For fall admission, 4/1 for domestic and international students; for spring admission, 9/1 for domestic and international students; for summer admission, 1/2 for domestic and international students. Application fee: $50. Electronic applications accepted. *Expenses: Tuition:* Full-time $44,580; part-time $1394 per credit hour. *Required fees:* $492. *Financial support:* In 2013–14, 41 students received support, including 2 fellowships with full and partial tuition reimbursements available (averaging $30,200 per year); scholarships/grants, traineeships, health care benefits, tuition waivers (partial), and unspecified assistantships also available. Support available to part-time students. Financial award application deadline: 6/30. *Faculty research:* Symptom assessment and self-management, illness prevention, nursing intervention research with vulnerable populations, palliative care, aging. *Total annual research expenditures:* $3.5 million. *Unit head:* Dr. Kathy H. Rideout, Dean, 585-273-8902, Fax: 585-273-1268, E-mail: kathy_rideout@urmc.rochester.edu. *Application contact:* Elaine Andolina, Director of Admissions, 585-275-2375, Fax: 585-756-8299, E-mail: elaine_andolina@urmc.rochester.edu.
Website: http://www.son.rochester.edu

University of South Africa, College of Human Sciences, Pretoria, South Africa. Offers adult education (M Ed); African languages (MA, PhD); African politics (MA, PhD); Afrikaans (MA, PhD); ancient history (MA, PhD); ancient Near Eastern studies (MA, PhD); anthropology (MA, PhD); applied linguistics (MA); Arabic (MA, PhD); archaeology (MA); art history (MA); Biblical archaeology (MA); Biblical studies (M Th, D Th, PhD); Christian spirituality (M Th, D Th); church history (M Th, D Th); classical studies (MA, PhD); clinical psychology (MA); communication (MA, PhD); comparative education (M Ed, Ed D); consulting psychology (D Admin, D Com, PhD); curriculum studies (M Ed, Ed D); development studies (M Admin, MA, D Admin, PhD); didactics (M Ed, Ed D); education (M Tech); education management (M Ed, Ed D); educational psychology (M Ed); English (MA); environmental education (M Ed); French (MA, PhD); German (MA, PhD); Greek (MA); guidance and counseling (M Ed); health studies (MA, PhD), including health sciences education (MA), health services management (MA), medical and surgical nursing science (critical care general) (MA), midwifery and neonatal nursing science (MA), trauma and emergency care (MA); history (MA, PhD); history of education (Ed D); inclusive education (M Ed, Ed D); information and communications technology policy and regulation (MA); information science (MA, MIS, PhD); international politics (MA, PhD); Islamic studies (MA, PhD); Italian (MA, PhD); Judaica (MA, PhD); linguistics (MA, PhD); mathematical education (M Ed); mathematics education (MA); missiology (M Th, D Th); modern Hebrew (MA, PhD); musicology (MA, MMus, D Mus, PhD); natural science education (M Ed); New Testament (M Th, D Th); Old Testament (D Th); pastoral therapy (M Th, D Th); philosophy (MA); philosophy of education (M Ed, Ed D); politics (MA, PhD); Portuguese (MA, PhD); practical theology (M Th, D Th); psychology (MA, MS, PhD); psychology of education (M Ed, Ed D); public health (MA); religious studies (MA, D Th, PhD); Romance languages (MA); Russian (MA, PhD); Semitic languages (MA, PhD); social behavior studies in HIV/AIDS (MA); social science (mental health) (MA); social science in development studies (MA); social science in psychology (MA); social science in social work (MA); social science in sociology (MA); social work (MSW, DSW, PhD); socio-education (M Ed, Ed D); sociolinguistics (MA); sociology (MA, PhD); Spanish (MA, PhD); systematic theology (M Th, D Th); TESOL (teaching English to speakers of other languages) (MA); theological ethics (M Th, D Th); theory of literature (MA, PhD); urban ministries (D Th); urban ministry (M Th).

University of South Carolina, The Graduate School, College of Nursing, Program in Advanced Practice Clinical Nursing, Columbia, SC 29208. Offers acute care nurse practitioner (Certificate); advanced practice clinical nursing (MSN). *Accreditation:* AACN. Part-time programs available. Postbaccalaureate distance learning degree programs offered (minimal on-campus study). *Entrance requirements:* For master's, master's degree in nursing, RN license; for Certificate, MSN. Additional exam requirements/recommendations for international students: Required—TOEFL (minimum score 570 paper-based). Electronic applications accepted. *Faculty research:* Systems research, evidence based practice, breast cancer, violence.

University of South Carolina, The Graduate School, College of Nursing, Program in Clinical Nursing, Columbia, SC 29208. Offers acute care clinical specialist (MSN); acute care nurse practitioner (MSN); women's health nurse practitioner (MSN). *Accreditation:* AACN. Part-time programs available. *Degree requirements:* For master's, thesis or alternative. *Entrance requirements:* For master's, GRE General Test or MAT, BS in nursing, RN licensure. Additional exam requirements/recommendations for international students: Required—TOEFL (minimum score 570 paper-based). Electronic applications accepted. *Faculty research:* Systems research, evidence based practice, breast cancer, violence.

University of South Florida, College of Nursing, Tampa, FL 33612. Offers adult gerontology acute care (DNP, PhD); adult gerontology acute care nursing (MS); adult gerontology primary care (DNP, PhD); adult gerontology primary care nursing (MS); adult gerontology primary care/occupational health nursing (MS); adult gerontology primary care/oncology nursing (MS, PhD); clinical nurse leader (MS); family health (DNP, PhD); family nurse practitioner (MS); nurse anesthesia (MS); nursing education (MS); nursing practice (DNP); nursing science (PhD), including nursing education; occupational health/adult-gerontology (DNP); oncology/adult-gerontology primary care (DNP); pediatric health (DNP, PhD); pediatric nurse practitioner (MS). *Accreditation:* AACN; AANA/CANAEP. Part-time programs available. *Faculty:* 46 full-time (40 women), 15 part-time/adjunct (11 women). *Students:* 177 full-time (150 women), 700 part-time (622 women); includes 272 minority (116 Black or African American, non-Hispanic/Latino; 2 American Indian or Alaska Native, non-Hispanic/Latino; 45 Asian, non-Hispanic/Latino; 93 Hispanic/Latino; 2 Native Hawaiian or other Pacific Islander, non-Hispanic/Latino; 14 Two or more races, non-Hispanic/Latino), 12 international. Average age 35. 656 applicants, 43% accepted, 224 enrolled. In 2013, 224 master's, 14 doctorates awarded. *Degree requirements:* For master's, comprehensive exam, thesis optional; for doctorate, comprehensive exam, thesis/dissertation. *Entrance requirements:* For master's, GRE General Test, bachelor's degree from accredited program with minimum GPA of 3.0 in all upper-division coursework; current license as Registered Nurse; 3 letters of recommendation; personal statement of goals; resume or curriculum vitae; personal interview; for doctorate, GRE General Test (recommended), bachelor's degree in nursing from a CCNA/NLNAC regionally-accredited institution with minimum GPA of 3.0 in all coursework or in all upper-division coursework; current license as Registered Nurse in Florida; undergraduate statistics course with minimum B grade; 3 letters of recommendation; statement of goals; resume; interview. Additional exam requirements/recommendations for international students: Required—TOEFL (minimum score 550 paper-based; 79 iBT). *Application deadline:* For fall admission, 2/15 for domestic students, 1/2 for international students; for spring admission, 10/1 for domestic students, 6/1 for international students. Application fee: $30. Electronic applications accepted. *Financial support:* In 2013–14, 36 students received support, including 7 research assistantships with tuition reimbursements available (averaging $18,935 per year), 29 teaching assistantships with tuition reimbursements available (averaging $30,814 per year); tuition waivers (partial) and unspecified assistantships also available. Financial award application deadline: 2/1; financial award applicants required to submit FAFSA. *Faculty research:* Women's health, palliative and end-of-life care, cardiac rehabilitation, complementary therapies for chronic illness and cancer. *Total annual research expenditures:* $3.4 million. *Unit head:* Dr. Dianne C. Morrison-Beedy, Dean and Professor, College of Nursing, 813-974-9091, Fax: 813-974-5418, E-mail: dmbeedy@health.usf.edu. *Application contact:* Dr. Connie Visovsky, Associate Professor and Associate Dean of Student Affairs, 813-396-9641, Fax: 813-974-5418, E-mail: cvisovsk@health.usf.edu.
Website: http://health.usf.edu/nursing/index.htm

The University of Texas Health Science Center at San Antonio, School of Nursing, San Antonio, TX 78229. Offers administrative management (MSN); adult-gerontology acute care nurse practitioner (PGC); clinical nurse leader (MSN); executive administrative management (DNP); family nurse practitioner (PGC); nurse practitioner (MSN), including adult-gerontology acute care nurse practitioner, family nurse practitioner, pediatric nurse practitioner primary care, psychiatric mental health nurse practitioner; nurse practitioner leadership (DNP); nursing (MSN, PhD); nursing education (MSN, PGC); pediatric nurse practitioner primary care (PGC); psychiatric mental health nurse practitioner (PGC); public health nurse leader (DNP). *Accreditation:* AACN. Part-time programs available. *Faculty:* 84 full-time (74 women), 42 part-time/adjunct (40 women). *Students:* 115 full-time (93 women), 140 part-time (123 women); includes 123 minority (24 Black or African American, non-Hispanic/Latino; 20 Asian, non-Hispanic/Latino; 74 Hispanic/Latino; 5 Two or more races, non-Hispanic/Latino), 7 international. Average age 37. 174 applicants, 59% accepted, 83 enrolled. In 2013, 67 master's, 6 doctorates, 5 other advanced degrees awarded. Terminal master's awarded for partial completion of doctoral program. *Degree requirements:* For master's, thesis optional; for doctorate, comprehensive exam, thesis/dissertation, final projects (for DNP). *Entrance requirements:* For master's, minimum GPA of 3.0, references, goal statement, BSN from accredited nursing school, RN licensure in Texas or compact state; for doctorate, GRE, MAT, minimum GPA of 3.0, personal interview, BSN and/or MSN from accredited nursing school, RN licensure in Texas or compact state, statistics course, references, curriculum vitae, goal statement; for PGC, minimum GPA of 3.0; references; goal statement; MSN from accredited nursing school; RN licensure in Texas or compact state; prerequisites in advanced health assessment, advanced pharmacotherapeutics, and advanced pathophysiology. Additional exam requirements/

recommendations for international students: Required—TOEFL (minimum score 550 paper-based; 68 iBT), IELTS (minimum score 6.5). *Application deadline:* For fall admission, 1/10 for domestic and international students; for spring admission, 7/1 for domestic students. Application fee: $65. Electronic applications accepted. *Financial support:* In 2013–14, 145 students received support, including 3 fellowships with full tuition reimbursements available (averaging $30,000 per year); institutionally sponsored loans and scholarships/grants also available. Financial award application deadline: 6/30; financial award applicants required to submit FAFSA. *Faculty research:* Pain, organizational structure, aging, quality and safety, health disparity, obesity and nutrition, women's and children's health. *Total annual research expenditures:* $500,265. *Unit head:* Dr. Eileen T. Breslin, Dean, 210-567-5800, Fax: 210-567-5929, E-mail: breslin@uthscsa.edu. *Application contact:* Brandy Finck, Interim Associate Dean for Admissions and Student Services, 210-567-5805, Fax: 210-567-6189, E-mail: finckb@uthscsa.edu.
Website: http://www.nursing.uthscsa.edu/

University of Virginia, School of Nursing, Charlottesville, VA 22903. Offers acute and specialty care (MSN); acute care nurse practitioner (MSN); clinical nurse leadership (MSN); community-public health leadership (MSN); nursing (DNP, PhD); psychiatric mental health counseling (MSN); MSN/MBA. *Accreditation:* AACN. Part-time programs available. *Faculty:* 45 full-time (41 women), 3 part-time/adjunct (all women). *Students:* 177 full-time (155 women), 147 part-time (133 women); includes 53 minority (27 Black or African American, non-Hispanic/Latino; 10 Asian, non-Hispanic/Latino; 11 Hispanic/Latino; 5 Two or more races, non-Hispanic/Latino), 4 international. Average age 36. 236 applicants, 61% accepted, 110 enrolled. In 2013, 94 master's, 14 doctorates awarded. *Degree requirements:* For doctorate, comprehensive exam (for some programs), capstone project (DNP), dissertation (PhD). *Entrance requirements:* For master's, GRE General Test, MAT; for doctorate, GRE General Test. Additional exam requirements/recommendations for international students: Required—TOEFL, IELTS. *Application deadline:* Applications are processed on a rolling basis. Application fee: $60. Electronic applications accepted. *Expenses:* Contact institution. *Financial support:* Fellowships, research assistantships, teaching assistantships, Federal Work-Study, and scholarships/grants available. Financial award applicants required to submit FAFSA. *Unit head:* Dorrie K. Fontaine, Dean, 434-924-0141, Fax: 434-982-1809, E-mail: dkf2u@virginia.edu. *Application contact:* Clay Hysell, Assistant Dean for Admissions and Financial Services, 434-924-0141, Fax: 434-982-1809, E-mail: nur-osa@virginia.edu.
Website: http://www.nursing.virginia.edu/

Vanderbilt University, Vanderbilt University School of Nursing, Nashville, TN 37240. Offers adult-gerontology acute care nurse practitioner (MSN), including hospitalist, intensivist; adult-gerontology primary care nurse practitioner (MSN); emergency nurse practitioner (MSN); family nurse practitioner (MSN); healthcare leadership (MSN); neonatal nurse practitioner (MSN); nurse midwifery (MSN); nurse midwifery/family nurse practitioner (MSN); nursing informatics (MSN); nursing practice (DNP); nursing science (PhD); pediatric acute care nurse practitioner (MSN); pediatric primary care nurse practitioner (MSN); psychiatric-mental health nurse practitioner (MSN); women's health nurse practitioner (MSN); women's health nurse practitioner/adult gerontology primary care nurse practitioner (MSN); MSN/M Div; MSN/MTS. *Accreditation:* ACNM/ACME (one or more programs are accredited). Part-time programs available. Postbaccalaureate distance learning degree programs offered (minimal on-campus study). *Faculty:* 139 full-time (124 women), 452 part-time/adjunct (319 women). *Students:* 527 full-time (463 women), 369 part-time (333 women); includes 120 minority (46 Black or African American, non-Hispanic/Latino; 8 American Indian or Alaska Native, non-Hispanic/Latino; 26 Asian, non-Hispanic/Latino; 24 Hispanic/Latino; 4 Native Hawaiian or other Pacific Islander, non-Hispanic/Latino; 12 Two or more races, non-Hispanic/Latino), 7 international. Average age 32. 1,257 applicants, 49% accepted, 457 enrolled. In 2013, 364 master's, 43 doctorates awarded. *Degree requirements:* For doctorate, comprehensive exam, thesis/dissertation. *Entrance requirements:* For master's, GRE General Test (within the past 5 years), minimum B average in undergraduate course work, 3 letters of recommendation; for doctorate, GRE General Test, interview, 3 letters of recommendation from doctorally-prepared faculty, MSN, essay. Additional exam requirements/recommendations for international students: Required—TOEFL (minimum score 570 paper-based), IELTS (minimum score 6.5). *Application deadline:* For fall admission, 12/1 priority date for domestic and international students. Applications are processed on a rolling basis. Application fee: $50. Electronic applications accepted. *Expenses:* Contact institution. *Financial support:* In 2013–14, 582 students received support. Scholarships/grants and health care benefits available. Support available to part-time students. Financial award application deadline: 3/15; financial award applicants required to submit FAFSA. *Faculty research:* Lymphedema, palliative care and bereavement, health services research including workforce, safety and quality of care, gerontology, better birth outcomes including nutrition. *Total annual research expenditures:* $2.5 million. *Unit head:* Dr. Linda Norman, Dean, 615-343-8876, Fax: 615-343-7711, E-mail: linda.norman@vanderbilt.edu. *Application contact:* Patricia Peerman, Assistant Dean for Enrollment Management, 615-322-3800, Fax: 615-343-0333, E-mail: vusn-admissions@vanderbilt.edu.
Website: http://www.nursing.vanderbilt.edu

Wayne State University, College of Nursing, Program in Advanced Practice Nursing with Women, Neonates and Children, Detroit, MI 48202. Offers neonatal nurse practitioner (MSN); nurse-midwife (MSN); pediatric nurse practitioner (MSN), including acute care, primary care; women's health nurse practitioner (MSN). *Accreditation:* AACN. Part-time programs available. *Students:* 59 full-time (53 women), 74 part-time (72 women); includes 17 minority (11 Black or African American, non-Hispanic/Latino; 2 Asian, non-Hispanic/Latino; 4 Hispanic/Latino), 6 international. Average age 32. 65 applicants, 55% accepted, 33 enrolled. In 2013, 40 degrees awarded. *Degree requirements:* For master's, thesis or alternative. *Entrance requirements:* For master's, minimum honor point average of 3.0 in upper-division course work; BA from NLN- or CCNE-accredited program; references; current RN license; personal statement. Additional exam requirements/recommendations for international students: Required—TOEFL (minimum score 550 paper-based; 79 iBT); Recommended—TWE (minimum score 6). *Application deadline:* For fall admission, 6/1 priority date for domestic students, 5/1 priority date for international students; for winter admission, 10/1 priority date for domestic students, 9/1 priority date for international students; for spring admission, 2/1 priority date for domestic students, 1/1 priority date for international students. Applications are processed on a rolling basis. Application fee: $50. Electronic applications accepted. *Expenses:* Contact institution. *Financial support:* In 2013–14, 17 students received support. Fellowships with tuition reimbursements available, research assistantships with tuition reimbursements available, teaching assistantships with tuition reimbursements available, scholarships/grants, and unspecified assistantships available. Financial award applicants required to submit FAFSA. *Faculty research:* Acculturation and parenting, domestic violence, evidence-based midwifery practice, pain in children, trauma and community violence. *Unit head:* Dr. Barbara Redman, Dean, 313-577-4070, Fax: 313-577-4571, E-mail: ae9080@wayne.edu. *Application contact:* Dr. Cynthia Redwine, Assistant Dean for the Office of Student Affairs, 313-577-4082, E-mail: nursinginfo@wayne.edu.
Website: http://nursing.wayne.edu/msn/specialty.php

Wright State University, School of Graduate Studies, College of Nursing and Health, Program in Nursing, Dayton, OH 45435. Offers acute care nurse practitioner (MS); administration of nursing and health care systems (MS); adult health (MS); child and adolescent health (MS); community health (MS); family nurse practitioner (MS); nurse practitioner (MS); school nurse (MS); MBA/MS. *Accreditation:* AACN. Part-time and evening/weekend programs available. *Degree requirements:* For master's, thesis or alternative. *Entrance requirements:* For master's, GRE General Test, BSN from NLN-accredited college, Ohio RN license. Additional exam requirements/recommendations for international students: Required—TOEFL. *Faculty research:* Clinical nursing and health, teaching, caring, pain administration, informatics and technology.

Adult Nursing

Adelphi University, College of Nursing and Public Health, Program in Adult/Geriatric Nurse Practitioner, Garden City, NY 11530-0701. Offers MS. *Students:* 88 part-time (82 women); includes 55 minority (27 Black or African American, non-Hispanic/Latino; 1 American Indian or Alaska Native, non-Hispanic/Latino; 19 Asian, non-Hispanic/Latino; 4 Hispanic/Latino; 1 Native Hawaiian or other Pacific Islander, non-Hispanic/Latino; 3 Two or more races, non-Hispanic/Latino). Average age 36. In 2013, 13 master's awarded. *Expenses: Tuition:* Full-time $32,530; part-time $1010 per credit. *Required fees:* $1150. Tuition and fees vary according to degree level and program. *Financial support:* Research assistantships, career-related internships or fieldwork, tuition waivers, and unspecified assistantships available. *Unit head:* Maryann Forbes, Chair, 516-877-3597, E-mail: forbes@adelphi.edu. *Application contact:* Christine Murphy, Director of Admissions, 516-877-3050, Fax: 516-877-3039, E-mail: graduateadmissions@adelphi.edu.

Allen College, Program in Nursing, Waterloo, IA 50703. Offers acute care nurse practitioner (MSN, Post-Master's Certificate); adult nurse practitioner (MSN, Post-Master's Certificate); adult psychiatric-mental health nurse practitioner (MSN, Post-Master's Certificate); community public health (MSN, Post-Master's Certificate); family nurse practitioner (MSN, Post-Master's Certificate); gerontological nurse practitioner (MSN, Post-Master's Certificate); health education (MSN); leadership in health care delivery (MSN, Post-Master's Certificate); nursing (DNP). Part-time programs available. Postbaccalaureate distance learning degree programs offered (minimal on-campus study). *Faculty:* 3 full-time (all women), 21 part-time/adjunct (20 women). *Students:* 21 full-time (19 women), 162 part-time (150 women); includes 5 minority (1 Black or African American, non-Hispanic/Latino; 2 Asian, non-Hispanic/Latino; 1 Hispanic/Latino; 1 Two or more races, non-Hispanic/Latino). Average age 34. 213 applicants, 57% accepted, 94 enrolled. In 2013, 41 master's, 4 other advanced degrees awarded. *Degree requirements:* For master's, thesis optional. *Entrance requirements:* For master's, minimum GPA of 3.0 in the last 60 hours of undergraduate coursework; for doctorate, minimum GPA of 3.25 in graduate coursework. Additional exam requirements/recommendations for international students: Recommended—TOEFL (minimum score 580 paper-based; 92 iBT), IELTS (minimum score 6). *Application deadline:* For fall admission, 2/1 priority date for domestic students; for spring admission, 9/1 priority date for domestic students. Applications are processed on a rolling basis. Application fee: $50. Electronic applications accepted. *Expenses: Tuition:* Full-time $14,534; part-time $755 per credit hour. *Required fees:* $935; $75 per credit hour. One-time fee: $275 part-time. Tuition and fees vary according to course load. *Financial support:* In 2013–14, 60 students received support. Institutionally sponsored loans, scholarships/grants, and traineeships available. Support available to part-time students. Financial award application deadline: 8/15; financial award applicants required to submit FAFSA. *Unit head:* Kendra Williams-Perez, Dean, School of Nursing, 319-226-2044, Fax: 319-226-2070, E-mail: kendra.williams-perez@allencollege.edu. *Application contact:* Molly Quinn, Admissions Counselor, 319-226-2001, Fax: 319-226-2010, E-mail: molly.quinn@allencollege.edu.
Website: http://www.allencollege.edu/

American University of Beirut, Graduate Programs, Rafic Hariri School of Nursing, Beirut, Lebanon. Offers adult care nursing (MSN); community and public health nursing (MSN); nursing administration (MSN); psychiatry mental health nursing (MSN). *Accreditation:* AACN. Part-time programs available. *Faculty:* 9 full-time (8 women), 12 part-time/adjunct (10 women). *Students:* 4 full-time (3 women), 56 part-time (44 women). Average age 29. 38 applicants, 87% accepted, 26 enrolled. In 2013, 17 master's awarded. *Degree requirements:* For master's, one foreign language, comprehensive exam, thesis optional. *Entrance requirements:* For master's, letter of recommendation. Additional exam requirements/recommendations for international students: Required—TOEFL (minimum score 600 paper-based); Recommended—IELTS. *Application deadline:* For fall admission, 4/1 for domestic and international students; for spring admission, 11/1 for domestic and international students. Applications are processed on a rolling basis. Application fee: $50. Electronic applications accepted. *Expenses: Tuition:* Full-time $14,724; part-time $818 per credit. *Required fees:* $692. Tuition and fees vary according to course load and program. *Financial support:* In 2013–14, 24 teaching assistantships with partial tuition reimbursements were awarded; unspecified assistantships also available. Financial award application deadline: 12/20. *Faculty research:* Pain management and palliative care, stress and post-traumatic stress disorder, health benefits and chronic illness, health promotion and community interventions. *Unit head:* Dr. Huda Huijer Abu-Saad, Director, 961-1374374 Ext. 5952, Fax: 961-1744476, E-mail: hh35@aub.edu.lb. *Application contact:* Dr. Salim Kanaan, Director, Admissions Office, 961-1-350000 Ext. 2594, Fax: 96-1-1750775, E-mail: sk00@aub.edu.lb.
Website: http://staff.aub.edu.lb/~webson

Angelo State University, College of Graduate Studies, College of Health and Human Services, Department of Nursing and Rehabilitation Sciences, San Angelo, TX 76909. Offers advanced practice registered nurse (MSN); nurse educator (MSN); registered nurse first assistant (MSN). Part-time and evening/weekend programs available. Postbaccalaureate distance learning degree programs offered (no on-campus study). *Degree requirements:* For master's, comprehensive exam. *Entrance requirements:* For master's, essay, three letters of recommendation. Additional exam requirements/

recommendations for international students: Required—TOEFL or IELTS. Electronic applications accepted.

Armstrong State University, School of Graduate Studies, Program in Nursing, Savannah, GA 31419-1997. Offers adult-gerontological acute care nurse practitioner (MSN); adult-gerontological clinical nurse specialist (MSN); adult-gerontological primary care nurse practitioner (MSN). *Accreditation:* AACN. Part-time and evening/weekend programs available. *Faculty:* 10 full-time (all women), 1 (woman) part-time/adjunct. *Students:* 24 full-time (21 women), 17 part-time (16 women); includes 5 minority (2 Black or African American, non-Hispanic/Latino; 1 Hispanic/Latino; 2 Two or more races, non-Hispanic/Latino). Average age 34. 17 applicants, 65% accepted, 10 enrolled. In 2013, 13 master's awarded. *Degree requirements:* For master's, comprehensive exam, project or thesis. *Entrance requirements:* For master's, GRE General Test or MAT, minimum GPA of 3.0, letter of recommendation, letter of intent. Additional exam requirements/recommendations for international students: Required—TOEFL (minimum score 523 paper-based; 70 iBT). *Application deadline:* For fall admission, 2/28 for domestic and international students; for spring admission, 11/15 for domestic students, 9/15 for international students. Applications are processed on a rolling basis. Application fee: $30. Electronic applications accepted. *Expenses:* Tuition, state resident: part-time $201 per credit hour. Tuition, nonresident: part-time $745 per credit hour. *Required fees:* $310 per semester. Tuition and fees vary according to course load, campus/location and program. *Financial support:* In 2013–14, research assistantships with full tuition reimbursements (averaging $5,000 per year) were awarded; Federal Work-Study, scholarships/grants, and unspecified assistantships also available. Support available to part-time students. Financial award application deadline: 3/1; financial award applicants required to submit FAFSA. *Faculty research:* Midwifery, mental health, nursing simulation, smoking cessation during pregnancy, asthma education, vulnerable populations, geriatrics, disaster nursing, complementary and alternative modalities, nephrology. *Unit head:* Dr. Catherine Gilbert, Department Head, 912-344-3145, E-mail: catherine.gilbert@armstrong.edu. *Application contact:* Jill Bell, Director/Graduate Enrollment Coordinator, 912-344-2798, Fax: 912-344-3488, E-mail: graduate@armstrong.edu.
Website: http://www.armstrong.edu/Health_professions/nursing/nursing_graduate_programs

Bloomsburg University of Pennsylvania, School of Graduate Studies, College of Science and Technology, Department of Nursing, Bloomsburg, PA 17815. Offers adult and family nurse practitioner (MSN); community health (MSN); nurse anesthesia (MSN); nursing (MSN); nursing administration (MSN). *Accreditation:* AACN; AANA/CANAEP. *Faculty:* 5 full-time (all women), 7 part-time/adjunct (all women). *Students:* 62 full-time (52 women), 26 part-time (17 women); includes 8 minority (6 Black or African American, non-Hispanic/Latino; 1 Asian, non-Hispanic/Latino; 1 Hispanic/Latino). Average age 35. 61 applicants, 84% accepted, 14 enrolled. In 2013, 36 master's awarded. *Degree requirements:* For master's, thesis (for some programs), clinical experience. *Entrance requirements:* For master's, minimum QPA of 3.0, personal statement, 2 letters of recommendation, nursing license. Additional exam requirements/recommendations for international students: Required—TOEFL. *Application deadline:* For fall admission, 1/1 for domestic students; for spring admission, 8/1 for domestic students. Applications are processed on a rolling basis. Application fee: $35 ($60 for international students). Electronic applications accepted. *Expenses:* Tuition, state resident: full-time $7956; part-time $442 per credit. Tuition, nonresident: full-time $11,934; part-time $663 per credit. *Required fees:* $95.50 per credit. $55 per semester. Tuition and fees vary according to course load. *Financial support:* Unspecified assistantships available. *Unit head:* Dr. Noreen Chikotas, Coordinator, 570-389-4609, Fax: 570-389-5008, E-mail: nchikota@bloomu.edu. *Application contact:* Jennifer Richard, Administrative Assistant, 570-389-4015, Fax: 570-389-3054, E-mail: jrichard@bloomu.edu.
Website: http://www.bloomu.edu/nursing

Boston College, William F. Connell School of Nursing, Chestnut Hill, MA 02467-3800. Offers adult-gerontology nursing (MS); community health nursing (MS); family health (MS); forensic nursing (MS); maternal/child health nursing (MS), including pediatric and women's health; nurse anesthesia (MS); nursing (PhD); palliative care (MS), including adult and pediatric; psychiatric-mental health nursing (MS); MBA/MS; MS/MA; MS/PhD. *Accreditation:* AACN; AANA/CANAEP (one or more programs are accredited). Part-time programs available. *Faculty:* 47 full-time (43 women), 42 part-time/adjunct (39 women). *Students:* 199 full-time (180 women), 79 part-time (73 women); includes 44 minority (14 Black or African American, non-Hispanic/Latino; 1 American Indian or Alaska Native, non-Hispanic/Latino; 13 Asian, non-Hispanic/Latino; 12 Hispanic/Latino; 4 Two or more races, non-Hispanic/Latino), 7 international. Average age 31. 502 applicants, 39% accepted, 87 enrolled. In 2013, 105 master's, 8 doctorates awarded. *Degree requirements:* For master's, comprehensive exam, research project; for doctorate, comprehensive exam, thesis/dissertation, computer literacy exam or foreign language. *Entrance requirements:* For master's, bachelor's degree in nursing; for doctorate, GRE General Test, MS in nursing. Additional exam requirements/recommendations for international students: Required—TOEFL (minimum score 600 paper-based; 100 iBT). *Application deadline:* For fall admission, 9/30 for domestic and international students; for winter admission, 1/15 for domestic and international students; for spring admission, 3/15 for domestic and international students. Applications are processed on a rolling basis. Application fee: $40. Electronic applications accepted. *Financial support:* In 2013–14, 174 students received support, including 7 fellowships with full tuition reimbursements available (averaging $20,000 per year), 21 teaching assistantships (averaging $4,800 per year); research assistantships, scholarships/grants, health care benefits, tuition waivers (partial), and unspecified assistantships also available. Support available to part-time students. Financial award application deadline: 3/1; financial award applicants required to submit FAFSA. *Faculty research:* Sexual and reproductive health, health promotion/illness prevention, eating disorders, violence, symptom management. *Total annual research expenditures:* $1.1 million. *Unit head:* Dr. Susan Gennaro, Dean, 617-552-4251, Fax: 617-552-0931, E-mail: susan.gennaro@bc.edu. *Application contact:* MaryBeth Crowley, Graduate Programs Assistant, 617-552-4928, Fax: 617-552-2121, E-mail: csongrad@bc.edu.
Website: http://www.bc.edu/schools/son/

California Baptist University, Program in Nursing, Riverside, CA 92504-3206. Offers clinical nurse specialist (MSN); family nurse practitioner (MSN); healthcare systems management (MSN); nursing (MSN); teaching-learning (MSN). Part-time programs available. *Faculty:* 15 full-time (all women), 7 part-time/adjunct (all women). *Students:* 49 full-time (41 women), 69 part-time (55 women); includes 61 minority (18 Black or African American, non-Hispanic/Latino; 1 American Indian or Alaska Native, non-Hispanic/Latino; 17 Asian, non-Hispanic/Latino; 22 Hispanic/Latino; 3 Two or more races, non-Hispanic/Latino). Average age 33. 48 applicants, 65% accepted, 20 enrolled. In 2013, 9 master's awarded. *Degree requirements:* For master's, comprehensive exam (for some programs), thesis or alternative, comprehensive exam or directed project thesis; capstone practicum. *Entrance requirements:* For master's, GRE or California Critical Thinking Skills Test; Test of Essential Academic Skills (TEAS), minimum undergraduate GPA of 3.25; Microsoft Office competency; health clearance; health insurance; CPR certification; vehicle insurance; random drug testing; background check clearance; passport photo; three recommendations; comprehensive essay; interview. Additional exam requirements/recommendations for international students: Required—TOEFL (minimum score 80 iBT). *Application deadline:* For fall admission, 8/1 priority date for domestic students, 7/1 for international students; for spring admission, 12/1 priority date for domestic students, 11/1 for international students. Applications are processed on a rolling basis. Application fee: $45. Electronic applications accepted. *Expenses: Tuition:* Full-time $10,080; part-time $560 per unit. *Required fees:* $175 per semester. One-time fee: $45. Tuition and fees vary according to course load and program. *Financial support:* Institutionally sponsored loans available. Financial award applicants required to submit CSS PROFILE or FAFSA. *Faculty research:* Qualitative research using Parse methodology, gerontology, disaster preparedness, medical-surgical nursing, maternal-child nursing. *Unit head:* Dr. Geneva Oaks, Dean, School of Nursing, 951-343-4702, E-mail: goaks@calbaptist.edu. *Application contact:* Dr. Rebecca Meyer, Director, Graduate Program in Nursing, 951-343-4952, Fax: 951-343-5095, E-mail: rmeyer@calbaptist.edu.
Website: http://www.calbaptist.edu/explore-cbu/schools-colleges/school-nursing/master-science-nursing/

Clarkson College, Master of Science in Nursing Program, Omaha, NE 68131. Offers adult nurse practitioner (MSN, Post-Master's Certificate); family nurse practitioner (MSN, Post-Master's Certificate); nursing education (MSN, Post-Master's Certificate); nursing health care leadership (MSN, Post-Master's Certificate). *Accreditation:* AANA/CANAEP. Part-time and evening/weekend programs available. Postbaccalaureate distance learning degree programs offered (minimal on-campus study). *Degree requirements:* For master's, on-campus skills assessment (family nurse practitioner, adult nurse practitioner), comprehensive exam or thesis. *Entrance requirements:* For master's, minimum GPA of 3.0, 2 references, resume. Additional exam requirements/recommendations for international students: Required—TOEFL (minimum score 600 paper-based; 100 iBT). Electronic applications accepted.

College of Mount Saint Vincent, School of Professional and Continuing Studies, Department of Nursing, Riverdale, NY 10471-1093. Offers adult nurse practitioner (MSN, PMC); family nurse practitioner (MSN, PMC); nurse educator (PMC); nursing administration (MSN); nursing for the adult and aged (MSN). *Accreditation:* AACN. Part-time programs available. *Entrance requirements:* For master's, BSN, interview, RN license, minimum GPA of 3.0, letters of reference. Additional exam requirements/recommendations for international students: Required—TOEFL. *Expenses:* Contact institution.

College of Staten Island of the City University of New York, Graduate Programs, Department of Nursing, Program in Adult Health Nursing, Staten Island, NY 10314-6600. Offers MS, Post-Master's Certificate. Part-time and evening/weekend programs available. *Faculty:* 3 full-time (all women), 5 part-time/adjunct (4 women). *Students:* 68 part-time (60 women). Average age 40. 40 applicants, 55% accepted, 14 enrolled. In 2013, 10 master's, 4 other advanced degrees awarded. *Degree requirements:* For master's, thesis optional; for Post-Master's Certificate, 12-21 credits with minimum of 500 supervised hours. *Entrance requirements:* For master's, bachelor's degree in nursing with minimum GPA of 3.0 in nursing major; 2 letters of recommendation; personal statement; current New York State RN license; minimum of one year of full-time experience or its equivalent as a registered nurse; for Post-Master's Certificate, master's degree in nursing; master's-level courses in pathophysiology, health assessment and pharmacology. Additional exam requirements/recommendations for international students: Required—TOEFL (minimum score 550 paper-based; 79 iBT), IELTS (minimum score 6.5). *Application deadline:* For fall admission, 5/1 priority date for domestic and international students; for spring admission, 12/2 priority date for domestic and international students. Applications are processed on a rolling basis. Application fee: $125. Electronic applications accepted. *Expenses:* Tuition, state resident: full-time $9240; part-time $385 per credit hour. Tuition, nonresident: full-time $17,040; part-time $710 per credit hour. *Required fees:* $428; $128 per term. *Financial support:* Career-related internships or fieldwork, Federal Work-Study, and scholarships/grants available. Support available to part-time students. Financial award applicants required to submit FAFSA. *Unit head:* Dr. June Como, Graduate Program Coordinator, 718-982-3818, Fax: 718-982-3813, E-mail: june.como@csi.cuny.edu. *Application contact:* Sasha Spence, Assistant Director for Graduate Admissions, 718-982-2019, Fax: 718-982-2500, E-mail: sasha.spence@.csi.cuny.edu.
Website: http://www.csi.cuny.edu/catalog/graduate/graduate-programs-in-nursing.htm

Columbia University, School of Nursing, Program in Adult-Gerontology Primary Care Nurse Practitioner, New York, NY 10032. Offers MS, Adv C. *Accreditation:* AACN. Part-time programs available. *Entrance requirements:* For master's, GRE General Test, NCLEX, BSN, 1 year of clinical experience (preferred); for Adv C, MSN. Additional exam requirements/recommendations for international students: Required—TOEFL (minimum score 100 iBT). Electronic applications accepted.

Daemen College, Department of Nursing, Amherst, NY 14226-3592. Offers adult nurse practitioner (MS, Post Master's Certificate); nurse executive leadership (Post Master's Certificate); nursing education (MS, Post Master's Certificate); nursing executive leadership (MS); nursing practice (DNP); palliative care nursing (Post Master's Certificate). Part-time programs available. *Degree requirements:* For master's, thesis or alternative, degree completed in 4 years; minimum GPA of 3.0; for doctorate, degree completed in 5 years; 500 post-master's clinical hours. *Entrance requirements:* For master's, BN, 1 year medical/surgical experience, RN license and state registration, statistics course with minimum C grade, 3 letters of recommendation, minimum GPA of 3.25, interview; for doctorate, MS in advance nursing practice; New York state RN license; goal statement; resume; interview; statistics course with minimum grade of 'C'; for Post Master's Certificate, master's degree in clinical area; RN license and current registration; one year of clinical experience; statistics course with minimum grade of 'C'; 3 letters of recommendation; interview; letter of intent. Additional exam requirements/recommendations for international students: Required—TOEFL (minimum score 500 paper-based; 63 iBT), IELTS (minimum score 5.5). Electronic applications accepted. *Faculty research:* Professional stress, client behavior, drug therapy, treatment modalities and pulmonary cancers, chemical dependency.

DeSales University, Graduate Division, Division of Healthcare and Natural Sciences, Center Valley, PA 18034-9568. Offers adult clinical nurse specialist (MSN); certified nurse midwives (MSN); certified nurse practitioners (MSN); clinical leadership (DNP); family nurse practitioner (MSN); information systems (MSIS); nurse educator (MSN); nurse practitioner (Post-Master's Certificate); physical therapy (DPT); physician assistant studies (MSPAS); MSN/MBA. Part-time programs available. In 2013, 5 doctorates awarded. *Degree requirements:* For master's, thesis optional. *Entrance requirements:* For master's, GRE General Test, MAT, minimum B average in undergraduate course work, health assessment course or equivalent, course work in statistics. Additional exam requirements/recommendations for international students: Required—TOEFL. *Application deadline:* Applications are processed on a rolling basis. Application fee: $35. Electronic applications accepted. *Expenses: Tuition:* Part-time $790 per credit. *Financial support:* Applicants required to submit FAFSA. *Unit head:* Dr. Mary Liz Doyle-Tadduni, Department Chair, Nursing, 610-282-1100 Ext. 1394, Fax: 610-282-2091, E-mail: carol.mest@desales.edu. *Application contact:* Abagail Wernicki, Director of Graduate Admissions, 610-282-1100 Ext. 1768, Fax: 610-282-2869, E-mail: abagail.wernicki@desales.edu.

Adult Nursing

Duke University, School of Nursing, Durham, NC 27708-0586. Offers acute care pediatric nurse practitioner (MSN); adult-gerontology nurse practitioner - acute care (MSN, Post Master's Certificate); adult-gerontology nurse practitioner - primary care (MSN, Post Master's Certificate), including adult-gerontology nurse practitioner (MSN), cardiology, oncology; family nurse practitioner (MSN); neonatal nurse practitioner (MSN); nurse anesthesia (MSN, DNP); nursing (PhD); nursing and health care leadership (MSN); nursing education (MSN); nursing informatics (MSN, Post Master's Certificate); pediatric nurse practitioner - primary care (MSN). *Accreditation:* AACN; AANA/CANAEP. Part-time and evening/weekend programs available. Postbaccalaureate distance learning degree programs offered (minimal on-campus study). *Faculty:* 74 full-time (64 women), 7 part-time/adjunct (4 women). *Students:* 127 full-time (113 women), 473 part-time (433 women); includes 131 minority (54 Black or African American, non-Hispanic/Latino; 9 American Indian or Alaska Native, non-Hispanic/Latino; 36 Asian, non-Hispanic/Latino; 27 Hispanic/Latino; 5 Native Hawaiian or other Pacific Islander, non-Hispanic/Latino), 14 international. Average age 34. 516 applicants, 50% accepted, 190 enrolled. In 2013, 179 master's, 49 doctorates, 23 other advanced degrees awarded. Terminal master's awarded for partial completion of doctoral program. *Degree requirements:* For master's, thesis optional; for doctorate, capstone project. *Entrance requirements:* For master's, GRE General Test (waived if undergraduate GPA of 3.4 or higher), 1 year of nursing experience (recommended), BSN, minimum GPA of 3.0, previous course work in statistics; for doctorate, GRE General Test (waived if undergraduate GPA of 3.4 or higher), BSN or MSN, minimum GPA of 3.0, portfolio, resume, personal statement, undergraduate statistics course, current licensure as a registered nurse, transcripts from all post-secondary institutions; for Post Master's Certificate, MSN, licensure or eligibility as a professional nurse, transcripts from all post-secondary institutions, previous course work in statistics. Additional exam requirements/recommendations for international students: Recommended—TOEFL (minimum score 550 paper-based; 83 iBT), IELTS (minimum score 7). *Application deadline:* For fall admission, 12/1 for domestic and international students; for spring admission, 5/1 for domestic and international students. Application fee: $50. Electronic applications accepted. *Expenses:* Contact institution. *Financial support:* Career-related internships or fieldwork, institutionally sponsored loans, scholarships/grants, traineeships, and tuition waivers (partial) available. Support available to part-time students. Financial award applicants required to submit FAFSA. *Faculty research:* Cardiovascular disease, caregiver skill training, data mining, prostate cancer, neonatal immune system. *Unit head:* Dr. Catherine L. Gilliss, Dean/Vice Chancellor for Nursing Affairs, 919-684-9444, Fax: 919-684-9414, E-mail: catherine.gilliss@duke.edu. *Application contact:* Ernie Rushing, Lead Admissions Processor/Admissions Officer, 919-668-6274, Fax: 919-668-4693, E-mail: stephen.rushing@dm.duke.edu.
Website: http://www.nursing.duke.edu/

Eastern Michigan University, Graduate School, College of Health and Human Services, School of Nursing, Ypsilanti, MI 48197. Offers nursing (MSN); quality improvement in health care systems (Graduate Certificate); teaching in health care systems (MSN, Graduate Certificate). *Accreditation:* AACN. Part-time and evening/weekend programs available. Postbaccalaureate distance learning degree programs offered (minimal on-campus study). *Faculty:* 23 full-time (21 women). *Students:* 3 full-time (all women), 32 part-time (26 women); includes 11 minority (6 Black or African American, non-Hispanic/Latino; 3 Asian, non-Hispanic/Latino; 2 Hispanic/Latino), 1 international. Average age 47. 31 applicants, 55% accepted, 10 enrolled. In 2013, 8 master's, 2 other advanced degrees awarded. *Degree requirements:* For master's, thesis optional. *Entrance requirements:* For master's, GRE General Test, Michigan RN license. Additional exam requirements/recommendations for international students: Required—TOEFL. *Application deadline:* Applications are processed on a rolling basis. Application fee: $35. *Expenses:* Tuition, state resident: full-time $12,300; part-time $466 per credit hour. Tuition, nonresident: full-time $23,159; part-time $918 per credit hour. *Required fees:* $71 per credit hour. $46 per semester. One-time fee: $100. Tuition and fees vary according to course level and degree level. *Financial support:* Fellowships, research assistantships with full tuition reimbursements, teaching assistantships with full tuition reimbursements, career-related internships or fieldwork, Federal Work-Study, institutionally sponsored loans, scholarships/grants, tuition waivers (partial), and unspecified assistantships available. Support available to part-time students. Financial award applicants required to submit FAFSA. *Unit head:* Dr. Michael Williams, Interim Director, 734-487-2310, Fax: 734-487-6946, E-mail: mwilliams@emich.edu. *Application contact:* Roberta Towns, Coordinator, School of Nursing, 734-487-2340, Fax: 734-487-6946, E-mail: rtowne1@emich.edu.
Website: http://www.emich.edu/nursing

Emory University, Nell Hodgson Woodruff School of Nursing, Atlanta, GA 30322-1100. Offers adult nurse practitioner (MSN); emergency nurse practitioner (MSN); family nurse practitioner (MSN); family nurse-midwife (MSN); health systems leadership (MSN); nurse-midwifery (MSN); pediatric nurse practitioner acute and primary care (MSN); women's health care (Title X) (MSN); women's health nurse practitioner (MSN); MSN/MPH. *Accreditation:* AACN; ACNM/ACME (one or more programs are accredited). Part-time programs available. *Entrance requirements:* For master's, GRE General Test or MAT, minimum GPA of 3.0, BS in nursing from an accredited institution, RN license and additional course work, 3 letters of recommendation. Additional exam requirements/recommendations for international students: Required—TOEFL (minimum score 600 paper-based; 100 iBT). Electronic applications accepted. *Expenses:* Contact institution. *Faculty research:* Older adult falls and injuries, minority health issues, cardiac symptoms and quality of life, bio-ethics and decision-making, menopausal issues.

Felician College, Program in Nursing, Lodi, NJ 07644-2117. Offers adult-gerontology nurse practitioner (MSN, PMC); executive leadership (MSN, PMC); family nurse practitioner (MSN, PMC); nursing education (MSN, PMC). *Accreditation:* AACN. Part-time and evening/weekend programs available. Postbaccalaureate distance learning degree programs offered (no on-campus study). *Students:* 5 full-time (4 women), 85 part-time (78 women); includes 50 minority (20 Black or African American, non-Hispanic/Latino; 14 Asian, non-Hispanic/Latino; 16 Hispanic/Latino). Average age 42. *Degree requirements:* For master's, scholarly project. *Entrance requirements:* For master's, BS in nursing or equivalent, minimum GPA of 3.0, 2 letters of recommendation, RN license; for PMC, RN license, minimum GPA of 2.75. Additional exam requirements/recommendations for international students: Recommended—TOEFL (minimum score 550 paper-based). *Application deadline:* Applications are processed on a rolling basis. Application fee: $40. *Expenses: Tuition:* Part-time $945 per credit. *Required fees:* $317.50 per semester. *Financial support:* In 2013–14, 10 students received support. Traineeships available. Financial award applicants required to submit FAFSA. *Faculty research:* Anxiety and fear, curriculum innovation, health promotion. *Unit head:* Dr. Muriel Shore, Dean, Division of Health Sciences, 201-559-6030, E-mail: shorem@felician.edu. *Application contact:* Elizabeth Barca, Senior Assistant Director, Graduate Admissions, 201-559-6077, Fax: 201-559-6138, E-mail: graduate@felician.edu.

Florida Atlantic University, Christine E. Lynn College of Nursing, Boca Raton, FL 33431-0991. Offers administrative and financial leadership in nursing and health care (Post Master's Certificate); adult/gerontological nurse practitioner (Post Master's Certificate); advanced holistic nursing (MS, Post Master's Certificate); clinical nurse leader (MS, Post Master's Certificate); family nurse practitioner (MS, Post Master's Certificate); nurse educator (MS, Post Master's Certificate); nursing (PhD); nursing administration and financial leadership (MS); nursing practice (DNP). *Accreditation:* AACN. Part-time programs available. *Faculty:* 30 full-time (27 women), 9 part-time/adjunct (8 women). *Students:* 29 full-time (27 women), 523 part-time (492 women); includes 254 minority (157 Black or African American, non-Hispanic/Latino; 2 American Indian or Alaska Native, non-Hispanic/Latino; 19 Asian, non-Hispanic/Latino; 62 Hispanic/Latino; 2 Native Hawaiian or other Pacific Islander, non-Hispanic/Latino; 12 Two or more races, non-Hispanic/Latino), 3 international. Average age 39. 463 applicants, 25% accepted, 111 enrolled. In 2013, 148 master's, 15 doctorates awarded. *Degree requirements:* For master's, thesis or alternative; for doctorate, comprehensive exam, thesis/dissertation. *Entrance requirements:* For master's, GRE General Test or MAT, bachelor's degree in nursing, Florida RN license, minimum GPA of 3.0, resume/curriculum vitae, letter of recommendation; for doctorate, GRE General Test or MAT, curriculum vitae, Florida RN license, minimum GPA of 3.5, master's degree in nursing, three letters of recommendation. *Application deadline:* For fall admission, 6/1 for domestic students, 2/15 for international students; for spring admission, 10/1 for domestic students, 7/15 for international students. Applications are processed on a rolling basis. Application fee: $30. *Expenses:* Tuition, state resident: full-time $6660; part-time $370 per credit hour. Tuition, nonresident: full-time $18,450; part-time $1025 per credit hour. Tuition and fees vary according to course load. *Financial support:* Research assistantships with partial tuition reimbursements, teaching assistantships with partial tuition reimbursements, career-related internships or fieldwork, Federal Work-Study, institutionally sponsored loans, scholarships/grants, and traineeships available. Support available to part-time students. *Faculty research:* Econometrics of nurse-patient relationship, Alzheimer's disease, community-based programs, falls, self-healing. *Unit head:* Dr. Marlaine Smith, Dean, 561-297-3206, Fax: 561-297-3687, E-mail: msmit230@fau.edu. *Application contact:* Carol Kruse, Graduate Coordinator, 561-297-3261, Fax: 561-297-0088, E-mail: ckruse@fau.edu.
Website: http://nursing.fau.edu/

Florida Southern College, Program in Nursing, Lakeland, FL 33801-5698. Offers adult gerontology clinical nurse specialist (MSN); adult gerontology primary care nurse practitioner (MSN); nurse educator (MSN); nursing administration (MSN). *Accreditation:* AACN. Part-time and evening/weekend programs available. *Entrance requirements:* For master's, Florida RN license, 3 letters of recommendation, personal statement, minimum GPA of 3.0, resume. Additional exam requirements/recommendations for international students: Required—TOEFL (minimum score 550 paper-based). *Expenses:* Contact institution. *Faculty research:* End of life care, dementia, health promotion.

The George Washington University, School of Nursing, Washington, DC 20052. Offers adult nurse practitioner (MSN, Post-Master's Certificate); clinical research administration (MSN); family nurse practitioner (MSN, Post-Master's Certificate); health care quality (MSN, Post-Master's Certificate); nursing (DNP); nursing leadership and management (MSN); palliative care nurse practitioner (Post-Master's Certificate). *Accreditation:* AACN. *Faculty:* 37 full-time (all women). *Students:* 36 full-time (33 women), 438 part-time (405 women); includes 114 minority (59 Black or African American, non-Hispanic/Latino; 7 American Indian or Alaska Native, non-Hispanic/Latino; 32 Asian, non-Hispanic/Latino; 15 Hispanic/Latino; 1 Two or more races, non-Hispanic/Latino), 8 international. Average age 38. 360 applicants, 83% accepted, 178 enrolled. In 2013, 79 master's, 26 doctorates awarded. *Unit head:* Jean E. Johnson, Dean, 202-994-3725, E-mail: sonjej@gwumc.edu. *Application contact:* Kristin Williams, Assistant Vice President for Graduate and Special Enrollment Management, 202-994-0467, Fax: 202-994-0371, E-mail: ksw@gwu.edu.
Website: http://nursing.gwumc.edu/

Georgia State University, Byrdine F. Lewis School of Nursing, Atlanta, GA 30303. Offers adult health clinical nurse specialist/nurse practitioner (MS, Certificate); child health clinical nurse specialist/pediatric nurse practitioner (MS, Certificate); family nurse practitioner (MS, Certificate); family psychiatric mental health nurse practitioner (MS, Certificate); nursing (PhD); nursing leadership in healthcare innovations (MS), including nursing administration, nursing informatics; nutrition (MS); perinatal clinical nurse specialist/women's health nurse practitioner (MS, Certificate); physical therapy (DPT); respiratory therapy (MS). *Accreditation:* AACN. Part-time programs available. Postbaccalaureate distance learning degree programs offered (minimal on-campus study). *Faculty:* 22 full-time (16 women). *Students:* 241 full-time (180 women), 262 part-time (236 women); includes 176 minority (120 Black or African American, non-Hispanic/Latino; 31 Asian, non-Hispanic/Latino; 13 Hispanic/Latino; 3 Native Hawaiian or other Pacific Islander, non-Hispanic/Latino; 9 Two or more races, non-Hispanic/Latino), 19 international. Average age 34. 583 applicants, 34% accepted, 160 enrolled. In 2013, 110 master's, 44 doctorates, 6 other advanced degrees awarded. *Degree requirements:* For doctorate, comprehensive exam, thesis/dissertation. *Entrance requirements:* For doctorate, GRE. Additional exam requirements/recommendations for international students: Required—TOEFL. *Application deadline:* For fall admission, 2/1 priority date for domestic and international students; for spring admission, 9/15 for domestic and international students. Applications are processed on a rolling basis. Application fee: $50. Electronic applications accepted. *Expenses:* Contact institution. *Financial support:* In 2013–14, research assistantships with full and partial tuition reimbursements (averaging $1,666 per year), teaching assistantships with full and partial tuition reimbursements (averaging $1,920 per year) were awarded; scholarships/grants, tuition waivers (full and partial), and unspecified assistantships also available. Support available to part-time students. Financial award application deadline: 8/1; financial award applicants required to submit FAFSA. *Faculty research:* Stroke intervention for caregivers, stroke prevention in African Americans; relationships between psychological distress and health outcomes in parents with a medically ill infant; medically fragile children; nursing expertise and patient outcomes. *Unit head:* Joan S. Cranford, Assistant Dean for Nursing, 404-413-1200, Fax: 404-413-1205, E-mail: jcranford2@gsu.edu. *Application contact:* Tiffany Norman, Senior Administrative Coordinator, 404-413-1190, Fax: 404-413-1205, E-mail: tnorman7@gsu.edu.
Website: http://nursing.gsu.edu/

Goldfarb School of Nursing at Barnes-Jewish College, Graduate Programs, St. Louis, MO 63110. Offers adult acute care nurse practitioner (MSN); adult nurse practitioner (MSN); nurse anesthesia (MSN); nurse educator (MSN); nurse executive (MSN); DNP/PhD. *Accreditation:* AACN; AANA/CANAEP. Part-time and evening/weekend programs available. Postbaccalaureate distance learning degree programs offered (minimal on-campus study). *Faculty:* 42 full-time (39 women), 6 part-time/adjunct (all women). *Students:* 81 full-time (67 women), 85 part-time (77 women); includes 28 minority (18 Black or African American, non-Hispanic/Latino; 2 Asian, non-Hispanic/Latino; 3 Hispanic/Latino; 3 Native Hawaiian or other Pacific Islander, non-Hispanic/Latino; 2 Two or more races, non-Hispanic/Latino). *Degree requirements:* For master's, thesis or alternative. *Entrance requirements:* For master's, 2 references, personal statement, curriculum vitae or resume. Additional exam requirements/recommendations for international students: Required—TOEFL (minimum score 575 paper-based; 85 iBT). *Application deadline:* For fall admission, 2/1 priority date for international students; for spring admission, 10/1 priority date for international students. Applications are processed on a rolling basis. Application fee: $50. *Expenses: Tuition:* Full-time $12,960; part-time $720 per credit hour. *Required fees:* $295; $720 per credit hour. Tuition and fees vary according to course load. *Financial support:* Fellowships, research assistantships, Federal Work-Study, institutionally sponsored loans, and scholarships/grants available. Support available to part-time students. Financial award applicants required to submit FAFSA. *Faculty research:* HIV stigma, HIV symptom management, palliative care with children and their families, heart disease prevention in Hispanic women, depression in the well elderly, alternative therapies in pre-term infants. *Unit head:* Dr. Michael Bleich, Dean, 314-362-0956, Fax: 314-362-0984, E-mail: mbleich@bjc.org. *Application contact:* Margaret Anne O'Connor, Program Officer, 314-454-7557, Fax: 314-362-0984, E-mail: maoconnor@bjc.org.

Gwynedd Mercy University, School of Nursing, Gwynedd Valley, PA 19437-0901. Offers clinical nurse specialist (MSN), including gerontology, oncology, pediatrics; nurse practitioner (MSN), including adult health, pediatric health. *Degree requirements:* For master's, thesis optional. *Entrance requirements:* For master's, GRE General Test or MAT, current nursing experience, physical assessment, course work in statistics, BSN from NLNAC-accredited program, 2 letters of recommendation, personal interview. Additional exam requirements/recommendations for international students: Required—TOEFL (minimum score 575 paper-based). Electronic applications accepted. *Expenses:* Contact institution. *Faculty research:* Critical thinking, primary care, domestic violence, multiculturalism, nursing centers.

Hampton University, Graduate College, School of Nursing, Hampton, VA 23668. Offers advanced adult nursing (MS); community health nursing (MS); community mental health/psychiatric nursing (MS); family nursing (MS); gerontological nursing for the nurse practitioner (MS); pediatric nursing (MS); women's health nursing (MS). *Accreditation:* AACN. Part-time and evening/weekend programs available. *Degree requirements:* For master's, thesis optional. *Entrance requirements:* For master's, GRE General Test. *Faculty research:* Curriculum development, physical and mental assessment.

Hunter College of the City University of New York, Graduate School, Schools of the Health Professions, Hunter-Bellevue School of Nursing, Program in Adult Nurse Practitioner, New York, NY 10065-5085. Offers MS. *Accreditation:* AACN. *Faculty:* 18 full-time (15 women), 25 part-time/adjunct (21 women). *Students:* 3 full-time (all women), 20 part-time (15 women); includes 7 minority (5 Asian, non-Hispanic/Latino; 2 Hispanic/Latino), 3 international. Average age 33. 28 applicants, 39% accepted, 10 enrolled. In 2013, 21 master's awarded. *Degree requirements:* For master's, practicum. *Entrance requirements:* For master's, minimum GPA of 3.0, New York RN license, 2 years of professional practice experience, BSN. Additional exam requirements/recommendations for international students: Required—TOEFL. *Application deadline:* For fall admission, 4/1 for domestic students, 2/1 for international students; for spring admission, 11/1 for domestic students, 9/1 for international students. Applications are processed on a rolling basis. Application fee: $125. *Financial support:* Federal Work-Study, scholarships/grants, and traineeships available. Support available to part-time students. Financial award application deadline: 5/1. *Unit head:* Dr. Anita Nirenberg, Interim Specialization Coordinator, 212-481-4359, Fax: 212-481-5078, E-mail: anirenbe@hunter.cuny.edu. *Application contact:* Milena Solo, Director for Graduate Admissions, 212-772-4480, E-mail: admissions@hunter.cuny.edu.
Website: http://www.hunter.cuny.edu/nursing/repository/files/graduate-fact-sheets/fsGNPANP8113.pdf

Indiana University–Purdue University Fort Wayne, College of Health and Human Services, Department of Nursing, Fort Wayne, IN 46805-1499. Offers adult-gerontology primary care nurse practitioner (MS); nurse executive (MS); nursing administration (Certificate); nursing education (MS); women's health nurse practitioner (MS). Part-time programs available. *Faculty:* 12 full-time (all women). *Students:* 5 full-time (all women), 63 part-time (60 women); includes 3 minority (2 Black or African American, non-Hispanic/Latino; 1 Asian, non-Hispanic/Latino). Average age 35. 34 applicants, 100% accepted, 25 enrolled. In 2013, 10 master's awarded. *Entrance requirements:* For master's, GRE Writing Test (if GPA below 3.0), BS in nursing, eligibility for Indiana RN license, minimum GPA of 3.0, essay, copy of resume, three references, undergraduate course work in research and statistics within last 5 years. Additional exam requirements/recommendations for international students: Required—TOEFL (minimum score 550 paper-based; 79 iBT); Recommended—TWE. *Application deadline:* For fall admission, 5/1 priority date for domestic and international students; for spring admission, 11/15 priority date for domestic students. Applications are processed on a rolling basis. Application fee: $55 ($60 for international students). Electronic applications accepted. *Financial support:* In 2013–14, 3 teaching assistantships with partial tuition reimbursements (averaging $13,322 per year) were awarded; scholarships/grants also available. Support available to part-time students. Financial award application deadline: 3/1; financial award applicants required to submit FAFSA. *Faculty research:* Pain management and substance abuse, high-risk alcohol use on campus, pediatric case management. *Unit head:* Dr. Lee-Ellen Kirkhorn, Chair/Professor, 260-481-6789, Fax: 260-481-5767, E-mail: kirkhorl@ipfw.edu. *Application contact:* Dr. Deborah Poling, Director of Graduate Program, 260-481-6276, Fax: 260-481-5767, E-mail: polingd@ipfw.edu.
Website: http://www.ipfw.edu/nursing/

Indiana University–Purdue University Indianapolis, School of Nursing, Indianapolis, IN 46202-2896. Offers acute care nurse practitioner (MSN); adult health clinical nurse specialist (MSN); adult health nursing (MSN), including adult clinical nurse specialist; adult nurse practitioner (MSN); adult psychiatric/mental health nursing (MSN); child psychiatric/mental health nursing (MSN); community health nursing (MSN); family nurse practitioner (MSN); neonatal nurse practitioner (MSN); nursing (MSN, DNP), including nursing administration (MSN), nursing education (MSN); nursing science (PhD); pediatric clinical nurse specialist (MSN); women's health nurse practitioner (MSN); MSN/MPA; MSN/MPH. Part-time programs available. *Faculty:* 85 full-time (82 women), 60 part-time/adjunct (all women). *Students:* 86 full-time (78 women), 371 part-time (351 women); includes 74 minority (39 Black or African American, non-Hispanic/Latino; 1 American Indian or Alaska Native, non-Hispanic/Latino; 14 Asian, non-Hispanic/Latino; 11 Hispanic/Latino; 9 Two or more races, non-Hispanic/Latino), 6 international. Average age 38. 224 applicants, 61% accepted, 102 enrolled. In 2013, 120 master's, 10 doctorates awarded. Terminal master's awarded for partial completion of doctoral program. *Degree requirements:* For master's, thesis; for doctorate, thesis/dissertation. *Entrance requirements:* For master's, minimum GPA of 3.0, RN license; for doctorate, GRE General Test, minimum GPA of 3.0, MSN, RN license, graduate statistics course with minimum B grade (not older than 3 years). Additional exam requirements/recommendations for international students: Required—TOEFL. *Application deadline:* For fall admission, 2/15 for domestic students; for spring admission, 9/15 for domestic students. Application fee: $55 ($65 for international students). *Financial support:* In 2013–14, 93 students received support. Fellowships with full tuition reimbursements available, research assistantships with full tuition reimbursements available, teaching assistantships with full tuition reimbursements available, Federal Work-Study, institutionally sponsored loans, scholarships/grants, and tuition waivers (full) available. Support available to part-time students. Financial award application deadline: 5/1. *Faculty research:* Clinical science, health systems. *Total annual research expenditures:* $3 million. *Unit head:* Dr. Patricia Ebright, Associate Dean for Graduate Programs, E-mail: nursing@iupui.edu. *Application contact:* Information Contact, 317-274-2806.
Website: http://nursing.iu.edu/

Kent State University, College of Nursing, Kent, OH 44242-0001. Offers acute care nurse practitioner (MSN); adult nurse practitioner (MSN); clinical nurse specialist (MSN); family nurse practitioner (MSN); geriatric nurse practitioner (MSN); health care management (MSN); nurse educator (MSN); nursing (PhD); nursing practice (DNP); pediatric nurse practitioner (MSN); psychiatric/mental health nurse practitioner (MSN); women's health nurse practitioner (MSN). PhD program offered jointly with The University of Akron. *Accreditation:* AACN. Part-time programs available. *Degree requirements:* For master's, thesis optional; for doctorate, comprehensive exam, thesis/dissertation. *Entrance requirements:* For master's, GRE (if undergraduate GPA less than 3.0), minimum GPA of 2.75; for doctorate, GRE, MSN. Additional exam requirements/recommendations for international students: Required—TOEFL. Electronic applications accepted. *Expenses:* Contact institution. *Faculty research:* Women and violence, methodological specialties, osteoporosis in women, new caregivers and the elderly.

La Salle University, School of Nursing and Health Sciences, Program in Nursing, Philadelphia, PA 19141-1199. Offers adult gerontology primary care nurse practitioner (MSN, Certificate); adult health and illness clinical nurse specialist (MSN); adult-gerontology clinical nurse specialist (MSN, Certificate); clinical nurse leader (MSN); family primary care nurse practitioner (MSN, Certificate); gerontology (Certificate); nurse anesthetist (MSN, Certificate); nursing (MSN, Certificate); nursing administration (MSN, Certificate); nursing education (Certificate); nursing practice (DNP); nursing service administration (MSN); public health nursing (MSN, Certificate); school nursing (Certificate); MSN/MBA; MSN/MPH. *Accreditation:* AANA/CANAEP. Part-time programs available. Postbaccalaureate distance learning degree programs offered (minimal on-campus study). *Faculty:* 13 full-time (12 women), 10 part-time/adjunct (8 women). *Students:* 4 full-time (all women), 379 part-time (331 women); includes 119 minority (70 Black or African American, non-Hispanic/Latino; 2 American Indian or Alaska Native, non-Hispanic/Latino; 31 Asian, non-Hispanic/Latino; 12 Hispanic/Latino; 4 Two or more races, non-Hispanic/Latino), 1 international. Average age 37. 133 applicants, 85% accepted, 63 enrolled. In 2013, 72 master's, 3 doctorates, 26 other advanced degrees awarded. *Degree requirements:* For doctorate, minimum of 1,000 hours of post baccalaureate clinical practice supervised by preceptors. *Entrance requirements:* For master's, GRE, MAT, or GMAT (for students with BSN GPA of less than 3.2), baccalaureate degree in nursing from an NLNAC- or CCNE-accredited program or an MSN Bridge program; Pennsylvania RN license; 2 letters of reference; resume; statement of philosophy articulating professional values and future educational goal; 1 year of work experience as a registered nurse; for doctorate, GRE (waived for applicants with MSN cumulative GPA of 3.7 or above), MSN from nationally-accredited program or master's degree, MBA or MHA from nationally-accredited program; resume or curriculum vitae; 2 letters of reference; interview; for Certificate, GRE, MAT, or GMAT (for students with BSN GPA of less than 3.2, baccalaureate degree in nursing from an NLNAC- or CCNE-accredited program or an MSN Bridge program; Pennsylvania RN license; 2 letters of reference; resume; statement of philosophy articulating professional values and future educational goal; 1 year of work experience as a registered nurse. Additional exam requirements/recommendations for international students: Required—TOEFL. *Application deadline:* For fall admission, 8/15 priority date for domestic students, 7/15 for international students; for spring admission, 12/15 priority date for domestic students, 11/15 for international students; for summer admission, 4/15 priority date for domestic students, 3/15 for international students. Applications are processed on a rolling basis. Application fee: $35. Electronic applications accepted. Application fee is waived when completed online. *Expenses:* Contact institution. *Financial support:* In 2013–14, 48 students received support. Teaching assistantships, scholarships/grants, and traineeships available. Support available to part-time students. Financial award application deadline: 8/31; financial award applicants required to submit FAFSA. *Unit head:* Dr. Patricia M. Dillon, Director, 215-951-1322, Fax: 215-951-1896, E-mail: msnapn@lasalle.edu. *Application contact:* Paul J. Reilly, Assistant Vice President, Enrollment Services, 215-951-1946, Fax: 215-951-1462, E-mail: reilly@lasalle.edu.

Lehman College of the City University of New York, School of Natural and Social Sciences, Department of Nursing, Bronx, NY 10468-1589. Offers adult health nursing (MS); nursing of older adults (MS); parent-child nursing (MS); pediatric nurse practitioner (MS). *Accreditation:* AACN. Part-time and evening/weekend programs available. *Entrance requirements:* For master's, bachelor's degree in nursing, New York RN license.

Lewis University, College of Nursing and Health Professions, Program in Nursing, Romeoville, IL 60446. Offers adult nurse practitioner (MSN); nursing administration (MSN); nursing education (MSN). *Accreditation:* AACN. Part-time and evening/weekend programs available. Postbaccalaureate distance learning degree programs offered (no on-campus study). *Students:* 23 full-time (22 women), 234 part-time (222 women); includes 72 minority (31 Black or African American, non-Hispanic/Latino; 23 Asian, non-Hispanic/Latino; 15 Hispanic/Latino; 1 Native Hawaiian or other Pacific Islander, non-Hispanic/Latino; 2 Two or more races, non-Hispanic/Latino). Average age 38. *Degree requirements:* For master's, clinical practicum. *Entrance requirements:* For master's, minimum undergraduate GPA of 3.0, degree in nursing, RN license, letter of recommendation, interview, resume or curriculum vitae. Additional exam requirements/recommendations for international students: Required—TOEFL (minimum score 550 paper-based; 80 iBT). *Application deadline:* For fall admission, 5/1 priority date for international students; for spring admission, 11/15 priority date for international students. Applications are processed on a rolling basis. Application fee: $40. Electronic applications accepted. *Financial support:* Federal Work-Study, scholarships/grants, tuition waivers (full and partial), and unspecified assistantships available. Financial award application deadline: 5/1; financial award applicants required to submit FAFSA. *Faculty research:* Cancer prevention, phenomenological methods, public policy analysis. *Total annual research expenditures:* $1,000. *Unit head:* 815-836-5610. *Application contact:* Nancy Wiksten, Adult Admission Counselor, 815-836-5628, Fax: 815-836-5578, E-mail: wikstena@lewisu.edu.
Website: http://www.lewisu.edu/

Loma Linda University, Department of Graduate Nursing, Program in Adult and Aging Family Nursing, Loma Linda, CA 92350. Offers MS. *Accreditation:* AACN. Part-time programs available. *Degree requirements:* For master's, thesis or alternative. *Entrance requirements:* For master's, GRE General Test, BSN, minimum GPA of 3.0, RN license. Additional exam requirements/recommendations for international students: Required—TOEFL. Electronic applications accepted. *Faculty research:* Coping, integration of research.

Long Island University–LIU Brooklyn, School of Nursing, Department of Adult Nurse Practitioner, Brooklyn, NY 11201-8423. Offers MS, Certificate. *Accreditation:* AACN. *Entrance requirements:* For master's, New York RN license, 2 letters of recommendation. Additional exam requirements/recommendations for international students: Required—TOEFL (minimum score 500 paper-based). Electronic applications accepted.

Adult Nursing

Louisiana State University Health Sciences Center, School of Nursing, New Orleans, LA 70112-2223. Offers advanced public/community health nursing (MN); clinical nurse specialist (MN); nurse anesthesia (MN); nurse practitioner (MN); nursing (DNS). *Accreditation:* AACN; AANA/CANAEP (one or more programs are accredited). Part-time programs available. *Degree requirements:* For master's, thesis optional; for doctorate, thesis/dissertation. *Entrance requirements:* For master's, GRE General Test, MAT, minimum GPA of 3.0; for doctorate, GRE General Test, minimum GPA of 3.5. Additional exam requirements/recommendations for international students: Required—TOEFL. Electronic applications accepted. *Faculty research:* Advanced clinical practice, nursing education, health, social support, nursing administration.

Loyola University Chicago, Graduate School, Marcella Niehoff School of Nursing, Adult Clinical Nurse Specialist Program, Chicago, IL 60660. Offers adult clinical nurse specialist (MSN, Certificate). Part-time and evening/weekend programs available. Postbaccalaureate distance learning degree programs offered (minimal on-campus study). *Students:* 2 full-time (both women), 29 part-time (all women); includes 3 minority (1 Black or African American, non-Hispanic/Latino; 1 Asian, non-Hispanic/Latino; 1 Hispanic/Latino). Average age 33. 17 applicants, 71% accepted, 9 enrolled. In 2013, 1 other advanced degree awarded. *Degree requirements:* For master's, comprehensive exam. *Entrance requirements:* For master's, Illinois nursing license, BSN, minimum nursing GPA of 3.0, 3 letters of recommendation, 1,000 hours of experience in area of specialty. *Expenses: Tuition:* Full-time $16,740; part-time $930 per credit. *Required fees:* $135 per semester. *Unit head:* Dr. Marijo Letizia, Associate Dean, 708-216-9325, Fax: 708-216-9555, E-mail: mletizi@luc.edu. *Application contact:* Amy Weatherford, Enrollment Advisor, School of Nursing, 773-508-3249, Fax: 773-508-3241, E-mail: aweatherford@luc.edu.
Website: http://www.luc.edu/nursing/

Loyola University Chicago, Graduate School, Marcella Niehoff School of Nursing, Adult Nurse Practitioner Program, Chicago, IL 60660. Offers adult clinical nurse practitioner (MSN); adult health (Certificate); adult nurse practitioner (MSN); cardiovascular nursing (Certificate). *Accreditation:* AACN. Part-time and evening/weekend programs available. Postbaccalaureate distance learning degree programs offered (minimal on-campus study). *Students:* 6 full-time (all women), 34 part-time (31 women); includes 8 minority (2 Black or African American, non-Hispanic/Latino; 5 Asian, non-Hispanic/Latino; 1 Hispanic/Latino). Average age 33. 41 applicants, 68% accepted, 21 enrolled. In 2013, 8 master's awarded. *Degree requirements:* For master's, comprehensive exam or oral thesis defense. *Entrance requirements:* For master's, BSN, minimum nursing GPA of 3.0, Illinois nursing license, 3 letters of recommendation, 1000 hours of experience before starting clinical. *Application deadline:* Applications are processed on a rolling basis. Application fee: $50. Electronic applications accepted. *Expenses: Tuition:* Full-time $16,740; part-time $930 per credit. *Required fees:* $135 per semester. *Financial support:* Traineeships available. *Faculty research:* Menopause. *Unit head:* Dr. Marijo Letizia, Associate Dean, 708-216-9325, Fax: 708-216-9555, E-mail: mletizi@luc.edu. *Application contact:* Amy Weatherford, Enrollment Advisor, School of Nursing, 773-508-3249, Fax: 773-508-3241, E-mail: aweatherford@luc.edu.
Website: http://www.luc.edu/nursing/index.shtml

Madonna University, Program in Nursing, Livonia, MI 48150-1173. Offers adult health: chronic health conditions (MSN); adult nurse practitioner (MSN); nursing administration (MSN); MSN/MSBA. *Accreditation:* AACN. Part-time programs available. *Degree requirements:* For master's, thesis or alternative. *Entrance requirements:* For master's, GRE General Test, Michigan nursing license. Electronic applications accepted. *Faculty research:* Coping, caring.

Marian University, School of Nursing and Health Professions, Fond du Lac, WI 54935-4699. Offers adult nurse practitioner (MSN); nurse educator (MSN). *Accreditation:* AACN. Part-time and evening/weekend programs available. *Faculty:* 5 full-time (all women), 10 part-time/adjunct (6 women). *Students:* 21 full-time (18 women), 77 part-time (71 women); includes 9 minority (3 Black or African American, non-Hispanic/Latino; 5 Hispanic/Latino; 1 Native Hawaiian or other Pacific Islander, non-Hispanic/Latino). Average age 37. In 2013, 24 master's awarded. *Degree requirements:* For master's, thesis, 675 clinical practicum hours. *Entrance requirements:* For master's, 3 letters of professional recommendation; undergraduate work in nursing research, statistics, health assessment. Additional exam requirements/recommendations for international students: Required—TOEFL (minimum score 525 paper-based; 70 iBT). *Application deadline:* Applications are processed on a rolling basis. Application fee: $50. Electronic applications accepted. *Expenses:* Contact institution. *Financial support:* In 2013–14, 3 students received support. Institutionally sponsored loans and scholarships/grants available. Support available to part-time students. Financial award application deadline: 3/1; financial award applicants required to submit FAFSA. *Unit head:* Dr. Julie Luetschwager, Dean, 920-923-8094, Fax: 920-923-8770, E-mail: jaluetschwager25@marianuniversity.edu. *Application contact:* Selina Scoles, Admissions Counselor, 920-923-8938, Fax: 920-923-8770, E-mail: sascoles30@marianuniversity.edu.
Website: http://www.marianuniversity.edu/nursing/

Marquette University, Graduate School, College of Nursing, Milwaukee, WI 53201-1881. Offers acute care nurse practitioner (Certificate); adult clinical nurse specialist (Certificate); adult nurse practitioner (Certificate); advanced practice nursing (MSN, DNP), including adult-older adult acute care (DNP), adults (MSN), adults-older adults (DNP), clinical nurse leader (MSN), health care systems leadership (DNP), nurse-midwifery (MSN), older adults (MSN), pediatrics acute care (MSN), pediatrics primary care (MSN), pediatrics-acute care (DNP), pediatrics-primary care (DNP), primary care (DNP), systems leadership and healthcare quality (MSN); family nurse practitioner (Certificate); nurse-midwifery (Certificate); nursing (PhD); pediatric acute care (Certificate); pediatric primary care (Certificate); systems leadership and healthcare quality (Certificate). *Accreditation:* AACN. *Faculty:* 35 full-time (34 women), 59 part-time/adjunct (58 women). *Students:* 105 full-time (96 women), 279 part-time (256 women); includes 28 minority (11 Black or African American, non-Hispanic/Latino; 7 Asian, non-Hispanic/Latino; 8 Hispanic/Latino; 2 Two or more races, non-Hispanic/Latino), 3 international. Average age 30. 322 applicants, 62% accepted, 98 enrolled. In 2013, 66 master's, 4 doctorates, 6 other advanced degrees awarded. Terminal master's awarded for partial completion of doctoral program. *Degree requirements:* For master's, comprehensive exam, thesis or alternative. *Entrance requirements:* For master's, GRE General Test, BSN, Wisconsin RN license, official transcripts from all current and previous colleges/universities except Marquette, three completed recommendation forms, resume, written statement of professional goals; for doctorate, GRE General Test, official transcripts from all current and previous colleges/universities except Marquette, three letters of recommendation, resume, written statement of professional goals, sample of scholarly writing. Additional exam requirements/recommendations for international students: Required—TOEFL (minimum score 530 paper-based). *Application deadline:* For fall admission, 2/15 for domestic and international students. Application fee: $50. Electronic applications accepted. *Financial support:* In 2013–14, 41 students received support, including 1 fellowship with partial tuition reimbursement available (averaging $17,500 per year), 2 research assistantships with full tuition reimbursements available (averaging $13,285 per year), 8 teaching assistantships with full tuition reimbursements available (averaging $13,912 per year); career-related internships or fieldwork, Federal Work-Study, scholarships/grants, health care benefits, tuition waivers (partial), and unspecified assistantships also available. Support available to part-time students. Financial award application deadline: 2/15. *Faculty research:* Psychosocial adjustment to chronic illness, gerontology, reminiscence, health policy: uninsured and access, hospital care delivery systems. *Total annual research expenditures:* $769,051. *Unit head:* Dr. Margaret Callahan, Dean, 414-288-3800, Fax: 414-288-1578. *Application contact:* Dr. Maureen O'Brien, Associate Dean/Clinical Associate Professor, 414-288-3823.
Website: http://www.marquette.edu/nursing/academicprograms-graduate.shtml

Maryville University of Saint Louis, College of Health Professions, The Catherine McAuley School of Nursing, St. Louis, MO 63141-7299. Offers adult nurse practitioner (MSN); advanced practice nursing (DNP); family nurse practitioner (MSN); geriatric nurse practitioner (MSN); nursing education (MSN). *Accreditation:* AACN. Postbaccalaureate distance learning degree programs offered. *Students:* 30 full-time (28 women), 1,551 part-time (1,416 women); includes 361 minority (181 Black or African American, non-Hispanic/Latino; 16 American Indian or Alaska Native, non-Hispanic/Latino; 59 Asian, non-Hispanic/Latino; 71 Hispanic/Latino; 5 Native Hawaiian or other Pacific Islander, non-Hispanic/Latino; 29 Two or more races, non-Hispanic/Latino), 3 international. Average age 36. In 2013, 37 master's awarded. *Degree requirements:* For master's, practicum. *Entrance requirements:* For master's, BSN, current licensure, minimum GPA of 3.0, 3 letters of recommendation, curriculum vitae. Additional exam requirements/recommendations for international students: Required—TOEFL (minimum score 550 paper-based). *Application deadline:* Applications are processed on a rolling basis. Application fee: $40 ($60 for international students). Electronic applications accepted. Application fee is waived when completed online. *Expenses: Tuition:* Full-time $23,812; part-time $728 per credit hour. *Required fees:* $395 per year. Tuition and fees vary according to course load, degree level and program. *Financial support:* Federal Work-Study and campus employment available. Support available to part-time students. Financial award application deadline: 3/1; financial award applicants required to submit FAFSA. *Unit head:* Dr. Elizabeth Buck, Director, 314-529-9453, Fax: 314-529-9139, E-mail: ebuck@maryville.edu. *Application contact:* Crystal Jacobsmeyer, Assistant Director, Graduate Enrollment Advising, 314-929-9654, Fax: 314-529-9927, E-mail: cjacobsmeyer@maryville.edu.
Website: http://www.maryville.edu/hp/nursing/

Medical University of South Carolina, College of Nursing, Adult-Gerontology Health Nurse Practitioner Program, Charleston, SC 29425. Offers MSN, DNP. Part-time programs available. Postbaccalaureate distance learning degree programs offered (minimal on-campus study). *Degree requirements:* For master's, comprehensive exam (for some programs), thesis optional; for doctorate, final project. *Entrance requirements:* For master's, BSN from nationally-accredited program, minimum nursing and cumulative GPA of 3.0, undergraduate-level statistics course, active RN License, 3 confidential references, current curriculum vitae or resume, essay; for doctorate, BSN from nationally-accredited program, minimum nursing and cumulative GPA of 3.0, undergraduate-level statistics course, active RN License, 3 confidential references, current curriculum vitae or resume, personal essay (for DNP). Additional exam requirements/recommendations for international students: Required—TOEFL (minimum score 550 paper-based; 80 iBT). Electronic applications accepted. *Faculty research:* Palliative care, dementia, hospital acquired infections, diabetes, advance practice nurse utilization.

Molloy College, Division of Nursing, Rockville Centre, NY 11571-5002. Offers adult nurse practitioner (Advanced Certificate); clinical nurse specialist: adult health (Advanced Certificate); family nurse practitioner (Advanced Certificate); nurse practitioner psychiatry (Advanced Certificate); nursing (MS, PhD); nursing administration (Advanced Certificate); nursing administration with informatics (Advanced Certificate); nursing education (Advanced Certificate); nursing informatics (Advanced Certificate); pediatric nurse practitioner (Advanced Certificate). *Accreditation:* AACN. Part-time and evening/weekend programs available. *Faculty:* 30 full-time (29 women), 10 part-time/adjunct (7 women). *Students:* 18 full-time (all women), 538 part-time (495 women); includes 289 minority (159 Black or African American, non-Hispanic/Latino; 1 American Indian or Alaska Native, non-Hispanic/Latino; 80 Asian, non-Hispanic/Latino; 43 Hispanic/Latino; 4 Native Hawaiian or other Pacific Islander, non-Hispanic/Latino; 2 Two or more races, non-Hispanic/Latino), 2 international. Average age 38. 241 applicants, 63% accepted, 122 enrolled. In 2013, 84 master's, 2 other advanced degrees awarded. *Degree requirements:* For master's, thesis optional. *Entrance requirements:* For master's, 3 letters of reference, BS in nursing, minimum undergraduate GPA of 3.0; for Advanced Certificate, 3 letters of reference, master's degree in nursing. *Application deadline:* For fall admission, 9/2 priority date for domestic students; for spring admission, 1/20 priority date for domestic students. Applications are processed on a rolling basis. Application fee: $60. *Expenses: Tuition:* Full-time $16,920; part-time $940 per credit. *Required fees:* $880. *Financial support:* Research assistantships with partial tuition reimbursements, teaching assistantships with partial tuition reimbursements, institutionally sponsored loans, scholarships/grants, and unspecified assistantships available. Support available to part-time students. Financial award application deadline: 4/1; financial award applicants required to submit FAFSA. *Unit head:* Dr. Jeannine Muldoon, Dean of Nursing, 516-323-3651, E-mail: jmuldoon@molloy.edu. *Application contact:* Alina Haitz, Assistant Director of Graduate Admissions, 516-323-4008, E-mail: ahaitz@molloy.edu.
Website: http://www.molloy.edu/academics/nursing-division

Monmouth University, The Graduate School, The Marjorie K. Unterberg School of Nursing and Health Studies, West Long Branch, NJ 07764-1898. Offers adult and gerontological nurse practitioner (MSN); adult-gerontological nurse practitioner (Post-Master's Certificate); family nurse practitioner (MSN, Post-Master's Certificate); family psychiatric and mental health advanced practice nursing (MSN); forensic nursing (MSN, Certificate); nursing (MSN); nursing administration (MSN, Post-Master's Certificate); nursing education (MSN, Post-Master's Certificate); nursing practice (DNP); physician assistant (MS); psychiatric-mental health nurse practitioner (Post-Master's Certificate); school nursing (MSN, Certificate). *Accreditation:* AACN. Part-time and evening/weekend programs available. *Faculty:* 14 full-time (all women), 4 part-time/adjunct (3 women). *Students:* 19 full-time (18 women), 269 part-time (252 women); includes 106 minority (35 Black or African American, non-Hispanic/Latino; 2 American Indian or Alaska Native, non-Hispanic/Latino; 51 Asian, non-Hispanic/Latino; 12 Hispanic/Latino; 3 Native Hawaiian or other Pacific Islander, non-Hispanic/Latino; 3 Two or more races, non-Hispanic/Latino), 2 international. Average age 39. 135 applicants, 98% accepted, 96 enrolled. In 2013, 54 master's, 7 doctorates awarded. *Degree requirements:* For master's, practicum (for some tracks). *Entrance requirements:* For master's, GRE General Test, BSN with minimum GPA of 2.75, current RN license, proof of liability and malpractice policy, personal statement, two letters of recommendation, college course work in health assessment, resume; minimum GPA of 3.0, minimum C grade in prerequisite courses, minimum 200 hours' clinical experience, 3 letters of recommendation, and interview (for MS); for doctorate, accredited master's nursing program degree with minimum GPA of 3.2, active RN license, national certification as Nurse Practitioner or Nurse Administrator, working knowledge of statistics, statement of goals and vision for change, 2 letters of recommendation, resume, interview. Additional exam requirements/recommendations for international students: Required—TOEFL (minimum score 550 paper-based; 79 iBT), IELTS (minimum score 6) or Michigan

English Language Assessment Battery (minimum score 77). *Application deadline:* For fall admission, 7/15 priority date for domestic students, 6/1 for international students; for spring admission, 11/15 priority date for domestic students, 11/1 for international students; for summer admission, 2/1 for domestic students. Applications are processed on a rolling basis. Application fee: $50. Electronic applications accepted. *Expenses: Tuition:* Part-time $1004 per credit hour. *Required fees:* $157 per semester. *Financial support:* In 2013–14, 163 students received support, including 113 fellowships (averaging $3,093 per year), 27 research assistantships (averaging $6,273 per year); career-related internships or fieldwork, scholarships/grants, and unspecified assistantships also available. Support available to part-time students. Financial award applicants required to submit FAFSA. *Faculty research:* Relationship of undergraduate GPA and GRE to succeeding in a graduate nursing program. *Unit head:* Dr. Janet Mahoney, Dean, 732-571-3443, Fax: 732-263-5131, E-mail: jmahoney@monmouth.edu. *Application contact:* Lauren Vento-Cifelli, Associate Vice President of Undergraduate and Graduate Admission, 732-571-3452, Fax: 732-263-5123, E-mail: gradadm@monmouth.edu.
Website: http://www.monmouth.edu/school-of-nursing-health/graduate-nursing-programs.aspx

Mount Carmel College of Nursing, Nursing Program, Columbus, OH 43222. Offers adult gerontology acute care nurse practitioner (MS); adult health clinical nurse specialist (MS); family nurse practitioner (MS); nursing administration (MS); nursing education (MS). *Accreditation:* AACN. Part-time programs available. *Faculty:* 8 full-time (7 women), 8 part-time/adjunct (7 women). *Students:* 94 full-time (89 women), 76 part-time (73 women); includes 35 minority (21 Black or African American, non-Hispanic/Latino; 2 American Indian or Alaska Native, non-Hispanic/Latino; 6 Asian, non-Hispanic/Latino; 2 Hispanic/Latino; 1 Native Hawaiian or other Pacific Islander, non-Hispanic/Latino; 3 Two or more races, non-Hispanic/Latino). Average age 38. 123 applicants, 50% accepted, 47 enrolled. In 2013, 41 master's awarded. *Degree requirements:* For master's, professional manuscript. *Entrance requirements:* For master's, letters of recommendation, statement of purpose, current resume, baccalaureate degree in nursing, current Ohio RN license, minimum cumulative GPA of 3.0. Additional exam requirements/recommendations for international students: Required—TOEFL (minimum score 550 paper-based; 80 iBT). *Application deadline:* For fall admission, 6/1 priority date for domestic students; for winter admission, 11/1 for domestic students; for spring admission, 10/1 priority date for domestic students; for summer admission, 3/1 for domestic students. Applications are processed on a rolling basis. Application fee: $30. *Expenses: Tuition:* Full-time $8560; part-time $428 per credit. *Required fees:* $75. *Financial support:* In 2013–14, 9 students received support. Institutionally sponsored loans and scholarships/grants available. Financial award application deadline: 3/15; financial award applicants required to submit FAFSA. *Unit head:* Dr. Angela Phillips-Lowe, Associate Dean, 614-234-5717, Fax: 614-234-2875, E-mail: aphillips-lowe@mccn.edu. *Application contact:* Kathleen Walters, Program Coordinator, 614-234-5408, Fax: 614-234-2875, E-mail: kwalters@mccn.edu.
Website: http://www.mccn.edu/

Mount Saint Mary College, Division of Nursing, Newburgh, NY 12550-3494. Offers adult nurse practitioner (MS, Advanced Certificate), including nursing education (MS), nursing management (MS); clinical nurse specialist-adult health (MS), including nursing education, nursing management; family nurse practitioner (Advanced Certificate). *Accreditation:* AACN. Part-time and evening/weekend programs available. *Faculty:* 4 full-time (all women). *Students:* 79 part-time (72 women); includes 19 minority (12 Black or African American, non-Hispanic/Latino; 1 Asian, non-Hispanic/Latino; 5 Hispanic/Latino; 1 Native Hawaiian or other Pacific Islander, non-Hispanic/Latino). Average age 39. 45 applicants, 47% accepted, 9 enrolled. In 2013, 13 master's, 3 other advanced degrees awarded. *Degree requirements:* For master's, research utilization project. *Entrance requirements:* For master's, BSN, minimum GPA of 3.0, RN license. *Application deadline:* For fall admission, 6/3 priority date for domestic students; for spring admission, 10/31 priority date for domestic students. Applications are processed on a rolling basis. Application fee: $45. Application fee is waived when completed online. *Expenses: Tuition:* Full-time $13,356; part-time $742 per credit. *Required fees:* $70 per semester. *Financial support:* In 2013–14, 8 students received support. Unspecified assistantships available. Financial award application deadline: 4/15; financial award applicants required to submit FAFSA. *Unit head:* Linda Ruta, Graduate Coordinator, 845-569-3512, Fax: 845-562-6762, E-mail: linda.ruta@msmc.edu. *Application contact:* Lisa Gallina, Director of Admissions for Graduate Programs and Adult Degree Completion, 845-569-3166, Fax: 845-569-3450, E-mail: lisa.gallina@msmc.edu.
Website: http://www.msmc.edu/Academics/Graduate_Programs/Master_of_Science_in_Nursing

New Mexico State University, Graduate School, College of Health and Social Services, School of Nursing, Las Cruces, NM 88003. Offers adult/gerontology nurse practitioner (DNP); family nurse practitioner (DNP); nursing (MSN, PhD); public/community health (DNP). *Accreditation:* AACN. Postbaccalaureate distance learning degree programs offered (minimal on-campus study). *Faculty:* 15 full-time (14 women). *Students:* 42 full-time (33 women), 64 part-time (56 women); includes 50 minority (11 Black or African American, non-Hispanic/Latino; 1 American Indian or Alaska Native, non-Hispanic/Latino; 1 Asian, non-Hispanic/Latino; 36 Hispanic/Latino; 1 Two or more races, non-Hispanic/Latino), 1 international. Average age 42. 50 applicants, 86% accepted, 36 enrolled. In 2013, 12 master's, 6 doctorates awarded. *Degree requirements:* For master's, comprehensive exam, thesis optional, clinical practice; for doctorate, comprehensive exam, thesis/dissertation. *Entrance requirements:* For master's, NCLEX exam, BSN, minimum GPA of 3.0, course work in statistics, 3 letters of reference, writing sample, RN license, CPR certification, proof of liability, immunizations, criminal background check; for doctorate, NCLEX exam, MSN, minimum GPA of 3.0, 3 letters of reference, writing sample, RN license, CPR certification, proof of liability, immunizations, criminal background check, statistics course. Additional exam requirements/recommendations for international students: Required—TOEFL (minimum score 550 paper-based; 79 iBT), IELTS (minimum score 6.5). *Application deadline:* For spring admission, 10/1 priority date for domestic students. Application fee: $40 ($50 for international students). Electronic applications accepted. *Expenses:* Tuition, state resident: full-time $5398; part-time $224.90 per credit. Tuition, nonresident: full-time $18,821; part-time $784.20 per credit. *Required fees:* $1310; $54.60 per credit. *Financial support:* In 2013–14, 31 students received support. Career-related internships or fieldwork, Federal Work-Study, scholarships/grants, traineeships, health care benefits, and unspecified assistantships available. Financial award application deadline: 3/1. *Faculty research:* Public policy, community health, health disparities, self efficacy and self management, psychiatric mental health. *Total annual research expenditures:* $3,424. *Unit head:* Dr. Pamela Schultz, Director, 575-646-3812, Fax: 575-646-2167, E-mail: pschultz@nmsu.edu. *Application contact:* Dr. Kathleen Huttlinger, Associate Director for Graduate Studies, 575-646-4387, Fax: 575-646-2167.
Website: http://schoolofnursing.nmsu.edu

New York University, College of Nursing, Doctor of Nursing Practice Program, New York, NY 10012-1019. Offers advanced practice nursing (DNP), including adult acute care, adult nurse practitioner/holistic nursing, adult nurse practitioner/palliative care nursing, adult primary care, adult primary care/geriatrics, family, geriatrics, mental health nursing, nurse-midwifery, pediatrics. Part-time and evening/weekend programs available. *Faculty:* 3 full-time (all women), 1 part-time/adjunct (0 women). *Students:* 1 (woman) full-time, 33 part-time (30 women); includes 7 minority (3 Black or African American, non-Hispanic/Latino; 3 Asian, non-Hispanic/Latino; 1 Hispanic/Latino). Average age 39. 18 applicants, 100% accepted, 12 enrolled. In 2013, 4 doctorates awarded. *Degree requirements:* For doctorate, thesis/dissertation, capstone. *Entrance requirements:* For doctorate, MAT or GRE (either taken within past 5 years), MS, RN license, interview, Nurse Practitioner Certification. Additional exam requirements/recommendations for international students: Required—TOEFL (minimum score 90 iBT), IELTS (minimum score 7). *Application deadline:* For fall admission, 3/1 for domestic students, 4/1 for international students. Applications are processed on a rolling basis. Application fee: $80. Electronic applications accepted. *Expenses: Tuition:* Full-time $35,856; part-time $1494 per unit. *Required fees:* $1408; $64 per unit. $473 per term. Tuition and fees vary according to course load and program. *Financial support:* Scholarships/grants available. Support available to part-time students. Financial award application deadline: 2/1. *Faculty research:* Geriatrics, HIV, elderly black diabetics, families and illness, oral systemic connection. *Unit head:* Dr. Rona Levin, Director, 212-998-5319, Fax: 212-995-3143, E-mail: rfl2039@nyu.edu. *Application contact:* Elizabeth Ensweiler, Assistant Director, Graduate Student Affairs and Admissions, 212-992-7653, Fax: 212-995-4302, E-mail: ee39@nyu.edu.

New York University, College of Nursing, Programs in Advanced Practice Nursing, New York, NY 10012-1019. Offers advanced practice nursing: adult acute care (MS, Advanced Certificate); advanced practice nursing: adult nurse practitioner/holistic nurse practitioner (Advanced Certificate); advanced practice nursing: adult nurse practitioner/palliative care nurse practitioner (Advanced Certificate); advanced practice nursing: adult primary care (MS, Advanced Certificate); advanced practice nursing: family (MS, Advanced Certificate); advanced practice nursing: geriatrics (Advanced Certificate); advanced practice nursing: mental health (MS); advanced practice nursing: mental health nursing (Advanced Certificate); advanced practice nursing: pediatrics (MS, Advanced Certificate); nurse midwifery (MS, Advanced Certificate); nursing administration (MS, Advanced Certificate); nursing education (MS, Advanced Certificate); nursing informatics (MS, Advanced Certificate); MS/MPA; MS/MPH. *Accreditation:* AACN; ACNM/ACME. Part-time programs available. *Faculty:* 22 full-time (all women), 54 part-time/adjunct (46 women). *Students:* 36 full-time (31 women), 622 part-time (549 women); includes 239 minority (73 Black or African American, non-Hispanic/Latino; 1 American Indian or Alaska Native, non-Hispanic/Latino; 116 Asian, non-Hispanic/Latino; 36 Hispanic/Latino; 6 Native Hawaiian or other Pacific Islander, non-Hispanic/Latino; 7 Two or more races, non-Hispanic/Latino), 16 international. Average age 37. 395 applicants, 67% accepted, 156 enrolled. In 2013, 186 master's, 8 other advanced degrees awarded. *Degree requirements:* For master's, thesis (for some programs). *Entrance requirements:* For master's, BS in nursing, AS in nursing with another BS/BA, interview, RN license, 1 year of clinical experience (3 for nursing education program); for Advanced Certificate, master's degree. Additional exam requirements/recommendations for international students: Required—TOEFL (minimum score 90 iBT), IELTS (minimum score 7). *Application deadline:* For fall admission, 7/1 for domestic and international students; for spring admission, 12/1 for domestic and international students. Application fee: $80. Electronic applications accepted. *Expenses: Tuition:* Full-time $35,856; part-time $1494 per unit. *Required fees:* $1408; $64 per unit. $473 per term. Tuition and fees vary according to course load and program. *Financial support:* In 2013–14, 182 students received support. Research assistantships, career-related internships or fieldwork, Federal Work-Study, scholarships/grants, traineeships, and unspecified assistantships available. Support available to part-time students. Financial award application deadline: 2/1; financial award applicants required to submit FAFSA. *Faculty research:* Geriatrics, HIV, elderly black diabetics, families and illness, oral systemic connection. *Unit head:* Dr. Judith Haber, Associate Dean, Graduate Programs, 212-998-9020, Fax: 212-995-3143, E-mail: jh33@nyu.edu. *Application contact:* Elizabeth Ensweiler, Assistant Director, Graduate Student Affairs and Admissions, 212-992-7653, Fax: 212-995-4302, E-mail: ee39@nyu.edu.

North Park University, School of Nursing, Chicago, IL 60625-4895. Offers advanced practice nursing (MS); leadership and management (MS); MBA/MS; MM/MSN; MS/MHR; MS/MNA. *Accreditation:* AACN. Part-time and evening/weekend programs available. *Degree requirements:* For master's, thesis. *Entrance requirements:* For master's, GMAT, MAT. *Faculty research:* Aging, consultation roles, critical thinking skills, family breakdown, science of caring.

Oakland University, Graduate Study and Lifelong Learning, School of Nursing, Program in Adult Health, Rochester, MI 48309-4401. Offers MSN. *Accreditation:* AACN. *Students:* 1 (woman) part-time; minority (Asian, non-Hispanic/Latino). Average age 43. *Degree requirements:* For master's, thesis (for some programs). *Entrance requirements:* For master's, GRE General Test, minimum GPA of 3.0. *Application deadline:* For fall admission, 8/1 for domestic students; for winter admission, 11/15 for domestic students. Applications are processed on a rolling basis. Application fee: $30. Electronic applications accepted. *Financial support:* Federal Work-Study, institutionally sponsored loans, and tuition waivers (full) available. Financial award application deadline: 3/1; financial award applicants required to submit FAFSA. *Unit head:* Dr. Linda Thompson, Dean, 248-370-4081, Fax: 248-370-4279. *Application contact:* Mary Bray, Graduate Program Coordinator, 248-370-4482.

Purdue University Calumet, Graduate Studies Office, School of Nursing, Hammond, IN 46323-2094. Offers adult health clinical nurse specialist (MS); critical care clinical nurse specialist (MS); family nurse practitioner (MS); nurse executive (MS). Part-time programs available. Postbaccalaureate distance learning degree programs offered (minimal on-campus study). *Entrance requirements:* For master's, BSN. Additional exam requirements/recommendations for international students: Required—TOEFL. Electronic applications accepted. *Faculty research:* Adult health, cardiovascular and pulmonary nursing.

Quinnipiac University, School of Nursing, Adult Nurse Practitioner Track, Hamden, CT 06518-1940. Offers MSN, DNP. Part-time programs available. *Faculty:* 14 full-time (13 women), 5 part-time/adjunct (3 women). *Students:* 25 full-time (23 women), 27 part-time (23 women); includes 12 minority (4 Black or African American, non-Hispanic/Latino; 5 Asian, non-Hispanic/Latino; 3 Hispanic/Latino), 1 international. 29 applicants, 76% accepted, 20 enrolled. In 2013, 25 master's awarded. *Degree requirements:* For master's, thesis optional, clinical practicum. *Entrance requirements:* For master's, RN license, minimum GPA of 3.0. Additional exam requirements/recommendations for international students: Required—TOEFL (minimum score 575 paper-based; 90 iBT), IELTS (minimum score 6.5). *Application deadline:* For fall admission, 6/1 priority date for domestic students, 4/30 for international students. Applications are processed on a rolling basis. Application fee: $45. Electronic applications accepted. *Expenses: Tuition:* Part-time $920 per credit. *Required fees:* $37 per credit. *Financial support:* In 2013–14, 3 students received support. Career-related internships or fieldwork, Federal Work-Study, scholarships/grants, tuition waivers (partial), and unspecified assistantships available. Support available to part-time students. Financial award application deadline: 6/1; financial award applicants required to submit FAFSA. *Unit head:* Dr. Lynn Price, Program Director, E-mail: lynn.price@quinnipiac.edu. *Application contact:* Office of

Adult Nursing

Graduate Admissions, 800-462-1944, Fax: 203-582-3443, E-mail: graduate@quinnipiac.edu.
Website: http://www.quinnipiac.edu/gradnursing

Research College of Nursing, Nursing Program, Kansas City, MO 64132. Offers adult-gerontological nurse practitioner (MSN); clinical nurse leader (MSN); executive practice and healthcare leadership (MSN); family nurse practitioner (MSN); nurse educator (MSN); nursing (MSN). *Accreditation:* AACN. Part-time programs available. Postbaccalaureate distance learning degree programs offered (no on-campus study). *Faculty:* 9 full-time (all women), 5 part-time/adjunct (2 women). *Students:* 19 full-time (18 women), 101 part-time (94 women). *Degree requirements:* For master's, research project. *Entrance requirements:* For master's, 3 letters of recommendation, official transcripts, resume. Additional exam requirements/recommendations for international students: Required—TOEFL (minimum score 550 paper-based), TWE. *Application deadline:* Applications are processed on a rolling basis. Application fee: $50. *Expenses: Tuition:* Part-time $445 per credit hour. *Required fees:* $25 per credit hour. Part-time tuition and fees vary according to course load. *Financial support:* Applicants required to submit FAFSA. *Unit head:* Dr. Nancy O. DeBasio, President and Dean, 816-995-2815, Fax: 816-995-2817, E-mail: nancy.debasio@researchcollege.edu. *Application contact:* Leslie Mendenhall, Director of Transfer and Graduate Recruitment, 816-995-2820, Fax: 816-995-2813, E-mail: leslie.mendenhall@researchcollege.edu.

Rush University, College of Nursing, Department of Adult Health and Gerontological Nursing, Chicago, IL 60612. Offers adult gerontology acute care clinical nurse specialist (DNP); adult gerontology acute care nurse practitioner (DNP); adult gerontology primary care clinical nurse specialist (DNP); adult gerontology primary care nurse practitioner (DNP); nurse anesthesia (DNP); nursing science (PhD); systems leadership (DNP). *Accreditation:* AACN; AANA/CANAEP (one or more programs are accredited). Part-time programs available. Postbaccalaureate distance learning degree programs offered (minimal on-campus study). *Students:* 89 full-time (69 women), 109 part-time (100 women); includes 40 minority (11 Black or African American, non-Hispanic/Latino; 1 American Indian or Alaska Native, non-Hispanic/Latino; 22 Asian, non-Hispanic/Latino; 5 Hispanic/Latino; 1 Native Hawaiian or other Pacific Islander, non-Hispanic/Latino). Average age 33. 170 applicants, 56% accepted, 78 enrolled. *Degree requirements:* For doctorate, capstone project (for DNP); dissertation (for PhD). *Entrance requirements:* For doctorate, GRE General Test (for DNP in nurse anesthesia; waived if cumulative GPA is 3.25 or greater, nursing GPA is 3.0 or greater, or a completed graduate program GPA is 3.5 or greater), interview, 3 letters of recommendation, personal statement, current resume. Additional exam requirements/recommendations for international students: Required—TOEFL. *Application deadline:* For fall admission, 1/2 for domestic students; for winter admission, 10/15 for domestic students; for spring admission, 8/1 for domestic students; for summer admission, 12/1 for domestic students. Applications are processed on a rolling basis. Application fee: $100. Electronic applications accepted. *Financial support:* Fellowships, research assistantships, teaching assistantships, Federal Work-Study, institutionally sponsored loans, scholarships/grants, traineeships, and health care benefits available. Support available to part-time students. Financial award application deadline: 3/1; financial award applicants required to submit FAFSA. *Faculty research:* Physical activity adherence in African-American women; reduction of health disparities; evidence-based interventions for caregivers; fish oil for HIV-related immunosenescence; BAILA: Being Active, Increasing Latinos Health Aging. *Total annual research expenditures:* $3.8 million. *Unit head:* Dr. Elizabeth Carlson, Chairperson, 312-942-7117, E-mail: elizabeth_carlson@rush.edu. *Application contact:* Jennifer Thorndyke, Admissions Specialist, 312-563-7526, E-mail: jennifer_thorndyke@rush.edu.
Website: http://www.rushu.rush.edu/servlet/Satellite?c=RushUnivLevel1Page&cid=1204497838852&pagename=Rush%2FRushUnivLevel1Page%2FLevel_1_College_Home_Page

Rutgers, The State University of New Jersey, Newark, Rutgers School of Nursing, Newark, NJ 07107-3001. Offers adult health (MSN); adult occupational health (MSN); advanced practice nursing (MSN, Post Master's Certificate); family nurse practitioner (MSN); nurse anesthesia (MSN); nursing (MSN); nursing informatics (MSN); urban health (PhD); women's health practitioner (MSN). *Accreditation:* AANA/CANAEP. Part-time programs available. *Entrance requirements:* For master's, GRE, RN license; basic life support, statistics, and health assessment experience. Additional exam requirements/recommendations for international students: Required—TOEFL. Electronic applications accepted. *Expenses:* Contact institution. *Faculty research:* HIV/AIDS, diabetes education, learned helplessness, nursing science, psychoeducation.

Sage Graduate School, School of Health Sciences, Department of Nursing, Program in Adult Health, Troy, NY 12180-4115. Offers MS, Post Master's Certificate. *Accreditation:* AACN. Part-time and evening/weekend programs available. *Faculty:* 5 full-time (all women), 9 part-time/adjunct (all women). *Students:* 5 full-time (all women), 13 part-time (all women); includes 1 minority (Asian, non-Hispanic/Latino), 2 international. Average age 38. 36 applicants, 39% accepted, 3 enrolled. In 2013, 15 master's, 8 other advanced degrees awarded. *Degree requirements:* For master's, thesis or alternative. *Entrance requirements:* For master's, BS in nursing, minimum GPA of 2.75, resume, 2 letters of recommendation. Additional exam requirements/recommendations for international students: Required—TOEFL (minimum score 550 paper-based). *Application deadline:* Applications are processed on a rolling basis. Application fee: $40. *Expenses: Tuition:* Full-time $11,880; part-time $660 per credit hour. *Financial support:* Fellowships, research assistantships, Federal Work-Study, scholarships/grants, and unspecified assistantships available. Support available to part-time students. Financial award application deadline: 3/1; financial award applicants required to submit FAFSA. *Unit head:* Dr. Esther Haskevitz, Dean, School of Health Sciences, 518-244-2296, Fax: 518-244-4571, E-mail: haskve@sage.edu. *Application contact:* Madeline Cafiero, Director of Graduate Programs in Nursing, 518-244-4574, Fax: 518-244-2009, E-mail: cafiem@sage.edu.

Sage Graduate School, School of Health Sciences, Department of Nursing, Program in Adult Nurse Practitioner, Troy, NY 12180-4115. Offers MS, Post Master's Certificate. *Accreditation:* AACN. Part-time and evening/weekend programs available. *Faculty:* 5 full-time (all women), 9 part-time/adjunct (all women). *Students:* 8 full-time (7 women), 44 part-time (36 women); includes 12 minority (6 Black or African American, non-Hispanic/Latino; 4 Asian, non-Hispanic/Latino; 2 Two or more races, non-Hispanic/Latino). Average age 39. 29 applicants, 41% accepted, 4 enrolled. In 2013, 14 master's awarded. *Degree requirements:* For master's, thesis or alternative. *Entrance requirements:* For master's, BS in nursing, minimum GPA of 2.75, resume, 2 letters of recommendation. Additional exam requirements/recommendations for international students: Required—TOEFL (minimum score 550 paper-based). *Application deadline:* Applications are processed on a rolling basis. Application fee: $40. *Expenses: Tuition:* Full-time $11,880; part-time $660 per credit hour. *Financial support:* Fellowships, research assistantships, Federal Work-Study, scholarships/grants, and unspecified assistantships available. Support available to part-time students. Financial award application deadline: 3/1; financial award applicants required to submit FAFSA. *Unit head:* Dr. Esther Haskevitz, Dean, School of Health Sciences, 518-244-2296, Fax: 518-244-4571, E-mail: haskve@sage.edu. *Application contact:* Madeline Cafiero, Director, 518-244-4574, Fax: 518-244-2009, E-mail: cafiem@sage.edu.

St. Catherine University, Graduate Programs, Program in Nursing, St. Paul, MN 55105. Offers adult gerontological nurse practitioner (MA); neonatal nurse practitioner (MA); nurse educator (MA); nursing (DNP); nursing: entry-level (MA); pediatric nurse practitioner (MA). Part-time and evening/weekend programs available. *Degree requirements:* For master's, thesis; for doctorate, portfolio, systems change project. *Entrance requirements:* For master's, GRE General Test, bachelor's degree in nursing, current nursing license, 2 years of recent clinical practice; for doctorate, master's degree in nursing, RN license, advanced nursing position. Additional exam requirements/recommendations for international students: Required—TOEFL (minimum score 600 paper-based; 100 iBT).

Saint Peter's University, School of Nursing, Nursing Program, Jersey City, NJ 07306-5997. Offers adult nurse practitioner (MSN, Certificate); advanced practice (DNP); case management (MSN, DNP). *Accreditation:* AACN. Part-time and evening/weekend programs available. *Entrance requirements:* Additional exam requirements/recommendations for international students: Required—TOEFL. Electronic applications accepted.

Seattle Pacific University, MS in Nursing Program, Seattle, WA 98119-1997. Offers administration (MSN); adult/gerontology nurse practitioner (MSN); clinical nurse specialist (MSN); family nurse practitioner (MSN, Certificate); informatics (MSN); nurse educator (MSN). *Accreditation:* AACN. Part-time programs available. *Students:* 9 full-time (7 women), 37 part-time (33 women); includes 8 minority (2 Black or African American, non-Hispanic/Latino; 5 Asian, non-Hispanic/Latino; 1 Hispanic/Latino), 1 international. Average age 41. 70 applicants, 30% accepted, 21 enrolled. In 2013, 27 master's awarded. *Degree requirements:* For master's, thesis. *Entrance requirements:* For master's, personal statement, transcripts, undergraduate nursing degree, proof of undergraduate statistics course with minimum GPA of 2.0, 2 recommendations. *Application deadline:* For fall admission, 1/15 priority date for domestic students; for spring admission, 1/15 for domestic students. Applications are processed on a rolling basis. Application fee: $50. Electronic applications accepted. *Expenses:* Contact institution. *Financial support:* Fellowships and scholarships/grants available. Financial award applicants required to submit FAFSA. *Unit head:* Dr. Susan Casey, Associate Dean, 206-281-2649, E-mail: caseys@spu.edu.
Website: http://www.spu.edu/depts/health-sciences/grad/index.asp

Seattle University, College of Nursing, Program in Advanced Practice Nursing Immersion, Seattle, WA 98122-1090. Offers adult/gerontological nurse practitioner (MSN); advanced community public health nursing (MSN); family nurse practitioner (MSN); family psychiatric mental health nurse practitioner (MSN); nurse midwifery (MSN). *Faculty:* 17 full-time (15 women), 9 part-time/adjunct (6 women). *Students:* 109 full-time (94 women), 6 part-time (5 women); includes 25 minority (3 Black or African American, non-Hispanic/Latino; 11 Asian, non-Hispanic/Latino; 2 Hispanic/Latino; 9 Two or more races, non-Hispanic/Latino). Average age 31. In 2013, 48 master's awarded. *Degree requirements:* For master's, thesis or scholarly project. *Entrance requirements:* For master's, GRE, bachelor's degree, minimum GPA of 3.0, professional resume, two recommendations, letter of intent. Additional exam requirements/recommendations for international students: Required—TOEFL (minimum score 92 iBT), IELTS. *Application deadline:* For fall admission, 12/1 for domestic and international students. Application fee: $55. Electronic applications accepted. *Financial support:* In 2013–14, 3 students received support. Scholarships/grants and traineeships available. Financial award applicants required to submit FAFSA. *Unit head:* Dr. Janiece DeSocio, Interim Dean, 206-296-5660, E-mail: desocioj@seattleu.edu. *Application contact:* Janet Shandley, Associate Dean of Graduate Admissions, 206-296-5900, Fax: 206-298-5656, E-mail: grad_admissions@seattleu.edu.
Website: http://www.seattleu.edu/nursing/msn/apni/

Seattle University, College of Nursing, Program in Nursing, Seattle, WA 98122-1090. Offers adult/gerontological nurse practitioner (MSN); advanced community public health (MSN); psychiatric mental health nurse practitioner (MSN). *Students:* 11 full-time (10 women), 4 part-time (all women); includes 2 minority (both Hispanic/Latino). Average age 36. 39 applicants, 36% accepted, 8 enrolled. In 2013, 7 master's awarded. *Degree requirements:* For master's, thesis or scholarly project. *Entrance requirements:* For master's, GRE, bachelor's degree in nursing or associate degree in nursing with baccalaureate in different major, 5-quarter statistics course, minimum cumulative GPA of 3.0, professional resume, two recommendations, letter of intent, copy of current RN license or ability to obtain RN license in WA state. Additional exam requirements/recommendations for international students: Required—TOEFL (minimum score 92 iBT), IELTS. *Application deadline:* For fall admission, 12/1 for domestic and international students. Application fee: $55. Electronic applications accepted. *Financial support:* In 2013–14, 1 student received support, including 2 teaching assistantships; scholarships/grants and traineeships also available. Financial award applicants required to submit FAFSA. *Unit head:* Dr. Azita Emami, Dean, 206-296-5660. *Application contact:* Janet Shandley, Associate Dean of Graduate Admissions, 206-296-5900, Fax: 206-298-5656, E-mail: grad_admissions@seattleu.edu.
Website: https://www.seattleu.edu/nursing/msn/

Seton Hall University, College of Nursing, South Orange, NJ 07079-2697. Offers advanced practice in primary health care (MSN, DNP), including adult/gerontological nurse practitioner, pediatric nurse practitioner; entry into practice (MSN); health systems administration (MSN, DNP); nursing (PhD); nursing case management (MSN); nursing education (MA); school nurse (MSN); MSN/MA. *Accreditation:* AACN. Part-time programs available. Postbaccalaureate distance learning degree programs offered (minimal on-campus study). *Degree requirements:* For master's, research project; for doctorate, dissertation or scholarly project. *Entrance requirements:* For doctorate, GRE (waived for students with GPA of 3.5 or higher). Additional exam requirements/recommendations for international students: Required—TOEFL. Electronic applications accepted. *Faculty research:* Parent/child, adult, and gerontological nursing; breast cancer; families of children with HIV; parish nursing.

Southeastern Louisiana University, College of Nursing and Health Sciences, School of Nursing, Hammond, LA 70402. Offers adult psychiatric/mental health nurse practitioner/clinical nurse specialist (MSN); education (MSN); nurse executive (MSN); nurse practice (DNP); nurse practitioner (MSN). *Accreditation:* AACN. Part-time and evening/weekend programs available. *Faculty:* 14 full-time (13 women), 5 part-time/adjunct (4 women). *Students:* 21 full-time (19 women), 138 part-time (121 women); includes 27 minority (17 Black or African American, non-Hispanic/Latino; 4 Asian, non-Hispanic/Latino; 5 Hispanic/Latino; 1 Two or more races, non-Hispanic/Latino). Average age 34. 72 applicants, 68% accepted, 19 enrolled. In 2013, 29 master's awarded. *Degree requirements:* For master's, thesis. *Entrance requirements:* For master's, GRE (verbal and quantitative), baccalaureate degree in nursing from accredited undergraduate nursing program; minimum GPA of 2.7; all transcripts from undergraduate school and any work attempted at the graduate level; curriculum vitae; valid Louisiana Registered Nurse license; letters of recommendation; letter of intent/statement of purpose. Additional exam requirements/recommendations for international students: Required—TOEFL (minimum score 500 paper-based; 61 iBT). *Application deadline:* For fall admission, 7/15 priority date for domestic students, 6/1 priority date for international students; for spring admission, 12/1 priority date for domestic students, 10/1 priority date for international students. Applications are processed on a rolling basis.

Application fee: $20 ($30 for international students). Electronic applications accepted. *Expenses:* Tuition, state resident: full-time $5047. Tuition, nonresident: full-time $17,066. *Required fees:* $1213. Tuition and fees vary according to degree level. *Financial support:* Federal Work-Study, institutionally sponsored loans, scholarships/grants, traineeships, and unspecified assistantships available. Support available to part-time students. Financial award application deadline: 5/1; financial award applicants required to submit FAFSA. *Faculty research:* Gender issues, LGBT issues, occupational health/safety, accelerated students, caring development. *Total annual research expenditures:* $103,409. *Unit head:* Dr. Lorinda J. Sealey, Graduate Nursing Program Director, 985-549-5045, Fax: 985-549-5087, E-mail: vjohnson@selu.edu. *Application contact:* Sandra Meyers, Graduate Admissions Analyst, 985-549-5620, Fax: 985-549-5632, E-mail: admissions@selu.edu.
Website: http://www.selu.edu/acad_research/depts/nurs

Southern Adventist University, School of Nursing, Collegedale, TN 37315-0370. Offers acute care nurse practitioner (MSN); adult nurse practitioner (MSN); family nurse practitioner (MSN); nurse educator (MSN); MSN/MSBA. Part-time programs available. *Degree requirements:* For master's, thesis or project. *Entrance requirements:* For master's, RN license. Additional exam requirements/recommendations for international students: Required—TOEFL (minimum score 600 paper-based). Electronic applications accepted. *Faculty research:* Pain management, ethics, corporate wellness, caring spirituality, stress.

South University, Program in Nursing, Tampa, FL 33614. Offers adult health nurse practitioner (MS); family nurse practitioner (MS); nurse educator (MS).

Spalding University, Graduate Studies, Kosair College of Health and Natural Sciences, School of Nursing, Louisville, KY 40203-2188. Offers adult nurse practitioner (MSN, PMC); family nurse practitioner (MSN, PMC); leadership in nursing and healthcare (MSN, PMC); pediatric nurse practitioner (MSN, PMC). *Accreditation:* AACN. Part-time and evening/weekend programs available. *Faculty:* 6 full-time (all women), 6 part-time/adjunct (5 women). *Students:* 98 full-time (85 women), 13 part-time (all women); includes 23 minority (19 Black or African American, non-Hispanic/Latino; 2 Asian, non-Hispanic/Latino; 1 Hispanic/Latino; 1 Two or more races, non-Hispanic/Latino). Average age 36. 136 applicants, 31% accepted, 39 enrolled. In 2013, 48 master's, 5 other advanced degrees awarded. *Degree requirements:* For master's, comprehensive exam (for some programs), thesis. *Entrance requirements:* For master's, GRE General Test, BSN or bachelor's degree, RN licensure, autobiographical statement, transcripts, letters of recommendation. Additional exam requirements/recommendations for international students: Required—TOEFL (minimum score 535 paper-based). *Application deadline:* For fall admission, 2/1 priority date for domestic students. Application fee: $30. *Expenses: Tuition:* Full-time $21,450. *Required fees:* $810. Tuition and fees vary according to course load, degree level, program and student level. *Financial support:* Career-related internships or fieldwork, scholarships/grants, and traineeships available. Support available to part-time students. Financial award application deadline: 3/30; financial award applicants required to submit FAFSA. *Faculty research:* Nurse educational administration, gerontology, bioterrorism, healthcare ethics, leadership. *Unit head:* Dr. Paula Travis, Chair, 502-873-4298, E-mail: clewis@spalding.edu. *Application contact:* Dr. Pam King, Assistant Professor, 502-873-4292, E-mail: pking@spalding.edu.
Website: http://www.spalding.edu/nursing/

Stony Brook University, State University of New York, Stony Brook University Medical Center, Health Sciences Center, School of Nursing, Program in Adult Health/Primary Care Nursing, Stony Brook, NY 11794. Offers adult health nurse practitioner (Certificate); adult health/primary care nursing (MS, DNP). *Accreditation:* AACN. Postbaccalaureate distance learning degree programs offered. *Students:* 3 full-time (2 women), 290 part-time (258 women); includes 90 minority (31 Black or African American, non-Hispanic/Latino; 37 Asian, non-Hispanic/Latino; 18 Hispanic/Latino; 4 Two or more races, non-Hispanic/Latino), 3 international. In 2013, 83 master's, 3 other advanced degrees awarded. *Degree requirements:* For master's, thesis. *Entrance requirements:* For master's, BSN, minimum GPA of 3.0, course work in statistics. Additional exam requirements/recommendations for international students: Required—TOEFL. *Application deadline:* For fall admission, 1/15 for domestic students. Application fee: $100. *Expenses:* Tuition, state resident: full-time $9870; part-time $411 per credit. Tuition, nonresident: full-time $18,350; part-time $765 per credit. *Financial support:* Application deadline: 3/15. *Unit head:* Dr. Diane K. Pastor, Chair, 631-444-6190, Fax: 631-444-3136, E-mail: diane.pastor@stonybrook.edu. *Application contact:* Dolores C. Bilges, Senior Staff Assistant, 631-444-2644, Fax: 631-444-3136, E-mail: dolores.bilges@stonybrook.edu.
Website: http://www.nursing.stonybrookmedicine.edu/about

Temple University, College of Health Professions and Social Work, Department of Nursing, Philadelphia, PA 19140. Offers adult-gerontology primary care (DNP); clinical nurse leader (MSN); family-individual across the lifespan (DNP); nurse educator (MSN); nursing (MSN, DNP). *Accreditation:* AACN. Part-time programs available. *Faculty:* 9 full-time (8 women), 3 part-time/adjunct (all women). *Students:* 6 full-time (5 women), 92 part-time (78 women); includes 51 minority (34 Black or African American, non-Hispanic/Latino; 9 Asian, non-Hispanic/Latino; 8 Hispanic/Latino), 1 international. 48 applicants, 58% accepted, 23 enrolled. In 2013, 12 master's, 9 doctorates awarded. *Degree requirements:* For master's and doctorate, evidence based practice project. *Entrance requirements:* For master's and doctorate, GRE General Test or MAT, 2 letters of reference, RN license, interview, statement of purpose, resume. Additional exam requirements/recommendations for international students: Required—TOEFL (minimum score 550 paper-based; 79 iBT). *Application deadline:* For fall admission, 2/15 priority date for domestic students, 1/15 for international students; for spring admission, 10/15 for domestic students, 9/15 for international students. Applications are processed on a rolling basis. Application fee: $60. Electronic applications accepted. *Financial support:* Federal Work-Study, scholarships/grants, traineeships, and tuition waivers available. Support available to part-time students. Financial award application deadline: 1/15. *Faculty research:* Health promotion, chronic illness, family support systems, primary care, health policy, community health services, evidence-based practice. *Total annual research expenditures:* $741,567. *Unit head:* Dr. Jane Kurz, RN, Chair, 215-707-8327, E-mail: jane.kurz@temple.edu. *Application contact:* Naseem Lodhi, Student Services Coordinator, 215-204-4618, E-mail: tunurse@temple.edu.

Texas Christian University, Harris College of Nursing and Health Sciences, Program in Nursing, Fort Worth, TX 76129-0002. Offers advanced practice registered nurse (DNP); clinical nurse leader (MSN); clinical nurse specialist: adult/gerontology nursing (MSN); clinical nurse specialist: pediatric nursing (MSN); nursing administration (DNP); nursing education (MSN). *Accreditation:* AACN; AANA/CANAEP (one or more programs are accredited). Part-time programs available. Postbaccalaureate distance learning degree programs offered (no on-campus study). *Faculty:* 18 full-time (16 women), 1 (woman) part-time/adjunct. *Students:* 44 full-time (35 women), 46 part-time (42 women); includes 8 minority (3 Black or African American, non-Hispanic/Latino; 2 Asian, non-Hispanic/Latino; 3 Hispanic/Latino), 1 international. Average age 43. 72 applicants, 63% accepted, 36 enrolled. In 2013, 19 master's, 17 doctorates awarded. *Degree requirements:* For master's, professional project; for doctorate, capstone project. *Entrance requirements:* For master's, GRE General Test, 3 letters of reference, essay, resume, two official transcripts from every institution attended; for doctorate, APRN recognition (national certification) or master's and experience in nursing administration; 3 letters of reference; essay; resume; two official transcripts from every institution attended. Additional exam requirements/recommendations for international students: Recommended—TOEFL. *Application deadline:* For fall admission, 4/1 for domestic students; for spring admission, 9/1 for domestic students; for summer admission, 2/1 for domestic students. Applications are processed on a rolling basis. Application fee: $60. Electronic applications accepted. *Expenses: Tuition:* Part-time $1270 per credit hour. Tuition and fees vary according to course load and program. *Financial support:* In 2013–14, 4 teaching assistantships (averaging $2,500 per year) were awarded. Financial award applicants required to submit FAFSA. *Unit head:* Dr. Kathy A. Baker, Director, Division of Nursing Graduate Studies and Scholarship, 817-257-6726, Fax: 817-257-8383, E-mail: kathy.baker@tcu.edu. *Application contact:* Mary Jane Allred, Administrative Program Specialist, 817-257-6726, Fax: 817-257-8383, E-mail: m.allred@tcu.edu.
Website: http://www.nursing.tcu.edu/graduate.asp

Texas Woman's University, Graduate School, College of Nursing, Denton, TX 76201. Offers acute care nurse practitioner (MS); adult health clinical nurse specialist (MS); adult health nurse practitioner (MS); child health clinical nurse specialist (MS); clinical nurse leader (MS); family nurse practitioner (MS); health systems management (MS); nursing education (MS); nursing practice (DNP); nursing science (PhD); pediatric nurse practitioner (MS); women's health clinical nurse specialist (MS); women's health nurse practitioner (MS). *Accreditation:* AACN. Part-time programs available. Postbaccalaureate distance learning degree programs offered. *Faculty:* 60 full-time (59 women), 46 part-time/adjunct (39 women). *Students:* 54 full-time (49 women), 910 part-time (848 women); includes 489 minority (221 Black or African American, non-Hispanic/Latino; 11 American Indian or Alaska Native, non-Hispanic/Latino; 184 Asian, non-Hispanic/Latino; 70 Hispanic/Latino; 3 Native Hawaiian or other Pacific Islander, non-Hispanic/Latino), 16 international. Average age 38. 430 applicants, 65% accepted, 193 enrolled. In 2013, 258 master's, 22 doctorates awarded. *Degree requirements:* For master's, comprehensive exam, thesis or alternative; for doctorate, comprehensive exam, thesis/dissertation. *Entrance requirements:* For master's, GRE or MAT, minimum GPA of 3.0 on last 60 hours in undergraduate nursing degree and overall, RN license, BS in nursing, basic statistics course; for doctorate, GRE (preferred minimum score 153 [500 old version] Verbal, 144 [500 old version] Quantitative, 4 Analytical), MS in nursing, minimum preferred GPA of 3.5, RN license, statistics, 2 letters of reference, curriculum vitae, graduate nursing-theory course, graduate research course, statement of professional goals and research interests. Additional exam requirements/recommendations for international students: Required—TOEFL (minimum score 550 paper-based; 79 iBT). *Application deadline:* For fall admission, 5/1 priority date for domestic students, 3/1 for international students; for spring admission, 9/15 priority date for domestic students, 7/1 for international students. Applications are processed on a rolling basis. Application fee: $50 ($75 for international students). Electronic applications accepted. *Expenses:* Tuition, state resident: full-time $4182; part-time $233.32 per credit hour. Tuition, nonresident: full-time $10,716; part-time $595.32 per credit hour. *Financial support:* In 2013–14, 149 students received support, including 10 research assistantships (averaging $5,600 per year), 1 teaching assistantship (averaging $5,600 per year); career-related internships or fieldwork, Federal Work-Study, institutionally sponsored loans, scholarships/grants, traineeships, health care benefits, and unspecified assistantships also available. Support available to part-time students. Financial award application deadline: 3/1; financial award applicants required to submit FAFSA. *Faculty research:* Screening, prevention, and treatment for intimate partner violence; needs of adolescents during childbirth intervention; a network analysis decision tool for nurse managers (social network analysis); support for adolescents with implantable cardioverter defibrillators; informatics: nurse staffing, safety, quality, and financial data as they relate to patient care outcomes; prevention and treatment of obesity; improving infant outcomes related to premature birth. *Total annual research expenditures:* $1.7 million. *Unit head:* Dr. Gayle Roux, Interim Dean and Associate Dean for Research and Clinical Scholarship, 940-898-2401, Fax: 940-898-2437, E-mail: nursing@twu.edu. *Application contact:* Dr. Samuel Wheeler, Assistant Director of Admissions, 940-898-3188, Fax: 940-898-3081, E-mail: wheelersr@twu.edu.
Website: http://www.twu.edu/nursing/

Troy University, Graduate School, College of Health and Human Services, Program in Nursing, Troy, AL 36082. Offers adult health (MSN); clinical nurse specialist adult health (DNP); clinical nurse specialist maternal infant (DNP); family nurse practitioner (MSN, DNP, PMC); informatics specialist (MSN); maternal infant (MSN). Part-time and evening/weekend programs available. *Faculty:* 15 full-time (8 women), 3 part-time/adjunct (1 woman). *Students:* 61 full-time (56 women), 228 part-time (193 women); includes 97 minority (77 Black or African American, non-Hispanic/Latino; 4 American Indian or Alaska Native, non-Hispanic/Latino; 2 Asian, non-Hispanic/Latino; 5 Hispanic/Latino; 9 Two or more races, non-Hispanic/Latino). Average age 34. 138 applicants, 80% accepted, 39 enrolled. In 2013, 81 master's, 9 doctorates awarded. *Degree requirements:* For master's, comprehensive exam, minimum GPA of 3.0, candidacy; for doctorate, minimum GPA of 3.0, submission of approved comprehensive e-portfolio, completion of residency synthesis project, minimum of 1000 hours of clinical practice, score of 80% or better on qualifying exam. *Entrance requirements:* For master's, GRE (minimum score of 850 on old exam or 294 on new exam) or GMAT (minimum score of 500), minimum GPA of 3.0, BSN, current RN licensure; 2 letters of reference, undergraduate health assessment course; for doctorate, GRE (minimum score of 850 on old exam or 294 on new exam) or GMAT (minimum score of 500), BSN or MSN, minimum GPA of 3.0, 2 letters of reference, current RN licensure, essay. Additional exam requirements/recommendations for international students: Required—TOEFL (minimum score 523 paper-based; 70 iBT), IELTS (minimum score 6). *Application deadline:* Applications are processed on a rolling basis. Application fee: $50. Electronic applications accepted. *Expenses:* Tuition, state resident: full-time $6084; part-time $338 per credit hour. Tuition, nonresident: full-time $12,168; part-time $676 per credit hour. *Required fees:* $630; $35 per credit hour. $50 per semester. *Financial support:* Available to part-time students. Applicants required to submit FAFSA. *Unit head:* Dr. Diane Weed, Director, School of Nursing, 334-670-5864, Fax: 334-670-3745, E-mail: lweed@troy.edu. *Application contact:* Brenda K. Campbell, Director of Graduate Admissions, 334-670-3178, Fax: 334-670-3733, E-mail: bcamp@troy.edu.

Universidad del Turabo, Graduate Programs, School of Health Sciences, Programs in Nursing, Program in Family Nurse Practitioner - Adult Nursing, Gurabo, PR 00778-3030. Offers MSN, Certificate.

University at Buffalo, the State University of New York, Graduate School, School of Nursing, Buffalo, NY 14214. Offers adult gerontology nurse practitioner (DNP); family nurse practitioner (DNP); health care systems and leadership (MS); nurse anesthetist (DNP); nursing (PhD); nursing education (Certificate); psychiatric/mental health nurse practitioner (DNP). *Accreditation:* AACN; AANA/CANAEP (one or more programs are accredited). Part-time programs available. Postbaccalaureate distance learning degree programs offered (no on-campus study). *Faculty:* 24 full-time (21 women), 2 part-time/adjunct (1 woman). *Students:* 80 full-time (60 women), 97 part-time (84 women); includes 35 minority (20 Black or African American, non-Hispanic/Latino; 2 American Indian or Alaska Native, non-Hispanic/Latino; 9 Asian, non-Hispanic/Latino; 1 Hispanic/Latino; 3 Native Hawaiian or other Pacific Islander, non-Hispanic/Latino). 118

applicants, 67% accepted, 58 enrolled. In 2013, 41 master's, 15 doctorates awarded. *Degree requirements:* For master's, thesis optional; for doctorate, comprehensive exam (for some programs), capstone (for DNP), dissertation (for PhD). *Entrance requirements:* For doctorate, GRE or MAT, minimum GPA of 3.0 (3.25 for PhD), RN license, BS or MS in nursing, 3 references, writing sample; for Certificate, interview, minimum GPA of 3.0 or GRE General Test, RN license, MS in nursing. Additional exam requirements/recommendations for international students: Required—TOEFL (minimum score 550 paper-based; 79 iBT), IELTS (minimum score 6.5). *Application deadline:* For fall admission, 7/1 for domestic students, 4/1 for international students; for spring admission, 12/1 for domestic students, 10/1 for international students; for summer admission, 4/1 for domestic students. Application fee: $75. Electronic applications accepted. *Financial support:* In 2013–14, 80 students received support, including 2 fellowships with full and partial tuition reimbursements available (averaging $17,000 per year), 7 research assistantships with full and partial tuition reimbursements available (averaging $10,600 per year), 7 teaching assistantships with full and partial tuition reimbursements available (averaging $10,600 per year); scholarships/grants, traineeships, health care benefits, and unspecified assistantships also available. Financial award application deadline: 3/15; financial award applicants required to submit FAFSA. *Faculty research:* Oncology, palliative care, gerontology, addictions, mental health, community wellness, sleep, workforce, care of underserved populations, quality and safety, person-centered care, adolescent health. *Total annual research expenditures:* $1.1 million. *Unit head:* Dr. Marsha L. Lewis, Dean and Professor, 716-829-2533, Fax: 716-829-2566, E-mail: ubnursingdean@buffalo.edu. *Application contact:* Dr. David J. Lang, Director of Student Affairs, 716-829-2537, Fax: 716-829-2067, E-mail: nursing@buffalo.edu.
Website: http://nursing.buffalo.edu/

University of Central Arkansas, Graduate School, College of Health and Behavioral Sciences, Department of Nursing, Conway, AR 72035-0001. Offers adult nurse practitioner (PMC); clinical nurse leader (PMC); clinical nurse specialist (MSN); family nurse practitioner (PMC); nurse educator (PMC); nurse practitioner (MSN). *Accreditation:* AACN. Part-time and evening/weekend programs available. Postbaccalaureate distance learning degree programs offered (minimal on-campus study). *Degree requirements:* For master's, comprehensive exam, thesis optional, clinicals. *Entrance requirements:* For master's, GRE General Test, minimum GPA of 2.7. Additional exam requirements/recommendations for international students: Required—TOEFL (minimum score 550 paper-based; 80 iBT). Electronic applications accepted. *Expenses:* Contact institution.

University of Central Florida, College of Nursing, Orlando, FL 32816. Offers adult-gerontology nurse practitioner (Post-Master's Certificate); family nurse practitioner (Post-Master's Certificate); nursing (MSN, PhD); nursing education (Post-Master's Certificate); nursing practice (DNP). *Accreditation:* AACN. Part-time and evening/weekend programs available. *Faculty:* 47 full-time (41 women), 78 part-time/adjunct (75 women). *Students:* 54 full-time (49 women), 264 part-time (239 women); includes 72 minority (35 Black or African American, non-Hispanic/Latino; 7 Asian, non-Hispanic/Latino; 25 Hispanic/Latino; 1 Native Hawaiian or other Pacific Islander, non-Hispanic/Latino; 4 Two or more races, non-Hispanic/Latino), 1 international. Average age 39. 179 applicants, 55% accepted, 71 enrolled. In 2013, 96 master's, 12 doctorates, 3 other advanced degrees awarded. *Degree requirements:* For master's, thesis or alternative. *Entrance requirements:* For master's, GRE General Test, minimum GPA of 3.0 in last 60 hours. Additional exam requirements/recommendations for international students: Required—TOEFL. *Application deadline:* For fall admission, 2/15 for domestic students; for spring admission, 9/15 for domestic students. Application fee: $30. Electronic applications accepted. *Financial support:* In 2013–14, 2 students received support, including 3 teaching assistantships with partial tuition reimbursements available (averaging $6,300 per year); fellowships with partial tuition reimbursements available, research assistantships with partial tuition reimbursements available, career-related internships or fieldwork, Federal Work-Study, institutionally sponsored loans, traineeships, and unspecified assistantships also available. Financial award application deadline: 3/1; financial award applicants required to submit FAFSA. *Unit head:* Dr. Mary Lou Sole, Interim Dean, 407-823-5496, Fax: 407-823-5675, E-mail: mary.sole@ucf.edu. *Application contact:* Barbara Rodriguez Lamas, Director, Admissions and Student Services, 407-823-2766, Fax: 407-823-6442, E-mail: gradadmissions@ucf.edu.
Website: http://nursing.ucf.edu/

University of Cincinnati, Graduate School, College of Nursing, Cincinnati, OH 45221-0038. Offers clinical nurse specialist (MSN), including adult health, community health, neonatal, nursing administration, occupational health, pediatric health, psychiatric nursing, women's health; nurse anesthesia (MSN); nurse midwifery (MSN); nurse practitioner (MSN), including acute care, ambulatory care, family, family/psychiatric, women's health; nursing (PhD); MBA/MSN. *Accreditation:* AACN; AANA/CANAEP (one or more programs are accredited); ACNM/ACME. Part-time programs available. Postbaccalaureate distance learning degree programs offered (no on-campus study). Terminal master's awarded for partial completion of doctoral program. *Degree requirements:* For master's, thesis or alternative; for doctorate, comprehensive exam, thesis/dissertation. *Entrance requirements:* For master's and doctorate, GRE General Test. Additional exam requirements/recommendations for international students: Required—TOEFL (minimum score 520 paper-based). Electronic applications accepted. *Faculty research:* Substance abuse, injury and violence, symptom management.

University of Colorado Colorado Springs, Beth-El College of Nursing and Health Sciences, Colorado Springs, CO 80933-7150. Offers nursing education (MSN); nursing practice (DNP); primary care nurse practitioner (MSN). *Accreditation:* AACN. Part-time programs available. Postbaccalaureate distance learning degree programs offered (minimal on-campus study). *Faculty:* 5 full-time (all women), 1 part-time/adjunct (0 women). *Students:* 14 full-time (13 women), 160 part-time (149 women); includes 32 minority (2 Black or African American, non-Hispanic/Latino; 2 American Indian or Alaska Native, non-Hispanic/Latino; 5 Asian, non-Hispanic/Latino; 21 Hispanic/Latino; 2 Two or more races, non-Hispanic/Latino). Average age 37. 125 applicants, 38% accepted, 42 enrolled. In 2013, 31 master's, 3 doctorates awarded. *Degree requirements:* For master's, comprehensive exam, thesis optional; for doctorate, capstone project. *Entrance requirements:* For master's, GRE General Test or MAT, BSN, minimum GPA of 3.0, unrestricted RN license; for doctorate, interview; active RN license; MA; minimum GPA of 3.3; National Certification as nurse practitioner or clinical nurse specialist; portfolio. Additional exam requirements/recommendations for international students: Required—TOEFL. *Application deadline:* For fall admission, 6/15 priority date for domestic students, 6/15 for international students; for spring admission, 9/15 for domestic and international students. Application fee: $60 ($75 for international students). Electronic applications accepted. *Expenses:* Contact institution. *Financial support:* In 2013–14, 17 students received support, including 17 fellowships (averaging $2,500 per year); career-related internships or fieldwork, Federal Work-Study, and scholarships/grants also available. Support available to part-time students. Financial award application deadline: 3/1; financial award applicants required to submit FAFSA. *Faculty research:* Women's health, uncertainty, empowerment, family experience in chronic illness. *Total annual research expenditures:* $2,568. *Unit head:* Dr. Amy Silva-Smith, Graduate Department Chairperson, 719-255-4490, Fax: 719-255-4416, E-mail: asilvasm@uccs.edu. *Application contact:* Diane Busch, Director, 719-255-4424, Fax: 719-255-4416, E-mail: dbusch@uccs.edu.
Website: http://www.uccs.edu/~bethel/

University of Colorado Denver, College of Nursing, Aurora, CO 80045. Offers adult clinical nurse specialist (MS); adult nurse practitioner (MS); family nurse practitioner (MS); family psychiatric mental health nurse practitioner (MS); health care informatics (MS); nurse-midwifery (MS); nursing (DNP, PhD); nursing leadership and health care systems (MS); pediatric nurse practitioner (MS); special studies (MS); women's health (MS); MS/PhD. *Accreditation:* ACNM/ACME (one or more programs are accredited). Part-time and evening/weekend programs available. Postbaccalaureate distance learning degree programs offered (minimal on-campus study). *Faculty:* 74 full-time (65 women), 58 part-time/adjunct (56 women). *Students:* 351 full-time (327 women), 138 part-time (125 women); includes 79 minority (12 Black or African American, non-Hispanic/Latino; 9 American Indian or Alaska Native, non-Hispanic/Latino; 13 Asian, non-Hispanic/Latino; 32 Hispanic/Latino; 2 Native Hawaiian or other Pacific Islander, non-Hispanic/Latino; 11 Two or more races, non-Hispanic/Latino), 7 international. Average age 33. 354 applicants, 43% accepted, 109 enrolled. In 2013, 108 master's, 28 doctorates awarded. Terminal master's awarded for partial completion of doctoral program. *Degree requirements:* For master's, thesis optional; for doctorate, comprehensive exam, thesis/dissertation, 42 credits of coursework. *Entrance requirements:* For master's, GRE if cumulative undergraduate GPA is less than 3.0, undergraduate nursing degree from NLNAC- or CCNE-accredited school or university; completion of research and statistics courses with minimum grade of C; copy of current and unencumbered nursing license; for doctorate, GRE, bachelor's and/or master's degrees in nursing from NLN- or CCNE-accredited institution; portfolio; minimum undergraduate GPA of 3.0, graduate 3.5; graduate-level intermediate statistics and master's-level nursing theory courses with minimum B grade; interview. Additional exam requirements/recommendations for international students: Required—TOEFL (minimum score 560 paper-based; 83 iBT). *Application deadline:* For fall admission, 2/15 for domestic students, 1/15 for international students; for spring admission, 7/1 for domestic students, 6/1 for international students. Application fee: $50 ($75 for international students). Electronic applications accepted. *Expenses:* Contact institution. *Financial support:* In 2013–14, 113 students received support. Fellowships, research assistantships, teaching assistantships, Federal Work-Study, institutionally sponsored loans, scholarships/grants, traineeships, and unspecified assistantships available. Support available to part-time students. Financial award application deadline: 4/1; financial award applicants required to submit FAFSA. *Faculty research:* Biological and behavioral phenomena in pregnancy and postpartum; patterns of glycemia during the insulin resistance of pregnancy; obesity, gestational diabetes, and relationship to neonatal adiposity; men's awareness and knowledge of male breast cancer; cognitive-behavioral therapy for chronic insomnia after breast cancer treatment; massage therapy for the treatment of tension-type headaches. *Total annual research expenditures:* $5.9 million. *Unit head:* Dr. Sarah Thompson, Dean, 303-724-1679, E-mail: sarah.a.thompson@ucdenver.edu. *Application contact:* Judy Campbell, Graduate Programs Coordinator, 303-724-8503, E-mail: judy.campbell@ucdenver.edu.
Website: http://www.ucdenver.edu/academics/colleges/nursing/Pages/default.aspx

University of Delaware, College of Health Sciences, School of Nursing, Newark, DE 19716. Offers adult nurse practitioner (MSN, PMC); cardiopulmonary clinical nurse specialist (MSN, PMC); cardiopulmonary clinical nurse specialist/adult nurse practitioner (MSN, PMC); family nurse practitioner (MSN, PMC); gerontology clinical nurse specialist (MSN, PMC); gerontology clinical nurse specialist geriatric nurse practitioner (PMC); gerontology clinical nurse specialist/geriatric nurse practitioner (MSN); health services administration (MSN, PMC); nursing of children clinical nurse specialist (MSN, PMC); nursing of children clinical nurse specialist/pediatric nurse practitioner (MSN, PMC); oncology/immune deficiency clinical nurse specialist (MSN, PMC); oncology/immune deficiency clinical nurse specialist/adult nurse practitioner (MSN, PMC); perinatal/women's health clinical nurse specialist (MSN, PMC); perinatal/women's health clinical nurse specialist/women's health nurse practitioner (MSN, PMC); psychiatric nursing clinical nurse specialist (MSN, PMC). *Accreditation:* AACN. Part-time and evening/weekend programs available. Postbaccalaureate distance learning degree programs offered (minimal on-campus study). *Degree requirements:* For master's, thesis optional. *Entrance requirements:* For master's, BSN, interview, RN license. Electronic applications accepted. *Faculty research:* Marriage and chronic illness, health promotion, congestive heart failure patient outcomes, school nursing, diabetes in children, culture, health disparities, cardiovascular, prison nursing, oncology, public policy, child obesity, smoking and teen pregnancy, blood pressure measurements, men's health.

University of Hawaii at Manoa, Graduate Division, School of Nursing and Dental Hygiene, Honolulu, HI 96822. Offers clinical nurse specialist (MS), including adult health, community mental health; nurse practitioner (MS), including adult health, community mental health, family nurse practitioner; nursing (PhD, Graduate Certificate); nursing administration (MS). *Accreditation:* AACN. Part-time programs available. Postbaccalaureate distance learning degree programs offered (minimal on-campus study). *Degree requirements:* For master's, thesis optional; for doctorate, comprehensive exam, thesis/dissertation. *Entrance requirements:* For master's, Hawaii RN license. Additional exam requirements/recommendations for international students: Required—TOEFL (minimum score 580 paper-based; 92 iBT), IELTS (minimum score 5). *Expenses:* Contact institution.

University of Illinois at Chicago, Graduate College, College of Nursing, Program in Nursing, Chicago, IL 60607-7128. Offers acute care clinical nurse specialist (MS); acute care nurse practitioner (MS); administrative nursing leadership (Certificate); administrative studies in nursing (MS); adult nurse practitioner (MS); adult/geriatric nurse practitioner (MS); advanced community health nurse specialist (MS); family nurse practitioner (MS); geriatric clinical nurse specialist (MS); geriatric nurse practitioner (MS); mental health clinical nurse specialist (MS); mental health nurse practitioner (MS); nurse midwifery (MS); occupational health/advanced community health nurse specialist (MS); occupational health/family nurse practitioner (MS); pediatric clinical nurse specialist (MS); pediatric nurse practitioner (MS); perinatal clinical nurse specialist (MS); school/advanced community health nurse specialist (MS); school/family nurse practitioner (MS); women's health nurse practitioner (MS). *Accreditation:* AACN. Part-time programs available. *Faculty:* 16 full-time (14 women). *Students:* 393 full-time (361 women), 410 part-time (367 women); includes 198 minority (48 Black or African American, non-Hispanic/Latino; 1 American Indian or Alaska Native, non-Hispanic/Latino; 64 Asian, non-Hispanic/Latino; 71 Hispanic/Latino; 2 Native Hawaiian or other Pacific Islander, non-Hispanic/Latino; 12 Two or more races, non-Hispanic/Latino), 29 international. Average age 32. 396 applicants, 62% accepted, 177 enrolled. In 2013, 184 master's awarded. *Degree requirements:* For master's, thesis or alternative. *Entrance requirements:* For master's, GRE General Test, minimum GPA of 2.75. Additional exam requirements/recommendations for international students: Required—TOEFL. *Application deadline:* For fall admission, 5/15 for domestic students, 2/15 for international students; for spring admission, 11/1 for domestic students, 7/15 for international students. Applications are processed on a rolling basis. Application fee: $40 ($50 for international students). Electronic applications accepted. *Expenses:* Tuition, state resident: full-time $11,066; part-time $3689 per term. Tuition, nonresident: full-time $23,064; part-time $7688 per term. *Required fees:* $3004; $1190 per term.

Tuition and fees vary according to course level and program. *Financial support:* Fellowships with full tuition reimbursements, research assistantships with full tuition reimbursements, teaching assistantships with full tuition reimbursements, career-related internships or fieldwork, Federal Work-Study, institutionally sponsored loans, scholarships/grants, traineeships, tuition waivers (full and partial), and unspecified assistantships available. Support available to part-time students. Financial award application deadline: 3/1; financial award applicants required to submit FAFSA. *Unit head:* Dr. Terri E. Weaver, Dean, 312-996-7808, E-mail: teweaver@uic.edu. *Application contact:* Receptionist, 312-413-2550, E-mail: gradcoll@uic.edu.

The University of Kansas, University of Kansas Medical Center, School of Nursing, Kansas City, KS 66160. Offers adult/gerontological clinical nurse specialist (PMC); adult/gerontological nurse practitioner (PMC); clinical research management (PMC); health care informatics (PMC); health professions educator (PMC); nurse midwife (PMC); nursing (MS, DNP, PhD); organizational leadership (PMC); psychiatric/mental health nurse practitioner (PMC); public health nursing (PMC). *Accreditation:* AACN; ACNM/ACME. Part-time programs available. Postbaccalaureate distance learning degree programs offered (minimal on-campus study). *Faculty:* 59. *Students:* 55 full-time (53 women), 323 part-time (303 women); includes 57 minority (23 Black or African American, non-Hispanic/Latino; 14 Asian, non-Hispanic/Latino; 16 Hispanic/Latino; 1 Native Hawaiian or other Pacific Islander, non-Hispanic/Latino; 3 Two or more races, non-Hispanic/Latino), 1 international. Average age 38. 113 applicants, 59% accepted, 61 enrolled. In 2013, 77 master's, 18 doctorates, 11 other advanced degrees awarded. Terminal master's awarded for partial completion of doctoral program. *Degree requirements:* For master's, comprehensive exam, thesis (for some programs), general oral exam; for doctorate, variable foreign language requirement, thesis/dissertation, comprehensive oral exam (for DNP); comprehensive written and oral exam (for PhD). *Entrance requirements:* For master's, bachelor's degree in nursing, minimum GPA of 3.0, 1 year of clinical experience, RN license in KS and MO; for doctorate, GRE General Test, bachelor's degree in nursing, minimum GPA of 3.5, RN license in KS and MO. Additional exam requirements/recommendations for international students: Required—TOEFL. *Application deadline:* For fall admission, 4/1 for domestic and international students; for spring admission, 9/1 for domestic and international students. Application fee: $60. Electronic applications accepted. *Financial support:* Research assistantships with full and partial tuition reimbursements, teaching assistantships with full and partial tuition reimbursements, scholarships/grants, and traineeships available. Financial award application deadline: 3/1; financial award applicants required to submit FAFSA. *Faculty research:* Breastfeeding practices of teen mothers, national database of nursing quality indicators, caregiving of families of patients using technology in the home, simulation in nursing education, diaphragm fatigue. *Total annual research expenditures:* $6.4 million. *Unit head:* Dr. Karen L. Miller, Dean, 913-588-1601, Fax: 913-588-1660, E-mail: kmiller@kumc.edu. *Application contact:* Dr. Pamela K. Barnes, Associate Dean, Student Affairs, 913-588-1619, Fax: 913-588-1615, E-mail: pbarnes2@kumc.edu.
Website: http://nursing.kumc.edu

University of Louisville, Graduate School, School of Nursing, Louisville, KY 40202. Offers adult nurse practitioner (MSN); family nurse practitioner (MSN); health professions education (MSN); neonatal nurse practitioner (MSN); nursing research (PhD); psychiatric mental health nurse practitioner (MSN). *Accreditation:* AACN. Part-time programs available. *Students:* 91 full-time (81 women), 47 part-time (42 women); includes 16 minority (8 Black or African American, non-Hispanic/Latino; 3 Asian, non-Hispanic/Latino; 3 Hispanic/Latino; 2 Two or more races, non-Hispanic/Latino), 6 international. Average age 36. 58 applicants, 74% accepted, 36 enrolled. In 2013, 33 master's, 3 doctorates awarded. Terminal master's awarded for partial completion of doctoral program. *Degree requirements:* For master's, thesis optional; for doctorate, comprehensive exam, thesis/dissertation. *Entrance requirements:* For master's, GRE General Test, bachelor's degree in nursing, minimum GPA of 3.0, RN license; for doctorate, GRE General Test, BSN or MSN with recommended minimum GPA of 3.0. Additional exam requirements/recommendations for international students: Required—TOEFL. *Application deadline:* For fall admission, 4/1 priority date for domestic students, 4/1 for international students. Applications are processed on a rolling basis. Application fee: $60. Electronic applications accepted. *Expenses:* Tuition, state resident: full-time $10,788; part-time $599 per credit hour. Tuition, nonresident: full-time $22,446; part-time $1247 per credit hour. *Required fees:* $196. Tuition and fees vary according to program and reciprocity agreements. *Financial support:* Fellowships with full tuition reimbursements, research assistantships with full tuition reimbursements, teaching assistantships with full tuition reimbursements, institutionally sponsored loans, scholarships/grants, traineeships, health care benefits, and unspecified assistantships available. Support available to part-time students. Financial award application deadline: 4/15; financial award applicants required to submit FAFSA. *Faculty research:* Maternal-child/family stress after pregnancy loss, postpartum depression, access to healthcare (underserved populations), quality of life issues, physical activity (impact on chronic/acute conditions). *Total annual research expenditures:* $718,934. *Unit head:* Dr. Marcia J. Hern, Dean, 502-852-8300, Fax: 502-852-5044, E-mail: m.hern@gwise.louisville.edu. *Application contact:* Dr. Lee Ridner, Interim Associate Dean for Academic Affairs and Director of MSN Programs, 502-852-8518, Fax: 502-852-0704, E-mail: romain01@louisville.edu.
Website: http://www.louisville.edu/nursing/

University of Massachusetts Amherst, Graduate School, School of Nursing, Amherst, MA 01003. Offers adult gerontology primary care (DNP); clinical nurse leader (MS); family nurse practitioner (DNP); nursing (PhD); public health nurse leader (DNP). *Accreditation:* AACN. Part-time programs available. Postbaccalaureate distance learning degree programs offered (minimal on-campus study). *Faculty:* 16 full-time (15 women). *Students:* 74 full-time (61 women), 161 part-time (149 women); includes 62 minority (31 Black or African American, non-Hispanic/Latino; 9 Asian, non-Hispanic/Latino; 19 Hispanic/Latino; 3 Two or more races, non-Hispanic/Latino), 6 international. Average age 40. 133 applicants, 80% accepted, 68 enrolled. In 2013, 9 master's, 32 doctorates awarded. Terminal master's awarded for partial completion of doctoral program. *Degree requirements:* For master's, thesis optional; for doctorate, comprehensive exam, thesis/dissertation. *Entrance requirements:* Additional exam requirements/recommendations for international students: Required—TOEFL (minimum score 550 paper-based; 80 iBT), IELTS (minimum score 6.5). *Application deadline:* For fall admission, 12/15 for domestic and international students. Applications are processed on a rolling basis. Application fee: $75. Electronic applications accepted. *Financial support:* Fellowships with full and partial tuition reimbursements, research assistantships with full and partial tuition reimbursements, teaching assistantships with full and partial tuition reimbursements, career-related internships or fieldwork, Federal Work-Study, scholarships/grants, traineeships, health care benefits, tuition waivers (full and partial), and unspecified assistantships available. Support available to part-time students. Financial award application deadline: 2/1. *Faculty research:* Health of older adults and their caretakers, mental health of individuals and families, health of children and adolescents, power and decision-making, transcultural health. *Unit head:* Dr. Stephen J. Cavanagh, Dean, 413-545-2703, Fax: 413-577-2550, E-mail: dean@nursing.umass.edu. *Application contact:* Lindsay DeSantis, Supervisor of Admissions, 413-545-0722, Fax: 413-577-0010, E-mail: gradadm@grad.umass.edu.
Website: http://www.umass.edu/nursing/

University of Massachusetts Dartmouth, Graduate School, College of Nursing, Programs in Nursing, North Dartmouth, MA 02747-2300. Offers adult gerontology primary care nurse practitioner (DNP); adult health clinical nurse specialist (DNP); adult health/adult nurse practitioner (MS); adult health/advanced practice (MS); adult health/nurse educator (MS); adult health/nurse manager (MS); adult nurse practitioner (PMC); community health nurse specialist (DNP); community nursing/advanced practice (MS); community nursing/nurse educator (MS); community nursing/nurse manager (MS); individualized nursing (PMC); nursing (MS, PhD); nursing practice (DNP). Part-time programs available. *Faculty:* 25 full-time (all women), 45 part-time/adjunct (44 women). *Students:* 103 part-time (95 women); includes 10 minority (4 Black or African American, non-Hispanic/Latino; 2 Asian, non-Hispanic/Latino; 4 Hispanic/Latino). Average age 40. 49 applicants, 92% accepted, 33 enrolled. In 2013, 25 master's, 1 doctorate, 2 other advanced degrees awarded. *Degree requirements:* For master's, thesis; for doctorate, comprehensive exam, thesis/dissertation, project (for DNP only). *Entrance requirements:* For master's, statement of purpose (minimum of 300 words), resume, 3 letters of recommendation, official transcripts, copy of RN license; for doctorate, GRE (for PhD), statement of purpose (minimum of 300 words), resume, 3 letters of recommendation, official transcripts, copy of RN license, scholarly writing sample (minimum 10 pages for PhD). Additional exam requirements/recommendations for international students: Required—TOEFL (minimum score 533 paper-based; 72 iBT). *Application deadline:* For fall admission, 2/15 priority date for domestic and international students. Applications are processed on a rolling basis. Application fee: $60. Electronic applications accepted. *Expenses:* Tuition, state resident: full-time $2071; part-time $86.29 per credit. Tuition, nonresident: full-time $8099; part-time $337.46 per credit. Tuition and fees vary according to course load and reciprocity agreements. *Financial support:* In 2013–14, 5 teaching assistantships with full and partial tuition reimbursements (averaging $7,500 per year) were awarded; Federal Work-Study and unspecified assistantships also available. Support available to part-time students. Financial award application deadline: 3/1; financial award applicants required to submit FAFSA. *Faculty research:* Pathophysiology, aging with spinal cord injury, relational ontology, severe mental illness, patient care. *Total annual research expenditures:* $1,000. *Unit head:* Kerry Fater, Graduate Program Director for Nursing Master's Programs, 508-999-8525, Fax: 508-999-9127, E-mail: kfater@umassd.edu. *Application contact:* Steven Briggs, Director of Marketing and Recruitment for Graduate Studies, 508-999-8604, Fax: 508-999-8183, E-mail: graduate@umassd.edu.
Website: http://www.umassd.edu/nursing/graduateprograms

University of Massachusetts Worcester, Graduate School of Nursing, Worcester, MA 01655-0115. Offers advanced practice nursing (DNP); family nurse practitioner (MS); gerontological adult acute care nurse practitioner (MS, Post Master's Certificate); gerontological adult primary care nurse practitioner (Post Master's Certificate); gerontological primary care nurse practitioner (MS); leadership (DNP); nurse educator (MS, Post Master's Certificate); nursing (PhD). *Accreditation:* AACN. *Faculty:* 19 full-time (17 women), 40 part-time/adjunct (33 women). *Students:* 153 full-time (129 women), 35 part-time (28 women); includes 30 minority (18 Black or African American, non-Hispanic/Latino; 7 Asian, non-Hispanic/Latino; 5 Hispanic/Latino). Average age 34. 254 applicants, 31% accepted, 57 enrolled. In 2013, 50 master's, 4 doctorates, 2 other advanced degrees awarded. *Degree requirements:* For doctorate, thesis/dissertation (for some programs), comprehensive exam (for PhD); capstone project and manuscript (for DNP). *Entrance requirements:* For master's, GRE General Test, bachelor's degree in nursing, course work in statistics, unrestricted Massachusetts license as registered nurse; for doctorate, GRE General Test, bachelor's or master's degree; for Post Master's Certificate, GRE General Test, MS in nursing. Additional exam requirements/recommendations for international students: Required—TOEFL. *Application deadline:* For fall admission, 12/1 priority date for domestic students. Applications are processed on a rolling basis. Application fee: $60. Electronic applications accepted. *Expenses:* Contact institution. *Financial support:* In 2013–14, 43 students received support. Institutionally sponsored loans, scholarships/grants, traineeships, and tuition waivers available. Support available to part-time students. Financial award application deadline: 5/16; financial award applicants required to submit FAFSA. *Faculty research:* Decision-making of partners and men with prostate cancer, coinfection (HIV and Hepatitis C) and treatment decisions, parent management of children with Type 1 diabetes, health literacy and discharge planning, Ghanaian women and self-care. *Total annual research expenditures:* $1.5 million. *Unit head:* Dr. Paulette Seymour-Route, Dean, 508-856-5801, Fax: 508-856-6552, E-mail: paulette.seymour-route@umassmed.edu. *Application contact:* Diane Brescia, Admissions Coordinator, 508-856-3488, Fax: 508-856-5851, E-mail: diane.brescia@umassmed.edu.
Website: http://www.umassmed.edu/gsn/

University of Miami, Graduate School, School of Nursing and Health Studies, Coral Gables, FL 33124. Offers acute care (MSN), including acute care nurse practitioner, nurse anesthesia; nursing (PhD); primary care (MSN), including adult nurse practitioner, family nurse practitioner, nurse midwifery, women's health practitioner. *Accreditation:* AACN; AANA/CANAEP; ACNM/ACME (one or more programs are accredited). Part-time programs available. *Degree requirements:* For master's, thesis optional; for doctorate, thesis/dissertation. *Entrance requirements:* For master's, GRE General Test, BSN, minimum GPA of 3.0, Florida RN license; for doctorate, GRE General Test, BSN or MSN, minimum GPA of 3.0. Additional exam requirements/recommendations for international students: Required—TOEFL (minimum score 550 paper-based). Electronic applications accepted. *Faculty research:* Transcultural nursing, exercise and depression in Alzheimer's disease, infectious diseases/HIV–AIDS, postpartum depression, outcomes assessment.

University of Michigan, Rackham Graduate School, School of Nursing, Ann Arbor, MI 48109. Offers acute care pediatric nurse practitioner (MS); adult-gerontology acute care clinical nurse specialist (MS); adult-gerontology acute care nurse practitioner (MS); adult-gerontology primary care nurse practitioner (MS); health systems, nursing leadership, and effectiveness science (MS); nurse midwife (MS); nurse midwife and family nurse practitioner (MS); nurse midwife and primary care pediatric nurse practitioner (MS); nursing (DNP, PhD, Post Master's Certificate); primary care family nurse practitioner (MS); primary care pediatric nurse practitioner (MS). *Accreditation:* AACN; ACNM/ACME (one or more programs are accredited). Part-time programs available. Postbaccalaureate distance learning degree programs offered (minimal on-campus study). Terminal master's awarded for partial completion of doctoral program. *Degree requirements:* For doctorate, thesis/dissertation. *Application deadline:* For fall admission, 2/1 for domestic students; for winter admission, 5/1 for domestic students; for spring admission, 11/1 for domestic students. Applications are processed on a rolling basis. Electronic applications accepted. Tuition and fees vary according to course level, course load, degree level, program and student level. *Financial support:* Fellowships with full and partial tuition reimbursements, research assistantships with full and partial tuition reimbursements, teaching assistantships with full tuition reimbursements, Federal Work-Study, institutionally sponsored loans, scholarships/grants, traineeships, and tuition waivers (partial) available. Support available to part-time students. *Faculty research:* Preparation of clinical nurse researchers, biobehavior, women's health, health promotion, substance abuse, psychobiology of menopause, fertility, obesity, health care systems. *Unit head:* Dr. Kathleen Potempa, Dean, 734-764-7185, Fax: 734-764-7186.

Application contact: James Diesing, Graduate Recruiting and Admissions Coordinator, 734-615-4739, E-mail: sn-osams@umich.edu.
Website: http://www.nursing.umich.edu/

University of Minnesota, Twin Cities Campus, Graduate School, School of Nursing, Program in Adult Health Clinical Nurse Specialist, Minneapolis, MN 55455-0213. Offers MS. *Accreditation:* AACN. *Degree requirements:* For master's, final oral exam, project or thesis. *Entrance requirements:* Additional exam requirements/recommendations for international students: Required—TOEFL (minimum score 586 paper-based).

University of Missouri, Graduate School, Sinclair School of Nursing, Columbia, MO 65211. Offers adult-gerontology clinical nurse specialist (DNP, Certificate); family nurse practitioner (DNP); family psychiatric and mental health nurse practitioner (DNP); nursing (MS, PhD); nursing leadership and innovations in health care (DNP); pediatric clinical nurse specialist (DNP, Certificate); pediatric nurse practitioner (DNP). *Accreditation:* AACN. Part-time programs available. *Faculty:* 20 full-time (18 women), 6 part-time/adjunct (all women). *Students:* 60 full-time (58 women), 232 part-time (211 women); includes 24 minority (9 Black or African American, non-Hispanic/Latino; 4 American Indian or Alaska Native, non-Hispanic/Latino; 2 Asian, non-Hispanic/Latino; 6 Hispanic/Latino; 3 Two or more races, non-Hispanic/Latino), 4 international. Average age 37. 131 applicants, 62% accepted, 61 enrolled. In 2013, 42 master's, 2 doctorates, 7 other advanced degrees awarded. *Degree requirements:* For master's, thesis optional, oral exam; for doctorate, thesis/dissertation. *Entrance requirements:* For master's, GRE General Test, BSN, minimum GPA of 3.0 during last 60 hours, nursing license. Additional exam requirements/recommendations for international students: Required—TOEFL (minimum score 550 paper-based; 79 iBT). *Application deadline:* For fall admission, 2/1 priority date for domestic and international students. Applications are processed on a rolling basis. Application fee: $55 ($75 for international students). Electronic applications accepted. *Financial support:* Fellowships, research assistantships, teaching assistantships, career-related internships or fieldwork, institutionally sponsored loans, scholarships/grants, traineeships, health care benefits, tuition waivers (full), and unspecified assistantships available. Support available to part-time students. *Faculty research:* Pain, stepfamilies, chemotherapy-related nausea and vomiting, stress management, self-care deficit theory. *Unit head:* Dr. Judith F. Miller, Dean, 573-882-0278, E-mail: millerjud@missouri.edu. *Application contact:* Laura Anderson, Senior Academic Advisor, 573-882-0294, E-mail: andersonla@missouri.edu.
Website: http://nursing.missouri.edu/

University of Missouri–Kansas City, School of Nursing and Health Studies, Kansas City, MO 64110-2499. Offers adult clinical nurse specialist (MSN), including adult nurse practitioner, women's health nurse practitioner (MSN, DNP); adult clinical nursing practice (DNP), including adult gerontology nurse practitioner, women's health nurse practitioner (MSN, DNP); clinical nursing practice (DNP), including family nurse practitioner; family nurse practitioner (MSN); neonatal nurse practitioner (MSN); nurse educator (MSN); nurse executive (MSN); nursing (PhD); nursing practice (DNP); pediatric clinical nursing practice (DNP), including pediatric nurse practitioner; pediatric nurse practitioner (MSN). *Accreditation:* AACN. Part-time programs available. Postbaccalaureate distance learning degree programs offered (minimal on-campus study). *Faculty:* 44 full-time (38 women), 55 part-time/adjunct (52 women). *Students:* 44 full-time (33 women), 401 part-time (370 women); includes 59 minority (25 Black or African American, non-Hispanic/Latino; 2 American Indian or Alaska Native, non-Hispanic/Latino; 12 Asian, non-Hispanic/Latino; 15 Hispanic/Latino; 5 Two or more races, non-Hispanic/Latino). Average age 37. 182 applicants, 68% accepted, 124 enrolled. In 2013, 106 master's, 15 doctorates awarded. *Degree requirements:* For master's, thesis or alternative. *Entrance requirements:* For master's, minimum undergraduate GPA of 3.2; for doctorate, GRE, 3 letters of reference. Additional exam requirements/recommendations for international students: Required—TOEFL (minimum score 550 paper-based; 80 iBT). *Application deadline:* For fall admission, 2/1 priority date for domestic and international students; for spring admission, 9/1 priority date for domestic and international students. Application fee: $45 ($50 for international students). *Expenses:* Tuition, state resident: full-time $6073; part-time $337.40 per credit hour. Tuition, nonresident: full-time $15,680; part-time $871.10 per credit hour. *Required fees:* $97.59 per credit hour. Full-time tuition and fees vary according to program. *Financial support:* In 2013–14, 13 teaching assistantships with partial tuition reimbursements (averaging $9,470 per year) were awarded; fellowships, research assistantships, career-related internships or fieldwork, Federal Work-Study, institutionally sponsored loans, and tuition waivers (full and partial) also available. Support available to part-time students. Financial award application deadline: 3/1; financial award applicants required to submit FAFSA. *Faculty research:* Geriatrics/gerontology, children's pain, neonatology, Alzheimer's care, cancer caregivers. *Unit head:* Dr. Ann Cary, Dean, 816-235-1723, Fax: 816-235-1701, E-mail: caryah@umkc.edu. *Application contact:* Judy Jellison, Coordinator for Admissions and Recruitment, 816-235-1740, Fax: 816-235-1701, E-mail: jellisonj@umkc.edu.
Website: http://nursing.umkc.edu/

University of Missouri–St. Louis, College of Nursing, St. Louis, MO 63121-4400. Offers adult nurse practitioner (DNP, Post Master's Certificate); clinical nurse specialist (DNP); family mental health nurse practitioner (DNP); family nurse practitioner (MSN, DNP, Post Master's Certificate); neonatal nurse practitioner (MSN); nurse educator (MSN); nurse leader (MSN); nurse practitioner (Post Master's Certificate); nursing (PhD); pediatric clinical nurse specialist (DNP); pediatric nurse practitioner (MSN, DNP, Post Master's Certificate); women's health nurse practitioner (MSN, Post Master's Certificate). *Accreditation:* AACN. Part-time programs available. *Faculty:* 14 full-time (13 women), 14 part-time/adjunct (13 women). *Students:* 227 part-time (217 women); includes 40 minority (35 Black or African American, non-Hispanic/Latino; 1 American Indian or Alaska Native, non-Hispanic/Latino; 1 Asian, non-Hispanic/Latino; 1 Hispanic/Latino; 2 Two or more races, non-Hispanic/Latino). Average age 35. 190 applicants, 51% accepted, 76 enrolled. In 2013, 80 master's, 8 doctorates, 2 other advanced degrees awarded. *Degree requirements:* For doctorate, comprehensive exam, thesis/dissertation; for Post Master's Certificate, thesis. *Entrance requirements:* For master's, 2 recommendation letters; minimum GPA of 3.0; BSN; nursing licensure; statement of purpose; course in differential/inferential statistics; for doctorate, GRE, 2 letters of recommendation, MSN, minimum GPA of 3.2, course in differential/inferential statistics; for Post Master's Certificate, 2 recommendation letters; MSN; advanced practice certificate; minimum GPA of 3.0; essay. Additional exam requirements/recommendations for international students: Recommended—TOEFL (minimum score 550 paper-based; 79 iBT), IELTS (minimum score 6.5). *Application deadline:* For fall admission, 2/15 for domestic and international students. Application fee: $50 ($40 for international students). Electronic applications accepted. *Expenses:* Tuition, state resident: full-time $7364; part-time $409.10 per credit hour. Tuition, nonresident: full-time $19,162; part-time $1008.50 per credit hour. *Financial support:* Application deadline: 4/1; applicants required to submit FAFSA. *Faculty research:* Health promotion and restoration, family disruption, violence, abuse, battered women, health survey methods. *Unit head:* Dr. Nancy Magnuson, Director, 314-516-6066. *Application contact:* 314-516-5458, Fax: 314-516-6996, E-mail: gradadm@umsl.edu.
Website: http://www.umsl.edu/divisions/nursing/

The University of North Carolina at Chapel Hill, School of Nursing, Chapel Hill, NC 27599-7460. Offers nursing (MSN, DNP, PhD, PMC), including adult nurse practitioner (MSN, PMC), children's health advanced practice (MSN, PMC), family nurse practitioner (MSN, PMC), health care systems (MSN, PMC), psychiatric/mental health nursing (MSN, PMC). Part-time programs available. *Degree requirements:* For master's, comprehensive exam, thesis; for doctorate, thesis/dissertation, 3 exams. *Entrance requirements:* For master's and doctorate, GRE General Test. Additional exam requirements/recommendations for international students: Required—TOEFL (minimum score 550 paper-based; 79 iBT), IELTS (minimum score 7). Electronic applications accepted. *Faculty research:* Preventing and managing chronic illness, reducing health disparities, Improving healthcare quality and patient outcomes, understanding biobehavioral and genetic bases of health and illness, developing innovative ways to enhance science and its clinical translation.

The University of North Carolina at Charlotte, The Graduate School, College of Health and Human Services, School of Nursing, Charlotte, NC 28223-0001. Offers administration (Post-Master's Certificate); advanced clinical (MSN, Post-Master's Certificate); anesthesia (MSN, Post-Master's Certificate); community health (MSN); family nurse practitioner (MSN, Post-Master's Certificate); health administration (MSN); mental health (MSN); nurse educator (MSN, Post-Master's Certificate); nursing (DNP); systems population (MSN). *Accreditation:* AACN. Part-time programs available. *Faculty:* 17 full-time (16 women), 6 part-time/adjunct (5 women). *Students:* 96 full-time (80 women), 124 part-time (119 women); includes 45 minority (30 Black or African American, non-Hispanic/Latino; 1 American Indian or Alaska Native, non-Hispanic/Latino; 8 Asian, non-Hispanic/Latino; 4 Hispanic/Latino; 2 Two or more races, non-Hispanic/Latino), 1 international. Average age 34. 216 applicants, 38% accepted, 72 enrolled. In 2013, 70 master's, 8 other advanced degrees awarded. Terminal master's awarded for partial completion of doctoral program. *Degree requirements:* For master's, thesis or alternative, practicum; for doctorate, thesis/dissertation or alternative, residency. *Entrance requirements:* For master's, GRE General Test, minimum GPA of 3.0 in undergraduate major; for doctorate, GRE, MAT, or GMAT, minimum GPA of 3.5. Additional exam requirements/recommendations for international students: Required—TOEFL (minimum score 570 paper-based; 83 iBT). *Application deadline:* For fall admission, 5/1 priority date for domestic students, 5/1 for international students; for spring admission, 10/1 priority date for domestic students, 10/1 for international students. Application fee: $75. Electronic applications accepted. *Expenses:* Tuition, state resident: full-time $3522. Tuition, nonresident: full-time $16,051. *Required fees:* $2585. Tuition and fees vary according to course load and program. *Financial support:* In 2013–14, 5 students received support, including 5 teaching assistantships (averaging $4,785 per year); research assistantships, career-related internships or fieldwork, institutionally sponsored loans, scholarships/grants, traineeships, and unspecified assistantships also available. Support available to part-time students. Financial award application deadline: 4/1; financial award applicants required to submit FAFSA. *Faculty research:* Improving care outcomes for the elderly; vulnerable populations; symptom management; self management/health promotion strategies of older adults; migration and maternal child health; health disparities, health literacy, and access to healthcare in Latino adults with diabetes; psychiatric nursing. *Total annual research expenditures:* $572,410. *Unit head:* Dr. Dee Baldwin, Associate Dean, 704-687-7952, Fax: 704-687-6017, E-mail: dbaldwi5@uncc.edu. *Application contact:* Kathy B. Giddings, Director of Graduate Admissions, 704-687-5503, Fax: 704-687-1668, E-mail: gradadm@uncc.edu.
Website: http://nursing.uncc.edu/

The University of North Carolina at Greensboro, Graduate School, School of Nursing, Greensboro, NC 27412-5001. Offers adult clinical nurse specialist (MSN, PMC); adult/gerontological nurse practitioner (MSN, PMC); nurse anesthesia (MSN, PMC); nursing (PhD); nursing administration (MSN); nursing education (MSN); MSN/MBA. *Accreditation:* AACN; AANA/CANAEP. *Degree requirements:* For master's, thesis or alternative. *Entrance requirements:* For master's, GRE General Test or MAT, BSN, clinical experience, liability insurance, RN license; for PMC, liability insurance, MSN, RN license. Additional exam requirements/recommendations for international students: Required—TOEFL. Electronic applications accepted.

University of North Florida, Brooks College of Health, School of Nursing, Jacksonville, FL 32224. Offers clinical nurse leader (MSN); clinical nurse specialist (MSN); family nurse practitioner (Certificate); nurse anesthetist (CRNA) (MSN); nursing practice (DNP); primary care nurse practitioner (MSN). *Accreditation:* AACN; AANA/CANAEP. Part-time programs available. *Faculty:* 29 full-time (23 women), 1 part-time/adjunct (0 women). *Students:* 93 full-time (70 women), 74 part-time (61 women); includes 33 minority (11 Black or African American, non-Hispanic/Latino; 1 American Indian or Alaska Native, non-Hispanic/Latino; 6 Asian, non-Hispanic/Latino; 12 Hispanic/Latino; 3 Two or more races, non-Hispanic/Latino), 2 international. Average age 34. 133 applicants, 40% accepted, 32 enrolled. In 2013, 45 master's, 3 doctorates awarded. *Degree requirements:* For master's, thesis optional. *Entrance requirements:* For master's, GRE General Test, minimum GPA of 3.0 in last 60 hours of course work, BSN, clinical experience, resume; for doctorate, GRE, master's degree in nursing specialty from nationally-accredited program; national certification in one of the following APRN roles: CNE, CNM, CNS, CRNA, CNP; minimum graduate GPA of 3.3; three letters of reference which address academic ability and clinical skills; active license as registered nurse or advanced practice registered nurse. Additional exam requirements/recommendations for international students: Required—TOEFL (minimum score 500 paper-based; 61 iBT). *Application deadline:* For fall admission, 3/15 for domestic students, 4/1 for international students. Application fee: $30. Electronic applications accepted. *Expenses:* Tuition, state resident: full-time $9794; part-time $408.10 per credit hour. Tuition, nonresident: full-time $22,383; part-time $932.61 per credit hour. *Required fees:* $2020; $84.20 per credit hour. Tuition and fees vary according to course load and program. *Financial support:* In 2013–14, 26 students received support. Research assistantships available. Financial award application deadline: 4/1; financial award applicants required to submit FAFSA. *Faculty research:* Teen pregnancy, diabetes, ethical decision-making, family caregivers. *Total annual research expenditures:* $66,739. *Unit head:* Dr. Li Loriz, Chair, 904-620-1053, E-mail: lloriz@unf.edu. *Application contact:* Beth Dibble, Assistant Director of Admissions for Nursing and Physical Therapy, 904-620-2684, Fax: 904-620-1832, E-mail: nursingadmissions@unf.edu.
Website: http://www.unf.edu/brooks/nursing

University of Pennsylvania, School of Nursing, Adult Acute Care Nurse Practitioner Program, Philadelphia, PA 19104. Offers acute care nurse practitioner (MSN). *Accreditation:* AACN. Part-time programs available. *Students:* 59 full-time (55 women), 124 part-time (110 women); includes 32 minority (11 Black or African American, non-Hispanic/Latino; 17 Asian, non-Hispanic/Latino; 1 Hispanic/Latino; 3 Two or more races, non-Hispanic/Latino), 5 international. 50 applicants, 54% accepted, 25 enrolled. In 2013, 69 master's awarded. *Entrance requirements:* For master's, GRE General Test, BSN, minimum GPA of 3.0, previous course work in statistics. *Application deadline:* For fall admission, 2/15 priority date for domestic students. Applications are processed on a rolling basis. Application fee: $70. *Expenses:* Contact institution. *Financial support:* Fellowships, research assistantships, teaching assistantships, Federal Work-Study, and institutionally sponsored loans available. Support available to part-time students. Financial award application deadline: 4/1. *Faculty research:* Post-injury disability,

bereavement and attributions in fire survivors, stress in staff nurses. *Unit head:* Assistant Dean of Admissions and Financial Aid, 866-867-6877, Fax: 215-573-8439, E-mail: admissions@nursing.upenn.edu. *Application contact:* Deborah Becker, Program Director, 215-898-0432, E-mail: debecker@nursing.upenn.edu.
Website: http://www.nursing.upenn.edu/

University of Pittsburgh, School of Nursing, Clinical Nurse Specialist Program, Pittsburgh, PA 15260. Offers adult-gerontology clinical nurse specialist (DNP); psychiatric mental health clinical nurse specialist (DNP). *Accreditation:* AACN. Part-time programs available. *Students:* 4 full-time (all women), 16 part-time (14 women); includes 2 minority (both Black or African American, non-Hispanic/Latino), 1 international. Average age 41. 4 applicants, 75% accepted, 2 enrolled. In 2013, 5 doctorates awarded. *Entrance requirements:* Additional exam requirements/recommendations for international students: Required—TOEFL (minimum score 550 paper-based; 80 iBT). *Application deadline:* For fall admission, 6/1 priority date for domestic and international students. Applications are processed on a rolling basis. Application fee: $50. Electronic applications accepted. *Expenses:* Tuition, state resident: full-time $19,964; part-time $807 per credit. Tuition, nonresident: full-time $32,686; part-time $1337 per credit. *Required fees:* $740; $200. Tuition and fees vary according to program. *Financial support:* In 2013–14, 4 students received support, including 1 fellowship with full tuition reimbursement available (averaging $24,108 per year), 3 teaching assistantships with full and partial tuition reimbursements available (averaging $21,884 per year); scholarships/grants, traineeships, health care benefits, and unspecified assistantships also available. Support available to part-time students. *Unit head:* Dr. Sandra Engberg, Associate Dean for Clinical Education, 412-624-3835, Fax: 412-624-8521, E-mail: sje1@pitt.edu. *Application contact:* Laurie Lapsley, Administrator of Graduate Student Services, 412-624-9670, Fax: 412-624-2409, E-mail: lapsleyl@pitt.edu.

University of Pittsburgh, School of Nursing, Nurse Practitioner Program, Pittsburgh, PA 15261. Offers adult-gerontology acute care nurse practitioner (DNP); adult-gerontology primary care nurse practitioner (DNP); family (individual across the lifespan) nurse practitioner (DNP); neonatal nurse practitioner (MSN, DNP); pediatric primary care nurse practitioner (DNP); psychiatric mental health nurse practitioner (DNP). *Accreditation:* AACN. Part-time programs available. *Students:* 66 full-time (59 women), 84 part-time (75 women); includes 11 minority (5 Black or African American, non-Hispanic/Latino; 2 American Indian or Alaska Native, non-Hispanic/Latino; 3 Asian, non-Hispanic/Latino; 1 Hispanic/Latino), 2 international. Average age 31. 95 applicants, 74% accepted, 57 enrolled. In 2013, 53 master's, 4 doctorates awarded. *Degree requirements:* For master's, comprehensive exam, thesis optional. *Entrance requirements:* For master's, GRE General Test or MAT, BSN, RN license, letters of recommendation, resume, course work in statistics, 1-3 years of nursing experience; for doctorate, GRE General Test, BSN, RN license, minimum GPA of 3.5, 3 letters of recommendation. Additional exam requirements/recommendations for international students: Required—TOEFL (minimum score 550 paper-based; 80 iBT). *Application deadline:* Applications are processed on a rolling basis. Application fee: $50. Electronic applications accepted. *Expenses:* Tuition, state resident: full-time $19,964; part-time $807 per credit. Tuition, nonresident: full-time $32,686; part-time $1337 per credit. *Required fees:* $740; $200. Tuition and fees vary according to program. *Financial support:* In 2013–14, 18 students received support, including 4 fellowships with full and partial tuition reimbursements available (averaging $22,521 per year), 3 research assistantships with full and partial tuition reimbursements available (averaging $21,884 per year), 15 teaching assistantships with full and partial tuition reimbursements available (averaging $13,535 per year); scholarships/grants, traineeships, health care benefits, and unspecified assistantships also available. Support available to part-time students. *Unit head:* Dr. Sandra Engberg, Associate Dean for Clinical Education, 412-624-3835, Fax: 412-624-8521, E-mail: sje1@pitt.edu. *Application contact:* Laurie Lapsley, Administrator of Graduate Student Services, 412-624-9670, Fax: 412-624-2409, E-mail: lapsleyl@pitt.edu.
Website: http://www.nursing.pitt.edu

University of Puerto Rico, Medical Sciences Campus, School of Nursing, San Juan, PR 00936-5067. Offers adult and elderly nursing (MSN); child and adolescent nursing (MSN); critical care nursing (MSN); family and community nursing (MSN); family nurse practitioner (MSN); maternity nursing (MSN); mental health and psychiatric nursing (MSN). *Accreditation:* AACN. *Entrance requirements:* For master's, GRE or EXADEP, interview, Puerto Rico RN license or professional license for international students, general and specific point average, article analysis. Electronic applications accepted. *Faculty research:* HIV, health disparities, teen violence, women and violence, neurological disorders.

University of Rochester, School of Nursing, Rochester, NY 14642. Offers acute care nurse practitioner (MS); adult nurse practitioner (MS); adult/geriatric nurse practitioner (MS); clinical nurse leader (MS); clinical research coordinator (MS); family nurse practitioner (MS); family psychiatric mental health nurse practitioner (MS); health care organization management and leadership (MS); health practice research (PhD); nursing (DNP); pediatric nurse practitioner (MS); pediatric nurse practitioner/neonatal nurse practitioner (MS). *Accreditation:* AACN. Part-time programs available. Postbaccalaureate distance learning degree programs offered (minimal on-campus study). *Faculty:* 60 full-time (52 women), 61 part-time/adjunct (47 women). *Students:* 33 full-time (29 women), 213 part-time (195 women); includes 32 minority (8 Black or African American, non-Hispanic/Latino; 10 Asian, non-Hispanic/Latino; 8 Hispanic/Latino; 6 Two or more races, non-Hispanic/Latino), 4 international. Average age 34. 41 applicants, 54% accepted, 16 enrolled. In 2013, 58 master's, 11 doctorates awarded. Terminal master's awarded for partial completion of doctoral program. *Degree requirements:* For master's, comprehensive exam (for some programs); for doctorate, thesis/dissertation. *Entrance requirements:* For master's, BS in nursing, minimum GPA of 3.0, course work in statistics; for doctorate, GRE General Test, MS in nursing, minimum GPA of 3.5. Additional exam requirements/recommendations for international students: Required—TOEFL (minimum score 560 paper-based; 88 iBT) or IELTS (minimum score 6.5) recommended. *Application deadline:* For fall admission, 4/1 for domestic and international students; for spring admission, 9/1 for domestic and international students; for summer admission, 1/2 for domestic and international students. Application fee: $50. Electronic applications accepted. *Expenses: Tuition:* Full-time $44,580; part-time $1394 per credit hour. *Required fees:* $492. *Financial support:* In 2013–14, 41 students received support, including 2 fellowships with full and partial tuition reimbursements available (averaging $30,200 per year); scholarships/grants, traineeships, health care benefits, tuition waivers (partial), and unspecified assistantships also available. Support available to part-time students. Financial award application deadline: 6/30. *Faculty research:* Symptom assessment and self-management, illness prevention, nursing intervention research with vulnerable populations, palliative care, aging. *Total annual research expenditures:* $3.5 million. *Unit head:* Dr. Kathy H. Rideout, Dean, 585-273-8902, Fax: 585-273-1268, E-mail: kathy_rideout@urmc.rochester.edu. *Application contact:* Elaine Andolina, Director of Admissions, 585-275-2375, Fax: 585-756-8299, E-mail: elaine_andolina@urmc.rochester.edu.
Website: http://www.son.rochester.edu

University of San Diego, Hahn School of Nursing and Health Science, San Diego, CA 92110. Offers adult-gerontology clinical nurse specialist (MSN); adult-gerontology nurse practitioner/family nurse practitioner (MSN); clinical nursing (MSN); executive nurse leader (MSN); family nurse practitioner (MSN); family/lifespan psychiatric-mental health nurse practitioner (MSN); healthcare informatics (MS, MSN); nursing (PhD); nursing practice (DNP); pediatric nurse practitioner/family nurse practitioner (MSN). *Accreditation:* AACN. Part-time and evening/weekend programs available. *Faculty:* 23 full-time (19 women), 48 part-time/adjunct (43 women). *Students:* 204 full-time (170 women), 166 part-time (144 women); includes 133 minority (26 Black or African American, non-Hispanic/Latino; 8 American Indian or Alaska Native, non-Hispanic/Latino; 50 Asian, non-Hispanic/Latino; 42 Hispanic/Latino; 1 Native Hawaiian or other Pacific Islander, non-Hispanic/Latino; 6 Two or more races, non-Hispanic/Latino), 7 international. Average age 36. 483 applicants, 58% accepted, 154 enrolled. In 2013, 91 master's, 33 doctorates awarded. *Degree requirements:* For doctorate, thesis/dissertation (for some programs), residency (DNP). *Entrance requirements:* For master's, GRE General Test (for entry-level nursing), BSN, current California RN licensure (except for entry-level nursing); minimum GPA of 3.0; for doctorate, minimum GPA of 3.5, MSN, current California RN licensure. Additional exam requirements/recommendations for international students: Required—TOEFL (minimum score 580 paper-based; 83 iBT), TWE. *Application deadline:* For fall admission, 3/1 priority date for domestic students, 3/1 for international students; for spring admission, 11/1 priority date for domestic students, 11/1 for international students. Applications are processed on a rolling basis. Application fee: $45. Electronic applications accepted. *Expenses: Tuition:* Full-time $23,580; part-time $1310 per credit. *Required fees:* $350. *Financial support:* In 2013–14, 250 students received support. Scholarships/grants and traineeships available. Support available to part-time students. Financial award application deadline: 4/1; financial award applicants required to submit FAFSA. *Faculty research:* Palliative and end of life care, maternal/child health, childhood obesity, health care disparities, cognitive functioning. *Unit head:* Dr. Sally Hardin, Dean, 619-260-4550, Fax: 619-260-6814. *Application contact:* Monica Mahon, Associate Director of Graduate Admissions, 619-260-4524, Fax: 619-260-4158, E-mail: grads@sandiego.edu.
Website: http://www.sandiego.edu/nursing/

The University of Scranton, College of Graduate and Continuing Education, Department of Nursing, Scranton, PA 18510-4595. Offers adult health nursing (MSN); family nurse practitioner (MSN, PMC); nurse anesthesia (MSN, PMC). Applicants accepted in odd-numbered years only. *Accreditation:* AACN; AANA/CANAEP. Part-time and evening/weekend programs available. *Faculty:* 13 full-time (all women), 2 part-time/adjunct (both women). *Students:* 42 full-time (37 women), 28 part-time (16 women); includes 9 minority (4 Black or African American, non-Hispanic/Latino; 3 Hispanic/Latino; 2 Two or more races, non-Hispanic/Latino). Average age 34. 58 applicants, 62% accepted. In 2013, 34 master's awarded. *Degree requirements:* For master's, thesis (for some programs), capstone experience. *Entrance requirements:* For master's, BSN, minimum GPA of 3.0, Pennsylvania RN license. Additional exam requirements/recommendations for international students: Required—TOEFL (minimum score 500 paper-based), IELTS (minimum score 5.5). *Application deadline:* For fall admission, 9/1 for domestic students. Applications are processed on a rolling basis. Application fee: $0. *Financial support:* In 2013–14, 6 students received support, including 6 teaching assistantships with full and partial tuition reimbursements available (averaging $6,600 per year); career-related internships or fieldwork, Federal Work-Study, and unspecified assistantships also available. Support available to part-time students. Financial award application deadline: 3/1. *Faculty research:* Home care, doctoral education, health care of women and children, pain, health promotion and adolescence. *Unit head:* Dr. Patricia Harrington, Chair, 570-941-7673, Fax: 570-941-4201, E-mail: harringtonp1@uofs.edu. *Application contact:* Dr. Mary Jane Hanson, Director, 570-941-4060, Fax: 570-941-4201, E-mail: hansonm2@scranton.edu.
Website: http://www.scranton.edu/academics/pcps/nursing/index.shtml

University of South Alabama, Graduate School, College of Nursing, Mobile, AL 36688. Offers adult health nursing (MSN); community/mental health nursing (MSN); maternal/child nursing (MSN); nursing (DNP). *Accreditation:* AACN. *Faculty:* 50 full-time (46 women), 31 part-time/adjunct (30 women). *Students:* 1,878 full-time (1,680 women), 241 part-time (208 women); includes 523 minority (341 Black or African American, non-Hispanic/Latino; 18 American Indian or Alaska Native, non-Hispanic/Latino; 76 Asian, non-Hispanic/Latino; 54 Hispanic/Latino; 7 Native Hawaiian or other Pacific Islander, non-Hispanic/Latino; 27 Two or more races, non-Hispanic/Latino), 10 international. 1,308 applicants, 64% accepted, 602 enrolled. In 2013, 332 master's, 44 doctorates awarded. *Degree requirements:* For master's, thesis optional. *Entrance requirements:* For master's, BSN, RN licensure, minimum GPA of 3.0, resume documenting clinical experience, background check, drug screening; for doctorate, GRE. *Application deadline:* For fall admission, 7/15 for domestic students; for spring admission, 12/1 for domestic students. Application fee: $35. *Expenses:* Tuition, state resident: full-time $8976; part-time $374 per credit hour. Tuition, nonresident: full-time $17,952; part-time $748 per credit hour. *Unit head:* Dr. Debra Davis, Dean, 251-445-9409, Fax: 251-445-9416. *Application contact:* Dr. Rosemary Rhodes, Director of Graduate Education, 251-445-9409, Fax: 251-445-9416, E-mail: kharriso@usouthal.edu.
Website: http://www.southalabama.edu/nursing

University of South Carolina, The Graduate School, College of Nursing, Program in Health Nursing, Columbia, SC 29208. Offers adult nurse practitioner (MSN); community/public health clinical nurse specialist (MSN); family nurse practitioner (MSN); pediatric nurse practitioner (MSN). *Accreditation:* AACN. Part-time programs available. *Degree requirements:* For master's, thesis or alternative. *Entrance requirements:* For master's, GRE General Test or MAT, BS in nursing, nursing license. Additional exam requirements/recommendations for international students: Required—TOEFL (minimum score 570 paper-based). Electronic applications accepted. *Faculty research:* System research, evidence based practice, breast cancer, violence.

University of Southern Maine, College of Science, Technology, and Health, School of Nursing, Portland, ME 04104-9300. Offers adult-gerontology primary care nurse practitioner (MS, PMC); clinical nurse leader (MS); education (MS); family nurse practitioner (MS, PMC); family psychiatric/mental health nurse practitioner (MS); management (MS); nursing (DNP); psychiatric-mental health nurse practitioner (PMC); MBA/MSN. *Accreditation:* AACN. Part-time programs available. *Faculty:* 11 full-time (all women), 10 part-time/adjunct (8 women). *Students:* 57 full-time (47 women), 53 part-time (46 women); includes 5 minority (1 American Indian or Alaska Native, non-Hispanic/Latino; 2 Asian, non-Hispanic/Latino; 1 Hispanic/Latino; 1 Two or more races, non-Hispanic/Latino). Average age 36. 140 applicants, 44% accepted, 29 enrolled. In 2013, 33 master's, 11 other advanced degrees awarded. *Degree requirements:* For master's, thesis optional. *Entrance requirements:* For master's, GRE General Test or MAT, minimum GPA of 3.0; for doctorate, GRE. Additional exam requirements/recommendations for international students: Required—TOEFL (minimum score 550 paper-based). *Application deadline:* For fall admission, 4/1 for domestic and international students; for spring admission, 10/1 for domestic and international students. Application fee: $65. Electronic applications accepted. *Expenses:* Tuition, state resident: part-time $380 per credit. Tuition, nonresident: part-time $1026 per credit. Part-time tuition and fees vary according to program. *Financial support:* Research assistantships, teaching assistantships, career-related internships or

fieldwork, Federal Work-Study, scholarships/grants, traineeships, tuition waivers (full and partial), and unspecified assistantships available. Support available to part-time students. Financial award application deadline: 2/15; financial award applicants required to submit FAFSA. *Faculty research:* Women's health, nursing history, weight control, community services, substance abuse. *Unit head:* Krista M. Meinersmann, Director of Nursing Program, 207-780-4993, E-mail: kmeinersmann@usm.maine.edu. *Application contact:* Mary Sloan, Assistant Dean of Graduate Studies and Director of Graduate Admissions, 207-780-4812, E-mail: gradstudies@usm.maine.edu.
Website: http://www.usm.maine.edu/nursing/

University of South Florida, College of Nursing, Tampa, FL 33612. Offers adult gerontology acute care (DNP, PhD); adult gerontology acute care nursing (MS); adult gerontology primary care (DNP, PhD); adult gerontology primary care nursing (MS); adult gerontology primary care/occupational health nursing (MS); adult gerontology primary care/oncology nursing (MS, PhD); clinical nurse leader (MS); family health (DNP, PhD); family nurse practitioner (MS); nurse anesthesia (MS); nursing education (MS); nursing practice (DNP); nursing science (PhD), including nursing education; occupational health/adult-gerontology (DNP); oncology/adult-gerontology primary care (DNP); pediatric health (DNP, PhD); pediatric nurse practitioner (MS). *Accreditation:* AACN; AANA/CANAEP. Part-time programs available. *Faculty:* 46 full-time (40 women), 15 part-time/adjunct (11 women). *Students:* 177 full-time (150 women), 700 part-time (622 women); includes 272 minority (116 Black or African American, non-Hispanic/Latino; 2 American Indian or Alaska Native, non-Hispanic/Latino; 45 Asian, non-Hispanic/Latino; 93 Hispanic/Latino; 2 Native Hawaiian or other Pacific Islander, non-Hispanic/Latino; 14 Two or more races, non-Hispanic/Latino), 12 international. Average age 35. 656 applicants, 43% accepted, 224 enrolled. In 2013, 224 master's, 14 doctorates awarded. *Degree requirements:* For master's, comprehensive exam, thesis optional; for doctorate, comprehensive exam, thesis/dissertation. *Entrance requirements:* For master's, GRE General Test, bachelor's degree from accredited program with minimum GPA of 3.0 in all upper-division coursework; current license as Registered Nurse; 3 letters of recommendation; personal statement of goals; resume or curriculum vitae; personal interview; for doctorate, GRE General Test (recommended), bachelor's degree in nursing from a CCNA/NLNAC regionally-accredited institution with minimum GPA of 3.0 in all coursework or in all upper-division coursework; current license as Registered Nurse in Florida; undergraduate statistics course with minimum B grade; 3 letters of recommendation; statement of goals; resume; interview. Additional exam requirements/recommendations for international students: Required—TOEFL (minimum score 550 paper-based; 79 iBT). *Application deadline:* For fall admission, 2/15 for domestic students, 1/2 for international students; for spring admission, 10/1 for domestic students, 6/1 for international students. Application fee: $30. Electronic applications accepted. *Financial support:* In 2013–14, 36 students received support, including 7 research assistantships with tuition reimbursements available (averaging $18,935 per year), 29 teaching assistantships with tuition reimbursements available (averaging $30,814 per year); tuition waivers (partial) and unspecified assistantships also available. Financial award application deadline: 2/1; financial award applicants required to submit FAFSA. *Faculty research:* Women's health, palliative and end-of-life care, cardiac rehabilitation, complementary therapies for chronic illness and cancer. *Total annual research expenditures:* $3.4 million. *Unit head:* Dr. Dianne C. Morrison-Beedy, Dean and Professor, College of Nursing, 813-974-9091, Fax: 813-974-5418, E-mail: dmbeedy@health.usf.edu. *Application contact:* Dr. Connie Visovsky, Associate Professor and Associate Dean of Student Affairs, 813-396-9641, Fax: 813-974-5418, E-mail: cvisovsk@health.usf.edu.
Website: http://health.usf.edu/nursing/index.htm

The University of Tampa, Nursing Programs, Tampa, FL 33606-1490. Offers adult nurse practitioner (MSN); family nurse practitioner (MSN). Part-time programs available. *Faculty:* 15 full-time (all women), 15 part-time/adjunct (14 women). *Students:* 2 full-time (both women), 134 part-time (119 women); includes 37 minority (10 Black or African American, non-Hispanic/Latino; 1 American Indian or Alaska Native, non-Hispanic/Latino; 6 Asian, non-Hispanic/Latino; 19 Hispanic/Latino; 1 Two or more races, non-Hispanic/Latino). Average age 34. 79 applicants, 51% accepted, 28 enrolled. In 2013, 39 master's awarded. *Degree requirements:* For master's, comprehensive exam, oral exam, practicum. *Entrance requirements:* For master's, GRE (minimum score of 1000, 4.0 on Analytical Writing portion), bachelor's degree in nursing, current Florida RN license, minimum GPA of 3.0. Additional exam requirements/recommendations for international students: Required—TOEFL or IELTS. *Application deadline:* Applications are processed on a rolling basis. Application fee: $40. Electronic applications accepted. *Expenses: Tuition:* Full-time $8928; part-time $558 per credit hour. *Required fees:* $80; $80 $40 per term. Tuition and fees vary according to program. *Financial support:* In 2013–14, 9 students received support. Unspecified assistantships available. Financial award applicants required to submit FAFSA. *Faculty research:* Vaccinations and public health, osteoporosis, cultural diversity, ethics, nursing practice. *Unit head:* Dr. Maria Warda, Director/Chair, 813-257-3302, Fax: 813-258-7214, E-mail: mwarda@ut.edu. *Application contact:* Brent Benner, Director of Admissions, 813-257-3642, E-mail: bbenner@ut.edu.

The University of Texas at Austin, Graduate School, School of Nursing, Austin, TX 78712-1111. Offers adult - gerontology clinical nurse specialist (MSN); child health (MSN), including administration, public health nursing, teaching; family nurse practitioner (MSN); family psychiatric/mental health nurse practitioner (MSN); holistic adult health (MSN), including administration, teaching; maternity (MSN), including administration, public health nursing, teaching; nursing (PhD); nursing administration and healthcare systems management (MSN); pediatric nurse practitioner (MSN); public health nursing (MSN). *Accreditation:* AACN. Part-time programs available. *Degree requirements:* For master's, thesis optional; for doctorate, thesis/dissertation. *Entrance requirements:* For master's and doctorate, GRE General Test. Additional exam requirements/recommendations for international students: Required—TOEFL (minimum score 550 paper-based). Electronic applications accepted. *Faculty research:* Chronic illness management, memory and aging, health promotion, women's health, adolescent health.

The University of Texas–Pan American, College of Health Sciences and Human Services, Department of Nursing, Edinburg, TX 78539. Offers adult health nursing (MSN); family nurse practitioner (MSN). *Accreditation:* AACN. Part-time and evening/weekend programs available. *Degree requirements:* For master's, thesis optional. *Entrance requirements:* For master's, Texas RN licensure, undergraduate physical statistic course. Additional exam requirements/recommendations for international students: Required—TOEFL (minimum score 550 paper-based). Electronic applications accepted. *Expenses:* Contact institution. *Faculty research:* Health promotion, adolescent pregnancy, herbal and nontraditional approaches, healing touch stress.

University of Wisconsin–Eau Claire, College of Nursing and Health Sciences, Program in Nursing, Eau Claire, WI 54702-4004. Offers adult-gerontological administration (DNP); adult-gerontological clinical nurse specialist (DNP); adult-gerontological education (MSN); adult-gerontological primary care nurse practitioner (DNP); family health administration (DNP); family health in education (MSN); family health nurse practitioner (DNP); nursing (MSN); nursing practice (DNP). Part-time programs available. *Faculty:* 8 full-time (all women), 2 part-time/adjunct (both women). *Students:* 33 full-time (30 women), 40 part-time (36 women); includes 1 minority (Asian, non-Hispanic/Latino). Average age 37. 48 applicants, 85% accepted, 24 enrolled. In 2013, 31 master's, 9 doctorates awarded. Terminal master's awarded for partial completion of doctoral program. *Degree requirements:* For master's, thesis optional, 500-600 hours clinical practicum, oral and written exams. *Entrance requirements:* For master's, Wisconsin RN license, minimum GPA of 3.0, undergraduate statistics, course work in health assessment. Additional exam requirements/recommendations for international students: Required—TOEFL (minimum score 79 iBT). *Application deadline:* For fall admission, 1/15 priority date for domestic and international students. Applications are processed on a rolling basis. Application fee: $86. *Expenses:* Contact institution. *Financial support:* In 2013–14, 10 students received support. Federal Work-Study and unspecified assistantships available. Financial award application deadline: 3/1; financial award applicants required to submit FAFSA. *Unit head:* Dr. Linda Young, Dean, 715-836-4904, Fax: 715-836-5925, E-mail: younglk@uwec.edu. *Application contact:* Dr. Mary Zwygart-Stauffacher, Director, 715-836-5287, E-mail: zwygarmc@uwec.edu.
Website: http://www.uwec.edu/conhs/programs/grad/index.htm

University of Wisconsin–Madison, School of Nursing, Madison, WI 53706-1380. Offers adult/gerontology (DNP); nursing (PhD); pediatrics (DNP); psychiatric mental health (DNP); MS/MPH. *Accreditation:* AACN. Part-time programs available. *Degree requirements:* For doctorate, comprehensive exam, thesis/dissertation. *Entrance requirements:* For doctorate, GRE General Test, 2 samples of scholarly written work, BS in nursing from an accredited program, minimum undergraduate GPA of 3.0 in last 60 credits (for PhD); licensure as professional nurse (for DNP). Additional exam requirements/recommendations for international students: Required—TOEFL (minimum score 600 paper-based; 100 iBT). Electronic applications accepted. *Expenses:* Tuition, state resident: full-time $10,728; part-time $790 per credit. Tuition, nonresident: full-time $24,054; part-time $1623 per credit. *Required fees:* $1130; $119 per credit. *Faculty research:* Nursing informatics to promote self-care and disease management skills among patients and caregivers; quality of care to frail, vulnerable, and chronically ill populations; study of health-related and health-seeking behaviors; eliminating health disparities; pain and symptom management for patients with cancer.

University of Wisconsin–Oshkosh, Graduate Studies, College of Nursing, Oshkosh, WI 54901. Offers adult health and illness (MSN); family nurse practitioner (MSN). *Accreditation:* AACN. Part-time programs available. *Degree requirements:* For master's, thesis or alternative, clinical paper. *Entrance requirements:* For master's, RN license, BSN, previous course work in statistics and health assessment, minimum undergraduate GPA of 3.0, letters of recommendation. Additional exam requirements/recommendations for international students: Required—TOEFL (minimum score 550 paper-based; 79 iBT). Electronic applications accepted. *Faculty research:* Adult health and illness, nurse practitioners practice, health care service, advanced practitioner roles, natural alternative complementary healthcare.

Vanderbilt University, Vanderbilt University School of Nursing, Nashville, TN 37240. Offers adult-gerontology acute care nurse practitioner (MSN), including hospitalist, intensivist; adult-gerontology primary care nurse practitioner (MSN); emergency nurse practitioner (MSN); family nurse practitioner (MSN); healthcare leadership (MSN); neonatal nurse practitioner (MSN); nurse midwifery (MSN); nurse midwifery/family nurse practitioner (MSN); nursing informatics (MSN); nursing practice (DNP); nursing science (PhD); pediatric acute care nurse practitioner (MSN); pediatric primary care nurse practitioner (MSN); psychiatric-mental health nurse practitioner (MSN); women's health nurse practitioner (MSN); women's health nurse practitioner/adult gerontology primary care nurse practitioner (MSN); MSN/M Div; MSN/MTS. *Accreditation:* ACNM/ACME (one or more programs are accredited). Part-time programs available. Postbaccalaureate distance learning degree programs offered (minimal on-campus study). *Faculty:* 139 full-time (124 women), 452 part-time/adjunct (319 women). *Students:* 527 full-time (463 women), 369 part-time (333 women); includes 120 minority (46 Black or African American, non-Hispanic/Latino; 8 American Indian or Alaska Native, non-Hispanic/Latino; 26 Asian, non-Hispanic/Latino; 24 Hispanic/Latino; 4 Native Hawaiian or other Pacific Islander, non-Hispanic/Latino; 12 Two or more races, non-Hispanic/Latino), 7 international. Average age 32. 1,257 applicants, 49% accepted, 457 enrolled. In 2013, 364 master's, 43 doctorates awarded. *Degree requirements:* For doctorate, comprehensive exam, thesis/dissertation. *Entrance requirements:* For master's, GRE General Test (within the past 5 years), minimum B average in undergraduate course work, 3 letters of recommendation; for doctorate, GRE General Test, interview, 3 letters of recommendation from doctorally-prepared faculty, MSN, essay. Additional exam requirements/recommendations for international students: Required—TOEFL (minimum score 570 paper-based), IELTS (minimum score 6.5). *Application deadline:* For fall admission, 12/1 priority date for domestic and international students. Applications are processed on a rolling basis. Application fee: $50. Electronic applications accepted. *Expenses:* Contact institution. *Financial support:* In 2013–14, 582 students received support. Scholarships/grants and health care benefits available. Support available to part-time students. Financial award application deadline: 3/15; financial award applicants required to submit FAFSA. *Faculty research:* Lymphedema, palliative care and bereavement, health services research including workforce, safety and quality of care, gerontology, better birth outcomes including nutrition. *Total annual research expenditures:* $2.5 million. *Unit head:* Dr. Linda Norman, Dean, 615-343-8876, Fax: 615-343-7711, E-mail: linda.norman@vanderbilt.edu. *Application contact:* Patricia Peerman, Assistant Dean for Enrollment Management, 615-322-3800, Fax: 615-343-0333, E-mail: vusn-admissions@vanderbilt.edu.
Website: http://www.nursing.vanderbilt.edu

Villanova University, College of Nursing, Villanova, PA 19085-1699. Offers adult nurse practitioner (MSN, Post Master's Certificate); family nurse practitioner (MSN, Post Master's Certificate); health care administration (MSN, Post Master's Certificate); nurse anesthetist (MSN, Post Master's Certificate); nursing (PhD); nursing education (MSN, Post Master's Certificate); nursing practice (DNP); pediatric nurse practitioner (MSN, Post Master's Certificate). *Accreditation:* AACN; AANA/CANAEP. Part-time programs available. Postbaccalaureate distance learning degree programs offered (minimal on-campus study). *Faculty:* 17 full-time (all women), 4 part-time/adjunct (all women). *Students:* 28 full-time (26 women), 191 part-time (161 women); includes 22 minority (2 Black or African American, non-Hispanic/Latino; 6 Asian, non-Hispanic/Latino; 7 Hispanic/Latino; 7 Two or more races, non-Hispanic/Latino), 18 international. Average age 30. 176 applicants, 65% accepted, 82 enrolled. In 2013, 64 master's, 7 doctorates, 5 other advanced degrees awarded. *Degree requirements:* For master's, independent study project; for doctorate, comprehensive exam, thesis/dissertation. *Entrance requirements:* For master's, GRE or MAT, BSN, 1 year of recent nursing experience, physical assessment, course work in statistics; for doctorate, GRE, MSN. Additional exam requirements/recommendations for international students: Required—TOEFL (minimum score 540 paper-based; 83 iBT), IELTS (minimum score 6.5). *Application deadline:* For fall admission, 7/1 priority date for domestic students, 7/1 for international students; for spring admission, 11/1 priority date for domestic students, 11/1 for international students. Applications are processed on a rolling basis. Application fee: $50. Electronic applications accepted. *Expenses:* Contact institution. *Financial support:* In 2013–14, 39 students received support, including 5 teaching assistantships with full tuition reimbursements available (averaging $14,475 per year); institutionally sponsored

loans, scholarships/grants, traineeships, tuition waivers (full), and unspecified assistantships also available. Financial award application deadline: 7/1; financial award applicants required to submit FAFSA. *Faculty research:* Genetics, ethics, cognitive development of students, women with disabilities, nursing leadership. *Unit head:* Dr. Marguerite K. Schlag, Assistant Dean/Director, Graduate Programs, 610-519-4907, Fax: 610-519-7650, E-mail: marguerite.schlag@villanova.edu.
Website: http://www.nursing.villanova.edu/

Virginia Commonwealth University, Graduate School, School of Nursing, Richmond, VA 23284-9005. Offers adult health acute nursing (MS); adult health primary nursing (MS); biobehavioral clinical research (PhD); child health nursing (MS); clinical nurse leader (MS); family health nursing (MS); nurse educator (MS); nurse practitioner (MS); nursing (Certificate); nursing administration (MS), including clinical nurse manager; psychiatric-mental health nursing (MS); women's health nursing (MS). Part-time and evening/weekend programs available. *Degree requirements:* For master's, thesis optional; for doctorate, thesis/dissertation. *Entrance requirements:* For master's, GRE General Test, BSN, minimum GPA of 2.8; for doctorate, GRE General Test. Additional exam requirements/recommendations for international students: Required—TOEFL (minimum score 600 paper-based; 100 iBT). Electronic applications accepted.

Walden University, Graduate Programs, School of Nursing, Minneapolis, MN 55401. Offers adult-gerontology acute care nurse practitioner (MSN); adult-gerontology nurse practitioner (MSN); education (MSN); family nurse practitioner (MSN); informatics (MSN); leadership and management (MSN); nursing (DNP, PhD, Post-Master's Certificate), including education (PhD), healthcare administration (PhD), interdisciplinary health (PhD), leadership (PhD), nursing education (Post-Master's Certificate), nursing informatics (Post-Master's Certificate), nursing leadership and management (Post-Master's Certificate), public health policy (PhD). *Accreditation:* AACN. Part-time and evening/weekend programs available. Postbaccalaureate distance learning degree programs offered (no on-campus study). *Faculty:* 22 full-time (19 women), 343 part-time/adjunct (301 women). *Students:* 5,828 full-time (5,240 women), 2,803 part-time (2,578 women); includes 2,920 minority (1,893 Black or African American, non-Hispanic/Latino; 40 American Indian or Alaska Native, non-Hispanic/Latino; 438 Asian, non-Hispanic/Latino; 391 Hispanic/Latino; 35 Native Hawaiian or other Pacific Islander, non-Hispanic/Latino; 123 Two or more races, non-Hispanic/Latino), 147 international. Average age 41. 1,795 applicants, 95% accepted, 1375 enrolled. In 2013, 1,879 master's, 1 doctorate, 36 other advanced degrees awarded. *Degree requirements:* For doctorate, thesis/dissertation (for some programs), residency (for some programs), field experience (for some programs). *Entrance requirements:* For master's, bachelor's degree or equivalent in related field or RN; minimum GPA of 2.5; official transcripts; goal statement (for some programs); access to computer and Internet; for doctorate, master's degree or higher, three years of related professional or academic experience, RN, goal statement (for some programs); access to computer and Internet; for Post-Master's Certificate, relevant work experience; access to computer and Internet. Additional exam requirements/recommendations for international students: Required—TOEFL (minimum score 550 paper-based; 79 iBT), IELTS (minimum score 6.5), Michigan English Language Assessment Battery (minimum score 82), or PTE. *Application deadline:* Applications are processed on a rolling basis. Application fee: $0. Electronic applications accepted. *Expenses: Tuition:* Full-time $11,813.55; part-time $500 per credit. *Required fees:* $618.76. *Financial support:* Fellowships, Federal Work-Study, scholarships/grants, unspecified assistantships, and family tuition reduction, active duty/veteran tuition reduction, group tuition reduction, interest-free payment plans, employee tuition reduction available. Support available to part-time students. Financial award applicants required to submit FAFSA. *Unit head:* Dr. Andrea Lindell, Associate Dean, 800-925-3368. *Application contact:* Jennifer Hall, Vice President of Enrollment Management, 866-4-WALDEN, E-mail: info@waldenu.edu.
Website: http://www.waldenu.edu/programs/colleges-schools/nursing

Wayne State University, College of Nursing, Area of Adult Health, Detroit, MI 48202. Offers MSN, Graduate Certificate. *Accreditation:* AACN. Part-time programs available. *Faculty:* 18 full-time (17 women). *Students:* 1 (woman) full-time, 59 part-time (51 women); includes 20 minority (9 Black or African American, non-Hispanic/Latino; 9 Asian, non-Hispanic/Latino; 2 Hispanic/Latino), 1 international. Average age 38. In 2013, 67 master's awarded. *Degree requirements:* For master's, thesis or alternative. *Entrance requirements:* For master's, bachelor's degree in nursing from an NLN- or CCNE-accredited program with minimum upper-division GPA of 3.0, three references, current Michigan RN, personal statement, interview; for Graduate Certificate, MS or MSN and/or DNP from nationally-accredited institution, minimum GPA of 3.0, eligible for licensure as a registered nurse in the State of Michigan. Additional exam requirements/recommendations for international students: Required—TOEFL (minimum score 550 paper-based; 79 iBT), TWE (minimum score 6), Michigan English Language Assessment Battery (minimum score 85); Recommended—IELTS (minimum score 6.5). *Application deadline:* For fall admission, 7/1 for domestic students, 5/1 priority date for international students; for winter admission, 11/1 for domestic students, 9/1 priority date for international students; for spring admission, 3/1 for domestic students, 1/1 priority date for international students. Applications are processed on a rolling basis. Application fee: $0. Electronic applications accepted. *Expenses:* Contact institution. *Financial support:* Institutionally sponsored loans, scholarships/grants, traineeships, and unspecified assistantships available. Financial award application deadline: 3/31; financial award applicants required to submit FAFSA. *Faculty research:* Hospice and palliative care, sleep promotion across the lifespan, chronic wound care in adults, patient health literacy and health disparities, improving heart failure outcomes. *Unit head:* Dr. Janet Harden, Interim Assistant Dean, Adult Health, 313-577-2221, E-mail: jharden@wayne.edu. *Application contact:* Eric Brown, Director, Office of Student Affairs for College of Nursing, 313-577-4082, E-mail: nursinginfo@wayne.edu.
Website: https://nursing.wayne.edu/

Wayne State University, College of Nursing, Program in Adult Primary Care Nursing, Detroit, MI 48202. Offers adult primary care nursing (MSN); gerontological nurse practitioner (MSN). *Accreditation:* AACN. Part-time programs available. *Students:* 3 full-time (all women), 94 part-time (81 women); includes 33 minority (15 Black or African American, non-Hispanic/Latino; 10 Asian, non-Hispanic/Latino; 5 Hispanic/Latino; 3 Two or more races, non-Hispanic/Latino), 2 international. Average age 36. In 2013, 26 master's awarded. *Degree requirements:* For master's, thesis or alternative. *Entrance requirements:* For master's, minimum honor point average of 3.0 in upper-division course work; BA from NLN- or CCNE-accredited program; references; current RN license; personal statement. Additional exam requirements/recommendations for international students: Required—TOEFL (minimum score 550 paper-based; 79 iBT); Recommended—TWE (minimum score 6). *Application deadline:* For fall admission, 6/1 priority date for domestic students, 5/1 priority date for international students; for winter admission, 10/1 priority date for domestic students, 9/1 priority date for international students; for spring admission, 2/1 priority date for domestic students, 1/1 priority date for international students. Applications are processed on a rolling basis. Application fee: $50. Electronic applications accepted. *Expenses:* Contact institution. *Financial support:* In 2013–14, 6 students received support. Fellowships with tuition reimbursements available, research assistantships with tuition reimbursements available, teaching assistantships with tuition reimbursements available, scholarships/grants, traineeships, and unspecified assistantships available. Support available to part-time students. Financial award applicants required to submit FAFSA. *Faculty research:* Smoking risk behaviors in adolescents, sleep disturbances in postmenopausal women, health disparities in urban environments, nurse practitioner interventions, care giving and pain management. *Unit head:* Dr. Barbara Redman, Dean, 313-577-4070, Fax: 313-577-4571, E-mail: ae9080@wayne.edu. *Application contact:* Dr. Cynthia Redwine, Assistant Dean for the Office of Student Affairs, 313-577-4082, E-mail: nursinginfo@wayne.edu.
Website: http://www.nursing.wayne.edu/msn/APCNPCurriculum.php

Western Connecticut State University, Division of Graduate Studies, School of Professional Studies, Nursing Department, Danbury, CT 06810-6885. Offers adult nurse practitioner (MSN); clinical nurse specialist (MSN). *Accreditation:* AACN. Part-time programs available. *Degree requirements:* For master's, clinical component, thesis or research project, completion of program in 6 years. *Entrance requirements:* For master's, MAT (if GPA less than 3.0), bachelor's degree in nursing, minimum GPA of 3.0, previous course work in statistics and nursing research, RN license. Additional exam requirements/recommendations for international students: Recommended—TOEFL (minimum score 550 paper-based; 79 iBT), IELTS (minimum score 6). *Expenses:* Contact institution. *Faculty research:* Evaluating effectiveness of Reiki and acupressure on stress reduction.

Wilmington University, College of Health Professions, New Castle, DE 19720-6491. Offers adult nurse practitioner (MSN); family nurse practitioner (MSN); gerontology nurse practitioner (MSN); nursing (MSN); nursing leadership (MSN); nursing practice (DNP). *Accreditation:* AACN. Part-time programs available. *Degree requirements:* For master's, thesis. *Entrance requirements:* For master's, BSN, RN license, interview, 3 letters of recommendation. Additional exam requirements/recommendations for international students: Required—TOEFL (minimum score 500 paper-based). Electronic applications accepted. *Faculty research:* Outcomes assessment, student writing ability.

Winona State University, College of Nursing and Health Sciences, Winona, MN 55987. Offers adult nurse practitioner (MS, Post Master's Certificate); clinical nurse specialist (MS, Post Master's Certificate); family nurse practitioner (MS, Post Master's Certificate); nurse administrator (MS); nurse educator (MS, Post Master's Certificate); nursing (DNP). *Accreditation:* AACN. Part-time programs available. Postbaccalaureate distance learning degree programs offered (no on-campus study). *Degree requirements:* For master's, thesis; for doctorate, capstone. *Entrance requirements:* For master's, GRE (if GPA less than 3.0). Additional exam requirements/recommendations for international students: Required—TOEFL (minimum score 550 paper-based).

Wright State University, School of Graduate Studies, College of Nursing and Health, Program in Nursing, Dayton, OH 45435. Offers acute care nurse practitioner (MS); administration of nursing and health care systems (MS); adult health (MS); child and adolescent health (MS); community health (MS); family nurse practitioner (MS); nurse practitioner (MS); school nurse (MS); MBA/MS. *Accreditation:* AACN. Part-time and evening/weekend programs available. *Degree requirements:* For master's, thesis or alternative. *Entrance requirements:* For master's, GRE General Test, BSN from NLN-accredited college, Ohio RN license. Additional exam requirements/recommendations for international students: Required—TOEFL. *Faculty research:* Clinical nursing and health, teaching, caring, pain administration, informatics and technology.

York College of Pennsylvania, Department of Nursing, York, PA 17405-7199. Offers adult gerontology clinical nurse specialist (MS), including administration, education; adult gerontology nurse practitioner (MS); certified nurse anesthetist (MS); nurse educator (MS); nursing (DNP). *Accreditation:* AACN; AANA/CANAEP. Part-time and evening/weekend programs available. *Faculty:* 10 full-time (all women), 4 part-time/adjunct (1 woman). *Students:* 33 full-time (26 women), 61 part-time (53 women); includes 12 minority (7 Black or African American, non-Hispanic/Latino; 2 American Indian or Alaska Native, non-Hispanic/Latino; 3 Asian, non-Hispanic/Latino), 1 international. Average age 37. 87 applicants, 31% accepted, 24 enrolled. In 2013, 26 master's, 4 doctorates awarded. *Entrance requirements:* For master's, GRE General Test, minimum GPA of 3.0 from CCNE- or NLNAC-accredited institution; for doctorate, master's degree in nursing from a CCNE- or NLNAC-accredited institution; minimum GPA of 3.0. Additional exam requirements/recommendations for international students: Required—TOEFL (minimum score 530 paper-based; 72 iBT). *Application deadline:* For fall admission, 7/15 priority date for domestic students; for spring admission, 11/15 priority date for domestic students. Applications are processed on a rolling basis. Application fee: $50. Electronic applications accepted. *Expenses: Tuition:* Full-time $12,870; part-time $715 per credit. *Required fees:* $1660; $360 per semester. Tuition and fees vary according to degree level. *Financial support:* Federal Work-Study available. *Faculty research:* Student stress response to simulation versus clinical, evidence-based practice in all clinical settings. *Unit head:* Dr. Richard Haas, Graduate Program Director, 717-815-1243, E-mail: rhaas@ycp.edu. *Application contact:* Diane Dube, Administrative Assistant, Graduate Programs in Nursing, 717-815-1462, E-mail: ddube@ycp.edu.
Website: http://www.ycp.edu/academics/academic-departments/nursing/

Community Health Nursing

Allen College, Program in Nursing, Waterloo, IA 50703. Offers acute care nurse practitioner (MSN, Post-Master's Certificate); adult nurse practitioner (MSN, Post-Master's Certificate); adult psychiatric-mental health nurse practitioner (MSN, Post-Master's Certificate); community public health (MSN, Post-Master's Certificate); family nurse practitioner (MSN, Post-Master's Certificate); gerontological nurse practitioner (MSN, Post-Master's Certificate); health education (MSN); leadership in health care delivery (MSN, Post-Master's Certificate); nursing (DNP). Part-time programs available. Postbaccalaureate distance learning degree programs offered (minimal on-campus study). *Faculty:* 3 full-time (all women), 21 part-time/adjunct (20 women). *Students:* 21 full-time (19 women), 162 part-time (150 women); includes 5 minority (1 Black or African

Community Health Nursing

American, non-Hispanic/Latino; 2 Asian, non-Hispanic/Latino; 1 Hispanic/Latino; 1 Two or more races, non-Hispanic/Latino). Average age 34. 213 applicants, 57% accepted, 94 enrolled. In 2013, 41 master's, 4 other advanced degrees awarded. *Degree requirements:* For master's, thesis optional. *Entrance requirements:* For master's, minimum GPA of 3.0 in the last 60 hours of undergraduate coursework; for doctorate, minimum GPA of 3.25 in graduate coursework. Additional exam requirements/recommendations for international students: Recommended—TOEFL (minimum score 580 paper-based; 92 iBT), IELTS (minimum score 6). *Application deadline:* For fall admission, 2/1 priority date for domestic students; for spring admission, 9/1 priority date for domestic students. Applications are processed on a rolling basis. Application fee: $50. Electronic applications accepted. *Expenses: Tuition:* Full-time $14,534; part-time $755 per credit hour. *Required fees:* $935; $75 per credit hour. One-time fee: $275 part-time. Tuition and fees vary according to course load. *Financial support:* In 2013–14, 60 students received support. Institutionally sponsored loans, scholarships/grants, and traineeships available. Support available to part-time students. Financial award application deadline: 8/15; financial award applicants required to submit FAFSA. *Unit head:* Kendra Williams-Perez, Dean, School of Nursing, 319-226-2044, Fax: 319-226-2070, E-mail: kendra.williams-perez@allencollege.edu. *Application contact:* Molly Quinn, Admissions Counselor, 319-226-2001, Fax: 319-226-2010, E-mail: molly.quinn@allencollege.edu.
Website: http://www.allencollege.edu/

American University of Beirut, Graduate Programs, Rafic Hariri School of Nursing, Beirut, Lebanon. Offers adult care nursing (MSN); community and public health nursing (MSN); nursing administration (MSN); psychiatry mental health nursing (MSN). *Accreditation:* AACN. Part-time programs available. *Faculty:* 9 full-time (8 women), 12 part-time/adjunct (10 women). *Students:* 4 full-time (3 women), 56 part-time (44 women). Average age 29. 38 applicants, 87% accepted, 26 enrolled. In 2013, 17 master's awarded. *Degree requirements:* For master's, one foreign language, comprehensive exam, thesis optional. *Entrance requirements:* For master's, letter of recommendation. Additional exam requirements/recommendations for international students: Required—TOEFL (minimum score 600 paper-based); Recommended—IELTS. *Application deadline:* For fall admission, 4/1 for domestic and international students; for spring admission, 11/1 for domestic and international students. Applications are processed on a rolling basis. Application fee: $50. Electronic applications accepted. *Expenses: Tuition:* Full-time $14,724; part-time $818 per credit. *Required fees:* $692. Tuition and fees vary according to course load and program. *Financial support:* In 2013–14, 24 teaching assistantships with partial tuition reimbursements were awarded; unspecified assistantships also available. Financial award application deadline: 12/20. *Faculty research:* Pain management and palliative care, stress and post-traumatic stress disorder, health benefits and chronic illness, health promotion and community interventions. *Unit head:* Dr. Huda Huijer Abu-Saad, Director, 961-1374374 Ext. 5952, Fax: 961-1744476, E-mail: hh35@aub.edu.lb. *Application contact:* Dr. Salim Kanaan, Director, Admissions Office, 961-1-350000 Ext. 2594, Fax: 96-1-1750775, E-mail: sk00@aub.edu.lb.
Website: http://staff.aub.edu.lb/~webson

Arizona State University at the Tempe campus, College of Nursing and Health Innovation, Phoenix, AZ 85004. Offers advanced nursing practice (DNP); child/family mental health nurse practitioner (Graduate Certificate); clinical research management (MS); community and public health practice (Graduate Certificate); community health (MS); exercise and wellness (MS), including exercise and wellness; family nurse practitioner (Graduate Certificate); healthcare innovation (MHI); international health for healthcare (Graduate Certificate); kinesiology (MS, PhD); nursing (MS, Graduate Certificate); nursing and healthcare innovation (PhD); nutrition (MS); physical activity nutrition and wellness (PhD), including physical activity, nutrition and wellness; public health (MPH); regulatory science and health safety (MS). *Accreditation:* AACN. Postbaccalaureate distance learning degree programs offered (minimal on-campus study). *Degree requirements:* For master's, comprehensive exam (for some programs), thesis (for some programs), interactive Program of Study (iPOS) submitted before completing 50 percent of required credit hours; for doctorate, comprehensive exam, thesis/dissertation, interactive Program of Study (iPOS) submitted before completing 50 percent of required credit hours. *Entrance requirements:* For master's and doctorate, GRE, minimum GPA of 3.0 or equivalent in last 2 years of work leading to bachelor's degree. Additional exam requirements/recommendations for international students: Required—TOEFL (minimum score 80 iBT), TOEFL, IELTS, or PTE. Electronic applications accepted. *Expenses:* Contact institution.

Augsburg College, Program in Transcultural Community Health Nursing, Minneapolis, MN 55454-1351. Offers MA. *Accreditation:* AACN. *Degree requirements:* For master's, thesis or alternative.

Boston College, William F. Connell School of Nursing, Chestnut Hill, MA 02467-3800. Offers adult-gerontology nursing (MS); community health nursing (MS); family health (MS); forensic nursing (MS); maternal/child health nursing (MS), including pediatric and women's health; nurse anesthesia (MS); nursing (PhD); palliative care (MS), including adult and pediatric; psychiatric-mental health nursing (MS); MBA/MS; MS/MA; MS/PhD. *Accreditation:* AACN; AANA/CANAEP (one or more programs are accredited). Part-time programs available. *Faculty:* 47 full-time (43 women), 42 part-time/adjunct (39 women). *Students:* 199 full-time (180 women), 79 part-time (73 women); includes 44 minority (14 Black or African American, non-Hispanic/Latino; 1 American Indian or Alaska Native, non-Hispanic/Latino; 13 Asian, non-Hispanic/Latino; 12 Hispanic/Latino; 4 Two or more races, non-Hispanic/Latino), 7 international. Average age 31. 502 applicants, 39% accepted, 87 enrolled. In 2013, 105 master's, 8 doctorates awarded. *Degree requirements:* For master's, comprehensive exam, research project; for doctorate, comprehensive exam, thesis/dissertation, computer literacy exam or foreign language. *Entrance requirements:* For master's, bachelor's degree in nursing; for doctorate, GRE General Test, MS in nursing. Additional exam requirements/recommendations for international students: Required—TOEFL (minimum score 600 paper-based; 100 iBT). *Application deadline:* For fall admission, 9/30 for domestic and international students; for winter admission, 1/15 for domestic and international students; for spring admission, 3/15 for domestic and international students. Applications are processed on a rolling basis. Application fee: $40. Electronic applications accepted. *Financial support:* In 2013–14, 174 students received support, including 7 fellowships with full tuition reimbursements available (averaging $20,000 per year), 21 teaching assistantships (averaging $4,800 per year); research assistantships, scholarships/grants, health care benefits, tuition waivers (partial), and unspecified assistantships also available. Support available to part-time students. Financial award application deadline: 3/1; financial award applicants required to submit FAFSA. *Faculty research:* Sexual and reproductive health, health promotion/illness prevention, eating disorders, violence, symptom management. *Total annual research expenditures:* $1.1 million. *Unit head:* Dr. Susan Gennaro, Dean, 617-552-4251, Fax: 617-552-0931, E-mail: susan.gennaro@bc.edu. *Application contact:* MaryBeth Crowley, Graduate Programs Assistant, 617-552-4928, Fax: 617-552-2121, E-mail: csongrad@bc.edu.
Website: http://www.bc.edu/schools/son/

Cleveland State University, College of Graduate Studies, School of Nursing, Cleveland, OH 44115. Offers clinical nurse leader (MSN); forensic nursing (MSN); nursing education (MSN); specialized population (MSN); urban education (PhD), including nursing education; MSN/MBA. *Accreditation:* AACN. Part-time programs available. Postbaccalaureate distance learning degree programs offered (no on-campus study). *Faculty:* 6 full-time (all women), 1 (woman) part-time/adjunct. *Students:* 20 full-time (all women), 28 part-time (26 women); includes 12 minority (8 Black or African American, non-Hispanic/Latino; 3 Hispanic/Latino; 1 Two or more races, non-Hispanic/Latino), 1 international. Average age 38. 65 applicants, 62% accepted, 20 enrolled. In 2013, 6 master's awarded. *Degree requirements:* For master's, thesis optional, portfolio, capstone practicum project; for doctorate, comprehensive exam, thesis/dissertation. *Entrance requirements:* For master's, RN license, BSN with minimum cumulative GPA of 3.0, recent (5 years) course work in statistics; for doctorate, GRE, MSN with minimum cumulative GPA of 3.25. Additional exam requirements/recommendations for international students: Required—TOEFL (minimum score 525 paper-based; 65 iBT), IELTS (minimum score 6). *Application deadline:* For fall admission, 3/1 priority date for domestic and international students. Application fee: $55. Electronic applications accepted. *Expenses:* Tuition, state resident: full-time $8335; part-time $521 per credit hour. Tuition, nonresident: full-time $15,670; part-time $979 per credit hour. *Required fees:* $50; $25 per semester. *Financial support:* In 2013–14, 4 students received support. Tuition waivers (full) and unspecified assistantships available. Financial award application deadline: 3/1; financial award applicants required to submit FAFSA. *Faculty research:* Diabetes management, African-American elders medication compliance, risk in home visiting, suffering, COPD and stress, nursing education, disaster health preparedness. *Total annual research expenditures:* $330,000. *Unit head:* Dr. Vida Lock, Dean, 216-523-7237, Fax: 216-687-3556, E-mail: v.lock@csuohio.edu. *Application contact:* Maureen Mitchell, Assistant Professor and Graduate Program Director, 216-523-7128, Fax: 216-687-3556, E-mail: m.m.mitchell1@csuohio.edu.
Website: http://www.csuohio.edu/nursing/

D'Youville College, School of Nursing, Buffalo, NY 14201-1084. Offers advanced practice nursing (DNP); community health nursing/education (MSN); community health nursing/management (MSN); family nurse practitioner (MSN, Certificate); nursing and health-related professions education (Certificate). *Accreditation:* AACN. Part-time programs available. *Students:* 51 full-time (45 women), 136 part-time (115 women); includes 25 minority (17 Black or African American, non-Hispanic/Latino; 1 American Indian or Alaska Native, non-Hispanic/Latino; 1 Asian, non-Hispanic/Latino; 6 Hispanic/Latino), 76 international. Average age 35. 261 applicants, 36% accepted, 73 enrolled. In 2013, 51 master's, 3 other advanced degrees awarded. *Degree requirements:* For master's, thesis or alternative, membership on board of community agency, publishable paper. *Entrance requirements:* For master's, BS in nursing, minimum GPA of 3.0, course work in statistics and computers. Additional exam requirements/recommendations for international students: Required—TOEFL (minimum score 500 paper-based). *Application deadline:* For fall admission, 5/1 priority date for international students; for spring admission, 9/1 priority date for international students. Applications are processed on a rolling basis. Application fee: $25. Electronic applications accepted. *Financial support:* Federal Work-Study, scholarships/grants, traineeships, and unspecified assistantships available. Support available to part-time students. Financial award application deadline: 3/1; financial award applicants required to submit FAFSA. *Faculty research:* Nursing curriculum, nursing theory-testing, wellness research, communication and socialization patterns. *Unit head:* Dr. Ann Caughill, Chair, 716-829-7892, Fax: 716-829-8159. *Application contact:* Mark Pavone, Graduate Admissions Director, 716-829-8400, Fax: 716-829-7900, E-mail: graduateadmissions@dyc.edu.
Website: http://www.dyc.edu/academics/nursing/

See Display on page 632 and Close-Up on page 815.

Hampton University, Graduate College, School of Nursing, Hampton, VA 23668. Offers advanced adult nursing (MS); community health nursing (MS); community mental health/psychiatric nursing (MS); family nursing (MS); gerontological nursing for the nurse practitioner (MS); pediatric nursing (MS); women's health nursing (MS). *Accreditation:* AACN. Part-time and evening/weekend programs available. *Degree requirements:* For master's, thesis optional. *Entrance requirements:* For master's, GRE General Test. *Faculty research:* Curriculum development, physical and mental assessment.

Hawai`i Pacific University, College of Nursing and Health Sciences, Honolulu, HI 96813. Offers community clinical nurse specialist (MSN); family nurse practitioner (MSN). Part-time and evening/weekend programs available. *Faculty:* 6 full-time (all women), 2 part-time/adjunct (both women). *Students:* 39 full-time (33 women), 16 part-time (11 women); includes 40 minority (2 Black or African American, non-Hispanic/Latino; 22 Asian, non-Hispanic/Latino; 7 Hispanic/Latino; 2 Native Hawaiian or other Pacific Islander, non-Hispanic/Latino; 7 Two or more races, non-Hispanic/Latino). Average age 38. 32 applicants, 75% accepted, 15 enrolled. In 2013, 7 master's awarded. *Degree requirements:* For master's, practicum, professional paper. *Entrance requirements:* For master's, bachelor's degree in nursing, minimum GPA of 3.0. Additional exam requirements/recommendations for international students: Recommended—TOEFL (minimum score 550 paper-based; 80 iBT), TWE (minimum score 5). *Application deadline:* Applications are processed on a rolling basis. Application fee: $50. Electronic applications accepted. *Financial support:* In 2013–14, 11 students received support. Career-related internships or fieldwork, Federal Work-Study, scholarships/grants, traineeships, and tuition waivers available. Financial award application deadline: 3/1; financial award applicants required to submit FAFSA. *Faculty research:* Hawaiian elders, traditional healing and nursing center. *Unit head:* Dr. Lynette Landry, Dean, 808-236-5811, E-mail: llandry@hpu.edu. *Application contact:* Rumi Yoshida, Associate Director of Graduate Admissions, 808-543-8034, Fax: 808-544-0280, E-mail: grad@hpu.edu.
Website: http://www.hpu.edu/CNHS/index.html

Holy Family University, Graduate School, School of Nursing, Philadelphia, PA 19114. Offers community health nursing (MSN); nursing administration (MSN); nursing education (MSN). *Accreditation:* AACN. Part-time and evening/weekend programs available. *Faculty:* 7 full-time (all women). *Students:* 42 part-time (39 women); includes 9 minority (4 Black or African American, non-Hispanic/Latino; 4 Asian, non-Hispanic/Latino; 1 Hispanic/Latino). Average age 36. 17 applicants, 82% accepted, 6 enrolled. In 2013, 12 master's awarded. *Degree requirements:* For master's, thesis or alternative, comprehensive portfolio, clinical practicum. *Entrance requirements:* For master's, BSN or RN from appropriately-accredited program, minimum GPA of 3.0, professional references, official transcripts of all college or university work, essay/personal statement, current resume, completion of one undergraduate statistics course with minimum grade of C. Additional exam requirements/recommendations for international students: Required—TOEFL (minimum score 550 paper-based; 79 iBT), IELTS (minimum score 6), or PTE (minimum score 54). *Application deadline:* For fall admission, 7/1 priority date for domestic and international students; for winter admission, 1/1 for domestic students; for spring admission, 11/1 priority date for domestic and international students; for summer admission, 4/1 priority date for domestic and international students. Applications are processed on a rolling basis. Application fee: $25. Electronic applications accepted. *Expenses: Tuition:* Full-time $12,060. *Required fees:* $250. Tuition and fees vary according to degree level. *Financial support:* In 2013–14, 1 student received support. Available to part-time students. Application deadline: 2/

15; applicants required to submit FAFSA. *Unit head:* Dr. Ana Maria Catanzaro, Dean, 267-341-3292, Fax: 215-637-6598, E-mail: acatanzaro@holyfamily.edu. *Application contact:* Gidget Matie Montelibano, Associate Director of Graduate Admissions, 267-341-3558, Fax: 215-637-1478, E-mail: gmontelibano@holyfamily.edu.
Website: http://www.holyfamily.edu/choosing-holy-family-u/academics/schools-of-study/school-of-nursing

Holy Names University, Graduate Division, Department of Nursing, Oakland, CA 94619-1699. Offers administration/management (MSN, PMC); clinical faculty (MSN, PMC); community health nursing/case manager (MSN); family nurse practitioner (MSN, PMC); MSN/MA; MSN/MBA. *Accreditation:* AACN. Part-time and evening/weekend programs available. *Faculty:* 3 full-time, 22 part-time/adjunct. *Students:* 31 full-time (26 women), 78 part-time (67 women); includes 66 minority (27 Black or African American, non-Hispanic/Latino; 25 Asian, non-Hispanic/Latino; 13 Hispanic/Latino; 1 Two or more races, non-Hispanic/Latino), 5 international. Average age 38. 97 applicants, 61% accepted, 49 enrolled. In 2013, 66 master's, 3 other advanced degrees awarded. *Entrance requirements:* For master's, bachelor's degree in nursing or related field; California RN license or eligibility; minimum cumulative GPA of 2.8, 3.0 in nursing courses from baccalaureate program; courses in pathophysiology, statistics, and research at the undergraduate level. Additional exam requirements/recommendations for international students: Required—TOEFL (minimum score 500 paper-based; 79 iBT). *Application deadline:* For fall admission, 8/1 priority date for domestic students, 7/15 priority date for international students; for spring admission, 12/1 priority date for domestic and international students; for summer admission, 5/1 priority date for domestic and international students. Applications are processed on a rolling basis. Application fee: $65. Electronic applications accepted. Application fee is waived when completed online. *Expenses: Tuition:* Part-time $866 per unit. *Financial support:* Career-related internships or fieldwork, Federal Work-Study, scholarships/grants, and unspecified assistantships available. Support available to part-time students. Financial award application deadline: 3/2; financial award applicants required to submit FAFSA. *Faculty research:* Women's reproductive health, gerontology, attitudes about aging, schizophrenic families, international health issues. *Unit head:* Dr. Miki Goodwin, Associate Professor/Chair of Nursing, 510-436-1374, E-mail: goodwin@hnu.edu. *Application contact:* Graduate Admission Office, 800-430-1321, E-mail: graduateadmissions@hnu.edu.

Hunter College of the City University of New York, Graduate School, Schools of the Health Professions, Hunter-Bellevue School of Nursing, Community Health Nursing Program, New York, NY 10065-5085. Offers MS. *Accreditation:* AACN. Part-time programs available. *Faculty:* 18 full-time (15 women), 25 part-time/adjunct (21 women). *Students:* 1 (woman) full-time, 33 part-time (29 women); includes 23 minority (19 Black or African American, non-Hispanic/Latino; 2 Asian, non-Hispanic/Latino; 2 Hispanic/Latino), 4 international. Average age 33. 18 applicants, 50% accepted, 7 enrolled. In 2013, 6 master's awarded. *Degree requirements:* For master's, practicum. *Entrance requirements:* For master's, minimum GPA of 3.0, New York RN license, BSN. Additional exam requirements/recommendations for international students: Required—TOEFL. *Application deadline:* For fall admission, 4/1 for domestic students, 2/1 for international students; for spring admission, 11/1 for domestic students, 9/1 for international students. Applications are processed on a rolling basis. Application fee: $125. *Financial support:* Federal Work-Study, scholarships/grants, traineeships, and tuition waivers (partial) available. Support available to part-time students. Financial award application deadline: 5/1; financial award applicants required to submit FAFSA. *Faculty research:* HIV/AIDS, health promotion with vulnerable populations. *Unit head:* Judith Aponte, Specialization Coordinator, 212-481-7568, E-mail: jap@hunter.cuny.edu. *Application contact:* Milena Solo, Director for Graduate Admissions, 212-772-4480, E-mail: admissions@hunter.cuny.edu.

Hunter College of the City University of New York, Graduate School, Schools of the Health Professions, Hunter-Bellevue School of Nursing, Community/Public Health Nursing/Urban Public Health Program, New York, NY 10065-5085. Offers MS/MPH. *Accreditation:* AACN. Part-time programs available. *Faculty:* 18 full-time (15 women), 25 part-time/adjunct (21 women). *Students:* 1 (woman) full-time, 33 part-time (29 women); includes 20 minority (15 Black or African American, non-Hispanic/Latino; 3 Asian, non-Hispanic/Latino; 2 Hispanic/Latino), 2 international. Average age 34. 18 applicants, 50% accepted, 7 enrolled. *Entrance requirements:* Additional exam requirements/recommendations for international students: Required—TOEFL. *Application deadline:* For fall admission, 4/1 for domestic students, 2/1 for international students; for spring admission, 11/1 for domestic students, 9/1 for international students. Applications are processed on a rolling basis. Application fee: $125. *Financial support:* Federal Work-Study, scholarships/grants, traineeships, and tuition waivers (partial) available. Support available to part-time students. Financial award application deadline: 5/1; financial award applicants required to submit FAFSA. *Faculty research:* HIV/AIDS, health promotion with vulnerable populations, immigrant health. *Unit head:* Judith Aponte, Specialization Coordinator, 212-481-7568, Fax: 212-481-5078, E-mail: jap@hunter.cuny.edu. *Application contact:* Milena Solo, Director for Graduate Admissions, 212-772-4288, E-mail: admissions@hunter.cuny.edu.
Website: http://www.hunter.cuny.edu/nursing/admissions/graduate

Husson University, Graduate Nursing Program, Bangor, ME 04401-2999. Offers advanced practice psychiatric nursing (MSN, PMC); family and community nurse practitioner (MSN, PMC); nursing education (MSN, PMC). *Accreditation:* AACN. Part-time programs available. *Faculty:* 3 full-time (all women), 3 part-time/adjunct (all women). *Students:* 10 full-time (8 women), 15 part-time (14 women); includes 1 minority (Two or more races, non-Hispanic/Latino). 29 applicants, 76% accepted, 21 enrolled. In 2013, 16 master's awarded. *Degree requirements:* For master's, comprehensive exam (for some programs). *Entrance requirements:* For master's, MAT or GRE, BSN. Additional exam requirements/recommendations for international students: Required—TOEFL (minimum score 550 paper-based). *Application deadline:* For fall admission, 6/30 for domestic students; for spring admission, 10/30 for domestic students. Application fee: $40. *Expenses:* Contact institution. *Financial support:* In 2013–14, 16 students received support. Federal Work-Study, institutionally sponsored loans, traineeships, and unspecified assistantships available. Financial award application deadline: 4/15; financial award applicants required to submit FAFSA. *Unit head:* Prof. Chrystal Adams, Director, Nurse Practitioner Program, 207-941-7080, E-mail: adamsc@husson.edu. *Application contact:* Kristen Card, Director of Graduate Admissions, 207-404-5660, Fax: 207-941-7935, E-mail: cardk@husson.edu.

Independence University, Program in Nursing, Salt Lake City, UT 84107. Offers community health (MSN); gerontology (MSN); nursing administration (MSN); wellness promotion (MSN).

Indiana University–Purdue University Indianapolis, School of Nursing, Indianapolis, IN 46202-2896. Offers acute care nurse practitioner (MSN); adult health clinical nurse specialist (MSN); adult health nursing (MSN), including adult clinical nurse specialist; adult nurse practitioner (MSN); adult psychiatric/mental health nursing (MSN); child psychiatric/mental health nursing (MSN); community health nursing (MSN); family nurse practitioner (MSN); neonatal nurse practitioner (MSN); nursing (MSN, DNP), including nursing administration (MSN), nursing education (MSN); nursing science (PhD); pediatric clinical nurse specialist (MSN); women's health nurse practitioner (MSN); MSN/MPA; MSN/MPH. Part-time programs available. *Faculty:* 85 full-time (82 women), 60 part-time/adjunct (all women). *Students:* 86 full-time (78 women), 371 part-time (351 women); includes 74 minority (39 Black or African American, non-Hispanic/Latino; 1 American Indian or Alaska Native, non-Hispanic/Latino; 14 Asian, non-Hispanic/Latino; 11 Hispanic/Latino; 9 Two or more races, non-Hispanic/Latino), 6 international. Average age 38. 224 applicants, 61% accepted, 102 enrolled. In 2013, 120 master's, 10 doctorates awarded. Terminal master's awarded for partial completion of doctoral program. *Degree requirements:* For master's, thesis; for doctorate, thesis/dissertation. *Entrance requirements:* For master's, minimum GPA of 3.0, RN license; for doctorate, GRE General Test, minimum GPA of 3.0, MSN, RN license, graduate statistics course with minimum B grade (not older than 3 years). Additional exam requirements/recommendations for international students: Required—TOEFL. *Application deadline:* For fall admission, 2/15 for domestic students; for spring admission, 9/15 for domestic students. Application fee: $55 ($65 for international students). *Financial support:* In 2013–14, 93 students received support. Fellowships with full tuition reimbursements available, research assistantships with full tuition reimbursements available, teaching assistantships with full tuition reimbursements available, Federal Work-Study, institutionally sponsored loans, scholarships/grants, and tuition waivers (full) available. Support available to part-time students. Financial award application deadline: 5/1. *Faculty research:* Clinical science, health systems. *Total annual research expenditures:* $3 million. *Unit head:* Dr. Patricia Ebright, Associate Dean for Graduate Programs, E-mail: nursing@iupui.edu. *Application contact:* Information Contact, 317-274-2806.
Website: http://nursing.iu.edu/

Kean University, College of Natural, Applied and Health Sciences, Program in Nursing, Union, NJ 07083. Offers clinical management with transcultural focus (MSN); community health nursing (MSN); school nursing (MSN). Part-time programs available. *Faculty:* 8 full-time (all women). *Students:* 14 full-time (12 women), 121 part-time (117 women); includes 62 minority (43 Black or African American, non-Hispanic/Latino; 11 Asian, non-Hispanic/Latino; 7 Hispanic/Latino; 1 Two or more races, non-Hispanic/Latino), 2 international. Average age 42. 72 applicants, 94% accepted, 49 enrolled. In 2013, 35 master's awarded. *Degree requirements:* For master's, thesis or alternative, clinical field experience. *Entrance requirements:* For master's, minimum GPA of 3.0; BS in nursing; RN license; 2 letters of recommendation; interview. Additional exam requirements/recommendations for international students: Required—TOEFL. *Application deadline:* For fall admission, 6/1 for domestic and international students; for spring admission, 12/1 for domestic and international students. Applications are processed on a rolling basis. Application fee: $75 ($150 for international students). Electronic applications accepted. *Expenses:* Tuition, state resident: full-time $12,099; part-time $589 per credit. Tuition, nonresident: full-time $16,399; part-time $722 per credit. *Required fees:* $3050; $139 per credit. Part-time tuition and fees vary according to course level, course load, degree level and program. *Financial support:* In 2013–14, 2 research assistantships with full tuition reimbursements (averaging $3,713 per year) were awarded; unspecified assistantships also available. Financial award applicants required to submit FAFSA. *Unit head:* Dr. Virginia Fitzsimons, Program Coordinator, 908-527-3396, E-mail: vfitzsim@kean.edu. *Application contact:* Ann-Marie Kay, Assistant Director of Graduate Admissions, 908-737-5922, Fax: 908-737-5925, E-mail: akay@kean.edu.
Website: http://grad.kean.edu/masters-programs/nursing-clinical-management

La Salle University, School of Nursing and Health Sciences, Program in Nursing, Philadelphia, PA 19141-1199. Offers adult gerontology primary care nurse practitioner (MSN, Certificate); adult health and illness clinical nurse specialist (MSN); adult-gerontology clinical nurse specialist (MSN, Certificate); clinical nurse leader (MSN); family primary care nurse practitioner (MSN, Certificate); gerontology (Certificate); nurse anesthetist (MSN, Certificate); nursing (MSN, Certificate); nursing administration (MSN, Certificate); nursing education (Certificate); nursing practice (DNP); nursing service administration (MSN); public health nursing (MSN, Certificate); school nursing (Certificate); MSN/MBA; MSN/MPH. *Accreditation:* AANA/CANAEP. Part-time programs available. Postbaccalaureate distance learning degree programs offered (minimal on-campus study). *Faculty:* 13 full-time (12 women), 10 part-time/adjunct (8 women). *Students:* 4 full-time (all women), 379 part-time (331 women); includes 119 minority (70 Black or African American, non-Hispanic/Latino; 2 American Indian or Alaska Native, non-Hispanic/Latino; 31 Asian, non-Hispanic/Latino; 12 Hispanic/Latino; 4 Two or more races, non-Hispanic/Latino), 1 international. Average age 37. 133 applicants, 85% accepted, 63 enrolled. In 2013, 72 master's, 3 doctorates, 26 other advanced degrees awarded. *Degree requirements:* For doctorate, minimum of 1,000 hours of post baccalaureate clinical practice supervised by preceptors. *Entrance requirements:* For master's, GRE, MAT, or GMAT (for students with BSN GPA of less than 3.2), baccalaureate degree in nursing from an NLNAC- or CCNE-accredited program or an MSN Bridge program; Pennsylvania RN license; 2 letters of reference; resume; statement of philosophy articulating professional values and future educational goal; 1 year of work experience as a registered nurse; for doctorate, GRE (waived for applicants with MSN cumulative GPA of 3.7 or above), MSN from nationally-accredited program or master's degree, MBA or MHA from nationally-accredited program; resume or curriculum vitae; 2 letters of reference; interview; for Certificate, GRE, MAT, or GMAT (for students with BSN GPA of less than 3.2, baccalaureate degree in nursing from an NLNAC- or CCNE-accredited program or an MSN Bridge program; Pennsylvania RN license; 2 letters of reference; resume; statement of philosophy articulating professional values and future educational goal; 1 year of work experience as a registered nurse. Additional exam requirements/recommendations for international students: Required—TOEFL. *Application deadline:* For fall admission, 8/15 priority date for domestic students, 7/15 for international students; for spring admission, 12/15 priority date for domestic students, 11/15 for international students; for summer admission, 4/15 priority date for domestic students, 3/15 for international students. Applications are processed on a rolling basis. Application fee: $35. Electronic applications accepted. Application fee is waived when completed online. *Expenses:* Contact institution. *Financial support:* In 2013–14, 48 students received support. Teaching assistantships, scholarships/grants, and traineeships available. Support available to part-time students. Financial award application deadline: 8/31; financial award applicants required to submit FAFSA. *Unit head:* Dr. Patricia M. Dillon, Director, 215-951-1322, Fax: 215-951-1896, E-mail: msnapn@lasalle.edu. *Application contact:* Paul J. Reilly, Assistant Vice President, Enrollment Services, 215-951-1946, Fax: 215-951-1462, E-mail: reilly@lasalle.edu.

Louisiana State University Health Sciences Center, School of Nursing, New Orleans, LA 70112-2223. Offers advanced public/community health nursing (MN); clinical nurse specialist (MN); nurse anesthesia (MN); nurse practitioner (MN); nursing (DNS). *Accreditation:* AACN; AANA/CANAEP (one or more programs are accredited). Part-time programs available. *Degree requirements:* For master's, thesis optional; for doctorate, thesis/dissertation. *Entrance requirements:* For master's, GRE General Test, MAT, minimum GPA of 3.0; for doctorate, GRE General Test, minimum GPA of 3.5. Additional exam requirements/recommendations for international students: Required—TOEFL. Electronic applications accepted. *Faculty research:* Advanced clinical practice, nursing education, health, social support, nursing administration.

New Mexico State University, Graduate School, College of Health and Social Services, School of Nursing, Las Cruces, NM 88003. Offers adult/gerontology nurse practitioner (DNP); family nurse practitioner (DNP); nursing (MSN, PhD); public/

community health (DNP). *Accreditation:* AACN. Postbaccalaureate distance learning degree programs offered (minimal on-campus study). *Faculty:* 15 full-time (14 women). *Students:* 42 full-time (33 women), 64 part-time (56 women); includes 50 minority (11 Black or African American, non-Hispanic/Latino; 1 American Indian or Alaska Native, non-Hispanic/Latino; 1 Asian, non-Hispanic/Latino; 36 Hispanic/Latino; 1 Two or more races, non-Hispanic/Latino), 1 international. Average age 42. 50 applicants, 86% accepted, 36 enrolled. In 2013, 12 master's, 6 doctorates awarded. *Degree requirements:* For master's, comprehensive exam, thesis optional, clinical practice; for doctorate, comprehensive exam, thesis/dissertation. *Entrance requirements:* For master's, NCLEX exam, BSN, minimum GPA of 3.0, course work in statistics, 3 letters of reference, writing sample, RN license, CPR certification, proof of liability, immunizations, criminal background check; for doctorate, NCLEX exam, MSN, minimum GPA of 3.0, 3 letters of reference, writing sample, RN license, CPR certification, proof of liability, immunizations, criminal background check, statistics course. Additional exam requirements/recommendations for international students: Required—TOEFL (minimum score 550 paper-based; 79 iBT), IELTS (minimum score 6.5). *Application deadline:* For spring admission, 10/1 priority date for domestic students. Application fee: $40 ($50 for international students). Electronic applications accepted. *Expenses:* Tuition, state resident: full-time $5398; part-time $224.90 per credit. Tuition, nonresident: full-time $18,821; part-time $784.20 per credit. *Required fees:* $1310; $54.60 per credit. *Financial support:* In 2013–14, 31 students received support. Career-related internships or fieldwork, Federal Work-Study, scholarships/grants, traineeships, health care benefits, and unspecified assistantships available. Financial award application deadline: 3/1. *Faculty research:* Public policy, community health, health disparities, self efficacy and self management, psychiatric mental health. *Total annual research expenditures:* $3,424. *Unit head:* Dr. Pamela Schultz, Director, 575-646-3812, Fax: 575-646-2167, E-mail: pschultz@nmsu.edu. *Application contact:* Dr. Kathleen Huttlinger, Associate Director for Graduate Studies, 575-646-4387, Fax: 575-646-2167.
Website: http://schoolofnursing.nmsu.edu

Oregon Health & Science University, School of Nursing, Program in Nursing Education, Portland, OR 97239-3098. Offers MN, MS, Post Master's Certificate.

Oregon Health & Science University, School of Nursing, Program in Public Health Nursing, Portland, OR 97239-3098. Offers primary care and disparities (MPH); public health (MPH, Post Master's Certificate). *Accreditation:* AACN. *Degree requirements:* For master's, thesis optional. *Entrance requirements:* For master's, GRE General Test, bachelor's degree in nursing, minimum undergraduate GPA of 3.0, previous course work in statistics.

Rush University, College of Nursing, Department of Community, Systems, and Mental Health Nursing, Chicago, IL 60612. Offers advanced public health nursing (DNP); family nurse practitioner (DNP); leadership to enhance population health outcomes (DNP); nursing science (PhD); psychiatric mental health nurse practitioner (DNP, Post-Graduate Certificate); systems leadership (DNP). *Accreditation:* AACN. Part-time programs available. Postbaccalaureate distance learning degree programs offered (minimal on-campus study). *Students:* 190 part-time (174 women); includes 41 minority (13 Black or African American, non-Hispanic/Latino; 4 American Indian or Alaska Native, non-Hispanic/Latino; 12 Asian, non-Hispanic/Latino; 11 Hispanic/Latino; 1 Native Hawaiian or other Pacific Islander, non-Hispanic/Latino). Average age 35. 170 applicants, 77% accepted, 118 enrolled. *Degree requirements:* For doctorate, capstone project (for DNP); dissertation (for PhD). *Entrance requirements:* For doctorate, GRE General Test (waived for DNP if cumulative GPA is 3.25 or greater, nursing GPA is 3.0 or greater, or a completed graduate program GPA is 3.5 or greater), interview, 3 letters of recommendation, personal statement, current resume; for Post-Graduate Certificate, interview, 3 letters of recommendation, personal statement, current resume. Additional exam requirements/recommendations for international students: Required—TOEFL. *Application deadline:* For fall admission, 1/2 for domestic students; for winter admission, 10/15 for domestic students; for spring admission, 8/4 for domestic students. Applications are processed on a rolling basis. Application fee: $100. Electronic applications accepted. *Financial support:* Fellowships, research assistantships, teaching assistantships, Federal Work-Study, scholarships/grants, traineeships, and health care benefits available. Support available to part-time students. Financial award application deadline: 3/1; financial award applicants required to submit FAFSA. *Faculty research:* Reduction of health disparities; evidence-based interventions for caregivers; patient-centered quality assessment of psychiatric inpatient environments; digital delivery of a parent-training program for urban, low-income parents; patient-centered predictors and outcomes of inter-professional care coordination. *Total annual research expenditures:* $3.8 million. *Unit head:* Dr. Arlene Miller, Chairperson, 312-942-7117, E-mail: arlene_miller@rush.edu. *Application contact:* Jennifer Thorndyke, Admissions Specialist, 312-563-7526, E-mail: jennifer_thorndyke@rush.edu.
Website: http://www.rushu.rush.edu/servlet/Satellite?c=RushUnivLevel1Page&cid=1204497838852&pagename=Rush%2FRushUnivLevel1Page%2FLevel_1_College_Home_Page

Sage Graduate School, School of Health Sciences, Department of Nursing, Program in Community Health, Troy, NY 12180-4115. Offers MS, Post Master's Certificate. *Accreditation:* AACN. Part-time programs available. *Faculty:* 5 full-time (all women), 9 part-time/adjunct (all women). *Students:* 2 part-time (both women). Average age 35. 3 applicants, 33% accepted. In 2013, 1 master's awarded. *Degree requirements:* For master's, thesis or alternative. *Entrance requirements:* For master's, BS in nursing, minimum GPA of 2.75, resume, 2 letters of recommendation. Additional exam requirements/recommendations for international students: Required—TOEFL (minimum score 550 paper-based). *Application deadline:* Applications are processed on a rolling basis. Application fee: $40. *Expenses: Tuition:* Full-time $11,880; part-time $660 per credit hour. *Financial support:* Fellowships, research assistantships, Federal Work-Study, scholarships/grants, and unspecified assistantships available. Support available to part-time students. Financial award application deadline: 3/1; financial award applicants required to submit FAFSA. *Unit head:* Dr. Esther Haskevitz, Dean, School of Health Sciences, 518-244-2296, Fax: 518-244-4571, E-mail: haskve@sage.edu. *Application contact:* Madeline Cafiero, Director, 518-244-4574, Fax: 518-244-2009, E-mail: cafiem@sage.edu.

San Francisco State University, Division of Graduate Studies, College of Health and Social Sciences, School of Nursing, San Francisco, CA 94132-1722. Offers adult acute care (MS); clinical nurse specialist (MS); community/public health nursing (MS); family nurse practitioner (MS, Certificate); nursing administration (MS); nursing education (MS); pediatrics (MS); women's health (MS). *Accreditation:* AACN. Part-time programs available. *Application deadline:* Applications are processed on a rolling basis. *Financial support:* Career-related internships or fieldwork available. *Unit head:* Dr. Mary-Ann van Dam, Director, 415-338-1802, E-mail: vandam@sfsu.edu. *Application contact:* Robert Strachan, Admission and Student Services Coordinator, 415-338-1802, E-mail: strachan@sfsu.edu.
Website: http://nursing.sfsu.edu

Seattle University, College of Nursing, Program in Advanced Practice Nursing Immersion, Seattle, WA 98122-1090. Offers adult/gerontological nurse practitioner (MSN); advanced community public health nursing (MSN); family nurse practitioner (MSN); family psychiatric mental health nurse practitioner (MSN); nurse midwifery (MSN). *Faculty:* 17 full-time (15 women), 9 part-time/adjunct (6 women). *Students:* 109 full-time (94 women), 6 part-time (5 women); includes 25 minority (3 Black or African American, non-Hispanic/Latino; 11 Asian, non-Hispanic/Latino; 2 Hispanic/Latino; 9 Two or more races, non-Hispanic/Latino). Average age 31. In 2013, 48 master's awarded. *Degree requirements:* For master's, thesis or scholarly project. *Entrance requirements:* For master's, GRE, bachelor's degree, minimum GPA of 3.0, professional resume, two recommendations, letter of intent. Additional exam requirements/recommendations for international students: Required—TOEFL (minimum score 92 iBT), IELTS. *Application deadline:* For fall admission, 12/1 for domestic and international students. Application fee: $55. Electronic applications accepted. *Financial support:* In 2013–14, 3 students received support. Scholarships/grants and traineeships available. Financial award applicants required to submit FAFSA. *Unit head:* Dr. Janiece DeSocio, Interim Dean, 206-296-5660, E-mail: desocioj@seattleu.edu. *Application contact:* Janet Shandley, Associate Dean of Graduate Admissions, 206-296-5900, Fax: 206-298-5656, E-mail: grad_admissions@seattleu.edu.
Website: http://www.seattleu.edu/nursing/msn/apni/

Seattle University, College of Nursing, Program in Nursing, Seattle, WA 98122-1090. Offers adult/gerontological nurse practitioner (MSN); advanced community public health (MSN); psychiatric mental health nurse practitioner (MSN). *Students:* 11 full-time (10 women), 4 part-time (all women); includes 2 minority (both Hispanic/Latino). Average age 36. 39 applicants, 36% accepted, 8 enrolled. In 2013, 7 master's awarded. *Degree requirements:* For master's, thesis or scholarly project. *Entrance requirements:* For master's, GRE, bachelor's degree in nursing or associate degree in nursing with baccalaureate in different major, 5-quarter statistics course, minimum cumulative GPA of 3.0, professional resume, two recommendations, letter of intent, copy of current RN license or ability to obtain RN license in WA state. Additional exam requirements/recommendations for international students: Required—TOEFL (minimum score 92 iBT), IELTS. *Application deadline:* For fall admission, 12/1 for domestic and international students. Application fee: $55. Electronic applications accepted. *Financial support:* In 2013–14, 1 student received support, including 2 teaching assistantships; scholarships/grants and traineeships also available. Financial award applicants required to submit FAFSA. *Unit head:* Dr. Azita Emami, Dean, 206-296-5660. *Application contact:* Janet Shandley, Associate Dean of Graduate Admissions, 206-296-5900, Fax: 206-298-5656, E-mail: grad_admissions@seattleu.edu.
Website: https://www.seattleu.edu/nursing/msn/

University of Cincinnati, Graduate School, College of Nursing, Cincinnati, OH 45221-0038. Offers clinical nurse specialist (MSN), including adult health, community health, neonatal, nursing administration, occupational health, pediatric health, psychiatric nursing, women's health; nurse anesthesia (MSN); nurse midwifery (MSN); nurse practitioner (MSN), including acute care, ambulatory care, family, family/psychiatric, women's health; nursing (PhD); MBA/MSN. *Accreditation:* AACN; AANA/CANAEP (one or more programs are accredited); ACNM/ACME. Part-time programs available. Postbaccalaureate distance learning degree programs offered (no on-campus study). Terminal master's awarded for partial completion of doctoral program. *Degree requirements:* For master's, thesis or alternative; for doctorate, comprehensive exam, thesis/dissertation. *Entrance requirements:* For master's and doctorate, GRE General Test. Additional exam requirements/recommendations for international students: Required—TOEFL (minimum score 520 paper-based). Electronic applications accepted. *Faculty research:* Substance abuse, injury and violence, symptom management.

University of Hartford, College of Education, Nursing, and Health Professions, Program in Nursing, West Hartford, CT 06117-1599. Offers community/public health nursing (MSN); nursing education (MSN); nursing management (MSN). *Accreditation:* AACN. Part-time and evening/weekend programs available. *Degree requirements:* For master's, research project. *Entrance requirements:* For master's, BSN, Connecticut RN license. Additional exam requirements/recommendations for international students: Required—TOEFL (minimum score 550 paper-based). Electronic applications accepted. *Expenses:* Contact institution. *Faculty research:* Child development, women in doctoral study, applying feminist theory in teaching methods, near death experience, grandmothers as primary care providers.

University of Hawaii at Manoa, Graduate Division, School of Nursing and Dental Hygiene, Honolulu, HI 96822. Offers clinical nurse specialist (MS), including adult health, community mental health; nurse practitioner (MS), including adult health, community mental health, family nurse practitioner; nursing (PhD, Graduate Certificate); nursing administration (MS). *Accreditation:* AACN. Part-time programs available. Postbaccalaureate distance learning degree programs offered (minimal on-campus study). *Degree requirements:* For master's, thesis optional; for doctorate, comprehensive exam, thesis/dissertation. *Entrance requirements:* For master's, Hawaii RN license. Additional exam requirements/recommendations for international students: Required—TOEFL (minimum score 580 paper-based; 92 iBT), IELTS (minimum score 5). *Expenses:* Contact institution.

University of Illinois at Chicago, Graduate College, College of Nursing, Program in Nursing, Chicago, IL 60607-7128. Offers acute care clinical nurse specialist (MS); acute care nurse practitioner (MS); administrative nursing leadership (Certificate); administrative studies in nursing (MS); adult nurse practitioner (MS); adult/geriatric nurse practitioner (MS); advanced community health nurse specialist (MS); family nurse practitioner (MS); geriatric clinical nurse specialist (MS); geriatric nurse practitioner (MS); mental health clinical nurse specialist (MS); mental health nurse practitioner (MS); nurse midwifery (MS); occupational health/advanced community health nurse specialist (MS); occupational health/family nurse practitioner (MS); pediatric clinical nurse specialist (MS); pediatric nurse practitioner (MS); perinatal clinical nurse specialist (MS); school/advanced community health nurse specialist (MS); school/family nurse practitioner (MS); women's health nurse practitioner (MS). *Accreditation:* AACN. Part-time programs available. *Faculty:* 16 full-time (14 women). *Students:* 393 full-time (361 women), 410 part-time (367 women); includes 198 minority (48 Black or African American, non-Hispanic/Latino; 1 American Indian or Alaska Native, non-Hispanic/Latino; 64 Asian, non-Hispanic/Latino; 71 Hispanic/Latino; 2 Native Hawaiian or other Pacific Islander, non-Hispanic/Latino; 12 Two or more races, non-Hispanic/Latino), 29 international. Average age 32. 396 applicants, 62% accepted, 177 enrolled. In 2013, 184 master's awarded. *Degree requirements:* For master's, thesis or alternative. *Entrance requirements:* For master's, GRE General Test, minimum GPA of 2.75. Additional exam requirements/recommendations for international students: Required—TOEFL. *Application deadline:* For fall admission, 5/15 for domestic students, 2/15 for international students; for spring admission, 11/1 for domestic students, 7/15 for international students. Applications are processed on a rolling basis. Application fee: $40 ($50 for international students). Electronic applications accepted. *Expenses:* Tuition, state resident: full-time $11,066; part-time $3689 per term. Tuition, nonresident: full-time $23,064; part-time $7688 per term. *Required fees:* $3004; $1190 per term. Tuition and fees vary according to course level and program. *Financial support:* Fellowships with full tuition reimbursements, research assistantships with full tuition reimbursements, teaching assistantships with full tuition reimbursements, career-related internships or fieldwork, Federal Work-Study, institutionally sponsored loans, scholarships/grants, traineeships, tuition waivers (full and partial), and unspecified assistantships available. Support available to part-time students. Financial award application deadline: 3/1; financial award applicants required to submit FAFSA. *Unit head:* Dr. Terri E. Weaver, Dean, 312-996-7808, E-mail: teweaver@uic.edu. *Application contact:* Receptionist, 312-413-2550, E-mail: gradcoll@uic.edu.

The University of Kansas, University of Kansas Medical Center, School of Nursing, Kansas City, KS 66160. Offers adult/gerontological clinical nurse specialist (PMC); adult/gerontological nurse practitioner (PMC); clinical research management (PMC); health care informatics (PMC); health professions educator (PMC); nurse midwife (PMC); nursing (MS, DNP, PhD); organizational leadership (PMC); psychiatric/mental health nurse practitioner (PMC); public health nursing (PMC). *Accreditation:* AACN; ACNM/ACME. Part-time programs available. Postbaccalaureate distance learning degree programs offered (minimal on-campus study). *Faculty:* 59. *Students:* 55 full-time (53 women), 323 part-time (303 women); includes 57 minority (23 Black or African American, non-Hispanic/Latino; 14 Asian, non-Hispanic/Latino; 16 Hispanic/Latino; 1 Native Hawaiian or other Pacific Islander, non-Hispanic/Latino; 3 Two or more races, non-Hispanic/Latino), 1 international. Average age 38. 113 applicants, 59% accepted, 61 enrolled. In 2013, 77 master's, 18 doctorates, 11 other advanced degrees awarded. Terminal master's awarded for partial completion of doctoral program. *Degree requirements:* For master's, comprehensive exam, thesis (for some programs), general oral exam; for doctorate, variable foreign language requirement, thesis/dissertation, comprehensive oral exam (for DNP); comprehensive written and oral exam (for PhD). *Entrance requirements:* For master's, bachelor's degree in nursing, minimum GPA of 3.0, 1 year of clinical experience, RN license in KS and MO; for doctorate, GRE General Test, bachelor's degree in nursing, minimum GPA of 3.5, RN license in KS and MO. Additional exam requirements/recommendations for international students: Required—TOEFL. *Application deadline:* For fall admission, 4/1 for domestic and international students; for spring admission, 9/1 for domestic and international students. Application fee: $60. Electronic applications accepted. *Financial support:* Research assistantships with full and partial tuition reimbursements, teaching assistantships with full and partial tuition reimbursements, scholarships/grants, and traineeships available. Financial award application deadline: 3/1; financial award applicants required to submit FAFSA. *Faculty research:* Breastfeeding practices of teen mothers, national database of nursing quality indicators, caregiving of families of patients using technology in the home, simulation in nursing education, diaphragm fatigue. *Total annual research expenditures:* $6.4 million. *Unit head:* Dr. Karen L. Miller, Dean, 913-588-1601, Fax: 913-588-1660, E-mail: kmiller@kumc.edu. *Application contact:* Dr. Pamela K. Barnes, Associate Dean, Student Affairs, 913-588-1619, Fax: 913-588-1615, E-mail: pbarnes2@kumc.edu.
Website: http://nursing.kumc.edu

University of Maryland, Baltimore, Graduate School, School of Nursing, Master's Program in Nursing, Baltimore, MD 21201. Offers community health nursing (MS); gerontological nursing (MS); maternal-child nursing (MS); medical-surgical nursing (MS); nurse-midwifery education (MS); nursing administration (MS); nursing education (MS); nursing health policy (MS); primary care nursing (MS); psychiatric nursing (MS); MS/MBA. MS/MBA offered jointly with University of Baltimore. *Accreditation:* AACN; AANA/CANAEP. Part-time programs available. *Students:* 345 full-time (297 women), 508 part-time (469 women); includes 288 minority (152 Black or African American, non-Hispanic/Latino; 2 American Indian or Alaska Native, non-Hispanic/Latino; 72 Asian, non-Hispanic/Latino; 32 Hispanic/Latino; 1 Native Hawaiian or other Pacific Islander, non-Hispanic/Latino; 29 Two or more races, non-Hispanic/Latino), 13 international. Average age 33. 971 applicants, 34% accepted, 253 enrolled. In 2013, 308 master's awarded. *Degree requirements:* For master's, comprehensive exam (for some programs), thesis or alternative. *Entrance requirements:* For master's, minimum GPA of 2.75, course work in statistics, BS in nursing. Additional exam requirements/recommendations for international students: Required—TOEFL (minimum score 550 paper-based; 80 iBT) or IELTS (minimum score 7). *Application deadline:* For fall admission, 2/1 for domestic students, 1/15 for international students. Application fee: $75. Electronic applications accepted. *Financial support:* Fellowships, research assistantships, teaching assistantships, career-related internships or fieldwork, and traineeships available. Support available to part-time students. Financial award application deadline: 2/15; financial award applicants required to submit FAFSA. *Unit head:* Dr. Jane Kapustin, Assistant Dean, 410-706-6741, Fax: 410-706-4231. *Application contact:* Marjorie Fass, Admissions Director, 410-706-0501, Fax: 410-706-7238.

University of Massachusetts Amherst, Graduate School, School of Nursing, Amherst, MA 01003. Offers adult gerontology primary care (DNP); clinical nurse leader (MS); family nurse practitioner (DNP); nursing (PhD); public health nurse leader (DNP). *Accreditation:* AACN. Part-time programs available. Postbaccalaureate distance learning degree programs offered (minimal on-campus study). *Faculty:* 16 full-time (15 women). *Students:* 74 full-time (61 women), 161 part-time (149 women); includes 62 minority (31 Black or African American, non-Hispanic/Latino; 9 Asian, non-Hispanic/Latino; 19 Hispanic/Latino; 3 Two or more races, non-Hispanic/Latino), 6 international. Average age 40. 133 applicants, 80% accepted, 68 enrolled. In 2013, 9 master's, 32 doctorates awarded. Terminal master's awarded for partial completion of doctoral program. *Degree requirements:* For master's, thesis optional; for doctorate, comprehensive exam, thesis/dissertation. *Entrance requirements:* Additional exam requirements/recommendations for international students: Required—TOEFL (minimum score 550 paper-based; 80 iBT), IELTS (minimum score 6.5). *Application deadline:* For fall admission, 12/15 for domestic and international students. Applications are processed on a rolling basis. Application fee: $75. Electronic applications accepted. *Financial support:* Fellowships with full and partial tuition reimbursements, research assistantships with full and partial tuition reimbursements, teaching assistantships with full and partial tuition reimbursements, career-related internships or fieldwork, Federal Work-Study, scholarships/grants, traineeships, health care benefits, tuition waivers (full and partial), and unspecified assistantships available. Support available to part-time students. Financial award application deadline: 2/1. *Faculty research:* Health of older adults and their caretakers, mental health of individuals and families, health of children and adolescents, power and decision-making, transcultural health. *Unit head:* Dr. Stephen J. Cavanagh, Dean, 413-545-2703, Fax: 413-577-2550, E-mail: dean@nursing.umass.edu. *Application contact:* Lindsay DeSantis, Supervisor of Admissions, 413-545-0722, Fax: 413-577-0010, E-mail: gradadm@grad.umass.edu.
Website: http://www.umass.edu/nursing/

University of Massachusetts Dartmouth, Graduate School, College of Nursing, Programs in Nursing, North Dartmouth, MA 02747-2300. Offers adult gerontology primary care nurse practitioner (DNP); adult health clinical nurse specialist (DNP); adult health/adult nurse practitioner (MS); adult health/advanced practice (MS); adult health/nurse educator (MS); adult health/nurse manager (MS); adult nurse practitioner (PMC); community health nurse specialist (DNP); community nursing/advanced practice (MS); community nursing/nurse educator (MS); community nursing/nurse manager (MS); individualized nursing (PMC); nursing (MS, PhD); nursing practice (DNP). Part-time programs available. *Faculty:* 25 full-time (all women), 45 part-time/adjunct (44 women). *Students:* 103 part-time (95 women); includes 10 minority (4 Black or African American, non-Hispanic/Latino; 2 Asian, non-Hispanic/Latino; 4 Hispanic/Latino). Average age 40. 49 applicants, 92% accepted, 33 enrolled. In 2013, 25 master's, 1 doctorate, 2 other advanced degrees awarded. *Degree requirements:* For master's, thesis; for doctorate, comprehensive exam, thesis/dissertation, project (for DNP only). *Entrance requirements:* For master's, statement of purpose (minimum of 300 words), resume, 3 letters of recommendation, official transcripts, copy of RN license; for doctorate, GRE (for PhD), statement of purpose (minimum of 300 words), resume, 3 letters of recommendation, official transcripts, copy of RN license, scholarly writing sample (minimum 10 pages for PhD). Additional exam requirements/recommendations for international students: Required—TOEFL (minimum score 533 paper-based; 72 iBT). *Application deadline:* For fall admission, 2/15 priority date for domestic and international students. Applications are processed on a rolling basis. Application fee: $60. Electronic applications accepted. *Expenses:* Tuition, state resident: full-time $2071; part-time $86.29 per credit. Tuition, nonresident: full-time $8099; part-time $337.46 per credit. Tuition and fees vary according to course load and reciprocity agreements. *Financial support:* In 2013–14, 5 teaching assistantships with full and partial tuition reimbursements (averaging $7,500 per year) were awarded; Federal Work-Study and unspecified assistantships also available. Support available to part-time students. Financial award application deadline: 3/1; financial award applicants required to submit FAFSA. *Faculty research:* Pathophysiology, aging with spinal cord injury, relational ontology, severe mental illness, patient care. *Total annual research expenditures:* $1,000. *Unit head:* Kerry Fater, Graduate Program Director for Nursing Master's Programs, 508-999-8525, Fax: 508-999-9127, E-mail: kfater@umassd.edu. *Application contact:* Steven Briggs, Director of Marketing and Recruitment for Graduate Studies, 508-999-8604, Fax: 508-999-8183, E-mail: graduate@umassd.edu.
Website: http://www.umassd.edu/nursing/graduateprograms

University of Minnesota, Twin Cities Campus, Graduate School, School of Nursing, Program in Public Health Nursing, Minneapolis, MN 55455-0213. Offers MS. *Accreditation:* AACN. Part-time programs available. Postbaccalaureate distance learning degree programs offered (minimal on-campus study). *Degree requirements:* For master's, final oral exam, project or thesis. *Entrance requirements:* Additional exam requirements/recommendations for international students: Required—TOEFL (minimum score 586 paper-based).

University of North Dakota, Graduate School, College of Nursing, Grand Forks, ND 58202. Offers advanced public health nursing (MS); family nurse practitioner (MS); gerontological nursing (MS); nurse anesthesia (MS); nursing (MS, PhD); nursing education (MS); psychiatric and mental health (MS). *Accreditation:* AACN; AANA/CANAEP (one or more programs are accredited). Part-time and evening/weekend programs available. Postbaccalaureate distance learning degree programs offered (minimal on-campus study). *Degree requirements:* For master's, thesis or alternative. *Entrance requirements:* For master's, minimum GPA of 3.0; for doctorate, GRE or MAT, minimum GPA of 3.0. Additional exam requirements/recommendations for international students: Required—TOEFL (minimum score 550 paper-based; 79 iBT), IELTS (minimum score 6.5). Electronic applications accepted. *Faculty research:* Adult health, anesthesia, rural health, health administration, family nurse practitioner.

University of Puerto Rico, Medical Sciences Campus, School of Nursing, San Juan, PR 00936-5067. Offers adult and elderly nursing (MSN); child and adolescent nursing (MSN); critical care nursing (MSN); family and community nursing (MSN); family nurse practitioner (MSN); maternity nursing (MSN); mental health and psychiatric nursing (MSN). *Accreditation:* AACN. *Entrance requirements:* For master's, GRE or EXADEP, interview, Puerto Rico RN license or professional license for international students, general and specific point average, article analysis. Electronic applications accepted. *Faculty research:* HIV, health disparities, teen violence, women and violence, neurological disorders.

University of South Alabama, Graduate School, College of Nursing, Mobile, AL 36688. Offers adult health nursing (MSN); community/mental health nursing (MSN); maternal/child nursing (MSN); nursing (DNP). *Accreditation:* AACN. *Faculty:* 50 full-time (46 women), 31 part-time/adjunct (30 women). *Students:* 1,878 full-time (1,680 women), 241 part-time (208 women); includes 523 minority (341 Black or African American, non-Hispanic/Latino; 18 American Indian or Alaska Native, non-Hispanic/Latino; 76 Asian, non-Hispanic/Latino; 54 Hispanic/Latino; 7 Native Hawaiian or other Pacific Islander, non-Hispanic/Latino; 27 Two or more races, non-Hispanic/Latino), 10 international. 1,308 applicants, 64% accepted, 602 enrolled. In 2013, 332 master's, 44 doctorates awarded. *Degree requirements:* For master's, thesis optional. *Entrance requirements:* For master's, BSN, RN licensure, minimum GPA of 3.0, resume documenting clinical experience, background check, drug screening; for doctorate, GRE. *Application deadline:* For fall admission, 7/15 for domestic students; for spring admission, 12/1 for domestic students. Application fee: $35. *Expenses:* Tuition, state resident: full-time $8976; part-time $374 per credit hour. Tuition, nonresident: full-time $17,952; part-time $748 per credit hour. *Unit head:* Dr. Debra Davis, Dean, 251-445-9409, Fax: 251-445-9416. *Application contact:* Dr. Rosemary Rhodes, Director of Graduate Education, 251-445-9409, Fax: 251-445-9416, E-mail: kharriso@usouthal.edu.
Website: http://www.southalabama.edu/nursing

University of South Carolina, The Graduate School, College of Nursing, Program in Health Nursing, Columbia, SC 29208. Offers adult nurse practitioner (MSN); community/public health clinical nurse specialist (MSN); family nurse practitioner (MSN); pediatric nurse practitioner (MSN). *Accreditation:* AACN. Part-time programs available. *Degree requirements:* For master's, thesis or alternative. *Entrance requirements:* For master's, GRE General Test or MAT, BS in nursing, nursing license. Additional exam requirements/recommendations for international students: Required—TOEFL (minimum score 570 paper-based). Electronic applications accepted. *Faculty research:* System research, evidence based practice, breast cancer, violence.

University of South Carolina, The Graduate School, College of Nursing, Program in Nursing and Public Health, Columbia, SC 29208. Offers MPH/MSN. *Accreditation:* AACN; CEPH. Part-time programs available. *Entrance requirements:* Additional exam requirements/recommendations for international students: Required—TOEFL (minimum score 570 paper-based). Electronic applications accepted. *Faculty research:* System research, evidence based practice, breast cancer, violence.

The University of Texas at Austin, Graduate School, School of Nursing, Austin, TX 78712-1111. Offers adult - gerontology clinical nurse specialist (MSN); child health (MSN), including administration, public health nursing, teaching; family nurse practitioner (MSN); family psychiatric/mental health nurse practitioner (MSN); holistic adult health (MSN), including administration, teaching; maternity (MSN), including administration, public health nursing, teaching; nursing (PhD); nursing administration and healthcare systems management (MSN); pediatric nurse practitioner (MSN); public health nursing (MSN). *Accreditation:* AACN. Part-time programs available. *Degree requirements:* For master's, thesis optional; for doctorate, thesis/dissertation. *Entrance requirements:* For master's and doctorate, GRE General Test. Additional exam requirements/recommendations for international students: Required—TOEFL (minimum score 550 paper-based). Electronic applications accepted. *Faculty research:* Chronic illness management, memory and aging, health promotion, women's health, adolescent health.

The University of Texas at Brownsville, Graduate Studies, College of Nursing, Brownsville, TX 78520-4991. Offers MSN. Part-time and evening/weekend programs available. Postbaccalaureate distance learning degree programs offered (no on-campus study). *Faculty:* 8 full-time (all women). *Students:* 26 full-time (21 women), 24 part-time

(17 women); includes 43 minority (7 Black or African American, non-Hispanic/Latino; 6 Asian, non-Hispanic/Latino; 30 Hispanic/Latino), 1 international. 32 applicants, 44% accepted, 11 enrolled. In 2013, 12 master's awarded. *Degree requirements:* For master's, comprehensive exam, thesis optional, capstone course. *Entrance requirements:* Additional exam requirements/recommendations for international students: Required—TOEFL (minimum score 550 paper-based; 77 iBT). *Application deadline:* For fall admission, 7/1 priority date for domestic students, 7/1 for international students; for spring admission, 12/1 priority date for domestic students, 12/1 for international students. Applications are processed on a rolling basis. Application fee: $30. Electronic applications accepted. *Expenses:* Tuition, state resident: full-time $3444; part-time $1148 per semester. Tuition, nonresident: full-time $9816. *Required fees:* $1018; $221 per credit hour. $401 per semester. *Financial support:* In 2013–14, 7 students received support, including 1 research assistantship (averaging $10,000 per year); Federal Work-Study, scholarships/grants, and unspecified assistantships also available. Financial award application deadline: 3/1; financial award applicants required to submit FAFSA. *Unit head:* Dr. Anne Rentfro, Associate Professor, 956-882-5070, Fax: 956-882-5100, E-mail: anne.rentfro@utb.edu. *Application contact:* Mari Montelongo, Graduate Studies Specialist, 956-882-7787, Fax: 956-882-7279, E-mail: mari.montelongo@utb.edu.
Website: http://www.utb.edu/vpaa/nursing/msn/Pages/default.aspx

The University of Texas Health Science Center at San Antonio, School of Nursing, San Antonio, TX 78229. Offers administrative management (MSN); adult-gerontology acute care nurse practitioner (PGC); clinical nurse leader (MSN); executive administrative management (DNP); family nurse practitioner (PGC); nurse practitioner (MSN), including adult-gerontology acute care nurse practitioner, family nurse practitioner, pediatric nurse practitioner primary care, psychiatric mental health nurse practitioner; nurse practitioner leadership (DNP); nursing (MSN, PhD); nursing education (MSN, PGC); pediatric nurse practitioner primary care (PGC); psychiatric mental health nurse practitioner (PGC); public health nurse leader (DNP). *Accreditation:* AACN. Part-time programs available. *Faculty:* 84 full-time (74 women), 42 part-time/adjunct (40 women). *Students:* 115 full-time (93 women), 140 part-time (123 women); includes 123 minority (24 Black or African American, non-Hispanic/Latino; 20 Asian, non-Hispanic/Latino; 74 Hispanic/Latino; 5 Two or more races, non-Hispanic/Latino), 7 international. Average age 37. 174 applicants, 59% accepted, 83 enrolled. In 2013, 67 master's, 6 doctorates, 5 other advanced degrees awarded. Terminal master's awarded for partial completion of doctoral program. *Degree requirements:* For master's, thesis optional; for doctorate, comprehensive exam, thesis/dissertation, final projects (for DNP). *Entrance requirements:* For master's, minimum GPA of 3.0, references, goal statement, BSN from accredited nursing school, RN licensure in Texas or compact state; for doctorate, GRE, MAT, minimum GPA of 3.0, personal interview, BSN and/or MSN from accredited nursing school, RN licensure in Texas or compact state, statistics course, references, curriculum vitae, goal statement; for PGC, minimum GPA of 3.0; references; goal statement; MSN from accredited nursing school; RN licensure in Texas or compact state; prerequisites in advanced health assessment, advanced pharmacotherapeutics, and advanced pathophysiology. Additional exam requirements/recommendations for international students: Required—TOEFL (minimum score 550 paper-based; 68 iBT), IELTS (minimum score 6.5). *Application deadline:* For fall admission, 1/10 for domestic and international students; for spring admission, 7/1 for domestic students. Application fee: $65. Electronic applications accepted. *Financial support:* In 2013–14, 145 students received support, including 3 fellowships with full tuition reimbursements available (averaging $30,000 per year); institutionally sponsored loans and scholarships/grants also available. Financial award application deadline: 6/30; financial award applicants required to submit FAFSA. *Faculty research:* Pain, organizational structure, aging, quality and safety, health disparity, obesity and nutrition, women's and children's health. *Total annual research expenditures:* $500,265. *Unit head:* Dr. Eileen T. Breslin, Dean, 210-567-5800, Fax: 210-567-5929, E-mail: breslin@uthscsa.edu. *Application contact:* Brandy Finck, Interim Associate Dean for Admissions and Student Services, 210-567-5805, Fax: 210-567-6189, E-mail: finckb@uthscsa.edu.
Website: http://www.nursing.uthscsa.edu/

The University of Toledo, College of Graduate Studies, College of Nursing, Department of Population and Community Care, Toledo, OH 43606-3390. Offers clinical nurse leader (MSN); family nurse practitioner (MSN, Certificate); nurse educator (MSN, Certificate); pediatric nurse practitioner (MSN, Certificate). Part-time programs available. *Students:* 70 full-time (60 women), 212 part-time (186 women); includes 27 minority (12 Black or African American, non-Hispanic/Latino; 1 American Indian or Alaska Native, non-Hispanic/Latino; 3 Asian, non-Hispanic/Latino; 7 Hispanic/Latino; 4 Two or more races, non-Hispanic/Latino), 1 international. Average age 32. 127 applicants, 81% accepted, 78 enrolled. In 2013, 82 master's, 10 other advanced degrees awarded. *Degree requirements:* For master's, thesis or alternative. *Entrance requirements:* For master's, GRE, BS in nursing, minimum undergraduate GPA of 3.0, statement of purpose, three letters of recommendation, transcripts from all prior institutions attended, Nursing CAS application, UT supplemental application; for Certificate, BS in nursing, minimum undergraduate GPA of 3.0, statement of purpose, three letters of recommendation, transcripts from all prior institutions attended. Additional exam requirements/recommendations for international students: Required—TOEFL (minimum score 550 paper-based; 80 iBT). Application fee: $45 ($75 for international students). Electronic applications accepted. *Financial support:* Research assistantships with full and partial tuition reimbursements, Federal Work-Study, scholarships/grants, traineeships, and tuition waivers (full and partial) available. *Unit head:* Dr. Kelley Phillips, Chair, 419-383-5892. *Application contact:* Joan Mulligan, Admissions Analyst, 419-383-4168, Fax: 419-383-6140, E-mail: joan.mulligan@utoledo.edu.
Website: http://www.utoledo.edu/nursing/

University of Washington, Tacoma, Graduate Programs, Program in Nursing, Tacoma, WA 98402-3100. Offers communities, populations and health (MN); leadership in healthcare (MN); nurse educator (MN). Part-time programs available. *Degree requirements:* For master's, thesis (for some programs), advance fieldwork. *Entrance requirements:* For master's, Washington State NCLEX exam, minimum GPA of 3.0. Additional exam requirements/recommendations for international students: Required—TOEFL (minimum score 580 paper-based; 70 iBT); Recommended—IELTS (minimum score 7). *Faculty research:* Hospice and palliative care; clinical trial decision-making; minority nurse retention; asthma and public health; injustice, suffering, difference: Linking Them to Us; adolescent health.

Wayne State University, College of Nursing, Area of Family Community Mental Health, Detroit, MI 48202. Offers MSN. *Accreditation:* AACN. Part-time programs available. *Faculty:* 15 full-time (all women). *Students:* 61 full-time (59 women), 108 part-time (100 women); includes 38 minority (26 Black or African American, non-Hispanic/Latino; 1 American Indian or Alaska Native, non-Hispanic/Latino; 9 Asian, non-Hispanic/Latino; 1 Hispanic/Latino; 1 Two or more races, non-Hispanic/Latino), 11 international. Average age 35. 66 applicants, 56% accepted, 33 enrolled. In 2013, 51 master's awarded. *Degree requirements:* For master's, thesis or alternative. *Entrance requirements:* For master's, minimum honor point average of 3.0 in upper-division course work; BA from NLN- or CCNE-accredited program; references; current RN license; personal statement. Additional exam requirements/recommendations for international students: Required—TOEFL (minimum score 550 paper-based; 79 iBT), TWE (minimum score 6), Michigan English Language Assessment Battery (minimum score 85); Recommended—IELTS (minimum score 6.5). *Application deadline:* For fall admission, 7/1 for domestic students, 5/1 priority date for international students; for winter admission, 11/1 for domestic students, 9/1 priority date for international students; for spring admission, 3/1 for domestic students, 1/1 priority date for international students. Applications are processed on a rolling basis. Application fee: $0. Electronic applications accepted. *Expenses:* Contact institution. *Financial support:* In 2013–14, 1 student received support. Fellowships with tuition reimbursements available, research assistantships with tuition reimbursements available, teaching assistantships with tuition reimbursements available, institutionally sponsored loans, scholarships/grants, traineeships, and unspecified assistantships available. Support available to part-time students. Financial award application deadline: 3/31; financial award applicants required to submit FAFSA. *Faculty research:* Cultural competence in the home care nursing community; prevention and management of depression in women (including caregivers and perinatal women); breastfeeding in low-income populations; promotion of mental health of vulnerable women, infants, and young children; palliative and end-of-life care for newborns and families. *Unit head:* Dr. Stephanie Schim, Assistant Dean, Family Community Mental Health, 313-577-5137. *Application contact:* Eric Brown, Director, Office of Student Affairs, 313-577-4082, E-mail: nursinginfo@wayne.edu.
Website: https://nursing.wayne.edu/

West Chester University of Pennsylvania, College of Health Sciences, Department of Nursing, West Chester, PA 19383. Offers nursing (DNP); public health nursing (MSN), including administration, education, integrative health. *Accreditation:* AACN. Part-time and evening/weekend programs available. Postbaccalaureate distance learning degree programs offered (minimal on-campus study). *Faculty:* 4 full-time (3 women). *Students:* 12 full-time (11 women), 17 part-time (15 women); includes 9 minority (7 Black or African American, non-Hispanic/Latino; 1 Asian, non-Hispanic/Latino; 1 Hispanic/Latino), 2 international. Average age 42. 11 applicants, 91% accepted, 7 enrolled. In 2013, 17 master's awarded. *Entrance requirements:* For master's, RN license, BSN or RN with bachelor's degree in another discipline, minimum GPA of 2.8, experience as a nurse providing direct clinical care, two letters of recommendation; for doctorate, minimum graduate GPA of 3.0, two letters of reference, interview. Additional exam requirements/recommendations for international students: Required—TOEFL (minimum score 550 paper-based; 80 iBT). *Application deadline:* For fall admission, 4/15 priority date for domestic students, 3/15 for international students; for spring admission, 10/15 priority date for domestic students, 9/1 for international students. Applications are processed on a rolling basis. Application fee: $45. Electronic applications accepted. *Expenses:* Tuition, state resident: full-time $7956; part-time $442 per credit. Tuition, nonresident: full-time $11,934; part-time $663 per credit. *Required fees:* $2134.20; $106.24 per credit. Tuition and fees vary according to campus/location and program. *Financial support:* Unspecified assistantships available. Support available to part-time students. Financial award application deadline: 2/15; financial award applicants required to submit FAFSA. *Unit head:* Dr. Charlotte Mackey, Chair and Graduate Coordinator, 610-436-3474, Fax: 610-436-3083, E-mail: cmackey@wcupa.edu.
Website: http://www.wcupa.edu/_ACADEMICS/HealthSciences/nursing/

Worcester State University, Graduate Studies, Department of Nursing, Program in Community and Public Health Nursing, Worcester, MA 01602-2597. Offers MSN. *Accreditation:* AACN. Part-time programs available. *Faculty:* 3 full-time (all women), 3 part-time/adjunct (all women). *Students:* 17 full-time (12 women), 20 part-time (19 women); includes 3 minority (all Black or African American, non-Hispanic/Latino), 2 international. Average age 42. 43 applicants, 72% accepted, 12 enrolled. In 2013, 6 master's awarded. *Degree requirements:* For master's, final project, practicum. *Entrance requirements:* For master's, GRE, MAT, unencumbered license to practice as a Registered Nurse in Massachusetts. Additional exam requirements/recommendations for international students: Required—TOEFL (minimum score 500 paper-based; 61 iBT). *Application deadline:* For fall admission, 6/15 for domestic and international students; for spring admission, 4/1 for domestic and international students. Applications are processed on a rolling basis. Application fee: $40. Electronic applications accepted. *Expenses: Tuition, area resident:* Part-time $150 per credit. Tuition, state resident: part-time $150 per credit. Tuition, nonresident: part-time $150 per credit. *Required fees:* $114.50 per credit. *Financial support:* In 2013–14, 2 students received support, including 2 research assistantships (averaging $4,800 per year). Financial award application deadline: 3/1; financial award applicants required to submit FAFSA. *Unit head:* Dr. Stephanie Chalupka, Coordinator, 508-929-8680, E-mail: schalupka@worcester.edu. *Application contact:* Sara Grady, Assistant Dean of Continuing Education, 508-929-8787, Fax: 508-929-8100, E-mail: sara.grady@worcester.edu.

Wright State University, School of Graduate Studies, College of Nursing and Health, Program in Nursing, Dayton, OH 45435. Offers acute care nurse practitioner (MS); administration of nursing and health care systems (MS); adult health (MS); child and adolescent health (MS); community health (MS); family nurse practitioner (MS); nurse practitioner (MS); school nurse (MS); MBA/MS. *Accreditation:* AACN. Part-time and evening/weekend programs available. *Degree requirements:* For master's, thesis or alternative. *Entrance requirements:* For master's, GRE General Test, BSN from NLN-accredited college, Ohio RN license. Additional exam requirements/recommendations for international students: Required—TOEFL. *Faculty research:* Clinical nursing and health, teaching, caring, pain administration, informatics and technology.

Family Nurse Practitioner Studies

Abilene Christian University, Graduate School, School of Nursing, Abilene, TX 79699-9100. Offers education and administration (MSN); family nurse practitioner (MSN); nursing (Certificate). *Accreditation:* AACN. Part-time programs available. *Faculty:* 7 part-time/adjunct (all women). *Students:* 1 (woman) part-time. 11 applicants. In 2013, 3 master's awarded. *Degree requirements:* For master's, practicum. *Entrance requirements:* For master's, GRE General Test. Additional exam requirements/

recommendations for international students: Required—TOEFL (minimum score 550 paper-based; 90 iBT), IELTS (minimum score 6.5). *Application deadline:* For fall admission, 4/1 priority date for domestic students; for spring admission, 11/1 for domestic students. Applications are processed on a rolling basis. Application fee: $50. Electronic applications accepted. *Expenses: Tuition:* Full-time $17,100; part-time $950 per credit hour. *Financial support:* Application deadline: 4/1; applicants required to submit FAFSA. *Unit head:* Dr. Becky Hammack, Graduate Director, 325-674-2265, Fax: 325-674-6256, E-mail: rsh12a@acu.edu. *Application contact:* Corey Patterson, Director of Graduate Admission and Recruiting, 325-674-6566, Fax: 325-674-6717, E-mail: gradinfo@acu.edu.

Albany State University, College of Sciences and Health Professions, Albany, GA 31705-2717. Offers criminal justice (MS), including corrections, forensic science, law enforcement, public administration; mathematics education (M Ed); nursing (MSN), including RN to MSN family nurse practitioner, RN to MSN nurse educator; science education (M Ed). Part-time and evening/weekend programs available. Postbaccalaureate distance learning degree programs offered. *Degree requirements:* For master's, comprehensive exam, thesis. *Entrance requirements:* For master's, GRE or MAT, official transcript, letters of recommendations, pre-medical/certificate of immunizations. Electronic applications accepted.

Allen College, Program in Nursing, Waterloo, IA 50703. Offers acute care nurse practitioner (MSN, Post-Master's Certificate); adult nurse practitioner (MSN, Post-Master's Certificate); adult psychiatric-mental health nurse practitioner (MSN, Post-Master's Certificate); community public health (MSN, Post-Master's Certificate); family nurse practitioner (MSN, Post-Master's Certificate); gerontological nurse practitioner (MSN, Post-Master's Certificate); health education (MSN); leadership in health care delivery (MSN, Post-Master's Certificate); nursing (DNP). Part-time programs available. Postbaccalaureate distance learning degree programs offered (minimal on-campus study). *Faculty:* 3 full-time (all women), 21 part-time/adjunct (20 women). *Students:* 21 full-time (19 women), 162 part-time (150 women); includes 5 minority (1 Black or African American, non-Hispanic/Latino; 2 Asian, non-Hispanic/Latino; 1 Hispanic/Latino; 1 Two or more races, non-Hispanic/Latino). Average age 34. 213 applicants, 57% accepted, 94 enrolled. In 2013, 41 master's, 4 other advanced degrees awarded. *Degree requirements:* For master's, thesis optional. *Entrance requirements:* For master's, minimum GPA of 3.0 in the last 60 hours of undergraduate coursework; for doctorate, minimum GPA of 3.25 in graduate coursework. Additional exam requirements/recommendations for international students: Recommended—TOEFL (minimum score 580 paper-based; 92 iBT), IELTS (minimum score 6). *Application deadline:* For fall admission, 2/1 priority date for domestic students; for spring admission, 9/1 priority date for domestic students. Applications are processed on a rolling basis. Application fee: $50. Electronic applications accepted. *Expenses: Tuition:* Full-time $14,534; part-time $755 per credit hour. *Required fees:* $935; $75 per credit hour. One-time fee: $275 part-time. Tuition and fees vary according to course load. *Financial support:* In 2013–14, 60 students received support. Institutionally sponsored loans, scholarships/grants, and traineeships available. Support available to part-time students. Financial award application deadline: 8/15; financial award applicants required to submit FAFSA. *Unit head:* Kendra Williams-Perez, Dean, School of Nursing, 319-226-2044, Fax: 319-226-2070, E-mail: kendra.williams-perez@allencollege.edu. *Application contact:* Molly Quinn, Admissions Counselor, 319-226-2001, Fax: 319-226-2010, E-mail: molly.quinn@allencollege.edu.
Website: http://www.allencollege.edu/

Alverno College, School of Nursing, Milwaukee, WI 53234-3922. Offers family nurse practitioner (MSN); mental health nurse practitioner (MSN); nursing education (MSN). *Accreditation:* AACN. Part-time and evening/weekend programs available. *Faculty:* 7 full-time (all women), 8 part-time/adjunct (4 women). *Students:* 82 full-time (79 women), 84 part-time (79 women); includes 48 minority (24 Black or African American, non-Hispanic/Latino; 1 American Indian or Alaska Native, non-Hispanic/Latino; 6 Asian, non-Hispanic/Latino; 11 Hispanic/Latino; 6 Two or more races, non-Hispanic/Latino), 1 international. Average age 36. 59 applicants, 100% accepted, 47 enrolled. In 2013, 33 master's awarded. *Degree requirements:* For master's, 500 clinical hours, capstone. *Entrance requirements:* For master's, BSN, current license. Additional exam requirements/recommendations for international students: Required—TOEFL. *Application deadline:* For fall admission, 7/15 priority date for domestic and international students; for spring admission, 12/15 priority date for domestic and international students. Applications are processed on a rolling basis. Application fee: $0. Electronic applications accepted. Application fee is waived when completed online. *Expenses:* Contact institution. *Financial support:* In 2013–14, 4 students received support. Federal Work-Study and scholarships/grants available. Support available to part-time students. Financial award application deadline: 4/15; financial award applicants required to submit FAFSA. *Faculty research:* Impact of stroke on sexuality, children's asthma management, factors affecting baccalaureate student success. *Unit head:* Dr. Carol Sabel, Associate Dean for MSN Program, 414-382-6309, Fax: 414-382-6354, E-mail: carol.sabel@alverno.edu. *Application contact:* Janet Stikel, Associate Director of Admissions - Adult and Graduate, 414-382-6112, Fax: 414-382-6354, E-mail: janet.stikel@alverno.edu.

Arizona State University at the Tempe campus, College of Nursing and Health Innovation, Phoenix, AZ 85004. Offers advanced nursing practice (DNP); child/family mental health nurse practitioner (Graduate Certificate); clinical research management (MS); community and public health practice (Graduate Certificate); community health (MS); exercise and wellness (MS), including exercise and wellness; family nurse practitioner (Graduate Certificate); healthcare innovation (MHI); international health for healthcare (Graduate Certificate); kinesiology (MS, PhD); nursing (MS, Graduate Certificate); nursing and healthcare innovation (PhD); nutrition (MS); physical activity nutrition and wellness (PhD), including physical activity, nutrition and wellness; public health (MPH); regulatory science and health safety (MS). *Accreditation:* AACN. Postbaccalaureate distance learning degree programs offered (minimal on-campus study). *Degree requirements:* For master's, comprehensive exam (for some programs), thesis (for some programs), interactive Program of Study (iPOS) submitted before completing 50 percent of required credit hours; for doctorate, comprehensive exam, thesis/dissertation, interactive Program of Study (iPOS) submitted before completing 50 percent of required credit hours. *Entrance requirements:* For master's and doctorate, GRE, minimum GPA of 3.0 or equivalent in last 2 years of work leading to bachelor's degree. Additional exam requirements/recommendations for international students: Required—TOEFL (minimum score 80 iBT), TOEFL, IELTS, or PTE. Electronic applications accepted. *Expenses:* Contact institution.

Barry University, School of Adult and Continuing Education, Division of Nursing, Program in Nurse Practitioner, Miami Shores, FL 33161-6695. Offers acute care nurse practitioner (MSN); family nurse practitioner (MSN); nurse practitioner (Certificate). *Accreditation:* AACN. Part-time and evening/weekend programs available. *Degree requirements:* For master's, research project or thesis. *Entrance requirements:* For master's, GRE General Test or MAT, BSN, minimum GPA of 3.0, course work in statistics. Electronic applications accepted. *Faculty research:* Child abuse, health beliefs, teenage pregnancy, cultural and clinical studies across the lifespan.

Baylor University, Graduate School, Louise Herrington School of Nursing, Dallas, TX 75246. Offers family nurse practitioner (MSN); neonatal nurse practitioner (MSN); nurse-midwifery (DNP). *Accreditation:* AACN. Part-time programs available. Postbaccalaureate distance learning degree programs offered (minimal on-campus study). *Faculty:* 11 full-time (all women), 3 part-time/adjunct (2 women). *Students:* 25 full-time (24 women), 41 part-time (37 women); includes 15 minority (5 Black or African American, non-Hispanic/Latino; 5 Asian, non-Hispanic/Latino; 4 Hispanic/Latino; 1 Two or more races, non-Hispanic/Latino). Average age 35. 47 applicants, 70% accepted, 26 enrolled. In 2013, 25 master's, 5 doctorates awarded. *Degree requirements:* For doctorate, comprehensive exam (for some programs), capstone project. *Entrance requirements:* For master's, GRE General Test or MAT; for doctorate, GRE General Test. Additional exam requirements/recommendations for international students: Required—TOEFL. *Application deadline:* For fall admission, 2/1 for domestic students. Application fee: $50. Electronic applications accepted. *Expenses: Tuition:* Full-time $25,866; part-time $1437 per credit hour. *Required fees:* $2736; $152 per credit hour. Tuition and fees vary according to course load and program. *Financial support:* In 2013–14, 66 students received support, including 1 teaching assistantship (averaging $4,167 per year); Federal Work-Study, scholarships/grants, and unspecified assistantships also available. Support available to part-time students. Financial award application deadline: 6/30; financial award applicants required to submit FAFSA. *Faculty research:* Women and strokes, obesity and pregnancy, educational environmental factors, international undeserved populations, midwifery. *Total annual research expenditures:* $5,000. *Unit head:* Dr. Barbara Camune, Graduate Program Director, 214-367-3754, Fax: 214-820-3375, E-mail: barbara_camune@baylor.edu. *Application contact:* Elaine Lark, Coordinator of Recruitment and Enrollment, 214-818-7839, Fax: 214-820-3835, E-mail: elaine_lark@baylor.edu.
Website: http://www.baylor.edu/nursing/

Bellarmine University, Donna and Allan Lansing School of Nursing and Health Sciences, Louisville, KY 40205. Offers family nurse practitioner (MSN); health science (MHS); nursing administration (MSN); nursing education (MSN); nursing practice (DNP); physical therapy (DPT). *Accreditation:* AACN; APTA. Part-time and evening/weekend programs available. *Faculty:* 21 full-time (19 women), 8 part-time/adjunct (5 women). *Students:* 162 full-time (111 women), 120 part-time (113 women); includes 16 minority (6 Black or African American, non-Hispanic/Latino; 1 American Indian or Alaska Native, non-Hispanic/Latino; 3 Asian, non-Hispanic/Latino; 3 Hispanic/Latino; 3 Two or more races, non-Hispanic/Latino). Average age 29. In 2013, 30 master's, 54 doctorates awarded. *Degree requirements:* For doctorate, comprehensive exam, thesis/dissertation. *Entrance requirements:* For master's, GRE General Test, RN license; for doctorate, GRE General Test, Physical Therapist Centralized Application Service (for DPT). Additional exam requirements/recommendations for international students: Required—TOEFL (minimum score 550 paper-based; 80 iBT). Application fee: $25. Electronic applications accepted. *Expenses:* Contact institution. *Financial support:* Career-related internships or fieldwork and scholarships/grants available. *Faculty research:* Nursing: pain, empathy, leadership styles, control; physical therapy: service-learning; exercise in chronic and pre-operative conditions, athletes; women's health; aging. *Unit head:* Dr. Mark Wiegand, Dean, 800-274-4723 Ext. 8368, E-mail: mwiegand@bellarmine.edu. *Application contact:* Julie Armstrong-Binnix, Health Science Recruiter, 800-274-4723 Ext. 8364, E-mail: julieab@bellarmine.edu.
Website: http://www.bellarmine.edu/lansing

Bellin College, School of Nursing, Green Bay, WI 54305. Offers family nurse practitioner (MSN); nurse educator (MSN). *Accreditation:* AACN. *Faculty:* 1 (woman) full-time, 3 part-time/adjunct (2 women). *Students:* 37 part-time (all women). *Expenses: Tuition:* Part-time $714 per credit. *Required fees:* $100 per year. *Unit head:* Dr. Kimberly Udlis, Graduate Program Director, 920-433-6624, Fax: 920-433-1921, E-mail: kimberly.udlis@bellincollege.edu.

Bloomsburg University of Pennsylvania, School of Graduate Studies, College of Science and Technology, Department of Nursing, Bloomsburg, PA 17815. Offers adult and family nurse practitioner (MSN); community health (MSN); nurse anesthesia (MSN); nursing (MSN); nursing administration (MSN). *Accreditation:* AACN; AANA/CANAEP. *Faculty:* 5 full-time (all women), 7 part-time/adjunct (all women). *Students:* 62 full-time (52 women), 26 part-time (17 women); includes 8 minority (6 Black or African American, non-Hispanic/Latino; 1 Asian, non-Hispanic/Latino; 1 Hispanic/Latino). Average age 35. 61 applicants, 84% accepted, 14 enrolled. In 2013, 36 master's awarded. *Degree requirements:* For master's, thesis (for some programs), clinical experience. *Entrance requirements:* For master's, minimum QPA of 3.0, personal statement, 2 letters of recommendation, nursing license. Additional exam requirements/recommendations for international students: Required—TOEFL. *Application deadline:* For fall admission, 1/1 for domestic students; for spring admission, 8/1 for domestic students. Applications are processed on a rolling basis. Application fee: $35 ($60 for international students). Electronic applications accepted. *Expenses:* Tuition, state resident: full-time $7956; part-time $442 per credit. Tuition, nonresident: full-time $11,934; part-time $663 per credit. *Required fees:* $95.50 per credit. $55 per semester. Tuition and fees vary according to course load. *Financial support:* Unspecified assistantships available. *Unit head:* Dr. Noreen Chikotas, Coordinator, 570-389-4609, Fax: 570-389-5008, E-mail: nchikota@bloomu.edu. *Application contact:* Jennifer Richard, Administrative Assistant, 570-389-4015, Fax: 570-389-3054, E-mail: jrichard@bloomu.edu.
Website: http://www.bloomu.edu/nursing

Bowie State University, Graduate Programs, Department of Nursing, Bowie, MD 20715-9465. Offers administration of nursing services (MS); family nurse practitioner (MS); nursing education (MS). Part-time programs available. *Degree requirements:* For master's, comprehensive exam, thesis, research paper. *Entrance requirements:* For master's, minimum GPA of 2.5. Electronic applications accepted. *Expenses:* Tuition, state resident: full-time $8665. Tuition, nonresident: full-time $16,007. *Required fees:* $1927. *Faculty research:* Minority health, women's health, gerontology, leadership management.

Brenau University, Sydney O. Smith Graduate School, College of Health and Science, Gainesville, GA 30501. Offers family nurse practitioner (MSN); nurse educator (MSN); nursing management (MSN); occupational therapy (MS); psychology (MS). *Accreditation:* AOTA. Part-time and evening/weekend programs available. *Degree requirements:* For master's, comprehensive exam (for some programs), thesis (for some programs), clinical practicum hours. *Entrance requirements:* For master's, GRE General Test or MAT (for some programs), interview, writing sample, references (for some programs). Additional exam requirements/recommendations for international students: Required—TOEFL (minimum score 500 paper-based; 61 iBT); Recommended—IELTS (minimum score 5). Electronic applications accepted. *Expenses:* Contact institution.

Brigham Young University, Graduate Studies, College of Nursing, Provo, UT 84602. Offers family nurse practitioner (MS). *Accreditation:* AACN. *Faculty:* 10 full-time (7 women), 1 part-time/adjunct (0 women). *Students:* 28 full-time (11 women). Average age 34. 44 applicants, 34% accepted, 15 enrolled. In 2013, 15 master's awarded. *Degree requirements:* For master's, thesis. *Entrance requirements:* For master's, GRE, minimum GPA of 3.0 in last 60 hours, interview, BS in nursing, pathophysiology class within undergraduate program, course work in basic statistics. Additional exam requirements/recommendations for international students: Required—TOEFL;

Recommended—IELTS. *Application deadline:* For spring admission, 12/1 for domestic students. Applications are processed on a rolling basis. Application fee: $50. Electronic applications accepted. *Expenses: Tuition:* Full-time $6130; part-time $340 per credit hour. Tuition and fees vary according to program and student's religious affiliation. *Financial support:* In 2013–14, 28 students received support, including 2 research assistantships with full and partial tuition reimbursements available (averaging $10,000 per year), 3 teaching assistantships with full and partial tuition reimbursements available (averaging $10,000 per year); institutionally sponsored loans, scholarships/grants, tuition waivers (full), and unspecified assistantships also available. Support available to part-time students. Financial award application deadline: 2/1; financial award applicants required to submit FAFSA. *Faculty research:* Critical care issues, end of life, childhood immunizations, children with diabetes, global health. *Total annual research expenditures:* $1,200. *Unit head:* Dr. Patricia Ravert, Dean, 801-422-1167, Fax: 801-422-0536, E-mail: patricia_ravert@byu.edu. *Application contact:* Lynette Jakins, Graduate Secretary, 801-422-4142, Fax: 801-422-0538, E-mail: lynette-jakins@byu.edu.
Website: http://nursing.byu.edu/

California Baptist University, Program in Nursing, Riverside, CA 92504-3206. Offers clinical nurse specialist (MSN); family nurse practitioner (MSN); healthcare systems management (MSN); nursing (MSN); teaching-learning (MSN). Part-time programs available. *Faculty:* 15 full-time (all women), 7 part-time/adjunct (all women). *Students:* 49 full-time (41 women), 69 part-time (55 women); includes 61 minority (18 Black or African American, non-Hispanic/Latino; 1 American Indian or Alaska Native, non-Hispanic/Latino; 17 Asian, non-Hispanic/Latino; 22 Hispanic/Latino; 3 Two or more races, non-Hispanic/Latino). Average age 33. 48 applicants, 65% accepted, 20 enrolled. In 2013, 9 master's awarded. *Degree requirements:* For master's, comprehensive exam (for some programs), thesis or alternative, comprehensive exam or directed project thesis; capstone practicum. *Entrance requirements:* For master's, GRE or California Critical Thinking Skills Test; Test of Essential Academic Skills (TEAS), minimum undergraduate GPA of 3.25; Microsoft Office competency; health clearance; health insurance; CPR certification; vehicle insurance; random drug testing; background check clearance; passport photo; three recommendations; comprehensive essay; interview. Additional exam requirements/recommendations for international students: Required—TOEFL (minimum score 80 iBT). *Application deadline:* For fall admission, 8/1 priority date for domestic students, 7/1 for international students; for spring admission, 12/1 priority date for domestic students, 11/1 for international students. Applications are processed on a rolling basis. Application fee: $45. Electronic applications accepted. *Expenses: Tuition:* Full-time $10,080; part-time $560 per unit. *Required fees:* $175 per semester. One-time fee: $45. Tuition and fees vary according to course load and program. *Financial support:* Institutionally sponsored loans available. Financial award applicants required to submit CSS PROFILE or FAFSA. *Faculty research:* Qualitative research using Parse methodology, gerontology, disaster preparedness, medical-surgical nursing, maternal-child nursing. *Unit head:* Dr. Geneva Oaks, Dean, School of Nursing, 951-343-4702, E-mail: goaks@calbaptist.edu. *Application contact:* Dr. Rebecca Meyer, Director, Graduate Program in Nursing, 951-343-4952, Fax: 951-343-5095, E-mail: rmeyer@calbaptist.edu.
Website: http://www.calbaptist.edu/explore-cbu/schools-colleges/school-nursing/master-science-nursing/

California State University, Fresno, Division of Graduate Studies, College of Health and Human Services, Department of Nursing, Fresno, CA 93740-8027. Offers nursing (MS), including clinical nurse, primary care nurse practitioner, specialist/nurse educator. *Accreditation:* AACN. Part-time and evening/weekend programs available. *Degree requirements:* For master's, thesis or alternative. *Entrance requirements:* For master's, GRE General Test, 1 year of clinical practice, previous course work in statistics, BSN, minimum GPA of 3.0 in nursing. Additional exam requirements/recommendations for international students: Required—TOEFL. Electronic applications accepted. *Faculty research:* Training grant, HIV assessment.

Carlow University, School of Nursing, Program in Family Nurse Practitioner, Pittsburgh, PA 15213-3165. Offers MSN, Certificate. Part-time programs available. *Students:* 185 full-time (173 women), 29 part-time (24 women); includes 13 minority (5 Black or African American, non-Hispanic/Latino; 4 Asian, non-Hispanic/Latino; 3 Hispanic/Latino; 1 Two or more races, non-Hispanic/Latino). Average age 34. 88 applicants, 93% accepted, 56 enrolled. In 2013, 62 master's, 2 other advanced degrees awarded. *Entrance requirements:* For master's, minimum undergraduate GPA of 3.0 from accredited BSN program; current license as RN in Pennsylvania; at least one year of recent clinical (bedside) nursing experience; course in statistics in past 6 years; two recommendations; personal statement; personal interview. Additional exam requirements/recommendations for international students: Required—TOEFL (minimum score 550 paper-based). *Application deadline:* Applications are processed on a rolling basis. Application fee: $20. Application fee is waived when completed online. *Expenses: Tuition:* Full-time $9523; part-time $744 per credit. Tuition and fees vary according to course load, degree level and program. *Unit head:* Dr. Karen A. Cummins, Director, Family Nurse Practitioner Program, 412-578-6112, Fax: 412-578-6114, E-mail: kacummins@carlow.edu. *Application contact:* Jo Danhires, Administrative Assistant, Admissions, 412-578-6059, Fax: 412-578-6321, E-mail: gradstudies@carlow.edu.
Website: http://www.carlow.edu/Master_of_Science_in_Nursing_Family_Nurse_Practitioner.aspx

Carson-Newman University, Department of Nursing, Jefferson City, TN 37760. Offers family nurse practitioner (MSN); nurse educator (MSN). *Accreditation:* AACN. *Faculty:* 2 full-time (both women), 10 part-time/adjunct (9 women). *Students:* 4 full-time (2 women), 55 part-time (45 women); includes 2 minority (1 Black or African American, non-Hispanic/Latino; 1 Two or more races, non-Hispanic/Latino), 1 international. Average age 32. In 2013, 20 master's awarded. *Application deadline:* For fall admission, 7/15 priority date for domestic students. Applications are processed on a rolling basis. Application fee: $50. *Expenses: Tuition:* Part-time $390 per credit hour. *Unit head:* Dr. Gregory A. Casalenuovo, Dean, 865-471-3426. *Application contact:* Graduate Admissions and Services Adviser, 865-473-3468, Fax: 865-472-3475.

Case Western Reserve University, Frances Payne Bolton School of Nursing, Doctor of Nursing Practice Program, Cleveland, OH 44106. Offers acute care nurse practitioner (DNP); adult gerontology nurse practitioner (DNP); educational leadership (DNP); family nurse practitioner (DNP); family systems psychiatric mental health nursing (DNP); midwifery/family nursing (DNP); neonatal nurse practitioner (DNP); pediatric nurse practitioner (DNP); practice leadership (DNP); women's health nurse practitioner (DNP). *Accreditation:* AACN. Part-time programs available. Postbaccalaureate distance learning degree programs offered (minimal on-campus study). *Students:* 169 full-time, 9 part-time; includes 10 minority (6 Black or African American, non-Hispanic/Latino; 1 Asian, non-Hispanic/Latino; 2 Hispanic/Latino; 1 Two or more races, non-Hispanic/Latino). 76 applicants, 97% accepted, 59 enrolled. In 2013, 38 doctorates awarded. Terminal master's awarded for partial completion of doctoral program. *Degree requirements:* For doctorate, thesis/dissertation. *Entrance requirements:* For doctorate, GRE General Test or MAT. Additional exam requirements/recommendations for international students: Required—TOEFL (minimum score 577 paper-based; 90 iBT), IELTS (minimum score 7). *Application deadline:* For fall admission, 6/1 priority date for domestic students, 6/1 for international students; for spring admission, 10/1 for domestic and international students. Applications are processed on a rolling basis. Application fee: $75. *Financial support:* In 2013–14, 90 students received support, including 9 fellowships with full tuition reimbursements available (averaging $31,325 per year), 1 research assistantship with partial tuition reimbursement available (averaging $14,472 per year); teaching assistantships, Federal Work-Study, institutionally sponsored loans, scholarships/grants, and tuition waivers (partial) also available. Support available to part-time students. Financial award application deadline: 5/15; financial award applicants required to submit FAFSA. *Faculty research:* Symptom science, family/community care, aging across the lifespan, self-management of health and illness, neuroscience. *Unit head:* Dr. Donna Dowling, Director, 216-368-1869, Fax: 216-368-3542, E-mail: dad10@case.edu. *Application contact:* Donna Hassik, Admissions Coordinator, 216-368-5253, Fax: 216-368-0124, E-mail: dmh7@case.edu.
Website: http://fpb.case.edu/DNP/

Case Western Reserve University, Frances Payne Bolton School of Nursing, Master's Programs in Nursing, Nurse Practitioner Program, Cleveland, OH 44106. Offers acute care cardiovascular nursing (MSN); acute care nurse practitioner (MSN); acute care/flight nurse (MSN); adult gerontology acute care nurse practitioner (MSN); adult gerontology nurse practitioner (MSN); adult gerontology oncology and palliative care (MSN); family nurse practitioner (MSN); family systems psychiatric mental health nursing (MSN); neonatal nurse practitioner (MSN); pediatric nurse practitioner (MSN); women's health nurse practitioner (MSN). Part-time programs available. Postbaccalaureate distance learning degree programs offered (minimal on-campus study). *Faculty:* 54 full-time (50 women), 5 part-time/adjunct (3 women). *Students:* 56 full-time, 145 part-time; includes 9 minority (6 Black or African American, non-Hispanic/Latino; 2 Asian, non-Hispanic/Latino; 1 Hispanic/Latino), 5 international. Average age 35. 70 applicants, 71% accepted, 33 enrolled. In 2013, 79 master's awarded. *Degree requirements:* For master's, thesis optional. *Entrance requirements:* For master's, GRE General Test or MAT. Additional exam requirements/recommendations for international students: Required—TOEFL (minimum score 577 paper-based; 90 iBT), IELTS (minimum score 7). *Application deadline:* For fall admission, 6/1 for domestic students; for spring admission, 10/1 for domestic students. Applications are processed on a rolling basis. Application fee: $75. *Financial support:* In 2013–14, 25 teaching assistantships (averaging $15,120 per year) were awarded; research assistantships, institutionally sponsored loans, and tuition waivers (partial) also available. Support available to part-time students. Financial award application deadline: 6/30; financial award applicants required to submit FAFSA. *Faculty research:* Symptom science, family/community care, aging across the lifespan, self-management of health and illness, neuroscience. *Unit head:* Dr. Carol Savrin, Director, 216-368-5304, Fax: 216-368-3542, E-mail: cls18@case.edu. *Application contact:* Donna Hassik, Admissions Coordinator, 216-368-5253, Fax: 216-368-0124, E-mail: dmh7@case.edu.
Website: http://fpb.cwru.edu/MSN/majors.shtm

Cedarville University, Graduate Programs, Cedarville, OH 45314-0601. Offers business administration (MBA); curriculum (M Ed); educational administration (M Ed); family nurse practitioner (MSN); global health ministries (MSN); instruction (M Ed); pharmacy (Pharm D). Part-time programs available. Postbaccalaureate distance learning degree programs offered (no on-campus study). *Faculty:* 23 full-time (12 women), 12 part-time/adjunct (5 women). *Students:* 119 full-time (74 women), 103 part-time (73 women); includes 16 minority (11 Black or African American, non-Hispanic/Latino; 4 Asian, non-Hispanic/Latino; 1 Native Hawaiian or other Pacific Islander, non-Hispanic/Latino), 4 international. Average age 31. In 2013, 26 master's awarded. *Degree requirements:* For master's, thesis. *Entrance requirements:* For master's, GRE, 2 professional recommendations; for doctorate, PCAT, professional recommendation from a practicing pharmacist or current employer/supervisor, resume, essay, interview. Additional exam requirements/recommendations for international students: Required—TOEFL (minimum score 550 paper-based; 80 iBT). *Application deadline:* For fall admission, 5/1 priority date for domestic and international students; for spring admission, 11/1 priority date for domestic and international students. Applications are processed on a rolling basis. Application fee: $30. Electronic applications accepted. *Financial support:* Scholarships/grants and unspecified assistantships available. Support available to part-time students. Financial award applicants required to submit FAFSA. *Unit head:* Dr. Mark McClain, Dean of Graduate Studies, 937-766-7700, E-mail: mcclain@cedarville.edu. *Application contact:* Roscoe F. Smith, Associate Vice-President of Enrollment, 937-766-7700, Fax: 937-766-7575, E-mail: smithr@cedarville.edu.
Website: http://www.cedarville.edu/academics/graduate/

Clarion University of Pennsylvania, Office of Transfer, Adult and Graduate Admissions, Master of Science in Nursing Program, Clarion, PA 16214. Offers family nurse practitioner (MSN); nurse educator (MSN). Program offered jointly with Slippery Rock University of Pennsylvania. Part-time programs available. Postbaccalaureate distance learning degree programs offered (no on-campus study). *Faculty:* 4 full-time (all women). *Students:* 36 part-time (33 women); includes 2 minority (1 Asian, non-Hispanic/Latino; 1 Two or more races, non-Hispanic/Latino). Average age 39. 64 applicants, 41% accepted, 26 enrolled. In 2013, 21 master's awarded. *Degree requirements:* For master's, comprehensive exam, thesis. *Entrance requirements:* For master's, minimum QPA of 2.75. Additional exam requirements/recommendations for international students: Required—TOEFL (minimum score 550 paper-based; 80 iBT). *Application deadline:* For fall admission, 6/1 for domestic students, 4/15 priority date for international students; for spring admission, 11/1 for domestic students, 9/15 priority date for international students. Application fee: $40. Electronic applications accepted. *Expenses:* Tuition, state resident: part-time $442 per credit. Tuition, nonresident: part-time $451 per credit. *Required fees:* $142.40 per semester. One-time fee: $150 part-time. *Financial support:* In 2013–14, 1 research assistantship with full and partial tuition reimbursement (averaging $9,420 per year) was awarded; career-related internships or fieldwork and unspecified assistantships also available. Financial award application deadline: 3/1. *Unit head:* Dr. Debbie Ciesielka, Graduate Coordinator, 412-578-7277, E-mail: dciesielka@clarion.edu. *Application contact:* Michelle Ritzler, Graduate Programs, 814-393-2337, E-mail: gradstudies@clarion.edu.
Website: http://www.clarion.edu/991/

Clarion University of Pennsylvania, Office of Transfer, Adult and Graduate Admissions, Online Certificate Programs, Clarion, PA 16214. Offers family nurse practitioner (Post-Master's Certificate); library science (CAS); nurse educator (Post-Master's Certificate); public relations (Certificate). *Accreditation:* ALA (one or more programs are accredited at the [master's] level). Part-time programs available. Postbaccalaureate distance learning degree programs offered (no on-campus study). *Faculty:* 34 full-time (20 women). *Students:* 15 part-time (12 women); includes 1 minority (Black or African American, non-Hispanic/Latino). Average age 35. 16 applicants, 100% accepted, 7 enrolled. In 2013, 12 CASs awarded. *Entrance requirements:* Additional exam requirements/recommendations for international students: Required—TOEFL (minimum score 550 paper-based; 80 iBT), IELTS (minimum score 7). *Application deadline:* For fall admission, 8/1 priority date for domestic students, 4/15 priority date for international students; for spring admission, 12/1 priority date for domestic students, 9/15 priority date for international students. Applications are processed on a rolling basis. Application fee: $40. Electronic applications accepted. *Expenses:* Tuition, state

resident: part-time $442 per credit. Tuition, nonresident: part-time $451 per credit. *Required fees:* $142.40 per semester. One-time fee: $150 part-time. *Financial support:* Research assistantships available. Financial award application deadline: 3/1. *Unit head:* Dr. William Buchanan, Chair, Library Science, 814-393-2271, Fax: 814-393-2150. *Application contact:* Michelle Ritzler, Assistant Director, Graduate Programs, 814-393-2337, Fax: 814-393-2722, E-mail: gradstudies@clarion.edu.
Website: http://www.clarion.edu/991/

Clarke University, Department of Nursing and Health, Dubuque, IA 52001-3198. Offers administration of nursing systems (MSN); advanced practice nursing (MSN); education (MSN); family nurse practitioner (MSN, PMC); nursing (DNP). *Accreditation:* AACN. Part-time programs available. *Faculty:* 10 full-time (9 women). *Students:* 42 full-time (41 women), 16 part-time (15 women). In 2013, 13 master's awarded. *Entrance requirements:* For master's, GRE General Test or MAT, BSN, minimum GPA of 3.0. *Application deadline:* For fall admission, 2/15 priority date for domestic students; for spring admission, 12/15 priority date for domestic students. Applications are processed on a rolling basis. Application fee: $25. Electronic applications accepted. *Expenses: Tuition:* Part-time $660 per credit. *Required fees:* $15 per credit. *Financial support:* In 2013–14, 6 students received support. Career-related internships or fieldwork available. Support available to part-time students. Financial award applicants required to submit FAFSA. *Faculty research:* Narrative pedagogy, ethics, end-of-life care, pedagogy, family systems. *Unit head:* Dr. Jan Lee, Chair, 800-224-2736, Fax: 319-584-8684. *Application contact:* Kara Shroeder, Information Contact, 563-588-6635, Fax: 563-588-6789, E-mail: graduate@clarke.edu.
Website: http://www.clarke.edu/

Clarkson College, Master of Science in Nursing Program, Omaha, NE 68131. Offers adult nurse practitioner (MSN, Post-Master's Certificate); family nurse practitioner (MSN, Post-Master's Certificate); nursing education (MSN, Post-Master's Certificate); nursing health care leadership (MSN, Post-Master's Certificate). *Accreditation:* AANA/CANAEP. Part-time and evening/weekend programs available. Postbaccalaureate distance learning degree programs offered (minimal on-campus study). *Degree requirements:* For master's, on-campus skills assessment (family nurse practitioner, adult nurse practitioner), comprehensive exam or thesis. *Entrance requirements:* For master's, minimum GPA of 3.0, 2 references, resume. Additional exam requirements/recommendations for international students: Required—TOEFL (minimum score 600 paper-based; 100 iBT). Electronic applications accepted.

College of Mount Saint Vincent, School of Professional and Continuing Studies, Department of Nursing, Riverdale, NY 10471-1093. Offers adult nurse practitioner (MSN, PMC); family nurse practitioner (MSN, PMC); nurse educator (PMC); nursing administration (MSN); nursing for the adult and aged (MSN). *Accreditation:* AACN. Part-time programs available. *Entrance requirements:* For master's, BSN, interview, RN license, minimum GPA of 3.0, letters of reference. Additional exam requirements/recommendations for international students: Required—TOEFL. *Expenses:* Contact institution.

The College of New Rochelle, Graduate School, Program in Nursing, New Rochelle, NY 10805-2308. Offers acute care nurse practitioner (MS, Certificate); clinical specialist in holistic nursing (MS, Certificate); family nurse practitioner (MS, Certificate); nursing and health care management (MS); nursing education (Certificate). *Accreditation:* AACN. Part-time programs available. *Faculty:* 6 full-time (5 women), 5 part-time/adjunct (4 women). *Students:* 113 part-time (104 women); includes 56 minority (44 Black or African American, non-Hispanic/Latino; 3 Asian, non-Hispanic/Latino; 9 Hispanic/Latino). Average age 40. In 2013, 17 master's awarded. *Entrance requirements:* For master's, GRE General Test or MAT, BSN, malpractice insurance, minimum GPA of 3.0, RN license. *Application deadline:* For fall admission, 8/15 priority date for domestic students; for spring admission, 12/1 priority date for domestic students. Applications are processed on a rolling basis. Application fee: $35. Electronic applications accepted. *Expenses:* Contact institution. *Financial support:* Traineeships available. Support available to part-time students. Financial award application deadline: 8/15. *Unit head:* Dr. Mary McGuinness, Acting Dean, School of Nursing, 914-654-5441, E-mail: mmcguiness@cnr.edu.

Columbia University, School of Nursing, Program in Family Nurse Practitioner, New York, NY 10032. Offers MS, Adv C. *Accreditation:* AACN. Part-time programs available. *Entrance requirements:* For master's, GRE General Test, NCLEX, BSN, 1 year of clinical experience (preferred); for Adv C, MSN. Additional exam requirements/recommendations for international students: Required—TOEFL (minimum score 100 iBT). Electronic applications accepted.

Concordia University Wisconsin, Graduate Programs, School of Human Services, Program in Nursing, Mequon, WI 53097-2402. Offers family nurse practitioner (MSN); geriatric nurse practitioner (MSN); nurse educator (MSN). *Accreditation:* AACN. Postbaccalaureate distance learning degree programs offered (minimal on-campus study). *Degree requirements:* For master's, comprehensive exam, thesis or alternative. *Entrance requirements:* Additional exam requirements/recommendations for international students: Required—TOEFL. *Expenses:* Contact institution.

Coppin State University, Division of Graduate Studies, Helene Fuld School of Nursing, Baltimore, MD 21216-3698. Offers family nurse practitioner (PMC); nursing (MSN). Part-time and evening/weekend programs available. *Degree requirements:* For master's, comprehensive exam, thesis, clinical internship. *Entrance requirements:* For master's, GRE, bachelor's degree in nursing, interview, minimum GPA of 3.0, RN license. Additional exam requirements/recommendations for international students: Required—TOEFL (minimum score 550 paper-based).

Cox College, Programs in Nursing, Springfield, MO 65802. Offers clinical nurse leader (MSN); family nurse practitioner (MSN); nurse educator (MSN). *Accreditation:* AACN. *Entrance requirements:* For master's, RN license, essay, 2 letters of recommendation, official transcripts. Electronic applications accepted.

Delta State University, Graduate Programs, School of Nursing, Cleveland, MS 38733. Offers family nurse practitioner (MSN); nurse administrator (MSN); nurse educator (MSN). *Accreditation:* AACN. Part-time programs available. *Faculty:* 5 full-time (all women), 1 (woman) part-time/adjunct. *Students:* 35 full-time (31 women), 8 part-time (7 women); includes 10 minority (all Black or African American, non-Hispanic/Latino). Average age 41. 23 applicants, 100% accepted, 19 enrolled. In 2013, 13 master's awarded. *Degree requirements:* For master's, thesis optional. *Entrance requirements:* For master's, GRE General Test. *Application deadline:* For fall admission, 8/1 priority date for domestic students; for spring admission, 12/1 priority date for domestic students. Applications are processed on a rolling basis. Application fee: $0. Electronic applications accepted. *Expenses:* Tuition, state resident: full-time $3006; part-time $334 per credit hour. Tuition, nonresident: full-time $3006; part-time $334 per credit hour. *Financial support:* Research assistantships, career-related internships or fieldwork, Federal Work-Study, and institutionally sponsored loans available. Financial award application deadline: 6/1. *Unit head:* Dr. Lizabeth Carlson, Dean, 662-846-4268, Fax: 662-846-4267, E-mail: lcarlson@deltastate.edu. *Application contact:* Dr. Albert Nylander, Dean of Graduate Studies, 662-846-4875, Fax: 662-846-4313, E-mail: grad-info@deltastate.edu.
Website: http://www.deltastate.edu/pages/252.asp

DePaul University, College of Science and Health, Chicago, IL 60614. Offers applied mathematics (MS); applied statistics (MS); biological sciences (MA, MS); chemistry (MS); mathematics education (MA); mathematics for teaching (MS); nursing (MS); nursing practice (DNP); physics (MS); psychology (MS); pure mathematics (MS); science education (MS); MA/PhD. *Faculty:* 66 full-time (40 women), 23 part-time/adjunct (21 women). *Students:* 485 full-time (338 women), 207 part-time (132 women); includes 198 minority (55 Black or African American, non-Hispanic/Latino; 1 American Indian or Alaska Native, non-Hispanic/Latino; 64 Asian, non-Hispanic/Latino; 53 Hispanic/Latino; 2 Native Hawaiian or other Pacific Islander, non-Hispanic/Latino; 23 Two or more races, non-Hispanic/Latino), 48 international. Average age 29. In 2013, 244 master's, 20 doctorates awarded. *Application deadline:* Applications are processed on a rolling basis. Application fee: $40. Electronic applications accepted. Tuition and fees vary according to course level, course load and degree level. *Financial support:* Applicants required to submit FAFSA. *Application contact:* Ann Spittle, Director of Graduate Admission, 773-325-7315, Fax: 312-476-3244, E-mail: graddepaul@depaul.edu.
Website: http://csh.depaul.edu/

DeSales University, Graduate Division, Division of Healthcare and Natural Sciences, Center Valley, PA 18034-9568. Offers adult clinical nurse specialist (MSN); certified nurse midwives (MSN); certified nurse practitioners (MSN); clinical leadership (DNP); family nurse practitioner (MSN); information systems (MSIS); nurse educator (MSN); nurse practitioner (Post-Master's Certificate); physical therapy (DPT); physician assistant studies (MSPAS); MSN/MBA. Part-time programs available. In 2013, 5 doctorates awarded. *Degree requirements:* For master's, thesis optional. *Entrance requirements:* For master's, GRE General Test, MAT, minimum B average in undergraduate course work, health assessment course or equivalent, course work in statistics. Additional exam requirements/recommendations for international students: Required—TOEFL. *Application deadline:* Applications are processed on a rolling basis. Application fee: $35. Electronic applications accepted. *Expenses: Tuition:* Part-time $790 per credit. *Financial support:* Applicants required to submit FAFSA. *Unit head:* Dr. Mary Liz Doyle-Tadduni, Department Chair, Nursing, 610-282-1100 Ext. 1394, Fax: 610-282-2091, E-mail: carol.mest@desales.edu. *Application contact:* Abagail Wernicki, Director of Graduate Admissions, 610-282-1100 Ext. 1768, Fax: 610-282-2869, E-mail: abagail.wernicki@desales.edu.

Dominican College, Division of Nursing, Orangeburg, NY 10962-1210. Offers MSN. Part-time and evening/weekend programs available. *Faculty:* 1 (woman) full-time, 6 part-time/adjunct (4 women). *Students:* 48 full-time (30 women), 3 part-time (all women). In 2013, 13 master's awarded. *Degree requirements:* For master's, guided research project, 750 hours of clinical practice with a final written project. *Entrance requirements:* For master's, RN license with 1 year of experience; minimum undergraduate GPA of 3.0; 3 letters of recommendation. Additional exam requirements/recommendations for international students: Required—TOEFL (minimum score 550 paper-based). *Application deadline:* Applications are processed on a rolling basis. Application fee: $50. *Expenses: Tuition:* Part-time $815 per credit. *Required fees:* $180 per semester. *Financial support:* Applicants required to submit FAFSA. *Unit head:* Dr. Nancy DiDona, Director, 845-848-6051, Fax: 845-398-4891, E-mail: nancydidona@dc.edu. *Application contact:* Joyce Elbe, Director of Admissions, 845-848-7896 Ext. 15, Fax: 845-365-3150, E-mail: admissions@dc.edu.

Drexel University, College of Nursing and Health Professions, Division of Graduate Nursing, Philadelphia, PA 19104-2875. Offers adult acute care (MSN); adult psychiatric/mental health (MSN); advanced practice nursing (MSN); clinical trials research (MSN); family nurse practitioner (MSN); leadership in health systems management (MSN); nursing education (MSN); pediatric primary care (MSN); women's health (MSN). *Accreditation:* AACN. Electronic applications accepted.

Duke University, School of Nursing, Durham, NC 27708-0586. Offers acute care pediatric nurse practitioner (MSN); adult-gerontology nurse practitioner - acute care (MSN, Post Master's Certificate); adult-gerontology nurse practitioner - primary care (MSN, Post Master's Certificate), including adult-gerontology nurse practitioner (MSN), cardiology, oncology; family nurse practitioner (MSN); neonatal nurse practitioner (MSN); nurse anesthesia (MSN, DNP); nursing (PhD); nursing and health care leadership (MSN); nursing education (MSN); nursing informatics (MSN, Post Master's Certificate); pediatric nurse practitioner - primary care (MSN). *Accreditation:* AACN; AANA/CANAEP. Part-time and evening/weekend programs available. Postbaccalaureate distance learning degree programs offered (minimal on-campus study). *Faculty:* 74 full-time (64 women), 7 part-time/adjunct (4 women). *Students:* 127 full-time (113 women), 473 part-time (433 women); includes 131 minority (54 Black or African American, non-Hispanic/Latino; 9 American Indian or Alaska Native, non-Hispanic/Latino; 36 Asian, non-Hispanic/Latino; 27 Hispanic/Latino; 5 Native Hawaiian or other Pacific Islander, non-Hispanic/Latino), 14 international. Average age 34. 516 applicants, 50% accepted, 190 enrolled. In 2013, 179 master's, 49 doctorates, 23 other advanced degrees awarded. Terminal master's awarded for partial completion of doctoral program. *Degree requirements:* For master's, thesis optional; for doctorate, capstone project. *Entrance requirements:* For master's, GRE General Test (waived if undergraduate GPA of 3.4 or higher), 1 year of nursing experience (recommended), BSN, minimum GPA of 3.0, previous course work in statistics; for doctorate, GRE General Test (waived if undergraduate GPA of 3.4 or higher), BSN or MSN, minimum GPA of 3.0, portfolio, resume, personal statement, undergraduate statistics course, current licensure as a registered nurse, transcripts from all post-secondary institutions; for Post Master's Certificate, MSN, licensure or eligibility as a professional nurse, transcripts from all post-secondary institutions, previous course work in statistics. Additional exam requirements/recommendations for international students: Recommended—TOEFL (minimum score 550 paper-based; 83 iBT), IELTS (minimum score 7). *Application deadline:* For fall admission, 12/1 for domestic and international students; for spring admission, 5/1 for domestic and international students. Application fee: $50. Electronic applications accepted. *Expenses:* Contact institution. *Financial support:* Career-related internships or fieldwork, institutionally sponsored loans, scholarships/grants, traineeships, and tuition waivers (partial) available. Support available to part-time students. Financial award applicants required to submit FAFSA. *Faculty research:* Cardiovascular disease, caregiver skill training, data mining, prostate cancer, neonatal immune system. *Unit head:* Dr. Catherine L. Gilliss, Dean/Vice Chancellor for Nursing Affairs, 919-684-9444, Fax: 919-684-9414, E-mail: catherine.gilliss@duke.edu. *Application contact:* Ernie Rushing, Lead Admissions Processor/Admissions Officer, 919-668-6274, Fax: 919-668-4693, E-mail: stephen.rushing@dm.duke.edu.
Website: http://www.nursing.duke.edu/

Duquesne University, School of Nursing, Master of Science in Nursing Program, Pittsburgh, PA 15282-0001. Offers family (individual across the life span) nurse practitioner (MSN); forensic nursing (MSN); nursing education (MSN). *Accreditation:* AACN. Part-time and evening/weekend programs available. Postbaccalaureate distance learning degree programs offered (minimal on-campus study). *Faculty:* 20 full-time (18 women), 4 part-time/adjunct (all women). *Students:* 73 full-time (67 women), 54 part-time (53 women); includes 23 minority (8 Black or African American, non-Hispanic/Latino; 1 American Indian or Alaska Native, non-Hispanic/Latino; 4 Asian, non-Hispanic/Latino; 5 Hispanic/Latino; 5 Two or more races, non-Hispanic/Latino), 1 international.

Average age 35. 206 applicants, 35% accepted, 55 enrolled. In 2013, 28 master's awarded. *Degree requirements:* For master's, culminating paper. *Entrance requirements:* For master's, current RN license; BSN with minimum GPA of 3.0; minimum of 1 year full-time work experience as RN prior to registration in clinical or specialty course. Additional exam requirements/recommendations for international students: Required—TOEFL (minimum score 600 paper-based; 80 iBT). *Application deadline:* For fall admission, 3/1 for domestic and international students. Application fee: $0. Electronic applications accepted. *Expenses: Tuition:* Full-time $18,162; part-time $1009 per credit. *Required fees:* $1728; $96 per credit. Tuition and fees vary according to program. *Financial support:* In 2013–14, 5 students received support, including 3 teaching assistantships with partial tuition reimbursements available (averaging $1,285 per year); research assistantships with partial tuition reimbursements available, scholarships/grants, traineeships, and tuition waivers (partial) also available. Support available to part-time students. Financial award application deadline: 7/1; financial award applicants required to submit FAFSA. *Faculty research:* Vulnerable populations, social justice, cultural competence, health disparities, wellness within chronic illness. *Unit head:* Dr. Joan Such Lockhart, Professor and Associate Dean of Academic Affairs, 412-396-6540, Fax: 412-396-1821, E-mail: lockhart@duq.edu. *Application contact:* Susan Hardner, Nurse Recruiter, 412-396-4945, Fax: 412-396-6346, E-mail: nursing@duq.edu.
Website: http://www.duq.edu/academics/schools/nursing/graduate-programs/master-science-nursing

Duquesne University, School of Nursing, Post Master's Certificate Program, Pittsburgh, PA 15282-0001. Offers family (individual across the life span) nurse practitioner (Post-Master's Certificate); forensic nursing (Post-Master's Certificate). Part-time and evening/weekend programs available. Postbaccalaureate distance learning degree programs offered (minimal on-campus study). *Faculty:* 10 full-time (9 women), 4 part-time/adjunct (all women). *Students:* 11 part-time (all women); includes 2 minority (1 Black or African American, non-Hispanic/Latino; 1 Hispanic/Latino). Average age 41. 19 applicants, 26% accepted, 4 enrolled. In 2013, 1 Post-Master's Certificate awarded. *Entrance requirements:* For degree, current RN license, BSN, MSN. Additional exam requirements/recommendations for international students: Required—TOEFL (minimum score 600 paper-based; 80 iBT). *Application deadline:* For fall admission, 3/1 for domestic and international students. Application fee: $0. *Expenses: Tuition:* Full-time $18,162; part-time $1009 per credit. *Required fees:* $1728; $96 per credit. Tuition and fees vary according to program. *Financial support:* Teaching assistantships with partial tuition reimbursements, scholarships/grants, traineeships, and tuition waivers (partial) available. Support available to part-time students. Financial award application deadline: 7/1; financial award applicants required to submit FAFSA. *Faculty research:* Vulnerable populations, social justice, cultural competence, health disparities, wellness within chronic illness. *Unit head:* Dr. Joan Such Lockhart, Professor and Associate Dean of Academic Affairs, 412-396-6540, Fax: 412-396-1821, E-mail: lockhart@duq.edu. *Application contact:* Susan Hardner, Nurse Recruiter, 412-396-4945, Fax: 412-396-6346, E-mail: nursing@duq.edu.
Website: http://www.duq.edu/academics/schools/nursing/graduate-programs/post-masters-certificates

D'Youville College, School of Nursing, Buffalo, NY 14201-1084. Offers advanced practice nursing (DNP); community health nursing/education (MSN); community health nursing/management (MSN); family nurse practitioner (MSN, Certificate); nursing and health-related professions education (Certificate). *Accreditation:* AACN. Part-time programs available. *Students:* 51 full-time (45 women), 136 part-time (115 women); includes 25 minority (17 Black or African American, non-Hispanic/Latino; 1 American Indian or Alaska Native, non-Hispanic/Latino; 1 Asian, non-Hispanic/Latino; 6 Hispanic/Latino), 76 international. Average age 35. 261 applicants, 36% accepted, 73 enrolled. In 2013, 51 master's, 3 other advanced degrees awarded. *Degree requirements:* For master's, thesis or alternative, membership on board of community agency, publishable paper. *Entrance requirements:* For master's, BS in nursing, minimum GPA of 3.0, course work in statistics and computers. Additional exam requirements/recommendations for international students: Required—TOEFL (minimum score 500 paper-based). *Application deadline:* For fall admission, 5/1 priority date for international students; for spring admission, 9/1 priority date for international students. Applications are processed on a rolling basis. Application fee: $25. Electronic applications accepted. *Financial support:* Federal Work-Study, scholarships/grants, traineeships, and unspecified assistantships available. Support available to part-time students. Financial award application deadline: 3/1; financial award applicants required to submit FAFSA. *Faculty research:* Nursing curriculum, nursing theory-testing, wellness research, communication and socialization patterns. *Unit head:* Dr. Ann Caughill, Chair, 716-829-7892, Fax: 716-829-8159. *Application contact:* Mark Pavone, Graduate Admissions Director, 716-829-8400, Fax: 716-829-7900, E-mail: graduateadmissions@dyc.edu.
Website: http://www.dyc.edu/academics/nursing/

See Display on page 632 and Close-Up on page 815.

Eastern Kentucky University, The Graduate School, College of Health Sciences, Department of Nursing, Richmond, KY 40475-3102. Offers rural community health care (MSN); rural health family nurse practitioner (MSN). *Accreditation:* AACN. *Entrance requirements:* For master's, GRE General Test, minimum GPA of 2.75.

Edinboro University of Pennsylvania, Department of Nursing, Edinboro, PA 16444. Offers advanced practice nursing (DNP); family nurse practitioner (MSN); nurse educator (MSN). Part-time and evening/weekend programs available. *Degree requirements:* For master's, thesis, competency exam. *Entrance requirements:* For master's, GRE or MAT, minimum QPA of 2.5. *Application deadline:* Applications are processed on a rolling basis. Application fee: $30. Electronic applications accepted. *Expenses:* Tuition, state resident: part-time $454 per credit hour. Tuition, nonresident: part-time $681 per credit hour. *Required fees:* $143.55 per credit hour. Part-time tuition and fees vary according to campus/location and program. *Financial support:* Research assistantships with full and partial tuition reimbursements, career-related internships or fieldwork, Federal Work-Study, scholarships/grants, and unspecified assistantships available. Support available to part-time students. Financial award application deadline: 2/15; financial award applicants required to submit FAFSA. *Unit head:* Dr. Thomas White, Chairperson, 814-732-2900, E-mail: twhite@edinboro.edu. *Application contact:* Dr. Thomas White, Chairperson, 814-732-2900, E-mail: twhite@edinboro.edu.
Website: http://www.edinboro.edu/departments/nursing/nursing.dot

Emory University, Nell Hodgson Woodruff School of Nursing, Atlanta, GA 30322-1100. Offers adult nurse practitioner (MSN); emergency nurse practitioner (MSN); family nurse practitioner (MSN); family nurse-midwife (MSN); health systems leadership (MSN); nurse-midwifery (MSN); pediatric nurse practitioner acute and primary care (MSN); women's health care (Title X) (MSN); women's health nurse practitioner (MSN); MSN/MPH. *Accreditation:* AACN; ACNM/ACME (one or more programs are accredited). Part-time programs available. *Entrance requirements:* For master's, GRE General Test or MAT, minimum GPA of 3.0, BS in nursing from an accredited institution, RN license and additional course work, 3 letters of recommendation. Additional exam requirements/recommendations for international students: Required—TOEFL (minimum score 600 paper-based; 100 iBT). Electronic applications accepted. *Expenses:* Contact institution. *Faculty research:* Older adult falls and injuries, minority health issues, cardiac symptoms and quality of life, bio-ethics and decision-making, menopausal issues.

Fairfield University, School of Nursing, Fairfield, CT 06824-5195. Offers advanced practice (DNP); executive (DNP); family nurse practitioner (MSN, DNP); nurse anesthesia (DNP); nursing leadership (MSN); psychiatric nurse practitioner (MSN, DNP). *Accreditation:* AACN; AANA/CANAEP. Part-time programs available. *Faculty:* 22 full-time (all women), 28 part-time/adjunct (23 women). *Students:* 27 full-time (23 women), 157 part-time (136 women); includes 37 minority (15 Black or African American, non-Hispanic/Latino; 10 Asian, non-Hispanic/Latino; 8 Hispanic/Latino; 2 Native Hawaiian or other Pacific Islander, non-Hispanic/Latino; 2 Two or more races, non-Hispanic/Latino), 8 international. Average age 37. 132 applicants, 52% accepted, 59 enrolled. In 2013, 39 master's, 3 doctorates awarded. *Degree requirements:* For master's, capstone project. *Entrance requirements:* For master's, minimum QPA of 3.0, RN license, resume, 2 recommendations; for doctorate, GRE (nurse anesthesia applicants only), MSN (minimum QPA of 3.2) or BSN (minimum QPA of 3.0); critical care nursing experience (for nurse anesthesia DNP candidates). Additional exam requirements/recommendations for international students: Required—TOEFL (minimum score 550 paper-based; 80 iBT) or IELTS (minimum score 6.5). *Application deadline:* For fall admission, 5/15 for international students; for spring admission, 10/15 for international students. Applications are processed on a rolling basis. Application fee: $60. Electronic applications accepted. *Expenses:* Contact institution. *Financial support:* In 2013–14, 4 students received support. Unspecified assistantships available. Financial award applicants required to submit FAFSA. *Faculty research:* Aging and sexual health, psychosocial needs of men with prostate cancer, nurse practitioner education, mentoring, psychiatric and mental health, incarceration of the mentally ill, recovery in schizophrenia, palliative and end of life care, maternal and child health, breastfeeding and lactation consultant, stress and emotional eating, care of veterans and their families, falls prevention and the elderly, health care leadership, interprofessional education, academic partnerships. *Total annual research expenditures:* $775,000. *Unit head:* Dr. Lynn Babington, Dean, 203-254-4000 Ext. 2701, Fax: 203-254-4126, E-mail: lbabington@fairfield.edu. *Application contact:* Marianne Gumpper, Director of Graduate and Continuing Studies Admission, 203-254-4184, Fax: 203-254-4073, E-mail: gradadmis@fairfield.edu.
Website: http://fairfield.edu/son

Felician College, Program in Nursing, Lodi, NJ 07644-2117. Offers adult-gerontology nurse practitioner (MSN, PMC); executive leadership (MSN, PMC); family nurse practitioner (MSN, PMC); nursing education (MSN, PMC). *Accreditation:* AACN. Part-time and evening/weekend programs available. Postbaccalaureate distance learning degree programs offered (no on-campus study). *Students:* 5 full-time (4 women), 85 part-time (78 women); includes 50 minority (20 Black or African American, non-Hispanic/Latino; 14 Asian, non-Hispanic/Latino; 16 Hispanic/Latino). Average age 42. *Degree requirements:* For master's, scholarly project. *Entrance requirements:* For master's, BS in nursing or equivalent, minimum GPA of 3.0, 2 letters of recommendation, RN license; for PMC, RN license, minimum GPA of 2.75. Additional exam requirements/recommendations for international students: Recommended—TOEFL (minimum score 550 paper-based). *Application deadline:* Applications are processed on a rolling basis. Application fee: $40. *Expenses: Tuition:* Part-time $945 per credit. *Required fees:* $317.50 per semester. *Financial support:* In 2013–14, 10 students received support. Traineeships available. Financial award applicants required to submit FAFSA. *Faculty research:* Anxiety and fear, curriculum innovation, health promotion. *Unit head:* Dr. Muriel Shore, Dean, Division of Health Sciences, 201-559-6030, E-mail: shorem@felician.edu. *Application contact:* Elizabeth Barca, Senior Assistant Director, Graduate Admissions, 201-559-6077, Fax: 201-559-6138, E-mail: graduate@felician.edu.

Florida Atlantic University, Christine E. Lynn College of Nursing, Boca Raton, FL 33431-0991. Offers administrative and financial leadership in nursing and health care (Post Master's Certificate); adult/gerontological nurse practitioner (Post Master's Certificate); advanced holistic nursing (MS, Post Master's Certificate); clinical nurse leader (MS, Post Master's Certificate); family nurse practitioner (MS, Post Master's Certificate); nurse educator (MS, Post Master's Certificate); nursing (PhD); nursing administration and financial leadership (MS); nursing practice (DNP). *Accreditation:* AACN. Part-time programs available. *Faculty:* 30 full-time (27 women), 9 part-time/adjunct (8 women). *Students:* 29 full-time (27 women), 523 part-time (492 women); includes 254 minority (157 Black or African American, non-Hispanic/Latino; 2 American Indian or Alaska Native, non-Hispanic/Latino; 19 Asian, non-Hispanic/Latino; 62 Hispanic/Latino; 2 Native Hawaiian or other Pacific Islander, non-Hispanic/Latino; 12 Two or more races, non-Hispanic/Latino), 3 international. Average age 39. 463 applicants, 25% accepted, 111 enrolled. In 2013, 148 master's, 15 doctorates awarded. *Degree requirements:* For master's, thesis or alternative; for doctorate, comprehensive exam, thesis/dissertation. *Entrance requirements:* For master's, GRE General Test or MAT, bachelor's degree in nursing, Florida RN license, minimum GPA of 3.0, resume/curriculum vitae, letter of recommendation; for doctorate, GRE General Test or MAT, curriculum vitae, Florida RN license, minimum GPA of 3.5, master's degree in nursing, three letters of recommendation. *Application deadline:* For fall admission, 6/1 for domestic students, 2/15 for international students; for spring admission, 10/1 for domestic students, 7/15 for international students. Applications are processed on a rolling basis. Application fee: $30. *Expenses:* Tuition, state resident: full-time $6660; part-time $370 per credit hour. Tuition, nonresident: full-time $18,450; part-time $1025 per credit hour. Tuition and fees vary according to course load. *Financial support:* Research assistantships with partial tuition reimbursements, teaching assistantships with partial tuition reimbursements, career-related internships or fieldwork, Federal Work-Study, institutionally sponsored loans, scholarships/grants, and traineeships available. Support available to part-time students. *Faculty research:* Econometrics of nurse-patient relationship, Alzheimer's disease, community-based programs, falls, self-healing. *Unit head:* Dr. Marlaine Smith, Dean, 561-297-3206, Fax: 561-297-3687, E-mail: msmit230@fau.edu. *Application contact:* Carol Kruse, Graduate Coordinator, 561-297-3261, Fax: 561-297-0088, E-mail: ckruse@fau.edu.
Website: http://nursing.fau.edu/

Florida State University, The Graduate School, College of Nursing, Tallahassee, FL 32312. Offers family nurse practitioner (DNP); health systems leadership (DNP); nurse educator (MSN, Certificate); nurse leader (MSN); nursing leadership (Certificate, Post-Graduate Certificate). *Accreditation:* AACN. Part-time programs available. Postbaccalaureate distance learning degree programs offered (minimal on-campus study). *Faculty:* 13 full-time (12 women). *Students:* 53 full-time (49 women), 26 part-time (all women); includes 16 minority (4 Black or African American, non-Hispanic/Latino; 1 Asian, non-Hispanic/Latino; 9 Hispanic/Latino; 2 Two or more races, non-Hispanic/Latino). Average age 38. 56 applicants, 61% accepted, 25 enrolled. In 2013, 5 master's, 18 doctorates awarded. *Degree requirements:* For master's, thesis optional. *Entrance requirements:* For master's, GRE General Test, MAT, minimum GPA of 3.0, BSN, Florida RN license; for doctorate, GRE General Test, MAT, minimum GPA of 3.0, BSN or MSN, Florida RN license. Additional exam requirements/recommendations for international students: Required—TOEFL (minimum score 550 paper-based). *Application deadline:* For fall admission, 7/1 for domestic and international students. Application fee: $30. Electronic applications accepted. *Expenses:* Tuition, state resident: part-time $403.51 per credit hour. Tuition, nonresident: part-time $1004.85 per

credit hour. *Required fees:* $75.81 per credit hour. One-time fee: $20 part-time. Tuition and fees vary according to course load, campus/location and student level. *Financial support:* In 2013–14, 75 students received support, including fellowships with partial tuition reimbursements available (averaging $6,300 per year), research assistantships with partial tuition reimbursements available (averaging $3,000 per year), 3 teaching assistantships with partial tuition reimbursements available (averaging $3,000 per year); career-related internships or fieldwork, Federal Work-Study, institutionally sponsored loans, scholarships/grants, traineeships, and tuition waivers (partial) also available. Financial award application deadline: 4/15; financial award applicants required to submit FAFSA. *Faculty research:* Distance learning, gerontology, health promotion, educational strategies, rehabilitation of brain injured patients. *Unit head:* Dr. Judith McFetridge-Durdle, Dean, 850-644-6846, Fax: 850-644-7660, E-mail: jdurdle@nursing.fsu.edu. *Application contact:* Carlos G. Urrutia, Director of Student Services, 850-644-5638, Fax: 850-645-7249, E-mail: currutia@fsu.edu.
Website: http://nursing.fsu.edu/

Francis Marion University, Graduate Programs, Department of Nursing, Florence, SC 29502-0547. Offers family nurse practitioner (MSN); nurse educator (MSN). Part-time programs available. *Faculty:* 8 full-time (all women). *Students:* 40 full-time (37 women), 7 part-time (4 women); includes 14 minority (12 Black or African American, non-Hispanic/Latino; 1 Asian, non-Hispanic/Latino; 1 Two or more races, non-Hispanic/Latino). Average age 34. 20 applicants, 80% accepted, 16 enrolled. *Entrance requirements:* For master's, GRE, official transcripts, two letters of recommendation, written statement, current SC nursing license. *Application deadline:* For fall admission, 3/15 for domestic students; for spring admission, 10/15 for domestic students. Applications are processed on a rolling basis. Application fee: $33. Electronic applications accepted. *Expenses:* Tuition, state resident: full-time $9184; part-time $459.20 per credit hour. Tuition, nonresident: full-time $18,368; part-time $918.40 per credit hour. *Required fees:* $13.50 per credit hour. $92 per semester. Tuition and fees vary according to program. *Financial support:* Available to part-time students. Application deadline: 3/1; applicants required to submit FAFSA. *Unit head:* Dr. Ruth Wittmann-Price, Chair, 843-661-4625, E-mail: rwittmannprice@fmarion.edu. *Application contact:* Rannie Gamble, Administrative Manager, 843-661-1286, Fax: 843-661-4688, E-mail: rgamble@fmarion.edu.

Frontier Nursing University, Graduate Programs, Hyden, KY 41749. Offers family nurse practitioner (MSN, DNP, Post Master's Certificate); nurse-midwifery (MSN, DNP, Post Master's Certificate); women's health care nurse practitioner (MSN, DNP, Post Master's Certificate). *Accreditation:* ACNM. *Degree requirements:* For doctorate, capstone project, practicum.

Gannon University, School of Graduate Studies, Morosky College of Health Professions and Sciences, Villa Maria School of Nursing, Program in Family Nurse Practitioner, Erie, PA 16541-0001. Offers MSN, Certificate. Part-time and evening/weekend programs available. *Students:* 1 (woman) part-time. Average age 47. 2 applicants, 100% accepted, 1 enrolled. *Degree requirements:* For master's, thesis (for some programs), practicum. *Entrance requirements:* For degree, GRE, interview. Additional exam requirements/recommendations for international students: Required—TOEFL (minimum score 79 iBT). *Application deadline:* Applications are processed on a rolling basis. Application fee: $25. Electronic applications accepted. *Expenses: Tuition:* Full-time $15,930; part-time $885 per credit. *Required fees:* $430; $18 per credit. Tuition and fees vary according to course load, degree level and program. *Unit head:* Dr. Kathleen Patterson, Director, 814-871-5547, E-mail: patterso018@gannon.edu. *Application contact:* Kara Morgan, Director of Graduate Admissions, 814-871-5831, Fax: 814-871-5827, E-mail: graduate@gannon.edu.

Georgetown University, Graduate School of Arts and Sciences, School of Nursing and Health Studies, Washington, DC 20057. Offers acute care nurse practitioner (MS); clinical nurse specialist (MS); family nurse practitioner (MS); nurse anesthesia (MS); nurse-midwifery (MS); nursing (DNP); nursing education (MS). *Accreditation:* AACN; AANA/CANAEP (one or more programs are accredited); ACNM/ACME (one or more programs are accredited). *Degree requirements:* For master's, thesis optional. *Entrance requirements:* For master's, GRE General Test or MAT, bachelor's degree in nursing from NLN-accredited school, minimum undergraduate GPA of 3.0. Additional exam requirements/recommendations for international students: Required—TOEFL. Application fee: $50 ($55 for international students). *Financial support:* Scholarships/grants and traineeships available. Financial award applicants required to submit FAFSA. *Unit head:* Dr. Patricia Ann Cloonan, Dean, 202-687-7318. *Application contact:* Graduate School Admissions Office, 202-687-5568.

The George Washington University, School of Nursing, Washington, DC 20052. Offers adult nurse practitioner (MSN, Post-Master's Certificate); clinical research administration (MSN); family nurse practitioner (MSN, Post-Master's Certificate); health care quality (MSN, Post-Master's Certificate); nursing (DNP); nursing leadership and management (MSN); palliative care nurse practitioner (Post-Master's Certificate). *Accreditation:* AACN. *Faculty:* 37 full-time (all women). *Students:* 36 full-time (33 women), 438 part-time (405 women); includes 114 minority (59 Black or African American, non-Hispanic/Latino; 7 American Indian or Alaska Native, non-Hispanic/Latino; 32 Asian, non-Hispanic/Latino; 15 Hispanic/Latino; 1 Two or more races, non-Hispanic/Latino), 8 international. Average age 38. 360 applicants, 83% accepted, 178 enrolled. In 2013, 79 master's, 26 doctorates awarded. *Unit head:* Jean E. Johnson, Dean, 202-994-3725, E-mail: sonjej@gwumc.edu. *Application contact:* Kristin Williams, Assistant Vice President for Graduate and Special Enrollment Management, 202-994-0467, Fax: 202-994-0371, E-mail: ksw@gwu.edu.
Website: http://nursing.gwumc.edu/

Georgia College & State University, Graduate School, College of Health Sciences, Graduate Nursing Program, Milledgeville, GA 31061. Offers family nurse practitioner (MSN); nursing practice (DNP). Part-time and evening/weekend programs available. *Students:* 87 part-time (80 women); includes 17 minority (all Black or African American, non-Hispanic/Latino). Average age 35. In 2013, 19 master's awarded. *Degree requirements:* For master's, comprehensive exam, thesis optional; for doctorate, capstone project, complete all required courses within a period of 7 years. *Entrance requirements:* For master's, GRE (taken within last 5 years), bachelor's degree in nursing, RN license, 1 year of clinical experience, minimum GPA of 2.75, statistics course; for doctorate, master's degree in nursing or anesthesia, minimum graduate GPA of 3.2, unencumbered RN licensure, 500 faculty-supervised clinical hours in master's program. Additional exam requirements/recommendations for international students: Recommended—TOEFL (minimum score 550 paper-based; 79 iBT). *Application deadline:* For fall admission, 7/1 priority date for domestic students; for spring admission, 4/1 priority date for domestic students. Applications are processed on a rolling basis. Application fee: $40. Electronic applications accepted. *Financial support:* In 2013–14, 2 research assistantships were awarded; unspecified assistantships also available. Financial award applicants required to submit FAFSA. *Unit head:* Dr. Deborah MacMillan, Assistant Director, Graduate Program, 478-751-1074, Fax: 478-757-1077, E-mail: debby.macmillan@gcsu.edu.

Georgia Regents University, The Graduate School, Family Nurse Practitioner Program, Augusta, GA 30912. Offers MSN, Post-Master's Certificate. *Students:* 19 full-time (17 women), 38 part-time (34 women); includes 15 minority (10 Black or African American, non-Hispanic/Latino; 1 Asian, non-Hispanic/Latino; 3 Hispanic/Latino; 1 Two or more races, non-Hispanic/Latino). Average age 32. 29 applicants, 52% accepted, 13 enrolled. In 2013, 16 master's awarded. *Entrance requirements:* For master's, GRE General Test or MAT, Georgia registered professional nurse license. Additional exam requirements/recommendations for international students: Required—TOEFL (minimum score 550 paper-based; 79 iBT). *Application deadline:* For fall admission, 2/1 for domestic and international students; for spring admission, 10/1 for domestic and international students. Application fee: $50. Electronic applications accepted. *Unit head:* Dr. Lucy Marion, Dean, 706-721-3771, Fax: 706-721-8169, E-mail: lumarion@georgiahealth.edu. *Application contact:* Karen Sturgill, Program Coordinator, 706-721-3676, Fax: 706-721-8169, E-mail: ksturgillt@georgiahealth.edu.
Website: http://www.gru.edu/nursing/programs.php

Georgia Southern University, Jack N. Averitt College of Graduate Studies, College of Health and Human Sciences, School of Nursing, Program in Nurse Practitioner, Statesboro, GA 30460. Offers MSN. Part-time programs available. Postbaccalaureate distance learning degree programs offered. *Students:* 22 full-time (21 women), 42 part-time (39 women); includes 10 minority (5 Black or African American, non-Hispanic/Latino; 1 American Indian or Alaska Native, non-Hispanic/Latino; 1 Asian, non-Hispanic/Latino; 1 Hispanic/Latino; 2 Two or more races, non-Hispanic/Latino). Average age 32. 55 applicants, 56% accepted, 21 enrolled. In 2013, 14 master's awarded. *Entrance requirements:* For master's, GRE General Test or MAT, minimum GPA of 3.0, Georgia nursing license, 2 years of clinical experience, CPR certification. Additional exam requirements/recommendations for international students: Required—TOEFL (minimum score 550 paper-based; 80 iBT), IELTS (minimum score 6). *Application deadline:* For fall admission, 3/1 priority date for domestic and international students; for spring admission, 10/1 priority date for domestic students, 10/1 for international students. Applications are processed on a rolling basis. Application fee: $50. Electronic applications accepted. *Expenses:* Tuition, state resident: full-time $7068; part-time $270 per semester hour. Tuition, nonresident: full-time $26,446; part-time $1077 per semester hour. *Required fees:* $2092. *Financial support:* In 2013–14, 20 students received support, including research assistantships with partial tuition reimbursements available (averaging $7,200 per year), teaching assistantships with partial tuition reimbursements available (averaging $7,200 per year); career-related internships or fieldwork, Federal Work-Study, scholarships/grants, traineeships, tuition waivers (partial), and unspecified assistantships also available. Support available to part-time students. Financial award application deadline: 4/15. *Faculty research:* Vulnerable populations, breast cancer, diabetes, mellitus, advanced practice nursing issues. *Unit head:* Dr. Deborah Allen, Graduate Program Director, 912-478-5056, Fax: 912-478-5036, E-mail: debbieallen@georgiasouthern.edu. *Application contact:* Amanda Gilliland, Coordinator for Graduate Student Recruitment, 912-478-5384, Fax: 912-478-0740, E-mail: gradadmissions@georgiasouthern.edu.

Georgia State University, Byrdine F. Lewis School of Nursing, Atlanta, GA 30303. Offers adult health clinical nurse specialist/nurse practitioner (MS, Certificate); child health clinical nurse specialist/pediatric nurse practitioner (MS, Certificate); family nurse practitioner (MS, Certificate); family psychiatric mental health nurse practitioner (MS, Certificate); nursing (PhD); nursing leadership in healthcare innovations (MS), including nursing administration, nursing informatics; nutrition (MS); perinatal clinical nurse specialist/women's health nurse practitioner (MS, Certificate); physical therapy (DPT); respiratory therapy (MS). *Accreditation:* AACN. Part-time programs available. Postbaccalaureate distance learning degree programs offered (minimal on-campus study). *Faculty:* 22 full-time (16 women). *Students:* 241 full-time (180 women), 262 part-time (236 women); includes 176 minority (120 Black or African American, non-Hispanic/Latino; 31 Asian, non-Hispanic/Latino; 13 Hispanic/Latino; 3 Native Hawaiian or other Pacific Islander, non-Hispanic/Latino; 9 Two or more races, non-Hispanic/Latino), 19 international. Average age 34. 583 applicants, 34% accepted, 160 enrolled. In 2013, 110 master's, 44 doctorates, 6 other advanced degrees awarded. *Degree requirements:* For doctorate, comprehensive exam, thesis/dissertation. *Entrance requirements:* For doctorate, GRE. Additional exam requirements/recommendations for international students: Required—TOEFL. *Application deadline:* For fall admission, 2/1 priority date for domestic and international students; for spring admission, 9/15 for domestic and international students. Applications are processed on a rolling basis. Application fee: $50. Electronic applications accepted. *Expenses:* Contact institution. *Financial support:* In 2013–14, research assistantships with full and partial tuition reimbursements (averaging $1,666 per year), teaching assistantships with full and partial tuition reimbursements (averaging $1,920 per year) were awarded; scholarships/grants, tuition waivers (full and partial), and unspecified assistantships also available. Support available to part-time students. Financial award application deadline: 8/1; financial award applicants required to submit FAFSA. *Faculty research:* Stroke intervention for caregivers, stroke prevention in African Americans; relationships between psychological distress and health outcomes in parents with a medically ill infant; medically fragile children; nursing expertise and patient outcomes. *Unit head:* Joan S. Cranford, Assistant Dean for Nursing, 404-413-1200, Fax: 404-413-1205, E-mail: jcranford2@gsu.edu. *Application contact:* Tiffany Norman, Senior Administrative Coordinator, 404-413-1190, Fax: 404-413-1205, E-mail: tnorman7@gsu.edu.
Website: http://nursing.gsu.edu/

Goshen College, Program in Nursing, Goshen, IN 46526-4794. Offers family nurse practitioner (MSN). *Accreditation:* AACN. Part-time and evening/weekend programs available. *Faculty:* 6 full-time (all women), 2 part-time/adjunct (both women). *Students:* 43 part-time (40 women), 3 international. *Degree requirements:* For master's, comprehensive exam (for some programs). *Entrance requirements:* For master's, minimum GPA of 3.0, curriculum vitae, bachelor's degree in nursing, active RN license, three professional recommendations, essay, one year of clinical nursing experience, statistics course, interview. Additional exam requirements/recommendations for international students: Required—TOEFL (minimum score 600 paper-based; 100 iBT). *Application deadline:* For fall admission, 3/14 for domestic students. Applications are processed on a rolling basis. Application fee: $50. Electronic applications accepted. *Expenses:* Contact institution. *Financial support:* Scholarships/grants available. Financial award applicants required to submit FAFSA. *Unit head:* Dr. Ruth Stoltzfus, RN, Director, 574-535-7973, E-mail: ruthas@goshen.edu. *Application contact:* Nina Mishler, Associate Director of Admissions, 574-535-7527, Fax: 574-535-7609, E-mail: ninajm@goshen.edu.
Website: http://www.goshen.edu/nursing/masters

Graceland University, School of Nursing, Independence, MO 64050-3434. Offers family nurse practitioner (MSN, PMC); nurse educator (MSN, PMC); organizational leadership (DNP). Part-time programs available. Postbaccalaureate distance learning degree programs offered (minimal on-campus study). *Faculty:* 13 full-time (all women), 9 part-time/adjunct (7 women). *Students:* 215 full-time (197 women), 339 part-time (303 women); includes 95 minority (37 Black or African American, non-Hispanic/Latino; 11 American Indian or Alaska Native, non-Hispanic/Latino; 15 Asian, non-Hispanic/Latino; 18 Hispanic/Latino; 2 Native Hawaiian or other Pacific Islander, non-Hispanic/Latino; 12 Two or more races, non-Hispanic/Latino), 4 international. Average age 44. 84 applicants, 89% accepted, 63 enrolled. In 2013, 71 master's awarded. *Degree requirements:* For master's, comprehensive exam (for some programs), thesis optional, scholarly project; for doctorate, capstone project. *Entrance requirements:* For master's,

BSN from nationally-accredited program, RN license, minimum GPA of 3.0; satisfactory criminal background check; for doctorate, MSN from nationally-accredited program, RN license, minimum GPA of 3.2; satisfactory criminal background check. Additional exam requirements/recommendations for international students: Recommended—TOEFL. *Application deadline:* For fall admission, 6/1 priority date for domestic students; for winter admission, 10/1 priority date for domestic students; for spring admission, 3/1 priority date for domestic students. Application fee: $50. Electronic applications accepted. *Expenses:* Contact institution. *Financial support:* Institutionally sponsored loans available. Support available to part-time students. Financial award applicants required to submit FAFSA. *Faculty research:* International nursing, family care-giving, health promotion. *Unit head:* Dr. Claudia D. Horton, Dean, 816-423-4670, Fax: 816-423-4753, E-mail: horton@graceland.edu. *Application contact:* Nick Walker, Program Consultant, 816-423-4717, Fax: 816-833-2990, E-mail: nowalker@graceland.edu.
Website: http://www.graceland.edu/nursing

Grambling State University, School of Graduate Studies and Research, College of Professional Studies, School of Nursing, Grambling, LA 71245. Offers family nurse practitioner (PMC); nursing (MSN). Part-time programs available. *Faculty:* 5 full-time (all women), 2 part-time/adjunct (both women). *Students:* 43 full-time (40 women), 23 part-time (20 women); includes 41 minority (39 Black or African American, non-Hispanic/Latino; 1 Asian, non-Hispanic/Latino; 1 Hispanic/Latino), 1 international. Average age 36. In 2013, 33 master's awarded. *Degree requirements:* For master's, comprehensive exam (for some programs), thesis (for some programs). *Entrance requirements:* For master's, GRE, minimum GPA of 3.0 on last degree, interview, 2 years of experience as RN. Additional exam requirements/recommendations for international students: Required—TOEFL (minimum score 500 paper-based; 62 iBT). *Application deadline:* For fall admission, 7/1 for domestic and international students; for spring admission, 12/1 for domestic and international students; for summer admission, 5/1 for domestic and international students. Applications are processed on a rolling basis. Application fee: $20 ($30 for international students). Electronic applications accepted. *Financial support:* Health care benefits and tuition waivers (full and partial) available. Financial award application deadline: 5/31; financial award applicants required to submit FAFSA. *Unit head:* Dr. Danita R. Potter, Interim Associate Dean, 318-274-2632, E-mail: potterd@gram.edu. *Application contact:* Dr. Rhonda Hensley, MSN Program Director, 318-274-2897, Fax: 318-274-3491, E-mail: hensleyr@gram.edu.
Website: http://www.gram.edu/academics/majors/professional%20studies/departments/nursing/

Grand Canyon University, College of Nursing, Phoenix, AZ 85017-1097. Offers acute care nurse practitioner (MS, PMC); clinical nurse specialist (PMC), including clinical nurse specialist, education; family nurse practitioner (MS); leadership in health care systems (MS); nurse education (MS). *Accreditation:* AACN. Part-time and evening/weekend programs available. Postbaccalaureate distance learning degree programs offered (no on-campus study). *Degree requirements:* For master's and PMC, comprehensive exam (for some programs). *Entrance requirements:* For master's, minimum cumulative and science course undergraduate GPA of 3.0. Additional exam requirements/recommendations for international students: Required—TOEFL (minimum score 575 paper-based; 90 iBT), IELTS (minimum score 7).

Gwynedd Mercy University, School of Nursing, Gwynedd Valley, PA 19437-0901. Offers clinical nurse specialist (MSN), including gerontology, oncology, pediatrics; nurse practitioner (MSN), including adult health, pediatric health. *Degree requirements:* For master's, thesis optional. *Entrance requirements:* For master's, GRE General Test or MAT, current nursing experience, physical assessment, course work in statistics, BSN from NLNAC-accredited program, 2 letters of recommendation, personal interview. Additional exam requirements/recommendations for international students: Required—TOEFL (minimum score 575 paper-based). Electronic applications accepted. *Expenses:* Contact institution. *Faculty research:* Critical thinking, primary care, domestic violence, multiculturalism, nursing centers.

Hardin-Simmons University, Graduate School, Patty Hanks Shelton School of Nursing, Abilene, TX 79698-0001. Offers advanced healthcare delivery (MSN); family nurse practitioner (MSN). Programs offered jointly with Abilene Christian University and McMurry University. *Accreditation:* AACN. Part-time programs available. *Faculty:* 6 full-time (all women), 2 part-time/adjunct (both women). *Students:* 4 full-time (all women), 7 part-time (4 women); includes 4 minority (3 Black or African American, non-Hispanic/Latino; 1 Hispanic/Latino), 1 international. Average age 37. 7 applicants, 100% accepted, 6 enrolled. In 2013, 8 master's awarded. *Degree requirements:* For master's, comprehensive exam, thesis or alternative. *Entrance requirements:* For master's, GRE, minimum undergraduate GPA of 3.0 in major, 2.8 overall; interview; upper-level course work in statistics; CPR certification; letters of recommendation. Additional exam requirements/recommendations for international students: Required—TOEFL (minimum score 550 paper-based; 75 iBT). *Application deadline:* For fall admission, 8/15 priority date for domestic students, 4/1 for international students; for spring admission, 1/5 priority date for domestic students, 9/1 for international students. Applications are processed on a rolling basis. Application fee: $50. *Expenses:* Contact institution. *Financial support:* In 2013–14, 1 student received support. Career-related internships or fieldwork and scholarships/grants available. Support available to part-time students. Financial award application deadline: 6/30; financial award applicants required to submit FAFSA. *Faculty research:* Child abuse, alternative medicine, pediatric chronic disease, health promotion. *Unit head:* Dr. Indira Tyler, Interim Director, 325-671-2367, Fax: 325-671-2386, E-mail: atoone@phssn.edu. *Application contact:* Dr. Nancy Kucinski, Dean of Graduate Studies, 325-670-1298, Fax: 325-670-1564, E-mail: gradoff@hsutx.edu.
Website: http://www.phssn.edu/

Hawai`i Pacific University, College of Nursing and Health Sciences, Honolulu, HI 96813. Offers community clinical nurse specialist (MSN); family nurse practitioner (MSN). Part-time and evening/weekend programs available. *Faculty:* 6 full-time (all women), 2 part-time/adjunct (both women). *Students:* 39 full-time (33 women), 16 part-time (11 women); includes 40 minority (2 Black or African American, non-Hispanic/Latino; 22 Asian, non-Hispanic/Latino; 7 Hispanic/Latino; 2 Native Hawaiian or other Pacific Islander, non-Hispanic/Latino; 7 Two or more races, non-Hispanic/Latino). Average age 38. 32 applicants, 75% accepted, 15 enrolled. In 2013, 7 master's awarded. *Degree requirements:* For master's, practicum, professional paper. *Entrance requirements:* For master's, bachelor's degree in nursing, minimum GPA of 3.0. Additional exam requirements/recommendations for international students: Recommended—TOEFL (minimum score 550 paper-based; 80 iBT), TWE (minimum score 5). *Application deadline:* Applications are processed on a rolling basis. Application fee: $50. Electronic applications accepted. *Financial support:* In 2013–14, 11 students received support. Career-related internships or fieldwork, Federal Work-Study, scholarships/grants, traineeships, and tuition waivers available. Financial award application deadline: 3/1; financial award applicants required to submit FAFSA. *Faculty research:* Hawaiian elders, traditional healing and nursing center. *Unit head:* Dr. Lynette Landry, Dean, 808-236-5811, E-mail: llandry@hpu.edu. *Application contact:* Rumi Yoshida, Associate Director of Graduate Admissions, 808-543-8034, Fax: 808-544-0280, E-mail: grad@hpu.edu.
Website: http://www.hpu.edu/CNHS/index.html

Holy Names University, Graduate Division, Department of Nursing, Oakland, CA 94619-1699. Offers administration/management (MSN, PMC); clinical faculty (MSN, PMC); community health nursing/case manager (MSN); family nurse practitioner (MSN, PMC); MSN/MA; MSN/MBA. *Accreditation:* AACN. Part-time and evening/weekend programs available. *Faculty:* 3 full-time, 22 part-time/adjunct. *Students:* 31 full-time (26 women), 78 part-time (67 women); includes 66 minority (27 Black or African American, non-Hispanic/Latino; 25 Asian, non-Hispanic/Latino; 13 Hispanic/Latino; 1 Two or more races, non-Hispanic/Latino), 5 international. Average age 38. 97 applicants, 61% accepted, 49 enrolled. In 2013, 66 master's, 3 other advanced degrees awarded. *Entrance requirements:* For master's, bachelor's degree in nursing or related field; California RN license or eligibility; minimum cumulative GPA of 2.8, 3.0 in nursing courses from baccalaureate program; courses in pathophysiology, statistics, and research at the undergraduate level. Additional exam requirements/recommendations for international students: Required—TOEFL (minimum score 500 paper-based; 79 iBT). *Application deadline:* For fall admission, 8/1 priority date for domestic students, 7/15 priority date for international students; for spring admission, 12/1 priority date for domestic and international students; for summer admission, 5/1 priority date for domestic and international students. Applications are processed on a rolling basis. Application fee: $65. Electronic applications accepted. Application fee is waived when completed online. *Expenses: Tuition:* Part-time $866 per unit. *Financial support:* Career-related internships or fieldwork, Federal Work-Study, scholarships/grants, and unspecified assistantships available. Support available to part-time students. Financial award application deadline: 3/2; financial award applicants required to submit FAFSA. *Faculty research:* Women's reproductive health, gerontology, attitudes about aging, schizophrenic families, international health issues. *Unit head:* Dr. Miki Goodwin, Associate Professor/Chair of Nursing, 510-436-1374, E-mail: goodwin@hnu.edu. *Application contact:* Graduate Admission Office, 800-430-1321, E-mail: graduateadmissions@hnu.edu.

Howard University, College of Nursing and Allied Health Sciences, Division of Nursing, Washington, DC 20059-0002. Offers nurse practitioner (Certificate); primary family health nursing (MSN). *Accreditation:* AACN. Part-time programs available. *Degree requirements:* For master's, comprehensive exam, thesis optional. *Entrance requirements:* For master's, RN license, minimum GPA of 3.0, BS in nursing. *Faculty research:* Urinary incontinence, breast cancer prevention, depression in the elderly, adolescent pregnancy.

Husson University, Graduate Nursing Program, Bangor, ME 04401-2999. Offers advanced practice psychiatric nursing (MSN, PMC); family and community nurse practitioner (MSN, PMC); nursing education (MSN, PMC). *Accreditation:* AACN. Part-time programs available. *Faculty:* 3 full-time (all women), 3 part-time/adjunct (all women). *Students:* 10 full-time (8 women), 15 part-time (14 women); includes 1 minority (Two or more races, non-Hispanic/Latino). 29 applicants, 76% accepted, 21 enrolled. In 2013, 16 master's awarded. *Degree requirements:* For master's, comprehensive exam (for some programs). *Entrance requirements:* For master's, MAT or GRE, BSN. Additional exam requirements/recommendations for international students: Required—TOEFL (minimum score 550 paper-based). *Application deadline:* For fall admission, 6/30 for domestic students; for spring admission, 10/30 for domestic students. Application fee: $40. *Expenses:* Contact institution. *Financial support:* In 2013–14, 16 students received support. Federal Work-Study, institutionally sponsored loans, traineeships, and unspecified assistantships available. Financial award application deadline: 4/15; financial award applicants required to submit FAFSA. *Unit head:* Prof. Chrystal Adams, Director, Nurse Practitioner Program, 207-941-7080, E-mail: adamsc@husson.edu. *Application contact:* Kristen Card, Director of Graduate Admissions, 207-404-5660, Fax: 207-941-7935, E-mail: cardk@husson.edu.

Illinois State University, Graduate School, Mennonite College of Nursing, Normal, IL 61790. Offers family nurse practitioner (PMC); nursing (MSN, PhD). *Accreditation:* AACN. *Faculty research:* Expanding the teaching-nursing home culture in the state of Illinois, advanced education nursing traineeship program, collaborative doctoral program-caring for older adults.

Indiana University–Purdue University Indianapolis, School of Nursing, Indianapolis, IN 46202-2896. Offers acute care nurse practitioner (MSN); adult health clinical nurse specialist (MSN); adult health nursing (MSN), including adult clinical nurse specialist; adult nurse practitioner (MSN); adult psychiatric/mental health nursing (MSN); child psychiatric/mental health nursing (MSN); community health nursing (MSN); family nurse practitioner (MSN); neonatal nurse practitioner (MSN); nursing (MSN, DNP), including nursing administration (MSN), nursing education (MSN); nursing science (PhD); pediatric clinical nurse specialist (MSN); women's health nurse practitioner (MSN); MSN/MPA; MSN/MPH. Part-time programs available. *Faculty:* 85 full-time (82 women), 60 part-time/adjunct (all women). *Students:* 86 full-time (78 women), 371 part-time (351 women); includes 74 minority (39 Black or African American, non-Hispanic/Latino; 1 American Indian or Alaska Native, non-Hispanic/Latino; 14 Asian, non-Hispanic/Latino; 11 Hispanic/Latino; 9 Two or more races, non-Hispanic/Latino), 6 international. Average age 38. 224 applicants, 61% accepted, 102 enrolled. In 2013, 120 master's, 10 doctorates awarded. Terminal master's awarded for partial completion of doctoral program. *Degree requirements:* For master's, thesis; for doctorate, thesis/dissertation. *Entrance requirements:* For master's, minimum GPA of 3.0, RN license; for doctorate, GRE General Test, minimum GPA of 3.0, MSN, RN license, graduate statistics course with minimum B grade (not older than 3 years). Additional exam requirements/recommendations for international students: Required—TOEFL. *Application deadline:* For fall admission, 2/15 for domestic students; for spring admission, 9/15 for domestic students. Application fee: $55 ($65 for international students). *Financial support:* In 2013–14, 93 students received support. Fellowships with full tuition reimbursements available, research assistantships with full tuition reimbursements available, teaching assistantships with full tuition reimbursements available, Federal Work-Study, institutionally sponsored loans, scholarships/grants, and tuition waivers (full) available. Support available to part-time students. Financial award application deadline: 5/1. *Faculty research:* Clinical science, health systems. *Total annual research expenditures:* $3 million. *Unit head:* Dr. Patricia Ebright, Associate Dean for Graduate Programs, E-mail: nursing@iupui.edu. *Application contact:* Information Contact, 317-274-2806.
Website: http://nursing.iu.edu/

Indiana University South Bend, School of Nursing, South Bend, IN 46634-7111. Offers family nurse practitioner (MSN). Part-time and evening/weekend programs available. *Faculty:* 4 full-time (all women). *Students:* 46 part-time (39 women); includes 9 minority (3 Black or African American, non-Hispanic/Latino; 2 Asian, non-Hispanic/Latino; 2 Hispanic/Latino; 2 Two or more races, non-Hispanic/Latino). Average age 43. 33 applicants, 48% accepted, 15 enrolled. In 2013, 10 master's awarded. *Entrance requirements:* For master's, GRE General Test, minimum GPA of 3.0. *Application deadline:* For fall admission, 4/1 for domestic students. *Financial support:* Teaching assistantships and Federal Work-Study available. Support available to part-time students. Financial award application deadline: 3/1; financial award applicants required to submit FAFSA. *Application contact:* Admissions Counselor, 574-520-4839, Fax: 574-520-4834, E-mail: graduate@iusb.edu.
Website: https://www.iusb.edu/nursing/msn.php

Kent State University, College of Nursing, Kent, OH 44242-0001. Offers acute care nurse practitioner (MSN); adult nurse practitioner (MSN); clinical nurse specialist (MSN); family nurse practitioner (MSN); geriatric nurse practitioner (MSN); health care management (MSN); nurse educator (MSN); nursing (PhD); nursing practice (DNP); pediatric nurse practitioner (MSN); psychiatric/mental health nurse practitioner (MSN); women's health nurse practitioner (MSN). PhD program offered jointly with The University of Akron. *Accreditation:* AACN. Part-time programs available. *Degree requirements:* For master's, thesis optional; for doctorate, comprehensive exam, thesis/dissertation. *Entrance requirements:* For master's, GRE (if undergraduate GPA less than 3.0), minimum GPA of 2.75; for doctorate, GRE, MSN. Additional exam requirements/recommendations for international students: Required—TOEFL. Electronic applications accepted. *Expenses:* Contact institution. *Faculty research:* Women and violence, methodological specialties, osteoporosis in women, new caregivers and the elderly.

La Salle University, School of Nursing and Health Sciences, Program in Nursing, Philadelphia, PA 19141-1199. Offers adult gerontology primary care nurse practitioner (MSN, Certificate); adult health and illness clinical nurse specialist (MSN); adult-gerontology clinical nurse specialist (MSN, Certificate); clinical nurse leader (MSN); family primary care nurse practitioner (MSN, Certificate); gerontology (Certificate); nurse anesthetist (MSN, Certificate); nursing (MSN, Certificate); nursing administration (MSN, Certificate); nursing education (Certificate); nursing practice (DNP); nursing service administration (MSN); public health nursing (MSN, Certificate); school nursing (Certificate); MSN/MBA; MSN/MPH. *Accreditation:* AANA/CANAEP. Part-time programs available. Postbaccalaureate distance learning degree programs offered (minimal on-campus study). *Faculty:* 13 full-time (12 women), 10 part-time/adjunct (8 women). *Students:* 4 full-time (all women), 379 part-time (331 women); includes 119 minority (70 Black or African American, non-Hispanic/Latino; 2 American Indian or Alaska Native, non-Hispanic/Latino; 31 Asian, non-Hispanic/Latino; 12 Hispanic/Latino; 4 Two or more races, non-Hispanic/Latino), 1 international. Average age 37. 133 applicants, 85% accepted, 63 enrolled. In 2013, 72 master's, 3 doctorates, 26 other advanced degrees awarded. *Degree requirements:* For doctorate, minimum of 1,000 hours of post baccalaureate clinical practice supervised by preceptors. *Entrance requirements:* For master's, GRE, MAT, or GMAT (for students with BSN GPA of less than 3.2), baccalaureate degree in nursing from an NLNAC- or CCNE-accredited program or an MSN Bridge program; Pennsylvania RN license; 2 letters of reference; resume; statement of philosophy articulating professional values and future educational goal; 1 year of work experience as a registered nurse; for doctorate, GRE (waived for applicants with MSN cumulative GPA of 3.7 or above), MSN from nationally-accredited program or master's degree, MBA or MHA from nationally-accredited program; resume or curriculum vitae; 2 letters of reference; interview; for Certificate, GRE, MAT, or GMAT (for students with BSN GPA of less than 3.2, baccalaureate degree in nursing from an NLNAC- or CCNE-accredited program or an MSN Bridge program; Pennsylvania RN license; 2 letters of reference; resume; statement of philosophy articulating professional values and future educational goal; 1 year of work experience as a registered nurse. Additional exam requirements/recommendations for international students: Required—TOEFL. *Application deadline:* For fall admission, 8/15 priority date for domestic students, 7/15 for international students; for spring admission, 12/15 priority date for domestic students, 11/15 for international students; for summer admission, 4/15 priority date for domestic students, 3/15 for international students. Applications are processed on a rolling basis. Application fee: $35. Electronic applications accepted. Application fee is waived when completed online. *Expenses:* Contact institution. *Financial support:* In 2013–14, 48 students received support. Teaching assistantships, scholarships/grants, and traineeships available. Support available to part-time students. Financial award application deadline: 8/31; financial award applicants required to submit FAFSA. *Unit head:* Dr. Patricia M. Dillon, Director, 215-951-1322, Fax: 215-951-1896, E-mail: msnapn@lasalle.edu. *Application contact:* Paul J. Reilly, Assistant Vice President, Enrollment Services, 215-951-1946, Fax: 215-951-1462, E-mail: reilly@lasalle.edu.

Lincoln Memorial University, Caylor School of Nursing, Harrogate, TN 37752-1901. Offers family nurse practitioner (MSN); nurse anesthesia (MSN); psychiatric mental health nurse practitioner (MSN). *Accreditation:* AANA/CANAEP. Part-time programs available. *Entrance requirements:* For master's, GRE.

Long Island University–LIU Post, School of Health Professions and Nursing, Department of Nursing, Brookville, NY 11548-1300. Offers clinical nurse specialist (MS); family nurse practitioner (MS, Certificate). *Accreditation:* AACN. Part-time and evening/weekend programs available. *Degree requirements:* For master's, thesis. *Entrance requirements:* For master's, minimum GPA of 3.0 in major, bachelor's degree in nursing, NYS registered nurse, interview. Electronic applications accepted. *Faculty research:* Lactation/breast cancer, early discharge in maternity.

Loyola University Chicago, Graduate School, Marcella Niehoff School of Nursing, Family Nurse Practitioner Program, Chicago, IL 60660. Offers emergency nurse (MSN). Part-time and evening/weekend programs available. Postbaccalaureate distance learning degree programs offered (minimal on-campus study). *Faculty:* 45 full-time (44 women). *Students:* 13 full-time (12 women), 110 part-time (101 women); includes 25 minority (5 Black or African American, non-Hispanic/Latino; 11 Asian, non-Hispanic/Latino; 8 Hispanic/Latino; 1 Two or more races, non-Hispanic/Latino), 1 international. Average age 32. 61 applicants, 66% accepted, 25 enrolled. In 2013, 21 master's awarded. *Degree requirements:* For master's, comprehensive exam. *Entrance requirements:* For master's, BSN, Illinois nursing license, minimum nursing GPA of 3.0, 1000 hours of experience before starting clinical. *Application deadline:* Applications are processed on a rolling basis. Application fee: $50. Electronic applications accepted. *Expenses: Tuition:* Full-time $16,740; part-time $930 per credit. *Required fees:* $135 per semester. *Financial support:* Traineeships available. Financial award applicants required to submit FAFSA. *Unit head:* Dr. Marijo Letizia, Associate Dean, 708-216-9325, Fax: 708-216-9555, E-mail: mletizi@luc.edu. *Application contact:* Amy Weatherford, Enrollment Advisor, School of Nursing, 773-508-3249, Fax: 773-508-3241, E-mail: aweatherford@luc.edu.
Website: http://www.luc.edu/nursing/

Malone University, Graduate Program in Nursing, Canton, OH 44709. Offers family nurse practitioner (MSN). *Accreditation:* AACN. Part-time and evening/weekend programs available. *Faculty:* 10 full-time (all women), 14 part-time/adjunct (13 women). *Students:* 65 part-time (62 women); includes 5 minority (2 Black or African American, non-Hispanic/Latino; 1 American Indian or Alaska Native, non-Hispanic/Latino; 1 Asian, non-Hispanic/Latino; 1 Hispanic/Latino). Average age 34. In 2013, 26 master's awarded. *Degree requirements:* For master's, thesis. *Entrance requirements:* For master's, minimum GPA of 3.0 from BSN program, interview, Ohio RN license. Additional exam requirements/recommendations for international students: Required—TOEFL (minimum score 550 paper-based; 79 iBT). *Application deadline:* Applications are processed on a rolling basis. *Expenses:* Contact institution. *Financial support:* Tuition waivers (partial) available. Support available to part-time students. Financial award application deadline: 6/30. *Faculty research:* Home heath care and geriatrics, community settings, culture, Hispanics, tuberculosis, geriatrics, Neuman Systems Model, nursing education. *Unit head:* Dr. Kathleen M. Flaherty, Director, 330-471-8330, Fax: 330-471-8607, E-mail: kflaherty@malone.edu. *Application contact:* Natalie D. Denholm, Recruiter/Adviser, 330-471-8207, Fax: 330-471-8570, E-mail: ndenholm@malone.edu.
Website: http://www.malone.edu/admissions/graduate/nursing/

Marquette University, Graduate School, College of Nursing, Milwaukee, WI 53201-1881. Offers acute care nurse practitioner (Certificate); adult clinical nurse specialist (Certificate); adult nurse practitioner (Certificate); advanced practice nursing (MSN, DNP), including adult-older adult acute care (DNP), adults (MSN), adults-older adults (DNP), clinical nurse leader (MSN), health care systems leadership (DNP), nurse-midwifery (MSN), older adults (MSN), pediatrics acute care (MSN), pediatrics primary care (MSN), pediatrics-acute care (DNP), pediatrics-primary care (DNP), primary care (DNP), systems leadership and healthcare quality (MSN); family nurse practitioner (Certificate); nurse-midwifery (Certificate); nursing (PhD); pediatric acute care (Certificate); pediatric primary care (Certificate); systems leadership and healthcare quality (Certificate). *Accreditation:* AACN. *Faculty:* 35 full-time (34 women), 59 part-time/adjunct (58 women). *Students:* 105 full-time (96 women), 279 part-time (256 women); includes 28 minority (11 Black or African American, non-Hispanic/Latino; 7 Asian, non-Hispanic/Latino; 8 Hispanic/Latino; 2 Two or more races, non-Hispanic/Latino), 3 international. Average age 30. 322 applicants, 62% accepted, 98 enrolled. In 2013, 66 master's, 4 doctorates, 6 other advanced degrees awarded. Terminal master's awarded for partial completion of doctoral program. *Degree requirements:* For master's, comprehensive exam, thesis or alternative. *Entrance requirements:* For master's, GRE General Test, BSN, Wisconsin RN license, official transcripts from all current and previous colleges/universities except Marquette, three completed recommendation forms, resume, written statement of professional goals; for doctorate, GRE General Test, official transcripts from all current and previous colleges/universities except Marquette, three letters of recommendation, resume, written statement of professional goals, sample of scholarly writing. Additional exam requirements/recommendations for international students: Required—TOEFL (minimum score 530 paper-based). *Application deadline:* For fall admission, 2/15 for domestic and international students. Application fee: $50. Electronic applications accepted. *Financial support:* In 2013–14, 41 students received support, including 1 fellowship with partial tuition reimbursement available (averaging $17,500 per year), 2 research assistantships with full tuition reimbursements available (averaging $13,285 per year), 8 teaching assistantships with full tuition reimbursements available (averaging $13,912 per year); career-related internships or fieldwork, Federal Work-Study, scholarships/grants, health care benefits, tuition waivers (partial), and unspecified assistantships also available. Support available to part-time students. Financial award application deadline: 2/15. *Faculty research:* Psychosocial adjustment to chronic illness, gerontology, reminiscence, health policy: uninsured and access, hospital care delivery systems. *Total annual research expenditures:* $769,051. *Unit head:* Dr. Margaret Callahan, Dean, 414-288-3800, Fax: 414-288-1578. *Application contact:* Dr. Maureen O'Brien, Associate Dean/Clinical Associate Professor, 414-288-3823.
Website: http://www.marquette.edu/nursing/academicprograms-graduate.shtml

Marymount University, School of Health Professions, Program in Nursing, Arlington, VA 22207-4299. Offers family nurse practitioner (MSN, Certificate); nursing (DNP). *Accreditation:* AACN. Part-time and evening/weekend programs available. *Faculty:* 6 full-time (all women), 2 part-time/adjunct (both women). *Students:* 11 full-time (all women), 58 part-time (54 women); includes 32 minority (17 Black or African American, non-Hispanic/Latino; 2 American Indian or Alaska Native, non-Hispanic/Latino; 5 Asian, non-Hispanic/Latino; 5 Hispanic/Latino; 2 Native Hawaiian or other Pacific Islander, non-Hispanic/Latino; 1 Two or more races, non-Hispanic/Latino), 2 international. Average age 38. 54 applicants, 31% accepted, 11 enrolled. In 2013, 18 master's, 2 doctorates, 1 other advanced degree awarded. *Degree requirements:* For master's, comprehensive exam; for doctorate, thesis/dissertation or alternative. *Entrance requirements:* For master's, 2 letters of recommendation, interview, resume, RN license, personal statement; for doctorate, 2 letters of recommendation, interview, resume, RN license, minimum MSN GPA of 3.5 or BSN 3.3; for Certificate, interview, master's degree in nursing. Additional exam requirements/recommendations for international students: Required—TOEFL (minimum score 600 paper-based; 96 iBT), IELTS (minimum score 6.5). *Application deadline:* For fall admission, 5/1 for domestic students, 7/1 for international students; for spring admission, 11/1 for domestic students, 9/16 for international students. Application fee: $40. Electronic applications accepted. *Expenses: Tuition:* Part-time $850 per credit. *Required fees:* $10 per credit. One-time fee: $200 part-time. Tuition and fees vary according to program. *Financial support:* In 2013–14, 7 students received support, including 2 teaching assistantships with partial tuition reimbursements available; research assistantships with partial tuition reimbursements available, career-related internships or fieldwork, Federal Work-Study, scholarships/grants, and unspecified assistantships also available. Support available to part-time students. Financial award applicants required to submit FAFSA. *Unit head:* Dr. Shelli Wolfe Mayer, Chair, 703-284-6886, Fax: 703-284-3819, E-mail: michelle.wolfe@marymount.edu. *Application contact:* Francesca Reed, Director, Graduate Admissions, 703-284-5901, Fax: 703-527-3815, E-mail: grad.admissions@marymount.edu.

Maryville University of Saint Louis, College of Health Professions, The Catherine McAuley School of Nursing, St. Louis, MO 63141-7299. Offers adult nurse practitioner (MSN); advanced practice nursing (DNP); family nurse practitioner (MSN); geriatric nurse practitioner (MSN); nursing education (MSN). *Accreditation:* AACN. Postbaccalaureate distance learning degree programs offered. *Students:* 30 full-time (28 women), 1,551 part-time (1,416 women); includes 361 minority (181 Black or African American, non-Hispanic/Latino; 16 American Indian or Alaska Native, non-Hispanic/Latino; 59 Asian, non-Hispanic/Latino; 71 Hispanic/Latino; 5 Native Hawaiian or other Pacific Islander, non-Hispanic/Latino; 29 Two or more races, non-Hispanic/Latino), 3 international. Average age 36. In 2013, 37 master's awarded. *Degree requirements:* For master's, practicum. *Entrance requirements:* For master's, BSN, current licensure, minimum GPA of 3.0, 3 letters of recommendation, curriculum vitae. Additional exam requirements/recommendations for international students: Required—TOEFL (minimum score 550 paper-based). *Application deadline:* Applications are processed on a rolling basis. Application fee: $40 ($60 for international students). Electronic applications accepted. Application fee is waived when completed online. *Expenses: Tuition:* Full-time $23,812; part-time $728 per credit hour. *Required fees:* $395 per year. Tuition and fees vary according to course load, degree level and program. *Financial support:* Federal Work-Study and campus employment available. Support available to part-time students. Financial award application deadline: 3/1; financial award applicants required to submit FAFSA. *Unit head:* Dr. Elizabeth Buck, Director, 314-529-9453, Fax: 314-529-9139, E-mail: ebuck@maryville.edu. *Application contact:* Crystal Jacobsmeyer, Assistant Director, Graduate Enrollment Advising, 314-929-9654, Fax: 314-529-9927, E-mail: cjacobsmeyer@maryville.edu.
Website: http://www.maryville.edu/hp/nursing/

McGill University, Faculty of Graduate and Postdoctoral Studies, Faculty of Medicine, School of Nursing, Montréal, QC H3A 2T5, Canada. Offers nurse practitioner (Graduate Diploma); nursing (M Sc A, PhD). PhD offered jointly with Université du Québec à Montréal.

McMurry University, Graduate Studies, Abilene, TX 79697. Offers education (MSN); family nurse practitioner (MSN).

Family Nurse Practitioner Studies

McNeese State University, Doré School of Graduate Studies, College of Nursing, Department of Graduate Nursing, Family Nurse Practitioner Program, Lake Charles, LA 70609. Offers PMC. *Degree requirements:* For PMC, thesis. *Entrance requirements:* For degree, GRE, MSN, eligible for unencumbered licensure as RN in Louisiana.

McNeese State University, Doré School of Graduate Studies, College of Nursing, Department of Graduate Nursing, Nursing Program, Lake Charles, LA 70609. Offers family nurse practitioner (MSN); family psychiatric/mental health nurse practitioner (MSN); nurse educator (MSN); nurse executive (MSN). *Degree requirements:* For master's, comprehensive exam. *Entrance requirements:* For master's, GRE, baccalaureate degree in nursing, minimum overall GPA of 2.7 for all undergraduate coursework, eligibility for unencumbered licensure as Registered Nurse in Louisiana or Texas, course in introductory statistics with minimum C grade, physical assessment skills, two letters of professional reference, 500-word essay, current resume.

Medical University of South Carolina, College of Nursing, Family Nurse Practitioner Program, Charleston, SC 29425. Offers MSN, DNP. Part-time programs available. Postbaccalaureate distance learning degree programs offered (minimal on-campus study). *Degree requirements:* For master's, thesis optional; for doctorate, final project. *Entrance requirements:* For master's, BSN from nationally-accredited program, minimum nursing and cumulative GPA of 3.0, undergraduate-level statistics course, active RN License, 3 confidential references, current curriculum vitae or resume, essay; for doctorate, BSN from nationally-accredited program, minimum nursing and cumulative GPA of 3.0, undergraduate-level statistics course, active RN License, 3 confidential references, current curriculum vitae or resume, personal essay (for DNP). Additional exam requirements/recommendations for international students: Required—TOEFL (minimum score 550 paper-based; 80 iBT). Electronic applications accepted. *Faculty research:* Primary care, smoking cessation, patient navigation, informatics, depression.

Middle Tennessee State University, College of Graduate Studies, College of Behavioral and Health Sciences, School of Nursing, Program in Family Nurse Practitioner, Murfreesboro, TN 37132. Offers MSN, Graduate Certificate. Part-time and evening/weekend programs available. Postbaccalaureate distance learning degree programs offered. *Students:* 52 full-time (47 women), 196 part-time (177 women); includes 35 minority (22 Black or African American, non-Hispanic/Latino; 2 American Indian or Alaska Native, non-Hispanic/Latino; 4 Asian, non-Hispanic/Latino; 3 Hispanic/Latino; 4 Two or more races, non-Hispanic/Latino). 139 applicants, 89% accepted. In 2013, 32 master's awarded. *Entrance requirements:* Additional exam requirements/recommendations for international students: Required—TOEFL (minimum score 525 paper-based; 71 iBT) or IELTS (minimum score 6). *Financial support:* Institutionally sponsored loans available. Support available to part-time students. Financial award application deadline: 5/1. *Unit head:* Dr. Jenny Sauls, Director, 615-898-2446, Fax: 615-898-5441, E-mail: jenny.sauls@mtsu.edu. *Application contact:* Dr. Michael D. Allen, Vice Provost for Research/Dean, 615-898-2840, Fax: 615-904-8020, E-mail: michael.allen@mtsu.edu.

Midwestern State University, Graduate School, Robert D. and Carol Gunn College of Health Sciences and Human Services, Wilson School of Nursing, Wichita Falls, TX 76308. Offers family nurse practitioner (MSN); family psychiatric mental health nurse practitioner (MSN); nurse educator (MSN). *Accreditation:* AACN. Part-time and evening/weekend programs available. *Degree requirements:* For master's, comprehensive exam, thesis optional. *Entrance requirements:* For master's, GRE General Test or MAT. Additional exam requirements/recommendations for international students: Required—TOEFL (minimum score 550 paper-based). *Application deadline:* For fall admission, 7/1 priority date for domestic students, 4/1 for international students; for spring admission, 11/1 priority date for domestic students, 8/1 for international students. Applications are processed on a rolling basis. Application fee: $35 ($50 for international students). Electronic applications accepted. *Expenses:* Tuition, state resident: full-time $3627; part-time $201.50 per credit hour. Tuition, nonresident: full-time $10,899; part-time $605.50 per credit hour. *Required fees:* $1357. *Financial support:* Teaching assistantships with partial tuition reimbursements, career-related internships or fieldwork, Federal Work-Study, institutionally sponsored loans, scholarships/grants, tuition waivers (partial), and unspecified assistantships available. Support available to part-time students. Financial award application deadline: 3/1; financial award applicants required to submit FAFSA. *Faculty research:* Infant feeding, musculoskeletal disorders, diabetes, community health education, water quality reporting. *Unit head:* Robin Lockhart, RN, Interim Chair, 940-397-4614, Fax: 940-397-4513, E-mail: robin.lockhart@mwsu.edu.
Website: http://www.mwsu.edu/academics/hs2/nursing/

Millersville University of Pennsylvania, College of Graduate and Professional Studies, School of Science and Mathematics, Department of Nursing, Millersville, PA 17551-0302. Offers family nurse practitioner (MSN); nursing education (MSN). Part-time and evening/weekend programs available. *Faculty:* 5 full-time (all women), 5 part-time/adjunct (all women). *Students:* 5 full-time (all women), 78 part-time (72 women); includes 10 minority (8 Black or African American, non-Hispanic/Latino; 2 Hispanic/Latino). Average age 38. 43 applicants, 67% accepted, 24 enrolled. In 2013, 25 master's awarded. *Degree requirements:* For master's, internship, scholarly project. *Entrance requirements:* For master's, 3 letters of recommendation; interview; resume; copy of RN license, goal statement, official transcripts. Additional exam requirements/recommendations for international students: Required—TOEFL (minimum score 550 paper-based, 79 iBT) or IELTS (minimum score 6). *Application deadline:* For fall admission, 1/15 for domestic and international students; for winter admission, 10/1 for domestic and international students; for spring admission, 10/1 for domestic and international students. Application fee: $40. Electronic applications accepted. *Expenses:* Tuition, state resident: full-time $7956; part-time $442 per credit. Tuition, nonresident: full-time $11,934; part-time $663 per credit. *Required fees:* $2196; $122 per credit. Tuition and fees vary according to course load. *Financial support:* In 2013–14, 3 students received support, including 3 research assistantships with full tuition reimbursements available (averaging $2,117 per year); institutionally sponsored loans and unspecified assistantships also available. Support available to part-time students. Financial award application deadline: 3/15; financial award applicants required to submit FAFSA. *Faculty research:* Family nurse practitioner, nurse educator. *Unit head:* Dr. Barbara J. Zimmerman, Chair, 717-872-3376, Fax: 717-871-4877, E-mail: barbara.zimmerman@millersville.edu. *Application contact:* Dr. Victor S. DeSantis, Dean of College of Graduate and Professional Studies/Associate Provost for Civic and Community Engagement, 717-872-3099, Fax: 717-872-3453, E-mail: victor.desantis@millersville.edu.
Website: http://www.millersville.edu/nursing/msn/

Minnesota State University Mankato, College of Graduate Studies and Research, College of Allied Health and Nursing, School of Nursing, Mankato, MN 56001. Offers family nursing (MSN), including family nurse practitioner; nursing (DNP). MSN offered jointly with Metropolitan State University; DNP with Metropolitan State University, Minnesota State University Moorhead, Winona State University. *Accreditation:* AACN. *Students:* 54 part-time (51 women). *Degree requirements:* For master's, comprehensive exam, internships, research project or thesis; for doctorate, capstone project. *Entrance requirements:* For master's, GRE General Test or on-campus essay, minimum GPA of 3.0 during previous 2 years, BSN or equivalent references; for doctorate, master's degree in nursing. Additional exam requirements/recommendations for international students: Required—TOEFL. *Application deadline:* For fall admission, 2/15 priority date for domestic students, 2/15 for international students. Applications are processed on a rolling basis. Application fee: $40. Electronic applications accepted. *Financial support:* Research assistantships with full tuition reimbursements and teaching assistantships with full tuition reimbursements available. Financial award application deadline: 3/15; financial award applicants required to submit FAFSA. *Faculty research:* Psychosocial nursing, computers in nursing, family adaptation. *Unit head:* Dr. Sue Ellen Bell, Graduate Coordinator, 507-389-6814. *Application contact:* Collaborative MSN Program Admissions, 507-389-6022.
Website: http://www.mnsu.edu/nursing/

Missouri State University, Graduate College, College of Health and Human Services, Department of Nursing, Springfield, MO 65897. Offers nursing (MSN), including family nurse practitioner, nurse educator. *Accreditation:* AACN. *Faculty:* 14 full-time (all women), 12 part-time/adjunct (9 women). *Students:* 18 full-time (17 women), 29 part-time (27 women); includes 5 minority (all Black or African American, non-Hispanic/Latino). Average age 37. 11 applicants, 91% accepted, 6 enrolled. In 2013, 17 master's awarded. *Degree requirements:* For master's, comprehensive exam, thesis or alternative. *Entrance requirements:* For master's, GRE General Test, minimum GPA of 3.0, RN license (for MSN), 1 year of work experience (for MPH). Additional exam requirements/recommendations for international students: Required—TOEFL (minimum score 550 paper-based; 79 iBT). *Application deadline:* For fall admission, 7/20 priority date for domestic students, 5/1 for international students; for spring admission, 12/20 priority date for domestic students, 9/1 for international students. Applications are processed on a rolling basis. Application fee: $35 ($50 for international students). Electronic applications accepted. *Expenses:* Tuition, state resident: full-time $4500; part-time $250 per credit hour. Tuition, nonresident: full-time $9018; part-time $501 per credit hour. *Required fees:* $361 per semester. Tuition and fees vary according to course level, course load and program. *Financial support:* In 2013–14, 2 research assistantships with full tuition reimbursements (averaging $8,324 per year) were awarded; Federal Work-Study, institutionally sponsored loans, scholarships/grants, and unspecified assistantships also available. Financial award application deadline: 3/31; financial award applicants required to submit FAFSA. *Faculty research:* Preconceptual health, women's health, nursing satisfaction, nursing education. *Unit head:* Dr. Kathryn Hope, Head, 417-836-5310, Fax: 417-836-5484, E-mail: nursing@missouristate.edu. *Application contact:* Misty Stewart, Coordinator of Admissions and Recruitment, 417-836-6079, Fax: 417-836-6200, E-mail: mistystewart@missouristate.edu.
Website: http://www.missouristate.edu/nursing/

Molloy College, Division of Nursing, Rockville Centre, NY 11571-5002. Offers adult nurse practitioner (Advanced Certificate); clinical nurse specialist: adult health (Advanced Certificate); family nurse practitioner (Advanced Certificate); nurse practitioner psychiatry (Advanced Certificate); nursing (MS, PhD); nursing administration (Advanced Certificate); nursing administration with informatics (Advanced Certificate); nursing education (Advanced Certificate); nursing informatics (Advanced Certificate); pediatric nurse practitioner (Advanced Certificate). *Accreditation:* AACN. Part-time and evening/weekend programs available. *Faculty:* 30 full-time (29 women), 10 part-time/adjunct (7 women). *Students:* 18 full-time (all women), 538 part-time (495 women); includes 289 minority (159 Black or African American, non-Hispanic/Latino; 1 American Indian or Alaska Native, non-Hispanic/Latino; 80 Asian, non-Hispanic/Latino; 43 Hispanic/Latino; 4 Native Hawaiian or other Pacific Islander, non-Hispanic/Latino; 2 Two or more races, non-Hispanic/Latino), 2 international. Average age 38. 241 applicants, 63% accepted, 122 enrolled. In 2013, 84 master's, 2 other advanced degrees awarded. *Degree requirements:* For master's, thesis optional. *Entrance requirements:* For master's, 3 letters of reference, BS in nursing, minimum undergraduate GPA of 3.0; for Advanced Certificate, 3 letters of reference, master's degree in nursing. *Application deadline:* For fall admission, 9/2 priority date for domestic students; for spring admission, 1/20 priority date for domestic students. Applications are processed on a rolling basis. Application fee: $60. *Expenses: Tuition:* Full-time $16,920; part-time $940 per credit. *Required fees:* $880. *Financial support:* Research assistantships with partial tuition reimbursements, teaching assistantships with partial tuition reimbursements, institutionally sponsored loans, scholarships/grants, and unspecified assistantships available. Support available to part-time students. Financial award application deadline: 4/1; financial award applicants required to submit FAFSA. *Unit head:* Dr. Jeannine Muldoon, Dean of Nursing, 516-323-3651, E-mail: jmuldoon@molloy.edu. *Application contact:* Alina Haitz, Assistant Director of Graduate Admissions, 516-323-4008, E-mail: ahaitz@molloy.edu.
Website: http://www.molloy.edu/academics/nursing-division

Monmouth University, The Graduate School, The Marjorie K. Unterberg School of Nursing and Health Studies, West Long Branch, NJ 07764-1898. Offers adult and gerontological nurse practitioner (MSN); adult-gerontological nurse practitioner (Post-Master's Certificate); family nurse practitioner (MSN, Post-Master's Certificate); family psychiatric and mental health advanced practice nursing (MSN); forensic nursing (MSN, Certificate); nursing (MSN); nursing administration (MSN, Post-Master's Certificate); nursing education (MSN, Post-Master's Certificate); nursing practice (DNP); physician assistant (MS); psychiatric-mental health nurse practitioner (Post-Master's Certificate); school nursing (MSN, Certificate). *Accreditation:* AACN. Part-time and evening/weekend programs available. *Faculty:* 14 full-time (all women), 4 part-time/adjunct (3 women). *Students:* 19 full-time (18 women), 269 part-time (252 women); includes 106 minority (35 Black or African American, non-Hispanic/Latino; 2 American Indian or Alaska Native, non-Hispanic/Latino; 51 Asian, non-Hispanic/Latino; 12 Hispanic/Latino; 3 Native Hawaiian or other Pacific Islander, non-Hispanic/Latino; 3 Two or more races, non-Hispanic/Latino), 2 international. Average age 39. 135 applicants, 98% accepted, 96 enrolled. In 2013, 54 master's, 7 doctorates awarded. *Degree requirements:* For master's, practicum (for some tracks). *Entrance requirements:* For master's, GRE General Test, BSN with minimum GPA of 2.75, current RN license, proof of liability and malpractice policy, personal statement, two letters of recommendation, college course work in health assessment, resume; minimum GPA of 3.0, minimum C grade in prerequisite courses, minimum 200 hours' clinical experience, 3 letters of recommendation, and interview (for MS); for doctorate, accredited master's nursing program degree with minimum GPA of 3.2, active RN license, national certification as Nurse Practitioner or Nurse Administrator, working knowledge of statistics, statement of goals and vision for change, 2 letters of recommendation, resume, interview. Additional exam requirements/recommendations for international students: Required—TOEFL (minimum score 550 paper-based; 79 iBT), IELTS (minimum score 6) or Michigan English Language Assessment Battery (minimum score 77). *Application deadline:* For fall admission, 7/15 priority date for domestic students, 6/1 for international students; for spring admission, 11/15 priority date for domestic students, 11/1 for international students; for summer admission, 2/1 for domestic students. Applications are processed on a rolling basis. Application fee: $50. Electronic applications accepted. *Expenses: Tuition:* Part-time $1004 per credit hour. *Required fees:* $157 per semester. *Financial support:* In 2013–14, 163 students received support, including 113 fellowships (averaging $3,093 per year), 27 research assistantships (averaging $6,273 per year); career-related internships or fieldwork, scholarships/grants, and unspecified

assistantships also available. Support available to part-time students. Financial award applicants required to submit FAFSA. *Faculty research:* Relationship of undergraduate GPA and GRE to succeeding in a graduate nursing program. *Unit head:* Dr. Janet Mahoney, Dean, 732-571-3443, Fax: 732-263-5131, E-mail: jmahoney@monmouth.edu. *Application contact:* Lauren Vento-Cifelli, Associate Vice President of Undergraduate and Graduate Admission, 732-571-3452, Fax: 732-263-5123, E-mail: gradadm@monmouth.edu.
Website: http://www.monmouth.edu/school-of-nursing-health/graduate-nursing-programs.aspx

Montana State University, College of Graduate Studies, College of Nursing, Bozeman, MT 59717. Offers clinical nurse leader (MN); family nurse practitioner (MN, Post-Master's Certificate); nursing education (Certificate, Post-Master's Certificate); psychiatric mental health nurse practitioner (MN). *Accreditation:* AACN. Part-time programs available. Postbaccalaureate distance learning degree programs offered (minimal on-campus study). *Degree requirements:* For master's, comprehensive exam, thesis (for some programs). *Entrance requirements:* For master's, GRE General Test, minimum GPA of 3.0 for undergraduate and post-baccalaureate work. Additional exam requirements/recommendations for international students: Required—TOEFL (minimum score 580 paper-based). Electronic applications accepted. *Faculty research:* Rural nursing, health disparities, environmental/public health, oral health, resilience.

Mount Carmel College of Nursing, Nursing Program, Columbus, OH 43222. Offers adult gerontology acute care nurse practitioner (MS); adult health clinical nurse specialist (MS); family nurse practitioner (MS); nursing administration (MS); nursing education (MS). *Accreditation:* AACN. Part-time programs available. *Faculty:* 8 full-time (7 women), 8 part-time/adjunct (7 women). *Students:* 94 full-time (89 women), 76 part-time (73 women); includes 35 minority (21 Black or African American, non-Hispanic/Latino; 2 American Indian or Alaska Native, non-Hispanic/Latino; 6 Asian, non-Hispanic/Latino; 2 Hispanic/Latino; 1 Native Hawaiian or other Pacific Islander, non-Hispanic/Latino; 3 Two or more races, non-Hispanic/Latino). Average age 38. 123 applicants, 50% accepted, 47 enrolled. In 2013, 41 master's awarded. *Degree requirements:* For master's, professional manuscript. *Entrance requirements:* For master's, letters of recommendation, statement of purpose, current resume, baccalaureate degree in nursing, current Ohio RN license, minimum cumulative GPA of 3.0. Additional exam requirements/recommendations for international students: Required—TOEFL (minimum score 550 paper-based; 80 iBT). *Application deadline:* For fall admission, 6/1 priority date for domestic students; for winter admission, 11/1 for domestic students; for spring admission, 10/1 priority date for domestic students; for summer admission, 3/1 for domestic students. Applications are processed on a rolling basis. Application fee: $30. *Expenses: Tuition:* Full-time $8560; part-time $428 per credit. *Required fees:* $75. *Financial support:* In 2013–14, 9 students received support. Institutionally sponsored loans and scholarships/grants available. Financial award application deadline: 3/15; financial award applicants required to submit FAFSA. *Unit head:* Dr. Angela Phillips-Lowe, Associate Dean, 614-234-5717, Fax: 614-234-2875, E-mail: aphillips-lowe@mccn.edu. *Application contact:* Kathleen Walters, Program Coordinator, 614-234-5408, Fax: 614-234-2875, E-mail: kwalters@mccn.edu.
Website: http://www.mccn.edu/

Mount Saint Mary College, Division of Nursing, Newburgh, NY 12550-3494. Offers adult nurse practitioner (MS, Advanced Certificate), including nursing education (MS), nursing management (MS); clinical nurse specialist-adult health (MS), including nursing education, nursing management; family nurse practitioner (Advanced Certificate). *Accreditation:* AACN. Part-time and evening/weekend programs available. *Faculty:* 4 full-time (all women). *Students:* 79 part-time (72 women); includes 19 minority (12 Black or African American, non-Hispanic/Latino; 1 Asian, non-Hispanic/Latino; 5 Hispanic/Latino; 1 Native Hawaiian or other Pacific Islander, non-Hispanic/Latino). Average age 39. 45 applicants, 47% accepted, 9 enrolled. In 2013, 13 master's, 3 other advanced degrees awarded. *Degree requirements:* For master's, research utilization project. *Entrance requirements:* For master's, BSN, minimum GPA of 3.0, RN license. *Application deadline:* For fall admission, 6/3 priority date for domestic students; for spring admission, 10/31 priority date for domestic students. Applications are processed on a rolling basis. Application fee: $45. Application fee is waived when completed online. *Expenses: Tuition:* Full-time $13,356; part-time $742 per credit. *Required fees:* $70 per semester. *Financial support:* In 2013–14, 8 students received support. Unspecified assistantships available. Financial award application deadline: 4/15; financial award applicants required to submit FAFSA. *Unit head:* Linda Ruta, Graduate Coordinator, 845-569-3512, Fax: 845-562-6762, E-mail: linda.ruta@msmc.edu. *Application contact:* Lisa Gallina, Director of Admissions for Graduate Programs and Adult Degree Completion, 845-569-3166, Fax: 845-569-3450, E-mail: lisa.gallina@msmc.edu.
Website: http://www.msmc.edu/Academics/Graduate_Programs/Master_of_Science_in_Nursing

Murray State University, College of Health Sciences and Human Services, Program in Nursing, Murray, KY 42071. Offers clinical nurse specialist (MSN); family nurse practitioner (MSN); nurse anesthesia (MSN). *Accreditation:* AACN; AANA/CANAEP. *Degree requirements:* For master's, research project. *Entrance requirements:* For master's, GRE General Test, BSN, interview, RN licensure. Additional exam requirements/recommendations for international students: Required—TOEFL (minimum score 550 paper-based). *Faculty research:* Fibromyalgis, primary care, rural health.

New Mexico State University, Graduate School, College of Health and Social Services, School of Nursing, Las Cruces, NM 88003. Offers adult/gerontology nurse practitioner (DNP); family nurse practitioner (DNP); nursing (MSN, PhD); public/community health (DNP). *Accreditation:* AACN. Postbaccalaureate distance learning degree programs offered (minimal on-campus study). *Faculty:* 15 full-time (14 women). *Students:* 42 full-time (33 women), 64 part-time (56 women); includes 50 minority (11 Black or African American, non-Hispanic/Latino; 1 American Indian or Alaska Native, non-Hispanic/Latino; 1 Asian, non-Hispanic/Latino; 36 Hispanic/Latino; 1 Two or more races, non-Hispanic/Latino), 1 international. Average age 42. 50 applicants, 86% accepted, 36 enrolled. In 2013, 12 master's, 6 doctorates awarded. *Degree requirements:* For master's, comprehensive exam, thesis optional, clinical practice; for doctorate, comprehensive exam, thesis/dissertation. *Entrance requirements:* For master's, NCLEX exam, BSN, minimum GPA of 3.0, course work in statistics, 3 letters of reference, writing sample, RN license, CPR certification, proof of liability, immunizations, criminal background check; for doctorate, NCLEX exam, MSN, minimum GPA of 3.0, 3 letters of reference, writing sample, RN license, CPR certification, proof of liability, immunizations, criminal background check, statistics course. Additional exam requirements/recommendations for international students: Required—TOEFL (minimum score 550 paper-based; 79 iBT), IELTS (minimum score 6.5). *Application deadline:* For spring admission, 10/1 priority date for domestic students. Application fee: $40 ($50 for international students). Electronic applications accepted. *Expenses:* Tuition, state resident: full-time $5398; part-time $224.90 per credit. Tuition, nonresident: full-time $18,821; part-time $784.20 per credit. *Required fees:* $1310; $54.60 per credit. *Financial support:* In 2013–14, 31 students received support. Career-related internships or fieldwork, Federal Work-Study, scholarships/grants, traineeships, health care benefits, and unspecified assistantships available. Financial award application deadline: 3/1. *Faculty research:* Public policy, community health, health disparities, self efficacy and self management, psychiatric mental health. *Total annual research expenditures:* $3,424. *Unit head:* Dr. Pamela Schultz, Director, 575-646-3812, Fax: 575-646-2167, E-mail: pschultz@nmsu.edu. *Application contact:* Dr. Kathleen Huttlinger, Associate Director for Graduate Studies, 575-646-4387, Fax: 575-646-2167.
Website: http://schoolofnursing.nmsu.edu

New York University, College of Nursing, Doctor of Nursing Practice Program, New York, NY 10012-1019. Offers advanced practice nursing (DNP), including adult acute care, adult nurse practitioner/holistic nursing, adult nurse practitioner/palliative care nursing, adult primary care, adult primary care/geriatrics, family, geriatrics, mental health nursing, nurse-midwifery, pediatrics. Part-time and evening/weekend programs available. *Faculty:* 3 full-time (all women), 1 part-time/adjunct (0 women). *Students:* 1 (woman) full-time, 33 part-time (30 women); includes 7 minority (3 Black or African American, non-Hispanic/Latino; 3 Asian, non-Hispanic/Latino; 1 Hispanic/Latino). Average age 39. 18 applicants, 100% accepted, 12 enrolled. In 2013, 4 doctorates awarded. *Degree requirements:* For doctorate, thesis/dissertation, capstone. *Entrance requirements:* For doctorate, MAT or GRE (either taken within past 5 years), MS, RN license, interview, Nurse Practitioner Certification. Additional exam requirements/recommendations for international students: Required—TOEFL (minimum score 90 iBT), IELTS (minimum score 7). *Application deadline:* For fall admission, 3/1 for domestic students, 4/1 for international students. Applications are processed on a rolling basis. Application fee: $80. Electronic applications accepted. *Expenses: Tuition:* Full-time $35,856; part-time $1494 per unit. *Required fees:* $1408; $64 per unit. $473 per term. Tuition and fees vary according to course load and program. *Financial support:* Scholarships/grants available. Support available to part-time students. Financial award application deadline: 2/1. *Faculty research:* Geriatrics, HIV, elderly black diabetics, families and illness, oral systemic connection. *Unit head:* Dr. Rona Levin, Director, 212-998-5319, Fax: 212-995-3143, E-mail: rfl2039@nyu.edu. *Application contact:* Elizabeth Ensweiler, Assistant Director, Graduate Student Affairs and Admissions, 212-992-7653, Fax: 212-995-4302, E-mail: ee39@nyu.edu.

New York University, College of Nursing, Programs in Advanced Practice Nursing, New York, NY 10012-1019. Offers advanced practice nursing: adult acute care (MS, Advanced Certificate); advanced practice nursing: adult nurse practitioner/holistic nurse practitioner (Advanced Certificate); advanced practice nursing: adult nurse practitioner/palliative care nurse practitioner (Advanced Certificate); advanced practice nursing: adult primary care (MS, Advanced Certificate); advanced practice nursing: family (MS, Advanced Certificate); advanced practice nursing: geriatrics (Advanced Certificate); advanced practice nursing: mental health (MS); advanced practice nursing: mental health nursing (Advanced Certificate); advanced practice nursing: pediatrics (MS, Advanced Certificate); nurse midwifery (MS, Advanced Certificate); nursing administration (MS, Advanced Certificate); nursing education (MS, Advanced Certificate); nursing informatics (MS, Advanced Certificate); MS/MPA; MS/MPH. *Accreditation:* AACN; ACNM/ACME. Part-time programs available. *Faculty:* 22 full-time (all women), 54 part-time/adjunct (46 women). *Students:* 36 full-time (31 women), 622 part-time (549 women); includes 239 minority (73 Black or African American, non-Hispanic/Latino; 1 American Indian or Alaska Native, non-Hispanic/Latino; 116 Asian, non-Hispanic/Latino; 36 Hispanic/Latino; 6 Native Hawaiian or other Pacific Islander, non-Hispanic/Latino; 7 Two or more races, non-Hispanic/Latino), 16 international. Average age 37. 395 applicants, 67% accepted, 156 enrolled. In 2013, 186 master's, 8 other advanced degrees awarded. *Degree requirements:* For master's, thesis (for some programs). *Entrance requirements:* For master's, BS in nursing, AS in nursing with another BS/BA, interview, RN license, 1 year of clinical experience (3 for nursing education program); for Advanced Certificate, master's degree. Additional exam requirements/recommendations for international students: Required—TOEFL (minimum score 90 iBT), IELTS (minimum score 7). *Application deadline:* For fall admission, 7/1 for domestic and international students; for spring admission, 12/1 for domestic and international students. Application fee: $80. Electronic applications accepted. *Expenses: Tuition:* Full-time $35,856; part-time $1494 per unit. *Required fees:* $1408; $64 per unit. $473 per term. Tuition and fees vary according to course load and program. *Financial support:* In 2013–14, 182 students received support. Research assistantships, career-related internships or fieldwork, Federal Work-Study, scholarships/grants, traineeships, and unspecified assistantships available. Support available to part-time students. Financial award application deadline: 2/1; financial award applicants required to submit FAFSA. *Faculty research:* Geriatrics, HIV, elderly black diabetics, families and illness, oral systemic connection. *Unit head:* Dr. Judith Haber, Associate Dean, Graduate Programs, 212-998-9020, Fax: 212-995-3143, E-mail: jh33@nyu.edu. *Application contact:* Elizabeth Ensweiler, Assistant Director, Graduate Student Affairs and Admissions, 212-992-7653, Fax: 212-995-4302, E-mail: ee39@nyu.edu.

Nicholls State University, Graduate Studies, College of Nursing and Allied Health, Thibodaux, LA 70310. Offers family nurse practitioner (MSN); family psychiatric/mental health nurse practitioner (MSN); nurse executive (MSN).

Northern Arizona University, Graduate College, College of Health and Human Services, School of Nursing, Flagstaff, AZ 86011. Offers family nurse practitioner (MSN, Certificate); nurse generalist (MSN); nursing practice (DNP). *Accreditation:* AACN. Part-time programs available. *Faculty:* 37 full-time (33 women), 7 part-time/adjunct (all women). *Students:* 30 full-time (22 women), 108 part-time (95 women); includes 32 minority (3 Black or African American, non-Hispanic/Latino; 5 American Indian or Alaska Native, non-Hispanic/Latino; 6 Asian, non-Hispanic/Latino; 15 Hispanic/Latino; 1 Native Hawaiian or other Pacific Islander, non-Hispanic/Latino; 2 Two or more races, non-Hispanic/Latino). Average age 42. 105 applicants, 57% accepted, 46 enrolled. In 2013, 34 master's, 5 other advanced degrees awarded. *Degree requirements:* For master's, thesis (for some programs), project or thesis. *Entrance requirements:* For master's, GRE General Test or minimum GPA of 3.0, undergraduate statistics or health assessment with minimum grade of B in last 5 years or 3 years of RN experience (nursing education). Additional exam requirements/recommendations for international students: Required—TOEFL (minimum score 550 paper-based; 80 iBT), IELTS (minimum score 7). *Application deadline:* For fall admission, 1/15 priority date for domestic and international students. Applications are processed on a rolling basis. Application fee: $65. Electronic applications accepted. *Financial support:* Career-related internships or fieldwork, Federal Work-Study, scholarships/grants, traineeships, health care benefits, tuition waivers, and unspecified assistantships available. Financial award applicants required to submit FAFSA. *Unit head:* Dr. Debera Thomas, Chair, 928-523-2656, Fax: 928-523-7171, E-mail: debera.thomas@nau.edu. *Application contact:* Penny Susan Walior, Student Academic Specialist, 928-523-6717, Fax: 928-523-9155, E-mail: graduatenursing@nau.edu.
Website: http://nau.edu/CHHS/Nursing/Welcome/

Northern Michigan University, College of Graduate Studies, College of Health Sciences and Professional Studies, School of Nursing, Marquette, MI 49855-5301. Offers DNP. *Accreditation:* AACN. Part-time programs available. Postbaccalaureate distance learning degree programs offered (minimal on-campus study). *Faculty:* 18 full-time (all women). *Students:* 17 part-time (14 women). Average age 35. *Entrance requirements:* For doctorate, Michigan RN license; minimum undergraduate GPA of 3.0; 3 letters of recommendation; written personal goal statement. Additional exam requirements/recommendations for international students: Required—TOEFL (minimum

score 550 paper-based; 79 iBT), IELTS (minimum score 6.5). *Application deadline:* For fall admission, 4/15 for domestic and international students; for winter admission, 11/15 for domestic students; for spring admission, 3/17 for domestic students. Application fee: $50. Electronic applications accepted. *Expenses:* Tuition, state resident: part-time $427 per credit. Tuition, nonresident: part-time $614.50 per credit. *Required fees:* $325 per semester. Tuition and fees vary according to course load and program. *Financial support:* In 2013–14, 3 students received support, including 3 teaching assistantships with full tuition reimbursements available (averaging $8,898 per year); Federal Work-Study, institutionally sponsored loans, and unspecified assistantships also available. Financial award application deadline: 3/1; financial award applicants required to submit FAFSA. *Faculty research:* Grief experiences in Alzheimer's caregivers, nursing students attitudes towards the elderly, using Facebook as a means of simulation and educational means for pediatric undergraduate nursing students, use of a nurse practitioner student educational intervention to reduce sugar sweetened beverage consumption in rural adolescents. *Unit head:* Dr. Brian Cherry, Assistant Provost of Graduate Education and Research, 906-227-2300, E-mail: graduate@nmu.edu. *Application contact:* Dr. Melissa Romero, Associate Professor and Graduate Program Coordinator, 906-227-2488, Fax: 906-227-1658, E-mail: mromero@nmu.edu.
Website: http://www.nmu.edu/nursing/

Oakland University, Graduate Study and Lifelong Learning, School of Nursing, Program in Family Nurse Practitioner, Rochester, MI 48309-4401. Offers MSN, Certificate. *Accreditation:* AACN. *Students:* 31 full-time (all women), 66 part-time (63 women); includes 9 minority (5 Black or African American, non-Hispanic/Latino; 3 Asian, non-Hispanic/Latino; 1 Hispanic/Latino), 1 international. Average age 38. 95 applicants, 12% accepted, 11 enrolled. In 2013, 9 master's, 1 other advanced degree awarded. *Degree requirements:* For master's, thesis. *Entrance requirements:* For master's, GRE General Test, minimum GPA of 3.0. Additional exam requirements/recommendations for international students: Required—TOEFL (minimum score 550 paper-based). *Application deadline:* For fall admission, 8/1 for domestic students, 5/1 priority date for international students; for winter admission, 11/15 for domestic students, 9/1 priority date for international students. Applications are processed on a rolling basis. Application fee: $0. Electronic applications accepted. *Expenses:* Contact institution. *Financial support:* Federal Work-Study, institutionally sponsored loans, and tuition waivers (full) available. Financial award application deadline: 3/1; financial award applicants required to submit FAFSA. *Unit head:* Mary Bray, Graduate Program Coordinator, 248-370-4482. *Application contact:* Mary Bray, Graduate Program Coordinator, 248-370-4482.

Ohio University, Graduate College, College of Health Sciences and Professions, School of Nursing, Athens, OH 45701-2979. Offers acute care nurse practitioner (MSN); acute care nurse practitioner and family nurse practitioner (MSN); acute care nurse practitioner and nurse administrator (MSN); acute care nurse practitioner and nurse educator (MSN); family nurse practitioner (MSN); nurse administrator (MSN); nurse administrator and family nurse practitioner (MSN); nurse educator (MSN); nurse educator and family nurse practitioner (MSN); nurse educator and nurse administrator (MSN). *Accreditation:* AACN. *Degree requirements:* For master's, capstone project. *Entrance requirements:* For master's, GRE, bachelor's degree in nursing from an accredited college or university, minimum overall undergraduate GPA of 3.0, official transcripts, statement of goals and objectives, resume, 3 letters of recommendation. Additional exam requirements/recommendations for international students: Required—TOEFL (minimum score 550 paper-based; 80 iBT) or IELTS (minimum score 6.5). Electronic applications accepted.

Old Dominion University, College of Health Sciences, Doctor of Nursing Practice Program, Norfolk, VA 23529. Offers advance practice (DNP); nurse executive (DNP). Part-time programs available. Postbaccalaureate distance learning degree programs offered (minimal on-campus study). *Faculty:* 4 full-time (all women), 3 part-time/adjunct (2 women). *Students:* 15 full-time (13 women), 40 part-time (35 women); includes 13 minority (11 Black or African American, non-Hispanic/Latino; 2 Asian, non-Hispanic/Latino). Average age 46. 54 applicants, 85% accepted, 37 enrolled. In 2013, 29 doctorates awarded. *Degree requirements:* For doctorate, thesis/dissertation, capstone project. *Entrance requirements:* Additional exam requirements/recommendations for international students: Required—TOEFL. *Application deadline:* For spring admission, 9/15 priority date for domestic students. Applications are processed on a rolling basis. Application fee: $50. Electronic applications accepted. *Expenses:* Tuition, state resident: full-time $9888; part-time $412 per credit. Tuition, nonresident: full-time $25,152; part-time $1048 per credit. *Required fees:* $59 per semester. One-time fee: $50. *Financial support:* In 2013–14, 2 students received support, including 2 fellowships with full tuition reimbursements available (averaging $15,000 per year), 1 teaching assistantship with full tuition reimbursement available (averaging $15,000 per year); scholarships/grants, traineeships, and unspecified assistantships also available. *Faculty research:* Cultural competency, sleep disorders, self-care in HIV positive African-American women, ethical decision-making in pediatric cases. *Unit head:* Dr. Carolyn M. Rutledge, Director, 757-683-5009, Fax: 757-683-5253, E-mail: crutledg@odu.edu. *Application contact:* Sue Parker, Coordinator, Graduate Student Services, 757-683-4298, Fax: 757-683-5253, E-mail: sparker@odu.edu.
Website: http://www.odu.edu/dnp

Old Dominion University, College of Health Sciences, School of Nursing, Family Nurse Practitioner Emphasis, Norfolk, VA 23529. Offers MSN. Part-time programs available. Postbaccalaureate distance learning degree programs offered (minimal on-campus study). *Faculty:* 3 full-time (all women), 9 part-time/adjunct (all women). *Students:* 46 full-time (43 women), 56 part-time (53 women); includes 16 minority (12 Black or African American, non-Hispanic/Latino; 3 Asian, non-Hispanic/Latino; 1 Hispanic/Latino). Average age 36. 114 applicants, 48% accepted, 41 enrolled. In 2013, 48 master's awarded. *Degree requirements:* For master's, comprehensive exam. *Entrance requirements:* For master's, GRE or MAT. Additional exam requirements/recommendations for international students: Required—TOEFL. *Application deadline:* For fall admission, 3/1 for domestic students, 4/15 for international students. Application fee: $50. *Expenses:* Tuition, state resident: full-time $9888; part-time $412 per credit. Tuition, nonresident: full-time $25,152; part-time $1048 per credit. *Required fees:* $59 per semester. One-time fee: $50. *Financial support:* In 2013–14, 2 research assistantships with partial tuition reimbursements (averaging $10,000 per year) were awarded; career-related internships or fieldwork, scholarships/grants, and traineeships also available. Support available to part-time students. *Faculty research:* Military families, nurse practitioner student reaching modalities, gerontology, pediatrics, ethics. *Unit head:* Dr. Micah Scott, Graduate Program Director, 757-683-5255, E-mail: mscott@odu.edu. *Application contact:* Sue Parker, Coordinator, Graduate Student Services, 757-683-4298, Fax: 757-683-5253, E-mail: sparker@odu.edu.
Website: http://hs.odu.edu/nursing/academics/family_nurse/family_nurse.shtml

Oregon Health & Science University, School of Nursing, Family Nurse Practitioner Program, Portland, OR 97239-3098. Offers MN, MS, Post Master's Certificate.

Otterbein University, Department of Nursing, Westerville, OH 43081. Offers advanced practice nurse educator (Certificate); clinical nurse leader (MSN); family nurse practitioner (MSN, Certificate); nurse anesthesia (MSN, Certificate); nursing (DNP); nursing service administration (MSN). *Accreditation:* AACN; AANA/CANAEP. Part-time and evening/weekend programs available. Postbaccalaureate distance learning degree programs offered (minimal on-campus study). *Degree requirements:* For master's, comprehensive exam (for some programs), thesis (for some programs). *Entrance requirements:* For master's, 2 reference forms, resume; for Certificate, official transcripts, 2 reference forms, essay, resumé. Additional exam requirements/recommendations for international students: Required—TOEFL (minimum score 550 paper-based; 79 iBT). *Faculty research:* Patient education, women's health, trauma curriculum development, administration.

Pace University, College of Health Professions, Lienhard School of Nursing, New York, NY 10038. Offers family nurse practitioner (MS); nurse practitioner (Advanced Certificate); nursing education (MA); nursing leadership (Advanced Certificate); nursing practice (DNP). *Accreditation:* AACN. Part-time and evening/weekend programs available. Postbaccalaureate distance learning degree programs offered. *Faculty:* 13 full-time (12 women), 36 part-time/adjunct (29 women). *Students:* 3 full-time (2 women), 427 part-time (390 women); includes 202 minority (98 Black or African American, non-Hispanic/Latino; 2 American Indian or Alaska Native, non-Hispanic/Latino; 68 Asian, non-Hispanic/Latino; 28 Hispanic/Latino; 1 Native Hawaiian or other Pacific Islander, non-Hispanic/Latino; 5 Two or more races, non-Hispanic/Latino), 2 international. Average age 35. 274 applicants, 69% accepted, 131 enrolled. In 2013, 120 master's, 15 doctorates, 3 other advanced degrees awarded. *Degree requirements:* For master's, thesis. *Entrance requirements:* For master's, GRE General Test or MAT, RN license, resume, personal statement, 2 letters of recommendation, official transcripts; for doctorate, RN license, resume, personal statement, 2 letters of recommendation, official transcripts, accredited master's degree in nursing, minimum GPA of 3.3, state certification; for Advanced Certificate, RN license, completion of 2nd degree in nursing. Additional exam requirements/recommendations for international students: Required—TOEFL. *Application deadline:* For fall admission, 3/1 priority date for domestic and international students; for spring admission, 10/14 for domestic students, 9/14 for international students. Applications are processed on a rolling basis. Application fee: $70. Electronic applications accepted. *Expenses:* Contact institution. *Financial support:* Research assistantships, career-related internships or fieldwork, Federal Work-Study, and tuition waivers (partial) available. Support available to part-time students. Financial award applicants required to submit FAFSA. *Unit head:* Dr. Harriet Feldman, Dean, College of Health Professions, 914-773-3245, E-mail: hfeldman@pace.edu. *Application contact:* Susan Ford-Goldschein, Director of Graduate Admissions, 914-422-4283, Fax: 914-422-4287, E-mail: gradwp@pace.edu.
Website: http://www.pace.edu/lienhard

Pacific Lutheran University, Graduate Programs and Continuing Education, School of Nursing, Program in Family Nurse Practitioner, Tacoma, WA 98447. Offers MSN. Program designed for the working nurse; classes typically held Thursday evenings and all day Friday. *Accreditation:* AACN. *Faculty:* 5 full-time (4 women), 2 part-time/adjunct (1 woman). *Students:* 12 full-time (all women), 1 (woman) part-time; includes 1 minority (Hispanic/Latino). Average age 34. 16 applicants, 63% accepted, 8 enrolled. In 2013, 8 master's awarded. *Degree requirements:* For master's, thesis or alternative. *Entrance requirements:* For master's, GRE General Test, minimum undergraduate GPA of 3.0. Additional exam requirements/recommendations for international students: Required—TOEFL (minimum score 550 paper-based; 86 iBT). *Application deadline:* For fall admission, 11/15 priority date for domestic and international students. Applications are processed on a rolling basis. Application fee: $40. Electronic applications accepted. *Expenses:* Contact institution. *Financial support:* In 2013–14, 2 students received support. Fellowships, Federal Work-Study, and scholarships/grants available. Financial award application deadline: 3/1; financial award applicants required to submit FAFSA. *Unit head:* Dr. Teri Woo, Associate Dean of Graduate Nursing Programs/Associate Professor of Nursing, 253-535-7686, E-mail: gradnurs@plu.edu. *Application contact:* Rachel Christopherson, Director, Graduate Admission, 253-535-8570, Fax: 253-536-5136, E-mail: gradadmission@plu.edu.

Point Loma Nazarene University, School of Nursing, San Diego, CA 92106-2899. Offers adult/gerontology nursing (MSN); family/individual health (MSN); general nursing (MSN); nursing (Post-MSN Certificate); pediatric nursing (MSN); psychiatric mental health (MSN). *Accreditation:* AACN. Part-time programs available. *Faculty:* 9 full-time (8 women). *Students:* 1 (woman) full-time, 82 part-time (70 women); includes 43 minority (9 Black or African American, non-Hispanic/Latino; 1 American Indian or Alaska Native, non-Hispanic/Latino; 26 Asian, non-Hispanic/Latino; 3 Hispanic/Latino; 3 Native Hawaiian or other Pacific Islander, non-Hispanic/Latino; 1 Two or more races, non-Hispanic/Latino). Average age 36. 32 applicants, 94% accepted, 24 enrolled. In 2013, 26 master's awarded. *Entrance requirements:* For master's, NCLEX, ADN or BSN in nursing, interview, RN license, essay, letters of recommendation, interview. *Application deadline:* For fall admission, 7/18 priority date for domestic students; for spring admission, 10/26 priority date for domestic students; for summer admission, 3/23 priority date for domestic students. Applications are processed on a rolling basis. Application fee: $50. *Expenses:* *Tuition:* Full-time $6900; part-time $567 per credit hour. *Financial support:* Applicants required to submit FAFSA. *Unit head:* Dr. Barb Taylor, Dean of the School of Nursing, 619-849-2766, E-mail: bataylor@pointloma.edu. *Application contact:* Laura Leinweber, Director of Graduate Admissions, 866-692-4723, E-mail: lauraleinweber@pointloma.edu.
Website: http://www.pointloma.edu/discover/graduate-school/graduate-programs/master-science-nursing-and-post-msn-certification

Prairie View A&M University, College of Nursing, Houston, TX 77030. Offers family nurse practitioner (MSN); nursing administration (MSN); nursing education (MSN). Part-time programs available. *Faculty:* 9 full-time (8 women), 13 part-time/adjunct (11 women). *Students:* 74 full-time (61 women), 107 part-time (99 women); includes 65 minority (63 Black or African American, non-Hispanic/Latino; 2 Hispanic/Latino), 4 international. Average age 37. 121 applicants, 42% accepted, 45 enrolled. In 2013, 46 master's awarded. *Degree requirements:* For master's, comprehensive exam, thesis. *Entrance requirements:* For master's, MAT or GRE, BS in nursing; 2 years of experience as a registered nurse; 1 course each in statistics, basic health and assessment. *Application deadline:* For fall admission, 7/1 priority date for domestic students, 7/1 for international students; for spring admission, 11/1 priority date for domestic students, 11/1 for international students. Applications are processed on a rolling basis. Application fee: $50. *Expenses:* Tuition, state resident: full-time $3776; part-time $209.77 per credit hour. Tuition, nonresident: full-time $10,183; part-time $565.77 per credit hour. *Required fees:* $2037; $446.50 per credit hour. *Financial support:* In 2013–14, 17 students received support. Career-related internships or fieldwork, Federal Work-Study, institutionally sponsored loans, scholarships/grants, and traineeships available. Support available to part-time students. Financial award application deadline: 4/1; financial award applicants required to submit FAFSA. *Faculty research:* Software development and violence prevention, health promotion and disease prevention. *Total annual research expenditures:* $350,000. *Unit head:* Dr. Betty N. Adams, Dean, 713-797-7009, Fax: 713-797-7013, E-mail: bnadams@pvamu.edu. *Application contact:* Dr. Forest Smith, Director of Student Services and Admissions, 713-797-7031, Fax: 713-797-7012, E-mail: fdsmith@pvamu.edu.
Website: http://www.pvamu.edu/nursing/

Purdue University Calumet, Graduate Studies Office, School of Nursing, Hammond, IN 46323-2094. Offers adult health clinical nurse specialist (MS); critical care clinical nurse specialist (MS); family nurse practitioner (MS); nurse executive (MS). Part-time programs available. Postbaccalaureate distance learning degree programs offered (minimal on-campus study). *Entrance requirements:* For master's, BSN. Additional exam requirements/recommendations for international students: Required—TOEFL. Electronic applications accepted. *Faculty research:* Adult health, cardiovascular and pulmonary nursing.

Queen's University at Kingston, School of Graduate Studies, Faculty of Health Sciences, School of Nursing, Kingston, ON K7L 3N6, Canada. Offers health and chronic illness (M Sc); nurse scientist (PhD); primary health care nurse practitioner (Certificate); women's and children's health (M Sc). *Degree requirements:* For master's, thesis. *Entrance requirements:* For master's, RN license. Additional exam requirements/recommendations for international students: Required—TOEFL. *Faculty research:* Women and children's health, health and chronic illness.

Quinnipiac University, School of Nursing, Family Nurse Practitioner Track, Hamden, CT 06518-1940. Offers MSN, DNP. Part-time programs available. *Faculty:* 14 full-time (13 women), 5 part-time/adjunct (3 women). *Students:* 19 full-time (all women), 32 part-time (30 women); includes 9 minority (4 Black or African American, non-Hispanic/Latino; 3 Asian, non-Hispanic/Latino; 2 Hispanic/Latino), 1 international. 30 applicants, 80% accepted, 17 enrolled. In 2013, 25 master's awarded. *Degree requirements:* For master's, thesis optional, clinical practicum. *Entrance requirements:* For master's, RN license, minimum GPA of 3.0. Additional exam requirements/recommendations for international students: Required—TOEFL (minimum score 575 paper-based; 90 iBT), IELTS (minimum score 6.5). *Application deadline:* For fall admission, 6/1 priority date for domestic students, 4/30 priority date for international students; for spring admission, 9/15 for international students. Applications are processed on a rolling basis. Application fee: $45. Electronic applications accepted. *Expenses: Tuition:* Part-time $920 per credit. *Required fees:* $37 per credit. *Financial support:* In 2013–14, 4 students received support. Career-related internships or fieldwork, Federal Work-Study, scholarships/grants, tuition waivers (partial), and unspecified assistantships available. Support available to part-time students. Financial award application deadline: 6/1. *Unit head:* Dr. Lynn Price, Program Director, E-mail: lynn.price@quinnipiac.edu. *Application contact:* Office of Graduate Admissions, 800-462-1944, Fax: 203-582-3443, E-mail: graduate@quinnipiac.edu.
Website: http://www.quinnipiac.edu/gradnursing

Regis College, School of Nursing, Science and Health Professions, Weston, MA 02493. Offers applied behavior analysis (MS); biomedical sciences (MS); health administration (MS); nurse practitioner (Certificate); nursing (MS, DNP); nursing education (Certificate). Part-time and evening/weekend programs available. *Degree requirements:* For master's, thesis. *Entrance requirements:* For master's, GRE General Test or MAT, minimum GPA of 3.0; for doctorate, MAT or GRE if GPA from master's lower than 3.5. Additional exam requirements/recommendations for international students: Required—TOEFL (minimum score 550 paper-based). Electronic applications accepted. *Faculty research:* Health policy, education, aging, job satisfaction, psychiatric nursing, critical thinking.

Research College of Nursing, Nursing Program, Kansas City, MO 64132. Offers adult-gerontological nurse practitioner (MSN); clinical nurse leader (MSN); executive practice and healthcare leadership (MSN); family nurse practitioner (MSN); nurse educator (MSN); nursing (MSN). *Accreditation:* AACN. Part-time programs available. Postbaccalaureate distance learning degree programs offered (no on-campus study). *Faculty:* 9 full-time (all women), 5 part-time/adjunct (2 women). *Students:* 19 full-time (18 women), 101 part-time (94 women). *Degree requirements:* For master's, research project. *Entrance requirements:* For master's, 3 letters of recommendation, official transcripts, resume. Additional exam requirements/recommendations for international students: Required—TOEFL (minimum score 550 paper-based), TWE. *Application deadline:* Applications are processed on a rolling basis. Application fee: $50. *Expenses: Tuition:* Part-time $445 per credit hour. *Required fees:* $25 per credit hour. Part-time tuition and fees vary according to course load. *Financial support:* Applicants required to submit FAFSA. *Unit head:* Dr. Nancy O. DeBasio, President and Dean, 816-995-2815, Fax: 816-995-2817, E-mail: nancy.debasio@researchcollege.edu. *Application contact:* Leslie Mendenhall, Director of Transfer and Graduate Recruitment, 816-995-2820, Fax: 816-995-2813, E-mail: leslie.mendenhall@researchcollege.edu.

Rivier University, School of Graduate Studies, Division of Nursing, Nashua, NH 03060. Offers adult psychiatric/mental health practitioner (MS); family nurse practitioner (MS); nursing education (MS). Part-time and evening/weekend programs available. *Entrance requirements:* For master's, GRE, MAT. Electronic applications accepted.

Rocky Mountain University of Health Professions, Doctor of Nursing Practice Program, Provo, UT 84606. Offers DNP. *Faculty:* 2 full-time (both women), 10 part-time/adjunct (8 women). *Students:* 34 full-time (24 women), 16 part-time (15 women); includes 20 minority (15 Black or African American, non-Hispanic/Latino; 3 Asian, non-Hispanic/Latino; 2 Hispanic/Latino). Average age 47. In 2013, 18 doctorates awarded. Application fee: $150. *Unit head:* Dr. Marie-Eileen Onieal, Program Director, 801-375-5125, E-mail: monieal@rmuohp.edu. *Application contact:* Bryce Greenberg, Director of Admissions, 801-734-6832, Fax: 801-734-6833, E-mail: bgreenberg@rmuohp.edu.
Website: http://rmuohp.edu/academics/nursing/

Rush University, College of Nursing, Department of Community, Systems, and Mental Health Nursing, Chicago, IL 60612. Offers advanced public health nursing (DNP); family nurse practitioner (DNP); leadership to enhance population health outcomes (DNP); nursing science (PhD); psychiatric mental health nurse practitioner (DNP, Post-Graduate Certificate); systems leadership (DNP). *Accreditation:* AACN. Part-time programs available. Postbaccalaureate distance learning degree programs offered (minimal on-campus study). *Students:* 190 part-time (174 women); includes 41 minority (13 Black or African American, non-Hispanic/Latino; 4 American Indian or Alaska Native, non-Hispanic/Latino; 12 Asian, non-Hispanic/Latino; 11 Hispanic/Latino; 1 Native Hawaiian or other Pacific Islander, non-Hispanic/Latino). Average age 35. 170 applicants, 77% accepted, 118 enrolled. *Degree requirements:* For doctorate, capstone project (for DNP); dissertation (for PhD). *Entrance requirements:* For doctorate, GRE General Test (waived for DNP if cumulative GPA is 3.25 or greater, nursing GPA is 3.0 or greater, or a completed graduate program GPA is 3.5 or greater), interview, 3 letters of recommendation, personal statement, current resume; for Post-Graduate Certificate, interview, 3 letters of recommendation, personal statement, current resume. Additional exam requirements/recommendations for international students: Required—TOEFL. *Application deadline:* For fall admission, 1/2 for domestic students; for winter admission, 10/15 for domestic students; for spring admission, 8/4 for domestic students. Applications are processed on a rolling basis. Application fee: $100. Electronic applications accepted. *Financial support:* Fellowships, research assistantships, teaching assistantships, Federal Work-Study, scholarships/grants, traineeships, and health care benefits available. Support available to part-time students. Financial award application deadline: 3/1; financial award applicants required to submit FAFSA. *Faculty research:* Reduction of health disparities; evidence-based interventions for caregivers; patient-centered quality assessment of psychiatric inpatient environments; digital delivery of a parent-training program for urban, low-income parents; patient-centered predictors and outcomes of inter-professional care coordination. *Total annual research expenditures:* $3.8 million. *Unit head:* Dr. Arlene Miller, Chairperson, 312-942-7117, E-mail: arlene_miller@rush.edu. *Application contact:* Jennifer Thorndyke, Admissions Specialist, 312-563-7526, E-mail: jennifer_thorndyke@rush.edu.
Website: http://www.rushu.rush.edu/servlet/Satellite?c=RushUnivLevel1Page&cid=1204497838852&pagename=Rush%2FRushUnivLevel1Page%2FLevel_1_College_Home_Page

Rutgers, The State University of New Jersey, Newark, Rutgers School of Nursing, Newark, NJ 07107-3001. Offers adult health (MSN); adult occupational health (MSN); advanced practice nursing (MSN, Post Master's Certificate); family nurse practitioner (MSN); nurse anesthesia (MSN); nursing (MSN); nursing informatics (MSN); urban health (PhD); women's health practitioner (MSN). *Accreditation:* AANA/CANAEP. Part-time programs available. *Entrance requirements:* For master's, GRE, RN license; basic life support, statistics, and health assessment experience. Additional exam requirements/recommendations for international students: Required—TOEFL. Electronic applications accepted. *Expenses:* Contact institution. *Faculty research:* HIV/AIDS, diabetes education, learned helplessness, nursing science, psychoeducation.

Sacred Heart University, Graduate Programs, College of Health Professions, Department of Nursing, Fairfield, CT 06825-1000. Offers clinical nurse leader (MSN); clinical practice in health care (DNP); family nurse practitioner (MSN); leadership in health care (DNP); nursing (DN Sc); nursing educator (MSN); patient care services administration (MSN). *Accreditation:* AACN. Part-time and evening/weekend programs available. Postbaccalaureate distance learning degree programs offered (no on-campus study). *Faculty:* 7 full-time (all women), 5 part-time/adjunct (all women). *Students:* 34 full-time (32 women), 645 part-time (595 women); includes 117 minority (50 Black or African American, non-Hispanic/Latino; 1 American Indian or Alaska Native, non-Hispanic/Latino; 26 Asian, non-Hispanic/Latino; 29 Hispanic/Latino; 1 Native Hawaiian or other Pacific Islander, non-Hispanic/Latino; 10 Two or more races, non-Hispanic/Latino). Average age 39. 110 applicants, 58% accepted, 46 enrolled. In 2013, 67 master's, 11 doctorates awarded. *Entrance requirements:* For master's, minimum GPA of 3.0, BSN or RN plus BS (for MSN); for doctorate, minimum GPA of 3.0, MSN or BSN plus MS (for DNP). Additional exam requirements/recommendations for international students: Required—PTE; Recommended—TOEFL (minimum score 570 paper-based; 80 iBT), IELTS (minimum score 6.5). *Application deadline:* Applications are processed on a rolling basis. Application fee: $60. Electronic applications accepted. *Expenses:* Contact institution. *Financial support:* Career-related internships or fieldwork and institutionally sponsored loans available. Support available to part-time students. Financial award applicants required to submit FAFSA. *Unit head:* Dr. Sue DeNisco, Chair, 203-365-7661, Fax: 203-365-7662, E-mail: deniscos@sacredheart.edu. *Application contact:* Kathy Dilks, Executive Director of Graduate Admissions, 203-365-4716, Fax: 203-365-4732, E-mail: gradstudies@sacredheart.edu.
Website: http://www.sacredheart.edu/graduate/nursing/

Sage Graduate School, School of Health Sciences, Department of Nursing, Program in Family Nurse Practitioner, Troy, NY 12180-4115. Offers MS, Post Master's Certificate. *Accreditation:* AACN. Part-time and evening/weekend programs available. *Faculty:* 5 full-time (all women), 9 part-time/adjunct (all women). *Students:* 16 full-time (all women), 60 part-time (55 women); includes 10 minority (4 Black or African American, non-Hispanic/Latino; 1 American Indian or Alaska Native, non-Hispanic/Latino; 2 Asian, non-Hispanic/Latino; 3 Hispanic/Latino), 1 international. Average age 35. 67 applicants, 46% accepted, 19 enrolled. In 2013, 14 master's, 3 other advanced degrees awarded. *Degree requirements:* For master's, thesis or alternative. *Entrance requirements:* For master's, BS in nursing, minimum GPA of 2.75, resume, 2 letters of recommendation. Additional exam requirements/recommendations for international students: Required—TOEFL (minimum score 550 paper-based). *Application deadline:* Applications are processed on a rolling basis. Application fee: $40. *Expenses: Tuition:* Full-time $11,880; part-time $660 per credit hour. *Financial support:* Fellowships, research assistantships, teaching assistantships, Federal Work-Study, scholarships/grants, and unspecified assistantships available. Support available to part-time students. Financial award application deadline: 3/1; financial award applicants required to submit FAFSA. *Unit head:* Dr. Esther Haskevitz, Dean, School of Health Sciences, 518-244-2296, Fax: 518-244-4571, E-mail: haskve@sage.edu. *Application contact:* Madeline Cafiero, Director, Graduate Programs in Nursing, 518-244-4574, Fax: 518-244-2009, E-mail: cafiem@sage.edu.

Saginaw Valley State University, Crystal M. Lange College of Nursing and Health Sciences, Program in Nurse Practitioner, University Center, MI 48710. Offers MSN, DNP. *Accreditation:* AACN. Part-time and evening/weekend programs available. Postbaccalaureate distance learning degree programs offered (minimal on-campus study). *Students:* 10 full-time (9 women), 64 part-time (56 women); includes 6 minority (4 Black or African American, non-Hispanic/Latino; 1 Asian, non-Hispanic/Latino; 1 Hispanic/Latino), 1 international. Average age 36. 3 applicants, 67% accepted, 12 enrolled. In 2013, 25 master's awarded. *Degree requirements:* For master's, thesis optional. *Entrance requirements:* For master's, GRE, minimum GPA of 3.0, license to practice nursing in MI; for doctorate, GRE, minimum GPA of 3.3, college chemistry with minimum C grade, college statistics with minimum B grade, employed as RN with current license in MI. Additional exam requirements/recommendations for international students: Required—TOEFL (minimum score 580 paper-based; 92 iBT). *Application deadline:* For fall admission, 7/15 for international students; for winter admission, 11/15 for international students; for spring admission, 4/15 for international students. Applications are processed on a rolling basis. Application fee: $30 ($80 for international students). Electronic applications accepted. *Expenses:* Tuition, state resident: full-time $8933; part-time $496.30 per credit hour. Tuition, nonresident: full-time $16,806; part-time $933.65 per credit hour. *Required fees:* $263; $14.60 per credit hour. Tuition and fees vary according to degree level. *Financial support:* Federal Work-Study and scholarships/grants available. Support available to part-time students. Financial award application deadline: 4/1; financial award applicants required to submit FAFSA. *Unit head:* Dr. Karen Brown-Fackler, Coordinator, 989-964-7112, Fax: 989-964-4925, E-mail: kmbrown4@svsu.edu. *Application contact:* Jenna Briggs, Director, Graduate and International Admissions, 989-964-6096, Fax: 989-964-2788, E-mail: gradadm@svsu.edu.

Saint Francis Medical Center College of Nursing, Graduate Programs, Peoria, IL 61603-3783. Offers adult gerontology (MSN); clinical nurse leader (MSN); family nurse practitioner (MSN); family psychiatric mental health nurse practitioner (MSN); neonatal nurse practitioner (MSN); nurse clinician (Post-Graduate Certificate); nurse educator (MSN, Post-Graduate Certificate); nursing (DNP); nursing management leadership (MSN). Part-time programs available. Postbaccalaureate distance learning degree programs offered (minimal on-campus study). *Faculty:* 4 full-time (all women), 4 part-time/adjunct (all women). *Students:* 13 full-time (12 women), 268 part-time (245 women); includes 17 minority (10 Black or African American, non-Hispanic/Latino; 2 Asian, non-Hispanic/Latino; 5 Hispanic/Latino), 2 international. Average age 37. 115 applicants, 89% accepted, 42 enrolled. In 2013, 17 master's, 2 doctorates awarded. *Degree requirements:* For master's, research experience, portfolio, practicum; for doctorate, practicum hours. *Entrance requirements:* For master's, nursing research, health assessment, graduate course work in statistics, RN license; for doctorate, master's degree in nursing, professional portfolio, graduate statistics, transcripts, RN license. Additional exam requirements/recommendations for international students:

Required—TOEFL. *Application deadline:* For fall admission, 6/1 priority date for domestic and international students; for spring admission, 11/15 priority date for domestic and international students. Applications are processed on a rolling basis. Application fee: $50. Electronic applications accepted. *Expenses: Tuition:* Full-time $6336; part-time $528 per semester hour. *Required fees:* $436. *Financial support:* In 2013–14, 8 students received support. Scholarships/grants and tuition waivers (partial) available. Support available to part-time students. Financial award application deadline: 6/15; financial award applicants required to submit FAFSA. *Faculty research:* Outcome and curriculum planning, health promotion, NCLEX-RN results, decision-making program evaluation. *Unit head:* Dr. Patti A. Stockert, President of the College, 309-655-4124, Fax: 309-624-8973, E-mail: patricia.a.stockert@osfhealthcare.org. *Application contact:* Dr. Janice F. Boundy, Dean, 309-655-2230, Fax: 309-624-8973, E-mail: jan.f.boundy@osfhealthcare.org.
Website: http://www.sfmccon.edu/graduate-programs/

St. John Fisher College, Wegmans School of Nursing, Advanced Practice Nursing Program, Rochester, NY 14618-3597. Offers advanced practice nursing (MS); clinical nurse specialist (Certificate); family nurse practitioner (Certificate); nurse educator (Certificate). *Accreditation:* AACN. Part-time and evening/weekend programs available. *Faculty:* 13 full-time (12 women). *Students:* 2 full-time (1 woman), 114 part-time (104 women); includes 15 minority (7 Black or African American, non-Hispanic/Latino; 4 Asian, non-Hispanic/Latino; 4 Hispanic/Latino), 2 international. Average age 33. 61 applicants, 49% accepted, 19 enrolled. In 2013, 23 master's awarded. *Degree requirements:* For master's, clinical practice, project; for Certificate, clinical practice. *Entrance requirements:* For master's, BSN; undergraduate course work in statistics, health assessment, and nursing research; current New York State RN license; 2 letters of recommendation; current resume. Additional exam requirements/recommendations for international students: Required—TOEFL (minimum score 575 paper-based; 80 iBT). *Application deadline:* Applications are processed on a rolling basis. Application fee: $30. Electronic applications accepted. *Expenses: Tuition:* Part-time $795 per credit hour. *Required fees:* $10 per credit hour. Tuition and fees vary according to course load, degree level and program. *Financial support:* In 2013–14, 29 students received support. Scholarships/grants and traineeships available. Financial award applicants required to submit FAFSA. *Faculty research:* Chronic illness, pediatric injury, women's health, public health policy, health care teams. *Unit head:* Dr. Cynthia McCloskey, Graduate Director, 585-385-8471, Fax: 585-385-8466, E-mail: cmccloskey@sjfc.edu. *Application contact:* Jose Perales, Director of Graduate Admissions, 585-385-8067, E-mail: jperales@sjfc.edu.

Saint Joseph's College of Maine, Master of Science in Nursing Program, Standish, ME 04084. Offers administration (MSN); education (MSN); family nurse practitioner (MSN); nursing administration and leadership (Certificate); nursing and health care education (Certificate). *Accreditation:* AACN. Part-time programs available. Postbaccalaureate distance learning degree programs offered (no on-campus study). *Entrance requirements:* For master's, MAT. Electronic applications accepted.

Samford University, Ida V. Moffett School of Nursing, Birmingham, AL 35229. Offers administration (DNP); advanced practice (DNP); family nurse practitioner (MSN); health systems management and leadership (MSN); nurse anesthesia (MSN); nurse educator (MSN). *Accreditation:* AACN; AANA/CANAEP (one or more programs are accredited). Part-time programs available. Postbaccalaureate distance learning degree programs offered (minimal on-campus study). *Faculty:* 16 full-time (all women), 4 part-time/adjunct (2 women). *Students:* 249 full-time (191 women), 25 part-time (17 women); includes 48 minority (23 Black or African American, non-Hispanic/Latino; 1 American Indian or Alaska Native, non-Hispanic/Latino; 13 Asian, non-Hispanic/Latino; 7 Hispanic/Latino; 4 Two or more races, non-Hispanic/Latino), 1 international. Average age 36. 89 applicants, 53% accepted, 45 enrolled. In 2013, 107 master's, 29 doctorates awarded. *Degree requirements:* For master's and doctorate, capstone project with oral presentation. *Entrance requirements:* For master's, MAT; GRE (for nurse anesthesia). Additional exam requirements/recommendations for international students: Required—TOEFL (minimum score 550 paper-based; 80 iBT). *Application deadline:* For fall admission, 6/1 priority date for domestic and international students; for spring admission, 9/1 priority date for domestic and international students. Application fee: $65. Electronic applications accepted. *Expenses:* Contact institution. *Financial support:* In 2013–14, 48 students received support. Institutionally sponsored loans, scholarships/grants, and traineeships available. Financial award application deadline: 3/1; financial award applicants required to submit FAFSA. *Faculty research:* Issues in rural health care, vulnerable populations, genetics and disabilities in pediatrics, geriatrics, parish nursing research, interprofessional education, global health disparities. *Unit head:* Dr. Nena F. Sanders, Dean, 205-726-2629, E-mail: nfsander@samford.edu. *Application contact:* Allyson Maddox, Director of Graduate Student Services, 205-726-2047, Fax: 205-726-4179, E-mail: amaddox@samford.edu.
Website: http://samford.edu/nursing

Samuel Merritt University, School of Nursing, Oakland, CA 94609-3108. Offers case management (MSN); family nurse practitioner (MSN, Certificate); nurse anesthetist (MSN, Certificate); nursing (MSN, DNP). *Accreditation:* AACN; AANA/CANAEP (one or more programs are accredited). Part-time and evening/weekend programs available. *Degree requirements:* For master's, thesis or alternative. *Entrance requirements:* For master's, minimum GPA of 2.5 in science, 3.0 overall; previous course work in statistics; current RN license. Additional exam requirements/recommendations for international students: Required—TOEFL. *Faculty research:* Gerontology, community health, maternal-child health, sexually transmitted diseases, substance abuse, oncology.

San Francisco State University, Division of Graduate Studies, College of Health and Social Sciences, School of Nursing, San Francisco, CA 94132-1722. Offers adult acute care (MS); clinical nurse specialist (MS); community/public health nursing (MS); family nurse practitioner (MS, Certificate); nursing administration (MS); nursing education (MS); pediatrics (MS); women's health (MS). *Accreditation:* AACN. Part-time programs available. *Application deadline:* Applications are processed on a rolling basis. *Financial support:* Career-related internships or fieldwork available. *Unit head:* Dr. Mary-Ann van Dam, Director, 415-338-1802, E-mail: vandam@sfsu.edu. *Application contact:* Robert Strachan, Admission and Student Services Coordinator, 415-338-1802, E-mail: strachan@sfsu.edu.
Website: http://nursing.sfsu.edu

Seattle Pacific University, MS in Nursing Program, Seattle, WA 98119-1997. Offers administration (MSN); adult/gerontology nurse practitioner (MSN); clinical nurse specialist (MSN); family nurse practitioner (MSN, Certificate); informatics (MSN); nurse educator (MSN). *Accreditation:* AACN. Part-time programs available. *Students:* 9 full-time (7 women), 37 part-time (33 women); includes 8 minority (2 Black or African American, non-Hispanic/Latino; 5 Asian, non-Hispanic/Latino; 1 Hispanic/Latino), 1 international. Average age 41. 70 applicants, 30% accepted, 21 enrolled. In 2013, 27 master's awarded. *Degree requirements:* For master's, thesis. *Entrance requirements:* For master's, personal statement, transcripts, undergraduate nursing degree, proof of undergraduate statistics course with minimum GPA of 2.0, 2 recommendations. *Application deadline:* For fall admission, 1/15 priority date for domestic students; for spring admission, 1/15 for domestic students. Applications are processed on a rolling basis. Application fee: $50. Electronic applications accepted. *Expenses:* Contact institution. *Financial support:* Fellowships and scholarships/grants available. Financial award applicants required to submit FAFSA. *Unit head:* Dr. Susan Casey, Associate Dean, 206-281-2649, E-mail: caseys@spu.edu.
Website: http://www.spu.edu/depts/health-sciences/grad/index.asp

Seattle University, College of Nursing, Program in Advanced Practice Nursing Immersion, Seattle, WA 98122-1090. Offers adult/gerontological nurse practitioner (MSN); advanced community public health nursing (MSN); family nurse practitioner (MSN); family psychiatric mental health nurse practitioner (MSN); nurse midwifery (MSN). *Faculty:* 17 full-time (15 women), 9 part-time/adjunct (6 women). *Students:* 109 full-time (94 women), 6 part-time (5 women); includes 25 minority (3 Black or African American, non-Hispanic/Latino; 11 Asian, non-Hispanic/Latino; 2 Hispanic/Latino; 9 Two or more races, non-Hispanic/Latino). Average age 31. In 2013, 48 master's awarded. *Degree requirements:* For master's, thesis or scholarly project. *Entrance requirements:* For master's, GRE, bachelor's degree, minimum GPA of 3.0, professional resume, two recommendations, letter of intent. Additional exam requirements/recommendations for international students: Required—TOEFL (minimum score 92 iBT), IELTS. *Application deadline:* For fall admission, 12/1 for domestic and international students. Application fee: $55. Electronic applications accepted. *Financial support:* In 2013–14, 3 students received support. Scholarships/grants and traineeships available. Financial award applicants required to submit FAFSA. *Unit head:* Dr. Janiece DeSocio, Interim Dean, 206-296-5660, E-mail: desocioj@seattleu.edu. *Application contact:* Janet Shandley, Associate Dean of Graduate Admissions, 206-296-5900, Fax: 206-298-5656, E-mail: grad_admissions@seattleu.edu.
Website: http://www.seattleu.edu/nursing/msn/apni/

Shenandoah University, Eleanor Wade Custer School of Nursing, Winchester, VA 22601-5195. Offers family nurse practitioner (Certificate); health informatics (Certificate); nursing (MSN, DNP); nursing education (Certificate); psychiatric mental health nurse practitioner (Certificate). *Accreditation:* AACN; ACNM/ACME. Part-time programs available. *Faculty:* 14 full-time (all women), 7 part-time/adjunct (6 women). *Students:* 39 full-time (35 women), 76 part-time (74 women); includes 23 minority (13 Black or African American, non-Hispanic/Latino; 2 American Indian or Alaska Native, non-Hispanic/Latino; 4 Asian, non-Hispanic/Latino; 4 Hispanic/Latino), 1 international. Average age 38. 56 applicants, 77% accepted, 32 enrolled. In 2013, 28 master's, 4 doctorates, 11 other advanced degrees awarded. *Degree requirements:* For master's, research project, clinical hours; for doctorate, scholarly project, clinical hours; for Certificate, clinical hours. *Entrance requirements:* For master's, United States RN license; minimum GPA of 3.0; appropriate clinical experience; curriculum vitae; 3 letters of recommendation; for doctorate, MSN, minimum GPA of 3.0, 3 letters of recommendation, essay, interview, BSN; for Certificate, MSN, minimum GPA of 3.0, 2 letters of recommendation, minimum of one year (2,080 hours) clinical nursing experience, interview. Additional exam requirements/recommendations for international students: Required—TOEFL (minimum score 610 paper-based; 83 iBT), IELTS (minimum score 7.5). *Application deadline:* For fall admission, 5/1 priority date for domestic and international students; for spring admission, 11/1 priority date for domestic and international students. Applications are processed on a rolling basis. Application fee: $30. Electronic applications accepted. *Expenses: Tuition:* Full-time $19,176; part-time $799 per credit. *Required fees:* $365 per term. Tuition and fees vary according to course level, course load and program. *Financial support:* In 2013–14, 13 students received support, including 3 teaching assistantships with partial tuition reimbursements available (averaging $4,912 per year); career-related internships or fieldwork, scholarships/grants, and unspecified assistantships also available. Support available to part-time students. Financial award application deadline: 3/15; financial award applicants required to submit FAFSA. *Faculty research:* Moral reasoning in nurses, improving health care access to underserved rural women, screening for depression and anxiety in the obese in a rural free clinic, health care outcomes among patients in a free clinic setting cared for by nurse practitioners, effects of depression on diabetes as evidenced by the relationship between the patient healthcare questionnaire (PHQ-9) scores and the patient's glycohemoglobin (HbA1c), policy development, research on a Virginia Nurses Hall of Fame inductee. *Unit head:* Dr. Kathryn Ganske, Director, 540-678-4374, Fax: 540-665-5519, E-mail: kganske@su.edu. *Application contact:* Andrew Woodall, Executive Director of Recruitment and Admissions, 540-665-4581, Fax: 540-665-4627, E-mail: admit@su.edu.
Website: http://www.nursing.su.edu

Sonoma State University, School of Science and Technology, Master's in Nursing Program, Rohnert Park, CA 94928. Offers family nurse practitioner (MSN). Part-time programs available. *Faculty:* 3 full-time (all women), 3 part-time/adjunct (all women). *Students:* 20 full-time (15 women), 111 part-time (91 women); includes 44 minority (6 Black or African American, non-Hispanic/Latino; 3 American Indian or Alaska Native, non-Hispanic/Latino; 22 Asian, non-Hispanic/Latino; 8 Hispanic/Latino; 5 Two or more races, non-Hispanic/Latino), 2 international. Average age 36. 91 applicants, 77% accepted, 21 enrolled. In 2013, 51 master's awarded. *Degree requirements:* For master's, comprehensive exam, thesis or alternative, oral exams. *Entrance requirements:* For master's, GRE General Test, BSN, minimum GPA of 3.0, course work in statistics, physical assessment, RN license. Additional exam requirements/recommendations for international students: Required—TOEFL (minimum score 500 paper-based). *Application deadline:* For fall admission, 11/30 for domestic students. Application fee: $55. *Expenses:* Tuition, state resident: full-time $8500. Tuition, nonresident: full-time $12,964. *Required fees:* $1762. *Financial support:* Traineeships available. Financial award applicants required to submit FAFSA. *Faculty research:* Neonatal ethics. *Unit head:* Dr. Deborah A. Roberts, Chair, 707-664-2465, E-mail: deborah.roberts@sonoma.edu. *Application contact:* Dr. Wendy Smith, Director, 707-664-2276, E-mail: wendy.smith@sonoma.edu.
Website: http://www.sonoma.edu/nursing/

Southeastern Louisiana University, College of Nursing and Health Sciences, School of Nursing, Hammond, LA 70402. Offers adult psychiatric/mental health nurse practitioner/clinical nurse specialist (MSN); education (MSN); nurse executive (MSN); nurse practice (DNP); nurse practitioner (MSN). *Accreditation:* AACN. Part-time and evening/weekend programs available. *Faculty:* 14 full-time (13 women), 5 part-time/adjunct (4 women). *Students:* 21 full-time (19 women), 138 part-time (121 women); includes 27 minority (17 Black or African American, non-Hispanic/Latino; 4 Asian, non-Hispanic/Latino; 5 Hispanic/Latino; 1 Two or more races, non-Hispanic/Latino). Average age 34. 72 applicants, 68% accepted, 19 enrolled. In 2013, 29 master's awarded. *Degree requirements:* For master's, thesis. *Entrance requirements:* For master's, GRE (verbal and quantitative), baccalaureate degree in nursing from accredited undergraduate nursing program; minimum GPA of 2.7; all transcripts from undergraduate school and any work attempted at the graduate level; curriculum vitae; valid Louisiana Registered Nurse license; letters of recommendation; letter of intent/statement of purpose. Additional exam requirements/recommendations for international students: Required—TOEFL (minimum score 500 paper-based; 61 iBT). *Application deadline:* For fall admission, 7/15 priority date for domestic students, 6/1 priority date for international students; for spring admission, 12/1 priority date for domestic students, 10/1 priority date for international students. Applications are processed on a rolling basis. Application fee: $20 ($30 for international students). Electronic applications accepted. *Expenses:* Tuition, state resident: full-time $5047. Tuition, nonresident: full-time

$17,066. *Required fees:* $1213. Tuition and fees vary according to degree level. *Financial support:* Federal Work-Study, institutionally sponsored loans, scholarships/grants, traineeships, and unspecified assistantships available. Support available to part-time students. Financial award application deadline: 5/1; financial award applicants required to submit FAFSA. *Faculty research:* Gender issues, LGBT issues, occupational health/safety, accelerated students, caring development. *Total annual research expenditures:* $103,409. *Unit head:* Dr. Lorinda J. Sealey, Graduate Nursing Program Director, 985-549-5045, Fax: 985-549-5087, E-mail: vjohnson@selu.edu. *Application contact:* Sandra Meyers, Graduate Admissions Analyst, 985-549-5620, Fax: 985-549-5632, E-mail: admissions@selu.edu.
Website: http://www.selu.edu/acad_research/depts/nurs

Southern Adventist University, School of Nursing, Collegedale, TN 37315-0370. Offers acute care nurse practitioner (MSN); adult nurse practitioner (MSN); family nurse practitioner (MSN); nurse educator (MSN); MSN/MSBA. Part-time programs available. *Degree requirements:* For master's, thesis or project. *Entrance requirements:* For master's, RN license. Additional exam requirements/recommendations for international students: Required—TOEFL (minimum score 600 paper-based). Electronic applications accepted. *Faculty research:* Pain management, ethics, corporate wellness, caring spirituality, stress.

Southern Illinois University Edwardsville, Graduate School, School of Nursing, Program in Family Nurse Practitioner, Edwardsville, IL 62026. Offers MS, Post-Master's Certificate. *Accreditation:* AACN. Part-time programs available. *Students:* 108 part-time (103 women); includes 8 minority (2 Black or African American, non-Hispanic/Latino; 5 Asian, non-Hispanic/Latino; 1 Two or more races, non-Hispanic/Latino). 93 applicants, 42% accepted. In 2013, 22 master's, 2 other advanced degrees awarded. *Degree requirements:* For master's, comprehensive exam. *Entrance requirements:* For master's, appropriate bachelor's degree, RN license. Additional exam requirements/recommendations for international students: Required—TOEFL (minimum score 550 paper-based, 79 iBT), IELTS (minimum score 6.5), Michigan Test of English Language Proficiency or PTE. *Application deadline:* For fall admission, 3/1 for domestic and international students. Application fee: $30. Electronic applications accepted. *Expenses:* Tuition, state resident: full-time $3551. Tuition, nonresident: full-time $8378. *Financial support:* Fellowships with full tuition reimbursements, research assistantships, teaching assistantships, institutionally sponsored loans, scholarships/grants, and unspecified assistantships available. Financial award application deadline: 3/1; financial award applicants required to submit FAFSA. *Unit head:* Dr. Kathy Ketchum, Associate Dean for Graduate Programs, 618-650-3936, Fax: 618-650-3864, E-mail: kketchu@siue.edu. *Application contact:* Melissa K. Mace, Assistant Director of Graduate and International Recruitment, 618-650-2756, Fax: 618-650-3618, E-mail: mmace@siue.edu.
Website: http://www.siue.edu/nursing/graduate

Southern Illinois University Edwardsville, Graduate School, School of Nursing, Program in Nursing Doctoral Practice, Edwardsville, IL 62026. Offers DNP. Part-time programs available. *Students:* 1 (woman) full-time, 25 part-time (24 women); includes 3 minority (2 Black or African American, non-Hispanic/Latino; 1 Asian, non-Hispanic/Latino). 6 applicants, 100% accepted. In 2013, 12 doctorates awarded. *Degree requirements:* For doctorate, thesis/dissertation or alternative, project. *Entrance requirements:* Additional exam requirements/recommendations for international students: Required—TOEFL (minimum score 550 paper-based, 79 iBT), IELTS (minimum score 6.5), Michigan Test of English Language Proficiency or PTE. *Application deadline:* For spring admission, 3/1 for domestic and international students; for summer admission, 3/1 for domestic and international students. Application fee: $30. Electronic applications accepted. *Expenses:* Tuition, state resident: full-time $3551. Tuition, nonresident: full-time $8378. *Financial support:* Institutionally sponsored loans, scholarships/grants, and unspecified assistantships available. Financial award application deadline: 3/1; financial award applicants required to submit FAFSA. *Unit head:* Dr. Kathy Ketchum, Assistant Dean for Graduate Programs, 618-650-3975, Fax: 618-650-3854, E-mail: kketchu@siue.edu. *Application contact:* Melissa K. Mace, Assistant Director of Graduate and International Programs, 618-650-2756, Fax: 618-650-3618, E-mail: mmace@siue.edu.
Website: http://www.siue.edu/nursing/graduate/dnp/

Southern University and Agricultural and Mechanical College, School of Nursing, Baton Rouge, LA 70813. Offers educator/administrator (PhD); family health nursing (MSN); family nurse practitioner (Post Master's Certificate); geriatric nurse practitioner/gerontology (PhD). *Accreditation:* AACN. Part-time programs available. *Degree requirements:* For master's, comprehensive exam, thesis; for doctorate, comprehensive exam, thesis/dissertation. *Entrance requirements:* For master's, GRE General Test, BSN, minimum GPA of 2.7; for doctorate, GRE General Test; for Post Master's Certificate, MSN. Additional exam requirements/recommendations for international students: Required—TOEFL (minimum score 525 paper-based). *Faculty research:* Health promotions, vulnerable populations, (community-based) cardiovascular participating research, health disparities chronic diseases, care of the elderly.

South University, Program in Nursing, Tampa, FL 33614. Offers adult health nurse practitioner (MS); family nurse practitioner (MS); nurse educator (MS).

South University, Program in Nursing, Royal Palm Beach, FL 33411. Offers family nurse practitioner (MS).

Spalding University, Graduate Studies, Kosair College of Health and Natural Sciences, School of Nursing, Louisville, KY 40203-2188. Offers adult nurse practitioner (MSN, PMC); family nurse practitioner (MSN, PMC); leadership in nursing and healthcare (MSN, PMC); pediatric nurse practitioner (MSN, PMC). *Accreditation:* AACN. Part-time and evening/weekend programs available. *Faculty:* 6 full-time (all women), 6 part-time/adjunct (5 women). *Students:* 98 full-time (85 women), 13 part-time (all women); includes 23 minority (19 Black or African American, non-Hispanic/Latino; 2 Asian, non-Hispanic/Latino; 1 Hispanic/Latino; 1 Two or more races, non-Hispanic/Latino). Average age 36. 136 applicants, 31% accepted, 39 enrolled. In 2013, 48 master's, 5 other advanced degrees awarded. *Degree requirements:* For master's, comprehensive exam (for some programs), thesis. *Entrance requirements:* For master's, GRE General Test, BSN or bachelor's degree, RN licensure, autobiographical statement, transcripts, letters of recommendation. Additional exam requirements/recommendations for international students: Required—TOEFL (minimum score 535 paper-based). *Application deadline:* For fall admission, 2/1 priority date for domestic students. Application fee: $30. *Expenses: Tuition:* Full-time $21,450. *Required fees:* $810. Tuition and fees vary according to course load, degree level, program and student level. *Financial support:* Career-related internships or fieldwork, scholarships/grants, and traineeships available. Support available to part-time students. Financial award application deadline: 3/30; financial award applicants required to submit FAFSA. *Faculty research:* Nurse educational administration, gerontology, bioterrorism, healthcare ethics, leadership. *Unit head:* Dr. Paula Travis, Chair, 502-873-4298, E-mail: clewis@spalding.edu. *Application contact:* Dr. Pam King, Assistant Professor, 502-873-4292, E-mail: pking@spalding.edu.
Website: http://www.spalding.edu/nursing/

State University of New York Downstate Medical Center, College of Nursing, Graduate Program in Nursing, Nurse Practitioner Program, Brooklyn, NY 11203-2098. Offers MS, Post Master's Certificate. *Accreditation:* AACN. Part-time programs available. *Degree requirements:* For master's, thesis optional. *Entrance requirements:* For master's, GRE, BSN; minimum GPA of 3.0; previous undergraduate course work in statistics, health assessment, and nursing research; RN license; for Post Master's Certificate, BSN; minimum GPA of 3.0; RN license; previous undergraduate course work in statistics, health assessment, and nursing research. *Faculty research:* Women's health.

State University of New York Institute of Technology, Program in Family Nurse Practitioner, Utica, NY 13504-3050. Offers MS, CAS. *Accreditation:* AACN. Part-time programs available. Postbaccalaureate distance learning degree programs offered (minimal on-campus study). *Faculty:* 7 full-time (all women), 12 part-time/adjunct (10 women). *Students:* 61 full-time (53 women), 86 part-time (81 women); includes 22 minority (11 Black or African American, non-Hispanic/Latino; 2 American Indian or Alaska Native, non-Hispanic/Latino; 5 Asian, non-Hispanic/Latino; 4 Hispanic/Latino), 1 international. Average age 38. 95 applicants, 56% accepted, 44 enrolled. In 2013, 29 master's awarded. *Degree requirements:* For master's, culminating seminar. *Entrance requirements:* For master's, minimum GPA of 3.0 in last 30 undergraduate hours, bachelor's degree in nursing, 1 year of professional experience, RN license, 2 letters of reference, resume, educational objective; for CAS, master's degree in nursing. Additional exam requirements/recommendations for international students: Required—TOEFL (minimum score 550 paper-based; 79 iBT), IELTS (minimum score 6.5). *Application deadline:* For fall admission, 8/1 for domestic students, 7/1 for international students; for spring admission, 12/1 for domestic students, 11/1 for international students. Applications are processed on a rolling basis. Application fee: $60. Electronic applications accepted. *Expenses:* Tuition, state resident: full-time $9870; part-time $411 per credit hour. Tuition, nonresident: full-time $20,150; part-time $765 per credit hour. *Required fees:* $1180; $50.73 per credit hour. *Financial support:* In 2013–14, 7 students received support, including 1 fellowship with full tuition reimbursement available (averaging $10,631 per year); scholarships/grants also available. Financial award application deadline: 6/1; financial award applicants required to submit FAFSA. *Faculty research:* Adult and family healthcare, critical thinking, epidemiology, refugee and women's health, child obesity. *Unit head:* Dr. Jennifer Klimek-Yingling, Program Coordinator, 315-792-7295, Fax: 315-792-7555, E-mail: klimekj@sunyit.edu. *Application contact:* Maryrose Raab, Coordinator of Graduate Center, 315-792-7347, Fax: 315-792-7221, E-mail: maryrose.raab@sunyit.edu.
Website: http://www.sunyit.edu/programs/graduate/nur/family_nurse_prac

State University of New York Upstate Medical University, College of Nursing, Syracuse, NY 13210-2334. Offers nurse practitioner (Post Master's Certificate); nursing (MS). *Accreditation:* AACN. Part-time programs available. Postbaccalaureate distance learning degree programs offered (no on-campus study). *Degree requirements:* For master's, thesis or alternative. *Entrance requirements:* For master's, 3 years of work experience. Electronic applications accepted.

Stony Brook University, State University of New York, Stony Brook University Medical Center, Health Sciences Center, School of Nursing, Program in Family Nurse Practitioner, Stony Brook, NY 11794. Offers MS, Certificate. *Accreditation:* AACN. Postbaccalaureate distance learning degree programs offered. *Students:* 14 part-time (all women); includes 8 minority (5 Black or African American, non-Hispanic/Latino; 1 Asian, non-Hispanic/Latino; 2 Hispanic/Latino). *Degree requirements:* For master's, thesis. *Entrance requirements:* For master's, BSN, minimum GPA of 3.0, course work in statistics. Additional exam requirements/recommendations for international students: Required—TOEFL. *Application deadline:* For fall admission, 1/15 for domestic students. Application fee: $60. *Expenses:* Tuition, state resident: full-time $9870; part-time $411 per credit. Tuition, nonresident: full-time $18,350; part-time $765 per credit. *Financial support:* Application deadline: 3/15. *Unit head:* Dr. Lee Anne Xippolitos, Dean, 631-444-3200, Fax: 631-444-6628, E-mail: lee.xippolitos@stonybrook.edu. *Application contact:* 631-444-2644, E-mail: dolores.bilges@stonybrook.edu.
Website: http://www.nursing.stonybrookmedicine.edu/about

Stony Brook University, State University of New York, Stony Brook University Medical Center, Health Sciences Center, School of Nursing, Program in Perinatal Women's Health Nursing, Stony Brook, NY 11794. Offers MS, DNP, Certificate. *Accreditation:* AACN. Postbaccalaureate distance learning degree programs offered. *Students:* 35 part-time (all women); includes 10 minority (5 Black or African American, non-Hispanic/Latino; 1 American Indian or Alaska Native, non-Hispanic/Latino; 1 Asian, non-Hispanic/Latino; 3 Hispanic/Latino). In 2013, 7 master's awarded. *Degree requirements:* For master's, thesis. *Entrance requirements:* For master's, BSN, minimum GPA of 3.0, course work in statistics. Additional exam requirements/recommendations for international students: Required—TOEFL. *Application deadline:* For fall admission, 1/15 for domestic students. Application fee: $100. *Expenses:* Tuition, state resident: full-time $9870; part-time $411 per credit. Tuition, nonresident: full-time $18,350; part-time $765 per credit. *Financial support:* Application deadline: 3/15. *Unit head:* Prof. Elizabeth Collins, Director, 631-444-3296, Fax: 631-444-3136, E-mail: elizabeth.collins@stonybrook.edu. *Application contact:* 631-632-2644, Fax: 631-632-3136, E-mail: dolores.bilges@stonybrook.edu.
Website: http://www.nursing.stonybrookmedicine.edu/

Temple University, College of Health Professions and Social Work, Department of Nursing, Philadelphia, PA 19140. Offers adult-gerontology primary care (DNP); clinical nurse leader (MSN); family-individual across the lifespan (DNP); nurse educator (MSN); nursing (MSN, DNP). *Accreditation:* AACN. Part-time programs available. *Faculty:* 9 full-time (8 women), 3 part-time/adjunct (all women). *Students:* 6 full-time (5 women), 92 part-time (78 women); includes 51 minority (34 Black or African American, non-Hispanic/Latino; 9 Asian, non-Hispanic/Latino; 8 Hispanic/Latino), 1 international. 48 applicants, 58% accepted, 23 enrolled. In 2013, 12 master's, 9 doctorates awarded. *Degree requirements:* For master's and doctorate, evidence based practice project. *Entrance requirements:* For master's and doctorate, GRE General Test or MAT, 2 letters of reference, RN license, interview, statement of purpose, resume. Additional exam requirements/recommendations for international students: Required—TOEFL (minimum score 550 paper-based; 79 iBT). *Application deadline:* For fall admission, 2/15 priority date for domestic students, 1/15 for international students; for spring admission, 10/15 for domestic students, 9/15 for international students. Applications are processed on a rolling basis. Application fee: $60. Electronic applications accepted. *Financial support:* Federal Work-Study, scholarships/grants, traineeships, and tuition waivers available. Support available to part-time students. Financial award application deadline: 1/15. *Faculty research:* Health promotion, chronic illness, family support systems, primary care, health policy, community health services, evidence-based practice. *Total annual research expenditures:* $741,567. *Unit head:* Dr. Jane Kurz, RN, Chair, 215-707-8327, E-mail: jane.kurz@temple.edu. *Application contact:* Naseem Lodhi, Student Services Coordinator, 215-204-4618, E-mail: tunurse@temple.edu.

Tennessee State University, The School of Graduate Studies and Research, College of Health Sciences, Division of Nursing, Nashville, TN 37209-1561. Offers family nurse practitioner (MSN); holistic nurse practitioner (MSN); nursing education (MSN). *Entrance requirements:* For master's, GRE General Test or MAT, BSN, current RN license, minimum GPA of 3.0.

Tennessee Technological University, Whitson-Hester School of Nursing, Cookeville, TN 38505. Offers family nurse practitioner (MSN); informatics (MSN); nursing administration (MSN); nursing education (MSN). Part-time and evening/weekend programs available. Postbaccalaureate distance learning degree programs offered (no on-campus study). *Students:* 22 full-time (19 women), 101 part-time (94 women); includes 11 minority (5 Black or African American, non-Hispanic/Latino; 2 Asian, non-Hispanic/Latino; 1 Hispanic/Latino; 3 Two or more races, non-Hispanic/Latino). 79 applicants, 65% accepted, 38 enrolled. In 2013, 14 master's awarded. *Degree requirements:* For master's, comprehensive exam, thesis or alternative. *Entrance requirements:* Additional exam requirements/recommendations for international students: Required—TOEFL (minimum score 600 paper-based; 100 iBT), IELTS (minimum score 5.5), PTE, or TOEIC (Test of English as an International Communication). *Application deadline:* For fall admission, 8/1 for domestic students, 5/1 for international students; for spring admission, 12/1 for domestic students, 10/1 for international students. Applications are processed on a rolling basis. Application fee: $35 ($40 for international students). Electronic applications accepted. *Expenses:* Tuition, state resident: full-time $9347; part-time $465 per credit hour. Tuition, nonresident: full-time $23,635; part-time $1152 per credit hour. *Financial support:* Application deadline: 4/1. *Unit head:* Dr. Bedelia Russell, Director, 931-372-3203, Fax: 931-372-6244, E-mail: bhrussell@tntech.edu. *Application contact:* Shelia K. Kendrick, Coordinator of Graduate Studies, 931-372-3808, Fax: 931-372-3497, E-mail: skendrick@tntech.edu.

Texas A&M International University, Office of Graduate Studies and Research, College of Nursing and Health Sciences, Laredo, TX 78041-1900. Offers family nurse practitioner (MSN). *Faculty:* 2 full-time (both women), 2 part-time/adjunct (both women). *Students:* 39 part-time (32 women); includes 37 minority (2 Asian, non-Hispanic/Latino; 35 Hispanic/Latino), 1 international. Average age 36. 43 applicants, 67% accepted, 23 enrolled. In 2013, 15 master's awarded. *Entrance requirements:* Additional exam requirements/recommendations for international students: Required—TOEFL (minimum score 550 paper-based; 79 iBT). *Application deadline:* For fall admission, 4/30 for domestic and international students; for spring admission, 11/30 for domestic students, 10/1 for international students. Applications are processed on a rolling basis. Application fee: $35 ($50 for international students). *Expenses:* Tuition, state resident: full-time $5184. *International tuition:* $11,556 full-time. *Unit head:* Glenda Walker, Dean, 956-326-2574, E-mail: glenda.walker@tamiu.edu. *Application contact:* Suzanne Hansen-Alford, Director of Graduate Recruiting, 956-326-3023, Fax: 956-326-3021, E-mail: enroll@tamiu.edu.
Website: http://www.tamiu.edu/cson/

Texas A&M University–Corpus Christi, Graduate Studies and Research, College of Nursing and Health Sciences, Corpus Christi, TX 78412-5503. Offers clinical nurse specialist (MSN); family nurse practitioner (MSN); health care administration (MSN); leadership in nursing systems (MSN). *Accreditation:* AACN. Part-time and evening/weekend programs available. *Degree requirements:* For master's, comprehensive exam, thesis (for some programs). *Entrance requirements:* For master's, GRE General Test. Additional exam requirements/recommendations for international students: Required—TOEFL. Electronic applications accepted.

Texas Tech University Health Sciences Center, School of Nursing, Lubbock, TX 79430. Offers acute care nurse practitioner (MSN, Certificate); administration (MSN); advanced practice (DNP); education (MSN); executive leadership (DNP); family nurse practitioner (MSN, Certificate); geriatric nurse practitioner (MSN, Certificate); pediatric nurse practitioner (MSN, Certificate). *Accreditation:* AACN. Part-time programs available. Postbaccalaureate distance learning degree programs offered (minimal on-campus study). *Degree requirements:* For master's, thesis optional. *Entrance requirements:* For master's, minimum GPA of 3.0, 3 letters of reference, BSN, RN license; for Certificate, minimum GPA of 3.0, 3 letters of reference, RN license. Additional exam requirements/recommendations for international students: Required—TOEFL (minimum score 550 paper-based). *Faculty research:* Diabetes/obesity, nurse competency, disease management, intervention and measurements, health disparities.

Texas Woman's University, Graduate School, College of Nursing, Denton, TX 76201. Offers acute care nurse practitioner (MS); adult health clinical nurse specialist (MS); adult health nurse practitioner (MS); child health clinical nurse specialist (MS); clinical nurse leader (MS); family nurse practitioner (MS); health systems management (MS); nursing education (MS); nursing practice (DNP); nursing science (PhD); pediatric nurse practitioner (MS); women's health clinical nurse specialist (MS); women's health nurse practitioner (MS). *Accreditation:* AACN. Part-time programs available. Postbaccalaureate distance learning degree programs offered. *Faculty:* 60 full-time (59 women), 46 part-time/adjunct (39 women). *Students:* 54 full-time (49 women), 910 part-time (848 women); includes 489 minority (221 Black or African American, non-Hispanic/Latino; 11 American Indian or Alaska Native, non-Hispanic/Latino; 184 Asian, non-Hispanic/Latino; 70 Hispanic/Latino; 3 Native Hawaiian or other Pacific Islander, non-Hispanic/Latino), 16 international. Average age 38. 430 applicants, 65% accepted, 193 enrolled. In 2013, 258 master's, 22 doctorates awarded. *Degree requirements:* For master's, comprehensive exam, thesis or alternative; for doctorate, comprehensive exam, thesis/dissertation. *Entrance requirements:* For master's, GRE or MAT, minimum GPA of 3.0 on last 60 hours in undergraduate nursing degree and overall, RN license, BS in nursing, basic statistics course; for doctorate, GRE (preferred minimum score 153 [500 old version] Verbal, 144 [500 old version] Quantitative, 4 Analytical), MS in nursing, minimum preferred GPA of 3.5, RN license, statistics, 2 letters of reference, curriculum vitae, graduate nursing-theory course, graduate research course, statement of professional goals and research interests. Additional exam requirements/recommendations for international students: Required—TOEFL (minimum score 550 paper-based; 79 iBT). *Application deadline:* For fall admission, 5/1 priority date for domestic students, 3/1 for international students; for spring admission, 9/15 priority date for domestic students, 7/1 for international students. Applications are processed on a rolling basis. Application fee: $50 ($75 for international students). Electronic applications accepted. *Expenses:* Tuition, state resident: full-time $4182; part-time $233.32 per credit hour. Tuition, nonresident: full-time $10,716; part-time $595.32 per credit hour. *Financial support:* In 2013–14, 149 students received support, including 10 research assistantships (averaging $5,600 per year), 1 teaching assistantship (averaging $5,600 per year); career-related internships or fieldwork, Federal Work-Study, institutionally sponsored loans, scholarships/grants, traineeships, health care benefits, and unspecified assistantships also available. Support available to part-time students. Financial award application deadline: 3/1; financial award applicants required to submit FAFSA. *Faculty research:* Screening, prevention, and treatment for intimate partner violence; needs of adolescents during childbirth intervention; a network analysis decision tool for nurse managers (social network analysis); support for adolescents with implantable cardioverter defibrillators; informatics: nurse staffing, safety, quality, and financial data as they relate to patient care outcomes; prevention and treatment of obesity; improving infant outcomes related to premature birth. *Total annual research expenditures:* $1.7 million. *Unit head:* Dr. Gayle Roux, Interim Dean and Associate Dean for Research and Clinical Scholarship, 940-898-2401, Fax: 940-898-2437, E-mail: nursing@twu.edu. *Application contact:* Dr. Samuel Wheeler, Assistant Director of Admissions, 940-898-3188, Fax: 940-898-3081, E-mail: wheelersr@twu.edu.
Website: http://www.twu.edu/nursing/

Troy University, Graduate School, College of Health and Human Services, Program in Nursing, Troy, AL 36082. Offers adult health (MSN); clinical nurse specialist adult health (DNP); clinical nurse specialist maternal infant (DNP); family nurse practitioner (MSN, DNP, PMC); informatics specialist (MSN); maternal infant (MSN). Part-time and evening/weekend programs available. *Faculty:* 15 full-time (8 women), 3 part-time/adjunct (1 woman). *Students:* 61 full-time (56 women), 228 part-time (193 women); includes 97 minority (77 Black or African American, non-Hispanic/Latino; 4 American Indian or Alaska Native, non-Hispanic/Latino; 2 Asian, non-Hispanic/Latino; 5 Hispanic/Latino; 9 Two or more races, non-Hispanic/Latino). Average age 34. 138 applicants, 80% accepted, 39 enrolled. In 2013, 81 master's, 9 doctorates awarded. *Degree requirements:* For master's, comprehensive exam, minimum GPA of 3.0, candidacy; for doctorate, minimum GPA of 3.0, submission of approved comprehensive e-portfolio, completion of residency synthesis project, minimum of 1000 hours of clinical practice, score of 80% or better on qualifying exam. *Entrance requirements:* For master's, GRE (minimum score of 850 on old exam or 294 on new exam) or GMAT (minimum score of 500), minimum GPA of 3.0, BSN, current RN licensure; 2 letters of reference, undergraduate health assessment course; for doctorate, GRE (minimum score of 850 on old exam or 294 on new exam) or GMAT (minimum score of 500), BSN or MSN, minimum GPA of 3.0, 2 letters of reference, current RN licensure, essay. Additional exam requirements/recommendations for international students: Required—TOEFL (minimum score 523 paper-based; 70 iBT), IELTS (minimum score 6). *Application deadline:* Applications are processed on a rolling basis. Application fee: $50. Electronic applications accepted. *Expenses:* Tuition, state resident: full-time $6084; part-time $338 per credit hour. Tuition, nonresident: full-time $12,168; part-time $676 per credit hour. *Required fees:* $630; $35 per credit hour. $50 per semester. *Financial support:* Available to part-time students. Applicants required to submit FAFSA. *Unit head:* Dr. Diane Weed, Director, School of Nursing, 334-670-5864, Fax: 334-670-3745, E-mail: lweed@troy.edu. *Application contact:* Brenda K. Campbell, Director of Graduate Admissions, 334-670-3178, Fax: 334-670-3733, E-mail: bcamp@troy.edu.

Uniformed Services University of the Health Sciences, Graduate School of Nursing, Bethesda, MD 20814-4799. Offers family nurse practitioner (MSN, DNP); nurse anesthesia (MSN); nursing science (PhD); perioperative clinical nurse specialist (MSN); psychiatric nurse practitioner (MSN, DNP). Program available to military officers only. *Accreditation:* AACN; AANA/CANAEP. *Faculty:* 42 full-time (24 women), 5 part-time/adjunct (4 women). *Students:* 62 full-time (31 women); includes 13 minority (7 Black or African American, non-Hispanic/Latino; 5 Asian, non-Hispanic/Latino; 1 Hispanic/Latino). Average age 34. 100 applicants, 62% accepted, 62 enrolled. In 2013, 57 master's, 1 doctorate awarded. *Degree requirements:* For master's, thesis or alternative; for doctorate, thesis/dissertation or alternative. *Entrance requirements:* For master's, GRE, BSN, clinical experience, minimum GPA of 3.0, previous course work in science; for doctorate, GRE. *Application deadline:* For fall admission, 7/1 for domestic students; for winter admission, 2/15 for domestic students. Application fee: $0. Electronic applications accepted. *Faculty research:* Prenatal care, military health care, military readiness, distance learning. *Unit head:* Dr. Carol A. Romano, Associate Dean for Academic Affairs, 301-295-1180, Fax: 301-295-1707, E-mail: carol.romano@usuhs.edu. *Application contact:* Terry Lynn Malavakis, Recording Secretary for Admissions Committee, 301-295-1055, Fax: 301-295-1707, E-mail: terry.malavakis@usuhs.edu.
Website: http://www.usuhs.mil/gsn/

Union University, School of Nursing, Jackson, TN 38305-3697. Offers executive leadership (DNP); nurse anesthesia (DNP); nurse anesthetist (PMC); nurse practitioner (DNP); nursing education (MSN, PMC). *Accreditation:* AACN; AANA/CANAEP. *Degree requirements:* For master's, thesis or alternative. *Entrance requirements:* For master's, GRE, 3 letters of reference, bachelor's degree in nursing, minimum GPA of 3.0. Additional exam requirements/recommendations for international students: Required—TOEFL (minimum score 560 paper-based). Electronic applications accepted. *Faculty research:* Children's health, occupational rehabilitation, informatics, health promotion.

United States University, Family Nurse Practitioner Program, Chula Vista, CA 91911. Offers MSN. *Degree requirements:* For master's, project. *Entrance requirements:* For master's, RN license, minimum cumulative undergraduate GPA of 2.5, background check, official transcripts, personal goal statement. Additional exam requirements/recommendations for international students: Required—TOEFL (minimum score 550 paper-based; 80 iBT).

Universidad del Turabo, Graduate Programs, School of Health Sciences, Programs in Nursing, Program in Family Nurse Practitioner, Gurabo, PR 00778-3030. Offers MSN.

University at Buffalo, the State University of New York, Graduate School, School of Nursing, Buffalo, NY 14214. Offers adult gerontology nurse practitioner (DNP); family nurse practitioner (DNP); health care systems and leadership (MS); nurse anesthetist (DNP); nursing (PhD); nursing education (Certificate); psychiatric/mental health nurse practitioner (DNP). *Accreditation:* AACN; AANA/CANAEP (one or more programs are accredited). Part-time programs available. Postbaccalaureate distance learning degree programs offered (no on-campus study). *Faculty:* 24 full-time (21 women), 2 part-time/adjunct (1 woman). *Students:* 80 full-time (60 women), 97 part-time (84 women); includes 35 minority (20 Black or African American, non-Hispanic/Latino; 2 American Indian or Alaska Native, non-Hispanic/Latino; 9 Asian, non-Hispanic/Latino; 1 Hispanic/Latino; 3 Native Hawaiian or other Pacific Islander, non-Hispanic/Latino). 118 applicants, 67% accepted, 58 enrolled. In 2013, 41 master's, 15 doctorates awarded. *Degree requirements:* For master's, thesis optional; for doctorate, comprehensive exam (for some programs), capstone (for DNP), dissertation (for PhD). *Entrance requirements:* For doctorate, GRE or MAT, minimum GPA of 3.0 (3.25 for PhD), RN license, BS or MS in nursing, 3 references, writing sample; for Certificate, interview, minimum GPA of 3.0 or GRE General Test, RN license, MS in nursing. Additional exam requirements/recommendations for international students: Required—TOEFL (minimum score 550 paper-based; 79 iBT), IELTS (minimum score 6.5). *Application deadline:* For fall admission, 7/1 for domestic students, 4/1 for international students; for spring admission, 12/1 for domestic students, 10/1 for international students; for summer admission, 4/1 for domestic students. Application fee: $75. Electronic applications accepted. *Financial support:* In 2013–14, 80 students received support, including 2 fellowships with full and partial tuition reimbursements available (averaging $17,000 per year), 7 research assistantships with full and partial tuition reimbursements available (averaging $10,600 per year), 7 teaching assistantships with full and partial tuition reimbursements available (averaging $10,600 per year); scholarships/grants, traineeships, health care benefits, and unspecified assistantships also available. Financial award application deadline: 3/15; financial award applicants required to submit FAFSA. *Faculty research:* Oncology, palliative care, gerontology, addictions, mental health, community wellness, sleep, workforce, care of underserved populations, quality and safety, person-centered care, adolescent health. *Total annual research expenditures:* $1.1 million. *Unit head:* Dr. Marsha L. Lewis, Dean and Professor, 716-829-2533, Fax: 716-829-2566, E-mail: ubnursingdean@buffalo.edu. *Application contact:* Dr. David J. Lang, Director of Student Affairs, 716-829-2537, Fax: 716-829-2067, E-mail: nursing@buffalo.edu.
Website: http://nursing.buffalo.edu/

The University of Alabama in Huntsville, School of Graduate Studies, College of Nursing, Huntsville, AL 35899. Offers family nurse practitioner (Certificate); nursing

(MSN, DNP), including acute care nurse practitioner (MSN), adult clinical nurse specialist (MSN), clinical nurse leader (MSN), family nurse practitioner (MSN), leadership in health care systems (MSN); nursing education (Certificate). DNP offered jointly with The University of Alabama at Birmingham. *Accreditation:* AACN. Part-time and evening/weekend programs available. Postbaccalaureate distance learning degree programs offered (minimal on-campus study). *Faculty:* 16 full-time (15 women), 4 part-time/adjunct (all women). *Students:* 67 full-time (63 women), 235 part-time (192 women); includes 40 minority (27 Black or African American, non-Hispanic/Latino; 5 American Indian or Alaska Native, non-Hispanic/Latino; 4 Asian, non-Hispanic/Latino; 3 Hispanic/Latino; 1 Two or more races, non-Hispanic/Latino), 10 international. Average age 36. 265 applicants, 59% accepted, 128 enrolled. In 2013, 75 master's, 10 doctorates, 5 other advanced degrees awarded. *Degree requirements:* For master's, comprehensive exam, thesis or alternative, oral and written exams. *Entrance requirements:* For master's, MAT or GRE, Alabama RN license, BSN, minimum GPA of 3.0; for doctorate, master's degree in nursing in an advanced practice area; for Certificate, MAT or GRE, minimum GPA of 3.0. Additional exam requirements/recommendations for international students: Required—TOEFL (minimum score 500 paper-based; 80 iBT), IELTS (minimum score 6.5). *Application deadline:* For fall admission, 7/15 for domestic students, 4/1 for international students; for spring admission, 11/30 for domestic students, 9/1 for international students. Applications are processed on a rolling basis. Application fee: $50. Electronic applications accepted. *Expenses:* Tuition, state resident: full-time $8912; part-time $540 per credit hour. Tuition, nonresident: full-time $20,774; part-time $1252 per credit hour. *Required fees:* $148 per semester. One-time fee: $150. *Financial support:* In 2013–14, 19 students received support, including 19 teaching assistantships with full tuition reimbursements available (averaging $7,876 per year); career-related internships or fieldwork, Federal Work-Study, institutionally sponsored loans, scholarships/grants, traineeships, health care benefits, and unspecified assistantships also available. Support available to part-time students. Financial award application deadline: 4/1; financial award applicants required to submit FAFSA. *Faculty research:* Health care informatics, chronic illness management, maternal and child health, genetics/genomics, technology and health care. *Total annual research expenditures:* $557,830. *Unit head:* Dr. Fay Raines, Dean, 256-824-6345, Fax: 256-824-6026, E-mail: rainesc@uah.edu. *Application contact:* Charles Davis, Director of Graduate Nursing Admissions and Advising, 256-824-2433, Fax: 256-824-6026, E-mail: charles.davis@uah.edu.
Website: http://www.uah.edu/nursing/welcome

The University of Arizona, College of Nursing, Tucson, AZ 85721. Offers health care informatics (Certificate); nurse practitioner (MS, Certificate); nursing (DNP, PhD); rural health (Certificate). *Accreditation:* AACN. Part-time programs available. Postbaccalaureate distance learning degree programs offered (minimal on-campus study). *Faculty:* 20 full-time (18 women). *Students:* 352 full-time (298 women), 202 part-time (169 women); includes 152 minority (36 Black or African American, non-Hispanic/Latino; 2 American Indian or Alaska Native, non-Hispanic/Latino; 29 Asian, non-Hispanic/Latino; 54 Hispanic/Latino; 3 Native Hawaiian or other Pacific Islander, non-Hispanic/Latino; 28 Two or more races, non-Hispanic/Latino). Average age 39. 629 applicants, 59% accepted, 266 enrolled. In 2013, 159 master's, 23 doctorates awarded. Terminal master's awarded for partial completion of doctoral program. *Degree requirements:* For master's, thesis optional; for doctorate, comprehensive exam, thesis/dissertation. *Entrance requirements:* For master's, BSN, eligibility for RN license; for doctorate, BSN; for Certificate, GRE General Test, Arizona RN license, BSN, minimum GPA of 3.0. Additional exam requirements/recommendations for international students: Required—TOEFL (minimum score 550 paper-based; 79 iBT). *Application deadline:* For fall admission, 1/15 for domestic and international students. Applications are processed on a rolling basis. Application fee: $75. Electronic applications accepted. *Expenses:* Contact institution. *Financial support:* In 2013–14, 11 research assistantships with full tuition reimbursements (averaging $18,220 per year), 3 teaching assistantships (averaging $18,327 per year) were awarded; career-related internships or fieldwork, institutionally sponsored loans, scholarships/grants, traineeships, health care benefits, tuition waivers (full), and unspecified assistantships also available. Financial award application deadline: 6/1. *Faculty research:* Vulnerable populations, injury mechanisms and biobehavioral responses, health care systems, informatics, rural health. *Total annual research expenditures:* $4.4 million. *Unit head:* Dr. Joan Shaver, Dean, 520-626-7124, Fax: 520-626-6424, E-mail: cmurdaugh@nursing.arizona.edu. *Application contact:* Oscar Parra, Assistant Dean, Student Affairs, 520-626-6154, Fax: 520-626-2211, E-mail: info@nursing.arizona.edu.
Website: http://www.nursing.arizona.edu/

University of Central Arkansas, Graduate School, College of Health and Behavioral Sciences, Department of Nursing, Conway, AR 72035-0001. Offers adult nurse practitioner (PMC); clinical nurse leader (PMC); clinical nurse specialist (MSN); family nurse practitioner (PMC); nurse educator (PMC); nurse practitioner (MSN). *Accreditation:* AACN. Part-time and evening/weekend programs available. Postbaccalaureate distance learning degree programs offered (minimal on-campus study). *Degree requirements:* For master's, comprehensive exam, thesis optional, clinicals. *Entrance requirements:* For master's, GRE General Test, minimum GPA of 2.7. Additional exam requirements/recommendations for international students: Required—TOEFL (minimum score 550 paper-based; 80 iBT). Electronic applications accepted. *Expenses:* Contact institution.

University of Central Florida, College of Nursing, Orlando, FL 32816. Offers adult-gerontology nurse practitioner (Post-Master's Certificate); family nurse practitioner (Post-Master's Certificate); nursing (MSN, PhD); nursing education (Post-Master's Certificate); nursing practice (DNP). *Accreditation:* AACN. Part-time and evening/weekend programs available. *Faculty:* 47 full-time (41 women), 78 part-time/adjunct (75 women). *Students:* 54 full-time (49 women), 264 part-time (239 women); includes 72 minority (35 Black or African American, non-Hispanic/Latino; 7 Asian, non-Hispanic/Latino; 25 Hispanic/Latino; 1 Native Hawaiian or other Pacific Islander, non-Hispanic/Latino; 4 Two or more races, non-Hispanic/Latino), 1 international. Average age 39. 179 applicants, 55% accepted, 71 enrolled. In 2013, 96 master's, 12 doctorates, 3 other advanced degrees awarded. *Degree requirements:* For master's, thesis or alternative. *Entrance requirements:* For master's, GRE General Test, minimum GPA of 3.0 in last 60 hours. Additional exam requirements/recommendations for international students: Required—TOEFL. *Application deadline:* For fall admission, 2/15 for domestic students; for spring admission, 9/15 for domestic students. Application fee: $30. Electronic applications accepted. *Financial support:* In 2013–14, 2 students received support, including 3 teaching assistantships with partial tuition reimbursements available (averaging $6,300 per year); fellowships with partial tuition reimbursements available, research assistantships with partial tuition reimbursements available, career-related internships or fieldwork, Federal Work-Study, institutionally sponsored loans, traineeships, and unspecified assistantships also available. Financial award application deadline: 3/1; financial award applicants required to submit FAFSA. *Unit head:* Dr. Mary Lou Sole, Interim Dean, 407-823-5496, Fax: 407-823-5675, E-mail: mary.sole@ucf.edu. *Application contact:* Barbara Rodriguez Lamas, Director, Admissions and Student Services, 407-823-2766, Fax: 407-823-6442, E-mail: gradadmissions@ucf.edu.
Website: http://nursing.ucf.edu/

University of Colorado Denver, College of Nursing, Aurora, CO 80045. Offers adult clinical nurse specialist (MS); adult nurse practitioner (MS); family nurse practitioner (MS); family psychiatric mental health nurse practitioner (MS); health care informatics (MS); nurse-midwifery (MS); nursing (DNP, PhD); nursing leadership and health care systems (MS); pediatric nurse practitioner (MS); special studies (MS); women's health (MS); MS/PhD. *Accreditation:* ACNM/ACME (one or more programs are accredited). Part-time and evening/weekend programs available. Postbaccalaureate distance learning degree programs offered (minimal on-campus study). *Faculty:* 74 full-time (65 women), 58 part-time/adjunct (56 women). *Students:* 351 full-time (327 women), 138 part-time (125 women); includes 79 minority (12 Black or African American, non-Hispanic/Latino; 9 American Indian or Alaska Native, non-Hispanic/Latino; 13 Asian, non-Hispanic/Latino; 32 Hispanic/Latino; 2 Native Hawaiian or other Pacific Islander, non-Hispanic/Latino; 11 Two or more races, non-Hispanic/Latino), 7 international. Average age 33. 354 applicants, 43% accepted, 109 enrolled. In 2013, 108 master's, 28 doctorates awarded. Terminal master's awarded for partial completion of doctoral program. *Degree requirements:* For master's, thesis optional; for doctorate, comprehensive exam, thesis/dissertation, 42 credits of coursework. *Entrance requirements:* For master's, GRE if cumulative undergraduate GPA is less than 3.0, undergraduate nursing degree from NLNAC- or CCNE-accredited school or university; completion of research and statistics courses with minimum grade of C; copy of current and unencumbered nursing license; for doctorate, GRE, bachelor's and/or master's degrees in nursing from NLN- or CCNE-accredited institution; portfolio; minimum undergraduate GPA of 3.0, graduate 3.5; graduate-level intermediate statistics and master's-level nursing theory courses with minimum B grade; interview. Additional exam requirements/recommendations for international students: Required—TOEFL (minimum score 560 paper-based; 83 iBT). *Application deadline:* For fall admission, 2/15 for domestic students, 1/15 for international students; for spring admission, 7/1 for domestic students, 6/1 for international students. Application fee: $50 ($75 for international students). Electronic applications accepted. *Expenses:* Contact institution. *Financial support:* In 2013–14, 113 students received support. Fellowships, research assistantships, teaching assistantships, Federal Work-Study, institutionally sponsored loans, scholarships/grants, traineeships, and unspecified assistantships available. Support available to part-time students. Financial award application deadline: 4/1; financial award applicants required to submit FAFSA. *Faculty research:* Biological and behavioral phenomena in pregnancy and postpartum; patterns of glycemia during the insulin resistance of pregnancy; obesity, gestational diabetes, and relationship to neonatal adiposity; men's awareness and knowledge of male breast cancer; cognitive-behavioral therapy for chronic insomnia after breast cancer treatment; massage therapy for the treatment of tension-type headaches. *Total annual research expenditures:* $5.9 million. *Unit head:* Dr. Sarah Thompson, Dean, 303-724-1679, E-mail: sarah.a.thompson@ucdenver.edu. *Application contact:* Judy Campbell, Graduate Programs Coordinator, 303-724-8503, E-mail: judy.campbell@ucdenver.edu.
Website: http://www.ucdenver.edu/academics/colleges/nursing/Pages/default.aspx

University of Delaware, College of Health Sciences, School of Nursing, Newark, DE 19716. Offers adult nurse practitioner (MSN, PMC); cardiopulmonary clinical nurse specialist (MSN, PMC); cardiopulmonary clinical nurse specialist/adult nurse practitioner (MSN, PMC); family nurse practitioner (MSN, PMC); gerontology clinical nurse specialist (MSN, PMC); gerontology clinical nurse specialist geriatric nurse practitioner (PMC); gerontology clinical nurse specialist/geriatric nurse practitioner (MSN); health services administration (MSN, PMC); nursing of children clinical nurse specialist (MSN, PMC); nursing of children clinical nurse specialist/pediatric nurse practitioner (MSN, PMC); oncology/immune deficiency clinical nurse specialist (MSN, PMC); oncology/immune deficiency clinical nurse specialist/adult nurse practitioner (MSN, PMC); perinatal/women's health clinical nurse specialist (MSN, PMC); perinatal/women's health clinical nurse specialist/women's health nurse practitioner (MSN, PMC); psychiatric nursing clinical nurse specialist (MSN, PMC). *Accreditation:* AACN. Part-time and evening/weekend programs available. Postbaccalaureate distance learning degree programs offered (minimal on-campus study). *Degree requirements:* For master's, thesis optional. *Entrance requirements:* For master's, BSN, interview, RN license. Electronic applications accepted. *Faculty research:* Marriage and chronic illness, health promotion, congestive heart failure patient outcomes, school nursing, diabetes in children, culture, health disparities, cardiovascular, prison nursing, oncology, public policy, child obesity, smoking and teen pregnancy, blood pressure measurements, men's health.

University of Detroit Mercy, College of Health Professions, Program in Family Nurse Practitioner, Detroit, MI 48221. Offers MSN, Certificate. *Accreditation:* AACN.

University of Hawaii at Manoa, Graduate Division, School of Nursing and Dental Hygiene, Honolulu, HI 96822. Offers clinical nurse specialist (MS), including adult health, community mental health; nurse practitioner (MS), including adult health, community mental health, family nurse practitioner; nursing (PhD, Graduate Certificate); nursing administration (MS). *Accreditation:* AACN. Part-time programs available. Postbaccalaureate distance learning degree programs offered (minimal on-campus study). *Degree requirements:* For master's, thesis optional; for doctorate, comprehensive exam, thesis/dissertation. *Entrance requirements:* For master's, Hawaii RN license. Additional exam requirements/recommendations for international students: Required—TOEFL (minimum score 580 paper-based; 92 iBT), IELTS (minimum score 5). *Expenses:* Contact institution.

University of Houston–Victoria, School of Nursing, Victoria, TX 77901-4450. Offers family nurse practitioner (MSN); nursing administration (MSN); nursing education (MSN). *Accreditation:* AACN. *Faculty:* 13 full-time (12 women). *Students:* 27 full-time (23 women), 42 part-time (35 women); includes 33 minority (18 Black or African American, non-Hispanic/Latino; 8 Asian, non-Hispanic/Latino; 7 Hispanic/Latino), 7 international. *Entrance requirements:* For master's, GRE or MAT, minimum GPA of 3.0 in last 60 hours of academic course work, valid Texas RN licensure, 2 letters of recommendation. *Application deadline:* For fall admission, 7/15 for domestic students, 6/1 for international students. Applications are processed on a rolling basis. Electronic applications accepted. *Expenses:* Tuition, state resident: full-time $4534; part-time $251 per credit hour. Tuition, nonresident: full-time $10,906; part-time $606 per contact hour. *Required fees:* $68 per semester hour. Tuition and fees vary according to course load. *Financial support:* Federal Work-Study, scholarships/grants, and unspecified assistantships available. Support available to part-time students. Financial award application deadline: 4/15. *Unit head:* Dr. Kathryn Tart, Dean, 361-570-4295, E-mail: neilld@uhv.edu. *Application contact:* Tammy Whatley, Senior Recruitment Coordinator, 361-570-4297, E-mail: whatleyt@uhv.edu.
Website: http://www.uhv.edu/nursing/

University of Illinois at Chicago, Graduate College, College of Nursing, Program in Nursing, Chicago, IL 60607-7128. Offers acute care clinical nurse specialist (MS); acute care nurse practitioner (MS); administrative nursing leadership (Certificate); administrative studies in nursing (MS); adult nurse practitioner (MS); adult/geriatric nurse practitioner (MS); advanced community health nurse specialist (MS); family nurse practitioner (MS); geriatric clinical nurse specialist (MS); geriatric nurse practitioner (MS); mental health clinical nurse specialist (MS); mental health nurse practitioner (MS); nurse midwifery (MS); occupational health/advanced community health nurse specialist (MS); occupational health/family nurse practitioner (MS); pediatric clinical nurse specialist (MS); pediatric nurse practitioner (MS); perinatal clinical nurse specialist (MS); school/advanced community health nurse specialist (MS); school/family nurse practitioner (MS); women's health nurse practitioner (MS). *Accreditation:* AACN. Part-time programs available. *Faculty:* 16 full-time (14 women). *Students:* 393 full-time (361 women), 410 part-time (367 women); includes 198 minority (48 Black or African American, non-Hispanic/Latino; 1 American Indian or Alaska Native, non-Hispanic/Latino; 64 Asian, non-Hispanic/Latino; 71 Hispanic/Latino; 2 Native Hawaiian or other Pacific Islander, non-Hispanic/Latino; 12 Two or more races, non-Hispanic/Latino), 29 international. Average age 32. 396 applicants, 62% accepted, 177 enrolled. In 2013, 184 master's awarded. *Degree requirements:* For master's, thesis or alternative. *Entrance requirements:* For master's, GRE General Test, minimum GPA of 2.75. Additional exam requirements/recommendations for international students: Required—TOEFL. *Application deadline:* For fall admission, 5/15 for domestic students, 2/15 for international students; for spring admission, 11/1 for domestic students, 7/15 for international students. Applications are processed on a rolling basis. Application fee: $40 ($50 for international students). Electronic applications accepted. *Expenses:* Tuition, state resident: full-time $11,066; part-time $3689 per term. Tuition, nonresident: full-time $23,064; part-time $7688 per term. *Required fees:* $3004; $1190 per term. Tuition and fees vary according to course level and program. *Financial support:* Fellowships with full tuition reimbursements, research assistantships with full tuition reimbursements, teaching assistantships with full tuition reimbursements, career-related internships or fieldwork, Federal Work-Study, institutionally sponsored loans, scholarships/grants, traineeships, tuition waivers (full and partial), and unspecified assistantships available. Support available to part-time students. Financial award application deadline: 3/1; financial award applicants required to submit FAFSA. *Unit head:* Dr. Terri E. Weaver, Dean, 312-996-7808, E-mail: teweaver@uic.edu. *Application contact:* Receptionist, 312-413-2550, E-mail: gradcoll@uic.edu.

University of Indianapolis, Graduate Programs, School of Nursing, Indianapolis, IN 46227-3697. Offers advanced practice nursing (DNP); family nurse practitioner (MSN); gerontological nurse practitioner (MSN); neonatal nurse practitioner (MSN); nurse-midwifery (MSN); nursing (MSN); nursing and health systems leadership (MSN); nursing education (MSN); women's health nurse practitioner (MSN); MBA/MSN. *Accreditation:* AACN; ACNM. *Faculty:* 5 full-time (4 women), 1 part-time/adjunct (0 women). *Students:* 15 full-time (14 women), 285 part-time (270 women); includes 42 minority (24 Black or African American, non-Hispanic/Latino; 6 Asian, non-Hispanic/Latino; 3 Hispanic/Latino; 9 Two or more races, non-Hispanic/Latino), 2 international. Average age 35. In 2013, 46 master's awarded. *Entrance requirements:* For master's, minimum GPA of 3.0, interview, letters of recommendation, resume, IN nursing license, 1 year of professional practice; for doctorate, graduate of NLNAC- or CCNE-accredited nursing program; MSN or MA with nursing major and minimum cumulative GPA of 3.25; unencumbered RN license with eligibility for licensure in Indiana; completion of graduate-level statistics course within last 5 years with minimum grade of B; resume; essay; official transcripts from all academic institutions. Additional exam requirements/recommendations for international students: Required—TOEFL (minimum score 550 paper-based). *Application deadline:* For fall admission, 8/1 for domestic students; for winter admission, 12/15 for domestic students; for spring admission, 4/15 for domestic students. Applications are processed on a rolling basis. Application fee: $60. Electronic applications accepted. *Expenses: Tuition:* Full-time $5436; part-time $810 per credit hour. *Financial support:* Federal Work-Study available. *Unit head:* Dr. Anne Thomas, Dean, 317-788-3206, E-mail: athomas@uindy.edu. *Application contact:* Sueann Meagher, Graduate Administrative Assistant, 317-788-8005, Fax: 317-788-3542, E-mail: meaghers@uindy.edu.
Website: http://nursing.uindy.edu/

University of Louisville, Graduate School, School of Nursing, Louisville, KY 40202. Offers adult nurse practitioner (MSN); family nurse practitioner (MSN); health professions education (MSN); neonatal nurse practitioner (MSN); nursing research (PhD); psychiatric mental health nurse practitioner (MSN). *Accreditation:* AACN. Part-time programs available. *Students:* 91 full-time (81 women), 47 part-time (42 women); includes 16 minority (8 Black or African American, non-Hispanic/Latino; 3 Asian, non-Hispanic/Latino; 3 Hispanic/Latino; 2 Two or more races, non-Hispanic/Latino), 6 international. Average age 36. 58 applicants, 74% accepted, 36 enrolled. In 2013, 33 master's, 3 doctorates awarded. Terminal master's awarded for partial completion of doctoral program. *Degree requirements:* For master's, thesis optional; for doctorate, comprehensive exam, thesis/dissertation. *Entrance requirements:* For master's, GRE General Test, bachelor's degree in nursing, minimum GPA of 3.0, RN license; for doctorate, GRE General Test, BSN or MSN with recommended minimum GPA of 3.0. Additional exam requirements/recommendations for international students: Required—TOEFL. *Application deadline:* For fall admission, 4/1 priority date for domestic students, 4/1 for international students. Applications are processed on a rolling basis. Application fee: $60. Electronic applications accepted. *Expenses:* Tuition, state resident: full-time $10,788; part-time $599 per credit hour. Tuition, nonresident: full-time $22,446; part-time $1247 per credit hour. *Required fees:* $196. Tuition and fees vary according to program and reciprocity agreements. *Financial support:* Fellowships with full tuition reimbursements, research assistantships with full tuition reimbursements, teaching assistantships with full tuition reimbursements, institutionally sponsored loans, scholarships/grants, traineeships, health care benefits, and unspecified assistantships available. Support available to part-time students. Financial award application deadline: 4/15; financial award applicants required to submit FAFSA. *Faculty research:* Maternal-child/family stress after pregnancy loss, postpartum depression, access to healthcare (underserved populations), quality of life issues, physical activity (impact on chronic/acute conditions). *Total annual research expenditures:* $718,934. *Unit head:* Dr. Marcia J. Hern, Dean, 502-852-8300, Fax: 502-852-5044, E-mail: m.hern@gwise.louisville.edu. *Application contact:* Dr. Lee Ridner, Interim Associate Dean for Academic Affairs and Director of MSN Programs, 502-852-8518, Fax: 502-852-0704, E-mail: romain01@louisville.edu.
Website: http://www.louisville.edu/nursing/

University of Maine, Graduate School, College of Natural Sciences, Forestry, and Agriculture, School of Nursing, Orono, ME 04469. Offers individualized (MS, CAS); nursing education (CGS); rural health family nurse practitioner (MS, CAS). *Accreditation:* AACN. *Faculty:* 17 full-time (13 women), 7 part-time/adjunct (3 women). *Students:* 10 full-time (8 women), 12 part-time (all women); includes 3 minority (2 American Indian or Alaska Native, non-Hispanic/Latino; 1 Hispanic/Latino), 1 international. Average age 38. 12 applicants, 50% accepted, 5 enrolled. In 2013, 8 master's, 2 other advanced degrees awarded. *Entrance requirements:* For master's, GRE General Test; for other advanced degree, master's degree. Additional exam requirements/recommendations for international students: Required—TOEFL. *Application deadline:* For fall admission, 2/1 for domestic students. Applications are processed on a rolling basis. Application fee: $65. Electronic applications accepted. *Expenses:* Tuition, state resident: full-time $7524. Tuition, nonresident: full-time $23,112. *Required fees:* $1970. *Financial support:* In 2013–14, 4 students received support. Career-related internships or fieldwork, Federal Work-Study, institutionally sponsored loans, and tuition waivers (full and partial) available. Support available to part-time students. Financial award application deadline: 3/1. *Unit head:* Dr. Nancy Fishwick, Director, 207-581-2505, Fax: 207-581-2585. *Application contact:* Scott G. Delcourt, Associate Dean of the Graduate School, 207-581-3291, Fax: 207-581-3232, E-mail: graduate@maine.edu.
Website: http://umaine.edu/nursing/

University of Mary, School of Health Sciences, Division of Nursing, Bismarck, ND 58504-9652. Offers family nurse practitioner (MSN); nurse administrator (MSN); nursing educator (MSN). *Accreditation:* AACN. Part-time and evening/weekend programs available. Postbaccalaureate distance learning degree programs offered (minimal on-campus study). *Degree requirements:* For master's, comprehensive exam (for some programs), thesis (for some programs), internship (family nurse practitioner), teaching practice. *Entrance requirements:* For master's, minimum GPA of 2.75 in nursing, interview, letters of recommendation, criminal background check, immunizations, statement of professional goals. Additional exam requirements/recommendations for international students: Required—TOEFL (minimum score 500 paper-based; 71 iBT). Electronic applications accepted. *Faculty research:* Gerontology issues, rural nursing, health policy, primary care, women's health.

University of Mary Hardin-Baylor, Graduate Studies in Nursing, Belton, TX 76513. Offers clinical nurse leader (MSN); family nurse practitioner (MSN, Post-Master's Certificate); nurse educator (Post-Master's Certificate); nursing education (MSN). *Accreditation:* AACN. Part-time and evening/weekend programs available. *Faculty:* 6 full-time (all women), 4 part-time/adjunct (3 women). *Students:* 44 full-time (all women), 6 part-time (all women); includes 13 minority (5 Black or African American, non-Hispanic/Latino; 2 Asian, non-Hispanic/Latino; 6 Hispanic/Latino). Average age 33. 57 applicants, 67% accepted, 31 enrolled. In 2013, 17 master's awarded. *Degree requirements:* For master's, practicum. *Entrance requirements:* For master's, full-time RN for 1 year, BSN, minimum GPA of 3.0 in last 60 hours of undergraduate program, two letters of recommendation. Additional exam requirements/recommendations for international students: Required—TOEFL (minimum score 550 paper-based; 80 iBT), IELTS (minimum score 6). *Application deadline:* For fall admission, 4/15 for domestic students, 4/15 priority date for international students; for spring admission, 11/1 for domestic students, 10/15 priority date for international students. Applications are processed on a rolling basis. Application fee: $35 ($135 for international students). Electronic applications accepted. *Expenses: Tuition:* Full-time $14,130; part-time $785 per credit hour. *Required fees:* $1350; $75 per credit hour. $50 per term. *Financial support:* Applicants required to submit FAFSA. *Unit head:* Dr. Carrie Johnson, Associate Professor/Director, Master of Science in Nursing Programs, 254-295-4178, E-mail: cjohnson@umhb.edu. *Application contact:* Melissa Ford, Director of Graduate Admissions, 254-295-4020, Fax: 254-295-5038, E-mail: mford@umhb.edu.
Website: http://graduate.umhb.edu/nursing/

University of Massachusetts Amherst, Graduate School, School of Nursing, Amherst, MA 01003. Offers adult gerontology primary care (DNP); clinical nurse leader (MS); family nurse practitioner (DNP); nursing (PhD); public health nurse leader (DNP). *Accreditation:* AACN. Part-time programs available. Postbaccalaureate distance learning degree programs offered (minimal on-campus study). *Faculty:* 16 full-time (15 women). *Students:* 74 full-time (61 women), 161 part-time (149 women); includes 62 minority (31 Black or African American, non-Hispanic/Latino; 9 Asian, non-Hispanic/Latino; 19 Hispanic/Latino; 3 Two or more races, non-Hispanic/Latino), 6 international. Average age 40. 133 applicants, 80% accepted, 68 enrolled. In 2013, 9 master's, 32 doctorates awarded. Terminal master's awarded for partial completion of doctoral program. *Degree requirements:* For master's, thesis optional; for doctorate, comprehensive exam, thesis/dissertation. *Entrance requirements:* Additional exam requirements/recommendations for international students: Required—TOEFL (minimum score 550 paper-based; 80 iBT), IELTS (minimum score 6.5). *Application deadline:* For fall admission, 12/15 for domestic and international students. Applications are processed on a rolling basis. Application fee: $75. Electronic applications accepted. *Financial support:* Fellowships with full and partial tuition reimbursements, research assistantships with full and partial tuition reimbursements, teaching assistantships with full and partial tuition reimbursements, career-related internships or fieldwork, Federal Work-Study, scholarships/grants, traineeships, health care benefits, tuition waivers (full and partial), and unspecified assistantships available. Support available to part-time students. Financial award application deadline: 2/1. *Faculty research:* Health of older adults and their caretakers, mental health of individuals and families, health of children and adolescents, power and decision-making, transcultural health. *Unit head:* Dr. Stephen J. Cavanagh, Dean, 413-545-2703, Fax: 413-577-2550, E-mail: dean@nursing.umass.edu. *Application contact:* Lindsay DeSantis, Supervisor of Admissions, 413-545-0722, Fax: 413-577-0010, E-mail: gradadm@grad.umass.edu.
Website: http://www.umass.edu/nursing/

University of Massachusetts Lowell, College of Health Sciences, School of Nursing, Program in Family Health Nursing, Lowell, MA 01854-2881. Offers MS. *Accreditation:* AACN. *Degree requirements:* For master's, thesis optional. *Entrance requirements:* For master's, GRE General Test, minimum GPA of 3.0, MA nursing license, interview, 3 letters of recommendation.

University of Massachusetts Worcester, Graduate School of Nursing, Worcester, MA 01655-0115. Offers advanced practice nursing (DNP); family nurse practitioner (MS); gerontological adult acute care nurse practitioner (MS, Post Master's Certificate); gerontological adult primary care nurse practitioner (Post Master's Certificate); gerontological primary care nurse practitioner (MS); leadership (DNP); nurse educator (MS, Post Master's Certificate); nursing (PhD). *Accreditation:* AACN. *Faculty:* 19 full-time (17 women), 40 part-time/adjunct (33 women). *Students:* 153 full-time (129 women), 35 part-time (28 women); includes 30 minority (18 Black or African American, non-Hispanic/Latino; 7 Asian, non-Hispanic/Latino; 5 Hispanic/Latino). Average age 34. 254 applicants, 31% accepted, 57 enrolled. In 2013, 50 master's, 4 doctorates, 2 other advanced degrees awarded. *Degree requirements:* For doctorate, thesis/dissertation (for some programs), comprehensive exam (for PhD); capstone project and manuscript (for DNP). *Entrance requirements:* For master's, GRE General Test, bachelor's degree in nursing, course work in statistics, unrestricted Massachusetts license as registered nurse; for doctorate, GRE General Test, bachelor's or master's degree; for Post Master's Certificate, GRE General Test, MS in nursing. Additional exam requirements/recommendations for international students: Required—TOEFL. *Application deadline:* For fall admission, 12/1 priority date for domestic students. Applications are processed on a rolling basis. Application fee: $60. Electronic applications accepted. *Expenses:* Contact institution. *Financial support:* In 2013–14, 43 students received support. Institutionally sponsored loans, scholarships/grants, traineeships, and tuition waivers available. Support available to part-time students. Financial award application deadline: 5/16; financial award applicants required to submit FAFSA. *Faculty research:* Decision-making of partners and men with prostate cancer, coinfection (HIV and Hepatitis C) and treatment decisions, parent management of children with Type 1 diabetes, health literacy and discharge planning, Ghanaian women and self-care. *Total annual research expenditures:* $1.5 million. *Unit head:* Dr. Paulette Seymour-Route, Dean, 508-856-5801, Fax: 508-856-6552, E-mail: paulette.seymour-route@umassmed.edu. *Application contact:* Diane Brescia, Admissions Coordinator, 508-856-3488, Fax: 508-856-5851, E-mail: diane.brescia@umassmed.edu.
Website: http://www.umassmed.edu/gsn/

University of Memphis, Loewenberg School of Nursing, Memphis, TN 38152. Offers advance practice-family nurse practitioner (MSN); executive nursing leadership (MSN); nursing (Graduate Certificate); nursing administration (MSN); nursing education (MSN); nursing informatics (MSN). *Accreditation:* AACN. Part-time and evening/weekend programs available. Postbaccalaureate distance learning degree programs offered. *Faculty:* 18 full-time (16 women), 5 part-time/adjunct (0 women). *Students:* 23 full-time (21 women), 240 part-time (214 women); includes 112 minority (100 Black or African American, non-Hispanic/Latino; 9 Asian, non-Hispanic/Latino; 1 Hispanic/Latino; 2 Two or more races, non-Hispanic/Latino), 1 international. Average age 35. 176 applicants, 38% accepted, 25 enrolled. In 2013, 47 master's, 2 other advanced degrees awarded. *Degree requirements:* For master's, comprehensive exam, thesis optional, scholarly project; completion of clinical practicum hours. *Entrance requirements:* For master's, NCLEX Exam, interview. Additional exam requirements/recommendations for international students: Required—TOEFL (minimum score 550 paper-based; 79 iBT). *Application deadline:* For fall admission, 2/15 for domestic and international students; for spring admission, 10/1 for domestic and international students. Application fee: $35 ($60 for international students). *Financial support:* In 2013–14, 147 students received support. Federal Work-Study and scholarships/grants available. Financial award application deadline: 2/15; financial award applicants required to submit FAFSA. *Faculty research:* Technology in nursing, nurse retention, cultural competence, health policy, health access. *Total annual research expenditures:* $560,619. *Unit head:* Dr. Robert Koch, Associate Dean, 901-678-3908, Fax: 901-678-4907, E-mail: rakoch@memphis.edu. *Application contact:* Dr. Karen Weddle-West, Information Contact, 901-678-2531, Fax: 901-678-5023, E-mail: gradsch@memphis.edu.
Website: http://www.memphis.edu/nursing

University of Miami, Graduate School, School of Nursing and Health Studies, Coral Gables, FL 33124. Offers acute care (MSN), including acute care nurse practitioner, nurse anesthesia; nursing (PhD); primary care (MSN), including adult nurse practitioner, family nurse practitioner, nurse midwifery, women's health practitioner. *Accreditation:* AACN; AANA/CANAEP; ACNM/ACME (one or more programs are accredited). Part-time programs available. *Degree requirements:* For master's, thesis optional; for doctorate, thesis/dissertation. *Entrance requirements:* For master's, GRE General Test, BSN, minimum GPA of 3.0, Florida RN license; for doctorate, GRE General Test, BSN or MSN, minimum GPA of 3.0. Additional exam requirements/recommendations for international students: Required—TOEFL (minimum score 550 paper-based). Electronic applications accepted. *Faculty research:* Transcultural nursing, exercise and depression in Alzheimer's disease, infectious diseases/HIV–AIDS, postpartum depression, outcomes assessment.

University of Michigan, Rackham Graduate School, School of Nursing, Ann Arbor, MI 48109. Offers acute care pediatric nurse practitioner (MS); adult-gerontology acute care clinical nurse specialist (MS); adult-gerontology acute care nurse practitioner (MS); adult-gerontology primary care nurse practitioner (MS); health systems, nursing leadership, and effectiveness science (MS); nurse midwife (MS); nurse midwife and family nurse practitioner (MS); nurse midwife and primary care pediatric nurse practitioner (MS); nursing (DNP, PhD, Post Master's Certificate); primary care family nurse practitioner (MS); primary care pediatric nurse practitioner (MS). *Accreditation:* AACN; ACNM/ACME (one or more programs are accredited). Part-time programs available. Postbaccalaureate distance learning degree programs offered (minimal on-campus study). Terminal master's awarded for partial completion of doctoral program. *Degree requirements:* For doctorate, thesis/dissertation. *Application deadline:* For fall admission, 2/1 for domestic students; for winter admission, 5/1 for domestic students; for spring admission, 11/1 for domestic students. Applications are processed on a rolling basis. Electronic applications accepted. Tuition and fees vary according to course level, course load, degree level, program and student level. *Financial support:* Fellowships with full and partial tuition reimbursements, research assistantships with full and partial tuition reimbursements, teaching assistantships with full tuition reimbursements, Federal Work-Study, institutionally sponsored loans, scholarships/grants, traineeships, and tuition waivers (partial) available. Support available to part-time students. *Faculty research:* Preparation of clinical nurse researchers, biobehavior, women's health, health promotion, substance abuse, psychobiology of menopause, fertility, obesity, health care systems. *Unit head:* Dr. Kathleen Potempa, Dean, 734-764-7185, Fax: 734-764-7186. *Application contact:* James Diesing, Graduate Recruiting and Admissions Coordinator, 734-615-4739, E-mail: sn-osams@umich.edu.
Website: http://www.nursing.umich.edu/

University of Michigan–Flint, School of Health Professions and Studies, Program in Nursing, Flint, MI 48502-1950. Offers family nurse practitioner (MSN); nursing (Certificate); nursing practice (DNP). *Accreditation:* AACN. Part-time programs available. *Faculty:* 9 full-time (all women), 6 part-time/adjunct (5 women). *Students:* 98 full-time (85 women), 80 part-time (71 women); includes 35 minority (15 Black or African American, non-Hispanic/Latino; 3 American Indian or Alaska Native, non-Hispanic/Latino; 6 Asian, non-Hispanic/Latino; 4 Hispanic/Latino; 1 Native Hawaiian or other Pacific Islander, non-Hispanic/Latino; 6 Two or more races, non-Hispanic/Latino), 3 international. Average age 39. 157 applicants, 38% accepted, 55 enrolled. In 2013, 15 master's, 18 doctorates awarded. *Degree requirements:* For master's, thesis. *Entrance requirements:* For master's, current Michigan RN license, minimum GPA of 3.2, three or more credits in college-level chemistry with minimum C grade, three or more credits in college-level statistics with minimum C grade. Additional exam requirements/recommendations for international students: Required—TOEFL (minimum score 560 paper-based; 84 iBT), IELTS (minimum score 6.5). *Application deadline:* For fall admission, 8/1 priority date for domestic students, 5/1 priority date for international students; for winter admission, 11/15 priority date for domestic students, 9/1 priority date for international students; for spring admission, 3/15 priority date for domestic students, 1/1 priority date for international students. Application fee: $55. Electronic applications accepted. *Expenses:* Contact institution. *Financial support:* Federal Work-Study, scholarships/grants, and unspecified assistantships available. Support available to part-time students. Financial award application deadline: 3/1; financial award applicants required to submit FAFSA. *Faculty research:* Family system stress, self breast exam, family roads evaluation, causal model testing for psychosocial development, basic needs. *Unit head:* Dr. Constance J. Creech, Director, 810-762-3420, Fax: 810-766-6851, E-mail: ccreech@umflint.edu. *Application contact:* Bradley T. Maki, Director of Graduate Admissions, 810-762-3171, Fax: 810-766-6789, E-mail: bmaki@umflint.edu.
Website: http://www.umflint.edu/graduateprograms/nursing.htm

University of Minnesota, Twin Cities Campus, Graduate School, School of Nursing, Family Nurse Practitioner Program, Minneapolis, MN 55455-0213. Offers MS. *Accreditation:* AACN. *Degree requirements:* For master's, final oral exam, project or thesis. *Entrance requirements:* Additional exam requirements/recommendations for international students: Required—TOEFL (minimum score 586 paper-based).

University of Missouri, Graduate School, Sinclair School of Nursing, Columbia, MO 65211. Offers adult-gerontology clinical nurse specialist (DNP, Certificate); family nurse practitioner (DNP); family psychiatric and mental health nurse practitioner (DNP); nursing (MS, PhD); nursing leadership and innovations in health care (DNP); pediatric clinical nurse specialist (DNP, Certificate); pediatric nurse practitioner (DNP). *Accreditation:* AACN. Part-time programs available. *Faculty:* 20 full-time (18 women), 6 part-time/adjunct (all women). *Students:* 60 full-time (58 women), 232 part-time (211 women); includes 24 minority (9 Black or African American, non-Hispanic/Latino; 4 American Indian or Alaska Native, non-Hispanic/Latino; 2 Asian, non-Hispanic/Latino; 6 Hispanic/Latino; 3 Two or more races, non-Hispanic/Latino), 4 international. Average age 37. 131 applicants, 62% accepted, 61 enrolled. In 2013, 42 master's, 2 doctorates, 7 other advanced degrees awarded. *Degree requirements:* For master's, thesis optional, oral exam; for doctorate, thesis/dissertation. *Entrance requirements:* For master's, GRE General Test, BSN, minimum GPA of 3.0 during last 60 hours, nursing license. Additional exam requirements/recommendations for international students: Required—TOEFL (minimum score 550 paper-based; 79 iBT). *Application deadline:* For fall admission, 2/1 priority date for domestic and international students. Applications are processed on a rolling basis. Application fee: $55 ($75 for international students). Electronic applications accepted. *Financial support:* Fellowships, research assistantships, teaching assistantships, career-related internships or fieldwork, institutionally sponsored loans, scholarships/grants, traineeships, health care benefits, tuition waivers (full), and unspecified assistantships available. Support available to part-time students. *Faculty research:* Pain, stepfamilies, chemotherapy-related nausea and vomiting, stress management, self-care deficit theory. *Unit head:* Dr. Judith F. Miller, Dean, 573-882-0278, E-mail: millerjud@missouri.edu. *Application contact:* Laura Anderson, Senior Academic Advisor, 573-882-0294, E-mail: andersonla@missouri.edu.
Website: http://nursing.missouri.edu/

University of Missouri–Kansas City, School of Nursing and Health Studies, Kansas City, MO 64110-2499. Offers adult clinical nurse specialist (MSN), including adult nurse practitioner, women's health nurse practitioner (MSN, DNP); adult clinical nursing practice (DNP), including adult gerontology nurse practitioner, women's health nurse practitioner (MSN, DNP); clinical nursing practice (DNP), including family nurse practitioner; family nurse practitioner (MSN); neonatal nurse practitioner (MSN); nurse educator (MSN); nurse executive (MSN); nursing (PhD); nursing practice (DNP); pediatric clinical nursing practice (DNP), including pediatric nurse practitioner; pediatric nurse practitioner (MSN). *Accreditation:* AACN. Part-time programs available. Postbaccalaureate distance learning degree programs offered (minimal on-campus study). *Faculty:* 44 full-time (38 women), 55 part-time/adjunct (52 women). *Students:* 44 full-time (33 women), 401 part-time (370 women); includes 59 minority (25 Black or African American, non-Hispanic/Latino; 2 American Indian or Alaska Native, non-Hispanic/Latino; 12 Asian, non-Hispanic/Latino; 15 Hispanic/Latino; 5 Two or more races, non-Hispanic/Latino). Average age 37. 182 applicants, 68% accepted, 124 enrolled. In 2013, 106 master's, 15 doctorates awarded. *Degree requirements:* For master's, thesis or alternative. *Entrance requirements:* For master's, minimum undergraduate GPA of 3.2; for doctorate, GRE, 3 letters of reference. Additional exam requirements/recommendations for international students: Required—TOEFL (minimum score 550 paper-based; 80 iBT). *Application deadline:* For fall admission, 2/1 priority date for domestic and international students; for spring admission, 9/1 priority date for domestic and international students. Application fee: $45 ($50 for international students). *Expenses:* Tuition, state resident: full-time $6073; part-time $337.40 per credit hour. Tuition, nonresident: full-time $15,680; part-time $871.10 per credit hour. *Required fees:* $97.59 per credit hour. Full-time tuition and fees vary according to program. *Financial support:* In 2013–14, 13 teaching assistantships with partial tuition reimbursements (averaging $9,470 per year) were awarded; fellowships, research assistantships, career-related internships or fieldwork, Federal Work-Study, institutionally sponsored loans, and tuition waivers (full and partial) also available. Support available to part-time students. Financial award application deadline: 3/1; financial award applicants required to submit FAFSA. *Faculty research:* Geriatrics/gerontology, children's pain, neonatology, Alzheimer's care, cancer caregivers. *Unit head:* Dr. Ann Cary, Dean, 816-235-1723, Fax: 816-235-1701, E-mail: caryah@umkc.edu. *Application contact:* Judy Jellison, Coordinator for Admissions and Recruitment, 816-235-1740, Fax: 816-235-1701, E-mail: jellisonj@umkc.edu.
Website: http://nursing.umkc.edu/

University of Missouri–St. Louis, College of Nursing, St. Louis, MO 63121-4400. Offers adult nurse practitioner (DNP, Post Master's Certificate); clinical nurse specialist (DNP); family mental health nurse practitioner (DNP); family nurse practitioner (MSN, DNP, Post Master's Certificate); neonatal nurse practitioner (MSN); nurse educator (MSN); nurse leader (MSN); nurse practitioner (Post Master's Certificate); nursing (PhD); pediatric clinical nurse specialist (DNP); pediatric nurse practitioner (MSN, DNP, Post Master's Certificate); women's health nurse practitioner (MSN, Post Master's Certificate). *Accreditation:* AACN. Part-time programs available. *Faculty:* 14 full-time (13 women), 14 part-time/adjunct (13 women). *Students:* 227 part-time (217 women); includes 40 minority (35 Black or African American, non-Hispanic/Latino; 1 American Indian or Alaska Native, non-Hispanic/Latino; 1 Asian, non-Hispanic/Latino; 1 Hispanic/Latino; 2 Two or more races, non-Hispanic/Latino). Average age 35. 190 applicants, 51% accepted, 76 enrolled. In 2013, 80 master's, 8 doctorates, 2 other advanced degrees awarded. *Degree requirements:* For doctorate, comprehensive exam, thesis/dissertation; for Post Master's Certificate, thesis. *Entrance requirements:* For master's, 2 recommendation letters; minimum GPA of 3.0; BSN; nursing licensure; statement of purpose; course in differential/inferential statistics; for doctorate, GRE, 2 letters of recommendation, MSN, minimum GPA of 3.2, course in differential/inferential statistics; for Post Master's Certificate, 2 recommendation letters; MSN; advanced practice certificate; minimum GPA of 3.0; essay. Additional exam requirements/recommendations for international students: Recommended—TOEFL (minimum score 550 paper-based; 79 iBT), IELTS (minimum score 6.5). *Application deadline:* For fall admission, 2/15 for domestic and international students. Application fee: $50 ($40 for international students). Electronic applications accepted. *Expenses:* Tuition, state resident: full-time $7364; part-time $409.10 per credit hour. Tuition, nonresident: full-time $19,162; part-time $1008.50 per credit hour. *Financial support:* Application deadline: 4/1; applicants required to submit FAFSA. *Faculty research:* Health promotion and restoration, family disruption, violence, abuse, battered women, health survey methods. *Unit head:* Dr. Nancy Magnuson, Director, 314-516-6066. *Application contact:* 314-516-5458, Fax: 314-516-6996, E-mail: gradadm@umsl.edu.
Website: http://www.umsl.edu/divisions/nursing/

University of Nevada, Las Vegas, Graduate College, School of Nursing, Las Vegas, NV 89154-3018. Offers family nurse practitioner (Advanced Certificate); nursing (MS, DNP); nursing education (Advanced Certificate); pediatric nurse practitioner (PhD, Post-Master's Certificate). *Accreditation:* AACN. Part-time programs available. Postbaccalaureate distance learning degree programs offered (minimal on-campus study). *Faculty:* 11 full-time (10 women), 9 part-time/adjunct (6 women). *Students:* 48 full-time (40 women), 74 part-time (65 women); includes 30 minority (5 Black or African American, non-Hispanic/Latino; 10 Asian, non-Hispanic/Latino; 6 Hispanic/Latino; 9 Two or more races, non-Hispanic/Latino), 4 international. Average age 41. 114 applicants, 54% accepted, 48 enrolled. In 2013, 16 master's, 8 doctorates, 1 other advanced degree awarded. *Entrance requirements:* For doctorate, GRE General Test. Additional exam requirements/recommendations for international students: Recommended—TOEFL (minimum score 550 paper-based; 80 iBT), IELTS (minimum score 7). *Application deadline:* For fall admission, 2/1 for domestic students, 5/1 for international students; for spring admission, 10/1 for international students. Application fee: $60 ($95 for international students). Electronic applications accepted. *Expenses:* Tuition, state

resident: full-time $4752; part-time $264 per credit. Tuition, nonresident: full-time $18,662; part-time $554.50 per credit. *International tuition:* $18,952 full-time. *Required fees:* $532; $12 per credit. $266 per semester. One-time fee: $35. Tuition and fees vary according to course load and program. *Financial support:* In 2013–14, 5 students received support, including 5 teaching assistantships with partial tuition reimbursements available (averaging $9,500 per year); institutionally sponsored loans, scholarships/grants, health care benefits, and unspecified assistantships also available. Financial award application deadline: 3/1. *Faculty research:* Health promotion issues such as obesity and exercise, dance and cardiovascular disease, informal caregiver stress and risk factors for depression, clinical management of hypertension and chronic obstructive pulmonary disease (COPD), childhood obesity and activity. *Total annual research expenditures:* $896,934. *Unit head:* Dr. Carolyn Yucha, Chair, 702-895-5307, E-mail: carolyn.yucha@unlv.edu. *Application contact:* Graduate College Admissions Evaluator, 702-895-3320, Fax: 702-895-4180, E-mail: gradcollege@unlv.edu.
Website: http://nursing.unlv.edu/

University of New Hampshire, Graduate School, School of Health and Human Services, Department of Nursing, Durham, NH 03824. Offers family practitioner (Postbaccalaureate Certificate); nursing (MS, DNP). *Accreditation:* AACN. Part-time programs available. *Faculty:* 11 full-time (9 women). *Students:* 57 full-time (46 women), 53 part-time (49 women); includes 11 minority (3 Black or African American, non-Hispanic/Latino; 1 American Indian or Alaska Native, non-Hispanic/Latino; 5 Asian, non-Hispanic/Latino; 2 Hispanic/Latino). Average age 33. 70 applicants, 47% accepted, 19 enrolled. In 2013, 48 master's, 1 other advanced degree awarded. *Degree requirements:* For master's, thesis or alternative. *Entrance requirements:* For master's, GRE General Test or MAT. Additional exam requirements/recommendations for international students: Required—TOEFL (minimum score 550 paper-based; 80 iBT). *Application deadline:* For fall admission, 4/1 priority date for domestic students, 4/1 for international students; for spring admission, 11/1 for domestic students. Applications are processed on a rolling basis. Application fee: $65. Electronic applications accepted. *Expenses:* Tuition, state resident: full-time $13,500; part-time $750 per credit hour. Tuition, nonresident: full-time $26,200; part-time $1100 per credit hour. *Required fees:* $1741; $435.25 per term. Tuition and fees vary according to course level, course load, campus/location and program. *Financial support:* In 2013–14, 2 students received support, including 2 teaching assistantships; fellowships, research assistantships, Federal Work-Study, scholarships/grants, and tuition waivers (full and partial) also available. Financial award application deadline: 2/15. *Faculty research:* Adult health, nursing administration, family nurse practitioner. *Unit head:* Dr. Gene Harkless, Chairperson, 603-862-2285. *Application contact:* Jane Dufresne, Administrative Assistant, 603-862-2299, E-mail: nursing.department@unh.edu.
Website: http://www.chhs.unh.edu/nursing/graduate-programs

The University of North Carolina at Chapel Hill, School of Nursing, Chapel Hill, NC 27599-7460. Offers nursing (MSN, DNP, PhD, PMC), including adult nurse practitioner (MSN, PMC), children's health advanced practice (MSN, PMC), family nurse practitioner (MSN, PMC), health care systems (MSN, PMC), psychiatric/mental health nursing (MSN, PMC). Part-time programs available. *Degree requirements:* For master's, comprehensive exam, thesis; for doctorate, thesis/dissertation, 3 exams. *Entrance requirements:* For master's and doctorate, GRE General Test. Additional exam requirements/recommendations for international students: Required—TOEFL (minimum score 550 paper-based; 79 iBT), IELTS (minimum score 7). Electronic applications accepted. *Faculty research:* Preventing and managing chronic illness, reducing health disparities, Improving healthcare quality and patient outcomes, understanding biobehavioral and genetic bases of health and illness, developing innovative ways to enhance science and its clinical translation.

The University of North Carolina at Charlotte, The Graduate School, College of Health and Human Services, School of Nursing, Charlotte, NC 28223-0001. Offers administration (Post-Master's Certificate); advanced clinical (MSN, Post-Master's Certificate); anesthesia (MSN, Post-Master's Certificate); community health (MSN); family nurse practitioner (MSN, Post-Master's Certificate); health administration (MSN); mental health (MSN); nurse educator (MSN, Post-Master's Certificate); nursing (DNP); systems population (MSN). *Accreditation:* AACN. Part-time programs available. *Faculty:* 17 full-time (16 women), 6 part-time/adjunct (5 women). *Students:* 96 full-time (80 women), 124 part-time (119 women); includes 45 minority (30 Black or African American, non-Hispanic/Latino; 1 American Indian or Alaska Native, non-Hispanic/Latino; 8 Asian, non-Hispanic/Latino; 4 Hispanic/Latino; 2 Two or more races, non-Hispanic/Latino), 1 international. Average age 34. 216 applicants, 38% accepted, 72 enrolled. In 2013, 70 master's, 8 other advanced degrees awarded. Terminal master's awarded for partial completion of doctoral program. *Degree requirements:* For master's, thesis or alternative, practicum; for doctorate, thesis/dissertation or alternative, residency. *Entrance requirements:* For master's, GRE General Test, minimum GPA of 3.0 in undergraduate major; for doctorate, GRE, MAT, or GMAT, minimum GPA of 3.5. Additional exam requirements/recommendations for international students: Required—TOEFL (minimum score 570 paper-based; 83 iBT). *Application deadline:* For fall admission, 5/1 priority date for domestic students, 5/1 for international students; for spring admission, 10/1 priority date for domestic students, 10/1 for international students. Application fee: $75. Electronic applications accepted. *Expenses:* Tuition, state resident: full-time $3522. Tuition, nonresident: full-time $16,051. *Required fees:* $2585. Tuition and fees vary according to course load and program. *Financial support:* In 2013–14, 5 students received support, including 5 teaching assistantships (averaging $4,785 per year); research assistantships, career-related internships or fieldwork, institutionally sponsored loans, scholarships/grants, traineeships, and unspecified assistantships also available. Support available to part-time students. Financial award application deadline: 4/1; financial award applicants required to submit FAFSA. *Faculty research:* Improving care outcomes for the elderly; vulnerable populations; symptom management; self management/health promotion strategies of older adults; migration and maternal child health; health disparities, health literacy, and access to healthcare in Latino adults with diabetes; psychiatric nursing. *Total annual research expenditures:* $572,410. *Unit head:* Dr. Dee Baldwin, Associate Dean, 704-687-7952, Fax: 704-687-6017, E-mail: dbaldwi5@uncc.edu. *Application contact:* Kathy B. Giddings, Director of Graduate Admissions, 704-687-5503, Fax: 704-687-1668, E-mail: gradadm@uncc.edu.
Website: http://nursing.uncc.edu/

The University of North Carolina Wilmington, School of Nursing, Wilmington, NC 28403-5995. Offers clinical research and product development (MS); family nurse practitioner (MSN). *Faculty:* 10 full-time (9 women), 1 (woman) part-time/adjunct. *Students:* 59 full-time (54 women), 61 part-time (53 women); includes 17 minority (6 Black or African American, non-Hispanic/Latino; 5 American Indian or Alaska Native, non-Hispanic/Latino; 5 Hispanic/Latino; 1 Two or more races, non-Hispanic/Latino). Average age 32. 134 applicants, 44% accepted, 43 enrolled. In 2013, 13 master's awarded. *Degree requirements:* For master's, comprehensive exam, thesis or project. *Entrance requirements:* For master's, GRE General Test, bachelor's degree in nursing. Additional exam requirements/recommendations for international students: Required—TOEFL (minimum score 550 paper-based; 79 iBT), IELTS (minimum score 6.5). *Application deadline:* For fall admission, 3/1 for domestic students. Applications are processed on a rolling basis. Application fee: $60. Electronic applications accepted. *Expenses:* Tuition, state resident: full-time $4163. Tuition, nonresident: full-time $16,098. *Financial support:* In 2013–14, 2 teaching assistantships with full and partial tuition reimbursements (averaging $9,500 per year) were awarded. Financial award application deadline: 3/15. *Unit head:* Dr. Deborah Pollard, Interim Director, 910-962-7410, E-mail: pollardd@uncw.edu. *Application contact:* Dr. Julie Taylor, Graduate Coordinator, 910-962-7927, E-mail: taylorjs@uncw.edu.
Website: http://www.uncw.edu/son/

University of North Dakota, Graduate School, College of Nursing, Department of Nursing, Grand Forks, ND 58202. Offers adult-gerontological nurse practitioner (MSN); advanced public health nurse (MSN); family nurse practitioner (MSN); nurse anesthesia (MSN); nurse educator (MSN); nursing (DNP, PhD); psychiatric and mental health nurse practitioner (MSN).

University of Northern Colorado, Graduate School, College of Natural and Health Sciences, School of Nursing, Greeley, CO 80639. Offers clinical nurse specialist in chronic illness (MS); family nurse practitioner (MS); nursing education (MS, PhD). *Accreditation:* AACN. Postbaccalaureate distance learning degree programs offered. *Degree requirements:* For master's, comprehensive exam, thesis or alternative; for doctorate, comprehensive exam, thesis/dissertation. *Entrance requirements:* For master's and doctorate, GRE General Test, minimum GPA of 3.0 in last 60 hours, BS in nursing, 2 letters of recommendation. Electronic applications accepted.

University of North Florida, Brooks College of Health, School of Nursing, Jacksonville, FL 32224. Offers clinical nurse leader (MSN); clinical nurse specialist (MSN); family nurse practitioner (Certificate); nurse anesthetist (CRNA) (MSN); nursing practice (DNP); primary care nurse practitioner (MSN). *Accreditation:* AACN; AANA/CANAEP. Part-time programs available. *Faculty:* 29 full-time (23 women), 1 part-time/adjunct (0 women). *Students:* 93 full-time (70 women), 74 part-time (61 women); includes 33 minority (11 Black or African American, non-Hispanic/Latino; 1 American Indian or Alaska Native, non-Hispanic/Latino; 6 Asian, non-Hispanic/Latino; 12 Hispanic/Latino; 3 Two or more races, non-Hispanic/Latino), 2 international. Average age 34. 133 applicants, 40% accepted, 32 enrolled. In 2013, 45 master's, 3 doctorates awarded. *Degree requirements:* For master's, thesis optional. *Entrance requirements:* For master's, GRE General Test, minimum GPA of 3.0 in last 60 hours of course work, BSN, clinical experience, resume; for doctorate, GRE, master's degree in nursing specialty from nationally-accredited program; national certification in one of the following APRN roles: CNE, CNM, CNS, CRNA, CNP; minimum graduate GPA of 3.3; three letters of reference which address academic ability and clinical skills; active license as registered nurse or advanced practice registered nurse. Additional exam requirements/recommendations for international students: Required—TOEFL (minimum score 500 paper-based; 61 iBT). *Application deadline:* For fall admission, 3/15 for domestic students, 4/1 for international students. Application fee: $30. Electronic applications accepted. *Expenses:* Tuition, state resident: full-time $9794; part-time $408.10 per credit hour. Tuition, nonresident: full-time $22,383; part-time $932.61 per credit hour. *Required fees:* $2020; $84.20 per credit hour. Tuition and fees vary according to course load and program. *Financial support:* In 2013–14, 26 students received support. Research assistantships available. Financial award application deadline: 4/1; financial award applicants required to submit FAFSA. *Faculty research:* Teen pregnancy, diabetes, ethical decision-making, family caregivers. *Total annual research expenditures:* $66,739. *Unit head:* Dr. Li Loriz, Chair, 904-620-1053, E-mail: lloriz@unf.edu. *Application contact:* Beth Dibble, Assistant Director of Admissions for Nursing and Physical Therapy, 904-620-2684, Fax: 904-620-1832, E-mail: nursingadmissions@unf.edu.
Website: http://www.unf.edu/brooks/nursing

University of North Georgia, Department of Nursing, Dahlonega, GA 30597. Offers family nurse practitioner (MS); nursing education (MS). Part-time programs available. *Degree requirements:* For master's, one foreign language, comprehensive exam, thesis. *Entrance requirements:* For master's, GRE General Test or MAT, minimum GPA of 2.5, 3 letters of recommendation, essay, current Georgia RN license, 1 year of post-licensure work, BSN, ASN. Additional exam requirements/recommendations for international students: Required—TOEFL (minimum score 550 paper-based; 79 iBT), IELTS (minimum score 6.5). Electronic applications accepted. *Faculty research:* Diabetes, hypertension, access to woman's health screening, simulation in nursing education, health care of undeserved populations.

University of Pennsylvania, School of Nursing, Family Health Nurse Practitioner Program, Philadelphia, PA 19104. Offers MSN, Certificate. *Accreditation:* AACN. Part-time programs available. *Students:* 28 full-time (25 women), 21 part-time (20 women); includes 12 minority (2 Black or African American, non-Hispanic/Latino; 7 Asian, non-Hispanic/Latino; 2 Hispanic/Latino; 1 Two or more races, non-Hispanic/Latino), 1 international. 21 applicants, 57% accepted, 11 enrolled. In 2013, 25 master's awarded. *Entrance requirements:* For master's, GRE General Test, 1 year of clinical experience in area of interest, BSN, minimum GPA of 3.0, previous course work in statistics. Additional exam requirements/recommendations for international students: Required—TOEFL. *Application deadline:* For fall admission, 2/15 priority date for domestic students. Applications are processed on a rolling basis. Application fee: $70. *Expenses:* Contact institution. *Financial support:* Research assistantships, teaching assistantships, career-related internships or fieldwork, Federal Work-Study, and institutionally sponsored loans available. Support available to part-time students. Financial award application deadline: 4/1. *Faculty research:* Evaluation of primary care practitioner practice, access to primary care. *Unit head:* Assistant Dean of Admissions and Financial Aid, 866-867-6877, Fax: 215-573-8439, E-mail: admissions@nursing.upenn.edu. *Application contact:* Ann O'Sullivan, Program Director, 215-898-4272, E-mail: osull@nursing.upenn.edu.
Website: http://www.nursing.upenn.edu/fnp/

University of Phoenix–Hawaii Campus, College of Nursing, Honolulu, HI 96813-4317. Offers education (MHA); family nurse practitioner (MSN); gerontology (MHA); health administration (MHA); nursing (MSN); nursing/health care education (MSN); MSN/MBA. Evening/weekend programs available. *Degree requirements:* For master's, thesis (for some programs). *Entrance requirements:* For master's, minimum undergraduate GPA of 2.5, 3 years of work experience, RN license. Additional exam requirements/recommendations for international students: Required—TOEFL (minimum score 550 paper-based; 79 iBT). Electronic applications accepted.

University of Phoenix–Online Campus, College of Health Sciences and Nursing, Phoenix, AZ 85034-7209. Offers family nurse practitioner (Certificate); health care (Certificate); health care education (Certificate); health care informatics (Certificate); informatics (MSN); nursing (MSN); nursing and health care education (MSN); MSN/MBA; MSN/MHA. *Accreditation:* AACN. Evening/weekend programs available. Postbaccalaureate distance learning degree programs offered. *Entrance requirements:* Additional exam requirements/recommendations for international students: Required—TOEFL, TOEIC (Test of English as an International Communication), Berlitz Online English Proficiency Exam, PTE, or IELTS. Electronic applications accepted. *Expenses:* Contact institution.

University of Phoenix–Phoenix Campus, College of Health Sciences and Nursing, Tempe, AZ 85282-2371. Offers family nurse practitioner (MSN, Certificate); gerontology health care (Certificate); health care education (MSN, Certificate); health care informatics (Certificate); informatics (MSN); nursing (MSN); MSN/MHA. Evening/

weekend programs available. Postbaccalaureate distance learning degree programs offered. *Entrance requirements:* Additional exam requirements/recommendations for international students: Required—TOEFL, TOEIC (Test of English as an International Communication), Berlitz Online English Proficiency Exam, PTE, or IELTS. Electronic applications accepted. *Expenses:* Contact institution.

University of Phoenix–Sacramento Valley Campus, College of Nursing, Sacramento, CA 95833-3632. Offers family nurse practitioner (MSN); health administration (MHA); health care education (MSN); nursing (MSN); MSN/MBA. Evening/weekend programs available. *Degree requirements:* For master's, thesis (for some programs). *Entrance requirements:* For master's, RN license, minimum undergraduate GPA of 2.5, 3 years work experience. Additional exam requirements/recommendations for international students: Required—TOEFL (minimum score 550 paper-based; 79 iBT). Electronic applications accepted.

University of Phoenix–Southern California Campus, College of Health Sciences and Nursing, Costa Mesa, CA 92626. Offers family nurse practitioner (MSN, Certificate); health care (Certificate); informatics (MSN); nursing (MSN); nursing/health care education (MSN, Certificate); MSN/MBA; MSN/MHA. Evening/weekend programs available. Postbaccalaureate distance learning degree programs offered. *Entrance requirements:* Additional exam requirements/recommendations for international students: Required—TOEFL, TOEIC (Test of English as an International Communication), Berlitz Online English Proficiency Exam, PTE, or IELTS. Electronic applications accepted. *Expenses:* Contact institution.

University of Pittsburgh, School of Nursing, Nurse Practitioner Program, Pittsburgh, PA 15261. Offers adult-gerontology acute care nurse practitioner (DNP); adult-gerontology primary care nurse practitioner (DNP); family (individual across the lifespan) nurse practitioner (DNP); neonatal nurse practitioner (MSN, DNP); pediatric primary care nurse practitioner (DNP); psychiatric mental health nurse practitioner (DNP). *Accreditation:* AACN. Part-time programs available. *Students:* 66 full-time (59 women), 84 part-time (75 women); includes 11 minority (5 Black or African American, non-Hispanic/Latino; 2 American Indian or Alaska Native, non-Hispanic/Latino; 3 Asian, non-Hispanic/Latino; 1 Hispanic/Latino), 2 international. Average age 31. 95 applicants, 74% accepted, 57 enrolled. In 2013, 53 master's, 4 doctorates awarded. *Degree requirements:* For master's, comprehensive exam, thesis optional. *Entrance requirements:* For master's, GRE General Test or MAT, BSN, RN license, letters of recommendation, resume, course work in statistics, 1-3 years of nursing experience; for doctorate, GRE General Test, BSN, RN license, minimum GPA of 3.5, 3 letters of recommendation. Additional exam requirements/recommendations for international students: Required—TOEFL (minimum score 550 paper-based; 80 iBT). *Application deadline:* Applications are processed on a rolling basis. Application fee: $50. Electronic applications accepted. *Expenses:* Tuition, state resident: full-time $19,964; part-time $807 per credit. Tuition, nonresident: full-time $32,686; part-time $1337 per credit. *Required fees:* $740; $200. Tuition and fees vary according to program. *Financial support:* In 2013–14, 18 students received support, including 4 fellowships with full and partial tuition reimbursements available (averaging $22,521 per year), 3 research assistantships with full and partial tuition reimbursements available (averaging $21,884 per year), 15 teaching assistantships with full and partial tuition reimbursements available (averaging $13,535 per year); scholarships/grants, traineeships, health care benefits, and unspecified assistantships also available. Support available to part-time students. *Unit head:* Dr. Sandra Engberg, Associate Dean for Clinical Education, 412-624-3835, Fax: 412-624-8521, E-mail: sje1@pitt.edu. *Application contact:* Laurie Lapsley, Administrator of Graduate Student Services, 412-624-9670, Fax: 412-624-2409, E-mail: lapsleyl@pitt.edu.
Website: http://www.nursing.pitt.edu

University of Puerto Rico, Medical Sciences Campus, School of Nursing, San Juan, PR 00936-5067. Offers adult and elderly nursing (MSN); child and adolescent nursing (MSN); critical care nursing (MSN); family and community nursing (MSN); family nurse practitioner (MSN); maternity nursing (MSN); mental health and psychiatric nursing (MSN). *Accreditation:* AACN. *Entrance requirements:* For master's, GRE or EXADEP, interview, Puerto Rico RN license or professional license for international students, general and specific point average, article analysis. Electronic applications accepted. *Faculty research:* HIV, health disparities, teen violence, women and violence, neurological disorders.

University of Rhode Island, Graduate School, College of Nursing, Kingston, RI 02881. Offers administration (MS); clinical nurse leader (MS); clinical specialist in gerontology (MS); clinical specialist in psychiatric/mental health (MS); family nurse practitioner (MS); gerontological nurse practitioner (MS); nursing (DNP, PhD); nursing education (MS). *Accreditation:* AACN; ACNM/ACME (one or more programs are accredited). Part-time programs available. *Faculty:* 26 full-time (25 women), 3 part-time/adjunct (2 women). *Students:* 46 full-time (42 women), 78 part-time (70 women); includes 11 minority (7 Black or African American, non-Hispanic/Latino; 1 Asian, non-Hispanic/Latino; 3 Hispanic/Latino), 4 international. In 2013, 38 master's, 4 doctorates awarded. *Degree requirements:* For master's, comprehensive exam; for doctorate, comprehensive exam, thesis/dissertation. *Entrance requirements:* For master's, GRE or MAT, 2 letters of recommendation, scholarly papers; for doctorate, GRE, 3 letters of recommendation, scholarly papers. Additional exam requirements/recommendations for international students: Required—TOEFL (minimum score 550 paper-based). *Application deadline:* For fall admission, 2/15 for domestic students, 2/1 for international students; for spring admission, 10/15 for domestic students, 7/15 for international students. Application fee: $65. Electronic applications accepted. *Expenses:* Tuition, state resident: full-time $11,532; part-time $641 per credit. Tuition, nonresident: full-time $23,606; part-time $1311 per credit. *Required fees:* $1388; $36 per credit. $35 per semester. One-time fee: $130. *Financial support:* In 2013–14, 4 teaching assistantships with full and partial tuition reimbursements (averaging $8,383 per year) were awarded. Financial award application deadline: 2/15; financial award applicants required to submit FAFSA. *Faculty research:* Group intervention for grieving women in prison, translating best practice in non-drug interventions for postoperative pain management, further development and testing of the pain assessment inventory, preschool motor and functional performance of two cohorts, neuroactivation of brain motor areas in preterm children. *Total annual research expenditures:* $1.2 million. *Unit head:* Dr. Mary Sullivan, Interim Dean, 401-874-5339, Fax: 401-874-2061, E-mail: mcsullivan@uri.edu. *Application contact:* Graduate Admission, 401-874-2872, E-mail: gradadm@etal.uri.edu.
Website: http://www.uri.edu/nursing/

University of Rochester, School of Nursing, Rochester, NY 14642. Offers acute care nurse practitioner (MS); adult nurse practitioner (MS); adult/geriatric nurse practitioner (MS); clinical nurse leader (MS); clinical research coordinator (MS); family nurse practitioner (MS); family psychiatric mental health nurse practitioner (MS); health care organization management and leadership (MS); health practice research (PhD); nursing (DNP); pediatric nurse practitioner (MS); pediatric nurse practitioner/neonatal nurse practitioner (MS). *Accreditation:* AACN. Part-time programs available. Postbaccalaureate distance learning degree programs offered (minimal on-campus study). *Faculty:* 60 full-time (52 women), 61 part-time/adjunct (47 women). *Students:* 33 full-time (29 women), 213 part-time (195 women); includes 32 minority (8 Black or African American, non-Hispanic/Latino; 10 Asian, non-Hispanic/Latino; 8 Hispanic/Latino; 6 Two or more races, non-Hispanic/Latino), 4 international. Average age 34. 41 applicants, 54% accepted, 16 enrolled. In 2013, 58 master's, 11 doctorates awarded. Terminal master's awarded for partial completion of doctoral program. *Degree requirements:* For master's, comprehensive exam (for some programs); for doctorate, thesis/dissertation. *Entrance requirements:* For master's, BS in nursing, minimum GPA of 3.0, course work in statistics; for doctorate, GRE General Test, MS in nursing, minimum GPA of 3.5. Additional exam requirements/recommendations for international students: Required—TOEFL (minimum score 560 paper-based; 88 iBT) or IELTS (minimum score 6.5) recommended. *Application deadline:* For fall admission, 4/1 for domestic and international students; for spring admission, 9/1 for domestic and international students; for summer admission, 1/2 for domestic and international students. Application fee: $50. Electronic applications accepted. *Expenses: Tuition:* Full-time $44,580; part-time $1394 per credit hour. *Required fees:* $492. *Financial support:* In 2013–14, 41 students received support, including 2 fellowships with full and partial tuition reimbursements available (averaging $30,200 per year); scholarships/grants, traineeships, health care benefits, tuition waivers (partial), and unspecified assistantships also available. Support available to part-time students. Financial award application deadline: 6/30. *Faculty research:* Symptom assessment and self-management, illness prevention, nursing intervention research with vulnerable populations, palliative care, aging. *Total annual research expenditures:* $3.5 million. *Unit head:* Dr. Kathy H. Rideout, Dean, 585-273-8902, Fax: 585-273-1268, E-mail: kathy_rideout@urmc.rochester.edu. *Application contact:* Elaine Andolina, Director of Admissions, 585-275-2375, Fax: 585-756-8299, E-mail: elaine_andolina@urmc.rochester.edu.
Website: http://www.son.rochester.edu

University of Saint Francis, Graduate School, Department of Nursing, Fort Wayne, IN 46808. Offers family nurse practitioner (MSN, Post Master's Certificate). *Accreditation:* AACN. Part-time and evening/weekend programs available. Postbaccalaureate distance learning degree programs offered (minimal on-campus study). *Faculty:* 9. *Students:* 33 full-time (30 women), 69 part-time (65 women); includes 7 minority (3 Black or African American, non-Hispanic/Latino; 3 Hispanic/Latino; 1 Two or more races, non-Hispanic/Latino). Average age 33. 10 applicants, 100% accepted, 10 enrolled. In 2013, 33 master's awarded. *Degree requirements:* For master's, research project. *Entrance requirements:* For master's, GRE (if undergraduate GPA is less than 3.0), minimum undergraduate GPA of 3.2; Indiana RN license; graduate or undergraduate statistics course within the last five years. *Application deadline:* For fall admission, 7/1 priority date for domestic students; for spring admission, 11/1 priority date for domestic students. Applications are processed on a rolling basis. Application fee: $20. Application fee is waived when completed online. *Financial support:* Federal Work-Study, scholarships/grants, and unspecified assistantships available. Support available to part-time students. Financial award application deadline: 3/10; financial award applicants required to submit FAFSA. *Unit head:* Dr. Wendy Clark, Assistant Professor/Director of the MSN Program, 260-399-7700 Ext. 8534, Fax: 260-399-8167, E-mail: wclark@sf.edu. *Application contact:* James Cashdollar, Admissions Counselor, 260-399-7700 Ext. 6302, Fax: 260-399-8152, E-mail: jcashdollar@sf.edu.
Website: http://www.sf.edu/sf/graduate/sohs/nursing

University of St. Francis, Leach College of Nursing, Joliet, IL 60435-6169. Offers family nurse practitioner (MSN, Post-Master's Certificate); family psychology/mental health nurse practitioner (MSN, Post-Master's Certificate); nursing administration (MSN); nursing education (MSN); nursing practice (DNP); teaching in nursing (Certificate). *Accreditation:* AACN. Part-time and evening/weekend programs available. Postbaccalaureate distance learning degree programs offered (no on-campus study). *Faculty:* 11 full-time (all women), 12 part-time/adjunct (11 women). *Students:* 90 full-time (76 women), 332 part-time (305 women); includes 122 minority (43 Black or African American, non-Hispanic/Latino; 1 American Indian or Alaska Native, non-Hispanic/Latino; 19 Asian, non-Hispanic/Latino; 45 Hispanic/Latino; 3 Native Hawaiian or other Pacific Islander, non-Hispanic/Latino; 11 Two or more races, non-Hispanic/Latino), 4 international. Average age 42. 343 applicants, 43% accepted, 111 enrolled. In 2013, 82 master's, 6 doctorates, 17 other advanced degrees awarded. *Entrance requirements:* For master's, minimum undergraduate GPA of 3.0, 2 years of full-time clinical experience, 3 letters recommendation, resume, nursing license, interview; for doctorate, MSN with minimum GPA of 3.0, national certification, interview, computer competency, medical/physical requirements, background check, liability insurance, resume, recommendation, graduate-level statistics course. Additional exam requirements/recommendations for international students: Required—TOEFL (minimum score 550 paper-based; 79 iBT), IELTS (minimum score 6.5). *Application deadline:* Applications are processed on a rolling basis. Application fee: $30. Electronic applications accepted. Application fee is waived when completed online. *Expenses:* Contact institution. *Financial support:* In 2013–14, 109 students received support. Scholarships/grants and tuition waivers (partial) available. Support available to part-time students. Financial award applicants required to submit FAFSA. *Unit head:* Dr. Carol Wilson, Dean, 815-740-3840, Fax: 815-740-4243, E-mail: cwilson@stfrancis.edu. *Application contact:* Sandra Sloka, Director of Admissions for Graduate and Degree Completion Programs, 800-735-7500, Fax: 815-740-3431, E-mail: ssloka@stfrancis.edu.
Website: http://www.stfrancis.edu/academics/college-of-nursing/

University of Saint Joseph, Department of Nursing, West Hartford, CT 06117-2700. Offers family nurse practitioner (MS); family psychiatric/mental health nurse practitioner (MS); nurse educator (MS); nursing practice (DNP). *Accreditation:* AACN. Part-time and evening/weekend programs available. *Degree requirements:* For master's, thesis. *Entrance requirements:* For master's, 2 letters of recommendation. *Application deadline:* Applications are processed on a rolling basis. Application fee: $50. Electronic applications accepted. Application fee is waived when completed online. *Financial support:* Career-related internships or fieldwork and unspecified assistantships available. Support available to part-time students. Financial award applicants required to submit FAFSA. *Unit head:* Dr. Patricia Padula Morgan, RN, Chair, 860-231-5591, E-mail: pmorgan@usj.edu. *Application contact:* Graduate Admissions Office, 860-231-5261, E-mail: graduate@usj.edu.
Website: http://www.usj.edu/academics/schools/school-of-health-natural-sciences/nursing/

University of San Diego, Hahn School of Nursing and Health Science, San Diego, CA 92110. Offers adult-gerontology clinical nurse specialist (MSN); adult-gerontology nurse practitioner/family nurse practitioner (MSN); clinical nursing (MSN); executive nurse leader (MSN); family nurse practitioner (MSN); family/lifespan psychiatric-mental health nurse practitioner (MSN); healthcare informatics (MS, MSN); nursing (PhD); nursing practice (DNP); pediatric nurse practitioner/family nurse practitioner (MSN). *Accreditation:* AACN. Part-time and evening/weekend programs available. *Faculty:* 23 full-time (19 women), 48 part-time/adjunct (43 women). *Students:* 204 full-time (170 women), 166 part-time (144 women); includes 133 minority (26 Black or African American, non-Hispanic/Latino; 8 American Indian or Alaska Native, non-Hispanic/Latino; 50 Asian, non-Hispanic/Latino; 42 Hispanic/Latino; 1 Native Hawaiian or other Pacific Islander, non-Hispanic/Latino; 6 Two or more races, non-Hispanic/Latino), 7 international. Average age 36. 483 applicants, 58% accepted, 154 enrolled. In 2013, 91 master's, 33 doctorates awarded. *Degree requirements:* For doctorate, thesis/dissertation (for some programs), residency (DNP). *Entrance requirements:* For

master's, GRE General Test (for entry-level nursing), BSN, current California RN licensure (except for entry-level nursing); minimum GPA of 3.0; for doctorate, minimum GPA of 3.5, MSN, current California RN licensure. Additional exam requirements/recommendations for international students: Required—TOEFL (minimum score 580 paper-based; 83 iBT), TWE. *Application deadline:* For fall admission, 3/1 priority date for domestic students, 3/1 for international students; for spring admission, 11/1 priority date for domestic students, 11/1 for international students. Applications are processed on a rolling basis. Application fee: $45. Electronic applications accepted. *Expenses: Tuition:* Full-time $23,580; part-time $1310 per credit. *Required fees:* $350. *Financial support:* In 2013–14, 250 students received support. Scholarships/grants and traineeships available. Support available to part-time students. Financial award application deadline: 4/1; financial award applicants required to submit FAFSA. *Faculty research:* Palliative and end of life care, maternal/child health, childhood obesity, health care disparities, cognitive functioning. *Unit head:* Dr. Sally Hardin, Dean, 619-260-4550, Fax: 619-260-6814. *Application contact:* Monica Mahon, Associate Director of Graduate Admissions, 619-260-4524, Fax: 619-260-4158, E-mail: grads@sandiego.edu.
Website: http://www.sandiego.edu/nursing/

University of San Francisco, School of Nursing and Health Professions, Doctoral Programs, San Francisco, CA 94117-1080. Offers clinical psychology (Psy D); executive leadership (DNP); family nurse practitioner (DNP); healthcare systems leadership (DNP); psychiatric mental health nurse practitioner (DNP). *Faculty:* 15 full-time (12 women), 10 part-time/adjunct (7 women). *Students:* 118 full-time (92 women), 34 part-time (31 women); includes 74 minority (13 Black or African American, non-Hispanic/Latino; 1 American Indian or Alaska Native, non-Hispanic/Latino; 32 Asian, non-Hispanic/Latino; 15 Hispanic/Latino; 1 Native Hawaiian or other Pacific Islander, non-Hispanic/Latino; 12 Two or more races, non-Hispanic/Latino), 2 international. Average age 41. 98 applicants, 70% accepted, 49 enrolled. In 2013, 39 doctorates awarded. *Entrance requirements:* For doctorate, nursing bachelor's degree, valid RN license in California. *Expenses: Tuition:* Full-time $21,150; part-time $1175 per unit. Tuition and fees vary according to course load, campus/location and program. *Financial support:* In 2013–14, 7 students received support. *Unit head:* Dr. Judith Karshmer, Dean, 415-422-6681, Fax: 415-422-6877, E-mail: nursing@usfca.edu. *Application contact:* Ingrid McVanner, Information Contact, 415-422-2746, Fax: 415-422-2217.

The University of Scranton, College of Graduate and Continuing Education, Department of Nursing, Scranton, PA 18510-4595. Offers adult health nursing (MSN); family nurse practitioner (MSN, PMC); nurse anesthesia (MSN, PMC). Applicants accepted in odd-numbered years only. *Accreditation:* AACN; AANA/CANAEP. Part-time and evening/weekend programs available. *Faculty:* 13 full-time (all women), 2 part-time/adjunct (both women). *Students:* 42 full-time (37 women), 28 part-time (16 women); includes 9 minority (4 Black or African American, non-Hispanic/Latino; 3 Hispanic/Latino; 2 Two or more races, non-Hispanic/Latino). Average age 34. 58 applicants, 62% accepted. In 2013, 34 master's awarded. *Degree requirements:* For master's, thesis (for some programs), capstone experience. *Entrance requirements:* For master's, BSN, minimum GPA of 3.0, Pennsylvania RN license. Additional exam requirements/recommendations for international students: Required—TOEFL (minimum score 500 paper-based), IELTS (minimum score 5.5). *Application deadline:* For fall admission, 9/1 for domestic students. Applications are processed on a rolling basis. Application fee: $0. *Financial support:* In 2013–14, 6 students received support, including 6 teaching assistantships with full and partial tuition reimbursements available (averaging $6,600 per year); career-related internships or fieldwork, Federal Work-Study, and unspecified assistantships also available. Support available to part-time students. Financial award application deadline: 3/1. *Faculty research:* Home care, doctoral education, health care of women and children, pain, health promotion and adolescence. *Unit head:* Dr. Patricia Harrington, Chair, 570-941-7673, Fax: 570-941-4201, E-mail: harringtonp1@uofs.edu. *Application contact:* Dr. Mary Jane Hanson, Director, 570-941-4060, Fax: 570-941-4201, E-mail: hansonm2@scranton.edu.
Website: http://www.scranton.edu/academics/pcps/nursing/index.shtml

University of South Carolina, The Graduate School, College of Nursing, Program in Health Nursing, Columbia, SC 29208. Offers adult nurse practitioner (MSN); community/public health clinical nurse specialist (MSN); family nurse practitioner (MSN); pediatric nurse practitioner (MSN). *Accreditation:* AACN. Part-time programs available. *Degree requirements:* For master's, thesis or alternative. *Entrance requirements:* For master's, GRE General Test or MAT, BS in nursing, nursing license. Additional exam requirements/recommendations for international students: Required—TOEFL (minimum score 570 paper-based). Electronic applications accepted. *Faculty research:* System research, evidence based practice, breast cancer, violence.

University of Southern Maine, College of Science, Technology, and Health, School of Nursing, Portland, ME 04104-9300. Offers adult-gerontology primary care nurse practitioner (MS, PMC); clinical nurse leader (MS); education (MS); family nurse practitioner (MS, PMC); family psychiatric/mental health nurse practitioner (MS); management (MS); nursing (DNP); psychiatric-mental health nurse practitioner (PMC); MBA/MSN. *Accreditation:* AACN. Part-time programs available. *Faculty:* 11 full-time (all women), 10 part-time/adjunct (8 women). *Students:* 57 full-time (47 women), 53 part-time (46 women); includes 5 minority (1 American Indian or Alaska Native, non-Hispanic/Latino; 2 Asian, non-Hispanic/Latino; 1 Hispanic/Latino; 1 Two or more races, non-Hispanic/Latino). Average age 36. 140 applicants, 44% accepted, 29 enrolled. In 2013, 33 master's, 11 other advanced degrees awarded. *Degree requirements:* For master's, thesis optional. *Entrance requirements:* For master's, GRE General Test or MAT, minimum GPA of 3.0; for doctorate, GRE. Additional exam requirements/recommendations for international students: Required—TOEFL (minimum score 550 paper-based). *Application deadline:* For fall admission, 4/1 for domestic and international students; for spring admission, 10/1 for domestic and international students. Application fee: $65. Electronic applications accepted. *Expenses:* Tuition, state resident: part-time $380 per credit. Tuition, nonresident: part-time $1026 per credit. Part-time tuition and fees vary according to program. *Financial support:* Research assistantships, teaching assistantships, career-related internships or fieldwork, Federal Work-Study, scholarships/grants, traineeships, tuition waivers (full and partial), and unspecified assistantships available. Support available to part-time students. Financial award application deadline: 2/15; financial award applicants required to submit FAFSA. *Faculty research:* Women's health, nursing history, weight control, community services, substance abuse. *Unit head:* Krista M. Meinersmann, Director of Nursing Program, 207-780-4993, E-mail: kmeinersmann@usm.maine.edu. *Application contact:* Mary Sloan, Assistant Dean of Graduate Studies and Director of Graduate Admissions, 207-780-4812, E-mail: gradstudies@usm.maine.edu.
Website: http://www.usm.maine.edu/nursing/

University of Southern Mississippi, Graduate School, College of Health, School of Nursing, Hattiesburg, MS 39406-0001. Offers family nurse practitioner (MSN); nursing (DNP, PhD); nursing executive (MSN); psychiatric nurse practitioner (MSN). *Accreditation:* AACN. Part-time and evening/weekend programs available. *Faculty:* 17 full-time (16 women), 1 part-time/adjunct (0 women). *Students:* 133 full-time (104 women), 42 part-time (40 women); includes 45 minority (33 Black or African American, non-Hispanic/Latino; 1 American Indian or Alaska Native, non-Hispanic/Latino; 1 Asian, non-Hispanic/Latino; 1 Hispanic/Latino; 9 Two or more races, non-Hispanic/Latino). Average age 37. 118 applicants, 61% accepted, 62 enrolled. In 2013, 45 master's, 9 doctorates awarded. *Degree requirements:* For master's, comprehensive exam, thesis optional; for doctorate, comprehensive exam, thesis/dissertation. *Entrance requirements:* For master's, GRE General Test, minimum GPA of 2.75 during last 60 hours, nursing license, BS in nursing; for doctorate, GRE General Test, master's degree in nursing, minimum GPA of 3.5. Additional exam requirements/recommendations for international students: Required—TOEFL, IELTS. *Application deadline:* For fall admission, 3/15 priority date for domestic students, 5/1 for international students; for spring admission, 1/10 priority date for domestic and international students. Applications are processed on a rolling basis. Application fee: $50. Electronic applications accepted. *Financial support:* In 2013–14, 14 research assistantships with full tuition reimbursements (averaging $12,577 per year), teaching assistantships (averaging $12,000 per year) were awarded; Federal Work-Study, institutionally sponsored loans, scholarships/grants, traineeships, health care benefits, and unspecified assistantships also available. Financial award application deadline: 3/15; financial award applicants required to submit FAFSA. *Faculty research:* Gerontology, caregivers, HIV, bereavement, pain, nursing leadership. *Unit head:* Dr. Katherine Nugent, Director and Associate Dean, 601-266-5500, Fax: 601-266-5927. *Application contact:* Dr. Sandra Bishop, Graduate Coordinator, 601-266-5500, Fax: 601-266-5927.
Website: http://www.usm.edu/graduateschool/table.php

University of South Florida, College of Nursing, Tampa, FL 33612. Offers adult gerontology acute care (DNP, PhD); adult gerontology acute care nursing (MS); adult gerontology primary care (DNP, PhD); adult gerontology primary care nursing (MS); adult gerontology primary care/occupational health nursing (MS); adult gerontology primary care/oncology nursing (MS, PhD); clinical nurse leader (MS); family health (DNP, PhD); family nurse practitioner (MS); nurse anesthesia (MS); nursing education (MS); nursing practice (DNP); nursing science (PhD), including nursing education; occupational health/adult-gerontology (DNP); oncology/adult-gerontology primary care (DNP); pediatric health (DNP, PhD); pediatric nurse practitioner (MS). *Accreditation:* AACN; AANA/CANAEP. Part-time programs available. *Faculty:* 46 full-time (40 women), 15 part-time/adjunct (11 women). *Students:* 177 full-time (150 women), 700 part-time (622 women); includes 272 minority (116 Black or African American, non-Hispanic/Latino; 2 American Indian or Alaska Native, non-Hispanic/Latino; 45 Asian, non-Hispanic/Latino; 93 Hispanic/Latino; 2 Native Hawaiian or other Pacific Islander, non-Hispanic/Latino; 14 Two or more races, non-Hispanic/Latino), 12 international. Average age 35. 656 applicants, 43% accepted, 224 enrolled. In 2013, 224 master's, 14 doctorates awarded. *Degree requirements:* For master's, comprehensive exam, thesis optional; for doctorate, comprehensive exam, thesis/dissertation. *Entrance requirements:* For master's, GRE General Test, bachelor's degree from accredited program with minimum GPA of 3.0 in all upper-division coursework; current license as Registered Nurse; 3 letters of recommendation; personal statement of goals; resume or curriculum vitae; personal interview; for doctorate, GRE General Test (recommended), bachelor's degree in nursing from a CCNA/NLNAC regionally-accredited institution with minimum GPA of 3.0 in all coursework or in all upper-division coursework; current license as Registered Nurse in Florida; undergraduate statistics course with minimum B grade; 3 letters of recommendation; statement of goals; resume; interview. Additional exam requirements/recommendations for international students: Required—TOEFL (minimum score 550 paper-based; 79 iBT). *Application deadline:* For fall admission, 2/15 for domestic students, 1/2 for international students; for spring admission, 10/1 for domestic students, 6/1 for international students. Application fee: $30. Electronic applications accepted. *Financial support:* In 2013–14, 36 students received support, including 7 research assistantships with tuition reimbursements available (averaging $18,935 per year), 29 teaching assistantships with tuition reimbursements available (averaging $30,814 per year); tuition waivers (partial) and unspecified assistantships also available. Financial award application deadline: 2/1; financial award applicants required to submit FAFSA. *Faculty research:* Women's health, palliative and end-of-life care, cardiac rehabilitation, complementary therapies for chronic illness and cancer. *Total annual research expenditures:* $3.4 million. *Unit head:* Dr. Dianne C. Morrison-Beedy, Dean and Professor, College of Nursing, 813-974-9091, Fax: 813-974-5418, E-mail: dmbeedy@health.usf.edu. *Application contact:* Dr. Connie Visovsky, Associate Professor and Associate Dean of Student Affairs, 813-396-9641, Fax: 813-974-5418, E-mail: cvisovsk@health.usf.edu.
Website: http://health.usf.edu/nursing/index.htm

The University of Tampa, Nursing Programs, Tampa, FL 33606-1490. Offers adult nurse practitioner (MSN); family nurse practitioner (MSN). Part-time programs available. *Faculty:* 15 full-time (all women), 15 part-time/adjunct (14 women). *Students:* 2 full-time (both women), 134 part-time (119 women); includes 37 minority (10 Black or African American, non-Hispanic/Latino; 1 American Indian or Alaska Native, non-Hispanic/Latino; 6 Asian, non-Hispanic/Latino; 19 Hispanic/Latino; 1 Two or more races, non-Hispanic/Latino). Average age 34. 79 applicants, 51% accepted, 28 enrolled. In 2013, 39 master's awarded. *Degree requirements:* For master's, comprehensive exam, oral exam, practicum. *Entrance requirements:* For master's, GRE (minimum score of 1000, 4.0 on Analytical Writing portion), bachelor's degree in nursing, current Florida RN license, minimum GPA of 3.0. Additional exam requirements/recommendations for international students: Required—TOEFL or IELTS. *Application deadline:* Applications are processed on a rolling basis. Application fee: $40. Electronic applications accepted. *Expenses: Tuition:* Full-time $8928; part-time $558 per credit hour. *Required fees:* $80; $80 $40 per term. Tuition and fees vary according to program. *Financial support:* In 2013–14, 9 students received support. Unspecified assistantships available. Financial award applicants required to submit FAFSA. *Faculty research:* Vaccinations and public health, osteoporosis, cultural diversity, ethics, nursing practice. *Unit head:* Dr. Maria Warda, Director/Chair, 813-257-3302, Fax: 813-258-7214, E-mail: mwarda@ut.edu. *Application contact:* Brent Benner, Director of Admissions, 813-257-3642, E-mail: bbenner@ut.edu.

The University of Tennessee at Chattanooga, Graduate School, College of Health, Education and Professional Studies, School of Nursing, Chattanooga, TN 37403. Offers administration (MSN); certified nurse anesthetist (Post-Master's Certificate); education (MSN); family nurse practitioner (MSN, Post-Master's Certificate); health care informatics (Post-Master's Certificate); nurse anesthesia (MSN); nurse education (Post-Master's Certificate); nursing (DNP). *Accreditation:* AACN; AANA/CANAEP (one or more programs are accredited). *Faculty:* 9 full-time (7 women), 2 part-time/adjunct (1 woman). *Students:* 72 full-time (39 women), 53 part-time (43 women); includes 11 minority (6 Black or African American, non-Hispanic/Latino; 1 Asian, non-Hispanic/Latino; 3 Hispanic/Latino; 1 Two or more races, non-Hispanic/Latino). Average age 33. 3 applicants, 100% accepted, 1 enrolled. In 2013, 35 master's, 10 doctorates, 2 other advanced degrees awarded. *Degree requirements:* For master's, thesis optional, qualifying exams, professional project; for Post-Master's Certificate, thesis or alternative, practicum, seminar. *Entrance requirements:* For master's, GRE General Test, MAT, BSN, minimum GPA of 3.0, eligibility for Tennessee RN license, 1 year of direct patient care experience; for Post-Master's Certificate, GRE General Test, MAT, MSN, minimum GPA of 3.0, eligibility for Tennessee RN license, one year of direct patient care experience. Additional exam requirements/recommendations for international students: Required—TOEFL (minimum score 550 paper-based; 79 iBT), IELTS (minimum score 6). *Application deadline:* For fall admission, 6/13 priority date for domestic students, 6/1

for international students; for spring admission, 10/15 priority date for domestic students, 10/1 for international students. Applications are processed on a rolling basis. Application fee: $30 ($35 for international students). Electronic applications accepted. *Financial support:* Career-related internships or fieldwork and scholarships/grants available. Support available to part-time students. *Faculty research:* Diabetes in women, health care for elderly, alternative medicine, hypertension, nurse anesthesia. *Total annual research expenditures:* $3.4 million. *Unit head:* Dr. Chris Smith, Interim Director, 423-425-1741, Fax: 423-425-4668, E-mail: chris-smith@utc.edu. *Application contact:* Dr. J. Randy Walker, Interim Dean of Graduate Studies, 423-425-4478, Fax: 423-425-5223, E-mail: randy-walker@utc.edu.
Website: http://www.utc.edu/Academic/Nursing/

The University of Texas at Arlington, Graduate School, College of Nursing, Arlington, TX 76019. Offers nurse practitioner (MSN); nursing administration (MSN); nursing education (MSN); nursing practice (DNP); nursing science (PhD). *Accreditation:* AACN. Part-time and evening/weekend programs available. Postbaccalaureate distance learning degree programs offered (no on-campus study). *Degree requirements:* For master's, practicum course; for doctorate, comprehensive exam (for some programs), thesis/dissertation (for some programs), proposal defense dissertation (for PhD); scholarship project (for DNP). *Entrance requirements:* For master's, GRE General Test if GPA less than 3.0, minimum GPA of 3.0, Texas nursing license, minimum C grade in undergraduate statistics course; for doctorate, GRE General Test (waived for MSN-to-PhD applicants), minimum undergraduate, graduate and statistics GPA of 3.0; Texas RN license; interview; written statement of goals. Additional exam requirements/recommendations for international students: Required—TOEFL (minimum score 550 paper-based), IELTS (minimum score 7). *Faculty research:* Simulation in clinical education and practice, cultural diversity, vulnerable populations, substance abuse.

The University of Texas at Austin, Graduate School, School of Nursing, Austin, TX 78712-1111. Offers adult - gerontology clinical nurse specialist (MSN); child health (MSN), including administration, public health nursing, teaching; family nurse practitioner (MSN); family psychiatric/mental health nurse practitioner (MSN); holistic adult health (MSN), including administration, teaching; maternity (MSN), including administration, public health nursing, teaching; nursing (PhD); nursing administration and healthcare systems management (MSN); pediatric nurse practitioner (MSN); public health nursing (MSN). *Accreditation:* AACN. Part-time programs available. *Degree requirements:* For master's, thesis optional; for doctorate, thesis/dissertation. *Entrance requirements:* For master's and doctorate, GRE General Test. Additional exam requirements/recommendations for international students: Required—TOEFL (minimum score 550 paper-based). Electronic applications accepted. *Faculty research:* Chronic illness management, memory and aging, health promotion, women's health, adolescent health.

The University of Texas at El Paso, Graduate School, School of Nursing, El Paso, TX 79968-0001. Offers family nurse practitioner (MSN); health care leadership and management (Certificate); interdisciplinary health sciences (PhD); nursing (DNP); nursing education (MSN, Certificate); nursing systems management (MSN). *Accreditation:* AACN. Postbaccalaureate distance learning degree programs offered (minimal on-campus study). *Degree requirements:* For master's, thesis optional; for doctorate, thesis/dissertation. *Entrance requirements:* For master's, minimum GPA of 3.0, resume; for doctorate, GRE, letters of reference, relevant personal/professional experience; master's degree in nursing (for DNP); for Certificate, bachelor's degree in nursing. Additional exam requirements/recommendations for international students: Required—TOEFL; Recommended—IELTS. Electronic applications accepted.

The University of Texas at Tyler, College of Nursing and Health Sciences, Program in Nursing, Tyler, TX 75799-0001. Offers nurse practitioner (MSN); nursing (PhD); nursing administration (MSN); nursing education (MSN); MSN/MBA. *Accreditation:* AACN. Part-time and evening/weekend programs available. Postbaccalaureate distance learning degree programs offered (no on-campus study). *Degree requirements:* For master's, comprehensive exam (for some programs), thesis (for some programs); for doctorate, thesis/dissertation. *Entrance requirements:* For master's, GRE General Test or MAT, GMAT, minimum undergraduate GPA of 3.0, course work in statistics, RN license, BSN. Additional exam requirements/recommendations for international students: Required—TOEFL. Electronic applications accepted. *Faculty research:* Psychosocial adjustment, aging, support/commitment of caregivers, psychological abuse and violence, hope/hopelessness, professional values, end of life care, suicidology, clinical supervision, workforce retention and issues, global health issues, health promotion.

The University of Texas Health Science Center at San Antonio, School of Nursing, San Antonio, TX 78229. Offers administrative management (MSN); adult-gerontology acute care nurse practitioner (PGC); clinical nurse leader (MSN); executive administrative management (DNP); family nurse practitioner (PGC); nurse practitioner (MSN), including adult-gerontology acute care nurse practitioner, family nurse practitioner, pediatric nurse practitioner primary care, psychiatric mental health nurse practitioner; nurse practitioner leadership (DNP); nursing (MSN, PhD); nursing education (MSN, PGC); pediatric nurse practitioner primary care (PGC); psychiatric mental health nurse practitioner (PGC); public health nurse leader (DNP). *Accreditation:* AACN. Part-time programs available. *Faculty:* 84 full-time (74 women), 42 part-time/adjunct (40 women). *Students:* 115 full-time (93 women), 140 part-time (123 women); includes 123 minority (24 Black or African American, non-Hispanic/Latino; 20 Asian, non-Hispanic/Latino; 74 Hispanic/Latino; 5 Two or more races, non-Hispanic/Latino), 7 international. Average age 37. 174 applicants, 59% accepted, 83 enrolled. In 2013, 67 master's, 6 doctorates, 5 other advanced degrees awarded. Terminal master's awarded for partial completion of doctoral program. *Degree requirements:* For master's, thesis optional; for doctorate, comprehensive exam, thesis/dissertation, final projects (for DNP). *Entrance requirements:* For master's, minimum GPA of 3.0, references, goal statement, BSN from accredited nursing school, RN licensure in Texas or compact state; for doctorate, GRE, MAT, minimum GPA of 3.0, personal interview, BSN and/or MSN from accredited nursing school, RN licensure in Texas or compact state, statistics course, references, curriculum vitae, goal statement; for PGC, minimum GPA of 3.0; references; goal statement; MSN from accredited nursing school; RN licensure in Texas or compact state; prerequisites in advanced health assessment, advanced pharmacotherapeutics, and advanced pathophysiology. Additional exam requirements/recommendations for international students: Required—TOEFL (minimum score 550 paper-based; 68 iBT), IELTS (minimum score 6.5). *Application deadline:* For fall admission, 1/10 for domestic and international students; for spring admission, 7/1 for domestic students. Application fee: $65. Electronic applications accepted. *Financial support:* In 2013–14, 145 students received support, including 3 fellowships with full tuition reimbursements available (averaging $30,000 per year); institutionally sponsored loans and scholarships/grants also available. Financial award application deadline: 6/30; financial award applicants required to submit FAFSA. *Faculty research:* Pain, organizational structure, aging, quality and safety, health disparity, obesity and nutrition, women's and children's health. *Total annual research expenditures:* $500,265. *Unit head:* Dr. Eileen T. Breslin, Dean, 210-567-5800, Fax: 210-567-5929, E-mail: breslin@uthscsa.edu. *Application contact:* Brandy Finck, Interim Associate Dean for Admissions and Student Services, 210-567-5805, Fax: 210-567-6189, E-mail: finckb@uthscsa.edu.
Website: http://www.nursing.uthscsa.edu/

The University of Texas–Pan American, College of Health Sciences and Human Services, Department of Nursing, Edinburg, TX 78539. Offers adult health nursing (MSN); family nurse practitioner (MSN). *Accreditation:* AACN. Part-time and evening/weekend programs available. *Degree requirements:* For master's, thesis optional. *Entrance requirements:* For master's, Texas RN licensure, undergraduate physical statistic course. Additional exam requirements/recommendations for international students: Required—TOEFL (minimum score 550 paper-based). Electronic applications accepted. *Expenses:* Contact institution. *Faculty research:* Health promotion, adolescent pregnancy, herbal and nontraditional approaches, healing touch stress.

The University of Toledo, College of Graduate Studies, College of Nursing, Department of Population and Community Care, Toledo, OH 43606-3390. Offers clinical nurse leader (MSN); family nurse practitioner (MSN, Certificate); nurse educator (MSN, Certificate); pediatric nurse practitioner (MSN, Certificate). Part-time programs available. *Students:* 70 full-time (60 women), 212 part-time (186 women); includes 27 minority (12 Black or African American, non-Hispanic/Latino; 1 American Indian or Alaska Native, non-Hispanic/Latino; 3 Asian, non-Hispanic/Latino; 7 Hispanic/Latino; 4 Two or more races, non-Hispanic/Latino), 1 international. Average age 32. 127 applicants, 81% accepted, 78 enrolled. In 2013, 82 master's, 10 other advanced degrees awarded. *Degree requirements:* For master's, thesis or alternative. *Entrance requirements:* For master's, GRE, BS in nursing, minimum undergraduate GPA of 3.0, statement of purpose, three letters of recommendation, transcripts from all prior institutions attended, Nursing CAS application, UT supplemental application; for Certificate, BS in nursing, minimum undergraduate GPA of 3.0, statement of purpose, three letters of recommendation, transcripts from all prior institutions attended. Additional exam requirements/recommendations for international students: Required—TOEFL (minimum score 550 paper-based; 80 iBT). Application fee: $45 ($75 for international students). Electronic applications accepted. *Financial support:* Research assistantships with full and partial tuition reimbursements, Federal Work-Study, scholarships/grants, traineeships, and tuition waivers (full and partial) available. *Unit head:* Dr. Kelley Phillips, Chair, 419-383-5892. *Application contact:* Joan Mulligan, Admissions Analyst, 419-383-4168, Fax: 419-383-6140, E-mail: joan.mulligan@utoledo.edu.
Website: http://www.utoledo.edu/nursing/

University of Victoria, Faculty of Graduate Studies, Faculty of Human and Social Development, School of Nursing, Victoria, BC V8W 2Y2, Canada. Offers advanced nursing practice (advanced practice leadership option) (MN); advanced nursing practice (nurse educator option) (MN); advanced nursing practice (nurse practitioner option) (MN); nursing (PhD). Part-time programs available. Postbaccalaureate distance learning degree programs offered (no on-campus study). *Entrance requirements:* Additional exam requirements/recommendations for international students: Required—TOEFL (minimum score 575 paper-based), IELTS (minimum score 7). Electronic applications accepted.

University of Wisconsin–Eau Claire, College of Nursing and Health Sciences, Program in Nursing, Eau Claire, WI 54702-4004. Offers adult-gerontological administration (DNP); adult-gerontological clinical nurse specialist (DNP); adult-gerontological education (MSN); adult-gerontological primary care nurse practitioner (DNP); family health administration (DNP); family health in education (MSN); family health nurse practitioner (DNP); nursing (MSN); nursing practice (DNP). Part-time programs available. *Faculty:* 8 full-time (all women), 2 part-time/adjunct (both women). *Students:* 33 full-time (30 women), 40 part-time (36 women); includes 1 minority (Asian, non-Hispanic/Latino). Average age 37. 48 applicants, 85% accepted, 24 enrolled. In 2013, 31 master's, 9 doctorates awarded. Terminal master's awarded for partial completion of doctoral program. *Degree requirements:* For master's, thesis optional, 500-600 hours clinical practicum, oral and written exams. *Entrance requirements:* For master's, Wisconsin RN license, minimum GPA of 3.0, undergraduate statistics, course work in health assessment. Additional exam requirements/recommendations for international students: Required—TOEFL (minimum score 79 iBT). *Application deadline:* For fall admission, 1/15 priority date for domestic and international students. Applications are processed on a rolling basis. Application fee: $86. *Expenses:* Contact institution. *Financial support:* In 2013–14, 10 students received support. Federal Work-Study and unspecified assistantships available. Financial award application deadline: 3/1; financial award applicants required to submit FAFSA. *Unit head:* Dr. Linda Young, Dean, 715-836-4904, Fax: 715-836-5925, E-mail: younglk@uwec.edu. *Application contact:* Dr. Mary Zwygart-Stauffacher, Director, 715-836-5287, E-mail: zwygarmc@uwec.edu.
Website: http://www.uwec.edu/conhs/programs/grad/index.htm

University of Wisconsin–Milwaukee, Graduate School, College of Nursing, Milwaukee, WI 53201. Offers family nursing practitioner (Post Master's Certificate); health professional education (Certificate); nursing (MN, PhD); public health (Certificate). *Accreditation:* AACN. Part-time programs available. *Faculty:* 30 full-time (29 women), 2 part-time/adjunct (both women). *Students:* 157 full-time (142 women), 90 part-time (79 women); includes 32 minority (13 Black or African American, non-Hispanic/Latino; 10 Asian, non-Hispanic/Latino; 1 Hispanic/Latino; 8 Two or more races, non-Hispanic/Latino), 7 international. Average age 38. 160 applicants, 57% accepted, 51 enrolled. In 2013, 42 master's, 8 doctorates awarded. *Degree requirements:* For master's, thesis; for doctorate, thesis/dissertation. *Entrance requirements:* For master's, GRE General Test or MAT, autobiographical sketch; for doctorate, GRE, minimum GPA of 3.2. Additional exam requirements/recommendations for international students: Required—TOEFL (minimum score 550 paper-based; 79 iBT), IELTS (minimum score 6.5). *Application deadline:* For fall admission, 1/1 priority date for domestic students; for spring admission, 9/1 for domestic students. Applications are processed on a rolling basis. Application fee: $56 ($96 for international students). Electronic applications accepted. *Financial support:* In 2013–14, 3 fellowships, 1 research assistantship, 9 teaching assistantships were awarded; career-related internships or fieldwork, Federal Work-Study, health care benefits, unspecified assistantships, and project assistantships also available. Support available to part-time students. Financial award application deadline: 4/15; financial award applicants required to submit FAFSA. *Total annual research expenditures:* $3.2 million. *Unit head:* Dr. Sally Lundeen, Dean, 414-229-4189, E-mail: slundeen@uwm.edu. *Application contact:* Kim Litwack, Representative, 414-229-5098.
Website: http://www.uwm.edu/Dept/Nursing/

University of Wisconsin–Oshkosh, Graduate Studies, College of Nursing, Oshkosh, WI 54901. Offers adult health and illness (MSN); family nurse practitioner (MSN). *Accreditation:* AACN. Part-time programs available. *Degree requirements:* For master's, thesis or alternative, clinical paper. *Entrance requirements:* For master's, RN license, BSN, previous course work in statistics and health assessment, minimum undergraduate GPA of 3.0, letters of recommendation. Additional exam requirements/recommendations for international students: Required—TOEFL (minimum score 550 paper-based; 79 iBT). Electronic applications accepted. *Faculty research:* Adult health and illness, nurse practitioners practice, health care service, advanced practitioner roles, natural alternative complementary healthcare.

Vanderbilt University, Vanderbilt University School of Nursing, Nashville, TN 37240. Offers adult-gerontology acute care nurse practitioner (MSN), including hospitalist, intensivist; adult-gerontology primary care nurse practitioner (MSN); emergency nurse

practitioner (MSN); family nurse practitioner (MSN); healthcare leadership (MSN); neonatal nurse practitioner (MSN); nurse midwifery (MSN); nurse midwifery/family nurse practitioner (MSN); nursing informatics (MSN); nursing practice (DNP); nursing science (PhD); pediatric acute care nurse practitioner (MSN); pediatric primary care nurse practitioner (MSN); psychiatric-mental health nurse practitioner (MSN); women's health nurse practitioner (MSN); women's health nurse practitioner/adult gerontology primary care nurse practitioner (MSN); MSN/M Div; MSN/MTS. *Accreditation:* ACNM/ACME (one or more programs are accredited). Part-time programs available. Postbaccalaureate distance learning degree programs offered (minimal on-campus study). *Faculty:* 139 full-time (124 women), 452 part-time/adjunct (319 women). *Students:* 527 full-time (463 women), 369 part-time (333 women); includes 120 minority (46 Black or African American, non-Hispanic/Latino; 8 American Indian or Alaska Native, non-Hispanic/Latino; 26 Asian, non-Hispanic/Latino; 24 Hispanic/Latino; 4 Native Hawaiian or other Pacific Islander, non-Hispanic/Latino; 12 Two or more races, non-Hispanic/Latino), 7 international. Average age 32. 1,257 applicants, 49% accepted, 457 enrolled. In 2013, 364 master's, 43 doctorates awarded. *Degree requirements:* For doctorate, comprehensive exam, thesis/dissertation. *Entrance requirements:* For master's, GRE General Test (within the past 5 years), minimum B average in undergraduate course work, 3 letters of recommendation; for doctorate, GRE General Test, interview, 3 letters of recommendation from doctorally-prepared faculty, MSN, essay. Additional exam requirements/recommendations for international students: Required—TOEFL (minimum score 570 paper-based), IELTS (minimum score 6.5). *Application deadline:* For fall admission, 12/1 priority date for domestic and international students. Applications are processed on a rolling basis. Application fee: $50. Electronic applications accepted. *Expenses:* Contact institution. *Financial support:* In 2013–14, 582 students received support. Scholarships/grants and health care benefits available. Support available to part-time students. Financial award application deadline: 3/15; financial award applicants required to submit FAFSA. *Faculty research:* Lymphedema, palliative care and bereavement, health services research including workforce, safety and quality of care, gerontology, better birth outcomes including nutrition. *Total annual research expenditures:* $2.5 million. *Unit head:* Dr. Linda Norman, Dean, 615-343-8876, Fax: 615-343-7711, E-mail: linda.norman@vanderbilt.edu. *Application contact:* Patricia Peerman, Assistant Dean for Enrollment Management, 615-322-3800, Fax: 615-343-0333, E-mail: vusn-admissions@vanderbilt.edu.
Website: http://www.nursing.vanderbilt.edu

Villanova University, College of Nursing, Villanova, PA 19085-1699. Offers adult nurse practitioner (MSN, Post Master's Certificate); family nurse practitioner (MSN, Post Master's Certificate); health care administration (MSN, Post Master's Certificate); nurse anesthetist (MSN, Post Master's Certificate); nursing (PhD); nursing education (MSN, Post Master's Certificate); nursing practice (DNP); pediatric nurse practitioner (MSN, Post Master's Certificate). *Accreditation:* AACN; AANA/CANAEP. Part-time programs available. Postbaccalaureate distance learning degree programs offered (minimal on-campus study). *Faculty:* 17 full-time (all women), 4 part-time/adjunct (all women). *Students:* 28 full-time (26 women), 191 part-time (161 women); includes 22 minority (2 Black or African American, non-Hispanic/Latino; 6 Asian, non-Hispanic/Latino; 7 Hispanic/Latino; 7 Two or more races, non-Hispanic/Latino), 18 international. Average age 30. 176 applicants, 65% accepted, 82 enrolled. In 2013, 64 master's, 7 doctorates, 5 other advanced degrees awarded. *Degree requirements:* For master's, independent study project; for doctorate, comprehensive exam, thesis/dissertation. *Entrance requirements:* For master's, GRE or MAT, BSN, 1 year of recent nursing experience, physical assessment, course work in statistics; for doctorate, GRE, MSN. Additional exam requirements/recommendations for international students: Required—TOEFL (minimum score 540 paper-based; 83 iBT), IELTS (minimum score 6.5). *Application deadline:* For fall admission, 7/1 priority date for domestic students, 7/1 for international students; for spring admission, 11/1 priority date for domestic students, 11/1 for international students. Applications are processed on a rolling basis. Application fee: $50. Electronic applications accepted. *Expenses:* Contact institution. *Financial support:* In 2013–14, 39 students received support, including 5 teaching assistantships with full tuition reimbursements available (averaging $14,475 per year); institutionally sponsored loans, scholarships/grants, traineeships, tuition waivers (full), and unspecified assistantships also available. Financial award application deadline: 7/1; financial award applicants required to submit FAFSA. *Faculty research:* Genetics, ethics, cognitive development of students, women with disabilities, nursing leadership. *Unit head:* Dr. Marguerite K. Schlag, Assistant Dean/Director, Graduate Programs, 610-519-4907, Fax: 610-519-7650, E-mail: marguerite.schlag@villanova.edu.
Website: http://www.nursing.villanova.edu/

Virginia Commonwealth University, Graduate School, School of Nursing, Nurse Practitioner Program, Richmond, VA 23284-9005. Offers MS, Certificate. Part-time programs available. *Entrance requirements:* For master's, GRE General Test, minimum GPA of 2.8. Additional exam requirements/recommendations for international students: Required—TOEFL (minimum score 600 paper-based; 100 iBT). Electronic applications accepted.

Wagner College, Division of Graduate Studies, Department of Nursing, Program in Family Nurse Practitioner, Staten Island, NY 10301-4495. Offers Certificate. Part-time and evening/weekend programs available. *Faculty:* 2 part-time/adjunct (both women). *Students:* 2 full-time (1 woman), 43 part-time (37 women); includes 9 minority (3 Black or African American, non-Hispanic/Latino; 2 Asian, non-Hispanic/Latino; 4 Hispanic/Latino), 1 international. Average age 33. 8 applicants, 100% accepted, 7 enrolled. *Entrance requirements:* For degree, master's degree in nursing from an NLN-accredited program, minimum GPA of 3.0, current NY State licensure as Professional Registered Nurse, malpractice insurance coverage, current immunization and physical exam. *Application deadline:* For fall admission, 5/1 priority date for domestic students; for spring admission, 12/1 for domestic students. Applications are processed on a rolling basis. Application fee: $50. *Expenses: Tuition:* Full-time $17,496; part-time $972 per credit. Tuition and fees vary according to course load. *Financial support:* In 2013–14, 1 student received support. Unspecified assistantships and alumni fellowship grants available. Financial award applicants required to submit FAFSA. *Unit head:* Dr. Paula Tropello, Associate Professor/Chairman, Department of Nursing, 718-390-3452, Fax: 718-420-4009, E-mail: ptropell@wagner.edu. *Application contact:* Patricia Clancy, Administrative Assistant, 718-420-4464, Fax: 718-390-3105, E-mail: patricia.clancy@wagner.edu.

Walden University, Graduate Programs, School of Nursing, Minneapolis, MN 55401. Offers adult-gerontology acute care nurse practitioner (MSN); adult-gerontology nurse practitioner (MSN); education (MSN); family nurse practitioner (MSN); informatics (MSN); leadership and management (MSN); nursing (DNP, PhD, Post-Master's Certificate), including education (PhD), healthcare administration (PhD), interdisciplinary health (PhD), leadership (PhD), nursing education (Post-Master's Certificate), nursing informatics (Post-Master's Certificate), nursing leadership and management (Post-Master's Certificate), public health policy (PhD). *Accreditation:* AACN. Part-time and evening/weekend programs available. Postbaccalaureate distance learning degree programs offered (no on-campus study). *Faculty:* 22 full-time (19 women), 343 part-time/adjunct (301 women). *Students:* 5,828 full-time (5,240 women), 2,803 part-time (2,578 women); includes 2,920 minority (1,893 Black or African American, non-Hispanic/Latino; 40 American Indian or Alaska Native, non-Hispanic/Latino; 438 Asian, non-Hispanic/Latino; 391 Hispanic/Latino; 35 Native Hawaiian or other Pacific Islander, non-Hispanic/Latino; 123 Two or more races, non-Hispanic/Latino), 147 international. Average age 41. 1,795 applicants, 95% accepted, 1375 enrolled. In 2013, 1,879 master's, 1 doctorate, 36 other advanced degrees awarded. *Degree requirements:* For doctorate, thesis/dissertation (for some programs), residency (for some programs), field experience (for some programs). *Entrance requirements:* For master's, bachelor's degree or equivalent in related field or RN; minimum GPA of 2.5; official transcripts; goal statement (for some programs); access to computer and Internet; for doctorate, master's degree or higher, three years of related professional or academic experience, RN, goal statement (for some programs); access to computer and Internet; for Post-Master's Certificate, relevant work experience; access to computer and Internet. Additional exam requirements/recommendations for international students: Required—TOEFL (minimum score 550 paper-based; 79 iBT), IELTS (minimum score 6.5), Michigan English Language Assessment Battery (minimum score 82), or PTE. *Application deadline:* Applications are processed on a rolling basis. Application fee: $0. Electronic applications accepted. *Expenses: Tuition:* Full-time $11,813.55; part-time $500 per credit. *Required fees:* $618.76. *Financial support:* Fellowships, Federal Work-Study, scholarships/grants, unspecified assistantships, and family tuition reduction, active duty/veteran tuition reduction, group tuition reduction, interest-free payment plans, employee tuition reduction available. Support available to part-time students. Financial award applicants required to submit FAFSA. *Unit head:* Dr. Andrea Lindell, Associate Dean, 800-925-3368. *Application contact:* Jennifer Hall, Vice President of Enrollment Management, 866-4-WALDEN, E-mail: info@waldenu.edu.
Website: http://www.waldenu.edu/programs/colleges-schools/nursing

Washington State University Spokane, Graduate Programs, College of Nursing, Spokane, WA 99210-1495. Offers advanced population health (MN, DNP); family nurse practitioner (MN, DNP); nursing (PhD); psychiatric/mental health nurse practitioner (DNP); psychiatric/mental health practitioner (MN). *Accreditation:* AACN. *Degree requirements:* For master's, comprehensive exam (for some programs), thesis (for some programs), oral exam, research project. *Entrance requirements:* For master's, minimum GPA of 3.0, Washington state RN license, physical assessment skills, course work in statistics, recommendations, written interview (for nurse practitioner). *Faculty research:* Cardiovascular and Type 2 diabetes in children, evaluation of strategies to increase physical activity in sedentary people.

Wayne State University, College of Nursing, Detroit, MI 48202. Offers adult health (MSN); adult primary care nursing (MSN), including adult primary care nursing, gerontological nurse practitioner; advanced practice nursing with women, neonates and children (MSN), including neonatal nurse practitioner, nurse-midwife, pediatric nurse practitioner, women's health nurse practitioner; community health nursing (MSN); complementary therapies in healthcare (Graduate Certificate); family community mental health (MSN); nurse practitioner (DNP), including infant mental health (DNP, PhD); nurse-midwifery (Graduate Certificate); nursing (PhD), including infant mental health (DNP, PhD), nursing; nursing education (Graduate Certificate); nursing practice (DNP); pediatric acute care nursing (Graduate Certificate); pediatric primary care nursing (Graduate Certificate); psychiatric mental health nurse practitioner (MSN); transcultural nursing (Graduate Certificate). *Accreditation:* AACN. Part-time programs available. *Faculty:* 36 full-time (35 women). *Students:* 113 full-time (107 women), 228 part-time (207 women); includes 93 minority (61 Black or African American, non-Hispanic/Latino; 1 American Indian or Alaska Native, non-Hispanic/Latino; 22 Asian, non-Hispanic/Latino; 6 Hispanic/Latino; 3 Two or more races, non-Hispanic/Latino), 21 international. Average age 37. 194 applicants, 44% accepted, 59 enrolled. In 2013, 118 master's, 22 doctorates, 9 other advanced degrees awarded. Terminal master's awarded for partial completion of doctoral program. *Degree requirements:* For master's, thesis or alternative; for doctorate, thesis/dissertation (for some programs). *Entrance requirements:* For master's, admission to Graduate School; minimum GPA of 3.0 in upper-division course work; BA from NLN- or CCNE-accredited program; three references; current RN license; personal statement; additional requirements in each of the clinical major areas; for doctorate, GRE General Test (for applicants without a master's degree), current RN license; interview; goals statement; bachelor's degree with minimum upper-division GPA of 3.5 or master's degree with minimum GPA of 3.3 (for PhD); master's degree in nursing with minimum GPA of 3.0 and writing sample (for DNP); reference letters (3 for PhD, 2 for DNP); for Graduate Certificate, graduate degree in nursing, current Michigan RN license, three letters of reference, personal goal statement. Additional exam requirements/recommendations for international students: Required—TOEFL (minimum score 550 paper-based; 79 iBT), TWE (minimum score 6), Michigan English Language Assessment Battery (minimum score 85); Recommended—IELTS (minimum score 6.5). *Application deadline:* For fall admission, 7/1 for domestic students, 5/1 for international students; for winter admission, 11/1 for domestic students, 9/1 for international students; for spring admission, 3/1 for domestic students, 1/1 for international students. Application fee: $0. Electronic applications accepted. *Expenses:* Contact institution. *Financial support:* In 2013–14, 67 students received support, including 47 fellowships with tuition reimbursements available, 1 research assistantship with tuition reimbursement available (averaging $18,071 per year), 5 teaching assistantships with tuition reimbursements available (averaging $27,990 per year); Federal Work-Study, institutionally sponsored loans, scholarships/grants, traineeships, and unspecified assistantships also available. Support available to part-time students. Financial award application deadline: 3/31; financial award applicants required to submit FAFSA. *Faculty research:* Diet-induced obesity in adults; environmental and physiological factors of asthma; high-risk families for child maltreatment; identifying non-invasive biomarkers of necrotizing enterocolotis; pain management and reduction of pain-related disparities. *Total annual research expenditures:* $823,339. *Unit head:* Dr. Nancy T. Artinian, Interim Dean, College of Nursing, 313-577-4071. *Application contact:* Dr. Eric Brown, Director, Office of Student Affairs for College of Nursing, 313-577-4082, Fax: 313-577-6949, E-mail: nursinginfo@wayne.edu.
Website: http://nursing.wayne.edu/

Western University of Health Sciences, College of Graduate Nursing, Master of Science in Nursing Program, Pomona, CA 91766-1854. Offers administrative nurse leader (MSN); ambulatory care (MSN); clinical nurse leader (MSN); family nurse practitioner (MSN); nursing (MSN). *Faculty:* 14 full-time (all women), 11 part-time/adjunct (10 women). *Students:* 255 full-time (218 women), 10 part-time (all women); includes 163 minority (20 Black or African American, non-Hispanic/Latino; 1 American Indian or Alaska Native, non-Hispanic/Latino; 88 Asian, non-Hispanic/Latino; 40 Hispanic/Latino; 1 Native Hawaiian or other Pacific Islander, non-Hispanic/Latino; 13 Two or more races, non-Hispanic/Latino), 2 international. Average age 31. 739 applicants, 23% accepted, 114 enrolled. In 2013, 73 master's awarded. *Degree requirements:* For master's, thesis. *Entrance requirements:* For master's, BSN, minimum GPA of 3.0, 3 letters of recommendation, resume/curriculum vitae. Additional exam requirements/recommendations for international students: Required—TOEFL. *Application deadline:* For fall admission, 10/1 for domestic students. Application fee: $60. Electronic applications accepted. *Unit head:* Dr. Karen J. Hanford, Dean, 909-469-5523, Fax: 909-469-5521, E-mail: khanford@westernu.edu. *Application contact:* Kathryn Ford, Director of Admissions/International Student Advisor, 909-469-5335, Fax: 909-469-5570, E-mail: admissions@westernu.edu.

Westminster College, School of Nursing and Health Sciences, Salt Lake City, UT 84105-3697. Offers family nurse practitioner (MSN); nurse anesthesia (MSNA); nurse education (MSNED); nursing (MSN); public health (MPH). *Accreditation:* AACN; AANA/CANAEP. *Faculty:* 11 full-time (5 women), 7 part-time/adjunct (4 women). *Students:* 119 full-time (75 women), 5 part-time (2 women); includes 21 minority (5 Black or African American, non-Hispanic/Latino; 1 American Indian or Alaska Native, non-Hispanic/Latino; 4 Asian, non-Hispanic/Latino; 7 Hispanic/Latino; 1 Native Hawaiian or other Pacific Islander, non-Hispanic/Latino; 3 Two or more races, non-Hispanic/Latino), 4 international. Average age 32. 246 applicants, 35% accepted, 56 enrolled. In 2013, 49 master's awarded. *Degree requirements:* For master's, clinical practicum, 504 clinical practice hours. *Entrance requirements:* For master's, GRE, resume, Utah RN license in good standing, minimum GPA of 3.0, 3 letters of reference, BSN from accredited nursing program, proof of clear state and federal background check, drug test results, personal interview, current PALS certification, current ACLS certification, document of current immunizations, physical and mental health certificate. Additional exam requirements/recommendations for international students: Required—TOEFL (minimum score 600 paper-based; 100 iBT), IELTS (minimum score 7.5). *Application deadline:* Applications are processed on a rolling basis. Application fee: $50. Electronic applications accepted. *Expenses:* Contact institution. *Financial support:* In 2013–14, 9 students received support. Career-related internships or fieldwork, unspecified assistantships, and tuition reimbursements, tuition remission available. Support available to part-time students. Financial award applicants required to submit FAFSA. *Faculty research:* Collaborative testing in nursing: student outcomes and perspectives, implementing new educational paradigms into pre-licensure nursing curricula. *Unit head:* Dr. Sheryl Steadman, Dean, 801-832-2164, Fax: 801-832-3110, E-mail: ssteadman@westminstercollege.edu. *Application contact:* Dr. John Baworowsky, Vice President of Enrollment Management, 801-832-2200, Fax: 801-832-3101, E-mail: admission@westminstercollege.edu.
Website: http://www.westminstercollege.edu/msn

West Texas A&M University, College of Nursing and Health Sciences, Department of Nursing, Canyon, TX 79016-0001. Offers family nurse practitioner (MSN); nursing (MSN). *Accreditation:* AACN. Part-time programs available. Postbaccalaureate distance learning degree programs offered (minimal on-campus study). *Degree requirements:* For master's, comprehensive exam, thesis optional. *Entrance requirements:* For master's, GRE General Test, bachelor's degree in nursing, minimum GPA of 3.0 in last 60 hours. Additional exam requirements/recommendations for international students: Required—TOEFL (minimum score 550 paper-based). Electronic applications accepted. *Faculty research:* Family-focused nursing, nursing traineeship, professional nursing.

West Virginia Wesleyan College, Department of Nursing, Buckhannon, WV 26201. Offers family nurse practitioner (Post Master's Certificate); family nurse practitoner (MS); nurse administrator (MS); nurse educator (MS); nurse-midwifery (MS); nursing administration (Post Master's Certificate); nursing education (Post Master's Certificate); psychiatric mental health nurse practitioner (MS); MSN/MBA.

Wilmington University, College of Health Professions, New Castle, DE 19720-6491. Offers adult nurse practitioner (MSN); family nurse practitioner (MSN); gerontology nurse practitioner (MSN); nursing (MSN); nursing leadership (MSN); nursing practice (DNP). *Accreditation:* AACN. Part-time programs available. *Degree requirements:* For master's, thesis. *Entrance requirements:* For master's, BSN, RN license, interview, 3 letters of recommendation. Additional exam requirements/recommendations for international students: Required—TOEFL (minimum score 500 paper-based). Electronic applications accepted. *Faculty research:* Outcomes assessment, student writing ability.

Winona State University, College of Nursing and Health Sciences, Winona, MN 55987. Offers adult nurse practitioner (MS, Post Master's Certificate); clinical nurse specialist (MS, Post Master's Certificate); family nurse practitioner (MS, Post Master's Certificate); nurse administrator (MS); nurse educator (MS, Post Master's Certificate); nursing (DNP). *Accreditation:* AACN. Part-time programs available. Postbaccalaureate distance learning degree programs offered (no on-campus study). *Degree requirements:* For master's, thesis; for doctorate, capstone. *Entrance requirements:* For master's, GRE (if GPA less than 3.0). Additional exam requirements/recommendations for international students: Required—TOEFL (minimum score 550 paper-based).

Wright State University, School of Graduate Studies, College of Nursing and Health, Program in Nursing, Dayton, OH 45435. Offers acute care nurse practitioner (MS); administration of nursing and health care systems (MS); adult health (MS); child and adolescent health (MS); community health (MS); family nurse practitioner (MS); nurse practitioner (MS); school nurse (MS); MBA/MS. *Accreditation:* AACN. Part-time and evening/weekend programs available. *Degree requirements:* For master's, thesis or alternative. *Entrance requirements:* For master's, GRE General Test, BSN from NLN-accredited college, Ohio RN license. Additional exam requirements/recommendations for international students: Required—TOEFL. *Faculty research:* Clinical nursing and health, teaching, caring, pain administration, informatics and technology.

Xavier University, College of Social Sciences, Health and Education, School of Nursing, Family Nurse Practitioner Program, Cincinnati, OH 45207. Offers MSN. Part-time programs available. *Faculty:* 3 full-time (all women). *Students:* 10 full-time (7 women), 22 part-time (all women); includes 11 minority (4 Black or African American, non-Hispanic/Latino; 4 Asian, non-Hispanic/Latino; 3 Hispanic/Latino). Average age 35. 14 applicants, 100% accepted, 14 enrolled. *Degree requirements:* For master's, capstone course. *Application deadline:* Applications are processed on a rolling basis. Electronic applications accepted. *Expenses: Tuition:* Part-time $594 per credit hour. *Required fees:* $3 per semester. *Financial support:* In 2013–14, 1 student received support. Scholarships/grants available. Financial award applicants required to submit FAFSA. *Unit head:* Dr. Susan M. Schmidt, Director, 513-745-3815, Fax: 513-745-1087, E-mail: schmidt@xavier.edu. *Application contact:* Marilyn Volk Gomez, Director of Nursing Student Services, 513-745-4392, Fax: 513-745-1087, E-mail: gomez@xavier.edu.
Website: http://www.xavier.edu/MSN/MSN-FNP.cfm

Forensic Nursing

Boston College, William F. Connell School of Nursing, Chestnut Hill, MA 02467-3800. Offers adult-gerontology nursing (MS); community health nursing (MS); family health (MS); forensic nursing (MS); maternal/child health nursing (MS), including pediatric and women's health; nurse anesthesia (MS); nursing (PhD); palliative care (MS), including adult and pediatric; psychiatric-mental health nursing (MS); MBA/MS; MS/MA; MS/PhD. *Accreditation:* AACN; AANA/CANAEP (one or more programs are accredited). Part-time programs available. *Faculty:* 47 full-time (43 women), 42 part-time/adjunct (39 women). *Students:* 199 full-time (180 women), 79 part-time (73 women); includes 44 minority (14 Black or African American, non-Hispanic/Latino; 1 American Indian or Alaska Native, non-Hispanic/Latino; 13 Asian, non-Hispanic/Latino; 12 Hispanic/Latino; 4 Two or more races, non-Hispanic/Latino), 7 international. Average age 31. 502 applicants, 39% accepted, 87 enrolled. In 2013, 105 master's, 8 doctorates awarded. *Degree requirements:* For master's, comprehensive exam, research project; for doctorate, comprehensive exam, thesis/dissertation, computer literacy exam or foreign language. *Entrance requirements:* For master's, bachelor's degree in nursing; for doctorate, GRE General Test, MS in nursing. Additional exam requirements/recommendations for international students: Required—TOEFL (minimum score 600 paper-based; 100 iBT). *Application deadline:* For fall admission, 9/30 for domestic and international students; for winter admission, 1/15 for domestic and international students; for spring admission, 3/15 for domestic and international students. Applications are processed on a rolling basis. Application fee: $40. Electronic applications accepted. *Financial support:* In 2013–14, 174 students received support, including 7 fellowships with full tuition reimbursements available (averaging $20,000 per year), 21 teaching assistantships (averaging $4,800 per year); research assistantships, scholarships/grants, health care benefits, tuition waivers (partial), and unspecified assistantships also available. Support available to part-time students. Financial award application deadline: 3/1; financial award applicants required to submit FAFSA. *Faculty research:* Sexual and reproductive health, health promotion/illness prevention, eating disorders, violence, symptom management. *Total annual research expenditures:* $1.1 million. *Unit head:* Dr. Susan Gennaro, Dean, 617-552-4251, Fax: 617-552-0931, E-mail: susan.gennaro@bc.edu. *Application contact:* MaryBeth Crowley, Graduate Programs Assistant, 617-552-4928, Fax: 617-552-2121, E-mail: csongrad@bc.edu.
Website: http://www.bc.edu/schools/son/

Cleveland State University, College of Graduate Studies, School of Nursing, Cleveland, OH 44115. Offers clinical nurse leader (MSN); forensic nursing (MSN); nursing education (MSN); specialized population (MSN); urban education (PhD), including nursing education; MSN/MBA. *Accreditation:* AACN. Part-time programs available. Postbaccalaureate distance learning degree programs offered (no on-campus study). *Faculty:* 6 full-time (all women), 1 (woman) part-time/adjunct. *Students:* 20 full-time (all women), 28 part-time (26 women); includes 12 minority (8 Black or African American, non-Hispanic/Latino; 3 Hispanic/Latino; 1 Two or more races, non-Hispanic/Latino), 1 international. Average age 38. 65 applicants, 62% accepted, 20 enrolled. In 2013, 6 master's awarded. *Degree requirements:* For master's, thesis optional, portfolio, capstone practicum project; for doctorate, comprehensive exam, thesis/dissertation. *Entrance requirements:* For master's, RN license, BSN with minimum cumulative GPA of 3.0, recent (5 years) course work in statistics; for doctorate, GRE, MSN with minimum cumulative GPA of 3.25. Additional exam requirements/recommendations for international students: Required—TOEFL (minimum score 525 paper-based; 65 iBT), IELTS (minimum score 6). *Application deadline:* For fall admission, 3/1 priority date for domestic and international students. Application fee: $55. Electronic applications accepted. *Expenses:* Tuition, state resident: full-time $8335; part-time $521 per credit hour. Tuition, nonresident: full-time $15,670; part-time $979 per credit hour. *Required fees:* $50; $25 per semester. *Financial support:* In 2013–14, 4 students received support. Tuition waivers (full) and unspecified assistantships available. Financial award application deadline: 3/1; financial award applicants required to submit FAFSA. *Faculty research:* Diabetes management, African-American elders medication compliance, risk in home visiting, suffering, COPD and stress, nursing education, disaster health preparedness. *Total annual research expenditures:* $330,000. *Unit head:* Dr. Vida Lock, Dean, 216-523-7237, Fax: 216-687-3556, E-mail: v.lock@csuohio.edu. *Application contact:* Maureen Mitchell, Assistant Professor and Graduate Program Director, 216-523-7128, Fax: 216-687-3556, E-mail: m.m.mitchell1@csuohio.edu.
Website: http://www.csuohio.edu/nursing/

Duquesne University, School of Nursing, Master of Science in Nursing Program, Pittsburgh, PA 15282-0001. Offers family (individual across the life span) nurse practitioner (MSN); forensic nursing (MSN); nursing education (MSN). *Accreditation:* AACN. Part-time and evening/weekend programs available. Postbaccalaureate distance learning degree programs offered (minimal on-campus study). *Faculty:* 20 full-time (18 women), 4 part-time/adjunct (all women). *Students:* 73 full-time (67 women), 54 part-time (53 women); includes 23 minority (8 Black or African American, non-Hispanic/Latino; 1 American Indian or Alaska Native, non-Hispanic/Latino; 4 Asian, non-Hispanic/Latino; 5 Hispanic/Latino; 5 Two or more races, non-Hispanic/Latino), 1 international. Average age 35. 206 applicants, 35% accepted, 55 enrolled. In 2013, 28 master's awarded. *Degree requirements:* For master's, culminating paper. *Entrance requirements:* For master's, current RN license; BSN with minimum GPA of 3.0; minimum of 1 year full-time work experience as RN prior to registration in clinical or specialty course. Additional exam requirements/recommendations for international students: Required—TOEFL (minimum score 600 paper-based; 80 iBT). *Application deadline:* For fall admission, 3/1 for domestic and international students. Application fee: $0. Electronic applications accepted. *Expenses: Tuition:* Full-time $18,162; part-time $1009 per credit. *Required fees:* $1728; $96 per credit. Tuition and fees vary according to program. *Financial support:* In 2013–14, 5 students received support, including 3 teaching assistantships with partial tuition reimbursements available (averaging $1,285 per year); research assistantships with partial tuition reimbursements available, scholarships/grants, traineeships, and tuition waivers (partial) also available. Support available to part-time students. Financial award application deadline: 7/1; financial award applicants required to submit FAFSA. *Faculty research:* Vulnerable populations, social justice, cultural competence, health disparities, wellness within chronic illness. *Unit head:* Dr. Joan Such Lockhart, Professor and Associate Dean of Academic Affairs, 412-396-6540, Fax: 412-396-1821, E-mail: lockhart@duq.edu. *Application contact:* Susan Hardner, Nurse Recruiter, 412-396-4945, Fax: 412-396-6346, E-mail: nursing@duq.edu.
Website: http://www.duq.edu/academics/schools/nursing/graduate-programs/master-science-nursing

Duquesne University, School of Nursing, Post Master's Certificate Program, Pittsburgh, PA 15282-0001. Offers family (individual across the life span) nurse practitioner (Post-Master's Certificate); forensic nursing (Post-Master's Certificate). Part-time and evening/weekend programs available. Postbaccalaureate distance learning degree programs offered (minimal on-campus study). *Faculty:* 10 full-time (9 women), 4 part-time/adjunct (all women). *Students:* 11 part-time (all women); includes 2 minority (1 Black or African American, non-Hispanic/Latino; 1 Hispanic/Latino). Average age 41. 19 applicants, 26% accepted, 4 enrolled. In 2013, 1 Post-Master's Certificate awarded. *Entrance requirements:* For degree, current RN license, BSN, MSN. Additional exam

requirements/recommendations for international students: Required—TOEFL (minimum score 600 paper-based; 80 iBT). *Application deadline:* For fall admission, 3/1 for domestic and international students. Application fee: $0. *Expenses: Tuition:* Full-time $18,162; part-time $1009 per credit. *Required fees:* $1728; $96 per credit. Tuition and fees vary according to program. *Financial support:* Teaching assistantships with partial tuition reimbursements, scholarships/grants, traineeships, and tuition waivers (partial) available. Support available to part-time students. Financial award application deadline: 7/1; financial award applicants required to submit FAFSA. *Faculty research:* Vulnerable populations, social justice, cultural competence, health disparities, wellness within chronic illness. *Unit head:* Dr. Joan Such Lockhart, Professor and Associate Dean of Academic Affairs, 412-396-6540, Fax: 412-396-1821, E-mail: lockhart@duq.edu. *Application contact:* Susan Hardner, Nurse Recruiter, 412-396-4945, Fax: 412-396-6346, E-mail: nursing@duq.edu.
Website: http://www.duq.edu/academics/schools/nursing/graduate-programs/post-masters-certificates

Fitchburg State University, Division of Graduate and Continuing Education, Program in Forensic Nursing, Fitchburg, MA 01420-2697. Offers MS, Certificate. *Accreditation:* AACN. Part-time and evening/weekend programs available. Postbaccalaureate distance learning degree programs offered (no on-campus study). *Entrance requirements:* Additional exam requirements/recommendations for international students: Required—TOEFL (minimum score 550 paper-based; 79 iBT). Electronic applications accepted.

Monmouth University, The Graduate School, The Marjorie K. Unterberg School of Nursing and Health Studies, West Long Branch, NJ 07764-1898. Offers adult and gerontological nurse practitioner (MSN); adult-gerontological nurse practitioner (Post-Master's Certificate); family nurse practitioner (MSN, Post-Master's Certificate); family psychiatric and mental health advanced practice nursing (MSN); forensic nursing (MSN, Certificate); nursing (MSN); nursing administration (MSN, Post-Master's Certificate); nursing education (MSN, Post-Master's Certificate); nursing practice (DNP); physician assistant (MS); psychiatric-mental health nurse practitioner (Post-Master's Certificate); school nursing (MSN, Certificate). *Accreditation:* AACN. Part-time and evening/weekend programs available. *Faculty:* 14 full-time (all women), 4 part-time/adjunct (3 women). *Students:* 19 full-time (18 women), 269 part-time (252 women); includes 106 minority (35 Black or African American, non-Hispanic/Latino; 2 American Indian or Alaska Native, non-Hispanic/Latino; 51 Asian, non-Hispanic/Latino; 12 Hispanic/Latino; 3 Native Hawaiian or other Pacific Islander, non-Hispanic/Latino; 3 Two or more races, non-Hispanic/Latino), 2 international. Average age 39. 135 applicants, 98% accepted, 96 enrolled. In 2013, 54 master's, 7 doctorates awarded. *Degree requirements:* For master's, practicum (for some tracks). *Entrance requirements:* For master's, GRE General Test, BSN with minimum GPA of 2.75, current RN license, proof of liability and malpractice policy, personal statement, two letters of recommendation, college course work in health assessment, resume; minimum GPA of 3.0, minimum C grade in prerequisite courses, minimum 200 hours' clinical experience, 3 letters of recommendation, and interview (for MS); for doctorate, accredited master's nursing program degree with minimum GPA of 3.2, active RN license, national certification as Nurse Practitioner or Nurse Administrator, working knowledge of statistics, statement of goals and vision for change, 2 letters of recommendation, resume, interview. Additional exam requirements/recommendations for international students: Required—TOEFL (minimum score 550 paper-based; 79 iBT), IELTS (minimum score 6) or Michigan English Language Assessment Battery (minimum score 77). *Application deadline:* For fall admission, 7/15 priority date for domestic students, 6/1 for international students; for spring admission, 11/15 priority date for domestic students, 11/1 for international students; for summer admission, 2/1 for domestic students. Applications are processed on a rolling basis. Application fee: $50. Electronic applications accepted. *Expenses: Tuition:* Part-time $1004 per credit hour. *Required fees:* $157 per semester. *Financial support:* In 2013–14, 163 students received support, including 113 fellowships (averaging $3,093 per year), 27 research assistantships (averaging $6,273 per year); career-related internships or fieldwork, scholarships/grants, and unspecified assistantships also available. Support available to part-time students. Financial award applicants required to submit FAFSA. *Faculty research:* Relationship of undergraduate GPA and GRE to succeeding in a graduate nursing program. *Unit head:* Dr. Janet Mahoney, Dean, 732-571-3443, Fax: 732-263-5131, E-mail: jmahoney@monmouth.edu. *Application contact:* Lauren Vento-Cifelli, Associate Vice President of Undergraduate and Graduate Admission, 732-571-3452, Fax: 732-263-5123, E-mail: gradadm@monmouth.edu.
Website: http://www.monmouth.edu/school-of-nursing-health/graduate-nursing-programs.aspx

National University, Academic Affairs, School of Health and Human Services, La Jolla, CA 92037-1011. Offers clinical affairs (MS); clinical informatics (Certificate); clinical regulatory affairs (MS); health and life science analytics (MS); health coaching (Certificate); health informatics (MS); healthcare administration (MHA); nurse anesthesia (MS); nursing (MS), including forensic nursing, nursing administration, nursing informatics; nursing administration (Certificate); nursing informatics (Certificate); nursing practice (DNP); public health (MPH), including health promotion, healthcare administration, mental health. Part-time and evening/weekend programs available. Postbaccalaureate distance learning degree programs offered (no on-campus study). *Faculty:* 20 full-time (12 women), 27 part-time/adjunct (16 women). *Students:* 229 full-time (176 women), 89 part-time (52 women); includes 215 minority (58 Black or African American, non-Hispanic/Latino; 1 American Indian or Alaska Native, non-Hispanic/Latino; 68 Asian, non-Hispanic/Latino; 63 Hispanic/Latino; 8 Native Hawaiian or other Pacific Islander, non-Hispanic/Latino; 17 Two or more races, non-Hispanic/Latino), 18 international. Average age 33. 118 applicants, 100% accepted, 92 enrolled. In 2013, 29 master's awarded. *Degree requirements:* For master's, thesis (for some programs). *Entrance requirements:* For master's, interview, minimum GPA of 2.5. Additional exam requirements/recommendations for international students: Required—TOEFL (minimum score 550 paper-based; 79 iBT), IELTS (minimum score 6). *Application deadline:* Applications are processed on a rolling basis. Application fee: $60 ($65 for international students). Electronic applications accepted. *Expenses: Tuition:* Full-time $13,824; part-time $1728 per course. One-time fee: $160. *Financial support:* Career-related internships or fieldwork, institutionally sponsored loans, scholarships/grants, and tuition waivers (partial) available. Support available to part-time students. Financial award application deadline: 6/30; financial award applicants required to submit FAFSA. *Faculty research:* Nursing education, obesity prevention, workforce diversity. *Unit head:* School of Health and Human Services, 800-628-8648, E-mail: shhs@nu.edu. *Application contact:* Louis Cruz, Interim Vice President for Enrollment Services, 800-628-8648, E-mail: advisor@nu.edu.
Website: http://www.nu.edu/OurPrograms/SchoolOfHealthAndHumanServices.html

Xavier University, College of Social Sciences, Health and Education, School of Nursing, Nursing Program, Cincinnati, OH 45207. Offers clinical nurse leader (MSN); education (MSN); forensic nursing (MSN); healthcare law (MSN); informatics (MSN); nursing administration (MSN); school nursing (MSN); MSN/M Ed; MSN/MBA; MSN/MS. *Faculty:* 16 full-time (15 women), 9 part-time/adjunct (all women). *Students:* 66 full-time (56 women), 170 part-time (162 women); includes 35 minority (17 Black or African American, non-Hispanic/Latino; 2 American Indian or Alaska Native, non-Hispanic/Latino; 5 Asian, non-Hispanic/Latino; 10 Hispanic/Latino; 1 Native Hawaiian or other Pacific Islander, non-Hispanic/Latino). Average age 37. 103 applicants, 66% accepted, 86 enrolled. In 2013, 78 master's awarded. *Expenses: Tuition:* Part-time $594 per credit hour. *Required fees:* $3 per semester. *Financial support:* In 2013–14, 68 students received support. *Unit head:* Dr. Susan M. Schmidt, Director, School of Nursing, 513-745-3814, E-mail: schmidt@xavier.edu. *Application contact:* Marilyn Volk Gomez, Director of Nursing Student Services, 513-745-4392, Fax: 513-745-1087, E-mail: gomez@xavier.edu.
Website: http://www.xavier.edu/msn/

Gerontological Nursing

Adelphi University, College of Nursing and Public Health, Program in Adult/Geriatric Nurse Practitioner, Garden City, NY 11530-0701. Offers MS. *Students:* 88 part-time (82 women); includes 55 minority (27 Black or African American, non-Hispanic/Latino; 1 American Indian or Alaska Native, non-Hispanic/Latino; 19 Asian, non-Hispanic/Latino; 4 Hispanic/Latino; 1 Native Hawaiian or other Pacific Islander, non-Hispanic/Latino; 3 Two or more races, non-Hispanic/Latino). Average age 36. In 2013, 13 master's awarded. *Expenses: Tuition:* Full-time $32,530; part-time $1010 per credit. *Required fees:* $1150. Tuition and fees vary according to degree level and program. *Financial support:* Research assistantships, career-related internships or fieldwork, tuition waivers, and unspecified assistantships available. *Unit head:* Maryann Forbes, Chair, 516-877-3597, E-mail: forbes@adelphi.edu. *Application contact:* Christine Murphy, Director of Admissions, 516-877-3050, Fax: 516-877-3039, E-mail: graduateadmissions@adelphi.edu.

Allen College, Program in Nursing, Waterloo, IA 50703. Offers acute care nurse practitioner (MSN, Post-Master's Certificate); adult nurse practitioner (MSN, Post-Master's Certificate); adult psychiatric-mental health nurse practitioner (MSN, Post-Master's Certificate); community public health (MSN, Post-Master's Certificate); family nurse practitioner (MSN, Post-Master's Certificate); gerontological nurse practitioner (MSN, Post-Master's Certificate); health education (MSN); leadership in health care delivery (MSN, Post-Master's Certificate); nursing (DNP). Part-time programs available. Postbaccalaureate distance learning degree programs offered (minimal on-campus study). *Faculty:* 3 full-time (all women), 21 part-time/adjunct (20 women). *Students:* 21 full-time (19 women), 162 part-time (150 women); includes 5 minority (1 Black or African American, non-Hispanic/Latino; 2 Asian, non-Hispanic/Latino; 1 Hispanic/Latino; 1 Two or more races, non-Hispanic/Latino). Average age 34. 213 applicants, 57% accepted, 94 enrolled. In 2013, 41 master's, 4 other advanced degrees awarded. *Degree requirements:* For master's, thesis optional. *Entrance requirements:* For master's, minimum GPA of 3.0 in the last 60 hours of undergraduate coursework; for doctorate, minimum GPA of 3.25 in graduate coursework. Additional exam requirements/recommendations for international students: Recommended—TOEFL (minimum score 580 paper-based; 92 iBT), IELTS (minimum score 6). *Application deadline:* For fall admission, 2/1 priority date for domestic students; for spring admission, 9/1 priority date for domestic students. Applications are processed on a rolling basis. Application fee: $50. Electronic applications accepted. *Expenses: Tuition:* Full-time $14,534; part-time $755 per credit hour. *Required fees:* $935; $75 per credit hour. One-time fee: $275 part-time. Tuition and fees vary according to course load. *Financial support:* In 2013–14, 60 students received support. Institutionally sponsored loans, scholarships/grants, and traineeships available. Support available to part-time students. Financial award application deadline: 8/15; financial award applicants required to submit FAFSA. *Unit head:* Kendra Williams-Perez, Dean, School of Nursing, 319-226-2044, Fax: 319-226-2070, E-mail: kendra.williams-perez@allencollege.edu. *Application contact:* Molly Quinn, Admissions Counselor, 319-226-2001, Fax: 319-226-2010, E-mail: molly.quinn@allencollege.edu.
Website: http://www.allencollege.edu/

Armstrong State University, School of Graduate Studies, Program in Nursing, Savannah, GA 31419-1997. Offers adult-gerontological acute care nurse practitioner (MSN); adult-gerontological clinical nurse specialist (MSN); adult-gerontological primary care nurse practitioner (MSN). *Accreditation:* AACN. Part-time and evening/weekend programs available. *Faculty:* 10 full-time (all women), 1 (woman) part-time/adjunct. *Students:* 24 full-time (21 women), 17 part-time (16 women); includes 5 minority (2 Black or African American, non-Hispanic/Latino; 1 Hispanic/Latino; 2 Two or more races, non-Hispanic/Latino). Average age 34. 17 applicants, 65% accepted, 10 enrolled. In 2013, 13 master's awarded. *Degree requirements:* For master's, comprehensive exam, project or thesis. *Entrance requirements:* For master's, GRE General Test or MAT, minimum GPA of 3.0, letter of recommendation, letter of intent. Additional exam requirements/recommendations for international students: Required—TOEFL (minimum score 523 paper-based; 70 iBT). *Application deadline:* For fall admission, 2/28 for domestic and international students; for spring admission, 11/15 for domestic students, 9/15 for international students. Applications are processed on a rolling basis. Application fee: $30. Electronic applications accepted. *Expenses:* Tuition, state resident: part-time $201 per credit hour. Tuition, nonresident: part-time $745 per credit hour. *Required fees:* $310 per semester. Tuition and fees vary according to course load, campus/location and program. *Financial support:* In 2013–14, research assistantships with full tuition reimbursements (averaging $5,000 per year) were awarded; Federal Work-Study, scholarships/grants, and unspecified assistantships also available. Support available to part-time students. Financial award application deadline: 3/1; financial award applicants required to submit FAFSA. *Faculty research:* Midwifery, mental health, nursing simulation, smoking cessation during pregnancy, asthma education, vulnerable populations, geriatrics, disaster nursing, complementary and alternative modalities, nephrology. *Unit head:* Dr. Catherine Gilbert, Department Head, 912-344-3145, E-mail: catherine.gilbert@armstrong.edu. *Application contact:* Jill Bell, Director/Graduate Enrollment Coordinator, 912-344-2798, Fax: 912-344-3488, E-mail: graduate@armstrong.edu.
Website: http://www.armstrong.edu/Health_professions/nursing/nursing_graduate_programs

Boston College, William F. Connell School of Nursing, Chestnut Hill, MA 02467-3800. Offers adult-gerontology nursing (MS); community health nursing (MS); family health (MS); forensic nursing (MS); maternal/child health nursing (MS), including pediatric and women's health; nurse anesthesia (MS); nursing (PhD); palliative care (MS), including adult and pediatric; psychiatric-mental health nursing (MS); MBA/MS; MS/MA; MS/PhD. *Accreditation:* AACN; AANA/CANAEP (one or more programs are accredited). Part-time programs available. *Faculty:* 47 full-time (43 women), 42 part-time/adjunct (39 women). *Students:* 199 full-time (180 women), 79 part-time (73 women); includes 44 minority (14 Black or African American, non-Hispanic/Latino; 1 American Indian or Alaska Native, non-Hispanic/Latino; 13 Asian, non-Hispanic/Latino; 12 Hispanic/Latino; 4 Two or more races, non-Hispanic/Latino), 7 international. Average age 31. 502 applicants, 39% accepted, 87 enrolled. In 2013, 105 master's, 8 doctorates awarded. *Degree requirements:* For master's, comprehensive exam, research project; for doctorate, comprehensive exam, thesis/dissertation, computer literacy exam or foreign language. *Entrance requirements:* For master's, bachelor's degree in nursing; for doctorate, GRE General Test, MS in nursing. Additional exam requirements/recommendations for international students: Required—TOEFL (minimum score 600 paper-based; 100 iBT). *Application deadline:* For fall admission, 9/30 for domestic and international students; for winter admission, 1/15 for domestic and international students; for spring admission, 3/15 for domestic and international students. Applications are processed on a rolling basis. Application fee: $40. Electronic applications accepted. *Financial support:* In 2013–14, 174 students received support, including 7 fellowships with full tuition reimbursements available (averaging $20,000 per year), 21 teaching assistantships (averaging $4,800 per year); research assistantships, scholarships/grants, health care benefits, tuition waivers (partial), and unspecified assistantships also available. Support available to part-time students. Financial award application deadline: 3/1; financial award applicants required to submit FAFSA. *Faculty research:* Sexual and reproductive health, health promotion/illness prevention, eating disorders, violence, symptom management. *Total annual research expenditures:* $1.1 million. *Unit head:* Dr. Susan Gennaro, Dean, 617-552-4251, Fax: 617-552-0931, E-mail: susan.gennaro@bc.edu. *Application contact:* MaryBeth Crowley, Graduate Programs Assistant, 617-552-4928, Fax: 617-552-2121, E-mail: csongrad@bc.edu.
Website: http://www.bc.edu/schools/son/

California State University, Stanislaus, College of Human and Health Sciences, Program in Nursing (MS), Turlock, CA 95382. Offers gerontological nursing (MS); nursing education (MS). *Accreditation:* AACN. Part-time programs available. *Degree requirements:* For master's, comprehensive exam, thesis or alternative. *Entrance requirements:* For master's, GRE or MAT, minimum GPA of 3.0, 3 letters of reference, RN. Additional exam requirements/recommendations for international students: Required—TOEFL (minimum score 550 paper-based). Electronic applications accepted.

Capella University, School of Public Service Leadership, Master's Programs in Nursing, Minneapolis, MN 55402. Offers diabetes nursing (MSN); general nursing (MSN); gerontology nursing (MSN); health information management (MS); nurse educator (MSN); nursing leadership and administration (MSN).

Caribbean University, Graduate School, Bayamón, PR 00960-0493. Offers administration and supervision (MA Ed); criminal justice (MA); curriculum and instruction (MA Ed, PhD), including elementary education (MA Ed), English education (MA Ed), history education (MA Ed), mathematics education (MA Ed), primary education (MA Ed), science education (MA Ed), Spanish education (MA Ed); educational technology in instructional systems (MA Ed); gerontology (MSN); human resources (MBA); museology, archiving and art history (MA Ed); neonatal pediatrics (MSN); physical education (MA Ed); special education (MA Ed). *Entrance requirements:* For master's, interview, minimum GPA of 2.5.

Case Western Reserve University, Frances Payne Bolton School of Nursing, Doctor of Nursing Practice Program, Cleveland, OH 44106. Offers acute care nurse practitioner (DNP); adult gerontology nurse practitioner (DNP); educational leadership (DNP); family nurse practitioner (DNP); family systems psychiatric mental health nursing (DNP); midwifery/family nursing (DNP); neonatal nurse practitioner (DNP); pediatric nurse practitioner (DNP); practice leadership (DNP); women's health nurse practitioner (DNP). *Accreditation:* AACN. Part-time programs available. Postbaccalaureate distance learning degree programs offered (minimal on-campus study). *Students:* 169 full-time, 9 part-time; includes 10 minority (6 Black or African American, non-Hispanic/Latino; 1 Asian, non-Hispanic/Latino; 2 Hispanic/Latino; 1 Two or more races, non-Hispanic/Latino). 76 applicants, 97% accepted, 59 enrolled. In 2013, 38 doctorates awarded. Terminal master's awarded for partial completion of doctoral program. *Degree requirements:* For doctorate, thesis/dissertation. *Entrance requirements:* For doctorate, GRE General Test or MAT. Additional exam requirements/recommendations for international students: Required—TOEFL (minimum score 577 paper-based; 90 iBT), IELTS (minimum score 7). *Application deadline:* For fall admission, 6/1 priority date for domestic students, 6/1 for international students; for spring admission, 10/1 for domestic and international students. Applications are processed on a rolling basis. Application fee: $75. *Financial support:* In 2013–14, 90 students received support, including 9 fellowships with full tuition reimbursements available (averaging $31,325 per year), 1 research assistantship with partial tuition reimbursement available (averaging $14,472 per year); teaching assistantships, Federal Work-Study, institutionally sponsored loans, scholarships/grants, and tuition waivers (partial) also available. Support available to part-time students. Financial award application deadline: 5/15; financial award applicants required to submit FAFSA. *Faculty research:* Symptom science, family/community care, aging across the lifespan, self-management of health and illness, neuroscience. *Unit head:* Dr. Donna Dowling, Director, 216-368-1869, Fax: 216-368-3542, E-mail: dad10@case.edu. *Application contact:* Donna Hassik, Admissions Coordinator, 216-368-5253, Fax: 216-368-0124, E-mail: dmh7@case.edu.
Website: http://fpb.case.edu/DNP/

Case Western Reserve University, Frances Payne Bolton School of Nursing, Master's Programs in Nursing, Nurse Practitioner Program, Cleveland, OH 44106. Offers acute care cardiovascular nursing (MSN); acute care nurse practitioner (MSN); acute care/flight nurse (MSN); adult gerontology acute care nurse practitioner (MSN); adult gerontology nurse practitioner (MSN); adult gerontology oncology and palliative care (MSN); family nurse practitioner (MSN); family systems psychiatric mental health nursing (MSN); neonatal nurse practitioner (MSN); pediatric nurse practitioner (MSN); women's health nurse practitioner (MSN). Part-time programs available. Postbaccalaureate distance learning degree programs offered (minimal on-campus study). *Faculty:* 54 full-time (50 women), 5 part-time/adjunct (3 women). *Students:* 56 full-time, 145 part-time; includes 9 minority (6 Black or African American, non-Hispanic/Latino; 2 Asian, non-Hispanic/Latino; 1 Hispanic/Latino), 5 international. Average age 35. 70 applicants, 71% accepted, 33 enrolled. In 2013, 79 master's awarded. *Degree requirements:* For master's, thesis optional. *Entrance requirements:* For master's, GRE General Test or MAT. Additional exam requirements/recommendations for international students: Required—TOEFL (minimum score 577 paper-based; 90 iBT), IELTS (minimum score 7). *Application deadline:* For fall admission, 6/1 for domestic students; for spring admission, 10/1 for domestic students. Applications are processed on a rolling basis. Application fee: $75. *Financial support:* In 2013–14, 25 teaching assistantships (averaging $15,120 per year) were awarded; research assistantships, institutionally sponsored loans, and tuition waivers (partial) also available. Support available to part-time students. Financial award application deadline: 6/30; financial award applicants required to submit FAFSA. *Faculty research:* Symptom science, family/community care, aging across the lifespan, self-management of health and illness, neuroscience. *Unit head:* Dr. Carol Savrin, Director, 216-368-5304, Fax: 216-368-3542, E-mail: cls18@case.edu. *Application contact:* Donna Hassik, Admissions Coordinator, 216-368-5253, Fax: 216-368-0124, E-mail: dmh7@case.edu.
Website: http://fpb.cwru.edu/MSN/majors.shtm

College of Mount Saint Vincent, School of Professional and Continuing Studies, Department of Nursing, Riverdale, NY 10471-1093. Offers adult nurse practitioner (MSN, PMC); family nurse practitioner (MSN, PMC); nurse educator (PMC); nursing administration (MSN); nursing for the adult and aged (MSN). *Accreditation:* AACN. Part-time programs available. *Entrance requirements:* For master's, BSN, interview, RN license, minimum GPA of 3.0, letters of reference. Additional exam requirements/recommendations for international students: Required—TOEFL. *Expenses:* Contact institution.

College of Staten Island of the City University of New York, Graduate Programs, Department of Nursing, Program in Gerontological Nursing, Staten Island, NY 10314-6600. Offers MS, Post-Master's Certificate. Part-time programs available. *Faculty:* 3 full-time (all women), 5 part-time/adjunct (4 women). *Students:* 6 part-time (all women). Average age 43. 2 applicants, 0% accepted, 2 enrolled. *Degree requirements:* For master's, thesis optional. *Entrance requirements:* For master's, bachelor's degree in nursing with minimum GPA of 3.0, RN license, 2 letters of reference, 1 year of full-time experience as a nurse or its equivalent, personal statement; for Post-Master's Certificate, master's degree in nursing. Additional exam requirements/recommendations for international students: Required—TOEFL (minimum score 550 paper-based; 79 iBT), IELTS (minimum score 6.5). *Application deadline:* For fall admission, 5/1 priority date for domestic and international students; for spring admission, 11/19 priority date for domestic and international students. Applications are processed on a rolling basis. Application fee: $125. Electronic applications accepted. *Expenses:* Tuition, state resident: full-time $9240; part-time $385 per credit hour. Tuition, nonresident: full-time $17,040; part-time $710 per credit hour. *Required fees:* $428; $128 per term. *Financial support:* Career-related internships or fieldwork, Federal Work-Study, scholarships/grants, and traineeships available. Support available to part-time students. Financial award applicants required to submit FAFSA. *Unit head:* Dr. June Como, Interim Director of Graduate Nursing Programs, 718-982-3818, Fax: 718-982-3813, E-mail: june.como@csi.cuny.edu. *Application contact:* Sasha Spence, Assistant Director for Graduate Admissions, 718-982-2019, Fax: 718-982-2500, E-mail: spence@mail.csi.cuny.edu.
Website: http://www.csi.cuny.edu/nursing/graduate.html

Columbia University, School of Nursing, Program in Adult-Gerontology Primary Care Nurse Practitioner, New York, NY 10032. Offers MS, Adv C. *Accreditation:* AACN. Part-time programs available. *Entrance requirements:* For master's, GRE General Test, NCLEX, BSN, 1 year of clinical experience (preferred); for Adv C, MSN. Additional exam requirements/recommendations for international students: Required—TOEFL (minimum score 100 iBT). Electronic applications accepted.

Concordia University Wisconsin, Graduate Programs, School of Human Services, Program in Nursing, Mequon, WI 53097-2402. Offers family nurse practitioner (MSN); geriatric nurse practitioner (MSN); nurse educator (MSN). *Accreditation:* AACN. Postbaccalaureate distance learning degree programs offered (minimal on-campus study). *Degree requirements:* For master's, comprehensive exam, thesis or alternative. *Entrance requirements:* Additional exam requirements/recommendations for international students: Required—TOEFL. *Expenses:* Contact institution.

Duke University, School of Nursing, Durham, NC 27708-0586. Offers acute care pediatric nurse practitioner (MSN); adult-gerontology nurse practitioner - acute care (MSN, Post Master's Certificate); adult-gerontology nurse practitioner - primary care (MSN, Post Master's Certificate), including adult-gerontology nurse practitioner (MSN), cardiology, oncology; family nurse practitioner (MSN); neonatal nurse practitioner (MSN); nurse anesthesia (MSN, DNP); nursing (PhD); nursing and health care leadership (MSN); nursing education (MSN); nursing informatics (MSN, Post Master's Certificate); pediatric nurse practitioner - primary care (MSN). *Accreditation:* AACN; AANA/CANAEP. Part-time and evening/weekend programs available. Postbaccalaureate distance learning degree programs offered (minimal on-campus study). *Faculty:* 74 full-time (64 women), 7 part-time/adjunct (4 women). *Students:* 127 full-time (113 women), 473 part-time (433 women); includes 131 minority (54 Black or African American, non-Hispanic/Latino; 9 American Indian or Alaska Native, non-Hispanic/Latino; 36 Asian, non-Hispanic/Latino; 27 Hispanic/Latino; 5 Native Hawaiian or other Pacific Islander, non-Hispanic/Latino), 14 international. Average age 34. 516 applicants, 50% accepted, 190 enrolled. In 2013, 179 master's, 49 doctorates, 23 other advanced degrees awarded. Terminal master's awarded for partial completion of doctoral program. *Degree requirements:* For master's, thesis optional; for doctorate, capstone project. *Entrance requirements:* For master's, GRE General Test (waived if undergraduate GPA of 3.4 or higher), 1 year of nursing experience (recommended), BSN, minimum GPA of 3.0, previous course work in statistics; for doctorate, GRE General Test (waived if undergraduate GPA of 3.4 or higher), BSN or MSN, minimum GPA of 3.0, portfolio, resume, personal statement, undergraduate statistics course, current licensure as a registered nurse, transcripts from all post-secondary institutions; for Post Master's Certificate, MSN, licensure or eligibility as a professional nurse, transcripts from all post-secondary institutions, previous course work in statistics. Additional exam requirements/recommendations for international students: Recommended—TOEFL (minimum score 550 paper-based; 83 iBT), IELTS (minimum score 7). *Application deadline:* For fall admission, 12/1 for domestic and international students; for spring admission, 5/1 for domestic and international students. Application fee: $50. Electronic applications accepted. *Expenses:* Contact institution. *Financial support:* Career-related internships or fieldwork, institutionally sponsored loans, scholarships/grants, traineeships, and tuition waivers (partial) available. Support available to part-time students. Financial award applicants required to submit FAFSA. *Faculty research:* Cardiovascular disease, caregiver skill training, data mining, prostate cancer, neonatal immune system. *Unit head:* Dr. Catherine L. Gilliss, Dean/Vice Chancellor for Nursing Affairs, 919-684-9444, Fax: 919-684-9414, E-mail: catherine.gilliss@duke.edu. *Application contact:* Ernie Rushing, Lead Admissions Processor/Admissions Officer, 919-668-6274, Fax: 919-668-4693, E-mail: stephen.rushing@dm.duke.edu.
Website: http://www.nursing.duke.edu/

Felician College, Program in Nursing, Lodi, NJ 07644-2117. Offers adult-gerontology nurse practitioner (MSN, PMC); executive leadership (MSN, PMC); family nurse practitioner (MSN, PMC); nursing education (MSN, PMC). *Accreditation:* AACN. Part-time and evening/weekend programs available. Postbaccalaureate distance learning degree programs offered (no on-campus study). *Students:* 5 full-time (4 women), 85 part-time (78 women); includes 50 minority (20 Black or African American, non-Hispanic/Latino; 14 Asian, non-Hispanic/Latino; 16 Hispanic/Latino). Average age 42. *Degree requirements:* For master's, scholarly project. *Entrance requirements:* For master's, BS in nursing or equivalent, minimum GPA of 3.0, 2 letters of recommendation, RN license; for PMC, RN license, minimum GPA of 2.75. Additional exam requirements/

recommendations for international students: Recommended—TOEFL (minimum score 550 paper-based). *Application deadline:* Applications are processed on a rolling basis. Application fee: $40. *Expenses: Tuition:* Part-time $945 per credit. *Required fees:* $317.50 per semester. *Financial support:* In 2013–14, 10 students received support. Traineeships available. Financial award applicants required to submit FAFSA. *Faculty research:* Anxiety and fear, curriculum innovation, health promotion. *Unit head:* Dr. Muriel Shore, Dean, Division of Health Sciences, 201-559-6030, E-mail: shorem@felician.edu. *Application contact:* Elizabeth Barca, Senior Assistant Director, Graduate Admissions, 201-559-6077, Fax: 201-559-6138, E-mail: graduate@felician.edu.

Florida Atlantic University, Christine E. Lynn College of Nursing, Boca Raton, FL 33431-0991. Offers administrative and financial leadership in nursing and health care (Post Master's Certificate); adult/gerontological nurse practitioner (Post Master's Certificate); advanced holistic nursing (MS, Post Master's Certificate); clinical nurse leader (MS, Post Master's Certificate); family nurse practitioner (MS, Post Master's Certificate); nurse educator (MS, Post Master's Certificate); nursing (PhD); nursing administration and financial leadership (MS); nursing practice (DNP). *Accreditation:* AACN. Part-time programs available. *Faculty:* 30 full-time (27 women), 9 part-time/adjunct (8 women). *Students:* 29 full-time (27 women), 523 part-time (492 women); includes 254 minority (157 Black or African American, non-Hispanic/Latino; 2 American Indian or Alaska Native, non-Hispanic/Latino; 19 Asian, non-Hispanic/Latino; 62 Hispanic/Latino; 2 Native Hawaiian or other Pacific Islander, non-Hispanic/Latino; 12 Two or more races, non-Hispanic/Latino), 3 international. Average age 39. 463 applicants, 25% accepted, 111 enrolled. In 2013, 148 master's, 15 doctorates awarded. *Degree requirements:* For master's, thesis or alternative; for doctorate, comprehensive exam, thesis/dissertation. *Entrance requirements:* For master's, GRE General Test or MAT, bachelor's degree in nursing, Florida RN license, minimum GPA of 3.0, resume/curriculum vitae, letter of recommendation; for doctorate, GRE General Test or MAT, curriculum vitae, Florida RN license, minimum GPA of 3.5, master's degree in nursing, three letters of recommendation. *Application deadline:* For fall admission, 6/1 for domestic students, 2/15 for international students; for spring admission, 10/1 for domestic students, 7/15 for international students. Applications are processed on a rolling basis. Application fee: $30. *Expenses:* Tuition, state resident: full-time $6660; part-time $370 per credit hour. Tuition, nonresident: full-time $18,450; part-time $1025 per credit hour. Tuition and fees vary according to course load. *Financial support:* Research assistantships with partial tuition reimbursements, teaching assistantships with partial tuition reimbursements, career-related internships or fieldwork, Federal Work-Study, institutionally sponsored loans, scholarships/grants, and traineeships available. Support available to part-time students. *Faculty research:* Econometrics of nurse-patient relationship, Alzheimer's disease, community-based programs, falls, self-healing. *Unit head:* Dr. Marlaine Smith, Dean, 561-297-3206, Fax: 561-297-3687, E-mail: msmit230@fau.edu. *Application contact:* Carol Kruse, Graduate Coordinator, 561-297-3261, Fax: 561-297-0088, E-mail: ckruse@fau.edu.
Website: http://nursing.fau.edu/

Florida Southern College, Program in Nursing, Lakeland, FL 33801-5698. Offers adult gerontology clinical nurse specialist (MSN); adult gerontology primary care nurse practitioner (MSN); nurse educator (MSN); nursing administration (MSN). *Accreditation:* AACN. Part-time and evening/weekend programs available. *Entrance requirements:* For master's, Florida RN license, 3 letters of recommendation, personal statement, minimum GPA of 3.0, resume. Additional exam requirements/recommendations for international students: Required—TOEFL (minimum score 550 paper-based). *Expenses:* Contact institution. *Faculty research:* End of life care, dementia, health promotion.

Gwynedd Mercy University, School of Nursing, Gwynedd Valley, PA 19437-0901. Offers clinical nurse specialist (MSN), including gerontology, oncology, pediatrics; nurse practitioner (MSN), including adult health, pediatric health. *Degree requirements:* For master's, thesis optional. *Entrance requirements:* For master's, GRE General Test or MAT, current nursing experience, physical assessment, course work in statistics, BSN from NLNAC-accredited program, 2 letters of recommendation, personal interview. Additional exam requirements/recommendations for international students: Required—TOEFL (minimum score 575 paper-based). Electronic applications accepted. *Expenses:* Contact institution. *Faculty research:* Critical thinking, primary care, domestic violence, multiculturalism, nursing centers.

Hampton University, Graduate College, School of Nursing, Hampton, VA 23668. Offers advanced adult nursing (MS); community health nursing (MS); community mental health/psychiatric nursing (MS); family nursing (MS); gerontological nursing for the nurse practitioner (MS); pediatric nursing (MS); women's health nursing (MS). *Accreditation:* AACN. Part-time and evening/weekend programs available. *Degree requirements:* For master's, thesis optional. *Entrance requirements:* For master's, GRE General Test. *Faculty research:* Curriculum development, physical and mental assessment.

Hunter College of the City University of New York, Graduate School, Schools of the Health Professions, Hunter-Bellevue School of Nursing, Gerontological Nurse Practitioner Program, New York, NY 10065-5085. Offers MS. *Accreditation:* AACN. Part-time programs available. *Faculty:* 18 full-time (15 women), 25 part-time/adjunct (21 women). *Students:* 1 (woman) full-time, 224 part-time (194 women); includes 94 minority (32 Black or African American, non-Hispanic/Latino; 43 Asian, non-Hispanic/Latino; 19 Hispanic/Latino), 14 international. Average age 33. 146 applicants, 27% accepted, 32 enrolled. In 2013, 52 master's awarded. *Degree requirements:* For master's, practicum. *Entrance requirements:* For master's, minimum GPA of 3.0, New York RN license, 2 years of professional practice experience, BSN. Additional exam requirements/recommendations for international students: Required—TOEFL. *Application deadline:* For fall admission, 4/1 for domestic students, 2/1 for international students; for spring admission, 11/1 for domestic students, 9/1 for international students. Applications are processed on a rolling basis. Application fee: $125. *Financial support:* Federal Work-Study, scholarships/grants, traineeships, and tuition waivers (partial) available. Support available to part-time students. Financial award application deadline: 5/1; financial award applicants required to submit FAFSA. *Unit head:* Dr. Anita Nerenberg, Interim Specialization Coordinator, 212-481-4359, Fax: 212-481-5078, E-mail: anerenbe@hunter.cuny.edu. *Application contact:* Milena Solo, Director for Graduate Admissions, 212-772-4482, E-mail: admissions@hunter.cuny.edu.
Website: http://www.hunter.cuny.edu/nursing/admissions/graduate

Independence University, Program in Nursing, Salt Lake City, UT 84107. Offers community health (MSN); gerontology (MSN); nursing administration (MSN); wellness promotion (MSN).

Indiana University–Purdue University Fort Wayne, College of Health and Human Services, Department of Nursing, Fort Wayne, IN 46805-1499. Offers adult-gerontology primary care nurse practitioner (MS); nurse executive (MS); nursing administration (Certificate); nursing education (MS); women's health nurse practitioner (MS). Part-time programs available. *Faculty:* 12 full-time (all women). *Students:* 5 full-time (all women), 63 part-time (60 women); includes 3 minority (2 Black or African American, non-Hispanic/Latino; 1 Asian, non-Hispanic/Latino). Average age 35. 34 applicants, 100% accepted, 25 enrolled. In 2013, 10 master's awarded. *Entrance requirements:* For master's, GRE Writing Test (if GPA below 3.0), BS in nursing, eligibility for Indiana RN license, minimum GPA of 3.0, essay, copy of resume, three references, undergraduate course work in research and statistics within last 5 years. Additional exam requirements/recommendations for international students: Required—TOEFL (minimum score 550 paper-based; 79 iBT); Recommended—TWE. *Application deadline:* For fall admission, 5/1 priority date for domestic and international students; for spring admission, 11/15 priority date for domestic students. Applications are processed on a rolling basis. Application fee: $55 ($60 for international students). Electronic applications accepted. *Financial support:* In 2013–14, 3 teaching assistantships with partial tuition reimbursements (averaging $13,322 per year) were awarded; scholarships/grants also available. Support available to part-time students. Financial award application deadline: 3/1; financial award applicants required to submit FAFSA. *Faculty research:* Pain management and substance abuse, high-risk alcohol use on campus, pediatric case management. *Unit head:* Dr. Lee-Ellen Kirkhorn, Chair/Professor, 260-481-6789, Fax: 260-481-5767, E-mail: kirkhorl@ipfw.edu. *Application contact:* Dr. Deborah Poling, Director of Graduate Program, 260-481-6276, Fax: 260-481-5767, E-mail: polingd@ipfw.edu.
Website: http://www.ipfw.edu/nursing/

Kent State University, College of Nursing, Kent, OH 44242-0001. Offers acute care nurse practitioner (MSN); adult nurse practitioner (MSN); clinical nurse specialist (MSN); family nurse practitioner (MSN); geriatric nurse practitioner (MSN); health care management (MSN); nurse educator (MSN); nursing (PhD); nursing practice (DNP); pediatric nurse practitioner (MSN); psychiatric/mental health nurse practitioner (MSN); women's health nurse practitioner (MSN). PhD program offered jointly with The University of Akron. *Accreditation:* AACN. Part-time programs available. *Degree requirements:* For master's, thesis optional; for doctorate, comprehensive exam, thesis/dissertation. *Entrance requirements:* For master's, GRE (if undergraduate GPA less than 3.0), minimum GPA of 2.75; for doctorate, GRE, MSN. Additional exam requirements/recommendations for international students: Required—TOEFL. Electronic applications accepted. *Expenses:* Contact institution. *Faculty research:* Women and violence, methodological specialties, osteoporosis in women, new caregivers and the elderly.

La Salle University, School of Nursing and Health Sciences, Program in Nursing, Philadelphia, PA 19141-1199. Offers adult gerontology primary care nurse practitioner (MSN, Certificate); adult health and illness clinical nurse specialist (MSN); adult-gerontology clinical nurse specialist (MSN, Certificate); clinical nurse leader (MSN); family primary care nurse practitioner (MSN, Certificate); gerontology (Certificate); nurse anesthetist (MSN, Certificate); nursing (MSN, Certificate); nursing administration (MSN, Certificate); nursing education (Certificate); nursing practice (DNP); nursing service administration (MSN); public health nursing (MSN, Certificate); school nursing (Certificate); MSN/MBA; MSN/MPH. *Accreditation:* AANA/CANAEP. Part-time programs available. Postbaccalaureate distance learning degree programs offered (minimal on-campus study). *Faculty:* 13 full-time (12 women), 10 part-time/adjunct (8 women). *Students:* 4 full-time (all women), 379 part-time (331 women); includes 119 minority (70 Black or African American, non-Hispanic/Latino; 2 American Indian or Alaska Native, non-Hispanic/Latino; 31 Asian, non-Hispanic/Latino; 12 Hispanic/Latino; 4 Two or more races, non-Hispanic/Latino), 1 international. Average age 37. 133 applicants, 85% accepted, 63 enrolled. In 2013, 72 master's, 3 doctorates, 26 other advanced degrees awarded. *Degree requirements:* For doctorate, minimum of 1,000 hours of post baccalaureate clinical practice supervised by preceptors. *Entrance requirements:* For master's, GRE, MAT, or GMAT (for students with BSN GPA of less than 3.2), baccalaureate degree in nursing from an NLNAC- or CCNE-accredited program or an MSN Bridge program; Pennsylvania RN license; 2 letters of reference; resume; statement of philosophy articulating professional values and future educational goal; 1 year of work experience as a registered nurse; for doctorate, GRE (waived for applicants with MSN cumulative GPA of 3.7 or above), MSN from nationally-accredited program or master's degree, MBA or MHA from nationally-accredited program; resume or curriculum vitae; 2 letters of reference; interview; for Certificate, GRE, MAT, or GMAT (for students with BSN GPA of less than 3.2, baccalaureate degree in nursing from an NLNAC- or CCNE-accredited program or an MSN Bridge program; Pennsylvania RN license; 2 letters of reference; resume; statement of philosophy articulating professional values and future educational goal; 1 year of work experience as a registered nurse. Additional exam requirements/recommendations for international students: Required—TOEFL. *Application deadline:* For fall admission, 8/15 priority date for domestic students, 7/15 for international students; for spring admission, 12/15 priority date for domestic students, 11/15 for international students; for summer admission, 4/15 priority date for domestic students, 3/15 for international students. Applications are processed on a rolling basis. Application fee: $35. Electronic applications accepted. Application fee is waived when completed online. *Expenses:* Contact institution. *Financial support:* In 2013–14, 48 students received support. Teaching assistantships, scholarships/grants, and traineeships available. Support available to part-time students. Financial award application deadline: 8/31; financial award applicants required to submit FAFSA. *Unit head:* Dr. Patricia M. Dillon, Director, 215-951-1322, Fax: 215-951-1896, E-mail: msnapn@lasalle.edu. *Application contact:* Paul J. Reilly, Assistant Vice President, Enrollment Services, 215-951-1946, Fax: 215-951-1462, E-mail: reilly@lasalle.edu.

Lehman College of the City University of New York, School of Natural and Social Sciences, Department of Nursing, Bronx, NY 10468-1589. Offers adult health nursing (MS); nursing of older adults (MS); parent-child nursing (MS); pediatric nurse practitioner (MS). *Accreditation:* AACN. Part-time and evening/weekend programs available. *Entrance requirements:* For master's, bachelor's degree in nursing, New York RN license.

Le Moyne College, Department of Nursing, Syracuse, NY 13214. Offers informatics (MS, CAS); nursing administration (MS, CAS); nursing education (MS, CAS); nursing gerontology (MS, CAS); palliative care (MS, CAS). *Accreditation:* AACN. Part-time and evening/weekend programs available. *Faculty:* 4 full-time (all women), 3 part-time/adjunct (2 women). *Students:* 13 part-time (12 women); includes 2 minority (both Black or African American, non-Hispanic/Latino). Average age 41. 14 applicants, 86% accepted, 5 enrolled. In 2013, 6 master's, 6 other advanced degrees awarded. *Degree requirements:* For master's, scholarly project. *Entrance requirements:* For master's, bachelor's degree, interview, minimum GPA of 3.0, New York RN license, 2 letters of recommendation, writing sample, transcripts. Additional exam requirements/recommendations for international students: Required—TOEFL (minimum score 550 paper-based; 79 iBT). *Application deadline:* For fall admission, 8/1 priority date for domestic and international students; for spring admission, 12/15 priority date for domestic and international students; for summer admission, 5/1 priority date for domestic and international students. Applications are processed on a rolling basis. Application fee: $50. *Expenses:* Contact institution. *Financial support:* In 2013–14, 2 students received support. Career-related internships or fieldwork, scholarships/grants, health care benefits, and unspecified assistantships available. Support available to part-time students. Financial award applicants required to submit FAFSA. *Faculty research:* Inter-profession education, gerontology, utilization of free healthcare services by the insured, health promotion education, innovative undergraduate nursing education models, patient and family education, horizontal violence. *Unit head:* Dr. Susan B. Bastable, Chair and Professor, Department of Nursing, 315-445-5436, Fax: 315-445-6024, E-mail: bastabsb@lemoyne.edu. *Application contact:* Kristen P. Trapasso, Senior

Director of Enrollment Management, 315-445-4265, Fax: 315-445-6092, E-mail: trapaskp@lemoyne.edu.
Website: http://www.lemoyne.edu/nursing

Loma Linda University, Department of Graduate Nursing, Program in Adult and Aging Family Nursing, Loma Linda, CA 92350. Offers MS. *Accreditation:* AACN. Part-time programs available. *Degree requirements:* For master's, thesis or alternative. *Entrance requirements:* For master's, GRE General Test, BSN, minimum GPA of 3.0, RN license. Additional exam requirements/recommendations for international students: Required—TOEFL. Electronic applications accepted. *Faculty research:* Coping, integration of research.

Marquette University, Graduate School, College of Nursing, Milwaukee, WI 53201-1881. Offers acute care nurse practitioner (Certificate); adult clinical nurse specialist (Certificate); adult nurse practitioner (Certificate); advanced practice nursing (MSN, DNP), including adult-older adult acute care (DNP), adults (MSN), adults-older adults (DNP), clinical nurse leader (MSN), health care systems leadership (DNP), nurse-midwifery (MSN), older adults (MSN), pediatrics acute care (MSN), pediatrics primary care (MSN), pediatrics-acute care (DNP), pediatrics-primary care (DNP), primary care (DNP), systems leadership and healthcare quality (MSN); family nurse practitioner (Certificate); nurse-midwifery (Certificate); nursing (PhD); pediatric acute care (Certificate); pediatric primary care (Certificate); systems leadership and healthcare quality (Certificate). *Accreditation:* AACN. *Faculty:* 35 full-time (34 women), 59 part-time/adjunct (58 women). *Students:* 105 full-time (96 women), 279 part-time (256 women); includes 28 minority (11 Black or African American, non-Hispanic/Latino; 7 Asian, non-Hispanic/Latino; 8 Hispanic/Latino; 2 Two or more races, non-Hispanic/Latino), 3 international. Average age 30. 322 applicants, 62% accepted, 98 enrolled. In 2013, 66 master's, 4 doctorates, 6 other advanced degrees awarded. Terminal master's awarded for partial completion of doctoral program. *Degree requirements:* For master's, comprehensive exam, thesis or alternative. *Entrance requirements:* For master's, GRE General Test, BSN, Wisconsin RN license, official transcripts from all current and previous colleges/universities except Marquette, three completed recommendation forms, resume, written statement of professional goals; for doctorate, GRE General Test, official transcripts from all current and previous colleges/universities except Marquette, three letters of recommendation, resume, written statement of professional goals, sample of scholarly writing. Additional exam requirements/recommendations for international students: Required—TOEFL (minimum score 530 paper-based). *Application deadline:* For fall admission, 2/15 for domestic and international students. Application fee: $50. Electronic applications accepted. *Financial support:* In 2013–14, 41 students received support, including 1 fellowship with partial tuition reimbursement available (averaging $17,500 per year), 2 research assistantships with full tuition reimbursements available (averaging $13,285 per year), 8 teaching assistantships with full tuition reimbursements available (averaging $13,912 per year); career-related internships or fieldwork, Federal Work-Study, scholarships/grants, health care benefits, tuition waivers (partial), and unspecified assistantships also available. Support available to part-time students. Financial award application deadline: 2/15. *Faculty research:* Psychosocial adjustment to chronic illness, gerontology, reminiscence, health policy: uninsured and access, hospital care delivery systems. *Total annual research expenditures:* $769,051. *Unit head:* Dr. Margaret Callahan, Dean, 414-288-3800, Fax: 414-288-1578. *Application contact:* Dr. Maureen O'Brien, Associate Dean/Clinical Associate Professor, 414-288-3823.
Website: http://www.marquette.edu/nursing/academicprograms-graduate.shtml

Maryville University of Saint Louis, College of Health Professions, The Catherine McAuley School of Nursing, St. Louis, MO 63141-7299. Offers adult nurse practitioner (MSN); advanced practice nursing (DNP); family nurse practitioner (MSN); geriatric nurse practitioner (MSN); nursing education (MSN). *Accreditation:* AACN. Postbaccalaureate distance learning degree programs offered. *Students:* 30 full-time (28 women), 1,551 part-time (1,416 women); includes 361 minority (181 Black or African American, non-Hispanic/Latino; 16 American Indian or Alaska Native, non-Hispanic/Latino; 59 Asian, non-Hispanic/Latino; 71 Hispanic/Latino; 5 Native Hawaiian or other Pacific Islander, non-Hispanic/Latino; 29 Two or more races, non-Hispanic/Latino), 3 international. Average age 36. In 2013, 37 master's awarded. *Degree requirements:* For master's, practicum. *Entrance requirements:* For master's, BSN, current licensure, minimum GPA of 3.0, 3 letters of recommendation, curriculum vitae. Additional exam requirements/recommendations for international students: Required—TOEFL (minimum score 550 paper-based). *Application deadline:* Applications are processed on a rolling basis. Application fee: $40 ($60 for international students). Electronic applications accepted. Application fee is waived when completed online. *Expenses: Tuition:* Full-time $23,812; part-time $728 per credit hour. *Required fees:* $395 per year. Tuition and fees vary according to course load, degree level and program. *Financial support:* Federal Work-Study and campus employment available. Support available to part-time students. Financial award application deadline: 3/1; financial award applicants required to submit FAFSA. *Unit head:* Dr. Elizabeth Buck, Director, 314-529-9453, Fax: 314-529-9139, E-mail: ebuck@maryville.edu. *Application contact:* Crystal Jacobsmeyer, Assistant Director, Graduate Enrollment Advising, 314-929-9654, Fax: 314-529-9927, E-mail: cjacobsmeyer@maryville.edu.
Website: http://www.maryville.edu/hp/nursing/

Medical University of South Carolina, College of Nursing, Adult-Gerontology Health Nurse Practitioner Program, Charleston, SC 29425. Offers MSN, DNP. Part-time programs available. Postbaccalaureate distance learning degree programs offered (minimal on-campus study). *Degree requirements:* For master's, comprehensive exam (for some programs), thesis optional; for doctorate, final project. *Entrance requirements:* For master's, BSN from nationally-accredited program, minimum nursing and cumulative GPA of 3.0, undergraduate-level statistics course, active RN License, 3 confidential references, current curriculum vitae or resume, essay; for doctorate, BSN from nationally-accredited program, minimum nursing and cumulative GPA of 3.0, undergraduate-level statistics course, active RN License, 3 confidential references, current curriculum vitae or resume, personal essay (for DNP). Additional exam requirements/recommendations for international students: Required—TOEFL (minimum score 550 paper-based; 80 iBT). Electronic applications accepted. *Faculty research:* Palliative care, dementia, hospital acquired infections, diabetes, advance practice nurse utilization.

MGH Institute of Health Professions, School of Nursing, Boston, MA 02129-4557. Offers advanced practice nursing (MSN); gerontological nursing (MSN); nursing (DNP); pediatric nursing (MSN); psychiatric nursing (MSN); teaching and learning for health care education (Certificate); women's health nursing (MSN). *Accreditation:* AACN. *Faculty:* 41 full-time (36 women), 14 part-time/adjunct (13 women). *Students:* 494 full-time (428 women), 85 part-time (77 women); includes 108 minority (32 Black or African American, non-Hispanic/Latino; 2 American Indian or Alaska Native, non-Hispanic/Latino; 38 Asian, non-Hispanic/Latino; 33 Hispanic/Latino; 3 Native Hawaiian or other Pacific Islander, non-Hispanic/Latino). Average age 32. 470 applicants, 52% accepted, 133 enrolled. In 2013, 85 master's, 12 doctorates, 98 other advanced degrees awarded. *Degree requirements:* For master's, thesis or alternative. *Entrance requirements:* For master's, GRE General Test, bachelor's degree from regionally-accredited college or university. Additional exam requirements/recommendations for international students: Required—TOEFL (minimum score 550 paper-based; 80 iBT). *Application deadline:* For fall admission, 12/1 for domestic and international students; for spring admission, 10/1 for domestic and international students. Application fee: $100. Electronic applications accepted. *Expenses: Tuition:* Part-time $1114 per credit. *Required fees:* $620 per term. One-time fee: $475 part-time. *Financial support:* In 2013–14, 75 students received support, including 4 research assistantships (averaging $1,200 per year), 17 teaching assistantships (averaging $1,200 per year); career-related internships or fieldwork, scholarships/grants, traineeships, and unspecified assistantships also available. Support available to part-time students. Financial award application deadline: 4/1; financial award applicants required to submit FAFSA. *Faculty research:* Biobehavioral nursing, HIV/AIDS, gerontological nursing, women's health, vulnerable populations, health systems. *Unit head:* Dr. Laurie Lauzon-Clabo, Dean, 617-643-0605, Fax: 617-726-8022, E-mail: llauzonclabo@mghihp.edu. *Application contact:* Lauren Putnam, Assistant Director of Admission, 617-726-3140, Fax: 617-726-8010, E-mail: admissions@mghihp.edu.
Website: http://www.mghihp.edu/academics/nursing/

Monmouth University, The Graduate School, The Marjorie K. Unterberg School of Nursing and Health Studies, West Long Branch, NJ 07764-1898. Offers adult and gerontological nurse practitioner (MSN); adult-gerontological nurse practitioner (Post-Master's Certificate); family nurse practitioner (MSN, Post-Master's Certificate); family psychiatric and mental health advanced practice nursing (MSN); forensic nursing (MSN, Certificate); nursing (MSN); nursing administration (MSN, Post-Master's Certificate); nursing education (MSN, Post-Master's Certificate); nursing practice (DNP); physician assistant (MS); psychiatric-mental health nurse practitioner (Post-Master's Certificate); school nursing (MSN, Certificate). *Accreditation:* AACN. Part-time and evening/weekend programs available. *Faculty:* 14 full-time (all women), 4 part-time/adjunct (3 women). *Students:* 19 full-time (18 women), 269 part-time (252 women); includes 106 minority (35 Black or African American, non-Hispanic/Latino; 2 American Indian or Alaska Native, non-Hispanic/Latino; 51 Asian, non-Hispanic/Latino; 12 Hispanic/Latino; 3 Native Hawaiian or other Pacific Islander, non-Hispanic/Latino; 3 Two or more races, non-Hispanic/Latino), 2 international. Average age 39. 135 applicants, 98% accepted, 96 enrolled. In 2013, 54 master's, 7 doctorates awarded. *Degree requirements:* For master's, practicum (for some tracks). *Entrance requirements:* For master's, GRE General Test, BSN with minimum GPA of 2.75, current RN license, proof of liability and malpractice policy, personal statement, two letters of recommendation, college course work in health assessment, resume; minimum GPA of 3.0, minimum C grade in prerequisite courses, minimum 200 hours' clinical experience, 3 letters of recommendation, and interview (for MS); for doctorate, accredited master's nursing program degree with minimum GPA of 3.2, active RN license, national certification as Nurse Practitioner or Nurse Administrator, working knowledge of statistics, statement of goals and vision for change, 2 letters of recommendation, resume, interview. Additional exam requirements/recommendations for international students: Required—TOEFL (minimum score 550 paper-based; 79 iBT), IELTS (minimum score 6) or Michigan English Language Assessment Battery (minimum score 77). *Application deadline:* For fall admission, 7/15 priority date for domestic students, 6/1 for international students; for spring admission, 11/15 priority date for domestic students, 11/1 for international students; for summer admission, 2/1 for domestic students. Applications are processed on a rolling basis. Application fee: $50. Electronic applications accepted. *Expenses: Tuition:* Part-time $1004 per credit hour. *Required fees:* $157 per semester. *Financial support:* In 2013–14, 163 students received support, including 113 fellowships (averaging $3,093 per year), 27 research assistantships (averaging $6,273 per year); career-related internships or fieldwork, scholarships/grants, and unspecified assistantships also available. Support available to part-time students. Financial award applicants required to submit FAFSA. *Faculty research:* Relationship of undergraduate GPA and GRE to succeeding in a graduate nursing program. *Unit head:* Dr. Janet Mahoney, Dean, 732-571-3443, Fax: 732-263-5131, E-mail: jmahoney@monmouth.edu. *Application contact:* Lauren Vento-Cifelli, Associate Vice President of Undergraduate and Graduate Admission, 732-571-3452, Fax: 732-263-5123, E-mail: gradadm@monmouth.edu.
Website: http://www.monmouth.edu/school-of-nursing-health/graduate-nursing-programs.aspx

Mount Carmel College of Nursing, Nursing Program, Columbus, OH 43222. Offers adult gerontology acute care nurse practitioner (MS); adult health clinical nurse specialist (MS); family nurse practitioner (MS); nursing administration (MS); nursing education (MS). *Accreditation:* AACN. Part-time programs available. *Faculty:* 8 full-time (7 women), 8 part-time/adjunct (7 women). *Students:* 94 full-time (89 women), 76 part-time (73 women); includes 35 minority (21 Black or African American, non-Hispanic/Latino; 2 American Indian or Alaska Native, non-Hispanic/Latino; 6 Asian, non-Hispanic/Latino; 2 Hispanic/Latino; 1 Native Hawaiian or other Pacific Islander, non-Hispanic/Latino; 3 Two or more races, non-Hispanic/Latino). Average age 38. 123 applicants, 50% accepted, 47 enrolled. In 2013, 41 master's awarded. *Degree requirements:* For master's, professional manuscript. *Entrance requirements:* For master's, letters of recommendation, statement of purpose, current resume, baccalaureate degree in nursing, current Ohio RN license, minimum cumulative GPA of 3.0. Additional exam requirements/recommendations for international students: Required—TOEFL (minimum score 550 paper-based; 80 iBT). *Application deadline:* For fall admission, 6/1 priority date for domestic students; for winter admission, 11/1 for domestic students; for spring admission, 10/1 priority date for domestic students; for summer admission, 3/1 for domestic students. Applications are processed on a rolling basis. Application fee: $30. *Expenses: Tuition:* Full-time $8560; part-time $428 per credit. *Required fees:* $75. *Financial support:* In 2013–14, 9 students received support. Institutionally sponsored loans and scholarships/grants available. Financial award application deadline: 3/15; financial award applicants required to submit FAFSA. *Unit head:* Dr. Angela Phillips-Lowe, Associate Dean, 614-234-5717, Fax: 614-234-2875, E-mail: aphillips-lowe@mccn.edu. *Application contact:* Kathleen Walters, Program Coordinator, 614-234-5408, Fax: 614-234-2875, E-mail: kwalters@mccn.edu.
Website: http://www.mccn.edu/

Nazareth College of Rochester, Graduate Studies, Department of Nursing, Gerontological Nurse Practitioner Program, Rochester, NY 14618-3790. Offers MS. *Accreditation:* AACN. Part-time programs available. *Entrance requirements:* For master's, minimum GPA of 3.0, RN license.

New Mexico State University, Graduate School, College of Health and Social Services, School of Nursing, Las Cruces, NM 88003. Offers adult/gerontology nurse practitioner (DNP); family nurse practitioner (DNP); nursing (MSN, PhD); public/community health (DNP). *Accreditation:* AACN. Postbaccalaureate distance learning degree programs offered (minimal on-campus study). *Faculty:* 15 full-time (14 women). *Students:* 42 full-time (33 women), 64 part-time (56 women); includes 50 minority (11 Black or African American, non-Hispanic/Latino; 1 American Indian or Alaska Native, non-Hispanic/Latino; 1 Asian, non-Hispanic/Latino; 36 Hispanic/Latino; 1 Two or more races, non-Hispanic/Latino), 1 international. Average age 42. 50 applicants, 86% accepted, 36 enrolled. In 2013, 12 master's, 6 doctorates awarded. *Degree requirements:* For master's, comprehensive exam, thesis optional, clinical practice; for doctorate, comprehensive exam, thesis/dissertation. *Entrance requirements:* For master's, NCLEX exam, BSN, minimum GPA of 3.0, course work in statistics, 3 letters of

reference, writing sample, RN license, CPR certification, proof of liability, immunizations, criminal background check; for doctorate, NCLEX exam, MSN, minimum GPA of 3.0, 3 letters of reference, writing sample, RN license, CPR certification, proof of liability, immunizations, criminal background check, statistics course. Additional exam requirements/recommendations for international students: Required—TOEFL (minimum score 550 paper-based; 79 iBT), IELTS (minimum score 6.5). *Application deadline:* For spring admission, 10/1 priority date for domestic students. Application fee: $40 ($50 for international students). Electronic applications accepted. *Expenses:* Tuition, state resident: full-time $5398; part-time $224.90 per credit. Tuition, nonresident: full-time $18,821; part-time $784.20 per credit. *Required fees:* $1310; $54.60 per credit. *Financial support:* In 2013–14, 31 students received support. Career-related internships or fieldwork, Federal Work-Study, scholarships/grants, traineeships, health care benefits, and unspecified assistantships available. Financial award application deadline: 3/1. *Faculty research:* Public policy, community health, health disparities, self efficacy and self management, psychiatric mental health. *Total annual research expenditures:* $3,424. *Unit head:* Dr. Pamela Schultz, Director, 575-646-3812, Fax: 575-646-2167, E-mail: pschultz@nmsu.edu. *Application contact:* Dr. Kathleen Huttlinger, Associate Director for Graduate Studies, 575-646-4387, Fax: 575-646-2167.
Website: http://schoolofnursing.nmsu.edu

New York University, College of Nursing, Doctor of Nursing Practice Program, New York, NY 10012-1019. Offers advanced practice nursing (DNP), including adult acute care, adult nurse practitioner/holistic nursing, adult nurse practitioner/palliative care nursing, adult primary care, adult primary care/geriatrics, family, geriatrics, mental health nursing, nurse-midwifery, pediatrics. Part-time and evening/weekend programs available. *Faculty:* 3 full-time (all women), 1 part-time/adjunct (0 women). *Students:* 1 (woman) full-time, 33 part-time (30 women); includes 7 minority (3 Black or African American, non-Hispanic/Latino; 3 Asian, non-Hispanic/Latino; 1 Hispanic/Latino). Average age 39. 18 applicants, 100% accepted, 12 enrolled. In 2013, 4 doctorates awarded. *Degree requirements:* For doctorate, thesis/dissertation, capstone. *Entrance requirements:* For doctorate, MAT or GRE (either taken within past 5 years), MS, RN license, interview, Nurse Practitioner Certification. Additional exam requirements/recommendations for international students: Required—TOEFL (minimum score 90 iBT), IELTS (minimum score 7). *Application deadline:* For fall admission, 3/1 for domestic students, 4/1 for international students. Applications are processed on a rolling basis. Application fee: $80. Electronic applications accepted. *Expenses: Tuition:* Full-time $35,856; part-time $1494 per unit. *Required fees:* $1408; $64 per unit. $473 per term. Tuition and fees vary according to course load and program. *Financial support:* Scholarships/grants available. Support available to part-time students. Financial award application deadline: 2/1. *Faculty research:* Geriatrics, HIV, elderly black diabetics, families and illness, oral systemic connection. *Unit head:* Dr. Rona Levin, Director, 212-998-5319, Fax: 212-995-3143, E-mail: rfl2039@nyu.edu. *Application contact:* Elizabeth Ensweiler, Assistant Director, Graduate Student Affairs and Admissions, 212-992-7653, Fax: 212-995-4302, E-mail: ee39@nyu.edu.

New York University, College of Nursing, Programs in Advanced Practice Nursing, New York, NY 10012-1019. Offers advanced practice nursing: adult acute care (MS, Advanced Certificate); advanced practice nursing: adult nurse practitioner/holistic nurse practitioner (Advanced Certificate); advanced practice nursing: adult nurse practitioner/palliative care nurse practitioner (Advanced Certificate); advanced practice nursing: adult primary care (MS, Advanced Certificate); advanced practice nursing: family (MS, Advanced Certificate); advanced practice nursing: geriatrics (Advanced Certificate); advanced practice nursing: mental health (MS); advanced practice nursing: mental health nursing (Advanced Certificate); advanced practice nursing: pediatrics (MS, Advanced Certificate); nurse midwifery (MS, Advanced Certificate); nursing administration (MS, Advanced Certificate); nursing education (MS, Advanced Certificate); nursing informatics (MS, Advanced Certificate); MS/MPA; MS/MPH. *Accreditation:* AACN; ACNM/ACME. Part-time programs available. *Faculty:* 22 full-time (all women), 54 part-time/adjunct (46 women). *Students:* 36 full-time (31 women), 622 part-time (549 women); includes 239 minority (73 Black or African American, non-Hispanic/Latino; 1 American Indian or Alaska Native, non-Hispanic/Latino; 116 Asian, non-Hispanic/Latino; 36 Hispanic/Latino; 6 Native Hawaiian or other Pacific Islander, non-Hispanic/Latino; 7 Two or more races, non-Hispanic/Latino), 16 international. Average age 37. 395 applicants, 67% accepted, 156 enrolled. In 2013, 186 master's, 8 other advanced degrees awarded. *Degree requirements:* For master's, thesis (for some programs). *Entrance requirements:* For master's, BS in nursing, AS in nursing with another BS/BA, interview, RN license, 1 year of clinical experience (3 for nursing education program); for Advanced Certificate, master's degree. Additional exam requirements/recommendations for international students: Required—TOEFL (minimum score 90 iBT), IELTS (minimum score 7). *Application deadline:* For fall admission, 7/1 for domestic and international students; for spring admission, 12/1 for domestic and international students. Application fee: $80. Electronic applications accepted. *Expenses: Tuition:* Full-time $35,856; part-time $1494 per unit. *Required fees:* $1408; $64 per unit. $473 per term. Tuition and fees vary according to course load and program. *Financial support:* In 2013–14, 182 students received support. Research assistantships, career-related internships or fieldwork, Federal Work-Study, scholarships/grants, traineeships, and unspecified assistantships available. Support available to part-time students. Financial award application deadline: 2/1; financial award applicants required to submit FAFSA. *Faculty research:* Geriatrics, HIV, elderly black diabetics, families and illness, oral systemic connection. *Unit head:* Dr. Judith Haber, Associate Dean, Graduate Programs, 212-998-9020, Fax: 212-995-3143, E-mail: jh33@nyu.edu. *Application contact:* Elizabeth Ensweiler, Assistant Director, Graduate Student Affairs and Admissions, 212-992-7653, Fax: 212-995-4302, E-mail: ee39@nyu.edu.

Oakland University, Graduate Study and Lifelong Learning, School of Nursing, Adult Gerontological Nurse Practitioner Program, Rochester, MI 48309-4401. Offers MSN, Certificate. *Students:* 14 full-time (all women), 30 part-time (26 women); includes 6 minority (3 Black or African American, non-Hispanic/Latino; 1 Asian, non-Hispanic/Latino; 1 Hispanic/Latino; 1 Two or more races, non-Hispanic/Latino), 2 international. Average age 43. 46 applicants, 24% accepted, 11 enrolled. In 2013, 3 master's, 1 other advanced degree awarded. Application fee: $0. *Unit head:* Dr. Linda Thompson, Dean, 248-370-4081, Fax: 248-370-4279. *Application contact:* Mary Bray, Graduate Program Coordinator, 248-370-4482.

Oregon Health & Science University, School of Nursing, Program in Gerontological Nursing, Portland, OR 97239-3098. Offers Post Master's Certificate. *Accreditation:* AACN. *Entrance requirements:* For degree, master's or associate's degree in nursing.

Point Loma Nazarene University, School of Nursing, San Diego, CA 92106-2899. Offers adult/gerontology nursing (MSN); family/individual health (MSN); general nursing (MSN); nursing (Post-MSN Certificate); pediatric nursing (MSN); psychiatric mental health (MSN). *Accreditation:* AACN. Part-time programs available. *Faculty:* 9 full-time (8 women). *Students:* 1 (woman) full-time, 82 part-time (70 women); includes 43 minority (9 Black or African American, non-Hispanic/Latino; 1 American Indian or Alaska Native, non-Hispanic/Latino; 26 Asian, non-Hispanic/Latino; 3 Hispanic/Latino; 3 Native Hawaiian or other Pacific Islander, non-Hispanic/Latino; 1 Two or more races, non-Hispanic/Latino). Average age 36. 32 applicants, 94% accepted, 24 enrolled. In 2013, 26 master's awarded. *Entrance requirements:* For master's, NCLEX, ADN or BSN in nursing, interview, RN license, essay, letters of recommendation, interview. *Application deadline:* For fall admission, 7/18 priority date for domestic students; for spring admission, 10/26 priority date for domestic students; for summer admission, 3/23 priority date for domestic students. Applications are processed on a rolling basis. Application fee: $50. *Expenses: Tuition:* Full-time $6900; part-time $567 per credit hour. *Financial support:* Applicants required to submit FAFSA. *Unit head:* Dr. Barb Taylor, Dean of the School of Nursing, 619-849-2766, E-mail: bataylor@pointloma.edu. *Application contact:* Laura Leinweber, Director of Graduate Admissions, 866-692-4723, E-mail: lauraleinweber@pointloma.edu.
Website: http://www.pointloma.edu/discover/graduate-school/graduate-programs/master-science-nursing-and-post-msn-certification

Research College of Nursing, Nursing Program, Kansas City, MO 64132. Offers adult-gerontological nurse practitioner (MSN); clinical nurse leader (MSN); executive practice and healthcare leadership (MSN); family nurse practitioner (MSN); nurse educator (MSN); nursing (MSN). *Accreditation:* AACN. Part-time programs available. Postbaccalaureate distance learning degree programs offered (no on-campus study). *Faculty:* 9 full-time (all women), 5 part-time/adjunct (2 women). *Students:* 19 full-time (18 women), 101 part-time (94 women). *Degree requirements:* For master's, research project. *Entrance requirements:* For master's, 3 letters of recommendation, official transcripts, resume. Additional exam requirements/recommendations for international students: Required—TOEFL (minimum score 550 paper-based), TWE. *Application deadline:* Applications are processed on a rolling basis. Application fee: $50. *Expenses: Tuition:* Part-time $445 per credit hour. *Required fees:* $25 per credit hour. Part-time tuition and fees vary according to course load. *Financial support:* Applicants required to submit FAFSA. *Unit head:* Dr. Nancy O. DeBasio, President and Dean, 816-995-2815, Fax: 816-995-2817, E-mail: nancy.debasio@researchcollege.edu. *Application contact:* Leslie Mendenhall, Director of Transfer and Graduate Recruitment, 816-995-2820, Fax: 816-995-2813, E-mail: leslie.mendenhall@researchcollege.edu.

Rush University, College of Nursing, Department of Adult Health and Gerontological Nursing, Chicago, IL 60612. Offers adult gerontology acute care clinical nurse specialist (DNP); adult gerontology acute care nurse practitioner (DNP); adult gerontology primary care clinical nurse specialist (DNP); adult gerontology primary care nurse practitioner (DNP); nurse anesthesia (DNP); nursing science (PhD); systems leadership (DNP). *Accreditation:* AACN; AANA/CANAEP (one or more programs are accredited). Part-time programs available. Postbaccalaureate distance learning degree programs offered (minimal on-campus study). *Students:* 89 full-time (69 women), 109 part-time (100 women); includes 40 minority (11 Black or African American, non-Hispanic/Latino; 1 American Indian or Alaska Native, non-Hispanic/Latino; 22 Asian, non-Hispanic/Latino; 5 Hispanic/Latino; 1 Native Hawaiian or other Pacific Islander, non-Hispanic/Latino). Average age 33. 170 applicants, 56% accepted, 78 enrolled. *Degree requirements:* For doctorate, capstone project (for DNP); dissertation (for PhD). *Entrance requirements:* For doctorate, GRE General Test (for DNP in nurse anesthesia; waived if cumulative GPA is 3.25 or greater, nursing GPA is 3.0 or greater, or a completed graduate program GPA is 3.5 or greater), interview, 3 letters of recommendation, personal statement, current resume. Additional exam requirements/recommendations for international students: Required—TOEFL. *Application deadline:* For fall admission, 1/2 for domestic students; for winter admission, 10/15 for domestic students; for spring admission, 8/1 for domestic students; for summer admission, 12/1 for domestic students. Applications are processed on a rolling basis. Application fee: $100. Electronic applications accepted. *Financial support:* Fellowships, research assistantships, teaching assistantships, Federal Work-Study, institutionally sponsored loans, scholarships/grants, traineeships, and health care benefits available. Support available to part-time students. Financial award application deadline: 3/1; financial award applicants required to submit FAFSA. *Faculty research:* Physical activity adherence in African-American women; reduction of health disparities; evidence-based interventions for caregivers; fish oil for HIV-related immunosenescence; BAILA: Being Active, Increasing Latinos Health Aging. *Total annual research expenditures:* $3.8 million. *Unit head:* Dr. Elizabeth Carlson, Chairperson, 312-942-7117, E-mail: elizabeth_carlson@rush.edu. *Application contact:* Jennifer Thorndyke, Admissions Specialist, 312-563-7526, E-mail: jennifer_thorndyke@rush.edu.
Website: http://www.rushu.rush.edu/servlet/Satellite?c=RushUnivLevel1Page&cid=1204497838852&pagename=Rush%2FRushUnivLevel1Page%2FLevel_1_College_Home_Page

Sage Graduate School, School of Health Sciences, Department of Nursing, Troy, NY 12180-4115. Offers adult geriatric advanced nursing (MS); adult gerontology nurse practitioner (MS); adult health (MS); adult nurse practitioner (MS, Post Master's Certificate); clinical nurse leader/specialist (Post Master's Certificate); community health (MS); counseling for nursing (Postbaccalaureate Certificate); education and leadership (DNS); family nurse practitioner (MS, Post Master's Certificate); gerontological nurse practitioner (Post Master's Certificate); nurse administrator/executive (Post Master's Certificate); nurse education (Post Master's Certificate); nursing (Post Master's Certificate); psychiatric mental health nurse clinical nurse specialist (MS); psychiatric mental health nurse practitioner (MS, Post Master's Certificate), including psychiatric mental health. *Accreditation:* AACN. Part-time and evening/weekend programs available. *Faculty:* 5 full-time (all women), 10 part-time/adjunct (all women). *Students:* 32 full-time (30 women), 174 part-time (161 women); includes 28 minority (12 Black or African American, non-Hispanic/Latino; 2 American Indian or Alaska Native, non-Hispanic/Latino; 8 Asian, non-Hispanic/Latino; 4 Hispanic/Latino; 2 Two or more races, non-Hispanic/Latino), 3 international. Average age 40. 171 applicants, 43% accepted, 35 enrolled. In 2013, 53 master's, 5 doctorates, 11 other advanced degrees awarded. *Degree requirements:* For master's, thesis or alternative. *Entrance requirements:* For master's, BS in nursing, minimum GPA of 2.75, resume, 2 letters of recommendation. Additional exam requirements/recommendations for international students: Required—TOEFL (minimum score 550 paper-based). *Application deadline:* Applications are processed on a rolling basis. Application fee: $40. *Expenses: Tuition:* Full-time $11,880; part-time $660 per credit hour. *Financial support:* Fellowships, research assistantships, Federal Work-Study, scholarships/grants, and unspecified assistantships available. Support available to part-time students. Financial award application deadline: 3/1; financial award applicants required to submit FAFSA. *Unit head:* Dr. Esther Haskevitz, Dean, School of Health Sciences, 518-244-2296, Fax: 518-244-4571, E-mail: haskve@sage.edu. *Application contact:* Dr. Glenda Kelman, Director, 518-244-2001, Fax: 518-244-2009, E-mail: kelmag@sage.edu.

St. Catherine University, Graduate Programs, Program in Nursing, St. Paul, MN 55105. Offers adult gerontological nurse practitioner (MA); neonatal nurse practitioner (MA); nurse educator (MA); nursing (DNP); nursing: entry-level (MA); pediatric nurse practitioner (MA). Part-time and evening/weekend programs available. *Degree requirements:* For master's, thesis; for doctorate, portfolio, systems change project. *Entrance requirements:* For master's, GRE General Test, bachelor's degree in nursing, current nursing license, 2 years of recent clinical practice; for doctorate, master's degree in nursing, RN license, advanced nursing position. Additional exam requirements/recommendations for international students: Required—TOEFL (minimum score 600 paper-based; 100 iBT).

Saint Francis Medical Center College of Nursing, Graduate Programs, Peoria, IL 61603-3783. Offers adult gerontology (MSN); clinical nurse leader (MSN); family nurse practitioner (MSN); family psychiatric mental health nurse practitioner (MSN); neonatal nurse practitioner (MSN); nurse clinician (Post-Graduate Certificate); nurse educator (MSN, Post-Graduate Certificate); nursing (DNP); nursing management leadership (MSN). Part-time programs available. Postbaccalaureate distance learning degree programs offered (minimal on-campus study). *Faculty:* 4 full-time (all women), 4 part-time/adjunct (all women). *Students:* 13 full-time (12 women), 268 part-time (245 women); includes 17 minority (10 Black or African American, non-Hispanic/Latino; 2 Asian, non-Hispanic/Latino; 5 Hispanic/Latino), 2 international. Average age 37. 115 applicants, 89% accepted, 42 enrolled. In 2013, 17 master's, 2 doctorates awarded. *Degree requirements:* For master's, research experience, portfolio, practicum; for doctorate, practicum hours. *Entrance requirements:* For master's, nursing research, health assessment, graduate course work in statistics, RN license; for doctorate, master's degree in nursing, professional portfolio, graduate statistics, transcripts, RN license. Additional exam requirements/recommendations for international students: Required—TOEFL. *Application deadline:* For fall admission, 6/1 priority date for domestic and international students; for spring admission, 11/15 priority date for domestic and international students. Applications are processed on a rolling basis. Application fee: $50. Electronic applications accepted. *Expenses: Tuition:* Full-time $6336; part-time $528 per semester hour. *Required fees:* $436. *Financial support:* In 2013–14, 8 students received support. Scholarships/grants and tuition waivers (partial) available. Support available to part-time students. Financial award application deadline: 6/15; financial award applicants required to submit FAFSA. *Faculty research:* Outcome and curriculum planning, health promotion, NCLEX-RN results, decision-making program evaluation. *Unit head:* Dr. Patti A. Stockert, President of the College, 309-655-4124, Fax: 309-624-8973, E-mail: patricia.a.stockert@osfhealthcare.org. *Application contact:* Dr. Janice F. Boundy, Dean, 309-655-2230, Fax: 309-624-8973, E-mail: jan.f.boundy@osfhealthcare.org.
Website: http://www.sfmccon.edu/graduate-programs/

Salem State University, School of Graduate Studies, Program in Nursing, Salem, MA 01970-5353. Offers adult-gerontology primary care nursing (MSN); nursing administration (MSN); nursing education (MSN); MBA/MSN. *Accreditation:* AACN. Part-time and evening/weekend programs available. *Students:* 31 full-time (24 women), 79 part-time (70 women); includes 12 minority (4 Black or African American, non-Hispanic/Latino; 4 Asian, non-Hispanic/Latino; 3 Hispanic/Latino; 1 Native Hawaiian or other Pacific Islander, non-Hispanic/Latino), 5 international. 18 applicants, 94% accepted, 16 enrolled. In 2013, 15 master's awarded. *Entrance requirements:* For master's, GRE or MAT. Additional exam requirements/recommendations for international students: Required—TOEFL (minimum score 550 paper-based; 80 iBT) or IELTS (minimum score 5.5). *Application deadline:* For fall admission, 5/1 for domestic students; for spring admission, 10/1 for domestic students. Applications are processed on a rolling basis. Application fee: $50. *Financial support:* Career-related internships or fieldwork, Federal Work-Study, scholarships/grants, and unspecified assistantships available. Support available to part-time students. Financial award application deadline: 5/1; financial award applicants required to submit FAFSA. *Application contact:* Dr. Lee A. Brossoit, Assistant Dean of Graduate Admissions, 978-542-6675, Fax: 978-542-7215, E-mail: lbrossoit@salemstate.edu.
Website: http://www.salemstate.edu/academics/schools/1819.php

San Jose State University, Graduate Studies and Research, College of Applied Sciences and Arts, School of Nursing, San Jose, CA 95192-0001. Offers gerontology nurse practitioner (MS); nursing (Certificate); nursing administration (MS); nursing education (MS). *Accreditation:* AACN. Part-time and evening/weekend programs available. *Degree requirements:* For master's, thesis. *Entrance requirements:* For master's, BS in nursing, RN license. Electronic applications accepted. *Faculty research:* Nurse-managed clinics, computers in nursing.

Seattle Pacific University, MS in Nursing Program, Seattle, WA 98119-1997. Offers administration (MSN); adult/gerontology nurse practitioner (MSN); clinical nurse specialist (MSN); family nurse practitioner (MSN, Certificate); informatics (MSN); nurse educator (MSN). *Accreditation:* AACN. Part-time programs available. *Students:* 9 full-time (7 women), 37 part-time (33 women); includes 8 minority (2 Black or African American, non-Hispanic/Latino; 5 Asian, non-Hispanic/Latino; 1 Hispanic/Latino), 1 international. Average age 41. 70 applicants, 30% accepted, 21 enrolled. In 2013, 27 master's awarded. *Degree requirements:* For master's, thesis. *Entrance requirements:* For master's, personal statement, transcripts, undergraduate nursing degree, proof of undergraduate statistics course with minimum GPA of 2.0, 2 recommendations. *Application deadline:* For fall admission, 1/15 priority date for domestic students; for spring admission, 1/15 for domestic students. Applications are processed on a rolling basis. Application fee: $50. Electronic applications accepted. *Expenses:* Contact institution. *Financial support:* Fellowships and scholarships/grants available. Financial award applicants required to submit FAFSA. *Unit head:* Dr. Susan Casey, Associate Dean, 206-281-2649, E-mail: caseys@spu.edu.
Website: http://www.spu.edu/depts/health-sciences/grad/index.asp

Seattle University, College of Nursing, Program in Advanced Practice Nursing Immersion, Seattle, WA 98122-1090. Offers adult/gerontological nurse practitioner (MSN); advanced community public health nursing (MSN); family nurse practitioner (MSN); family psychiatric mental health nurse practitioner (MSN); nurse midwifery (MSN). *Faculty:* 17 full-time (15 women), 9 part-time/adjunct (6 women). *Students:* 109 full-time (94 women), 6 part-time (5 women); includes 25 minority (3 Black or African American, non-Hispanic/Latino; 11 Asian, non-Hispanic/Latino; 2 Hispanic/Latino; 9 Two or more races, non-Hispanic/Latino). Average age 31. In 2013, 48 master's awarded. *Degree requirements:* For master's, thesis or scholarly project. *Entrance requirements:* For master's, GRE, bachelor's degree, minimum GPA of 3.0, professional resume, two recommendations, letter of intent. Additional exam requirements/recommendations for international students: Required—TOEFL (minimum score 92 iBT), IELTS. *Application deadline:* For fall admission, 12/1 for domestic and international students. Application fee: $55. Electronic applications accepted. *Financial support:* In 2013–14, 3 students received support. Scholarships/grants and traineeships available. Financial award applicants required to submit FAFSA. *Unit head:* Dr. Janiece DeSocio, Interim Dean, 206-296-5660, E-mail: desocioj@seattleu.edu. *Application contact:* Janet Shandley, Associate Dean of Graduate Admissions, 206-296-5900, Fax: 206-298-5656, E-mail: grad_admissions@seattleu.edu.
Website: http://www.seattleu.edu/nursing/msn/apni/

Seattle University, College of Nursing, Program in Nursing, Seattle, WA 98122-1090. Offers adult/gerontological nurse practitioner (MSN); advanced community public health (MSN); psychiatric mental health nurse practitioner (MSN). *Students:* 11 full-time (10 women), 4 part-time (all women); includes 2 minority (both Hispanic/Latino). Average age 36. 39 applicants, 36% accepted, 8 enrolled. In 2013, 7 master's awarded. *Degree requirements:* For master's, thesis or scholarly project. *Entrance requirements:* For master's, GRE, bachelor's degree in nursing or associate degree in nursing with baccalaureate in different major, 5-quarter statistics course, minimum cumulative GPA of 3.0, professional resume, two recommendations, letter of intent, copy of current RN license or ability to obtain RN license in WA state. Additional exam requirements/recommendations for international students: Required—TOEFL (minimum score 92 iBT), IELTS. *Application deadline:* For fall admission, 12/1 for domestic and international students. Application fee: $55. Electronic applications accepted. *Financial support:* In 2013–14, 1 student received support, including 2 teaching assistantships; scholarships/grants and traineeships also available. Financial award applicants required to submit FAFSA. *Unit head:* Dr. Azita Emami, Dean, 206-296-5660. *Application contact:* Janet Shandley, Associate Dean of Graduate Admissions, 206-296-5900, Fax: 206-298-5656, E-mail: grad_admissions@seattleu.edu.
Website: https://www.seattleu.edu/nursing/msn/

Seton Hall University, College of Nursing, South Orange, NJ 07079-2697. Offers advanced practice in primary health care (MSN, DNP), including adult/gerontological nurse practitioner, pediatric nurse practitioner; entry into practice (MSN); health systems administration (MSN, DNP); nursing (PhD); nursing case management (MSN); nursing education (MA); school nurse (MSN); MSN/MA. *Accreditation:* AACN. Part-time programs available. Postbaccalaureate distance learning degree programs offered (minimal on-campus study). *Degree requirements:* For master's, research project; for doctorate, dissertation or scholarly project. *Entrance requirements:* For doctorate, GRE (waived for students with GPA of 3.5 or higher). Additional exam requirements/recommendations for international students: Required—TOEFL. Electronic applications accepted. *Faculty research:* Parent/child, adult, and gerontological nursing; breast cancer; families of children with HIV; parish nursing.

Southern University and Agricultural and Mechanical College, School of Nursing, Baton Rouge, LA 70813. Offers educator/administrator (PhD); family health nursing (MSN); family nurse practitioner (Post Master's Certificate); geriatric nurse practitioner/gerontology (PhD). *Accreditation:* AACN. Part-time programs available. *Degree requirements:* For master's, comprehensive exam, thesis; for doctorate, comprehensive exam, thesis/dissertation. *Entrance requirements:* For master's, GRE General Test, BSN, minimum GPA of 2.7; for doctorate, GRE General Test; for Post Master's Certificate, MSN. Additional exam requirements/recommendations for international students: Required—TOEFL (minimum score 525 paper-based). *Faculty research:* Health promotions, vulnerable populations, (community-based) cardiovascular participating research, health disparities chronic diseases, care of the elderly.

Texas Christian University, Harris College of Nursing and Health Sciences, Program in Nursing, Fort Worth, TX 76129-0002. Offers advanced practice registered nurse (DNP); clinical nurse leader (MSN); clinical nurse specialist: adult/gerontology nursing (MSN); clinical nurse specialist: pediatric nursing (MSN); nursing administration (DNP); nursing education (MSN). *Accreditation:* AACN; AANA/CANAEP (one or more programs are accredited). Part-time programs available. Postbaccalaureate distance learning degree programs offered (no on-campus study). *Faculty:* 18 full-time (16 women), 1 (woman) part-time/adjunct. *Students:* 44 full-time (35 women), 46 part-time (42 women); includes 8 minority (3 Black or African American, non-Hispanic/Latino; 2 Asian, non-Hispanic/Latino; 3 Hispanic/Latino), 1 international. Average age 43. 72 applicants, 63% accepted, 36 enrolled. In 2013, 19 master's, 17 doctorates awarded. *Degree requirements:* For master's, professional project; for doctorate, capstone project. *Entrance requirements:* For master's, GRE General Test, 3 letters of reference, essay, resume, two official transcripts from every institution attended; for doctorate, APRN recognition (national certification) or master's and experience in nursing administration; 3 letters of reference; essay; resume; two official transcripts from every institution attended. Additional exam requirements/recommendations for international students: Recommended—TOEFL. *Application deadline:* For fall admission, 4/1 for domestic students; for spring admission, 9/1 for domestic students; for summer admission, 2/1 for domestic students. Applications are processed on a rolling basis. Application fee: $60. Electronic applications accepted. *Expenses: Tuition:* Part-time $1270 per credit hour. Tuition and fees vary according to course load and program. *Financial support:* In 2013–14, 4 teaching assistantships (averaging $2,500 per year) were awarded. Financial award applicants required to submit FAFSA. *Unit head:* Dr. Kathy A. Baker, Director, Division of Nursing Graduate Studies and Scholarship, 817-257-6726, Fax: 817-257-8383, E-mail: kathy.baker@tcu.edu. *Application contact:* Mary Jane Allred, Administrative Program Specialist, 817-257-6726, Fax: 817-257-8383, E-mail: m.allred@tcu.edu.
Website: http://www.nursing.tcu.edu/graduate.asp

Texas Tech University Health Sciences Center, School of Nursing, Lubbock, TX 79430. Offers acute care nurse practitioner (MSN, Certificate); administration (MSN); advanced practice (DNP); education (MSN); executive leadership (DNP); family nurse practitioner (MSN, Certificate); geriatric nurse practitioner (MSN, Certificate); pediatric nurse practitioner (MSN, Certificate). *Accreditation:* AACN. Part-time programs available. Postbaccalaureate distance learning degree programs offered (minimal on-campus study). *Degree requirements:* For master's, thesis optional. *Entrance requirements:* For master's, minimum GPA of 3.0, 3 letters of reference, BSN, RN license; for Certificate, minimum GPA of 3.0, 3 letters of reference, RN license. Additional exam requirements/recommendations for international students: Required—TOEFL (minimum score 550 paper-based). *Faculty research:* Diabetes/obesity, nurse competency, disease management, intervention and measurements, health disparities.

University at Buffalo, the State University of New York, Graduate School, School of Nursing, Buffalo, NY 14214. Offers adult gerontology nurse practitioner (DNP); family nurse practitioner (DNP); health care systems and leadership (MS); nurse anesthetist (DNP); nursing (PhD); nursing education (Certificate); psychiatric/mental health nurse practitioner (DNP). *Accreditation:* AACN; AANA/CANAEP (one or more programs are accredited). Part-time programs available. Postbaccalaureate distance learning degree programs offered (no on-campus study). *Faculty:* 24 full-time (21 women), 2 part-time/adjunct (1 woman). *Students:* 80 full-time (60 women), 97 part-time (84 women); includes 35 minority (20 Black or African American, non-Hispanic/Latino; 2 American Indian or Alaska Native, non-Hispanic/Latino; 9 Asian, non-Hispanic/Latino; 1 Hispanic/Latino; 3 Native Hawaiian or other Pacific Islander, non-Hispanic/Latino). 118 applicants, 67% accepted, 58 enrolled. In 2013, 41 master's, 15 doctorates awarded. *Degree requirements:* For master's, thesis optional; for doctorate, comprehensive exam (for some programs), capstone (for DNP), dissertation (for PhD). *Entrance requirements:* For doctorate, GRE or MAT, minimum GPA of 3.0 (3.25 for PhD), RN license, BS or MS in nursing, 3 references, writing sample; for Certificate, interview, minimum GPA of 3.0 or GRE General Test, RN license, MS in nursing. Additional exam requirements/recommendations for international students: Required—TOEFL (minimum score 550 paper-based; 79 iBT), IELTS (minimum score 6.5). *Application deadline:* For fall admission, 7/1 for domestic students, 4/1 for international students; for spring admission, 12/1 for domestic students, 10/1 for international students; for summer admission, 4/1 for domestic students. Application fee: $75. Electronic applications accepted. *Financial support:* In 2013–14, 80 students received support, including 2 fellowships with full and partial tuition reimbursements available (averaging $17,000 per year), 7 research assistantships with full and partial tuition reimbursements available (averaging $10,600 per year), 7 teaching assistantships with full and partial tuition reimbursements available (averaging $10,600 per year); scholarships/grants, traineeships, health care benefits, and unspecified assistantships also available. Financial award application deadline: 3/15; financial award applicants required to submit FAFSA. *Faculty research:* Oncology, palliative care, gerontology, addictions, mental

health, community wellness, sleep, workforce, care of underserved populations, quality and safety, person-centered care, adolescent health. *Total annual research expenditures:* $1.1 million. *Unit head:* Dr. Marsha L. Lewis, Dean and Professor, 716-829-2533, Fax: 716-829-2566, E-mail: ubnursingdean@buffalo.edu. *Application contact:* Dr. David J. Lang, Director of Student Affairs, 716-829-2537, Fax: 716-829-2067, E-mail: nursing@buffalo.edu.
Website: http://nursing.buffalo.edu/

University of Central Florida, College of Nursing, Orlando, FL 32816. Offers adult-gerontology nurse practitioner (Post-Master's Certificate); family nurse practitioner (Post-Master's Certificate); nursing (MSN, PhD); nursing education (Post-Master's Certificate); nursing practice (DNP). *Accreditation:* AACN. Part-time and evening/weekend programs available. *Faculty:* 47 full-time (41 women), 78 part-time/adjunct (75 women). *Students:* 54 full-time (49 women), 264 part-time (239 women); includes 72 minority (35 Black or African American, non-Hispanic/Latino; 7 Asian, non-Hispanic/Latino; 25 Hispanic/Latino; 1 Native Hawaiian or other Pacific Islander, non-Hispanic/Latino; 4 Two or more races, non-Hispanic/Latino), 1 international. Average age 39. 179 applicants, 55% accepted, 71 enrolled. In 2013, 96 master's, 12 doctorates, 3 other advanced degrees awarded. *Degree requirements:* For master's, thesis or alternative. *Entrance requirements:* For master's, GRE General Test, minimum GPA of 3.0 in last 60 hours. Additional exam requirements/recommendations for international students: Required—TOEFL. *Application deadline:* For fall admission, 2/15 for domestic students; for spring admission, 9/15 for domestic students. Application fee: $30. Electronic applications accepted. *Financial support:* In 2013–14, 2 students received support, including 3 teaching assistantships with partial tuition reimbursements available (averaging $6,300 per year); fellowships with partial tuition reimbursements available, research assistantships with partial tuition reimbursements available, career-related internships or fieldwork, Federal Work-Study, institutionally sponsored loans, traineeships, and unspecified assistantships also available. Financial award application deadline: 3/1; financial award applicants required to submit FAFSA. *Unit head:* Dr. Mary Lou Sole, Interim Dean, 407-823-5496, Fax: 407-823-5675, E-mail: mary.sole@ucf.edu. *Application contact:* Barbara Rodriguez Lamas, Director, Admissions and Student Services, 407-823-2766, Fax: 407-823-6442, E-mail: gradadmissions@ucf.edu.
Website: http://nursing.ucf.edu/

University of Colorado Colorado Springs, Beth-El College of Nursing and Health Sciences, Colorado Springs, CO 80933-7150. Offers nursing education (MSN); nursing practice (DNP); primary care nurse practitioner (MSN). *Accreditation:* AACN. Part-time programs available. Postbaccalaureate distance learning degree programs offered (minimal on-campus study). *Faculty:* 5 full-time (all women), 1 part-time/adjunct (0 women). *Students:* 14 full-time (13 women), 160 part-time (149 women); includes 32 minority (2 Black or African American, non-Hispanic/Latino; 2 American Indian or Alaska Native, non-Hispanic/Latino; 5 Asian, non-Hispanic/Latino; 21 Hispanic/Latino; 2 Two or more races, non-Hispanic/Latino). Average age 37. 125 applicants, 38% accepted, 42 enrolled. In 2013, 31 master's, 3 doctorates awarded. *Degree requirements:* For master's, comprehensive exam, thesis optional; for doctorate, capstone project. *Entrance requirements:* For master's, GRE General Test or MAT, BSN, minimum GPA of 3.0, unrestricted RN license; for doctorate, interview; active RN license; MA; minimum GPA of 3.3; National Certification as nurse practitioner or clinical nurse specialist; portfolio. Additional exam requirements/recommendations for international students: Required—TOEFL. *Application deadline:* For fall admission, 6/15 priority date for domestic students, 6/15 for international students; for spring admission, 9/15 for domestic and international students. Application fee: $60 ($75 for international students). Electronic applications accepted. *Expenses:* Contact institution. *Financial support:* In 2013–14, 17 students received support, including 17 fellowships (averaging $2,500 per year); career-related internships or fieldwork, Federal Work-Study, and scholarships/grants also available. Support available to part-time students. Financial award application deadline: 3/1; financial award applicants required to submit FAFSA. *Faculty research:* Women's health, uncertainty, empowerment, family experience in chronic illness. *Total annual research expenditures:* $2,568. *Unit head:* Dr. Amy Silva-Smith, Graduate Department Chairperson, 719-255-4490, Fax: 719-255-4416, E-mail: asilvasm@uccs.edu. *Application contact:* Diane Busch, Director, 719-255-4424, Fax: 719-255-4416, E-mail: dbusch@uccs.edu.
Website: http://www.uccs.edu/~bethel/

University of Delaware, College of Health Sciences, School of Nursing, Newark, DE 19716. Offers adult nurse practitioner (MSN, PMC); cardiopulmonary clinical nurse specialist (MSN, PMC); cardiopulmonary clinical nurse specialist/adult nurse practitioner (MSN, PMC); family nurse practitioner (MSN, PMC); gerontology clinical nurse specialist (MSN, PMC); gerontology clinical nurse specialist geriatric nurse practitioner (PMC); gerontology clinical nurse specialist/geriatric nurse practitioner (MSN); health services administration (MSN, PMC); nursing of children clinical nurse specialist (MSN, PMC); nursing of children clinical nurse specialist/pediatric nurse practitioner (MSN, PMC); oncology/immune deficiency clinical nurse specialist (MSN, PMC); oncology/immune deficiency clinical nurse specialist/adult nurse practitioner (MSN, PMC); perinatal/women's health clinical nurse specialist (MSN, PMC); perinatal/women's health clinical nurse specialist/women's health nurse practitioner (MSN, PMC); psychiatric nursing clinical nurse specialist (MSN, PMC). *Accreditation:* AACN. Part-time and evening/weekend programs available. Postbaccalaureate distance learning degree programs offered (minimal on-campus study). *Degree requirements:* For master's, thesis optional. *Entrance requirements:* For master's, BSN, interview, RN license. Electronic applications accepted. *Faculty research:* Marriage and chronic illness, health promotion, congestive heart failure patient outcomes, school nursing, diabetes in children, culture, health disparities, cardiovascular, prison nursing, oncology, public policy, child obesity, smoking and teen pregnancy, blood pressure measurements, men's health.

University of Illinois at Chicago, Graduate College, College of Nursing, Program in Nursing, Chicago, IL 60607-7128. Offers acute care clinical nurse specialist (MS); acute care nurse practitioner (MS); administrative nursing leadership (Certificate); administrative studies in nursing (MS); adult nurse practitioner (MS); adult/geriatric nurse practitioner (MS); advanced community health nurse specialist (MS); family nurse practitioner (MS); geriatric clinical nurse specialist (MS); geriatric nurse practitioner (MS); mental health clinical nurse specialist (MS); mental health nurse practitioner (MS); nurse midwifery (MS); occupational health/advanced community health nurse specialist (MS); occupational health/family nurse practitioner (MS); pediatric clinical nurse specialist (MS); pediatric nurse practitioner (MS); perinatal clinical nurse specialist (MS); school/advanced community health nurse specialist (MS); school/family nurse practitioner (MS); women's health nurse practitioner (MS). *Accreditation:* AACN. Part-time programs available. *Faculty:* 16 full-time (14 women). *Students:* 393 full-time (361 women), 410 part-time (367 women); includes 198 minority (48 Black or African American, non-Hispanic/Latino; 1 American Indian or Alaska Native, non-Hispanic/Latino; 64 Asian, non-Hispanic/Latino; 71 Hispanic/Latino; 2 Native Hawaiian or other Pacific Islander, non-Hispanic/Latino; 12 Two or more races, non-Hispanic/Latino), 29 international. Average age 32. 396 applicants, 62% accepted, 177 enrolled. In 2013, 184 master's awarded. *Degree requirements:* For master's, thesis or alternative. *Entrance requirements:* For master's, GRE General Test, minimum GPA of 2.75. Additional exam requirements/recommendations for international students: Required—TOEFL. *Application deadline:* For fall admission, 5/15 for domestic students, 2/15 for international students; for spring admission, 11/1 for domestic students, 7/15 for international students. Applications are processed on a rolling basis. Application fee: $40 ($50 for international students). Electronic applications accepted. *Expenses:* Tuition, state resident: full-time $11,066; part-time $3689 per term. Tuition, nonresident: full-time $23,064; part-time $7688 per term. *Required fees:* $3004; $1190 per term. Tuition and fees vary according to course level and program. *Financial support:* Fellowships with full tuition reimbursements, research assistantships with full tuition reimbursements, teaching assistantships with full tuition reimbursements, career-related internships or fieldwork, Federal Work-Study, institutionally sponsored loans, scholarships/grants, traineeships, tuition waivers (full and partial), and unspecified assistantships available. Support available to part-time students. Financial award application deadline: 3/1; financial award applicants required to submit FAFSA. *Unit head:* Dr. Terri E. Weaver, Dean, 312-996-7808, E-mail: teweaver@uic.edu. *Application contact:* Receptionist, 312-413-2550, E-mail: gradcoll@uic.edu.

The University of Kansas, University of Kansas Medical Center, School of Nursing, Kansas City, KS 66160. Offers adult/gerontological clinical nurse specialist (PMC); adult/gerontological nurse practitioner (PMC); clinical research management (PMC); health care informatics (PMC); health professions educator (PMC); nurse midwife (PMC); nursing (MS, DNP, PhD); organizational leadership (PMC); psychiatric/mental health nurse practitioner (PMC); public health nursing (PMC). *Accreditation:* AACN; ACNM/ACME. Part-time programs available. Postbaccalaureate distance learning degree programs offered (minimal on-campus study). *Faculty:* 59. *Students:* 55 full-time (53 women), 323 part-time (303 women); includes 57 minority (23 Black or African American, non-Hispanic/Latino; 14 Asian, non-Hispanic/Latino; 16 Hispanic/Latino; 1 Native Hawaiian or other Pacific Islander, non-Hispanic/Latino; 3 Two or more races, non-Hispanic/Latino), 1 international. Average age 38. 113 applicants, 59% accepted, 61 enrolled. In 2013, 77 master's, 18 doctorates, 11 other advanced degrees awarded. Terminal master's awarded for partial completion of doctoral program. *Degree requirements:* For master's, comprehensive exam, thesis (for some programs), general oral exam; for doctorate, variable foreign language requirement, thesis/dissertation, comprehensive oral exam (for DNP); comprehensive written and oral exam (for PhD). *Entrance requirements:* For master's, bachelor's degree in nursing, minimum GPA of 3.0, 1 year of clinical experience, RN license in KS and MO; for doctorate, GRE General Test, bachelor's degree in nursing, minimum GPA of 3.5, RN license in KS and MO. Additional exam requirements/recommendations for international students: Required—TOEFL. *Application deadline:* For fall admission, 4/1 for domestic and international students; for spring admission, 9/1 for domestic and international students. Application fee: $60. Electronic applications accepted. *Financial support:* Research assistantships with full and partial tuition reimbursements, teaching assistantships with full and partial tuition reimbursements, scholarships/grants, and traineeships available. Financial award application deadline: 3/1; financial award applicants required to submit FAFSA. *Faculty research:* Breastfeeding practices of teen mothers, national database of nursing quality indicators, caregiving of families of patients using technology in the home, simulation in nursing education, diaphragm fatigue. *Total annual research expenditures:* $6.4 million. *Unit head:* Dr. Karen L. Miller, Dean, 913-588-1601, Fax: 913-588-1660, E-mail: kmiller@kumc.edu. *Application contact:* Dr. Pamela K. Barnes, Associate Dean, Student Affairs, 913-588-1619, Fax: 913-588-1615, E-mail: pbarnes2@kumc.edu.
Website: http://nursing.kumc.edu

University of Maryland, Baltimore, Graduate School, School of Nursing, Master's Program in Nursing, Baltimore, MD 21201. Offers community health nursing (MS); gerontological nursing (MS); maternal-child nursing (MS); medical-surgical nursing (MS); nurse-midwifery education (MS); nursing administration (MS); nursing education (MS); nursing health policy (MS); primary care nursing (MS); psychiatric nursing (MS); MS/MBA. MS/MBA offered jointly with University of Baltimore. *Accreditation:* AACN; AANA/CANAEP. Part-time programs available. *Students:* 345 full-time (297 women), 508 part-time (469 women); includes 288 minority (152 Black or African American, non-Hispanic/Latino; 2 American Indian or Alaska Native, non-Hispanic/Latino; 72 Asian, non-Hispanic/Latino; 32 Hispanic/Latino; 1 Native Hawaiian or other Pacific Islander, non-Hispanic/Latino; 29 Two or more races, non-Hispanic/Latino), 13 international. Average age 33. 971 applicants, 34% accepted, 253 enrolled. In 2013, 308 master's awarded. *Degree requirements:* For master's, comprehensive exam (for some programs), thesis or alternative. *Entrance requirements:* For master's, minimum GPA of 2.75, course work in statistics, BS in nursing. Additional exam requirements/recommendations for international students: Required—TOEFL (minimum score 550 paper-based; 80 iBT) or IELTS (minimum score 7). *Application deadline:* For fall admission, 2/1 for domestic students, 1/15 for international students. Application fee: $75. Electronic applications accepted. *Financial support:* Fellowships, research assistantships, teaching assistantships, career-related internships or fieldwork, and traineeships available. Support available to part-time students. Financial award application deadline: 2/15; financial award applicants required to submit FAFSA. *Unit head:* Dr. Jane Kapustin, Assistant Dean, 410-706-6741, Fax: 410-706-4231. *Application contact:* Marjorie Fass, Admissions Director, 410-706-0501, Fax: 410-706-7238.

University of Massachusetts Amherst, Graduate School, School of Nursing, Amherst, MA 01003. Offers adult gerontology primary care (DNP); clinical nurse leader (MS); family nurse practitioner (DNP); nursing (PhD); public health nurse leader (DNP). *Accreditation:* AACN. Part-time programs available. Postbaccalaureate distance learning degree programs offered (minimal on-campus study). *Faculty:* 16 full-time (15 women). *Students:* 74 full-time (61 women), 161 part-time (149 women); includes 62 minority (31 Black or African American, non-Hispanic/Latino; 9 Asian, non-Hispanic/Latino; 19 Hispanic/Latino; 3 Two or more races, non-Hispanic/Latino), 6 international. Average age 40. 133 applicants, 80% accepted, 68 enrolled. In 2013, 9 master's, 32 doctorates awarded. Terminal master's awarded for partial completion of doctoral program. *Degree requirements:* For master's, thesis optional; for doctorate, comprehensive exam, thesis/dissertation. *Entrance requirements:* Additional exam requirements/recommendations for international students: Required—TOEFL (minimum score 550 paper-based; 80 iBT), IELTS (minimum score 6.5). *Application deadline:* For fall admission, 12/15 for domestic and international students. Applications are processed on a rolling basis. Application fee: $75. Electronic applications accepted. *Financial support:* Fellowships with full and partial tuition reimbursements, research assistantships with full and partial tuition reimbursements, teaching assistantships with full and partial tuition reimbursements, career-related internships or fieldwork, Federal Work-Study, scholarships/grants, traineeships, health care benefits, tuition waivers (full and partial), and unspecified assistantships available. Support available to part-time students. Financial award application deadline: 2/1. *Faculty research:* Health of older adults and their caretakers, mental health of individuals and families, health of children and adolescents, power and decision-making, transcultural health. *Unit head:* Dr. Stephen J. Cavanagh, Dean, 413-545-2703, Fax: 413-577-2550, E-mail: dean@nursing.umass.edu. *Application contact:* Lindsay DeSantis, Supervisor of Admissions, 413-545-0722, Fax: 413-577-0010, E-mail: gradadm@grad.umass.edu.
Website: http://www.umass.edu/nursing/

University of Massachusetts Dartmouth, Graduate School, College of Nursing, Programs in Nursing, North Dartmouth, MA 02747-2300. Offers adult gerontology primary care nurse practitioner (DNP); adult health clinical nurse specialist (DNP); adult

health/adult nurse practitioner (MS); adult health/advanced practice (MS); adult health/nurse educator (MS); adult health/nurse manager (MS); adult nurse practitioner (PMC); community health nurse specialist (DNP); community nursing/advanced practice (MS); community nursing/nurse educator (MS); community nursing/nurse manager (MS); individualized nursing (PMC); nursing (MS, PhD); nursing practice (DNP). Part-time programs available. *Faculty:* 25 full-time (all women), 45 part-time/adjunct (44 women). *Students:* 103 part-time (95 women); includes 10 minority (4 Black or African American, non-Hispanic/Latino; 2 Asian, non-Hispanic/Latino; 4 Hispanic/Latino). Average age 40. 49 applicants, 92% accepted, 33 enrolled. In 2013, 25 master's, 1 doctorate, 2 other advanced degrees awarded. *Degree requirements:* For master's, thesis; for doctorate, comprehensive exam, thesis/dissertation, project (for DNP only). *Entrance requirements:* For master's, statement of purpose (minimum of 300 words), resume, 3 letters of recommendation, official transcripts, copy of RN license; for doctorate, GRE (for PhD), statement of purpose (minimum of 300 words), resume, 3 letters of recommendation, official transcripts, copy of RN license, scholarly writing sample (minimum 10 pages for PhD). Additional exam requirements/recommendations for international students: Required—TOEFL (minimum score 533 paper-based; 72 iBT). *Application deadline:* For fall admission, 2/15 priority date for domestic and international students. Applications are processed on a rolling basis. Application fee: $60. Electronic applications accepted. *Expenses:* Tuition, state resident: full-time $2071; part-time $86.29 per credit. Tuition, nonresident: full-time $8099; part-time $337.46 per credit. Tuition and fees vary according to course load and reciprocity agreements. *Financial support:* In 2013–14, 5 teaching assistantships with full and partial tuition reimbursements (averaging $7,500 per year) were awarded; Federal Work-Study and unspecified assistantships also available. Support available to part-time students. Financial award application deadline: 3/1; financial award applicants required to submit FAFSA. *Faculty research:* Pathophysiology, aging with spinal cord injury, relational ontology, severe mental illness, patient care. *Total annual research expenditures:* $1,000. *Unit head:* Kerry Fater, Graduate Program Director for Nursing Master's Programs, 508-999-8525, Fax: 508-999-9127, E-mail: kfater@umassd.edu. *Application contact:* Steven Briggs, Director of Marketing and Recruitment for Graduate Studies, 508-999-8604, Fax: 508-999-8183, E-mail: graduate@umassd.edu.
Website: http://www.umassd.edu/nursing/graduateprograms

University of Massachusetts Lowell, College of Health Sciences, School of Nursing, Program in Adult/Gerontological Nursing, Lowell, MA 01854-2881. Offers MS, Graduate Certificate. *Accreditation:* AACN. *Degree requirements:* For master's, thesis optional. *Entrance requirements:* For master's, GRE General Test, minimum GPA of 3.0, MA nursing license, interview, 3 letters of recommendation.

University of Massachusetts Worcester, Graduate School of Nursing, Worcester, MA 01655-0115. Offers advanced practice nursing (DNP); family nurse practitioner (MS); gerontological adult acute care nurse practitioner (MS, Post Master's Certificate); gerontological adult primary care nurse practitioner (Post Master's Certificate); gerontological primary care nurse practitioner (MS); leadership (DNP); nurse educator (MS, Post Master's Certificate); nursing (PhD). *Accreditation:* AACN. *Faculty:* 19 full-time (17 women), 40 part-time/adjunct (33 women). *Students:* 153 full-time (129 women), 35 part-time (28 women); includes 30 minority (18 Black or African American, non-Hispanic/Latino; 7 Asian, non-Hispanic/Latino; 5 Hispanic/Latino). Average age 34. 254 applicants, 31% accepted, 57 enrolled. In 2013, 50 master's, 4 doctorates, 2 other advanced degrees awarded. *Degree requirements:* For doctorate, thesis/dissertation (for some programs), comprehensive exam (for PhD); capstone project and manuscript (for DNP). *Entrance requirements:* For master's, GRE General Test, bachelor's degree in nursing, course work in statistics, unrestricted Massachusetts license as registered nurse; for doctorate, GRE General Test, bachelor's or master's degree; for Post Master's Certificate, GRE General Test, MS in nursing. Additional exam requirements/recommendations for international students: Required—TOEFL. *Application deadline:* For fall admission, 12/1 priority date for domestic students. Applications are processed on a rolling basis. Application fee: $60. Electronic applications accepted. *Expenses:* Contact institution. *Financial support:* In 2013–14, 43 students received support. Institutionally sponsored loans, scholarships/grants, traineeships, and tuition waivers available. Support available to part-time students. Financial award application deadline: 5/16; financial award applicants required to submit FAFSA. *Faculty research:* Decision-making of partners and men with prostate cancer, coinfection (HIV and Hepatitis C) and treatment decisions, parent management of children with Type 1 diabetes, health literacy and discharge planning, Ghanaian women and self-care. *Total annual research expenditures:* $1.5 million. *Unit head:* Dr. Paulette Seymour-Route, Dean, 508-856-5801, Fax: 508-856-6552, E-mail: paulette.seymour-route@umassmed.edu. *Application contact:* Diane Brescia, Admissions Coordinator, 508-856-3488, Fax: 508-856-5851, E-mail: diane.brescia@umassmed.edu.
Website: http://www.umassmed.edu/gsn/

University of Michigan, Rackham Graduate School, School of Nursing, Ann Arbor, MI 48109. Offers acute care pediatric nurse practitioner (MS); adult-gerontology acute care clinical nurse specialist (MS); adult-gerontology acute care nurse practitioner (MS); adult-gerontology primary care nurse practitioner (MS); health systems, nursing leadership, and effectiveness science (MS); nurse midwife (MS); nurse midwife and family nurse practitioner (MS); nurse midwife and primary care pediatric nurse practitioner (MS); nursing (DNP, PhD, Post Master's Certificate); primary care family nurse practitioner (MS); primary care pediatric nurse practitioner (MS). *Accreditation:* AACN; ACNM/ACME (one or more programs are accredited). Part-time programs available. Postbaccalaureate distance learning degree programs offered (minimal on-campus study). Terminal master's awarded for partial completion of doctoral program. *Degree requirements:* For doctorate, thesis/dissertation. *Application deadline:* For fall admission, 2/1 for domestic students; for winter admission, 5/1 for domestic students; for spring admission, 11/1 for domestic students. Applications are processed on a rolling basis. Electronic applications accepted. Tuition and fees vary according to course level, course load, degree level, program and student level. *Financial support:* Fellowships with full and partial tuition reimbursements, research assistantships with full and partial tuition reimbursements, teaching assistantships with full tuition reimbursements, Federal Work-Study, institutionally sponsored loans, scholarships/grants, traineeships, and tuition waivers (partial) available. Support available to part-time students. *Faculty research:* Preparation of clinical nurse researchers, biobehavior, women's health, health promotion, substance abuse, psychobiology of menopause, fertility, obesity, health care systems. *Unit head:* Dr. Kathleen Potempa, Dean, 734-764-7185, Fax: 734-764-7186. *Application contact:* James Diesing, Graduate Recruiting and Admissions Coordinator, 734-615-4739, E-mail: sn-osams@umich.edu.
Website: http://www.nursing.umich.edu/

University of Minnesota, Twin Cities Campus, Graduate School, School of Nursing, Gerontological Nurse Practitioner Program, Minneapolis, MN 55455-0213. Offers MS. *Accreditation:* AACN. *Degree requirements:* For master's, final oral exam, project or thesis. *Entrance requirements:* Additional exam requirements/recommendations for international students: Required—TOEFL (minimum score 586 paper-based).

University of Minnesota, Twin Cities Campus, Graduate School, School of Nursing, Program in Gerontological Clinical Nurse Specialist, Minneapolis, MN 55455-0213. Offers advanced clinical specialist in gerontology (MS). *Accreditation:* AACN. Part-time programs available. *Degree requirements:* For master's, final oral exam, project or thesis. *Entrance requirements:* Additional exam requirements/recommendations for international students: Required—TOEFL (minimum score 586 paper-based).

University of Missouri, Graduate School, Sinclair School of Nursing, Columbia, MO 65211. Offers adult-gerontology clinical nurse specialist (DNP, Certificate); family nurse practitioner (DNP); family psychiatric and mental health nurse practitioner (DNP); nursing (MS, PhD); nursing leadership and innovations in health care (DNP); pediatric clinical nurse specialist (DNP, Certificate); pediatric nurse practitioner (DNP). *Accreditation:* AACN. Part-time programs available. *Faculty:* 20 full-time (18 women), 6 part-time/adjunct (all women). *Students:* 60 full-time (58 women), 232 part-time (211 women); includes 24 minority (9 Black or African American, non-Hispanic/Latino; 4 American Indian or Alaska Native, non-Hispanic/Latino; 2 Asian, non-Hispanic/Latino; 6 Hispanic/Latino; 3 Two or more races, non-Hispanic/Latino), 4 international. Average age 37. 131 applicants, 62% accepted, 61 enrolled. In 2013, 42 master's, 2 doctorates, 7 other advanced degrees awarded. *Degree requirements:* For master's, thesis optional, oral exam; for doctorate, thesis/dissertation. *Entrance requirements:* For master's, GRE General Test, BSN, minimum GPA of 3.0 during last 60 hours, nursing license. Additional exam requirements/recommendations for international students: Required—TOEFL (minimum score 550 paper-based; 79 iBT). *Application deadline:* For fall admission, 2/1 priority date for domestic and international students. Applications are processed on a rolling basis. Application fee: $55 ($75 for international students). Electronic applications accepted. *Financial support:* Fellowships, research assistantships, teaching assistantships, career-related internships or fieldwork, institutionally sponsored loans, scholarships/grants, traineeships, health care benefits, tuition waivers (full), and unspecified assistantships available. Support available to part-time students. *Faculty research:* Pain, stepfamilies, chemotherapy-related nausea and vomiting, stress management, self-care deficit theory. *Unit head:* Dr. Judith F. Miller, Dean, 573-882-0278, E-mail: millerjud@missouri.edu. *Application contact:* Laura Anderson, Senior Academic Advisor, 573-882-0294, E-mail: andersonla@missouri.edu.
Website: http://nursing.missouri.edu/

University of Missouri–Kansas City, School of Nursing and Health Studies, Kansas City, MO 64110-2499. Offers adult clinical nurse specialist (MSN), including adult nurse practitioner, women's health nurse practitioner (MSN, DNP); adult clinical nursing practice (DNP), including adult gerontology nurse practitioner, women's health nurse practitioner (MSN, DNP); clinical nursing practice (DNP), including family nurse practitioner; family nurse practitioner (MSN); neonatal nurse practitioner (MSN); nurse educator (MSN); nurse executive (MSN); nursing (PhD); nursing practice (DNP); pediatric clinical nursing practice (DNP), including pediatric nurse practitioner; pediatric nurse practitioner (MSN). *Accreditation:* AACN. Part-time programs available. Postbaccalaureate distance learning degree programs offered (minimal on-campus study). *Faculty:* 44 full-time (38 women), 55 part-time/adjunct (52 women). *Students:* 44 full-time (33 women), 401 part-time (370 women); includes 59 minority (25 Black or African American, non-Hispanic/Latino; 2 American Indian or Alaska Native, non-Hispanic/Latino; 12 Asian, non-Hispanic/Latino; 15 Hispanic/Latino; 5 Two or more races, non-Hispanic/Latino). Average age 37. 182 applicants, 68% accepted, 124 enrolled. In 2013, 106 master's, 15 doctorates awarded. *Degree requirements:* For master's, thesis or alternative. *Entrance requirements:* For master's, minimum undergraduate GPA of 3.2; for doctorate, GRE, 3 letters of reference. Additional exam requirements/recommendations for international students: Required—TOEFL (minimum score 550 paper-based; 80 iBT). *Application deadline:* For fall admission, 2/1 priority date for domestic and international students; for spring admission, 9/1 priority date for domestic and international students. Application fee: $45 ($50 for international students). *Expenses:* Tuition, state resident: full-time $6073; part-time $337.40 per credit hour. Tuition, nonresident: full-time $15,680; part-time $871.10 per credit hour. *Required fees:* $97.59 per credit hour. Full-time tuition and fees vary according to program. *Financial support:* In 2013–14, 13 teaching assistantships with partial tuition reimbursements (averaging $9,470 per year) were awarded; fellowships, research assistantships, career-related internships or fieldwork, Federal Work-Study, institutionally sponsored loans, and tuition waivers (full and partial) also available. Support available to part-time students. Financial award application deadline: 3/1; financial award applicants required to submit FAFSA. *Faculty research:* Geriatrics/gerontology, children's pain, neonatology, Alzheimer's care, cancer caregivers. *Unit head:* Dr. Ann Cary, Dean, 816-235-1723, Fax: 816-235-1701, E-mail: caryah@umkc.edu. *Application contact:* Judy Jellison, Coordinator for Admissions and Recruitment, 816-235-1740, Fax: 816-235-1701, E-mail: jellisonj@umkc.edu.
Website: http://nursing.umkc.edu/

The University of North Carolina at Greensboro, Graduate School, School of Nursing, Greensboro, NC 27412-5001. Offers adult clinical nurse specialist (MSN, PMC); adult/gerontological nurse practitioner (MSN, PMC); nurse anesthesia (MSN, PMC); nursing (PhD); nursing administration (MSN); nursing education (MSN); MSN/MBA. *Accreditation:* AACN; AANA/CANAEP. *Degree requirements:* For master's, thesis or alternative. *Entrance requirements:* For master's, GRE General Test or MAT, BSN, clinical experience, liability insurance, RN license; for PMC, liability insurance, MSN, RN license. Additional exam requirements/recommendations for international students: Required—TOEFL. Electronic applications accepted.

University of North Dakota, Graduate School, College of Nursing, Department of Nursing, Grand Forks, ND 58202. Offers adult-gerontological nurse practitioner (MSN); advanced public health nurse (MSN); family nurse practitioner (MSN); nurse anesthesia (MSN); nurse educator (MSN); nursing (DNP, PhD); psychiatric and mental health nurse practitioner (MSN).

University of Phoenix–Bay Area Campus, College of Nursing, San Jose, CA 95134-1805. Offers education (MHA); gerontology (MHA); health administration (MHA, DHA); informatics (MHA, MSN); nursing (MSN, PhD); nursing/health care education (MSN); MSN/MBA. Evening/weekend programs available. Postbaccalaureate distance learning degree programs offered (no on-campus study). *Degree requirements:* For master's, thesis (for some programs). *Entrance requirements:* For master's, minimum undergraduate GPA of 2.5, 3 years of work experience, RN license. Additional exam requirements/recommendations for international students: Required—TOEFL (minimum score 550 paper-based; 79 iBT). Electronic applications accepted.

University of Phoenix–Phoenix Campus, College of Health Sciences and Nursing, Tempe, AZ 85282-2371. Offers family nurse practitioner (MSN, Certificate); gerontology health care (Certificate); health care education (MSN, Certificate); health care informatics (Certificate); informatics (MSN); nursing (MSN); MSN/MHA. Evening/weekend programs available. Postbaccalaureate distance learning degree programs offered. *Entrance requirements:* Additional exam requirements/recommendations for international students: Required—TOEFL, TOEIC (Test of English as an International Communication), Berlitz Online English Proficiency Exam, PTE, or IELTS. Electronic applications accepted. *Expenses:* Contact institution.

University of Pittsburgh, School of Nursing, Clinical Nurse Specialist Program, Pittsburgh, PA 15260. Offers adult-gerontology clinical nurse specialist (DNP); psychiatric mental health clinical nurse specialist (DNP). *Accreditation:* AACN. Part-time programs available. *Students:* 4 full-time (all women), 16 part-time (14 women); includes 2 minority (both Black or African American, non-Hispanic/Latino), 1 international.

Average age 41. 4 applicants, 75% accepted, 2 enrolled. In 2013, 5 doctorates awarded. *Entrance requirements:* Additional exam requirements/recommendations for international students: Required—TOEFL (minimum score 550 paper-based; 80 iBT). *Application deadline:* For fall admission, 6/1 priority date for domestic and international students. Applications are processed on a rolling basis. Application fee: $50. Electronic applications accepted. *Expenses:* Tuition, state resident: full-time $19,964; part-time $807 per credit. Tuition, nonresident: full-time $32,686; part-time $1337 per credit. *Required fees:* $740; $200. Tuition and fees vary according to program. *Financial support:* In 2013–14, 4 students received support, including 1 fellowship with full tuition reimbursement available (averaging $24,108 per year), 3 teaching assistantships with full and partial tuition reimbursements available (averaging $21,884 per year); scholarships/grants, traineeships, health care benefits, and unspecified assistantships also available. Support available to part-time students. *Unit head:* Dr. Sandra Engberg, Associate Dean for Clinical Education, 412-624-3835, Fax: 412-624-8521, E-mail: sje1@pitt.edu. *Application contact:* Laurie Lapsley, Administrator of Graduate Student Services, 412-624-9670, Fax: 412-624-2409, E-mail: lapsleyl@pitt.edu.

University of Pittsburgh, School of Nursing, Nurse Practitioner Program, Pittsburgh, PA 15261. Offers adult-gerontology acute care nurse practitioner (DNP); adult-gerontology primary care nurse practitioner (DNP); family (individual across the lifespan) nurse practitioner (DNP); neonatal nurse practitioner (MSN, DNP); pediatric primary care nurse practitioner (DNP); psychiatric mental health nurse practitioner (DNP). *Accreditation:* AACN. Part-time programs available. *Students:* 66 full-time (59 women), 84 part-time (75 women); includes 11 minority (5 Black or African American, non-Hispanic/Latino; 2 American Indian or Alaska Native, non-Hispanic/Latino; 3 Asian, non-Hispanic/Latino; 1 Hispanic/Latino), 2 international. Average age 31. 95 applicants, 74% accepted, 57 enrolled. In 2013, 53 master's, 4 doctorates awarded. *Degree requirements:* For master's, comprehensive exam, thesis optional. *Entrance requirements:* For master's, GRE General Test or MAT, BSN, RN license, letters of recommendation, resume, course work in statistics, 1-3 years of nursing experience; for doctorate, GRE General Test, BSN, RN license, minimum GPA of 3.5, 3 letters of recommendation. Additional exam requirements/recommendations for international students: Required—TOEFL (minimum score 550 paper-based; 80 iBT). *Application deadline:* Applications are processed on a rolling basis. Application fee: $50. Electronic applications accepted. *Expenses:* Tuition, state resident: full-time $19,964; part-time $807 per credit. Tuition, nonresident: full-time $32,686; part-time $1337 per credit. *Required fees:* $740; $200. Tuition and fees vary according to program. *Financial support:* In 2013–14, 18 students received support, including 4 fellowships with full and partial tuition reimbursements available (averaging $22,521 per year), 3 research assistantships with full and partial tuition reimbursements available (averaging $21,884 per year), 15 teaching assistantships with full and partial tuition reimbursements available (averaging $13,535 per year); scholarships/grants, traineeships, health care benefits, and unspecified assistantships also available. Support available to part-time students. *Unit head:* Dr. Sandra Engberg, Associate Dean for Clinical Education, 412-624-3835, Fax: 412-624-8521, E-mail: sje1@pitt.edu. *Application contact:* Laurie Lapsley, Administrator of Graduate Student Services, 412-624-9670, Fax: 412-624-2409, E-mail: lapsleyl@pitt.edu.
Website: http://www.nursing.pitt.edu

University of Puerto Rico, Medical Sciences Campus, School of Nursing, San Juan, PR 00936-5067. Offers adult and elderly nursing (MSN); child and adolescent nursing (MSN); critical care nursing (MSN); family and community nursing (MSN); family nurse practitioner (MSN); maternity nursing (MSN); mental health and psychiatric nursing (MSN). *Accreditation:* AACN. *Entrance requirements:* For master's, GRE or EXADEP, interview, Puerto Rico RN license or professional license for international students, general and specific point average, article analysis. Electronic applications accepted. *Faculty research:* HIV, health disparities, teen violence, women and violence, neurological disorders.

University of Rhode Island, Graduate School, College of Nursing, Kingston, RI 02881. Offers administration (MS); clinical nurse leader (MS); clinical specialist in gerontology (MS); clinical specialist in psychiatric/mental health (MS); family nurse practitioner (MS); gerontological nurse practitioner (MS); nursing (DNP, PhD); nursing education (MS). *Accreditation:* AACN; ACNM/ACME (one or more programs are accredited). Part-time programs available. *Faculty:* 26 full-time (25 women), 3 part-time/adjunct (2 women). *Students:* 46 full-time (42 women), 78 part-time (70 women); includes 11 minority (7 Black or African American, non-Hispanic/Latino; 1 Asian, non-Hispanic/Latino; 3 Hispanic/Latino), 4 international. In 2013, 38 master's, 4 doctorates awarded. *Degree requirements:* For master's, comprehensive exam; for doctorate, comprehensive exam, thesis/dissertation. *Entrance requirements:* For master's, GRE or MAT, 2 letters of recommendation, scholarly papers; for doctorate, GRE, 3 letters of recommendation, scholarly papers. Additional exam requirements/recommendations for international students: Required—TOEFL (minimum score 550 paper-based). *Application deadline:* For fall admission, 2/15 for domestic students, 2/1 for international students; for spring admission, 10/15 for domestic students, 7/15 for international students. Application fee: $65. Electronic applications accepted. *Expenses:* Tuition, state resident: full-time $11,532; part-time $641 per credit. Tuition, nonresident: full-time $23,606; part-time $1311 per credit. *Required fees:* $1388; $36 per credit. $35 per semester. One-time fee: $130. *Financial support:* In 2013–14, 4 teaching assistantships with full and partial tuition reimbursements (averaging $8,383 per year) were awarded. Financial award application deadline: 2/15; financial award applicants required to submit FAFSA. *Faculty research:* Group intervention for grieving women in prison, translating best practice in non-drug interventions for postoperative pain management, further development and testing of the pain assessment inventory, preschool motor and functional performance of two cohorts, neuroactivation of brain motor areas in preterm children. *Total annual research expenditures:* $1.2 million. *Unit head:* Dr. Mary Sullivan, Interim Dean, 401-874-5339, Fax: 401-874-2061, E-mail: mcsullivan@uri.edu. *Application contact:* Graduate Admission, 401-874-2872, E-mail: gradadm@etal.uri.edu.
Website: http://www.uri.edu/nursing/

University of Rochester, School of Nursing, Rochester, NY 14642. Offers acute care nurse practitioner (MS); adult nurse practitioner (MS); adult/geriatric nurse practitioner (MS); clinical nurse leader (MS); clinical research coordinator (MS); family nurse practitioner (MS); family psychiatric mental health nurse practitioner (MS); health care organization management and leadership (MS); health practice research (PhD); nursing (DNP); pediatric nurse practitioner (MS); pediatric nurse practitioner/neonatal nurse practitioner (MS). *Accreditation:* AACN. Part-time programs available. Postbaccalaureate distance learning degree programs offered (minimal on-campus study). *Faculty:* 60 full-time (52 women), 61 part-time/adjunct (47 women). *Students:* 33 full-time (29 women), 213 part-time (195 women); includes 32 minority (8 Black or African American, non-Hispanic/Latino; 10 Asian, non-Hispanic/Latino; 8 Hispanic/Latino; 6 Two or more races, non-Hispanic/Latino), 4 international. Average age 34. 41 applicants, 54% accepted, 16 enrolled. In 2013, 58 master's, 11 doctorates awarded. Terminal master's awarded for partial completion of doctoral program. *Degree requirements:* For master's, comprehensive exam (for some programs); for doctorate, thesis/dissertation. *Entrance requirements:* For master's, BS in nursing, minimum GPA of 3.0, course work in statistics; for doctorate, GRE General Test, MS in nursing, minimum GPA of 3.5. Additional exam requirements/recommendations for international students: Required—TOEFL (minimum score 560 paper-based; 88 iBT) or IELTS (minimum score 6.5) recommended. *Application deadline:* For fall admission, 4/1 for domestic and international students; for spring admission, 9/1 for domestic and international students; for summer admission, 1/2 for domestic and international students. Application fee: $50. Electronic applications accepted. *Expenses: Tuition:* Full-time $44,580; part-time $1394 per credit hour. *Required fees:* $492. *Financial support:* In 2013–14, 41 students received support, including 2 fellowships with full and partial tuition reimbursements available (averaging $30,200 per year); scholarships/grants, traineeships, health care benefits, tuition waivers (partial), and unspecified assistantships also available. Support available to part-time students. Financial award application deadline: 6/30. *Faculty research:* Symptom assessment and self-management, illness prevention, nursing intervention research with vulnerable populations, palliative care, aging. *Total annual research expenditures:* $3.5 million. *Unit head:* Dr. Kathy H. Rideout, Dean, 585-273-8902, Fax: 585-273-1268, E-mail: kathy_rideout@urmc.rochester.edu. *Application contact:* Elaine Andolina, Director of Admissions, 585-275-2375, Fax: 585-756-8299, E-mail: elaine_andolina@urmc.rochester.edu.
Website: http://www.son.rochester.edu

University of San Diego, Hahn School of Nursing and Health Science, San Diego, CA 92110. Offers adult-gerontology clinical nurse specialist (MSN); adult-gerontology nurse practitioner/family nurse practitioner (MSN); clinical nursing (MSN); executive nurse leader (MSN); family nurse practitioner (MSN); family/lifespan psychiatric-mental health nurse practitioner (MSN); healthcare informatics (MS, MSN); nursing (PhD); nursing practice (DNP); pediatric nurse practitioner/family nurse practitioner (MSN). *Accreditation:* AACN. Part-time and evening/weekend programs available. *Faculty:* 23 full-time (19 women), 48 part-time/adjunct (43 women). *Students:* 204 full-time (170 women), 166 part-time (144 women); includes 133 minority (26 Black or African American, non-Hispanic/Latino; 8 American Indian or Alaska Native, non-Hispanic/Latino; 50 Asian, non-Hispanic/Latino; 42 Hispanic/Latino; 1 Native Hawaiian or other Pacific Islander, non-Hispanic/Latino; 6 Two or more races, non-Hispanic/Latino), 7 international. Average age 36. 483 applicants, 58% accepted, 154 enrolled. In 2013, 91 master's, 33 doctorates awarded. *Degree requirements:* For doctorate, thesis/dissertation (for some programs), residency (DNP). *Entrance requirements:* For master's, GRE General Test (for entry-level nursing), BSN, current California RN licensure (except for entry-level nursing); minimum GPA of 3.0; for doctorate, minimum GPA of 3.5, MSN, current California RN licensure. Additional exam requirements/recommendations for international students: Required—TOEFL (minimum score 580 paper-based; 83 iBT), TWE. *Application deadline:* For fall admission, 3/1 priority date for domestic students, 3/1 for international students; for spring admission, 11/1 priority date for domestic students, 11/1 for international students. Applications are processed on a rolling basis. Application fee: $45. Electronic applications accepted. *Expenses: Tuition:* Full-time $23,580; part-time $1310 per credit. *Required fees:* $350. *Financial support:* In 2013–14, 250 students received support. Scholarships/grants and traineeships available. Support available to part-time students. Financial award application deadline: 4/1; financial award applicants required to submit FAFSA. *Faculty research:* Palliative and end of life care, maternal/child health, childhood obesity, health care disparities, cognitive functioning. *Unit head:* Dr. Sally Hardin, Dean, 619-260-4550, Fax: 619-260-6814. *Application contact:* Monica Mahon, Associate Director of Graduate Admissions, 619-260-4524, Fax: 619-260-4158, E-mail: grads@sandiego.edu.
Website: http://www.sandiego.edu/nursing/

University of Southern Maine, College of Science, Technology, and Health, School of Nursing, Portland, ME 04104-9300. Offers adult-gerontology primary care nurse practitioner (MS, PMC); clinical nurse leader (MS); education (MS); family nurse practitioner (MS, PMC); family psychiatric/mental health nurse practitioner (MS); management (MS); nursing (DNP); psychiatric-mental health nurse practitioner (PMC); MBA/MSN. *Accreditation:* AACN. Part-time programs available. *Faculty:* 11 full-time (all women), 10 part-time/adjunct (8 women). *Students:* 57 full-time (47 women), 53 part-time (46 women); includes 5 minority (1 American Indian or Alaska Native, non-Hispanic/Latino; 2 Asian, non-Hispanic/Latino; 1 Hispanic/Latino; 1 Two or more races, non-Hispanic/Latino). Average age 36. 140 applicants, 44% accepted, 29 enrolled. In 2013, 33 master's, 11 other advanced degrees awarded. *Degree requirements:* For master's, thesis optional. *Entrance requirements:* For master's, GRE General Test or MAT, minimum GPA of 3.0; for doctorate, GRE. Additional exam requirements/recommendations for international students: Required—TOEFL (minimum score 550 paper-based). *Application deadline:* For fall admission, 4/1 for domestic and international students; for spring admission, 10/1 for domestic and international students. Application fee: $65. Electronic applications accepted. *Expenses:* Tuition, state resident: part-time $380 per credit. Tuition, nonresident: part-time $1026 per credit. Part-time tuition and fees vary according to program. *Financial support:* Research assistantships, teaching assistantships, career-related internships or fieldwork, Federal Work-Study, scholarships/grants, traineeships, tuition waivers (full and partial), and unspecified assistantships available. Support available to part-time students. Financial award application deadline: 2/15; financial award applicants required to submit FAFSA. *Faculty research:* Women's health, nursing history, weight control, community services, substance abuse. *Unit head:* Krista M. Meinersmann, Director of Nursing Program, 207-780-4993, E-mail: kmeinersmann@usm.maine.edu. *Application contact:* Mary Sloan, Assistant Dean of Graduate Studies and Director of Graduate Admissions, 207-780-4812, E-mail: gradstudies@usm.maine.edu.
Website: http://www.usm.maine.edu/nursing/

University of South Florida, College of Nursing, Tampa, FL 33612. Offers adult gerontology acute care (DNP, PhD); adult gerontology acute care nursing (MS); adult gerontology primary care (DNP, PhD); adult gerontology primary care nursing (MS); adult gerontology primary care/occupational health nursing (MS); adult gerontology primary care/oncology nursing (MS, PhD); clinical nurse leader (MS); family health (DNP, PhD); family nurse practitioner (MS); nurse anesthesia (MS); nursing education (MS); nursing practice (DNP); nursing science (PhD), including nursing education; occupational health/adult-gerontology (DNP); oncology/adult-gerontology primary care (DNP); pediatric health (DNP, PhD); pediatric nurse practitioner (MS). *Accreditation:* AACN; AANA/CANAEP. Part-time programs available. *Faculty:* 46 full-time (40 women), 15 part-time/adjunct (11 women). *Students:* 177 full-time (150 women), 700 part-time (622 women); includes 272 minority (116 Black or African American, non-Hispanic/Latino; 2 American Indian or Alaska Native, non-Hispanic/Latino; 45 Asian, non-Hispanic/Latino; 93 Hispanic/Latino; 2 Native Hawaiian or other Pacific Islander, non-Hispanic/Latino; 14 Two or more races, non-Hispanic/Latino), 12 international. Average age 35. 656 applicants, 43% accepted, 224 enrolled. In 2013, 224 master's, 14 doctorates awarded. *Degree requirements:* For master's, comprehensive exam, thesis optional; for doctorate, comprehensive exam, thesis/dissertation. *Entrance requirements:* For master's, GRE General Test, bachelor's degree from accredited program with minimum GPA of 3.0 in all upper-division coursework; current license as Registered Nurse; 3 letters of recommendation; personal statement of goals; resume or curriculum vitae; personal interview; for doctorate, GRE General Test (recommended), bachelor's degree in nursing from a CCNA/NLNAC regionally-accredited institution with minimum GPA of 3.0 in all coursework or in all upper-division coursework; current license as Registered Nurse in Florida; undergraduate statistics course with minimum B

grade; 3 letters of recommendation; statement of goals; resume; interview. Additional exam requirements/recommendations for international students: Required—TOEFL (minimum score 550 paper-based; 79 iBT). *Application deadline:* For fall admission, 2/15 for domestic students, 1/2 for international students; for spring admission, 10/1 for domestic students, 6/1 for international students. Application fee: $30. Electronic applications accepted. *Financial support:* In 2013–14, 36 students received support, including 7 research assistantships with tuition reimbursements available (averaging $18,935 per year), 29 teaching assistantships with tuition reimbursements available (averaging $30,814 per year); tuition waivers (partial) and unspecified assistantships also available. Financial award application deadline: 2/1; financial award applicants required to submit FAFSA. *Faculty research:* Women's health, palliative and end-of-life care, cardiac rehabilitation, complementary therapies for chronic illness and cancer. *Total annual research expenditures:* $3.4 million. *Unit head:* Dr. Dianne C. Morrison-Beedy, Dean and Professor, College of Nursing, 813-974-9091, Fax: 813-974-5418, E-mail: dmbeedy@health.usf.edu. *Application contact:* Dr. Connie Visovsky, Associate Professor and Associate Dean of Student Affairs, 813-396-9641, Fax: 813-974-5418, E-mail: cvisovsk@health.usf.edu.
Website: http://health.usf.edu/nursing/index.htm

The University of Texas at Austin, Graduate School, School of Nursing, Austin, TX 78712-1111. Offers adult - gerontology clinical nurse specialist (MSN); child health (MSN), including administration, public health nursing, teaching; family nurse practitioner (MSN); family psychiatric/mental health nurse practitioner (MSN); holistic adult health (MSN), including administration, teaching; maternity (MSN), including administration, public health nursing, teaching; nursing (PhD); nursing administration and healthcare systems management (MSN); pediatric nurse practitioner (MSN); public health nursing (MSN). *Accreditation:* AACN. Part-time programs available. *Degree requirements:* For master's, thesis optional; for doctorate, thesis/dissertation. *Entrance requirements:* For master's and doctorate, GRE General Test. Additional exam requirements/recommendations for international students: Required—TOEFL (minimum score 550 paper-based). Electronic applications accepted. *Faculty research:* Chronic illness management, memory and aging, health promotion, women's health, adolescent health.

The University of Texas Health Science Center at San Antonio, School of Nursing, San Antonio, TX 78229. Offers administrative management (MSN); adult-gerontology acute care nurse practitioner (PGC); clinical nurse leader (MSN); executive administrative management (DNP); family nurse practitioner (PGC); nurse practitioner (MSN), including adult-gerontology acute care nurse practitioner, family nurse practitioner, pediatric nurse practitioner primary care, psychiatric mental health nurse practitioner; nurse practitioner leadership (DNP); nursing (MSN, PhD); nursing education (MSN, PGC); pediatric nurse practitioner primary care (PGC); psychiatric mental health nurse practitioner (PGC); public health nurse leader (DNP). *Accreditation:* AACN. Part-time programs available. *Faculty:* 84 full-time (74 women), 42 part-time/adjunct (40 women). *Students:* 115 full-time (93 women), 140 part-time (123 women); includes 123 minority (24 Black or African American, non-Hispanic/Latino; 20 Asian, non-Hispanic/Latino; 74 Hispanic/Latino; 5 Two or more races, non-Hispanic/Latino), 7 international. Average age 37. 174 applicants, 59% accepted, 83 enrolled. In 2013, 67 master's, 6 doctorates, 5 other advanced degrees awarded. Terminal master's awarded for partial completion of doctoral program. *Degree requirements:* For master's, thesis optional; for doctorate, comprehensive exam, thesis/dissertation, final projects (for DNP). *Entrance requirements:* For master's, minimum GPA of 3.0, references, goal statement, BSN from accredited nursing school, RN licensure in Texas or compact state; for doctorate, GRE, MAT, minimum GPA of 3.0, personal interview, BSN and/or MSN from accredited nursing school, RN licensure in Texas or compact state, statistics course, references, curriculum vitae, goal statement; for PGC, minimum GPA of 3.0; references; goal statement; MSN from accredited nursing school; RN licensure in Texas or compact state; prerequisites in advanced health assessment, advanced pharmacotherapeutics, and advanced pathophysiology. Additional exam requirements/recommendations for international students: Required—TOEFL (minimum score 550 paper-based; 68 iBT), IELTS (minimum score 6.5). *Application deadline:* For fall admission, 1/10 for domestic and international students; for spring admission, 7/1 for domestic students. Application fee: $65. Electronic applications accepted. *Financial support:* In 2013–14, 145 students received support, including 3 fellowships with full tuition reimbursements available (averaging $30,000 per year); institutionally sponsored loans and scholarships/grants also available. Financial award application deadline: 6/30; financial award applicants required to submit FAFSA. *Faculty research:* Pain, organizational structure, aging, quality and safety, health disparity, obesity and nutrition, women's and children's health. *Total annual research expenditures:* $500,265. *Unit head:* Dr. Eileen T. Breslin, Dean, 210-567-5800, Fax: 210-567-5929, E-mail: breslin@uthscsa.edu. *Application contact:* Brandy Finck, Interim Associate Dean for Admissions and Student Services, 210-567-5805, Fax: 210-567-6189, E-mail: finckb@uthscsa.edu.
Website: http://www.nursing.uthscsa.edu/

University of Utah, Graduate School, College of Nursing, Gerontology Interdisciplinary Program, Salt Lake City, UT 84112. Offers MS, Certificate. *Accreditation:* AACN. Part-time and evening/weekend programs available. Postbaccalaureate distance learning degree programs offered (no on-campus study). *Students:* 8 full-time (7 women), 7 part-time (6 women); includes 3 minority (1 Black or African American, non-Hispanic/Latino; 1 American Indian or Alaska Native, non-Hispanic/Latino; 1 Hispanic/Latino), 1 international. Average age 44. 11 applicants, 91% accepted, 10 enrolled. In 2013, 7 master's awarded. *Degree requirements:* For master's, thesis or project. *Entrance requirements:* For master's, GRE General Test (if cumulative GPA is less than 3.2), minimum undergraduate GPA of 3.0. Additional exam requirements/recommendations for international students: Required—TOEFL (minimum score 500 paper-based; 85 iBT). *Application deadline:* For fall admission, 1/15 for domestic and international students. Applications are processed on a rolling basis. Application fee: $55 ($65 for international students). Electronic applications accepted. *Expenses:* Contact institution. *Financial support:* In 2013–14, 4 students received support, including 4 fellowships with partial tuition reimbursements available (averaging $3,500 per year); scholarships/grants and health care benefits also available. Support available to part-time students. Financial award application deadline: 1/15; financial award applicants required to submit FAFSA. *Faculty research:* Spousal bereavement, family caregiving, health promotion and self-care, geriatric care management, technology and aging. *Unit head:* Kara Dassel, Director, 801-585-7438, Fax: 801-587-7697, E-mail: kara.dassel@nurs.utah.edu. *Application contact:* Arminka Zeljkovic, Program Manager, 801-581-8198, Fax: 801-585-9705, E-mail: arminka.zeljkovic@nurs.utah.edu.
Website: http://www.nursing.utah.edu/gerontology/

University of Wisconsin–Eau Claire, College of Nursing and Health Sciences, Program in Nursing, Eau Claire, WI 54702-4004. Offers adult-gerontological administration (DNP); adult-gerontological clinical nurse specialist (DNP); adult-gerontological education (MSN); adult-gerontological primary care nurse practitioner (DNP); family health administration (DNP); family health in education (MSN); family health nurse practitioner (DNP); nursing (MSN); nursing practice (DNP). Part-time programs available. *Faculty:* 8 full-time (all women), 2 part-time/adjunct (both women). *Students:* 33 full-time (30 women); 40 part-time (36 women); includes 1 minority (Asian, non-Hispanic/Latino). Average age 37. 48 applicants, 85% accepted, 24 enrolled. In 2013, 31 master's, 9 doctorates awarded. Terminal master's awarded for partial completion of doctoral program. *Degree requirements:* For master's, thesis optional, 500-600 hours clinical practicum, oral and written exams. *Entrance requirements:* For master's, Wisconsin RN license, minimum GPA of 3.0, undergraduate statistics, course work in health assessment. Additional exam requirements/recommendations for international students: Required—TOEFL (minimum score 79 iBT). *Application deadline:* For fall admission, 1/15 priority date for domestic and international students. Applications are processed on a rolling basis. Application fee: $86. *Expenses:* Contact institution. *Financial support:* In 2013–14, 10 students received support. Federal Work-Study and unspecified assistantships available. Financial award application deadline: 3/1; financial award applicants required to submit FAFSA. *Unit head:* Dr. Linda Young, Dean, 715-836-4904, Fax: 715-836-5925, E-mail: younglk@uwec.edu. *Application contact:* Dr. Mary Zwygart-Stauffacher, Director, 715-836-5287, E-mail: zwygarmc@uwec.edu.
Website: http://www.uwec.edu/conhs/programs/grad/index.htm

University of Wisconsin–Madison, School of Nursing, Madison, WI 53706-1380. Offers adult/gerontology (DNP); nursing (PhD); pediatrics (DNP); psychiatric mental health (DNP); MS/MPH. *Accreditation:* AACN. Part-time programs available. *Degree requirements:* For doctorate, comprehensive exam, thesis/dissertation. *Entrance requirements:* For doctorate, GRE General Test, 2 samples of scholarly written work, BS in nursing from an accredited program, minimum undergraduate GPA of 3.0 in last 60 credits (for PhD); licensure as professional nurse (for DNP). Additional exam requirements/recommendations for international students: Required—TOEFL (minimum score 600 paper-based; 100 iBT). Electronic applications accepted. *Expenses:* Tuition, state resident: full-time $10,728; part-time $790 per credit. Tuition, nonresident: full-time $24,054; part-time $1623 per credit. *Required fees:* $1130; $119 per credit. *Faculty research:* Nursing informatics to promote self-care and disease management skills among patients and caregivers; quality of care to frail, vulnerable, and chronically ill populations; study of health-related and health-seeking behaviors; eliminating health disparities; pain and symptom management for patients with cancer.

Vanderbilt University, Vanderbilt University School of Nursing, Nashville, TN 37240. Offers adult-gerontology acute care nurse practitioner (MSN), including hospitalist, intensivist; adult-gerontology primary care nurse practitioner (MSN); emergency nurse practitioner (MSN); family nurse practitioner (MSN); healthcare leadership (MSN); neonatal nurse practitioner (MSN); nurse midwifery (MSN); nurse midwifery/family nurse practitioner (MSN); nursing informatics (MSN); nursing practice (DNP); nursing science (PhD); pediatric acute care nurse practitioner (MSN); pediatric primary care nurse practitioner (MSN); psychiatric-mental health nurse practitioner (MSN); women's health nurse practitioner (MSN); women's health nurse practitioner/adult gerontology primary care nurse practitioner (MSN); MSN/M Div; MSN/MTS. *Accreditation:* ACNM/ACME (one or more programs are accredited). Part-time programs available. Postbaccalaureate distance learning degree programs offered (minimal on-campus study). *Faculty:* 139 full-time (124 women), 452 part-time/adjunct (319 women). *Students:* 527 full-time (463 women), 369 part-time (333 women); includes 120 minority (46 Black or African American, non-Hispanic/Latino; 8 American Indian or Alaska Native, non-Hispanic/Latino; 26 Asian, non-Hispanic/Latino; 24 Hispanic/Latino; 4 Native Hawaiian or other Pacific Islander, non-Hispanic/Latino; 12 Two or more races, non-Hispanic/Latino), 7 international. Average age 32. 1,257 applicants, 49% accepted, 457 enrolled. In 2013, 364 master's, 43 doctorates awarded. *Degree requirements:* For doctorate, comprehensive exam, thesis/dissertation. *Entrance requirements:* For master's, GRE General Test (within the past 5 years), minimum B average in undergraduate course work, 3 letters of recommendation; for doctorate, GRE General Test, interview, 3 letters of recommendation from doctorally-prepared faculty, MSN, essay. Additional exam requirements/recommendations for international students: Required—TOEFL (minimum score 570 paper-based), IELTS (minimum score 6.5). *Application deadline:* For fall admission, 12/1 priority date for domestic and international students. Applications are processed on a rolling basis. Application fee: $50. Electronic applications accepted. *Expenses:* Contact institution. *Financial support:* In 2013–14, 582 students received support. Scholarships/grants and health care benefits available. Support available to part-time students. Financial award application deadline: 3/15; financial award applicants required to submit FAFSA. *Faculty research:* Lymphedema, palliative care and bereavement, health services research including workforce, safety and quality of care, gerontology, better birth outcomes including nutrition. *Total annual research expenditures:* $2.5 million. *Unit head:* Dr. Linda Norman, Dean, 615-343-8876, Fax: 615-343-7711, E-mail: linda.norman@vanderbilt.edu. *Application contact:* Patricia Peerman, Assistant Dean for Enrollment Management, 615-322-3800, Fax: 615-343-0333, E-mail: vusn-admissions@vanderbilt.edu.
Website: http://www.nursing.vanderbilt.edu

Walden University, Graduate Programs, School of Nursing, Minneapolis, MN 55401. Offers adult-gerontology acute care nurse practitioner (MSN); adult-gerontology nurse practitioner (MSN); education (MSN); family nurse practitioner (MSN); informatics (MSN); leadership and management (MSN); nursing (DNP, PhD, Post-Master's Certificate), including education (PhD), healthcare administration (PhD), interdisciplinary health (PhD), leadership (PhD), nursing education (Post-Master's Certificate), nursing informatics (Post-Master's Certificate), nursing leadership and management (Post-Master's Certificate), public health policy (PhD). *Accreditation:* AACN. Part-time and evening/weekend programs available. Postbaccalaureate distance learning degree programs offered (no on-campus study). *Faculty:* 22 full-time (19 women), 343 part-time/adjunct (301 women). *Students:* 5,828 full-time (5,240 women), 2,803 part-time (2,578 women); includes 2,920 minority (1,893 Black or African American, non-Hispanic/Latino; 40 American Indian or Alaska Native, non-Hispanic/Latino; 438 Asian, non-Hispanic/Latino; 391 Hispanic/Latino; 35 Native Hawaiian or other Pacific Islander, non-Hispanic/Latino; 123 Two or more races, non-Hispanic/Latino), 147 international. Average age 41. 1,795 applicants, 95% accepted, 1375 enrolled. In 2013, 1,879 master's, 1 doctorate, 36 other advanced degrees awarded. *Degree requirements:* For doctorate, thesis/dissertation (for some programs), residency (for some programs), field experience (for some programs). *Entrance requirements:* For master's, bachelor's degree or equivalent in related field or RN; minimum GPA of 2.5; official transcripts; goal statement (for some programs); access to computer and Internet; for doctorate, master's degree or higher, three years of related professional or academic experience, RN, goal statement (for some programs); access to computer and Internet; for Post-Master's Certificate, relevant work experience; access to computer and Internet. Additional exam requirements/recommendations for international students: Required—TOEFL (minimum score 550 paper-based; 79 iBT), IELTS (minimum score 6.5), Michigan English Language Assessment Battery (minimum score 82), or PTE. *Application deadline:* Applications are processed on a rolling basis. Application fee: $0. Electronic applications accepted. *Expenses: Tuition:* Full-time $11,813.55; part-time $500 per credit. *Required fees:* $618.76. *Financial support:* Fellowships, Federal Work-Study, scholarships/grants, unspecified assistantships, and family tuition reduction, active duty/veteran tuition reduction, group tuition reduction, interest-free payment plans, employee tuition reduction available. Support available to part-time students. Financial award applicants required to submit FAFSA. *Unit head:* Dr. Andrea Lindell, Associate Dean, 800-925-

3368. *Application contact:* Jennifer Hall, Vice President of Enrollment Management, 866-4-WALDEN, E-mail: info@waldenu.edu.
Website: http://www.waldenu.edu/programs/colleges-schools/nursing

Wayne State University, College of Nursing, Program in Adult Primary Care Nursing, Detroit, MI 48202. Offers adult primary care nursing (MSN); gerontological nurse practitioner (MSN). *Accreditation:* AACN. Part-time programs available. *Students:* 3 full-time (all women), 94 part-time (81 women); includes 33 minority (15 Black or African American, non-Hispanic/Latino; 10 Asian, non-Hispanic/Latino; 5 Hispanic/Latino; 3 Two or more races, non-Hispanic/Latino), 2 international. Average age 36. In 2013, 26 master's awarded. *Degree requirements:* For master's, thesis or alternative. *Entrance requirements:* For master's, minimum honor point average of 3.0 in upper-division course work; BA from NLN- or CCNE-accredited program; references; current RN license; personal statement. Additional exam requirements/recommendations for international students: Required—TOEFL (minimum score 550 paper-based; 79 iBT); Recommended—TWE (minimum score 6). *Application deadline:* For fall admission, 6/1 priority date for domestic students, 5/1 priority date for international students; for winter admission, 10/1 priority date for domestic students, 9/1 priority date for international students; for spring admission, 2/1 priority date for domestic students, 1/1 priority date for international students. Applications are processed on a rolling basis. Application fee: $50. Electronic applications accepted. *Expenses:* Contact institution. *Financial support:* In 2013–14, 6 students received support. Fellowships with tuition reimbursements available, research assistantships with tuition reimbursements available, teaching assistantships with tuition reimbursements available, scholarships/grants, traineeships, and unspecified assistantships available. Support available to part-time students. Financial award applicants required to submit FAFSA. *Faculty research:* Smoking risk behaviors in adolescents, sleep disturbances in postmenopausal women, health disparities in urban environments, nurse practitioner interventions, care giving and pain management. *Unit head:* Dr. Barbara Redman, Dean, 313-577-4070, Fax: 313-577-4571, E-mail: ae9080@wayne.edu. *Application contact:* Dr. Cynthia Redwine, Assistant Dean for the Office of Student Affairs, 313-577-4082, E-mail: nursinginfo@wayne.edu.
Website: http://www.nursing.wayne.edu/msn/APCNPCurriculum.php

Wilmington University, College of Health Professions, New Castle, DE 19720-6491. Offers adult nurse practitioner (MSN); family nurse practitioner (MSN); gerontology nurse practitioner (MSN); nursing (MSN); nursing leadership (MSN); nursing practice (DNP). *Accreditation:* AACN. Part-time programs available. *Degree requirements:* For master's, thesis. *Entrance requirements:* For master's, BSN, RN license, interview, 3 letters of recommendation. Additional exam requirements/recommendations for international students: Required—TOEFL (minimum score 500 paper-based). Electronic applications accepted. *Faculty research:* Outcomes assessment, student writing ability.

York College of Pennsylvania, Department of Nursing, York, PA 17405-7199. Offers adult gerontology clinical nurse specialist (MS), including administration, education; adult gerontology nurse practitioner (MS); certified nurse anesthetist (MS); nurse educator (MS); nursing (DNP). *Accreditation:* AACN; AANA/CANAEP. Part-time and evening/weekend programs available. *Faculty:* 10 full-time (all women), 4 part-time/adjunct (1 woman). *Students:* 33 full-time (26 women), 61 part-time (53 women); includes 12 minority (7 Black or African American, non-Hispanic/Latino; 2 American Indian or Alaska Native, non-Hispanic/Latino; 3 Asian, non-Hispanic/Latino), 1 international. Average age 37. 87 applicants, 31% accepted, 24 enrolled. In 2013, 26 master's, 4 doctorates awarded. *Entrance requirements:* For master's, GRE General Test, minimum GPA of 3.0 from CCNE- or NLNAC-accredited institution; for doctorate, master's degree in nursing from a CCNE- or NLNAC-accredited institution; minimum GPA of 3.0. Additional exam requirements/recommendations for international students: Required—TOEFL (minimum score 530 paper-based; 72 iBT). *Application deadline:* For fall admission, 7/15 priority date for domestic students; for spring admission, 11/15 priority date for domestic students. Applications are processed on a rolling basis. Application fee: $50. Electronic applications accepted. *Expenses: Tuition:* Full-time $12,870; part-time $715 per credit. *Required fees:* $1660; $360 per semester. Tuition and fees vary according to degree level. *Financial support:* Federal Work-Study available. *Faculty research:* Student stress response to simulation versus clinical, evidence-based practice in all clinical settings. *Unit head:* Dr. Richard Haas, Graduate Program Director, 717-815-1243, E-mail: rhaas@ycp.edu. *Application contact:* Diane Dube, Administrative Assistant, Graduate Programs in Nursing, 717-815-1462, E-mail: ddube@ycp.edu.
Website: http://www.ycp.edu/academics/academic-departments/nursing/

HIV/AIDS Nursing

University of Delaware, College of Health Sciences, School of Nursing, Newark, DE 19716. Offers adult nurse practitioner (MSN, PMC); cardiopulmonary clinical nurse specialist (MSN, PMC); cardiopulmonary clinical nurse specialist/adult nurse practitioner (MSN, PMC); family nurse practitioner (MSN, PMC); gerontology clinical nurse specialist (MSN, PMC); gerontology clinical nurse specialist geriatric nurse practitioner (PMC); gerontology clinical nurse specialist/geriatric nurse practitioner (MSN); health services administration (MSN, PMC); nursing of children clinical nurse specialist (MSN, PMC); nursing of children clinical nurse specialist/pediatric nurse practitioner (MSN, PMC); oncology/immune deficiency clinical nurse specialist (MSN, PMC); oncology/immune deficiency clinical nurse specialist/adult nurse practitioner (MSN, PMC); perinatal/women's health clinical nurse specialist (MSN, PMC); perinatal/women's health clinical nurse specialist/women's health nurse practitioner (MSN, PMC); psychiatric nursing clinical nurse specialist (MSN, PMC). *Accreditation:* AACN. Part-time and evening/weekend programs available. Postbaccalaureate distance learning degree programs offered (minimal on-campus study). *Degree requirements:* For master's, thesis optional. *Entrance requirements:* For master's, BSN, interview, RN license. Electronic applications accepted. *Faculty research:* Marriage and chronic illness, health promotion, congestive heart failure patient outcomes, school nursing, diabetes in children, culture, health disparities, cardiovascular, prison nursing, oncology, public policy, child obesity, smoking and teen pregnancy, blood pressure measurements, men's health.

Hospice Nursing

Madonna University, Program in Hospice, Livonia, MI 48150-1173. Offers MSH. Part-time and evening/weekend programs available. *Degree requirements:* For master's, thesis or alternative. *Entrance requirements:* For master's, GRE General Test, minimum undergraduate GPA of 3.0, 2 letters of recommendation, interview. Electronic applications accepted.

Maternal and Child/Neonatal Nursing

Baylor University, Graduate School, Louise Herrington School of Nursing, Dallas, TX 75246. Offers family nurse practitioner (MSN); neonatal nurse practitioner (MSN); nurse-midwifery (DNP). *Accreditation:* AACN. Part-time programs available. Postbaccalaureate distance learning degree programs offered (minimal on-campus study). *Faculty:* 11 full-time (all women), 3 part-time/adjunct (2 women). *Students:* 25 full-time (24 women), 41 part-time (37 women); includes 15 minority (5 Black or African American, non-Hispanic/Latino; 5 Asian, non-Hispanic/Latino; 4 Hispanic/Latino; 1 Two or more races, non-Hispanic/Latino). Average age 35. 47 applicants, 70% accepted, 26 enrolled. In 2013, 25 master's, 5 doctorates awarded. *Degree requirements:* For doctorate, comprehensive exam (for some programs), capstone project. *Entrance requirements:* For master's, GRE General Test or MAT; for doctorate, GRE General Test. Additional exam requirements/recommendations for international students: Required—TOEFL. *Application deadline:* For fall admission, 2/1 for domestic students. Application fee: $50. Electronic applications accepted. *Expenses: Tuition:* Full-time $25,866; part-time $1437 per credit hour. *Required fees:* $2736; $152 per credit hour. Tuition and fees vary according to course load and program. *Financial support:* In 2013–14, 66 students received support, including 1 teaching assistantship (averaging $4,167 per year); Federal Work-Study, scholarships/grants, and unspecified assistantships also available. Support available to part-time students. Financial award application deadline: 6/30; financial award applicants required to submit FAFSA. *Faculty research:* Women and strokes, obesity and pregnancy, educational environmental factors, international undeserved populations, midwifery. *Total annual research expenditures:* $5,000. *Unit head:* Dr. Barbara Camune, Graduate Program Director, 214-367-3754, Fax: 214-820-3375, E-mail: barbara_camune@baylor.edu. *Application contact:* Elaine Lark, Coordinator of Recruitment and Enrollment, 214-818-7839, Fax: 214-820-3835, E-mail: elaine_lark@baylor.edu.
Website: http://www.baylor.edu/nursing/

Boston College, William F. Connell School of Nursing, Chestnut Hill, MA 02467-3800. Offers adult-gerontology nursing (MS); community health nursing (MS); family health (MS); forensic nursing (MS); maternal/child health nursing (MS), including pediatric and women's health; nurse anesthesia (MS); nursing (PhD); palliative care (MS), including adult and pediatric; psychiatric-mental health nursing (MS); MBA/MS; MS/MA; MS/PhD. *Accreditation:* AACN; AANA/CANAEP (one or more programs are accredited). Part-time programs available. *Faculty:* 47 full-time (43 women), 42 part-time/adjunct (39 women). *Students:* 199 full-time (180 women), 79 part-time (73 women); includes 44 minority (14 Black or African American, non-Hispanic/Latino; 1 American Indian or Alaska Native, non-Hispanic/Latino; 13 Asian, non-Hispanic/Latino; 12 Hispanic/Latino; 4 Two or more races, non-Hispanic/Latino), 7 international. Average age 31. 502 applicants, 39% accepted, 87 enrolled. In 2013, 105 master's, 8 doctorates awarded. *Degree requirements:* For master's, comprehensive exam, research project; for doctorate, comprehensive exam, thesis/dissertation, computer literacy exam or foreign language. *Entrance requirements:* For master's, bachelor's degree in nursing; for doctorate, GRE General Test, MS in nursing. Additional exam requirements/recommendations for international students: Required—TOEFL (minimum score 600 paper-based; 100 iBT). *Application deadline:* For fall admission, 9/30 for domestic and international students; for winter admission, 1/15 for domestic and international students; for spring admission, 3/15 for domestic and international students. Applications are processed on a rolling basis. Application fee: $40. Electronic applications accepted. *Financial support:* In 2013–14, 174 students received support, including 7 fellowships with full tuition reimbursements available (averaging $20,000 per year), 21 teaching assistantships (averaging $4,800 per year); research assistantships, scholarships/grants, health care benefits, tuition waivers (partial), and unspecified assistantships also available. Support available to part-time students. Financial award application deadline: 3/1; financial award applicants required to submit FAFSA. *Faculty research:* Sexual and reproductive health, health promotion/illness prevention, eating disorders, violence, symptom

management. *Total annual research expenditures:* $1.1 million. *Unit head:* Dr. Susan Gennaro, Dean, 617-552-4251, Fax: 617-552-0931, E-mail: susan.gennaro@bc.edu. *Application contact:* MaryBeth Crowley, Graduate Programs Assistant, 617-552-4928, Fax: 617-552-2121, E-mail: csongrad@bc.edu.
Website: http://www.bc.edu/schools/son/

Case Western Reserve University, Frances Payne Bolton School of Nursing, Doctor of Nursing Practice Program, Cleveland, OH 44106. Offers acute care nurse practitioner (DNP); adult gerontology nurse practitioner (DNP); educational leadership (DNP); family nurse practitioner (DNP); family systems psychiatric mental health nursing (DNP); midwifery/family nursing (DNP); neonatal nurse practitioner (DNP); pediatric nurse practitioner (DNP); practice leadership (DNP); women's health nurse practitioner (DNP). *Accreditation:* AACN. Part-time programs available. Postbaccalaureate distance learning degree programs offered (minimal on-campus study). *Students:* 169 full-time, 9 part-time; includes 10 minority (6 Black or African American, non-Hispanic/Latino; 1 Asian, non-Hispanic/Latino; 2 Hispanic/Latino; 1 Two or more races, non-Hispanic/ Latino). 76 applicants, 97% accepted, 59 enrolled. In 2013, 38 doctorates awarded. Terminal master's awarded for partial completion of doctoral program. *Degree requirements:* For doctorate, thesis/dissertation. *Entrance requirements:* For doctorate, GRE General Test or MAT. Additional exam requirements/recommendations for international students: Required—TOEFL (minimum score 577 paper-based; 90 iBT), IELTS (minimum score 7). *Application deadline:* For fall admission, 6/1 priority date for domestic students, 6/1 for international students; for spring admission, 10/1 for domestic and international students. Applications are processed on a rolling basis. Application fee: $75. *Financial support:* In 2013–14, 90 students received support, including 9 fellowships with full tuition reimbursements available (averaging $31,325 per year), 1 research assistantship with partial tuition reimbursement available (averaging $14,472 per year); teaching assistantships, Federal Work-Study, institutionally sponsored loans, scholarships/grants, and tuition waivers (partial) also available. Support available to part-time students. Financial award application deadline: 5/15; financial award applicants required to submit FAFSA. *Faculty research:* Symptom science, family/ community care, aging across the lifespan, self-management of health and illness, neuroscience. *Unit head:* Dr. Donna Dowling, Director, 216-368-1869, Fax: 216-368-3542, E-mail: dad10@case.edu. *Application contact:* Donna Hassik, Admissions Coordinator, 216-368-5253, Fax: 216-368-0124, E-mail: dmh7@case.edu.
Website: http://fpb.case.edu/DNP/

Case Western Reserve University, Frances Payne Bolton School of Nursing, Master's Programs in Nursing, Nurse Practitioner Program, Cleveland, OH 44106. Offers acute care cardiovascular nursing (MSN); acute care nurse practitioner (MSN); acute care/ flight nurse (MSN); adult gerontology acute care nurse practitioner (MSN); adult gerontology nurse practitioner (MSN); adult gerontology oncology and palliative care (MSN); family nurse practitioner (MSN); family systems psychiatric mental health nursing (MSN); neonatal nurse practitioner (MSN); pediatric nurse practitioner (MSN); women's health nurse practitioner (MSN). Part-time programs available. Postbaccalaureate distance learning degree programs offered (minimal on-campus study). *Faculty:* 54 full-time (50 women), 5 part-time/adjunct (3 women). *Students:* 56 full-time, 145 part-time; includes 9 minority (6 Black or African American, non-Hispanic/ Latino; 2 Asian, non-Hispanic/Latino; 1 Hispanic/Latino), 5 international. Average age 35. 70 applicants, 71% accepted, 33 enrolled. In 2013, 79 master's awarded. *Degree requirements:* For master's, thesis optional. *Entrance requirements:* For master's, GRE General Test or MAT. Additional exam requirements/recommendations for international students: Required—TOEFL (minimum score 577 paper-based; 90 iBT), IELTS (minimum score 7). *Application deadline:* For fall admission, 6/1 for domestic students; for spring admission, 10/1 for domestic students. Applications are processed on a rolling basis. Application fee: $75. *Financial support:* In 2013–14, 25 teaching assistantships (averaging $15,120 per year) were awarded; research assistantships, institutionally sponsored loans, and tuition waivers (partial) also available. Support available to part-time students. Financial award application deadline: 6/30; financial award applicants required to submit FAFSA. *Faculty research:* Symptom science, family/community care, aging across the lifespan, self-management of health and illness, neuroscience. *Unit head:* Dr. Carol Savrin, Director, 216-368-5304, Fax: 216-368-3542, E-mail: cls18@ case.edu. *Application contact:* Donna Hassik, Admissions Coordinator, 216-368-5253, Fax: 216-368-0124, E-mail: dmh7@case.edu.
Website: http://fpb.cwru.edu/MSN/majors.shtm

Duke University, School of Nursing, Durham, NC 27708-0586. Offers acute care pediatric nurse practitioner (MSN); adult-gerontology nurse practitioner - acute care (MSN, Post Master's Certificate); adult-gerontology nurse practitioner - primary care (MSN, Post Master's Certificate), including adult-gerontology nurse practitioner (MSN), cardiology, oncology; family nurse practitioner (MSN); neonatal nurse practitioner (MSN); nurse anesthesia (MSN, DNP); nursing (PhD); nursing and health care leadership (MSN); nursing education (MSN); nursing informatics (MSN, Post Master's Certificate); pediatric nurse practitioner - primary care (MSN). *Accreditation:* AACN; AANA/CANAEP. Part-time and evening/weekend programs available. Postbaccalaureate distance learning degree programs offered (minimal on-campus study). *Faculty:* 74 full-time (64 women), 7 part-time/adjunct (4 women). *Students:* 127 full-time (113 women), 473 part-time (433 women); includes 131 minority (54 Black or African American, non-Hispanic/Latino; 9 American Indian or Alaska Native, non-Hispanic/Latino; 36 Asian, non-Hispanic/Latino; 27 Hispanic/Latino; 5 Native Hawaiian or other Pacific Islander, non-Hispanic/Latino), 14 international. Average age 34. 516 applicants, 50% accepted, 190 enrolled. In 2013, 179 master's, 49 doctorates, 23 other advanced degrees awarded. Terminal master's awarded for partial completion of doctoral program. *Degree requirements:* For master's, thesis optional; for doctorate, capstone project. *Entrance requirements:* For master's, GRE General Test (waived if undergraduate GPA of 3.4 or higher), 1 year of nursing experience (recommended), BSN, minimum GPA of 3.0, previous course work in statistics; for doctorate, GRE General Test (waived if undergraduate GPA of 3.4 or higher), BSN or MSN, minimum GPA of 3.0, portfolio, resume, personal statement, undergraduate statistics course, current licensure as a registered nurse, transcripts from all post-secondary institutions; for Post Master's Certificate, MSN, licensure or eligibility as a professional nurse, transcripts from all post-secondary institutions, previous course work in statistics. Additional exam requirements/recommendations for international students: Recommended—TOEFL (minimum score 550 paper-based; 83 iBT), IELTS (minimum score 7). *Application deadline:* For fall admission, 12/1 for domestic and international students; for spring admission, 5/1 for domestic and international students. Application fee: $50. Electronic applications accepted. *Expenses:* Contact institution. *Financial support:* Career-related internships or fieldwork, institutionally sponsored loans, scholarships/grants, traineeships, and tuition waivers (partial) available. Support available to part-time students. Financial award applicants required to submit FAFSA. *Faculty research:* Cardiovascular disease, caregiver skill training, data mining, prostate cancer, neonatal immune system. *Unit head:* Dr. Catherine L. Gilliss, Dean/Vice Chancellor for Nursing Affairs, 919-684-9444, Fax: 919-684-9414, E-mail: catherine.gilliss@duke.edu. *Application contact:* Ernie Rushing, Lead Admissions Processor/Admissions Officer, 919-668-6274, Fax: 919-668-4693, E-mail: stephen.rushing@dm.duke.edu.
Website: http://www.nursing.duke.edu/

Hardin-Simmons University, Graduate School, Patty Hanks Shelton School of Nursing, Abilene, TX 79698-0001. Offers advanced healthcare delivery (MSN); family nurse practitioner (MSN). Programs offered jointly with Abilene Christian University and McMurry University. *Accreditation:* AACN. Part-time programs available. *Faculty:* 6 full-time (all women), 2 part-time/adjunct (both women). *Students:* 4 full-time (all women), 7 part-time (4 women); includes 4 minority (3 Black or African American, non-Hispanic/ Latino; 1 Hispanic/Latino), 1 international. Average age 37. 7 applicants, 100% accepted, 6 enrolled. In 2013, 8 master's awarded. *Degree requirements:* For master's, comprehensive exam, thesis or alternative. *Entrance requirements:* For master's, GRE, minimum undergraduate GPA of 3.0 in major, 2.8 overall; interview; upper-level course work in statistics; CPR certification; letters of recommendation. Additional exam requirements/recommendations for international students: Required—TOEFL (minimum score 550 paper-based; 75 iBT). *Application deadline:* For fall admission, 8/15 priority date for domestic students, 4/1 for international students; for spring admission, 1/5 priority date for domestic students, 9/1 for international students. Applications are processed on a rolling basis. Application fee: $50. *Expenses:* Contact institution. *Financial support:* In 2013–14, 1 student received support. Career-related internships or fieldwork and scholarships/grants available. Support available to part-time students. Financial award application deadline: 6/30; financial award applicants required to submit FAFSA. *Faculty research:* Child abuse, alternative medicine, pediatric chronic disease, health promotion. *Unit head:* Dr. Indira Tyler, Interim Director, 325-671-2367, Fax: 325-671-2386, E-mail: atoone@phssn.edu. *Application contact:* Dr. Nancy Kucinski, Dean of Graduate Studies, 325-670-1298, Fax: 325-670-1564, E-mail: gradoff@hsutx.edu.
Website: http://www.phssn.edu/

Indiana University–Purdue University Indianapolis, School of Nursing, Indianapolis, IN 46202-2896. Offers acute care nurse practitioner (MSN); adult health clinical nurse specialist (MSN); adult health nursing (MSN), including adult clinical nurse specialist; adult nurse practitioner (MSN); adult psychiatric/mental health nursing (MSN); child psychiatric/mental health nursing (MSN); community health nursing (MSN); family nurse practitioner (MSN); neonatal nurse practitioner (MSN); nursing (MSN, DNP), including nursing administration (MSN), nursing education (MSN); nursing science (PhD); pediatric clinical nurse specialist (MSN); women's health nurse practitioner (MSN); MSN/MPA; MSN/MPH. Part-time programs available. *Faculty:* 85 full-time (82 women), 60 part-time/adjunct (all women). *Students:* 86 full-time (78 women), 371 part-time (351 women); includes 74 minority (39 Black or African American, non-Hispanic/Latino; 1 American Indian or Alaska Native, non-Hispanic/Latino; 14 Asian, non-Hispanic/Latino; 11 Hispanic/Latino; 9 Two or more races, non-Hispanic/Latino), 6 international. Average age 38. 224 applicants, 61% accepted, 102 enrolled. In 2013, 120 master's, 10 doctorates awarded. Terminal master's awarded for partial completion of doctoral program. *Degree requirements:* For master's, thesis; for doctorate, thesis/dissertation. *Entrance requirements:* For master's, minimum GPA of 3.0, RN license; for doctorate, GRE General Test, minimum GPA of 3.0, MSN, RN license, graduate statistics course with minimum B grade (not older than 3 years). Additional exam requirements/ recommendations for international students: Required—TOEFL. *Application deadline:* For fall admission, 2/15 for domestic students; for spring admission, 9/15 for domestic students. Application fee: $55 ($65 for international students). *Financial support:* In 2013–14, 93 students received support. Fellowships with full tuition reimbursements available, research assistantships with full tuition reimbursements available, teaching assistantships with full tuition reimbursements available, Federal Work-Study, institutionally sponsored loans, scholarships/grants, and tuition waivers (full) available. Support available to part-time students. Financial award application deadline: 5/1. *Faculty research:* Clinical science, health systems. *Total annual research expenditures:* $3 million. *Unit head:* Dr. Patricia Ebright, Associate Dean for Graduate Programs, E-mail: nursing@iupui.edu. *Application contact:* Information Contact, 317-274-2806.
Website: http://nursing.iu.edu/

Lehman College of the City University of New York, School of Natural and Social Sciences, Department of Nursing, Bronx, NY 10468-1589. Offers adult health nursing (MS); nursing of older adults (MS); parent-child nursing (MS); pediatric nurse practitioner (MS). *Accreditation:* AACN. Part-time and evening/weekend programs available. *Entrance requirements:* For master's, bachelor's degree in nursing, New York RN license.

Medical University of South Carolina, College of Nursing, Pediatric Nurse Practitioner Program, Charleston, SC 29425. Offers MSN, DNP. *Accreditation:* AACN. Part-time programs available. Postbaccalaureate distance learning degree programs offered (minimal on-campus study). *Degree requirements:* For master's, comprehensive exam (for some programs), thesis optional; for doctorate, final project. *Entrance requirements:* For master's, BSN from nationally-accredited program, minimum nursing and cumulative GPA of 3.0, undergraduate-level statistics course, active RN License, 3 confidential references, current curriculum vitae or resume, essay; for doctorate, BSN from nationally-accredited program, minimum nursing and cumulative GPA of 3.0, undergraduate-level statistics course, active RN License, 3 confidential references, current curriculum vitae or resume, personal essay (for DNP). Additional exam requirements/recommendations for international students: Required—TOEFL (minimum score 550 paper-based; 80 iBT). Electronic applications accepted. *Faculty research:* School based clinics, epilepsy, caregiver burden, ADD/ADHD, developmental disorders.

Point Loma Nazarene University, School of Nursing, San Diego, CA 92106-2899. Offers adult/gerontology nursing (MSN); family/individual health (MSN); general nursing (MSN); nursing (Post-MSN Certificate); pediatric nursing (MSN); psychiatric mental health (MSN). *Accreditation:* AACN. Part-time programs available. *Faculty:* 9 full-time (8 women). *Students:* 1 (woman) full-time, 82 part-time (70 women); includes 43 minority (9 Black or African American, non-Hispanic/Latino; 1 American Indian or Alaska Native, non-Hispanic/Latino; 26 Asian, non-Hispanic/Latino; 3 Hispanic/Latino; 3 Native Hawaiian or other Pacific Islander, non-Hispanic/Latino; 1 Two or more races, non-Hispanic/Latino). Average age 36. 32 applicants, 94% accepted, 24 enrolled. In 2013, 26 master's awarded. *Entrance requirements:* For master's, NCLEX, ADN or BSN in nursing, interview, RN license, essay, letters of recommendation, interview. *Application deadline:* For fall admission, 7/18 priority date for domestic students; for spring admission, 10/26 priority date for domestic students; for summer admission, 3/23 priority date for domestic students. Applications are processed on a rolling basis. Application fee: $50. *Expenses: Tuition:* Full-time $6900; part-time $567 per credit hour. *Financial support:* Applicants required to submit FAFSA. *Unit head:* Dr. Barb Taylor, Dean of the School of Nursing, 619-849-2766, E-mail: bataylor@pointloma.edu. *Application contact:* Laura Leinweber, Director of Graduate Admissions, 866-692-4723, E-mail: lauraleinweber@pointloma.edu.
Website: http://www.pointloma.edu/discover/graduate-school/graduate-programs/master-science-nursing-and-post-msn-certification

Rush University, College of Nursing, Department of Women, Children and Family Nursing, Chicago, IL 60612. Offers neonatal clinical nurse specialist (DNP); neonatal nurse practitioner (DNP, Post-Graduate Certificate); nursing science (PhD); pediatric acute care nurse practitioner (DNP, Post-Graduate Certificate); pediatric clinical nurse specialist (DNP); pediatric primary care nurse practitioner (DNP); pediatric primary nurse practitioner (Post-Graduate Certificate); systems leadership (DNP). *Accreditation:* AACN. Part-time programs available. Postbaccalaureate distance learning degree

programs offered (minimal on-campus study). *Students:* 83 part-time (81 women); includes 9 minority (3 Black or African American, non-Hispanic/Latino; 3 Asian, non-Hispanic/Latino; 2 Hispanic/Latino; 1 Native Hawaiian or other Pacific Islander, non-Hispanic/Latino). Average age 32. 83 applicants, 81% accepted, 65 enrolled. *Degree requirements:* For doctorate, leadership project (for DNP); dissertation (for PhD). *Entrance requirements:* For doctorate, GRE General Test (waived for DNP if cumulative GPA is 3.25 or greater, nursing GPA is 3.0 or greater, or a completed graduate program GPA is 3.5 or greater), interview, 3 letters of recommendation, personal statement, current resume; for Post-Graduate Certificate, MSN in a clinical discipline, 3 letters of recommendation, personal statement, current resume, interview. Additional exam requirements/recommendations for international students: Required—TOEFL. *Application deadline:* For fall admission, 1/2 for domestic students; for winter admission, 10/15 for domestic students; for spring admission, 8/4 for domestic students; for summer admission, 2/17 for domestic students. Applications are processed on a rolling basis. Application fee: $100. Electronic applications accepted. *Financial support:* Fellowships, research assistantships, teaching assistantships with tuition reimbursements, Federal Work-Study, scholarships/grants, traineeships, and health care benefits available. Support available to part-time students. Financial award application deadline: 3/1; financial award applicants required to submit FAFSA. *Faculty research:* Reduction of health disparities; benefit of human milk feedings for low birth weight infants; decision-making when living with a BRCA mutation over 5-8 year time period; accelerating adoption of comparative effectiveness research in premature infants. *Total annual research expenditures:* $3.8 million. *Unit head:* Dr. Jan Engstrom, Acting Chairperson, 312-942-7117, E-mail: janet_l_engstrom@rush.edu. *Application contact:* Jennifer Thorndyke, Admissions Specialist, 312-563-7526, E-mail: jennifer_thorndyke@rush.edu.
Website: http://www.rushu.rush.edu/servlet/Satellite?c=RushUnivLevel1Page&cid=1204497838852&pagename=Rush%2FRushUnivLevel1Page%2FLevel_1_College_Home_Page

St. Catherine University, Graduate Programs, Program in Nursing, St. Paul, MN 55105. Offers adult gerontological nurse practitioner (MA); neonatal nurse practitioner (MA); nurse educator (MA); nursing (DNP); nursing: entry-level (MA); pediatric nurse practitioner (MA). Part-time and evening/weekend programs available. *Degree requirements:* For master's, thesis; for doctorate, portfolio, systems change project. *Entrance requirements:* For master's, GRE General Test, bachelor's degree in nursing, current nursing license, 2 years of recent clinical practice; for doctorate, master's degree in nursing, RN license, advanced nursing position. Additional exam requirements/recommendations for international students: Required—TOEFL (minimum score 600 paper-based; 100 iBT).

Saint Francis Medical Center College of Nursing, Graduate Programs, Peoria, IL 61603-3783. Offers adult gerontology (MSN); clinical nurse leader (MSN); family nurse practitioner (MSN); family psychiatric mental health nurse practitioner (MSN); neonatal nurse practitioner (MSN); nurse clinician (Post-Graduate Certificate); nurse educator (MSN, Post-Graduate Certificate); nursing (DNP); nursing management leadership (MSN). Part-time programs available. Postbaccalaureate distance learning degree programs offered (minimal on-campus study). *Faculty:* 4 full-time (all women), 4 part-time/adjunct (all women). *Students:* 13 full-time (12 women), 268 part-time (245 women); includes 17 minority (10 Black or African American, non-Hispanic/Latino; 2 Asian, non-Hispanic/Latino; 5 Hispanic/Latino), 2 international. Average age 37. 115 applicants, 89% accepted, 42 enrolled. In 2013, 17 master's, 2 doctorates awarded. *Degree requirements:* For master's, research experience, portfolio, practicum; for doctorate, practicum hours. *Entrance requirements:* For master's, nursing research, health assessment, graduate course work in statistics, RN license; for doctorate, master's degree in nursing, professional portfolio, graduate statistics, transcripts, RN license. Additional exam requirements/recommendations for international students: Required—TOEFL. *Application deadline:* For fall admission, 6/1 priority date for domestic and international students; for spring admission, 11/15 priority date for domestic and international students. Applications are processed on a rolling basis. Application fee: $50. Electronic applications accepted. *Expenses: Tuition:* Full-time $6336; part-time $528 per semester hour. *Required fees:* $436. *Financial support:* In 2013–14, 8 students received support. Scholarships/grants and tuition waivers (partial) available. Support available to part-time students. Financial award application deadline: 6/15; financial award applicants required to submit FAFSA. *Faculty research:* Outcome and curriculum planning, health promotion, NCLEX-RN results, decision-making program evaluation. *Unit head:* Dr. Patti A. Stockert, President of the College, 309-655-4124, Fax: 309-624-8973, E-mail: patricia.a.stockert@osfhealthcare.org. *Application contact:* Dr. Janice F. Boundy, Dean, 309-655-2230, Fax: 309-624-8973, E-mail: jan.f.boundy@osfhealthcare.org.
Website: http://www.sfmccon.edu/graduate-programs/

Stony Brook University, State University of New York, Stony Brook University Medical Center, Health Sciences Center, School of Nursing, Program in Neonatal Nursing, Stony Brook, NY 11794. Offers neonatal nurse practitioner (Certificate); neonatal nursing (MS, DNP). *Accreditation:* AACN. Postbaccalaureate distance learning degree programs offered. *Students:* 9 full-time (all women), 36 part-time (all women); includes 15 minority (3 Black or African American, non-Hispanic/Latino; 8 Asian, non-Hispanic/Latino; 2 Hispanic/Latino; 1 Native Hawaiian or other Pacific Islander, non-Hispanic/Latino; 1 Two or more races, non-Hispanic/Latino), 2 international. In 2013, 20 master's, 3 other advanced degrees awarded. *Degree requirements:* For master's, thesis. *Entrance requirements:* For master's, BSN, minimum GPA of 3.0, course work in statistics. Additional exam requirements/recommendations for international students: Required—TOEFL. *Application deadline:* For fall admission, 1/15 for domestic students. Application fee: $100. *Expenses:* Tuition, state resident: full-time $9870; part-time $411 per credit. Tuition, nonresident: full-time $18,350; part-time $765 per credit. *Financial support:* Application deadline: 3/15. *Unit head:* Dr. Paula M. Timoney, Clinical Associate Professor/Director, 631-444-3298, Fax: 631-444-3136, E-mail: paula.timoney@stonybrook.edu. *Application contact:* Director, 631-632-3298, Fax: 631-444-3136, E-mail: paula.timoney@stonybrook.edu.
Website: http://www.nursing.stonybrookmedicine.edu/

Stony Brook University, State University of New York, Stony Brook University Medical Center, Health Sciences Center, School of Nursing, Program in Perinatal Women's Health Nursing, Stony Brook, NY 11794. Offers MS, DNP, Certificate. *Accreditation:* AACN. Postbaccalaureate distance learning degree programs offered. *Students:* 35 part-time (all women); includes 10 minority (5 Black or African American, non-Hispanic/Latino; 1 American Indian or Alaska Native, non-Hispanic/Latino; 1 Asian, non-Hispanic/Latino; 3 Hispanic/Latino). In 2013, 7 master's awarded. *Degree requirements:* For master's, thesis. *Entrance requirements:* For master's, BSN, minimum GPA of 3.0, course work in statistics. Additional exam requirements/recommendations for international students: Required—TOEFL. *Application deadline:* For fall admission, 1/15 for domestic students. Application fee: $100. *Expenses:* Tuition, state resident: full-time $9870; part-time $411 per credit. Tuition, nonresident: full-time $18,350; part-time $765 per credit. *Financial support:* Application deadline: 3/15. *Unit head:* Prof. Elizabeth Collins, Director, 631-444-3296, Fax: 631-444-3136, E-mail: elizabeth.collins@stonybrook.edu. *Application contact:* 631-632-2644, Fax: 631-632-3136, E-mail: dolores.bilges@stonybrook.edu.
Website: http://www.nursing.stonybrookmedicine.edu/

University of Alberta, Faculty of Medicine and Dentistry and Faculty of Graduate Studies and Research, Graduate Programs in Medicine, Department of Obstetrics and Gynecology, Edmonton, AB T6G 2E1, Canada. Offers MD. *Entrance requirements:* Additional exam requirements/recommendations for international students: Required—TOEFL. *Faculty research:* Parturition, fetal/neonatal lung development, nitric oxide, vascular reactivity, pre-eclampsia gestational diabetes.

University of Cincinnati, Graduate School, College of Nursing, Cincinnati, OH 45221-0038. Offers clinical nurse specialist (MSN), including adult health, community health, neonatal, nursing administration, occupational health, pediatric health, psychiatric nursing, women's health; nurse anesthesia (MSN); nurse midwifery (MSN); nurse practitioner (MSN), including acute care, ambulatory care, family, family/psychiatric, women's health; nursing (PhD); MBA/MSN. *Accreditation:* AACN; AANA/CANAEP (one or more programs are accredited); ACNM/ACME. Part-time programs available. Postbaccalaureate distance learning degree programs offered (no on-campus study). Terminal master's awarded for partial completion of doctoral program. *Degree requirements:* For master's, thesis or alternative; for doctorate, comprehensive exam, thesis/dissertation. *Entrance requirements:* For master's and doctorate, GRE General Test. Additional exam requirements/recommendations for international students: Required—TOEFL (minimum score 520 paper-based). Electronic applications accepted. *Faculty research:* Substance abuse, injury and violence, symptom management.

University of Delaware, College of Health Sciences, School of Nursing, Newark, DE 19716. Offers adult nurse practitioner (MSN, PMC); cardiopulmonary clinical nurse specialist (MSN, PMC); cardiopulmonary clinical nurse specialist/adult nurse practitioner (MSN, PMC); family nurse practitioner (MSN, PMC); gerontology clinical nurse specialist (MSN, PMC); gerontology clinical nurse specialist geriatric nurse practitioner (PMC); gerontology clinical nurse specialist/geriatric nurse practitioner (MSN); health services administration (MSN, PMC); nursing of children clinical nurse specialist (MSN, PMC); nursing of children clinical nurse specialist/pediatric nurse practitioner (MSN, PMC); oncology/immune deficiency clinical nurse specialist (MSN, PMC); oncology/immune deficiency clinical nurse specialist/adult nurse practitioner (MSN, PMC); perinatal/women's health clinical nurse specialist (MSN, PMC); perinatal/women's health clinical nurse specialist/women's health nurse practitioner (MSN, PMC); psychiatric nursing clinical nurse specialist (MSN, PMC). *Accreditation:* AACN. Part-time and evening/weekend programs available. Postbaccalaureate distance learning degree programs offered (minimal on-campus study). *Degree requirements:* For master's, thesis optional. *Entrance requirements:* For master's, BSN, interview, RN license. Electronic applications accepted. *Faculty research:* Marriage and chronic illness, health promotion, congestive heart failure patient outcomes, school nursing, diabetes in children, culture, health disparities, cardiovascular, prison nursing, oncology, public policy, child obesity, smoking and teen pregnancy, blood pressure measurements, men's health.

University of Illinois at Chicago, Graduate College, College of Nursing, Program in Nursing, Chicago, IL 60607-7128. Offers acute care clinical nurse specialist (MS); acute care nurse practitioner (MS); administrative nursing leadership (Certificate); administrative studies in nursing (MS); adult nurse practitioner (MS); adult/geriatric nurse practitioner (MS); advanced community health nurse specialist (MS); family nurse practitioner (MS); geriatric clinical nurse specialist (MS); geriatric nurse practitioner (MS); mental health clinical nurse specialist (MS); mental health nurse practitioner (MS); nurse midwifery (MS); occupational health/advanced community health nurse specialist (MS); occupational health/family nurse practitioner (MS); pediatric clinical nurse specialist (MS); pediatric nurse practitioner (MS); perinatal clinical nurse specialist (MS); school/advanced community health nurse specialist (MS); school/family nurse practitioner (MS); women's health nurse practitioner (MS). *Accreditation:* AACN. Part-time programs available. *Faculty:* 16 full-time (14 women). *Students:* 393 full-time (361 women), 410 part-time (367 women); includes 198 minority (48 Black or African American, non-Hispanic/Latino; 1 American Indian or Alaska Native, non-Hispanic/Latino; 64 Asian, non-Hispanic/Latino; 71 Hispanic/Latino; 2 Native Hawaiian or other Pacific Islander, non-Hispanic/Latino; 12 Two or more races, non-Hispanic/Latino), 29 international. Average age 32. 396 applicants, 62% accepted, 177 enrolled. In 2013, 184 master's awarded. *Degree requirements:* For master's, thesis or alternative. *Entrance requirements:* For master's, GRE General Test, minimum GPA of 2.75. Additional exam requirements/recommendations for international students: Required—TOEFL. *Application deadline:* For fall admission, 5/15 for domestic students, 2/15 for international students; for spring admission, 11/1 for domestic students, 7/15 for international students. Applications are processed on a rolling basis. Application fee: $40 ($50 for international students). Electronic applications accepted. *Expenses:* Tuition, state resident: full-time $11,066; part-time $3689 per term. Tuition, nonresident: full-time $23,064; part-time $7688 per term. *Required fees:* $3004; $1190 per term. Tuition and fees vary according to course level and program. *Financial support:* Fellowships with full tuition reimbursements, research assistantships with full tuition reimbursements, teaching assistantships with full tuition reimbursements, career-related internships or fieldwork, Federal Work-Study, institutionally sponsored loans, scholarships/grants, traineeships, tuition waivers (full and partial), and unspecified assistantships available. Support available to part-time students. Financial award application deadline: 3/1; financial award applicants required to submit FAFSA. *Unit head:* Dr. Terri E. Weaver, Dean, 312-996-7808, E-mail: teweaver@uic.edu. *Application contact:* Receptionist, 312-413-2550, E-mail: gradcoll@uic.edu.

University of Indianapolis, Graduate Programs, School of Nursing, Indianapolis, IN 46227-3697. Offers advanced practice nursing (DNP); family nurse practitioner (MSN); gerontological nurse practitioner (MSN); neonatal nurse practitioner (MSN); nurse-midwifery (MSN); nursing (MSN); nursing and health systems leadership (MSN); nursing education (MSN); women's health nurse practitioner (MSN); MBA/MSN. *Accreditation:* AACN; ACNM. *Faculty:* 5 full-time (4 women), 1 part-time/adjunct (0 women). *Students:* 15 full-time (14 women), 285 part-time (270 women); includes 42 minority (24 Black or African American, non-Hispanic/Latino; 6 Asian, non-Hispanic/Latino; 3 Hispanic/Latino; 9 Two or more races, non-Hispanic/Latino), 2 international. Average age 35. In 2013, 46 master's awarded. *Entrance requirements:* For master's, minimum GPA of 3.0, interview, letters of recommendation, resume, IN nursing license, 1 year of professional practice; for doctorate, graduate of NLNAC- or CCNE-accredited nursing program; MSN or MA with nursing major and minimum cumulative GPA of 3.25; unencumbered RN license with eligibility for licensure in Indiana; completion of graduate-level statistics course within last 5 years with minimum grade of B; resume; essay; official transcripts from all academic institutions. Additional exam requirements/recommendations for international students: Required—TOEFL (minimum score 550 paper-based). *Application deadline:* For fall admission, 8/1 for domestic students; for winter admission, 12/15 for domestic students; for spring admission, 4/15 for domestic students. Applications are processed on a rolling basis. Application fee: $60. Electronic applications accepted. *Expenses: Tuition:* Full-time $5436; part-time $810 per credit hour. *Financial support:* Federal Work-Study available. *Unit head:* Dr. Anne Thomas, Dean, 317-788-3206, E-mail: athomas@uindy.edu. *Application contact:* Sueann

Meagher, Graduate Administrative Assistant, 317-788-8005, Fax: 317-788-3542, E-mail: meaghers@uindy.edu.
Website: http://nursing.uindy.edu/

University of Louisville, Graduate School, School of Nursing, Louisville, KY 40202. Offers adult nurse practitioner (MSN); family nurse practitioner (MSN); health professions education (MSN); neonatal nurse practitioner (MSN); nursing research (PhD); psychiatric mental health nurse practitioner (MSN). *Accreditation:* AACN. Part-time programs available. *Students:* 91 full-time (81 women), 47 part-time (42 women); includes 16 minority (8 Black or African American, non-Hispanic/Latino; 3 Asian, non-Hispanic/Latino; 3 Hispanic/Latino; 2 Two or more races, non-Hispanic/Latino), 6 international. Average age 36. 58 applicants, 74% accepted, 36 enrolled. In 2013, 33 master's, 3 doctorates awarded. Terminal master's awarded for partial completion of doctoral program. *Degree requirements:* For master's, thesis optional; for doctorate, comprehensive exam, thesis/dissertation. *Entrance requirements:* For master's, GRE General Test, bachelor's degree in nursing, minimum GPA of 3.0, RN license; for doctorate, GRE General Test, BSN or MSN with recommended minimum GPA of 3.0. Additional exam requirements/recommendations for international students: Required—TOEFL. *Application deadline:* For fall admission, 4/1 priority date for domestic students, 4/1 for international students. Applications are processed on a rolling basis. Application fee: $60. Electronic applications accepted. *Expenses:* Tuition, state resident: full-time $10,788; part-time $599 per credit hour. Tuition, nonresident: full-time $22,446; part-time $1247 per credit hour. *Required fees:* $196. Tuition and fees vary according to program and reciprocity agreements. *Financial support:* Fellowships with full tuition reimbursements, research assistantships with full tuition reimbursements, teaching assistantships with full tuition reimbursements, institutionally sponsored loans, scholarships/grants, traineeships, health care benefits, and unspecified assistantships available. Support available to part-time students. Financial award application deadline: 4/15; financial award applicants required to submit FAFSA. *Faculty research:* Maternal-child/family stress after pregnancy loss, postpartum depression, access to healthcare (underserved populations), quality of life issues, physical activity (impact on chronic/acute conditions). *Total annual research expenditures:* $718,934. *Unit head:* Dr. Marcia J. Hern, Dean, 502-852-8300, Fax: 502-852-5044, E-mail: m.hern@gwise.louisville.edu. *Application contact:* Dr. Lee Ridner, Interim Associate Dean for Academic Affairs and Director of MSN Programs, 502-852-8518, Fax: 502-852-0704, E-mail: romain01@louisville.edu.
Website: http://www.louisville.edu/nursing/

University of Maryland, Baltimore, Graduate School, School of Nursing, Master's Program in Nursing, Baltimore, MD 21201. Offers community health nursing (MS); gerontological nursing (MS); maternal-child nursing (MS); medical-surgical nursing (MS); nurse-midwifery education (MS); nursing administration (MS); nursing education (MS); nursing health policy (MS); primary care nursing (MS); psychiatric nursing (MS); MS/MBA. MS/MBA offered jointly with University of Baltimore. *Accreditation:* AACN; AANA/CANAEP. Part-time programs available. *Students:* 345 full-time (297 women), 508 part-time (469 women); includes 288 minority (152 Black or African American, non-Hispanic/Latino; 2 American Indian or Alaska Native, non-Hispanic/Latino; 72 Asian, non-Hispanic/Latino; 32 Hispanic/Latino; 1 Native Hawaiian or other Pacific Islander, non-Hispanic/Latino; 29 Two or more races, non-Hispanic/Latino), 13 international. Average age 33. 971 applicants, 34% accepted, 253 enrolled. In 2013, 308 master's awarded. *Degree requirements:* For master's, comprehensive exam (for some programs), thesis or alternative. *Entrance requirements:* For master's, minimum GPA of 2.75, course work in statistics, BS in nursing. Additional exam requirements/recommendations for international students: Required—TOEFL (minimum score 550 paper-based; 80 iBT) or IELTS (minimum score 7). *Application deadline:* For fall admission, 2/1 for domestic students, 1/15 for international students. Application fee: $75. Electronic applications accepted. *Financial support:* Fellowships, research assistantships, teaching assistantships, career-related internships or fieldwork, and traineeships available. Support available to part-time students. Financial award application deadline: 2/15; financial award applicants required to submit FAFSA. *Unit head:* Dr. Jane Kapustin, Assistant Dean, 410-706-6741, Fax: 410-706-4231. *Application contact:* Marjorie Fass, Admissions Director, 410-706-0501, Fax: 410-706-7238.

University of Missouri–Kansas City, School of Nursing and Health Studies, Kansas City, MO 64110-2499. Offers adult clinical nurse specialist (MSN), including adult nurse practitioner, women's health nurse practitioner (MSN, DNP); adult clinical nursing practice (DNP), including adult gerontology nurse practitioner, women's health nurse practitioner (MSN, DNP); clinical nursing practice (DNP), including family nurse practitioner; family nurse practitioner (MSN); neonatal nurse practitioner (MSN); nurse educator (MSN); nurse executive (MSN); nursing (PhD); nursing practice (DNP); pediatric clinical nursing practice (DNP), including pediatric nurse practitioner; pediatric nurse practitioner (MSN). *Accreditation:* AACN. Part-time programs available. Postbaccalaureate distance learning degree programs offered (minimal on-campus study). *Faculty:* 44 full-time (38 women), 55 part-time/adjunct (52 women). *Students:* 44 full-time (33 women), 401 part-time (370 women); includes 59 minority (25 Black or African American, non-Hispanic/Latino; 2 American Indian or Alaska Native, non-Hispanic/Latino; 12 Asian, non-Hispanic/Latino; 15 Hispanic/Latino; 5 Two or more races, non-Hispanic/Latino). Average age 37. 182 applicants, 68% accepted, 124 enrolled. In 2013, 106 master's, 15 doctorates awarded. *Degree requirements:* For master's, thesis or alternative. *Entrance requirements:* For master's, minimum undergraduate GPA of 3.2; for doctorate, GRE, 3 letters of reference. Additional exam requirements/recommendations for international students: Required—TOEFL (minimum score 550 paper-based; 80 iBT). *Application deadline:* For fall admission, 2/1 priority date for domestic and international students; for spring admission, 9/1 priority date for domestic and international students. Application fee: $45 ($50 for international students). *Expenses:* Tuition, state resident: full-time $6073; part-time $337.40 per credit hour. Tuition, nonresident: full-time $15,680; part-time $871.10 per credit hour. *Required fees:* $97.59 per credit hour. Full-time tuition and fees vary according to program. *Financial support:* In 2013–14, 13 teaching assistantships with partial tuition reimbursements (averaging $9,470 per year) were awarded; fellowships, research assistantships, career-related internships or fieldwork, Federal Work-Study, institutionally sponsored loans, and tuition waivers (full and partial) also available. Support available to part-time students. Financial award application deadline: 3/1; financial award applicants required to submit FAFSA. *Faculty research:* Geriatrics/gerontology, children's pain, neonatology, Alzheimer's care, cancer caregivers. *Unit head:* Dr. Ann Cary, Dean, 816-235-1723, Fax: 816-235-1701, E-mail: caryah@umkc.edu. *Application contact:* Judy Jellison, Coordinator for Admissions and Recruitment, 816-235-1740, Fax: 816-235-1701, E-mail: jellisonj@umkc.edu.
Website: http://nursing.umkc.edu/

University of Missouri–St. Louis, College of Nursing, St. Louis, MO 63121-4400. Offers adult nurse practitioner (DNP, Post Master's Certificate); clinical nurse specialist (DNP); family mental health nurse practitioner (DNP); family nurse practitioner (MSN, DNP, Post Master's Certificate); neonatal nurse practitioner (MSN); nurse educator (MSN); nurse leader (MSN); nurse practitioner (Post Master's Certificate); nursing (PhD); pediatric clinical nurse specialist (DNP); pediatric nurse practitioner (MSN, DNP, Post Master's Certificate); women's health nurse practitioner (MSN, Post Master's Certificate). *Accreditation:* AACN. Part-time programs available. *Faculty:* 14 full-time (13 women), 14 part-time/adjunct (13 women). *Students:* 227 part-time (217 women); includes 40 minority (35 Black or African American, non-Hispanic/Latino; 1 American Indian or Alaska Native, non-Hispanic/Latino; 1 Asian, non-Hispanic/Latino; 1 Hispanic/Latino; 2 Two or more races, non-Hispanic/Latino). Average age 35. 190 applicants, 51% accepted, 76 enrolled. In 2013, 80 master's, 8 doctorates, 2 other advanced degrees awarded. *Degree requirements:* For doctorate, comprehensive exam, thesis/dissertation; for Post Master's Certificate, thesis. *Entrance requirements:* For master's, 2 recommendation letters; minimum GPA of 3.0; BSN; nursing licensure; statement of purpose; course in differential/inferential statistics; for doctorate, GRE, 2 letters of recommendation, MSN, minimum GPA of 3.2, course in differential/inferential statistics; for Post Master's Certificate, 2 recommendation letters; MSN; advanced practice certificate; minimum GPA of 3.0; essay. Additional exam requirements/recommendations for international students: Recommended—TOEFL (minimum score 550 paper-based; 79 iBT), IELTS (minimum score 6.5). *Application deadline:* For fall admission, 2/15 for domestic and international students. Application fee: $50 ($40 for international students). Electronic applications accepted. *Expenses:* Tuition, state resident: full-time $7364; part-time $409.10 per credit hour. Tuition, nonresident: full-time $19,162; part-time $1008.50 per credit hour. *Financial support:* Application deadline: 4/1; applicants required to submit FAFSA. *Faculty research:* Health promotion and restoration, family disruption, violence, abuse, battered women, health survey methods. *Unit head:* Dr. Nancy Magnuson, Director, 314-516-6066. *Application contact:* 314-516-5458, Fax: 314-516-6996, E-mail: gradadm@umsl.edu.
Website: http://www.umsl.edu/divisions/nursing/

University of Pennsylvania, School of Nursing, Family Health Nurse Practitioner Program, Philadelphia, PA 19104. Offers MSN, Certificate. *Accreditation:* AACN. Part-time programs available. *Students:* 28 full-time (25 women), 21 part-time (20 women); includes 12 minority (2 Black or African American, non-Hispanic/Latino; 7 Asian, non-Hispanic/Latino; 2 Hispanic/Latino; 1 Two or more races, non-Hispanic/Latino), 1 international. 21 applicants, 57% accepted, 11 enrolled. In 2013, 25 master's awarded. *Entrance requirements:* For master's, GRE General Test, 1 year of clinical experience in area of interest, BSN, minimum GPA of 3.0, previous course work in statistics. Additional exam requirements/recommendations for international students: Required—TOEFL. *Application deadline:* For fall admission, 2/15 priority date for domestic students. Applications are processed on a rolling basis. Application fee: $70. *Expenses:* Contact institution. *Financial support:* Research assistantships, teaching assistantships, career-related internships or fieldwork, Federal Work-Study, and institutionally sponsored loans available. Support available to part-time students. Financial award application deadline: 4/1. *Faculty research:* Evaluation of primary care practitioner practice, access to primary care. *Unit head:* Assistant Dean of Admissions and Financial Aid, 866-867-6877, Fax: 215-573-8439, E-mail: admissions@nursing.upenn.edu. *Application contact:* Ann O'Sullivan, Program Director, 215-898-4272, E-mail: osull@nursing.upenn.edu.
Website: http://www.nursing.upenn.edu/fnp/

University of Pennsylvania, School of Nursing, Neonatal Nurse Practitioner Program, Philadelphia, PA 19104. Offers MSN. *Accreditation:* AACN. Part-time programs available. *Students:* 3 full-time (all women), 8 part-time (all women); includes 2 minority (1 Black or African American, non-Hispanic/Latino; 1 Two or more races, non-Hispanic/Latino), 1 international. 1 applicant, 100% accepted, 1 enrolled. In 2013, 5 master's awarded. *Entrance requirements:* For master's, GRE General Test, BSN, minimum GPA of 3.0, previous course work in statistics, 1 year of experience in a neonatal intensive care unit. Additional exam requirements/recommendations for international students: Required—TOEFL. *Application deadline:* For fall admission, 2/15 priority date for domestic students. Applications are processed on a rolling basis. Application fee: $70. *Expenses:* Contact institution. *Financial support:* Fellowships, research assistantships, teaching assistantships, career-related internships or fieldwork, Federal Work-Study, and institutionally sponsored loans available. Support available to part-time students. Financial award application deadline: 4/1. *Faculty research:* Neurobehavioral development, temperament, newborn sucking behaviors, parenting pre-term infants. *Unit head:* Assistant Dean of Admissions and Financial Aid, 866-867-6877, Fax: 215-573-8439, E-mail: admissions@nursing.upenn.edu. *Application contact:* Judy Verger, Program Director, 215-898-4271, E-mail: jtv@nursing.upenn.edu.
Website: http://www.nursing.upenn.edu/

University of Pennsylvania, School of Nursing, Perinatal Advanced Practice Nurse Specialist Program, Philadelphia, PA 19104. Offers MSN. *Accreditation:* AACN. Part-time programs available. *Students:* 20 full-time (all women), 23 part-time (22 women); includes 9 minority (5 Black or African American, non-Hispanic/Latino; 3 Asian, non-Hispanic/Latino; 1 Hispanic/Latino). 16 applicants, 44% accepted, 6 enrolled. In 2013, 9 master's awarded. *Entrance requirements:* For master's, GRE General Test, BSN, minimum GPA of 3.0, previous course work in statistics. Additional exam requirements/recommendations for international students: Required—TOEFL. *Application deadline:* For fall admission, 2/15 priority date for domestic students. Applications are processed on a rolling basis. Application fee: $70. *Expenses:* Contact institution. *Financial support:* Fellowships, research assistantships, teaching assistantships, career-related internships or fieldwork, Federal Work-Study, and institutionally sponsored loans available. Support available to part-time students. Financial award application deadline: 4/1. *Unit head:* Assistant Dean of Admissions and Financial Aid, 866-867-6877, Fax: 215-573-8439, E-mail: admissions@nursing.upenn.edu. *Application contact:* Sylvia V. J. English, Enrollment Management Coordinator, 866-867-6877, Fax: 215-573-8439, E-mail: admissions@nursing.upenn.edu.

University of Pittsburgh, School of Nursing, Nurse Practitioner Program, Pittsburgh, PA 15261. Offers adult-gerontology acute care nurse practitioner (DNP); adult-gerontology primary care nurse practitioner (DNP); family (individual across the lifespan) nurse practitioner (DNP); neonatal nurse practitioner (MSN, DNP); pediatric primary care nurse practitioner (DNP); psychiatric mental health nurse practitioner (DNP). *Accreditation:* AACN. Part-time programs available. *Students:* 66 full-time (59 women), 84 part-time (75 women); includes 11 minority (5 Black or African American, non-Hispanic/Latino; 2 American Indian or Alaska Native, non-Hispanic/Latino; 3 Asian, non-Hispanic/Latino; 1 Hispanic/Latino), 2 international. Average age 31. 95 applicants, 74% accepted, 57 enrolled. In 2013, 53 master's, 4 doctorates awarded. *Degree requirements:* For master's, comprehensive exam, thesis optional. *Entrance requirements:* For master's, GRE General Test or MAT, BSN, RN license, letters of recommendation, resume, course work in statistics, 1-3 years of nursing experience; for doctorate, GRE General Test, BSN, RN license, minimum GPA of 3.5, 3 letters of recommendation. Additional exam requirements/recommendations for international students: Required—TOEFL (minimum score 550 paper-based; 80 iBT). *Application deadline:* Applications are processed on a rolling basis. Application fee: $50. Electronic applications accepted. *Expenses:* Tuition, state resident: full-time $19,964; part-time $807 per credit. Tuition, nonresident: full-time $32,686; part-time $1337 per credit. *Required fees:* $740; $200. Tuition and fees vary according to program. *Financial support:* In 2013–14, 18 students received support, including 4 fellowships with full and partial tuition reimbursements available (averaging $22,521 per year), 3 research assistantships with full and partial tuition reimbursements available (averaging $21,884 per year), 15 teaching assistantships with full and partial tuition reimbursements available (averaging $13,535 per year); scholarships/grants, traineeships, health care

benefits, and unspecified assistantships also available. Support available to part-time students. *Unit head:* Dr. Sandra Engberg, Associate Dean for Clinical Education, 412-624-3835, Fax: 412-624-8521, E-mail: sje1@pitt.edu. *Application contact:* Laurie Lapsley, Administrator of Graduate Student Services, 412-624-9670, Fax: 412-624-2409, E-mail: lapsleyl@pitt.edu.
Website: http://www.nursing.pitt.edu

University of Puerto Rico, Medical Sciences Campus, School of Nursing, San Juan, PR 00936-5067. Offers adult and elderly nursing (MSN); child and adolescent nursing (MSN); critical care nursing (MSN); family and community nursing (MSN); family nurse practitioner (MSN); maternity nursing (MSN); mental health and psychiatric nursing (MSN). *Accreditation:* AACN. *Entrance requirements:* For master's, GRE or EXADEP, interview, Puerto Rico RN license or professional license for international students, general and specific point average, article analysis. Electronic applications accepted. *Faculty research:* HIV, health disparities, teen violence, women and violence, neurological disorders.

University of Rochester, School of Nursing, Rochester, NY 14642. Offers acute care nurse practitioner (MS); adult nurse practitioner (MS); adult/geriatric nurse practitioner (MS); clinical nurse leader (MS); clinical research coordinator (MS); family nurse practitioner (MS); family psychiatric mental health nurse practitioner (MS); health care organization management and leadership (MS); health practice research (PhD); nursing (DNP); pediatric nurse practitioner (MS); pediatric nurse practitioner/neonatal nurse practitioner (MS). *Accreditation:* AACN. Part-time programs available. Postbaccalaureate distance learning degree programs offered (minimal on-campus study). *Faculty:* 60 full-time (52 women), 61 part-time/adjunct (47 women). *Students:* 33 full-time (29 women), 213 part-time (195 women); includes 32 minority (8 Black or African American, non-Hispanic/Latino; 10 Asian, non-Hispanic/Latino; 8 Hispanic/Latino; 6 Two or more races, non-Hispanic/Latino), 4 international. Average age 34. 41 applicants, 54% accepted, 16 enrolled. In 2013, 58 master's, 11 doctorates awarded. Terminal master's awarded for partial completion of doctoral program. *Degree requirements:* For master's, comprehensive exam (for some programs); for doctorate, thesis/dissertation. *Entrance requirements:* For master's, BS in nursing, minimum GPA of 3.0, course work in statistics; for doctorate, GRE General Test, MS in nursing, minimum GPA of 3.5. Additional exam requirements/recommendations for international students: Required—TOEFL (minimum score 560 paper-based; 88 iBT) or IELTS (minimum score 6.5) recommended. *Application deadline:* For fall admission, 4/1 for domestic and international students; for spring admission, 9/1 for domestic and international students; for summer admission, 1/2 for domestic and international students. Application fee: $50. Electronic applications accepted. *Expenses: Tuition:* Full-time $44,580; part-time $1394 per credit hour. *Required fees:* $492. *Financial support:* In 2013–14, 41 students received support, including 2 fellowships with full and partial tuition reimbursements available (averaging $30,200 per year); scholarships/grants, traineeships, health care benefits, tuition waivers (partial), and unspecified assistantships also available. Support available to part-time students. Financial award application deadline: 6/30. *Faculty research:* Symptom assessment and self-management, illness prevention, nursing intervention research with vulnerable populations, palliative care, aging. *Total annual research expenditures:* $3.5 million. *Unit head:* Dr. Kathy H. Rideout, Dean, 585-273-8902, Fax: 585-273-1268, E-mail: kathy_rideout@urmc.rochester.edu. *Application contact:* Elaine Andolina, Director of Admissions, 585-275-2375, Fax: 585-756-8299, E-mail: elaine_andolina@urmc.rochester.edu.
Website: http://www.son.rochester.edu

University of South Africa, College of Human Sciences, Pretoria, South Africa. Offers adult education (M Ed); African languages (MA, PhD); African politics (MA, PhD); Afrikaans (MA, PhD); ancient history (MA, PhD); ancient Near Eastern studies (MA, PhD); anthropology (MA, PhD); applied linguistics (MA); Arabic (MA, PhD); archaeology (MA); art history (MA); Biblical archaeology (MA); Biblical studies (M Th, D Th, PhD); Christian spirituality (M Th, D Th); church history (M Th, D Th); classical studies (MA, PhD); clinical psychology (MA); communication (MA, PhD); comparative education (M Ed, Ed D); consulting psychology (D Admin, D Com, PhD); curriculum studies (M Ed, Ed D); development studies (M Admin, MA, D Admin, PhD); didactics (M Ed, Ed D); education (M Tech); education management (M Ed, Ed D); educational psychology (M Ed); English (MA); environmental education (M Ed); French (MA, PhD); German (MA, PhD); Greek (MA); guidance and counseling (M Ed); health studies (MA, PhD), including health sciences education (MA), health services management (MA), medical and surgical nursing science (critical care general) (MA), midwifery and neonatal nursing science (MA), trauma and emergency care (MA); history (MA, PhD); history of education (Ed D); inclusive education (M Ed, Ed D); information and communications technology policy and regulation (MA); information science (MA, MIS, PhD); international politics (MA, PhD); Islamic studies (MA, PhD); Italian (MA, PhD); Judaica (MA, PhD); linguistics (MA, PhD); mathematical education (M Ed); mathematics education (MA); missiology (M Th, D Th); modern Hebrew (MA, PhD); musicology (MA, MMus, D Mus, PhD); natural science education (M Ed); New Testament (M Th, D Th); Old Testament (D Th); pastoral therapy (M Th, D Th); philosophy (MA); philosophy of education (M Ed, Ed D); politics (MA, PhD); Portuguese (MA, PhD); practical theology (M Th, D Th); psychology (MA, MS, PhD); psychology of education (M Ed, Ed D); public health (MA); religious studies (MA, D Th, PhD); Romance languages (MA); Russian (MA, PhD); Semitic languages (MA, PhD); social behavior studies in HIV/AIDS (MA); social science (mental health) (MA); social science in development studies (MA); social science in psychology (MA); social science in social work (MA); social science in sociology (MA); social work (MSW, DSW, PhD); socio-education (M Ed, Ed D); sociolinguistics (MA); sociology (MA, PhD); Spanish (MA, PhD); systematic theology (M Th, D Th); TESOL (teaching English to speakers of other languages) (MA); theological ethics (M Th, D Th); theory of literature (MA, PhD); urban ministries (D Th); urban ministry (M Th).

University of South Alabama, Graduate School, College of Nursing, Mobile, AL 36688. Offers adult health nursing (MSN); community/mental health nursing (MSN); maternal/child nursing (MSN); nursing (DNP). *Accreditation:* AACN. *Faculty:* 50 full-time (46 women), 31 part-time/adjunct (30 women). *Students:* 1,878 full-time (1,680 women), 241 part-time (208 women); includes 523 minority (341 Black or African American, non-Hispanic/Latino; 18 American Indian or Alaska Native, non-Hispanic/Latino; 76 Asian, non-Hispanic/Latino; 54 Hispanic/Latino; 7 Native Hawaiian or other Pacific Islander, non-Hispanic/Latino; 27 Two or more races, non-Hispanic/Latino), 10 international. 1,308 applicants, 64% accepted, 602 enrolled. In 2013, 332 master's, 44 doctorates awarded. *Degree requirements:* For master's, thesis optional. *Entrance requirements:* For master's, BSN, RN licensure, minimum GPA of 3.0, resume documenting clinical experience, background check, drug screening; for doctorate, GRE. *Application deadline:* For fall admission, 7/15 for domestic students; for spring admission, 12/1 for domestic students. Application fee: $35. *Expenses:* Tuition, state resident: full-time $8976; part-time $374 per credit hour. Tuition, nonresident: full-time $17,952; part-time $748 per credit hour. *Unit head:* Dr. Debra Davis, Dean, 251-445-9409, Fax: 251-445-9416. *Application contact:* Dr. Rosemary Rhodes, Director of Graduate Education, 251-445-9409, Fax: 251-445-9416, E-mail: kharriso@usouthal.edu.
Website: http://www.southalabama.edu/nursing

University of Southern Mississippi, Graduate School, College of Health, School of Nursing, Hattiesburg, MS 39406-0001. Offers family nurse practitioner (MSN); nursing (DNP, PhD); nursing executive (MSN); psychiatric nurse practitioner (MSN). *Accreditation:* AACN. Part-time and evening/weekend programs available. *Faculty:* 17 full-time (16 women), 1 part-time/adjunct (0 women). *Students:* 133 full-time (104 women), 42 part-time (40 women); includes 45 minority (33 Black or African American, non-Hispanic/Latino; 1 American Indian or Alaska Native, non-Hispanic/Latino; 1 Asian, non-Hispanic/Latino; 1 Hispanic/Latino; 9 Two or more races, non-Hispanic/Latino). Average age 37. 118 applicants, 61% accepted, 62 enrolled. In 2013, 45 master's, 9 doctorates awarded. *Degree requirements:* For master's, comprehensive exam, thesis optional; for doctorate, comprehensive exam, thesis/dissertation. *Entrance requirements:* For master's, GRE General Test, minimum GPA of 2.75 during last 60 hours, nursing license, BS in nursing; for doctorate, GRE General Test, master's degree in nursing, minimum GPA of 3.5. Additional exam requirements/recommendations for international students: Required—TOEFL, IELTS. *Application deadline:* For fall admission, 3/15 priority date for domestic students, 5/1 for international students; for spring admission, 1/10 priority date for domestic and international students. Applications are processed on a rolling basis. Application fee: $50. Electronic applications accepted. *Financial support:* In 2013–14, 14 research assistantships with full tuition reimbursements (averaging $12,577 per year), teaching assistantships (averaging $12,000 per year) were awarded; Federal Work-Study, institutionally sponsored loans, scholarships/grants, traineeships, health care benefits, and unspecified assistantships also available. Financial award application deadline: 3/15; financial award applicants required to submit FAFSA. *Faculty research:* Gerontology, caregivers, HIV, bereavement, pain, nursing leadership. *Unit head:* Dr. Katherine Nugent, Director and Associate Dean, 601-266-5500, Fax: 601-266-5927. *Application contact:* Dr. Sandra Bishop, Graduate Coordinator, 601-266-5500, Fax: 601-266-5927.
Website: http://www.usm.edu/graduateschool/table.php

The University of Texas at Austin, Graduate School, School of Nursing, Austin, TX 78712-1111. Offers adult - gerontology clinical nurse specialist (MSN); child health (MSN), including administration, public health nursing, teaching; family nurse practitioner (MSN); family psychiatric/mental health nurse practitioner (MSN); holistic adult health (MSN), including administration, teaching; maternity (MSN), including administration, public health nursing, teaching; nursing (PhD); nursing administration and healthcare systems management (MSN); pediatric nurse practitioner (MSN); public health nursing (MSN). *Accreditation:* AACN. Part-time programs available. *Degree requirements:* For master's, thesis optional; for doctorate, thesis/dissertation. *Entrance requirements:* For master's and doctorate, GRE General Test. Additional exam requirements/recommendations for international students: Required—TOEFL (minimum score 550 paper-based). Electronic applications accepted. *Faculty research:* Chronic illness management, memory and aging, health promotion, women's health, adolescent health.

Vanderbilt University, Vanderbilt University School of Nursing, Nashville, TN 37240. Offers adult-gerontology acute care nurse practitioner (MSN), including hospitalist, intensivist; adult-gerontology primary care nurse practitioner (MSN); emergency nurse practitioner (MSN); family nurse practitioner (MSN); healthcare leadership (MSN); neonatal nurse practitioner (MSN); nurse midwifery (MSN); nurse midwifery/family nurse practitioner (MSN); nursing informatics (MSN); nursing practice (DNP); nursing science (PhD); pediatric acute care nurse practitioner (MSN); pediatric primary care nurse practitioner (MSN); psychiatric-mental health nurse practitioner (MSN); women's health nurse practitioner (MSN); women's health nurse practitioner/adult gerontology primary care nurse practitioner (MSN); MSN/M Div; MSN/MTS. *Accreditation:* ACNM/ACME (one or more programs are accredited). Part-time programs available. Postbaccalaureate distance learning degree programs offered (minimal on-campus study). *Faculty:* 139 full-time (124 women), 452 part-time/adjunct (319 women). *Students:* 527 full-time (463 women), 369 part-time (333 women); includes 120 minority (46 Black or African American, non-Hispanic/Latino; 8 American Indian or Alaska Native, non-Hispanic/Latino; 26 Asian, non-Hispanic/Latino; 24 Hispanic/Latino; 4 Native Hawaiian or other Pacific Islander, non-Hispanic/Latino; 12 Two or more races, non-Hispanic/Latino), 7 international. Average age 32. 1,257 applicants, 49% accepted, 457 enrolled. In 2013, 364 master's, 43 doctorates awarded. *Degree requirements:* For doctorate, comprehensive exam, thesis/dissertation. *Entrance requirements:* For master's, GRE General Test (within the past 5 years), minimum B average in undergraduate course work, 3 letters of recommendation; for doctorate, GRE General Test, interview, 3 letters of recommendation from doctorally-prepared faculty, MSN, essay. Additional exam requirements/recommendations for international students: Required—TOEFL (minimum score 570 paper-based), IELTS (minimum score 6.5). *Application deadline:* For fall admission, 12/1 priority date for domestic and international students. Applications are processed on a rolling basis. Application fee: $50. Electronic applications accepted. *Expenses:* Contact institution. *Financial support:* In 2013–14, 582 students received support. Scholarships/grants and health care benefits available. Support available to part-time students. Financial award application deadline: 3/15; financial award applicants required to submit FAFSA. *Faculty research:* Lymphedema, palliative care and bereavement, health services research including workforce, safety and quality of care, gerontology, better birth outcomes including nutrition. *Total annual research expenditures:* $2.5 million. *Unit head:* Dr. Linda Norman, Dean, 615-343-8876, Fax: 615-343-7711, E-mail: linda.norman@vanderbilt.edu. *Application contact:* Patricia Peerman, Assistant Dean for Enrollment Management, 615-322-3800, Fax: 615-343-0333, E-mail: vusn-admissions@vanderbilt.edu.
Website: http://www.nursing.vanderbilt.edu

Wayne State University, College of Nursing, Program in Advanced Practice Nursing with Women, Neonates and Children, Detroit, MI 48202. Offers neonatal nurse practitioner (MSN); nurse-midwife (MSN); pediatric nurse practitioner (MSN), including acute care, primary care; women's health nurse practitioner (MSN). *Accreditation:* AACN. Part-time programs available. *Students:* 59 full-time (53 women), 74 part-time (72 women); includes 17 minority (11 Black or African American, non-Hispanic/Latino; 2 Asian, non-Hispanic/Latino; 4 Hispanic/Latino), 6 international. Average age 32. 65 applicants, 55% accepted, 33 enrolled. In 2013, 40 degrees awarded. *Degree requirements:* For master's, thesis or alternative. *Entrance requirements:* For master's, minimum honor point average of 3.0 in upper-division course work; BA from NLN- or CCNE-accredited program; references; current RN license; personal statement. Additional exam requirements/recommendations for international students: Required—TOEFL (minimum score 550 paper-based; 79 iBT); Recommended—TWE (minimum score 6). *Application deadline:* For fall admission, 6/1 priority date for domestic students, 5/1 priority date for international students; for winter admission, 10/1 priority date for domestic students, 9/1 priority date for international students; for spring admission, 2/1 priority date for domestic students, 1/1 priority date for international students. Applications are processed on a rolling basis. Application fee: $50. Electronic applications accepted. *Expenses:* Contact institution. *Financial support:* In 2013–14, 17 students received support. Fellowships with tuition reimbursements available, research assistantships with tuition reimbursements available, teaching assistantships with tuition reimbursements available, scholarships/grants, and unspecified assistantships available. Financial award applicants required to submit FAFSA. *Faculty research:* Acculturation and parenting, domestic violence, evidence-based midwifery practice, pain

in children, trauma and community violence. *Unit head:* Dr. Barbara Redman, Dean, 313-577-4070, Fax: 313-577-4571, E-mail: ae9080@wayne.edu. *Application contact:* Dr. Cynthia Redwine, Assistant Dean for the Office of Student Affairs, 313-577-4082, E-mail: nursinginfo@wayne.edu.
Website: http://nursing.wayne.edu/msn/specialty.php

Medical/Surgical Nursing

Angelo State University, College of Graduate Studies, College of Health and Human Services, Department of Nursing and Rehabilitation Sciences, San Angelo, TX 76909. Offers advanced practice registered nurse (MSN); nurse educator (MSN); registered nurse first assistant (MSN). Part-time and evening/weekend programs available. Postbaccalaureate distance learning degree programs offered (no on-campus study). *Degree requirements:* For master's, comprehensive exam. *Entrance requirements:* For master's, essay, three letters of recommendation. Additional exam requirements/recommendations for international students: Required—TOEFL or IELTS. Electronic applications accepted.

Boston College, William F. Connell School of Nursing, Chestnut Hill, MA 02467-3800. Offers adult-gerontology nursing (MS); community health nursing (MS); family health (MS); forensic nursing (MS); maternal/child health nursing (MS), including pediatric and women's health; nurse anesthesia (MS); nursing (PhD); palliative care (MS), including adult and pediatric; psychiatric-mental health nursing (MS); MBA/MS; MS/MA; MS/PhD. *Accreditation:* AACN; AANA/CANAEP (one or more programs are accredited). Part-time programs available. *Faculty:* 47 full-time (43 women), 42 part-time/adjunct (39 women). *Students:* 199 full-time (180 women), 79 part-time (73 women); includes 44 minority (14 Black or African American, non-Hispanic/Latino; 1 American Indian or Alaska Native, non-Hispanic/Latino; 13 Asian, non-Hispanic/Latino; 12 Hispanic/Latino; 4 Two or more races, non-Hispanic/Latino), 7 international. Average age 31. 502 applicants, 39% accepted, 87 enrolled. In 2013, 105 master's, 8 doctorates awarded. *Degree requirements:* For master's, comprehensive exam, research project; for doctorate, comprehensive exam, thesis/dissertation, computer literacy exam or foreign language. *Entrance requirements:* For master's, bachelor's degree in nursing; for doctorate, GRE General Test, MS in nursing. Additional exam requirements/recommendations for international students: Required—TOEFL (minimum score 600 paper-based; 100 iBT). *Application deadline:* For fall admission, 9/30 for domestic and international students; for winter admission, 1/15 for domestic and international students; for spring admission, 3/15 for domestic and international students. Applications are processed on a rolling basis. Application fee: $40. Electronic applications accepted. *Financial support:* In 2013–14, 174 students received support, including 7 fellowships with full tuition reimbursements available (averaging $20,000 per year), 21 teaching assistantships (averaging $4,800 per year); research assistantships, scholarships/grants, health care benefits, tuition waivers (partial), and unspecified assistantships also available. Support available to part-time students. Financial award application deadline: 3/1; financial award applicants required to submit FAFSA. *Faculty research:* Sexual and reproductive health, health promotion/illness prevention, eating disorders, violence, symptom management. *Total annual research expenditures:* $1.1 million. *Unit head:* Dr. Susan Gennaro, Dean, 617-552-4251, Fax: 617-552-0931, E-mail: susan.gennaro@bc.edu. *Application contact:* MaryBeth Crowley, Graduate Programs Assistant, 617-552-4928, Fax: 617-552-2121, E-mail: csongrad@bc.edu.
Website: http://www.bc.edu/schools/son/

Daemen College, Department of Nursing, Amherst, NY 14226-3592. Offers adult nurse practitioner (MS, Post Master's Certificate); nurse executive leadership (Post Master's Certificate); nursing education (MS, Post Master's Certificate); nursing executive leadership (MS); nursing practice (DNP); palliative care nursing (Post Master's Certificate). Part-time programs available. *Degree requirements:* For master's, thesis or alternative, degree completed in 4 years; minimum GPA of 3.0; for doctorate, degree completed in 5 years; 500 post-master's clinical hours. *Entrance requirements:* For master's, BN, 1 year medical/surgical experience, RN license and state registration, statistics course with minimum C grade, 3 letters of recommendation, minimum GPA of 3.25, interview; for doctorate, MS in advance nursing practice; New York state RN license; goal statement; resume; interview; statistics course with minimum grade of 'C'; for Post Master's Certificate, master's degree in clinical area; RN license and current registration; one year of clinical experience; statistics course with minimum grade of 'C'; 3 letters of recommendation; interview; letter of intent. Additional exam requirements/recommendations for international students: Required—TOEFL (minimum score 500 paper-based; 63 iBT), IELTS (minimum score 5.5). Electronic applications accepted. *Faculty research:* Professional stress, client behavior, drug therapy, treatment modalities and pulmonary cancers, chemical dependency.

Eastern Virginia Medical School, Master of Surgical Assisting Program, Norfolk, VA 23501-1980. Offers MSA. *Faculty:* 1 full-time (0 women), 7 part-time/adjunct (3 women). *Students:* 38 full-time (31 women); includes 14 minority (7 Black or African American, non-Hispanic/Latino; 5 Asian, non-Hispanic/Latino; 2 Two or more races, non-Hispanic/Latino). 45 applicants, 24 enrolled. In 2013, 13 master's awarded. *Application deadline:* For fall admission, 4/15 for domestic students. Applications are processed on a rolling basis. Application fee: $60. Electronic applications accepted. *Expenses:* Contact institution. *Financial support:* Applicants required to submit FAFSA. *Unit head:* R. Clinton Crews, Program Director, 757-446-8961, Fax: 757-446-6179, E-mail: crewsrc@evms.edu. *Application contact:* Jennifer Land, Administrative Support Coordinator, 757-446-5779, Fax: 757-446-6179, E-mail: landjj@evms.edu.
Website: http://evms.edu/education/masters_programs/surgical_assistant_program/

Inter American University of Puerto Rico, Arecibo Campus, Program in Nursing, Arecibo, PR 00614-4050. Offers critical care nursing (MSN); surgical nursing (MSN). *Entrance requirements:* For master's, EXADEP or GRE General Test or MAT, 2 letters of recommendation, bachelor's degree in nursing, minimum GPA of 2.5 in last 60 credits, minimum 1 year nursing experience, nursing license.

Pontifical Catholic University of Puerto Rico, College of Sciences, Department of Nursing, Program in Medical-Surgical Nursing, Ponce, PR 00717-0777. Offers MSN. Part-time and evening/weekend programs available. *Degree requirements:* For master's, comprehensive exam (for some programs), thesis, clinical research paper. *Entrance requirements:* For master's, GRE General Test, 2 letters of recommendation, interview, minimum GPA of 2.75. Electronic applications accepted.

Saint Francis Medical Center College of Nursing, Graduate Programs, Peoria, IL 61603-3783. Offers adult gerontology (MSN); clinical nurse leader (MSN); family nurse practitioner (MSN); family psychiatric mental health nurse practitioner (MSN); neonatal nurse practitioner (MSN); nurse clinician (Post-Graduate Certificate); nurse educator (MSN, Post-Graduate Certificate); nursing (DNP); nursing management leadership (MSN). Part-time programs available. Postbaccalaureate distance learning degree programs offered (minimal on-campus study). *Faculty:* 4 full-time (all women), 4 part-time/adjunct (all women). *Students:* 13 full-time (12 women), 268 part-time (245 women); includes 17 minority (10 Black or African American, non-Hispanic/Latino; 2 Asian, non-Hispanic/Latino; 5 Hispanic/Latino), 2 international. Average age 37. 115 applicants, 89% accepted, 42 enrolled. In 2013, 17 master's, 2 doctorates awarded. *Degree requirements:* For master's, research experience, portfolio, practicum; for doctorate, practicum hours. *Entrance requirements:* For master's, nursing research, health assessment, graduate course work in statistics, RN license; for doctorate, master's degree in nursing, professional portfolio, graduate statistics, transcripts, RN license. Additional exam requirements/recommendations for international students: Required—TOEFL. *Application deadline:* For fall admission, 6/1 priority date for domestic and international students; for spring admission, 11/15 priority date for domestic and international students. Applications are processed on a rolling basis. Application fee: $50. Electronic applications accepted. *Expenses: Tuition:* Full-time $6336; part-time $528 per semester hour. *Required fees:* $436. *Financial support:* In 2013–14, 8 students received support. Scholarships/grants and tuition waivers (partial) available. Support available to part-time students. Financial award application deadline: 6/15; financial award applicants required to submit FAFSA. *Faculty research:* Outcome and curriculum planning, health promotion, NCLEX-RN results, decision-making program evaluation. *Unit head:* Dr. Patti A. Stockert, President of the College, 309-655-4124, Fax: 309-624-8973, E-mail: patricia.a.stockert@osfhealthcare.org. *Application contact:* Dr. Janice F. Boundy, Dean, 309-655-2230, Fax: 309-624-8973, E-mail: jan.f.boundy@osfhealthcare.org.
Website: http://www.sfmccon.edu/graduate-programs/

State University of New York Downstate Medical Center, College of Nursing, Graduate Program in Nursing, Program in Clinical Nurse Specialist, Brooklyn, NY 11203-2098. Offers MS, Post Master's Certificate.

Uniformed Services University of the Health Sciences, Graduate School of Nursing, Bethesda, MD 20814-4799. Offers family nurse practitioner (MSN, DNP); nurse anesthesia (MSN); nursing science (PhD); perioperative clinical nurse specialist (MSN); psychiatric nurse practitioner (MSN, DNP). Program available to military officers only. *Accreditation:* AACN; AANA/CANAEP. *Faculty:* 42 full-time (24 women), 5 part-time/adjunct (4 women). *Students:* 62 full-time (31 women); includes 13 minority (7 Black or African American, non-Hispanic/Latino; 5 Asian, non-Hispanic/Latino; 1 Hispanic/Latino). Average age 34. 100 applicants, 62% accepted, 62 enrolled. In 2013, 57 master's, 1 doctorate awarded. *Degree requirements:* For master's, thesis or alternative; for doctorate, thesis/dissertation or alternative. *Entrance requirements:* For master's, GRE, BSN, clinical experience, minimum GPA of 3.0, previous course work in science; for doctorate, GRE. *Application deadline:* For fall admission, 7/1 for domestic students; for winter admission, 2/15 for domestic students. Application fee: $0. Electronic applications accepted. *Faculty research:* Prenatal care, military health care, military readiness, distance learning. *Unit head:* Dr. Carol A. Romano, Associate Dean for Academic Affairs, 301-295-1180, Fax: 301-295-1707, E-mail: carol.romano@usuhs.edu. *Application contact:* Terry Lynn Malavakis, Recording Secretary for Admissions Committee, 301-295-1055, Fax: 301-295-1707, E-mail: terry.malavakis@usuhs.edu.
Website: http://www.usuhs.mil/gsn/

Universidad Adventista de las Antillas, EGECED Department, Mayagüez, PR 00681-0118. Offers curriculum and instruction (M Ed); health education (M Ed); medical surgical nursing (MN); school administration and supervision (M Ed). *Degree requirements:* For master's, comprehensive exam (for some programs), thesis (for some programs). *Entrance requirements:* For master's, EXADEP or GRE General Test, recommendations. Application fee: $175. Electronic applications accepted. *Expenses: Tuition:* Full-time $2400; part-time $200 per credit. *Required fees:* $235 per semester. One-time fee: $30. Tuition and fees vary according to course load. *Financial support:* Fellowships and Federal Work-Study available. *Unit head:* Director, 787-834-9595 Ext. 2282, Fax: 787-834-9595. *Application contact:* Prof. Yolanda Ferrer, Director of Admission, 787-834-9595 Ext. 2261, Fax: 787-834-9597, E-mail: admissions@uaa.edu.
Website: http://www.uaa.edu

University of Maryland, Baltimore, Graduate School, School of Nursing, Master's Program in Nursing, Baltimore, MD 21201. Offers community health nursing (MS); gerontological nursing (MS); maternal-child nursing (MS); medical-surgical nursing (MS); nurse-midwifery education (MS); nursing administration (MS); nursing education (MS); nursing health policy (MS); primary care nursing (MS); psychiatric nursing (MS); MS/MBA. MS/MBA offered jointly with University of Baltimore. *Accreditation:* AACN; AANA/CANAEP. Part-time programs available. *Students:* 345 full-time (297 women), 508 part-time (469 women); includes 288 minority (152 Black or African American, non-Hispanic/Latino; 2 American Indian or Alaska Native, non-Hispanic/Latino; 72 Asian, non-Hispanic/Latino; 32 Hispanic/Latino; 1 Native Hawaiian or other Pacific Islander, non-Hispanic/Latino; 29 Two or more races, non-Hispanic/Latino), 13 international. Average age 33. 971 applicants, 34% accepted, 253 enrolled. In 2013, 308 master's awarded. *Degree requirements:* For master's, comprehensive exam (for some programs), thesis or alternative. *Entrance requirements:* For master's, minimum GPA of 2.75, course work in statistics, BS in nursing. Additional exam requirements/recommendations for international students: Required—TOEFL (minimum score 550 paper-based; 80 iBT) or IELTS (minimum score 7). *Application deadline:* For fall admission, 2/1 for domestic students, 1/15 for international students. Application fee: $75. Electronic applications accepted. *Financial support:* Fellowships, research assistantships, teaching assistantships, career-related internships or fieldwork, and traineeships available. Support available to part-time students. Financial award application deadline: 2/15; financial award applicants required to submit FAFSA. *Unit head:* Dr. Jane Kapustin, Assistant Dean, 410-706-6741, Fax: 410-706-4231. *Application contact:* Marjorie Fass, Admissions Director, 410-706-0501, Fax: 410-706-7238.

University of South Africa, College of Human Sciences, Pretoria, South Africa. Offers adult education (M Ed); African languages (MA, PhD); African politics (MA, PhD); Afrikaans (MA, PhD); ancient history (MA, PhD); ancient Near Eastern studies (MA, PhD); anthropology (MA, PhD); applied linguistics (MA); Arabic (MA, PhD); archaeology (MA); art history (MA); Biblical archaeology (MA); Biblical studies (M Th, D Th, PhD); Christian spirituality (M Th, D Th); church history (M Th, D Th); classical studies (MA, PhD); clinical psychology (MA); communication (MA, PhD); comparative education (M Ed, Ed D); consulting psychology (D Admin, D Com, PhD); curriculum studies (M Ed,

Ed D); development studies (M Admin, MA, D Admin, PhD); didactics (M Ed, Ed D); education (M Tech); education management (M Ed, Ed D); educational psychology (M Ed); English (MA); environmental education (M Ed); French (MA, PhD); German (MA, PhD); Greek (MA); guidance and counseling (M Ed); health studies (MA, PhD), including health sciences education (MA), health services management (MA), medical and surgical nursing science (critical care general) (MA), midwifery and neonatal nursing science (MA), trauma and emergency care (MA); history (MA, PhD); history of education (Ed D); inclusive education (M Ed, Ed D); information and communications technology policy and regulation (MA); information science (MA, MIS, PhD); international politics (MA, PhD); Islamic studies (MA, PhD); Italian (MA, PhD); Judaica (MA, PhD); linguistics (MA, PhD); mathematical education (M Ed); mathematics education (MA); missiology (M Th, D Th); modern Hebrew (MA, PhD); musicology (MA, MMus, D Mus, PhD); natural science education (M Ed); New Testament (M Th, D Th); Old Testament (D Th); pastoral therapy (M Th, D Th); philosophy (MA); philosophy of education (M Ed, Ed D); politics (MA, PhD); Portuguese (MA, PhD); practical theology (M Th, D Th); psychology (MA, MS, PhD); psychology of education (M Ed, Ed D); public health (MA); religious studies (MA, D Th, PhD); Romance languages (MA); Russian (MA, PhD); Semitic languages (MA, PhD); social behavior studies in HIV/AIDS (MA); social science (mental health) (MA); social science in development studies (MA); social science in psychology (MA); social science in social work (MA); social science in sociology (MA); social work (MSW, DSW, PhD); socio-education (M Ed, Ed D); sociolinguistics (MA); sociology (MA, PhD); Spanish (MA, PhD); systematic theology (M Th, D Th); TESOL (teaching English to speakers of other languages) (MA); theological ethics (M Th, D Th); theory of literature (MA, PhD); urban ministries (D Th); urban ministry (M Th).

University of South Carolina, The Graduate School, College of Nursing, Program in Clinical Nursing, Columbia, SC 29208. Offers acute care clinical specialist (MSN); acute care nurse practitioner (MSN); women's health nurse practitioner (MSN). *Accreditation:* AACN. Part-time programs available. *Degree requirements:* For master's, thesis or alternative. *Entrance requirements:* For master's, GRE General Test or MAT, BS in nursing, RN licensure. Additional exam requirements/recommendations for international students: Required—TOEFL (minimum score 570 paper-based). Electronic applications accepted. *Faculty research:* Systems research, evidence based practice, breast cancer, violence.

Ursuline College, School of Graduate Studies, Programs in Nursing, Pepper Pike, OH 44124-4398. Offers care management (MSN); nurse practitioner (MSN); nursing (DNP); nursing education (MSN); palliative care (MSN). *Accreditation:* AACN. Part-time programs available. *Faculty:* 6 full-time (all women), 13 part-time/adjunct (10 women). *Students:* 9 full-time (7 women), 245 part-time (235 women); includes 69 minority (58 Black or African American, non-Hispanic/Latino; 6 Asian, non-Hispanic/Latino; 2 Hispanic/Latino; 3 Two or more races, non-Hispanic/Latino), 1 international. Average age 36. 91 applicants, 79% accepted, 60 enrolled. In 2013, 57 master's, 2 doctorates awarded. *Degree requirements:* For master's, comprehensive exam. *Entrance requirements:* For master's, minimum undergraduate GPA of 3.0, bachelor's degree in nursing, eligibility for or current Ohio RN license. Additional exam requirements/recommendations for international students: Required—TOEFL (minimum score 500 paper-based). *Application deadline:* For fall admission, 8/1 priority date for domestic students. Applications are processed on a rolling basis. Application fee: $25. *Expenses: Tuition:* Full-time $16,920; part-time $940 per credit. *Required fees:* $270. *Financial support:* In 2013–14, 9 students received support. Federal Work-Study available. Financial award application deadline: 3/1. *Unit head:* Dr. Janet Baker, Director, 440-864-8172, Fax: 440-684-6053, E-mail: jbaker@ursuline.edu. *Application contact:* Stephanie Pratt, Graduate Admission Coordinator, 440-646-8119, Fax: 440-684-6138, E-mail: graduateadmissions@ursuline.edu.

Nurse Anesthesia

Adventist University of Health Sciences, Program in Nurse Anesthesia, Orlando, FL 32803. Offers MS. *Accreditation:* AANA/CANAEP. *Entrance requirements:* For master's, GRE or MAT, minimum undergraduate cumulative GPA of 3.0, 1 year of intensive critical care nursing experience, 3 recommendations, interview.

Albany Medical College, Center for Nurse Anesthesiology, Albany, NY 12208. Offers anesthesia (MS). *Accreditation:* AANA/CANAEP. *Degree requirements:* For master's, thesis, thesis proposal/clinical research. *Entrance requirements:* For master's, GRE General Test, BSN or appropriate bachelor's degree, current RN license, critical care experience, organic chemistry, research methods. Electronic applications accepted. *Expenses:* Contact institution.

Arkansas State University, Graduate School, College of Nursing and Health Professions, School of Nursing, State University, AR 72467. Offers aging studies (Certificate); health care management (Certificate); health communications (Certificate); health sciences (MS); health sciences education (Certificate); nurse anesthesia (MSN); nursing (MSN); nursing practice (DNP). *Accreditation:* AANA/CANAEP (one or more programs are accredited). Part-time programs available. *Faculty:* 16 full-time (14 women). *Students:* 96 full-time (34 women), 120 part-time (108 women); includes 38 minority (26 Black or African American, non-Hispanic/Latino; 3 American Indian or Alaska Native, non-Hispanic/Latino; 2 Asian, non-Hispanic/Latino; 4 Hispanic/Latino; 3 Two or more races, non-Hispanic/Latino). Average age 33. 153 applicants, 32% accepted, 44 enrolled. In 2013, 103 master's awarded. *Degree requirements:* For master's, comprehensive exam, thesis or alternative; for doctorate, comprehensive exam, thesis/dissertation. *Entrance requirements:* For master's, GRE General Test or MAT, appropriate bachelor's degree, current Arkansas nursing license, CPR certification, physical examination, professional liability insurance, critical care experience, ACLS Certification, PALS Certification, interview, immunization records, personal goal statement, health assessment; for doctorate, GRE or MAT, appropriate master's degree, current Arkansas nursing license, CPR certification, physical examination, professional liability insurance, critical care experience, ACLS Certification, PALS Certification, interview, immunization records, personal goal statement, health assessment, TB skin test, NCLEX-RN Exam, background check. Additional exam requirements/recommendations for international students: Required—TOEFL (minimum score 550 paper-based; 79 iBT), IELTS (minimum score 6), PTE (minimum score 56). *Application deadline:* Applications are processed on a rolling basis. Electronic applications accepted. *Expenses:* Contact institution. *Financial support:* In 2013–14, 9 students received support. Fellowships, career-related internships or fieldwork, scholarships/grants, and unspecified assistantships available. Financial award application deadline: 7/1; financial award applicants required to submit FAFSA. *Unit head:* Dr. Marilyn Duran, Chair, 870-972-3074, Fax: 870-972-2954, E-mail: mduran@astate.edu. *Application contact:* Vickey Ring, Graduate Admissions Coordinator, 870-972-3029, Fax: 870-972-3857, E-mail: vickeyring@astate.edu.
Website: http://www.astate.edu/college/conhp/departments/nursing/

Barry University, College of Health Sciences, Program in Anesthesiology, Miami Shores, FL 33161-6695. Offers MS. *Accreditation:* AANA/CANAEP. *Degree requirements:* For master's, comprehensive exam. *Entrance requirements:* For master's, GRE General Test, minimum GPA of 3.0; 2 courses in chemistry (1 with lab); minimum 1 year critical care experience; BSN or RN; 4-year bachelor's degree in health sciences, nursing, biology, or chemistry. Electronic applications accepted. *Faculty research:* Use of computers in education, psychological well-bring of health care providers.

Baylor College of Medicine, School of Allied Health Sciences, Graduate Program in Nurse Anesthesia, Houston, TX 77030-3498. Offers DNP. *Accreditation:* AANA/CANAEP. *Degree requirements:* For doctorate, comprehensive exam, thesis/dissertation. *Entrance requirements:* For doctorate, GRE General Test, Texas nursing license, 1 year of work experience in critical care nursing, minimum GPA of 3.0, BSN, statistics, organic chemistry. Electronic applications accepted. *Expenses:* Contact institution. *Faculty research:* Education, simulation.

Bloomsburg University of Pennsylvania, School of Graduate Studies, College of Science and Technology, Department of Nursing, Bloomsburg, PA 17815. Offers adult and family nurse practitioner (MSN); community health (MSN); nurse anesthesia (MSN); nursing (MSN); nursing administration (MSN). *Accreditation:* AACN; AANA/CANAEP. *Faculty:* 5 full-time (all women), 7 part-time/adjunct (all women). *Students:* 62 full-time (52 women), 26 part-time (17 women); includes 8 minority (6 Black or African American, non-Hispanic/Latino; 1 Asian, non-Hispanic/Latino; 1 Hispanic/Latino). Average age 35. 61 applicants, 84% accepted, 14 enrolled. In 2013, 36 master's awarded. *Degree requirements:* For master's, thesis (for some programs), clinical experience. *Entrance requirements:* For master's, minimum QPA of 3.0, personal statement, 2 letters of recommendation, nursing license. Additional exam requirements/recommendations for international students: Required—TOEFL. *Application deadline:* For fall admission, 1/1 for domestic students; for spring admission, 8/1 for domestic students. Applications are processed on a rolling basis. Application fee: $35 ($60 for international students). Electronic applications accepted. *Expenses:* Tuition, state resident: full-time $7956; part-time $442 per credit. Tuition, nonresident: full-time $11,934; part-time $663 per credit. *Required fees:* $95.50 per credit. $55 per semester. Tuition and fees vary according to course load. *Financial support:* Unspecified assistantships available. *Unit head:* Dr. Noreen Chikotas, Coordinator, 570-389-4609, Fax: 570-389-5008, E-mail: nchikota@bloomu.edu. *Application contact:* Jennifer Richard, Administrative Assistant, 570-389-4015, Fax: 570-389-3054, E-mail: jrichard@bloomu.edu.
Website: http://www.bloomu.edu/nursing

Boston College, William F. Connell School of Nursing, Chestnut Hill, MA 02467-3800. Offers adult-gerontology nursing (MS); community health nursing (MS); family health (MS); forensic nursing (MS); maternal/child health nursing (MS), including pediatric and women's health; nurse anesthesia (MS); nursing (PhD); palliative care (MS), including adult and pediatric; psychiatric-mental health nursing (MS); MBA/MS; MS/MA; MS/PhD. *Accreditation:* AACN; AANA/CANAEP (one or more programs are accredited). Part-time programs available. *Faculty:* 47 full-time (43 women), 42 part-time/adjunct (39 women). *Students:* 199 full-time (180 women), 79 part-time (73 women); includes 44 minority (14 Black or African American, non-Hispanic/Latino; 1 American Indian or Alaska Native, non-Hispanic/Latino; 13 Asian, non-Hispanic/Latino; 12 Hispanic/Latino; 4 Two or more races, non-Hispanic/Latino), 7 international. Average age 31. 502 applicants, 39% accepted, 87 enrolled. In 2013, 105 master's, 8 doctorates awarded. *Degree requirements:* For master's, comprehensive exam, research project; for doctorate, comprehensive exam, thesis/dissertation, computer literacy exam or foreign language. *Entrance requirements:* For master's, bachelor's degree in nursing; for doctorate, GRE General Test, MS in nursing. Additional exam requirements/recommendations for international students: Required—TOEFL (minimum score 600 paper-based; 100 iBT). *Application deadline:* For fall admission, 9/30 for domestic and international students; for winter admission, 1/15 for domestic and international students; for spring admission, 3/15 for domestic and international students. Applications are processed on a rolling basis. Application fee: $40. Electronic applications accepted. *Financial support:* In 2013–14, 174 students received support, including 7 fellowships with full tuition reimbursements available (averaging $20,000 per year), 21 teaching assistantships (averaging $4,800 per year); research assistantships, scholarships/grants, health care benefits, tuition waivers (partial), and unspecified assistantships also available. Support available to part-time students. Financial award application deadline: 3/1; financial award applicants required to submit FAFSA. *Faculty research:* Sexual and reproductive health, health promotion/illness prevention, eating disorders, violence, symptom management. *Total annual research expenditures:* $1.1 million. *Unit head:* Dr. Susan Gennaro, Dean, 617-552-4251, Fax: 617-552-0931, E-mail: susan.gennaro@bc.edu. *Application contact:* MaryBeth Crowley, Graduate Programs Assistant, 617-552-4928, Fax: 617-552-2121, E-mail: csongrad@bc.edu.
Website: http://www.bc.edu/schools/son/

Bradley University, Graduate School, College of Education and Health Sciences, Department of Nursing, Peoria, IL 61625-0002. Offers nurse administered anesthesia (MSN); nursing administration (MSN). Part-time and evening/weekend programs available. *Degree requirements:* For master's, comprehensive exam, thesis optional. *Entrance requirements:* For master's, GRE General Test or MAT, interview, Illinois RN license, advanced cardiac life support certification, pediatric advanced life support certification, 3 letters of recommendation. Additional exam requirements/recommendations for international students: Required—TOEFL (minimum score 550 paper-based; 79 iBT). *Expenses: Tuition:* Full-time $14,580; part-time $810 per credit hour. Tuition and fees vary according to course load and program.

Bryan College of Health Sciences, School of Nurse Anesthesia, Lincoln, NE 68506-1398. Offers MS. *Accreditation:* AANA/CANAEP.

California State University, Fullerton, Graduate Studies, College of Health and Human Development, Department of Nursing, Fullerton, CA 92834-9480. Offers leadership (MSN); nurse anesthesia (MSN); nurse educator (MSN); nursing (DNP); women's health care (MSN). *Accreditation:* AACN; AANA/CANAEP. Part-time programs available. *Students:* 186 full-time (138 women), 134 part-time (120 women); includes 174 minority (15 Black or African American, non-Hispanic/Latino; 3 American Indian or Alaska Native, non-Hispanic/Latino; 92 Asian, non-Hispanic/Latino; 50 Hispanic/Latino; 2 Native Hawaiian or other Pacific Islander, non-Hispanic/Latino; 12 Two or more races,

non-Hispanic/Latino), 3 international. Average age 35. 431 applicants, 38% accepted, 131 enrolled. In 2013, 117 master's awarded. Application fee: $55. *Financial support:* Career-related internships or fieldwork, Federal Work-Study, institutionally sponsored loans, scholarships/grants, and traineeships available. Support available to part-time students. Financial award application deadline: 3/1; financial award applicants required to submit FAFSA. *Unit head:* Dr. Cindy Greenberg, Chair, 657-278-3336. *Application contact:* Admissions/Applications, 657-278-2371.
Website: http://nursing.fullerton.edu/

Case Western Reserve University, Frances Payne Bolton School of Nursing, Master's Programs in Nursing, Program in Nurse Anesthesia, Cleveland, OH 44106. Offers MSN. *Accreditation:* AANA/CANAEP. *Students:* 51 (13 women); includes 3 minority (1 Black or African American, non-Hispanic/Latino; 1 Asian, non-Hispanic/Latino; 1 Hispanic/Latino). 145 applicants, 23% accepted, 27 enrolled. In 2013, 26 master's awarded. *Degree requirements:* For master's, thesis optional. *Entrance requirements:* For master's, GRE General Test or MAT. *Application deadline:* For fall admission, 1/15 for domestic students. Application fee: $75. *Financial support:* Research assistantships, teaching assistantships, institutionally sponsored loans, and tuition waivers (partial) available. Support available to part-time students. Financial award application deadline: 6/30. *Faculty research:* Mechanical ventilation antioxidant trial, intravenous function and mechanical ventilation, impact of taxane on peripheral nerve function. *Unit head:* Maryanne McDowell, Head, 216-368-0221, E-mail: mxm861@case.edu. *Application contact:* Donna Hassik, Admissions Coordinator, 216-368-5253, Fax: 216-368-0124, E-mail: dmh7@case.edu.
Website: http://fpb.cwru.edu/MSN/anesthesia.shtm

Central Connecticut State University, School of Graduate Studies, School of Arts and Sciences, Department of Biology, New Britain, CT 06050-4010. Offers biological sciences (MA, MS), including anesthesia (MS), ecology and environmental sciences (MA), general biology (MA), health sciences (MS), professional education (MS); biology (Certificate). Part-time and evening/weekend programs available. *Faculty:* 4 full-time (0 women), 2 part-time/adjunct (both women). *Students:* 130 full-time (85 women), 34 part-time (23 women); includes 25 minority (9 Black or African American, non-Hispanic/Latino; 11 Asian, non-Hispanic/Latino; 3 Hispanic/Latino; 2 Two or more races, non-Hispanic/Latino), 1 international. Average age 30. 30 applicants, 67% accepted, 11 enrolled. In 2013, 46 master's, 10 other advanced degrees awarded. *Degree requirements:* For master's, comprehensive exam, thesis or alternative; for Certificate, qualifying exam. *Entrance requirements:* For master's and Certificate, minimum undergraduate GPA of 2.7, essay, letters of recommendation. Additional exam requirements/recommendations for international students: Required—TOEFL (minimum score 550 paper-based; 79 iBT). *Application deadline:* For fall admission, 6/1 for domestic students, 5/1 for international students; for spring admission, 11/1 for domestic and international students. Applications are processed on a rolling basis. Application fee: $50. Electronic applications accepted. Part-time tuition and fees vary according to degree level. *Financial support:* In 2013–14, 2 students received support, including 2 research assistantships; career-related internships or fieldwork, Federal Work-Study, scholarships/grants, and unspecified assistantships also available. Support available to part-time students. Financial award application deadline: 3/1; financial award applicants required to submit FAFSA. *Faculty research:* Environmental science, anesthesia, health sciences, zoology, animal behavior. *Unit head:* Dr. Douglas Carter, Chair, 860-832-2645, E-mail: carterd@ccsu.edu. *Application contact:* Patricia Gardner, Associate Director of Graduate Studies, 860-832-2350, Fax: 860-832-2362, E-mail: graduateadmissions@ccsu.edu.
Website: http://www.ccsu.edu/page.cfm?p=14516

Columbia University, School of Nursing, Program in Nurse Anesthesia, New York, NY 10032. Offers MS, Adv C. *Accreditation:* AACN; AANA/CANAEP. *Entrance requirements:* For master's, GRE General Test, NCLEX, BSN, 1 year of intensive care unit experience; for Adv C, MSN, 1 year of intensive care unit experience. Additional exam requirements/recommendations for international students: Required—TOEFL (minimum score 100 iBT). Electronic applications accepted.

Drexel University, College of Nursing and Health Professions, Department of Nurse Anesthesia, Philadelphia, PA 19104-2875. Offers MSN. *Accreditation:* AACN; AANA/CANAEP. Electronic applications accepted.

Duke University, School of Nursing, Durham, NC 27708-0586. Offers acute care pediatric nurse practitioner (MSN); adult-gerontology nurse practitioner - acute care (MSN, Post Master's Certificate); adult-gerontology nurse practitioner - primary care (MSN, Post Master's Certificate), including adult-gerontology nurse practitioner (MSN), cardiology, oncology; family nurse practitioner (MSN); neonatal nurse practitioner (MSN); nurse anesthesia (MSN, DNP); nursing (PhD); nursing and health care leadership (MSN); nursing education (MSN); nursing informatics (MSN, Post Master's Certificate); pediatric nurse practitioner - primary care (MSN). *Accreditation:* AACN; AANA/CANAEP. Part-time and evening/weekend programs available. Postbaccalaureate distance learning degree programs offered (minimal on-campus study). *Faculty:* 74 full-time (64 women), 7 part-time/adjunct (4 women). *Students:* 127 full-time (113 women), 473 part-time (433 women); includes 131 minority (54 Black or African American, non-Hispanic/Latino; 9 American Indian or Alaska Native, non-Hispanic/Latino; 36 Asian, non-Hispanic/Latino; 27 Hispanic/Latino; 5 Native Hawaiian or other Pacific Islander, non-Hispanic/Latino), 14 international. Average age 34. 516 applicants, 50% accepted, 190 enrolled. In 2013, 179 master's, 49 doctorates, 23 other advanced degrees awarded. Terminal master's awarded for partial completion of doctoral program. *Degree requirements:* For master's, thesis optional; for doctorate, capstone project. *Entrance requirements:* For master's, GRE General Test (waived if undergraduate GPA of 3.4 or higher), 1 year of nursing experience (recommended), BSN, minimum GPA of 3.0, previous course work in statistics; for doctorate, GRE General Test (waived if undergraduate GPA of 3.4 or higher), BSN or MSN, minimum GPA of 3.0, portfolio, resume, personal statement, undergraduate statistics course, current licensure as a registered nurse, transcripts from all post-secondary institutions; for Post Master's Certificate, MSN, licensure or eligibility as a professional nurse, transcripts from all post-secondary institutions, previous course work in statistics. Additional exam requirements/recommendations for international students: Recommended—TOEFL (minimum score 550 paper-based; 83 iBT), IELTS (minimum score 7). *Application deadline:* For fall admission, 12/1 for domestic and international students; for spring admission, 5/1 for domestic and international students. Application fee: $50. Electronic applications accepted. *Expenses:* Contact institution. *Financial support:* Career-related internships or fieldwork, institutionally sponsored loans, scholarships/grants, traineeships, and tuition waivers (partial) available. Support available to part-time students. Financial award applicants required to submit FAFSA. *Faculty research:* Cardiovascular disease, caregiver skill training, data mining, prostate cancer, neonatal immune system. *Unit head:* Dr. Catherine L. Gilliss, Dean/Vice Chancellor for Nursing Affairs, 919-684-9444, Fax: 919-684-9414, E-mail: catherine.gilliss@duke.edu. *Application contact:* Ernie Rushing, Lead Admissions Processor/Admissions Officer, 919-668-6274, Fax: 919-668-4693, E-mail: stephen.rushing@dm.duke.edu.
Website: http://www.nursing.duke.edu/

Fairfield University, School of Nursing, Fairfield, CT 06824-5195. Offers advanced practice (DNP); executive (DNP); family nurse practitioner (MSN, DNP); nurse anesthesia (DNP); nursing leadership (MSN); psychiatric nurse practitioner (MSN, DNP). *Accreditation:* AACN; AANA/CANAEP. Part-time programs available. *Faculty:* 22 full-time (all women), 28 part-time/adjunct (23 women). *Students:* 27 full-time (23 women), 157 part-time (136 women); includes 37 minority (15 Black or African American, non-Hispanic/Latino; 10 Asian, non-Hispanic/Latino; 8 Hispanic/Latino; 2 Native Hawaiian or other Pacific Islander, non-Hispanic/Latino; 2 Two or more races, non-Hispanic/Latino), 8 international. Average age 37. 132 applicants, 52% accepted, 59 enrolled. In 2013, 39 master's, 3 doctorates awarded. *Degree requirements:* For master's, capstone project. *Entrance requirements:* For master's, minimum QPA of 3.0, RN license, resume, 2 recommendations; for doctorate, GRE (nurse anesthesia applicants only), MSN (minimum QPA of 3.2) or BSN (minimum QPA of 3.0); critical care nursing experience (for nurse anesthesia DNP candidates). Additional exam requirements/recommendations for international students: Required—TOEFL (minimum score 550 paper-based; 80 iBT) or IELTS (minimum score 6.5). *Application deadline:* For fall admission, 5/15 for international students; for spring admission, 10/15 for international students. Applications are processed on a rolling basis. Application fee: $60. Electronic applications accepted. *Expenses:* Contact institution. *Financial support:* In 2013–14, 4 students received support. Unspecified assistantships available. Financial award applicants required to submit FAFSA. *Faculty research:* Aging and sexual health, psychosocial needs of men with prostate cancer, nurse practitioner education, mentoring, psychiatric and mental health, incarceration of the mentally ill, recovery in schizophrenia, palliative and end of life care, maternal and child health, breastfeeding and lactation consultant, stress and emotional eating, care of veterans and their families, falls prevention and the elderly, health care leadership, interprofessional education, academic partnerships. *Total annual research expenditures:* $775,000. *Unit head:* Dr. Lynn Babington, Dean, 203-254-4000 Ext. 2701, Fax: 203-254-4126, E-mail: lbabington@fairfield.edu. *Application contact:* Marianne Gumpper, Director of Graduate and Continuing Studies Admission, 203-254-4184, Fax: 203-254-4073, E-mail: gradadmis@fairfield.edu.
Website: http://fairfield.edu/son

Florida Gulf Coast University, College of Health Professions, Program in Nurse Anesthesia, Fort Myers, FL 33965-6565. Offers MSN. *Accreditation:* AACN; AANA/CANAEP. Part-time programs available. *Degree requirements:* For master's, thesis or alternative. *Entrance requirements:* For master's, GRE General Test, MAT, minimum GPA of 3.0. Additional exam requirements/recommendations for international students: Required—TOEFL (minimum score 550 paper-based). Electronic applications accepted. *Faculty research:* Gerontology, community health, ethical and legal aspects of health care, critical care.

Gannon University, School of Graduate Studies, Morosky College of Health Professions and Sciences, Villa Maria School of Nursing, Program in Nurse Anesthesia, Erie, PA 16541-0001. Offers MSN, Certificate. Part-time and evening/weekend programs available. *Students:* 1 part-time (0 women). Average age 41. *Degree requirements:* For master's, thesis (for some programs), practicum. *Entrance requirements:* For degree, completion of statistics and research courses, minimum GPA of 3.0, 4 letters of recommendation, 2 years of clinical experience, interview. Additional exam requirements/recommendations for international students: Required—TOEFL (minimum score 79 iBT). *Application deadline:* For winter admission, 5/1 for domestic students. Application fee: $25. Electronic applications accepted. *Expenses: Tuition:* Full-time $15,930; part-time $885 per credit. *Required fees:* $430; $18 per credit. Tuition and fees vary according to course load, degree level and program. *Unit head:* Dr. Kathleen Patterson, Director, 814-871-5547, E-mail: patterso018@gannon.edu. *Application contact:* Kara Morgan, Director of Graduate Admissions, 814-871-5831, Fax: 814-871-5827, E-mail: graduate@gannon.edu.

Georgetown University, Graduate School of Arts and Sciences, School of Nursing and Health Studies, Washington, DC 20057. Offers acute care nurse practitioner (MS); clinical nurse specialist (MS); family nurse practitioner (MS); nurse anesthesia (MS); nurse-midwifery (MS); nursing (DNP); nursing education (MS). *Accreditation:* AACN; AANA/CANAEP (one or more programs are accredited); ACNM/ACME (one or more programs are accredited). *Degree requirements:* For master's, thesis optional. *Entrance requirements:* For master's, GRE General Test or MAT, bachelor's degree in nursing from NLN-accredited school, minimum undergraduate GPA of 3.0. Additional exam requirements/recommendations for international students: Required—TOEFL. Application fee: $50 ($55 for international students). *Financial support:* Scholarships/grants and traineeships available. Financial award applicants required to submit FAFSA. *Unit head:* Dr. Patricia Ann Cloonan, Dean, 202-687-7318. *Application contact:* Graduate School Admissions Office, 202-687-5568.

Georgia Regents University, The Graduate School, Nursing Anesthesia Program, Augusta, GA 30912. Offers MSN. *Accreditation:* AACN; AANA/CANAEP. *Students:* 68 full-time (48 women), 1 (woman) part-time; includes 14 minority (6 Black or African American, non-Hispanic/Latino; 2 Asian, non-Hispanic/Latino; 5 Hispanic/Latino; 1 Two or more races, non-Hispanic/Latino). Average age 29. 108 applicants, 24% accepted, 18 enrolled. In 2013, 15 master's awarded. *Entrance requirements:* For master's, GRE General Test, Georgia RN license, at least 1 year of critical care RN experience. Additional exam requirements/recommendations for international students: Required—TOEFL (minimum score 550 paper-based; 79 iBT). *Application deadline:* For fall admission, 11/1 for domestic and international students. Application fee: $50. Electronic applications accepted. *Unit head:* Dr. Lucy Marion, Dean, 706-721-3771, Fax: 706-721-8169, E-mail: lumarion@georgiahealth.edu. *Application contact:* Melvenia Blanchard, Office Specialist, 706-721-9558, Fax: 706-721-8169, E-mail: mblanchard@georgiahealth.edu.
Website: http://www.gru.edu/nursing/nap.php

Goldfarb School of Nursing at Barnes-Jewish College, Graduate Programs, St. Louis, MO 63110. Offers adult acute care nurse practitioner (MSN); adult nurse practitioner (MSN); nurse anesthesia (MSN); nurse educator (MSN); nurse executive (MSN); DNP/PhD. *Accreditation:* AACN; AANA/CANAEP. Part-time and evening/weekend programs available. Postbaccalaureate distance learning degree programs offered (minimal on-campus study). *Faculty:* 42 full-time (39 women), 6 part-time/adjunct (all women). *Students:* 81 full-time (67 women), 85 part-time (77 women); includes 28 minority (18 Black or African American, non-Hispanic/Latino; 2 Asian, non-Hispanic/Latino; 3 Hispanic/Latino; 3 Native Hawaiian or other Pacific Islander, non-Hispanic/Latino; 2 Two or more races, non-Hispanic/Latino). *Degree requirements:* For master's, thesis or alternative. *Entrance requirements:* For master's, 2 references, personal statement, curriculum vitae or resume. Additional exam requirements/recommendations for international students: Required—TOEFL (minimum score 575 paper-based; 85 iBT). *Application deadline:* For fall admission, 2/1 priority date for international students; for spring admission, 10/1 priority date for international students. Applications are processed on a rolling basis. Application fee: $50. *Expenses: Tuition:* Full-time $12,960; part-time $720 per credit hour. *Required fees:* $295; $720 per credit hour. Tuition and fees vary according to course load. *Financial support:* Fellowships, research assistantships, Federal Work-Study, institutionally sponsored loans, and scholarships/grants available. Support available to part-time students. Financial award applicants required to submit FAFSA. *Faculty research:* HIV stigma, HIV symptom management, palliative care with children and their families, heart disease prevention in Hispanic women, depression in the well elderly, alternative therapies in pre-term infants. *Unit head:* Dr. Michael Bleich, Dean, 314-362-0956, Fax: 314-362-0984, E-mail: mbleich@bjc.org. *Application contact:* Margaret Anne O'Connor, Program Officer, 314-454-7557, Fax: 314-362-0984, E-mail: maoconnor@bjc.org.

Gonzaga University, School of Education, Program in Anesthesiology Education, Spokane, WA 99258. Offers M Anesth Ed. *Accreditation:* AANA/CANAEP. Part-time programs available. *Students:* 8 full-time (3 women), 8 part-time (2 women); includes 7 minority (1 Black or African American, non-Hispanic/Latino; 2 American Indian or Alaska Native, non-Hispanic/Latino; 3 Asian, non-Hispanic/Latino; 1 Two or more races, non-Hispanic/Latino). Average age 34. In 2013, 8 master's awarded. *Degree requirements:* For master's, comprehensive exam. *Entrance requirements:* For master's, GRE General Test or MAT. Additional exam requirements/recommendations for international students: Required—TOEFL. *Application deadline:* For fall admission, 12/1 for domestic students. Application fee: $50. Electronic applications accepted. *Expenses:* Contact institution. *Financial support:* Application deadline: 2/1; applicants required to submit FAFSA. *Unit head:* Dr. Dan Mahoney, University Program Director, 509-328-4220 Ext. 3584. *Application contact:* Julie McCulloh, Dean of Admissions, 509-313-6592, Fax: 509-313-5780, E-mail: mcculloh@gu.gonzaga.edu.

Gooding Institute of Nurse Anesthesia, Program in Nurse Anesthesia, Panama City, FL 32401. Offers MS. *Accreditation:* AANA/CANAEP. *Degree requirements:* For master's, comprehensive exam, thesis. *Entrance requirements:* For master's, GRE General Test, BSN or BA, RN license.

Inter American University of Puerto Rico, Arecibo Campus, Program in Anesthesia, Arecibo, PR 00614-4050. Offers MS. *Accreditation:* AANA/CANAEP. *Degree requirements:* For master's, comprehensive exam, thesis optional. *Entrance requirements:* For master's, GRE, EXADEP, 2 letters of recommendation, bachelor's degree in nursing, interview, minimum GPA of 3.0 in last 60 credits, minimum 1 year experience.

La Roche College, School of Graduate Studies and Adult Education, Program in Health Sciences, Pittsburgh, PA 15237-5898. Offers nurse anesthesia (MS). *Accreditation:* AANA/CANAEP. *Faculty:* 2 full-time (0 women), 4 part-time/adjunct (2 women). *Students:* 37 full-time (27 women), 1 (woman) part-time, 2 international. Average age 30. 18 applicants, 100% accepted, 18 enrolled. In 2013, 13 master's awarded. *Degree requirements:* For master's, thesis optional. *Entrance requirements:* For master's, GRE General Test, prior acceptance to the Allegheny Valley School of Anesthesia. *Application deadline:* For fall admission, 12/31 for domestic students. Application fee: $50. Electronic applications accepted. *Expenses: Tuition:* Full-time $15,360. *Financial support:* Application deadline: 3/31; applicants required to submit FAFSA. *Unit head:* Dr. Don Fujito, Coordinator, 412-536-1157, Fax: 412-536-1175, E-mail: fujitod1@laroche.edu. *Application contact:* Hope Schiffgens, Director of Graduate Studies and Adult Education, 412-536-1266, Fax: 412-536-1283, E-mail: schombh1@laroche.edu.

La Salle University, School of Nursing and Health Sciences, Program in Nursing, Philadelphia, PA 19141-1199. Offers adult gerontology primary care nurse practitioner (MSN, Certificate); adult health and illness clinical nurse specialist (MSN); adult-gerontology clinical nurse specialist (MSN, Certificate); clinical nurse leader (MSN); family primary care nurse practitioner (MSN, Certificate); gerontology (Certificate); nurse anesthetist (MSN, Certificate); nursing (MSN, Certificate); nursing administration (MSN, Certificate); nursing education (Certificate); nursing practice (DNP); nursing service administration (MSN); public health nursing (MSN, Certificate); school nursing (Certificate); MSN/MBA; MSN/MPH. *Accreditation:* AANA/CANAEP. Part-time programs available. Postbaccalaureate distance learning degree programs offered (minimal on-campus study). *Faculty:* 13 full-time (12 women), 10 part-time/adjunct (8 women). *Students:* 4 full-time (all women), 379 part-time (331 women); includes 119 minority (70 Black or African American, non-Hispanic/Latino; 2 American Indian or Alaska Native, non-Hispanic/Latino; 31 Asian, non-Hispanic/Latino; 12 Hispanic/Latino; 4 Two or more races, non-Hispanic/Latino), 1 international. Average age 37. 133 applicants, 85% accepted, 63 enrolled. In 2013, 72 master's, 3 doctorates, 26 other advanced degrees awarded. *Degree requirements:* For doctorate, minimum of 1,000 hours of post baccalaureate clinical practice supervised by preceptors. *Entrance requirements:* For master's, GRE, MAT, or GMAT (for students with BSN GPA of less than 3.2), baccalaureate degree in nursing from an NLNAC- or CCNE-accredited program or an MSN Bridge program; Pennsylvania RN license; 2 letters of reference; resume; statement of philosophy articulating professional values and future educational goal; 1 year of work experience as a registered nurse; for doctorate, GRE (waived for applicants with MSN cumulative GPA of 3.7 or above), MSN from nationally-accredited program or master's degree, MBA or MHA from nationally-accredited program; resume or curriculum vitae; 2 letters of reference; interview; for Certificate, GRE, MAT, or GMAT (for students with BSN GPA of less than 3.2, baccalaureate degree in nursing from an NLNAC- or CCNE-accredited program or an MSN Bridge program; Pennsylvania RN license; 2 letters of reference; resume; statement of philosophy articulating professional values and future educational goal; 1 year of work experience as a registered nurse. Additional exam requirements/recommendations for international students: Required—TOEFL. *Application deadline:* For fall admission, 8/15 priority date for domestic students, 7/15 for international students; for spring admission, 12/15 priority date for domestic students, 11/15 for international students; for summer admission, 4/15 priority date for domestic students, 3/15 for international students. Applications are processed on a rolling basis. Application fee: $35. Electronic applications accepted. Application fee is waived when completed online. *Expenses:* Contact institution. *Financial support:* In 2013–14, 48 students received support. Teaching assistantships, scholarships/grants, and traineeships available. Support available to part-time students. Financial award application deadline: 8/31; financial award applicants required to submit FAFSA. *Unit head:* Dr. Patricia M. Dillon, Director, 215-951-1322, Fax: 215-951-1896, E-mail: msnapn@lasalle.edu. *Application contact:* Paul J. Reilly, Assistant Vice President, Enrollment Services, 215-951-1946, Fax: 215-951-1462, E-mail: reilly@lasalle.edu.

Lincoln Memorial University, Caylor School of Nursing, Harrogate, TN 37752-1901. Offers family nurse practitioner (MSN); nurse anesthesia (MSN); psychiatric mental health nurse practitioner (MSN). *Accreditation:* AANA/CANAEP. Part-time programs available. *Entrance requirements:* For master's, GRE.

Louisiana State University Health Sciences Center, School of Nursing, New Orleans, LA 70112-2223. Offers advanced public/community health nursing (MN); clinical nurse specialist (MN); nurse anesthesia (MN); nurse practitioner (MN); nursing (DNS). *Accreditation:* AACN; AANA/CANAEP (one or more programs are accredited). Part-time programs available. *Degree requirements:* For master's, thesis optional; for doctorate, thesis/dissertation. *Entrance requirements:* For master's, GRE General Test, MAT, minimum GPA of 3.0; for doctorate, GRE General Test, minimum GPA of 3.5. Additional exam requirements/recommendations for international students: Required—TOEFL. Electronic applications accepted. *Faculty research:* Advanced clinical practice, nursing education, health, social support, nursing administration.

Lourdes University, Graduate School, Sylvania, OH 43560-2898. Offers business (MBA); leadership (M Ed); nurse anesthesia (MSN); nurse educator (MSN); nurse leader (MSN); organizational leadership (MOL); reading (M Ed); teaching and curriculum (M Ed); theology (MA). Evening/weekend programs available. *Entrance requirements:* Additional exam requirements/recommendations for international students: Required—TOEFL. *Application deadline:* For fall admission, 6/15 priority date for domestic students; for spring admission, 11/1 priority date for domestic students. Application fee: $25. *Application contact:* Melissa Bergfeld, Administrative Assistant, 419-824-3517, Fax: 419-824-3510, E-mail: mbergfeld2@lourdes.edu.
Website: http://www.lourdes.edu/gradschool.aspx

Marshall University, Academic Affairs Division, College of Business, Program in Nurse Anesthesia, Huntington, WV 25755. Offers DMPNA. Program offered jointly with Charleston Area Medical Center. *Students:* 78 full-time (46 women); includes 5 minority (1 Black or African American, non-Hispanic/Latino; 3 Asian, non-Hispanic/Latino; 1 Hispanic/Latino). Average age 31. In 2013, 26 doctorates awarded. *Unit head:* Dr. Nancy Tierney, Director, 304-388-9950, E-mail: nancy.tierney@camc.org. *Application contact:* Information Contact, Graduate Admissions, 304-746-1900, Fax: 304-746-1902, E-mail: services@marshall.edu.
Website: http://camcinstitute.org/anesthesia/

Mayo School of Health Sciences, Doctor of Nurse Anesthesia Practice Program, Rochester, MN 55905. Offers DNAP. *Accreditation:* AANA/CANAEP. *Faculty:* 5 part-time/adjunct (3 women). *Students:* 25 full-time (14 women); includes 3 minority (2 Black or African American, non-Hispanic/Latino; 1 Asian, non-Hispanic/Latino). 127 applicants, 22% accepted, 25 enrolled. In 2013, 25 doctorates awarded. *Degree requirements:* For doctorate, comprehensive exam, research project. *Entrance requirements:* For doctorate, GRE General Test, minimum GPA of 3.0; minimum 1 year of critical care experience. Additional exam requirements/recommendations for international students: Required—TOEFL. *Application deadline:* For fall admission, 9/1 for domestic students. Application fee: $50. Electronic applications accepted. *Expenses:* Contact institution. *Financial support:* Scholarships/grants, health care benefits, and stipends available. Financial award applicants required to submit FAFSA. *Unit head:* Mary Shirk Marienau, Director, 507-284-8331, Fax: 507-284-2818, E-mail: marienau.mary@mayo.edu. *Application contact:* Julie Predmore, Administrative Assistant, 507-286-4163, Fax: 507-284-2818, E-mail: predmore.julie@mayo.edu.
Website: http://www.mayo.edu/mshs

Medical University of South Carolina, College of Health Professions, Anesthesia for Nurses Program, Charleston, SC 29425. Offers MSNA. *Accreditation:* AANA/CANAEP. *Degree requirements:* For master's, comprehensive exam, research project, clinical practica. *Entrance requirements:* For master's, GRE General Test, interview, minimum GPA of 3.0, 2 years of RN (ICU) experience, RN license. Additional exam requirements/recommendations for international students: Required—TOEFL (minimum score 600 paper-based). Electronic applications accepted. *Faculty research:* Stress in nurse anesthesia, economic changes and continuing education.

Middle Tennessee School of Anesthesia, Graduate Programs, Madison, TN 37116. Offers anesthesia (MS); anesthesia practice (DNAP). *Accreditation:* AANA/CANAEP. *Students:* 211 full-time (123 women). *Degree requirements:* For master's, project; for doctorate, capstone project. *Entrance requirements:* For master's, GRE General Test, RN license, 1 year of critical-care nursing experience, BSN, general chemistry (minimum of 3 semester hours). *Application deadline:* For fall admission, 10/31 for domestic students. Applications are processed on a rolling basis. *Financial support:* Traineeships available. *Unit head:* Dr. Chris Hulin, Dean and Program Administrator, 615-868-6503, Fax: 615-732-7676, E-mail: chris@mtsa.edu. *Application contact:* Pam Nimmo, Admissions and Financial Aid Assistant, 615-868-6503, Fax: 615-732-7662, E-mail: pam@mtsa.edu.
Website: http://www.mtsa.edu/

Midwestern University, Glendale Campus, College of Health Sciences, Arizona Campus, Program in Nurse Anesthesia, Glendale, AZ 85308. Offers MS. *Accreditation:* AANA/CANAEP. *Expenses:* Contact institution.

Millikin University, School of Nursing, Decatur, IL 62522-2084. Offers clinical nurse leader (MSN); entry into nursing practice: pre-licensure (MSN); nurse anesthesia (DNP); nurse educator (MSN); nursing practice (DNP). *Accreditation:* AACN; AANA/CANAEP. Part-time programs available. *Faculty:* 17 full-time (15 women), 5 part-time/adjunct (4 women). *Students:* 41 full-time (30 women), 26 part-time (19 women); includes 7 minority (2 Black or African American, non-Hispanic/Latino; 1 American Indian or Alaska Native, non-Hispanic/Latino; 1 Asian, non-Hispanic/Latino; 3 Hispanic/Latino). Average age 32. 69 applicants, 51% accepted, 21 enrolled. In 2013, 8 master's awarded. *Degree requirements:* For master's, thesis or alternative, research project. *Entrance requirements:* For master's, GRE, official academic transcript(s), essay, immunizations, statistics course, 3 letters of recommendation, CPR certification, professional liability/malpractice insurance; for doctorate, GRE (if undergraduate cumulative GPA is below 3.0), official academic transcript(s); undergraduate courses: nursing research, health assessment, inorganic and organic chemistry, intro to statistics; graduate-level statistics; 3 written recommendations; Assessment of Critical Care Skills form; written statement; resume or curriculum vita. Additional exam requirements/recommendations for international students: Required—TOEFL (minimum score 550 paper-based; 79 iBT). *Application deadline:* For spring admission, 11/1 for domestic students. Applications are processed on a rolling basis. Application fee: $0. Electronic applications accepted. *Expenses: Tuition:* Full-time $20,300; part-time $700 per credit hour. Tuition and fees vary according to program. *Financial support:* In 2013–14, 13 students received support. Institutionally sponsored loans available. Financial award applicants required to submit FAFSA. *Faculty research:* Congestive heart failure, quality of life, transcultural nursing issues, teaching/learning strategies, maternal - newborn. *Unit head:* Dr. Kathy Booker, Director, 217-424-6348, Fax: 217-420-6731, E-mail: kbooker@millikin.edu. *Application contact:* Marianne Taylor, Administrative Assistant, 800-373-7733 Ext. 5034, Fax: 217-420-6677, E-mail: mgtaylor@millikin.edu.
Website: http://www.millikin.edu/academics/cps/nursing/programs

Missouri State University, Graduate College, College of Health and Human Services, Department of Biomedical Sciences, Program in Nurse Anesthesia, Springfield, MO 65897. Offers MS. *Accreditation:* AANA/CANAEP. *Students:* 34 full-time (18 women), 1 part-time (0 women); includes 2 minority (1 Asian, non-Hispanic/Latino; 1 Hispanic/Latino). Average age 33. 7 applicants, 100% accepted, 7 enrolled. In 2013, 12 master's awarded. *Degree requirements:* For master's, comprehensive exam, thesis or alternative, oral exams. *Entrance requirements:* For master's, GRE General Test, 1 year of experience in acute care nursing, current RN license, interview, minimum GPA of 3.0 during final 60 hours of course work. Additional exam requirements/recommendations for international students: Required—TOEFL (minimum score 550 paper-based; 79 iBT). *Application deadline:* For fall admission, 11/1 priority date for domestic students, 11/1 for international students; for spring admission, 7/1 priority date for domestic students, 7/1 for international students. Application fee: $35. *Expenses:* Tuition, state resident: full-time $4500; part-time $250 per credit hour. Tuition, nonresident: full-time $9018; part-time $501 per credit hour. *Required fees:* $361 per semester. Tuition and fees vary according to course level, course load and program. *Financial support:* Career-related internships or fieldwork and institutionally sponsored loans available. Support available to part-time students. Financial award application deadline: 3/31; financial award applicants required to submit FAFSA. *Unit head:* Monika Feeney, Program Director,

417-838-5603, Fax: 417-836-5588, E-mail: monikafeeney@missouristate.edu. *Application contact:* Monika Feeney, Program Director, 417-836-5603, Fax: 417-836-5588, E-mail: monikafeeneyt@missouristate.edu.

Mount Marty College, Graduate Studies Division, Yankton, SD 57078-3724. Offers business administration (MBA); nurse anesthesia (MS); nursing (MSN); pastoral ministries (MPM). *Accreditation:* AANA/CANAEP (one or more programs are accredited). *Degree requirements:* For master's, thesis or alternative. *Entrance requirements:* For master's, GRE General Test, minimum GPA of 3.0. Electronic applications accepted. *Faculty research:* Clinical anesthesia, professional characteristics, motivations of applicants.

Murray State University, College of Health Sciences and Human Services, Program in Nursing, Murray, KY 42071. Offers clinical nurse specialist (MSN); family nurse practitioner (MSN); nurse anesthesia (MSN). *Accreditation:* AACN; AANA/CANAEP. *Degree requirements:* For master's, research project. *Entrance requirements:* For master's, GRE General Test, BSN, interview, RN licensure. Additional exam requirements/recommendations for international students: Required—TOEFL (minimum score 550 paper-based). *Faculty research:* Fibromyalgis, primary care, rural health.

National University, Academic Affairs, School of Health and Human Services, La Jolla, CA 92037-1011. Offers clinical affairs (MS); clinical informatics (Certificate); clinical regulatory affairs (MS); health and life science analytics (MS); health coaching (Certificate); health informatics (MS); healthcare administration (MHA); nurse anesthesia (MS); nursing (MS), including forensic nursing, nursing administration, nursing informatics; nursing administration (Certificate); nursing informatics (Certificate); nursing practice (DNP); public health (MPH), including health promotion, healthcare administration, mental health. Part-time and evening/weekend programs available. Postbaccalaureate distance learning degree programs offered (no on-campus study). *Faculty:* 20 full-time (12 women), 27 part-time/adjunct (16 women). *Students:* 229 full-time (176 women), 89 part-time (52 women); includes 215 minority (58 Black or African American, non-Hispanic/Latino; 1 American Indian or Alaska Native, non-Hispanic/Latino; 68 Asian, non-Hispanic/Latino; 63 Hispanic/Latino; 8 Native Hawaiian or other Pacific Islander, non-Hispanic/Latino; 17 Two or more races, non-Hispanic/Latino), 18 international. Average age 33. 118 applicants, 100% accepted, 92 enrolled. In 2013, 29 master's awarded. *Degree requirements:* For master's, thesis (for some programs). *Entrance requirements:* For master's, interview, minimum GPA of 2.5. Additional exam requirements/recommendations for international students: Required—TOEFL (minimum score 550 paper-based; 79 iBT), IELTS (minimum score 6). *Application deadline:* Applications are processed on a rolling basis. Application fee: $60 ($65 for international students). Electronic applications accepted. *Expenses: Tuition:* Full-time $13,824; part-time $1728 per course. One-time fee: $160. *Financial support:* Career-related internships or fieldwork, institutionally sponsored loans, scholarships/grants, and tuition waivers (partial) available. Support available to part-time students. Financial award application deadline: 6/30; financial award applicants required to submit FAFSA. *Faculty research:* Nursing education, obesity prevention, workforce diversity. *Unit head:* School of Health and Human Services, 800-628-8648, E-mail: shhs@nu.edu. *Application contact:* Louis Cruz, Interim Vice President for Enrollment Services, 800-628-8648, E-mail: advisor@nu.edu.
Website: http://www.nu.edu/OurPrograms/SchoolOfHealthAndHumanServices.html

Newman University, School of Nursing and Allied Health, Wichita, KS 67213-2097. Offers nurse anesthesia (MS). *Accreditation:* AANA/CANAEP. *Faculty:* 1 (woman) full-time, 5 part-time/adjunct (2 women). *Students:* 47 full-time (28 women), 29 part-time (17 women); includes 12 minority (3 Black or African American, non-Hispanic/Latino; 3 Asian, non-Hispanic/Latino; 3 Hispanic/Latino; 2 Native Hawaiian or other Pacific Islander, non-Hispanic/Latino; 1 Two or more races, non-Hispanic/Latino). Average age 31. 134 applicants, 19% accepted, 25 enrolled. In 2013, 22 master's awarded. *Degree requirements:* For master's, thesis optional. *Entrance requirements:* For master's, GRE General Test, registered professional nursing license in Kansas, 3 professional recommendations, 1-page letter detailing professional and educational goals, BSN, statistics course, 1 year of employment, interview. Additional exam requirements/recommendations for international students: Required—TOEFL (minimum score 600 paper-based; 100 iBT). *Application deadline:* For fall admission, 11/15 for domestic and international students. Applications are processed on a rolling basis. Application fee: $25 ($40 for international students). Electronic applications accepted. *Expenses:* Contact institution. *Financial support:* Application deadline: 8/15; applicants required to submit FAFSA. *Unit head:* Prof. Sharon Niemann, Director of the Master of Science in Nurse Anesthesia Program, 316-942-4291 Ext. 2272, Fax: 316-942-4483, E-mail: niemanns@newmanu.edu. *Application contact:* Linda Kay Sabala, Director of Graduate Admissions, 316-942-4291 Ext. 2230, Fax: 316-942-4483.

Oakland University, Graduate Study and Lifelong Learning, School of Nursing, Program in Nurse Anesthetist, Rochester, MI 48309-4401. Offers MSN, Certificate. Programs offered jointly with Beaumont Hospital Corporation. *Accreditation:* AACN; AANA/CANAEP. *Students:* 60 full-time (37 women), 3 part-time (1 woman); includes 4 minority (1 Black or African American, non-Hispanic/Latino; 2 Asian, non-Hispanic/Latino; 1 Hispanic/Latino), 2 international. Average age 35. 173 applicants, 14% accepted, 23 enrolled. In 2013, 15 master's, 1 other advanced degree awarded. *Degree requirements:* For master's, thesis (for some programs). *Entrance requirements:* For master's, GRE General Test. Additional exam requirements/recommendations for international students: Required—TOEFL (minimum score 550 paper-based). *Application deadline:* For fall admission, 10/15 for domestic and international students. Application fee: $0. Electronic applications accepted. *Expenses:* Contact institution. *Financial support:* Federal Work-Study, institutionally sponsored loans, and tuition waivers (full) available. Financial award application deadline: 3/1; financial award applicants required to submit FAFSA. *Unit head:* Mary Bray, Graduate Program Coordinator, 248-370-4482. *Application contact:* Mary Bray, Graduate Program Coordinator, 248-370-4482.

Old Dominion University, College of Health Sciences, School of Nursing, Nurse Anesthesia Program, Virginia Beach, VA 23453. Offers MSN. *Faculty:* 1 full-time (0 women), 3 part-time/adjunct (2 women). *Students:* 38 full-time (32 women), 1 (woman) part-time; includes 9 minority (6 Black or African American, non-Hispanic/Latino; 1 Asian, non-Hispanic/Latino; 1 Hispanic/Latino; 1 Two or more races, non-Hispanic/Latino). Average age 33. 70 applicants, 21% accepted, 9 enrolled. *Degree requirements:* For master's, comprehensive exam, statistics, organic chemistry. *Entrance requirements:* For master's, GRE. *Application deadline:* For fall admission, 10/15 priority date for domestic students; for spring admission, 3/15 for domestic and international students. Applications are processed on a rolling basis. Application fee: $50. Electronic applications accepted. *Expenses:* Tuition, state resident: full-time $9888; part-time $412 per credit. Tuition, nonresident: full-time $25,152; part-time $1048 per credit. *Required fees:* $59 per semester. One-time fee: $50. *Unit head:* Dr. Nathaniel Michael Apatov, Graduate Program Director, 757-368-4174, Fax: 757-386-4176, E-mail: napatov@odu.edu. *Application contact:* Sue Parker, Coordinator, Graduate Student Services, 757-683-4298, Fax: 757-683-5253, E-mail: sparker@odu.edu.
Website: http://hs.odu.edu/nursing/academics/nurse_anesthesia/nurse_anesthesia.shtml

Oregon Health & Science University, School of Nursing, Program in Nurse Anesthesia, Portland, OR 97239-3098. Offers MN, MS. *Accreditation:* AANA/CANAEP.

Otterbein University, Department of Nursing, Westerville, OH 43081. Offers advanced practice nurse educator (Certificate); clinical nurse leader (MSN); family nurse practitioner (MSN, Certificate); nurse anesthesia (MSN, Certificate); nursing (DNP); nursing service administration (MSN). *Accreditation:* AACN; AANA/CANAEP. Part-time and evening/weekend programs available. Postbaccalaureate distance learning degree programs offered (minimal on-campus study). *Degree requirements:* For master's, comprehensive exam (for some programs), thesis (for some programs). *Entrance requirements:* For master's, 2 reference forms, resume; for Certificate, official transcripts, 2 reference forms, essay, resumé. Additional exam requirements/recommendations for international students: Required—TOEFL (minimum score 550 paper-based; 79 iBT). *Faculty research:* Patient education, women's health, trauma curriculum development, administration.

Our Lady of the Lake College, School of Nursing, Program in Nurse Anesthesia, Baton Rouge, LA 70808. Offers MS. *Accreditation:* AANA/CANAEP. *Degree requirements:* For master's, clinical practicum. *Entrance requirements:* For master's, GRE, current RN license; baccalaureate degree in nursing; 1 year of full-time experience (2 years preferred) as RN in adult critical care setting (adult intensive care unit preferred); minimum cumulative GPA of 3.0; one undergraduate or graduate chemistry course. Additional exam requirements/recommendations for international students: Required—TOEFL.

Rosalind Franklin University of Medicine and Science, College of Health Professions, Nurse Anesthesia Department, North Chicago, IL 60064-3095. Offers MS. *Accreditation:* AANA/CANAEP. *Entrance requirements:* For master's, GRE, RN license, ICU experience. Additional exam requirements/recommendations for international students: Required—TOEFL. Electronic applications accepted. *Faculty research:* Patient safety, pediatric anesthesia, instructional technology.

Rush University, College of Nursing, Department of Adult Health and Gerontological Nursing, Chicago, IL 60612. Offers adult gerontology acute care clinical nurse specialist (DNP); adult gerontology acute care nurse practitioner (DNP); adult gerontology primary care clinical nurse specialist (DNP); adult gerontology primary care nurse practitioner (DNP); nurse anesthesia (DNP); nursing science (PhD); systems leadership (DNP). *Accreditation:* AACN; AANA/CANAEP (one or more programs are accredited). Part-time programs available. Postbaccalaureate distance learning degree programs offered (minimal on-campus study). *Students:* 89 full-time (69 women), 109 part-time (100 women); includes 40 minority (11 Black or African American, non-Hispanic/Latino; 1 American Indian or Alaska Native, non-Hispanic/Latino; 22 Asian, non-Hispanic/Latino; 5 Hispanic/Latino; 1 Native Hawaiian or other Pacific Islander, non-Hispanic/Latino). Average age 33. 170 applicants, 56% accepted, 78 enrolled. *Degree requirements:* For doctorate, capstone project (for DNP); dissertation (for PhD). *Entrance requirements:* For doctorate, GRE General Test (for DNP in nurse anesthesia; waived if cumulative GPA is 3.25 or greater, nursing GPA is 3.0 or greater, or a completed graduate program GPA is 3.5 or greater), interview, 3 letters of recommendation, personal statement, current resume. Additional exam requirements/recommendations for international students: Required—TOEFL. *Application deadline:* For fall admission, 1/2 for domestic students; for winter admission, 10/15 for domestic students; for spring admission, 8/1 for domestic students; for summer admission, 12/1 for domestic students. Applications are processed on a rolling basis. Application fee: $100. Electronic applications accepted. *Financial support:* Fellowships, research assistantships, teaching assistantships, Federal Work-Study, institutionally sponsored loans, scholarships/grants, traineeships, and health care benefits available. Support available to part-time students. Financial award application deadline: 3/1; financial award applicants required to submit FAFSA. *Faculty research:* Physical activity adherence in African-American women; reduction of health disparities; evidence-based interventions for caregivers; fish oil for HIV-related immunosenescence; BAILA: Being Active, Increasing Latinos Health Aging. *Total annual research expenditures:* $3.8 million. *Unit head:* Dr. Elizabeth Carlson, Chairperson, 312-942-7117, E-mail: elizabeth_carlson@rush.edu. *Application contact:* Jennifer Thorndyke, Admissions Specialist, 312-563-7526, E-mail: jennifer_thorndyke@rush.edu.
Website: http://www.rushu.rush.edu/servlet/Satellite?c=RushUnivLevel1Page&cid=1204497838852&pagename=Rush%2FRushUnivLevel1Page%2FLevel_1_College_Home_Page

Rutgers, The State University of New Jersey, Newark, Rutgers School of Nursing, Newark, NJ 07107-3001. Offers adult health (MSN); adult occupational health (MSN); advanced practice nursing (MSN, Post Master's Certificate); family nurse practitioner (MSN); nurse anesthesia (MSN); nursing (MSN); nursing informatics (MSN); urban health (PhD); women's health practitioner (MSN). *Accreditation:* AANA/CANAEP. Part-time programs available. *Entrance requirements:* For master's, GRE, RN license; basic life support, statistics, and health assessment experience. Additional exam requirements/recommendations for international students: Required—TOEFL. Electronic applications accepted. *Expenses:* Contact institution. *Faculty research:* HIV/AIDS, diabetes education, learned helplessness, nursing science, psychoeducation.

Saint Joseph's University, College of Arts and Sciences, Department of Health Services, Philadelphia, PA 19131-1395. Offers health administration (MS, Post-Master's Certificate); health care ethics (Post-Master's Certificate); health education (MS, Post-Master's Certificate); health informatics (Post-Master's Certificate); healthcare ethics (MS); long-term care administration (MS); nurse anesthesia (MS); school nurse certification (MS). Part-time and evening/weekend programs available. *Faculty:* 5 full-time (1 woman), 16 part-time/adjunct (6 women). *Students:* 46 full-time (25 women), 431 part-time (315 women); includes 168 minority (120 Black or African American, non-Hispanic/Latino; 29 Asian, non-Hispanic/Latino; 15 Hispanic/Latino; 2 Native Hawaiian or other Pacific Islander, non-Hispanic/Latino; 2 Two or more races, non-Hispanic/Latino), 14 international. Average age 34. 234 applicants, 74% accepted, 135 enrolled. In 2013, 83 master's awarded. *Entrance requirements:* For master's, GRE (if GPA less than 3.0), 2 letters of recommendation, resume, personal statement, official transcripts. Additional exam requirements/recommendations for international students: Required—TOEFL (minimum score 550 paper-based; 80 iBT), IELTS (minimum score 6.5). *Application deadline:* For fall admission, 7/15 priority date for domestic students, 4/15 for international students; for winter admission, 1/15 for international students; for spring admission, 11/15 priority date for domestic students, 10/15 for international students. Applications are processed on a rolling basis. Application fee: $35. Electronic applications accepted. *Expenses: Tuition:* Part-time $786 per credit hour. Tuition and fees vary according to degree level and program. *Financial support:* Career-related internships or fieldwork and unspecified assistantships available. Financial award applicants required to submit FAFSA. *Unit head:* Nakia Henderson, Director, 610-660-3131, E-mail: gradstudies@sju.edu. *Application contact:* Elisabeth Woodward, Director of Marketing and Admissions, Graduate Arts and Sciences, 610-660-3131, Fax: 610-660-3230, E-mail: gradstudies@sju.edu.
Website: http://sju.edu/majors-programs/graduate-arts-sciences/masters/health-administration-ms

Saint Mary's University of Minnesota, Schools of Graduate and Professional Programs, Graduate School of Health and Human Services, Nurse Anesthesia Program,

Winona, MN 55987-1399. Offers MS. Offered jointly with the Minneapolis School of Anesthesia. *Accreditation:* AANA/CANAEP. *Unit head:* Merri Moody, Director, 612-728-5133. *Application contact:* Russell Kreager, Director of Admissions for Graduate and Professional Programs, 612-728-5207, Fax: 612-728-5121, E-mail: rkreager@smumn.edu.
Website: http://www.smumn.edu/graduate-home/areas-of-study/graduate-school-of-health-human-services/ms-in-nurse-anesthesia

Saint Vincent College, Program in Health Services, Latrobe, PA 15650-2690. Offers nurse anesthesia (MS).

Samford University, Ida V. Moffett School of Nursing, Birmingham, AL 35229. Offers administration (DNP); advanced practice (DNP); family nurse practitioner (MSN); health systems management and leadership (MSN); nurse anesthesia (MSN); nurse educator (MSN). *Accreditation:* AACN; AANA/CANAEP (one or more programs are accredited). Part-time programs available. Postbaccalaureate distance learning degree programs offered (minimal on-campus study). *Faculty:* 16 full-time (all women), 4 part-time/adjunct (2 women). *Students:* 249 full-time (191 women), 25 part-time (17 women); includes 48 minority (23 Black or African American, non-Hispanic/Latino; 1 American Indian or Alaska Native, non-Hispanic/Latino; 13 Asian, non-Hispanic/Latino; 7 Hispanic/Latino; 4 Two or more races, non-Hispanic/Latino), 1 international. Average age 36. 89 applicants, 53% accepted, 45 enrolled. In 2013, 107 master's, 29 doctorates awarded. *Degree requirements:* For master's and doctorate, capstone project with oral presentation. *Entrance requirements:* For master's, MAT; GRE (for nurse anesthesia). Additional exam requirements/recommendations for international students: Required—TOEFL (minimum score 550 paper-based; 80 iBT). *Application deadline:* For fall admission, 6/1 priority date for domestic and international students; for spring admission, 9/1 priority date for domestic and international students. Application fee: $65. Electronic applications accepted. *Expenses:* Contact institution. *Financial support:* In 2013–14, 48 students received support. Institutionally sponsored loans, scholarships/grants, and traineeships available. Financial award application deadline: 3/1; financial award applicants required to submit FAFSA. *Faculty research:* Issues in rural health care, vulnerable populations, genetics and disabilities in pediatrics, geriatrics, parish nursing research, interprofessional education, global health disparities. *Unit head:* Dr. Nena F. Sanders, Dean, 205-726-2629, E-mail: nfsander@samford.edu. *Application contact:* Allyson Maddox, Director of Graduate Student Services, 205-726-2047, Fax: 205-726-4179, E-mail: amaddox@samford.edu.
Website: http://samford.edu/nursing

Samuel Merritt University, School of Nursing, Oakland, CA 94609-3108. Offers case management (MSN); family nurse practitioner (MSN, Certificate); nurse anesthetist (MSN, Certificate); nursing (MSN, DNP). *Accreditation:* AACN; AANA/CANAEP (one or more programs are accredited). Part-time and evening/weekend programs available. *Degree requirements:* For master's, thesis or alternative. *Entrance requirements:* For master's, minimum GPA of 2.5 in science, 3.0 overall; previous course work in statistics; current RN license. Additional exam requirements/recommendations for international students: Required—TOEFL. *Faculty research:* Gerontology, community health, maternal-child health, sexually transmitted diseases, substance abuse, oncology.

Southern Illinois University Edwardsville, Graduate School, School of Nursing, Program in Nurse Anesthesia, Edwardsville, IL 62026-0001. Offers MS, Post-Master's Certificate. *Accreditation:* AANA/CANAEP. Part-time programs available. *Students:* 71 full-time (47 women), 3 part-time (1 woman); includes 10 minority (3 Black or African American, non-Hispanic/Latino; 5 Asian, non-Hispanic/Latino; 1 Hispanic/Latino; 1 Two or more races, non-Hispanic/Latino). In 2013, 24 master's, 2 other advanced degrees awarded. *Degree requirements:* For master's, comprehensive exam. *Entrance requirements:* For master's, appropriate bachelor's degree, RN license, minimum undergraduate nursing GPA of 3.0. Additional exam requirements/recommendations for international students: Required—TOEFL (minimum score 550 paper-based, 79 iBT), IELTS (minimum score 6.5), Michigan Test of English Language Proficiency or PTE. *Application deadline:* For spring admission, 6/1 for domestic and international students. Application fee: $30. Electronic applications accepted. *Expenses:* Tuition, state resident: full-time $3551. Tuition, nonresident: full-time $8378. *Financial support:* Fellowships, research assistantships, teaching assistantships, institutionally sponsored loans, scholarships/grants, and unspecified assistantships available. Financial award application deadline: 3/1; financial award applicants required to submit FAFSA. *Unit head:* Dr. Kathy Ketchum, Associate Dean for Graduate Programs, 618-650-3936, E-mail: kketchu@siue.edu. *Application contact:* Melissa K. Mace, Assistant Director of Graduate and International Recruitment, 618-650-2756, Fax: 618-650-3618, E-mail: mmace@siue.edu.
Website: http://www.siue.edu/nursing/graduate

State University of New York Downstate Medical Center, College of Nursing, Graduate Program in Nursing, Program in Nurse Anesthesia, Brooklyn, NY 11203-2098. Offers MS. *Accreditation:* AACN; AANA/CANAEP. *Degree requirements:* For master's, thesis optional. *Entrance requirements:* For master's, GRE, BSN; minimum GPA of 3.0; previous undergraduate course work in statistics, health assessment, and nursing research; RN license.

Texas Christian University, Harris College of Nursing and Health Sciences, School of Nurse Anesthesia, Fort Worth, TX 76129. Offers MSNA, DNP-A. Postbaccalaureate distance learning degree programs offered (minimal on-campus study). *Faculty:* 10 full-time (4 women), 1 (woman) part-time/adjunct. *Students:* 123 full-time (77 women), 43 part-time (25 women); includes 31 minority (5 Black or African American, non-Hispanic/Latino; 1 American Indian or Alaska Native, non-Hispanic/Latino; 9 Asian, non-Hispanic/Latino; 12 Hispanic/Latino; 4 Two or more races, non-Hispanic/Latino), 1 international. Average age 29. 63 applicants, 100% accepted, 63 enrolled. In 2013, 59 master's, 16 doctorates awarded. *Entrance requirements:* For master's and doctorate, GRE, RN license, CCRN Certification. Additional exam requirements/recommendations for international students: Required—TOEFL (minimum score 600 paper-based). *Application deadline:* For fall admission, 7/1 for domestic and international students. Application fee: $50. *Expenses:* Contact institution. *Financial support:* Traineeships available. Financial award applicants required to submit FAFSA. *Unit head:* Dr. Kay K. Sanders, Director, 817-257-7887, E-mail: k.sanders@tcu.edu. *Application contact:* 817-257-7515, Fax: 817-257-7484, E-mail: frogmail@tcu.edu.
Website: http://www.crna.tcu.edu/

Texas Wesleyan University, Graduate Programs, Programs in Nurse Anesthesia, Fort Worth, TX 76105-1536. Offers MHS, MSNA, DNAP. *Accreditation:* AANA/CANAEP (one or more programs are accredited). *Entrance requirements:* For master's, GRE General Test, master's degree; copy of current Council on Certification/Recertification card (all applicants must be Certified RN Anesthetists); minimum GPA of 3.0, science 2.75; undergraduate statistics course with minimum C grade; graduate statistics course with minimum B grade; graduate-level research course; current curriculum vitae; 3 letters of support; for doctorate, master's degree; copy of current Council on Certification/Recertification card (all applicants must be Certified RN Anesthetists); minimum GPA of 3.0, science 2.75; undergraduate statistics course with minimum C grade; graduate statistics course with minimum B grade, graduate-level research course; current curriculum vitae; 3 letters of support. *Expenses:* Contact institution.

Uniformed Services University of the Health Sciences, Graduate School of Nursing, Bethesda, MD 20814-4799. Offers family nurse practitioner (MSN, DNP); nurse anesthesia (MSN); nursing science (PhD); perioperative clinical nurse specialist (MSN); psychiatric nurse practitioner (MSN, DNP). Program available to military officers only. *Accreditation:* AACN; AANA/CANAEP. *Faculty:* 42 full-time (24 women), 5 part-time/adjunct (4 women). *Students:* 62 full-time (31 women); includes 13 minority (7 Black or African American, non-Hispanic/Latino; 5 Asian, non-Hispanic/Latino; 1 Hispanic/Latino). Average age 34. 100 applicants, 62% accepted, 62 enrolled. In 2013, 57 master's, 1 doctorate awarded. *Degree requirements:* For master's, thesis or alternative; for doctorate, thesis/dissertation or alternative. *Entrance requirements:* For master's, GRE, BSN, clinical experience, minimum GPA of 3.0, previous course work in science; for doctorate, GRE. *Application deadline:* For fall admission, 7/1 for domestic students; for winter admission, 2/15 for domestic students. Application fee: $0. Electronic applications accepted. *Faculty research:* Prenatal care, military health care, military readiness, distance learning. *Unit head:* Dr. Carol A. Romano, Associate Dean for Academic Affairs, 301-295-1180, Fax: 301-295-1707, E-mail: carol.romano@usuhs.edu. *Application contact:* Terry Lynn Malavakis, Recording Secretary for Admissions Committee, 301-295-1055, Fax: 301-295-1707, E-mail: terry.malavakis@usuhs.edu.
Website: http://www.usuhs.mil/gsn/

Union University, School of Nursing, Jackson, TN 38305-3697. Offers executive leadership (DNP); nurse anesthesia (DNP); nurse anesthetist (PMC); nurse practitioner (DNP); nursing education (MSN, PMC). *Accreditation:* AACN; AANA/CANAEP. *Degree requirements:* For master's, thesis or alternative. *Entrance requirements:* For master's, GRE, 3 letters of reference, bachelor's degree in nursing, minimum GPA of 3.0. Additional exam requirements/recommendations for international students: Required—TOEFL (minimum score 560 paper-based). Electronic applications accepted. *Faculty research:* Children's health, occupational rehabilitation, informatics, health promotion.

University at Buffalo, the State University of New York, Graduate School, School of Nursing, Buffalo, NY 14214. Offers adult gerontology nurse practitioner (DNP); family nurse practitioner (DNP); health care systems and leadership (MS); nurse anesthetist (DNP); nursing (PhD); nursing education (Certificate); psychiatric/mental health nurse practitioner (DNP). *Accreditation:* AACN; AANA/CANAEP (one or more programs are accredited). Part-time programs available. Postbaccalaureate distance learning degree programs offered (no on-campus study). *Faculty:* 24 full-time (21 women), 2 part-time/adjunct (1 woman). *Students:* 80 full-time (60 women), 97 part-time (84 women); includes 35 minority (20 Black or African American, non-Hispanic/Latino; 2 American Indian or Alaska Native, non-Hispanic/Latino; 9 Asian, non-Hispanic/Latino; 1 Hispanic/Latino; 3 Native Hawaiian or other Pacific Islander, non-Hispanic/Latino). 118 applicants, 67% accepted, 58 enrolled. In 2013, 41 master's, 15 doctorates awarded. *Degree requirements:* For master's, thesis optional; for doctorate, comprehensive exam (for some programs), capstone (for DNP), dissertation (for PhD). *Entrance requirements:* For doctorate, GRE or MAT, minimum GPA of 3.0 (3.25 for PhD), RN license, BS or MS in nursing, 3 references, writing sample; for Certificate, interview, minimum GPA of 3.0 or GRE General Test, RN license, MS in nursing. Additional exam requirements/recommendations for international students: Required—TOEFL (minimum score 550 paper-based; 79 iBT), IELTS (minimum score 6.5). *Application deadline:* For fall admission, 7/1 for domestic students, 4/1 for international students; for spring admission, 12/1 for domestic students, 10/1 for international students; for summer admission, 4/1 for domestic students. Application fee: $75. Electronic applications accepted. *Financial support:* In 2013–14, 80 students received support, including 2 fellowships with full and partial tuition reimbursements available (averaging $17,000 per year), 7 research assistantships with full and partial tuition reimbursements available (averaging $10,600 per year), 7 teaching assistantships with full and partial tuition reimbursements available (averaging $10,600 per year); scholarships/grants, traineeships, health care benefits, and unspecified assistantships also available. Financial award application deadline: 3/15; financial award applicants required to submit FAFSA. *Faculty research:* Oncology, palliative care, gerontology, addictions, mental health, community wellness, sleep, workforce, care of underserved populations, quality and safety, person-centered care, adolescent health. *Total annual research expenditures:* $1.1 million. *Unit head:* Dr. Marsha L. Lewis, Dean and Professor, 716-829-2533, Fax: 716-829-2566, E-mail: ubnursingdean@buffalo.edu. *Application contact:* Dr. David J. Lang, Director of Student Affairs, 716-829-2537, Fax: 716-829-2067, E-mail: nursing@buffalo.edu.
Website: http://nursing.buffalo.edu/

The University of Alabama at Birmingham, School of Nursing, Birmingham, AL 35294. Offers nurse anesthesia (MSN); nursing (MSN, DNP, PhD). *Accreditation:* AACN. Part-time programs available. Terminal master's awarded for partial completion of doctoral program. *Degree requirements:* For doctorate, thesis/dissertation, research mentorship experience. *Entrance requirements:* For master's, GRE, GMAT, or MAT, BS in nursing, interview; for doctorate, GRE General Test, computer literacy, course work in statistics, interview, minimum GPA of 3.0, MS in nursing, references, writing sample. Additional exam requirements/recommendations for international students: Required—TOEFL. Electronic applications accepted. *Expenses:* Contact institution.

The University of British Columbia, Faculty of Medicine, Department of Anesthesiology, Pharmacology and Therapeutics, Vancouver, BC V6T 1Z3, Canada. Offers M Sc, PhD. *Faculty:* 20 full-time (4 women), 2 part-time/adjunct (0 women). *Students:* 29 full-time (12 women); includes 11 minority (10 Asian, non-Hispanic/Latino; 1 Hispanic/Latino), 8 international. Average age 28. 29 applicants, 17% accepted, 5 enrolled. In 2013, 2 master's, 1 doctorate awarded. Terminal master's awarded for partial completion of doctoral program. *Degree requirements:* For master's, thesis; for doctorate, comprehensive exam, thesis/dissertation. *Entrance requirements:* For master's, MD or appropriate bachelor's degree; for doctorate, MD or M Sc. Additional exam requirements/recommendations for international students: Required—TOEFL (minimum score 600 paper-based; 100 iBT). *Application deadline:* For fall admission, 4/1 for domestic students, 3/1 for international students; for winter admission, 8/1 for domestic students, 7/1 for international students; for spring admission, 12/1 for domestic students, 11/1 for international students. Application fee: $90 Canadian dollars ($150 Canadian dollars for international students). Electronic applications accepted. *Expenses: Tuition, area resident:* Full-time $8000 Canadian dollars. *Financial support:* In 2013–14, 10 students received support, including 10 fellowships (averaging $21,409 per year), 16 research assistantships with full and partial tuition reimbursements available (averaging $20,576 per year); institutionally sponsored loans, scholarships/grants, and unspecified assistantships also available. Financial award application deadline: 10/15. *Faculty research:* Cellular, biochemical, autonomic, and cardiovascular pharmacology; neuropharmacology and pulmonary pharmacology. *Total annual research expenditures:* $406,074 Canadian dollars. *Unit head:* Dr. C. B. Warriner, Head, 604-822-2575, Fax: 604-822-2281, E-mail: brian.warriner@vch.ca. *Application contact:* Wynne Leung, Graduate Secretary, 604-827-3289, Fax: 604-822-6012, E-mail: wynne.leung@ubc.ca.
Website: http://www.apt.ubc.ca/

University of Cincinnati, Graduate School, College of Nursing, Cincinnati, OH 45221-0038. Offers clinical nurse specialist (MSN), including adult health, community health, neonatal, nursing administration, occupational health, pediatric health, psychiatric nursing, women's health; nurse anesthesia (MSN); nurse midwifery (MSN); nurse practitioner (MSN), including acute care, ambulatory care, family, family/psychiatric, women's health; nursing (PhD); MBA/MSN. *Accreditation:* AACN; AANA/CANAEP (one or more programs are accredited); ACNM/ACME. Part-time programs available. Postbaccalaureate distance learning degree programs offered (no on-campus study). Terminal master's awarded for partial completion of doctoral program. *Degree requirements:* For master's, thesis or alternative; for doctorate, comprehensive exam, thesis/dissertation. *Entrance requirements:* For master's and doctorate, GRE General Test. Additional exam requirements/recommendations for international students: Required—TOEFL (minimum score 520 paper-based). Electronic applications accepted. *Faculty research:* Substance abuse, injury and violence, symptom management.

University of Detroit Mercy, College of Health Professions, Program in Nurse Anesthesiology, Detroit, MI 48221. Offers MS. *Accreditation:* AANA/CANAEP. *Entrance requirements:* For master's, GRE General Test, minimum GPA of 3.0. *Expenses:* Contact institution.

The University of Kansas, University of Kansas Medical Center, School of Health Professions, Department of Nurse Anesthesia Education, Kansas City, KS 66160. Offers MS, DNP. *Accreditation:* AANA/CANAEP. *Faculty:* 7 full-time (5 women), 25 part-time/adjunct (18 women). *Students:* 68 full-time (48 women); includes 8 minority (5 Black or African American, non-Hispanic/Latino; 1 American Indian or Alaska Native, non-Hispanic/Latino; 1 Asian, non-Hispanic/Latino; 1 Two or more races, non-Hispanic/Latino). Average age 30. 83 applicants, 36% accepted, 23 enrolled. In 2013, 21 master's awarded. *Degree requirements:* For master's, comprehensive exam, thesis or alternative; for doctorate, comprehensive exam, thesis/dissertation or alternative. *Entrance requirements:* For master's and doctorate, bachelor's degree in nursing or related field, RN license, 2 years of experience as an RN including 1 year of experience in ICU; five science classes (anatomy, physiology, microbiology and 2 chemistry) and statistics. Additional exam requirements/recommendations for international students: Required—TOEFL. *Application deadline:* For fall admission, 7/15 for domestic and international students. Application fee: $60. Electronic applications accepted. *Expenses:* Contact institution. *Financial support:* Traineeships available. Financial award application deadline: 3/1; financial award applicants required to submit FAFSA. *Faculty research:* Simulation training. *Total annual research expenditures:* $27,000. *Unit head:* Dr. Donna S. Nyght, Chair, 913-588-6612, Fax: 913-588-3334, E-mail: dnyght@kumc.edu. *Application contact:* Carrie Hewitt, Administrative Officer, 913-588-6612, Fax: 913-588-3334, E-mail: na@kumc.edu.
Website: http://www.kumc.edu/school-of-health-professions/nurse-anesthesia-education.html

University of Miami, Graduate School, School of Nursing and Health Studies, Coral Gables, FL 33124. Offers acute care (MSN), including acute care nurse practitioner, nurse anesthesia; nursing (PhD); primary care (MSN), including adult nurse practitioner, family nurse practitioner, nurse midwifery, women's health practitioner. *Accreditation:* AACN; AANA/CANAEP; ACNM/ACME (one or more programs are accredited). Part-time programs available. *Degree requirements:* For master's, thesis optional; for doctorate, thesis/dissertation. *Entrance requirements:* For master's, GRE General Test, BSN, minimum GPA of 3.0, Florida RN license; for doctorate, GRE General Test, BSN or MSN, minimum GPA of 3.0. Additional exam requirements/recommendations for international students: Required—TOEFL (minimum score 550 paper-based). Electronic applications accepted. *Faculty research:* Transcultural nursing, exercise and depression in Alzheimer's disease, infectious diseases/HIV–AIDS, postpartum depression, outcomes assessment.

University of Michigan–Flint, School of Health Professions and Studies, Program in Anesthesia, Flint, MI 48502-1950. Offers MS, DrAP. *Accreditation:* AACN; AANA/CANAEP. Part-time programs available. *Faculty:* 3 full-time (2 women), 7 part-time/adjunct (5 women). *Students:* 37 full-time (26 women), 37 part-time (23 women); includes 8 minority (2 Black or African American, non-Hispanic/Latino; 4 Asian, non-Hispanic/Latino; 2 Two or more races, non-Hispanic/Latino), 1 international. Average age 36. 146 applicants, 25% accepted, 37 enrolled. In 2013, 15 master's, 3 doctorates awarded. *Degree requirements:* For master's, thesis. *Entrance requirements:* For master's, GRE, BSN or BS in science, minimum 1 year of critical care RN experience, RN license, minimum GPA of 3.0 in prerequisites, current certification as an advanced cardiac life support provider (ACLS), current certification as a pediatric advanced life support provider (PALS). Additional exam requirements/recommendations for international students: Required—TOEFL (minimum score 560 paper-based; 84 iBT), IELTS (minimum score 6.5). *Application deadline:* For fall admission, 8/1 priority date for domestic students, 5/1 priority date for international students; for winter admission, 11/15 priority date for domestic students, 9/1 priority date for international students; for spring admission, 3/15 priority date for domestic students, 1/1 priority date for international students. Application fee: $55. Electronic applications accepted. *Expenses:* Contact institution. *Financial support:* Career-related internships or fieldwork, scholarships/grants, traineeships, and unspecified assistantships available. Support available to part-time students. Financial award application deadline: 3/1; financial award applicants required to submit FAFSA. *Faculty research:* CRNA expected retirement patterns, factors of importance in CENA selection of first job, lidocaine 4% in ETT cuff and reducing in coughing on emergence, orientation of spinal needle benel, length of time to discharge outpatients. *Unit head:* Dr. Shawn Fryzel, Director, 810-257-9264, Fax: 810-760-0839, E-mail: sfryzel@hurleymc.com. *Application contact:* Bradley T. Maki, Director of Graduate Admissions, 810-762-3171, Fax: 810-766-6789, E-mail: bmaki@umflint.edu.
Website: http://www.umflint.edu/graduateprograms/anesthesia.htm

University of Minnesota, Twin Cities Campus, Graduate School, School of Nursing, Program in Nurse Anesthetist, Minneapolis, MN 55455-0213. Offers MS. *Accreditation:* AANA/CANAEP. *Entrance requirements:* Additional exam requirements/recommendations for international students: Required—TOEFL (minimum score 586 paper-based).

University of New England, Westbrook College of Health Professions, Program in Nurse Anesthesia, Biddeford, ME 04005-9526. Offers MS. Program affiliated with St. Joseph's Hospital School of Anesthesia for Nurses, RI. *Accreditation:* AANA/CANAEP. *Faculty:* 2 full-time (both women), 3 part-time/adjunct (2 women). *Students:* 94 full-time (63 women); includes 14 minority (6 Black or African American, non-Hispanic/Latino; 5 Asian, non-Hispanic/Latino; 2 Hispanic/Latino; 1 Two or more races, non-Hispanic/Latino). Average age 33. 66 applicants, 58% accepted, 30 enrolled. In 2013, 34 master's awarded. *Degree requirements:* For master's, thesis, clinical practicum. *Entrance requirements:* For master's, GRE, RN license, 1 year of acute care experience, 3 letters of reference, Advanced Cardiac Life Support Certification, Pediatric Advanced Life Support Certification. *Application deadline:* For fall admission, 11/1 for domestic and international students. Applications are processed on a rolling basis. Electronic applications accepted. *Financial support:* Application deadline: 5/1; applicants required to submit FAFSA. *Unit head:* Maribeth Massie, Program Director and Assistant Clinical Professor, MSNA Program, 207-221-4519, Fax: 207-523-1900, E-mail: mmassie@une.edu. *Application contact:* Dr. Cynthia Forrest, Vice President for Student Affairs, 207-221-4225, Fax: 207-523-1925, E-mail: gradadmissions@une.edu.
Website: http://www.une.edu/wchp/sna

The University of North Carolina at Charlotte, The Graduate School, College of Health and Human Services, School of Nursing, Charlotte, NC 28223-0001. Offers administration (Post-Master's Certificate); advanced clinical (MSN, Post-Master's Certificate); anesthesia (MSN, Post-Master's Certificate); community health (MSN); family nurse practitioner (MSN, Post-Master's Certificate); health administration (MSN); mental health (MSN); nurse educator (MSN, Post-Master's Certificate); nursing (DNP); systems population (MSN). *Accreditation:* AACN. Part-time programs available. *Faculty:* 17 full-time (16 women), 6 part-time/adjunct (5 women). *Students:* 96 full-time (80 women), 124 part-time (119 women); includes 45 minority (30 Black or African American, non-Hispanic/Latino; 1 American Indian or Alaska Native, non-Hispanic/Latino; 8 Asian, non-Hispanic/Latino; 4 Hispanic/Latino; 2 Two or more races, non-Hispanic/Latino), 1 international. Average age 34. 216 applicants, 38% accepted, 72 enrolled. In 2013, 70 master's, 8 other advanced degrees awarded. Terminal master's awarded for partial completion of doctoral program. *Degree requirements:* For master's, thesis or alternative, practicum; for doctorate, thesis/dissertation or alternative, residency. *Entrance requirements:* For master's, GRE General Test, minimum GPA of 3.0 in undergraduate major; for doctorate, GRE, MAT, or GMAT, minimum GPA of 3.5. Additional exam requirements/recommendations for international students: Required—TOEFL (minimum score 570 paper-based; 83 iBT). *Application deadline:* For fall admission, 5/1 priority date for domestic students, 5/1 for international students; for spring admission, 10/1 priority date for domestic students, 10/1 for international students. Application fee: $75. Electronic applications accepted. *Expenses:* Tuition, state resident: full-time $3522. Tuition, nonresident: full-time $16,051. *Required fees:* $2585. Tuition and fees vary according to course load and program. *Financial support:* In 2013–14, 5 students received support, including 5 teaching assistantships (averaging $4,785 per year); research assistantships, career-related internships or fieldwork, institutionally sponsored loans, scholarships/grants, traineeships, and unspecified assistantships also available. Support available to part-time students. Financial award application deadline: 4/1; financial award applicants required to submit FAFSA. *Faculty research:* Improving care outcomes for the elderly; vulnerable populations; symptom management; self management/health promotion strategies of older adults; migration and maternal child health; health disparities, health literacy, and access to healthcare in Latino adults with diabetes; psychiatric nursing. *Total annual research expenditures:* $572,410. *Unit head:* Dr. Dee Baldwin, Associate Dean, 704-687-7952, Fax: 704-687-6017, E-mail: dbaldwi5@uncc.edu. *Application contact:* Kathy B. Giddings, Director of Graduate Admissions, 704-687-5503, Fax: 704-687-1668, E-mail: gradadm@uncc.edu.
Website: http://nursing.uncc.edu/

The University of North Carolina at Greensboro, Graduate School, School of Nursing, Greensboro, NC 27412-5001. Offers adult clinical nurse specialist (MSN, PMC); adult/gerontological nurse practitioner (MSN, PMC); nurse anesthesia (MSN, PMC); nursing (PhD); nursing administration (MSN); nursing education (MSN); MSN/MBA. *Accreditation:* AACN; AANA/CANAEP. *Degree requirements:* For master's, thesis or alternative. *Entrance requirements:* For master's, GRE General Test or MAT, BSN, clinical experience, liability insurance, RN license; for PMC, liability insurance, MSN, RN license. Additional exam requirements/recommendations for international students: Required—TOEFL. Electronic applications accepted.

University of North Dakota, Graduate School, College of Nursing, Department of Nursing, Grand Forks, ND 58202. Offers adult-gerontological nurse practitioner (MSN); advanced public health nurse (MSN); family nurse practitioner (MSN); nurse anesthesia (MSN); nurse educator (MSN); nursing (DNP, PhD); psychiatric and mental health nurse practitioner (MSN).

University of North Florida, Brooks College of Health, School of Nursing, Jacksonville, FL 32224. Offers clinical nurse leader (MSN); clinical nurse specialist (MSN); family nurse practitioner (Certificate); nurse anesthetist (CRNA) (MSN); nursing practice (DNP); primary care nurse practitioner (MSN). *Accreditation:* AACN; AANA/CANAEP. Part-time programs available. *Faculty:* 29 full-time (23 women), 1 part-time/adjunct (0 women). *Students:* 93 full-time (70 women), 74 part-time (61 women); includes 33 minority (11 Black or African American, non-Hispanic/Latino; 1 American Indian or Alaska Native, non-Hispanic/Latino; 6 Asian, non-Hispanic/Latino; 12 Hispanic/Latino; 3 Two or more races, non-Hispanic/Latino), 2 international. Average age 34. 133 applicants, 40% accepted, 32 enrolled. In 2013, 45 master's, 3 doctorates awarded. *Degree requirements:* For master's, thesis optional. *Entrance requirements:* For master's, GRE General Test, minimum GPA of 3.0 in last 60 hours of course work, BSN, clinical experience, resume; for doctorate, GRE, master's degree in nursing specialty from nationally-accredited program; national certification in one of the following APRN roles: CNE, CNM, CNS, CRNA, CNP; minimum graduate GPA of 3.3; three letters of reference which address academic ability and clinical skills; active license as registered nurse or advanced practice registered nurse. Additional exam requirements/recommendations for international students: Required—TOEFL (minimum score 500 paper-based; 61 iBT). *Application deadline:* For fall admission, 3/15 for domestic students, 4/1 for international students. Application fee: $30. Electronic applications accepted. *Expenses:* Tuition, state resident: full-time $9794; part-time $408.10 per credit hour. Tuition, nonresident: full-time $22,383; part-time $932.61 per credit hour. *Required fees:* $2020; $84.20 per credit hour. Tuition and fees vary according to course load and program. *Financial support:* In 2013–14, 26 students received support. Research assistantships available. Financial award application deadline: 4/1; financial award applicants required to submit FAFSA. *Faculty research:* Teen pregnancy, diabetes, ethical decision-making, family caregivers. *Total annual research expenditures:* $66,739. *Unit head:* Dr. Li Loriz, Chair, 904-620-1053, E-mail: lloriz@unf.edu. *Application contact:* Beth Dibble, Assistant Director of Admissions for Nursing and Physical Therapy, 904-620-2684, Fax: 904-620-1832, E-mail: nursingadmissions@unf.edu.
Website: http://www.unf.edu/brooks/nursing

University of Pennsylvania, School of Nursing, Nurse Anesthetist Program, Philadelphia, PA 19104. Offers MSN. *Accreditation:* AANA/CANAEP. *Students:* 47 full-time (29 women), 7 part-time (6 women); includes 9 minority (3 Black or African American, non-Hispanic/Latino; 4 Asian, non-Hispanic/Latino; 2 Two or more races, non-Hispanic/Latino). 10 applicants, 50% accepted, 5 enrolled. In 2013, 22 master's awarded. Application fee: $70. *Unit head:* Assistant Dean of Admissions and Financial Aid, 866-867-6877, Fax: 215-573-8439, E-mail: admissions@nursing.upenn.edu. *Application contact:* Maria Magro, Program Director, 215-898-8292, E-mail: magro@nursing.upenn.edu.

University of Pittsburgh, School of Nursing, Nurse Anesthesia Program, Pittsburgh, PA 15260. Offers MSN, DNP. *Accreditation:* AACN; AANA/CANAEP. *Students:* 107 full-time (74 women), 18 part-time (16 women); includes 13 minority (6 Black or African American, non-Hispanic/Latino; 6 Asian, non-Hispanic/Latino; 1 Hispanic/Latino), 1 international. Average age 28. 217 applicants, 24% accepted, 49 enrolled. In 2013, 42 master's, 1 doctorate awarded. *Degree requirements:* For master's, comprehensive exam, thesis optional. *Entrance requirements:* For master's, GRE General Test, BSN, RN license, 1-3 years of nursing experience, letters of recommendation, resume, course work in statistics. Additional exam requirements/recommendations for international students: Required—TOEFL (minimum score 550 paper-based; 80 iBT). *Application deadline:* For fall admission, 1/5 for domestic and international students. Application fee:

$50. Electronic applications accepted. *Expenses:* Tuition, state resident: full-time $19,964; part-time $807 per credit. Tuition, nonresident: full-time $32,686; part-time $1337 per credit. *Required fees:* $740; $200. Tuition and fees vary according to program. *Unit head:* John O'Donnell, Director, 412-624-4860, Fax: 412-624-2401, E-mail: jod01@pitt.edu. *Application contact:* Laurie Lapsley, Administrator of Graduate Student Services, 412-624-9670, Fax: 412-624-2409, E-mail: lapsleyl@pitt.edu.
Website: http://www.nursing.pitt.edu/

The University of Scranton, College of Graduate and Continuing Education, Department of Nursing, Scranton, PA 18510-4595. Offers adult health nursing (MSN); family nurse practitioner (MSN, PMC); nurse anesthesia (MSN, PMC). Applicants accepted in odd-numbered years only. *Accreditation:* AACN; AANA/CANAEP. Part-time and evening/weekend programs available. *Faculty:* 13 full-time (all women), 2 part-time/adjunct (both women). *Students:* 42 full-time (37 women), 28 part-time (16 women); includes 9 minority (4 Black or African American, non-Hispanic/Latino; 3 Hispanic/Latino; 2 Two or more races, non-Hispanic/Latino). Average age 34. 58 applicants, 62% accepted. In 2013, 34 master's awarded. *Degree requirements:* For master's, thesis (for some programs), capstone experience. *Entrance requirements:* For master's, BSN, minimum GPA of 3.0, Pennsylvania RN license. Additional exam requirements/recommendations for international students: Required—TOEFL (minimum score 500 paper-based), IELTS (minimum score 5.5). *Application deadline:* For fall admission, 9/1 for domestic students. Applications are processed on a rolling basis. Application fee: $0. *Financial support:* In 2013–14, 6 students received support, including 6 teaching assistantships with full and partial tuition reimbursements available (averaging $6,600 per year); career-related internships or fieldwork, Federal Work-Study, and unspecified assistantships also available. Support available to part-time students. Financial award application deadline: 3/1. *Faculty research:* Home care, doctoral education, health care of women and children, pain, health promotion and adolescence. *Unit head:* Dr. Patricia Harrington, Chair, 570-941-7673, Fax: 570-941-4201, E-mail: harringtonp1@uofs.edu. *Application contact:* Dr. Mary Jane Hanson, Director, 570-941-4060, Fax: 570-941-4201, E-mail: hansonm2@scranton.edu.
Website: http://www.scranton.edu/academics/pcps/nursing/index.shtml

University of South Carolina, School of Medicine and The Graduate School, Graduate Programs in Medicine, Program in Nurse Anesthesia, Columbia, SC 29208. Offers MNA. *Accreditation:* AACN; AANA/CANAEP. *Degree requirements:* For master's, comprehensive exam, practicum. *Entrance requirements:* For master's, GRE, 1 year of critical care experience, RN license. Electronic applications accepted. *Expenses:* Contact institution. *Faculty research:* Neuroscience, cardiovascular, hormones, stress, homeostasis.

University of South Florida, College of Nursing, Tampa, FL 33612. Offers adult gerontology acute care (DNP, PhD); adult gerontology acute care nursing (MS); adult gerontology primary care (DNP, PhD); adult gerontology primary care nursing (MS); adult gerontology primary care/occupational health nursing (MS); adult gerontology primary care/oncology nursing (MS, PhD); clinical nurse leader (MS); family health (DNP, PhD); family nurse practitioner (MS); nurse anesthesia (MS); nursing education (MS); nursing practice (DNP); nursing science (PhD), including nursing education; occupational health/adult-gerontology (DNP); oncology/adult-gerontology primary care (DNP); pediatric health (DNP, PhD); pediatric nurse practitioner (MS). *Accreditation:* AACN; AANA/CANAEP. Part-time programs available. *Faculty:* 46 full-time (40 women), 15 part-time/adjunct (11 women). *Students:* 177 full-time (150 women), 700 part-time (622 women); includes 272 minority (116 Black or African American, non-Hispanic/Latino; 2 American Indian or Alaska Native, non-Hispanic/Latino; 45 Asian, non-Hispanic/Latino; 93 Hispanic/Latino; 2 Native Hawaiian or other Pacific Islander, non-Hispanic/Latino; 14 Two or more races, non-Hispanic/Latino), 12 international. Average age 35. 656 applicants, 43% accepted, 224 enrolled. In 2013, 224 master's, 14 doctorates awarded. *Degree requirements:* For master's, comprehensive exam, thesis optional; for doctorate, comprehensive exam, thesis/dissertation. *Entrance requirements:* For master's, GRE General Test, bachelor's degree from accredited program with minimum GPA of 3.0 in all upper-division coursework; current license as Registered Nurse; 3 letters of recommendation; personal statement of goals; resume or curriculum vitae; personal interview; for doctorate, GRE General Test (recommended), bachelor's degree in nursing from a CCNA/NLNAC regionally-accredited institution with minimum GPA of 3.0 in all coursework or in all upper-division coursework; current license as Registered Nurse in Florida; undergraduate statistics course with minimum B grade; 3 letters of recommendation; statement of goals; resume; interview. Additional exam requirements/recommendations for international students: Required—TOEFL (minimum score 550 paper-based; 79 iBT). *Application deadline:* For fall admission, 2/15 for domestic students, 1/2 for international students; for spring admission, 10/1 for domestic students, 6/1 for international students. Application fee: $30. Electronic applications accepted. *Financial support:* In 2013–14, 36 students received support, including 7 research assistantships with tuition reimbursements available (averaging $18,935 per year), 29 teaching assistantships with tuition reimbursements available (averaging $30,814 per year); tuition waivers (partial) and unspecified assistantships also available. Financial award application deadline: 2/1; financial award applicants required to submit FAFSA. *Faculty research:* Women's health, palliative and end-of-life care, cardiac rehabilitation, complementary therapies for chronic illness and cancer. *Total annual research expenditures:* $3.4 million. *Unit head:* Dr. Dianne C. Morrison-Beedy, Dean and Professor, College of Nursing, 813-974-9091, Fax: 813-974-5418, E-mail: dmbeedy@health.usf.edu. *Application contact:* Dr. Connie Visovsky, Associate Professor and Associate Dean of Student Affairs, 813-396-9641, Fax: 813-974-5418, E-mail: cvisovsk@health.usf.edu.
Website: http://health.usf.edu/nursing/index.htm

The University of Tennessee at Chattanooga, Graduate School, College of Health, Education and Professional Studies, School of Nursing, Chattanooga, TN 37403. Offers administration (MSN); certified nurse anesthetist (Post-Master's Certificate); education (MSN); family nurse practitioner (MSN, Post-Master's Certificate); health care informatics (Post-Master's Certificate); nurse anesthesia (MSN); nurse education (Post-Master's Certificate); nursing (DNP). *Accreditation:* AACN; AANA/CANAEP (one or more programs are accredited). *Faculty:* 9 full-time (7 women), 2 part-time/adjunct (1 woman). *Students:* 72 full-time (39 women), 53 part-time (43 women); includes 11 minority (6 Black or African American, non-Hispanic/Latino; 1 Asian, non-Hispanic/Latino; 3 Hispanic/Latino; 1 Two or more races, non-Hispanic/Latino). Average age 33. 3 applicants, 100% accepted, 1 enrolled. In 2013, 35 master's, 10 doctorates, 2 other advanced degrees awarded. *Degree requirements:* For master's, thesis optional, qualifying exams, professional project; for Post-Master's Certificate, thesis or alternative, practicum, seminar. *Entrance requirements:* For master's, GRE General Test, MAT, BSN, minimum GPA of 3.0, eligibility for Tennessee RN license, 1 year of direct patient care experience; for Post-Master's Certificate, GRE General Test, MAT, MSN, minimum GPA of 3.0, eligibility for Tennessee RN license, one year of direct patient care experience. Additional exam requirements/recommendations for international students: Required—TOEFL (minimum score 550 paper-based; 79 iBT), IELTS (minimum score 6). *Application deadline:* For fall admission, 6/13 priority date for domestic students, 6/1 for international students; for spring admission, 10/15 priority date for domestic students, 10/1 for international students. Applications are processed on a rolling basis. Application fee: $30 ($35 for international students). Electronic applications accepted. *Financial support:* Career-related internships or fieldwork and scholarships/grants available. Support available to part-time students. *Faculty research:* Diabetes in women, health care for elderly, alternative medicine, hypertension, nurse anesthesia. *Total annual research expenditures:* $3.4 million. *Unit head:* Dr. Chris Smith, Interim Director, 423-425-1741, Fax: 423-425-4668, E-mail: chris-smith@utc.edu. *Application contact:* Dr. J. Randy Walker, Interim Dean of Graduate Studies, 423-425-4478, Fax: 423-425-5223, E-mail: randy-walker@utc.edu.
Website: http://www.utc.edu/Academic/Nursing/

University of Wisconsin–La Crosse, Graduate Studies, College of Science and Health, Department of Biology, La Crosse, WI 54601-3742. Offers aquatic sciences (MS); biology (MS); cellular and molecular biology (MS); clinical microbiology (MS); microbiology (MS); nurse anesthesia (MS); physiology (MS). Part-time programs available. *Faculty:* 22 full-time (8 women), 3 part-time/adjunct (1 woman). *Students:* 21 full-time (13 women), 37 part-time (24 women); includes 7 minority (2 Asian, non-Hispanic/Latino; 4 Hispanic/Latino; 1 Two or more races, non-Hispanic/Latino), 5 international. Average age 28. 107 applicants, 26% accepted, 25 enrolled. In 2013, 16 master's awarded. *Degree requirements:* For master's, comprehensive exam, thesis. *Entrance requirements:* For master's, GRE General Test, minimum GPA of 2.85. Additional exam requirements/recommendations for international students: Required—TOEFL (minimum score 550 paper-based; 79 iBT). *Application deadline:* For fall admission, 2/1 priority date for domestic and international students; for spring admission, 1/4 priority date for domestic and international students. Applications are processed on a rolling basis. Electronic applications accepted. *Financial support:* Research assistantships with partial tuition reimbursements, Federal Work-Study, scholarships/grants, health care benefits, and tuition waivers (partial) available. Support available to part-time students. Financial award application deadline: 3/15; financial award applicants required to submit FAFSA. *Unit head:* Dr. Thomas Volk, Coordinator of Graduate Studies, 608-785-6972, Fax: 608-785-6959, E-mail: volk.thom@uwlax.edu. *Application contact:* Corey Sjoquist, Director of Admissions, 608-785-8939, E-mail: admissions@uwlax.edu.
Website: http://uwlax.edu/biology/

Villanova University, College of Nursing, Villanova, PA 19085-1699. Offers adult nurse practitioner (MSN, Post Master's Certificate); family nurse practitioner (MSN, Post Master's Certificate); health care administration (MSN, Post Master's Certificate); nurse anesthetist (MSN, Post Master's Certificate); nursing (PhD); nursing education (MSN, Post Master's Certificate); nursing practice (DNP); pediatric nurse practitioner (MSN, Post Master's Certificate). *Accreditation:* AACN; AANA/CANAEP. Part-time programs available. Postbaccalaureate distance learning degree programs offered (minimal on-campus study). *Faculty:* 17 full-time (all women), 4 part-time/adjunct (all women). *Students:* 28 full-time (26 women), 191 part-time (161 women); includes 22 minority (2 Black or African American, non-Hispanic/Latino; 6 Asian, non-Hispanic/Latino; 7 Hispanic/Latino; 7 Two or more races, non-Hispanic/Latino), 18 international. Average age 30. 176 applicants, 65% accepted, 82 enrolled. In 2013, 64 master's, 7 doctorates, 5 other advanced degrees awarded. *Degree requirements:* For master's, independent study project; for doctorate, comprehensive exam, thesis/dissertation. *Entrance requirements:* For master's, GRE or MAT, BSN, 1 year of recent nursing experience, physical assessment, course work in statistics; for doctorate, GRE, MSN. Additional exam requirements/recommendations for international students: Required—TOEFL (minimum score 540 paper-based; 83 iBT), IELTS (minimum score 6.5). *Application deadline:* For fall admission, 7/1 priority date for domestic students, 7/1 for international students; for spring admission, 11/1 priority date for domestic students, 11/1 for international students. Applications are processed on a rolling basis. Application fee: $50. Electronic applications accepted. *Expenses:* Contact institution. *Financial support:* In 2013–14, 39 students received support, including 5 teaching assistantships with full tuition reimbursements available (averaging $14,475 per year); institutionally sponsored loans, scholarships/grants, traineeships, tuition waivers (full), and unspecified assistantships also available. Financial award application deadline: 7/1; financial award applicants required to submit FAFSA. *Faculty research:* Genetics, ethics, cognitive development of students, women with disabilities, nursing leadership. *Unit head:* Dr. Marguerite K. Schlag, Assistant Dean/Director, Graduate Programs, 610-519-4907, Fax: 610-519-7650, E-mail: marguerite.schlag@villanova.edu.
Website: http://www.nursing.villanova.edu/

Virginia Commonwealth University, Graduate School, School of Allied Health Professions, Department of Nurse Anesthesia, Richmond, VA 23284-9005. Offers MSNA, DNAP. *Accreditation:* AANA/CANAEP. *Degree requirements:* For master's, thesis. *Entrance requirements:* For master's, GRE General Test, 1 year experience in acute critical care nursing, current state RN license, minimum GPA of 3.0; for doctorate, GRE General Test, accredited MSNA, CCNA certification, minimum GPA of 3.0. Additional exam requirements/recommendations for international students: Required—TOEFL (minimum score 600 paper-based; 100 iBT); Recommended—IELTS (minimum score 6.5). Electronic applications accepted. *Faculty research:* Obstetrical anesthesia, ambulatory anesthesia, regional anesthesia, practice profiles, clinical practice.

Virginia Commonwealth University, Graduate School, School of Allied Health Professions, Doctoral Program in Health Related Sciences, Richmond, VA 23284-9005. Offers clinical laboratory sciences (PhD); gerontology (PhD); health administration (PhD); nurse anesthesia (PhD); occupational therapy (PhD); physical therapy (PhD); radiation sciences (PhD); rehabilitation leadership (PhD). *Entrance requirements:* For doctorate, GRE General Test or MAT, minimum GPA of 3.3 in master's degree. Additional exam requirements/recommendations for international students: Required—TOEFL (minimum score 600 paper-based; 100 iBT); Recommended—IELTS (minimum score 6.5). Electronic applications accepted.

Wayne State University, Eugene Applebaum College of Pharmacy and Health Sciences, Department of Health Care Sciences, Program in Nursing Anesthesia, Detroit, MI 48202. Offers nurse anesthesia (MS); pediatric nurse anesthesia (Certificate). *Accreditation:* AACN; AANA/CANAEP. *Faculty:* 1 (woman) full-time, 4 part-time/adjunct (2 women). *Students:* 36 full-time (22 women); includes 11 minority (1 Black or African American, non-Hispanic/Latino; 8 Asian, non-Hispanic/Latino; 2 Two or more races, non-Hispanic/Latino). Average age 32. In 2013, 11 master's, 1 other advanced degree awarded. *Entrance requirements:* For master's, GRE General Test, bachelor's degree in nursing or related science with minimum GPA of 3.0 overall and in science, current RN license, CCRN certification, one year of full-time experience in adult ICU, ACLS certification, hospital shadow experience (arranged by department); for Certificate, MS in anesthesia from accredited program, meeting with course coordinators from Children's Hospital of Michigan. Additional exam requirements/recommendations for international students: Required—TOEFL (minimum score 550 paper-based; 79 iBT), Michigan English Language Assessment Battery (minimum score 85); Recommended—IELTS (minimum score 6.5), TWE (minimum score 5.5). *Application deadline:* For fall admission, 7/1 for domestic students, 5/1 priority date for international students. Application fee: $0. Electronic applications accepted. *Expenses:* Contact institution. *Financial support:* Scholarships/grants available. Financial award application deadline: 3/31; financial award applicants required to submit FAFSA. *Faculty research:* Music therapy in pain management; student success/students perspective; pace maker

management-safety, airway devices, IV Tylenol for pain. *Unit head:* Dr. Prudentia A. Worth, Program Director, 313-993-7168, E-mail: aa1635@wayne.edu.
Website: http://www.cphs.wayne.edu/anesth/

Webster University, College of Arts and Sciences, Department of Biological Sciences, Program in Nurse Anesthesia, St. Louis, MO 63119-3194. Offers MS. *Accreditation:* AANA/CANAEP. Postbaccalaureate distance learning degree programs offered. *Degree requirements:* For master's, thesis. *Entrance requirements:* For master's, 1 year of work-related experience, 75 hours of graduate course work, BSN, interview, minimum GPA of 3.0. Additional exam requirements/recommendations for international students: Required—TOEFL. *Expenses: Tuition:* Full-time $11,610; part-time $645 per credit hour. Tuition and fees vary according to campus/location and program. *Faculty research:* Clinical anesthesia, substance abuse education in the health professions, technology and education, clinical pharmacology.

Westminster College, School of Nursing and Health Sciences, Salt Lake City, UT 84105-3697. Offers family nurse practitioner (MSN); nurse anesthesia (MSNA); nurse education (MSNED); nursing (MSN); public health (MPH). *Accreditation:* AACN; AANA/CANAEP. *Faculty:* 11 full-time (5 women), 7 part-time/adjunct (4 women). *Students:* 119 full-time (75 women), 5 part-time (2 women); includes 21 minority (5 Black or African American, non-Hispanic/Latino; 1 American Indian or Alaska Native, non-Hispanic/Latino; 4 Asian, non-Hispanic/Latino; 7 Hispanic/Latino; 1 Native Hawaiian or other Pacific Islander, non-Hispanic/Latino; 3 Two or more races, non-Hispanic/Latino), 4 international. Average age 32. 246 applicants, 35% accepted, 56 enrolled. In 2013, 49 master's awarded. *Degree requirements:* For master's, clinical practicum, 504 clinical practice hours. *Entrance requirements:* For master's, GRE, resume, Utah RN license in good standing, minimum GPA of 3.0, 3 letters of reference, BSN from accredited nursing program, proof of clear state and federal background check, drug test results, personal interview, current PALS certification, current ACLS certification, document of current immunizations, physical and mental health certificate. Additional exam requirements/recommendations for international students: Required—TOEFL (minimum score 600 paper-based; 100 iBT), IELTS (minimum score 7.5). *Application deadline:* Applications are processed on a rolling basis. Application fee: $50. Electronic applications accepted. *Expenses:* Contact institution. *Financial support:* In 2013–14, 9 students received support. Career-related internships or fieldwork, unspecified assistantships, and tuition reimbursements, tuition remission available. Support available to part-time students. Financial award applicants required to submit FAFSA. *Faculty research:* Collaborative testing in nursing: student outcomes and perspectives, implementing new educational paradigms into pre-licensure nursing curricula. *Unit head:* Dr. Sheryl Steadman, Dean, 801-832-2164, Fax: 801-832-3110, E-mail: ssteadman@westminstercollege.edu. *Application contact:* Dr. John Baworowsky, Vice President of Enrollment Management, 801-832-2200, Fax: 801-832-3101, E-mail: admission@westminstercollege.edu.
Website: http://www.westminstercollege.edu/msn

York College of Pennsylvania, Department of Nursing, York, PA 17405-7199. Offers adult gerontology clinical nurse specialist (MS), including administration, education; adult gerontology nurse practitioner (MS); certified nurse anesthetist (MS); nurse educator (MS); nursing (DNP). *Accreditation:* AACN; AANA/CANAEP. Part-time and evening/weekend programs available. *Faculty:* 10 full-time (all women), 4 part-time/adjunct (1 woman). *Students:* 33 full-time (26 women), 61 part-time (53 women); includes 12 minority (7 Black or African American, non-Hispanic/Latino; 2 American Indian or Alaska Native, non-Hispanic/Latino; 3 Asian, non-Hispanic/Latino), 1 international. Average age 37. 87 applicants, 31% accepted, 24 enrolled. In 2013, 26 master's, 4 doctorates awarded. *Entrance requirements:* For master's, GRE General Test, minimum GPA of 3.0 from CCNE- or NLNAC-accredited institution; for doctorate, master's degree in nursing from a CCNE- or NLNAC-accredited institution; minimum GPA of 3.0. Additional exam requirements/recommendations for international students: Required—TOEFL (minimum score 530 paper-based; 72 iBT). *Application deadline:* For fall admission, 7/15 priority date for domestic students; for spring admission, 11/15 priority date for domestic students. Applications are processed on a rolling basis. Application fee: $50. Electronic applications accepted. *Expenses: Tuition:* Full-time $12,870; part-time $715 per credit. *Required fees:* $1660; $360 per semester. Tuition and fees vary according to degree level. *Financial support:* Federal Work-Study available. *Faculty research:* Student stress response to simulation versus clinical, evidence-based practice in all clinical settings. *Unit head:* Dr. Richard Haas, Graduate Program Director, 717-815-1243, E-mail: rhaas@ycp.edu. *Application contact:* Diane Dube, Administrative Assistant, Graduate Programs in Nursing, 717-815-1462, E-mail: ddube@ycp.edu.
Website: http://www.ycp.edu/academics/academic-departments/nursing/

Nurse Midwifery

Bastyr University, School of Natural Health Arts and Sciences, Kenmore, WA 98028-4966. Offers counseling psychology (MA); holistic landscape design (Certificate); midwifery (MS); nutrition (MS); nutrition and clinical health psychology (MS). *Accreditation:* AND. Part-time programs available. *Students:* 328 full-time (295 women), 40 part-time (38 women); includes 74 minority (5 Black or African American, non-Hispanic/Latino; 1 American Indian or Alaska Native, non-Hispanic/Latino; 28 Asian, non-Hispanic/Latino; 13 Hispanic/Latino; 27 Two or more races, non-Hispanic/Latino), 21 international. Average age 30. *Degree requirements:* For master's, thesis optional. *Entrance requirements:* For master's, 1-2 years' basic sciences course work (depending on program). Additional exam requirements/recommendations for international students: Required—TOEFL (minimum score 550 paper-based; 79 iBT). *Application deadline:* For fall admission, 3/15 priority date for domestic and international students. Applications are processed on a rolling basis. Application fee: $75. *Financial support:* In 2013–14, 47 students received support. Career-related internships or fieldwork, Federal Work-Study, and scholarships/grants available. Support available to part-time students. Financial award application deadline: 4/15; financial award applicants required to submit FAFSA. *Faculty research:* Whole-food nutrition for type 2 diabetes; meditation in end-of-life care; stress management; Qi Gong, Tai Chi and yoga for older adults; Echinacea and immunology. *Unit head:* Dr. Timothy Callahan, Vice President and Provost, 425-602-3110, Fax: 425-823-6222. *Application contact:* Admissions Office, 425-602-3330, Fax: 425-602-3090, E-mail: admissions@bastyr.edu.
Website: http://www.bastyr.edu/academics/schools-departments/school-natural-health-arts-sciences

Baylor University, Graduate School, Louise Herrington School of Nursing, Dallas, TX 75246. Offers family nurse practitioner (MSN); neonatal nurse practitioner (MSN); nurse-midwifery (DNP). *Accreditation:* AACN. Part-time programs available. Postbaccalaureate distance learning degree programs offered (minimal on-campus study). *Faculty:* 11 full-time (all women), 3 part-time/adjunct (2 women). *Students:* 25 full-time (24 women), 41 part-time (37 women); includes 15 minority (5 Black or African American, non-Hispanic/Latino; 5 Asian, non-Hispanic/Latino; 4 Hispanic/Latino; 1 Two or more races, non-Hispanic/Latino). Average age 35. 47 applicants, 70% accepted, 26 enrolled. In 2013, 25 master's, 5 doctorates awarded. *Degree requirements:* For doctorate, comprehensive exam (for some programs), capstone project. *Entrance requirements:* For master's, GRE General Test or MAT; for doctorate, GRE General Test. Additional exam requirements/recommendations for international students: Required—TOEFL. *Application deadline:* For fall admission, 2/1 for domestic students. Application fee: $50. Electronic applications accepted. *Expenses: Tuition:* Full-time $25,866; part-time $1437 per credit hour. *Required fees:* $2736; $152 per credit hour. Tuition and fees vary according to course load and program. *Financial support:* In 2013–14, 66 students received support, including 1 teaching assistantship (averaging $4,167 per year); Federal Work-Study, scholarships/grants, and unspecified assistantships also available. Support available to part-time students. Financial award application deadline: 6/30; financial award applicants required to submit FAFSA. *Faculty research:* Women and strokes, obesity and pregnancy, educational environmental factors, international undeserved populations, midwifery. *Total annual research expenditures:* $5,000. *Unit head:* Dr. Barbara Camune, Graduate Program Director, 214-367-3754, Fax: 214-820-3375, E-mail: barbara_camune@baylor.edu. *Application contact:* Elaine Lark, Coordinator of Recruitment and Enrollment, 214-818-7839, Fax: 214-820-3835, E-mail: elaine_lark@baylor.edu.
Website: http://www.baylor.edu/nursing/

Bethel University, Graduate School, St. Paul, MN 55112-6999. Offers autism spectrum disorders (Certificate); business administration (MBA); communication (MA); counseling psychology (MA); educational leadership (Ed D); gerontology (MA); international baccalaureate education (Certificate); K-12 education (MA); literacy education (MA, Certificate); nurse educator (Certificate); nurse leader (Certificate); nurse-midwifery (MS); nursing (MS); physician assistant (MS); postsecondary teaching (Certificate); special education (MA); strategic leadership (MA); teaching (MA). Part-time and evening/weekend programs available. Postbaccalaureate distance learning degree programs offered (no on-campus study). *Faculty:* 13 full-time (7 women), 89 part-time/adjunct (43 women). *Students:* 692 full-time (457 women), 573 part-time (371 women); includes 170 minority (86 Black or African American, non-Hispanic/Latino; 1 American Indian or Alaska Native, non-Hispanic/Latino; 49 Asian, non-Hispanic/Latino; 20 Hispanic/Latino; 1 Native Hawaiian or other Pacific Islander, non-Hispanic/Latino; 13 Two or more races, non-Hispanic/Latino), 21 international. Average age 37. In 2013, 166 master's, 9 doctorates, 11 other advanced degrees awarded. *Degree requirements:* For master's, comprehensive exam (for some programs), thesis (for some programs); for doctorate, comprehensive exam, thesis/dissertation. *Entrance requirements:* Additional exam requirements/recommendations for international students: Required—TOEFL (minimum score 550 paper-based; 80 iBT). *Application deadline:* Applications are processed on a rolling basis. Electronic applications accepted. Tuition and fees vary according to course load, degree level and program. *Financial support:* Teaching assistantships, career-related internships or fieldwork, and scholarships/grants available. Support available to part-time students. Financial award applicants required to submit FAFSA. *Unit head:* Dick Crombie, Vice-President/Dean, 651-635-8000, Fax: 651-635-8004, E-mail: gs@bethel.edu. *Application contact:* Director of Admissions, 651-635-8000, Fax: 651-635-8004, E-mail: gs@bethel.edu.
Website: http://gs.bethel.edu/

Case Western Reserve University, Frances Payne Bolton School of Nursing, Doctor of Nursing Practice Program, Cleveland, OH 44106. Offers acute care nurse practitioner (DNP); adult gerontology nurse practitioner (DNP); educational leadership (DNP); family nurse practitioner (DNP); family systems psychiatric mental health nursing (DNP); midwifery/family nursing (DNP); neonatal nurse practitioner (DNP); pediatric nurse practitioner (DNP); practice leadership (DNP); women's health nurse practitioner (DNP). *Accreditation:* AACN. Part-time programs available. Postbaccalaureate distance learning degree programs offered (minimal on-campus study). *Students:* 169 full-time, 9 part-time; includes 10 minority (6 Black or African American, non-Hispanic/Latino; 1 Asian, non-Hispanic/Latino; 2 Hispanic/Latino; 1 Two or more races, non-Hispanic/Latino). 76 applicants, 97% accepted, 59 enrolled. In 2013, 38 doctorates awarded. Terminal master's awarded for partial completion of doctoral program. *Degree requirements:* For doctorate, thesis/dissertation. *Entrance requirements:* For doctorate, GRE General Test or MAT. Additional exam requirements/recommendations for international students: Required—TOEFL (minimum score 577 paper-based; 90 iBT), IELTS (minimum score 7). *Application deadline:* For fall admission, 6/1 priority date for domestic students, 6/1 for international students; for spring admission, 10/1 for domestic and international students. Applications are processed on a rolling basis. Application fee: $75. *Financial support:* In 2013–14, 90 students received support, including 9 fellowships with full tuition reimbursements available (averaging $31,325 per year), 1 research assistantship with partial tuition reimbursement available (averaging $14,472 per year); teaching assistantships, Federal Work-Study, institutionally sponsored loans, scholarships/grants, and tuition waivers (partial) also available. Support available to part-time students. Financial award application deadline: 5/15; financial award applicants required to submit FAFSA. *Faculty research:* Symptom science, family/community care, aging across the lifespan, self-management of health and illness, neuroscience. *Unit head:* Dr. Donna Dowling, Director, 216-368-1869, Fax: 216-368-3542, E-mail: dad10@case.edu. *Application contact:* Donna Hassik, Admissions Coordinator, 216-368-5253, Fax: 216-368-0124, E-mail: dmh7@case.edu.
Website: http://fpb.case.edu/DNP/

Case Western Reserve University, Frances Payne Bolton School of Nursing, Master's Programs in Nursing, Program in Nurse Midwifery, Cleveland, OH 44106. Offers MSN. *Accreditation:* ACNM/ACME. *Students:* 10; includes 1 minority (Black or African American, non-Hispanic/Latino). 4 applicants, 75% accepted, 3 enrolled. In 2013, 2 master's awarded. *Degree requirements:* For master's, thesis optional. *Entrance requirements:* For master's, GRE General Test or MAT. Additional exam requirements/recommendations for international students: Required—TOEFL (minimum score 577 paper-based; 90 iBT), IELTS (minimum score 7). *Application deadline:* For fall admission, 6/1 for domestic and international students; for spring admission, 10/1 for domestic and international students. Applications are processed on a rolling basis. Application fee: $75. *Financial support:* Fellowships, research assistantships, teaching assistantships, institutionally sponsored loans, and tuition waivers (partial) available. Support available to part-time students. Financial award application deadline: 6/30;

financial award applicants required to submit FAFSA. *Faculty research:* Clinical nursing, normal childbearing, descriptive studies of care, high risk pregnancy side effects of bed rest, strengthening and expanding nursing services. *Unit head:* Dr. Gretchen Mettler, Head, 216-368-0671, E-mail: ggm@case.edu. *Application contact:* Donna Hassik, Admissions Coordinator, 216-368-5253, Fax: 216-368-0124, E-mail: dmh7@case.edu. Website: http://fpb.case.edu/MSN/midwifery.shtm

Columbia University, School of Nursing, Program in Nurse Midwifery, New York, NY 10032. Offers MS. *Accreditation:* AACN; ACNM/ACME. Part-time programs available. *Entrance requirements:* For master's, GRE General Test, NCLEX, BSN, 1 year of clinical experience (preferred). Additional exam requirements/recommendations for international students: Required—TOEFL (minimum score 100 iBT). Electronic applications accepted.

DeSales University, Graduate Division, Division of Healthcare and Natural Sciences, Center Valley, PA 18034-9568. Offers adult clinical nurse specialist (MSN); certified nurse midwives (MSN); certified nurse practitioners (MSN); clinical leadership (DNP); family nurse practitioner (MSN); information systems (MSIS); nurse educator (MSN); nurse practitioner (Post-Master's Certificate); physical therapy (DPT); physician assistant studies (MSPAS); MSN/MBA. Part-time programs available. In 2013, 5 doctorates awarded. *Degree requirements:* For master's, thesis optional. *Entrance requirements:* For master's, GRE General Test, MAT, minimum B average in undergraduate course work, health assessment course or equivalent, course work in statistics. Additional exam requirements/recommendations for international students: Required—TOEFL. *Application deadline:* Applications are processed on a rolling basis. Application fee: $35. Electronic applications accepted. *Expenses: Tuition:* Part-time $790 per credit. *Financial support:* Applicants required to submit FAFSA. *Unit head:* Dr. Mary Liz Doyle-Tadduni, Department Chair, Nursing, 610-282-1100 Ext. 1394, Fax: 610-282-2091, E-mail: carol.mest@desales.edu. *Application contact:* Abagail Wernicki, Director of Graduate Admissions, 610-282-1100 Ext. 1768, Fax: 610-282-2869, E-mail: abagail.wernicki@desales.edu.

Emory University, Nell Hodgson Woodruff School of Nursing, Atlanta, GA 30322-1100. Offers adult nurse practitioner (MSN); emergency nurse practitioner (MSN); family nurse practitioner (MSN); family nurse-midwife (MSN); health systems leadership (MSN); nurse-midwifery (MSN); pediatric nurse practitioner acute and primary care (MSN); women's health care (Title X) (MSN); women's health nurse practitioner (MSN); MSN/MPH. *Accreditation:* AACN; ACNM/ACME (one or more programs are accredited). Part-time programs available. *Entrance requirements:* For master's, GRE General Test or MAT, minimum GPA of 3.0, BS in nursing from an accredited institution, RN license and additional course work, 3 letters of recommendation. Additional exam requirements/recommendations for international students: Required—TOEFL (minimum score 600 paper-based; 100 iBT). Electronic applications accepted. *Expenses:* Contact institution. *Faculty research:* Older adult falls and injuries, minority health issues, cardiac symptoms and quality of life, bio-ethics and decision-making, menopausal issues.

Frontier Nursing University, Graduate Programs, Hyden, KY 41749. Offers family nurse practitioner (MSN, DNP, Post Master's Certificate); nurse-midwifery (MSN, DNP, Post Master's Certificate); women's health care nurse practitioner (MSN, DNP, Post Master's Certificate). *Accreditation:* ACNM. *Degree requirements:* For doctorate, capstone project, practicum.

Georgetown University, Graduate School of Arts and Sciences, School of Nursing and Health Studies, Washington, DC 20057. Offers acute care nurse practitioner (MS); clinical nurse specialist (MS); family nurse practitioner (MS); nurse anesthesia (MS); nurse-midwifery (MS); nursing (DNP); nursing education (MS). *Accreditation:* AACN; AANA/CANAEP (one or more programs are accredited); ACNM/ACME (one or more programs are accredited). *Degree requirements:* For master's, thesis optional. *Entrance requirements:* For master's, GRE General Test or MAT, bachelor's degree in nursing from NLN-accredited school, minimum undergraduate GPA of 3.0. Additional exam requirements/recommendations for international students: Required—TOEFL. Application fee: $50 ($55 for international students). *Financial support:* Scholarships/grants and traineeships available. Financial award applicants required to submit FAFSA. *Unit head:* Dr. Patricia Ann Cloonan, Dean, 202-687-7318. *Application contact:* Graduate School Admissions Office, 202-687-5568.

Marquette University, Graduate School, College of Nursing, Milwaukee, WI 53201-1881. Offers acute care nurse practitioner (Certificate); adult clinical nurse specialist (Certificate); adult nurse practitioner (Certificate); advanced practice nursing (MSN, DNP), including adult-older adult acute care (DNP), adults (MSN), adults-older adults (DNP), clinical nurse leader (MSN), health care systems leadership (DNP), nurse-midwifery (MSN), older adults (MSN), pediatrics acute care (MSN), pediatrics primary care (MSN), pediatrics-acute care (DNP), pediatrics-primary care (DNP), primary care (DNP), systems leadership and healthcare quality (MSN); family nurse practitioner (Certificate); nurse-midwifery (Certificate); nursing (PhD); pediatric acute care (Certificate); pediatric primary care (Certificate); systems leadership and healthcare quality (Certificate). *Accreditation:* AACN. *Faculty:* 35 full-time (34 women), 59 part-time/adjunct (58 women). *Students:* 105 full-time (96 women), 279 part-time (256 women); includes 28 minority (11 Black or African American, non-Hispanic/Latino; 7 Asian, non-Hispanic/Latino; 8 Hispanic/Latino; 2 Two or more races, non-Hispanic/Latino), 3 international. Average age 30. 322 applicants, 62% accepted, 98 enrolled. In 2013, 66 master's, 4 doctorates, 6 other advanced degrees awarded. Terminal master's awarded for partial completion of doctoral program. *Degree requirements:* For master's, comprehensive exam, thesis or alternative. *Entrance requirements:* For master's, GRE General Test, BSN, Wisconsin RN license, official transcripts from all current and previous colleges/universities except Marquette, three completed recommendation forms, resume, written statement of professional goals; for doctorate, GRE General Test, official transcripts from all current and previous colleges/universities except Marquette, three letters of recommendation, resume, written statement of professional goals, sample of scholarly writing. Additional exam requirements/recommendations for international students: Required—TOEFL (minimum score 530 paper-based). *Application deadline:* For fall admission, 2/15 for domestic and international students. Application fee: $50. Electronic applications accepted. *Financial support:* In 2013–14, 41 students received support, including 1 fellowship with partial tuition reimbursement available (averaging $17,500 per year), 2 research assistantships with full tuition reimbursements available (averaging $13,285 per year), 8 teaching assistantships with full tuition reimbursements available (averaging $13,912 per year); career-related internships or fieldwork, Federal Work-Study, scholarships/grants, health care benefits, tuition waivers (partial), and unspecified assistantships also available. Support available to part-time students. Financial award application deadline: 2/15. *Faculty research:* Psychosocial adjustment to chronic illness, gerontology, reminiscence, health policy: uninsured and access, hospital care delivery systems. *Total annual research expenditures:* $769,051. *Unit head:* Dr. Margaret Callahan, Dean, 414-288-3800, Fax: 414-288-1578. *Application contact:* Dr. Maureen O'Brien, Associate Dean/Clinical Associate Professor, 414-288-3823.
Website: http://www.marquette.edu/nursing/academicprograms-graduate.shtml

Midwives College of Utah, Graduate Program, Salt Lake City, UT 84106. Offers MS. *Accreditation:* MEAC. *Degree requirements:* For master's, comprehensive exam (for some programs), thesis.

National College of Midwifery, Graduate Programs, Taos, NM 87571. Offers MS, PhD. *Accreditation:* MEAC. Part-time and evening/weekend programs available. Postbaccalaureate distance learning degree programs offered (no on-campus study). *Degree requirements:* For master's, thesis, publication; for doctorate, thesis/dissertation, presentation, publication. *Entrance requirements:* For master's and doctorate, midwifery license or certification. Electronic applications accepted.

New York University, College of Nursing, Doctor of Nursing Practice Program, New York, NY 10012-1019. Offers advanced practice nursing (DNP), including adult acute care, adult nurse practitioner/holistic nursing, adult nurse practitioner/palliative care nursing, adult primary care, adult primary care/geriatrics, family, geriatrics, mental health nursing, nurse-midwifery, pediatrics. Part-time and evening/weekend programs available. *Faculty:* 3 full-time (all women), 1 part-time/adjunct (0 women). *Students:* 1 (woman) full-time, 33 part-time (30 women); includes 7 minority (3 Black or African American, non-Hispanic/Latino; 3 Asian, non-Hispanic/Latino; 1 Hispanic/Latino). Average age 39. 18 applicants, 100% accepted, 12 enrolled. In 2013, 4 doctorates awarded. *Degree requirements:* For doctorate, thesis/dissertation, capstone. *Entrance requirements:* For doctorate, MAT or GRE (either taken within past 5 years), MS, RN license, interview, Nurse Practitioner Certification. Additional exam requirements/recommendations for international students: Required—TOEFL (minimum score 90 iBT), IELTS (minimum score 7). *Application deadline:* For fall admission, 3/1 for domestic students, 4/1 for international students. Applications are processed on a rolling basis. Application fee: $80. Electronic applications accepted. *Expenses: Tuition:* Full-time $35,856; part-time $1494 per unit. *Required fees:* $1408; $64 per unit. $473 per term. Tuition and fees vary according to course load and program. *Financial support:* Scholarships/grants available. Support available to part-time students. Financial award application deadline: 2/1. *Faculty research:* Geriatrics, HIV, elderly black diabetics, families and illness, oral systemic connection. *Unit head:* Dr. Rona Levin, Director, 212-998-5319, Fax: 212-995-3143, E-mail: rfl2039@nyu.edu. *Application contact:* Elizabeth Ensweiler, Assistant Director, Graduate Student Affairs and Admissions, 212-992-7653, Fax: 212-995-4302, E-mail: ee39@nyu.edu.

New York University, College of Nursing, Programs in Advanced Practice Nursing, New York, NY 10012-1019. Offers advanced practice nursing: adult acute care (MS, Advanced Certificate); advanced practice nursing: adult nurse practitioner/holistic nurse practitioner (Advanced Certificate); advanced practice nursing: adult nurse practitioner/palliative care nurse practitioner (Advanced Certificate); advanced practice nursing: adult primary care (MS, Advanced Certificate); advanced practice nursing: family (MS, Advanced Certificate); advanced practice nursing: geriatrics (Advanced Certificate); advanced practice nursing: mental health (MS); advanced practice nursing: mental health nursing (Advanced Certificate); advanced practice nursing: pediatrics (MS, Advanced Certificate); nurse midwifery (MS, Advanced Certificate); nursing administration (MS, Advanced Certificate); nursing education (MS, Advanced Certificate); nursing informatics (MS, Advanced Certificate); MS/MPA; MS/MPH. *Accreditation:* AACN; ACNM/ACME. Part-time programs available. *Faculty:* 22 full-time (all women), 54 part-time/adjunct (46 women). *Students:* 36 full-time (31 women), 622 part-time (549 women); includes 239 minority (73 Black or African American, non-Hispanic/Latino; 1 American Indian or Alaska Native, non-Hispanic/Latino; 116 Asian, non-Hispanic/Latino; 36 Hispanic/Latino; 6 Native Hawaiian or other Pacific Islander, non-Hispanic/Latino; 7 Two or more races, non-Hispanic/Latino), 16 international. Average age 37. 395 applicants, 67% accepted, 156 enrolled. In 2013, 186 master's, 8 other advanced degrees awarded. *Degree requirements:* For master's, thesis (for some programs). *Entrance requirements:* For master's, BS in nursing, AS in nursing with another BS/BA, interview, RN license, 1 year of clinical experience (3 for nursing education program); for Advanced Certificate, master's degree. Additional exam requirements/recommendations for international students: Required—TOEFL (minimum score 90 iBT), IELTS (minimum score 7). *Application deadline:* For fall admission, 7/1 for domestic and international students; for spring admission, 12/1 for domestic and international students. Application fee: $80. Electronic applications accepted. *Expenses: Tuition:* Full-time $35,856; part-time $1494 per unit. *Required fees:* $1408; $64 per unit. $473 per term. Tuition and fees vary according to course load and program. *Financial support:* In 2013–14, 182 students received support. Research assistantships, career-related internships or fieldwork, Federal Work-Study, scholarships/grants, traineeships, and unspecified assistantships available. Support available to part-time students. Financial award application deadline: 2/1; financial award applicants required to submit FAFSA. *Faculty research:* Geriatrics, HIV, elderly black diabetics, families and illness, oral systemic connection. *Unit head:* Dr. Judith Haber, Associate Dean, Graduate Programs, 212-998-9020, Fax: 212-995-3143, E-mail: jh33@nyu.edu. *Application contact:* Elizabeth Ensweiler, Assistant Director, Graduate Student Affairs and Admissions, 212-992-7653, Fax: 212-995-4302, E-mail: ee39@nyu.edu.

Old Dominion University, College of Health Sciences, School of Nursing, Norfolk, VA 23529. Offers family nurse practitioner (MSN); nurse administrator (MSN); nurse anesthesia (MSN); nurse educator (MSN); nurse midwifery (MSN); nursing practice (DNP); women's health nurse practitioner (MSN). *Accreditation:* AACN; AANA/CANAEP (one or more programs are accredited). Part-time programs available. Postbaccalaureate distance learning degree programs offered (no on-campus study). *Faculty:* 6 full-time (5 women), 17 part-time/adjunct (15 women). *Students:* 111 full-time (100 women), 123 part-time (115 women); includes 45 minority (34 Black or African American, non-Hispanic/Latino; 7 Asian, non-Hispanic/Latino; 2 Hispanic/Latino; 2 Two or more races, non-Hispanic/Latino). Average age 38. 258 applicants, 61% accepted, 117 enrolled. In 2013, 60 master's, 29 doctorates awarded. *Degree requirements:* For master's, comprehensive exam; for doctorate, capstone project. *Entrance requirements:* For master's, GRE or MAT, BSN, minimum GPA of 3.0 in nursing and overall. Additional exam requirements/recommendations for international students: Required—TOEFL. *Application deadline:* For fall admission, 5/1 for domestic students, 4/15 for international students. Applications are processed on a rolling basis. Application fee: $50. Electronic applications accepted. *Expenses:* Tuition, state resident: full-time $9888; part-time $412 per credit. Tuition, nonresident: full-time $25,152; part-time $1048 per credit. *Required fees:* $59 per semester. One-time fee: $50. *Financial support:* In 2013–14, 18 students received support, including 2 research assistantships with partial tuition reimbursements available (averaging $10,000 per year), 1 teaching assistantship (averaging $2,500 per year); career-related internships or fieldwork, scholarships/grants, traineeships, and tuition waivers (partial) also available. Support available to part-time students. Financial award application deadline: 2/15; financial award applicants required to submit FAFSA. *Faculty research:* Health and culture, cardiovascular health, transition of military families, genetics, cultural diversity. *Total annual research expenditures:* $231,117. *Unit head:* Dr. Karen Karlowicz, Chair, 757-683-5262, Fax: 757-683-5253, E-mail: nursgpd@odu.edu. *Application contact:* Sue Parker, Coordinator, Graduate Student Services, 757-683-4298, Fax: 757-683-5253, E-mail: sparker@odu.edu.
Website: http://www.odu.edu/nursing

Oregon Health & Science University, School of Nursing, Program in Nurse Midwifery, Portland, OR 97239-3098. Offers MN, MS, Post Master's Certificate. *Accreditation:* AACN; ACNM/ACME (one or more programs are accredited). *Degree requirements:* For master's, thesis optional. *Entrance requirements:* For master's, GRE General Test, bachelor's degree in nursing, minimum undergraduate GPA of 3.0, previous course work in statistics; for Post Master's Certificate, master's degree in nursing.

Philadelphia University, College of Science, Health and the Liberal Arts, Program in Midwifery, Philadelphia, PA 19144. Offers midwifery (MS); nurse midwifery (Postbaccalaureate Certificate). *Accreditation:* ACNM/ACME. Part-time and evening/weekend programs available. Postbaccalaureate distance learning degree programs offered (minimal on-campus study). *Entrance requirements:* For master's, GRE or MAT. Additional exam requirements/recommendations for international students: Required—TOEFL (minimum score 550 paper-based; 79 iBT). Electronic applications accepted.

Seattle University, College of Nursing, Program in Advanced Practice Nursing Immersion, Seattle, WA 98122-1090. Offers adult/gerontological nurse practitioner (MSN); advanced community public health nursing (MSN); family nurse practitioner (MSN); family psychiatric mental health nurse practitioner (MSN); nurse midwifery (MSN). *Faculty:* 17 full-time (15 women), 9 part-time/adjunct (6 women). *Students:* 109 full-time (94 women), 6 part-time (5 women); includes 25 minority (3 Black or African American, non-Hispanic/Latino; 11 Asian, non-Hispanic/Latino; 2 Hispanic/Latino; 9 Two or more races, non-Hispanic/Latino). Average age 31. In 2013, 48 master's awarded. *Degree requirements:* For master's, thesis or scholarly project. *Entrance requirements:* For master's, GRE, bachelor's degree, minimum GPA of 3.0, professional resume, two recommendations, letter of intent. Additional exam requirements/recommendations for international students: Required—TOEFL (minimum score 92 iBT), IELTS. *Application deadline:* For fall admission, 12/1 for domestic and international students. Application fee: $55. Electronic applications accepted. *Financial support:* In 2013–14, 3 students received support. Scholarships/grants and traineeships available. Financial award applicants required to submit FAFSA. *Unit head:* Dr. Janiece DeSocio, Interim Dean, 206-296-5660, E-mail: desocioj@seattleu.edu. *Application contact:* Janet Shandley, Associate Dean of Graduate Admissions, 206-296-5900, Fax: 206-298-5656, E-mail: grad_admissions@seattleu.edu.
Website: http://www.seattleu.edu/nursing/msn/apni/

State University of New York Downstate Medical Center, College of Nursing, Graduate Program in Nursing, Program in Nurse Midwifery, Brooklyn, NY 11203-2098. Offers MS, Post Master's Certificate. *Accreditation:* ACNM.

Stony Brook University, State University of New York, Stony Brook University Medical Center, Health Sciences Center, School of Nursing, Program in Nurse Midwifery, Stony Brook, NY 11794. Offers MS, Certificate. *Accreditation:* AACN; ACNM/ACME. Postbaccalaureate distance learning degree programs offered. *Students:* 17 part-time (all women); includes 8 minority (6 Black or African American, non-Hispanic/Latino; 1 Asian, non-Hispanic/Latino; 1 Hispanic/Latino). In 2013, 6 master's, 1 other advanced degree awarded. *Degree requirements:* For master's, thesis. *Entrance requirements:* For master's, BSN, minimum GPA of 3.0, course work in statistics. Additional exam requirements/recommendations for international students: Required—TOEFL. *Application deadline:* For fall admission, 1/15 for domestic students. Application fee: $100. *Expenses:* Tuition, state resident: full-time $9870; part-time $411 per credit. Tuition, nonresident: full-time $18,350; part-time $765 per credit. *Financial support:* Fellowships, research assistantships, and teaching assistantships available. Financial award application deadline: 3/15. *Unit head:* Dr. Kelly Caramore Walker, Director, 631-444-3299, Fax: 631-444-3136, E-mail: kelly.walker@stonybrook.edu. *Application contact:* Assistant Dean, Admissions and Records, 631-632-2644, Fax: 631-444-3136, E-mail: dolores.bilges@stonybrook.edu.
Website: http://www.nursing.stonybrookmedicine.edu/

University of Cincinnati, Graduate School, College of Nursing, Cincinnati, OH 45221-0038. Offers clinical nurse specialist (MSN), including adult health, community health, neonatal, nursing administration, occupational health, pediatric health, psychiatric nursing, women's health; nurse anesthesia (MSN); nurse midwifery (MSN); nurse practitioner (MSN), including acute care, ambulatory care, family, family/psychiatric, women's health; nursing (PhD); MBA/MSN. *Accreditation:* AACN; AANA/CANAEP (one or more programs are accredited); ACNM/ACME. Part-time programs available. Postbaccalaureate distance learning degree programs offered (no on-campus study). Terminal master's awarded for partial completion of doctoral program. *Degree requirements:* For master's, thesis or alternative; for doctorate, comprehensive exam, thesis/dissertation. *Entrance requirements:* For master's and doctorate, GRE General Test. Additional exam requirements/recommendations for international students: Required—TOEFL (minimum score 520 paper-based). Electronic applications accepted. *Faculty research:* Substance abuse, injury and violence, symptom management.

University of Colorado Denver, College of Nursing, Aurora, CO 80045. Offers adult clinical nurse specialist (MS); adult nurse practitioner (MS); family nurse practitioner (MS); family psychiatric mental health nurse practitioner (MS); health care informatics (MS); nurse-midwifery (MS); nursing (DNP, PhD); nursing leadership and health care systems (MS); pediatric nurse practitioner (MS); special studies (MS); women's health (MS); MS/PhD. *Accreditation:* ACNM/ACME (one or more programs are accredited). Part-time and evening/weekend programs available. Postbaccalaureate distance learning degree programs offered (minimal on-campus study). *Faculty:* 74 full-time (65 women), 58 part-time/adjunct (56 women). *Students:* 351 full-time (327 women), 138 part-time (125 women); includes 79 minority (12 Black or African American, non-Hispanic/Latino; 9 American Indian or Alaska Native, non-Hispanic/Latino; 13 Asian, non-Hispanic/Latino; 32 Hispanic/Latino; 2 Native Hawaiian or other Pacific Islander, non-Hispanic/Latino; 11 Two or more races, non-Hispanic/Latino), 7 international. Average age 33. 354 applicants, 43% accepted, 109 enrolled. In 2013, 108 master's, 28 doctorates awarded. Terminal master's awarded for partial completion of doctoral program. *Degree requirements:* For master's, thesis optional; for doctorate, comprehensive exam, thesis/dissertation, 42 credits of coursework. *Entrance requirements:* For master's, GRE if cumulative undergraduate GPA is less than 3.0, undergraduate nursing degree from NLNAC- or CCNE-accredited school or university; completion of research and statistics courses with minimum grade of C; copy of current and unencumbered nursing license; for doctorate, GRE, bachelor's and/or master's degrees in nursing from NLN- or CCNE-accredited institution; portfolio; minimum undergraduate GPA of 3.0, graduate 3.5; graduate-level intermediate statistics and master's-level nursing theory courses with minimum B grade; interview. Additional exam requirements/recommendations for international students: Required—TOEFL (minimum score 560 paper-based; 83 iBT). *Application deadline:* For fall admission, 2/15 for domestic students, 1/15 for international students; for spring admission, 7/1 for domestic students, 6/1 for international students. Application fee: $50 ($75 for international students). Electronic applications accepted. *Expenses:* Contact institution. *Financial support:* In 2013–14, 113 students received support. Fellowships, research assistantships, teaching assistantships, Federal Work-Study, institutionally sponsored loans, scholarships/grants, traineeships, and unspecified assistantships available. Support available to part-time students. Financial award application deadline: 4/1; financial award applicants required to submit FAFSA. *Faculty research:* Biological and behavioral phenomena in pregnancy and postpartum; patterns of glycemia during the insulin resistance of pregnancy; obesity, gestational diabetes, and relationship to neonatal adiposity; men's awareness and knowledge of male breast cancer; cognitive-behavioral therapy for chronic insomnia after breast cancer treatment; massage therapy for the treatment of tension-type headaches. *Total annual research expenditures:* $5.9 million. *Unit head:* Dr. Sarah Thompson, Dean, 303-724-1679, E-mail: sarah.a.thompson@ucdenver.edu. *Application contact:* Judy Campbell, Graduate Programs Coordinator, 303-724-8503, E-mail: judy.campbell@ucdenver.edu.
Website: http://www.ucdenver.edu/academics/colleges/nursing/Pages/default.aspx

University of Illinois at Chicago, Graduate College, College of Nursing, Program in Nursing, Chicago, IL 60607-7128. Offers acute care clinical nurse specialist (MS); acute care nurse practitioner (MS); administrative nursing leadership (Certificate); administrative studies in nursing (MS); adult nurse practitioner (MS); adult/geriatric nurse practitioner (MS); advanced community health nurse specialist (MS); family nurse practitioner (MS); geriatric clinical nurse specialist (MS); geriatric nurse practitioner (MS); mental health clinical nurse specialist (MS); mental health nurse practitioner (MS); nurse midwifery (MS); occupational health/advanced community health nurse specialist (MS); occupational health/family nurse practitioner (MS); pediatric clinical nurse specialist (MS); pediatric nurse practitioner (MS); perinatal clinical nurse specialist (MS); school/advanced community health nurse specialist (MS); school/family nurse practitioner (MS); women's health nurse practitioner (MS). *Accreditation:* AACN. Part-time programs available. *Faculty:* 16 full-time (14 women). *Students:* 393 full-time (361 women), 410 part-time (367 women); includes 198 minority (48 Black or African American, non-Hispanic/Latino; 1 American Indian or Alaska Native, non-Hispanic/Latino; 64 Asian, non-Hispanic/Latino; 71 Hispanic/Latino; 2 Native Hawaiian or other Pacific Islander, non-Hispanic/Latino; 12 Two or more races, non-Hispanic/Latino), 29 international. Average age 32. 396 applicants, 62% accepted, 177 enrolled. In 2013, 184 master's awarded. *Degree requirements:* For master's, thesis or alternative. *Entrance requirements:* For master's, GRE General Test, minimum GPA of 2.75. Additional exam requirements/recommendations for international students: Required—TOEFL. *Application deadline:* For fall admission, 5/15 for domestic students, 2/15 for international students; for spring admission, 11/1 for domestic students, 7/15 for international students. Applications are processed on a rolling basis. Application fee: $40 ($50 for international students). Electronic applications accepted. *Expenses:* Tuition, state resident: full-time $11,066; part-time $3689 per term. Tuition, nonresident: full-time $23,064; part-time $7688 per term. *Required fees:* $3004; $1190 per term. Tuition and fees vary according to course level and program. *Financial support:* Fellowships with full tuition reimbursements, research assistantships with full tuition reimbursements, teaching assistantships with full tuition reimbursements, career-related internships or fieldwork, Federal Work-Study, institutionally sponsored loans, scholarships/grants, traineeships, tuition waivers (full and partial), and unspecified assistantships available. Support available to part-time students. Financial award application deadline: 3/1; financial award applicants required to submit FAFSA. *Unit head:* Dr. Terri E. Weaver, Dean, 312-996-7808, E-mail: teweaver@uic.edu. *Application contact:* Receptionist, 312-413-2550, E-mail: gradcoll@uic.edu.

University of Indianapolis, Graduate Programs, School of Nursing, Indianapolis, IN 46227-3697. Offers advanced practice nursing (DNP); family nurse practitioner (MSN); gerontological nurse practitioner (MSN); neonatal nurse practitioner (MSN); nurse-midwifery (MSN); nursing (MSN); nursing and health systems leadership (MSN); nursing education (MSN); women's health nurse practitioner (MSN); MBA/MSN. *Accreditation:* AACN; ACNM. *Faculty:* 5 full-time (4 women), 1 part-time/adjunct (0 women). *Students:* 15 full-time (14 women), 285 part-time (270 women); includes 42 minority (24 Black or African American, non-Hispanic/Latino; 6 Asian, non-Hispanic/Latino; 3 Hispanic/Latino; 9 Two or more races, non-Hispanic/Latino), 2 international. Average age 35. In 2013, 46 master's awarded. *Entrance requirements:* For master's, minimum GPA of 3.0, interview, letters of recommendation, resume, IN nursing license, 1 year of professional practice; for doctorate, graduate of NLNAC- or CCNE-accredited nursing program; MSN or MA with nursing major and minimum cumulative GPA of 3.25; unencumbered RN license with eligibility for licensure in Indiana; completion of graduate-level statistics course within last 5 years with minimum grade of B; resume; essay; official transcripts from all academic institutions. Additional exam requirements/recommendations for international students: Required—TOEFL (minimum score 550 paper-based). *Application deadline:* For fall admission, 8/1 for domestic students; for winter admission, 12/15 for domestic students; for spring admission, 4/15 for domestic students. Applications are processed on a rolling basis. Application fee: $60. Electronic applications accepted. *Expenses: Tuition:* Full-time $5436; part-time $810 per credit hour. *Financial support:* Federal Work-Study available. *Unit head:* Dr. Anne Thomas, Dean, 317-788-3206, E-mail: athomas@uindy.edu. *Application contact:* Sueann Meagher, Graduate Administrative Assistant, 317-788-8005, Fax: 317-788-3542, E-mail: meaghers@uindy.edu.
Website: http://nursing.uindy.edu/

The University of Kansas, University of Kansas Medical Center, School of Nursing, Kansas City, KS 66160. Offers adult/gerontological clinical nurse specialist (PMC); adult/gerontological nurse practitioner (PMC); clinical research management (PMC); health care informatics (PMC); health professions educator (PMC); nurse midwife (PMC); nursing (MS, DNP, PhD); organizational leadership (PMC); psychiatric/mental health nurse practitioner (PMC); public health nursing (PMC). *Accreditation:* AACN; ACNM/ACME. Part-time programs available. Postbaccalaureate distance learning degree programs offered (minimal on-campus study). *Faculty:* 59. *Students:* 55 full-time (53 women), 323 part-time (303 women); includes 57 minority (23 Black or African American, non-Hispanic/Latino; 14 Asian, non-Hispanic/Latino; 16 Hispanic/Latino; 1 Native Hawaiian or other Pacific Islander, non-Hispanic/Latino; 3 Two or more races, non-Hispanic/Latino), 1 international. Average age 38. 113 applicants, 59% accepted, 61 enrolled. In 2013, 77 master's, 18 doctorates, 11 other advanced degrees awarded. Terminal master's awarded for partial completion of doctoral program. *Degree requirements:* For master's, comprehensive exam, thesis (for some programs), general oral exam; for doctorate, variable foreign language requirement, thesis/dissertation, comprehensive oral exam (for DNP); comprehensive written and oral exam (for PhD). *Entrance requirements:* For master's, bachelor's degree in nursing, minimum GPA of 3.0, 1 year of clinical experience, RN license in KS and MO; for doctorate, GRE General Test, bachelor's degree in nursing, minimum GPA of 3.5, RN license in KS and MO. Additional exam requirements/recommendations for international students: Required—TOEFL. *Application deadline:* For fall admission, 4/1 for domestic and international students; for spring admission, 9/1 for domestic and international students. Application fee: $60. Electronic applications accepted. *Financial support:* Research assistantships with full and partial tuition reimbursements, teaching assistantships with full and partial tuition reimbursements, scholarships/grants, and traineeships available. Financial award application deadline: 3/1; financial award applicants required to submit FAFSA. *Faculty research:* Breastfeeding practices of teen mothers, national database of nursing quality indicators, caregiving of families of patients using technology in the home, simulation in nursing education, diaphragm fatigue. *Total annual research expenditures:* $6.4 million. *Unit head:* Dr. Karen L. Miller, Dean, 913-588-1601, Fax: 913-588-1660, E-mail: kmiller@kumc.edu. *Application contact:* Dr. Pamela K. Barnes, Associate Dean, Student Affairs, 913-588-1619, Fax: 913-588-1615, E-mail: pbarnes2@kumc.edu.
Website: http://nursing.kumc.edu

The University of Manchester, School of Nursing, Midwifery and Social Work, Manchester, United Kingdom. Offers nursing (M Phil, PhD); social work (M Phil, PhD).

University of Maryland, Baltimore, Graduate School, School of Nursing, Master's Program in Nursing, Baltimore, MD 21201. Offers community health nursing (MS);

gerontological nursing (MS); maternal-child nursing (MS); medical-surgical nursing (MS); nurse-midwifery education (MS); nursing administration (MS); nursing education (MS); nursing health policy (MS); primary care nursing (MS); psychiatric nursing (MS); MS/MBA. MS/MBA offered jointly with University of Baltimore. *Accreditation:* AACN; AANA/CANAEP. Part-time programs available. *Students:* 345 full-time (297 women), 508 part-time (469 women); includes 288 minority (152 Black or African American, non-Hispanic/Latino; 2 American Indian or Alaska Native, non-Hispanic/Latino; 72 Asian, non-Hispanic/Latino; 32 Hispanic/Latino; 1 Native Hawaiian or other Pacific Islander, non-Hispanic/Latino; 29 Two or more races, non-Hispanic/Latino), 13 international. Average age 33. 971 applicants, 34% accepted, 253 enrolled. In 2013, 308 master's awarded. *Degree requirements:* For master's, comprehensive exam (for some programs), thesis or alternative. *Entrance requirements:* For master's, minimum GPA of 2.75, course work in statistics, BS in nursing. Additional exam requirements/recommendations for international students: Required—TOEFL (minimum score 550 paper-based; 80 iBT) or IELTS (minimum score 7). *Application deadline:* For fall admission, 2/1 for domestic students, 1/15 for international students. Application fee: $75. Electronic applications accepted. *Financial support:* Fellowships, research assistantships, teaching assistantships, career-related internships or fieldwork, and traineeships available. Support available to part-time students. Financial award application deadline: 2/15; financial award applicants required to submit FAFSA. *Unit head:* Dr. Jane Kapustin, Assistant Dean, 410-706-6741, Fax: 410-706-4231. *Application contact:* Marjorie Fass, Admissions Director, 410-706-0501, Fax: 410-706-7238.

University of Miami, Graduate School, School of Nursing and Health Studies, Coral Gables, FL 33124. Offers acute care (MSN), including acute care nurse practitioner, nurse anesthesia; nursing (PhD); primary care (MSN), including adult nurse practitioner, family nurse practitioner, nurse midwifery, women's health practitioner. *Accreditation:* AACN; AANA/CANAEP; ACNM/ACME (one or more programs are accredited). Part-time programs available. *Degree requirements:* For master's, thesis optional; for doctorate, thesis/dissertation. *Entrance requirements:* For master's, GRE General Test, BSN, minimum GPA of 3.0, Florida RN license; for doctorate, GRE General Test, BSN or MSN, minimum GPA of 3.0. Additional exam requirements/recommendations for international students: Required—TOEFL (minimum score 550 paper-based). Electronic applications accepted. *Faculty research:* Transcultural nursing, exercise and depression in Alzheimer's disease, infectious diseases/HIV–AIDS, postpartum depression, outcomes assessment.

University of Michigan, Rackham Graduate School, School of Nursing, Ann Arbor, MI 48109. Offers acute care pediatric nurse practitioner (MS); adult-gerontology acute care clinical nurse specialist (MS); adult-gerontology acute care nurse practitioner (MS); adult-gerontology primary care nurse practitioner (MS); health systems, nursing leadership, and effectiveness science (MS); nurse midwife (MS); nurse midwife and family nurse practitioner (MS); nurse midwife and primary care pediatric nurse practitioner (MS); nursing (DNP, PhD, Post Master's Certificate); primary care family nurse practitioner (MS); primary care pediatric nurse practitioner (MS). *Accreditation:* AACN; ACNM/ACME (one or more programs are accredited). Part-time programs available. Postbaccalaureate distance learning degree programs offered (minimal on-campus study). Terminal master's awarded for partial completion of doctoral program. *Degree requirements:* For doctorate, thesis/dissertation. *Application deadline:* For fall admission, 2/1 for domestic students; for winter admission, 5/1 for domestic students; for spring admission, 11/1 for domestic students. Applications are processed on a rolling basis. Electronic applications accepted. Tuition and fees vary according to course level, course load, degree level, program and student level. *Financial support:* Fellowships with full and partial tuition reimbursements, research assistantships with full and partial tuition reimbursements, teaching assistantships with full tuition reimbursements, Federal Work-Study, institutionally sponsored loans, scholarships/grants, traineeships, and tuition waivers (partial) available. Support available to part-time students. *Faculty research:* Preparation of clinical nurse researchers, biobehavior, women's health, health promotion, substance abuse, psychobiology of menopause, fertility, obesity, health care systems. *Unit head:* Dr. Kathleen Potempa, Dean, 734-764-7185, Fax: 734-764-7186. *Application contact:* James Diesing, Graduate Recruiting and Admissions Coordinator, 734-615-4739, E-mail: sn-osams@umich.edu.
Website: http://www.nursing.umich.edu/

University of Minnesota, Twin Cities Campus, Graduate School, School of Nursing, Nurse Midwifery Program, Minneapolis, MN 55455-0213. Offers MS. *Accreditation:* ACNM/ACME. Postbaccalaureate distance learning degree programs offered (minimal on-campus study). *Degree requirements:* For master's, final oral exam, project or thesis. *Entrance requirements:* Additional exam requirements/recommendations for international students: Required—TOEFL (minimum score 586 paper-based).

University of Pennsylvania, School of Nursing, Program in Nurse Midwifery, Philadelphia, PA 19104. Offers MSN. *Accreditation:* AACN; ACNM/ACME. Part-time programs available. *Students:* 25 full-time (24 women), 11 part-time (all women); includes 14 minority (10 Black or African American, non-Hispanic/Latino; 1 Asian, non-Hispanic/Latino; 1 Hispanic/Latino; 2 Two or more races, non-Hispanic/Latino). 9 applicants, 56% accepted, 4 enrolled. In 2013, 16 master's awarded. *Entrance requirements:* For master's, GRE General Test, BSN, minimum GPA of 3.0, previous course work in statistics, physical assessment. Additional exam requirements/recommendations for international students: Required—TOEFL. *Application deadline:* For fall admission, 2/15 priority date for domestic students. Applications are processed on a rolling basis. Application fee: $70. *Expenses:* Contact institution. *Financial support:* Fellowships, research assistantships, teaching assistantships, career-related internships or fieldwork, Federal Work-Study, and institutionally sponsored loans available. Support available to part-time students. Financial award application deadline: 4/1. *Faculty research:* Breast-feeding protocols, history of midwifery, hydrotherapy in labor, cocaine abuse during pregnancy, stress in pregnancy. *Unit head:* Assistant Dean of Admissions and Financial Aid, 866-867-6877, Fax: 215-573-8439, E-mail: admissions@nursing.upenn.edu. *Application contact:* William McCool, Program Director, 215-573-7679, E-mail: mccoolwf@nursing.upenn.edu.
Website: http://www.nursing.upenn.edu

University of Puerto Rico, Medical Sciences Campus, Graduate School of Public Health, Department of Human Development, Program in Nurse Midwifery, San Juan, PR 00936-5067. Offers MPH, Certificate. *Accreditation:* ACNM/ACME. Part-time programs available. *Entrance requirements:* For master's, GRE, previous course work in algebra.

University of South Africa, College of Human Sciences, Pretoria, South Africa. Offers adult education (M Ed); African languages (MA, PhD); African politics (MA, PhD); Afrikaans (MA, PhD); ancient history (MA, PhD); ancient Near Eastern studies (MA, PhD); anthropology (MA, PhD); applied linguistics (MA); Arabic (MA, PhD); archaeology (MA); art history (MA); Biblical archaeology (MA); Biblical studies (M Th, D Th, PhD); Christian spirituality (M Th, D Th); church history (M Th, D Th); classical studies (MA, PhD); clinical psychology (MA); communication (MA, PhD); comparative education (M Ed, Ed D); consulting psychology (D Admin, D Com, PhD); curriculum studies (M Ed, Ed D); development studies (M Admin, MA, D Admin, PhD); didactics (M Ed, Ed D); education (M Tech); education management (M Ed, Ed D); educational psychology (M Ed); English (MA); environmental education (M Ed); French (MA, PhD); German (MA, PhD); Greek (MA); guidance and counseling (M Ed); health studies (MA, PhD), including health sciences education (MA), health services management (MA), medical and surgical nursing science (critical care general) (MA), midwifery and neonatal nursing science (MA), trauma and emergency care (MA); history (MA, PhD); history of education (Ed D); inclusive education (M Ed, Ed D); information and communications technology policy and regulation (MA); information science (MA, MIS, PhD); international politics (MA, PhD); Islamic studies (MA, PhD); Italian (MA, PhD); Judaica (MA, PhD); linguistics (MA, PhD); mathematical education (M Ed); mathematics education (MA); missiology (M Th, D Th); modern Hebrew (MA, PhD); musicology (MA, MMus, D Mus, PhD); natural science education (M Ed); New Testament (M Th, D Th); Old Testament (D Th); pastoral therapy (M Th, D Th); philosophy (MA); philosophy of education (M Ed, Ed D); politics (MA, PhD); Portuguese (MA, PhD); practical theology (M Th, D Th); psychology (MA, MS, PhD); psychology of education (M Ed, Ed D); public health (MA); religious studies (MA, D Th, PhD); Romance languages (MA); Russian (MA, PhD); Semitic languages (MA, PhD); social behavior studies in HIV/AIDS (MA); social science (mental health) (MA); social science in development studies (MA); social science in psychology (MA); social science in social work (MA); social science in sociology (MA); social work (MSW, DSW, PhD); socio-education (M Ed, Ed D); sociolinguistics (MA); sociology (MA, PhD); Spanish (MA, PhD); systematic theology (M Th, D Th); TESOL (teaching English to speakers of other languages) (MA); theological ethics (M Th, D Th); theory of literature (MA, PhD); urban ministries (D Th); urban ministry (M Th).

Vanderbilt University, Vanderbilt University School of Nursing, Nashville, TN 37240. Offers adult-gerontology acute care nurse practitioner (MSN), including hospitalist, intensivist; adult-gerontology primary care nurse practitioner (MSN); emergency nurse practitioner (MSN); family nurse practitioner (MSN); healthcare leadership (MSN); neonatal nurse practitioner (MSN); nurse midwifery (MSN); nurse midwifery/family nurse practitioner (MSN); nursing informatics (MSN); nursing practice (DNP); nursing science (PhD); pediatric acute care nurse practitioner (MSN); pediatric primary care nurse practitioner (MSN); psychiatric-mental health nurse practitioner (MSN); women's health nurse practitioner (MSN); women's health nurse practitioner/adult gerontology primary care nurse practitioner (MSN); MSN/M Div; MSN/MTS. *Accreditation:* ACNM/ACME (one or more programs are accredited). Part-time programs available. Postbaccalaureate distance learning degree programs offered (minimal on-campus study). *Faculty:* 139 full-time (124 women), 452 part-time/adjunct (319 women). *Students:* 527 full-time (463 women), 369 part-time (333 women); includes 120 minority (46 Black or African American, non-Hispanic/Latino; 8 American Indian or Alaska Native, non-Hispanic/Latino; 26 Asian, non-Hispanic/Latino; 24 Hispanic/Latino; 4 Native Hawaiian or other Pacific Islander, non-Hispanic/Latino; 12 Two or more races, non-Hispanic/Latino), 7 international. Average age 32. 1,257 applicants, 49% accepted, 457 enrolled. In 2013, 364 master's, 43 doctorates awarded. *Degree requirements:* For doctorate, comprehensive exam, thesis/dissertation. *Entrance requirements:* For master's, GRE General Test (within the past 5 years), minimum B average in undergraduate course work, 3 letters of recommendation; for doctorate, GRE General Test, interview, 3 letters of recommendation from doctorally-prepared faculty, MSN, essay. Additional exam requirements/recommendations for international students: Required—TOEFL (minimum score 570 paper-based), IELTS (minimum score 6.5). *Application deadline:* For fall admission, 12/1 priority date for domestic and international students. Applications are processed on a rolling basis. Application fee: $50. Electronic applications accepted. *Expenses:* Contact institution. *Financial support:* In 2013–14, 582 students received support. Scholarships/grants and health care benefits available. Support available to part-time students. Financial award application deadline: 3/15; financial award applicants required to submit FAFSA. *Faculty research:* Lymphedema, palliative care and bereavement, health services research including workforce, safety and quality of care, gerontology, better birth outcomes including nutrition. *Total annual research expenditures:* $2.5 million. *Unit head:* Dr. Linda Norman, Dean, 615-343-8876, Fax: 615-343-7711, E-mail: linda.norman@vanderbilt.edu. *Application contact:* Patricia Peerman, Assistant Dean for Enrollment Management, 615-322-3800, Fax: 615-343-0333, E-mail: vusn-admissions@vanderbilt.edu.
Website: http://www.nursing.vanderbilt.edu

Wayne State University, College of Nursing, Program in Advanced Practice Nursing with Women, Neonates and Children, Detroit, MI 48202. Offers neonatal nurse practitioner (MSN); nurse-midwife (MSN); pediatric nurse practitioner (MSN), including acute care, primary care; women's health nurse practitioner (MSN). *Accreditation:* AACN. Part-time programs available. *Students:* 59 full-time (53 women), 74 part-time (72 women); includes 17 minority (11 Black or African American, non-Hispanic/Latino; 2 Asian, non-Hispanic/Latino; 4 Hispanic/Latino), 6 international. Average age 32. 65 applicants, 55% accepted, 33 enrolled. In 2013, 40 degrees awarded. *Degree requirements:* For master's, thesis or alternative. *Entrance requirements:* For master's, minimum honor point average of 3.0 in upper-division course work; BA from NLN- or CCNE-accredited program; references; current RN license; personal statement. Additional exam requirements/recommendations for international students: Required—TOEFL (minimum score 550 paper-based; 79 iBT); Recommended—TWE (minimum score 6). *Application deadline:* For fall admission, 6/1 priority date for domestic students, 5/1 priority date for international students; for winter admission, 10/1 priority date for domestic students, 9/1 priority date for international students; for spring admission, 2/1 priority date for domestic students, 1/1 priority date for international students. Applications are processed on a rolling basis. Application fee: $50. Electronic applications accepted. *Expenses:* Contact institution. *Financial support:* In 2013–14, 17 students received support. Fellowships with tuition reimbursements available, research assistantships with tuition reimbursements available, teaching assistantships with tuition reimbursements available, scholarships/grants, and unspecified assistantships available. Financial award applicants required to submit FAFSA. *Faculty research:* Acculturation and parenting, domestic violence, evidence-based midwifery practice, pain in children, trauma and community violence. *Unit head:* Dr. Barbara Redman, Dean, 313-577-4070, Fax: 313-577-4571, E-mail: ae9080@wayne.edu. *Application contact:* Dr. Cynthia Redwine, Assistant Dean for the Office of Student Affairs, 313-577-4082, E-mail: nursinginfo@wayne.edu.
Website: http://nursing.wayne.edu/msn/specialty.php

West Virginia Wesleyan College, Department of Nursing, Buckhannon, WV 26201. Offers family nurse practitioner (Post Master's Certificate); family nurse practitoner (MS); nurse administrator (MS); nurse educator (MS); nurse-midwifery (MS); nursing administration (Post Master's Certificate); nursing education (Post Master's Certificate); psychiatric mental health nurse practitioner (MS); MSN/MBA.

Nursing and Healthcare Administration

Abilene Christian University, Graduate School, School of Nursing, Abilene, TX 79699-9100. Offers education and administration (MSN); family nurse practitioner (MSN); nursing (Certificate). *Accreditation:* AACN. Part-time programs available. *Faculty:* 7 part-time/adjunct (all women). *Students:* 1 (woman) part-time. 11 applicants. In 2013, 3 master's awarded. *Degree requirements:* For master's, practicum. *Entrance requirements:* For master's, GRE General Test. Additional exam requirements/recommendations for international students: Required—TOEFL (minimum score 550 paper-based; 90 iBT), IELTS (minimum score 6.5). *Application deadline:* For fall admission, 4/1 priority date for domestic students; for spring admission, 11/1 for domestic students. Applications are processed on a rolling basis. Application fee: $50. Electronic applications accepted. *Expenses: Tuition:* Full-time $17,100; part-time $950 per credit hour. *Financial support:* Application deadline: 4/1; applicants required to submit FAFSA. *Unit head:* Dr. Becky Hammack, Graduate Director, 325-674-2265, Fax: 325-674-6256, E-mail: rsh12a@acu.edu. *Application contact:* Corey Patterson, Director of Graduate Admission and Recruiting, 325-674-6566, Fax: 325-674-6717, E-mail: gradinfo@acu.edu.

Adelphi University, College of Nursing and Public Health, Program in Nursing Administration, Garden City, NY 11530-0701. Offers MS, Certificate. *Students:* 14 part-time (13 women); includes 8 minority (6 Black or African American, non-Hispanic/Latino; 2 Hispanic/Latino). Average age 44. In 2013, 7 master's awarded. *Expenses: Tuition:* Full-time $32,530; part-time $1010 per credit. *Required fees:* $1150. Tuition and fees vary according to degree level and program. *Financial support:* Research assistantships, career-related internships or fieldwork, Federal Work-Study, tuition waivers, and unspecified assistantships available. *Unit head:* Joan Valas, Director, 516-877-4571, E-mail: valas@adelphi.edu. *Application contact:* Christine Murphy, Director of Admissions, 516-877-3050, Fax: 516-877-3039, E-mail: graduateadmissions@adelphi.edu.

Allen College, Program in Nursing, Waterloo, IA 50703. Offers acute care nurse practitioner (MSN, Post-Master's Certificate); adult nurse practitioner (MSN, Post-Master's Certificate); adult psychiatric-mental health nurse practitioner (MSN, Post-Master's Certificate); community public health (MSN, Post-Master's Certificate); family nurse practitioner (MSN, Post-Master's Certificate); gerontological nurse practitioner (MSN, Post-Master's Certificate); health education (MSN); leadership in health care delivery (MSN, Post-Master's Certificate); nursing (DNP). Part-time programs available. Postbaccalaureate distance learning degree programs offered (minimal on-campus study). *Faculty:* 3 full-time (all women), 21 part-time/adjunct (20 women). *Students:* 21 full-time (19 women), 162 part-time (150 women); includes 5 minority (1 Black or African American, non-Hispanic/Latino; 2 Asian, non-Hispanic/Latino; 1 Hispanic/Latino; 1 Two or more races, non-Hispanic/Latino). Average age 34. 213 applicants, 57% accepted, 94 enrolled. In 2013, 41 master's, 4 other advanced degrees awarded. *Degree requirements:* For master's, thesis optional. *Entrance requirements:* For master's, minimum GPA of 3.0 in the last 60 hours of undergraduate coursework; for doctorate, minimum GPA of 3.25 in graduate coursework. Additional exam requirements/recommendations for international students: Recommended—TOEFL (minimum score 580 paper-based; 92 iBT), IELTS (minimum score 6). *Application deadline:* For fall admission, 2/1 priority date for domestic students; for spring admission, 9/1 priority date for domestic students. Applications are processed on a rolling basis. Application fee: $50. Electronic applications accepted. *Expenses: Tuition:* Full-time $14,534; part-time $755 per credit hour. *Required fees:* $935; $75 per credit hour. One-time fee: $275 part-time. Tuition and fees vary according to course load. *Financial support:* In 2013–14, 60 students received support. Institutionally sponsored loans, scholarships/grants, and traineeships available. Support available to part-time students. Financial award application deadline: 8/15; financial award applicants required to submit FAFSA. *Unit head:* Kendra Williams-Perez, Dean, School of Nursing, 319-226-2044, Fax: 319-226-2070, E-mail: kendra.williams-perez@allencollege.edu. *Application contact:* Molly Quinn, Admissions Counselor, 319-226-2001, Fax: 319-226-2010, E-mail: molly.quinn@allencollege.edu.
Website: http://www.allencollege.edu/

American International College, School of Health Sciences, Department of Nursing, Springfield, MA 01109-3189. Offers nursing administration (MSN); nursing education (MSN). *Accreditation:* AACN. Part-time and evening/weekend programs available. Postbaccalaureate distance learning degree programs offered (minimal on-campus study). *Faculty:* 1 (woman) full-time, 1 (woman) part-time/adjunct. *Students:* 12 full-time (all women), 11 part-time (9 women); includes 4 minority (all Black or African American, non-Hispanic/Latino). Average age 39. 17 applicants, 94% accepted, 12 enrolled. In 2013, 10 master's awarded. *Entrance requirements:* For master's, BSN, minimum GPA of 3.0. Additional exam requirements/recommendations for international students: Required—TOEFL or IELTS. *Application deadline:* For fall admission, 7/1 for domestic and international students; for spring admission, 12/1 for domestic and international students. Applications are processed on a rolling basis. Application fee: $50. Electronic applications accepted. *Expenses: Tuition:* Full-time $14,040; part-time $780 per credit. Tuition and fees vary according to course load, degree level and program. *Financial support:* Applicants required to submit FAFSA. *Unit head:* Dr. Ellen Furman, Associate Director of Graduate Nursing, 413-205-3918, Fax: 413-654-1430, E-mail: ellen.furman@aic.edu. *Application contact:* Kerry Barnes, Director of Graduate Admissions, 413-205-3703, Fax: 413-205-3051, E-mail: kerry.barnes@aic.edu.
Website: http://www.aic.edu/academics/hs/nursing

American University of Beirut, Graduate Programs, Rafic Hariri School of Nursing, Beirut, Lebanon. Offers adult care nursing (MSN); community and public health nursing (MSN); nursing administration (MSN); psychiatry mental health nursing (MSN). *Accreditation:* AACN. Part-time programs available. *Faculty:* 9 full-time (8 women), 12 part-time/adjunct (10 women). *Students:* 4 full-time (3 women), 56 part-time (44 women). Average age 29. 38 applicants, 87% accepted, 26 enrolled. In 2013, 17 master's awarded. *Degree requirements:* For master's, one foreign language, comprehensive exam, thesis optional. *Entrance requirements:* For master's, letter of recommendation. Additional exam requirements/recommendations for international students: Required—TOEFL (minimum score 600 paper-based); Recommended—IELTS. *Application deadline:* For fall admission, 4/1 for domestic and international students; for spring admission, 11/1 for domestic and international students. Applications are processed on a rolling basis. Application fee: $50. Electronic applications accepted. *Expenses: Tuition:* Full-time $14,724; part-time $818 per credit. *Required fees:* $692. Tuition and fees vary according to course load and program. *Financial support:* In 2013–14, 24 teaching assistantships with partial tuition reimbursements were awarded; unspecified assistantships also available. Financial award application deadline: 12/20. *Faculty research:* Pain management and palliative care, stress and post-traumatic stress disorder, health benefits and chronic illness, health promotion and community interventions. *Unit head:* Dr. Huda Huijer Abu-Saad, Director, 961-1374374 Ext. 5952, Fax: 961-1744476, E-mail: hh35@aub.edu.lb. *Application contact:* Dr. Salim Kanaan, Director, Admissions Office, 961-1-350000 Ext. 2594, Fax: 96-1-1750775, E-mail: sk00@aub.edu.lb.
Website: http://staff.aub.edu.lb/~webson

Arizona State University at the Tempe campus, College of Nursing and Health Innovation, Phoenix, AZ 85004. Offers advanced nursing practice (DNP); child/family mental health nurse practitioner (Graduate Certificate); clinical research management (MS); community and public health practice (Graduate Certificate); community health (MS); exercise and wellness (MS), including exercise and wellness; family nurse practitioner (Graduate Certificate); healthcare innovation (MHI); international health for healthcare (Graduate Certificate); kinesiology (MS, PhD); nursing (MS, Graduate Certificate); nursing and healthcare innovation (PhD); nutrition (MS); physical activity nutrition and wellness (PhD), including physical activity, nutrition and wellness; public health (MPH); regulatory science and health safety (MS). *Accreditation:* AACN. Postbaccalaureate distance learning degree programs offered (minimal on-campus study). *Degree requirements:* For master's, comprehensive exam (for some programs), thesis (for some programs), interactive Program of Study (iPOS) submitted before completing 50 percent of required credit hours; for doctorate, comprehensive exam, thesis/dissertation, interactive Program of Study (iPOS) submitted before completing 50 percent of required credit hours. *Entrance requirements:* For master's and doctorate, GRE, minimum GPA of 3.0 or equivalent in last 2 years of work leading to bachelor's degree. Additional exam requirements/recommendations for international students: Required—TOEFL (minimum score 80 iBT), TOEFL, IELTS, or PTE. Electronic applications accepted. *Expenses:* Contact institution.

Athabasca University, Centre for Nursing and Health Studies, Athabasca, AB T9S 3A3, Canada. Offers advanced nursing practice (MN, Advanced Diploma); generalist (MN); health studies-leadership (MHS). Part-time programs available. Postbaccalaureate distance learning degree programs offered. *Degree requirements:* For master's, comprehensive exam (for some programs). *Entrance requirements:* For master's, bachelor's degree in health-related field, 2 years professional health service experience (MHS), bachelor's degree in nursing, 2 years nursing experience (MN), minimum GPA of 3.0 in final 30 credits; for Advanced Diploma, RN license, 2 years health care experience. Electronic applications accepted. *Expenses:* Contact institution.

Austin Peay State University, College of Graduate Studies, College of Behavioral and Health Sciences, School of Nursing, Clarksville, TN 37044. Offers advanced practice (MSN); nursing administration (MSN); nursing education (MSN); nursing informatics (MSN). Part-time programs available. Postbaccalaureate distance learning degree programs offered. *Faculty:* 9 full-time (all women), 7 part-time/adjunct (all women). *Students:* 47 full-time (43 women), 136 part-time (129 women); includes 30 minority (18 Black or African American, non-Hispanic/Latino; 4 Asian, non-Hispanic/Latino; 4 Hispanic/Latino; 4 Two or more races, non-Hispanic/Latino). Average age 35. 47 applicants, 85% accepted, 37 enrolled. In 2013, 39 master's awarded. *Degree requirements:* For master's, comprehensive exam. *Entrance requirements:* For master's, GRE General Test, minimum GPA of 3.0, RN license eligibility, 3 letters of recommendation. Additional exam requirements/recommendations for international students: Required—TOEFL (minimum score 600 paper-based). *Application deadline:* For fall admission, 8/5 priority date for domestic students. Applications are processed on a rolling basis. Application fee: $25. Electronic applications accepted. *Expenses:* Tuition, state resident: full-time $7500; part-time $375 per credit hour. Tuition, nonresident: full-time $20,800; part-time $1040 per credit hour. *Required fees:* $1284; $64.20 per credit hour. *Financial support:* In 2013–14, research assistantships with full tuition reimbursements (averaging $6,500 per year) were awarded; career-related internships or fieldwork, Federal Work-Study, institutionally sponsored loans, scholarships/grants, and unspecified assistantships also available. Support available to part-time students. *Unit head:* Dr. Patty Orr, Director, 931-221-7710, Fax: 931-221-7595, E-mail: orrp@apsu.edu. *Application contact:* June D. Lee, Graduate Coordinator, 800-859-4723, Fax: 931-221-7641, E-mail: gradadmissions@apsu.edu.
Website: http://www.apsu.edu/nursing

Barry University, School of Adult and Continuing Education, Division of Nursing, Program in Nursing Administration, Miami Shores, FL 33161-6695. Offers MSN, PhD, Certificate. *Accreditation:* AACN. Part-time and evening/weekend programs available. *Degree requirements:* For master's, research project or thesis. *Entrance requirements:* For master's, GRE General Test or MAT, BSN, minimum GPA of 3.0, course work in statistics. Electronic applications accepted. *Faculty research:* Power/empowerment, health delivery systems, managed care, employee health and well being.

Barry University, School of Adult and Continuing Education, Division of Nursing and Andreas School of Business, Program in Nursing Administration and Business Administration, Miami Shores, FL 33161-6695. Offers MSN/MBA. *Accreditation:* AACN. Part-time and evening/weekend programs available. Electronic applications accepted. *Faculty research:* Power/empowerment, health delivery systems, managed care, employee health well-being.

Bellarmine University, Donna and Allan Lansing School of Nursing and Health Sciences, Louisville, KY 40205. Offers family nurse practitioner (MSN); health science (MHS); nursing administration (MSN); nursing education (MSN); nursing practice (DNP); physical therapy (DPT). *Accreditation:* AACN; APTA. Part-time and evening/weekend programs available. *Faculty:* 21 full-time (19 women), 8 part-time/adjunct (5 women). *Students:* 162 full-time (111 women), 120 part-time (113 women); includes 16 minority (6 Black or African American, non-Hispanic/Latino; 1 American Indian or Alaska Native, non-Hispanic/Latino; 3 Asian, non-Hispanic/Latino; 3 Hispanic/Latino; 3 Two or more races, non-Hispanic/Latino). Average age 29. In 2013, 30 master's, 54 doctorates awarded. *Degree requirements:* For doctorate, comprehensive exam, thesis/dissertation. *Entrance requirements:* For master's, GRE General Test, RN license; for doctorate, GRE General Test, Physical Therapist Centralized Application Service (for DPT). Additional exam requirements/recommendations for international students: Required—TOEFL (minimum score 550 paper-based; 80 iBT). Application fee: $25. Electronic applications accepted. *Expenses:* Contact institution. *Financial support:* Career-related internships or fieldwork and scholarships/grants available. *Faculty research:* Nursing: pain, empathy, leadership styles, control; physical therapy: service-learning; exercise in chronic and pre-operative conditions, athletes; women's health; aging. *Unit head:* Dr. Mark Wiegand, Dean, 800-274-4723 Ext. 8368, E-mail: mwiegand@bellarmine.edu. *Application contact:* Julie Armstrong-Binnix, Health Science Recruiter, 800-274-4723 Ext. 8364, E-mail: julieab@bellarmine.edu.
Website: http://www.bellarmine.edu/lansing

Bethel University, Graduate School, St. Paul, MN 55112-6999. Offers autism spectrum disorders (Certificate); business administration (MBA); communication (MA); counseling psychology (MA); educational leadership (Ed D); gerontology (MA); international

baccalaureate education (Certificate); K-12 education (MA); literacy education (MA, Certificate); nurse educator (Certificate); nurse leader (Certificate); nurse-midwifery (MS); nursing (MS); physician assistant (MS); postsecondary teaching (Certificate); special education (MA); strategic leadership (MA); teaching (MA). Part-time and evening/weekend programs available. Postbaccalaureate distance learning degree programs offered (no on-campus study). *Faculty:* 13 full-time (7 women), 89 part-time/adjunct (43 women). *Students:* 692 full-time (457 women), 573 part-time (371 women); includes 170 minority (86 Black or African American, non-Hispanic/Latino; 1 American Indian or Alaska Native, non-Hispanic/Latino; 49 Asian, non-Hispanic/Latino; 20 Hispanic/Latino; 1 Native Hawaiian or other Pacific Islander, non-Hispanic/Latino; 13 Two or more races, non-Hispanic/Latino), 21 international. Average age 37. In 2013, 166 master's, 9 doctorates, 11 other advanced degrees awarded. *Degree requirements:* For master's, comprehensive exam (for some programs), thesis (for some programs); for doctorate, comprehensive exam, thesis/dissertation. *Entrance requirements:* Additional exam requirements/recommendations for international students: Required—TOEFL (minimum score 550 paper-based; 80 iBT). *Application deadline:* Applications are processed on a rolling basis. Electronic applications accepted. Tuition and fees vary according to course load, degree level and program. *Financial support:* Teaching assistantships, career-related internships or fieldwork, and scholarships/grants available. Support available to part-time students. Financial award applicants required to submit FAFSA. *Unit head:* Dick Crombie, Vice-President/Dean, 651-635-8000, Fax: 651-635-8004, E-mail: gs@bethel.edu. *Application contact:* Director of Admissions, 651-635-8000, Fax: 651-635-8004, E-mail: gs@bethel.edu.
Website: http://gs.bethel.edu/

Bloomsburg University of Pennsylvania, School of Graduate Studies, College of Science and Technology, Department of Nursing, Bloomsburg, PA 17815. Offers adult and family nurse practitioner (MSN); community health (MSN); nurse anesthesia (MSN); nursing (MSN); nursing administration (MSN). *Accreditation:* AACN; AANA/CANAEP. *Faculty:* 5 full-time (all women), 7 part-time/adjunct (all women). *Students:* 62 full-time (52 women), 26 part-time (17 women); includes 8 minority (6 Black or African American, non-Hispanic/Latino; 1 Asian, non-Hispanic/Latino; 1 Hispanic/Latino). Average age 35. 61 applicants, 84% accepted, 14 enrolled. In 2013, 36 master's awarded. *Degree requirements:* For master's, thesis (for some programs), clinical experience. *Entrance requirements:* For master's, minimum QPA of 3.0, personal statement, 2 letters of recommendation, nursing license. Additional exam requirements/recommendations for international students: Required—TOEFL. *Application deadline:* For fall admission, 1/1 for domestic students; for spring admission, 8/1 for domestic students. Applications are processed on a rolling basis. Application fee: $35 ($60 for international students). Electronic applications accepted. *Expenses:* Tuition, state resident: full-time $7956; part-time $442 per credit. Tuition, nonresident: full-time $11,934; part-time $663 per credit. *Required fees:* $95.50 per credit. $55 per semester. Tuition and fees vary according to course load. *Financial support:* Unspecified assistantships available. *Unit head:* Dr. Noreen Chikotas, Coordinator, 570-389-4609, Fax: 570-389-5008, E-mail: nchikota@bloomu.edu. *Application contact:* Jennifer Richard, Administrative Assistant, 570-389-4015, Fax: 570-389-3054, E-mail: jrichard@bloomu.edu.
Website: http://www.bloomu.edu/nursing

Bowie State University, Graduate Programs, Department of Nursing, Bowie, MD 20715-9465. Offers administration of nursing services (MS); family nurse practitioner (MS); nursing education (MS). Part-time programs available. *Degree requirements:* For master's, comprehensive exam, thesis, research paper. *Entrance requirements:* For master's, minimum GPA of 2.5. Electronic applications accepted. *Expenses:* Tuition, state resident: full-time $8665. Tuition, nonresident: full-time $16,007. *Required fees:* $1927. *Faculty research:* Minority health, women's health, gerontology, leadership management.

Bradley University, Graduate School, College of Education and Health Sciences, Department of Nursing, Peoria, IL 61625-0002. Offers nurse administered anesthesia (MSN); nursing administration (MSN). Part-time and evening/weekend programs available. *Degree requirements:* For master's, comprehensive exam, thesis optional. *Entrance requirements:* For master's, GRE General Test or MAT, interview, Illinois RN license, advanced cardiac life support certification, pediatric advanced life support certification, 3 letters of recommendation. Additional exam requirements/recommendations for international students: Required—TOEFL (minimum score 550 paper-based; 79 iBT). *Expenses: Tuition:* Full-time $14,580; part-time $810 per credit hour. Tuition and fees vary according to course load and program.

Brenau University, Sydney O. Smith Graduate School, College of Health and Science, Gainesville, GA 30501. Offers family nurse practitioner (MSN); nurse educator (MSN); nursing management (MSN); occupational therapy (MS); psychology (MS). *Accreditation:* AOTA. Part-time and evening/weekend programs available. *Degree requirements:* For master's, comprehensive exam (for some programs), thesis (for some programs), clinical practicum hours. *Entrance requirements:* For master's, GRE General Test or MAT (for some programs), interview, writing sample, references (for some programs). Additional exam requirements/recommendations for international students: Required—TOEFL (minimum score 500 paper-based; 61 iBT); Recommended—IELTS (minimum score 5). Electronic applications accepted. *Expenses:* Contact institution.

California State University, Fullerton, Graduate Studies, College of Health and Human Development, Department of Nursing, Fullerton, CA 92834-9480. Offers leadership (MSN); nurse anesthesia (MSN); nurse educator (MSN); nursing (DNP); women's health care (MSN). *Accreditation:* AACN; AANA/CANAEP. Part-time programs available. *Students:* 186 full-time (138 women), 134 part-time (120 women); includes 174 minority (15 Black or African American, non-Hispanic/Latino; 3 American Indian or Alaska Native, non-Hispanic/Latino; 92 Asian, non-Hispanic/Latino; 50 Hispanic/Latino; 2 Native Hawaiian or other Pacific Islander, non-Hispanic/Latino; 12 Two or more races, non-Hispanic/Latino), 3 international. Average age 35. 431 applicants, 38% accepted, 131 enrolled. In 2013, 117 master's awarded. Application fee: $55. *Financial support:* Career-related internships or fieldwork, Federal Work-Study, institutionally sponsored loans, scholarships/grants, and traineeships available. Support available to part-time students. Financial award application deadline: 3/1; financial award applicants required to submit FAFSA. *Unit head:* Dr. Cindy Greenberg, Chair, 657-278-3336. *Application contact:* Admissions/Applications, 657-278-2371.
Website: http://nursing.fullerton.edu/

Capella University, School of Public Service Leadership, Master's Programs in Nursing, Minneapolis, MN 55402. Offers diabetes nursing (MSN); general nursing (MSN); gerontology nursing (MSN); health information management (MS); nurse educator (MSN); nursing leadership and administration (MSN).

Capital University, School of Nursing, Columbus, OH 43209-2394. Offers administration (MSN); legal studies (MSN); theological studies (MSN); JD/MSN; MBA/MSN; MSN/MTS. *Accreditation:* AACN. Part-time and evening/weekend programs available. *Degree requirements:* For master's, thesis or alternative. *Entrance requirements:* For master's, BSN, current RN license, minimum GPA of 3.0, undergraduate courses in statistics and research. Additional exam requirements/recommendations for international students: Required—TOEFL (minimum score 550 paper-based). *Expenses:* Contact institution. *Faculty research:* Bereavement, wellness/health promotion, emergency cardiac care, critical thinking, complementary and alternative healthcare.

Carlow University, School of Nursing, Program in Nursing Leadership and Education, Pittsburgh, PA 15213-3165. Offers MSN. Part-time and evening/weekend programs available. Postbaccalaureate distance learning degree programs offered (minimal on-campus study). *Students:* 27 full-time (26 women), 20 part-time (19 women); includes 5 minority (2 Black or African American, non-Hispanic/Latino; 1 American Indian or Alaska Native, non-Hispanic/Latino; 1 Hispanic/Latino; 1 Two or more races, non-Hispanic/Latino), 2 international. Average age 34. 26 applicants, 100% accepted, 19 enrolled. In 2013, 25 master's awarded. *Degree requirements:* For master's, internship. *Entrance requirements:* For master's, minimum undergraduate GPA of 3.0 from accredited BSN program; current license as RN in Pennsylvania; course in statistics in past 6 years; two recommendations; personal statement; personal interview. Additional exam requirements/recommendations for international students: Required—TOEFL (minimum score 550 paper-based). Application fee: $20. Application fee is waived when completed online. *Expenses: Tuition:* Full-time $9523; part-time $744 per credit. Tuition and fees vary according to course load, degree level and program. *Unit head:* Dr. Peggy Slota, Director, Nursing Leadership and DNP Programs, 412-578-6102, Fax: 412-578-6114, E-mail: mmslota@carlow.edu. *Application contact:* Jo Danhires, Administrative Assistant, Admissions, 412-578-6059, Fax: 412-578-6321, E-mail: gradstudies@carlow.edu.
Website: http://www.carlow.edu/Master_of_Science_in_Nursing_Concentration_in_Education_and_Leadership.aspx

Case Western Reserve University, Frances Payne Bolton School of Nursing, Doctor of Nursing Practice Program, Cleveland, OH 44106. Offers acute care nurse practitioner (DNP); adult gerontology nurse practitioner (DNP); educational leadership (DNP); family nurse practitioner (DNP); family systems psychiatric mental health nursing (DNP); midwifery/family nursing (DNP); neonatal nurse practitioner (DNP); pediatric nurse practitioner (DNP); practice leadership (DNP); women's health nurse practitioner (DNP). *Accreditation:* AACN. Part-time programs available. Postbaccalaureate distance learning degree programs offered (minimal on-campus study). *Students:* 169 full-time, 9 part-time; includes 10 minority (6 Black or African American, non-Hispanic/Latino; 1 Asian, non-Hispanic/Latino; 2 Hispanic/Latino; 1 Two or more races, non-Hispanic/Latino). 76 applicants, 97% accepted, 59 enrolled. In 2013, 38 doctorates awarded. Terminal master's awarded for partial completion of doctoral program. *Degree requirements:* For doctorate, thesis/dissertation. *Entrance requirements:* For doctorate, GRE General Test or MAT. Additional exam requirements/recommendations for international students: Required—TOEFL (minimum score 577 paper-based; 90 iBT), IELTS (minimum score 7). *Application deadline:* For fall admission, 6/1 priority date for domestic students, 6/1 for international students; for spring admission, 10/1 for domestic and international students. Applications are processed on a rolling basis. Application fee: $75. *Financial support:* In 2013–14, 90 students received support, including 9 fellowships with full tuition reimbursements available (averaging $31,325 per year), 1 research assistantship with partial tuition reimbursement available (averaging $14,472 per year); teaching assistantships, Federal Work-Study, institutionally sponsored loans, scholarships/grants, and tuition waivers (partial) also available. Support available to part-time students. Financial award application deadline: 5/15; financial award applicants required to submit FAFSA. *Faculty research:* Symptom science, family/community care, aging across the lifespan, self-management of health and illness, neuroscience. *Unit head:* Dr. Donna Dowling, Director, 216-368-1869, Fax: 216-368-3542, E-mail: dad10@case.edu. *Application contact:* Donna Hassik, Admissions Coordinator, 216-368-5253, Fax: 216-368-0124, E-mail: dmh7@case.edu.
Website: http://fpb.case.edu/DNP/

Cedar Crest College, Program in Nursing, Allentown, PA 18104-6196. Offers nursing administration (MS); nursing education (MS). Part-time programs available. *Faculty:* 6 full-time (all women). *Students:* 34 part-time (31 women); includes 3 minority (1 Asian, non-Hispanic/Latino; 2 Hispanic/Latino). Average age 44. In 2013, 9 master's awarded. *Expenses: Tuition:* Part-time $661 per credit. *Unit head:* Dr. Wendy Robb, Director, 610-606-4666, E-mail: wjrobb@cedarcrest.edu. *Application contact:* Mary Ellen Hickes, Director of School of Adult and Graduate Education, 610-606-4666, E-mail: sage@cedarcrest.edu.
Website: http://sage.cedarcrest.edu/degrees/graduate/nursing-science/

Central Methodist University, College of Graduate and Extended Studies, Fayette, MO 65248-1198. Offers clinical counseling (MS); clinical nurse leader (MSN); education (M Ed); music education (MME); nurse educator (MSN). Part-time and evening/weekend programs available. Postbaccalaureate distance learning degree programs offered (no on-campus study). *Degree requirements:* For master's, thesis. *Entrance requirements:* For master's, GRE General Test, minimum GPA of 2.75. *Application deadline:* Applications are processed on a rolling basis. Application fee: $25. Electronic applications accepted. *Expenses: Tuition:* Part-time $360 per credit hour. Part-time tuition and fees vary according to campus/location and program. *Financial support:* Tuition waivers available. Support available to part-time students. Financial award application deadline: 6/5; financial award applicants required to submit FAFSA. *Unit head:* Dr. Rita Gulstad, Provost, 660-248-6212, Fax: 660-248-6392, E-mail: rgulstad@centralmethodist.edu. *Application contact:* Aimee Sage, Director of Graduate Admissions, 660-248-6651, Fax: 660-248-6392, E-mail: asage@centralmethodist.edu.
Website: http://www.centralmethodist.edu/graduate/

Chatham University, Nursing Programs, Pittsburgh, PA 15232-2826. Offers education/leadership (MSN); nursing (DNP). *Accreditation:* AACN. Postbaccalaureate distance learning degree programs offered (minimal on-campus study). *Faculty:* 9 full-time (8 women), 8 part-time/adjunct (5 women). *Students:* 38 full-time (31 women), 71 part-time (61 women); includes 28 minority (19 Black or African American, non-Hispanic/Latino; 6 Asian, non-Hispanic/Latino; 3 Hispanic/Latino), 1 international. Average age 46. 186 applicants, 47% accepted, 50 enrolled. In 2013, 27 master's, 51 doctorates awarded. *Entrance requirements:* For master's, RN license, BSN, minimum GPA of 3.0; for doctorate, RN license, MSN. Additional exam requirements/recommendations for international students: Required—TOEFL (minimum score 600 paper-based; 100 iBT), IELTS (minimum score 6.5), TWE. *Application deadline:* For fall admission, 5/1 priority date for domestic and international students. Applications are processed on a rolling basis. Application fee: $0. Electronic applications accepted. Application fee is waived when completed online. *Expenses: Tuition:* Full-time $14,886; part-time $827 per credit hour. One-time fee: $396 full-time. *Financial support:* Applicants required to submit FAFSA. *Unit head:* Dr. Diane Hunker, Director, 412-365-1738, E-mail: dhunker@chatham.edu. *Application contact:* David Vey, Admissions Support Specialist, 412-365-1498, Fax: 412-365-1720, E-mail: dvey@chatham.edu.
Website: http://www.chatham.edu/nursing

Clarke University, Department of Nursing and Health, Dubuque, IA 52001-3198. Offers administration of nursing systems (MSN); advanced practice nursing (MSN); education (MSN); family nurse practitioner (MSN, PMC); nursing (DNP). *Accreditation:* AACN. Part-time programs available. *Faculty:* 10 full-time (9 women). *Students:* 42 full-time (41 women), 16 part-time (15 women). In 2013, 13 master's awarded. *Entrance requirements:* For master's, GRE General Test or MAT, BSN, minimum GPA of 3.0. *Application deadline:* For fall admission, 2/15 priority date for domestic students; for

spring admission, 12/15 priority date for domestic students. Applications are processed on a rolling basis. Application fee: $25. Electronic applications accepted. *Expenses: Tuition:* Part-time $660 per credit. *Required fees:* $15 per credit. *Financial support:* In 2013–14, 6 students received support. Career-related internships or fieldwork available. Support available to part-time students. Financial award applicants required to submit FAFSA. *Faculty research:* Narrative pedagogy, ethics, end-of-life care, pedagogy, family systems. *Unit head:* Dr. Jan Lee, Chair, 800-224-2736, Fax: 319-584-8684. *Application contact:* Kara Shroeder, Information Contact, 563-588-6635, Fax: 563-588-6789, E-mail: graduate@clarke.edu.
Website: http://www.clarke.edu/

Clarkson College, Master of Science In Nursing Program, Omaha, NE 68131. Offers adult nurse practitioner (MSN, Post-Master's Certificate); family nurse practitioner (MSN, Post-Master's Certificate); nursing education (MSN, Post-Master's Certificate); nursing health care leadership (MSN, Post-Master's Certificate). *Accreditation:* AANA/CANAEP. Part-time and evening/weekend programs available. Postbaccalaureate distance learning degree programs offered (minimal on-campus study). *Degree requirements:* For master's, on-campus skills assessment (family nurse practitioner, adult nurse practitioner), comprehensive exam or thesis. *Entrance requirements:* For master's, minimum GPA of 3.0, 2 references, resume. Additional exam requirements/recommendations for international students: Required—TOEFL (minimum score 600 paper-based; 100 iBT). Electronic applications accepted.

Clarkson College, Program in Health Care Administration, Omaha, NE 68131-2739. Offers MHCA. Part-time and evening/weekend programs available. Postbaccalaureate distance learning degree programs offered (no on-campus study). *Entrance requirements:* For master's, minimum GPA of 3.0, resume, references. Additional exam requirements/recommendations for international students: Required—TOEFL (minimum score 600 paper-based; 100 iBT). Electronic applications accepted.

College of Mount Saint Vincent, School of Professional and Continuing Studies, Department of Nursing, Riverdale, NY 10471-1093. Offers adult nurse practitioner (MSN, PMC); family nurse practitioner (MSN, PMC); nurse educator (PMC); nursing administration (MSN); nursing for the adult and aged (MSN). *Accreditation:* AACN. Part-time programs available. *Entrance requirements:* For master's, BSN, interview, RN license, minimum GPA of 3.0, letters of reference. Additional exam requirements/recommendations for international students: Required—TOEFL. *Expenses:* Contact institution.

The College of New Rochelle, Graduate School, Program in Nursing, New Rochelle, NY 10805-2308. Offers acute care nurse practitioner (MS, Certificate); clinical specialist in holistic nursing (MS, Certificate); family nurse practitioner (MS, Certificate); nursing and health care management (MS); nursing education (Certificate). *Accreditation:* AACN. Part-time programs available. *Faculty:* 6 full-time (5 women), 5 part-time/adjunct (4 women). *Students:* 113 part-time (104 women); includes 56 minority (44 Black or African American, non-Hispanic/Latino; 3 Asian, non-Hispanic/Latino; 9 Hispanic/Latino). Average age 40. In 2013, 17 master's awarded. *Entrance requirements:* For master's, GRE General Test or MAT, BSN, malpractice insurance, minimum GPA of 3.0, RN license. *Application deadline:* For fall admission, 8/15 priority date for domestic students; for spring admission, 12/1 priority date for domestic students. Applications are processed on a rolling basis. Application fee: $35. Electronic applications accepted. *Expenses:* Contact institution. *Financial support:* Traineeships available. Support available to part-time students. Financial award application deadline: 8/15. *Unit head:* Dr. Mary McGuinness, Acting Dean, School of Nursing, 914-654-5441, E-mail: mmcguiness@cnr.edu.

Cox College, Programs in Nursing, Springfield, MO 65802. Offers clinical nurse leader (MSN); family nurse practitioner (MSN); nurse educator (MSN). *Accreditation:* AACN. *Entrance requirements:* For master's, RN license, essay, 2 letters of recommendation, official transcripts. Electronic applications accepted.

Daemen College, Department of Nursing, Amherst, NY 14226-3592. Offers adult nurse practitioner (MS, Post Master's Certificate); nurse executive leadership (Post Master's Certificate); nursing education (MS, Post Master's Certificate); nursing executive leadership (MS); nursing practice (DNP); palliative care nursing (Post Master's Certificate). Part-time programs available. *Degree requirements:* For master's, thesis or alternative, degree completed in 4 years; minimum GPA of 3.0; for doctorate, degree completed in 5 years; 500 post-master's clinical hours. *Entrance requirements:* For master's, BN, 1 year medical/surgical experience, RN license and state registration, statistics course with minimum C grade, 3 letters of recommendation, minimum GPA of 3.25, interview; for doctorate, MS in advance nursing practice; New York state RN license; goal statement; resume; interview; statistics course with minimum grade of 'C'; for Post Master's Certificate, master's degree in clinical area; RN license and current registration; one year of clinical experience; statistics course with minimum grade of 'C'; 3 letters of recommendation; interview; letter of intent. Additional exam requirements/recommendations for international students: Required—TOEFL (minimum score 500 paper-based; 63 iBT), IELTS (minimum score 5.5). Electronic applications accepted. *Faculty research:* Professional stress, client behavior, drug therapy, treatment modalities and pulmonary cancers, chemical dependency.

DeSales University, Graduate Division, Division of Healthcare and Natural Sciences, Center Valley, PA 18034-9568. Offers adult clinical nurse specialist (MSN); certified nurse midwives (MSN); certified nurse practitioners (MSN); clinical leadership (DNP); family nurse practitioner (MSN); information systems (MSIS); nurse educator (MSN); nurse practitioner (Post-Master's Certificate); physical therapy (DPT); physician assistant studies (MSPAS); MSN/MBA. Part-time programs available. In 2013, 5 doctorates awarded. *Degree requirements:* For master's, thesis optional. *Entrance requirements:* For master's, GRE General Test, MAT, minimum B average in undergraduate course work, health assessment course or equivalent, course work in statistics. Additional exam requirements/recommendations for international students: Required—TOEFL. *Application deadline:* Applications are processed on a rolling basis. Application fee: $35. Electronic applications accepted. *Expenses: Tuition:* Part-time $790 per credit. *Financial support:* Applicants required to submit FAFSA. *Unit head:* Dr. Mary Liz Doyle-Tadduni, Department Chair, Nursing, 610-282-1100 Ext. 1394, Fax: 610-282-2091, E-mail: carol.mest@desales.edu. *Application contact:* Abagail Wernicki, Director of Graduate Admissions, 610-282-1100 Ext. 1768, Fax: 610-282-2869, E-mail: abagail.wernicki@desales.edu.

Drexel University, College of Nursing and Health Professions, Division of Graduate Nursing, Philadelphia, PA 19104-2875. Offers adult acute care (MSN); adult psychiatric/mental health (MSN); advanced practice nursing (MSN); clinical trials research (MSN); family nurse practitioner (MSN); leadership in health systems management (MSN); nursing education (MSN); pediatric primary care (MSN); women's health (MSN). *Accreditation:* AACN. Electronic applications accepted.

Duke University, School of Nursing, Durham, NC 27708-0586. Offers acute care pediatric nurse practitioner (MSN); adult-gerontology nurse practitioner - acute care (MSN, Post Master's Certificate); adult-gerontology nurse practitioner - primary care (MSN, Post Master's Certificate), including adult-gerontology nurse practitioner (MSN), cardiology, oncology; family nurse practitioner (MSN); neonatal nurse practitioner (MSN); nurse anesthesia (MSN, DNP); nursing (PhD); nursing and health care leadership (MSN); nursing education (MSN); nursing informatics (MSN, Post Master's Certificate); pediatric nurse practitioner - primary care (MSN). *Accreditation:* AACN; AANA/CANAEP. Part-time and evening/weekend programs available. Postbaccalaureate distance learning degree programs offered (minimal on-campus study). *Faculty:* 74 full-time (64 women), 7 part-time/adjunct (4 women). *Students:* 127 full-time (113 women), 473 part-time (433 women); includes 131 minority (54 Black or African American, non-Hispanic/Latino; 9 American Indian or Alaska Native, non-Hispanic/Latino; 36 Asian, non-Hispanic/Latino; 27 Hispanic/Latino; 5 Native Hawaiian or other Pacific Islander, non-Hispanic/Latino), 14 international. Average age 34. 516 applicants, 50% accepted, 190 enrolled. In 2013, 179 master's, 49 doctorates, 23 other advanced degrees awarded. Terminal master's awarded for partial completion of doctoral program. *Degree requirements:* For master's, thesis optional; for doctorate, capstone project. *Entrance requirements:* For master's, GRE General Test (waived if undergraduate GPA of 3.4 or higher), 1 year of nursing experience (recommended), BSN, minimum GPA of 3.0, previous course work in statistics; for doctorate, GRE General Test (waived if undergraduate GPA of 3.4 or higher), BSN or MSN, minimum GPA of 3.0, portfolio, resume, personal statement, undergraduate statistics course, current licensure as a registered nurse, transcripts from all post-secondary institutions; for Post Master's Certificate, MSN, licensure or eligibility as a professional nurse, transcripts from all post-secondary institutions, previous course work in statistics. Additional exam requirements/recommendations for international students: Recommended—TOEFL (minimum score 550 paper-based; 83 iBT), IELTS (minimum score 7). *Application deadline:* For fall admission, 12/1 for domestic and international students; for spring admission, 5/1 for domestic and international students. Application fee: $50. Electronic applications accepted. *Expenses:* Contact institution. *Financial support:* Career-related internships or fieldwork, institutionally sponsored loans, scholarships/grants, traineeships, and tuition waivers (partial) available. Support available to part-time students. Financial award applicants required to submit FAFSA. *Faculty research:* Cardiovascular disease, caregiver skill training, data mining, prostate cancer, neonatal immune system. *Unit head:* Dr. Catherine L. Gilliss, Dean/Vice Chancellor for Nursing Affairs, 919-684-9444, Fax: 919-684-9414, E-mail: catherine.gilliss@duke.edu. *Application contact:* Ernie Rushing, Lead Admissions Processor/Admissions Officer, 919-668-6274, Fax: 919-668-4693, E-mail: stephen.rushing@dm.duke.edu.
Website: http://www.nursing.duke.edu/

D'Youville College, School of Nursing, Buffalo, NY 14201-1084. Offers advanced practice nursing (DNP); community health nursing/education (MSN); community health nursing/management (MSN); family nurse practitioner (MSN, Certificate); nursing and health-related professions education (Certificate). *Accreditation:* AACN. Part-time programs available. *Students:* 51 full-time (45 women), 136 part-time (115 women); includes 25 minority (17 Black or African American, non-Hispanic/Latino; 1 American Indian or Alaska Native, non-Hispanic/Latino; 1 Asian, non-Hispanic/Latino; 6 Hispanic/Latino), 76 international. Average age 35. 261 applicants, 36% accepted, 73 enrolled. In 2013, 51 master's, 3 other advanced degrees awarded. *Degree requirements:* For master's, thesis or alternative, membership on board of community agency, publishable paper. *Entrance requirements:* For master's, BS in nursing, minimum GPA of 3.0, course work in statistics and computers. Additional exam requirements/recommendations for international students: Required—TOEFL (minimum score 500 paper-based). *Application deadline:* For fall admission, 5/1 priority date for international students; for spring admission, 9/1 priority date for international students. Applications are processed on a rolling basis. Application fee: $25. Electronic applications accepted. *Financial support:* Federal Work-Study, scholarships/grants, traineeships, and unspecified assistantships available. Support available to part-time students. Financial award application deadline: 3/1; financial award applicants required to submit FAFSA. *Faculty research:* Nursing curriculum, nursing theory-testing, wellness research, communication and socialization patterns. *Unit head:* Dr. Ann Caughill, Chair, 716-829-7892, Fax: 716-829-8159. *Application contact:* Mark Pavone, Graduate Admissions Director, 716-829-8400, Fax: 716-829-7900, E-mail: graduateadmissions@dyc.edu.
Website: http://www.dyc.edu/academics/nursing/

See Display on page 632 and Close-Up on page 815.

Eastern Mennonite University, Program in Nursing, Harrisonburg, VA 22802-2462. Offers leadership and management (MSN); leadership/school nursing (MSN). *Accreditation:* AACN. Part-time programs available. Postbaccalaureate distance learning degree programs offered (minimal on-campus study). *Degree requirements:* For master's, leadership project. *Entrance requirements:* For master's, RN license, one year of full-time work experience as RN, minimum GPA of 3.0. Additional exam requirements/recommendations for international students: Required—TOEFL. *Faculty research:* Community health, international health, effectiveness of the nursing school environment, development of caring ability in nursing students, international nursing students.

Eastern Michigan University, Graduate School, College of Health and Human Services, School of Health Sciences, Program in Clinical Research Administration, Ypsilanti, MI 48197. Offers MS, Graduate Certificate. Part-time and evening/weekend programs available. Postbaccalaureate distance learning degree programs offered (minimal on-campus study). *Students:* 14 full-time (8 women), 21 part-time (14 women); includes 4 minority (2 Black or African American, non-Hispanic/Latino; 2 Two or more races, non-Hispanic/Latino), 17 international. Average age 30. 51 applicants, 53% accepted, 17 enrolled. In 2013, 18 master's, 2 other advanced degrees awarded. *Entrance requirements:* Additional exam requirements/recommendations for international students: Required—TOEFL. *Application deadline:* Applications are processed on a rolling basis. Application fee: $35. *Expenses:* Tuition, state resident: full-time $12,300; part-time $466 per credit hour. Tuition, nonresident: full-time $23,159; part-time $918 per credit hour. *Required fees:* $71 per credit hour. $46 per semester. One-time fee: $100. Tuition and fees vary according to course level and degree level. *Financial support:* Fellowships, research assistantships with full tuition reimbursements, teaching assistantships with full tuition reimbursements, career-related internships or fieldwork, Federal Work-Study, institutionally sponsored loans, scholarships/grants, tuition waivers (partial), and unspecified assistantships available. Support available to part-time students. Financial award applicants required to submit FAFSA. *Unit head:* Dr. Colleen Croxall, Director, 734-487-4096, Fax: 734-487-4095, E-mail: ccroxall@emich.edu. *Application contact:* Dr. Stephen Sonstein, Program Director, 734-487-1238, Fax: 734-487-4095, E-mail: stephen.sonstein@emich.edu.

Elms College, Division of Nursing, Chicopee, MA 01013-2839. Offers nursing and health services management (MSN); nursing education (MSN). *Accreditation:* AACN. Part-time and evening/weekend programs available. *Entrance requirements:* Additional exam requirements/recommendations for international students: Required—TOEFL.

Emmanuel College, Graduate Studies, Graduate Program in Nursing, Boston, MA 02115. Offers nursing education (MSN); nursing management/administration (MSN). Part-time and evening/weekend programs available. *Faculty:* 4 full-time (all women), 4 part-time/adjunct (all women). *Students:* 51 part-time (47 women); includes 9 minority (6 Black or African American, non-Hispanic/Latino; 1 American Indian or Alaska Native, non-Hispanic/Latino; 1 Asian, non-Hispanic/Latino; 1 Hispanic/Latino). Average age 49. *Degree requirements:* For master's, 36 credits, including 6-credit practicum. *Entrance*

requirements: For master's, transcripts from all regionally-accredited institutions attended (showing proof of bachelor's degree completion), proof of RN license, 2 letters of recommendation, essay, resume, interview. Additional exam requirements/recommendations for international students: Required—TOEFL (minimum score 600 paper-based; 106 iBT) or IELTS (minimum score 6.5). *Application deadline:* For fall admission, 4/30 for domestic students. Applications are processed on a rolling basis. Application fee: $0. Electronic applications accepted. *Financial support:* Applicants required to submit FAFSA. *Unit head:* Sandy Robbins, Dean of Enrollment, 617-735-9700, Fax: 617-507-0434, E-mail: graduatestudies@emmanuel.edu. *Application contact:* Enrollment Counselor, 617-735-9700, Fax: 617-507-0434, E-mail: graduatestudies@emmanuel.edu.
Website: http://www.emmanuel.edu/graduate-studies-nursing/academics/nursing.html

Emory University, Nell Hodgson Woodruff School of Nursing, Atlanta, GA 30322-1100. Offers adult nurse practitioner (MSN); emergency nurse practitioner (MSN); family nurse practitioner (MSN); family nurse-midwife (MSN); health systems leadership (MSN); nurse-midwifery (MSN); pediatric nurse practitioner acute and primary care (MSN); women's health care (Title X) (MSN); women's health nurse practitioner (MSN); MSN/MPH. *Accreditation:* AACN; ACNM/ACME (one or more programs are accredited). Part-time programs available. *Entrance requirements:* For master's, GRE General Test or MAT, minimum GPA of 3.0, BS in nursing from an accredited institution, RN license and additional course work, 3 letters of recommendation. Additional exam requirements/recommendations for international students: Required—TOEFL (minimum score 600 paper-based; 100 iBT). Electronic applications accepted. *Expenses:* Contact institution. *Faculty research:* Older adult falls and injuries, minority health issues, cardiac symptoms and quality of life, bio-ethics and decision-making, menopausal issues.

Fairfield University, School of Nursing, Fairfield, CT 06824-5195. Offers advanced practice (DNP); executive (DNP); family nurse practitioner (MSN, DNP); nurse anesthesia (DNP); nursing leadership (MSN); psychiatric nurse practitioner (MSN, DNP). *Accreditation:* AACN; AANA/CANAEP. Part-time programs available. *Faculty:* 22 full-time (all women), 28 part-time/adjunct (23 women). *Students:* 27 full-time (23 women), 157 part-time (136 women); includes 37 minority (15 Black or African American, non-Hispanic/Latino; 10 Asian, non-Hispanic/Latino; 8 Hispanic/Latino; 2 Native Hawaiian or other Pacific Islander, non-Hispanic/Latino; 2 Two or more races, non-Hispanic/Latino), 8 international. Average age 37. 132 applicants, 52% accepted, 59 enrolled. In 2013, 39 master's, 3 doctorates awarded. *Degree requirements:* For master's, capstone project. *Entrance requirements:* For master's, minimum QPA of 3.0, RN license, resume, 2 recommendations; for doctorate, GRE (nurse anesthesia applicants only), MSN (minimum QPA of 3.2) or BSN (minimum QPA of 3.0); critical care nursing experience (for nurse anesthesia DNP candidates). Additional exam requirements/recommendations for international students: Required—TOEFL (minimum score 550 paper-based; 80 iBT) or IELTS (minimum score 6.5). *Application deadline:* For fall admission, 5/15 for international students; for spring admission, 10/15 for international students. Applications are processed on a rolling basis. Application fee: $60. Electronic applications accepted. *Expenses:* Contact institution. *Financial support:* In 2013–14, 4 students received support. Unspecified assistantships available. Financial award applicants required to submit FAFSA. *Faculty research:* Aging and sexual health, psychosocial needs of men with prostate cancer, nurse practitioner education, mentoring, psychiatric and mental health, incarceration of the mentally ill, recovery in schizophrenia, palliative and end of life care, maternal and child health, breastfeeding and lactation consultant, stress and emotional eating, care of veterans and their families, falls prevention and the elderly, health care leadership, interprofessional education, academic partnerships. *Total annual research expenditures:* $775,000. *Unit head:* Dr. Lynn Babington, Dean, 203-254-4000 Ext. 2701, Fax: 203-254-4126, E-mail: lbabington@fairfield.edu. *Application contact:* Marianne Gumpper, Director of Graduate and Continuing Studies Admission, 203-254-4184, Fax: 203-254-4073, E-mail: gradadmis@fairfield.edu.
Website: http://fairfield.edu/son

Felician College, Doctor of Nursing Practice Program, Lodi, NJ 07644-2117. Offers advanced practice (DNP); executive leadership (DNP). Postbaccalaureate distance learning degree programs offered (no on-campus study). *Students:* 14 part-time (11 women); includes 10 minority (7 Black or African American, non-Hispanic/Latino; 1 American Indian or Alaska Native, non-Hispanic/Latino; 1 Asian, non-Hispanic/Latino; 1 Native Hawaiian or other Pacific Islander, non-Hispanic/Latino). *Degree requirements:* For doctorate, project, residency. *Expenses: Tuition:* Part-time $945 per credit. *Required fees:* $317.50 per semester. *Application contact:* Nicole Vitale, Assistant Director of Graduate Admissions, 201-559-6077, Fax: 201-559-6138, E-mail: graduate@felician.edu.

Felician College, Program in Nursing, Lodi, NJ 07644-2117. Offers adult-gerontology nurse practitioner (MSN, PMC); executive leadership (MSN, PMC); family nurse practitioner (MSN, PMC); nursing education (MSN, PMC). *Accreditation:* AACN. Part-time and evening/weekend programs available. Postbaccalaureate distance learning degree programs offered (no on-campus study). *Students:* 5 full-time (4 women), 85 part-time (78 women); includes 50 minority (20 Black or African American, non-Hispanic/Latino; 14 Asian, non-Hispanic/Latino; 16 Hispanic/Latino). Average age 42. *Degree requirements:* For master's, scholarly project. *Entrance requirements:* For master's, BS in nursing or equivalent, minimum GPA of 3.0, 2 letters of recommendation, RN license; for PMC, RN license, minimum GPA of 2.75. Additional exam requirements/recommendations for international students: Recommended—TOEFL (minimum score 550 paper-based). *Application deadline:* Applications are processed on a rolling basis. Application fee: $40. *Expenses: Tuition:* Part-time $945 per credit. *Required fees:* $317.50 per semester. *Financial support:* In 2013–14, 10 students received support. Traineeships available. Financial award applicants required to submit FAFSA. *Faculty research:* Anxiety and fear, curriculum innovation, health promotion. *Unit head:* Dr. Muriel Shore, Dean, Division of Health Sciences, 201-559-6030, E-mail: shorem@felician.edu. *Application contact:* Elizabeth Barca, Senior Assistant Director, Graduate Admissions, 201-559-6077, Fax: 201-559-6138, E-mail: graduate@felician.edu.

Ferris State University, College of Health Professions, School of Nursing, Big Rapids, MI 49307. Offers nursing (MSN); nursing administration (MSN); nursing education (MSN); nursing informatics (MSN). Part-time and evening/weekend programs available. Postbaccalaureate distance learning degree programs offered (minimal on-campus study). *Faculty:* 5 full-time (all women), 1 (woman) part-time/adjunct. *Students:* 1 (woman) full-time, 103 part-time (91 women); includes 5 minority (2 Black or African American, non-Hispanic/Latino; 1 American Indian or Alaska Native, non-Hispanic/Latino; 1 Native Hawaiian or other Pacific Islander, non-Hispanic/Latino; 1 Two or more races, non-Hispanic/Latino). Average age 40. 25 applicants, 92% accepted, 21 enrolled. In 2013, 20 master's awarded. *Degree requirements:* For master's, comprehensive exam, practicum, practicum project. *Entrance requirements:* For master's, BS in nursing or related field with registered nurse license, writing sample, letters of reference, 2 years' clinical experience. Additional exam requirements/recommendations for international students: Required—TOEFL (minimum score 550 paper-based; 61 iBT). *Application deadline:* For fall admission, 4/15 priority date for domestic students; for spring admission, 10/15 for domestic students. Applications are processed on a rolling basis. Application fee: $30. Electronic applications accepted. Application fee is waived when completed online. *Financial support:* In 2013–14, 3 students received support. Fellowships, research assistantships, teaching assistantships, career-related internships or fieldwork, and scholarships/grants available. Financial award application deadline: 4/15. *Faculty research:* Nursing education-minority student focus, student attitudes toward aging. *Unit head:* Dr. Susan Owens, Program Coordinator, 231-591-2267, Fax: 231-591-2325, E-mail: owenss3@ferris.edu. *Application contact:* Debby Buck, Off-Campus Program Secretary, 231-591-2270, Fax: 231-591-3788, E-mail: buckd@ferris.edu.
Website: http://www.ferris.edu/htmls/colleges/alliedhe/Nursing/homepage.htm

Florida Agricultural and Mechanical University, Division of Graduate Studies, Research, and Continuing Education, School of Allied Health Sciences, Tallahassee, FL 32307-3200. Offers health administration (MS); occupational therapy (MOT); physical therapy (MPT). *Degree requirements:* For master's, thesis (for some programs). *Entrance requirements:* For master's, GRE General Test or GMAT, minimum GPA of 3.0. Additional exam requirements/recommendations for international students: Required—TOEFL (minimum score 550 paper-based).

Florida Atlantic University, Christine E. Lynn College of Nursing, Boca Raton, FL 33431-0991. Offers administrative and financial leadership in nursing and health care (Post Master's Certificate); adult/gerontological nurse practitioner (Post Master's Certificate); advanced holistic nursing (MS, Post Master's Certificate); clinical nurse leader (MS, Post Master's Certificate); family nurse practitioner (MS, Post Master's Certificate); nurse educator (MS, Post Master's Certificate); nursing (PhD); nursing administration and financial leadership (MS); nursing practice (DNP). *Accreditation:* AACN. Part-time programs available. *Faculty:* 30 full-time (27 women), 9 part-time/adjunct (8 women). *Students:* 29 full-time (27 women), 523 part-time (492 women); includes 254 minority (157 Black or African American, non-Hispanic/Latino; 2 American Indian or Alaska Native, non-Hispanic/Latino; 19 Asian, non-Hispanic/Latino; 62 Hispanic/Latino; 2 Native Hawaiian or other Pacific Islander, non-Hispanic/Latino; 12 Two or more races, non-Hispanic/Latino), 3 international. Average age 39. 463 applicants, 25% accepted, 111 enrolled. In 2013, 148 master's, 15 doctorates awarded. *Degree requirements:* For master's, thesis or alternative; for doctorate, comprehensive exam, thesis/dissertation. *Entrance requirements:* For master's, GRE General Test or MAT, bachelor's degree in nursing, Florida RN license, minimum GPA of 3.0, resume/curriculum vitae, letter of recommendation; for doctorate, GRE General Test or MAT, curriculum vitae, Florida RN license, minimum GPA of 3.5, master's degree in nursing, three letters of recommendation. *Application deadline:* For fall admission, 6/1 for domestic students, 2/15 for international students; for spring admission, 10/1 for domestic students, 7/15 for international students. Applications are processed on a rolling basis. Application fee: $30. *Expenses:* Tuition, state resident: full-time $6660; part-time $370 per credit hour. Tuition, nonresident: full-time $18,450; part-time $1025 per credit hour. Tuition and fees vary according to course load. *Financial support:* Research assistantships with partial tuition reimbursements, teaching assistantships with partial tuition reimbursements, career-related internships or fieldwork, Federal Work-Study, institutionally sponsored loans, scholarships/grants, and traineeships available. Support available to part-time students. *Faculty research:* Econometrics of nurse-patient relationship, Alzheimer's disease, community-based programs, falls, self-healing. *Unit head:* Dr. Marlaine Smith, Dean, 561-297-3206, Fax: 561-297-3687, E-mail: msmit230@fau.edu. *Application contact:* Carol Kruse, Graduate Coordinator, 561-297-3261, Fax: 561-297-0088, E-mail: ckruse@fau.edu.
Website: http://nursing.fau.edu/

Florida Southern College, Program in Nursing, Lakeland, FL 33801-5698. Offers adult gerontology clinical nurse specialist (MSN); adult gerontology primary care nurse practitioner (MSN); nurse educator (MSN); nursing administration (MSN). *Accreditation:* AACN. Part-time and evening/weekend programs available. *Entrance requirements:* For master's, Florida RN license, 3 letters of recommendation, personal statement, minimum GPA of 3.0, resume. Additional exam requirements/recommendations for international students: Required—TOEFL (minimum score 550 paper-based). *Expenses:* Contact institution. *Faculty research:* End of life care, dementia, health promotion.

Florida State University, The Graduate School, College of Nursing, Tallahassee, FL 32312. Offers family nurse practitioner (DNP); health systems leadership (DNP); nurse educator (MSN, Certificate); nurse leader (MSN); nursing leadership (Certificate, Post-Graduate Certificate). *Accreditation:* AACN. Part-time programs available. Postbaccalaureate distance learning degree programs offered (minimal on-campus study). *Faculty:* 13 full-time (12 women). *Students:* 53 full-time (49 women), 26 part-time (all women); includes 16 minority (4 Black or African American, non-Hispanic/Latino; 1 Asian, non-Hispanic/Latino; 9 Hispanic/Latino; 2 Two or more races, non-Hispanic/Latino). Average age 38. 56 applicants, 61% accepted, 25 enrolled. In 2013, 5 master's, 18 doctorates awarded. *Degree requirements:* For master's, thesis optional. *Entrance requirements:* For master's, GRE General Test, MAT, minimum GPA of 3.0, BSN, Florida RN license; for doctorate, GRE General Test, MAT, minimum GPA of 3.0, BSN or MSN, Florida RN license. Additional exam requirements/recommendations for international students: Required—TOEFL (minimum score 550 paper-based). *Application deadline:* For fall admission, 7/1 for domestic and international students. Application fee: $30. Electronic applications accepted. *Expenses:* Tuition, state resident: part-time $403.51 per credit hour. Tuition, nonresident: part-time $1004.85 per credit hour. *Required fees:* $75.81 per credit hour. One-time fee: $20 part-time. Tuition and fees vary according to course load, campus/location and student level. *Financial support:* In 2013–14, 75 students received support, including fellowships with partial tuition reimbursements available (averaging $6,300 per year), research assistantships with partial tuition reimbursements available (averaging $3,000 per year), 3 teaching assistantships with partial tuition reimbursements available (averaging $3,000 per year); career-related internships or fieldwork, Federal Work-Study, institutionally sponsored loans, scholarships/grants, traineeships, and tuition waivers (partial) also available. Financial award application deadline: 4/15; financial award applicants required to submit FAFSA. *Faculty research:* Distance learning, gerontology, health promotion, educational strategies, rehabilitation of brain injured patients. *Unit head:* Dr. Judith McFetridge-Durdle, Dean, 850-644-6846, Fax: 850-644-7660, E-mail: jdurdle@nursing.fsu.edu. *Application contact:* Carlos G. Urrutia, Director of Student Services, 850-644-5638, Fax: 850-645-7249, E-mail: currutia@fsu.edu.
Website: http://nursing.fsu.edu/

Framingham State University, Continuing Education, Program in Nursing, Framingham, MA 01701-9101. Offers nursing education (MSN); nursing leadership (MSN). *Accreditation:* AACN. *Entrance requirements:* For master's, BSN; minimum cumulative undergraduate GPA of 3.0, 3.25 in nursing courses; coursework in statistics; 2 letters of recommendation; interview. Electronic applications accepted.

Gannon University, School of Graduate Studies, Morosky College of Health Professions and Sciences, Villa Maria School of Nursing, Program in Nursing Administration, Erie, PA 16541-0001. Offers MSN. Part-time and evening/weekend programs available. *Students:* 1 full-time (0 women), 83 part-time (61 women); includes 4 minority (2 Black or African American, non-Hispanic/Latino; 1 American Indian or Alaska Native, non-Hispanic/Latino; 1 Hispanic/Latino). Average age 36. 29 applicants, 76% accepted, 16 enrolled. In 2013, 16 master's awarded. *Degree requirements:* For master's, thesis (for some programs), practicum. *Entrance requirements:* For master's, GRE, RN, BSN, interview. Additional exam requirements/recommendations for international students: Required—TOEFL (minimum score 79 iBT). *Application deadline:* Applications are processed on a rolling basis. Application fee: $25. Electronic applications accepted. *Expenses: Tuition:* Full-time $15,930; part-time $885 per credit. *Required fees:* $430; $18 per credit. Tuition and fees vary according to course load, degree level and program. *Unit head:* Dr. Kathleen Patterson, Director, 814-871-5547, E-mail: patterso018@gannon.edu. *Application contact:* Kara Morgan, Director of Graduate Admissions, 814-871-5831, Fax: 814-871-5827, E-mail: graduate@gannon.edu.

George Mason University, College of Health and Human Services, School of Nursing, Fairfax, VA 22030. Offers nursing (MSN, DNP, PhD); nursing administration (Certificate); nursing education (Certificate). *Faculty:* 33 full-time (32 women), 44 part-time/adjunct (42 women). *Students:* 82 full-time (77 women), 187 part-time (175 women); includes 98 minority (47 Black or African American, non-Hispanic/Latino; 2 American Indian or Alaska Native, non-Hispanic/Latino; 26 Asian, non-Hispanic/Latino; 18 Hispanic/Latino; 1 Native Hawaiian or other Pacific Islander, non-Hispanic/Latino; 4 Two or more races, non-Hispanic/Latino), 9 international. Average age 40. 182 applicants, 55% accepted, 71 enrolled. In 2013, 78 master's, 16 doctorates, 3 other advanced degrees awarded. *Degree requirements:* For master's, comprehensive exam (for some programs), thesis in clinical classes; for doctorate, comprehensive exam (for some programs), thesis/dissertation (for some programs). *Entrance requirements:* For master's, 2 official transcripts; expanded goals statement; resume; BSN from accredited institution; minimum GPA of 3.0 in last 60 credits of undergraduate work; 2 letters of recommendation; completion of undergraduate statistics and graduate-level bivariate statistics; certification in professional CPR; for doctorate, 2 official transcripts; expanded goals statement; resume; 3 recommendation letters; nursing license; at least 1 year of work experience as an RN; interview; writing sample; evidence of graduate-level course in applied statistics; master's in nursing with minimum GPA of 3.5; for Certificate, 2 official transcripts; expanded goals statement; resume; master's degree from accredited institution or currently enrolled with minimum GPA of 3.0. Additional exam requirements/recommendations for international students: Required—TOEFL (minimum score 570 paper-based; 88 iBT), IELTS (minimum score 6.5), PTE. *Application deadline:* For fall admission, 2/1 priority date for domestic students; for spring admission, 11/1 for domestic students. Application fee: $65 ($80 for international students). Electronic applications accepted. *Expenses:* Contact institution. *Financial support:* In 2013–14, 14 students received support, including 11 fellowships (averaging $15,091 per year), 3 research assistantships with full and partial tuition reimbursements available (averaging $36,667 per year); career-related internships or fieldwork, Federal Work-Study, scholarships/grants, unspecified assistantships, and health care benefits (for full-time research or teaching assistantship recipients) also available. Financial award application deadline: 3/1; financial award applicants required to submit FAFSA. *Faculty research:* Research in health care, nursing science. *Total annual research expenditures:* $366,930. *Unit head:* Carol Urban, Acting Director, 703-993-2991, Fax: 703-993-3606, E-mail: curban@gmu.edu. *Application contact:* Janice Lee-Beverly, Program Support, 703-993-1947, Fax: 703-993-1943, E-mail: jleebev1@gmu.edu.
Website: http://chhs.gmu.edu/nursing

The George Washington University, School of Nursing, Washington, DC 20052. Offers adult nurse practitioner (MSN, Post-Master's Certificate); clinical research administration (MSN); family nurse practitioner (MSN, Post-Master's Certificate); health care quality (MSN, Post-Master's Certificate); nursing (DNP); nursing leadership and management (MSN); palliative care nurse practitioner (Post-Master's Certificate). *Accreditation:* AACN. *Faculty:* 37 full-time (all women). *Students:* 36 full-time (33 women), 438 part-time (405 women); includes 114 minority (59 Black or African American, non-Hispanic/Latino; 7 American Indian or Alaska Native, non-Hispanic/Latino; 32 Asian, non-Hispanic/Latino; 15 Hispanic/Latino; 1 Two or more races, non-Hispanic/Latino); 8 international. Average age 38. 360 applicants, 83% accepted, 178 enrolled. In 2013, 79 master's, 26 doctorates awarded. *Unit head:* Jean E. Johnson, Dean, 202-994-3725, E-mail: sonjej@gwumc.edu. *Application contact:* Kristin Williams, Assistant Vice President for Graduate and Special Enrollment Management, 202-994-0467, Fax: 202-994-0371, E-mail: ksw@gwu.edu.
Website: http://nursing.gwumc.edu/

Georgia Regents University, The Graduate School, Clinical Nurse Leader Program, Augusta, GA 30912. Offers MSN. *Students:* 188 full-time (163 women); includes 46 minority (30 Black or African American, non-Hispanic/Latino; 8 Asian, non-Hispanic/Latino; 5 Hispanic/Latino; 3 Two or more races, non-Hispanic/Latino), 1 international. Average age 27. 96 applicants, 49% accepted, 40 enrolled. In 2013, 13 master's awarded. *Entrance requirements:* For master's, GRE General Test or MAT, bachelor's degree or higher in a non-nursing discipline. Additional exam requirements/recommendations for international students: Required—TOEFL (minimum score 550 paper-based; 79 iBT). *Application deadline:* For fall admission, 4/1 for domestic and international students. Application fee: $50. Electronic applications accepted. *Unit head:* Dr. Lucy Marion, Dean, 706-721-3771, Fax: 706-721-8169, E-mail: lumarion@georgiahealth.edu. *Application contact:* Olivia Mitchell, Program Coordinator, 706-721-9767, Fax: 706-721-8169, E-mail: omitchel@georgiahealth.edu.
Website: http://www.gru.edu/nursing/cnl.php

Georgia State University, Byrdine F. Lewis School of Nursing, Atlanta, GA 30303. Offers adult health clinical nurse specialist/nurse practitioner (MS, Certificate); child health clinical nurse specialist/pediatric nurse practitioner (MS, Certificate); family nurse practitioner (MS, Certificate); family psychiatric mental health nurse practitioner (MS, Certificate); nursing (PhD); nursing leadership in healthcare innovations (MS), including nursing administration, nursing informatics; nutrition (MS); perinatal clinical nurse specialist/women's health nurse practitioner (MS, Certificate); physical therapy (DPT); respiratory therapy (MS). *Accreditation:* AACN. Part-time programs available. Postbaccalaureate distance learning degree programs offered (minimal on-campus study). *Faculty:* 22 full-time (16 women). *Students:* 241 full-time (180 women), 262 part-time (236 women); includes 176 minority (120 Black or African American, non-Hispanic/Latino; 31 Asian, non-Hispanic/Latino; 13 Hispanic/Latino; 3 Native Hawaiian or other Pacific Islander, non-Hispanic/Latino; 9 Two or more races, non-Hispanic/Latino), 19 international. Average age 34. 583 applicants, 34% accepted, 160 enrolled. In 2013, 110 master's, 44 doctorates, 6 other advanced degrees awarded. *Degree requirements:* For doctorate, comprehensive exam, thesis/dissertation. *Entrance requirements:* For doctorate, GRE. Additional exam requirements/recommendations for international students: Required—TOEFL. *Application deadline:* For fall admission, 2/1 priority date for domestic and international students; for spring admission, 9/15 for domestic and international students. Applications are processed on a rolling basis. Application fee: $50. Electronic applications accepted. *Expenses:* Contact institution. *Financial support:* In 2013–14, research assistantships with full and partial tuition reimbursements (averaging $1,666 per year), teaching assistantships with full and partial tuition reimbursements (averaging $1,920 per year) were awarded; scholarships/grants, tuition waivers (full and partial), and unspecified assistantships also available. Support available to part-time students. Financial award application deadline: 8/1; financial award applicants required to submit FAFSA. *Faculty research:* Stroke intervention for caregivers, stroke prevention in African Americans; relationships between psychological distress and health outcomes in parents with a medically ill infant; medically fragile children; nursing expertise and patient outcomes. *Unit head:* Joan S. Cranford, Assistant Dean for Nursing, 404-413-1200, Fax: 404-413-1205, E-mail: jcranford2@gsu.edu. *Application contact:* Tiffany Norman, Senior Administrative Coordinator, 404-413-1190, Fax: 404-413-1205, E-mail: tnorman7@gsu.edu.
Website: http://nursing.gsu.edu/

Grand Valley State University, Kirkhof College of Nursing, Allendale, MI 49401-9403. Offers advanced practice (MSN); case management (MSN); nursing administration (MSN); nursing education (MSN); nursing practice (DNP); MSN/MBA. *Accreditation:* AACN. Part-time programs available. *Degree requirements:* For master's, thesis optional. *Entrance requirements:* For master's, GRE, minimum GPA of 3.0 in upper-division course work, course work in statistics, Michigan RN license. Additional exam requirements/recommendations for international students: Required—TOEFL. Electronic applications accepted. *Faculty research:* Multigenerational health promotion, chronic disease prevention, end-of-life issues, nursing workload, family caregiver health.

Grantham University, College of Nursing and Allied Health, Lenexa, KS 66219. Offers case management (MSN); health systems management (MS); healthcare administration (MHA); nursing education (MSN); nursing informatics (MSN); nursing management and organizational leadership (MSN). Part-time and evening/weekend programs available. Postbaccalaureate distance learning degree programs offered (no on-campus study). *Faculty:* 1 (woman) full-time, 11 part-time/adjunct (5 women). *Students:* 64 full-time (43 women), 166 part-time (123 women); includes 116 minority (94 Black or African American, non-Hispanic/Latino; 4 Asian, non-Hispanic/Latino; 9 Hispanic/Latino; 1 Native Hawaiian or other Pacific Islander, non-Hispanic/Latino; 8 Two or more races, non-Hispanic/Latino). Average age 40. 230 applicants, 100% accepted, 230 enrolled. In 2013, 61 master's awarded. *Degree requirements:* For master's, thesis, major applied research paper and practicum (MSN). *Entrance requirements:* For master's, bachelor's degree from accredited degree-granting institution with minimum GPA of 2.5, BSN from an accredited nursing program, valid RN license. Additional exam requirements/recommendations for international students: Required—TOEFL (minimum score 530 paper-based; 71 iBT). *Application deadline:* Applications are processed on a rolling basis. Application fee: $30. Electronic applications accepted. *Expenses: Tuition:* Full-time $3900; part-time $325 per credit hour. *Required fees:* $35 per term. One-time fee: $100. *Financial support:* In 2013–14, 230 students received support. Scholarships/grants available. *Faculty research:* Pharmacy licensure, vaccination certification. *Unit head:* Dr. Susan Fairchild, Dean, School of Nursing, 800-955-2527, E-mail: admissions@grantham.edu. *Application contact:* Jared Parlette, Vice President of Admissions, 800-955-2527, E-mail: admissions@grantham.edu.
Website: http://www.grantham.edu/colleges-and-schools/college-of-nursing-and-allied-health/

Herzing University Online, Program in Nursing, Milwaukee, WI 53203. Offers nursing (MSN); nursing education (MSN); nursing management (MSN). *Accreditation:* AACN. Postbaccalaureate distance learning degree programs offered (no on-campus study).

Holy Family University, Graduate School, School of Nursing, Philadelphia, PA 19114. Offers community health nursing (MSN); nursing administration (MSN); nursing education (MSN). *Accreditation:* AACN. Part-time and evening/weekend programs available. *Faculty:* 7 full-time (all women). *Students:* 42 part-time (39 women); includes 9 minority (4 Black or African American, non-Hispanic/Latino; 4 Asian, non-Hispanic/Latino; 1 Hispanic/Latino). Average age 36. 17 applicants, 82% accepted, 6 enrolled. In 2013, 12 master's awarded. *Degree requirements:* For master's, thesis or alternative, comprehensive portfolio, clinical practicum. *Entrance requirements:* For master's, BSN or RN from appropriately-accredited program, minimum GPA of 3.0, professional references, official transcripts of all college or university work, essay/personal statement, current resume, completion of one undergraduate statistics course with minimum grade of C. Additional exam requirements/recommendations for international students: Required—TOEFL (minimum score 550 paper-based; 79 iBT), IELTS (minimum score 6), or PTE (minimum score 54). *Application deadline:* For fall admission, 7/1 priority date for domestic and international students; for winter admission, 1/1 for domestic students; for spring admission, 11/1 priority date for domestic and international students; for summer admission, 4/1 priority date for domestic and international students. Applications are processed on a rolling basis. Application fee: $25. Electronic applications accepted. *Expenses: Tuition:* Full-time $12,060. *Required fees:* $250. Tuition and fees vary according to degree level. *Financial support:* In 2013–14, 1 student received support. Available to part-time students. Application deadline: 2/15; applicants required to submit FAFSA. *Unit head:* Dr. Ana Maria Catanzaro, Dean, 267-341-3292, Fax: 215-637-6598, E-mail: acatanzaro@holyfamily.edu. *Application contact:* Gidget Matie Montelibano, Associate Director of Graduate Admissions, 267-341-3558, Fax: 215-637-1478, E-mail: gmontelibano@holyfamily.edu.
Website: http://www.holyfamily.edu/choosing-holy-family-u/academics/schools-of-study/school-of-nursing

Holy Names University, Graduate Division, Department of Nursing, Oakland, CA 94619-1699. Offers administration/management (MSN, PMC); clinical faculty (MSN, PMC); community health nursing/case manager (MSN); family nurse practitioner (MSN, PMC); MSN/MA; MSN/MBA. *Accreditation:* AACN. Part-time and evening/weekend programs available. *Faculty:* 3 full-time, 22 part-time/adjunct. *Students:* 31 full-time (26 women), 78 part-time (67 women); includes 66 minority (27 Black or African American, non-Hispanic/Latino; 25 Asian, non-Hispanic/Latino; 13 Hispanic/Latino; 1 Two or more races, non-Hispanic/Latino), 5 international. Average age 38. 97 applicants, 61% accepted, 49 enrolled. In 2013, 66 master's, 3 other advanced degrees awarded. *Entrance requirements:* For master's, bachelor's degree in nursing or related field; California RN license or eligibility; minimum cumulative GPA of 2.8, 3.0 in nursing courses from baccalaureate program; courses in pathophysiology, statistics, and research at the undergraduate level. Additional exam requirements/recommendations for international students: Required—TOEFL (minimum score 500 paper-based; 79 iBT). *Application deadline:* For fall admission, 8/1 priority date for domestic students, 7/15 priority date for international students; for spring admission, 12/1 priority date for domestic and international students; for summer admission, 5/1 priority date for domestic and international students. Applications are processed on a rolling basis. Application fee: $65. Electronic applications accepted. Application fee is waived when completed online. *Expenses: Tuition:* Part-time $866 per unit. *Financial support:* Career-related internships or fieldwork, Federal Work-Study, scholarships/grants, and unspecified assistantships available. Support available to part-time students. Financial award application deadline: 3/2; financial award applicants required to submit FAFSA. *Faculty research:* Women's reproductive health, gerontology, attitudes about aging, schizophrenic families, international health issues. *Unit head:* Dr. Miki Goodwin, Associate Professor/Chair of Nursing, 510-436-1374, E-mail: goodwin@hnu.edu. *Application contact:* Graduate Admission Office, 800-430-1321, E-mail: graduateadmissions@hnu.edu.

Immaculata University, College of Graduate Studies, Division of Nursing, Immaculata, PA 19345. Offers nursing administration (MSN); nursing education (MSN). *Accreditation:* AACN. Part-time and evening/weekend programs available. *Entrance requirements:* For master's, MAT or GRE, BSN, minimum undergraduate GPA of 3.0. Additional exam requirements/recommendations for international students: Required—

TOEFL. *Application deadline:* Applications are processed on a rolling basis. Application fee: $50. *Expenses: Tuition:* Part-time $660 per credit. Part-time tuition and fees vary according to degree level and program. *Financial support:* Application deadline: 5/1; applicants required to submit FAFSA. *Unit head:* Dr. Jane Tang, RN, Program Director, 610-647-4400 Ext. 3309, Fax: 610-993-8550, E-mail: jtang@immaculata.edu.
Website: http://www.immaculata.edu/nursing/

Independence University, Program in Nursing, Salt Lake City, UT 84107. Offers community health (MSN); gerontology (MSN); nursing administration (MSN); wellness promotion (MSN).

Indiana University Kokomo, School of Nursing, Kokomo, IN 46904-9003. Offers nurse administrator (MSN); nurse educator (MSN). *Students:* 3 full-time (all women), 35 part-time (all women), 1 international. 14 applicants, 93% accepted, 11 enrolled. *Unit head:* Dr. Mary P. Bourke, Assistant Dean of Graduate Programs, 765-455-9326, E-mail: mbourke@iuk.edu. *Application contact:* Admissions Office, 765-455-9326.
Website: http://www.iuk.edu/academics/majors/nursing/graduate-programs/index.shtml

Indiana University of Pennsylvania, School of Graduate Studies and Research, College of Health and Human Services, Department of Nursing and Allied Health, Program in Nursing Administration, Indiana, PA 15705-1087. Offers MS. *Accreditation:* AACN. Part-time programs available. *Faculty:* 7 full-time (6 women). *Students:* 10 part-time (8 women). Average age 37. 10 applicants, 50% accepted, 4 enrolled. In 2013, 1 master's awarded. *Degree requirements:* For master's, thesis optional, practicum. *Entrance requirements:* Additional exam requirements/recommendations for international students: Required—TOEFL (minimum score 540 paper-based). *Application deadline:* Applications are processed on a rolling basis. Application fee: $50. Electronic applications accepted. *Expenses:* Tuition, state resident: full-time $3978; part-time $442 per credit. Tuition, nonresident: full-time $5967; part-time $663 per credit. *Required fees:* $2080; $115.55 per credit. $93 per semester. Tuition and fees vary according to degree level and program. *Financial support:* In 2013–14, 1 research assistantship with full and partial tuition reimbursement (averaging $2,720 per year) was awarded; career-related internships or fieldwork, Federal Work-Study, scholarships/grants, and unspecified assistantships also available. Financial award application deadline: 4/15; financial award applicants required to submit FAFSA. *Unit head:* Dr. Nashat Zuraikat, Graduate Coordinator, 724-357-3262, E-mail: zuraikat@iup.edu.
Website: http://www.iup.edu/grad/nursing/default.aspx

Indiana University–Purdue University Fort Wayne, College of Health and Human Services, Department of Nursing, Fort Wayne, IN 46805-1499. Offers adult-gerontology primary care nurse practitioner (MS); nurse executive (MS); nursing administration (Certificate); nursing education (MS); women's health nurse practitioner (MS). Part-time programs available. *Faculty:* 12 full-time (all women). *Students:* 5 full-time (all women), 63 part-time (60 women); includes 3 minority (2 Black or African American, non-Hispanic/Latino; 1 Asian, non-Hispanic/Latino). Average age 35. 34 applicants, 100% accepted, 25 enrolled. In 2013, 10 master's awarded. *Entrance requirements:* For master's, GRE Writing Test (if GPA below 3.0), BS in nursing, eligibility for Indiana RN license, minimum GPA of 3.0, essay, copy of resume, three references, undergraduate course work in research and statistics within last 5 years. Additional exam requirements/recommendations for international students: Required—TOEFL (minimum score 550 paper-based; 79 iBT); Recommended—TWE. *Application deadline:* For fall admission, 5/1 priority date for domestic and international students; for spring admission, 11/15 priority date for domestic students. Applications are processed on a rolling basis. Application fee: $55 ($60 for international students). Electronic applications accepted. *Financial support:* In 2013–14, 3 teaching assistantships with partial tuition reimbursements (averaging $13,322 per year) were awarded; scholarships/grants also available. Support available to part-time students. Financial award application deadline: 3/1; financial award applicants required to submit FAFSA. *Faculty research:* Pain management and substance abuse, high-risk alcohol use on campus, pediatric case management. *Unit head:* Dr. Lee-Ellen Kirkhorn, Chair/Professor, 260-481-6789, Fax: 260-481-5767, E-mail: kirkhorl@ipfw.edu. *Application contact:* Dr. Deborah Poling, Director of Graduate Program, 260-481-6276, Fax: 260-481-5767, E-mail: polingd@ipfw.edu.
Website: http://www.ipfw.edu/nursing/

Indiana University–Purdue University Indianapolis, School of Nursing, Master of Science in Nursing Program, Indianapolis, IN 46202-2896. Offers nursing administration (MSN); nursing education (MSN). *Students:* 31 full-time (27 women), 303 part-time (284 women); includes 54 minority (27 Black or African American, non-Hispanic/Latino; 11 Asian, non-Hispanic/Latino; 8 Hispanic/Latino; 8 Two or more races, non-Hispanic/Latino), 3 international. 200 applicants, 59% accepted, 88 enrolled. In 2013, 120 master's awarded. *Entrance requirements:* For master's, background check, statistics. *Unit head:* Associate Dean for Graduate Programs, 317-274-2806, E-mail: nursing@iupui.edu. *Application contact:* Lisa Thompson, Graduate Advisor, 317-274-2806, E-mail: lisrthom@iu.edu.
Website: http://nursing.iu.edu/graduate/programs/msn/index.shtml

Indiana Wesleyan University, College of Adult and Professional Studies, Graduate Studies in Business, Marion, IN 46953. Offers accounting (MBA, Graduate Certificate); applied management (MBA); business administration (MBA); health care (MBA, Graduate Certificate); human resources (MBA, Graduate Certificate); management (MS); organizational leadership (MA). Part-time and evening/weekend programs available. Postbaccalaureate distance learning degree programs offered (no on-campus study). *Degree requirements:* For master's, applied business or management project. *Entrance requirements:* For master's, minimum GPA of 2.5, 2 years of related work experience. Additional exam requirements/recommendations for international students: Required—TOEFL (minimum score 550 paper-based). Electronic applications accepted. *Expenses: Tuition:* Full-time $8712; part-time $484 per credit hour. *Required fees:* $1673; $105 per credit hour. Tuition and fees vary according to course load, degree level, campus/location and program.

Indiana Wesleyan University, Graduate School, School of Nursing, Marion, IN 46953-4974. Offers nursing administration (MS); nursing education (MS); primary care nursing (MS); MSN/MBA. *Accreditation:* AACN. Part-time programs available. Postbaccalaureate distance learning degree programs offered (minimal on-campus study). *Degree requirements:* For master's, capstone project or thesis. *Entrance requirements:* For master's, writing sample, RN license, 1 year of related experience, graduate statistics course. Additional exam requirements/recommendations for international students: Required—TOEFL. *Expenses:* Contact institution. *Faculty research:* Primary health care with international emphasis, international nursing.

Jefferson College of Health Sciences, Program in Nursing, Roanoke, VA 24031-3186. Offers nursing education (MSN); nursing management (MSN). *Accreditation:* AACN. Part-time programs available. *Degree requirements:* For master's, project. *Entrance requirements:* For master's, MAT. Additional exam requirements/recommendations for international students: Required—TOEFL (minimum score 550 paper-based; 80 iBT). Electronic applications accepted. *Faculty research:* Nursing, teaching and learning techniques, cultural competence, spirituality and nursing.

Kaplan University, Davenport Campus, School of Nursing, Davenport, IA 52807-2095. Offers nurse administrator (MS); nurse educator (MS). Part-time and evening/weekend programs available. Postbaccalaureate distance learning degree programs offered (no on-campus study). *Entrance requirements:* For master's, RN. Additional exam requirements/recommendations for international students: Required—TOEFL (minimum score 550 paper-based).

Kean University, College of Natural, Applied and Health Sciences, Program in Nursing, Union, NJ 07083. Offers clinical management with transcultural focus (MSN); community health nursing (MSN); school nursing (MSN). Part-time programs available. *Faculty:* 8 full-time (all women). *Students:* 14 full-time (12 women), 121 part-time (117 women); includes 62 minority (43 Black or African American, non-Hispanic/Latino; 11 Asian, non-Hispanic/Latino; 7 Hispanic/Latino; 1 Two or more races, non-Hispanic/Latino), 2 international. Average age 42. 72 applicants, 94% accepted, 49 enrolled. In 2013, 35 master's awarded. *Degree requirements:* For master's, thesis or alternative, clinical field experience. *Entrance requirements:* For master's, minimum GPA of 3.0; BS in nursing; RN license; 2 letters of recommendation; interview. Additional exam requirements/recommendations for international students: Required—TOEFL. *Application deadline:* For fall admission, 6/1 for domestic and international students; for spring admission, 12/1 for domestic and international students. Applications are processed on a rolling basis. Application fee: $75 ($150 for international students). Electronic applications accepted. *Expenses:* Tuition, state resident: full-time $12,099; part-time $589 per credit. Tuition, nonresident: full-time $16,399; part-time $722 per credit. *Required fees:* $3050; $139 per credit. Part-time tuition and fees vary according to course level, course load, degree level and program. *Financial support:* In 2013–14, 2 research assistantships with full tuition reimbursements (averaging $3,713 per year) were awarded; unspecified assistantships also available. Financial award applicants required to submit FAFSA. *Unit head:* Dr. Virginia Fitzsimons, Program Coordinator, 908-527-3396, E-mail: vfitzsim@kean.edu. *Application contact:* Ann-Marie Kay, Assistant Director of Graduate Admissions, 908-737-5922, Fax: 908-737-5925, E-mail: akay@kean.edu.
Website: http://grad.kean.edu/masters-programs/nursing-clinical-management

Kent State University, College of Nursing, Kent, OH 44242-0001. Offers acute care nurse practitioner (MSN); adult nurse practitioner (MSN); clinical nurse specialist (MSN); family nurse practitioner (MSN); geriatric nurse practitioner (MSN); health care management (MSN); nurse educator (MSN); nursing (PhD); nursing practice (DNP); pediatric nurse practitioner (MSN); psychiatric/mental health nurse practitioner (MSN); women's health nurse practitioner (MSN). PhD program offered jointly with The University of Akron. *Accreditation:* AACN. Part-time programs available. *Degree requirements:* For master's, thesis optional; for doctorate, comprehensive exam, thesis/dissertation. *Entrance requirements:* For master's, GRE (if undergraduate GPA less than 3.0), minimum GPA of 2.75; for doctorate, GRE, MSN. Additional exam requirements/recommendations for international students: Required—TOEFL. Electronic applications accepted. *Expenses:* Contact institution. *Faculty research:* Women and violence, methodological specialties, osteoporosis in women, new caregivers and the elderly.

Lamar University, College of Graduate Studies, College of Arts and Sciences, Department of Nursing, Beaumont, TX 77710. Offers nursing administration (MSN); nursing education (MSN); MSN/MBA. Part-time and evening/weekend programs available. Postbaccalaureate distance learning degree programs offered. *Degree requirements:* For master's, comprehensive exam, practicum project presentation, evidence-based project. *Entrance requirements:* For master's, GRE General Test, MAT, criminal background check, RN license, NLN-accredited BSN, college course work in graduate statistics in past 5 years, letters of recommendation, minimum undergraduate GPA of 3.0. Additional exam requirements/recommendations for international students: Required—TOEFL. *Faculty research:* Student retention, theory, care giving, online course and research.

La Roche College, School of Graduate Studies and Adult Education, Program in Nursing, Pittsburgh, PA 15237-5898. Offers nursing education (MSN); nursing management (MSN). *Accreditation:* AANA/CANAEP. Part-time and evening/weekend programs available. Postbaccalaureate distance learning degree programs offered (minimal on-campus study). *Faculty:* 3 full-time (all women), 2 part-time/adjunct (1 woman). *Students:* 6 full-time (all women), 7 part-time (all women), 1 international. Average age 43. 6 applicants, 50% accepted, 1 enrolled. In 2013, 7 master's awarded. *Degree requirements:* For master's, thesis optional, internship, practicum. *Entrance requirements:* For master's, GRE General Test, BSN, nursing license, work experience. Additional exam requirements/recommendations for international students: Recommended—TOEFL (minimum score 550 paper-based). *Application deadline:* For fall admission, 8/15 priority date for domestic students, 8/15 for international students; for spring admission, 12/15 priority date for domestic students, 12/15 for international students. Applications are processed on a rolling basis. Application fee: $50. Electronic applications accepted. *Expenses:* Contact institution. *Financial support:* Application deadline: 3/31; applicants required to submit FAFSA. *Faculty research:* Patient education, perception. *Unit head:* Dr. Terri Liberto, Division Chair, 412-847-1813, Fax: 412-536-1175, E-mail: terri.liberto@laroche.edu. *Application contact:* Hope Schiffgens, Director of Graduate Studies and Adult Education, 412-536-1266, Fax: 412-536-1283, E-mail: schombh1@laroche.edu.

La Salle University, School of Nursing and Health Sciences, Program in Nursing, Philadelphia, PA 19141-1199. Offers adult gerontology primary care nurse practitioner (MSN, Certificate); adult health and illness clinical nurse specialist (MSN); adult-gerontology clinical nurse specialist (MSN, Certificate); clinical nurse leader (MSN); family primary care nurse practitioner (MSN, Certificate); gerontology (Certificate); nurse anesthetist (MSN, Certificate); nursing (MSN, Certificate); nursing administration (MSN, Certificate); nursing education (Certificate); nursing practice (DNP); nursing service administration (MSN); public health nursing (MSN, Certificate); school nursing (Certificate); MSN/MBA; MSN/MPH. *Accreditation:* AANA/CANAEP. Part-time programs available. Postbaccalaureate distance learning degree programs offered (minimal on-campus study). *Faculty:* 13 full-time (12 women), 10 part-time/adjunct (8 women). *Students:* 4 full-time (all women), 379 part-time (331 women); includes 119 minority (70 Black or African American, non-Hispanic/Latino; 2 American Indian or Alaska Native, non-Hispanic/Latino; 31 Asian, non-Hispanic/Latino; 12 Hispanic/Latino; 4 Two or more races, non-Hispanic/Latino), 1 international. Average age 37. 133 applicants, 85% accepted, 63 enrolled. In 2013, 72 master's, 3 doctorates, 26 other advanced degrees awarded. *Degree requirements:* For doctorate, minimum of 1,000 hours of post baccalaureate clinical practice supervised by preceptors. *Entrance requirements:* For master's, GRE, MAT, or GMAT (for students with BSN GPA of less than 3.2), baccalaureate degree in nursing from an NLNAC- or CCNE-accredited program or an MSN Bridge program; Pennsylvania RN license; 2 letters of reference; resume; statement of philosophy articulating professional values and future educational goal; 1 year of work experience as a registered nurse; for doctorate, GRE (waived for applicants with MSN cumulative GPA of 3.7 or above), MSN from nationally-accredited program or master's degree, MBA or MHA from nationally-accredited program; resume or curriculum vitae; 2 letters of reference; interview; for Certificate, GRE, MAT, or GMAT (for students with BSN GPA of less than 3.2, baccalaureate degree in nursing from an NLNAC- or CCNE-accredited program or an MSN Bridge program; Pennsylvania RN license; 2 letters of reference; resume; statement of philosophy articulating professional values and future educational goal; 1 year of work experience as a registered nurse. Additional exam requirements/recommendations for international students: Required—TOEFL. *Application deadline:* For fall admission, 8/15 priority date for domestic students, 7/15 for international students; for spring admission, 12/15 priority date for domestic students, 11/15 for international students; for summer admission, 4/15 priority date for domestic students, 3/15 for international students. Applications are processed on a rolling basis. Application fee: $35. Electronic applications accepted. Application fee is waived when completed online. *Expenses:* Contact institution. *Financial support:* In 2013–14, 48 students received support. Teaching assistantships, scholarships/grants, and traineeships available. Support available to part-time students. Financial award application deadline: 8/31; financial award applicants required to submit FAFSA. *Unit head:* Dr. Patricia M. Dillon, Director, 215-951-1322, Fax: 215-951-1896, E-mail: msnapn@lasalle.edu. *Application contact:* Paul J. Reilly, Assistant Vice President, Enrollment Services, 215-951-1946, Fax: 215-951-1462, E-mail: reilly@lasalle.edu.

Le Moyne College, Department of Nursing, Syracuse, NY 13214. Offers informatics (MS, CAS); nursing administration (MS, CAS); nursing education (MS, CAS); nursing gerontology (MS, CAS); palliative care (MS, CAS). *Accreditation:* AACN. Part-time and evening/weekend programs available. *Faculty:* 4 full-time (all women), 3 part-time/adjunct (2 women). *Students:* 13 part-time (12 women); includes 2 minority (both Black or African American, non-Hispanic/Latino). Average age 41. 14 applicants, 86% accepted, 5 enrolled. In 2013, 6 master's, 6 other advanced degrees awarded. *Degree requirements:* For master's, scholarly project. *Entrance requirements:* For master's, bachelor's degree, interview, minimum GPA of 3.0, New York RN license, 2 letters of recommendation, writing sample, transcripts. Additional exam requirements/recommendations for international students: Required—TOEFL (minimum score 550 paper-based; 79 iBT). *Application deadline:* For fall admission, 8/1 priority date for domestic and international students; for spring admission, 12/15 priority date for domestic and international students; for summer admission, 5/1 priority date for domestic and international students. Applications are processed on a rolling basis. Application fee: $50. *Expenses:* Contact institution. *Financial support:* In 2013–14, 2 students received support. Career-related internships or fieldwork, scholarships/grants, health care benefits, and unspecified assistantships available. Support available to part-time students. Financial award applicants required to submit FAFSA. *Faculty research:* Inter-profession education, gerontology, utilization of free healthcare services by the insured, health promotion education, innovative undergraduate nursing education models, patient and family education, horizontal violence. *Unit head:* Dr. Susan B. Bastable, Chair and Professor, Department of Nursing, 315-445-5436, Fax: 315-445-6024, E-mail: bastabsb@lemoyne.edu. *Application contact:* Kristen P. Trapasso, Senior Director of Enrollment Management, 315-445-4265, Fax: 315-445-6092, E-mail: trapaskp@lemoyne.edu.
Website: http://www.lemoyne.edu/nursing

Lewis University, College of Nursing and Health Professions, Program in Nursing, Romeoville, IL 60446. Offers adult nurse practitioner (MSN); nursing administration (MSN); nursing education (MSN). *Accreditation:* AACN. Part-time and evening/weekend programs available. Postbaccalaureate distance learning degree programs offered (no on-campus study). *Students:* 23 full-time (22 women), 234 part-time (222 women); includes 72 minority (31 Black or African American, non-Hispanic/Latino; 23 Asian, non-Hispanic/Latino; 15 Hispanic/Latino; 1 Native Hawaiian or other Pacific Islander, non-Hispanic/Latino; 2 Two or more races, non-Hispanic/Latino). Average age 38. *Degree requirements:* For master's, clinical practicum. *Entrance requirements:* For master's, minimum undergraduate GPA of 3.0, degree in nursing, RN license, letter of recommendation, interview, resume or curriculum vitae. Additional exam requirements/recommendations for international students: Required—TOEFL (minimum score 550 paper-based; 80 iBT). *Application deadline:* For fall admission, 5/1 priority date for international students; for spring admission, 11/15 priority date for international students. Applications are processed on a rolling basis. Application fee: $40. Electronic applications accepted. *Financial support:* Federal Work-Study, scholarships/grants, tuition waivers (full and partial), and unspecified assistantships available. Financial award application deadline: 5/1; financial award applicants required to submit FAFSA. *Faculty research:* Cancer prevention, phenomenological methods, public policy analysis. *Total annual research expenditures:* $1,000. *Unit head:* 815-836-5610. *Application contact:* Nancy Wiksten, Adult Admission Counselor, 815-836-5628, Fax: 815-836-5578, E-mail: wikstena@lewisu.edu.
Website: http://www.lewisu.edu/

Liberty University, School of Health Sciences, Lynchburg, VA 24515. Offers biomedical sciences (MS); clinical mental health counseling (MA); global health (MPH); health promotion (MPH); human services (MA), including addictions and recovery, business, Christian ministry, criminal justice, crisis response and trauma, executive leadership, health and wellness, life coaching, marriage and family, military resilience; marriage and family therapy (MA); nurse educator (MS); nursing (MSN); nursing administration (MSN); nutrition (MPH); pastoral care and counseling (PhD); professional counseling (MA, PhD). *Students:* 2,830 full-time (2,293 women), 6,275 part-time (5,051 women); includes 1,677 minority (1,178 Black or African American, non-Hispanic/Latino; 19 American Indian or Alaska Native, non-Hispanic/Latino; 36 Asian, non-Hispanic/Latino; 278 Hispanic/Latino; 7 Native Hawaiian or other Pacific Islander, non-Hispanic/Latino; 159 Two or more races, non-Hispanic/Latino), 177 international. Average age 37. 9,147 applicants, 50% accepted, 2939 enrolled. In 2013, 2,618 master's, 11 doctorates awarded. *Degree requirements:* For master's, thesis (for some programs); for doctorate, thesis/dissertation. *Entrance requirements:* For doctorate, MAT or GRE, minimum GPA of 3.25 in master's program, 2-3 recommendations, writing samples (for some programs), letter of intent, professional vitae. Additional exam requirements/recommendations for international students: Required—TOEFL (minimum score 600 paper-based; 100 iBT). Application fee: $50. *Expenses: Tuition:* Full-time $9630; part-time $535 per credit hour. *Required fees:* $175 per term. One-time fee: $50. Tuition and fees vary according to course load, degree level, campus/location and program. *Application contact:* Jay Bridge, Director of Admissions, 800-424-9595, Fax: 800-628-7977, E-mail: gradadmissions@liberty.edu.

Loma Linda University, Department of Graduate Nursing, Program in Nursing Administration, Loma Linda, CA 92350. Offers MS. *Accreditation:* AACN. Part-time programs available. *Degree requirements:* For master's, thesis or alternative. *Entrance requirements:* For master's, GRE General Test, BSN, minimum GPA of 3.0, RN license. Additional exam requirements/recommendations for international students: Required—TOEFL. Electronic applications accepted. *Faculty research:* Job aspects contributing to satisfaction among leaders in health care institutions, leadership content significant to RN graduates.

Long Island University–LIU Brooklyn, School of Nursing, Department of Nurse Executive, Brooklyn, NY 11201-8423. Offers MS. *Accreditation:* AACN. *Entrance requirements:* For master's, New York RN license, 2 letters of recommendation. Additional exam requirements/recommendations for international students: Required—TOEFL (minimum score 500 paper-based).

Lourdes University, Graduate School, Sylvania, OH 43560-2898. Offers business (MBA); leadership (M Ed); nurse anesthesia (MSN); nurse educator (MSN); nurse leader (MSN); organizational leadership (MOL); reading (M Ed); teaching and curriculum (M Ed); theology (MA). Evening/weekend programs available. *Entrance requirements:* Additional exam requirements/recommendations for international students: Required—TOEFL. *Application deadline:* For fall admission, 6/15 priority date for domestic students; for spring admission, 11/1 priority date for domestic students. Application fee: $25. *Application contact:* Melissa Bergfeld, Administrative Assistant, 419-824-3517, Fax: 419-824-3510, E-mail: mbergfeld2@lourdes.edu.
Website: http://www.lourdes.edu/gradschool.aspx

Loyola University Chicago, Graduate School, Marcella Niehoff School of Nursing, Nursing Administration Program, Chicago, IL 60660. Offers MSN. Part-time and evening/weekend programs available. Postbaccalaureate distance learning degree programs offered (minimal on-campus study). *Faculty:* 45 full-time (44 women). *Students:* 1 (woman) full-time, 35 part-time (31 women); includes 13 minority (3 Black or African American, non-Hispanic/Latino; 6 Asian, non-Hispanic/Latino; 2 Hispanic/Latino; 2 Native Hawaiian or other Pacific Islander, non-Hispanic/Latino). Average age 38. 16 applicants, 56% accepted, 6 enrolled. In 2013, 10 master's awarded. *Degree requirements:* For master's, comprehensive exam or oral thesis defense. *Entrance requirements:* For master's, BSN, minimum nursing GPA of 3.0, IL nursing license, 1000 hours of experience before starting clinical. *Application deadline:* Applications are processed on a rolling basis. Application fee: $50. Electronic applications accepted. *Expenses: Tuition:* Full-time $16,740; part-time $930 per credit. *Required fees:* $135 per semester. *Financial support:* Traineeships available. Financial award application deadline: 3/1. *Faculty research:* Patient classification systems, career/job mobility. *Unit head:* Dr. Marijo Letizia, Associate Dean, 708-216-9325, Fax: 708-216-9555, E-mail: mletizi@luc.edu. *Application contact:* Amy Weatherford, Enrollment Advisor, School of Nursing, 708-216-3751, Fax: 708-216-9555, E-mail: aweatherford@luc.edu.
Website: http://www.luc.edu/nursing/

Lynchburg College, Graduate Studies, School of Health Sciences and Human Performance, MS Program in Nursing, Lynchburg, VA 24501-3199. Offers clinical nurse leader (MS); nursing education (MS). *Accreditation:* AACN. Part-time and evening/weekend programs available. Postbaccalaureate distance learning degree programs offered (minimal on-campus study). *Faculty:* 4 full-time (all women), 1 (woman) part-time/adjunct. *Students:* 2 full-time (both women), 16 part-time (14 women); includes 2 minority (1 Black or African American, non-Hispanic/Latino; 1 Hispanic/Latino), 1 international. Average age 40. In 2013, 4 master's awarded. *Degree requirements:* For master's, practicum. *Entrance requirements:* For master's, GRE or 2 years of professional nursing experience, official transcripts, personal essay, 3 letters of recommendation, current unrestricted registered nurse license in Virginia. Additional exam requirements/recommendations for international students: Required—TOEFL (minimum score 550 paper-based; 79 iBT), IELTS (minimum score 6.5). *Application deadline:* For fall admission, 7/31 for domestic students, 6/1 for international students; for spring admission, 11/30 for domestic students, 10/15 for international students. Applications are processed on a rolling basis. Application fee: $30. Electronic applications accepted. Application fee is waived when completed online. *Financial support:* Fellowships, Federal Work-Study, scholarships/grants, health care benefits, and unspecified assistantships available. Support available to part-time students. Financial award application deadline: 7/31; financial award applicants required to submit FAFSA. *Unit head:* Dr. Nancy Overstreet, Associate Professor/Director of MSN Program, 434-544-8340, E-mail: overstreet.n@lynchburg.edu. *Application contact:* Anne Pingstock, Executive Assistant, Graduate Studies, 434-544-8383, E-mail: gradstudies@lynchburg.edu.
Website: http://www.lynchburg.edu/master-science-nursing

Madonna University, Program in Nursing, Livonia, MI 48150-1173. Offers adult health: chronic health conditions (MSN); adult nurse practitioner (MSN); nursing administration (MSN); MSN/MSBA. *Accreditation:* AACN. Part-time programs available. *Degree requirements:* For master's, thesis or alternative. *Entrance requirements:* For master's, GRE General Test, Michigan nursing license. Electronic applications accepted. *Faculty research:* Coping, caring.

Marquette University, Graduate School, College of Nursing, Milwaukee, WI 53201-1881. Offers acute care nurse practitioner (Certificate); adult clinical nurse specialist (Certificate); adult nurse practitioner (Certificate); advanced practice nursing (MSN, DNP), including adult-older adult acute care (DNP), adults (MSN), adults-older adults (DNP), clinical nurse leader (MSN), health care systems leadership (DNP), nurse-midwifery (MSN), older adults (MSN), pediatrics acute care (MSN), pediatrics primary care (MSN), pediatrics-acute care (DNP), pediatrics-primary care (DNP), primary care (DNP), systems leadership and healthcare quality (MSN); family nurse practitioner (Certificate); nurse-midwifery (Certificate); nursing (PhD); pediatric acute care (Certificate); pediatric primary care (Certificate); systems leadership and healthcare quality (Certificate). *Accreditation:* AACN. *Faculty:* 35 full-time (34 women), 59 part-time/adjunct (58 women). *Students:* 105 full-time (96 women), 279 part-time (256 women); includes 28 minority (11 Black or African American, non-Hispanic/Latino; 7 Asian, non-Hispanic/Latino; 8 Hispanic/Latino; 2 Two or more races, non-Hispanic/Latino), 3 international. Average age 30. 322 applicants, 62% accepted, 98 enrolled. In 2013, 66 master's, 4 doctorates, 6 other advanced degrees awarded. Terminal master's awarded for partial completion of doctoral program. *Degree requirements:* For master's, comprehensive exam, thesis or alternative. *Entrance requirements:* For master's, GRE General Test, BSN, Wisconsin RN license, official transcripts from all current and previous colleges/universities except Marquette, three completed recommendation forms, resume, written statement of professional goals; for doctorate, GRE General Test, official transcripts from all current and previous colleges/universities except Marquette, three letters of recommendation, resume, written statement of professional goals, sample of scholarly writing. Additional exam requirements/recommendations for international students: Required—TOEFL (minimum score 530 paper-based). *Application deadline:* For fall admission, 2/15 for domestic and international students. Application fee: $50. Electronic applications accepted. *Financial support:* In 2013–14, 41 students received support, including 1 fellowship with partial tuition reimbursement available (averaging $17,500 per year), 2 research assistantships with full tuition reimbursements available (averaging $13,285 per year), 8 teaching assistantships with full tuition reimbursements available (averaging $13,912 per year); career-related internships or fieldwork, Federal Work-Study, scholarships/grants, health care benefits, tuition waivers (partial), and unspecified assistantships also available. Support available to part-time students. Financial award application deadline: 2/15. *Faculty research:* Psychosocial adjustment to chronic illness, gerontology, reminiscence, health policy: uninsured and access, hospital care delivery systems. *Total annual research expenditures:* $769,051. *Unit head:* Dr. Margaret Callahan, Dean, 414-288-3800, Fax: 414-288-1578. *Application contact:* Dr. Maureen O'Brien, Associate Dean/Clinical Associate Professor, 414-288-3823.
Website: http://www.marquette.edu/nursing/academicprograms-graduate.shtml

McKendree University, Graduate Programs, Master of Science in Nursing Program, Lebanon, IL 62254-1299. Offers nursing education (MSN); nursing management/administration (MSN). *Accreditation:* AACN. Part-time and evening/weekend programs available. Postbaccalaureate distance learning degree programs offered (no on-campus study). *Degree requirements:* For master's, research project or thesis. *Entrance requirements:* For master's, resume, references, valid Professional Registered Nurse license. Additional exam requirements/recommendations for international students: Required—TOEFL. Electronic applications accepted.

McNeese State University, Doré School of Graduate Studies, College of Nursing, Department of Graduate Nursing, Nursing Case Management Program, Lake Charles, LA 70609. Offers Postbaccalaureate Certificate. *Degree requirements:* For Postbaccalaureate Certificate, thesis. *Entrance requirements:* For degree, GRE, MSN, eligible for unencumbered licensure as RN in Louisiana.

McNeese State University, Doré School of Graduate Studies, College of Nursing, Department of Graduate Nursing, Nursing Program, Lake Charles, LA 70609. Offers family nurse practitioner (MSN); family psychiatric/mental health nurse practitioner (MSN); nurse educator (MSN); nurse executive (MSN). *Degree requirements:* For master's, comprehensive exam. *Entrance requirements:* For master's, GRE, baccalaureate degree in nursing, minimum overall GPA of 2.7 for all undergraduate coursework, eligibility for unencumbered licensure as Registered Nurse in Louisiana or Texas, course in introductory statistics with minimum C grade, physical assessment skills, two letters of professional reference, 500-word essay, current resume.

Medical University of South Carolina, College of Nursing, Nurse Administrator Program, Charleston, SC 29425. Offers MSN. *Accreditation:* AACN. Part-time programs available. Postbaccalaureate distance learning degree programs offered (no on-campus study). *Degree requirements:* For master's, thesis optional. *Entrance requirements:* For master's, BSN, nursing license, minimum GPA of 3.0, current curriculum vitae, essay, three references. Additional exam requirements/recommendations for international students: Required—TOEFL (minimum score 600 paper-based). Electronic applications accepted. *Faculty research:* Hospital billing for nursing intensity.

Mercy College, School of Health and Natural Sciences, Programs in Nursing, Dobbs Ferry, NY 10522-1189. Offers nursing administration (MS); nursing education (MS). *Accreditation:* AACN. Part-time and evening/weekend programs available. Postbaccalaureate distance learning degree programs offered (no on-campus study). *Students:* 4 full-time (3 women), 167 part-time (151 women); includes 105 minority (77 Black or African American, non-Hispanic/Latino; 14 Asian, non-Hispanic/Latino; 14 Hispanic/Latino), 3 international. Average age 33. 82 applicants, 77% accepted, 35 enrolled. In 2013, 33 master's awarded. *Degree requirements:* For master's, comprehensive exam (for some programs), written comprehensive exam or the production of a comprehensive project. *Entrance requirements:* For master's, interview, two letters of reference, skills assessment, bachelor's degree, RN registration in the U.S. Additional exam requirements/recommendations for international students: Required—TOEFL (minimum score 600 paper-based; 100 iBT), IELTS (minimum score 8). *Application deadline:* For fall admission, 8/1 for international students. Applications are processed on a rolling basis. Application fee: $62. Electronic applications accepted. *Expenses: Tuition:* Full-time $19,344; part-time $806 per credit. *Required fees:* $580; $806 per credit. $145 per term. Tuition and fees vary according to course load, degree level and program. *Financial support:* Career-related internships or fieldwork, Federal Work-Study, scholarships/grants, and unspecified assistantships available. Support available to part-time students. Financial award applicants required to submit FAFSA. *Unit head:* Dr. Joan Toglia, Dean, School of Health and Natural Sciences, 914-674-7837, E-mail: jtoglia@mercy.edu. *Application contact:* Allison Gurdineer, Senior Director of Admissions, 877-637-2946, Fax: 914-674-7382, E-mail: admissions@mercy.edu.
Website: https://www.mercy.edu/academics/school-of-health-and-natural-sciences/graduate-programs/

Metropolitan State University, College of Health, Community and Professional Studies, St. Paul, MN 55106-5000. Offers advanced dental therapy (MS); leadership and management (MSN); nurse educator (MSN); nursing (DNP); psychology (MA). *Accreditation:* AACN. Part-time programs available. *Degree requirements:* For master's, thesis or alternative; for doctorate, thesis/dissertation or alternative. *Entrance requirements:* For master's, GRE General Test, minimum GPA of 3.0, RN license, BS/BA; for doctorate, minimum GPA of 3.0; RN license, MSN. Additional exam requirements/recommendations for international students: Required—TOEFL (minimum score 550 paper-based). *Expenses:* Tuition, state resident: full-time $5548. Tuition, nonresident: full-time $10,929. *Faculty research:* Women's health, gerontology.

Middle Tennessee State University, College of Graduate Studies, University College, Murfreesboro, TN 37132. Offers advanced studies in teaching and learning (M Ed); human resources leadership (MPS); nursing administration (MSN); nursing education (MSN); strategic leadership (MPS); training and development (MPS). Part-time and evening/weekend programs available. Postbaccalaureate distance learning degree programs offered. *Students:* 58 full-time (52 women), 263 part-time (222 women). *Entrance requirements:* Additional exam requirements/recommendations for international students: Required—TOEFL (minimum score 525 paper-based; 71 iBT) or IELTS (minimum score 6). *Application deadline:* For fall admission, 6/1 for domestic and international students. Applications are processed on a rolling basis. Application fee: $25 ($30 for international students). *Financial support:* In 2013–14, 2 students received support. Tuition waivers available. Support available to part-time students. Financial award application deadline: 5/1. *Unit head:* Dr. Mike Boyle, Dean, 615-494-8877, Fax: 615-896-7925, E-mail: mike.boyle@mtsu.edu. *Application contact:* Dr. Michael D. Allen, Dean and Vice Provost for Research, 615-898-2840, Fax: 615-904-8020, E-mail: michael.allen@mtsu.edu.
Website: http://www.mtsu.edu/universitycollege/

Millikin University, School of Nursing, Decatur, IL 62522-2084. Offers clinical nurse leader (MSN); entry into nursing practice: pre-licensure (MSN); nurse anesthesia (DNP); nurse educator (MSN); nursing practice (DNP). *Accreditation:* AACN; AANA/CANAEP. Part-time programs available. *Faculty:* 17 full-time (15 women), 5 part-time/adjunct (4 women). *Students:* 41 full-time (30 women), 26 part-time (19 women); includes 7 minority (2 Black or African American, non-Hispanic/Latino; 1 American Indian or Alaska Native, non-Hispanic/Latino; 1 Asian, non-Hispanic/Latino; 3 Hispanic/Latino). Average age 32. 69 applicants, 51% accepted, 21 enrolled. In 2013, 8 master's awarded. *Degree requirements:* For master's, thesis or alternative, research project. *Entrance requirements:* For master's, GRE, official academic transcript(s), essay, immunizations, statistics course, 3 letters of recommendation, CPR certification, professional liability/malpractice insurance; for doctorate, GRE (if undergraduate cumulative GPA is below 3.0), official academic transcript(s); undergraduate courses: nursing research, health assessment, inorganic and organic chemistry, intro to statistics; graduate-level statistics; 3 written recommendations; Assessment of Critical Care Skills form; written statement; resume or curriculum vita. Additional exam requirements/recommendations for international students: Required—TOEFL (minimum score 550 paper-based; 79 iBT). *Application deadline:* For spring admission, 11/1 for domestic students. Applications are processed on a rolling basis. Application fee: $0. Electronic applications accepted. *Expenses: Tuition:* Full-time $20,300; part-time $700 per credit hour. Tuition and fees vary according to program. *Financial support:* In 2013–14, 13 students received support. Institutionally sponsored loans available. Financial award applicants required to submit FAFSA. *Faculty research:* Congestive heart failure, quality of life, transcultural nursing issues, teaching/learning strategies, maternal - newborn. *Unit head:* Dr. Kathy Booker, Director, 217-424-6348, Fax: 217-420-6731, E-mail: kbooker@millikin.edu. *Application contact:* Marianne Taylor, Administrative Assistant, 800-373-7733 Ext. 5034, Fax: 217-420-6677, E-mail: mgtaylor@millikin.edu.
Website: http://www.millikin.edu/academics/cps/nursing/programs

Missouri Western State University, Program in Health Care Leadership, St. Joseph, MO 64507-2294. Offers MSN. Part-time programs available. *Students:* 13 part-time (all women). Average age 39. 3 applicants, 67% accepted, 2 enrolled. In 2013, 5 master's awarded. *Entrance requirements:* For master's, minimum GPA of 2.75, interview. Additional exam requirements/recommendations for international students: Recommended—TOEFL (minimum score 500 paper-based; 61 iBT), IELTS (minimum score 5.5). *Application deadline:* For fall admission, 7/15 for domestic students, 6/15 for international students; for spring admission, 10/1 for domestic students, 10/15 for international students. Applications are processed on a rolling basis. Application fee: $45 ($50 for international students). Electronic applications accepted. *Expenses:* Tuition, state resident: full-time $6019; part-time $300.96 per credit hour. Tuition, nonresident: full-time $11,194; part-time $559.71 per credit hour. *Required fees:* $542; $99 per credit hour. $176 per semester. Tuition and fees vary according to course load and program. *Financial support:* Scholarships/grants and unspecified assistantships available. Support available to part-time students. *Unit head:* Dr. Carolyn Brose, Coordinator, 816-271-5912, E-mail: brose@missouriwestern.edu. *Application contact:* Dr. Benjamin D. Caldwell, Dean of the Graduate School, 816-271-4394, Fax: 816-271-4525, E-mail: graduate@missouriwestern.edu.
Website: https://www.missouriwestern.edu/nursing/master-of-science-in-nursing/

Molloy College, Division of Nursing, Rockville Centre, NY 11571-5002. Offers adult nurse practitioner (Advanced Certificate); clinical nurse specialist: adult health (Advanced Certificate); family nurse practitioner (Advanced Certificate); nurse practitioner psychiatry (Advanced Certificate); nursing (MS, PhD); nursing administration (Advanced Certificate); nursing administration with informatics (Advanced Certificate); nursing education (Advanced Certificate); nursing informatics (Advanced Certificate); pediatric nurse practitioner (Advanced Certificate). *Accreditation:* AACN. Part-time and evening/weekend programs available. *Faculty:* 30 full-time (29 women), 10 part-time/adjunct (7 women). *Students:* 18 full-time (all women), 538 part-time (495 women); includes 289 minority (159 Black or African American, non-Hispanic/Latino; 1 American Indian or Alaska Native, non-Hispanic/Latino; 80 Asian, non-Hispanic/Latino; 43 Hispanic/Latino; 4 Native Hawaiian or other Pacific Islander, non-Hispanic/Latino; 2 Two or more races, non-Hispanic/Latino), 2 international. Average age 38. 241 applicants, 63% accepted, 122 enrolled. In 2013, 84 master's, 2 other advanced degrees awarded. *Degree requirements:* For master's, thesis optional. *Entrance requirements:* For master's, 3 letters of reference, BS in nursing, minimum undergraduate GPA of 3.0; for Advanced Certificate, 3 letters of reference, master's degree in nursing. *Application deadline:* For fall admission, 9/2 priority date for domestic students; for spring admission, 1/20 priority date for domestic students. Applications are processed on a rolling basis. Application fee: $60. *Expenses: Tuition:* Full-time $16,920; part-time $940 per credit. *Required fees:* $880. *Financial support:* Research assistantships with partial tuition reimbursements, teaching assistantships with partial tuition reimbursements, institutionally sponsored loans, scholarships/grants, and unspecified assistantships available. Support available to part-time students. Financial award application deadline: 4/1; financial award applicants required to submit FAFSA. *Unit head:* Dr. Jeannine Muldoon, Dean of Nursing, 516-323-3651, E-mail: jmuldoon@molloy.edu. *Application contact:* Alina Haitz, Assistant Director of Graduate Admissions, 516-323-4008, E-mail: ahaitz@molloy.edu.
Website: http://www.molloy.edu/academics/nursing-division

Monmouth University, The Graduate School, The Marjorie K. Unterberg School of Nursing and Health Studies, West Long Branch, NJ 07764-1898. Offers adult and gerontological nurse practitioner (MSN); adult-gerontological nurse practitioner (Post-Master's Certificate); family nurse practitioner (MSN, Post-Master's Certificate); family psychiatric and mental health advanced practice nursing (MSN); forensic nursing (MSN, Certificate); nursing (MSN); nursing administration (MSN, Post-Master's Certificate); nursing education (MSN, Post-Master's Certificate); nursing practice (DNP); physician assistant (MS); psychiatric-mental health nurse practitioner (Post-Master's Certificate); school nursing (MSN, Certificate). *Accreditation:* AACN. Part-time and evening/weekend programs available. *Faculty:* 14 full-time (all women), 4 part-time/adjunct (3 women). *Students:* 19 full-time (18 women), 269 part-time (252 women); includes 106 minority (35 Black or African American, non-Hispanic/Latino; 2 American Indian or Alaska Native, non-Hispanic/Latino; 51 Asian, non-Hispanic/Latino; 12 Hispanic/Latino; 3 Native Hawaiian or other Pacific Islander, non-Hispanic/Latino; 3 Two or more races, non-Hispanic/Latino), 2 international. Average age 39. 135 applicants, 98% accepted, 96 enrolled. In 2013, 54 master's, 7 doctorates awarded. *Degree requirements:* For master's, practicum (for some tracks). *Entrance requirements:* For master's, GRE General Test, BSN with minimum GPA of 2.75, current RN license, proof of liability and malpractice policy, personal statement, two letters of recommendation, college course work in health assessment, resume; minimum GPA of 3.0, minimum C grade in prerequisite courses, minimum 200 hours' clinical experience, 3 letters of recommendation, and interview (for MS); for doctorate, accredited master's nursing program degree with minimum GPA of 3.2, active RN license, national certification as Nurse Practitioner or Nurse Administrator, working knowledge of statistics, statement of goals and vision for change, 2 letters of recommendation, resume, interview. Additional exam requirements/recommendations for international students: Required—TOEFL (minimum score 550 paper-based; 79 iBT), IELTS (minimum score 6) or Michigan English Language Assessment Battery (minimum score 77). *Application deadline:* For fall admission, 7/15 priority date for domestic students, 6/1 for international students; for spring admission, 11/15 priority date for domestic students, 11/1 for international students; for summer admission, 2/1 for domestic students. Applications are processed on a rolling basis. Application fee: $50. Electronic applications accepted. *Expenses: Tuition:* Part-time $1004 per credit hour. *Required fees:* $157 per semester. *Financial support:* In 2013–14, 163 students received support, including 113 fellowships (averaging $3,093 per year), 27 research assistantships (averaging $6,273 per year); career-related internships or fieldwork, scholarships/grants, and unspecified assistantships also available. Support available to part-time students. Financial award applicants required to submit FAFSA. *Faculty research:* Relationship of undergraduate GPA and GRE to succeeding in a graduate nursing program. *Unit head:* Dr. Janet Mahoney, Dean, 732-571-3443, Fax: 732-263-5131, E-mail: jmahoney@monmouth.edu. *Application contact:* Lauren Vento-Cifelli, Associate Vice President of Undergraduate and Graduate Admission, 732-571-3452, Fax: 732-263-5123, E-mail: gradadm@monmouth.edu.
Website: http://www.monmouth.edu/school-of-nursing-health/graduate-nursing-programs.aspx

Montana State University, College of Graduate Studies, College of Nursing, Bozeman, MT 59717. Offers clinical nurse leader (MN); family nurse practitioner (MN, Post-Master's Certificate); nursing education (Certificate, Post-Master's Certificate); psychiatric mental health nurse practitioner (MN). *Accreditation:* AACN. Part-time programs available. Postbaccalaureate distance learning degree programs offered (minimal on-campus study). *Degree requirements:* For master's, comprehensive exam, thesis (for some programs). *Entrance requirements:* For master's, GRE General Test, minimum GPA of 3.0 for undergraduate and post-baccalaureate work. Additional exam requirements/recommendations for international students: Required—TOEFL (minimum score 580 paper-based). Electronic applications accepted. *Faculty research:* Rural nursing, health disparities, environmental/public health, oral health, resilience.

Moravian College, Moravian College Comenius Center, St. Luke's School of Nursing, Bethlehem, PA 18018-6650. Offers clinical nurse leader (MS); nurse administrator (MS); nurse educator (MS). *Accreditation:* AACN. Part-time and evening/weekend programs available. *Degree requirements:* For master's, comprehensive exam (for some programs), evidence-based practice project. *Entrance requirements:* For master's, GRE or MAT. Additional exam requirements/recommendations for international students: Required—TOEFL (minimum score 550 paper-based; 90 iBT).

Mount Carmel College of Nursing, Nursing Program, Columbus, OH 43222. Offers adult gerontology acute care nurse practitioner (MS); adult health clinical nurse specialist (MS); family nurse practitioner (MS); nursing administration (MS); nursing education (MS). *Accreditation:* AACN. Part-time programs available. *Faculty:* 8 full-time (7 women), 8 part-time/adjunct (7 women). *Students:* 94 full-time (89 women), 76 part-time (73 women); includes 35 minority (21 Black or African American, non-Hispanic/Latino; 2 American Indian or Alaska Native, non-Hispanic/Latino; 6 Asian, non-Hispanic/Latino; 2 Hispanic/Latino; 1 Native Hawaiian or other Pacific Islander, non-Hispanic/Latino; 3 Two or more races, non-Hispanic/Latino). Average age 38. 123 applicants, 50% accepted, 47 enrolled. In 2013, 41 master's awarded. *Degree requirements:* For master's, professional manuscript. *Entrance requirements:* For master's, letters of recommendation, statement of purpose, current resume, baccalaureate degree in nursing, current Ohio RN license, minimum cumulative GPA of 3.0. Additional exam requirements/recommendations for international students: Required—TOEFL (minimum score 550 paper-based; 80 iBT). *Application deadline:* For fall admission, 6/1 priority date for domestic students; for winter admission, 11/1 for domestic students; for spring admission, 10/1 priority date for domestic students; for summer admission, 3/1 for domestic students. Applications are processed on a rolling basis. Application fee: $30. *Expenses: Tuition:* Full-time $8560; part-time $428 per credit. *Required fees:* $75. *Financial support:* In 2013–14, 9 students received support. Institutionally sponsored loans and scholarships/grants available. Financial award application deadline: 3/15; financial award applicants required to submit FAFSA. *Unit head:* Dr. Angela Phillips-Lowe, Associate Dean, 614-234-5717, Fax: 614-234-2875, E-mail: aphillips-lowe@mccn.edu. *Application contact:* Kathleen Walters, Program Coordinator, 614-234-5408, Fax: 614-234-2875, E-mail: kwalters@mccn.edu.
Website: http://www.mccn.edu/

Mount Mary University, Graduate Division, Program in Business Administration, Milwaukee, WI 53222-4597. Offers general management (MBA); health systems leadership (MBA). Part-time and evening/weekend programs available. *Faculty:* 1 (woman) full-time, 5 part-time/adjunct (1 woman). *Students:* 28 full-time (23 women), 11 part-time (9 women); includes 11 minority (5 Black or African American, non-Hispanic/Latino; 1 Asian, non-Hispanic/Latino; 4 Hispanic/Latino; 1 Two or more races, non-Hispanic/Latino). Average age 35. 12 applicants, 92% accepted, 5 enrolled. In 2013, 9 master's awarded. *Degree requirements:* For master's, terminal project. *Entrance requirements:* For master's, minimum GPA of 2.75. Additional exam requirements/recommendations for international students: Required—TOEFL (minimum score 80 iBT) or IELTS (minimum score 6.5). *Application deadline:* For fall admission, 7/15 for domestic and international students; for spring admission, 12/1 for domestic and international students. Applications are processed on a rolling basis. Application fee: $45 ($100 for international students). Electronic applications accepted. *Expenses:* Contact institution. *Financial support:* Career-related internships or fieldwork and Federal Work-Study available. Support available to part-time students. Financial award application deadline: 5/1; financial award applicants required to submit FAFSA. *Unit head:* Dr. Kristen Roche, Director, 414-258-4810, E-mail: rochek@mtmary.edu. *Application contact:* Dr. Douglas J. Mickelson, Dean for Graduate Education, 414-256-1252, Fax: 414-256-0167, E-mail: mickelsd@mtmary.edu.
Website: http://www.mtmary.edu/majors-programs/graduate/mba/index.html

Mount St. Joseph University, Master of Science in Nursing Program, Cincinnati, OH 45233-1670. Offers administration (MSN); clinical nurse leader (MSN); education (MSN). Part-time programs available. *Faculty:* 10 full-time (9 women), 23 part-time/adjunct (all women). *Students:* 33 part-time (31 women); includes 3 minority (all Black or African American, non-Hispanic/Latino). Average age 45. 24 applicants, 67% accepted, 16 enrolled. *Entrance requirements:* For master's, essay; BSN from regionally-accredited university; minimum undergraduate GPA of 3.25 or GRE; professional resume; three professional references; interview; 2 years of clinical nursing experience; active RN license; criminal background check. Additional exam requirements/recommendations for international students: Required—TOEFL (minimum score 560 paper-based; 83 iBT). Application fee: $50. Electronic applications accepted. *Expenses: Tuition:* Full-time $18,400; part-time $575 per credit hour. *Required fees:* $450; $450 per year. Part-time tuition and fees vary according to course load, degree level and program. *Financial support:* Application deadline: 3/1; applicants required to submit FAFSA. *Unit head:* Dr. Nancy Hinzman, MSN/DNP Director, 513-244-4325, E-mail: nancy_hinzman@mail.msj.edu. *Application contact:* Mary Brigham, Assistant Director for Graduate Recruitment, 513-244-4233, Fax: 513-244-4629, E-mail: mary_brigham@mail.msj.edu.
Website: http://www.msj.edu/academics/graduate-programs/master-of-science-in-nursing/

Mount Saint Mary College, Division of Nursing, Newburgh, NY 12550-3494. Offers adult nurse practitioner (MS, Advanced Certificate), including nursing education (MS), nursing management (MS); clinical nurse specialist-adult health (MS), including nursing education, nursing management; family nurse practitioner (Advanced Certificate). *Accreditation:* AACN. Part-time and evening/weekend programs available. *Faculty:* 4 full-time (all women). *Students:* 79 part-time (72 women); includes 19 minority (12 Black or African American, non-Hispanic/Latino; 1 Asian, non-Hispanic/Latino; 5 Hispanic/Latino; 1 Native Hawaiian or other Pacific Islander, non-Hispanic/Latino). Average age 39. 45 applicants, 47% accepted, 9 enrolled. In 2013, 13 master's, 3 other advanced degrees awarded. *Degree requirements:* For master's, research utilization project. *Entrance requirements:* For master's, BSN, minimum GPA of 3.0, RN license. *Application deadline:* For fall admission, 6/3 priority date for domestic students; for spring admission, 10/31 priority date for domestic students. Applications are processed on a rolling basis. Application fee: $45. Application fee is waived when completed online. *Expenses: Tuition:* Full-time $13,356; part-time $742 per credit. *Required fees:* $70 per semester. *Financial support:* In 2013–14, 8 students received support. Unspecified assistantships available. Financial award application deadline: 4/15; financial award applicants required to submit FAFSA. *Unit head:* Linda Ruta, Graduate Coordinator, 845-569-3512, Fax: 845-562-6762, E-mail: linda.ruta@msmc.edu. *Application contact:* Lisa Gallina, Director of Admissions for Graduate Programs and Adult Degree Completion, 845-569-3166, Fax: 845-569-3450, E-mail: lisa.gallina@msmc.edu.
Website: http://www.msmc.edu/Academics/Graduate_Programs/Master_of_Science_in_Nursing

National University, Academic Affairs, School of Health and Human Services, La Jolla, CA 92037-1011. Offers clinical affairs (MS); clinical informatics (Certificate); clinical regulatory affairs (MS); health and life science analytics (MS); health coaching (Certificate); health informatics (MS); healthcare administration (MHA); nurse anesthesia (MS); nursing (MS), including forensic nursing, nursing administration, nursing informatics; nursing administration (Certificate); nursing informatics (Certificate); nursing practice (DNP); public health (MPH), including health promotion, healthcare administration, mental health. Part-time and evening/weekend programs available. Postbaccalaureate distance learning degree programs offered (no on-campus study). *Faculty:* 20 full-time (12 women), 27 part-time/adjunct (16 women). *Students:* 229 full-time (176 women), 89 part-time (52 women); includes 215 minority (58 Black or African American, non-Hispanic/Latino; 1 American Indian or Alaska Native, non-Hispanic/Latino; 68 Asian, non-Hispanic/Latino; 63 Hispanic/Latino; 8 Native Hawaiian or other Pacific Islander, non-Hispanic/Latino; 17 Two or more races, non-Hispanic/Latino), 18 international. Average age 33. 118 applicants, 100% accepted, 92 enrolled. In 2013, 29 master's awarded. *Degree requirements:* For master's, thesis (for some programs). *Entrance requirements:* For master's, interview, minimum GPA of 2.5. Additional exam requirements/recommendations for international students: Required—TOEFL (minimum score 550 paper-based; 79 iBT), IELTS (minimum score 6). *Application deadline:* Applications are processed on a rolling basis. Application fee: $60 ($65 for international students). Electronic applications accepted. *Expenses: Tuition:* Full-time $13,824; part-time $1728 per course. One-time fee: $160. *Financial support:* Career-related internships or fieldwork, institutionally sponsored loans, scholarships/grants, and tuition waivers (partial) available. Support available to part-time students. Financial award application deadline: 6/30; financial award applicants required to submit FAFSA. *Faculty research:* Nursing education, obesity prevention, workforce diversity. *Unit head:* School of Health and Human Services, 800-628-8648, E-mail: shhs@nu.edu. *Application contact:* Louis Cruz, Interim Vice President for Enrollment Services, 800-628-8648, E-mail: advisor@nu.edu.
Website: http://www.nu.edu/OurPrograms/SchoolOfHealthAndHumanServices.html

Nebraska Methodist College, Program in Nursing, Omaha, NE 68114. Offers nurse educator (MSN); nurse executive (MSN). *Accreditation:* AACN. Evening/weekend programs available. Postbaccalaureate distance learning degree programs offered (no on-campus study). *Faculty:* 2 full-time (both women), 5 part-time/adjunct (all women). *Students:* 82 full-time (81 women), 39 part-time (36 women); includes 5 minority (4 Black or African American, non-Hispanic/Latino; 1 Asian, non-Hispanic/Latino). Average age 37. 156 applicants, 21% accepted, 28 enrolled. In 2013, 20 master's awarded. *Degree requirements:* For master's, thesis or alternative, Evidence Based Practice (EBP) project. *Entrance requirements:* For master's, interview. Additional exam requirements/recommendations for international students: Required—TOEFL (minimum score 550 paper-based; 80 iBT). *Application deadline:* For spring admission, 11/1 for domestic and international students. Applications are processed on a rolling basis. Application fee: $25. *Expenses: Tuition:* Full-time $12,258; part-time $681 per credit hour. *Required fees:* $450; $450 per year. *Financial support:* Research assistantships with full and partial tuition reimbursements and scholarships/grants available. Financial award applicants required to submit FAFSA. *Faculty research:* Spirituality, student outcomes, service-learning, leadership and administration, women's issues. *Unit head:* Dr. Linda Foley, Director, Graduate Nursing, 402-354-7050, Fax: 402-354-7020, E-mail: linda.foley@methodistcollege.edu. *Application contact:* Laurel Zentner, Recruitment and Admissions Coordinator, 402-354-7170, Fax: 402-354-7020, E-mail: admissions@methodistcollege.edu.
Website: http://www.methodistcollege.edu/nursing-online

Nicholls State University, Graduate Studies, College of Nursing and Allied Health, Thibodaux, LA 70310. Offers family nurse practitioner (MSN); family psychiatric/mental health nurse practitioner (MSN); nurse executive (MSN).

Northeastern University, Bouvé College of Health Sciences, Boston, MA 02115-5096. Offers audiology (Au D); biotechnology (MS); counseling psychology (MS, PhD, CAGS); counseling/school psychology (PhD); exercise physiology (MS), including exercise physiology, public health; health informatics (MS); nursing (MS, PhD, CAGS), including acute care (MS), administration (MS), anesthesia (MS), primary care (MS), psychiatric mental health (MS); pharmaceutical sciences (PhD); pharmaceutics and drug delivery systems (MS); pharmacology (MS); physical therapy (DPT); physician assistant (MS); school psychology (PhD, CAGS); school/counseling psychology (PhD); speech language pathology (MS); urban public health (MPH); MS/MBA. *Accreditation:* ACPE (one or more programs are accredited). Part-time and evening/weekend programs available. *Degree requirements:* For doctorate, thesis/dissertation (for some programs); for CAGS, comprehensive exam.

North Park University, School of Nursing, Chicago, IL 60625-4895. Offers advanced practice nursing (MS); leadership and management (MS); MBA/MS; MM/MSN; MS/MHR; MS/MNA. *Accreditation:* AACN. Part-time and evening/weekend programs available. *Degree requirements:* For master's, thesis. *Entrance requirements:* For master's, GMAT, MAT. *Faculty research:* Aging, consultation roles, critical thinking skills, family breakdown, science of caring.

Northwest Nazarene University, Graduate Studies, Program in Nursing, Nampa, ID 83686-5897. Offers MSN. *Accreditation:* AACN. Postbaccalaureate distance learning degree programs offered (no on-campus study). *Faculty:* 1 (woman) full-time, 6 part-time/adjunct (all women). *Students:* 17 full-time (16 women). Average age 40. 24 applicants, 88% accepted, 12 enrolled. In 2013, 6 master's awarded. *Degree requirements:* For master's, internship. Application fee: $50. *Expenses: Tuition:* Part-time $565 per credit. *Unit head:* Dr. Barbara Lester, Director, 208-467-8679, E-mail: balester@nnu.edu. *Application contact:* Sandy Blom, Graduate Nursing Coordinator, 208-467-8642, Fax: 208-467-8651, E-mail: sblom@nnu.edu.
Website: http://www.nnu.edu/msn

Norwich University, College of Graduate and Continuing Studies, Master of Science in Nursing Program, Northfield, VT 05663. Offers nursing administration (MSN); nursing education (MSN). *Accreditation:* AACN. Evening/weekend programs available. Postbaccalaureate distance learning degree programs offered (minimal on-campus study). *Faculty:* 9 part-time/adjunct (5 women). *Students:* 82 full-time (78 women); includes 7 minority (4 Black or African American, non-Hispanic/Latino; 3 Asian, non-Hispanic/Latino). Average age 43. 114 applicants, 28% accepted, 31 enrolled. In 2013, 37 master's awarded. *Entrance requirements:* For master's, minimum undergraduate GPA of 2.75. Additional exam requirements/recommendations for international students: Required—TOEFL (minimum score 600 paper-based; 94 iBT). *Application deadline:* For fall admission, 8/1 for domestic and international students; for winter admission, 11/1 for domestic and international students; for spring admission, 2/1 for domestic and international students; for summer admission, 5/1 for domestic and international students. Applications are processed on a rolling basis. Application fee: $50. Electronic applications accepted. *Expenses:* Contact institution. *Financial support:* In 2013–14, 20 students received support. Scholarships/grants available. Financial award applicants required to submit FAFSA. *Unit head:* Dr. Sharon Richie-Melvan, Director, 802-485-2600, E-mail: srichiem@norwich.edu. *Application contact:* Rija Ramahatra, Associate Program Director, 802-485-2892, Fax: 802-485-2533, E-mail: rramahatr@norwich.edu.
Website: http://online.norwich.edu/degree-programs/masters/master-science-nursing/overview

Ohio University, Graduate College, College of Health Sciences and Professions, School of Nursing, Athens, OH 45701-2979. Offers acute care nurse practitioner (MSN);

acute care nurse practitioner and family nurse practitioner (MSN); acute care nurse practitioner and nurse administrator (MSN); acute care nurse practitioner and nurse educator (MSN); family nurse practitioner (MSN); nurse administrator (MSN); nurse administrator and family nurse practitioner (MSN); nurse educator (MSN); nurse educator and family nurse practitioner (MSN); nurse educator and nurse administrator (MSN). *Accreditation:* AACN. *Degree requirements:* For master's, capstone project. *Entrance requirements:* For master's, GRE, bachelor's degree in nursing from an accredited college or university, minimum overall undergraduate GPA of 3.0, official transcripts, statement of goals and objectives, resume, 3 letters of recommendation. Additional exam requirements/recommendations for international students: Required—TOEFL (minimum score 550 paper-based; 80 iBT) or IELTS (minimum score 6.5). Electronic applications accepted.

Old Dominion University, College of Health Sciences, Doctor of Nursing Practice Program, Norfolk, VA 23529. Offers advance practice (DNP); nurse executive (DNP). Part-time programs available. Postbaccalaureate distance learning degree programs offered (minimal on-campus study). *Faculty:* 4 full-time (all women), 3 part-time/adjunct (2 women). *Students:* 15 full-time (13 women), 40 part-time (35 women); includes 13 minority (11 Black or African American, non-Hispanic/Latino; 2 Asian, non-Hispanic/Latino). Average age 46. 54 applicants, 85% accepted, 37 enrolled. In 2013, 29 doctorates awarded. *Degree requirements:* For doctorate, thesis/dissertation, capstone project. *Entrance requirements:* Additional exam requirements/recommendations for international students: Required—TOEFL. *Application deadline:* For spring admission, 9/15 priority date for domestic students. Applications are processed on a rolling basis. Application fee: $50. Electronic applications accepted. *Expenses:* Tuition, state resident: full-time $9888; part-time $412 per credit. Tuition, nonresident: full-time $25,152; part-time $1048 per credit. *Required fees:* $59 per semester. One-time fee: $50. *Financial support:* In 2013–14, 2 students received support, including 2 fellowships with full tuition reimbursements available (averaging $15,000 per year), 1 teaching assistantship with full tuition reimbursement available (averaging $15,000 per year); scholarships/grants, traineeships, and unspecified assistantships also available. *Faculty research:* Cultural competency, sleep disorders, self-care in HIV positive African-American women, ethical decision-making in pediatric cases. *Unit head:* Dr. Carolyn M. Rutledge, Director, 757-683-5009, Fax: 757-683-5253, E-mail: crutledg@odu.edu. *Application contact:* Sue Parker, Coordinator, Graduate Student Services, 757-683-4298, Fax: 757-683-5253, E-mail: sparker@odu.edu.
Website: http://www.odu.edu/dnp

Old Dominion University, College of Health Sciences, School of Nursing, Nurse Administrator Emphasis, Norfolk, VA 23529. Offers MSN. Part-time programs available. Postbaccalaureate distance learning degree programs offered. *Faculty:* 1 (woman) full-time, 3 part-time/adjunct (2 women). *Students:* 5 full-time (all women), 3 part-time (all women); includes 2 minority (both Black or African American, non-Hispanic/Latino). Average age 41. 15 applicants, 47% accepted, 5 enrolled. In 2013, 9 master's awarded. *Degree requirements:* For master's, comprehensive exam. *Entrance requirements:* Additional exam requirements/recommendations for international students: Required—TOEFL. *Application deadline:* For fall admission, 5/1 priority date for domestic students, 4/15 for international students. Applications are processed on a rolling basis. Application fee: $50. Electronic applications accepted. *Expenses:* Tuition, state resident: full-time $9888; part-time $412 per credit. Tuition, nonresident: full-time $25,152; part-time $1048 per credit. *Required fees:* $59 per semester. One-time fee: $50. *Faculty research:* Telehealth, vulnerable populations. *Unit head:* Dr. Carolyn M. Rutledge, Graduate Program Director, 757-683-5009, Fax: 757-683-5253, E-mail: crutledg@odu.edu. *Application contact:* Sue Parker, Coordinator, Graduate Student Services, 757-683-4298, Fax: 757-683-5253, E-mail: sparker@odu.edu.
Website: http://hs.odu.edu/nursing/academics/nurse_admin/nurse_admin.shtml

Otterbein University, Department of Nursing, Westerville, OH 43081. Offers advanced practice nurse educator (Certificate); clinical nurse leader (MSN); family nurse practitioner (MSN, Certificate); nurse anesthesia (MSN, Certificate); nursing (DNP); nursing service administration (MSN). *Accreditation:* AACN; AANA/CANAEP. Part-time and evening/weekend programs available. Postbaccalaureate distance learning degree programs offered (minimal on-campus study). *Degree requirements:* For master's, comprehensive exam (for some programs), thesis (for some programs). *Entrance requirements:* For master's, 2 reference forms, resume; for Certificate, official transcripts, 2 reference forms, essay, resumé. Additional exam requirements/recommendations for international students: Required—TOEFL (minimum score 550 paper-based; 79 iBT). *Faculty research:* Patient education, women's health, trauma curriculum development, administration.

Our Lady of the Lake College, School of Nursing, Program in Nursing, Baton Rouge, LA 70808. Offers administration (MS); education (MS). Part-time programs available. *Degree requirements:* For master's, capstone project. *Entrance requirements:* For master's, BSN with minimum GPA of 3.0 during the last 60 hours of undergraduate work, 1 year of clinical nursing experience as a registered nurse, current licensure or eligibility to practice as registered nurse in Louisiana, 3 professional references, 3 credit hours of undergraduate statistics with minimum C average.

Our Lady of the Lake University of San Antonio, School of Professional Studies, Program in Nursing, San Antonio, TX 78207-4689. Offers nurse administration (MSN); nurse education (MSN). Postbaccalaureate distance learning degree programs offered (no on-campus study). *Faculty:* 1 (woman) full-time, 1 (woman) part-time/adjunct. *Students:* 17 full-time (16 women), 4 part-time (all women); includes 12 minority (3 Black or African American, non-Hispanic/Latino; 1 American Indian or Alaska Native, non-Hispanic/Latino; 8 Hispanic/Latino). Average age 43. 20 applicants, 100% accepted, 15 enrolled. *Degree requirements:* For master's, comprehensive exam. *Entrance requirements:* For master's, GRE General Test or MAT. Additional exam requirements/recommendations for international students: Required—TOEFL. *Application deadline:* For fall admission, 4/1 priority date for domestic and international students; for spring admission, 11/1 priority date for domestic and international students; for summer admission, 2/1 priority date for domestic and international students. Applications are processed on a rolling basis. Application fee: $25 ($50 for international students). Electronic applications accepted. *Expenses: Tuition:* Full-time $9120; part-time $760 per credit. *Required fees:* $698; $334 per trimester. Tuition and fees vary according to course load, degree level, campus/location and program. *Financial support:* Career-related internships or fieldwork, institutionally sponsored loans, scholarships/grants, and tuition waivers (partial) available. Support available to part-time students. Financial award application deadline: 4/15. *Unit head:* Dr. Wanda Sparks, Chair, 210-431-4162, E-mail: wrsparks@lake.ollusa.edu. *Application contact:* Graduate Admission, 210-431-3961, Fax: 210-431-4013, E-mail: gradadm@lake.ollusa.edu.

Pace University, College of Health Professions, Lienhard School of Nursing, New York, NY 10038. Offers family nurse practitioner (MS); nurse practitioner (Advanced Certificate); nursing education (MA); nursing leadership (Advanced Certificate); nursing practice (DNP). *Accreditation:* AACN. Part-time and evening/weekend programs available. Postbaccalaureate distance learning degree programs offered. *Faculty:* 13 full-time (12 women), 36 part-time/adjunct (29 women). *Students:* 3 full-time (2 women), 427 part-time (390 women); includes 202 minority (98 Black or African American, non-Hispanic/Latino; 2 American Indian or Alaska Native, non-Hispanic/Latino; 68 Asian, non-Hispanic/Latino; 28 Hispanic/Latino; 1 Native Hawaiian or other Pacific Islander, non-Hispanic/Latino; 5 Two or more races, non-Hispanic/Latino), 2 international. Average age 35. 274 applicants, 69% accepted, 131 enrolled. In 2013, 120 master's, 15 doctorates, 3 other advanced degrees awarded. *Degree requirements:* For master's, thesis. *Entrance requirements:* For master's, GRE General Test or MAT, RN license, resume, personal statement, 2 letters of recommendation, official transcripts; for doctorate, RN license, resume, personal statement, 2 letters of recommendation, official transcripts, accredited master's degree in nursing, minimum GPA of 3.3, state certification; for Advanced Certificate, RN license, completion of 2nd degree in nursing. Additional exam requirements/recommendations for international students: Required—TOEFL. *Application deadline:* For fall admission, 3/1 priority date for domestic and international students; for spring admission, 10/14 for domestic students, 9/14 for international students. Applications are processed on a rolling basis. Application fee: $70. Electronic applications accepted. *Expenses:* Contact institution. *Financial support:* Research assistantships, career-related internships or fieldwork, Federal Work-Study, and tuition waivers (partial) available. Support available to part-time students. Financial award applicants required to submit FAFSA. *Unit head:* Dr. Harriet Feldman, Dean, College of Health Professions, 914-773-3245, E-mail: hfeldman@pace.edu. *Application contact:* Susan Ford-Goldschein, Director of Graduate Admissions, 914-422-4283, Fax: 914-422-4287, E-mail: gradwp@pace.edu.
Website: http://www.pace.edu/lienhard

Pacific Lutheran University, Graduate Programs and Continuing Education, School of Nursing, Program in Care and Outcomes Manager, Tacoma, WA 98447. Offers client systems management (MSN); health care systems management (MSN). *Accreditation:* AACN. In 2013, 13 master's awarded. *Degree requirements:* For master's, thesis or alternative. *Entrance requirements:* For master's, GRE General Test, minimum undergraduate GPA of 3.0. Additional exam requirements/recommendations for international students: Required—TOEFL (minimum score 550 paper-based; 86 iBT). *Application deadline:* For fall admission, 11/15 priority date for domestic and international students. Applications are processed on a rolling basis. Application fee: $40. Electronic applications accepted. *Expenses:* Contact institution. *Financial support:* Federal Work-Study and scholarships/grants available. Financial award application deadline: 3/1; financial award applicants required to submit FAFSA. *Unit head:* Dr. Teri Woo, Associate Dean of Graduate Nursing Programs/Associate Professor of Nursing, 253-535-7686, E-mail: gradnurs@plu.edu. *Application contact:* Rachel Christopherson, Director of Graduate Admission, 253-535-8570, Fax: 253-536-5136, E-mail: gradadmission@plu.edu.

Piedmont College, School of Nursing and Health Sciences, Demorest, GA 30535-0010. Offers nursing administration (MSN); nursing education (MSN). *Expenses: Tuition:* Full-time $7992; part-time $444 per credit hour.

Prairie View A&M University, College of Nursing, Houston, TX 77030. Offers family nurse practitioner (MSN); nursing administration (MSN); nursing education (MSN). Part-time programs available. *Faculty:* 9 full-time (8 women), 13 part-time/adjunct (11 women). *Students:* 74 full-time (61 women), 107 part-time (99 women); includes 65 minority (63 Black or African American, non-Hispanic/Latino; 2 Hispanic/Latino), 4 international. Average age 37. 121 applicants, 42% accepted, 45 enrolled. In 2013, 46 master's awarded. *Degree requirements:* For master's, comprehensive exam, thesis. *Entrance requirements:* For master's, MAT or GRE, BS in nursing; 2 years of experience as a registered nurse; 1 course each in statistics, basic health and assessment. *Application deadline:* For fall admission, 7/1 priority date for domestic students, 7/1 for international students; for spring admission, 11/1 priority date for domestic students, 11/1 for international students. Applications are processed on a rolling basis. Application fee: $50. *Expenses:* Tuition, state resident: full-time $3776; part-time $209.77 per credit hour. Tuition, nonresident: full-time $10,183; part-time $565.77 per credit hour. *Required fees:* $2037; $446.50 per credit hour. *Financial support:* In 2013–14, 17 students received support. Career-related internships or fieldwork, Federal Work-Study, institutionally sponsored loans, scholarships/grants, and traineeships available. Support available to part-time students. Financial award application deadline: 4/1; financial award applicants required to submit FAFSA. *Faculty research:* Software development and violence prevention, health promotion and disease prevention. *Total annual research expenditures:* $350,000. *Unit head:* Dr. Betty N. Adams, Dean, 713-797-7009, Fax: 713-797-7013, E-mail: bnadams@pvamu.edu. *Application contact:* Dr. Forest Smith, Director of Student Services and Admissions, 713-797-7031, Fax: 713-797-7012, E-mail: fdsmith@pvamu.edu.
Website: http://www.pvamu.edu/nursing/

Purdue University Calumet, Graduate Studies Office, School of Nursing, Hammond, IN 46323-2094. Offers adult health clinical nurse specialist (MS); critical care clinical nurse specialist (MS); family nurse practitioner (MS); nurse executive (MS). Part-time programs available. Postbaccalaureate distance learning degree programs offered (minimal on-campus study). *Entrance requirements:* For master's, BSN. Additional exam requirements/recommendations for international students: Required—TOEFL. Electronic applications accepted. *Faculty research:* Adult health, cardiovascular and pulmonary nursing.

Queens University of Charlotte, Presbyterian School of Nursing, Charlotte, NC 28274-0002. Offers nursing management (MSN). *Accreditation:* AACN. *Degree requirements:* For master's, research project. *Entrance requirements:* For master's, minimum GPA of 3.0. Additional exam requirements/recommendations for international students: Required—TOEFL. Electronic applications accepted. *Expenses:* Contact institution.

Research College of Nursing, Nursing Program, Kansas City, MO 64132. Offers adult-gerontological nurse practitioner (MSN); clinical nurse leader (MSN); executive practice and healthcare leadership (MSN); family nurse practitioner (MSN); nurse educator (MSN); nursing (MSN). *Accreditation:* AACN. Part-time programs available. Postbaccalaureate distance learning degree programs offered (no on-campus study). *Faculty:* 9 full-time (all women), 5 part-time/adjunct (2 women). *Students:* 19 full-time (18 women), 101 part-time (94 women). *Degree requirements:* For master's, research project. *Entrance requirements:* For master's, 3 letters of recommendation, official transcripts, resume. Additional exam requirements/recommendations for international students: Required—TOEFL (minimum score 550 paper-based), TWE. *Application deadline:* Applications are processed on a rolling basis. Application fee: $50. *Expenses: Tuition:* Part-time $445 per credit hour. *Required fees:* $25 per credit hour. Part-time tuition and fees vary according to course load. *Financial support:* Applicants required to submit FAFSA. *Unit head:* Dr. Nancy O. DeBasio, President and Dean, 816-995-2815, Fax: 816-995-2817, E-mail: nancy.debasio@researchcollege.edu. *Application contact:* Leslie Mendenhall, Director of Transfer and Graduate Recruitment, 816-995-2820, Fax: 816-995-2813, E-mail: leslie.mendenhall@researchcollege.edu.

Roberts Wesleyan College, Department of Nursing, Rochester, NY 14624-1997. Offers nursing administration (MSN); nursing education (MSN). *Accreditation:* AACN. Evening/weekend programs available. Postbaccalaureate distance learning degree programs offered (no on-campus study). *Faculty:* 13 full-time (all women), 6 part-time/adjunct (4 women). *Students:* 67 full-time (63 women); includes 10 minority (5 Black or African American, non-Hispanic/Latino; 2 American Indian or Alaska Native, non-Hispanic/Latino; 1 Asian, non-Hispanic/Latino; 2 Hispanic/Latino), 7 international. Average age 39. 53 applicants, 100% accepted, 36 enrolled. In 2013, 2 master's

awarded. *Degree requirements:* For master's, thesis. *Entrance requirements:* For master's, minimum GPA of 3.0; BS in nursing; interview; RN license; resume; course work in statistics. Additional exam requirements/recommendations for international students: Required—TOEFL (minimum score 90 iBT), IELTS (minimum score 6.5). *Application deadline:* Applications are processed on a rolling basis. Application fee: $0. *Expenses: Tuition:* Full-time $12,816; part-time $712 per credit hour. One-time fee: $300. Tuition and fees vary according to course load and program. *Financial support:* In 2013–14, 21 students received support. Scholarships/grants available. Financial award applicants required to submit FAFSA. *Unit head:* Dr. Cheryl B. Crotser, Chairperson and Director of Graduate Program, 585-594-6668, E-mail: crotser_cheryl@roberts.edu. *Application contact:* Brenda Mutton, Admissions Coordinator, 585-594-6686, E-mail: mutton_brenda@roberts.edu.
Website: http://www.roberts.edu/gradnursing

Rush University, College of Nursing, Direct Entry Master's for Non-Nurses: Generalist Entry Master's Clinical Nurse Leader Program, Chicago, IL 60612. Offers MSN. *Students:* 190 full-time (165 women); includes 50 minority (15 Black or African American, non-Hispanic/Latino; 18 Asian, non-Hispanic/Latino; 17 Hispanic/Latino). Average age 27. 103 applicants, 57% accepted, 46 enrolled. *Degree requirements:* For master's, comprehensive exam, capstone project. *Entrance requirements:* For master's, GRE General Test (waived if cumulative GPA is 3.25 or greater), interview, 3 letters of recommendation, personal statement, current resume. Additional exam requirements/recommendations for international students: Required—TOEFL. *Application deadline:* For fall admission, 1/5 for domestic students; for spring admission, 8/4 for domestic students; for summer admission, 12/1 for domestic students. Application fee: $100. Electronic applications accepted. *Financial support:* Research assistantships, Federal Work-Study, scholarships/grants, and health care benefits available. Support available to part-time students. Financial award application deadline: 3/1; financial award applicants required to submit FAFSA. *Unit head:* Dr. Frank Hicks, Director for Generalist Education/Assistant Dean for Academic Affairs, 312-942-7117, Fax: 312-942-3043. *Application contact:* Molly Spurlock, Manager for Admissions and Social Media, 312-942-6222, E-mail: molly_spurlock@rush.edu.
Website: http://www.rushu.rush.edu/servlet/Satellite?MetaAttrName=meta_university&ParentId=1320160850241&ParentType=RushUnivLevel3Page&c=content_block&cid=1211

Rush University, College of Nursing, MSN for RN's: Clinical Nurse Leader (CNL) Program, Chicago, IL 60612. Offers MSN. Part-time programs available. Postbaccalaureate distance learning degree programs offered (no on-campus study). *Students:* 53 part-time (46 women); includes 17 minority (2 Black or African American, non-Hispanic/Latino; 3 American Indian or Alaska Native, non-Hispanic/Latino; 5 Asian, non-Hispanic/Latino; 7 Hispanic/Latino). Average age 35. 50 applicants, 76% accepted, 37 enrolled. *Degree requirements:* For master's, thesis, clinical residency, capstone project. *Entrance requirements:* For master's, GRE (waived if cumulative GPA is 3.25 or greater or if nursing GPA is 3.0 or greater), interview, 3 letters of recommendation, personal statement, current resume. Additional exam requirements/recommendations for international students: Required—TOEFL. *Application deadline:* For fall admission, 5/1 for domestic students; for spring admission, 8/4 for domestic students; for summer admission, 12/1 for domestic students. Applications are processed on a rolling basis. Application fee: $100. Electronic applications accepted. *Financial support:* Research assistantships, Federal Work-Study, scholarships/grants, and health care benefits available. Support available to part-time students. Financial award application deadline: 3/1; financial award applicants required to submit FAFSA. *Unit head:* Dr. Frank Hicks, Director of Generalist Education/Assistant Dean for Academic Affairs, 312-942-5587, E-mail: frank_d_hicks@rush.edu. *Application contact:* Jennifer Thorndyke, Admissions Specialist, 312-563-7526, E-mail: jennifer_thorndyke@rush.edu.
Website: http://www.rushu.rush.edu/servlet/Satellite?MetaAttrName=meta_university&ParentId=1320160849834&ParentType=RushUnivLevel2Page&c=content_block&cid=1221

Sacred Heart University, Graduate Programs, College of Health Professions, Department of Nursing, Fairfield, CT 06825-1000. Offers clinical nurse leader (MSN); clinical practice in health care (DNP); family nurse practitioner (MSN); leadership in health care (DNP); nursing (DN Sc); nursing educator (MSN); patient care services administration (MSN). *Accreditation:* AACN. Part-time and evening/weekend programs available. Postbaccalaureate distance learning degree programs offered (no on-campus study). *Faculty:* 7 full-time (all women), 5 part-time/adjunct (all women). *Students:* 34 full-time (32 women), 645 part-time (595 women); includes 117 minority (50 Black or African American, non-Hispanic/Latino; 1 American Indian or Alaska Native, non-Hispanic/Latino; 26 Asian, non-Hispanic/Latino; 29 Hispanic/Latino; 1 Native Hawaiian or other Pacific Islander, non-Hispanic/Latino; 10 Two or more races, non-Hispanic/Latino). Average age 39. 110 applicants, 58% accepted, 46 enrolled. In 2013, 67 master's, 11 doctorates awarded. *Entrance requirements:* For master's, minimum GPA of 3.0, BSN or RN plus BS (for MSN); for doctorate, minimum GPA of 3.0, MSN or BSN plus MS (for DNP). Additional exam requirements/recommendations for international students: Required—PTE; Recommended—TOEFL (minimum score 570 paper-based; 80 iBT), IELTS (minimum score 6.5). *Application deadline:* Applications are processed on a rolling basis. Application fee: $60. Electronic applications accepted. *Expenses:* Contact institution. *Financial support:* Career-related internships or fieldwork and institutionally sponsored loans available. Support available to part-time students. Financial award applicants required to submit FAFSA. *Unit head:* Dr. Sue DeNisco, Chair, 203-365-7661, Fax: 203-365-7662, E-mail: deniscos@sacredheart.edu. *Application contact:* Kathy Dilks, Executive Director of Graduate Admissions, 203-365-4716, Fax: 203-365-4732, E-mail: gradstudies@sacredheart.edu.
Website: http://www.sacredheart.edu/graduate/nursing/

Sage Graduate School, School of Health Sciences, Department of Nursing, Troy, NY 12180-4115. Offers adult geriatric advanced nursing (MS); adult gerontology nurse practitioner (MS); adult health (MS); adult nurse practitioner (MS, Post Master's Certificate); clinical nurse leader/specialist (Post Master's Certificate); community health (MS); counseling for nursing (Postbaccalaureate Certificate); education and leadership (DNS); family nurse practitioner (MS, Post Master's Certificate); gerontological nurse practitioner (Post Master's Certificate); nurse administrator/executive (Post Master's Certificate); nurse education (Post Master's Certificate); nursing (Post Master's Certificate); psychiatric mental health nurse clinical nurse specialist (MS); psychiatric mental health nurse practitioner (MS, Post Master's Certificate), including psychiatric mental health. *Accreditation:* AACN. Part-time and evening/weekend programs available. *Faculty:* 5 full-time (all women), 10 part-time/adjunct (all women). *Students:* 32 full-time (30 women), 174 part-time (161 women); includes 28 minority (12 Black or African American, non-Hispanic/Latino; 2 American Indian or Alaska Native, non-Hispanic/Latino; 8 Asian, non-Hispanic/Latino; 4 Hispanic/Latino; 2 Two or more races, non-Hispanic/Latino), 3 international. Average age 40. 171 applicants, 43% accepted, 35 enrolled. In 2013, 53 master's, 5 doctorates, 11 other advanced degrees awarded. *Degree requirements:* For master's, thesis or alternative. *Entrance requirements:* For master's, BS in nursing, minimum GPA of 2.75, resume, 2 letters of recommendation. Additional exam requirements/recommendations for international students: Required—TOEFL (minimum score 550 paper-based). *Application deadline:* Applications are processed on a rolling basis. Application fee: $40. *Expenses: Tuition:* Full-time $11,880; part-time $660 per credit hour. *Financial support:* Fellowships, research assistantships, Federal Work-Study, scholarships/grants, and unspecified assistantships available. Support available to part-time students. Financial award application deadline: 3/1; financial award applicants required to submit FAFSA. *Unit head:* Dr. Esther Haskevitz, Dean, School of Health Sciences, 518-244-2296, Fax: 518-244-4571, E-mail: haskve@sage.edu. *Application contact:* Dr. Glenda Kelman, Director, 518-244-2001, Fax: 518-244-2009, E-mail: kelmag@sage.edu.

Saginaw Valley State University, Crystal M. Lange College of Nursing and Health Sciences, Program in Health System Nurse Specialist, University Center, MI 48710. Offers MSN. *Accreditation:* AACN. Part-time and evening/weekend programs available. *Students:* 9 part-time (all women); includes 1 minority (Black or African American, non-Hispanic/Latino). Average age 39. 2 applicants, 50% accepted, 1 enrolled. In 2013, 4 master's awarded. *Degree requirements:* For master's, thesis optional. *Entrance requirements:* For master's, GRE, minimum GPA of 3.0. Additional exam requirements/recommendations for international students: Required—TOEFL (minimum score 580 paper-based; 92 iBT). *Application deadline:* For fall admission, 7/15 for international students; for winter admission, 11/15 for international students; for spring admission, 4/15 for international students. Applications are processed on a rolling basis. Application fee: $30 ($80 for international students). Electronic applications accepted. *Expenses:* Tuition, state resident: full-time $8933; part-time $496.30 per credit hour. Tuition, nonresident: full-time $16,806; part-time $933.65 per credit hour. *Required fees:* $263; $14.60 per credit hour. Tuition and fees vary according to degree level. *Financial support:* Federal Work-Study and scholarships/grants available. Support available to part-time students. Financial award application deadline: 4/1; financial award applicants required to submit FAFSA. *Unit head:* Dr. Sally Decker, Department Chair, 989-964-4098, E-mail: decker@svsu.edu. *Application contact:* Jenna Briggs, Director, Graduate and International Admissions, 989-964-6096, Fax: 989-964-2788, E-mail: gradadm@svsu.edu.

Saint Francis Medical Center College of Nursing, Graduate Programs, Peoria, IL 61603-3783. Offers adult gerontology (MSN); clinical nurse leader (MSN); family nurse practitioner (MSN); family psychiatric mental health nurse practitioner (MSN); neonatal nurse practitioner (MSN); nurse clinician (Post-Graduate Certificate); nurse educator (MSN, Post-Graduate Certificate); nursing (DNP); nursing management leadership (MSN). Part-time programs available. Postbaccalaureate distance learning degree programs offered (minimal on-campus study). *Faculty:* 4 full-time (all women), 4 part-time/adjunct (all women). *Students:* 13 full-time (12 women), 268 part-time (245 women); includes 17 minority (10 Black or African American, non-Hispanic/Latino; 2 Asian, non-Hispanic/Latino; 5 Hispanic/Latino), 2 international. Average age 37. 115 applicants, 89% accepted, 42 enrolled. In 2013, 17 master's, 2 doctorates awarded. *Degree requirements:* For master's, research experience, portfolio, practicum; for doctorate, practicum hours. *Entrance requirements:* For master's, nursing research, health assessment, graduate course work in statistics, RN license; for doctorate, master's degree in nursing, professional portfolio, graduate statistics, transcripts, RN license. Additional exam requirements/recommendations for international students: Required—TOEFL. *Application deadline:* For fall admission, 6/1 priority date for domestic and international students; for spring admission, 11/15 priority date for domestic and international students. Applications are processed on a rolling basis. Application fee: $50. Electronic applications accepted. *Expenses: Tuition:* Full-time $6336; part-time $528 per semester hour. *Required fees:* $436. *Financial support:* In 2013–14, 8 students received support. Scholarships/grants and tuition waivers (partial) available. Support available to part-time students. Financial award application deadline: 6/15; financial award applicants required to submit FAFSA. *Faculty research:* Outcome and curriculum planning, health promotion, NCLEX-RN results, decision-making program evaluation. *Unit head:* Dr. Patti A. Stockert, President of the College, 309-655-4124, Fax: 309-624-8973, E-mail: patricia.a.stockert@osfhealthcare.org. *Application contact:* Dr. Janice F. Boundy, Dean, 309-655-2230, Fax: 309-624-8973, E-mail: jan.f.boundy@osfhealthcare.org.
Website: http://www.sfmccon.edu/graduate-programs/

Saint Joseph's College of Maine, Master of Science in Nursing Program, Standish, ME 04084. Offers administration (MSN); education (MSN); family nurse practitioner (MSN); nursing administration and leadership (Certificate); nursing and health care education (Certificate). *Accreditation:* AACN. Part-time programs available. Postbaccalaureate distance learning degree programs offered (no on-campus study). *Entrance requirements:* For master's, MAT. Electronic applications accepted.

Saint Joseph's University, College of Arts and Sciences, Department of Health Services, Philadelphia, PA 19131-1395. Offers health administration (MS, Post-Master's Certificate); health care ethics (Post-Master's Certificate); health education (MS, Post-Master's Certificate); health informatics (Post-Master's Certificate); healthcare ethics (MS); long-term care administration (MS); nurse anesthesia (MS); school nurse certification (MS). Part-time and evening/weekend programs available. *Faculty:* 5 full-time (1 woman), 16 part-time/adjunct (6 women). *Students:* 46 full-time (25 women), 431 part-time (315 women); includes 168 minority (120 Black or African American, non-Hispanic/Latino; 29 Asian, non-Hispanic/Latino; 15 Hispanic/Latino; 2 Native Hawaiian or other Pacific Islander, non-Hispanic/Latino; 2 Two or more races, non-Hispanic/Latino), 14 international. Average age 34. 234 applicants, 74% accepted, 135 enrolled. In 2013, 83 master's awarded. *Entrance requirements:* For master's, GRE (if GPA less than 3.0), 2 letters of recommendation, resume, personal statement, official transcripts. Additional exam requirements/recommendations for international students: Required—TOEFL (minimum score 550 paper-based; 80 iBT), IELTS (minimum score 6.5). *Application deadline:* For fall admission, 7/15 priority date for domestic students, 4/15 for international students; for winter admission, 1/15 for international students; for spring admission, 11/15 priority date for domestic students, 10/15 for international students. Applications are processed on a rolling basis. Application fee: $35. Electronic applications accepted. *Expenses: Tuition:* Part-time $786 per credit hour. Tuition and fees vary according to degree level and program. *Financial support:* Career-related internships or fieldwork and unspecified assistantships available. Financial award applicants required to submit FAFSA. *Unit head:* Nakia Henderson, Director, 610-660-3131, E-mail: gradstudies@sju.edu. *Application contact:* Elisabeth Woodward, Director of Marketing and Admissions, Graduate Arts and Sciences, 610-660-3131, Fax: 610-660-3230, E-mail: gradstudies@sju.edu.
Website: http://sju.edu/majors-programs/graduate-arts-sciences/masters/health-administration-ms

Saint Joseph's University, College of Arts and Sciences, Program in Gerontological Services, Philadelphia, PA 19131-1395. Offers gerontological services (MS, Post-Master's Certificate); long-term care administration (MS). Part-time and evening/weekend programs available. *Faculty:* 1 (woman) full-time, 2 part-time/adjunct (both women). *Students:* 2 full-time (1 woman), 17 part-time (14 women); includes 8 minority (6 Black or African American, non-Hispanic/Latino; 2 Asian, non-Hispanic/Latino), 1 international. Average age 36. 12 applicants, 75% accepted, 8 enrolled. In 2013, 2 master's awarded. *Entrance requirements:* For master's, 2 letters of recommendation, personal statement, resume. Additional exam requirements/recommendations for international students: Required—TOEFL (minimum score 550 paper-based; 80 iBT). *Application deadline:* For fall admission, 7/15 priority date for domestic students, 4/15 for

international students; for winter admission, 1/15 for international students; for spring admission, 11/15 priority date for domestic students, 10/15 for international students. Applications are processed on a rolling basis. Application fee: $35. Electronic applications accepted. *Expenses: Tuition:* Part-time $786 per credit hour. Tuition and fees vary according to degree level and program. *Financial support:* Fellowships available. Financial award applicants required to submit FAFSA. *Unit head:* Dr. Catherine Murray, Director, 610-660-1805, E-mail: cmurray@sju.edu. *Application contact:* Elisabeth Woodward, Director of Marketing and Admissions, Graduate Arts and Sciences, 610-660-3131, Fax: 610-660-3230, E-mail: gradstudies@sju.edu.
Website: http://www.sju.edu/majors-programs/graduate-arts-sciences/masters/gerontological-services-ms

Saint Peter's University, School of Nursing, Nursing Program, Jersey City, NJ 07306-5997. Offers adult nurse practitioner (MSN, Certificate); advanced practice (DNP); case management (MSN, DNP). *Accreditation:* AACN. Part-time and evening/weekend programs available. *Entrance requirements:* Additional exam requirements/recommendations for international students: Required—TOEFL. Electronic applications accepted.

Saint Vincent College, Program in Health Services Leadership, Latrobe, PA 15650-2690. Offers MS.

Salem State University, School of Graduate Studies, Program in Nursing, Salem, MA 01970-5353. Offers adult-gerontology primary care nursing (MSN); nursing administration (MSN); nursing education (MSN); MBA/MSN. *Accreditation:* AACN. Part-time and evening/weekend programs available. *Students:* 31 full-time (24 women), 79 part-time (70 women); includes 12 minority (4 Black or African American, non-Hispanic/Latino; 4 Asian, non-Hispanic/Latino; 3 Hispanic/Latino; 1 Native Hawaiian or other Pacific Islander, non-Hispanic/Latino), 5 international. 18 applicants, 94% accepted, 16 enrolled. In 2013, 15 master's awarded. *Entrance requirements:* For master's, GRE or MAT. Additional exam requirements/recommendations for international students: Required—TOEFL (minimum score 550 paper-based; 80 iBT) or IELTS (minimum score 5.5). *Application deadline:* For fall admission, 5/1 for domestic students; for spring admission, 10/1 for domestic students. Applications are processed on a rolling basis. Application fee: $50. *Financial support:* Career-related internships or fieldwork, Federal Work-Study, scholarships/grants, and unspecified assistantships available. Support available to part-time students. Financial award application deadline: 5/1; financial award applicants required to submit FAFSA. *Application contact:* Dr. Lee A. Brossoit, Assistant Dean of Graduate Admissions, 978-542-6675, Fax: 978-542-7215, E-mail: lbrossoit@salemstate.edu.
Website: http://www.salemstate.edu/academics/schools/1819.php

Salisbury University, Program in Nursing, Salisbury, MD 21801-6837. Offers health care leadership (MS); nurse educator (MS); nursing (MS). Part-time programs available. Postbaccalaureate distance learning degree programs offered. *Faculty:* 5 full-time (4 women). *Students:* 1 (woman) full-time, 18 part-time (all women); includes 6 minority (all Black or African American, non-Hispanic/Latino). Average age 36. 18 applicants, 28% accepted, 3 enrolled. In 2013, 17 master's awarded. *Entrance requirements:* For master's, GRE, minimum undergraduate GPA of 3.0, 2 letters of recommendation, resume, personal statement, current and active RN license, interview, CPR certification, personal statement. Additional exam requirements/recommendations for international students: Required—TOEFL (minimum score 550 paper-based; 79 iBT), IELTS (minimum score 6.5). *Application deadline:* For fall admission, 4/15 priority date for domestic and international students. Applications are processed on a rolling basis. Application fee: $50. Electronic applications accepted. *Expenses:* Tuition, state resident: part-time $342 per credit hour. Tuition, nonresident: part-time $631 per credit hour. *Required fees:* $76 per credit hour. Tuition and fees vary according to program. *Financial support:* In 2013–14, 7 students received support. Institutionally sponsored loans, scholarships/grants, and unspecified assistantships available. Support available to part-time students. Financial award application deadline: 3/1; financial award applicants required to submit FAFSA. *Faculty research:* Geriatrics, dementia, adolescent health, domestic violence. *Unit head:* Dr. Lisa Seldomridge, Chair of Department of Nursing, 410-543-6413, E-mail: laseldomridge@salisbury.edu. *Application contact:* Carmel Boger, Administrative Assistant for Graduate and Second Degree Nursing Program, 410-543-6420, E-mail: ciboger@salisbury.edu.
Website: http://www.salisbury.edu/Nursing/MS.html

Samford University, Ida V. Moffett School of Nursing, Birmingham, AL 35229. Offers administration (DNP); advanced practice (DNP); family nurse practitioner (MSN); health systems management and leadership (MSN); nurse anesthesia (MSN); nurse educator (MSN). *Accreditation:* AACN; AANA/CANAEP (one or more programs are accredited). Part-time programs available. Postbaccalaureate distance learning degree programs offered (minimal on-campus study). *Faculty:* 16 full-time (all women), 4 part-time/adjunct (2 women). *Students:* 249 full-time (191 women), 25 part-time (17 women); includes 48 minority (23 Black or African American, non-Hispanic/Latino; 1 American Indian or Alaska Native, non-Hispanic/Latino; 13 Asian, non-Hispanic/Latino; 7 Hispanic/Latino; 4 Two or more races, non-Hispanic/Latino), 1 international. Average age 36. 89 applicants, 53% accepted, 45 enrolled. In 2013, 107 master's, 29 doctorates awarded. *Degree requirements:* For master's and doctorate, capstone project with oral presentation. *Entrance requirements:* For master's, MAT; GRE (for nurse anesthesia). Additional exam requirements/recommendations for international students: Required—TOEFL (minimum score 550 paper-based; 80 iBT). *Application deadline:* For fall admission, 6/1 priority date for domestic and international students; for spring admission, 9/1 priority date for domestic and international students. Application fee: $65. Electronic applications accepted. *Expenses:* Contact institution. *Financial support:* In 2013–14, 48 students received support. Institutionally sponsored loans, scholarships/grants, and traineeships available. Financial award application deadline: 3/1; financial award applicants required to submit FAFSA. *Faculty research:* Issues in rural health care, vulnerable populations, genetics and disabilities in pediatrics, geriatrics, parish nursing research, interprofessional education, global health disparities. *Unit head:* Dr. Nena F. Sanders, Dean, 205-726-2629, E-mail: nfsander@samford.edu. *Application contact:* Allyson Maddox, Director of Graduate Student Services, 205-726-2047, Fax: 205-726-4179, E-mail: amaddox@samford.edu.
Website: http://samford.edu/nursing

Samuel Merritt University, School of Nursing, Oakland, CA 94609-3108. Offers case management (MSN); family nurse practitioner (MSN, Certificate); nurse anesthetist (MSN, Certificate); nursing (MSN, DNP). *Accreditation:* AACN; AANA/CANAEP (one or more programs are accredited). Part-time and evening/weekend programs available. *Degree requirements:* For master's, thesis or alternative. *Entrance requirements:* For master's, minimum GPA of 2.5 in science, 3.0 overall; previous course work in statistics; current RN license. Additional exam requirements/recommendations for international students: Required—TOEFL. *Faculty research:* Gerontology, community health, maternal-child health, sexually transmitted diseases, substance abuse, oncology.

San Francisco State University, Division of Graduate Studies, College of Health and Social Sciences, School of Nursing, San Francisco, CA 94132-1722. Offers adult acute care (MS); clinical nurse specialist (MS); community/public health nursing (MS); family nurse practitioner (MS, Certificate); nursing administration (MS); nursing education (MS); pediatrics (MS); women's health (MS). *Accreditation:* AACN. Part-time programs available. *Application deadline:* Applications are processed on a rolling basis. *Financial support:* Career-related internships or fieldwork available. *Unit head:* Dr. Mary-Ann van Dam, Director, 415-338-1802, E-mail: vandam@sfsu.edu. *Application contact:* Robert Strachan, Admission and Student Services Coordinator, 415-338-1802, E-mail: strachan@sfsu.edu.
Website: http://nursing.sfsu.edu

San Jose State University, Graduate Studies and Research, College of Applied Sciences and Arts, School of Nursing, San Jose, CA 95192-0001. Offers gerontology nurse practitioner (MS); nursing (Certificate); nursing administration (MS); nursing education (MS). *Accreditation:* AACN. Part-time and evening/weekend programs available. *Degree requirements:* For master's, thesis. *Entrance requirements:* For master's, BS in nursing, RN license. Electronic applications accepted. *Faculty research:* Nurse-managed clinics, computers in nursing.

Seattle Pacific University, MS in Nursing Program, Seattle, WA 98119-1997. Offers administration (MSN); adult/gerontology nurse practitioner (MSN); clinical nurse specialist (MSN); family nurse practitioner (MSN, Certificate); informatics (MSN); nurse educator (MSN). *Accreditation:* AACN. Part-time programs available. *Students:* 9 full-time (7 women), 37 part-time (33 women); includes 8 minority (2 Black or African American, non-Hispanic/Latino; 5 Asian, non-Hispanic/Latino; 1 Hispanic/Latino), 1 international. Average age 41. 70 applicants, 30% accepted, 21 enrolled. In 2013, 27 master's awarded. *Degree requirements:* For master's, thesis. *Entrance requirements:* For master's, personal statement, transcripts, undergraduate nursing degree, proof of undergraduate statistics course with minimum GPA of 2.0, 2 recommendations. *Application deadline:* For fall admission, 1/15 priority date for domestic students; for spring admission, 1/15 for domestic students. Applications are processed on a rolling basis. Application fee: $50. Electronic applications accepted. *Expenses:* Contact institution. *Financial support:* Fellowships and scholarships/grants available. Financial award applicants required to submit FAFSA. *Unit head:* Dr. Susan Casey, Associate Dean, 206-281-2649, E-mail: caseys@spu.edu.
Website: http://www.spu.edu/depts/health-sciences/grad/index.asp

Seton Hall University, College of Nursing, South Orange, NJ 07079-2697. Offers advanced practice in primary health care (MSN, DNP), including adult/gerontological nurse practitioner, pediatric nurse practitioner; entry into practice (MSN); health systems administration (MSN, DNP); nursing (PhD); nursing case management (MSN); nursing education (MA); school nurse (MSN); MSN/MA. *Accreditation:* AACN. Part-time programs available. Postbaccalaureate distance learning degree programs offered (minimal on-campus study). *Degree requirements:* For master's, research project; for doctorate, dissertation or scholarly project. *Entrance requirements:* For doctorate, GRE (waived for students with GPA of 3.5 or higher). Additional exam requirements/recommendations for international students: Required—TOEFL. Electronic applications accepted. *Faculty research:* Parent/child, adult, and gerontological nursing; breast cancer; families of children with HIV; parish nursing.

Southeastern Louisiana University, College of Nursing and Health Sciences, School of Nursing, Hammond, LA 70402. Offers adult psychiatric/mental health nurse practitioner/clinical nurse specialist (MSN); education (MSN); nurse executive (MSN); nurse practice (DNP); nurse practitioner (MSN). *Accreditation:* AACN. Part-time and evening/weekend programs available. *Faculty:* 14 full-time (13 women), 5 part-time/adjunct (4 women). *Students:* 21 full-time (19 women), 138 part-time (121 women); includes 27 minority (17 Black or African American, non-Hispanic/Latino; 4 Asian, non-Hispanic/Latino; 5 Hispanic/Latino; 1 Two or more races, non-Hispanic/Latino). Average age 34. 72 applicants, 68% accepted, 19 enrolled. In 2013, 29 master's awarded. *Degree requirements:* For master's, thesis. *Entrance requirements:* For master's, GRE (verbal and quantitative), baccalaureate degree in nursing from accredited undergraduate nursing program; minimum GPA of 2.7; all transcripts from undergraduate school and any work attempted at the graduate level; curriculum vitae; valid Louisiana Registered Nurse license; letters of recommendation; letter of intent/statement of purpose. Additional exam requirements/recommendations for international students: Required—TOEFL (minimum score 500 paper-based; 61 iBT). *Application deadline:* For fall admission, 7/15 priority date for domestic students, 6/1 priority date for international students; for spring admission, 12/1 priority date for domestic students, 10/1 priority date for international students. Applications are processed on a rolling basis. Application fee: $20 ($30 for international students). Electronic applications accepted. *Expenses:* Tuition, state resident: full-time $5047. Tuition, nonresident: full-time $17,066. *Required fees:* $1213. Tuition and fees vary according to degree level. *Financial support:* Federal Work-Study, institutionally sponsored loans, scholarships/grants, traineeships, and unspecified assistantships available. Support available to part-time students. Financial award application deadline: 5/1; financial award applicants required to submit FAFSA. *Faculty research:* Gender issues, LGBT issues, occupational health/safety, accelerated students, caring development. *Total annual research expenditures:* $103,409. *Unit head:* Dr. Lorinda J. Sealey, Graduate Nursing Program Director, 985-549-5045, Fax: 985-549-5087, E-mail: vjohnson@selu.edu. *Application contact:* Sandra Meyers, Graduate Admissions Analyst, 985-549-5620, Fax: 985-549-5632, E-mail: admissions@selu.edu.
Website: http://www.selu.edu/acad_research/depts/nurs

Southern Adventist University, School of Nursing, Collegedale, TN 37315-0370. Offers acute care nurse practitioner (MSN); adult nurse practitioner (MSN); family nurse practitioner (MSN); nurse educator (MSN); MSN/MSBA. Part-time programs available. *Degree requirements:* For master's, thesis or project. *Entrance requirements:* For master's, RN license. Additional exam requirements/recommendations for international students: Required—TOEFL (minimum score 600 paper-based). Electronic applications accepted. *Faculty research:* Pain management, ethics, corporate wellness, caring spirituality, stress.

Southern Connecticut State University, School of Graduate Studies, School of Health and Human Services, Department of Nursing, New Haven, CT 06515-1355. Offers nursing administration (MSN); nursing education (MSN). *Accreditation:* AACN. Part-time and evening/weekend programs available. *Degree requirements:* For master's, thesis. *Entrance requirements:* For master's, GRE, MAT, interview, minimum QPA of 2.8, RN license, minimum 1 year of professional nursing experience. Electronic applications accepted.

Southern Illinois University Edwardsville, Graduate School, School of Nursing, Program in Health Care and Nursing Administration, Edwardsville, IL 62026-0001. Offers MS, Post-Master's Certificate. Part-time programs available. *Students:* 23 part-time (22 women); includes 2 minority (both Black or African American, non-Hispanic/Latino). 13 applicants, 85% accepted. In 2013, 1 master's awarded. *Degree requirements:* For master's, comprehensive exam. *Entrance requirements:* For master's, RN licensure, minimum undergraduate nursing GPA of 3.0, BS from CCNE- or NLNAC-accredited program. Additional exam requirements/recommendations for international students: Required—TOEFL (minimum score 550 paper-based, 79 iBT), IELTS (minimum score 6.5), Michigan Test of English Language Proficiency or PTE. *Application deadline:* For fall admission, 3/1 for domestic and international students. Application fee: $30. Electronic applications accepted. *Expenses:* Tuition, state resident: full-time $3551. Tuition, nonresident: full-time $8378. *Financial support:* Institutionally sponsored loans, scholarships/grants, and unspecified assistantships

available. Financial award application deadline: 3/1; financial award applicants required to submit FAFSA. *Unit head:* Dr. Kathy Ketchum, Associate Dean for Graduate Programs, 618-650-3936, E-mail: kketchu@siue.edu. *Application contact:* Melissa K. Mace, Assistant Director of Graduate and International Recruitment, 618-650-2756, Fax: 618-650-3618, E-mail: mmace@siue.edu.
Website: http://www.siue.edu/nursing/graduate

Southern Nazarene University, College of Professional and Graduate Studies, School of Nursing, Bethany, OK 73008. Offers nursing education (MS); nursing leadership (MS). *Accreditation:* AACN. Part-time and evening/weekend programs available. *Degree requirements:* For master's, thesis. *Entrance requirements:* For master's, minimum undergraduate cumulative GPA of 3.0; baccalaureate degree in nursing from nationally-accredited program; current unencumbered registered nurse licensure in Oklahoma or eligibility for same; documentation of basic computer skills; basic statistics course; statement of professional goals; three letters of recommendation. Additional exam requirements/recommendations for international students: Required—TOEFL (minimum score 550 paper-based). *Unit head:* Dr. Katie Sigler, Chair, 405-717-6217, E-mail: ksigler@snu.edu.
Website: http://snu.edu/school-of-nursing

Southern University and Agricultural and Mechanical College, School of Nursing, Baton Rouge, LA 70813. Offers educator/administrator (PhD); family health nursing (MSN); family nurse practitioner (Post Master's Certificate); geriatric nurse practitioner/ gerontology (PhD). *Accreditation:* AACN. Part-time programs available. *Degree requirements:* For master's, comprehensive exam, thesis; for doctorate, comprehensive exam, thesis/dissertation. *Entrance requirements:* For master's, GRE General Test, BSN, minimum GPA of 2.7; for doctorate, GRE General Test; for Post Master's Certificate, MSN. Additional exam requirements/recommendations for international students: Required—TOEFL (minimum score 525 paper-based). *Faculty research:* Health promotions, vulnerable populations, (community-based) cardiovascular participating research, health disparities chronic diseases, care of the elderly.

Spalding University, Graduate Studies, Kosair College of Health and Natural Sciences, School of Nursing, Louisville, KY 40203-2188. Offers adult nurse practitioner (MSN, PMC); family nurse practitioner (MSN, PMC); leadership in nursing and healthcare (MSN, PMC); pediatric nurse practitioner (MSN, PMC). *Accreditation:* AACN. Part-time and evening/weekend programs available. *Faculty:* 6 full-time (all women), 6 part-time/ adjunct (5 women). *Students:* 98 full-time (85 women), 13 part-time (all women); includes 23 minority (19 Black or African American, non-Hispanic/Latino; 2 Asian, non-Hispanic/Latino; 1 Hispanic/Latino; 1 Two or more races, non-Hispanic/Latino). Average age 36. 136 applicants, 31% accepted, 39 enrolled. In 2013, 48 master's, 5 other advanced degrees awarded. *Degree requirements:* For master's, comprehensive exam (for some programs), thesis. *Entrance requirements:* For master's, GRE General Test, BSN or bachelor's degree, RN licensure, autobiographical statement, transcripts, letters of recommendation. Additional exam requirements/recommendations for international students: Required—TOEFL (minimum score 535 paper-based). *Application deadline:* For fall admission, 2/1 priority date for domestic students. Application fee: $30. *Expenses: Tuition:* Full-time $21,450. *Required fees:* $810. Tuition and fees vary according to course load, degree level, program and student level. *Financial support:* Career-related internships or fieldwork, scholarships/grants, and traineeships available. Support available to part-time students. Financial award application deadline: 3/30; financial award applicants required to submit FAFSA. *Faculty research:* Nurse educational administration, gerontology, bioterrorism, healthcare ethics, leadership. *Unit head:* Dr. Paula Travis, Chair, 502-873-4298, E-mail: clewis@spalding.edu. *Application contact:* Dr. Pam King, Assistant Professor, 502-873-4292, E-mail: pking@spalding.edu.
Website: http://www.spalding.edu/nursing/

Spring Hill College, Graduate Programs, Program in Nursing, Mobile, AL 36608-1791. Offers clinical nurse leader (MSN, Post-Master's Certificate). *Accreditation:* AACN. Part-time and evening/weekend programs available. Postbaccalaureate distance learning degree programs offered (no on-campus study). *Faculty:* 2 full-time (both women). *Students:* 20 part-time (17 women); includes 13 minority (10 Black or African American, non-Hispanic/Latino; 3 Asian, non-Hispanic/Latino). Average age 43. In 2013, 9 master's, 2 other advanced degrees awarded. *Degree requirements:* For master's, comprehensive exam, capstone courses, completion of program within 6 calendar years; for Post-Master's Certificate, 460 clinical integration hours. *Entrance requirements:* For master's, RN license in state where practicing nursing; 1 year of clinical nursing experience; work in clinical setting or access to health care facility for clinical integration/research; 3 written references; employer verification; resume; 500-word essay explaining how becoming a CNL will help applicant achieve personal and professional goals; for Post-Master's Certificate, RN license; master's degree in nursing. Additional exam requirements/recommendations for international students: Required—TOEFL (minimum score 550 paper-based; 80 iBT), IELTS (minimum score 6.5), CPE or CAE (minimum score C), Michigan English Language Assessment Battery (minimum score 90). *Application deadline:* For fall admission, 8/1 priority date for domestic and international students; for spring admission, 12/1 priority date for domestic and international students. Applications are processed on a rolling basis. Application fee: $25 ($35 for international students). Electronic applications accepted. *Expenses:* Contact institution. *Financial support:* Applicants required to submit FAFSA. *Unit head:* Dr. Ola H. Fox, Director, 251-380-4486, Fax: 251-460-4495, E-mail: ofox@shc.edu. *Application contact:* Donna B. Tarasavage, Associate Director, Academic Affairs, 251-380-3067, Fax: 251-460-2182, E-mail: dtarasavage@shc.edu.
Website: http://www.shc.edu/page/master-science-nursing

State University of New York Institute of Technology, Program in Business Administration in Technology Management, Utica, NY 13504-3050. Offers accounting and finance (MBA); business management (MBA); health services management (MBA); human resource management (MBA); marketing management (MBA). Part-time programs available. Postbaccalaureate distance learning degree programs offered (no on-campus study). *Faculty:* 10 full-time (2 women), 2 part-time/adjunct (1 woman). *Students:* 29 full-time (13 women), 89 part-time (26 women); includes 17 minority (5 Black or African American, non-Hispanic/Latino; 8 Asian, non-Hispanic/Latino; 3 Hispanic/Latino; 1 Two or more races, non-Hispanic/Latino), 1 international. Average age 33. 78 applicants, 54% accepted, 29 enrolled. In 2013, 57 master's awarded. *Degree requirements:* For master's, capstone course. *Entrance requirements:* For master's, GMAT, resume, one letter of reference. Additional exam requirements/ recommendations for international students: Required—TOEFL (minimum score 550 paper-based; 79 iBT), IELTS (minimum score 6.5). *Application deadline:* For fall admission, 8/1 priority date for domestic students, 7/1 for international students; for spring admission, 12/1 for domestic students, 11/1 for international students. Applications are processed on a rolling basis. Application fee: $60. Electronic applications accepted. *Expenses:* Tuition, state resident: full-time $9870; part-time $411 per credit hour. Tuition, nonresident: full-time $20,150; part-time $765 per credit hour. *Required fees:* $1180; $50.73 per credit hour. *Financial support:* In 2013–14, 3 students received support, including 1 fellowship with full tuition reimbursement available (averaging $5,545 per year), 2 research assistantships with partial tuition reimbursements available (averaging $4,000 per year); unspecified assistantships also available. Financial award application deadline: 6/1; financial award applicants required to submit FAFSA. *Faculty research:* Technology management, writing schools, leadership, new products. *Unit head:* Dr. Rafael Romero, Program Coordinator and Associate Professor, 315-792-7337, Fax: 315-792-7138, E-mail: rafael.romero@sunyit.edu. *Application contact:* Maryrose Raab, Coordinator of Graduate Center, 315-792-7347, Fax: 315-792-7221, E-mail: maryrose.raab@sunyit.edu.
Website: http://www.sunyit.edu/programs/graduate/mbatm/

Teachers College, Columbia University, Graduate Faculty of Education, Department of Organization and Leadership, Program in Nurse Executive, New York, NY 10027. Offers administration studies (MA); nurse executive (Ed D); professorial studies (MA). *Faculty:* 1 full-time, 2 part-time/adjunct. *Students:* 12 full-time (11 women), 17 part-time (15 women); includes 13 minority (6 Black or African American, non-Hispanic/Latino; 5 Asian, non-Hispanic/Latino; 2 Hispanic/Latino). Average age 54. 19 applicants, 79% accepted, 11 enrolled. In 2013, 12 master's, 2 doctorates awarded. *Degree requirements:* For master's, capstone project; for doctorate, thesis/dissertation. *Entrance requirements:* For master's, BSN, minimum cumulative GPA of 3.0 from the undergraduate program, one year of continuous post-baccalaureate full-time clinical nursing practice experience in a particular area; for doctorate, GRE General Test or MAT, BSN, nursing license, graduate degree and/or minimum of 36 graduate points/ credits, one year of continuous post-baccalaureate full-time nursing or healthcare management experience. Additional exam requirements/recommendations for international students: Required—TOEFL (minimum score 600 paper-based). *Application deadline:* For fall admission, 1/15 for domestic students. Applications are processed on a rolling basis. Application fee: $65. Electronic applications accepted. *Financial support:* Career-related internships or fieldwork, Federal Work-Study, institutionally sponsored loans, traineeships, and tuition waivers (full and partial) available. Support available to part-time students. Financial award application deadline: 2/1. *Faculty research:* Health care administration, health care law, nursing administration and education, consumer satisfaction with health care. *Unit head:* Prof. Elaine La Monica Rigolosi, Coordinator, 212-678-4004, E-mail: ell9@columbia.edu. *Application contact:* Debbie Lesperance, Assistant Director of Admission, 212-678-3710, Fax: 212-678-4171.
Website: http://www.tc.edu/o%26l/NurseExec/

Temple University, College of Health Professions and Social Work, Department of Nursing, Philadelphia, PA 19140. Offers adult-gerontology primary care (DNP); clinical nurse leader (MSN); family-individual across the lifespan (DNP); nurse educator (MSN); nursing (MSN, DNP). *Accreditation:* AACN. Part-time programs available. *Faculty:* 9 full-time (8 women), 3 part-time/adjunct (all women). *Students:* 6 full-time (5 women), 92 part-time (78 women); includes 51 minority (34 Black or African American, non-Hispanic/ Latino; 9 Asian, non-Hispanic/Latino; 8 Hispanic/Latino), 1 international. 48 applicants, 58% accepted, 23 enrolled. In 2013, 12 master's, 9 doctorates awarded. *Degree requirements:* For master's and doctorate, evidence based practice project. *Entrance requirements:* For master's and doctorate, GRE General Test or MAT, 2 letters of reference, RN license, interview, statement of purpose, resume. Additional exam requirements/recommendations for international students: Required—TOEFL (minimum score 550 paper-based; 79 iBT). *Application deadline:* For fall admission, 2/15 priority date for domestic students, 1/15 for international students; for spring admission, 10/15 for domestic students, 9/15 for international students. Applications are processed on a rolling basis. Application fee: $60. Electronic applications accepted. *Financial support:* Federal Work-Study, scholarships/grants, traineeships, and tuition waivers available. Support available to part-time students. Financial award application deadline: 1/15. *Faculty research:* Health promotion, chronic illness, family support systems, primary care, health policy, community health services, evidence-based practice. *Total annual research expenditures:* $741,567. *Unit head:* Dr. Jane Kurz, RN, Chair, 215-707-8327, E-mail: jane.kurz@temple.edu. *Application contact:* Naseem Lodhi, Student Services Coordinator, 215-204-4618, E-mail: tunurse@temple.edu.

Tennessee Technological University, Whitson-Hester School of Nursing, Cookeville, TN 38505. Offers family nurse practitioner (MSN); informatics (MSN); nursing administration (MSN); nursing education (MSN). Part-time and evening/weekend programs available. Postbaccalaureate distance learning degree programs offered (no on-campus study). *Students:* 22 full-time (19 women), 101 part-time (94 women); includes 11 minority (5 Black or African American, non-Hispanic/Latino; 2 Asian, non-Hispanic/Latino; 1 Hispanic/Latino; 3 Two or more races, non-Hispanic/Latino). 79 applicants, 65% accepted, 38 enrolled. In 2013, 14 master's awarded. *Degree requirements:* For master's, comprehensive exam, thesis or alternative. *Entrance requirements:* Additional exam requirements/recommendations for international students: Required—TOEFL (minimum score 600 paper-based; 100 iBT), IELTS (minimum score 5.5), PTE, or TOEIC (Test of English as an International Communication). *Application deadline:* For fall admission, 8/1 for domestic students, 5/1 for international students; for spring admission, 12/1 for domestic students, 10/1 for international students. Applications are processed on a rolling basis. Application fee: $35 ($40 for international students). Electronic applications accepted. *Expenses:* Tuition, state resident: full-time $9347; part-time $465 per credit hour. Tuition, nonresident: full-time $23,635; part-time $1152 per credit hour. *Financial support:* Application deadline: 4/1. *Unit head:* Dr. Bedelia Russell, Director, 931-372-3203, Fax: 931-372-6244, E-mail: bhrussell@tntech.edu. *Application contact:* Shelia K. Kendrick, Coordinator of Graduate Studies, 931-372-3808, Fax: 931-372-3497, E-mail: skendrick@tntech.edu.

Texas A&M University–Corpus Christi, Graduate Studies and Research, College of Nursing and Health Sciences, Corpus Christi, TX 78412-5503. Offers clinical nurse specialist (MSN); family nurse practitioner (MSN); health care administration (MSN); leadership in nursing systems (MSN). *Accreditation:* AACN. Part-time and evening/ weekend programs available. *Degree requirements:* For master's, comprehensive exam, thesis (for some programs). *Entrance requirements:* For master's, GRE General Test. Additional exam requirements/recommendations for international students: Required—TOEFL. Electronic applications accepted.

Texas Christian University, Harris College of Nursing and Health Sciences, Program in Nursing, Fort Worth, TX 76129-0002. Offers advanced practice registered nurse (DNP); clinical nurse leader (MSN); clinical nurse specialist: adult/gerontology nursing (MSN); clinical nurse specialist: pediatric nursing (MSN); nursing administration (DNP); nursing education (MSN). *Accreditation:* AACN; AANA/CANAEP (one or more programs are accredited). Part-time programs available. Postbaccalaureate distance learning degree programs offered (no on-campus study). *Faculty:* 18 full-time (16 women), 1 (woman) part-time/adjunct. *Students:* 44 full-time (35 women), 46 part-time (42 women); includes 8 minority (3 Black or African American, non-Hispanic/Latino; 2 Asian, non-Hispanic/Latino; 3 Hispanic/Latino), 1 international. Average age 43. 72 applicants, 63% accepted, 36 enrolled. In 2013, 19 master's, 17 doctorates awarded. *Degree requirements:* For master's, professional project; for doctorate, capstone project. *Entrance requirements:* For master's, GRE General Test, 3 letters of reference, essay, resume, two official transcripts from every institution attended; for doctorate, APRN recognition (national certification) or master's and experience in nursing administration; 3 letters of reference; essay; resume; two official transcripts from every institution attended. Additional exam requirements/recommendations for international students: Recommended—TOEFL. *Application deadline:* For fall admission, 4/1 for domestic

students; for spring admission, 9/1 for domestic students; for summer admission, 2/1 for domestic students. Applications are processed on a rolling basis. Application fee: $60. Electronic applications accepted. *Expenses: Tuition:* Part-time $1270 per credit hour. Tuition and fees vary according to course load and program. *Financial support:* In 2013–14, 4 teaching assistantships (averaging $2,500 per year) were awarded. Financial award applicants required to submit FAFSA. *Unit head:* Dr. Kathy A. Baker, Director, Division of Nursing Graduate Studies and Scholarship, 817-257-6726, Fax: 817-257-8383, E-mail: kathy.baker@tcu.edu. *Application contact:* Mary Jane Allred, Administrative Program Specialist, 817-257-6726, Fax: 817-257-8383, E-mail: m.allred@tcu.edu.
Website: http://www.nursing.tcu.edu/graduate.asp

Texas Tech University Health Sciences Center, School of Nursing, Lubbock, TX 79430. Offers acute care nurse practitioner (MSN, Certificate); administration (MSN); advanced practice (DNP); education (MSN); executive leadership (DNP); family nurse practitioner (MSN, Certificate); geriatric nurse practitioner (MSN, Certificate); pediatric nurse practitioner (MSN, Certificate). *Accreditation:* AACN. Part-time programs available. Postbaccalaureate distance learning degree programs offered (minimal on-campus study). *Degree requirements:* For master's, thesis optional. *Entrance requirements:* For master's, minimum GPA of 3.0, 3 letters of reference, BSN, RN license; for Certificate, minimum GPA of 3.0, 3 letters of reference, RN license. Additional exam requirements/recommendations for international students: Required—TOEFL (minimum score 550 paper-based). *Faculty research:* Diabetes/obesity, nurse competency, disease management, intervention and measurements, health disparities.

Texas Woman's University, Graduate School, College of Nursing, Denton, TX 76201. Offers acute care nurse practitioner (MS); adult health clinical nurse specialist (MS); adult health nurse practitioner (MS); child health clinical nurse specialist (MS); clinical nurse leader (MS); family nurse practitioner (MS); health systems management (MS); nursing education (MS); nursing practice (DNP); nursing science (PhD); pediatric nurse practitioner (MS); women's health clinical nurse specialist (MS); women's health nurse practitioner (MS). *Accreditation:* AACN. Part-time programs available. Postbaccalaureate distance learning degree programs offered. *Faculty:* 60 full-time (59 women), 46 part-time/adjunct (39 women). *Students:* 54 full-time (49 women), 910 part-time (848 women); includes 489 minority (221 Black or African American, non-Hispanic/Latino; 11 American Indian or Alaska Native, non-Hispanic/Latino; 184 Asian, non-Hispanic/Latino; 70 Hispanic/Latino; 3 Native Hawaiian or other Pacific Islander, non-Hispanic/Latino), 16 international. Average age 38. 430 applicants, 65% accepted, 193 enrolled. In 2013, 258 master's, 22 doctorates awarded. *Degree requirements:* For master's, comprehensive exam, thesis or alternative; for doctorate, comprehensive exam, thesis/dissertation. *Entrance requirements:* For master's, GRE or MAT, minimum GPA of 3.0 on last 60 hours in undergraduate nursing degree and overall, RN license, BS in nursing, basic statistics course; for doctorate, GRE (preferred minimum score 153 [500 old version] Verbal, 144 [500 old version] Quantitative, 4 Analytical), MS in nursing, minimum preferred GPA of 3.5, RN license, statistics, 2 letters of reference, curriculum vitae, graduate nursing-theory course, graduate research course, statement of professional goals and research interests. Additional exam requirements/recommendations for international students: Required—TOEFL (minimum score 550 paper-based; 79 iBT). *Application deadline:* For fall admission, 5/1 priority date for domestic students, 3/1 for international students; for spring admission, 9/15 priority date for domestic students, 7/1 for international students. Applications are processed on a rolling basis. Application fee: $50 ($75 for international students). Electronic applications accepted. *Expenses:* Tuition, state resident: full-time $4182; part-time $233.32 per credit hour. Tuition, nonresident: full-time $10,716; part-time $595.32 per credit hour. *Financial support:* In 2013–14, 149 students received support, including 10 research assistantships (averaging $5,600 per year), 1 teaching assistantship (averaging $5,600 per year); career-related internships or fieldwork, Federal Work-Study, institutionally sponsored loans, scholarships/grants, traineeships, health care benefits, and unspecified assistantships also available. Support available to part-time students. Financial award application deadline: 3/1; financial award applicants required to submit FAFSA. *Faculty research:* Screening, prevention, and treatment for intimate partner violence; needs of adolescents during childbirth intervention; a network analysis decision tool for nurse managers (social network analysis); support for adolescents with implantable cardioverter defibrillators; informatics: nurse staffing, safety, quality, and financial data as they relate to patient care outcomes; prevention and treatment of obesity; improving infant outcomes related to premature birth. *Total annual research expenditures:* $1.7 million. *Unit head:* Dr. Gayle Roux, Interim Dean and Associate Dean for Research and Clinical Scholarship, 940-898-2401, Fax: 940-898-2437, E-mail: nursing@twu.edu. *Application contact:* Dr. Samuel Wheeler, Assistant Director of Admissions, 940-898-3188, Fax: 940-898-3081, E-mail: wheelersr@twu.edu.
Website: http://www.twu.edu/nursing/

Trident University International, College of Health Sciences, Program in Health Sciences, Cypress, CA 90630. Offers clinical research administration (MS, Certificate); emergency and disaster management (MS, Certificate); environmental health science (Certificate); health care administration (PhD); health care management (MS), including health informatics; health education (MS, Certificate); health informatics (Certificate); health sciences (PhD); international health (MS); international health: educator or researcher option (PhD); international health: practitioner option (PhD); law and expert witness studies (MS, Certificate); public health (MS); quality assurance (Certificate). Part-time and evening/weekend programs available. Postbaccalaureate distance learning degree programs offered (no on-campus study). *Degree requirements:* For doctorate, comprehensive exam, thesis/dissertation, defense of dissertation. *Entrance requirements:* For master's, minimum GPA of 2.5 (students with GPA 3.0 or greater may transfer up to 30% of graduate level credits); for doctorate, minimum GPA of 3.4, curriculum vitae, course work in research methods or statistics. Additional exam requirements/recommendations for international students: Required—TOEFL. Electronic applications accepted.

Union University, School of Nursing, Jackson, TN 38305-3697. Offers executive leadership (DNP); nurse anesthesia (DNP); nurse anesthetist (PMC); nurse practitioner (DNP); nursing education (MSN, PMC). *Accreditation:* AACN; AANA/CANAEP. *Degree requirements:* For master's, thesis or alternative. *Entrance requirements:* For master's, GRE, 3 letters of reference, bachelor's degree in nursing, minimum GPA of 3.0. Additional exam requirements/recommendations for international students: Required—TOEFL (minimum score 560 paper-based). Electronic applications accepted. *Faculty research:* Children's health, occupational rehabilitation, informatics, health promotion.

United States University, School of Nursing, Cypress, CA 90630. Offers administrator (MSN); educator (MSN).

Universidad Metropolitana, School of Health Sciences, Department of Nursing, San Juan, PR 00928-1150. Offers case management (Certificate); nursing (MSN); oncology nursing (Certificate).

University at Buffalo, the State University of New York, Graduate School, School of Nursing, Buffalo, NY 14214. Offers adult gerontology nurse practitioner (DNP); family nurse practitioner (DNP); health care systems and leadership (MS); nurse anesthetist (DNP); nursing (PhD); nursing education (Certificate); psychiatric/mental health nurse practitioner (DNP). *Accreditation:* AACN; AANA/CANAEP (one or more programs are accredited). Part-time programs available. Postbaccalaureate distance learning degree programs offered (no on-campus study). *Faculty:* 24 full-time (21 women), 2 part-time/adjunct (1 woman). *Students:* 80 full-time (60 women), 97 part-time (84 women); includes 35 minority (20 Black or African American, non-Hispanic/Latino; 2 American Indian or Alaska Native, non-Hispanic/Latino; 9 Asian, non-Hispanic/Latino; 1 Hispanic/Latino; 3 Native Hawaiian or other Pacific Islander, non-Hispanic/Latino). 118 applicants, 67% accepted, 58 enrolled. In 2013, 41 master's, 15 doctorates awarded. *Degree requirements:* For master's, thesis optional; for doctorate, comprehensive exam (for some programs), capstone (for DNP), dissertation (for PhD). *Entrance requirements:* For doctorate, GRE or MAT, minimum GPA of 3.0 (3.25 for PhD), RN license, BS or MS in nursing, 3 references, writing sample; for Certificate, interview, minimum GPA of 3.0 or GRE General Test, RN license, MS in nursing. Additional exam requirements/recommendations for international students: Required—TOEFL (minimum score 550 paper-based; 79 iBT), IELTS (minimum score 6.5). *Application deadline:* For fall admission, 7/1 for domestic students, 4/1 for international students; for spring admission, 12/1 for domestic students, 10/1 for international students; for summer admission, 4/1 for domestic students. Application fee: $75. Electronic applications accepted. *Financial support:* In 2013–14, 80 students received support, including 2 fellowships with full and partial tuition reimbursements available (averaging $17,000 per year), 7 research assistantships with full and partial tuition reimbursements available (averaging $10,600 per year), 7 teaching assistantships with full and partial tuition reimbursements available (averaging $10,600 per year); scholarships/grants, traineeships, health care benefits, and unspecified assistantships also available. Financial award application deadline: 3/15; financial award applicants required to submit FAFSA. *Faculty research:* Oncology, palliative care, gerontology, addictions, mental health, community wellness, sleep, workforce, care of underserved populations, quality and safety, person-centered care, adolescent health. *Total annual research expenditures:* $1.1 million. *Unit head:* Dr. Marsha L. Lewis, Dean and Professor, 716-829-2533, Fax: 716-829-2566, E-mail: ubnursingdean@buffalo.edu. *Application contact:* Dr. David J. Lang, Director of Student Affairs, 716-829-2537, Fax: 716-829-2067, E-mail: nursing@buffalo.edu.
Website: http://nursing.buffalo.edu/

University of Central Arkansas, Graduate School, College of Health and Behavioral Sciences, Department of Nursing, Conway, AR 72035-0001. Offers adult nurse practitioner (PMC); clinical nurse leader (PMC); clinical nurse specialist (MSN); family nurse practitioner (PMC); nurse educator (PMC); nurse practitioner (MSN). *Accreditation:* AACN. Part-time and evening/weekend programs available. Postbaccalaureate distance learning degree programs offered (minimal on-campus study). *Degree requirements:* For master's, comprehensive exam, thesis optional, clinicals. *Entrance requirements:* For master's, GRE General Test, minimum GPA of 2.7. Additional exam requirements/recommendations for international students: Required—TOEFL (minimum score 550 paper-based; 80 iBT). Electronic applications accepted. *Expenses:* Contact institution.

University of Cincinnati, Graduate School, College of Nursing, Cincinnati, OH 45221-0038. Offers clinical nurse specialist (MSN), including adult health, community health, neonatal, nursing administration, occupational health, pediatric health, psychiatric nursing, women's health; nurse anesthesia (MSN); nurse midwifery (MSN); nurse practitioner (MSN), including acute care, ambulatory care, family, family/psychiatric, women's health; nursing (PhD); MBA/MSN. *Accreditation:* AACN; AANA/CANAEP (one or more programs are accredited); ACNM/ACME. Part-time programs available. Postbaccalaureate distance learning degree programs offered (no on-campus study). Terminal master's awarded for partial completion of doctoral program. *Degree requirements:* For master's, thesis or alternative; for doctorate, comprehensive exam, thesis/dissertation. *Entrance requirements:* For master's and doctorate, GRE General Test. Additional exam requirements/recommendations for international students: Required—TOEFL (minimum score 520 paper-based). Electronic applications accepted. *Faculty research:* Substance abuse, injury and violence, symptom management.

University of Colorado Denver, College of Nursing, Aurora, CO 80045. Offers adult clinical nurse specialist (MS); adult nurse practitioner (MS); family nurse practitioner (MS); family psychiatric mental health nurse practitioner (MS); health care informatics (MS); nurse-midwifery (MS); nursing (DNP, PhD); nursing leadership and health care systems (MS); pediatric nurse practitioner (MS); special studies (MS); women's health (MS); MS/PhD. *Accreditation:* ACNM/ACME (one or more programs are accredited). Part-time and evening/weekend programs available. Postbaccalaureate distance learning degree programs offered (minimal on-campus study). *Faculty:* 74 full-time (65 women), 58 part-time/adjunct (56 women). *Students:* 351 full-time (327 women), 138 part-time (125 women); includes 79 minority (12 Black or African American, non-Hispanic/Latino; 9 American Indian or Alaska Native, non-Hispanic/Latino; 13 Asian, non-Hispanic/Latino; 32 Hispanic/Latino; 2 Native Hawaiian or other Pacific Islander, non-Hispanic/Latino; 11 Two or more races, non-Hispanic/Latino), 7 international. Average age 33. 354 applicants, 43% accepted, 109 enrolled. In 2013, 108 master's, 28 doctorates awarded. Terminal master's awarded for partial completion of doctoral program. *Degree requirements:* For master's, thesis optional; for doctorate, comprehensive exam, thesis/dissertation, 42 credits of coursework. *Entrance requirements:* For master's, GRE if cumulative undergraduate GPA is less than 3.0, undergraduate nursing degree from NLNAC- or CCNE-accredited school or university; completion of research and statistics courses with minimum grade of C; copy of current and unencumbered nursing license; for doctorate, GRE, bachelor's and/or master's degrees in nursing from NLN- or CCNE-accredited institution; portfolio; minimum undergraduate GPA of 3.0, graduate 3.5; graduate-level intermediate statistics and master's-level nursing theory courses with minimum B grade; interview. Additional exam requirements/recommendations for international students: Required—TOEFL (minimum score 560 paper-based; 83 iBT). *Application deadline:* For fall admission, 2/15 for domestic students, 1/15 for international students; for spring admission, 7/1 for domestic students, 6/1 for international students. Application fee: $50 ($75 for international students). Electronic applications accepted. *Expenses:* Contact institution. *Financial support:* In 2013–14, 113 students received support. Fellowships, research assistantships, teaching assistantships, Federal Work-Study, institutionally sponsored loans, scholarships/grants, traineeships, and unspecified assistantships available. Support available to part-time students. Financial award application deadline: 4/1; financial award applicants required to submit FAFSA. *Faculty research:* Biological and behavioral phenomena in pregnancy and postpartum; patterns of glycemia during the insulin resistance of pregnancy; obesity, gestational diabetes, and relationship to neonatal adiposity; men's awareness and knowledge of male breast cancer; cognitive-behavioral therapy for chronic insomnia after breast cancer treatment; massage therapy for the treatment of tension-type headaches. *Total annual research expenditures:* $5.9 million. *Unit head:* Dr. Sarah Thompson, Dean, 303-724-1679, E-mail: sarah.a.thompson@ucdenver.edu. *Application contact:* Judy Campbell, Graduate Programs Coordinator, 303-724-8503, E-mail: judy.campbell@ucdenver.edu.
Website: http://www.ucdenver.edu/academics/colleges/nursing/Pages/default.aspx

University of Delaware, College of Health Sciences, School of Nursing, Newark, DE 19716. Offers adult nurse practitioner (MSN, PMC); cardiopulmonary clinical nurse specialist (MSN, PMC); cardiopulmonary clinical nurse specialist/adult nurse practitioner (MSN, PMC); family nurse practitioner (MSN, PMC); gerontology clinical nurse specialist

(MSN, PMC); gerontology clinical nurse specialist geriatric nurse practitioner (PMC); gerontology clinical nurse specialist/geriatric nurse practitioner (MSN); health services administration (MSN, PMC); nursing of children clinical nurse specialist (MSN, PMC); nursing of children clinical nurse specialist/pediatric nurse practitioner (MSN, PMC); oncology/immune deficiency clinical nurse specialist (MSN, PMC); oncology/immune deficiency clinical nurse specialist/adult nurse practitioner (MSN, PMC); perinatal/women's health clinical nurse specialist (MSN, PMC); perinatal/women's health clinical nurse specialist/women's health nurse practitioner (MSN, PMC); psychiatric nursing clinical nurse specialist (MSN, PMC). *Accreditation:* AACN. Part-time and evening/weekend programs available. Postbaccalaureate distance learning degree programs offered (minimal on-campus study). *Degree requirements:* For master's, thesis optional. *Entrance requirements:* For master's, BSN, interview, RN license. Electronic applications accepted. *Faculty research:* Marriage and chronic illness, health promotion, congestive heart failure patient outcomes, school nursing, diabetes in children, culture, health disparities, cardiovascular, prison nursing, oncology, public policy, child obesity, smoking and teen pregnancy, blood pressure measurements, men's health.

University of Hawaii at Manoa, Graduate Division, School of Nursing and Dental Hygiene, Honolulu, HI 96822. Offers clinical nurse specialist (MS), including adult health, community mental health; nurse practitioner (MS), including adult health, community mental health, family nurse practitioner; nursing (PhD, Graduate Certificate); nursing administration (MS). *Accreditation:* AACN. Part-time programs available. Postbaccalaureate distance learning degree programs offered (minimal on-campus study). *Degree requirements:* For master's, thesis optional; for doctorate, comprehensive exam, thesis/dissertation. *Entrance requirements:* For master's, Hawaii RN license. Additional exam requirements/recommendations for international students: Required—TOEFL (minimum score 580 paper-based; 92 iBT), IELTS (minimum score 5). *Expenses:* Contact institution.

University of Houston–Victoria, School of Nursing, Victoria, TX 77901-4450. Offers family nurse practitioner (MSN); nursing administration (MSN); nursing education (MSN). *Accreditation:* AACN. *Faculty:* 13 full-time (12 women). *Students:* 27 full-time (23 women), 42 part-time (35 women); includes 33 minority (18 Black or African American, non-Hispanic/Latino; 8 Asian, non-Hispanic/Latino; 7 Hispanic/Latino), 7 international. *Entrance requirements:* For master's, GRE or MAT, minimum GPA of 3.0 in last 60 hours of academic course work, valid Texas RN licensure, 2 letters of recommendation. *Application deadline:* For fall admission, 7/15 for domestic students, 6/1 for international students. Applications are processed on a rolling basis. Electronic applications accepted. *Expenses:* Tuition, state resident: full-time $4534; part-time $251 per credit hour. Tuition, nonresident: full-time $10,906; part-time $606 per contact hour. *Required fees:* $68 per semester hour. Tuition and fees vary according to course load. *Financial support:* Federal Work-Study, scholarships/grants, and unspecified assistantships available. Support available to part-time students. Financial award application deadline: 4/15. *Unit head:* Dr. Kathryn Tart, Dean, 361-570-4295, E-mail: neilld@uhv.edu. *Application contact:* Tammy Whatley, Senior Recruitment Coordinator, 361-570-4297, E-mail: whatleyt@uhv.edu.
Website: http://www.uhv.edu/nursing/

University of Illinois at Chicago, Graduate College, College of Nursing, Program in Nursing, Chicago, IL 60607-7128. Offers acute care clinical nurse specialist (MS); acute care nurse practitioner (MS); administrative nursing leadership (Certificate); administrative studies in nursing (MS); adult nurse practitioner (MS); adult/geriatric nurse practitioner (MS); advanced community health nurse specialist (MS); family nurse practitioner (MS); geriatric clinical nurse specialist (MS); geriatric nurse practitioner (MS); mental health clinical nurse specialist (MS); mental health nurse practitioner (MS); nurse midwifery (MS); occupational health/advanced community health nurse specialist (MS); occupational health/family nurse practitioner (MS); pediatric clinical nurse specialist (MS); pediatric nurse practitioner (MS); perinatal clinical nurse specialist (MS); school/advanced community health nurse specialist (MS); school/family nurse practitioner (MS); women's health nurse practitioner (MS). *Accreditation:* AACN. Part-time programs available. *Faculty:* 16 full-time (14 women). *Students:* 393 full-time (361 women), 410 part-time (367 women); includes 198 minority (48 Black or African American, non-Hispanic/Latino; 1 American Indian or Alaska Native, non-Hispanic/Latino; 64 Asian, non-Hispanic/Latino; 71 Hispanic/Latino; 2 Native Hawaiian or other Pacific Islander, non-Hispanic/Latino; 12 Two or more races, non-Hispanic/Latino), 29 international. Average age 32. 396 applicants, 62% accepted, 177 enrolled. In 2013, 184 master's awarded. *Degree requirements:* For master's, thesis or alternative. *Entrance requirements:* For master's, GRE General Test, minimum GPA of 2.75. Additional exam requirements/recommendations for international students: Required—TOEFL. *Application deadline:* For fall admission, 5/15 for domestic students, 2/15 for international students; for spring admission, 11/1 for domestic students, 7/15 for international students. Applications are processed on a rolling basis. Application fee: $40 ($50 for international students). Electronic applications accepted. *Expenses:* Tuition, state resident: full-time $11,066; part-time $3689 per term. Tuition, nonresident: full-time $23,064; part-time $7688 per term. *Required fees:* $3004; $1190 per term. Tuition and fees vary according to course level and program. *Financial support:* Fellowships with full tuition reimbursements, research assistantships with full tuition reimbursements, teaching assistantships with full tuition reimbursements, career-related internships or fieldwork, Federal Work-Study, institutionally sponsored loans, scholarships/grants, traineeships, tuition waivers (full and partial), and unspecified assistantships available. Support available to part-time students. Financial award application deadline: 3/1; financial award applicants required to submit FAFSA. *Unit head:* Dr. Terri E. Weaver, Dean, 312-996-7808, E-mail: teweaver@uic.edu. *Application contact:* Receptionist, 312-413-2550, E-mail: gradcoll@uic.edu.

University of Indianapolis, Graduate Programs, School of Nursing, Indianapolis, IN 46227-3697. Offers advanced practice nursing (DNP); family nurse practitioner (MSN); gerontological nurse practitioner (MSN); neonatal nurse practitioner (MSN); nurse-midwifery (MSN); nursing (MSN); nursing and health systems leadership (MSN); nursing education (MSN); women's health nurse practitioner (MSN); MBA/MSN. *Accreditation:* AACN; ACNM. *Faculty:* 5 full-time (4 women), 1 part-time/adjunct (0 women). *Students:* 15 full-time (14 women), 285 part-time (270 women); includes 42 minority (24 Black or African American, non-Hispanic/Latino; 6 Asian, non-Hispanic/Latino; 3 Hispanic/Latino; 9 Two or more races, non-Hispanic/Latino), 2 international. Average age 35. In 2013, 46 master's awarded. *Entrance requirements:* For master's, minimum GPA of 3.0, interview, letters of recommendation, resume, IN nursing license, 1 year of professional practice; for doctorate, graduate of NLNAC- or CCNE-accredited nursing program; MSN or MA with nursing major and minimum cumulative GPA of 3.25; unencumbered RN license with eligibility for licensure in Indiana; completion of graduate-level statistics course within last 5 years with minimum grade of B; resume; essay; official transcripts from all academic institutions. Additional exam requirements/recommendations for international students: Required—TOEFL (minimum score 550 paper-based). *Application deadline:* For fall admission, 8/1 for domestic students; for winter admission, 12/15 for domestic students; for spring admission, 4/15 for domestic students. Applications are processed on a rolling basis. Application fee: $60. Electronic applications accepted. *Expenses: Tuition:* Full-time $5436; part-time $810 per credit hour. *Financial support:* Federal Work-Study available. *Unit head:* Dr. Anne Thomas, Dean, 317-788-3206, E-mail: athomas@uindy.edu. *Application contact:* Sueann Meagher, Graduate Administrative Assistant, 317-788-8005, Fax: 317-788-3542, E-mail: meaghers@uindy.edu.
Website: http://nursing.uindy.edu/

The University of Kansas, University of Kansas Medical Center, School of Nursing, Kansas City, KS 66160. Offers adult/gerontological clinical nurse specialist (PMC); adult/gerontological nurse practitioner (PMC); clinical research management (PMC); health care informatics (PMC); health professions educator (PMC); nurse midwife (PMC); nursing (MS, DNP, PhD); organizational leadership (PMC); psychiatric/mental health nurse practitioner (PMC); public health nursing (PMC). *Accreditation:* AACN; ACNM/ACME. Part-time programs available. Postbaccalaureate distance learning degree programs offered (minimal on-campus study). *Faculty:* 59. *Students:* 55 full-time (53 women), 323 part-time (303 women); includes 57 minority (23 Black or African American, non-Hispanic/Latino; 14 Asian, non-Hispanic/Latino; 16 Hispanic/Latino; 1 Native Hawaiian or other Pacific Islander, non-Hispanic/Latino; 3 Two or more races, non-Hispanic/Latino), 1 international. Average age 38. 113 applicants, 59% accepted, 61 enrolled. In 2013, 77 master's, 18 doctorates, 11 other advanced degrees awarded. Terminal master's awarded for partial completion of doctoral program. *Degree requirements:* For master's, comprehensive exam, thesis (for some programs), general oral exam; for doctorate, variable foreign language requirement, thesis/dissertation, comprehensive oral exam (for DNP); comprehensive written and oral exam (for PhD). *Entrance requirements:* For master's, bachelor's degree in nursing, minimum GPA of 3.0, 1 year of clinical experience, RN license in KS and MO; for doctorate, GRE General Test, bachelor's degree in nursing, minimum GPA of 3.5, RN license in KS and MO. Additional exam requirements/recommendations for international students: Required—TOEFL. *Application deadline:* For fall admission, 4/1 for domestic and international students; for spring admission, 9/1 for domestic and international students. Application fee: $60. Electronic applications accepted. *Financial support:* Research assistantships with full and partial tuition reimbursements, teaching assistantships with full and partial tuition reimbursements, scholarships/grants, and traineeships available. Financial award application deadline: 3/1; financial award applicants required to submit FAFSA. *Faculty research:* Breastfeeding practices of teen mothers, national database of nursing quality indicators, caregiving of families of patients using technology in the home, simulation in nursing education, diaphragm fatigue. *Total annual research expenditures:* $6.4 million. *Unit head:* Dr. Karen L. Miller, Dean, 913-588-1601, Fax: 913-588-1660, E-mail: kmiller@kumc.edu. *Application contact:* Dr. Pamela K. Barnes, Associate Dean, Student Affairs, 913-588-1619, Fax: 913-588-1615, E-mail: pbarnes2@kumc.edu.
Website: http://nursing.kumc.edu

University of Mary, School of Health Sciences, Division of Nursing, Bismarck, ND 58504-9652. Offers family nurse practitioner (MSN); nurse administrator (MSN); nursing educator (MSN). *Accreditation:* AACN. Part-time and evening/weekend programs available. Postbaccalaureate distance learning degree programs offered (minimal on-campus study). *Degree requirements:* For master's, comprehensive exam (for some programs), thesis (for some programs), internship (family nurse practitioner), teaching practice. *Entrance requirements:* For master's, minimum GPA of 2.75 in nursing, interview, letters of recommendation, criminal background check, immunizations, statement of professional goals. Additional exam requirements/recommendations for international students: Required—TOEFL (minimum score 500 paper-based; 71 iBT). Electronic applications accepted. *Faculty research:* Gerontology issues, rural nursing, health policy, primary care, women's health.

University of Mary Hardin-Baylor, Graduate Studies in Nursing, Belton, TX 76513. Offers clinical nurse leader (MSN); family nurse practitioner (MSN, Post-Master's Certificate); nurse educator (Post-Master's Certificate); nursing education (MSN). *Accreditation:* AACN. Part-time and evening/weekend programs available. *Faculty:* 6 full-time (all women), 4 part-time/adjunct (3 women). *Students:* 44 full-time (all women), 6 part-time (all women); includes 13 minority (5 Black or African American, non-Hispanic/Latino; 2 Asian, non-Hispanic/Latino; 6 Hispanic/Latino). Average age 33. 57 applicants, 67% accepted, 31 enrolled. In 2013, 17 master's awarded. *Degree requirements:* For master's, practicum. *Entrance requirements:* For master's, full-time RN for 1 year, BSN, minimum GPA of 3.0 in last 60 hours of undergraduate program, two letters of recommendation. Additional exam requirements/recommendations for international students: Required—TOEFL (minimum score 550 paper-based; 80 iBT), IELTS (minimum score 6). *Application deadline:* For fall admission, 4/15 for domestic students, 4/15 priority date for international students; for spring admission, 11/1 for domestic students, 10/15 priority date for international students. Applications are processed on a rolling basis. Application fee: $35 ($135 for international students). Electronic applications accepted. *Expenses: Tuition:* Full-time $14,130; part-time $785 per credit hour. *Required fees:* $1350; $75 per credit hour. $50 per term. *Financial support:* Applicants required to submit FAFSA. *Unit head:* Dr. Carrie Johnson, Associate Professor/Director, Master of Science in Nursing Programs, 254-295-4178, E-mail: cjohnson@umhb.edu. *Application contact:* Melissa Ford, Director of Graduate Admissions, 254-295-4020, Fax: 254-295-5038, E-mail: mford@umhb.edu.
Website: http://graduate.umhb.edu/nursing/

University of Maryland, Baltimore, Graduate School, School of Nursing, Master's Program in Nursing, Baltimore, MD 21201. Offers community health nursing (MS); gerontological nursing (MS); maternal-child nursing (MS); medical-surgical nursing (MS); nurse-midwifery education (MS); nursing administration (MS); nursing education (MS); nursing health policy (MS); primary care nursing (MS); psychiatric nursing (MS); MS/MBA. MS/MBA offered jointly with University of Baltimore. *Accreditation:* AACN; AANA/CANAEP. Part-time programs available. *Students:* 345 full-time (297 women), 508 part-time (469 women); includes 288 minority (152 Black or African American, non-Hispanic/Latino; 2 American Indian or Alaska Native, non-Hispanic/Latino; 72 Asian, non-Hispanic/Latino; 32 Hispanic/Latino; 1 Native Hawaiian or other Pacific Islander, non-Hispanic/Latino; 29 Two or more races, non-Hispanic/Latino), 13 international. Average age 33. 971 applicants, 34% accepted, 253 enrolled. In 2013, 308 master's awarded. *Degree requirements:* For master's, comprehensive exam (for some programs), thesis or alternative. *Entrance requirements:* For master's, minimum GPA of 2.75, course work in statistics, BS in nursing. Additional exam requirements/recommendations for international students: Required—TOEFL (minimum score 550 paper-based; 80 iBT) or IELTS (minimum score 7). *Application deadline:* For fall admission, 2/1 for domestic students, 1/15 for international students. Application fee: $75. Electronic applications accepted. *Financial support:* Fellowships, research assistantships, teaching assistantships, career-related internships or fieldwork, and traineeships available. Support available to part-time students. Financial award application deadline: 2/15; financial award applicants required to submit FAFSA. *Unit head:* Dr. Jane Kapustin, Assistant Dean, 410-706-6741, Fax: 410-706-4231. *Application contact:* Marjorie Fass, Admissions Director, 410-706-0501, Fax: 410-706-7238.

University of Massachusetts Amherst, Graduate School, School of Nursing, Amherst, MA 01003. Offers adult gerontology primary care (DNP); clinical nurse leader (MS); family nurse practitioner (DNP); nursing (PhD); public health nurse leader (DNP). *Accreditation:* AACN. Part-time programs available. Postbaccalaureate distance learning degree programs offered (minimal on-campus study). *Faculty:* 16 full-time (15 women). *Students:* 74 full-time (61 women), 161 part-time (149 women); includes 62

minority (31 Black or African American, non-Hispanic/Latino; 9 Asian, non-Hispanic/Latino; 19 Hispanic/Latino; 3 Two or more races, non-Hispanic/Latino), 6 international. Average age 40. 133 applicants, 80% accepted, 68 enrolled. In 2013, 9 master's, 32 doctorates awarded. Terminal master's awarded for partial completion of doctoral program. *Degree requirements:* For master's, thesis optional; for doctorate, comprehensive exam, thesis/dissertation. *Entrance requirements:* Additional exam requirements/recommendations for international students: Required—TOEFL (minimum score 550 paper-based; 80 iBT), IELTS (minimum score 6.5). *Application deadline:* For fall admission, 12/15 for domestic and international students. Applications are processed on a rolling basis. Application fee: $75. Electronic applications accepted. *Financial support:* Fellowships with full and partial tuition reimbursements, research assistantships with full and partial tuition reimbursements, teaching assistantships with full and partial tuition reimbursements, career-related internships or fieldwork, Federal Work-Study, scholarships/grants, traineeships, health care benefits, tuition waivers (full and partial), and unspecified assistantships available. Support available to part-time students. Financial award application deadline: 2/1. *Faculty research:* Health of older adults and their caretakers, mental health of individuals and families, health of children and adolescents, power and decision-making, transcultural health. *Unit head:* Dr. Stephen J. Cavanagh, Dean, 413-545-2703, Fax: 413-577-2550, E-mail: dean@nursing.umass.edu. *Application contact:* Lindsay DeSantis, Supervisor of Admissions, 413-545-0722, Fax: 413-577-0010, E-mail: gradadm@grad.umass.edu.
Website: http://www.umass.edu/nursing/

University of Massachusetts Dartmouth, Graduate School, College of Nursing, Programs in Nursing, North Dartmouth, MA 02747-2300. Offers adult gerontology primary care nurse practitioner (DNP); adult health clinical nurse specialist (DNP); adult health/adult nurse practitioner (MS); adult health/advanced practice (MS); adult health/nurse educator (MS); adult health/nurse manager (MS); adult nurse practitioner (PMC); community health nurse specialist (DNP); community nursing/advanced practice (MS); community nursing/nurse educator (MS); community nursing/nurse manager (MS); individualized nursing (PMC); nursing (MS, PhD); nursing practice (DNP). Part-time programs available. *Faculty:* 25 full-time (all women), 45 part-time/adjunct (44 women). *Students:* 103 part-time (95 women); includes 10 minority (4 Black or African American, non-Hispanic/Latino; 2 Asian, non-Hispanic/Latino; 4 Hispanic/Latino). Average age 40. 49 applicants, 92% accepted, 33 enrolled. In 2013, 25 master's, 1 doctorate, 2 other advanced degrees awarded. *Degree requirements:* For master's, thesis; for doctorate, comprehensive exam, thesis/dissertation, project (for DNP only). *Entrance requirements:* For master's, statement of purpose (minimum of 300 words), resume, 3 letters of recommendation, official transcripts, copy of RN license; for doctorate, GRE (for PhD), statement of purpose (minimum of 300 words), resume, 3 letters of recommendation, official transcripts, copy of RN license, scholarly writing sample (minimum 10 pages for PhD). Additional exam requirements/recommendations for international students: Required—TOEFL (minimum score 533 paper-based; 72 iBT). *Application deadline:* For fall admission, 2/15 priority date for domestic and international students. Applications are processed on a rolling basis. Application fee: $60. Electronic applications accepted. *Expenses:* Tuition, state resident: full-time $2071; part-time $86.29 per credit. Tuition, nonresident: full-time $8099; part-time $337.46 per credit. Tuition and fees vary according to course load and reciprocity agreements. *Financial support:* In 2013–14, 5 teaching assistantships with full and partial tuition reimbursements (averaging $7,500 per year) were awarded; Federal Work-Study and unspecified assistantships also available. Support available to part-time students. Financial award application deadline: 3/1; financial award applicants required to submit FAFSA. *Faculty research:* Pathophysiology, aging with spinal cord injury, relational ontology, severe mental illness, patient care. *Total annual research expenditures:* $1,000. *Unit head:* Kerry Fater, Graduate Program Director for Nursing Master's Programs, 508-999-8525, Fax: 508-999-9127, E-mail: kfater@umassd.edu. *Application contact:* Steven Briggs, Director of Marketing and Recruitment for Graduate Studies, 508-999-8604, Fax: 508-999-8183, E-mail: graduate@umassd.edu.
Website: http://www.umassd.edu/nursing/graduateprograms

University of Massachusetts Lowell, College of Health Sciences, School of Nursing, DNP Program, Lowell, MA 01854-2881. Offers DNP.

University of Massachusetts Worcester, Graduate School of Nursing, Worcester, MA 01655-0115. Offers advanced practice nursing (DNP); family nurse practitioner (MS); gerontological adult acute care nurse practitioner (MS, Post Master's Certificate); gerontological adult primary care nurse practitioner (Post Master's Certificate); gerontological primary care nurse practitioner (MS); leadership (DNP); nurse educator (MS, Post Master's Certificate); nursing (PhD). *Accreditation:* AACN. *Faculty:* 19 full-time (17 women), 40 part-time/adjunct (33 women). *Students:* 153 full-time (129 women), 35 part-time (28 women); includes 30 minority (18 Black or African American, non-Hispanic/Latino; 7 Asian, non-Hispanic/Latino; 5 Hispanic/Latino). Average age 34. 254 applicants, 31% accepted, 57 enrolled. In 2013, 50 master's, 4 doctorates, 2 other advanced degrees awarded. *Degree requirements:* For doctorate, thesis/dissertation (for some programs), comprehensive exam (for PhD); capstone project and manuscript (for DNP). *Entrance requirements:* For master's, GRE General Test, bachelor's degree in nursing, course work in statistics, unrestricted Massachusetts license as registered nurse; for doctorate, GRE General Test, bachelor's or master's degree; for Post Master's Certificate, GRE General Test, MS in nursing. Additional exam requirements/recommendations for international students: Required—TOEFL. *Application deadline:* For fall admission, 12/1 priority date for domestic students. Applications are processed on a rolling basis. Application fee: $60. Electronic applications accepted. *Expenses:* Contact institution. *Financial support:* In 2013–14, 43 students received support. Institutionally sponsored loans, scholarships/grants, traineeships, and tuition waivers available. Support available to part-time students. Financial award application deadline: 5/16; financial award applicants required to submit FAFSA. *Faculty research:* Decision-making of partners and men with prostate cancer, coinfection (HIV and Hepatitis C) and treatment decisions, parent management of children with Type 1 diabetes, health literacy and discharge planning, Ghanaian women and self-care. *Total annual research expenditures:* $1.5 million. *Unit head:* Dr. Paulette Seymour-Route, Dean, 508-856-5801, Fax: 508-856-6552, E-mail: paulette.seymour-route@umassmed.edu. *Application contact:* Diane Brescia, Admissions Coordinator, 508-856-3488, Fax: 508-856-5851, E-mail: diane.brescia@umassmed.edu.
Website: http://www.umassmed.edu/gsn/

University of Memphis, Loewenberg School of Nursing, Memphis, TN 38152. Offers advance practice-family nurse practitioner (MSN); executive nursing leadership (MSN); nursing (Graduate Certificate); nursing administration (MSN); nursing education (MSN); nursing informatics (MSN). *Accreditation:* AACN. Part-time and evening/weekend programs available. Postbaccalaureate distance learning degree programs offered. *Faculty:* 18 full-time (16 women), 5 part-time/adjunct (0 women). *Students:* 23 full-time (21 women), 240 part-time (214 women); includes 112 minority (100 Black or African American, non-Hispanic/Latino; 9 Asian, non-Hispanic/Latino; 1 Hispanic/Latino; 2 Two or more races, non-Hispanic/Latino), 1 international. Average age 35. 176 applicants, 38% accepted, 25 enrolled. In 2013, 47 master's, 2 other advanced degrees awarded. *Degree requirements:* For master's, comprehensive exam, thesis optional, scholarly project; completion of clinical practicum hours. *Entrance requirements:* For master's, NCLEX Exam, interview. Additional exam requirements/recommendations for international students: Required—TOEFL (minimum score 550 paper-based; 79 iBT). *Application deadline:* For fall admission, 2/15 for domestic and international students; for spring admission, 10/1 for domestic and international students. Application fee: $35 ($60 for international students). *Financial support:* In 2013–14, 147 students received support. Federal Work-Study and scholarships/grants available. Financial award application deadline: 2/15; financial award applicants required to submit FAFSA. *Faculty research:* Technology in nursing, nurse retention, cultural competence, health policy, health access. *Total annual research expenditures:* $560,619. *Unit head:* Dr. Robert Koch, Associate Dean, 901-678-3908, Fax: 901-678-4907, E-mail: rakoch@memphis.edu. *Application contact:* Dr. Karen Weddle-West, Information Contact, 901-678-2531, Fax: 901-678-5023, E-mail: gradsch@memphis.edu.
Website: http://www.memphis.edu/nursing

University of Michigan, Rackham Graduate School, School of Nursing, Ann Arbor, MI 48109. Offers acute care pediatric nurse practitioner (MS); adult-gerontology acute care clinical nurse specialist (MS); adult-gerontology acute care nurse practitioner (MS); adult-gerontology primary care nurse practitioner (MS); health systems, nursing leadership, and effectiveness science (MS); nurse midwife (MS); nurse midwife and family nurse practitioner (MS); nurse midwife and primary care pediatric nurse practitioner (MS); nursing (DNP, PhD, Post Master's Certificate); primary care family nurse practitioner (MS); primary care pediatric nurse practitioner (MS). *Accreditation:* AACN; ACNM/ACME (one or more programs are accredited). Part-time programs available. Postbaccalaureate distance learning degree programs offered (minimal on-campus study). Terminal master's awarded for partial completion of doctoral program. *Degree requirements:* For doctorate, thesis/dissertation. *Application deadline:* For fall admission, 2/1 for domestic students; for winter admission, 5/1 for domestic students; for spring admission, 11/1 for domestic students. Applications are processed on a rolling basis. Electronic applications accepted. Tuition and fees vary according to course level, course load, degree level, program and student level. *Financial support:* Fellowships with full and partial tuition reimbursements, research assistantships with full and partial tuition reimbursements, teaching assistantships with full tuition reimbursements, Federal Work-Study, institutionally sponsored loans, scholarships/grants, traineeships, and tuition waivers (partial) available. Support available to part-time students. *Faculty research:* Preparation of clinical nurse researchers, biobehavior, women's health, health promotion, substance abuse, psychobiology of menopause, fertility, obesity, health care systems. *Unit head:* Dr. Kathleen Potempa, Dean, 734-764-7185, Fax: 734-764-7186. *Application contact:* James Diesing, Graduate Recruiting and Admissions Coordinator, 734-615-4739, E-mail: sn-osams@umich.edu.
Website: http://www.nursing.umich.edu/

University of Minnesota, Twin Cities Campus, Graduate School, School of Nursing, Program in Nursing and Health Care Systems Administration, Minneapolis, MN 55455-0213. Offers MS. *Accreditation:* AACN. Part-time programs available. *Degree requirements:* For master's, final oral exam, project or thesis. *Entrance requirements:* Additional exam requirements/recommendations for international students: Required—TOEFL (minimum score 586 paper-based).

University of Missouri, Graduate School, Sinclair School of Nursing, Columbia, MO 65211. Offers adult-gerontology clinical nurse specialist (DNP, Certificate); family nurse practitioner (DNP); family psychiatric and mental health nurse practitioner (DNP); nursing (MS, PhD); nursing leadership and innovations in health care (DNP); pediatric clinical nurse specialist (DNP, Certificate); pediatric nurse practitioner (DNP). *Accreditation:* AACN. Part-time programs available. *Faculty:* 20 full-time (18 women), 6 part-time/adjunct (all women). *Students:* 60 full-time (58 women), 232 part-time (211 women); includes 24 minority (9 Black or African American, non-Hispanic/Latino; 4 American Indian or Alaska Native, non-Hispanic/Latino; 2 Asian, non-Hispanic/Latino; 6 Hispanic/Latino; 3 Two or more races, non-Hispanic/Latino), 4 international. Average age 37. 131 applicants, 62% accepted, 61 enrolled. In 2013, 42 master's, 2 doctorates, 7 other advanced degrees awarded. *Degree requirements:* For master's, thesis optional, oral exam; for doctorate, thesis/dissertation. *Entrance requirements:* For master's, GRE General Test, BSN, minimum GPA of 3.0 during last 60 hours, nursing license. Additional exam requirements/recommendations for international students: Required—TOEFL (minimum score 550 paper-based; 79 iBT). *Application deadline:* For fall admission, 2/1 priority date for domestic and international students. Applications are processed on a rolling basis. Application fee: $55 ($75 for international students). Electronic applications accepted. *Financial support:* Fellowships, research assistantships, teaching assistantships, career-related internships or fieldwork, institutionally sponsored loans, scholarships/grants, traineeships, health care benefits, tuition waivers (full), and unspecified assistantships available. Support available to part-time students. *Faculty research:* Pain, stepfamilies, chemotherapy-related nausea and vomiting, stress management, self-care deficit theory. *Unit head:* Dr. Judith F. Miller, Dean, 573-882-0278, E-mail: millerjud@missouri.edu. *Application contact:* Laura Anderson, Senior Academic Advisor, 573-882-0294, E-mail: andersonla@missouri.edu.
Website: http://nursing.missouri.edu/

University of Missouri–Kansas City, School of Nursing and Health Studies, Kansas City, MO 64110-2499. Offers adult clinical nurse specialist (MSN), including adult nurse practitioner, women's health nurse practitioner (MSN, DNP); adult clinical nursing practice (DNP), including adult gerontology nurse practitioner, women's health nurse practitioner (MSN, DNP); clinical nursing practice (DNP), including family nurse practitioner; family nurse practitioner (MSN); neonatal nurse practitioner (MSN); nurse educator (MSN); nurse executive (MSN); nursing (PhD); nursing practice (DNP); pediatric clinical nursing practice (DNP), including pediatric nurse practitioner; pediatric nurse practitioner (MSN). *Accreditation:* AACN. Part-time programs available. Postbaccalaureate distance learning degree programs offered (minimal on-campus study). *Faculty:* 44 full-time (38 women), 55 part-time/adjunct (52 women). *Students:* 44 full-time (33 women), 401 part-time (370 women); includes 59 minority (25 Black or African American, non-Hispanic/Latino; 2 American Indian or Alaska Native, non-Hispanic/Latino; 12 Asian, non-Hispanic/Latino; 15 Hispanic/Latino; 5 Two or more races, non-Hispanic/Latino). Average age 37. 182 applicants, 68% accepted, 124 enrolled. In 2013, 106 master's, 15 doctorates awarded. *Degree requirements:* For master's, thesis or alternative. *Entrance requirements:* For master's, minimum undergraduate GPA of 3.2; for doctorate, GRE, 3 letters of reference. Additional exam requirements/recommendations for international students: Required—TOEFL (minimum score 550 paper-based; 80 iBT). *Application deadline:* For fall admission, 2/1 priority date for domestic and international students; for spring admission, 9/1 priority date for domestic and international students. Application fee: $45 ($50 for international students). *Expenses:* Tuition, state resident: full-time $6073; part-time $337.40 per credit hour. Tuition, nonresident: full-time $15,680; part-time $871.10 per credit hour. *Required fees:* $97.59 per credit hour. Full-time tuition and fees vary according to program. *Financial support:* In 2013–14, 13 teaching assistantships with partial tuition reimbursements (averaging $9,470 per year) were awarded; fellowships, research assistantships, career-related internships or fieldwork, Federal Work-Study, institutionally sponsored loans, and tuition waivers (full and partial) also available. Support available to part-time students. Financial award application deadline: 3/1; financial award applicants required to submit FAFSA. *Faculty research:* Geriatrics/gerontology, children's pain, neonatology, Alzheimer's care, cancer caregivers. *Unit head:* Dr. Ann Cary, Dean, 816-235-1723, Fax: 816-235-1701, E-mail: caryah@

umkc.edu. *Application contact:* Judy Jellison, Coordinator for Admissions and Recruitment, 816-235-1740, Fax: 816-235-1701, E-mail: jellisonj@umkc.edu.
Website: http://nursing.umkc.edu/

University of Missouri–St. Louis, College of Nursing, St. Louis, MO 63121-4400. Offers adult nurse practitioner (DNP, Post Master's Certificate); clinical nurse specialist (DNP); family mental health nurse practitioner (DNP); family nurse practitioner (MSN, DNP, Post Master's Certificate); neonatal nurse practitioner (MSN); nurse educator (MSN); nurse leader (MSN); nurse practitioner (Post Master's Certificate); nursing (PhD); pediatric clinical nurse specialist (DNP); pediatric nurse practitioner (MSN, DNP, Post Master's Certificate); women's health nurse practitioner (MSN, Post Master's Certificate). *Accreditation:* AACN. Part-time programs available. *Faculty:* 14 full-time (13 women), 14 part-time/adjunct (13 women). *Students:* 227 part-time (217 women); includes 40 minority (35 Black or African American, non-Hispanic/Latino; 1 American Indian or Alaska Native, non-Hispanic/Latino; 1 Asian, non-Hispanic/Latino; 1 Hispanic/Latino; 2 Two or more races, non-Hispanic/Latino). Average age 35. 190 applicants, 51% accepted, 76 enrolled. In 2013, 80 master's, 8 doctorates, 2 other advanced degrees awarded. *Degree requirements:* For doctorate, comprehensive exam, thesis/dissertation; for Post Master's Certificate, thesis. *Entrance requirements:* For master's, 2 recommendation letters; minimum GPA of 3.0; BSN; nursing licensure; statement of purpose; course in differential/inferential statistics; for doctorate, GRE, 2 letters of recommendation, MSN, minimum GPA of 3.2, course in differential/inferential statistics; for Post Master's Certificate, 2 recommendation letters; MSN; advanced practice certificate; minimum GPA of 3.0; essay. Additional exam requirements/recommendations for international students: Recommended—TOEFL (minimum score 550 paper-based; 79 iBT), IELTS (minimum score 6.5). *Application deadline:* For fall admission, 2/15 for domestic and international students. Application fee: $50 ($40 for international students). Electronic applications accepted. *Expenses:* Tuition, state resident: full-time $7364; part-time $409.10 per credit hour. Tuition, nonresident: full-time $19,162; part-time $1008.50 per credit hour. *Financial support:* Application deadline: 4/1; applicants required to submit FAFSA. *Faculty research:* Health promotion and restoration, family disruption, violence, abuse, battered women, health survey methods. *Unit head:* Dr. Nancy Magnuson, Director, 314-516-6066. *Application contact:* 314-516-5458, Fax: 314-516-6996, E-mail: gradadm@umsl.edu.
Website: http://www.umsl.edu/divisions/nursing/

The University of North Carolina at Chapel Hill, School of Nursing, Chapel Hill, NC 27599-7460. Offers nursing (MSN, DNP, PhD, PMC), including adult nurse practitioner (MSN, PMC), children's health advanced practice (MSN, PMC), family nurse practitioner (MSN, PMC), health care systems (MSN, PMC), psychiatric/mental health nursing (MSN, PMC). Part-time programs available. *Degree requirements:* For master's, comprehensive exam, thesis; for doctorate, thesis/dissertation, 3 exams. *Entrance requirements:* For master's and doctorate, GRE General Test. Additional exam requirements/recommendations for international students: Required—TOEFL (minimum score 550 paper-based; 79 iBT), IELTS (minimum score 7). Electronic applications accepted. *Faculty research:* Preventing and managing chronic illness, reducing health disparities, Improving healthcare quality and patient outcomes, understanding biobehavioral and genetic bases of health and illness, developing innovative ways to enhance science and its clinical translation.

The University of North Carolina at Greensboro, Graduate School, School of Nursing, Greensboro, NC 27412-5001. Offers adult clinical nurse specialist (MSN, PMC); adult/gerontological nurse practitioner (MSN, PMC); nurse anesthesia (MSN, PMC); nursing (PhD); nursing administration (MSN); nursing education (MSN); MSN/MBA. *Accreditation:* AACN; AANA/CANAEP. *Degree requirements:* For master's, thesis or alternative. *Entrance requirements:* For master's, GRE General Test or MAT, BSN, clinical experience, liability insurance, RN license; for PMC, liability insurance, MSN, RN license. Additional exam requirements/recommendations for international students: Required—TOEFL. Electronic applications accepted.

The University of North Carolina at Pembroke, Graduate Studies, Department of Nursing, Pembroke, NC 28372-1510. Offers clinical nurse leader (MSN); nurse educator (MSN); rural case manager (MSN). Part-time programs available.

University of North Florida, Brooks College of Health, School of Nursing, Jacksonville, FL 32224. Offers clinical nurse leader (MSN); clinical nurse specialist (MSN); family nurse practitioner (Certificate); nurse anesthetist (CRNA) (MSN); nursing practice (DNP); primary care nurse practitioner (MSN). *Accreditation:* AACN; AANA/CANAEP. Part-time programs available. *Faculty:* 29 full-time (23 women), 1 part-time/adjunct (0 women). *Students:* 93 full-time (70 women), 74 part-time (61 women); includes 33 minority (11 Black or African American, non-Hispanic/Latino; 1 American Indian or Alaska Native, non-Hispanic/Latino; 6 Asian, non-Hispanic/Latino; 12 Hispanic/Latino; 3 Two or more races, non-Hispanic/Latino), 2 international. Average age 34. 133 applicants, 40% accepted, 32 enrolled. In 2013, 45 master's, 3 doctorates awarded. *Degree requirements:* For master's, thesis optional. *Entrance requirements:* For master's, GRE General Test, minimum GPA of 3.0 in last 60 hours of course work, BSN, clinical experience, resume; for doctorate, GRE, master's degree in nursing specialty from nationally-accredited program; national certification in one of the following APRN roles: CNE, CNM, CNS, CRNA, CNP; minimum graduate GPA of 3.3; three letters of reference which address academic ability and clinical skills; active license as registered nurse or advanced practice registered nurse. Additional exam requirements/recommendations for international students: Required—TOEFL (minimum score 500 paper-based; 61 iBT). *Application deadline:* For fall admission, 3/15 for domestic students, 4/1 for international students. Application fee: $30. Electronic applications accepted. *Expenses:* Tuition, state resident: full-time $9794; part-time $408.10 per credit hour. Tuition, nonresident: full-time $22,383; part-time $932.61 per credit hour. *Required fees:* $2020; $84.20 per credit hour. Tuition and fees vary according to course load and program. *Financial support:* In 2013–14, 26 students received support. Research assistantships available. Financial award application deadline: 4/1; financial award applicants required to submit FAFSA. *Faculty research:* Teen pregnancy, diabetes, ethical decision-making, family caregivers. *Total annual research expenditures:* $66,739. *Unit head:* Dr. Li Loriz, Chair, 904-620-1053, E-mail: lloriz@unf.edu. *Application contact:* Beth Dibble, Assistant Director of Admissions for Nursing and Physical Therapy, 904-620-2684, Fax: 904-620-1832, E-mail: nursingadmissions@unf.edu.
Website: http://www.unf.edu/brooks/nursing

University of Pennsylvania, School of Nursing, Health Leadership Program, Philadelphia, PA 19104. Offers MSN. *Accreditation:* AACN. Part-time programs available. *Students:* 4 full-time (all women), 15 part-time (13 women); includes 5 minority (2 Black or African American, non-Hispanic/Latino; 2 Asian, non-Hispanic/Latino; 1 Hispanic/Latino). In 2013, 9 master's awarded. *Entrance requirements:* For master's, GRE General Test, BSN, minimum GPA of 3.0, previous course work in statistics, 1 year of clinical experience in area of interest. Additional exam requirements/recommendations for international students: Required—TOEFL. *Application deadline:* For fall admission, 2/15 priority date for domestic students. Applications are processed on a rolling basis. Application fee: $70. *Expenses:* Contact institution. *Financial support:* Teaching assistantships, career-related internships or fieldwork, Federal Work-Study, and institutionally sponsored loans available. Support available to part-time students. Financial award application deadline: 4/1. *Faculty research:* Payment structures for nurse practitioners, delirium in older adults. *Unit head:* Assistant Dean of Admissions and Financial Aid, 866-867-6877, Fax: 215-573-8439, E-mail: admissions@nursing.upenn.edu. *Application contact:* Susan Keim, Program Director, 215-573-9759, E-mail: skeim@nursing.upenn.edu.

University of Pennsylvania, School of Nursing, Program in Nursing and Health Care Administration, Philadelphia, PA 19104. Offers MSN, PhD, MBA/MSN. *Accreditation:* AACN. Part-time programs available. *Students:* 8 full-time (7 women), 19 part-time (14 women); includes 2 minority (1 Black or African American, non-Hispanic/Latino; 1 Two or more races, non-Hispanic/Latino), 1 international. 4 applicants, 25% accepted, 1 enrolled. In 2013, 12 master's awarded. Terminal master's awarded for partial completion of doctoral program. *Degree requirements:* For doctorate, thesis/dissertation. *Entrance requirements:* For master's, GRE General Test, BSN, minimum GPA of 3.0, previous course work in statistics; for doctorate, GRE General Test, BSN or MSN, minimum GPA of 3.0. Additional exam requirements/recommendations for international students: Required—TOEFL. *Application deadline:* For fall admission, 2/15 priority date for domestic students. Applications are processed on a rolling basis. Application fee: $70. *Expenses:* Contact institution. *Financial support:* Research assistantships, teaching assistantships, career-related internships or fieldwork, Federal Work-Study, and institutionally sponsored loans available. Support available to part-time students. Financial award application deadline: 12/15. *Faculty research:* Nursing services and policy, home health services utilization. *Unit head:* Assistant Dean of Admissions and Financial Aid, 866-867-6877, Fax: 215-573-8439, E-mail: admissions@nursing.upenn.edu. *Application contact:* Susan Keim, Program Director, 215-573-9759, E-mail: skeim@nursing.upenn.edu.
Website: http://www.nursing.upenn.edu/

University of Phoenix–Bay Area Campus, College of Nursing, San Jose, CA 95134-1805. Offers education (MHA); gerontology (MHA); health administration (MHA, DHA); informatics (MHA, MSN); nursing (MSN, PhD); nursing/health care education (MSN); MSN/MBA. Evening/weekend programs available. Postbaccalaureate distance learning degree programs offered (no on-campus study). *Degree requirements:* For master's, thesis (for some programs). *Entrance requirements:* For master's, minimum undergraduate GPA of 2.5, 3 years of work experience, RN license. Additional exam requirements/recommendations for international students: Required—TOEFL (minimum score 550 paper-based; 79 iBT). Electronic applications accepted.

University of Phoenix–Washington D.C. Campus, College of Nursing, Washington, DC 20001. Offers education (MHA); gerontology (MHA); health administration (MHA, DHA); informatics (MHA, MSN); nursing (MSN, PhD); nursing/health care education (MSN); MSN/MBA; MSN/MHA.

University of Pittsburgh, School of Nursing, Nurse Specialty Role Program, Pittsburgh, PA 15260. Offers clinical nurse leader (MSN); nursing (DNP); nursing administration (MSN); nursing informatics (MSN). *Accreditation:* AACN. Part-time programs available. *Students:* 11 full-time (9 women), 70 part-time (60 women); includes 6 minority (3 Black or African American, non-Hispanic/Latino; 3 Asian, non-Hispanic/Latino), 2 international. Average age 38. 43 applicants, 74% accepted, 26 enrolled. In 2013, 13 master's, 10 doctorates awarded. *Degree requirements:* For master's, comprehensive exam, thesis optional. *Entrance requirements:* For master's, GRE or MAT, BSN, RN license, letters of recommendation, resume, course work in statistics, 1-3 years of nursing experience. Additional exam requirements/recommendations for international students: Required—TOEFL (minimum score 550 paper-based; 80 iBT). *Application deadline:* For fall admission, 6/1 priority date for domestic students, 6/1 for international students; for spring admission, 2/15 priority date for domestic students, 2/15 for international students. Applications are processed on a rolling basis. Application fee: $50. Electronic applications accepted. *Expenses:* Tuition, state resident: full-time $19,964; part-time $807 per credit. Tuition, nonresident: full-time $32,686; part-time $1337 per credit. *Required fees:* $740; $200. Tuition and fees vary according to program. *Unit head:* Dr. Sandra Engberg, Associate Dean for Clinical Education, 412-624-3835, Fax: 412-624-8521, E-mail: sje1@pitt.edu. *Application contact:* Laurie Lapsley, Administrator of Graduate Student Services, 412-624-9670, Fax: 412-624-2409, E-mail: lapsleyl@pitt.edu.
Website: http://www.nursing.pitt.edu/

University of Rhode Island, Graduate School, College of Nursing, Kingston, RI 02881. Offers administration (MS); clinical nurse leader (MS); clinical specialist in gerontology (MS); clinical specialist in psychiatric/mental health (MS); family nurse practitioner (MS); gerontological nurse practitioner (MS); nursing (DNP, PhD); nursing education (MS). *Accreditation:* AACN; ACNM/ACME (one or more programs are accredited). Part-time programs available. *Faculty:* 26 full-time (25 women), 3 part-time/adjunct (2 women). *Students:* 46 full-time (42 women), 78 part-time (70 women); includes 11 minority (7 Black or African American, non-Hispanic/Latino; 1 Asian, non-Hispanic/Latino; 3 Hispanic/Latino), 4 international. In 2013, 38 master's, 4 doctorates awarded. *Degree requirements:* For master's, comprehensive exam; for doctorate, comprehensive exam, thesis/dissertation. *Entrance requirements:* For master's, GRE or MAT, 2 letters of recommendation, scholarly papers; for doctorate, GRE, 3 letters of recommendation, scholarly papers. Additional exam requirements/recommendations for international students: Required—TOEFL (minimum score 550 paper-based). *Application deadline:* For fall admission, 2/15 for domestic students, 2/1 for international students; for spring admission, 10/15 for domestic students, 7/15 for international students. Application fee: $65. Electronic applications accepted. *Expenses:* Tuition, state resident: full-time $11,532; part-time $641 per credit. Tuition, nonresident: full-time $23,606; part-time $1311 per credit. *Required fees:* $1388; $36 per credit. $35 per semester. One-time fee: $130. *Financial support:* In 2013–14, 4 teaching assistantships with full and partial tuition reimbursements (averaging $8,383 per year) were awarded. Financial award application deadline: 2/15; financial award applicants required to submit FAFSA. *Faculty research:* Group intervention for grieving women in prison, translating best practice in non-drug interventions for postoperative pain management, further development and testing of the pain assessment inventory, preschool motor and functional performance of two cohorts, neuroactivation of brain motor areas in preterm children. *Total annual research expenditures:* $1.2 million. *Unit head:* Dr. Mary Sullivan, Interim Dean, 401-874-5339, Fax: 401-874-2061, E-mail: mcsullivan@uri.edu. *Application contact:* Graduate Admission, 401-874-2872, E-mail: gradadm@etal.uri.edu.
Website: http://www.uri.edu/nursing/

University of Rochester, School of Nursing, Rochester, NY 14642. Offers acute care nurse practitioner (MS); adult nurse practitioner (MS); adult/geriatric nurse practitioner (MS); clinical nurse leader (MS); clinical research coordinator (MS); family nurse practitioner (MS); family psychiatric mental health nurse practitioner (MS); health care organization management and leadership (MS); health practice research (PhD); nursing (DNP); pediatric nurse practitioner (MS); pediatric nurse practitioner/neonatal nurse practitioner (MS). *Accreditation:* AACN. Part-time programs available. Postbaccalaureate distance learning degree programs offered (minimal on-campus study). *Faculty:* 60 full-time (52 women), 61 part-time/adjunct (47 women). *Students:* 33 full-time (29 women), 213 part-time (195 women); includes 32 minority (8 Black or African American, non-Hispanic/Latino; 10 Asian, non-Hispanic/Latino; 8 Hispanic/Latino; 6 Two or more races, non-Hispanic/Latino), 4 international. Average age 34. 41

applicants, 54% accepted, 16 enrolled. In 2013, 58 master's, 11 doctorates awarded. Terminal master's awarded for partial completion of doctoral program. *Degree requirements:* For master's, comprehensive exam (for some programs); for doctorate, thesis/dissertation. *Entrance requirements:* For master's, BS in nursing, minimum GPA of 3.0, course work in statistics; for doctorate, GRE General Test, MS in nursing, minimum GPA of 3.5. Additional exam requirements/recommendations for international students: Required—TOEFL (minimum score 560 paper-based; 88 iBT) or IELTS (minimum score 6.5) recommended. *Application deadline:* For fall admission, 4/1 for domestic and international students; for spring admission, 9/1 for domestic and international students; for summer admission, 1/2 for domestic and international students. Application fee: $50. Electronic applications accepted. *Expenses: Tuition:* Full-time $44,580; part-time $1394 per credit hour. *Required fees:* $492. *Financial support:* In 2013–14, 41 students received support, including 2 fellowships with full and partial tuition reimbursements available (averaging $30,200 per year); scholarships/grants, traineeships, health care benefits, tuition waivers (partial), and unspecified assistantships also available. Support available to part-time students. Financial award application deadline: 6/30. *Faculty research:* Symptom assessment and self-management, illness prevention, nursing intervention research with vulnerable populations, palliative care, aging. *Total annual research expenditures:* $3.5 million. *Unit head:* Dr. Kathy H. Rideout, Dean, 585-273-8902, Fax: 585-273-1268, E-mail: kathy_rideout@urmc.rochester.edu. *Application contact:* Elaine Andolina, Director of Admissions, 585-275-2375, Fax: 585-756-8299, E-mail: elaine_andolina@urmc.rochester.edu.
Website: http://www.son.rochester.edu

University of St. Francis, Leach College of Nursing, Joliet, IL 60435-6169. Offers family nurse practitioner (MSN, Post-Master's Certificate); family psychology/mental health nurse practitioner (MSN, Post-Master's Certificate); nursing administration (MSN); nursing education (MSN); nursing practice (DNP); teaching in nursing (Certificate). *Accreditation:* AACN. Part-time and evening/weekend programs available. Postbaccalaureate distance learning degree programs offered (no on-campus study). *Faculty:* 11 full-time (all women), 12 part-time/adjunct (11 women). *Students:* 90 full-time (76 women), 332 part-time (305 women); includes 122 minority (43 Black or African American, non-Hispanic/Latino; 1 American Indian or Alaska Native, non-Hispanic/Latino; 19 Asian, non-Hispanic/Latino; 45 Hispanic/Latino; 3 Native Hawaiian or other Pacific Islander, non-Hispanic/Latino; 11 Two or more races, non-Hispanic/Latino), 4 international. Average age 42. 343 applicants, 43% accepted, 111 enrolled. In 2013, 82 master's, 6 doctorates, 17 other advanced degrees awarded. *Entrance requirements:* For master's, minimum undergraduate GPA of 3.0, 2 years of full-time clinical experience, 3 letters recommendation, resume, nursing license, interview; for doctorate, MSN with minimum GPA of 3.0, national certification, interview, computer competency, medical/physical requirements, background check, liability insurance, resume, recommendation, graduate-level statistics course. Additional exam requirements/recommendations for international students: Required—TOEFL (minimum score 550 paper-based; 79 iBT), IELTS (minimum score 6.5). *Application deadline:* Applications are processed on a rolling basis. Application fee: $30. Electronic applications accepted. Application fee is waived when completed online. *Expenses:* Contact institution. *Financial support:* In 2013–14, 109 students received support. Scholarships/grants and tuition waivers (partial) available. Support available to part-time students. Financial award applicants required to submit FAFSA. *Unit head:* Dr. Carol Wilson, Dean, 815-740-3840, Fax: 815-740-4243, E-mail: cwilson@stfrancis.edu. *Application contact:* Sandra Sloka, Director of Admissions for Graduate and Degree Completion Programs, 800-735-7500, Fax: 815-740-3431, E-mail: ssloka@stfrancis.edu.
Website: http://www.stfrancis.edu/academics/college-of-nursing/

University of Saint Mary, Graduate Programs, Program in Nursing, Leavenworth, KS 66048-5082. Offers nurse administrator (MSN); nurse educator (MSN). Part-time programs available. Postbaccalaureate distance learning degree programs offered (no on-campus study). *Students:* 8 full-time (7 women), 4 part-time (all women). *Entrance requirements:* For master's, BSN from CCNE- or NLNAC-accredited baccalaureate nursing program at regionally-accredited institution. *Expenses: Tuition:* Part-time $550 per credit hour. *Unit head:* Dr. Glenna Mahoney, Department Chair, 877-307-4915, Fax: 913-345-2802. *Application contact:* Dr. Joyce Lasseter, Director, 877-307-4915, Fax: 913-345-2802.
Website: http://online.stmary.edu/MSN/master-science-nursing.asp

University of San Diego, Hahn School of Nursing and Health Science, San Diego, CA 92110. Offers adult-gerontology clinical nurse specialist (MSN); adult-gerontology nurse practitioner/family nurse practitioner (MSN); clinical nursing (MSN); executive nurse leader (MSN); family nurse practitioner (MSN); family/lifespan psychiatric-mental health nurse practitioner (MSN); healthcare informatics (MS, MSN); nursing (PhD); nursing practice (DNP); pediatric nurse practitioner/family nurse practitioner (MSN). *Accreditation:* AACN. Part-time and evening/weekend programs available. *Faculty:* 23 full-time (19 women), 48 part-time/adjunct (43 women). *Students:* 204 full-time (170 women), 166 part-time (144 women); includes 133 minority (26 Black or African American, non-Hispanic/Latino; 8 American Indian or Alaska Native, non-Hispanic/Latino; 50 Asian, non-Hispanic/Latino; 42 Hispanic/Latino; 1 Native Hawaiian or other Pacific Islander, non-Hispanic/Latino; 6 Two or more races, non-Hispanic/Latino), 7 international. Average age 36. 483 applicants, 58% accepted, 154 enrolled. In 2013, 91 master's, 33 doctorates awarded. *Degree requirements:* For doctorate, thesis/dissertation (for some programs), residency (DNP). *Entrance requirements:* For master's, GRE General Test (for entry-level nursing), BSN, current California RN licensure (except for entry-level nursing); minimum GPA of 3.0; for doctorate, minimum GPA of 3.5, MSN, current California RN licensure. Additional exam requirements/recommendations for international students: Required—TOEFL (minimum score 580 paper-based; 83 iBT), TWE. *Application deadline:* For fall admission, 3/1 priority date for domestic students, 3/1 for international students; for spring admission, 11/1 priority date for domestic students, 11/1 for international students. Applications are processed on a rolling basis. Application fee: $45. Electronic applications accepted. *Expenses: Tuition:* Full-time $23,580; part-time $1310 per credit. *Required fees:* $350. *Financial support:* In 2013–14, 250 students received support. Scholarships/grants and traineeships available. Support available to part-time students. Financial award application deadline: 4/1; financial award applicants required to submit FAFSA. *Faculty research:* Palliative and end of life care, maternal/child health, childhood obesity, health care disparities, cognitive functioning. *Unit head:* Dr. Sally Hardin, Dean, 619-260-4550, Fax: 619-260-6814. *Application contact:* Monica Mahon, Associate Director of Graduate Admissions, 619-260-4524, Fax: 619-260-4158, E-mail: grads@sandiego.edu.
Website: http://www.sandiego.edu/nursing/

University of San Francisco, School of Nursing and Health Professions, Doctoral Programs, San Francisco, CA 94117-1080. Offers clinical psychology (Psy D); executive leadership (DNP); family nurse practitioner (DNP); healthcare systems leadership (DNP); psychiatric mental health nurse practitioner (DNP). *Faculty:* 15 full-time (12 women), 10 part-time/adjunct (7 women). *Students:* 118 full-time (92 women), 34 part-time (31 women); includes 74 minority (13 Black or African American, non-Hispanic/Latino; 1 American Indian or Alaska Native, non-Hispanic/Latino; 32 Asian, non-Hispanic/Latino; 15 Hispanic/Latino; 1 Native Hawaiian or other Pacific Islander, non-Hispanic/Latino; 12 Two or more races, non-Hispanic/Latino), 2 international. Average age 41. 98 applicants, 70% accepted, 49 enrolled. In 2013, 39 doctorates awarded. *Entrance requirements:* For doctorate, nursing bachelor's degree, valid RN license in California. *Expenses: Tuition:* Full-time $21,150; part-time $1175 per unit. Tuition and fees vary according to course load, campus/location and program. *Financial support:* In 2013–14, 7 students received support. *Unit head:* Dr. Judith Karshmer, Dean, 415-422-6681, Fax: 415-422-6877, E-mail: nursing@usfca.edu. *Application contact:* Ingrid McVanner, Information Contact, 415-422-2746, Fax: 415-422-2217.

University of San Francisco, School of Nursing and Health Professions, Master's Programs, San Francisco, CA 94117-1080. Offers behavioral health (MSBH); clinical nurse leader (MS); public health (MPH). *Faculty:* 14 full-time (12 women), 30 part-time/adjunct (24 women). *Students:* 355 full-time (301 women), 108 part-time (97 women); includes 237 minority (26 Black or African American, non-Hispanic/Latino; 2 American Indian or Alaska Native, non-Hispanic/Latino; 122 Asian, non-Hispanic/Latino; 61 Hispanic/Latino; 5 Native Hawaiian or other Pacific Islander, non-Hispanic/Latino; 21 Two or more races, non-Hispanic/Latino), 4 international. Average age 33. 524 applicants, 52% accepted, 170 enrolled. In 2013, 106 master's awarded. *Application deadline:* For fall admission, 5/15 priority date for domestic students; for spring admission, 11/30 priority date for domestic students. *Expenses: Tuition:* Full-time $21,150; part-time $1175 per unit. Tuition and fees vary according to course load, campus/location and program. *Financial support:* In 2013–14, 50 students received support. *Unit head:* Dr. Michelle Montagno, Director, 415-422-4074, E-mail: mjmontagno@usfca.edu. *Application contact:* Ingrid McVanner, Information Contact, 415-422-2746, Fax: 415-422-2217.

University of South Carolina, The Graduate School, College of Nursing, Program in Nursing Administration, Columbia, SC 29208. Offers MSN. *Accreditation:* AACN. Part-time programs available. *Degree requirements:* For master's, thesis or alternative. *Entrance requirements:* For master's, GRE General Test or MAT, BS in nursing, nursing license. Additional exam requirements/recommendations for international students: Required—TOEFL (minimum score 570 paper-based). Electronic applications accepted. *Faculty research:* System research, evidence based practice, breast cancer, violence.

University of Southern Maine, College of Science, Technology, and Health, School of Nursing, Portland, ME 04104-9300. Offers adult-gerontology primary care nurse practitioner (MS, PMC); clinical nurse leader (MS); education (MS); family nurse practitioner (MS, PMC); family psychiatric/mental health nurse practitioner (MS); management (MS); nursing (DNP); psychiatric-mental health nurse practitioner (PMC); MBA/MSN. *Accreditation:* AACN. Part-time programs available. *Faculty:* 11 full-time (all women), 10 part-time/adjunct (8 women). *Students:* 57 full-time (47 women), 53 part-time (46 women); includes 5 minority (1 American Indian or Alaska Native, non-Hispanic/Latino; 2 Asian, non-Hispanic/Latino; 1 Hispanic/Latino; 1 Two or more races, non-Hispanic/Latino). Average age 36. 140 applicants, 44% accepted, 29 enrolled. In 2013, 33 master's, 11 other advanced degrees awarded. *Degree requirements:* For master's, thesis optional. *Entrance requirements:* For master's, GRE General Test or MAT, minimum GPA of 3.0; for doctorate, GRE. Additional exam requirements/recommendations for international students: Required—TOEFL (minimum score 550 paper-based). *Application deadline:* For fall admission, 4/1 for domestic and international students; for spring admission, 10/1 for domestic and international students. Application fee: $65. Electronic applications accepted. *Expenses:* Tuition, state resident: part-time $380 per credit. Tuition, nonresident: part-time $1026 per credit. Part-time tuition and fees vary according to program. *Financial support:* Research assistantships, teaching assistantships, career-related internships or fieldwork, Federal Work-Study, scholarships/grants, traineeships, tuition waivers (full and partial), and unspecified assistantships available. Support available to part-time students. Financial award application deadline: 2/15; financial award applicants required to submit FAFSA. *Faculty research:* Women's health, nursing history, weight control, community services, substance abuse. *Unit head:* Krista M. Meinersmann, Director of Nursing Program, 207-780-4993, E-mail: kmeinersmann@usm.maine.edu. *Application contact:* Mary Sloan, Assistant Dean of Graduate Studies and Director of Graduate Admissions, 207-780-4812, E-mail: gradstudies@usm.maine.edu.
Website: http://www.usm.maine.edu/nursing/

University of Southern Mississippi, Graduate School, College of Health, School of Nursing, Hattiesburg, MS 39406-0001. Offers family nurse practitioner (MSN); nursing (DNP, PhD); nursing executive (MSN); psychiatric nurse practitioner (MSN). *Accreditation:* AACN. Part-time and evening/weekend programs available. *Faculty:* 17 full-time (16 women), 1 part-time/adjunct (0 women). *Students:* 133 full-time (104 women), 42 part-time (40 women); includes 45 minority (33 Black or African American, non-Hispanic/Latino; 1 American Indian or Alaska Native, non-Hispanic/Latino; 1 Asian, non-Hispanic/Latino; 1 Hispanic/Latino; 9 Two or more races, non-Hispanic/Latino). Average age 37. 118 applicants, 61% accepted, 62 enrolled. In 2013, 45 master's, 9 doctorates awarded. *Degree requirements:* For master's, comprehensive exam, thesis optional; for doctorate, comprehensive exam, thesis/dissertation. *Entrance requirements:* For master's, GRE General Test, minimum GPA of 2.75 during last 60 hours, nursing license, BS in nursing; for doctorate, GRE General Test, master's degree in nursing, minimum GPA of 3.5. Additional exam requirements/recommendations for international students: Required—TOEFL, IELTS. *Application deadline:* For fall admission, 3/15 priority date for domestic students, 5/1 for international students; for spring admission, 1/10 priority date for domestic and international students. Applications are processed on a rolling basis. Application fee: $50. Electronic applications accepted. *Financial support:* In 2013–14, 14 research assistantships with full tuition reimbursements (averaging $12,577 per year), teaching assistantships (averaging $12,000 per year) were awarded; Federal Work-Study, institutionally sponsored loans, scholarships/grants, traineeships, health care benefits, and unspecified assistantships also available. Financial award application deadline: 3/15; financial award applicants required to submit FAFSA. *Faculty research:* Gerontology, caregivers, HIV, bereavement, pain, nursing leadership. *Unit head:* Dr. Katherine Nugent, Director and Associate Dean, 601-266-5500, Fax: 601-266-5927. *Application contact:* Dr. Sandra Bishop, Graduate Coordinator, 601-266-5500, Fax: 601-266-5927.
Website: http://www.usm.edu/graduateschool/table.php

University of South Florida, College of Nursing, Tampa, FL 33612. Offers adult gerontology acute care (DNP, PhD); adult gerontology acute care nursing (MS); adult gerontology primary care (DNP, PhD); adult gerontology primary care nursing (MS); adult gerontology primary care/occupational health nursing (MS); adult gerontology primary care/oncology nursing (MS, PhD); clinical nurse leader (MS); family health (DNP, PhD); family nurse practitioner (MS); nurse anesthesia (MS); nursing education (MS); nursing practice (DNP); nursing science (PhD), including nursing education; occupational health/adult-gerontology (DNP); oncology/adult-gerontology primary care (DNP); pediatric health (DNP, PhD); pediatric nurse practitioner (MS). *Accreditation:* AACN; AANA/CANAEP. Part-time programs available. *Faculty:* 46 full-time (40 women), 15 part-time/adjunct (11 women). *Students:* 177 full-time (150 women), 700 part-time (622 women); includes 272 minority (116 Black or African American, non-Hispanic/Latino; 2 American Indian or Alaska Native, non-Hispanic/Latino; 45 Asian, non-Hispanic/Latino; 93 Hispanic/Latino; 2 Native Hawaiian or other Pacific Islander, non-Hispanic/Latino; 14 Two or more races, non-Hispanic/Latino), 12 international. Average age 35. 656 applicants, 43% accepted, 224 enrolled. In 2013, 224 master's, 14

doctorates awarded. *Degree requirements:* For master's, comprehensive exam, thesis optional; for doctorate, comprehensive exam, thesis/dissertation. *Entrance requirements:* For master's, GRE General Test, bachelor's degree from accredited program with minimum GPA of 3.0 in all upper-division coursework; current license as Registered Nurse; 3 letters of recommendation; personal statement of goals; resume or curriculum vitae; personal interview; for doctorate, GRE General Test (recommended), bachelor's degree in nursing from a CCNA/NLNAC regionally-accredited institution with minimum GPA of 3.0 in all coursework or in all upper-division coursework; current license as Registered Nurse in Florida; undergraduate statistics course with minimum B grade; 3 letters of recommendation; statement of goals; resume; interview. Additional exam requirements/recommendations for international students: Required—TOEFL (minimum score 550 paper-based; 79 iBT). *Application deadline:* For fall admission, 2/15 for domestic students, 1/2 for international students; for spring admission, 10/1 for domestic students, 6/1 for international students. Application fee: $30. Electronic applications accepted. *Financial support:* In 2013–14, 36 students received support, including 7 research assistantships with tuition reimbursements available (averaging $18,935 per year), 29 teaching assistantships with tuition reimbursements available (averaging $30,814 per year); tuition waivers (partial) and unspecified assistantships also available. Financial award application deadline: 2/1; financial award applicants required to submit FAFSA. *Faculty research:* Women's health, palliative and end-of-life care, cardiac rehabilitation, complementary therapies for chronic illness and cancer. *Total annual research expenditures:* $3.4 million. *Unit head:* Dr. Dianne C. Morrison-Beedy, Dean and Professor, College of Nursing, 813-974-9091, Fax: 813-974-5418, E-mail: dmbeedy@health.usf.edu. *Application contact:* Dr. Connie Visovsky, Associate Professor and Associate Dean of Student Affairs, 813-396-9641, Fax: 813-974-5418, E-mail: cvisovsk@health.usf.edu.
Website: http://health.usf.edu/nursing/index.htm

The University of Tennessee at Chattanooga, Graduate School, College of Health, Education and Professional Studies, School of Nursing, Chattanooga, TN 37403. Offers administration (MSN); certified nurse anesthetist (Post-Master's Certificate); education (MSN); family nurse practitioner (MSN, Post-Master's Certificate); health care informatics (Post-Master's Certificate); nurse anesthesia (MSN); nurse education (Post-Master's Certificate); nursing (DNP). *Accreditation:* AACN; AANA/CANAEP (one or more programs are accredited). *Faculty:* 9 full-time (7 women), 2 part-time/adjunct (1 woman). *Students:* 72 full-time (39 women), 53 part-time (43 women); includes 11 minority (6 Black or African American, non-Hispanic/Latino; 1 Asian, non-Hispanic/Latino; 3 Hispanic/Latino; 1 Two or more races, non-Hispanic/Latino). Average age 33. 3 applicants, 100% accepted, 1 enrolled. In 2013, 35 master's, 10 doctorates, 2 other advanced degrees awarded. *Degree requirements:* For master's, thesis optional, qualifying exams, professional project; for Post-Master's Certificate, thesis or alternative, practicum, seminar. *Entrance requirements:* For master's, GRE General Test, MAT, BSN, minimum GPA of 3.0, eligibility for Tennessee RN license, 1 year of direct patient care experience; for Post-Master's Certificate, GRE General Test, MAT, MSN, minimum GPA of 3.0, eligibility for Tennessee RN license, one year of direct patient care experience. Additional exam requirements/recommendations for international students: Required—TOEFL (minimum score 550 paper-based; 79 iBT), IELTS (minimum score 6). *Application deadline:* For fall admission, 6/13 priority date for domestic students, 6/1 for international students; for spring admission, 10/15 priority date for domestic students, 10/1 for international students. Applications are processed on a rolling basis. Application fee: $30 ($35 for international students). Electronic applications accepted. *Financial support:* Career-related internships or fieldwork and scholarships/grants available. Support available to part-time students. *Faculty research:* Diabetes in women, health care for elderly, alternative medicine, hypertension, nurse anesthesia. *Total annual research expenditures:* $3.4 million. *Unit head:* Dr. Chris Smith, Interim Director, 423-425-1741, Fax: 423-425-4668, E-mail: chris-smith@utc.edu. *Application contact:* Dr. J. Randy Walker, Interim Dean of Graduate Studies, 423-425-4478, Fax: 423-425-5223, E-mail: randy-walker@utc.edu.
Website: http://www.utc.edu/Academic/Nursing/

The University of Tennessee Health Science Center, College of Nursing, Memphis, TN 38163-0002. Offers advanced practice nursing (DNP); clinical nurse leader (MSN). *Accreditation:* AACN; AANA/CANAEP. Postbaccalaureate distance learning degree programs offered (minimal on-campus study). *Degree requirements:* For master's, thesis; for doctorate, thesis/dissertation. *Entrance requirements:* For master's, GRE General Test, BSN, minimum GPA of 3.0; for doctorate, minimum GPA of 3.0. Additional exam requirements/recommendations for international students: Required—TOEFL. *Application deadline:* For fall admission, 2/1 for domestic students; for winter admission, 9/1 for domestic students. Application fee: $50. Electronic applications accepted. *Expenses:* Contact institution. *Financial support:* Fellowships with partial tuition reimbursements, teaching assistantships, Federal Work-Study, institutionally sponsored loans, scholarships/grants, and traineeships available. Support available to part-time students. Financial award application deadline: 2/28; financial award applicants required to submit FAFSA. *Unit head:* Dr. Wendy Likes, Interim Dean, 901-448-6135, Fax: 901-448-4121, E-mail: wlikes@uthsc.edu. *Application contact:* Dr. Wendy Likes, Interim Dean, 901-448-6135, Fax: 901-448-4121, E-mail: wlikes@uthsc.edu.
Website: http://uthsc.edu/nursing/

The University of Texas at Arlington, Graduate School, College of Nursing, Arlington, TX 76019. Offers nurse practitioner (MSN); nursing administration (MSN); nursing education (MSN); nursing practice (DNP); nursing science (PhD). *Accreditation:* AACN. Part-time and evening/weekend programs available. Postbaccalaureate distance learning degree programs offered (no on-campus study). *Degree requirements:* For master's, practicum course; for doctorate, comprehensive exam (for some programs), thesis/dissertation (for some programs), proposal defense dissertation (for PhD); scholarship project (for DNP). *Entrance requirements:* For master's, GRE General Test if GPA less than 3.0, minimum GPA of 3.0, Texas nursing license, minimum C grade in undergraduate statistics course; for doctorate, GRE General Test (waived for MSN-to-PhD applicants), minimum undergraduate, graduate and statistics GPA of 3.0; Texas RN license; interview; written statement of goals. Additional exam requirements/recommendations for international students: Required—TOEFL (minimum score 550 paper-based), IELTS (minimum score 7). *Faculty research:* Simulation in clinical education and practice, cultural diversity, vulnerable populations, substance abuse.

The University of Texas at Austin, Graduate School, School of Nursing, Austin, TX 78712-1111. Offers adult - gerontology clinical nurse specialist (MSN); child health (MSN), including administration, public health nursing, teaching; family nurse practitioner (MSN); family psychiatric/mental health nurse practitioner (MSN); holistic adult health (MSN), including administration, teaching; maternity (MSN), including administration, public health nursing, teaching; nursing (PhD); nursing administration and healthcare systems management (MSN); pediatric nurse practitioner (MSN); public health nursing (MSN). *Accreditation:* AACN. Part-time programs available. *Degree requirements:* For master's, thesis optional; for doctorate, thesis/dissertation. *Entrance requirements:* For master's and doctorate, GRE General Test. Additional exam requirements/recommendations for international students: Required—TOEFL (minimum score 550 paper-based). Electronic applications accepted. *Faculty research:* Chronic illness management, memory and aging, health promotion, women's health, adolescent health.

The University of Texas at El Paso, Graduate School, School of Nursing, El Paso, TX 79968-0001. Offers family nurse practitioner (MSN); health care leadership and management (Certificate); interdisciplinary health sciences (PhD); nursing (DNP); nursing education (MSN, Certificate); nursing systems management (MSN). *Accreditation:* AACN. Postbaccalaureate distance learning degree programs offered (minimal on-campus study). *Degree requirements:* For master's, thesis optional; for doctorate, thesis/dissertation. *Entrance requirements:* For master's, minimum GPA of 3.0, resume; for doctorate, GRE, letters of reference, relevant personal/professional experience; master's degree in nursing (for DNP); for Certificate, bachelor's degree in nursing. Additional exam requirements/recommendations for international students: Required—TOEFL; Recommended—IELTS. Electronic applications accepted.

The University of Texas at Tyler, College of Nursing and Health Sciences, Program in Nursing, Tyler, TX 75799-0001. Offers nurse practitioner (MSN); nursing (PhD); nursing administration (MSN); nursing education (MSN); MSN/MBA. *Accreditation:* AACN. Part-time and evening/weekend programs available. Postbaccalaureate distance learning degree programs offered (no on-campus study). *Degree requirements:* For master's, comprehensive exam (for some programs), thesis (for some programs); for doctorate, thesis/dissertation. *Entrance requirements:* For master's, GRE General Test or MAT, GMAT, minimum undergraduate GPA of 3.0, course work in statistics, RN license, BSN. Additional exam requirements/recommendations for international students: Required—TOEFL. Electronic applications accepted. *Faculty research:* Psychosocial adjustment, aging, support/commitment of caregivers, psychological abuse and violence, hope/hopelessness, professional values, end of life care, suicidology, clinical supervision, workforce retention and issues, global health issues, health promotion.

The University of Texas Health Science Center at San Antonio, School of Nursing, San Antonio, TX 78229. Offers administrative management (MSN); adult-gerontology acute care nurse practitioner (PGC); clinical nurse leader (MSN); executive administrative management (DNP); family nurse practitioner (PGC); nurse practitioner (MSN), including adult-gerontology acute care nurse practitioner, family nurse practitioner, pediatric nurse practitioner primary care, psychiatric mental health nurse practitioner; nurse practitioner leadership (DNP); nursing (MSN, PhD); nursing education (MSN, PGC); pediatric nurse practitioner primary care (PGC); psychiatric mental health nurse practitioner (PGC); public health nurse leader (DNP). *Accreditation:* AACN. Part-time programs available. *Faculty:* 84 full-time (74 women), 42 part-time/adjunct (40 women). *Students:* 115 full-time (93 women), 140 part-time (123 women); includes 123 minority (24 Black or African American, non-Hispanic/Latino; 20 Asian, non-Hispanic/Latino; 74 Hispanic/Latino; 5 Two or more races, non-Hispanic/Latino), 7 international. Average age 37. 174 applicants, 59% accepted, 83 enrolled. In 2013, 67 master's, 6 doctorates, 5 other advanced degrees awarded. Terminal master's awarded for partial completion of doctoral program. *Degree requirements:* For master's, thesis optional; for doctorate, comprehensive exam, thesis/dissertation, final projects (for DNP). *Entrance requirements:* For master's, minimum GPA of 3.0, references, goal statement, BSN from accredited nursing school, RN licensure in Texas or compact state; for doctorate, GRE, MAT, minimum GPA of 3.0, personal interview, BSN and/or MSN from accredited nursing school, RN licensure in Texas or compact state, statistics course, references, curriculum vitae, goal statement; for PGC, minimum GPA of 3.0; references; goal statement; MSN from accredited nursing school; RN licensure in Texas or compact state; prerequisites in advanced health assessment, advanced pharmacotherapeutics, and advanced pathophysiology. Additional exam requirements/recommendations for international students: Required—TOEFL (minimum score 550 paper-based; 68 iBT), IELTS (minimum score 6.5). *Application deadline:* For fall admission, 1/10 for domestic and international students; for spring admission, 7/1 for domestic students. Application fee: $65. Electronic applications accepted. *Financial support:* In 2013–14, 145 students received support, including 3 fellowships with full tuition reimbursements available (averaging $30,000 per year); institutionally sponsored loans and scholarships/grants also available. Financial award application deadline: 6/30; financial award applicants required to submit FAFSA. *Faculty research:* Pain, organizational structure, aging, quality and safety, health disparity, obesity and nutrition, women's and children's health. *Total annual research expenditures:* $500,265. *Unit head:* Dr. Eileen T. Breslin, Dean, 210-567-5800, Fax: 210-567-5929, E-mail: breslin@uthscsa.edu. *Application contact:* Brandy Finck, Interim Associate Dean for Admissions and Student Services, 210-567-5805, Fax: 210-567-6189, E-mail: finckb@uthscsa.edu.
Website: http://www.nursing.uthscsa.edu/

University of the Incarnate Word, School of Graduate Studies and Research, School of Nursing and Health Professions, Program in Nursing, San Antonio, TX 78209-6397. Offers clinical nursing leader (MSN); clinical nursing specialist (MSN); nursing (DNP). *Accreditation:* AACN. Part-time and evening/weekend programs available. *Faculty:* 14 full-time (all women), 1 part-time/adjunct (0 women). *Students:* 12 full-time (8 women), 50 part-time (34 women); includes 54 minority (8 Black or African American, non-Hispanic/Latino; 6 Asian, non-Hispanic/Latino; 39 Hispanic/Latino; 1 Two or more races, non-Hispanic/Latino), 11 international. Average age 41. 44 applicants, 70% accepted, 17 enrolled. In 2013, 14 master's, 2 doctorates awarded. *Degree requirements:* For master's, capstone, clinical hours. *Entrance requirements:* For master's, baccalaureate degree in nursing from CCNE- or NLN-accredited program including courses in statistics and health assessment; minimum undergraduate cumulative GPA of 2.5, 3.0 in upper-division nursing courses; three professional references; license to practice nursing in Texas or recognized state. Additional exam requirements/recommendations for international students: Required—TOEFL (minimum score 560 paper-based; 83 iBT). *Application deadline:* Applications are processed on a rolling basis. Application fee: $20. Electronic applications accepted. *Expenses: Tuition:* Part-time $815 per credit hour. *Required fees:* $86 per credit hour. One-time fee: $40 part-time. Tuition and fees vary according to degree level and program. *Financial support:* Federal Work-Study, scholarships/grants, and traineeships available. Support available to part-time students. Financial award applicants required to submit FAFSA. *Unit head:* Dr. Holly Cassells, Chair, Graduate Programs, 210-829-3977, Fax: 210-829-3174, E-mail: cassells@uiwtx.edu. *Application contact:* Andrea Cyterski-Acosta, Dean of Enrollment, 210-829-6005, Fax: 210-829-3921, E-mail: admis@uiwtx.edu.
Website: http://www.uiw.edu/msn/

The University of Toledo, College of Graduate Studies, College of Nursing, Department of Population and Community Care, Toledo, OH 43606-3390. Offers clinical nurse leader (MSN); family nurse practitioner (MSN, Certificate); nurse educator (MSN, Certificate); pediatric nurse practitioner (MSN, Certificate). Part-time programs available. *Students:* 70 full-time (60 women), 212 part-time (186 women); includes 27 minority (12 Black or African American, non-Hispanic/Latino; 1 American Indian or Alaska Native, non-Hispanic/Latino; 3 Asian, non-Hispanic/Latino; 7 Hispanic/Latino; 4 Two or more races, non-Hispanic/Latino), 1 international. Average age 32. 127 applicants, 81% accepted, 78 enrolled. In 2013, 82 master's, 10 other advanced degrees awarded. *Degree requirements:* For master's, thesis or alternative. *Entrance requirements:* For master's, GRE, BS in nursing, minimum undergraduate GPA of 3.0, statement of purpose, three letters of recommendation, transcripts from all prior institutions attended, Nursing CAS application, UT supplemental application; for Certificate, BS in nursing, minimum undergraduate GPA of 3.0, statement of purpose, three letters of recommendation, transcripts from all prior institutions attended. Additional exam requirements/recommendations for international students: Required—TOEFL (minimum

score 550 paper-based; 80 iBT). Application fee: $45 ($75 for international students). Electronic applications accepted. *Financial support:* Research assistantships with full and partial tuition reimbursements, Federal Work-Study, scholarships/grants, traineeships, and tuition waivers (full and partial) available. *Unit head:* Dr. Kelley Phillips, Chair, 419-383-5892. *Application contact:* Joan Mulligan, Admissions Analyst, 419-383-4168, Fax: 419-383-6140, E-mail: joan.mulligan@utoledo.edu.
Website: http://www.utoledo.edu/nursing/

University of Victoria, Faculty of Graduate Studies, Faculty of Human and Social Development, School of Nursing, Victoria, BC V8W 2Y2, Canada. Offers advanced nursing practice (advanced practice leadership option) (MN); advanced nursing practice (nurse educator option) (MN); advanced nursing practice (nurse practitioner option) (MN); nursing (PhD). Part-time programs available. Postbaccalaureate distance learning degree programs offered (no on-campus study). *Entrance requirements:* Additional exam requirements/recommendations for international students: Required—TOEFL (minimum score 575 paper-based), IELTS (minimum score 7). Electronic applications accepted.

University of Virginia, School of Nursing, Charlottesville, VA 22903. Offers acute and specialty care (MSN); acute care nurse practitioner (MSN); clinical nurse leadership (MSN); community-public health leadership (MSN); nursing (DNP, PhD); psychiatric mental health counseling (MSN); MSN/MBA. *Accreditation:* AACN. Part-time programs available. *Faculty:* 45 full-time (41 women), 3 part-time/adjunct (all women). *Students:* 177 full-time (155 women), 147 part-time (133 women); includes 53 minority (27 Black or African American, non-Hispanic/Latino; 10 Asian, non-Hispanic/Latino; 11 Hispanic/Latino; 5 Two or more races, non-Hispanic/Latino), 4 international. Average age 36. 236 applicants, 61% accepted, 110 enrolled. In 2013, 94 master's, 14 doctorates awarded. *Degree requirements:* For doctorate, comprehensive exam (for some programs), capstone project (DNP), dissertation (PhD). *Entrance requirements:* For master's, GRE General Test, MAT; for doctorate, GRE General Test. Additional exam requirements/recommendations for international students: Required—TOEFL, IELTS. *Application deadline:* Applications are processed on a rolling basis. Application fee: $60. Electronic applications accepted. *Expenses:* Contact institution. *Financial support:* Fellowships, research assistantships, teaching assistantships, Federal Work-Study, and scholarships/grants available. Financial award applicants required to submit FAFSA. *Unit head:* Dorrie K. Fontaine, Dean, 434-924-0141, Fax: 434-982-1809, E-mail: dkf2u@virginia.edu. *Application contact:* Clay Hysell, Assistant Dean for Admissions and Financial Services, 434-924-0141, Fax: 434-982-1809, E-mail: nur-osa@virginia.edu.
Website: http://www.nursing.virginia.edu/

University of Washington, Tacoma, Graduate Programs, Program in Nursing, Tacoma, WA 98402-3100. Offers communities, populations and health (MN); leadership in healthcare (MN); nurse educator (MN). Part-time programs available. *Degree requirements:* For master's, thesis (for some programs), advance fieldwork. *Entrance requirements:* For master's, Washington State NCLEX exam, minimum GPA of 3.0. Additional exam requirements/recommendations for international students: Required—TOEFL (minimum score 580 paper-based; 70 iBT); Recommended—IELTS (minimum score 7). *Faculty research:* Hospice and palliative care; clinical trial decision-making; minority nurse retention; asthma and public health; injustice, suffering, difference: Linking Them to Us; adolescent health.

University of West Florida, College of Professional Studies, Department of Research and Advanced Studies, Pensacola, FL 32514-5750. Offers administration (MSA), including acquisition and contract administration, biomedical/pharmaceutical, criminal justice administration, database administration, education leadership, healthcare administration, human performance technology, leadership, nursing administration, public administration, software engineering and administration; college student personnel administration (M Ed), including college personnel administration, guidance and counseling; curriculum and instruction (M Ed, Ed S); educational leadership (M Ed); middle and secondary level education and ESOL (M Ed). Part-time and evening/weekend programs available. *Entrance requirements:* For master's, GRE or MAT, official transcripts; minimum undergraduate GPA of 3.0; letter of intent; three letters of recommendation; resume. Additional exam requirements/recommendations for international students: Required—TOEFL (minimum score 550 paper-based).

University of West Florida, College of Professional Studies, Program in Administration, Pensacola, FL 32514-5750. Offers acquisition and contract administration (MSA); database administration (MSA); health care administration (MSA); human performance technology (MSA); leadership (MSA); public administration (MSA); software engineering administration (MSA). Part-time and evening/weekend programs available. Postbaccalaureate distance learning degree programs offered (no on-campus study). *Entrance requirements:* For master's, GRE General Test, letter of intent, names of references. Additional exam requirements/recommendations for international students: Required—TOEFL (minimum score 550 paper-based).

University of Wisconsin–Eau Claire, College of Nursing and Health Sciences, Program in Nursing, Eau Claire, WI 54702-4004. Offers adult-gerontological administration (DNP); adult-gerontological clinical nurse specialist (DNP); adult-gerontological education (MSN); adult-gerontological primary care nurse practitioner (DNP); family health administration (DNP); family health in education (MSN); family health nurse practitioner (DNP); nursing (MSN); nursing practice (DNP). Part-time programs available. *Faculty:* 8 full-time (all women), 2 part-time/adjunct (both women). *Students:* 33 full-time (30 women), 40 part-time (36 women); includes 1 minority (Asian, non-Hispanic/Latino). Average age 37. 48 applicants, 85% accepted, 24 enrolled. In 2013, 31 master's, 9 doctorates awarded. Terminal master's awarded for partial completion of doctoral program. *Degree requirements:* For master's, thesis optional, 500-600 hours clinical practicum, oral and written exams. *Entrance requirements:* For master's, Wisconsin RN license, minimum GPA of 3.0, undergraduate statistics, course work in health assessment. Additional exam requirements/recommendations for international students: Required—TOEFL (minimum score 79 iBT). *Application deadline:* For fall admission, 1/15 priority date for domestic and international students. Applications are processed on a rolling basis. Application fee: $86. *Expenses:* Contact institution. *Financial support:* In 2013–14, 10 students received support. Federal Work-Study and unspecified assistantships available. Financial award application deadline: 3/1; financial award applicants required to submit FAFSA. *Unit head:* Dr. Linda Young, Dean, 715-836-4904, Fax: 715-836-5925, E-mail: youngLk@uwec.edu. *Application contact:* Dr. Mary Zwygart-Stauffacher, Director, 715-836-5287, E-mail: zwygarmc@uwec.edu.
Website: http://www.uwec.edu/conhs/programs/grad/index.htm

University of Wisconsin–Green Bay, Graduate Studies, Program in Nursing Leadership and Management in Health Systems, Green Bay, WI 54311-7001. Offers MS. Part-time programs available. Postbaccalaureate distance learning degree programs offered (no on-campus study). *Faculty:* 3 full-time (all women), 2 part-time/adjunct (both women). *Students:* 18 part-time (16 women); includes 1 minority (Black or African American, non-Hispanic/Latino). Average age 43. 24 applicants, 92% accepted, 15 enrolled. *Degree requirements:* For master's, 9-credit practicum. *Entrance requirements:* For master's, baccalaureate degree in nursing with minimum GPA of 3.0; college-level inferential statistics course with minimum C grade (within past 5 years); statement of interest; official undergraduate and graduate transcripts; three letters of evaluation; curriculum vitae or resume; copy of current, unencumbered RN license; background check. Additional exam requirements/recommendations for international students: Required—TOEFL. *Application deadline:* Applications are processed on a rolling basis. Application fee: $56. *Expenses:* Tuition, state resident: full-time $7640; part-time $424 per credit. Tuition, nonresident: full-time $16,772; part-time $932 per credit. *Required fees:* $1378. Full-time tuition and fees vary according to course load and reciprocity agreements. *Unit head:* Dr. Janet Reilly, Director, 920-465-2826, E-mail: reillyj@uwgb.edu. *Application contact:* Mary Valitchka, Graduate Studies Coordinator, 920-465-2123, Fax: 920-465-5043, E-mail: valitchm@uwgb.edu.
Website: http://www.uwgb.edu/nursing/msn/overview.asp

Ursuline College, School of Graduate Studies, Programs in Nursing, Pepper Pike, OH 44124-4398. Offers care management (MSN); nurse practitioner (MSN); nursing (DNP); nursing education (MSN); palliative care (MSN). *Accreditation:* AACN. Part-time programs available. *Faculty:* 6 full-time (all women), 13 part-time/adjunct (10 women). *Students:* 9 full-time (7 women), 245 part-time (235 women); includes 69 minority (58 Black or African American, non-Hispanic/Latino; 6 Asian, non-Hispanic/Latino; 2 Hispanic/Latino; 3 Two or more races, non-Hispanic/Latino), 1 international. Average age 36. 91 applicants, 79% accepted, 60 enrolled. In 2013, 57 master's, 2 doctorates awarded. *Degree requirements:* For master's, comprehensive exam. *Entrance requirements:* For master's, minimum undergraduate GPA of 3.0, bachelor's degree in nursing, eligibility for or current Ohio RN license. Additional exam requirements/recommendations for international students: Required—TOEFL (minimum score 500 paper-based). *Application deadline:* For fall admission, 8/1 priority date for domestic students. Applications are processed on a rolling basis. Application fee: $25. *Expenses: Tuition:* Full-time $16,920; part-time $940 per credit. *Required fees:* $270. *Financial support:* In 2013–14, 9 students received support. Federal Work-Study available. Financial award application deadline: 3/1. *Unit head:* Dr. Janet Baker, Director, 440-864-8172, Fax: 440-684-6053, E-mail: jbaker@ursuline.edu. *Application contact:* Stephanie Pratt, Graduate Admission Coordinator, 440-646-8119, Fax: 440-684-6138, E-mail: graduateadmissions@ursuline.edu.

Vanderbilt University, Vanderbilt University School of Nursing, Nashville, TN 37240. Offers adult-gerontology acute care nurse practitioner (MSN), including hospitalist, intensivist; adult-gerontology primary care nurse practitioner (MSN); emergency nurse practitioner (MSN); family nurse practitioner (MSN); healthcare leadership (MSN); neonatal nurse practitioner (MSN); nurse midwifery (MSN); nurse midwifery/family nurse practitioner (MSN); nursing informatics (MSN); nursing practice (DNP); nursing science (PhD); pediatric acute care nurse practitioner (MSN); pediatric primary care nurse practitioner (MSN); psychiatric-mental health nurse practitioner (MSN); women's health nurse practitioner (MSN); women's health nurse practitioner/adult gerontology primary care nurse practitioner (MSN); MSN/M Div; MSN/MTS. *Accreditation:* ACNM/ACME (one or more programs are accredited). Part-time programs available. Postbaccalaureate distance learning degree programs offered (minimal on-campus study). *Faculty:* 139 full-time (124 women), 452 part-time/adjunct (319 women). *Students:* 527 full-time (463 women), 369 part-time (333 women); includes 120 minority (46 Black or African American, non-Hispanic/Latino; 8 American Indian or Alaska Native, non-Hispanic/Latino; 26 Asian, non-Hispanic/Latino; 24 Hispanic/Latino; 4 Native Hawaiian or other Pacific Islander, non-Hispanic/Latino; 12 Two or more races, non-Hispanic/Latino), 7 international. Average age 32. 1,257 applicants, 49% accepted, 457 enrolled. In 2013, 364 master's, 43 doctorates awarded. *Degree requirements:* For doctorate, comprehensive exam, thesis/dissertation. *Entrance requirements:* For master's, GRE General Test (within the past 5 years), minimum B average in undergraduate course work, 3 letters of recommendation; for doctorate, GRE General Test, interview, 3 letters of recommendation from doctorally-prepared faculty, MSN, essay. Additional exam requirements/recommendations for international students: Required—TOEFL (minimum score 570 paper-based), IELTS (minimum score 6.5). *Application deadline:* For fall admission, 12/1 priority date for domestic and international students. Applications are processed on a rolling basis. Application fee: $50. Electronic applications accepted. *Expenses:* Contact institution. *Financial support:* In 2013–14, 582 students received support. Scholarships/grants and health care benefits available. Support available to part-time students. Financial award application deadline: 3/15; financial award applicants required to submit FAFSA. *Faculty research:* Lymphedema, palliative care and bereavement, health services research including workforce, safety and quality of care, gerontology, better birth outcomes including nutrition. *Total annual research expenditures:* $2.5 million. *Unit head:* Dr. Linda Norman, Dean, 615-343-8876, Fax: 615-343-7711, E-mail: linda.norman@vanderbilt.edu. *Application contact:* Patricia Peerman, Assistant Dean for Enrollment Management, 615-322-3800, Fax: 615-343-0333, E-mail: vusn-admissions@vanderbilt.edu.
Website: http://www.nursing.vanderbilt.edu

Villanova University, College of Nursing, Villanova, PA 19085-1699. Offers adult nurse practitioner (MSN, Post Master's Certificate); family nurse practitioner (MSN, Post Master's Certificate); health care administration (MSN, Post Master's Certificate); nurse anesthetist (MSN, Post Master's Certificate); nursing (PhD); nursing education (MSN, Post Master's Certificate); nursing practice (DNP); pediatric nurse practitioner (MSN, Post Master's Certificate). *Accreditation:* AACN; AANA/CANAEP. Part-time programs available. Postbaccalaureate distance learning degree programs offered (minimal on-campus study). *Faculty:* 17 full-time (all women), 4 part-time/adjunct (all women). *Students:* 28 full-time (26 women), 191 part-time (161 women); includes 22 minority (2 Black or African American, non-Hispanic/Latino; 6 Asian, non-Hispanic/Latino; 7 Hispanic/Latino; 7 Two or more races, non-Hispanic/Latino), 18 international. Average age 30. 176 applicants, 65% accepted, 82 enrolled. In 2013, 64 master's, 7 doctorates, 5 other advanced degrees awarded. *Degree requirements:* For master's, independent study project; for doctorate, comprehensive exam, thesis/dissertation. *Entrance requirements:* For master's, GRE or MAT, BSN, 1 year of recent nursing experience, physical assessment, course work in statistics; for doctorate, GRE, MSN. Additional exam requirements/recommendations for international students: Required—TOEFL (minimum score 540 paper-based; 83 iBT), IELTS (minimum score 6.5). *Application deadline:* For fall admission, 7/1 priority date for domestic students, 7/1 for international students; for spring admission, 11/1 priority date for domestic students, 11/1 for international students. Applications are processed on a rolling basis. Application fee: $50. Electronic applications accepted. *Expenses:* Contact institution. *Financial support:* In 2013–14, 39 students received support, including 5 teaching assistantships with full tuition reimbursements available (averaging $14,475 per year); institutionally sponsored loans, scholarships/grants, traineeships, tuition waivers (full), and unspecified assistantships also available. Financial award application deadline: 7/1; financial award applicants required to submit FAFSA. *Faculty research:* Genetics, ethics, cognitive development of students, women with disabilities, nursing leadership. *Unit head:* Dr. Marguerite K. Schlag, Assistant Dean/Director, Graduate Programs, 610-519-4907, Fax: 610-519-7650, E-mail: marguerite.schlag@villanova.edu.
Website: http://www.nursing.villanova.edu/

Virginia Commonwealth University, Graduate School, School of Nursing, Richmond, VA 23284-9005. Offers adult health acute nursing (MS); adult health primary nursing (MS); biobehavioral clinical research (PhD); child health nursing (MS); clinical nurse leader (MS); family health nursing (MS); nurse educator (MS); nurse practitioner (MS); nursing (Certificate); nursing administration (MS), including clinical nurse manager;

psychiatric-mental health nursing (MS); women's health nursing (MS). Part-time and evening/weekend programs available. *Degree requirements:* For master's, thesis optional; for doctorate, thesis/dissertation. *Entrance requirements:* For master's, GRE General Test, BSN, minimum GPA of 2.8; for doctorate, GRE General Test. Additional exam requirements/recommendations for international students: Required—TOEFL (minimum score 600 paper-based; 100 iBT). Electronic applications accepted.

Walden University, Graduate Programs, School of Nursing, Minneapolis, MN 55401. Offers adult-gerontology acute care nurse practitioner (MSN); adult-gerontology nurse practitioner (MSN); education (MSN); family nurse practitioner (MSN); informatics (MSN); leadership and management (MSN); nursing (DNP, PhD, Post-Master's Certificate), including education (PhD), healthcare administration (PhD), interdisciplinary health (PhD), leadership (PhD), nursing education (Post-Master's Certificate), nursing informatics (Post-Master's Certificate), nursing leadership and management (Post-Master's Certificate), public health policy (PhD). *Accreditation:* AACN. Part-time and evening/weekend programs available. Postbaccalaureate distance learning degree programs offered (no on-campus study). *Faculty:* 22 full-time (19 women), 343 part-time/adjunct (301 women). *Students:* 5,828 full-time (5,240 women), 2,803 part-time (2,578 women); includes 2,920 minority (1,893 Black or African American, non-Hispanic/Latino; 40 American Indian or Alaska Native, non-Hispanic/Latino; 438 Asian, non-Hispanic/Latino; 391 Hispanic/Latino; 35 Native Hawaiian or other Pacific Islander, non-Hispanic/Latino; 123 Two or more races, non-Hispanic/Latino), 147 international. Average age 41. 1,795 applicants, 95% accepted, 1375 enrolled. In 2013, 1,879 master's, 1 doctorate, 36 other advanced degrees awarded. *Degree requirements:* For doctorate, thesis/dissertation (for some programs), residency (for some programs), field experience (for some programs). *Entrance requirements:* For master's, bachelor's degree or equivalent in related field or RN; minimum GPA of 2.5; official transcripts; goal statement (for some programs); access to computer and Internet; for doctorate, master's degree or higher, three years of related professional or academic experience, RN, goal statement (for some programs); access to computer and Internet; for Post-Master's Certificate, relevant work experience; access to computer and Internet. Additional exam requirements/recommendations for international students: Required—TOEFL (minimum score 550 paper-based; 79 iBT), IELTS (minimum score 6.5), Michigan English Language Assessment Battery (minimum score 82), or PTE. *Application deadline:* Applications are processed on a rolling basis. Application fee: $0. Electronic applications accepted. *Expenses: Tuition:* Full-time $11,813.55; part-time $500 per credit. *Required fees:* $618.76. *Financial support:* Fellowships, Federal Work-Study, scholarships/grants, unspecified assistantships, and family tuition reduction, active duty/veteran tuition reduction, group tuition reduction, interest-free payment plans, employee tuition reduction available. Support available to part-time students. Financial award applicants required to submit FAFSA. *Unit head:* Dr. Andrea Lindell, Associate Dean, 800-925-3368. *Application contact:* Jennifer Hall, Vice President of Enrollment Management, 866-4-WALDEN, E-mail: info@waldenu.edu.
Website: http://www.waldenu.edu/programs/colleges-schools/nursing

Walsh University, Graduate Studies, School of Nursing, North Canton, OH 44720-3396. Offers academic nurse educator (MSN); clinical nurse leader (MSN); nursing practice (DNP). Part-time and evening/weekend programs available. Postbaccalaureate distance learning degree programs offered (minimal on-campus study). *Faculty:* 6 full-time (all women), 6 part-time/adjunct (5 women). *Students:* 13 full-time (10 women), 29 part-time (all women); includes 2 minority (1 Black or African American, non-Hispanic/Latino; 1 Hispanic/Latino). Average age 39. 27 applicants, 89% accepted, 19 enrolled. *Degree requirements:* For doctorate, scholarly project; residency practicum. *Entrance requirements:* For master's, undergraduate nursing degree, current unencumbered RN license, completion of an undergraduate or graduate statistics course, essay, interview, recommendations; for doctorate, BSN; master's degree; statistics and research courses; essay; interview. Additional exam requirements/recommendations for international students: Required—TOEFL. *Application deadline:* Applications are processed on a rolling basis. Electronic applications accepted. *Expenses: Tuition:* Full-time $10,890; part-time $605 per credit hour. *Required fees:* $100; $100. *Financial support:* In 2013–14, 32 students received support. Research assistantships, tuition waivers (partial), and tuition discounts available. Financial award application deadline: 12/31; financial award applicants required to submit FAFSA. *Faculty research:* Faith community nursing, gerontology, women's health, global nursing education, nursing assessment, grief and reconstitution, health needs of psychiatric patients, psychometric testing. *Unit head:* Dr. Karen Gehrling, Director, Graduate Program in Nursing, 330-244-4649, Fax: 330-490-7371, E-mail: kgehrling@walsh.edu. *Application contact:* Audra Dice, Graduate and Transfer Admissions Counselor, 330-490-7181, Fax: 330-244-4680, E-mail: adice@walsh.edu.
Website: http://www.walsh.edu/master-of-science-in-nursing

Washburn University, School of Nursing, Topeka, KS 66621. Offers clinical nurse leader (MSN); nursing (DNP). *Accreditation:* AACN. Part-time programs available. *Entrance requirements:* Additional exam requirements/recommendations for international students: Required—TOEFL. *Application deadline:* For fall admission, 3/15 for international students. Application fee: $35. *Expenses:* Tuition, state resident: full-time $5850; part-time $325 per credit hour. Tuition, nonresident: full-time $11,916; part-time $662 per credit hour. *Required fees:* $86; $43 per semester. Tuition and fees vary according to program. *Financial support:* Application deadline: 2/15. *Unit head:* Dr. Monica S. Scheibmeir, Dean, 785-670-1526, E-mail: monica.scheibmeir@washburn.edu. *Application contact:* Mary V. Allen, Director of Student Services, 785-670-1533, E-mail: mary.allen@washburn.edu.
Website: http://www.washburn.edu/sonu

Washington Adventist University, Program in Nursing - Business Leadership, Takoma Park, MD 20912. Offers MSN. Part-time programs available. *Entrance requirements:* Additional exam requirements/recommendations for international students: Required—TOEFL (minimum score 550 paper-based), IELTS (minimum score 5).

Waynesburg University, Graduate and Professional Studies, Canonsburg, PA 15370. Offers business (MBA), including energy management, finance, health systems, human resources, leadership, market development; counseling (MA), including addictions counseling, clinical mental health; education (M Ed, MAT), including autism (M Ed), curriculum and instruction (M Ed), educational leadership (M Ed), online teaching (M Ed); nursing (MSN), including administration, education, informatics; nursing practice (DNP); special education (M Ed); technology (M Ed); MSN/MBA. *Accreditation:* AACN. Part-time and evening/weekend programs available. *Faculty:* 11 full-time (5 women), 136 part-time/adjunct (80 women). *Students:* 146 full-time (99 women), 419 part-time (268 women). In 2013, 290 master's, 7 doctorates awarded. *Degree requirements:* For doctorate, thesis/dissertation. *Entrance requirements:* Additional exam requirements/recommendations for international students: Required—TOEFL. *Application deadline:* For fall admission, 8/1 priority date for domestic students. Applications are processed on a rolling basis. Electronic applications accepted. *Financial support:* Available to part-time students. Application deadline: 5/1. *Unit head:* David Mariner, Dean, 724-743-4420, Fax: 724-743-4425, E-mail: dmariner@waynesburg.edu. *Application contact:* Dr. Michael Bednarski, Director of Enrollment, 724-743-4420, Fax: 724-743-4425, E-mail: mbednars@waynesburg.edu.
Website: http://www.waynesburg.edu/

West Chester University of Pennsylvania, College of Health Sciences, Department of Nursing, West Chester, PA 19383. Offers nursing (DNP); public health nursing (MSN), including administration, education, integrative health. *Accreditation:* AACN. Part-time and evening/weekend programs available. Postbaccalaureate distance learning degree programs offered (minimal on-campus study). *Faculty:* 4 full-time (3 women). *Students:* 12 full-time (11 women), 17 part-time (15 women); includes 9 minority (7 Black or African American, non-Hispanic/Latino; 1 Asian, non-Hispanic/Latino; 1 Hispanic/Latino), 2 international. Average age 42. 11 applicants, 91% accepted, 7 enrolled. In 2013, 17 master's awarded. *Entrance requirements:* For master's, RN license, BSN or RN with bachelor's degree in another discipline, minimum GPA of 2.8, experience as a nurse providing direct clinical care, two letters of recommendation; for doctorate, minimum graduate GPA of 3.0, two letters of reference, interview. Additional exam requirements/recommendations for international students: Required—TOEFL (minimum score 550 paper-based; 80 iBT). *Application deadline:* For fall admission, 4/15 priority date for domestic students, 3/15 for international students; for spring admission, 10/15 priority date for domestic students, 9/1 for international students. Applications are processed on a rolling basis. Application fee: $45. Electronic applications accepted. *Expenses:* Tuition, state resident: full-time $7956; part-time $442 per credit. Tuition, nonresident: full-time $11,934; part-time $663 per credit. *Required fees:* $2134.20; $106.24 per credit. Tuition and fees vary according to campus/location and program. *Financial support:* Unspecified assistantships available. Support available to part-time students. Financial award application deadline: 2/15; financial award applicants required to submit FAFSA. *Unit head:* Dr. Charlotte Mackey, Chair and Graduate Coordinator, 610-436-3474, Fax: 610-436-3083, E-mail: cmackey@wcupa.edu.
Website: http://www.wcupa.edu/_ACADEMICS/HealthSciences/nursing/

Western Governors University, College of Health Professions, Salt Lake City, UT 84107. Offers healthcare management (MBA); leadership and management (MSN); nursing education (MSN). Evening/weekend programs available. *Degree requirements:* For master's, capstone project. *Entrance requirements:* For master's, Readiness Assessment, transcripts. Additional exam requirements/recommendations for international students: Required—TOEFL (minimum score 450 paper-based; 80 iBT). Electronic applications accepted.

Western University of Health Sciences, College of Graduate Nursing, Master of Science in Nursing Program, Pomona, CA 91766-1854. Offers administrative nurse leader (MSN); ambulatory care (MSN); clinical nurse leader (MSN); family nurse practitioner (MSN); nursing (MSN). *Faculty:* 14 full-time (all women), 11 part-time/adjunct (10 women). *Students:* 255 full-time (218 women), 10 part-time (all women); includes 163 minority (20 Black or African American, non-Hispanic/Latino; 1 American Indian or Alaska Native, non-Hispanic/Latino; 88 Asian, non-Hispanic/Latino; 40 Hispanic/Latino; 1 Native Hawaiian or other Pacific Islander, non-Hispanic/Latino; 13 Two or more races, non-Hispanic/Latino), 2 international. Average age 31. 739 applicants, 23% accepted, 114 enrolled. In 2013, 73 master's awarded. *Degree requirements:* For master's, thesis. *Entrance requirements:* For master's, BSN, minimum GPA of 3.0, 3 letters of recommendation, resume/curriculum vitae. Additional exam requirements/recommendations for international students: Required—TOEFL. *Application deadline:* For fall admission, 10/1 for domestic students. Application fee: $60. Electronic applications accepted. *Unit head:* Dr. Karen J. Hanford, Dean, 909-469-5523, Fax: 909-469-5521, E-mail: khanford@westernu.edu. *Application contact:* Kathryn Ford, Director of Admissions/International Student Advisor, 909-469-5335, Fax: 909-469-5570, E-mail: admissions@westernu.edu.

West Virginia Wesleyan College, Department of Nursing, Buckhannon, WV 26201. Offers family nurse practitioner (Post Master's Certificate); family nurse practitoner (MS); nurse administrator (MS); nurse educator (MS); nurse-midwifery (MS); nursing administration (Post Master's Certificate); nursing education (Post Master's Certificate); psychiatric mental health nurse practitioner (MS); MSN/MBA.

Wilmington University, College of Health Professions, New Castle, DE 19720-6491. Offers adult nurse practitioner (MSN); family nurse practitioner (MSN); gerontology nurse practitioner (MSN); nursing (MSN); nursing leadership (MSN); nursing practice (DNP). *Accreditation:* AACN. Part-time programs available. *Degree requirements:* For master's, thesis. *Entrance requirements:* For master's, BSN, RN license, interview, 3 letters of recommendation. Additional exam requirements/recommendations for international students: Required—TOEFL (minimum score 500 paper-based). Electronic applications accepted. *Faculty research:* Outcomes assessment, student writing ability.

Winona State University, College of Nursing and Health Sciences, Winona, MN 55987. Offers adult nurse practitioner (MS, Post Master's Certificate); clinical nurse specialist (MS, Post Master's Certificate); family nurse practitioner (MS, Post Master's Certificate); nurse administrator (MS); nurse educator (MS, Post Master's Certificate); nursing (DNP). *Accreditation:* AACN. Part-time programs available. Postbaccalaureate distance learning degree programs offered (no on-campus study). *Degree requirements:* For master's, thesis; for doctorate, capstone. *Entrance requirements:* For master's, GRE (if GPA less than 3.0). Additional exam requirements/recommendations for international students: Required—TOEFL (minimum score 550 paper-based).

Wright State University, School of Graduate Studies, College of Nursing and Health, Program in Nursing, Dayton, OH 45435. Offers acute care nurse practitioner (MS); administration of nursing and health care systems (MS); adult health (MS); child and adolescent health (MS); community health (MS); family nurse practitioner (MS); nurse practitioner (MS); school nurse (MS); MBA/MS. *Accreditation:* AACN. Part-time and evening/weekend programs available. *Degree requirements:* For master's, thesis or alternative. *Entrance requirements:* For master's, GRE General Test, BSN from NLN-accredited college, Ohio RN license. Additional exam requirements/recommendations for international students: Required—TOEFL. *Faculty research:* Clinical nursing and health, teaching, caring, pain administration, informatics and technology.

Xavier University, College of Social Sciences, Health and Education, School of Nursing, Nursing Program, Cincinnati, OH 45207. Offers clinical nurse leader (MSN); education (MSN); forensic nursing (MSN); healthcare law (MSN); informatics (MSN); nursing administration (MSN); school nursing (MSN); MSN/M Ed; MSN/MBA; MSN/MS. *Faculty:* 16 full-time (15 women), 9 part-time/adjunct (all women). *Students:* 66 full-time (56 women), 170 part-time (162 women); includes 35 minority (17 Black or African American, non-Hispanic/Latino; 2 American Indian or Alaska Native, non-Hispanic/Latino; 5 Asian, non-Hispanic/Latino; 10 Hispanic/Latino; 1 Native Hawaiian or other Pacific Islander, non-Hispanic/Latino). Average age 37. 103 applicants, 66% accepted, 86 enrolled. In 2013, 78 master's awarded. *Expenses: Tuition:* Part-time $594 per credit hour. *Required fees:* $3 per semester. *Financial support:* In 2013–14, 68 students received support. *Unit head:* Dr. Susan M. Schmidt, Director, School of Nursing, 513-745-3814, E-mail: schmidt@xavier.edu. *Application contact:* Marilyn Volk Gomez, Director of Nursing Student Services, 513-745-4392, Fax: 513-745-1087, E-mail: gomez@xavier.edu.
Website: http://www.xavier.edu/msn/

Nursing and Healthcare Administration

York College of Pennsylvania, Department of Nursing, York, PA 17405-7199. Offers adult gerontology clinical nurse specialist (MS), including administration, education; adult gerontology nurse practitioner (MS); certified nurse anesthetist (MS); nurse educator (MS); nursing (DNP). *Accreditation:* AACN; AANA/CANAEP. Part-time and evening/weekend programs available. *Faculty:* 10 full-time (all women), 4 part-time/adjunct (1 woman). *Students:* 33 full-time (26 women), 61 part-time (53 women); includes 12 minority (7 Black or African American, non-Hispanic/Latino; 2 American Indian or Alaska Native, non-Hispanic/Latino; 3 Asian, non-Hispanic/Latino), 1 international. Average age 37. 87 applicants, 31% accepted, 24 enrolled. In 2013, 26 master's, 4 doctorates awarded. *Entrance requirements:* For master's, GRE General Test, minimum GPA of 3.0 from CCNE- or NLNAC-accredited institution; for doctorate, master's degree in nursing from a CCNE- or NLNAC-accredited institution; minimum GPA of 3.0. Additional exam requirements/recommendations for international students: Required—TOEFL (minimum score 530 paper-based; 72 iBT). *Application deadline:* For fall admission, 7/15 priority date for domestic students; for spring admission, 11/15 priority date for domestic students. Applications are processed on a rolling basis. Application fee: $50. Electronic applications accepted. *Expenses: Tuition:* Full-time $12,870; part-time $715 per credit. *Required fees:* $1660; $360 per semester. Tuition and fees vary according to degree level. *Financial support:* Federal Work-Study available. *Faculty research:* Student stress response to simulation versus clinical, evidence-based practice in all clinical settings. *Unit head:* Dr. Richard Haas, Graduate Program Director, 717-815-1243, E-mail: rhaas@ycp.edu. *Application contact:* Diane Dube, Administrative Assistant, Graduate Programs in Nursing, 717-815-1462, E-mail: ddube@ycp.edu.
Website: http://www.ycp.edu/academics/academic-departments/nursing/

Nursing Education

Abilene Christian University, Graduate School, School of Nursing, Abilene, TX 79699-9100. Offers education and administration (MSN); family nurse practitioner (MSN); nursing (Certificate). *Accreditation:* AACN. Part-time programs available. *Faculty:* 7 part-time/adjunct (all women). *Students:* 1 (woman) part-time. 11 applicants. In 2013, 3 master's awarded. *Degree requirements:* For master's, practicum. *Entrance requirements:* For master's, GRE General Test. Additional exam requirements/recommendations for international students: Required—TOEFL (minimum score 550 paper-based; 90 iBT), IELTS (minimum score 6.5). *Application deadline:* For fall admission, 4/1 priority date for domestic students; for spring admission, 11/1 for domestic students. Applications are processed on a rolling basis. Application fee: $50. Electronic applications accepted. *Expenses: Tuition:* Full-time $17,100; part-time $950 per credit hour. *Financial support:* Application deadline: 4/1; applicants required to submit FAFSA. *Unit head:* Dr. Becky Hammack, Graduate Director, 325-674-2265, Fax: 325-674-6256, E-mail: rsh12a@acu.edu. *Application contact:* Corey Patterson, Director of Graduate Admission and Recruiting, 325-674-6566, Fax: 325-674-6717, E-mail: gradinfo@acu.edu.

Adelphi University, College of Nursing and Public Health, Program in Nursing Education, Garden City, NY 11530-0701. Offers MS, Certificate. *Students:* 13 part-time (12 women); includes 7 minority (6 Black or African American, non-Hispanic/Latino; 1 Asian, non-Hispanic/Latino). Average age 44. In 2013, 5 master's awarded. *Expenses: Tuition:* Full-time $32,530; part-time $1010 per credit. *Required fees:* $1150. Tuition and fees vary according to degree level and program. *Financial support:* Teaching assistantships, career-related internships or fieldwork, Federal Work-Study, tuition waivers, and unspecified assistantships available. *Unit head:* Joan Valas, Director, 516-877-4571, E-mail: valas@adelphi.edu. *Application contact:* Christine Murphy, Director of Admissions, 516-877-3050, Fax: 516-877-3039, E-mail: graduateadmissions@adelphi.edu.

Albany State University, College of Sciences and Health Professions, Albany, GA 31705-2717. Offers criminal justice (MS), including corrections, forensic science, law enforcement, public administration; mathematics education (M Ed); nursing (MSN), including RN to MSN family nurse practitioner, RN to MSN nurse educator; science education (M Ed). Part-time and evening/weekend programs available. Postbaccalaureate distance learning degree programs offered. *Degree requirements:* For master's, comprehensive exam, thesis. *Entrance requirements:* For master's, GRE or MAT, official transcript, letters of recommendations, pre-medical/certificate of immunizations. Electronic applications accepted.

Alverno College, School of Nursing, Milwaukee, WI 53234-3922. Offers family nurse practitioner (MSN); mental health nurse practitioner (MSN); nursing education (MSN). *Accreditation:* AACN. Part-time and evening/weekend programs available. *Faculty:* 7 full-time (all women), 8 part-time/adjunct (4 women). *Students:* 82 full-time (79 women), 84 part-time (79 women); includes 48 minority (24 Black or African American, non-Hispanic/Latino; 1 American Indian or Alaska Native, non-Hispanic/Latino; 6 Asian, non-Hispanic/Latino; 11 Hispanic/Latino; 6 Two or more races, non-Hispanic/Latino), 1 international. Average age 36. 59 applicants, 100% accepted, 47 enrolled. In 2013, 33 master's awarded. *Degree requirements:* For master's, 500 clinical hours, capstone. *Entrance requirements:* For master's, BSN, current license. Additional exam requirements/recommendations for international students: Required—TOEFL. *Application deadline:* For fall admission, 7/15 priority date for domestic and international students; for spring admission, 12/15 priority date for domestic and international students. Applications are processed on a rolling basis. Application fee: $0. Electronic applications accepted. Application fee is waived when completed online. *Expenses:* Contact institution. *Financial support:* In 2013–14, 4 students received support. Federal Work-Study and scholarships/grants available. Support available to part-time students. Financial award application deadline: 4/15; financial award applicants required to submit FAFSA. *Faculty research:* Impact of stroke on sexuality, children's asthma management, factors affecting baccalaureate student success. *Unit head:* Dr. Carol Sabel, Associate Dean for MSN Program, 414-382-6309, Fax: 414-382-6354, E-mail: carol.sabel@alverno.edu. *Application contact:* Janet Stikel, Associate Director of Admissions - Adult and Graduate, 414-382-6112, Fax: 414-382-6354, E-mail: janet.stikel@alverno.edu.

American International College, School of Health Sciences, Department of Nursing, Springfield, MA 01109-3189. Offers nursing administration (MSN); nursing education (MSN). *Accreditation:* AACN. Part-time and evening/weekend programs available. Postbaccalaureate distance learning degree programs offered (minimal on-campus study). *Faculty:* 1 (woman) full-time, 1 (woman) part-time/adjunct. *Students:* 12 full-time (all women), 11 part-time (9 women); includes 4 minority (all Black or African American, non-Hispanic/Latino). Average age 39. 17 applicants, 94% accepted, 12 enrolled. In 2013, 10 master's awarded. *Entrance requirements:* For master's, BSN, minimum GPA of 3.0. Additional exam requirements/recommendations for international students: Required—TOEFL or IELTS. *Application deadline:* For fall admission, 7/1 for domestic and international students; for spring admission, 12/1 for domestic and international students. Applications are processed on a rolling basis. Application fee: $50. Electronic applications accepted. *Expenses: Tuition:* Full-time $14,040; part-time $780 per credit. Tuition and fees vary according to course load, degree level and program. *Financial support:* Applicants required to submit FAFSA. *Unit head:* Dr. Ellen Furman, Associate Director of Graduate Nursing, 413-205-3918, Fax: 413-654-1430, E-mail: ellen.furman@aic.edu. *Application contact:* Kerry Barnes, Director of Graduate Admissions, 413-205-3703, Fax: 413-205-3051, E-mail: kerry.barnes@aic.edu.
Website: http://www.aic.edu/academics/hs/nursing

Angelo State University, College of Graduate Studies, College of Health and Human Services, Department of Nursing and Rehabilitation Sciences, San Angelo, TX 76909. Offers advanced practice registered nurse (MSN); nurse educator (MSN); registered nurse first assistant (MSN). Part-time and evening/weekend programs available. Postbaccalaureate distance learning degree programs offered (no on-campus study). *Degree requirements:* For master's, comprehensive exam. *Entrance requirements:* For master's, essay, three letters of recommendation. Additional exam requirements/recommendations for international students: Required—TOEFL or IELTS. Electronic applications accepted.

Auburn University, Graduate School, School of Nursing, Auburn University, AL 36849. Offers nursing educator (MSN); primary care practitioner (MSN). *Accreditation:* AACN. *Faculty:* 17 full-time (15 women). *Students:* 2 full-time (both women), 77 part-time (72 women); includes 12 minority (9 Black or African American, non-Hispanic/Latino; 1 American Indian or Alaska Native, non-Hispanic/Latino; 1 Asian, non-Hispanic/Latino; 1 Hispanic/Latino), 1 international. Average age 31. 87 applicants, 79% accepted, 47 enrolled. In 2013, 29 master's awarded. *Expenses:* Tuition, state resident: full-time $8262; part-time $459 per credit hour. Tuition, nonresident: full-time $24,786; part-time $1377 per credit hour. Tuition and fees vary according to degree level and program. *Unit head:* Dr. Gregg Newschwander, Dean, 334-844-3658, E-mail: gen0002@auburn.edu. *Application contact:* Dr. George Flowers, Dean of the Graduate School, 334-844-4700, E-mail: gradadm@auburn.edu.
Website: http://www.auburn.edu/academic/nursing/

Austin Peay State University, College of Graduate Studies, College of Behavioral and Health Sciences, School of Nursing, Clarksville, TN 37044. Offers advanced practice (MSN); nursing administration (MSN); nursing education (MSN); nursing informatics (MSN). Part-time programs available. Postbaccalaureate distance learning degree programs offered. *Faculty:* 9 full-time (all women), 7 part-time/adjunct (all women). *Students:* 47 full-time (43 women), 136 part-time (129 women); includes 30 minority (18 Black or African American, non-Hispanic/Latino; 4 Asian, non-Hispanic/Latino; 4 Hispanic/Latino; 4 Two or more races, non-Hispanic/Latino). Average age 35. 47 applicants, 85% accepted, 37 enrolled. In 2013, 39 master's awarded. *Degree requirements:* For master's, comprehensive exam. *Entrance requirements:* For master's, GRE General Test, minimum GPA of 3.0, RN license eligibility, 3 letters of recommendation. Additional exam requirements/recommendations for international students: Required—TOEFL (minimum score 600 paper-based). *Application deadline:* For fall admission, 8/5 priority date for domestic students. Applications are processed on a rolling basis. Application fee: $25. Electronic applications accepted. *Expenses:* Tuition, state resident: full-time $7500; part-time $375 per credit hour. Tuition, nonresident: full-time $20,800; part-time $1040 per credit hour. *Required fees:* $1284; $64.20 per credit hour. *Financial support:* In 2013–14, research assistantships with full tuition reimbursements (averaging $6,500 per year) were awarded; career-related internships or fieldwork, Federal Work-Study, institutionally sponsored loans, scholarships/grants, and unspecified assistantships also available. Support available to part-time students. *Unit head:* Dr. Patty Orr, Director, 931-221-7710, Fax: 931-221-7595, E-mail: orrp@apsu.edu. *Application contact:* June D. Lee, Graduate Coordinator, 800-859-4723, Fax: 931-221-7641, E-mail: gradadmissions@apsu.edu.
Website: http://www.apsu.edu/nursing

Azusa Pacific University, School of Nursing, Azusa, CA 91702-7000. Offers nursing (MSN); nursing education (PhD). *Accreditation:* AACN. Part-time and evening/weekend programs available. *Degree requirements:* For master's, thesis optional. *Entrance requirements:* For master's, BSN.

Barry University, School of Adult and Continuing Education, Division of Nursing, Program in Nursing Education, Miami Shores, FL 33161-6695. Offers MSN, Certificate. *Accreditation:* AACN. Part-time and evening/weekend programs available. *Degree requirements:* For master's, research project or thesis. *Entrance requirements:* For master's, GRE General Test or MAT, BSN, minimum GPA of 3.0, course work in statistics. Electronic applications accepted. *Faculty research:* HIV/AIDS, gerontology.

Bellarmine University, Donna and Allan Lansing School of Nursing and Health Sciences, Louisville, KY 40205. Offers family nurse practitioner (MSN); health science (MHS); nursing administration (MSN); nursing education (MSN); nursing practice (DNP); physical therapy (DPT). *Accreditation:* AACN; APTA. Part-time and evening/weekend programs available. *Faculty:* 21 full-time (19 women), 8 part-time/adjunct (5 women). *Students:* 162 full-time (111 women), 120 part-time (113 women); includes 16 minority (6 Black or African American, non-Hispanic/Latino; 1 American Indian or Alaska Native, non-Hispanic/Latino; 3 Asian, non-Hispanic/Latino; 3 Hispanic/Latino; 3 Two or more races, non-Hispanic/Latino). Average age 29. In 2013, 30 master's, 54 doctorates awarded. *Degree requirements:* For doctorate, comprehensive exam, thesis/dissertation. *Entrance requirements:* For master's, GRE General Test, RN license; for doctorate, GRE General Test, Physical Therapist Centralized Application Service (for DPT). Additional exam requirements/recommendations for international students: Required—TOEFL (minimum score 550 paper-based; 80 iBT). Application fee: $25. Electronic applications accepted. *Expenses:* Contact institution. *Financial support:* Career-related internships or fieldwork and scholarships/grants available. *Faculty research:* Nursing: pain, empathy, leadership styles, control; physical therapy: service-learning; exercise in chronic and pre-operative conditions, athletes; women's health; aging. *Unit head:* Dr. Mark Wiegand, Dean, 800-274-4723 Ext. 8368, E-mail: mwiegand@bellarmine.edu. *Application contact:* Julie Armstrong-Binnix, Health Science Recruiter, 800-274-4723 Ext. 8364, E-mail: julieab@bellarmine.edu.
Website: http://www.bellarmine.edu/lansing

Bellin College, School of Nursing, Green Bay, WI 54305. Offers family nurse practitioner (MSN); nurse educator (MSN). *Accreditation:* AACN. *Faculty:* 1 (woman) full-time, 3 part-time/adjunct (2 women). *Students:* 37 part-time (all women). *Expenses: Tuition:* Part-time $714 per credit. *Required fees:* $100 per year. *Unit head:* Dr. Kimberly Udlis, Graduate Program Director, 920-433-6624, Fax: 920-433-1921, E-mail: kimberly.udlis@bellincollege.edu.

Bethel University, Graduate School, St. Paul, MN 55112-6999. Offers autism spectrum disorders (Certificate); business administration (MBA); communication (MA); counseling psychology (MA); educational leadership (Ed D); gerontology (MA); international baccalaureate education (Certificate); K-12 education (MA); literacy education (MA, Certificate); nurse educator (Certificate); nurse leader (Certificate); nurse-midwifery (MS); nursing (MS); physician assistant (MS); postsecondary teaching (Certificate); special education (MA); strategic leadership (MA); teaching (MA). Part-time and evening/weekend programs available. Postbaccalaureate distance learning degree programs offered (no on-campus study). *Faculty:* 13 full-time (7 women), 89 part-time/adjunct (43 women). *Students:* 692 full-time (457 women), 573 part-time (371 women); includes 170 minority (86 Black or African American, non-Hispanic/Latino; 1 American Indian or Alaska Native, non-Hispanic/Latino; 49 Asian, non-Hispanic/Latino; 20 Hispanic/Latino; 1 Native Hawaiian or other Pacific Islander, non-Hispanic/Latino; 13 Two or more races, non-Hispanic/Latino), 21 international. Average age 37. In 2013, 166 master's, 9 doctorates, 11 other advanced degrees awarded. *Degree requirements:* For master's, comprehensive exam (for some programs), thesis (for some programs); for doctorate, comprehensive exam, thesis/dissertation. *Entrance requirements:* Additional exam requirements/recommendations for international students: Required—TOEFL (minimum score 550 paper-based; 80 iBT). *Application deadline:* Applications are processed on a rolling basis. Electronic applications accepted. Tuition and fees vary according to course load, degree level and program. *Financial support:* Teaching assistantships, career-related internships or fieldwork, and scholarships/grants available. Support available to part-time students. Financial award applicants required to submit FAFSA. *Unit head:* Dick Crombie, Vice-President/Dean, 651-635-8000, Fax: 651-635-8004, E-mail: gs@bethel.edu. *Application contact:* Director of Admissions, 651-635-8000, Fax: 651-635-8004, E-mail: gs@bethel.edu.
Website: http://gs.bethel.edu/

Bowie State University, Graduate Programs, Department of Nursing, Bowie, MD 20715-9465. Offers administration of nursing services (MS); family nurse practitioner (MS); nursing education (MS). Part-time programs available. *Degree requirements:* For master's, comprehensive exam, thesis, research paper. *Entrance requirements:* For master's, minimum GPA of 2.5. Electronic applications accepted. *Expenses:* Tuition, state resident: full-time $8665. Tuition, nonresident: full-time $16,007. *Required fees:* $1927. *Faculty research:* Minority health, women's health, gerontology, leadership management.

Brenau University, Sydney O. Smith Graduate School, College of Health and Science, Gainesville, GA 30501. Offers family nurse practitioner (MSN); nurse educator (MSN); nursing management (MSN); occupational therapy (MS); psychology (MS). *Accreditation:* AOTA. Part-time and evening/weekend programs available. *Degree requirements:* For master's, comprehensive exam (for some programs), thesis (for some programs), clinical practicum hours. *Entrance requirements:* For master's, GRE General Test or MAT (for some programs), interview, writing sample, references (for some programs). Additional exam requirements/recommendations for international students: Required—TOEFL (minimum score 500 paper-based; 61 iBT); Recommended—IELTS (minimum score 5). Electronic applications accepted. *Expenses:* Contact institution.

California Baptist University, Program in Nursing, Riverside, CA 92504-3206. Offers clinical nurse specialist (MSN); family nurse practitioner (MSN); healthcare systems management (MSN); nursing (MSN); teaching-learning (MSN). Part-time programs available. *Faculty:* 15 full-time (all women), 7 part-time/adjunct (all women). *Students:* 49 full-time (41 women), 69 part-time (55 women); includes 61 minority (18 Black or African American, non-Hispanic/Latino; 1 American Indian or Alaska Native, non-Hispanic/Latino; 17 Asian, non-Hispanic/Latino; 22 Hispanic/Latino; 3 Two or more races, non-Hispanic/Latino). Average age 33. 48 applicants, 65% accepted, 20 enrolled. In 2013, 9 master's awarded. *Degree requirements:* For master's, comprehensive exam (for some programs), thesis or alternative, comprehensive exam or directed project thesis; capstone practicum. *Entrance requirements:* For master's, GRE or California Critical Thinking Skills Test; Test of Essential Academic Skills (TEAS), minimum undergraduate GPA of 3.25; Microsoft Office competency; health clearance; health insurance; CPR certification; vehicle insurance; random drug testing; background check clearance; passport photo; three recommendations; comprehensive essay; interview. Additional exam requirements/recommendations for international students: Required—TOEFL (minimum score 80 iBT). *Application deadline:* For fall admission, 8/1 priority date for domestic students, 7/1 for international students; for spring admission, 12/1 priority date for domestic students, 11/1 for international students. Applications are processed on a rolling basis. Application fee: $45. Electronic applications accepted. *Expenses: Tuition:* Full-time $10,080; part-time $560 per unit. *Required fees:* $175 per semester. One-time fee: $45. Tuition and fees vary according to course load and program. *Financial support:* Institutionally sponsored loans available. Financial award applicants required to submit CSS PROFILE or FAFSA. *Faculty research:* Qualitative research using Parse methodology, gerontology, disaster preparedness, medical-surgical nursing, maternal-child nursing. *Unit head:* Dr. Geneva Oaks, Dean, School of Nursing, 951-343-4702, E-mail: goaks@calbaptist.edu. *Application contact:* Dr. Rebecca Meyer, Director, Graduate Program in Nursing, 951-343-4952, Fax: 951-343-5095, E-mail: rmeyer@calbaptist.edu.
Website: http://www.calbaptist.edu/explore-cbu/schools-colleges/school-nursing/master-science-nursing/

California State University, Fresno, Division of Graduate Studies, College of Health and Human Services, Department of Nursing, Fresno, CA 93740-8027. Offers nursing (MS), including clinical nurse, primary care nurse practitioner, specialist/nurse educator. *Accreditation:* AACN. Part-time and evening/weekend programs available. *Degree requirements:* For master's, thesis or alternative. *Entrance requirements:* For master's, GRE General Test, 1 year of clinical practice, previous course work in statistics, BSN, minimum GPA of 3.0 in nursing. Additional exam requirements/recommendations for international students: Required—TOEFL. Electronic applications accepted. *Faculty research:* Training grant, HIV assessment.

California State University, Fullerton, Graduate Studies, College of Health and Human Development, Department of Nursing, Fullerton, CA 92834-9480. Offers leadership (MSN); nurse anesthesia (MSN); nurse educator (MSN); nursing (DNP); women's health care (MSN). *Accreditation:* AACN; AANA/CANAEP. Part-time programs available. *Students:* 186 full-time (138 women), 134 part-time (120 women); includes 174 minority (15 Black or African American, non-Hispanic/Latino; 3 American Indian or Alaska Native, non-Hispanic/Latino; 92 Asian, non-Hispanic/Latino; 50 Hispanic/Latino; 2 Native Hawaiian or other Pacific Islander, non-Hispanic/Latino; 12 Two or more races, non-Hispanic/Latino), 3 international. Average age 35. 431 applicants, 38% accepted, 131 enrolled. In 2013, 117 master's awarded. Application fee: $55. *Financial support:* Career-related internships or fieldwork, Federal Work-Study, institutionally sponsored loans, scholarships/grants, and traineeships available. Support available to part-time students. Financial award application deadline: 3/1; financial award applicants required to submit FAFSA. *Unit head:* Dr. Cindy Greenberg, Chair, 657-278-3336. *Application contact:* Admissions/Applications, 657-278-2371.
Website: http://nursing.fullerton.edu/

California State University, Stanislaus, College of Human and Health Sciences, Program in Nursing (MS), Turlock, CA 95382. Offers gerontological nursing (MS); nursing education (MS). *Accreditation:* AACN. Part-time programs available. *Degree requirements:* For master's, comprehensive exam, thesis or alternative. *Entrance requirements:* For master's, GRE or MAT, minimum GPA of 3.0, 3 letters of reference, RN. Additional exam requirements/recommendations for international students: Required—TOEFL (minimum score 550 paper-based). Electronic applications accepted.

Capella University, School of Public Service Leadership, Doctoral Programs in Nursing, Minneapolis, MN 55402. Offers nursing education (PhD); nursing practice (DNP).

Capella University, School of Public Service Leadership, Master's Programs in Nursing, Minneapolis, MN 55402. Offers diabetes nursing (MSN); general nursing (MSN); gerontology nursing (MSN); health information management (MS); nurse educator (MSN); nursing leadership and administration (MSN).

Carlow University, School of Nursing, Program in Nursing Leadership and Education, Pittsburgh, PA 15213-3165. Offers MSN. Part-time and evening/weekend programs available. Postbaccalaureate distance learning degree programs offered (minimal on-campus study). *Students:* 27 full-time (26 women), 20 part-time (19 women); includes 5 minority (2 Black or African American, non-Hispanic/Latino; 1 American Indian or Alaska Native, non-Hispanic/Latino; 1 Hispanic/Latino; 1 Two or more races, non-Hispanic/Latino), 2 international. Average age 34. 26 applicants, 100% accepted, 19 enrolled. In 2013, 25 master's awarded. *Degree requirements:* For master's, internship. *Entrance requirements:* For master's, minimum undergraduate GPA of 3.0 from accredited BSN program; current license as RN in Pennsylvania; course in statistics in past 6 years; two recommendations; personal statement; personal interview. Additional exam requirements/recommendations for international students: Required—TOEFL (minimum score 550 paper-based). Application fee: $20. Application fee is waived when completed online. *Expenses: Tuition:* Full-time $9523; part-time $744 per credit. Tuition and fees vary according to course load, degree level and program. *Unit head:* Dr. Peggy Slota, Director, Nursing Leadership and DNP Programs, 412-578-6102, Fax: 412-578-6114, E-mail: mmslota@carlow.edu. *Application contact:* Jo Danhires, Administrative Assistant, Admissions, 412-578-6059, Fax: 412-578-6321, E-mail: gradstudies@carlow.edu.
Website: http://www.carlow.edu/Master_of_Science_in_Nursing_Concentration_in_Education_and_Leadership.aspx

Carson-Newman University, Department of Nursing, Jefferson City, TN 37760. Offers family nurse practitioner (MSN); nurse educator (MSN). *Accreditation:* AACN. *Faculty:* 2 full-time (both women), 10 part-time/adjunct (9 women). *Students:* 4 full-time (2 women), 55 part-time (45 women); includes 2 minority (1 Black or African American, non-Hispanic/Latino; 1 Two or more races, non-Hispanic/Latino), 1 international. Average age 32. In 2013, 20 master's awarded. *Application deadline:* For fall admission, 7/15 priority date for domestic students. Applications are processed on a rolling basis. Application fee: $50. *Expenses: Tuition:* Part-time $390 per credit hour. *Unit head:* Dr. Gregory A. Casalenuovo, Dean, 865-471-3426. *Application contact:* Graduate Admissions and Services Adviser, 865-473-3468, Fax: 865-472-3475.

Case Western Reserve University, Frances Payne Bolton School of Nursing, Doctor of Nursing Practice Program, Cleveland, OH 44106. Offers acute care nurse practitioner (DNP); adult gerontology nurse practitioner (DNP); educational leadership (DNP); family nurse practitioner (DNP); family systems psychiatric mental health nursing (DNP); midwifery/family nursing (DNP); neonatal nurse practitioner (DNP); pediatric nurse practitioner (DNP); practice leadership (DNP); women's health nurse practitioner (DNP). *Accreditation:* AACN. Part-time programs available. Postbaccalaureate distance learning degree programs offered (minimal on-campus study). *Students:* 169 full-time, 9 part-time; includes 10 minority (6 Black or African American, non-Hispanic/Latino; 1 Asian, non-Hispanic/Latino; 2 Hispanic/Latino; 1 Two or more races, non-Hispanic/Latino). 76 applicants, 97% accepted, 59 enrolled. In 2013, 38 doctorates awarded. Terminal master's awarded for partial completion of doctoral program. *Degree requirements:* For doctorate, thesis/dissertation. *Entrance requirements:* For doctorate, GRE General Test or MAT. Additional exam requirements/recommendations for international students: Required—TOEFL (minimum score 577 paper-based; 90 iBT), IELTS (minimum score 7). *Application deadline:* For fall admission, 6/1 priority date for domestic students, 6/1 for international students; for spring admission, 10/1 for domestic and international students. Applications are processed on a rolling basis. Application fee: $75. *Financial support:* In 2013–14, 90 students received support, including 9 fellowships with full tuition reimbursements available (averaging $31,325 per year), 1 research assistantship with partial tuition reimbursement available (averaging $14,472 per year); teaching assistantships, Federal Work-Study, institutionally sponsored loans, scholarships/grants, and tuition waivers (partial) also available. Support available to part-time students. Financial award application deadline: 5/15; financial award applicants required to submit FAFSA. *Faculty research:* Symptom science, family/community care, aging across the lifespan, self-management of health and illness, neuroscience. *Unit head:* Dr. Donna Dowling, Director, 216-368-1869, Fax: 216-368-3542, E-mail: dad10@case.edu. *Application contact:* Donna Hassik, Admissions Coordinator, 216-368-5253, Fax: 216-368-0124, E-mail: dmh7@case.edu.
Website: http://fpb.case.edu/DNP/

Case Western Reserve University, Frances Payne Bolton School of Nursing, Master's Programs in Nursing, Cleveland, OH 44106. Offers nurse anesthesia (MSN); nurse educator (MSN); nurse midwifery (MSN); nurse practitioner (MSN), including acute care cardiovascular nursing, acute care nurse practitioner, acute care/flight nurse, adult gerontology acute care nurse practitioner, adult gerontology nurse practitioner, adult gerontology oncology and palliative care, family nurse practitioner, family systems psychiatric mental health nursing, neonatal nurse practitioner, pediatric nurse practitioner, women's health nurse practitioner; nursing (MN). Part-time programs available. Postbaccalaureate distance learning degree programs offered (minimal on-campus study). *Faculty:* 54 full-time (50 women), 5 part-time/adjunct (3 women). *Students:* 169 (148 women); includes 12 minority (6 Black or African American, non-Hispanic/Latino; 3 Asian, non-Hispanic/Latino; 3 Hispanic/Latino). Average age 35. 70 applicants, 90% accepted, 33 enrolled. In 2013, 119 master's awarded. *Degree requirements:* For master's, thesis optional. *Entrance requirements:* For master's, GRE General Test or MAT. Additional exam requirements/recommendations for international students: Required—TOEFL (minimum score 577 paper-based; 90 iBT), IELTS (minimum score 7). *Application deadline:* For fall admission, 6/1 for domestic and international students; for spring admission, 10/1 for domestic and international students. Applications are processed on a rolling basis. Application fee: $75. *Financial support:* In 2013–14, 25 teaching assistantships with tuition reimbursements (averaging $15,120 per year) were awarded; fellowships, research assistantships, institutionally sponsored loans, traineeships, and tuition waivers (partial) also available. Support available to part-time students. Financial award application deadline: 6/30; financial award applicants required to submit FAFSA. *Faculty research:* Symptom science,

family/community care, aging across the lifespan, self-management of health and illness, neuroscience. *Unit head:* Dr. Carol Savrin, Director, 216-368-5304, Fax: 215-368-3542, E-mail: cls18@case.edu. *Application contact:* Donna Hassik, Admissions Coordinator, 216-368-5253, Fax: 216-368-0124, E-mail: dmh7@case.edu.
Website: http://fpb.case.edu/MSN/

Cedar Crest College, Program in Nursing, Allentown, PA 18104-6196. Offers nursing administration (MS); nursing education (MS). Part-time programs available. *Faculty:* 6 full-time (all women). *Students:* 34 part-time (31 women); includes 3 minority (1 Asian, non-Hispanic/Latino; 2 Hispanic/Latino). Average age 44. In 2013, 9 master's awarded. *Expenses: Tuition:* Part-time $661 per credit. *Unit head:* Dr. Wendy Robb, Director, 610-606-4666, E-mail: wjrobb@cedarcrest.edu. *Application contact:* Mary Ellen Hickes, Director of School of Adult and Graduate Education, 610-606-4666, E-mail: sage@cedarcrest.edu.
Website: http://sage.cedarcrest.edu/degrees/graduate/nursing-science/

Central Methodist University, College of Graduate and Extended Studies, Fayette, MO 65248-1198. Offers clinical counseling (MS); clinical nurse leader (MSN); education (M Ed); music education (MME); nurse educator (MSN). Part-time and evening/weekend programs available. Postbaccalaureate distance learning degree programs offered (no on-campus study). *Degree requirements:* For master's, thesis. *Entrance requirements:* For master's, GRE General Test, minimum GPA of 2.75. *Application deadline:* Applications are processed on a rolling basis. Application fee: $25. Electronic applications accepted. *Expenses: Tuition:* Part-time $360 per credit hour. Part-time tuition and fees vary according to campus/location and program. *Financial support:* Tuition waivers available. Support available to part-time students. Financial award application deadline: 6/5; financial award applicants required to submit FAFSA. *Unit head:* Dr. Rita Gulstad, Provost, 660-248-6212, Fax: 660-248-6392, E-mail: rgulstad@centralmethodist.edu. *Application contact:* Aimee Sage, Director of Graduate Admissions, 660-248-6651, Fax: 660-248-6392, E-mail: asage@centralmethodist.edu.
Website: http://www.centralmethodist.edu/graduate/

Chatham University, Nursing Programs, Pittsburgh, PA 15232-2826. Offers education/leadership (MSN); nursing (DNP). *Accreditation:* AACN. Postbaccalaureate distance learning degree programs offered (minimal on-campus study). *Faculty:* 9 full-time (8 women), 8 part-time/adjunct (5 women). *Students:* 38 full-time (31 women), 71 part-time (61 women); includes 28 minority (19 Black or African American, non-Hispanic/Latino; 6 Asian, non-Hispanic/Latino; 3 Hispanic/Latino), 1 international. Average age 46. 186 applicants, 47% accepted, 50 enrolled. In 2013, 27 master's, 51 doctorates awarded. *Entrance requirements:* For master's, RN license, BSN, minimum GPA of 3.0; for doctorate, RN license, MSN. Additional exam requirements/recommendations for international students: Required—TOEFL (minimum score 600 paper-based; 100 iBT), IELTS (minimum score 6.5), TWE. *Application deadline:* For fall admission, 5/1 priority date for domestic and international students. Applications are processed on a rolling basis. Application fee: $0. Electronic applications accepted. Application fee is waived when completed online. *Expenses: Tuition:* Full-time $14,886; part-time $827 per credit hour. One-time fee: $396 full-time. *Financial support:* Applicants required to submit FAFSA. *Unit head:* Dr. Diane Hunker, Director, 412-365-1738, E-mail: dhunker@chatham.edu. *Application contact:* David Vey, Admissions Support Specialist, 412-365-1498, Fax: 412-365-1720, E-mail: dvey@chatham.edu.
Website: http://www.chatham.edu/nursing

Clarion University of Pennsylvania, Office of Transfer, Adult and Graduate Admissions, Master of Science in Nursing Program, Clarion, PA 16214. Offers family nurse practitioner (MSN); nurse educator (MSN). Program offered jointly with Slippery Rock University of Pennsylvania. Part-time programs available. Postbaccalaureate distance learning degree programs offered (no on-campus study). *Faculty:* 4 full-time (all women). *Students:* 36 part-time (33 women); includes 2 minority (1 Asian, non-Hispanic/Latino; 1 Two or more races, non-Hispanic/Latino). Average age 39. 64 applicants, 41% accepted, 26 enrolled. In 2013, 21 master's awarded. *Degree requirements:* For master's, comprehensive exam, thesis. *Entrance requirements:* For master's, minimum QPA of 2.75. Additional exam requirements/recommendations for international students: Required—TOEFL (minimum score 550 paper-based; 80 iBT). *Application deadline:* For fall admission, 6/1 for domestic students, 4/15 priority date for international students; for spring admission, 11/1 for domestic students, 9/15 priority date for international students. Application fee: $40. Electronic applications accepted. *Expenses:* Tuition, state resident: part-time $442 per credit. Tuition, nonresident: part-time $451 per credit. *Required fees:* $142.40 per semester. One-time fee: $150 part-time. *Financial support:* In 2013–14, 1 research assistantship with full and partial tuition reimbursement (averaging $9,420 per year) was awarded; career-related internships or fieldwork and unspecified assistantships also available. Financial award application deadline: 3/1. *Unit head:* Dr. Debbie Ciesielka, Graduate Coordinator, 412-578-7277, E-mail: dciesielka@clarion.edu. *Application contact:* Michelle Ritzler, Graduate Programs, 814-393-2337, E-mail: gradstudies@clarion.edu.
Website: http://www.clarion.edu/991/

Clarion University of Pennsylvania, Office of Transfer, Adult and Graduate Admissions, Online Certificate Programs, Clarion, PA 16214. Offers family nurse practitioner (Post-Master's Certificate); library science (CAS); nurse educator (Post-Master's Certificate); public relations (Certificate). *Accreditation:* ALA (one or more programs are accredited at the [master's] level). Part-time programs available. Postbaccalaureate distance learning degree programs offered (no on-campus study). *Faculty:* 34 full-time (20 women). *Students:* 15 part-time (12 women); includes 1 minority (Black or African American, non-Hispanic/Latino). Average age 35. 16 applicants, 100% accepted, 7 enrolled. In 2013, 12 CASs awarded. *Entrance requirements:* Additional exam requirements/recommendations for international students: Required—TOEFL (minimum score 550 paper-based; 80 iBT), IELTS (minimum score 7). *Application deadline:* For fall admission, 8/1 priority date for domestic students, 4/15 priority date for international students; for spring admission, 12/1 priority date for domestic students, 9/15 priority date for international students. Applications are processed on a rolling basis. Application fee: $40. Electronic applications accepted. *Expenses:* Tuition, state resident: part-time $442 per credit. Tuition, nonresident: part-time $451 per credit. *Required fees:* $142.40 per semester. One-time fee: $150 part-time. *Financial support:* Research assistantships available. Financial award application deadline: 3/1. *Unit head:* Dr. William Buchanan, Chair, Library Science, 814-393-2271, Fax: 814-393-2150. *Application contact:* Michelle Ritzler, Assistant Director, Graduate Programs, 814-393-2337, Fax: 814-393-2722, E-mail: gradstudies@clarion.edu.
Website: http://www.clarion.edu/991/

Clarke University, Department of Nursing and Health, Dubuque, IA 52001-3198. Offers administration of nursing systems (MSN); advanced practice nursing (MSN); education (MSN); family nurse practitioner (MSN, PMC); nursing (DNP). *Accreditation:* AACN. Part-time programs available. *Faculty:* 10 full-time (9 women). *Students:* 42 full-time (41 women), 16 part-time (15 women). In 2013, 13 master's awarded. *Entrance requirements:* For master's, GRE General Test or MAT, BSN, minimum GPA of 3.0. *Application deadline:* For fall admission, 2/15 priority date for domestic students; for spring admission, 12/15 priority date for domestic students. Applications are processed on a rolling basis. Application fee: $25. Electronic applications accepted. *Expenses: Tuition:* Part-time $660 per credit. *Required fees:* $15 per credit. *Financial support:* In 2013–14, 6 students received support. Career-related internships or fieldwork available. Support available to part-time students. Financial award applicants required to submit FAFSA. *Faculty research:* Narrative pedagogy, ethics, end-of-life care, pedagogy, family systems. *Unit head:* Dr. Jan Lee, Chair, 800-224-2736, Fax: 319-584-8684. *Application contact:* Kara Shroeder, Information Contact, 563-588-6635, Fax: 563-588-6789, E-mail: graduate@clarke.edu.
Website: http://www.clarke.edu/

Clarkson College, Master of Science in Nursing Program, Omaha, NE 68131. Offers adult nurse practitioner (MSN, Post-Master's Certificate); family nurse practitioner (MSN, Post-Master's Certificate); nursing education (MSN, Post-Master's Certificate); nursing health care leadership (MSN, Post-Master's Certificate). *Accreditation:* AANA/CANAEP. Part-time and evening/weekend programs available. Postbaccalaureate distance learning degree programs offered (minimal on-campus study). *Degree requirements:* For master's, on-campus skills assessment (family nurse practitioner, adult nurse practitioner), comprehensive exam or thesis. *Entrance requirements:* For master's, minimum GPA of 3.0, 2 references, resume. Additional exam requirements/recommendations for international students: Required—TOEFL (minimum score 600 paper-based; 100 iBT). Electronic applications accepted.

Cleveland State University, College of Graduate Studies, College of Education and Human Services, Program in Urban Education, Specialization in Nursing Education, Cleveland, OH 44115. Offers PhD. Part-time programs available. *Faculty:* 6 full-time (all women). *Students:* 1 full-time (0 women), 1 (woman) part-time. Average age 54. *Degree requirements:* For doctorate, one foreign language, comprehensive exam, thesis/dissertation. *Entrance requirements:* For doctorate, General GRE Test (minimum score of 297 for combined Verbal and Quantitative exams, 4.0 preferred for Analytical Writing), minimum GPA of 3.25 for MSN, curriculum vitae or resume, personal statement, 2 letters of recommendation. Additional exam requirements/recommendations for international students: Required—TOEFL (minimum score 525 paper-based), IELTS (minimum score 6). *Expenses:* Tuition, state resident: full-time $8335; part-time $521 per credit hour. Tuition, nonresident: full-time $15,670; part-time $979 per credit hour. *Required fees:* $50; $25 per semester. *Faculty research:* Aspects of educating individuals to function in a complex applied discipline, educating nurses. *Unit head:* Dr. Graham Stead, Program Coordinator, 216-875-9869, E-mail: g.b.stead@csuohio.edu. *Application contact:* Rita M. Grabowski, Administrative Coordinator, 216-687-4697, Fax: 216-875-9697, E-mail: r.grabowski@csuohio.edu.
Website: http://www.csuohio.edu/cehs/departments/DOC/ne_doc.html

Cleveland State University, College of Graduate Studies, School of Nursing, Cleveland, OH 44115. Offers clinical nurse leader (MSN); forensic nursing (MSN); nursing education (MSN); specialized population (MSN); urban education (PhD), including nursing education; MSN/MBA. *Accreditation:* AACN. Part-time programs available. Postbaccalaureate distance learning degree programs offered (no on-campus study). *Faculty:* 6 full-time (all women), 1 (woman) part-time/adjunct. *Students:* 20 full-time (all women), 28 part-time (26 women); includes 12 minority (8 Black or African American, non-Hispanic/Latino; 3 Hispanic/Latino; 1 Two or more races, non-Hispanic/Latino), 1 international. Average age 38. 65 applicants, 62% accepted, 20 enrolled. In 2013, 6 master's awarded. *Degree requirements:* For master's, thesis optional, portfolio, capstone practicum project; for doctorate, comprehensive exam, thesis/dissertation. *Entrance requirements:* For master's, RN license, BSN with minimum cumulative GPA of 3.0, recent (5 years) course work in statistics; for doctorate, GRE, MSN with minimum cumulative GPA of 3.25. Additional exam requirements/recommendations for international students: Required—TOEFL (minimum score 525 paper-based; 65 iBT), IELTS (minimum score 6). *Application deadline:* For fall admission, 3/1 priority date for domestic and international students. Application fee: $55. Electronic applications accepted. *Expenses:* Tuition, state resident: full-time $8335; part-time $521 per credit hour. Tuition, nonresident: full-time $15,670; part-time $979 per credit hour. *Required fees:* $50; $25 per semester. *Financial support:* In 2013–14, 4 students received support. Tuition waivers (full) and unspecified assistantships available. Financial award application deadline: 3/1; financial award applicants required to submit FAFSA. *Faculty research:* Diabetes management, African-American elders medication compliance, risk in home visiting, suffering, COPD and stress, nursing education, disaster health preparedness. *Total annual research expenditures:* $330,000. *Unit head:* Dr. Vida Lock, Dean, 216-523-7237, Fax: 216-687-3556, E-mail: v.lock@csuohio.edu. *Application contact:* Maureen Mitchell, Assistant Professor and Graduate Program Director, 216-523-7128, Fax: 216-687-3556, E-mail: m.m.mitchell1@csuohio.edu.
Website: http://www.csuohio.edu/nursing/

College of Mount Saint Vincent, School of Professional and Continuing Studies, Department of Nursing, Riverdale, NY 10471-1093. Offers adult nurse practitioner (MSN, PMC); family nurse practitioner (MSN, PMC); nurse educator (PMC); nursing administration (MSN); nursing for the adult and aged (MSN). *Accreditation:* AACN. Part-time programs available. *Entrance requirements:* For master's, BSN, interview, RN license, minimum GPA of 3.0, letters of reference. Additional exam requirements/recommendations for international students: Required—TOEFL. *Expenses:* Contact institution.

The College of New Rochelle, Graduate School, Program in Nursing, New Rochelle, NY 10805-2308. Offers acute care nurse practitioner (MS, Certificate); clinical specialist in holistic nursing (MS, Certificate); family nurse practitioner (MS, Certificate); nursing and health care management (MS); nursing education (Certificate). *Accreditation:* AACN. Part-time programs available. *Faculty:* 6 full-time (5 women), 5 part-time/adjunct (4 women). *Students:* 113 part-time (104 women); includes 56 minority (44 Black or African American, non-Hispanic/Latino; 3 Asian, non-Hispanic/Latino; 9 Hispanic/Latino). Average age 40. In 2013, 17 master's awarded. *Entrance requirements:* For master's, GRE General Test or MAT, BSN, malpractice insurance, minimum GPA of 3.0, RN license. *Application deadline:* For fall admission, 8/15 priority date for domestic students; for spring admission, 12/1 priority date for domestic students. Applications are processed on a rolling basis. Application fee: $35. Electronic applications accepted. *Expenses:* Contact institution. *Financial support:* Traineeships available. Support available to part-time students. Financial award application deadline: 8/15. *Unit head:* Dr. Mary McGuinness, Acting Dean, School of Nursing, 914-654-5441, E-mail: mmcguiness@cnr.edu.

College of Staten Island of the City University of New York, Graduate Programs, Department of Nursing, Program in Nursing Education, Staten Island, NY 10314-6600. Offers Post-Master's Certificate. In 2013, 1 Post-Master's Certificate awarded. *Degree requirements:* For Post-Master's Certificate, 12 credits. *Entrance requirements:* For degree, master's degree in nursing or acceptance into the master's nursing program of the College of Staten Island; current NY State RN license. Additional exam requirements/recommendations for international students: Required—TOEFL (minimum score 550 paper-based; 79 iBT), IELTS (minimum score 6.5). *Application deadline:* For fall admission, 5/1 priority date for domestic and international students; for spring admission, 11/19 priority date for domestic and international students. Application fee: $125. *Expenses:* Tuition, state resident: full-time $9240; part-time $385 per credit hour. Tuition, nonresident: full-time $17,040; part-time $710 per credit hour. *Required fees:* $428; $128 per term. *Financial support:* Career-related internships or fieldwork, Federal Work-Study, and scholarships/grants available. Support available to part-time students.

Financial award applicants required to submit FAFSA. *Unit head:* Dr. June Como, Coordinator, 718-982-3818, Fax: 718-982-3813, E-mail: june.como@csi.cuny.edu. *Application contact:* Sasha Spence, Assistant Director for Graduate Admissions, 718-982-2019, Fax: 718-982-2500, E-mail: sasha.spence@csi.cuny.edu.
Website: http://www.csi.cuny.edu/nursing/graduate.html

Concordia University Wisconsin, Graduate Programs, School of Human Services, Program in Nursing, Mequon, WI 53097-2402. Offers family nurse practitioner (MSN); geriatric nurse practitioner (MSN); nurse educator (MSN). *Accreditation:* AACN. Postbaccalaureate distance learning degree programs offered (minimal on-campus study). *Degree requirements:* For master's, comprehensive exam, thesis or alternative. *Entrance requirements:* Additional exam requirements/recommendations for international students: Required—TOEFL. *Expenses:* Contact institution.

Cox College, Programs in Nursing, Springfield, MO 65802. Offers clinical nurse leader (MSN); family nurse practitioner (MSN); nurse educator (MSN). *Accreditation:* AACN. *Entrance requirements:* For master's, RN license, essay, 2 letters of recommendation, official transcripts. Electronic applications accepted.

Daemen College, Department of Nursing, Amherst, NY 14226-3592. Offers adult nurse practitioner (MS, Post Master's Certificate); nurse executive leadership (Post Master's Certificate); nursing education (MS, Post Master's Certificate); nursing executive leadership (MS); nursing practice (DNP); palliative care nursing (Post Master's Certificate). Part-time programs available. *Degree requirements:* For master's, thesis or alternative, degree completed in 4 years; minimum GPA of 3.0; for doctorate, degree completed in 5 years; 500 post-master's clinical hours. *Entrance requirements:* For master's, BN, 1 year medical/surgical experience, RN license and state registration, statistics course with minimum C grade, 3 letters of recommendation, minimum GPA of 3.25, interview; for doctorate, MS in advance nursing practice; New York state RN license; goal statement; resume; interview; statistics course with minimum grade of 'C'; for Post Master's Certificate, master's degree in clinical area; RN license and current registration; one year of clinical experience; statistics course with minimum grade of 'C'; 3 letters of recommendation; interview; letter of intent. Additional exam requirements/recommendations for international students: Required—TOEFL (minimum score 500 paper-based; 63 iBT), IELTS (minimum score 5.5). Electronic applications accepted. *Faculty research:* Professional stress, client behavior, drug therapy, treatment modalities and pulmonary cancers, chemical dependency.

Delta State University, Graduate Programs, School of Nursing, Cleveland, MS 38733. Offers family nurse practitioner (MSN); nurse administrator (MSN); nurse educator (MSN). *Accreditation:* AACN. Part-time programs available. *Faculty:* 5 full-time (all women), 1 (woman) part-time/adjunct. *Students:* 35 full-time (31 women), 8 part-time (7 women); includes 10 minority (all Black or African American, non-Hispanic/Latino). Average age 41. 23 applicants, 100% accepted, 19 enrolled. In 2013, 13 master's awarded. *Degree requirements:* For master's, thesis optional. *Entrance requirements:* For master's, GRE General Test. *Application deadline:* For fall admission, 8/1 priority date for domestic students; for spring admission, 12/1 priority date for domestic students. Applications are processed on a rolling basis. Application fee: $0. Electronic applications accepted. *Expenses:* Tuition, state resident: full-time $3006; part-time $334 per credit hour. Tuition, nonresident: full-time $3006; part-time $334 per credit hour. *Financial support:* Research assistantships, career-related internships or fieldwork, Federal Work-Study, and institutionally sponsored loans available. Financial award application deadline: 6/1. *Unit head:* Dr. Lizabeth Carlson, Dean, 662-846-4268, Fax: 662-846-4267, E-mail: lcarlson@deltastate.edu. *Application contact:* Dr. Albert Nylander, Dean of Graduate Studies, 662-846-4875, Fax: 662-846-4313, E-mail: grad-info@deltastate.edu.
Website: http://www.deltastate.edu/pages/252.asp

DeSales University, Graduate Division, Division of Healthcare and Natural Sciences, Center Valley, PA 18034-9568. Offers adult clinical nurse specialist (MSN); certified nurse midwives (MSN); certified nurse practitioners (MSN); clinical leadership (DNP); family nurse practitioner (MSN); information systems (MSIS); nurse educator (MSN); nurse practitioner (Post-Master's Certificate); physical therapy (DPT); physician assistant studies (MSPAS); MSN/MBA. Part-time programs available. In 2013, 5 doctorates awarded. *Degree requirements:* For master's, thesis optional. *Entrance requirements:* For master's, GRE General Test, MAT, minimum B average in undergraduate course work, health assessment course or equivalent, course work in statistics. Additional exam requirements/recommendations for international students: Required—TOEFL. *Application deadline:* Applications are processed on a rolling basis. Application fee: $35. Electronic applications accepted. *Expenses:* *Tuition:* Part-time $790 per credit. *Financial support:* Applicants required to submit FAFSA. *Unit head:* Dr. Mary Liz Doyle-Tadduni, Department Chair, Nursing, 610-282-1100 Ext. 1394, Fax: 610-282-2091, E-mail: carol.mest@desales.edu. *Application contact:* Abagail Wernicki, Director of Graduate Admissions, 610-282-1100 Ext. 1768, Fax: 610-282-2869, E-mail: abagail.wernicki@desales.edu.

Drexel University, College of Nursing and Health Professions, Division of Graduate Nursing, Philadelphia, PA 19104-2875. Offers adult acute care (MSN); adult psychiatric/mental health (MSN); advanced practice nursing (MSN); clinical trials research (MSN); family nurse practitioner (MSN); leadership in health systems management (MSN); nursing education (MSN); pediatric primary care (MSN); women's health (MSN). *Accreditation:* AACN. Electronic applications accepted.

Duke University, School of Nursing, Durham, NC 27708-0586. Offers acute care pediatric nurse practitioner (MSN); adult-gerontology nurse practitioner - acute care (MSN, Post Master's Certificate); adult-gerontology nurse practitioner - primary care (MSN, Post Master's Certificate), including adult-gerontology nurse practitioner (MSN), cardiology, oncology; family nurse practitioner (MSN); neonatal nurse practitioner (MSN); nurse anesthesia (MSN, DNP); nursing (PhD); nursing and health care leadership (MSN); nursing education (MSN); nursing informatics (MSN, Post Master's Certificate); pediatric nurse practitioner - primary care (MSN). *Accreditation:* AACN; AANA/CANAEP. Part-time and evening/weekend programs available. Postbaccalaureate distance learning degree programs offered (minimal on-campus study). *Faculty:* 74 full-time (64 women), 7 part-time/adjunct (4 women). *Students:* 127 full-time (113 women), 473 part-time (433 women); includes 131 minority (54 Black or African American, non-Hispanic/Latino; 9 American Indian or Alaska Native, non-Hispanic/Latino; 36 Asian, non-Hispanic/Latino; 27 Hispanic/Latino; 5 Native Hawaiian or other Pacific Islander, non-Hispanic/Latino), 14 international. Average age 34. 516 applicants, 50% accepted, 190 enrolled. In 2013, 179 master's, 49 doctorates, 23 other advanced degrees awarded. Terminal master's awarded for partial completion of doctoral program. *Degree requirements:* For master's, thesis optional; for doctorate, capstone project. *Entrance requirements:* For master's, GRE General Test (waived if undergraduate GPA of 3.4 or higher), 1 year of nursing experience (recommended), BSN, minimum GPA of 3.0, previous course work in statistics; for doctorate, GRE General Test (waived if undergraduate GPA of 3.4 or higher), BSN or MSN, minimum GPA of 3.0, portfolio, resume, personal statement, undergraduate statistics course, current licensure as a registered nurse, transcripts from all post-secondary institutions; for Post Master's Certificate, MSN, licensure or eligibility as a professional nurse, transcripts from all post-secondary institutions, previous course work in statistics. Additional exam requirements/recommendations for international students: Recommended—TOEFL (minimum score 550 paper-based; 83 iBT), IELTS (minimum score 7). *Application deadline:* For fall admission, 12/1 for domestic and international students; for spring admission, 5/1 for domestic and international students. Application fee: $50. Electronic applications accepted. *Expenses:* Contact institution. *Financial support:* Career-related internships or fieldwork, institutionally sponsored loans, scholarships/grants, traineeships, and tuition waivers (partial) available. Support available to part-time students. Financial award applicants required to submit FAFSA. *Faculty research:* Cardiovascular disease, caregiver skill training, data mining, prostate cancer, neonatal immune system. *Unit head:* Dr. Catherine L. Gilliss, Dean/Vice Chancellor for Nursing Affairs, 919-684-9444, Fax: 919-684-9414, E-mail: catherine.gilliss@duke.edu. *Application contact:* Ernie Rushing, Lead Admissions Processor/Admissions Officer, 919-668-6274, Fax: 919-668-4693, E-mail: stephen.rushing@dm.duke.edu.
Website: http://www.nursing.duke.edu/

Duquesne University, School of Nursing, Master of Science in Nursing Program, Pittsburgh, PA 15282-0001. Offers family (individual across the life span) nurse practitioner (MSN); forensic nursing (MSN); nursing education (MSN). *Accreditation:* AACN. Part-time and evening/weekend programs available. Postbaccalaureate distance learning degree programs offered (minimal on-campus study). *Faculty:* 20 full-time (18 women), 4 part-time/adjunct (all women). *Students:* 73 full-time (67 women), 54 part-time (53 women); includes 23 minority (8 Black or African American, non-Hispanic/Latino; 1 American Indian or Alaska Native, non-Hispanic/Latino; 4 Asian, non-Hispanic/Latino; 5 Hispanic/Latino; 5 Two or more races, non-Hispanic/Latino), 1 international. Average age 35. 206 applicants, 35% accepted, 55 enrolled. In 2013, 28 master's awarded. *Degree requirements:* For master's, culminating paper. *Entrance requirements:* For master's, current RN license; BSN with minimum GPA of 3.0; minimum of 1 year full-time work experience as RN prior to registration in clinical or specialty course. Additional exam requirements/recommendations for international students: Required—TOEFL (minimum score 600 paper-based; 80 iBT). *Application deadline:* For fall admission, 3/1 for domestic and international students. Application fee: $0. Electronic applications accepted. *Expenses:* *Tuition:* Full-time $18,162; part-time $1009 per credit. *Required fees:* $1728; $96 per credit. Tuition and fees vary according to program. *Financial support:* In 2013–14, 5 students received support, including 3 teaching assistantships with partial tuition reimbursements available (averaging $1,285 per year); research assistantships with partial tuition reimbursements available, scholarships/grants, traineeships, and tuition waivers (partial) also available. Support available to part-time students. Financial award application deadline: 7/1; financial award applicants required to submit FAFSA. *Faculty research:* Vulnerable populations, social justice, cultural competence, health disparities, wellness within chronic illness. *Unit head:* Dr. Joan Such Lockhart, Professor and Associate Dean of Academic Affairs, 412-396-6540, Fax: 412-396-1821, E-mail: lockhart@duq.edu. *Application contact:* Susan Hardner, Nurse Recruiter, 412-396-4945, Fax: 412-396-6346, E-mail: nursing@duq.edu.
Website: http://www.duq.edu/academics/schools/nursing/graduate-programs/master-science-nursing

D'Youville College, School of Nursing, Buffalo, NY 14201-1084. Offers advanced practice nursing (DNP); community health nursing/education (MSN); community health nursing/management (MSN); family nurse practitioner (MSN, Certificate); nursing and health-related professions education (Certificate). *Accreditation:* AACN. Part-time programs available. *Students:* 51 full-time (45 women), 136 part-time (115 women); includes 25 minority (17 Black or African American, non-Hispanic/Latino; 1 American Indian or Alaska Native, non-Hispanic/Latino; 1 Asian, non-Hispanic/Latino; 6 Hispanic/Latino), 76 international. Average age 35. 261 applicants, 36% accepted, 73 enrolled. In 2013, 51 master's, 3 other advanced degrees awarded. *Degree requirements:* For master's, thesis or alternative, membership on board of community agency, publishable paper. *Entrance requirements:* For master's, BS in nursing, minimum GPA of 3.0, course work in statistics and computers. Additional exam requirements/recommendations for international students: Required—TOEFL (minimum score 500 paper-based). *Application deadline:* For fall admission, 5/1 priority date for international students; for spring admission, 9/1 priority date for international students. Applications are processed on a rolling basis. Application fee: $25. Electronic applications accepted. *Financial support:* Federal Work-Study, scholarships/grants, traineeships, and unspecified assistantships available. Support available to part-time students. Financial award application deadline: 3/1; financial award applicants required to submit FAFSA. *Faculty research:* Nursing curriculum, nursing theory-testing, wellness research, communication and socialization patterns. *Unit head:* Dr. Ann Caughill, Chair, 716-829-7892, Fax: 716-829-8159. *Application contact:* Mark Pavone, Graduate Admissions Director, 716-829-8400, Fax: 716-829-7900, E-mail: graduateadmissions@dyc.edu.
Website: http://www.dyc.edu/academics/nursing/

See Display on page 632 and Close-Up on page 815.

Eastern Michigan University, Graduate School, College of Health and Human Services, School of Nursing, Ypsilanti, MI 48197. Offers nursing (MSN); quality improvement in health care systems (Graduate Certificate); teaching in health care systems (MSN, Graduate Certificate). *Accreditation:* AACN. Part-time and evening/weekend programs available. Postbaccalaureate distance learning degree programs offered (minimal on-campus study). *Faculty:* 23 full-time (21 women). *Students:* 3 full-time (all women), 32 part-time (26 women); includes 11 minority (6 Black or African American, non-Hispanic/Latino; 3 Asian, non-Hispanic/Latino; 2 Hispanic/Latino), 1 international. Average age 47. 31 applicants, 55% accepted, 10 enrolled. In 2013, 8 master's, 2 other advanced degrees awarded. *Degree requirements:* For master's, thesis optional. *Entrance requirements:* For master's, GRE General Test, Michigan RN license. Additional exam requirements/recommendations for international students: Required—TOEFL. *Application deadline:* Applications are processed on a rolling basis. Application fee: $35. *Expenses:* Tuition, state resident: full-time $12,300; part-time $466 per credit hour. Tuition, nonresident: full-time $23,159; part-time $918 per credit hour. *Required fees:* $71 per credit hour. $46 per semester. One-time fee: $100. Tuition and fees vary according to course level and degree level. *Financial support:* Fellowships, research assistantships with full tuition reimbursements, teaching assistantships with full tuition reimbursements, career-related internships or fieldwork, Federal Work-Study, institutionally sponsored loans, scholarships/grants, tuition waivers (partial), and unspecified assistantships available. Support available to part-time students. Financial award applicants required to submit FAFSA. *Unit head:* Dr. Michael Williams, Interim Director, 734-487-2310, Fax: 734-487-6946, E-mail: mwilliams@emich.edu. *Application contact:* Roberta Towns, Coordinator, School of Nursing, 734-487-2340, Fax: 734-487-6946, E-mail: rtowne1@emich.edu.
Website: http://www.emich.edu/nursing

Edinboro University of Pennsylvania, Department of Nursing, Edinboro, PA 16444. Offers advanced practice nursing (DNP); family nurse practitioner (MSN); nurse educator (MSN). Part-time and evening/weekend programs available. *Degree requirements:* For master's, thesis, competency exam. *Entrance requirements:* For master's, GRE or MAT, minimum QPA of 2.5. *Application deadline:* Applications are processed on a rolling basis. Application fee: $30. Electronic applications accepted. *Expenses:* Tuition, state resident: part-time $454 per credit hour. Tuition, nonresident:

part-time $681 per credit hour. *Required fees:* $143.55 per credit hour. Part-time tuition and fees vary according to campus/location and program. *Financial support:* Research assistantships with full and partial tuition reimbursements, career-related internships or fieldwork, Federal Work-Study, scholarships/grants, and unspecified assistantships available. Support available to part-time students. Financial award application deadline: 2/15; financial award applicants required to submit FAFSA. *Unit head:* Dr. Thomas White, Chairperson, 814-732-2900, E-mail: twhite@edinboro.edu. *Application contact:* Dr. Thomas White, Chairperson, 814-732-2900, E-mail: twhite@edinboro.edu.
Website: http://www.edinboro.edu/departments/nursing/nursing.dot

Elms College, Division of Nursing, Chicopee, MA 01013-2839. Offers nursing and health services management (MSN); nursing education (MSN). *Accreditation:* AACN. Part-time and evening/weekend programs available. *Entrance requirements:* Additional exam requirements/recommendations for international students: Required—TOEFL.

Emmanuel College, Graduate Studies, Graduate Program in Nursing, Boston, MA 02115. Offers nursing education (MSN); nursing management/administration (MSN). Part-time and evening/weekend programs available. *Faculty:* 4 full-time (all women), 4 part-time/adjunct (all women). *Students:* 51 part-time (47 women); includes 9 minority (6 Black or African American, non-Hispanic/Latino; 1 American Indian or Alaska Native, non-Hispanic/Latino; 1 Asian, non-Hispanic/Latino; 1 Hispanic/Latino). Average age 49. *Degree requirements:* For master's, 36 credits, including 6-credit practicum. *Entrance requirements:* For master's, transcripts from all regionally-accredited institutions attended (showing proof of bachelor's degree completion), proof of RN license, 2 letters of recommendation, essay, resume, interview. Additional exam requirements/recommendations for international students: Required—TOEFL (minimum score 600 paper-based; 106 iBT) or IELTS (minimum score 6.5). *Application deadline:* For fall admission, 4/30 for domestic students. Applications are processed on a rolling basis. Application fee: $0. Electronic applications accepted. *Financial support:* Applicants required to submit FAFSA. *Unit head:* Sandy Robbins, Dean of Enrollment, 617-735-9700, Fax: 617-507-0434, E-mail: graduatestudies@emmanuel.edu. *Application contact:* Enrollment Counselor, 617-735-9700, Fax: 617-507-0434, E-mail: graduatestudies@emmanuel.edu.
Website: http://www.emmanuel.edu/graduate-studies-nursing/academics/nursing.html

Excelsior College, School of Nursing, Albany, NY 12203-5159. Offers clinical systems management (MS); nursing (MS); nursing education (MS); nursing informatics (MS). Part-time and evening/weekend programs available. Postbaccalaureate distance learning degree programs offered (no on-campus study). *Faculty:* 13 part-time/adjunct (all women). *Students:* 550 part-time (448 women); includes 184 minority (106 Black or African American, non-Hispanic/Latino; 4 American Indian or Alaska Native, non-Hispanic/Latino; 30 Asian, non-Hispanic/Latino; 29 Hispanic/Latino; 5 Native Hawaiian or other Pacific Islander, non-Hispanic/Latino; 10 Two or more races, non-Hispanic/Latino). Average age 46. In 2013, 124 master's awarded. *Entrance requirements:* For master's, RN license. *Application deadline:* Applications are processed on a rolling basis. Application fee: $100. Electronic applications accepted. *Expenses: Tuition:* Part-time $565 per credit. *Financial support:* Scholarships/grants and traineeships available. Support available to part-time students. Financial award application deadline: 8/21. *Faculty research:* Leadership development, test anxiety, use of technology in online learning. *Unit head:* Dr. Barbara Pieper, Associate Dean, Graduate Program in Nursing, 518-464-8500, Fax: 518-464-8777, E-mail: msn@excelsior.edu. *Application contact:* Christine McIlwraith, Graduate Advisor, 518-464-8500, Fax: 518-464-8777, E-mail: nursingmasters@excelsior.edu.

Felician College, Program in Nursing, Lodi, NJ 07644-2117. Offers adult-gerontology nurse practitioner (MSN, PMC); executive leadership (MSN, PMC); family nurse practitioner (MSN, PMC); nursing education (MSN, PMC). *Accreditation:* AACN. Part-time and evening/weekend programs available. Postbaccalaureate distance learning degree programs offered (no on-campus study). *Students:* 5 full-time (4 women), 85 part-time (78 women); includes 50 minority (20 Black or African American, non-Hispanic/Latino; 14 Asian, non-Hispanic/Latino; 16 Hispanic/Latino). Average age 42. *Degree requirements:* For master's, scholarly project. *Entrance requirements:* For master's, BS in nursing or equivalent, minimum GPA of 3.0, 2 letters of recommendation, RN license; for PMC, RN license, minimum GPA of 2.75. Additional exam requirements/recommendations for international students: Recommended—TOEFL (minimum score 550 paper-based). *Application deadline:* Applications are processed on a rolling basis. Application fee: $40. *Expenses: Tuition:* Part-time $945 per credit. *Required fees:* $317.50 per semester. *Financial support:* In 2013–14, 10 students received support. Traineeships available. Financial award applicants required to submit FAFSA. *Faculty research:* Anxiety and fear, curriculum innovation, health promotion. *Unit head:* Dr. Muriel Shore, Dean, Division of Health Sciences, 201-559-6030, E-mail: shorem@felician.edu. *Application contact:* Elizabeth Barca, Senior Assistant Director, Graduate Admissions, 201-559-6077, Fax: 201-559-6138, E-mail: graduate@felician.edu.

Ferris State University, College of Health Professions, School of Nursing, Big Rapids, MI 49307. Offers nursing (MSN); nursing administration (MSN); nursing education (MSN); nursing informatics (MSN). Part-time and evening/weekend programs available. Postbaccalaureate distance learning degree programs offered (minimal on-campus study). *Faculty:* 5 full-time (all women), 1 (woman) part-time/adjunct. *Students:* 1 (woman) full-time, 103 part-time (91 women); includes 5 minority (2 Black or African American, non-Hispanic/Latino; 1 American Indian or Alaska Native, non-Hispanic/Latino; 1 Native Hawaiian or other Pacific Islander, non-Hispanic/Latino; 1 Two or more races, non-Hispanic/Latino). Average age 40. 25 applicants, 92% accepted, 21 enrolled. In 2013, 20 master's awarded. *Degree requirements:* For master's, comprehensive exam, practicum, practicum project. *Entrance requirements:* For master's, BS in nursing or related field with registered nurse license, writing sample, letters of reference, 2 years' clinical experience. Additional exam requirements/recommendations for international students: Required—TOEFL (minimum score 550 paper-based; 61 iBT). *Application deadline:* For fall admission, 4/15 priority date for domestic students; for spring admission, 10/15 for domestic students. Applications are processed on a rolling basis. Application fee: $30. Electronic applications accepted. Application fee is waived when completed online. *Financial support:* In 2013–14, 3 students received support. Fellowships, research assistantships, teaching assistantships, career-related internships or fieldwork, and scholarships/grants available. Financial award application deadline: 4/15. *Faculty research:* Nursing education-minority student focus, student attitudes toward aging. *Unit head:* Dr. Susan Owens, Program Coordinator, 231-591-2267, Fax: 231-591-2325, E-mail: owenss3@ferris.edu. *Application contact:* Debby Buck, Off-Campus Program Secretary, 231-591-2270, Fax: 231-591-3788, E-mail: buckd@ferris.edu.
Website: http://www.ferris.edu/htmls/colleges/alliedhe/Nursing/homepage.htm

Florida Atlantic University, Christine E. Lynn College of Nursing, Boca Raton, FL 33431-0991. Offers administrative and financial leadership in nursing and health care (Post Master's Certificate); adult/gerontological nurse practitioner (Post Master's Certificate); advanced holistic nursing (MS, Post Master's Certificate); clinical nurse leader (MS, Post Master's Certificate); family nurse practitioner (MS, Post Master's Certificate); nurse educator (MS, Post Master's Certificate); nursing (PhD); nursing administration and financial leadership (MS); nursing practice (DNP). *Accreditation:* AACN. Part-time programs available. *Faculty:* 30 full-time (27 women), 9 part-time/adjunct (8 women). *Students:* 29 full-time (27 women), 523 part-time (492 women); includes 254 minority (157 Black or African American, non-Hispanic/Latino; 2 American Indian or Alaska Native, non-Hispanic/Latino; 19 Asian, non-Hispanic/Latino; 62 Hispanic/Latino; 2 Native Hawaiian or other Pacific Islander, non-Hispanic/Latino; 12 Two or more races, non-Hispanic/Latino), 3 international. Average age 39. 463 applicants, 25% accepted, 111 enrolled. In 2013, 148 master's, 15 doctorates awarded. *Degree requirements:* For master's, thesis or alternative; for doctorate, comprehensive exam, thesis/dissertation. *Entrance requirements:* For master's, GRE General Test or MAT, bachelor's degree in nursing, Florida RN license, minimum GPA of 3.0, resume/curriculum vitae, letter of recommendation; for doctorate, GRE General Test or MAT, curriculum vitae, Florida RN license, minimum GPA of 3.5, master's degree in nursing, three letters of recommendation. *Application deadline:* For fall admission, 6/1 for domestic students, 2/15 for international students; for spring admission, 10/1 for domestic students, 7/15 for international students. Applications are processed on a rolling basis. Application fee: $30. *Expenses:* Tuition, state resident: full-time $6660; part-time $370 per credit hour. Tuition, nonresident: full-time $18,450; part-time $1025 per credit hour. Tuition and fees vary according to course load. *Financial support:* Research assistantships with partial tuition reimbursements, teaching assistantships with partial tuition reimbursements, career-related internships or fieldwork, Federal Work-Study, institutionally sponsored loans, scholarships/grants, and traineeships available. Support available to part-time students. *Faculty research:* Econometrics of nurse-patient relationship, Alzheimer's disease, community-based programs, falls, self-healing. *Unit head:* Dr. Marlaine Smith, Dean, 561-297-3206, Fax: 561-297-3687, E-mail: msmit230@fau.edu. *Application contact:* Carol Kruse, Graduate Coordinator, 561-297-3261, Fax: 561-297-0088, E-mail: ckruse@fau.edu.
Website: http://nursing.fau.edu/

Florida Southern College, Program in Nursing, Lakeland, FL 33801-5698. Offers adult gerontology clinical nurse specialist (MSN); adult gerontology primary care nurse practitioner (MSN); nurse educator (MSN); nursing administration (MSN). *Accreditation:* AACN. Part-time and evening/weekend programs available. *Entrance requirements:* For master's, Florida RN license, 3 letters of recommendation, personal statement, minimum GPA of 3.0, resume. Additional exam requirements/recommendations for international students: Required—TOEFL (minimum score 550 paper-based). *Expenses:* Contact institution. *Faculty research:* End of life care, dementia, health promotion.

Florida State University, The Graduate School, College of Nursing, Tallahassee, FL 32312. Offers family nurse practitioner (DNP); health systems leadership (DNP); nurse educator (MSN, Certificate); nurse leader (MSN); nursing leadership (Certificate, Post-Graduate Certificate). *Accreditation:* AACN. Part-time programs available. Postbaccalaureate distance learning degree programs offered (minimal on-campus study). *Faculty:* 13 full-time (12 women). *Students:* 53 full-time (49 women), 26 part-time (all women); includes 16 minority (4 Black or African American, non-Hispanic/Latino; 1 Asian, non-Hispanic/Latino; 9 Hispanic/Latino; 2 Two or more races, non-Hispanic/Latino). Average age 38. 56 applicants, 61% accepted, 25 enrolled. In 2013, 5 master's, 18 doctorates awarded. *Degree requirements:* For master's, thesis optional. *Entrance requirements:* For master's, GRE General Test, MAT, minimum GPA of 3.0, BSN, Florida RN license; for doctorate, GRE General Test, MAT, minimum GPA of 3.0, BSN or MSN, Florida RN license. Additional exam requirements/recommendations for international students: Required—TOEFL (minimum score 550 paper-based). *Application deadline:* For fall admission, 7/1 for domestic and international students. Application fee: $30. Electronic applications accepted. *Expenses:* Tuition, state resident: part-time $403.51 per credit hour. Tuition, nonresident: part-time $1004.85 per credit hour. *Required fees:* $75.81 per credit hour. One-time fee: $20 part-time. Tuition and fees vary according to course load, campus/location and student level. *Financial support:* In 2013–14, 75 students received support, including fellowships with partial tuition reimbursements available (averaging $6,300 per year), research assistantships with partial tuition reimbursements available (averaging $3,000 per year), 3 teaching assistantships with partial tuition reimbursements available (averaging $3,000 per year); career-related internships or fieldwork, Federal Work-Study, institutionally sponsored loans, scholarships/grants, traineeships, and tuition waivers (partial) also available. Financial award application deadline: 4/15; financial award applicants required to submit FAFSA. *Faculty research:* Distance learning, gerontology, health promotion, educational strategies, rehabilitation of brain injured patients. *Unit head:* Dr. Judith McFetridge-Durdle, Dean, 850-644-6846, Fax: 850-644-7660, E-mail: jdurdle@nursing.fsu.edu. *Application contact:* Carlos G. Urrutia, Director of Student Services, 850-644-5638, Fax: 850-645-7249, E-mail: currutia@fsu.edu.
Website: http://nursing.fsu.edu/

Framingham State University, Continuing Education, Program in Nursing, Framingham, MA 01701-9101. Offers nursing education (MSN); nursing leadership (MSN). *Accreditation:* AACN. *Entrance requirements:* For master's, BSN; minimum cumulative undergraduate GPA of 3.0, 3.25 in nursing courses; coursework in statistics; 2 letters of recommendation; interview. Electronic applications accepted.

Francis Marion University, Graduate Programs, Department of Nursing, Florence, SC 29502-0547. Offers family nurse practitioner (MSN); nurse educator (MSN). Part-time programs available. *Faculty:* 8 full-time (all women). *Students:* 40 full-time (37 women), 7 part-time (4 women); includes 14 minority (12 Black or African American, non-Hispanic/Latino; 1 Asian, non-Hispanic/Latino; 1 Two or more races, non-Hispanic/Latino). Average age 34. 20 applicants, 80% accepted, 16 enrolled. *Entrance requirements:* For master's, GRE, official transcripts, two letters of recommendation, written statement, current SC nursing license. *Application deadline:* For fall admission, 3/15 for domestic students; for spring admission, 10/15 for domestic students. Applications are processed on a rolling basis. Application fee: $33. Electronic applications accepted. *Expenses:* Tuition, state resident: full-time $9184; part-time $459.20 per credit hour. Tuition, nonresident: full-time $18,368; part-time $918.40 per credit hour. *Required fees:* $13.50 per credit hour. $92 per semester. Tuition and fees vary according to program. *Financial support:* Available to part-time students. Application deadline: 3/1; applicants required to submit FAFSA. *Unit head:* Dr. Ruth Wittmann-Price, Chair, 843-661-4625, E-mail: rwittmannprice@fmarion.edu. *Application contact:* Rannie Gamble, Administrative Manager, 843-661-1286, Fax: 843-661-4688, E-mail: rgamble@fmarion.edu.

George Mason University, College of Health and Human Services, School of Nursing, Fairfax, VA 22030. Offers nursing (MSN, DNP, PhD); nursing administration (Certificate); nursing education (Certificate). *Faculty:* 33 full-time (32 women), 44 part-time/adjunct (42 women). *Students:* 82 full-time (77 women), 187 part-time (175 women); includes 98 minority (47 Black or African American, non-Hispanic/Latino; 2 American Indian or Alaska Native, non-Hispanic/Latino; 26 Asian, non-Hispanic/Latino; 18 Hispanic/Latino; 1 Native Hawaiian or other Pacific Islander, non-Hispanic/Latino; 4 Two or more races, non-Hispanic/Latino), 9 international. Average age 40. 182 applicants, 55% accepted, 71 enrolled. In 2013, 78 master's, 16 doctorates, 3 other advanced degrees awarded. *Degree requirements:* For master's, comprehensive exam (for some programs), thesis in clinical classes; for doctorate, comprehensive exam (for some programs), thesis/dissertation (for some programs). *Entrance requirements:* For master's, 2 official transcripts; expanded goals statement; resume; BSN from accredited

institution; minimum GPA of 3.0 in last 60 credits of undergraduate work; 2 letters of recommendation; completion of undergraduate statistics and graduate-level bivariate statistics; certification in professional CPR; for doctorate, 2 official transcripts; expanded goals statement; resume; 3 recommendation letters; nursing license; at least 1 year of work experience as an RN; interview; writing sample; evidence of graduate-level course in applied statistics; master's in nursing with minimum GPA of 3.5; for Certificate, 2 official transcripts; expanded goals statement; resume; master's degree from accredited institution or currently enrolled with minimum GPA of 3.0. Additional exam requirements/recommendations for international students: Required—TOEFL (minimum score 570 paper-based; 88 iBT), IELTS (minimum score 6.5), PTE. *Application deadline:* For fall admission, 2/1 priority date for domestic students; for spring admission, 11/1 for domestic students. Application fee: $65 ($80 for international students). Electronic applications accepted. *Expenses:* Contact institution. *Financial support:* In 2013–14, 14 students received support, including 11 fellowships (averaging $15,091 per year), 3 research assistantships with full and partial tuition reimbursements available (averaging $36,667 per year); career-related internships or fieldwork, Federal Work-Study, scholarships/grants, unspecified assistantships, and health care benefits (for full-time research or teaching assistantship recipients) also available. Financial award application deadline: 3/1; financial award applicants required to submit FAFSA. *Faculty research:* Research in health care, nursing science. *Total annual research expenditures:* $366,930. *Unit head:* Carol Urban, Acting Director, 703-993-2991, Fax: 703-993-3606, E-mail: curban@gmu.edu. *Application contact:* Janice Lee-Beverly, Program Support, 703-993-1947, Fax: 703-993-1943, E-mail: jleebev1@gmu.edu.
Website: http://chhs.gmu.edu/nursing

Georgetown University, Graduate School of Arts and Sciences, School of Nursing and Health Studies, Washington, DC 20057. Offers acute care nurse practitioner (MS); clinical nurse specialist (MS); family nurse practitioner (MS); nurse anesthesia (MS); nurse-midwifery (MS); nursing (DNP); nursing education (MS). *Accreditation:* AACN; AANA/CANAEP (one or more programs are accredited); ACNM/ACME (one or more programs are accredited). *Degree requirements:* For master's, thesis optional. *Entrance requirements:* For master's, GRE General Test or MAT, bachelor's degree in nursing from NLN-accredited school, minimum undergraduate GPA of 3.0. Additional exam requirements/recommendations for international students: Required—TOEFL. Application fee: $50 ($55 for international students). *Financial support:* Scholarships/grants and traineeships available. Financial award applicants required to submit FAFSA. *Unit head:* Dr. Patricia Ann Cloonan, Dean, 202-687-7318. *Application contact:* Graduate School Admissions Office, 202-687-5568.

Goldfarb School of Nursing at Barnes-Jewish College, Graduate Programs, St. Louis, MO 63110. Offers adult acute care nurse practitioner (MSN); adult nurse practitioner (MSN); nurse anesthesia (MSN); nurse educator (MSN); nurse executive (MSN); DNP/PhD. *Accreditation:* AACN; AANA/CANAEP. Part-time and evening/weekend programs available. Postbaccalaureate distance learning degree programs offered (minimal on-campus study). *Faculty:* 42 full-time (39 women), 6 part-time/adjunct (all women). *Students:* 81 full-time (67 women), 85 part-time (77 women); includes 28 minority (18 Black or African American, non-Hispanic/Latino; 2 Asian, non-Hispanic/Latino; 3 Hispanic/Latino; 3 Native Hawaiian or other Pacific Islander, non-Hispanic/Latino; 2 Two or more races, non-Hispanic/Latino). *Degree requirements:* For master's, thesis or alternative. *Entrance requirements:* For master's, 2 references, personal statement, curriculum vitae or resume. Additional exam requirements/recommendations for international students: Required—TOEFL (minimum score 575 paper-based; 85 iBT). *Application deadline:* For fall admission, 2/1 priority date for international students; for spring admission, 10/1 priority date for international students. Applications are processed on a rolling basis. Application fee: $50. *Expenses: Tuition:* Full-time $12,960; part-time $720 per credit hour. *Required fees:* $295; $720 per credit hour. Tuition and fees vary according to course load. *Financial support:* Fellowships, research assistantships, Federal Work-Study, institutionally sponsored loans, and scholarships/grants available. Support available to part-time students. Financial award applicants required to submit FAFSA. *Faculty research:* HIV stigma, HIV symptom management, palliative care with children and their families, heart disease prevention in Hispanic women, depression in the well elderly, alternative therapies in pre-term infants. *Unit head:* Dr. Michael Bleich, Dean, 314-362-0956, Fax: 314-362-0984, E-mail: mbleich@bjc.org. *Application contact:* Margaret Anne O'Connor, Program Officer, 314-454-7557, Fax: 314-362-0984, E-mail: maoconnor@bjc.org.

Graceland University, School of Nursing, Independence, MO 64050-3434. Offers family nurse practitioner (MSN, PMC); nurse educator (MSN, PMC); organizational leadership (DNP). Part-time programs available. Postbaccalaureate distance learning degree programs offered (minimal on-campus study). *Faculty:* 13 full-time (all women), 9 part-time/adjunct (7 women). *Students:* 215 full-time (197 women), 339 part-time (303 women); includes 95 minority (37 Black or African American, non-Hispanic/Latino; 11 American Indian or Alaska Native, non-Hispanic/Latino; 15 Asian, non-Hispanic/Latino; 18 Hispanic/Latino; 2 Native Hawaiian or other Pacific Islander, non-Hispanic/Latino; 12 Two or more races, non-Hispanic/Latino), 4 international. Average age 44. 84 applicants, 89% accepted, 63 enrolled. In 2013, 71 master's awarded. *Degree requirements:* For master's, comprehensive exam (for some programs), thesis optional, scholarly project; for doctorate, capstone project. *Entrance requirements:* For master's, BSN from nationally-accredited program, RN license, minimum GPA of 3.0; satisfactory criminal background check; for doctorate, MSN from nationally-accredited program, RN license, minimum GPA of 3.2; satisfactory criminal background check. Additional exam requirements/recommendations for international students: Recommended—TOEFL. *Application deadline:* For fall admission, 6/1 priority date for domestic students; for winter admission, 10/1 priority date for domestic students; for spring admission, 3/1 priority date for domestic students. Application fee: $50. Electronic applications accepted. *Expenses:* Contact institution. *Financial support:* Institutionally sponsored loans available. Support available to part-time students. Financial award applicants required to submit FAFSA. *Faculty research:* International nursing, family care-giving, health promotion. *Unit head:* Dr. Claudia D. Horton, Dean, 816-423-4670, Fax: 816-423-4753, E-mail: horton@graceland.edu. *Application contact:* Nick Walker, Program Consultant, 816-423-4717, Fax: 816-833-2990, E-mail: nowalker@graceland.edu.
Website: http://www.graceland.edu/nursing

Grand Canyon University, College of Nursing, Phoenix, AZ 85017-1097. Offers acute care nurse practitioner (MS, PMC); clinical nurse specialist (PMC), including clinical nurse specialist, education; family nurse practitioner (MS); leadership in health care systems (MS); nurse education (MS). *Accreditation:* AACN. Part-time and evening/weekend programs available. Postbaccalaureate distance learning degree programs offered (no on-campus study). *Degree requirements:* For master's and PMC, comprehensive exam (for some programs). *Entrance requirements:* For master's, minimum cumulative and science course undergraduate GPA of 3.0. Additional exam requirements/recommendations for international students: Required—TOEFL (minimum score 575 paper-based; 90 iBT), IELTS (minimum score 7).

Grand Valley State University, Kirkhof College of Nursing, Allendale, MI 49401-9403. Offers advanced practice (MSN); case management (MSN); nursing administration (MSN); nursing education (MSN); nursing practice (DNP); MSN/MBA. *Accreditation:* AACN. Part-time programs available. *Degree requirements:* For master's, thesis optional. *Entrance requirements:* For master's, GRE, minimum GPA of 3.0 in upper-division course work, course work in statistics, Michigan RN license. Additional exam requirements/recommendations for international students: Required—TOEFL. Electronic applications accepted. *Faculty research:* Multigenerational health promotion, chronic disease prevention, end-of-life issues, nursing workload, family caregiver health.

Grantham University, College of Nursing and Allied Health, Lenexa, KS 66219. Offers case management (MSN); health systems management (MS); healthcare administration (MHA); nursing education (MSN); nursing informatics (MSN); nursing management and organizational leadership (MSN). Part-time and evening/weekend programs available. Postbaccalaureate distance learning degree programs offered (no on-campus study). *Faculty:* 1 (woman) full-time, 11 part-time/adjunct (5 women). *Students:* 64 full-time (43 women), 166 part-time (123 women); includes 116 minority (94 Black or African American, non-Hispanic/Latino; 4 Asian, non-Hispanic/Latino; 9 Hispanic/Latino; 1 Native Hawaiian or other Pacific Islander, non-Hispanic/Latino; 8 Two or more races, non-Hispanic/Latino). Average age 40. 230 applicants, 100% accepted, 230 enrolled. In 2013, 61 master's awarded. *Degree requirements:* For master's, thesis, major applied research paper and practicum (MSN). *Entrance requirements:* For master's, bachelor's degree from accredited degree-granting institution with minimum GPA of 2.5, BSN from an accredited nursing program, valid RN license. Additional exam requirements/recommendations for international students: Required—TOEFL (minimum score 530 paper-based; 71 iBT). *Application deadline:* Applications are processed on a rolling basis. Application fee: $30. Electronic applications accepted. *Expenses: Tuition:* Full-time $3900; part-time $325 per credit hour. *Required fees:* $35 per term. One-time fee: $100. *Financial support:* In 2013–14, 230 students received support. Scholarships/grants available. *Faculty research:* Pharmacy licensure, vaccination certification. *Unit head:* Dr. Susan Fairchild, Dean, School of Nursing, 800-955-2527, E-mail: admissions@grantham.edu. *Application contact:* Jared Parlette, Vice President of Admissions, 800-955-2527, E-mail: admissions@grantham.edu.
Website: http://www.grantham.edu/colleges-and-schools/college-of-nursing-and-allied-health/

Herzing University Online, Program in Nursing, Milwaukee, WI 53203. Offers nursing (MSN); nursing education (MSN); nursing management (MSN). *Accreditation:* AACN. Postbaccalaureate distance learning degree programs offered (no on-campus study).

Holy Family University, Graduate School, School of Nursing, Philadelphia, PA 19114. Offers community health nursing (MSN); nursing administration (MSN); nursing education (MSN). *Accreditation:* AACN. Part-time and evening/weekend programs available. *Faculty:* 7 full-time (all women). *Students:* 42 part-time (39 women); includes 9 minority (4 Black or African American, non-Hispanic/Latino; 4 Asian, non-Hispanic/Latino; 1 Hispanic/Latino). Average age 36. 17 applicants, 82% accepted, 6 enrolled. In 2013, 12 master's awarded. *Degree requirements:* For master's, thesis or alternative, comprehensive portfolio, clinical practicum. *Entrance requirements:* For master's, BSN or RN from appropriately-accredited program, minimum GPA of 3.0, professional references, official transcripts of all college or university work, essay/personal statement, current resume, completion of one undergraduate statistics course with minimum grade of C. Additional exam requirements/recommendations for international students: Required—TOEFL (minimum score 550 paper-based; 79 iBT), IELTS (minimum score 6), or PTE (minimum score 54). *Application deadline:* For fall admission, 7/1 priority date for domestic and international students; for winter admission, 1/1 for domestic students; for spring admission, 11/1 priority date for domestic and international students; for summer admission, 4/1 priority date for domestic and international students. Applications are processed on a rolling basis. Application fee: $25. Electronic applications accepted. *Expenses: Tuition:* Full-time $12,060. *Required fees:* $250. Tuition and fees vary according to degree level. *Financial support:* In 2013–14, 1 student received support. Available to part-time students. Application deadline: 2/15; applicants required to submit FAFSA. *Unit head:* Dr. Ana Maria Catanzaro, Dean, 267-341-3292, Fax: 215-637-6598, E-mail: acatanzaro@holyfamily.edu. *Application contact:* Gidget Matie Montelibano, Associate Director of Graduate Admissions, 267-341-3558, Fax: 215-637-1478, E-mail: gmontelibano@holyfamily.edu.
Website: http://www.holyfamily.edu/choosing-holy-family-u/academics/schools-of-study/school-of-nursing

Holy Names University, Graduate Division, Department of Nursing, Oakland, CA 94619-1699. Offers administration/management (MSN, PMC); clinical faculty (MSN, PMC); community health nursing/case manager (MSN); family nurse practitioner (MSN, PMC); MSN/MA; MSN/MBA. *Accreditation:* AACN. Part-time and evening/weekend programs available. *Faculty:* 3 full-time, 22 part-time/adjunct. *Students:* 31 full-time (26 women), 78 part-time (67 women); includes 66 minority (27 Black or African American, non-Hispanic/Latino; 25 Asian, non-Hispanic/Latino; 13 Hispanic/Latino; 1 Two or more races, non-Hispanic/Latino), 5 international. Average age 38. 97 applicants, 61% accepted, 49 enrolled. In 2013, 66 master's, 3 other advanced degrees awarded. *Entrance requirements:* For master's, bachelor's degree in nursing or related field; California RN license or eligibility; minimum cumulative GPA of 2.8, 3.0 in nursing courses from baccalaureate program; courses in pathophysiology, statistics, and research at the undergraduate level. Additional exam requirements/recommendations for international students: Required—TOEFL (minimum score 500 paper-based; 79 iBT). *Application deadline:* For fall admission, 8/1 priority date for domestic students, 7/15 priority date for international students; for spring admission, 12/1 priority date for domestic and international students; for summer admission, 5/1 priority date for domestic and international students. Applications are processed on a rolling basis. Application fee: $65. Electronic applications accepted. Application fee is waived when completed online. *Expenses: Tuition:* Part-time $866 per unit. *Financial support:* Career-related internships or fieldwork, Federal Work-Study, scholarships/grants, and unspecified assistantships available. Support available to part-time students. Financial award application deadline: 3/2; financial award applicants required to submit FAFSA. *Faculty research:* Women's reproductive health, gerontology, attitudes about aging, schizophrenic families, international health issues. *Unit head:* Dr. Miki Goodwin, Associate Professor/Chair of Nursing, 510-436-1374, E-mail: goodwin@hnu.edu. *Application contact:* Graduate Admission Office, 800-430-1321, E-mail: graduateadmissions@hnu.edu.

Husson University, Graduate Nursing Program, Bangor, ME 04401-2999. Offers advanced practice psychiatric nursing (MSN, PMC); family and community nurse practitioner (MSN, PMC); nursing education (MSN, PMC). *Accreditation:* AACN. Part-time programs available. *Faculty:* 3 full-time (all women), 3 part-time/adjunct (all women). *Students:* 10 full-time (8 women), 15 part-time (14 women); includes 1 minority (Two or more races, non-Hispanic/Latino). 29 applicants, 76% accepted, 21 enrolled. In 2013, 16 master's awarded. *Degree requirements:* For master's, comprehensive exam (for some programs). *Entrance requirements:* For master's, MAT or GRE, BSN. Additional exam requirements/recommendations for international students: Required—TOEFL (minimum score 550 paper-based). *Application deadline:* For fall admission, 6/30 for domestic students; for spring admission, 10/30 for domestic students. Application fee: $40. *Expenses:* Contact institution. *Financial support:* In 2013–14, 16 students received support. Federal Work-Study, institutionally sponsored loans, traineeships, and unspecified assistantships available. Financial award application deadline: 4/15; financial award applicants required to submit FAFSA. *Unit head:* Prof. Chrystal Adams,

Director, Nurse Practitioner Program, 207-941-7080, E-mail: adamsc@husson.edu. *Application contact:* Kristen Card, Director of Graduate Admissions, 207-404-5660, Fax: 207-941-7935, E-mail: cardk@husson.edu.

Immaculata University, College of Graduate Studies, Division of Nursing, Immaculata, PA 19345. Offers nursing administration (MSN); nursing education (MSN). *Accreditation:* AACN. Part-time and evening/weekend programs available. *Entrance requirements:* For master's, MAT or GRE, BSN, minimum undergraduate GPA of 3.0. Additional exam requirements/recommendations for international students: Required—TOEFL. *Application deadline:* Applications are processed on a rolling basis. Application fee: $50. *Expenses: Tuition:* Part-time $660 per credit. Part-time tuition and fees vary according to degree level and program. *Financial support:* Application deadline: 5/1; applicants required to submit FAFSA. *Unit head:* Dr. Jane Tang, RN, Program Director, 610-647-4400 Ext. 3309, Fax: 610-993-8550, E-mail: jtang@immaculata.edu.
Website: http://www.immaculata.edu/nursing/

Indiana University Kokomo, School of Nursing, Kokomo, IN 46904-9003. Offers nurse administrator (MSN); nurse educator (MSN). *Students:* 3 full-time (all women), 35 part-time (all women), 1 international. 14 applicants, 93% accepted, 11 enrolled. *Unit head:* Dr. Mary P. Bourke, Assistant Dean of Graduate Programs, 765-455-9326, E-mail: mbourke@iuk.edu. *Application contact:* Admissions Office, 765-455-9326.
Website: http://www.iuk.edu/academics/majors/nursing/graduate-programs/index.shtml

Indiana University of Pennsylvania, School of Graduate Studies and Research, College of Health and Human Services, Department of Nursing and Allied Health, Program in Nursing Education, Indiana, PA 15705-1087. Offers MS. Part-time programs available. *Faculty:* 7 full-time (6 women). *Students:* 1 (woman) full-time, 22 part-time (20 women). Average age 40. 19 applicants, 74% accepted, 11 enrolled. In 2013, 20 master's awarded. *Degree requirements:* For master's, thesis optional, practicum. *Entrance requirements:* Additional exam requirements/recommendations for international students: Required—TOEFL (minimum score 540 paper-based). *Application deadline:* Applications are processed on a rolling basis. Application fee: $50. Electronic applications accepted. *Expenses:* Tuition, state resident: full-time $3978; part-time $442 per credit. Tuition, nonresident: full-time $5967; part-time $663 per credit. *Required fees:* $2080; $115.55 per credit. $93 per semester. Tuition and fees vary according to degree level and program. *Financial support:* In 2013–14, 4 research assistantships with full and partial tuition reimbursements (averaging $2,078 per year) were awarded; career-related internships or fieldwork, Federal Work-Study, scholarships/grants, and unspecified assistantships also available. Financial award application deadline: 4/15; financial award applicants required to submit FAFSA. *Unit head:* Dr. Nashat Zuraikat, Graduate Coordinator, 724-357-3262, E-mail: zuraikat@iup.edu.
Website: http://www.iup.edu/grad/nursing/default.aspx

Indiana University–Purdue University Fort Wayne, College of Health and Human Services, Department of Nursing, Fort Wayne, IN 46805-1499. Offers adult-gerontology primary care nurse practitioner (MS); nurse executive (MS); nursing administration (Certificate); nursing education (MS); women's health nurse practitioner (MS). Part-time programs available. *Faculty:* 12 full-time (all women). *Students:* 5 full-time (all women), 63 part-time (60 women); includes 3 minority (2 Black or African American, non-Hispanic/Latino; 1 Asian, non-Hispanic/Latino). Average age 35. 34 applicants, 100% accepted, 25 enrolled. In 2013, 10 master's awarded. *Entrance requirements:* For master's, GRE Writing Test (if GPA below 3.0), BS in nursing, eligibility for Indiana RN license, minimum GPA of 3.0, essay, copy of resume, three references, undergraduate course work in research and statistics within last 5 years. Additional exam requirements/recommendations for international students: Required—TOEFL (minimum score 550 paper-based; 79 iBT); Recommended—TWE. *Application deadline:* For fall admission, 5/1 priority date for domestic and international students; for spring admission, 11/15 priority date for domestic students. Applications are processed on a rolling basis. Application fee: $55 ($60 for international students). Electronic applications accepted. *Financial support:* In 2013–14, 3 teaching assistantships with partial tuition reimbursements (averaging $13,322 per year) were awarded; scholarships/grants also available. Support available to part-time students. Financial award application deadline: 3/1; financial award applicants required to submit FAFSA. *Faculty research:* Pain management and substance abuse, high-risk alcohol use on campus, pediatric case management. *Unit head:* Dr. Lee-Ellen Kirkhorn, Chair/Professor, 260-481-6789, Fax: 260-481-5767, E-mail: kirkhorl@ipfw.edu. *Application contact:* Dr. Deborah Poling, Director of Graduate Program, 260-481-6276, Fax: 260-481-5767, E-mail: polingd@ipfw.edu.
Website: http://www.ipfw.edu/nursing/

Indiana University–Purdue University Indianapolis, School of Nursing, Master of Science in Nursing Program, Indianapolis, IN 46202-2896. Offers nursing administration (MSN); nursing education (MSN). *Students:* 31 full-time (27 women), 303 part-time (284 women); includes 54 minority (27 Black or African American, non-Hispanic/Latino; 11 Asian, non-Hispanic/Latino; 8 Hispanic/Latino; 8 Two or more races, non-Hispanic/Latino), 3 international. 200 applicants, 59% accepted, 88 enrolled. In 2013, 120 master's awarded. *Entrance requirements:* For master's, background check, statistics. *Unit head:* Associate Dean for Graduate Programs, 317-274-2806, E-mail: nursing@iupui.edu. *Application contact:* Lisa Thompson, Graduate Advisor, 317-274-2806, E-mail: lisrthom@iu.edu.
Website: http://nursing.iu.edu/graduate/programs/msn/index.shtml

Indiana Wesleyan University, Graduate School, School of Nursing, Marion, IN 46953-4974. Offers nursing administration (MS); nursing education (MS); primary care nursing (MS); MSN/MBA. *Accreditation:* AACN. Part-time programs available. Postbaccalaureate distance learning degree programs offered (minimal on-campus study). *Degree requirements:* For master's, capstone project or thesis. *Entrance requirements:* For master's, writing sample, RN license, 1 year of related experience, graduate statistics course. Additional exam requirements/recommendations for international students: Required—TOEFL. *Expenses:* Contact institution. *Faculty research:* Primary health care with international emphasis, international nursing.

Jefferson College of Health Sciences, Program in Nursing, Roanoke, VA 24031-3186. Offers nursing education (MSN); nursing management (MSN). *Accreditation:* AACN. Part-time programs available. *Degree requirements:* For master's, project. *Entrance requirements:* For master's, MAT. Additional exam requirements/recommendations for international students: Required—TOEFL (minimum score 550 paper-based; 80 iBT). Electronic applications accepted. *Faculty research:* Nursing, teaching and learning techniques, cultural competence, spirituality and nursing.

Kaplan University, Davenport Campus, School of Nursing, Davenport, IA 52807-2095. Offers nurse administrator (MS); nurse educator (MS). Part-time and evening/weekend programs available. Postbaccalaureate distance learning degree programs offered (no on-campus study). *Entrance requirements:* For master's, RN. Additional exam requirements/recommendations for international students: Required—TOEFL (minimum score 550 paper-based).

Kent State University, College of Nursing, Kent, OH 44242-0001. Offers acute care nurse practitioner (MSN); adult nurse practitioner (MSN); clinical nurse specialist (MSN); family nurse practitioner (MSN); geriatric nurse practitioner (MSN); health care management (MSN); nurse educator (MSN); nursing (PhD); nursing practice (DNP); pediatric nurse practitioner (MSN); psychiatric/mental health nurse practitioner (MSN); women's health nurse practitioner (MSN). PhD program offered jointly with The University of Akron. *Accreditation:* AACN. Part-time programs available. *Degree requirements:* For master's, thesis optional; for doctorate, comprehensive exam, thesis/dissertation. *Entrance requirements:* For master's, GRE (if undergraduate GPA less than 3.0), minimum GPA of 2.75; for doctorate, GRE, MSN. Additional exam requirements/recommendations for international students: Required—TOEFL. Electronic applications accepted. *Expenses:* Contact institution. *Faculty research:* Women and violence, methodological specialties, osteoporosis in women, new caregivers and the elderly.

Lamar University, College of Graduate Studies, College of Arts and Sciences, Department of Nursing, Beaumont, TX 77710. Offers nursing administration (MSN); nursing education (MSN); MSN/MBA. Part-time and evening/weekend programs available. Postbaccalaureate distance learning degree programs offered. *Degree requirements:* For master's, comprehensive exam, practicum project presentation, evidence-based project. *Entrance requirements:* For master's, GRE General Test, MAT, criminal background check, RN license, NLN-accredited BSN, college course work in graduate statistics in past 5 years, letters of recommendation, minimum undergraduate GPA of 3.0. Additional exam requirements/recommendations for international students: Required—TOEFL. *Faculty research:* Student retention, theory, care giving, online course and research.

La Roche College, School of Graduate Studies and Adult Education, Program in Nursing, Pittsburgh, PA 15237-5898. Offers nursing education (MSN); nursing management (MSN). *Accreditation:* AANA/CANAEP. Part-time and evening/weekend programs available. Postbaccalaureate distance learning degree programs offered (minimal on-campus study). *Faculty:* 3 full-time (all women), 2 part-time/adjunct (1 woman). *Students:* 6 full-time (all women), 7 part-time (all women), 1 international. Average age 43. 6 applicants, 50% accepted, 1 enrolled. In 2013, 7 master's awarded. *Degree requirements:* For master's, thesis optional, internship, practicum. *Entrance requirements:* For master's, GRE General Test, BSN, nursing license, work experience. Additional exam requirements/recommendations for international students: Recommended—TOEFL (minimum score 550 paper-based). *Application deadline:* For fall admission, 8/15 priority date for domestic students, 8/15 for international students; for spring admission, 12/15 priority date for domestic students, 12/15 for international students. Applications are processed on a rolling basis. Application fee: $50. Electronic applications accepted. *Expenses:* Contact institution. *Financial support:* Application deadline: 3/31; applicants required to submit FAFSA. *Faculty research:* Patient education, perception. *Unit head:* Dr. Terri Liberto, Division Chair, 412-847-1813, Fax: 412-536-1175, E-mail: terri.liberto@laroche.edu. *Application contact:* Hope Schiffgens, Director of Graduate Studies and Adult Education, 412-536-1266, Fax: 412-536-1283, E-mail: schombh1@laroche.edu.

La Salle University, School of Nursing and Health Sciences, Program in Nursing, Philadelphia, PA 19141-1199. Offers adult gerontology primary care nurse practitioner (MSN, Certificate); adult health and illness clinical nurse specialist (MSN); adult-gerontology clinical nurse specialist (MSN, Certificate); clinical nurse leader (MSN); family primary care nurse practitioner (MSN, Certificate); gerontology (Certificate); nurse anesthetist (MSN, Certificate); nursing (MSN, Certificate); nursing administration (MSN, Certificate); nursing education (Certificate); nursing practice (DNP); nursing service administration (MSN); public health nursing (MSN, Certificate); school nursing (Certificate); MSN/MBA; MSN/MPH. *Accreditation:* AANA/CANAEP. Part-time programs available. Postbaccalaureate distance learning degree programs offered (minimal on-campus study). *Faculty:* 13 full-time (12 women), 10 part-time/adjunct (8 women). *Students:* 4 full-time (all women), 379 part-time (331 women); includes 119 minority (70 Black or African American, non-Hispanic/Latino; 2 American Indian or Alaska Native, non-Hispanic/Latino; 31 Asian, non-Hispanic/Latino; 12 Hispanic/Latino; 4 Two or more races, non-Hispanic/Latino), 1 international. Average age 37. 133 applicants, 85% accepted, 63 enrolled. In 2013, 72 master's, 3 doctorates, 26 other advanced degrees awarded. *Degree requirements:* For doctorate, minimum of 1,000 hours of post baccalaureate clinical practice supervised by preceptors. *Entrance requirements:* For master's, GRE, MAT, or GMAT (for students with BSN GPA of less than 3.2), baccalaureate degree in nursing from an NLNAC- or CCNE-accredited program or an MSN Bridge program; Pennsylvania RN license; 2 letters of reference; resume; statement of philosophy articulating professional values and future educational goal; 1 year of work experience as a registered nurse; for doctorate, GRE (waived for applicants with MSN cumulative GPA of 3.7 or above), MSN from nationally-accredited program or master's degree, MBA or MHA from nationally-accredited program; resume or curriculum vitae; 2 letters of reference; interview; for Certificate, GRE, MAT, or GMAT (for students with BSN GPA of less than 3.2, baccalaureate degree in nursing from an NLNAC- or CCNE-accredited program or an MSN Bridge program; Pennsylvania RN license; 2 letters of reference; resume; statement of philosophy articulating professional values and future educational goal; 1 year of work experience as a registered nurse. Additional exam requirements/recommendations for international students: Required—TOEFL. *Application deadline:* For fall admission, 8/15 priority date for domestic students, 7/15 for international students; for spring admission, 12/15 priority date for domestic students, 11/15 for international students; for summer admission, 4/15 priority date for domestic students, 3/15 for international students. Applications are processed on a rolling basis. Application fee: $35. Electronic applications accepted. Application fee is waived when completed online. *Expenses:* Contact institution. *Financial support:* In 2013–14, 48 students received support. Teaching assistantships, scholarships/grants, and traineeships available. Support available to part-time students. Financial award application deadline: 8/31; financial award applicants required to submit FAFSA. *Unit head:* Dr. Patricia M. Dillon, Director, 215-951-1322, Fax: 215-951-1896, E-mail: msnapn@lasalle.edu. *Application contact:* Paul J. Reilly, Assistant Vice President, Enrollment Services, 215-951-1946, Fax: 215-951-1462, E-mail: reilly@lasalle.edu.

Le Moyne College, Department of Nursing, Syracuse, NY 13214. Offers informatics (MS, CAS); nursing administration (MS, CAS); nursing education (MS, CAS); nursing gerontology (MS, CAS); palliative care (MS, CAS). *Accreditation:* AACN. Part-time and evening/weekend programs available. *Faculty:* 4 full-time (all women), 3 part-time/adjunct (2 women). *Students:* 13 part-time (12 women); includes 2 minority (both Black or African American, non-Hispanic/Latino). Average age 41. 14 applicants, 86% accepted, 5 enrolled. In 2013, 6 master's, 6 other advanced degrees awarded. *Degree requirements:* For master's, scholarly project. *Entrance requirements:* For master's, bachelor's degree, interview, minimum GPA of 3.0, New York RN license, 2 letters of recommendation, writing sample, transcripts. Additional exam requirements/recommendations for international students: Required—TOEFL (minimum score 550 paper-based; 79 iBT). *Application deadline:* For fall admission, 8/1 priority date for domestic and international students; for spring admission, 12/15 priority date for domestic and international students; for summer admission, 5/1 priority date for domestic and international students. Applications are processed on a rolling basis. Application fee: $50. *Expenses:* Contact institution. *Financial support:* In 2013–14, 2 students received support. Career-related internships or fieldwork, scholarships/grants, health care benefits, and unspecified assistantships available. Support available to part-time students. Financial award applicants required to submit FAFSA. *Faculty research:*

Inter-profession education, gerontology, utilization of free healthcare services by the insured, health promotion education, innovative undergraduate nursing education models, patient and family education, horizontal violence. *Unit head:* Dr. Susan B. Bastable, Chair and Professor, Department of Nursing, 315-445-5436, Fax: 315-445-6024, E-mail: bastabsb@lemoyne.edu. *Application contact:* Kristen P. Trapasso, Senior Director of Enrollment Management, 315-445-4265, Fax: 315-445-6092, E-mail: trapaskp@lemoyne.edu.
Website: http://www.lemoyne.edu/nursing

Lewis University, College of Nursing and Health Professions, Program in Nursing, Romeoville, IL 60446. Offers adult nurse practitioner (MSN); nursing administration (MSN); nursing education (MSN). *Accreditation:* AACN. Part-time and evening/weekend programs available. Postbaccalaureate distance learning degree programs offered (no on-campus study). *Students:* 23 full-time (22 women), 234 part-time (222 women); includes 72 minority (31 Black or African American, non-Hispanic/Latino; 23 Asian, non-Hispanic/Latino; 15 Hispanic/Latino; 1 Native Hawaiian or other Pacific Islander, non-Hispanic/Latino; 2 Two or more races, non-Hispanic/Latino). Average age 38. *Degree requirements:* For master's, clinical practicum. *Entrance requirements:* For master's, minimum undergraduate GPA of 3.0, degree in nursing, RN license, letter of recommendation, interview, resume or curriculum vitae. Additional exam requirements/recommendations for international students: Required—TOEFL (minimum score 550 paper-based; 80 iBT). *Application deadline:* For fall admission, 5/1 priority date for international students; for spring admission, 11/15 priority date for international students. Applications are processed on a rolling basis. Application fee: $40. Electronic applications accepted. *Financial support:* Federal Work-Study, scholarships/grants, tuition waivers (full and partial), and unspecified assistantships available. Financial award application deadline: 5/1; financial award applicants required to submit FAFSA. *Faculty research:* Cancer prevention, phenomenological methods, public policy analysis. *Total annual research expenditures:* $1,000. *Unit head:* 815-836-5610. *Application contact:* Nancy Wiksten, Adult Admission Counselor, 815-836-5628, Fax: 815-836-5578, E-mail: wikstena@lewisu.edu.
Website: http://www.lewisu.edu/

Liberty University, School of Health Sciences, Lynchburg, VA 24515. Offers biomedical sciences (MS); clinical mental health counseling (MA); global health (MPH); health promotion (MPH); human services (MA), including addictions and recovery, business, Christian ministry, criminal justice, crisis response and trauma, executive leadership, health and wellness, life coaching, marriage and family, military resilience; marriage and family therapy (MA); nurse educator (MS); nursing (MSN); nursing administration (MSN); nutrition (MPH); pastoral care and counseling (PhD); professional counseling (MA, PhD). *Students:* 2,830 full-time (2,293 women), 6,275 part-time (5,051 women); includes 1,677 minority (1,178 Black or African American, non-Hispanic/Latino; 19 American Indian or Alaska Native, non-Hispanic/Latino; 36 Asian, non-Hispanic/Latino; 278 Hispanic/Latino; 7 Native Hawaiian or other Pacific Islander, non-Hispanic/Latino; 159 Two or more races, non-Hispanic/Latino), 177 international. Average age 37. 9,147 applicants, 50% accepted, 2939 enrolled. In 2013, 2,618 master's, 11 doctorates awarded. *Degree requirements:* For master's, thesis (for some programs); for doctorate, thesis/dissertation. *Entrance requirements:* For doctorate, MAT or GRE, minimum GPA of 3.25 in master's program, 2-3 recommendations, writing samples (for some programs), letter of intent, professional vitae. Additional exam requirements/recommendations for international students: Required—TOEFL (minimum score 600 paper-based; 100 iBT). Application fee: $50. *Expenses: Tuition:* Full-time $9630; part-time $535 per credit hour. *Required fees:* $175 per term. One-time fee: $50. Tuition and fees vary according to course load, degree level, campus/location and program. *Application contact:* Jay Bridge, Director of Admissions, 800-424-9595, Fax: 800-628-7977, E-mail: gradadmissions@liberty.edu.

Lourdes University, Graduate School, Sylvania, OH 43560-2898. Offers business (MBA); leadership (M Ed); nurse anesthesia (MSN); nurse educator (MSN); nurse leader (MSN); organizational leadership (MOL); reading (M Ed); teaching and curriculum (M Ed); theology (MA). Evening/weekend programs available. *Entrance requirements:* Additional exam requirements/recommendations for international students: Required—TOEFL. *Application deadline:* For fall admission, 6/15 priority date for domestic students; for spring admission, 11/1 priority date for domestic students. Application fee: $25. *Application contact:* Melissa Bergfeld, Administrative Assistant, 419-824-3517, Fax: 419-824-3510, E-mail: mbergfeld2@lourdes.edu.
Website: http://www.lourdes.edu/gradschool.aspx

Lynchburg College, Graduate Studies, School of Health Sciences and Human Performance, MS Program in Nursing, Lynchburg, VA 24501-3199. Offers clinical nurse leader (MS); nursing education (MS). *Accreditation:* AACN. Part-time and evening/weekend programs available. Postbaccalaureate distance learning degree programs offered (minimal on-campus study). *Faculty:* 4 full-time (all women), 1 (woman) part-time/adjunct. *Students:* 2 full-time (both women), 16 part-time (14 women); includes 2 minority (1 Black or African American, non-Hispanic/Latino; 1 Hispanic/Latino), 1 international. Average age 40. In 2013, 4 master's awarded. *Degree requirements:* For master's, practicum. *Entrance requirements:* For master's, GRE or 2 years of professional nursing experience, official transcripts, personal essay, 3 letters of recommendation, current unrestricted registered nurse license in Virginia. Additional exam requirements/recommendations for international students: Required—TOEFL (minimum score 550 paper-based; 79 iBT), IELTS (minimum score 6.5). *Application deadline:* For fall admission, 7/31 for domestic students, 6/1 for international students; for spring admission, 11/30 for domestic students, 10/15 for international students. Applications are processed on a rolling basis. Application fee: $30. Electronic applications accepted. Application fee is waived when completed online. *Financial support:* Fellowships, Federal Work-Study, scholarships/grants, health care benefits, and unspecified assistantships available. Support available to part-time students. Financial award application deadline: 7/31; financial award applicants required to submit FAFSA. *Unit head:* Dr. Nancy Overstreet, Associate Professor/Director of MSN Program, 434-544-8340, E-mail: overstreet.n@lynchburg.edu. *Application contact:* Anne Pingstock, Executive Assistant, Graduate Studies, 434-544-8383, E-mail: gradstudies@lynchburg.edu.
Website: http://www.lynchburg.edu/master-science-nursing

Marian University, School of Nursing and Health Professions, Fond du Lac, WI 54935-4699. Offers adult nurse practitioner (MSN); nurse educator (MSN). *Accreditation:* AACN. Part-time and evening/weekend programs available. *Faculty:* 5 full-time (all women), 10 part-time/adjunct (6 women). *Students:* 21 full-time (18 women), 77 part-time (71 women); includes 9 minority (3 Black or African American, non-Hispanic/Latino; 5 Hispanic/Latino; 1 Native Hawaiian or other Pacific Islander, non-Hispanic/Latino). Average age 37. In 2013, 24 master's awarded. *Degree requirements:* For master's, thesis, 675 clinical practicum hours. *Entrance requirements:* For master's, 3 letters of professional recommendation; undergraduate work in nursing research, statistics, health assessment. Additional exam requirements/recommendations for international students: Required—TOEFL (minimum score 525 paper-based; 70 iBT). *Application deadline:* Applications are processed on a rolling basis. Application fee: $50. Electronic applications accepted. *Expenses:* Contact institution. *Financial support:* In 2013–14, 3 students received support. Institutionally sponsored loans and scholarships/grants available. Support available to part-time students. Financial award application deadline: 3/1; financial award applicants required to submit FAFSA. *Unit head:* Dr. Julie Luetschwager, Dean, 920-923-8094, Fax: 920-923-8770, E-mail: jaluetschwager25@marianuniversity.edu. *Application contact:* Selina Scoles, Admissions Counselor, 920-923-8938, Fax: 920-923-8770, E-mail: sascoles30@marianuniversity.edu.
Website: http://www.marianuniversity.edu/nursing/

Maryville University of Saint Louis, College of Health Professions, The Catherine McAuley School of Nursing, St. Louis, MO 63141-7299. Offers adult nurse practitioner (MSN); advanced practice nursing (DNP); family nurse practitioner (MSN); geriatric nurse practitioner (MSN); nursing education (MSN). *Accreditation:* AACN. Postbaccalaureate distance learning degree programs offered. *Students:* 30 full-time (28 women), 1,551 part-time (1,416 women); includes 361 minority (181 Black or African American, non-Hispanic/Latino; 16 American Indian or Alaska Native, non-Hispanic/Latino; 59 Asian, non-Hispanic/Latino; 71 Hispanic/Latino; 5 Native Hawaiian or other Pacific Islander, non-Hispanic/Latino; 29 Two or more races, non-Hispanic/Latino), 3 international. Average age 36. In 2013, 37 master's awarded. *Degree requirements:* For master's, practicum. *Entrance requirements:* For master's, BSN, current licensure, minimum GPA of 3.0, 3 letters of recommendation, curriculum vitae. Additional exam requirements/recommendations for international students: Required—TOEFL (minimum score 550 paper-based). *Application deadline:* Applications are processed on a rolling basis. Application fee: $40 ($60 for international students). Electronic applications accepted. Application fee is waived when completed online. *Expenses: Tuition:* Full-time $23,812; part-time $728 per credit hour. *Required fees:* $395 per year. Tuition and fees vary according to course load, degree level and program. *Financial support:* Federal Work-Study and campus employment available. Support available to part-time students. Financial award application deadline: 3/1; financial award applicants required to submit FAFSA. *Unit head:* Dr. Elizabeth Buck, Director, 314-529-9453, Fax: 314-529-9139, E-mail: ebuck@maryville.edu. *Application contact:* Crystal Jacobsmeyer, Assistant Director, Graduate Enrollment Advising, 314-929-9654, Fax: 314-529-9927, E-mail: cjacobsmeyer@maryville.edu.
Website: http://www.maryville.edu/hp/nursing/

McKendree University, Graduate Programs, Master of Science in Nursing Program, Lebanon, IL 62254-1299. Offers nursing education (MSN); nursing management/administration (MSN). *Accreditation:* AACN. Part-time and evening/weekend programs available. Postbaccalaureate distance learning degree programs offered (no on-campus study). *Degree requirements:* For master's, research project or thesis. *Entrance requirements:* For master's, resume, references, valid Professional Registered Nurse license. Additional exam requirements/recommendations for international students: Required—TOEFL. Electronic applications accepted.

McMurry University, Graduate Studies, Abilene, TX 79697. Offers education (MSN); family nurse practitioner (MSN).

McNeese State University, Doré School of Graduate Studies, College of Nursing, Department of Graduate Nursing, Nursing Program, Lake Charles, LA 70609. Offers family nurse practitioner (MSN); family psychiatric/mental health nurse practitioner (MSN); nurse educator (MSN); nurse executive (MSN). *Degree requirements:* For master's, comprehensive exam. *Entrance requirements:* For master's, GRE, baccalaureate degree in nursing, minimum overall GPA of 2.7 for all undergraduate coursework, eligibility for unencumbered licensure as Registered Nurse in Louisiana or Texas, course in introductory statistics with minimum C grade, physical assessment skills, two letters of professional reference, 500-word essay, current resume.

Medical University of South Carolina, College of Nursing, Nurse Educator Program, Charleston, SC 29425. Offers MSN. Part-time and evening/weekend programs available. Postbaccalaureate distance learning degree programs offered (no on-campus study). *Degree requirements:* For master's, thesis optional. *Entrance requirements:* For master's, BSN, course work in statistics, nursing license, minimum GPA of 3.0, current curriculum vitae, essay, three references. Additional exam requirements/recommendations for international students: Required—TOEFL (minimum score 600 paper-based). Electronic applications accepted. *Faculty research:* Prenatal care outcomes, perinatal wellness in Hispanic women, use of personal digital assistants (PDAs) in clinical practice.

Mercy College, School of Health and Natural Sciences, Programs in Nursing, Dobbs Ferry, NY 10522-1189. Offers nursing administration (MS); nursing education (MS). *Accreditation:* AACN. Part-time and evening/weekend programs available. Postbaccalaureate distance learning degree programs offered (no on-campus study). *Students:* 4 full-time (3 women), 167 part-time (151 women); includes 105 minority (77 Black or African American, non-Hispanic/Latino; 14 Asian, non-Hispanic/Latino; 14 Hispanic/Latino), 3 international. Average age 33. 82 applicants, 77% accepted, 35 enrolled. In 2013, 33 master's awarded. *Degree requirements:* For master's, comprehensive exam (for some programs), written comprehensive exam or the production of a comprehensive project. *Entrance requirements:* For master's, interview, two letters of reference, skills assessment, bachelor's degree, RN registration in the U.S. Additional exam requirements/recommendations for international students: Required—TOEFL (minimum score 600 paper-based; 100 iBT), IELTS (minimum score 8). *Application deadline:* For fall admission, 8/1 for international students. Applications are processed on a rolling basis. Application fee: $62. Electronic applications accepted. *Expenses: Tuition:* Full-time $19,344; part-time $806 per credit. *Required fees:* $580; $806 per credit. $145 per term. Tuition and fees vary according to course load, degree level and program. *Financial support:* Career-related internships or fieldwork, Federal Work-Study, scholarships/grants, and unspecified assistantships available. Support available to part-time students. Financial award applicants required to submit FAFSA. *Unit head:* Dr. Joan Toglia, Dean, School of Health and Natural Sciences, 914-674-7837, E-mail: jtoglia@mercy.edu. *Application contact:* Allison Gurdineer, Senior Director of Admissions, 877-637-2946, Fax: 914-674-7382, E-mail: admissions@mercy.edu.
Website: https://www.mercy.edu/academics/school-of-health-and-natural-sciences/graduate-programs/

Messiah College, Program in Nursing, Mechanicsburg, PA 17055. Offers nurse educator (MSN). *Expenses: Tuition:* Part-time $595 per credit hour. *Required fees:* $30 per course.

Metropolitan State University, College of Health, Community and Professional Studies, St. Paul, MN 55106-5000. Offers advanced dental therapy (MS); leadership and management (MSN); nurse educator (MSN); nursing (DNP); psychology (MA). *Accreditation:* AACN. Part-time programs available. *Degree requirements:* For master's, thesis or alternative; for doctorate, thesis/dissertation or alternative. *Entrance requirements:* For master's, GRE General Test, minimum GPA of 3.0, RN license, BS/BA; for doctorate, minimum GPA of 3.0; RN license, MSN. Additional exam requirements/recommendations for international students: Required—TOEFL (minimum score 550 paper-based). *Expenses:* Tuition, state resident: full-time $5548. Tuition, nonresident: full-time $10,929. *Faculty research:* Women's health, gerontology.

MGH Institute of Health Professions, School of Nursing, Boston, MA 02129-4557. Offers advanced practice nursing (MSN); gerontological nursing (MSN); nursing (DNP); pediatric nursing (MSN); psychiatric nursing (MSN); teaching and learning for health care education (Certificate); women's health nursing (MSN). *Accreditation:* AACN.

Faculty: 41 full-time (36 women), 14 part-time/adjunct (13 women). *Students:* 494 full-time (428 women), 85 part-time (77 women); includes 108 minority (32 Black or African American, non-Hispanic/Latino; 2 American Indian or Alaska Native, non-Hispanic/Latino; 38 Asian, non-Hispanic/Latino; 33 Hispanic/Latino; 3 Native Hawaiian or other Pacific Islander, non-Hispanic/Latino). Average age 32. 470 applicants, 52% accepted, 133 enrolled. In 2013, 85 master's, 12 doctorates, 98 other advanced degrees awarded. *Degree requirements:* For master's, thesis or alternative. *Entrance requirements:* For master's, GRE General Test, bachelor's degree from regionally-accredited college or university. Additional exam requirements/recommendations for international students: Required—TOEFL (minimum score 550 paper-based; 80 iBT). *Application deadline:* For fall admission, 12/1 for domestic and international students; for spring admission, 10/1 for domestic and international students. Application fee: $100. Electronic applications accepted. *Expenses: Tuition:* Part-time $1114 per credit. *Required fees:* $620 per term. One-time fee: $475 part-time. *Financial support:* In 2013–14, 75 students received support, including 4 research assistantships (averaging $1,200 per year), 17 teaching assistantships (averaging $1,200 per year); career-related internships or fieldwork, scholarships/grants, traineeships, and unspecified assistantships also available. Support available to part-time students. Financial award application deadline: 4/1; financial award applicants required to submit FAFSA. *Faculty research:* Biobehavioral nursing, HIV/AIDS, gerontological nursing, women's health, vulnerable populations, health systems. *Unit head:* Dr. Laurie Lauzon-Clabo, Dean, 617-643-0605, Fax: 617-726-8022, E-mail: llauzonclabo@mghihp.edu. *Application contact:* Lauren Putnam, Assistant Director of Admission, 617-726-3140, Fax: 617-726-8010, E-mail: admissions@mghihp.edu.
Website: http://www.mghihp.edu/academics/nursing/

Middle Tennessee State University, College of Graduate Studies, University College, Murfreesboro, TN 37132. Offers advanced studies in teaching and learning (M Ed); human resources leadership (MPS); nursing administration (MSN); nursing education (MSN); strategic leadership (MPS); training and development (MPS). Part-time and evening/weekend programs available. Postbaccalaureate distance learning degree programs offered. *Students:* 58 full-time (52 women), 263 part-time (222 women). *Entrance requirements:* Additional exam requirements/recommendations for international students: Required—TOEFL (minimum score 525 paper-based; 71 iBT) or IELTS (minimum score 6). *Application deadline:* For fall admission, 6/1 for domestic and international students. Applications are processed on a rolling basis. Application fee: $25 ($30 for international students). *Financial support:* In 2013–14, 2 students received support. Tuition waivers available. Support available to part-time students. Financial award application deadline: 5/1. *Unit head:* Dr. Mike Boyle, Dean, 615-494-8877, Fax: 615-896-7925, E-mail: mike.boyle@mtsu.edu. *Application contact:* Dr. Michael D. Allen, Dean and Vice Provost for Research, 615-898-2840, Fax: 615-904-8020, E-mail: michael.allen@mtsu.edu.
Website: http://www.mtsu.edu/universitycollege/

Midwestern State University, Graduate School, Robert D. and Carol Gunn College of Health Sciences and Human Services, Wilson School of Nursing, Wichita Falls, TX 76308. Offers family nurse practitioner (MSN); family psychiatric mental health nurse practitioner (MSN); nurse educator (MSN). *Accreditation:* AACN. Part-time and evening/weekend programs available. *Degree requirements:* For master's, comprehensive exam, thesis optional. *Entrance requirements:* For master's, GRE General Test or MAT. Additional exam requirements/recommendations for international students: Required—TOEFL (minimum score 550 paper-based). *Application deadline:* For fall admission, 7/1 priority date for domestic students, 4/1 for international students; for spring admission, 11/1 priority date for domestic students, 8/1 for international students. Applications are processed on a rolling basis. Application fee: $35 ($50 for international students). Electronic applications accepted. *Expenses:* Tuition, state resident: full-time $3627; part-time $201.50 per credit hour. Tuition, nonresident: full-time $10,899; part-time $605.50 per credit hour. *Required fees:* $1357. *Financial support:* Teaching assistantships with partial tuition reimbursements, career-related internships or fieldwork, Federal Work-Study, institutionally sponsored loans, scholarships/grants, tuition waivers (partial), and unspecified assistantships available. Support available to part-time students. Financial award application deadline: 3/1; financial award applicants required to submit FAFSA. *Faculty research:* Infant feeding, musculoskeletal disorders, diabetes, community health education, water quality reporting. *Unit head:* Robin Lockhart, RN, Interim Chair, 940-397-4614, Fax: 940-397-4513, E-mail: robin.lockhart@mwsu.edu.
Website: http://www.mwsu.edu/academics/hs2/nursing/

Millersville University of Pennsylvania, College of Graduate and Professional Studies, School of Science and Mathematics, Department of Nursing, Millersville, PA 17551-0302. Offers family nurse practitioner (MSN); nursing education (MSN). Part-time and evening/weekend programs available. *Faculty:* 5 full-time (all women), 5 part-time/adjunct (all women). *Students:* 5 full-time (all women), 78 part-time (72 women); includes 10 minority (8 Black or African American, non-Hispanic/Latino; 2 Hispanic/Latino). Average age 38. 43 applicants, 67% accepted, 24 enrolled. In 2013, 25 master's awarded. *Degree requirements:* For master's, internship, scholarly project. *Entrance requirements:* For master's, 3 letters of recommendation; interview; resume; copy of RN license, goal statement, official transcripts. Additional exam requirements/recommendations for international students: Required—TOEFL (minimum score 550 paper-based, 79 iBT) or IELTS (minimum score 6). *Application deadline:* For fall admission, 1/15 for domestic and international students; for winter admission, 10/1 for domestic and international students; for spring admission, 10/1 for domestic and international students. Application fee: $40. Electronic applications accepted. *Expenses:* Tuition, state resident: full-time $7956; part-time $442 per credit. Tuition, nonresident: full-time $11,934; part-time $663 per credit. *Required fees:* $2196; $122 per credit. Tuition and fees vary according to course load. *Financial support:* In 2013–14, 3 students received support, including 3 research assistantships with full tuition reimbursements available (averaging $2,117 per year); institutionally sponsored loans and unspecified assistantships also available. Support available to part-time students. Financial award application deadline: 3/15; financial award applicants required to submit FAFSA. *Faculty research:* Family nurse practitioner, nurse educator. *Unit head:* Dr. Barbara J. Zimmerman, Chair, 717-872-3376, Fax: 717-871-4877, E-mail: barbara.zimmerman@millersville.edu. *Application contact:* Dr. Victor S. DeSantis, Dean of College of Graduate and Professional Studies/Associate Provost for Civic and Community Engagement, 717-872-3099, Fax: 717-872-3453, E-mail: victor.desantis@millersville.edu.
Website: http://www.millersville.edu/nursing/msn/

Millikin University, School of Nursing, Decatur, IL 62522-2084. Offers clinical nurse leader (MSN); entry into nursing practice: pre-licensure (MSN); nurse anesthesia (DNP); nurse educator (MSN); nursing practice (DNP). *Accreditation:* AACN; AANA/CANAEP. Part-time programs available. *Faculty:* 17 full-time (15 women), 5 part-time/adjunct (4 women). *Students:* 41 full-time (30 women), 26 part-time (19 women); includes 7 minority (2 Black or African American, non-Hispanic/Latino; 1 American Indian or Alaska Native, non-Hispanic/Latino; 1 Asian, non-Hispanic/Latino; 3 Hispanic/Latino). Average age 32. 69 applicants, 51% accepted, 21 enrolled. In 2013, 8 master's awarded. *Degree requirements:* For master's, thesis or alternative, research project. *Entrance requirements:* For master's, GRE, official academic transcript(s), essay, immunizations, statistics course, 3 letters of recommendation, CPR certification, professional liability/malpractice insurance; for doctorate, GRE (if undergraduate cumulative GPA is below 3.0), official academic transcript(s); undergraduate courses: nursing research, health assessment, inorganic and organic chemistry, intro to statistics; graduate-level statistics; 3 written recommendations; Assessment of Critical Care Skills form; written statement; resume or curriculum vita. Additional exam requirements/recommendations for international students: Required—TOEFL (minimum score 550 paper-based; 79 iBT). *Application deadline:* For spring admission, 11/1 for domestic students. Applications are processed on a rolling basis. Application fee: $0. Electronic applications accepted. *Expenses: Tuition:* Full-time $20,300; part-time $700 per credit hour. Tuition and fees vary according to program. *Financial support:* In 2013–14, 13 students received support. Institutionally sponsored loans available. Financial award applicants required to submit FAFSA. *Faculty research:* Congestive heart failure, quality of life, transcultural nursing issues, teaching/learning strategies, maternal - newborn. *Unit head:* Dr. Kathy Booker, Director, 217-424-6348, Fax: 217-420-6731, E-mail: kbooker@millikin.edu. *Application contact:* Marianne Taylor, Administrative Assistant, 800-373-7733 Ext. 5034, Fax: 217-420-6677, E-mail: mgtaylor@millikin.edu.
Website: http://www.millikin.edu/academics/cps/nursing/programs

Minnesota State University Moorhead, Graduate Studies, College of Education and Human Services, Tri-College University Nursing Consortium, Moorhead, MN 56563-0002. Offers MS. Program offered jointly with North Dakota State University and Concordia College. *Accreditation:* AACN. *Degree requirements:* For master's, thesis or alternative, final oral exam. *Entrance requirements:* For master's, 3 letters of recommendation, minimum GPA of 3.0, RN licensure, bachelor's degree with nursing major. Additional exam requirements/recommendations for international students: Required—TOEFL (minimum score 550 paper-based). Electronic applications accepted. *Expenses:* Contact institution.

Missouri State University, Graduate College, College of Health and Human Services, Department of Nursing, Springfield, MO 65897. Offers nursing (MSN), including family nurse practitioner, nurse educator. *Accreditation:* AACN. *Faculty:* 14 full-time (all women), 12 part-time/adjunct (9 women). *Students:* 18 full-time (17 women), 29 part-time (27 women); includes 5 minority (all Black or African American, non-Hispanic/Latino). Average age 37. 11 applicants, 91% accepted, 6 enrolled. In 2013, 17 master's awarded. *Degree requirements:* For master's, comprehensive exam, thesis or alternative. *Entrance requirements:* For master's, GRE General Test, minimum GPA of 3.0, RN license (for MSN), 1 year of work experience (for MPH). Additional exam requirements/recommendations for international students: Required—TOEFL (minimum score 550 paper-based; 79 iBT). *Application deadline:* For fall admission, 7/20 priority date for domestic students, 5/1 for international students; for spring admission, 12/20 priority date for domestic students, 9/1 for international students. Applications are processed on a rolling basis. Application fee: $35 ($50 for international students). Electronic applications accepted. *Expenses:* Tuition, state resident: full-time $4500; part-time $250 per credit hour. Tuition, nonresident: full-time $9018; part-time $501 per credit hour. *Required fees:* $361 per semester. Tuition and fees vary according to course level, course load and program. *Financial support:* In 2013–14, 2 research assistantships with full tuition reimbursements (averaging $8,324 per year) were awarded; Federal Work-Study, institutionally sponsored loans, scholarships/grants, and unspecified assistantships also available. Financial award application deadline: 3/31; financial award applicants required to submit FAFSA. *Faculty research:* Preconceptual health, women's health, nursing satisfaction, nursing education. *Unit head:* Dr. Kathryn Hope, Head, 417-836-5310, Fax: 417-836-5484, E-mail: nursing@missouristate.edu. *Application contact:* Misty Stewart, Coordinator of Admissions and Recruitment, 417-836-6079, Fax: 417-836-6200, E-mail: mistystewart@missouristate.edu.
Website: http://www.missouristate.edu/nursing/

Molloy College, Division of Nursing, Rockville Centre, NY 11571-5002. Offers adult nurse practitioner (Advanced Certificate); clinical nurse specialist: adult health (Advanced Certificate); family nurse practitioner (Advanced Certificate); nurse practitioner psychiatry (Advanced Certificate); nursing (MS, PhD); nursing administration (Advanced Certificate); nursing administration with informatics (Advanced Certificate); nursing education (Advanced Certificate); nursing informatics (Advanced Certificate); pediatric nurse practitioner (Advanced Certificate). *Accreditation:* AACN. Part-time and evening/weekend programs available. *Faculty:* 30 full-time (29 women), 10 part-time/adjunct (7 women). *Students:* 18 full-time (all women), 538 part-time (495 women); includes 289 minority (159 Black or African American, non-Hispanic/Latino; 1 American Indian or Alaska Native, non-Hispanic/Latino; 80 Asian, non-Hispanic/Latino; 43 Hispanic/Latino; 4 Native Hawaiian or other Pacific Islander, non-Hispanic/Latino; 2 Two or more races, non-Hispanic/Latino), 2 international. Average age 38. 241 applicants, 63% accepted, 122 enrolled. In 2013, 84 master's, 2 other advanced degrees awarded. *Degree requirements:* For master's, thesis optional. *Entrance requirements:* For master's, 3 letters of reference, BS in nursing, minimum undergraduate GPA of 3.0; for Advanced Certificate, 3 letters of reference, master's degree in nursing. *Application deadline:* For fall admission, 9/2 priority date for domestic students; for spring admission, 1/20 priority date for domestic students. Applications are processed on a rolling basis. Application fee: $60. *Expenses: Tuition:* Full-time $16,920; part-time $940 per credit. *Required fees:* $880. *Financial support:* Research assistantships with partial tuition reimbursements, teaching assistantships with partial tuition reimbursements, institutionally sponsored loans, scholarships/grants, and unspecified assistantships available. Support available to part-time students. Financial award application deadline: 4/1; financial award applicants required to submit FAFSA. *Unit head:* Dr. Jeannine Muldoon, Dean of Nursing, 516-323-3651, E-mail: jmuldoon@molloy.edu. *Application contact:* Alina Haitz, Assistant Director of Graduate Admissions, 516-323-4008, E-mail: ahaitz@molloy.edu.
Website: http://www.molloy.edu/academics/nursing-division

Monmouth University, The Graduate School, The Marjorie K. Unterberg School of Nursing and Health Studies, West Long Branch, NJ 07764-1898. Offers adult and gerontological nurse practitioner (MSN); adult-gerontological nurse practitioner (Post-Master's Certificate); family nurse practitioner (MSN, Post-Master's Certificate); family psychiatric and mental health advanced practice nursing (MSN); forensic nursing (MSN, Certificate); nursing (MSN); nursing administration (MSN, Post-Master's Certificate); nursing education (MSN, Post-Master's Certificate); nursing practice (DNP); physician assistant (MS); psychiatric-mental health nurse practitioner (Post-Master's Certificate); school nursing (MSN, Certificate). *Accreditation:* AACN. Part-time and evening/weekend programs available. *Faculty:* 14 full-time (all women), 4 part-time/adjunct (3 women). *Students:* 19 full-time (18 women), 269 part-time (252 women); includes 106 minority (35 Black or African American, non-Hispanic/Latino; 2 American Indian or Alaska Native, non-Hispanic/Latino; 51 Asian, non-Hispanic/Latino; 12 Hispanic/Latino; 3 Native Hawaiian or other Pacific Islander, non-Hispanic/Latino; 3 Two or more races, non-Hispanic/Latino), 2 international. Average age 39. 135 applicants, 98% accepted, 96 enrolled. In 2013, 54 master's, 7 doctorates awarded. *Degree requirements:* For master's, practicum (for some tracks). *Entrance requirements:* For master's, GRE General Test, BSN with minimum GPA of 2.75, current RN license, proof of liability and malpractice policy, personal statement, two letters of recommendation, college course work in health assessment, resume; minimum GPA of 3.0, minimum C grade in prerequisite courses, minimum 200 hours' clinical experience, 3 letters of

recommendation, and interview (for MS); for doctorate, accredited master's nursing program degree with minimum GPA of 3.2, active RN license, national certification as Nurse Practitioner or Nurse Administrator, working knowledge of statistics, statement of goals and vision for change, 2 letters of recommendation, resume, interview. Additional exam requirements/recommendations for international students: Required—TOEFL (minimum score 550 paper-based; 79 iBT), IELTS (minimum score 6) or Michigan English Language Assessment Battery (minimum score 77). *Application deadline:* For fall admission, 7/15 priority date for domestic students, 6/1 for international students; for spring admission, 11/15 priority date for domestic students, 11/1 for international students; for summer admission, 2/1 for domestic students. Applications are processed on a rolling basis. Application fee: $50. Electronic applications accepted. *Expenses: Tuition:* Part-time $1004 per credit hour. *Required fees:* $157 per semester. *Financial support:* In 2013–14, 163 students received support, including 113 fellowships (averaging $3,093 per year), 27 research assistantships (averaging $6,273 per year); career-related internships or fieldwork, scholarships/grants, and unspecified assistantships also available. Support available to part-time students. Financial award applicants required to submit FAFSA. *Faculty research:* Relationship of undergraduate GPA and GRE to succeeding in a graduate nursing program. *Unit head:* Dr. Janet Mahoney, Dean, 732-571-3443, Fax: 732-263-5131, E-mail: jmahoney@monmouth.edu. *Application contact:* Lauren Vento-Cifelli, Associate Vice President of Undergraduate and Graduate Admission, 732-571-3452, Fax: 732-263-5123, E-mail: gradadm@monmouth.edu.
Website: http://www.monmouth.edu/school-of-nursing-health/graduate-nursing-programs.aspx

Montana State University, College of Graduate Studies, College of Nursing, Bozeman, MT 59717. Offers clinical nurse leader (MN); family nurse practitioner (MN, Post-Master's Certificate); nursing education (Certificate, Post-Master's Certificate); psychiatric mental health nurse practitioner (MN). *Accreditation:* AACN. Part-time programs available. Postbaccalaureate distance learning degree programs offered (minimal on-campus study). *Degree requirements:* For master's, comprehensive exam, thesis (for some programs). *Entrance requirements:* For master's, GRE General Test, minimum GPA of 3.0 for undergraduate and post-baccalaureate work. Additional exam requirements/recommendations for international students: Required—TOEFL (minimum score 580 paper-based). Electronic applications accepted. *Faculty research:* Rural nursing, health disparities, environmental/public health, oral health, resilience.

Moravian College, Moravian College Comenius Center, St. Luke's School of Nursing, Bethlehem, PA 18018-6650. Offers clinical nurse leader (MS); nurse administrator (MS); nurse educator (MS). *Accreditation:* AACN. Part-time and evening/weekend programs available. *Degree requirements:* For master's, comprehensive exam (for some programs), evidence-based practice project. *Entrance requirements:* For master's, GRE or MAT. Additional exam requirements/recommendations for international students: Required—TOEFL (minimum score 550 paper-based; 90 iBT).

Mount Carmel College of Nursing, Nursing Program, Columbus, OH 43222. Offers adult gerontology acute care nurse practitioner (MS); adult health clinical nurse specialist (MS); family nurse practitioner (MS); nursing administration (MS); nursing education (MS). *Accreditation:* AACN. Part-time programs available. *Faculty:* 8 full-time (7 women), 8 part-time/adjunct (7 women). *Students:* 94 full-time (89 women), 76 part-time (73 women); includes 35 minority (21 Black or African American, non-Hispanic/Latino; 2 American Indian or Alaska Native, non-Hispanic/Latino; 6 Asian, non-Hispanic/Latino; 2 Hispanic/Latino; 1 Native Hawaiian or other Pacific Islander, non-Hispanic/Latino; 3 Two or more races, non-Hispanic/Latino). Average age 38. 123 applicants, 50% accepted, 47 enrolled. In 2013, 41 master's awarded. *Degree requirements:* For master's, professional manuscript. *Entrance requirements:* For master's, letters of recommendation, statement of purpose, current resume, baccalaureate degree in nursing, current Ohio RN license, minimum cumulative GPA of 3.0. Additional exam requirements/recommendations for international students: Required—TOEFL (minimum score 550 paper-based; 80 iBT). *Application deadline:* For fall admission, 6/1 priority date for domestic students; for winter admission, 11/1 for domestic students; for spring admission, 10/1 priority date for domestic students; for summer admission, 3/1 for domestic students. Applications are processed on a rolling basis. Application fee: $30. *Expenses: Tuition:* Full-time $8560; part-time $428 per credit. *Required fees:* $75. *Financial support:* In 2013–14, 9 students received support. Institutionally sponsored loans and scholarships/grants available. Financial award application deadline: 3/15; financial award applicants required to submit FAFSA. *Unit head:* Dr. Angela Phillips-Lowe, Associate Dean, 614-234-5717, Fax: 614-234-2875, E-mail: aphillips-lowe@mccn.edu. *Application contact:* Kathleen Walters, Program Coordinator, 614-234-5408, Fax: 614-234-2875, E-mail: kwalters@mccn.edu.
Website: http://www.mccn.edu/

Mount St. Joseph University, Master of Science in Nursing Program, Cincinnati, OH 45233-1670. Offers administration (MSN); clinical nurse leader (MSN); education (MSN). Part-time programs available. *Faculty:* 10 full-time (9 women), 23 part-time/adjunct (all women). *Students:* 33 part-time (31 women); includes 3 minority (all Black or African American, non-Hispanic/Latino). Average age 45. 24 applicants, 67% accepted, 16 enrolled. *Entrance requirements:* For master's, essay; BSN from regionally-accredited university; minimum undergraduate GPA of 3.25 or GRE; professional resume; three professional references; interview; 2 years of clinical nursing experience; active RN license; criminal background check. Additional exam requirements/recommendations for international students: Required—TOEFL (minimum score 560 paper-based; 83 iBT). Application fee: $50. Electronic applications accepted. *Expenses: Tuition:* Full-time $18,400; part-time $575 per credit hour. *Required fees:* $450; $450 per year. Part-time tuition and fees vary according to course load, degree level and program. *Financial support:* Application deadline: 3/1; applicants required to submit FAFSA. *Unit head:* Dr. Nancy Hinzman, MSN/DNP Director, 513-244-4325, E-mail: nancy_hinzman@mail.msj.edu. *Application contact:* Mary Brigham, Assistant Director for Graduate Recruitment, 513-244-4233, Fax: 513-244-4629, E-mail: mary_brigham@mail.msj.edu.
Website: http://www.msj.edu/academics/graduate-programs/master-of-science-in-nursing/

Mount Saint Mary College, Division of Nursing, Newburgh, NY 12550-3494. Offers adult nurse practitioner (MS, Advanced Certificate), including nursing education (MS), nursing management (MS); clinical nurse specialist-adult health (MS), including nursing education, nursing management; family nurse practitioner (Advanced Certificate). *Accreditation:* AACN. Part-time and evening/weekend programs available. *Faculty:* 4 full-time (all women). *Students:* 79 part-time (72 women); includes 19 minority (12 Black or African American, non-Hispanic/Latino; 1 Asian, non-Hispanic/Latino; 5 Hispanic/Latino; 1 Native Hawaiian or other Pacific Islander, non-Hispanic/Latino). Average age 39. 45 applicants, 47% accepted, 9 enrolled. In 2013, 13 master's, 3 other advanced degrees awarded. *Degree requirements:* For master's, research utilization project. *Entrance requirements:* For master's, BSN, minimum GPA of 3.0, RN license. *Application deadline:* For fall admission, 6/3 priority date for domestic students; for spring admission, 10/31 priority date for domestic students. Applications are processed on a rolling basis. Application fee: $45. Application fee is waived when completed online. *Expenses: Tuition:* Full-time $13,356; part-time $742 per credit. *Required fees:* $70 per semester. *Financial support:* In 2013–14, 8 students received support. Unspecified assistantships available. Financial award application deadline: 4/15; financial award applicants required to submit FAFSA. *Unit head:* Linda Ruta, Graduate Coordinator, 845-569-3512, Fax: 845-562-6762, E-mail: linda.ruta@msmc.edu. *Application contact:* Lisa Gallina, Director of Admissions for Graduate Programs and Adult Degree Completion, 845-569-3166, Fax: 845-569-3450, E-mail: lisa.gallina@msmc.edu.
Website: http://www.msmc.edu/Academics/Graduate_Programs/Master_of_Science_in_Nursing

Nebraska Methodist College, Program in Nursing, Omaha, NE 68114. Offers nurse educator (MSN); nurse executive (MSN). *Accreditation:* AACN. Evening/weekend programs available. Postbaccalaureate distance learning degree programs offered (no on-campus study). *Faculty:* 2 full-time (both women), 5 part-time/adjunct (all women). *Students:* 82 full-time (81 women), 39 part-time (36 women); includes 5 minority (4 Black or African American, non-Hispanic/Latino; 1 Asian, non-Hispanic/Latino). Average age 37. 156 applicants, 21% accepted, 28 enrolled. In 2013, 20 master's awarded. *Degree requirements:* For master's, thesis or alternative, Evidence Based Practice (EBP) project. *Entrance requirements:* For master's, interview. Additional exam requirements/recommendations for international students: Required—TOEFL (minimum score 550 paper-based; 80 iBT). *Application deadline:* For spring admission, 11/1 for domestic and international students. Applications are processed on a rolling basis. Application fee: $25. *Expenses: Tuition:* Full-time $12,258; part-time $681 per credit hour. *Required fees:* $450; $450 per year. *Financial support:* Research assistantships with full and partial tuition reimbursements and scholarships/grants available. Financial award applicants required to submit FAFSA. *Faculty research:* Spirituality, student outcomes, service-learning, leadership and administration, women's issues. *Unit head:* Dr. Linda Foley, Director, Graduate Nursing, 402-354-7050, Fax: 402-354-7020, E-mail: linda.foley@methodistcollege.edu. *Application contact:* Laurel Zentner, Recruitment and Admissions Coordinator, 402-354-7170, Fax: 402-354-7020, E-mail: admissions@methodistcollege.edu.
Website: http://www.methodistcollege.edu/nursing-online

New York University, College of Nursing, Programs in Advanced Practice Nursing, New York, NY 10012-1019. Offers advanced practice nursing: adult acute care (MS, Advanced Certificate); advanced practice nursing: adult nurse practitioner/holistic nurse practitioner (Advanced Certificate); advanced practice nursing: adult nurse practitioner/palliative care nurse practitioner (Advanced Certificate); advanced practice nursing: adult primary care (MS, Advanced Certificate); advanced practice nursing: family (MS, Advanced Certificate); advanced practice nursing: geriatrics (Advanced Certificate); advanced practice nursing: mental health (MS); advanced practice nursing: mental health nursing (Advanced Certificate); advanced practice nursing: pediatrics (MS, Advanced Certificate); nurse midwifery (MS, Advanced Certificate); nursing administration (MS, Advanced Certificate); nursing education (MS, Advanced Certificate); nursing informatics (MS, Advanced Certificate); MS/MPA; MS/MPH. *Accreditation:* AACN; ACNM/ACME. Part-time programs available. *Faculty:* 22 full-time (all women), 54 part-time/adjunct (46 women). *Students:* 36 full-time (31 women), 622 part-time (549 women); includes 239 minority (73 Black or African American, non-Hispanic/Latino; 1 American Indian or Alaska Native, non-Hispanic/Latino; 116 Asian, non-Hispanic/Latino; 36 Hispanic/Latino; 6 Native Hawaiian or other Pacific Islander, non-Hispanic/Latino; 7 Two or more races, non-Hispanic/Latino), 16 international. Average age 37. 395 applicants, 67% accepted, 156 enrolled. In 2013, 186 master's, 8 other advanced degrees awarded. *Degree requirements:* For master's, thesis (for some programs). *Entrance requirements:* For master's, BS in nursing, AS in nursing with another BS/BA, interview, RN license, 1 year of clinical experience (3 for nursing education program); for Advanced Certificate, master's degree. Additional exam requirements/recommendations for international students: Required—TOEFL (minimum score 90 iBT), IELTS (minimum score 7). *Application deadline:* For fall admission, 7/1 for domestic and international students; for spring admission, 12/1 for domestic and international students. Application fee: $80. Electronic applications accepted. *Expenses: Tuition:* Full-time $35,856; part-time $1494 per unit. *Required fees:* $1408; $64 per unit. $473 per term. Tuition and fees vary according to course load and program. *Financial support:* In 2013–14, 182 students received support. Research assistantships, career-related internships or fieldwork, Federal Work-Study, scholarships/grants, traineeships, and unspecified assistantships available. Support available to part-time students. Financial award application deadline: 2/1; financial award applicants required to submit FAFSA. *Faculty research:* Geriatrics, HIV, elderly black diabetics, families and illness, oral systemic connection. *Unit head:* Dr. Judith Haber, Associate Dean, Graduate Programs, 212-998-9020, Fax: 212-995-3143, E-mail: jh33@nyu.edu. *Application contact:* Elizabeth Ensweiler, Assistant Director, Graduate Student Affairs and Admissions, 212-992-7653, Fax: 212-995-4302, E-mail: ee39@nyu.edu.

Northeastern State University, College of Science and Health Professions, Program in Nursing Education, Muskogee, OK 74401. Offers MSN. *Faculty:* 3 full-time (all women). *Students:* 3 full-time (all women), 21 part-time (all women); includes 8 minority (1 Black or African American, non-Hispanic/Latino; 4 American Indian or Alaska Native, non-Hispanic/Latino; 1 Asian, non-Hispanic/Latino; 2 Two or more races, non-Hispanic/Latino). Average age 43. In 2013, 7 master's awarded. Application fee: $25. *Expenses:* Tuition, state resident: full-time $3029; part-time $168.25 per credit hour. Tuition, nonresident: full-time $7709; part-time $428.25 per credit hour. *Required fees:* $35.90 per credit hour. *Unit head:* Dr. Joyce Van Nostrand, Department Chair, 918-456-5511 Ext. 5410, E-mail: vannostr@nsuok.edu. *Application contact:* Margie Railey, Administrative Assistant, 918-456-5511 Ext. 2093, Fax: 918-458-2061, E-mail: railey@nsouk.edu.
Website: http://academics.nsuok.edu/healthprofessions/DegreePrograms/Graduate/NursingEducationMSN.aspx

Norwich University, College of Graduate and Continuing Studies, Master of Science in Nursing Program, Northfield, VT 05663. Offers nursing administration (MSN); nursing education (MSN). *Accreditation:* AACN. Evening/weekend programs available. Postbaccalaureate distance learning degree programs offered (minimal on-campus study). *Faculty:* 9 part-time/adjunct (5 women). *Students:* 82 full-time (78 women); includes 7 minority (4 Black or African American, non-Hispanic/Latino; 3 Asian, non-Hispanic/Latino). Average age 43. 114 applicants, 28% accepted, 31 enrolled. In 2013, 37 master's awarded. *Entrance requirements:* For master's, minimum undergraduate GPA of 2.75. Additional exam requirements/recommendations for international students: Required—TOEFL (minimum score 600 paper-based; 94 iBT). *Application deadline:* For fall admission, 8/1 for domestic and international students; for winter admission, 11/1 for domestic and international students; for spring admission, 2/1 for domestic and international students; for summer admission, 5/1 for domestic and international students. Applications are processed on a rolling basis. Application fee: $50. Electronic applications accepted. *Expenses:* Contact institution. *Financial support:* In 2013–14, 20 students received support. Scholarships/grants available. Financial award applicants required to submit FAFSA. *Unit head:* Dr. Sharon Richie-Melvan, Director, 802-485-2600, E-mail: srichiem@norwich.edu. *Application contact:* Rija Ramahatra, Associate Program Director, 802-485-2892, Fax: 802-485-2533, E-mail: rramahatr@norwich.edu.
Website: http://online.norwich.edu/degree-programs/masters/master-science-nursing/overview

Nursing Education

Nova Southeastern University, College of Nursing, Fort Lauderdale, FL 33314-7796. Offers advanced practice registered nurse (APRN) (MSN); nursing (MSN); nursing education (PhD); nursing practice (DNP). *Accreditation:* AACN. Part-time and evening/weekend programs available. Postbaccalaureate distance learning degree programs offered (no on-campus study). *Faculty:* 12 full-time (all women), 25 part-time/adjunct (all women). *Students:* 3 full-time (all women), 374 part-time (336 women); includes 215 minority (114 Black or African American, non-Hispanic/Latino; 23 Asian, non-Hispanic/Latino; 76 Hispanic/Latino; 2 Two or more races, non-Hispanic/Latino), 3 international. Average age 41. In 2013, 34 master's, 3 doctorates awarded. *Degree requirements:* For doctorate, comprehensive exam, thesis/dissertation. *Entrance requirements:* For doctorate, minimum GPA of 3.5, BSN, RN. Additional exam requirements/recommendations for international students: Recommended—TOEFL. *Application deadline:* For fall admission, 3/1 priority date for domestic students, 3/1 for international students; for winter admission, 11/1 for domestic and international students. Applications are processed on a rolling basis. Application fee: $50. Electronic applications accepted. *Faculty research:* Nursing education, curriculum, clinical research, interdisciplinary research. *Unit head:* Dr. Marcella Rutherford, Dean, 954-262-1963, E-mail: rmarcell@nova.edu. *Application contact:* Keatta Jerry, E-mail: keatta@nova.edu.
Website: http://www.nova.edu/nursing/

Oakland University, Graduate Study and Lifelong Learning, School of Nursing, Program in Nursing Education, Rochester, MI 48309-4401. Offers MSN, Certificate. *Students:* 4 full-time (3 women), 10 part-time (all women); includes 3 minority (2 Black or African American, non-Hispanic/Latino; 1 Hispanic/Latino). Average age 40. In 2013, 12 master's awarded. Application fee: $0. *Unit head:* Dr. Linda Thompson, Dean, 248-370-4081, Fax: 248-370-4279. *Application contact:* Mary Bray, Graduate Program Coordinator, 248-370-4482.

Ohio University, Graduate College, College of Health Sciences and Professions, School of Nursing, Athens, OH 45701-2979. Offers acute care nurse practitioner (MSN); acute care nurse practitioner and family nurse practitioner (MSN); acute care nurse practitioner and nurse administrator (MSN); acute care nurse practitioner and nurse educator (MSN); family nurse practitioner (MSN); nurse administrator (MSN); nurse administrator and family nurse practitioner (MSN); nurse educator (MSN); nurse educator and family nurse practitioner (MSN); nurse educator and nurse administrator (MSN). *Accreditation:* AACN. *Degree requirements:* For master's, capstone project. *Entrance requirements:* For master's, GRE, bachelor's degree in nursing from an accredited college or university, minimum overall undergraduate GPA of 3.0, official transcripts, statement of goals and objectives, resume, 3 letters of recommendation. Additional exam requirements/recommendations for international students: Required—TOEFL (minimum score 550 paper-based; 80 iBT) or IELTS (minimum score 6.5). Electronic applications accepted.

Oklahoma Baptist University, Program in Nursing, Shawnee, OK 74804. Offers global nursing (MSN); nursing education (MSN). *Accreditation:* AACN.

Oklahoma City University, Kramer School of Nursing, Oklahoma City, OK 73106-1402. Offers health care systems leadership and administration (MSN); nursing (PhD); nursing education (MSN); nursing practice (DNP). Part-time and evening/weekend programs available. *Faculty:* 14 full-time (12 women), 5 part-time/adjunct (3 women). *Students:* 78 full-time (51 women), 116 part-time (101 women); includes 43 minority (10 Black or African American, non-Hispanic/Latino; 16 American Indian or Alaska Native, non-Hispanic/Latino; 9 Asian, non-Hispanic/Latino; 3 Hispanic/Latino; 5 Two or more races, non-Hispanic/Latino), 55 international. Average age 36. 97 applicants, 69% accepted, 37 enrolled. In 2013, 14 master's, 8 doctorates awarded. *Degree requirements:* For master's, thesis, minimum GPA of 3.0; for doctorate, comprehensive exam, thesis/dissertation, minimum GPA of 3.0. *Entrance requirements:* For master's, registered nurse licensure, minimum undergraduate GPA of 3.0, BSN from nationally-accredited nursing program, completion of courses in health assessment and statistics; for doctorate, GRE, approved scholarly paper, or published article/paper in a refereed journal, current RN licensure, bachelor's and master's degrees from accredited programs (at least one of which must be in nursing), minimum graduate GPA of 3.5, personal essay. Additional exam requirements/recommendations for international students: Required—TOEFL (minimum score 550 paper-based; 80 iBT), IELTS (minimum score 6). *Application deadline:* Applications are processed on a rolling basis. Application fee: $50. Electronic applications accepted. *Expenses: Tuition:* Full-time $16,848; part-time $936 per credit hour. Tuition and fees vary according to course load, degree level and program. *Financial support:* Federal Work-Study, institutionally sponsored loans, scholarships/grants, and tuition waivers available. Support available to part-time students. Financial award applicants required to submit FAFSA. *Unit head:* Dr. Lois Salmeron, Dean, Kramer School of Nursing, 405-208-5900, Fax: 405-208-5914, E-mail: lsalmeron@okcu.edu. *Application contact:* Heidi Puckett, Director of Graduate Admissions, 800-633-7242, Fax: 405-208-5916, E-mail: gadmissions@okcu.edu.
Website: http://www.okcu.edu/nursing/

Old Dominion University, College of Health Sciences, School of Nursing, Nurse Educator Emphasis, Norfolk, VA 23529. Offers MSN. Part-time programs available. Postbaccalaureate distance learning degree programs offered (minimal on-campus study). *Faculty:* 1 (woman) full-time, 2 part-time/adjunct (both women). In 2013, 12 master's awarded. *Degree requirements:* For master's, comprehensive exam, thesis optional. *Entrance requirements:* For master's, GRE/MAT. *Application deadline:* For spring admission, 5/5 for domestic students. Application fee: $50. *Expenses:* Tuition, state resident: full-time $9888; part-time $412 per credit. Tuition, nonresident: full-time $25,152; part-time $1048 per credit. *Required fees:* $59 per semester. One-time fee: $50. *Financial support:* In 2013–14, 1 teaching assistantship (averaging $2,500 per year) was awarded. *Faculty research:* Technology in nursing education, evidence-based instructional strategies, clinical judgment and decision-making. *Total annual research expenditures:* $35,726. *Unit head:* Dr. Kim Curry-Lourenco, Graduate Program Director, 757-683-5261, E-mail: kcurrylo@odu.edu. *Application contact:* Sue Parker, Coordinator, Graduate Student Services, 757-683-4298, Fax: 757-683-5253, E-mail: sparker@odu.edu.
Website: http://hs.odu.edu/nursing/academics/nurse_educator/nurse_educator.shtml

Oregon Health & Science University, School of Nursing, Program in Nursing Education, Portland, OR 97239-3098. Offers MN, MS, Post Master's Certificate.

Otterbein University, Department of Nursing, Westerville, OH 43081. Offers advanced practice nurse educator (Certificate); clinical nurse leader (MSN); family nurse practitioner (MSN, Certificate); nurse anesthesia (MSN, Certificate); nursing (DNP); nursing service administration (MSN). *Accreditation:* AACN; AANA/CANAEP. Part-time and evening/weekend programs available. Postbaccalaureate distance learning degree programs offered (minimal on-campus study). *Degree requirements:* For master's, comprehensive exam (for some programs), thesis (for some programs). *Entrance requirements:* For master's, 2 reference forms, resume; for Certificate, official transcripts, 2 reference forms, essay, resumé. Additional exam requirements/recommendations for international students: Required—TOEFL (minimum score 550 paper-based; 79 iBT). *Faculty research:* Patient education, women's health, trauma curriculum development, administration.

Our Lady of the Lake College, School of Nursing, Program in Nursing, Baton Rouge, LA 70808. Offers administration (MS); education (MS). Part-time programs available. *Degree requirements:* For master's, capstone project. *Entrance requirements:* For master's, BSN with minimum GPA of 3.0 during the last 60 hours of undergraduate work, 1 year of clinical nursing experience as a registered nurse, current licensure or eligibility to practice as registered nurse in Louisiana, 3 professional references, 3 credit hours of undergraduate statistics with minimum C average.

Our Lady of the Lake University of San Antonio, School of Professional Studies, Program in Nursing, San Antonio, TX 78207-4689. Offers nurse administration (MSN); nurse education (MSN). Postbaccalaureate distance learning degree programs offered (no on-campus study). *Faculty:* 1 (woman) full-time, 1 (woman) part-time/adjunct. *Students:* 17 full-time (16 women), 4 part-time (all women); includes 12 minority (3 Black or African American, non-Hispanic/Latino; 1 American Indian or Alaska Native, non-Hispanic/Latino; 8 Hispanic/Latino). Average age 43. 20 applicants, 100% accepted, 15 enrolled. *Degree requirements:* For master's, comprehensive exam. *Entrance requirements:* For master's, GRE General Test or MAT. Additional exam requirements/recommendations for international students: Required—TOEFL. *Application deadline:* For fall admission, 4/1 priority date for domestic and international students; for spring admission, 11/1 priority date for domestic and international students; for summer admission, 2/1 priority date for domestic and international students. Applications are processed on a rolling basis. Application fee: $25 ($50 for international students). Electronic applications accepted. *Expenses: Tuition:* Full-time $9120; part-time $760 per credit. *Required fees:* $698; $334 per trimester. Tuition and fees vary according to course load, degree level, campus/location and program. *Financial support:* Career-related internships or fieldwork, institutionally sponsored loans, scholarships/grants, and tuition waivers (partial) available. Support available to part-time students. Financial award application deadline: 4/15. *Unit head:* Dr. Wanda Sparks, Chair, 210-431-4162, E-mail: wrsparks@lake.ollusa.edu. *Application contact:* Graduate Admission, 210-431-3961, Fax: 210-431-4013, E-mail: gradadm@lake.ollusa.edu.

Pace University, College of Health Professions, Lienhard School of Nursing, New York, NY 10038. Offers family nurse practitioner (MS); nurse practitioner (Advanced Certificate); nursing education (MA); nursing leadership (Advanced Certificate); nursing practice (DNP). *Accreditation:* AACN. Part-time and evening/weekend programs available. Postbaccalaureate distance learning degree programs offered. *Faculty:* 13 full-time (12 women), 36 part-time/adjunct (29 women). *Students:* 3 full-time (2 women), 427 part-time (390 women); includes 202 minority (98 Black or African American, non-Hispanic/Latino; 2 American Indian or Alaska Native, non-Hispanic/Latino; 68 Asian, non-Hispanic/Latino; 28 Hispanic/Latino; 1 Native Hawaiian or other Pacific Islander, non-Hispanic/Latino; 5 Two or more races, non-Hispanic/Latino), 2 international. Average age 35. 274 applicants, 69% accepted, 131 enrolled. In 2013, 120 master's, 15 doctorates, 3 other advanced degrees awarded. *Degree requirements:* For master's, thesis. *Entrance requirements:* For master's, GRE General Test or MAT, RN license, resume, personal statement, 2 letters of recommendation, official transcripts; for doctorate, RN license, resume, personal statement, 2 letters of recommendation, official transcripts, accredited master's degree in nursing, minimum GPA of 3.3, state certification; for Advanced Certificate, RN license, completion of 2nd degree in nursing. Additional exam requirements/recommendations for international students: Required—TOEFL. *Application deadline:* For fall admission, 3/1 priority date for domestic and international students; for spring admission, 10/14 for domestic students, 9/14 for international students. Applications are processed on a rolling basis. Application fee: $70. Electronic applications accepted. *Expenses:* Contact institution. *Financial support:* Research assistantships, career-related internships or fieldwork, Federal Work-Study, and tuition waivers (partial) available. Support available to part-time students. Financial award applicants required to submit FAFSA. *Unit head:* Dr. Harriet Feldman, Dean, College of Health Professions, 914-773-3245, E-mail: hfeldman@pace.edu. *Application contact:* Susan Ford-Goldschein, Director of Graduate Admissions, 914-422-4283, Fax: 914-422-4287, E-mail: gradwp@pace.edu.
Website: http://www.pace.edu/lienhard

Piedmont College, School of Nursing and Health Sciences, Demorest, GA 30535-0010. Offers nursing administration (MSN); nursing education (MSN). *Expenses: Tuition:* Full-time $7992; part-time $444 per credit hour.

Prairie View A&M University, College of Nursing, Houston, TX 77030. Offers family nurse practitioner (MSN); nursing administration (MSN); nursing education (MSN). Part-time programs available. *Faculty:* 9 full-time (8 women), 13 part-time/adjunct (11 women). *Students:* 74 full-time (61 women), 107 part-time (99 women); includes 65 minority (63 Black or African American, non-Hispanic/Latino; 2 Hispanic/Latino), 4 international. Average age 37. 121 applicants, 42% accepted, 45 enrolled. In 2013, 46 master's awarded. *Degree requirements:* For master's, comprehensive exam, thesis. *Entrance requirements:* For master's, MAT or GRE, BS in nursing; 2 years of experience as a registered nurse; 1 course each in statistics, basic health and assessment. *Application deadline:* For fall admission, 7/1 priority date for domestic students, 7/1 for international students; for spring admission, 11/1 priority date for domestic students, 11/1 for international students. Applications are processed on a rolling basis. Application fee: $50. *Expenses:* Tuition, state resident: full-time $3776; part-time $209.77 per credit hour. Tuition, nonresident: full-time $10,183; part-time $565.77 per credit hour. *Required fees:* $2037; $446.50 per credit hour. *Financial support:* In 2013–14, 17 students received support. Career-related internships or fieldwork, Federal Work-Study, institutionally sponsored loans, scholarships/grants, and traineeships available. Support available to part-time students. Financial award application deadline: 4/1; financial award applicants required to submit FAFSA. *Faculty research:* Software development and violence prevention, health promotion and disease prevention. *Total annual research expenditures:* $350,000. *Unit head:* Dr. Betty N. Adams, Dean, 713-797-7009, Fax: 713-797-7013, E-mail: bnadams@pvamu.edu. *Application contact:* Dr. Forest Smith, Director of Student Services and Admissions, 713-797-7031, Fax: 713-797-7012, E-mail: fdsmith@pvamu.edu.
Website: http://www.pvamu.edu/nursing/

Ramapo College of New Jersey, Master of Science in Nursing Program, Mahwah, NJ 07430. Offers nursing education (MSN). Part-time programs available. *Faculty:* 1 (woman) full-time, 2 part-time/adjunct (1 woman). *Students:* 3 full-time (2 women), 37 part-time (34 women); includes 6 minority (1 Black or African American, non-Hispanic/Latino; 4 Asian, non-Hispanic/Latino; 1 Hispanic/Latino), 2 international. Average age 43. In 2013, 15 master's awarded. *Entrance requirements:* For master's, official transcript; personal statement; 2 letters of recommendation; resume; current licensure as a Registered Nurse, or eligibility for licensure; evidence of one year recent experience as a Registered Nurse prior to entry into clinical practicum courses; evidence of undergraduate statistics course; satisfactory completion of criminal background. Additional exam requirements/recommendations for international students: Required—TOEFL (minimum score 550 paper-based; 90 iBT); Recommended—IELTS (minimum score 6). *Application deadline:* Applications are processed on a rolling basis. Application fee: $60. Electronic applications accepted. *Expenses: Tuition, area resident:* Part-time $582.45 per credit. Tuition, nonresident: part-time $748.70 per credit. *Required fees:* $127.05 per credit. *Financial support:* In 2013–14, 10 students received support, including 10 fellowships with partial tuition reimbursements available (averaging $1,992

per year); traineeships also available. Financial award applicants required to submit FAFSA. *Faculty research:* Learning styles and critical thinking, evidence-based education, outcomes measurement. *Unit head:* Dr. Kathleen M. Burke, Assistant Dean, Master of Science in Nursing Program, 201-684-7737, E-mail: kmburke@ramapo.edu. *Application contact:* Ulysses Simpkins, Program Assistant, 201-684-7749, E-mail: usimpkin@ramapo.edu.
Website: http://www.ramapo.edu/msn/

Regis College, School of Nursing, Science and Health Professions, Weston, MA 02493. Offers applied behavior analysis (MS); biomedical sciences (MS); health administration (MS); nurse practitioner (Certificate); nursing (MS, DNP); nursing education (Certificate). Part-time and evening/weekend programs available. *Degree requirements:* For master's, thesis. *Entrance requirements:* For master's, GRE General Test or MAT, minimum GPA of 3.0; for doctorate, MAT or GRE if GPA from master's lower than 3.5. Additional exam requirements/recommendations for international students: Required—TOEFL (minimum score 550 paper-based). Electronic applications accepted. *Faculty research:* Health policy, education, aging, job satisfaction, psychiatric nursing, critical thinking.

Research College of Nursing, Nursing Program, Kansas City, MO 64132. Offers adult-gerontological nurse practitioner (MSN); clinical nurse leader (MSN); executive practice and healthcare leadership (MSN); family nurse practitioner (MSN); nurse educator (MSN); nursing (MSN). *Accreditation:* AACN. Part-time programs available. Postbaccalaureate distance learning degree programs offered (no on-campus study). *Faculty:* 9 full-time (all women), 5 part-time/adjunct (2 women). *Students:* 19 full-time (18 women), 101 part-time (94 women). *Degree requirements:* For master's, research project. *Entrance requirements:* For master's, 3 letters of recommendation, official transcripts, resume. Additional exam requirements/recommendations for international students: Required—TOEFL (minimum score 550 paper-based), TWE. *Application deadline:* Applications are processed on a rolling basis. Application fee: $50. *Expenses: Tuition:* Part-time $445 per credit hour. *Required fees:* $25 per credit hour. Part-time tuition and fees vary according to course load. *Financial support:* Applicants required to submit FAFSA. *Unit head:* Dr. Nancy O. DeBasio, President and Dean, 816-995-2815, Fax: 816-995-2817, E-mail: nancy.debasio@researchcollege.edu. *Application contact:* Leslie Mendenhall, Director of Transfer and Graduate Recruitment, 816-995-2820, Fax: 816-995-2813, E-mail: leslie.mendenhall@researchcollege.edu.

Rivier University, School of Graduate Studies, Division of Nursing, Nashua, NH 03060. Offers adult psychiatric/mental health practitioner (MS); family nurse practitioner (MS); nursing education (MS). Part-time and evening/weekend programs available. *Entrance requirements:* For master's, GRE, MAT. Electronic applications accepted.

Roberts Wesleyan College, Department of Nursing, Rochester, NY 14624-1997. Offers nursing administration (MSN); nursing education (MSN). *Accreditation:* AACN. Evening/weekend programs available. Postbaccalaureate distance learning degree programs offered (no on-campus study). *Faculty:* 13 full-time (all women), 6 part-time/adjunct (4 women). *Students:* 67 full-time (63 women); includes 10 minority (5 Black or African American, non-Hispanic/Latino; 2 American Indian or Alaska Native, non-Hispanic/Latino; 1 Asian, non-Hispanic/Latino; 2 Hispanic/Latino), 7 international. Average age 39. 53 applicants, 100% accepted, 36 enrolled. In 2013, 2 master's awarded. *Degree requirements:* For master's, thesis. *Entrance requirements:* For master's, minimum GPA of 3.0; BS in nursing; interview; RN license; resume; course work in statistics. Additional exam requirements/recommendations for international students: Required—TOEFL (minimum score 90 iBT), IELTS (minimum score 6.5). *Application deadline:* Applications are processed on a rolling basis. Application fee: $0. *Expenses: Tuition:* Full-time $12,816; part-time $712 per credit hour. One-time fee: $300. Tuition and fees vary according to course load and program. *Financial support:* In 2013–14, 21 students received support. Scholarships/grants available. Financial award applicants required to submit FAFSA. *Unit head:* Dr. Cheryl B. Crotser, Chairperson and Director of Graduate Program, 585-594-6668, E-mail: crotser_cheryl@roberts.edu. *Application contact:* Brenda Mutton, Admissions Coordinator, 585-594-6686, E-mail: mutton_brenda@roberts.edu.
Website: http://www.roberts.edu/gradnursing

Sacred Heart University, Graduate Programs, College of Health Professions, Department of Nursing, Fairfield, CT 06825-1000. Offers clinical nurse leader (MSN); clinical practice in health care (DNP); family nurse practitioner (MSN); leadership in health care (DNP); nursing (DN Sc); nursing educator (MSN); patient care services administration (MSN). *Accreditation:* AACN. Part-time and evening/weekend programs available. Postbaccalaureate distance learning degree programs offered (no on-campus study). *Faculty:* 7 full-time (all women), 5 part-time/adjunct (all women). *Students:* 34 full-time (32 women), 645 part-time (595 women); includes 117 minority (50 Black or African American, non-Hispanic/Latino; 1 American Indian or Alaska Native, non-Hispanic/Latino; 26 Asian, non-Hispanic/Latino; 29 Hispanic/Latino; 1 Native Hawaiian or other Pacific Islander, non-Hispanic/Latino; 10 Two or more races, non-Hispanic/Latino). Average age 39. 110 applicants, 58% accepted, 46 enrolled. In 2013, 67 master's, 11 doctorates awarded. *Entrance requirements:* For master's, minimum GPA of 3.0, BSN or RN plus BS (for MSN); for doctorate, minimum GPA of 3.0, MSN or BSN plus MS (for DNP). Additional exam requirements/recommendations for international students: Required—PTE; Recommended—TOEFL (minimum score 570 paper-based; 80 iBT), IELTS (minimum score 6.5). *Application deadline:* Applications are processed on a rolling basis. Application fee: $60. Electronic applications accepted. *Expenses:* Contact institution. *Financial support:* Career-related internships or fieldwork and institutionally sponsored loans available. Support available to part-time students. Financial award applicants required to submit FAFSA. *Unit head:* Dr. Sue DeNisco, Chair, 203-365-7661, Fax: 203-365-7662, E-mail: deniscos@sacredheart.edu. *Application contact:* Kathy Dilks, Executive Director of Graduate Admissions, 203-365-4716, Fax: 203-365-4732, E-mail: gradstudies@sacredheart.edu.
Website: http://www.sacredheart.edu/graduate/nursing/

Sage Graduate School, School of Health Sciences, Department of Nursing, Program in Education and Leadership, Troy, NY 12180-4115. Offers DNS. *Faculty:* 5 full-time (all women), 2 part-time/adjunct (both women). *Students:* 43 part-time (all women); includes 3 minority (1 Black or African American, non-Hispanic/Latino; 1 Asian, non-Hispanic/Latino; 1 Hispanic/Latino). Average age 51. 23 applicants, 39% accepted, 6 enrolled. In 2013, 5 doctorates awarded. *Degree requirements:* For doctorate, thesis/dissertation. *Entrance requirements:* For doctorate, master's degree in nursing from accredited institution; minimum GPA of 3.5; official transcripts; academic curriculum vitae; 3 letters of recommendation; 1-2 page personal essay; interview; current registered nurse license. Additional exam requirements/recommendations for international students: Required—TOEFL (minimum score 550 paper-based). Application fee: $40. *Expenses: Tuition:* Full-time $11,880; part-time $660 per credit hour. *Financial support:* Fellowships, research assistantships, Federal Work-Study, scholarships/grants, and unspecified assistantships available. Support available to part-time students. *Unit head:* Dr. Esther Haskevitz, Dean, School of Health Sciences, 518-244-2296, Fax: 518-244-4571, E-mail: haskve@sage.edu. *Application contact:* Dr. Joan Dacher, Professor/Director, 518-244-2042, Fax: 518-244-2009, E-mail: dachej@sage.edu.

St. Catherine University, Graduate Programs, Program in Nursing, St. Paul, MN 55105. Offers adult gerontological nurse practitioner (MA); neonatal nurse practitioner (MA); nurse educator (MA); nursing (DNP); nursing: entry-level (MA); pediatric nurse practitioner (MA). Part-time and evening/weekend programs available. *Degree requirements:* For master's, thesis; for doctorate, portfolio, systems change project. *Entrance requirements:* For master's, GRE General Test, bachelor's degree in nursing, current nursing license, 2 years of recent clinical practice; for doctorate, master's degree in nursing, RN license, advanced nursing position. Additional exam requirements/recommendations for international students: Required—TOEFL (minimum score 600 paper-based; 100 iBT).

Saint Francis Medical Center College of Nursing, Graduate Programs, Peoria, IL 61603-3783. Offers adult gerontology (MSN); clinical nurse leader (MSN); family nurse practitioner (MSN); family psychiatric mental health nurse practitioner (MSN); neonatal nurse practitioner (MSN); nurse clinician (Post-Graduate Certificate); nurse educator (MSN, Post-Graduate Certificate); nursing (DNP); nursing management leadership (MSN). Part-time programs available. Postbaccalaureate distance learning degree programs offered (minimal on-campus study). *Faculty:* 4 full-time (all women), 4 part-time/adjunct (all women). *Students:* 13 full-time (12 women), 268 part-time (245 women); includes 17 minority (10 Black or African American, non-Hispanic/Latino; 2 Asian, non-Hispanic/Latino; 5 Hispanic/Latino), 2 international. Average age 37. 115 applicants, 89% accepted, 42 enrolled. In 2013, 17 master's, 2 doctorates awarded. *Degree requirements:* For master's, research experience, portfolio, practicum; for doctorate, practicum hours. *Entrance requirements:* For master's, nursing research, health assessment, graduate course work in statistics, RN license; for doctorate, master's degree in nursing, professional portfolio, graduate statistics, transcripts, RN license. Additional exam requirements/recommendations for international students: Required—TOEFL. *Application deadline:* For fall admission, 6/1 priority date for domestic and international students; for spring admission, 11/15 priority date for domestic and international students. Applications are processed on a rolling basis. Application fee: $50. Electronic applications accepted. *Expenses: Tuition:* Full-time $6336; part-time $528 per semester hour. *Required fees:* $436. *Financial support:* In 2013–14, 8 students received support. Scholarships/grants and tuition waivers (partial) available. Support available to part-time students. Financial award application deadline: 6/15; financial award applicants required to submit FAFSA. *Faculty research:* Outcome and curriculum planning, health promotion, NCLEX-RN results, decision-making program evaluation. *Unit head:* Dr. Patti A. Stockert, President of the College, 309-655-4124, Fax: 309-624-8973, E-mail: patricia.a.stockert@osfhealthcare.org. *Application contact:* Dr. Janice F. Boundy, Dean, 309-655-2230, Fax: 309-624-8973, E-mail: jan.f.boundy@osfhealthcare.org.
Website: http://www.sfmccon.edu/graduate-programs/

St. John Fisher College, Wegmans School of Nursing, Advanced Practice Nursing Program, Rochester, NY 14618-3597. Offers advanced practice nursing (MS); clinical nurse specialist (Certificate); family nurse practitioner (Certificate); nurse educator (Certificate). *Accreditation:* AACN. Part-time and evening/weekend programs available. *Faculty:* 13 full-time (12 women). *Students:* 2 full-time (1 woman), 114 part-time (104 women); includes 15 minority (7 Black or African American, non-Hispanic/Latino; 4 Asian, non-Hispanic/Latino; 4 Hispanic/Latino), 2 international. Average age 33. 61 applicants, 49% accepted, 19 enrolled. In 2013, 23 master's awarded. *Degree requirements:* For master's, clinical practice, project; for Certificate, clinical practice. *Entrance requirements:* For master's, BSN; undergraduate course work in statistics, health assessment, and nursing research; current New York State RN license; 2 letters of recommendation; current resume. Additional exam requirements/recommendations for international students: Required—TOEFL (minimum score 575 paper-based; 80 iBT). *Application deadline:* Applications are processed on a rolling basis. Application fee: $30. Electronic applications accepted. *Expenses: Tuition:* Part-time $795 per credit hour. *Required fees:* $10 per credit hour. Tuition and fees vary according to course load, degree level and program. *Financial support:* In 2013–14, 29 students received support. Scholarships/grants and traineeships available. Financial award applicants required to submit FAFSA. *Faculty research:* Chronic illness, pediatric injury, women's health, public health policy, health care teams. *Unit head:* Dr. Cynthia McCloskey, Graduate Director, 585-385-8471, Fax: 585-385-8466, E-mail: cmccloskey@sjfc.edu. *Application contact:* Jose Perales, Director of Graduate Admissions, 585-385-8067, E-mail: jperales@sjfc.edu.

Saint Joseph's College of Maine, Master of Science in Nursing Program, Standish, ME 04084. Offers administration (MSN); education (MSN); family nurse practitioner (MSN); nursing administration and leadership (Certificate); nursing and health care education (Certificate). *Accreditation:* AACN. Part-time programs available. Postbaccalaureate distance learning degree programs offered (no on-campus study). *Entrance requirements:* For master's, MAT. Electronic applications accepted.

Salem State University, School of Graduate Studies, Program in Nursing, Salem, MA 01970-5353. Offers adult-gerontology primary care nursing (MSN); nursing administration (MSN); nursing education (MSN); MBA/MSN. *Accreditation:* AACN. Part-time and evening/weekend programs available. *Students:* 31 full-time (24 women), 79 part-time (70 women); includes 12 minority (4 Black or African American, non-Hispanic/Latino; 4 Asian, non-Hispanic/Latino; 3 Hispanic/Latino; 1 Native Hawaiian or other Pacific Islander, non-Hispanic/Latino), 5 international. 18 applicants, 94% accepted, 16 enrolled. In 2013, 15 master's awarded. *Entrance requirements:* For master's, GRE or MAT. Additional exam requirements/recommendations for international students: Required—TOEFL (minimum score 550 paper-based; 80 iBT) or IELTS (minimum score 5.5). *Application deadline:* For fall admission, 5/1 for domestic students; for spring admission, 10/1 for domestic students. Applications are processed on a rolling basis. Application fee: $50. *Financial support:* Career-related internships or fieldwork, Federal Work-Study, scholarships/grants, and unspecified assistantships available. Support available to part-time students. Financial award application deadline: 5/1; financial award applicants required to submit FAFSA. *Application contact:* Dr. Lee A. Brossoit, Assistant Dean of Graduate Admissions, 978-542-6675, Fax: 978-542-7215, E-mail: lbrossoit@salemstate.edu.
Website: http://www.salemstate.edu/academics/schools/1819.php

Salisbury University, Program in Nursing, Salisbury, MD 21801-6837. Offers health care leadership (MS); nurse educator (MS); nursing (MS). Part-time programs available. Postbaccalaureate distance learning degree programs offered. *Faculty:* 5 full-time (4 women). *Students:* 1 (woman) full-time, 18 part-time (all women); includes 6 minority (all Black or African American, non-Hispanic/Latino). Average age 36. 18 applicants, 28% accepted, 3 enrolled. In 2013, 17 master's awarded. *Entrance requirements:* For master's, GRE, minimum undergraduate GPA of 3.0, 2 letters of recommendation, resume, personal statement, current and active RN license, interview, CPR certification, personal statement. Additional exam requirements/recommendations for international students: Required—TOEFL (minimum score 550 paper-based; 79 iBT), IELTS (minimum score 6.5). *Application deadline:* For fall admission, 4/15 priority date for domestic and international students. Applications are processed on a rolling basis. Application fee: $50. Electronic applications accepted. *Expenses:* Tuition, state resident: part-time $342 per credit hour. Tuition, nonresident: part-time $631 per credit hour. *Required fees:* $76 per credit hour. Tuition and fees vary according to program. *Financial support:* In 2013–14, 7 students received support. Institutionally sponsored loans, scholarships/grants, and unspecified assistantships available. Support available

to part-time students. Financial award application deadline: 3/1; financial award applicants required to submit FAFSA. *Faculty research:* Geriatrics, dementia, adolescent health, domestic violence. *Unit head:* Dr. Lisa Seldomridge, Chair of Department of Nursing, 410-543-6413, E-mail: laseldomridge@salisbury.edu. *Application contact:* Carmel Boger, Administrative Assistant for Graduate and Second Degree Nursing Program, 410-543-6420, E-mail: ciboger@salisbury.edu.
Website: http://www.salisbury.edu/Nursing/MS.html

Samford University, Ida V. Moffett School of Nursing, Birmingham, AL 35229. Offers administration (DNP); advanced practice (DNP); family nurse practitioner (MSN); health systems management and leadership (MSN); nurse anesthesia (MSN); nurse educator (MSN). *Accreditation:* AACN; AANA/CANAEP (one or more programs are accredited). Part-time programs available. Postbaccalaureate distance learning degree programs offered (minimal on-campus study). *Faculty:* 16 full-time (all women), 4 part-time/adjunct (2 women). *Students:* 249 full-time (191 women), 25 part-time (17 women); includes 48 minority (23 Black or African American, non-Hispanic/Latino; 1 American Indian or Alaska Native, non-Hispanic/Latino; 13 Asian, non-Hispanic/Latino; 7 Hispanic/Latino; 4 Two or more races, non-Hispanic/Latino), 1 international. Average age 36. 89 applicants, 53% accepted, 45 enrolled. In 2013, 107 master's, 29 doctorates awarded. *Degree requirements:* For master's and doctorate, capstone project with oral presentation. *Entrance requirements:* For master's, MAT; GRE (for nurse anesthesia). Additional exam requirements/recommendations for international students: Required—TOEFL (minimum score 550 paper-based; 80 iBT). *Application deadline:* For fall admission, 6/1 priority date for domestic and international students; for spring admission, 9/1 priority date for domestic and international students. Application fee: $65. Electronic applications accepted. *Expenses:* Contact institution. *Financial support:* In 2013–14, 48 students received support. Institutionally sponsored loans, scholarships/grants, and traineeships available. Financial award application deadline: 3/1; financial award applicants required to submit FAFSA. *Faculty research:* Issues in rural health care, vulnerable populations, genetics and disabilities in pediatrics, geriatrics, parish nursing research, interprofessional education, global health disparities. *Unit head:* Dr. Nena F. Sanders, Dean, 205-726-2629, E-mail: nfsander@samford.edu. *Application contact:* Allyson Maddox, Director of Graduate Student Services, 205-726-2047, Fax: 205-726-4179, E-mail: amaddox@samford.edu.
Website: http://samford.edu/nursing

San Francisco State University, Division of Graduate Studies, College of Health and Social Sciences, School of Nursing, San Francisco, CA 94132-1722. Offers adult acute care (MS); clinical nurse specialist (MS); community/public health nursing (MS); family nurse practitioner (MS, Certificate); nursing administration (MS); nursing education (MS); pediatrics (MS); women's health (MS). *Accreditation:* AACN. Part-time programs available. *Application deadline:* Applications are processed on a rolling basis. *Financial support:* Career-related internships or fieldwork available. *Unit head:* Dr. Mary-Ann van Dam, Director, 415-338-1802, E-mail: vandam@sfsu.edu. *Application contact:* Robert Strachan, Admission and Student Services Coordinator, 415-338-1802, E-mail: strachan@sfsu.edu.
Website: http://nursing.sfsu.edu

San Jose State University, Graduate Studies and Research, College of Applied Sciences and Arts, School of Nursing, San Jose, CA 95192-0001. Offers gerontology nurse practitioner (MS); nursing (Certificate); nursing administration (MS); nursing education (MS). *Accreditation:* AACN. Part-time and evening/weekend programs available. *Degree requirements:* For master's, thesis. *Entrance requirements:* For master's, BS in nursing, RN license. Electronic applications accepted. *Faculty research:* Nurse-managed clinics, computers in nursing.

Seattle Pacific University, MS in Nursing Program, Seattle, WA 98119-1997. Offers administration (MSN); adult/gerontology nurse practitioner (MSN); clinical nurse specialist (MSN); family nurse practitioner (MSN, Certificate); informatics (MSN); nurse educator (MSN). *Accreditation:* AACN. Part-time programs available. *Students:* 9 full-time (7 women), 37 part-time (33 women); includes 8 minority (2 Black or African American, non-Hispanic/Latino; 5 Asian, non-Hispanic/Latino; 1 Hispanic/Latino), 1 international. Average age 41. 70 applicants, 30% accepted, 21 enrolled. In 2013, 27 master's awarded. *Degree requirements:* For master's, thesis. *Entrance requirements:* For master's, personal statement, transcripts, undergraduate nursing degree, proof of undergraduate statistics course with minimum GPA of 2.0, 2 recommendations. *Application deadline:* For fall admission, 1/15 priority date for domestic students; for spring admission, 1/15 for domestic students. Applications are processed on a rolling basis. Application fee: $50. Electronic applications accepted. *Expenses:* Contact institution. *Financial support:* Fellowships and scholarships/grants available. Financial award applicants required to submit FAFSA. *Unit head:* Dr. Susan Casey, Associate Dean, 206-281-2649, E-mail: caseys@spu.edu.
Website: http://www.spu.edu/depts/health-sciences/grad/index.asp

Seton Hall University, College of Nursing, South Orange, NJ 07079-2697. Offers advanced practice in primary health care (MSN, DNP), including adult/gerontological nurse practitioner, pediatric nurse practitioner; entry into practice (MSN); health systems administration (MSN, DNP); nursing (PhD); nursing case management (MSN); nursing education (MA); school nurse (MSN); MSN/MA. *Accreditation:* AACN. Part-time programs available. Postbaccalaureate distance learning degree programs offered (minimal on-campus study). *Degree requirements:* For master's, research project; for doctorate, dissertation or scholarly project. *Entrance requirements:* For doctorate, GRE (waived for students with GPA of 3.5 or higher). Additional exam requirements/recommendations for international students: Required—TOEFL. Electronic applications accepted. *Faculty research:* Parent/child, adult, and gerontological nursing; breast cancer; families of children with HIV; parish nursing.

Shenandoah University, Eleanor Wade Custer School of Nursing, Winchester, VA 22601-5195. Offers family nurse practitioner (Certificate); health informatics (Certificate); nursing (MSN, DNP); nursing education (Certificate); psychiatric mental health nurse practitioner (Certificate). *Accreditation:* AACN; ACNM/ACME. Part-time programs available. *Faculty:* 14 full-time (all women), 7 part-time/adjunct (6 women). *Students:* 39 full-time (35 women), 76 part-time (74 women); includes 23 minority (13 Black or African American, non-Hispanic/Latino; 2 American Indian or Alaska Native, non-Hispanic/Latino; 4 Asian, non-Hispanic/Latino; 4 Hispanic/Latino), 1 international. Average age 38. 56 applicants, 77% accepted, 32 enrolled. In 2013, 28 master's, 4 doctorates, 11 other advanced degrees awarded. *Degree requirements:* For master's, research project, clinical hours; for doctorate, scholarly project, clinical hours; for Certificate, clinical hours. *Entrance requirements:* For master's, United States RN license; minimum GPA of 3.0; appropriate clinical experience; curriculum vitae; 3 letters of recommendation; for doctorate, MSN, minimum GPA of 3.0, 3 letters of recommendation, essay, interview, BSN; for Certificate, MSN, minimum GPA of 3.0, 2 letters of recommendation, minimum of one year (2,080 hours) clinical nursing experience, interview. Additional exam requirements/recommendations for international students: Required—TOEFL (minimum score 610 paper-based; 83 iBT), IELTS (minimum score 7.5). *Application deadline:* For fall admission, 5/1 priority date for domestic and international students; for spring admission, 11/1 priority date for domestic and international students. Applications are processed on a rolling basis. Application fee: $30. Electronic applications accepted. *Expenses: Tuition:* Full-time $19,176; part-time $799 per credit. *Required fees:* $365 per term. Tuition and fees vary according to course level, course load and program. *Financial support:* In 2013–14, 13 students received support, including 3 teaching assistantships with partial tuition reimbursements available (averaging $4,912 per year); career-related internships or fieldwork, scholarships/grants, and unspecified assistantships also available. Support available to part-time students. Financial award application deadline: 3/15; financial award applicants required to submit FAFSA. *Faculty research:* Moral reasoning in nurses, improving health care access to underserved rural women, screening for depression and anxiety in the obese in a rural free clinic, health care outcomes among patients in a free clinic setting cared for by nurse practitioners, effects of depression on diabetes as evidenced by the relationship between the patient healthcare questionnaire (PHQ-9) scores and the patient's glycohemoglobin (HbA1c), policy development, research on a Virginia Nurses Hall of Fame inductee. *Unit head:* Dr. Kathryn Ganske, Director, 540-678-4374, Fax: 540-665-5519, E-mail: kganske@su.edu. *Application contact:* Andrew Woodall, Executive Director of Recruitment and Admissions, 540-665-4581, Fax: 540-665-4627, E-mail: admit@su.edu.
Website: http://www.nursing.su.edu

Southeastern Louisiana University, College of Nursing and Health Sciences, School of Nursing, Hammond, LA 70402. Offers adult psychiatric/mental health nurse practitioner/clinical nurse specialist (MSN); education (MSN); nurse executive (MSN); nurse practice (DNP); nurse practitioner (MSN). *Accreditation:* AACN. Part-time and evening/weekend programs available. *Faculty:* 14 full-time (13 women), 5 part-time/adjunct (4 women). *Students:* 21 full-time (19 women), 138 part-time (121 women); includes 27 minority (17 Black or African American, non-Hispanic/Latino; 4 Asian, non-Hispanic/Latino; 5 Hispanic/Latino; 1 Two or more races, non-Hispanic/Latino). Average age 34. 72 applicants, 68% accepted, 19 enrolled. In 2013, 29 master's awarded. *Degree requirements:* For master's, thesis. *Entrance requirements:* For master's, GRE (verbal and quantitative), baccalaureate degree in nursing from accredited undergraduate nursing program; minimum GPA of 2.7; all transcripts from undergraduate school and any work attempted at the graduate level; curriculum vitae; valid Louisiana Registered Nurse license; letters of recommendation; letter of intent/statement of purpose. Additional exam requirements/recommendations for international students: Required—TOEFL (minimum score 500 paper-based; 61 iBT). *Application deadline:* For fall admission, 7/15 priority date for domestic students, 6/1 priority date for international students; for spring admission, 12/1 priority date for domestic students, 10/1 priority date for international students. Applications are processed on a rolling basis. Application fee: $20 ($30 for international students). Electronic applications accepted. *Expenses:* Tuition, state resident: full-time $5047. Tuition, nonresident: full-time $17,066. *Required fees:* $1213. Tuition and fees vary according to degree level. *Financial support:* Federal Work-Study, institutionally sponsored loans, scholarships/grants, traineeships, and unspecified assistantships available. Support available to part-time students. Financial award application deadline: 5/1; financial award applicants required to submit FAFSA. *Faculty research:* Gender issues, LGBT issues, occupational health/safety, accelerated students, caring development. *Total annual research expenditures:* $103,409. *Unit head:* Dr. Lorinda J. Sealey, Graduate Nursing Program Director, 985-549-5045, Fax: 985-549-5087, E-mail: vjohnson@selu.edu. *Application contact:* Sandra Meyers, Graduate Admissions Analyst, 985-549-5620, Fax: 985-549-5632, E-mail: admissions@selu.edu.
Website: http://www.selu.edu/acad_research/depts/nurs

Southern Connecticut State University, School of Graduate Studies, School of Health and Human Services, Department of Nursing, New Haven, CT 06515-1355. Offers nursing administration (MSN); nursing education (MSN). *Accreditation:* AACN. Part-time and evening/weekend programs available. *Degree requirements:* For master's, thesis. *Entrance requirements:* For master's, GRE, MAT, interview, minimum QPA of 2.8, RN license, minimum 1 year of professional nursing experience. Electronic applications accepted.

Southern Illinois University Edwardsville, Graduate School, School of Nursing, Program in Nurse Educator, Edwardsville, IL 62026-0001. Offers MS, Post-Master's Certificate. Part-time programs available. *Students:* 37 part-time (36 women); includes 3 minority (2 Black or African American, non-Hispanic/Latino; 1 Hispanic/Latino). 16 applicants, 100% accepted. In 2013, 13 master's awarded. *Degree requirements:* For master's, comprehensive exam. *Entrance requirements:* For master's, RN licensure, minimum undergraduate nursing GPA of 3.0. Additional exam requirements/recommendations for international students: Required—TOEFL (minimum score 550 paper-based, 79 iBT), IELTS (minimum score 6.5), Michigan Test of English Language Proficiency or PTE. *Application deadline:* For fall admission, 3/1 for domestic and international students. Application fee: $30. Electronic applications accepted. *Expenses:* Tuition, state resident: full-time $3551. Tuition, nonresident: full-time $8378. *Financial support:* Institutionally sponsored loans, scholarships/grants, and unspecified assistantships available. Financial award application deadline: 3/1; financial award applicants required to submit FAFSA. *Unit head:* Dr. Kathy Ketchum, Associate Dean for Graduate Programs, 618-650-3936, E-mail: kketchu@siue.edu. *Application contact:* Melissa K. Mace, Assistant Director of Graduate and International Recruitment, 618-650-2756, Fax: 618-650-3618, E-mail: mmace@siue.edu.
Website: http://www.siue.edu/nursing/graduate

Southern Nazarene University, College of Professional and Graduate Studies, School of Nursing, Bethany, OK 73008. Offers nursing education (MS); nursing leadership (MS). *Accreditation:* AACN. Part-time and evening/weekend programs available. *Degree requirements:* For master's, thesis. *Entrance requirements:* For master's, minimum undergraduate cumulative GPA of 3.0; baccalaureate degree in nursing from nationally-accredited program; current unencumbered registered nurse licensure in Oklahoma or eligibility for same; documentation of basic computer skills; basic statistics course; statement of professional goals; three letters of recommendation. Additional exam requirements/recommendations for international students: Required—TOEFL (minimum score 550 paper-based). *Unit head:* Dr. Katie Sigler, Chair, 405-717-6217, E-mail: ksigler@snu.edu.
Website: http://snu.edu/school-of-nursing

Southern University and Agricultural and Mechanical College, School of Nursing, Baton Rouge, LA 70813. Offers educator/administrator (PhD); family health nursing (MSN); family nurse practitioner (Post Master's Certificate); geriatric nurse practitioner/gerontology (PhD). *Accreditation:* AACN. Part-time programs available. *Degree requirements:* For master's, comprehensive exam, thesis; for doctorate, comprehensive exam, thesis/dissertation. *Entrance requirements:* For master's, GRE General Test, BSN, minimum GPA of 2.7; for doctorate, GRE General Test; for Post Master's Certificate, MSN. Additional exam requirements/recommendations for international students: Required—TOEFL (minimum score 525 paper-based). *Faculty research:* Health promotions, vulnerable populations, (community-based) cardiovascular participating research, health disparities chronic diseases, care of the elderly.

South University, Graduate Programs, College of Nursing, Savannah, GA 31406. Offers nurse educator (MS).

South University, Program in Nursing, Tampa, FL 33614. Offers adult health nurse practitioner (MS); family nurse practitioner (MS); nurse educator (MS).

State University of New York Empire State College, School for Graduate Studies, Program in Nursing Education, Saratoga Springs, NY 12866-4391. Offers MSN. Postbaccalaureate distance learning degree programs offered. *Degree requirements:* For master's, capstone.

State University of New York Institute of Technology, Program in Nursing Education, Utica, NY 13504-3050. Offers MS, CAS. Part-time programs available. Postbaccalaureate distance learning degree programs offered (no on-campus study). *Faculty:* 5 full-time (all women), 5 part-time/adjunct (4 women). *Students:* 7 full-time (6 women), 59 part-time (56 women); includes 15 minority (11 Black or African American, non-Hispanic/Latino; 4 Asian, non-Hispanic/Latino). Average age 44. 49 applicants, 69% accepted, 25 enrolled. In 2013, 13 master's awarded. *Degree requirements:* For master's, culminating internship. *Entrance requirements:* For master's, minimum GPA of 3.0 in last 30 hours of undergraduate work, bachelor's in nursing, 1 year of RN experience, RN license, 2 letters of reference, resume, educational objective; for CAS, master's degree in nursing. Additional exam requirements/recommendations for international students: Required—TOEFL (minimum score 550 paper-based; 79 iBT), IELTS (minimum score 6.5). *Application deadline:* For fall admission, 8/1 for domestic students, 7/1 for international students; for spring admission, 12/1 for domestic students, 11/1 for international students. Applications are processed on a rolling basis. Application fee: $60. Electronic applications accepted. *Expenses:* Tuition, state resident: full-time $9870; part-time $411 per credit hour. Tuition, nonresident: full-time $20,150; part-time $765 per credit hour. *Required fees:* $1180; $50.73 per credit hour. *Financial support:* In 2013–14, 1 student received support. Scholarships/grants available. Financial award application deadline: 6/1; financial award applicants required to submit FAFSA. *Faculty research:* Nursing faculty shortages, curriculum enhancements, measurement and assessment, evidence-based practice. *Unit head:* Francia Reed, Program Coordinator and Clinical Assistant Professor, 315-792-7295, Fax: 315-792-7555, E-mail: francia.reed@sunyit.edu. *Application contact:* Maryrose Raab, Coordinator of Graduate Center, 315-792-7347, Fax: 315-792-7221, E-mail: maryrose.raab@sunyit.edu.
Website: http://www.sunyit.edu/programs/graduate/nur/nursing_education

Stony Brook University, State University of New York, Stony Brook University Medical Center, Health Sciences Center, School of Nursing, Program in Nursing Education, Stony Brook, NY 11794. Offers MS, Certificate. Postbaccalaureate distance learning degree programs offered (minimal on-campus study). *Students:* 31 part-time (30 women); includes 11 minority (7 Black or African American, non-Hispanic/Latino; 3 Hispanic/Latino; 1 Two or more races, non-Hispanic/Latino). *Entrance requirements:* For master's, baccalaureate degree with major in nursing, minimum cumulative GPA of 3.0, current professional RN license, three letters of recommendation. *Application deadline:* For fall admission, 2/19 for domestic students. Electronic applications accepted. *Expenses:* Tuition, state resident: full-time $9870; part-time $411 per credit. Tuition, nonresident: full-time $18,350; part-time $765 per credit. *Unit head:* Dr. Lee Anne Xippolitos, Dean, 631-444-3200, Fax: 631-444-6628, E-mail: lee.xippolitos@stonybrook.edu. *Application contact:* Dr. Kathleen Shurpin, Professor/Director, Doctor of Nursing Practice Program, 631-444-3267, Fax: 631-444-3136, E-mail: kathleen.shurpin@stonybrook.edu.
Website: http://www.nursing.stonybrookmedicine.edu/nursingeducationmaster

Temple University, College of Health Professions and Social Work, Department of Nursing, Philadelphia, PA 19140. Offers adult-gerontology primary care (DNP); clinical nurse leader (MSN); family-individual across the lifespan (DNP); nurse educator (MSN); nursing (MSN, DNP). *Accreditation:* AACN. Part-time programs available. *Faculty:* 9 full-time (8 women), 3 part-time/adjunct (all women). *Students:* 6 full-time (5 women), 92 part-time (78 women); includes 51 minority (34 Black or African American, non-Hispanic/Latino; 9 Asian, non-Hispanic/Latino; 8 Hispanic/Latino), 1 international. 48 applicants, 58% accepted, 23 enrolled. In 2013, 12 master's, 9 doctorates awarded. *Degree requirements:* For master's and doctorate, evidence based practice project. *Entrance requirements:* For master's and doctorate, GRE General Test or MAT, 2 letters of reference, RN license, interview, statement of purpose, resume. Additional exam requirements/recommendations for international students: Required—TOEFL (minimum score 550 paper-based; 79 iBT). *Application deadline:* For fall admission, 2/15 priority date for domestic students, 1/15 for international students; for spring admission, 10/15 for domestic students, 9/15 for international students. Applications are processed on a rolling basis. Application fee: $60. Electronic applications accepted. *Financial support:* Federal Work-Study, scholarships/grants, traineeships, and tuition waivers available. Support available to part-time students. Financial award application deadline: 1/15. *Faculty research:* Health promotion, chronic illness, family support systems, primary care, health policy, community health services, evidence-based practice. *Total annual research expenditures:* $741,567. *Unit head:* Dr. Jane Kurz, RN, Chair, 215-707-8327, E-mail: jane.kurz@temple.edu. *Application contact:* Naseem Lodhi, Student Services Coordinator, 215-204-4618, E-mail: tunurse@temple.edu.

Tennessee Technological University, Whitson-Hester School of Nursing, Cookeville, TN 38505. Offers family nurse practitioner (MSN); informatics (MSN); nursing administration (MSN); nursing education (MSN). Part-time and evening/weekend programs available. Postbaccalaureate distance learning degree programs offered (no on-campus study). *Students:* 22 full-time (19 women), 101 part-time (94 women); includes 11 minority (5 Black or African American, non-Hispanic/Latino; 2 Asian, non-Hispanic/Latino; 1 Hispanic/Latino; 3 Two or more races, non-Hispanic/Latino). 79 applicants, 65% accepted, 38 enrolled. In 2013, 14 master's awarded. *Degree requirements:* For master's, comprehensive exam, thesis or alternative. *Entrance requirements:* Additional exam requirements/recommendations for international students: Required—TOEFL (minimum score 600 paper-based; 100 iBT), IELTS (minimum score 5.5), PTE, or TOEIC (Test of English as an International Communication). *Application deadline:* For fall admission, 8/1 for domestic students, 5/1 for international students; for spring admission, 12/1 for domestic students, 10/1 for international students. Applications are processed on a rolling basis. Application fee: $35 ($40 for international students). Electronic applications accepted. *Expenses:* Tuition, state resident: full-time $9347; part-time $465 per credit hour. Tuition, nonresident: full-time $23,635; part-time $1152 per credit hour. *Financial support:* Application deadline: 4/1. *Unit head:* Dr. Bedelia Russell, Director, 931-372-3203, Fax: 931-372-6244, E-mail: bhrussell@tntech.edu. *Application contact:* Shelia K. Kendrick, Coordinator of Graduate Studies, 931-372-3808, Fax: 931-372-3497, E-mail: skendrick@tntech.edu.

Texas Christian University, Harris College of Nursing and Health Sciences, Program in Nursing, Fort Worth, TX 76129-0002. Offers advanced practice registered nurse (DNP); clinical nurse leader (MSN); clinical nurse specialist: adult/gerontology nursing (MSN); clinical nurse specialist: pediatric nursing (MSN); nursing administration (DNP); nursing education (MSN). *Accreditation:* AACN; AANA/CANAEP (one or more programs are accredited). Part-time programs available. Postbaccalaureate distance learning degree programs offered (no on-campus study). *Faculty:* 18 full-time (16 women), 1 (woman) part-time/adjunct. *Students:* 44 full-time (35 women), 46 part-time (42 women); includes 8 minority (3 Black or African American, non-Hispanic/Latino; 2 Asian, non-Hispanic/Latino; 3 Hispanic/Latino), 1 international. Average age 43. 72 applicants, 63% accepted, 36 enrolled. In 2013, 19 master's, 17 doctorates awarded. *Degree requirements:* For master's, professional project; for doctorate, capstone project. *Entrance requirements:* For master's, GRE General Test, 3 letters of reference, essay, resume, two official transcripts from every institution attended; for doctorate, APRN recognition (national certification) or master's and experience in nursing administration; 3 letters of reference; essay; resume; two official transcripts from every institution attended. Additional exam requirements/recommendations for international students: Recommended—TOEFL. *Application deadline:* For fall admission, 4/1 for domestic students; for spring admission, 9/1 for domestic students; for summer admission, 2/1 for domestic students. Applications are processed on a rolling basis. Application fee: $60. Electronic applications accepted. *Expenses: Tuition:* Part-time $1270 per credit hour. Tuition and fees vary according to course load and program. *Financial support:* In 2013–14, 4 teaching assistantships (averaging $2,500 per year) were awarded. Financial award applicants required to submit FAFSA. *Unit head:* Dr. Kathy A. Baker, Director, Division of Nursing Graduate Studies and Scholarship, 817-257-6726, Fax: 817-257-8383, E-mail: kathy.baker@tcu.edu. *Application contact:* Mary Jane Allred, Administrative Program Specialist, 817-257-6726, Fax: 817-257-8383, E-mail: m.allred@tcu.edu.
Website: http://www.nursing.tcu.edu/graduate.asp

Texas Tech University Health Sciences Center, School of Nursing, Lubbock, TX 79430. Offers acute care nurse practitioner (MSN, Certificate); administration (MSN); advanced practice (DNP); education (MSN); executive leadership (DNP); family nurse practitioner (MSN, Certificate); geriatric nurse practitioner (MSN, Certificate); pediatric nurse practitioner (MSN, Certificate). *Accreditation:* AACN. Part-time programs available. Postbaccalaureate distance learning degree programs offered (minimal on-campus study). *Degree requirements:* For master's, thesis optional. *Entrance requirements:* For master's, minimum GPA of 3.0, 3 letters of reference, BSN, RN license; for Certificate, minimum GPA of 3.0, 3 letters of reference, RN license. Additional exam requirements/recommendations for international students: Required—TOEFL (minimum score 550 paper-based). *Faculty research:* Diabetes/obesity, nurse competency, disease management, intervention and measurements, health disparities.

Texas Woman's University, Graduate School, College of Nursing, Denton, TX 76201. Offers acute care nurse practitioner (MS); adult health clinical nurse specialist (MS); adult health nurse practitioner (MS); child health clinical nurse specialist (MS); clinical nurse leader (MS); family nurse practitioner (MS); health systems management (MS); nursing education (MS); nursing practice (DNP); nursing science (PhD); pediatric nurse practitioner (MS); women's health clinical nurse specialist (MS); women's health nurse practitioner (MS). *Accreditation:* AACN. Part-time programs available. Postbaccalaureate distance learning degree programs offered. *Faculty:* 60 full-time (59 women), 46 part-time/adjunct (39 women). *Students:* 54 full-time (49 women), 910 part-time (848 women); includes 489 minority (221 Black or African American, non-Hispanic/Latino; 11 American Indian or Alaska Native, non-Hispanic/Latino; 184 Asian, non-Hispanic/Latino; 70 Hispanic/Latino; 3 Native Hawaiian or other Pacific Islander, non-Hispanic/Latino), 16 international. Average age 38. 430 applicants, 65% accepted, 193 enrolled. In 2013, 258 master's, 22 doctorates awarded. *Degree requirements:* For master's, comprehensive exam, thesis or alternative; for doctorate, comprehensive exam, thesis/dissertation. *Entrance requirements:* For master's, GRE or MAT, minimum GPA of 3.0 on last 60 hours in undergraduate nursing degree and overall, RN license, BS in nursing, basic statistics course; for doctorate, GRE (preferred minimum score 153 [500 old version] Verbal, 144 [500 old version] Quantitative, 4 Analytical), MS in nursing, minimum preferred GPA of 3.5, RN license, statistics, 2 letters of reference, curriculum vitae, graduate nursing-theory course, graduate research course, statement of professional goals and research interests. Additional exam requirements/recommendations for international students: Required—TOEFL (minimum score 550 paper-based; 79 iBT). *Application deadline:* For fall admission, 5/1 priority date for domestic students, 3/1 for international students; for spring admission, 9/15 priority date for domestic students, 7/1 for international students. Applications are processed on a rolling basis. Application fee: $50 ($75 for international students). Electronic applications accepted. *Expenses:* Tuition, state resident: full-time $4182; part-time $233.32 per credit hour. Tuition, nonresident: full-time $10,716; part-time $595.32 per credit hour. *Financial support:* In 2013–14, 149 students received support, including 10 research assistantships (averaging $5,600 per year), 1 teaching assistantship (averaging $5,600 per year); career-related internships or fieldwork, Federal Work-Study, institutionally sponsored loans, scholarships/grants, traineeships, health care benefits, and unspecified assistantships also available. Support available to part-time students. Financial award application deadline: 3/1; financial award applicants required to submit FAFSA. *Faculty research:* Screening, prevention, and treatment for intimate partner violence; needs of adolescents during childbirth intervention; a network analysis decision tool for nurse managers (social network analysis); support for adolescents with implantable cardioverter defibrillators; informatics: nurse staffing, safety, quality, and financial data as they relate to patient care outcomes; prevention and treatment of obesity; improving infant outcomes related to premature birth. *Total annual research expenditures:* $1.7 million. *Unit head:* Dr. Gayle Roux, Interim Dean and Associate Dean for Research and Clinical Scholarship, 940-898-2401, Fax: 940-898-2437, E-mail: nursing@twu.edu. *Application contact:* Dr. Samuel Wheeler, Assistant Director of Admissions, 940-898-3188, Fax: 940-898-3081, E-mail: wheelersr@twu.edu.
Website: http://www.twu.edu/nursing/

Thomas Edison State College, School of Nursing, Program in Nurse Educator, Trenton, NJ 08608-1176. Offers Post-Master's Certificate. *Accreditation:* AACN. Part-time programs available. Postbaccalaureate distance learning degree programs offered (no on-campus study). *Degree requirements:* For Post-Master's Certificate, nursing education seminar and online practicum. *Entrance requirements:* For degree, master's degree in nursing, RN. Additional exam requirements/recommendations for international students: Required—TOEFL (minimum score 550 paper-based; 79 iBT). Electronic applications accepted.

Towson University, Program in Nursing, Towson, MD 21252-0001. Offers nursing (MS); nursing education (Postbaccalaureate Certificate). *Accreditation:* AACN. Part-time programs available. *Students:* 28 full-time (24 women), 56 part-time (55 women); includes 24 minority (20 Black or African American, non-Hispanic/Latino; 1 American Indian or Alaska Native, non-Hispanic/Latino; 1 Asian, non-Hispanic/Latino; 2 Two or more races, non-Hispanic/Latino), 1 international. *Degree requirements:* For master's, thesis optional. *Entrance requirements:* For master's, minimum GPA of 3.0, copy of current nursing license, bachelor's degree in nursing, current resume or curriculum vitae, completion of an elementary statistics and/or nursing research course, completion of an approved physical assessment course; for Postbaccalaureate Certificate, minimum GPA of 3.0, copy of current nursing license, current resume or curriculum vitae, bachelor's degree, completion of an elementary statistics and/or nursing research course, completion of an approved physical assessment course, personal statement. *Application deadline:* Applications are processed on a rolling basis. Application fee: $45. Electronic applications accepted. *Financial support:* Application deadline: 4/1. *Unit head:* Dr. Kathleen Ogle, Graduate Program Director, 410-704-4389, E-mail: kogle@towson.edu. *Application contact:* Alicia Arkell-Kleis, Information Contact, 410-704-6004, E-mail: grads@towson.edu.

Union University, School of Nursing, Jackson, TN 38305-3697. Offers executive leadership (DNP); nurse anesthesia (DNP); nurse anesthetist (PMC); nurse practitioner

(DNP); nursing education (MSN, PMC). *Accreditation:* AACN; AANA/CANAEP. *Degree requirements:* For master's, thesis or alternative. *Entrance requirements:* For master's, GRE, 3 letters of reference, bachelor's degree in nursing, minimum GPA of 3.0. Additional exam requirements/recommendations for international students: Required—TOEFL (minimum score 560 paper-based). Electronic applications accepted. *Faculty research:* Children's health, occupational rehabilitation, informatics, health promotion.

United States University, School of Nursing, Cypress, CA 90630. Offers administrator (MSN); educator (MSN).

The University of Alabama in Huntsville, School of Graduate Studies, College of Nursing, Huntsville, AL 35899. Offers family nurse practitioner (Certificate); nursing (MSN, DNP), including acute care nurse practitioner (MSN), adult clinical nurse specialist (MSN), clinical nurse leader (MSN), family nurse practitioner (MSN), leadership in health care systems (MSN); nursing education (Certificate). DNP offered jointly with The University of Alabama at Birmingham. *Accreditation:* AACN. Part-time and evening/weekend programs available. Postbaccalaureate distance learning degree programs offered (minimal on-campus study). *Faculty:* 16 full-time (15 women), 4 part-time/adjunct (all women). *Students:* 67 full-time (63 women), 235 part-time (192 women); includes 40 minority (27 Black or African American, non-Hispanic/Latino; 5 American Indian or Alaska Native, non-Hispanic/Latino; 4 Asian, non-Hispanic/Latino; 3 Hispanic/Latino; 1 Two or more races, non-Hispanic/Latino), 10 international. Average age 36. 265 applicants, 59% accepted, 128 enrolled. In 2013, 75 master's, 10 doctorates, 5 other advanced degrees awarded. *Degree requirements:* For master's, comprehensive exam, thesis or alternative, oral and written exams. *Entrance requirements:* For master's, MAT or GRE, Alabama RN license, BSN, minimum GPA of 3.0; for doctorate, master's degree in nursing in an advanced practice area; for Certificate, MAT or GRE, minimum GPA of 3.0. Additional exam requirements/recommendations for international students: Required—TOEFL (minimum score 500 paper-based; 80 iBT), IELTS (minimum score 6.5). *Application deadline:* For fall admission, 7/15 for domestic students, 4/1 for international students; for spring admission, 11/30 for domestic students, 9/1 for international students. Applications are processed on a rolling basis. Application fee: $50. Electronic applications accepted. *Expenses:* Tuition, state resident: full-time $8912; part-time $540 per credit hour. Tuition, nonresident: full-time $20,774; part-time $1252 per credit hour. *Required fees:* $148 per semester. One-time fee: $150. *Financial support:* In 2013–14, 19 students received support, including 19 teaching assistantships with full tuition reimbursements available (averaging $7,876 per year); career-related internships or fieldwork, Federal Work-Study, institutionally sponsored loans, scholarships/grants, traineeships, health care benefits, and unspecified assistantships also available. Support available to part-time students. Financial award application deadline: 4/1; financial award applicants required to submit FAFSA. *Faculty research:* Health care informatics, chronic illness management, maternal and child health, genetics/genomics, technology and health care. *Total annual research expenditures:* $557,830. *Unit head:* Dr. Fay Raines, Dean, 256-824-6345, Fax: 256-824-6026, E-mail: rainesc@uah.edu. *Application contact:* Charles Davis, Director of Graduate Nursing Admissions and Advising, 256-824-2433, Fax: 256-824-6026, E-mail: charles.davis@uah.edu.
Website: http://www.uah.edu/nursing/welcome

University of Central Arkansas, Graduate School, College of Health and Behavioral Sciences, Department of Nursing, Conway, AR 72035-0001. Offers adult nurse practitioner (PMC); clinical nurse leader (PMC); clinical nurse specialist (MSN); family nurse practitioner (PMC); nurse educator (PMC); nurse practitioner (MSN). *Accreditation:* AACN. Part-time and evening/weekend programs available. Postbaccalaureate distance learning degree programs offered (minimal on-campus study). *Degree requirements:* For master's, comprehensive exam, thesis optional, clinicals. *Entrance requirements:* For master's, GRE General Test, minimum GPA of 2.7. Additional exam requirements/recommendations for international students: Required—TOEFL (minimum score 550 paper-based; 80 iBT). Electronic applications accepted. *Expenses:* Contact institution.

University of Central Florida, College of Nursing, Orlando, FL 32816. Offers adult-gerontology nurse practitioner (Post-Master's Certificate); family nurse practitioner (Post-Master's Certificate); nursing (MSN, PhD); nursing education (Post-Master's Certificate); nursing practice (DNP). *Accreditation:* AACN. Part-time and evening/weekend programs available. *Faculty:* 47 full-time (41 women), 78 part-time/adjunct (75 women). *Students:* 54 full-time (49 women), 264 part-time (239 women); includes 72 minority (35 Black or African American, non-Hispanic/Latino; 7 Asian, non-Hispanic/Latino; 25 Hispanic/Latino; 1 Native Hawaiian or other Pacific Islander, non-Hispanic/Latino; 4 Two or more races, non-Hispanic/Latino), 1 international. Average age 39. 179 applicants, 55% accepted, 71 enrolled. In 2013, 96 master's, 12 doctorates, 3 other advanced degrees awarded. *Degree requirements:* For master's, thesis or alternative. *Entrance requirements:* For master's, GRE General Test, minimum GPA of 3.0 in last 60 hours. Additional exam requirements/recommendations for international students: Required—TOEFL. *Application deadline:* For fall admission, 2/15 for domestic students; for spring admission, 9/15 for domestic students. Application fee: $30. Electronic applications accepted. *Financial support:* In 2013–14, 2 students received support, including 3 teaching assistantships with partial tuition reimbursements available (averaging $6,300 per year); fellowships with partial tuition reimbursements available, research assistantships with partial tuition reimbursements available, career-related internships or fieldwork, Federal Work-Study, institutionally sponsored loans, traineeships, and unspecified assistantships also available. Financial award application deadline: 3/1; financial award applicants required to submit FAFSA. *Unit head:* Dr. Mary Lou Sole, Interim Dean, 407-823-5496, Fax: 407-823-5675, E-mail: mary.sole@ucf.edu. *Application contact:* Barbara Rodriguez Lamas, Director, Admissions and Student Services, 407-823-2766, Fax: 407-823-6442, E-mail: gradadmissions@ucf.edu.
Website: http://nursing.ucf.edu/

University of Colorado Colorado Springs, Beth-El College of Nursing and Health Sciences, Colorado Springs, CO 80933-7150. Offers nursing education (MSN); nursing practice (DNP); primary care nurse practitioner (MSN). *Accreditation:* AACN. Part-time programs available. Postbaccalaureate distance learning degree programs offered (minimal on-campus study). *Faculty:* 5 full-time (all women), 1 part-time/adjunct (0 women). *Students:* 14 full-time (13 women), 160 part-time (149 women); includes 32 minority (2 Black or African American, non-Hispanic/Latino; 2 American Indian or Alaska Native, non-Hispanic/Latino; 5 Asian, non-Hispanic/Latino; 21 Hispanic/Latino; 2 Two or more races, non-Hispanic/Latino). Average age 37. 125 applicants, 38% accepted, 42 enrolled. In 2013, 31 master's, 3 doctorates awarded. *Degree requirements:* For master's, comprehensive exam, thesis optional; for doctorate, capstone project. *Entrance requirements:* For master's, GRE General Test or MAT, BSN, minimum GPA of 3.0, unrestricted RN license; for doctorate, interview; active RN license; MA; minimum GPA of 3.3; National Certification as nurse practitioner or clinical nurse specialist; portfolio. Additional exam requirements/recommendations for international students: Required—TOEFL. *Application deadline:* For fall admission, 6/15 priority date for domestic students, 6/15 for international students; for spring admission, 9/15 for domestic and international students. Application fee: $60 ($75 for international students). Electronic applications accepted. *Expenses:* Contact institution. *Financial support:* In 2013–14, 17 students received support, including 17 fellowships (averaging $2,500 per year); career-related internships or fieldwork, Federal Work-Study, and scholarships/grants also available. Support available to part-time students. Financial award application deadline: 3/1; financial award applicants required to submit FAFSA. *Faculty research:* Women's health, uncertainty, empowerment, family experience in chronic illness. *Total annual research expenditures:* $2,568. *Unit head:* Dr. Amy Silva-Smith, Graduate Department Chairperson, 719-255-4490, Fax: 719-255-4416, E-mail: asilvasm@uccs.edu. *Application contact:* Diane Busch, Director, 719-255-4424, Fax: 719-255-4416, E-mail: dbusch@uccs.edu.
Website: http://www.uccs.edu/~bethel/

University of Hartford, College of Education, Nursing, and Health Professions, Program in Nursing, West Hartford, CT 06117-1599. Offers community/public health nursing (MSN); nursing education (MSN); nursing management (MSN). *Accreditation:* AACN. Part-time and evening/weekend programs available. *Degree requirements:* For master's, research project. *Entrance requirements:* For master's, BSN, Connecticut RN license. Additional exam requirements/recommendations for international students: Required—TOEFL (minimum score 550 paper-based). Electronic applications accepted. *Expenses:* Contact institution. *Faculty research:* Child development, women in doctoral study, applying feminist theory in teaching methods, near death experience, grandmothers as primary care providers.

University of Houston–Victoria, School of Nursing, Victoria, TX 77901-4450. Offers family nurse practitioner (MSN); nursing administration (MSN); nursing education (MSN). *Accreditation:* AACN. *Faculty:* 13 full-time (12 women). *Students:* 27 full-time (23 women), 42 part-time (35 women); includes 33 minority (18 Black or African American, non-Hispanic/Latino; 8 Asian, non-Hispanic/Latino; 7 Hispanic/Latino), 7 international. *Entrance requirements:* For master's, GRE or MAT, minimum GPA of 3.0 in last 60 hours of academic course work, valid Texas RN licensure, 2 letters of recommendation. *Application deadline:* For fall admission, 7/15 for domestic students, 6/1 for international students. Applications are processed on a rolling basis. Electronic applications accepted. *Expenses:* Tuition, state resident: full-time $4534; part-time $251 per credit hour. Tuition, nonresident: full-time $10,906; part-time $606 per contact hour. *Required fees:* $68 per semester hour. Tuition and fees vary according to course load. *Financial support:* Federal Work-Study, scholarships/grants, and unspecified assistantships available. Support available to part-time students. Financial award application deadline: 4/15. *Unit head:* Dr. Kathryn Tart, Dean, 361-570-4295, E-mail: neilld@uhv.edu. *Application contact:* Tammy Whatley, Senior Recruitment Coordinator, 361-570-4297, E-mail: whatleyt@uhv.edu.
Website: http://www.uhv.edu/nursing/

University of Indianapolis, Graduate Programs, School of Nursing, Indianapolis, IN 46227-3697. Offers advanced practice nursing (DNP); family nurse practitioner (MSN); gerontological nurse practitioner (MSN); neonatal nurse practitioner (MSN); nurse-midwifery (MSN); nursing (MSN); nursing and health systems leadership (MSN); nursing education (MSN); women's health nurse practitioner (MSN); MBA/MSN. *Accreditation:* AACN; ACNM. *Faculty:* 5 full-time (4 women), 1 part-time/adjunct (0 women). *Students:* 15 full-time (14 women), 285 part-time (270 women); includes 42 minority (24 Black or African American, non-Hispanic/Latino; 6 Asian, non-Hispanic/Latino; 3 Hispanic/Latino; 9 Two or more races, non-Hispanic/Latino), 2 international. Average age 35. In 2013, 46 master's awarded. *Entrance requirements:* For master's, minimum GPA of 3.0, interview, letters of recommendation, resume, IN nursing license, 1 year of professional practice; for doctorate, graduate of NLNAC- or CCNE-accredited nursing program; MSN or MA with nursing major and minimum cumulative GPA of 3.25; unencumbered RN license with eligibility for licensure in Indiana; completion of graduate-level statistics course within last 5 years with minimum grade of B; resume; essay; official transcripts from all academic institutions. Additional exam requirements/recommendations for international students: Required—TOEFL (minimum score 550 paper-based). *Application deadline:* For fall admission, 8/1 for domestic students; for winter admission, 12/15 for domestic students; for spring admission, 4/15 for domestic students. Applications are processed on a rolling basis. Application fee: $60. Electronic applications accepted. *Expenses: Tuition:* Full-time $5436; part-time $810 per credit hour. *Financial support:* Federal Work-Study available. *Unit head:* Dr. Anne Thomas, Dean, 317-788-3206, E-mail: athomas@uindy.edu. *Application contact:* Sueann Meagher, Graduate Administrative Assistant, 317-788-8005, Fax: 317-788-3542, E-mail: meaghers@uindy.edu.
Website: http://nursing.uindy.edu/

University of Maine, Graduate School, College of Natural Sciences, Forestry, and Agriculture, School of Nursing, Orono, ME 04469. Offers individualized (MS, CAS); nursing education (CGS); rural health family nurse practitioner (MS, CAS). *Accreditation:* AACN. *Faculty:* 17 full-time (13 women), 7 part-time/adjunct (3 women). *Students:* 10 full-time (8 women), 12 part-time (all women); includes 3 minority (2 American Indian or Alaska Native, non-Hispanic/Latino; 1 Hispanic/Latino), 1 international. Average age 38. 12 applicants, 50% accepted, 5 enrolled. In 2013, 8 master's, 2 other advanced degrees awarded. *Entrance requirements:* For master's, GRE General Test; for other advanced degree, master's degree. Additional exam requirements/recommendations for international students: Required—TOEFL. *Application deadline:* For fall admission, 2/1 for domestic students. Applications are processed on a rolling basis. Application fee: $65. Electronic applications accepted. *Expenses:* Tuition, state resident: full-time $7524. Tuition, nonresident: full-time $23,112. *Required fees:* $1970. *Financial support:* In 2013–14, 4 students received support. Career-related internships or fieldwork, Federal Work-Study, institutionally sponsored loans, and tuition waivers (full and partial) available. Support available to part-time students. Financial award application deadline: 3/1. *Unit head:* Dr. Nancy Fishwick, Director, 207-581-2505, Fax: 207-581-2585. *Application contact:* Scott G. Delcourt, Associate Dean of the Graduate School, 207-581-3291, Fax: 207-581-3232, E-mail: graduate@maine.edu.
Website: http://umaine.edu/nursing/

University of Mary, School of Health Sciences, Division of Nursing, Bismarck, ND 58504-9652. Offers family nurse practitioner (MSN); nurse administrator (MSN); nursing educator (MSN). *Accreditation:* AACN. Part-time and evening/weekend programs available. Postbaccalaureate distance learning degree programs offered (minimal on-campus study). *Degree requirements:* For master's, comprehensive exam (for some programs), thesis (for some programs), internship (family nurse practitioner), teaching practice. *Entrance requirements:* For master's, minimum GPA of 2.75 in nursing, interview, letters of recommendation, criminal background check, immunizations, statement of professional goals. Additional exam requirements/recommendations for international students: Required—TOEFL (minimum score 500 paper-based; 71 iBT). Electronic applications accepted. *Faculty research:* Gerontology issues, rural nursing, health policy, primary care, women's health.

University of Mary Hardin-Baylor, Graduate Studies in Education, Belton, TX 76513. Offers administration of intervention programs (M Ed); curriculum and instruction (M Ed); educational administration (M Ed, Ed D), including higher education (Ed D), leadership in nursing education (Ed D), P-12 (Ed D). Part-time and evening/weekend programs available. *Faculty:* 13 full-time (10 women), 6 part-time/adjunct (2 women). *Students:* 46 full-time (33 women), 61 part-time (40 women); includes 35 minority (15 Black or African American, non-Hispanic/Latino; 1 American Indian or Alaska Native, non-Hispanic/

Latino; 19 Hispanic/Latino), 1 international. Average age 38. 72 applicants, 88% accepted, 47 enrolled. In 2013, 13 master's, 30 doctorates awarded. *Degree requirements:* For master's, comprehensive exam; for doctorate, thesis/dissertation. *Entrance requirements:* For master's, minimum GPA of 3.0, interview; for doctorate, minimum GPA of 3.5, interview, essay, resume, employment verification, employer letter of support, 3 letters of recommendation. Additional exam requirements/recommendations for international students: Required—TOEFL (minimum score 550 paper-based; 80 iBT), IELTS (minimum score 6). *Application deadline:* For fall admission, 6/1 for domestic students, 6/15 priority date for international students; for spring admission, 11/1 for domestic students, 10/15 priority date for international students. Applications are processed on a rolling basis. Application fee: $35 ($135 for international students). Electronic applications accepted. *Expenses: Tuition:* Full-time $14,130; part-time $785 per credit hour. *Required fees:* $1350; $75 per credit hour. $50 per term. *Financial support:* Federal Work-Study and scholarships (for some active duty military personnel only) available. Support available to part-time students. Financial award application deadline: 6/1; financial award applicants required to submit FAFSA. *Unit head:* Dr. Marlene Zipperlen, Dean, College of Education/Director, Doctor of Education Program, 254-295-4572, Fax: 254-295-4480, E-mail: mzipperlen@umhb.edu. *Application contact:* Melissa Ford, Director of Graduate Admissions, 254-295-4020, Fax: 254-295-5038, E-mail: mford@umhb.edu.
Website: http://graduate.umhb.edu/education/

University of Mary Hardin-Baylor, Graduate Studies in Nursing, Belton, TX 76513. Offers clinical nurse leader (MSN); family nurse practitioner (MSN, Post-Master's Certificate); nurse educator (Post-Master's Certificate); nursing education (MSN). *Accreditation:* AACN. Part-time and evening/weekend programs available. *Faculty:* 6 full-time (all women), 4 part-time/adjunct (3 women). *Students:* 44 full-time (all women), 6 part-time (all women); includes 13 minority (5 Black or African American, non-Hispanic/Latino; 2 Asian, non-Hispanic/Latino; 6 Hispanic/Latino). Average age 33. 57 applicants, 67% accepted, 31 enrolled. In 2013, 17 master's awarded. *Degree requirements:* For master's, practicum. *Entrance requirements:* For master's, full-time RN for 1 year, BSN, minimum GPA of 3.0 in last 60 hours of undergraduate program, two letters of recommendation. Additional exam requirements/recommendations for international students: Required—TOEFL (minimum score 550 paper-based; 80 iBT), IELTS (minimum score 6). *Application deadline:* For fall admission, 4/15 for domestic students, 4/15 priority date for international students; for spring admission, 11/1 for domestic students, 10/15 priority date for international students. Applications are processed on a rolling basis. Application fee: $35 ($135 for international students). Electronic applications accepted. *Expenses: Tuition:* Full-time $14,130; part-time $785 per credit hour. *Required fees:* $1350; $75 per credit hour. $50 per term. *Financial support:* Applicants required to submit FAFSA. *Unit head:* Dr. Carrie Johnson, Associate Professor/Director, Master of Science in Nursing Programs, 254-295-4178, E-mail: cjohnson@umhb.edu. *Application contact:* Melissa Ford, Director of Graduate Admissions, 254-295-4020, Fax: 254-295-5038, E-mail: mford@umhb.edu.
Website: http://graduate.umhb.edu/nursing/

University of Maryland, Baltimore, Graduate School, School of Nursing, Master's Program in Nursing, Baltimore, MD 21201. Offers community health nursing (MS); gerontological nursing (MS); maternal-child nursing (MS); medical-surgical nursing (MS); nurse-midwifery education (MS); nursing administration (MS); nursing education (MS); nursing health policy (MS); primary care nursing (MS); psychiatric nursing (MS); MS/MBA. MS/MBA offered jointly with University of Baltimore. *Accreditation:* AACN; AANA/CANAEP. Part-time programs available. *Students:* 345 full-time (297 women), 508 part-time (469 women); includes 288 minority (152 Black or African American, non-Hispanic/Latino; 2 American Indian or Alaska Native, non-Hispanic/Latino; 72 Asian, non-Hispanic/Latino; 32 Hispanic/Latino; 1 Native Hawaiian or other Pacific Islander, non-Hispanic/Latino; 29 Two or more races, non-Hispanic/Latino), 13 international. Average age 33. 971 applicants, 34% accepted, 253 enrolled. In 2013, 308 master's awarded. *Degree requirements:* For master's, comprehensive exam (for some programs), thesis or alternative. *Entrance requirements:* For master's, minimum GPA of 2.75, course work in statistics, BS in nursing. Additional exam requirements/recommendations for international students: Required—TOEFL (minimum score 550 paper-based; 80 iBT) or IELTS (minimum score 7). *Application deadline:* For fall admission, 2/1 for domestic students, 1/15 for international students. Application fee: $75. Electronic applications accepted. *Financial support:* Fellowships, research assistantships, teaching assistantships, career-related internships or fieldwork, and traineeships available. Support available to part-time students. Financial award application deadline: 2/15; financial award applicants required to submit FAFSA. *Unit head:* Dr. Jane Kapustin, Assistant Dean, 410-706-6741, Fax: 410-706-4231. *Application contact:* Marjorie Fass, Admissions Director, 410-706-0501, Fax: 410-706-7238.

University of Massachusetts Dartmouth, Graduate School, College of Nursing, Programs in Nursing, North Dartmouth, MA 02747-2300. Offers adult gerontology primary care nurse practitioner (DNP); adult health clinical nurse specialist (DNP); adult health/adult nurse practitioner (MS); adult health/advanced practice (MS); adult health/nurse educator (MS); adult health/nurse manager (MS); adult nurse practitioner (PMC); community health nurse specialist (DNP); community nursing/advanced practice (MS); community nursing/nurse educator (MS); community nursing/nurse manager (MS); individualized nursing (PMC); nursing (MS, PhD); nursing practice (DNP). Part-time programs available. *Faculty:* 25 full-time (all women), 45 part-time/adjunct (44 women). *Students:* 103 part-time (95 women); includes 10 minority (4 Black or African American, non-Hispanic/Latino; 2 Asian, non-Hispanic/Latino; 4 Hispanic/Latino). Average age 40. 49 applicants, 92% accepted, 33 enrolled. In 2013, 25 master's, 1 doctorate, 2 other advanced degrees awarded. *Degree requirements:* For master's, thesis; for doctorate, comprehensive exam, thesis/dissertation, project (for DNP only). *Entrance requirements:* For master's, statement of purpose (minimum of 300 words), resume, 3 letters of recommendation, official transcripts, copy of RN license; for doctorate, GRE (for PhD), statement of purpose (minimum of 300 words), resume, 3 letters of recommendation, official transcripts, copy of RN license, scholarly writing sample (minimum 10 pages for PhD). Additional exam requirements/recommendations for international students: Required—TOEFL (minimum score 533 paper-based; 72 iBT). *Application deadline:* For fall admission, 2/15 priority date for domestic and international students. Applications are processed on a rolling basis. Application fee: $60. Electronic applications accepted. *Expenses:* Tuition, state resident: full-time $2071; part-time $86.29 per credit. Tuition, nonresident: full-time $8099; part-time $337.46 per credit. Tuition and fees vary according to course load and reciprocity agreements. *Financial support:* In 2013–14, 5 teaching assistantships with full and partial tuition reimbursements (averaging $7,500 per year) were awarded; Federal Work-Study and unspecified assistantships also available. Support available to part-time students. Financial award application deadline: 3/1; financial award applicants required to submit FAFSA. *Faculty research:* Pathophysiology, aging with spinal cord injury, relational ontology, severe mental illness, patient care. *Total annual research expenditures:* $1,000. *Unit head:* Kerry Fater, Graduate Program Director for Nursing Master's Programs, 508-999-8525, Fax: 508-999-9127, E-mail: kfater@umassd.edu. *Application contact:* Steven Briggs, Director of Marketing and Recruitment for Graduate Studies, 508-999-8604, Fax: 508-999-8183, E-mail: graduate@umassd.edu.
Website: http://www.umassd.edu/nursing/graduateprograms

University of Massachusetts Worcester, Graduate School of Nursing, Worcester, MA 01655-0115. Offers advanced practice nursing (DNP); family nurse practitioner (MS); gerontological adult acute care nurse practitioner (MS, Post Master's Certificate); gerontological adult primary care nurse practitioner (Post Master's Certificate); gerontological primary care nurse practitioner (MS); leadership (DNP); nurse educator (MS, Post Master's Certificate); nursing (PhD). *Accreditation:* AACN. *Faculty:* 19 full-time (17 women), 40 part-time/adjunct (33 women). *Students:* 153 full-time (129 women), 35 part-time (28 women); includes 30 minority (18 Black or African American, non-Hispanic/Latino; 7 Asian, non-Hispanic/Latino; 5 Hispanic/Latino). Average age 34. 254 applicants, 31% accepted, 57 enrolled. In 2013, 50 master's, 4 doctorates, 2 other advanced degrees awarded. *Degree requirements:* For doctorate, thesis/dissertation (for some programs), comprehensive exam (for PhD); capstone project and manuscript (for DNP). *Entrance requirements:* For master's, GRE General Test, bachelor's degree in nursing, course work in statistics, unrestricted Massachusetts license as registered nurse; for doctorate, GRE General Test, bachelor's or master's degree; for Post Master's Certificate, GRE General Test, MS in nursing. Additional exam requirements/recommendations for international students: Required—TOEFL. *Application deadline:* For fall admission, 12/1 priority date for domestic students. Applications are processed on a rolling basis. Application fee: $60. Electronic applications accepted. *Expenses:* Contact institution. *Financial support:* In 2013–14, 43 students received support. Institutionally sponsored loans, scholarships/grants, traineeships, and tuition waivers available. Support available to part-time students. Financial award application deadline: 5/16; financial award applicants required to submit FAFSA. *Faculty research:* Decision-making of partners and men with prostate cancer, coinfection (HIV and Hepatitis C) and treatment decisions, parent management of children with Type 1 diabetes, health literacy and discharge planning, Ghanaian women and self-care. *Total annual research expenditures:* $1.5 million. *Unit head:* Dr. Paulette Seymour-Route, Dean, 508-856-5801, Fax: 508-856-6552, E-mail: paulette.seymour-route@umassmed.edu. *Application contact:* Diane Brescia, Admissions Coordinator, 508-856-3488, Fax: 508-856-5851, E-mail: diane.brescia@umassmed.edu.
Website: http://www.umassmed.edu/gsn/

University of Memphis, Loewenberg School of Nursing, Memphis, TN 38152. Offers advance practice-family nurse practitioner (MSN); executive nursing leadership (MSN); nursing (Graduate Certificate); nursing administration (MSN); nursing education (MSN); nursing informatics (MSN). *Accreditation:* AACN. Part-time and evening/weekend programs available. Postbaccalaureate distance learning degree programs offered. *Faculty:* 18 full-time (16 women), 5 part-time/adjunct (0 women). *Students:* 23 full-time (21 women), 240 part-time (214 women); includes 112 minority (100 Black or African American, non-Hispanic/Latino; 9 Asian, non-Hispanic/Latino; 1 Hispanic/Latino; 2 Two or more races, non-Hispanic/Latino), 1 international. Average age 35. 176 applicants, 38% accepted, 25 enrolled. In 2013, 47 master's, 2 other advanced degrees awarded. *Degree requirements:* For master's, comprehensive exam, thesis optional, scholarly project; completion of clinical practicum hours. *Entrance requirements:* For master's, NCLEX Exam, interview. Additional exam requirements/recommendations for international students: Required—TOEFL (minimum score 550 paper-based; 79 iBT). *Application deadline:* For fall admission, 2/15 for domestic and international students; for spring admission, 10/1 for domestic and international students. Application fee: $35 ($60 for international students). *Financial support:* In 2013–14, 147 students received support. Federal Work-Study and scholarships/grants available. Financial award application deadline: 2/15; financial award applicants required to submit FAFSA. *Faculty research:* Technology in nursing, nurse retention, cultural competence, health policy, health access. *Total annual research expenditures:* $560,619. *Unit head:* Dr. Robert Koch, Associate Dean, 901-678-3908, Fax: 901-678-4907, E-mail: rakoch@memphis.edu. *Application contact:* Dr. Karen Weddle-West, Information Contact, 901-678-2531, Fax: 901-678-5023, E-mail: gradsch@memphis.edu.
Website: http://www.memphis.edu/nursing

University of Missouri–Kansas City, School of Nursing and Health Studies, Kansas City, MO 64110-2499. Offers adult clinical nurse specialist (MSN), including adult nurse practitioner, women's health nurse practitioner (MSN, DNP); adult clinical nursing practice (DNP), including adult gerontology nurse practitioner, women's health nurse practitioner (MSN, DNP); clinical nursing practice (DNP), including family nurse practitioner; family nurse practitioner (MSN); neonatal nurse practitioner (MSN); nurse educator (MSN); nurse executive (MSN); nursing (PhD); nursing practice (DNP); pediatric clinical nursing practice (DNP), including pediatric nurse practitioner; pediatric nurse practitioner (MSN). *Accreditation:* AACN. Part-time programs available. Postbaccalaureate distance learning degree programs offered (minimal on-campus study). *Faculty:* 44 full-time (38 women), 55 part-time/adjunct (52 women). *Students:* 44 full-time (33 women), 401 part-time (370 women); includes 59 minority (25 Black or African American, non-Hispanic/Latino; 2 American Indian or Alaska Native, non-Hispanic/Latino; 12 Asian, non-Hispanic/Latino; 15 Hispanic/Latino; 5 Two or more races, non-Hispanic/Latino). Average age 37. 182 applicants, 68% accepted, 124 enrolled. In 2013, 106 master's, 15 doctorates awarded. *Degree requirements:* For master's, thesis or alternative. *Entrance requirements:* For master's, minimum undergraduate GPA of 3.2; for doctorate, GRE, 3 letters of reference. Additional exam requirements/recommendations for international students: Required—TOEFL (minimum score 550 paper-based; 80 iBT). *Application deadline:* For fall admission, 2/1 priority date for domestic and international students; for spring admission, 9/1 priority date for domestic and international students. Application fee: $45 ($50 for international students). *Expenses:* Tuition, state resident: full-time $6073; part-time $337.40 per credit hour. Tuition, nonresident: full-time $15,680; part-time $871.10 per credit hour. *Required fees:* $97.59 per credit hour. Full-time tuition and fees vary according to program. *Financial support:* In 2013–14, 13 teaching assistantships with partial tuition reimbursements (averaging $9,470 per year) were awarded; fellowships, research assistantships, career-related internships or fieldwork, Federal Work-Study, institutionally sponsored loans, and tuition waivers (full and partial) also available. Support available to part-time students. Financial award application deadline: 3/1; financial award applicants required to submit FAFSA. *Faculty research:* Geriatrics/gerontology, children's pain, neonatology, Alzheimer's care, cancer caregivers. *Unit head:* Dr. Ann Cary, Dean, 816-235-1723, Fax: 816-235-1701, E-mail: caryah@umkc.edu. *Application contact:* Judy Jellison, Coordinator for Admissions and Recruitment, 816-235-1740, Fax: 816-235-1701, E-mail: jellisonj@umkc.edu.
Website: http://nursing.umkc.edu/

University of Missouri–St. Louis, College of Nursing, St. Louis, MO 63121-4400. Offers adult nurse practitioner (DNP, Post Master's Certificate); clinical nurse specialist (DNP); family mental health nurse practitioner (DNP); family nurse practitioner (MSN, DNP, Post Master's Certificate); neonatal nurse practitioner (MSN); nurse educator (MSN); nurse leader (MSN); nurse practitioner (Post Master's Certificate); nursing (PhD); pediatric clinical nurse specialist (DNP); pediatric nurse practitioner (MSN, DNP, Post Master's Certificate); women's health nurse practitioner (MSN, Post Master's Certificate). *Accreditation:* AACN. Part-time programs available. *Faculty:* 14 full-time (13 women), 14 part-time/adjunct (13 women). *Students:* 227 part-time (217 women);

includes 40 minority (35 Black or African American, non-Hispanic/Latino; 1 American Indian or Alaska Native, non-Hispanic/Latino; 1 Asian, non-Hispanic/Latino; 1 Hispanic/Latino; 2 Two or more races, non-Hispanic/Latino). Average age 35. 190 applicants, 51% accepted, 76 enrolled. In 2013, 80 master's, 8 doctorates, 2 other advanced degrees awarded. *Degree requirements:* For doctorate, comprehensive exam, thesis/dissertation; for Post Master's Certificate, thesis. *Entrance requirements:* For master's, 2 recommendation letters; minimum GPA of 3.0; BSN; nursing licensure; statement of purpose; course in differential/inferential statistics; for doctorate, GRE, 2 letters of recommendation, MSN, minimum GPA of 3.2, course in differential/inferential statistics; for Post Master's Certificate, 2 recommendation letters; MSN; advanced practice certificate; minimum GPA of 3.0; essay. Additional exam requirements/recommendations for international students: Recommended—TOEFL (minimum score 550 paper-based; 79 iBT), IELTS (minimum score 6.5). *Application deadline:* For fall admission, 2/15 for domestic and international students. Application fee: $50 ($40 for international students). Electronic applications accepted. *Expenses:* Tuition, state resident: full-time $7364; part-time $409.10 per credit hour. Tuition, nonresident: full-time $19,162; part-time $1008.50 per credit hour. *Financial support:* Application deadline: 4/1; applicants required to submit FAFSA. *Faculty research:* Health promotion and restoration, family disruption, violence, abuse, battered women, health survey methods. *Unit head:* Dr. Nancy Magnuson, Director, 314-516-6066. *Application contact:* 314-516-5458, Fax: 314-516-6996, E-mail: gradadm@umsl.edu.
Website: http://www.umsl.edu/divisions/nursing/

University of Nevada, Las Vegas, Graduate College, School of Nursing, Las Vegas, NV 89154-3018. Offers family nurse practitioner (Advanced Certificate); nursing (MS, DNP); nursing education (Advanced Certificate); pediatric nurse practitioner (PhD, Post-Master's Certificate). *Accreditation:* AACN. Part-time programs available. Postbaccalaureate distance learning degree programs offered (minimal on-campus study). *Faculty:* 11 full-time (10 women), 9 part-time/adjunct (6 women). *Students:* 48 full-time (40 women), 74 part-time (65 women); includes 30 minority (5 Black or African American, non-Hispanic/Latino; 10 Asian, non-Hispanic/Latino; 6 Hispanic/Latino; 9 Two or more races, non-Hispanic/Latino), 4 international. Average age 41. 114 applicants, 54% accepted, 48 enrolled. In 2013, 16 master's, 8 doctorates, 1 other advanced degree awarded. *Entrance requirements:* For doctorate, GRE General Test. Additional exam requirements/recommendations for international students: Recommended—TOEFL (minimum score 550 paper-based; 80 iBT), IELTS (minimum score 7). *Application deadline:* For fall admission, 2/1 for domestic students, 5/1 for international students; for spring admission, 10/1 for international students. Application fee: $60 ($95 for international students). Electronic applications accepted. *Expenses:* Tuition, state resident: full-time $4752; part-time $264 per credit. Tuition, nonresident: full-time $18,662; part-time $554.50 per credit. *International tuition:* $18,952 full-time. *Required fees:* $532; $12 per credit. $266 per semester. One-time fee: $35. Tuition and fees vary according to course load and program. *Financial support:* In 2013–14, 5 students received support, including 5 teaching assistantships with partial tuition reimbursements available (averaging $9,500 per year); institutionally sponsored loans, scholarships/grants, health care benefits, and unspecified assistantships also available. Financial award application deadline: 3/1. *Faculty research:* Health promotion issues such as obesity and exercise, dance and cardiovascular disease, informal caregiver stress and risk factors for depression, clinical management of hypertension and chronic obstructive pulmonary disease (COPD), childhood obesity and activity. *Total annual research expenditures:* $896,934. *Unit head:* Dr. Carolyn Yucha, Chair, 702-895-5307, E-mail: carolyn.yucha@unlv.edu. *Application contact:* Graduate College Admissions Evaluator, 702-895-3320, Fax: 702-895-4180, E-mail: gradcollege@unlv.edu.
Website: http://nursing.unlv.edu/

University of New Brunswick Fredericton, School of Graduate Studies, Faculty of Nursing, Fredericton, NB E3B 5A3, Canada. Offers nurse educator (MN); nurse practitioner (MN); nursing (thesis/report) (MN). Part-time programs available. Postbaccalaureate distance learning degree programs offered. *Faculty:* 22 full-time (all women). *Students:* 11 full-time (10 women), 22 part-time (all women). In 2013, 8 master's awarded. *Degree requirements:* For master's, comprehensive exam (for some programs), thesis (for some programs). *Entrance requirements:* For master's, undergraduate coursework in statistics and nursing research, minimum GPA of 3.3, registration as a nurse (or eligibility) in New Brunswick. Additional exam requirements/recommendations for international students: Required—TOEFL (minimum score 600 paper-based). *Application deadline:* For winter admission, 1/2 priority date for domestic students. Application fee: $50 Canadian dollars. Electronic applications accepted. *Financial support:* In 2013–14, 7 fellowships, 2 research assistantships were awarded. *Faculty research:* Violence and abuse; healthy child development, chronic illness and addiction; rural populations' access to health care and primary healthcare; teaching and learning in the classroom, clinical lab, and by distance; Aboriginal nursing. *Unit head:* Kathy Wilson, Assistant Dean of Graduate and Advanced RN Studies, 506-458-7640, Fax: 506-447-3057, E-mail: kewilson@unb.ca. *Application contact:* Francis Perry, Graduate Secretary, 506-451-6844, Fax: 506-447-3057, E-mail: fperry@unb.ca.
Website: http://www.unb.ca/fredericton/nursing/graduate/

The University of North Carolina at Charlotte, The Graduate School, College of Health and Human Services, School of Nursing, Charlotte, NC 28223-0001. Offers administration (Post-Master's Certificate); advanced clinical (MSN, Post-Master's Certificate); anesthesia (MSN, Post-Master's Certificate); community health (MSN); family nurse practitioner (MSN, Post-Master's Certificate); health administration (MSN); mental health (MSN); nurse educator (MSN, Post-Master's Certificate); nursing (DNP); systems population (MSN). *Accreditation:* AACN. Part-time programs available. *Faculty:* 17 full-time (16 women), 6 part-time/adjunct (5 women). *Students:* 96 full-time (80 women), 124 part-time (119 women); includes 45 minority (30 Black or African American, non-Hispanic/Latino; 1 American Indian or Alaska Native, non-Hispanic/Latino; 8 Asian, non-Hispanic/Latino; 4 Hispanic/Latino; 2 Two or more races, non-Hispanic/Latino), 1 international. Average age 34. 216 applicants, 38% accepted, 72 enrolled. In 2013, 70 master's, 8 other advanced degrees awarded. Terminal master's awarded for partial completion of doctoral program. *Degree requirements:* For master's, thesis or alternative, practicum; for doctorate, thesis/dissertation or alternative, residency. *Entrance requirements:* For master's, GRE General Test, minimum GPA of 3.0 in undergraduate major; for doctorate, GRE, MAT, or GMAT, minimum GPA of 3.5. Additional exam requirements/recommendations for international students: Required—TOEFL (minimum score 570 paper-based; 83 iBT). *Application deadline:* For fall admission, 5/1 priority date for domestic students, 5/1 for international students; for spring admission, 10/1 priority date for domestic students, 10/1 for international students. Application fee: $75. Electronic applications accepted. *Expenses:* Tuition, state resident: full-time $3522. Tuition, nonresident: full-time $16,051. *Required fees:* $2585. Tuition and fees vary according to course load and program. *Financial support:* In 2013–14, 5 students received support, including 5 teaching assistantships (averaging $4,785 per year); research assistantships, career-related internships or fieldwork, institutionally sponsored loans, scholarships/grants, traineeships, and unspecified assistantships also available. Support available to part-time students. Financial award application deadline: 4/1; financial award applicants required to submit FAFSA. *Faculty research:* Improving care outcomes for the elderly; vulnerable populations; symptom management; self management/health promotion strategies of older adults; migration and maternal child health; health disparities, health literacy, and access to healthcare in Latino adults with diabetes; psychiatric nursing. *Total annual research expenditures:* $572,410. *Unit head:* Dr. Dee Baldwin, Associate Dean, 704-687-7952, Fax: 704-687-6017, E-mail: dbaldwi5@uncc.edu. *Application contact:* Kathy B. Giddings, Director of Graduate Admissions, 704-687-5503, Fax: 704-687-1668, E-mail: gradadm@uncc.edu.
Website: http://nursing.uncc.edu/

The University of North Carolina at Greensboro, Graduate School, School of Nursing, Greensboro, NC 27412-5001. Offers adult clinical nurse specialist (MSN, PMC); adult/gerontological nurse practitioner (MSN, PMC); nurse anesthesia (MSN, PMC); nursing (PhD); nursing administration (MSN); nursing education (MSN); MSN/MBA. *Accreditation:* AACN; AANA/CANAEP. *Degree requirements:* For master's, thesis or alternative. *Entrance requirements:* For master's, GRE General Test or MAT, BSN, clinical experience, liability insurance, RN license; for PMC, liability insurance, MSN, RN license. Additional exam requirements/recommendations for international students: Required—TOEFL. Electronic applications accepted.

The University of North Carolina at Pembroke, Graduate Studies, Department of Nursing, Pembroke, NC 28372-1510. Offers clinical nurse leader (MSN); nurse educator (MSN); rural case manager (MSN). Part-time programs available.

University of North Dakota, Graduate School, College of Nursing, Department of Nursing, Grand Forks, ND 58202. Offers adult-gerontological nurse practitioner (MSN); advanced public health nurse (MSN); family nurse practitioner (MSN); nurse anesthesia (MSN); nurse educator (MSN); nursing (DNP, PhD); psychiatric and mental health nurse practitioner (MSN).

University of Northern Colorado, Graduate School, College of Natural and Health Sciences, School of Nursing, Greeley, CO 80639. Offers clinical nurse specialist in chronic illness (MS); family nurse practitioner (MS); nursing education (MS, PhD). *Accreditation:* AACN. Postbaccalaureate distance learning degree programs offered. *Degree requirements:* For master's, comprehensive exam, thesis or alternative; for doctorate, comprehensive exam, thesis/dissertation. *Entrance requirements:* For master's and doctorate, GRE General Test, minimum GPA of 3.0 in last 60 hours, BS in nursing, 2 letters of recommendation. Electronic applications accepted.

University of North Georgia, Department of Nursing, Dahlonega, GA 30597. Offers family nurse practitioner (MS); nursing education (MS). Part-time programs available. *Degree requirements:* For master's, one foreign language, comprehensive exam, thesis. *Entrance requirements:* For master's, GRE General Test or MAT, minimum GPA of 2.5, 3 letters of recommendation, essay, current Georgia RN license, 1 year of post-licensure work, BSN, ASN. Additional exam requirements/recommendations for international students: Required—TOEFL (minimum score 550 paper-based; 79 iBT), IELTS (minimum score 6.5). Electronic applications accepted. *Faculty research:* Diabetes, hypertension, access to woman's health screening, simulation in nursing education, health care of undeserved populations.

University of Phoenix–Atlanta Campus, College of Nursing, Sandy Springs, GA 30350-4153. Offers health administration (MHA); nursing (MSN); nursing/health care education (MSN); MSN/MBA; MSN/MHA. Evening/weekend programs available. Postbaccalaureate distance learning degree programs offered. *Degree requirements:* For master's, thesis (for some programs). *Entrance requirements:* For master's, minimum undergraduate GPA of 2.5, 3 years of work experience. Additional exam requirements/recommendations for international students: Required—TOEFL (minimum score 550 paper-based; 79 iBT). Electronic applications accepted.

University of Phoenix–Augusta Campus, College of Nursing, Augusta, GA 30909-4583. Offers health administration (MHA); nursing (MSN); nursing/health care education (MSN); MSN/MBA; MSN/MHA. Postbaccalaureate distance learning degree programs offered.

University of Phoenix–Bay Area Campus, College of Nursing, San Jose, CA 95134-1805. Offers education (MHA); gerontology (MHA); health administration (MHA, DHA); informatics (MHA, MSN); nursing (MSN, PhD); nursing/health care education (MSN); MSN/MBA. Evening/weekend programs available. Postbaccalaureate distance learning degree programs offered (no on-campus study). *Degree requirements:* For master's, thesis (for some programs). *Entrance requirements:* For master's, minimum undergraduate GPA of 2.5, 3 years of work experience, RN license. Additional exam requirements/recommendations for international students: Required—TOEFL (minimum score 550 paper-based; 79 iBT). Electronic applications accepted.

University of Phoenix–Birmingham Campus, College of Health and Human Services, Birmingham, AL 35242. Offers education (MHA); gerontology (MHA); health administration (MHA); health care management (MBA); informatics (MHA); nursing (MSN); nursing/health care education (MSN); MSN/MBA; MSN/MHA.

University of Phoenix–Charlotte Campus, College of Nursing, Charlotte, NC 28273-3409. Offers education (MHA); gerontology (MHA); health administration (MHA); informatics (MHA, MSN); nursing (MSN); nursing/health care education (MSN). Evening/weekend programs available. *Degree requirements:* For master's, thesis (for some programs). *Entrance requirements:* For master's, minimum undergraduate GPA of 2.5, 3 years work experience. Additional exam requirements/recommendations for international students: Required—TOEFL (minimum score 550 paper-based; 79 iBT). Electronic applications accepted.

University of Phoenix–Cheyenne Campus, College of Nursing, Cheyenne, WY 82009. Offers health administration (MHA); nursing (MSN); nursing/health care education (MSN); MSN/MBA; MSN/MHA. Postbaccalaureate distance learning degree programs offered.

University of Phoenix–Des Moines Campus, College of Nursing, Des Moines, IA 50309. Offers education (MHA); gerontology (MHA); health administration (MHA, DHA); informatics (MHA, MSN); nursing (MSN, PhD); nursing/health care education (MSN).

University of Phoenix–Hawaii Campus, College of Nursing, Honolulu, HI 96813-4317. Offers education (MHA); family nurse practitioner (MSN); gerontology (MHA); health administration (MHA); nursing (MSN); nursing/health care education (MSN); MSN/MBA. Evening/weekend programs available. *Degree requirements:* For master's, thesis (for some programs). *Entrance requirements:* For master's, minimum undergraduate GPA of 2.5, 3 years of work experience, RN license. Additional exam requirements/recommendations for international students: Required—TOEFL (minimum score 550 paper-based; 79 iBT). Electronic applications accepted.

University of Phoenix–Idaho Campus, College of Nursing, Meridian, ID 83642-5114. Offers health administration (MHA); nursing (MSN); nursing/health care education (MSN); MSN/MBA. Evening/weekend programs available. Postbaccalaureate distance learning degree programs offered. *Degree requirements:* For master's, thesis (for some programs). *Entrance requirements:* For master's, minimum undergraduate GPA of 2.5, 3 years of work experience. Additional exam requirements/recommendations for international students: Required—TOEFL (minimum score 550 paper-based). Electronic applications accepted.

University of Phoenix–Indianapolis Campus, College of Nursing, Indianapolis, IN 46250-932. Offers health administration (MHA); nursing (MSN); nursing/health care education (MSN); MSN/MBA; MSN/MHA. Evening/weekend programs available.

Postbaccalaureate distance learning degree programs offered. *Degree requirements:* For master's, thesis. *Entrance requirements:* For master's, 3 years work experience, minimum undergraduate GPA of 2.5. Additional exam requirements/recommendations for international students: Required—TOEFL (minimum score 500 paper-based). Electronic applications accepted.

University of Phoenix–New Mexico Campus, College of Nursing, Albuquerque, NM 87113-1570. Offers health administration (MHA); health care education (MSN); nursing (MSN); MSN/MBA. Evening/weekend programs available. *Degree requirements:* For master's, thesis (for some programs). *Entrance requirements:* For master's, minimum undergraduate GPA of 2.5, 3 years of work experience, RN license. Additional exam requirements/recommendations for international students: Required—TOEFL (minimum score 550 paper-based; 79 iBT). Electronic applications accepted.

University of Phoenix–North Florida Campus, College of Nursing, Jacksonville, FL 32216-0959. Offers health administration (MHA); health care education (MSN); nursing (MSN); MSN/MBA; MSN/MHA. Evening/weekend programs available. *Degree requirements:* For master's, thesis (for some programs). *Entrance requirements:* For master's, minimum undergraduate GPA of 2.5, 3 years work experience, RN license. Additional exam requirements/recommendations for international students: Required—TOEFL (minimum score 550 paper-based; 79 iBT). Electronic applications accepted.

University of Phoenix–Northwest Arkansas Campus, College of Nursing, Rogers, AR 72756-9615. Offers health administration (MHA); health care education (MSN); nursing (MSN); MSN/MBA.

University of Phoenix–Online Campus, College of Health Sciences and Nursing, Phoenix, AZ 85034-7209. Offers family nurse practitioner (Certificate); health care (Certificate); health care education (Certificate); health care informatics (Certificate); informatics (MSN); nursing (MSN); nursing and health care education (MSN); MSN/MBA; MSN/MHA. *Accreditation:* AACN. Evening/weekend programs available. Postbaccalaureate distance learning degree programs offered. *Entrance requirements:* Additional exam requirements/recommendations for international students: Required—TOEFL, TOEIC (Test of English as an International Communication), Berlitz Online English Proficiency Exam, PTE, or IELTS. Electronic applications accepted. *Expenses:* Contact institution.

University of Phoenix–Phoenix Campus, College of Health Sciences and Nursing, Tempe, AZ 85282-2371. Offers family nurse practitioner (MSN, Certificate); gerontology health care (Certificate); health care education (MSN, Certificate); health care informatics (Certificate); informatics (MSN); nursing (MSN); MSN/MHA. Evening/weekend programs available. Postbaccalaureate distance learning degree programs offered. *Entrance requirements:* Additional exam requirements/recommendations for international students: Required—TOEFL, TOEIC (Test of English as an International Communication), Berlitz Online English Proficiency Exam, PTE, or IELTS. Electronic applications accepted. *Expenses:* Contact institution.

University of Phoenix–Pittsburgh Campus, College of Nursing, Pittsburgh, PA 15276. Offers health administration (MHA); health care education (MSN); nursing (MSN); MSN/MBA; MSN/MHA. Evening/weekend programs available. *Degree requirements:* For master's, thesis (for some programs). *Entrance requirements:* For master's, minimum undergraduate GPA of 2.5, 3 years work experience, current RN license (nursing). Additional exam requirements/recommendations for international students: Required—TOEFL (minimum score 550 paper-based; 79 iBT). Electronic applications accepted.

University of Phoenix–Richmond-Virginia Beach Campus, College of Nursing, Glen Allen, VA 23060. Offers health administration (MHA); health care education (MSN); nursing (MSN); MSN/MBA; MSN/MHA. Evening/weekend programs available. *Degree requirements:* For master's, thesis (for some programs). *Entrance requirements:* For master's, minimum undergraduate GPA of 2.5, 3 years work experience, current RN license for nursing programs. Additional exam requirements/recommendations for international students: Required—TOEFL (minimum score 500 paper-based; 79 iBT). Electronic applications accepted.

University of Phoenix–Sacramento Valley Campus, College of Nursing, Sacramento, CA 95833-3632. Offers family nurse practitioner (MSN); health administration (MHA); health care education (MSN); nursing (MSN); MSN/MBA. Evening/weekend programs available. *Degree requirements:* For master's, thesis (for some programs). *Entrance requirements:* For master's, RN license, minimum undergraduate GPA of 2.5, 3 years work experience. Additional exam requirements/recommendations for international students: Required—TOEFL (minimum score 550 paper-based; 79 iBT). Electronic applications accepted.

University of Phoenix–San Diego Campus, College of Nursing, San Diego, CA 92123. Offers health care education (MSN); nursing (MSN); MSN/MBA. Evening/weekend programs available. *Degree requirements:* For master's, thesis (for some programs). *Entrance requirements:* For master's, minimum undergraduate GPA of 2.5, 3 years work experience, RN license. Additional exam requirements/recommendations for international students: Required—TOEFL (minimum score 550 paper-based; 79 iBT). Electronic applications accepted.

University of Phoenix–Savannah Campus, College of Nursing, Savannah, GA 31405-7400. Offers health administration (MHA); nursing (MSN); nursing/health care education (MSN); MSN/MBA; MSN/MHA.

University of Phoenix–Southern California Campus, College of Health Sciences and Nursing, Costa Mesa, CA 92626. Offers family nurse practitioner (MSN, Certificate); health care (Certificate); informatics (MSN); nursing (MSN); nursing/health care education (MSN, Certificate); MSN/MBA; MSN/MHA. Evening/weekend programs available. Postbaccalaureate distance learning degree programs offered. *Entrance requirements:* Additional exam requirements/recommendations for international students: Required—TOEFL, TOEIC (Test of English as an International Communication), Berlitz Online English Proficiency Exam, PTE, or IELTS. Electronic applications accepted. *Expenses:* Contact institution.

University of Phoenix–South Florida Campus, College of Nursing, Miramar, FL 33030. Offers health administration (MHA); health care education (MSN); nursing (MSN); MSN/MBA; MSN/MHA. Evening/weekend programs available. *Degree requirements:* For master's, thesis (for some programs). *Entrance requirements:* For master's, minimum undergraduate GPA of 2.5, 3 years work experience, RN license. Additional exam requirements/recommendations for international students: Required—TOEFL (minimum score 550 paper-based; 79 iBT). Electronic applications accepted.

University of Phoenix–Utah Campus, College of Nursing, Salt Lake City, UT 84123-4617. Offers health care education (MSN); nursing (MSN); MSN/MBA. Evening/weekend programs available. *Degree requirements:* For master's, thesis (for some programs). *Entrance requirements:* For master's, minimum undergraduate GPA of 2.5, 3 years work experience, RN license. Additional exam requirements/recommendations for international students: Required—TOEFL (minimum score 550 paper-based; 79 iBT). Electronic applications accepted.

University of Phoenix–Washington D.C. Campus, College of Nursing, Washington, DC 20001. Offers education (MHA); gerontology (MHA); health administration (MHA, DHA); informatics (MHA, MSN); nursing (MSN, PhD); nursing/health care education (MSN); MSN/MBA; MSN/MHA.

University of Phoenix–West Florida Campus, College of Nursing, Temple Terrace, FL 33637. Offers health administration (MHA); health care education (MSN); nursing (MSN); MSN/MBA; MSN/MHA. Evening/weekend programs available. Postbaccalaureate distance learning degree programs offered. *Degree requirements:* For master's, thesis (for some programs). *Entrance requirements:* For master's, minimum undergraduate GPA of 2.5, RN license, 3 years work experience. Additional exam requirements/recommendations for international students: Required—TOEFL (minimum score 550 paper-based; 79 iBT). Electronic applications accepted.

University of Portland, School of Nursing, Portland, OR 97203. Offers clinical nurse leader (MS); nurse educator (MS); nursing (DNP). *Accreditation:* AACN. Part-time and evening/weekend programs available. Postbaccalaureate distance learning degree programs offered (minimal on-campus study). *Faculty:* 16 full-time (15 women), 10 part-time/adjunct (8 women). *Students:* 57 part-time (48 women); includes 4 minority (2 Asian, non-Hispanic/Latino; 1 Hispanic/Latino; 1 Two or more races, non-Hispanic/Latino), 2 international. Average age 36. In 2013, 12 master's, 6 doctorates awarded. *Entrance requirements:* For master's, GRE General Test or MAT, Oregon RN license, BSN, course work in statistics, resume, letters of recommendation, writing sample; for doctorate, GRE General Test or MAT, Oregon RN license, BSN or MSN, 2 letters of recommendation, resume, writing sample, official transcripts. Additional exam requirements/recommendations for international students: Required—TOEFL (minimum score 550 paper-based; 80 iBT), IELTS (minimum score 7). *Application deadline:* For fall admission, 11/2 priority date for domestic and international students; for spring admission, 1/7 priority date for domestic and international students. Applications are processed on a rolling basis. Application fee: $50. *Expenses:* Contact institution. *Financial support:* Fellowships, research assistantships, Federal Work-Study, and scholarships/grants available. Support available to part-time students. Financial award application deadline: 3/1; financial award applicants required to submit FAFSA. *Unit head:* Dr. Katherine Crabtree, Associate Dean, 503-943-7211, E-mail: nursing@up.edu. *Application contact:* Chris Olinger, Assistant to the Provost and Dean of the Graduate School, 503-943-7107, Fax: 503-943-7315, E-mail: olingerc@up.edu.
Website: http://nursing.up.edu/default.aspx?cid-7047&pid-207

University of Rhode Island, Graduate School, College of Nursing, Kingston, RI 02881. Offers administration (MS); clinical nurse leader (MS); clinical specialist in gerontology (MS); clinical specialist in psychiatric/mental health (MS); family nurse practitioner (MS); gerontological nurse practitioner (MS); nursing (DNP, PhD); nursing education (MS). *Accreditation:* AACN; ACNM/ACME (one or more programs are accredited). Part-time programs available. *Faculty:* 26 full-time (25 women), 3 part-time/adjunct (2 women). *Students:* 46 full-time (42 women), 78 part-time (70 women); includes 11 minority (7 Black or African American, non-Hispanic/Latino; 1 Asian, non-Hispanic/Latino; 3 Hispanic/Latino), 4 international. In 2013, 38 master's, 4 doctorates awarded. *Degree requirements:* For master's, comprehensive exam; for doctorate, comprehensive exam, thesis/dissertation. *Entrance requirements:* For master's, GRE or MAT, 2 letters of recommendation, scholarly papers; for doctorate, GRE, 3 letters of recommendation, scholarly papers. Additional exam requirements/recommendations for international students: Required—TOEFL (minimum score 550 paper-based). *Application deadline:* For fall admission, 2/15 for domestic students, 2/1 for international students; for spring admission, 10/15 for domestic students, 7/15 for international students. Application fee: $65. Electronic applications accepted. *Expenses:* Tuition, state resident: full-time $11,532; part-time $641 per credit. Tuition, nonresident: full-time $23,606; part-time $1311 per credit. *Required fees:* $1388; $36 per credit. $35 per semester. One-time fee: $130. *Financial support:* In 2013–14, 4 teaching assistantships with full and partial tuition reimbursements (averaging $8,383 per year) were awarded. Financial award application deadline: 2/15; financial award applicants required to submit FAFSA. *Faculty research:* Group intervention for grieving women in prison, translating best practice in non-drug interventions for postoperative pain management, further development and testing of the pain assessment inventory, preschool motor and functional performance of two cohorts, neuroactivation of brain motor areas in preterm children. *Total annual research expenditures:* $1.2 million. *Unit head:* Dr. Mary Sullivan, Interim Dean, 401-874-5339, Fax: 401-874-2061, E-mail: mcsullivan@uri.edu. *Application contact:* Graduate Admission, 401-874-2872, E-mail: gradadm@etal.uri.edu.
Website: http://www.uri.edu/nursing/

University of St. Francis, Leach College of Nursing, Joliet, IL 60435-6169. Offers family nurse practitioner (MSN, Post-Master's Certificate); family psychology/mental health nurse practitioner (MSN, Post-Master's Certificate); nursing administration (MSN); nursing education (MSN); nursing practice (DNP); teaching in nursing (Certificate). *Accreditation:* AACN. Part-time and evening/weekend programs available. Postbaccalaureate distance learning degree programs offered (no on-campus study). *Faculty:* 11 full-time (all women), 12 part-time/adjunct (11 women). *Students:* 90 full-time (76 women), 332 part-time (305 women); includes 122 minority (43 Black or African American, non-Hispanic/Latino; 1 American Indian or Alaska Native, non-Hispanic/Latino; 19 Asian, non-Hispanic/Latino; 45 Hispanic/Latino; 3 Native Hawaiian or other Pacific Islander, non-Hispanic/Latino; 11 Two or more races, non-Hispanic/Latino), 4 international. Average age 42. 343 applicants, 43% accepted, 111 enrolled. In 2013, 82 master's, 6 doctorates, 17 other advanced degrees awarded. *Entrance requirements:* For master's, minimum undergraduate GPA of 3.0, 2 years of full-time clinical experience, 3 letters recommendation, resume, nursing license, interview; for doctorate, MSN with minimum GPA of 3.0, national certification, interview, computer competency, medical/physical requirements, background check, liability insurance, resume, recommendation, graduate-level statistics course. Additional exam requirements/recommendations for international students: Required—TOEFL (minimum score 550 paper-based; 79 iBT), IELTS (minimum score 6.5). *Application deadline:* Applications are processed on a rolling basis. Application fee: $30. Electronic applications accepted. Application fee is waived when completed online. *Expenses:* Contact institution. *Financial support:* In 2013–14, 109 students received support. Scholarships/grants and tuition waivers (partial) available. Support available to part-time students. Financial award applicants required to submit FAFSA. *Unit head:* Dr. Carol Wilson, Dean, 815-740-3840, Fax: 815-740-4243, E-mail: cwilson@stfrancis.edu. *Application contact:* Sandra Sloka, Director of Admissions for Graduate and Degree Completion Programs, 800-735-7500, Fax: 815-740-3431, E-mail: ssloka@stfrancis.edu.
Website: http://www.stfrancis.edu/academics/college-of-nursing/

University of Saint Joseph, Department of Nursing, West Hartford, CT 06117-2700. Offers family nurse practitioner (MS); family psychiatric/mental health nurse practitioner (MS); nurse educator (MS); nursing practice (DNP). *Accreditation:* AACN. Part-time and evening/weekend programs available. *Degree requirements:* For master's, thesis. *Entrance requirements:* For master's, 2 letters of recommendation. *Application deadline:* Applications are processed on a rolling basis. Application fee: $50. Electronic applications accepted. Application fee is waived when completed online. *Financial support:* Career-related internships or fieldwork and unspecified assistantships available. Support available to part-time students. Financial award applicants required to submit FAFSA. *Unit head:* Dr. Patricia Padula Morgan, RN, Chair, 860-231-5591,

E-mail: pmorgan@usj.edu. *Application contact:* Graduate Admissions Office, 860-231-5261, E-mail: graduate@usj.edu.
Website: http://www.usj.edu/academics/schools/school-of-health-natural-sciences/nursing/

University of Saint Mary, Graduate Programs, Program in Nursing, Leavenworth, KS 66048-5082. Offers nurse administrator (MSN); nurse educator (MSN). Part-time programs available. Postbaccalaureate distance learning degree programs offered (no on-campus study). *Students:* 8 full-time (7 women), 4 part-time (all women). *Entrance requirements:* For master's, BSN from CCNE- or NLNAC-accredited baccalaureate nursing program at regionally-accredited institution. *Expenses: Tuition:* Part-time $550 per credit hour. *Unit head:* Dr. Glenna Mahoney, Department Chair, 877-307-4915, Fax: 913-345-2802. *Application contact:* Dr. Joyce Lasseter, Director, 877-307-4915, Fax: 913-345-2802.
Website: http://online.stmary.edu/MSN/master-science-nursing.asp

University of Southern Maine, College of Science, Technology, and Health, School of Nursing, Portland, ME 04104-9300. Offers adult-gerontology primary care nurse practitioner (MS, PMC); clinical nurse leader (MS); education (MS); family nurse practitioner (MS, PMC); family psychiatric/mental health nurse practitioner (MS); management (MS); nursing (DNP); psychiatric-mental health nurse practitioner (PMC); MBA/MSN. *Accreditation:* AACN. Part-time programs available. *Faculty:* 11 full-time (all women), 10 part-time/adjunct (8 women). *Students:* 57 full-time (47 women), 53 part-time (46 women); includes 5 minority (1 American Indian or Alaska Native, non-Hispanic/Latino; 2 Asian, non-Hispanic/Latino; 1 Hispanic/Latino; 1 Two or more races, non-Hispanic/Latino). Average age 36. 140 applicants, 44% accepted, 29 enrolled. In 2013, 33 master's, 11 other advanced degrees awarded. *Degree requirements:* For master's, thesis optional. *Entrance requirements:* For master's, GRE General Test or MAT, minimum GPA of 3.0; for doctorate, GRE. Additional exam requirements/recommendations for international students: Required—TOEFL (minimum score 550 paper-based). *Application deadline:* For fall admission, 4/1 for domestic and international students; for spring admission, 10/1 for domestic and international students. Application fee: $65. Electronic applications accepted. *Expenses:* Tuition, state resident: part-time $380 per credit. Tuition, nonresident: part-time $1026 per credit. Part-time tuition and fees vary according to program. *Financial support:* Research assistantships, teaching assistantships, career-related internships or fieldwork, Federal Work-Study, scholarships/grants, traineeships, tuition waivers (full and partial), and unspecified assistantships available. Support available to part-time students. Financial award application deadline: 2/15; financial award applicants required to submit FAFSA. *Faculty research:* Women's health, nursing history, weight control, community services, substance abuse. *Unit head:* Krista M. Meinersmann, Director of Nursing Program, 207-780-4993, E-mail: kmeinersmann@usm.maine.edu. *Application contact:* Mary Sloan, Assistant Dean of Graduate Studies and Director of Graduate Admissions, 207-780-4812, E-mail: gradstudies@usm.maine.edu.
Website: http://www.usm.maine.edu/nursing/

University of South Florida, College of Nursing, Tampa, FL 33612. Offers adult gerontology acute care (DNP, PhD); adult gerontology acute care nursing (MS); adult gerontology primary care (DNP, PhD); adult gerontology primary care nursing (MS); adult gerontology primary care/occupational health nursing (MS); adult gerontology primary care/oncology nursing (MS, PhD); clinical nurse leader (MS); family health (DNP, PhD); family nurse practitioner (MS); nurse anesthesia (MS); nursing education (MS); nursing practice (DNP); nursing science (PhD), including nursing education; occupational health/adult-gerontology (DNP); oncology/adult-gerontology primary care (DNP); pediatric health (DNP, PhD); pediatric nurse practitioner (MS). *Accreditation:* AACN; AANA/CANAEP. Part-time programs available. *Faculty:* 46 full-time (40 women), 15 part-time/adjunct (11 women). *Students:* 177 full-time (150 women), 700 part-time (622 women); includes 272 minority (116 Black or African American, non-Hispanic/Latino; 2 American Indian or Alaska Native, non-Hispanic/Latino; 45 Asian, non-Hispanic/Latino; 93 Hispanic/Latino; 2 Native Hawaiian or other Pacific Islander, non-Hispanic/Latino; 14 Two or more races, non-Hispanic/Latino), 12 international. Average age 35. 656 applicants, 43% accepted, 224 enrolled. In 2013, 224 master's, 14 doctorates awarded. *Degree requirements:* For master's, comprehensive exam, thesis optional; for doctorate, comprehensive exam, thesis/dissertation. *Entrance requirements:* For master's, GRE General Test, bachelor's degree from accredited program with minimum GPA of 3.0 in all upper-division coursework; current license as Registered Nurse; 3 letters of recommendation; personal statement of goals; resume or curriculum vitae; personal interview; for doctorate, GRE General Test (recommended), bachelor's degree in nursing from a CCNA/NLNAC regionally-accredited institution with minimum GPA of 3.0 in all coursework or in all upper-division coursework; current license as Registered Nurse in Florida; undergraduate statistics course with minimum B grade; 3 letters of recommendation; statement of goals; resume; interview. Additional exam requirements/recommendations for international students: Required—TOEFL (minimum score 550 paper-based; 79 iBT). *Application deadline:* For fall admission, 2/15 for domestic students, 1/2 for international students; for spring admission, 10/1 for domestic students, 6/1 for international students. Application fee: $30. Electronic applications accepted. *Financial support:* In 2013–14, 36 students received support, including 7 research assistantships with tuition reimbursements available (averaging $18,935 per year), 29 teaching assistantships with tuition reimbursements available (averaging $30,814 per year); tuition waivers (partial) and unspecified assistantships also available. Financial award application deadline: 2/1; financial award applicants required to submit FAFSA. *Faculty research:* Women's health, palliative and end-of-life care, cardiac rehabilitation, complementary therapies for chronic illness and cancer. *Total annual research expenditures:* $3.4 million. *Unit head:* Dr. Dianne C. Morrison-Beedy, Dean and Professor, College of Nursing, 813-974-9091, Fax: 813-974-5418, E-mail: dmbeedy@health.usf.edu. *Application contact:* Dr. Connie Visovsky, Associate Professor and Associate Dean of Student Affairs, 813-396-9641, Fax: 813-974-5418, E-mail: cvisovsk@health.usf.edu.
Website: http://health.usf.edu/nursing/index.htm

The University of Tennessee at Chattanooga, Graduate School, College of Health, Education and Professional Studies, School of Nursing, Chattanooga, TN 37403. Offers administration (MSN); certified nurse anesthetist (Post-Master's Certificate); education (MSN); family nurse practitioner (MSN, Post-Master's Certificate); health care informatics (Post-Master's Certificate); nurse anesthesia (MSN); nurse education (Post-Master's Certificate); nursing (DNP). *Accreditation:* AACN; AANA/CANAEP (one or more programs are accredited). *Faculty:* 9 full-time (7 women), 2 part-time/adjunct (1 woman). *Students:* 72 full-time (39 women), 53 part-time (43 women); includes 11 minority (6 Black or African American, non-Hispanic/Latino; 1 Asian, non-Hispanic/Latino; 3 Hispanic/Latino; 1 Two or more races, non-Hispanic/Latino). Average age 33. 3 applicants, 100% accepted, 1 enrolled. In 2013, 35 master's, 10 doctorates, 2 other advanced degrees awarded. *Degree requirements:* For master's, thesis optional, qualifying exams, professional project; for Post-Master's Certificate, thesis or alternative, practicum, seminar. *Entrance requirements:* For master's, GRE General Test, MAT, BSN, minimum GPA of 3.0, eligibility for Tennessee RN license, 1 year of direct patient care experience; for Post-Master's Certificate, GRE General Test, MAT, MSN, minimum GPA of 3.0, eligibility for Tennessee RN license, one year of direct patient care experience. Additional exam requirements/recommendations for international students: Required—TOEFL (minimum score 550 paper-based; 79 iBT), IELTS (minimum score 6). *Application deadline:* For fall admission, 6/13 priority date for domestic students, 6/1 for international students; for spring admission, 10/15 priority date for domestic students, 10/1 for international students. Applications are processed on a rolling basis. Application fee: $30 ($35 for international students). Electronic applications accepted. *Financial support:* Career-related internships or fieldwork and scholarships/grants available. Support available to part-time students. *Faculty research:* Diabetes in women, health care for elderly, alternative medicine, hypertension, nurse anesthesia. *Total annual research expenditures:* $3.4 million. *Unit head:* Dr. Chris Smith, Interim Director, 423-425-1741, Fax: 423-425-4668, E-mail: chris-smith@utc.edu. *Application contact:* Dr. J. Randy Walker, Interim Dean of Graduate Studies, 423-425-4478, Fax: 423-425-5223, E-mail: randy-walker@utc.edu.
Website: http://www.utc.edu/Academic/Nursing/

The University of Texas at Arlington, Graduate School, College of Nursing, Arlington, TX 76019. Offers nurse practitioner (MSN); nursing administration (MSN); nursing education (MSN); nursing practice (DNP); nursing science (PhD). *Accreditation:* AACN. Part-time and evening/weekend programs available. Postbaccalaureate distance learning degree programs offered (no on-campus study). *Degree requirements:* For master's, practicum course; for doctorate, comprehensive exam (for some programs), thesis/dissertation (for some programs), proposal defense dissertation (for PhD); scholarship project (for DNP). *Entrance requirements:* For master's, GRE General Test if GPA less than 3.0, minimum GPA of 3.0, Texas nursing license, minimum C grade in undergraduate statistics course; for doctorate, GRE General Test (waived for MSN-to-PhD applicants), minimum undergraduate, graduate and statistics GPA of 3.0; Texas RN license; interview; written statement of goals. Additional exam requirements/recommendations for international students: Required—TOEFL (minimum score 550 paper-based), IELTS (minimum score 7). *Faculty research:* Simulation in clinical education and practice, cultural diversity, vulnerable populations, substance abuse.

The University of Texas at Austin, Graduate School, School of Nursing, Austin, TX 78712-1111. Offers adult - gerontology clinical nurse specialist (MSN); child health (MSN), including administration, public health nursing, teaching; family nurse practitioner (MSN); family psychiatric/mental health nurse practitioner (MSN); holistic adult health (MSN), including administration, teaching; maternity (MSN), including administration, public health nursing, teaching; nursing (PhD); nursing administration and healthcare systems management (MSN); pediatric nurse practitioner (MSN); public health nursing (MSN). *Accreditation:* AACN. Part-time programs available. *Degree requirements:* For master's, thesis optional; for doctorate, thesis/dissertation. *Entrance requirements:* For master's and doctorate, GRE General Test. Additional exam requirements/recommendations for international students: Required—TOEFL (minimum score 550 paper-based). Electronic applications accepted. *Faculty research:* Chronic illness management, memory and aging, health promotion, women's health, adolescent health.

The University of Texas at El Paso, Graduate School, School of Nursing, El Paso, TX 79968-0001. Offers family nurse practitioner (MSN); health care leadership and management (Certificate); interdisciplinary health sciences (PhD); nursing (DNP); nursing education (MSN, Certificate); nursing systems management (MSN). *Accreditation:* AACN. Postbaccalaureate distance learning degree programs offered (minimal on-campus study). *Degree requirements:* For master's, thesis optional; for doctorate, thesis/dissertation. *Entrance requirements:* For master's, minimum GPA of 3.0, resume; for doctorate, GRE, letters of reference, relevant personal/professional experience; master's degree in nursing (for DNP); for Certificate, bachelor's degree in nursing. Additional exam requirements/recommendations for international students: Required—TOEFL; Recommended—IELTS. Electronic applications accepted.

The University of Texas at Tyler, College of Nursing and Health Sciences, Program in Nursing, Tyler, TX 75799-0001. Offers nurse practitioner (MSN); nursing (PhD); nursing administration (MSN); nursing education (MSN); MSN/MBA. *Accreditation:* AACN. Part-time and evening/weekend programs available. Postbaccalaureate distance learning degree programs offered (no on-campus study). *Degree requirements:* For master's, comprehensive exam (for some programs), thesis (for some programs); for doctorate, thesis/dissertation. *Entrance requirements:* For master's, GRE General Test or MAT, GMAT, minimum undergraduate GPA of 3.0, course work in statistics, RN license, BSN. Additional exam requirements/recommendations for international students: Required—TOEFL. Electronic applications accepted. *Faculty research:* Psychosocial adjustment, aging, support/commitment of caregivers, psychological abuse and violence, hope/hopelessness, professional values, end of life care, suicidology, clinical supervision, workforce retention and issues, global health issues, health promotion.

The University of Texas Health Science Center at San Antonio, School of Nursing, San Antonio, TX 78229. Offers administrative management (MSN); adult-gerontology acute care nurse practitioner (PGC); clinical nurse leader (MSN); executive administrative management (DNP); family nurse practitioner (PGC); nurse practitioner (MSN), including adult-gerontology acute care nurse practitioner, family nurse practitioner, pediatric nurse practitioner primary care, psychiatric mental health nurse practitioner; nurse practitioner leadership (DNP); nursing (MSN, PhD); nursing education (MSN, PGC); pediatric nurse practitioner primary care (PGC); psychiatric mental health nurse practitioner (PGC); public health nurse leader (DNP). *Accreditation:* AACN. Part-time programs available. *Faculty:* 84 full-time (74 women), 42 part-time/adjunct (40 women). *Students:* 115 full-time (93 women), 140 part-time (123 women); includes 123 minority (24 Black or African American, non-Hispanic/Latino; 20 Asian, non-Hispanic/Latino; 74 Hispanic/Latino; 5 Two or more races, non-Hispanic/Latino), 7 international. Average age 37. 174 applicants, 59% accepted, 83 enrolled. In 2013, 67 master's, 6 doctorates, 5 other advanced degrees awarded. Terminal master's awarded for partial completion of doctoral program. *Degree requirements:* For master's, thesis optional; for doctorate, comprehensive exam, thesis/dissertation, final projects (for DNP). *Entrance requirements:* For master's, minimum GPA of 3.0, references, goal statement, BSN from accredited nursing school, RN licensure in Texas or compact state; for doctorate, GRE, MAT, minimum GPA of 3.0, personal interview, BSN and/or MSN from accredited nursing school, RN licensure in Texas or compact state, statistics course, references, curriculum vitae, goal statement; for PGC, minimum GPA of 3.0; references; goal statement; MSN from accredited nursing school; RN licensure in Texas or compact state; prerequisites in advanced health assessment, advanced pharmacotherapeutics, and advanced pathophysiology. Additional exam requirements/recommendations for international students: Required—TOEFL (minimum score 550 paper-based; 68 iBT), IELTS (minimum score 6.5). *Application deadline:* For fall admission, 1/10 for domestic and international students; for spring admission, 7/1 for domestic students. Application fee: $65. Electronic applications accepted. *Financial support:* In 2013–14, 145 students received support, including 3 fellowships with full tuition reimbursements available (averaging $30,000 per year); institutionally sponsored loans and scholarships/grants also available. Financial award application deadline: 6/30; financial award applicants required to submit FAFSA. *Faculty research:* Pain, organizational structure, aging, quality and safety, health disparity, obesity and nutrition, women's and children's health. *Total annual research expenditures:* $500,265. *Unit head:* Dr. Eileen T. Breslin, Dean, 210-567-5800, Fax: 210-567-5929, E-mail: breslin@

uthscsa.edu. *Application contact:* Brandy Finck, Interim Associate Dean for Admissions and Student Services, 210-567-5805, Fax: 210-567-6189, E-mail: finckb@uthscsa.edu. Website: http://www.nursing.uthscsa.edu/

The University of Toledo, College of Graduate Studies, College of Nursing, Department of Population and Community Care, Toledo, OH 43606-3390. Offers clinical nurse leader (MSN); family nurse practitioner (MSN, Certificate); nurse educator (MSN, Certificate); pediatric nurse practitioner (MSN, Certificate). Part-time programs available. *Students:* 70 full-time (60 women), 212 part-time (186 women); includes 27 minority (12 Black or African American, non-Hispanic/Latino; 1 American Indian or Alaska Native, non-Hispanic/Latino; 3 Asian, non-Hispanic/Latino; 7 Hispanic/Latino; 4 Two or more races, non-Hispanic/Latino), 1 international. Average age 32. 127 applicants, 81% accepted, 78 enrolled. In 2013, 82 master's, 10 other advanced degrees awarded. *Degree requirements:* For master's, thesis or alternative. *Entrance requirements:* For master's, GRE, BS in nursing, minimum undergraduate GPA of 3.0, statement of purpose, three letters of recommendation, transcripts from all prior institutions attended, Nursing CAS application, UT supplemental application; for Certificate, BS in nursing, minimum undergraduate GPA of 3.0, statement of purpose, three letters of recommendation, transcripts from all prior institutions attended. Additional exam requirements/recommendations for international students: Required—TOEFL (minimum score 550 paper-based; 80 iBT). Application fee: $45 ($75 for international students). Electronic applications accepted. *Financial support:* Research assistantships with full and partial tuition reimbursements, Federal Work-Study, scholarships/grants, traineeships, and tuition waivers (full and partial) available. *Unit head:* Dr. Kelley Phillips, Chair, 419-383-5892. *Application contact:* Joan Mulligan, Admissions Analyst, 419-383-4168, Fax: 419-383-6140, E-mail: joan.mulligan@utoledo.edu. Website: http://www.utoledo.edu/nursing/

University of Victoria, Faculty of Graduate Studies, Faculty of Human and Social Development, School of Nursing, Victoria, BC V8W 2Y2, Canada. Offers advanced nursing practice (advanced practice leadership option) (MN); advanced nursing practice (nurse educator option) (MN); advanced nursing practice (nurse practitioner option) (MN); nursing (PhD). Part-time programs available. Postbaccalaureate distance learning degree programs offered (no on-campus study). *Entrance requirements:* Additional exam requirements/recommendations for international students: Required—TOEFL (minimum score 575 paper-based), IELTS (minimum score 7). Electronic applications accepted.

University of Washington, Tacoma, Graduate Programs, Program in Nursing, Tacoma, WA 98402-3100. Offers communities, populations and health (MN); leadership in healthcare (MN); nurse educator (MN). Part-time programs available. *Degree requirements:* For master's, thesis (for some programs), advance fieldwork. *Entrance requirements:* For master's, Washington State NCLEX exam, minimum GPA of 3.0. Additional exam requirements/recommendations for international students: Required—TOEFL (minimum score 580 paper-based; 70 iBT); Recommended—IELTS (minimum score 7). *Faculty research:* Hospice and palliative care; clinical trial decision-making; minority nurse retention; asthma and public health; injustice, suffering, difference: Linking Them to Us; adolescent health.

University of West Georgia, Tanner Health System School of Nursing, Carrollton, GA 30118. Offers health systems leadership (Post-Master's Certificate); nursing (MSN); nursing education (Ed D, Post-Master's Certificate). *Accreditation:* AACN. Part-time programs available. Postbaccalaureate distance learning degree programs offered (no on-campus study). *Faculty:* 11 full-time (10 women), 1 (woman) part-time/adjunct. *Students:* 70 full-time (67 women), 52 part-time (48 women); includes 35 minority (31 Black or African American, non-Hispanic/Latino; 4 Hispanic/Latino). Average age 42. 96 applicants, 83% accepted, 56 enrolled. In 2013, 23 master's awarded. *Degree requirements:* For master's, comprehensive exam, thesis optional; for doctorate, comprehensive exam, thesis/dissertation. *Entrance requirements:* For master's, BSN, RN license, minimum GPA of 3.0 for upper-division nursing courses, two letters of recommendation, resume, official transcript, undergraduate statistics course with minimum C grade; for doctorate, GRE, MSN, minimum GPA of 3.0 in graduate nursing program, three letters of recommendation, 5-page sample of academic writing, RN license, resume or curriculum vitae, official transcripts; for Post-Master's Certificate, MSN, official transcripts, curriculum vitae/resume, two letters of recommendation. Additional exam requirements/recommendations for international students: Required—TOEFL (minimum score 523 paper-based; 69 iBT); Recommended—IELTS (minimum score 6.5). *Application deadline:* For fall admission, 6/1 for domestic and international students. Applications are processed on a rolling basis. Application fee: $40. Electronic applications accepted. *Expenses:* Contact institution. *Financial support:* In 2013–14, 8 students received support, including 1 research assistantship with full tuition reimbursement available (averaging $6,000 per year); scholarships/grants and unspecified assistantships also available. Financial award application deadline: 4/1; financial award applicants required to submit FAFSA. *Faculty research:* Caring in nursing education, pain assessment in older adults, pain outcomes. *Unit head:* Dr. Kathryn Mary Grams, Dean, 678-839-5642, Fax: 678-839-6553, E-mail: kgrams@westga.edu. *Application contact:* Embry Ice, Graduate Studies Associate, 678-839-5115, Fax: 678-839-6553, E-mail: eice@westga.edu.
Website: http://nursing.westga.edu

University of Wisconsin–Eau Claire, College of Nursing and Health Sciences, Program in Nursing, Eau Claire, WI 54702-4004. Offers adult-gerontological administration (DNP); adult-gerontological clinical nurse specialist (DNP); adult-gerontological education (MSN); adult-gerontological primary care nurse practitioner (DNP); family health administration (DNP); family health in education (MSN); family health nurse practitioner (DNP); nursing (MSN); nursing practice (DNP). Part-time programs available. *Faculty:* 8 full-time (all women), 2 part-time/adjunct (both women). *Students:* 33 full-time (30 women), 40 part-time (36 women); includes 1 minority (Asian, non-Hispanic/Latino). Average age 37. 48 applicants, 85% accepted, 24 enrolled. In 2013, 31 master's, 9 doctorates awarded. Terminal master's awarded for partial completion of doctoral program. *Degree requirements:* For master's, thesis optional, 500-600 hours clinical practicum, oral and written exams. *Entrance requirements:* For master's, Wisconsin RN license, minimum GPA of 3.0, undergraduate statistics, course work in health assessment. Additional exam requirements/recommendations for international students: Required—TOEFL (minimum score 79 iBT). *Application deadline:* For fall admission, 1/15 priority date for domestic and international students. Applications are processed on a rolling basis. Application fee: $86. *Expenses:* Contact institution. *Financial support:* In 2013–14, 10 students received support. Federal Work-Study and unspecified assistantships available. Financial award application deadline: 3/1; financial award applicants required to submit FAFSA. *Unit head:* Dr. Linda Young, Dean, 715-836-4904, Fax: 715-836-5925, E-mail: younglk@uwec.edu. *Application contact:* Dr. Mary Zwygart-Stauffacher, Director, 715-836-5287, E-mail: zwygarmc@uwec.edu.
Website: http://www.uwec.edu/conhs/programs/grad/index.htm

Ursuline College, School of Graduate Studies, Programs in Nursing, Pepper Pike, OH 44124-4398. Offers care management (MSN); nurse practitioner (MSN); nursing (DNP); nursing education (MSN); palliative care (MSN). *Accreditation:* AACN. Part-time programs available. *Faculty:* 6 full-time (all women), 13 part-time/adjunct (10 women). *Students:* 9 full-time (7 women), 245 part-time (235 women); includes 69 minority (58 Black or African American, non-Hispanic/Latino; 6 Asian, non-Hispanic/Latino; 2 Hispanic/Latino; 3 Two or more races, non-Hispanic/Latino), 1 international. Average age 36. 91 applicants, 79% accepted, 60 enrolled. In 2013, 57 master's, 2 doctorates awarded. *Degree requirements:* For master's, comprehensive exam. *Entrance requirements:* For master's, minimum undergraduate GPA of 3.0, bachelor's degree in nursing, eligibility for or current Ohio RN license. Additional exam requirements/recommendations for international students: Required—TOEFL (minimum score 500 paper-based). *Application deadline:* For fall admission, 8/1 priority date for domestic students. Applications are processed on a rolling basis. Application fee: $25. *Expenses:* *Tuition:* Full-time $16,920; part-time $940 per credit. *Required fees:* $270. *Financial support:* In 2013–14, 9 students received support. Federal Work-Study available. Financial award application deadline: 3/1. *Unit head:* Dr. Janet Baker, Director, 440-864-8172, Fax: 440-684-6053, E-mail: jbaker@ursuline.edu. *Application contact:* Stephanie Pratt, Graduate Admission Coordinator, 440-646-8119, Fax: 440-684-6138, E-mail: graduateadmissions@ursuline.edu.

Valparaiso University, Graduate School, College of Nursing and Health Professions, Valparaiso, IN 46383. Offers management (Certificate); nursing education (MSN, Certificate); MSN/MBA. *Accreditation:* AACN. Part-time and evening/weekend programs available. Postbaccalaureate distance learning degree programs offered (minimal on-campus study). *Faculty:* 11 part-time/adjunct (all women). *Students:* 36 full-time (30 women), 55 part-time (51 women); includes 13 minority (8 Black or African American, non-Hispanic/Latino; 5 Hispanic/Latino), 15 international. Average age 37. In 2013, 7 master's awarded. *Entrance requirements:* For master's, minimum GPA of 3.0, undergraduate major in nursing, Indiana registered nursing license, undergraduate courses in research and statistics. Additional exam requirements/recommendations for international students: Required—TOEFL (minimum score 550 paper-based; 80 iBT), IELTS (minimum score 6). *Application deadline:* Applications are processed on a rolling basis. Application fee: $30 ($50 for international students). Electronic applications accepted. *Expenses:* Contact institution. *Financial support:* Available to part-time students. Applicants required to submit FAFSA. *Unit head:* Dr. Janet Brown, Dean, 219-464-5289, Fax: 219-464-5425, E-mail: janet.brown@valpo.edu. *Application contact:* Jessica Choquette, Graduate Admissions Specialist, 219-464-5313, Fax: 219-464-5381, E-mail: jessica.choquette@valpo.edu.
Website: http://www.valpo.edu/nursing/

Villanova University, College of Nursing, Villanova, PA 19085-1699. Offers adult nurse practitioner (MSN, Post Master's Certificate); family nurse practitioner (MSN, Post Master's Certificate); health care administration (MSN, Post Master's Certificate); nurse anesthetist (MSN, Post Master's Certificate); nursing (PhD); nursing education (MSN, Post Master's Certificate); nursing practice (DNP); pediatric nurse practitioner (MSN, Post Master's Certificate). *Accreditation:* AACN; AANA/CANAEP. Part-time programs available. Postbaccalaureate distance learning degree programs offered (minimal on-campus study). *Faculty:* 17 full-time (all women), 4 part-time/adjunct (all women). *Students:* 28 full-time (26 women), 191 part-time (161 women); includes 22 minority (2 Black or African American, non-Hispanic/Latino; 6 Asian, non-Hispanic/Latino; 7 Hispanic/Latino; 7 Two or more races, non-Hispanic/Latino), 18 international. Average age 30. 176 applicants, 65% accepted, 82 enrolled. In 2013, 64 master's, 7 doctorates, 5 other advanced degrees awarded. *Degree requirements:* For master's, independent study project; for doctorate, comprehensive exam, thesis/dissertation. *Entrance requirements:* For master's, GRE or MAT, BSN, 1 year of recent nursing experience, physical assessment, course work in statistics; for doctorate, GRE, MSN. Additional exam requirements/recommendations for international students: Required—TOEFL (minimum score 540 paper-based; 83 iBT), IELTS (minimum score 6.5). *Application deadline:* For fall admission, 7/1 priority date for domestic students, 7/1 for international students; for spring admission, 11/1 priority date for domestic students, 11/1 for international students. Applications are processed on a rolling basis. Application fee: $50. Electronic applications accepted. *Expenses:* Contact institution. *Financial support:* In 2013–14, 39 students received support, including 5 teaching assistantships with full tuition reimbursements available (averaging $14,475 per year); institutionally sponsored loans, scholarships/grants, traineeships, tuition waivers (full), and unspecified assistantships also available. Financial award application deadline: 7/1; financial award applicants required to submit FAFSA. *Faculty research:* Genetics, ethics, cognitive development of students, women with disabilities, nursing leadership. *Unit head:* Dr. Marguerite K. Schlag, Assistant Dean/Director, Graduate Programs, 610-519-4907, Fax: 610-519-7650, E-mail: marguerite.schlag@villanova.edu.
Website: http://www.nursing.villanova.edu/

Virginia Commonwealth University, Graduate School, School of Nursing, Richmond, VA 23284-9005. Offers adult health acute nursing (MS); adult health primary nursing (MS); biobehavioral clinical research (PhD); child health nursing (MS); clinical nurse leader (MS); family health nursing (MS); nurse educator (MS); nurse practitioner (MS); nursing (Certificate); nursing administration (MS), including clinical nurse manager; psychiatric-mental health nursing (MS); women's health nursing (MS). Part-time and evening/weekend programs available. *Degree requirements:* For master's, thesis optional; for doctorate, thesis/dissertation. *Entrance requirements:* For master's, GRE General Test, BSN, minimum GPA of 2.8; for doctorate, GRE General Test. Additional exam requirements/recommendations for international students: Required—TOEFL (minimum score 600 paper-based; 100 iBT). Electronic applications accepted.

Walden University, Graduate Programs, School of Nursing, Minneapolis, MN 55401. Offers adult-gerontology acute care nurse practitioner (MSN); adult-gerontology nurse practitioner (MSN); education (MSN); family nurse practitioner (MSN); informatics (MSN); leadership and management (MSN); nursing (DNP, PhD, Post-Master's Certificate), including education (PhD), healthcare administration (PhD), interdisciplinary health (PhD), leadership (PhD), nursing education (Post-Master's Certificate), nursing informatics (Post-Master's Certificate), nursing leadership and management (Post-Master's Certificate), public health policy (PhD). *Accreditation:* AACN. Part-time and evening/weekend programs available. Postbaccalaureate distance learning degree programs offered (no on-campus study). *Faculty:* 22 full-time (19 women), 343 part-time/adjunct (301 women). *Students:* 5,828 full-time (5,240 women), 2,803 part-time (2,578 women); includes 2,920 minority (1,893 Black or African American, non-Hispanic/Latino; 40 American Indian or Alaska Native, non-Hispanic/Latino; 438 Asian, non-Hispanic/Latino; 391 Hispanic/Latino; 35 Native Hawaiian or other Pacific Islander, non-Hispanic/Latino; 123 Two or more races, non-Hispanic/Latino), 147 international. Average age 41. 1,795 applicants, 95% accepted, 1375 enrolled. In 2013, 1,879 master's, 1 doctorate, 36 other advanced degrees awarded. *Degree requirements:* For doctorate, thesis/dissertation (for some programs), residency (for some programs), field experience (for some programs). *Entrance requirements:* For master's, bachelor's degree or equivalent in related field or RN; minimum GPA of 2.5; official transcripts; goal statement (for some programs); access to computer and Internet; for doctorate, master's degree or higher, three years of related professional or academic experience, RN, goal statement (for some programs); access to computer and Internet; for Post-Master's Certificate, relevant work experience; access to computer and Internet. Additional exam requirements/recommendations for international students: Required—TOEFL (minimum score 550 paper-based; 79 iBT), IELTS (minimum score 6.5), Michigan English Language Assessment Battery (minimum score 82), or PTE. *Application deadline:*

Nursing Education

Applications are processed on a rolling basis. Application fee: $0. Electronic applications accepted. *Expenses: Tuition:* Full-time $11,813.55; part-time $500 per credit. *Required fees:* $618.76. *Financial support:* Fellowships, Federal Work-Study, scholarships/grants, unspecified assistantships, and family tuition reduction, active duty/veteran tuition reduction, group tuition reduction, interest-free payment plans, employee tuition reduction available. Support available to part-time students. Financial award applicants required to submit FAFSA. *Unit head:* Dr. Andrea Lindell, Associate Dean, 800-925-3368. *Application contact:* Jennifer Hall, Vice President of Enrollment Management, 866-4-WALDEN, E-mail: info@waldenu.edu.
Website: http://www.waldenu.edu/programs/colleges-schools/nursing

Walsh University, Graduate Studies, School of Nursing, North Canton, OH 44720-3396. Offers academic nurse educator (MSN); clinical nurse leader (MSN); nursing practice (DNP). Part-time and evening/weekend programs available. Postbaccalaureate distance learning degree programs offered (minimal on-campus study). *Faculty:* 6 full-time (all women), 6 part-time/adjunct (5 women). *Students:* 13 full-time (10 women), 29 part-time (all women); includes 2 minority (1 Black or African American, non-Hispanic/Latino; 1 Hispanic/Latino). Average age 39. 27 applicants, 89% accepted, 19 enrolled. *Degree requirements:* For doctorate, scholarly project; residency practicum. *Entrance requirements:* For master's, undergraduate nursing degree, current unencumbered RN license, completion of an undergraduate or graduate statistics course, essay, interview, recommendations; for doctorate, BSN; master's degree; statistics and research courses; essay; interview. Additional exam requirements/recommendations for international students: Required—TOEFL. *Application deadline:* Applications are processed on a rolling basis. Electronic applications accepted. *Expenses: Tuition:* Full-time $10,890; part-time $605 per credit hour. *Required fees:* $100; $100. *Financial support:* In 2013–14, 32 students received support. Research assistantships, tuition waivers (partial), and tuition discounts available. Financial award application deadline: 12/31; financial award applicants required to submit FAFSA. *Faculty research:* Faith community nursing, gerontology, women's health, global nursing education, nursing assessment, grief and reconstitution, health needs of psychiatric patients, psychometric testing. *Unit head:* Dr. Karen Gehrling, Director, Graduate Program in Nursing, 330-244-4649, Fax: 330-490-7371, E-mail: kgehrling@walsh.edu. *Application contact:* Audra Dice, Graduate and Transfer Admissions Counselor, 330-490-7181, Fax: 330-244-4680, E-mail: adice@walsh.edu.
Website: http://www.walsh.edu/master-of-science-in-nursing

Washington Adventist University, Program in Nursing - Education, Takoma Park, MD 20912. Offers MS. Part-time programs available. *Entrance requirements:* Additional exam requirements/recommendations for international students: Required—TOEFL (minimum score 550 paper-based), IELTS (minimum score 5).

Waynesburg University, Graduate and Professional Studies, Canonsburg, PA 15370. Offers business (MBA), including energy management, finance, health systems, human resources, leadership, market development; counseling (MA), including addictions counseling, clinical mental health; education (M Ed, MAT), including autism (M Ed), curriculum and instruction (M Ed), educational leadership (M Ed), online teaching (M Ed); nursing (MSN), including administration, education, informatics; nursing practice (DNP); special education (M Ed); technology (M Ed); MSN/MBA. *Accreditation:* AACN. Part-time and evening/weekend programs available. *Faculty:* 11 full-time (5 women), 136 part-time/adjunct (80 women). *Students:* 146 full-time (99 women), 419 part-time (268 women). In 2013, 290 master's, 7 doctorates awarded. *Degree requirements:* For doctorate, thesis/dissertation. *Entrance requirements:* Additional exam requirements/recommendations for international students: Required—TOEFL. *Application deadline:* For fall admission, 8/1 priority date for domestic students. Applications are processed on a rolling basis. Electronic applications accepted. *Financial support:* Available to part-time students. Application deadline: 5/1. *Unit head:* David Mariner, Dean, 724-743-4420, Fax: 724-743-4425, E-mail: dmariner@waynesburg.edu. *Application contact:* Dr. Michael Bednarski, Director of Enrollment, 724-743-4420, Fax: 724-743-4425, E-mail: mbednars@waynesburg.edu.
Website: http://www.waynesburg.edu/

Wayne State University, College of Nursing, Program in Nursing Education, Detroit, MI 48202. Offers Graduate Certificate. *Students:* 1 (woman) full-time, 1 (woman) part-time. 1 applicant. In 2013, 13 degrees awarded. *Entrance requirements:* For degree, GRE General Test, MSN or concurrent enrollment in master's program, current RN license, statement of purpose, three letters of reference. Additional exam requirements/recommendations for international students: Required—TOEFL (minimum score 550 paper-based; 79 iBT); Recommended—TWE (minimum score 6). *Application deadline:* For fall admission, 6/1 priority date for domestic students, 5/1 priority date for international students; for winter admission, 10/1 priority date for domestic students, 9/1 priority date for international students; for spring admission, 2/1 priority date for domestic students, 1/1 priority date for international students. Applications are processed on a rolling basis. Application fee: $50. Electronic applications accepted. *Expenses:* Contact institution. *Financial support:* Scholarships/grants and traineeships available. Financial award application deadline: 7/1. *Unit head:* Dr. Barbara Redman, Dean, 313-577-4070, Fax: 313-577-4571, E-mail: ae9080@wayne.edu. *Application contact:* Nancy Artinian, Professor, 313-577-4143, E-mail: n.artinian@wayne.edu.
Website: http://www.nursing.wayne.edu/certificate/gcnecurriculum.php

West Chester University of Pennsylvania, College of Health Sciences, Department of Nursing, West Chester, PA 19383. Offers nursing (DNP); public health nursing (MSN), including administration, education, integrative health. *Accreditation:* AACN. Part-time and evening/weekend programs available. Postbaccalaureate distance learning degree programs offered (minimal on-campus study). *Faculty:* 4 full-time (3 women). *Students:* 12 full-time (11 women), 17 part-time (15 women); includes 9 minority (7 Black or African American, non-Hispanic/Latino; 1 Asian, non-Hispanic/Latino; 1 Hispanic/Latino), 2 international. Average age 42. 11 applicants, 91% accepted, 7 enrolled. In 2013, 17 master's awarded. *Entrance requirements:* For master's, RN license, BSN or RN with bachelor's degree in another discipline, minimum GPA of 2.8, experience as a nurse providing direct clinical care, two letters of recommendation; for doctorate, minimum graduate GPA of 3.0, two letters of reference, interview. Additional exam requirements/recommendations for international students: Required—TOEFL (minimum score 550 paper-based; 80 iBT). *Application deadline:* For fall admission, 4/15 priority date for domestic students, 3/15 for international students; for spring admission, 10/15 priority date for domestic students, 9/1 for international students. Applications are processed on a rolling basis. Application fee: $45. Electronic applications accepted. *Expenses:* Tuition, state resident: full-time $7956; part-time $442 per credit. Tuition, nonresident: full-time $11,934; part-time $663 per credit. *Required fees:* $2134.20; $106.24 per credit. Tuition and fees vary according to campus/location and program. *Financial support:* Unspecified assistantships available. Support available to part-time students. Financial award application deadline: 2/15; financial award applicants required to submit FAFSA. *Unit head:* Dr. Charlotte Mackey, Chair and Graduate Coordinator, 610-436-3474, Fax: 610-436-3083, E-mail: cmackey@wcupa.edu.
Website: http://www.wcupa.edu/_ACADEMICS/HealthSciences/nursing/

Western Carolina University, Graduate School, College of Health and Human Sciences, School of Nursing, Cullowhee, NC 28723. Offers nurse educator (PMC); nursing (MSN). *Accreditation:* AACN; AANA/CANAEP. Part-time and evening/weekend programs available. *Degree requirements:* For master's, comprehensive exam, thesis or alternative. *Entrance requirements:* For master's, GRE General Test, BSN with minimum GPA of 3.0, 3 references, 1 year of clinical experience. Additional exam requirements/recommendations for international students: Required—TOEFL (minimum score 550 paper-based; 79 iBT).

Western Connecticut State University, Division of Graduate Studies, School of Professional Studies, Ed D in Nursing Education Program (Online), Danbury, CT 06810-6885. Offers Ed D. Offered in collaboration with Southern Connecticut State University. Postbaccalaureate distance learning degree programs offered (no on-campus study). *Degree requirements:* For doctorate, thesis/dissertation. *Entrance requirements:* For doctorate, GRE or MAT, official transcripts, current copy of RN license, three letters of reference, curriculum vitae or resume, personal statement.

Western Governors University, College of Health Professions, Salt Lake City, UT 84107. Offers healthcare management (MBA); leadership and management (MSN); nursing education (MSN). Evening/weekend programs available. *Degree requirements:* For master's, capstone project. *Entrance requirements:* For master's, Readiness Assessment, transcripts. Additional exam requirements/recommendations for international students: Required—TOEFL (minimum score 450 paper-based; 80 iBT). Electronic applications accepted.

Westminster College, School of Nursing and Health Sciences, Salt Lake City, UT 84105-3697. Offers family nurse practitioner (MSN); nurse anesthesia (MSNA); nurse education (MSNED); nursing (MSN); public health (MPH). *Accreditation:* AACN; AANA/CANAEP. *Faculty:* 11 full-time (5 women), 7 part-time/adjunct (4 women). *Students:* 119 full-time (75 women), 5 part-time (2 women); includes 21 minority (5 Black or African American, non-Hispanic/Latino; 1 American Indian or Alaska Native, non-Hispanic/Latino; 4 Asian, non-Hispanic/Latino; 7 Hispanic/Latino; 1 Native Hawaiian or other Pacific Islander, non-Hispanic/Latino; 3 Two or more races, non-Hispanic/Latino), 4 international. Average age 32. 246 applicants, 35% accepted, 56 enrolled. In 2013, 49 master's awarded. *Degree requirements:* For master's, clinical practicum, 504 clinical practice hours. *Entrance requirements:* For master's, GRE, resume, Utah RN license in good standing, minimum GPA of 3.0, 3 letters of reference, BSN from accredited nursing program, proof of clear state and federal background check, drug test results, personal interview, current PALS certification, current ACLS certification, document of current immunizations, physical and mental health certificate. Additional exam requirements/recommendations for international students: Required—TOEFL (minimum score 600 paper-based; 100 iBT), IELTS (minimum score 7.5). *Application deadline:* Applications are processed on a rolling basis. Application fee: $50. Electronic applications accepted. *Expenses:* Contact institution. *Financial support:* In 2013–14, 9 students received support. Career-related internships or fieldwork, unspecified assistantships, and tuition reimbursements, tuition remission available. Support available to part-time students. Financial award applicants required to submit FAFSA. *Faculty research:* Collaborative testing in nursing: student outcomes and perspectives, implementing new educational paradigms into pre-licensure nursing curricula. *Unit head:* Dr. Sheryl Steadman, Dean, 801-832-2164, Fax: 801-832-3110, E-mail: ssteadman@westminstercollege.edu. *Application contact:* Dr. John Baworowsky, Vice President of Enrollment Management, 801-832-2200, Fax: 801-832-3101, E-mail: admission@westminstercollege.edu.
Website: http://www.westminstercollege.edu/msn

West Virginia Wesleyan College, Department of Nursing, Buckhannon, WV 26201. Offers family nurse practitioner (Post Master's Certificate); family nurse practitoner (MS); nurse administrator (MS); nurse educator (MS); nurse-midwifery (MS); nursing administration (Post Master's Certificate); nursing education (Post Master's Certificate); psychiatric mental health nurse practitioner (MS); MSN/MBA.

Winona State University, College of Nursing and Health Sciences, Winona, MN 55987. Offers adult nurse practitioner (MS, Post Master's Certificate); clinical nurse specialist (MS, Post Master's Certificate); family nurse practitioner (MS, Post Master's Certificate); nurse administrator (MS); nurse educator (MS, Post Master's Certificate); nursing (DNP). *Accreditation:* AACN. Part-time programs available. Postbaccalaureate distance learning degree programs offered (no on-campus study). *Degree requirements:* For master's, thesis; for doctorate, capstone. *Entrance requirements:* For master's, GRE (if GPA less than 3.0). Additional exam requirements/recommendations for international students: Required—TOEFL (minimum score 550 paper-based).

Worcester State University, Graduate Studies, Department of Nursing, Program in Nurse Educator, Worcester, MA 01602-2597. Offers MSN. *Accreditation:* AACN. Part-time programs available. *Faculty:* 3 full-time (all women), 3 part-time/adjunct (all women). *Students:* 1 (woman) full-time, 21 part-time (20 women); includes 2 minority (1 Black or African American, non-Hispanic/Latino; 1 Hispanic/Latino). Average age 45. 43 applicants, 72% accepted, 6 enrolled. *Degree requirements:* For master's, practicum. *Entrance requirements:* For master's, GRE, MAT, unencumbered license to practice as a Registered Nurse in Massachusetts. Additional exam requirements/recommendations for international students: Required—TOEFL (minimum score 500 paper-based; 61 iBT). *Application deadline:* For fall admission, 6/15 for domestic and international students; for spring admission, 4/1 for domestic and international students. Applications are processed on a rolling basis. Application fee: $40. Electronic applications accepted. *Expenses: Tuition, area resident:* Part-time $150 per credit. Tuition, state resident: part-time $150 per credit. Tuition, nonresident: part-time $150 per credit. *Required fees:* $114.50 per credit. *Financial support:* Application deadline: 3/1; applicants required to submit FAFSA. *Unit head:* Dr. Stephanie Chalupka, Coordinator, 508-929-8680, E-mail: schalupka@worcester.edu. *Application contact:* Sara Grady, Assistant Dean of Continuing Education, 508-929-8787, Fax: 508-929-8100, E-mail: sara.grady@worcester.edu.

Xavier University, College of Social Sciences, Health and Education, School of Nursing, Nursing Program, Cincinnati, OH 45207. Offers clinical nurse leader (MSN); education (MSN); forensic nursing (MSN); healthcare law (MSN); informatics (MSN); nursing administration (MSN); school nursing (MSN); MSN/M Ed; MSN/MBA; MSN/MS. *Faculty:* 16 full-time (15 women), 9 part-time/adjunct (all women). *Students:* 66 full-time (56 women), 170 part-time (162 women); includes 35 minority (17 Black or African American, non-Hispanic/Latino; 2 American Indian or Alaska Native, non-Hispanic/Latino; 5 Asian, non-Hispanic/Latino; 10 Hispanic/Latino; 1 Native Hawaiian or other Pacific Islander, non-Hispanic/Latino). Average age 37. 103 applicants, 66% accepted, 86 enrolled. In 2013, 78 master's awarded. *Expenses: Tuition:* Part-time $594 per credit hour. *Required fees:* $3 per semester. *Financial support:* In 2013–14, 68 students received support. *Unit head:* Dr. Susan M. Schmidt, Director, School of Nursing, 513-745-3814, E-mail: schmidt@xavier.edu. *Application contact:* Marilyn Volk Gomez, Director of Nursing Student Services, 513-745-4392, Fax: 513-745-1087, E-mail: gomez@xavier.edu.
Website: http://www.xavier.edu/msn/

York College of Pennsylvania, Department of Nursing, York, PA 17405-7199. Offers adult gerontology clinical nurse specialist (MS), including administration, education; adult gerontology nurse practitioner (MS); certified nurse anesthetist (MS); nurse educator (MS); nursing (DNP). *Accreditation:* AACN; AANA/CANAEP. Part-time and evening/weekend programs available. *Faculty:* 10 full-time (all women), 4 part-time/adjunct (1 woman). *Students:* 33 full-time (26 women), 61 part-time (53 women);

includes 12 minority (7 Black or African American, non-Hispanic/Latino; 2 American Indian or Alaska Native, non-Hispanic/Latino; 3 Asian, non-Hispanic/Latino), 1 international. Average age 37. 87 applicants, 31% accepted, 24 enrolled. In 2013, 26 master's, 4 doctorates awarded. *Entrance requirements:* For master's, GRE General Test, minimum GPA of 3.0 from CCNE- or NLNAC-accredited institution; for doctorate, master's degree in nursing from a CCNE- or NLNAC-accredited institution; minimum GPA of 3.0. Additional exam requirements/recommendations for international students: Required—TOEFL (minimum score 530 paper-based; 72 iBT). *Application deadline:* For fall admission, 7/15 priority date for domestic students; for spring admission, 11/15 priority date for domestic students. Applications are processed on a rolling basis. Application fee: $50. Electronic applications accepted. *Expenses: Tuition:* Full-time $12,870; part-time $715 per credit. *Required fees:* $1660; $360 per semester. Tuition and fees vary according to degree level. *Financial support:* Federal Work-Study available. *Faculty research:* Student stress response to simulation versus clinical, evidence-based practice in all clinical settings. *Unit head:* Dr. Richard Haas, Graduate Program Director, 717-815-1243, E-mail: rhaas@ycp.edu. *Application contact:* Diane Dube, Administrative Assistant, Graduate Programs in Nursing, 717-815-1462, E-mail: ddube@ycp.edu.
Website: http://www.ycp.edu/academics/academic-departments/nursing/

Nursing Informatics

Austin Peay State University, College of Graduate Studies, College of Behavioral and Health Sciences, School of Nursing, Clarksville, TN 37044. Offers advanced practice (MSN); nursing administration (MSN); nursing education (MSN); nursing informatics (MSN). Part-time programs available. Postbaccalaureate distance learning degree programs offered. *Faculty:* 9 full-time (all women), 7 part-time/adjunct (all women). *Students:* 47 full-time (43 women), 136 part-time (129 women); includes 30 minority (18 Black or African American, non-Hispanic/Latino; 4 Asian, non-Hispanic/Latino; 4 Hispanic/Latino; 4 Two or more races, non-Hispanic/Latino). Average age 35. 47 applicants, 85% accepted, 37 enrolled. In 2013, 39 master's awarded. *Degree requirements:* For master's, comprehensive exam. *Entrance requirements:* For master's, GRE General Test, minimum GPA of 3.0, RN license eligibility, 3 letters of recommendation. Additional exam requirements/recommendations for international students: Required—TOEFL (minimum score 600 paper-based). *Application deadline:* For fall admission, 8/5 priority date for domestic students. Applications are processed on a rolling basis. Application fee: $25. Electronic applications accepted. *Expenses:* Tuition, state resident: full-time $7500; part-time $375 per credit hour. Tuition, nonresident: full-time $20,800; part-time $1040 per credit hour. *Required fees:* $1284; $64.20 per credit hour. *Financial support:* In 2013–14, research assistantships with full tuition reimbursements (averaging $6,500 per year) were awarded; career-related internships or fieldwork, Federal Work-Study, institutionally sponsored loans, scholarships/grants, and unspecified assistantships also available. Support available to part-time students. *Unit head:* Dr. Patty Orr, Director, 931-221-7710, Fax: 931-221-7595, E-mail: orrp@apsu.edu. *Application contact:* June D. Lee, Graduate Coordinator, 800-859-4723, Fax: 931-221-7641, E-mail: gradadmissions@apsu.edu.
Website: http://www.apsu.edu/nursing

Duke University, School of Nursing, Durham, NC 27708-0586. Offers acute care pediatric nurse practitioner (MSN); adult-gerontology nurse practitioner - acute care (MSN, Post Master's Certificate); adult-gerontology nurse practitioner - primary care (MSN, Post Master's Certificate), including adult-gerontology nurse practitioner (MSN), cardiology, oncology; family nurse practitioner (MSN); neonatal nurse practitioner (MSN); nurse anesthesia (MSN, DNP); nursing (PhD); nursing and health care leadership (MSN); nursing education (MSN); nursing informatics (MSN, Post Master's Certificate); pediatric nurse practitioner - primary care (MSN). *Accreditation:* AACN; AANA/CANAEP. Part-time and evening/weekend programs available. Postbaccalaureate distance learning degree programs offered (minimal on-campus study). *Faculty:* 74 full-time (64 women), 7 part-time/adjunct (4 women). *Students:* 127 full-time (113 women), 473 part-time (433 women); includes 131 minority (54 Black or African American, non-Hispanic/Latino; 9 American Indian or Alaska Native, non-Hispanic/Latino; 36 Asian, non-Hispanic/Latino; 27 Hispanic/Latino; 5 Native Hawaiian or other Pacific Islander, non-Hispanic/Latino), 14 international. Average age 34. 516 applicants, 50% accepted, 190 enrolled. In 2013, 179 master's, 49 doctorates, 23 other advanced degrees awarded. Terminal master's awarded for partial completion of doctoral program. *Degree requirements:* For master's, thesis optional; for doctorate, capstone project. *Entrance requirements:* For master's, GRE General Test (waived if undergraduate GPA of 3.4 or higher), 1 year of nursing experience (recommended), BSN, minimum GPA of 3.0, previous course work in statistics; for doctorate, GRE General Test (waived if undergraduate GPA of 3.4 or higher), BSN or MSN, minimum GPA of 3.0, portfolio, resume, personal statement, undergraduate statistics course, current licensure as a registered nurse, transcripts from all post-secondary institutions; for Post Master's Certificate, MSN, licensure or eligibility as a professional nurse, transcripts from all post-secondary institutions, previous course work in statistics. Additional exam requirements/recommendations for international students: Recommended—TOEFL (minimum score 550 paper-based; 83 iBT), IELTS (minimum score 7). *Application deadline:* For fall admission, 12/1 for domestic and international students; for spring admission, 5/1 for domestic and international students. Application fee: $50. Electronic applications accepted. *Expenses:* Contact institution. *Financial support:* Career-related internships or fieldwork, institutionally sponsored loans, scholarships/grants, traineeships, and tuition waivers (partial) available. Support available to part-time students. Financial award applicants required to submit FAFSA. *Faculty research:* Cardiovascular disease, caregiver skill training, data mining, prostate cancer, neonatal immune system. *Unit head:* Dr. Catherine L. Gilliss, Dean/Vice Chancellor for Nursing Affairs, 919-684-9444, Fax: 919-684-9414, E-mail: catherine.gilliss@duke.edu. *Application contact:* Ernie Rushing, Lead Admissions Processor/Admissions Officer, 919-668-6274, Fax: 919-668-4693, E-mail: stephen.rushing@dm.duke.edu.
Website: http://www.nursing.duke.edu/

Excelsior College, School of Nursing, Albany, NY 12203-5159. Offers clinical systems management (MS); nursing (MS); nursing education (MS); nursing informatics (MS). Part-time and evening/weekend programs available. Postbaccalaureate distance learning degree programs offered (no on-campus study). *Faculty:* 13 part-time/adjunct (all women). *Students:* 550 part-time (448 women); includes 184 minority (106 Black or African American, non-Hispanic/Latino; 4 American Indian or Alaska Native, non-Hispanic/Latino; 30 Asian, non-Hispanic/Latino; 29 Hispanic/Latino; 5 Native Hawaiian or other Pacific Islander, non-Hispanic/Latino; 10 Two or more races, non-Hispanic/Latino). Average age 46. In 2013, 124 master's awarded. *Entrance requirements:* For master's, RN license. *Application deadline:* Applications are processed on a rolling basis. Application fee: $100. Electronic applications accepted. *Expenses: Tuition:* Part-time $565 per credit. *Financial support:* Scholarships/grants and traineeships available. Support available to part-time students. Financial award application deadline: 8/21. *Faculty research:* Leadership development, test anxiety, use of technology in online learning. *Unit head:* Dr. Barbara Pieper, Associate Dean, Graduate Program in Nursing, 518-464-8500, Fax: 518-464-8777, E-mail: msn@excelsior.edu. *Application contact:* Christine McIlwraith, Graduate Advisor, 518-464-8500, Fax: 518-464-8777, E-mail: nursingmasters@excelsior.edu.

Ferris State University, College of Health Professions, School of Nursing, Big Rapids, MI 49307. Offers nursing (MSN); nursing administration (MSN); nursing education (MSN); nursing informatics (MSN). Part-time and evening/weekend programs available. Postbaccalaureate distance learning degree programs offered (minimal on-campus study). *Faculty:* 5 full-time (all women), 1 (woman) part-time/adjunct. *Students:* 1 (woman) full-time, 103 part-time (91 women); includes 5 minority (2 Black or African American, non-Hispanic/Latino; 1 American Indian or Alaska Native, non-Hispanic/Latino; 1 Native Hawaiian or other Pacific Islander, non-Hispanic/Latino; 1 Two or more races, non-Hispanic/Latino). Average age 40. 25 applicants, 92% accepted, 21 enrolled. In 2013, 20 master's awarded. *Degree requirements:* For master's, comprehensive exam, practicum, practicum project. *Entrance requirements:* For master's, BS in nursing or related field with registered nurse license, writing sample, letters of reference, 2 years' clinical experience. Additional exam requirements/recommendations for international students: Required—TOEFL (minimum score 550 paper-based; 61 iBT). *Application deadline:* For fall admission, 4/15 priority date for domestic students; for spring admission, 10/15 for domestic students. Applications are processed on a rolling basis. Application fee: $30. Electronic applications accepted. Application fee is waived when completed online. *Financial support:* In 2013–14, 3 students received support. Fellowships, research assistantships, teaching assistantships, career-related internships or fieldwork, and scholarships/grants available. Financial award application deadline: 4/15. *Faculty research:* Nursing education-minority student focus, student attitudes toward aging. *Unit head:* Dr. Susan Owens, Program Coordinator, 231-591-2267, Fax: 231-591-2325, E-mail: owenss3@ferris.edu. *Application contact:* Debby Buck, Off-Campus Program Secretary, 231-591-2270, Fax: 231-591-3788, E-mail: buckd@ferris.edu.
Website: http://www.ferris.edu/htmls/colleges/alliedhe/Nursing/homepage.htm

Georgia State University, Byrdine F. Lewis School of Nursing, Atlanta, GA 30303. Offers adult health clinical nurse specialist/nurse practitioner (MS, Certificate); child health clinical nurse specialist/pediatric nurse practitioner (MS, Certificate); family nurse practitioner (MS, Certificate); family psychiatric mental health nurse practitioner (MS, Certificate); nursing (PhD); nursing leadership in healthcare innovations (MS), including nursing administration, nursing informatics; nutrition (MS); perinatal clinical nurse specialist/women's health nurse practitioner (MS, Certificate); physical therapy (DPT); respiratory therapy (MS). *Accreditation:* AACN. Part-time programs available. Postbaccalaureate distance learning degree programs offered (minimal on-campus study). *Faculty:* 22 full-time (16 women). *Students:* 241 full-time (180 women), 262 part-time (236 women); includes 176 minority (120 Black or African American, non-Hispanic/Latino; 31 Asian, non-Hispanic/Latino; 13 Hispanic/Latino; 3 Native Hawaiian or other Pacific Islander, non-Hispanic/Latino; 9 Two or more races, non-Hispanic/Latino), 19 international. Average age 34. 583 applicants, 34% accepted, 160 enrolled. In 2013, 110 master's, 44 doctorates, 6 other advanced degrees awarded. *Degree requirements:* For doctorate, comprehensive exam, thesis/dissertation. *Entrance requirements:* For doctorate, GRE. Additional exam requirements/recommendations for international students: Required—TOEFL. *Application deadline:* For fall admission, 2/1 priority date for domestic and international students; for spring admission, 9/15 for domestic and international students. Applications are processed on a rolling basis. Application fee: $50. Electronic applications accepted. *Expenses:* Contact institution. *Financial support:* In 2013–14, research assistantships with full and partial tuition reimbursements (averaging $1,666 per year), teaching assistantships with full and partial tuition reimbursements (averaging $1,920 per year) were awarded; scholarships/grants, tuition waivers (full and partial), and unspecified assistantships also available. Support available to part-time students. Financial award application deadline: 8/1; financial award applicants required to submit FAFSA. *Faculty research:* Stroke intervention for caregivers, stroke prevention in African Americans; relationships between psychological distress and health outcomes in parents with a medically ill infant; medically fragile children; nursing expertise and patient outcomes. *Unit head:* Joan S. Cranford, Assistant Dean for Nursing, 404-413-1200, Fax: 404-413-1205, E-mail: jcranford2@gsu.edu. *Application contact:* Tiffany Norman, Senior Administrative Coordinator, 404-413-1190, Fax: 404-413-1205, E-mail: tnorman7@gsu.edu.
Website: http://nursing.gsu.edu/

Grantham University, College of Nursing and Allied Health, Lenexa, KS 66219. Offers case management (MSN); health systems management (MS); healthcare administration (MHA); nursing education (MSN); nursing informatics (MSN); nursing management and organizational leadership (MSN). Part-time and evening/weekend programs available. Postbaccalaureate distance learning degree programs offered (no on-campus study). *Faculty:* 1 (woman) full-time, 11 part-time/adjunct (5 women). *Students:* 64 full-time (43 women), 166 part-time (123 women); includes 116 minority (94 Black or African American, non-Hispanic/Latino; 4 Asian, non-Hispanic/Latino; 9 Hispanic/Latino; 1 Native Hawaiian or other Pacific Islander, non-Hispanic/Latino; 8 Two or more races, non-Hispanic/Latino). Average age 40. 230 applicants, 100% accepted, 230 enrolled. In 2013, 61 master's awarded. *Degree requirements:* For master's, thesis, major applied research paper and practicum (MSN). *Entrance requirements:* For master's, bachelor's degree from accredited degree-granting institution with minimum GPA of 2.5, BSN from an accredited nursing program, valid RN license. Additional exam requirements/recommendations for international students: Required—TOEFL (minimum score 530 paper-based; 71 iBT). *Application deadline:* Applications are processed on a rolling basis. Application fee: $30. Electronic applications accepted. *Expenses: Tuition:* Full-time $3900; part-time $325 per credit hour. *Required fees:* $35 per term. One-time fee: $100. *Financial support:* In 2013–14, 230 students received support. Scholarships/grants available. *Faculty research:* Pharmacy licensure, vaccination certification. *Unit head:* Dr. Susan Fairchild, Dean, School of Nursing, 800-955-2527, E-mail:

admissions@grantham.edu. *Application contact:* Jared Parlette, Vice President of Admissions, 800-955-2527, E-mail: admissions@grantham.edu.
Website: http://www.grantham.edu/colleges-and-schools/college-of-nursing-and-allied-health/

Le Moyne College, Department of Nursing, Syracuse, NY 13214. Offers informatics (MS, CAS); nursing administration (MS, CAS); nursing education (MS, CAS); nursing gerontology (MS, CAS); palliative care (MS, CAS). *Accreditation:* AACN. Part-time and evening/weekend programs available. *Faculty:* 4 full-time (all women), 3 part-time/adjunct (2 women). *Students:* 13 part-time (12 women); includes 2 minority (both Black or African American, non-Hispanic/Latino). Average age 41. 14 applicants, 86% accepted, 5 enrolled. In 2013, 6 master's, 6 other advanced degrees awarded. *Degree requirements:* For master's, scholarly project. *Entrance requirements:* For master's, bachelor's degree, interview, minimum GPA of 3.0, New York RN license, 2 letters of recommendation, writing sample, transcripts. Additional exam requirements/recommendations for international students: Required—TOEFL (minimum score 550 paper-based; 79 iBT). *Application deadline:* For fall admission, 8/1 priority date for domestic and international students; for spring admission, 12/15 priority date for domestic and international students; for summer admission, 5/1 priority date for domestic and international students. Applications are processed on a rolling basis. Application fee: $50. *Expenses:* Contact institution. *Financial support:* In 2013–14, 2 students received support. Career-related internships or fieldwork, scholarships/grants, health care benefits, and unspecified assistantships available. Support available to part-time students. Financial award applicants required to submit FAFSA. *Faculty research:* Inter-profession education, gerontology, utilization of free healthcare services by the insured, health promotion education, innovative undergraduate nursing education models, patient and family education, horizontal violence. *Unit head:* Dr. Susan B. Bastable, Chair and Professor, Department of Nursing, 315-445-5436, Fax: 315-445-6024, E-mail: bastabsb@lemoyne.edu. *Application contact:* Kristen P. Trapasso, Senior Director of Enrollment Management, 315-445-4265, Fax: 315-445-6092, E-mail: trapaskp@lemoyne.edu.
Website: http://www.lemoyne.edu/nursing

Loyola University Chicago, Graduate School, Marcella Niehoff School of Nursing, Doctor of Nursing Practice Program, Maywood, IL 60153. Offers infection prevention (DNP); informatics and outcomes (DNP). Evening/weekend programs available. Postbaccalaureate distance learning degree programs offered (minimal on-campus study). *Faculty:* 45 full-time (44 women). *Students:* 4 full-time (all women), 27 part-time (24 women); includes 9 minority (3 Black or African American, non-Hispanic/Latino; 2 Asian, non-Hispanic/Latino; 4 Hispanic/Latino). Average age 46. 26 applicants, 62% accepted, 12 enrolled. In 2013, 8 doctorates awarded. *Degree requirements:* For doctorate, capstone project. *Entrance requirements:* For doctorate, BSN or MSN, minimum GPA of 3.25, Illinois nursing license, 3 letters of recommendation, 1000 hours of experience and certification in area of specialty, curriculum vitae. Additional exam requirements/recommendations for international students: Required—TOEFL. *Expenses: Tuition:* Full-time $16,740; part-time $930 per credit. *Required fees:* $135 per semester. *Unit head:* Dr. Marijo Letizia, Associate Dean, 708-216-9325, Fax: 708-216-9555, E-mail: mletizi@luc.edu. *Application contact:* Amy Weatherford, Enrollment Advisor, School of Nursing, 773-508-3249, Fax: 773-508-3241, E-mail: aweatherford@luc.edu.
Website: http://www.luc.edu/nursing/dnp/

Molloy College, Division of Nursing, Rockville Centre, NY 11571-5002. Offers adult nurse practitioner (Advanced Certificate); clinical nurse specialist: adult health (Advanced Certificate); family nurse practitioner (Advanced Certificate); nurse practitioner psychiatry (Advanced Certificate); nursing (MS, PhD); nursing administration (Advanced Certificate); nursing administration with informatics (Advanced Certificate); nursing education (Advanced Certificate); nursing informatics (Advanced Certificate); pediatric nurse practitioner (Advanced Certificate). *Accreditation:* AACN. Part-time and evening/weekend programs available. *Faculty:* 30 full-time (29 women), 10 part-time/adjunct (7 women). *Students:* 18 full-time (all women), 538 part-time (495 women); includes 289 minority (159 Black or African American, non-Hispanic/Latino; 1 American Indian or Alaska Native, non-Hispanic/Latino; 80 Asian, non-Hispanic/Latino; 43 Hispanic/Latino; 4 Native Hawaiian or other Pacific Islander, non-Hispanic/Latino; 2 Two or more races, non-Hispanic/Latino), 2 international. Average age 38. 241 applicants, 63% accepted, 122 enrolled. In 2013, 84 master's, 2 other advanced degrees awarded. *Degree requirements:* For master's, thesis optional. *Entrance requirements:* For master's, 3 letters of reference, BS in nursing, minimum undergraduate GPA of 3.0; for Advanced Certificate, 3 letters of reference, master's degree in nursing. *Application deadline:* For fall admission, 9/2 priority date for domestic students; for spring admission, 1/20 priority date for domestic students. Applications are processed on a rolling basis. Application fee: $60. *Expenses: Tuition:* Full-time $16,920; part-time $940 per credit. *Required fees:* $880. *Financial support:* Research assistantships with partial tuition reimbursements, teaching assistantships with partial tuition reimbursements, institutionally sponsored loans, scholarships/grants, and unspecified assistantships available. Support available to part-time students. Financial award application deadline: 4/1; financial award applicants required to submit FAFSA. *Unit head:* Dr. Jeannine Muldoon, Dean of Nursing, 516-323-3651, E-mail: jmuldoon@molloy.edu. *Application contact:* Alina Haitz, Assistant Director of Graduate Admissions, 516-323-4008, E-mail: ahaitz@molloy.edu.
Website: http://www.molloy.edu/academics/nursing-division

National University, Academic Affairs, School of Health and Human Services, La Jolla, CA 92037-1011. Offers clinical affairs (MS); clinical informatics (Certificate); clinical regulatory affairs (MS); health and life science analytics (MS); health coaching (Certificate); health informatics (MS); healthcare administration (MHA); nurse anesthesia (MS); nursing (MS), including forensic nursing, nursing administration, nursing informatics; nursing administration (Certificate); nursing informatics (Certificate); nursing practice (DNP); public health (MPH), including health promotion, healthcare administration, mental health. Part-time and evening/weekend programs available. Postbaccalaureate distance learning degree programs offered (no on-campus study). *Faculty:* 20 full-time (12 women), 27 part-time/adjunct (16 women). *Students:* 229 full-time (176 women), 89 part-time (52 women); includes 215 minority (58 Black or African American, non-Hispanic/Latino; 1 American Indian or Alaska Native, non-Hispanic/Latino; 68 Asian, non-Hispanic/Latino; 63 Hispanic/Latino; 8 Native Hawaiian or other Pacific Islander, non-Hispanic/Latino; 17 Two or more races, non-Hispanic/Latino), 18 international. Average age 33. 118 applicants, 100% accepted, 92 enrolled. In 2013, 29 master's awarded. *Degree requirements:* For master's, thesis (for some programs). *Entrance requirements:* For master's, interview, minimum GPA of 2.5. Additional exam requirements/recommendations for international students: Required—TOEFL (minimum score 550 paper-based; 79 iBT), IELTS (minimum score 6). *Application deadline:* Applications are processed on a rolling basis. Application fee: $60 ($65 for international students). Electronic applications accepted. *Expenses: Tuition:* Full-time $13,824; part-time $1728 per course. One-time fee: $160. *Financial support:* Career-related internships or fieldwork, institutionally sponsored loans, scholarships/grants, and tuition waivers (partial) available. Support available to part-time students. Financial award application deadline: 6/30; financial award applicants required to submit FAFSA. *Faculty research:* Nursing education, obesity prevention, workforce diversity. *Unit head:* School of Health and Human Services, 800-628-8648, E-mail: shhs@nu.edu. *Application contact:* Louis Cruz, Interim Vice President for Enrollment Services, 800-628-8648, E-mail: advisor@nu.edu.
Website: http://www.nu.edu/OurPrograms/SchoolOfHealthAndHumanServices.html

New York University, College of Nursing, Programs in Advanced Practice Nursing, New York, NY 10012-1019. Offers advanced practice nursing: adult acute care (MS, Advanced Certificate); advanced practice nursing: adult nurse practitioner/holistic nurse practitioner (Advanced Certificate); advanced practice nursing: adult nurse practitioner/palliative care nurse practitioner (Advanced Certificate); advanced practice nursing: adult primary care (MS, Advanced Certificate); advanced practice nursing: family (MS, Advanced Certificate); advanced practice nursing: geriatrics (Advanced Certificate); advanced practice nursing: mental health (MS); advanced practice nursing: mental health nursing (Advanced Certificate); advanced practice nursing: pediatrics (MS, Advanced Certificate); nurse midwifery (MS, Advanced Certificate); nursing administration (MS, Advanced Certificate); nursing education (MS, Advanced Certificate); nursing informatics (MS, Advanced Certificate); MS/MPA; MS/MPH. *Accreditation:* AACN; ACNM/ACME. Part-time programs available. *Faculty:* 22 full-time (all women), 54 part-time/adjunct (46 women). *Students:* 36 full-time (31 women), 622 part-time (549 women); includes 239 minority (73 Black or African American, non-Hispanic/Latino; 1 American Indian or Alaska Native, non-Hispanic/Latino; 116 Asian, non-Hispanic/Latino; 36 Hispanic/Latino; 6 Native Hawaiian or other Pacific Islander, non-Hispanic/Latino; 7 Two or more races, non-Hispanic/Latino), 16 international. Average age 37. 395 applicants, 67% accepted, 156 enrolled. In 2013, 186 master's, 8 other advanced degrees awarded. *Degree requirements:* For master's, thesis (for some programs). *Entrance requirements:* For master's, BS in nursing, AS in nursing with another BS/BA, interview, RN license, 1 year of clinical experience (3 for nursing education program); for Advanced Certificate, master's degree. Additional exam requirements/recommendations for international students: Required—TOEFL (minimum score 90 iBT), IELTS (minimum score 7). *Application deadline:* For fall admission, 7/1 for domestic and international students; for spring admission, 12/1 for domestic and international students. Application fee: $80. Electronic applications accepted. *Expenses: Tuition:* Full-time $35,856; part-time $1494 per unit. *Required fees:* $1408; $64 per unit. $473 per term. Tuition and fees vary according to course load and program. *Financial support:* In 2013–14, 182 students received support. Research assistantships, career-related internships or fieldwork, Federal Work-Study, scholarships/grants, traineeships, and unspecified assistantships available. Support available to part-time students. Financial award application deadline: 2/1; financial award applicants required to submit FAFSA. *Faculty research:* Geriatrics, HIV, elderly black diabetics, families and illness, oral systemic connection. *Unit head:* Dr. Judith Haber, Associate Dean, Graduate Programs, 212-998-9020, Fax: 212-995-3143, E-mail: jh33@nyu.edu. *Application contact:* Elizabeth Ensweiler, Assistant Director, Graduate Student Affairs and Admissions, 212-992-7653, Fax: 212-995-4302, E-mail: ee39@nyu.edu.

Rutgers, The State University of New Jersey, Newark, Rutgers School of Nursing, Program in Nursing Informatics - Newark, Newark, NJ 07102. Offers MSN. Program offered jointly with New Jersey Institute of Technology. *Entrance requirements:* Additional exam requirements/recommendations for international students: Required—TOEFL. Electronic applications accepted.

Rutgers, The State University of New Jersey, Newark, Rutgers School of Nursing, Program in Nursing Informatics - Stratford, Newark, NJ 07102. Offers MSN. Program offered jointly with New Jersey Institute of Technology. *Entrance requirements:* Additional exam requirements/recommendations for international students: Required—TOEFL. Electronic applications accepted.

Seattle Pacific University, MS in Nursing Program, Seattle, WA 98119-1997. Offers administration (MSN); adult/gerontology nurse practitioner (MSN); clinical nurse specialist (MSN); family nurse practitioner (MSN, Certificate); informatics (MSN); nurse educator (MSN). *Accreditation:* AACN. Part-time programs available. *Students:* 9 full-time (7 women), 37 part-time (33 women); includes 8 minority (2 Black or African American, non-Hispanic/Latino; 5 Asian, non-Hispanic/Latino; 1 Hispanic/Latino), 1 international. Average age 41. 70 applicants, 30% accepted, 21 enrolled. In 2013, 27 master's awarded. *Degree requirements:* For master's, thesis. *Entrance requirements:* For master's, personal statement, transcripts, undergraduate nursing degree, proof of undergraduate statistics course with minimum GPA of 2.0, 2 recommendations. *Application deadline:* For fall admission, 1/15 priority date for domestic students; for spring admission, 1/15 for domestic students. Applications are processed on a rolling basis. Application fee: $50. Electronic applications accepted. *Expenses:* Contact institution. *Financial support:* Fellowships and scholarships/grants available. Financial award applicants required to submit FAFSA. *Unit head:* Dr. Susan Casey, Associate Dean, 206-281-2649, E-mail: caseys@spu.edu.
Website: http://www.spu.edu/depts/health-sciences/grad/index.asp

Tennessee Technological University, Whitson-Hester School of Nursing, Cookeville, TN 38505. Offers family nurse practitioner (MSN); informatics (MSN); nursing administration (MSN); nursing education (MSN). Part-time and evening/weekend programs available. Postbaccalaureate distance learning degree programs offered (no on-campus study). *Students:* 22 full-time (19 women), 101 part-time (94 women); includes 11 minority (5 Black or African American, non-Hispanic/Latino; 2 Asian, non-Hispanic/Latino; 1 Hispanic/Latino; 3 Two or more races, non-Hispanic/Latino). 79 applicants, 65% accepted, 38 enrolled. In 2013, 14 master's awarded. *Degree requirements:* For master's, comprehensive exam, thesis or alternative. *Entrance requirements:* Additional exam requirements/recommendations for international students: Required—TOEFL (minimum score 600 paper-based; 100 iBT), IELTS (minimum score 5.5), PTE, or TOEIC (Test of English as an International Communication). *Application deadline:* For fall admission, 8/1 for domestic students, 5/1 for international students; for spring admission, 12/1 for domestic students, 10/1 for international students. Applications are processed on a rolling basis. Application fee: $35 ($40 for international students). Electronic applications accepted. *Expenses:* Tuition, state resident: full-time $9347; part-time $465 per credit hour. Tuition, nonresident: full-time $23,635; part-time $1152 per credit hour. *Financial support:* Application deadline: 4/1. *Unit head:* Dr. Bedelia Russell, Director, 931-372-3203, Fax: 931-372-6244, E-mail: bhrussell@tntech.edu. *Application contact:* Shelia K. Kendrick, Coordinator of Graduate Studies, 931-372-3808, Fax: 931-372-3497, E-mail: skendrick@tntech.edu.

Troy University, Graduate School, College of Health and Human Services, Program in Nursing, Troy, AL 36082. Offers adult health (MSN); clinical nurse specialist adult health (DNP); clinical nurse specialist maternal infant (DNP); family nurse practitioner (MSN, DNP, PMC); informatics specialist (MSN); maternal infant (MSN). Part-time and evening/weekend programs available. *Faculty:* 15 full-time (8 women), 3 part-time/adjunct (1 woman). *Students:* 61 full-time (56 women), 228 part-time (193 women); includes 97 minority (77 Black or African American, non-Hispanic/Latino; 4 American Indian or Alaska Native, non-Hispanic/Latino; 2 Asian, non-Hispanic/Latino; 5 Hispanic/Latino; 9 Two or more races, non-Hispanic/Latino). Average age 34. 138 applicants, 80% accepted, 39 enrolled. In 2013, 81 master's, 9 doctorates awarded. *Degree requirements:* For master's, comprehensive exam, minimum GPA of 3.0, candidacy; for doctorate, minimum GPA of 3.0, submission of approved comprehensive e-portfolio, completion of residency synthesis project, minimum of 1000 hours of clinical practice, score of 80% or better on qualifying exam. *Entrance requirements:* For master's, GRE (minimum score of 850 on old exam or 294 on new exam) or GMAT (minimum score of 500), minimum GPA of 3.0, BSN, current RN licensure; 2 letters of reference, undergraduate health assessment course; for doctorate, GRE (minimum score of 850 on old exam or 294 on new exam) or GMAT (minimum score of 500), BSN or MSN, minimum GPA of 3.0, 2 letters of reference, current RN licensure, essay. Additional exam requirements/recommendations for international students: Required—TOEFL (minimum score 523 paper-based; 70 iBT), IELTS (minimum score 6). *Application deadline:* Applications are processed on a rolling basis. Application fee: $50. Electronic applications accepted. *Expenses:* Tuition, state resident: full-time $6084; part-time $338 per credit hour. Tuition, nonresident: full-time $12,168; part-time $676 per credit hour. *Required fees:* $630; $35 per credit hour. $50 per semester. *Financial support:* Available to part-time students. Applicants required to submit FAFSA. *Unit head:* Dr. Diane Weed, Director, School of Nursing, 334-670-5864, Fax: 334-670-3745, E-mail: lweed@troy.edu. *Application contact:* Brenda K. Campbell, Director of Graduate Admissions, 334-670-3178, Fax: 334-670-3733, E-mail: bcamp@troy.edu.

University of Memphis, Loewenberg School of Nursing, Memphis, TN 38152. Offers advance practice-family nurse practitioner (MSN); executive nursing leadership (MSN); nursing (Graduate Certificate); nursing administration (MSN); nursing education (MSN); nursing informatics (MSN). *Accreditation:* AACN. Part-time and evening/weekend programs available. Postbaccalaureate distance learning degree programs offered. *Faculty:* 18 full-time (16 women), 5 part-time/adjunct (0 women). *Students:* 23 full-time (21 women), 240 part-time (214 women); includes 112 minority (100 Black or African American, non-Hispanic/Latino; 9 Asian, non-Hispanic/Latino; 1 Hispanic/Latino; 2 Two or more races, non-Hispanic/Latino), 1 international. Average age 35. 176 applicants, 38% accepted, 25 enrolled. In 2013, 47 master's, 2 other advanced degrees awarded. *Degree requirements:* For master's, comprehensive exam, thesis optional, scholarly project; completion of clinical practicum hours. *Entrance requirements:* For master's, NCLEX Exam, interview. Additional exam requirements/recommendations for international students: Required—TOEFL (minimum score 550 paper-based; 79 iBT). *Application deadline:* For fall admission, 2/15 for domestic and international students; for spring admission, 10/1 for domestic and international students. Application fee: $35 ($60 for international students). *Financial support:* In 2013–14, 147 students received support. Federal Work-Study and scholarships/grants available. Financial award application deadline: 2/15; financial award applicants required to submit FAFSA. *Faculty research:* Technology in nursing, nurse retention, cultural competence, health policy, health access. *Total annual research expenditures:* $560,619. *Unit head:* Dr. Robert Koch, Associate Dean, 901-678-3908, Fax: 901-678-4907, E-mail: rakoch@memphis.edu. *Application contact:* Dr. Karen Weddle-West, Information Contact, 901-678-2531, Fax: 901-678-5023, E-mail: gradsch@memphis.edu.
Website: http://www.memphis.edu/nursing

University of Phoenix–Bay Area Campus, College of Nursing, San Jose, CA 95134-1805. Offers education (MHA); gerontology (MHA); health administration (MHA, DHA); informatics (MHA, MSN); nursing (MSN, PhD); nursing/health care education (MSN); MSN/MBA. Evening/weekend programs available. Postbaccalaureate distance learning degree programs offered (no on-campus study). *Degree requirements:* For master's, thesis (for some programs). *Entrance requirements:* For master's, minimum undergraduate GPA of 2.5, 3 years of work experience, RN license. Additional exam requirements/recommendations for international students: Required—TOEFL (minimum score 550 paper-based; 79 iBT). Electronic applications accepted.

University of Phoenix–Charlotte Campus, College of Nursing, Charlotte, NC 28273-3409. Offers education (MHA); gerontology (MHA); health administration (MHA); informatics (MHA, MSN); nursing (MSN); nursing/health care education (MSN). Evening/weekend programs available. *Degree requirements:* For master's, thesis (for some programs). *Entrance requirements:* For master's, minimum undergraduate GPA of 2.5, 3 years work experience. Additional exam requirements/recommendations for international students: Required—TOEFL (minimum score 550 paper-based; 79 iBT). Electronic applications accepted.

University of Phoenix–Des Moines Campus, College of Nursing, Des Moines, IA 50309. Offers education (MHA); gerontology (MHA); health administration (MHA, DHA); informatics (MHA, MSN); nursing (MSN, PhD); nursing/health care education (MSN).

University of Phoenix–Phoenix Campus, College of Health Sciences and Nursing, Tempe, AZ 85282-2371. Offers family nurse practitioner (MSN, Certificate); gerontology health care (Certificate); health care education (MSN, Certificate); health care informatics (Certificate); informatics (MSN); nursing (MSN); MSN/MHA. Evening/weekend programs available. Postbaccalaureate distance learning degree programs offered. *Entrance requirements:* Additional exam requirements/recommendations for international students: Required—TOEFL, TOEIC (Test of English as an International Communication), Berlitz Online English Proficiency Exam, PTE, or IELTS. Electronic applications accepted. *Expenses:* Contact institution.

University of Phoenix–Southern California Campus, College of Health Sciences and Nursing, Costa Mesa, CA 92626. Offers family nurse practitioner (MSN, Certificate); health care (Certificate); informatics (MSN); nursing (MSN); nursing/health care education (MSN, Certificate); MSN/MBA; MSN/MHA. Evening/weekend programs available. Postbaccalaureate distance learning degree programs offered. *Entrance requirements:* Additional exam requirements/recommendations for international students: Required—TOEFL, TOEIC (Test of English as an International Communication), Berlitz Online English Proficiency Exam, PTE, or IELTS. Electronic applications accepted. *Expenses:* Contact institution.

University of Phoenix–Washington D.C. Campus, College of Nursing, Washington, DC 20001. Offers education (MHA); gerontology (MHA); health administration (MHA, DHA); informatics (MHA, MSN); nursing (MSN, PhD); nursing/health care education (MSN); MSN/MBA; MSN/MHA.

University of Pittsburgh, School of Nursing, Nurse Specialty Role Program, Pittsburgh, PA 15260. Offers clinical nurse leader (MSN); nursing (DNP); nursing administration (MSN); nursing informatics (MSN). *Accreditation:* AACN. Part-time programs available. *Students:* 11 full-time (9 women), 70 part-time (60 women); includes 6 minority (3 Black or African American, non-Hispanic/Latino; 3 Asian, non-Hispanic/Latino), 2 international. Average age 38. 43 applicants, 74% accepted, 26 enrolled. In 2013, 13 master's, 10 doctorates awarded. *Degree requirements:* For master's, comprehensive exam, thesis optional. *Entrance requirements:* For master's, GRE or MAT, BSN, RN license, letters of recommendation, resume, course work in statistics, 1-3 years of nursing experience. Additional exam requirements/recommendations for international students: Required—TOEFL (minimum score 550 paper-based; 80 iBT). *Application deadline:* For fall admission, 6/1 priority date for domestic students, 6/1 for international students; for spring admission, 2/15 priority date for domestic students, 2/15 for international students. Applications are processed on a rolling basis. Application fee: $50. Electronic applications accepted. *Expenses:* Tuition, state resident: full-time $19,964; part-time $807 per credit. Tuition, nonresident: full-time $32,686; part-time $1337 per credit. *Required fees:* $740; $200. Tuition and fees vary according to program. *Unit head:* Dr. Sandra Engberg, Associate Dean for Clinical Education, 412-624-3835, Fax: 412-624-8521, E-mail: sje1@pitt.edu. *Application contact:* Laurie Lapsley, Administrator of Graduate Student Services, 412-624-9670, Fax: 412-624-2409, E-mail: lapsleyl@pitt.edu.
Website: http://www.nursing.pitt.edu/

Vanderbilt University, Vanderbilt University School of Nursing, Nashville, TN 37240. Offers adult-gerontology acute care nurse practitioner (MSN), including hospitalist, intensivist; adult-gerontology primary care nurse practitioner (MSN); emergency nurse practitioner (MSN); family nurse practitioner (MSN); healthcare leadership (MSN); neonatal nurse practitioner (MSN); nurse midwifery (MSN); nurse midwifery/family nurse practitioner (MSN); nursing informatics (MSN); nursing practice (DNP); nursing science (PhD); pediatric acute care nurse practitioner (MSN); pediatric primary care nurse practitioner (MSN); psychiatric-mental health nurse practitioner (MSN); women's health nurse practitioner (MSN); women's health nurse practitioner/adult gerontology primary care nurse practitioner (MSN); MSN/M Div; MSN/MTS. *Accreditation:* ACNM/ACME (one or more programs are accredited). Part-time programs available. Postbaccalaureate distance learning degree programs offered (minimal on-campus study). *Faculty:* 139 full-time (124 women), 452 part-time/adjunct (319 women). *Students:* 527 full-time (463 women), 369 part-time (333 women); includes 120 minority (46 Black or African American, non-Hispanic/Latino; 8 American Indian or Alaska Native, non-Hispanic/Latino; 26 Asian, non-Hispanic/Latino; 24 Hispanic/Latino; 4 Native Hawaiian or other Pacific Islander, non-Hispanic/Latino; 12 Two or more races, non-Hispanic/Latino), 7 international. Average age 32. 1,257 applicants, 49% accepted, 457 enrolled. In 2013, 364 master's, 43 doctorates awarded. *Degree requirements:* For doctorate, comprehensive exam, thesis/dissertation. *Entrance requirements:* For master's, GRE General Test (within the past 5 years), minimum B average in undergraduate course work, 3 letters of recommendation; for doctorate, GRE General Test, interview, 3 letters of recommendation from doctorally-prepared faculty, MSN, essay. Additional exam requirements/recommendations for international students: Required—TOEFL (minimum score 570 paper-based), IELTS (minimum score 6.5). *Application deadline:* For fall admission, 12/1 priority date for domestic and international students. Applications are processed on a rolling basis. Application fee: $50. Electronic applications accepted. *Expenses:* Contact institution. *Financial support:* In 2013–14, 582 students received support. Scholarships/grants and health care benefits available. Support available to part-time students. Financial award application deadline: 3/15; financial award applicants required to submit FAFSA. *Faculty research:* Lymphedema, palliative care and bereavement, health services research including workforce, safety and quality of care, gerontology, better birth outcomes including nutrition. *Total annual research expenditures:* $2.5 million. *Unit head:* Dr. Linda Norman, Dean, 615-343-8876, Fax: 615-343-7711, E-mail: linda.norman@vanderbilt.edu. *Application contact:* Patricia Peerman, Assistant Dean for Enrollment Management, 615-322-3800, Fax: 615-343-0333, E-mail: vusn-admissions@vanderbilt.edu.
Website: http://www.nursing.vanderbilt.edu

Walden University, Graduate Programs, School of Nursing, Minneapolis, MN 55401. Offers adult-gerontology acute care nurse practitioner (MSN); adult-gerontology nurse practitioner (MSN); education (MSN); family nurse practitioner (MSN); informatics (MSN); leadership and management (MSN); nursing (DNP, PhD, Post-Master's Certificate), including education (PhD), healthcare administration (PhD), interdisciplinary health (PhD), leadership (PhD), nursing education (Post-Master's Certificate), nursing informatics (Post-Master's Certificate), nursing leadership and management (Post-Master's Certificate), public health policy (PhD). *Accreditation:* AACN. Part-time and evening/weekend programs available. Postbaccalaureate distance learning degree programs offered (no on-campus study). *Faculty:* 22 full-time (19 women), 343 part-time/adjunct (301 women). *Students:* 5,828 full-time (5,240 women), 2,803 part-time (2,578 women); includes 2,920 minority (1,893 Black or African American, non-Hispanic/Latino; 40 American Indian or Alaska Native, non-Hispanic/Latino; 438 Asian, non-Hispanic/Latino; 391 Hispanic/Latino; 35 Native Hawaiian or other Pacific Islander, non-Hispanic/Latino; 123 Two or more races, non-Hispanic/Latino), 147 international. Average age 41. 1,795 applicants, 95% accepted, 1375 enrolled. In 2013, 1,879 master's, 1 doctorate, 36 other advanced degrees awarded. *Degree requirements:* For doctorate, thesis/dissertation (for some programs), residency (for some programs), field experience (for some programs). *Entrance requirements:* For master's, bachelor's degree or equivalent in related field or RN; minimum GPA of 2.5; official transcripts; goal statement (for some programs); access to computer and Internet; for doctorate, master's degree or higher, three years of related professional or academic experience, RN, goal statement (for some programs); access to computer and Internet; for Post-Master's Certificate, relevant work experience; access to computer and Internet. Additional exam requirements/recommendations for international students: Required—TOEFL (minimum score 550 paper-based; 79 iBT), IELTS (minimum score 6.5), Michigan English Language Assessment Battery (minimum score 82), or PTE. *Application deadline:* Applications are processed on a rolling basis. Application fee: $0. Electronic applications accepted. *Expenses: Tuition:* Full-time $11,813.55; part-time $500 per credit. *Required fees:* $618.76. *Financial support:* Fellowships, Federal Work-Study, scholarships/grants, unspecified assistantships, and family tuition reduction, active duty/veteran tuition reduction, group tuition reduction, interest-free payment plans, employee tuition reduction available. Support available to part-time students. Financial award applicants required to submit FAFSA. *Unit head:* Dr. Andrea Lindell, Associate Dean, 800-925-3368. *Application contact:* Jennifer Hall, Vice President of Enrollment Management, 866-4-WALDEN, E-mail: info@waldenu.edu.
Website: http://www.waldenu.edu/programs/colleges-schools/nursing

Waynesburg University, Graduate and Professional Studies, Canonsburg, PA 15370. Offers business (MBA), including energy management, finance, health systems, human resources, leadership, market development; counseling (MA), including addictions counseling, clinical mental health; education (M Ed, MAT), including autism (M Ed), curriculum and instruction (M Ed), educational leadership (M Ed), online teaching (M Ed); nursing (MSN), including administration, education, informatics; nursing practice (DNP); special education (M Ed); technology (M Ed); MSN/MBA. *Accreditation:* AACN. Part-time and evening/weekend programs available. *Faculty:* 11 full-time (5 women), 136 part-time/adjunct (80 women). *Students:* 146 full-time (99 women), 419 part-time (268 women). In 2013, 290 master's, 7 doctorates awarded. *Degree requirements:* For doctorate, thesis/dissertation. *Entrance requirements:* Additional exam requirements/recommendations for international students: Required—TOEFL. *Application deadline:* For fall admission, 8/1 priority date for domestic students. Applications are processed on a rolling basis. Electronic applications accepted. *Financial support:* Available to part-time students. Application deadline: 5/1. *Unit head:* David Mariner, Dean, 724-743-4420, Fax: 724-743-4425, E-mail: dmariner@waynesburg.edu. *Application contact:* Dr. Michael Bednarski, Director of Enrollment, 724-743-4420, Fax: 724-743-4425, E-mail: mbednars@waynesburg.edu.
Website: http://www.waynesburg.edu/

Occupational Health Nursing

Rutgers, The State University of New Jersey, Newark, Rutgers School of Nursing, Newark, NJ 07107-3001. Offers adult health (MSN); adult occupational health (MSN); advanced practice nursing (MSN, Post Master's Certificate); family nurse practitioner (MSN); nurse anesthesia (MSN); nursing (MSN); nursing informatics (MSN); urban health (PhD); women's health practitioner (MSN). *Accreditation:* AANA/CANAEP. Part-time programs available. *Entrance requirements:* For master's, GRE, RN license; basic life support, statistics, and health assessment experience. Additional exam requirements/recommendations for international students: Required—TOEFL. Electronic applications accepted. *Expenses:* Contact institution. *Faculty research:* HIV/AIDS, diabetes education, learned helplessness, nursing science, psychoeducation.

University of Cincinnati, Graduate School, College of Nursing, Cincinnati, OH 45221-0038. Offers clinical nurse specialist (MSN), including adult health, community health, neonatal, nursing administration, occupational health, pediatric health, psychiatric nursing, women's health; nurse anesthesia (MSN); nurse midwifery (MSN); nurse practitioner (MSN), including acute care, ambulatory care, family, family/psychiatric, women's health; nursing (PhD); MBA/MSN. *Accreditation:* AACN; AANA/CANAEP (one or more programs are accredited); ACNM/ACME. Part-time programs available. Postbaccalaureate distance learning degree programs offered (no on-campus study). Terminal master's awarded for partial completion of doctoral program. *Degree requirements:* For master's, thesis or alternative; for doctorate, comprehensive exam, thesis/dissertation. *Entrance requirements:* For master's and doctorate, GRE General Test. Additional exam requirements/recommendations for international students: Required—TOEFL (minimum score 520 paper-based). Electronic applications accepted. *Faculty research:* Substance abuse, injury and violence, symptom management.

University of Illinois at Chicago, Graduate College, College of Nursing, Program in Nursing, Chicago, IL 60607-7128. Offers acute care clinical nurse specialist (MS); acute care nurse practitioner (MS); administrative nursing leadership (Certificate); administrative studies in nursing (MS); adult nurse practitioner (MS); adult/geriatric nurse practitioner (MS); advanced community health nurse specialist (MS); family nurse practitioner (MS); geriatric clinical nurse specialist (MS); geriatric nurse practitioner (MS); mental health clinical nurse specialist (MS); mental health nurse practitioner (MS); nurse midwifery (MS); occupational health/advanced community health nurse specialist (MS); occupational health/family nurse practitioner (MS); pediatric clinical nurse specialist (MS); pediatric nurse practitioner (MS); perinatal clinical nurse specialist (MS); school/advanced community health nurse specialist (MS); school/family nurse practitioner (MS); women's health nurse practitioner (MS). *Accreditation:* AACN. Part-time programs available. *Faculty:* 16 full-time (14 women). *Students:* 393 full-time (361 women), 410 part-time (367 women); includes 198 minority (48 Black or African American, non-Hispanic/Latino; 1 American Indian or Alaska Native, non-Hispanic/Latino; 64 Asian, non-Hispanic/Latino; 71 Hispanic/Latino; 2 Native Hawaiian or other Pacific Islander, non-Hispanic/Latino; 12 Two or more races, non-Hispanic/Latino), 29 international. Average age 32. 396 applicants, 62% accepted, 177 enrolled. In 2013, 184 master's awarded. *Degree requirements:* For master's, thesis or alternative. *Entrance requirements:* For master's, GRE General Test, minimum GPA of 2.75. Additional exam requirements/recommendations for international students: Required—TOEFL. *Application deadline:* For fall admission, 5/15 for domestic students, 2/15 for international students; for spring admission, 11/1 for domestic students, 7/15 for international students. Applications are processed on a rolling basis. Application fee: $40 ($50 for international students). Electronic applications accepted. *Expenses:* Tuition, state resident: full-time $11,066; part-time $3689 per term. Tuition, nonresident: full-time $23,064; part-time $7688 per term. *Required fees:* $3004; $1190 per term. Tuition and fees vary according to course level and program. *Financial support:* Fellowships with full tuition reimbursements, research assistantships with full tuition reimbursements, teaching assistantships with full tuition reimbursements, career-related internships or fieldwork, Federal Work-Study, institutionally sponsored loans, scholarships/grants, traineeships, tuition waivers (full and partial), and unspecified assistantships available. Support available to part-time students. Financial award application deadline: 3/1; financial award applicants required to submit FAFSA. *Unit head:* Dr. Terri E. Weaver, Dean, 312-996-7808, E-mail: teweaver@uic.edu. *Application contact:* Receptionist, 312-413-2550, E-mail: gradcoll@uic.edu.

University of Minnesota, Twin Cities Campus, School of Public Health, Division of Environmental Health Sciences, Area in Occupational Health Nursing, Minneapolis, MN 55455-0213. Offers MPH, MS, PhD, MPH/MS. *Accreditation:* AACN. *Degree requirements:* For doctorate, thesis/dissertation. *Entrance requirements:* For master's and doctorate, GRE General Test. Electronic applications accepted.

The University of North Carolina at Chapel Hill, Graduate School, Gillings School of Global Public Health, Public Health Leadership Program, Chapel Hill, NC 27599. Offers health care and prevention (MPH); leadership (MPH); occupational health nursing (MPH). Part-time programs available. Postbaccalaureate distance learning degree programs offered (minimal on-campus study). *Degree requirements:* For master's, comprehensive exam, thesis (MS), paper (MPH). *Entrance requirements:* For master's, GRE General Test, minimum GPA of 3.0 (recommended), public health experience. Additional exam requirements/recommendations for international students: Required—TOEFL. Electronic applications accepted. *Faculty research:* Occupational health issues, clinical outcomes, prenatal and early childcare, adolescent health, effectiveness of home visiting, issues in occupational health nursing, community-based interventions.

University of South Florida, College of Nursing, Tampa, FL 33612. Offers adult gerontology acute care (DNP, PhD); adult gerontology acute care nursing (MS); adult gerontology primary care (DNP, PhD); adult gerontology primary care nursing (MS); adult gerontology primary care/occupational health nursing (MS); adult gerontology primary care/oncology nursing (MS, PhD); clinical nurse leader (MS); family health (DNP, PhD); family nurse practitioner (MS); nurse anesthesia (MS); nursing education (MS); nursing practice (DNP); nursing science (PhD), including nursing education; occupational health/adult-gerontology (DNP); oncology/adult-gerontology primary care (DNP); pediatric health (DNP, PhD); pediatric nurse practitioner (MS). *Accreditation:* AACN; AANA/CANAEP. Part-time programs available. *Faculty:* 46 full-time (40 women), 15 part-time/adjunct (11 women). *Students:* 177 full-time (150 women), 700 part-time (622 women); includes 272 minority (116 Black or African American, non-Hispanic/Latino; 2 American Indian or Alaska Native, non-Hispanic/Latino; 45 Asian, non-Hispanic/Latino; 93 Hispanic/Latino; 2 Native Hawaiian or other Pacific Islander, non-Hispanic/Latino; 14 Two or more races, non-Hispanic/Latino), 12 international. Average age 35. 656 applicants, 43% accepted, 224 enrolled. In 2013, 224 master's, 14 doctorates awarded. *Degree requirements:* For master's, comprehensive exam, thesis optional; for doctorate, comprehensive exam, thesis/dissertation. *Entrance requirements:* For master's, GRE General Test, bachelor's degree from accredited program with minimum GPA of 3.0 in all upper-division coursework; current license as Registered Nurse; 3 letters of recommendation; personal statement of goals; resume or curriculum vitae; personal interview; for doctorate, GRE General Test (recommended), bachelor's degree in nursing from a CCNA/NLNAC regionally-accredited institution with minimum GPA of 3.0 in all coursework or in all upper-division coursework; current license as Registered Nurse in Florida; undergraduate statistics course with minimum B grade; 3 letters of recommendation; statement of goals; resume; interview. Additional exam requirements/recommendations for international students: Required—TOEFL (minimum score 550 paper-based; 79 iBT). *Application deadline:* For fall admission, 2/15 for domestic students, 1/2 for international students; for spring admission, 10/1 for domestic students, 6/1 for international students. Application fee: $30. Electronic applications accepted. *Financial support:* In 2013–14, 36 students received support, including 7 research assistantships with tuition reimbursements available (averaging $18,935 per year), 29 teaching assistantships with tuition reimbursements available (averaging $30,814 per year); tuition waivers (partial) and unspecified assistantships also available. Financial award application deadline: 2/1; financial award applicants required to submit FAFSA. *Faculty research:* Women's health, palliative and end-of-life care, cardiac rehabilitation, complementary therapies for chronic illness and cancer. *Total annual research expenditures:* $3.4 million. *Unit head:* Dr. Dianne C. Morrison-Beedy, Dean and Professor, College of Nursing, 813-974-9091, Fax: 813-974-5418, E-mail: dmbeedy@health.usf.edu. *Application contact:* Dr. Connie Visovsky, Associate Professor and Associate Dean of Student Affairs, 813-396-9641, Fax: 813-974-5418, E-mail: cvisovsk@health.usf.edu.
Website: http://health.usf.edu/nursing/index.htm

University of the Sacred Heart, Graduate Programs, Department of Natural Sciences, San Juan, PR 00914-0383. Offers occupational health and safety (MS); occupational nursing (MSN). Part-time and evening/weekend programs available.

Oncology Nursing

Case Western Reserve University, Frances Payne Bolton School of Nursing, Master's Programs in Nursing, Nurse Practitioner Program, Cleveland, OH 44106. Offers acute care cardiovascular nursing (MSN); acute care nurse practitioner (MSN); acute care/flight nurse (MSN); adult gerontology acute care nurse practitioner (MSN); adult gerontology nurse practitioner (MSN); adult gerontology oncology and palliative care (MSN); family nurse practitioner (MSN); family systems psychiatric mental health nursing (MSN); neonatal nurse practitioner (MSN); pediatric nurse practitioner (MSN); women's health nurse practitioner (MSN). Part-time programs available. Postbaccalaureate distance learning degree programs offered (minimal on-campus study). *Faculty:* 54 full-time (50 women), 5 part-time/adjunct (3 women). *Students:* 56 full-time, 145 part-time; includes 9 minority (6 Black or African American, non-Hispanic/Latino; 2 Asian, non-Hispanic/Latino; 1 Hispanic/Latino), 5 international. Average age 35. 70 applicants, 71% accepted, 33 enrolled. In 2013, 79 master's awarded. *Degree requirements:* For master's, thesis optional. *Entrance requirements:* For master's, GRE General Test or MAT. Additional exam requirements/recommendations for international students: Required—TOEFL (minimum score 577 paper-based; 90 iBT), IELTS (minimum score 7). *Application deadline:* For fall admission, 6/1 for domestic students; for spring admission, 10/1 for domestic students. Applications are processed on a rolling basis. Application fee: $75. *Financial support:* In 2013–14, 25 teaching assistantships (averaging $15,120 per year) were awarded; research assistantships, institutionally sponsored loans, and tuition waivers (partial) also available. Support available to part-time students. Financial award application deadline: 6/30; financial award applicants required to submit FAFSA. *Faculty research:* Symptom science, family/community care, aging across the lifespan, self-management of health and illness, neuroscience. *Unit head:* Dr. Carol Savrin, Director, 216-368-5304, Fax: 216-368-3542, E-mail: cls18@case.edu. *Application contact:* Donna Hassik, Admissions Coordinator, 216-368-5253, Fax: 216-368-0124, E-mail: dmh7@case.edu.
Website: http://fpb.cwru.edu/MSN/majors.shtm

Duke University, School of Nursing, Durham, NC 27708-0586. Offers acute care pediatric nurse practitioner (MSN); adult-gerontology nurse practitioner - acute care (MSN, Post Master's Certificate); adult-gerontology nurse practitioner - primary care (MSN, Post Master's Certificate), including adult-gerontology nurse practitioner (MSN), cardiology, oncology; family nurse practitioner (MSN); neonatal nurse practitioner (MSN); nurse anesthesia (MSN, DNP); nursing (PhD); nursing and health care leadership (MSN); nursing education (MSN); nursing informatics (MSN, Post Master's Certificate); pediatric nurse practitioner - primary care (MSN). *Accreditation:* AACN; AANA/CANAEP. Part-time and evening/weekend programs available. Postbaccalaureate distance learning degree programs offered (minimal on-campus study). *Faculty:* 74 full-time (64 women), 7 part-time/adjunct (4 women). *Students:* 127 full-time (113 women), 473 part-time (433 women); includes 131 minority (54 Black or African American, non-Hispanic/Latino; 9 American Indian or Alaska Native, non-Hispanic/Latino; 36 Asian, non-Hispanic/Latino; 27 Hispanic/Latino; 5 Native Hawaiian or other Pacific Islander, non-Hispanic/Latino), 14 international. Average age 34. 516 applicants, 50% accepted, 190 enrolled. In 2013, 179 master's, 49 doctorates, 23 other advanced degrees awarded. Terminal master's awarded for partial completion of doctoral program. *Degree requirements:* For master's, thesis optional; for doctorate, capstone project. *Entrance requirements:* For master's, GRE General Test (waived if undergraduate GPA of 3.4 or higher), 1 year of nursing experience (recommended), BSN, minimum GPA of 3.0, previous course work in statistics; for doctorate, GRE General Test (waived if undergraduate GPA of 3.4 or higher), BSN or MSN, minimum

GPA of 3.0, portfolio, resume, personal statement, undergraduate statistics course, current licensure as a registered nurse, transcripts from all post-secondary institutions; for Post Master's Certificate, MSN, licensure or eligibility as a professional nurse, transcripts from all post-secondary institutions, previous course work in statistics. Additional exam requirements/recommendations for international students: Recommended—TOEFL (minimum score 550 paper-based; 83 iBT), IELTS (minimum score 7). *Application deadline:* For fall admission, 12/1 for domestic and international students; for spring admission, 5/1 for domestic and international students. Application fee: $50. Electronic applications accepted. *Expenses:* Contact institution. *Financial support:* Career-related internships or fieldwork, institutionally sponsored loans, scholarships/grants, traineeships, and tuition waivers (partial) available. Support available to part-time students. Financial award applicants required to submit FAFSA. *Faculty research:* Cardiovascular disease, caregiver skill training, data mining, prostate cancer, neonatal immune system. *Unit head:* Dr. Catherine L. Gilliss, Dean/Vice Chancellor for Nursing Affairs, 919-684-9444, Fax: 919-684-9414, E-mail: catherine.gilliss@duke.edu. *Application contact:* Ernie Rushing, Lead Admissions Processor/Admissions Officer, 919-668-6274, Fax: 919-668-4693, E-mail: stephen.rushing@dm.duke.edu.
Website: http://www.nursing.duke.edu/

Goldfarb School of Nursing at Barnes-Jewish College, Graduate Programs, St. Louis, MO 63110. Offers adult acute care nurse practitioner (MSN); adult nurse practitioner (MSN); nurse anesthesia (MSN); nurse educator (MSN); nurse executive (MSN); DNP/PhD. *Accreditation:* AACN; AANA/CANAEP. Part-time and evening/weekend programs available. Postbaccalaureate distance learning degree programs offered (minimal on-campus study). *Faculty:* 42 full-time (39 women), 6 part-time/adjunct (all women). *Students:* 81 full-time (67 women), 85 part-time (77 women); includes 28 minority (18 Black or African American, non-Hispanic/Latino; 2 Asian, non-Hispanic/Latino; 3 Hispanic/Latino; 3 Native Hawaiian or other Pacific Islander, non-Hispanic/Latino; 2 Two or more races, non-Hispanic/Latino). *Degree requirements:* For master's, thesis or alternative. *Entrance requirements:* For master's, 2 references, personal statement, curriculum vitae or resume. Additional exam requirements/recommendations for international students: Required—TOEFL (minimum score 575 paper-based; 85 iBT). *Application deadline:* For fall admission, 2/1 priority date for international students; for spring admission, 10/1 priority date for international students. Applications are processed on a rolling basis. Application fee: $50. *Expenses: Tuition:* Full-time $12,960; part-time $720 per credit hour. *Required fees:* $295; $720 per credit hour. Tuition and fees vary according to course load. *Financial support:* Fellowships, research assistantships, Federal Work-Study, institutionally sponsored loans, and scholarships/grants available. Support available to part-time students. Financial award applicants required to submit FAFSA. *Faculty research:* HIV stigma, HIV symptom management, palliative care with children and their families, heart disease prevention in Hispanic women, depression in the well elderly, alternative therapies in pre-term infants. *Unit head:* Dr. Michael Bleich, Dean, 314-362-0956, Fax: 314-362-0984, E-mail: mbleich@bjc.org. *Application contact:* Margaret Anne O'Connor, Program Officer, 314-454-7557, Fax: 314-362-0984, E-mail: maoconnor@bjc.org.

Gwynedd Mercy University, School of Nursing, Gwynedd Valley, PA 19437-0901. Offers clinical nurse specialist (MSN), including gerontology, oncology, pediatrics; nurse practitioner (MSN), including adult health, pediatric health. *Degree requirements:* For master's, thesis optional. *Entrance requirements:* For master's, GRE General Test or MAT, current nursing experience, physical assessment, course work in statistics, BSN from NLNAC-accredited program, 2 letters of recommendation, personal interview. Additional exam requirements/recommendations for international students: Required—TOEFL (minimum score 575 paper-based). Electronic applications accepted. *Expenses:* Contact institution. *Faculty research:* Critical thinking, primary care, domestic violence, multiculturalism, nursing centers.

Loyola University Chicago, Graduate School, Marcella Niehoff School of Nursing, Oncology Clinical Nurse Specialist Program, Chicago, IL 60660. Offers MSN, Certificate. *Accreditation:* AACN. Part-time and evening/weekend programs available. Postbaccalaureate distance learning degree programs offered (minimal on-campus study). *Faculty:* 45 full-time (44 women). *Students:* 1 (woman) full-time, 10 part-time (all women); includes 2 minority (both Asian, non-Hispanic/Latino). Average age 40. 6 applicants, 83% accepted, 5 enrolled. In 2013, 5 other advanced degrees awarded. *Degree requirements:* For master's, comprehensive exam or oral thesis defense. *Entrance requirements:* For master's, Illinois nursing license, BSN, minimum nursing GPA of 3.0, 3 letters of recommendation, 1000 hours of experience before starting clinical. *Application deadline:* Applications are processed on a rolling basis. Application fee: $50. Electronic applications accepted. *Expenses: Tuition:* Full-time $16,740; part-time $930 per credit. *Required fees:* $135 per semester. *Financial support:* Teaching assistantships, traineeships, and unspecified assistantships available. Financial award application deadline: 3/1. *Faculty research:* Breast cancer, coping with cancer, pain. *Unit head:* Dr. Marijo Letizia, Associate Dean, 708-216-9325, Fax: 708-216-9555, E-mail: mletizi@luc.edu. *Application contact:* Amy Weatherford, Enrollment Advisor, School of Nursing, 708-216-3751, Fax: 708-216-9555, E-mail: aweatherford@luc.edu.
Website: http://www.luc.edu/nursing/

Universidad Metropolitana, School of Health Sciences, Department of Nursing, San Juan, PR 00928-1150. Offers case management (Certificate); nursing (MSN); oncology nursing (Certificate).

University of Delaware, College of Health Sciences, School of Nursing, Newark, DE 19716. Offers adult nurse practitioner (MSN, PMC); cardiopulmonary clinical nurse specialist (MSN, PMC); cardiopulmonary clinical nurse specialist/adult nurse practitioner (MSN, PMC); family nurse practitioner (MSN, PMC); gerontology clinical nurse specialist (MSN, PMC); gerontology clinical nurse specialist geriatric nurse practitioner (PMC); gerontology clinical nurse specialist/geriatric nurse practitioner (MSN); health services administration (MSN, PMC); nursing of children clinical nurse specialist (MSN, PMC); nursing of children clinical nurse specialist/pediatric nurse practitioner (MSN, PMC); oncology/immune deficiency clinical nurse specialist (MSN, PMC); oncology/immune deficiency clinical nurse specialist/adult nurse practitioner (MSN, PMC); perinatal/women's health clinical nurse specialist (MSN, PMC); perinatal/women's health clinical nurse specialist/women's health nurse practitioner (MSN, PMC); psychiatric nursing clinical nurse specialist (MSN, PMC). *Accreditation:* AACN. Part-time and evening/weekend programs available. Postbaccalaureate distance learning degree programs offered (minimal on-campus study). *Degree requirements:* For master's, thesis optional. *Entrance requirements:* For master's, BSN, interview, RN license. Electronic applications accepted. *Faculty research:* Marriage and chronic illness, health promotion, congestive heart failure patient outcomes, school nursing, diabetes in children, culture, health disparities, cardiovascular, prison nursing, oncology, public policy, child obesity, smoking and teen pregnancy, blood pressure measurements, men's health.

University of South Florida, College of Nursing, Tampa, FL 33612. Offers adult gerontology acute care (DNP, PhD); adult gerontology acute care nursing (MS); adult gerontology primary care (DNP, PhD); adult gerontology primary care nursing (MS); adult gerontology primary care/occupational health nursing (MS); adult gerontology primary care/oncology nursing (MS, PhD); clinical nurse leader (MS); family health (DNP, PhD); family nurse practitioner (MS); nurse anesthesia (MS); nursing education (MS); nursing practice (DNP); nursing science (PhD), including nursing education; occupational health/adult-gerontology (DNP); oncology/adult-gerontology primary care (DNP); pediatric health (DNP, PhD); pediatric nurse practitioner (MS). *Accreditation:* AACN; AANA/CANAEP. Part-time programs available. *Faculty:* 46 full-time (40 women), 15 part-time/adjunct (11 women). *Students:* 177 full-time (150 women), 700 part-time (622 women); includes 272 minority (116 Black or African American, non-Hispanic/Latino; 2 American Indian or Alaska Native, non-Hispanic/Latino; 45 Asian, non-Hispanic/Latino; 93 Hispanic/Latino; 2 Native Hawaiian or other Pacific Islander, non-Hispanic/Latino; 14 Two or more races, non-Hispanic/Latino), 12 international. Average age 35. 656 applicants, 43% accepted, 224 enrolled. In 2013, 224 master's, 14 doctorates awarded. *Degree requirements:* For master's, comprehensive exam, thesis optional; for doctorate, comprehensive exam, thesis/dissertation. *Entrance requirements:* For master's, GRE General Test, bachelor's degree from accredited program with minimum GPA of 3.0 in all upper-division coursework; current license as Registered Nurse; 3 letters of recommendation; personal statement of goals; resume or curriculum vitae; personal interview; for doctorate, GRE General Test (recommended), bachelor's degree in nursing from a CCNA/NLNAC regionally-accredited institution with minimum GPA of 3.0 in all coursework or in all upper-division coursework; current license as Registered Nurse in Florida; undergraduate statistics course with minimum B grade; 3 letters of recommendation; statement of goals; resume; interview. Additional exam requirements/recommendations for international students: Required—TOEFL (minimum score 550 paper-based; 79 iBT). *Application deadline:* For fall admission, 2/15 for domestic students, 1/2 for international students; for spring admission, 10/1 for domestic students, 6/1 for international students. Application fee: $30. Electronic applications accepted. *Financial support:* In 2013–14, 36 students received support, including 7 research assistantships with tuition reimbursements available (averaging $18,935 per year), 29 teaching assistantships with tuition reimbursements available (averaging $30,814 per year); tuition waivers (partial) and unspecified assistantships also available. Financial award application deadline: 2/1; financial award applicants required to submit FAFSA. *Faculty research:* Women's health, palliative and end-of-life care, cardiac rehabilitation, complementary therapies for chronic illness and cancer. *Total annual research expenditures:* $3.4 million. *Unit head:* Dr. Dianne C. Morrison-Beedy, Dean and Professor, College of Nursing, 813-974-9091, Fax: 813-974-5418, E-mail: dmbeedy@health.usf.edu. *Application contact:* Dr. Connie Visovsky, Associate Professor and Associate Dean of Student Affairs, 813-396-9641, Fax: 813-974-5418, E-mail: cvisovsk@health.usf.edu.
Website: http://health.usf.edu/nursing/index.htm

Pediatric Nursing

Boston College, William F. Connell School of Nursing, Chestnut Hill, MA 02467-3800. Offers adult-gerontology nursing (MS); community health nursing (MS); family health (MS); forensic nursing (MS); maternal/child health nursing (MS), including pediatric and women's health; nurse anesthesia (MS); nursing (PhD); palliative care (MS), including adult and pediatric; psychiatric-mental health nursing (MS); MBA/MS; MS/MA; MS/PhD. *Accreditation:* AACN; AANA/CANAEP (one or more programs are accredited). Part-time programs available. *Faculty:* 47 full-time (43 women), 42 part-time/adjunct (39 women). *Students:* 199 full-time (180 women), 79 part-time (73 women); includes 44 minority (14 Black or African American, non-Hispanic/Latino; 1 American Indian or Alaska Native, non-Hispanic/Latino; 13 Asian, non-Hispanic/Latino; 12 Hispanic/Latino; 4 Two or more races, non-Hispanic/Latino), 7 international. Average age 31. 502 applicants, 39% accepted, 87 enrolled. In 2013, 105 master's, 8 doctorates awarded. *Degree requirements:* For master's, comprehensive exam, research project; for doctorate, comprehensive exam, thesis/dissertation, computer literacy exam or foreign language. *Entrance requirements:* For master's, bachelor's degree in nursing; for doctorate, GRE General Test, MS in nursing. Additional exam requirements/recommendations for international students: Required—TOEFL (minimum score 600 paper-based; 100 iBT). *Application deadline:* For fall admission, 9/30 for domestic and international students; for winter admission, 1/15 for domestic and international students; for spring admission, 3/15 for domestic and international students. Applications are processed on a rolling basis. Application fee: $40. Electronic applications accepted. *Financial support:* In 2013–14, 174 students received support, including 7 fellowships with full tuition reimbursements available (averaging $20,000 per year), 21 teaching assistantships (averaging $4,800 per year); research assistantships, scholarships/grants, health care benefits, tuition waivers (partial), and unspecified assistantships also available. Support available to part-time students. Financial award application deadline: 3/1; financial award applicants required to submit FAFSA. *Faculty research:* Sexual and reproductive health, health promotion/illness prevention, eating disorders, violence, symptom management. *Total annual research expenditures:* $1.1 million. *Unit head:* Dr. Susan Gennaro, Dean, 617-552-4251, Fax: 617-552-0931, E-mail: susan.gennaro@bc.edu. *Application contact:* MaryBeth Crowley, Graduate Programs Assistant, 617-552-4928, Fax: 617-552-2121, E-mail: csongrad@bc.edu.
Website: http://www.bc.edu/schools/son/

Caribbean University, Graduate School, Bayamón, PR 00960-0493. Offers administration and supervision (MA Ed); criminal justice (MA); curriculum and instruction (MA Ed, PhD), including elementary education (MA Ed), English education (MA Ed), history education (MA Ed), mathematics education (MA Ed), primary education (MA Ed), science education (MA Ed), Spanish education (MA Ed); educational technology in instructional systems (MA Ed); gerontology (MSN); human resources (MBA); museology, archiving and art history (MA Ed); neonatal pediatrics (MSN); physical education (MA Ed); special education (MA Ed). *Entrance requirements:* For master's, interview, minimum GPA of 2.5.

Case Western Reserve University, Frances Payne Bolton School of Nursing, Doctor of Nursing Practice Program, Cleveland, OH 44106. Offers acute care nurse practitioner (DNP); adult gerontology nurse practitioner (DNP); educational leadership (DNP); family nurse practitioner (DNP); family systems psychiatric mental health nursing (DNP); midwifery/family nursing (DNP); neonatal nurse practitioner (DNP); pediatric nurse

practitioner (DNP); practice leadership (DNP); women's health nurse practitioner (DNP). *Accreditation:* AACN. Part-time programs available. Postbaccalaureate distance learning degree programs offered (minimal on-campus study). *Students:* 169 full-time, 9 part-time; includes 10 minority (6 Black or African American, non-Hispanic/Latino; 1 Asian, non-Hispanic/Latino; 2 Hispanic/Latino; 1 Two or more races, non-Hispanic/Latino). 76 applicants, 97% accepted, 59 enrolled. In 2013, 38 doctorates awarded. Terminal master's awarded for partial completion of doctoral program. *Degree requirements:* For doctorate, thesis/dissertation. *Entrance requirements:* For doctorate, GRE General Test or MAT. Additional exam requirements/recommendations for international students: Required—TOEFL (minimum score 577 paper-based; 90 iBT), IELTS (minimum score 7). *Application deadline:* For fall admission, 6/1 priority date for domestic students, 6/1 for international students; for spring admission, 10/1 for domestic and international students. Applications are processed on a rolling basis. Application fee: $75. *Financial support:* In 2013–14, 90 students received support, including 9 fellowships with full tuition reimbursements available (averaging $31,325 per year), 1 research assistantship with partial tuition reimbursement available (averaging $14,472 per year); teaching assistantships, Federal Work-Study, institutionally sponsored loans, scholarships/grants, and tuition waivers (partial) also available. Support available to part-time students. Financial award application deadline: 5/15; financial award applicants required to submit FAFSA. *Faculty research:* Symptom science, family/community care, aging across the lifespan, self-management of health and illness, neuroscience. *Unit head:* Dr. Donna Dowling, Director, 216-368-1869, Fax: 216-368-3542, E-mail: dad10@case.edu. *Application contact:* Donna Hassik, Admissions Coordinator, 216-368-5253, Fax: 216-368-0124, E-mail: dmh7@case.edu.
Website: http://fpb.case.edu/DNP/

Case Western Reserve University, Frances Payne Bolton School of Nursing, Master's Programs in Nursing, Nurse Practitioner Program, Cleveland, OH 44106. Offers acute care cardiovascular nursing (MSN); acute care nurse practitioner (MSN); acute care/flight nurse (MSN); adult gerontology acute care nurse practitioner (MSN); adult gerontology nurse practitioner (MSN); adult gerontology oncology and palliative care (MSN); family nurse practitioner (MSN); family systems psychiatric mental health nursing (MSN); neonatal nurse practitioner (MSN); pediatric nurse practitioner (MSN); women's health nurse practitioner (MSN). Part-time programs available. Postbaccalaureate distance learning degree programs offered (minimal on-campus study). *Faculty:* 54 full-time (50 women), 5 part-time/adjunct (3 women). *Students:* 56 full-time, 145 part-time; includes 9 minority (6 Black or African American, non-Hispanic/Latino; 2 Asian, non-Hispanic/Latino; 1 Hispanic/Latino), 5 international. Average age 35. 70 applicants, 71% accepted, 33 enrolled. In 2013, 79 master's awarded. *Degree requirements:* For master's, thesis optional. *Entrance requirements:* For master's, GRE General Test or MAT. Additional exam requirements/recommendations for international students: Required—TOEFL (minimum score 577 paper-based; 90 iBT), IELTS (minimum score 7). *Application deadline:* For fall admission, 6/1 for domestic students; for spring admission, 10/1 for domestic students. Applications are processed on a rolling basis. Application fee: $75. *Financial support:* In 2013–14, 25 teaching assistantships (averaging $15,120 per year) were awarded; research assistantships, institutionally sponsored loans, and tuition waivers (partial) also available. Support available to part-time students. Financial award application deadline: 6/30; financial award applicants required to submit FAFSA. *Faculty research:* Symptom science, family/community care, aging across the lifespan, self-management of health and illness, neuroscience. *Unit head:* Dr. Carol Savrin, Director, 216-368-5304, Fax: 216-368-3542, E-mail: cls18@case.edu. *Application contact:* Donna Hassik, Admissions Coordinator, 216-368-5253, Fax: 216-368-0124, E-mail: dmh7@case.edu.
Website: http://fpb.cwru.edu/MSN/majors.shtm

Columbia University, School of Nursing, Program in Pediatric Nurse Practitioner, New York, NY 10032. Offers MS, Adv C. *Accreditation:* AACN. Part-time programs available. *Entrance requirements:* For master's, GRE General Test, NCLEX, BSN, 1 year of clinical experience (preferred); for Adv C, MSN. Additional exam requirements/recommendations for international students: Required—TOEFL. Electronic applications accepted.

Drexel University, College of Nursing and Health Professions, Division of Graduate Nursing, Philadelphia, PA 19104-2875. Offers adult acute care (MSN); adult psychiatric/mental health (MSN); advanced practice nursing (MSN); clinical trials research (MSN); family nurse practitioner (MSN); leadership in health systems management (MSN); nursing education (MSN); pediatric primary care (MSN); women's health (MSN). *Accreditation:* AACN. Electronic applications accepted.

Duke University, School of Nursing, Durham, NC 27708-0586. Offers acute care pediatric nurse practitioner (MSN); adult-gerontology nurse practitioner - acute care (MSN, Post Master's Certificate); adult-gerontology nurse practitioner - primary care (MSN, Post Master's Certificate), including adult-gerontology nurse practitioner (MSN), cardiology, oncology; family nurse practitioner (MSN); neonatal nurse practitioner (MSN); nurse anesthesia (MSN, DNP); nursing (PhD); nursing and health care leadership (MSN); nursing education (MSN); nursing informatics (MSN, Post Master's Certificate); pediatric nurse practitioner - primary care (MSN). *Accreditation:* AACN; AANA/CANAEP. Part-time and evening/weekend programs available. Postbaccalaureate distance learning degree programs offered (minimal on-campus study). *Faculty:* 74 full-time (64 women), 7 part-time/adjunct (4 women). *Students:* 127 full-time (113 women), 473 part-time (433 women); includes 131 minority (54 Black or African American, non-Hispanic/Latino; 9 American Indian or Alaska Native, non-Hispanic/Latino; 36 Asian, non-Hispanic/Latino; 27 Hispanic/Latino; 5 Native Hawaiian or other Pacific Islander, non-Hispanic/Latino), 14 international. Average age 34. 516 applicants, 50% accepted, 190 enrolled. In 2013, 179 master's, 49 doctorates, 23 other advanced degrees awarded. Terminal master's awarded for partial completion of doctoral program. *Degree requirements:* For master's, thesis optional; for doctorate, capstone project. *Entrance requirements:* For master's, GRE General Test (waived if undergraduate GPA of 3.4 or higher), 1 year of nursing experience (recommended), BSN, minimum GPA of 3.0, previous course work in statistics; for doctorate, GRE General Test (waived if undergraduate GPA of 3.4 or higher), BSN or MSN, minimum GPA of 3.0, portfolio, resume, personal statement, undergraduate statistics course, current licensure as a registered nurse, transcripts from all post-secondary institutions; for Post Master's Certificate, MSN, licensure or eligibility as a professional nurse, transcripts from all post-secondary institutions, previous course work in statistics. Additional exam requirements/recommendations for international students: Recommended—TOEFL (minimum score 550 paper-based; 83 iBT), IELTS (minimum score 7). *Application deadline:* For fall admission, 12/1 for domestic and international students; for spring admission, 5/1 for domestic and international students. Application fee: $50. Electronic applications accepted. *Expenses:* Contact institution. *Financial support:* Career-related internships or fieldwork, institutionally sponsored loans, scholarships/grants, traineeships, and tuition waivers (partial) available. Support available to part-time students. Financial award applicants required to submit FAFSA. *Faculty research:* Cardiovascular disease, caregiver skill training, data mining, prostate cancer, neonatal immune system. *Unit head:* Dr. Catherine L. Gilliss, Dean/Vice Chancellor for Nursing Affairs, 919-684-9444, Fax: 919-684-9414, E-mail: catherine.gilliss@duke.edu. *Application contact:* Ernie Rushing, Lead Admissions Processor/Admissions Officer, 919-668-6274, Fax: 919-668-4693, E-mail: stephen.rushing@dm.duke.edu.
Website: http://www.nursing.duke.edu/

Emory University, Nell Hodgson Woodruff School of Nursing, Atlanta, GA 30322-1100. Offers adult nurse practitioner (MSN); emergency nurse practitioner (MSN); family nurse practitioner (MSN); family nurse-midwife (MSN); health systems leadership (MSN); nurse-midwifery (MSN); pediatric nurse practitioner acute and primary care (MSN); women's health care (Title X) (MSN); women's health nurse practitioner (MSN); MSN/MPH. *Accreditation:* AACN; ACNM/ACME (one or more programs are accredited). Part-time programs available. *Entrance requirements:* For master's, GRE General Test or MAT, minimum GPA of 3.0, BS in nursing from an accredited institution, RN license and additional course work, 3 letters of recommendation. Additional exam requirements/recommendations for international students: Required—TOEFL (minimum score 600 paper-based; 100 iBT). Electronic applications accepted. *Expenses:* Contact institution. *Faculty research:* Older adult falls and injuries, minority health issues, cardiac symptoms and quality of life, bio-ethics and decision-making, menopausal issues.

Georgia Regents University, The Graduate School, Pediatric Nurse Practitioner Program, Augusta, GA 30912. Offers MSN, Post-Master's Certificate. *Students:* 1 (woman) full-time, 7 part-time (6 women). Average age 29. 4 applicants, 50% accepted, 2 enrolled. In 2013, 3 master's awarded. *Entrance requirements:* For master's, GRE General Test or MAT, Georgia license as a registered professional nurse. Additional exam requirements/recommendations for international students: Required—TOEFL (minimum score 550 paper-based; 79 iBT). *Application deadline:* For fall admission, 2/1 for domestic and international students; for spring admission, 10/1 for domestic and international students. Application fee: $50. Electronic applications accepted. *Unit head:* Dr. Lucy Marion, Dean, 706-721-3771, Fax: 706-721-8169, E-mail: lumarion@georgiahealth.edu. *Application contact:* Karen Sturgill, Program Coordinator, 706-721-3676, Fax: 706-721-8169, E-mail: ksturgillt@georgiahealth.edu.
Website: http://www.gru.edu/nursing/programs.php

Georgia State University, Byrdine F. Lewis School of Nursing, Atlanta, GA 30303. Offers adult health clinical nurse specialist/nurse practitioner (MS, Certificate); child health clinical nurse specialist/pediatric nurse practitioner (MS, Certificate); family nurse practitioner (MS, Certificate); family psychiatric mental health nurse practitioner (MS, Certificate); nursing (PhD); nursing leadership in healthcare innovations (MS), including nursing administration, nursing informatics; nutrition (MS); perinatal clinical nurse specialist/women's health nurse practitioner (MS, Certificate); physical therapy (DPT); respiratory therapy (MS). *Accreditation:* AACN. Part-time programs available. Postbaccalaureate distance learning degree programs offered (minimal on-campus study). *Faculty:* 22 full-time (16 women). *Students:* 241 full-time (180 women), 262 part-time (236 women); includes 176 minority (120 Black or African American, non-Hispanic/Latino; 31 Asian, non-Hispanic/Latino; 13 Hispanic/Latino; 3 Native Hawaiian or other Pacific Islander, non-Hispanic/Latino; 9 Two or more races, non-Hispanic/Latino), 19 international. Average age 34. 583 applicants, 34% accepted, 160 enrolled. In 2013, 110 master's, 44 doctorates, 6 other advanced degrees awarded. *Degree requirements:* For doctorate, comprehensive exam, thesis/dissertation. *Entrance requirements:* For doctorate, GRE. Additional exam requirements/recommendations for international students: Required—TOEFL. *Application deadline:* For fall admission, 2/1 priority date for domestic and international students; for spring admission, 9/15 for domestic and international students. Applications are processed on a rolling basis. Application fee: $50. Electronic applications accepted. *Expenses:* Contact institution. *Financial support:* In 2013–14, research assistantships with full and partial tuition reimbursements (averaging $1,666 per year), teaching assistantships with full and partial tuition reimbursements (averaging $1,920 per year) were awarded; scholarships/grants, tuition waivers (full and partial), and unspecified assistantships also available. Support available to part-time students. Financial award application deadline: 8/1; financial award applicants required to submit FAFSA. *Faculty research:* Stroke intervention for caregivers, stroke prevention in African Americans; relationships between psychological distress and health outcomes in parents with a medically ill infant; medically fragile children; nursing expertise and patient outcomes. *Unit head:* Joan S. Cranford, Assistant Dean for Nursing, 404-413-1200, Fax: 404-413-1205, E-mail: jcranford2@gsu.edu. *Application contact:* Tiffany Norman, Senior Administrative Coordinator, 404-413-1190, Fax: 404-413-1205, E-mail: tnorman7@gsu.edu.
Website: http://nursing.gsu.edu/

Gwynedd Mercy University, School of Nursing, Gwynedd Valley, PA 19437-0901. Offers clinical nurse specialist (MSN), including gerontology, oncology, pediatrics; nurse practitioner (MSN), including adult health, pediatric health. *Degree requirements:* For master's, thesis optional. *Entrance requirements:* For master's, GRE General Test or MAT, current nursing experience, physical assessment, course work in statistics, BSN from NLNAC-accredited program, 2 letters of recommendation, personal interview. Additional exam requirements/recommendations for international students: Required—TOEFL (minimum score 575 paper-based). Electronic applications accepted. *Expenses:* Contact institution. *Faculty research:* Critical thinking, primary care, domestic violence, multiculturalism, nursing centers.

Hampton University, Graduate College, School of Nursing, Hampton, VA 23668. Offers advanced adult nursing (MS); community health nursing (MS); community mental health/psychiatric nursing (MS); family nursing (MS); gerontological nursing for the nurse practitioner (MS); pediatric nursing (MS); women's health nursing (MS). *Accreditation:* AACN. Part-time and evening/weekend programs available. *Degree requirements:* For master's, thesis optional. *Entrance requirements:* For master's, GRE General Test. *Faculty research:* Curriculum development, physical and mental assessment.

Indiana University–Purdue University Indianapolis, School of Nursing, Indianapolis, IN 46202-2896. Offers acute care nurse practitioner (MSN); adult health clinical nurse specialist (MSN); adult health nursing (MSN), including adult clinical nurse specialist; adult nurse practitioner (MSN); adult psychiatric/mental health nursing (MSN); child psychiatric/mental health nursing (MSN); community health nursing (MSN); family nurse practitioner (MSN); neonatal nurse practitioner (MSN); nursing (MSN, DNP), including nursing administration (MSN), nursing education (MSN); nursing science (PhD); pediatric clinical nurse specialist (MSN); women's health nurse practitioner (MSN); MSN/MPA; MSN/MPH. Part-time programs available. *Faculty:* 85 full-time (82 women), 60 part-time/adjunct (all women). *Students:* 86 full-time (78 women), 371 part-time (351 women); includes 74 minority (39 Black or African American, non-Hispanic/Latino; 1 American Indian or Alaska Native, non-Hispanic/Latino; 14 Asian, non-Hispanic/Latino; 11 Hispanic/Latino; 9 Two or more races, non-Hispanic/Latino), 6 international. Average age 38. 224 applicants, 61% accepted, 102 enrolled. In 2013, 120 master's, 10 doctorates awarded. Terminal master's awarded for partial completion of doctoral program. *Degree requirements:* For master's, thesis; for doctorate, thesis/dissertation. *Entrance requirements:* For master's, minimum GPA of 3.0, RN license; for doctorate, GRE General Test, minimum GPA of 3.0, MSN, RN license, graduate statistics course with minimum B grade (not older than 3 years). Additional exam requirements/recommendations for international students: Required—TOEFL. *Application deadline:* For fall admission, 2/15 for domestic students; for spring admission, 9/15 for domestic students. Application fee: $55 ($65 for international students). *Financial support:* In

2013–14, 93 students received support. Fellowships with full tuition reimbursements available, research assistantships with full tuition reimbursements available, teaching assistantships with full tuition reimbursements available, Federal Work-Study, institutionally sponsored loans, scholarships/grants, and tuition waivers (full) available. Support available to part-time students. Financial award application deadline: 5/1. *Faculty research:* Clinical science, health systems. *Total annual research expenditures:* $3 million. *Unit head:* Dr. Patricia Ebright, Associate Dean for Graduate Programs, E-mail: nursing@iupui.edu. *Application contact:* Information Contact, 317-274-2806.
Website: http://nursing.iu.edu/

Kent State University, College of Nursing, Kent, OH 44242-0001. Offers acute care nurse practitioner (MSN); adult nurse practitioner (MSN); clinical nurse specialist (MSN); family nurse practitioner (MSN); geriatric nurse practitioner (MSN); health care management (MSN); nurse educator (MSN); nursing (PhD); nursing practice (DNP); pediatric nurse practitioner (MSN); psychiatric/mental health nurse practitioner (MSN); women's health nurse practitioner (MSN). PhD program offered jointly with The University of Akron. *Accreditation:* AACN. Part-time programs available. *Degree requirements:* For master's, thesis optional; for doctorate, comprehensive exam, thesis/dissertation. *Entrance requirements:* For master's, GRE (if undergraduate GPA less than 3.0), minimum GPA of 2.75; for doctorate, GRE, MSN. Additional exam requirements/recommendations for international students: Required—TOEFL. Electronic applications accepted. *Expenses:* Contact institution. *Faculty research:* Women and violence, methodological specialties, osteoporosis in women, new caregivers and the elderly.

Lehman College of the City University of New York, School of Natural and Social Sciences, Department of Nursing, Bronx, NY 10468-1589. Offers adult health nursing (MS); nursing of older adults (MS); parent-child nursing (MS); pediatric nurse practitioner (MS). *Accreditation:* AACN. Part-time and evening/weekend programs available. *Entrance requirements:* For master's, bachelor's degree in nursing, New York RN license.

Loma Linda University, Department of Graduate Nursing, Program in Growing Family Nursing, Loma Linda, CA 92350. Offers MS. *Accreditation:* AACN. Part-time programs available. *Degree requirements:* For master's, thesis or alternative. *Entrance requirements:* For master's, GRE General Test, BSN, minimum GPA of 3.0, RN license. Additional exam requirements/recommendations for international students: Required—TOEFL. Electronic applications accepted. *Faculty research:* Family coping in chronic illness; women, identity, and career/family issues.

Marquette University, Graduate School, College of Nursing, Milwaukee, WI 53201-1881. Offers acute care nurse practitioner (Certificate); adult clinical nurse specialist (Certificate); adult nurse practitioner (Certificate); advanced practice nursing (MSN, DNP), including adult-older adult acute care (DNP), adults (MSN), adults-older adults (DNP), clinical nurse leader (MSN), health care systems leadership (DNP), nurse-midwifery (MSN), older adults (MSN), pediatrics acute care (MSN), pediatrics primary care (MSN), pediatrics-acute care (DNP), pediatrics-primary care (DNP), primary care (DNP), systems leadership and healthcare quality (MSN); family nurse practitioner (Certificate); nurse-midwifery (Certificate); nursing (PhD); pediatric acute care (Certificate); pediatric primary care (Certificate); systems leadership and healthcare quality (Certificate). *Accreditation:* AACN. *Faculty:* 35 full-time (34 women), 59 part-time/adjunct (58 women). *Students:* 105 full-time (96 women), 279 part-time (256 women); includes 28 minority (11 Black or African American, non-Hispanic/Latino; 7 Asian, non-Hispanic/Latino; 8 Hispanic/Latino; 2 Two or more races, non-Hispanic/Latino), 3 international. Average age 30. 322 applicants, 62% accepted, 98 enrolled. In 2013, 66 master's, 4 doctorates, 6 other advanced degrees awarded. Terminal master's awarded for partial completion of doctoral program. *Degree requirements:* For master's, comprehensive exam, thesis or alternative. *Entrance requirements:* For master's, GRE General Test, BSN, Wisconsin RN license, official transcripts from all current and previous colleges/universities except Marquette, three completed recommendation forms, resume, written statement of professional goals; for doctorate, GRE General Test, official transcripts from all current and previous colleges/universities except Marquette, three letters of recommendation, resume, written statement of professional goals, sample of scholarly writing. Additional exam requirements/recommendations for international students: Required—TOEFL (minimum score 530 paper-based). *Application deadline:* For fall admission, 2/15 for domestic and international students. Application fee: $50. Electronic applications accepted. *Financial support:* In 2013–14, 41 students received support, including 1 fellowship with partial tuition reimbursement available (averaging $17,500 per year), 2 research assistantships with full tuition reimbursements available (averaging $13,285 per year), 8 teaching assistantships with full tuition reimbursements available (averaging $13,912 per year); career-related internships or fieldwork, Federal Work-Study, scholarships/grants, health care benefits, tuition waivers (partial), and unspecified assistantships also available. Support available to part-time students. Financial award application deadline: 2/15. *Faculty research:* Psychosocial adjustment to chronic illness, gerontology, reminiscence, health policy: uninsured and access, hospital care delivery systems. *Total annual research expenditures:* $769,051. *Unit head:* Dr. Margaret Callahan, Dean, 414-288-3800, Fax: 414-288-1578. *Application contact:* Dr. Maureen O'Brien, Associate Dean/Clinical Associate Professor, 414-288-3823.
Website: http://www.marquette.edu/nursing/academicprograms-graduate.shtml

MGH Institute of Health Professions, School of Nursing, Boston, MA 02129-4557. Offers advanced practice nursing (MSN); gerontological nursing (MSN); nursing (DNP); pediatric nursing (MSN); psychiatric nursing (MSN); teaching and learning for health care education (Certificate); women's health nursing (MSN). *Accreditation:* AACN. *Faculty:* 41 full-time (36 women), 14 part-time/adjunct (13 women). *Students:* 494 full-time (428 women), 85 part-time (77 women); includes 108 minority (32 Black or African American, non-Hispanic/Latino; 2 American Indian or Alaska Native, non-Hispanic/Latino; 38 Asian, non-Hispanic/Latino; 33 Hispanic/Latino; 3 Native Hawaiian or other Pacific Islander, non-Hispanic/Latino). Average age 32. 470 applicants, 52% accepted, 133 enrolled. In 2013, 85 master's, 12 doctorates, 98 other advanced degrees awarded. *Degree requirements:* For master's, thesis or alternative. *Entrance requirements:* For master's, GRE General Test, bachelor's degree from regionally-accredited college or university. Additional exam requirements/recommendations for international students: Required—TOEFL (minimum score 550 paper-based; 80 iBT). *Application deadline:* For fall admission, 12/1 for domestic and international students; for spring admission, 10/1 for domestic and international students. Application fee: $100. Electronic applications accepted. *Expenses: Tuition:* Part-time $1114 per credit. *Required fees:* $620 per term. One-time fee: $475 part-time. *Financial support:* In 2013–14, 75 students received support, including 4 research assistantships (averaging $1,200 per year), 17 teaching assistantships (averaging $1,200 per year); career-related internships or fieldwork, scholarships/grants, traineeships, and unspecified assistantships also available. Support available to part-time students. Financial award application deadline: 4/1; financial award applicants required to submit FAFSA. *Faculty research:* Biobehavioral nursing, HIV/AIDS, gerontological nursing, women's health, vulnerable populations, health systems. *Unit head:* Dr. Laurie Lauzon-Clabo, Dean, 617-643-0605, Fax: 617-726-8022, E-mail: llauzonclabo@mghihp.edu. *Application contact:* Lauren Putnam, Assistant Director of Admission, 617-726-3140, Fax: 617-726-8010, E-mail: admissions@mghihp.edu.
Website: http://www.mghihp.edu/academics/nursing/

Molloy College, Division of Nursing, Rockville Centre, NY 11571-5002. Offers adult nurse practitioner (Advanced Certificate); clinical nurse specialist: adult health (Advanced Certificate); family nurse practitioner (Advanced Certificate); nurse practitioner psychiatry (Advanced Certificate); nursing (MS, PhD); nursing administration (Advanced Certificate); nursing administration with informatics (Advanced Certificate); nursing education (Advanced Certificate); nursing informatics (Advanced Certificate); pediatric nurse practitioner (Advanced Certificate). *Accreditation:* AACN. Part-time and evening/weekend programs available. *Faculty:* 30 full-time (29 women), 10 part-time/adjunct (7 women). *Students:* 18 full-time (all women), 538 part-time (495 women); includes 289 minority (159 Black or African American, non-Hispanic/Latino; 1 American Indian or Alaska Native, non-Hispanic/Latino; 80 Asian, non-Hispanic/Latino; 43 Hispanic/Latino; 4 Native Hawaiian or other Pacific Islander, non-Hispanic/Latino; 2 Two or more races, non-Hispanic/Latino), 2 international. Average age 38. 241 applicants, 63% accepted, 122 enrolled. In 2013, 84 master's, 2 other advanced degrees awarded. *Degree requirements:* For master's, thesis optional. *Entrance requirements:* For master's, 3 letters of reference, BS in nursing, minimum undergraduate GPA of 3.0; for Advanced Certificate, 3 letters of reference, master's degree in nursing. *Application deadline:* For fall admission, 9/2 priority date for domestic students; for spring admission, 1/20 priority date for domestic students. Applications are processed on a rolling basis. Application fee: $60. *Expenses: Tuition:* Full-time $16,920; part-time $940 per credit. *Required fees:* $880. *Financial support:* Research assistantships with partial tuition reimbursements, teaching assistantships with partial tuition reimbursements, institutionally sponsored loans, scholarships/grants, and unspecified assistantships available. Support available to part-time students. Financial award application deadline: 4/1; financial award applicants required to submit FAFSA. *Unit head:* Dr. Jeannine Muldoon, Dean of Nursing, 516-323-3651, E-mail: jmuldoon@molloy.edu. *Application contact:* Alina Haitz, Assistant Director of Graduate Admissions, 516-323-4008, E-mail: ahaitz@molloy.edu.
Website: http://www.molloy.edu/academics/nursing-division

New York University, College of Nursing, Doctor of Nursing Practice Program, New York, NY 10012-1019. Offers advanced practice nursing (DNP), including adult acute care, adult nurse practitioner/holistic nursing, adult nurse practitioner/palliative care nursing, adult primary care, adult primary care/geriatrics, family, geriatrics, mental health nursing, nurse-midwifery, pediatrics. Part-time and evening/weekend programs available. *Faculty:* 3 full-time (all women), 1 part-time/adjunct (0 women). *Students:* 1 (woman) full-time, 33 part-time (30 women); includes 7 minority (3 Black or African American, non-Hispanic/Latino; 3 Asian, non-Hispanic/Latino; 1 Hispanic/Latino). Average age 39. 18 applicants, 100% accepted, 12 enrolled. In 2013, 4 doctorates awarded. *Degree requirements:* For doctorate, thesis/dissertation, capstone. *Entrance requirements:* For doctorate, MAT or GRE (either taken within past 5 years), MS, RN license, interview, Nurse Practitioner Certification. Additional exam requirements/recommendations for international students: Required—TOEFL (minimum score 90 iBT), IELTS (minimum score 7). *Application deadline:* For fall admission, 3/1 for domestic students, 4/1 for international students. Applications are processed on a rolling basis. Application fee: $80. Electronic applications accepted. *Expenses: Tuition:* Full-time $35,856; part-time $1494 per unit. *Required fees:* $1408; $64 per unit. $473 per term. Tuition and fees vary according to course load and program. *Financial support:* Scholarships/grants available. Support available to part-time students. Financial award application deadline: 2/1. *Faculty research:* Geriatrics, HIV, elderly black diabetics, families and illness, oral systemic connection. *Unit head:* Dr. Rona Levin, Director, 212-998-5319, Fax: 212-995-3143, E-mail: rfl2039@nyu.edu. *Application contact:* Elizabeth Ensweiler, Assistant Director, Graduate Student Affairs and Admissions, 212-992-7653, Fax: 212-995-4302, E-mail: ee39@nyu.edu.

New York University, College of Nursing, Programs in Advanced Practice Nursing, New York, NY 10012-1019. Offers advanced practice nursing: adult acute care (MS, Advanced Certificate); advanced practice nursing: adult nurse practitioner/holistic nurse practitioner (Advanced Certificate); advanced practice nursing: adult nurse practitioner/palliative care nurse practitioner (Advanced Certificate); advanced practice nursing: adult primary care (MS, Advanced Certificate); advanced practice nursing: family (MS, Advanced Certificate); advanced practice nursing: geriatrics (Advanced Certificate); advanced practice nursing: mental health (MS); advanced practice nursing: mental health nursing (Advanced Certificate); advanced practice nursing: pediatrics (MS, Advanced Certificate); nurse midwifery (MS, Advanced Certificate); nursing administration (MS, Advanced Certificate); nursing education (MS, Advanced Certificate); nursing informatics (MS, Advanced Certificate); MS/MPA; MS/MPH. *Accreditation:* AACN; ACNM/ACME. Part-time programs available. *Faculty:* 22 full-time (all women), 54 part-time/adjunct (46 women). *Students:* 36 full-time (31 women), 622 part-time (549 women); includes 239 minority (73 Black or African American, non-Hispanic/Latino; 1 American Indian or Alaska Native, non-Hispanic/Latino; 116 Asian, non-Hispanic/Latino; 36 Hispanic/Latino; 6 Native Hawaiian or other Pacific Islander, non-Hispanic/Latino; 7 Two or more races, non-Hispanic/Latino), 16 international. Average age 37. 395 applicants, 67% accepted, 156 enrolled. In 2013, 186 master's, 8 other advanced degrees awarded. *Degree requirements:* For master's, thesis (for some programs). *Entrance requirements:* For master's, BS in nursing, AS in nursing with another BS/BA, interview, RN license, 1 year of clinical experience (3 for nursing education program); for Advanced Certificate, master's degree. Additional exam requirements/recommendations for international students: Required—TOEFL (minimum score 90 iBT), IELTS (minimum score 7). *Application deadline:* For fall admission, 7/1 for domestic and international students; for spring admission, 12/1 for domestic and international students. Application fee: $80. Electronic applications accepted. *Expenses: Tuition:* Full-time $35,856; part-time $1494 per unit. *Required fees:* $1408; $64 per unit. $473 per term. Tuition and fees vary according to course load and program. *Financial support:* In 2013–14, 182 students received support. Research assistantships, career-related internships or fieldwork, Federal Work-Study, scholarships/grants, traineeships, and unspecified assistantships available. Support available to part-time students. Financial award application deadline: 2/1; financial award applicants required to submit FAFSA. *Faculty research:* Geriatrics, HIV, elderly black diabetics, families and illness, oral systemic connection. *Unit head:* Dr. Judith Haber, Associate Dean, Graduate Programs, 212-998-9020, Fax: 212-995-3143, E-mail: jh33@nyu.edu. *Application contact:* Elizabeth Ensweiler, Assistant Director, Graduate Student Affairs and Admissions, 212-992-7653, Fax: 212-995-4302, E-mail: ee39@nyu.edu.

Queen's University at Kingston, School of Graduate Studies, Faculty of Health Sciences, School of Nursing, Kingston, ON K7L 3N6, Canada. Offers health and chronic illness (M Sc); nurse scientist (PhD); primary health care nurse practitioner (Certificate); women's and children's health (M Sc). *Degree requirements:* For master's, thesis. *Entrance requirements:* For master's, RN license. Additional exam requirements/recommendations for international students: Required—TOEFL. *Faculty research:* Women and children's health, health and chronic illness.

Rush University, College of Nursing, Department of Women, Children and Family Nursing, Chicago, IL 60612. Offers neonatal clinical nurse specialist (DNP); neonatal

nurse practitioner (DNP, Post-Graduate Certificate); nursing science (PhD); pediatric acute care nurse practitioner (DNP, Post-Graduate Certificate); pediatric clinical nurse specialist (DNP); pediatric primary care nurse practitioner (DNP); pediatric primary nurse practitioner (Post-Graduate Certificate); systems leadership (DNP). *Accreditation:* AACN. Part-time programs available. Postbaccalaureate distance learning degree programs offered (minimal on-campus study). *Students:* 83 part-time (81 women); includes 9 minority (3 Black or African American, non-Hispanic/Latino; 3 Asian, non-Hispanic/Latino; 2 Hispanic/Latino; 1 Native Hawaiian or other Pacific Islander, non-Hispanic/Latino). Average age 32. 83 applicants, 81% accepted, 65 enrolled. *Degree requirements:* For doctorate, leadership project (for DNP); dissertation (for PhD). *Entrance requirements:* For doctorate, GRE General Test (waived for DNP if cumulative GPA is 3.25 or greater, nursing GPA is 3.0 or greater, or a completed graduate program GPA is 3.5 or greater), interview, 3 letters of recommendation, personal statement, current resume; for Post-Graduate Certificate, MSN in a clinical discipline, 3 letters of recommendation, personal statement, current resume, interview. Additional exam requirements/recommendations for international students: Required—TOEFL. *Application deadline:* For fall admission, 1/2 for domestic students; for winter admission, 10/15 for domestic students; for spring admission, 8/4 for domestic students; for summer admission, 2/17 for domestic students. Applications are processed on a rolling basis. Application fee: $100. Electronic applications accepted. *Financial support:* Fellowships, research assistantships, teaching assistantships with tuition reimbursements, Federal Work-Study, scholarships/grants, traineeships, and health care benefits available. Support available to part-time students. Financial award application deadline: 3/1; financial award applicants required to submit FAFSA. *Faculty research:* Reduction of health disparities; benefit of human milk feedings for low birth weight infants; decision-making when living with a BRCA mutation over 5-8 year time period; accelerating adoption of comparative effectiveness research in premature infants. *Total annual research expenditures:* $3.8 million. *Unit head:* Dr. Jan Engstrom, Acting Chairperson, 312-942-7117, E-mail: janet_l_engstrom@rush.edu. *Application contact:* Jennifer Thorndyke, Admissions Specialist, 312-563-7526, E-mail: jennifer_thorndyke@rush.edu.
Website: http://www.rushu.rush.edu/servlet/Satellite?c=RushUnivLevel1Page&cid=1204497838852&pagename=Rush%2FRushUnivLevel1Page%2FLevel_1_College_Home_Page

St. Catherine University, Graduate Programs, Program in Nursing, St. Paul, MN 55105. Offers adult gerontological nurse practitioner (MA); neonatal nurse practitioner (MA); nurse educator (MA); nursing (DNP); nursing: entry-level (MA); pediatric nurse practitioner (MA). Part-time and evening/weekend programs available. *Degree requirements:* For master's, thesis; for doctorate, portfolio, systems change project. *Entrance requirements:* For master's, GRE General Test, bachelor's degree in nursing, current nursing license, 2 years of recent clinical practice; for doctorate, master's degree in nursing, RN license, advanced nursing position. Additional exam requirements/recommendations for international students: Required—TOEFL (minimum score 600 paper-based; 100 iBT).

San Francisco State University, Division of Graduate Studies, College of Health and Social Sciences, School of Nursing, San Francisco, CA 94132-1722. Offers adult acute care (MS); clinical nurse specialist (MS); community/public health nursing (MS); family nurse practitioner (MS, Certificate); nursing administration (MS); nursing education (MS); pediatrics (MS); women's health (MS). *Accreditation:* AACN. Part-time programs available. *Application deadline:* Applications are processed on a rolling basis. *Financial support:* Career-related internships or fieldwork available. *Unit head:* Dr. Mary-Ann van Dam, Director, 415-338-1802, E-mail: vandam@sfsu.edu. *Application contact:* Robert Strachan, Admission and Student Services Coordinator, 415-338-1802, E-mail: strachan@sfsu.edu.
Website: http://nursing.sfsu.edu

Seton Hall University, College of Nursing, South Orange, NJ 07079-2697. Offers advanced practice in primary health care (MSN, DNP), including adult/gerontological nurse practitioner, pediatric nurse practitioner; entry into practice (MSN); health systems administration (MSN, DNP); nursing (PhD); nursing case management (MSN); nursing education (MA); school nurse (MSN); MSN/MA. *Accreditation:* AACN. Part-time programs available. Postbaccalaureate distance learning degree programs offered (minimal on-campus study). *Degree requirements:* For master's, research project; for doctorate, dissertation or scholarly project. *Entrance requirements:* For doctorate, GRE (waived for students with GPA of 3.5 or higher). Additional exam requirements/recommendations for international students: Required—TOEFL. Electronic applications accepted. *Faculty research:* Parent/child, adult, and gerontological nursing; breast cancer; families of children with HIV; parish nursing.

Spalding University, Graduate Studies, Kosair College of Health and Natural Sciences, School of Nursing, Louisville, KY 40203-2188. Offers adult nurse practitioner (MSN, PMC); family nurse practitioner (MSN, PMC); leadership in nursing and healthcare (MSN, PMC); pediatric nurse practitioner (MSN, PMC). *Accreditation:* AACN. Part-time and evening/weekend programs available. *Faculty:* 6 full-time (all women), 6 part-time/adjunct (5 women). *Students:* 98 full-time (85 women), 13 part-time (all women); includes 23 minority (19 Black or African American, non-Hispanic/Latino; 2 Asian, non-Hispanic/Latino; 1 Hispanic/Latino; 1 Two or more races, non-Hispanic/Latino). Average age 36. 136 applicants, 31% accepted, 39 enrolled. In 2013, 48 master's, 5 other advanced degrees awarded. *Degree requirements:* For master's, comprehensive exam (for some programs), thesis. *Entrance requirements:* For master's, GRE General Test, BSN or bachelor's degree, RN licensure, autobiographical statement, transcripts, letters of recommendation. Additional exam requirements/recommendations for international students: Required—TOEFL (minimum score 535 paper-based). *Application deadline:* For fall admission, 2/1 priority date for domestic students. Application fee: $30. *Expenses: Tuition:* Full-time $21,450. *Required fees:* $810. Tuition and fees vary according to course load, degree level, program and student level. *Financial support:* Career-related internships or fieldwork, scholarships/grants, and traineeships available. Support available to part-time students. Financial award application deadline: 3/30; financial award applicants required to submit FAFSA. *Faculty research:* Nurse educational administration, gerontology, bioterrorism, healthcare ethics, leadership. *Unit head:* Dr. Paula Travis, Chair, 502-873-4298, E-mail: clewis@spalding.edu. *Application contact:* Dr. Pam King, Assistant Professor, 502-873-4292, E-mail: pking@spalding.edu.
Website: http://www.spalding.edu/nursing/

Stony Brook University, State University of New York, Stony Brook University Medical Center, Health Sciences Center, School of Nursing, Program in Child Health Nursing, Stony Brook, NY 11794. Offers child health nurse practitioner (Certificate); child health nursing (MS, DNP). *Accreditation:* AACN. Postbaccalaureate distance learning degree programs offered. *Students:* 4 full-time (all women), 57 part-time (all women); includes 11 minority (3 Black or African American, non-Hispanic/Latino; 3 Asian, non-Hispanic/Latino; 4 Hispanic/Latino; 1 Two or more races, non-Hispanic/Latino), 8 international. In 2013, 10 master's, 2 other advanced degrees awarded. *Degree requirements:* For master's, thesis. *Entrance requirements:* For master's, BSN, minimum GPA of 3.0, course work in statistics. Additional exam requirements/recommendations for international students: Required—TOEFL. *Application deadline:* For fall admission, 1/15 for domestic students. Application fee: $100. *Expenses:* Tuition, state resident: full-time $9870; part-time $411 per credit. Tuition, nonresident: full-time $18,350; part-time $765 per credit. *Financial support:* Application deadline: 3/15. *Unit head:* Prof. Arleen Steckel, Chair, 631-444-3264, Fax: 631-444-3136, E-mail: arleen.steckel@stonybrook.edu. *Application contact:* Dolores C. Bilges, Assistant Dean, Admissions and Records, 631-444-2644, Fax: 631-444-3136, E-mail: dolores.bilges@stonybrook.edu.
Website: http://www.stonybrook.edu/sb/departments/nursing.shtml

Texas Christian University, Harris College of Nursing and Health Sciences, Program in Nursing, Fort Worth, TX 76129-0002. Offers advanced practice registered nurse (DNP); clinical nurse leader (MSN); clinical nurse specialist: adult/gerontology nursing (MSN); clinical nurse specialist: pediatric nursing (MSN); nursing administration (DNP); nursing education (MSN). *Accreditation:* AACN; AANA/CANAEP (one or more programs are accredited). Part-time programs available. Postbaccalaureate distance learning degree programs offered (no on-campus study). *Faculty:* 18 full-time (16 women), 1 (woman) part-time/adjunct. *Students:* 44 full-time (35 women), 46 part-time (42 women); includes 8 minority (3 Black or African American, non-Hispanic/Latino; 2 Asian, non-Hispanic/Latino; 3 Hispanic/Latino), 1 international. Average age 43. 72 applicants, 63% accepted, 36 enrolled. In 2013, 19 master's, 17 doctorates awarded. *Degree requirements:* For master's, professional project; for doctorate, capstone project. *Entrance requirements:* For master's, GRE General Test, 3 letters of reference, essay, resume, two official transcripts from every institution attended; for doctorate, APRN recognition (national certification) or master's and experience in nursing administration; 3 letters of reference; essay; resume; two official transcripts from every institution attended. Additional exam requirements/recommendations for international students: Recommended—TOEFL. *Application deadline:* For fall admission, 4/1 for domestic students; for spring admission, 9/1 for domestic students; for summer admission, 2/1 for domestic students. Applications are processed on a rolling basis. Application fee: $60. Electronic applications accepted. *Expenses: Tuition:* Part-time $1270 per credit hour. Tuition and fees vary according to course load and program. *Financial support:* In 2013–14, 4 teaching assistantships (averaging $2,500 per year) were awarded. Financial award applicants required to submit FAFSA. *Unit head:* Dr. Kathy A. Baker, Director, Division of Nursing Graduate Studies and Scholarship, 817-257-6726, Fax: 817-257-8383, E-mail: kathy.baker@tcu.edu. *Application contact:* Mary Jane Allred, Administrative Program Specialist, 817-257-6726, Fax: 817-257-8383, E-mail: m.allred@tcu.edu.
Website: http://www.nursing.tcu.edu/graduate.asp

Texas Tech University Health Sciences Center, School of Nursing, Lubbock, TX 79430. Offers acute care nurse practitioner (MSN, Certificate); administration (MSN); advanced practice (DNP); education (MSN); executive leadership (DNP); family nurse practitioner (MSN, Certificate); geriatric nurse practitioner (MSN, Certificate); pediatric nurse practitioner (MSN, Certificate). *Accreditation:* AACN. Part-time programs available. Postbaccalaureate distance learning degree programs offered (minimal on-campus study). *Degree requirements:* For master's, thesis optional. *Entrance requirements:* For master's, minimum GPA of 3.0, 3 letters of reference, BSN, RN license; for Certificate, minimum GPA of 3.0, 3 letters of reference, RN license. Additional exam requirements/recommendations for international students: Required—TOEFL (minimum score 550 paper-based). *Faculty research:* Diabetes/obesity, nurse competency, disease management, intervention and measurements, health disparities.

Texas Woman's University, Graduate School, College of Nursing, Denton, TX 76201. Offers acute care nurse practitioner (MS); adult health clinical nurse specialist (MS); adult health nurse practitioner (MS); child health clinical nurse specialist (MS); clinical nurse leader (MS); family nurse practitioner (MS); health systems management (MS); nursing education (MS); nursing practice (DNP); nursing science (PhD); pediatric nurse practitioner (MS); women's health clinical nurse specialist (MS); women's health nurse practitioner (MS). *Accreditation:* AACN. Part-time programs available. Postbaccalaureate distance learning degree programs offered. *Faculty:* 60 full-time (59 women), 46 part-time/adjunct (39 women). *Students:* 54 full-time (49 women), 910 part-time (848 women); includes 489 minority (221 Black or African American, non-Hispanic/Latino; 11 American Indian or Alaska Native, non-Hispanic/Latino; 184 Asian, non-Hispanic/Latino; 70 Hispanic/Latino; 3 Native Hawaiian or other Pacific Islander, non-Hispanic/Latino), 16 international. Average age 38. 430 applicants, 65% accepted, 193 enrolled. In 2013, 258 master's, 22 doctorates awarded. *Degree requirements:* For master's, comprehensive exam, thesis or alternative; for doctorate, comprehensive exam, thesis/dissertation. *Entrance requirements:* For master's, GRE or MAT, minimum GPA of 3.0 on last 60 hours in undergraduate nursing degree and overall, RN license, BS in nursing, basic statistics course; for doctorate, GRE (preferred minimum score 153 [500 old version] Verbal, 144 [500 old version] Quantitative, 4 Analytical), MS in nursing, minimum preferred GPA of 3.5, RN license, statistics, 2 letters of reference, curriculum vitae, graduate nursing-theory course, graduate research course, statement of professional goals and research interests. Additional exam requirements/recommendations for international students: Required—TOEFL (minimum score 550 paper-based; 79 iBT). *Application deadline:* For fall admission, 5/1 priority date for domestic students, 3/1 for international students; for spring admission, 9/15 priority date for domestic students, 7/1 for international students. Applications are processed on a rolling basis. Application fee: $50 ($75 for international students). Electronic applications accepted. *Expenses:* Tuition, state resident: full-time $4182; part-time $233.32 per credit hour. Tuition, nonresident: full-time $10,716; part-time $595.32 per credit hour. *Financial support:* In 2013–14, 149 students received support, including 10 research assistantships (averaging $5,600 per year), 1 teaching assistantship (averaging $5,600 per year); career-related internships or fieldwork, Federal Work-Study, institutionally sponsored loans, scholarships/grants, traineeships, health care benefits, and unspecified assistantships also available. Support available to part-time students. Financial award application deadline: 3/1; financial award applicants required to submit FAFSA. *Faculty research:* Screening, prevention, and treatment for intimate partner violence; needs of adolescents during childbirth intervention; a network analysis decision tool for nurse managers (social network analysis); support for adolescents with implantable cardioverter defibrillators; informatics: nurse staffing, safety, quality, and financial data as they relate to patient care outcomes; prevention and treatment of obesity; improving infant outcomes related to premature birth. *Total annual research expenditures:* $1.7 million. *Unit head:* Dr. Gayle Roux, Interim Dean and Associate Dean for Research and Clinical Scholarship, 940-898-2401, Fax: 940-898-2437, E-mail: nursing@twu.edu. *Application contact:* Dr. Samuel Wheeler, Assistant Director of Admissions, 940-898-3188, Fax: 940-898-3081, E-mail: wheelersr@twu.edu.
Website: http://www.twu.edu/nursing/

University of Cincinnati, Graduate School, College of Nursing, Cincinnati, OH 45221-0038. Offers clinical nurse specialist (MSN), including adult health, community health, neonatal, nursing administration, occupational health, pediatric health, psychiatric nursing, women's health; nurse anesthesia (MSN); nurse midwifery (MSN); nurse practitioner (MSN), including acute care, ambulatory care, family, family/psychiatric, women's health; nursing (PhD); MBA/MSN. *Accreditation:* AACN; AANA/CANAEP (one or more programs are accredited); ACNM/ACME. Part-time programs available. Postbaccalaureate distance learning degree programs offered (no on-campus study). Terminal master's awarded for partial completion of doctoral program. *Degree requirements:* For master's, thesis or alternative; for doctorate, comprehensive exam,

624-3835, Fax: 412-624-8521, E-mail: sje1@pitt.edu. *Application contact:* Laurie Lapsley, Administrator of Graduate Student Services, 412-624-9670, Fax: 412-624-2409, E-mail: lapsleyl@pitt.edu.
Website: http://www.nursing.pitt.edu

University of Puerto Rico, Medical Sciences Campus, School of Nursing, San Juan, PR 00936-5067. Offers adult and elderly nursing (MSN); child and adolescent nursing (MSN); critical care nursing (MSN); family and community nursing (MSN); family nurse practitioner (MSN); maternity nursing (MSN); mental health and psychiatric nursing (MSN). *Accreditation:* AACN. *Entrance requirements:* For master's, GRE or EXADEP, interview, Puerto Rico RN license or professional license for international students, general and specific point average, article analysis. Electronic applications accepted. *Faculty research:* HIV, health disparities, teen violence, women and violence, neurological disorders.

University of Rochester, School of Nursing, Rochester, NY 14642. Offers acute care nurse practitioner (MS); adult nurse practitioner (MS); adult/geriatric nurse practitioner (MS); clinical nurse leader (MS); clinical research coordinator (MS); family nurse practitioner (MS); family psychiatric mental health nurse practitioner (MS); health care organization management and leadership (MS); health practice research (PhD); nursing (DNP); pediatric nurse practitioner (MS); pediatric nurse practitioner/neonatal nurse practitioner (MS). *Accreditation:* AACN. Part-time programs available. Postbaccalaureate distance learning degree programs offered (minimal on-campus study). *Faculty:* 60 full-time (52 women), 61 part-time/adjunct (47 women). *Students:* 33 full-time (29 women), 213 part-time (195 women); includes 32 minority (8 Black or African American, non-Hispanic/Latino; 10 Asian, non-Hispanic/Latino; 8 Hispanic/Latino; 6 Two or more races, non-Hispanic/Latino), 4 international. Average age 34. 41 applicants, 54% accepted, 16 enrolled. In 2013, 58 master's, 11 doctorates awarded. Terminal master's awarded for partial completion of doctoral program. *Degree requirements:* For master's, comprehensive exam (for some programs); for doctorate, thesis/dissertation. *Entrance requirements:* For master's, BS in nursing, minimum GPA of 3.0, course work in statistics; for doctorate, GRE General Test, MS in nursing, minimum GPA of 3.5. Additional exam requirements/recommendations for international students: Required—TOEFL (minimum score 560 paper-based; 88 iBT) or IELTS (minimum score 6.5) recommended. *Application deadline:* For fall admission, 4/1 for domestic and international students; for spring admission, 9/1 for domestic and international students; for summer admission, 1/2 for domestic and international students. Application fee: $50. Electronic applications accepted. *Expenses: Tuition:* Full-time $44,580; part-time $1394 per credit hour. *Required fees:* $492. *Financial support:* In 2013–14, 41 students received support, including 2 fellowships with full and partial tuition reimbursements available (averaging $30,200 per year); scholarships/grants, traineeships, health care benefits, tuition waivers (partial), and unspecified assistantships also available. Support available to part-time students. Financial award application deadline: 6/30. *Faculty research:* Symptom assessment and self-management, illness prevention, nursing intervention research with vulnerable populations, palliative care, aging. *Total annual research expenditures:* $3.5 million. *Unit head:* Dr. Kathy H. Rideout, Dean, 585-273-8902, Fax: 585-273-1268, E-mail: kathy_rideout@urmc.rochester.edu. *Application contact:* Elaine Andolina, Director of Admissions, 585-275-2375, Fax: 585-756-8299, E-mail: elaine_andolina@urmc.rochester.edu.
Website: http://www.son.rochester.edu

University of San Diego, Hahn School of Nursing and Health Science, San Diego, CA 92110. Offers adult-gerontology clinical nurse specialist (MSN); adult-gerontology nurse practitioner/family nurse practitioner (MSN); clinical nursing (MSN); executive nurse leader (MSN); family nurse practitioner (MSN); family/lifespan psychiatric-mental health nurse practitioner (MSN); healthcare informatics (MS, MSN); nursing (PhD); nursing practice (DNP); pediatric nurse practitioner/family nurse practitioner (MSN). *Accreditation:* AACN. Part-time and evening/weekend programs available. *Faculty:* 23 full-time (19 women), 48 part-time/adjunct (43 women). *Students:* 204 full-time (170 women), 166 part-time (144 women); includes 133 minority (26 Black or African American, non-Hispanic/Latino; 8 American Indian or Alaska Native, non-Hispanic/Latino; 50 Asian, non-Hispanic/Latino; 42 Hispanic/Latino; 1 Native Hawaiian or other Pacific Islander, non-Hispanic/Latino; 6 Two or more races, non-Hispanic/Latino), 7 international. Average age 36. 483 applicants, 58% accepted, 154 enrolled. In 2013, 91 master's, 33 doctorates awarded. *Degree requirements:* For doctorate, thesis/dissertation (for some programs), residency (DNP). *Entrance requirements:* For master's, GRE General Test (for entry-level nursing), BSN, current California RN licensure (except for entry-level nursing); minimum GPA of 3.0; for doctorate, minimum GPA of 3.5, MSN, current California RN licensure. Additional exam requirements/recommendations for international students: Required—TOEFL (minimum score 580 paper-based; 83 iBT), TWE. *Application deadline:* For fall admission, 3/1 priority date for domestic students, 3/1 for international students; for spring admission, 11/1 priority date for domestic students, 11/1 for international students. Applications are processed on a rolling basis. Application fee: $45. Electronic applications accepted. *Expenses: Tuition:* Full-time $23,580; part-time $1310 per credit. *Required fees:* $350. *Financial support:* In 2013–14, 250 students received support. Scholarships/grants and traineeships available. Support available to part-time students. Financial award application deadline: 4/1; financial award applicants required to submit FAFSA. *Faculty research:* Palliative and end of life care, maternal/child health, childhood obesity, health care disparities, cognitive functioning. *Unit head:* Dr. Sally Hardin, Dean, 619-260-4550, Fax: 619-260-6814. *Application contact:* Monica Mahon, Associate Director of Graduate Admissions, 619-260-4524, Fax: 619-260-4158, E-mail: grads@sandiego.edu.
Website: http://www.sandiego.edu/nursing/

University of South Carolina, The Graduate School, College of Nursing, Program in Health Nursing, Columbia, SC 29208. Offers adult nurse practitioner (MSN); community/public health clinical nurse specialist (MSN); family nurse practitioner (MSN); pediatric nurse practitioner (MSN). *Accreditation:* AACN. Part-time programs available. *Degree requirements:* For master's, thesis or alternative. *Entrance requirements:* For master's, GRE General Test or MAT, BS in nursing, nursing license. Additional exam requirements/recommendations for international students: Required—TOEFL (minimum score 570 paper-based). Electronic applications accepted. *Faculty research:* System research, evidence based practice, breast cancer, violence.

University of South Florida, College of Nursing, Tampa, FL 33612. Offers adult gerontology acute care (DNP, PhD); adult gerontology acute care nursing (MS); adult gerontology primary care (DNP, PhD); adult gerontology primary care nursing (MS); adult gerontology primary care/occupational health nursing (MS); adult gerontology primary care/oncology nursing (MS, PhD); clinical nurse leader (MS); family health (DNP, PhD); family nurse practitioner (MS); nurse anesthesia (MS); nursing education (MS); nursing practice (DNP); nursing science (PhD), including nursing education; occupational health/adult-gerontology (DNP); oncology/adult-gerontology primary care (DNP); pediatric health (DNP, PhD); pediatric nurse practitioner (MS). *Accreditation:* AACN; AANA/CANAEP. Part-time programs available. *Faculty:* 46 full-time (40 women), 15 part-time/adjunct (11 women). *Students:* 177 full-time (150 women), 700 part-time (622 women); includes 272 minority (116 Black or African American, non-Hispanic/Latino; 2 American Indian or Alaska Native, non-Hispanic/Latino; 45 Asian, non-Hispanic/Latino; 93 Hispanic/Latino; 2 Native Hawaiian or other Pacific Islander, non-Hispanic/Latino; 14 Two or more races, non-Hispanic/Latino), 12 international. Average age 35. 656 applicants, 43% accepted, 224 enrolled. In 2013, 224 master's, 14 doctorates awarded. *Degree requirements:* For master's, comprehensive exam, thesis optional; for doctorate, comprehensive exam, thesis/dissertation. *Entrance requirements:* For master's, GRE General Test, bachelor's degree from accredited program with minimum GPA of 3.0 in all upper-division coursework; current license as Registered Nurse; 3 letters of recommendation; personal statement of goals; resume or curriculum vitae; personal interview; for doctorate, GRE General Test (recommended), bachelor's degree in nursing from a CCNA/NLNAC regionally-accredited institution with minimum GPA of 3.0 in all coursework or in all upper-division coursework; current license as Registered Nurse in Florida; undergraduate statistics course with minimum B grade; 3 letters of recommendation; statement of goals; resume; interview. Additional exam requirements/recommendations for international students: Required—TOEFL (minimum score 550 paper-based; 79 iBT). *Application deadline:* For fall admission, 2/15 for domestic students, 1/2 for international students; for spring admission, 10/1 for domestic students, 6/1 for international students. Application fee: $30. Electronic applications accepted. *Financial support:* In 2013–14, 36 students received support, including 7 research assistantships with tuition reimbursements available (averaging $18,935 per year), 29 teaching assistantships with tuition reimbursements available (averaging $30,814 per year); tuition waivers (partial) and unspecified assistantships also available. Financial award application deadline: 2/1; financial award applicants required to submit FAFSA. *Faculty research:* Women's health, palliative and end-of-life care, cardiac rehabilitation, complementary therapies for chronic illness and cancer. *Total annual research expenditures:* $3.4 million. *Unit head:* Dr. Dianne C. Morrison-Beedy, Dean and Professor, College of Nursing, 813-974-9091, Fax: 813-974-5418, E-mail: dmbeedy@health.usf.edu. *Application contact:* Dr. Connie Visovsky, Associate Professor and Associate Dean of Student Affairs, 813-396-9641, Fax: 813-974-5418, E-mail: cvisovsk@health.usf.edu.
Website: http://health.usf.edu/nursing/index.htm

The University of Texas at Austin, Graduate School, School of Nursing, Austin, TX 78712-1111. Offers adult - gerontology clinical nurse specialist (MSN); child health (MSN), including administration, public health nursing, teaching; family nurse practitioner (MSN); family psychiatric/mental health nurse practitioner (MSN); holistic adult health (MSN), including administration, teaching; maternity (MSN), including administration, public health nursing, teaching; nursing (PhD); nursing administration and healthcare systems management (MSN); pediatric nurse practitioner (MSN); public health nursing (MSN). *Accreditation:* AACN. Part-time programs available. *Degree requirements:* For master's, thesis optional; for doctorate, thesis/dissertation. *Entrance requirements:* For master's and doctorate, GRE General Test. Additional exam requirements/recommendations for international students: Required—TOEFL (minimum score 550 paper-based). Electronic applications accepted. *Faculty research:* Chronic illness management, memory and aging, health promotion, women's health, adolescent health.

The University of Texas Health Science Center at San Antonio, School of Nursing, San Antonio, TX 78229. Offers administrative management (MSN); adult-gerontology acute care nurse practitioner (PGC); clinical nurse leader (MSN); executive administrative management (DNP); family nurse practitioner (PGC); nurse practitioner (MSN), including adult-gerontology acute care nurse practitioner, family nurse practitioner, pediatric nurse practitioner primary care, psychiatric mental health nurse practitioner; nurse practitioner leadership (DNP); nursing (MSN, PhD); nursing education (MSN, PGC); pediatric nurse practitioner primary care (PGC); psychiatric mental health nurse practitioner (PGC); public health nurse leader (DNP). *Accreditation:* AACN. Part-time programs available. *Faculty:* 84 full-time (74 women), 42 part-time/adjunct (40 women). *Students:* 115 full-time (93 women), 140 part-time (123 women); includes 123 minority (24 Black or African American, non-Hispanic/Latino; 20 Asian, non-Hispanic/Latino; 74 Hispanic/Latino; 5 Two or more races, non-Hispanic/Latino), 7 international. Average age 37. 174 applicants, 59% accepted, 83 enrolled. In 2013, 67 master's, 6 doctorates, 5 other advanced degrees awarded. Terminal master's awarded for partial completion of doctoral program. *Degree requirements:* For master's, thesis optional; for doctorate, comprehensive exam, thesis/dissertation, final projects (for DNP). *Entrance requirements:* For master's, minimum GPA of 3.0, references, goal statement, BSN from accredited nursing school, RN licensure in Texas or compact state; for doctorate, GRE, MAT, minimum GPA of 3.0, personal interview, BSN and/or MSN from accredited nursing school, RN licensure in Texas or compact state, statistics course, references, curriculum vitae, goal statement; for PGC, minimum GPA of 3.0; references; goal statement; MSN from accredited nursing school; RN licensure in Texas or compact state; prerequisites in advanced health assessment, advanced pharmacotherapeutics, and advanced pathophysiology. Additional exam requirements/recommendations for international students: Required—TOEFL (minimum score 550 paper-based; 68 iBT), IELTS (minimum score 6.5). *Application deadline:* For fall admission, 1/10 for domestic and international students; for spring admission, 7/1 for domestic students. Application fee: $65. Electronic applications accepted. *Financial support:* In 2013–14, 145 students received support, including 3 fellowships with full tuition reimbursements available (averaging $30,000 per year); institutionally sponsored loans and scholarships/grants also available. Financial award application deadline: 6/30; financial award applicants required to submit FAFSA. *Faculty research:* Pain, organizational structure, aging, quality and safety, health disparity, obesity and nutrition, women's and children's health. *Total annual research expenditures:* $500,265. *Unit head:* Dr. Eileen T. Breslin, Dean, 210-567-5800, Fax: 210-567-5929, E-mail: breslin@uthscsa.edu. *Application contact:* Brandy Finck, Interim Associate Dean for Admissions and Student Services, 210-567-5805, Fax: 210-567-6189, E-mail: finckb@uthscsa.edu.
Website: http://www.nursing.uthscsa.edu/

The University of Toledo, College of Graduate Studies, College of Nursing, Department of Population and Community Care, Toledo, OH 43606-3390. Offers clinical nurse leader (MSN); family nurse practitioner (MSN, Certificate); nurse educator (MSN, Certificate); pediatric nurse practitioner (MSN, Certificate). Part-time programs available. *Students:* 70 full-time (60 women), 212 part-time (186 women); includes 27 minority (12 Black or African American, non-Hispanic/Latino; 1 American Indian or Alaska Native, non-Hispanic/Latino; 3 Asian, non-Hispanic/Latino; 7 Hispanic/Latino; 4 Two or more races, non-Hispanic/Latino), 1 international. Average age 32. 127 applicants, 81% accepted, 78 enrolled. In 2013, 82 master's, 10 other advanced degrees awarded. *Degree requirements:* For master's, thesis or alternative. *Entrance requirements:* For master's, GRE, BS in nursing, minimum undergraduate GPA of 3.0, statement of purpose, three letters of recommendation, transcripts from all prior institutions attended, Nursing CAS application, UT supplemental application; for Certificate, BS in nursing, minimum undergraduate GPA of 3.0, statement of purpose, three letters of recommendation, transcripts from all prior institutions attended. Additional exam requirements/recommendations for international students: Required—TOEFL (minimum score 550 paper-based; 80 iBT). Application fee: $45 ($75 for international students). Electronic applications accepted. *Financial support:* Research assistantships with full and partial tuition reimbursements, Federal Work-Study, scholarships/grants, traineeships, and tuition waivers (full and partial) available. *Unit head:* Dr. Kelley

Phillips, Chair, 419-383-5892. *Application contact:* Joan Mulligan, Admissions Analyst, 419-383-4168, Fax: 419-383-6140, E-mail: joan.mulligan@utoledo.edu.
Website: http://www.utoledo.edu/nursing/

University of Wisconsin–Madison, School of Nursing, Madison, WI 53706-1380. Offers adult/gerontology (DNP); nursing (PhD); pediatrics (DNP); psychiatric mental health (DNP); MS/MPH. *Accreditation:* AACN. Part-time programs available. *Degree requirements:* For doctorate, comprehensive exam, thesis/dissertation. *Entrance requirements:* For doctorate, GRE General Test, 2 samples of scholarly written work, BS in nursing from an accredited program, minimum undergraduate GPA of 3.0 in last 60 credits (for PhD); licensure as professional nurse (for DNP). Additional exam requirements/recommendations for international students: Required—TOEFL (minimum score 600 paper-based; 100 iBT). Electronic applications accepted. *Expenses:* Tuition, state resident: full-time $10,728; part-time $790 per credit. Tuition, nonresident: full-time $24,054; part-time $1623 per credit. *Required fees:* $1130; $119 per credit. *Faculty research:* Nursing informatics to promote self-care and disease management skills among patients and caregivers; quality of care to frail, vulnerable, and chronically ill populations; study of health-related and health-seeking behaviors; eliminating health disparities; pain and symptom management for patients with cancer.

Vanderbilt University, Vanderbilt University School of Nursing, Nashville, TN 37240. Offers adult-gerontology acute care nurse practitioner (MSN), including hospitalist, intensivist; adult-gerontology primary care nurse practitioner (MSN); emergency nurse practitioner (MSN); family nurse practitioner (MSN); healthcare leadership (MSN); neonatal nurse practitioner (MSN); nurse midwifery (MSN); nurse midwifery/family nurse practitioner (MSN); nursing informatics (MSN); nursing practice (DNP); nursing science (PhD); pediatric acute care nurse practitioner (MSN); pediatric primary care nurse practitioner (MSN); psychiatric-mental health nurse practitioner (MSN); women's health nurse practitioner (MSN); women's health nurse practitioner/adult gerontology primary care nurse practitioner (MSN); MSN/M Div; MSN/MTS. *Accreditation:* ACNM/ACME (one or more programs are accredited). Part-time programs available. Postbaccalaureate distance learning degree programs offered (minimal on-campus study). *Faculty:* 139 full-time (124 women), 452 part-time/adjunct (319 women). *Students:* 527 full-time (463 women), 369 part-time (333 women); includes 120 minority (46 Black or African American, non-Hispanic/Latino; 8 American Indian or Alaska Native, non-Hispanic/Latino; 26 Asian, non-Hispanic/Latino; 24 Hispanic/Latino; 4 Native Hawaiian or other Pacific Islander, non-Hispanic/Latino; 12 Two or more races, non-Hispanic/Latino), 7 international. Average age 32. 1,257 applicants, 49% accepted, 457 enrolled. In 2013, 364 master's, 43 doctorates awarded. *Degree requirements:* For doctorate, comprehensive exam, thesis/dissertation. *Entrance requirements:* For master's, GRE General Test (within the past 5 years), minimum B average in undergraduate course work, 3 letters of recommendation; for doctorate, GRE General Test, interview, 3 letters of recommendation from doctorally-prepared faculty, MSN, essay. Additional exam requirements/recommendations for international students: Required—TOEFL (minimum score 570 paper-based), IELTS (minimum score 6.5). *Application deadline:* For fall admission, 12/1 priority date for domestic and international students. Applications are processed on a rolling basis. Application fee: $50. Electronic applications accepted. *Expenses:* Contact institution. *Financial support:* In 2013–14, 582 students received support. Scholarships/grants and health care benefits available. Support available to part-time students. Financial award application deadline: 3/15; financial award applicants required to submit FAFSA. *Faculty research:* Lymphedema, palliative care and bereavement, health services research including workforce, safety and quality of care, gerontology, better birth outcomes including nutrition. *Total annual research expenditures:* $2.5 million. *Unit head:* Dr. Linda Norman, Dean, 615-343-8876, Fax: 615-343-7711, E-mail: linda.norman@vanderbilt.edu. *Application contact:* Patricia Peerman, Assistant Dean for Enrollment Management, 615-322-3800, Fax: 615-343-0333, E-mail: vusn-admissions@vanderbilt.edu.
Website: http://www.nursing.vanderbilt.edu

Villanova University, College of Nursing, Villanova, PA 19085-1699. Offers adult nurse practitioner (MSN, Post Master's Certificate); family nurse practitioner (MSN, Post Master's Certificate); health care administration (MSN, Post Master's Certificate); nurse anesthetist (MSN, Post Master's Certificate); nursing (PhD); nursing education (MSN, Post Master's Certificate); nursing practice (DNP); pediatric nurse practitioner (MSN, Post Master's Certificate). *Accreditation:* AACN; AANA/CANAEP. Part-time programs available. Postbaccalaureate distance learning degree programs offered (minimal on-campus study). *Faculty:* 17 full-time (all women), 4 part-time/adjunct (all women). *Students:* 28 full-time (26 women), 191 part-time (161 women); includes 22 minority (2 Black or African American, non-Hispanic/Latino; 6 Asian, non-Hispanic/Latino; 7 Hispanic/Latino; 7 Two or more races, non-Hispanic/Latino), 18 international. Average age 30. 176 applicants, 65% accepted, 82 enrolled. In 2013, 64 master's, 7 doctorates, 5 other advanced degrees awarded. *Degree requirements:* For master's, independent study project; for doctorate, comprehensive exam, thesis/dissertation. *Entrance requirements:* For master's, GRE or MAT, BSN, 1 year of recent nursing experience, physical assessment, course work in statistics; for doctorate, GRE, MSN. Additional exam requirements/recommendations for international students: Required—TOEFL (minimum score 540 paper-based; 83 iBT), IELTS (minimum score 6.5). *Application deadline:* For fall admission, 7/1 priority date for domestic students, 7/1 for international students; for spring admission, 11/1 priority date for domestic students, 11/1 for international students. Applications are processed on a rolling basis. Application fee: $50. Electronic applications accepted. *Expenses:* Contact institution. *Financial support:* In 2013–14, 39 students received support, including 5 teaching assistantships with full tuition reimbursements available (averaging $14,475 per year); institutionally sponsored loans, scholarships/grants, traineeships, tuition waivers (full), and unspecified assistantships also available. Financial award application deadline: 7/1; financial award applicants required to submit FAFSA. *Faculty research:* Genetics, ethics, cognitive development of students, women with disabilities, nursing leadership. *Unit head:* Dr. Marguerite K. Schlag, Assistant Dean/Director, Graduate Programs, 610-519-4907, Fax: 610-519-7650, E-mail: marguerite.schlag@villanova.edu.
Website: http://www.nursing.villanova.edu/

Virginia Commonwealth University, Graduate School, School of Nursing, Richmond, VA 23284-9005. Offers adult health acute nursing (MS); adult health primary nursing (MS); biobehavioral clinical research (PhD); child health nursing (MS); clinical nurse leader (MS); family health nursing (MS); nurse educator (MS); nurse practitioner (MS); nursing (Certificate); nursing administration (MS), including clinical nurse manager; psychiatric-mental health nursing (MS); women's health nursing (MS). Part-time and evening/weekend programs available. *Degree requirements:* For master's, thesis optional; for doctorate, thesis/dissertation. *Entrance requirements:* For master's, GRE General Test, BSN, minimum GPA of 2.8; for doctorate, GRE General Test. Additional exam requirements/recommendations for international students: Required—TOEFL (minimum score 600 paper-based; 100 iBT). Electronic applications accepted.

Wayne State University, College of Nursing, Program in Advanced Practice Nursing with Women, Neonates and Children, Detroit, MI 48202. Offers neonatal nurse practitioner (MSN); nurse-midwife (MSN); pediatric nurse practitioner (MSN), including acute care, primary care; women's health nurse practitioner (MSN). *Accreditation:* AACN. Part-time programs available. *Students:* 59 full-time (53 women), 74 part-time (72 women); includes 17 minority (11 Black or African American, non-Hispanic/Latino; 2 Asian, non-Hispanic/Latino; 4 Hispanic/Latino), 6 international. Average age 32. 65 applicants, 55% accepted, 33 enrolled. In 2013, 40 degrees awarded. *Degree requirements:* For master's, thesis or alternative. *Entrance requirements:* For master's, minimum honor point average of 3.0 in upper-division course work; BA from NLN- or CCNE-accredited program; references; current RN license; personal statement. Additional exam requirements/recommendations for international students: Required—TOEFL (minimum score 550 paper-based; 79 iBT); Recommended—TWE (minimum score 6). *Application deadline:* For fall admission, 6/1 priority date for domestic students, 5/1 priority date for international students; for winter admission, 10/1 priority date for domestic students, 9/1 priority date for international students; for spring admission, 2/1 priority date for domestic students, 1/1 priority date for international students. Applications are processed on a rolling basis. Application fee: $50. Electronic applications accepted. *Expenses:* Contact institution. *Financial support:* In 2013–14, 17 students received support. Fellowships with tuition reimbursements available, research assistantships with tuition reimbursements available, teaching assistantships with tuition reimbursements available, scholarships/grants, and unspecified assistantships available. Financial award applicants required to submit FAFSA. *Faculty research:* Acculturation and parenting, domestic violence, evidence-based midwifery practice, pain in children, trauma and community violence. *Unit head:* Dr. Barbara Redman, Dean, 313-577-4070, Fax: 313-577-4571, E-mail: ae9080@wayne.edu. *Application contact:* Dr. Cynthia Redwine, Assistant Dean for the Office of Student Affairs, 313-577-4082, E-mail: nursinginfo@wayne.edu.
Website: http://nursing.wayne.edu/msn/specialty.php

Wright State University, School of Graduate Studies, College of Nursing and Health, Program in Nursing, Dayton, OH 45435. Offers acute care nurse practitioner (MS); administration of nursing and health care systems (MS); adult health (MS); child and adolescent health (MS); community health (MS); family nurse practitioner (MS); nurse practitioner (MS); school nurse (MS); MBA/MS. *Accreditation:* AACN. Part-time and evening/weekend programs available. *Degree requirements:* For master's, thesis or alternative. *Entrance requirements:* For master's, GRE General Test, BSN from NLN-accredited college, Ohio RN license. Additional exam requirements/recommendations for international students: Required—TOEFL. *Faculty research:* Clinical nursing and health, teaching, caring, pain administration, informatics and technology.

Psychiatric Nursing

Allen College, Program in Nursing, Waterloo, IA 50703. Offers acute care nurse practitioner (MSN, Post-Master's Certificate); adult nurse practitioner (MSN, Post-Master's Certificate); adult psychiatric-mental health nurse practitioner (MSN, Post-Master's Certificate); community public health (MSN, Post-Master's Certificate); family nurse practitioner (MSN, Post-Master's Certificate); gerontological nurse practitioner (MSN, Post-Master's Certificate); health education (MSN); leadership in health care delivery (MSN, Post-Master's Certificate); nursing (DNP). Part-time programs available. Postbaccalaureate distance learning degree programs offered (minimal on-campus study). *Faculty:* 3 full-time (all women), 21 part-time/adjunct (20 women). *Students:* 21 full-time (19 women), 162 part-time (150 women); includes 5 minority (1 Black or African American, non-Hispanic/Latino; 2 Asian, non-Hispanic/Latino; 1 Hispanic/Latino; 1 Two or more races, non-Hispanic/Latino). Average age 34. 213 applicants, 57% accepted, 94 enrolled. In 2013, 41 master's, 4 other advanced degrees awarded. *Degree requirements:* For master's, thesis optional. *Entrance requirements:* For master's, minimum GPA of 3.0 in the last 60 hours of undergraduate coursework; for doctorate, minimum GPA of 3.25 in graduate coursework. Additional exam requirements/recommendations for international students: Recommended—TOEFL (minimum score 580 paper-based; 92 iBT), IELTS (minimum score 6). *Application deadline:* For fall admission, 2/1 priority date for domestic students; for spring admission, 9/1 priority date for domestic students. Applications are processed on a rolling basis. Application fee: $50. Electronic applications accepted. *Expenses: Tuition:* Full-time $14,534; part-time $755 per credit hour. *Required fees:* $935; $75 per credit hour. One-time fee: $275 part-time. Tuition and fees vary according to course load. *Financial support:* In 2013–14, 60 students received support. Institutionally sponsored loans, scholarships/grants, and traineeships available. Support available to part-time students. Financial award application deadline: 8/15; financial award applicants required to submit FAFSA. *Unit head:* Kendra Williams-Perez, Dean, School of Nursing, 319-226-2044, Fax: 319-226-2070, E-mail: kendra.williams-perez@allencollege.edu. *Application contact:* Molly Quinn, Admissions Counselor, 319-226-2001, Fax: 319-226-2010, E-mail: molly.quinn@allencollege.edu.
Website: http://www.allencollege.edu/

Alverno College, School of Nursing, Milwaukee, WI 53234-3922. Offers family nurse practitioner (MSN); mental health nurse practitioner (MSN); nursing education (MSN). *Accreditation:* AACN. Part-time and evening/weekend programs available. *Faculty:* 7 full-time (all women), 8 part-time/adjunct (4 women). *Students:* 82 full-time (79 women), 84 part-time (79 women); includes 48 minority (24 Black or African American, non-Hispanic/Latino; 1 American Indian or Alaska Native, non-Hispanic/Latino; 6 Asian, non-Hispanic/Latino; 11 Hispanic/Latino; 6 Two or more races, non-Hispanic/Latino), 1 international. Average age 36. 59 applicants, 100% accepted, 47 enrolled. In 2013, 33 master's awarded. *Degree requirements:* For master's, 500 clinical hours, capstone. *Entrance requirements:* For master's, BSN, current license. Additional exam requirements/recommendations for international students: Required—TOEFL. *Application deadline:* For fall admission, 7/15 priority date for domestic and international students; for spring admission, 12/15 priority date for domestic and international students. Applications are processed on a rolling basis. Application fee: $0. Electronic applications accepted. Application fee is waived when completed online. *Expenses:* Contact institution. *Financial support:* In 2013–14, 4 students received support. Federal Work-Study and scholarships/grants available. Support available to part-time students. Financial award application deadline: 4/15; financial award applicants required to submit

FAFSA. *Faculty research:* Impact of stroke on sexuality, children's asthma management, factors affecting baccalaureate student success. *Unit head:* Dr. Carol Sabel, Associate Dean for MSN Program, 414-382-6309, Fax: 414-382-6354, E-mail: carol.sabel@alverno.edu. *Application contact:* Janet Stikel, Associate Director of Admissions - Adult and Graduate, 414-382-6112, Fax: 414-382-6354, E-mail: janet.stikel@alverno.edu.

American University of Beirut, Graduate Programs, Rafic Hariri School of Nursing, Beirut, Lebanon. Offers adult care nursing (MSN); community and public health nursing (MSN); nursing administration (MSN); psychiatry mental health nursing (MSN). *Accreditation:* AACN. Part-time programs available. *Faculty:* 9 full-time (8 women), 12 part-time/adjunct (10 women). *Students:* 4 full-time (3 women), 56 part-time (44 women). Average age 29. 38 applicants, 87% accepted, 26 enrolled. In 2013, 17 master's awarded. *Degree requirements:* For master's, one foreign language, comprehensive exam, thesis optional. *Entrance requirements:* For master's, letter of recommendation. Additional exam requirements/recommendations for international students: Required—TOEFL (minimum score 600 paper-based); Recommended—IELTS. *Application deadline:* For fall admission, 4/1 for domestic and international students; for spring admission, 11/1 for domestic and international students. Applications are processed on a rolling basis. Application fee: $50. Electronic applications accepted. *Expenses: Tuition:* Full-time $14,724; part-time $818 per credit. *Required fees:* $692. Tuition and fees vary according to course load and program. *Financial support:* In 2013–14, 24 teaching assistantships with partial tuition reimbursements were awarded; unspecified assistantships also available. Financial award application deadline: 12/20. *Faculty research:* Pain management and palliative care, stress and post-traumatic stress disorder, health benefits and chronic illness, health promotion and community interventions. *Unit head:* Dr. Huda Huijer Abu-Saad, Director, 961-1374374 Ext. 5952, Fax: 961-1744476, E-mail: hh35@aub.edu.lb. *Application contact:* Dr. Salim Kanaan, Director, Admissions Office, 961-1-350000 Ext. 2594, Fax: 96-1-1750775, E-mail: sk00@aub.edu.lb.
Website: http://staff.aub.edu.lb/~webson

Arizona State University at the Tempe campus, College of Nursing and Health Innovation, Phoenix, AZ 85004. Offers advanced nursing practice (DNP); child/family mental health nurse practitioner (Graduate Certificate); clinical research management (MS); community and public health practice (Graduate Certificate); community health (MS); exercise and wellness (MS), including exercise and wellness; family nurse practitioner (Graduate Certificate); healthcare innovation (MHI); international health for healthcare (Graduate Certificate); kinesiology (MS, PhD); nursing (MS, Graduate Certificate); nursing and healthcare innovation (PhD); nutrition (MS); physical activity nutrition and wellness (PhD), including physical activity, nutrition and wellness; public health (MPH); regulatory science and health safety (MS). *Accreditation:* AACN. Postbaccalaureate distance learning degree programs offered (minimal on-campus study). *Degree requirements:* For master's, comprehensive exam (for some programs), thesis (for some programs), interactive Program of Study (iPOS) submitted before completing 50 percent of required credit hours; for doctorate, comprehensive exam, thesis/dissertation, interactive Program of Study (iPOS) submitted before completing 50 percent of required credit hours. *Entrance requirements:* For master's and doctorate, GRE, minimum GPA of 3.0 or equivalent in last 2 years of work leading to bachelor's degree. Additional exam requirements/recommendations for international students: Required—TOEFL (minimum score 80 iBT), TOEFL, IELTS, or PTE. Electronic applications accepted. *Expenses:* Contact institution.

Boston College, William F. Connell School of Nursing, Chestnut Hill, MA 02467-3800. Offers adult-gerontology nursing (MS); community health nursing (MS); family health (MS); forensic nursing (MS); maternal/child health nursing (MS), including pediatric and women's health; nurse anesthesia (MS); nursing (PhD); palliative care (MS), including adult and pediatric; psychiatric-mental health nursing (MS); MBA/MS; MS/MA; MS/PhD. *Accreditation:* AACN; AANA/CANAEP (one or more programs are accredited). Part-time programs available. *Faculty:* 47 full-time (43 women), 42 part-time/adjunct (39 women). *Students:* 199 full-time (180 women), 79 part-time (73 women); includes 44 minority (14 Black or African American, non-Hispanic/Latino; 1 American Indian or Alaska Native, non-Hispanic/Latino; 13 Asian, non-Hispanic/Latino; 12 Hispanic/Latino; 4 Two or more races, non-Hispanic/Latino), 7 international. Average age 31. 502 applicants, 39% accepted, 87 enrolled. In 2013, 105 master's, 8 doctorates awarded. *Degree requirements:* For master's, comprehensive exam, research project; for doctorate, comprehensive exam, thesis/dissertation, computer literacy exam or foreign language. *Entrance requirements:* For master's, bachelor's degree in nursing; for doctorate, GRE General Test, MS in nursing. Additional exam requirements/recommendations for international students: Required—TOEFL (minimum score 600 paper-based; 100 iBT). *Application deadline:* For fall admission, 9/30 for domestic and international students; for winter admission, 1/15 for domestic and international students; for spring admission, 3/15 for domestic and international students. Applications are processed on a rolling basis. Application fee: $40. Electronic applications accepted. *Financial support:* In 2013–14, 174 students received support, including 7 fellowships with full tuition reimbursements available (averaging $20,000 per year), 21 teaching assistantships (averaging $4,800 per year); research assistantships, scholarships/grants, health care benefits, tuition waivers (partial), and unspecified assistantships also available. Support available to part-time students. Financial award application deadline: 3/1; financial award applicants required to submit FAFSA. *Faculty research:* Sexual and reproductive health, health promotion/illness prevention, eating disorders, violence, symptom management. *Total annual research expenditures:* $1.1 million. *Unit head:* Dr. Susan Gennaro, Dean, 617-552-4251, Fax: 617-552-0931, E-mail: susan.gennaro@bc.edu. *Application contact:* MaryBeth Crowley, Graduate Programs Assistant, 617-552-4928, Fax: 617-552-2121, E-mail: csongrad@bc.edu.
Website: http://www.bc.edu/schools/son/

Case Western Reserve University, Frances Payne Bolton School of Nursing, Doctor of Nursing Practice Program, Cleveland, OH 44106. Offers acute care nurse practitioner (DNP); adult gerontology nurse practitioner (DNP); educational leadership (DNP); family nurse practitioner (DNP); family systems psychiatric mental health nursing (DNP); midwifery/family nursing (DNP); neonatal nurse practitioner (DNP); pediatric nurse practitioner (DNP); practice leadership (DNP); women's health nurse practitioner (DNP). *Accreditation:* AACN. Part-time programs available. Postbaccalaureate distance learning degree programs offered (minimal on-campus study). *Students:* 169 full-time, 9 part-time; includes 10 minority (6 Black or African American, non-Hispanic/Latino; 1 Asian, non-Hispanic/Latino; 2 Hispanic/Latino; 1 Two or more races, non-Hispanic/Latino). 76 applicants, 97% accepted, 59 enrolled. In 2013, 38 doctorates awarded. Terminal master's awarded for partial completion of doctoral program. *Degree requirements:* For doctorate, thesis/dissertation. *Entrance requirements:* For doctorate, GRE General Test or MAT. Additional exam requirements/recommendations for international students: Required—TOEFL (minimum score 577 paper-based; 90 iBT), IELTS (minimum score 7). *Application deadline:* For fall admission, 6/1 priority date for domestic students, 6/1 for international students; for spring admission, 10/1 for domestic and international students. Applications are processed on a rolling basis. Application fee: $75. *Financial support:* In 2013–14, 90 students received support, including 9 fellowships with full tuition reimbursements available (averaging $31,325 per year), 1 research assistantship with partial tuition reimbursement available (averaging $14,472 per year); teaching assistantships, Federal Work-Study, institutionally sponsored loans, scholarships/grants, and tuition waivers (partial) also available. Support available to part-time students. Financial award application deadline: 5/15; financial award applicants required to submit FAFSA. *Faculty research:* Symptom science, family/community care, aging across the lifespan, self-management of health and illness, neuroscience. *Unit head:* Dr. Donna Dowling, Director, 216-368-1869, Fax: 216-368-3542, E-mail: dad10@case.edu. *Application contact:* Donna Hassik, Admissions Coordinator, 216-368-5253, Fax: 216-368-0124, E-mail: dmh7@case.edu.
Website: http://fpb.case.edu/DNP/

Case Western Reserve University, Frances Payne Bolton School of Nursing, Master's Programs in Nursing, Nurse Practitioner Program, Cleveland, OH 44106. Offers acute care cardiovascular nursing (MSN); acute care nurse practitioner (MSN); acute care/flight nurse (MSN); adult gerontology acute care nurse practitioner (MSN); adult gerontology nurse practitioner (MSN); adult gerontology oncology and palliative care (MSN); family nurse practitioner (MSN); family systems psychiatric mental health nursing (MSN); neonatal nurse practitioner (MSN); pediatric nurse practitioner (MSN); women's health nurse practitioner (MSN). Part-time programs available. Postbaccalaureate distance learning degree programs offered (minimal on-campus study). *Faculty:* 54 full-time (50 women), 5 part-time/adjunct (3 women). *Students:* 56 full-time, 145 part-time; includes 9 minority (6 Black or African American, non-Hispanic/Latino; 2 Asian, non-Hispanic/Latino; 1 Hispanic/Latino), 5 international. Average age 35. 70 applicants, 71% accepted, 33 enrolled. In 2013, 79 master's awarded. *Degree requirements:* For master's, thesis optional. *Entrance requirements:* For master's, GRE General Test or MAT. Additional exam requirements/recommendations for international students: Required—TOEFL (minimum score 577 paper-based; 90 iBT), IELTS (minimum score 7). *Application deadline:* For fall admission, 6/1 for domestic students; for spring admission, 10/1 for domestic students. Applications are processed on a rolling basis. Application fee: $75. *Financial support:* In 2013–14, 25 teaching assistantships (averaging $15,120 per year) were awarded; research assistantships, institutionally sponsored loans, and tuition waivers (partial) also available. Support available to part-time students. Financial award application deadline: 6/30; financial award applicants required to submit FAFSA. *Faculty research:* Symptom science, family/community care, aging across the lifespan, self-management of health and illness, neuroscience. *Unit head:* Dr. Carol Savrin, Director, 216-368-5304, Fax: 216-368-3542, E-mail: cls18@case.edu. *Application contact:* Donna Hassik, Admissions Coordinator, 216-368-5253, Fax: 216-368-0124, E-mail: dmh7@case.edu.
Website: http://fpb.cwru.edu/MSN/majors.shtm

Columbia University, School of Nursing, Program in Psychiatric Mental Health Nursing, New York, NY 10032. Offers MS, Adv C. *Accreditation:* AACN. Part-time programs available. *Entrance requirements:* For master's, GRE General Test, NCLEX, BSN, 1 year of clinical experience (preferred); for Adv C, MSN. Additional exam requirements/recommendations for international students: Required—TOEFL (minimum score 100 iBT). Electronic applications accepted.

Drexel University, College of Nursing and Health Professions, Division of Graduate Nursing, Philadelphia, PA 19104-2875. Offers adult acute care (MSN); adult psychiatric/mental health (MSN); advanced practice nursing (MSN); clinical trials research (MSN); family nurse practitioner (MSN); leadership in health systems management (MSN); nursing education (MSN); pediatric primary care (MSN); women's health (MSN). *Accreditation:* AACN. Electronic applications accepted.

Fairfield University, School of Nursing, Fairfield, CT 06824-5195. Offers advanced practice (DNP); executive (DNP); family nurse practitioner (MSN, DNP); nurse anesthesia (DNP); nursing leadership (MSN); psychiatric nurse practitioner (MSN, DNP). *Accreditation:* AACN; AANA/CANAEP. Part-time programs available. *Faculty:* 22 full-time (all women), 28 part-time/adjunct (23 women). *Students:* 27 full-time (23 women), 157 part-time (136 women); includes 37 minority (15 Black or African American, non-Hispanic/Latino; 10 Asian, non-Hispanic/Latino; 8 Hispanic/Latino; 2 Native Hawaiian or other Pacific Islander, non-Hispanic/Latino; 2 Two or more races, non-Hispanic/Latino), 8 international. Average age 37. 132 applicants, 52% accepted, 59 enrolled. In 2013, 39 master's, 3 doctorates awarded. *Degree requirements:* For master's, capstone project. *Entrance requirements:* For master's, minimum QPA of 3.0, RN license, resume, 2 recommendations; for doctorate, GRE (nurse anesthesia applicants only), MSN (minimum QPA of 3.2) or BSN (minimum QPA of 3.0); critical care nursing experience (for nurse anesthesia DNP candidates). Additional exam requirements/recommendations for international students: Required—TOEFL (minimum score 550 paper-based; 80 iBT) or IELTS (minimum score 6.5). *Application deadline:* For fall admission, 5/15 for international students; for spring admission, 10/15 for international students. Applications are processed on a rolling basis. Application fee: $60. Electronic applications accepted. *Expenses:* Contact institution. *Financial support:* In 2013–14, 4 students received support. Unspecified assistantships available. Financial award applicants required to submit FAFSA. *Faculty research:* Aging and sexual health, psychosocial needs of men with prostate cancer, nurse practitioner education, mentoring, psychiatric and mental health, incarceration of the mentally ill, recovery in schizophrenia, palliative and end of life care, maternal and child health, breastfeeding and lactation consultant, stress and emotional eating, care of veterans and their families, falls prevention and the elderly, health care leadership, interprofessional education, academic partnerships. *Total annual research expenditures:* $775,000. *Unit head:* Dr. Lynn Babington, Dean, 203-254-4000 Ext. 2701, Fax: 203-254-4126, E-mail: lbabington@fairfield.edu. *Application contact:* Marianne Gumpper, Director of Graduate and Continuing Studies Admission, 203-254-4184, Fax: 203-254-4073, E-mail: gradadmis@fairfield.edu.
Website: http://fairfield.edu/son

Georgia State University, Byrdine F. Lewis School of Nursing, Atlanta, GA 30303. Offers adult health clinical nurse specialist/nurse practitioner (MS, Certificate); child health clinical nurse specialist/pediatric nurse practitioner (MS, Certificate); family nurse practitioner (MS, Certificate); family psychiatric mental health nurse practitioner (MS, Certificate); nursing (PhD); nursing leadership in healthcare innovations (MS), including nursing administration, nursing informatics; nutrition (MS); perinatal clinical nurse specialist/women's health nurse practitioner (MS, Certificate); physical therapy (DPT); respiratory therapy (MS). *Accreditation:* AACN. Part-time programs available. Postbaccalaureate distance learning degree programs offered (minimal on-campus study). *Faculty:* 22 full-time (16 women). *Students:* 241 full-time (180 women), 262 part-time (236 women); includes 176 minority (120 Black or African American, non-Hispanic/Latino; 31 Asian, non-Hispanic/Latino; 13 Hispanic/Latino; 3 Native Hawaiian or other Pacific Islander, non-Hispanic/Latino; 9 Two or more races, non-Hispanic/Latino), 19 international. Average age 34. 583 applicants, 34% accepted, 160 enrolled. In 2013, 110 master's, 44 doctorates, 6 other advanced degrees awarded. *Degree requirements:* For doctorate, comprehensive exam, thesis/dissertation. *Entrance requirements:* For doctorate, GRE. Additional exam requirements/recommendations for international students: Required—TOEFL. *Application deadline:* For fall admission, 2/1 priority date for domestic and international students; for spring admission, 9/15 for domestic and international students. Applications are processed on a rolling basis. Application fee: $50. Electronic applications accepted. *Expenses:* Contact institution. *Financial support:* In 2013–14, research assistantships with full and partial tuition reimbursements

(averaging $1,666 per year), teaching assistantships with full and partial tuition reimbursements (averaging $1,920 per year) were awarded; scholarships/grants, tuition waivers (full and partial), and unspecified assistantships also available. Support available to part-time students. Financial award application deadline: 8/1; financial award applicants required to submit FAFSA. *Faculty research:* Stroke intervention for caregivers, stroke prevention in African Americans; relationships between psychological distress and health outcomes in parents with a medically ill infant; medically fragile children; nursing expertise and patient outcomes. *Unit head:* Joan S. Cranford, Assistant Dean for Nursing, 404-413-1200, Fax: 404-413-1205, E-mail: jcranford2@gsu.edu. *Application contact:* Tiffany Norman, Senior Administrative Coordinator, 404-413-1190, Fax: 404-413-1205, E-mail: tnorman7@gsu.edu.
Website: http://nursing.gsu.edu/

Hampton University, Graduate College, School of Nursing, Hampton, VA 23668. Offers advanced adult nursing (MS); community health nursing (MS); community mental health/psychiatric nursing (MS); family nursing (MS); gerontological nursing for the nurse practitioner (MS); pediatric nursing (MS); women's health nursing (MS). *Accreditation:* AACN. Part-time and evening/weekend programs available. *Degree requirements:* For master's, thesis optional. *Entrance requirements:* For master's, GRE General Test. *Faculty research:* Curriculum development, physical and mental assessment.

Hunter College of the City University of New York, Graduate School, Schools of the Health Professions, Hunter-Bellevue School of Nursing, Program in Psychiatric Nursing, New York, NY 10065-5085. Offers MS, AC. *Accreditation:* AACN. Part-time programs available. *Faculty:* 18 full-time (15 women), 25 part-time/adjunct (21 women). *Students:* 2 full-time (1 woman), 92 part-time (69 women); includes 50 minority (26 Black or African American, non-Hispanic/Latino; 16 Asian, non-Hispanic/Latino; 8 Hispanic/Latino), 1 international. Average age 38. 38 applicants, 68% accepted, 21 enrolled. In 2013, 19 master's, 4 other advanced degrees awarded. *Degree requirements:* For master's, practicum. *Entrance requirements:* For master's, minimum GPA of 3.0, New York RN license, BSN. Additional exam requirements/recommendations for international students: Required—TOEFL. *Application deadline:* For fall admission, 4/1 for domestic students, 2/1 for international students; for spring admission, 11/1 for domestic students, 9/1 for international students. Applications are processed on a rolling basis. Application fee: $125. *Financial support:* Federal Work-Study, scholarships/grants, traineeships, and tuition waivers (partial) available. Support available to part-time students. Financial award application deadline: 5/1; financial award applicants required to submit FAFSA. *Faculty research:* Nursing approaches with the homeless, chronic mentally ill, and depressed; power and empathy. *Unit head:* Dr. Kunsook Bernstein, Coordinator, 212-481-4346, Fax: 212-481-5078, E-mail: kbernst@hunter.cuny.edu. *Application contact:* Milena Solo, Director for Graduate Admissions, 212-772-4288, E-mail: admissions@hunter.cuny.edu.
Website: http://www.hunter.cuny.edu/nursing/repository/files/graduate-fact-sheets/FactPsych.NP.Jan.%2026-2012.FINAL.pdf

Husson University, Graduate Nursing Program, Bangor, ME 04401-2999. Offers advanced practice psychiatric nursing (MSN, PMC); family and community nurse practitioner (MSN, PMC); nursing education (MSN, PMC). *Accreditation:* AACN. Part-time programs available. *Faculty:* 3 full-time (all women), 3 part-time/adjunct (all women). *Students:* 10 full-time (8 women), 15 part-time (14 women); includes 1 minority (Two or more races, non-Hispanic/Latino). 29 applicants, 76% accepted, 21 enrolled. In 2013, 16 master's awarded. *Degree requirements:* For master's, comprehensive exam (for some programs). *Entrance requirements:* For master's, MAT or GRE, BSN. Additional exam requirements/recommendations for international students: Required—TOEFL (minimum score 550 paper-based). *Application deadline:* For fall admission, 6/30 for domestic students; for spring admission, 10/30 for domestic students. Application fee: $40. *Expenses:* Contact institution. *Financial support:* In 2013–14, 16 students received support. Federal Work-Study, institutionally sponsored loans, traineeships, and unspecified assistantships available. Financial award application deadline: 4/15; financial award applicants required to submit FAFSA. *Unit head:* Prof. Chrystal Adams, Director, Nurse Practitioner Program, 207-941-7080, E-mail: adamsc@husson.edu. *Application contact:* Kristen Card, Director of Graduate Admissions, 207-404-5660, Fax: 207-941-7935, E-mail: cardk@husson.edu.

Indiana University–Purdue University Indianapolis, School of Nursing, Indianapolis, IN 46202-2896. Offers acute care nurse practitioner (MSN); adult health clinical nurse specialist (MSN); adult health nursing (MSN), including adult clinical nurse specialist; adult nurse practitioner (MSN); adult psychiatric/mental health nursing (MSN); child psychiatric/mental health nursing (MSN); community health nursing (MSN); family nurse practitioner (MSN); neonatal nurse practitioner (MSN); nursing (MSN, DNP), including nursing administration (MSN), nursing education (MSN); nursing science (PhD); pediatric clinical nurse specialist (MSN); women's health nurse practitioner (MSN); MSN/MPA; MSN/MPH. Part-time programs available. *Faculty:* 85 full-time (82 women), 60 part-time/adjunct (all women). *Students:* 86 full-time (78 women), 371 part-time (351 women); includes 74 minority (39 Black or African American, non-Hispanic/Latino; 1 American Indian or Alaska Native, non-Hispanic/Latino; 14 Asian, non-Hispanic/Latino; 11 Hispanic/Latino; 9 Two or more races, non-Hispanic/Latino), 6 international. Average age 38. 224 applicants, 61% accepted, 102 enrolled. In 2013, 120 master's, 10 doctorates awarded. Terminal master's awarded for partial completion of doctoral program. *Degree requirements:* For master's, thesis; for doctorate, thesis/dissertation. *Entrance requirements:* For master's, minimum GPA of 3.0, RN license; for doctorate, GRE General Test, minimum GPA of 3.0, MSN, RN license, graduate statistics course with minimum B grade (not older than 3 years). Additional exam requirements/recommendations for international students: Required—TOEFL. *Application deadline:* For fall admission, 2/15 for domestic students; for spring admission, 9/15 for domestic students. Application fee: $55 ($65 for international students). *Financial support:* In 2013–14, 93 students received support. Fellowships with full tuition reimbursements available, research assistantships with full tuition reimbursements available, teaching assistantships with full tuition reimbursements available, Federal Work-Study, institutionally sponsored loans, scholarships/grants, and tuition waivers (full) available. Support available to part-time students. Financial award application deadline: 5/1. *Faculty research:* Clinical science, health systems. *Total annual research expenditures:* $3 million. *Unit head:* Dr. Patricia Ebright, Associate Dean for Graduate Programs, E-mail: nursing@iupui.edu. *Application contact:* Information Contact, 317-274-2806.
Website: http://nursing.iu.edu/

Kent State University, College of Nursing, Kent, OH 44242-0001. Offers acute care nurse practitioner (MSN); adult nurse practitioner (MSN); clinical nurse specialist (MSN); family nurse practitioner (MSN); geriatric nurse practitioner (MSN); health care management (MSN); nurse educator (MSN); nursing (PhD); nursing practice (DNP); pediatric nurse practitioner (MSN); psychiatric/mental health nurse practitioner (MSN); women's health nurse practitioner (MSN). PhD program offered jointly with The University of Akron. *Accreditation:* AACN. Part-time programs available. *Degree requirements:* For master's, thesis optional; for doctorate, comprehensive exam, thesis/dissertation. *Entrance requirements:* For master's, GRE (if undergraduate GPA less than 3.0), minimum GPA of 2.75; for doctorate, GRE, MSN. Additional exam requirements/recommendations for international students: Required—TOEFL. Electronic applications accepted. *Expenses:* Contact institution. *Faculty research:* Women and violence, methodological specialties, osteoporosis in women, new caregivers and the elderly.

Lincoln Memorial University, Caylor School of Nursing, Harrogate, TN 37752-1901. Offers family nurse practitioner (MSN); nurse anesthesia (MSN); psychiatric mental health nurse practitioner (MSN). *Accreditation:* AANA/CANAEP. Part-time programs available. *Entrance requirements:* For master's, GRE.

McNeese State University, Doré School of Graduate Studies, College of Nursing, Department of Graduate Nursing, Family Psychiatric/Mental Health Nurse Practitioner Program, Lake Charles, LA 70609. Offers PMC. *Degree requirements:* For PMC, thesis. *Entrance requirements:* For degree, GRE, MSN, eligible for unencumbered licensure as RN in Louisiana.

McNeese State University, Doré School of Graduate Studies, College of Nursing, Department of Graduate Nursing, Nursing Program, Lake Charles, LA 70609. Offers family nurse practitioner (MSN); family psychiatric/mental health nurse practitioner (MSN); nurse educator (MSN); nurse executive (MSN). *Degree requirements:* For master's, comprehensive exam. *Entrance requirements:* For master's, GRE, baccalaureate degree in nursing, minimum overall GPA of 2.7 for all undergraduate coursework, eligibility for unencumbered licensure as Registered Nurse in Louisiana or Texas, course in introductory statistics with minimum C grade, physical assessment skills, two letters of professional reference, 500-word essay, current resume.

MGH Institute of Health Professions, School of Nursing, Boston, MA 02129-4557. Offers advanced practice nursing (MSN); gerontological nursing (MSN); nursing (DNP); pediatric nursing (MSN); psychiatric nursing (MSN); teaching and learning for health care education (Certificate); women's health nursing (MSN). *Accreditation:* AACN. *Faculty:* 41 full-time (36 women), 14 part-time/adjunct (13 women). *Students:* 494 full-time (428 women), 85 part-time (77 women); includes 108 minority (32 Black or African American, non-Hispanic/Latino; 2 American Indian or Alaska Native, non-Hispanic/Latino; 38 Asian, non-Hispanic/Latino; 33 Hispanic/Latino; 3 Native Hawaiian or other Pacific Islander, non-Hispanic/Latino). Average age 32. 470 applicants, 52% accepted, 133 enrolled. In 2013, 85 master's, 12 doctorates, 98 other advanced degrees awarded. *Degree requirements:* For master's, thesis or alternative. *Entrance requirements:* For master's, GRE General Test, bachelor's degree from regionally-accredited college or university. Additional exam requirements/recommendations for international students: Required—TOEFL (minimum score 550 paper-based; 80 iBT). *Application deadline:* For fall admission, 12/1 for domestic and international students; for spring admission, 10/1 for domestic and international students. Application fee: $100. Electronic applications accepted. *Expenses: Tuition:* Part-time $1114 per credit. *Required fees:* $620 per term. One-time fee: $475 part-time. *Financial support:* In 2013–14, 75 students received support, including 4 research assistantships (averaging $1,200 per year), 17 teaching assistantships (averaging $1,200 per year); career-related internships or fieldwork, scholarships/grants, traineeships, and unspecified assistantships also available. Support available to part-time students. Financial award application deadline: 4/1; financial award applicants required to submit FAFSA. *Faculty research:* Biobehavioral nursing, HIV/AIDS, gerontological nursing, women's health, vulnerable populations, health systems. *Unit head:* Dr. Laurie Lauzon-Clabo, Dean, 617-643-0605, Fax: 617-726-8022, E-mail: llauzonclabo@mghihp.edu. *Application contact:* Lauren Putnam, Assistant Director of Admission, 617-726-3140, Fax: 617-726-8010, E-mail: admissions@mghihp.edu.
Website: http://www.mghihp.edu/academics/nursing/

Midwestern State University, Graduate School, Robert D. and Carol Gunn College of Health Sciences and Human Services, Wilson School of Nursing, Wichita Falls, TX 76308. Offers family nurse practitioner (MSN); family psychiatric mental health nurse practitioner (MSN); nurse educator (MSN). *Accreditation:* AACN. Part-time and evening/weekend programs available. *Degree requirements:* For master's, comprehensive exam, thesis optional. *Entrance requirements:* For master's, GRE General Test or MAT. Additional exam requirements/recommendations for international students: Required—TOEFL (minimum score 550 paper-based). *Application deadline:* For fall admission, 7/1 priority date for domestic students, 4/1 for international students; for spring admission, 11/1 priority date for domestic students, 8/1 for international students. Applications are processed on a rolling basis. Application fee: $35 ($50 for international students). Electronic applications accepted. *Expenses:* Tuition, state resident: full-time $3627; part-time $201.50 per credit hour. Tuition, nonresident: full-time $10,899; part-time $605.50 per credit hour. *Required fees:* $1357. *Financial support:* Teaching assistantships with partial tuition reimbursements, career-related internships or fieldwork, Federal Work-Study, institutionally sponsored loans, scholarships/grants, tuition waivers (partial), and unspecified assistantships available. Support available to part-time students. Financial award application deadline: 3/1; financial award applicants required to submit FAFSA. *Faculty research:* Infant feeding, musculoskeletal disorders, diabetes, community health education, water quality reporting. *Unit head:* Robin Lockhart, RN, Interim Chair, 940-397-4614, Fax: 940-397-4513, E-mail: robin.lockhart@mwsu.edu.
Website: http://www.mwsu.edu/academics/hs2/nursing/

Molloy College, Division of Nursing, Rockville Centre, NY 11571-5002. Offers adult nurse practitioner (Advanced Certificate); clinical nurse specialist: adult health (Advanced Certificate); family nurse practitioner (Advanced Certificate); nurse practitioner psychiatry (Advanced Certificate); nursing (MS, PhD); nursing administration (Advanced Certificate); nursing administration with informatics (Advanced Certificate); nursing education (Advanced Certificate); nursing informatics (Advanced Certificate); pediatric nurse practitioner (Advanced Certificate). *Accreditation:* AACN. Part-time and evening/weekend programs available. *Faculty:* 30 full-time (29 women), 10 part-time/adjunct (7 women). *Students:* 18 full-time (all women), 538 part-time (495 women); includes 289 minority (159 Black or African American, non-Hispanic/Latino; 1 American Indian or Alaska Native, non-Hispanic/Latino; 80 Asian, non-Hispanic/Latino; 43 Hispanic/Latino; 4 Native Hawaiian or other Pacific Islander, non-Hispanic/Latino; 2 Two or more races, non-Hispanic/Latino), 2 international. Average age 38. 241 applicants, 63% accepted, 122 enrolled. In 2013, 84 master's, 2 other advanced degrees awarded. *Degree requirements:* For master's, thesis optional. *Entrance requirements:* For master's, 3 letters of reference, BS in nursing, minimum undergraduate GPA of 3.0; for Advanced Certificate, 3 letters of reference, master's degree in nursing. *Application deadline:* For fall admission, 9/2 priority date for domestic students; for spring admission, 1/20 priority date for domestic students. Applications are processed on a rolling basis. Application fee: $60. *Expenses: Tuition:* Full-time $16,920; part-time $940 per credit. *Required fees:* $880. *Financial support:* Research assistantships with partial tuition reimbursements, teaching assistantships with partial tuition reimbursements, institutionally sponsored loans, scholarships/grants, and unspecified assistantships available. Support available to part-time students. Financial award application deadline: 4/1; financial award applicants required to submit FAFSA. *Unit head:* Dr. Jeannine Muldoon, Dean of Nursing, 516-323-3651, E-mail: jmuldoon@molloy.edu. *Application contact:* Alina Haitz, Assistant Director of Graduate Admissions, 516-323-4008, E-mail: ahaitz@molloy.edu.
Website: http://www.molloy.edu/academics/nursing-division

Monmouth University, The Graduate School, The Marjorie K. Unterberg School of Nursing and Health Studies, West Long Branch, NJ 07764-1898. Offers adult and gerontological nurse practitioner (MSN); adult-gerontological nurse practitioner (Post-Master's Certificate); family nurse practitioner (MSN, Post-Master's Certificate); family psychiatric and mental health advanced practice nursing (MSN); forensic nursing (MSN, Certificate); nursing (MSN); nursing administration (MSN, Post-Master's Certificate); nursing education (MSN, Post-Master's Certificate); nursing practice (DNP); physician assistant (MS); psychiatric-mental health nurse practitioner (Post-Master's Certificate); school nursing (MSN, Certificate). *Accreditation:* AACN. Part-time and evening/weekend programs available. *Faculty:* 14 full-time (all women), 4 part-time/adjunct (3 women). *Students:* 19 full-time (18 women), 269 part-time (252 women); includes 106 minority (35 Black or African American, non-Hispanic/Latino; 2 American Indian or Alaska Native, non-Hispanic/Latino; 51 Asian, non-Hispanic/Latino; 12 Hispanic/Latino; 3 Native Hawaiian or other Pacific Islander, non-Hispanic/Latino; 3 Two or more races, non-Hispanic/Latino), 2 international. Average age 39. 135 applicants, 98% accepted, 96 enrolled. In 2013, 54 master's, 7 doctorates awarded. *Degree requirements:* For master's, practicum (for some tracks). *Entrance requirements:* For master's, GRE General Test, BSN with minimum GPA of 2.75, current RN license, proof of liability and malpractice policy, personal statement, two letters of recommendation, college course work in health assessment, resume; minimum GPA of 3.0, minimum C grade in prerequisite courses, minimum 200 hours' clinical experience, 3 letters of recommendation, and interview (for MS); for doctorate, accredited master's nursing program degree with minimum GPA of 3.2, active RN license, national certification as Nurse Practitioner or Nurse Administrator, working knowledge of statistics, statement of goals and vision for change, 2 letters of recommendation, resume, interview. Additional exam requirements/recommendations for international students: Required—TOEFL (minimum score 550 paper-based; 79 iBT), IELTS (minimum score 6) or Michigan English Language Assessment Battery (minimum score 77). *Application deadline:* For fall admission, 7/15 priority date for domestic students, 6/1 for international students; for spring admission, 11/15 priority date for domestic students, 11/1 for international students; for summer admission, 2/1 for domestic students. Applications are processed on a rolling basis. Application fee: $50. Electronic applications accepted. *Expenses: Tuition:* Part-time $1004 per credit hour. *Required fees:* $157 per semester. *Financial support:* In 2013–14, 163 students received support, including 113 fellowships (averaging $3,093 per year), 27 research assistantships (averaging $6,273 per year); career-related internships or fieldwork, scholarships/grants, and unspecified assistantships also available. Support available to part-time students. Financial award applicants required to submit FAFSA. *Faculty research:* Relationship of undergraduate GPA and GRE to succeeding in a graduate nursing program. *Unit head:* Dr. Janet Mahoney, Dean, 732-571-3443, Fax: 732-263-5131, E-mail: jmahoney@monmouth.edu. *Application contact:* Lauren Vento-Cifelli, Associate Vice President of Undergraduate and Graduate Admission, 732-571-3452, Fax: 732-263-5123, E-mail: gradadm@monmouth.edu.
Website: http://www.monmouth.edu/school-of-nursing-health/graduate-nursing-programs.aspx

Montana State University, College of Graduate Studies, College of Nursing, Bozeman, MT 59717. Offers clinical nurse leader (MN); family nurse practitioner (MN, Post-Master's Certificate); nursing education (Certificate, Post-Master's Certificate); psychiatric mental health nurse practitioner (MN). *Accreditation:* AACN. Part-time programs available. Postbaccalaureate distance learning degree programs offered (minimal on-campus study). *Degree requirements:* For master's, comprehensive exam, thesis (for some programs). *Entrance requirements:* For master's, GRE General Test, minimum GPA of 3.0 for undergraduate and post-baccalaureate work. Additional exam requirements/recommendations for international students: Required—TOEFL (minimum score 580 paper-based). Electronic applications accepted. *Faculty research:* Rural nursing, health disparities, environmental/public health, oral health, resilience.

New York University, College of Nursing, Doctor of Nursing Practice Program, New York, NY 10012-1019. Offers advanced practice nursing (DNP), including adult acute care, adult nurse practitioner/holistic nursing, adult nurse practitioner/palliative care nursing, adult primary care, adult primary care/geriatrics, family, geriatrics, mental health nursing, nurse-midwifery, pediatrics. Part-time and evening/weekend programs available. *Faculty:* 3 full-time (all women), 1 part-time/adjunct (0 women). *Students:* 1 (woman) full-time, 33 part-time (30 women); includes 7 minority (3 Black or African American, non-Hispanic/Latino; 3 Asian, non-Hispanic/Latino; 1 Hispanic/Latino). Average age 39. 18 applicants, 100% accepted, 12 enrolled. In 2013, 4 doctorates awarded. *Degree requirements:* For doctorate, thesis/dissertation, capstone. *Entrance requirements:* For doctorate, MAT or GRE (either taken within past 5 years), MS, RN license, interview, Nurse Practitioner Certification. Additional exam requirements/recommendations for international students: Required—TOEFL (minimum score 90 iBT), IELTS (minimum score 7). *Application deadline:* For fall admission, 3/1 for domestic students, 4/1 for international students. Applications are processed on a rolling basis. Application fee: $80. Electronic applications accepted. *Expenses: Tuition:* Full-time $35,856; part-time $1494 per unit. *Required fees:* $1408; $64 per unit. $473 per term. Tuition and fees vary according to course load and program. *Financial support:* Scholarships/grants available. Support available to part-time students. Financial award application deadline: 2/1. *Faculty research:* Geriatrics, HIV, elderly black diabetics, families and illness, oral systemic connection. *Unit head:* Dr. Rona Levin, Director, 212-998-5319, Fax: 212-995-3143, E-mail: rfl2039@nyu.edu. *Application contact:* Elizabeth Ensweiler, Assistant Director, Graduate Student Affairs and Admissions, 212-992-7653, Fax: 212-995-4302, E-mail: ee39@nyu.edu.

New York University, College of Nursing, Programs in Advanced Practice Nursing, New York, NY 10012-1019. Offers advanced practice nursing: adult acute care (MS, Advanced Certificate); advanced practice nursing: adult nurse practitioner/holistic nurse practitioner (Advanced Certificate); advanced practice nursing: adult nurse practitioner/palliative care nurse practitioner (Advanced Certificate); advanced practice nursing: adult primary care (MS, Advanced Certificate); advanced practice nursing: family (MS, Advanced Certificate); advanced practice nursing: geriatrics (Advanced Certificate); advanced practice nursing: mental health (MS); advanced practice nursing: mental health nursing (Advanced Certificate); advanced practice nursing: pediatrics (MS, Advanced Certificate); nurse midwifery (MS, Advanced Certificate); nursing administration (MS, Advanced Certificate); nursing education (MS, Advanced Certificate); nursing informatics (MS, Advanced Certificate); MS/MPA; MS/MPH. *Accreditation:* AACN; ACNM/ACME. Part-time programs available. *Faculty:* 22 full-time (all women), 54 part-time/adjunct (46 women). *Students:* 36 full-time (31 women), 622 part-time (549 women); includes 239 minority (73 Black or African American, non-Hispanic/Latino; 1 American Indian or Alaska Native, non-Hispanic/Latino; 116 Asian, non-Hispanic/Latino; 36 Hispanic/Latino; 6 Native Hawaiian or other Pacific Islander, non-Hispanic/Latino; 7 Two or more races, non-Hispanic/Latino), 16 international. Average age 37. 395 applicants, 67% accepted, 156 enrolled. In 2013, 186 master's, 8 other advanced degrees awarded. *Degree requirements:* For master's, thesis (for some programs). *Entrance requirements:* For master's, BS in nursing, AS in nursing with another BS/BA, interview, RN license, 1 year of clinical experience (3 for nursing education program); for Advanced Certificate, master's degree. Additional exam requirements/recommendations for international students: Required—TOEFL (minimum score 90 iBT), IELTS (minimum score 7). *Application deadline:* For fall admission, 7/1 for domestic and international students; for spring admission, 12/1 for domestic and international students. Application fee: $80. Electronic applications accepted. *Expenses: Tuition:* Full-time $35,856; part-time $1494 per unit. *Required fees:* $1408; $64 per unit. $473 per term. Tuition and fees vary according to course load and program. *Financial support:* In 2013–14, 182 students received support. Research assistantships, career-related internships or fieldwork, Federal Work-Study, scholarships/grants, traineeships, and unspecified assistantships available. Support available to part-time students. Financial award application deadline: 2/1; financial award applicants required to submit FAFSA. *Faculty research:* Geriatrics, HIV, elderly black diabetics, families and illness, oral systemic connection. *Unit head:* Dr. Judith Haber, Associate Dean, Graduate Programs, 212-998-9020, Fax: 212-995-3143, E-mail: jh33@nyu.edu. *Application contact:* Elizabeth Ensweiler, Assistant Director, Graduate Student Affairs and Admissions, 212-992-7653, Fax: 212-995-4302, E-mail: ee39@nyu.edu.

Nicholls State University, Graduate Studies, College of Nursing and Allied Health, Thibodaux, LA 70310. Offers family nurse practitioner (MSN); family psychiatric/mental health nurse practitioner (MSN); nurse executive (MSN).

Northeastern University, Bouvé College of Health Sciences, Boston, MA 02115-5096. Offers audiology (Au D); biotechnology (MS); counseling psychology (MS, PhD, CAGS); counseling/school psychology (PhD); exercise physiology (MS), including exercise physiology, public health; health informatics (MS); nursing (MS, PhD, CAGS), including acute care (MS), administration (MS), anesthesia (MS), primary care (MS), psychiatric mental health (MS); pharmaceutical sciences (PhD); pharmaceutics and drug delivery systems (MS); pharmacology (MS); physical therapy (DPT); physician assistant (MS); school psychology (PhD, CAGS); school/counseling psychology (PhD); speech language pathology (MS); urban public health (MPH); MS/MBA. *Accreditation:* ACPE (one or more programs are accredited). Part-time and evening/weekend programs available. *Degree requirements:* For doctorate, thesis/dissertation (for some programs); for CAGS, comprehensive exam.

Oregon Health & Science University, School of Nursing, Program in Mental Health Nursing, Portland, OR 97239-3098. Offers MN, MS, Post Master's Certificate. *Accreditation:* AACN. *Degree requirements:* For master's, thesis optional. *Entrance requirements:* For master's, GRE General Test, bachelor's degree in nursing, minimum undergraduate GPA of 3.0, previous course work in statistics; for Post Master's Certificate, master's degree in nursing.

Point Loma Nazarene University, School of Nursing, San Diego, CA 92106-2899. Offers adult/gerontology nursing (MSN); family/individual health (MSN); general nursing (MSN); nursing (Post-MSN Certificate); pediatric nursing (MSN); psychiatric mental health (MSN). *Accreditation:* AACN. Part-time programs available. *Faculty:* 9 full-time (8 women). *Students:* 1 (woman) full-time, 82 part-time (70 women); includes 43 minority (9 Black or African American, non-Hispanic/Latino; 1 American Indian or Alaska Native, non-Hispanic/Latino; 26 Asian, non-Hispanic/Latino; 3 Hispanic/Latino; 3 Native Hawaiian or other Pacific Islander, non-Hispanic/Latino; 1 Two or more races, non-Hispanic/Latino). Average age 36. 32 applicants, 94% accepted, 24 enrolled. In 2013, 26 master's awarded. *Entrance requirements:* For master's, NCLEX, ADN or BSN in nursing, interview, RN license, essay, letters of recommendation, interview. *Application deadline:* For fall admission, 7/18 priority date for domestic students; for spring admission, 10/26 priority date for domestic students; for summer admission, 3/23 priority date for domestic students. Applications are processed on a rolling basis. Application fee: $50. *Expenses: Tuition:* Full-time $6900; part-time $567 per credit hour. *Financial support:* Applicants required to submit FAFSA. *Unit head:* Dr. Barb Taylor, Dean of the School of Nursing, 619-849-2766, E-mail: bataylor@pointloma.edu. *Application contact:* Laura Leinweber, Director of Graduate Admissions, 866-692-4723, E-mail: lauraleinweber@pointloma.edu.
Website: http://www.pointloma.edu/discover/graduate-school/graduate-programs/master-science-nursing-and-post-msn-certification

Pontifical Catholic University of Puerto Rico, College of Sciences, Department of Nursing, Program in Mental Health and Psychiatric Nursing, Ponce, PR 00717-0777. Offers MSN. Part-time and evening/weekend programs available. *Degree requirements:* For master's, comprehensive exam (for some programs), thesis, clinical research paper. *Entrance requirements:* For master's, GRE General Test, 2 letters of recommendation, interview, minimum GPA of 2.75. Electronic applications accepted.

Rivier University, School of Graduate Studies, Division of Nursing, Nashua, NH 03060. Offers adult psychiatric/mental health practitioner (MS); family nurse practitioner (MS); nursing education (MS). Part-time and evening/weekend programs available. *Entrance requirements:* For master's, GRE, MAT. Electronic applications accepted.

Rush University, College of Nursing, Department of Community, Systems, and Mental Health Nursing, Chicago, IL 60612. Offers advanced public health nursing (DNP); family nurse practitioner (DNP); leadership to enhance population health outcomes (DNP); nursing science (PhD); psychiatric mental health nurse practitioner (DNP, Post-Graduate Certificate); systems leadership (DNP). *Accreditation:* AACN. Part-time programs available. Postbaccalaureate distance learning degree programs offered (minimal on-campus study). *Students:* 190 part-time (174 women); includes 41 minority (13 Black or African American, non-Hispanic/Latino; 4 American Indian or Alaska Native, non-Hispanic/Latino; 12 Asian, non-Hispanic/Latino; 11 Hispanic/Latino; 1 Native Hawaiian or other Pacific Islander, non-Hispanic/Latino). Average age 35. 170 applicants, 77% accepted, 118 enrolled. *Degree requirements:* For doctorate, capstone project (for DNP); dissertation (for PhD). *Entrance requirements:* For doctorate, GRE General Test (waived for DNP if cumulative GPA is 3.25 or greater, nursing GPA is 3.0 or greater, or a completed graduate program GPA is 3.5 or greater), interview, 3 letters of recommendation, personal statement, current resume; for Post-Graduate Certificate, interview, 3 letters of recommendation, personal statement, current resume. Additional exam requirements/recommendations for international students: Required—TOEFL. *Application deadline:* For fall admission, 1/2 for domestic students; for winter admission, 10/15 for domestic students; for spring admission, 8/4 for domestic students. Applications are processed on a rolling basis. Application fee: $100. Electronic applications accepted. *Financial support:* Fellowships, research assistantships, teaching assistantships, Federal Work-Study, scholarships/grants, traineeships, and health care benefits available. Support available to part-time students. Financial award application deadline: 3/1; financial award applicants required to submit FAFSA. *Faculty research:* Reduction of health disparities; evidence-based interventions for caregivers; patient-centered quality assessment of psychiatric inpatient environments; digital delivery of a parent-training program for urban, low-income parents; patient-centered predictors and outcomes of inter-professional care coordination. *Total annual research expenditures:* $3.8 million. *Unit head:* Dr. Arlene Miller, Chairperson, 312-942-7117, E-mail: arlene_miller@rush.edu. *Application contact:* Jennifer Thorndyke, Admissions Specialist, 312-563-7526, E-mail: jennifer_thorndyke@rush.edu.
Website: http://www.rushu.rush.edu/servlet/Satellite?c=RushUnivLevel1Page&cid=1204497838852&pagename=Rush%2FRushUnivLevel1Page%2FLevel_1_College_Home_Page

Sage Graduate School, School of Health Sciences, Department of Nursing, Program in Psychiatric Mental Health Nurse Practitioner, Troy, NY 12180-4115. Offers MS, Post

Master's Certificate. *Accreditation:* AACN. Part-time and evening/weekend programs available. *Faculty:* 5 full-time (all women), 9 part-time/adjunct (all women). *Students:* 3 full-time (2 women), 12 part-time (all women); includes 2 minority (1 Black or African American, non-Hispanic/Latino; 1 American Indian or Alaska Native, non-Hispanic/Latino). Average age 42. 13 applicants, 46% accepted, 3 enrolled. In 2013, 9 master's awarded. *Degree requirements:* For master's, thesis or alternative. *Entrance requirements:* For master's, BS in nursing, minimum GPA of 2.75, resume, 2 letters of recommendation. Additional exam requirements/recommendations for international students: Required—TOEFL (minimum score 550 paper-based). *Application deadline:* Applications are processed on a rolling basis. Application fee: $40. *Expenses: Tuition:* Full-time $11,880; part-time $660 per credit hour. *Financial support:* Fellowships, research assistantships, teaching assistantships, Federal Work-Study, scholarships/grants, and unspecified assistantships available. Support available to part-time students. Financial award application deadline: 3/1; financial award applicants required to submit FAFSA. *Unit head:* Dr. Esther Haskevitz, Dean, School of Health Sciences, 518-244-2296, Fax: 518-244-4571, E-mail: haskve@sage.edu. *Application contact:* Madeline Cafiero, Director, 518-244-4574, Fax: 518-244-2009, E-mail: cafiem@sage.edu.

Saint Francis Medical Center College of Nursing, Graduate Programs, Peoria, IL 61603-3783. Offers adult gerontology (MSN); clinical nurse leader (MSN); family nurse practitioner (MSN); family psychiatric mental health nurse practitioner (MSN); neonatal nurse practitioner (MSN); nurse clinician (Post-Graduate Certificate); nurse educator (MSN, Post-Graduate Certificate); nursing (DNP); nursing management leadership (MSN). Part-time programs available. Postbaccalaureate distance learning degree programs offered (minimal on-campus study). *Faculty:* 4 full-time (all women), 4 part-time/adjunct (all women). *Students:* 13 full-time (12 women), 268 part-time (245 women); includes 17 minority (10 Black or African American, non-Hispanic/Latino; 2 Asian, non-Hispanic/Latino; 5 Hispanic/Latino), 2 international. Average age 37. 115 applicants, 89% accepted, 42 enrolled. In 2013, 17 master's, 2 doctorates awarded. *Degree requirements:* For master's, research experience, portfolio, practicum; for doctorate, practicum hours. *Entrance requirements:* For master's, nursing research, health assessment, graduate course work in statistics, RN license; for doctorate, master's degree in nursing, professional portfolio, graduate statistics, transcripts, RN license. Additional exam requirements/recommendations for international students: Required—TOEFL. *Application deadline:* For fall admission, 6/1 priority date for domestic and international students; for spring admission, 11/15 priority date for domestic and international students. Applications are processed on a rolling basis. Application fee: $50. Electronic applications accepted. *Expenses: Tuition:* Full-time $6336; part-time $528 per semester hour. *Required fees:* $436. *Financial support:* In 2013–14, 8 students received support. Scholarships/grants and tuition waivers (partial) available. Support available to part-time students. Financial award application deadline: 6/15; financial award applicants required to submit FAFSA. *Faculty research:* Outcome and curriculum planning, health promotion, NCLEX-RN results, decision-making program evaluation. *Unit head:* Dr. Patti A. Stockert, President of the College, 309-655-4124, Fax: 309-624-8973, E-mail: patricia.a.stockert@osfhealthcare.org. *Application contact:* Dr. Janice F. Boundy, Dean, 309-655-2230, Fax: 309-624-8973, E-mail: jan.f.boundy@osfhealthcare.org.
Website: http://www.sfmccon.edu/graduate-programs/

Seattle University, College of Nursing, Program in Advanced Practice Nursing Immersion, Seattle, WA 98122-1090. Offers adult/gerontological nurse practitioner (MSN); advanced community public health nursing (MSN); family nurse practitioner (MSN); family psychiatric mental health nurse practitioner (MSN); nurse midwifery (MSN). *Faculty:* 17 full-time (15 women), 9 part-time/adjunct (6 women). *Students:* 109 full-time (94 women), 6 part-time (5 women); includes 25 minority (3 Black or African American, non-Hispanic/Latino; 11 Asian, non-Hispanic/Latino; 2 Hispanic/Latino; 9 Two or more races, non-Hispanic/Latino). Average age 31. In 2013, 48 master's awarded. *Degree requirements:* For master's, thesis or scholarly project. *Entrance requirements:* For master's, GRE, bachelor's degree, minimum GPA of 3.0, professional resume, two recommendations, letter of intent. Additional exam requirements/recommendations for international students: Required—TOEFL (minimum score 92 iBT), IELTS. *Application deadline:* For fall admission, 12/1 for domestic and international students. Application fee: $55. Electronic applications accepted. *Financial support:* In 2013–14, 3 students received support. Scholarships/grants and traineeships available. Financial award applicants required to submit FAFSA. *Unit head:* Dr. Janiece DeSocio, Interim Dean, 206-296-5660, E-mail: desocioj@seattleu.edu. *Application contact:* Janet Shandley, Associate Dean of Graduate Admissions, 206-296-5900, Fax: 206-298-5656, E-mail: grad_admissions@seattleu.edu.
Website: http://www.seattleu.edu/nursing/msn/apni/

Seattle University, College of Nursing, Program in Nursing, Seattle, WA 98122-1090. Offers adult/gerontological nurse practitioner (MSN); advanced community public health (MSN); psychiatric mental health nurse practitioner (MSN). *Students:* 11 full-time (10 women), 4 part-time (all women); includes 2 minority (both Hispanic/Latino). Average age 36. 39 applicants, 36% accepted, 8 enrolled. In 2013, 7 master's awarded. *Degree requirements:* For master's, thesis or scholarly project. *Entrance requirements:* For master's, GRE, bachelor's degree in nursing or associate degree in nursing with baccalaureate in different major, 5-quarter statistics course, minimum cumulative GPA of 3.0, professional resume, two recommendations, letter of intent, copy of current RN license or ability to obtain RN license in WA state. Additional exam requirements/recommendations for international students: Required—TOEFL (minimum score 92 iBT), IELTS. *Application deadline:* For fall admission, 12/1 for domestic and international students. Application fee: $55. Electronic applications accepted. *Financial support:* In 2013–14, 1 student received support, including 2 teaching assistantships; scholarships/grants and traineeships also available. Financial award applicants required to submit FAFSA. *Unit head:* Dr. Azita Emami, Dean, 206-296-5660. *Application contact:* Janet Shandley, Associate Dean of Graduate Admissions, 206-296-5900, Fax: 206-298-5656, E-mail: grad_admissions@seattleu.edu.
Website: https://www.seattleu.edu/nursing/msn/

Shenandoah University, Eleanor Wade Custer School of Nursing, Winchester, VA 22601-5195. Offers family nurse practitioner (Certificate); health informatics (Certificate); nursing (MSN, DNP); nursing education (Certificate); psychiatric mental health nurse practitioner (Certificate). *Accreditation:* AACN; ACNM/ACME. Part-time programs available. *Faculty:* 14 full-time (all women), 7 part-time/adjunct (6 women). *Students:* 39 full-time (35 women), 76 part-time (74 women); includes 23 minority (13 Black or African American, non-Hispanic/Latino; 2 American Indian or Alaska Native, non-Hispanic/Latino; 4 Asian, non-Hispanic/Latino; 4 Hispanic/Latino), 1 international. Average age 38. 56 applicants, 77% accepted, 32 enrolled. In 2013, 28 master's, 4 doctorates, 11 other advanced degrees awarded. *Degree requirements:* For master's, research project, clinical hours; for doctorate, scholarly project, clinical hours; for Certificate, clinical hours. *Entrance requirements:* For master's, United States RN license; minimum GPA of 3.0; appropriate clinical experience; curriculum vitae; 3 letters of recommendation; for doctorate, MSN, minimum GPA of 3.0, 3 letters of recommendation, essay, interview, BSN; for Certificate, MSN, minimum GPA of 3.0, 2 letters of recommendation, minimum of one year (2,080 hours) clinical nursing experience, interview. Additional exam requirements/recommendations for international students: Required—TOEFL (minimum score 610 paper-based; 83 iBT), IELTS (minimum score 7.5). *Application deadline:* For fall admission, 5/1 priority date for domestic and international students; for spring admission, 11/1 priority date for domestic and international students. Applications are processed on a rolling basis. Application fee: $30. Electronic applications accepted. *Expenses: Tuition:* Full-time $19,176; part-time $799 per credit. *Required fees:* $365 per term. Tuition and fees vary according to course level, course load and program. *Financial support:* In 2013–14, 13 students received support, including 3 teaching assistantships with partial tuition reimbursements available (averaging $4,912 per year); career-related internships or fieldwork, scholarships/grants, and unspecified assistantships also available. Support available to part-time students. Financial award application deadline: 3/15; financial award applicants required to submit FAFSA. *Faculty research:* Moral reasoning in nurses, improving health care access to underserved rural women, screening for depression and anxiety in the obese in a rural free clinic, health care outcomes among patients in a free clinic setting cared for by nurse practitioners, effects of depression on diabetes as evidenced by the relationship between the patient healthcare questionnaire (PHQ-9) scores and the patient's glycohemoglobin (HbA1c), policy development, research on a Virginia Nurses Hall of Fame inductee. *Unit head:* Dr. Kathryn Ganske, Director, 540-678-4374, Fax: 540-665-5519, E-mail: kganske@su.edu. *Application contact:* Andrew Woodall, Executive Director of Recruitment and Admissions, 540-665-4581, Fax: 540-665-4627, E-mail: admit@su.edu.
Website: http://www.nursing.su.edu

Southeastern Louisiana University, College of Nursing and Health Sciences, School of Nursing, Hammond, LA 70402. Offers adult psychiatric/mental health nurse practitioner/clinical nurse specialist (MSN); education (MSN); nurse executive (MSN); nurse practice (DNP); nurse practitioner (MSN). *Accreditation:* AACN. Part-time and evening/weekend programs available. *Faculty:* 14 full-time (13 women), 5 part-time/adjunct (4 women). *Students:* 21 full-time (19 women), 138 part-time (121 women); includes 27 minority (17 Black or African American, non-Hispanic/Latino; 4 Asian, non-Hispanic/Latino; 5 Hispanic/Latino; 1 Two or more races, non-Hispanic/Latino). Average age 34. 72 applicants, 68% accepted, 19 enrolled. In 2013, 29 master's awarded. *Degree requirements:* For master's, thesis. *Entrance requirements:* For master's, GRE (verbal and quantitative), baccalaureate degree in nursing from accredited undergraduate nursing program; minimum GPA of 2.7; all transcripts from undergraduate school and any work attempted at the graduate level; curriculum vitae; valid Louisiana Registered Nurse license; letters of recommendation; letter of intent/statement of purpose. Additional exam requirements/recommendations for international students: Required—TOEFL (minimum score 500 paper-based; 61 iBT). *Application deadline:* For fall admission, 7/15 priority date for domestic students, 6/1 priority date for international students; for spring admission, 12/1 priority date for domestic students, 10/1 priority date for international students. Applications are processed on a rolling basis. Application fee: $20 ($30 for international students). Electronic applications accepted. *Expenses:* Tuition, state resident: full-time $5047. Tuition, nonresident: full-time $17,066. *Required fees:* $1213. Tuition and fees vary according to degree level. *Financial support:* Federal Work-Study, institutionally sponsored loans, scholarships/grants, traineeships, and unspecified assistantships available. Support available to part-time students. Financial award application deadline: 5/1; financial award applicants required to submit FAFSA. *Faculty research:* Gender issues, LGBT issues, occupational health/safety, accelerated students, caring development. *Total annual research expenditures:* $103,409. *Unit head:* Dr. Lorinda J. Sealey, Graduate Nursing Program Director, 985-549-5045, Fax: 985-549-5087, E-mail: vjohnson@selu.edu. *Application contact:* Sandra Meyers, Graduate Admissions Analyst, 985-549-5620, Fax: 985-549-5632, E-mail: admissions@selu.edu.
Website: http://www.selu.edu/acad_research/depts/nurs

Southern Arkansas University–Magnolia, Graduate Programs, Magnolia, AR 71753. Offers agriculture (MS); business administration (MBA); computer and information sciences (MS); education (M Ed), including counseling and development, curriculum and instruction, educational administration and supervision, elementary education, reading, secondary education, TESOL; kinesiology (M Ed); library media and information specialist (M Ed); mental health and clinical counseling (MS); public administration (MPA); school counseling (M Ed); teaching (MAT). *Accreditation:* NCATE. Part-time and evening/weekend programs available. Postbaccalaureate distance learning degree programs offered. *Faculty:* 34 full-time (15 women), 8 part-time/adjunct (5 women). *Students:* 48 full-time (22 women), 269 part-time (167 women); includes 85 minority (78 Black or African American, non-Hispanic/Latino; 2 Asian, non-Hispanic/Latino; 2 Hispanic/Latino; 1 Native Hawaiian or other Pacific Islander, non-Hispanic/Latino; 2 Two or more races, non-Hispanic/Latino), 5 international. Average age 33. 149 applicants, 73% accepted, 109 enrolled. In 2013, 149 master's awarded. *Degree requirements:* For master's, comprehensive exam (for some programs), thesis optional. *Entrance requirements:* For master's, GRE, MAT or GMAT, minimum GPA of 2.5. Additional exam requirements/recommendations for international students: Required—TOEFL, IELTS. *Application deadline:* For fall admission, 7/10 for domestic and international students; for winter admission, 12/1 for domestic and international students; for spring admission, 12/1 for domestic and international students; for summer admission, 4/1 for domestic students. Applications are processed on a rolling basis. Application fee: $25 ($50 for international students). Electronic applications accepted. *Expenses:* Tuition, state resident: part-time $254 per credit hour. Tuition, nonresident: part-time $370 per credit hour. *Required fees:* $136 per credit hour. $259 per semester. Tuition and fees vary according to course load and program. *Financial support:* Career-related internships or fieldwork, Federal Work-Study, scholarships/grants, tuition waivers (full), and unspecified assistantships available. Financial award applicants required to submit FAFSA. *Faculty research:* Alternative certification for teachers, supervision of instruction, instructional leadership, counseling. *Unit head:* Dr. Kim Bloss, Dean, School of Graduate Studies, 870-235-4150, Fax: 870-235-5227, E-mail: kkbloss@saumag.edu. *Application contact:* Shrijana Malaka, Admissions Specialist, 870-235-4150, Fax: 870-235-5227, E-mail: smalakar@saumag.edu.
Website: http://www.saumag.edu/graduate

Stony Brook University, State University of New York, Stony Brook University Medical Center, Health Sciences Center, School of Nursing, Program in Mental Health/Psychiatric Nursing, Stony Brook, NY 11794. Offers MS, Certificate. *Accreditation:* AACN. *Students:* 14 full-time (13 women), 73 part-time (60 women); includes 29 minority (12 Black or African American, non-Hispanic/Latino; 7 Asian, non-Hispanic/Latino; 5 Hispanic/Latino; 5 Two or more races, non-Hispanic/Latino). In 2013, 14 master's, 3 other advanced degrees awarded. *Degree requirements:* For master's, thesis. *Entrance requirements:* For master's, BSN, minimum GPA of 3.0, course work in statistics. Additional exam requirements/recommendations for international students: Required—TOEFL. *Application deadline:* For fall admission, 1/15 for domestic students. Application fee: $100. *Expenses:* Tuition, state resident: full-time $9870; part-time $411 per credit. Tuition, nonresident: full-time $18,350; part-time $765 per credit. *Financial support:* Application deadline: 3/15. *Unit head:* Dr. Michael A. Chiarello, Clinical Associate Professor/Director, 631-444-3271, Fax: 631-444-3136, E-mail: michael.chiarello@stonybrook.edu. *Application contact:* Director, 631-444-3271, Fax: 631-444-3136.
Website: http://www.nursing.stonybrookmedicine.edu/

Uniformed Services University of the Health Sciences, Graduate School of Nursing, Bethesda, MD 20814-4799. Offers family nurse practitioner (MSN, DNP); nurse

anesthesia (MSN); nursing science (PhD); perioperative clinical nurse specialist (MSN); psychiatric nurse practitioner (MSN, DNP). Program available to military officers only. *Accreditation:* AACN; AANA/CANAEP. *Faculty:* 42 full-time (24 women), 5 part-time/adjunct (4 women). *Students:* 62 full-time (31 women); includes 13 minority (7 Black or African American, non-Hispanic/Latino; 5 Asian, non-Hispanic/Latino; 1 Hispanic/Latino). Average age 34. 100 applicants, 62% accepted, 62 enrolled. In 2013, 57 master's, 1 doctorate awarded. *Degree requirements:* For master's, thesis or alternative; for doctorate, thesis/dissertation or alternative. *Entrance requirements:* For master's, GRE, BSN, clinical experience, minimum GPA of 3.0, previous course work in science; for doctorate, GRE. *Application deadline:* For fall admission, 7/1 for domestic students; for winter admission, 2/15 for domestic students. Application fee: $0. Electronic applications accepted. *Faculty research:* Prenatal care, military health care, military readiness, distance learning. *Unit head:* Dr. Carol A. Romano, Associate Dean for Academic Affairs, 301-295-1180, Fax: 301-295-1707, E-mail: carol.romano@usuhs.edu. *Application contact:* Terry Lynn Malavakis, Recording Secretary for Admissions Committee, 301-295-1055, Fax: 301-295-1707, E-mail: terry.malavakis@usuhs.edu.
Website: http://www.usuhs.mil/gsn/

University at Buffalo, the State University of New York, Graduate School, School of Nursing, Buffalo, NY 14214. Offers adult gerontology nurse practitioner (DNP); family nurse practitioner (DNP); health care systems and leadership (MS); nurse anesthetist (DNP); nursing (PhD); nursing education (Certificate); psychiatric/mental health nurse practitioner (DNP). *Accreditation:* AACN; AANA/CANAEP (one or more programs are accredited). Part-time programs available. Postbaccalaureate distance learning degree programs offered (no on-campus study). *Faculty:* 24 full-time (21 women), 2 part-time/adjunct (1 woman). *Students:* 80 full-time (60 women), 97 part-time (84 women); includes 35 minority (20 Black or African American, non-Hispanic/Latino; 2 American Indian or Alaska Native, non-Hispanic/Latino; 9 Asian, non-Hispanic/Latino; 1 Hispanic/Latino; 3 Native Hawaiian or other Pacific Islander, non-Hispanic/Latino). 118 applicants, 67% accepted, 58 enrolled. In 2013, 41 master's, 15 doctorates awarded. *Degree requirements:* For master's, thesis optional; for doctorate, comprehensive exam (for some programs), capstone (for DNP), dissertation (for PhD). *Entrance requirements:* For doctorate, GRE or MAT, minimum GPA of 3.0 (3.25 for PhD), RN license, BS or MS in nursing, 3 references, writing sample; for Certificate, interview, minimum GPA of 3.0 or GRE General Test, RN license, MS in nursing. Additional exam requirements/recommendations for international students: Required—TOEFL (minimum score 550 paper-based; 79 iBT), IELTS (minimum score 6.5). *Application deadline:* For fall admission, 7/1 for domestic students, 4/1 for international students; for spring admission, 12/1 for domestic students, 10/1 for international students; for summer admission, 4/1 for domestic students. Application fee: $75. Electronic applications accepted. *Financial support:* In 2013–14, 80 students received support, including 2 fellowships with full and partial tuition reimbursements available (averaging $17,000 per year), 7 research assistantships with full and partial tuition reimbursements available (averaging $10,600 per year), 7 teaching assistantships with full and partial tuition reimbursements available (averaging $10,600 per year); scholarships/grants, traineeships, health care benefits, and unspecified assistantships also available. Financial award application deadline: 3/15; financial award applicants required to submit FAFSA. *Faculty research:* Oncology, palliative care, gerontology, addictions, mental health, community wellness, sleep, workforce, care of underserved populations, quality and safety, person-centered care, adolescent health. *Total annual research expenditures:* $1.1 million. *Unit head:* Dr. Marsha L. Lewis, Dean and Professor, 716-829-2533, Fax: 716-829-2566, E-mail: ubnursingdean@buffalo.edu. *Application contact:* Dr. David J. Lang, Director of Student Affairs, 716-829-2537, Fax: 716-829-2067, E-mail: nursing@buffalo.edu.
Website: http://nursing.buffalo.edu/

University of Cincinnati, Graduate School, College of Nursing, Cincinnati, OH 45221-0038. Offers clinical nurse specialist (MSN), including adult health, community health, neonatal, nursing administration, occupational health, pediatric health, psychiatric nursing, women's health; nurse anesthesia (MSN); nurse midwifery (MSN); nurse practitioner (MSN), including acute care, ambulatory care, family, family/psychiatric, women's health; nursing (PhD); MBA/MSN. *Accreditation:* AACN; AANA/CANAEP (one or more programs are accredited); ACNM/ACME. Part-time programs available. Postbaccalaureate distance learning degree programs offered (no on-campus study). Terminal master's awarded for partial completion of doctoral program. *Degree requirements:* For master's, thesis or alternative; for doctorate, comprehensive exam, thesis/dissertation. *Entrance requirements:* For master's and doctorate, GRE General Test. Additional exam requirements/recommendations for international students: Required—TOEFL (minimum score 520 paper-based). Electronic applications accepted. *Faculty research:* Substance abuse, injury and violence, symptom management.

University of Colorado Denver, College of Nursing, Aurora, CO 80045. Offers adult clinical nurse specialist (MS); adult nurse practitioner (MS); family nurse practitioner (MS); family psychiatric mental health nurse practitioner (MS); health care informatics (MS); nurse-midwifery (MS); nursing (DNP, PhD); nursing leadership and health care systems (MS); pediatric nurse practitioner (MS); special studies (MS); women's health (MS); MS/PhD. *Accreditation:* ACNM/ACME (one or more programs are accredited). Part-time and evening/weekend programs available. Postbaccalaureate distance learning degree programs offered (minimal on-campus study). *Faculty:* 74 full-time (65 women), 58 part-time/adjunct (56 women). *Students:* 351 full-time (327 women), 138 part-time (125 women); includes 79 minority (12 Black or African American, non-Hispanic/Latino; 9 American Indian or Alaska Native, non-Hispanic/Latino; 13 Asian, non-Hispanic/Latino; 32 Hispanic/Latino; 2 Native Hawaiian or other Pacific Islander, non-Hispanic/Latino; 11 Two or more races, non-Hispanic/Latino), 7 international. Average age 33. 354 applicants, 43% accepted, 109 enrolled. In 2013, 108 master's, 28 doctorates awarded. Terminal master's awarded for partial completion of doctoral program. *Degree requirements:* For master's, thesis optional; for doctorate, comprehensive exam, thesis/dissertation, 42 credits of coursework. *Entrance requirements:* For master's, GRE if cumulative undergraduate GPA is less than 3.0, undergraduate nursing degree from NLNAC- or CCNE-accredited school or university; completion of research and statistics courses with minimum grade of C; copy of current and unencumbered nursing license; for doctorate, GRE, bachelor's and/or master's degrees in nursing from NLN- or CCNE-accredited institution; portfolio; minimum undergraduate GPA of 3.0, graduate 3.5; graduate-level intermediate statistics and master's-level nursing theory courses with minimum B grade; interview. Additional exam requirements/recommendations for international students: Required—TOEFL (minimum score 560 paper-based; 83 iBT). *Application deadline:* For fall admission, 2/15 for domestic students, 1/15 for international students; for spring admission, 7/1 for domestic students, 6/1 for international students. Application fee: $50 ($75 for international students). Electronic applications accepted. *Expenses:* Contact institution. *Financial support:* In 2013–14, 113 students received support. Fellowships, research assistantships, teaching assistantships, Federal Work-Study, institutionally sponsored loans, scholarships/grants, traineeships, and unspecified assistantships available. Support available to part-time students. Financial award application deadline: 4/1; financial award applicants required to submit FAFSA. *Faculty research:* Biological and behavioral phenomena in pregnancy and postpartum; patterns of glycemia during the insulin resistance of pregnancy; obesity, gestational diabetes, and relationship to neonatal adiposity; men's awareness and knowledge of male breast cancer; cognitive-behavioral therapy for chronic insomnia after breast cancer treatment; massage therapy for the treatment of tension-type headaches. *Total annual research expenditures:* $5.9 million. *Unit head:* Dr. Sarah Thompson, Dean, 303-724-1679, E-mail: sarah.a.thompson@ucdenver.edu. *Application contact:* Judy Campbell, Graduate Programs Coordinator, 303-724-8503, E-mail: judy.campbell@ucdenver.edu.
Website: http://www.ucdenver.edu/academics/colleges/nursing/Pages/default.aspx

University of Delaware, College of Health Sciences, School of Nursing, Newark, DE 19716. Offers adult nurse practitioner (MSN, PMC); cardiopulmonary clinical nurse specialist (MSN, PMC); cardiopulmonary clinical nurse specialist/adult nurse practitioner (MSN, PMC); family nurse practitioner (MSN, PMC); gerontology clinical nurse specialist (MSN, PMC); gerontology clinical nurse specialist geriatric nurse practitioner (PMC); gerontology clinical nurse specialist/geriatric nurse practitioner (MSN); health services administration (MSN, PMC); nursing of children clinical nurse specialist (MSN, PMC); nursing of children clinical nurse specialist/pediatric nurse practitioner (MSN, PMC); oncology/immune deficiency clinical nurse specialist (MSN, PMC); oncology/immune deficiency clinical nurse specialist/adult nurse practitioner (MSN, PMC); perinatal/women's health clinical nurse specialist (MSN, PMC); perinatal/women's health clinical nurse specialist/women's health nurse practitioner (MSN, PMC); psychiatric nursing clinical nurse specialist (MSN, PMC). *Accreditation:* AACN. Part-time and evening/weekend programs available. Postbaccalaureate distance learning degree programs offered (minimal on-campus study). *Degree requirements:* For master's, thesis optional. *Entrance requirements:* For master's, BSN, interview, RN license. Electronic applications accepted. *Faculty research:* Marriage and chronic illness, health promotion, congestive heart failure patient outcomes, school nursing, diabetes in children, culture, health disparities, cardiovascular, prison nursing, oncology, public policy, child obesity, smoking and teen pregnancy, blood pressure measurements, men's health.

University of Illinois at Chicago, Graduate College, College of Nursing, Program in Nursing, Chicago, IL 60607-7128. Offers acute care clinical nurse specialist (MS); acute care nurse practitioner (MS); administrative nursing leadership (Certificate); administrative studies in nursing (MS); adult nurse practitioner (MS); adult/geriatric nurse practitioner (MS); advanced community health nurse specialist (MS); family nurse practitioner (MS); geriatric clinical nurse specialist (MS); geriatric nurse practitioner (MS); mental health clinical nurse specialist (MS); mental health nurse practitioner (MS); nurse midwifery (MS); occupational health/advanced community health nurse specialist (MS); occupational health/family nurse practitioner (MS); pediatric clinical nurse specialist (MS); pediatric nurse practitioner (MS); perinatal clinical nurse specialist (MS); school/advanced community health nurse specialist (MS); school/family nurse practitioner (MS); women's health nurse practitioner (MS). *Accreditation:* AACN. Part-time programs available. *Faculty:* 16 full-time (14 women). *Students:* 393 full-time (361 women), 410 part-time (367 women); includes 198 minority (48 Black or African American, non-Hispanic/Latino; 1 American Indian or Alaska Native, non-Hispanic/Latino; 64 Asian, non-Hispanic/Latino; 71 Hispanic/Latino; 2 Native Hawaiian or other Pacific Islander, non-Hispanic/Latino; 12 Two or more races, non-Hispanic/Latino), 29 international. Average age 32. 396 applicants, 62% accepted, 177 enrolled. In 2013, 184 master's awarded. *Degree requirements:* For master's, thesis or alternative. *Entrance requirements:* For master's, GRE General Test, minimum GPA of 2.75. Additional exam requirements/recommendations for international students: Required—TOEFL. *Application deadline:* For fall admission, 5/15 for domestic students, 2/15 for international students; for spring admission, 11/1 for domestic students, 7/15 for international students. Applications are processed on a rolling basis. Application fee: $40 ($50 for international students). Electronic applications accepted. *Expenses:* Tuition, state resident: full-time $11,066; part-time $3689 per term. Tuition, nonresident: full-time $23,064; part-time $7688 per term. *Required fees:* $3004; $1190 per term. Tuition and fees vary according to course level and program. *Financial support:* Fellowships with full tuition reimbursements, research assistantships with full tuition reimbursements, teaching assistantships with full tuition reimbursements, career-related internships or fieldwork, Federal Work-Study, institutionally sponsored loans, scholarships/grants, traineeships, tuition waivers (full and partial), and unspecified assistantships available. Support available to part-time students. Financial award application deadline: 3/1; financial award applicants required to submit FAFSA. *Unit head:* Dr. Terri E. Weaver, Dean, 312-996-7808, E-mail: teweaver@uic.edu. *Application contact:* Receptionist, 312-413-2550, E-mail: gradcoll@uic.edu.

The University of Kansas, University of Kansas Medical Center, School of Nursing, Kansas City, KS 66160. Offers adult/gerontological clinical nurse specialist (PMC); adult/gerontological nurse practitioner (PMC); clinical research management (PMC); health care informatics (PMC); health professions educator (PMC); nurse midwife (PMC); nursing (MS, DNP, PhD); organizational leadership (PMC); psychiatric/mental health nurse practitioner (PMC); public health nursing (PMC). *Accreditation:* AACN; ACNM/ACME. Part-time programs available. Postbaccalaureate distance learning degree programs offered (minimal on-campus study). *Faculty:* 59. *Students:* 55 full-time (53 women), 323 part-time (303 women); includes 57 minority (23 Black or African American, non-Hispanic/Latino; 14 Asian, non-Hispanic/Latino; 16 Hispanic/Latino; 1 Native Hawaiian or other Pacific Islander, non-Hispanic/Latino; 3 Two or more races, non-Hispanic/Latino), 1 international. Average age 38. 113 applicants, 59% accepted, 61 enrolled. In 2013, 77 master's, 18 doctorates, 11 other advanced degrees awarded. Terminal master's awarded for partial completion of doctoral program. *Degree requirements:* For master's, comprehensive exam, thesis (for some programs), general oral exam; for doctorate, variable foreign language requirement, thesis/dissertation, comprehensive oral exam (for DNP); comprehensive written and oral exam (for PhD). *Entrance requirements:* For master's, bachelor's degree in nursing, minimum GPA of 3.0, 1 year of clinical experience, RN license in KS and MO; for doctorate, GRE General Test, bachelor's degree in nursing, minimum GPA of 3.5, RN license in KS and MO. Additional exam requirements/recommendations for international students: Required—TOEFL. *Application deadline:* For fall admission, 4/1 for domestic and international students; for spring admission, 9/1 for domestic and international students. Application fee: $60. Electronic applications accepted. *Financial support:* Research assistantships with full and partial tuition reimbursements, teaching assistantships with full and partial tuition reimbursements, scholarships/grants, and traineeships available. Financial award application deadline: 3/1; financial award applicants required to submit FAFSA. *Faculty research:* Breastfeeding practices of teen mothers, national database of nursing quality indicators, caregiving of families of patients using technology in the home, simulation in nursing education, diaphragm fatigue. *Total annual research expenditures:* $6.4 million. *Unit head:* Dr. Karen L. Miller, Dean, 913-588-1601, Fax: 913-588-1660, E-mail: kmiller@kumc.edu. *Application contact:* Dr. Pamela K. Barnes, Associate Dean, Student Affairs, 913-588-1619, Fax: 913-588-1615, E-mail: pbarnes2@kumc.edu.
Website: http://nursing.kumc.edu

University of Louisville, Graduate School, School of Nursing, Louisville, KY 40202. Offers adult nurse practitioner (MSN); family nurse practitioner (MSN); health professions education (MSN); neonatal nurse practitioner (MSN); nursing research (PhD); psychiatric mental health nurse practitioner (MSN). *Accreditation:* AACN. Part-time programs available. *Students:* 91 full-time (81 women), 47 part-time (42 women); includes 16 minority (8 Black or African American, non-Hispanic/Latino; 3 Asian, non-Hispanic/Latino; 3 Hispanic/Latino; 2 Two or more races, non-Hispanic/Latino), 6

international. Average age 36. 58 applicants, 74% accepted, 36 enrolled. In 2013, 33 master's, 3 doctorates awarded. Terminal master's awarded for partial completion of doctoral program. *Degree requirements:* For master's, thesis optional; for doctorate, comprehensive exam, thesis/dissertation. *Entrance requirements:* For master's, GRE General Test, bachelor's degree in nursing, minimum GPA of 3.0, RN license; for doctorate, GRE General Test, BSN or MSN with recommended minimum GPA of 3.0. Additional exam requirements/recommendations for international students: Required—TOEFL. *Application deadline:* For fall admission, 4/1 priority date for domestic students, 4/1 for international students. Applications are processed on a rolling basis. Application fee: $60. Electronic applications accepted. *Expenses:* Tuition, state resident: full-time $10,788; part-time $599 per credit hour. Tuition, nonresident: full-time $22,446; part-time $1247 per credit hour. *Required fees:* $196. Tuition and fees vary according to program and reciprocity agreements. *Financial support:* Fellowships with full tuition reimbursements, research assistantships with full tuition reimbursements, teaching assistantships with full tuition reimbursements, institutionally sponsored loans, scholarships/grants, traineeships, health care benefits, and unspecified assistantships available. Support available to part-time students. Financial award application deadline: 4/15; financial award applicants required to submit FAFSA. *Faculty research:* Maternal-child/family stress after pregnancy loss, postpartum depression, access to healthcare (underserved populations), quality of life issues, physical activity (impact on chronic/acute conditions). *Total annual research expenditures:* $718,934. *Unit head:* Dr. Marcia J. Hern, Dean, 502-852-8300, Fax: 502-852-5044, E-mail: m.hern@gwise.louisville.edu. *Application contact:* Dr. Lee Ridner, Interim Associate Dean for Academic Affairs and Director of MSN Programs, 502-852-8518, Fax: 502-852-0704, E-mail: romain01@louisville.edu.
Website: http://www.louisville.edu/nursing/

University of Maryland, Baltimore, Graduate School, School of Nursing, Master's Program in Nursing, Baltimore, MD 21201. Offers community health nursing (MS); gerontological nursing (MS); maternal-child nursing (MS); medical-surgical nursing (MS); nurse-midwifery education (MS); nursing administration (MS); nursing education (MS); nursing health policy (MS); primary care nursing (MS); psychiatric nursing (MS); MS/MBA. MS/MBA offered jointly with University of Baltimore. *Accreditation:* AACN; AANA/CANAEP. Part-time programs available. *Students:* 345 full-time (297 women), 508 part-time (469 women); includes 288 minority (152 Black or African American, non-Hispanic/Latino; 2 American Indian or Alaska Native, non-Hispanic/Latino; 72 Asian, non-Hispanic/Latino; 32 Hispanic/Latino; 1 Native Hawaiian or other Pacific Islander, non-Hispanic/Latino; 29 Two or more races, non-Hispanic/Latino), 13 international. Average age 33. 971 applicants, 34% accepted, 253 enrolled. In 2013, 308 master's awarded. *Degree requirements:* For master's, comprehensive exam (for some programs), thesis or alternative. *Entrance requirements:* For master's, minimum GPA of 2.75, course work in statistics, BS in nursing. Additional exam requirements/recommendations for international students: Required—TOEFL (minimum score 550 paper-based; 80 iBT) or IELTS (minimum score 7). *Application deadline:* For fall admission, 2/1 for domestic students, 1/15 for international students. Application fee: $75. Electronic applications accepted. *Financial support:* Fellowships, research assistantships, teaching assistantships, career-related internships or fieldwork, and traineeships available. Support available to part-time students. Financial award application deadline: 2/15; financial award applicants required to submit FAFSA. *Unit head:* Dr. Jane Kapustin, Assistant Dean, 410-706-6741, Fax: 410-706-4231. *Application contact:* Marjorie Fass, Admissions Director, 410-706-0501, Fax: 410-706-7238.

University of Massachusetts Lowell, College of Health Sciences, School of Nursing, Program in Psychiatric and Mental Health Nursing, Lowell, MA 01854-2881. Offers MS, Graduate Certificate. *Accreditation:* AACN. Part-time programs available. *Degree requirements:* For master's, thesis optional. *Entrance requirements:* For master's, GRE General Test, minimum GPA of 3.0, MA nursing license, interview, 3 letters of recommendation.

University of Minnesota, Twin Cities Campus, Graduate School, School of Nursing, Program in Psychiatric Mental Health Clinical Nurse Specialist, Minneapolis, MN 55455-0213. Offers MS. *Accreditation:* AACN. Part-time programs available. *Entrance requirements:* Additional exam requirements/recommendations for international students: Required—TOEFL (minimum score 586 paper-based).

University of Missouri, Graduate School, Sinclair School of Nursing, Columbia, MO 65211. Offers adult-gerontology clinical nurse specialist (DNP, Certificate); family nurse practitioner (DNP); family psychiatric and mental health nurse practitioner (DNP); nursing (MS, PhD); nursing leadership and innovations in health care (DNP); pediatric clinical nurse specialist (DNP, Certificate); pediatric nurse practitioner (DNP). *Accreditation:* AACN. Part-time programs available. *Faculty:* 20 full-time (18 women), 6 part-time/adjunct (all women). *Students:* 60 full-time (58 women), 232 part-time (211 women); includes 24 minority (9 Black or African American, non-Hispanic/Latino; 4 American Indian or Alaska Native, non-Hispanic/Latino; 2 Asian, non-Hispanic/Latino; 6 Hispanic/Latino; 3 Two or more races, non-Hispanic/Latino), 4 international. Average age 37. 131 applicants, 62% accepted, 61 enrolled. In 2013, 42 master's, 2 doctorates, 7 other advanced degrees awarded. *Degree requirements:* For master's, thesis optional, oral exam; for doctorate, thesis/dissertation. *Entrance requirements:* For master's, GRE General Test, BSN, minimum GPA of 3.0 during last 60 hours, nursing license. Additional exam requirements/recommendations for international students: Required—TOEFL (minimum score 550 paper-based; 79 iBT). *Application deadline:* For fall admission, 2/1 priority date for domestic and international students. Applications are processed on a rolling basis. Application fee: $55 ($75 for international students). Electronic applications accepted. *Financial support:* Fellowships, research assistantships, teaching assistantships, career-related internships or fieldwork, institutionally sponsored loans, scholarships/grants, traineeships, health care benefits, tuition waivers (full), and unspecified assistantships available. Support available to part-time students. *Faculty research:* Pain, stepfamilies, chemotherapy-related nausea and vomiting, stress management, self-care deficit theory. *Unit head:* Dr. Judith F. Miller, Dean, 573-882-0278, E-mail: millerjud@missouri.edu. *Application contact:* Laura Anderson, Senior Academic Advisor, 573-882-0294, E-mail: andersonla@missouri.edu.
Website: http://nursing.missouri.edu/

University of Missouri–St. Louis, College of Nursing, St. Louis, MO 63121-4400. Offers adult nurse practitioner (DNP, Post Master's Certificate); clinical nurse specialist (DNP); family mental health nurse practitioner (DNP); family nurse practitioner (MSN, DNP, Post Master's Certificate); neonatal nurse practitioner (MSN); nurse educator (MSN); nurse leader (MSN); nurse practitioner (Post Master's Certificate); nursing (PhD); pediatric clinical nurse specialist (DNP); pediatric nurse practitioner (MSN, DNP, Post Master's Certificate); women's health nurse practitioner (MSN, Post Master's Certificate). *Accreditation:* AACN. Part-time programs available. *Faculty:* 14 full-time (13 women), 14 part-time/adjunct (13 women). *Students:* 227 part-time (217 women); includes 40 minority (35 Black or African American, non-Hispanic/Latino; 1 American Indian or Alaska Native, non-Hispanic/Latino; 1 Asian, non-Hispanic/Latino; 1 Hispanic/Latino; 2 Two or more races, non-Hispanic/Latino). Average age 35. 190 applicants, 51% accepted, 76 enrolled. In 2013, 80 master's, 8 doctorates, 2 other advanced degrees awarded. *Degree requirements:* For doctorate, comprehensive exam, thesis/dissertation; for Post Master's Certificate, thesis. *Entrance requirements:* For master's, 2 recommendation letters; minimum GPA of 3.0; BSN; nursing licensure; statement of purpose; course in differential/inferential statistics; for doctorate, GRE, 2 letters of recommendation, MSN, minimum GPA of 3.2, course in differential/inferential statistics; for Post Master's Certificate, 2 recommendation letters; MSN; advanced practice certificate; minimum GPA of 3.0; essay. Additional exam requirements/recommendations for international students: Recommended—TOEFL (minimum score 550 paper-based; 79 iBT), IELTS (minimum score 6.5). *Application deadline:* For fall admission, 2/15 for domestic and international students. Application fee: $50 ($40 for international students). Electronic applications accepted. *Expenses:* Tuition, state resident: full-time $7364; part-time $409.10 per credit hour. Tuition, nonresident: full-time $19,162; part-time $1008.50 per credit hour. *Financial support:* Application deadline: 4/1; applicants required to submit FAFSA. *Faculty research:* Health promotion and restoration, family disruption, violence, abuse, battered women, health survey methods. *Unit head:* Dr. Nancy Magnuson, Director, 314-516-6066. *Application contact:* 314-516-5458, Fax: 314-516-6996, E-mail: gradadm@umsl.edu.
Website: http://www.umsl.edu/divisions/nursing/

The University of North Carolina at Chapel Hill, School of Nursing, Chapel Hill, NC 27599-7460. Offers nursing (MSN, DNP, PhD, PMC), including adult nurse practitioner (MSN, PMC), children's health advanced practice (MSN, PMC), family nurse practitioner (MSN, PMC), health care systems (MSN, PMC), psychiatric/mental health nursing (MSN, PMC). Part-time programs available. *Degree requirements:* For master's, comprehensive exam, thesis; for doctorate, thesis/dissertation, 3 exams. *Entrance requirements:* For master's and doctorate, GRE General Test. Additional exam requirements/recommendations for international students: Required—TOEFL (minimum score 550 paper-based; 79 iBT), IELTS (minimum score 7). Electronic applications accepted. *Faculty research:* Preventing and managing chronic illness, reducing health disparities, Improving healthcare quality and patient outcomes, understanding biobehavioral and genetic bases of health and illness, developing innovative ways to enhance science and its clinical translation.

The University of North Carolina at Charlotte, The Graduate School, College of Health and Human Services, School of Nursing, Charlotte, NC 28223-0001. Offers administration (Post-Master's Certificate); advanced clinical (MSN, Post-Master's Certificate); anesthesia (MSN, Post-Master's Certificate); community health (MSN); family nurse practitioner (MSN, Post-Master's Certificate); health administration (MSN); mental health (MSN); nurse educator (MSN, Post-Master's Certificate); nursing (DNP); systems population (MSN). *Accreditation:* AACN. Part-time programs available. *Faculty:* 17 full-time (16 women), 6 part-time/adjunct (5 women). *Students:* 96 full-time (80 women), 124 part-time (119 women); includes 45 minority (30 Black or African American, non-Hispanic/Latino; 1 American Indian or Alaska Native, non-Hispanic/Latino; 8 Asian, non-Hispanic/Latino; 4 Hispanic/Latino; 2 Two or more races, non-Hispanic/Latino), 1 international. Average age 34. 216 applicants, 38% accepted, 72 enrolled. In 2013, 70 master's, 8 other advanced degrees awarded. Terminal master's awarded for partial completion of doctoral program. *Degree requirements:* For master's, thesis or alternative, practicum; for doctorate, thesis/dissertation or alternative, residency. *Entrance requirements:* For master's, GRE General Test, minimum GPA of 3.0 in undergraduate major; for doctorate, GRE, MAT, or GMAT, minimum GPA of 3.5. Additional exam requirements/recommendations for international students: Required—TOEFL (minimum score 570 paper-based; 83 iBT). *Application deadline:* For fall admission, 5/1 priority date for domestic students, 5/1 for international students; for spring admission, 10/1 priority date for domestic students, 10/1 for international students. Application fee: $75. Electronic applications accepted. *Expenses:* Tuition, state resident: full-time $3522. Tuition, nonresident: full-time $16,051. *Required fees:* $2585. Tuition and fees vary according to course load and program. *Financial support:* In 2013–14, 5 students received support, including 5 teaching assistantships (averaging $4,785 per year); research assistantships, career-related internships or fieldwork, institutionally sponsored loans, scholarships/grants, traineeships, and unspecified assistantships also available. Support available to part-time students. Financial award application deadline: 4/1; financial award applicants required to submit FAFSA. *Faculty research:* Improving care outcomes for the elderly; vulnerable populations; symptom management; self management/health promotion strategies of older adults; migration and maternal child health; health disparities, health literacy, and access to healthcare in Latino adults with diabetes; psychiatric nursing. *Total annual research expenditures:* $572,410. *Unit head:* Dr. Dee Baldwin, Associate Dean, 704-687-7952, Fax: 704-687-6017, E-mail: dbaldwi5@uncc.edu. *Application contact:* Kathy B. Giddings, Director of Graduate Admissions, 704-687-5503, Fax: 704-687-1668, E-mail: gradadm@uncc.edu.
Website: http://nursing.uncc.edu/

University of North Dakota, Graduate School, College of Nursing, Department of Nursing, Grand Forks, ND 58202. Offers adult-gerontological nurse practitioner (MSN); advanced public health nurse (MSN); family nurse practitioner (MSN); nurse anesthesia (MSN); nurse educator (MSN); nursing (DNP, PhD); psychiatric and mental health nurse practitioner (MSN).

University of Pennsylvania, School of Nursing, Psychiatric Mental Health Advanced Practice Nurse Program, Philadelphia, PA 19104. Offers adult and special populations (MSN); child and family (MSN); geropsychiatrics (MSN). *Accreditation:* AACN. Part-time programs available. *Students:* 8 full-time (all women), 21 part-time (16 women); includes 8 minority (3 Black or African American, non-Hispanic/Latino; 3 Hispanic/Latino; 2 Two or more races, non-Hispanic/Latino), 2 international. 8 applicants, 38% accepted, 3 enrolled. In 2013, 13 master's awarded. *Entrance requirements:* For master's, GRE General Test, BSN, minimum GPA of 3.0, previous course work in statistics. Additional exam requirements/recommendations for international students: Required—TOEFL. *Application deadline:* For fall admission, 2/15 priority date for domestic students. Applications are processed on a rolling basis. Application fee: $70. *Expenses:* Contact institution. *Financial support:* Fellowships, research assistantships, teaching assistantships, career-related internships or fieldwork, Federal Work-Study, and institutionally sponsored loans available. Support available to part-time students. Financial award application deadline: 4/1. *Faculty research:* Use of restraints in psychiatry, victims of trauma, spiritual use of prayer by cancer patients, coping strategies of African-Americans, urban health care. *Unit head:* Assistant Dean of Admissions and Financial Aid, 866-867-6877, Fax: 215-573-8439, E-mail: admissions@nursing.upenn.edu. *Application contact:* Laura Leahy, Associate Director, 215-746-5469, E-mail: leahylgl@nursing.upenn.edu.
Website: http://www.nursing.upenn.edu/psych/Pages/default.aspx

University of Pittsburgh, School of Nursing, Clinical Nurse Specialist Program, Pittsburgh, PA 15260. Offers adult-gerontology clinical nurse specialist (DNP); psychiatric mental health clinical nurse specialist (DNP). *Accreditation:* AACN. Part-time programs available. *Students:* 4 full-time (all women), 16 part-time (14 women); includes 2 minority (both Black or African American, non-Hispanic/Latino), 1 international. Average age 41. 4 applicants, 75% accepted, 2 enrolled. In 2013, 5 doctorates awarded. *Entrance requirements:* Additional exam requirements/recommendations for international students: Required—TOEFL (minimum score 550 paper-based; 80 iBT). *Application deadline:* For fall admission, 6/1 priority date for domestic and international students. Applications are processed on a rolling basis. Application fee: $50. Electronic applications accepted. *Expenses:* Tuition, state resident: full-time $19,964; part-time $807 per credit. Tuition, nonresident: full-time $32,686; part-time $1337 per credit. *Required fees:* $740; $200. Tuition and fees vary according to program. *Financial support:* In 2013–14, 4 students received support, including 1 fellowship with full tuition reimbursement available (averaging $24,108 per year), 3 teaching assistantships with full and partial tuition reimbursements available (averaging $21,884 per year); scholarships/grants, traineeships, health care benefits, and unspecified assistantships also available. Support available to part-time students. *Unit head:* Dr. Sandra Engberg, Associate Dean for Clinical Education, 412-624-3835, Fax: 412-624-8521, E-mail: sje1@pitt.edu. *Application contact:* Laurie Lapsley, Administrator of Graduate Student Services, 412-624-9670, Fax: 412-624-2409, E-mail: lapsleyl@pitt.edu.

University of Pittsburgh, School of Nursing, Nurse Practitioner Program, Pittsburgh, PA 15261. Offers adult-gerontology acute care nurse practitioner (DNP); adult-gerontology primary care nurse practitioner (DNP); family (individual across the lifespan) nurse practitioner (DNP); neonatal nurse practitioner (MSN, DNP); pediatric primary care nurse practitioner (DNP); psychiatric mental health nurse practitioner (DNP). *Accreditation:* AACN. Part-time programs available. *Students:* 66 full-time (59 women), 84 part-time (75 women); includes 11 minority (5 Black or African American, non-Hispanic/Latino; 2 American Indian or Alaska Native, non-Hispanic/Latino; 3 Asian, non-Hispanic/Latino; 1 Hispanic/Latino), 2 international. Average age 31. 95 applicants, 74% accepted, 57 enrolled. In 2013, 53 master's, 4 doctorates awarded. *Degree requirements:* For master's, comprehensive exam, thesis optional. *Entrance requirements:* For master's, GRE General Test or MAT, BSN, RN license, letters of recommendation, resume, course work in statistics, 1-3 years of nursing experience; for doctorate, GRE General Test, BSN, RN license, minimum GPA of 3.5, 3 letters of recommendation. Additional exam requirements/recommendations for international students: Required—TOEFL (minimum score 550 paper-based; 80 iBT). *Application deadline:* Applications are processed on a rolling basis. Application fee: $50. Electronic applications accepted. *Expenses:* Tuition, state resident: full-time $19,964; part-time $807 per credit. Tuition, nonresident: full-time $32,686; part-time $1337 per credit. *Required fees:* $740; $200. Tuition and fees vary according to program. *Financial support:* In 2013–14, 18 students received support, including 4 fellowships with full and partial tuition reimbursements available (averaging $22,521 per year), 3 research assistantships with full and partial tuition reimbursements available (averaging $21,884 per year), 15 teaching assistantships with full and partial tuition reimbursements available (averaging $13,535 per year); scholarships/grants, traineeships, health care benefits, and unspecified assistantships also available. Support available to part-time students. *Unit head:* Dr. Sandra Engberg, Associate Dean for Clinical Education, 412-624-3835, Fax: 412-624-8521, E-mail: sje1@pitt.edu. *Application contact:* Laurie Lapsley, Administrator of Graduate Student Services, 412-624-9670, Fax: 412-624-2409, E-mail: lapsleyl@pitt.edu.
Website: http://www.nursing.pitt.edu

University of Puerto Rico, Medical Sciences Campus, School of Nursing, San Juan, PR 00936-5067. Offers adult and elderly nursing (MSN); child and adolescent nursing (MSN); critical care nursing (MSN); family and community nursing (MSN); family nurse practitioner (MSN); maternity nursing (MSN); mental health and psychiatric nursing (MSN). *Accreditation:* AACN. *Entrance requirements:* For master's, GRE or EXADEP, interview, Puerto Rico RN license or professional license for international students, general and specific point average, article analysis. Electronic applications accepted. *Faculty research:* HIV, health disparities, teen violence, women and violence, neurological disorders.

University of Rhode Island, Graduate School, College of Nursing, Kingston, RI 02881. Offers administration (MS); clinical nurse leader (MS); clinical specialist in gerontology (MS); clinical specialist in psychiatric/mental health (MS); family nurse practitioner (MS); gerontological nurse practitioner (MS); nursing (DNP, PhD); nursing education (MS). *Accreditation:* AACN; ACNM/ACME (one or more programs are accredited). Part-time programs available. *Faculty:* 26 full-time (25 women), 3 part-time/adjunct (2 women). *Students:* 46 full-time (42 women), 78 part-time (70 women); includes 11 minority (7 Black or African American, non-Hispanic/Latino; 1 Asian, non-Hispanic/Latino; 3 Hispanic/Latino), 4 international. In 2013, 38 master's, 4 doctorates awarded. *Degree requirements:* For master's, comprehensive exam; for doctorate, comprehensive exam, thesis/dissertation. *Entrance requirements:* For master's, GRE or MAT, 2 letters of recommendation, scholarly papers; for doctorate, GRE, 3 letters of recommendation, scholarly papers. Additional exam requirements/recommendations for international students: Required—TOEFL (minimum score 550 paper-based). *Application deadline:* For fall admission, 2/15 for domestic students, 2/1 for international students; for spring admission, 10/15 for domestic students, 7/15 for international students. Application fee: $65. Electronic applications accepted. *Expenses:* Tuition, state resident: full-time $11,532; part-time $641 per credit. Tuition, nonresident: full-time $23,606; part-time $1311 per credit. *Required fees:* $1388; $36 per credit. $35 per semester. One-time fee: $130. *Financial support:* In 2013–14, 4 teaching assistantships with full and partial tuition reimbursements (averaging $8,383 per year) were awarded. Financial award application deadline: 2/15; financial award applicants required to submit FAFSA. *Faculty research:* Group intervention for grieving women in prison, translating best practice in non-drug interventions for postoperative pain management, further development and testing of the pain assessment inventory, preschool motor and functional performance of two cohorts, neuroactivation of brain motor areas in preterm children. *Total annual research expenditures:* $1.2 million. *Unit head:* Dr. Mary Sullivan, Interim Dean, 401-874-5339, Fax: 401-874-2061, E-mail: mcsullivan@uri.edu. *Application contact:* Graduate Admission, 401-874-2872, E-mail: gradadm@etal.uri.edu.
Website: http://www.uri.edu/nursing/

University of Rochester, School of Nursing, Rochester, NY 14642. Offers acute care nurse practitioner (MS); adult nurse practitioner (MS); adult/geriatric nurse practitioner (MS); clinical nurse leader (MS); clinical research coordinator (MS); family nurse practitioner (MS); family psychiatric mental health nurse practitioner (MS); health care organization management and leadership (MS); health practice research (PhD); nursing (DNP); pediatric nurse practitioner (MS); pediatric nurse practitioner/neonatal nurse practitioner (MS). *Accreditation:* AACN. Part-time programs available. Postbaccalaureate distance learning degree programs offered (minimal on-campus study). *Faculty:* 60 full-time (52 women), 61 part-time/adjunct (47 women). *Students:* 33 full-time (29 women), 213 part-time (195 women); includes 32 minority (8 Black or African American, non-Hispanic/Latino; 10 Asian, non-Hispanic/Latino; 8 Hispanic/Latino; 6 Two or more races, non-Hispanic/Latino), 4 international. Average age 34. 41 applicants, 54% accepted, 16 enrolled. In 2013, 58 master's, 11 doctorates awarded. Terminal master's awarded for partial completion of doctoral program. *Degree requirements:* For master's, comprehensive exam (for some programs); for doctorate, thesis/dissertation. *Entrance requirements:* For master's, BS in nursing, minimum GPA of 3.0, course work in statistics; for doctorate, GRE General Test, MS in nursing, minimum GPA of 3.5. Additional exam requirements/recommendations for international students: Required—TOEFL (minimum score 560 paper-based; 88 iBT) or IELTS (minimum score 6.5) recommended. *Application deadline:* For fall admission, 4/1 for domestic and international students; for spring admission, 9/1 for domestic and international students; for summer admission, 1/2 for domestic and international students. Application fee: $50. Electronic applications accepted. *Expenses: Tuition:* Full-time $44,580; part-time $1394 per credit hour. *Required fees:* $492. *Financial support:* In 2013–14, 41 students received support, including 2 fellowships with full and partial tuition reimbursements available (averaging $30,200 per year); scholarships/grants, traineeships, health care benefits, tuition waivers (partial), and unspecified assistantships also available. Support available to part-time students. Financial award application deadline: 6/30. *Faculty research:* Symptom assessment and self-management, illness prevention, nursing intervention research with vulnerable populations, palliative care, aging. *Total annual research expenditures:* $3.5 million. *Unit head:* Dr. Kathy H. Rideout, Dean, 585-273-8902, Fax: 585-273-1268, E-mail: kathy_rideout@urmc.rochester.edu. *Application contact:* Elaine Andolina, Director of Admissions, 585-275-2375, Fax: 585-756-8299, E-mail: elaine_andolina@urmc.rochester.edu.
Website: http://www.son.rochester.edu

University of St. Francis, Leach College of Nursing, Joliet, IL 60435-6169. Offers family nurse practitioner (MSN, Post-Master's Certificate); family psychology/mental health nurse practitioner (MSN, Post-Master's Certificate); nursing administration (MSN); nursing education (MSN); nursing practice (DNP); teaching in nursing (Certificate). *Accreditation:* AACN. Part-time and evening/weekend programs available. Postbaccalaureate distance learning degree programs offered (no on-campus study). *Faculty:* 11 full-time (all women), 12 part-time/adjunct (11 women). *Students:* 90 full-time (76 women), 332 part-time (305 women); includes 122 minority (43 Black or African American, non-Hispanic/Latino; 1 American Indian or Alaska Native, non-Hispanic/Latino; 19 Asian, non-Hispanic/Latino; 45 Hispanic/Latino; 3 Native Hawaiian or other Pacific Islander, non-Hispanic/Latino; 11 Two or more races, non-Hispanic/Latino), 4 international. Average age 42. 343 applicants, 43% accepted, 111 enrolled. In 2013, 82 master's, 6 doctorates, 17 other advanced degrees awarded. *Entrance requirements:* For master's, minimum undergraduate GPA of 3.0, 2 years of full-time clinical experience, 3 letters recommendation, resume, nursing license, interview; for doctorate, MSN with minimum GPA of 3.0, national certification, interview, computer competency, medical/physical requirements, background check, liability insurance, resume, recommendation, graduate-level statistics course. Additional exam requirements/recommendations for international students: Required—TOEFL (minimum score 550 paper-based; 79 iBT), IELTS (minimum score 6.5). *Application deadline:* Applications are processed on a rolling basis. Application fee: $30. Electronic applications accepted. Application fee is waived when completed online. *Expenses:* Contact institution. *Financial support:* In 2013–14, 109 students received support. Scholarships/grants and tuition waivers (partial) available. Support available to part-time students. Financial award applicants required to submit FAFSA. *Unit head:* Dr. Carol Wilson, Dean, 815-740-3840, Fax: 815-740-4243, E-mail: cwilson@stfrancis.edu. *Application contact:* Sandra Sloka, Director of Admissions for Graduate and Degree Completion Programs, 800-735-7500, Fax: 815-740-3431, E-mail: ssloka@stfrancis.edu.
Website: http://www.stfrancis.edu/academics/college-of-nursing/

University of Saint Joseph, Department of Nursing, West Hartford, CT 06117-2700. Offers family nurse practitioner (MS); family psychiatric/mental health nurse practitioner (MS); nurse educator (MS); nursing practice (DNP). *Accreditation:* AACN. Part-time and evening/weekend programs available. *Degree requirements:* For master's, thesis. *Entrance requirements:* For master's, 2 letters of recommendation. *Application deadline:* Applications are processed on a rolling basis. Application fee: $50. Electronic applications accepted. Application fee is waived when completed online. *Financial support:* Career-related internships or fieldwork and unspecified assistantships available. Support available to part-time students. Financial award applicants required to submit FAFSA. *Unit head:* Dr. Patricia Padula Morgan, RN, Chair, 860-231-5591, E-mail: pmorgan@usj.edu. *Application contact:* Graduate Admissions Office, 860-231-5261, E-mail: graduate@usj.edu.
Website: http://www.usj.edu/academics/schools/school-of-health-natural-sciences/nursing/

University of San Diego, Hahn School of Nursing and Health Science, San Diego, CA 92110. Offers adult-gerontology clinical nurse specialist (MSN); adult-gerontology nurse practitioner/family nurse practitioner (MSN); clinical nursing (MSN); executive nurse leader (MSN); family nurse practitioner (MSN); family/lifespan psychiatric-mental health nurse practitioner (MSN); healthcare informatics (MS, MSN); nursing (PhD); nursing practice (DNP); pediatric nurse practitioner/family nurse practitioner (MSN). *Accreditation:* AACN. Part-time and evening/weekend programs available. *Faculty:* 23 full-time (19 women), 48 part-time/adjunct (43 women). *Students:* 204 full-time (170 women), 166 part-time (144 women); includes 133 minority (26 Black or African American, non-Hispanic/Latino; 8 American Indian or Alaska Native, non-Hispanic/Latino; 50 Asian, non-Hispanic/Latino; 42 Hispanic/Latino; 1 Native Hawaiian or other Pacific Islander, non-Hispanic/Latino; 6 Two or more races, non-Hispanic/Latino), 7 international. Average age 36. 483 applicants, 58% accepted, 154 enrolled. In 2013, 91 master's, 33 doctorates awarded. *Degree requirements:* For doctorate, thesis/dissertation (for some programs), residency (DNP). *Entrance requirements:* For master's, GRE General Test (for entry-level nursing), BSN, current California RN licensure (except for entry-level nursing); minimum GPA of 3.0; for doctorate, minimum GPA of 3.5, MSN, current California RN licensure. Additional exam requirements/recommendations for international students: Required—TOEFL (minimum score 580 paper-based; 83 iBT), TWE. *Application deadline:* For fall admission, 3/1 priority date for domestic students, 3/1 for international students; for spring admission, 11/1 priority date for domestic students, 11/1 for international students. Applications are processed on a rolling basis. Application fee: $45. Electronic applications accepted. *Expenses: Tuition:* Full-time $23,580; part-time $1310 per credit. *Required fees:* $350. *Financial support:* In 2013–14, 250 students received support. Scholarships/grants and traineeships available. Support available to part-time students. Financial award application deadline: 4/1; financial award applicants required to submit FAFSA. *Faculty research:* Palliative and end of life care, maternal/child health, childhood obesity, health care disparities, cognitive functioning. *Unit head:* Dr. Sally Hardin, Dean, 619-260-4550, Fax: 619-260-6814. *Application contact:* Monica Mahon, Associate Director of Graduate Admissions, 619-260-4524, Fax: 619-260-4158, E-mail: grads@sandiego.edu.
Website: http://www.sandiego.edu/nursing/

University of San Francisco, School of Nursing and Health Professions, Doctoral Programs, San Francisco, CA 94117-1080. Offers clinical psychology (Psy D); executive leadership (DNP); family nurse practitioner (DNP); healthcare systems leadership (DNP); psychiatric mental health nurse practitioner (DNP). *Faculty:* 15 full-time (12 women), 10 part-time/adjunct (7 women). *Students:* 118 full-time (92 women), 34 part-time (31 women); includes 74 minority (13 Black or African American, non-Hispanic/Latino; 1 American Indian or Alaska Native, non-Hispanic/Latino; 32 Asian, non-Hispanic/Latino; 15 Hispanic/Latino; 1 Native Hawaiian or other Pacific Islander, non-Hispanic/Latino; 12 Two or more races, non-Hispanic/Latino), 2 international. Average age 41. 98 applicants, 70% accepted, 49 enrolled. In 2013, 39 doctorates awarded. *Entrance requirements:* For doctorate, nursing bachelor's degree, valid RN license in California. *Expenses: Tuition:* Full-time $21,150; part-time $1175 per unit. Tuition and fees vary according to course load, campus/location and program. *Financial support:* In 2013–14, 7 students received support. *Unit head:* Dr. Judith Karshmer, Dean, 415-422-6681, Fax: 415-422-6877, E-mail: nursing@usfca.edu. *Application contact:* Ingrid McVanner, Information Contact, 415-422-2746, Fax: 415-422-2217.

Psychiatric Nursing

University of South Carolina, The Graduate School, College of Nursing, Program in Advanced Practice Nursing in Psychiatric Mental Health, Columbia, SC 29208. Offers MSN, Certificate. Part-time programs available. Postbaccalaureate distance learning degree programs offered (minimal on-campus study). *Entrance requirements:* For master's, master's degree in nursing, RN license; for Certificate, MSN. Additional exam requirements/recommendations for international students: Required—TOEFL (minimum score 570 paper-based). Electronic applications accepted. *Faculty research:* Systems research, evidence based practice, breast cancer, violence.

University of South Carolina, The Graduate School, College of Nursing, Program in Community Mental Health and Psychiatric Health Nursing, Columbia, SC 29208. Offers psychiatric/mental health nurse practitioner (MSN); psychiatric/mental health specialist (MSN). *Accreditation:* AACN. Part-time programs available. *Degree requirements:* For master's, thesis or alternative. *Entrance requirements:* For master's, GRE General Test, MAT, BS in nursing, nursing license. Additional exam requirements/recommendations for international students: Required—TOEFL (minimum score 570 paper-based). Electronic applications accepted. *Faculty research:* Systems research, evidence based practice, breast cancer, violence.

University of Southern Maine, College of Science, Technology, and Health, School of Nursing, Portland, ME 04104-9300. Offers adult-gerontology primary care nurse practitioner (MS, PMC); clinical nurse leader (MS); education (MS); family nurse practitioner (MS, PMC); family psychiatric/mental health nurse practitioner (MS); management (MS); nursing (DNP); psychiatric-mental health nurse practitioner (PMC); MBA/MSN. *Accreditation:* AACN. Part-time programs available. *Faculty:* 11 full-time (all women), 10 part-time/adjunct (8 women). *Students:* 57 full-time (47 women), 53 part-time (46 women); includes 5 minority (1 American Indian or Alaska Native, non-Hispanic/Latino; 2 Asian, non-Hispanic/Latino; 1 Hispanic/Latino; 1 Two or more races, non-Hispanic/Latino). Average age 36. 140 applicants, 44% accepted, 29 enrolled. In 2013, 33 master's, 11 other advanced degrees awarded. *Degree requirements:* For master's, thesis optional. *Entrance requirements:* For master's, GRE General Test or MAT, minimum GPA of 3.0; for doctorate, GRE. Additional exam requirements/recommendations for international students: Required—TOEFL (minimum score 550 paper-based). *Application deadline:* For fall admission, 4/1 for domestic and international students; for spring admission, 10/1 for domestic and international students. Application fee: $65. Electronic applications accepted. *Expenses:* Tuition, state resident: part-time $380 per credit. Tuition, nonresident: part-time $1026 per credit. Part-time tuition and fees vary according to program. *Financial support:* Research assistantships, teaching assistantships, career-related internships or fieldwork, Federal Work-Study, scholarships/grants, traineeships, tuition waivers (full and partial), and unspecified assistantships available. Support available to part-time students. Financial award application deadline: 2/15; financial award applicants required to submit FAFSA. *Faculty research:* Women's health, nursing history, weight control, community services, substance abuse. *Unit head:* Krista M. Meinersmann, Director of Nursing Program, 207-780-4993, E-mail: kmeinersmann@usm.maine.edu. *Application contact:* Mary Sloan, Assistant Dean of Graduate Studies and Director of Graduate Admissions, 207-780-4812, E-mail: gradstudies@usm.maine.edu.
Website: http://www.usm.maine.edu/nursing/

University of Southern Mississippi, Graduate School, College of Health, School of Nursing, Hattiesburg, MS 39406-0001. Offers family nurse practitioner (MSN); nursing (DNP, PhD); nursing executive (MSN); psychiatric nurse practitioner (MSN). *Accreditation:* AACN. Part-time and evening/weekend programs available. *Faculty:* 17 full-time (16 women), 1 part-time/adjunct (0 women). *Students:* 133 full-time (104 women), 42 part-time (40 women); includes 45 minority (33 Black or African American, non-Hispanic/Latino; 1 American Indian or Alaska Native, non-Hispanic/Latino; 1 Asian, non-Hispanic/Latino; 1 Hispanic/Latino; 9 Two or more races, non-Hispanic/Latino). Average age 37. 118 applicants, 61% accepted, 62 enrolled. In 2013, 45 master's, 9 doctorates awarded. *Degree requirements:* For master's, comprehensive exam, thesis optional; for doctorate, comprehensive exam, thesis/dissertation. *Entrance requirements:* For master's, GRE General Test, minimum GPA of 2.75 during last 60 hours, nursing license, BS in nursing; for doctorate, GRE General Test, master's degree in nursing, minimum GPA of 3.5. Additional exam requirements/recommendations for international students: Required—TOEFL, IELTS. *Application deadline:* For fall admission, 3/15 priority date for domestic students, 5/1 for international students; for spring admission, 1/10 priority date for domestic and international students. Applications are processed on a rolling basis. Application fee: $50. Electronic applications accepted. *Financial support:* In 2013–14, 14 research assistantships with full tuition reimbursements (averaging $12,577 per year), teaching assistantships (averaging $12,000 per year) were awarded; Federal Work-Study, institutionally sponsored loans, scholarships/grants, traineeships, health care benefits, and unspecified assistantships also available. Financial award application deadline: 3/15; financial award applicants required to submit FAFSA. *Faculty research:* Gerontology, caregivers, HIV, bereavement, pain, nursing leadership. *Unit head:* Dr. Katherine Nugent, Director and Associate Dean, 601-266-5500, Fax: 601-266-5927. *Application contact:* Dr. Sandra Bishop, Graduate Coordinator, 601-266-5500, Fax: 601-266-5927.
Website: http://www.usm.edu/graduateschool/table.php

The University of Texas at Austin, Graduate School, School of Nursing, Austin, TX 78712-1111. Offers adult - gerontology clinical nurse specialist (MSN); child health (MSN), including administration, public health nursing, teaching; family nurse practitioner (MSN); family psychiatric/mental health nurse practitioner (MSN); holistic adult health (MSN), including administration, teaching; maternity (MSN), including administration, public health nursing, teaching; nursing (PhD); nursing administration and healthcare systems management (MSN); pediatric nurse practitioner (MSN); public health nursing (MSN). *Accreditation:* AACN. Part-time programs available. *Degree requirements:* For master's, thesis optional; for doctorate, thesis/dissertation. *Entrance requirements:* For master's and doctorate, GRE General Test. Additional exam requirements/recommendations for international students: Required—TOEFL (minimum score 550 paper-based). Electronic applications accepted. *Faculty research:* Chronic illness management, memory and aging, health promotion, women's health, adolescent health.

The University of Texas Health Science Center at San Antonio, School of Nursing, San Antonio, TX 78229. Offers administrative management (MSN); adult-gerontology acute care nurse practitioner (PGC); clinical nurse leader (MSN); executive administrative management (DNP); family nurse practitioner (PGC); nurse practitioner (MSN), including adult-gerontology acute care nurse practitioner, family nurse practitioner, pediatric nurse practitioner primary care, psychiatric mental health nurse practitioner; nurse practitioner leadership (DNP); nursing (MSN, PhD); nursing education (MSN, PGC); pediatric nurse practitioner primary care (PGC); psychiatric mental health nurse practitioner (PGC); public health nurse leader (DNP). *Accreditation:* AACN. Part-time programs available. *Faculty:* 84 full-time (74 women), 42 part-time/adjunct (40 women). *Students:* 115 full-time (93 women), 140 part-time (123 women); includes 123 minority (24 Black or African American, non-Hispanic/Latino; 20 Asian, non-Hispanic/Latino; 74 Hispanic/Latino; 5 Two or more races, non-Hispanic/Latino), 7 international. Average age 37. 174 applicants, 59% accepted, 83 enrolled. In 2013, 67 master's, 6 doctorates, 5 other advanced degrees awarded. Terminal master's awarded for partial completion of doctoral program. *Degree requirements:* For master's, thesis optional; for doctorate, comprehensive exam, thesis/dissertation, final projects (for DNP). *Entrance requirements:* For master's, minimum GPA of 3.0, references, goal statement, BSN from accredited nursing school, RN licensure in Texas or compact state; for doctorate, GRE, MAT, minimum GPA of 3.0, personal interview, BSN and/or MSN from accredited nursing school, RN licensure in Texas or compact state, statistics course, references, curriculum vitae, goal statement; for PGC, minimum GPA of 3.0; references; goal statement; MSN from accredited nursing school; RN licensure in Texas or compact state; prerequisites in advanced health assessment, advanced pharmacotherapeutics, and advanced pathophysiology. Additional exam requirements/recommendations for international students: Required—TOEFL (minimum score 550 paper-based; 68 iBT), IELTS (minimum score 6.5). *Application deadline:* For fall admission, 1/10 for domestic and international students; for spring admission, 7/1 for domestic students. Application fee: $65. Electronic applications accepted. *Financial support:* In 2013–14, 145 students received support, including 3 fellowships with full tuition reimbursements available (averaging $30,000 per year); institutionally sponsored loans and scholarships/grants also available. Financial award application deadline: 6/30; financial award applicants required to submit FAFSA. *Faculty research:* Pain, organizational structure, aging, quality and safety, health disparity, obesity and nutrition, women's and children's health. *Total annual research expenditures:* $500,265. *Unit head:* Dr. Eileen T. Breslin, Dean, 210-567-5800, Fax: 210-567-5929, E-mail: breslin@uthscsa.edu. *Application contact:* Brandy Finck, Interim Associate Dean for Admissions and Student Services, 210-567-5805, Fax: 210-567-6189, E-mail: finckb@uthscsa.edu.
Website: http://www.nursing.uthscsa.edu/

University of Virginia, School of Nursing, Charlottesville, VA 22903. Offers acute and specialty care (MSN); acute care nurse practitioner (MSN); clinical nurse leadership (MSN); community-public health leadership (MSN); nursing (DNP, PhD); psychiatric mental health counseling (MSN); MSN/MBA. *Accreditation:* AACN. Part-time programs available. *Faculty:* 45 full-time (41 women), 3 part-time/adjunct (all women). *Students:* 177 full-time (155 women), 147 part-time (133 women); includes 53 minority (27 Black or African American, non-Hispanic/Latino; 10 Asian, non-Hispanic/Latino; 11 Hispanic/Latino; 5 Two or more races, non-Hispanic/Latino), 4 international. Average age 36. 236 applicants, 61% accepted, 110 enrolled. In 2013, 94 master's, 14 doctorates awarded. *Degree requirements:* For doctorate, comprehensive exam (for some programs), capstone project (DNP), dissertation (PhD). *Entrance requirements:* For master's, GRE General Test, MAT; for doctorate, GRE General Test. Additional exam requirements/recommendations for international students: Required—TOEFL, IELTS. *Application deadline:* Applications are processed on a rolling basis. Application fee: $60. Electronic applications accepted. *Expenses:* Contact institution. *Financial support:* Fellowships, research assistantships, teaching assistantships, Federal Work-Study, and scholarships/grants available. Financial award applicants required to submit FAFSA. *Unit head:* Dorrie K. Fontaine, Dean, 434-924-0141, Fax: 434-982-1809, E-mail: dkf2u@virginia.edu. *Application contact:* Clay Hysell, Assistant Dean for Admissions and Financial Services, 434-924-0141, Fax: 434-982-1809, E-mail: nur-osa@virginia.edu.
Website: http://www.nursing.virginia.edu/

University of Wisconsin–Madison, School of Nursing, Madison, WI 53706-1380. Offers adult/gerontology (DNP); nursing (PhD); pediatrics (DNP); psychiatric mental health (DNP); MS/MPH. *Accreditation:* AACN. Part-time programs available. *Degree requirements:* For doctorate, comprehensive exam, thesis/dissertation. *Entrance requirements:* For doctorate, GRE General Test, 2 samples of scholarly written work, BS in nursing from an accredited program, minimum undergraduate GPA of 3.0 in last 60 credits (for PhD); licensure as professional nurse (for DNP). Additional exam requirements/recommendations for international students: Required—TOEFL (minimum score 600 paper-based; 100 iBT). Electronic applications accepted. *Expenses:* Tuition, state resident: full-time $10,728; part-time $790 per credit. Tuition, nonresident: full-time $24,054; part-time $1623 per credit. *Required fees:* $1130; $119 per credit. *Faculty research:* Nursing informatics to promote self-care and disease management skills among patients and caregivers; quality of care to frail, vulnerable, and chronically ill populations; study of health-related and health-seeking behaviors; eliminating health disparities; pain and symptom management for patients with cancer.

Vanderbilt University, Vanderbilt University School of Nursing, Nashville, TN 37240. Offers adult-gerontology acute care nurse practitioner (MSN), including hospitalist, intensivist; adult-gerontology primary care nurse practitioner (MSN); emergency nurse practitioner (MSN); family nurse practitioner (MSN); healthcare leadership (MSN); neonatal nurse practitioner (MSN); nurse midwifery (MSN); nurse midwifery/family nurse practitioner (MSN); nursing informatics (MSN); nursing practice (DNP); nursing science (PhD); pediatric acute care nurse practitioner (MSN); pediatric primary care nurse practitioner (MSN); psychiatric-mental health nurse practitioner (MSN); women's health nurse practitioner (MSN); women's health nurse practitioner/adult gerontology primary care nurse practitioner (MSN); MSN/M Div; MSN/MTS. *Accreditation:* ACNM/ACME (one or more programs are accredited). Part-time programs available. Postbaccalaureate distance learning degree programs offered (minimal on-campus study). *Faculty:* 139 full-time (124 women), 452 part-time/adjunct (319 women). *Students:* 527 full-time (463 women), 369 part-time (333 women); includes 120 minority (46 Black or African American, non-Hispanic/Latino; 8 American Indian or Alaska Native, non-Hispanic/Latino; 26 Asian, non-Hispanic/Latino; 24 Hispanic/Latino; 4 Native Hawaiian or other Pacific Islander, non-Hispanic/Latino; 12 Two or more races, non-Hispanic/Latino), 7 international. Average age 32. 1,257 applicants, 49% accepted, 457 enrolled. In 2013, 364 master's, 43 doctorates awarded. *Degree requirements:* For doctorate, comprehensive exam, thesis/dissertation. *Entrance requirements:* For master's, GRE General Test (within the past 5 years), minimum B average in undergraduate course work, 3 letters of recommendation; for doctorate, GRE General Test, interview, 3 letters of recommendation from doctorally-prepared faculty, MSN, essay. Additional exam requirements/recommendations for international students: Required—TOEFL (minimum score 570 paper-based), IELTS (minimum score 6.5). *Application deadline:* For fall admission, 12/1 priority date for domestic and international students. Applications are processed on a rolling basis. Application fee: $50. Electronic applications accepted. *Expenses:* Contact institution. *Financial support:* In 2013–14, 582 students received support. Scholarships/grants and health care benefits available. Support available to part-time students. Financial award application deadline: 3/15; financial award applicants required to submit FAFSA. *Faculty research:* Lymphedema, palliative care and bereavement, health services research including workforce, safety and quality of care, gerontology, better birth outcomes including nutrition. *Total annual research expenditures:* $2.5 million. *Unit head:* Dr. Linda Norman, Dean, 615-343-8876, Fax: 615-343-7711, E-mail: linda.norman@vanderbilt.edu. *Application contact:* Patricia Peerman, Assistant Dean for Enrollment Management, 615-322-3800, Fax: 615-343-0333, E-mail: vusn-admissions@vanderbilt.edu.
Website: http://www.nursing.vanderbilt.edu

Virginia Commonwealth University, Graduate School, School of Nursing, Richmond, VA 23284-9005. Offers adult health acute nursing (MS); adult health primary nursing (MS); biobehavioral clinical research (PhD); child health nursing (MS); clinical nurse leader (MS); family health nursing (MS); nurse educator (MS); nurse practitioner (MS); nursing (Certificate); nursing administration (MS), including clinical nurse manager; psychiatric-mental health nursing (MS); women's health nursing (MS). Part-time and evening/weekend programs available. *Degree requirements:* For master's, thesis optional; for doctorate, thesis/dissertation. *Entrance requirements:* For master's, GRE General Test, BSN, minimum GPA of 2.8; for doctorate, GRE General Test. Additional exam requirements/recommendations for international students: Required—TOEFL (minimum score 600 paper-based; 100 iBT). Electronic applications accepted.

Washington State University Spokane, Graduate Programs, College of Nursing, Spokane, WA 99210-1495. Offers advanced population health (MN, DNP); family nurse practitioner (MN, DNP); nursing (PhD); psychiatric/mental health nurse practitioner (DNP); psychiatric/mental health practitioner (MN). *Accreditation:* AACN. *Degree requirements:* For master's, comprehensive exam (for some programs), thesis (for some programs), oral exam, research project. *Entrance requirements:* For master's, minimum GPA of 3.0, Washington state RN license, physical assessment skills, course work in statistics, recommendations, written interview (for nurse practitioner). *Faculty research:* Cardiovascular and Type 2 diabetes in children, evaluation of strategies to increase physical activity in sedentary people.

Wayne State University, College of Nursing, Area of Family Community Mental Health, Detroit, MI 48202. Offers MSN. *Accreditation:* AACN. Part-time programs available. *Faculty:* 15 full-time (all women). *Students:* 61 full-time (59 women), 108 part-time (100 women); includes 38 minority (26 Black or African American, non-Hispanic/Latino; 1 American Indian or Alaska Native, non-Hispanic/Latino; 9 Asian, non-Hispanic/Latino; 1 Hispanic/Latino; 1 Two or more races, non-Hispanic/Latino), 11 international. Average age 35. 66 applicants, 56% accepted, 33 enrolled. In 2013, 51 master's awarded. *Degree requirements:* For master's, thesis or alternative. *Entrance requirements:* For master's, minimum honor point average of 3.0 in upper-division course work; BA from NLN- or CCNE-accredited program; references; current RN license; personal statement. Additional exam requirements/recommendations for international students: Required—TOEFL (minimum score 550 paper-based; 79 iBT), TWE (minimum score 6), Michigan English Language Assessment Battery (minimum score 85); Recommended—IELTS (minimum score 6.5). *Application deadline:* For fall admission, 7/1 for domestic students, 5/1 priority date for international students; for winter admission, 11/1 for domestic students, 9/1 priority date for international students; for spring admission, 3/1 for domestic students, 1/1 priority date for international students. Applications are processed on a rolling basis. Application fee: $0. Electronic applications accepted. *Expenses:* Contact institution. *Financial support:* In 2013–14, 1 student received support. Fellowships with tuition reimbursements available, research assistantships with tuition reimbursements available, teaching assistantships with tuition reimbursements available, institutionally sponsored loans, scholarships/grants, traineeships, and unspecified assistantships available. Support available to part-time students. Financial award application deadline: 3/31; financial award applicants required to submit FAFSA. *Faculty research:* Cultural competence in the home care nursing community; prevention and management of depression in women (including caregivers and perinatal women); breastfeeding in low-income populations; promotion of mental health of vulnerable women, infants, and young children; palliative and end-of-life care for newborns and families. *Unit head:* Dr. Stephanie Schim, Assistant Dean, Family Community Mental Health, 313-577-5137. *Application contact:* Eric Brown, Director, Office of Student Affairs, 313-577-4082, E-mail: nursinginfo@wayne.edu.
Website: https://nursing.wayne.edu/

Wayne State University, College of Nursing, Program in Psychiatric Mental Health Nurse Practitioner, Detroit, MI 48202. Offers MSN. *Accreditation:* AACN. Part-time programs available. *Students:* 9 full-time (6 women), 37 part-time (34 women); includes 13 minority (10 Black or African American, non-Hispanic/Latino; 3 Asian, non-Hispanic/Latino), 2 international. Average age 42. 29 applicants, 62% accepted, 16 enrolled. In 2013, 8 degrees awarded. *Degree requirements:* For master's, thesis or alternative. *Entrance requirements:* For master's, bachelor's degree in nursing from an NLN- or CCNE-accredited program with minimum upper-division GPA of 3.0, three references, current Michigan RN, personal statement, interview. Additional exam requirements/recommendations for international students: Required—TOEFL (minimum score 550 paper-based; 79 iBT); Recommended—TWE (minimum score 6). *Application deadline:* For fall admission, 6/1 priority date for domestic students, 5/1 priority date for international students; for winter admission, 10/1 priority date for domestic students, 9/1 priority date for international students; for spring admission, 2/1 priority date for domestic students, 1/1 priority date for international students. Applications are processed on a rolling basis. Application fee: $50. Electronic applications accepted. *Expenses:* Contact institution. *Financial support:* In 2013–14, 3 students received support. Research assistantships, institutionally sponsored loans, and scholarships/grants available. Support available to part-time students. Financial award applicants required to submit FAFSA. *Faculty research:* Immigrant and minority health, homelessness, HIV/AIDS, promotion of sleep, substance abuse. *Unit head:* Dr. Barbara Redman, Dean, 313-577-4070, Fax: 313-577-4571, E-mail: ae9080@wayne.edu. *Application contact:* Dr. Cynthia Redwine, Assistant Dean for the Office of Student Affairs, 313-577-4082, E-mail: nursinginfo@wayne.edu.
Website: http://www.nursing.wayne.edu/msn/pmhcurriculum.php

West Virginia Wesleyan College, Department of Nursing, Buckhannon, WV 26201. Offers family nurse practitioner (Post Master's Certificate); family nurse practitoner (MS); nurse administrator (MS); nurse educator (MS); nurse-midwifery (MS); nursing administration (Post Master's Certificate); nursing education (Post Master's Certificate); psychiatric mental health nurse practitioner (MS); MSN/MBA.

School Nursing

Cambridge College, School of Education, Cambridge, MA 02138-5304. Offers autism specialist (M Ed); autism/behavior analyst (M Ed); behavior analyst (Post-Master's Certificate); behavioral management (M Ed); early childhood teacher (M Ed); education specialist in curriculum and instruction (CAGS); educational leadership (Ed D); elementary teacher (M Ed); English as a second language (M Ed, Certificate); general science (M Ed); health education (Post-Master's Certificate); health/family and consumer sciences (M Ed); history (M Ed); individualized (M Ed); information technology literacy (M Ed); instructional technology (M Ed); interdisciplinary studies (M Ed); library teacher (M Ed); literacy education (M Ed); mathematics (M Ed); mathematics specialist (Certificate); middle school mathematics and science (M Ed); school administration (M Ed, CAGS); school guidance counselor (M Ed); school nurse education (M Ed); school social worker/school adjustment counselor (M Ed); special education administrator (CAGS); special education/moderate disabilities (M Ed); teaching skills and methodologies (M Ed). Part-time and evening/weekend programs available. Postbaccalaureate distance learning degree programs offered (minimal on-campus study). *Degree requirements:* For master's, thesis, internship/practicum (licensure program only); for doctorate, thesis/dissertation; for other advanced degree, thesis. *Entrance requirements:* For master's, interview, resume, documentation of licensure, 2 professional references; for doctorate, official transcripts, interview, resume, documentation of licensure (if any), written personal statement/essay, portfolio of scholarly and professional work, qualifying assessment, 2 professional references, health insurance, immunizations form; for other advanced degree, official transcripts, interview, resume, documentation of licensure (if any), written personal statement/essay, 2 professional references, health insurance, immunizations form. Additional exam requirements/recommendations for international students: Required—TOEFL (minimum score 550 paper-based; 79 iBT), Michigan English Language Assessment Battery (minimum score 85); Recommended—IELTS (minimum score 6). Electronic applications accepted. *Expenses:* Contact institution. *Faculty research:* Adult education, accelerated learning, mathematics education, brain compatible learning, special education and law.

Eastern Mennonite University, Program in Nursing, Harrisonburg, VA 22802-2462. Offers leadership and management (MSN); leadership/school nursing (MSN). *Accreditation:* AACN. Part-time programs available. Postbaccalaureate distance learning degree programs offered (minimal on-campus study). *Degree requirements:* For master's, leadership project. *Entrance requirements:* For master's, RN license, one year of full-time work experience as RN, minimum GPA of 3.0. Additional exam requirements/recommendations for international students: Required—TOEFL. *Faculty research:* Community health, international health, effectiveness of the nursing school environment, development of caring ability in nursing students, international nursing students.

Eastern University, Graduate Education Programs, St. Davids, PA 19087-3696. Offers ESL program specialist (K-12) (Certificate); general supervisor (PreK-12) (Certificate); health and physical education (K-12) (Certificate); middle level (4-8) (Certificate); multicultural education (M Ed); pre K-4 (Certificate); pre K-4 with special education (Certificate); reading (M Ed); reading specialist (K-12) (Certificate); reading supervisor (K-12) (Certificate); school health services (M Ed); school health supervisor (Certificate); school nurse (Certificate); school principalship (K-12) (Certificate); secondary biology education (7-12) (Certificate); secondary chemistry education (7-12) (Certificate); secondary communication education (7-12) (Certificate); secondary education (7-12) (Certificate); secondary English education (7-12) (Certificate); secondary math education (7-12) (Certificate); secondary social studies education (7-12) (Certificate); special education (M Ed); special education (7-12) (Certificate); special education (Pre K-8) (Certificate); special education supervisor (N-12) (Certificate); TESOL (M Ed); world language (Certificate), including French, Mandarin Chinese, Spanish. Part-time and evening/weekend programs available. Postbaccalaureate distance learning degree programs offered (no on-campus study). *Faculty:* 22 full-time (11 women), 26 part-time/adjunct (18 women). *Students:* 77 full-time (58 women), 223 part-time (149 women); includes 112 minority (81 Black or African American, non-Hispanic/Latino; 1 American Indian or Alaska Native, non-Hispanic/Latino; 9 Asian, non-Hispanic/Latino; 18 Hispanic/Latino; 1 Native Hawaiian or other Pacific Islander, non-Hispanic/Latino; 2 Two or more races, non-Hispanic/Latino), 7 international. Average age 34. 94 applicants, 100% accepted, 81 enrolled. In 2013, 120 master's awarded. *Entrance requirements:* For master's, minimum GPA of 2.5; for Certificate, minimum GPA of 3.0. Additional exam requirements/recommendations for international students: Required—TOEFL. *Application deadline:* For fall admission, 8/14 for domestic students; for spring admission, 12/20 for domestic students. Applications are processed on a rolling basis. Application fee: $35. Application fee is waived when completed online. *Expenses: Tuition:* Full-time $15,600; part-time $650 per credit. *Required fees:* $27.50 per semester. One-time fee: $50. Tuition and fees vary according to course load, degree level and program. *Financial support:* In 2013–14, 84 students received support, including 6 research assistantships with partial tuition reimbursements available (averaging $7,710 per year); scholarships/grants and unspecified assistantships also available. Financial award application deadline: 3/15; financial award applicants required to submit FAFSA. *Unit head:* Harry Gutelius, Associate Dean, 610-341-1729. *Application contact:* Michael Perpiglia, Associate Director of Enrollment, 610-341-5947, Fax: 484-581-1276, E-mail: mperpigl@eastern.edu.
Website: http://www.eastern.edu/academics/programs/loeb-school-education-0/graduateprograms

Felician College, Program in Education, Lodi, NJ 07644-2117. Offers education (MA); educational leadership (principal/supervision) (MA); educational supervision (PMC); principal (PMC); school nursing and health education (MA, Certificate). *Accreditation:* Teacher Education Accreditation Council. Part-time and evening/weekend programs available. *Students:* 10 full-time (8 women), 58 part-time (52 women); includes 23 minority (7 Black or African American, non-Hispanic/Latino; 7 Asian, non-Hispanic/Latino; 6 Hispanic/Latino; 3 Two or more races, non-Hispanic/Latino), 3 international. Average age 37. *Degree requirements:* For master's, project. *Entrance requirements:* For master's, MAT, minimum GPA of 3.0, 3 letters of recommendation. Additional exam requirements/recommendations for international students: Recommended—TOEFL (minimum score 550 paper-based). *Application deadline:* Applications are processed on a rolling basis. Application fee: $40. *Expenses: Tuition:* Part-time $945 per credit. *Required fees:* $317.50 per semester. *Financial support:* Federal Work-Study available. *Unit head:* Dr. Rosemarie Liebmann, Associate Dean, 201-559-3537, E-mail: liebmannr@felician.edu. *Application contact:* Dr. Margaret Smolin, Associate Director, Graduate Admissions, 201-559-6077, Fax: 201-559-6138, E-mail: graduate@felician.edu.

Kean University, College of Natural, Applied and Health Sciences, Program in Nursing, Union, NJ 07083. Offers clinical management with transcultural focus (MSN); community health nursing (MSN); school nursing (MSN). Part-time programs available. *Faculty:* 8 full-time (all women). *Students:* 14 full-time (12 women), 121 part-time (117 women); includes 62 minority (43 Black or African American, non-Hispanic/Latino; 11 Asian, non-Hispanic/Latino; 7 Hispanic/Latino; 1 Two or more races, non-Hispanic/Latino), 2 international. Average age 42. 72 applicants, 94% accepted, 49 enrolled. In 2013, 35 master's awarded. *Degree requirements:* For master's, thesis or alternative, clinical field experience. *Entrance requirements:* For master's, minimum GPA of 3.0; BS in nursing; RN license; 2 letters of recommendation; interview. Additional exam requirements/recommendations for international students: Required—TOEFL. *Application deadline:* For fall admission, 6/1 for domestic and international students; for spring admission, 12/1 for domestic and international students. Applications are

processed on a rolling basis. Application fee: $75 ($150 for international students). Electronic applications accepted. *Expenses:* Tuition, state resident: full-time $12,099; part-time $589 per credit. Tuition, nonresident: full-time $16,399; part-time $722 per credit. *Required fees:* $3050; $139 per credit. Part-time tuition and fees vary according to course level, course load, degree level and program. *Financial support:* In 2013–14, 2 research assistantships with full tuition reimbursements (averaging $3,713 per year) were awarded; unspecified assistantships also available. Financial award applicants required to submit FAFSA. *Unit head:* Dr. Virginia Fitzsimons, Program Coordinator, 908-527-3396, E-mail: vfitzsim@kean.edu. *Application contact:* Ann-Marie Kay, Assistant Director of Graduate Admissions, 908-737-5922, Fax: 908-737-5925, E-mail: akay@kean.edu.
Website: http://grad.kean.edu/masters-programs/nursing-clinical-management

La Salle University, School of Nursing and Health Sciences, Program in Nursing, Philadelphia, PA 19141-1199. Offers adult gerontology primary care nurse practitioner (MSN, Certificate); adult health and illness clinical nurse specialist (MSN); adult-gerontology clinical nurse specialist (MSN, Certificate); clinical nurse leader (MSN); family primary care nurse practitioner (MSN, Certificate); gerontology (Certificate); nurse anesthetist (MSN, Certificate); nursing (MSN, Certificate); nursing administration (MSN, Certificate); nursing education (Certificate); nursing practice (DNP); nursing service administration (MSN); public health nursing (MSN, Certificate); school nursing (Certificate); MSN/MBA; MSN/MPH. *Accreditation:* AANA/CANAEP. Part-time programs available. Postbaccalaureate distance learning degree programs offered (minimal on-campus study). *Faculty:* 13 full-time (12 women), 10 part-time/adjunct (8 women). *Students:* 4 full-time (all women), 379 part-time (331 women); includes 119 minority (70 Black or African American, non-Hispanic/Latino; 2 American Indian or Alaska Native, non-Hispanic/Latino; 31 Asian, non-Hispanic/Latino; 12 Hispanic/Latino; 4 Two or more races, non-Hispanic/Latino), 1 international. Average age 37. 133 applicants, 85% accepted, 63 enrolled. In 2013, 72 master's, 3 doctorates, 26 other advanced degrees awarded. *Degree requirements:* For doctorate, minimum of 1,000 hours of post baccalaureate clinical practice supervised by preceptors. *Entrance requirements:* For master's, GRE, MAT, or GMAT (for students with BSN GPA of less than 3.2), baccalaureate degree in nursing from an NLNAC- or CCNE-accredited program or an MSN Bridge program; Pennsylvania RN license; 2 letters of reference; resume; statement of philosophy articulating professional values and future educational goal; 1 year of work experience as a registered nurse; for doctorate, GRE (waived for applicants with MSN cumulative GPA of 3.7 or above), MSN from nationally-accredited program or master's degree, MBA or MHA from nationally-accredited program; resume or curriculum vitae; 2 letters of reference; interview; for Certificate, GRE, MAT, or GMAT (for students with BSN GPA of less than 3.2, baccalaureate degree in nursing from an NLNAC- or CCNE-accredited program or an MSN Bridge program; Pennsylvania RN license; 2 letters of reference; resume; statement of philosophy articulating professional values and future educational goal; 1 year of work experience as a registered nurse. Additional exam requirements/recommendations for international students: Required—TOEFL. *Application deadline:* For fall admission, 8/15 priority date for domestic students, 7/15 for international students; for spring admission, 12/15 priority date for domestic students, 11/15 for international students; for summer admission, 4/15 priority date for domestic students, 3/15 for international students. Applications are processed on a rolling basis. Application fee: $35. Electronic applications accepted. Application fee is waived when completed online. *Expenses:* Contact institution. *Financial support:* In 2013–14, 48 students received support. Teaching assistantships, scholarships/grants, and traineeships available. Support available to part-time students. Financial award application deadline: 8/31; financial award applicants required to submit FAFSA. *Unit head:* Dr. Patricia M. Dillon, Director, 215-951-1322, Fax: 215-951-1896, E-mail: msnapn@lasalle.edu. *Application contact:* Paul J. Reilly, Assistant Vice President, Enrollment Services, 215-951-1946, Fax: 215-951-1462, E-mail: reilly@lasalle.edu.

Monmouth University, The Graduate School, The Marjorie K. Unterberg School of Nursing and Health Studies, West Long Branch, NJ 07764-1898. Offers adult and gerontological nurse practitioner (MSN); adult-gerontological nurse practitioner (Post-Master's Certificate); family nurse practitioner (MSN, Post-Master's Certificate); family psychiatric and mental health advanced practice nursing (MSN); forensic nursing (MSN, Certificate); nursing (MSN); nursing administration (MSN, Post-Master's Certificate); nursing education (MSN, Post-Master's Certificate); nursing practice (DNP); physician assistant (MS); psychiatric-mental health nurse practitioner (Post-Master's Certificate); school nursing (MSN, Certificate). *Accreditation:* AACN. Part-time and evening/weekend programs available. *Faculty:* 14 full-time (all women), 4 part-time/adjunct (3 women). *Students:* 19 full-time (18 women), 269 part-time (252 women); includes 106 minority (35 Black or African American, non-Hispanic/Latino; 2 American Indian or Alaska Native, non-Hispanic/Latino; 51 Asian, non-Hispanic/Latino; 12 Hispanic/Latino; 3 Native Hawaiian or other Pacific Islander, non-Hispanic/Latino; 3 Two or more races, non-Hispanic/Latino), 2 international. Average age 39. 135 applicants, 98% accepted, 96 enrolled. In 2013, 54 master's, 7 doctorates awarded. *Degree requirements:* For master's, practicum (for some tracks). *Entrance requirements:* For master's, GRE General Test, BSN with minimum GPA of 2.75, current RN license, proof of liability and malpractice policy, personal statement, two letters of recommendation, college course work in health assessment, resume; minimum GPA of 3.0, minimum C grade in prerequisite courses, minimum 200 hours' clinical experience, 3 letters of recommendation, and interview (for MS); for doctorate, accredited master's nursing program degree with minimum GPA of 3.2, active RN license, national certification as Nurse Practitioner or Nurse Administrator, working knowledge of statistics, statement of goals and vision for change, 2 letters of recommendation, resume, interview. Additional exam requirements/recommendations for international students: Required—TOEFL (minimum score 550 paper-based; 79 iBT), IELTS (minimum score 6) or Michigan English Language Assessment Battery (minimum score 77). *Application deadline:* For fall admission, 7/15 priority date for domestic students, 6/1 for international students; for spring admission, 11/15 priority date for domestic students, 11/1 for international students; for summer admission, 2/1 for domestic students. Applications are processed on a rolling basis. Application fee: $50. Electronic applications accepted. *Expenses: Tuition:* Part-time $1004 per credit hour. *Required fees:* $157 per semester. *Financial support:* In 2013–14, 163 students received support, including 113 fellowships (averaging $3,093 per year), 27 research assistantships (averaging $6,273 per year); career-related internships or fieldwork, scholarships/grants, and unspecified assistantships also available. Support available to part-time students. Financial award applicants required to submit FAFSA. *Faculty research:* Relationship of undergraduate GPA and GRE to succeeding in a graduate nursing program. *Unit head:* Dr. Janet Mahoney, Dean, 732-571-3443, Fax: 732-263-5131, E-mail: jmahoney@monmouth.edu. *Application contact:* Lauren Vento-Cifelli, Associate Vice President of Undergraduate and Graduate Admission, 732-571-3452, Fax: 732-263-5123, E-mail: gradadm@monmouth.edu.
Website: http://www.monmouth.edu/school-of-nursing-health/graduate-nursing-programs.aspx

Rowan University, Graduate School, College of Education, Department of Special Educational Services/Instruction, Glassboro, NJ 08028-1701. Offers counseling in educational settings (MA); educational services (Ed S); higher education administration (MA); principal preparation (CAGS); school administration (MA); school and public librarianship (MA); school nursing (Postbaccalaureate Certificate); school psychology (MA, Ed S); supervisor (CAGS). *Accreditation:* NCATE. Part-time and evening/weekend programs available. *Faculty:* 22 full-time (15 women), 18 part-time/adjunct (12 women). *Students:* 117 full-time (93 women), 211 part-time (154 women); includes 64 minority (42 Black or African American, non-Hispanic/Latino; 1 American Indian or Alaska Native, non-Hispanic/Latino; 5 Asian, non-Hispanic/Latino; 14 Hispanic/Latino; 2 Two or more races, non-Hispanic/Latino), 3 international. Average age 31. 127 applicants, 94% accepted, 76 enrolled. In 2013, 109 master's, 31 other advanced degrees awarded. *Degree requirements:* For master's, comprehensive exam, thesis; for other advanced degree, thesis or alternative. *Entrance requirements:* For master's and other advanced degree, GRE General Test. Additional exam requirements/recommendations for international students: Required—TOEFL. *Application deadline:* Applications are processed on a rolling basis. Application fee: $65. Electronic applications accepted. *Expenses: Tuition, area resident:* Part-time $638 per credit. Tuition, state resident: full-time $5742. *Required fees:* $142 per credit. Tuition and fees vary according to course level and program. *Financial support:* Career-related internships or fieldwork, Federal Work-Study, scholarships/grants, and unspecified assistantships available. Support available to part-time students. *Unit head:* Dr. Horacio Sosa, Dean, College of Graduate and Continuing Education, 856-256-4747, Fax: 856-256-5638, E-mail: sosa@rowan.edu. *Application contact:* Admissions and Enrollment Services, 856-256-5145, Fax: 856-256-5637, E-mail: haynes@rowan.edu.

Saint Joseph's University, College of Arts and Sciences, Department of Health Services, Philadelphia, PA 19131-1395. Offers health administration (MS, Post-Master's Certificate); health care ethics (Post-Master's Certificate); health education (MS, Post-Master's Certificate); health informatics (Post-Master's Certificate); healthcare ethics (MS); long-term care administration (MS); nurse anesthesia (MS); school nurse certification (MS). Part-time and evening/weekend programs available. *Faculty:* 5 full-time (1 woman), 16 part-time/adjunct (6 women). *Students:* 46 full-time (25 women), 431 part-time (315 women); includes 168 minority (120 Black or African American, non-Hispanic/Latino; 29 Asian, non-Hispanic/Latino; 15 Hispanic/Latino; 2 Native Hawaiian or other Pacific Islander, non-Hispanic/Latino; 2 Two or more races, non-Hispanic/Latino), 14 international. Average age 34. 234 applicants, 74% accepted, 135 enrolled. In 2013, 83 master's awarded. *Entrance requirements:* For master's, GRE (if GPA less than 3.0), 2 letters of recommendation, resume, personal statement, official transcripts. Additional exam requirements/recommendations for international students: Required—TOEFL (minimum score 550 paper-based; 80 iBT), IELTS (minimum score 6.5). *Application deadline:* For fall admission, 7/15 priority date for domestic students, 4/15 for international students; for winter admission, 1/15 for international students; for spring admission, 11/15 priority date for domestic students, 10/15 for international students. Applications are processed on a rolling basis. Application fee: $35. Electronic applications accepted. *Expenses: Tuition:* Part-time $786 per credit hour. Tuition and fees vary according to degree level and program. *Financial support:* Career-related internships or fieldwork and unspecified assistantships available. Financial award applicants required to submit FAFSA. *Unit head:* Nakia Henderson, Director, 610-660-3131, E-mail: gradstudies@sju.edu. *Application contact:* Elisabeth Woodward, Director of Marketing and Admissions, Graduate Arts and Sciences, 610-660-3131, Fax: 610-660-3230, E-mail: gradstudies@sju.edu.
Website: http://sju.edu/majors-programs/graduate-arts-sciences/masters/health-administration-ms

Seton Hall University, College of Nursing, South Orange, NJ 07079-2697. Offers advanced practice in primary health care (MSN, DNP), including adult/gerontological nurse practitioner, pediatric nurse practitioner; entry into practice (MSN); health systems administration (MSN, DNP); nursing (PhD); nursing case management (MSN); nursing education (MA); school nurse (MSN); MSN/MA. *Accreditation:* AACN. Part-time programs available. Postbaccalaureate distance learning degree programs offered (minimal on-campus study). *Degree requirements:* For master's, research project; for doctorate, dissertation or scholarly project. *Entrance requirements:* For doctorate, GRE (waived for students with GPA of 3.5 or higher). Additional exam requirements/recommendations for international students: Required—TOEFL. Electronic applications accepted. *Faculty research:* Parent/child, adult, and gerontological nursing; breast cancer; families of children with HIV; parish nursing.

University of Illinois at Chicago, Graduate College, College of Nursing, Program in Nursing, Chicago, IL 60607-7128. Offers acute care clinical nurse specialist (MS); acute care nurse practitioner (MS); administrative nursing leadership (Certificate); administrative studies in nursing (MS); adult nurse practitioner (MS); adult/geriatric nurse practitioner (MS); advanced community health nurse specialist (MS); family nurse practitioner (MS); geriatric clinical nurse specialist (MS); geriatric nurse practitioner (MS); mental health clinical nurse specialist (MS); mental health nurse practitioner (MS); nurse midwifery (MS); occupational health/advanced community health nurse specialist (MS); occupational health/family nurse practitioner (MS); pediatric clinical nurse specialist (MS); pediatric nurse practitioner (MS); perinatal clinical nurse specialist (MS); school/advanced community health nurse specialist (MS); school/family nurse practitioner (MS); women's health nurse practitioner (MS). *Accreditation:* AACN. Part-time programs available. *Faculty:* 16 full-time (14 women). *Students:* 393 full-time (361 women), 410 part-time (367 women); includes 198 minority (48 Black or African American, non-Hispanic/Latino; 1 American Indian or Alaska Native, non-Hispanic/Latino; 64 Asian, non-Hispanic/Latino; 71 Hispanic/Latino; 2 Native Hawaiian or other Pacific Islander, non-Hispanic/Latino; 12 Two or more races, non-Hispanic/Latino), 29 international. Average age 32. 396 applicants, 62% accepted, 177 enrolled. In 2013, 184 master's awarded. *Degree requirements:* For master's, thesis or alternative. *Entrance requirements:* For master's, GRE General Test, minimum GPA of 2.75. Additional exam requirements/recommendations for international students: Required—TOEFL. *Application deadline:* For fall admission, 5/15 for domestic students, 2/15 for international students; for spring admission, 11/1 for domestic students, 7/15 for international students. Applications are processed on a rolling basis. Application fee: $40 ($50 for international students). Electronic applications accepted. *Expenses:* Tuition, state resident: full-time $11,066; part-time $3689 per term. Tuition, nonresident: full-time $23,064; part-time $7688 per term. *Required fees:* $3004; $1190 per term. Tuition and fees vary according to course level and program. *Financial support:* Fellowships with full tuition reimbursements, research assistantships with full tuition reimbursements, teaching assistantships with full tuition reimbursements, career-related internships or fieldwork, Federal Work-Study, institutionally sponsored loans, scholarships/grants, traineeships, tuition waivers (full and partial), and unspecified assistantships available. Support available to part-time students. Financial award application deadline: 3/1; financial award applicants required to submit FAFSA. *Unit head:* Dr. Terri E. Weaver, Dean, 312-996-7808, E-mail: teweaver@uic.edu. *Application contact:* Receptionist, 312-413-2550, E-mail: gradcoll@uic.edu.

Wright State University, School of Graduate Studies, College of Nursing and Health, Program in Nursing, Dayton, OH 45435. Offers acute care nurse practitioner (MS); administration of nursing and health care systems (MS); adult health (MS); child and adolescent health (MS); community health (MS); family nurse practitioner (MS); nurse practitioner (MS); school nurse (MS); MBA/MS. *Accreditation:* AACN. Part-time and evening/weekend programs available. *Degree requirements:* For master's, thesis or alternative. *Entrance requirements:* For master's, GRE General Test, BSN from NLN-accredited college, Ohio RN license. Additional exam requirements/recommendations for international students: Required—TOEFL. *Faculty research:* Clinical nursing and health, teaching, caring, pain administration, informatics and technology.

Xavier University, College of Social Sciences, Health and Education, School of Nursing, Nursing Program, Cincinnati, OH 45207. Offers clinical nurse leader (MSN); education (MSN); forensic nursing (MSN); healthcare law (MSN); informatics (MSN); nursing administration (MSN); school nursing (MSN); MSN/M Ed; MSN/MBA; MSN/MS. *Faculty:* 16 full-time (15 women), 9 part-time/adjunct (all women). *Students:* 66 full-time (56 women), 170 part-time (162 women); includes 35 minority (17 Black or African American, non-Hispanic/Latino; 2 American Indian or Alaska Native, non-Hispanic/Latino; 5 Asian, non-Hispanic/Latino; 10 Hispanic/Latino; 1 Native Hawaiian or other Pacific Islander, non-Hispanic/Latino). Average age 37. 103 applicants, 66% accepted, 86 enrolled. In 2013, 78 master's awarded. *Expenses: Tuition:* Part-time $594 per credit hour. *Required fees:* $3 per semester. *Financial support:* In 2013–14, 68 students received support. *Unit head:* Dr. Susan M. Schmidt, Director, School of Nursing, 513-745-3814, E-mail: schmidt@xavier.edu. *Application contact:* Marilyn Volk Gomez, Director of Nursing Student Services, 513-745-4392, Fax: 513-745-1087, E-mail: gomez@xavier.edu.
Website: http://www.xavier.edu/msn/

Transcultural Nursing

Augsburg College, Program in Transcultural Community Health Nursing, Minneapolis, MN 55454-1351. Offers MA. *Accreditation:* AACN. *Degree requirements:* For master's, thesis or alternative.

Rutgers, The State University of New Jersey, Newark, Rutgers School of Nursing, Newark, NJ 07107-3001. Offers adult health (MSN); adult occupational health (MSN); advanced practice nursing (MSN, Post Master's Certificate); family nurse practitioner (MSN); nurse anesthesia (MSN); nursing (MSN); nursing informatics (MSN); urban health (PhD); women's health practitioner (MSN). *Accreditation:* AANA/CANAEP. Part-time programs available. *Entrance requirements:* For master's, GRE, RN license; basic life support, statistics, and health assessment experience. Additional exam requirements/recommendations for international students: Required—TOEFL. Electronic applications accepted. *Expenses:* Contact institution. *Faculty research:* HIV/AIDS, diabetes education, learned helplessness, nursing science, psychoeducation.

Women's Health Nursing

California State University, Fullerton, Graduate Studies, College of Health and Human Development, Department of Nursing, Fullerton, CA 92834-9480. Offers leadership (MSN); nurse anesthesia (MSN); nurse educator (MSN); nursing (DNP); women's health care (MSN). *Accreditation:* AACN; AANA/CANAEP. Part-time programs available. *Students:* 186 full-time (138 women), 134 part-time (120 women); includes 174 minority (15 Black or African American, non-Hispanic/Latino; 3 American Indian or Alaska Native, non-Hispanic/Latino; 92 Asian, non-Hispanic/Latino; 50 Hispanic/Latino; 2 Native Hawaiian or other Pacific Islander, non-Hispanic/Latino; 12 Two or more races, non-Hispanic/Latino), 3 international. Average age 35. 431 applicants, 38% accepted, 131 enrolled. In 2013, 117 master's awarded. Application fee: $55. *Financial support:* Career-related internships or fieldwork, Federal Work-Study, institutionally sponsored loans, scholarships/grants, and traineeships available. Support available to part-time students. Financial award application deadline: 3/1; financial award applicants required to submit FAFSA. *Unit head:* Dr. Cindy Greenberg, Chair, 657-278-3336. *Application contact:* Admissions/Applications, 657-278-2371.
Website: http://nursing.fullerton.edu/

Case Western Reserve University, Frances Payne Bolton School of Nursing, Doctor of Nursing Practice Program, Cleveland, OH 44106. Offers acute care nurse practitioner (DNP); adult gerontology nurse practitioner (DNP); educational leadership (DNP); family nurse practitioner (DNP); family systems psychiatric mental health nursing (DNP); midwifery/family nursing (DNP); neonatal nurse practitioner (DNP); pediatric nurse practitioner (DNP); practice leadership (DNP); women's health nurse practitioner (DNP). *Accreditation:* AACN. Part-time programs available. Postbaccalaureate distance learning degree programs offered (minimal on-campus study). *Students:* 169 full-time, 9 part-time; includes 10 minority (6 Black or African American, non-Hispanic/Latino; 1 Asian, non-Hispanic/Latino; 2 Hispanic/Latino; 1 Two or more races, non-Hispanic/Latino). 76 applicants, 97% accepted, 59 enrolled. In 2013, 38 doctorates awarded. Terminal master's awarded for partial completion of doctoral program. *Degree requirements:* For doctorate, thesis/dissertation. *Entrance requirements:* For doctorate, GRE General Test or MAT. Additional exam requirements/recommendations for international students: Required—TOEFL (minimum score 577 paper-based; 90 iBT), IELTS (minimum score 7). *Application deadline:* For fall admission, 6/1 priority date for domestic students, 6/1 for international students; for spring admission, 10/1 for domestic and international students. Applications are processed on a rolling basis. Application fee: $75. *Financial support:* In 2013–14, 90 students received support, including 9 fellowships with full tuition reimbursements available (averaging $31,325 per year), 1 research assistantship with partial tuition reimbursement available (averaging $14,472 per year); teaching assistantships, Federal Work-Study, institutionally sponsored loans, scholarships/grants, and tuition waivers (partial) also available. Support available to part-time students. Financial award application deadline: 5/15; financial award applicants required to submit FAFSA. *Faculty research:* Symptom science, family/community care, aging across the lifespan, self-management of health and illness, neuroscience. *Unit head:* Dr. Donna Dowling, Director, 216-368-1869, Fax: 216-368-3542, E-mail: dad10@case.edu. *Application contact:* Donna Hassik, Admissions Coordinator, 216-368-5253, Fax: 216-368-0124, E-mail: dmh7@case.edu.
Website: http://fpb.case.edu/DNP/

Case Western Reserve University, Frances Payne Bolton School of Nursing, Master's Programs in Nursing, Nurse Practitioner Program, Cleveland, OH 44106. Offers acute care cardiovascular nursing (MSN); acute care nurse practitioner (MSN); acute care/flight nurse (MSN); adult gerontology acute care nurse practitioner (MSN); adult gerontology nurse practitioner (MSN); adult gerontology oncology and palliative care (MSN); family nurse practitioner (MSN); family systems psychiatric mental health nursing (MSN); neonatal nurse practitioner (MSN); pediatric nurse practitioner (MSN); women's health nurse practitioner (MSN). Part-time programs available. Postbaccalaureate distance learning degree programs offered (minimal on-campus study). *Faculty:* 54 full-time (50 women), 5 part-time/adjunct (3 women). *Students:* 56 full-time, 145 part-time; includes 9 minority (6 Black or African American, non-Hispanic/Latino; 2 Asian, non-Hispanic/Latino; 1 Hispanic/Latino), 5 international. Average age 35. 70 applicants, 71% accepted, 33 enrolled. In 2013, 79 master's awarded. *Degree requirements:* For master's, thesis optional. *Entrance requirements:* For master's, GRE General Test or MAT. Additional exam requirements/recommendations for international students: Required—TOEFL (minimum score 577 paper-based; 90 iBT), IELTS (minimum score 7). *Application deadline:* For fall admission, 6/1 for domestic students; for spring admission, 10/1 for domestic students. Applications are processed on a rolling basis. Application fee: $75. *Financial support:* In 2013–14, 25 teaching assistantships (averaging $15,120 per year) were awarded; research assistantships, institutionally sponsored loans, and tuition waivers (partial) also available. Support available to part-time students. Financial award application deadline: 6/30; financial award applicants required to submit FAFSA. *Faculty research:* Symptom science, family/community care, aging across the lifespan, self-management of health and illness, neuroscience. *Unit head:* Dr. Carol Savrin, Director, 216-368-5304, Fax: 216-368-3542, E-mail: cls18@case.edu. *Application contact:* Donna Hassik, Admissions Coordinator, 216-368-5253, Fax: 216-368-0124, E-mail: dmh7@case.edu.
Website: http://fpb.cwru.edu/MSN/majors.shtm

Drexel University, College of Nursing and Health Professions, Division of Graduate Nursing, Philadelphia, PA 19104-2875. Offers adult acute care (MSN); adult psychiatric/mental health (MSN); advanced practice nursing (MSN); clinical trials research (MSN); family nurse practitioner (MSN); leadership in health systems management (MSN); nursing education (MSN); pediatric primary care (MSN); women's health (MSN). *Accreditation:* AACN. Electronic applications accepted.

Emory University, Nell Hodgson Woodruff School of Nursing, Atlanta, GA 30322-1100. Offers adult nurse practitioner (MSN); emergency nurse practitioner (MSN); family nurse practitioner (MSN); family nurse-midwife (MSN); health systems leadership (MSN); nurse-midwifery (MSN); pediatric nurse practitioner acute and primary care (MSN); women's health care (Title X) (MSN); women's health nurse practitioner (MSN); MSN/MPH. *Accreditation:* AACN; ACNM/ACME (one or more programs are accredited). Part-time programs available. *Entrance requirements:* For master's, GRE General Test or MAT, minimum GPA of 3.0, BS in nursing from an accredited institution, RN license and additional course work, 3 letters of recommendation. Additional exam requirements/recommendations for international students: Required—TOEFL (minimum score 600 paper-based; 100 iBT). Electronic applications accepted. *Expenses:* Contact institution. *Faculty research:* Older adult falls and injuries, minority health issues, cardiac symptoms and quality of life, bio-ethics and decision-making, menopausal issues.

Frontier Nursing University, Graduate Programs, Hyden, KY 41749. Offers family nurse practitioner (MSN, DNP, Post Master's Certificate); nurse-midwifery (MSN, DNP, Post Master's Certificate); women's health care nurse practitioner (MSN, DNP, Post Master's Certificate). *Accreditation:* ACNM. *Degree requirements:* For doctorate, capstone project, practicum.

Georgia State University, Byrdine F. Lewis School of Nursing, Atlanta, GA 30303. Offers adult health clinical nurse specialist/nurse practitioner (MS, Certificate); child health clinical nurse specialist/pediatric nurse practitioner (MS, Certificate); family nurse practitioner (MS, Certificate); family psychiatric mental health nurse practitioner (MS, Certificate); nursing (PhD); nursing leadership in healthcare innovations (MS), including nursing administration, nursing informatics; nutrition (MS); perinatal clinical nurse specialist/women's health nurse practitioner (MS, Certificate); physical therapy (DPT); respiratory therapy (MS). *Accreditation:* AACN. Part-time programs available. Postbaccalaureate distance learning degree programs offered (minimal on-campus study). *Faculty:* 22 full-time (16 women). *Students:* 241 full-time (180 women), 262 part-time (236 women); includes 176 minority (120 Black or African American, non-Hispanic/Latino; 31 Asian, non-Hispanic/Latino; 13 Hispanic/Latino; 3 Native Hawaiian or other Pacific Islander, non-Hispanic/Latino; 9 Two or more races, non-Hispanic/Latino), 19 international. Average age 34. 583 applicants, 34% accepted, 160 enrolled. In 2013, 110 master's, 44 doctorates, 6 other advanced degrees awarded. *Degree requirements:* For doctorate, comprehensive exam, thesis/dissertation. *Entrance requirements:* For doctorate, GRE. Additional exam requirements/recommendations for international students: Required—TOEFL. *Application deadline:* For fall admission, 2/1 priority date for domestic and international students; for spring admission, 9/15 for domestic and international students. Applications are processed on a rolling basis. Application fee: $50. Electronic applications accepted. *Expenses:* Contact institution. *Financial support:* In 2013–14, research assistantships with full and partial tuition reimbursements (averaging $1,666 per year), teaching assistantships with full and partial tuition reimbursements (averaging $1,920 per year) were awarded; scholarships/grants, tuition waivers (full and partial), and unspecified assistantships also available. Support available to part-time students. Financial award application deadline: 8/1; financial award applicants required to submit FAFSA. *Faculty research:* Stroke intervention for caregivers, stroke prevention in African Americans; relationships between psychological distress and health outcomes in parents with a medically ill infant; medically fragile children; nursing expertise and patient outcomes. *Unit head:* Joan S. Cranford, Assistant Dean for Nursing, 404-413-1200, Fax: 404-413-1205, E-mail: jcranford2@gsu.edu.

Women's Health Nursing

Application contact: Tiffany Norman, Senior Administrative Coordinator, 404-413-1190, Fax: 404-413-1205, E-mail: tnorman7@gsu.edu.
Website: http://nursing.gsu.edu/

Hampton University, Graduate College, School of Nursing, Hampton, VA 23668. Offers advanced adult nursing (MS); community health nursing (MS); community mental health/psychiatric nursing (MS); family nursing (MS); gerontological nursing for the nurse practitioner (MS); pediatric nursing (MS); women's health nursing (MS). *Accreditation:* AACN. Part-time and evening/weekend programs available. *Degree requirements:* For master's, thesis optional. *Entrance requirements:* For master's, GRE General Test. *Faculty research:* Curriculum development, physical and mental assessment.

Indiana University–Purdue University Fort Wayne, College of Health and Human Services, Department of Nursing, Fort Wayne, IN 46805-1499. Offers adult-gerontology primary care nurse practitioner (MS); nurse executive (MS); nursing administration (Certificate); nursing education (MS); women's health nurse practitioner (MS). Part-time programs available. *Faculty:* 12 full-time (all women). *Students:* 5 full-time (all women), 63 part-time (60 women); includes 3 minority (2 Black or African American, non-Hispanic/Latino; 1 Asian, non-Hispanic/Latino). Average age 35. 34 applicants, 100% accepted, 25 enrolled. In 2013, 10 master's awarded. *Entrance requirements:* For master's, GRE Writing Test (if GPA below 3.0), BS in nursing, eligibility for Indiana RN license, minimum GPA of 3.0, essay, copy of resume, three references, undergraduate course work in research and statistics within last 5 years. Additional exam requirements/recommendations for international students: Required—TOEFL (minimum score 550 paper-based; 79 iBT); Recommended—TWE. *Application deadline:* For fall admission, 5/1 priority date for domestic and international students; for spring admission, 11/15 priority date for domestic students. Applications are processed on a rolling basis. Application fee: $55 ($60 for international students). Electronic applications accepted. *Financial support:* In 2013–14, 3 teaching assistantships with partial tuition reimbursements (averaging $13,322 per year) were awarded; scholarships/grants also available. Support available to part-time students. Financial award application deadline: 3/1; financial award applicants required to submit FAFSA. *Faculty research:* Pain management and substance abuse, high-risk alcohol use on campus, pediatric case management. *Unit head:* Dr. Lee-Ellen Kirkhorn, Chair/Professor, 260-481-6789, Fax: 260-481-5767, E-mail: kirkhorl@ipfw.edu. *Application contact:* Dr. Deborah Poling, Director of Graduate Program, 260-481-6276, Fax: 260-481-5767, E-mail: polingd@ipfw.edu.
Website: http://www.ipfw.edu/nursing/

Indiana University–Purdue University Indianapolis, School of Nursing, Indianapolis, IN 46202-2896. Offers acute care nurse practitioner (MSN); adult health clinical nurse specialist (MSN); adult health nursing (MSN), including adult clinical nurse specialist; adult nurse practitioner (MSN); adult psychiatric/mental health nursing (MSN); child psychiatric/mental health nursing (MSN); community health nursing (MSN); family nurse practitioner (MSN); neonatal nurse practitioner (MSN); nursing (MSN, DNP), including nursing administration (MSN), nursing education (MSN); nursing science (PhD); pediatric clinical nurse specialist (MSN); women's health nurse practitioner (MSN); MSN/MPA; MSN/MPH. Part-time programs available. *Faculty:* 85 full-time (82 women), 60 part-time/adjunct (all women). *Students:* 86 full-time (78 women), 371 part-time (351 women); includes 74 minority (39 Black or African American, non-Hispanic/Latino; 1 American Indian or Alaska Native, non-Hispanic/Latino; 14 Asian, non-Hispanic/Latino; 11 Hispanic/Latino; 9 Two or more races, non-Hispanic/Latino), 6 international. Average age 38. 224 applicants, 61% accepted, 102 enrolled. In 2013, 120 master's, 10 doctorates awarded. Terminal master's awarded for partial completion of doctoral program. *Degree requirements:* For master's, thesis; for doctorate, thesis/dissertation. *Entrance requirements:* For master's, minimum GPA of 3.0, RN license; for doctorate, GRE General Test, minimum GPA of 3.0, MSN, RN license, graduate statistics course with minimum B grade (not older than 3 years). Additional exam requirements/recommendations for international students: Required—TOEFL. *Application deadline:* For fall admission, 2/15 for domestic students; for spring admission, 9/15 for domestic students. Application fee: $55 ($65 for international students). *Financial support:* In 2013–14, 93 students received support. Fellowships with full tuition reimbursements available, research assistantships with full tuition reimbursements available, teaching assistantships with full tuition reimbursements available, Federal Work-Study, institutionally sponsored loans, scholarships/grants, and tuition waivers (full) available. Support available to part-time students. Financial award application deadline: 5/1. *Faculty research:* Clinical science, health systems. *Total annual research expenditures:* $3 million. *Unit head:* Dr. Patricia Ebright, Associate Dean for Graduate Programs, E-mail: nursing@iupui.edu. *Application contact:* Information Contact, 317-274-2806.
Website: http://nursing.iu.edu/

Kent State University, College of Nursing, Kent, OH 44242-0001. Offers acute care nurse practitioner (MSN); adult nurse practitioner (MSN); clinical nurse specialist (MSN); family nurse practitioner (MSN); geriatric nurse practitioner (MSN); health care management (MSN); nurse educator (MSN); nursing (PhD); nursing practice (DNP); pediatric nurse practitioner (MSN); psychiatric/mental health nurse practitioner (MSN); women's health nurse practitioner (MSN). PhD program offered jointly with The University of Akron. *Accreditation:* AACN. Part-time programs available. *Degree requirements:* For master's, thesis optional; for doctorate, comprehensive exam, thesis/dissertation. *Entrance requirements:* For master's, GRE (if undergraduate GPA less than 3.0), minimum GPA of 2.75; for doctorate, GRE, MSN. Additional exam requirements/recommendations for international students: Required—TOEFL. Electronic applications accepted. *Expenses:* Contact institution. *Faculty research:* Women and violence, methodological specialties, osteoporosis in women, new caregivers and the elderly.

Loyola University Chicago, Graduate School, Marcella Niehoff School of Nursing, Women's Health Nurse Practitioner Program, Chicago, IL 60660. Offers MSN, Certificate. *Accreditation:* AACN. Part-time and evening/weekend programs available. *Faculty:* 45 full-time (44 women). *Students:* 12 part-time (all women); includes 2 minority (1 Black or African American, non-Hispanic/Latino; 1 Hispanic/Latino), 1 international. Average age 34. 6 applicants, 83% accepted, 3 enrolled. In 2013, 3 master's awarded. *Degree requirements:* For master's, comprehensive exam or oral thesis defense. *Entrance requirements:* For master's, BSN, minimum nursing GPA of 3.0, 1000 hours of experience before starting clinical, Illinois nursing license, 3 letters of reference. *Application deadline:* Applications are processed on a rolling basis. Application fee: $50. Electronic applications accepted. *Expenses: Tuition:* Full-time $16,740; part-time $930 per credit. *Required fees:* $135 per semester. *Financial support:* Teaching assistantships and traineeships available. Financial award application deadline: 3/1. *Faculty research:* Breast feeding, postpartum depression, pre-term labor toxicity. *Unit head:* Dr. Marijo Letizia, Associate Dean, 708-216-9325, Fax: 708-216-9555, E-mail: mletizi@luc.edu. *Application contact:* Amy Weatherford, Enrollment Advisor, School of Nursing, 708-216-3751, Fax: 708-216-9555, E-mail: aweatherford@luc.edu.
Website: http://www.luc.edu/nursing/

MGH Institute of Health Professions, School of Nursing, Boston, MA 02129-4557. Offers advanced practice nursing (MSN); gerontological nursing (MSN); nursing (DNP); pediatric nursing (MSN); psychiatric nursing (MSN); teaching and learning for health care education (Certificate); women's health nursing (MSN). *Accreditation:* AACN. *Faculty:* 41 full-time (36 women), 14 part-time/adjunct (13 women). *Students:* 494 full-time (428 women), 85 part-time (77 women); includes 108 minority (32 Black or African American, non-Hispanic/Latino; 2 American Indian or Alaska Native, non-Hispanic/Latino; 38 Asian, non-Hispanic/Latino; 33 Hispanic/Latino; 3 Native Hawaiian or other Pacific Islander, non-Hispanic/Latino). Average age 32. 470 applicants, 52% accepted, 133 enrolled. In 2013, 85 master's, 12 doctorates, 98 other advanced degrees awarded. *Degree requirements:* For master's, thesis or alternative. *Entrance requirements:* For master's, GRE General Test, bachelor's degree from regionally-accredited college or university. Additional exam requirements/recommendations for international students: Required—TOEFL (minimum score 550 paper-based; 80 iBT). *Application deadline:* For fall admission, 12/1 for domestic and international students; for spring admission, 10/1 for domestic and international students. Application fee: $100. Electronic applications accepted. *Expenses: Tuition:* Part-time $1114 per credit. *Required fees:* $620 per term. One-time fee: $475 part-time. *Financial support:* In 2013–14, 75 students received support, including 4 research assistantships (averaging $1,200 per year), 17 teaching assistantships (averaging $1,200 per year); career-related internships or fieldwork, scholarships/grants, traineeships, and unspecified assistantships also available. Support available to part-time students. Financial award application deadline: 4/1; financial award applicants required to submit FAFSA. *Faculty research:* Biobehavioral nursing, HIV/AIDS, gerontological nursing, women's health, vulnerable populations, health systems. *Unit head:* Dr. Laurie Lauzon-Clabo, Dean, 617-643-0605, Fax: 617-726-8022, E-mail: llauzonclabo@mghihp.edu. *Application contact:* Lauren Putnam, Assistant Director of Admission, 617-726-3140, Fax: 617-726-8010, E-mail: admissions@mghihp.edu.
Website: http://www.mghihp.edu/academics/nursing/

Old Dominion University, College of Health Sciences, School of Nursing, Norfolk, VA 23529. Offers family nurse practitioner (MSN); nurse administrator (MSN); nurse anesthesia (MSN); nurse educator (MSN); nurse midwifery (MSN); nursing practice (DNP); women's health nurse practitioner (MSN). *Accreditation:* AACN; AANA/CANAEP (one or more programs are accredited). Part-time programs available. Postbaccalaureate distance learning degree programs offered (no on-campus study). *Faculty:* 6 full-time (5 women), 17 part-time/adjunct (15 women). *Students:* 111 full-time (100 women), 123 part-time (115 women); includes 45 minority (34 Black or African American, non-Hispanic/Latino; 7 Asian, non-Hispanic/Latino; 2 Hispanic/Latino; 2 Two or more races, non-Hispanic/Latino). Average age 38. 258 applicants, 61% accepted, 117 enrolled. In 2013, 60 master's, 29 doctorates awarded. *Degree requirements:* For master's, comprehensive exam; for doctorate, capstone project. *Entrance requirements:* For master's, GRE or MAT, BSN, minimum GPA of 3.0 in nursing and overall. Additional exam requirements/recommendations for international students: Required—TOEFL. *Application deadline:* For fall admission, 5/1 for domestic students, 4/15 for international students. Applications are processed on a rolling basis. Application fee: $50. Electronic applications accepted. *Expenses:* Tuition, state resident: full-time $9888; part-time $412 per credit. Tuition, nonresident: full-time $25,152; part-time $1048 per credit. *Required fees:* $59 per semester. One-time fee: $50. *Financial support:* In 2013–14, 18 students received support, including 2 research assistantships with partial tuition reimbursements available (averaging $10,000 per year), 1 teaching assistantship (averaging $2,500 per year); career-related internships or fieldwork, scholarships/grants, traineeships, and tuition waivers (partial) also available. Support available to part-time students. Financial award application deadline: 2/15; financial award applicants required to submit FAFSA. *Faculty research:* Health and culture, cardiovascular health, transition of military families, genetics, cultural diversity. *Total annual research expenditures:* $231,117. *Unit head:* Dr. Karen Karlowicz, Chair, 757-683-5262, Fax: 757-683-5253, E-mail: nursgpd@odu.edu. *Application contact:* Sue Parker, Coordinator, Graduate Student Services, 757-683-4298, Fax: 757-683-5253, E-mail: sparker@odu.edu.
Website: http://www.odu.edu/nursing

Queen's University at Kingston, School of Graduate Studies, Faculty of Health Sciences, School of Nursing, Kingston, ON K7L 3N6, Canada. Offers health and chronic illness (M Sc); nurse scientist (PhD); primary health care nurse practitioner (Certificate); women's and children's health (M Sc). *Degree requirements:* For master's, thesis. *Entrance requirements:* For master's, RN license. Additional exam requirements/recommendations for international students: Required—TOEFL. *Faculty research:* Women and children's health, health and chronic illness.

Rosalind Franklin University of Medicine and Science, College of Health Professions, Department of Interprofessional Healthcare Studies, Women's Healthcare Studies Program, North Chicago, IL 60064-3095. Offers MS, Certificate. Part-time and evening/weekend programs available. Postbaccalaureate distance learning degree programs offered (minimal on-campus study). *Degree requirements:* For master's, thesis optional, project. *Entrance requirements:* For master's, licensure/registration/certification in clinical health field, minimum GPA of 3.0, BS or BA. Additional exam requirements/recommendations for international students: Required—TOEFL.

Rutgers, The State University of New Jersey, Newark, Rutgers School of Nursing, Newark, NJ 07107-3001. Offers adult health (MSN); adult occupational health (MSN); advanced practice nursing (MSN, Post Master's Certificate); family nurse practitioner (MSN); nurse anesthesia (MSN); nursing (MSN); nursing informatics (MSN); urban health (PhD); women's health practitioner (MSN). *Accreditation:* AANA/CANAEP. Part-time programs available. *Entrance requirements:* For master's, GRE, RN license; basic life support, statistics, and health assessment experience. Additional exam requirements/recommendations for international students: Required—TOEFL. Electronic applications accepted. *Expenses:* Contact institution. *Faculty research:* HIV/AIDS, diabetes education, learned helplessness, nursing science, psychoeducation.

San Francisco State University, Division of Graduate Studies, College of Health and Social Sciences, School of Nursing, San Francisco, CA 94132-1722. Offers adult acute care (MS); clinical nurse specialist (MS); community/public health nursing (MS); family nurse practitioner (MS, Certificate); nursing administration (MS); nursing education (MS); pediatrics (MS); women's health (MS). *Accreditation:* AACN. Part-time programs available. *Application deadline:* Applications are processed on a rolling basis. *Financial support:* Career-related internships or fieldwork available. *Unit head:* Dr. Mary-Ann van Dam, Director, 415-338-1802, E-mail: vandam@sfsu.edu. *Application contact:* Robert Strachan, Admission and Student Services Coordinator, 415-338-1802, E-mail: strachan@sfsu.edu.
Website: http://nursing.sfsu.edu

Stony Brook University, State University of New York, Stony Brook University Medical Center, Health Sciences Center, School of Nursing, Program in Perinatal Women's Health Nursing, Stony Brook, NY 11794. Offers MS, DNP, Certificate. *Accreditation:* AACN. Postbaccalaureate distance learning degree programs offered. *Students:* 35 part-time (all women); includes 10 minority (5 Black or African American, non-Hispanic/Latino; 1 American Indian or Alaska Native, non-Hispanic/Latino; 1 Asian, non-Hispanic/Latino; 3 Hispanic/Latino). In 2013, 7 master's awarded. *Degree requirements:* For master's, thesis. *Entrance requirements:* For master's, BSN, minimum GPA of 3.0, course work in statistics. Additional exam requirements/recommendations for international students: Required—TOEFL. *Application deadline:* For fall admission, 1/15 for domestic students. Application fee: $100. *Expenses:* Tuition,

state resident: full-time $9870; part-time $411 per credit. Tuition, nonresident: full-time $18,350; part-time $765 per credit. *Financial support:* Application deadline: 3/15. *Unit head:* Prof. Elizabeth Collins, Director, 631-444-3296, Fax: 631-444-3136, E-mail: elizabeth.collins@stonybrook.edu. *Application contact:* 631-632-2644, Fax: 631-632-3136, E-mail: dolores.bilges@stonybrook.edu.
Website: http://www.nursing.stonybrookmedicine.edu/

Texas Woman's University, Graduate School, College of Nursing, Denton, TX 76201. Offers acute care nurse practitioner (MS); adult health clinical nurse specialist (MS); adult health nurse practitioner (MS); child health clinical nurse specialist (MS); clinical nurse leader (MS); family nurse practitioner (MS); health systems management (MS); nursing education (MS); nursing practice (DNP); nursing science (PhD); pediatric nurse practitioner (MS); women's health clinical nurse specialist (MS); women's health nurse practitioner (MS). *Accreditation:* AACN. Part-time programs available. Postbaccalaureate distance learning degree programs offered. *Faculty:* 60 full-time (59 women), 46 part-time/adjunct (39 women). *Students:* 54 full-time (49 women), 910 part-time (848 women); includes 489 minority (221 Black or African American, non-Hispanic/Latino; 11 American Indian or Alaska Native, non-Hispanic/Latino; 184 Asian, non-Hispanic/Latino; 70 Hispanic/Latino; 3 Native Hawaiian or other Pacific Islander, non-Hispanic/Latino), 16 international. Average age 38. 430 applicants, 65% accepted, 193 enrolled. In 2013, 258 master's, 22 doctorates awarded. *Degree requirements:* For master's, comprehensive exam, thesis or alternative; for doctorate, comprehensive exam, thesis/dissertation. *Entrance requirements:* For master's, GRE or MAT, minimum GPA of 3.0 on last 60 hours in undergraduate nursing degree and overall, RN license, BS in nursing, basic statistics course; for doctorate, GRE (preferred minimum score 153 [500 old version] Verbal, 144 [500 old version] Quantitative, 4 Analytical), MS in nursing, minimum preferred GPA of 3.5, RN license, statistics, 2 letters of reference, curriculum vitae, graduate nursing-theory course, graduate research course, statement of professional goals and research interests. Additional exam requirements/recommendations for international students: Required—TOEFL (minimum score 550 paper-based; 79 iBT). *Application deadline:* For fall admission, 5/1 priority date for domestic students, 3/1 for international students; for spring admission, 9/15 priority date for domestic students, 7/1 for international students. Applications are processed on a rolling basis. Application fee: $50 ($75 for international students). Electronic applications accepted. *Expenses:* Tuition, state resident: full-time $4182; part-time $233.32 per credit hour. Tuition, nonresident: full-time $10,716; part-time $595.32 per credit hour. *Financial support:* In 2013–14, 149 students received support, including 10 research assistantships (averaging $5,600 per year), 1 teaching assistantship (averaging $5,600 per year); career-related internships or fieldwork, Federal Work-Study, institutionally sponsored loans, scholarships/grants, traineeships, health care benefits, and unspecified assistantships also available. Support available to part-time students. Financial award application deadline: 3/1; financial award applicants required to submit FAFSA. *Faculty research:* Screening, prevention, and treatment for intimate partner violence; needs of adolescents during childbirth intervention; a network analysis decision tool for nurse managers (social network analysis); support for adolescents with implantable cardioverter defibrillators; informatics: nurse staffing, safety, quality, and financial data as they relate to patient care outcomes; prevention and treatment of obesity; improving infant outcomes related to premature birth. *Total annual research expenditures:* $1.7 million. *Unit head:* Dr. Gayle Roux, Interim Dean and Associate Dean for Research and Clinical Scholarship, 940-898-2401, Fax: 940-898-2437, E-mail: nursing@twu.edu. *Application contact:* Dr. Samuel Wheeler, Assistant Director of Admissions, 940-898-3188, Fax: 940-898-3081, E-mail: wheelersr@twu.edu.
Website: http://www.twu.edu/nursing/

University of Cincinnati, Graduate School, College of Nursing, Cincinnati, OH 45221-0038. Offers clinical nurse specialist (MSN), including adult health, community health, neonatal, nursing administration, occupational health, pediatric health, psychiatric nursing, women's health; nurse anesthesia (MSN); nurse midwifery (MSN); nurse practitioner (MSN), including acute care, ambulatory care, family, family/psychiatric, women's health; nursing (PhD); MBA/MSN. *Accreditation:* AACN; AANA/CANAEP (one or more programs are accredited); ACNM/ACME. Part-time programs available. Postbaccalaureate distance learning degree programs offered (no on-campus study). Terminal master's awarded for partial completion of doctoral program. *Degree requirements:* For master's, thesis or alternative; for doctorate, comprehensive exam, thesis/dissertation. *Entrance requirements:* For master's and doctorate, GRE General Test. Additional exam requirements/recommendations for international students: Required—TOEFL (minimum score 520 paper-based). Electronic applications accepted. *Faculty research:* Substance abuse, injury and violence, symptom management.

University of Colorado Denver, College of Nursing, Aurora, CO 80045. Offers adult clinical nurse specialist (MS); adult nurse practitioner (MS); family nurse practitioner (MS); family psychiatric mental health nurse practitioner (MS); health care informatics (MS); nurse-midwifery (MS); nursing (DNP, PhD); nursing leadership and health care systems (MS); pediatric nurse practitioner (MS); special studies (MS); women's health (MS); MS/PhD. *Accreditation:* ACNM/ACME (one or more programs are accredited). Part-time and evening/weekend programs available. Postbaccalaureate distance learning degree programs offered (minimal on-campus study). *Faculty:* 74 full-time (65 women), 58 part-time/adjunct (56 women). *Students:* 351 full-time (327 women), 138 part-time (125 women); includes 79 minority (12 Black or African American, non-Hispanic/Latino; 9 American Indian or Alaska Native, non-Hispanic/Latino; 13 Asian, non-Hispanic/Latino; 32 Hispanic/Latino; 2 Native Hawaiian or other Pacific Islander, non-Hispanic/Latino; 11 Two or more races, non-Hispanic/Latino), 7 international. Average age 33. 354 applicants, 43% accepted, 109 enrolled. In 2013, 108 master's, 28 doctorates awarded. Terminal master's awarded for partial completion of doctoral program. *Degree requirements:* For master's, thesis optional; for doctorate, comprehensive exam, thesis/dissertation, 42 credits of coursework. *Entrance requirements:* For master's, GRE if cumulative undergraduate GPA is less than 3.0, undergraduate nursing degree from NLNAC- or CCNE-accredited school or university; completion of research and statistics courses with minimum grade of C; copy of current and unencumbered nursing license; for doctorate, GRE, bachelor's and/or master's degrees in nursing from NLN- or CCNE-accredited institution; portfolio; minimum undergraduate GPA of 3.0, graduate 3.5; graduate-level intermediate statistics and master's-level nursing theory courses with minimum B grade; interview. Additional exam requirements/recommendations for international students: Required—TOEFL (minimum score 560 paper-based; 83 iBT). *Application deadline:* For fall admission, 2/15 for domestic students, 1/15 for international students; for spring admission, 7/1 for domestic students, 6/1 for international students. Application fee: $50 ($75 for international students). Electronic applications accepted. *Expenses:* Contact institution. *Financial support:* In 2013–14, 113 students received support. Fellowships, research assistantships, teaching assistantships, Federal Work-Study, institutionally sponsored loans, scholarships/grants, traineeships, and unspecified assistantships available. Support available to part-time students. Financial award application deadline: 4/1; financial award applicants required to submit FAFSA. *Faculty research:* Biological and behavioral phenomena in pregnancy and postpartum; patterns of glycemia during the insulin resistance of pregnancy; obesity, gestational diabetes, and relationship to neonatal adiposity; men's awareness and knowledge of male breast cancer; cognitive-behavioral therapy for chronic insomnia after breast cancer treatment; massage therapy for the treatment of tension-type headaches. *Total annual research expenditures:* $5.9 million. *Unit head:* Dr. Sarah Thompson, Dean, 303-724-1679, E-mail: sarah.a.thompson@ucdenver.edu. *Application contact:* Judy Campbell, Graduate Programs Coordinator, 303-724-8503, E-mail: judy.campbell@ucdenver.edu.
Website: http://www.ucdenver.edu/academics/colleges/nursing/Pages/default.aspx

University of Delaware, College of Health Sciences, School of Nursing, Newark, DE 19716. Offers adult nurse practitioner (MSN, PMC); cardiopulmonary clinical nurse specialist (MSN, PMC); cardiopulmonary clinical nurse specialist/adult nurse practitioner (MSN, PMC); family nurse practitioner (MSN, PMC); gerontology clinical nurse specialist (MSN, PMC); gerontology clinical nurse specialist geriatric nurse practitioner (PMC); gerontology clinical nurse specialist/geriatric nurse practitioner (MSN); health services administration (MSN, PMC); nursing of children clinical nurse specialist (MSN, PMC); nursing of children clinical nurse specialist/pediatric nurse practitioner (MSN, PMC); oncology/immune deficiency clinical nurse specialist (MSN, PMC); oncology/immune deficiency clinical nurse specialist/adult nurse practitioner (MSN, PMC); perinatal/women's health clinical nurse specialist (MSN, PMC); perinatal/women's health clinical nurse specialist/women's health nurse practitioner (MSN, PMC); psychiatric nursing clinical nurse specialist (MSN, PMC). *Accreditation:* AACN. Part-time and evening/weekend programs available. Postbaccalaureate distance learning degree programs offered (minimal on-campus study). *Degree requirements:* For master's, thesis optional. *Entrance requirements:* For master's, BSN, interview, RN license. Electronic applications accepted. *Faculty research:* Marriage and chronic illness, health promotion, congestive heart failure patient outcomes, school nursing, diabetes in children, culture, health disparities, cardiovascular, prison nursing, oncology, public policy, child obesity, smoking and teen pregnancy, blood pressure measurements, men's health.

University of Illinois at Chicago, Graduate College, College of Nursing, Program in Nursing, Chicago, IL 60607-7128. Offers acute care clinical nurse specialist (MS); acute care nurse practitioner (MS); administrative nursing leadership (Certificate); administrative studies in nursing (MS); adult nurse practitioner (MS); adult/geriatric nurse practitioner (MS); advanced community health nurse specialist (MS); family nurse practitioner (MS); geriatric clinical nurse specialist (MS); geriatric nurse practitioner (MS); mental health clinical nurse specialist (MS); mental health nurse practitioner (MS); nurse midwifery (MS); occupational health/advanced community health nurse specialist (MS); occupational health/family nurse practitioner (MS); pediatric clinical nurse specialist (MS); pediatric nurse practitioner (MS); perinatal clinical nurse specialist (MS); school/advanced community health nurse specialist (MS); school/family nurse practitioner (MS); women's health nurse practitioner (MS). *Accreditation:* AACN. Part-time programs available. *Faculty:* 16 full-time (14 women). *Students:* 393 full-time (361 women), 410 part-time (367 women); includes 198 minority (48 Black or African American, non-Hispanic/Latino; 1 American Indian or Alaska Native, non-Hispanic/Latino; 64 Asian, non-Hispanic/Latino; 71 Hispanic/Latino; 2 Native Hawaiian or other Pacific Islander, non-Hispanic/Latino; 12 Two or more races, non-Hispanic/Latino), 29 international. Average age 32. 396 applicants, 62% accepted, 177 enrolled. In 2013, 184 master's awarded. *Degree requirements:* For master's, thesis or alternative. *Entrance requirements:* For master's, GRE General Test, minimum GPA of 2.75. Additional exam requirements/recommendations for international students: Required—TOEFL. *Application deadline:* For fall admission, 5/15 for domestic students, 2/15 for international students; for spring admission, 11/1 for domestic students, 7/15 for international students. Applications are processed on a rolling basis. Application fee: $40 ($50 for international students). Electronic applications accepted. *Expenses:* Tuition, state resident: full-time $11,066; part-time $3689 per term. Tuition, nonresident: full-time $23,064; part-time $7688 per term. *Required fees:* $3004; $1190 per term. Tuition and fees vary according to course level and program. *Financial support:* Fellowships with full tuition reimbursements, research assistantships with full tuition reimbursements, teaching assistantships with full tuition reimbursements, career-related internships or fieldwork, Federal Work-Study, institutionally sponsored loans, scholarships/grants, traineeships, tuition waivers (full and partial), and unspecified assistantships available. Support available to part-time students. Financial award application deadline: 3/1; financial award applicants required to submit FAFSA. *Unit head:* Dr. Terri E. Weaver, Dean, 312-996-7808, E-mail: teweaver@uic.edu. *Application contact:* Receptionist, 312-413-2550, E-mail: gradcoll@uic.edu.

University of Indianapolis, Graduate Programs, School of Nursing, Indianapolis, IN 46227-3697. Offers advanced practice nursing (DNP); family nurse practitioner (MSN); gerontological nurse practitioner (MSN); neonatal nurse practitioner (MSN); nurse-midwifery (MSN); nursing (MSN); nursing and health systems leadership (MSN); nursing education (MSN); women's health nurse practitioner (MSN); MBA/MSN. *Accreditation:* AACN; ACNM. *Faculty:* 5 full-time (4 women), 1 part-time/adjunct (0 women). *Students:* 15 full-time (14 women), 285 part-time (270 women); includes 42 minority (24 Black or African American, non-Hispanic/Latino; 6 Asian, non-Hispanic/Latino; 3 Hispanic/Latino; 9 Two or more races, non-Hispanic/Latino), 2 international. Average age 35. In 2013, 46 master's awarded. *Entrance requirements:* For master's, minimum GPA of 3.0, interview, letters of recommendation, resume, IN nursing license, 1 year of professional practice; for doctorate, graduate of NLNAC- or CCNE-accredited nursing program; MSN or MA with nursing major and minimum cumulative GPA of 3.25; unencumbered RN license with eligibility for licensure in Indiana; completion of graduate-level statistics course within last 5 years with minimum grade of B; resume; essay; official transcripts from all academic institutions. Additional exam requirements/recommendations for international students: Required—TOEFL (minimum score 550 paper-based). *Application deadline:* For fall admission, 8/1 for domestic students; for winter admission, 12/15 for domestic students; for spring admission, 4/15 for domestic students. Applications are processed on a rolling basis. Application fee: $60. Electronic applications accepted. *Expenses: Tuition:* Full-time $5436; part-time $810 per credit hour. *Financial support:* Federal Work-Study available. *Unit head:* Dr. Anne Thomas, Dean, 317-788-3206, E-mail: athomas@uindy.edu. *Application contact:* Sueann Meagher, Graduate Administrative Assistant, 317-788-8005, Fax: 317-788-3542, E-mail: meaghers@uindy.edu.
Website: http://nursing.uindy.edu/

University of Minnesota, Twin Cities Campus, Graduate School, School of Nursing, Program in Women's Health Nurse Practitioner, Minneapolis, MN 55455-0213. Offers MS. *Accreditation:* AACN. Postbaccalaureate distance learning degree programs offered (minimal on-campus study). *Entrance requirements:* Additional exam requirements/recommendations for international students: Required—TOEFL (minimum score 586 paper-based).

University of Missouri–Kansas City, School of Nursing and Health Studies, Kansas City, MO 64110-2499. Offers adult clinical nurse specialist (MSN), including adult nurse practitioner, women's health nurse practitioner (MSN, DNP); adult clinical nursing practice (DNP), including adult gerontology nurse practitioner, women's health nurse practitioner (MSN, DNP); clinical nursing practice (DNP), including family nurse practitioner; family nurse practitioner (MSN); neonatal nurse practitioner (MSN); nurse educator (MSN); nurse executive (MSN); nursing (PhD); nursing practice (DNP); pediatric clinical nursing practice (DNP), including pediatric nurse practitioner; pediatric nurse practitioner (MSN). *Accreditation:* AACN. Part-time programs available. Postbaccalaureate distance learning degree programs offered (minimal on-campus

study). *Faculty:* 44 full-time (38 women), 55 part-time/adjunct (52 women). *Students:* 44 full-time (33 women), 401 part-time (370 women); includes 59 minority (25 Black or African American, non-Hispanic/Latino; 2 American Indian or Alaska Native, non-Hispanic/Latino; 12 Asian, non-Hispanic/Latino; 15 Hispanic/Latino; 5 Two or more races, non-Hispanic/Latino). Average age 37. 182 applicants, 68% accepted, 124 enrolled. In 2013, 106 master's, 15 doctorates awarded. *Degree requirements:* For master's, thesis or alternative. *Entrance requirements:* For master's, minimum undergraduate GPA of 3.2; for doctorate, GRE, 3 letters of reference. Additional exam requirements/recommendations for international students: Required—TOEFL (minimum score 550 paper-based; 80 iBT). *Application deadline:* For fall admission, 2/1 priority date for domestic and international students; for spring admission, 9/1 priority date for domestic and international students. Application fee: $45 ($50 for international students). *Expenses:* Tuition, state resident: full-time $6073; part-time $337.40 per credit hour. Tuition, nonresident: full-time $15,680; part-time $871.10 per credit hour. *Required fees:* $97.59 per credit hour. Full-time tuition and fees vary according to program. *Financial support:* In 2013–14, 13 teaching assistantships with partial tuition reimbursements (averaging $9,470 per year) were awarded; fellowships, research assistantships, career-related internships or fieldwork, Federal Work-Study, institutionally sponsored loans, and tuition waivers (full and partial) also available. Support available to part-time students. Financial award application deadline: 3/1; financial award applicants required to submit FAFSA. *Faculty research:* Geriatrics/gerontology, children's pain, neonatology, Alzheimer's care, cancer caregivers. *Unit head:* Dr. Ann Cary, Dean, 816-235-1723, Fax: 816-235-1701, E-mail: caryah@umkc.edu. *Application contact:* Judy Jellison, Coordinator for Admissions and Recruitment, 816-235-1740, Fax: 816-235-1701, E-mail: jellisonj@umkc.edu.
Website: http://nursing.umkc.edu/

University of Missouri–St. Louis, College of Nursing, St. Louis, MO 63121-4400. Offers adult nurse practitioner (DNP, Post Master's Certificate); clinical nurse specialist (DNP); family mental health nurse practitioner (DNP); family nurse practitioner (MSN, DNP, Post Master's Certificate); neonatal nurse practitioner (MSN); nurse educator (MSN); nurse leader (MSN); nurse practitioner (Post Master's Certificate); nursing (PhD); pediatric clinical nurse specialist (DNP); pediatric nurse practitioner (MSN, DNP, Post Master's Certificate); women's health nurse practitioner (MSN, Post Master's Certificate). *Accreditation:* AACN. Part-time programs available. *Faculty:* 14 full-time (13 women), 14 part-time/adjunct (13 women). *Students:* 227 part-time (217 women); includes 40 minority (35 Black or African American, non-Hispanic/Latino; 1 American Indian or Alaska Native, non-Hispanic/Latino; 1 Asian, non-Hispanic/Latino; 1 Hispanic/Latino; 2 Two or more races, non-Hispanic/Latino). Average age 35. 190 applicants, 51% accepted, 76 enrolled. In 2013, 80 master's, 8 doctorates, 2 other advanced degrees awarded. *Degree requirements:* For doctorate, comprehensive exam, thesis/dissertation; for Post Master's Certificate, thesis. *Entrance requirements:* For master's, 2 recommendation letters; minimum GPA of 3.0; BSN; nursing licensure; statement of purpose; course in differential/inferential statistics; for doctorate, GRE, 2 letters of recommendation, MSN, minimum GPA of 3.2, course in differential/inferential statistics; for Post Master's Certificate, 2 recommendation letters; MSN; advanced practice certificate; minimum GPA of 3.0; essay. Additional exam requirements/recommendations for international students: Recommended—TOEFL (minimum score 550 paper-based; 79 iBT), IELTS (minimum score 6.5). *Application deadline:* For fall admission, 2/15 for domestic and international students. Application fee: $50 ($40 for international students). Electronic applications accepted. *Expenses:* Tuition, state resident: full-time $7364; part-time $409.10 per credit hour. Tuition, nonresident: full-time $19,162; part-time $1008.50 per credit hour. *Financial support:* Application deadline: 4/1; applicants required to submit FAFSA. *Faculty research:* Health promotion and restoration, family disruption, violence, abuse, battered women, health survey methods. *Unit head:* Dr. Nancy Magnuson, Director, 314-516-6066. *Application contact:* 314-516-5458, Fax: 314-516-6996, E-mail: gradadm@umsl.edu.
Website: http://www.umsl.edu/divisions/nursing/

University of Pennsylvania, School of Nursing, Women's Healthcare Nurse Practitioner Program, Philadelphia, PA 19104. Offers MSN. *Accreditation:* AACN. Part-time programs available. Postbaccalaureate distance learning degree programs offered (minimal on-campus study). *Students:* 12 full-time (all women), 9 part-time (all women); includes 5 minority (2 Black or African American, non-Hispanic/Latino; 2 Asian, non-Hispanic/Latino; 1 Hispanic/Latino). In 2013, 9 master's awarded. *Entrance requirements:* For master's, GRE General Test, BSN, minimum GPA of 3.0, previous course work in statistics, physical assessment experience. Additional exam requirements/recommendations for international students: Required—TOEFL. *Application deadline:* For fall admission, 2/15 priority date for domestic students. Applications are processed on a rolling basis. Application fee: $70. *Expenses:* Contact institution. *Financial support:* Fellowships, research assistantships, teaching assistantships, career-related internships or fieldwork, Federal Work-Study, and institutionally sponsored loans available. Support available to part-time students. Financial award application deadline: 4/1. *Faculty research:* New mother and infant healthcare follow-up, adequacy of antepartum care, models of healthcare. *Unit head:* Assistant Dean of Admissions and Financial Aid, 866-867-6877, Fax: 215-573-8439, E-mail: admissions@nursing.upenn.edu. *Application contact:* Wendy Grube, Program Director, 215-898-1169, E-mail: wgrube@nursing.upenn.edu.
Website: http://www.nursing.upenn.edu/

University of South Carolina, The Graduate School, College of Nursing, Program in Clinical Nursing, Columbia, SC 29208. Offers acute care clinical specialist (MSN); acute care nurse practitioner (MSN); women's health nurse practitioner (MSN). *Accreditation:* AACN. Part-time programs available. *Degree requirements:* For master's, thesis or alternative. *Entrance requirements:* For master's, GRE General Test or MAT, BS in nursing, RN licensure. Additional exam requirements/recommendations for international students: Required—TOEFL (minimum score 570 paper-based). Electronic applications accepted. *Faculty research:* Systems research, evidence based practice, breast cancer, violence.

Vanderbilt University, Vanderbilt University School of Nursing, Nashville, TN 37240. Offers adult-gerontology acute care nurse practitioner (MSN), including hospitalist, intensivist; adult-gerontology primary care nurse practitioner (MSN); emergency nurse practitioner (MSN); family nurse practitioner (MSN); healthcare leadership (MSN); neonatal nurse practitioner (MSN); nurse midwifery (MSN); nurse midwifery/family nurse practitioner (MSN); nursing informatics (MSN); nursing practice (DNP); nursing science (PhD); pediatric acute care nurse practitioner (MSN); pediatric primary care nurse practitioner (MSN); psychiatric-mental health nurse practitioner (MSN); women's health nurse practitioner (MSN); women's health nurse practitioner/adult gerontology primary care nurse practitioner (MSN); MSN/M Div; MSN/MTS. *Accreditation:* ACNM/ACME (one or more programs are accredited). Part-time programs available. Postbaccalaureate distance learning degree programs offered (minimal on-campus study). *Faculty:* 139 full-time (124 women), 452 part-time/adjunct (319 women). *Students:* 527 full-time (463 women), 369 part-time (333 women); includes 120 minority (46 Black or African American, non-Hispanic/Latino; 8 American Indian or Alaska Native, non-Hispanic/Latino; 26 Asian, non-Hispanic/Latino; 24 Hispanic/Latino; 4 Native Hawaiian or other Pacific Islander, non-Hispanic/Latino; 12 Two or more races, non-Hispanic/Latino), 7 international. Average age 32. 1,257 applicants, 49% accepted, 457 enrolled. In 2013, 364 master's, 43 doctorates awarded. *Degree requirements:* For doctorate, comprehensive exam, thesis/dissertation. *Entrance requirements:* For master's, GRE General Test (within the past 5 years), minimum B average in undergraduate course work, 3 letters of recommendation; for doctorate, GRE General Test, interview, 3 letters of recommendation from doctorally-prepared faculty, MSN, essay. Additional exam requirements/recommendations for international students: Required—TOEFL (minimum score 570 paper-based), IELTS (minimum score 6.5). *Application deadline:* For fall admission, 12/1 priority date for domestic and international students. Applications are processed on a rolling basis. Application fee: $50. Electronic applications accepted. *Expenses:* Contact institution. *Financial support:* In 2013–14, 582 students received support. Scholarships/grants and health care benefits available. Support available to part-time students. Financial award application deadline: 3/15; financial award applicants required to submit FAFSA. *Faculty research:* Lymphedema, palliative care and bereavement, health services research including workforce, safety and quality of care, gerontology, better birth outcomes including nutrition. *Total annual research expenditures:* $2.5 million. *Unit head:* Dr. Linda Norman, Dean, 615-343-8876, Fax: 615-343-7711, E-mail: linda.norman@vanderbilt.edu. *Application contact:* Patricia Peerman, Assistant Dean for Enrollment Management, 615-322-3800, Fax: 615-343-0333, E-mail: vusn-admissions@vanderbilt.edu.
Website: http://www.nursing.vanderbilt.edu

Virginia Commonwealth University, Graduate School, School of Nursing, Richmond, VA 23284-9005. Offers adult health acute nursing (MS); adult health primary nursing (MS); biobehavioral clinical research (PhD); child health nursing (MS); clinical nurse leader (MS); family health nursing (MS); nurse educator (MS); nurse practitioner (MS); nursing (Certificate); nursing administration (MS), including clinical nurse manager; psychiatric-mental health nursing (MS); women's health nursing (MS). Part-time and evening/weekend programs available. *Degree requirements:* For master's, thesis optional; for doctorate, thesis/dissertation. *Entrance requirements:* For master's, GRE General Test, BSN, minimum GPA of 2.8; for doctorate, GRE General Test. Additional exam requirements/recommendations for international students: Required—TOEFL (minimum score 600 paper-based; 100 iBT). Electronic applications accepted.

Wayne State University, College of Nursing, Program in Advanced Practice Nursing with Women, Neonates and Children, Detroit, MI 48202. Offers neonatal nurse practitioner (MSN); nurse-midwife (MSN); pediatric nurse practitioner (MSN), including acute care, primary care; women's health nurse practitioner (MSN). *Accreditation:* AACN. Part-time programs available. *Students:* 59 full-time (53 women), 74 part-time (72 women); includes 17 minority (11 Black or African American, non-Hispanic/Latino; 2 Asian, non-Hispanic/Latino; 4 Hispanic/Latino), 6 international. Average age 32. 65 applicants, 55% accepted, 33 enrolled. In 2013, 40 degrees awarded. *Degree requirements:* For master's, thesis or alternative. *Entrance requirements:* For master's, minimum honor point average of 3.0 in upper-division course work; BA from NLN- or CCNE-accredited program; references; current RN license; personal statement. Additional exam requirements/recommendations for international students: Required—TOEFL (minimum score 550 paper-based; 79 iBT); Recommended—TWE (minimum score 6). *Application deadline:* For fall admission, 6/1 priority date for domestic students, 5/1 priority date for international students; for winter admission, 10/1 priority date for domestic students, 9/1 priority date for international students; for spring admission, 2/1 priority date for domestic students, 1/1 priority date for international students. Applications are processed on a rolling basis. Application fee: $50. Electronic applications accepted. *Expenses:* Contact institution. *Financial support:* In 2013–14, 17 students received support. Fellowships with tuition reimbursements available, research assistantships with tuition reimbursements available, teaching assistantships with tuition reimbursements available, scholarships/grants, and unspecified assistantships available. Financial award applicants required to submit FAFSA. *Faculty research:* Acculturation and parenting, domestic violence, evidence-based midwifery practice, pain in children, trauma and community violence. *Unit head:* Dr. Barbara Redman, Dean, 313-577-4070, Fax: 313-577-4571, E-mail: ae9080@wayne.edu. *Application contact:* Dr. Cynthia Redwine, Assistant Dean for the Office of Student Affairs, 313-577-4082, E-mail: nursinginfo@wayne.edu.
Website: http://nursing.wayne.edu/msn/specialty.php

ADELPHI UNIVERSITY

College of Nursing and Public Health

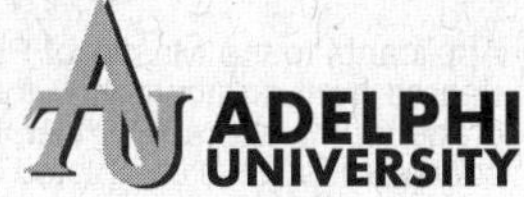

Programs of Study

The College of Nursing and Public Health, renamed in June 2013, focuses on public health issues and has combined Adelphi's hallmark nursing programs with relevant healthcare programs to address today's health issues and those of the future. Students benefit from a holistic approach that focuses on community intervention, health maintenance and management, and environmental health.

More than 90,000 Adelphi alumni have embraced its small class sizes and strong collaboration with faculty. Adelphi graduates are working as nurses in private and hospital settings; as administrators and educators; and in organizations as managers, researchers, educators, advocates, and directors.

The College offers Master of Science (M.S.) programs in Adult/Geriatric Nurse Practitioner, Nursing Administration, and Nursing Education; a Ph.D. in Nursing; a Master of Public Health (M.P.H.); a fully online M.S. in Nutrition program; a fully online and traditional M.S. in Healthcare Informatics program; and post-master's certificate programs in adult health practitioner, nursing administration, and nursing education.

The M.S. in Adult/Geriatric Nurse Practitioner program (52 credits) entails in-depth study of adult health nursing. The curriculum integrates theoretical knowledge and practical skills while exploring the issues and forces within the healthcare delivery system that affect the roles of the advanced practice nurse. The program emphasizes scientific inquiry as a tool for building clinical knowledge and testing the validity of the theoretical assumptions underlying nursing practice. Students have opportunities to work with advanced practice nurses and other health professionals in a variety of clinical settings.

The M.S. in Nursing Administration program (45 credits) prepares nurse managers who can function in a variety of healthcare settings. Topics include nursing theories, group dynamics, communication, and professional issues and trends. To prepare to serve as leaders in improving healthcare services, students study leadership roles in the healthcare field. Through the program's research component, students gain practice in analyzing and implementing research findings.

The M.S. in Nursing Education program (46 credits) prepares nurse educators who are competent to function in a variety of educational and healthcare settings. Students will acquire knowledge, skills, and values related to teaching and learning, instructional design, assessment and measurement strategies, curriculum development implementation, and evaluation in nursing education. Seminar and practicum is an opportunity for students to be guided by expert nurse educators and apply their knowledge as nurse educators.

The multidisciplinary M.P.H. program's goal is to provide society with knowledgeable, professionally educated people to enhance the public health infrastructure and the health of populations. The program provides students with a wide range of skills and tools necessary to work in the public health arena. The emphasis is on early action and prevention in the healthcare system, rather than on the traditional approach of treating illnesses.

The 34-credit—and 100 percent online—M.S. in Nutrition program is designed to prepare students to help improve patient health through nutrition. This program is geared for professionals who have bachelor's or graduate degrees in healthcare and are licensed and practicing in their field, such as nurses, physicians, podiatrists, and chiropractors.

The M.S. in Healthcare Informatics combines concepts in healthcare, information technology, and leadership practice to provide students with the knowledge and skills needed to be a valuable developer and manager of health information systems.

The Ph.D. in Nursing program is an innovative 54-credit program designed to advance healthcare teaching, research, and leadership by educating nurses with a master's degree to become nursing scholars and educators. The plan of study offers strong core courses in both nursing science and research. The program may be taken on a full-time (9–12 credits) or part-time basis following a progressive program plan. Most of the courses are offered one day a week. Students are admitted only in the fall semester and proceed through the program in cohorts, taking classes together.

The post-master's certificate programs in nursing administration, adult health nurse practitioner, and nursing education are designed for students who already hold a master's degree in nursing and want to specialize in another discipline. The programs aim to strengthen the administrative or clinical capability of master's-prepared nurses who are planning or are already involved in a role expansion or role change. The program is a part-time course of study.

Research Facilities

The Nursing Resource Center features learning laboratories that simulate hospital and clinical settings. A clinical coordinator provides supervision as students gain invaluable practice. One laboratory is set up with all appropriate hospital supplies and equipment, including advanced patient-care mannequins and simulators. The second laboratory is equipped with state-of-the-art nursing tools for complete assessment practice. The computer laboratory offers online learning and practice programs.

The University's primary research holdings are at Swirbul Library and include 603,000 volumes (including bound periodicals and government publications); 786,000 items in microformats; 35,000 audiovisual items; and online access to more than 80,000 e-book titles, 76,000 electronic journal titles, and 265 research databases.

Value

Earning an Adelphi degree means joining a growing network of more than 90,000 alumni. For the eighth straight year, Adelphi was designated a Best Buy by the *Fiske Guide to Colleges*, one of only twenty private universities nationwide to earn that distinction. *The Princeton Review* also named Adelphi a Best College in the Northeast, and *Forbes* magazine named Adelphi a Top College. According to payscale.com's 2013 College Education ROI rankings, Adelphi ranks in the top 15 percent of colleges and universities nationwide for return on investment. The numbers speak for themselves—91 percent of Adelphi undergraduates receive financial aid or scholarships.

Financial Aid

Adelphi University offers a wide variety of federal aid programs, state grants, scholarship and fellowship programs, on- and off-campus employment, and teaching and research assistantships. More information is available online at ecampus.adelphi.edu/sfs.

Cost of Study

For the 2014–15 academic year, the tuition rate is $1,055 per credit for nursing master's programs and $1,170 for the Ph.D. program. University fees range from $330 to $575 per semester.

Living and Housing Costs

The University assists single and married students in finding suitable accommodations whenever possible. The cost of living depends on the location and number of rooms rented.

Location

Located in historic Garden City, New York, just 23 miles from Manhattan, where students can take advantage of numerous cultural and internship opportunities, Adelphi's 75-acre suburban campus is known for the beauty of its landscape and architecture. The campus is a short walk from the Long Island Rail Road and is convenient to New York's major airports and several major highways. Off-campus centers are located in Manhattan, the Hudson Valley, and Suffolk County.

The University and The College

Founded in 1896, Adelphi is a fully accredited, private university with nearly 8,000 undergraduate, graduate, and returning-adult students in the arts and sciences, business, clinical psychology, education, nursing, and social work. Students come from forty states and forty-five countries.

The College of Nursing and Public Health is dedicated to providing students with the skills, knowledge, and specialized training to succeed as qualified caregivers and leaders in the nursing profession. The course of study combines theory, research, clinical practice, and community service. Adelphi's extensive school and community partnerships provide wide-ranging opportunities to gain fieldwork experience. The curricula of the College of Nursing and Public Health are registered by the New York State Education Department and Division of Professional Education, and are accredited by the Commission on Collegiate Nursing Education (CCNE).

Applying

Each master's degree applicant should have a bachelor's degree in nursing, with a course in basic statistics, and be licensed as a professional registered nurse. Students must submit a completed application, a $50 application fee, official college transcripts, and two letters of recommendation. Applications are processed on a rolling basis.

Adelphi University

Applicants to the Master of Public Health program should have a bachelor's degree from an accredited four-year institution; a minimum 2.75 cumulative grade point average; must have completed an undergraduate statistics course; must have completed an M.P.H. program admissions form; completed a 500-word (typed) essay on reasons for applying to the program; and submit two letters of recommendation.

Applicants to the M.S. in Nutrition program should have a bachelor's degree from an accredited four-year institution; a minimum 2.75 cumulative grade point average; completed an undergraduate introductory nutrition course, an introductory statistics course, a human anatomy and physiology two-course sequence with laboratory, and a minimum 4-credit chemistry course with laboratory; completed the Master of Science in Nutrition degree program application form; completed a 500-word essay on reasons for applying to the program; completed a personal interview (not required to be on campus, can be via electronic technology); and submitted two letters of recommendation.

Applicants for the Ph.D. program must have an M.S. or M.S.N. from an accredited nursing program (CCNE or National League for Nursing Accrediting Commission [NLNAC] approved) and submit a completed application, three professional letters of reference (from a supervisor, committee chair, former professor, etc.), satisfactory GRE scores (taken within the last five years), licensure as an RN in New York State, a professional writing sample, and an interview with at least 2 members of the College of Nursing and Public Health. All application materials must be received by March 15 to be considered for the following fall semester for the Ph.D. program.

Correspondence and Information

800-ADELPHI (toll-free)
nursing.adelphi.edu/

THE FACULTY AND THEIR RESEARCH

Judith Ackerhalt, Ed.D., Columbia. Therapeutic communication.
Deborah Ambrosio-Mawhirter, Ed.D., Dowling. Human assessment: a holistic approach.
Helen Ballestas, Ph.D., Capella. Patient-centered nursing care.
Stefni Bogard, M.S.N., Pennsylvania. Health assessment throughout the lifespan; adult health nursing.
Jacqueline Brandwein, M.A., NYU. Alterations in the holistic integrity of the childbearing family; alterations of holistic integrity of children.
Nancy Cole, M.S., Adelphi. Holistic approach to alterations in physiological integrity; nursing care of adults; professionalism in the provision of holistic care.
Patrick R. Coonan, Ed.D., Columbia Teachers College.
Christine Coughlin, Ed.D., Columbia Teachers College. Patient/family perception of care; leadership qualities of frontline nursing leaders.
Diane Dembicki, Ph.D., Colorado State. Public health/community nutrition; international health and nutrition; cultural diversity; developmental education.
Margo DeSevo, Ph.D., NYU. Genetics and maternity.
Patricia Donohue-Porter, Ph.D. Adelphi. Quality improvement; patient safety; leadership.
Patricia Facquet, Ed.D., Cambridge College. Pediatric palliative care; adolescent medicine; simulation.
Darylann Ficken, D.N.P., Columbia.
Maryann Forbes, Ph.D., Adelphi. Effects of long-term mechanical ventilation on patients and families; nursing care of the COPD patient; simulation in nursing education; gerontology.
Yvonne Gray, M.S., SUNY Downstate. Technology information literacy; professionalism in the provision of holistic care.
Clarilee Hauser, Ph.D., California, San Francisco. Alterations in holistic integrity managed in community; community health nursing; professionalism in the provision of holistic care.
Beth Heydemann, M.S., Columbia. Cardiovascular and thoracic surgery; adult primary care; case management; patient-centered nursing care.
Stephen Holzemer, Ph.D., Adelphi. Community health; health policy; critical thinking.
William Jacobowitz, Ed.D., Columbia Teachers College. Mental health nursing.
Marilyn Klainberg, Ed.D., Columbia Teachers College. Use of computers to enhance nursing practice and nursing education.
Elizabeth Lee, Ph.D., Connecticut. Adult health nursing; health promotion and disease prevention; health assessment.
Seonah Lee, Ph.D., Illinois. Clinical decision support systems and evaluation criteria for mixed-method research.
Shan Liu, Ph.D., Yale. Pharmacology.
Teresa L. Mascitti, M.S.N., Molloy. Pathophysiology for nurse practitioners; adult health nursing; health assessment.
Andrea McCrink, Ed.D., Dowling. Pediatric nursing; high-risk behaviors in teens and college students.
Ditsapelo McFarland, Ph.D., Boston College. Women's health; cultural diversities in healthcare.
Deborah J. Murphy, M.S., Columbia. Holistic healthcare.
Anne Peirce, Ph.D., Maryland. Professional nursing practice; philosophical foundations of nursing science; dissertation guidance.
Janet Raman, Ed.D., Dowling. Pharmacology; academic success of the nursing student.
Maureen Roller, D.N.P., Case Western Reserve. Adult internal medicine; older adults; relationship to exercise adherence.
K. C. Rondello, M.D., St. George's (Grenada). Health management in times of disaster; hospital and healthcare policy and management.
Bayla Samter, M.S., Columbia. Physical assessment of the adult; adult health nursing; health assessment.
Holly K. Shaw, Ph.D., Adelphi. Advanced nursing practice; communication in nursing.
Margaret Silver, M.Ed., Columbia Teachers College. Aging and chronic mental illness.
Yiyuan Sun, D.N.Sc., Yale. Cancer prevention and early detection; symptom management (oncology).
Arlene Trolman, Ed.D., Columbia. Alterations in holistic integrity managed in the community.
Joan Valas, Ph.D., Columbia. Technology and information; ethics; chronic illness; social inequalities.
Thomas J. Virgona, Ph.D., Long Island University, C.W. Post. Disaster recovery; information security; healthcare informatics.
Jane White, Ph.D., Catholic University. Research (qualitative and quantitative approaches); nursing science and epidemiology.

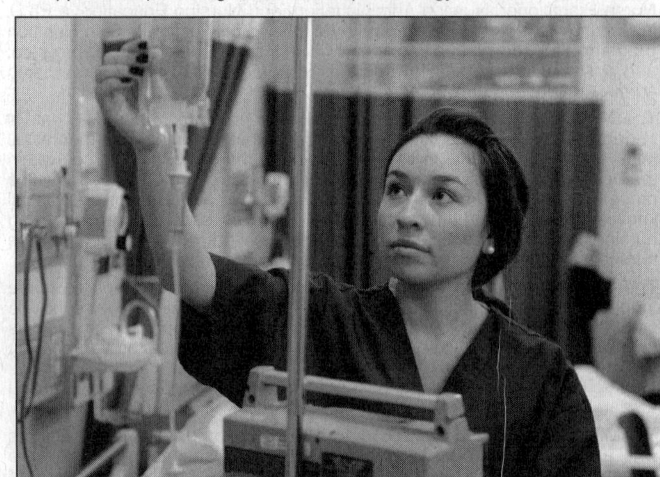

The College of Nursing and Public Health prepares qualified caregivers and leaders who are ready to make an impact in their communities.

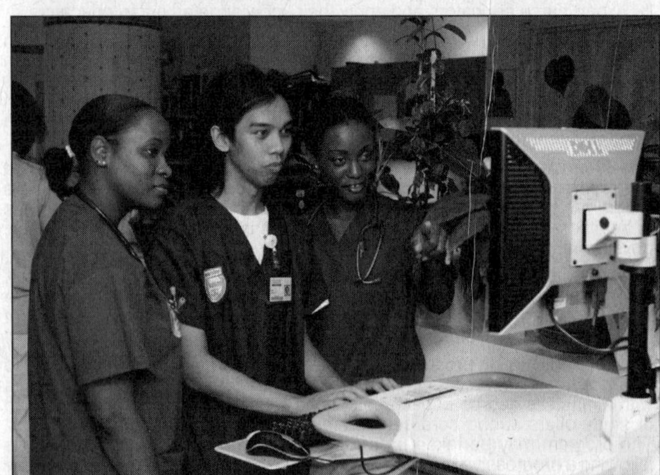

The comprehensive education in the College of Nursing and Public Health is grounded in practice, delivery, innovation, and efficiency.

D'YOUVILLE COLLEGE

Department of Nursing

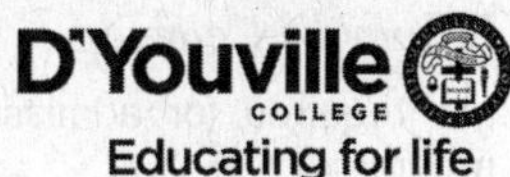

Programs of Study

At the graduate level, nursing programs include a Doctor of Nursing Practice (D.N.P.); Master of Science (M.S.) in community health nursing with concentrations in advanced clinical nursing, nursing management, and nursing education; and Master of Science in family nurse practitioner studies as well as a post-master's certificate in family nurse practitioner and nursing and health-related professions education studies.

Innovative class scheduling provides working professionals the opportunity to study full-time by attending one to two days per week. This alternative scheduling allows students to continue working in their professions while earning their degrees.

Research Facilities

The Montante Family Library contains over 100,000 volumes and provides access to over 50,000 unique journals, newspapers, and magazines. The library provides state-of-the-art computer reference facilities for both in-house and off-site users, including access to over 90 online databases. The multimillion-dollar Health Science Building houses state-of-the-art robotic simulation labs, as well as laboratories for anatomy, organic chemistry, quantitative analysis, and computer science. It also houses classrooms, faculty member offices, and development centers, including one for career development.

Financial Aid

D'Youville attempts to provide financial aid for students who would not otherwise be able to attend. Determination of aid is based on the Free Application for Federal Student Aid. Aid is available in the form of grants, loans, and employment on campus. In addition, D'Youville offers scholarships for academic achievement to incoming students.

Graduate students must be matriculated for 6 or more credits in a degree program. Nurse traineeship assistance is available to students enrolled for a minimum of 9 credit hours per semester in the graduate nursing program. Canadian students (citizens and landed immigrants) are offered a 20 percent net tuition reduction and may also apply for the Ontario Student Assistance Program (OSAP).

Cost of Study

Graduate tuition for 2014–15 is $850 per credit hour for master's and advanced certificate programs and $924 per credit hour for doctoral programs. A general College fee of between $65 and $185 is required, based on credit hours taken.

Living and Housing Costs

Marguerite Hall, the residence facility, houses men and women on separate floors and includes a coed floor for graduate and adult students. For 2014–15, room and board costs $5,400 per semester. Overnight accommodation is available, space permitting. A residence-apartment complex houses 175 junior, senior, and graduate students in one- and four-bedroom apartments. The resident apartment complex rates range from $4,416 for a single room within a four-bedroom apartment per semester.

Student Group

Graduate degree programs are enhanced by a 13:1 student-faculty ratio. The current enrollment is 334 full-time and 266 part-time graduate students. Seventy percent of the students are women, 15 percent are members of minority groups, and 16 percent are internationals students.

Location

D'Youville is situated on Buffalo's residential west side. The College is within minutes of many social attractions, including the downtown shopping center, the Kleinhans Music hall, the Albright-Knox Art Gallery, two museums, and several theaters that offer stage productions. Seasonal changes in the area offer a variety of recreational opportunities. Buffalo is only 90 minutes from Toronto and 25 minutes from Niagara Falls, making it a gateway to recreation areas in western New York and Ontario.

D'Youville enjoys a diversified interchange with the community due to its affiliations with schools, hospitals, and social agencies in the area. College students in the Buffalo area number more than 60,000.

The College

Commencing in 1942, D'Youville College was the first private college in New York State to offer a four-year Bachelor of Science in Nursing degree program. The College offers six doctoral, thirteen master's-level, and six postbaccalaureate programs as well as baccalaureate and advanced certificate programs. Graduate programs, in addition to nursing, include education (childhood, adolescence, special, curriculum and instruction, and TESOL), health services administration, international business, M.B.A., and occupational therapy. Doctoral programs include chiropractic, educational leadership, health administration, nursing practice, pharmacy, and physical therapy. D'Youville offers the undergraduate degrees of Bachelor of Arts (B.A.), Bachelor of Science (B.S.), and Bachelor of Science in Nursing (B.S.N.). Majors include accounting, accounting information systems, biology, business management, chemistry, chiropractic (seven-year B.S./D.C.), dietetics, education (childhood, adolescence, and special), English, exercise and sports studies, global studies, health services, health analytics, history, mathematics, nursing, nursing RN to B.S.N. (online and hybrid), occupational therapy, philosophy, physical therapy (six-year sequential degree program), pre-professional studies (dental, law, medicine, pharmacy, and veterinary studies), psychology, and sociology. Five-year combined bachelor's/master's (B.S./M.S.) programs are offered in dietetics, education, and human occupation/occupational therapy, and physician assistant studies.

Applying

A master's degree in advanced practice nursing from an approved or accredited college or university and RN licensure are required for admission to the Doctor of Nursing Practice program.

A baccalaureate degree in nursing from an approved or accredited college or university and RN licensure are required for admission to the graduate nursing programs. Licensure as a registered nurse in New York State or Ontario and a minimum of one year of experience as a registered nurse are required of candidates applying to the nurse practitioner programs. Admission to graduate programs is based on an overall evaluation of credentials, including the applicant's undergraduate record, with a minimum 3.0 overall GPA (on a 4.0 scale) and 3.25 for the DNP program. Applicants whose native language is not English must submit a minimum TOEFL score of 500. Graduate applications are reviewed on a rolling basis.

Correspondence and Information

Mark A. Pavone
Director of Graduate Admission
D'Youville College
One D'Youville Square
320 Porter Avenue
Buffalo, New York 14201
Phone: 716-829-8400
800-777-3921 (toll-free)
E-mail: graduateadmissions@dyc.edu
Website: http://www.dyc.edu

THE FACULTY

Denise Dunford, Associate Professor and Director of Family Nurse Practitioner Program; D.N.S., SUNY at Buffalo.
Judith Lewis, Dean, School of Nursing; Ed.D., Cincinnati.
Kathleen Mariano, Associate Professor; D.N.S., SUNY at Buffalo.
Abigail Mitchell; Assistant Professor; D.H.Ed., A. T. Still.
Eileen Nahigian, Assistant Professor; D.N.S., SUNY at Buffalo.
Sharon Mang, Assistant Professor; D.N.P., Chatham.
Shannon McCrory-Churchill, Assistant Professor; D.H.Ed., A. T. Still.
Tina Sinatra-Wilhelm; Assistant Professor; DNP, Chatham.

Section 24
Public Health

This section contains a directory of institutions offering graduate work in public health, followed by an in-depth entry submitted by an institution that chose to prepare a detailed program description. Additional information about programs listed in the directory but not augmented by an in-depth entry may be obtained by writing directly to the dean of a graduate school or chair of a department at the address given in the directory.

For programs offering related work, see also in this book *Allied Health; Biological and Biomedical Sciences; Ecology, Environmental Biology, and Evolutionary Biology; Health Services; Microbiological Sciences; Nursing;* and *Nutrition.* In the other guides in this series:

Graduate Programs in the Humanities, Arts & Social Sciences

See *Family and Consumer Sciences (Gerontology)* and *Sociology, Anthropology, and Archaeology (Demography and Population Studies)*

Graduate Programs in the Physical Sciences, Mathematics, Agricultural Sciences, the Environment & Natural Resources

See *Mathematical Sciences* and *Environmental Sciences and Management*

Graduate Programs in Engineering & Applied Sciences

See *Biomedical Engineering and Biotechnology, Civil and Environmental Engineering, Industrial Engineering, Energy and Power Engineering (Nuclear Engineering),* and *Management of Engineering and Technology*

Graduate Programs in Business, Education, Information Studies, Law & Social Work

See *Education.*

CONTENTS

Program Directories

Display and Close-Up

Public Health—General

Adelphi University, College of Nursing and Public Health, Program in Public Health, Garden City, NY 11530-0701. Offers MPH. *Students:* 2 full-time (1 woman), 22 part-time (17 women); includes 14 minority (8 Black or African American, non-Hispanic/Latino; 2 Asian, non-Hispanic/Latino; 2 Hispanic/Latino; 2 Two or more races, non-Hispanic/Latino). Average age 33. *Expenses: Tuition:* Full-time $32,530; part-time $1010 per credit. *Required fees:* $1150. Tuition and fees vary according to degree level and program. *Financial support:* Research assistantships, career-related internships or fieldwork, Federal Work-Study, tuition waivers, and unspecified assistantships available. *Unit head:* Philip Alcabes, Director, 516-237-8668, E-mail: palcabes@adelphi.edu. *Application contact:* Christine Murphy, Director of Admissions, 516-877-3050, Fax: 516-877-3039, E-mail: graduateadmissions@adelphi.edu.

Adelphi University, University College, Graduate Certificate in Emergency Management Program, Garden City, NY 11530-0701. Offers Certificate. Part-time and evening/weekend programs available. *Students:* 8 full-time (3 women), 17 part-time (9 women); includes 7 minority (4 Black or African American, non-Hispanic/Latino; 1 Asian, non-Hispanic/Latino; 1 Hispanic/Latino; 1 Native Hawaiian or other Pacific Islander, non-Hispanic/Latino). Average age 38. In 2013, 2 Certificates awarded. *Application deadline:* For fall admission, 5/1 for international students; for spring admission, 12/1 for international students. Applications are processed on a rolling basis. Application fee: $50. Electronic applications accepted. *Expenses: Tuition:* Full-time $32,530; part-time $1010 per credit. *Required fees:* $1150. Tuition and fees vary according to degree level and program. *Faculty research:* Emergency nursing, disaster management, disaster preparedness. *Unit head:* Shawn O'Riley, Dean, 516-877-3412, E-mail: ucinfo@adelphi.edu. *Application contact:* Christine Murphy, Director of Admissions, 516-877-3050, Fax: 516-877-3039, E-mail: graduateadmissions@adelphi.edu.
Website: http://academics.adelphi.edu/universitycollege/emergency-management-certificate.php

Allen College, Program in Nursing, Waterloo, IA 50703. Offers acute care nurse practitioner (MSN, Post-Master's Certificate); adult nurse practitioner (MSN, Post-Master's Certificate); adult psychiatric-mental health nurse practitioner (MSN, Post-Master's Certificate); community public health (MSN, Post-Master's Certificate); family nurse practitioner (MSN, Post-Master's Certificate); gerontological nurse practitioner (MSN, Post-Master's Certificate); health education (MSN); leadership in health care delivery (MSN, Post-Master's Certificate); nursing (DNP). Part-time programs available. Postbaccalaureate distance learning degree programs offered (minimal on-campus study). *Faculty:* 3 full-time (all women), 21 part-time/adjunct (20 women). *Students:* 21 full-time (19 women), 162 part-time (150 women); includes 5 minority (1 Black or African American, non-Hispanic/Latino; 2 Asian, non-Hispanic/Latino; 1 Hispanic/Latino; 1 Two or more races, non-Hispanic/Latino). Average age 34. 213 applicants, 57% accepted, 94 enrolled. In 2013, 41 master's, 4 other advanced degrees awarded. *Degree requirements:* For master's, thesis optional. *Entrance requirements:* For master's, minimum GPA of 3.0 in the last 60 hours of undergraduate coursework; for doctorate, minimum GPA of 3.25 in graduate coursework. Additional exam requirements/recommendations for international students: Recommended—TOEFL (minimum score 580 paper-based; 92 iBT), IELTS (minimum score 6). *Application deadline:* For fall admission, 2/1 priority date for domestic students; for spring admission, 9/1 priority date for domestic students. Applications are processed on a rolling basis. Application fee: $50. Electronic applications accepted. *Expenses: Tuition:* Full-time $14,534; part-time $755 per credit hour. *Required fees:* $935; $75 per credit hour. One-time fee: $275 part-time. Tuition and fees vary according to course load. *Financial support:* In 2013–14, 60 students received support. Institutionally sponsored loans, scholarships/grants, and traineeships available. Support available to part-time students. Financial award application deadline: 8/15; financial award applicants required to submit FAFSA. *Unit head:* Kendra Williams-Perez, Dean, School of Nursing, 319-226-2044, Fax: 319-226-2070, E-mail: kendra.williams-perez@allencollege.edu. *Application contact:* Molly Quinn, Admissions Counselor, 319-226-2001, Fax: 319-226-2010, E-mail: molly.quinn@allencollege.edu.
Website: http://www.allencollege.edu/

American Public University System, AMU/APU Graduate Programs, Charles Town, WV 25414. Offers accounting (MBA, MS); criminal justice (MA), including business administration, emergency and disaster management, general (MA, MS); educational leadership (M Ed); emergency and disaster management (MA); entrepreneurship (MBA); environmental policy and management (MS), including environmental planning, environmental sustainability, fish and wildlife management, general (MA, MS), global environmental management; finance (MBA); general (MBA); global business management (MBA); history (MA), including American history, ancient and classical history, European history, global history, public history; homeland security (MA), including business administration, counter-terrorism studies, criminal justice, cyber, emergency management and public health, intelligence studies, transportation security; homeland security resource allocation (MBA); humanities (MA); information technology (MS), including digital forensics, enterprise software development, information assurance and security, IT project management; information technology management (MBA); intelligence studies (MA), including criminal intelligence, cyber, general (MA, MS), homeland security, intelligence analysis, intelligence collection, intelligence management, intelligence operations, terrorism studies; international relations and conflict resolution (MA), including comparative and security issues, conflict resolution, international and transnational security issues, peacekeeping; legal studies (MA); management (MA), including defense management, general (MA, MS), human resource management, organizational leadership, public administration; marketing (MBA); military history (MA), including American military history, American Revolution, civil war, war since 1945, World War II; military studies (MA), including joint warfare, strategic leadership; national security studies (MA), including general (MA, MS), homeland security, regional security studies, security and intelligence analysis, terrorism studies; nonprofit management (MBA); political science (MA), including American politics and government, comparative government and development, general (MA, MS), international relations, public policy; psychology (MA); public administration (MPA), including disaster management, environmental policy, health policy, human resources, national security, organizational management, security management; public health (MPH); reverse logistics management (MA); school counseling (M Ed); security management (MA); space studies (MS), including aerospace science, general (MA, MS), planetary science; sports and health sciences (MS); teaching (M Ed), including curriculum and instruction for elementary teachers, elementary reading, English language learners, instructional leadership, online learning, special education; transportation and logistics management (MA), including general (MA, MS), maritime engineering management, reverse logistics management. Programs offered via distance learning only. Part-time and evening/weekend programs available. Postbaccalaureate distance learning degree programs offered (no on-campus study). *Faculty:* 432 full-time (242 women), 1,722 part-time/adjunct (829 women). *Students:* 511 full-time (241 women), 10,947 part-time (4,294 women); includes 3,760 minority (2,058 Black or African American, non-Hispanic/Latino; 88 American Indian or Alaska Native, non-Hispanic/Latino; 293 Asian, non-Hispanic/Latino; 876 Hispanic/Latino; 91 Native Hawaiian or other Pacific Islander, non-Hispanic/Latino; 354 Two or more races, non-Hispanic/Latino), 134 international. Average age 36. In 2013, 3,323 master's awarded. *Degree requirements:* For master's, comprehensive exam or practicum. *Entrance requirements:* For master's, official transcript showing earned bachelor's degree from institution accredited by recognized accrediting body. Additional exam requirements/recommendations for international students: Required—TOEFL (minimum score 550 paper-based), IELTS (minimum score 6.5). *Application deadline:* Applications are processed on a rolling basis. Application fee: $0. Electronic applications accepted. *Expenses: Tuition:* Part-time $325 per semester hour. *Financial support:* Applicants required to submit FAFSA. *Faculty research:* Military history, criminal justice, management performance, national security. *Unit head:* Dr. Karan Powell, Executive Vice President and Provost, 877-468-6268, Fax: 304-724-3780. *Application contact:* Terry Grant, Vice President of Enrollment Management, 877-468-6268, Fax: 304-724-3780, E-mail: info@apus.edu.
Website: http://www.apus.edu

American University of Armenia, Graduate Programs, Yerevan, Armenia. Offers business administration (MBA); computer and information science (MS), including business management, design and manufacturing, energy (ME, MS), industrial engineering and systems management; economics (MS); industrial engineering and systems management (ME), including business, computer aided design/manufacturing, energy (ME, MS), information technology; law (LL M); political science and international affairs (MPSIA); public health (MPH); teaching English as a foreign language (MA). Part-time and evening/weekend programs available. *Faculty:* 30 full-time (10 women), 42 part-time/adjunct (13 women). *Students:* 398 full-time (272 women), 138 part-time (84 women). Average age 24. 351 applicants, 77% accepted, 247 enrolled. In 2013, 215 master's awarded. *Degree requirements:* For master's, thesis (for some programs), capstone/project. *Entrance requirements:* For master's, GRE, GMAT, or LSAT. Additional exam requirements/recommendations for international students: Recommended—TOEFL (minimum score 79 iBT), IELTS (minimum score 6.5). *Application deadline:* For fall admission, 3/31 for domestic and international students; for spring admission, 12/20 for domestic and international students. Applications are processed on a rolling basis. Application fee: $30 ($70 for international students). *Expenses: Tuition:* Full-time $2683; part-time $122 per credit. Full-time tuition and fees vary according to program. *Financial support:* In 2013–14, 199 students received support. Teaching assistantships with partial tuition reimbursements available, career-related internships or fieldwork, institutionally sponsored loans, scholarships/grants, unspecified assistantships, and tuition assistance, institutionally-sponsored work study available. Support available to part-time students. Financial award application deadline: 6/30. *Faculty research:* Microfinance, finance (rural/development, international, corporate), firm life cycle theory, TESOL, language proficiency testing, public policy, administrative law, economic development, cryptography, artificial intelligence, energy efficiency/renewable energy, computer-aided design/manufacturing, health financing, tuberculosis control, mother/child health, preventive ophthalmology, post-earthquake psychopathological investigations, tobacco control, environmental health risk assessments. *Total annual research expenditures:* $465,763. *Unit head:* Dr. Dennis Leavens, Provost, 374 10512526, E-mail: provost@aua.am. *Application contact:* Karine Satamyan, Admissions Coordinator, 374-10324040, E-mail: grad@aua.am.
Website: http://www.aua.am

American University of Beirut, Graduate Programs, Faculty of Health Sciences, Beirut, Lebanon. Offers environmental sciences (MS), including environmental health; epidemiology (MS); epidemiology and biostatistics (MPH); health management and policy (MPH); health promotion and community health (MPH); population health (MS). Part-time programs available. *Faculty:* 26 full-time (18 women), 7 part-time/adjunct (4 women). *Students:* 42 full-time (37 women), 103 part-time (84 women). Average age 25. 132 applicants, 65% accepted, 48 enrolled. In 2013, 52 master's awarded. *Degree requirements:* For master's, one foreign language, comprehensive exam, thesis (for some programs). *Entrance requirements:* For master's, 2 letters of recommendation, personal statement, transcripts. Additional exam requirements/recommendations for international students: Required—TOEFL (minimum score 583 paper-based; 97 iBT), IELTS (minimum score 7). *Application deadline:* For fall admission, 2/7 priority date for domestic and international students; for spring admission, 11/1 for domestic and international students. Application fee: $50. Electronic applications accepted. *Expenses: Tuition:* Full-time $14,724; part-time $818 per credit. *Required fees:* $692. Tuition and fees vary according to course load and program. *Financial support:* In 2013–14, 56 students received support. Scholarships/grants, health care benefits, and unspecified assistantships available. Financial award application deadline: 4/1. *Faculty research:* Tobacco control; health of the elderly; youth health; mental health; women's health; reproductive and sexual health, including HIV/AIDS; water quality; health systems; quality in health care delivery; health human resources; health policy; occupational and environmental health; social inequality; social determinants of health; non-communicable diseases. *Total annual research expenditures:* $1 million. *Unit head:* Iman Adel Nuwayhid, Dean, 961-1759683, Fax: 961-1744470, E-mail: nuwayhid@aub.edu.lb. *Application contact:* Mitra Tauk, Administrative Coordinator, 961-1-350000 Ext. 4687, Fax: 96-1-1744470, E-mail: mt12@aub.edu.lb.

Argosy University, Atlanta, College of Health Sciences, Atlanta, GA 30328. Offers public health (MPH).

Argosy University, Chicago, College of Health Sciences, Chicago, IL 60601. Offers public health (MPH).

Argosy University, Dallas, College of Health Sciences, Farmers Branch, TX 75244. Offers public health (MPH).

Argosy University, Denver, College of Health Sciences, Denver, CO 80231. Offers public health (MPH).

Argosy University, Hawai`i, College of Health Sciences, Honolulu, HI 96813. Offers public health (MPH).

Argosy University, Inland Empire, College of Health Sciences, Ontario, CA 91761. Offers public health (MPH).

Argosy University, Los Angeles, College of Health Sciences, Santa Monica, CA 90045. Offers public health (MPH).

Argosy University, Nashville, College of Health Sciences, Nashville, TN 37214. Offers public health (MPH).

Argosy University, Orange County, College of Health Sciences, Orange, CA 92868. Offers public health (MPH).

Argosy University, Phoenix, College of Health Sciences, Phoenix, AZ 85021. Offers public health (MPH).

Argosy University, Salt Lake City, College of Health Sciences, Draper, UT 84020. Offers public health (MPH).

Argosy University, San Diego, College of Health Sciences, San Diego, CA 92108. Offers public health (MPH).

Argosy University, San Francisco Bay Area, College of Health Sciences, Alameda, CA 94501. Offers public health (MPH).

Argosy University, Sarasota, College of Health Sciences, Sarasota, FL 34235. Offers public health (MPH).

Argosy University, Schaumburg, College of Health Sciences, Schaumburg, IL 60173-5403. Offers public health (MPH).

Argosy University, Seattle, College of Health Sciences, Seattle, WA 98121. Offers public health (MPH).

Argosy University, Tampa, College of Health Sciences, Tampa, FL 33607. Offers public health (MPH).

Argosy University, Twin Cities, College of Health Sciences, Eagan, MN 55121. Offers health services management (MS); public health (MPH).

Argosy University, Washington DC, College of Health Sciences, Arlington, VA 22209. Offers public health (MPH).

Arizona State University at the Tempe campus, College of Nursing and Health Innovation, Phoenix, AZ 85004. Offers advanced nursing practice (DNP); child/family mental health nurse practitioner (Graduate Certificate); clinical research management (MS); community and public health practice (Graduate Certificate); community health (MS); exercise and wellness (MS), including exercise and wellness; family nurse practitioner (Graduate Certificate); healthcare innovation (MHI); international health for healthcare (Graduate Certificate); kinesiology (MS, PhD); nursing (MS, Graduate Certificate); nursing and healthcare innovation (PhD); nutrition (MS); physical activity nutrition and wellness (PhD), including physical activity, nutrition and wellness; public health (MPH); regulatory science and health safety (MS). *Accreditation:* AACN. Postbaccalaureate distance learning degree programs offered (minimal on-campus study). *Degree requirements:* For master's, comprehensive exam (for some programs), thesis (for some programs), interactive Program of Study (iPOS) submitted before completing 50 percent of required credit hours; for doctorate, comprehensive exam, thesis/dissertation, interactive Program of Study (iPOS) submitted before completing 50 percent of required credit hours. *Entrance requirements:* For master's and doctorate, GRE, minimum GPA of 3.0 or equivalent in last 2 years of work leading to bachelor's degree. Additional exam requirements/recommendations for international students: Required—TOEFL (minimum score 80 iBT), TOEFL, IELTS, or PTE. Electronic applications accepted. *Expenses:* Contact institution.

Armstrong State University, School of Graduate Studies, Program in Public Health, Savannah, GA 31419-1997. Offers MPH. *Accreditation:* CEPH. Part-time and evening/weekend programs available. Postbaccalaureate distance learning degree programs offered (no on-campus study). *Faculty:* 5 full-time (3 women), 1 part-time/adjunct (0 women). *Students:* 20 full-time (15 women), 44 part-time (32 women); includes 32 minority (27 Black or African American, non-Hispanic/Latino; 2 Asian, non-Hispanic/Latino; 1 Hispanic/Latino; 2 Two or more races, non-Hispanic/Latino), 4 international. Average age 38. 34 applicants, 59% accepted, 20 enrolled. In 2013, 31 master's awarded. *Degree requirements:* For master's, comprehensive exam, thesis optional, internship. *Entrance requirements:* For master's, GMAT or GRE General Test, MAT, letters of recommendation, letter of intent, minimum undergraduate GPA of 2.8. Additional exam requirements/recommendations for international students: Required—TOEFL. *Application deadline:* For fall admission, 6/1 priority date for domestic students, 5/1 priority date for international students; for spring admission, 11/15 priority date for domestic students, 9/15 priority date for international students; for summer admission, 4/15 for domestic students, 9/15 priority date for international students. Applications are processed on a rolling basis. Application fee: $30. Electronic applications accepted. *Expenses:* Tuition, state resident: part-time $201 per credit hour. Tuition, nonresident: part-time $745 per credit hour. *Required fees:* $310 per semester. Tuition and fees vary according to course load, campus/location and program. *Financial support:* In 2013–14, research assistantships with full tuition reimbursements (averaging $5,000 per year) were awarded; career-related internships or fieldwork, Federal Work-Study, scholarships/grants, tuition waivers (full), and unspecified assistantships also available. Support available to part-time students. Financial award application deadline: 3/15; financial award applicants required to submit FAFSA. *Unit head:* Dr. Sandy Streater, Department Chair, Health Sciences, 912-344-2798, Fax: 912-344-3477, E-mail: sandy.streater@armstrong.edu. *Application contact:* Jill Bell, Director, Graduate Enrollment Services, 912-344-2798, Fax: 912-344-3477, E-mail: graduate@armstrong.edu.
Website: http://www.armstrong.edu/Health_Professions/Health_Sciences/healthsciences_master_of_public_health

A.T. Still University, School of Health Management, Kirksville, MO 63501. Offers dental public health (MPH); health administration (MHA, DHA); health education (DH Ed); public health (MPH). Part-time and evening/weekend programs available. Postbaccalaureate distance learning degree programs offered (no on-campus study). *Faculty:* 20 full-time (10 women), 49 part-time/adjunct (27 women). *Students:* 164 full-time (123 women), 256 part-time (144 women); includes 143 minority (61 Black or African American, non-Hispanic/Latino; 4 American Indian or Alaska Native, non-Hispanic/Latino; 46 Asian, non-Hispanic/Latino; 25 Hispanic/Latino; 3 Native Hawaiian or other Pacific Islander, non-Hispanic/Latino; 4 Two or more races, non-Hispanic/Latino), 12 international. Average age 34. 154 applicants, 93% accepted, 114 enrolled. In 2013, 132 master's, 13 doctorates awarded. *Degree requirements:* For master's, thesis, integrated terminal project, practicum; for doctorate, thesis/dissertation. *Entrance requirements:* For master's, minimum GPA of 3.0, bachelor's degree or equivalent, background check, essay, three references; for doctorate, minimum GPA of 3.0, master's or terminal degree, background check, essay, three references. Additional exam requirements/recommendations for international students: Required—TOEFL (minimum score 550 paper-based; 80 iBT). *Application deadline:* For fall admission, 5/31 for domestic and international students; for winter admission, 8/2 for domestic and international students; for spring admission, 11/8 for domestic and international students; for summer admission, 1/24 for domestic and international students. Application fee: $70. Electronic applications accepted. *Expenses:* Contact institution. *Financial support:* Scholarships/grants available. Financial award application deadline: 5/1; financial award applicants required to submit FAFSA. *Faculty research:* Public health: influence of availability of comprehensive wellness resources online, student wellness, oral health care needs assessment of community, oral health knowledge and behaviors of Medicaid-eligible pregnant women and mothers of young children in relations to early childhood caries and tooth decay, alcohol use and alcohol related problems among college students. *Unit head:* Dr. Donald Altman, Interim Dean, 660-626-2820, Fax: 660-626-2826, E-mail: daltman@atsu.edu. *Application contact:* Sarah Spencer, Associate Director, Admissions, 660-626-2820 Ext. 2669, Fax: 660-626-2826, E-mail: sspencer@atsu.edu.
Website: http://www.atsu.edu/shm

Auburn University at Montgomery, School of Sciences, Department of Public Administration and Political Science, Montgomery, AL 36124-4023. Offers international relations (MIR); nonprofit management and leadership (Certificate); political science (MPS); public administration (MPA); public administration and public policy (PhD); public health care administration and policy (Certificate). PhD offered jointly with Auburn University. *Accreditation:* NASPAA (one or more programs are accredited). Part-time and evening/weekend programs available. *Faculty:* 3 full-time (1 woman), 1 part-time/adjunct (0 women). *Students:* 11 full-time (7 women), 66 part-time (44 women); includes 31 minority (29 Black or African American, non-Hispanic/Latino; 2 Hispanic/Latino), 1 international. Average age 37. In 2013, 24 master's awarded. *Degree requirements:* For master's, comprehensive exam; for doctorate, thesis/dissertation. *Entrance requirements:* For master's, GRE General Test or MAT; for doctorate, GRE General Test. *Application deadline:* Applications are processed on a rolling basis. Electronic applications accepted. *Expenses:* Tuition, state resident: full-time $5994; part-time $333 per credit hour. Tuition, nonresident: full-time $17,982; part-time $999 per credit hour. *Financial support:* Research assistantships, career-related internships or fieldwork, and scholarships/grants available. Support available to part-time students. Financial award application deadline: 3/1; financial award applicants required to submit FAFSA. *Unit head:* Dr. Andrew Cortell, Department Head, 334-244-3622, E-mail: acortell@aum.edu. *Application contact:* Dr. William Ellis, Graduate Coordinator, 334-244-3177, Fax: 334-244-3992, E-mail: wellis3@aum.edu.
Website: http://sciences.aum.edu/departments/political-science-and-public-administration

Austin Peay State University, College of Graduate Studies, College of Behavioral and Health Sciences, Department of Health and Human Performance, Clarksville, TN 37044. Offers health leadership (MS). Part-time and evening/weekend programs available. Postbaccalaureate distance learning degree programs offered (no on-campus study). *Faculty:* 6 full-time (3 women). *Students:* 15 full-time (6 women), 30 part-time (21 women); includes 14 minority (13 Black or African American, non-Hispanic/Latino; 1 Hispanic/Latino). Average age 27. 41 applicants, 90% accepted, 32 enrolled. In 2013, 32 master's awarded. *Degree requirements:* For master's, comprehensive exam, thesis optional. *Entrance requirements:* For master's, GRE General Test, 3 letters of recommendation, minimum undergraduate GPA of 2.5. Additional exam requirements/recommendations for international students: Required—TOEFL (minimum score 500 paper-based). *Application deadline:* For fall admission, 8/5 priority date for domestic students. Applications are processed on a rolling basis. Application fee: $25. Electronic applications accepted. *Expenses:* Tuition, state resident: full-time $7500; part-time $375 per credit hour. Tuition, nonresident: full-time $20,800; part-time $1040 per credit hour. *Required fees:* $1284; $64.20 per credit hour. *Financial support:* In 2013–14, research assistantships with full tuition reimbursements (averaging $6,500 per year) were awarded; career-related internships or fieldwork, Federal Work-Study, institutionally sponsored loans, scholarships/grants, and unspecified assistantships also available. Support available to part-time students. Financial award application deadline: 3/1; financial award applicants required to submit FAFSA. *Unit head:* Dr. Marcy Maurer, Chair, 931-221-6105, Fax: 931-221-7040, E-mail: maurerm@apsu.edu. *Application contact:* June D. Lee, Graduate Coordinator, 800-859-4723, Fax: 931-221-7641, E-mail: gradadmissions@apsu.edu.
Website: http://www.apsu.edu/hhp/

Barry University, School of Podiatric Medicine, Podiatric Medicine and Surgery Program, Podiatric Medicine/Public Health Option, Miami Shores, FL 33161-6695. Offers DPM/MPH.

Benedictine University, Graduate Programs, Program in Public Health, Lisle, IL 60532-0900. Offers administration of health care institutions (MPH); dietetics (MPH); disaster management (MPH); health education (MPH); health information systems (MPH); MBA/MPH; MPH/MS. Part-time and evening/weekend programs available. Postbaccalaureate distance learning degree programs offered. *Students:* 78 full-time (62 women), 340 part-time (254 women); includes 159 minority (97 Black or African American, non-Hispanic/Latino; 3 American Indian or Alaska Native, non-Hispanic/Latino; 47 Asian, non-Hispanic/Latino; 11 Hispanic/Latino; 1 Native Hawaiian or other Pacific Islander, non-Hispanic/Latino), 14 international. Average age 33. 195 applicants, 86% accepted, 143 enrolled. In 2013, 207 master's awarded. *Entrance requirements:* For master's, MAT, GRE, or GMAT. Additional exam requirements/recommendations for international students: Required—TOEFL (minimum score 550 paper-based). *Application deadline:* For fall admission, 9/1 for domestic students; for winter admission, 12/1 for domestic students; for spring admission, 2/15 for domestic students. Application fee: $40. *Expenses: Tuition:* Part-time $590 per credit hour. *Financial support:* Career-related internships or fieldwork and health care benefits available. Support available to part-time students. *Unit head:* Dr. Georgeen Polyak, Director, 630-829-6217, E-mail: gpolyak@ben.edu. *Application contact:* Kari Gibbons, Associate Vice President, Enrollment Center, 630-829-6200, Fax: 630-829-6584, E-mail: kgibbons@ben.edu.

Boise State University, College of Health Sciences, Boise, ID 83725-0399. Offers MHS, MN, MSN, Graduate Certificate. Part-time programs available. *Degree requirements:* For master's, thesis. *Entrance requirements:* For master's, GRE General Test, GMAT or MAT, minimum GPA of 3.0. Electronic applications accepted.

Boston University, Henry M. Goldman School of Dental Medicine, Boston, MA 02118. Offers advanced general dentistry (CAGS); dental public health (MS, MSD, D Sc D, CAGS); dentistry (DMD); endodontics (MSD, D Sc D, CAGS); operative dentistry (MSD, D Sc D, CAGS); oral and maxillofacial surgery (MSD, D Sc D, CAGS); oral biology (MSD, D Sc, D Sc D, PhD); orthodontics (MSD, D Sc D, CAGS); pediatric dentistry (MSD, D Sc D, CAGS); periodontology (MSD, D Sc D, CAGS); prosthodontics (MSD, D Sc D, CAGS). *Accreditation:* ADA (one or more programs are accredited). *Faculty:* 119 full-time (53 women), 83 part-time/adjunct (24 women). *Students:* 818 full-time (423 women); includes 158 minority (8 Black or African American, non-Hispanic/Latino; 1 American Indian or Alaska Native, non-Hispanic/Latino; 102 Asian, non-Hispanic/Latino; 40 Hispanic/Latino; 7 Two or more races, non-Hispanic/Latino), 359 international. Average age 28. 6,681 applicants, 8% accepted, 263 enrolled. In 2013, 14 master's, 199 doctorates, 55 other advanced degrees awarded. *Degree requirements:* For master's and CAGS, thesis; for doctorate, thesis/dissertation (for some programs). *Entrance requirements:* For doctorate, DAT (for DMD), minimum recommended GPA of 3.0 (for DMD); for CAGS, National Board Dental Exam Part 1, dental degree. Additional exam requirements/recommendations for international students: Required—TOEFL. *Application deadline:* For fall admission, 12/1 for domestic and international students. Applications are processed on a rolling basis. Application fee: $75 ($105 for international students). Electronic applications accepted. *Expenses:* Contact institution. *Financial support:* In 2013–14, 480 students received support. Career-related internships or fieldwork, institutionally sponsored loans, and stipends and scholarships (for Advanced Education in General Dentistry and Oral and Maxillofacial Surgery residents) available. Financial award application deadline: 4/15; financial award applicants required to submit FAFSA. *Faculty research:* Defense mechanisms, bone-cell regulation, protein

biochemistry, molecular biology, biomaterials. *Unit head:* Dr. Jeffrey W. Hutter, Dean, 617-638-4780. *Application contact:* Admissions Representative, 617-638-4787, Fax: 617-638-4798, E-mail: sdmadmis@bu.edu.
Website: http://www.bu.edu/dental

Boston University, School of Public Health, Boston, MA 02118. Offers MA, MPH, MS, Dr PH, PhD, JD/MPH, MBA/MPH, MD/MPH, MPH/MA, MSW/MPH. *Accreditation:* CEPH. Part-time and evening/weekend programs available. *Faculty:* 153 full-time, 271 part-time/adjunct. *Students:* 642 full-time (511 women), 384 part-time (307 women); includes 234 minority (47 Black or African American, non-Hispanic/Latino; 1 American Indian or Alaska Native, non-Hispanic/Latino; 102 Asian, non-Hispanic/Latino; 59 Hispanic/Latino; 25 Two or more races, non-Hispanic/Latino), 129 international. Average age 27. 2,439 applicants, 48% accepted, 337 enrolled. In 2013, 370 master's, 17 doctorates awarded. *Degree requirements:* For master's, comprehensive exam (for some programs), thesis optional, culminating experience, practicum; for doctorate, thesis/dissertation, comprehensive written and oral exams. *Entrance requirements:* For master's, GRE, MCAT, GMAT, LSAT, DAT, U.S. bachelor's degree or international equivalent; for doctorate, GRE, MCAT, GMAT, LSAT, MPH or equivalent. Additional exam requirements/recommendations for international students: Required—TOEFL (minimum score 600 paper-based; 100 iBT), IELTS (minimum score 6). *Application deadline:* For fall admission, 2/1 priority date for domestic and international students; for spring admission, 10/15 priority date for domestic and international students. Applications are processed on a rolling basis. Application fee: $115. Electronic applications accepted. *Expenses:* Contact institution. *Financial support:* In 2013–14, 357 students received support. Fellowships, career-related internships or fieldwork, Federal Work-Study, institutionally sponsored loans, scholarships/grants, traineeships, and tuition waivers (partial) available. Support available to part-time students. Financial award application deadline: 5/31; financial award applicants required to submit FAFSA. *Faculty research:* Clinical trials, observational studies, environmental epidemiology, global ecology, environmental sustainability, community health, environmental justice, infectious disease, non-infectious disease, research methods, pharmaceutical assessment, bioethics, health law, human rights, health policy, management, finance and management, family health, disease control in developing countries, child and adolescent health, women's health, health disparities. *Unit head:* Dr. Robert F. Meenan, Dean, 617-638-4640, Fax: 617-638-5299, E-mail: asksph@bu.edu. *Application contact:* LePhan Quan, Associate Director of Admissions, 617-638-4640, Fax: 617-638-5299, E-mail: asksph@bu.edu.
Website: http://sph.bu.edu

Bowling Green State University, Graduate College, College of Health and Human Services, Program in Public Health, Bowling Green, OH 43403. Offers MPH. *Accreditation:* CEPH. Part-time programs available. *Degree requirements:* For master's, thesis or alternative. *Entrance requirements:* For master's, GRE General Test, minimum GPA of 3.0. Additional exam requirements/recommendations for international students: Required—TOEFL. Electronic applications accepted.

Brooklyn College of the City University of New York, School of Natural and Behavioral Sciences, Department of Health and Nutrition Sciences, Program in Public Health, Brooklyn, NY 11210-2889. Offers general public health (MPH); health care policy and administration (MPH). *Accreditation:* CEPH. *Degree requirements:* For master's, thesis or alternative, 46 credits. *Entrance requirements:* For master's, GRE, 2 letters of recommendation, essay, interview. *Application deadline:* For fall admission, 3/1 priority date for domestic students, 2/1 priority date for international students; for spring admission, 11/1 priority date for domestic students, 10/1 priority date for international students. Applications are processed on a rolling basis. Application fee: $125. Electronic applications accepted. *Expenses: Tuition, area resident:* Full-time $4585; part-time $385 per credit. Tuition, state resident: full-time $4585; part-time $385 per credit. Tuition, nonresident: part-time $710 per credit. *Required fees:* $430; $153 per semester. Tuition and fees vary according to course load. *Financial support:* Application deadline: 5/1. *Unit head:* Jean Grassman, Graduate Deputy Chairperson, 718-951-5026, Fax: 718-951-4670. *Application contact:* Jean Grassman, Graduate Deputy Chairperson, 718-951-5026, Fax: 718-951-4670.

Brown University, Graduate School, Division of Biology and Medicine, School of Public Health, Program in Public Health, Providence, RI 02912. Offers MPH. *Accreditation:* CEPH. *Entrance requirements:* For master's, GRE General Test or MCAT. Additional exam requirements/recommendations for international students: Required—TOEFL.

California Baptist University, Program in Public Health, Riverside, CA 92504-3206. Offers food, nutrition and health (MPH); health policy and administration (MPH); physical activity (MPH). Part-time and evening/weekend programs available. *Degree requirements:* For master's, capstone project; practicum. *Entrance requirements:* For master's, minimum undergraduate GPA of 2.75, bachelor's degree transcripts, three recommendations, 500-word essay, resume, interview. Additional exam requirements/recommendations for international students: Required—TOEFL (minimum score 80 iBT). *Application deadline:* For fall admission, 8/1 priority date for domestic students, 7/1 for international students; for spring admission, 12/1 priority date for domestic students, 11/1 for international students. Applications are processed on a rolling basis. Application fee: $45. Electronic applications accepted. *Expenses:* Contact institution. *Financial support:* Applicants required to submit CSS PROFILE or FAFSA. *Unit head:* Dr. Chuck Sands, Dean, College of Allied Health, 951-343-4619, E-mail: csands@calbaptist.edu. *Application contact:* Dr. Wayne Fletcher, Chair, Department of Health Sciences, 951-552-8724, E-mail: wfletcher@calbaptist.edu.
Website: http://www.calbaptist.edu/explore-cbu/schools-colleges/college-allied-health/health-sciences/master-public-health/

California State University, Fresno, Division of Graduate Studies, College of Health and Human Services, Department of Public Health, Fresno, CA 93740-8027. Offers health policy and management (MPH); health promotion (MPH). *Accreditation:* CEPH. Part-time and evening/weekend programs available. *Degree requirements:* For master's, thesis or alternative. *Entrance requirements:* For master's, GRE General Test, minimum GPA of 2.5. Additional exam requirements/recommendations for international students: Required—TOEFL. Electronic applications accepted. *Faculty research:* Foster parent training, geriatrics, tobacco control.

California State University, Fullerton, Graduate Studies, College of Health and Human Development, Department of Health Science, Fullerton, CA 92834-9480. Offers public health (MPH). *Accreditation:* CEPH. Part-time programs available. *Students:* 32 full-time (24 women), 29 part-time (19 women); includes 41 minority (3 Black or African American, non-Hispanic/Latino; 12 Asian, non-Hispanic/Latino; 24 Hispanic/Latino; 1 Native Hawaiian or other Pacific Islander, non-Hispanic/Latino; 1 Two or more races, non-Hispanic/Latino), 1 international. Average age 32. 162 applicants, 23% accepted, 25 enrolled. In 2013, 41 master's awarded. *Entrance requirements:* For master's, minimum GPA of 3.0 in last 60 units attempted. Application fee: $55. *Financial support:* Career-related internships or fieldwork, Federal Work-Study, institutionally sponsored loans, and scholarships/grants available. Support available to part-time students. Financial award application deadline: 3/1; financial award applicants required to submit FAFSA. *Unit head:* Dr. Jessie Jones, Department Head, 657-278-2620. *Application contact:* Admissions/Applications, 657-278-2371.

California State University, Northridge, Graduate Studies, College of Health and Human Development, Department of Health Sciences, Northridge, CA 91330. Offers health administration (MS); public health (MPH). *Accreditation:* CEPH. *Entrance requirements:* For master's, GRE General Test or minimum GPA of 3.0. Additional exam requirements/recommendations for international students: Required—TOEFL. *Faculty research:* Labor market needs assessment, health education products, dental hygiene, independent practice prototype.

California State University, San Bernardino, Graduate Studies, College of Natural Sciences, Program in Health Science, San Bernardino, CA 92407-2397. Offers health science (MS); public health (MPH). *Students:* 8 full-time (7 women), 12 part-time (9 women); includes 12 minority (1 Black or African American, non-Hispanic/Latino; 3 Asian, non-Hispanic/Latino; 6 Hispanic/Latino; 2 Two or more races, non-Hispanic/Latino), 2 international. Average age 28. 3 applicants. In 2013, 18 master's awarded. *Unit head:* Dr. Marsha Greer, Chair, 909-537-5339, Fax: 909-537-7037, E-mail: mgreer@csusb.edu. *Application contact:* Dr. Jeffrey Thompson, Dean of Graduate Studies, 909-537-5058, E-mail: jthompso@csusb.edu.

Case Western Reserve University, School of Medicine and School of Graduate Studies, Graduate Programs in Medicine, Department of Epidemiology and Biostatistics, Program in Public Health, Cleveland, OH 44106. Offers MPH. *Accreditation:* CEPH. Part-time programs available. *Degree requirements:* For master's, essay, field experience, presentation. *Entrance requirements:* For master's, GRE General Test or MCAT, 3 letters of recommendation. Additional exam requirements/recommendations for international students: Required—TOEFL. Electronic applications accepted. *Faculty research:* Public policy and aging, statistical modeling, behavioral medicine and evaluation, continuous quality improvement; tobacco cessation and prevention.

Charles Drew University of Medicine and Science, College of Science and Health, Los Angeles, CA 90059. Offers urban public health (MPH).

Chicago State University, School of Graduate and Professional Studies, College of Health Sciences, Department of Health Studies, Chicago, IL 60628. Offers public health (MPH).

Claremont Graduate University, Graduate Programs, School of Community and Global Health, Claremont, CA 91773. Offers health promotion science (PhD); public health (MPH). *Accreditation:* CEPH. *Faculty:* 12 full-time (5 women). *Students:* 36 full-time (23 women), 29 part-time (23 women); includes 42 minority (5 Black or African American, non-Hispanic/Latino; 17 Asian, non-Hispanic/Latino; 16 Hispanic/Latino; 4 Two or more races, non-Hispanic/Latino), 4 international. Average age 30. In 2013, 21 master's awarded. *Entrance requirements:* For master's and doctorate, GRE. Additional exam requirements/recommendations for international students: Required—TOEFL (minimum score 550 paper-based; 80 iBT). *Application deadline:* For fall admission, 2/1 priority date for domestic and international students; for spring admission, 11/1 priority date for domestic students. Applications are processed on a rolling basis. Application fee: $80. Electronic applications accepted. *Expenses: Tuition:* Full-time $40,560; part-time $1690 per credit. *Required fees:* $275 per semester. Tuition and fees vary according to program. *Financial support:* Fellowships, research assistantships, teaching assistantships, Federal Work-Study, institutionally sponsored loans, and scholarships/grants available. Support available to part-time students. Financial award application deadline: 2/15; financial award applicants required to submit FAFSA. *Unit head:* Stewart Donaldson, Dean, 909-607-8235, E-mail: stewart.donaldson@cgu.edu. *Application contact:* Admissions Office, 909-607-7811, E-mail: information@cgu.edu.
Website: http://www.cgu.edu/pages/5644.asp

Cleveland State University, College of Graduate Studies, College of Education and Human Services, Department of Health, Physical Education, Recreation and Dance, Cleveland, OH 44115. Offers community health education (M Ed); exercise science (M Ed); human performance (M Ed); physical education pedagogy (M Ed); public health (MPH); school health education (M Ed); sport and exercise psychology (M Ed); sports management (M Ed). Part-time programs available. *Faculty:* 7 full-time (4 women), 3 part-time/adjunct (2 women). *Students:* 49 full-time (31 women), 79 part-time (46 women); includes 32 minority (25 Black or African American, non-Hispanic/Latino; 2 Asian, non-Hispanic/Latino; 5 Hispanic/Latino), 7 international. Average age 35. 103 applicants, 72% accepted, 35 enrolled. In 2013, 40 master's awarded. *Degree requirements:* For master's, comprehensive exam, thesis optional. *Entrance requirements:* For master's, GRE General Test or MAT (if undergraduate GPA less than 2.75), minimum undergraduate GPA of 2.75. Additional exam requirements/recommendations for international students: Required—TOEFL (minimum score 525 paper-based), IELTS (minimum score 6). *Application deadline:* For fall admission, 7/15 priority date for domestic students; for spring admission, 12/15 priority date for domestic students. Applications are processed on a rolling basis. Application fee: $30. Electronic applications accepted. *Expenses:* Tuition, state resident: full-time $8335; part-time $521 per credit hour. Tuition, nonresident: full-time $15,670; part-time $979 per credit hour. *Required fees:* $50; $25 per semester. *Financial support:* In 2013–14, 6 research assistantships with full and partial tuition reimbursements (averaging $3,480 per year), 1 teaching assistantship with full and partial tuition reimbursement (averaging $3,480 per year) were awarded; career-related internships or fieldwork, tuition waivers (full), and unspecified assistantships also available. Financial award application deadline: 3/15. *Faculty research:* Bone density, marketing fitness centers, motor development of disabled, online learning and survey research. *Unit head:* Dr. Sheila M. Patterson, Chairperson, 216-687-4870, Fax: 216-687-5410, E-mail: s.m.patterson@csuohio.edu. *Application contact:* Deborah L. Brown, Interim Assistant Director, Graduate Admissions, 216-523-7572, Fax: 216-687-5400, E-mail: d.l.brown@csuohio.edu.
Website: http://www.csuohio.edu/cehs/departments/HPERD/hperd_dept.html

Columbia University, Columbia University Mailman School of Public Health, New York, NY 10032. Offers Exec MPH, MPH, MS, Dr PH, PhD, DDS/MPH, MBA/MPH, MD/MPH, MPA/MPH, MPH/MIA, MPH/MOT, MPH/MS, MPH/MSN, MPH/MSSW. PhD offered in cooperation with the Graduate School of Arts and Sciences. *Accreditation:* CEPH (one or more programs are accredited). Part-time and evening/weekend programs available. *Faculty:* 251 full-time (120 women), 215 part-time/adjunct (96 women). *Students:* 988 full-time (784 women), 336 part-time (221 women); includes 467 minority (94 Black or African American, non-Hispanic/Latino; 2 American Indian or Alaska Native, non-Hispanic/Latino; 206 Asian, non-Hispanic/Latino; 129 Hispanic/Latino; 1 Native Hawaiian or other Pacific Islander, non-Hispanic/Latino; 35 Two or more races, non-Hispanic/Latino), 193 international. Average age 28. 2,846 applicants, 57% accepted, 616 enrolled. In 2013, 525 master's, 20 doctorates awarded. *Degree requirements:* For master's, thesis (for some programs); for doctorate, comprehensive exam, thesis/dissertation. *Entrance requirements:* For master's, GRE General Test; for doctorate, GRE General Test, MPH or equivalent (Dr PH). Additional exam requirements/recommendations for international students: Required—TOEFL (minimum score 600 paper-based; 100 iBT). *Application deadline:* For fall admission, 12/1 priority date for domestic and international students. Application fee: $120. Electronic applications accepted. *Expenses:* Contact institution. *Financial support:* In 2013–14, 651 students received support. Fellowships, research assistantships, teaching assistantships, career-related internships or fieldwork, Federal Work-Study, and traineeships available. Support available to part-time students. Financial award application deadline: 2/1; financial award applicants required to submit FAFSA. *Unit head:* Dr. Linda P. Fried,

Dean/Professor, 212-305-9300, Fax: 212-305-9342, E-mail: lpfried@columbia.edu. *Application contact:* Dr. Joseph Korevec, Director of Admissions and Financial Aid, 212-305-8698, Fax: 212-342-1861, E-mail: ph-admit@columbia.edu.
Website: http://www.mailman.hs.columbia.edu/

Dartmouth College, The Dartmouth Institute, Program in Public Health, Hanover, NH 03755. Offers MPH. Degree awarded through Medical School. *Accreditation:* CEPH. Part-time programs available. *Degree requirements:* For master's, research project or practicum. *Entrance requirements:* For master's, GRE or MCAT, 3 letters of recommendation. Additional exam requirements/recommendations for international students: Required—TOEFL.

Davenport University, Sneden Graduate School, Grand Rapids, MI 49512. Offers accounting (MBA); business administration (EMBA); finance (MBA); health care management (MBA); human resources (MBA); information assurance (MS); public health (MPH); strategic management (MBA). Evening/weekend programs available. *Entrance requirements:* For master's, GMAT, minimum undergraduate GPA of 2.75. Additional exam requirements/recommendations for international students: Required—TOEFL. Electronic applications accepted. *Faculty research:* Leadership, management, marketing, organizational culture.

DePaul University, College of Liberal Arts and Social Sciences, Chicago, IL 60614. Offers Arabic (MA); Chinese (MA); English (MA); French (MA); German (MA); history (MA); interdisciplinary studies (MA, MS); international public service (MS); international studies (MA); Italian (MA); Japanese (MA); leadership and policy studies (MS); liberal studies (MA); new media studies (MA); nonprofit management (MNM); public administration (MPA); public health (MPH); public service management (MS); social work (MSW); sociology (MA); Spanish (MA); sustainable urban development (MA); women and gender studies (MA); writing and publishing (MA); writing, rhetoric, and discourse (MA); MA/PhD. Part-time and evening/weekend programs available. Postbaccalaureate distance learning degree programs offered (no on-campus study). *Faculty:* 75 full-time (38 women), 26 part-time/adjunct (15 women). *Students:* 539 full-time (382 women), 391 part-time (255 women); includes 302 minority (150 Black or African American, non-Hispanic/Latino; 30 Asian, non-Hispanic/Latino; 91 Hispanic/Latino; 1 Native Hawaiian or other Pacific Islander, non-Hispanic/Latino; 30 Two or more races, non-Hispanic/Latino), 33 international. Average age 29. In 2013, 419 master's awarded. Terminal master's awarded for partial completion of doctoral program. *Degree requirements:* For master's, variable foreign language requirement, comprehensive exam (for some programs), thesis (for some programs). *Application deadline:* Applications are processed on a rolling basis. Application fee: $40. Electronic applications accepted. Tuition and fees vary according to course level, course load and degree level. *Financial support:* Applicants required to submit FAFSA. *Unit head:* Dr. Charles Suchar, Dean, 773-325-7305. *Application contact:* Ann Spittle, Director of Graduate Admission, 773-325-7315, Fax: 312-476-3244, E-mail: graddepaul@depaul.edu.
Website: http://las.depaul.edu/

Des Moines University, College of Health Sciences, Program in Public Health, Des Moines, IA 50312-4104. Offers MPH. *Accreditation:* CEPH. Part-time and evening/weekend programs available. *Entrance requirements:* For master's, minimum GPA of 3.0. Additional exam requirements/recommendations for international students: Required—TOEFL (minimum score 600 paper-based). Electronic applications accepted. *Expenses:* Contact institution. *Faculty research:* Quality improvement, women's health, health promotion, patient education.

Drexel University, School of Public Health, Philadelphia, PA 19104-2875. Offers MPH, MS, PhD, Certificate. *Accreditation:* CEPH. *Entrance requirements:* For master's, GMAT, GRE, LSAT, or MCAT, previous course work in statistics and word processing. Additional exam requirements/recommendations for international students: Required—TOEFL. Electronic applications accepted. *Expenses:* Contact institution. *Faculty research:* Epidemiology, behavioral and social sciences, problem-based learning.

East Carolina University, Brody School of Medicine, Program in Public Health, Greenville, NC 27858-4353. Offers MPH, MD/MPH. *Accreditation:* CEPH. Part-time programs available. *Degree requirements:* For master's, field placement professional paper. *Entrance requirements:* For master's, GRE or MCAT. Additional exam requirements/recommendations for international students: Required—TOEFL (minimum score 550 paper-based). *Application deadline:* For fall admission, 4/15 for domestic and international students; for spring admission, 10/15 for domestic and international students. Application fee: $50. Electronic applications accepted. *Expenses:* Tuition, state resident: full-time $4223. Tuition, nonresident: full-time $16,540. *Required fees:* $2184. *Financial support:* Research assistantships with full tuition reimbursements and unspecified assistantships available. Financial award applicants required to submit FAFSA. *Faculty research:* Public health, disparities in public health. *Unit head:* Dr. Lloyd F. Novick, Chairman, Family Medicine, 252-744-4079, Fax: 252-744-2987, E-mail: novickl@ecu.edu. *Application contact:* Dr. Lloyd F. Novick, Chairman, Family Medicine, 252-744-4079, Fax: 252-744-2987, E-mail: novickl@ecu.edu.

East Carolina University, Graduate School, College of Fine Arts and Communication, School of Communication, Greenville, NC 27858-4353. Offers health communication (MA). *Entrance requirements:* For master's, GRE. *Expenses:* Tuition, state resident: full-time $4223. Tuition, nonresident: full-time $16,540. *Required fees:* $2184. *Financial support:* Teaching assistantships available. *Unit head:* Dr. Linda Kean, Director, 252-328-4227, E-mail: keanl@ecu.edu. *Application contact:* Dean of Graduate School, 252-328-6012, Fax: 252-328-6071, E-mail: gradschool@ecu.edu.
Website: http://www.ecu.edu/cs-cfac/comm/graduate/index.cfm

Eastern Virginia Medical School, Master of Public Health Program, Norfolk, VA 23501-1980. Offers MPH. Program offered jointly with Old Dominion University. *Accreditation:* CEPH. Evening/weekend programs available. *Faculty:* 5 full-time (3 women), 31 part-time/adjunct (17 women). *Students:* 83 full-time (65 women), 13 part-time (12 women); includes 45 minority (33 Black or African American, non-Hispanic/Latino; 6 Asian, non-Hispanic/Latino; 6 Two or more races, non-Hispanic/Latino). 116 applicants, 48 enrolled. In 2013, 57 master's awarded. *Degree requirements:* For master's, field practicum. *Entrance requirements:* For master's, GRE General Test. Additional exam requirements/recommendations for international students: Required—TOEFL (minimum score 650 paper-based). *Application deadline:* For fall admission, 4/30 for domestic and international students. Applications are processed on a rolling basis. Application fee: $60. Electronic applications accepted. *Expenses:* Contact institution. *Financial support:* Applicants required to submit FAFSA. *Unit head:* Dr. Brian C. Martin, Program Director, 757-466-6120, Fax: 757-446-6121, E-mail: martinbc@evms.edu. *Application contact:* Aileen Litwin, Instructional Technology Support Analyst, 757-446-6029, Fax: 757-446-6121, E-mail: litwinam@evms.edu.
Website: http://evms.edu/education/masters_programs/graduate_program_in_public_health/

East Tennessee State University, School of Graduate Studies, College of Public Health, Department of Public Health, Johnson City, TN 37614. Offers MPH, DPH, PhD, Postbaccalaureate Certificate. *Expenses:* Tuition, state resident: full-time $7900; part-time $395 per credit hour. Tuition, nonresident: full-time $21,960; part-time $1098 per credit hour. *Required fees:* $1345; $84 per credit hour. *Unit head:* Dr. Randy Wykoff, Dean, 423-439-4243, Fax: 423-439-5238, E-mail: wykoff@etsu.edu. *Application contact:* Mary Duncan, Graduate Specialist, 423-439-4302, Fax: 423-439-5624, E-mail: duncanm@etsu.edu.

Elmhurst College, Graduate Programs, Program in Public Health, Elmhurst, IL 60126-3296. Offers MPH. Part-time and evening/weekend programs available. Postbaccalaureate distance learning degree programs offered (no on-campus study). *Faculty:* 3 full-time (1 woman), 1 part-time/adjunct (0 women). *Students:* 13 full-time (11 women), 4 part-time (all women); includes 10 minority (8 Black or African American, non-Hispanic/Latino; 2 Asian, non-Hispanic/Latino), 1 international. Average age 28. 32 applicants, 66% accepted, 17 enrolled. *Degree requirements:* For master's, practicum. *Entrance requirements:* For master's, 3 recommendations, resume, statement of purpose. Additional exam requirements/recommendations for international students: Required—TOEFL (minimum score 550 paper-based; 79 iBT). *Application deadline:* Applications are processed on a rolling basis. Application fee: $0. Electronic applications accepted. *Expenses:* Contact institution. *Financial support:* In 2013–14, 4 students received support. Federal Work-Study and scholarships/grants available. Support available to part-time students. Financial award application deadline: 6/1; financial award applicants required to submit FAFSA. *Application contact:* Timothy J. Panfil, Director of Enrollment Management, School for Professional Studies, 630-617-3300 Ext. 3256, Fax: 630-617-6471, E-mail: panfilt@elmhurst.edu.
Website: http://public.elmhurst.edu/master_public_health

Emory University, Rollins School of Public Health, Atlanta, GA 30322. Offers MPH, MSPH, PhD, JD/MPH, MBA/MPH, MD/MPH, MM Sc/MPH, MSN/MPH. *Accreditation:* CEPH (one or more programs are accredited). Part-time and evening/weekend programs available. Postbaccalaureate distance learning degree programs offered (minimal on-campus study). *Degree requirements:* For master's, variable foreign language requirement, comprehensive exam (for some programs), thesis (for some programs), practicum. *Entrance requirements:* For master's, GRE General Test. Additional exam requirements/recommendations for international students: Required—TOEFL (minimum score 550 paper-based; 80 iBT). Electronic applications accepted. *Expenses:* Contact institution. *Faculty research:* HIV/AIDS prevention, infectious disease, minority health, health disparities, bioterrorism.

Excelsior College, School of Health Sciences, Albany, NY 12203-5159. Offers health care informatics (Certificate); health professions education (MSHS); public health (MSHS). Part-time and evening/weekend programs available. Postbaccalaureate distance learning degree programs offered (no on-campus study). *Faculty:* 12 part-time/adjunct (9 women). *Students:* 35 part-time (24 women); includes 14 minority (9 Black or African American, non-Hispanic/Latino; 2 American Indian or Alaska Native, non-Hispanic/Latino; 1 Hispanic/Latino; 1 Native Hawaiian or other Pacific Islander, non-Hispanic/Latino; 1 Two or more races, non-Hispanic/Latino). Average age 46. *Entrance requirements:* For degree, bachelor's degree in applicable field. *Application deadline:* Applications are processed on a rolling basis. Application fee: $50. Electronic applications accepted. *Expenses: Tuition:* Part-time $565 per credit. *Financial support:* In 2013–14, 1 student received support. Scholarships/grants available. Support available to part-time students. *Faculty research:* Use of technology in online learning. *Unit head:* Dr. Deborah Sopczyk, Dean, 518-464-8500, Fax: 518-464-8777, E-mail: informatics@excelsior.edu. *Application contact:* Laura Goff, Director of Advisement and Evaluation, 518-464-8500, Fax: 518-464-8777, E-mail: lgoff@excelsior.edu.

Florida Agricultural and Mechanical University, Division of Graduate Studies, Research, and Continuing Education, College of Pharmacy and Pharmaceutical Sciences, Institute of Public Health, Tallahassee, FL 32307-3200. Offers MPH. *Accreditation:* CEPH. *Entrance requirements:* Additional exam requirements/recommendations for international students: Required—TOEFL.

Florida International University, Robert Stempel College of Public Health and Social Work, Programs in Public Health, Miami, FL 33199. Offers biostatistics (MPH); environmental and occupational health (MPH, PhD); epidemiology (MPH, PhD); health policy and management (MPH); health promotion and disease prevention (PhD); health promotion and diseases prevention (MPH). Ph D program has fall admissions only; MPH offered jointly with University of Miami. *Accreditation:* CEPH. Part-time and evening/weekend programs available. Postbaccalaureate distance learning degree programs offered (no on-campus study). *Degree requirements:* For master's, thesis optional; for doctorate, comprehensive exam, thesis/dissertation. *Entrance requirements:* For master's, minimum GPA of 3.0, letters of recommendation; for doctorate, GRE, resume, minimum GPA of 3.0, letters of recommendation, letter of intent. Additional exam requirements/recommendations for international students: Required—TOEFL (minimum score 550 paper-based; 80 iBT). Electronic applications accepted. *Expenses:* Contact institution. *Faculty research:* Drugs/AIDS intervention among migrant workers, provision of services for active/recovering drug users with HIV.

Florida State University, The Graduate School, College of Social Sciences and Public Policy, Public Health Program, Tallahassee, FL 32306. Offers MPH. Part-time programs available. *Faculty:* 6 full-time (1 woman), 2 part-time/adjunct (0 women). *Students:* 25 full-time (13 women), 16 part-time (12 women); includes 24 minority (18 Black or African American, non-Hispanic/Latino; 1 American Indian or Alaska Native, non-Hispanic/Latino; 4 Asian, non-Hispanic/Latino; 1 Hispanic/Latino). Average age 26. 70 applicants, 59% accepted, 13 enrolled. In 2013, 18 master's awarded. *Degree requirements:* For master's, internship, research paper. *Entrance requirements:* For master's, GRE General Test, minimum GPA of 3.0. Additional exam requirements/recommendations for international students: Required—TOEFL (minimum score 550 paper-based; 80 iBT). *Application deadline:* For fall admission, 7/1 priority date for domestic students, 7/1 for international students; for spring admission, 11/1 for domestic and international students. Applications are processed on a rolling basis. Application fee: $30. Electronic applications accepted. *Expenses:* Tuition, state resident: part-time $403.51 per credit hour. Tuition, nonresident: part-time $1004.85 per credit hour. *Required fees:* $75.81 per credit hour. One-time fee: $20 part-time. Tuition and fees vary according to course load, campus/location and student level. *Financial support:* In 2013–14, 3 students received support, including 3 research assistantships with full tuition reimbursements available (averaging $5,000 per year); fellowships with tuition reimbursements available, career-related internships or fieldwork, Federal Work-Study, institutionally sponsored loans, and unspecified assistantships also available. Financial award application deadline: 2/15. *Faculty research:* Health behavior surveillance, long term care policy, long term care evaluation, HMOs, Medicaid. *Total annual research expenditures:* $1 million. *Unit head:* Dr. William G. Weissert, Director, 850-644-4418, Fax: 850-644-1367, E-mail: william.weissert@fsu.edu. *Application contact:* Kaley Boggs, Academic Program Specialist, 850-644-4418, E-mail: kboggs@fsu.edu.
Website: http://www.coss.fsu.edu/publichealth/

Fort Valley State University, College of Graduate Studies and Extended Education, Program in Public Health, Fort Valley, GA 31030. Offers environmental health (MPH). *Degree requirements:* For master's, thesis. *Entrance requirements:* For master's, GRE General Test. Additional exam requirements/recommendations for international students: Recommended—TOEFL.

George Mason University, College of Health and Human Services, Department of Global and Community Health, Fairfax, VA 22030. Offers global health (MS); public

health (MPH, Certificate). *Accreditation:* CEPH. *Faculty:* 12 full-time (8 women), 16 part-time/adjunct (13 women). *Students:* 70 full-time (58 women), 62 part-time (55 women); includes 58 minority (21 Black or African American, non-Hispanic/Latino; 22 Asian, non-Hispanic/Latino; 11 Hispanic/Latino; 1 Native Hawaiian or other Pacific Islander, non-Hispanic/Latino; 3 Two or more races, non-Hispanic/Latino), 9 international. Average age 29. 144 applicants, 69% accepted, 51 enrolled. In 2013, 54 master's, 1 other advanced degree awarded. *Degree requirements:* For master's, comprehensive exam (for some programs), thesis or practicum. *Entrance requirements:* For master's, GRE, 2 official transcripts; expanded goals statement; 3 letters of recommendation; resume; 1 completed course in health science, statistics, natural sciences and social science (for MPH); 6 credits of foreign language if not fluent (for MS in global health); for Certificate, 2 official transcripts; expanded goals statement; 3 letters of recommendation; resume; bachelor's degree from regionally-accredited institution with minimum GPA of 3.0; statistics and college-level algebra with minimum B grade (for Certificate in biostatistics). Additional exam requirements/recommendations for international students: Required—TOEFL (minimum score 570 paper-based; 88 iBT), IELTS (minimum score 6.5), PTE. *Application deadline:* For fall admission, 4/1 priority date for domestic students; for spring admission, 11/1 priority date for domestic students. Applications are processed on a rolling basis. Application fee: $65 ($80 for international students). Electronic applications accepted. *Expenses:* Contact institution. *Financial support:* In 2013–14, 4 students received support, including 4 research assistantships with full and partial tuition reimbursements available (averaging $14,250 per year); career-related internships or fieldwork, Federal Work-Study, scholarships/grants, unspecified assistantships, and health care benefits (for full-time research or teaching assistantship recipients) also available. Financial award application deadline: 3/1; financial award applicants required to submit FAFSA. *Faculty research:* Health issues and the needs of affected populations at the regional and global level. *Total annual research expenditures:* $21,323. *Unit head:* Keith Howell, Interim Chair, 703-993-9633, Fax: 703-993-1943, E-mail: khowell@gmu.edu. *Application contact:* Ali Weinstein, Graduate Coordinator, 703-993-9632, Fax: 703-993-1908, E-mail: aweinst2@gmu.edu.
Website: http://chhs.gmu.edu/gch/index

George Mason University, College of Health and Human Services, Department of Health Administration and Policy, Fairfax, VA 22030. Offers health and medical policy (MS); health informatics (MS); health informatics and data analytics (Certificate); health policy (Certificate); health systems management (MHA); physician practice management (Certificate); public health leadership and management (Certificate); quality improvement and outcomes management in health care systems (Certificate); senior housing administration (Certificate). *Accreditation:* CAHME. *Faculty:* 17 full-time (5 women), 17 part-time/adjunct (7 women). *Students:* 78 full-time (55 women), 105 part-time (74 women); includes 85 minority (37 Black or African American, non-Hispanic/Latino; 33 Asian, non-Hispanic/Latino; 12 Hispanic/Latino; 1 Native Hawaiian or other Pacific Islander, non-Hispanic/Latino; 2 Two or more races, non-Hispanic/Latino), 21 international. Average age 33. 140 applicants, 66% accepted, 58 enrolled. In 2013, 45 master's, 4 other advanced degrees awarded. *Degree requirements:* For master's, comprehensive exam,, internship. *Entrance requirements:* For master's, GRE recommended if undergraduate GPA is below 3.0 (for senior housing administration MS only), 2 official transcripts; expanded goals statement; 3 letters of recommendation; resume; 1 year of work experience (for MHA in health systems management); for Certificate, 2 official transcripts; expanded goals statement; 3 letters of recommendation; resume. Additional exam requirements/recommendations for international students: Required—TOEFL (minimum score 570 paper-based; 88 iBT), IELTS (minimum score 6.5), PTE. *Application deadline:* For fall admission, 4/1 priority date for domestic students; for spring admission, 11/1 priority date for domestic students. Applications are processed on a rolling basis. Application fee: $65 ($80 for international students). Electronic applications accepted. *Expenses:* Contact institution. *Financial support:* In 2013–14, 3 students received support, including 3 research assistantships with full and partial tuition reimbursements available (averaging $16,333 per year); career-related internships or fieldwork, Federal Work-Study, scholarships/grants, unspecified assistantships, and health care benefits (for full-time research or teaching assistantship recipients) also available. Support available to part-time students. Financial award application deadline: 3/1; financial award applicants required to submit FAFSA. *Faculty research:* Universal health care, publications, relationships between malpractice pressure and rates of Cesarean section and VBAC, seniors and Wii gaming, relationships between changes in physician's incomes and practice settings and their care to Medicaid and charity patients. *Total annual research expenditures:* $306,284. *Unit head:* Dr. P. J. Maddox, Chair, 703-993-1982, Fax: 703-993-1953, E-mail: pmaddox@gmu.edu. *Application contact:* Valerie Bartush, Office Manager, 703-993-1929, Fax: 703-993-1953, E-mail: vbartush@gmu.edu.
Website: http://chhs.gmu.edu/hap/index

Georgetown University, Graduate School of Arts and Sciences, Programs in Biomedical Sciences, Department of Microbiology and Immunology, Washington, DC 20057. Offers biohazardous threat agents and emerging infectious diseases (MS); biomedical science policy and advocacy (MS); general microbiology and immunology (MS); global infectious diseases (PhD); microbiology and immunology (PhD). Part-time programs available. *Degree requirements:* For master's, 30 credit hours of coursework; for doctorate, comprehensive exam, thesis/dissertation. *Entrance requirements:* For master's, GRE General Test, 3 letters of reference, bachelor's degree in related field; for doctorate, GRE General Test, 3 letters of reference, MS/BS in related field. Additional exam requirements/recommendations for international students: Required—TOEFL (minimum score 505 paper-based). *Application deadline:* For fall admission, 7/1 for domestic students, 6/1 priority date for international students; for winter admission, 2/2 priority date for domestic students, 1/2 priority date for international students; for spring admission, 11/1 for domestic students, 10/1 priority date for international students. Applications are processed on a rolling basis. Application fee: $75. Electronic applications accepted. *Financial support:* Fellowships with full tuition reimbursements available. *Faculty research:* Pathogenesis and basic biology of the fungus Candida albicans, molecular biology of viral immunopathological mechanisms in Multiple Sclerosis. *Unit head:* Dr. Richard A. Calderone, Chair, 202-687-1513, E-mail: calderor@georgetown.edu. *Application contact:* Kimberly Bassalian, Graduate Program Coordinator, 202-687-3422, Fax: 202-687-1800, E-mail: kdb70@georgetown.edu.
Website: http://microbiology.georgetown.edu/

The George Washington University, School of Public Health and Health Services, Department of Global Health, Washington, DC 20052. Offers MPH, JD/MPH, LL M/MPH, MD/MPH. *Accreditation:* CEPH. *Faculty:* 14 full-time (8 women). *Students:* 60 full-time (53 women), 90 part-time (79 women); includes 47 minority (22 Black or African American, non-Hispanic/Latino; 2 American Indian or Alaska Native, non-Hispanic/Latino; 11 Asian, non-Hispanic/Latino; 11 Hispanic/Latino; 1 Two or more races, non-Hispanic/Latino), 7 international. Average age 29. 260 applicants, 82% accepted. In 2013, 61 master's awarded. *Degree requirements:* For master's, case study or special project. *Entrance requirements:* For master's, GMAT, GRE General Test, or MCAT. Additional exam requirements/recommendations for international students: Required—TOEFL. *Application deadline:* For fall admission, 4/15 priority date for domestic students, 4/15 for international students; for spring admission, 11/1 for domestic and international students. Applications are processed on a rolling basis. Application fee: $75. *Financial support:* In 2013–14, 24 students received support. Tuition waivers available. Financial award application deadline: 2/15. *Unit head:* Dr. James Tielsch, Chair, 202-994-0270, Fax: 202-994-1955, E-mail: jtielsch@gwu.edu. *Application contact:* Jane Smith, Director of Admissions, 202-994-0248, Fax: 202-994-1860, E-mail: sphhsinfo@gwumc.edu.

The George Washington University, School of Public Health and Health Services, Department of Health Services Management and Leadership, Washington, DC 20052. Offers health management and leadership (MHSA); health policy (MHSA); health services administration (Specialist); public health management (MPH). *Accreditation:* CAHME (one or more programs are accredited). *Faculty:* 7 full-time (3 women). *Degree requirements:* For master's, internship or residency. *Entrance requirements:* For master's, GMAT or GRE; for Specialist, GMAT or GRE, master's degree in related field. Additional exam requirements/recommendations for international students: Required—TOEFL. *Application deadline:* For fall admission, 5/15 priority date for domestic students; for winter admission, 11/15 for domestic students; for spring admission, 4/1 for domestic students. Applications are processed on a rolling basis. Application fee: $75. *Financial support:* Career-related internships or fieldwork, Federal Work-Study, and institutionally sponsored loans available. Financial award application deadline: 6/1. *Faculty research:* Hospital administration, ambulatory health care, social gerontology, health care financing, health care ethics. *Unit head:* Dr. Robert Burke, Chair, 202-994-5560, Fax: 202-416-0075, E-mail: bobburke@gwu.edu. *Application contact:* Jane Smith, Director of Admissions, 202-994-0248, Fax: 202-994-1860, E-mail: sphhsinfo@gwumc.edu.
Website: http://publichealth.gwu.edu/departments/health-services-management-and-leadership

Georgia Regents University, The Graduate School, Program in Public Health–Informatics, Augusta, GA 30912. Offers health informatics (MPH); health management (MPH). Part-time programs available. *Faculty:* 7 full-time (5 women). *Students:* 11 full-time (8 women), 22 part-time (14 women); includes 17 minority (12 Black or African American, non-Hispanic/Latino; 3 Asian, non-Hispanic/Latino; 1 Hispanic/Latino; 1 Two or more races, non-Hispanic/Latino). Average age 34. 28 applicants, 39% accepted, 7 enrolled. In 2013, 5 master's awarded. *Degree requirements:* For master's, thesis (for some programs). *Entrance requirements:* For master's, GRE General Test. Additional exam requirements/recommendations for international students: Required—TOEFL. *Application deadline:* For fall admission, 6/1 for domestic and international students. Application fee: $50. Electronic applications accepted. *Financial support:* Federal Work-Study available. Financial award application deadline: 5/31; financial award applicants required to submit FAFSA. *Unit head:* Dr. Douglas Keskula, Interim Dean, 706-721-2621, Fax: 706-721-7312, E-mail: dkeskula@georgiahealth.edu. *Application contact:* Lori Prince, Interim Chair, 706-721-3436, E-mail: lprince@georgiahealth.edu.
Website: http://www.gru.edu/alliedhealth/hmi/mph/

Georgia Southern University, Jack N. Averitt College of Graduate Studies, Jiann-Ping Hsu College of Public Health, Program in Public Health, Statesboro, GA 30460. Offers biostatistics (MPH, Dr PH); community health behavior and education (Dr PH); community health education (MPH); environmental health sciences (MPH); epidemiology (MPH); health policy and management (MPH, Dr PH). *Accreditation:* CEPH. Part-time programs available. *Students:* 130 full-time (96 women), 50 part-time (39 women); includes 95 minority (80 Black or African American, non-Hispanic/Latino; 5 Asian, non-Hispanic/Latino; 4 Hispanic/Latino; 1 Native Hawaiian or other Pacific Islander, non-Hispanic/Latino; 5 Two or more races, non-Hispanic/Latino), 32 international. Average age 30. 213 applicants, 68% accepted, 61 enrolled. In 2013, 29 master's, 9 doctorates awarded. *Degree requirements:* For master's, thesis optional, practicum; for doctorate, comprehensive exam, thesis/dissertation, practicum. *Entrance requirements:* For master's, GRE General Test, minimum GPA of 2.75, resume, 3 letters of reference; for doctorate, GRE, GMAT, MCAT, LSAT, 3 letters of reference, statement of purpose, resume or curriculum vitae. Additional exam requirements/recommendations for international students: Required—TOEFL (minimum score 550 paper-based; 80 iBT), IELTS (minimum score 6). *Application deadline:* For fall admission, 3/1 priority date for domestic and international students; for spring admission, 10/1 priority date for domestic students, 10/1 for international students. Applications are processed on a rolling basis. Application fee: $50. Electronic applications accepted. *Expenses:* Contact institution. *Financial support:* In 2013–14, 54 students received support, including research assistantships with partial tuition reimbursements available (averaging $7,200 per year), teaching assistantships with partial tuition reimbursements available (averaging $7,200 per year); career-related internships or fieldwork, Federal Work-Study, scholarships/grants, tuition waivers (partial), and unspecified assistantships also available. Support available to part-time students. Financial award application deadline: 4/15; financial award applicants required to submit FAFSA. *Faculty research:* Rural public health best practices, health disparity elimination, community initiatives to enhance public health, cost effectiveness analysis, epidemiology of rural public health, environmental health issues, health care system assessment, rural health care, health policy and healthcare financing, survival analysis, nonparametric statistics and resampling methods, micro-arrays and genomics, data imputation techniques and clinical trial methodology. *Total annual research expenditures:* $281,707. *Unit head:* Sarah Peterson, Student Services Coordinator, 912-478-2413, Fax: 912-478-5811, E-mail: speterson@georgiasouthern.edu. *Application contact:* Amanda Gilliland, Coordinator for Graduate Student Recruitment, 912-478-5384, Fax: 912-478-0740, E-mail: gradadmissions@georgiasouthern.edu.
Website: http://chhs.georgiasouthern.edu/health/

Georgia State University, Andrew Young School of Policy Studies, Department of Public Management and Policy, Atlanta, GA 30303. Offers criminal justice (MPA); disaster management (Certificate); disaster policy (MPA); environmental policy (PhD); health policy (PhD); management and finance (MPA); nonprofit management (MPA, Certificate); nonprofit policy (MPA); planning and economic development (MPP, Certificate); policy analysis and evaluation (MPA), including planning and economic development; public and nonprofit management (PhD); public finance and budgeting (PhD), including science and technology policy, urban and regional economic development; public finance policy (MPA), including social policy; public health (MPA). *Accreditation:* NASPAA (one or more programs are accredited). Part-time programs available. *Faculty:* 17 full-time (8 women), 3 part-time/adjunct (0 women). *Students:* 139 full-time (76 women), 95 part-time (59 women); includes 98 minority (69 Black or African American, non-Hispanic/Latino; 9 Asian, non-Hispanic/Latino; 11 Hispanic/Latino; 9 Two or more races, non-Hispanic/Latino), 19 international. Average age 29. 310 applicants, 55% accepted, 68 enrolled. In 2013, 68 master's, 9 other advanced degrees awarded. Terminal master's awarded for partial completion of doctoral program. *Degree requirements:* For master's, thesis optional; for doctorate, comprehensive exam, thesis/dissertation. *Entrance requirements:* For master's and doctorate, GRE. Additional exam requirements/recommendations for international students: Required—TOEFL (minimum score 603 paper-based; 100 iBT) or IELTS (minimum score 7). *Application deadline:* For fall admission, 2/15 for domestic and international students; for spring admission, 10/1 for domestic and international students. Application fee: $50. Electronic applications accepted. *Expenses: Tuition, area resident:* Full-time $4176; part-time $348 per credit hour. Tuition, state resident: full-time $14,544; part-time $1212 per credit hour. Tuition, nonresident: full-time $14,544; part-time $1212 per credit hour. Tuition and fees vary

according to course load and program. *Financial support:* In 2013–14, fellowships (averaging $8,194 per year), research assistantships (averaging $8,068 per year), teaching assistantships (averaging $3,600 per year) were awarded; institutionally sponsored loans, scholarships/grants, health care benefits, and unspecified assistantships also available. Financial award application deadline: 2/1. *Faculty research:* Public budgeting and finance, public management, nonprofit management, performance measurement and management, urban development. *Unit head:* Dr. Gregory Burr Lewis, Chair and Professor, 404-413-0114, Fax: 404-413-0104, E-mail: glewis@gsu.edu. *Application contact:* Charisma Parker, Admissions Coordinator, 404-413-0030, Fax: 404-413-0023, E-mail: cparker28@gsu.edu.
Website: http://aysps.gsu.edu/pmap/

Georgia State University, Institute of Public Health, Atlanta, GA 30302-3995. Offers MPH, PhD, Certificate. *Accreditation:* CEPH. Part-time programs available. *Faculty:* 18 full-time (12 women). *Students:* 169 full-time (126 women), 70 part-time (57 women); includes 112 minority (76 Black or African American, non-Hispanic/Latino; 22 Asian, non-Hispanic/Latino; 7 Hispanic/Latino; 7 Two or more races, non-Hispanic/Latino), 28 international. Average age 31. 279 applicants, 52% accepted, 90 enrolled. In 2013, 60 master's, 7 doctorates awarded. *Degree requirements:* For master's, thesis, statistics and research methods; applied practicum; for doctorate, comprehensive exam, thesis/dissertation, basic/advanced statistics and research methods; applied, research or teaching practicum. *Entrance requirements:* For master's, doctorate, and Certificate, GRE or GMAT. Additional exam requirements/recommendations for international students: Required—TOEFL (minimum score 550 paper-based; 80 iBT). *Application deadline:* For fall admission, 2/1 for domestic and international students; for spring admission, 10/1 for domestic and international students. Application fee: $50. Electronic applications accepted. *Expenses:* Contact institution. *Financial support:* In 2013–14, fellowships (averaging $2,500 per year), research assistantships with full tuition reimbursements (averaging $22,000 per year), teaching assistantships with full tuition reimbursements (averaging $22,000 per year) were awarded; career-related internships or fieldwork, scholarships/grants, health care benefits, unspecified assistantships, and out-of-state tuition waivers also available. *Faculty research:* Infectious and chronic disease epidemiology; environmental health and the built environment; adolescent risk behaviors: tobacco use, alcohol and drug use, and risky sexual behaviors; reduction of health disparities especially among minority populations in urban areas; program evaluation, evidence-based interventions and implementation. *Unit head:* Dr. Michael P. Eriksen, Dean, 404-413-1132, Fax: 404-413-1140, E-mail: meriksen@gsu.edu. *Application contact:* Courtney M. Burton, Graduate Coordinator, 404-413-1143, E-mail: cmburton@gsu.edu.
Website: http://publichealth.gsu.edu/

The Graduate Center, City University of New York, Graduate Studies, Program in Public Health, New York, NY 10016-4039. Offers DPH. *Accreditation:* CEPH. Part-time programs available. *Degree requirements:* For doctorate, thesis/dissertation, exams, research seminars. *Entrance requirements:* For doctorate, GRE General Test, MPH, 2 letters of recommendation, curriculum vitae or resume.

Grand Canyon University, College of Nursing and Health Sciences, Phoenix, AZ 85017-1097. Offers addiction counseling (MS); health care administration (MS); health care informatics (MS); marriage and family therapy (MS); professional counseling (MS); public health (MS). Part-time and evening/weekend programs available. Postbaccalaureate distance learning degree programs offered (no on-campus study). *Entrance requirements:* For master's, undergraduate degree with minimum GPA of 2.8. Additional exam requirements/recommendations for international students: Required—TOEFL (minimum score 575 paper-based; 90 iBT), IELTS (minimum score 7).

Harvard University, Cyprus International Institute for the Environment and Public Health in Association with Harvard School of Public Health, Cambridge, MA 02138. Offers environmental health (MS); environmental/public health (PhD); epidemiology and biostatistics (MS). *Entrance requirements:* For master's and doctorate, GRE, resume/curriculum vitae, 3 letters of recommendation, BA or BS (including diploma and official transcripts). Additional exam requirements/recommendations for international students: Required—TOEFL, IELTS (minimum score 7). Electronic applications accepted. *Expenses: Tuition:* Full-time $38,888. *Required fees:* $958. Tuition and fees vary according to campus/location, program and student level. *Faculty research:* Air pollution, climate change, biostatistics, sustainable development, environmental management.

Harvard University, Harvard School of Public Health, Master of Public Health Program, Boston, MA 02115-6096. Offers clinical effectiveness (MPH); global health (MPH); health and social behavior (MPH); health management (MPH); health policy (MPH); occupational and environmental health (MPH); quantitative methods (MPH); JD/MPH; MD/MPH. Part-time programs available. *Students:* 163 full-time, 223 part-time; includes 106 minority (22 Black or African American, non-Hispanic/Latino; 56 Asian, non-Hispanic/Latino; 21 Hispanic/Latino; 7 Two or more races, non-Hispanic/Latino), 144 international. Average age 32. 696 applicants, 48% accepted, 254 enrolled. In 2013, 280 master's awarded. *Entrance requirements:* For master's, GRE, MCAT, GMAT, DAT, LSAT. Additional exam requirements/recommendations for international students: Required—TOEFL (minimum score 600 paper-based; 100 iBT); Recommended—IELTS (minimum score 7). *Application deadline:* For fall admission, 12/15 priority date for domestic and international students. Applications are processed on a rolling basis. Application fee: $120. Electronic applications accepted. *Expenses: Tuition:* Full-time $38,888. *Required fees:* $958. Tuition and fees vary according to campus/location, program and student level. *Financial support:* Federal Work-Study, scholarships/grants, and unspecified assistantships available. Support available to part-time students. Financial award application deadline: 2/15; financial award applicants required to submit FAFSA. *Faculty research:* Clinical effectiveness, global health, health and social behavior, health care management and policy, law and public health, occupational and environmental health, quantitative methods. *Unit head:* Dr. Murray Mittleman, Chair of the MPH Steering Committee, 617-432-0090, Fax: 617-432-3365, E-mail: mmittlem@hsph.harvard.edu. *Application contact:* Vincent W. James, Director of Admissions, 617-432-1031, Fax: 617-432-7080, E-mail: admissions@hsph.harvard.edu.
Website: http://www.hsph.harvard.edu/master-of-public-health-program/

See Display below and Close-Up on page 887,

Harvard University, Harvard School of Public Health, PhD Program in Biological Sciences in Public Health, Boston, MA 02115. Offers PhD. *Faculty:* 22 full-time (9 women), 28 part-time/adjunct (6 women). *Students:* 55 full-time (39 women); includes 13 minority (4 Black or African American, non-Hispanic/Latino; 3 Asian, non-Hispanic/Latino; 3 Hispanic/Latino; 3 Two or more races, non-Hispanic/Latino), 15 international. Average age 27. 438 applicants, 12% accepted, 40 enrolled. In 2013, 32 doctorates awarded. *Degree requirements:* For doctorate, qualifying examination, dissertation/defense. *Entrance requirements:* For doctorate, GRE General Test. Additional exam requirements/recommendations for international students: Required—TOEFL. *Application deadline:* For fall admission, 12/8 for domestic students. *Expenses: Tuition:* Full-time $38,888. *Required fees:* $958. Tuition and fees vary according to campus/location, program and student level. *Financial support:* Fellowships, research assistantships, teaching assistantships, institutionally sponsored loans, and tuition waivers (full) available. Financial award application deadline: 1/1. *Faculty research:* Nutrition biochemistry, molecular and cellular toxicology, cardiovascular disease, cancer biology, immunology and infectious diseases, environmental health physiology. *Unit head:* Carole Knapp, Administrator, 617-432-2932.

See Display below and Close-Up on page 887,

Public Health—General

Hofstra University, School of Health Sciences and Human Services, Programs in Health, Hempstead, NY 11549. Offers community health (MS); health administration (MHA); public health (MPH).

Howard University, College of Medicine, Program in Public Health, Washington, DC 20059-0002. Offers MPH.

Hunter College of the City University of New York, Graduate School, Schools of the Health Professions, School of Health Sciences, Programs in Urban Public Health, New York, NY 10065-5085. Offers community health education (MPH); environmental and occupational health sciences (MPH, MS); epidemiology and biostatistics (MPH); health policy management (MPH); nutrition (MPH); MS/MPH. *Accreditation:* CEPH. Part-time programs available. *Faculty:* 21 full-time (17 women), 11 part-time/adjunct (6 women). *Students:* 39 full-time (30 women), 232 part-time (176 women); includes 101 minority (41 Black or African American, non-Hispanic/Latino; 2 American Indian or Alaska Native, non-Hispanic/Latino; 30 Asian, non-Hispanic/Latino; 28 Hispanic/Latino), 10 international. Average age 31. 428 applicants, 52% accepted, 123 enrolled. In 2013, 95 master's awarded. *Degree requirements:* For master's, comprehensive exam. *Entrance requirements:* For master's, GRE General Test, undergraduate major in natural or social sciences, health studies, nutrition or related field; 1 year of work or volunteer experience related to public health, nutrition, environmental health, social services, or community organization. Additional exam requirements/recommendations for international students: Required—TOEFL. *Application deadline:* For fall admission, 4/1 for domestic students, 2/1 for international students; for spring admission, 11/1 for domestic students, 9/1 for international students. Application fee: $125. *Financial support:* Application deadline: 3/1. *Unit head:* Jack Caravanos, Director, 212-396-7780, Fax: 212-481-5260, E-mail: jcaravan@hunter.cuny.edu. *Application contact:* Milena Solo, Director for Graduate Admissions, 212-772-4288, E-mail: admissions@hunter.cuny.edu.
Website: http://cuny.edu/site/sph/hunter-college/a-programs/graduate.html

Idaho State University, Office of Graduate Studies, College of Education, Department of Educational Foundations, Pocatello, ID 83209-8059. Offers child and family studies (M Ed); curriculum leadership (M Ed); education (M Ed); educational administration (M Ed); educational foundations (5th Year Certificate); elementary education (M Ed), including K-12 education, literacy, secondary education. Part-time programs available. *Degree requirements:* For master's, comprehensive exam, thesis optional, oral exam, written exam; for 5th Year Certificate, comprehensive exam, thesis (for some programs), oral exam, written exam. *Entrance requirements:* For master's, GRE General Test or MAT, minimum undergraduate GPA of 3.0; for 5th Year Certificate, GRE General Test, minimum undergraduate GPA of 3.0, master's degree. Additional exam requirements/recommendations for international students: Required—TOEFL (minimum score 550 paper-based; 80 iBT). Electronic applications accepted. *Faculty research:* Child and families studies; business education; special education; math, science, and technology education.

Idaho State University, Office of Graduate Studies, Kasiska College of Health Professions, Department of Health and Nutrition Sciences, Program in Public Health, Pocatello, ID 83209-8109. Offers MPH. *Accreditation:* CEPH. Part-time programs available. *Degree requirements:* For master's, comprehensive exam, thesis. *Entrance requirements:* For master's, GRE General Test, minimum GPA of 3.0 for upper division classes, 2 letters of recommendation. Additional exam requirements/recommendations for international students: Required—TOEFL (minimum score 600 paper-based). Electronic applications accepted.

Independence University, Program in Public Health, Salt Lake City, UT 84107. Offers MPH. Part-time and evening/weekend programs available. Postbaccalaureate distance learning degree programs offered (no on-campus study). *Degree requirements:* For master's, final project or thesis.

Indiana University Bloomington, School of Public Health, Department of Applied Health Science, Bloomington, IN 47405. Offers behavioral, social, and community health (MPH); family health (MPH); health behavior (PhD); nutrition science (MS); professional health education (MPH); public health administration (MPH); safety management (MS); school and college health education (MS). *Accreditation:* CEPH (one or more programs are accredited). *Faculty:* 30 full-time (19 women). *Students:* 144 full-time (104 women), 26 part-time (16 women); includes 46 minority (23 Black or African American, non-Hispanic/Latino; 1 American Indian or Alaska Native, non-Hispanic/Latino; 8 Asian, non-Hispanic/Latino; 10 Hispanic/Latino; 4 Two or more races, non-Hispanic/Latino), 32 international. Average age 30. 129 applicants, 71% accepted, 58 enrolled. In 2013, 53 master's, 6 doctorates awarded. *Degree requirements:* For master's, thesis optional; for doctorate, comprehensive exam, thesis/dissertation. *Entrance requirements:* For master's, GRE (for MS in nutrition science), 3 recommendations; for doctorate, GRE, 3 recommendations. Additional exam requirements/recommendations for international students: Required—TOEFL (minimum score 550 paper-based; 80 iBT). *Application deadline:* For fall admission, 2/1 priority date for domestic students, 12/1 priority date for international students; for spring admission, 11/15 priority date for domestic students, 9/1 priority date for international students. Application fee: $55 ($65 for international students). Electronic applications accepted. *Financial support:* Fellowships, research assistantships with full and partial tuition reimbursements, teaching assistantships with full and partial tuition reimbursements, career-related internships or fieldwork, Federal Work-Study, institutionally sponsored loans, scholarships/grants, health care benefits, tuition waivers (partial), unspecified assistantships, and fee remissions available. Financial award application deadline: 3/1; financial award applicants required to submit FAFSA. *Faculty research:* Cancer education, HIV/AIDS and drug education, public health, parent-child interactions, safety education, obesity, public health policy, public health administration, school health, health education, human development, nutrition, human sexuality, chronic disease, early childhood health. *Total annual research expenditures:* $1.4 million. *Unit head:* Dr. David K. Lohrmann, Chair, 812-856-5101, Fax: 812-855-3936, E-mail: dlohrman@indiana.edu. *Application contact:* Dr. Susan Middlestadt, Associate Professor and Graduate Coordinator, 812-856-5768, Fax: 812-855-3936, E-mail: semiddle@indiana.edu.
Website: http://www.publichealth.indiana.edu/departments/applied-health-science/index.shtml

Indiana University Kokomo, Division of Allied Health Sciences, Kokomo, IN 46904-9003. Offers public health management (MPH). *Students:* 2 full-time (both women), 25 part-time (17 women); includes 2 minority (1 Black or African American, non-Hispanic/Latino; 1 Two or more races, non-Hispanic/Latino). 9 applicants, 100% accepted, 3 enrolled. In 2013, 4 master's awarded. *Application contact:* Admissions Office, 765-455-9357.
Website: http://www.iuk.edu/academics/majors/allied-health-sciences/index.shtml

Indiana University–Purdue University Indianapolis, School of Public Health, Indianapolis, IN 46202-2896. Offers biostatistics (MPH); environmental health science (MPH); epidemiology (MPH, PhD); health administration (MHA); health policy and management (MPH, PhD); social and behavioral sciences (MPH). *Accreditation:* CEPH. *Students:* 121 full-time (87 women), 161 part-time (111 women); includes 66 minority (32 Black or African American, non-Hispanic/Latino; 19 Asian, non-Hispanic/Latino; 13 Hispanic/Latino; 1 Native Hawaiian or other Pacific Islander, non-Hispanic/Latino; 1 Two or more races, non-Hispanic/Latino), 10 international. Average age 30. 185 applicants, 70% accepted, 95 enrolled. In 2013, 25 master's awarded. Application fee: $55 ($65 for international students). *Expenses:* Contact institution. *Financial support:* In 2013–14, 1 fellowship (averaging $17,650 per year), 4 research assistantships (averaging $22,000 per year), 8 teaching assistantships (averaging $24,000 per year) were awarded. *Unit head:* Dr. Paul Halverson, Dean, 317-274-4242. *Application contact:* Shawne Mathis, Student Services Coordinator, 317-278-0337, E-mail: snmathis@iupui.edu.
Website: http://www.pbhealth.iupui.edu/

Johns Hopkins University, Bloomberg School of Public Health, Baltimore, MD 21205. Offers MHA, MHS, MPH, MPP, MSPH, Sc M, Dr PH, PhD, Sc D, JD/MPH, MBA/MPH, MHS/MA, MSN/MPH, MSW/MPH. *Accreditation:* CEPH (one or more programs are accredited). Part-time programs available. Postbaccalaureate distance learning degree programs offered (minimal on-campus study). *Faculty:* 633 full-time (348 women), 793 part-time/adjunct (433 women). *Students:* 1,419 full-time (1,019 women), 463 part-time (303 women); includes 520 minority (108 Black or African American, non-Hispanic/Latino; 6 American Indian or Alaska Native, non-Hispanic/Latino; 260 Asian, non-Hispanic/Latino; 82 Hispanic/Latino; 1 Native Hawaiian or other Pacific Islander, non-Hispanic/Latino; 63 Two or more races, non-Hispanic/Latino), 487 international. Average age 30. 2,650 applicants, 41% accepted, 561 enrolled. In 2013, 694 master's, 146 doctorates awarded. *Degree requirements:* For master's, comprehensive exam (for some programs), thesis (for some programs); for doctorate, comprehensive exam, thesis/dissertation. *Entrance requirements:* For master's and doctorate, GRE General Test, 3 letters of recommendation, resume/curriculum vitae. Additional exam requirements/recommendations for international students: Required—TOEFL. *Application deadline:* Applications are processed on a rolling basis. Application fee: $45. Electronic applications accepted. *Financial support:* In 2013–14, 1,256 students received support, including 38 fellowships (averaging $34,333 per year), 59 research assistantships (averaging $23,525 per year), 11 teaching assistantships (averaging $3,126 per year); career-related internships or fieldwork, Federal Work-Study, institutionally sponsored loans, scholarships/grants, traineeships, health care benefits, and stipends also available. Support available to part-time students. Financial award application deadline: 3/15; financial award applicants required to submit FAFSA. *Faculty research:* Biodefense studies, infectious/chronic disease, human nutrition, environmental hazards, genetics. *Total annual research expenditures:* $372.9 million. *Unit head:* Dr. Michael J. Klag, Dean, 410-955-3540, Fax: 410-955-0121, E-mail: mklag@jhu.edu. *Application contact:* Leslie K. Vink, Director of Recruitment, Communications and Events, 410-955-3543, Fax: 410-955-0464, E-mail: leslie.vink@jhu.edu.
Website: http://www.jhsph.edu/

Kansas State University, College of Veterinary Medicine, Department of Clinical Sciences, Manhattan, KS 66506. Offers MPH. *Faculty:* 58 full-time (21 women), 16 part-time/adjunct (10 women). *Students:* 47 full-time (34 women), 27 part-time (18 women); includes 5 minority (2 Black or African American, non-Hispanic/Latino; 2 Asian, non-Hispanic/Latino; 1 Hispanic/Latino), 5 international. Average age 32. 42 applicants, 50% accepted, 16 enrolled. In 2013, 26 master's awarded. *Degree requirements:* For master's, thesis. *Entrance requirements:* For master's, GRE, DVM. Additional exam requirements/recommendations for international students: Required—TOEFL (minimum score 550 paper-based). *Application deadline:* For fall admission, 2/1 priority date for domestic and international students; for spring admission, 8/1 priority date for domestic and international students. Applications are processed on a rolling basis. Application fee: $50 ($75 for international students). Electronic applications accepted. *Financial support:* In 2013–14, 11 research assistantships (averaging $30,118 per year) were awarded; institutionally sponsored loans and scholarships/grants also available. Financial award application deadline: 3/1; financial award applicants required to submit FAFSA. *Faculty research:* Clinical trials, equine gastrointestinal ulceration, leptospirosis, food animal pharmacology, equine immunology, diabetes. *Total annual research expenditures:* $1.2 million. *Unit head:* Dr. Michael Cates, Director and Professor, 785-532-2042, E-mail: cates@ksu.edu. *Application contact:* Barta Stevenson, Program Assistant, 785-532-2042, E-mail: bstevens@vet.k-state.edu.
Website: http://www.vet.k-state.edu/depts/ClinicalSciences/

Kansas State University, Graduate School, College of Human Ecology, Department of Human Nutrition, Manhattan, KS 66506. Offers human nutrition (MS, PhD); nutritional sciences (PhD); public health nutrition (PhD); public health physical activity (PhD); sensory analysis and consumer behavior (PhD). Part-time programs available. *Faculty:* 17 full-time (10 women), 11 part-time/adjunct (3 women). *Students:* 19 full-time (11 women), 5 part-time (3 women); includes 3 minority (2 Asian, non-Hispanic/Latino; 1 Hispanic/Latino), 13 international. Average age 30. 34 applicants, 21% accepted, 5 enrolled. In 2013, 3 doctorates awarded. *Degree requirements:* For master's, thesis or alternative, residency; for doctorate, thesis/dissertation, residency. *Entrance requirements:* For master's, GRE General Test, minimum undergraduate GPA of 3.0; for doctorate, GRE General Test, minimum graduate GPA of 3.0. Additional exam requirements/recommendations for international students: Required—TOEFL (minimum score 550 paper-based; 79 iBT), IELTS (minimum score 6.5). *Application deadline:* For fall admission, 2/1 priority date for domestic and international students; for spring admission, 8/1 priority date for domestic and international students. Applications are processed on a rolling basis. Application fee: $50 ($75 for international students). Electronic applications accepted. *Financial support:* In 2013–14, 15 students received support, including 18 research assistantships (averaging $20,000 per year), 4 teaching assistantships with tuition reimbursements available (averaging $11,671 per year); career-related internships or fieldwork, Federal Work-Study, institutionally sponsored loans, scholarships/grants, health care benefits, and tuition waivers (full) also available. Support available to part-time students. Financial award application deadline: 3/1; financial award applicants required to submit FAFSA. *Faculty research:* Biochemical and molecular nutrition, public health nutrition, human and clinical nutrition, sensory analysis and consumer behavior. *Total annual research expenditures:* $809,805. *Unit head:* Dr. Mark Haub, Head, 785-532-5508, Fax: 785-532-3132, E-mail: nutrgrad@ksu.edu. *Application contact:* Janet Finney, Senior Administrative Specialist, 785-532-5508, Fax: 785-532-3132, E-mail: nutrgrad@ksu.edu.
Website: http://www.he.k-state.edu/hn/

La Salle University, School of Nursing and Health Sciences, Program in Public Health, Philadelphia, PA 19141-1199. Offers MPH, MPH/MSN. Part-time and evening/weekend programs available. *Faculty:* 3 full-time (all women), 1 part-time/adjunct (0 women). *Students:* 1 (woman) full-time, 22 part-time (16 women); includes 19 minority (14 Black or African American, non-Hispanic/Latino; 3 Asian, non-Hispanic/Latino; 1 Hispanic/Latino; 1 Two or more races, non-Hispanic/Latino), 1 international. Average age 30. 31 applicants, 55% accepted, 4 enrolled. In 2013, 8 master's awarded. *Degree requirements:* For master's, capstone project. *Entrance requirements:* For master's, minimum undergraduate GPA of 3.0; curriculum vitae/resume; personal statement; 2 letters of reference; interview; prior academic and professional experience in healthcare (recommended). Additional exam requirements/recommendations for international students: Required—TOEFL. *Application deadline:* For fall admission, 8/15 priority date for domestic students, 8/15 for international students; for spring admission, 12/15 priority date for domestic students, 11/15 for international students; for summer admission, 4/14 priority date for domestic students, 3/15 for international students. Application fee: $35. Electronic applications accepted. Application fee is waived when completed online.

Expenses: Tuition: Full-time $20,750; part-time $695 per credit hour. *Required fees:* $300; $200 per year. Tuition and fees vary according to program. *Financial support:* In 2013–14, 1 student received support. Federal Work-Study and scholarships/grants available. Support available to part-time students. Financial award applicants required to submit FAFSA. *Unit head:* Dr. Holly Harner, Director, 215-951-1865, Fax: 215-951-1896, E-mail: mph@lasalle.edu. *Application contact:* Paul J. Reilly, Assistant Vice President, Enrollment Services, 215-951-1940 Ext. 215, Fax: 215-951-1462, E-mail: roszkows@lasalle.edu.
Website: http://www.lasalle.edu/grad/index.php?section-snhs&group-mph&page-index

Laurentian University, School of Graduate Studies and Research, Interdisciplinary Program in Rural and Northern Health, Sudbury, ON P3E 2C6, Canada. Offers PhD.

Loma Linda University, School of Public Health, Loma Linda, CA 92350. Offers MBA, MHA, MPH, MSPH, Dr PH, Postbaccalaureate Certificate. *Accreditation:* CEPH (one or more programs are accredited). Part-time programs available. *Degree requirements:* For doctorate, thesis/dissertation. *Entrance requirements:* For master's, GRE General Test, baccalaureate degree, minimum 3.0 GPA; for doctorate, GRE General Test, minimum GPA of 3.2. Additional exam requirements/recommendations for international students: Required—TOEFL (minimum score 550 paper-based) or Michigan English Language Assessment Battery. Electronic applications accepted. *Faculty research:* Lifestyle and health, nutrition and cancer, nutrition and cardiovascular disease, smoking and health, aging and longevity.

Louisiana State University Health Sciences Center, School of Public Health, New Orleans, LA 70112. Offers behavioral and community health sciences (MPH); biostatistics (MPH, MS, PhD); community health sciences (PhD); environmental and occupational health sciences (MPH); epidemiology (MPH, PhD); health policy and systems management (MPH). *Accreditation:* CEPH. Part-time programs available. *Entrance requirements:* For master's, GRE General Test.

Louisiana State University in Shreveport, College of Business, Education, and Human Development, Program in Public Health, Shreveport, LA 71115-2399. Offers MPH. Program offered jointly with Louisiana State University Health Sciences Center at Shreveport. Part-time and evening/weekend programs available. *Students:* 9 full-time (7 women), 6 part-time (5 women); includes 1 minority (Hispanic/Latino), 2 international. Average age 34. 14 applicants, 100% accepted, 3 enrolled. In 2013, 12 master's awarded. *Entrance requirements:* For master's, GRE or MCAT, 3 letters of recommendation, professional statement, personal interview. Additional exam requirements/recommendations for international students: Required—TOEFL (minimum score 550 paper-based; 80 iBT). *Application deadline:* For fall admission, 6/30 for domestic and international students; for spring admission, 11/30 for domestic and international students. Application fee: $10 ($20 for international students). *Expenses: Tuition, area resident:* Part-time $182 per credit hour. *Required fees:* $51. *Unit head:* Dr. Timothy Winter, Program Director, 318-797-5218, E-mail: timothy.winter@lsus.edu. *Application contact:* Christianne Wojcik, Director of Academic Services, 318-797-5247, Fax: 318-798-4120, E-mail: christianne.wojcik@lsus.edu.

Loyola University Chicago, Graduate School, Public Health Program, Chicago, IL 60660. Offers MPH. Part-time programs available. Postbaccalaureate distance learning degree programs offered (minimal on-campus study). *Faculty:* 7 full-time (3 women), 1 part-time/adjunct (0 women). *Students:* 24 full-time (18 women), 22 part-time (15 women); includes 13 minority (4 Black or African American, non-Hispanic/Latino; 5 Asian, non-Hispanic/Latino; 2 Hispanic/Latino; 1 Native Hawaiian or other Pacific Islander, non-Hispanic/Latino; 1 Two or more races, non-Hispanic/Latino). Average age 32. 81 applicants, 41% accepted, 9 enrolled. In 2013, 16 master's awarded. *Degree requirements:* For master's, comprehensive exam. *Entrance requirements:* For master's, GRE, MCAT. *Application deadline:* For fall admission, 5/15 for domestic and international students; for spring admission, 11/15 for domestic and international students. Application fee is waived when completed online. *Expenses: Tuition:* Full-time $16,740; part-time $930 per credit. *Required fees:* $135 per semester. *Financial support:* Career-related internships or fieldwork available. Financial award applicants required to submit FAFSA. *Faculty research:* Genetics of hypertension and obesity, Vitamin D metabolism, kidney diseases. *Unit head:* Dr. Samuel Attoh, Dean, 773-508-3459, Fax: 773-508-2460, E-mail: sattoh@luc.edu. *Application contact:* Izlze Berzins, Administrative Coordinator, 708-327-9224, Fax: 708-327-9090, E-mail: iberzin@lumc.edu.

Marshall University, Academic Affairs Division, College of Health Professions, Department of Public Health, Huntington, WV 25755. Offers MPH. *Faculty:* 1 full-time (0 women). *Unit head:* William Pewen, Chair, 304-696-3743, E-mail: pewen@marshall.edu. *Application contact:* Information Contact, 304-746-1900, Fax: 304-746-1902, E-mail: services@marshall.edu.
Website: http://www.marshall.edu/cohp/index.php/departments/public-health/

Medical College of Wisconsin, Graduate School of Biomedical Sciences, Department of Population Health, Program in Public Health, Milwaukee, WI 53226-0509. Offers public and community health (PhD); public health (MPH, Graduate Certificate). *Accreditation:* CEPH. *Entrance requirements:* For master's, doctorate, and Graduate Certificate, GRE, official transcripts, three letters of recommendation. Additional exam requirements/recommendations for international students: Required—TOEFL.

Medical College of Wisconsin, Graduate School of Biomedical Sciences, Program in Public and Community Health, Milwaukee, WI 53226-0509. Offers PhD, MD/PhD. *Accreditation:* CEPH. *Degree requirements:* For doctorate, comprehensive exam, thesis/dissertation. *Entrance requirements:* For doctorate, GRE, official transcripts, three letters of recommendation. Additional exam requirements/recommendations for international students: Required—TOEFL (minimum score 580 paper-based; 100 iBT). Electronic applications accepted. *Expenses:* Contact institution. *Faculty research:* Community-academic partnerships, community-based participatory research, injury prevention, health policy, women's health, emergency medical services.

Mercer University, Graduate Studies, Cecil B. Day Campus, College of Health Professions, Atlanta, GA 30341. Offers physical therapy (DPT); physician assistant (MM Sc); public health (MPH). *Faculty:* 23 full-time (17 women), 3 part-time/adjunct (2 women). *Students:* 281 full-time (208 women), 3 part-time (1 woman); includes 105 minority (70 Black or African American, non-Hispanic/Latino; 17 Asian, non-Hispanic/Latino; 6 Hispanic/Latino; 12 Two or more races, non-Hispanic/Latino), 3 international. Average age 26. In 2013, 42 master's, 26 doctorates awarded. *Unit head:* Richard V. Swindle, Senior Vice President, 678-547-6397, E-mail: swindle_rv@mercer.edu. *Application contact:* Tracey M. Wofford, Associate Director of Admissions, 678-547-6422, E-mail: wofford_tm@mercer.edu.
Website: http://chp.mercer.edu/

Michigan State University, College of Human Medicine and The Graduate School, Graduate Programs in Human Medicine, Program in Public Health, East Lansing, MI 48824. Offers MPH.

Missouri State University, Graduate College, College of Health and Human Services, Program in Public Health, Springfield, MO 65897. Offers MPH. *Accreditation:* CEPH. *Faculty:* 3 full-time (1 woman). *Students:* 13 full-time (10 women), 19 part-time (10 women); includes 5 minority (2 Black or African American, non-Hispanic/Latino; 2 Asian, non-Hispanic/Latino; 1 Hispanic/Latino), 7 international. Average age 29. 25 applicants, 68% accepted, 9 enrolled. In 2013, 7 master's awarded. *Degree requirements:* For master's, comprehensive exam, thesis or alternative. *Entrance requirements:* For master's, GRE, minimum GPA of 3.0, 1 year of work experience. Additional exam requirements/recommendations for international students: Required—TOEFL (minimum score 550 paper-based; 79 iBT). *Application deadline:* For fall admission, 7/20 priority date for domestic students, 5/1 for international students; for spring admission, 12/20 priority date for domestic students, 9/1 for international students. Applications are processed on a rolling basis. Application fee: $35 ($50 for international students). Electronic applications accepted. *Expenses:* Tuition, state resident: full-time $4500; part-time $250 per credit hour. Tuition, nonresident: full-time $9018; part-time $501 per credit hour. *Required fees:* $361 per semester. Tuition and fees vary according to course level, course load and program. *Financial support:* In 2013–14, 1 research assistantship with full tuition reimbursement (averaging $8,324 per year) was awarded; Federal Work-Study, institutionally sponsored loans, scholarships/grants, and unspecified assistantships also available. Financial award application deadline: 3/31; financial award applicants required to submit FAFSA. *Unit head:* Dr. David Claborn, Program Director, 417-836-8945, E-mail: davidclaborn@missouristate.edu. *Application contact:* Misty Stewart, Coordinator of Graduate Recruitment, 417-836-6079, Fax: 417-836-6200, E-mail: mistystewart@missouristate.edu.
Website: http://www.missouristate.edu/mph/

Monroe College, King Graduate School, Bronx, NY 10468-5407. Offers business management (MBA); criminal justice (MS); executive leadership in hospitality management (MS); public health (MPH). Program also offered in New Rochelle, NY. Postbaccalaureate distance learning degree programs offered.

Montclair State University, The Graduate School, College of Education and Human Services, Department of Health and Nutrition Sciences, Program in Public Health, Montclair, NJ 07043-1624. Offers MPH. Part-time and evening/weekend programs available. *Degree requirements:* For master's, comprehensive exam, thesis or alternative. *Entrance requirements:* For master's, GRE General Test, essay, 2 letters of recommendation. Additional exam requirements/recommendations for international students: Required—TOEFL (minimum score 83 iBT), IELTS (minimum score 6.5). Electronic applications accepted.

Morehouse School of Medicine, Master of Public Health Program, Atlanta, GA 30310-1495. Offers epidemiology (MPH); health administration, management and policy (MPH); health education/health promotion (MPH); international health (MPH). *Accreditation:* CEPH. Part-time programs available. *Students:* 37 full-time (27 women), 5 part-time (3 women); includes 33 minority (32 Black or African American, non-Hispanic/Latino; 1 American Indian or Alaska Native, non-Hispanic/Latino). Average age 28. In 2013, 13 master's awarded. *Degree requirements:* For master's, thesis, practicum, public health leadership seminar. *Entrance requirements:* For master's, GRE General Test, writing test, public health or human service experience. Additional exam requirements/recommendations for international students: Required—TOEFL (minimum score 550 paper-based). *Application deadline:* For fall admission, 3/1 for domestic and international students. Application fee: $50. Electronic applications accepted. *Expenses:* Contact institution. *Financial support:* Fellowships, research assistantships with partial tuition reimbursements, teaching assistantships, career-related internships or fieldwork, Federal Work-Study, institutionally sponsored loans, scholarships/grants, and unspecified assistantships available. Support available to part-time students. Financial award application deadline: 5/1; financial award applicants required to submit FAFSA. *Faculty research:* Women's and adolescent health, violence prevention, cancer epidemiology/disparities, substance abuse prevention. *Unit head:* Dr. Stephanie Miles-Richardson, Interim Director, 404-752-1944, Fax: 404-752-1051, E-mail: smiles-richardson@msm.edu. *Application contact:* Brandon Hunter, Director of Admissions, 404-752-1650, Fax: 404-752-1512, E-mail: mphadmissions@msm.edu.
Website: http://www.msm.edu/educationTraining/degreePrograms/mph.aspx

Morgan State University, School of Graduate Studies, School of Community Health and Policy, Baltimore, MD 21251. Offers nursing (MS); public health (MPH, Dr PH). *Accreditation:* CEPH. *Degree requirements:* For doctorate, thesis/dissertation. *Entrance requirements:* For doctorate, GRE, minimum GPA of 3.0. Additional exam requirements/recommendations for international students: Required—TOEFL (minimum score 550 paper-based).

National University, Academic Affairs, School of Health and Human Services, La Jolla, CA 92037-1011. Offers clinical affairs (MS); clinical informatics (Certificate); clinical regulatory affairs (MS); health and life science analytics (MS); health coaching (Certificate); health informatics (MS); healthcare administration (MHA); nurse anesthesia (MS); nursing (MS), including forensic nursing, nursing administration, nursing informatics; nursing administration (Certificate); nursing informatics (Certificate); nursing practice (DNP); public health (MPH), including health promotion, healthcare administration, mental health. Part-time and evening/weekend programs available. Postbaccalaureate distance learning degree programs offered (no on-campus study). *Faculty:* 20 full-time (12 women), 27 part-time/adjunct (16 women). *Students:* 229 full-time (176 women), 89 part-time (52 women); includes 215 minority (58 Black or African American, non-Hispanic/Latino; 1 American Indian or Alaska Native, non-Hispanic/Latino; 68 Asian, non-Hispanic/Latino; 63 Hispanic/Latino; 8 Native Hawaiian or other Pacific Islander, non-Hispanic/Latino; 17 Two or more races, non-Hispanic/Latino), 18 international. Average age 33. 118 applicants, 100% accepted, 92 enrolled. In 2013, 29 master's awarded. *Degree requirements:* For master's, thesis (for some programs). *Entrance requirements:* For master's, interview, minimum GPA of 2.5. Additional exam requirements/recommendations for international students: Required—TOEFL (minimum score 550 paper-based; 79 iBT), IELTS (minimum score 6). *Application deadline:* Applications are processed on a rolling basis. Application fee: $60 ($65 for international students). Electronic applications accepted. *Expenses: Tuition:* Full-time $13,824; part-time $1728 per course. One-time fee: $160. *Financial support:* Career-related internships or fieldwork, institutionally sponsored loans, scholarships/grants, and tuition waivers (partial) available. Support available to part-time students. Financial award application deadline: 6/30; financial award applicants required to submit FAFSA. *Faculty research:* Nursing education, obesity prevention, workforce diversity. *Unit head:* School of Health and Human Services, 800-628-8648, E-mail: shhs@nu.edu. *Application contact:* Louis Cruz, Interim Vice President for Enrollment Services, 800-628-8648, E-mail: advisor@nu.edu.
Website: http://www.nu.edu/OurPrograms/SchoolOfHealthAndHumanServices.html

New Mexico State University, Graduate School, College of Health and Social Services, Department of Public Health Sciences, Las Cruces, NM 88003-8001. Offers community health education (MPH); health management, administration and policy (MPH). Part-time programs available. Postbaccalaureate distance learning degree programs offered (minimal on-campus study). *Faculty:* 11 full-time (6 women), 2 part-time/adjunct (1 woman). *Students:* 32 full-time (30 women), 28 part-time (21 women); includes 24 minority (3 Black or African American, non-Hispanic/Latino; 4 American Indian or Alaska Native, non-Hispanic/Latino; 2 Asian, non-Hispanic/Latino; 14 Hispanic/Latino; 1 Two or more races, non-Hispanic/Latino), 1 international. Average age 34. 37 applicants, 68% accepted, 18 enrolled. In 2013, 25 master's awarded. *Degree requirements:* For master's, thesis optional. *Entrance requirements:* For master's, GRE.

Additional exam requirements/recommendations for international students: Required—TOEFL (minimum score 550 paper-based; 79 iBT), IELTS (minimum score 6.5). *Application deadline:* For fall admission, 2/15 for domestic and international students. Application fee: $40 ($50 for international students). Electronic applications accepted. *Expenses:* Tuition, state resident: full-time $5398; part-time $224.90 per credit. Tuition, nonresident: full-time $18,821; part-time $784.20 per credit. *Required fees:* $1310; $54.60 per credit. *Financial support:* In 2013–14, 19 students received support, including 8 teaching assistantships (averaging $8,131 per year); career-related internships or fieldwork, Federal Work-Study, health care benefits, and unspecified assistantships also available. Financial award application deadline: 4/1. *Faculty research:* Community health education, health issues of U.S.-Mexico border, health policy and management, victims of violence, environmental and occupational health issues. *Total annual research expenditures:* $79,183. *Unit head:* Dr. Mark J. Kittleson, Head, 575-646-4300, Fax: 575-646-4343, E-mail: kittle@nmsu.edu. *Application contact:* Dr. James Robinson, III, Graduate Coordinator, 575-646-7431, E-mail: jrobin3@nmsu.edu.
Website: http://publichealth.nmsu.edu

New York Medical College, School of Health Sciences and Practice, Valhalla, NY 10595-1691. Offers MPH, MS, DPT, Dr PH, Graduate Certificate. *Accreditation:* CEPH. Part-time and evening/weekend programs available. Postbaccalaureate distance learning degree programs offered (no on-campus study). *Faculty:* 26 full-time, 77 part-time/adjunct. *Students:* 285 full-time, 230 part-time. Average age 29. 950 applicants, 41% accepted, 264 enrolled. In 2013, 189 master's, 50 doctorates awarded. *Degree requirements:* For master's, thesis, capstone; for doctorate, comprehensive exam, thesis/dissertation, project (for DPT only). *Entrance requirements:* For master's, minimum undergraduate GPA of 3.0; for doctorate, GRE, minimum graduate GPA of 3.2. Additional exam requirements/recommendations for international students: Required—TOEFL (minimum score 637 paper-based; 96 iBT), IELTS (minimum score 7). *Application deadline:* For fall admission, 8/1 priority date for domestic students, 5/15 for international students; for spring admission, 12/1 priority date for domestic students, 10/15 for international students. Applications are processed on a rolling basis. Electronic applications accepted. *Expenses:* Contact institution. *Financial support:* Research assistantships with full and partial tuition reimbursements, teaching assistantships with full and partial tuition reimbursements, career-related internships or fieldwork, Federal Work-Study, institutionally sponsored loans, health care benefits, and tuition waivers (partial) available. Support available to part-time students. Financial award applicants required to submit FAFSA. *Faculty research:* Disaster preparedness, autism, health literacy, adolescent HIV, health disparities, women's health issues, tobacco control, sexual trauma, homelessness, workplace health promotion and stress management. *Unit head:* Dr. Robert W. Amler, Dean, 914-594-4843, Fax: 914-594-4292. *Application contact:* Pamela Suett, Director of Recruitment, 914-594-4510, Fax: 914-594-4292, E-mail: shsp_admissions@nymc.edu.
Website: http://www.nymc.edu/shsp

New York Medical College, School of Health Sciences and Practice, Department of Epidemiology and Community Health, Program in Behavioral Sciences and Health Promotion, Valhalla, NY 10595-1691. Offers advanced public health (Graduate Certificate); behavioral sciences and health promotion (MPH). Part-time and evening/weekend programs available. *Faculty:* 5 full-time, 16 part-time/adjunct. *Students:* 40 full-time, 53 part-time. Average age 32. 40 applicants, 78% accepted, 30 enrolled. In 2013, 25 master's awarded. *Degree requirements:* For master's, thesis. *Entrance requirements:* For master's, minimum undergraduate GPA of 3.0. Additional exam requirements/recommendations for international students: Required—TOEFL (minimum score 637 paper-based; 110 iBT), IELTS (minimum score 7). *Application deadline:* For fall admission, 8/1 priority date for domestic students, 5/15 for international students; for spring admission, 12/1 priority date for domestic students, 10/15 for international students. Applications are processed on a rolling basis. Application fee: $50 ($100 for international students). Electronic applications accepted. *Expenses: Tuition:* Full-time $49,170; part-time $910 per credit. Tuition and fees vary according to program. *Financial support:* Career-related internships or fieldwork, Federal Work-Study, institutionally sponsored loans, health care benefits, and tuition reimbursements available. Support available to part-time students. Financial award applicants required to submit FAFSA. *Unit head:* Dr. Penny Liberatos, Assistant Professor, 914-594-4804, Fax: 914-594-3481, E-mail: penny_liberatos@nymc.edu. *Application contact:* Pamela Suett, Director of Recruitment, 914-594-4510, Fax: 914-594-4292, E-mail: shsp_admissions@nymc.edu.
Website: http://www.nymc.edu/shsp

New York University, Steinhardt School of Culture, Education, and Human Development, Department of Nutrition, Food Studies, and Public Health, Program in Public Health, New York, NY 10003. Offers community and international health (MPH); global health leadership (MPH); public health nutrition (MPH). *Accreditation:* CEPH. Part-time programs available. *Faculty:* 7 full-time (5 women). *Students:* 6 full-time (all women), 2 part-time (both women); includes 3 minority (2 Asian, non-Hispanic/Latino; 1 Hispanic/Latino). Average age 32. 44 applicants, 7% accepted, 2 enrolled. In 2013, 1 degree awarded. *Degree requirements:* For master's, thesis (for some programs). *Entrance requirements:* For master's, GRE General Test. Additional exam requirements/recommendations for international students: Required—TOEFL. *Application deadline:* For fall admission, 12/1 priority date for domestic and international students; for spring admission, 11/1 for domestic and international students. Applications are processed on a rolling basis. Application fee: $75. Electronic applications accepted. *Expenses: Tuition:* Full-time $35,856; part-time $1494 per unit. *Required fees:* $1408; $64 per unit. $473 per term. Tuition and fees vary according to course load and program. *Financial support:* Fellowships with full and partial tuition reimbursements, career-related internships or fieldwork, Federal Work-Study, institutionally sponsored loans, scholarships/grants, and tuition waivers (partial) available. Support available to part-time students. Financial award application deadline: 2/1; financial award applicants required to submit FAFSA. *Faculty research:* Social epidemiology, primary health care, global health, immigrants and health, infectious disease prevention, HIV/AIDS. *Unit head:* Prof. James Macinko, Director, 212-998-5592, Fax: 212-995-4192, E-mail: james.macinko@nyu.edu. *Application contact:* 212-998-5030, Fax: 212-995-4328, E-mail: steinhardt.gradadmissions@nyu.edu.
Website: http://steinhardt.nyu.edu/nutrition/public_health

North Dakota State University, College of Graduate and Interdisciplinary Studies, College of Pharmacy, Nursing and Allied Sciences, Fargo, ND 58108. Offers MPH, MS, DNP, PhD. Part-time programs available. *Faculty:* 20 full-time (10 women), 3 part-time/adjunct (2 women). *Students:* 82 full-time (62 women), 22 part-time (17 women); includes 13 minority (1 Black or African American, non-Hispanic/Latino; 4 American Indian or Alaska Native, non-Hispanic/Latino; 3 Asian, non-Hispanic/Latino; 5 Two or more races, non-Hispanic/Latino), 24 international. Average age 32. 131 applicants, 44% accepted, 48 enrolled. In 2013, 2 master's, 17 doctorates awarded. Terminal master's awarded for partial completion of doctoral program. *Degree requirements:* For master's, thesis; for doctorate, thesis/dissertation. *Entrance requirements:* For master's and doctorate, GRE General Test. Additional exam requirements/recommendations for international students: Required—TOEFL. *Application deadline:* Applications are processed on a rolling basis. Application fee: $35. Electronic applications accepted. *Financial support:* Research assistantships with full tuition reimbursements, career-related internships or fieldwork, Federal Work-Study, institutionally sponsored loans, and scholarships/grants available. Financial award application deadline: 4/1. *Unit head:* Dr. Charles D. Peterson, Dean, 701-231-7456, Fax: 701-231-7606. *Application contact:* Dr. Jonathan Sheng, Assistant Professor, 701-231-6140, Fax: 701-231-8333, E-mail: jonathan.sheng@ndsu.edu.

Northeastern University, Bouvé College of Health Sciences, Boston, MA 02115-5096. Offers audiology (Au D); biotechnology (MS); counseling psychology (MS, PhD, CAGS); counseling/school psychology (PhD); exercise physiology (MS), including exercise physiology, public health; health informatics (MS); nursing (MS, PhD, CAGS), including acute care (MS), administration (MS), anesthesia (MS), primary care (MS), psychiatric mental health (MS); pharmaceutical sciences (PhD); pharmaceutics and drug delivery systems (MS); pharmacology (MS); physical therapy (DPT); physician assistant (MS); school psychology (PhD, CAGS); school/counseling psychology (PhD); speech language pathology (MS); urban public health (MPH); MS/MBA. *Accreditation:* ACPE (one or more programs are accredited). Part-time and evening/weekend programs available. *Degree requirements:* For doctorate, thesis/dissertation (for some programs); for CAGS, comprehensive exam.

Northeast Ohio Medical University, College of Graduate Studies, Rootstown, OH 44272-0095. Offers bioethics (Certificate); health-system pharmacy administration (MS); integrated pharmaceutical medicine (MS, PhD); public health (MS). *Faculty:* 80 part-time/adjunct (26 women). *Students:* 38 full-time (21 women); includes 4 minority (3 Asian, non-Hispanic/Latino; 1 Hispanic/Latino). Average age 28. 45 applicants, 84% accepted, 38 enrolled. In 2013, 9 master's, 1 doctorate awarded. *Application deadline:* For fall admission, 9/1 priority date for domestic students; for winter admission, 1/5 priority date for domestic students. Applications are processed on a rolling basis. Application fee: $45. Electronic applications accepted. Full-time tuition and fees vary according to program. Part-time tuition and fees vary according to degree level. *Unit head:* Dr. Walter E. Horton, Jr., Dean of the College of Graduate Studies. *Application contact:* Luke Gloeckner, Associate Director for Enrollment Services and Registration, 330-325-6274, E-mail: lgloeckner@gmail.com.
Website: http://www.neomed.edu/academics/graduatestudies

Northern Arizona University, Graduate College, College of Health and Human Services, Program in Clinical and Translational Science, Flagstaff, AZ 86011. Offers Certificate. *Entrance requirements:* Additional exam requirements/recommendations for international students: Required—TOEFL (minimum score 550 paper-based; 80 iBT), IELTS (minimum score 7). Application fee: $65. *Financial support:* Applicants required to submit FAFSA.

Northern Illinois University, Graduate School, College of Health and Human Sciences, School of Nursing and Health Studies, De Kalb, IL 60115-2854. Offers nursing (MS); public health (MPH). *Accreditation:* AACN. Part-time programs available. *Faculty:* 12 full-time (11 women), 1 (woman) part-time/adjunct. *Students:* 39 full-time (34 women), 257 part-time (236 women); includes 64 minority (17 Black or African American, non-Hispanic/Latino; 23 Asian, non-Hispanic/Latino; 21 Hispanic/Latino; 3 Two or more races, non-Hispanic/Latino), 7 international. Average age 35. 148 applicants, 40% accepted, 29 enrolled. In 2013, 75 master's awarded. *Degree requirements:* For master's, thesis optional, internship. *Entrance requirements:* For master's, minimum GPA of 3.0 in last 60 hours, BA in nursing, nursing license. Additional exam requirements/recommendations for international students: Required—TOEFL (minimum score 550 paper-based). *Application deadline:* For fall admission, 6/1 for domestic students, 5/1 for international students; for spring admission, 11/1 for domestic students, 10/1 for international students. Applications are processed on a rolling basis. Application fee: $40. Electronic applications accepted. *Financial support:* In 2013–14, 1 research assistantship with full tuition reimbursement, 23 teaching assistantships with full tuition reimbursements were awarded; fellowships with full tuition reimbursements, career-related internships or fieldwork, Federal Work-Study, scholarships/grants, tuition waivers (full), and unspecified assistantships also available. Support available to part-time students. Financial award applicants required to submit FAFSA. *Faculty research:* Neonatal intensive care, stress and coping, refugee and immigrant issues, older adults, autoimmune disorders. *Unit head:* Dr. Janice Strom, Chair, 815-753-6550, Fax: 815-753-0814, E-mail: jstrom@niu.edu. *Application contact:* Graduate School Office, 815-753-0395, E-mail: gradsch@niu.edu.
Website: http://www.chhs.niu.edu/nursing/

Northwestern University, Fienberg School of Medicine, Program in Public Health, Evanston, IL 60208. Offers MPH. *Accreditation:* CEPH. Part-time and evening/weekend programs available. *Entrance requirements:* For master's, GRE General Test. Additional exam requirements/recommendations for international students: Required—TOEFL. *Faculty research:* Cardiovascular epidemiology, cancer epidemiology, nutritional interventions for the prevention of cardiovascular disease and cancer, women's health, outcomes research.

Nova Southeastern University, College of Osteopathic Medicine, Fort Lauderdale, FL 33328. Offers biomedical informatics (MS, Graduate Certificate), including biomedical informatics (MS), clinical informatics (Graduate Certificate), public health informatics (Graduate Certificate); disaster and emergency preparedness (MS); osteopathic medicine (DO); public health (MPH). *Accreditation:* AOsA. *Faculty:* 107 full-time (55 women), 1,235 part-time/adjunct (297 women). *Students:* 1,036 full-time (439 women), 171 part-time (101 women); includes 537 minority (81 Black or African American, non-Hispanic/Latino; 247 Asian, non-Hispanic/Latino; 168 Hispanic/Latino; 41 Two or more races, non-Hispanic/Latino), 31 international. Average age 28. 4,012 applicants, 12% accepted, 246 enrolled. In 2013, 70 master's, 215 doctorates, 1 other advanced degree awarded. *Entrance requirements:* For master's, GRE, licensed healthcare professional or GRE; for doctorate, MCAT, biology, chemistry, organic chemistry, physics (all with labs), and English. *Application deadline:* For fall admission, 1/15 for domestic students. Applications are processed on a rolling basis. Application fee: $50. Electronic applications accepted. *Expenses:* Contact institution. *Financial support:* In 2013–14, 39 students received support, including 24 fellowships (averaging $45,593 per year); research assistantships, teaching assistantships, Federal Work-Study, and scholarships/grants also available. Financial award application deadline: 6/1; financial award applicants required to submit FAFSA. *Faculty research:* Teaching strategies, simulated patient use, HIV/AIDS education, minority health issues, managed care education. *Unit head:* Anthony J. Silavgni, DO, Dean, 954-262-1407, E-mail: silvagni@hpd.nova.edu. *Application contact:* Monica Sanchez, Admissions Counselor, College of Osteopathic Medicine, 954-262-1110, Fax: 954-262-2282, E-mail: mh1156@nova.edu.
Website: http://www.medicine.nova.edu/

The Ohio State University, College of Public Health, Columbus, OH 43210. Offers MHA, MPH, MS, PhD, JD/MHA, MHA/MBA, MHA/MD, MHA/MPA, MHA/MS, MPH/JD, MPH/MD, OD/MPH. *Accreditation:* CAHME; CEPH. Part-time programs available. *Faculty:* 40. *Students:* 244 full-time (180 women), 59 part-time (40 women); includes 56 minority (24 Black or African American, non-Hispanic/Latino; 1 American Indian or Alaska Native, non-Hispanic/Latino; 19 Asian, non-Hispanic/Latino; 8 Hispanic/Latino; 4 Two or more races, non-Hispanic/Latino), 20 international. Average age 29. In 2013, 106 master's, 7 doctorates awarded. Terminal master's awarded for partial completion of doctoral program. *Degree requirements:* For master's, thesis optional, practicum.

Entrance requirements: For master's and doctorate, GRE. Additional exam requirements/recommendations for international students: Required—TOEFL (minimum score 600 paper-based; 100 iBT); Recommended—IELTS (minimum score 8). *Application deadline:* For fall admission, 11/15 for domestic and international students. Applications are processed on a rolling basis. Application fee: $60 ($70 for international students). Electronic applications accepted. *Financial support:* Fellowships with tuition reimbursements and research assistantships with tuition reimbursements available. *Unit head:* Dr. William J. Martin, II, Dean, 614-292-8350, E-mail: martin.3047@osu.edu. *Application contact:* 614-292-8350, Fax: 614-247-1846, E-mail: cph@cph.osu.edu. Website: http://cph.osu.edu/

Ohio University, Graduate College, College of Health Sciences and Professions, Department of Social and Public Health, Athens, OH 45701-2979. Offers early child development and family life (MS); family studies (MS); health administration (MHA); public health (MPH); social work (MSW). *Accreditation:* CEPH. Part-time and evening/weekend programs available. Postbaccalaureate distance learning degree programs offered (no on-campus study). *Degree requirements:* For master's, capstone (MPH). *Entrance requirements:* For master's, GMAT, GRE General Test, previous course work in accounting, management, and statistics, previous public health background (MHA, MPH). Additional exam requirements/recommendations for international students: Required—TOEFL (minimum score 550 paper-based; 80 iBT) or IELTS (minimum score 6.5). Electronic applications accepted. *Expenses:* Contact institution. *Faculty research:* Health care management, health policy, managed care, health behavior, disease prevention.

Old Dominion University, College of Health Sciences, Program in Community Health and Environmental Health, Norfolk, VA 23529. Offers MS. Part-time and evening/weekend programs available. Postbaccalaureate distance learning degree programs offered (no on-campus study). *Faculty:* 5 full-time (2 women), 3 part-time/adjunct (1 woman). *Students:* 3 full-time (1 woman), 15 part-time (8 women); includes 6 minority (3 Black or African American, non-Hispanic/Latino; 1 Asian, non-Hispanic/Latino; 2 Hispanic/Latino), 1 international. Average age 33. 10 applicants, 80% accepted, 7 enrolled. In 2013, 4 master's awarded. *Degree requirements:* For master's, comprehensive exam, oral exam, written exam, practicum or thesis. *Entrance requirements:* For master's, GRE General Test, minimum GPA of 2.75. Additional exam requirements/recommendations for international students: Required—TOEFL (minimum score 650 paper-based). *Application deadline:* For fall admission, 8/1 priority date for domestic students, 7/1 priority date for international students; for winter admission, 11/1 priority date for domestic students, 10/1 priority date for international students; for spring admission, 4/1 priority date for domestic students, 3/1 priority date for international students. Applications are processed on a rolling basis. Application fee: $50. Electronic applications accepted. *Expenses:* Tuition, state resident: full-time $9888; part-time $412 per credit. Tuition, nonresident: full-time $25,152; part-time $1048 per credit. *Required fees:* $59 per semester. One-time fee: $50. *Financial support:* In 2013–14, 5 research assistantships with tuition reimbursements (averaging $14,000 per year), 2 teaching assistantships with partial tuition reimbursements (averaging $10,000 per year) were awarded; career-related internships or fieldwork, institutionally sponsored loans, scholarships/grants, and tuition waivers (partial) also available. Financial award applicants required to submit FAFSA. *Faculty research:* Toxicology, occupational health, environmental hazards. *Total annual research expenditures:* $150,133. *Unit head:* Dr. Anna Jeng, Graduate Program Director, 757-683-4594, Fax: 757-683-4410, E-mail: hjeng@odu.edu. *Application contact:* William Heffelfinger, Director of Graduate Admissions, 757-683-5554, Fax: 757-683-3255, E-mail: gradadmit@odu.edu. Website: http://hs.odu.edu/commhealth/

Oregon State University, College of Public Health and Human Sciences, Program in Public Health, Corvallis, OR 97331. Offers biostatistics (MPH); environmental and occupational health and safety (MPH, PhD); epidemiology (MPH); health management and policy (MPH); health policy (PhD); health promotion and health behavior (MPH, PhD); international health (MPH). *Accreditation:* CEPH. Part-time programs available. *Faculty:* 29 full-time (16 women), 4 part-time/adjunct (3 women). *Students:* 137 full-time (102 women), 29 part-time (18 women); includes 37 minority (4 Black or African American, non-Hispanic/Latino; 7 Asian, non-Hispanic/Latino; 17 Hispanic/Latino; 9 Two or more races, non-Hispanic/Latino), 15 international. Average age 32. 163 applicants, 58% accepted, 48 enrolled. In 2013, 39 master's, 3 doctorates awarded. Terminal master's awarded for partial completion of doctoral program. *Degree requirements:* For doctorate, one foreign language, thesis/dissertation. *Entrance requirements:* For master's and doctorate, GRE, minimum GPA of 3.0 in last 90 hours. Additional exam requirements/recommendations for international students: Required—TOEFL (minimum score 80 iBT), IELTS (minimum score 6.5). *Application deadline:* For fall admission, 12/1 for domestic students. Applications are processed on a rolling basis. Application fee: $60. *Expenses:* Contact institution. *Financial support:* Fellowships, research assistantships, teaching assistantships, career-related internships or fieldwork, Federal Work-Study, and institutionally sponsored loans available. Support available to part-time students. Financial award application deadline: 2/1. *Faculty research:* Traffic safety, health safety, injury control, health promotion. *Unit head:* Dr. Sheryl Thorburn, Professor/Co-Director, 541-737-9493. *Application contact:* Eileen Kaspar, Public Health Graduate Programs Manager, 541-737-3825, E-mail: eileen.kaspar@oregonstate.edu.

Penn State Hershey Medical Center, College of Medicine, Graduate School Programs in the Biomedical Sciences, Graduate Program in Public Health, Hershey, PA 17033. Offers MPH. Part-time and evening/weekend programs available. *Students:* 32 full-time (23 women); includes 9 minority (3 Black or African American, non-Hispanic/Latino; 5 Asian, non-Hispanic/Latino; 1 Hispanic/Latino), 3 international. 56 applicants, 73% accepted, 22 enrolled. *Degree requirements:* For master's, thesis or alternative. *Entrance requirements:* Additional exam requirements/recommendations for international students: Required—TOEFL (minimum score 550 paper-based; 80 iBT). *Application deadline:* For fall admission, 1/31 for domestic students, 2/1 for international students. Applications are processed on a rolling basis. Application fee: $65. Electronic applications accepted. *Financial support:* Fellowships available. Financial award applicants required to submit FAFSA. *Unit head:* Dr. Roger T. Anderson, Director, 717-531-7178, E-mail: rta11@psu.edu. *Application contact:* Amanda Perry, Program Coordinator, 717-531-1502, Fax: 717-531-4359, E-mail: mphprogram@phs.psu.edu. Website: http://www2.med.psu.edu/phs/graduate-programs/

Penn State Hershey Medical Center, College of Medicine, Graduate School Programs in the Biomedical Sciences, Graduate Program in Public Health Sciences, Hershey, PA 17033. Offers MS. Part-time programs available. *Students:* 10 full-time (7 women); includes 1 minority (Asian, non-Hispanic/Latino), 3 international. 26 applicants, 12% accepted, 3 enrolled. In 2013, 9 master's awarded. *Degree requirements:* For master's, thesis or alternative. *Entrance requirements:* Additional exam requirements/recommendations for international students: Required—TOEFL (minimum score 550 paper-based). *Application deadline:* For fall admission, 1/31 priority date for domestic students, 2/1 priority date for international students. Applications are processed on a rolling basis. Application fee: $65. Electronic applications accepted. *Financial support:* Fellowships available. Financial award applicants required to submit FAFSA. *Faculty research:* Clinical trials, statistical methods in genetic epidemiology, genetic factors in nicotine dependence and dementia syndromes, health economics, cancer. *Unit head:* Dr. Douglas Leslie, Chair, 717-531-7178, Fax: 717-531-5779, E-mail: hes-grad-hmc@psu.edu. *Application contact:* Mardi Sawyer, Program Administrator, 717-531-7178, Fax: 717-531-5779, E-mail: hes-grad-hmc@psu.edu. Website: http://www.pennstatehershey.org/web/phs/programs

Ponce School of Medicine & Health Sciences, Program in Public Health, Ponce, PR 00732-7004. Offers epidemiology (Dr PH); public health (MPH). *Accreditation:* CEPH. *Faculty:* 4 full-time (all women), 11 part-time/adjunct (4 women). *Students:* 135 full-time (101 women); all minorities (134 Hispanic/Latino; 1 Two or more races, non-Hispanic/Latino). Average age 34. 57 applicants, 88% accepted, 46 enrolled. In 2013, 22 master's, 1 doctorate awarded. *Degree requirements:* For master's, one foreign language, comprehensive exam, thesis. *Entrance requirements:* For master's, GRE General Test or EXADEP, proficiency in Spanish and English, minimum GPA of 2.7, 3 letters of recommendation; for doctorate, GRE, proficiency in Spanish and English, minimum GPA of 3.0, letter of recommendation. *Application deadline:* For fall admission, 5/15 for domestic students. Application fee: $150. *Financial support:* In 2013–14, 73 students received support. Scholarships/grants available. Financial award application deadline: 5/30; financial award applicants required to submit FAFSA. *Unit head:* Dr. Elizabeth Anne Peterson, Head, 787-840-2575 Ext. 2232, E-mail: apeterson@psm.edu. *Application contact:* Maria Colon, Admissions Officer, 787-840-2575 Ext. 2143, E-mail: mcolon@psm.edu.

Portland State University, Graduate Studies, College of Urban and Public Affairs, School of Community Health, Portland, OR 97207-0751. Offers aging (Certificate); health education (MA, MS); health education and health promotion (MPH); health studies (MPA, MPH), including health administration. MPH offered jointly with Oregon Health & Science University. *Accreditation:* CEPH. Part-time programs available. *Faculty:* 21 full-time (16 women), 28 part-time/adjunct (13 women). *Students:* 39 full-time (33 women), 28 part-time (27 women); includes 13 minority (2 Black or African American, non-Hispanic/Latino; 1 American Indian or Alaska Native, non-Hispanic/Latino; 2 Asian, non-Hispanic/Latino; 4 Hispanic/Latino; 4 Two or more races, non-Hispanic/Latino), 3 international. Average age 30. 127 applicants, 40% accepted, 45 enrolled. In 2013, 45 master's awarded. *Degree requirements:* For master's, oral and written exams. *Entrance requirements:* For master's, GRE General Test, 3 letters of recommendation, minimum GPA of 3.0. Additional exam requirements/recommendations for international students: Required—TOEFL (minimum score 550 paper-based). *Application deadline:* For fall admission, 2/1 for domestic and international students. Application fee: $50. *Expenses:* Tuition, state resident: full-time $9207; part-time $341 per credit. Tuition, nonresident: full-time $14,391; part-time $533 per credit. *Required fees:* $1263; $22 per credit. $98 per quarter. One-time fee: $150. Tuition and fees vary according to program. *Financial support:* In 2013–14, 7 research assistantships with full and partial tuition reimbursements (averaging $5,695 per year), 1 teaching assistantship with full tuition reimbursement (averaging $3,186 per year) were awarded; career-related internships or fieldwork, Federal Work-Study, scholarships/grants, and unspecified assistantships also available. Support available to part-time students. Financial award application deadline: 3/1; financial award applicants required to submit FAFSA. *Total annual research expenditures:* $1.2 million. *Unit head:* Dr. Carlos J. Crespo, Director, 503-725-5120, Fax: 503-725-5100. *Application contact:* Elizabeth Bull, Assistant to the Director, 503-725-4592, Fax: 503-725-5100, E-mail: bulle@pdx.edu. Website: http://www.healthed.pdx.edu/

Purdue University, Graduate School, College of Health and Human Sciences, Department of Nutrition Science, West Lafayette, IN 47907. Offers animal health (MS, PhD); biochemical and molecular nutrition (MS, PhD); growth and development (MS, PhD); human and clinical nutrition (MS, PhD); public health and education (MS, PhD). *Faculty:* 22 full-time (14 women), 10 part-time/adjunct (all women). *Students:* 44 full-time (37 women), 2 part-time (both women); includes 5 minority (2 Black or African American, non-Hispanic/Latino; 1 Asian, non-Hispanic/Latino; 1 Hispanic/Latino; 1 Two or more races, non-Hispanic/Latino), 20 international. Average age 27. 78 applicants, 21% accepted, 10 enrolled. In 2013, 2 master's, 4 doctorates awarded. *Degree requirements:* For master's, thesis; for doctorate, thesis/dissertation. *Entrance requirements:* For master's and doctorate, GRE General Test (minimum scores in verbal and quantitative areas of 1000 or 300 on new scoring), minimum undergraduate GPA of 3.0 or equivalent. Additional exam requirements/recommendations for international students: Required—TOEFL (minimum score 600 paper-based; 77 iBT). *Application deadline:* For fall admission, 1/10 for domestic and international students. Applications are processed on a rolling basis. Application fee: $60 ($75 for international students). Electronic applications accepted. *Financial support:* Fellowships, research assistantships, and teaching assistantships available. Support available to part-time students. Financial award applicants required to submit FAFSA. *Faculty research:* Nutrient requirements, nutrient metabolism, nutrition and disease prevention. *Unit head:* Dr. Connie M. Weaver, Head, 765-494-8237, Fax: 765-494-0674, E-mail: weavercm@purdue.edu. *Application contact:* James C. Smith, Chair of the Graduate Committee, 765-494-0302, E-mail: fleet@purdue.edu. Website: http://www.cfs.purdue.edu/fn/

Purdue University, School of Veterinary Medicine and Graduate School, Graduate Programs in Veterinary Medicine, Department of Comparative Pathobiology, West Lafayette, IN 47907-2027. Offers comparative epidemiology and public health (MS); comparative epidemiology and public heath (PhD); comparative microbiology and immunology (MS, PhD); comparative pathobiology (MS, PhD); interdisciplinary studies (PhD), including microbial pathogenesis, molecular signaling and cancer biology, molecular virology; lab animal medicine (MS); veterinary anatomic pathology (MS); veterinary clinical pathology (MS). Terminal master's awarded for partial completion of doctoral program. *Degree requirements:* For master's, thesis (for some programs); for doctorate, thesis/dissertation. *Entrance requirements:* For master's and doctorate, GRE General Test. Additional exam requirements/recommendations for international students: Required—TOEFL (minimum score 575 paper-based), IELTS (minimum score 6.5), TWE (minimum score 4). Electronic applications accepted.

Queen's University at Kingston, School of Graduate Studies, Faculty of Health Sciences, Department of Community Health and Epidemiology, Kingston, ON K7L 3N6, Canada. Offers epidemiology (PhD); epidemiology and population health (M Sc); health services (M Sc); policy research and clinical epidemiology (M Sc); public health (MPH). Part-time programs available. *Degree requirements:* For master's, thesis. *Entrance requirements:* For master's, GRE General Test (strongly recommended). Additional exam requirements/recommendations for international students: Required—TOEFL (minimum score 600 paper-based). *Faculty research:* Cancer epidemiology, clinical trials, biostatistics health services research, health policy.

Rutgers, The State University of New Jersey, Camden, School of Public Health, Stratford, NJ 08084. Offers general public health (Certificate); health systems and policy (MPH); DO/MPH. *Accreditation:* CEPH. Part-time and evening/weekend programs available. *Degree requirements:* For master's, thesis, internship. *Entrance requirements:* For master's, GRE General Test. Additional exam requirements/recommendations for international students: Required—TOEFL. Electronic applications accepted.

Rutgers, The State University of New Jersey, Newark, School of Public Health, Newark, NJ 07107-1709. Offers clinical epidemiology (Certificate); dental public health

(MPH); general public health (Certificate); public policy and oral health services administration (Certificate); quantitative methods (MPH); urban health (MPH); DMD/MPH; MD/MPH; MS/MPH. *Accreditation:* CEPH. Part-time and evening/weekend programs available. *Degree requirements:* For master's, thesis, internship. *Entrance requirements:* For master's, GRE General Test. Additional exam requirements/recommendations for international students: Required—TOEFL. Electronic applications accepted.

Rutgers, The State University of New Jersey, New Brunswick, Edward J. Bloustein School of Planning and Public Policy, Program in Public Health, Piscataway, NJ 08854-8097. Offers MPH, Dr PH, PhD, MBA/MPH, MD/MPH. MPH, Dr PH, PhD, MD/MPH, MBA/MPH offered jointly wtih University of Medicine and Dentistry of New Jersey. *Accreditation:* CEPH. Part-time and evening/weekend programs available. *Degree requirements:* For master's, internship; for doctorate, thesis/dissertation. *Entrance requirements:* For master's, GMAT, GRE General Test; for doctorate, GRE General Test, MPH (Dr PH). Additional exam requirements/recommendations for international students: Required—TOEFL. *Expenses:* Contact institution. *Faculty research:* Epidemiology, risk perception, statistical research design, health care utilization, health promotion.

Rutgers, The State University of New Jersey, New Brunswick, School of Public Health, Piscataway, NJ 08854. Offers biostatistics (MPH, MS, Dr PH, PhD); clinical epidemiology (Certificate); environmental and occupational health (MPH, Dr PH, PhD, Certificate); epidemiology (MPH, Dr PH, PhD); general public health (Certificate); health education and behavioral science (MPH, Dr PH, PhD); health systems and policy (MPH, PhD); public health preparedness (Certificate); DO/MPH; JD/MPH; MD/MPH; MPH/MBA; MPH/MSPA; MS/MPH; Psy D/MPH. *Accreditation:* CEPH. Part-time and evening/weekend programs available. *Degree requirements:* For master's, thesis, internship; for doctorate, comprehensive exam, thesis/dissertation. *Entrance requirements:* For master's, GRE General Test; for doctorate, GRE General Test, MPH (Dr PH); MA, MPH, or MS (PhD). Additional exam requirements/recommendations for international students: Required—TOEFL. Electronic applications accepted.

St. Catherine University, Graduate Programs, Program in Holistic Health Studies, St. Paul, MN 55105. Offers MA. Part-time programs available. *Degree requirements:* For master's, thesis optional. *Entrance requirements:* For master's, 1 course in anatomy, physiology and psychology. Additional exam requirements/recommendations for international students: Required—TOEFL (minimum score 600 paper-based; 100 iBT). *Expenses:* Contact institution.

St. John's University, College of Pharmacy and Health Sciences, Graduate Programs in Pharmaceutical Sciences and Division of Library and Information Science, Master of Public Health Program, Queens, NY 11439. Offers MPH. Part-time and evening/weekend programs available. *Students:* 5 full-time (4 women), 1 (woman) part-time; includes 5 minority (2 Black or African American, non-Hispanic/Latino; 2 Asian, non-Hispanic/Latino; 1 Hispanic/Latino). Average age 33. 28 applicants, 39% accepted, 6 enrolled. *Degree requirements:* For master's, comprehensive exam, thesis optional, fieldwork. *Entrance requirements:* For master's, GRE, bachelor's degree with pharmacy or related major, minimum GPA of 3.0, 3 letters of recommendation, personal statement. Additional exam requirements/recommendations for international students: Required—TOEFL (minimum score 600 paper-based; 100 iBT), IELTS (minimum score 5.5). *Application deadline:* For fall admission, 3/1 priority date for domestic students, 5/1 priority date for international students; for spring admission, 11/1 priority date for domestic and international students. Applications are processed on a rolling basis. Application fee: $70. Electronic applications accepted. *Expenses:* Contact institution. *Financial support:* Research assistantships, career-related internships or fieldwork, and scholarships/grants available. Support available to part-time students. Financial award application deadline: 3/1; financial award applicants required to submit FAFSA. *Unit head:* Dr. Wenchen Wu, Chair, 718-990-6640, E-mail: wuw@stjohns.edu. *Application contact:* Robert Medrano, Director of Graduate Admissions, 718-990-1601, Fax: 718-990-5686, E-mail: gradhelp@stjohns.edu.
Website: http://www.stjohns.edu/academics/schools-and-colleges/college-pharmacy-and-health-sciences/programs-and-majors

Saint Louis University, Graduate Education, School of Public Health and Graduate Education, Department of Health Management and Policy, St. Louis, MO 63103-2097. Offers health administration (MHA); health policy (MPH); public health studies (PhD). *Accreditation:* CAHME. Part-time programs available. *Degree requirements:* For master's, comprehensive exam, internship. *Entrance requirements:* For master's, GMAT or GRE General Test, LSAT, MCAT, letters of recommendation, resume. Additional exam requirements/recommendations for international students: Required—TOEFL (minimum score 525 paper-based). *Faculty research:* Management of HIV/AIDS, rural health services, prevention of asthma, genetics and health services use, health insurance and access to care.

Salus University, College of Health Sciences, Elkins Park, PA 19027-1598. Offers physician assistant (MMS); public health (MPH). *Accreditation:* ARC-PA. *Entrance requirements:* For master's, GRE (recommended). Additional exam requirements/recommendations for international students: Required—TOEFL. Electronic applications accepted.

San Diego State University, Graduate and Research Affairs, College of Health and Human Services, Graduate School of Public Health, San Diego, CA 92182. Offers environmental health (MPH); epidemiology (MPH, PhD), including biostatistics (MPH); global emergency preparedness and response (MS); global health (PhD); health behavior (PhD); health promotion (MPH); health services administration (MPH); toxicology (MS); MPH/MA; MSW/MPH. *Accreditation:* CAHME (one or more programs are accredited); CEPH (one or more programs are accredited). Part-time programs available. *Degree requirements:* For master's, comprehensive exam (for some programs), thesis (for some programs); for doctorate, thesis/dissertation. *Entrance requirements:* For master's, GMAT (MPH in health services administration), GRE General Test; for doctorate, GRE General Test. Additional exam requirements/recommendations for international students: Required—TOEFL. *Faculty research:* Evaluation of tobacco, AIDS prevalence and prevention, mammography, infant death project, Alzheimer's in elderly Chinese.

San Francisco State University, Division of Graduate Studies, College of Health and Social Sciences, Department of Health Education, San Francisco, CA 94132-1722. Offers MPH. *Accreditation:* CEPH. Part-time programs available. *Students:* Average age 36. *Application deadline:* Applications are processed on a rolling basis. *Unit head:* Dr. Mary Beth Love, Chair and Graduate Program Coordinator, 415-338-1413, E-mail: love@sfsu.edu. *Application contact:* Prof. Sally Geisse, Graduate Co-Coordinator, 415-338-1413, E-mail: sgeisse@sfsu.edu.
Website: http://healthed.sfsu.edu/

San Jose State University, Graduate Studies and Research, College of Applied Sciences and Arts, Department of Health Science, San Jose, CA 95192-0001. Offers applied social gerontology (Certificate); community health education (MPH). *Accreditation:* CEPH (one or more programs are accredited). Postbaccalaureate distance learning degree programs offered. *Entrance requirements:* For master's, GRE General Test. Electronic applications accepted. *Faculty research:* Behavioral science in occupational and health care settings, epidemiology in health care settings.

Sarah Lawrence College, Graduate Studies, Program in Health Advocacy, Bronxville, NY 10708-5999. Offers MA. Part-time programs available. *Faculty:* 11 part-time/adjunct (8 women). *Students:* 18 full-time (all women), 11 part-time (all women); includes 7 minority (2 Black or African American, non-Hispanic/Latino; 3 Hispanic/Latino; 2 Two or more races, non-Hispanic/Latino), 1 international. In 2013, 18 master's awarded. *Degree requirements:* For master's, thesis, fieldwork. *Entrance requirements:* For master's, previous course work in biology and microeconomics, minimum B average in undergraduate course work. Additional exam requirements/recommendations for international students: Required—TOEFL (minimum score 600 paper-based). *Application deadline:* For fall admission, 2/1 priority date for domestic students. Applications are processed on a rolling basis. Application fee: $60. Electronic applications accepted. *Financial support:* In 2013–14, 14 fellowships (averaging $4,448 per year) were awarded; career-related internships or fieldwork and scholarships/grants also available. Support available to part-time students. Financial award application deadline: 3/1; financial award applicants required to submit FAFSA. *Unit head:* Vicki Breitbart, Director, 914-395-2371, E-mail: vbreitbart@sarahlawrence.edu. *Application contact:* Emanual Lomax, Director of Graduate Admission, 914-395-2371, E-mail: elomax@sarahlawrence.edu.

Seattle University, Albers School of Business and Economics, Center for Leadership Formation, Seattle, WA 98122-1090. Offers health leadership (EMBA); leadership (EMBA, Certificate). Evening/weekend programs available. *Faculty:* 16 full-time (5 women), 6 part-time/adjunct (all women). *Students:* 52 full-time (26 women); includes 14 minority (5 Black or African American, non-Hispanic/Latino; 6 Asian, non-Hispanic/Latino; 1 Hispanic/Latino; 2 Two or more races, non-Hispanic/Latino). Average age 41. 46 applicants, 80% accepted, 31 enrolled. In 2013, 37 master's awarded. *Entrance requirements:* For master's, GMAT, 7 years of continuous professional experience, undergraduate degree with minimum GPA of 3.0, resume, writing sample, statement of intent/interest; for Certificate, 7 years of continuous professional experience, undergraduate degree with minimum GPA of 3.0. *Application deadline:* Applications are processed on a rolling basis. Application fee: $55. Electronic applications accepted. *Expenses:* Contact institution. *Financial support:* In 2013–14, 10 students received support. *Unit head:* Dr. Marilyn Gist, Executive Director, 206-296-5374, E-mail: gistm@seattleu.edu. *Application contact:* Sommer Harrison, Recruiting Coordinator, 206-296-2529, Fax: 206-296-2374, E-mail: emba@seattleu.edu.
Website: http://www.seattleu.edu/albers/executiveeducation/

Simon Fraser University, Office of Graduate Studies, Faculty of Health Sciences, Burnaby, BC V5A 1S6, Canada. Offers global health (Graduate Diploma); health sciences (M Sc, PhD); public health (MPH). *Students:* 177 full-time (138 women), 4 part-time (2 women). 373 applicants, 39% accepted, 53 enrolled. In 2013, 66 master's, 1 other advanced degree awarded. *Degree requirements:* For master's, thesis (for some programs); for doctorate, comprehensive exam, thesis/dissertation. *Entrance requirements:* For master's, minimum GPA of 3.0 (on scale of 4.33), or 3.33 based on last 60 credits of undergraduate courses; for doctorate, minimum GPA of 3.5 (on scale of 4.33); for Graduate Diploma, minimum GPA of 2.5 (on scale of 4.33), or 2.67 based on the last 60 credits of undergraduate courses. Additional exam requirements/recommendations for international students: Recommended—TOEFL (minimum score 580 paper-based; 93 iBT), IELTS (minimum score 7), TWE (minimum score 5). Application fee: $90 ($125 for international students). Electronic applications accepted. *Expenses: Tuition, area resident:* Full-time $5084 Canadian dollars. *Required fees:* $840 Canadian dollars. *Financial support:* In 2013–14, 42 students received support, including 39 fellowships (averaging $6,250 per year), teaching assistantships (averaging $5,608 per year); research assistantships, career-related internships or fieldwork, and scholarships/grants also available. *Unit head:* Dr. Jamie Scott, Graduate Chair, 778-782-7189, Fax: 778-782-5927, E-mail: msc-phd-grad-chair@sfu.ca. *Application contact:* Jennifer Van Rassel, Graduate Secretary, 778-782-7036, Fax: 778-782-5927, E-mail: fhsgrads@sfu.ca.
Website: http://www.fhs.sfu.ca/

Southern Connecticut State University, School of Graduate Studies, School of Health and Human Services, Department of Public Health, New Haven, CT 06515-1355. Offers MPH. *Accreditation:* CEPH. Part-time and evening/weekend programs available. *Degree requirements:* For master's, thesis or alternative. *Entrance requirements:* For master's, minimum undergraduate QPA of 3.0 in graduate major field or 2.5 overall, interview. Electronic applications accepted.

State University of New York Downstate Medical Center, College of Medicine, Program in Public Health, Brooklyn, NY 11203-2098. Offers urban and immigrant health (MPH); MD/MPH. *Accreditation:* CEPH. Part-time programs available. *Degree requirements:* For master's, practicum. *Entrance requirements:* For master's, GRE, MCAT or OAT, 2 letters of recommendation, minimum undergraduate GPA of 3.0. Additional exam requirements/recommendations for international students: Required—TOEFL (minimum score 550 paper-based).

Stony Brook University, State University of New York, Stony Brook University Medical Center, Health Sciences Center, School of Medicine, Program in Public Health, Stony Brook, NY 11794. Offers community health (MPH); evaluation sciences (MPH); family violence (MPH); health communication (Certificate); health economics (MPH); population health (MPH); substance abuse (MPH). *Accreditation:* CEPH. *Students:* 36 full-time (28 women), 20 part-time (15 women); includes 22 minority (1 Black or African American, non-Hispanic/Latino; 13 Asian, non-Hispanic/Latino; 8 Hispanic/Latino), 6 international. Average age 39. 84 applicants, 62% accepted, 40 enrolled. In 2013, 22 master's awarded. *Entrance requirements:* For master's, GRE, 3 references, bachelor's degree from accredited college or university with minimum GPA of 3.0, essays, interview. Additional exam requirements/recommendations for international students: Required—TOEFL (minimum score 85 iBT). *Application deadline:* For fall admission, 6/1 for domestic students, 3/15 for international students. Application fee: $100. Electronic applications accepted. *Expenses:* Tuition, state resident: full-time $9870; part-time $411 per credit. Tuition, nonresident: full-time $18,350; part-time $765 per credit. *Financial support:* In 2013–14, 1 fellowship was awarded. *Faculty research:* Population health, health service research, health economics. *Unit head:* Dr. Lisa A. Benz Scott, Director, 631-444-9396, Fax: 631-444-3480, E-mail: lisa.benzscott@stonybrook.edu. *Application contact:* Dr. Jack Fuhrer, 631-444-2113, Fax: 631-444-6032, E-mail: somadmissions@stonybrook.edu.
Website: http://www.stonybrookmedicalcenter.org/publichealth/

Syracuse University, Maxwell School of Citizenship and Public Affairs, Program in Public Health, Syracuse, NY 13244. Offers MPH, CAS. *Students:* 11 full-time (9 women), 4 part-time (3 women), 1 international. Average age 38. In 2013, 7 master's awarded. *Unit head:* Dr. Thomas H. Dennison, Associate Director, 315-443-9060, Fax: 315-443-3385, E-mail: dennis@maxwell.syr.edu. *Application contact:* Dr. Thomas H. Dennison, Associate Director, 315-443-9060, Fax: 315-443-3385, E-mail: dennis@maxwell.syr.edu.

Temple University, College of Health Professions and Social Work, Department of Public Health, Philadelphia, PA 19122. Offers clinical research and translational

medicine (MS); environmental health (MPH); epidemiology (MS); epidemiology and biostatistics (MPH); health policy (PhD); health policy and management (MPH); school health education (Ed M); social and behavioral sciences (MPH, PhD). *Accreditation:* CEPH (one or more programs are accredited). Part-time and evening/weekend programs available. *Faculty:* 27 full-time (18 women). *Students:* 47 full-time (30 women), 45 part-time (37 women); includes 27 minority (9 Black or African American, non-Hispanic/Latino; 10 Asian, non-Hispanic/Latino; 7 Hispanic/Latino; 1 Two or more races, non-Hispanic/Latino), 9 international. 188 applicants, 45% accepted, 29 enrolled. In 2013, 29 master's, 3 doctorates awarded. Terminal master's awarded for partial completion of doctoral program. *Degree requirements:* For master's, thesis (for some programs), capstone project; for doctorate, comprehensive exam, thesis/dissertation. *Entrance requirements:* For master's, GRE General Test (for MS only); DAT, GMAT, MCAT, OAT, PCAT (alternates for MPH, Ed M), minimum undergraduate GPA of 3.0, letters of reference, statement of goals, writing sample, resume, interview (only for MS); for doctorate, GRE General Test, minimum undergraduate GPA of 3.0, 3 letters of reference, statement of goals, writing sample, resume. Additional exam requirements/recommendations for international students: Required—TOEFL (minimum score 550 paper-based; 79 iBT). *Application deadline:* For fall admission, 3/1 for domestic students, 2/1 for international students; for spring admission, 10/15 for domestic students, 8/1 for international students. Applications are processed on a rolling basis. Application fee: $60. Electronic applications accepted. *Financial support:* In 2013–14, 1 fellowship with tuition reimbursement, 4 research assistantships with tuition reimbursements, 8 teaching assistantships with tuition reimbursements were awarded; career-related internships or fieldwork, Federal Work-Study, scholarships/grants, tuition waivers (partial), and unspecified assistantships also available. Financial award application deadline: 1/15. *Faculty research:* Smoking cessation, obesity prevention, tobacco policy, community engagement, health communication. *Total annual research expenditures:* $3.9 million. *Unit head:* Dr. Alice J. Hausman, Chair, 215-204-5112, Fax: 215-204-1854, E-mail: hausman@temple.edu. *Application contact:* Joyce Hankins, 215-204-7213, E-mail: joyce.hankins@temple.edu.
Website: http://chpsw.temple.edu/publichealth/home

Tennessee State University, The School of Graduate Studies and Research, College of Health Sciences, Department of Public Health, Health Administration and Health Sciences, Nashville, TN 37209-1561. Offers public health (MPH). *Degree requirements:* For master's, capstone project.

Texas A&M Health Science Center, School of Rural Public Health, College Station, TX 77840. Offers environmental/occupational health (MPH); epidemiology/biostatistics (MPH); health policy/management (MPH); social and behavioral health (MPH). *Accreditation:* CEPH. Part-time programs available. Postbaccalaureate distance learning degree programs offered (no on-campus study). *Degree requirements:* For master's, thesis optional. *Entrance requirements:* For master's, GRE General Test, minimum undergraduate GPA of 3.0. Electronic applications accepted. *Faculty research:* Tobacco cessation, youth health risk.

Texas A&M University, College of Veterinary Medicine and Biomedical Sciences, Department of Veterinary Integrative Biosciences, College Station, TX 77843. Offers veterinary public health (MS), including epidemiology. *Faculty:* 29. *Students:* 51 full-time (27 women), 13 part-time (10 women); includes 11 minority (1 Black or African American, non-Hispanic/Latino; 5 Asian, non-Hispanic/Latino; 3 Hispanic/Latino; 2 Two or more races, non-Hispanic/Latino), 16 international. Average age 27. 16 applicants, 50% accepted, 8 enrolled. In 2013, 19 master's awarded. Terminal master's awarded for partial completion of doctoral program. *Degree requirements:* For master's, comprehensive exam, thesis. *Entrance requirements:* For master's, GRE General Test, minimum undergraduate GPA of 3.0. Additional exam requirements/recommendations for international students: Required—TOEFL. *Application deadline:* For fall admission, 7/15 priority date for domestic students, 4/1 priority date for international students; for spring admission, 10/1 priority date for domestic students, 9/15 priority date for international students. Applications are processed on a rolling basis. Application fee: $50 ($75 for international students). Electronic applications accepted. *Expenses:* Tuition, state resident: full-time $4078; part-time $226.55 per credit hour. Tuition, nonresident: full-time $10,450; part-time $580.55 per credit hour. *Required fees:* $2328; $278.50 per credit hour. $642.45 per semester. *Financial support:* In 2013–14, fellowships (averaging $18,000 per year), research assistantships (averaging $15,600 per year), teaching assistantships (averaging $15,600 per year) were awarded; institutionally sponsored loans, unspecified assistantships, and clinical associateships also available. Financial award application deadline: 7/15; financial award applicants required to submit FAFSA. *Faculty research:* Metal toxicology, reproductive biology, genetics of neural development, developmental biology, environmental toxicology. *Unit head:* Dr. Evelyn Tiffany-Castiglioni, Head, 979-458-1077, E-mail: c-tiffany@tamu.edu. *Application contact:* Graduate Admissions, 979-845-1044, E-mail: admissions@tamu.edu.
Website: http://vetmed.tamu.edu/vibs

Thomas Jefferson University, Jefferson School of Population Health, Program in Public Health, Philadelphia, PA 19107. Offers MPH, Certificate. *Accreditation:* CEPH. Part-time and evening/weekend programs available. Postbaccalaureate distance learning degree programs offered (minimal on-campus study). Terminal master's awarded for partial completion of doctoral program. *Degree requirements:* For master's, capstone project or thesis. *Entrance requirements:* For master's, GRE or other graduate examination, 2 letters of recommendation, interview, curriculum vitae. Additional exam requirements/recommendations for international students: Required—TOEFL (minimum score 100 iBT). Electronic applications accepted.

Touro University, Graduate Programs, Vallejo, CA 94592. Offers education (MA); medical health sciences (MS); osteopathic medicine (DO); pharmacy (Pharm D); public health (MPH). *Accreditation:* AOsA; ARC-PA. Part-time and evening/weekend programs available. *Faculty:* 103 full-time (54 women), 57 part-time/adjunct (33 women). *Students:* 1,390 full-time (841 women), 27 part-time (20 women). *Degree requirements:* For master's, comprehensive exam, thesis; for doctorate, comprehensive exam. *Entrance requirements:* For doctorate, BS/BA. *Application deadline:* For fall admission, 3/15 for domestic students; for winter admission, 12/1 for domestic students. Applications are processed on a rolling basis. Application fee: $100. Electronic applications accepted. *Financial support:* Fellowships, research assistantships, teaching assistantships, Federal Work-Study, and scholarships/grants available. Support available to part-time students. Financial award applicants required to submit FAFSA. *Faculty research:* Cancer, heart disease. *Application contact:* Steve Davis, Director of Admissions, 707-638-5270, Fax: 707-638-5250, E-mail: steven.davis@tu.edu.

Trident University International, College of Health Sciences, Cypress, CA 90630. Offers MS, PhD, Certificate. Part-time and evening/weekend programs available. Postbaccalaureate distance learning degree programs offered (no on-campus study). *Degree requirements:* For doctorate, comprehensive exam, thesis/dissertation. *Entrance requirements:* For master's, minimum GPA of 2.5 (students with GPA 3.0 or greater may transfer up to 30% of graduate level credits); for doctorate, minimum GPA of 3.4. Additional exam requirements/recommendations for international students: Required—TOEFL. Electronic applications accepted.

Trinity Washington University, School of Business and Graduate Studies, Washington, DC 20017-1094. Offers business administration (MBA); communication (MA); international security studies (MA); organizational management (MSA), including federal program management, human resource management, nonprofit management, organizational development, public and community health. Part-time and evening/weekend programs available. *Degree requirements:* For master's, thesis (for some programs), capstone project (MSA). *Entrance requirements:* For master's, minimum GPA of 2.5. Additional exam requirements/recommendations for international students: Required—TOEFL (minimum score 550 paper-based). *Application deadline:* For fall admission, 4/1 priority date for domestic students; for winter admission, 11/1 priority date for domestic students; for spring admission, 11/1 priority date for domestic students. Applications are processed on a rolling basis. Application fee: $40. *Expenses: Tuition:* Part-time $715 per credit. *Financial support:* Career-related internships or fieldwork and unspecified assistantships available. Support available to part-time students. Financial award application deadline: 4/1; financial award applicants required to submit FAFSA. *Unit head:* Dr. Peggy Lewis, Associate Dean, 202-884-9204, E-mail: lewisp@trinitydc.edu. *Application contact:* Alesha Tyson, Director of Admissions for School of Business and Graduate Studies, 202-884-9400, Fax: 202-884-9229, E-mail: tysona@trinitydc.edu.
Website: http://www.trinitydc.edu/bgs/

Tufts University, School of Medicine, Public Health and Professional Degree Programs, Boston, MA 02111. Offers biomedical sciences (MS); development and regulation of medicines and devices (MS); health communication (MS); pain research, education and policy (MS); physician assistant (MS); public health (MPH, Dr PH). MS programs offered jointly with Emerson College. *Accreditation:* CEPH (one or more programs are accredited). Part-time and evening/weekend programs available. *Faculty:* 77 full-time (26 women), 44 part-time/adjunct (22 women). *Students:* 324 full-time (189 women), 80 part-time (61 women); includes 137 minority (13 Black or African American, non-Hispanic/Latino; 87 Asian, non-Hispanic/Latino; 17 Hispanic/Latino; 20 Two or more races, non-Hispanic/Latino), 24 international. Average age 27. 1,267 applicants, 52% accepted, 245 enrolled. In 2013, 171 master's awarded. *Degree requirements:* For master's, thesis (for some programs); for doctorate, thesis/dissertation. *Entrance requirements:* For master's, GRE General Test, MCAT, GMAT. Additional exam requirements/recommendations for international students: Required—TOEFL (minimum score 96 iBT). *Application deadline:* For fall admission, 1/15 priority date for domestic students, 1/15 for international students; for spring admission, 10/25 priority date for domestic students, 10/25 for international students. Applications are processed on a rolling basis. Application fee: $70. Electronic applications accepted. *Expenses:* Contact institution. *Financial support:* In 2013–14, 17 students received support, including 1 fellowship (averaging $3,000 per year), 21 research assistantships (averaging $500 per year), 35 teaching assistantships (averaging $2,000 per year); Federal Work-Study and scholarships/grants also available. Support available to part-time students. Financial award application deadline: 2/4; financial award applicants required to submit FAFSA. *Faculty research:* Environmental and occupational health, nutrition, epidemiology, health communication, health services management and policy, biostatics, protein interaction, mRNA processing, vascular pathology. *Unit head:* Dr. Aviva Must, Dean, 617-636-0935, Fax: 617-636-0898, E-mail: aviva.must@tufts.edu. *Application contact:* Emily Keily, Director of Admissions, 617-636-0935, Fax: 617-636-0898, E-mail: med-phpd@tufts.edu.
Website: http://publichealth.tufts.edu

Tulane University, School of Public Health and Tropical Medicine, New Orleans, LA 70118-5669. Offers MHA, MMM, MPH, MPHTM, MS, MSPH, Dr PH, PhD, Sc D, Diploma, JD/MHA, JD/MSPH, MD/MPH, MD/MPHTM, MD/MSPH, MD/PhD, MSW/MPH. MS, PhD offered through the Graduate School. *Accreditation:* CAHME (one or more programs are accredited); CEPH (one or more programs are accredited). Part-time and evening/weekend programs available. Postbaccalaureate distance learning degree programs offered (no on-campus study). Terminal master's awarded for partial completion of doctoral program. *Degree requirements:* For master's, comprehensive exam (for some programs); for doctorate, comprehensive exam, thesis/dissertation. *Entrance requirements:* For master's and doctorate, GRE General Test. Additional exam requirements/recommendations for international students: Required—TOEFL. Electronic applications accepted. *Expenses:* Contact institution.

Uniformed Services University of the Health Sciences, School of Medicine, Graduate Programs in the Biomedical Sciences and Public Health, Bethesda, MD 20814. Offers emerging infectious diseases (PhD); medical and clinical psychology (PhD), including clinical psychology, medical psychology; molecular and cell biology (MS, PhD); neuroscience (PhD); preventive medicine and biometrics (MPH, MS, MSPH, MTMH, Dr PH, PhD), including environmental health sciences (PhD), healthcare administration and policy (MS), medical zoology (PhD), public health (MPH, MSPH, Dr PH), tropical medicine and hygiene (MTMH). *Faculty:* 372 full-time (119 women), 4,044 part-time/adjunct (908 women). *Students:* 240 full-time (133 women); includes 40 minority (15 Black or African American, non-Hispanic/Latino; 13 Asian, non-Hispanic/Latino; 12 Hispanic/Latino), 30 international. Average age 25. 598 applicants, 17% accepted, 77 enrolled. In 2013, 19 master's, 50 doctorates awarded. Terminal master's awarded for partial completion of doctoral program. *Degree requirements:* For master's, comprehensive exam, thesis or alternative; for doctorate, comprehensive exam, thesis/dissertation, qualifying exam. *Entrance requirements:* For master's, GRE General Test; for doctorate, GRE General Test, minimum GPA of 3.0. Additional exam requirements/recommendations for international students: Required—TOEFL. *Application deadline:* For fall admission, 1/1 priority date for domestic and international students. Applications are processed on a rolling basis. Application fee: $0. Electronic applications accepted. *Financial support:* In 2013–14, fellowships with full tuition reimbursements (averaging $27,000 per year), research assistantships with full tuition reimbursements (averaging $27,000 per year) were awarded; career-related internships or fieldwork, scholarships/grants, health care benefits, and tuition waivers (full) also available. *Unit head:* Dr. Eleanor S. Metcalf, Associate Dean, 301-295-1104, E-mail: emetcalf@usuhs.edu. *Application contact:* Tina Finley, Administrative Officer, 301-295-3642, Fax: 301-295-6772, E-mail: netina.finley@usuhs.edu.
Website: http://www.usuhs.mil/graded

Uniformed Services University of the Health Sciences, School of Medicine, Graduate Programs in the Biomedical Sciences and Public Health, Department of Preventive Medicine and Biometrics, Program in Public Health, Bethesda, MD 20814-4799. Offers MPH, MSPH, Dr PH. *Accreditation:* CEPH (one or more programs are accredited). *Degree requirements:* For master's, comprehensive exam; for doctorate, thesis/dissertation, qualifying exam. *Entrance requirements:* For master's, GRE General Test; for doctorate, GRE General Test, minimum GPA of 3.0. Additional exam requirements/recommendations for international students: Required—TOEFL. *Application deadline:* For fall admission, 1/1 priority date for domestic students. Applications are processed on a rolling basis. Application fee: $0. *Financial support:* Fellowships with full tuition reimbursements, scholarships/grants, health care benefits, and tuition waivers (full) available. *Faculty research:* Epidemiology, biostatistics, health services administration, environmental and occupational health, tropical public health. *Unit head:* Dr. David Cruess, Director, 301-295-3465, Fax: 301-295-1933, E-mail: dcruess@usuhs.edu. *Application contact:* Elena Marina Sherman, Program

Administrative Specialist, 301-295-3913, Fax: 301-295-6772, E-mail: elena.sherman@usuhs.edu.
Website: http://www.usuhs.mil/pmb

Université de Montréal, Faculty of Arts and Sciences, Program in Societies, Public Policies and Health, Montréal, QC H3C 3J7, Canada. Offers DESS.

Université de Montréal, Faculty of Medicine, Program in Communal and Public Health, Montréal, QC H3C 3J7, Canada. Offers community health (M Sc, DESS); public health (PhD). *Accreditation:* CEPH. Part-time programs available. Terminal master's awarded for partial completion of doctoral program. *Degree requirements:* For master's, thesis; for doctorate, thesis/dissertation, general exam. *Entrance requirements:* For master's and doctorate, proficiency in French, knowledge of English; for DESS, proficiency in French. Electronic applications accepted. *Faculty research:* Epidemiology, health services utilization, health promotion and education, health behaviors, poverty and child health.

University at Albany, State University of New York, School of Public Health, Program in Public Health, Rensselaer, NY 12144. Offers MPH, Dr PH. *Degree requirements:* For master's, thesis; for doctorate, thesis/dissertation. *Entrance requirements:* For master's and doctorate, GRE General Test. Additional exam requirements/recommendations for international students: Required—TOEFL (minimum score 550 paper-based). Electronic applications accepted.

University at Buffalo, the State University of New York, Graduate School, School of Public Health and Health Professions, Department of Epidemiology and Environmental Health, Buffalo, NY 14214. Offers epidemiology (MS, PhD); public health (MPH). *Accreditation:* CEPH. Part-time programs available. *Faculty:* 13 full-time (7 women), 6 part-time/adjunct (3 women). *Students:* 46 full-time (29 women), 14 part-time (11 women); includes 7 minority (2 Black or African American, non-Hispanic/Latino; 5 Asian, non-Hispanic/Latino), 8 international. Average age 29. 147 applicants, 46% accepted, 39 enrolled. In 2013, 15 master's awarded. Terminal master's awarded for partial completion of doctoral program. *Degree requirements:* For master's, comprehensive exam, thesis; for doctorate, comprehensive exam, thesis/dissertation. *Entrance requirements:* For master's and doctorate, GRE General Test. Additional exam requirements/recommendations for international students: Required—TOEFL (minimum score 600 paper-based; 100 iBT). *Application deadline:* For fall admission, 1/15 priority date for domestic and international students. Applications are processed on a rolling basis. Application fee: $50. Electronic applications accepted. *Financial support:* In 2013–14, 17 students received support, including 4 fellowships with full tuition reimbursements available (averaging $22,000 per year), 5 research assistantships with full tuition reimbursements available (averaging $20,000 per year); teaching assistantships with full tuition reimbursements available, career-related internships or fieldwork, Federal Work-Study, institutionally sponsored loans, health care benefits, and unspecified assistantships also available. Financial award application deadline: 2/1; financial award applicants required to submit FAFSA. *Faculty research:* Epidemiology of cancer, nutrition, infectious diseases, epidemiology of environmental, women's health and cardiovascular disease research. *Unit head:* Dr. Youfa Yang, Chair, 716-829-5375, Fax: 716-829-2979, E-mail: phhpadv@buffalo.edu. *Application contact:* Dr. Carl Li, Director of Graduate Studies, 716-829-5382, Fax: 716-829-2979, E-mail: carlli@buffalo.edu.
Website: http://sphhp.buffalo.edu/spm/

The University of Akron, Graduate School, College of Health Professions, School of Nursing, Akron, OH 44325-3701. Offers nursing (MSN, PhD); nursing practice (DNP); public health (MPH). PhD offered jointly with Kent State University. *Accreditation:* AACN; AANA/CANAEP (one or more programs are accredited). Part-time programs available. *Faculty:* 16 full-time (all women), 42 part-time/adjunct (39 women). *Students:* 46 full-time (34 women), 362 part-time (300 women); includes 59 minority (35 Black or African American, non-Hispanic/Latino; 5 Asian, non-Hispanic/Latino; 12 Hispanic/Latino; 1 Native Hawaiian or other Pacific Islander, non-Hispanic/Latino; 6 Two or more races, non-Hispanic/Latino), 3 international. Average age 34. 117 applicants, 75% accepted, 59 enrolled. In 2013, 75 master's awarded. *Degree requirements:* For doctorate, one foreign language, thesis/dissertation, qualifying exam. *Entrance requirements:* For master's, current Ohio state license as registered nurse, three letters of reference, 300-word essay, interview with program coordinator; for doctorate, GRE, minimum GPA of 3.0, MSN, nursing license or eligibility for licensure, writing sample, letters of recommendation, interview, resume, personal statement of research interests and career goals. Additional exam requirements/recommendations for international students: Required—TOEFL (minimum score 550 paper-based; 79 iBT). *Application deadline:* For fall admission, 7/15 for domestic and international students. Applications are processed on a rolling basis. Application fee: $40 ($60 for international students). Electronic applications accepted. *Expenses:* Tuition, state resident: full-time $7430; part-time $412.80 per credit hour. Tuition, nonresident: full-time $12,722; part-time $706.80 per credit hour. *Required fees:* $53 per credit hour. $12 per semester. Tuition and fees vary according to course load and program. *Financial support:* In 2013–14, 11 teaching assistantships with full tuition reimbursements were awarded; career-related internships or fieldwork and Federal Work-Study also available. *Faculty research:* Health promotion and chronic disease prevention, mental health and psychosocial resilience, gerontological health, trauma and violence, gut oxygenation during shock and trauma, simulation and the pedagogy of teaching and learning. *Total annual research expenditures:* $596,812. *Unit head:* Dr. Elaine Fisher, Director, 330-972-6125, E-mail: efisher@uakron.edu. *Application contact:* Dr. Marlene Huff, Graduate Director, 330-972-7555, E-mail: mhuff@uakron.edu.
Website: http://www.uakron.edu/nursing/

The University of Alabama at Birmingham, School of Public Health, Program in Public Health, Birmingham, AL 35294. Offers accelerated industrial hygiene (MPH); applied epidemiology (MSPH); biostatistics (MPH); clinical and translational science (MSPH); environmental health (MPH); environmental health and toxicology (MSPH); epidemiology (MPH); general theory and practice (MPH); health behavior (MPH); health care organization (MPH); health policy quantitative policy analysis (MPH); industrial hygiene (MPH, MSPH); maternal and child health policy (Dr PH); maternal and child health policy and leadership (MPH); occupational health and safety (MPH); outcomes research (MSPH, Dr PH); pharmacoepidemiology and comparative effectiveness research (MSPH); public health (PhD); public health management (Dr PH); public health preparedness management (MPH). *Accreditation:* CEPH. *Entrance requirements:* For master's and doctorate, GRE, evaluations. Additional exam requirements/recommendations for international students: Recommended—TOEFL (minimum score 550 paper-based; 79 iBT), IELTS (minimum score 6.5).

University of Alaska Anchorage, College of Health, Department of Health Sciences, Anchorage, AK 99508. Offers public health practice (MPH). *Accreditation:* CEPH. Part-time programs available. *Degree requirements:* For master's, comprehensive exam, thesis. *Entrance requirements:* For master's, writing sample. Additional exam requirements/recommendations for international students: Required—TOEFL (minimum score 550 paper-based).

University of Alberta, School of Public Health, Department of Public Health Sciences, Edmonton, AB T6G 2E1, Canada. Offers clinical epidemiology (M Sc, MPH); environmental and occupational health (MPH); environmental health sciences (M Sc); epidemiology (M Sc); global health (M Sc, MPH); health policy and management (MPH); health policy research (M Sc); health technology assessment (MPH); occupational health (M Sc); population health (M Sc); public health leadership (MPH); public health sciences (PhD); quantitative methods (MPH). *Accreditation:* CEPH (one or more programs are accredited). Terminal master's awarded for partial completion of doctoral program. *Degree requirements:* For master's, thesis (for some programs); for doctorate, thesis/dissertation. *Entrance requirements:* For master's, GMAT or GRE General Test. Additional exam requirements/recommendations for international students: Required—TOEFL (minimum score 550 paper-based) or IELTS (minimum score 6). Electronic applications accepted. *Faculty research:* Biostatistics, health promotion and socio-behavioral health science.

The University of Arizona, Mel and Enid Zuckerman College of Public Health, Program in Public Health, Tucson, AZ 85721. Offers MPH, Dr PH, PhD. *Faculty:* 30 full-time (17 women), 6 part-time/adjunct (4 women). *Students:* 196 full-time (140 women), 71 part-time (49 women); includes 93 minority (7 Black or African American, non-Hispanic/Latino; 7 American Indian or Alaska Native, non-Hispanic/Latino; 16 Asian, non-Hispanic/Latino; 30 Hispanic/Latino; 33 Two or more races, non-Hispanic/Latino), 10 international. Average age 33. 376 applicants, 53% accepted, 66 enrolled. In 2013, 90 master's, 2 doctorates awarded. *Entrance requirements:* Additional exam requirements/recommendations for international students: Required—TOEFL (minimum score 550 paper-based; 79 iBT). *Application deadline:* For fall admission, 1/1 for domestic and international students. Applications are processed on a rolling basis. Application fee: $75. Electronic applications accepted. *Expenses:* Tuition, state resident: full-time $11,526. Tuition, nonresident: full-time $27,398. *Financial support:* In 2013–14, 40 research assistantships with tuition reimbursements (averaging $23,856 per year), 7 teaching assistantships (averaging $24,265 per year) were awarded. *Total annual research expenditures:* $12.7 million. *Unit head:* Dr. Iman Hakim, Dean, 520-626-7083, E-mail: ihakim@email.arizona.edu. *Application contact:* Amy Clicken, Senior Program Coordinator, 520-626-3201, E-mail: coph-admit@email.arizona.edu.

University of Arkansas for Medical Sciences, College of Public Health, Little Rock, AR 72205-7199. Offers biostatistics (MPH); environmental and occupational health (MPH, Certificate); epidemiology (MPH, PhD); health behavior and health education (MPH); health policy and management (MPH); health promotion and prevention research (PhD); health services administration (MHSA); health systems research (PhD); public health (Certificate); public health leadership (Dr PH). Part-time programs available. *Faculty:* 37 full-time (19 women), 9 part-time/adjunct (5 women). *Students:* 56 full-time (35 women), 85 part-time (58 women); includes 54 minority (38 Black or African American, non-Hispanic/Latino; 1 American Indian or Alaska Native, non-Hispanic/Latino; 8 Asian, non-Hispanic/Latino; 3 Hispanic/Latino; 1 Native Hawaiian or other Pacific Islander, non-Hispanic/Latino; 3 Two or more races, non-Hispanic/Latino), 5 international. Average age 30. 70 applicants, 91% accepted, 33 enrolled. In 2013, 2 master's, 1 doctorate, 2 other advanced degrees awarded. *Degree requirements:* For master's, preceptorship, culminating experience, internship; for doctorate, comprehensive exam, capstone. *Entrance requirements:* For master's, GRE, GMAT, LSAT, PCAT, MCAT, DAT; for doctorate, GRE. Additional exam requirements/recommendations for international students: Required—TOEFL (minimum score 80 iBT), IELTS. *Application deadline:* For fall admission, 3/1 for domestic students, 2/1 for international students; for spring admission, 8/1 for domestic and international students; for summer admission, 2/1 for domestic and international students. Application fee: $25 ($50 for international students). Electronic applications accepted. *Expenses:* Contact institution. *Financial support:* In 2013–14, 8 research assistantships with full tuition reimbursements (averaging $13,000 per year) were awarded; scholarships/grants and tuition waivers (full and partial) also available. *Faculty research:* Health systems, tobacco prevention control, obesity prevention, environmental and occupational exposure, cancer prevention. *Unit head:* Dr. James M. Raczynski, Dean, 501-526-6600, E-mail: raczynskijameson@uams.edu. *Application contact:* Angie Choi, Director of Admission, 501-526-4620, Fax: 501-526-6750, E-mail: anchoi@uams.edu.
Website: http://publichealth.uams.edu/

The University of British Columbia, Faculty of Medicine, School of Population and Public Health, Vancouver, BC V6T 1Z3, Canada. Offers health administration (MHA); health care and epidemiology (MH Sc, PhD); public health (MPH). *Accreditation:* CEPH (one or more programs are accredited). Postbaccalaureate distance learning degree programs offered (minimal on-campus study). *Degree requirements:* For master's, thesis (for some programs), major paper (MH Sc), research project (MHA); for doctorate, thesis/dissertation. *Entrance requirements:* For master's, GRE General Test or GMAT, PCAT, MCAT (MHA), MD or equivalent (for MH Sc); 4-year undergraduate degree from accredited university with minimum B+ overall academic average and in math or statistics course at undergraduate level (for MPH); 4-year undergraduate degree from accredited university with minimum B+ overall academic average plus work experience (for MHA); for doctorate, master's degree from accredited university with minimum B+ overall academic average and in math or statistics course at undergraduate level. Additional exam requirements/recommendations for international students: Required—TOEFL. Electronic applications accepted. *Expenses: Tuition, area resident:* Full-time $8000 Canadian dollars. *Faculty research:* Population and public health, clinical epidemiology, epidemiology and biostatistics, global health and vulnerable populations, health care services and systems, occupational and environmental health, public health emerging threats and rapid response, social and life course determinants of health, health administration.

University of California, Berkeley, Graduate Division, Haas School of Business and School of Public Health, Concurrent MBA/MPH Program, Berkeley, CA 94720-1500. Offers MBA/MPH. *Accreditation:* AACSB; CEPH. *Students:* 35 full-time (22 women); includes 9 minority (8 Asian, non-Hispanic/Latino; 1 Hispanic/Latino), 9 international. Average age 28. *Entrance requirements:* Additional exam requirements/recommendations for international students: Required—TOEFL. *Application deadline:* For fall admission, 10/16 for domestic and international students; for winter admission, 1/8 for domestic and international students; for spring admission, 3/12 for domestic and international students. Application fee: $200. Electronic applications accepted. *Financial support:* Fellowships with tuition reimbursements, teaching assistantships with tuition reimbursements, career-related internships or fieldwork, scholarships/grants, and unspecified assistantships available. Financial award application deadline: 6/12. *Faculty research:* Accounting, business and public policy, economic analysis and public policy, entrepreneurship, finance, management of organizations, marketing, operations and information technology management, real estate. *Unit head:* Prof. Kristi Raube, Director, Health Services Management Program, 510-642-5023, Fax: 510-643-6659, E-mail: raube@haas.berkeley.edu. *Application contact:* Lee Forgue, Student Affairs Officer, 510-642-5023, Fax: 510-643-6659, E-mail: eilis@haas.berkeley.edu.
Website: http://www.haas.berkeley.edu/

University of California, Berkeley, Graduate Division, School of Public Health, Group in Environmental Health Sciences, Berkeley, CA 94720-1500. Offers MPH, MS, Dr PH, PhD. *Degree requirements:* For master's, comprehensive exam (MPH), project or thesis (MS); for doctorate, thesis/dissertation, departmental and qualifying exams. *Entrance requirements:* For master's, GRE General Test, minimum GPA of 3.0; previous course work in biology, calculus, and chemistry; 3 letters of recommendation; for doctorate, GRE General Test, master's degree in relevant scientific discipline or engineering; minimum GPA of 3.0; previous course work in biology, calculus, and chemistry; 3 letters of recommendation. Additional exam requirements/recommendations for international students: Required—TOEFL. *Faculty research:* Toxicology, industrial hygiene, exposure assessment, risk assessment, ergonomics.

University of California, Berkeley, Graduate Division, School of Public Health, Group in Epidemiology, Berkeley, CA 94720-1500. Offers epidemiology (MS, PhD); infectious diseases (MPH, PhD). *Accreditation:* CEPH (one or more programs are accredited). *Degree requirements:* For master's, comprehensive exam; for doctorate, thesis/dissertation, oral and written exam. *Entrance requirements:* For master's, GRE General Test, minimum GPA of 3.0; MD, DDS, DVM, or PhD in biomedical science (MPH); for doctorate, GRE General Test, minimum GPA of 3.0.

University of California, Berkeley, Graduate Division, School of Public Health, Programs in Public Health, Berkeley, CA 94720-1500. Offers MPH, Dr PH. *Accreditation:* CEPH. Postbaccalaureate distance learning degree programs offered (minimal on-campus study). *Degree requirements:* For doctorate, thesis/dissertation, exam. *Entrance requirements:* For doctorate, GRE General Test, minimum GPA of 3.0.

University of California, Irvine, College of Health Sciences, Program in Public Health, Irvine, CA 92697. Offers MPH, PhD. *Students:* 36 full-time (31 women), 2 part-time (both women); includes 24 minority (1 Black or African American, non-Hispanic/Latino; 13 Asian, non-Hispanic/Latino; 6 Hispanic/Latino; 4 Two or more races, non-Hispanic/Latino), 3 international. Average age 27. 163 applicants, 41% accepted, 22 enrolled. In 2013, 13 master's awarded. Application fee: $80 ($100 for international students). *Unit head:* Oladele A. Ogunseitan, Chair, 949-824-6350, Fax: 949-824-2056, E-mail: oladele.ogunseitan@uci.edu. *Application contact:* Stephanie Uiga, Graduate Student Affairs Officer, 949-824-7095, E-mail: suiga@uci.edu.
Website: http://publichealth.uci.edu/

University of California, Irvine, School of Social Ecology, Programs in Social Ecology, Irvine, CA 92697. Offers environmental analysis and design (PhD); epidemiology and public health (PhD); social ecology (PhD). *Students:* 9 full-time (8 women), 2 part-time (0 women); includes 2 minority (1 Asian, non-Hispanic/Latino; 1 Hispanic/Latino), 1 international. Average age 33. 32 applicants, 13% accepted, 2 enrolled. In 2013, 3 doctorates awarded. Application fee: $80 ($100 for international students). *Unit head:* Valerie Jenness, Dean, 949-824-6094, Fax: 949-824-1845, E-mail: jenness@uci.edu. *Application contact:* Adriana Collins, Director of Graduate Student Services, 949-824-5918, Fax: 949-824-1845, E-mail: ajcollins@uci.edu.
Website: http://socialecology.uci.edu/core/graduate-se-core-programs

University of California, Los Angeles, Graduate Division, School of Public Health, Los Angeles, CA 90095. Offers MPH, MS, D Env, Dr PH, PhD, JD/MPH, MA/MPH, MBA/MPH, MD/MPH, MD/PhD, MSW/MPH. *Accreditation:* CAHME (one or more programs are accredited); CEPH (one or more programs are accredited). *Degree requirements:* For doctorate, thesis/dissertation, oral and written qualifying exams. *Entrance requirements:* For master's, GRE General Test, minimum GPA of 3.0; for doctorate, GRE General Test, minimum undergraduate GPA of 3.0. Electronic applications accepted.

University of California, San Diego, Office of Graduate Studies, Program in Public Health, La Jolla, CA 92093-0901. Offers public health and epidemiology (PhD); public health and global health (PhD); public health and health behavior (PhD). Program offered jointly with San Diego State University. *Students:* 35 (25 women); includes 11 minority (3 Black or African American, non-Hispanic/Latino; 4 Asian, non-Hispanic/Latino; 4 Hispanic/Latino), 4 international. In 2013, 11 doctorates awarded. *Degree requirements:* For doctorate, thesis/dissertation, 2 semesters/quarters of teaching assistantship. *Entrance requirements:* For doctorate, GRE General Test, minimum GPA of 3.0. Additional exam requirements/recommendations for international students: Required—TOEFL, IELTS. *Application deadline:* For fall admission, 12/14 for domestic students. Application fee: $55. Electronic applications accepted. *Expenses:* Tuition, state resident: full-time $11,220; part-time $1870 per quarter. Tuition, nonresident: full-time $26,322; part-time $4387 per quarter. *Required fees:* $519.50 per quarter. Part-time tuition and fees vary according to course load and program. *Faculty research:* Maternal and pediatric HIV/AIDS; healthy aging and gender differences; non-parametric and semi-parametric regression, resampling, and the analysis of high-dimensional data; neighborhood correlates of physical activity in children, teens, adults and older adults; medication safety and medication therapy management through practice-based research networks. *Unit head:* John Pierce, Program Director, 858-822-2380, E-mail: jppierce@ucsd.edu. *Application contact:* Hollie Ward, Graduate Coordinator, 858-822-2382, E-mail: hward@ucsd.edu.
Website: http://publichealth.ucsd.edu/jdp/

University of Colorado Denver, Colorado School of Public Health, Program in Public Health, Aurora, CO 80045. Offers community and behavioral health (MPH, Dr PH); environmental and occupational health (MPH); epidemiology (MPH); health systems, management and policy (MPH). *Accreditation:* CEPH. Part-time and evening/weekend programs available. *Faculty:* 14 full-time (13 women). *Students:* 295 full-time (247 women), 49 part-time (39 women); includes 77 minority (17 Black or African American, non-Hispanic/Latino; 3 American Indian or Alaska Native, non-Hispanic/Latino; 16 Asian, non-Hispanic/Latino; 31 Hispanic/Latino; 10 Two or more races, non-Hispanic/Latino), 5 international. Average age 30. 657 applicants, 71% accepted, 132 enrolled. In 2013, 106 master's awarded. *Degree requirements:* For master's, thesis or alternative, 42 credit hours; for doctorate, comprehensive exam, thesis/dissertation, 67 credit hours. *Entrance requirements:* For master's, GRE, MCAT, DAT, LSAT, PCAT, GMAT or master's degree from accredited institution, baccalaureate degree or equivalent; minimum GPA of 3.0; transcripts; references; resume; essay; for doctorate, GRE, MCAT, DAT, LSAT, PCAT or GMAT, MPH or master's or higher degree in related field or equivalent; 2 years of previous work experience in public health; essay; resume. Additional exam requirements/recommendations for international students: Required—TOEFL (minimum score 550 paper-based; 80 iBT). *Application deadline:* For fall admission, 12/15 priority date for domestic students, 12/1 priority date for international students. Application fee: $65. Electronic applications accepted. *Expenses:* Contact institution. *Financial support:* In 2013–14, 125 students received support. Fellowships, research assistantships, teaching assistantships, Federal Work-Study, institutionally sponsored loans, scholarships/grants, traineeships, and unspecified assistantships available. Financial award application deadline: 3/15; financial award applicants required to submit FAFSA. *Faculty research:* Cancer prevention by nutrition, cancer survivorship outcomes, social and cultural factors related to health. *Unit head:* Dr. Lori Crane, Chair, 303-724-4385, E-mail: lori.crane@ucdenver.edu. *Application contact:* Carla Denerstein, Departmental Assistant, 303-724-4446, E-mail: carla.denerstein@ucdenver.edu.
Website: http://www.ucdenver.edu/academics/colleges/PublicHealth/departments/CommunityBehavioralHealth/Pages/CommunityBehavioralHealth.aspx

University of Connecticut, Graduate School, University of Connecticut Health Center, Field of Public Health, Storrs, CT 06269. Offers MPH, JD/MPH. *Degree requirements:* For master's, comprehensive exam. *Entrance requirements:* Additional exam requirements/recommendations for international students: Required—TOEFL (minimum score 550 paper-based). Electronic applications accepted.

University of Connecticut Health Center, Graduate School, Program in Public Health, Farmington, CT 06030. Offers MPH, DMD/MPH, MD/MPH. *Accreditation:* CEPH. Part-time and evening/weekend programs available. *Degree requirements:* For master's, thesis optional. *Entrance requirements:* For master's, GRE. Additional exam requirements/recommendations for international students: Required—TOEFL (minimum score 600 paper-based). Electronic applications accepted. *Faculty research:* Cancer epidemiology, birth defects, gerontology, health manpower, health services.

University of Florida, College of Medicine, Program in Clinical Investigation, Gainesville, FL 32611. Offers clinical investigation (MS); epidemiology (MS); public health (MPH). Part-time programs available. *Entrance requirements:* For master's, GRE, MD, PhD, DMD/DDS or Pharm D. *Expenses:* Tuition, state resident: full-time $12,640. Tuition, nonresident: full-time $30,000.

University of Florida, Graduate School, College of Public Health and Health Professions, Programs in Public Health, Gainesville, FL 32611. Offers biostatistics (MPH); environmental and global health (PhD); environmental health (MPH); epidemiology (MPH); one health (PhD); public health (MPH, PhD, Certificate); public health management and policy (MPH); public health practice (MPH); social and behavioral sciences (MPH); DPT/MPH; DVM/MPH; JD/MPH; MD/MPH; Pharm D/MPH. *Accreditation:* CEPH. Postbaccalaureate distance learning degree programs offered. *Students:* 152 full-time (115 women), 63 part-time (36 women); includes 70 minority (26 Black or African American, non-Hispanic/Latino; 3 American Indian or Alaska Native, non-Hispanic/Latino; 21 Asian, non-Hispanic/Latino; 20 Hispanic/Latino), 18 international. Average age 30. 380 applicants, 41% accepted, 63 enrolled. In 2013, 85 master's, 1 doctorate awarded. *Degree requirements:* For master's, internship. *Entrance requirements:* For master's, GRE General Test, minimum GPA of 3.0. Additional exam requirements/recommendations for international students: Required—TOEFL (minimum score 550 paper-based; 80 iBT), IELTS (minimum score 6). *Application deadline:* For fall admission, 7/1 for domestic students, 4/1 for international students. Application fee: $30. *Expenses:* Tuition, state resident: full-time $12,640. Tuition, nonresident: full-time $30,000. *Financial support:* In 2013–14, 29 students received support, including 2 fellowships (averaging $17,022 per year), 8 research assistantships (averaging $16,662 per year), 19 teaching assistantships (averaging $12,380 per year). Financial award applicants required to submit FAFSA. *Unit head:* Sarah L. McKune, PhD, Program Director, 352-328-0615, Fax: 352-273-6448, E-mail: smckune@ufl.edu. *Application contact:* Telisha Martin, PhD, Associate Director, MPH Program, 352-273-6444, E-mail: martints@ufl.edu.
Website: http://www.mph.ufl.edu/

University of Georgia, College of Public Health, Doctor of Public Health Program, Athens, GA 30602. Offers Dr PH.

University of Hawaii at Manoa, John A. Burns School of Medicine, Department of Public Health Sciences and Epidemiology, Honolulu, HI 96822. Offers epidemiology (PhD); global health and population studies (Graduate Certificate); public health (MPH, MS, Dr PH). *Accreditation:* CEPH. Part-time programs available. *Entrance requirements:* Additional exam requirements/recommendations for international students: Required—TOEFL (minimum score 550 paper-based; 79 iBT), IELTS (minimum score 5).

University of Illinois at Chicago, Graduate College, School of Public Health, Chicago, IL 60607-7128. Offers MHA, MPH, MS, Dr PH, PhD, DDS/MPH, MBA/MPH, MD/PhD, MPH/MS. *Accreditation:* CEPH (one or more programs are accredited). Part-time programs available. *Faculty:* 69 full-time (36 women), 52 part-time/adjunct (21 women). *Students:* 392 full-time (290 women), 295 part-time (211 women); includes 267 minority (98 Black or African American, non-Hispanic/Latino; 102 Asian, non-Hispanic/Latino; 63 Hispanic/Latino; 4 Native Hawaiian or other Pacific Islander, non-Hispanic/Latino), 59 international. Average age 32. 1,288 applicants, 60% accepted, 236 enrolled. In 2013, 226 master's, 14 doctorates awarded. Terminal master's awarded for partial completion of doctoral program. *Degree requirements:* For master's, thesis, field practicum; for doctorate, thesis/dissertation, independent research, internship. *Entrance requirements:* For master's and doctorate, GRE General Test, minimum GPA of 2.75. Additional exam requirements/recommendations for international students: Required—TOEFL. *Application deadline:* For fall admission, 2/1 for domestic students, 1/1 priority date for international students. Applications are processed on a rolling basis. Application fee: $40 ($50 for international students). Electronic applications accepted. *Expenses:* Tuition, state resident: full-time $11,066; part-time $3689 per term. Tuition, nonresident: full-time $23,064; part-time $7688 per term. *Required fees:* $3004; $1190 per term. Tuition and fees vary according to course level and program. *Financial support:* In 2013–14, 4 fellowships with full tuition reimbursements were awarded; research assistantships with full tuition reimbursements, teaching assistantships with full tuition reimbursements, career-related internships or fieldwork, Federal Work-Study, institutionally sponsored loans, scholarships/grants, traineeships, tuition waivers (full), and unspecified assistantships also available. Support available to part-time students. Financial award application deadline: 3/1; financial award applicants required to submit FAFSA. *Faculty research:* Global health, community health, environmental and occupational health, epidemiology and biostatistics, health policy and administration. *Total annual research expenditures:* $34.1 million. *Unit head:* Dr. Paul Brandt-Rauf, Dean, 312-996-6620. *Application contact:* Prof. Babette Neuberger, Associate Dean and Director of Graduate Studies, 312-996-5381, Fax: 312-996-1734, E-mail: bjn@uic.edu.
Website: http://publichealth.uic.edu/

University of Illinois at Springfield, Graduate Programs, College of Public Affairs and Administration, Program in Public Health, Springfield, IL 62703-5407. Offers community health (Graduate Certificate); emergency preparedness and homeland security (Graduate Certificate); epidemiology (Graduate Certificate); public health (MPH). Part-time and evening/weekend programs available. Postbaccalaureate distance learning degree programs offered (no on-campus study). *Faculty:* 5 full-time (3 women), 3 part-time/adjunct (2 women). *Students:* 32 full-time (21 women), 57 part-time (43 women); includes 32 minority (24 Black or African American, non-Hispanic/Latino; 6 Asian, non-Hispanic/Latino; 2 Hispanic/Latino), 10 international. Average age 32. 70 applicants, 47% accepted, 24 enrolled. In 2013, 22 master's, 6 other advanced degrees awarded. *Degree requirements:* For master's, comprehensive exam, internship. *Entrance requirements:* For master's, GRE, minimum undergraduate GPA of 3.0, 3 letters of recommendation, statement of personal goals. Additional exam requirements/recommendations for international students: Required—TOEFL (minimum score 500 paper-based; 61 iBT). *Application deadline:* Applications are processed on a rolling basis. Application fee: $60 ($75 for international students). Electronic applications accepted. *Expenses:* Tuition, state resident: full-time $7440. Tuition, nonresident: full-time $15,744. *Required fees:* $2985.60. *Financial support:* In 2013–14, fellowships with full tuition reimbursements (averaging $9,900 per year), research assistantships with full tuition reimbursements (averaging $9,550 per year), teaching assistantships with full tuition reimbursements (averaging $9,700 per year) were awarded; career-related internships or fieldwork, Federal Work-Study, scholarships/grants, health care benefits, and unspecified assistantships also available. Support available to part-time students. Financial award application deadline: 11/15; financial award applicants required to

submit FAFSA. *Unit head:* Dr. Sharron Lafollette, Program Administrator, 217-206-7894, Fax: 217-206-7279, E-mail: slafo1@uis.edu. *Application contact:* Dr. Lynn Pardie, Office of Graduate Studies, 800-252-8533, Fax: 217-206-7623, E-mail: lpard1@uis.edu.
Website: http://www.uis.edu/publichealth/

University of Illinois at Urbana–Champaign, Graduate College, College of Applied Health Sciences, Department of Kinesiology and Community Health, Champaign, IL 61820. Offers community health (MS, MSPH, PhD); kinesiology (MS, PhD); public health (MPH); rehabilitation (MS); PhD/MPH. *Students:* 138 (83 women). Application fee: $75 ($90 for international students). *Unit head:* Wojciech Chodzko-Zajko, Head, 217-244-0823, Fax: 217-244-7322, E-mail: wojtek@illinois.edu. *Application contact:* Julie Jenkins, Office Administrator, 217-333-1083, Fax: 217-244-7322, E-mail: jjenkns@illinois.edu.
Website: http://www.kch.illinois.edu/

University of Indianapolis, Graduate Programs, College of Health Sciences, Indianapolis, IN 46227-3697. Offers MHS, MOT, MPH, MS, DHS, DPT, OTD. *Students:* 217 full-time (176 women), 165 part-time (137 women); includes 25 minority (10 Black or African American, non-Hispanic/Latino; 8 Asian, non-Hispanic/Latino; 3 Hispanic/Latino; 1 Native Hawaiian or other Pacific Islander, non-Hispanic/Latino; 3 Two or more races, non-Hispanic/Latino), 46 international. Average age 27. In 2013, 82 master's, 49 doctorates awarded. *Expenses: Tuition:* Full-time $5436; part-time $810 per credit hour. *Unit head:* Dr. E. John McIlvried, Associate Provost and Dean of the Graduate School, 317-788-3477, E-mail: jmcilvried@uindy.edu. *Application contact:* Dr. E. John McIlvried, Associate Provost and Dean of the Graduate School, 317-788-3477, E-mail: jmcilvried@uindy.edu.
Website: http://www.uindy.edu/health-sciences

The University of Iowa, College of Dentistry and Graduate College, Graduate Programs in Dentistry, Department of Preventive and Community Dentistry, Iowa City, IA 52242-1316. Offers dental public health (MS). *Degree requirements:* For master's, thesis. *Entrance requirements:* For master's, GRE, DDS. Additional exam requirements/recommendations for international students: Required—TOEFL.

The University of Iowa, Graduate College, College of Public Health, Iowa City, IA 52242-1316. Offers MHA, MPH, MS, PhD, Certificate, DVM/MPH, JD/MHA, JD/MPH, MBA/MHA, MD/MPH, MHA/MA, MS/MA, MS/MS, Pharm D/MPH. *Accreditation:* CEPH. *Degree requirements:* For master's, exam; for doctorate, comprehensive exam, thesis/dissertation. *Entrance requirements:* For master's and doctorate, GRE General Test, minimum GPA of 3.0. Additional exam requirements/recommendations for international students: Required—TOEFL. Electronic applications accepted. *Expenses:* Contact institution.

The University of Kansas, University of Kansas Medical Center, School of Medicine, Department of Preventive Medicine and Public Health, Kansas City, KS 66160. Offers clinical research (MS); environmental health sciences (MPH); epidemiology (MPH); public health management (MPH); social and behavioral health (MPH); MD/MPH; PhD/MPH. Part-time programs available. *Faculty:* 69. *Students:* 30 full-time (23 women), 60 part-time (41 women); includes 27 minority (6 Black or African American, non-Hispanic/Latino; 2 American Indian or Alaska Native, non-Hispanic/Latino; 11 Asian, non-Hispanic/Latino; 3 Hispanic/Latino; 5 Two or more races, non-Hispanic/Latino), 7 international. Average age 34. 62 applicants, 52% accepted, 24 enrolled. In 2013, 37 master's awarded. *Degree requirements:* For master's, thesis, capstone practicum defense. *Entrance requirements:* For master's, GRE, MCAT, LSAT, GMAT or other equivalent graduate professional exam. Additional exam requirements/recommendations for international students: Required—TOEFL. *Application deadline:* For fall admission, 3/1 for domestic and international students. Applications are processed on a rolling basis. Application fee: $60. Electronic applications accepted. *Financial support:* Research assistantships, career-related internships or fieldwork, Federal Work-Study, scholarships/grants, and unspecified assistantships available. Financial award application deadline: 3/1; financial award applicants required to submit FAFSA. *Faculty research:* Cancer screening and prevention, smoking cessation, obesity and physical activity, health services/outcomes research, health disparities. *Total annual research expenditures:* $6.9 million. *Unit head:* Dr. Edward F. Ellerbeck, Chairman, 913-588-2774, Fax: 913-588-2780, E-mail: eellerbe@kumc.edu. *Application contact:* Tanya Honderick, MPH Director, 913-588-2720, Fax: 913-588-8505, E-mail: thonderick@kumc.edu.
Website: http://www.kumc.edu/school-of-medicine/preventive-medicine-and-public-health.html

University of Kentucky, Graduate School, College of Public Health, Program in Public Health, Lexington, KY 40506-0032. Offers MPH. *Accreditation:* CEPH. *Entrance requirements:* For master's, GRE General Test, minimum undergraduate GPA of 2.75. Additional exam requirements/recommendations for international students: Required—TOEFL (minimum score 550 paper-based). Electronic applications accepted.

University of Louisville, Graduate School, School of Public Health and Information Sciences, Department of Environmental and Occupational Health Sciences, Louisville, KY 40202. Offers environmental and occupational health sciences (MPH); public health (PhD), including environmental health. *Accreditation:* CEPH. *Degree requirements:* For master's, thesis optional; for doctorate, comprehensive exam, thesis/dissertation. *Entrance requirements:* For master's and doctorate, GRE General Test. Additional exam requirements/recommendations for international students: Required—TOEFL (minimum score 600 paper-based; 100 iBT). *Application deadline:* For fall admission, 5/1 for domestic and international students. Application fee: $60. Electronic applications accepted. *Expenses:* Tuition, state resident: full-time $10,788; part-time $599 per credit hour. Tuition, nonresident: full-time $22,446; part-time $1247 per credit hour. *Required fees:* $196. Tuition and fees vary according to program and reciprocity agreements. *Financial support:* Research assistantships with full tuition reimbursements, health care benefits, and unspecified assistantships available. Financial award applicants required to submit FAFSA. *Faculty research:* Breast cancer in minority populations, health policy, clinical trials, chronic disease, genetic epidemiology, program evaluation, electronic medical records, children's environmental health, lung injury. *Unit head:* Dr. David J. Tollerud, Department Chair, 502-852-3290, Fax: 502-852-3291, E-mail: david.tollerud@louisville.edu.
Website: http://louisville.edu/sphis/departments/environmental-occupational-health-sciences

The University of Manchester, School of Dentistry, Manchester, United Kingdom. Offers basic dental sciences (cancer studies) (M Phil, PhD); basic dental sciences (molecular genetics) (M Phil, PhD); basic dental sciences (stem cell biology) (M Phil, PhD); biomaterials sciences and dental technology (M Phil, PhD); dental public health/community dentistry (M Phil, PhD); dental science (clinical) (PhD); endodontology (M Phil, PhD); fixed and removable prosthodontics (M Phil, PhD); operative dentistry (M Phil, PhD); oral and maxillofacial surgery (M Phil, PhD); oral radiology (M Phil, PhD); orthodontics (M Phil, PhD); restorative dentistry (M Phil, PhD).

University of Maryland, College Park, Academic Affairs, School of Public Health, College Park, MD 20742. Offers MA, MHA, MPH, MS, PhD. Part-time and evening/weekend programs available. *Faculty:* 109 full-time (63 women), 71 part-time/adjunct (45 women). *Students:* 196 full-time (145 women), 74 part-time (59 women); includes 102 minority (54 Black or African American, non-Hispanic/Latino; 1 American Indian or Alaska Native, non-Hispanic/Latino; 28 Asian, non-Hispanic/Latino; 13 Hispanic/Latino; 6 Two or more races, non-Hispanic/Latino), 31 international. 713 applicants, 24% accepted, 89 enrolled. In 2013, 42 master's, 16 doctorates awarded. *Degree requirements:* For doctorate, thesis/dissertation. *Entrance requirements:* For master's and doctorate, GRE General Test, minimum GPA of 3.0, 3 letters of recommendation. Additional exam requirements/recommendations for international students: Required—TOEFL. *Application deadline:* For fall admission, 1/15 for domestic students, 2/1 for international students; for spring admission, 6/1 for international students. Applications are processed on a rolling basis. Application fee: $75. Electronic applications accepted. *Expenses:* Tuition, state resident: full-time $10,314; part-time $573 per credit hour. Tuition, nonresident: full-time $22,248; part-time $1236 per credit. *Required fees:* $1446; $403.15 per semester. Tuition and fees vary according to program. *Financial support:* In 2013–14, 22 fellowships with full and partial tuition reimbursements (averaging $26,966 per year), 12 research assistantships (averaging $16,059 per year), 88 teaching assistantships (averaging $15,959 per year) were awarded; career-related internships or fieldwork, Federal Work-Study, and scholarships/grants also available. Support available to part-time students. Financial award applicants required to submit FAFSA. *Total annual research expenditures:* $12.6 million. *Unit head:* Dr. Jane E. Clark, Dean, 301-405-2438, Fax: 301-314-9167, E-mail: jeclark@umd.edu. *Application contact:* Dr. Charles A. Caramello, Dean of Graduate School, 301-405-0358, Fax: 301-314-9305, E-mail: ccaramel@umd.edu.

University of Massachusetts Amherst, Graduate School, Interdisciplinary Programs, Dual Degree Program in Public Health and Public Policy and Administration, Amherst, MA 01003. Offers MPH/MPPA. *Students:* 1 (woman) full-time, 1 (woman) part-time. Average age 35. *Entrance requirements:* Additional exam requirements/recommendations for international students: Required—TOEFL (minimum score 550 paper-based; 80 iBT), IELTS (minimum score 6.5). *Application deadline:* For fall admission, 2/1 for domestic and international students. Applications are processed on a rolling basis. Application fee: $75. Electronic applications accepted. *Financial support:* Career-related internships or fieldwork, Federal Work-Study, scholarships/grants, traineeships, health care benefits, tuition waivers, and unspecified assistantships available. Support available to part-time students. Financial award application deadline: 2/1. *Unit head:* Dr. Kathryn McDermott, Director, 413-545-2714, E-mail: szoller@pubpol.umass.edu. *Application contact:* Lindsay DeSantis, Supervisor of Admissions, 413-545-0722, Fax: 413-577-0010, E-mail: gradadm@grad.umass.edu.
Website: http://www.masspolicy.org/acad_mppa_health.html

University of Massachusetts Amherst, Graduate School, School of Public Health and Health Sciences, Department of Public Health, Amherst, MA 01003. Offers biostatistics (MPH, MS, PhD); community health education (MPH, MS, PhD); environmental health sciences (MPH, MS, PhD); epidemiology (MPH, MS, PhD); health policy and management (MPH, MS, PhD); nutrition (MPH, PhD); public health practice (MPH); MPH/MPPA. *Accreditation:* CEPH (one or more programs are accredited). Part-time and evening/weekend programs available. Postbaccalaureate distance learning degree programs offered (no on-campus study). *Faculty:* 53 full-time (29 women). *Students:* 117 full-time (83 women), 271 part-time (213 women); includes 89 minority (34 Black or African American, non-Hispanic/Latino; 23 Asian, non-Hispanic/Latino; 25 Hispanic/Latino; 7 Two or more races, non-Hispanic/Latino), 45 international. Average age 36. 359 applicants, 69% accepted, 94 enrolled. In 2013, 120 master's, 1 doctorate awarded. Terminal master's awarded for partial completion of doctoral program. *Degree requirements:* For master's, thesis (for some programs); for doctorate, comprehensive exam, thesis/dissertation. *Entrance requirements:* For master's and doctorate, GRE General Test. Additional exam requirements/recommendations for international students: Required—TOEFL (minimum score 550 paper-based; 80 iBT), IELTS (minimum score 6.5). *Application deadline:* For fall admission, 2/1 for domestic and international students. Applications are processed on a rolling basis. Application fee: $75. Electronic applications accepted. *Financial support:* Fellowships with full and partial tuition reimbursements, research assistantships with full and partial tuition reimbursements, teaching assistantships with full and partial tuition reimbursements, career-related internships or fieldwork, Federal Work-Study, scholarships/grants, traineeships, health care benefits, tuition waivers (full and partial), and unspecified assistantships available. Support available to part-time students. Financial award application deadline: 2/1; financial award applicants required to submit FAFSA. *Unit head:* Dr. Paula Stamps, Graduate Program Director, 413-545-2861, Fax: 413-545-1645. *Application contact:* Lindsay DeSantis, Supervisor of Admissions, 413-545-0722, Fax: 413-577-0010, E-mail: gradadm@grad.umass.edu.
Website: http://www.umass.edu/sphhs/public_health/

University of Massachusetts Lowell, College of Health Sciences, Department of Clinical Laboratory and Nutritional Sciences, Lowell, MA 01854-2881. Offers clinical laboratory sciences (MS); clinical pathology (Graduate Certificate); nutritional sciences (Graduate Certificate); public health laboratory sciences (Graduate Certificate). *Accreditation:* NAACLS. Part-time programs available. Postbaccalaureate distance learning degree programs offered. *Degree requirements:* For master's, thesis optional. *Entrance requirements:* For master's, GRE General Test, minimum GPA of 3.0, letters of recommendation. *Faculty research:* Cardiovascular disease, lipoprotein metabolism, micronutrient evaluation, alcohol metabolism, mycobacterial drug resistance.

University of Memphis, Graduate School, School of Public Health, Memphis, TN 38152. Offers biostatistics (MPH); environmental health (MPH); epidemiology (MPH); health systems management (MPH); public health (MHA); social and behavioral sciences (MPH). Part-time and evening/weekend programs available. Postbaccalaureate distance learning degree programs offered. *Faculty:* 14 full-time (2 women), 5 part-time/adjunct (1 woman). *Students:* 64 full-time (42 women), 36 part-time (24 women); includes 34 minority (21 Black or African American, non-Hispanic/Latino; 6 Asian, non-Hispanic/Latino; 5 Hispanic/Latino; 2 Two or more races, non-Hispanic/Latino), 15 international. Average age 32. 102 applicants, 51% accepted, 24 enrolled. In 2013, 17 master's awarded. *Degree requirements:* For master's, comprehensive exam, thesis. *Entrance requirements:* For master's, GRE, letters of recommendation. Additional exam requirements/recommendations for international students: Required—TOEFL. *Application deadline:* For fall admission, 4/1 for domestic students; for spring admission, 11/1 for domestic students. Application fee: $35 ($60 for international students). Electronic applications accepted. *Financial support:* In 2013–14, 46 students received support. Research assistantships with full tuition reimbursements available, Federal Work-Study, scholarships/grants, and unspecified assistantships available. Financial award application deadline: 2/15; financial award applicants required to submit FAFSA. *Faculty research:* Health and medical savings accounts, adoption rates, health informatics, Telehealth technologies, biostatistics, environmental health, epidemiology, health systems management, social and behavioral sciences. *Unit head:* Dr. Lisa M. Klesges, Director, 901-678-4637, E-mail: lmklsges@memphis.edu. *Application contact:* Dr. Karen Weddle-West, Information Contact, 901-678-2531, Fax: 901-678-5023, E-mail: gradsch@memphis.edu.
Website: http://www.memphis.edu/sph/

University of Miami, Graduate School, Miller School of Medicine, Graduate Programs in Medicine, Department of Epidemiology and Public Health, Coral Gables, FL 33124.

Offers epidemiology (PhD); public health (MPH, MSPH); JD/MPH; MD/MPH; MD/PhD; MPA/MPH; MPH/MAIA. *Accreditation:* CEPH (one or more programs are accredited). Part-time programs available. *Degree requirements:* For master's, thesis (for some programs), project, practicum; for doctorate, comprehensive exam, thesis/dissertation. *Entrance requirements:* For master's, GRE General Test, minimum GPA of 3.0, 3 letters of recommendation; for doctorate, GRE General Test, minimum GPA of 3.0, course work in epidemiology and statistics, 3 letters of recommendation. Additional exam requirements/recommendations for international students: Required—TOEFL (minimum score 550 paper-based; 59 iBT). Electronic applications accepted. *Faculty research:* Behavioral epidemiology, substance abuse, AIDS, cardiovascular diseases, women's health.

University of Michigan, School of Public Health, Ann Arbor, MI 48109. Offers MHSA, MPH, MS, PhD, JD/MHSA, MD/MPH, MHSA/MBA, MHSA/MNA, MHSA/MPP, MHSA/MSIOE, MPH/JD, MPH/MA, MPH/MBA, MPH/MPP, MPH/MS, MPH/MSW. MS and PhD offered through the Horace H. Rackham School of Graduate Studies. *Accreditation:* CAHME (one or more programs are accredited); CEPH (one or more programs are accredited). Part-time and evening/weekend programs available. Terminal master's awarded for partial completion of doctoral program. *Degree requirements:* For doctorate, oral defense of dissertation, preliminary exam. *Entrance requirements:* For master's and doctorate, GRE General Test. Additional exam requirements/recommendations for international students: Required—TOEFL (minimum score 560 paper-based; 100 iBT). Electronic applications accepted. Tuition and fees vary according to course level, course load, degree level, program and student level.

University of Michigan–Flint, School of Health Professions and Studies, Flint, MI 48502-1950. Offers anesthesia (MS, DrAP); health education (MS); nursing (MSN, DNP, Certificate), including family nurse practitioner (MSN), nursing (Certificate), nursing practice (DNP); physical therapy (DPT, PhD), including entry-level (DPT), physical therapy (PhD), transitional (DPT); public health (MPH), including health administration, health education. Part-time programs available. *Faculty:* 30 full-time (25 women), 23 part-time/adjunct (17 women). *Students:* 338 full-time (243 women), 204 part-time (155 women); includes 86 minority (37 Black or African American, non-Hispanic/Latino; 3 American Indian or Alaska Native, non-Hispanic/Latino; 21 Asian, non-Hispanic/Latino; 13 Hispanic/Latino; 1 Native Hawaiian or other Pacific Islander, non-Hispanic/Latino; 11 Two or more races, non-Hispanic/Latino), 34 international. Average age 33. 711 applicants, 30% accepted, 198 enrolled. In 2013, 40 master's, 73 doctorates awarded. *Entrance requirements:* Additional exam requirements/recommendations for international students: Required—TOEFL (minimum score 560 paper-based; 84 iBT), IELTS (minimum score 6.5). *Application deadline:* For fall admission, 8/1 priority date for domestic students, 5/1 priority date for international students; for winter admission, 11/15 priority date for domestic students, 9/1 priority date for international students; for spring admission, 3/15 priority date for domestic students, 1/1 priority date for international students. Application fee: $55. Electronic applications accepted. *Expenses:* Contact institution. *Financial support:* Career-related internships or fieldwork, Federal Work-Study, scholarships/grants, and traineeships available. Support available to part-time students. Financial award application deadline: 3/1; financial award applicants required to submit FAFSA. *Faculty research:* Male colorectal cancer, Flint health careers, auditory stimulation, nurse preparation training, healthy aging and physical therapy. *Unit head:* Dr. David Gordon, Dean, 810-237-6503, Fax: 810-237-6532, E-mail: dgordon@umflint.edu. *Application contact:* Brad T. Maki, Executive Secretary, 810-762-3171, Fax: 810-766-6789, E-mail: bmaki@umflint.edu.
Website: http://www.umflint.edu/shps/

University of Minnesota, Twin Cities Campus, School of Public Health, Minneapolis, MN 55455. Offers MHA, MPH, MS, PhD, Certificate, DVM/MPH, JD/MS, JD/PhD, MD/MPH, MD/PhD, MPH/JD, MPH/MS, MPH/MSN, MPP/MS. *Accreditation:* CEPH (one or more programs are accredited). Part-time programs available. Postbaccalaureate distance learning degree programs offered (minimal on-campus study). Terminal master's awarded for partial completion of doctoral program. *Degree requirements:* For doctorate, thesis/dissertation. *Entrance requirements:* For master's and doctorate, GRE General Test. Additional exam requirements/recommendations for international students: Required—TOEFL. Electronic applications accepted. *Expenses:* Contact institution.

University of Missouri, Graduate School, Master of Public Health Program, Columbia, MO 65211. Offers global public health (Graduate Certificate); health promotion and policy (MPH); public health (Graduate Certificate); veterinary public health (MPH); DVM/MPH; MPH/MA; MPH/MPA. *Accreditation:* CEPH. *Students:* 88 full-time (67 women), 104 part-time (83 women); includes 43 minority (19 Black or African American, non-Hispanic/Latino; 9 Asian, non-Hispanic/Latino; 10 Hispanic/Latino; 5 Two or more races, non-Hispanic/Latino), 16 international. Average age 30. 133 applicants, 84% accepted, 79 enrolled. In 2013, 40 master's, 49 other advanced degrees awarded. *Entrance requirements:* Additional exam requirements/recommendations for international students: Required—TOEFL (minimum score 550 paper-based; 80 iBT). *Application deadline:* For fall admission, 6/30 priority date for domestic and international students. Applications are processed on a rolling basis. Application fee: $55 ($75 for international students). Electronic applications accepted. *Financial support:* Fellowships with tuition reimbursements, research assistantships with tuition reimbursements, teaching assistantships with tuition reimbursements, scholarships/grants, traineeships, health care benefits, and unspecified assistantships available. Support available to part-time students. *Faculty research:* Health professions, health care equality, global health, communicable diseases, public health; zoonosis and infectious diseases, medical education, inquiry-based learning, social determinants of health, violence against women, health disparities, breast cancer screening, epigenetic, nursing, environmental health, cancer and chronic diseases, environmental exposures with metals, geographical information systems, substance use disorders/addictions, mental health. *Unit head:* Lise Saffran, Interim Director, 573-884-6835, E-mail: saffranl@health.missouri.edu. *Application contact:* Sandra Gummersheimer, Academic Advisor, 573-884-6836, E-mail: gummersheimers@health.missouri.edu.
Website: http://publichealth.missouri.edu/

University of Missouri, School of Medicine, Program in Public Health, Columbia, MO 65211. Offers MS. *Accreditation:* CEPH. *Students:* 1 full-time (0 women), 1 part-time (0 women), 1 international. Average age 35. *Entrance requirements:* For master's, 3 letters of recommendation; personal statement; curriculum vitae or resume; verification from medical school and residency program; official transcripts. Additional exam requirements/recommendations for international students: Required—TOEFL (minimum score 500 paper-based). *Unit head:* Dr. Steven C. Zweig, Chair, Department of Family and Community Medicine, 573-884-7411. *Application contact:* Ashley Granger, Administrative Assistant, 573-884-7060, E-mail: grangeran@health.missouri.edu.
Website: http://www.fcm.missouri.edu

The University of Montana, Graduate School, College of Health Professions and Biomedical Sciences, School of Public and Community Health Sciences, Missoula, MT 59812-0002. Offers public health (MPH, CPH). *Accreditation:* CEPH. Part-time programs available. Postbaccalaureate distance learning degree programs offered. *Unit head:* Craig Molgaard, Chair, 406-243-4445, Fax: 406-243-4209, E-mail: craig.molgaard@umontana.edu. *Application contact:* Information Contact, E-mail: gradschl@mso.umt.edu.
Website: http://www.health.umt.edu/schools/pch/

University of Nebraska Medical Center, College of Public Health, Omaha, NE 68198-4355. Offers MPH. *Accreditation:* CEPH. Part-time programs available. Postbaccalaureate distance learning degree programs offered (minimal on-campus study). *Degree requirements:* For master's, service-learning capstone course. *Entrance requirements:* Additional exam requirements/recommendations for international students: Required—TOEFL (minimum score 550 paper-based). Electronic applications accepted. *Expenses: Required fees:* $300 per semester. Tuition and fees vary according to program. *Faculty research:* Ethics, environmental health, cultural influence on health, rural health policy, cancer prevention.

University of Nevada, Las Vegas, Graduate College, School of Community Health Sciences, Department of Environmental and Occupational Health, Las Vegas, NV 89154-3064. Offers public health (MPH, PhD). *Faculty:* 12 full-time (6 women), 3 part-time/adjunct (all women). *Students:* 37 full-time (26 women), 50 part-time (36 women); includes 33 minority (4 Black or African American, non-Hispanic/Latino; 4 American Indian or Alaska Native, non-Hispanic/Latino; 6 Asian, non-Hispanic/Latino; 9 Hispanic/Latino; 2 Native Hawaiian or other Pacific Islander, non-Hispanic/Latino; 8 Two or more races, non-Hispanic/Latino), 5 international. Average age 35. 29 applicants, 59% accepted, 8 enrolled. In 2013, 26 master's awarded. *Entrance requirements:* Additional exam requirements/recommendations for international students: Required—TOEFL (minimum score 550 paper-based; 80 iBT), IELTS (minimum score 7). *Application deadline:* For fall admission, 4/1 for domestic students, 5/1 for international students; for spring admission, 11/1 for domestic students, 10/1 for international students. Application fee: $60 ($95 for international students). Electronic applications accepted. *Expenses:* Tuition, state resident: full-time $4752; part-time $264 per credit. Tuition, nonresident: full-time $18,662; part-time $554.50 per credit. *International tuition:* $18,952 full-time. *Required fees:* $532; $12 per credit. $266 per semester. One-time fee: $35. Tuition and fees vary according to course load and program. *Financial support:* In 2013–14, 20 students received support, including 20 research assistantships with partial tuition reimbursements available (averaging $10,295 per year); institutionally sponsored loans, scholarships/grants, health care benefits, and unspecified assistantships also available. Financial award application deadline: 3/1. *Faculty research:* Environmental health: micro (mold) to macro (Lake Mead ecosystem). *Total annual research expenditures:* $1.8 million. *Unit head:* Chris Cochran, Chair/Associate Professor, 702-895-1400, E-mail: chris.cochran@unlv.edu. *Application contact:* Graduate College Admissions Evaluator, 702-895-3320, Fax: 702-895-4180, E-mail: gradcollege@unlv.edu.
Website: http://publichealth.unlv.edu/EOH_welcome.html

University of Nevada, Reno, Graduate School, Division of Health Sciences, Department of Public Health, Reno, NV 89557. Offers MPH, PhD, MPH/MSN. *Accreditation:* CEPH. Terminal master's awarded for partial completion of doctoral program. *Degree requirements:* For master's, thesis optional, culminating experience; for doctorate, thesis/dissertation. *Entrance requirements:* For master's, GRE General Test, GMAT, LSAT, MCAT or DAT, minimum GPA of 2.75; for doctorate, GRE General Test, GMAT, LSAT, MCAT or DAT, minimum GPA of 3.0. Additional exam requirements/recommendations for international students: Required—TOEFL (minimum score 500 paper-based; 61 iBT), IELTS (minimum score 6). Electronic applications accepted. *Faculty research:* Biomechanics and basic fundamentals of skiing, social psychology in sports and recreation, fitness and aging, elementary physical education, body fat evaluation.

University of New England, College of Graduate Studies–Public Health, Portland, ME 04103. Offers MPH, Certificate. Part-time and evening/weekend programs available. Postbaccalaureate distance learning degree programs offered (no on-campus study). *Faculty:* 3 full-time (2 women), 10 part-time/adjunct (5 women). *Students:* 211 full-time (152 women), 37 part-time (26 women); includes 22 minority (13 Black or African American, non-Hispanic/Latino; 2 American Indian or Alaska Native, non-Hispanic/Latino; 5 Asian, non-Hispanic/Latino; 2 Hispanic/Latino). Average age 33. 251 applicants, 69% accepted, 131 enrolled. In 2013, 27 master's, 4 other advanced degrees awarded. *Application deadline:* Applications are processed on a rolling basis. Application fee: $40. Electronic applications accepted. *Financial support:* Application deadline: 5/1; applicants required to submit FAFSA. *Unit head:* Dr. Denise Bisaillon, Director, Graduate Programs in Public Health/Associate Professor, 207-221-4464. *Application contact:* Dr. Cynthia Forrest, Vice President for Student Affairs, 207-221-4225, Fax: 207-523-1925, E-mail: gradadmissions@une.edu.
Website: http://www.une.edu/publichealth

University of New Hampshire, Graduate School Manchester Campus, Manchester, NH 03101. Offers business administration (MBA); counseling (M Ed); education (M Ed, MAT); educational administration and supervision (M Ed, Ed S); information technology (MS); management of technology (MS); public administration (MPA); public health (MPH, Certificate); social work (MSW); software systems engineering (Certificate). Part-time and evening/weekend programs available. *Students:* 2 full-time (0 women), 5 part-time (0 women), 2 international. Average age 38. 6 applicants, 17% accepted, 1 enrolled. In 2013, 1 master's awarded. *Degree requirements:* For master's, thesis or alternative. *Entrance requirements:* Additional exam requirements/recommendations for international students: Required—TOEFL (minimum score 550 paper-based; 80 iBT). *Application deadline:* For fall admission, 6/1 for domestic students, 4/1 for international students; for spring admission, 12/1 for domestic students. Applications are processed on a rolling basis. Application fee: $65. Electronic applications accepted. *Expenses:* Tuition, state resident: full-time $13,500; part-time $750 per credit hour. Tuition, nonresident: full-time $26,200; part-time $1100 per credit hour. *Required fees:* $1741; $435.25 per term. Tuition and fees vary according to course level, course load, campus/location and program. *Financial support:* Fellowships, research assistantships, teaching assistantships, Federal Work-Study, scholarships/grants, health care benefits, and unspecified assistantships available. Support available to part-time students. Financial award application deadline: 3/1; financial award applicants required to submit FAFSA. *Unit head:* Candice Brown, Director, 603-641-4313, E-mail: unhm.gradcenter@unh.edu. *Application contact:* Graduate Admissions Office, 603-862-3000, Fax: 603-862-0275, E-mail: grad.school@unh.edu.
Website: http://www.gradschool.unh.edu/manchester/

University of New Hampshire, Graduate School, School of Health and Human Services, Department of Health Management and Policy, Durham, NH 03824. Offers public health (MPH, Postbaccalaureate Certificate). Part-time and evening/weekend programs available. *Faculty:* 9 full-time (4 women). *Students:* 23 full-time (20 women), 23 part-time (18 women); includes 4 minority (all Black or African American, non-Hispanic/Latino), 2 international. Average age 33. 34 applicants, 71% accepted, 12 enrolled. In 2013, 15 master's, 2 other advanced degrees awarded. *Entrance requirements:* For master's, GMAT or GRE General Test. Additional exam requirements/recommendations for international students: Required—TOEFL (minimum score 550 paper-based; 80 iBT). *Application deadline:* For fall admission, 6/1 priority date for domestic students, 4/1 for international students; for spring admission, 12/1 for domestic students. Applications are processed on a rolling basis. Application fee: $65. Electronic applications accepted. *Expenses:* Contact institution. *Financial support:* In

2013–14, 1 student received support. Fellowships, research assistantships, teaching assistantships, and scholarships/grants available. Financial award application deadline: 2/15. *Unit head:* Bob McGrath, Chairperson, 603-862-5047. *Application contact:* Chris Hamann, Administrative Assistant, 603-862-2733, E-mail: masterof.publichealth@unh.edu.
Website: http://chhs.unh.edu/hmp/index

University of New Mexico, School of Medicine, Program in Public Health, Albuquerque, NM 87131-5196. Offers community health (MPH); epidemiology (MPH); health systems, services and policy (MPH). *Accreditation:* CEPH. Part-time programs available. Postbaccalaureate distance learning degree programs offered. *Faculty:* 11 full-time (7 women), 4 part-time/adjunct (3 women). *Students:* 17 full-time (15 women), 16 part-time (12 women); includes 16 minority (3 Black or African American, non-Hispanic/Latino; 2 American Indian or Alaska Native, non-Hispanic/Latino; 1 Asian, non-Hispanic/Latino; 9 Hispanic/Latino; 1 Two or more races, non-Hispanic/Latino), 1 international. Average age 36. 46 applicants, 59% accepted, 17 enrolled. In 2013, 15 master's awarded. *Degree requirements:* For master's, thesis. *Entrance requirements:* For master's, GRE, MCAT, 2 years of experience in health field. Additional exam requirements/recommendations for international students: Required—TOEFL. *Application deadline:* For fall admission, 2/1 for domestic students. Application fee: $50. *Financial support:* Fellowships, research assistantships with tuition reimbursements, and Federal Work-Study available. Financial award application deadline: 12/15; financial award applicants required to submit FAFSA. *Faculty research:* Epidemiology, rural health, environmental health, Native American health issues. *Total annual research expenditures:* $1 million. *Unit head:* Dr. Kristine Tollestrup, Director, 505-272-4173, Fax: 505-272-4494, E-mail: ktollestrup@salud.unm.edu. *Application contact:* Gayle Garcia, Education Coordinator, 505-272-3982, Fax: 505-272-4494, E-mail: garciag@salud.unm.edu.
Website: http://fcm.unm.edu/

The University of North Carolina at Chapel Hill, Graduate School, Gillings School of Global Public Health, Chapel Hill, NC 27499-7400. Offers MHA, MPH, MS, MSCR, MSEE, MSPH, Dr PH, PhD, DDS/MPH, JD/MPH, MBA/MHA, MBA/MSPH, MD/MPH, MD/MSPH, MHA/MBA, MHA/MCRP, MHA/MSIS, MHA/MSLS, MPH/MCRP, MPH/MSW, MSPH/M Ed, MSPH/MCRP, MSPH/MSIS, MSPH/MSLS, MSPH/MSW, MSPH/PhD. *Accreditation:* CAHME (one or more programs are accredited); CEPH (one or more programs are accredited). Part-time programs available. Postbaccalaureate distance learning degree programs offered (minimal on-campus study). Terminal master's awarded for partial completion of doctoral program. *Degree requirements:* For master's, comprehensive exam, thesis, paper, capstone; for doctorate, comprehensive exam, thesis/dissertation. *Entrance requirements:* For master's and doctorate, GRE General Test, minimum GPA of 3.0 (recommended). Additional exam requirements/recommendations for international students: Required—TOEFL. Electronic applications accepted. *Faculty research:* Infection disease, health promotion and disease prevention, injury prevention, international health, environmental studies, occupational health studies.

The University of North Carolina at Charlotte, The Graduate School, College of Health and Human Services, Department of Health Behavior and Administration, Charlotte, NC 28223-0001. Offers community health (Certificate); health administration (MHA); health services research (PhD); public health (MSPH). *Accreditation:* CAHME. Part-time programs available. *Degree requirements:* For master's, thesis or comprehensive exam; for doctorate, thesis/dissertation. *Entrance requirements:* For master's, GRE or MAT (public health), GRE or GMAT (health administration), minimum GPA of 3.0 during previous 2 years, 2.75 overall. Additional exam requirements/recommendations for international students: Required—TOEFL (minimum score 557 paper-based; 83 iBT). *Application deadline:* For fall admission, 7/1 for domestic students, 5/1 for international students; for spring admission, 11/1 for domestic students, 10/1 for international students. Applications are processed on a rolling basis. Application fee: $65 ($75 for international students). Electronic applications accepted. *Expenses:* Tuition, state resident: full-time $3522. Tuition, nonresident: full-time $16,051. *Required fees:* $2585. Tuition and fees vary according to course load and program. *Financial support:* Research assistantships, teaching assistantships, career-related internships or fieldwork, Federal Work-Study, institutionally sponsored loans, scholarships/grants, and unspecified assistantships available. Support available to part-time students. Financial award application deadline: 4/1; financial award applicants required to submit FAFSA. *Faculty research:* Pediatric asthma self-management, reproductive epidemiology, social aspects of injury prevention, chronic illness self-care, competency-based professional education, cognitive health, aging and dementia, infant health outcomes, policing and suicide, data mining for health executive decision support, segmentation analyses in identifying patient satisfaction problems in the primary care setting, enhancing community capacity through data sharing. *Unit head:* Dr. Gary S. Silverman, Chair, 704-687-7191, Fax: 704-687-6122, E-mail: arharver@uncc.edu. *Application contact:* Kathy B. Giddings, Director of Graduate Admissions, 704-687-5503, Fax: 704-687-1668, E-mail: gradadm@uncc.edu.
Website: http://publichealth.uncc.edu/degrees-and-programs/phs-graduate-programs

University of North Dakota, Graduate School, College of Nursing, Department of Nursing, Grand Forks, ND 58202. Offers adult-gerontological nurse practitioner (MSN); advanced public health nurse (MSN); family nurse practitioner (MSN); nurse anesthesia (MSN); nurse educator (MSN); nursing (DNP, PhD); psychiatric and mental health nurse practitioner (MSN).

University of Northern Colorado, Graduate School, College of Natural and Health Sciences, School of Human Sciences, Program in Public Health, Greeley, CO 80639. Offers public health education (MPH). *Accreditation:* CEPH. *Degree requirements:* For master's, comprehensive exam, thesis or alternative. *Entrance requirements:* For master's, GRE General Test, 2 letters of recommendation. Electronic applications accepted.

University of North Florida, Brooks College of Health, Department of Public Health, Jacksonville, FL 32224. Offers aging services (Certificate); community health (MPH); geriatric management (MSH); health administration (MHA); rehabilitation counseling (MS). *Accreditation:* CEPH. Part-time and evening/weekend programs available. *Faculty:* 16 full-time (9 women), 4 part-time/adjunct (3 women). *Students:* 119 full-time (79 women), 59 part-time (34 women); includes 52 minority (20 Black or African American, non-Hispanic/Latino; 2 American Indian or Alaska Native, non-Hispanic/Latino; 9 Asian, non-Hispanic/Latino; 18 Hispanic/Latino; 3 Two or more races, non-Hispanic/Latino), 6 international. Average age 30. 271 applicants, 40% accepted, 72 enrolled. In 2013, 57 master's awarded. *Degree requirements:* For master's, thesis optional. *Entrance requirements:* For master's, GRE General Test (MSH, MS, MPH); GMAT or GRE General Test (MHA), minimum GPA of 3.0 in last 60 hours. Additional exam requirements/recommendations for international students: Required—TOEFL (minimum score 500 paper-based). *Application deadline:* For fall admission, 7/1 for domestic students, 5/1 for international students; for spring admission, 11/1 for domestic students, 10/1 for international students. Application fee: $30. Electronic applications accepted. *Expenses:* Tuition, state resident: full-time $9794; part-time $408.10 per credit hour. Tuition, nonresident: full-time $22,383; part-time $932.61 per credit hour. *Required fees:* $2020; $84.20 per credit hour. Tuition and fees vary according to course load and program. *Financial support:* In 2013–14, 38 students received support, including 2 teaching assistantships (averaging $1,500 per year); research assistantships, career-related internships or fieldwork, Federal Work-Study, scholarships/grants, and tuition waivers (partial) also available. Support available to part-time students. Financial award application deadline: 4/1; financial award applicants required to submit FAFSA. *Faculty research:* Dietary supplements; alcohol, tobacco, and other drug use prevention; turnover among health professionals; aging; psychosocial aspects of disabilities. *Total annual research expenditures:* $21,747. *Unit head:* Dr. Jeffrey Harrison, Chair, 904-620-1440, Fax: 904-620-2848, E-mail: jeffrey.harrison@unf.edu. *Application contact:* Dr. Heather Kenney, Director of Advising, 904-620-2810, Fax: 904-620-1030, E-mail: heather.kenney@unf.edu.
Website: http://www.unf.edu/brooks/public_health/

University of North Texas Health Science Center at Fort Worth, School of Public Health, Fort Worth, TX 76107-2699. Offers biostatistics (MPH); community health (MPH); disease control and prevention (Dr PH); environmental and occupational health sciences (MPH); epidemiology (MPH); health administration (MHA); health policy and management (MPH, Dr PH); DO/MPH; MS/MPH; MSN/MPH. MPH offered jointly with University of North Texas; DO/MPH with Texas College of Osteopathic Medicine. *Accreditation:* CEPH. Part-time and evening/weekend programs available. *Degree requirements:* For master's, thesis or alternative, supervised internship; for doctorate, thesis/dissertation, supervised internship. *Entrance requirements:* For master's, GRE General Test. Additional exam requirements/recommendations for international students: Required—TOEFL. Electronic applications accepted.

University of Oklahoma Health Sciences Center, Graduate College, College of Public Health, Program in General Public Health, Oklahoma City, OK 73190. Offers MPH, Dr PH. *Faculty:* 7 full-time (3 women), 1 part-time/adjunct (0 women). *Students:* 78 full-time (55 women), 65 part-time (48 women); includes 66 minority (18 Black or African American, non-Hispanic/Latino; 11 American Indian or Alaska Native, non-Hispanic/Latino; 17 Asian, non-Hispanic/Latino; 7 Hispanic/Latino; 13 Two or more races, non-Hispanic/Latino), 18 international. Average age 30. 209 applicants, 71% accepted, 66 enrolled. In 2013, 20 master's, 2 doctorates awarded. *Expenses:* Tuition, state resident: full-time $3504; part-time $175.20 per credit hour. Tuition, nonresident: full-time $13,504; part-time $675.20 per credit hour. *Required fees:* $1545; $52.70 per credit hour. $245.25 per semester. Tuition and fees vary according to course load. *Unit head:* Dr. Gary Raskob, Dean, 405-271-2232. *Application contact:* Robin Howell, Information Contact, 405-271-2308, E-mail: robin_howell@ouhsc.edu.

University of Oklahoma Health Sciences Center, Graduate College, College of Public Health, Program in Preparedness and Terrorism, Oklahoma City, OK 73190. Offers MPH. *Faculty:* 16 full-time (8 women), 6 part-time/adjunct (4 women). *Students:* 2 full-time (both women), 1 part-time (0 women). Average age 54. In 2013, 2 master's awarded. *Expenses:* Tuition, state resident: full-time $3504; part-time $175.20 per credit hour. Tuition, nonresident: full-time $13,504; part-time $675.20 per credit hour. *Required fees:* $1545; $52.70 per credit hour. $245.25 per semester. Tuition and fees vary according to course load. *Unit head:* Dr. Gary Raskob, Dean, 405-271-2232. *Application contact:* Robin Howell, Information Contact, 405-271-2308, E-mail: robin_howell@ouhsc.edu.

University of Ottawa, Faculty of Graduate and Postdoctoral Studies, Interdisciplinary Programs, Program in Population Health, Ottawa, ON K1N 6N5, Canada. Offers PhD. *Degree requirements:* For doctorate, comprehensive exam, thesis/dissertation. Electronic applications accepted. *Faculty research:* Population health.

University of Pennsylvania, Perelman School of Medicine, Master of Public Health Program, Philadelphia, PA 19129. Offers generalist (MPH); global health (MPH); DMD/MPH; JD/MPH; MD/MPH; MPH/MBE; MSCE/MPH; MSN/MPH; MSSP/MPH; MSW/MPH; PhD/MPH. Part-time and evening/weekend programs available. *Faculty:* 33 full-time (19 women), 35 part-time/adjunct (19 women). *Students:* 44 full-time (33 women), 51 part-time (43 women); includes 30 minority (12 Black or African American, non-Hispanic/Latino; 14 Asian, non-Hispanic/Latino; 2 Hispanic/Latino; 2 Two or more races, non-Hispanic/Latino). 117 applicants, 62% accepted, 41 enrolled. In 2013, 24 master's awarded. *Entrance requirements:* For master's, GRE. Additional exam requirements/recommendations for international students: Recommended—TOEFL. *Application deadline:* For fall and spring admission, 4/30 for domestic and international students. Applications are processed on a rolling basis. Application fee: $70. *Financial support:* In 2013–14, 14 students received support, including 2 fellowships with partial tuition reimbursements available (averaging $1,000 per year), 14 teaching assistantships with partial tuition reimbursements available; scholarships/grants and tuition waivers (partial) also available. Financial award application deadline: 5/15. *Faculty research:* Health disparities, health behaviors, obesity, global health, epidemiology and prevention research. *Unit head:* Dr. Jennifer A. Pinto-Martin, Director, 215-898-4726, E-mail: pinto@nursing.upenn.edu. *Application contact:* Moriah Hall, MPH Program Coordinator, 215-573-8841, E-mail: moriahh@mail.med.upenn.edu.
Website: http://www.publichealth.med.upenn.edu/

University of Pittsburgh, Graduate School of Public Health, Pittsburgh, PA 15260. Offers MHA, MPH, MS, Dr PH, PhD, Certificate, JD/MPH, MD/MPH, MD/PhD, MID/MPH, MPH/MPA, MPH/MSW, MPH/PhD. *Accreditation:* CEPH (one or more programs are accredited). Part-time programs available. *Faculty:* 170 full-time (82 women), 117 part-time/adjunct (37 women). *Students:* 415 full-time (286 women), 216 part-time (155 women); includes 117 minority (32 Black or African American, non-Hispanic/Latino; 49 Asian, non-Hispanic/Latino; 22 Hispanic/Latino; 14 Two or more races, non-Hispanic/Latino), 150 international. Average age 29. 1,599 applicants, 53% accepted, 188 enrolled. In 2013, 166 master's, 47 doctorates awarded. Terminal master's awarded for partial completion of doctoral program. *Degree requirements:* For master's, comprehensive exam (for some programs), thesis; for doctorate, comprehensive exam, thesis/dissertation. *Entrance requirements:* For master's, doctorate, and Certificate, GRE, bachelor's degree, recommendations, professional statement, transcripts. Additional exam requirements/recommendations for international students: Required—TOEFL (minimum score 550 paper-based; 80 iBT) or IELTS (minimum score 6.5). *Application deadline:* For fall admission, 1/15 for domestic and international students; for winter admission, 10/15 for domestic students, 8/1 for international students; for spring admission, 10/14 for domestic students, 8/1 for international students; for summer admission, 12/1 for international students. Applications are processed on a rolling basis. Application fee: $120. Electronic applications accepted. *Expenses:* Tuition, state resident: full-time $19,964; part-time $807 per credit. Tuition, nonresident: full-time $32,686; part-time $1337 per credit. *Required fees:* $740; $200. Tuition and fees vary according to program. *Financial support:* Fellowships, research assistantships, teaching assistantships, career-related internships or fieldwork, scholarships/grants, traineeships, health care benefits, and unspecified assistantships available. Support available to part-time students. Financial award applicants required to submit FAFSA. *Faculty research:* Statistical genetics, genetic epidemiology, community-based participatory research, occupational and pulmonary medicine, Epstein-Barr virus. *Total annual research expenditures:* $73 million. *Unit head:* Dr. Donald S. Burke, Dean, 412-624-3001, E-mail: donburke@pitt.edu. *Application contact:* Karrie Lukin, Admissions Manager, 412-624-3003, E-mail: stuaff@pitt.edu.
Website: http://www.publichealth.pitt.edu/

University of Rochester, School of Medicine and Dentistry, Graduate Programs in Medicine and Dentistry, Department of Community and Preventive Medicine, Programs in Public Health and Clinical Investigation, Rochester, NY 14627. Offers clinical investigation (MS); public health (MPH); MBA/MPH; MD/MPH; MPH/MS; MPH/PhD. *Accreditation:* CEPH. *Entrance requirements:* For master's, GRE General Test. *Expenses: Tuition:* Full-time $44,580; part-time $1394 per credit hour. *Required fees:* $492.

University of San Francisco, School of Nursing and Health Professions, Master's Programs, San Francisco, CA 94117-1080. Offers behavioral health (MSBH); clinical nurse leader (MS); public health (MPH). *Faculty:* 14 full-time (12 women), 30 part-time/adjunct (24 women). *Students:* 355 full-time (301 women), 108 part-time (97 women); includes 237 minority (26 Black or African American, non-Hispanic/Latino; 2 American Indian or Alaska Native, non-Hispanic/Latino; 122 Asian, non-Hispanic/Latino; 61 Hispanic/Latino; 5 Native Hawaiian or other Pacific Islander, non-Hispanic/Latino; 21 Two or more races, non-Hispanic/Latino), 4 international. Average age 33. 524 applicants, 52% accepted, 170 enrolled. In 2013, 106 master's awarded. *Application deadline:* For fall admission, 5/15 priority date for domestic students; for spring admission, 11/30 priority date for domestic students. *Expenses: Tuition:* Full-time $21,150; part-time $1175 per unit. Tuition and fees vary according to course load, campus/location and program. *Financial support:* In 2013–14, 50 students received support. *Unit head:* Dr. Michelle Montagno, Director, 415-422-4074, E-mail: mjmontagno@usfca.edu. *Application contact:* Ingrid McVanner, Information Contact, 415-422-2746, Fax: 415-422-2217.

University of South Africa, College of Human Sciences, Pretoria, South Africa. Offers adult education (M Ed); African languages (MA, PhD); African politics (MA, PhD); Afrikaans (MA, PhD); ancient history (MA, PhD); ancient Near Eastern studies (MA, PhD); anthropology (MA, PhD); applied linguistics (MA); Arabic (MA, PhD); archaeology (MA); art history (MA); Biblical archaeology (MA); Biblical studies (M Th, D Th, PhD); Christian spirituality (M Th, D Th); church history (M Th, D Th); classical studies (MA, PhD); clinical psychology (MA); communication (MA, PhD); comparative education (M Ed, Ed D); consulting psychology (D Admin, D Com, PhD); curriculum studies (M Ed, Ed D); development studies (M Admin, MA, D Admin, PhD); didactics (M Ed, Ed D); education (M Tech); education management (M Ed, Ed D); educational psychology (M Ed); English (MA); environmental education (M Ed); French (MA, PhD); German (MA, PhD); Greek (MA); guidance and counseling (M Ed); health studies (MA, PhD), including health sciences education (MA), health services management (MA), medical and surgical nursing science (critical care general) (MA), midwifery and neonatal nursing science (MA), trauma and emergency care (MA); history (MA, PhD); history of education (Ed D); inclusive education (M Ed, Ed D); information and communications technology policy and regulation (MA); information science (MA, MIS, PhD); international politics (MA, PhD); Islamic studies (MA, PhD); Italian (MA, PhD); Judaica (MA, PhD); linguistics (MA, PhD); mathematical education (M Ed); mathematics education (MA); missiology (M Th, D Th); modern Hebrew (MA, PhD); musicology (MA, MMus, D Mus, PhD); natural science education (M Ed); New Testament (M Th, D Th); Old Testament (D Th); pastoral therapy (M Th, D Th); philosophy (MA); philosophy of education (M Ed, Ed D); politics (MA, PhD); Portuguese (MA, PhD); practical theology (M Th, D Th); psychology (MA, MS, PhD); psychology of education (M Ed, Ed D); public health (MA); religious studies (MA, D Th, PhD); Romance languages (MA); Russian (MA, PhD); Semitic languages (MA, PhD); social behavior studies in HIV/AIDS (MA); social science (mental health) (MA); social science in development studies (MA); social science in psychology (MA); social science in social work (MA); social science in sociology (MA); social work (MSW, DSW, PhD); socio-education (M Ed, Ed D); sociolinguistics (MA); sociology (MA, PhD); Spanish (MA, PhD); systematic theology (M Th, D Th); TESOL (teaching English to speakers of other languages) (MA); theological ethics (M Th, D Th); theory of literature (MA, PhD); urban ministries (D Th); urban ministry (M Th).

University of South Carolina, The Graduate School, Arnold School of Public Health, Program in General Public Health, Columbia, SC 29208. Offers MPH. *Accreditation:* CEPH. Part-time programs available. *Degree requirements:* For master's, comprehensive exam, practicum. *Entrance requirements:* For master's, DAT or MCAT, GRE General Test, previously earned MD or doctoral degree. Additional exam requirements/recommendations for international students: Required—TOEFL (minimum score 570 paper-based). Electronic applications accepted.

University of South Carolina, The Graduate School, Arnold School of Public Health, Program in Physical Activity and Public Health, Columbia, SC 29208. Offers MPH. *Accreditation:* CEPH. Part-time programs available. *Degree requirements:* For master's, comprehensive exam, practicum. *Entrance requirements:* For master's, GRE. Additional exam requirements/recommendations for international students: Required—TOEFL (minimum score 570 paper-based). Electronic applications accepted.

University of South Carolina, The Graduate School, College of Nursing, Program in Nursing and Public Health, Columbia, SC 29208. Offers MPH/MSN. *Accreditation:* AACN; CEPH. Part-time programs available. *Entrance requirements:* Additional exam requirements/recommendations for international students: Required—TOEFL (minimum score 570 paper-based). Electronic applications accepted. *Faculty research:* System research, evidence based practice, breast cancer, violence.

University of Southern California, Keck School of Medicine and Graduate School, Graduate Programs in Medicine, Department of Preventive Medicine, Master of Public Health Program, Los Angeles, CA 90032. Offers biostatistics-epidemiology (MPH); child and family health (MPH); environmental health (MPH); global health leadership (MPH); health communication (MPH); health education and promotion (MPH); public health policy (MPH). *Accreditation:* CEPH. Part-time and evening/weekend programs available. *Faculty:* 22 full-time (12 women), 3 part-time/adjunct (0 women). *Students:* 179 full-time (136 women), 31 part-time (24 women); includes 120 minority (19 Black or African American, non-Hispanic/Latino; 64 Asian, non-Hispanic/Latino; 37 Hispanic/Latino), 36 international. Average age 24. 205 applicants, 70% accepted, 73 enrolled. In 2013, 90 master's awarded. *Degree requirements:* For master's, practicum, final report, oral presentation. *Entrance requirements:* For master's, GRE General Test, MCAT, GMAT, minimum GPA of 3.0. Additional exam requirements/recommendations for international students: Required—TOEFL (minimum score 600 paper-based; 90 iBT). *Application deadline:* For fall admission, 6/1 priority date for domestic and international students; for spring admission, 10/1 priority date for domestic and international students; for summer admission, 3/1 for domestic and international students. Applications are processed on a rolling basis. Application fee: $85. Electronic applications accepted. *Financial support:* Career-related internships or fieldwork, Federal Work-Study, institutionally sponsored loans, and scholarships/grants available. Support available to part-time students. Financial award application deadline: 5/4; financial award applicants required to submit CSS PROFILE or FAFSA. *Faculty research:* Substance abuse prevention, cancer and heart disease prevention, mass media and health communication research, health promotion, treatment compliance. *Unit head:* Dr. Louise A. Rohrbach, Director, 323-442-8237, Fax: 323-442-8297, E-mail: rohrbac@usc.edu. *Application contact:* Valerie Burris, Admissions Counselor, 323-442-7257, Fax: 323-442-8297, E-mail: valeriem@usc.edu.
Website: http://mph.usc.edu/

University of Southern California, Keck School of Medicine and Graduate School, Graduate Programs in Medicine, Department of Preventive Medicine, Program in Health Behavior Research, Los Angeles, CA 90032. Offers PhD. *Faculty:* 19 full-time (12 women). *Students:* 27 full-time (14 women); includes 11 minority (2 Black or African American, non-Hispanic/Latino; 7 Asian, non-Hispanic/Latino; 2 Hispanic/Latino), 3 international. Average age 32. 43 applicants, 26% accepted, 7 enrolled. In 2013, 6 doctorates awarded. *Degree requirements:* For doctorate, comprehensive exam, thesis/dissertation. *Entrance requirements:* For doctorate, GRE General Test, minimum GPA of 3.0 (3.5 preferred). Additional exam requirements/recommendations for international students: Required—TOEFL (minimum score 600 paper-based; 100 iBT). *Application deadline:* For fall admission, 12/1 priority date for domestic and international students. Application fee: $85. Electronic applications accepted. *Financial support:* In 2013–14, 27 students received support, including 10 fellowships with full tuition reimbursements available (averaging $33,395 per year), 7 research assistantships with full and partial tuition reimbursements available (averaging $33,395 per year), 8 teaching assistantships with full and partial tuition reimbursements available (averaging $33,395 per year); institutionally sponsored loans, scholarships/grants, traineeships, health care benefits, and unspecified assistantships also available. Financial award application deadline: 5/4; financial award applicants required to submit CSS PROFILE or FAFSA. *Faculty research:* Obesity prevention; etiology and prevention of substance abuse, other addictive behaviors, and chronic diseases; health disparities; translational research. *Unit head:* Dr. Jennifer Unger, Director, 323-442-8234, E-mail: unger@usc.edu. *Application contact:* Marny Barovich, Program Manager, 323-442-8299, E-mail: barovich@hsc.usc.edu.
Website: http://phdhbr.usc.edu

University of Southern Maine, College of Management and Human Service, Muskie School of Public Service, Program in Health Policy and Management, Portland, ME 04104-9300. Offers public health (MPH, CGS); MBA/MPH. *Accreditation:* CAHME. Part-time and evening/weekend programs available. Postbaccalaureate distance learning degree programs offered (minimal on-campus study). *Faculty:* 7 full-time (2 women). *Students:* 20 full-time (14 women), 30 part-time (19 women); includes 3 minority (1 American Indian or Alaska Native, non-Hispanic/Latino; 1 Asian, non-Hispanic/Latino; 1 Two or more races, non-Hispanic/Latino), 1 international. Average age 34. 33 applicants, 79% accepted, 14 enrolled. In 2013, 11 master's awarded. *Degree requirements:* For master's, thesis, capstone project, field experience. *Entrance requirements:* For master's, GRE General Test. Additional exam requirements/recommendations for international students: Required—TOEFL. *Application deadline:* For fall admission, 2/1 priority date for domestic and international students; for spring admission, 12/1 for domestic and international students. Applications are processed on a rolling basis. Application fee: $65. Electronic applications accepted. *Expenses:* Tuition, state resident: part-time $380 per credit. Tuition, nonresident: part-time $1026 per credit. Part-time tuition and fees vary according to program. *Financial support:* Fellowships, research assistantships, career-related internships or fieldwork, Federal Work-Study, scholarships/grants, tuition waivers (partial), and unspecified assistantships available. Support available to part-time students. Financial award application deadline: 4/1; financial award applicants required to submit FAFSA. *Faculty research:* Public health systems, population health and health policy, rural health, patient safety, health services research, aging and disability policy, Medicare and Medicaid policy, mental health policy. *Unit head:* Dr. Elise Bolda, Chair, 207-780-4847, E-mail: eliseb@usm.maine.edu. *Application contact:* Mary Sloan, Assistant Dean of Graduate Studies and Director of Graduate Admissions, 207-780-4812, E-mail: gradstudies@usm.maine.edu.

University of Southern Mississippi, Graduate School, College of Health, Department of Community Health Sciences, Hattiesburg, MS 39406-0001. Offers epidemiology and biostatistics (MPH); health education (MPH); health policy/administration (MPH); occupational/environmental health (MPH); public health nutrition (MPH). *Accreditation:* CEPH. Part-time and evening/weekend programs available. *Faculty:* 8 full-time (4 women), 1 part-time/adjunct (0 women). *Students:* 92 full-time (60 women), 9 part-time (4 women); includes 38 minority (29 Black or African American, non-Hispanic/Latino; 1 American Indian or Alaska Native, non-Hispanic/Latino; 2 Asian, non-Hispanic/Latino; 6 Two or more races, non-Hispanic/Latino), 13 international. Average age 34. 71 applicants, 93% accepted, 45 enrolled. *Degree requirements:* For master's, comprehensive exam, thesis (for some programs). *Entrance requirements:* For master's, GRE General Test, minimum GPA of 2.75 in last 60 hours. Additional exam requirements/recommendations for international students: Required—TOEFL, IELTS. *Application deadline:* For fall admission, 3/1 priority date for domestic and international students; for spring admission, 1/10 priority date for domestic and international students. Applications are processed on a rolling basis. Application fee: $50. Electronic applications accepted. *Financial support:* In 2013–14, 5 research assistantships with full tuition reimbursements (averaging $7,000 per year), 1 teaching assistantship with full tuition reimbursement (averaging $8,263 per year) were awarded; career-related internships or fieldwork, Federal Work-Study, institutionally sponsored loans, scholarships/grants, health care benefits, and unspecified assistantships also available. Financial award application deadline: 3/15; financial award applicants required to submit FAFSA. *Faculty research:* Rural health care delivery, school health, nutrition of pregnant teens, risk factor reduction, sexually transmitted diseases. *Unit head:* Dr. Ray Newman, Interim Chair, 601-266-5437, Fax: 601-266-5043. *Application contact:* Shonna Breland, Manager of Graduate Admissions, 601-266-6563, Fax: 601-266-5138.
Website: http://www.usm.edu/chs

University of South Florida, College of Public Health, Tampa, FL 33612. Offers MHA, MPH, MSPH, Dr PH, PhD. *Accreditation:* CEPH (one or more programs are accredited). Part-time and evening/weekend programs available. Postbaccalaureate distance learning degree programs offered (minimal on-campus study). *Degree requirements:* For master's, comprehensive exam, thesis (for some programs); for doctorate, comprehensive exam, thesis/dissertation. *Entrance requirements:* For master's, GRE General Test, minimum GPA of 3.0 in upper-level course work, 3 professional letters of recommendation, resume/curriculum vitae; for doctorate, GRE General Test, minimum GPA of 3.0 in upper-level course work, goal statement letter, three professional letters of recommendation, resume/curriculum vitae, writing sample. Additional exam requirements/recommendations for international students: Required—TOEFL (minimum score 550 paper-based; 79 iBT). Electronic applications accepted.

University of South Florida, Innovative Education Graduate Certificate Programs, Tampa, FL 33620-9951. *Unit head:* Kathy Barnes, Interdisciplinary Programs Coordinator, 813-974-8031, Fax: 813-974-7061, E-mail: barnesk@usf.edu. *Application contact:* Karen Tylinski, Metro Initiatives, 813-974-9943, Fax: 813-974-7061, E-mail: ktylinsk@usf.edu.
Website: http://www.usf.edu/innovative-education/

The University of Tennessee, Graduate School, College of Education, Health and Human Sciences, Program in Public Health, Knoxville, TN 37996. Offers community health education (MPH); gerontology (MPH); health planning/administration (MPH); MS/MPH. *Accreditation:* CEPH. *Degree requirements:* For master's, thesis optional. *Entrance requirements:* For master's, minimum GPA of 2.7. Additional exam requirements/recommendations for international students: Required—TOEFL. Electronic applications accepted. *Expenses:* Tuition, state resident: full-time $9540;

part-time $531 per credit hour. Tuition, nonresident: full-time $27,728; part-time $1542 per credit hour. *Required fees:* $1404; $67 per credit hour.

The University of Texas Health Science Center at Houston, The University of Texas School of Public Health, Houston, TX 77030. Offers MPH, MS, Dr PH, PhD, Certificate, JD/MPH, MBA/MPH, MD/MPH, MGPS/MPH, MP Aff/MPH, MS/MPH, MSN/MPH, MSW/ MPH, PhD/MPH. Applications to dual degree programs are handled independently between the collaborating institutions. *Accreditation:* CEPH. Part-time programs available. *Faculty:* 158 full-time, 32 part-time/adjunct. *Students:* 610 full-time, 664 part-time; includes 444 minority (107 Black or African American, non-Hispanic/Latino; 3 American Indian or Alaska Native, non-Hispanic/Latino; 135 Asian, non-Hispanic/Latino; 183 Hispanic/Latino; 16 Two or more races, non-Hispanic/Latino), 301 international. Average age 28. 1,269 applicants, 58% accepted, 364 enrolled. In 2013, 330 master's, 55 doctorates awarded. *Degree requirements:* For master's, thesis (for some programs); for doctorate, comprehensive exam, thesis/dissertation. *Entrance requirements:* For master's and doctorate, GRE General Test. Additional exam requirements/ recommendations for international students: Required—TOEFL (minimum score 565 paper-based; 86 iBT). *Application deadline:* For fall admission, 3/1 for domestic and international students; for spring admission, 8/1 for domestic and international students. Applications are processed on a rolling basis. Application fee: $120. Electronic applications accepted. *Expenses:* Tuition, state resident: full-time $3474; part-time $193 per credit hour. Tuition, nonresident: full-time $13,644; part-time $758 per credit hour. *Required fees:* $226.30; $87 per credit hour. *Financial support:* Career-related internships or fieldwork, institutionally sponsored loans, scholarships/grants, traineeships, health care benefits, and unspecified assistantships available. Support available to part-time students. Financial award application deadline: 5/5; financial award applicants required to submit FAFSA. *Faculty research:* Chronic and infectious disease epidemiology; health promotion and health education; applied and theoretical biostatistics; health management, policy and economics; environmental and occupational health. *Total annual research expenditures:* $54.2 million. *Unit head:* Dr. Mary Ann Smith, Associate Dean for Student Affairs, 713-500-9236, Fax: 713-500-9068, E-mail: mary.a.smith@uth.tmc.edu. *Application contact:* Tiaresa E. Carter, Admissions Coordinator, 713-500-9035, Fax: 713-500-9068, E-mail: tiaresa.e.carter@uth.tmc.edu.
Website: https://sph.uth.edu

The University of Texas Medical Branch, Graduate School of Biomedical Sciences, Department of Preventive Medicine and Community Health, Program in Public Health, Galveston, TX 77555. Offers MPH. *Accreditation:* CEPH. *Degree requirements:* For master's, thesis. *Entrance requirements:* For master's, GRE, United States Medical Licensing Exam (USMLE) or NBE, preventive medicine residency. Additional exam requirements/recommendations for international students: Required—TOEFL (minimum score 550 paper-based). Electronic applications accepted.

University of the Sciences, College of Graduate Studies, Mayes College of Healthcare Business and Policy, Program in Public Health, Philadelphia, PA 19104-4495. Offers MPH. Part-time and evening/weekend programs available. Postbaccalaureate distance learning degree programs offered (no on-campus study). *Students:* 47. In 2013, 10 master's awarded. *Entrance requirements:* Additional exam requirements/ recommendations for international students: Required—TOEFL, TWE. *Expenses: Tuition:* Part-time $1447 per credit. Tuition and fees vary according to campus/location and program. *Unit head:* Dr. Glenn Beamer, Graduate Program Director, 267-295-3178, E-mail: g.beamer@usp.edu. *Application contact:* Joyce D'Angelo, Administrative Assistant, 215-596-8937, E-mail: j.dangel@usp.edu.

University of the Sciences, College of Graduate Studies, Program in Health Policy and Public Health, Philadelphia, PA 19104-4495. Offers health policy (MPH, MS, PhD); public health (MPH). Part-time and evening/weekend programs available. Postbaccalaureate distance learning degree programs offered (no on-campus study). *Faculty:* 11 full-time (5 women), 4 part-time/adjunct (2 women). *Students:* 18 full-time (10 women), 55 part-time (32 women); includes 13 minority (5 Black or African American, non-Hispanic/Latino; 6 Asian, non-Hispanic/Latino; 2 Hispanic/Latino), 6 international. Average age 40. 54 applicants, 61% accepted, 17 enrolled. In 2013, 12 master's, 1 doctorate awarded. *Degree requirements:* For doctorate, comprehensive exam, thesis/dissertation. *Entrance requirements:* For master's and doctorate, GRE General Test. Additional exam requirements/recommendations for international students: Required—TOEFL, TWE. *Application deadline:* For fall admission, 6/1 for domestic students, 5/1 for international students; for winter admission, 12/1 for domestic students, 10/1 for international students; for spring admission, 3/1 for international students. Applications are processed on a rolling basis. Application fee: $50. *Expenses:* Contact institution. *Financial support:* Tuition waivers (partial) and unspecified assistantships available. Support available to part-time students. Financial award application deadline: 5/1. *Faculty research:* Managed care, pharmacoeconomics, health law and regulation, rehabilitation, genetic technologies. *Unit head:* Dr. Shenaz Tejani-Butt, Associate Dean, Graduate Studies, E-mail: graduate@usciences.edu. *Application contact:* Christopher Miciek, Associate Director, Graduate Admissions, 215-596-8597, E-mail: c.miciek@usciences.edu.

The University of Toledo, College of Graduate Studies, College of Medicine and Life Sciences, Department of Public Health and Preventative Medicine, Toledo, OH 43606-3390. Offers biostatistics and epidemiology (Certificate); contemporary gerontological practice (Certificate); environmental and occupational health and safety (MPH); epidemiology (Certificate); global public health (Certificate); health promotion and education (MPH); industrial hygiene (MSOH); medical and health science teaching and learning (Certificate); occupational health (Certificate); public health administration (MPH); public health and emergency response (Certificate); public health epidemiology (MPH); public health nutrition (MPH); MD/MPH. Part-time and evening/weekend programs available. *Faculty:* 9. *Students:* 69 full-time (50 women), 88 part-time (66 women); includes 50 minority (35 Black or African American, non-Hispanic/Latino; 10 Asian, non-Hispanic/Latino; 4 Hispanic/Latino; 1 Two or more races, non-Hispanic/ Latino), 6 international. Average age 30. 92 applicants, 80% accepted, 52 enrolled. In 2013, 59 master's, 15 other advanced degrees awarded. *Degree requirements:* For master's, thesis or alternative. *Entrance requirements:* For master's, GRE, minimum undergraduate GPA of 3.0, three letters of recommendation, statement of purpose, transcripts from all prior institutions attended, resume; for Certificate, minimum undergraduate GPA of 3.0, three letters of recommendation, statement of purpose, transcripts from all prior institutions attended, resume. Additional exam requirements/ recommendations for international students: Required—TOEFL (minimum score 550 paper-based; 80 iBT), IELTS (minimum score 6.5). *Application deadline:* For fall admission, 6/15 for domestic students, 3/15 priority date for international students; for spring admission, 10/15 for domestic students, 6/15 for international students; for summer admission, 3/15 for domestic students, 10/15 for international students. Applications are processed on a rolling basis. Application fee: $45 ($75 for international students). Electronic applications accepted. *Financial support:* In 2013–14, 4 research assistantships with full tuition reimbursements (averaging $10,000 per year) were awarded; Federal Work-Study, institutionally sponsored loans, scholarships/grants, tuition waivers (full and partial), and unspecified assistantships also available. *Unit head:* Dr. Sheryl A. Milz, Chair, 419-383-3976, Fax: 419-383-6140, E-mail: sheryl.milz@utoledo.edu. *Application contact:* Admissions Analyst, 419-383-4112, Fax: 419-383-6140.
Website: http://nocphmph.org/

University of Toronto, School of Graduate Studies, Dalla Lana School of Public Health, Toronto, ON M5S 1A1, Canada. Offers biostatistics (M Sc, PhD); community health (M Sc); epidemiology (MPH, PhD); health and behavioral science (PhD); health promotion (MPH); social science and health (PhD). *Accreditation:* CAHME (one or more programs are accredited); CEPH (one or more programs are accredited). Part-time programs available. *Degree requirements:* For master's, thesis (for some programs), practicum; for doctorate, comprehensive exam, thesis/dissertation, oral thesis defense. *Entrance requirements:* For master's, 2 letters of reference, relevant professional/ research experience, minimum B average in final year; for doctorate, 2 letters of reference, relevant professional/research experience, minimum B+ average. Additional exam requirements/recommendations for international students: Required—TOEFL (minimum score 580 paper-based; 93 iBT), TWE (minimum score 5). Electronic applications accepted. *Expenses:* Contact institution.

University of Utah, School of Medicine and Graduate School, Graduate Programs in Medicine, Programs in Public Health, Salt Lake City, UT 84112-1107. Offers biostatistics (M Stat); public health (MPH, MSPH, PhD). *Accreditation:* CEPH (one or more programs are accredited). Part-time programs available. *Degree requirements:* For master's, comprehensive exam, thesis or project (MSPH); for doctorate, comprehensive exam, thesis/dissertation. *Entrance requirements:* For master's and doctorate, GRE General Test, 3 letters of reference, in-person interviews, minimum GPA of 3.0. Additional exam requirements/recommendations for international students: Required—TOEFL (minimum score 550 paper-based). Electronic applications accepted. *Expenses:* Tuition, state resident: full-time $5259. Tuition, nonresident: full-time $18,569. *Required fees:* $841. Tuition and fees vary according to course load. *Faculty research:* Health services, health policy, epidemiology of chronic disease, infectious disease epidemiology, cancer epidemiology.

University of Virginia, School of Medicine, Department of Public Health Sciences, Program in Public Health, Charlottesville, VA 22903. Offers MPH, MPP/MPH. *Accreditation:* CEPH. *Students:* 37 full-time (30 women), 4 part-time (3 women); includes 14 minority (4 Black or African American, non-Hispanic/Latino; 7 Asian, non-Hispanic/Latino; 3 Hispanic/Latino). Average age 26. 89 applicants, 65% accepted, 25 enrolled. In 2013, 26 master's awarded. *Degree requirements:* For master's, written or oral comprehensive exam or thesis. *Entrance requirements:* For master's, GRE, MCAT, LSAT or GMAT, 2 letters of recommendation. Additional exam requirements/ recommendations for international students: Required—TOEFL. *Application deadline:* For fall admission, 3/30 for domestic and international students. Applications are processed on a rolling basis. Application fee: $60. Electronic applications accepted. *Expenses:* Tuition, state resident: part-time $334 per credit hour. Tuition, nonresident: part-time $1224 per credit hour. *Financial support:* Applicants required to submit FAFSA. *Unit head:* Dr. Ruth Gaare Bernheim, Chair, 434-924-8430, Fax: 434-924-8437, E-mail: rg3r@virginia.edu. *Application contact:* Tracey L. Brookman, Academic Programs Administrator, 434-924-8430, Fax: 434-924-8437, E-mail: phsdegrees@virginia.edu.
Website: http://www.medicine.virginia.edu/clinical/departments/phs/degree_programs/mph

University of Virginia, School of Nursing, Charlottesville, VA 22903. Offers acute and specialty care (MSN); acute care nurse practitioner (MSN); clinical nurse leadership (MSN); community-public health leadership (MSN); nursing (DNP, PhD); psychiatric mental health counseling (MSN); MSN/MBA. *Accreditation:* AACN. Part-time programs available. *Faculty:* 45 full-time (41 women), 3 part-time/adjunct (all women). *Students:* 177 full-time (155 women), 147 part-time (133 women); includes 53 minority (27 Black or African American, non-Hispanic/Latino; 10 Asian, non-Hispanic/Latino; 11 Hispanic/ Latino; 5 Two or more races, non-Hispanic/Latino), 4 international. Average age 36. 236 applicants, 61% accepted, 110 enrolled. In 2013, 94 master's, 14 doctorates awarded. *Degree requirements:* For doctorate, comprehensive exam (for some programs), capstone project (DNP), dissertation (PhD). *Entrance requirements:* For master's, GRE General Test, MAT; for doctorate, GRE General Test. Additional exam requirements/ recommendations for international students: Required—TOEFL, IELTS. *Application deadline:* Applications are processed on a rolling basis. Application fee: $60. Electronic applications accepted. *Expenses:* Contact institution. *Financial support:* Fellowships, research assistantships, teaching assistantships, Federal Work-Study, and scholarships/grants available. Financial award applicants required to submit FAFSA. *Unit head:* Dorrie K. Fontaine, Dean, 434-924-0141, Fax: 434-982-1809, E-mail: dkf2u@virginia.edu. *Application contact:* Clay Hysell, Assistant Dean for Admissions and Financial Services, 434-924-0141, Fax: 434-982-1809, E-mail: nur-osa@virginia.edu.
Website: http://www.nursing.virginia.edu/

University of Washington, Graduate School, School of Public Health, Executive MPH Program, Seattle, WA 98195. Offers MPH. Evening/weekend programs available. Postbaccalaureate distance learning degree programs offered (minimal on-campus study). *Students:* 3 full-time (2 women), 38 part-time (31 women); includes 19 minority (3 Black or African American, non-Hispanic/Latino; 1 American Indian or Alaska Native, non-Hispanic/Latino; 15 Asian, non-Hispanic/Latino), 3 international. Average age 41. 46 applicants, 91% accepted, 34 enrolled. In 2013, 25 master's awarded. *Degree requirements:* For master's, capstone or thesis, practicum. *Entrance requirements:* For master's, GRE General Test or other comparable test scores (unless applicant already has graduate-level degree from accredited U.S. institution). Additional exam requirements/recommendations for international students: Required—TOEFL (minimum score 580 paper-based; 70 iBT). *Application deadline:* For fall admission, 12/1 for domestic students, 11/1 for international students. Application fee: $85. Electronic applications accepted. *Financial support:* In 2013–14, 1 student received support. *Unit head:* Dr. Gail Greenwood, Associate Director, Executive MPH Program, 206-616-2942, Fax: 206-543-3964, E-mail: gail1@uw.edu. *Application contact:* Cindy Moore, Student Services Coordinator, 206-685-7580, Fax: 206-543-3964, E-mail: uwedpapp@uw.edu.

University of Waterloo, Graduate Studies, Faculty of Applied Health Sciences, School of Public Health and Health Systems, Program in Public Health, Waterloo, ON N2L 3G1, Canada. Offers MPH. Part-time programs available. Postbaccalaureate distance learning degree programs offered (minimal on-campus study). *Degree requirements:* For master's, practicum. *Entrance requirements:* For master's, honour's degree, minimum B average, resume, 1 year work experience. Additional exam requirements/ recommendations for international students: Required—TOEFL, TWE. Electronic applications accepted. *Faculty research:* Public health, population health, health communication, health promotion and disease prevention, environmental health.

University of West Florida, College of Arts and Sciences: Sciences, School of Allied Health and Life Sciences, Program in Public Health, Pensacola, FL 32514-5750. Offers MPH. *Accreditation:* CEPH. Part-time and evening/weekend programs available. *Entrance requirements:* For master's, GRE (minimum score: verbal 450, quantitative 550), GMAT (minimum score 465), or MCAT (minimum score 25), official transcripts; two personal writing samples (e.g., written reports completed by applicant or other representative samples of professional writing skills); basic computer competency; three letters of recommendation. Additional exam requirements/recommendations for international students: Required—TOEFL (minimum score 550 paper-based).

University of Wisconsin–Milwaukee, Graduate School, College of Nursing, Milwaukee, WI 53201. Offers family nursing practitioner (Post Master's Certificate); health professional education (Certificate); nursing (MN, PhD); public health (Certificate). *Accreditation:* AACN. Part-time programs available. *Faculty:* 30 full-time (29 women), 2 part-time/adjunct (both women). *Students:* 157 full-time (142 women), 90 part-time (79 women); includes 32 minority (13 Black or African American, non-Hispanic/Latino; 10 Asian, non-Hispanic/Latino; 1 Hispanic/Latino; 8 Two or more races, non-Hispanic/Latino), 7 international. Average age 38. 160 applicants, 57% accepted, 51 enrolled. In 2013, 42 master's, 8 doctorates awarded. *Degree requirements:* For master's, thesis; for doctorate, thesis/dissertation. *Entrance requirements:* For master's, GRE General Test or MAT, autobiographical sketch; for doctorate, GRE, minimum GPA of 3.2. Additional exam requirements/recommendations for international students: Required—TOEFL (minimum score 550 paper-based; 79 iBT), IELTS (minimum score 6.5). *Application deadline:* For fall admission, 1/1 priority date for domestic students; for spring admission, 9/1 for domestic students. Applications are processed on a rolling basis. Application fee: $56 ($96 for international students). Electronic applications accepted. *Financial support:* In 2013–14, 3 fellowships, 1 research assistantship, 9 teaching assistantships were awarded; career-related internships or fieldwork, Federal Work-Study, health care benefits, unspecified assistantships, and project assistantships also available. Support available to part-time students. Financial award application deadline: 4/15; financial award applicants required to submit FAFSA. *Total annual research expenditures:* $3.2 million. *Unit head:* Dr. Sally Lundeen, Dean, 414-229-4189, E-mail: slundeen@uwm.edu. *Application contact:* Kim Litwack, Representative, 414-229-5098.
Website: http://www.uwm.edu/Dept/Nursing/

University of Wisconsin–Milwaukee, Graduate School, Zilber School of Public Health, Department of Public Health, Milwaukee, WI 53201-0413. Offers community and behavioral health promotion (PhD); public health (MPH, Graduate Certificate). *Students:* 31 full-time (23 women), 14 part-time (13 women); includes 12 minority (4 Black or African American, non-Hispanic/Latino; 6 Asian, non-Hispanic/Latino; 2 Two or more races, non-Hispanic/Latino), 4 international. Average age 31. 74 applicants, 46% accepted, 16 enrolled. *Unit head:* Amy Harley, Assistant Professor, 414-229-4342, E-mail: harley@uwm.edu. *Application contact:* Darcie K. G. Warren, Graduate Program Manager, 414-229-5633, E-mail: darcie@uwm.edu.

Vanderbilt University, Graduate School, Center for Medicine, Health, and Society, Nashville, TN 37240-1001. Offers MA, MD/MA. *Accreditation:* CEPH. *Faculty:* 3 full-time (1 woman). *Students:* 5 full-time (4 women). Average age 24. 13 applicants, 38% accepted, 5 enrolled. In 2013, 3 master's awarded. *Degree requirements:* For master's, comprehensive exam (for some programs), thesis (for some programs). *Entrance requirements:* Additional exam requirements/recommendations for international students: Required—TOEFL (minimum score 570 paper-based; 88 iBT). *Application deadline:* For fall admission, 1/15 for domestic and international students. Electronic applications accepted. *Financial support:* Federal Work-Study, scholarships/grants, and health care benefits available. Financial award application deadline: 1/15; financial award applicants required to submit CSS PROFILE or FAFSA. *Faculty research:* Cultural history of health and disease, the rise of scientific medicine, scientific and medical constructions of gender and sexuality, integrative medicine, domestic and international public health, healthcare administration. *Unit head:* Dr. Jonathan Metzl, Director for Center for Medicine, Health and Society/Director of Graduate Studies, 615-343-0916, Fax: 615-343-8889, E-mail: jonathan.metzl@vanderbilt.edu. *Application contact:* Lynn Lentz, Program Administrator, 615-343-0916, Fax: 615-322-2731, E-mail: lynn.lentz@vanderbilt.edu.
Website: http://www.vanderbilt.edu/mhs/

Vanderbilt University, School of Medicine, Program in Public Health, Nashville, TN 37240-1001. Offers MPH. *Degree requirements:* For master's, thesis, project. *Entrance requirements:* For master's, curriculum vitae.

Virginia Commonwealth University, Medical College of Virginia-Professional Programs, School of Medicine, School of Medicine Graduate Programs, Department of Epidemiology and Community Health, Richmond, VA 23284-9005. Offers epidemiology (MPH, PhD); public health practice (MPH); social and behavioral science (MPH); MD/MPH; MSW/MPH. *Accreditation:* CEPH. Part-time programs available. *Degree requirements:* For doctorate, comprehensive exam, thesis/dissertation. *Entrance requirements:* For master's, GRE; for doctorate, GRE General Test, interview, 3 letters of recommendation, minimum graduate GPA of 3.0, master's degree in public health or related field including epidemiology and biostatistics. Additional exam requirements/recommendations for international students: Required—TOEFL (minimum score 600 paper-based; 100 iBT). Electronic applications accepted. *Faculty research:* Sickle cell anemia, breast cancer, HIV/AIDS, hospital epidemiology, infectious diseases.

Virginia Polytechnic Institute and State University, Virginia-Maryland Regional College of Veterinary Medicine, Blacksburg, VA 24061. Offers biomedical and veterinary sciences (MS, PhD); public health (MPH); research in translational medicine (Certificate); veterinary medicine (DVM). *Accreditation:* AVMA (one or more programs are accredited). *Faculty:* 105 full-time (45 women), 1 (woman) part-time/adjunct. *Students:* 573 full-time (428 women), 44 part-time (35 women); includes 67 minority (17 Black or African American, non-Hispanic/Latino; 13 Asian, non-Hispanic/Latino; 13 Hispanic/Latino; 1 Native Hawaiian or other Pacific Islander, non-Hispanic/Latino; 23 Two or more races, non-Hispanic/Latino), 32 international. Average age 26. 102 applicants, 69% accepted, 47 enrolled. In 2013, 14 master's, 104 doctorates awarded. *Degree requirements:* For master's, comprehensive exam (for some programs), thesis (for some programs); for doctorate, comprehensive exam (for some programs), thesis/dissertation (for some programs). *Entrance requirements:* For master's and doctorate, GRE/GMAT (may vary by department). Additional exam requirements/recommendations for international students: Required—TOEFL (minimum score 550 paper-based). *Application deadline:* For fall admission, 8/1 for domestic students, 4/1 for international students; for spring admission, 1/1 for domestic students, 9/1 for international students. Applications are processed on a rolling basis. Application fee: $75. Electronic applications accepted. *Expenses:* Contact institution. *Financial support:* In 2013–14, 1 fellowship (averaging $39,777 per year), 14 research assistantships with full tuition reimbursements (averaging $23,189 per year), 44 teaching assistantships with full tuition reimbursements (averaging $21,977 per year) were awarded. Financial award application deadline: 3/1; financial award applicants required to submit FAFSA. *Total annual research expenditures:* $6.6 million. *Unit head:* Dr. Cyril R. Clark, Dean, 540-231-7666, Fax: 540-231-7367, E-mail: cvmdean@vt.edu. *Application contact:* Shelia Steele, Executive Assistant, 540-231-7910, Fax: 540-231-7367, E-mail: ssteele@vt.edu.
Website: http://www.vetmed.vt.edu

Walden University, Graduate Programs, School of Counseling, Minneapolis, MN 55401. Offers addiction counseling (MS), including addictions and public health, child and adolescent counseling, family studies and interventions, forensic counseling, general program (MS, PhD), trauma and crisis counseling; counselor education and supervision (PhD), including consultation, counseling and social change, forensic mental health counseling, general program (MS, PhD), nonprofit management and leadership, trauma and crisis; marriage, couple, and family counseling (MS), including forensic counseling, general program (MS, PhD), trauma and crisis counseling; mental health counseling (MS), including forensic counseling, general program (MS, PhD), trauma and crisis counseling; school counseling (MS), including addictions counseling, crisis and trauma, general program (MS, PhD), military. Part-time and evening/weekend programs available. Postbaccalaureate distance learning degree programs offered (minimal on-campus study). *Faculty:* 50 full-time (38 women), 238 part-time/adjunct (172 women). *Students:* 2,019 full-time (1,709 women), 1,566 part-time (1,345 women); includes 1,622 minority (1,223 Black or African American, non-Hispanic/Latino; 21 American Indian or Alaska Native, non-Hispanic/Latino; 36 Asian, non-Hispanic/Latino; 231 Hispanic/Latino; 8 Native Hawaiian or other Pacific Islander, non-Hispanic/Latino; 103 Two or more races, non-Hispanic/Latino), 19 international. Average age 38. 789 applicants, 90% accepted, 623 enrolled. In 2013, 410 master's awarded. *Degree requirements:* For master's, residency, field experience, professional development plan, licensure plan; for doctorate, thesis/dissertation, residency, practicum, internship. *Entrance requirements:* For master's, bachelor's degree or higher; minimum GPA of 2.5; official transcripts; goal statement (for some programs); access to computer and Internet; for doctorate, master's degree or higher; three years of related professional or academic experience (preferred); minimum GPA of 3.0; goal statement and current resume (select programs); official transcripts; access to computer and Internet. Additional exam requirements/recommendations for international students: Required—TOEFL (minimum score 550 paper-based; 79 iBT), IELTS (minimum score 6.5), Michigan English Language Assessment Battery (minimum score 82), or PTE. *Application deadline:* Applications are processed on a rolling basis. Application fee: $0. Electronic applications accepted. *Expenses: Tuition:* Full-time $11,813.55; part-time $500 per credit. *Required fees:* $618.76. *Financial support:* Federal Work-Study, scholarships/grants, unspecified assistantships, and family tuition reduction, active duty/veteran tuition reduction, group tuition reduction, interest-free payment plans, employee tuition reduction available. Support available to part-time students. Financial award applicants required to submit FAFSA. *Unit head:* Dr. Savitri Dixon-Saxon, Associate Dean, 800-925-3368. *Application contact:* Jennifer Hall, Vice President of Enrollment Management, 866-4-WALDEN, E-mail: info@waldenu.edu.

Walden University, Graduate Programs, School of Health Sciences, Minneapolis, MN 55401. Offers clinical research administration (MS, Graduate Certificate); health education and promotion (MS); health informatics (MS); health services (PhD), including community health, healthcare administration, leadership, public health policy, self-designed; healthcare administration (MHA); public health (MPH, Dr PH, PhD), including community health and education (PhD), epidemiology (PhD). Part-time and evening/weekend programs available. Postbaccalaureate distance learning degree programs offered (minimal on-campus study). *Faculty:* 18 full-time (12 women), 236 part-time/adjunct (120 women). *Students:* 2,563 full-time (1,867 women), 1,775 part-time (1,233 women); includes 2,532 minority (1,963 Black or African American, non-Hispanic/Latino; 29 American Indian or Alaska Native, non-Hispanic/Latino; 212 Asian, non-Hispanic/Latino; 238 Hispanic/Latino; 15 Native Hawaiian or other Pacific Islander, non-Hispanic/Latino; 75 Two or more races, non-Hispanic/Latino), 97 international. Average age 39. 1,191 applicants, 94% accepted, 861 enrolled. In 2013, 723 master's, 121 doctorates, 17 other advanced degrees awarded. *Degree requirements:* For doctorate, thesis/dissertation, residency. *Entrance requirements:* For master's, bachelor's degree or higher; minimum GPA of 2.5; official transcripts; goal statement (for some programs); access to computer and Internet; for doctorate, master's degree or higher; three years of related professional or academic experience (preferred); minimum GPA of 3.0; goal statement and current resume (select programs); official transcripts; access to computer and Internet; for Graduate Certificate, relevant work experience; access to computer and Internet. Additional exam requirements/recommendations for international students: Required—TOEFL (minimum score 550 paper-based; 79 iBT), IELTS (minimum score 6.5), Michigan English Language Assessment Battery (minimum score 82), or PTE. *Application deadline:* Applications are processed on a rolling basis. Application fee: $0. Electronic applications accepted. *Expenses: Tuition:* Full-time $11,813.55; part-time $500 per credit. *Required fees:* $618.76. *Financial support:* Fellowships, Federal Work-Study, scholarships/grants, unspecified assistantships, and family tuition reduction, active duty/veteran tuition reduction, group tuition reduction, interest-free payment plans, employee tuition reduction available. Support available to part-time students. Financial award applicants required to submit FAFSA. *Unit head:* Dr. Jorg Westermann, Associate Dean, 800-925-3368. *Application contact:* Jennifer Hall, Vice President of Enrollment Management, 866-4-WALDEN, E-mail: info@waldenu.edu.
Website: http://www.waldenu.edu/colleges-schools/school-of-health-sciences

Walden University, Graduate Programs, School of Nursing, Minneapolis, MN 55401. Offers adult-gerontology acute care nurse practitioner (MSN); adult-gerontology nurse practitioner (MSN); education (MSN); family nurse practitioner (MSN); informatics (MSN); leadership and management (MSN); nursing (DNP, PhD, Post-Master's Certificate), including education (PhD), healthcare administration (PhD), interdisciplinary health (PhD), leadership (PhD), nursing education (Post-Master's Certificate), nursing informatics (Post-Master's Certificate), nursing leadership and management (Post-Master's Certificate), public health policy (PhD). *Accreditation:* AACN. Part-time and evening/weekend programs available. Postbaccalaureate distance learning degree programs offered (no on-campus study). *Faculty:* 22 full-time (19 women), 343 part-time/adjunct (301 women). *Students:* 5,828 full-time (5,240 women), 2,803 part-time (2,578 women); includes 2,920 minority (1,893 Black or African American, non-Hispanic/Latino; 40 American Indian or Alaska Native, non-Hispanic/Latino; 438 Asian, non-Hispanic/Latino; 391 Hispanic/Latino; 35 Native Hawaiian or other Pacific Islander, non-Hispanic/Latino; 123 Two or more races, non-Hispanic/Latino), 147 international. Average age 41. 1,795 applicants, 95% accepted, 1375 enrolled. In 2013, 1,879 master's, 1 doctorate, 36 other advanced degrees awarded. *Degree requirements:* For doctorate, thesis/dissertation (for some programs), residency (for some programs), field experience (for some programs). *Entrance requirements:* For master's, bachelor's degree or equivalent in related field or RN; minimum GPA of 2.5; official transcripts; goal statement (for some programs); access to computer and Internet; for doctorate, master's degree or higher, three years of related professional or academic experience, RN, goal statement (for some programs); access to computer and Internet; for Post-Master's Certificate, relevant work experience; access to computer and Internet. Additional exam requirements/recommendations for international students: Required—TOEFL (minimum score 550 paper-based; 79 iBT), IELTS (minimum score 6.5), Michigan English Language Assessment Battery (minimum score 82), or PTE. *Application deadline:* Applications are processed on a rolling basis. Application fee: $0. Electronic applications accepted. *Expenses: Tuition:* Full-time $11,813.55; part-time $500 per credit. *Required fees:* $618.76. *Financial support:* Fellowships, Federal Work-Study, scholarships/grants, unspecified assistantships, and family tuition reduction, active duty/veteran tuition reduction, group tuition reduction, interest-free payment plans, employee tuition reduction available. Support available to part-time students. Financial award applicants required to submit FAFSA. *Unit head:* Dr. Andrea Lindell, Associate Dean, 800-925-3368. *Application contact:* Jennifer Hall, Vice President of Enrollment Management, 866-4-WALDEN, E-mail: info@waldenu.edu.
Website: http://www.waldenu.edu/programs/colleges-schools/nursing

Walden University, Graduate Programs, School of Social Work and Human Services, Minneapolis, MN 55401. Offers addictions (MSW); addictions and social work (DSW); children, families, and couples (MSW); clinical expertise (DSW); criminal justice (DSW); crisis and trauma (MSW); disaster, crisis, and intervention (DSW); forensic populations and settings (MSW); general program (MSW); human services (MS, PhD), including clinical social work (PhD), criminal justice, disaster, crisis and intervention, family studies and intervention strategies (PhD), family studies and interventions, general program, human services administration (PhD), human services and administration (MS), public health, social policy analysis and planning; medical social work (MSW, DSW); military families and culture (MSW); policy practice (DSW); social work (PhD), including addictions and social work, clinical expertise, disaster, crisis and intervention (MS, PhD), family studies and interventions (MS, PhD), medical social work, policy practice, social work administration; social work administration (DSW). Part-time and evening/weekend programs available. Postbaccalaureate distance learning degree programs offered (minimal on-campus study). *Faculty:* 11 full-time (7 women), 89 part-time/adjunct (60 women). *Students:* 906 full-time (794 women), 469 part-time (394 women); includes 930 minority (812 Black or African American, non-Hispanic/Latino; 14 American Indian or Alaska Native, non-Hispanic/Latino; 12 Asian, non-Hispanic/Latino; 61 Hispanic/Latino; 4 Native Hawaiian or other Pacific Islander, non-Hispanic/Latino; 27 Two or more races, non-Hispanic/Latino), 11 international. Average age 41. 673 applicants, 97% accepted, 555 enrolled. In 2013, 417 master's, 11 doctorates awarded. *Degree requirements:* For master's, residency (for some programs); for doctorate, thesis/dissertation, residency. *Entrance requirements:* For master's, bachelor's degree or higher; minimum GPA of 2.5; official transcripts; goal statement (for some programs); access to computer and Internet; for doctorate, master's degree or higher; three years of related professional or academic experience (preferred); minimum GPA of 3.0; goal statement and current resume (select programs); official transcripts; access to computer and Internet. Additional exam requirements/recommendations for international students: Required—TOEFL (minimum score 550 paper-based; 79 iBT), IELTS (minimum score 6.5), Michigan English Language Assessment Battery (minimum score 82), or PTE. *Application deadline:* Applications are processed on a rolling basis. Application fee: $0. Electronic applications accepted. *Expenses: Tuition:* Full-time $11,813.55; part-time $500 per credit. *Required fees:* $618.76. *Financial support:* Fellowships, Federal Work-Study, scholarships/grants, unspecified assistantships, and family tuition reduction, active duty/veteran tuition reduction, group tuition reduction, interest-free payment plans, employee tuition reduction available. Support available to part-time students. Financial award applicants required to submit FAFSA. *Unit head:* Dr. Savitri Dixon-Saxon, Associate Dean, 800-925-3368. *Application contact:* Jennifer Hall, Vice President of Enrollment Management, 866-4-WALDEN, E-mail: info@waldenu.edu.
Website: http://www.waldenu.edu/colleges-schools/school-of-social-work-and-human-services/academic-programs

Washington University in St. Louis, George Warren Brown School of Social Work, St. Louis, MO 63130. Offers Alaska native/American Indian studies (MSW); children, youth and families (MSW); gerontology (MSW); mental health (MSW); public health (MPA, MPH), including epidemiology/biostatistics (MPH), global health (MPA); social and economic development (MSW); social work (MSW, PhD), including health (MSW); JD/MSW; M Arch/MSW; MBA/MSW; MPH/MBA; MSW/M Div; MSW/MAPS; MSW/MJCS; MSW/MPH. MSW/M Div and MSW/MAPS offered jointly with Eden Theological Seminary. *Accreditation:* CSWE (one or more programs are accredited). *Faculty:* 42 full-time (24 women), 81 part-time/adjunct (49 women). *Students:* 298 full-time (263 women), 5 part-time (all women); includes 78 minority (32 Black or African American, non-Hispanic/Latino; 4 American Indian or Alaska Native, non-Hispanic/Latino; 18 Asian, non-Hispanic/Latino; 9 Hispanic/Latino; 2 Native Hawaiian or other Pacific Islander, non-Hispanic/Latino; 13 Two or more races, non-Hispanic/Latino), 47 international. Average age 26. 817 applicants, 62% accepted, 303 enrolled. In 2013, 239 master's, 5 doctorates awarded. *Degree requirements:* For master's, 60 credit hours (MSW), 52 credit hours (MPH); practicum; for doctorate, comprehensive exam, thesis/dissertation. *Entrance requirements:* For master's, GRE, GMAT, LSAT, or MCAT (public health), minimum GPA of 3.0; for doctorate, GRE, MA or MSW. Additional exam requirements/recommendations for international students: Required—TOEFL (minimum score 100 iBT). *Application deadline:* For fall admission, 3/1 priority date for domestic and international students. Applications are processed on a rolling basis. Application fee: $40. Electronic applications accepted. *Expenses:* Contact institution. *Financial support:* In 2013–14, 301 students received support. Fellowships, research assistantships, Federal Work-Study, institutionally sponsored loans, scholarships/grants, health care benefits, tuition waivers (partial), and unspecified assistantships available. Support available to part-time students. Financial award application deadline: 3/1; financial award applicants required to submit FAFSA. *Faculty research:* Mental health services, social development, child welfare, at-risk teens, autism, environmental health, health policy, health communications, obesity, violence and injury prevention, chronic disease prevention, poverty, public health, productive aging/gerontology, social work, civic engagement, school social work, program evaluation, health disparities. *Unit head:* Dr. Edward F. Lawlor, Dean/Professor, 314-935-6693, Fax: 314-935-8511, E-mail: elawlor@wustl.edu. *Application contact:* Leslie D. Duling, Admissions Counselor, 314-935-6694, Fax: 314-935-4859, E-mail: lduling@brownschool.wustl.edu.
Website: http://gwbweb.wustl.edu/

Washington University in St. Louis, School of Medicine, Master of Population Health Sciences Program, St. Louis, MO 63110. Offers clinical epidemiology (MPHS); health services (MPHS); psychiatric and behavioral health sciences (MPHS); quantitative methods (MPHS). Part-time programs available. *Faculty:* 31 part-time/adjunct (18 women). *Students:* 5 full-time (2 women), 8 part-time (3 women). Average age 31. In 2013, 10 master's awarded. *Entrance requirements:* For master's, clinical doctorate degree (or in pursuit of one). Additional exam requirements/recommendations for international students: Required—TOEFL. *Application deadline:* For fall admission, 1/9 priority date for domestic and international students. Applications are processed on a rolling basis. *Financial support:* In 2013–14, 5 students received support. Scholarships/grants available. *Faculty research:* Epidemiology, public health, biostatistics, cancer/chronic disease prevention, comparative effectiveness research. *Unit head:* Dr. Graham Colditz, Director, 314-454-7939, E-mail: colditzg@wustl.edu. *Application contact:* Joyce Linn, Program Coordinator, 314-362-5501, E-mail: linnj@wudosis.wustl.edu.
Website: http://www.mphs.wustl.edu/

Wayne State University, School of Medicine, Graduate Programs in Medicine, Department of Family Medicine and Public Health Sciences, Detroit, MI 48202. Offers public health (MPH), including occupational and environmental health, public health practice, quantitative health sciences; public health practice (Graduate Certificate). *Students:* 22 full-time (13 women), 30 part-time (15 women); includes 15 minority (5 Black or African American, non-Hispanic/Latino; 8 Asian, non-Hispanic/Latino; 1 Hispanic/Latino; 1 Two or more races, non-Hispanic/Latino), 13 international. Average age 32. 187 applicants, 21% accepted, 22 enrolled. In 2013, 14 master's, 3 other advanced degrees awarded. *Degree requirements:* For master's, thesis (for some programs), project or thesis. *Entrance requirements:* For master's, GRE, undergraduate work in mathematics, natural sciences, and social sciences; experience in health-related position, admission to graduate school, minimum undergraduate GPA of 3.0 overall and in mathematics, social sciences, and natural sciences, college-level mathematics, personal statement, three letters of recommendation; for Graduate Certificate, undergraduate work in mathematics, natural sciences, and social sciences; experience in health-related position, admission to graduate school, minimum undergraduate GPA of 3.0 overall and in mathematics, social sciences, and natural sciences, college-level mathematics, personal statement, three letters of recommendation. Additional exam requirements/recommendations for international students: Required—TOEFL (minimum score 550 paper-based; 100 iBT), TWE (minimum score 6); Recommended—IELTS (minimum score 6.5). *Application deadline:* For fall admission, 2/1 for domestic students, 1/1 priority date for international students. Application fee: $0. Electronic applications accepted. *Expenses:* Contact institution. *Financial support:* In 2013–14, 7 students received support. Scholarships/grants available. Financial award application deadline: 3/31; financial award applicants required to submit FAFSA. *Faculty research:* Urban health disparities, community health promotion, substance abuse etiology and prevention, HIV/AIDS, interpersonal violence. *Unit head:* Dr. Kimberly Campbell-Voytal, Program Director, 313-577-1051, E-mail: kvoytal@med.wayne.edu.
Website: http://gradprograms.med.wayne.edu/program-spotlight.php?id=26

West Chester University of Pennsylvania, College of Health Sciences, Department of Health, West Chester, PA 19383. Offers community health (MPH); emergency preparedness (Certificate); environmental health (MPH); health care management (MPH, Certificate); integrative health (MPH, Certificate); nutrition (MPH); school health (M Ed). *Accreditation:* CEPH. Part-time and evening/weekend programs available. *Faculty:* 17 full-time (13 women), 3 part-time/adjunct (all women). *Students:* 115 full-time (85 women), 95 part-time (73 women); includes 79 minority (66 Black or African American, non-Hispanic/Latino; 1 American Indian or Alaska Native, non-Hispanic/Latino; 5 Asian, non-Hispanic/Latino; 3 Hispanic/Latino; 4 Two or more races, non-Hispanic/Latino), 15 international. Average age 31. 156 applicants, 83% accepted, 76 enrolled. In 2013, 101 master's, 18 other advanced degrees awarded. *Degree requirements:* For master's, thesis or alternative, minimum GPA of 3.0; research report (for M Ed); major project and practicum (for MPH); for Certificate, minimum GPA of 3.0. *Entrance requirements:* For master's, goal statement, two letters of recommendation, undergraduate Introduction to Statistics course. Additional exam requirements/recommendations for international students: Required—TOEFL (minimum score 550 paper-based; 80 iBT). *Application deadline:* For fall admission, 4/15 priority date for domestic students, 3/15 for international students; for spring admission, 10/15 priority date for domestic students, 9/1 for international students. Applications are processed on a rolling basis. Application fee: $45. Electronic applications accepted. *Expenses:* Tuition, state resident: full-time $7956; part-time $442 per credit. Tuition, nonresident: full-time $11,934; part-time $663 per credit. *Required fees:* $2134.20; $106.24 per credit. Tuition and fees vary according to campus/location and program. *Financial support:* Unspecified assistantships available. Support available to part-time students. Financial award application deadline: 2/15; financial award applicants required to submit FAFSA. *Faculty research:* Healthy school communities, community health issues and evidence-based programs, environment and health, nutrition and health, integrative health. *Unit head:* Dr. Bethann Cinelli, Chair, 610-436-2267, E-mail: bcinelli@wcupa.edu. *Application contact:* Dr. Lynn Carson, Graduate Coordinator, 610-436-2138, E-mail: lcarson@wcupa.edu.
Website: http://www.wcupa.edu/_ACADEMICS/HealthSciences/health/

Western Kentucky University, Graduate Studies, College of Health and Human Services, Department of Public Health, Bowling Green, KY 42101. Offers healthcare administration (MHA); public health (MPH). *Accreditation:* CEPH. Part-time and evening/weekend programs available. *Degree requirements:* For master's, comprehensive exam, thesis or alternative. *Entrance requirements:* For master's, GRE General Test, minimum GPA of 2.75. Additional exam requirements/recommendations for international students: Required—TOEFL (minimum score 555 paper-based; 79 iBT). *Faculty research:* Health education training, driver traffic safety, community readiness, occupational injuries, local health departments.

Westminster College, School of Nursing and Health Sciences, Salt Lake City, UT 84105-3697. Offers family nurse practitioner (MSN); nurse anesthesia (MSNA); nurse education (MSNED); nursing (MSN); public health (MPH). *Accreditation:* AACN; AANA/CANAEP. *Faculty:* 11 full-time (5 women), 7 part-time/adjunct (4 women). *Students:* 119 full-time (75 women), 5 part-time (2 women); includes 21 minority (5 Black or African American, non-Hispanic/Latino; 1 American Indian or Alaska Native, non-Hispanic/Latino; 4 Asian, non-Hispanic/Latino; 7 Hispanic/Latino; 1 Native Hawaiian or other Pacific Islander, non-Hispanic/Latino; 3 Two or more races, non-Hispanic/Latino), 4 international. Average age 32. 246 applicants, 35% accepted, 56 enrolled. In 2013, 49 master's awarded. *Degree requirements:* For master's, clinical practicum, 504 clinical practice hours. *Entrance requirements:* For master's, GRE, resume, Utah RN license in good standing, minimum GPA of 3.0, 3 letters of reference, BSN from accredited nursing program, proof of clear state and federal background check, drug test results, personal interview, current PALS certification, current ACLS certification, document of current immunizations, physical and mental health certificate. Additional exam requirements/recommendations for international students: Required—TOEFL (minimum score 600 paper-based; 100 iBT), IELTS (minimum score 7.5). *Application deadline:* Applications are processed on a rolling basis. Application fee: $50. Electronic applications accepted. *Expenses:* Contact institution. *Financial support:* In 2013–14, 9 students received support. Career-related internships or fieldwork, unspecified assistantships, and tuition reimbursements, tuition remission available. Support available to part-time students. Financial award applicants required to submit FAFSA. *Faculty research:* Collaborative testing in nursing: student outcomes and perspectives, implementing new educational paradigms into pre-licensure nursing curricula. *Unit head:* Dr. Sheryl Steadman, Dean, 801-832-2164, Fax: 801-832-3110, E-mail: ssteadman@westminstercollege.edu. *Application contact:* Dr. John Baworowsky, Vice President of Enrollment Management, 801-832-2200, Fax: 801-832-3101, E-mail: admission@westminstercollege.edu.
Website: http://www.westminstercollege.edu/msn

West Virginia University, School of Medicine, Department of Community Medicine, Program in Public Health, Morgantown, WV 26506. Offers community health/preventative medicine (MPH). *Accreditation:* CEPH. Part-time programs available. Postbaccalaureate distance learning degree programs offered (minimal on-campus study). *Degree requirements:* For master's, practicum, project. *Entrance requirements:* For master's, GRE General Test, MCAT, medical degree, medical internship. *Expenses:* Contact institution. *Faculty research:* Occupational health, environmental health, clinical epidemiology, health care management, prevention.

Wright State University, School of Medicine, Program in Public Health, Dayton, OH 45435. Offers health promotion and education (MPH); public health management (MPH); public health nursing (MPH). *Accreditation:* CEPH.

Yale University, School of Medicine, Yale School of Public Health, New Haven, CT 06520. Offers applied biostatistics and epidemiology (APMPH); biostatistics (MPH, MS, PhD), including global health (MPH); chronic disease epidemiology (MPH, PhD), including global health (MPH); environmental health sciences (MPH, PhD), including global health (MPH); epidemiology of microbial diseases (MPH, PhD), including global health (MPH); global health (APMPH); health management (MPH), including global health; health policy (MPH), including global health; health policy and administration (APMPH, PhD); occupational and environmental medicine (APMPH); preventive medicine (APMPH); social and behavioral sciences (APMPH, MPH), including global health (MPH); JD/MPH; M Div/MPH; MBA/MPH; MD/MPH; MEM/MPH; MFS/MPH; MM Sc/MPH; MPH/MA; MSN/MPH. MS and PhD offered through the Graduate School. *Accreditation:* CEPH. Part-time programs available. Terminal master's awarded for partial completion of doctoral program. *Degree requirements:* For master's, thesis, summer internship; for doctorate, comprehensive exam, thesis/dissertation, residency. *Entrance requirements:* For master's, GMAT, GRE, or MCAT, two years of undergraduate coursework in math and science; for doctorate, GRE General Test. Additional exam requirements/recommendations for international students: Required—TOEFL (minimum score 100 iBT). Electronic applications accepted. *Expenses:* Contact institution. *Faculty research:* Genetic and emerging infections epidemiology, virology, cost/quality, vector biology, quantitative methods, aging, asthma, cancer.

Community Health

Adelphi University, Ruth S. Ammon School of Education, Program in Health Studies, Garden City, NY 11530-0701. Offers community health education (MA, Certificate); school health education (MA). Part-time and evening/weekend programs available. *Students:* 12 full-time (7 women), 34 part-time (18 women); includes 5 minority (2 Black or African American, non-Hispanic/Latino; 3 Hispanic/Latino), 1 international. Average age 26. In 2013, 13 master's awarded. *Degree requirements:* For master's, internship. *Entrance requirements:* For master's, 3 letters of recommendation, resume, minimum cumulative GPA of 2.75. Additional exam requirements/recommendations for international students: Required—TOEFL (minimum score 550 paper-based; 80 iBT). *Application deadline:* For fall admission, 4/1 for international students; for spring admission, 11/1 for international students. Applications are processed on a rolling basis. Application fee: $50. Electronic applications accepted. *Expenses: Tuition:* Full-time $32,530; part-time $1010 per credit. *Required fees:* $1150. Tuition and fees vary according to degree level and program. *Financial support:* Fellowships, research assistantships with partial tuition reimbursements, teaching assistantships, career-related internships or fieldwork, Federal Work-Study, institutionally sponsored loans, and tuition waivers (full) available. Support available to part-time students. Financial award application deadline: 2/15; financial award applicants required to submit FAFSA. *Faculty research:* Alcohol abuse, tobacco cessation, drug abuse, healthy family lives, healthy personal living. *Unit head:* Dr. Ronald Feingold, Director, 516-877-4764, E-mail: feingold@adelphi.edu. *Application contact:* Christine Murphy, Director of Admissions, 516-877-3050, Fax: 516-877-3039, E-mail: graduateadmissions@adelphi.edu.

American University of Beirut, Graduate Programs, Faculty of Health Sciences, Beirut, Lebanon. Offers environmental sciences (MS), including environmental health; epidemiology (MS); epidemiology and biostatistics (MPH); health management and policy (MPH); health promotion and community health (MPH); population health (MS). Part-time programs available. *Faculty:* 26 full-time (18 women), 7 part-time/adjunct (4 women). *Students:* 42 full-time (37 women), 103 part-time (84 women). Average age 25. 132 applicants, 65% accepted, 48 enrolled. In 2013, 52 master's awarded. *Degree requirements:* For master's, one foreign language, comprehensive exam, thesis (for some programs). *Entrance requirements:* For master's, 2 letters of recommendation, personal statement, transcripts. Additional exam requirements/recommendations for international students: Required—TOEFL (minimum score 583 paper-based; 97 iBT), IELTS (minimum score 7). *Application deadline:* For fall admission, 2/7 priority date for domestic and international students; for spring admission, 11/1 for domestic and international students. Application fee: $50. Electronic applications accepted. *Expenses: Tuition:* Full-time $14,724; part-time $818 per credit. *Required fees:* $692. Tuition and fees vary according to course load and program. *Financial support:* In 2013–14, 56 students received support. Scholarships/grants, health care benefits, and unspecified assistantships available. Financial award application deadline: 4/1. *Faculty research:* Tobacco control; health of the elderly; youth health; mental health; women's health; reproductive and sexual health, including HIV/AIDS; water quality; health systems; quality in health care delivery; health human resources; health policy; occupational and environmental health; social inequality; social determinants of health; non-communicable diseases. *Total annual research expenditures:* $1 million. *Unit head:* Iman Adel Nuwayhid, Dean, 961-1759683, Fax: 961-1744470, E-mail: nuwayhid@aub.edu.lb. *Application contact:* Mitra Tauk, Administrative Coordinator, 961-1-350000 Ext. 4687, Fax: 96-1-1744470, E-mail: mt12@aub.edu.lb.

Arcadia University, Graduate Studies, Department of Medical Science and Community Health, Glenside, PA 19038-3295. Offers health education (MA, MSHE); physician assistant (MM Sc); MM Sc/MAHE; MM Sc/MSPH. *Entrance requirements:* For master's, GRE General Test or MCAT. Additional exam requirements/recommendations for international students: Required—TOEFL. *Expenses:* Contact institution.

Arizona State University at the Tempe campus, College of Nursing and Health Innovation, Phoenix, AZ 85004. Offers advanced nursing practice (DNP); child/family mental health nurse practitioner (Graduate Certificate); clinical research management (MS); community and public health practice (Graduate Certificate); community health (MS); exercise and wellness (MS), including exercise and wellness; family nurse practitioner (Graduate Certificate); healthcare innovation (MHI); international health for healthcare (Graduate Certificate); kinesiology (MS, PhD); nursing (MS, Graduate Certificate); nursing and healthcare innovation (PhD); nutrition (MS); physical activity nutrition and wellness (PhD), including physical activity, nutrition and wellness; public health (MPH); regulatory science and health safety (MS). *Accreditation:* AACN. Postbaccalaureate distance learning degree programs offered (minimal on-campus study). *Degree requirements:* For master's, comprehensive exam (for some programs), thesis (for some programs), interactive Program of Study (iPOS) submitted before completing 50 percent of required credit hours; for doctorate, comprehensive exam, thesis/dissertation, interactive Program of Study (iPOS) submitted before completing 50 percent of required credit hours. *Entrance requirements:* For master's and doctorate, GRE, minimum GPA of 3.0 or equivalent in last 2 years of work leading to bachelor's degree. Additional exam requirements/recommendations for international students: Required—TOEFL (minimum score 80 iBT), TOEFL, IELTS, or PTE. Electronic applications accepted. *Expenses:* Contact institution.

Austin Peay State University, College of Graduate Studies, College of Behavioral and Health Sciences, Department of Health and Human Performance, Clarksville, TN 37044. Offers health leadership (MS). Part-time and evening/weekend programs available. Postbaccalaureate distance learning degree programs offered (no on-campus study). *Faculty:* 6 full-time (3 women). *Students:* 15 full-time (6 women), 30 part-time (21 women); includes 14 minority (13 Black or African American, non-Hispanic/Latino; 1 Hispanic/Latino). Average age 27. 41 applicants, 90% accepted, 32 enrolled. In 2013, 32 master's awarded. *Degree requirements:* For master's, comprehensive exam, thesis optional. *Entrance requirements:* For master's, GRE General Test, 3 letters of recommendation, minimum undergraduate GPA of 2.5. Additional exam requirements/recommendations for international students: Required—TOEFL (minimum score 500 paper-based). *Application deadline:* For fall admission, 8/5 priority date for domestic students. Applications are processed on a rolling basis. Application fee: $25. Electronic applications accepted. *Expenses:* Tuition, state resident: full-time $7500; part-time $375 per credit hour. Tuition, nonresident: full-time $20,800; part-time $1040 per credit hour. *Required fees:* $1284; $64.20 per credit hour. *Financial support:* In 2013–14, research assistantships with full tuition reimbursements (averaging $6,500 per year) were awarded; career-related internships or fieldwork, Federal Work-Study, institutionally sponsored loans, scholarships/grants, and unspecified assistantships also available. Support available to part-time students. Financial award application deadline: 3/1; financial award applicants required to submit FAFSA. *Unit head:* Dr. Marcy Maurer, Chair, 931-221-6105, Fax: 931-221-7040, E-mail: maurerm@apsu.edu. *Application contact:* June D. Lee, Graduate Coordinator, 800-859-4723, Fax: 931-221-7641, E-mail: gradadmissions@apsu.edu.
Website: http://www.apsu.edu/hhp/

Baylor University, Graduate School, School of Education, Department of Health, Human Performance and Recreation, Waco, TX 76798. Offers community health education (MPH); exercise physiology (MS Ed); kinesiology, exercise nutrition and health promotion (PhD); sport management (MS Ed); sport pedagogy (MS Ed). *Accreditation:* NCATE. Part-time programs available. *Faculty:* 13 full-time (5 women), 3 part-time/adjunct (1 woman). *Students:* 79 full-time (40 women), 28 part-time (14 women); includes 26 minority (9 Black or African American, non-Hispanic/Latino; 1 American Indian or Alaska Native, non-Hispanic/Latino; 3 Asian, non-Hispanic/Latino; 8 Hispanic/Latino; 5 Two or more races, non-Hispanic/Latino), 9 international. 30 applicants, 87% accepted. In 2013, 48 master's awarded. *Degree requirements:* For master's, comprehensive exam, thesis optional; for doctorate, comprehensive exam, thesis/dissertation. *Entrance requirements:* For master's and doctorate, GRE General Test. Additional exam requirements/recommendations for international students: Required—TOEFL. *Application deadline:* For fall admission, 2/1 priority date for domestic students, 2/1 for international students; for spring admission, 10/1 for domestic and international students. Applications are processed on a rolling basis. Application fee: $25. Electronic applications accepted. *Expenses: Tuition:* Full-time $25,866; part-time $1437 per credit hour. *Required fees:* $2736; $152 per credit hour. Tuition and fees vary according to course load and program. *Financial support:* In 2013–14, 35 students received support, including 1 research assistantship with tuition reimbursement available, 33 teaching assistantships with tuition reimbursements available; career-related internships or fieldwork, Federal Work-Study, institutionally sponsored loans, tuition waivers (partial), and unspecified assistantships also available. Financial award application deadline: 2/1. *Faculty research:* Behavior change theory, nutrition and enzyme therapy, exercise testing, health planning, sport management. *Unit head:* Dr. Jeffrey Petersen, Graduate Program Director, 254-710-4007, Fax: 254-710-3527, E-mail: jeffrey_petersen@baylor.edu. *Application contact:* Kathy Mirick, Administrative Assistant, 254-710-3526, Fax: 254-710-3527, E-mail: kathy_mirick@baylor.edu.
Website: http://www.baylor.edu/HHPR/

Bloomsburg University of Pennsylvania, School of Graduate Studies, College of Science and Technology, Department of Nursing, Bloomsburg, PA 17815. Offers adult and family nurse practitioner (MSN); community health (MSN); nurse anesthesia (MSN); nursing (MSN); nursing administration (MSN). *Accreditation:* AACN; AANA/CANAEP. *Faculty:* 5 full-time (all women), 7 part-time/adjunct (all women). *Students:* 62 full-time (52 women), 26 part-time (17 women); includes 8 minority (6 Black or African American, non-Hispanic/Latino; 1 Asian, non-Hispanic/Latino; 1 Hispanic/Latino). Average age 35. 61 applicants, 84% accepted, 14 enrolled. In 2013, 36 master's awarded. *Degree requirements:* For master's, thesis (for some programs), clinical experience. *Entrance requirements:* For master's, minimum QPA of 3.0, personal statement, 2 letters of recommendation, nursing license. Additional exam requirements/recommendations for international students: Required—TOEFL. *Application deadline:* For fall admission, 1/1 for domestic students; for spring admission, 8/1 for domestic students. Applications are processed on a rolling basis. Application fee: $35 ($60 for international students). Electronic applications accepted. *Expenses:* Tuition, state resident: full-time $7956; part-time $442 per credit. Tuition, nonresident: full-time $11,934; part-time $663 per credit. *Required fees:* $95.50 per credit. $55 per semester. Tuition and fees vary according to course load. *Financial support:* Unspecified assistantships available. *Unit head:* Dr. Noreen Chikotas, Coordinator, 570-389-4609, Fax: 570-389-5008, E-mail: nchikota@bloomu.edu. *Application contact:* Jennifer Richard, Administrative Assistant, 570-389-4015, Fax: 570-389-3054, E-mail: jrichard@bloomu.edu.
Website: http://www.bloomu.edu/nursing

Brooklyn College of the City University of New York, School of Natural and Behavioral Sciences, Department of Health and Nutrition Sciences, Program in Community Health, Brooklyn, NY 11210-2889. Offers community health education (MA); thanatology (MA). *Accreditation:* CEPH. *Degree requirements:* For master's, thesis or alternative. *Entrance requirements:* For master's, 2 letters of recommendation, essay. Additional exam requirements/recommendations for international students: Required—TOEFL. *Application deadline:* For fall admission, 3/1 priority date for domestic students, 2/1 priority date for international students; for spring admission, 11/1 priority date for domestic students, 10/1 priority date for international students. Applications are processed on a rolling basis. Application fee: $125. Electronic applications accepted. *Expenses: Tuition, area resident:* Full-time $4585; part-time $385 per credit. Tuition, state resident: full-time $4585; part-time $385 per credit. Tuition, nonresident: part-time $710 per credit. *Required fees:* $430; $153 per semester. Tuition and fees vary according to course load. *Financial support:* Federal Work-Study, institutionally sponsored loans, and scholarships/grants available. Support available to part-time students. Financial award application deadline: 5/1; financial award applicants required to submit FAFSA. *Faculty research:* Diet restriction, religious practices in bereavement, diabetes, stress management, palliative care. *Unit head:* Raymond Weston, Graduate Deputy Chairperson, 718-951-5026, Fax: 718-951-4670. *Application contact:* Raymond Weston, Graduate Deputy Chairperson, 718-951-5026, Fax: 718-951-4670.

Brown University, Graduate School, Division of Biology and Medicine, School of Public Health, Providence, RI 02912. Offers behavioral and social sciences intervention (M Sc); biostatistics (AM, Sc M, PhD); epidemiology (Sc M); health services, policy and practice (PhD); public health (MPH); MD/PhD. *Accreditation:* CEPH. *Degree requirements:* For doctorate, thesis/dissertation, preliminary exam. *Entrance* *requirements:* For master's and doctorate, GRE General Test. Additional exam requirements/recommendations for international students: Required—TOEFL.

Canisius College, Graduate Division, School of Education and Human Services, Office of Professional Studies, Buffalo, NY 14208-1098. Offers applied nutrition (MS, Certificate); community and school health (MS); health and human performance (MS); health information technology (MS); respiratory care (MS). Postbaccalaureate distance learning degree programs offered (no on-campus study). *Faculty:* 17 part-time/adjunct (11 women). *Students:* 51 full-time (35 women), 37 part-time (26 women); includes 16 minority (8 Black or African American, non-Hispanic/Latino; 1 American Indian or Alaska Native, non-Hispanic/Latino; 7 Hispanic/Latino), 2 international. Average age 32. 98 applicants, 57% accepted, 24 enrolled. In 2013, 29 master's awarded. *Entrance requirements:* Additional exam requirements/recommendations for international students: Required—TOEFL (minimum score 550 paper-based, 80 iBT), IELTS (minimum score 6.5), or CAEL (minimum score 70). *Application deadline:* Applications are processed on a rolling basis. Application fee: $25. Electronic applications accepted. Application fee is waived when completed online. *Expenses: Tuition:* Part-time $750 per credit hour. *Financial support:* Career-related internships or fieldwork, Federal Work-Study, scholarships/grants, and unspecified assistantships available. Support available to part-time students. Financial award application deadline: 4/30; financial award applicants required to submit FAFSA. *Faculty research:* Nutrition, community and school health; community and health; health and human performance applied; nutrition and respiratory care. *Unit head:* Dr. Khalid Bibi, Executive Director, 716-888-8296. *Application contact:* Julie A. Zulewski, Director of Graduate Admission, 716-888-2548, Fax: 716-888-3195, E-mail: zulewskj@canisius.edu.
Website: http://www.canisius.edu/graduate/

Clemson University, Graduate School, College of Health, Education, and Human Development, Eugene T. Moore School of Education, Program in Counselor Education, Clemson, SC 29634. Offers clinical mental health counseling (M Ed); community mental health (M Ed); school counseling (K-12) (M Ed); student affairs (higher education) (M Ed). *Accreditation:* ACA; NCATE. Part-time and evening/weekend programs available. *Students:* 135 full-time (109 women), 14 part-time (10 women); includes 29 minority (17 Black or African American, non-Hispanic/Latino; 3 Asian, non-Hispanic/Latino; 6 Hispanic/Latino; 1 Native Hawaiian or other Pacific Islander, non-Hispanic/Latino; 2 Two or more races, non-Hispanic/Latino), 1 international. Average age 24. 271 applicants, 43% accepted, 63 enrolled. In 2013, 47 master's awarded. *Degree requirements:* For master's, comprehensive exam. *Entrance requirements:* For master's, GRE General Test. Additional exam requirements/recommendations for international students: Required—TOEFL; Recommended—IELTS. *Application deadline:* For fall admission, 2/1 priority date for domestic students; for spring admission, 10/1 for domestic students. Applications are processed on a rolling basis. Application fee: $70 ($80 for international students). Electronic applications accepted. *Expenses:* Contact institution. *Financial support:* In 2013–14, 84 students received support, including 9 research assistantships with partial tuition reimbursements available (averaging $7,586 per year), 3 teaching assistantships with partial tuition reimbursements available (averaging $22,987 per year); institutionally sponsored loans, health care benefits, and unspecified assistantships also available. Financial award application deadline: 6/1; financial award applicants required to submit FAFSA. *Faculty research:* At-risk youth, ethnic identity development across the life span, postsecondary transitions and college readiness, distance and distributed learning environments, the student veteran experience in college, student development theory. *Unit head:* Dr. Michael J. Padilla, Director/Associate Dean, 864-656-4444, Fax: 864-656-0311, E-mail: padilla@clemson.edu. *Application contact:* Dr. David Fleming, Graduate Coordinator, 864-656-1881, Fax: 864-656-0311, E-mail: dflemin@clemson.edu.

The College at Brockport, State University of New York, School of Health and Human Performance, Department of Health Science, Brockport, NY 14420-2997. Offers health education (MS Ed), including community health education, health education K-12. *Faculty:* 4 full-time (1 woman), 5 part-time/adjunct (1 woman). *Students:* 9 full-time (4 women), 8 part-time (5 women); includes 1 minority (Hispanic/Latino). 13 applicants, 85% accepted, 8 enrolled. In 2013, 13 master's awarded. *Degree requirements:* For master's, thesis or alternative. *Entrance requirements:* For master's, minimum GPA of 3.0, letters of recommendation. Additional exam requirements/recommendations for international students: Required—TOEFL (minimum score 550 paper-based; 79 iBT), IELTS (minimum score 6.5). *Application deadline:* For fall admission, 3/1 priority date for domestic and international students; for spring admission, 10/1 priority date for domestic and international students; for summer admission, 3/1 priority date for domestic and international students. Application fee: $80. Electronic applications accepted. *Expenses:* Tuition, state resident: full-time $9870. Tuition, nonresident: full-time $18,350. *Required fees:* $1848. *Financial support:* In 2013–14, 1 teaching assistantship with full tuition reimbursement (averaging $6,000 per year) was awarded; Federal Work-Study, scholarships/grants, and unspecified assistantships also available. Support available to part-time students. Financial award application deadline: 3/15; financial award applicants required to submit FAFSA. *Faculty research:* Nutrition, substance use, HIV/AIDS, bioethics, worksite health. *Unit head:* Dr. Patti Follansbee, Chairperson, 585-395-5483, Fax: 585-395-5246, E-mail: pfollans@brockport.edu. *Application contact:* Danielle A. Welch, Graduate Admissions Counselor, 585-395-5465, Fax: 585-395-2515.
Website: http://www.brockport.edu/healthsci/graduate/

Columbia University, Columbia University Mailman School of Public Health, Division of Sociomedical Sciences, New York, NY 10032. Offers MPH, Dr PH, PhD. PhD offered in cooperation with the Graduate School of Arts and Sciences. *Accreditation:* CEPH (one or more programs are accredited). Part-time programs available. *Students:* 216 full-time (190 women), 29 part-time (21 women); includes 91 minority (23 Black or African American, non-Hispanic/Latino; 34 Asian, non-Hispanic/Latino; 25 Hispanic/Latino; 9 Two or more races, non-Hispanic/Latino), 18 international. Average age 27. 602 applicants, 56% accepted, 114 enrolled. In 2013, 88 master's, 8 doctorates awarded. *Degree requirements:* For master's, thesis; for doctorate, thesis/dissertation. *Entrance requirements:* For master's, GRE General Test; for doctorate, GRE General Test, MPH or equivalent (Dr PH). Additional exam requirements/recommendations for international students: Required—TOEFL (minimum score 600 paper-based; 100 iBT). *Application deadline:* For fall admission, 12/1 priority date for domestic and international students. Application fee: $120. Electronic applications accepted. *Financial support:* Research assistantships, teaching assistantships, career-related internships or fieldwork, and Federal Work-Study available. Support available to part-time students. Financial award application deadline: 2/1; financial award applicants required to submit FAFSA. *Faculty research:* Social and cultural factors in health and health care, health services delivery and utilization, health promotion and disease prevention, AIDS. *Unit head:* Dr. Lisa Metsch, Chair, 212-305-5656. *Application contact:* Dr. Joseph Korevec, Director of Admissions and Financial Aid, 212-305-8698, Fax: 212-342-1861, E-mail: ph-admit@columbia.edu.
Website: http://www.mailman.hs.columbia.edu/sms/index.html

Dalhousie University, Faculty of Medicine, Department of Community Health and Epidemiology, Halifax, NS B3H 4R2, Canada. Offers M Sc. *Degree requirements:* For master's, thesis. *Entrance requirements:* Additional exam requirements/recommendations for international students: Required—1 of 5 approved tests: TOEFL, IELTS, CANTEST, CAEL, Michigan English Language Assessment Battery. Electronic applications accepted. *Expenses:* Contact institution. *Faculty research:* Population health, health promotion and disease prevention, health services utilization, chronic disease epidemiology.

Duquesne University, School of Education, Department of Counseling, Psychology, and Special Education, Program in Special Education, Pittsburgh, PA 15282-0001. Offers cognitive, behavior, physical/health disabilities (MS Ed); community and special education support (MS Ed). Part-time and evening/weekend programs available. *Faculty:* 7 full-time (6 women). *Students:* 14 full-time (12 women), 1 (woman) part-time; includes 1 minority (Black or African American, non-Hispanic/Latino), 2 international. Average age 26. 23 applicants, 30% accepted, 5 enrolled. In 2013, 16 master's awarded. *Degree requirements:* For master's, thesis optional. *Entrance requirements:* For master's, bachelor's degree. Additional exam requirements/recommendations for international students: Required—TOEFL (minimum score 550 paper-based), IELTS (minimum score 7). *Application deadline:* For fall admission, 9/1 for domestic students; for spring admission, 1/1 for domestic students. Applications are processed on a rolling basis. Application fee: $0. Electronic applications accepted. Application fee is waived when completed online. *Expenses: Tuition:* Full-time $18,162; part-time $1009 per credit. *Required fees:* $1728; $96 per credit. Tuition and fees vary according to program. *Financial support:* In 2013–14, 1 research assistantship was awarded. Support available to part-time students. *Unit head:* Dr. Morgan Chitiyo, Associate Professor, 412-396-4036, Fax: 412-396-1340, E-mail: chitiyom@duq.edu. *Application contact:* Michael Dolinger, Director of Student and Academic Services, 412-396-6647, Fax: 412-396-5585, E-mail: dolingerm@duq.edu.
Website: http://www.duq.edu/academics/schools/education/graduate-programs-education/msed-special-education

East Carolina University, Graduate School, Thomas Harriot College of Arts and Sciences, Department of Political Science, Greenville, NC 27858-4353. Offers community health administration (Certificate); public administration (MPA); security studies (Certificate). *Accreditation:* NASPAA. Part-time and evening/weekend programs available. *Degree requirements:* For master's, one foreign language, comprehensive exam. *Entrance requirements:* For master's, GRE General Test. Additional exam requirements/recommendations for international students: Required—TOEFL. *Application deadline:* For fall admission, 6/1 priority date for domestic students; for spring admission, 10/15 for domestic students. Applications are processed on a rolling basis. Application fee: $50. *Expenses:* Tuition, state resident: full-time $4223. Tuition, nonresident: full-time $16,540. *Required fees:* $2184. *Financial support:* Research assistantships with partial tuition reimbursements, teaching assistantships with partial tuition reimbursements, and Federal Work-Study available. Support available to part-time students. Financial award application deadline: 6/1. *Unit head:* Dr. Robert Thompson, Interim Chair, 252-328-5686, E-mail: thompsonro@ecu.edu. *Application contact:* Dean of Graduate School, 252-328-6012, Fax: 252-328-6071, E-mail: gradschool@ecu.edu.
Website: http://www.ecu.edu/polsci/mpa/index.html

Eastern Kentucky University, The Graduate School, College of Health Sciences, Department of Health Promotion and Administration, Richmond, KY 40475-3102. Offers community health (MPH). *Degree requirements:* For master's, comprehensive exam, thesis optional. *Entrance requirements:* For master's, GRE or MAT, letters of recommendation. *Faculty research:* Risk behavior, health systems, injury control, nutrition.

George Mason University, College of Health and Human Services, Department of Global and Community Health, Fairfax, VA 22030. Offers global health (MS); public health (MPH, Certificate). *Accreditation:* CEPH. *Faculty:* 12 full-time (8 women), 16 part-time/adjunct (13 women). *Students:* 70 full-time (58 women), 62 part-time (55 women); includes 58 minority (21 Black or African American, non-Hispanic/Latino; 22 Asian, non-Hispanic/Latino; 11 Hispanic/Latino; 1 Native Hawaiian or other Pacific Islander, non-Hispanic/Latino; 3 Two or more races, non-Hispanic/Latino), 9 international. Average age 29. 144 applicants, 69% accepted, 51 enrolled. In 2013, 54 master's, 1 other advanced degree awarded. *Degree requirements:* For master's, comprehensive exam (for some programs), thesis or practicum. *Entrance requirements:* For master's, GRE, 2 official transcripts; expanded goals statement; 3 letters of recommendation; resume; 1 completed course in health science, statistics, natural sciences and social science (for MPH); 6 credits of foreign language if not fluent (for MS in global health); for Certificate, 2 official transcripts; expanded goals statement; 3 letters of recommendation; resume; bachelor's degree from regionally-accredited institution with minimum GPA of 3.0; statistics and college-level algebra with minimum B grade (for Certificate in biostatistics). Additional exam requirements/recommendations for international students: Required—TOEFL (minimum score 570 paper-based; 88 iBT), IELTS (minimum score 6.5), PTE. *Application deadline:* For fall admission, 4/1 priority date for domestic students; for spring admission, 11/1 priority date for domestic students. Applications are processed on a rolling basis. Application fee: $65 ($80 for international students). Electronic applications accepted. *Expenses:* Contact institution. *Financial support:* In 2013–14, 4 students received support, including 4 research assistantships with full and partial tuition reimbursements available (averaging $14,250 per year); career-related internships or fieldwork, Federal Work-Study, scholarships/grants, unspecified assistantships, and health care benefits (for full-time research or teaching assistantship recipients) also available. Financial award application deadline: 3/1; financial award applicants required to submit FAFSA. *Faculty research:* Health issues and the needs of affected populations at the regional and global level. *Total annual research expenditures:* $21,323. *Unit head:* Keith Howell, Interim Chair, 703-993-9633, Fax: 703-993-1943, E-mail: khowell@gmu.edu. *Application contact:* Ali Weinstein, Graduate Coordinator, 703-993-9632, Fax: 703-993-1908, E-mail: aweinst2@gmu.edu.
Website: http://chhs.gmu.edu/gch/index

Georgia Southern University, Jack N. Averitt College of Graduate Studies, Jiann-Ping Hsu College of Public Health, Program in Public Health, Statesboro, GA 30460. Offers biostatistics (MPH, Dr PH); community health behavior and education (Dr PH); community health education (MPH); environmental health sciences (MPH); epidemiology (MPH); health policy and management (MPH, Dr PH). *Accreditation:* CEPH. Part-time programs available. *Students:* 130 full-time (96 women), 50 part-time (39 women); includes 95 minority (80 Black or African American, non-Hispanic/Latino; 5 Asian, non-Hispanic/Latino; 4 Hispanic/Latino; 1 Native Hawaiian or other Pacific Islander, non-Hispanic/Latino; 5 Two or more races, non-Hispanic/Latino), 32 international. Average age 30. 213 applicants, 68% accepted, 61 enrolled. In 2013, 29 master's, 9 doctorates awarded. *Degree requirements:* For master's, thesis optional, practicum; for doctorate, comprehensive exam, thesis/dissertation, practicum. *Entrance requirements:* For master's, GRE General Test, minimum GPA of 2.75, resume, 3 letters of reference; for doctorate, GRE, GMAT, MCAT, LSAT, 3 letters of reference, statement of purpose, resume or curriculum vitae. Additional exam requirements/recommendations for international students: Required—TOEFL (minimum score 550 paper-based; 80 iBT), IELTS (minimum score 6). *Application deadline:* For fall admission, 3/1 priority date for domestic and international students; for spring admission, 10/1 priority date for domestic students, 10/1 for international students. Applications are processed on a rolling basis. Application fee: $50. Electronic

applications accepted. *Expenses:* Contact institution. *Financial support:* In 2013–14, 54 students received support, including research assistantships with partial tuition reimbursements available (averaging $7,200 per year), teaching assistantships with partial tuition reimbursements available (averaging $7,200 per year); career-related internships or fieldwork, Federal Work-Study, scholarships/grants, tuition waivers (partial), and unspecified assistantships also available. Support available to part-time students. Financial award application deadline: 4/15; financial award applicants required to submit FAFSA. *Faculty research:* Rural public health best practices, health disparity elimination, community initiatives to enhance public health, cost effectiveness analysis, epidemiology of rural public health, environmental health issues, health care system assessment, rural health care, health policy and healthcare financing, survival analysis, nonparametric statistics and resampling methods, micro-arrays and genomics, data imputation techniques and clinical trial methodology. *Total annual research expenditures:* $281,707. *Unit head:* Sarah Peterson, Student Services Coordinator, 912-478-2413, Fax: 912-478-5811, E-mail: speterson@georgiasouthern.edu. *Application contact:* Amanda Gilliland, Coordinator for Graduate Student Recruitment, 912-478-5384, Fax: 912-478-0740, E-mail: gradadmissions@georgiasouthern.edu.
Website: http://chhs.georgiasouthern.edu/health/

Hofstra University, School of Health Sciences and Human Services, Programs in Health, Hempstead, NY 11549. Offers community health (MS); health administration (MHA); public health (MPH).

Hunter College of the City University of New York, Graduate School, Schools of the Health Professions, School of Health Sciences, Programs in Urban Public Health, Program in Community Health Education, New York, NY 10065-5085. Offers MPH. *Accreditation:* CEPH. Part-time and evening/weekend programs available. *Faculty:* 1 (woman) full-time, 2 part-time/adjunct (both women). *Students:* 8 full-time (6 women), 65 part-time (51 women); includes 36 minority (15 Black or African American, non-Hispanic/Latino; 9 Asian, non-Hispanic/Latino; 12 Hispanic/Latino), 1 international. Average age 32. 111 applicants, 53% accepted, 28 enrolled. In 2013, 15 master's awarded. *Degree requirements:* For master's, comprehensive exam, thesis optional, internship. *Entrance requirements:* For master's, GRE General Test, previous course work in calculus and statistics. Additional exam requirements/recommendations for international students: Required—TOEFL. *Application deadline:* For fall admission, 4/1 for domestic students; for spring admission, 11/1 for domestic students. Application fee: $125. *Financial support:* In 2013–14, 6 fellowships were awarded; career-related internships or fieldwork, Federal Work-Study, institutionally sponsored loans, and tuition waivers (partial) also available. Support available to part-time students. Financial award application deadline: 3/1. *Unit head:* Nicholas Freudenberg, Director, Center of Community and Urban Health, 212-396-7738, Fax: 212-481-5260, E-mail: nfreuden@hunter.cuny.edu. *Application contact:* Milena Solo, Director of Graduate Admissions, 212-772-4482, Fax: 212-650-3336, E-mail: admissions@hunter.cuny.edu.
Website: http://www.hunter.cuny.edu/uph/grad-test/community-health-education-1

Icahn School of Medicine at Mount Sinai, Graduate School of Biological Sciences, New York, NY 10029-6504. Offers biomedical sciences (MS, PhD); clinical research education (MS, PhD); community medicine (MPH); genetic counseling (MS); neurosciences (PhD); MD/PhD. Terminal master's awarded for partial completion of doctoral program. *Degree requirements:* For master's, thesis; for doctorate, comprehensive exam, thesis/dissertation. *Entrance requirements:* For master's, GRE General Test; for doctorate, GRE General Test, GRE Subject Test, 3 years of college pre-med course work. Additional exam requirements/recommendations for international students: Required—TOEFL. Electronic applications accepted. *Faculty research:* Cancer, genetics and genomics, immunology, neuroscience, developmental and stem cell biology, translational research.

Idaho State University, Office of Graduate Studies, Kasiska College of Health Professions, Department of Family Medicine, Pocatello, ID 83209-8357. Offers Post-Master's Certificate. *Degree requirements:* For Post-Master's Certificate, comprehensive exam, thesis optional, 3 year residency program. *Entrance requirements:* For degree, GRE General Test, MD or DO. Additional exam requirements/recommendations for international students: Required—TOEFL (minimum score 600 paper-based). Electronic applications accepted. *Faculty research:* Health disparities in primary care, cardiovascular risk reduction (particularly in dyslipidemia, diabetes, hypertension), health application of geographic information systems, mechanisms for increasing quality in primary care, collaborative care models for improving health.

Independence University, Program in Health Services, Salt Lake City, UT 84107. Offers community health (MSHS); wellness promotion (MSHS). Part-time and evening/weekend programs available. Postbaccalaureate distance learning degree programs offered (no on-campus study). *Degree requirements:* For master's, fieldwork, internship, final project (wellness promotion). *Entrance requirements:* For master's, previous course work in psychology.

Indiana State University, College of Graduate and Professional Studies, College of Nursing, Health and Human Services, Department of Health, Safety, and Environmental Health Sciences, Terre Haute, IN 47809. Offers community health promotion (MA, MS); health and safety education (MA, MS); occupational safety management (MA, MS). *Accreditation:* NCATE (one or more programs are accredited). *Degree requirements:* For master's, thesis or alternative. *Entrance requirements:* For master's, GRE General Test. Electronic applications accepted.

Indiana University Bloomington, School of Public Health, Department of Applied Health Science, Bloomington, IN 47405. Offers behavioral, social, and community health (MPH); family health (MPH); health behavior (PhD); nutrition science (MS); professional health education (MPH); public health administration (MPH); safety management (MS); school and college health education (MS). *Accreditation:* CEPH (one or more programs are accredited). *Faculty:* 30 full-time (19 women). *Students:* 144 full-time (104 women), 26 part-time (16 women); includes 46 minority (23 Black or African American, non-Hispanic/Latino; 1 American Indian or Alaska Native, non-Hispanic/Latino; 8 Asian, non-Hispanic/Latino; 10 Hispanic/Latino; 4 Two or more races, non-Hispanic/Latino), 32 international. Average age 30. 129 applicants, 71% accepted, 58 enrolled. In 2013, 53 master's, 6 doctorates awarded. *Degree requirements:* For master's, thesis optional; for doctorate, comprehensive exam, thesis/dissertation. *Entrance requirements:* For master's, GRE (for MS in nutrition science), 3 recommendations; for doctorate, GRE, 3 recommendations. Additional exam requirements/recommendations for international students: Required—TOEFL (minimum score 550 paper-based; 80 iBT). *Application deadline:* For fall admission, 2/1 priority date for domestic students, 12/1 priority date for international students; for spring admission, 11/15 priority date for domestic students, 9/1 priority date for international students. Application fee: $55 ($65 for international students). Electronic applications accepted. *Financial support:* Fellowships, research assistantships with full and partial tuition reimbursements, teaching assistantships with full and partial tuition reimbursements, career-related internships or fieldwork, Federal Work-Study, institutionally sponsored loans, scholarships/grants, health care benefits, tuition waivers (partial), unspecified assistantships, and fee remissions available. Financial award application deadline: 3/1; financial award applicants required to submit FAFSA. *Faculty research:* Cancer education, HIV/AIDS and drug education, public health, parent-child interactions, safety education, obesity, public health policy, public health administration, school health, health education, human development, nutrition, human sexuality, chronic disease, early childhood health. *Total annual research expenditures:* $1.4 million. *Unit head:* Dr. David K. Lohrmann, Chair, 812-856-5101, Fax: 812-855-3936, E-mail: dlohrman@indiana.edu. *Application contact:* Dr. Susan Middlestadt, Associate Professor and Graduate Coordinator, 812-856-5768, Fax: 812-855-3936, E-mail: semiddle@indiana.edu.
Website: http://www.publichealth.indiana.edu/departments/applied-health-science/index.shtml

Indiana University–Purdue University Indianapolis, School of Public Health, Indianapolis, IN 46202-2896. Offers biostatistics (MPH); environmental health science (MPH); epidemiology (MPH, PhD); health administration (MHA); health policy and management (MPH, PhD); social and behavioral sciences (MPH). *Accreditation:* CEPH. *Students:* 121 full-time (87 women), 161 part-time (111 women); includes 66 minority (32 Black or African American, non-Hispanic/Latino; 19 Asian, non-Hispanic/Latino; 13 Hispanic/Latino; 1 Native Hawaiian or other Pacific Islander, non-Hispanic/Latino; 1 Two or more races, non-Hispanic/Latino), 10 international. Average age 30. 185 applicants, 70% accepted, 95 enrolled. In 2013, 25 master's awarded. Application fee: $55 ($65 for international students). *Expenses:* Contact institution. *Financial support:* In 2013–14, 1 fellowship (averaging $17,650 per year), 4 research assistantships (averaging $22,000 per year), 8 teaching assistantships (averaging $24,000 per year) were awarded. *Unit head:* Dr. Paul Halverson, Dean, 317-274-4242. *Application contact:* Shawne Mathis, Student Services Coordinator, 317-278-0337, E-mail: snmathis@iupui.edu.
Website: http://www.pbhealth.iupui.edu/

Johns Hopkins University, Bloomberg School of Public Health, Department of Health, Behavior and Society, Baltimore, MD 21218-2699. Offers genetic counseling (Sc M); health education and health communication (MSPH); social and behavioral sciences (Dr PH, PhD); social factors in health (MHS). *Faculty:* 43 full-time (30 women), 59 part-time/adjunct (40 women). *Students:* 107 full-time (97 women), 10 part-time (8 women); includes 33 minority (11 Black or African American, non-Hispanic/Latino; 11 Asian, non-Hispanic/Latino; 7 Hispanic/Latino; 4 Two or more races, non-Hispanic/Latino), 14 international. Average age 29. 241 applicants, 33% accepted, 35 enrolled. In 2013, 27 master's, 18 doctorates awarded. *Degree requirements:* For master's, comprehensive exam (for some programs), thesis (for some programs); for doctorate, comprehensive exam, thesis/dissertation. *Entrance requirements:* For master's, GRE, curriculum vitae, 3 letters of recommendation; for doctorate, GRE, transcripts, curriculum vitae, 3 recommendation letters. Additional exam requirements/recommendations for international students: Required—TOEFL (minimum score 600 paper-based; 100 iBT). *Application deadline:* For fall admission, 12/1 for domestic and international students. Applications are processed on a rolling basis. Application fee: $45. Electronic applications accepted. *Financial support:* Fellowships with tuition reimbursements, research assistantships, teaching assistantships, career-related internships or fieldwork, Federal Work-Study, scholarships/grants, traineeships, health care benefits, unspecified assistantships, and stipends available. Financial award application deadline: 3/15. *Faculty research:* Social determinants of health and structural and community-level inventions to improve health, communication and health education, behavioral and social aspects of genetic counseling. *Total annual research expenditures:* $6.3 million. *Unit head:* David R. Holtgrave, Department Chair, 410-502-4076, Fax: 410-502-4080, E-mail: dholtgra@jhsph.edu. *Application contact:* Barbara W. Diehl, Senior Academic Program Coordinator, 410-502-4415, Fax: 410-502-4333, E-mail: bdiehl@jhsph.edu.
Website: http://jhsph.edu/dept/hbs

Long Island University–LIU Brooklyn, School of Health Professions, Department of Community Health, Brooklyn, NY 11201-8423. Offers community mental health (MS); family health (MS); health management (MS). Part-time and evening/weekend programs available. *Entrance requirements:* For master's, 2 letters of recommendation. Additional exam requirements/recommendations for international students: Required—TOEFL (minimum score 500 paper-based). Electronic applications accepted.

Louisiana State University Health Sciences Center, School of Public Health, New Orleans, LA 70112. Offers behavioral and community health sciences (MPH); biostatistics (MPH, MS, PhD); community health sciences (PhD); environmental and occupational health sciences (MPH); epidemiology (MPH, PhD); health policy and systems management (MPH). *Accreditation:* CEPH. Part-time programs available. *Entrance requirements:* For master's, GRE General Test.

Massachusetts School of Professional Psychology, Graduate Programs, Boston, MA 02132. Offers applied psychology in higher education student personnel administration (MA); clinical psychology (Psy D); counseling psychology (MA); counseling psychology and community mental health (MA); counseling psychology and global mental health (MA); executive coaching (Graduate Certificate); forensic and counseling psychology (MA); leadership psychology (Psy D); organizational psychology (MA); primary care psychology (MA); respecialization in clinical psychology (Certificate); school psychology (Psy D); MA/CAGS. *Accreditation:* APA. *Degree requirements:* For master's, comprehensive exam (for some programs); for doctorate, thesis/dissertation (for some programs). Electronic applications accepted.

McGill University, Faculty of Graduate and Postdoctoral Studies, Faculty of Medicine, Department of Epidemiology and Biostatistics, Montréal, QC H3A 2T5, Canada. Offers community health (M Sc); environmental health (M Sc); epidemiology and biostatistics (M Sc, PhD, Diploma); health care evaluation (M Sc); medical statistics (M Sc). *Accreditation:* CEPH (one or more programs are accredited).

Medical College of Wisconsin, Graduate School of Biomedical Sciences, Department of Population Health, Program in Public Health, Milwaukee, WI 53226-0509. Offers public and community health (PhD); public health (MPH, Graduate Certificate). *Accreditation:* CEPH. *Entrance requirements:* For master's, doctorate, and Graduate Certificate, GRE, official transcripts, three letters of recommendation. Additional exam requirements/recommendations for international students: Required—TOEFL.

Medical College of Wisconsin, Graduate School of Biomedical Sciences, Program in Public and Community Health, Milwaukee, WI 53226-0509. Offers PhD, MD/PhD. *Accreditation:* CEPH. *Degree requirements:* For doctorate, comprehensive exam, thesis/dissertation. *Entrance requirements:* For doctorate, GRE, official transcripts, three letters of recommendation. Additional exam requirements/recommendations for international students: Required—TOEFL (minimum score 580 paper-based; 100 iBT). Electronic applications accepted. *Expenses:* Contact institution. *Faculty research:* Community-academic partnerships, community-based participatory research, injury prevention, health policy, women's health, emergency medical services.

Meharry Medical College, School of Graduate Studies, Division of Community Health Sciences, Nashville, TN 37208-9989. Offers occupational medicine (MSPH); public health administration (MSPH). *Accreditation:* CEPH. Part-time and evening/weekend programs available. *Degree requirements:* For master's, thesis, externship. *Entrance requirements:* For master's, GRE General Test, GMAT. *Expenses:* Contact institution. *Faculty research:* Policy and management, health care financing, health education and promotion.

Memorial University of Newfoundland, Faculty of Medicine and School of Graduate Studies, Graduate Programs in Medicine, Division of Community Health and Humanities, St. John's, NL A1C 5S7, Canada. Offers community health (M Sc, PhD,

Diploma). Part-time programs available. *Degree requirements:* For master's, thesis; for doctorate, comprehensive exam, thesis/dissertation, oral defense of thesis. *Entrance requirements:* For master's, MD or B Sc; for doctorate, MD or M Sc; for Diploma, bachelor's degree in health-related field. Additional exam requirements/ recommendations for international students: Required—TOEFL. *Faculty research:* Health care delivery and administration, health services, psychosocial, aging.

Midwestern State University, Graduate School, Robert D. and Carol Gunn College of Health Sciences and Human Services, Department of Criminal Justice and Health Services Administration, Wichita Falls, TX 76308. Offers criminal justice (MA); health information management (MHA); medical practice management (MHA); public and community sector health care management (MHA); rural and urban hospital management (MHA). Part-time and evening/weekend programs available. *Degree requirements:* For master's, comprehensive exam, thesis. *Entrance requirements:* For master's, GRE. Additional exam requirements/recommendations for international students: Required—TOEFL (minimum score 550 paper-based). *Application deadline:* For fall admission, 7/1 priority date for domestic students, 4/1 for international students; for spring admission, 11/1 priority date for domestic students, 8/1 for international students. Applications are processed on a rolling basis. Application fee: $35 ($50 for international students). Electronic applications accepted. *Expenses:* Tuition, state resident: full-time $3627; part-time $201.50 per credit hour. Tuition, nonresident: full-time $10,899; part-time $605.50 per credit hour. *Required fees:* $1357. *Financial support:* Teaching assistantships with partial tuition reimbursements, career-related internships or fieldwork, Federal Work-Study, institutionally sponsored loans, scholarships/grants, tuition waivers (partial), and unspecified assistantships available. Support available to part-time students. Financial award application deadline: 3/1; financial award applicants required to submit FAFSA. *Faculty research:* Universal service policy, telehealth, bullying, healthcare financial management, public health ethics. *Unit head:* Dr. Nathan R. Moran, Chair, 940-397-4752, Fax: 940-397-6291, E-mail: nathan.moran@mwsu.edu.
Website: http://www.mwsu.edu/academics/hs2/health-admin/

Minnesota State University Mankato, College of Graduate Studies and Research, College of Allied Health and Nursing, Department of Health Science, Mankato, MN 56001. Offers community health education (MS); school health education (MS, Postbaccalaureate Certificate). Part-time programs available. *Students:* 5 full-time (all women), 25 part-time (18 women). *Degree requirements:* For master's, comprehensive exam, thesis or alternative. *Entrance requirements:* For master's, minimum GPA of 3.0 during previous 2 years; for Postbaccalaureate Certificate, teaching license. Additional exam requirements/recommendations for international students: Required—TOEFL (minimum score 500 paper-based; 61 iBT). *Application deadline:* For fall admission, 7/1 for domestic students, 5/1 for international students; for spring admission, 11/1 for domestic students, 10/1 for international students. Applications are processed on a rolling basis. Application fee: $40. Electronic applications accepted. *Financial support:* Research assistantships with full tuition reimbursements, teaching assistantships with full tuition reimbursements, career-related internships or fieldwork, and Federal Work-Study available. Support available to part-time students. Financial award application deadline: 3/15; financial award applicants required to submit FAFSA. *Faculty research:* Teaching methods, stress prophylaxis and management, effects of alcohol. *Unit head:* Dr. Dawn Larsen, Graduate Coordinator, 507-389-2113. *Application contact:* 507-389-2321, E-mail: grad@mnsu.edu.
Website: http://ahn.mnsu.edu/health/

New Jersey City University, Graduate Studies and Continuing Education, College of Professional Studies, Department of Health Sciences, Jersey City, NJ 07305-1597. Offers community health education (MS); health administration (MS); school health education (MS). Part-time and evening/weekend programs available. *Faculty:* 5 full-time (all women), 7 part-time/adjunct (2 women). *Students:* 10 full-time (7 women), 58 part-time (50 women); includes 32 minority (15 Black or African American, non-Hispanic/ Latino; 7 Asian, non-Hispanic/Latino; 10 Hispanic/Latino), 2 international. Average age 40. In 2013, 18 master's awarded. *Degree requirements:* For master's, thesis or alternative, internship. *Entrance requirements:* Additional exam requirements/ recommendations for international students: Required—TOEFL (minimum score 61 iBT). *Application deadline:* For fall admission, 8/1 priority date for domestic students; for spring admission, 12/1 for domestic students. Applications are processed on a rolling basis. Application fee: $0. *Expenses: Tuition, area resident:* Part-time $527.90 per credit. Tuition, nonresident: part-time $947.75 per credit. *Financial support:* Career-related internships or fieldwork and unspecified assistantships available. *Unit head:* Dr. Lilliam Rosado, Chairperson, 201-200-3431, E-mail: lrosado@njcu.edu. *Application contact:* Dr. William Bajor, Dean of Graduate Studies, 201-200-3409, Fax: 201-200-3411, E-mail: wbajor@njcu.edu.

New Mexico State University, Graduate School, College of Health and Social Services, Department of Public Health Sciences, Las Cruces, NM 88003-8001. Offers community health education (MPH); health management, administration and policy (MPH). Part-time programs available. Postbaccalaureate distance learning degree programs offered (minimal on-campus study). *Faculty:* 11 full-time (6 women), 2 part-time/adjunct (1 woman). *Students:* 32 full-time (30 women), 28 part-time (21 women); includes 24 minority (3 Black or African American, non-Hispanic/Latino; 4 American Indian or Alaska Native, non-Hispanic/Latino; 2 Asian, non-Hispanic/Latino; 14 Hispanic/ Latino; 1 Two or more races, non-Hispanic/Latino), 1 international. Average age 34. 37 applicants, 68% accepted, 18 enrolled. In 2013, 25 master's awarded. *Degree requirements:* For master's, thesis optional. *Entrance requirements:* For master's, GRE. Additional exam requirements/recommendations for international students: Required—TOEFL (minimum score 550 paper-based; 79 iBT), IELTS (minimum score 6.5). *Application deadline:* For fall admission, 2/15 for domestic and international students. Application fee: $40 ($50 for international students). Electronic applications accepted. *Expenses:* Tuition, state resident: full-time $5398; part-time $224.90 per credit. Tuition, nonresident: full-time $18,821; part-time $784.20 per credit. *Required fees:* $1310; $54.60 per credit. *Financial support:* In 2013–14, 19 students received support, including 8 teaching assistantships (averaging $8,131 per year); career-related internships or fieldwork, Federal Work-Study, health care benefits, and unspecified assistantships also available. Financial award application deadline: 4/1. *Faculty research:* Community health education, health issues of U.S.-Mexico border, health policy and management, victims of violence, environmental and occupational health issues. *Total annual research expenditures:* $79,183. *Unit head:* Dr. Mark J. Kittleson, Head, 575-646-4300, Fax: 575-646-4343, E-mail: kittle@nmsu.edu. *Application contact:* Dr. James Robinson, III, Graduate Coordinator, 575-646-7431, E-mail: jrobin3@ nmsu.edu.
Website: http://publichealth.nmsu.edu

New York University, Steinhardt School of Culture, Education, and Human Development, Department of Nutrition, Food Studies, and Public Health, Program in Public Health, New York, NY 10003. Offers community and international health (MPH); global health leadership (MPH); public health nutrition (MPH). *Accreditation:* CEPH. Part-time programs available. *Faculty:* 7 full-time (5 women). *Students:* 6 full-time (all women), 2 part-time (both women); includes 3 minority (2 Asian, non-Hispanic/Latino; 1 Hispanic/Latino). Average age 32. 44 applicants, 7% accepted, 2 enrolled. In 2013, 1 degree awarded. *Degree requirements:* For master's, thesis (for some programs). *Entrance requirements:* For master's, GRE General Test. Additional exam requirements/ recommendations for international students: Required—TOEFL. *Application deadline:* For fall admission, 12/1 priority date for domestic and international students; for spring admission, 11/1 for domestic and international students. Applications are processed on a rolling basis. Application fee: $75. Electronic applications accepted. *Expenses: Tuition:* Full-time $35,856; part-time $1494 per unit. *Required fees:* $1408; $64 per unit. $473 per term. Tuition and fees vary according to course load and program. *Financial support:* Fellowships with full and partial tuition reimbursements, career-related internships or fieldwork, Federal Work-Study, institutionally sponsored loans, scholarships/grants, and tuition waivers (partial) available. Support available to part-time students. Financial award application deadline: 2/1; financial award applicants required to submit FAFSA. *Faculty research:* Social epidemiology, primary health care, global health, immigrants and health, infectious disease prevention, HIV/AIDS. *Unit head:* Prof. James Macinko, Director, 212-998-5592, Fax: 212-995-4192, E-mail: james.macinko@nyu.edu. *Application contact:* 212-998-5030, Fax: 212-995-4328, E-mail: steinhardt.gradadmissions@nyu.edu.
Website: http://steinhardt.nyu.edu/nutrition/public_health

Quinnipiac University, School of Nursing, Care of Populations Track, Hamden, CT 06518-1940. Offers DNP. Part-time programs available. *Faculty:* 14 full-time (13 women), 5 part-time/adjunct (3 women). *Students:* 16 part-time (14 women); includes 3 minority (2 Black or African American, non-Hispanic/Latino; 1 Hispanic/Latino). 14 applicants, 93% accepted, 11 enrolled. In 2013, 5 doctorates awarded. *Entrance requirements:* Additional exam requirements/recommendations for international students: Required—TOEFL (minimum score 575 paper-based; 90 iBT), IELTS (minimum score 6.5). *Application deadline:* For fall admission, 6/1 for domestic students, 4/30 for international students. Applications are processed on a rolling basis. Application fee: $45. Electronic applications accepted. *Expenses: Tuition:* Part-time $920 per credit. *Required fees:* $37 per credit. *Financial support:* Career-related internships or fieldwork, Federal Work-Study, scholarships/grants, tuition waivers (partial), and unspecified assistantships available. Support available to part-time students. Financial award application deadline: 6/1. *Unit head:* Dr. Lynn Price, Program Director, E-mail: lynn.price@quinnipiac.edu. *Application contact:* Office of Graduate Admissions, 800-462-1944, Fax: 203-582-3443, E-mail: graduate@quinnipiac.edu.
Website: http://www.quinnipiac.edu/gradnursing

Sage Graduate School, School of Health Sciences, Department of Psychology, Troy, NY 12180-4115. Offers community psychology (MA), including child care and children's services, community counseling, community health education, community psychology, general psychology; counseling and community psychology (MA); forensic mental health (MS, Certificate). Part-time and evening/weekend programs available. *Faculty:* 4 full-time (3 women), 4 part-time/adjunct (3 women). *Students:* 58 full-time (49 women), 60 part-time (54 women); includes 21 minority (9 Black or African American, non-Hispanic/ Latino; 1 American Indian or Alaska Native, non-Hispanic/Latino; 1 Asian, non-Hispanic/ Latino; 7 Hispanic/Latino; 3 Two or more races, non-Hispanic/Latino). Average age 28. 120 applicants, 49% accepted, 33 enrolled. In 2013, 44 master's, 2 other advanced degrees awarded. *Degree requirements:* For master's, thesis or alternative. *Entrance requirements:* For master's, GRE General Test. Additional exam requirements/ recommendations for international students: Required—TOEFL (minimum score 550 paper-based). *Application deadline:* Applications are processed on a rolling basis. Application fee: $40. *Expenses: Tuition:* Full-time $11,880; part-time $660 per credit hour. *Financial support:* Fellowships, research assistantships, Federal Work-Study, scholarships/grants, and unspecified assistantships available. Support available to part-time students. Financial award application deadline: 3/1; financial award applicants required to submit FAFSA. *Faculty research:* Effectiveness of arts integration programs in elementary/secondary schools, literacy-based substance abuse program, outcome evaluation of program to increase college entry among urban youth. *Unit head:* Dr. Esther Haskevitz, Interim Dean, School of Health Sciences, 518-244-2296, Fax: 518-244-4571, E-mail: haskve@sage.edu. *Application contact:* Dr. Bronna Romanoff, Director, 518-244-2260, Fax: 518-244-4545, E-mail: romanb@sage.edu.

Saint Louis University, Graduate Education, School of Public Health and Graduate Education, Department of Community Health, St. Louis, MO 63103-2097. Offers MPH, MS, MSPH. *Accreditation:* CEPH. Part-time programs available. Postbaccalaureate distance learning degree programs offered (no on-campus study). *Degree requirements:* For master's, comprehensive exam. *Entrance requirements:* For master's, GRE General Test, LSAT, GMAT or MCAT, letters of recommendation, resume. Additional exam requirements/recommendations for international students: Required—TOEFL (minimum score 525 paper-based). Electronic applications accepted. *Faculty research:* Obesity prevention, health disparities, health policy, child health.

Southern Illinois University Carbondale, Graduate School, College of Education and Human Services, Department of Health Education and Recreation, Program in Community Health Education, Carbondale, IL 62901-4701. Offers MPH. *Accreditation:* CEPH. *Faculty:* 7 full-time (4 women). *Students:* 38 full-time (28 women), 7 part-time (5 women); includes 17 minority (14 Black or African American, non-Hispanic/Latino; 2 Asian, non-Hispanic/Latino; 1 Hispanic/Latino), 3 international. 42 applicants, 50% accepted, 15 enrolled. In 2013, 13 master's awarded. *Entrance requirements:* Additional exam requirements/recommendations for international students: Required—TOEFL. Application fee: $50. *Unit head:* Dr. Stephen L. Brown, Chair, 618-453-2777, Fax: 618-453-1829, E-mail: slbrown@siu.edu. *Application contact:* Carol Reynolds, Administrative Assistant, 618-453-2415, Fax: 618-453-1829, E-mail: creynolds@ siu.edu.

Southern New Hampshire University, School of Arts and Sciences, Manchester, NH 03106-1045. Offers community mental health (Graduate Certificate); community mental health and mental health counseling (MS); fiction and nonfiction (MFA); teaching English as a foreign language (MS). Part-time and evening/weekend programs available. *Degree requirements:* For master's, one foreign language, thesis. *Entrance requirements:* For master's, minimum GPA of 2.75 (for MS in teaching English as a foreign language), 3.0 (for MFA). Additional exam requirements/recommendations for international students: Required—TOEFL (minimum score 550 paper-based; 79 iBT), IELTS (minimum score 6.5), TWE (minimum score 5). Electronic applications accepted. *Expenses:* Contact institution. *Faculty research:* Action research, state of the art practice in behavioral health services, wraparound approaches to working with youth, learning styles.

State University of New York Downstate Medical Center, College of Medicine, Program in Public Health, Brooklyn, NY 11203-2098. Offers urban and immigrant health (MPH); MD/MPH. *Accreditation:* CEPH. Part-time programs available. *Degree requirements:* For master's, practicum. *Entrance requirements:* For master's, GRE, MCAT or OAT, 2 letters of recommendation, minimum undergraduate GPA of 3.0. Additional exam requirements/recommendations for international students: Required—TOEFL (minimum score 550 paper-based).

Stony Brook University, State University of New York, Stony Brook University Medical Center, Health Sciences Center, School of Medicine, Program in Population Health and Clinical Outcomes Research, Stony Brook, NY 11794. Offers PhD. *Degree requirements:* For doctorate, thesis/dissertation. *Entrance requirements:* For doctorate,

GRE, personal or telephone interview, minimum GPA of 3.0 in undergraduate work. Additional exam requirements/recommendations for international students: Required—TOEFL (minimum score 600 paper-based; 90 iBT). *Application deadline:* For fall admission, 1/15 for domestic students. *Expenses:* Tuition, state resident: full-time $9870; part-time $411 per credit. Tuition, nonresident: full-time $18,350; part-time $765 per credit. *Unit head:* Dr. Annie Laurie Shroyer, Director, 631-444-7875, E-mail: annielaurie.shroyer@stonybrook.edu. *Application contact:* Jonathan Ragone, Program Coordinator, 631-632-4378, E-mail: jonathan.ragone@stonybrook.edu.
Website: http://stonybrook.edu/sb/phcor/index.html

Stony Brook University, State University of New York, Stony Brook University Medical Center, Health Sciences Center, School of Medicine, Program in Public Health, Stony Brook, NY 11794. Offers community health (MPH); evaluation sciences (MPH); family violence (MPH); health communication (Certificate); health economics (MPH); population health (MPH); substance abuse (MPH). *Accreditation:* CEPH. *Students:* 36 full-time (28 women), 20 part-time (15 women); includes 22 minority (1 Black or African American, non-Hispanic/Latino; 13 Asian, non-Hispanic/Latino; 8 Hispanic/Latino), 6 international. Average age 39. 84 applicants, 62% accepted, 40 enrolled. In 2013, 22 master's awarded. *Entrance requirements:* For master's, GRE, 3 references, bachelor's degree from accredited college or university with minimum GPA of 3.0, essays, interview. Additional exam requirements/recommendations for international students: Required—TOEFL (minimum score 85 iBT). *Application deadline:* For fall admission, 6/1 for domestic students, 3/15 for international students. Application fee: $100. Electronic applications accepted. *Expenses:* Tuition, state resident: full-time $9870; part-time $411 per credit. Tuition, nonresident: full-time $18,350; part-time $765 per credit. *Financial support:* In 2013–14, 1 fellowship was awarded. *Faculty research:* Population health, health service research, health economics. *Unit head:* Dr. Lisa A. Benz Scott, Director, 631-444-9396, Fax: 631-444-3480, E-mail: lisa.benzscott@stonybrook.edu. *Application contact:* Dr. Jack Fuhrer, 631-444-2113, Fax: 631-444-6032, E-mail: somadmissions@stonybrook.edu.
Website: http://www.stonybrookmedicalcenter.org/publichealth/

Syracuse University, Falk College of Sport and Human Dynamics, Program in Child and Family Health in the Global Community, Syracuse, NY 13244. Offers MS. Part-time programs available. *Students:* 7 full-time (6 women), 1 (woman) part-time. Average age 28. 11 applicants, 64% accepted, 3 enrolled. In 2013, 2 master's awarded. *Entrance requirements:* For master's, GRE. Additional exam requirements/recommendations for international students: Required—TOEFL (minimum score 100 iBT). *Application deadline:* For fall admission, 3/15 priority date for domestic students, 3/15 for international students; for spring admission, 11/15 priority date for domestic and international students. Application fee: $75. Electronic applications accepted. *Financial support:* Fellowships with full tuition reimbursements, research assistantships with partial tuition reimbursements, and teaching assistantships with partial tuition reimbursements available. Financial award application deadline: 1/15. *Unit head:* Dr. Brooks Gump, Graduate Program Director, 315-443-2206, Fax: 315-443-2562, E-mail: bbgump@syr.edu. *Application contact:* Felicia Otero, Director, College Relations, 315-443-5555, Fax: 315-443-2562, E-mail: falk@syr.edu.
Website: http://falk.syr.edu/

Temple University, College of Health Professions and Social Work, Department of Public Health, Philadelphia, PA 19122. Offers clinical research and translational medicine (MS); environmental health (MPH); epidemiology (MS); epidemiology and biostatistics (MPH); health policy (PhD); health policy and management (MPH); school health education (Ed M); social and behavioral sciences (MPH, PhD). *Accreditation:* CEPH (one or more programs are accredited). Part-time and evening/weekend programs available. *Faculty:* 27 full-time (18 women). *Students:* 47 full-time (30 women), 45 part-time (37 women); includes 27 minority (9 Black or African American, non-Hispanic/Latino; 10 Asian, non-Hispanic/Latino; 7 Hispanic/Latino; 1 Two or more races, non-Hispanic/Latino), 9 international. 188 applicants, 45% accepted, 29 enrolled. In 2013, 29 master's, 3 doctorates awarded. Terminal master's awarded for partial completion of doctoral program. *Degree requirements:* For master's, thesis (for some programs), capstone project; for doctorate, comprehensive exam, thesis/dissertation. *Entrance requirements:* For master's, GRE General Test (for MS only); DAT, GMAT, MCAT, OAT, PCAT (alternates for MPH, Ed M), minimum undergraduate GPA of 3.0, letters of reference, statement of goals, writing sample, resume, interview (only for MS); for doctorate, GRE General Test, minimum undergraduate GPA of 3.0, 3 letters of reference, statement of goals, writing sample, resume. Additional exam requirements/recommendations for international students: Required—TOEFL (minimum score 550 paper-based; 79 iBT). *Application deadline:* For fall admission, 3/1 for domestic students, 2/1 for international students; for spring admission, 10/15 for domestic students, 8/1 for international students. Applications are processed on a rolling basis. Application fee: $60. Electronic applications accepted. *Financial support:* In 2013–14, 1 fellowship with tuition reimbursement, 4 research assistantships with tuition reimbursements, 8 teaching assistantships with tuition reimbursements were awarded; career-related internships or fieldwork, Federal Work-Study, scholarships/grants, tuition waivers (partial), and unspecified assistantships also available. Financial award application deadline: 1/15. *Faculty research:* Smoking cessation, obesity prevention, tobacco policy, community engagement, health communication. *Total annual research expenditures:* $3.9 million. *Unit head:* Dr. Alice J. Hausman, Chair, 215-204-5112, Fax: 215-204-1854, E-mail: hausman@temple.edu. *Application contact:* Joyce Hankins, 215-204-7213, E-mail: joyce.hankins@temple.edu.
Website: http://chpsw.temple.edu/publichealth/home

Universidad de Ciencias Medicas, Graduate Programs, San Jose, Costa Rica. Offers dermatology (SP); family health (MS); health service center administration (MHA); human anatomy (MS); medical and surgery (MD); occupational medicine (MS); pharmacy (Pharm D). Part-time programs available. *Degree requirements:* For master's, thesis; for doctorate and SP, comprehensive exam. *Entrance requirements:* For master's, MD or bachelor's degree; for doctorate, admissions test; for SP, admissions test, MD.

Université de Montréal, Faculty of Medicine, Program in Communal and Public Health, Montréal, QC H3C 3J7, Canada. Offers community health (M Sc, DESS); public health (PhD). *Accreditation:* CEPH. Part-time programs available. Terminal master's awarded for partial completion of doctoral program. *Degree requirements:* For master's, thesis; for doctorate, thesis/dissertation, general exam. *Entrance requirements:* For master's and doctorate, proficiency in French, knowledge of English; for DESS, proficiency in French. Electronic applications accepted. *Faculty research:* Epidemiology, health services utilization, health promotion and education, health behaviors, poverty and child health.

Université Laval, Faculty of Medicine, Graduate Programs in Medicine, Department of Social and Preventive Medicine, Program in Community Health, Québec, QC G1K 7P4, Canada. Offers M Sc, PhD. Part-time programs available. Terminal master's awarded for partial completion of doctoral program. *Degree requirements:* For master's, thesis (for some programs); for doctorate, comprehensive exam, thesis/dissertation. *Entrance requirements:* For master's, knowledge of French, comprehension of written English; for doctorate, French exam, comprehension of French, written comprehension of English. Electronic applications accepted.

Université Laval, Faculty of Medicine, Post-Professional Programs in Medical Studies, Québec, QC G1K 7P4, Canada. Offers anatomy–pathology (DESS); anesthesiology (DESS); cardiology (DESS); care of older people (Diploma); clinical research (DESS); community health (DESS); dermatology (DESS); diagnostic radiology (DESS); emergency medicine (Diploma); family medicine (DESS); general surgery (DESS); geriatrics (DESS); hematology (DESS); internal medicine (DESS); maternal and fetal medicine (Diploma); medical biochemistry (DESS); medical microbiology and infectious diseases (DESS); medical oncology (DESS); nephrology (DESS); neurology (DESS); neurosurgery (DESS); obstetrics and gynecology (DESS); ophthalmology (DESS); orthopedic surgery (DESS); oto-rhino-laryngology (DESS); palliative medicine (Diploma); pediatrics (DESS); plastic surgery (DESS); psychiatry (DESS); pulmonary medicine (DESS); radiology–oncology (DESS); thoracic surgery (DESS); urology (DESS). *Degree requirements:* For other advanced degree, comprehensive exam. *Entrance requirements:* For degree, knowledge of French. Electronic applications accepted.

University at Buffalo, the State University of New York, Graduate School, School of Public Health and Health Professions, Department of Community Health and Health Behavior, Buffalo, NY 14214. Offers MPH, PhD. *Accreditation:* CEPH. Part-time programs available. *Faculty:* 7 full-time (4 women). *Students:* 30 full-time (23 women), 4 part-time (2 women); includes 7 minority (4 Black or African American, non-Hispanic/Latino; 3 Asian, non-Hispanic/Latino), 2 international. Average age 26. 109 applicants, 38% accepted, 19 enrolled. In 2013, 7 master's, 1 doctorate awarded. *Degree requirements:* For master's, thesis; for doctorate, comprehensive exam, thesis/dissertation. *Entrance requirements:* For master's and doctorate, GRE. Additional exam requirements/recommendations for international students: Required—TOEFL (minimum score 79 iBT). *Application deadline:* For fall admission, 1/15 priority date for domestic students, 2/1 priority date for international students. Applications are processed on a rolling basis. Application fee: $50. Electronic applications accepted. *Financial support:* In 2013–14, 6 students received support, including 2 fellowships with full tuition reimbursements available (averaging $4,000 per year), 2 research assistantships with full tuition reimbursements available (averaging $21,000 per year). Financial award application deadline: 3/15; financial award applicants required to submit FAFSA. *Unit head:* Dr. Gary A. Giovino, Chair, 716-829-6952, E-mail: ggiovino@buffalo.edu. *Application contact:* Barbara L. Sen, Graduate Program Coordinator, 716-829-6956, Fax: 716-829-6040, E-mail: bsen@buffalo.edu.
Website: http://sphhp.buffalo.edu/community-health-and-health-behavior.html

The University of Alabama, Graduate School, College of Human Environmental Sciences, Program in Human Environmental Science, Tuscaloosa, AL 35487. Offers family financial planning and counseling (MS); interactive technology (MS); quality management (MS); restaurant and meeting management (MS); rural community health (MS); sport management (MS). *Faculty:* 1 full-time (0 women). *Students:* 55 full-time (34 women), 98 part-time (48 women); includes 41 minority (30 Black or African American, non-Hispanic/Latino; 2 American Indian or Alaska Native, non-Hispanic/Latino; 2 Asian, non-Hispanic/Latino; 2 Hispanic/Latino; 5 Two or more races, non-Hispanic/Latino), 1 international. Average age 34. 102 applicants, 69% accepted, 60 enrolled. In 2013, 88 master's awarded. *Degree requirements:* For master's, comprehensive exam. *Entrance requirements:* For master's, GRE (for some specializations), minimum GPA of 3.0. Additional exam requirements/recommendations for international students: Required—TOEFL. *Application deadline:* Applications are processed on a rolling basis. Application fee: $50 ($60 for international students). Electronic applications accepted. *Expenses:* Tuition, state resident: full-time $9450. Tuition, nonresident: full-time $23,950. *Faculty research:* Hospitality management, sports medicine education, technology and education. *Unit head:* Dr. Milla D. Boschung, Dean, 205-348-6250, Fax: 205-348-1786, E-mail: mboschun@ches.ua.edu. *Application contact:* Dr. Stuart Usdan, Associate Dean, 205-348-6150, Fax: 205-348-3789, E-mail: susdan@ches.ua.edu.

University of Alberta, School of Public Health, Department of Public Health Sciences, Edmonton, AB T6G 2E1, Canada. Offers clinical epidemiology (M Sc, MPH); environmental and occupational health (MPH); environmental health sciences (M Sc); epidemiology (M Sc); global health (M Sc, MPH); health policy and management (MPH); health policy research (M Sc); health technology assessment (MPH); occupational health (M Sc); population health (M Sc); public health leadership (MPH); public health sciences (PhD); quantitative methods (MPH). *Accreditation:* CEPH (one or more programs are accredited). Terminal master's awarded for partial completion of doctoral program. *Degree requirements:* For master's, thesis (for some programs); for doctorate, thesis/dissertation. *Entrance requirements:* For master's, GMAT or GRE General Test. Additional exam requirements/recommendations for international students: Required—TOEFL (minimum score 550 paper-based) or IELTS (minimum score 6). Electronic applications accepted. *Faculty research:* Biostatistics, health promotion and socio-behavioral health science.

University of Arkansas, Graduate School, College of Education and Health Professions, Department of Health, Human Performance and Recreation, Program in Community Health Promotion, Fayetteville, AR 72701-1201. Offers MS, PhD.

University of Calgary, Cumming School of Medicine and Faculty of Graduate Studies, Department of Community Health Sciences, Calgary, AB T2N 1N4, Canada. Offers M Sc, PhD. *Degree requirements:* For master's, thesis; for doctorate, thesis/dissertation, candidacy exam. *Entrance requirements:* For master's and doctorate, minimum GPA of 3.2. Additional exam requirements/recommendations for international students: Required—TOEFL (minimum score 600 paper-based). Electronic applications accepted. *Faculty research:* Epidemiology, health research, biostatistics, health economics, health policy.

University of California, Los Angeles, Graduate Division, School of Public Health, Department of Community Health Sciences, Los Angeles, CA 90095. Offers public health (MPH, MS, Dr PH, PhD); JD/MPH; MA/MPH; MD/MPH; MSW/MPH. *Degree requirements:* For master's, comprehensive exam or thesis; for doctorate, thesis/dissertation, oral and written qualifying exams. *Entrance requirements:* For master's, GRE General Test, minimum GPA of 3.0; for doctorate, GRE General Test, minimum undergraduate GPA of 3.0. Electronic applications accepted.

University of Colorado Denver, College of Liberal Arts and Sciences, Program in Humanities, Denver, CO 80217. Offers community health science (MSS); humanities (MH); international studies (MSS); philosophy and theory (MH); social justice (MSS); society and the environment (MSS); visual studies (MH); women's and gender studies (MSS). Part-time and evening/weekend programs available. *Faculty:* 2 full-time (1 woman). *Students:* 45 full-time (38 women), 27 part-time (19 women); includes 13 minority (3 Black or African American, non-Hispanic/Latino; 1 American Indian or Alaska Native, non-Hispanic/Latino; 2 Asian, non-Hispanic/Latino; 4 Hispanic/Latino; 3 Two or more races, non-Hispanic/Latino). Average age 34. 24 applicants, 63% accepted, 10 enrolled. In 2013, 25 master's awarded. *Degree requirements:* For master's, 36 credit hours, project or thesis. *Entrance requirements:* For master's, writing sample, statement of purpose/letter of intent, three letters of recommendation. Additional exam requirements/recommendations for international students: Required—TOEFL (minimum score 537 paper-based; 75 iBT); Recommended—IELTS (minimum score 6.5). *Application deadline:* For fall admission, 5/15 for domestic students, 5/15 priority date for international students; for spring admission, 10/15 for domestic students, 10/15 priority

date for international students. Application fee: $50 ($75 for international students). Electronic applications accepted. *Financial support:* In 2013–14, 2 students received support. Fellowships, research assistantships, teaching assistantships, Federal Work-Study, institutionally sponsored loans, scholarships/grants, and traineeships available. Financial award application deadline: 4/1; financial award applicants required to submit FAFSA. *Faculty research:* Women and gender in the classical Mediterranean, communication theory and democracy, relationship between psychology and philosophy. *Unit head:* Myra Bookman, Associate Director of Humanities and Social Science, 303-556-2496, Fax: 303-556-8100, E-mail: myra.bookman@ucdenver.edu. *Application contact:* Catherine Osmundson, Program Assistant, 303-556-2305, E-mail: catherine.osmundson@ucdenver.edu.
Website: http://www.ucdenver.edu/academics/colleges/CLAS/Programs/HumanitiesSocialSciences/Programs/Pages/MasterofHumanities.aspx

University of Colorado Denver, Colorado School of Public Health, Program in Public Health, Aurora, CO 80045. Offers community and behavioral health (MPH, Dr PH); environmental and occupational health (MPH); epidemiology (MPH); health systems, management and policy (MPH). *Accreditation:* CEPH. Part-time and evening/weekend programs available. *Faculty:* 14 full-time (13 women). *Students:* 295 full-time (247 women), 49 part-time (39 women); includes 77 minority (17 Black or African American, non-Hispanic/Latino; 3 American Indian or Alaska Native, non-Hispanic/Latino; 16 Asian, non-Hispanic/Latino; 31 Hispanic/Latino; 10 Two or more races, non-Hispanic/Latino), 5 international. Average age 30. 657 applicants, 71% accepted, 132 enrolled. In 2013, 106 master's awarded. *Degree requirements:* For master's, thesis or alternative, 42 credit hours; for doctorate, comprehensive exam, thesis/dissertation, 67 credit hours. *Entrance requirements:* For master's, GRE, MCAT, DAT, LSAT, PCAT, GMAT or master's degree from accredited institution, baccalaureate degree or equivalent; minimum GPA of 3.0; transcripts; references; resume; essay; for doctorate, GRE, MCAT, DAT, LSAT, PCAT or GMAT, MPH or master's or higher degree in related field or equivalent; 2 years of previous work experience in public health; essay; resume. Additional exam requirements/recommendations for international students: Required—TOEFL (minimum score 550 paper-based; 80 iBT). *Application deadline:* For fall admission, 12/15 priority date for domestic students, 12/1 priority date for international students. Application fee: $65. Electronic applications accepted. *Expenses:* Contact institution. *Financial support:* In 2013–14, 125 students received support. Fellowships, research assistantships, teaching assistantships, Federal Work-Study, institutionally sponsored loans, scholarships/grants, traineeships, and unspecified assistantships available. Financial award application deadline: 3/15; financial award applicants required to submit FAFSA. *Faculty research:* Cancer prevention by nutrition, cancer survivorship outcomes, social and cultural factors related to health. *Unit head:* Dr. Lori Crane, Chair, 303-724-4385, E-mail: lori.crane@ucdenver.edu. *Application contact:* Carla Denerstein, Departmental Assistant, 303-724-4446, E-mail: carla.denerstein@ucdenver.edu.
Website: http://www.ucdenver.edu/academics/colleges/PublicHealth/departments/CommunityBehavioralHealth/Pages/CommunityBehavioralHealth.aspx

University of Colorado Denver, School of Medicine, Physician Assistant Program, Aurora, CO 80045. Offers child health associate (MPAS), including global health, leadership, education, advocacy, development, and scholarship, rural health, urban/underserved populations. *Accreditation:* ARC-PA. *Students:* 132 full-time (107 women); includes 15 minority (1 American Indian or Alaska Native, non-Hispanic/Latino; 6 Asian, non-Hispanic/Latino; 8 Hispanic/Latino). Average age 27. 1,313 applicants, 3% accepted, 44 enrolled. In 2013, 43 master's awarded. *Degree requirements:* For master's, comprehensive exam, successful completion of all coursework and rotations. *Entrance requirements:* For master's, GRE General Test, minimum GPA of 2.8, 3 letters of recommendation, prerequisite courses in chemistry, biology, general genetics, psychology and statistics, interviews. Additional exam requirements/recommendations for international students: Required—TOEFL (minimum score 550 paper-based; 80 iBT). *Application deadline:* For fall admission, 9/1 for domestic students, 8/15 for international students. Application fee: $170. Electronic applications accepted. *Expenses:* Contact institution. *Financial support:* In 2013–14, 85 students received support. Fellowships, research assistantships, teaching assistantships, career-related internships or fieldwork, Federal Work-Study, institutionally sponsored loans, scholarships/grants, traineeships, and unspecified assistantships available. Financial award application deadline: 3/15; financial award applicants required to submit FAFSA. *Faculty research:* Clinical genetics and genetic counseling, evidence-based medicine, pediatric allergy and asthma, childhood diabetes, standardized patient assessment. *Unit head:* Jonathan Bowser, Program Director, 303-724-1349, E-mail: jonathan.bowser@ucdenver.edu. *Application contact:* Kay Denler, Director of Admissions, 303-724-7963, E-mail: kay.denler@ucdenver.edu.
Website: http://www.ucdenver.edu/academics/colleges/medicalschool/education/degree_programs/PAProgram/Pages/Home.aspx

University of Illinois at Chicago, Graduate College, School of Public Health, Division of Community Health Sciences, Chicago, IL 60607-7128. Offers MPH, MS, Dr PH, PhD. *Accreditation:* CEPH (one or more programs are accredited). Part-time programs available. *Faculty:* 18 full-time (12 women), 10 part-time/adjunct (6 women). *Students:* 131 full-time (116 women), 71 part-time (64 women); includes 79 minority (32 Black or African American, non-Hispanic/Latino; 17 Asian, non-Hispanic/Latino; 18 Hispanic/Latino; 2 Native Hawaiian or other Pacific Islander, non-Hispanic/Latino; 10 Two or more races, non-Hispanic/Latino), 7 international. Average age 30. 379 applicants, 70% accepted, 75 enrolled. In 2013, 66 master's, 5 doctorates awarded. Terminal master's awarded for partial completion of doctoral program. *Degree requirements:* For master's, thesis, field practicum; for doctorate, thesis/dissertation, independent research, internship. *Entrance requirements:* For master's and doctorate, GRE General Test, minimum GPA of 2.75. Additional exam requirements/recommendations for international students: Required—TOEFL. *Application deadline:* For fall admission, 2/1 for domestic students, 1/1 priority date for international students. Applications are processed on a rolling basis. Application fee: $40 ($50 for international students). Electronic applications accepted. *Expenses:* Tuition, state resident: full-time $11,066; part-time $3689 per term. Tuition, nonresident: full-time $23,064; part-time $7688 per term. *Required fees:* $3004; $1190 per term. Tuition and fees vary according to course level and program. *Financial support:* Fellowships with full tuition reimbursements, research assistantships with full tuition reimbursements, teaching assistantships with full tuition reimbursements, career-related internships or fieldwork, Federal Work-Study, institutionally sponsored loans, scholarships/grants, traineeships, and unspecified assistantships available. Support available to part-time students. Financial award application deadline: 3/1; financial award applicants required to submit FAFSA. *Faculty research:* Promoting wellness, disease prevention; public health preparedness; public health security capabilities. *Total annual research expenditures:* $603,000. *Unit head:* Prof. Jesus Ramirez-Valles, Director, 312-996-6346, E-mail: valles@uic.edu. *Application contact:* David Brand, Academic Coordinator, 312-996-8940, Fax: 312-996-3551, E-mail: dbrand@uic.edu.
Website: http://publichealth.uic.edu/departments/communityhealthsciences/

University of Illinois at Springfield, Graduate Programs, College of Public Affairs and Administration, Program in Public Health, Springfield, IL 62703-5407. Offers community health (Graduate Certificate); emergency preparedness and homeland security (Graduate Certificate); epidemiology (Graduate Certificate); public health (MPH). Part-time and evening/weekend programs available. Postbaccalaureate distance learning degree programs offered (no on-campus study). *Faculty:* 5 full-time (3 women), 3 part-time/adjunct (2 women). *Students:* 32 full-time (21 women), 57 part-time (43 women); includes 32 minority (24 Black or African American, non-Hispanic/Latino; 6 Asian, non-Hispanic/Latino; 2 Hispanic/Latino), 10 international. Average age 32. 70 applicants, 47% accepted, 24 enrolled. In 2013, 22 master's, 6 other advanced degrees awarded. *Degree requirements:* For master's, comprehensive exam, internship. *Entrance requirements:* For master's, GRE, minimum undergraduate GPA of 3.0, 3 letters of recommendation, statement of personal goals. Additional exam requirements/recommendations for international students: Required—TOEFL (minimum score 500 paper-based; 61 iBT). *Application deadline:* Applications are processed on a rolling basis. Application fee: $60 ($75 for international students). Electronic applications accepted. *Expenses:* Tuition, state resident: full-time $7440. Tuition, nonresident: full-time $15,744. *Required fees:* $2985.60. *Financial support:* In 2013–14, fellowships with full tuition reimbursements (averaging $9,900 per year), research assistantships with full tuition reimbursements (averaging $9,550 per year), teaching assistantships with full tuition reimbursements (averaging $9,700 per year) were awarded; career-related internships or fieldwork, Federal Work-Study, scholarships/grants, health care benefits, and unspecified assistantships also available. Support available to part-time students. Financial award application deadline: 11/15; financial award applicants required to submit FAFSA. *Unit head:* Dr. Sharron Lafollette, Program Administrator, 217-206-7894, Fax: 217-206-7279, E-mail: slafo1@uis.edu. *Application contact:* Dr. Lynn Pardie, Office of Graduate Studies, 800-252-8533, Fax: 217-206-7623, E-mail: lpard1@uis.edu.
Website: http://www.uis.edu/publichealth/

University of Illinois at Urbana–Champaign, Graduate College, College of Applied Health Sciences, Department of Kinesiology and Community Health, Champaign, IL 61820. Offers community health (MS, MSPH, PhD); kinesiology (MS, PhD); public health (MPH); rehabilitation (MS); PhD/MPH. *Students:* 138 (83 women). Application fee: $75 ($90 for international students). *Unit head:* Wojciech Chodzko-Zajko, Head, 217-244-0823, Fax: 217-244-7322, E-mail: wojtek@illinois.edu. *Application contact:* Julie Jenkins, Office Administrator, 217-333-1083, Fax: 217-244-7322, E-mail: jjenkns@illinois.edu.
Website: http://www.kch.illinois.edu/

The University of Iowa, Graduate College, College of Public Health, Department of Community and Behavioral Health, Iowa City, IA 52242-1316. Offers MPH, MS, PhD. *Accreditation:* CEPH. *Degree requirements:* For master's, thesis; for doctorate, comprehensive exam, thesis/dissertation. *Entrance requirements:* For master's and doctorate, GRE General Test, minimum GPA of 3.0. Additional exam requirements/recommendations for international students: Required—TOEFL (minimum score 600 paper-based; 100 iBT). Electronic applications accepted.

University of Louisville, Graduate School, College of Education and Human Development, Department of Health and Sport Sciences, Louisville, KY 40292-0001. Offers community health education (M Ed); exercise physiology (MS); health and physical education (MAT); sport administration (MS). Part-time and evening/weekend programs available. *Students:* 54 full-time (22 women), 11 part-time (9 women); includes 12 minority (6 Black or African American, non-Hispanic/Latino; 1 American Indian or Alaska Native, non-Hispanic/Latino; 1 Asian, non-Hispanic/Latino; 3 Hispanic/Latino; 1 Two or more races, non-Hispanic/Latino), 3 international. Average age 27. 91 applicants, 70% accepted, 40 enrolled. In 2013, 16 master's awarded. *Entrance requirements:* For master's, GRE General Test. Additional exam requirements/recommendations for international students: Required—TOEFL (minimum score 560 paper-based; 83 iBT). Application fee: $60. Electronic applications accepted. *Expenses:* Tuition, state resident: full-time $10,788; part-time $599 per credit hour. Tuition, nonresident: full-time $22,446; part-time $1247 per credit hour. *Required fees:* $196. Tuition and fees vary according to program and reciprocity agreements. *Financial support:* Fellowships, research assistantships, teaching assistantships, career-related internships or fieldwork, Federal Work-Study, scholarships/grants, health care benefits, and unspecified assistantships available. Financial award application deadline: 6/1; financial award applicants required to submit FAFSA. *Faculty research:* Impact of sports and sport marketing on society, factors associated with school and community health, cardiac and pulmonary rehabilitation, impact of participation in activities on student retention and graduation, strength and conditioning. *Unit head:* Dr. Anita Moorman, Chair, 502-852-0553, Fax: 502-852-4534, E-mail: amm@louisville.edu. *Application contact:* Libby Leggett, Director, Graduate Admissions, 502-852-3101, Fax: 502-852-6536, E-mail: gradadm@louisville.edu.
Website: http://www.louisville.edu/education/departments/hss

University of Manitoba, Faculty of Medicine and Faculty of Graduate Studies, Graduate Programs in Medicine, Department of Community Health Sciences, Winnipeg, MB R3T 2N2, Canada. Offers M Sc, MPH, PhD, G Dip. Part-time programs available. *Degree requirements:* For master's, thesis; for doctorate, thesis/dissertation. *Entrance requirements:* For master's and doctorate, minimum GPA of 3.0. *Faculty research:* Health services, aboriginal health, health policy, epidemiology, international health.

University of Massachusetts Amherst, Graduate School, School of Public Health and Health Sciences, Department of Public Health, Amherst, MA 01003. Offers biostatistics (MPH, MS, PhD); community health education (MPH, MS, PhD); environmental health sciences (MPH, MS, PhD); epidemiology (MPH, MS, PhD); health policy and management (MPH, MS, PhD); nutrition (MPH, PhD); public health practice (MPH); MPH/MPPA. *Accreditation:* CEPH (one or more programs are accredited). Part-time and evening/weekend programs available. Postbaccalaureate distance learning degree programs offered (no on-campus study). *Faculty:* 53 full-time (29 women). *Students:* 117 full-time (83 women), 271 part-time (213 women); includes 89 minority (34 Black or African American, non-Hispanic/Latino; 23 Asian, non-Hispanic/Latino; 25 Hispanic/Latino; 7 Two or more races, non-Hispanic/Latino), 45 international. Average age 36. 359 applicants, 69% accepted, 94 enrolled. In 2013, 120 master's, 1 doctorate awarded. Terminal master's awarded for partial completion of doctoral program. *Degree requirements:* For master's, thesis (for some programs); for doctorate, comprehensive exam, thesis/dissertation. *Entrance requirements:* For master's and doctorate, GRE General Test. Additional exam requirements/recommendations for international students: Required—TOEFL (minimum score 550 paper-based; 80 iBT), IELTS (minimum score 6.5). *Application deadline:* For fall admission, 2/1 for domestic and international students. Applications are processed on a rolling basis. Application fee: $75. Electronic applications accepted. *Financial support:* Fellowships with full and partial tuition reimbursements, research assistantships with full and partial tuition reimbursements, teaching assistantships with full and partial tuition reimbursements, career-related internships or fieldwork, Federal Work-Study, scholarships/grants, traineeships, health care benefits, tuition waivers (full and partial), and unspecified assistantships available. Support available to part-time students. Financial award application deadline: 2/1; financial award applicants required to submit FAFSA. *Unit head:* Dr. Paula Stamps, Graduate Program Director, 413-545-2861, Fax: 413-545-1645. *Application contact:* Lindsay DeSantis, Supervisor of Admissions, 413-545-0722, Fax: 413-577-0010, E-mail: gradadm@grad.umass.edu.
Website: http://www.umass.edu/sphhs/public_health/

University of Miami, Graduate School, School of Education and Human Development, Department of Educational and Psychological Studies, Program in Community Well-Being, Coral Gables, FL 33124. Offers PhD. *Faculty:* 8 full-time (3 women). *Students:* 2 full-time (both women); includes 1 minority (Black or African American, non-Hispanic/Latino), 1 international. Average age 29. 12 applicants, 17% accepted, 2 enrolled. *Degree requirements:* For doctorate, thesis/dissertation. *Entrance requirements:* For doctorate, GRE General Test. Additional exam requirements/recommendations for international students: Required—TOEFL (minimum score 550 paper-based; 80 iBT); Recommended—IELTS. *Application deadline:* For fall admission, 1/15 for domestic students, 10/1 for international students. Application fee: $65. Electronic applications accepted. *Financial support:* In 2013–14, 2 students received support. Application deadline: 3/1; applicants required to submit FAFSA. *Unit head:* Dr. Dina Birman, Associate Professor and Program Director, 305-284-3001, E-mail: d.birman@miami.edu. *Application contact:* Lois Heffernan, Graduate Admissions Coordinator, 305-284-2167, Fax: 305-284-9395, E-mail: lheffernan@miami.edu.
Website: http://www.education.miami.edu/program/Programs.asp?Program_ID=148&Src=Graduate

University of Minnesota, Twin Cities Campus, School of Public Health, Major in Community Health Education, Minneapolis, MN 55455-0213. Offers MPH. *Accreditation:* CEPH. Part-time programs available. *Degree requirements:* For master's, fieldwork, project. *Entrance requirements:* For master's, GRE General Test. Additional exam requirements/recommendations for international students: Required—TOEFL. Electronic applications accepted. *Faculty research:* Assessing population behavior, designing community-wide prevention and treatment, preventing alcohol and drug abuse, influencing health policies.

University of Missouri, School of Medicine and Graduate School, Graduate Programs in Medicine, Columbia, MO 65211. Offers family and community medicine (MS); health administration (MS); medical pharmacology and physiology (MS, PhD); molecular microbiology and immunology (MS, PhD); pathology and anatomical sciences (MS). Part-time programs available. *Faculty:* 71 full-time (16 women), 12 part-time/adjunct (4 women). *Students:* 55 full-time (30 women), 3 part-time (all women); includes 6 minority (4 Black or African American, non-Hispanic/Latino; 1 American Indian or Alaska Native, non-Hispanic/Latino; 1 Hispanic/Latino), 25 international. Average age 28. 73 applicants, 16% accepted, 11 enrolled. In 2013, 1 master's, 13 doctorates awarded. *Degree requirements:* For doctorate, thesis/dissertation. *Entrance requirements:* For master's and doctorate, GRE General Test, minimum GPA of 3.0. Additional exam requirements/recommendations for international students: Required—TOEFL. *Application deadline:* Applications are processed on a rolling basis. Application fee: $55 ($75 for international students). *Expenses:* Contact institution. *Financial support:* Fellowships, research assistantships, teaching assistantships, career-related internships or fieldwork, and institutionally sponsored loans available. *Faculty research:* HIV enzymes, calcium and heart function, gene study and Muscular Dystrophy, military medical training using simulation technology, clinical and translational science. *Unit head:* William M. Crist, Dean Emeritus, 573-884-8733, E-mail: cristwm@missouri.edu. *Application contact:* Charles Rudkin, Graduate Programs Assistant, 573-882-4637, E-mail: rudkinc@health.missouri.edu.
Website: http://som.missouri.edu/departments.shtml

The University of Montana, Graduate School, Phyllis J. Washington College of Education and Human Sciences, Department of Health and Human Performance, Missoula, MT 59812-0002. Offers community health (MS); exercise science (MS); health and human performance generalist (MS). Part-time programs available. *Entrance requirements:* For master's, GRE General Test. Additional exam requirements/recommendations for international students: Required—TOEFL. *Application deadline:* For fall admission, 3/15 priority date for domestic students. Applications are processed on a rolling basis. Application fee: $45. *Financial support:* Teaching assistantships with full tuition reimbursements, Federal Work-Study, and unspecified assistantships available. Financial award application deadline: 3/1; financial award applicants required to submit FAFSA. *Faculty research:* Exercise physiology, performance psychology, nutrition, pre-employment physical screening, program evaluation. *Unit head:* Scott T. Richter, Chair, 406-243-5246, E-mail: scott.richter@umontana.edu. *Application contact:* Information Contact, E-mail: gradschl@mso.umt.edu.
Website: http://www.coehs.umt.edu/hhp/

University of Nevada, Las Vegas, Graduate College, School of Community Health Sciences, Las Vegas, NV 89154-3063. Offers MHA, MPH, PhD. *Faculty:* 15 full-time (6 women), 7 part-time/adjunct (6 women). *Students:* 65 full-time (44 women), 78 part-time (51 women); includes 52 minority (14 Black or African American, non-Hispanic/Latino; 4 American Indian or Alaska Native, non-Hispanic/Latino; 14 Asian, non-Hispanic/Latino; 10 Hispanic/Latino; 2 Native Hawaiian or other Pacific Islander, non-Hispanic/Latino; 8 Two or more races, non-Hispanic/Latino), 10 international. Average age 35. 59 applicants, 69% accepted, 21 enrolled. In 2013, 47 master's, 1 doctorate awarded. *Entrance requirements:* Additional exam requirements/recommendations for international students: Required—TOEFL, IELTS (minimum score 7). *Application deadline:* For fall admission, 5/1 for international students; for spring admission, 10/1 for international students. Application fee: $60 ($95 for international students). Electronic applications accepted. *Expenses:* Tuition, state resident: full-time $4752; part-time $264 per credit. Tuition, nonresident: full-time $18,662; part-time $554.50 per credit. *International tuition:* $18,952 full-time. *Required fees:* $532; $12 per credit. $266 per semester. One-time fee: $35. Tuition and fees vary according to course load and program. *Financial support:* In 2013–14, 23 students received support, including 23 research assistantships with partial tuition reimbursements available (averaging $10,039 per year); institutionally sponsored loans, scholarships/grants, health care benefits, and unspecified assistantships also available. Financial award application deadline: 3/1. *Faculty research:* Environmental health: micro (mold) to macro (Lake Mead ecosystem); health promotion and disease prevention: asthma, diabetes, cancer, HIV/AIDS, substance abuse, injury, hospital-acquired infections; health management and policy; health disparities/health equity; health information systems. *Total annual research expenditures:* $3.2 million. *Unit head:* Dr. Shawn Gerstenberger, Dean, 702-895-1565, Fax: 702-895-5184, E-mail: shawn.gerstenberger@unlv.edu. *Application contact:* Graduate College Admissions Evaluator, 702-895-3320, Fax: 702-895-4180, E-mail: gradcollege@unlv.edu.
Website: http://publichealth.unlv.edu/

University of New Mexico, Graduate School, College of Education, Department of Health, Exercise and Sports Sciences, Program in Health Education, Albuquerque, NM 87131-2039. Offers community health education (MS). *Accreditation:* NCATE. Part-time programs available. *Faculty:* 6 full-time (3 women). *Students:* 16 full-time (all women), 20 part-time (17 women); includes 21 minority (1 Black or African American, non-Hispanic/Latino; 6 American Indian or Alaska Native, non-Hispanic/Latino; 12 Hispanic/Latino; 1 Native Hawaiian or other Pacific Islander, non-Hispanic/Latino; 1 Two or more races, non-Hispanic/Latino), 4 international. Average age 30. 15 applicants, 60% accepted, 9 enrolled. In 2013, 14 master's awarded. *Degree requirements:* For master's, comprehensive exam, thesis optional. *Entrance requirements:* For master's, 3 letters of reference, resume, minimum cumulative GPA of 3.0 in last 2 years of bachelor's degree, letter of intent. Additional exam requirements/recommendations for international students: Required—TOEFL (minimum score 550 paper-based). *Application deadline:* For fall admission, 6/15 priority date for domestic students; for spring admission, 11/1 priority date for domestic students. Applications are processed on a rolling basis. Application fee: $50. Electronic applications accepted. *Financial support:* In 2013–14, 23 students received support, including 2 fellowships (averaging $2,290 per year), 3 teaching assistantships with full tuition reimbursements available (averaging $11,911 per year); career-related internships or fieldwork, institutionally sponsored loans, scholarships/grants, and health care benefits also available. Financial award application deadline: 3/1; financial award applicants required to submit FAFSA. *Faculty research:* Alcohol and families, health behaviors and sexuality, multicultural health behavior, health promotion policy, school/community-based prevention, health and aging. *Total annual research expenditures:* $91,910. *Unit head:* Dr. Elias Duryea, Coordinator, 505-277-5151, Fax: 505-277-6227, E-mail: duryea@unm.edu. *Application contact:* Carol Catania, Graduate Coordinator, 505-277-5151, Fax: 505-277-6227, E-mail: catania@unm.edu.
Website: http://coe.unm.edu/departments/hess/health-education/health-education-ms.html

University of New Mexico, School of Medicine, Program in Public Health, Albuquerque, NM 87131-5196. Offers community health (MPH); epidemiology (MPH); health systems, services and policy (MPH). *Accreditation:* CEPH. Part-time programs available. Postbaccalaureate distance learning degree programs offered. *Faculty:* 11 full-time (7 women), 4 part-time/adjunct (3 women). *Students:* 17 full-time (15 women), 16 part-time (12 women); includes 16 minority (3 Black or African American, non-Hispanic/Latino; 2 American Indian or Alaska Native, non-Hispanic/Latino; 1 Asian, non-Hispanic/Latino; 9 Hispanic/Latino; 1 Two or more races, non-Hispanic/Latino), 1 international. Average age 36. 46 applicants, 59% accepted, 17 enrolled. In 2013, 15 master's awarded. *Degree requirements:* For master's, thesis. *Entrance requirements:* For master's, GRE, MCAT, 2 years of experience in health field. Additional exam requirements/recommendations for international students: Required—TOEFL. *Application deadline:* For fall admission, 2/1 for domestic students. Application fee: $50. *Financial support:* Fellowships, research assistantships with tuition reimbursements, and Federal Work-Study available. Financial award application deadline: 12/15; financial award applicants required to submit FAFSA. *Faculty research:* Epidemiology, rural health, environmental health, Native American health issues. *Total annual research expenditures:* $1 million. *Unit head:* Dr. Kristine Tollestrup, Director, 505-272-4173, Fax: 505-272-4494, E-mail: ktollestrup@salud.unm.edu. *Application contact:* Gayle Garcia, Education Coordinator, 505-272-3982, Fax: 505-272-4494, E-mail: garciag@salud.unm.edu.
Website: http://fcm.unm.edu/

The University of North Carolina at Charlotte, The Graduate School, College of Health and Human Services, Department of Health Behavior and Administration, Charlotte, NC 28223-0001. Offers community health (Certificate); health administration (MHA); health services research (PhD); public health (MSPH). *Accreditation:* CAHME. Part-time programs available. *Degree requirements:* For master's, thesis or comprehensive exam; for doctorate, thesis/dissertation. *Entrance requirements:* For master's, GRE or MAT (public health), GRE or GMAT (health administration), minimum GPA of 3.0 during previous 2 years, 2.75 overall. Additional exam requirements/recommendations for international students: Required—TOEFL (minimum score 557 paper-based; 83 iBT). *Application deadline:* For fall admission, 7/1 for domestic students, 5/1 for international students; for spring admission, 11/1 for domestic students, 10/1 for international students. Applications are processed on a rolling basis. Application fee: $65 ($75 for international students). Electronic applications accepted. *Expenses:* Tuition, state resident: full-time $3522. Tuition, nonresident: full-time $16,051. *Required fees:* $2585. Tuition and fees vary according to course load and program. *Financial support:* Research assistantships, teaching assistantships, career-related internships or fieldwork, Federal Work-Study, institutionally sponsored loans, scholarships/grants, and unspecified assistantships available. Support available to part-time students. Financial award application deadline: 4/1; financial award applicants required to submit FAFSA. *Faculty research:* Pediatric asthma self-management, reproductive epidemiology, social aspects of injury prevention, chronic illness self-care, competency-based professional education, cognitive health, aging and dementia, infant health outcomes, policing and suicide, data mining for health executive decision support, segmentation analyses in identifying patient satisfaction problems in the primary care setting, enhancing community capacity through data sharing. *Unit head:* Dr. Gary S. Silverman, Chair, 704-687-7191, Fax: 704-687-6122, E-mail: arharver@uncc.edu. *Application contact:* Kathy B. Giddings, Director of Graduate Admissions, 704-687-5503, Fax: 704-687-1668, E-mail: gradadm@uncc.edu.
Website: http://publichealth.uncc.edu/degrees-and-programs/phs-graduate-programs

The University of North Carolina at Charlotte, The Graduate School, College of Health and Human Services, School of Nursing, Charlotte, NC 28223-0001. Offers administration (Post-Master's Certificate); advanced clinical (MSN, Post-Master's Certificate); anesthesia (MSN, Post-Master's Certificate); community health (MSN); family nurse practitioner (MSN, Post-Master's Certificate); health administration (MSN); mental health (MSN); nurse educator (MSN, Post-Master's Certificate); nursing (DNP); systems population (MSN). *Accreditation:* AACN. Part-time programs available. *Faculty:* 17 full-time (16 women), 6 part-time/adjunct (5 women). *Students:* 96 full-time (80 women), 124 part-time (119 women); includes 45 minority (30 Black or African American, non-Hispanic/Latino; 1 American Indian or Alaska Native, non-Hispanic/Latino; 8 Asian, non-Hispanic/Latino; 4 Hispanic/Latino; 2 Two or more races, non-Hispanic/Latino), 1 international. Average age 34. 216 applicants, 38% accepted, 72 enrolled. In 2013, 70 master's, 8 other advanced degrees awarded. Terminal master's awarded for partial completion of doctoral program. *Degree requirements:* For master's, thesis or alternative, practicum; for doctorate, thesis/dissertation or alternative, residency. *Entrance requirements:* For master's, GRE General Test, minimum GPA of 3.0 in undergraduate major; for doctorate, GRE, MAT, or GMAT, minimum GPA of 3.5. Additional exam requirements/recommendations for international students: Required—TOEFL (minimum score 570 paper-based; 83 iBT). *Application deadline:* For fall admission, 5/1 priority date for domestic students, 5/1 for international students; for spring admission, 10/1 priority date for domestic students, 10/1 for international students. Application fee: $75. Electronic applications accepted. *Expenses:* Tuition, state resident: full-time $3522. Tuition, nonresident: full-time $16,051. *Required fees:* $2585. Tuition and fees vary according to course load and program. *Financial support:* In 2013–14, 5 students received support, including 5 teaching assistantships (averaging $4,785 per year); research assistantships, career-related internships or fieldwork, institutionally sponsored loans, scholarships/grants, traineeships, and unspecified assistantships also available. Support available to part-time students. Financial award application deadline: 4/1; financial award applicants required to submit FAFSA. *Faculty research:* Improving care outcomes for the elderly; vulnerable populations; symptom management; self management/health promotion strategies of older adults; migration and maternal child health; health disparities, health literacy, and access to healthcare in Latino adults with diabetes; psychiatric nursing. *Total annual research expenditures:* $572,410. *Unit head:* Dr. Dee Baldwin, Associate Dean, 704-687-7952, Fax: 704-687-

6017, E-mail: dbaldwi5@uncc.edu. *Application contact:* Kathy B. Giddings, Director of Graduate Admissions, 704-687-5503, Fax: 704-687-1668, E-mail: gradadm@uncc.edu. Website: http://nursing.uncc.edu/

The University of North Carolina at Greensboro, Graduate School, School of Health and Human Performance, Department of Public Health Education, Greensboro, NC 27412-5001. Offers community health education (MPH, Dr PH). *Accreditation:* CEPH; NCATE. *Degree requirements:* For master's, comprehensive exam, thesis or alternative. *Entrance requirements:* For master's, GRE General Test or MAT. Additional exam requirements/recommendations for international students: Required—TOEFL. Electronic applications accepted. *Faculty research:* Peer facilitator training, innovative health education approaches.

University of Northern British Columbia, Office of Graduate Studies, Prince George, BC V2N 4Z9, Canada. Offers business administration (Diploma); community health science (M Sc); disability management (MA); education (M Ed); first nations studies (MA); gender studies (MA); history (MA); interdisciplinary studies (MA); international studies (MA); mathematical, computer and physical sciences (M Sc); natural resources and environmental studies (M Sc, MA, MNRES, PhD); political science (MA); psychology (M Sc, PhD); social work (MSW). Part-time and evening/weekend programs available. Postbaccalaureate distance learning degree programs offered (no on-campus study). *Degree requirements:* For master's, thesis; for doctorate, thesis/dissertation. *Entrance requirements:* For master's, GRE, minimum B average in undergraduate course work; for doctorate, candidacy exam, minimum A average in graduate course work.

University of North Florida, Brooks College of Health, Department of Public Health, Jacksonville, FL 32224. Offers aging services (Certificate); community health (MPH); geriatric management (MSH); health administration (MHA); rehabilitation counseling (MS). *Accreditation:* CEPH. Part-time and evening/weekend programs available. *Faculty:* 16 full-time (9 women), 4 part-time/adjunct (3 women). *Students:* 119 full-time (79 women), 59 part-time (34 women); includes 52 minority (20 Black or African American, non-Hispanic/Latino; 2 American Indian or Alaska Native, non-Hispanic/Latino; 9 Asian, non-Hispanic/Latino; 18 Hispanic/Latino; 3 Two or more races, non-Hispanic/Latino), 6 international. Average age 30. 271 applicants, 40% accepted, 72 enrolled. In 2013, 57 master's awarded. *Degree requirements:* For master's, thesis optional. *Entrance requirements:* For master's, GRE General Test (MSH, MS, MPH); GMAT or GRE General Test (MHA), minimum GPA of 3.0 in last 60 hours. Additional exam requirements/recommendations for international students: Required—TOEFL (minimum score 500 paper-based). *Application deadline:* For fall admission, 7/1 for domestic students, 5/1 for international students; for spring admission, 11/1 for domestic students, 10/1 for international students. Application fee: $30. Electronic applications accepted. *Expenses:* Tuition, state resident: full-time $9794; part-time $408.10 per credit hour. Tuition, nonresident: full-time $22,383; part-time $932.61 per credit hour. *Required fees:* $2020; $84.20 per credit hour. Tuition and fees vary according to course load and program. *Financial support:* In 2013–14, 38 students received support, including 2 teaching assistantships (averaging $1,500 per year); research assistantships, career-related internships or fieldwork, Federal Work-Study, scholarships/grants, and tuition waivers (partial) also available. Support available to part-time students. Financial award application deadline: 4/1; financial award applicants required to submit FAFSA. *Faculty research:* Dietary supplements; alcohol, tobacco, and other drug use prevention; turnover among health professionals; aging; psychosocial aspects of disabilities. *Total annual research expenditures:* $21,747. *Unit head:* Dr. Jeffrey Harrison, Chair, 904-620-1440, Fax: 904-620-2848, E-mail: jeffrey.harrison@unf.edu. *Application contact:* Dr. Heather Kenney, Director of Advising, 904-620-2810, Fax: 904-620-1030, E-mail: heather.kenney@unf.edu. Website: http://www.unf.edu/brooks/public_health/

University of North Texas Health Science Center at Fort Worth, School of Public Health, Fort Worth, TX 76107-2699. Offers biostatistics (MPH); community health (MPH); disease control and prevention (Dr PH); environmental and occupational health sciences (MPH); epidemiology (MPH); health administration (MHA); health policy and management (MPH, Dr PH); DO/MPH; MS/MPH; MSN/MPH. MPH offered jointly with University of North Texas; DO/MPH with Texas College of Osteopathic Medicine. *Accreditation:* CEPH. Part-time and evening/weekend programs available. *Degree requirements:* For master's, thesis or alternative, supervised internship; for doctorate, thesis/dissertation, supervised internship. *Entrance requirements:* For master's, GRE General Test. Additional exam requirements/recommendations for international students: Required—TOEFL. Electronic applications accepted.

University of Ottawa, Faculty of Graduate and Postdoctoral Studies, Faculty of Medicine, Department of Epidemiology and Community Medicine, Ottawa, ON K1N 6N5, Canada. Offers epidemiology (M Sc), including health technology assessment. *Degree requirements:* For master's, thesis. *Entrance requirements:* For master's, honors degree or equivalent, minimum B average. Electronic applications accepted. *Faculty research:* Epidemiologic concepts and methods, health technology assessment.

University of Ottawa, Faculty of Graduate and Postdoctoral Studies, Interdisciplinary Programs, Ottawa, ON K1N 6N5, Canada. Offers e-business (Certificate); e-commerce (Certificate); finance (Certificate); health services and policies research (Diploma); population health (PhD); population health risk assessment and management (Certificate); public management and governance (Certificate); systems science (Certificate).

University of Phoenix–Birmingham Campus, College of Health and Human Services, Birmingham, AL 35242. Offers education (MHA); gerontology (MHA); health administration (MHA); health care management (MBA); informatics (MHA); nursing (MSN); nursing/health care education (MSN); MSN/MBA; MSN/MHA.

University of Phoenix–Central Valley Campus, College of Nursing, Fresno, CA 93720-1562. Offers education (MHA); gerontology (MHA); health administration (MHA); nursing (MSN); MSN/MBA.

University of Phoenix–Chattanooga Campus, College of Nursing, Chattanooga, TN 37421-3707. Offers education (MHA); gerontology (MHA); health administration (MHA).

University of Phoenix–Hawaii Campus, College of Nursing, Honolulu, HI 96813-4317. Offers education (MHA); family nurse practitioner (MSN); gerontology (MHA); health administration (MHA); nursing (MSN); nursing/health care education (MSN); MSN/MBA. Evening/weekend programs available. *Degree requirements:* For master's, thesis (for some programs). *Entrance requirements:* For master's, minimum undergraduate GPA of 2.5, 3 years of work experience, RN license. Additional exam requirements/recommendations for international students: Required—TOEFL (minimum score 550 paper-based; 79 iBT). Electronic applications accepted.

University of Pittsburgh, Graduate School of Public Health, Department of Behavioral and Community Health Science, Pittsburgh, PA 15260. Offers behavioral and community health sciences (MPH, Dr PH); community-based participatory research and practice (Certificate); health equity (Certificate); lesbian, gay, bisexual and transgender health and wellness (Certificate); program evaluation (Certificate); MID/MPH; MPH/MPA; MPH/MSW; MPH/PhD. *Accreditation:* CAHME (one or more programs are accredited). Part-time programs available. *Faculty:* 14 full-time (7 women), 18 part-time/adjunct (6 women). *Students:* 61 full-time (47 women), 47 part-time (37 women); includes 27 minority (10 Black or African American, non-Hispanic/Latino; 9 Asian, non-Hispanic/Latino; 8 Hispanic/Latino), 5 international. Average age 29. 296 applicants, 58% accepted, 34 enrolled. In 2013, 34 master's, 6 doctorates awarded. *Degree requirements:* For master's, thesis; for doctorate, comprehensive exam, thesis/dissertation, preliminary exams. *Entrance requirements:* For master's and Certificate, GRE; for doctorate, GRE, master's degree in public health or related field. Additional exam requirements/recommendations for international students: Required—TOEFL (minimum score 550 paper-based; 80 iBT) or IELTS (minimum score 6.5). *Application deadline:* For fall admission, 1/15 for domestic and international students; for winter admission, 9/1 for international students; for spring admission, 10/15 for domestic students, 8/1 for international students; for summer admission, 12/1 for international students. Applications are processed on a rolling basis. Application fee: $120. Electronic applications accepted. *Expenses:* Tuition, state resident: full-time $19,964; part-time $807 per credit. Tuition, nonresident: full-time $32,686; part-time $1337 per credit. *Required fees:* $740; $200. Tuition and fees vary according to program. *Financial support:* In 2013–14, 11 students received support, including 2 fellowships with partial tuition reimbursements available (averaging $225 per year), 6 research assistantships with full and partial tuition reimbursements available (averaging $25,843 per year), 4 teaching assistantships with full and partial tuition reimbursements available (averaging $16,970 per year); unspecified assistantships also available. Financial award applicants required to submit FAFSA. *Faculty research:* Community-based participatory research, health equity, evaluation science, LGBT health, aging. *Total annual research expenditures:* $2.8 million. *Unit head:* Dr. Steven Albert, Chairman, 412-624-3102, Fax: 412-648-5975, E-mail: smalbert@pitt.edu. *Application contact:* Natalie C. Arnold, Recruitment and Academic Affairs Administrator, 412-624-3107, Fax: 412-624-5510, E-mail: narnold@pitt.edu.
Website: http://www.bchs.pitt.edu/

University of Pittsburgh, Graduate School of Public Health, Department of Infectious Diseases and Microbiology, Pittsburgh, PA 15260. Offers infectious disease management, intervention, and community practice (MPH); infectious disease pathogenesis, eradication, and laboratory practice (MPH); infectious diseases and microbiology (MS, PhD). Part-time programs available. *Faculty:* 19 full-time (6 women), 4 part-time/adjunct (1 woman). *Students:* 50 full-time (42 women), 15 part-time (10 women); includes 8 minority (2 Black or African American, non-Hispanic/Latino; 4 Asian, non-Hispanic/Latino; 1 Hispanic/Latino; 1 Two or more races, non-Hispanic/Latino), 11 international. Average age 27. 155 applicants, 63% accepted, 15 enrolled. In 2013, 25 master's, 4 doctorates awarded. Terminal master's awarded for partial completion of doctoral program. *Degree requirements:* For master's, one foreign language, comprehensive exam (for some programs), thesis; for doctorate, one foreign language, comprehensive exam, thesis/dissertation. *Entrance requirements:* For master's and doctorate, GRE General Test, MCAT, or DAT. Additional exam requirements/recommendations for international students: Required—TOEFL (minimum score 550 paper-based; 80 iBT) or IELTS (minimum score 6.5). *Application deadline:* For fall admission, 1/15 for domestic and international students; for spring admission, 10/15 for domestic students, 8/1 for international students; for summer admission, 12/1 for international students. Applications are processed on a rolling basis. Application fee: $120. Electronic applications accepted. *Expenses:* Tuition, state resident: full-time $19,964; part-time $807 per credit. Tuition, nonresident: full-time $32,686; part-time $1337 per credit. *Required fees:* $740; $200. Tuition and fees vary according to program. *Financial support:* In 2013–14, 12 research assistantships with full and partial tuition reimbursements (averaging $8,754 per year) were awarded. Financial award applicants required to submit FAFSA. *Faculty research:* HIV, Epstein-Barr virus, virology, immunology, malaria. *Total annual research expenditures:* $14.8 million. *Unit head:* Dr. Charles R. Rinaldo, Jr., Chairman, 412-624-3928, Fax: 412-624-4953, E-mail: rinaldo@pitt.edu. *Application contact:* Dr. Jeremy Martinson, Assistant Professor, 412-624-5646, Fax: 412-383-8926, E-mail: jmartins@pitt.edu.
Website: http://www.idm.pitt.edu/

University of Saskatchewan, College of Medicine, Department of Community Health and Epidemiology, Saskatoon, SK S7N 5A2, Canada. Offers M Sc, PhD. *Degree requirements:* For master's, thesis; for doctorate, thesis/dissertation. *Entrance requirements:* Additional exam requirements/recommendations for international students: Required—TOEFL. *Expenses: Tuition, area resident:* Full-time $3585 Canadian dollars; part-time $585 Canadian dollars per course. Tuition, nonresident: part-time $877 Canadian dollars per course. *International tuition:* $5377 Canadian dollars full-time. *Required fees:* $889.51 Canadian dollars.

University of South Florida, College of Public Health, Department of Community and Family Health, Tampa, FL 33620-9951. Offers MPH, MSPH, Dr PH, PhD. *Accreditation:* CEPH (one or more programs are accredited). Part-time and evening/weekend programs available. *Degree requirements:* For master's, comprehensive exam, thesis (for some programs); for doctorate, comprehensive exam, thesis/dissertation. *Entrance requirements:* For master's, GRE General Test, minimum GPA of 3.0 in upper-level course work, goal statement letter, two professional letters of recommendation, resume/curriculum vitae; for doctorate, GRE General Test, minimum GPA of 3.0 in upper-level course work, goal statement letter, three professional letters of recommendation, resume/curriculum vitae, writing sample. Additional exam requirements/recommendations for international students: Required—TOEFL (minimum score 550 paper-based; 79 iBT). Electronic applications accepted. *Faculty research:* Family violence, high-risk infants, medical material and child health, healthy start, social marketing, adolescent health, high-risk behaviors.

University of South Florida, Innovative Education Graduate Certificate Programs, Tampa, FL 33620-9951. *Unit head:* Kathy Barnes, Interdisciplinary Programs Coordinator, 813-974-8031, Fax: 813-974-7061, E-mail: barnesk@usf.edu. *Application contact:* Karen Tylinski, Metro Initiatives, 813-974-9943, Fax: 813-974-7061, E-mail: ktylinsk@usf.edu.
Website: http://www.usf.edu/innovative-education/

The University of Tennessee, Graduate School, College of Education, Health and Human Sciences, Program in Human Ecology, Knoxville, TN 37996. Offers child and family studies (PhD); community health (PhD); nutrition science (PhD); retailing and consumer sciences (PhD); textile science (PhD). *Degree requirements:* For doctorate, thesis/dissertation. *Entrance requirements:* For doctorate, GRE General Test, minimum GPA of 2.7. Additional exam requirements/recommendations for international students: Required—TOEFL. Electronic applications accepted. *Expenses:* Tuition, state resident: full-time $9540; part-time $531 per credit hour. Tuition, nonresident: full-time $27,728; part-time $1542 per credit hour. *Required fees:* $1404; $67 per credit hour.

The University of Tennessee, Graduate School, College of Education, Health and Human Sciences, Program in Public Health, Knoxville, TN 37996. Offers community health education (MPH); gerontology (MPH); health planning/administration (MPH); MS/MPH. *Accreditation:* CEPH. *Degree requirements:* For master's, thesis optional. *Entrance requirements:* For master's, minimum GPA of 2.7. Additional exam requirements/recommendations for international students: Required—TOEFL. Electronic applications accepted. *Expenses:* Tuition, state resident: full-time $9540;

part-time $531 per credit hour. Tuition, nonresident: full-time $27,728; part-time $1542 per credit hour. *Required fees:* $1404; $67 per credit hour.

The University of Texas Medical Branch, Graduate School of Biomedical Sciences, Department of Preventive Medicine and Community Health, Galveston, TX 77555. Offers population health sciences (MS, PhD); public health (MPH); rehabilitation sciences (PhD). *Accreditation:* CEPH. *Degree requirements:* For master's, thesis; for doctorate, thesis/dissertation. *Entrance requirements:* For master's, GRE General Test or MAT; for doctorate, GRE General Test. Additional exam requirements/recommendations for international students: Required—TOEFL (minimum score 550 paper-based). Electronic applications accepted.

University of Virginia, School of Nursing, Charlottesville, VA 22903. Offers acute and specialty care (MSN); acute care nurse practitioner (MSN); clinical nurse leadership (MSN); community-public health leadership (MSN); nursing (DNP, PhD); psychiatric mental health counseling (MSN); MSN/MBA. *Accreditation:* AACN. Part-time programs available. *Faculty:* 45 full-time (41 women), 3 part-time/adjunct (all women). *Students:* 177 full-time (155 women), 147 part-time (133 women); includes 53 minority (27 Black or African American, non-Hispanic/Latino; 10 Asian, non-Hispanic/Latino; 11 Hispanic/Latino; 5 Two or more races, non-Hispanic/Latino), 4 international. Average age 36. 236 applicants, 61% accepted, 110 enrolled. In 2013, 94 master's, 14 doctorates awarded. *Degree requirements:* For doctorate, comprehensive exam (for some programs), capstone project (DNP), dissertation (PhD). *Entrance requirements:* For master's, GRE General Test, MAT; for doctorate, GRE General Test. Additional exam requirements/recommendations for international students: Required—TOEFL, IELTS. *Application deadline:* Applications are processed on a rolling basis. Application fee: $60. Electronic applications accepted. *Expenses:* Contact institution. *Financial support:* Fellowships, research assistantships, teaching assistantships, Federal Work-Study, and scholarships/grants available. Financial award applicants required to submit FAFSA. *Unit head:* Dorrie K. Fontaine, Dean, 434-924-0141, Fax: 434-982-1809, E-mail: dkf2u@virginia.edu. *Application contact:* Clay Hysell, Assistant Dean for Admissions and Financial Services, 434-924-0141, Fax: 434-982-1809, E-mail: nur-osa@virginia.edu.
Website: http://www.nursing.virginia.edu/

University of Washington, Graduate School, School of Public Health, Department of Health Services, Seattle, WA 98195. Offers clinical research (MS); community-oriented public health practice (MPH); evaluative sciences and statistics (PhD); health behavior and social determinants of health (PhD); health economics (PhD); health informatics and health information management (MHIHIM); health services (MS, PhD); health services administration (EMHA, MHA); health systems and policy (MPH); health systems research (PhD); maternal and child health (MPH); social and behavioral sciences (MPH); JD/MHA; MHA/MBA; MHA/MD; MHA/MPA; MPH/JD; MPH/MD; MPH/MN; MPH/MPA; MPH/MS; MPH/MSD; MPH/MSW; MPH/PhD. *Faculty:* 63 full-time (30 women), 56 part-time/adjunct (25 women). *Students:* 121 full-time (101 women), 19 part-time (11 women); includes 28 minority (3 Black or African American, non-Hispanic/Latino; 2 American Indian or Alaska Native, non-Hispanic/Latino; 23 Asian, non-Hispanic/Latino), 5 international. Average age 30. 242 applicants, 48% accepted, 36 enrolled. In 2013, 43 master's, 9 doctorates awarded. Terminal master's awarded for partial completion of doctoral program. *Degree requirements:* For master's, thesis (for some programs), practicum (MPH); for doctorate, comprehensive exam, thesis/dissertation. *Entrance requirements:* For master's and doctorate, GRE General Test, minimum GPA of 3.0. Additional exam requirements/recommendations for international students: Required—TOEFL (minimum score 580 paper-based; 92 iBT), IELTS (minimum score 7). *Application deadline:* For fall admission, 1/1 for domestic students, 11/1 for international students. Application fee: 85 Albanian leks. Electronic applications accepted. *Financial support:* In 2013–14, 45 students received support, including 12 fellowships with full and partial tuition reimbursements available (averaging $22,000 per year), 9 research assistantships with full and partial tuition reimbursements available (averaging $18,700 per year), 9 teaching assistantships with full and partial tuition reimbursements available (averaging $4,575 per year); institutionally sponsored loans, traineeships, and health care benefits also available. Financial award application deadline: 2/28; financial award applicants required to submit FAFSA. *Faculty research:* Public health practice, health promotion and disease prevention, maternal and child health, organizational behavior and culture, health policy. *Unit head:* Dr. Larry Kessler, Chair, 206-543-2930. *Application contact:* Kitty A. Andert, MPH/MS/PhD Programs Manager, 206-616-2926, Fax: 206-543-3964, E-mail: hservmph@u.washington.edu.
Website: http://depts.washington.edu/hserv/

University of West Florida, College of Professional Studies, Department of Health, Leisure, and Exercise Science, Community Health Education Program, Pensacola, FL 32514-5750. Offers aging studies (MS); health promotion and worksite wellness (MS); psychosocial (MS). Part-time and evening/weekend programs available. *Degree requirements:* For master's, thesis or alternative. *Entrance requirements:* For master's, GRE or MAT, official transcripts; minimum GPA of 3.0; letter of intent; three personal references. Additional exam requirements/recommendations for international students: Required—TOEFL (minimum score 550 paper-based).

University of Wisconsin–La Crosse, Graduate Studies, College of Science and Health, Department of Health Education and Health Promotion, Program in Community Health Education, La Crosse, WI 54601-3742. Offers MPH, MS. *Accreditation:* CEPH. *Faculty:* 7 full-time (4 women), 1 (woman) part-time/adjunct. *Students:* 15 full-time (13 women), 8 part-time (6 women); includes 2 minority (1 Black or African American, non-Hispanic/Latino; 1 Hispanic/Latino), 1 international. Average age 30. 18 applicants, 94% accepted, 10 enrolled. In 2013, 7 master's awarded. *Degree requirements:* For master's, thesis. *Entrance requirements:* For master's, GRE General Test, GRE Subject Test (MPH), 3 letters of recommendation. Additional exam requirements/recommendations for international students: Required—TOEFL (minimum score 550 paper-based; 79 iBT). Electronic applications accepted. *Financial support:* Research assistantships with partial tuition reimbursements, Federal Work-Study, scholarships/grants, health care benefits, and tuition waivers (partial) available. Support available to part-time students. Financial award applicants required to submit FAFSA. *Unit head:* Dr. Gary Gilmore, Director, 608-785-8163, E-mail: gilmore.gary@uwlax.edu. *Application contact:* Corey Sjoquist, Director of Admissions, 608-785-8939, E-mail: admissions@uwlax.edu.
Website: http://www.uwlax.edu/sah/hehp/

University of Wisconsin–Madison, School of Medicine and Public Health and Graduate School, Graduate Programs in Medicine, Department of Population Health Sciences, Madison, WI 53726. Offers epidemiology (MS, PhD); population health (MS, PhD). *Accreditation:* CEPH. Part-time programs available. *Faculty:* 104 full-time (54 women), 2 part-time/adjunct (0 women). *Students:* 56 full-time (38 women), 14 part-time (9 women); includes 17 minority (8 Black or African American, non-Hispanic/Latino; 7 Asian, non-Hispanic/Latino; 2 Hispanic/Latino), 10 international. Average age 31. 97 applicants, 40% accepted, 20 enrolled. In 2013, 9 master's, 10 doctorates awarded. Terminal master's awarded for partial completion of doctoral program. *Degree requirements:* For master's, thesis, thesis defense; for doctorate, comprehensive exam, thesis/dissertation, qualifying exam, preliminary exam, dissertation defense. *Entrance requirements:* For master's and doctorate, GRE taken within the last 5 years (MCAT or LSAT acceptable for those with doctoral degrees), minimum GPA of 3.0, quantitative preparation (calculus, statistics, or other) with minimum B average. Additional exam requirements/recommendations for international students: Required—TOEFL (minimum score 580 paper-based; 92 iBT). *Application deadline:* For fall admission, 1/15 for domestic and international students. Application fee: $56. Electronic applications accepted. *Expenses:* Tuition, state resident: full-time $10,728; part-time $790 per credit. Tuition, nonresident: full-time $24,054; part-time $1623 per credit. *Required fees:* $1130; $119 per credit. *Financial support:* Fellowships with full tuition reimbursements, research assistantships with full tuition reimbursements, teaching assistantships with full tuition reimbursements, scholarships/grants, traineeships, health care benefits, and unspecified assistantships available. Support available to part-time students. *Faculty research:* Epidemiology (cancer, environmental, aging, infectious and genetic disease), determinants of population health, health services research, social and behavioral health sciences, biostatistics. *Total annual research expenditures:* $11.4 million. *Unit head:* Kathy Rutlin, MS/PhD Programs Coordinator, 608-265-8108, Fax: 608-263-2820, E-mail: karutlin@wisc.edu. *Application contact:* Quinn H. Fullenkamp, Assistant Programs Coordinator, 608-263-6583, Fax: 608-263-2820, E-mail: qhfullen@wisc.edu.
Website: http://www.pophealth.wisc.edu

University of Wyoming, College of Education, Programs in Counselor Education, Laramie, WY 82071. Offers community mental health (MS); counselor education and supervision (PhD); school counseling (MS); student affairs (MS). *Accreditation:* ACA (one or more programs are accredited). *Degree requirements:* For master's, comprehensive exam (for some programs), thesis optional; for doctorate, thesis/dissertation, video demonstration. *Entrance requirements:* For master's, interview, background check; for doctorate, video tape session, interview, writing sample, master's degree, background check. Additional exam requirements/recommendations for international students: Required—TOEFL. *Faculty research:* Wyoming SAGE photovoice project; accountable school counseling programs; GLBT issues; addictions; play therapy-early childhood mental health.

Virginia Commonwealth University, Medical College of Virginia-Professional Programs, School of Medicine, School of Medicine Graduate Programs, Department of Epidemiology and Community Health, Richmond, VA 23284-9005. Offers epidemiology (MPH, PhD); public health practice (MPH); social and behavioral science (MPH); MD/MPH; MSW/MPH. *Accreditation:* CEPH. Part-time programs available. *Degree requirements:* For doctorate, comprehensive exam, thesis/dissertation. *Entrance requirements:* For master's, GRE; for doctorate, GRE General Test, interview, 3 letters of recommendation, minimum graduate GPA of 3.0, master's degree in public health or related field including epidemiology and biostatistics. Additional exam requirements/recommendations for international students: Required—TOEFL (minimum score 600 paper-based; 100 iBT). Electronic applications accepted. *Faculty research:* Sickle cell anemia, breast cancer, HIV/AIDS, hospital epidemiology, infectious diseases.

Virginia State University, School of Graduate Studies, Research, and Outreach, School of Engineering, Science and Technology, Department of Psychology, Petersburg, VA 23806-0001. Offers behavioral and community health sciences (PhD); clinical health psychology (PhD); clinical psychology (MS); general psychology (MS). *Degree requirements:* For master's, one foreign language, thesis. *Entrance requirements:* For master's, GRE General Test.

Walden University, Graduate Programs, School of Health Sciences, Minneapolis, MN 55401. Offers clinical research administration (MS, Graduate Certificate); health education and promotion (MS); health informatics (MS); health services (PhD), including community health, healthcare administration, leadership, public health policy, self-designed; healthcare administration (MHA); public health (MPH, Dr PH, PhD), including community health and education (PhD), epidemiology (PhD). Part-time and evening/weekend programs available. Postbaccalaureate distance learning degree programs offered (minimal on-campus study). *Faculty:* 18 full-time (12 women), 236 part-time/adjunct (120 women). *Students:* 2,563 full-time (1,867 women), 1,775 part-time (1,233 women); includes 2,532 minority (1,963 Black or African American, non-Hispanic/Latino; 29 American Indian or Alaska Native, non-Hispanic/Latino; 212 Asian, non-Hispanic/Latino; 238 Hispanic/Latino; 15 Native Hawaiian or other Pacific Islander, non-Hispanic/Latino; 75 Two or more races, non-Hispanic/Latino), 97 international. Average age 39. 1,191 applicants, 94% accepted, 861 enrolled. In 2013, 723 master's, 121 doctorates, 17 other advanced degrees awarded. *Degree requirements:* For doctorate, thesis/dissertation, residency. *Entrance requirements:* For master's, bachelor's degree or higher; minimum GPA of 2.5; official transcripts; goal statement (for some programs); access to computer and Internet; for doctorate, master's degree or higher; three years of related professional or academic experience (preferred); minimum GPA of 3.0; goal statement and current resume (select programs); official transcripts; access to computer and Internet; for Graduate Certificate, relevant work experience; access to computer and Internet. Additional exam requirements/recommendations for international students: Required—TOEFL (minimum score 550 paper-based; 79 iBT), IELTS (minimum score 6.5), Michigan English Language Assessment Battery (minimum score 82), or PTE. *Application deadline:* Applications are processed on a rolling basis. Application fee: $0. Electronic applications accepted. *Expenses: Tuition:* Full-time $11,813.55; part-time $500 per credit. *Required fees:* $618.76. *Financial support:* Fellowships, Federal Work-Study, scholarships/grants, unspecified assistantships, and family tuition reduction, active duty/veteran tuition reduction, group tuition reduction, interest-free payment plans, employee tuition reduction available. Support available to part-time students. Financial award applicants required to submit FAFSA. *Unit head:* Dr. Jorg Westermann, Associate Dean, 800-925-3368. *Application contact:* Jennifer Hall, Vice President of Enrollment Management, 866-4-WALDEN, E-mail: info@waldenu.edu.
Website: http://www.waldenu.edu/colleges-schools/school-of-health-sciences

Washington State University Spokane, Graduate Programs, College of Nursing, Spokane, WA 99210-1495. Offers advanced population health (MN, DNP); family nurse practitioner (MN, DNP); nursing (PhD); psychiatric/mental health nurse practitioner (DNP); psychiatric/mental health practitioner (MN). *Accreditation:* AACN. *Degree requirements:* For master's, comprehensive exam (for some programs), thesis (for some programs), oral exam, research project. *Entrance requirements:* For master's, minimum GPA of 3.0, Washington state RN license, physical assessment skills, course work in statistics, recommendations, written interview (for nurse practitioner). *Faculty research:* Cardiovascular and Type 2 diabetes in children, evaluation of strategies to increase physical activity in sedentary people.

West Chester University of Pennsylvania, College of Health Sciences, Department of Health, West Chester, PA 19383. Offers community health (MPH); emergency preparedness (Certificate); environmental health (MPH); health care management (MPH, Certificate); integrative health (MPH, Certificate); nutrition (MPH); school health (M Ed). *Accreditation:* CEPH. Part-time and evening/weekend programs available. *Faculty:* 17 full-time (13 women), 3 part-time/adjunct (all women). *Students:* 115 full-time (85 women), 95 part-time (73 women); includes 79 minority (66 Black or African American, non-Hispanic/Latino; 1 American Indian or Alaska Native, non-Hispanic/Latino; 5 Asian, non-Hispanic/Latino; 3 Hispanic/Latino; 4 Two or more races, non-Hispanic/Latino), 15 international. Average age 31. 156 applicants, 83% accepted, 76 enrolled. In 2013, 101 master's, 18 other advanced degrees awarded. *Degree requirements:* For master's, thesis or alternative, minimum GPA of 3.0; research report (for M Ed); major project and practicum (for MPH); for Certificate, minimum GPA of 3.0. *Entrance requirements:* For master's, goal statement, two letters of recommendation,

undergraduate Introduction to Statistics course. Additional exam requirements/ recommendations for international students: Required—TOEFL (minimum score 550 paper-based; 80 iBT). *Application deadline:* For fall admission, 4/15 priority date for domestic students, 3/15 for international students; for spring admission, 10/15 priority date for domestic students, 9/1 for international students. Applications are processed on a rolling basis. Application fee: $45. Electronic applications accepted. *Expenses:* Tuition, state resident: full-time $7956; part-time $442 per credit. Tuition, nonresident: full-time $11,934; part-time $663 per credit. *Required fees:* $2134.20; $106.24 per credit. Tuition and fees vary according to campus/location and program. *Financial support:* Unspecified assistantships available. Support available to part-time students. Financial award application deadline: 2/15; financial award applicants required to submit FAFSA. *Faculty research:* Healthy school communities, community health issues and evidence-based programs, environment and health, nutrition and health, integrative health. *Unit head:* Dr. Bethann Cinelli, Chair, 610-436-2267, E-mail: bcinelli@wcupa.edu. *Application contact:* Dr. Lynn Carson, Graduate Coordinator, 610-436-2138, E-mail: lcarson@wcupa.edu.
Website: http://www.wcupa.edu/_ACADEMICS/HealthSciences/health/

West Virginia University, School of Medicine, Department of Community Medicine, Program in Public Health, Morgantown, WV 26506. Offers community health/ preventative medicine (MPH). *Accreditation:* CEPH. Part-time programs available. Postbaccalaureate distance learning degree programs offered (minimal on-campus study). *Degree requirements:* For master's, practicum, project. *Entrance requirements:* For master's, GRE General Test, MCAT, medical degree, medical internship. *Expenses:* Contact institution. *Faculty research:* Occupational health, environmental health, clinical epidemiology, health care management, prevention.

Environmental and Occupational Health

American University of Beirut, Graduate Programs, Faculty of Health Sciences, Beirut, Lebanon. Offers environmental sciences (MS), including environmental health; epidemiology (MS); epidemiology and biostatistics (MPH); health management and policy (MPH); health promotion and community health (MPH); population health (MS). Part-time programs available. *Faculty:* 26 full-time (18 women), 7 part-time/adjunct (4 women). *Students:* 42 full-time (37 women), 103 part-time (84 women). Average age 25. 132 applicants, 65% accepted, 48 enrolled. In 2013, 52 master's awarded. *Degree requirements:* For master's, one foreign language, comprehensive exam, thesis (for some programs). *Entrance requirements:* For master's, 2 letters of recommendation, personal statement, transcripts. Additional exam requirements/recommendations for international students: Required—TOEFL (minimum score 583 paper-based; 97 iBT), IELTS (minimum score 7). *Application deadline:* For fall admission, 2/7 priority date for domestic and international students; for spring admission, 11/1 for domestic and international students. Application fee: $50. Electronic applications accepted. *Expenses: Tuition:* Full-time $14,724; part-time $818 per credit. *Required fees:* $692. Tuition and fees vary according to course load and program. *Financial support:* In 2013–14, 56 students received support. Scholarships/grants, health care benefits, and unspecified assistantships available. Financial award application deadline: 4/1. *Faculty research:* Tobacco control; health of the elderly; youth health; mental health; women's health; reproductive and sexual health, including HIV/AIDS; water quality; health systems; quality in health care delivery; health human resources; health policy; occupational and environmental health; social inequality; social determinants of health; non-communicable diseases. *Total annual research expenditures:* $1 million. *Unit head:* Iman Adel Nuwayhid, Dean, 961-1759683, Fax: 961-1744470, E-mail: nuwayhid@aub.edu.lb. *Application contact:* Mitra Tauk, Administrative Coordinator, 961-1-350000 Ext. 4687, Fax: 96-1-1744470, E-mail: mt12@aub.edu.lb.

Anna Maria College, Graduate Division, Program in Occupational and Environmental Health and Safety, Paxton, MA 01612. Offers MS. Part-time and evening/weekend programs available. *Degree requirements:* For master's, thesis. *Entrance requirements:* For master's, minimum GPA of 2.7. Additional exam requirements/recommendations for international students: Required—TOEFL (minimum score 500 paper-based). Electronic applications accepted.

Boise State University, College of Health Sciences, Department of Community and Environmental Health, Boise, ID 83725-0399. Offers environmental health (MHS); evaluation and research (MHS); health policy (MHS); health promotion (MHS); health services leadership (MHS).

Boston University, School of Public Health, Environmental Health Department, Boston, MA 02215. Offers MPH, MS, PhD. *Accreditation:* CEPH (one or more programs are accredited). Part-time and evening/weekend programs available. *Faculty:* 14 full-time, 20 part-time/adjunct. *Students:* 29 full-time (23 women), 18 part-time (15 women); includes 11 minority (1 Black or African American, non-Hispanic/Latino; 6 Asian, non-Hispanic/Latino; 4 Hispanic/Latino), 5 international. Average age 26. 138 applicants, 45% accepted, 18 enrolled. In 2013, 12 master's, 3 doctorates awarded. *Degree requirements:* For master's, comprehensive exam (for some programs), thesis (for some programs); for doctorate, one foreign language, thesis/dissertation, comprehensive written and oral exams. *Entrance requirements:* For master's, GRE, LSAT, GMAT, DAT, or MCAT, U.S. bachelor's degree or foreign equivalent; for doctorate, GRE, MCAT, MPH or equivalent. Additional exam requirements/recommendations for international students: Required—TOEFL (minimum score 600 paper-based; 100 iBT) or IELTS (minimum score 6). *Application deadline:* For fall admission, 2/1 priority date for domestic and international students; for spring admission, 10/15 priority date for domestic and international students. Applications are processed on a rolling basis. Application fee: $115. Electronic applications accepted. *Expenses: Tuition:* Full-time $43,970; part-time $1374 per credit hour. *Required fees:* $60 per semester. Tuition and fees vary according to class time, course level and program. *Financial support:* Career-related internships or fieldwork, Federal Work-Study, institutionally sponsored loans, and scholarships/grants available. Support available to part-time students. Financial award application deadline: 3/1; financial award applicants required to submit FAFSA. *Unit head:* Dr. Roberta White, Chair, 617-638-4620, E-mail: envhlth@bu.edu. *Application contact:* LePhan Quan, Associate Director of Admissions, 617-638-4640, Fax: 617-638-5299, E-mail: asksph@bu.edu.

California State University, Northridge, Graduate Studies, College of Health and Human Development, Department of Environmental and Occupational Health, Northridge, CA 91330. Offers environmental and occupational health (MS); industrial hygiene (MS). *Degree requirements:* For master's, seminar, field experience, comprehensive exam or thesis. *Entrance requirements:* For master's, GRE General Test or minimum GPA of 3.0. Additional exam requirements/recommendations for international students: Required—TOEFL.

Capella University, School of Public Service Leadership, Doctoral Programs in Healthcare, Minneapolis, MN 55402. Offers criminal justice (PhD); emergency management (PhD); epidemiology (Dr PH); general health administration (DHA); general public administration (DPA); health advocacy and leadership (Dr PH); health care administration (PhD); health care leadership (DHA); health policy advocacy (DHA); multidisciplinary human services (PhD); nonprofit management and leadership (PhD); public safety leadership (PhD); social and community services (PhD).

Capella University, School of Public Service Leadership, Master's Programs in Healthcare, Minneapolis, MN 55402. Offers criminal justice (MS); emergency management (MS); general public health (MPH); gerontology (MS); health administration (MHA); health care operations (MHA); health management policy (MPH); health policy (MHA); homeland security (MS); multidisciplinary human sevrices (MS); public administration (MPA); public safety leadership (MS); social and community services (MS); social behavioral sciences (MPH); MS/MPA.

Clemson University, Graduate School, College of Engineering and Science, Department of Environmental Engineering and Earth Sciences, Program in Environmental Health Physics, Anderson, SC 29625-6510. Offers MS. *Entrance requirements:* Additional exam requirements/recommendations for international students: Required—TOEFL, IELTS. *Application deadline:* Applications are processed on a rolling basis. Application fee: $85 ($90 for international students). *Faculty research:* Nuclear forensics, environmental radiochemistry, actinide biogeochemistry, environmental mineralogy, computational materials science. *Unit head:* Dr. Tanju Karanfil, Chair, 864-656-1005, Fax: 864-656-0672, E-mail: tkaranf@clemson.edu. *Application contact:* Dr. Timothy A. Devol, Graduate Student Services Coordinator, 864-656-3278, Fax: 864-656-0672, E-mail: ehp-l@clemson.edu.
Website: http://www.clemson.edu/ces/eees/gradprog/ehp/

Colorado State University, College of Veterinary Medicine and Biomedical Sciences, Department of Environmental and Radiological Health Sciences, Fort Collins, CO 80523-1681. Offers environmental health (MS, PhD); radiological health sciences (MS, PhD). Part-time programs available. *Faculty:* 26 full-time (8 women), 1 part-time/adjunct (0 women). *Students:* 74 full-time (51 women), 38 part-time (22 women); includes 9 minority (2 American Indian or Alaska Native, non-Hispanic/Latino; 2 Asian, non-Hispanic/Latino; 4 Hispanic/Latino; 1 Two or more races, non-Hispanic/Latino), 7 international. Average age 31. 75 applicants, 72% accepted, 36 enrolled. In 2013, 56 master's, 2 doctorates awarded. Terminal master's awarded for partial completion of doctoral program. *Degree requirements:* For master's, comprehensive exam (for some programs), thesis (for some programs), publishable paper; for doctorate, comprehensive exam, thesis/dissertation, publishable paper. *Entrance requirements:* For master's, GRE General Test, 1 year of course work in biology lab and chemistry lab, 1 semester of course work in organic chemistry, course work in calculus, resume, 3 letters of recommendation, bachelor's degree, minimum GPA 3.0, transcripts, written statement; for doctorate, GRE General Test, 1 year of course work in biology lab and chemistry lab, 1 semester of course work in organic chemistry, course work in calculus, resume, 3 letters of recommendation, evidence of research capability, bachelor's degree, minimum GPA 3.0, transcripts, written statement. Additional exam requirements/ recommendations for international students: Required—TOEFL (minimum score 550 paper-based; 80 iBT), IELTS. *Application deadline:* For fall admission, 6/30 for domestic and international students; for spring admission, 11/1 for domestic and international students. Applications are processed on a rolling basis. Application fee: $50. Electronic applications accepted. *Expenses:* Tuition, state resident: full-time $9075.40; part-time $504 per credit. Tuition, nonresident: full-time $22,248; part-time $1236 per credit. *Required fees:* $1819; $60 per credit. *Financial support:* In 2013–14, 32 students received support, including 19 fellowships with tuition reimbursements available (averaging $35,529 per year), 12 research assistantships with tuition reimbursements available (averaging $21,110 per year), 1 teaching assistantship with tuition reimbursement available (averaging $14,875 per year); scholarships/grants, traineeships, and unspecified assistantships also available. Financial award application deadline: 4/30. *Faculty research:* Air pollution commuter study, dietary interventions for improved gut health and immunity, agricultural health and safety, impacts of space travel on the human body, radiation protection and Fukushima accident. *Total annual research expenditures:* $7.9 million. *Unit head:* Dr. Jac A. Nickoloff, Professor/Department Head, 970-491-6674, Fax: 970-491-0623, E-mail: j.nickoloff@colostate.edu. *Application contact:* Jeanne A. Brockway, Graduate Program Coordinator, 970-491-5003, Fax: 970-491-2940, E-mail: jeanne.brockway@colostate.edu.
Website: http://csu-cvmbs.colostate.edu/academics/erhs/Pages/graduate-studies.aspx

Columbia Southern University, College of Safety and Emergency Services, Orange Beach, AL 36561. Offers criminal justice administration (MS); emergency services management (MS); occupational safety and health (MS), including environmental management. Part-time and evening/weekend programs available. Postbaccalaureate distance learning degree programs offered (no on-campus study). *Entrance requirements:* For master's, bachelor's degree from accredited/approved institution. Additional exam requirements/recommendations for international students: Required—TOEFL. Electronic applications accepted.

Columbia University, Columbia University Mailman School of Public Health, Department of Environmental Health Sciences, New York, NY 10032. Offers MPH, Dr PH, PhD. PhD offered in cooperation with the Graduate School of Arts and Sciences. *Accreditation:* CEPH (one or more programs are accredited). Part-time programs available. *Students:* 65 full-time (57 women), 8 part-time (5 women); includes 24 minority (2 Black or African American, non-Hispanic/Latino; 12 Asian, non-Hispanic/ Latino; 8 Hispanic/Latino; 2 Two or more races, non-Hispanic/Latino), 8 international. Average age 27. 133 applicants, 56% accepted, 28 enrolled. In 2013, 22 master's, 2 doctorates awarded. *Degree requirements:* For master's, thesis optional; for doctorate, thesis/dissertation. *Entrance requirements:* For master's, GRE General Test, 1 year of course work in biology, general chemistry, organic chemistry, and mathematics; for doctorate, GRE General Test, MPH or equivalent (Dr PH). Additional exam requirements/recommendations for international students: Required—TOEFL (minimum score 600 paper-based; 100 iBT). *Application deadline:* For fall admission, 12/1 priority date for domestic and international students. Applications are processed on a rolling basis. Application fee: $120. Electronic applications accepted. *Financial support:* Research assistantships, teaching assistantships, career-related internships or fieldwork, and Federal Work-Study available. Support available to part-time students. Financial award application deadline: 2/1; financial award applicants required to submit

FAFSA. *Faculty research:* Health effects of environmental and occupational exposure to chemicals and radiation, molecular epidemiology, risk assessment, molecular toxicology, environmental policy. *Unit head:* Dr. Tomas Guilarte, Chair, 212-305-3466, Fax: 212-305-4012. *Application contact:* Dr. Joseph Korevec, Director of Admissions and Financial Aid, 212-305-8698, Fax: 212-342-1861, E-mail: ph-admit@columbia.edu.
Website: http://mailman.hs.columbia.edu/ehs/index.html

Duke University, Graduate School, Integrated Toxicology and Environmental Health Program, Durham, NC 27708. Offers Certificate. *Faculty:* 33. *Students:* 5 full-time (3 women); includes 1 minority (Black or African American, non-Hispanic/Latino), 1 international. 23 applicants, 13% accepted, 2 enrolled. *Entrance requirements:* Additional exam requirements/recommendations for international students: Required—TOEFL (minimum score 577 paper-based; 90 iBT) or IELTS (minimum score 7). *Application deadline:* For fall admission, 12/8 priority date for domestic and international students. Application fee: $80. Electronic applications accepted. *Financial support:* Fellowships available. Financial award application deadline: 12/8. *Unit head:* Cynthia Kuhn, Director, 919-613-8078, Fax: 919-668-1799, E-mail: emarion@duke.edu. *Application contact:* Elizabeth Hutton, Director of Admissions, 919-684-3913, Fax: 919-684-2277, E-mail: grad-admissions@duke.edu.
Website: http://sites.nicholas.duke.edu/envhealth/

East Carolina University, Graduate School, College of Health and Human Performance, Department of Health Education and Promotion, Greenville, NC 27858-4353. Offers environmental health (MS); health education (MA Ed); health education and promotion (MA). *Accreditation:* NCATE. *Degree requirements:* For master's, comprehensive exam, thesis optional. *Entrance requirements:* For master's, GRE General Test or MAT. Additional exam requirements/recommendations for international students: Required—TOEFL. *Application deadline:* For fall admission, 6/1 priority date for domestic students. Applications are processed on a rolling basis. Application fee: $50. *Expenses:* Tuition, state resident: full-time $4223. Tuition, nonresident: full-time $16,540. *Required fees:* $2184. *Financial support:* Fellowships, research assistantships, teaching assistantships, and career-related internships or fieldwork available. Support available to part-time students. Financial award application deadline: 6/1. *Faculty research:* Community health education, worksite health promotion, school health education, environmental health. *Unit head:* Dr. J. Don Chaney, Chair, 252-737-4942, E-mail: chaneyj@ecu.edu. *Application contact:* Dr. J. Don Chaney, Chair, 252-737-4942, E-mail: chaneyj@ecu.edu.
Website: http://www.ecu.edu/hlth/

East Carolina University, Graduate School, Thomas Harriot College of Arts and Sciences, Department of Psychology, Program in Health Psychology, Greenville, NC 27858-4353. Offers clinical health psychology (PhD); occupational health psychology (PhD); pediatric school psychology (PhD). *Entrance requirements:* For doctorate, GRE. *Expenses:* Tuition, state resident: full-time $4223. Tuition, nonresident: full-time $16,540. *Required fees:* $2184. *Financial support:* Fellowships, research assistantships, and teaching assistantships available. *Unit head:* Dr. Samuel F. Sears, Jr., Chair, 252-328-6118, Fax: 252-328-6283, E-mail: searss@ecu.edu. *Application contact:* Dean of Graduate School, 252-328-6012, Fax: 252-328-6071, E-mail: gradschool@ecu.edu.
Website: http://www.ecu.edu/psyc/Health-Psychology-Doctoral-Program.cfm

Eastern Kentucky University, The Graduate School, College of Health Sciences, Department of Clinical Laboratory Science/Environmental Health Science, Richmond, KY 40475-3102. Offers environmental health science (MPH). *Accreditation:* CEPH. *Degree requirements:* For master's, comprehensive exam, thesis optional, practicum, capstone course. *Entrance requirements:* For master's, GRE. *Faculty research:* Water quality, food safety, occupational health, air quality.

East Tennessee State University, School of Graduate Studies, College of Public Health, Department of Environmental Health, Johnson City, TN 37614. Offers MSEH, PhD. Part-time programs available. *Faculty:* 6 full-time (2 women), 4 part-time/adjunct (0 women). *Students:* 2 full-time (1 woman), 3 part-time (2 women). Average age 28. 3 applicants, 67% accepted, 2 enrolled. In 2013, 1 master's, 2 doctorates awarded. *Degree requirements:* For master's, comprehensive exam, research project or thesis; environmental health practice; seminar; for doctorate, comprehensive exam, thesis/dissertation, environmental health practice, seminar. *Entrance requirements:* For master's, GRE General Test, 30 hours of course work in natural and physical sciences, minimum GPA of 3.0, three letters of recommendation; for doctorate, GRE General Test, MPH or MS in related field of study with research-based thesis, three letters of recommendation, curriculum vitae or resume. Additional exam requirements/recommendations for international students: Required—TOEFL (minimum score 550 paper-based; 79 iBT). *Application deadline:* For fall admission, 6/1 for domestic students, 4/30 for international students; for spring admission, 11/1 for domestic students, 9/30 for international students. Application fee: $35 ($45 for international students). Electronic applications accepted. *Expenses:* Tuition, state resident: full-time $7900; part-time $395 per credit hour. Tuition, nonresident: full-time $21,960; part-time $1098 per credit hour. *Required fees:* $1345; $84 per credit hour. *Financial support:* In 2013–14, 5 students received support, including 5 research assistantships with full tuition reimbursements available (averaging $10,000 per year); career-related internships or fieldwork, institutionally sponsored loans, scholarships/grants, and unspecified assistantships also available. Financial award application deadline: 7/1; financial award applicants required to submit FAFSA. *Faculty research:* Water quality, ecotoxicology, occupational health, indoor air quality, community-focused environmental health. *Unit head:* Dr. Phillip R. Scheuerman, Chair, 423-439-7633, Fax: 423-439-5238, E-mail: philsche@etsu.edu. *Application contact:* Mary Duncan, Graduate Specialist, 423-439-4302, Fax: 423-439-5624, E-mail: duncanm@etsu.edu.
Website: http://www.etsu.edu/cph/eh/

Embry-Riddle Aeronautical University–Worldwide, Worldwide Headquarters - Graduate Programs, Program in Business Administration and Management, Daytona Beach, FL 32114-3900. Offers air transportation management (Graduate Certificate); airport planning design and development (Graduate Certificate); aviation (MBAA); aviation enterprises in the global environment (Graduate Certificate); aviation-aerospace industrial management (Graduate Certificate); engineering management (MSEM); integrated logistics management (Graduate Certificate); leadership (MSL); logistics and supply chain management (MSLSCM); management (MSM); modeling and simulation management (Graduate Certificate); occupational safety management (MSOSM); project management (MSPM, Graduate Certificate). Part-time and evening/weekend programs available. Postbaccalaureate distance learning degree programs offered (no on-campus study). *Degree requirements:* For master's, comprehensive exam (for some programs), thesis (for some programs). *Entrance requirements:* Additional exam requirements/recommendations for international students: Recommended—TOEFL (minimum score 550 paper-based; 79 iBT). Electronic applications accepted. *Faculty research:* Healthcare operations management, humanitarian logistics, supply chain risk management, collaborative supply chain management, intersection of collaborative supply chain management and the learning organization, development of assessment tool measuring supply chain collaborative capacity, teaching effectiveness, teaching quality, management style effectiveness, aeronautics, small/medium-sized business leadership study, leadership factors, critical thinking, efficacy of ePortfolio.

Emory University, Rollins School of Public Health, Department of Environmental Health, Atlanta, GA 30322-1100. Offers environmental health (MPH); environmental health and epidemiology (MSPH); environmental health sciences (PhD); global environmental health (MPH). *Accreditation:* CEPH. Part-time programs available. *Degree requirements:* For master's, thesis, practicum. *Entrance requirements:* For master's, GRE General Test. Additional exam requirements/recommendations for international students: Required—TOEFL. Electronic applications accepted.

Florida International University, Robert Stempel College of Public Health and Social Work, Programs in Public Health, Miami, FL 33199. Offers biostatistics (MPH); environmental and occupational health (MPH, PhD); epidemiology (MPH, PhD); health policy and management (MPH); health promotion and disease prevention (PhD); health promotion and diseases prevention (MPH). Ph D program has fall admissions only; MPH offered jointly with University of Miami. *Accreditation:* CEPH. Part-time and evening/weekend programs available. Postbaccalaureate distance learning degree programs offered (no on-campus study). *Degree requirements:* For master's, thesis optional; for doctorate, comprehensive exam, thesis/dissertation. *Entrance requirements:* For master's, minimum GPA of 3.0, letters of recommendation; for doctorate, GRE, resume, minimum GPA of 3.0, letters of recommendation, letter of intent. Additional exam requirements/recommendations for international students: Required—TOEFL (minimum score 550 paper-based; 80 iBT). Electronic applications accepted. *Expenses:* Contact institution. *Faculty research:* Drugs/AIDS intervention among migrant workers, provision of services for active/recovering drug users with HIV.

Fort Valley State University, College of Graduate Studies and Extended Education, Program in Public Health, Fort Valley, GA 31030. Offers environmental health (MPH). *Degree requirements:* For master's, thesis. *Entrance requirements:* For master's, GRE General Test. Additional exam requirements/recommendations for international students: Recommended—TOEFL.

Gannon University, School of Graduate Studies, College of Engineering and Business, School of Engineering and Computer Science, Program in Environmental Science and Engineering, Erie, PA 16541-0001. Offers environmental health and engineering (MS). Part-time and evening/weekend programs available. *Students:* 10 full-time (3 women), 2 part-time (1 woman); includes 1 minority (Black or African American, non-Hispanic/Latino), 4 international. Average age 27. 20 applicants, 50% accepted, 3 enrolled. In 2013, 4 master's awarded. *Degree requirements:* For master's, thesis (for some programs), research paper or project (for some programs). *Entrance requirements:* For master's, GRE, bachelor's degree in science or engineering. Additional exam requirements/recommendations for international students: Required—TOEFL (minimum score 79 iBT). *Application deadline:* Applications are processed on a rolling basis. Application fee: $25. Electronic applications accepted. *Expenses: Tuition:* Full-time $15,930; part-time $885 per credit. *Required fees:* $430; $18 per credit. Tuition and fees vary according to course load, degree level and program. *Financial support:* Scholarships/grants and unspecified assistantships available. Financial award application deadline: 7/1; financial award applicants required to submit FAFSA. *Unit head:* Dr. Harry Diz, Chair, 814-871-7633, E-mail: diz001@gannon.edu. *Application contact:* Kara Morgan, Director of Graduate Admissions, 814-871-5831, Fax: 814-871-5827, E-mail: graduate@gannon.edu.

The George Washington University, School of Public Health and Health Services, Department of Environmental and Occupational Health, Washington, DC 20052. Offers environmental health science and policy (MPH); public health (MPH). *Accreditation:* CEPH. *Faculty:* 10 full-time (6 women). *Students:* 1 (woman) full-time, 8 part-time (7 women); includes 2 minority (1 Black or African American, non-Hispanic/Latino; 1 Hispanic/Latino). Average age 36. *Degree requirements:* For master's, case study or special project. *Entrance requirements:* For master's, GMAT, GRE General Test, or MCAT. Additional exam requirements/recommendations for international students: Required—TOEFL. *Application deadline:* For fall admission, 4/15 priority date for domestic students, 4/15 for international students; for spring admission, 11/1 for domestic and international students. Applications are processed on a rolling basis. Application fee: $75. *Financial support:* In 2013–14, 7 students received support. Tuition waivers available. Financial award application deadline: 2/15. *Unit head:* Dr. Melissa Perry, Director, 202-994-1734, E-mail: mperry@gwu.edu. *Application contact:* Jane Smith, Director of Admissions, 202-994-0248, Fax: 202-994-1860, E-mail: sphhsinfo@gwumc.edu.

Georgia Southern University, Jack N. Averitt College of Graduate Studies, Allen E. Paulson College of Engineering and Information Technology, Department of Mechanical Engineering, Program in Occupational Safety and Environmental Compliance, Statesboro, GA 30460. Offers Graduate Certificate. *Students:* 1 part-time (0 women). Average age 24. 4 applicants, 100% accepted. *Expenses:* Tuition, state resident: full-time $7068; part-time $270 per semester hour. Tuition, nonresident: full-time $26,446; part-time $1077 per semester hour. *Required fees:* $2092. *Financial support:* In 2013–14, 1 student received support. *Unit head:* Dr. Brian Vlcek, Chair, 912-478-5721, Fax: 912-478-1455, E-mail: vlvlcek@georgiasouthern.edu. *Application contact:* Amanda Gilliland, Coordinator for Graduate Student Recruitment, 912-478-5384, Fax: 912-478-0740, E-mail: gradadmissions@georgiasouthern.edu.

Georgia Southern University, Jack N. Averitt College of Graduate Studies, Jiann-Ping Hsu College of Public Health, Program in Public Health, Statesboro, GA 30460. Offers biostatistics (MPH, Dr PH); community health behavior and education (Dr PH); community health education (MPH); environmental health sciences (MPH); epidemiology (MPH); health policy and management (MPH, Dr PH). *Accreditation:* CEPH. Part-time programs available. *Students:* 130 full-time (96 women), 50 part-time (39 women); includes 95 minority (80 Black or African American, non-Hispanic/Latino; 5 Asian, non-Hispanic/Latino; 4 Hispanic/Latino; 1 Native Hawaiian or other Pacific Islander, non-Hispanic/Latino; 5 Two or more races, non-Hispanic/Latino), 32 international. Average age 30. 213 applicants, 68% accepted, 61 enrolled. In 2013, 29 master's, 9 doctorates awarded. *Degree requirements:* For master's, thesis optional, practicum; for doctorate, comprehensive exam, thesis/dissertation, practicum. *Entrance requirements:* For master's, GRE General Test, minimum GPA of 2.75, resume, 3 letters of reference; for doctorate, GRE, GMAT, MCAT, LSAT, 3 letters of reference, statement of purpose, resume or curriculum vitae. Additional exam requirements/recommendations for international students: Required—TOEFL (minimum score 550 paper-based; 80 iBT), IELTS (minimum score 6). *Application deadline:* For fall admission, 3/1 priority date for domestic and international students; for spring admission, 10/1 priority date for domestic students, 10/1 for international students. Applications are processed on a rolling basis. Application fee: $50. Electronic applications accepted. *Expenses:* Contact institution. *Financial support:* In 2013–14, 54 students received support, including research assistantships with partial tuition reimbursements available (averaging $7,200 per year), teaching assistantships with partial tuition reimbursements available (averaging $7,200 per year); career-related internships or fieldwork, Federal Work-Study, scholarships/grants, tuition waivers (partial), and unspecified assistantships also available. Support available to part-time students. Financial award application deadline: 4/15; financial award applicants required to submit FAFSA. *Faculty research:* Rural public health best practices, health disparity elimination, community initiatives to enhance public health, cost effectiveness analysis, epidemiology of rural public health, environmental health issues, health care system

assessment, rural health care, health policy and healthcare financing, survival analysis, nonparametric statistics and resampling methods, micro-arrays and genomics, data imputation techniques and clinical trial methodology. *Total annual research expenditures:* $281,707. *Unit head:* Sarah Peterson, Student Services Coordinator, 912-478-2413, Fax: 912-478-5811, E-mail: speterson@georgiasouthern.edu. *Application contact:* Amanda Gilliland, Coordinator for Graduate Student Recruitment, 912-478-5384, Fax: 912-478-0740, E-mail: gradadmissions@georgiasouthern.edu.
Website: http://chhs.georgiasouthern.edu/health/

Harvard University, Cyprus International Institute for the Environment and Public Health in Association with Harvard School of Public Health, Cambridge, MA 02138. Offers environmental health (MS); environmental/public health (PhD); epidemiology and biostatistics (MS). *Entrance requirements:* For master's and doctorate, GRE, resume/curriculum vitae, 3 letters of recommendation, BA or BS (including diploma and official transcripts). Additional exam requirements/recommendations for international students: Required—TOEFL, IELTS (minimum score 7). Electronic applications accepted. *Expenses: Tuition:* Full-time $38,888. *Required fees:* $958. Tuition and fees vary according to campus/location, program and student level. *Faculty research:* Air pollution, climate change, biostatistics, sustainable development, environmental management.

Harvard University, Harvard School of Public Health, Department of Environmental Health, Boston, MA 02115-6096. Offers environmental health (SM, PhD, SD); exposure, epidemiology, and risk (SM, SD); occupational health (SM, SD); physiology (PhD, SD). Part-time programs available. *Faculty:* 24 full-time (3 women), 41 part-time/adjunct (10 women). *Students:* 86 full-time (55 women), 1 part-time (0 women); includes 15 minority (2 Black or African American, non-Hispanic/Latino; 8 Asian, non-Hispanic/Latino; 4 Hispanic/Latino; 1 Two or more races, non-Hispanic/Latino), 51 international. Average age 26. 86 applicants, 45% accepted, 25 enrolled. In 2013, 14 master's, 12 doctorates awarded. *Degree requirements:* For doctorate, thesis/dissertation, qualifying exam. *Entrance requirements:* For master's, GRE, MCAT; for doctorate, GRE. Additional exam requirements/recommendations for international students: Required—TOEFL (minimum score 600 paper-based; 100 iBT); Recommended—IELTS (minimum score 7). *Application deadline:* For fall admission, 12/15 for domestic and international students. Application fee: $120. Electronic applications accepted. *Expenses: Tuition:* Full-time $38,888. *Required fees:* $958. Tuition and fees vary according to campus/location, program and student level. *Financial support:* Fellowships, research assistantships, teaching assistantships, career-related internships or fieldwork, Federal Work-Study, scholarships/grants, traineeships, and unspecified assistantships available. Support available to part-time students. Financial award application deadline: 2/15; financial award applicants required to submit FAFSA. *Faculty research:* Exposure assessment, epidemiology, risk assessment, environmental epidemiology, ergonomics and safety, environmental exposure assessment, occupational hygiene, industrial hygiene and occupational safety, population genetics, indoor and outdoor air pollution, cell and molecular biology of the lungs, infectious diseases. *Unit head:* Dr. Douglas Dockery, Chairman, 617-432-1270, Fax: 617-432-6913. *Application contact:* Vincent W. James, Director of Admissions, 617-432-1031, Fax: 617-432-7080, E-mail: admissions@hsph.harvard.edu.
Website: http://www.hsph.harvard.edu/environmental-health/

Hunter College of the City University of New York, Graduate School, Schools of the Health Professions, School of Health Sciences, Programs in Urban Public Health, Program in Environmental and Occupational Health Sciences, New York, NY 10065-5085. Offers MPH, MS. *Accreditation:* ABET (one or more programs are accredited); CEPH. Part-time and evening/weekend programs available. *Faculty:* 3 full-time (2 women), 1 part-time/adjunct (0 women). *Students:* 3 full-time (all women), 45 part-time (29 women); includes 17 minority (5 Black or African American, non-Hispanic/Latino; 1 American Indian or Alaska Native, non-Hispanic/Latino; 8 Asian, non-Hispanic/Latino; 3 Hispanic/Latino), 3 international. Average age 30. 30 applicants, 90% accepted, 21 enrolled. In 2013, 11 master's awarded. *Degree requirements:* For master's, comprehensive exam, thesis optional, internship. *Entrance requirements:* For master's, GRE General Test, previous course work in calculus and statistics. Additional exam requirements/recommendations for international students: Required—TOEFL. *Application deadline:* For fall admission, 4/1 for domestic students, 2/1 for international students; for spring admission, 11/1 for domestic students, 9/1 for international students. Application fee: $125. *Financial support:* In 2013–14, 6 fellowships were awarded; career-related internships or fieldwork, Federal Work-Study, institutionally sponsored loans, and tuition waivers (partial) also available. Support available to part-time students. Financial award application deadline: 3/1. *Faculty research:* Hazardous waste, asbestos, lead exposures, worker training, public employees. *Unit head:* Jack Caravanos, Director, 212-396-7780. *Application contact:* Milena Solo, Director for Graduate Admissions, 212-772-4280, E-mail: admissions@hunter.cuny.edu.
Website: http://cuny.edu/site/sph/hunter-college/a-programs/graduate/eohs/eohs-mph.html

Indiana State University, College of Graduate and Professional Studies, College of Nursing, Health and Human Services, Department of Health, Safety, and Environmental Health Sciences, Terre Haute, IN 47809. Offers community health promotion (MA, MS); health and safety education (MA, MS); occupational safety management (MA, MS). *Accreditation:* NCATE (one or more programs are accredited). *Degree requirements:* For master's, thesis or alternative. *Entrance requirements:* For master's, GRE General Test. Electronic applications accepted.

Indiana University Bloomington, School of Public Health, Department of Environmental Health, Bloomington, IN 47405. Offers MPH, PhD. *Faculty:* 5 full-time (3 women). *Students:* 11 full-time (7 women), 1 (woman) part-time; includes 3 minority (all Black or African American, non-Hispanic/Latino), 2 international. 16 applicants, 81% accepted, 8 enrolled. In 2013, 1 master's awarded. *Degree requirements:* For doctorate, comprehensive exam, thesis/dissertation. *Entrance requirements:* For master's, GRE if cumulative GPA less than 2.8; for doctorate, GRE. Additional exam requirements/recommendations for international students: Required—TOEFL (minimum score 550 paper-based; 80 iBT). *Application deadline:* For fall admission, 2/1 priority date for domestic students, 12/1 priority date for international students. Application fee: $55 ($65 for international students). Electronic applications accepted. *Financial support:* In 2013–14, 10 students received support. Fellowships, research assistantships with partial tuition reimbursements available, teaching assistantships, Federal Work-Study, institutionally sponsored loans, health care benefits, and tuition waivers available. Financial award applicants required to submit FAFSA. *Faculty research:* Toxicology, environmental health, oxidative stress, cancer biology. *Total annual research expenditures:* $577,771. *Unit head:* Dr. Alan Ewert, Chair, 812-856-2448, E-mail: aewert@indiana.edu. *Application contact:* Julie Wilson, Assistant Director of Student Services, 812-856-2448, E-mail: jaw@indiana.edu.
Website: http://www.publichealth.indiana.edu/departments/environmental-health/index.shtml

Indiana University of Pennsylvania, School of Graduate Studies and Research, College of Health and Human Services, Department of Safety Sciences, Program in Safety Sciences, Indiana, PA 15705-1087. Offers MS. Part-time programs available. Postbaccalaureate distance learning degree programs offered (minimal on-campus study). *Faculty:* 6 full-time (1 woman). *Students:* 17 full-time (0 women), 43 part-time (12 women); includes 5 minority (1 Black or African American, non-Hispanic/Latino; 1 Asian, non-Hispanic/Latino; 2 Hispanic/Latino; 1 Two or more races, non-Hispanic/Latino), 3 international. Average age 33. 74 applicants, 35% accepted, 19 enrolled. In 2013, 25 master's awarded. *Degree requirements:* For master's, thesis optional. *Entrance requirements:* For master's, 2 letters of recommendation. Additional exam requirements/recommendations for international students: Required—TOEFL (minimum score 540 paper-based). *Application deadline:* For fall admission, 4/1 priority date for domestic students. Applications are processed on a rolling basis. Application fee: $50. Electronic applications accepted. *Expenses:* Tuition, state resident: full-time $3978; part-time $442 per credit. Tuition, nonresident: full-time $5967; part-time $663 per credit. *Required fees:* $2080; $115.55 per credit. $93 per semester. Tuition and fees vary according to degree level and program. *Financial support:* In 2013–14, 1 fellowship with full tuition reimbursement (averaging $1,250 per year), 7 research assistantships with full and partial tuition reimbursements (averaging $4,669 per year) were awarded; teaching assistantships, career-related internships or fieldwork, Federal Work-Study, scholarships/grants, and unspecified assistantships also available. Financial award application deadline: 4/15; financial award applicants required to submit FAFSA. *Unit head:* Dr. Helmut Paschold, Graduate Coordinator, 724-357-3017, E-mail: helmut.paschold@iup.edu.
Website: http://www.iup.edu/grad/safety/default.aspx

Indiana University–Purdue University Indianapolis, School of Public and Environmental Affairs, Indianapolis, IN 46202. Offers criminal justice and public safety (MS); homeland security and emergency management (Graduate Certificate); library management (Graduate Certificate); nonprofit management (Graduate Certificate); public affairs (MPA); public management (Graduate Certificate); social entrepreneurship: nonprofit and public benefit organizations (Graduate Certificate); JD/MPA; MLS/NMC; MLS/PMC; MPA/MA. *Accreditation:* CAHME (one or more programs are accredited); NASPAA. Part-time and evening/weekend programs available. Postbaccalaureate distance learning degree programs offered (no on-campus study). *Entrance requirements:* For master's, GRE General Test, GMAT or LSAT, minimum GPA of 3.0 (preferred). Additional exam requirements/recommendations for international students: Required—TOEFL (minimum score 93 iBT), IELTS (minimum score 6.5). Electronic applications accepted. *Faculty research:* Nonprofit and public management, public policy, urban policy, sustainability policy, disaster preparedness and recovery, vehicular safety, homicide, offender rehabilitation and re-entry.

Indiana University–Purdue University Indianapolis, School of Public Health, Indianapolis, IN 46202-2896. Offers biostatistics (MPH); environmental health science (MPH); epidemiology (MPH, PhD); health administration (MHA); health policy and management (MPH, PhD); social and behavioral sciences (MPH). *Accreditation:* CEPH. *Students:* 121 full-time (87 women), 161 part-time (111 women); includes 66 minority (32 Black or African American, non-Hispanic/Latino; 19 Asian, non-Hispanic/Latino; 13 Hispanic/Latino; 1 Native Hawaiian or other Pacific Islander, non-Hispanic/Latino; 1 Two or more races, non-Hispanic/Latino), 10 international. Average age 30. 185 applicants, 70% accepted, 95 enrolled. In 2013, 25 master's awarded. Application fee: $55 ($65 for international students). *Expenses:* Contact institution. *Financial support:* In 2013–14, 1 fellowship (averaging $17,650 per year), 4 research assistantships (averaging $22,000 per year), 8 teaching assistantships (averaging $24,000 per year) were awarded. *Unit head:* Dr. Paul Halverson, Dean, 317-274-4242. *Application contact:* Shawne Mathis, Student Services Coordinator, 317-278-0337, E-mail: snmathis@iupui.edu.
Website: http://www.pbhealth.iupui.edu/

Johns Hopkins University, Bloomberg School of Public Health, Department of Environmental Health Sciences, Baltimore, MD 21218-2699. Offers environmental health engineering (PhD); environmental health sciences (MHS, Dr PH); occupational and environmental health (PhD); occupational and environmental hygiene (MHS, MHS); physiology (PhD); toxicology (PhD). Postbaccalaureate distance learning degree programs offered (minimal on-campus study). *Faculty:* 71 full-time (27 women), 58 part-time/adjunct (26 women). *Students:* 67 full-time (42 women), 22 part-time (17 women); includes 30 minority (8 Black or African American, non-Hispanic/Latino; 14 Asian, non-Hispanic/Latino; 5 Hispanic/Latino; 3 Two or more races, non-Hispanic/Latino), 13 international. Average age 29. 112 applicants, 54% accepted, 40 enrolled. In 2013, 23 master's, 11 doctorates awarded. *Degree requirements:* For master's, essay, presentation; for doctorate, comprehensive exam, thesis/dissertation, 1-year full-time residency, oral and written exams. *Entrance requirements:* For master's, GRE General Test or MCAT, 3 letters of recommendation, transcripts; for doctorate, GRE General Test or MCAT, 3 letters of recommendation. Additional exam requirements/recommendations for international students: Required—TOEFL (minimum score 600 paper-based). *Application deadline:* For fall admission, 12/15 priority date for domestic and international students. Applications are processed on a rolling basis. Application fee: $45. Electronic applications accepted. *Financial support:* Fellowships with full tuition reimbursements, Federal Work-Study, institutionally sponsored loans, scholarships/grants, traineeships, health care benefits, and stipends available. Support available to part-time students. Financial award application deadline: 3/15; financial award applicants required to submit FAFSA. *Faculty research:* Chemical carcinogenesis/toxicology, lung disease, occupational and environmental health, nuclear imaging, molecular epidemiology. *Total annual research expenditures:* $23.7 million. *Unit head:* Dr. John Davis Groopman, Chair, 410-955-3720, Fax: 410-955-0617, E-mail: jgroopma@jhsph.edu. *Application contact:* Nina J. Kulacki, Academic Program Manager, 410-955-2212, Fax: 410-955-0617, E-mail: nkulacki@jhsph.edu.
Website: http://www.jhsph.edu/Dept/EHS/

Keene State College, School of Professional and Graduate Studies, Keene, NH 03435. Offers curriculum and instruction (M Ed); education leadership (PMC); educational leadership (M Ed); safety and occupational health applied science (MS); school counselor (M Ed, PMC); special education (M Ed); teacher certification (Postbaccalaureate Certificate). *Accreditation:* NCATE. Part-time and evening/weekend programs available. *Faculty:* 8 full-time (5 women), 12 part-time/adjunct (6 women). *Students:* 39 full-time (33 women), 46 part-time (32 women); includes 8 minority (1 American Indian or Alaska Native, non-Hispanic/Latino; 2 Asian, non-Hispanic/Latino; 5 Hispanic/Latino). Average age 30. 46 applicants, 61% accepted, 13 enrolled. In 2013, 26 master's, 1 other advanced degree awarded. *Entrance requirements:* For master's, PRAXIS I, 3 references; official transcripts; minimum GPA of 2.5; interview. Additional exam requirements/recommendations for international students: Required—TOEFL (minimum score 550 paper-based; 61 iBT). *Application deadline:* For fall admission, 4/1 for domestic students; for spring admission, 12/1 for domestic students. Applications are processed on a rolling basis. Application fee: $50. Electronic applications accepted. *Expenses:* Tuition, state resident: full-time $10,410; part-time $480 per credit. Tuition, nonresident: full-time $17,795; part-time $530 per credit. *Required fees:* $2366; $94 per credit. Full-time tuition and fees vary according to course load. *Financial support:* Career-related internships or fieldwork, Federal Work-Study, institutionally sponsored loans, scholarships/grants, and unspecified assistantships available. Support available to part-time students. Financial award application deadline: 3/1; financial award applicants required to submit FAFSA. *Unit head:* Dr. Wayne Hartz, Interim Dean of Professional and Graduate Studies, 603-358-2220, E-mail: whartz@keene.edu.

Application contact: Peggy Richmond, Director of Admissions, 603-358-2276, Fax: 603-358-2767, E-mail: admissions@keene.edu.
Website: http://www.keene.edu/gradstudies/

Lewis University, College of Arts and Sciences, Program in Public Safety Administration, Romeoville, IL 60446. Offers MS. Part-time and evening/weekend programs available. Postbaccalaureate distance learning degree programs offered (no on-campus study). *Students:* 9 full-time (3 women), 71 part-time (17 women); includes 20 minority (10 Black or African American, non-Hispanic/Latino; 2 Asian, non-Hispanic/Latino; 8 Hispanic/Latino). Average age 36. *Entrance requirements:* For master's, bachelor's degree, 2 letters of recommendation. Additional exam requirements/recommendations for international students: Required—TOEFL (minimum score 500 paper-based; 80 iBT). *Application deadline:* For fall admission, 5/1 priority date for international students; for spring admission, 11/15 priority date for international students. Applications are processed on a rolling basis. Application fee: $40. Electronic applications accepted. *Financial support:* Application deadline: 5/1; applicants required to submit FAFSA. *Unit head:* Dr. Calvin Edwards, Chair of Justice, Law and Public Safety Studies, 815-838-0500, Fax: 815-836-5870, E-mail: koloshsa@lewisu.edu. *Application contact:* Anne Czech, Graduate Admission Counselor, 815-838-0500 Ext. 5027, Fax: 815-836-5578, E-mail: czechan@lewisu.edu.

Loma Linda University, School of Public Health, Programs in Environmental and Occupational Health, Loma Linda, CA 92350. Offers MPH, MSPH. *Accreditation:* CEPH. *Entrance requirements:* Additional exam requirements/recommendations for international students: Required—Michigan English Language Assessment Battery or TOEFL. *Faculty research:* Human exposure to toxins, smog.

Louisiana State University Health Sciences Center, School of Public Health, New Orleans, LA 70112. Offers behavioral and community health sciences (MPH); biostatistics (MPH, MS, PhD); community health sciences (PhD); environmental and occupational health sciences (MPH); epidemiology (MPH, PhD); health policy and systems management (MPH). *Accreditation:* CEPH. Part-time programs available. *Entrance requirements:* For master's, GRE General Test.

Loyola University Chicago, Graduate School, Marcella Niehoff School of Nursing, Population-Based Infection Control and Environmental Safety Program, Chicago, IL 60660. Offers MSN, Certificate. Part-time and evening/weekend programs available. *Faculty:* 45 full-time (44 women). *Students:* 1 (woman) full-time, 7 part-time (all women); includes 1 minority (Black or African American, non-Hispanic/Latino). Average age 38. 1 applicant, 100% accepted. In 2013, 4 master's, 1 other advanced degree awarded. *Degree requirements:* For master's, comprehensive exam. *Entrance requirements:* For master's, Illinois nursing license, 3 letters of recommendation, minimum nursing GPA of 3.0, 1000 hours of experience before starting clinical. Application fee: $50. *Expenses: Tuition:* Full-time $16,740; part-time $930 per credit. *Required fees:* $135 per semester. *Financial support:* Traineeships available. *Unit head:* Dr. Marijo Letizia, Associate Dean, MSN and DNP Programs, 708-216-9325, Fax: 708-216-9555, E-mail: meltizi@luc.edu. *Application contact:* Amy Weatherford, Enrollment Advisor, School of Nursing, 708-216-3751, Fax: 708-216-9555, E-mail: aweatherford@luc.edu.
Website: http://www.luc.edu/nursing/

McGill University, Faculty of Graduate and Postdoctoral Studies, Faculty of Medicine, Department of Epidemiology and Biostatistics, Montréal, QC H3A 2T5, Canada. Offers community health (M Sc); environmental health (M Sc); epidemiology and biostatistics (M Sc, PhD, Diploma); health care evaluation (M Sc); medical statistics (M Sc). *Accreditation:* CEPH (one or more programs are accredited).

McGill University, Faculty of Graduate and Postdoctoral Studies, Faculty of Medicine and Department of Epidemiology and Biostatistics, Department of Occupational Health, Montréal, QC H3A 2T5, Canada. Offers M Sc, PhD.

Meharry Medical College, School of Graduate Studies, Division of Community Health Sciences, Nashville, TN 37208-9989. Offers occupational medicine (MSPH); public health administration (MSPH). *Accreditation:* CEPH. Part-time and evening/weekend programs available. *Degree requirements:* For master's, thesis, externship. *Entrance requirements:* For master's, GRE General Test, GMAT. *Expenses:* Contact institution. *Faculty research:* Policy and management, health care financing, health education and promotion.

Mercer University, Graduate Studies, Cecil B. Day Campus, Penfield College, Macon, GA 31207-0003. Offers clinical mental health (MS); counselor education and supervision (PhD); organizational leadership (MS); public safety leadership (MS); school counseling (MS). *Faculty:* 19 full-time (10 women), 16 part-time/adjunct (12 women). *Students:* 130 full-time (105 women), 233 part-time (188 women); includes 184 minority (159 Black or African American, non-Hispanic/Latino; 11 Asian, non-Hispanic/Latino; 11 Hispanic/Latino; 2 Native Hawaiian or other Pacific Islander, non-Hispanic/Latino; 1 Two or more races, non-Hispanic/Latino), 3 international. Average age 33. In 2013, 80 master's awarded. *Unit head:* Dr. Priscilla R. Danheiser, Dean, 678-547-6028, E-mail: danheiser_p@mercer.edu. *Application contact:* Tracey M. Wofford, Associate Director of Admissions, 678-547-6422, E-mail: wofford_tm@mercer.edu.
Website: http://ccps.mercer.edu/graduate/

Mississippi Valley State University, Department of Natural Science and Environmental Health, Program in Environmental Health, Itta Bena, MS 38941-1400. Offers MS. Evening/weekend programs available.

Murray State University, College of Health Sciences and Human Services, Program in Occupational Safety and Health, Murray, KY 42071. Offers environmental science (MS); industrial hygiene (MS); safety management (MS). *Accreditation:* ABET. Part-time programs available. *Degree requirements:* For master's, comprehensive exam, thesis optional, professional internship. Electronic applications accepted. *Faculty research:* Light effects on plant growth, ergonomics, toxic effects of pets' pesticides, traffic safety.

New York Medical College, School of Health Sciences and Practice, Department of Environmental Health Science, Valhalla, NY 10595-1691. Offers environmental health science (MPH); industrial hygiene (Graduate Certificate). *Accreditation:* CEPH. Part-time and evening/weekend programs available. Postbaccalaureate distance learning degree programs offered (no on-campus study). *Faculty:* 5 full-time, 9 part-time/adjunct. *Students:* 25 full-time, 35 part-time. Average age 32. 35 applicants, 71% accepted, 20 enrolled. In 2013, 15 master's awarded. *Degree requirements:* For master's, thesis, capstone. *Entrance requirements:* For master's, minimum undergraduate GPA of 3.0. Additional exam requirements/recommendations for international students: Required—TOEFL (minimum score 637 paper-based; 110 iBT), IELTS (minimum score 7). *Application deadline:* For fall admission, 8/1 priority date for domestic students, 5/15 for international students; for spring admission, 12/1 priority date for domestic students, 10/15 for international students. Applications are processed on a rolling basis. Application fee: $50 ($100 for international students). Electronic applications accepted. *Expenses: Tuition:* Full-time $49,170; part-time $910 per credit. Tuition and fees vary according to program. *Financial support:* Career-related internships or fieldwork, Federal Work-Study, institutionally sponsored loans, health care benefits, tuition waivers (partial), and tuition reimbursements available. Support available to part-time students. Financial award applicants required to submit FAFSA. *Unit head:* Dr. Diane E. Heck, Chair, 914-594-4804, Fax: 914-594-4292, E-mail: diane_heck@nymc.edu. *Application contact:* Pamela Suett, Director of Recruitment, 914-594-4510, Fax: 914-594-4292, E-mail: shsp_admissions@nymc.edu.
Website: http://www.nymc.edu/shsp

New York University, Graduate School of Arts and Science, Department of Environmental Medicine, New York, NY 10012-1019. Offers environmental health sciences (MS, PhD), including biostatistics (PhD), environmental hygiene (MS), epidemiology (PhD), ergonomics and biomechanics (PhD), exposure assessment and health effects (PhD), molecular toxicology/carcinogenesis (PhD), toxicology. Part-time programs available. *Faculty:* 26 full-time (7 women). *Students:* 55 full-time (34 women), 13 part-time (3 women); includes 16 minority (1 Black or African American, non-Hispanic/Latino; 8 Asian, non-Hispanic/Latino; 6 Hispanic/Latino; 1 Two or more races, non-Hispanic/Latino), 23 international. Average age 31. 69 applicants, 55% accepted, 18 enrolled. In 2013, 14 master's, 7 doctorates awarded. Terminal master's awarded for partial completion of doctoral program. *Degree requirements:* For master's, thesis or alternative; for doctorate, one foreign language, thesis/dissertation, oral and written exams. *Entrance requirements:* For master's and doctorate, GRE General Test, minimum GPA of 3.0; bachelor's degree in biological, physical, or engineering science. Additional exam requirements/recommendations for international students: Required—TOEFL. *Application deadline:* For fall admission, 12/18 for domestic and international students. Application fee: $95. *Expenses: Tuition:* Full-time $35,856; part-time $1494 per unit. *Required fees:* $1408; $64 per unit. $473 per term. Tuition and fees vary according to course load and program. *Financial support:* Fellowships with tuition reimbursements, teaching assistantships with tuition reimbursements, career-related internships or fieldwork, Federal Work-Study, institutionally sponsored loans, and health care benefits available. Financial award application deadline: 12/18; financial award applicants required to submit FAFSA. *Unit head:* Dr. Max Costa, Chair, 845-731-3661, Fax: 845-351-2058, E-mail: ehs@env.med.nyu.edu. *Application contact:* Dr. Jerome J. Solomon, Director of Graduate Studies, 845-731-3661, Fax: 845-351-2058, E-mail: ehs@env.med.nyu.edu.
Website: http://environmental-medicine.med.nyu.edu/

North Carolina Agricultural and Technical State University, School of Graduate Studies, School of Technology, Department of Construction Management and Occupational Safety and Health, Greensboro, NC 27411. Offers construction management (MSTM); environmental and occupational safety (MSTM); occupational safety and health (MSTM).

Northeastern State University, College of Business and Technology, Program in Environmental, Health, and Safety Management, Tahlequah, OK 74464-2399. Offers MEHS. Part-time and evening/weekend programs available. *Faculty:* 4 full-time (1 woman), 1 part-time/adjunct (0 women). *Students:* 15 full-time (1 woman), 11 part-time (5 women); includes 13 minority (1 Black or African American, non-Hispanic/Latino; 9 American Indian or Alaska Native, non-Hispanic/Latino; 1 Asian, non-Hispanic/Latino; 2 Two or more races, non-Hispanic/Latino), 1 international. Average age 34. In 2013, 1 master's awarded. *Degree requirements:* For master's, synergistic experience. *Entrance requirements:* For master's, GRE, MAT, minimum GPA of 2.5. Additional exam requirements/recommendations for international students: Required—TOEFL. *Application deadline:* For fall admission, 6/1 priority date for domestic students. Applications are processed on a rolling basis. Application fee: $25. Electronic applications accepted. *Expenses:* Tuition, state resident: full-time $3029; part-time $168.25 per credit hour. Tuition, nonresident: full-time $7709; part-time $428.25 per credit hour. *Required fees:* $35.90 per credit hour. *Financial support:* Teaching assistantships and Federal Work-Study available. Financial award application deadline: 3/1. *Unit head:* Dr. Michael Turner, Chair, 918-456-5511 Ext. 2970, Fax: 918-458-2337, E-mail: turne003@nsuok.edu. *Application contact:* Margie Railey, Administrative Assistant, 918-456-5511 Ext. 2093, Fax: 918-458-2061, E-mail: railey@nsouk.edu.
Website: http://academics.nsuok.edu/businesstechnology/Graduate/MEHS.aspx

Oakland University, Graduate Study and Lifelong Learning, School of Health Sciences, Program in Safety Management, Rochester, MI 48309-4401. Offers MS. *Faculty:* 1 part-time/adjunct (0 women). *Students:* 19 part-time (8 women); includes 7 minority (4 Black or African American, non-Hispanic/Latino; 1 American Indian or Alaska Native, non-Hispanic/Latino; 2 Hispanic/Latino). Average age 37. 113 applicants, 6% accepted, 6 enrolled. *Application deadline:* For fall admission, 8/1 for domestic students; for winter admission, 12/1 for domestic students; for spring admission, 4/1 for domestic students. Application fee: $35. *Unit head:* Dr. Charles McGlothlin, Director, 248-370-2664, E-mail: mcglothl@oakland.edu. *Application contact:* Christina J. Grabowski, Associate Director of Graduate Study and Lifelong Learning, 248-370-3167, Fax: 248-370-4114, E-mail: grabowsk@oakland.edu.

Old Dominion University, College of Health Sciences, Program in Community Health and Environmental Health, Norfolk, VA 23529. Offers MS. Part-time and evening/weekend programs available. Postbaccalaureate distance learning degree programs offered (no on-campus study). *Faculty:* 5 full-time (2 women), 3 part-time/adjunct (1 woman). *Students:* 3 full-time (1 woman), 15 part-time (8 women); includes 6 minority (3 Black or African American, non-Hispanic/Latino; 1 Asian, non-Hispanic/Latino; 2 Hispanic/Latino), 1 international. Average age 33. 10 applicants, 80% accepted, 7 enrolled. In 2013, 4 master's awarded. *Degree requirements:* For master's, comprehensive exam, oral exam, written exam, practicum or thesis. *Entrance requirements:* For master's, GRE General Test, minimum GPA of 2.75. Additional exam requirements/recommendations for international students: Required—TOEFL (minimum score 650 paper-based). *Application deadline:* For fall admission, 8/1 priority date for domestic students, 7/1 priority date for international students; for winter admission, 11/1 priority date for domestic students, 10/1 priority date for international students; for spring admission, 4/1 priority date for domestic students, 3/1 priority date for international students. Applications are processed on a rolling basis. Application fee: $50. Electronic applications accepted. *Expenses:* Tuition, state resident: full-time $9888; part-time $412 per credit. Tuition, nonresident: full-time $25,152; part-time $1048 per credit. *Required fees:* $59 per semester. One-time fee: $50. *Financial support:* In 2013–14, 5 research assistantships with tuition reimbursements (averaging $14,000 per year), 2 teaching assistantships with partial tuition reimbursements (averaging $10,000 per year) were awarded; career-related internships or fieldwork, institutionally sponsored loans, scholarships/grants, and tuition waivers (partial) also available. Financial award applicants required to submit FAFSA. *Faculty research:* Toxicology, occupational health, environmental hazards. *Total annual research expenditures:* $150,133. *Unit head:* Dr. Anna Jeng, Graduate Program Director, 757-683-4594, Fax: 757-683-4410, E-mail: hjeng@odu.edu. *Application contact:* William Heffelfinger, Director of Graduate Admissions, 757-683-5554, Fax: 757-683-3255, E-mail: gradadmit@odu.edu.
Website: http://hs.odu.edu/commhealth/

Oregon State University, College of Public Health and Human Sciences, Program in Public Health, Corvallis, OR 97331. Offers biostatistics (MPH); environmental and occupational health and safety (MPH, PhD); epidemiology (MPH); health management and policy (MPH); health policy (PhD); health promotion and health behavior (MPH, PhD); international health (MPH). *Accreditation:* CEPH. Part-time programs available. *Faculty:* 29 full-time (16 women), 4 part-time/adjunct (3 women). *Students:* 137 full-time (102 women), 29 part-time (18 women); includes 37 minority (4 Black or African American, non-Hispanic/Latino; 7 Asian, non-Hispanic/Latino; 17 Hispanic/Latino; 9 Two or more races, non-Hispanic/Latino), 15 international. Average age 32. 163 applicants, 58% accepted, 48 enrolled. In 2013, 39 master's, 3 doctorates awarded. Terminal master's awarded for partial completion of doctoral program. *Degree requirements:* For doctorate, one foreign language, thesis/dissertation. *Entrance requirements:* For master's and doctorate, GRE, minimum GPA of 3.0 in last 90 hours. Additional exam requirements/recommendations for international students: Required—TOEFL (minimum score 80 iBT), IELTS (minimum score 6.5). *Application deadline:* For fall admission, 12/1 for domestic students. Applications are processed on a rolling basis. Application fee: $60. *Expenses:* Contact institution. *Financial support:* Fellowships, research assistantships, teaching assistantships, career-related internships or fieldwork, Federal Work-Study, and institutionally sponsored loans available. Support available to part-time students. Financial award application deadline: 2/1. *Faculty research:* Traffic safety, health safety, injury control, health promotion. *Unit head:* Dr. Sheryl Thorburn, Professor/Co-Director, 541-737-9493. *Application contact:* Eileen Kaspar, Public Health Graduate Programs Manager, 541-737-3825, E-mail: eileen.kaspar@oregonstate.edu.

Purdue University, Graduate School, College of Health and Human Sciences, School of Health Sciences, West Lafayette, IN 47907. Offers health physics (MS, PhD); medical physics (MS, PhD); occupational and environmental health science (MS, PhD), including aerosol deposition and lung disease, ergonomics, exposure and risk assessment, indoor air quality and bioaerosols (PhD), liver/lung toxicology; radiation biology (PhD); toxicology (PhD); MS/PhD. Part-time programs available. *Faculty:* 11 full-time (5 women), 28 part-time/adjunct (5 women). *Students:* 28 full-time (8 women), 10 part-time (3 women); includes 6 minority (1 Black or African American, non-Hispanic/Latino; 3 Asian, non-Hispanic/Latino; 1 Hispanic/Latino; 1 Two or more races, non-Hispanic/Latino), 10 international. Average age 28. 77 applicants, 42% accepted, 13 enrolled. In 2013, 6 master's, 6 doctorates awarded. *Degree requirements:* For master's, thesis optional; for doctorate, one foreign language, thesis/dissertation. *Entrance requirements:* For master's and doctorate, GRE General Test, minimum undergraduate GPA of 3.0 or equivalent. Additional exam requirements/recommendations for international students: Required—TOEFL (minimum score 550 paper-based; 77 iBT); Recommended—TWE. *Application deadline:* For fall admission, 5/15 for domestic and international students; for spring admission, 10/15 for domestic and international students. Applications are processed on a rolling basis. Application fee: $60 ($75 for international students). Electronic applications accepted. *Financial support:* In 2013–14, fellowships with tuition reimbursements (averaging $14,400 per year), research assistantships with tuition reimbursements (averaging $12,000 per year), teaching assistantships with tuition reimbursements (averaging $12,000 per year) were awarded; career-related internships or fieldwork and traineeships also available. Support available to part-time students. Financial award applicants required to submit FAFSA. *Faculty research:* Environmental toxicology, industrial hygiene, radiation dosimetry. *Unit head:* Dr. Wei Zheng, Head, 765-494-1419, E-mail: wz18@purdue.edu. *Application contact:* Jennifer S. Franklin, Graduate Contact, 765-494-0248, E-mail: jfranklin@purdue.edu.
Website: http://www.healthsciences.purdue.edu/

Rochester Institute of Technology, Graduate Enrollment Services, College of Applied Science and Technology, School of Engineering Technology, Department of Civil Engineering Technology, Environmental Management and Safety, Program in Environmental Health and Safety Management, Rochester, NY 14623-5603. Offers MS. Part-time programs available. Postbaccalaureate distance learning degree programs offered (no on-campus study). *Students:* 24 full-time (10 women), 22 part-time (6 women); includes 7 minority (2 Black or African American, non-Hispanic/Latino; 1 Asian, non-Hispanic/Latino; 4 Hispanic/Latino), 10 international. Average age 31. 66 applicants, 30% accepted, 13 enrolled. In 2013, 36 master's awarded. *Degree requirements:* For master's, thesis or project. *Entrance requirements:* Additional exam requirements/recommendations for international students: Required—TOEFL (minimum score 550 paper-based; 79 iBT) or IELTS (minimum score 6). *Application deadline:* Applications are processed on a rolling basis. Application fee: $60. Electronic applications accepted. *Expenses: Tuition:* Full-time $37,236; part-time $1552 per credit hour. *Required fees:* $250. *Faculty research:* Design, implementation and effectiveness of integrated environmental health and safety management systems in industry. *Unit head:* Joseph Rosenbeck, Graduate Program Director, 585-475-6469, E-mail: jmrcem@rit.edu. *Application contact:* Diane Ellison, Assistant Vice President, Graduate Enrollment Services, 585-475-2229, Fax: 585-475-7164, E-mail: gradinfo@rit.edu.
Website: http://www.rit.edu/cast/cetems/ms-in-environmental-health-and-safety-management.php

Rutgers, The State University of New Jersey, New Brunswick, School of Public Health, Piscataway, NJ 08854. Offers biostatistics (MPH, MS, Dr PH, PhD); clinical epidemiology (Certificate); environmental and occupational health (MPH, Dr PH, PhD, Certificate); epidemiology (MPH, Dr PH, PhD); general public health (Certificate); health education and behavioral science (MPH, Dr PH, PhD); health systems and policy (MPH, PhD); public health preparedness (Certificate); DO/MPH; JD/MPH; MD/MPH; MPH/MBA; MPH/MSPA; MS/MPH; Psy D/MPH. *Accreditation:* CEPH. Part-time and evening/weekend programs available. *Degree requirements:* For master's, thesis, internship; for doctorate, comprehensive exam, thesis/dissertation. *Entrance requirements:* For master's, GRE General Test; for doctorate, GRE General Test, MPH (Dr PH); MA, MPH, or MS (PhD). Additional exam requirements/recommendations for international students: Required—TOEFL. Electronic applications accepted.

Saint Joseph's University, College of Arts and Sciences, Programs in Environmental Protection and Safety Management, Philadelphia, PA 19131-1395. Offers environmental protection and safety management (MS, Post-Master's Certificate). Part-time and evening/weekend programs available. *Faculty:* 9 part-time/adjunct (2 women). *Students:* 1 full-time (0 women), 15 part-time (2 women); includes 4 minority (all Black or African American, non-Hispanic/Latino). Average age 38. 10 applicants, 80% accepted, 3 enrolled. In 2013, 8 master's awarded. *Entrance requirements:* For master's, GRE (if GPA less than 2.75), minimum GPA of 2.75, 2 letters of recommendation, resume. Additional exam requirements/recommendations for international students: Required—TOEFL (minimum score 550 paper-based; 80 iBT). *Application deadline:* For fall admission, 7/15 priority date for domestic students, 4/15 for international students; for winter admission, 1/15 for international students; for spring admission, 11/15 priority date for domestic students, 10/15 for international students. Applications are processed on a rolling basis. Application fee: $35. Electronic applications accepted. *Expenses: Tuition:* Part-time $786 per credit hour. Tuition and fees vary according to degree level and program. *Financial support:* Applicants required to submit FAFSA. *Unit head:* Cheralynn Ewing, Director, Graduate Criminal Justice and Public Safety Institute, 610-660-3131, E-mail: gradstudies@sju.edu. *Application contact:* Elisabeth Woodward, Director of Marketing and Admissions, Graduate Arts and Sciences, 610-660-3131, Fax: 610-660-3230, E-mail: gradstudies@sju.edu.
Website: http://sju.edu/majors-programs/graduate-arts-sciences/masters/environmental-protection-and-safety-management-ms

Saint Joseph's University, College of Arts and Sciences, Programs in Public Safety and Management, Philadelphia, PA 19131-1395. Offers homeland security (MS, Certificate); public safety management (MS, Certificate). Part-time and evening/weekend programs available. Postbaccalaureate distance learning degree programs offered. *Faculty:* 9 part-time/adjunct (2 women). *Students:* 1 (woman) full-time, 27 part-time (2 women); includes 6 minority (5 Black or African American, non-Hispanic/Latino; 1 Two or more races, non-Hispanic/Latino). Average age 36. 4 applicants, 100% accepted, 2 enrolled. In 2013, 19 master's awarded. *Entrance requirements:* For master's, GRE (if GPA less than 3.0), 2 letters of recommendation, resume, personal statement, official transcripts. Additional exam requirements/recommendations for international students: Required—TOEFL (minimum score 550 paper-based; 80 iBT). *Application deadline:* For fall admission, 7/15 priority date for domestic students, 4/15 for international students; for winter admission, 1/15 for international students; for spring admission, 11/15 priority date for domestic students, 10/15 for international students. Applications are processed on a rolling basis. Application fee: $35. Electronic applications accepted. *Expenses: Tuition:* Part-time $786 per credit hour. Tuition and fees vary according to degree level and program. *Financial support:* Applicants required to submit FAFSA. *Unit head:* Cheralynn Ewing, Associate Dean and Executive Director, Graduate Arts and Sciences, 610-660-3131, E-mail: cewing@sju.edu. *Application contact:* Elisabeth Woodward, Director of Marketing and Admissions, Graduate Arts and Sciences, 610-660-3131, Fax: 610-660-3230, E-mail: gradstudies@sju.edu.
Website: http://www.sju.edu/majors-programs/graduate-arts-sciences/masters/public-safety-management

Saint Mary's University of Minnesota, Schools of Graduate and Professional Programs, Graduate School of Business and Technology, Public Safety Administration Program, Winona, MN 55987-1399. Offers MA. *Unit head:* Matthew Nowakowski, Dean, 612-728-5142, E-mail: mnowakow@smumn.edu. *Application contact:* Russell Kreager, Director of Admissions for Graduate and Professional Programs, 612-728-5207, Fax: 612-728-5121, E-mail: rkreager@smumn.edu.
Website: http://www.smumn.edu/graduate-home/areas-of-study/graduate-school-of-business-technology/ma-in-public-safety-administration

San Diego State University, Graduate and Research Affairs, College of Health and Human Services, Graduate School of Public Health, San Diego, CA 92182. Offers environmental health (MPH); epidemiology (MPH, PhD), including biostatistics (MPH); global emergency preparedness and response (MS); global health (PhD); health behavior (PhD); health promotion (MPH); health services administration (MPH); toxicology (MS); MPH/MA; MSW/MPH. *Accreditation:* CAHME (one or more programs are accredited); CEPH (one or more programs are accredited). Part-time programs available. *Degree requirements:* For master's, comprehensive exam (for some programs), thesis (for some programs); for doctorate, thesis/dissertation. *Entrance requirements:* For master's, GMAT (MPH in health services administration), GRE General Test; for doctorate, GRE General Test. Additional exam requirements/recommendations for international students: Required—TOEFL. *Faculty research:* Evaluation of tobacco, AIDS prevalence and prevention, mammography, infant death project, Alzheimer's in elderly Chinese.

Southeastern Oklahoma State University, School of Arts and Sciences, Durant, OK 74701-0609. Offers biology (MT); computer information systems (MT); occupational safety and health (MT). Part-time and evening/weekend programs available. *Degree requirements:* For master's, thesis optional. *Entrance requirements:* For master's, minimum GPA of 3.0 in last 60 hours or 2.75 overall. Additional exam requirements/recommendations for international students: Required—TOEFL (minimum score 550 paper-based; 79 iBT). Electronic applications accepted.

Temple University, College of Health Professions and Social Work, Department of Public Health, Philadelphia, PA 19122. Offers clinical research and translational medicine (MS); environmental health (MPH); epidemiology (MS); epidemiology and biostatistics (MPH); health policy (PhD); health policy and management (MPH); school health education (Ed M); social and behavioral sciences (MPH, PhD). *Accreditation:* CEPH (one or more programs are accredited). Part-time and evening/weekend programs available. *Faculty:* 27 full-time (18 women). *Students:* 47 full-time (30 women), 45 part-time (37 women); includes 27 minority (9 Black or African American, non-Hispanic/Latino; 10 Asian, non-Hispanic/Latino; 7 Hispanic/Latino; 1 Two or more races, non-Hispanic/Latino), 9 international. 188 applicants, 45% accepted, 29 enrolled. In 2013, 29 master's, 3 doctorates awarded. Terminal master's awarded for partial completion of doctoral program. *Degree requirements:* For master's, thesis (for some programs), capstone project; for doctorate, comprehensive exam, thesis/dissertation. *Entrance requirements:* For master's, GRE General Test (for MS only); DAT, GMAT, MCAT, OAT, PCAT (alternates for MPH, Ed M), minimum undergraduate GPA of 3.0, letters of reference, statement of goals, writing sample, resume, interview (only for MS); for doctorate, GRE General Test, minimum undergraduate GPA of 3.0, 3 letters of reference, statement of goals, writing sample, resume. Additional exam requirements/recommendations for international students: Required—TOEFL (minimum score 550 paper-based; 79 iBT). *Application deadline:* For fall admission, 3/1 for domestic students, 2/1 for international students; for spring admission, 10/15 for domestic students, 8/1 for international students. Applications are processed on a rolling basis. Application fee: $60. Electronic applications accepted. *Financial support:* In 2013–14, 1 fellowship with tuition reimbursement, 4 research assistantships with tuition reimbursements, 8 teaching assistantships with tuition reimbursements were awarded; career-related internships or fieldwork, Federal Work-Study, scholarships/grants, tuition waivers (partial), and unspecified assistantships also available. Financial award application deadline: 1/15. *Faculty research:* Smoking cessation, obesity prevention, tobacco policy, community engagement, health communication. *Total annual research expenditures:* $3.9 million. *Unit head:* Dr. Alice J. Hausman, Chair, 215-204-5112, Fax: 215-204-1854, E-mail: hausman@temple.edu. *Application contact:* Joyce Hankins, 215-204-7213, E-mail: joyce.hankins@temple.edu.
Website: http://chpsw.temple.edu/publichealth/home

Texas A&M Health Science Center, School of Rural Public Health, College Station, TX 77840. Offers environmental/occupational health (MPH); epidemiology/biostatistics (MPH); health policy/management (MPH); social and behavioral health (MPH). *Accreditation:* CEPH. Part-time programs available. Postbaccalaureate distance learning degree programs offered (no on-campus study). *Degree requirements:* For master's, thesis optional. *Entrance requirements:* For master's, GRE General Test, minimum undergraduate GPA of 3.0. Electronic applications accepted. *Faculty research:* Tobacco cessation, youth health risk.

Towson University, Program in Occupational Science, Towson, MD 21252-0001. Offers Sc D. Part-time and evening/weekend programs available. *Students:* 8 full-time (7 women), 6 part-time (2 women); includes 4 minority (2 Black or African American, non-Hispanic/Latino; 1 Asian, non-Hispanic/Latino; 1 Two or more races, non-Hispanic/Latino), 2 international. *Degree requirements:* For doctorate, thesis/dissertation. *Entrance requirements:* For doctorate, master's degree with minimum GPA of 3.25, interview, 3 letters of recommendation, letter of intent. Additional exam requirements/recommendations for international students: Required—TOEFL (minimum score 600 paper-based). *Application deadline:* For fall admission, 8/15 for domestic and international students; for winter admission, 11/15 for domestic and international students; for spring admission, 1/15 for domestic and international students. Applications are processed on a rolling basis. Application fee: $45. Electronic applications accepted. *Financial support:* Application deadline: 4/1. *Unit head:* Dr. Beth Merryman, Graduate Program Director, 410-704-2762, E-mail: bmerryman@

towson.edu. *Application contact:* Alicia Arkell-Kleis, Information Contact, 410-704-6004, E-mail: grads@towson.edu.
Website: http://grad.towson.edu/program/doctoral/osc-scd/

Trident University International, College of Health Sciences, Program in Health Sciences, Cypress, CA 90630. Offers clinical research administration (MS, Certificate); emergency and disaster management (MS, Certificate); environmental health science (Certificate); health care administration (PhD); health care management (MS), including health informatics; health education (MS, Certificate); health informatics (Certificate); health sciences (PhD); international health (MS); international health: educator or researcher option (PhD); international health: practitioner option (PhD); law and expert witness studies (MS, Certificate); public health (MS); quality assurance (Certificate). Part-time and evening/weekend programs available. Postbaccalaureate distance learning degree programs offered (no on-campus study). *Degree requirements:* For doctorate, comprehensive exam, thesis/dissertation, defense of dissertation. *Entrance requirements:* For master's, minimum GPA of 2.5 (students with GPA 3.0 or greater may transfer up to 30% of graduate level credits); for doctorate, minimum GPA of 3.4, curriculum vitae, course work in research methods or statistics. Additional exam requirements/recommendations for international students: Required—TOEFL. Electronic applications accepted.

Tufts University, Cummings School of Veterinary Medicine, Program in Conservation Medicine, Medford, MA 02155. Offers MS. *Degree requirements:* For master's, case study, preceptorship. *Entrance requirements:* For master's, GRE, official transcripts, curriculum vitae. Additional exam requirements/recommendations for international students: Required—TOEFL or IELTS. Electronic applications accepted. *Faculty research:* Non-invasive saliva collection techniques for free-ranging mountain gorillas and captive eastern gorillas, animal sentinels for infectious diseases.

Tufts University, School of Engineering, Department of Civil and Environmental Engineering, Medford, MA 02155. Offers bioengineering (ME, MS), including environmental technology; civil engineering (ME, MS, PhD), including geotechnical engineering, structural engineering, water diplomacy (PhD); environmental engineering (ME, MS, PhD), including environmental engineering and environmental sciences, environmental geotechnology, environmental health, environmental science and management, hazardous materials management, water diplomacy (PhD), water resources engineering. Part-time programs available. *Faculty:* 18 full-time, 5 part-time/adjunct. *Students:* 84 full-time (39 women); includes 5 minority (1 Asian, non-Hispanic/Latino; 2 Hispanic/Latino; 2 Two or more races, non-Hispanic/Latino), 24 international. Average age 27. 179 applicants, 51% accepted, 26 enrolled. In 2013, 25 master's, 7 doctorates awarded. Terminal master's awarded for partial completion of doctoral program. *Degree requirements:* For master's, thesis or alternative; for doctorate, thesis/dissertation. *Entrance requirements:* For master's and doctorate, GRE General Test. Additional exam requirements/recommendations for international students: Required—TOEFL (minimum score 550 paper-based; 80 iBT), IELTS (minimum score 6.5). *Application deadline:* For fall admission, 1/15 priority date for domestic students, 1/15 for international students; for spring admission, 9/15 for domestic and international students. Applications are processed on a rolling basis. Application fee: $75. Electronic applications accepted. *Financial support:* Fellowships with full tuition reimbursements, research assistantships with full and partial tuition reimbursements, teaching assistantships with full and partial tuition reimbursements, Federal Work-Study, scholarships/grants, tuition waivers (partial), and unspecified assistantships available. Financial award application deadline: 5/15; financial award applicants required to submit FAFSA. *Faculty research:* Environmental and water resources engineering, environmental health, geotechnical and geoenvironmental engineering, structural engineering and mechanics, water diplomacy. *Unit head:* Dr. Kurt Pennell, Chair, 617-627-3211, Fax: 617-627-3994. *Application contact:* Laura Sacco, Information Contact, 617-627-3211, E-mail: ceeinfo@tufts.edu.
Website: http://www.ase.tufts.edu/cee/

Tulane University, School of Public Health and Tropical Medicine, Department of Environmental Health Sciences, New Orleans, LA 70118-5669. Offers MPH, MSPH, Dr PH, PhD, JD/MSPH. *Accreditation:* ABET (one or more programs are accredited); CEPH (one or more programs are accredited). *Degree requirements:* For doctorate, comprehensive exam, thesis/dissertation. *Entrance requirements:* For master's and doctorate, GRE General Test. Additional exam requirements/recommendations for international students: Required—TOEFL. Electronic applications accepted.

Uniformed Services University of the Health Sciences, School of Medicine, Graduate Programs in the Biomedical Sciences and Public Health, Bethesda, MD 20814. Offers emerging infectious diseases (PhD); medical and clinical psychology (PhD), including clinical psychology, medical psychology; molecular and cell biology (MS, PhD); neuroscience (PhD); preventive medicine and biometrics (MPH, MS, MSPH, MTMH, Dr PH, PhD), including environmental health sciences (PhD), healthcare administration and policy (MS), medical zoology (PhD), public health (MPH, MSPH, Dr PH), tropical medicine and hygiene (MTMH). *Faculty:* 372 full-time (119 women), 4,044 part-time/adjunct (908 women). *Students:* 240 full-time (133 women); includes 40 minority (15 Black or African American, non-Hispanic/Latino; 13 Asian, non-Hispanic/Latino; 12 Hispanic/Latino), 30 international. Average age 25. 598 applicants, 17% accepted, 77 enrolled. In 2013, 19 master's, 50 doctorates awarded. Terminal master's awarded for partial completion of doctoral program. *Degree requirements:* For master's, comprehensive exam, thesis or alternative; for doctorate, comprehensive exam, thesis/dissertation, qualifying exam. *Entrance requirements:* For master's, GRE General Test; for doctorate, GRE General Test, minimum GPA of 3.0. Additional exam requirements/recommendations for international students: Required—TOEFL. *Application deadline:* For fall admission, 1/1 priority date for domestic and international students. Applications are processed on a rolling basis. Application fee: $0. Electronic applications accepted. *Financial support:* In 2013–14, fellowships with full tuition reimbursements (averaging $27,000 per year), research assistantships with full tuition reimbursements (averaging $27,000 per year) were awarded; career-related internships or fieldwork, scholarships/grants, health care benefits, and tuition waivers (full) also available. *Unit head:* Dr. Eleanor S. Metcalf, Associate Dean, 301-295-1104, E-mail: emetcalf@usuhs.edu. *Application contact:* Tina Finley, Administrative Officer, 301-295-3642, Fax: 301-295-6772, E-mail: netina.finley@usuhs.edu.
Website: http://www.usuhs.mil/graded

Uniformed Services University of the Health Sciences, School of Medicine, Graduate Programs in the Biomedical Sciences and Public Health, Department of Preventive Medicine and Biometrics, Program in Environmental Health Sciences, Bethesda, MD 20814-4799. Offers PhD. *Accreditation:* CEPH. *Degree requirements:* For doctorate, comprehensive exam, thesis/dissertation, qualifying exam. *Entrance requirements:* For doctorate, GRE, minimum GPA of 3.0. Additional exam requirements/recommendations for international students: Required—TOEFL. *Application deadline:* For fall admission, 1/1 priority date for domestic students. Applications are processed on a rolling basis. Application fee: $0. *Financial support:* Fellowships with full tuition reimbursements and tuition waivers (full) available. *Unit head:* Dr. David Cruess, Director, 301-295-3465, Fax: 301-295-1933, E-mail: dcruess@usuhs.edu. *Application contact:* Elena Marina Sherman, Program Administrative Specialist, 301-295-3913, Fax: 301-295-6772, E-mail: elena.sherman@usuhs.edu.

Universidad Autonoma de Guadalajara, Graduate Programs, Guadalajara, Mexico. Offers administrative law and justice (LL M); advertising and corporate communications (MA); architecture (M Arch); business (MBA); computational science (MCC); education (Ed M, Ed D); English-Spanish translation (MA); entrepreneurship and management (MBA); integrated management of digital animation (MA); international business (MIB); international corporate law (LL M); internet technologies (MS); manufacturing systems (MMS); occupational health (MS); philosophy (MA, PhD); power electronics (MS); quality systems (MQS); renewable energy (MS); social evaluation of projects (MBA); strategic market research (MBA); tax law (MA); teaching mathematics (MA).

Universidad de Ciencias Medicas, Graduate Programs, San Jose, Costa Rica. Offers dermatology (SP); family health (MS); health service center administration (MHA); human anatomy (MS); medical and surgery (MD); occupational medicine (MS); pharmacy (Pharm D). Part-time programs available. *Degree requirements:* For master's, thesis; for doctorate and SP, comprehensive exam. *Entrance requirements:* For master's, MD or bachelor's degree; for doctorate, admissions test; for SP, admissions test, MD.

Université de Montréal, Faculty of Medicine, Department of Environmental and Occupational Health, Montréal, QC H3C 3J7, Canada. Offers M Sc. *Accreditation:* CEPH. *Degree requirements:* For master's, thesis. *Entrance requirements:* For master's, proficiency in French, knowledge of English. Electronic applications accepted. *Faculty research:* Metabolism of chemical substances, toxicity, biological surveillance, risk analysis.

Université du Québec à Montréal, Graduate Programs, Program in Ergonomics in Occupational Health and Safety, Montréal, QC H3C 3P8, Canada. Offers Diploma. Part-time programs available. *Entrance requirements:* For degree, appropriate bachelor's degree or equivalent, proficiency in French.

Université Laval, Faculty of Medicine, Graduate Programs in Medicine, Department of Social and Preventive Medicine, Program in Accident Prevention and Occupational Health and Safety Management, Québec, QC G1K 7P4, Canada. Offers Diploma. Part-time programs available. *Entrance requirements:* For degree, knowledge of French. Electronic applications accepted.

University at Albany, State University of New York, School of Public Health, Department of Environmental Health Sciences, Albany, NY 12222-0001. Offers environmental and analytical chemistry (MS, PhD); environmental and occupational health (MS, PhD); toxicology (MS, PhD). *Degree requirements:* For master's, thesis; for doctorate, comprehensive exam, thesis/dissertation. *Entrance requirements:* For master's and doctorate, GRE General Test, GRE Subject Test, 3 letters of reference. Additional exam requirements/recommendations for international students: Required—TOEFL (minimum score 600 paper-based). Electronic applications accepted. *Faculty research:* Xenobiotic metabolism, neurotoxicity of halogenated hydrocarbons, pharmac/toxicogenomics, environmental analytical chemistry.

The University of Alabama at Birmingham, School of Public Health, Program in Environmental Health Sciences, Birmingham, AL 35294. Offers environmental health sciences research (PhD); industrial hygiene (PhD). *Degree requirements:* For doctorate, comprehensive exam, thesis/dissertation. *Entrance requirements:* For doctorate, GRE General Test, evaluation forms. Additional exam requirements/recommendations for international students: Recommended—TOEFL, IELTS. Electronic applications accepted. *Faculty research:* Aquatic toxicology, virology.

The University of Alabama at Birmingham, School of Public Health, Program in Public Health, Birmingham, AL 35294. Offers accelerated industrial hygiene (MPH); applied epidemiology (MSPH); biostatistics (MPH); clinical and translational science (MSPH); environmental health (MPH); environmental health and toxicology (MSPH); epidemiology (MPH); general theory and practice (MPH); health behavior (MPH); health care organization (MPH); health policy quantitative policy analysis (MPH); industrial hygiene (MPH, MSPH); maternal and child health policy (Dr PH); maternal and child health policy and leadership (MPH); occupational health and safety (MPH); outcomes research (MSPH, Dr PH); pharmacoepidemiology and comparative effectiveness research (MSPH); public health (PhD); public health management (Dr PH); public health preparedness management (MPH). *Accreditation:* CEPH. *Entrance requirements:* For master's and doctorate, GRE, evaluations. Additional exam requirements/recommendations for international students: Recommended—TOEFL (minimum score 550 paper-based; 79 iBT), IELTS (minimum score 6.5).

University of Alberta, School of Public Health, Department of Public Health Sciences, Edmonton, AB T6G 2E1, Canada. Offers clinical epidemiology (M Sc, MPH); environmental and occupational health (MPH); environmental health sciences (M Sc); epidemiology (M Sc); global health (M Sc, MPH); health policy and management (MPH); health policy research (M Sc); health technology assessment (MPH); occupational health (M Sc); population health (M Sc); public health leadership (MPH); public health sciences (PhD); quantitative methods (MPH). *Accreditation:* CEPH (one or more programs are accredited). Terminal master's awarded for partial completion of doctoral program. *Degree requirements:* For master's, thesis (for some programs); for doctorate, thesis/dissertation. *Entrance requirements:* For master's, GMAT or GRE General Test. Additional exam requirements/recommendations for international students: Required—TOEFL (minimum score 550 paper-based) or IELTS (minimum score 6). Electronic applications accepted. *Faculty research:* Biostatistics, health promotion and socio-behavioral health science.

University of Arkansas for Medical Sciences, College of Public Health, Little Rock, AR 72205-7199. Offers biostatistics (MPH); environmental and occupational health (MPH, Certificate); epidemiology (MPH, PhD); health behavior and health education (MPH); health policy and management (MPH); health promotion and prevention research (PhD); health services administration (MHSA); health systems research (PhD); public health (Certificate); public health leadership (Dr PH). Part-time programs available. *Faculty:* 37 full-time (19 women), 9 part-time/adjunct (5 women). *Students:* 56 full-time (35 women), 85 part-time (58 women); includes 54 minority (38 Black or African American, non-Hispanic/Latino; 1 American Indian or Alaska Native, non-Hispanic/Latino; 8 Asian, non-Hispanic/Latino; 3 Hispanic/Latino; 1 Native Hawaiian or other Pacific Islander, non-Hispanic/Latino; 3 Two or more races, non-Hispanic/Latino), 5 international. Average age 30. 70 applicants, 91% accepted, 33 enrolled. In 2013, 2 master's, 1 doctorate, 2 other advanced degrees awarded. *Degree requirements:* For master's, preceptorship, culminating experience, internship; for doctorate, comprehensive exam, capstone. *Entrance requirements:* For master's, GRE, GMAT, LSAT, PCAT, MCAT, DAT; for doctorate, GRE. Additional exam requirements/recommendations for international students: Required—TOEFL (minimum score 80 iBT), IELTS. *Application deadline:* For fall admission, 3/1 for domestic students, 2/1 for international students; for spring admission, 8/1 for domestic and international students; for summer admission, 2/1 for domestic and international students. Application fee: $25 ($50 for international students). Electronic applications accepted. *Expenses:* Contact institution. *Financial support:* In 2013–14, 8 research assistantships with full tuition reimbursements (averaging $13,000 per year) were awarded; scholarships/grants and tuition waivers (full and partial) also available. *Faculty research:* Health systems, tobacco prevention control, obesity prevention, environmental and occupational exposure, cancer prevention. *Unit head:* Dr. James M. Raczynski, Dean, 501-526-6600,

E-mail: raczynskijameson@uams.edu. *Application contact:* Angie Choi, Director of Admission, 501-526-4620, Fax: 501-526-6750, E-mail: anchoi@uams.edu.
Website: http://publichealth.uams.edu/

The University of British Columbia, School of Environmental Health, Vancouver, BC V6T 1Z1, Canada. Offers M Sc, PhD. Part-time programs available. *Degree requirements:* For master's, comprehensive exam (for some programs), thesis optional; for doctorate, comprehensive exam, thesis/dissertation. *Entrance requirements:* For master's and doctorate, GRE. Additional exam requirements/recommendations for international students: Required—TOEFL (minimum score 600 paper-based; 100 iBT); Recommended—TWE. Electronic applications accepted. *Expenses: Tuition, area resident:* Full-time $8000 Canadian dollars. *Faculty research:* Acoustics, exposure assessment and epidemiology, occupational and environmental respiratory disease, occupational and environmental policy.

University of California, Berkeley, Graduate Division, School of Public Health, Group in Environmental Health Sciences, Berkeley, CA 94720-1500. Offers MPH, MS, Dr PH, PhD. *Degree requirements:* For master's, comprehensive exam (MPH), project or thesis (MS); for doctorate, thesis/dissertation, departmental and qualifying exams. *Entrance requirements:* For master's, GRE General Test, minimum GPA of 3.0; previous course work in biology, calculus, and chemistry; 3 letters of recommendation; for doctorate, GRE General Test, master's degree in relevant scientific discipline or engineering; minimum GPA of 3.0; previous course work in biology, calculus, and chemistry; 3 letters of recommendation. Additional exam requirements/recommendations for international students: Required—TOEFL. *Faculty research:* Toxicology, industrial hygiene, exposure assessment, risk assessment, ergonomics.

University of California, Los Angeles, Graduate Division, School of Public Health, Department of Environmental Health Sciences, Los Angeles, CA 90095. Offers environmental health sciences (MS, PhD); environmental science and engineering (D Env); molecular toxicology (PhD); JD/MPH. *Accreditation:* ABET (one or more programs are accredited). *Degree requirements:* For master's, comprehensive exam or thesis; for doctorate, thesis/dissertation, oral and written qualifying exams. *Entrance requirements:* For master's, GRE General Test, minimum GPA of 3.0; for doctorate, GRE General Test, minimum undergraduate GPA of 3.0. Electronic applications accepted.

University of Central Missouri, The Graduate School, Warrensburg, MO 6409. Offers accountancy (MA); accounting (MBA); applied mathematics (MS); aviation safety (MA); biology (MS); business administration (MBA); career and technical education leadership (MS); college student personnel administration (MS); communication (MA); computer science (MS); counseling (MS); criminal justice (MS); educational leadership (Ed D); educational technology (MS); elementary and early childhood education (MSE); English (MA); environmental studies (MA); finance (MBA); history (MA); human services/educational technology (Ed S); human services/learning resources (Ed S); human services/professional counseling (Ed S); industrial hygiene (MS); industrial management (MS); information systems (MBA); information technology (MS); kinesiology (MS); library science and information services (MS); literacy education (MSE); marketing (MBA); mathematics (MS); music (MA); occupational safety management (MS); psychology (MS); rural family nursing (MS); school administration (MSE); social gerontology (MS); sociology (MA); special education (MSE); speech language pathology (MS); superintendency (Ed S); teaching (MAT); teaching English as a second language (MA); technology (MS); technology management (PhD); theatre (MA). Part-time programs available. *Faculty:* 233. *Students:* 890 full-time (396 women), 1,486 part-time (1,001 women); includes 192 minority (97 Black or African American, non-Hispanic/Latino; 9 American Indian or Alaska Native, non-Hispanic/Latino; 32 Asian, non-Hispanic/Latino; 40 Hispanic/Latino; 3 Native Hawaiian or other Pacific Islander, non-Hispanic/Latino; 11 Two or more races, non-Hispanic/Latino), 539 international. Average age 31. 1,953 applicants, 75% accepted. In 2013, 719 master's, 58 other advanced degrees awarded. *Degree requirements:* For master's and Ed S, comprehensive exam (for some programs), thesis (for some programs). *Entrance requirements:* Additional exam requirements/recommendations for international students: Required—TOEFL (minimum score 550 paper-based; 79 iBT). *Application deadline:* For fall admission, 6/1 for domestic students; for spring admission, 10/1 for domestic and international students. Applications are processed on a rolling basis. Application fee: $30 ($75 for international students). Electronic applications accepted. *Expenses:* Tuition, state resident: full-time $7326; part-time $276.25 per credit hour. Tuition, nonresident: full-time $13,956; part-time $552.50 per credit hour. *Required fees:* $29 per credit hour. *Financial support:* In 2013–14, 118 students received support, including 271 research assistantships with full and partial tuition reimbursements available (averaging $7,500 per year), 109 teaching assistantships with full and partial tuition reimbursements available (averaging $7,500 per year); career-related internships or fieldwork, Federal Work-Study, scholarships/grants, and administrative and laboratory assistantships also available. Support available to part-time students. Financial award application deadline: 3/1; financial award applicants required to submit FAFSA. *Unit head:* Dr. Joseph Vaughn, Assistant Provost for Research/Dean, 660-543-4092, Fax: 660-543-4778, E-mail: vaughn@ucmo.edu. *Application contact:* Brittany Lawrence, Graduate Student Services Coordinator, 660-543-4621, Fax: 660-543-4778, E-mail: gradinfo@ucmo.edu.
Website: http://www.ucmo.edu/graduate/

University of Cincinnati, Graduate School, College of Medicine, Graduate Programs in Biomedical Sciences, Department of Environmental Health, Cincinnati, OH 45221. Offers environmental and industrial hygiene (MS, PhD); environmental and occupational medicine (MS); environmental genetics and molecular toxicology (MS, PhD); epidemiology and biostatistics (MS, PhD); occupational safety and ergonomics (MS, PhD). *Accreditation:* ABET (one or more programs are accredited). Terminal master's awarded for partial completion of doctoral program. *Degree requirements:* For master's, thesis; for doctorate, thesis/dissertation, qualifying exam. *Entrance requirements:* For master's, GRE General Test, bachelor's degree in science; for doctorate, GRE General Test. Additional exam requirements/recommendations for international students: Required—TOEFL (minimum score 600 paper-based; 100 iBT). Electronic applications accepted. *Faculty research:* Carcinogens and mutagenesis, pulmonary studies, reproduction and development.

University of Colorado Denver, College of Liberal Arts and Sciences, Department of Geography and Environmental Sciences, Denver, CO 80217. Offers environmental sciences (MS), including air quality, ecosystems, environmental health, environmental science education, geo-spatial analysis, hazardous waste, water quality. Part-time and evening/weekend programs available. *Faculty:* 12 full-time (4 women), 6 part-time/adjunct (1 woman). *Students:* 35 full-time (26 women), 3 part-time (2 women); includes 7 minority (1 Asian, non-Hispanic/Latino; 5 Hispanic/Latino; 1 Two or more races, non-Hispanic/Latino), 7 international. Average age 29. 34 applicants, 74% accepted, 15 enrolled. In 2013, 16 master's awarded. *Degree requirements:* For master's, thesis or alternative, 30 credits including 21 of core requirements and 9 of environmental science electives. *Entrance requirements:* For master's, GRE General Test, BA in one of the natural/physical sciences or engineering (or equivalent background); prerequisite coursework in calculus and physics (one semester each), general chemistry with lab and general biology with lab (two semesters each), three letters of recommendation. Additional exam requirements/recommendations for international students: Required—TOEFL (minimum score 537 paper-based; 75 iBT); Recommended—IELTS (minimum score 6.5). *Application deadline:* For fall admission, 4/1 for domestic and international students; for spring admission, 10/1 for domestic and international students. Application fee: $50 ($75 for international students). Electronic applications accepted. *Financial support:* In 2013–14, 7 students received support. Fellowships, research assistantships, teaching assistantships, Federal Work-Study, institutionally sponsored loans, scholarships/grants, and traineeships available. Financial award application deadline: 4/1; financial award applicants required to submit FAFSA. *Faculty research:* Air quality, environmental health, ecosystems, hazardous waste, water quality, geo-spatial analysis and environmental science education. *Unit head:* Dr. Frederick Chambers, Director of MS in Environmental Sciences Program, 303-556-2619, Fax: 303-556-6197, E-mail: frederick.chambers@ucdenver.edu. *Application contact:* Sue Eddleman, Program Assistant, 303-556-2276, E-mail: sue.eddleman@ucdenver.edu.
Website: http://www.ucdenver.edu/academics/colleges/CLAS/Departments/ges/Programs/MasterofScience/Pages/MasterofScience.aspx

University of Colorado Denver, Colorado School of Public Health, Program in Public Health, Aurora, CO 80045. Offers community and behavioral health (MPH, Dr PH); environmental and occupational health (MPH); epidemiology (MPH); health systems, management and policy (MPH). *Accreditation:* CEPH. Part-time and evening/weekend programs available. *Faculty:* 14 full-time (13 women). *Students:* 295 full-time (247 women), 49 part-time (39 women); includes 77 minority (17 Black or African American, non-Hispanic/Latino; 3 American Indian or Alaska Native, non-Hispanic/Latino; 16 Asian, non-Hispanic/Latino; 31 Hispanic/Latino; 10 Two or more races, non-Hispanic/Latino), 5 international. Average age 30. 657 applicants, 71% accepted, 132 enrolled. In 2013, 106 master's awarded. *Degree requirements:* For master's, thesis or alternative, 42 credit hours; for doctorate, comprehensive exam, thesis/dissertation, 67 credit hours. *Entrance requirements:* For master's, GRE, MCAT, DAT, LSAT, PCAT, GMAT or master's degree from accredited institution, baccalaureate degree or equivalent; minimum GPA of 3.0; transcripts; references; resume; essay; for doctorate, GRE, MCAT, DAT, LSAT, PCAT or GMAT, MPH or master's or higher degree in related field or equivalent; 2 years of previous work experience in public health; essay; resume. Additional exam requirements/recommendations for international students: Required—TOEFL (minimum score 550 paper-based; 80 iBT). *Application deadline:* For fall admission, 12/15 priority date for domestic students, 12/1 priority date for international students. Application fee: $65. Electronic applications accepted. *Expenses:* Contact institution. *Financial support:* In 2013–14, 125 students received support. Fellowships, research assistantships, teaching assistantships, Federal Work-Study, institutionally sponsored loans, scholarships/grants, traineeships, and unspecified assistantships available. Financial award application deadline: 3/15; financial award applicants required to submit FAFSA. *Faculty research:* Cancer prevention by nutrition, cancer survivorship outcomes, social and cultural factors related to health. *Unit head:* Dr. Lori Crane, Chair, 303-724-4385, E-mail: lori.crane@ucdenver.edu. *Application contact:* Carla Denerstein, Departmental Assistant, 303-724-4446, E-mail: carla.denerstein@ucdenver.edu.
Website: http://www.ucdenver.edu/academics/colleges/PublicHealth/departments/CommunityBehavioralHealth/Pages/CommunityBehavioralHealth.aspx

University of Connecticut, Graduate School, Center for Continuing Studies, Program in Occupational Safety and Health Management, Storrs, CT 06269. Offers MPS.

University of Denver, University College, Denver, CO 80208. Offers arts and culture (MLS, Certificate), including art, literature, and culture, arts development and program management (Certificate), creative writing; environmental policy and management (MAS, Certificate), including energy and sustainability (Certificate), environmental assessment of nuclear power (Certificate), environmental health and safety (Certificate), environmental management, natural resource management (Certificate); geographic information systems (MAS, Certificate); global affairs (MLS, Certificate), including translation studies, world history and culture; healthcare leadership (MPH, Certificate), including healthcare policy, law, and ethics, medical and healthcare information technologies, strategic management of healthcare; information and communications technology (MCIS, Certificate), including database design and administration (Certificate), geographic information systems (MCIS), information security systems security (Certificate), information systems security (MCIS), project management (MCIS, MPS, Certificate), software design and administration (Certificate), software design and programming (MCIS), technology management, telecommunications technology (MCIS), Web design and development; leadership and organizations (MPS, Certificate), including human capital in organizations, philanthropic leadership, project management (MCIS, MPS, Certificate), strategic innovation and change; organizational and professional communication (MPS, Certificate), including alternative dispute resolution, organizational communication, organizational development and training, public relations and marketing; security management (MAS, Certificate), including emergency planning and response, information security (MAS), organizational security; strategic human resource management (MPS, Certificate), including global human resources (MPS), human resource management and development (MPS). Part-time and evening/weekend programs available. Postbaccalaureate distance learning degree programs offered (no on-campus study). *Faculty:* 139 part-time/adjunct (61 women). *Students:* 49 full-time (16 women), 1,297 part-time (732 women); includes 272 minority (92 Black or African American, non-Hispanic/Latino; 5 American Indian or Alaska Native, non-Hispanic/Latino; 30 Asian, non-Hispanic/Latino; 114 Hispanic/Latino; 3 Native Hawaiian or other Pacific Islander, non-Hispanic/Latino; 28 Two or more races, non-Hispanic/Latino), 92 international. Average age 35. 542 applicants, 95% accepted, 362 enrolled. In 2013, 374 master's, 128 other advanced degrees awarded. *Degree requirements:* For master's, capstone project. *Entrance requirements:* For master's, transcripts, two letters of recommendation, personal statement, resume. Additional exam requirements/recommendations for international students: Required—TOEFL (minimum score 550 paper-based; 80 iBT). *Application deadline:* For fall admission, 7/18 priority date for domestic students, 5/2 priority date for international students; for winter admission, 10/24 priority date for domestic students, 9/19 priority date for international students; for spring admission, 2/1 for domestic students, 12/14 for international students; for summer admission, 4/18 priority date for domestic students, 3/7 priority date for international students. Applications are processed on a rolling basis. Application fee: $75. Electronic applications accepted. *Expenses:* Contact institution. *Financial support:* In 2013–14, 28 students received support. Applicants required to submit FAFSA. *Unit head:* Dr. Michael McGuire, Interim Dean, 303-871-3518, E-mail: mmcguire@du.edu. *Application contact:* Information Contact, 303-871-2291, E-mail: ucoladm@du.edu.
Website: http://www.universitycollege.du.edu/

University of Florida, Graduate School, College of Public Health and Health Professions, Department of Environmental and Global Health, Gainesville, FL 32610. Offers one health (MHS). *Faculty:* 13 full-time (5 women), 5 part-time/adjunct (1 woman). *Students:* 5 full-time (4 women), 2 part-time (1 woman); includes 2 minority (both Black or African American, non-Hispanic/Latino), 1 international. Average age 32. 10 applicants, 40% accepted, 1 enrolled. *Entrance requirements:* For master's, GRE, minimum GPA of 3.0. Additional exam requirements/recommendations for international students: Required—TOEFL (minimum score 550 paper-based; 80 iBT), IELTS (minimum score 6). *Application deadline:* For fall admission, 1/1 for domestic students. Application fee: $30. *Expenses:* Tuition, state resident: full-time $12,640. Tuition, nonresident: full-time $30,000. *Financial support:* Applicants required to submit FAFSA.

Unit head: Dr. Gregory C. Gray, MD, Chair, 352-273-9449, E-mail: gcgray@phhp.ufl.edu. *Application contact:* Office of Admissions, 352-392-1365, E-mail: webrequests@admissions.ufl.edu.
Website: http://egh.phhp.ufl.edu/

University of Florida, Graduate School, College of Public Health and Health Professions, Programs in Public Health, Gainesville, FL 32611. Offers biostatistics (MPH); environmental and global health (PhD); environmental health (MPH); epidemiology (MPH); one health (PhD); public health (MPH, PhD, Certificate); public health management and policy (MPH); public health practice (MPH); social and behavioral sciences (MPH); DPT/MPH; DVM/MPH; JD/MPH; MD/MPH; Pharm D/MPH. *Accreditation:* CEPH. Postbaccalaureate distance learning degree programs offered. *Students:* 152 full-time (115 women), 63 part-time (36 women); includes 70 minority (26 Black or African American, non-Hispanic/Latino; 3 American Indian or Alaska Native, non-Hispanic/Latino; 21 Asian, non-Hispanic/Latino; 20 Hispanic/Latino), 18 international. Average age 30. 380 applicants, 41% accepted, 63 enrolled. In 2013, 85 master's, 1 doctorate awarded. *Degree requirements:* For master's, internship. *Entrance requirements:* For master's, GRE General Test, minimum GPA of 3.0. Additional exam requirements/recommendations for international students: Required—TOEFL (minimum score 550 paper-based; 80 iBT), IELTS (minimum score 6). *Application deadline:* For fall admission, 7/1 for domestic students, 4/1 for international students. Application fee: $30. *Expenses:* Tuition, state resident: full-time $12,640. Tuition, nonresident: full-time $30,000. *Financial support:* In 2013–14, 29 students received support, including 2 fellowships (averaging $17,022 per year), 8 research assistantships (averaging $16,662 per year), 19 teaching assistantships (averaging $12,380 per year). Financial award applicants required to submit FAFSA. *Unit head:* Sarah L. McKune, PhD, Program Director, 352-328-0615, Fax: 352-273-6448, E-mail: smckune@ufl.edu. *Application contact:* Telisha Martin, PhD, Associate Director, MPH Program, 352-273-6444, E-mail: martints@ufl.edu.
Website: http://www.mph.ufl.edu/

University of Georgia, College of Public Health, Department of Environmental Health Science, Athens, GA 30602. Offers MPH, MSEH. *Accreditation:* CEPH. Terminal master's awarded for partial completion of doctoral program. *Degree requirements:* For master's, thesis. *Entrance requirements:* For master's, GRE General Test. Additional exam requirements/recommendations for international students: Required—TOEFL. Electronic applications accepted. *Faculty research:* Risk assessment, environmental toxicology, water quality, air quality.

University of Illinois at Chicago, Graduate College, School of Public Health, Division of Environmental and Occupational Health Sciences, Chicago, IL 60607-7128. Offers MPH, MS, Dr PH, PhD. *Accreditation:* ABET (one or more programs are accredited); CEPH (one or more programs are accredited). Part-time programs available. *Faculty:* 11 full-time (7 women), 12 part-time/adjunct (6 women). *Students:* 55 full-time (39 women), 9 part-time (6 women); includes 30 minority (9 Black or African American, non-Hispanic/Latino; 15 Asian, non-Hispanic/Latino; 4 Hispanic/Latino; 1 Native Hawaiian or other Pacific Islander, non-Hispanic/Latino; 1 Two or more races, non-Hispanic/Latino), 11 international. Average age 30. 72 applicants, 79% accepted, 23 enrolled. In 2013, 17 master's, 2 doctorates awarded. Terminal master's awarded for partial completion of doctoral program. *Degree requirements:* For master's, thesis, field practicum; for doctorate, thesis/dissertation, independent research, internship. *Entrance requirements:* For master's and doctorate, GRE General Test, minimum GPA of 2.75. Additional exam requirements/recommendations for international students: Required—TOEFL. *Application deadline:* For fall admission, 2/1 for domestic students, 1/1 priority date for international students. Application fee: $40 ($50 for international students). Electronic applications accepted. *Expenses:* Tuition, state resident: full-time $11,066; part-time $3689 per term. Tuition, nonresident: full-time $23,064; part-time $7688 per term. *Required fees:* $3004; $1190 per term. Tuition and fees vary according to course level and program. *Financial support:* Fellowships with full tuition reimbursements, research assistantships with full tuition reimbursements, teaching assistantships with full tuition reimbursements, career-related internships or fieldwork, Federal Work-Study, institutionally sponsored loans, scholarships/grants, traineeships, and unspecified assistantships available. Support available to part-time students. Financial award application deadline: 3/1; financial award applicants required to submit FAFSA. *Faculty research:* Workers compensation, injury and illness surveillance, and disparities in occupational health; emergency/disaster management and continuity planning; water quality; air pollution; environmental chemistry; industrial hygiene; occupational medicine; hazardous substances management; toxicology; occupational safety, environmental epidemiology, and policy. *Total annual research expenditures:* $3.6 million. *Unit head:* Prof. Linda Forst, Director, 312-355-3826, E-mail: forst-l@uic.edu.
Website: http://publichealth.uic.edu/departments/environmentalandoccupationalhealthsciences/

The University of Iowa, Graduate College, College of Public Health, Department of Occupational and Environmental Health, Iowa City, IA 52242-1316. Offers agricultural safety and health (MS, PhD); ergonomics (MPH); industrial hygiene (MS, PhD); occupational and environmental health (MPH, MS, PhD, Certificate); MS/MA; MS/MS. *Accreditation:* ABET (one or more programs are accredited); CEPH. *Degree requirements:* For master's, thesis optional, exam; for doctorate, comprehensive exam, thesis/dissertation. *Entrance requirements:* For master's and doctorate, GRE General Test, minimum GPA of 3.0. Additional exam requirements/recommendations for international students: Required—TOEFL (minimum score 600 paper-based; 100 iBT). Electronic applications accepted.

The University of Kansas, University of Kansas Medical Center, School of Medicine, Department of Preventive Medicine and Public Health, Kansas City, KS 66160. Offers clinical research (MS); environmental health sciences (MPH); epidemiology (MPH); public health management (MPH); social and behavioral health (MPH); MD/MPH; PhD/MPH. Part-time programs available. *Faculty:* 69. *Students:* 30 full-time (23 women), 60 part-time (41 women); includes 27 minority (6 Black or African American, non-Hispanic/Latino; 2 American Indian or Alaska Native, non-Hispanic/Latino; 11 Asian, non-Hispanic/Latino; 3 Hispanic/Latino; 5 Two or more races, non-Hispanic/Latino), 7 international. Average age 34. 62 applicants, 52% accepted, 24 enrolled. In 2013, 37 master's awarded. *Degree requirements:* For master's, thesis, capstone practicum defense. *Entrance requirements:* For master's, GRE, MCAT, LSAT, GMAT or other equivalent graduate professional exam. Additional exam requirements/recommendations for international students: Required—TOEFL. *Application deadline:* For fall admission, 3/1 for domestic and international students. Applications are processed on a rolling basis. Application fee: $60. Electronic applications accepted. *Financial support:* Research assistantships, career-related internships or fieldwork, Federal Work-Study, scholarships/grants, and unspecified assistantships available. Financial award application deadline: 3/1; financial award applicants required to submit FAFSA. *Faculty research:* Cancer screening and prevention, smoking cessation, obesity and physical activity, health services/outcomes research, health disparities. *Total annual research expenditures:* $6.9 million. *Unit head:* Dr. Edward F. Ellerbeck, Chairman, 913-588-2774, Fax: 913-588-2780, E-mail: eellerbe@kumc.edu. *Application contact:* Tanya Honderick, MPH Director, 913-588-2720, Fax: 913-588-8505, E-mail: thonderick@kumc.edu.
Website: http://www.kumc.edu/school-of-medicine/preventive-medicine-and-public-health.html

University of Louisville, Graduate School, School of Public Health and Information Sciences, Department of Environmental and Occupational Health Sciences, Louisville, KY 40202. Offers environmental and occupational health sciences (MPH); public health (PhD), including environmental health. *Accreditation:* CEPH. *Degree requirements:* For master's, thesis optional; for doctorate, comprehensive exam, thesis/dissertation. *Entrance requirements:* For master's and doctorate, GRE General Test. Additional exam requirements/recommendations for international students: Required—TOEFL (minimum score 600 paper-based; 100 iBT). *Application deadline:* For fall admission, 5/1 for domestic and international students. Application fee: $60. Electronic applications accepted. *Expenses:* Tuition, state resident: full-time $10,788; part-time $599 per credit hour. Tuition, nonresident: full-time $22,446; part-time $1247 per credit hour. *Required fees:* $196. Tuition and fees vary according to program and reciprocity agreements. *Financial support:* Research assistantships with full tuition reimbursements, health care benefits, and unspecified assistantships available. Financial award applicants required to submit FAFSA. *Faculty research:* Breast cancer in minority populations, health policy, clinical trials, chronic disease, genetic epidemiology, program evaluation, electronic medical records, children's environmental health, lung injury. *Unit head:* Dr. David J. Tollerud, Department Chair, 502-852-3290, Fax: 502-852-3291, E-mail: david.tollerud@louisville.edu.
Website: http://louisville.edu/sphis/departments/environmental-occupational-health-sciences

University of Maryland, College Park, Academic Affairs, School of Public Health, Maryland Institute for Applied Environmental Health, College Park, MD 20742. Offers environmental health sciences (MPH). *Faculty:* 9 full-time (5 women), 7 part-time/adjunct (4 women). *Students:* 9 full-time (6 women), 9 part-time (8 women); includes 10 minority (6 Black or African American, non-Hispanic/Latino; 1 Asian, non-Hispanic/Latino; 2 Hispanic/Latino; 1 Two or more races, non-Hispanic/Latino), 1 international. 43 applicants, 51% accepted, 9 enrolled. In 2013, 7 master's awarded. *Entrance requirements:* For master's, GRE General Test, 3 letters of recommendation, minimum undergraduate GPA of 3.0, undergraduate transcripts, statement of goals and interests. *Application deadline:* For fall admission, 5/1 for domestic and international students. Applications are processed on a rolling basis. Application fee: $75. Electronic applications accepted. *Expenses:* Tuition, state resident: full-time $10,314; part-time $573 per credit hour. Tuition, nonresident: full-time $22,248; part-time $1236 per credit. *Required fees:* $1446; $403.15 per semester. Tuition and fees vary according to program. *Financial support:* In 2013–14, 4 teaching assistantships (averaging $16,448 per year) were awarded. Financial award applicants required to submit FAFSA. *Total annual research expenditures:* $2.5 million. *Unit head:* Donald Milton, Director, 301-405-0389, E-mail: dmilton@umd.edu. *Application contact:* Dr. Charles A. Caramello, Dean of Graduate School, 301-405-0358, Fax: 301-314-9305, E-mail: ccaramel@umd.edu.
Website: http://sph.umd.edu/miaeh/

University of Massachusetts Amherst, Graduate School, School of Public Health and Health Sciences, Department of Public Health, Amherst, MA 01003. Offers biostatistics (MPH, MS, PhD); community health education (MPH, MS, PhD); environmental health sciences (MPH, MS, PhD); epidemiology (MPH, MS, PhD); health policy and management (MPH, MS, PhD); nutrition (MPH, PhD); public health practice (MPH); MPH/MPPA. *Accreditation:* CEPH (one or more programs are accredited). Part-time and evening/weekend programs available. Postbaccalaureate distance learning degree programs offered (no on-campus study). *Faculty:* 53 full-time (29 women). *Students:* 117 full-time (83 women), 271 part-time (213 women); includes 89 minority (34 Black or African American, non-Hispanic/Latino; 23 Asian, non-Hispanic/Latino; 25 Hispanic/Latino; 7 Two or more races, non-Hispanic/Latino), 45 international. Average age 36. 359 applicants, 69% accepted, 94 enrolled. In 2013, 120 master's, 1 doctorate awarded. Terminal master's awarded for partial completion of doctoral program. *Degree requirements:* For master's, thesis (for some programs); for doctorate, comprehensive exam, thesis/dissertation. *Entrance requirements:* For master's and doctorate, GRE General Test. Additional exam requirements/recommendations for international students: Required—TOEFL (minimum score 550 paper-based; 80 iBT), IELTS (minimum score 6.5). *Application deadline:* For fall admission, 2/1 for domestic and international students. Applications are processed on a rolling basis. Application fee: $75. Electronic applications accepted. *Financial support:* Fellowships with full and partial tuition reimbursements, research assistantships with full and partial tuition reimbursements, teaching assistantships with full and partial tuition reimbursements, career-related internships or fieldwork, Federal Work-Study, scholarships/grants, traineeships, health care benefits, tuition waivers (full and partial), and unspecified assistantships available. Support available to part-time students. Financial award application deadline: 2/1; financial award applicants required to submit FAFSA. *Unit head:* Dr. Paula Stamps, Graduate Program Director, 413-545-2861, Fax: 413-545-1645. *Application contact:* Lindsay DeSantis, Supervisor of Admissions, 413-545-0722, Fax: 413-577-0010, E-mail: gradadm@grad.umass.edu.
Website: http://www.umass.edu/sphhs/public_health/

University of Memphis, Graduate School, School of Public Health, Memphis, TN 38152. Offers biostatistics (MPH); environmental health (MPH); epidemiology (MPH); health systems management (MPH); public health (MHA); social and behavioral sciences (MPH). Part-time and evening/weekend programs available. Postbaccalaureate distance learning degree programs offered. *Faculty:* 14 full-time (2 women), 5 part-time/adjunct (1 woman). *Students:* 64 full-time (42 women), 36 part-time (24 women); includes 34 minority (21 Black or African American, non-Hispanic/Latino; 6 Asian, non-Hispanic/Latino; 5 Hispanic/Latino; 2 Two or more races, non-Hispanic/Latino), 15 international. Average age 32. 102 applicants, 51% accepted, 24 enrolled. In 2013, 17 master's awarded. *Degree requirements:* For master's, comprehensive exam, thesis. *Entrance requirements:* For master's, GRE, letters of recommendation. Additional exam requirements/recommendations for international students: Required—TOEFL. *Application deadline:* For fall admission, 4/1 for domestic students; for spring admission, 11/1 for domestic students. Application fee: $35 ($60 for international students). Electronic applications accepted. *Financial support:* In 2013–14, 46 students received support. Research assistantships with full tuition reimbursements available, Federal Work-Study, scholarships/grants, and unspecified assistantships available. Financial award application deadline: 2/15; financial award applicants required to submit FAFSA. *Faculty research:* Health and medical savings accounts, adoption rates, health informatics, Telehealth technologies, biostatistics, environmental health, epidemiology, health systems management, social and behavioral sciences. *Unit head:* Dr. Lisa M. Klesges, Director, 901-678-4637, E-mail: lmklsges@memphis.edu. *Application contact:* Dr. Karen Weddle-West, Information Contact, 901-678-2531, Fax: 901-678-5023, E-mail: gradsch@memphis.edu.
Website: http://www.memphis.edu/sph/

University of Miami, Graduate School, College of Engineering, Department of Industrial Engineering, Program in Occupational Ergonomics and Safety, Coral Gables, FL 33124. Offers environmental health and safety (MS); occupational ergonomics and safety (MSOES). Part-time programs available. *Degree requirements:* For master's, thesis optional. *Entrance requirements:* For master's, GRE General Test, minimum GPA of 3.0. Additional exam requirements/recommendations for international students: Required—TOEFL (minimum score 550 paper-based). Electronic applications accepted. *Faculty research:* Noise, heat stress, water pollution.

University of Michigan, School of Public Health, Department of Environmental Health Sciences, Ann Arbor, MI 48109. Offers environmental health sciences (MS, PhD); environmental quality and health (MPH); human nutrition (MPH); industrial hygiene (MPH, MS); nutritional sciences (MS); occupational and environmental epidemiology (MPH); toxicology (MPH, MS, PhD). *Accreditation:* CEPH (one or more programs are accredited). Part-time programs available. Terminal master's awarded for partial completion of doctoral program. *Degree requirements:* For master's, thesis (for some programs); for doctorate, thesis/dissertation, preliminary exam, oral defense of dissertation. *Entrance requirements:* For master's and doctorate, GRE General Test and/or MCAT. Additional exam requirements/recommendations for international students: Required—TOEFL (minimum score 560 paper-based; 100 iBT). Electronic applications accepted. Tuition and fees vary according to course level, course load, degree level, program and student level. *Faculty research:* Toxicology, occupational hygiene, nutrition, environmental exposure sciences, environmental epidemiology.

University of Minnesota, Twin Cities Campus, School of Public Health, Division of Environmental Health Sciences, Area in Environmental Health Policy, Minneapolis, MN 55455-0213. Offers MPH, MS, PhD. *Accreditation:* CEPH (one or more programs are accredited). *Degree requirements:* For doctorate, thesis/dissertation. *Entrance requirements:* For master's and doctorate, GRE General Test. Electronic applications accepted.

University of Minnesota, Twin Cities Campus, School of Public Health, Division of Environmental Health Sciences, Area in Occupational Medicine, Minneapolis, MN 55455-0213. Offers MPH. *Accreditation:* CEPH. *Entrance requirements:* For master's, GRE General Test. Electronic applications accepted.

University of Minnesota, Twin Cities Campus, School of Public Health, Major in Public Health Practice, Minneapolis, MN 55455-0213. Offers core concepts (Certificate); food safety and biosecurity (Certificate); occupational health and safety (Certificate); preparedness, response and recovery (Certificate); public health practice (MPH); DVM/MPH; MD/MPH. Part-time programs available. Postbaccalaureate distance learning degree programs offered (no on-campus study). *Degree requirements:* For master's, thesis. *Entrance requirements:* For master's, GRE, MCAT, United States Medical Licensing Exam. Additional exam requirements/recommendations for international students: Required—TOEFL (minimum score 600 paper-based). Electronic applications accepted.

University of Nebraska Medical Center, Program in Environmental, Agricultural and Occupational Health, Omaha, NE 68198-4388. Offers MS, PhD. Terminal master's awarded for partial completion of doctoral program. *Degree requirements:* For master's, comprehensive exam (for some programs), thesis; for doctorate, comprehensive exam (for some programs), thesis/dissertation. *Entrance requirements:* For master's, GRE General Test, bachelor's degree in chemistry, biology, biochemistry or related area; for doctorate, GRE General Test, BS in chemistry, biology, biochemistry or related area. Additional exam requirements/recommendations for international students: Required—TOEFL (minimum score 550 paper-based). Electronic applications accepted. *Expenses: Required fees:* $300 per semester. Tuition and fees vary according to program. *Faculty research:* Mechanisms of carcinogenesis, alcohol and metal toxicity, DNA damage, human molecular genetics, agrochemicals in soil and water.

University of Nevada, Reno, Graduate School, Interdisciplinary Program in Environmental Sciences and Health, Reno, NV 89557. Offers MS, PhD. Terminal master's awarded for partial completion of doctoral program. *Degree requirements:* For master's, thesis; for doctorate, thesis/dissertation. *Entrance requirements:* For master's, GRE General Test, minimum GPA of 2.75; for doctorate, GRE General Test, minimum GPA of 3.0. Additional exam requirements/recommendations for international students: Required—TOEFL (minimum score 500 paper-based; 61 iBT), IELTS (minimum score 6). Electronic applications accepted. *Faculty research:* Environmental chemistry, environmental toxicology, ecological toxicology.

University of New Haven, Graduate School, College of Arts and Sciences, Program in Environmental Sciences, West Haven, CT 06516-1916. Offers environmental ecology (MS); environmental geoscience (MS); environmental health and management (MS); environmental science (MS); environmental science education (MS); geographical information systems (MS, Certificate). Part-time and evening/weekend programs available. *Students:* 25 full-time (12 women), 20 part-time (11 women); includes 8 minority (3 Black or African American, non-Hispanic/Latino; 2 Asian, non-Hispanic/Latino; 3 Hispanic/Latino), 8 international. 42 applicants, 90% accepted, 14 enrolled. In 2013, 11 master's, 3 other advanced degrees awarded. *Degree requirements:* For master's, thesis optional, research project. *Entrance requirements:* Additional exam requirements/recommendations for international students: Required—TOEFL (minimum score 80 iBT), IELTS, PTE (minimum score 53). *Application deadline:* For fall admission, 5/31 for international students; for winter admission, 10/15 for international students; for spring admission, 1/15 for international students. Applications are processed on a rolling basis. Application fee: $75. Electronic applications accepted. Application fee is waived when completed online. *Expenses: Tuition:* Full-time $21,600; part-time $800 per credit hour. *Required fees:* $45 per trimester. *Financial support:* Research assistantships with partial tuition reimbursements, teaching assistantships with partial tuition reimbursements, career-related internships or fieldwork, Federal Work-Study, scholarships/grants, and unspecified assistantships available. Support available to part-time students. Financial award applicants required to submit FAFSA. *Faculty research:* Mapping and assessing geological and living resources in Long Island Sound, geology, San Salvador Island, Bahamas. *Unit head:* Dr. Roman Zajac, Coordinator, 203-932-7114, E-mail: rzajac@newhaven.edu. *Application contact:* Eloise Gormley, Director of Graduate Admissions, 203-932-7440, E-mail: gradinfo@newhaven.edu.
Website: http://www.newhaven.edu/4728/

University of North Alabama, Office of Professional and Interdisciplinary Studies, Florence, AL 35632-0001. Offers community development (MPS); information technology (MPS); security and safety leadership (MPS). Part-time and evening/weekend programs available. *Students:* 9 full-time (4 women), 24 part-time (10 women); includes 9 minority (8 Black or African American, non-Hispanic/Latino; 1 Hispanic/Latino), 1 international. Average age 36. 28 applicants, 79% accepted, 17 enrolled. *Degree requirements:* For master's, comprehensive exam (for some programs), thesis optional. *Entrance requirements:* For master's, ETS PPI, baccalaureate degree from accredited institution; minimum cumulative GPA of 2.75 or 3.0 in last 60 hours of undergraduate study; personal statement. Additional exam requirements/recommendations for international students: Required—TOEFL (minimum score 550 paper-based; 79 iBT), IELTS (minimum score 6). *Application deadline:* For fall admission, 7/1 for domestic and international students; for spring admission, 12/1 for domestic and international students. Applications are processed on a rolling basis. Application fee: $25 ($50 for international students). Electronic applications accepted. *Expenses:* Tuition, state resident: full-time $4968; part-time $3312 per year. Tuition, nonresident: full-time $9936; part-time $6624 per year. *Required fees:* $970; $60.33 per credit. $362 per semester. *Financial support:* Applicants required to submit FAFSA. *Unit head:* Dr. Craig T. Robertson, Director, 256-765-5003, E-mail: ctrobertson@una.edu. *Application contact:* Russ Durracott, Graduate Admissions Counselor, 256-765-4447, E-mail: erdarracott@una.edu.
Website: http://www.una.edu/masters-professional-studies/index.html

The University of North Carolina at Chapel Hill, Graduate School, Gillings School of Global Public Health, Department of Environmental Sciences and Engineering, Chapel Hill, NC 27599. Offers air, radiation and industrial hygiene (MPH, MS, MSEE, MSPH, PhD); aquatic and atmospheric sciences (MPH, MS, MSPH, PhD); environmental engineering (MPH, MS, MSEE, MSPH, PhD); environmental health sciences (MPH, MS, MSPH, PhD); environmental management and policy (MPH, MS, MSPH, PhD). Terminal master's awarded for partial completion of doctoral program. *Degree requirements:* For master's, comprehensive exam, thesis (for some programs), research paper; for doctorate, comprehensive exam, thesis/dissertation. *Entrance requirements:* For master's and doctorate, GRE General Test, minimum GPA of 3.0 (recommended). Additional exam requirements/recommendations for international students: Required—TOEFL. Electronic applications accepted. *Faculty research:* Air, radiation and industrial hygiene, aquatic and atmospheric sciences, environmental health sciences, environmental management and policy, water resources engineering.

University of North Texas Health Science Center at Fort Worth, School of Public Health, Fort Worth, TX 76107-2699. Offers biostatistics (MPH); community health (MPH); disease control and prevention (Dr PH); environmental and occupational health sciences (MPH); epidemiology (MPH); health administration (MHA); health policy and management (MPH, Dr PH); DO/MPH; MS/MPH; MSN/MPH. MPH offered jointly with University of North Texas; DO/MPH with Texas College of Osteopathic Medicine. *Accreditation:* CEPH. Part-time and evening/weekend programs available. *Degree requirements:* For master's, thesis or alternative, supervised internship; for doctorate, thesis/dissertation, supervised internship. *Entrance requirements:* For master's, GRE General Test. Additional exam requirements/recommendations for international students: Required—TOEFL. Electronic applications accepted.

University of Oklahoma Health Sciences Center, Graduate College, College of Public Health, Department of Occupational and Environmental Health, Oklahoma City, OK 73190. Offers MPH, MS, Dr PH, PhD, JD/MPH, JD/MS. JD/MPH, JD/MS offered jointly with University of Oklahoma. *Accreditation:* ABET (one or more programs are accredited); CEPH (one or more programs are accredited). Part-time programs available. *Faculty:* 4 full-time (1 woman). *Students:* 13 full-time (6 women), 13 part-time (7 women); includes 10 minority (3 Black or African American, non-Hispanic/Latino; 2 American Indian or Alaska Native, non-Hispanic/Latino; 2 Asian, non-Hispanic/Latino; 3 Two or more races, non-Hispanic/Latino). Average age 30. 6 applicants, 50% accepted, 3 enrolled. In 2013, 7 master's awarded. *Degree requirements:* For master's, comprehensive exam, thesis (for some programs); for doctorate, comprehensive exam, thesis/dissertation. *Entrance requirements:* For master's, GRE General Test (for all except occupational medicine), 3 letters of recommendation, resume; for doctorate, GRE (for all except occupational medicine), 3 letters of recommendation, resume. Additional exam requirements/recommendations for international students: Required—TOEFL (minimum score 570 paper-based). *Application deadline:* For fall admission, 7/1 for domestic students; for winter admission, 4/1 for domestic students; for spring admission, 12/1 for domestic students. Applications are processed on a rolling basis. Application fee: $50. *Expenses:* Tuition, state resident: full-time $3504; part-time $175.20 per credit hour. Tuition, nonresident: full-time $13,504; part-time $675.20 per credit hour. *Required fees:* $1545; $52.70 per credit hour. $245.25 per semester. Tuition and fees vary according to course load. *Financial support:* In 2013–14, 6 research assistantships (averaging $15,000 per year) were awarded; career-related internships or fieldwork, institutionally sponsored loans, traineeships, and tuition waivers (partial) also available. Support available to part-time students. Financial award application deadline: 5/1. *Faculty research:* Environmental safety, accident prevention and injury control. *Unit head:* Dr. Margaret Phillips, Interim Chair, 405-271-2070, E-mail: margaret.phillips@ouhsc.edu. *Application contact:* Robin Howell, Information Contact, 405-271-2308, E-mail: robin_howell@ouhsc.edu.

University of Pittsburgh, Graduate School of Public Health, Department of Environmental and Occupational Health, Pittsburgh, PA 15260. Offers environmental and occupational health (MPH, MS, Dr PH, PhD); environmental health risk assessment (Certificate); public health preparedness (Certificate). *Accreditation:* CEPH (one or more programs are accredited). Part-time programs available. *Faculty:* 27 full-time (9 women), 25 part-time/adjunct (6 women). *Students:* 38 full-time (25 women), 10 part-time (7 women); includes 7 minority (3 Black or African American, non-Hispanic/Latino; 2 Asian, non-Hispanic/Latino; 1 Hispanic/Latino; 1 Two or more races, non-Hispanic/Latino), 16 international. Average age 29. 61 applicants, 57% accepted, 10 enrolled. In 2013, 8 master's, 2 doctorates awarded. Terminal master's awarded for partial completion of doctoral program. *Degree requirements:* For master's, comprehensive exam (for some programs), thesis; for doctorate, comprehensive exam, thesis/dissertation, preliminary exams. *Entrance requirements:* For master's and Certificate, GRE General Test; for doctorate, GRE General Test, minimum GPA of 3.4; background in biology, physics, chemistry and calculus. Additional exam requirements/recommendations for international students: Required—TOEFL (minimum score 550 paper-based; 80 iBT) or IELTS (minimum score 6.5). *Application deadline:* For fall admission, 6/1 for domestic students, 3/15 for international students; for winter admission, 11/1 for domestic students, 8/1 for international students; for spring admission, 10/15 for domestic students, 8/1 for international students; for summer admission, 12/1 for international students. Applications are processed on a rolling basis. Application fee: $120. Electronic applications accepted. *Expenses:* Tuition, state resident: full-time $19,964; part-time $807 per credit. Tuition, nonresident: full-time $32,686; part-time $1337 per credit. *Required fees:* $740; $200. Tuition and fees vary according to program. *Financial support:* In 2013–14, 16 students received support, including 16 research assistantships (averaging $17,683 per year), 1 teaching assistantship (averaging $2,500 per year); career-related internships or fieldwork, scholarships/grants, traineeships, health care benefits, and unspecified assistantships also available. Support available to part-time students. *Faculty research:* Molecular toxicology, redox signaling, gene environment interaction, progenitor-progeny lineage, occupational and pulmonary medicine. *Total annual research expenditures:* $7.3 million. *Unit head:* Dr. Bruce R. Pitt, Chairman, 412-383-8400, Fax: 412-383-7658, E-mail: brucep@pitt.edu. *Application contact:* Eileen Penny Weiss, Student Affairs Administrator, 412-383-7297, Fax: 412-383-7658, E-mail: pweiss@pitt.edu.
Website: http://www.eoh.pitt.edu/

University of Puerto Rico, Medical Sciences Campus, Graduate School of Public Health, Department of Environmental Health, Doctoral Program in Environmental Health, San Juan, PR 00936-5067. Offers MS, Dr PH. Part-time programs available. *Expenses:* Contact institution.

University of Saint Francis, Graduate School, Keith Busse School of Business and Entrepreneurial Leadership, Fort Wayne, IN 46808-3994. Offers business administration (MBA); environmental health (MEH); healthcare administration (MHA); sustainability (MBA). *Accreditation:* ACBSP. Part-time and evening/weekend programs available.

Postbaccalaureate distance learning degree programs offered (no on-campus study). *Faculty:* 8. *Students:* 74 full-time (38 women), 69 part-time (35 women); includes 22 minority (12 Black or African American, non-Hispanic/Latino; 2 Asian, non-Hispanic/Latino; 7 Hispanic/Latino; 1 Two or more races, non-Hispanic/Latino), 3 international. Average age 34. 73 applicants, 97% accepted, 71 enrolled. In 2013, 12 master's awarded. *Entrance requirements:* For master's, minimum undergraduate GPA of 2.75. *Application deadline:* For fall admission, 7/1 priority date for domestic students; for spring admission, 11/1 priority date for domestic students. Applications are processed on a rolling basis. Application fee: $20. Application fee is waived when completed online. *Financial support:* Federal Work-Study, scholarships/grants, and unspecified assistantships available. Support available to part-time students. Financial award application deadline: 3/10; financial award applicants required to submit FAFSA. *Unit head:* Dr. Karen Palumbo, Professor/Graduate Program Director, 260-399-7700 Ext. 8312, Fax: 260-399-8174, E-mail: kpalumbo@sf.edu. *Application contact:* James Cashdollar, Admissions Counselor, 260-399-7700 Ext. 6302, Fax: 260-399-8152, E-mail: jcashdollar@sf.edu.
Website: http://www.sf.edu/sf/graduate/business

University of Saint Francis, Graduate School, Program in Environmental Health, Fort Wayne, IN 46808-3994. Offers MEH. Part-time programs available. Postbaccalaureate distance learning degree programs offered (no on-campus study). *Degree requirements:* For master's, professional e-portfolio. *Entrance requirements:* For master's, bachelor's degree or higher from regionally-accredited institution, minimum cumulative GPA of 2.75, letter of recommendation. *Unit head:* Dr. Doug Barcalow, Director, 260-399-7700 Ext. 8400, Fax: 260-399-8170, E-mail: dbarcalow@sf.edu. *Application contact:* James Cashdollar, Admissions Counselor, 260-399-7700 Ext. 6302, E-mail: jcashdollar@sf.edu.
Website: http://www.sf.edu/sf/online/programs/online-environmental-health

University of South Alabama, Graduate School, Program in Environmental Toxicology, Mobile, AL 36688-0002. Offers MS. *Faculty:* 1 full-time (0 women). *Students:* 15 full-time (10 women), 4 part-time (1 woman); includes 2 minority (both Black or African American, non-Hispanic/Latino), 3 international. 12 applicants, 50% accepted, 6 enrolled. In 2013, 6 master's awarded. *Degree requirements:* For master's, thesis. *Entrance requirements:* For master's, GRE. *Application deadline:* For fall admission, 7/15 for domestic students, 6/15 for international students; for spring admission, 12/1 for domestic students, 11/1 for international students. Application fee: $35. *Expenses:* Tuition, state resident: full-time $8976; part-time $374 per credit hour. Tuition, nonresident: full-time $17,952; part-time $748 per credit hour. *Unit head:* Dr. B. Keith Harrison, Dean of the Graduate School, 251-460-6310, E-mail: kharrison@southalabama.edu. *Application contact:* Dr. David Forbes, Director of Graduate Studies, 251-460-6181, E-mail: dforbes@southalabama.edu.

University of South Carolina, The Graduate School, Arnold School of Public Health, Department of Environmental Health Sciences, Program in Environmental Quality, Columbia, SC 29208. Offers MPH, MS, MSPH, PhD. *Accreditation:* CEPH (one or more programs are accredited). Part-time programs available. *Degree requirements:* For master's, comprehensive exam, thesis (for some programs), practicum (MPH); for doctorate, one foreign language, comprehensive exam, thesis/dissertation. *Entrance requirements:* For master's and doctorate, GRE General Test. Additional exam requirements/recommendations for international students: Required—TOEFL (minimum score 570 paper-based). Electronic applications accepted. *Faculty research:* Environmental assessment and planning; environmental toxicology; ecosystems analysis; air quality monitoring and modeling.

University of Southern California, Keck School of Medicine and Graduate School, Graduate Programs in Medicine, Department of Preventive Medicine, Master of Public Health Program, Los Angeles, CA 90032. Offers biostatistics-epidemiology (MPH); child and family health (MPH); environmental health (MPH); global health leadership (MPH); health communication (MPH); health education and promotion (MPH); public health policy (MPH). *Accreditation:* CEPH. Part-time and evening/weekend programs available. *Faculty:* 22 full-time (12 women), 3 part-time/adjunct (0 women). *Students:* 179 full-time (136 women), 31 part-time (24 women); includes 120 minority (19 Black or African American, non-Hispanic/Latino; 64 Asian, non-Hispanic/Latino; 37 Hispanic/Latino), 36 international. Average age 24. 205 applicants, 70% accepted, 73 enrolled. In 2013, 90 master's awarded. *Degree requirements:* For master's, practicum, final report, oral presentation. *Entrance requirements:* For master's, GRE General Test, MCAT, GMAT, minimum GPA of 3.0. Additional exam requirements/recommendations for international students: Required—TOEFL (minimum score 600 paper-based; 90 iBT). *Application deadline:* For fall admission, 6/1 priority date for domestic and international students; for spring admission, 10/1 priority date for domestic and international students; for summer admission, 3/1 for domestic and international students. Applications are processed on a rolling basis. Application fee: $85. Electronic applications accepted. *Financial support:* Career-related internships or fieldwork, Federal Work-Study, institutionally sponsored loans, and scholarships/grants available. Support available to part-time students. Financial award application deadline: 5/4; financial award applicants required to submit CSS PROFILE or FAFSA. *Faculty research:* Substance abuse prevention, cancer and heart disease prevention, mass media and health communication research, health promotion, treatment compliance. *Unit head:* Dr. Louise A. Rohrbach, Director, 323-442-8237, Fax: 323-442-8297, E-mail: rohrbac@usc.edu. *Application contact:* Valerie Burris, Admissions Counselor, 323-442-7257, Fax: 323-442-8297, E-mail: valeriem@usc.edu.
Website: http://mph.usc.edu/

University of Southern Mississippi, Graduate School, College of Health, Department of Community Health Sciences, Hattiesburg, MS 39406-0001. Offers epidemiology and biostatistics (MPH); health education (MPH); health policy/administration (MPH); occupational/environmental health (MPH); public health nutrition (MPH). *Accreditation:* CEPH. Part-time and evening/weekend programs available. *Faculty:* 8 full-time (4 women), 1 part-time/adjunct (0 women). *Students:* 92 full-time (60 women), 9 part-time (4 women); includes 38 minority (29 Black or African American, non-Hispanic/Latino; 1 American Indian or Alaska Native, non-Hispanic/Latino; 2 Asian, non-Hispanic/Latino; 6 Two or more races, non-Hispanic/Latino), 13 international. Average age 34. 71 applicants, 93% accepted, 45 enrolled. *Degree requirements:* For master's, comprehensive exam, thesis (for some programs). *Entrance requirements:* For master's, GRE General Test, minimum GPA of 2.75 in last 60 hours. Additional exam requirements/recommendations for international students: Required—TOEFL, IELTS. *Application deadline:* For fall admission, 3/1 priority date for domestic and international students; for spring admission, 1/10 priority date for domestic and international students. Applications are processed on a rolling basis. Application fee: $50. Electronic applications accepted. *Financial support:* In 2013–14, 5 research assistantships with full tuition reimbursements (averaging $7,000 per year), 1 teaching assistantship with full tuition reimbursement (averaging $8,263 per year) were awarded; career-related internships or fieldwork, Federal Work-Study, institutionally sponsored loans, scholarships/grants, health care benefits, and unspecified assistantships also available. Financial award application deadline: 3/15; financial award applicants required to submit FAFSA. *Faculty research:* Rural health care delivery, school health, nutrition of pregnant teens, risk factor reduction, sexually transmitted diseases. *Unit head:* Dr. Ray Newman, Interim Chair, 601-266-5437, Fax: 601-266-5043. *Application contact:* Shonna Breland, Manager of Graduate Admissions, 601-266-6563, Fax: 601-266-5138.
Website: http://www.usm.edu/chs

University of South Florida, College of Public Health, Department of Environmental and Occupational Health, Tampa, FL 33620-9951. Offers MPH, MSPH, PhD. *Accreditation:* ABET (one or more programs are accredited); CEPH (one or more programs are accredited). Part-time and evening/weekend programs available. *Degree requirements:* For master's, comprehensive exam, thesis (for some programs); for doctorate, comprehensive exam, thesis/dissertation. *Entrance requirements:* For master's, GRE General Test, minimum GPA of 3.0 in upper-level course work, goal statement letter, two professional letters of recommendation, resume/curriculum vitae; for doctorate, GRE General Test, minimum GPA of 3.0 in upper-level course work, goal statement letter, three professional letters of recommendation, resume/curriculum vitae, writing sample. Additional exam requirements/recommendations for international students: Required—TOEFL (minimum score 550 paper-based; 79 iBT). Electronic applications accepted. *Faculty research:* Biomedical assessment/stress test, risk impact, nitrobenzes on mammalism glutathion transferases, lysimeter research management, independent hygiene development.

University of South Florida, Innovative Education Graduate Certificate Programs, Tampa, FL 33620-9951. *Unit head:* Kathy Barnes, Interdisciplinary Programs Coordinator, 813-974-8031, Fax: 813-974-7061, E-mail: barnesk@usf.edu. *Application contact:* Karen Tylinski, Metro Initiatives, 813-974-9943, Fax: 813-974-7061, E-mail: ktylinsk@usf.edu.
Website: http://www.usf.edu/innovative-education/

The University of Texas at Tyler, College of Engineering and Computer Science, Department of Civil Engineering, Tyler, TX 75799-0001. Offers environmental engineering (MS); industrial safety (MS); structural engineering (MS); transportation engineering (MS); water resources engineering (MS). Part-time and evening/weekend programs available. *Degree requirements:* For master's, thesis optional. *Entrance requirements:* For master's, GRE General Test, bachelor's degree in engineering, associated science degree. Additional exam requirements/recommendations for international students: Required—TOEFL. *Faculty research:* Non-destructive strength testing, indoor air quality, transportation routing and signaling, pavement replacement criteria, flood water routing, construction and long-term behavior of innovative geotechnical foundation and embankment construction used in highway construction, engineering education.

University of the Sacred Heart, Graduate Programs, Department of Natural Sciences, Program in Occupational Health and Safety, San Juan, PR 00914-0383. Offers MS.

The University of Toledo, College of Graduate Studies, College of Medicine and Life Sciences, Department of Public Health and Preventative Medicine, Toledo, OH 43606-3390. Offers biostatistics and epidemiology (Certificate); contemporary gerontological practice (Certificate); environmental and occupational health and safety (MPH); epidemiology (Certificate); global public health (Certificate); health promotion and education (MPH); industrial hygiene (MSOH); medical and health science teaching and learning (Certificate); occupational health (Certificate); public health administration (MPH); public health and emergency response (Certificate); public health epidemiology (MPH); public health nutrition (MPH); MD/MPH. Part-time and evening/weekend programs available. *Faculty:* 9. *Students:* 69 full-time (50 women), 88 part-time (66 women); includes 50 minority (35 Black or African American, non-Hispanic/Latino; 10 Asian, non-Hispanic/Latino; 4 Hispanic/Latino; 1 Two or more races, non-Hispanic/Latino), 6 international. Average age 30. 92 applicants, 80% accepted, 52 enrolled. In 2013, 59 master's, 15 other advanced degrees awarded. *Degree requirements:* For master's, thesis or alternative. *Entrance requirements:* For master's, GRE, minimum undergraduate GPA of 3.0, three letters of recommendation, statement of purpose, transcripts from all prior institutions attended, resume; for Certificate, minimum undergraduate GPA of 3.0, three letters of recommendation, statement of purpose, transcripts from all prior institutions attended, resume. Additional exam requirements/recommendations for international students: Required—TOEFL (minimum score 550 paper-based; 80 iBT), IELTS (minimum score 6.5). *Application deadline:* For fall admission, 6/15 for domestic students, 3/15 priority date for international students; for spring admission, 10/15 for domestic students, 6/15 for international students; for summer admission, 3/15 for domestic students, 10/15 for international students. Applications are processed on a rolling basis. Application fee: $45 ($75 for international students). Electronic applications accepted. *Financial support:* In 2013–14, 4 research assistantships with full tuition reimbursements (averaging $10,000 per year) were awarded; Federal Work-Study, institutionally sponsored loans, scholarships/grants, tuition waivers (full and partial), and unspecified assistantships also available. *Unit head:* Dr. Sheryl A. Milz, Chair, 419-383-3976, Fax: 419-383-6140, E-mail: sheryl.milz@utoledo.edu. *Application contact:* Admissions Analyst, 419-383-4112, Fax: 419-383-6140.
Website: http://nocphmph.org/

University of Washington, Graduate School, School of Public Health, Department of Environmental and Occupational Health Sciences, Seattle, WA 98195. Offers environmental and occupational health (MPH); environmental and occupational hygiene (PhD); environmental health (MS); occupational and environmental exposure sciences (MS); occupational and environmental medicine (MPH); toxicology (MS, PhD); MPH/MPA; MS/MPA. Part-time programs available. *Faculty:* 34 full-time (9 women), 7 part-time/adjunct (3 women). *Students:* 65 full-time (42 women), 9 part-time (6 women); includes 22 minority (3 Black or African American, non-Hispanic/Latino; 3 American Indian or Alaska Native, non-Hispanic/Latino; 16 Asian, non-Hispanic/Latino), 6 international. Average age 30. 114 applicants, 32% accepted, 22 enrolled. In 2013, 16 master's, 6 doctorates awarded. Terminal master's awarded for partial completion of doctoral program. *Degree requirements:* For master's, comprehensive exam, thesis (for some programs), project or thesis; for doctorate, comprehensive exam, thesis/dissertation. *Entrance requirements:* For master's, GRE General Test, one year each of physics, general chemistry, and biology; two quarters of organic chemistry; one quarter of calculus; for doctorate, GRE General Test, minimum GPA of 3.0, prerequisite course work in biology, chemistry, physics, calculus. Additional exam requirements/recommendations for international students: Required—TOEFL (minimum score 580 paper-based; 92 iBT). *Application deadline:* For fall admission, 12/1 for domestic and international students. Application fee: $85. Electronic applications accepted. *Financial support:* In 2013–14, 70 students received support, including 65 fellowships with full tuition reimbursements available (averaging $42,000 per year), 111 research assistantships with full tuition reimbursements available (averaging $42,000 per year), 19 teaching assistantships with full tuition reimbursements available (averaging $42,000 per year); career-related internships or fieldwork, institutionally sponsored loans, scholarships/grants, traineeships, health care benefits, and unspecified assistantships also available. Financial award application deadline: 12/1. *Faculty research:* Developmental and behavioral toxicology, biochemical toxicology, exposure assessment, hazardous waste, industrial chemistry. *Unit head:* Dr. David Kalman, Chair, 206-543-6991, Fax: 206-543-0477. *Application contact:* Rory A. Murphy, Manager,

Student Services, 206-543-6991, Fax: 206-543-0477, E-mail: ehgrad@u.washington.edu.
Website: http://depts.washington.edu/envhlth/

University of West Florida, College of Professional Studies, Department of Health, Leisure, and Exercise Science, Community Health Education Program, Pensacola, FL 32514-5750. Offers aging studies (MS); health promotion and worksite wellness (MS); psychosocial (MS). Part-time and evening/weekend programs available. *Degree requirements:* For master's, thesis or alternative. *Entrance requirements:* For master's, GRE or MAT, official transcripts; minimum GPA of 3.0; letter of intent; three personal references. Additional exam requirements/recommendations for international students: Required—TOEFL (minimum score 550 paper-based).

University of Wisconsin–Milwaukee, Graduate School, Zilber School of Public Health, Department of Environmental and Occupational Health, Milwaukee, WI 53201-0413. Offers PhD. *Students:* 6 full-time (2 women), 3 part-time (1 woman); includes 2 minority (1 Asian, non-Hispanic/Latino; 1 Two or more races, non-Hispanic/Latino). Average age 40. 4 applicants, 50% accepted, 2 enrolled. *Unit head:* Darcie Galowitch, Representative, 414-229-3264, E-mail: darcie@uwm.edu. *Application contact:* Darcie K. G. Warren, Graduate Program Manager, 414-229-5633, E-mail: darcie@uwm.edu.

University of Wisconsin–Whitewater, School of Graduate Studies, College of Education and Professional Studies, Department of Occupational and Environmental Safety, Whitewater, WI 53190-1790. Offers safety (MS). Part-time and evening/weekend programs available. Postbaccalaureate distance learning degree programs offered (no on-campus study). *Degree requirements:* For master's, thesis or alternative. *Entrance requirements:* For master's, 2 letters of recommendation. Additional exam requirements/recommendations for international students: Required—TOEFL (minimum score 550 paper-based; 80 iBT), IELTS (minimum score 6). Electronic applications accepted. *Faculty research:* Industrial ergonomics; work, measurement, and design; product design/evaluation.

Wayne State University, School of Medicine, Graduate Programs in Medicine, Department of Family Medicine and Public Health Sciences, Detroit, MI 48202. Offers public health (MPH), including occupational and environmental health, public health practice, quantitative health sciences; public health practice (Graduate Certificate). *Students:* 22 full-time (13 women), 30 part-time (15 women); includes 15 minority (5 Black or African American, non-Hispanic/Latino; 8 Asian, non-Hispanic/Latino; 1 Hispanic/Latino; 1 Two or more races, non-Hispanic/Latino), 13 international. Average age 32. 187 applicants, 21% accepted, 22 enrolled. In 2013, 14 master's, 3 other advanced degrees awarded. *Degree requirements:* For master's, thesis (for some programs), project or thesis. *Entrance requirements:* For master's, GRE, undergraduate work in mathematics, natural sciences, and social sciences; experience in health-related position, admission to graduate school, minimum undergraduate GPA of 3.0 overall and in mathematics, social sciences, and natural sciences, college-level mathematics, personal statement, three letters of recommendation; for Graduate Certificate, undergraduate work in mathematics, natural sciences, and social sciences; experience in health-related position, admission to graduate school, minimum undergraduate GPA of 3.0 overall and in mathematics, social sciences, and natural sciences, college-level mathematics, personal statement, three letters of recommendation. Additional exam requirements/recommendations for international students: Required—TOEFL (minimum score 550 paper-based; 100 iBT), TWE (minimum score 6); Recommended—IELTS (minimum score 6.5). *Application deadline:* For fall admission, 2/1 for domestic students, 1/1 priority date for international students. Application fee: $0. Electronic applications accepted. *Expenses:* Contact institution. *Financial support:* In 2013–14, 7 students received support. Scholarships/grants available. Financial award application deadline: 3/31; financial award applicants required to submit FAFSA. *Faculty research:* Urban health disparities, community health promotion, substance abuse etiology and prevention, HIV/AIDS, interpersonal violence. *Unit head:* Dr. Kimberly Campbell-Voytal, Program Director, 313-577-1051, E-mail: kvoytal@med.wayne.edu.
Website: http://gradprograms.med.wayne.edu/program-spotlight.php?id=26

West Chester University of Pennsylvania, College of Health Sciences, Department of Health, West Chester, PA 19383. Offers community health (MPH); emergency preparedness (Certificate); environmental health (MPH); health care management (MPH, Certificate); integrative health (MPH, Certificate); nutrition (MPH); school health (M Ed). *Accreditation:* CEPH. Part-time and evening/weekend programs available. *Faculty:* 17 full-time (13 women), 3 part-time/adjunct (all women). *Students:* 115 full-time (85 women), 95 part-time (73 women); includes 79 minority (66 Black or African American, non-Hispanic/Latino; 1 American Indian or Alaska Native, non-Hispanic/Latino; 5 Asian, non-Hispanic/Latino; 3 Hispanic/Latino; 4 Two or more races, non-Hispanic/Latino), 15 international. Average age 31. 156 applicants, 83% accepted, 76 enrolled. In 2013, 101 master's, 18 other advanced degrees awarded. *Degree requirements:* For master's, thesis or alternative, minimum GPA of 3.0; research report (for M Ed); major project and practicum (for MPH); for Certificate, minimum GPA of 3.0. *Entrance requirements:* For master's, goal statement, two letters of recommendation, undergraduate Introduction to Statistics course. Additional exam requirements/recommendations for international students: Required—TOEFL (minimum score 550 paper-based; 80 iBT). *Application deadline:* For fall admission, 4/15 priority date for domestic students, 3/15 for international students; for spring admission, 10/15 priority date for domestic students, 9/1 for international students. Applications are processed on a rolling basis. Application fee: $45. Electronic applications accepted. *Expenses:* Tuition, state resident: full-time $7956; part-time $442 per credit. Tuition, nonresident: full-time $11,934; part-time $663 per credit. *Required fees:* $2134.20; $106.24 per credit. Tuition and fees vary according to campus/location and program. *Financial support:* Unspecified assistantships available. Support available to part-time students. Financial award application deadline: 2/15; financial award applicants required to submit FAFSA. *Faculty research:* Healthy school communities, community health issues and evidence-based programs, environment and health, nutrition and health, integrative health. *Unit head:* Dr. Bethann Cinelli, Chair, 610-436-2267, E-mail: bcinelli@wcupa.edu. *Application contact:* Dr. Lynn Carson, Graduate Coordinator, 610-436-2138, E-mail: lcarson@wcupa.edu.
Website: http://www.wcupa.edu/_ACADEMICS/HealthSciences/health/

West Virginia University, College of Engineering and Mineral Resources, Department of Industrial and Management Systems Engineering, Program in Occupational Safety and Health, Morgantown, WV 26506. Offers PhD. Part-time programs available. Postbaccalaureate distance learning degree programs offered (minimal on-campus study). *Degree requirements:* For doctorate, comprehensive exam, thesis/dissertation. *Entrance requirements:* For doctorate, GRE General Test, Minimum GPA of 3.5. Additional exam requirements/recommendations for international students: Required—TOEFL. *Faculty research:* Safety management, ergonomics and workplace design, safety and health training, construction safety.

Yale University, School of Medicine, Yale School of Public Health, New Haven, CT 06520. Offers applied biostatistics and epidemiology (APMPH); biostatistics (MPH, MS, PhD), including global health (MPH); chronic disease epidemiology (MPH, PhD), including global health (MPH); environmental health sciences (MPH, PhD), including global health (MPH); epidemiology of microbial diseases (MPH, PhD), including global health (MPH); global health (APMPH); health management (MPH), including global health; health policy (MPH), including global health; health policy and administration (APMPH, PhD); occupational and environmental medicine (APMPH); preventive medicine (APMPH); social and behavioral sciences (APMPH, MPH), including global health (MPH); JD/MPH; M Div/MPH; MBA/MPH; MD/MPH; MEM/MPH; MFS/MPH; MM Sc/MPH; MPH/MA; MSN/MPH. MS and PhD offered through the Graduate School. *Accreditation:* CEPH. Part-time programs available. Terminal master's awarded for partial completion of doctoral program. *Degree requirements:* For master's, thesis, summer internship; for doctorate, comprehensive exam, thesis/dissertation, residency. *Entrance requirements:* For master's, GMAT, GRE, or MCAT, two years of undergraduate coursework in math and science; for doctorate, GRE General Test. Additional exam requirements/recommendations for international students: Required—TOEFL (minimum score 100 iBT). Electronic applications accepted. *Expenses:* Contact institution. *Faculty research:* Genetic and emerging infections epidemiology, virology, cost/quality, vector biology, quantitative methods, aging, asthma, cancer.

Epidemiology

American University of Beirut, Graduate Programs, Faculty of Health Sciences, Beirut, Lebanon. Offers environmental sciences (MS), including environmental health; epidemiology (MS); epidemiology and biostatistics (MPH); health management and policy (MPH); health promotion and community health (MPH); population health (MS). Part-time programs available. *Faculty:* 26 full-time (18 women), 7 part-time/adjunct (4 women). *Students:* 42 full-time (37 women), 103 part-time (84 women). Average age 25. 132 applicants, 65% accepted, 48 enrolled. In 2013, 52 master's awarded. *Degree requirements:* For master's, one foreign language, comprehensive exam, thesis (for some programs). *Entrance requirements:* For master's, 2 letters of recommendation, personal statement, transcripts. Additional exam requirements/recommendations for international students: Required—TOEFL (minimum score 583 paper-based; 97 iBT), IELTS (minimum score 7). *Application deadline:* For fall admission, 2/7 priority date for domestic and international students; for spring admission, 11/1 for domestic and international students. Application fee: $50. Electronic applications accepted. *Expenses: Tuition:* Full-time $14,724; part-time $818 per credit. *Required fees:* $692. Tuition and fees vary according to course load and program. *Financial support:* In 2013–14, 56 students received support. Scholarships/grants, health care benefits, and unspecified assistantships available. Financial award application deadline: 4/1. *Faculty research:* Tobacco control; health of the elderly; youth health; mental health; women's health; reproductive and sexual health, including HIV/AIDS; water quality; health systems; quality in health care delivery; health human resources; health policy; occupational and environmental health; social inequality; social determinants of health; non-communicable diseases. *Total annual research expenditures:* $1 million. *Unit head:* Iman Adel Nuwayhid, Dean, 961-1759683, Fax: 961-1744470, E-mail: nuwayhid@aub.edu.lb. *Application contact:* Mitra Tauk, Administrative Coordinator, 961-1-350000 Ext. 4687, Fax: 96-1-1744470, E-mail: mt12@aub.edu.lb.

Boston University, School of Public Health, Epidemiology Department, Boston, MA 02215. Offers MPH, MS, PhD. *Accreditation:* CEPH (one or more programs are accredited). Part-time and evening/weekend programs available. *Faculty:* 25 full-time, 60 part-time/adjunct. *Students:* 133 full-time (94 women), 101 part-time (74 women); includes 60 minority (8 Black or African American, non-Hispanic/Latino; 31 Asian, non-Hispanic/Latino; 16 Hispanic/Latino; 5 Two or more races, non-Hispanic/Latino), 33 international. Average age 28. 565 applicants, 36% accepted, 65 enrolled. In 2013, 86 master's, 5 doctorates awarded. *Degree requirements:* For master's, comprehensive exam (for some programs), thesis (for some programs); for doctorate, comprehensive exam, thesis/dissertation. *Entrance requirements:* For master's, GRE, LSAT, GMAT, DAT or MCAT, U.S. bachelor's degree or foreign equivalent; for doctorate, GRE, MCAT, GMAT, LSAT, MPH or equivalent. Additional exam requirements/recommendations for international students: Required—TOEFL (minimum score 600 paper-based; 100 iBT), IELTS (minimum score 6). *Application deadline:* For fall admission, 2/1 priority date for domestic and international students; for spring admission, 10/15 priority date for domestic and international students. Applications are processed on a rolling basis. Application fee: $115. Electronic applications accepted. *Expenses: Tuition:* Full-time $43,970; part-time $1374 per credit hour. *Required fees:* $60 per semester. Tuition and fees vary according to class time, course level and program. *Financial support:* Career-related internships or fieldwork, Federal Work-Study, institutionally sponsored loans, and scholarships/grants available. Support available to part-time students. Financial award application deadline: 3/1; financial award applicants required to submit FAFSA. *Unit head:* Dr. C. Robert Horsburgh, Jr., Chair, 617-638-7775, E-mail: epi@bu.edu. *Application contact:* LePhan Quan, Associate Director of Admissions, 617-638-4640, Fax: 617-638-5299, E-mail: asksph@bu.edu.
Website: http://sph.bu.edu/epi

Brown University, Graduate School, Division of Biology and Medicine, School of Public Health, Department of Epidemiology, Providence, RI 02912. Offers Sc M, PhD. *Degree requirements:* For doctorate, thesis/dissertation, preliminary exam. *Entrance requirements:* For master's and doctorate, GRE General Test.

Capella University, School of Public Service Leadership, Doctoral Programs in Healthcare, Minneapolis, MN 55402. Offers criminal justice (PhD); emergency management (PhD); epidemiology (Dr PH); general health administration (DHA); general public administration (DPA); health advocacy and leadership (Dr PH); health care administration (PhD); health care leadership (DHA); health policy advocacy (DHA); multidisciplinary human services (PhD); nonprofit management and leadership (PhD); public safety leadership (PhD); social and community services (PhD).

Case Western Reserve University, School of Medicine and School of Graduate Studies, Graduate Programs in Medicine, Department of Epidemiology and Biostatistics, Program in Epidemiology, Cleveland, OH 44106. Offers MS, PhD. *Accreditation:* CEPH. Part-time programs available. Terminal master's awarded for partial completion of doctoral program. *Degree requirements:* For master's, comprehensive exam, thesis; for doctorate, comprehensive exam, thesis/dissertation. *Entrance requirements:* For master's, GRE General Test or MCAT, 3 recommendations; for doctorate, GRE General Test, 3 recommendations. Additional exam requirements/recommendations for international students: Required—TOEFL (minimum score 550 paper-based). Electronic applications accepted. *Faculty research:* Cardiovascular epidemiology, cancer risk factors, HIV in underserved populations, effectiveness studies in Medicare patients.

Case Western Reserve University, School of Medicine and School of Graduate Studies, Graduate Programs in Medicine, Department of Epidemiology and Biostatistics, Program in Genetic and Molecular Epidemiology, Cleveland, OH 44106. Offers MS, PhD. *Degree requirements:* For master's, comprehensive exam, thesis; for doctorate, comprehensive exam, thesis/dissertation. *Entrance requirements:* For master's and doctorate, GRE. Additional exam requirements/recommendations for international students: Required—TOEFL (minimum score 550 paper-based).

Columbia University, Columbia University Mailman School of Public Health, Department of Epidemiology, New York, NY 10032. Offers MPH, MS, Dr PH, PhD. PhD offered in cooperation with the Graduate School of Arts and Sciences. *Accreditation:* CEPH (one or more programs are accredited). Part-time programs available. *Students:* 279 full-time (210 women), 95 part-time (70 women); includes 137 minority (25 Black or African American, non-Hispanic/Latino; 1 American Indian or Alaska Native, non-Hispanic/Latino; 60 Asian, non-Hispanic/Latino; 37 Hispanic/Latino; 14 Two or more races, non-Hispanic/Latino), 63 international. Average age 28. 708 applicants, 61% accepted, 174 enrolled. In 2013, 114 master's, 7 doctorates awarded. *Degree requirements:* For master's, thesis; for doctorate, thesis/dissertation. *Entrance requirements:* For master's, GRE General Test; for doctorate, GRE General Test, MPH or equivalent (Dr PH). Additional exam requirements/recommendations for international students: Required—TOEFL (minimum score 600 paper-based; 100 iBT). *Application deadline:* For fall admission, 12/1 priority date for domestic and international students. Application fee: $120. Electronic applications accepted. *Financial support:* Research assistantships, teaching assistantships, career-related internships or fieldwork, and Federal Work-Study available. Support available to part-time students. Financial award application deadline: 2/1; financial award applicants required to submit FAFSA. *Faculty research:* Infectious disease epidemiology, chronic disease epidemiology, social epidemiology, psychiatric epidemiology, neurological epidemiology. *Unit head:* Dr. Sandro Galeo, Chairperson, 212-305-9410. *Application contact:* Dr. Joseph Korevec, Director of Admissions and Financial Aid, 212-305-8698, Fax: 212-342-1861, E-mail: ph-admit@columbia.edu.
Website: http://www.mailman.hs.columbia.edu/epi/index.html

Cornell University, Graduate School, Graduate Fields of Comparative Biomedical Sciences, Field of Comparative Biomedical Sciences, Ithaca, NY 14853-0001. Offers cellular and molecular medicine (MS, PhD); developmental and reproductive biology (MS, PhD); infectious diseases (MS, PhD); population medicine and epidemiology (MS, PhD); structural and functional biology (MS, PhD). *Faculty:* 104 full-time (32 women). *Students:* 32 full-time (22 women); includes 3 minority (1 Asian, non-Hispanic/Latino; 2 Hispanic/Latino), 12 international. Average age 29. 47 applicants, 23% accepted, 6 enrolled. In 2013, 2 master's, 12 doctorates awarded. *Degree requirements:* For master's, thesis; for doctorate, comprehensive exam, thesis/dissertation. *Entrance requirements:* For master's and doctorate, GRE General Test, 2 letters of recommendation. Additional exam requirements/recommendations for international students: Required—TOEFL (minimum score 550 paper-based; 77 iBT). *Application deadline:* For fall admission, 12/15 for domestic students. Application fee: $95. Electronic applications accepted. *Financial support:* In 2013–14, 18 students received support, including 3 fellowships with full tuition reimbursements available, 14 research assistantships with full tuition reimbursements available, 1 teaching assistantship with full tuition reimbursement available; institutionally sponsored loans, scholarships/grants, health care benefits, tuition waivers (full and partial), and unspecified assistantships also available. Financial award applicants required to submit FAFSA. *Faculty research:* Receptors and signal transduction, viral and bacterial infectious diseases, tumor metastasis, clinical sciences/nutritional disease, developmental/neurological disorders. *Unit head:* Director of Graduate Studies, 607-253-3276, Fax: 607-253-3756. *Application contact:* Graduate Field Assistant, 607-253-3276, Fax: 607-253-3756, E-mail: graduate_edcvm@cornell.edu.
Website: http://www.gradschool.cornell.edu/fields.php?id-64&a-2

Dalhousie University, Faculty of Medicine, Department of Community Health and Epidemiology, Halifax, NS B3H 4R2, Canada. Offers M Sc. *Degree requirements:* For master's, thesis. *Entrance requirements:* Additional exam requirements/recommendations for international students: Required—1 of 5 approved tests: TOEFL, IELTS, CANTEST, CAEL, Michigan English Language Assessment Battery. Electronic applications accepted. *Expenses:* Contact institution. *Faculty research:* Population health, health promotion and disease prevention, health services utilization, chronic disease epidemiology.

Drexel University, School of Public Health, Department of Epidemiology and Biostatistics, Philadelphia, PA 19104-2875. Offers biostatistics (MS); epidemiology (PhD); epidemiology and biostatistics (Certificate).

Emory University, Rollins School of Public Health, Department of Environmental Health, Atlanta, GA 30322-1100. Offers environmental health (MPH); environmental health and epidemiology (MSPH); environmental health sciences (PhD); global environmental health (MPH). *Accreditation:* CEPH. Part-time programs available. *Degree requirements:* For master's, thesis, practicum. *Entrance requirements:* For master's, GRE General Test. Additional exam requirements/recommendations for international students: Required—TOEFL. Electronic applications accepted.

Emory University, Rollins School of Public Health, Department of Epidemiology, Atlanta, GA 30322-1100. Offers MPH, MSPH, PhD. *Accreditation:* CEPH. Part-time programs available. *Degree requirements:* For master's, thesis, practicum. *Entrance requirements:* For master's, GRE General Test. Additional exam requirements/recommendations for international students: Required—TOEFL (minimum score 550 paper-based; 80 iBT). Electronic applications accepted. *Expenses:* Contact institution. *Faculty research:* Cancer, infectious diseases, epidemiological methods, environmental/occupational health, women's and children's health.

Emory University, Rollins School of Public Health, Online Program in Public Health, Atlanta, GA 30322-1100. Offers applied epidemiology (MPH); applied public health informatics (MPH); prevention science (MPH). Part-time and evening/weekend programs available. Postbaccalaureate distance learning degree programs offered (minimal on-campus study). *Degree requirements:* For master's, thesis, practicum. *Entrance requirements:* For master's, GRE. Additional exam requirements/recommendations for international students: Required—TOEFL (minimum score 550 paper-based; 80 iBT). Electronic applications accepted.

Florida International University, Robert Stempel College of Public Health and Social Work, Programs in Public Health, Miami, FL 33199. Offers biostatistics (MPH); environmental and occupational health (MPH, PhD); epidemiology (MPH, PhD); health policy and management (MPH); health promotion and disease prevention (PhD); health promotion and diseases prevention (MPH). Ph D program has fall admissions only; MPH offered jointly with University of Miami. *Accreditation:* CEPH. Part-time and evening/weekend programs available. Postbaccalaureate distance learning degree programs offered (no on-campus study). *Degree requirements:* For master's, thesis optional; for doctorate, comprehensive exam, thesis/dissertation. *Entrance requirements:* For master's, minimum GPA of 3.0, letters of recommendation; for doctorate, GRE, resume, minimum GPA of 3.0, letters of recommendation, letter of intent. Additional exam requirements/recommendations for international students: Required—TOEFL (minimum score 550 paper-based; 80 iBT). Electronic applications accepted. *Expenses:* Contact institution. *Faculty research:* Drugs/AIDS intervention among migrant workers, provision of services for active/recovering drug users with HIV.

Georgetown University, Graduate School of Arts and Sciences, Programs in Biomedical Sciences, Department of Biostatistics, Bioinformatics and Biomathematics, Washington, DC 20057-1484. Offers biostatistics (MS, Graduate Certificate), including bioinformatics (MS), epidemiology (MS); epidemiology (Graduate Certificate). *Entrance requirements:* For master's, GRE General Test. Additional exam requirements/recommendations for international students: Required—TOEFL. *Application deadline:* Applications are processed on a rolling basis. Application fee: $50 ($55 for international students). *Financial support:* Career-related internships or fieldwork available. Financial award application deadline: 2/1. *Faculty research:* Occupation epidemiology, cancer. *Unit head:* Ming Tony Tan, Chair, 202-687-0824, E-mail: ming.tan@georgetown.edu. *Application contact:* Office of the Dean of Research and Graduate Education, 202-687-3690.

The George Washington University, Columbian College of Arts and Sciences, Program in Epidemiology, Washington, DC 20052. Offers MS, PhD. Part-time and evening/weekend programs available. *Students:* 10 part-time (6 women); includes 4 minority (1 Asian, non-Hispanic/Latino; 3 Hispanic/Latino). Average age 33. 43 applicants, 26% accepted. In 2013, 2 master's, 3 doctorates awarded. *Degree requirements:* For master's, comprehensive exam; for doctorate, thesis/dissertation, general exam. *Entrance requirements:* For master's and doctorate, GRE General Test, minimum GPA of 3.0. Additional exam requirements/recommendations for international students: Required—TOEFL (minimum score 550 paper-based; 80 iBT). *Application deadline:* For fall admission, 1/15 priority date for domestic and international students; for spring admission, 10/1 priority date for domestic students, 9/1 priority date for international students. Applications are processed on a rolling basis. Application fee: $75. Electronic applications accepted. *Financial support:* In 2013–14, 1 student received support. Fellowships with tuition reimbursements available, teaching assistantships, and tuition waivers available. *Unit head:* Dr. Sean D. Cleary, Director, 202-994-5757, Fax: 202-994-0082, E-mail: sphsdc@gwumc.edu. *Application contact:* 202-994-6210, Fax: 202-994-6213, E-mail: askccas@gwu.edu.

The George Washington University, School of Public Health and Health Services, Department of Epidemiology and Biostatistics, Washington, DC 20052. Offers biostatistics (MPH); epidemiology (MPH); microbiology and emerging infectious diseases (MSPH). *Faculty:* 29 full-time (20 women). *Students:* 54 full-time (43 women), 77 part-time (60 women); includes 37 minority (18 Black or African American, non-Hispanic/Latino; 16 Asian, non-Hispanic/Latino; 2 Hispanic/Latino; 1 Two or more races, non-Hispanic/Latino), 12 international. Average age 28. 342 applicants, 75% accepted. In 2013, 51 master's awarded. *Degree requirements:* For master's, case study or special project. *Entrance requirements:* For master's, GMAT, GRE General Test, or MCAT. Additional exam requirements/recommendations for international students: Required—TOEFL. *Application deadline:* For fall admission, 4/15 priority date for domestic students, 4/15 for international students; for spring admission, 11/1 for domestic and international students. Applications are processed on a rolling basis. Application fee: $75. *Financial support:* In 2013–14, 6 students received support. Tuition waivers available. Financial award application deadline: 2/15. *Unit head:* Dr. Alan E. Greenberg, Chair, 202-994-0612, E-mail: aeg1@gwu.edu. *Application contact:* Jane Smith, Director of Admissions, 202-994-0248, Fax: 202-994-1860, E-mail: sphhsinfo@gwumc.edu.

Georgia Southern University, Jack N. Averitt College of Graduate Studies, Jiann-Ping Hsu College of Public Health, Program in Public Health, Statesboro, GA 30460. Offers biostatistics (MPH, Dr PH); community health behavior and education (Dr PH); community health education (MPH); environmental health sciences (MPH); epidemiology (MPH); health policy and management (MPH, Dr PH). *Accreditation:* CEPH. Part-time programs available. *Students:* 130 full-time (96 women), 50 part-time (39 women); includes 95 minority (80 Black or African American, non-Hispanic/Latino; 5 Asian, non-Hispanic/Latino; 4 Hispanic/Latino; 1 Native Hawaiian or other Pacific Islander, non-Hispanic/Latino; 5 Two or more races, non-Hispanic/Latino), 32 international. Average age 30. 213 applicants, 68% accepted, 61 enrolled. In 2013, 29 master's, 9 doctorates awarded. *Degree requirements:* For master's, thesis optional, practicum; for doctorate, comprehensive exam, thesis/dissertation, practicum. *Entrance requirements:* For master's, GRE General Test, minimum GPA of 2.75, resume, 3 letters of reference; for doctorate, GRE, GMAT, MCAT, LSAT, 3 letters of reference, statement of purpose, resume or curriculum vitae. Additional exam requirements/recommendations for international students: Required—TOEFL (minimum score 550 paper-based; 80 iBT), IELTS (minimum score 6). *Application deadline:* For fall admission, 3/1 priority date for domestic and international students; for spring admission, 10/1 priority date for domestic students, 10/1 for international students. Applications are processed on a rolling basis. Application fee: $50. Electronic applications accepted. *Expenses:* Contact institution. *Financial support:* In 2013–14, 54 students received support, including research assistantships with partial tuition reimbursements available (averaging $7,200 per year), teaching assistantships with partial tuition reimbursements available (averaging $7,200 per year); career-related internships or fieldwork, Federal Work-Study, scholarships/grants, tuition waivers (partial), and unspecified assistantships also available. Support available to part-time students. Financial award application deadline: 4/15; financial award applicants required to submit FAFSA. *Faculty research:* Rural public health best practices, health disparity elimination, community initiatives to enhance public health, cost effectiveness analysis, epidemiology of rural public health, environmental health issues, health care system assessment, rural health care, health policy and healthcare financing, survival analysis, nonparametric statistics and resampling methods, micro-arrays and genomics, data imputation techniques and clinical trial methodology. *Total annual research expenditures:* $281,707. *Unit head:* Sarah Peterson, Student Services Coordinator, 912-478-2413, Fax: 912-478-5811, E-mail: speterson@georgiasouthern.edu. *Application contact:* Amanda Gilliland, Coordinator for Graduate Student Recruitment, 912-478-5384, Fax: 912-478-0740, E-mail: gradadmissions@georgiasouthern.edu.
Website: http://chhs.georgiasouthern.edu/health/

Harvard University, Cyprus International Institute for the Environment and Public Health in Association with Harvard School of Public Health, Cambridge, MA 02138. Offers environmental health (MS); environmental/public health (PhD); epidemiology and biostatistics (MS). *Entrance requirements:* For master's and doctorate, GRE, resume/curriculum vitae, 3 letters of recommendation, BA or BS (including diploma and official transcripts). Additional exam requirements/recommendations for international students: Required—TOEFL, IELTS (minimum score 7). Electronic applications accepted. *Expenses: Tuition:* Full-time $38,888. *Required fees:* $958. Tuition and fees vary according to campus/location, program and student level. *Faculty research:* Air pollution, climate change, biostatistics, sustainable development, environmental management.

Harvard University, Harvard School of Public Health, Department of Epidemiology, Boston, MA 02115-6096. Offers cancer epidemiology (SM); cardiovascular epidemiology (SM, SD); clinical epidemiology (SM, SD); environmental/occupational epidemiology (SM, SD); epidemiologic methods (SD); epidemiology of aging (SM, SD); infectious diseases (SM, SD); molecular/genetic epidemiology (SD); neuroepidemiology (SD); oral and dental health epidemiology (SM, SD); pharmacoepidemiology (SM, SD); psychiatric epidemiology (SM); reproductive epidemiology (SM, SD). Part-time programs available. *Faculty:* 20 full-time (6 women), 84 part-time/adjunct (37 women). *Students:* 133 full-time, 44 part-time; includes 44 minority (3 Black or African American, non-Hispanic/Latino; 29 Asian, non-Hispanic/Latino; 6 Hispanic/Latino; 6 Two or more races, non-Hispanic/Latino), 68 international. Average age 27. 459 applicants, 22% accepted, 64 enrolled. In 2013, 41 master's, 23 doctorates awarded. *Degree requirements:* For doctorate, thesis/dissertation, qualifying exam. *Entrance requirements:* For master's, GRE, MCAT; for doctorate, GRE. Additional exam requirements/recommendations for international students: Required—TOEFL (minimum score 600 paper-based; 100 iBT); Recommended—IELTS (minimum score 7). *Application deadline:* For fall admission, 12/15 for domestic and international students. Application fee: $120. Electronic applications accepted. *Expenses: Tuition:* Full-time $38,888. *Required fees:* $958. Tuition and fees vary according to campus/location, program and student level. *Financial support:* Fellowships, research assistantships, teaching assistantships, Federal Work-Study, scholarships/grants, traineeships, and unspecified assistantships available. Support available to part-time students. Financial award application deadline: 2/15; financial award applicants required to submit FAFSA. *Faculty research:* Cancer prevention and epidemiology; epidemiologic methods; epidemiology of aging; infectious diseases; pharmacoepidemiology; cardiovascular, clinical, environmental and occupational, molecular/genetic, neuropsychiatric, nutritional, psychiatric, reproductive, perinatal, and pediatric epidemiology. *Unit head:* Dr. Michelle A. Williams, Chair, 617-432-6477, Fax: 617-432-7805, E-mail: mawilliams@hsph.harvard.edu. *Application contact:* Vincent W. James, Director of Admissions, 617-432-1031, Fax: 617-432-7080, E-mail: admissions@hsph.harvard.edu.
Website: http://www.hsph.harvard.edu/epidemiology/

Harvard University, Harvard School of Public Health, Department of Nutrition, Boston, MA 02115-6096. Offers nutrition (PhD, SD); nutritional epidemiology (SD); public health nutrition (SD). *Faculty:* 11 full-time (5 women), 22 part-time/adjunct (6 women). *Students:* 29 full-time, 2 part-time; includes 6 minority (1 Asian, non-Hispanic/Latino; 2 Hispanic/Latino; 3 Two or more races, non-Hispanic/Latino), 17 international. Average age 29. 51 applicants, 16% accepted, 8 enrolled. In 2013, 6 doctorates awarded. *Degree requirements:* For doctorate, thesis/dissertation, qualifying exam. *Entrance requirements:* For doctorate, GRE. Additional exam requirements/recommendations for international students: Required—TOEFL (minimum score 600 paper-based; 100 iBT); Recommended—IELTS (minimum score 7). *Application deadline:* For fall admission, 12/15 for domestic and international students. Application fee: $120. Electronic applications accepted. *Expenses: Tuition:* Full-time $38,888. *Required fees:* $958. Tuition and fees vary according to campus/location, program and student level. *Financial support:* Fellowships, research assistantships, teaching assistantships, Federal Work-Study, scholarships/grants, traineeships, and unspecified assistantships available. Support available to part-time students. Financial award application deadline: 2/15; financial award applicants required to submit FAFSA. *Faculty research:* Dietary and genetic factors affecting heart diseases in humans; interactions among nutrition, immunity, and infection; role of diet and lifestyle in preventing macrovascular complications in diabetics. *Unit head:* Dr. Walter Willett, Chair, 617-432-1333, Fax: 617-432-2435, E-mail: walter.willett@channing.harvard.edu. *Application contact:* Vincent W. James, Director of Admissions, 617-432-1031, Fax: 617-432-7080, E-mail: admissions@hsph.harvard.edu.
Website: http://www.hsph.harvard.edu/nutrition/

Hunter College of the City University of New York, Graduate School, Schools of the Health Professions, School of Health Sciences, Programs in Urban Public Health, Program in Epidemiology and Biostatistics, New York, NY 10065-5085. Offers MPH. *Accreditation:* CEPH. Part-time and evening/weekend programs available. *Faculty:* 1 (woman) full-time. *Students:* 7 full-time (3 women), 37 part-time (23 women); includes 22 minority (11 Black or African American, non-Hispanic/Latino; 5 Asian, non-Hispanic/Latino; 6 Hispanic/Latino), 3 international. Average age 32. 85 applicants, 60% accepted, 27 enrolled. In 2013, 16 master's awarded. *Degree requirements:* For master's, comprehensive exam, thesis optional, internship. *Entrance requirements:* For master's, GRE General Test, previous course work in calculus and statistics. Additional exam requirements/recommendations for international students: Required—TOEFL. *Application deadline:* For fall admission, 4/1 for domestic students; for spring admission, 11/1 for domestic students. Application fee: $125. *Financial support:* In 2013–14, 6 fellowships were awarded; career-related internships or fieldwork, Federal Work-Study, institutionally sponsored loans, and tuition waivers (partial) also available. Support available to part-time students. Financial award application deadline: 3/1. *Unit head:* Prof. Lorna Thorpe, Program Director, 212-396-7746, Fax: 212-481-5260, E-mail: lthor@hunter.cuny.edu. *Application contact:* Milena Solo, Director for Graduate Admissions, 212-772-4288, Fax: 212-650-3336, E-mail: milena.solo@hunter.cuny.edu.
Website: http://www.hunter.cuny.edu/uph/grad-test/epidemiology-biostatistics

Indiana University Bloomington, School of Public Health, Department of Epidemiology and Biostatistics, Bloomington, IN 47405. Offers biostatistics (MPH); epidemiology (MPH, PhD). *Faculty:* 7 full-time (3 women), 3 part-time/adjunct (all women). *Students:* 26 full-time (18 women), 3 part-time (all women); includes 9 minority (6 Black or African American, non-Hispanic/Latino; 3 Hispanic/Latino), 8 international. 49 applicants, 51% accepted, 10 enrolled. In 2013, 5 master's awarded. *Degree requirements:* For master's, thesis or alternative; for doctorate, comprehensive exam, thesis/dissertation. *Entrance requirements:* For master's, GRE (for applicants with cumulative undergraduate GPA less than 2.8); for doctorate, GRE. Additional exam requirements/recommendations for international students: Required—TOEFL (minimum score 550 paper-based; 80 iBT). *Application deadline:* For fall admission, 2/1 priority date for domestic students, 12/1 priority date for international students. Application fee: $55 ($65 for international students). Electronic applications accepted. *Financial support:* In 2013–14, 15 students received support. Fellowships, research assistantships with partial tuition reimbursements available, Federal Work-Study, institutionally sponsored loans, and health care benefits available. Financial award application deadline: 3/15; financial award applicants required to submit FAFSA. *Faculty research:* Nutritional epidemiology, cancer epidemiology, global health, biostatistics. *Unit head:* Dr. Ka He, Chair, 812-856-2448, E-mail: kahe@indiana.edu. *Application contact:* Julie Wilson, Assistant Director of Student Services, 812-856-2448, E-mail: jaw@indiana.edu.
Website: http://www.publichealth.indiana.edu/departments/epidemiology/index.shtml

Indiana University–Purdue University Indianapolis, School of Public Health, Indianapolis, IN 46202-2896. Offers biostatistics (MPH); environmental health science (MPH); epidemiology (MPH, PhD); health administration (MHA); health policy and management (MPH, PhD); social and behavioral sciences (MPH). *Accreditation:* CEPH. *Students:* 121 full-time (87 women), 161 part-time (111 women); includes 66 minority (32 Black or African American, non-Hispanic/Latino; 19 Asian, non-Hispanic/Latino; 13 Hispanic/Latino; 1 Native Hawaiian or other Pacific Islander, non-Hispanic/Latino; 1 Two or more races, non-Hispanic/Latino), 10 international. Average age 30. 185 applicants, 70% accepted, 95 enrolled. In 2013, 25 master's awarded. Application fee: $55 ($65 for international students). *Expenses:* Contact institution. *Financial support:* In 2013–14, 1 fellowship (averaging $17,650 per year), 4 research assistantships (averaging $22,000 per year), 8 teaching assistantships (averaging $24,000 per year) were awarded. *Unit head:* Dr. Paul Halverson, Dean, 317-274-4242. *Application contact:* Shawne Mathis, Student Services Coordinator, 317-278-0337, E-mail: snmathis@iupui.edu.
Website: http://www.pbhealth.iupui.edu/

Johns Hopkins University, Bloomberg School of Public Health, Department of Epidemiology, Baltimore, MD 21205. Offers cancer etiology and prevention (MHS, Sc M, PhD, Sc D); cardiovascular diseases (MHS, Sc M, PhD, Sc D); clinical epidemiology (MHS, Sc M, PhD, Sc D); clinical trials (PhD, Sc D); epidemiology (MHS, Sc M, Dr PH, PhD, Sc D); epidemiology of aging (MHS, Sc M, PhD, Sc D); genetic epidemiology (MHS, Sc M, PhD, Sc D); infectious disease epidemiology (MHS, Sc M, PhD, Sc D); occupational and environmental epidemiology (MHS, Sc M, PhD, Sc D). Part-time programs available. *Faculty:* 80 full-time (44 women), 82 part-time/adjunct (36 women). *Students:* 141 full-time (106 women), 20 part-time (13 women); includes 32 minority (5 Black or African American, non-Hispanic/Latino; 1 American Indian or Alaska Native, non-Hispanic/Latino; 18 Asian, non-Hispanic/Latino; 6 Hispanic/Latino; 2 Two or more races, non-Hispanic/Latino), 49 international. Average age 29. 302 applicants, 35% accepted, 63 enrolled. In 2013, 26 master's, 23 doctorates awarded. *Degree requirements:* For master's, comprehensive exam, thesis, 1-year full-time residency; for doctorate, comprehensive exam, thesis/dissertation, 2 years' full-time residency, oral and written exams, student teaching. *Entrance requirements:* For master's, GRE General Test or MCAT, 3 letters of recommendation, curriculum vitae; for doctorate, GRE General Test, minimum 1 year of work experience, 3 letters of recommendation, curriculum vitae, academic records from all schools. Additional exam requirements/recommendations for international students: Required—TOEFL (minimum score 600 paper-based; 100 iBT); Recommended—IELTS (minimum score 7.5), TWE. *Application deadline:* For fall admission, 12/1 priority date for domestic students. Applications are processed on a rolling basis. Application fee: $45. Electronic applications accepted. *Financial support:* Fellowships, Federal Work-Study, institutionally sponsored loans, scholarships/grants, traineeships, tuition waivers (partial), and stipends available. Support available to part-time students. Financial award application deadline: 3/15; financial award applicants required to submit FAFSA. *Faculty research:* Cancer and congenital malformations, nutritional epidemiology, AIDS, tuberculosis, cardiovascular disease, risk assessment. *Total annual research expenditures:* $70.1 million. *Unit head:* Dr. David D. Celentano, Chair, 410-955-3286, Fax: 410-955-0863, E-mail: dcelenta@jhsph.edu. *Application contact:* Frances S. Burman, Academic Program Manager, 410-955-3926, Fax: 410-955-0863, E-mail: fburman@jhsph.edu.
Website: http://www.jhsph.edu/dept/epi/index.html

Johns Hopkins University, Bloomberg School of Public Health, Department of International Health, Baltimore, MD 21205. Offers global disease epidemiology and control (MHS, PhD); health systems (MHS, PhD); human nutrition (MHS, PhD); international health (MSPH, Dr PH); registered dietician (MSPH); social and behavioral interventions (MHS, PhD). *Faculty:* 137 full-time (82 women), 185 part-time/adjunct (63 women). *Students:* 284 full-time (212 women), 4 part-time (3 women); includes 70 minority (11 Black or African American, non-Hispanic/Latino; 1 American Indian or Alaska Native, non-Hispanic/Latino; 41 Asian, non-Hispanic/Latino; 6 Hispanic/Latino; 11 Two or more races, non-Hispanic/Latino), 73 international. Average age 28. 515 applicants, 44% accepted, 104 enrolled. In 2013, 78 master's, 24 doctorates awarded. *Degree requirements:* For master's, comprehensive exam, thesis (for some programs), 1-year full-time residency, 4-9 month internship; for doctorate, comprehensive exam, thesis/dissertation or alternative, 1.5 years' full-time residency, oral and written exams. *Entrance requirements:* For master's, GRE General Test or MCAT, 3 letters of recommendation, resume; for doctorate, GRE General Test or MCAT, 3 letters of recommendation, resume, transcripts. Additional exam requirements/recommendations for international students: Required—TOEFL (minimum score 600 paper-based; 100 iBT); Recommended—IELTS (minimum score 7). *Application deadline:* For fall admission, 1/2 priority date for domestic and international students. Applications are processed on a rolling basis. Application fee: $45. Electronic applications accepted. *Financial support:* Fellowships, Federal Work-Study, institutionally sponsored loans, scholarships/grants, traineeships, and stipends available. Financial award application deadline: 1/2. *Faculty research:* Nutrition, infectious diseases, health systems, health economics, humanitarian emergencies. *Total annual research expenditures:* $72 million. *Unit head:* Dr. David Peters, Chair, 410-955-3928, Fax: 410-955-7159, E-mail: dpeters@jhsph.edu. *Application contact:* Cristina G. Salazar, Academic Program Manager, 410-955-3734, Fax: 410-955-7159, E-mail: csalazar@jhsph.edu.
Website: http://www.jhsph.edu/dept/IH/

Loma Linda University, School of Public Health, Programs in Epidemiology and Biostatistics, Loma Linda, CA 92350. Offers MPH, MSPH, Dr PH, Postbaccalaureate Certificate. *Entrance requirements:* Additional exam requirements/recommendations for international students: Required—Michigan English Language Assessment Battery or TOEFL.

Louisiana State University Health Sciences Center, School of Public Health, New Orleans, LA 70112. Offers behavioral and community health sciences (MPH); biostatistics (MPH, MS, PhD); community health sciences (PhD); environmental and occupational health sciences (MPH); epidemiology (MPH, PhD); health policy and systems management (MPH). *Accreditation:* CEPH. Part-time programs available. *Entrance requirements:* For master's, GRE General Test.

McGill University, Faculty of Graduate and Postdoctoral Studies, Faculty of Medicine, Department of Epidemiology and Biostatistics, Montréal, QC H3A 2T5, Canada. Offers community health (M Sc); environmental health (M Sc); epidemiology and biostatistics (M Sc, PhD, Diploma); health care evaluation (M Sc); medical statistics (M Sc). *Accreditation:* CEPH (one or more programs are accredited).

Medical College of Wisconsin, Graduate School of Biomedical Sciences, Department of Population Health, Milwaukee, WI 53226-0509. Offers biostatistics (PhD); epidemiology (MS); public health (MPH, PhD, Graduate Certificate), including public and community health (PhD), public health (MPH, Graduate Certificate). *Entrance requirements:* For master's, doctorate, and Graduate Certificate, GRE, official transcripts, three letters of recommendation. Additional exam requirements/recommendations for international students: Required—TOEFL.

Medical University of South Carolina, College of Graduate Studies, Division of Biostatistics and Epidemiology, Charleston, SC 29425. Offers biostatistics (MS, PhD); epidemiology (MS, PhD); DMD/PhD; MD/PhD. Terminal master's awarded for partial completion of doctoral program. *Degree requirements:* For master's, comprehensive exam, thesis (for some programs); for doctorate, comprehensive exam, oral and written exams. *Entrance requirements:* For master's, GRE General Test, two semesters of college-level calculus; for doctorate, GRE General Test, interview, minimum GPA of 3.0, two semesters of college-level calculus. Additional exam requirements/recommendations for international students: Required—TOEFL (minimum score 600 paper-based; 100 iBT). Electronic applications accepted. *Faculty research:* Health disparities, central nervous system injuries, radiation exposure, analysis of clinical trial data, biomedical information.

Memorial University of Newfoundland, Faculty of Medicine and School of Graduate Studies, Graduate Programs in Medicine, Division of Clinical Epidemiology, St. John's, NL A1C 5S7, Canada. Offers M Sc, PhD, Diploma.

Michigan State University, College of Human Medicine and The Graduate School, Graduate Programs in Human Medicine, Department of Epidemiology, East Lansing, MI 48824. Offers MS, PhD. *Degree requirements:* For master's, oral thesis defense. *Entrance requirements:* Additional exam requirements/recommendations for international students: Required—TOEFL. Electronic applications accepted.

Morehouse School of Medicine, Master of Public Health Program, Atlanta, GA 30310-1495. Offers epidemiology (MPH); health administration, management and policy (MPH); health education/health promotion (MPH); international health (MPH). *Accreditation:* CEPH. Part-time programs available. *Students:* 37 full-time (27 women), 5 part-time (3 women); includes 33 minority (32 Black or African American, non-Hispanic/Latino; 1 American Indian or Alaska Native, non-Hispanic/Latino). Average age 28. In 2013, 13 master's awarded. *Degree requirements:* For master's, thesis, practicum, public health leadership seminar. *Entrance requirements:* For master's, GRE General Test, writing test, public health or human service experience. Additional exam requirements/recommendations for international students: Required—TOEFL (minimum score 550 paper-based). *Application deadline:* For fall admission, 3/1 for domestic and international students. Application fee: $50. Electronic applications accepted. *Expenses:* Contact institution. *Financial support:* Fellowships, research assistantships with partial tuition reimbursements, teaching assistantships, career-related internships or fieldwork, Federal Work-Study, institutionally sponsored loans, scholarships/grants, and unspecified assistantships available. Support available to part-time students. Financial award application deadline: 5/1; financial award applicants required to submit FAFSA. *Faculty research:* Women's and adolescent health, violence prevention, cancer epidemiology/disparities, substance abuse prevention. *Unit head:* Dr. Stephanie Miles-Richardson, Interim Director, 404-752-1944, Fax: 404-752-1051, E-mail: smiles-richardson@msm.edu. *Application contact:* Brandon Hunter, Director of Admissions, 404-752-1650, Fax: 404-752-1512, E-mail: mphadmissions@msm.edu.
Website: http://www.msm.edu/educationTraining/degreePrograms/mph.aspx

New York Medical College, School of Health Sciences and Practice, Department of Epidemiology and Community Health, Program in Epidemiology, Valhalla, NY 10595-1691. Offers MPH. *Accreditation:* CEPH. Part-time and evening/weekend programs available. *Faculty:* 4 full-time, 14 part-time/adjunct. *Students:* 25 full-time, 40 part-time. Average age 32. 37 applicants, 68% accepted, 18 enrolled. In 2013, 18 master's awarded. *Degree requirements:* For master's, thesis. *Entrance requirements:* For master's, minimum undergraduate GPA of 3.0. Additional exam requirements/recommendations for international students: Required—TOEFL (minimum score 600 paper-based; 100 iBT), IELTS (minimum score 7). *Application deadline:* For fall admission, 8/1 priority date for domestic students, 5/15 for international students; for spring admission, 12/1 priority date for domestic students, 12/1 for international students. Applications are processed on a rolling basis. Application fee: $50 ($100 for international students). Electronic applications accepted. *Expenses: Tuition:* Full-time $49,170; part-time $910 per credit. Tuition and fees vary according to program. *Financial support:* Career-related internships or fieldwork, Federal Work-Study, institutionally sponsored loans, health care benefits, tuition waivers (partial), and tuition reimbursements available. Support available to part-time students. Financial award applicants required to submit FAFSA. *Unit head:* Dr. Maureen Kennedy, Director of MPH Studies, 914-594-4804, Fax: 914-594-4292, E-mail: jennifer_calder@nymc.edu. *Application contact:* Pamela Suett, Director of Recruitment, 914-594-4510, Fax: 914-594-4292, E-mail: shsp_admissions@nymc.edu.
Website: http://www.nymc.edu/shsp

New York University, Graduate School of Arts and Science, Department of Environmental Medicine, New York, NY 10012-1019. Offers environmental health sciences (MS, PhD), including biostatistics (PhD), environmental hygiene (MS), epidemiology (PhD), ergonomics and biomechanics (PhD), exposure assessment and health effects (PhD), molecular toxicology/carcinogenesis (PhD), toxicology. Part-time programs available. *Faculty:* 26 full-time (7 women). *Students:* 55 full-time (34 women), 13 part-time (3 women); includes 16 minority (1 Black or African American, non-Hispanic/Latino; 8 Asian, non-Hispanic/Latino; 6 Hispanic/Latino; 1 Two or more races, non-Hispanic/Latino), 23 international. Average age 31. 69 applicants, 55% accepted, 18 enrolled. In 2013, 14 master's, 7 doctorates awarded. Terminal master's awarded for partial completion of doctoral program. *Degree requirements:* For master's, thesis or alternative; for doctorate, one foreign language, thesis/dissertation, oral and written exams. *Entrance requirements:* For master's and doctorate, GRE General Test, minimum GPA of 3.0; bachelor's degree in biological, physical, or engineering science. Additional exam requirements/recommendations for international students: Required—TOEFL. *Application deadline:* For fall admission, 12/18 for domestic and international students. Application fee: $95. *Expenses: Tuition:* Full-time $35,856; part-time $1494 per unit. *Required fees:* $1408; $64 per unit. $473 per term. Tuition and fees vary according to course load and program. *Financial support:* Fellowships with tuition reimbursements, teaching assistantships with tuition reimbursements, career-related internships or fieldwork, Federal Work-Study, institutionally sponsored loans, and health care benefits available. Financial award application deadline: 12/18; financial award applicants required to submit FAFSA. *Unit head:* Dr. Max Costa, Chair, 845-731-3661, Fax: 845-351-2058, E-mail: ehs@env.med.nyu.edu. *Application contact:* Dr. Jerome J. Solomon, Director of Graduate Studies, 845-731-3661, Fax: 845-351-2058, E-mail: ehs@env.med.nyu.edu.
Website: http://environmental-medicine.med.nyu.edu/

North Carolina State University, College of Veterinary Medicine, Program in Comparative Biomedical Sciences, Raleigh, NC 27695. Offers cell biology (MS, PhD); infectious disease (MS, PhD); pathology (MS, PhD); pharmacology (MS, PhD); population medicine (MS, PhD). Part-time programs available. *Degree requirements:* For master's, thesis; for doctorate, thesis/dissertation. *Entrance requirements:* For master's and doctorate, GRE General Test. Additional exam requirements/recommendations for international students: Required—TOEFL (minimum score 550 paper-based). Electronic applications accepted. *Expenses:* Contact institution. *Faculty research:* Infectious diseases, cell biology, pharmacology and toxicology, genomics, pathology and population medicine.

North Dakota State University, College of Graduate and Interdisciplinary Studies, College of Agriculture, Food Systems, and Natural Resources, Department of Veterinary and Microbiological Sciences, Fargo, ND 58108. Offers international infectious disease (MS); microbiology (MS); molecular pathogenesis (PhD). Part-time programs available. *Faculty:* 15 full-time (8 women). *Students:* 11 full-time (6 women), 6 part-time (4 women), 5 international. Average age 30. 2 applicants, 50% accepted, 1 enrolled. In 2013, 8 master's, 1 doctorate awarded. *Degree requirements:* For master's, thesis; for doctorate, thesis/dissertation, oral and written preliminary exams. *Entrance requirements:* For master's and doctorate, GRE. Additional exam requirements/recommendations for international students: Required—TOEFL (minimum score 525 paper-based; 71 iBT). *Application deadline:* For fall admission, 2/15 priority date for domestic students. Applications are processed on a rolling basis. Application fee: $35. *Financial support:* Fellowships with full tuition reimbursements, research assistantships with full tuition reimbursements, teaching assistantships with full tuition reimbursements, Federal Work-Study, and institutionally sponsored loans available. Financial award application deadline: 4/15. *Faculty research:* Bacterial gene regulation, antibiotic resistance, molecular virology, mechanisms of bacterial pathogenesis, immunology of animals. *Unit head:* Dr. Charlene Wolf-Hall, Head, 701-231-7667, E-mail: charlene.hall@ndsu.edu. *Application contact:* Dr. John McEvoy, Associate Professor, 701-231-8530, Fax: 701-231-7514, E-mail: eugene.berry@ndsu.edu.
Website: http://vetmicro.ndsu.nodak.edu/

Northwestern University, Fienberg School of Medicine and Interdepartmental Programs, Integrated Graduate Programs in the Life Sciences, Chicago, IL 60611. Offers biostatistics (PhD); epidemiology (PhD); health and biomedical informatics (PhD); health services and outcomes research (PhD); healthcare quality and patient safety (PhD); translational outcomes in science (PhD). *Degree requirements:* For doctorate, comprehensive exam, thesis/dissertation, written and oral qualifying exams. *Entrance requirements:* For doctorate, GRE General Test. Additional exam requirements/recommendations for international students: Required—TOEFL (minimum score 600 paper-based). Electronic applications accepted.

Oregon Health & Science University, School of Medicine, Graduate Programs in Medicine, Department of Public Health and Preventive Medicine, Portland, OR 97239-3098. Offers biostatistics (MBST, MS, Graduate Certificate); epidemiology and biostatistics (MPH). *Accreditation:* CEPH. Part-time programs available. *Faculty:* 7 full-time (5 women), 26 part-time/adjunct (8 women). *Students:* 30 full-time (19 women), 31 part-time (26 women); includes 11 minority (2 Black or African American, non-Hispanic/Latino; 1 American Indian or Alaska Native, non-Hispanic/Latino; 5 Asian, non-Hispanic/Latino; 1 Native Hawaiian or other Pacific Islander, non-Hispanic/Latino; 2 Two or more races, non-Hispanic/Latino). Average age 32. 52 applicants, 46% accepted, 16 enrolled. In 2013, 23 master's awarded. *Degree requirements:* For master's, thesis, fieldwork/internship. *Entrance requirements:* For master's, GRE General Test (minimum scores: 153 Verbal/148 Quantitative/4.5 Analytical), previous undergraduate course work in statistics. Additional exam requirements/recommendations for international students: Required—TOEFL (minimum score 550 paper-based; 87 iBT). *Application deadline:* For fall admission, 2/1 for domestic students. Application fee: $70. Electronic applications accepted. *Financial support:* Health care benefits available. *Faculty research:* Epidemiologic research, biostatistics, health services research, community-based research, health disparities. *Unit head:* Dr. Thomas M. Becker, Professor/Chair, 503-494-8257, Fax: 503-494-4981, E-mail: pmph@ohsu.edu. *Application contact:* Tree Triano, Education Manager, 503-494-2012, Fax: 503-494-4981, E-mail: pmph@ohsu.edu.
Website: http://www.ohsu.edu/public-health

Oregon State University, College of Public Health and Human Sciences, Program in Public Health, Corvallis, OR 97331. Offers biostatistics (MPH); environmental and occupational health and safety (MPH, PhD); epidemiology (MPH); health management and policy (MPH); health policy (PhD); health promotion and health behavior (MPH, PhD); international health (MPH). *Accreditation:* CEPH. Part-time programs available. *Faculty:* 29 full-time (16 women), 4 part-time/adjunct (3 women). *Students:* 137 full-time (102 women), 29 part-time (18 women); includes 37 minority (4 Black or African American, non-Hispanic/Latino; 7 Asian, non-Hispanic/Latino; 17 Hispanic/Latino; 9 Two or more races, non-Hispanic/Latino), 15 international. Average age 32. 163 applicants, 58% accepted, 48 enrolled. In 2013, 39 master's, 3 doctorates awarded. Terminal master's awarded for partial completion of doctoral program. *Degree requirements:* For doctorate, one foreign language, thesis/dissertation. *Entrance requirements:* For master's and doctorate, GRE, minimum GPA of 3.0 in last 90 hours. Additional exam requirements/recommendations for international students: Required—TOEFL (minimum score 80 iBT), IELTS (minimum score 6.5). *Application deadline:* For fall admission, 12/1 for domestic students. Applications are processed on a rolling basis. Application fee: $60. *Expenses:* Contact institution. *Financial support:* Fellowships, research assistantships, teaching assistantships, career-related internships or fieldwork, Federal Work-Study, and institutionally sponsored loans available. Support available to part-time students. Financial award application deadline: 2/1. *Faculty research:* Traffic safety, health safety, injury control, health promotion. *Unit head:* Dr. Sheryl Thorburn, Professor/Co-Director, 541-737-9493. *Application contact:* Eileen Kaspar, Public Health Graduate Programs Manager, 541-737-3825, E-mail: eileen.kaspar@oregonstate.edu.

Ponce School of Medicine & Health Sciences, Program in Public Health, Ponce, PR 00732-7004. Offers epidemiology (Dr PH); public health (MPH). *Accreditation:* CEPH. *Faculty:* 4 full-time (all women), 11 part-time/adjunct (4 women). *Students:* 135 full-time (101 women); all minorities (134 Hispanic/Latino; 1 Two or more races, non-Hispanic/Latino). Average age 34. 57 applicants, 88% accepted, 46 enrolled. In 2013, 22 master's, 1 doctorate awarded. *Degree requirements:* For master's, one foreign language, comprehensive exam, thesis. *Entrance requirements:* For master's, GRE General Test or EXADEP, proficiency in Spanish and English, minimum GPA of 2.7, 3 letters of recommendation; for doctorate, GRE, proficiency in Spanish and English, minimum GPA of 3.0, letter of recommendation. *Application deadline:* For fall admission, 5/15 for domestic students. Application fee: $150. *Financial support:* In 2013–14, 73 students received support. Scholarships/grants available. Financial award application deadline: 5/30; financial award applicants required to submit FAFSA. *Unit head:* Dr. Elizabeth Anne Peterson, Head, 787-840-2575 Ext. 2232, E-mail: apeterson@psm.edu. *Application contact:* Maria Colon, Admissions Officer, 787-840-2575 Ext. 2143, E-mail: mcolon@psm.edu.

Purdue University, School of Veterinary Medicine and Graduate School, Graduate Programs in Veterinary Medicine, Department of Comparative Pathobiology, West Lafayette, IN 47907-2027. Offers comparative epidemiology and public health (MS); comparative epidemiology and public heath (PhD); comparative microbiology and immunology (MS, PhD); comparative pathobiology (MS, PhD); interdisciplinary studies (PhD), including microbial pathogenesis, molecular signaling and cancer biology, molecular virology; lab animal medicine (MS); veterinary anatomic pathology (MS); veterinary clinical pathology (MS). Terminal master's awarded for partial completion of doctoral program. *Degree requirements:* For master's, thesis (for some programs); for doctorate, thesis/dissertation. *Entrance requirements:* For master's and doctorate, GRE General Test. Additional exam requirements/recommendations for international students: Required—TOEFL (minimum score 575 paper-based), IELTS (minimum score 6.5), TWE (minimum score 4). Electronic applications accepted.

Queen's University at Kingston, School of Graduate Studies, Faculty of Health Sciences, Department of Community Health and Epidemiology, Kingston, ON K7L 3N6, Canada. Offers epidemiology (PhD); epidemiology and population health (M Sc); health services (M Sc); policy research and clinical epidemiology (M Sc); public health (MPH). Part-time programs available. *Degree requirements:* For master's, thesis. *Entrance requirements:* For master's, GRE General Test (strongly recommended). Additional exam requirements/recommendations for international students: Required—TOEFL (minimum score 600 paper-based). *Faculty research:* Cancer epidemiology, clinical trials, biostatistics health services research, health policy.

Epidemiology

Rutgers, The State University of New Jersey, Newark, School of Public Health, Newark, NJ 07107-1709. Offers clinical epidemiology (Certificate); dental public health (MPH); general public health (Certificate); public policy and oral health services administration (Certificate); quantitative methods (MPH); urban health (MPH); DMD/MPH; MD/MPH; MS/MPH. *Accreditation:* CEPH. Part-time and evening/weekend programs available. *Degree requirements:* For master's, thesis, internship. *Entrance requirements:* For master's, GRE General Test. Additional exam requirements/recommendations for international students: Required—TOEFL. Electronic applications accepted.

Rutgers, The State University of New Jersey, New Brunswick, School of Public Health, Piscataway, NJ 08854. Offers biostatistics (MPH, MS, Dr PH, PhD); clinical epidemiology (Certificate); environmental and occupational health (MPH, Dr PH, PhD, Certificate); epidemiology (MPH, Dr PH, PhD); general public health (Certificate); health education and behavioral science (MPH, Dr PH, PhD); health systems and policy (MPH, PhD); public health preparedness (Certificate); DO/MPH; JD/MPH; MD/MPH; MPH/MBA; MPH/MSPA; MS/MPH; Psy D/MPH. *Accreditation:* CEPH. Part-time and evening/weekend programs available. *Degree requirements:* For master's, thesis, internship; for doctorate, comprehensive exam, thesis/dissertation. *Entrance requirements:* For master's, GRE General Test; for doctorate, GRE General Test, MPH (Dr PH); MA, MPH, or MS (PhD). Additional exam requirements/recommendations for international students: Required—TOEFL. Electronic applications accepted.

San Diego State University, Graduate and Research Affairs, College of Health and Human Services, Graduate School of Public Health, San Diego, CA 92182. Offers environmental health (MPH); epidemiology (MPH, PhD), including biostatistics (MPH); global emergency preparedness and response (MS); global health (PhD); health behavior (PhD); health promotion (MPH); health services administration (MPH); toxicology (MS); MPH/MA; MSW/MPH. *Accreditation:* CAHME (one or more programs are accredited); CEPH (one or more programs are accredited). Part-time programs available. *Degree requirements:* For master's, comprehensive exam (for some programs), thesis (for some programs); for doctorate, thesis/dissertation. *Entrance requirements:* For master's, GMAT (MPH in health services administration), GRE General Test; for doctorate, GRE General Test. Additional exam requirements/recommendations for international students: Required—TOEFL. *Faculty research:* Evaluation of tobacco, AIDS prevalence and prevention, mammography, infant death project, Alzheimer's in elderly Chinese.

Stanford University, School of Medicine, Graduate Programs in Medicine, Department of Health Research and Policy, Division of Epidemiology, Stanford, CA 94305-9991. Offers MS. *Degree requirements:* For master's, thesis. *Entrance requirements:* Additional exam requirements/recommendations for international students: Required—TOEFL. Electronic applications accepted. *Expenses: Tuition:* Full-time $42,690; part-time $949 per credit. *Required fees:* $185.

Temple University, College of Health Professions and Social Work, Department of Public Health, Philadelphia, PA 19122. Offers clinical research and translational medicine (MS); environmental health (MPH); epidemiology (MS); epidemiology and biostatistics (MPH); health policy (PhD); health policy and management (MPH); school health education (Ed M); social and behavioral sciences (MPH, PhD). *Accreditation:* CEPH (one or more programs are accredited). Part-time and evening/weekend programs available. *Faculty:* 27 full-time (18 women). *Students:* 47 full-time (30 women), 45 part-time (37 women); includes 27 minority (9 Black or African American, non-Hispanic/Latino; 10 Asian, non-Hispanic/Latino; 7 Hispanic/Latino; 1 Two or more races, non-Hispanic/Latino), 9 international. 188 applicants, 45% accepted, 29 enrolled. In 2013, 29 master's, 3 doctorates awarded. Terminal master's awarded for partial completion of doctoral program. *Degree requirements:* For master's, thesis (for some programs), capstone project; for doctorate, comprehensive exam, thesis/dissertation. *Entrance requirements:* For master's, GRE General Test (for MS only); DAT, GMAT, MCAT, OAT, PCAT (alternates for MPH, Ed M), minimum undergraduate GPA of 3.0, letters of reference, statement of goals, writing sample, resume, interview (only for MS); for doctorate, GRE General Test, minimum undergraduate GPA of 3.0, 3 letters of reference, statement of goals, writing sample, resume. Additional exam requirements/recommendations for international students: Required—TOEFL (minimum score 550 paper-based; 79 iBT). *Application deadline:* For fall admission, 3/1 for domestic students, 2/1 for international students; for spring admission, 10/15 for domestic students, 8/1 for international students. Applications are processed on a rolling basis. Application fee: $60. Electronic applications accepted. *Financial support:* In 2013–14, 1 fellowship with tuition reimbursement, 4 research assistantships with tuition reimbursements, 8 teaching assistantships with tuition reimbursements were awarded; career-related internships or fieldwork, Federal Work-Study, scholarships/grants, tuition waivers (partial), and unspecified assistantships also available. Financial award application deadline: 1/15. *Faculty research:* Smoking cessation, obesity prevention, tobacco policy, community engagement, health communication. *Total annual research expenditures:* $3.9 million. *Unit head:* Dr. Alice J. Hausman, Chair, 215-204-5112, Fax: 215-204-1854, E-mail: hausman@temple.edu. *Application contact:* Joyce Hankins, 215-204-7213, E-mail: joyce.hankins@temple.edu.
Website: http://chpsw.temple.edu/publichealth/home

Texas A&M Health Science Center, School of Rural Public Health, College Station, TX 77840. Offers environmental/occupational health (MPH); epidemiology/biostatistics (MPH); health policy/management (MPH); social and behavioral health (MPH). *Accreditation:* CEPH. Part-time programs available. Postbaccalaureate distance learning degree programs offered (no on-campus study). *Degree requirements:* For master's, thesis optional. *Entrance requirements:* For master's, GRE General Test, minimum undergraduate GPA of 3.0. Electronic applications accepted. *Faculty research:* Tobacco cessation, youth health risk.

Texas A&M University, College of Veterinary Medicine and Biomedical Sciences, Department of Veterinary Integrative Biosciences, College Station, TX 77843. Offers veterinary public health (MS), including epidemiology. *Faculty:* 29. *Students:* 51 full-time (27 women), 13 part-time (10 women); includes 11 minority (1 Black or African American, non-Hispanic/Latino; 5 Asian, non-Hispanic/Latino; 3 Hispanic/Latino; 2 Two or more races, non-Hispanic/Latino), 16 international. Average age 27. 16 applicants, 50% accepted, 8 enrolled. In 2013, 19 master's awarded. Terminal master's awarded for partial completion of doctoral program. *Degree requirements:* For master's, comprehensive exam, thesis. *Entrance requirements:* For master's, GRE General Test, minimum undergraduate GPA of 3.0. Additional exam requirements/recommendations for international students: Required—TOEFL. *Application deadline:* For fall admission, 7/15 priority date for domestic students, 4/1 priority date for international students; for spring admission, 10/1 priority date for domestic students, 9/15 priority date for international students. Applications are processed on a rolling basis. Application fee: $50 ($75 for international students). Electronic applications accepted. *Expenses:* Tuition, state resident: full-time $4078; part-time $226.55 per credit hour. Tuition, nonresident: full-time $10,450; part-time $580.55 per credit hour. *Required fees:* $2328; $278.50 per credit hour. $642.45 per semester. *Financial support:* In 2013–14, fellowships (averaging $18,000 per year), research assistantships (averaging $15,600 per year), teaching assistantships (averaging $15,600 per year) were awarded; institutionally sponsored loans, unspecified assistantships, and clinical associateships also available. Financial award application deadline: 7/15; financial award applicants required to submit FAFSA. *Faculty research:* Metal toxicology, reproductive biology, genetics of neural development, developmental biology, environmental toxicology. *Unit head:* Dr. Evelyn Tiffany-Castiglioni, Head, 979-458-1077, E-mail: c-tiffany@tamu.edu. *Application contact:* Graduate Admissions, 979-845-1044, E-mail: admissions@tamu.edu.
Website: http://vetmed.tamu.edu/vibs

Thomas Edison State College, School of Applied Science and Technology, Program in Clinical Trials Management, Trenton, NJ 08608-1176. Offers Graduate Certificate. Part-time programs available. Postbaccalaureate distance learning degree programs offered (no on-campus study). *Entrance requirements:* Additional exam requirements/recommendations for international students: Required—TOEFL (minimum score 550 paper-based; 79 iBT). Electronic applications accepted.

Tufts University, Graduate School of Arts and Sciences, Graduate Certificate Programs, Program in Epidemiology, Medford, MA 02155. Offers Certificate. Electronic applications accepted.

Tufts University, Sackler School of Graduate Biomedical Sciences, Clinical and Translational Science Program, Medford, MA 02155. Offers MS, PhD. *Faculty:* 34 full-time (10 women). *Students:* 24 full-time (11 women), 3 part-time (2 women); includes 3 minority (all Asian, non-Hispanic/Latino), 8 international. Average age 37. 20 applicants, 65% accepted, 10 enrolled. In 2013, 13 master's, 1 doctorate awarded. Terminal master's awarded for partial completion of doctoral program. *Degree requirements:* For master's, thesis; for doctorate, comprehensive exam, thesis/dissertation. *Entrance requirements:* For master's, MD or PhD, strong clinical research background. Additional exam requirements/recommendations for international students: Required—TOEFL (minimum score 600 paper-based; 100 iBT). *Application deadline:* For fall admission, 12/15 for domestic and international students. Application fee: $70. Electronic applications accepted. *Financial support:* Application deadline: 12/15. *Faculty research:* Clinical study design, mathematical modeling, meta analysis, epidemiologic research, coronary heart disease. *Unit head:* Dr. David Kent, Program Director, 617-636-3234, Fax: 617-636-8023, E-mail: dkent@tuftsmedicalcenter.edu. *Application contact:* Kellie Melchin, Associate Director of Admissions, 617-636-6767, Fax: 617-636-0375, E-mail: sackler-school@tufts.edu.
Website: http://sackler.tufts.edu/Academics/Degree-Programs/PhD-Programs/Clinical-and-Translational-Science

Tulane University, School of Public Health and Tropical Medicine, Department of Epidemiology, New Orleans, LA 70118-5669. Offers MPH, MS, Dr PH, PhD. MS and PhD offered through the Graduate School. *Accreditation:* CEPH (one or more programs are accredited). Part-time programs available. *Degree requirements:* For doctorate, comprehensive exam, thesis/dissertation. *Entrance requirements:* For master's and doctorate, GRE General Test. Additional exam requirements/recommendations for international students: Required—TOEFL. Electronic applications accepted. *Faculty research:* Environment, cancer, cardiovascular epidemiology, women's health.

Université Laval, Faculty of Medicine, Graduate Programs in Medicine, Department of Medicine, Programs in Epidemiology, Québec, QC G1K 7P4, Canada. Offers M Sc, PhD. Terminal master's awarded for partial completion of doctoral program. *Degree requirements:* For master's, thesis; for doctorate, comprehensive exam, thesis/dissertation. *Entrance requirements:* For master's and doctorate, knowledge of French, comprehension of written English. Electronic applications accepted.

University at Albany, State University of New York, School of Public Health, Department of Epidemiology and Biostatistics, Albany, NY 12222-0001. Offers MS, PhD. *Degree requirements:* For master's, thesis; for doctorate, thesis/dissertation. *Entrance requirements:* For master's and doctorate, GRE General Test. Additional exam requirements/recommendations for international students: Required—TOEFL (minimum score 550 paper-based). Electronic applications accepted.

University at Buffalo, the State University of New York, Graduate School, School of Public Health and Health Professions, Department of Epidemiology and Environmental Health, Buffalo, NY 14214. Offers epidemiology (MS, PhD); public health (MPH). *Accreditation:* CEPH. Part-time programs available. *Faculty:* 13 full-time (7 women), 6 part-time/adjunct (3 women). *Students:* 46 full-time (29 women), 14 part-time (11 women); includes 7 minority (2 Black or African American, non-Hispanic/Latino; 5 Asian, non-Hispanic/Latino), 8 international. Average age 29. 147 applicants, 46% accepted, 39 enrolled. In 2013, 15 master's awarded. Terminal master's awarded for partial completion of doctoral program. *Degree requirements:* For master's, comprehensive exam, thesis; for doctorate, comprehensive exam, thesis/dissertation. *Entrance requirements:* For master's and doctorate, GRE General Test. Additional exam requirements/recommendations for international students: Required—TOEFL (minimum score 600 paper-based; 100 iBT). *Application deadline:* For fall admission, 1/15 priority date for domestic and international students. Applications are processed on a rolling basis. Application fee: $50. Electronic applications accepted. *Financial support:* In 2013–14, 17 students received support, including 4 fellowships with full tuition reimbursements available (averaging $22,000 per year), 5 research assistantships with full tuition reimbursements available (averaging $20,000 per year); teaching assistantships with full tuition reimbursements available, career-related internships or fieldwork, Federal Work-Study, institutionally sponsored loans, health care benefits, and unspecified assistantships also available. Financial award application deadline: 2/1; financial award applicants required to submit FAFSA. *Faculty research:* Epidemiology of cancer, nutrition, infectious diseases, epidemiology of environmental, women's health and cardiovascular disease research. *Unit head:* Dr. Youfa Yang, Chair, 716-829-5375, Fax: 716-829-2979, E-mail: phhpadv@buffalo.edu. *Application contact:* Dr. Carl Li, Director of Graduate Studies, 716-829-5382, Fax: 716-829-2979, E-mail: carlli@buffalo.edu.
Website: http://sphhp.buffalo.edu/spm/

The University of Alabama at Birmingham, School of Public Health, Program in Epidemiology, Birmingham, AL 35294. Offers PhD. *Degree requirements:* For doctorate, thesis/dissertation, teaching practicum. *Entrance requirements:* For doctorate, GRE General Test, MPH or MSPH. Additional exam requirements/recommendations for international students: Recommended—TOEFL, IELTS. *Faculty research:* Biometry.

The University of Alabama at Birmingham, School of Public Health, Program in Public Health, Birmingham, AL 35294. Offers accelerated industrial hygiene (MPH); applied epidemiology (MSPH); biostatistics (MPH); clinical and translational science (MSPH); environmental health (MPH); environmental health and toxicology (MSPH); epidemiology (MPH); general theory and practice (MPH); health behavior (MPH); health care organization (MPH); health policy quantitative policy analysis (MPH); industrial hygiene (MPH, MSPH); maternal and child health policy (Dr PH); maternal and child health policy and leadership (MPH); occupational health and safety (MPH); outcomes research (MSPH, Dr PH); pharmacoepidemiology and comparative effectiveness research (MSPH); public health (PhD); public health management (Dr PH); public health preparedness management (MPH). *Accreditation:* CEPH. *Entrance requirements:* For master's and doctorate, GRE, evaluations. Additional exam requirements/recommendations for international students: Recommended—TOEFL (minimum score 550 paper-based; 79 iBT), IELTS (minimum score 6.5).

University of Alberta, School of Public Health, Department of Public Health Sciences, Edmonton, AB T6G 2E1, Canada. Offers clinical epidemiology (M Sc, MPH); environmental and occupational health (MPH); environmental health sciences (M Sc); epidemiology (M Sc); global health (M Sc, MPH); health policy and management (MPH); health policy research (M Sc); health technology assessment (MPH); occupational health (M Sc); population health (M Sc); public health leadership (MPH); public health sciences (PhD); quantitative methods (MPH). *Accreditation:* CEPH (one or more programs are accredited). Terminal master's awarded for partial completion of doctoral program. *Degree requirements:* For master's, thesis (for some programs); for doctorate, thesis/dissertation. *Entrance requirements:* For master's, GMAT or GRE General Test. Additional exam requirements/recommendations for international students: Required—TOEFL (minimum score 550 paper-based) or IELTS (minimum score 6). Electronic applications accepted. *Faculty research:* Biostatistics, health promotion and socio-behavioral health science.

The University of Arizona, Mel and Enid Zuckerman College of Public Health, Program in Epidemiology, Tucson, AZ 85721. Offers MS, PhD. *Faculty:* 13 full-time (8 women), 1 part-time/adjunct (0 women). *Students:* 14 full-time (9 women), 4 part-time (0 women); includes 6 minority (1 Black or African American, non-Hispanic/Latino; 2 Asian, non-Hispanic/Latino; 1 Hispanic/Latino; 2 Two or more races, non-Hispanic/Latino), 2 international. Average age 34. 53 applicants, 19% accepted, 2 enrolled. In 2013, 4 doctorates awarded. *Entrance requirements:* Additional exam requirements/recommendations for international students: Required—TOEFL (minimum score 550 paper-based; 79 iBT). *Application deadline:* For fall admission, 1/1 for domestic and international students. Applications are processed on a rolling basis. Application fee: $75. Electronic applications accepted. *Expenses:* Tuition, state resident: full-time $11,526. Tuition, nonresident: full-time $27,398. *Financial support:* In 2013–14, 7 research assistantships (averaging $19,034 per year), 13 teaching assistantships (averaging $27,146 per year) were awarded. *Total annual research expenditures:* $3.5 million. *Unit head:* Dr. Iman Hakim, Dean, 520-626-7083, E-mail: ihakim@email.arizona.edu. *Application contact:* Amy Glicken, Special Assistant to the Dean, 520-626-3201, E-mail: coph-admit@email.arizona.edu.

University of Arkansas for Medical Sciences, College of Public Health, Little Rock, AR 72205-7199. Offers biostatistics (MPH); environmental and occupational health (MPH, Certificate); epidemiology (MPH, PhD); health behavior and health education (MPH); health policy and management (MPH); health promotion and prevention research (PhD); health services administration (MHSA); health systems research (PhD); public health (Certificate); public health leadership (Dr PH). Part-time programs available. *Faculty:* 37 full-time (19 women), 9 part-time/adjunct (5 women). *Students:* 56 full-time (35 women), 85 part-time (58 women); includes 54 minority (38 Black or African American, non-Hispanic/Latino; 1 American Indian or Alaska Native, non-Hispanic/Latino; 8 Asian, non-Hispanic/Latino; 3 Hispanic/Latino; 1 Native Hawaiian or other Pacific Islander, non-Hispanic/Latino; 3 Two or more races, non-Hispanic/Latino), 5 international. Average age 30. 70 applicants, 91% accepted, 33 enrolled. In 2013, 2 master's, 1 doctorate, 2 other advanced degrees awarded. *Degree requirements:* For master's, preceptorship, culminating experience, internship; for doctorate, comprehensive exam, capstone. *Entrance requirements:* For master's, GRE, GMAT, LSAT, PCAT, MCAT, DAT; for doctorate, GRE. Additional exam requirements/recommendations for international students: Required—TOEFL (minimum score 80 iBT), IELTS. *Application deadline:* For fall admission, 3/1 for domestic students, 2/1 for international students; for spring admission, 8/1 for domestic and international students; for summer admission, 2/1 for domestic and international students. Application fee: $25 ($50 for international students). Electronic applications accepted. *Expenses:* Contact institution. *Financial support:* In 2013–14, 8 research assistantships with full tuition reimbursements (averaging $13,000 per year) were awarded; scholarships/grants and tuition waivers (full and partial) also available. *Faculty research:* Health systems, tobacco prevention control, obesity prevention, environmental and occupational exposure, cancer prevention. *Unit head:* Dr. James M. Raczynski, Dean, 501-526-6600, E-mail: raczynskijameson@uams.edu. *Application contact:* Angie Choi, Director of Admission, 501-526-4620, Fax: 501-526-6750, E-mail: anchoi@uams.edu.
Website: http://publichealth.uams.edu/

The University of British Columbia, Faculty of Medicine, School of Population and Public Health, Vancouver, BC V6T 1Z3, Canada. Offers health administration (MHA); health care and epidemiology (MH Sc, PhD); public health (MPH). *Accreditation:* CEPH (one or more programs are accredited). Postbaccalaureate distance learning degree programs offered (minimal on-campus study). *Degree requirements:* For master's, thesis (for some programs), major paper (MH Sc), research project (MHA); for doctorate, thesis/dissertation. *Entrance requirements:* For master's, GRE General Test or GMAT, PCAT, MCAT (MHA), MD or equivalent (for MH Sc); 4-year undergraduate degree from accredited university with minimum B+ overall academic average and in math or statistics course at undergraduate level (for MPH); 4-year undergraduate degree from accredited university with minimum B+ overall academic average plus work experience (for MHA); for doctorate, master's degree from accredited university with minimum B+ overall academic average and in math or statistics course at undergraduate level. Additional exam requirements/recommendations for international students: Required—TOEFL. Electronic applications accepted. *Expenses: Tuition, area resident:* Full-time $8000 Canadian dollars. *Faculty research:* Population and public health, clinical epidemiology, epidemiology and biostatistics, global health and vulnerable populations, health care services and systems, occupational and environmental health, public health emerging threats and rapid response, social and life course determinants of health, health administration.

University of California, Berkeley, Graduate Division, School of Public Health, Group in Epidemiology, Berkeley, CA 94720-1500. Offers epidemiology (MS, PhD); infectious diseases (MPH, PhD). *Accreditation:* CEPH (one or more programs are accredited). *Degree requirements:* For master's, comprehensive exam; for doctorate, thesis/dissertation, oral and written exam. *Entrance requirements:* For master's, GRE General Test, minimum GPA of 3.0; MD, DDS, DVM, or PhD in biomedical science (MPH); for doctorate, GRE General Test, minimum GPA of 3.0.

University of California, Davis, Graduate Studies, Graduate Group in Epidemiology, Davis, CA 95616. Offers MS, PhD. Terminal master's awarded for partial completion of doctoral program. *Degree requirements:* For master's, comprehensive exam (for some programs), thesis (for some programs); for doctorate, thesis/dissertation. *Entrance requirements:* For master's and doctorate, GRE General Test, GRE Subject Test (biology), minimum GPA of 3.25. Additional exam requirements/recommendations for international students: Required—TOEFL (minimum score 550 paper-based). Electronic applications accepted. *Faculty research:* Environmental/occupational wildlife, reproductive and veterinary epidemiology, infectious/chronic disease epidemiology, public health.

University of California, Irvine, School of Medicine, Department of Epidemiology, Irvine, CA 92697. Offers MS, PhD. *Students:* 10 full-time (6 women); includes 6 minority (3 Asian, non-Hispanic/Latino; 3 Hispanic/Latino). Average age 28. 38 applicants, 21% accepted, 5 enrolled. In 2013, 1 doctorate awarded. Terminal master's awarded for partial completion of doctoral program. *Degree requirements:* For master's, comprehensive exam, thesis; for doctorate, comprehensive exam, thesis/dissertation, 72 quarter units. *Entrance requirements:* For master's, GRE, minimum GPA of 3.0, letters of recommendation; for doctorate, GRE, minimum GPA of 3.0, personal statement, letters of recommendation. Additional exam requirements/recommendations for international students: Required—TOEFL (minimum score 550 paper-based; 80 iBT), IELTS (minimum score 7). *Application deadline:* For fall admission, 1/15 priority date for domestic and international students. Application fee: $80 ($100 for international students). Electronic applications accepted. *Financial support:* In 2013–14, fellowships with full tuition reimbursements (averaging $25,000 per year), research assistantships with full tuition reimbursements (averaging $46,000 per year), teaching assistantships with full tuition reimbursements (averaging $33,000 per year) were awarded; Federal Work-Study, institutionally sponsored loans, scholarships/grants, traineeships, health care benefits, and unspecified assistantships also available. Financial award application deadline: 1/15; financial award applicants required to submit FAFSA. *Faculty research:* Genetic/molecular epidemiology, cancer epidemiology, biostatistics, environmental health, occupational health. *Total annual research expenditures:* $15 million. *Unit head:* Dr. Hoda Anton-Culver, Chair, 949-824-7401, Fax: 949-824-4773, E-mail: hantoncu@uci.edu. *Application contact:* Julie Strope, Departmental Administrator, 949-824-0306, Fax: 949-824-4773, E-mail: jstrope@uci.edu.
Website: http://www.epi.uci.edu/

University of California, Irvine, School of Social Ecology, Programs in Social Ecology, Irvine, CA 92697. Offers environmental analysis and design (PhD); epidemiology and public health (PhD); social ecology (PhD). *Students:* 9 full-time (8 women), 2 part-time (0 women); includes 2 minority (1 Asian, non-Hispanic/Latino; 1 Hispanic/Latino), 1 international. Average age 33. 32 applicants, 13% accepted, 2 enrolled. In 2013, 3 doctorates awarded. Application fee: $80 ($100 for international students). *Unit head:* Valerie Jenness, Dean, 949-824-6094, Fax: 949-824-1845, E-mail: jenness@uci.edu. *Application contact:* Adriana Collins, Director of Graduate Student Services, 949-824-5918, Fax: 949-824-1845, E-mail: ajcollins@uci.edu.
Website: http://socialecology.uci.edu/core/graduate-se-core-programs

University of California, Los Angeles, Graduate Division, School of Public Health, Department of Epidemiology, Los Angeles, CA 90095. Offers MPH, MS, Dr PH, PhD, MD/MPH. *Degree requirements:* For master's, comprehensive exam or thesis; for doctorate, thesis/dissertation, oral and written qualifying exams. *Entrance requirements:* For master's, GRE General Test, minimum GPA of 3.0; for doctorate, GRE General Test, minimum undergraduate GPA of 3.0. Electronic applications accepted.

University of California, San Diego, Office of Graduate Studies, Program in Public Health, La Jolla, CA 92093-0901. Offers public health and epidemiology (PhD); public health and global health (PhD); public health and health behavior (PhD). Program offered jointly with San Diego State University. *Students:* 35 (25 women); includes 11 minority (3 Black or African American, non-Hispanic/Latino; 4 Asian, non-Hispanic/Latino; 4 Hispanic/Latino), 4 international. In 2013, 11 doctorates awarded. *Degree requirements:* For doctorate, thesis/dissertation, 2 semesters/quarters of teaching assistantship. *Entrance requirements:* For doctorate, GRE General Test, minimum GPA of 3.0. Additional exam requirements/recommendations for international students: Required—TOEFL, IELTS. *Application deadline:* For fall admission, 12/14 for domestic students. Application fee: $55. Electronic applications accepted. *Expenses:* Tuition, state resident: full-time $11,220; part-time $1870 per quarter. Tuition, nonresident: full-time $26,322; part-time $4387 per quarter. *Required fees:* $519.50 per quarter. Part-time tuition and fees vary according to course load and program. *Faculty research:* Maternal and pediatric HIV/AIDS; healthy aging and gender differences; non-parametric and semi-parametric regression, resampling, and the analysis of high-dimensional data; neighborhood correlates of physical activity in children, teens, adults and older adults; medication safety and medication therapy management through practice-based research networks. *Unit head:* John Pierce, Program Director, 858-822-2380, E-mail: jppierce@ucsd.edu. *Application contact:* Hollie Ward, Graduate Coordinator, 858-822-2382, E-mail: hward@ucsd.edu.
Website: http://publichealth.ucsd.edu/jdp/

University of Cincinnati, Graduate School, College of Medicine, Graduate Programs in Biomedical Sciences, Department of Environmental Health, Cincinnati, OH 45221. Offers environmental and industrial hygiene (MS, PhD); environmental and occupational medicine (MS); environmental genetics and molecular toxicology (MS, PhD); epidemiology and biostatistics (MS, PhD); occupational safety and ergonomics (MS, PhD). *Accreditation:* ABET (one or more programs are accredited). Terminal master's awarded for partial completion of doctoral program. *Degree requirements:* For master's, thesis; for doctorate, thesis/dissertation, qualifying exam. *Entrance requirements:* For master's, GRE General Test, bachelor's degree in science; for doctorate, GRE General Test. Additional exam requirements/recommendations for international students: Required—TOEFL (minimum score 600 paper-based; 100 iBT). Electronic applications accepted. *Faculty research:* Carcinogens and mutagenesis, pulmonary studies, reproduction and development.

University of Colorado Denver, Colorado School of Public Health, Department of Epidemiology, Aurora, CO 80045. Offers MS, PhD. Part-time programs available. *Faculty:* 14 full-time (12 women), 4 part-time/adjunct (3 women). *Students:* 19 full-time (11 women), 3 part-time (all women); includes 5 minority (1 Black or African American, non-Hispanic/Latino; 1 American Indian or Alaska Native, non-Hispanic/Latino; 2 Hispanic/Latino; 1 Two or more races, non-Hispanic/Latino), 1 international. Average age 30. 23 applicants, 26% accepted, 5 enrolled. In 2013, 2 master's, 1 doctorate awarded. *Degree requirements:* For master's, thesis, 38 credit hours; for doctorate, comprehensive exam, thesis/dissertation, 67 credit hours. *Entrance requirements:* For master's, GRE General Test, baccalaureate degree in scientific field, minimum GPA of 3.0, math course work through integral calculus, two official copies of all academic transcripts, four letters of recommendation/reference, essays describing the applicant's career goals and reasons for applying to the program, resume; for doctorate, GRE or MCAT, bachelor's, master's, or higher degree; minimum undergraduate and graduate GPA of 3.0; coursework in calculus, organic chemistry, epidemiology, biological sciences, and public health; 2 official copies of all academic transcripts; 4 letters of reference; essays. Additional exam requirements/recommendations for international students: Required—TOEFL (minimum score 550 paper-based; 80 iBT). *Application deadline:* For fall admission, 2/1 priority date for domestic students, 1/15 priority date for international students. Application fee: $65. Electronic applications accepted. *Expenses:* Contact institution. *Financial support:* In 2013–14, 11 students received support. Fellowships, research assistantships, teaching assistantships, Federal Work-Study, institutionally sponsored loans, scholarships/grants, traineeships, and unspecified assistantships available. Financial award application deadline: 3/1; financial award applicants required to submit FAFSA. *Faculty research:* Public health practice and practice-based research, reproductive and perinatal epidemiology, obesity, infectious disease epidemiology, diabetes. *Unit head:* Dr. Jill Norris, Chair, 303-724-4428, E-mail: jill.norris@ucdenver.edu. *Application contact:* Melodie Proffitt, Department Assistant, 303-724-4488, E-mail: melodie.proffitt@ucdenver.edu.
Website: http://www.ucdenver.edu/academics/colleges/PublicHealth/departments/Epidemiology/Pages/welcome.aspx

University of Colorado Denver, Colorado School of Public Health, Program in Public Health, Aurora, CO 80045. Offers community and behavioral health (MPH, Dr PH);

environmental and occupational health (MPH); epidemiology (MPH); health systems, management and policy (MPH). *Accreditation:* CEPH. Part-time and evening/weekend programs available. *Faculty:* 14 full-time (13 women). *Students:* 295 full-time (247 women), 49 part-time (39 women); includes 77 minority (17 Black or African American, non-Hispanic/Latino; 3 American Indian or Alaska Native, non-Hispanic/Latino; 16 Asian, non-Hispanic/Latino; 31 Hispanic/Latino; 10 Two or more races, non-Hispanic/Latino), 5 international. Average age 30. 657 applicants, 71% accepted, 132 enrolled. In 2013, 106 master's awarded. *Degree requirements:* For master's, thesis or alternative, 42 credit hours; for doctorate, comprehensive exam, thesis/dissertation, 67 credit hours. *Entrance requirements:* For master's, GRE, MCAT, DAT, LSAT, PCAT, GMAT or master's degree from accredited institution, baccalaureate degree or equivalent; minimum GPA of 3.0; transcripts; references; resume; essay; for doctorate, GRE, MCAT, DAT, LSAT, PCAT or GMAT, MPH or master's or higher degree in related field or equivalent; 2 years of previous work experience in public health; essay; resume. Additional exam requirements/recommendations for international students: Required—TOEFL (minimum score 550 paper-based; 80 iBT). *Application deadline:* For fall admission, 12/15 priority date for domestic students, 12/1 priority date for international students. Application fee: $65. Electronic applications accepted. *Expenses:* Contact institution. *Financial support:* In 2013–14, 125 students received support. Fellowships, research assistantships, teaching assistantships, Federal Work-Study, institutionally sponsored loans, scholarships/grants, traineeships, and unspecified assistantships available. Financial award application deadline: 3/15; financial award applicants required to submit FAFSA. *Faculty research:* Cancer prevention by nutrition, cancer survivorship outcomes, social and cultural factors related to health. *Unit head:* Dr. Lori Crane, Chair, 303-724-4385, E-mail: lori.crane@ucdenver.edu. *Application contact:* Carla Denerstein, Departmental Assistant, 303-724-4446, E-mail: carla.denerstein@ucdenver.edu.
Website: http://www.ucdenver.edu/academics/colleges/PublicHealth/departments/CommunityBehavioralHealth/Pages/CommunityBehavioralHealth.aspx

University of Florida, College of Medicine, Program in Clinical Investigation, Gainesville, FL 32611. Offers clinical investigation (MS); epidemiology (MS); public health (MPH). Part-time programs available. *Entrance requirements:* For master's, GRE, MD, PhD, DMD/DDS or Pharm D. *Expenses:* Tuition, state resident: full-time $12,640. Tuition, nonresident: full-time $30,000.

University of Florida, Graduate School, College of Public Health and Health Professions, Department of Epidemiology, Gainesville, FL 32610. Offers clinical and translational science (PhD); epidemiology (MS, PhD). *Faculty:* 10 full-time (5 women). *Students:* 23 full-time (13 women), 3 part-time (1 woman); includes 5 minority (2 Black or African American, non-Hispanic/Latino; 2 Asian, non-Hispanic/Latino; 1 Hispanic/Latino), 10 international. Average age 30. 50 applicants, 8% accepted, 4 enrolled. In 2013, 2 doctorates awarded. *Degree requirements:* For master's, thesis; for doctorate, thesis/dissertation. *Entrance requirements:* For master's and doctorate, GRE, minimum GPA of 3.0. Additional exam requirements/recommendations for international students: Required—TOEFL (minimum score 550 paper-based; 80 iBT), IELTS (minimum score 6). *Application deadline:* For fall admission, 2/1 for domestic students. Application fee: $30. *Expenses:* Tuition, state resident: full-time $12,640. Tuition, nonresident: full-time $30,000. *Financial support:* In 2013–14, 18 students received support, including 3 fellowships (averaging $18,695 per year), 8 research assistantships (averaging $15,010 per year), 10 teaching assistantships (averaging $19,220 per year). Financial award applicants required to submit FAFSA. *Unit head:* Linda Cottler, PhD, Chair, 352-273-5468, E-mail: lbcottler@ufl.edu. *Application contact:* Betsy Jones, Program Assistant, 352-273-5961, E-mail: bjcop@ufl.edu.
Website: http://epidemiology.phhp.ufl.edu/

University of Florida, Graduate School, College of Public Health and Health Professions, Programs in Public Health, Gainesville, FL 32611. Offers biostatistics (MPH); environmental and global health (PhD); environmental health (MPH); epidemiology (MPH); one health (PhD); public health (MPH, PhD, Certificate); public health management and policy (MPH); public health practice (MPH); social and behavioral sciences (MPH); DPT/MPH; DVM/MPH; JD/MPH; MD/MPH; Pharm D/MPH. *Accreditation:* CEPH. Postbaccalaureate distance learning degree programs offered. *Students:* 152 full-time (115 women), 63 part-time (36 women); includes 70 minority (26 Black or African American, non-Hispanic/Latino; 3 American Indian or Alaska Native, non-Hispanic/Latino; 21 Asian, non-Hispanic/Latino; 20 Hispanic/Latino), 18 international. Average age 30. 380 applicants, 41% accepted, 63 enrolled. In 2013, 85 master's, 1 doctorate awarded. *Degree requirements:* For master's, internship. *Entrance requirements:* For master's, GRE General Test, minimum GPA of 3.0. Additional exam requirements/recommendations for international students: Required—TOEFL (minimum score 550 paper-based; 80 iBT), IELTS (minimum score 6). *Application deadline:* For fall admission, 7/1 for domestic students, 4/1 for international students. Application fee: $30. *Expenses:* Tuition, state resident: full-time $12,640. Tuition, nonresident: full-time $30,000. *Financial support:* In 2013–14, 29 students received support, including 2 fellowships (averaging $17,022 per year), 8 research assistantships (averaging $16,662 per year), 19 teaching assistantships (averaging $12,380 per year). Financial award applicants required to submit FAFSA. *Unit head:* Sarah L. McKune, PhD, Program Director, 352-328-0615, Fax: 352-273-6448, E-mail: smckune@ufl.edu. *Application contact:* Telisha Martin, PhD, Associate Director, MPH Program, 352-273-6444, E-mail: martints@ufl.edu.
Website: http://www.mph.ufl.edu/

University of Guelph, Ontario Veterinary College and Graduate Studies, Graduate Programs in Veterinary Sciences, Department of Population Medicine, Guelph, ON N1G 2W1, Canada. Offers epidemiology (M Sc, DV Sc, PhD); health management (DV Sc); population medicine and health management (M Sc); swine health management (M Sc); theriogenology (M Sc, DV Sc). *Degree requirements:* For master's, thesis; for doctorate, comprehensive exam, thesis/dissertation. *Entrance requirements:* Additional exam requirements/recommendations for international students: Required—TOEFL.

University of Hawaii at Manoa, John A. Burns School of Medicine, Department of Public Health Sciences and Epidemiology, Program in Epidemiology, Honolulu, HI 96822. Offers PhD. Part-time programs available. *Degree requirements:* For doctorate, comprehensive exam, thesis/dissertation. *Entrance requirements:* For doctorate, GRE General Test. Additional exam requirements/recommendations for international students: Required—TOEFL (minimum score 600 paper-based; 100 iBT), IELTS (minimum score 7).

University of Illinois at Chicago, Graduate College, School of Public Health, Epidemiology and Biostatistics Division, Chicago, IL 60607-7128. Offers biostatistics (MPH, MS, PhD); epidemiology (MPH, MS, PhD). Part-time programs available. *Faculty:* 20 full-time (6 women), 8 part-time/adjunct (5 women). *Students:* 87 full-time (55 women), 54 part-time (37 women); includes 49 minority (7 Black or African American, non-Hispanic/Latino; 29 Asian, non-Hispanic/Latino; 9 Hispanic/Latino; 4 Two or more races, non-Hispanic/Latino), 23 international. Average age 31. 340 applicants, 55% accepted, 39 enrolled. In 2013, 46 master's, 2 doctorates awarded. Terminal master's awarded for partial completion of doctoral program. *Degree requirements:* For master's, thesis, field practicum; for doctorate, thesis/dissertation, independent research, internship. *Entrance requirements:* For master's and doctorate, GRE General Test, minimum GPA of 2.75. Additional exam requirements/recommendations for international students: Required—TOEFL. *Application deadline:* For fall admission, 2/1 for domestic students, 1/1 priority date for international students. Application fee: $40 ($50 for international students). Electronic applications accepted. *Expenses:* Tuition, state resident: full-time $11,066; part-time $3689 per term. Tuition, nonresident: full-time $23,064; part-time $7688 per term. *Required fees:* $3004; $1190 per term. Tuition and fees vary according to course level and program. *Financial support:* In 2013–14, 17 students received support. Fellowships with full tuition reimbursements available, research assistantships with full tuition reimbursements available, teaching assistantships with full tuition reimbursements available, career-related internships or fieldwork, Federal Work-Study, institutionally sponsored loans, scholarships/grants, traineeships, tuition waivers (full), and unspecified assistantships available. Support available to part-time students. Financial award application deadline: 3/1; financial award applicants required to submit FAFSA. *Faculty research:* Quantitative methods. *Total annual research expenditures:* $1.7 million. *Unit head:* Dr. Ronald Hershow, Division Director, 312-996-4759, E-mail: rchersho@uic.edu.
Website: http://publichealth.uic.edu/departments/epidemiologyandbiostatistics/

University of Illinois at Springfield, Graduate Programs, College of Public Affairs and Administration, Program in Public Health, Springfield, IL 62703-5407. Offers community health (Graduate Certificate); emergency preparedness and homeland security (Graduate Certificate); epidemiology (Graduate Certificate); public health (MPH). Part-time and evening/weekend programs available. Postbaccalaureate distance learning degree programs offered (no on-campus study). *Faculty:* 5 full-time (3 women), 3 part-time/adjunct (2 women). *Students:* 32 full-time (21 women), 57 part-time (43 women); includes 32 minority (24 Black or African American, non-Hispanic/Latino; 6 Asian, non-Hispanic/Latino; 2 Hispanic/Latino), 10 international. Average age 32. 70 applicants, 47% accepted, 24 enrolled. In 2013, 22 master's, 6 other advanced degrees awarded. *Degree requirements:* For master's, comprehensive exam, internship. *Entrance requirements:* For master's, GRE, minimum undergraduate GPA of 3.0, 3 letters of recommendation, statement of personal goals. Additional exam requirements/recommendations for international students: Required—TOEFL (minimum score 500 paper-based; 61 iBT). *Application deadline:* Applications are processed on a rolling basis. Application fee: $60 ($75 for international students). Electronic applications accepted. *Expenses:* Tuition, state resident: full-time $7440. Tuition, nonresident: full-time $15,744. *Required fees:* $2985.60. *Financial support:* In 2013–14, fellowships with full tuition reimbursements (averaging $9,900 per year), research assistantships with full tuition reimbursements (averaging $9,550 per year), teaching assistantships with full tuition reimbursements (averaging $9,700 per year) were awarded; career-related internships or fieldwork, Federal Work-Study, scholarships/grants, health care benefits, and unspecified assistantships also available. Support available to part-time students. Financial award application deadline: 11/15; financial award applicants required to submit FAFSA. *Unit head:* Dr. Sharron Lafollette, Program Administrator, 217-206-7894, Fax: 217-206-7279, E-mail: slafo1@uis.edu. *Application contact:* Dr. Lynn Pardie, Office of Graduate Studies, 800-252-8533, Fax: 217-206-7623, E-mail: lpard1@uis.edu.
Website: http://www.uis.edu/publichealth/

The University of Iowa, Graduate College, College of Public Health, Department of Epidemiology, Iowa City, IA 52242-1316. Offers clinical investigation (MS); epidemiology (MPH, MS, PhD). *Accreditation:* CEPH. *Degree requirements:* For master's, thesis optional, exam; for doctorate, comprehensive exam, thesis/dissertation. *Entrance requirements:* For master's and doctorate, GRE General Test, minimum GPA of 3.0. Additional exam requirements/recommendations for international students: Required—TOEFL (minimum score 600 paper-based; 100 iBT). Electronic applications accepted.

The University of Kansas, University of Kansas Medical Center, School of Medicine, Department of Preventive Medicine and Public Health, Kansas City, KS 66160. Offers clinical research (MS); environmental health sciences (MPH); epidemiology (MPH); public health management (MPH); social and behavioral health (MPH); MD/MPH; PhD/MPH. Part-time programs available. *Faculty:* 69. *Students:* 30 full-time (23 women), 60 part-time (41 women); includes 27 minority (6 Black or African American, non-Hispanic/Latino; 2 American Indian or Alaska Native, non-Hispanic/Latino; 11 Asian, non-Hispanic/Latino; 3 Hispanic/Latino; 5 Two or more races, non-Hispanic/Latino), 7 international. Average age 34. 62 applicants, 52% accepted, 24 enrolled. In 2013, 37 master's awarded. *Degree requirements:* For master's, thesis, capstone practicum defense. *Entrance requirements:* For master's, GRE, MCAT, LSAT, GMAT or other equivalent graduate professional exam. Additional exam requirements/recommendations for international students: Required—TOEFL. *Application deadline:* For fall admission, 3/1 for domestic and international students. Applications are processed on a rolling basis. Application fee: $60. Electronic applications accepted. *Financial support:* Research assistantships, career-related internships or fieldwork, Federal Work-Study, scholarships/grants, and unspecified assistantships available. Financial award application deadline: 3/1; financial award applicants required to submit FAFSA. *Faculty research:* Cancer screening and prevention, smoking cessation, obesity and physical activity, health services/outcomes research, health disparities. *Total annual research expenditures:* $6.9 million. *Unit head:* Dr. Edward F. Ellerbeck, Chairman, 913-588-2774, Fax: 913-588-2780, E-mail: eellerbe@kumc.edu. *Application contact:* Tanya Honderick, MPH Director, 913-588-2720, Fax: 913-588-8505, E-mail: thonderick@kumc.edu.
Website: http://www.kumc.edu/school-of-medicine/preventive-medicine-and-public-health.html

University of Kentucky, Graduate School, College of Public Health, Program in Epidemiology and Biostatistics, Lexington, KY 40506-0032. Offers PhD.

University of Louisville, Graduate School, School of Public Health and Information Sciences, Department of Epidemiology and Population Health, Louisville, KY 40292-0001. Offers epidemiology (MPH, MS, PhD). Part-time programs available. *Students:* 6 full-time (3 women), 16 part-time (11 women); includes 5 minority (1 Black or African American, non-Hispanic/Latino; 4 Asian, non-Hispanic/Latino), 5 international. Average age 33. 13 applicants, 62% accepted, 5 enrolled. In 2013, 10 master's awarded. Terminal master's awarded for partial completion of doctoral program. *Degree requirements:* For master's, thesis; for doctorate, comprehensive exam, thesis/dissertation. *Entrance requirements:* For master's, GRE General Test; for doctorate, GRE General Test, master's degree in related field. Additional exam requirements/recommendations for international students: Required—TOEFL. *Application deadline:* For fall admission, 2/1 for domestic students, 1/2 priority date for international students. Applications are processed on a rolling basis. Application fee: $60. Electronic applications accepted. *Expenses:* Tuition, state resident: full-time $10,788; part-time $599 per credit hour. Tuition, nonresident: full-time $22,446; part-time $1247 per credit hour. *Required fees:* $196. Tuition and fees vary according to program and reciprocity agreements. *Financial support:* In 2013–14, fellowships with full tuition reimbursements (averaging $20,000 per year), research assistantships with full tuition reimbursements (averaging $20,000 per year) were awarded; teaching assistantships, scholarships/grants, traineeships, health care benefits, and unspecified assistantships also available. Financial award applicants required to submit FAFSA. *Faculty research:* Breast cancer in minority populations, health policy, clinical trials, chronic disease, genetic epidemiology, Cystic Fibrosis, breast cancer and longevity, Alzheimer's, Parkinson's and microbiomes, lead exposure and Army work, autism and the environment. *Unit*

head: Dr. Richard Baumgartner, Professor and Chair, 502-852-2038, E-mail: rnbaum01@gwise.louisville.edu. *Application contact:* Vicki Lewis, Administrative Assistant, 502-852-1798, Fax: 502-852-3294, E-mail: vicki.lewis@louisville.edu.
Website: http://louisville.edu/sphis/departments/epidemiology-population-health

University of Maryland, Baltimore, Graduate School, Graduate Program in Life Sciences, Baltimore, MD 21201. Offers biochemistry and molecular biology (MS, PhD), including biochemistry; epidemiology (PhD); gerontology (PhD); molecular medicine (MS, PhD), including cancer biology (PhD), cell and molecular physiology (PhD), human genetics and genomic medicine (PhD), molecular medicine (MS), molecular toxicology and pharmacology (PhD); molecular microbiology and immunology (PhD); neuroscience (PhD); physical rehabilitation science (PhD); toxicology (MS, PhD); MD/MS; MD/PhD. *Students:* 287 full-time (156 women), 71 part-time (42 women); includes 91 minority (27 Black or African American, non-Hispanic/Latino; 39 Asian, non-Hispanic/Latino; 15 Hispanic/Latino; 10 Two or more races, non-Hispanic/Latino), 45 international. Average age 29. 633 applicants, 23% accepted, 71 enrolled. In 2013, 31 master's, 42 doctorates awarded. *Degree requirements:* For master's, comprehensive exam (for some programs), thesis (for some programs); for doctorate, comprehensive exam, thesis/dissertation. *Entrance requirements:* For master's and doctorate, GRE. Additional exam requirements/recommendations for international students: Required—TOEFL (minimum score 550 paper-based; 80 iBT); Recommended—IELTS (minimum score 7). *Application deadline:* For fall admission, 12/14 for domestic students, 1/15 for international students. Application fee: $75. Electronic applications accepted. *Financial support:* In 2013–14, research assistantships with partial tuition reimbursements (averaging $25,000 per year) were awarded; fellowships, scholarships/grants, health care benefits, and unspecified assistantships also available. Financial award application deadline: 3/1; financial award applicants required to submit FAFSA. *Faculty research:* Cancer, reproduction, cardiovascular, immunology. *Unit head:* Dr. Dudley Strickland, Assistant Dean for Graduate Studies, 410-706-8010. *Application contact:* Keith T. Brooks, Assistant Dean, 410-706-7131, Fax: 410-706-3473, E-mail: kbrooks@umaryland.edu.
Website: http://lifesciences.umaryland.edu

University of Maryland, Baltimore, Graduate School, Graduate Programs in Pharmacy, Department of Pharmaceutical Health Service Research, Baltimore, MD 21201. Offers epidemiology (MS); pharmacy administration (PhD); Pharm D/PhD. *Degree requirements:* For doctorate, comprehensive exam, thesis/dissertation. *Entrance requirements:* For doctorate, GRE General Test. Additional exam requirements/recommendations for international students: Required—TOEFL, IELTS. Electronic applications accepted. *Faculty research:* Pharmacoeconomics, outcomes research, public health policy, drug therapy and aging.

University of Maryland, Baltimore, School of Medicine, Department of Epidemiology and Public Health, Baltimore, MD 21201. Offers biostatistics (MS); clinical research (MS); epidemiology and preventive medicine (MPH, MS, PhD); gerontology (PhD); human genetics and genomic medicine (MS, PhD); molecular epidemiology (MS, PhD); toxicology (MS, PhD); JD/MS; MD/PhD; MS/PhD. *Accreditation:* CEPH. Part-time programs available. *Students:* 83 full-time (56 women), 76 part-time (51 women); includes 51 minority (26 Black or African American, non-Hispanic/Latino; 20 Asian, non-Hispanic/Latino; 5 Hispanic/Latino), 27 international. Average age 32. 225 applicants, 44% accepted, 37 enrolled. In 2013, 18 master's, 1 doctorate awarded. *Degree requirements:* For doctorate, comprehensive exam, thesis/dissertation. *Entrance requirements:* For master's and doctorate, GRE General Test. Additional exam requirements/recommendations for international students: Required—TOEFL (minimum score 550 paper-based; 80 iBT); Recommended—IELTS (minimum score 7). *Application deadline:* For fall admission, 1/15 for domestic and international students. Application fee: $75. Electronic applications accepted. *Expenses:* Contact institution. *Financial support:* In 2013–14, research assistantships with partial tuition reimbursements (averaging $25,000 per year) were awarded; fellowships, Federal Work-Study, scholarships/grants, and unspecified assistantships also available. Financial award application deadline: 3/1; financial award applicants required to submit FAFSA. *Unit head:* Dr. Laura Hungerford, Program Director, 410-706-8492, Fax: 410-706-4225. *Application contact:* Jessica Kelley, Program Coordinator, 410-706-8492, Fax: 410-706-4225, E-mail: jkelley@som.umaryland.edu.
Website: http://medschool.umaryland.edu/Epidemiology/

University of Maryland, Baltimore County, Graduate School, College of Arts, Humanities and Social Sciences, Department of Emergency Health Services, Baltimore, MD 21250. Offers administration, planning, and policy (MS); education (MS); emergency health services (MS); emergency management (Postbaccalaureate Certificate); preventive medicine and epidemiology (MS). Part-time and evening/weekend programs available. Postbaccalaureate distance learning degree programs offered (no on-campus study). *Faculty:* 1 full-time (0 women), 9 part-time/adjunct (1 woman). *Students:* 20 full-time (8 women), 21 part-time (10 women); includes 2 minority (both Black or African American, non-Hispanic/Latino), 6 international. Average age 32. 13 applicants, 85% accepted, 10 enrolled. In 2013, 13 master's awarded. *Degree requirements:* For master's, comprehensive exam, thesis (for some programs), capstone project. *Entrance requirements:* For master's, GRE General Test, minimum GPA of 3.0. Additional exam requirements/recommendations for international students: Required—TOEFL (minimum score 85 iBT). *Application deadline:* For fall admission, 7/1 for domestic students, 4/1 for international students; for spring admission, 10/15 for domestic students, 9/1 for international students. Applications are processed on a rolling basis. Application fee: $50. Electronic applications accepted. One-time fee: $200 full-time. *Financial support:* In 2013–14, 2 students received support, including 1 fellowship with tuition reimbursement available (averaging $70,000 per year), 1 research assistantship with tuition reimbursement available (averaging $21,000 per year); career-related internships or fieldwork, Federal Work-Study, scholarships/grants, health care benefits, and unspecified assistantships also available. Financial award application deadline: 5/30; financial award applicants required to submit FAFSA. *Faculty research:* EMS management, disaster health services, emergency management. *Total annual research expenditures:* $50,000. *Unit head:* Dr. Bruce Walz, Chairman, 410-455-3223. *Application contact:* Dr. Rick Bissell, Program Director, 410-455-3776, Fax: 410-455-3045, E-mail: bissell@umbc.edu.
Website: http://ehs.umbc.edu/

University of Maryland, College Park, Academic Affairs, School of Public Health, Department of Epidemiology and Biostatistics, College Park, MD 20742. Offers biostatistics (MPH); epidemiology (MPH, PhD). *Faculty:* 16 full-time (7 women), 7 part-time/adjunct (3 women). *Students:* 19 full-time (16 women), 16 part-time (12 women); includes 14 minority (2 Black or African American, non-Hispanic/Latino; 7 Asian, non-Hispanic/Latino; 2 Hispanic/Latino; 3 Two or more races, non-Hispanic/Latino), 4 international. 185 applicants, 8% accepted, 8 enrolled. In 2013, 6 master's, 2 doctorates awarded. *Application deadline:* For fall admission, 1/15 for domestic and international students. Application fee: $75. *Expenses:* Tuition, state resident: full-time $10,314; part-time $573 per credit hour. Tuition, nonresident: full-time $22,248; part-time $1236 per credit. *Required fees:* $1446; $403.15 per semester. Tuition and fees vary according to program. *Financial support:* In 2013–14, 3 fellowships with full tuition reimbursements (averaging $53,470 per year), 8 research assistantships (averaging $15,933 per year), 2 teaching assistantships (averaging $16,259 per year) were awarded. *Total annual research expenditures:* $708,269. *Unit head:* Dr. Mei-Ling Lee, Chair, 301-405-4581, E-mail: mltlee@umd.edu. *Application contact:* Dr. Charles A. Caramello, Dean of Graduate School, 301-405-0358, Fax: 301-314-9305, E-mail: ccaramel@umd.edu.
Website: http://www.sph.umd.edu/epib/

University of Massachusetts Amherst, Graduate School, School of Public Health and Health Sciences, Department of Public Health, Amherst, MA 01003. Offers biostatistics (MPH, MS, PhD); community health education (MPH, MS, PhD); environmental health sciences (MPH, MS, PhD); epidemiology (MPH, MS, PhD); health policy and management (MPH, MS, PhD); nutrition (MPH, PhD); public health practice (MPH); MPH/MPPA. *Accreditation:* CEPH (one or more programs are accredited). Part-time and evening/weekend programs available. Postbaccalaureate distance learning degree programs offered (no on-campus study). *Faculty:* 53 full-time (29 women). *Students:* 117 full-time (83 women), 271 part-time (213 women); includes 89 minority (34 Black or African American, non-Hispanic/Latino; 23 Asian, non-Hispanic/Latino; 25 Hispanic/Latino; 7 Two or more races, non-Hispanic/Latino), 45 international. Average age 36. 359 applicants, 69% accepted, 94 enrolled. In 2013, 120 master's, 1 doctorate awarded. Terminal master's awarded for partial completion of doctoral program. *Degree requirements:* For master's, thesis (for some programs); for doctorate, comprehensive exam, thesis/dissertation. *Entrance requirements:* For master's and doctorate, GRE General Test. Additional exam requirements/recommendations for international students: Required—TOEFL (minimum score 550 paper-based; 80 iBT), IELTS (minimum score 6.5). *Application deadline:* For fall admission, 2/1 for domestic and international students. Applications are processed on a rolling basis. Application fee: $75. Electronic applications accepted. *Financial support:* Fellowships with full and partial tuition reimbursements, research assistantships with full and partial tuition reimbursements, teaching assistantships with full and partial tuition reimbursements, career-related internships or fieldwork, Federal Work-Study, scholarships/grants, traineeships, health care benefits, tuition waivers (full and partial), and unspecified assistantships available. Support available to part-time students. Financial award application deadline: 2/1; financial award applicants required to submit FAFSA. *Unit head:* Dr. Paula Stamps, Graduate Program Director, 413-545-2861, Fax: 413-545-1645. *Application contact:* Lindsay DeSantis, Supervisor of Admissions, 413-545-0722, Fax: 413-577-0010, E-mail: gradadm@grad.umass.edu.
Website: http://www.umass.edu/sphhs/public_health/

University of Massachusetts Lowell, College of Health Sciences, Department of Work Environment, Lowell, MA 01854-2881. Offers cleaner production and pollution prevention (MS, Sc D); environmental risk assessment (Certificate); epidemiology (MS, Sc D); ergonomics and safety (MS, Sc D); identification and control of ergonomic hazards (Certificate); job stress and healthy job redesign (Certificate); occupational and environmental hygiene (MS, Sc D); radiological health physics and general work environment protection (Certificate); work environment policy (MS, Sc D). *Accreditation:* ABET (one or more programs are accredited). Part-time programs available. Terminal master's awarded for partial completion of doctoral program. *Degree requirements:* For master's, thesis optional; for doctorate, thesis/dissertation. *Entrance requirements:* For master's and doctorate, GRE General Test. Additional exam requirements/recommendations for international students: Required—TOEFL.

University of Memphis, Graduate School, School of Public Health, Memphis, TN 38152. Offers biostatistics (MPH); environmental health (MPH); epidemiology (MPH); health systems management (MPH); public health (MHA); social and behavioral sciences (MPH). Part-time and evening/weekend programs available. Postbaccalaureate distance learning degree programs offered. *Faculty:* 14 full-time (2 women), 5 part-time/adjunct (1 woman). *Students:* 64 full-time (42 women), 36 part-time (24 women); includes 34 minority (21 Black or African American, non-Hispanic/Latino; 6 Asian, non-Hispanic/Latino; 5 Hispanic/Latino; 2 Two or more races, non-Hispanic/Latino), 15 international. Average age 32. 102 applicants, 51% accepted, 24 enrolled. In 2013, 17 master's awarded. *Degree requirements:* For master's, comprehensive exam, thesis. *Entrance requirements:* For master's, GRE, letters of recommendation. Additional exam requirements/recommendations for international students: Required—TOEFL. *Application deadline:* For fall admission, 4/1 for domestic students; for spring admission, 11/1 for domestic students. Application fee: $35 ($60 for international students). Electronic applications accepted. *Financial support:* In 2013–14, 46 students received support. Research assistantships with full tuition reimbursements available, Federal Work-Study, scholarships/grants, and unspecified assistantships available. Financial award application deadline: 2/15; financial award applicants required to submit FAFSA. *Faculty research:* Health and medical savings accounts, adoption rates, health informatics, Telehealth technologies, biostatistics, environmental health, epidemiology, health systems management, social and behavioral sciences. *Unit head:* Dr. Lisa M. Klesges, Director, 901-678-4637, E-mail: lmklsges@memphis.edu. *Application contact:* Dr. Karen Weddle-West, Information Contact, 901-678-2531, Fax: 901-678-5023, E-mail: gradsch@memphis.edu.
Website: http://www.memphis.edu/sph/

University of Miami, Graduate School, Miller School of Medicine, Graduate Programs in Medicine, Department of Epidemiology and Public Health, Coral Gables, FL 33124. Offers epidemiology (PhD); public health (MPH, MSPH); JD/MPH; MD/MPH; MD/PhD; MPA/MPH; MPH/MAIA. *Accreditation:* CEPH (one or more programs are accredited). Part-time programs available. *Degree requirements:* For master's, thesis (for some programs), project, practicum; for doctorate, comprehensive exam, thesis/dissertation. *Entrance requirements:* For master's, GRE General Test, minimum GPA of 3.0, 3 letters of recommendation; for doctorate, GRE General Test, minimum GPA of 3.0, course work in epidemiology and statistics, 3 letters of recommendation. Additional exam requirements/recommendations for international students: Required—TOEFL (minimum score 550 paper-based; 59 iBT). Electronic applications accepted. *Faculty research:* Behavioral epidemiology, substance abuse, AIDS, cardiovascular diseases, women's health.

University of Michigan, School of Public Health, Department of Epidemiology, Ann Arbor, MI 48109-2029. Offers dental public health (MPH); epidemiological science (PhD); epidemiology (MS); general epidemiology (MPH); hospital and molecular epidemiology (MPH); international health (MPH). PhD and MS offered through the Horace H. Rackham School of Graduate Studies. *Accreditation:* CEPH (one or more programs are accredited). Part-time programs available. Terminal master's awarded for partial completion of doctoral program. *Degree requirements:* For master's, thesis (for some programs); for doctorate, comprehensive exam, thesis/dissertation, oral defense of dissertation, preliminary exam. *Entrance requirements:* For master's and doctorate, GRE General Test, MCAT. Additional exam requirements/recommendations for international students: Required—TOEFL (minimum score 560 paper-based; 100 iBT). Electronic applications accepted. Tuition and fees vary according to course level, course load, degree level, program and student level. *Faculty research:* Molecular virology, infectious diseases, women's health, genetics, social epidemiology.

University of Minnesota, Twin Cities Campus, School of Public Health, Division of Environmental Health Sciences, Area in Environmental and Occupational Epidemiology, Minneapolis, MN 55455-0213. Offers MPH, MS, PhD. *Accreditation:* CEPH (one or more programs are accredited). *Degree requirements:* For doctorate, thesis/dissertation.

Entrance requirements: For master's and doctorate, GRE General Test. Electronic applications accepted.

University of Minnesota, Twin Cities Campus, School of Public Health, Major in Epidemiology, Minneapolis, MN 55455-0213. Offers MPH, PhD. *Accreditation:* CEPH (one or more programs are accredited). Part-time programs available. Terminal master's awarded for partial completion of doctoral program. *Degree requirements:* For master's, fieldwork, project; for doctorate, comprehensive exam, thesis/dissertation. *Entrance requirements:* For master's, GRE General Test; for doctorate, GRE General Test, master's degree in related field. Additional exam requirements/recommendations for international students: Required—TOEFL. Electronic applications accepted. *Expenses:* Contact institution. *Faculty research:* Prevention of cardiovascular disease, nutrition, genetic epidemiology, behavioral interventions, research methods.

University of New Mexico, School of Medicine, Program in Public Health, Albuquerque, NM 87131-5196. Offers community health (MPH); epidemiology (MPH); health systems, services and policy (MPH). *Accreditation:* CEPH. Part-time programs available. Postbaccalaureate distance learning degree programs offered. *Faculty:* 11 full-time (7 women), 4 part-time/adjunct (3 women). *Students:* 17 full-time (15 women), 16 part-time (12 women); includes 16 minority (3 Black or African American, non-Hispanic/Latino; 2 American Indian or Alaska Native, non-Hispanic/Latino; 1 Asian, non-Hispanic/Latino; 9 Hispanic/Latino; 1 Two or more races, non-Hispanic/Latino), 1 international. Average age 36. 46 applicants, 59% accepted, 17 enrolled. In 2013, 15 master's awarded. *Degree requirements:* For master's, thesis. *Entrance requirements:* For master's, GRE, MCAT, 2 years of experience in health field. Additional exam requirements/recommendations for international students: Required—TOEFL. *Application deadline:* For fall admission, 2/1 for domestic students. Application fee: $50. *Financial support:* Fellowships, research assistantships with tuition reimbursements, and Federal Work-Study available. Financial award application deadline: 12/15; financial award applicants required to submit FAFSA. *Faculty research:* Epidemiology, rural health, environmental health, Native American health issues. *Total annual research expenditures:* $1 million. *Unit head:* Dr. Kristine Tollestrup, Director, 505-272-4173, Fax: 505-272-4494, E-mail: ktollestrup@salud.unm.edu. *Application contact:* Gayle Garcia, Education Coordinator, 505-272-3982, Fax: 505-272-4494, E-mail: garciag@salud.unm.edu.
Website: http://fcm.unm.edu/

The University of North Carolina at Chapel Hill, Graduate School, Gillings School of Global Public Health, Department of Epidemiology, Chapel Hill, NC 27599. Offers MPH, MSCR, PhD. *Accreditation:* CEPH (one or more programs are accredited). Terminal master's awarded for partial completion of doctoral program. *Degree requirements:* For master's, comprehensive exam, major paper; for doctorate, comprehensive exam, thesis/dissertation. *Entrance requirements:* For master's and doctorate, GRE General Test, minimum GPA of 3.0 (recommended). Additional exam requirements/recommendations for international students: Required—TOEFL. Electronic applications accepted. *Faculty research:* Chronic disease: cancer, cardiovascular, nutritional; environmental/occupational injury; infectious diseases; reproductive diseases; healthcare.

The University of North Carolina at Chapel Hill, School of Dentistry and Graduate School, Graduate Programs in Dentistry, Chapel Hill, NC 27599. Offers dental hygiene (MS); endodontics (MS); epidemiology (PhD); operative dentistry (MS); oral and maxillofacial pathology (MS); oral and maxillofacial radiology (MS); oral biology (PhD); orthodontics (MS); pediatric dentistry (MS); periodontology (MS); prosthodontics (MS). *Degree requirements:* For master's, thesis; for doctorate, thesis/dissertation. *Entrance requirements:* For master's, GRE General Test (for orthodontics and oral biology only); National Dental Board Part I (Part II if available), dental degree (for all except dental hygiene); for doctorate, GRE General Test. Additional exam requirements/recommendations for international students: Required—TOEFL (minimum score 550 paper-based; 79 iBT). Electronic applications accepted. *Expenses:* Contact institution. *Faculty research:* Clinical research, inflammation, immunology, neuroscience, molecular biology.

University of North Texas Health Science Center at Fort Worth, School of Public Health, Fort Worth, TX 76107-2699. Offers biostatistics (MPH); community health (MPH); disease control and prevention (Dr PH); environmental and occupational health sciences (MPH); epidemiology (MPH); health administration (MHA); health policy and management (MPH, Dr PH); DO/MPH; MS/MPH; MSN/MPH. MPH offered jointly with University of North Texas; DO/MPH with Texas College of Osteopathic Medicine. *Accreditation:* CEPH. Part-time and evening/weekend programs available. *Degree requirements:* For master's, thesis or alternative, supervised internship; for doctorate, thesis/dissertation, supervised internship. *Entrance requirements:* For master's, GRE General Test. Additional exam requirements/recommendations for international students: Required—TOEFL. Electronic applications accepted.

University of Oklahoma Health Sciences Center, Graduate College, College of Public Health, Program in Biostatistics and Epidemiology, Oklahoma City, OK 73190. Offers biostatistics (MPH, MS, Dr PH, PhD); epidemiology (MPH, MS, Dr PH, PhD). *Accreditation:* CEPH (one or more programs are accredited). Part-time programs available. *Faculty:* 10 full-time (7 women), 1 (woman) part-time/adjunct. *Students:* 24 full-time (13 women), 23 part-time (17 women); includes 14 minority (4 Black or African American, non-Hispanic/Latino; 5 Asian, non-Hispanic/Latino; 1 Hispanic/Latino; 4 Two or more races, non-Hispanic/Latino), 11 international. Average age 30. 40 applicants, 35% accepted, 9 enrolled. In 2013, 18 master's, 1 doctorate awarded. *Degree requirements:* For master's, comprehensive exam, thesis (for some programs); for doctorate, comprehensive exam, thesis/dissertation. *Entrance requirements:* For master's, 3 letters of recommendation, resume; for doctorate, GRE General Test, letters of recommendation. Additional exam requirements/recommendations for international students: Required—TOEFL (minimum score 570 paper-based), TWE. *Application deadline:* For fall admission, 7/1 for domestic students; for winter admission, 4/1 for domestic students; for spring admission, 12/1 for domestic students. Applications are processed on a rolling basis. Application fee: $50. *Expenses:* Tuition, state resident: full-time $3504; part-time $175.20 per credit hour. Tuition, nonresident: full-time $13,504; part-time $675.20 per credit hour. *Required fees:* $1545; $52.70 per credit hour. $245.25 per semester. Tuition and fees vary according to course load. *Financial support:* In 2013–14, 7 research assistantships (averaging $14,000 per year) were awarded; career-related internships or fieldwork, institutionally sponsored loans, and traineeships also available. Support available to part-time students. Financial award application deadline: 5/1. *Faculty research:* Statistical methodology, applied statistics, acute and chronic disease epidemiology. *Unit head:* Dr. Julie Stoner, Interim Chair, 405-271-2229, E-mail: julie-stoner@ouhsc.edu. *Application contact:* Robin Howell, Information Contact, 405-271-2308, E-mail: robin_howell@ouhsc.edu.

University of Ottawa, Faculty of Graduate and Postdoctoral Studies, Faculty of Medicine, Department of Epidemiology and Community Medicine, Ottawa, ON K1N 6N5, Canada. Offers epidemiology (M Sc), including health technology assessment. *Degree requirements:* For master's, thesis. *Entrance requirements:* For master's, honors degree or equivalent, minimum B average. Electronic applications accepted. *Faculty research:* Epidemiologic concepts and methods, health technology assessment.

University of Pennsylvania, Perelman School of Medicine, Center for Clinical Epidemiology and Biostatistics, Philadelphia, PA 19104. Offers clinical epidemiology (MSCE). *Accreditation:* CEPH. Part-time programs available. *Faculty:* 82 full-time (32 women), 90 part-time/adjunct (27 women). *Students:* 96 full-time (64 women), 2 part-time (1 woman); includes 35 minority (4 Black or African American, non-Hispanic/Latino; 16 Asian, non-Hispanic/Latino; 13 Hispanic/Latino; 2 Two or more races, non-Hispanic/Latino). Average age 34. 42 applicants, 93% accepted, 29 enrolled. In 2013, 30 master's awarded. *Degree requirements:* For master's, comprehensive exam, thesis. *Entrance requirements:* For master's, GRE General Test or MCAT, advanced degree, clinical experience. Additional exam requirements/recommendations for international students: Required—TOEFL. *Application deadline:* For fall admission, 12/1 priority date for domestic and international students. Application fee: $0. Electronic applications accepted. *Expenses:* Contact institution. *Financial support:* In 2013–14, 70 students received support, including 65 fellowships with full and partial tuition reimbursements available (averaging $45,500 per year); career-related internships or fieldwork, scholarships/grants, health care benefits, and unspecified assistantships also available. Financial award application deadline: 12/1. *Faculty research:* Health services research, pharmacoepidemiology, women's health, cancer epidemiology, genetic epidemiology. *Total annual research expenditures:* $46 million. *Unit head:* Dr. Harold I. Feldman, Director, 215-573-0901, Fax: 215-573-2265, E-mail: hfeldman@mail.med.upenn.edu. *Application contact:* Jennifer E. Kuklinski, Associate Director for Graduate Training in Epidemiology, 215-573-2382, Fax: 215-573-5315, E-mail: jkuklins@mail.med.upenn.edu.
Website: http://www.cceb.upenn.edu/

University of Pittsburgh, Graduate School of Public Health, Department of Epidemiology, Pittsburgh, PA 15260. Offers MPH, MS, Dr PH, PhD, MD/PhD. *Accreditation:* CEPH (one or more programs are accredited). Part-time programs available. *Faculty:* 49 full-time (34 women), 30 part-time/adjunct (12 women). *Students:* 83 full-time (60 women), 41 part-time (31 women); includes 16 minority (4 Black or African American, non-Hispanic/Latino; 6 Asian, non-Hispanic/Latino; 5 Hispanic/Latino; 1 Two or more races, non-Hispanic/Latino), 34 international. Average age 31. 513 applicants, 49% accepted, 33 enrolled. In 2013, 21 master's, 21 doctorates awarded. Terminal master's awarded for partial completion of doctoral program. *Degree requirements:* For master's, comprehensive exam (for some programs), thesis (for some programs), internship experience (MPH); for doctorate, comprehensive exam, thesis/dissertation, teaching practicum. *Entrance requirements:* For master's, GRE General Test, DAT, MCAT, 3 credits each of course work in human biology and algebra or higher mathematics, 6 in behavioral science (MPH); minimum GPA of 3.0; for doctorate, GRE General Test, DAT, MCAT, 3 credits of course work in biology and math, minimum GPA of 3.0. Additional exam requirements/recommendations for international students: Required—TOEFL (minimum score 550 paper-based; 80 iBT) or IELTS (minimum score 6.5). *Application deadline:* For fall admission, 6/1 priority date for domestic students, 3/15 priority date for international students; for spring admission, 8/15 priority date for domestic students, 8/1 for international students; for summer admission, 12/1 for international students. Applications are processed on a rolling basis. Application fee: $120. Electronic applications accepted. *Expenses:* Tuition, state resident: full-time $19,964; part-time $807 per credit. Tuition, nonresident: full-time $32,686; part-time $1337 per credit. *Required fees:* $740; $200. Tuition and fees vary according to program. *Financial support:* In 2013–14, 33 students received support, including 1 fellowship with full tuition reimbursement available (averaging $150 per year), 32 research assistantships with full tuition reimbursements available (averaging $24,204 per year), 1 teaching assistantship with full tuition reimbursement available (averaging $20,568 per year); career-related internships or fieldwork, scholarships/grants, and traineeships also available. Support available to part-time students. Financial award applicants required to submit FAFSA. *Faculty research:* Aging, cardiovascular, clinical trials, diabetes, psychiatric, women's health, genetics, alcohol. *Total annual research expenditures:* $33.8 million. *Unit head:* Dr. Anne B. Newman, Chair, 412-624-3056, Fax: 412-624-3737, E-mail: newmana@edc.pitt.edu. *Application contact:* Lori S. Smith, Student Affairs Manager, 412-383-5269, E-mail: smithl@edc.pitt.edu.
Website: http://www.epidemiology.pitt.edu/

University of Prince Edward Island, Atlantic Veterinary College, Graduate Program in Veterinary Medicine, Charlottetown, PE C1A 4P3, Canada. Offers anatomy (M Sc, PhD); bacteriology (M Sc, PhD); clinical pharmacology (M Sc, PhD); clinical sciences (M Sc, PhD); epidemiology (M Sc, PhD), including reproduction; fish health (M Sc, PhD); food animal nutrition (M Sc, PhD); immunology (M Sc, PhD); microanatomy (M Sc, PhD); parasitology (M Sc, PhD); pathology (M Sc, PhD); pharmacology (M Sc, PhD); physiology (M Sc, PhD); toxicology (M Sc, PhD); veterinary science (M Vet Sc); virology (M Sc, PhD). Part-time programs available. *Degree requirements:* For master's, thesis; for doctorate, thesis/dissertation. *Entrance requirements:* For master's, DVM, B Sc honors degree, or equivalent; for doctorate, M Sc. Additional exam requirements/recommendations for international students: Required—TOEFL (minimum score 550 paper-based; 80 iBT). *Expenses:* Contact institution. *Faculty research:* Animal health management, infectious diseases, fin fish and shellfish health, basic biomedical sciences, ecosystem health.

University of Puerto Rico, Medical Sciences Campus, Graduate School of Public Health, Department of Social Sciences, Program in Epidemiology, San Juan, PR 00936-5067. Offers MPH, MS. *Accreditation:* CEPH (one or more programs are accredited). Part-time programs available. *Entrance requirements:* For master's, GRE, previous course work in biology, chemistry, physics, mathematics, and social sciences. *Expenses:* Contact institution.

University of Rochester, School of Medicine and Dentistry, Graduate Programs in Medicine and Dentistry, Department of Community and Preventive Medicine, Program in Epidemiology, Rochester, NY 14627. Offers PhD. *Degree requirements:* For doctorate, thesis/dissertation, qualifying exam. *Entrance requirements:* For doctorate, GRE General Test. *Expenses: Tuition:* Full-time $44,580; part-time $1394 per credit hour. *Required fees:* $492.

University of Saskatchewan, College of Medicine, Department of Community Health and Epidemiology, Saskatoon, SK S7N 5A2, Canada. Offers M Sc, PhD. *Degree requirements:* For master's, thesis; for doctorate, thesis/dissertation. *Entrance requirements:* Additional exam requirements/recommendations for international students: Required—TOEFL. *Expenses: Tuition, area resident:* Full-time $3585 Canadian dollars; part-time $585 Canadian dollars per course. Tuition, nonresident: part-time $877 Canadian dollars per course. *International tuition:* $5377 Canadian dollars full-time. *Required fees:* $889.51 Canadian dollars.

University of South Carolina, The Graduate School, Arnold School of Public Health, Department of Epidemiology and Biostatistics, Program in Epidemiology, Columbia, SC 29208. Offers MPH, MSPH, Dr PH, PhD. *Accreditation:* CEPH (one or more programs are accredited). Part-time programs available. *Degree requirements:* For master's, comprehensive exam, thesis (for some programs), practicum (MPH); for doctorate, comprehensive exam, thesis/dissertation (for some programs), practicum. *Entrance requirements:* For master's, GRE General Test; for doctorate, GRE General Test, master's degree. Additional exam requirements/recommendations for international students: Required—TOEFL (minimum score 570 paper-based; 88 iBT). Electronic applications accepted. *Faculty research:* Cancer epidemiology, mental health epidemiology, health effects of physical activity, environmental epidemiology, genetic epidemiology, asthma epidemiology.

University of Southern California, Keck School of Medicine and Graduate School, Graduate Programs in Medicine, Department of Preventive Medicine, Division of Biostatistics, Los Angeles, CA 90089. Offers applied biostatistics and epidemiology (MS); biostatistics (MS, PhD); epidemiology (PhD); molecular epidemiology (MS). *Faculty:* 90 full-time (39 women), 4 part-time/adjunct (2 women). *Students:* 114 full-time (46 women); includes 24 minority (1 Black or African American, non-Hispanic/Latino; 1 American Indian or Alaska Native, non-Hispanic/Latino; 18 Asian, non-Hispanic/Latino; 3 Hispanic/Latino; 1 Native Hawaiian or other Pacific Islander, non-Hispanic/Latino), 69 international. Average age 29. 92 applicants, 60% accepted, 34 enrolled. In 2013, 9 master's, 10 doctorates awarded. Terminal master's awarded for partial completion of doctoral program. *Degree requirements:* For master's, thesis; for doctorate, thesis/dissertation. *Entrance requirements:* For master's, GRE General Test, GRE Subject Test, minimum GPA of 3.0; for doctorate, GRE General Test, GRE Subject Test, minimum GPA of 3.5. Additional exam requirements/recommendations for international students: Required—TOEFL (minimum score 600 paper-based; 100 iBT), IELTS (minimum score 7). *Application deadline:* For fall admission, 12/1 priority date for domestic and international students; for winter admission, 5/15 priority date for domestic and international students; for spring admission, 11/1 priority date for domestic and international students; for summer admission, 3/1 priority date for domestic and international students. Applications are processed on a rolling basis. Application fee: $85. Electronic applications accepted. *Financial support:* In 2013–14, 10 fellowships with full tuition reimbursements (averaging $30,000 per year), 49 research assistantships with full and partial tuition reimbursements (averaging $30,000 per year), 18 teaching assistantships with full and partial tuition reimbursements (averaging $30,000 per year) were awarded; career-related internships or fieldwork, Federal Work-Study, institutionally sponsored loans, scholarships/grants, traineeships, health care benefits, and unspecified assistantships also available. Financial award application deadline: 5/4; financial award applicants required to submit CSS PROFILE or FAFSA. *Faculty research:* Clinical trials in ophthalmology and cancer research, methods of analysis for epidemiological studies, genetic epidemiology. *Total annual research expenditures:* $1.3 million. *Unit head:* Dr. Kiros Berhane, Director, Graduate Programs in Biostatistics and Epidemiology, 323-442-1994, Fax: 323-442-2993, E-mail: kiros@usc.edu. *Application contact:* Mary L. Trujillo, Student Advisor, 323-442-2633, Fax: 323-442-2993, E-mail: mtrujill@usc.edu.
Website: http://keck.usc.edu/Education/Academic_Department_and_Divisions/Department_of_Preventive_Medicine/Divisions/Biostatistics.aspx

University of Southern California, Keck School of Medicine and Graduate School, Graduate Programs in Medicine, Department of Preventive Medicine, Master of Public Health Program, Los Angeles, CA 90032. Offers biostatistics-epidemiology (MPH); child and family health (MPH); environmental health (MPH); global health leadership (MPH); health communication (MPH); health education and promotion (MPH); public health policy (MPH). *Accreditation:* CEPH. Part-time and evening/weekend programs available. *Faculty:* 22 full-time (12 women), 3 part-time/adjunct (0 women). *Students:* 179 full-time (136 women), 31 part-time (24 women); includes 120 minority (19 Black or African American, non-Hispanic/Latino; 64 Asian, non-Hispanic/Latino; 37 Hispanic/Latino), 36 international. Average age 24. 205 applicants, 70% accepted, 73 enrolled. In 2013, 90 master's awarded. *Degree requirements:* For master's, practicum, final report, oral presentation. *Entrance requirements:* For master's, GRE General Test, MCAT, GMAT, minimum GPA of 3.0. Additional exam requirements/recommendations for international students: Required—TOEFL (minimum score 600 paper-based; 90 iBT). *Application deadline:* For fall admission, 6/1 priority date for domestic and international students; for spring admission, 10/1 priority date for domestic and international students; for summer admission, 3/1 for domestic and international students. Applications are processed on a rolling basis. Application fee: $85. Electronic applications accepted. *Financial support:* Career-related internships or fieldwork, Federal Work-Study, institutionally sponsored loans, and scholarships/grants available. Support available to part-time students. Financial award application deadline: 5/4; financial award applicants required to submit CSS PROFILE or FAFSA. *Faculty research:* Substance abuse prevention, cancer and heart disease prevention, mass media and health communication research, health promotion, treatment compliance. *Unit head:* Dr. Louise A. Rohrbach, Director, 323-442-8237, Fax: 323-442-8297, E-mail: rohrbac@usc.edu. *Application contact:* Valerie Burris, Admissions Counselor, 323-442-7257, Fax: 323-442-8297, E-mail: valeriem@usc.edu.
Website: http://mph.usc.edu/

University of Southern Mississippi, Graduate School, College of Health, Department of Community Health Sciences, Hattiesburg, MS 39406-0001. Offers epidemiology and biostatistics (MPH); health education (MPH); health policy/administration (MPH); occupational/environmental health (MPH); public health nutrition (MPH). *Accreditation:* CEPH. Part-time and evening/weekend programs available. *Faculty:* 8 full-time (4 women), 1 part-time/adjunct (0 women). *Students:* 92 full-time (60 women), 9 part-time (4 women); includes 38 minority (29 Black or African American, non-Hispanic/Latino; 1 American Indian or Alaska Native, non-Hispanic/Latino; 2 Asian, non-Hispanic/Latino; 6 Two or more races, non-Hispanic/Latino), 13 international. Average age 34. 71 applicants, 93% accepted, 45 enrolled. *Degree requirements:* For master's, comprehensive exam, thesis (for some programs). *Entrance requirements:* For master's, GRE General Test, minimum GPA of 2.75 in last 60 hours. Additional exam requirements/recommendations for international students: Required—TOEFL, IELTS. *Application deadline:* For fall admission, 3/1 priority date for domestic and international students; for spring admission, 1/10 priority date for domestic and international students. Applications are processed on a rolling basis. Application fee: $50. Electronic applications accepted. *Financial support:* In 2013–14, 5 research assistantships with full tuition reimbursements (averaging $7,000 per year), 1 teaching assistantship with full tuition reimbursement (averaging $8,263 per year) were awarded; career-related internships or fieldwork, Federal Work-Study, institutionally sponsored loans, scholarships/grants, health care benefits, and unspecified assistantships also available. Financial award application deadline: 3/15; financial award applicants required to submit FAFSA. *Faculty research:* Rural health care delivery, school health, nutrition of pregnant teens, risk factor reduction, sexually transmitted diseases. *Unit head:* Dr. Ray Newman, Interim Chair, 601-266-5437, Fax: 601-266-5043. *Application contact:* Shonna Breland, Manager of Graduate Admissions, 601-266-6563, Fax: 601-266-5138.
Website: http://www.usm.edu/chs

University of South Florida, College of Public Health, Department of Epidemiology and Biostatistics, Tampa, FL 33620-9951. Offers MPH, MSPH, PhD. *Accreditation:* CEPH (one or more programs are accredited). Part-time and evening/weekend programs available. *Degree requirements:* For master's, comprehensive exam, thesis (for some programs); for doctorate, comprehensive exam, thesis/dissertation. *Entrance requirements:* For master's, GRE General Test, minimum GPA of 3.0 in upper-level course work, goal statement letter, two professional letters of recommendation, resume/curriculum vitae; for doctorate, GRE General Test, minimum GPA of 3.0 in upper-level course work, 3 professional letters of recommendation, resume/curriculum vitae, writing sample. Additional exam requirements/recommendations for international students: Required—TOEFL (minimum score 550 paper-based; 79 iBT). Electronic applications accepted. *Faculty research:* Dementia, mental illness, mental health preventative trails, rural health outreach, clinical and administrative studies.

University of South Florida, Innovative Education Graduate Certificate Programs, Tampa, FL 33620-9951. *Unit head:* Kathy Barnes, Interdisciplinary Programs Coordinator, 813-974-8031, Fax: 813-974-7061, E-mail: barnesk@usf.edu. *Application contact:* Karen Tylinski, Metro Initiatives, 813-974-9943, Fax: 813-974-7061, E-mail: ktylinsk@usf.edu.
Website: http://www.usf.edu/innovative-education/

University of South Florida, Morsani College of Medicine and Graduate School, Graduate Programs in Medical Sciences, Tampa, FL 33620-9951. Offers aging and neuroscience (MSMS); allergy, immunology and infectious disease (PhD); anatomy (MSMS, PhD); athletic training (MSMS); bioinformatics and computational biology (MSBCB); biotechnology (MSB); clinical and translational research (MSMS, PhD); health informatics (MSHI, MSMS); health science (MSMS); interdisciplinary medical sciences (MSMS); medical microbiology and immunology (MSMS); metabolic and nutritional medicine (MSMS); molecular medicine (MSMS, PhD); molecular pharmacology and physiology (PhD); neurology (PhD); pathology and laboratory medicine (PhD); pharmacology and therapeutics (PhD); physiology and biophysics (PhD); women's health (MSMS). *Students:* 336 full-time (182 women), 39 part-time (21 women); includes 170 minority (45 Black or African American, non-Hispanic/Latino; 54 Asian, non-Hispanic/Latino; 59 Hispanic/Latino; 2 Native Hawaiian or other Pacific Islander, non-Hispanic/Latino; 10 Two or more races, non-Hispanic/Latino), 17 international. Average age 26. 1,066 applicants, 44% accepted, 250 enrolled. In 2013, 191 master's, 12 doctorates awarded. Terminal master's awarded for partial completion of doctoral program. *Degree requirements:* For master's, comprehensive exam, thesis; for doctorate, comprehensive exam, thesis/dissertation. *Entrance requirements:* For master's, GRE General Test or GMAT, bachelor's degree or equivalent from regionally-accredited university with minimum GPA of 3.0 in upper-division sciences coursework; prerequisites in general biology, general chemistry, general physics, organic chemistry, quantitative analysis, and integral and differential calculus; for doctorate, GRE General Test (minimum score of 600 quantitative), bachelor's degree from regionally-accredited university with minimum GPA of 3.0 in upper-division sciences coursework; 3 letters of recommendation; personal interview; 1-2 page personal statement; prerequisites in biology, chemistry, physics, organic chemistry, quantitative analysis, and integral/differential calculus. Additional exam requirements/recommendations for international students: Required—TOEFL (minimum score 550 paper-based; 79 iBT) or IELTS (minimum score 6.5). *Application deadline:* For fall admission, 2/15 for domestic students, 1/2 for international students. Application fee: $30. *Expenses:* Contact institution. *Faculty research:* Anatomy, biochemistry, cancer biology, cardiovascular disease, cell biology, immunology, microbiology, molecular biology, neuroscience, pharmacology, physiology. *Unit head:* Dr. Michael Barber, Professor and Associate Dean for Graduate and Postdoctoral Affairs, 813-974-9908, Fax: 813-974-4317, E-mail: mbarber@health.usf.edu. *Application contact:* Dr. Eric Bennett, Graduate Director, PhD Program in Medical Sciences, 813-974-1545, Fax: 813-974-4317, E-mail: esbennet@health.usf.edu.
Website: http://health.usf.edu/nocms/medicine/graduatestudies/

The University of Tennessee Health Science Center, College of Graduate Health Sciences, Memphis, TN 38163-0002. Offers biomedical engineering (MS, PhD); biomedical sciences (PhD); dental sciences (MDS); epidemiology (MS); health outcomes and policy research (PhD); laboratory research and management (MS); nursing science (PhD); pharmaceutical sciences (PhD); pharmacology (MS); speech and hearing science (PhD); DDS/PhD; DNP/PhD; MD/PhD; Pharm D/PhD. *Faculty:* 318 full-time (92 women), 59 part-time/adjunct (16 women). *Students:* 220 full-time (102 women), 22 part-time (13 women); includes 194 minority (22 Black or African American, non-Hispanic/Latino; 161 Asian, non-Hispanic/Latino; 7 Hispanic/Latino; 3 Native Hawaiian or other Pacific Islander, non-Hispanic/Latino; 1 Two or more races, non-Hispanic/Latino), 106 international. Average age 25. 404 applicants, 17% accepted, 64 enrolled. In 2013, 13 master's, 25 doctorates awarded. Terminal master's awarded for partial completion of doctoral program. *Degree requirements:* For master's, comprehensive exam, thesis; for doctorate, comprehensive exam, thesis/dissertation, oral and written preliminary and comprehensive exams. *Entrance requirements:* For master's and doctorate, GRE General Test, minimum GPA of 3.0. Additional exam requirements/recommendations for international students: Required—TOEFL (minimum score 79 iBT); Recommended—IELTS (minimum score 6.5). *Application deadline:* For fall admission, 5/15 priority date for domestic students. Applications are processed on a rolling basis. Application fee: $0. Electronic applications accepted. *Financial support:* In 2013–14, 125 students received support, including 125 research assistantships (averaging $23,000 per year); career-related internships or fieldwork, Federal Work-Study, institutionally sponsored loans, and tuition waivers (full and partial) also available. Support available to part-time students. Financial award application deadline: 2/25; financial award applicants required to submit FAFSA. *Unit head:* Dr. Donald B. Thomason, Dean, 901-448-5538, E-mail: dthomaso@uthsc.edu. *Application contact:* William Carter, Director for Admissions, 901-448-1687, E-mail: wcarte17@uthsc.edu.
Website: http://www.uthsc.edu/grad/

The University of Toledo, College of Graduate Studies, College of Medicine and Life Sciences, Department of Public Health and Preventative Medicine, Toledo, OH 43606-3390. Offers biostatistics and epidemiology (Certificate); contemporary gerontological practice (Certificate); environmental and occupational health and safety (MPH); epidemiology (Certificate); global public health (Certificate); health promotion and education (MPH); industrial hygiene (MSOH); medical and health science teaching and learning (Certificate); occupational health (Certificate); public health administration (MPH); public health and emergency response (Certificate); public health epidemiology (MPH); public health nutrition (MPH); MD/MPH. Part-time and evening/weekend programs available. *Faculty:* 9. *Students:* 69 full-time (50 women), 88 part-time (66 women); includes 50 minority (35 Black or African American, non-Hispanic/Latino; 10 Asian, non-Hispanic/Latino; 4 Hispanic/Latino; 1 Two or more races, non-Hispanic/Latino), 6 international. Average age 30. 92 applicants, 80% accepted, 52 enrolled. In 2013, 59 master's, 15 other advanced degrees awarded. *Degree requirements:* For master's, thesis or alternative. *Entrance requirements:* For master's, GRE, minimum undergraduate GPA of 3.0, three letters of recommendation, statement of purpose, transcripts from all prior institutions attended, resume; for Certificate, minimum undergraduate GPA of 3.0, three letters of recommendation, statement of purpose, transcripts from all prior institutions attended, resume. Additional exam requirements/recommendations for international students: Required—TOEFL (minimum score 550 paper-based; 80 iBT), IELTS (minimum score 6.5). *Application deadline:* For fall admission, 6/15 for domestic students, 3/15 priority date for international students; for spring admission, 10/15 for domestic students, 6/15 for international students; for summer admission, 3/15 for domestic students, 10/15 for international students. Applications are processed on a rolling basis. Application fee: $45 ($75 for international students). Electronic applications accepted. *Financial support:* In 2013–14, 4 research assistantships with full tuition reimbursements (averaging $10,000 per year) were awarded; Federal Work-Study, institutionally sponsored loans, scholarships/grants, tuition waivers (full and partial), and unspecified assistantships also available. *Unit head:* Dr. Sheryl A. Milz, Chair, 419-383-3976, Fax: 419-383-6140, E-mail: sheryl.milz@

utoledo.edu. *Application contact:* Admissions Analyst, 419-383-4112, Fax: 419-383-6140.
Website: http://nocphmph.org/

University of Toronto, School of Graduate Studies, Dalla Lana School of Public Health, Toronto, ON M5S 1A1, Canada. Offers biostatistics (M Sc, PhD); community health (M Sc); epidemiology (MPH, PhD); health and behavioral science (PhD); health promotion (MPH); social science and health (PhD). *Accreditation:* CAHME (one or more programs are accredited); CEPH (one or more programs are accredited). Part-time programs available. *Degree requirements:* For master's, thesis (for some programs), practicum; for doctorate, comprehensive exam, thesis/dissertation, oral thesis defense. *Entrance requirements:* For master's, 2 letters of reference, relevant professional/research experience, minimum B average in final year; for doctorate, 2 letters of reference, relevant professional/research experience, minimum B+ average. Additional exam requirements/recommendations for international students: Required—TOEFL (minimum score 580 paper-based; 93 iBT), TWE (minimum score 5). Electronic applications accepted. *Expenses:* Contact institution.

University of Washington, Graduate School, School of Public Health, Department of Epidemiology, Seattle, WA 98195. Offers clinical research (MS); epidemiology (MPH, MS, PhD); global health (MPH); maternal/child health (MPH); MPH/MPA. *Accreditation:* CEPH (one or more programs are accredited). *Faculty:* 65 full-time (38 women), 39 part-time/adjunct (17 women). *Students:* 120 full-time (84 women), 30 part-time (20 women); includes 19 minority (3 Black or African American, non-Hispanic/Latino; 2 American Indian or Alaska Native, non-Hispanic/Latino; 14 Asian, non-Hispanic/Latino), 12 international. Average age 32. 234 applicants, 37% accepted, 40 enrolled. In 2013, 41 master's, 18 doctorates awarded. *Degree requirements:* For master's, comprehensive exam (for some programs), thesis; for doctorate, comprehensive exam, thesis/dissertation, general exam, dissertation proposal, final exam (dissertation defense). *Entrance requirements:* For master's, GRE (except for those holding PhD, MD, DDS, DVM, DO or equivalent from U.S. institutions); for doctorate, GRE. Additional exam requirements/recommendations for international students: Required—TOEFL (minimum score 580 paper-based, 92 iBT), IELTS (minimum score 7), or PTE (minimum score of 65). *Application deadline:* For fall admission, 12/1 for domestic students, 11/1 for international students. Application fee: $85. Electronic applications accepted. *Expenses:* Contact institution. *Financial support:* In 2013–14, 138 students received support, including 70 fellowships with partial tuition reimbursements available, 40 research assistantships with partial tuition reimbursements available, 12 teaching assistantships with partial tuition reimbursements available; career-related internships or fieldwork, Federal Work-Study, traineeships, health care benefits, tuition waivers, and unspecified assistantships also available. Support available to part-time students. Financial award application deadline: 12/1; financial award applicants required to submit FAFSA. *Faculty research:* Chronic disease, health disparities and social determinants of health, aging and neuroepidemiology, maternal and child health, molecular and genetic epidemiology. *Unit head:* Dr. Scott Davis, Chair, 206-543-1065, E-mail: epiapply@uw.edu. *Application contact:* Kate O'Brien, Student Services Manager, 206-543-1065, E-mail: epiapply@uw.edu.
Website: http://depts.washington.edu/epidem/

The University of Western Ontario, Faculty of Graduate Studies, Biosciences Division, Department of Epidemiology and Biostatistics, London, ON N6A 5B8, Canada. Offers M Sc, PhD. *Accreditation:* CEPH (one or more programs are accredited). Part-time programs available. *Degree requirements:* For master's, thesis; for doctorate, comprehensive exam, thesis proposal defense. *Entrance requirements:* For master's, BA or B Sc honors degree, minimum B+ average in last 10 courses; for doctorate, M Sc or equivalent, minimum B+ average in last 10 courses. *Faculty research:* Chronic disease epidemiology, clinical epidemiology.

University of Wisconsin–Madison, School of Medicine and Public Health and Graduate School, Graduate Programs in Medicine, Department of Population Health Sciences, Madison, WI 53726. Offers epidemiology (MS, PhD); population health (MS, PhD). *Accreditation:* CEPH. Part-time programs available. *Faculty:* 104 full-time (54 women), 2 part-time/adjunct (0 women). *Students:* 56 full-time (38 women), 14 part-time (9 women); includes 17 minority (8 Black or African American, non-Hispanic/Latino; 7 Asian, non-Hispanic/Latino; 2 Hispanic/Latino), 10 international. Average age 31. 97 applicants, 40% accepted, 20 enrolled. In 2013, 9 master's, 10 doctorates awarded. Terminal master's awarded for partial completion of doctoral program. *Degree requirements:* For master's, thesis, thesis defense; for doctorate, comprehensive exam, thesis/dissertation, qualifying exam, preliminary exam, dissertation defense. *Entrance requirements:* For master's and doctorate, GRE taken within the last 5 years (MCAT or LSAT acceptable for those with doctoral degrees), minimum GPA of 3.0, quantitative preparation (calculus, statistics, or other) with minimum B average. Additional exam requirements/recommendations for international students: Required—TOEFL (minimum score 580 paper-based; 92 iBT). *Application deadline:* For fall admission, 1/15 for domestic and international students. Application fee: $56. Electronic applications accepted. *Expenses:* Tuition, state resident: full-time $10,728; part-time $790 per credit. Tuition, nonresident: full-time $24,054; part-time $1623 per credit. *Required fees:* $1130; $119 per credit. *Financial support:* Fellowships with full tuition reimbursements, research assistantships with full tuition reimbursements, teaching assistantships with full tuition reimbursements, scholarships/grants, traineeships, health care benefits, and unspecified assistantships available. Support available to part-time students. *Faculty research:* Epidemiology (cancer, environmental, aging, infectious and genetic disease), determinants of population health, health services research, social and behavioral health sciences, biostatistics. *Total annual research expenditures:* $11.4 million. *Unit head:* Kathy Rutlin, MS/PhD Programs Coordinator, 608-265-8108, Fax: 608-263-2820, E-mail: karutlin@wisc.edu. *Application contact:* Quinn H. Fullenkamp, Assistant Programs Coordinator, 608-263-6583, Fax: 608-263-2820, E-mail: qhfullen@wisc.edu.
Website: http://www.pophealth.wisc.edu

Virginia Commonwealth University, Medical College of Virginia-Professional Programs, School of Medicine, School of Medicine Graduate Programs, Department of Epidemiology and Community Health, Richmond, VA 23284-9005. Offers epidemiology (MPH, PhD); public health practice (MPH); social and behavioral science (MPH); MD/MPH; MSW/MPH. *Accreditation:* CEPH. Part-time programs available. *Degree requirements:* For doctorate, comprehensive exam, thesis/dissertation. *Entrance requirements:* For master's, GRE; for doctorate, GRE General Test, interview, 3 letters of recommendation, minimum graduate GPA of 3.0, master's degree in public health or related field including epidemiology and biostatistics. Additional exam requirements/recommendations for international students: Required—TOEFL (minimum score 600 paper-based; 100 iBT). Electronic applications accepted. *Faculty research:* Sickle cell anemia, breast cancer, HIV/AIDS, hospital epidemiology, infectious diseases.

Walden University, Graduate Programs, School of Health Sciences, Minneapolis, MN 55401. Offers clinical research administration (MS, Graduate Certificate); health education and promotion (MS); health informatics (MS); health services (PhD), including community health, healthcare administration, leadership, public health policy, self-designed; healthcare administration (MHA); public health (MPH, Dr PH, PhD), including community health and education (PhD), epidemiology (PhD). Part-time and evening/weekend programs available. Postbaccalaureate distance learning degree programs offered (minimal on-campus study). *Faculty:* 18 full-time (12 women), 236 part-time/adjunct (120 women). *Students:* 2,563 full-time (1,867 women), 1,775 part-time (1,233 women); includes 2,532 minority (1,963 Black or African American, non-Hispanic/Latino; 29 American Indian or Alaska Native, non-Hispanic/Latino; 212 Asian, non-Hispanic/Latino; 238 Hispanic/Latino; 15 Native Hawaiian or other Pacific Islander, non-Hispanic/Latino; 75 Two or more races, non-Hispanic/Latino), 97 international. Average age 39. 1,191 applicants, 94% accepted, 861 enrolled. In 2013, 723 master's, 121 doctorates, 17 other advanced degrees awarded. *Degree requirements:* For doctorate, thesis/dissertation, residency. *Entrance requirements:* For master's, bachelor's degree or higher; minimum GPA of 2.5; official transcripts; goal statement (for some programs); access to computer and Internet; for doctorate, master's degree or higher; three years of related professional or academic experience (preferred); minimum GPA of 3.0; goal statement and current resume (select programs); official transcripts; access to computer and Internet; for Graduate Certificate, relevant work experience; access to computer and Internet. Additional exam requirements/recommendations for international students: Required—TOEFL (minimum score 550 paper-based; 79 iBT), IELTS (minimum score 6.5), Michigan English Language Assessment Battery (minimum score 82), or PTE. *Application deadline:* Applications are processed on a rolling basis. Application fee: $0. Electronic applications accepted. *Expenses:* *Tuition:* Full-time $11,813.55; part-time $500 per credit. *Required fees:* $618.76. *Financial support:* Fellowships, Federal Work-Study, scholarships/grants, unspecified assistantships, and family tuition reduction, active duty/veteran tuition reduction, group tuition reduction, interest-free payment plans, employee tuition reduction available. Support available to part-time students. Financial award applicants required to submit FAFSA. *Unit head:* Dr. Jorg Westermann, Associate Dean, 800-925-3368. *Application contact:* Jennifer Hall, Vice President of Enrollment Management, 866-4-WALDEN, E-mail: info@waldenu.edu.
Website: http://www.waldenu.edu/colleges-schools/school-of-health-sciences

Washington University in St. Louis, George Warren Brown School of Social Work, St. Louis, MO 63130. Offers Alaska native/American Indian studies (MSW); children, youth and families (MSW); gerontology (MSW); mental health (MSW); public health (MPA, MPH), including epidemiology/biostatistics (MPH), global health (MPA); social and economic development (MSW); social work (MSW, PhD), including health (MSW); JD/MSW; M Arch/MSW; MBA/MSW; MPH/MBA; MSW/M Div; MSW/MAPS; MSW/MJCS; MSW/MPH. MSW/M Div and MSW/MAPS offered jointly with Eden Theological Seminary. *Accreditation:* CSWE (one or more programs are accredited). *Faculty:* 42 full-time (24 women), 81 part-time/adjunct (49 women). *Students:* 298 full-time (263 women), 5 part-time (all women); includes 78 minority (32 Black or African American, non-Hispanic/Latino; 4 American Indian or Alaska Native, non-Hispanic/Latino; 18 Asian, non-Hispanic/Latino; 9 Hispanic/Latino; 2 Native Hawaiian or other Pacific Islander, non-Hispanic/Latino; 13 Two or more races, non-Hispanic/Latino), 47 international. Average age 26. 817 applicants, 62% accepted, 303 enrolled. In 2013, 239 master's, 5 doctorates awarded. *Degree requirements:* For master's, 60 credit hours (MSW), 52 credit hours (MPH); practicum; for doctorate, comprehensive exam, thesis/dissertation. *Entrance requirements:* For master's, GRE, GMAT, LSAT, or MCAT (public health), minimum GPA of 3.0; for doctorate, GRE, MA or MSW. Additional exam requirements/recommendations for international students: Required—TOEFL (minimum score 100 iBT). *Application deadline:* For fall admission, 3/1 priority date for domestic and international students. Applications are processed on a rolling basis. Application fee: $40. Electronic applications accepted. *Expenses:* Contact institution. *Financial support:* In 2013–14, 301 students received support. Fellowships, research assistantships, Federal Work-Study, institutionally sponsored loans, scholarships/grants, health care benefits, tuition waivers (partial), and unspecified assistantships available. Support available to part-time students. Financial award application deadline: 3/1; financial award applicants required to submit FAFSA. *Faculty research:* Mental health services, social development, child welfare, at-risk teens, autism, environmental health, health policy, health communications, obesity, violence and injury prevention, chronic disease prevention, poverty, public health, productive aging/gerontology, social work, civic engagement, school social work, program evaluation, health disparities. *Unit head:* Dr. Edward F. Lawlor, Dean/Professor, 314-935-6693, Fax: 314-935-8511, E-mail: elawlor@wustl.edu. *Application contact:* Leslie D. Duling, Admissions Counselor, 314-935-6694, Fax: 314-935-4859, E-mail: lduling@brownschool.wustl.edu.
Website: http://gwbweb.wustl.edu/

Weill Cornell Medical College, Weill Cornell Graduate School of Medical Sciences, Program in Clinical Epidemiology and Health Services Research, New York, NY 10021. Offers MS. *Degree requirements:* For master's, thesis. *Entrance requirements:* For master's, 3 years of work experience, MD or RN certificate. *Faculty research:* Research methodology, biostatistical techniques, data management, decision analysis, health economics.

Yale University, School of Medicine, Yale School of Public Health, New Haven, CT 06520. Offers applied biostatistics and epidemiology (APMPH); biostatistics (MPH, MS, PhD), including global health (MPH); chronic disease epidemiology (MPH, PhD), including global health (MPH); environmental health sciences (MPH, PhD), including global health (MPH); epidemiology of microbial diseases (MPH, PhD), including global health (MPH); global health (APMPH); health management (MPH), including global health; health policy (MPH), including global health; health policy and administration (APMPH, PhD); occupational and environmental medicine (APMPH); preventive medicine (APMPH); social and behavioral sciences (APMPH, MPH), including global health (MPH); JD/MPH; M Div/MPH; MBA/MPH; MD/MPH; MEM/MPH; MFS/MPH; MM Sc/MPH; MPH/MA; MSN/MPH. MS and PhD offered through the Graduate School. *Accreditation:* CEPH. Part-time programs available. Terminal master's awarded for partial completion of doctoral program. *Degree requirements:* For master's, thesis, summer internship; for doctorate, comprehensive exam, thesis/dissertation, residency. *Entrance requirements:* For master's, GMAT, GRE, or MCAT, two years of undergraduate coursework in math and science; for doctorate, GRE General Test. Additional exam requirements/recommendations for international students: Required—TOEFL (minimum score 100 iBT). Electronic applications accepted. *Expenses:* Contact institution. *Faculty research:* Genetic and emerging infections epidemiology, virology, cost/quality, vector biology, quantitative methods, aging, asthma, cancer.

Health Promotion

American University, College of Arts and Sciences, Washington, DC 20016-8012. Offers addiction and addictive behavior (Certificate); anthropology (PhD); applied microeconomics (Certificate); applied statistics (Certificate); art history (MA); arts management (MA, Certificate); Asian studies (Certificate); audio production (Certificate); audio technology (MA); behavior, cognition, and neuroscience (PhD); bilingual education (MA, Certificate); biology (MA, MS); chemistry (MS); clinical psychology (PhD); computer science (MS, Certificate); creative writing (MFA); curriculum and instruction (M Ed, Certificate); economics (MA, PhD); environmental assessment (Certificate); environmental science (MS); ethics, peace, and global affairs (MA); gender analysis in economics (Certificate); health promotion management (MS); history (MA, PhD); international arts management (Certificate); international economic relations (Certificate); international economics (MA); international training and education (MA); literature (MA); mathematics (MA); North American studies (Certificate); nutrition education (MS, Certificate); philosophy (MA); professional science: biotechnology (MS); professional science: environmental assessment (MS); professional science: quantitative analysis (MS); psychobiology of healing (Certificate); psychology (MA); psychology: general (PhD); public anthropology (MA, Certificate); public sociology (Certificate); social research (Certificate); sociology (MA); Spanish: Latin American studies (MA); special education: learning disabilities (MA); statistics (MS); studio art (MFA); teaching (MAT); teaching English as a foreign language (MA); teaching: early childhood (Certificate); teaching: elementary (Certificate); teaching: ESOL (Certificate); teaching: secondary (Certificate); technology in arts management (Certificate); TESOL (MA); translation: French (Certificate); translation: Russian (Certificate); translation: Spanish (Certificate); women's, gender, and sexuality studies (Certificate). Part-time and evening/weekend programs available. Postbaccalaureate distance learning degree programs offered (no on-campus study). *Faculty:* 358 full-time (187 women), 254 part-time/adjunct (127 women). *Students:* 627 full-time (411 women), 416 part-time (300 women); includes 206 minority (91 Black or African American, non-Hispanic/Latino; 5 American Indian or Alaska Native, non-Hispanic/Latino; 32 Asian, non-Hispanic/Latino; 64 Hispanic/Latino; 1 Native Hawaiian or other Pacific Islander, non-Hispanic/Latino; 13 Two or more races, non-Hispanic/Latino), 124 international. Average age 29. 1,672 applicants, 52% accepted, 361 enrolled. In 2013, 382 master's, 38 doctorates, 33 other advanced degrees awarded. Terminal master's awarded for partial completion of doctoral program. *Degree requirements:* For master's, comprehensive exam (for some programs), thesis (for some programs); for doctorate, comprehensive exam (for some programs), thesis/dissertation. *Entrance requirements:* For master's, GRE, minimum GPA of 3.0 in last 60 credit hours, letter of recommendation, statement of purpose, resume, unofficial transcript; for doctorate, GRE, minimum GPA of 3.0 for all graduate work, letter of recommendation, statement of purpose, resume, unofficial transcript. Additional exam requirements/recommendations for international students: Required—TOEFL (minimum score 600 paper-based; 100 iBT), IELTS (minimum score 7). *Application deadline:* For fall admission, 2/1 for domestic students; for spring admission, 10/1 for domestic students. Applications are processed on a rolling basis. Application fee: $55. Electronic applications accepted. *Expenses: Tuition:* Full-time $25,920; part-time $1482 per credit hour. *Required fees:* $430. Tuition and fees vary according to course load and program. *Financial support:* Fellowships, research assistantships with full and partial tuition reimbursements, teaching assistantships with full and partial tuition reimbursements, career-related internships or fieldwork, Federal Work-Study, institutionally sponsored loans, scholarships/grants, traineeships, tuition waivers (full and partial), and unspecified assistantships available. Support available to part-time students. Financial award applicants required to submit FAFSA. *Unit head:* Dr. Peter Starr, Dean, 202-885-2446, Fax: 202-885-2429, E-mail: pstarr@american.edu. *Application contact:* Kathleen Clowery, Associate Director, Graduate Enrollment Management, 202-885-3621, Fax: 202-885-1505, E-mail: clowery@american.edu.
Website: http://www.american.edu/cas/

American University of Beirut, Graduate Programs, Faculty of Health Sciences, Beirut, Lebanon. Offers environmental sciences (MS), including environmental health; epidemiology (MS); epidemiology and biostatistics (MPH); health management and policy (MPH); health promotion and community health (MPH); population health (MS). Part-time programs available. *Faculty:* 26 full-time (18 women), 7 part-time/adjunct (4 women). *Students:* 42 full-time (37 women), 103 part-time (84 women). Average age 25. 132 applicants, 65% accepted, 48 enrolled. In 2013, 52 master's awarded. *Degree requirements:* For master's, one foreign language, comprehensive exam, thesis (for some programs). *Entrance requirements:* For master's, 2 letters of recommendation, personal statement, transcripts. Additional exam requirements/recommendations for international students: Required—TOEFL (minimum score 583 paper-based; 97 iBT), IELTS (minimum score 7). *Application deadline:* For fall admission, 2/7 priority date for domestic and international students; for spring admission, 11/1 for domestic and international students. Application fee: $50. Electronic applications accepted. *Expenses: Tuition:* Full-time $14,724; part-time $818 per credit. *Required fees:* $692. Tuition and fees vary according to course load and program. *Financial support:* In 2013–14, 56 students received support. Scholarships/grants, health care benefits, and unspecified assistantships available. Financial award application deadline: 4/1. *Faculty research:* Tobacco control; health of the elderly; youth health; mental health; women's health; reproductive and sexual health, including HIV/AIDS; water quality; health systems; quality in health care delivery; health human resources; health policy; occupational and environmental health; social inequality; social determinants of health; non-communicable diseases. *Total annual research expenditures:* $1 million. *Unit head:* Iman Adel Nuwayhid, Dean, 961-1759683, Fax: 961-1744470, E-mail: nuwayhid@aub.edu.lb. *Application contact:* Mitra Tauk, Administrative Coordinator, 961-1-350000 Ext. 4687, Fax: 96-1-1744470, E-mail: mt12@aub.edu.lb.

Auburn University, Graduate School, College of Education, Department of Kinesiology, Auburn University, AL 36849. Offers exercise science (M Ed, MS, PhD); health promotion (M Ed, MS); kinesiology (PhD); physical education/teacher education (M Ed, MS, Ed D, Ed S). *Accreditation:* NCATE. Part-time programs available. *Faculty:* 19 full-time (9 women). *Students:* 89 full-time (43 women), 21 part-time (9 women); includes 17 minority (15 Black or African American, non-Hispanic/Latino; 1 Asian, non-Hispanic/Latino; 1 Hispanic/Latino), 5 international. Average age 26. 136 applicants, 71% accepted, 60 enrolled. In 2013, 38 master's, 10 doctorates awarded. *Degree requirements:* For master's, thesis (for some programs); for doctorate, thesis/dissertation; for Ed S, exam, field project. *Entrance requirements:* For master's, GRE General Test; for doctorate and Ed S, GRE General Test, interview, master's degree. *Application deadline:* For fall admission, 7/7 for domestic students; for spring admission, 11/24 for domestic students. Applications are processed on a rolling basis. Application fee: $50 ($60 for international students). Electronic applications accepted. *Expenses:* Tuition, state resident: full-time $8262; part-time $459 per credit hour. Tuition, nonresident: full-time $24,786; part-time $1377 per credit hour. Tuition and fees vary according to degree level and program. *Financial support:* Research assistantships, teaching assistantships, and Federal Work-Study available. Support available to part-time students. Financial award application deadline: 3/15; financial award applicants required to submit FAFSA. *Faculty research:* Biomechanics, exercise physiology, motor skill learning, school health, curriculum development. *Unit head:* Dr. Mary E. Rudisill, Head, 334-844-1458. *Application contact:* Dr. George Flowers, Dean of the Graduate School, 334-844-2125.

Ball State University, Graduate School, College of Applied Science and Technology, Fisher Institute for Wellness and Gerontology, Interdepartmental Program in Wellness Management, Muncie, IN 47306-1099. Offers MA, MS. *Students:* 9 full-time (8 women), 2 part-time (1 woman); includes 2 minority (1 Black or African American, non-Hispanic/Latino; 1 Two or more races, non-Hispanic/Latino), 2 international. Average age 25. 8 applicants, 75% accepted, 1 enrolled. In 2013, 8 master's awarded. *Entrance requirements:* For master's, GRE General Test, interview. Application fee: $25 ($35 for international students). *Financial support:* In 2013–14, 11 students received support, including 11 teaching assistantships (averaging $8,873 per year); research assistantships with full tuition reimbursements available and career-related internships or fieldwork also available. Financial award application deadline: 3/1. *Unit head:* Dr. Jane Ellery, Head, 765-285-8119, E-mail: jellery@bsu.edu. *Application contact:* Dr. Robert Morris, Associate Provost for Research and Dean of the Graduate School, 765-285-5723, Fax: 765-285-1328, E-mail: rmorris@bsu.edu.
Website: http://www.bsu.edu/wellness/

Baylor University, Graduate School, School of Education, Department of Health, Human Performance and Recreation, Waco, TX 76798. Offers community health education (MPH); exercise physiology (MS Ed); kinesiology, exercise nutrition and health promotion (PhD); sport management (MS Ed); sport pedagogy (MS Ed). *Accreditation:* NCATE. Part-time programs available. *Faculty:* 13 full-time (5 women), 3 part-time/adjunct (1 woman). *Students:* 79 full-time (40 women), 28 part-time (14 women); includes 26 minority (9 Black or African American, non-Hispanic/Latino; 1 American Indian or Alaska Native, non-Hispanic/Latino; 3 Asian, non-Hispanic/Latino; 8 Hispanic/Latino; 5 Two or more races, non-Hispanic/Latino), 9 international. 30 applicants, 87% accepted. In 2013, 48 master's awarded. *Degree requirements:* For master's, comprehensive exam, thesis optional; for doctorate, comprehensive exam, thesis/dissertation. *Entrance requirements:* For master's and doctorate, GRE General Test. Additional exam requirements/recommendations for international students: Required—TOEFL. *Application deadline:* For fall admission, 2/1 priority date for domestic students, 2/1 for international students; for spring admission, 10/1 for domestic and international students. Applications are processed on a rolling basis. Application fee: $25. Electronic applications accepted. *Expenses: Tuition:* Full-time $25,866; part-time $1437 per credit hour. *Required fees:* $2736; $152 per credit hour. Tuition and fees vary according to course load and program. *Financial support:* In 2013–14, 35 students received support, including 1 research assistantship with tuition reimbursement available, 33 teaching assistantships with tuition reimbursements available; career-related internships or fieldwork, Federal Work-Study, institutionally sponsored loans, tuition waivers (partial), and unspecified assistantships also available. Financial award application deadline: 2/1. *Faculty research:* Behavior change theory, nutrition and enzyme therapy, exercise testing, health planning, sport management. *Unit head:* Dr. Jeffrey Petersen, Graduate Program Director, 254-710-4007, Fax: 254-710-3527, E-mail: jeffrey_petersen@baylor.edu. *Application contact:* Kathy Mirick, Administrative Assistant, 254-710-3526, Fax: 254-710-3527, E-mail: kathy_mirick@baylor.edu.
Website: http://www.baylor.edu/HHPR/

Benedictine University, Graduate Programs, Program in Nutrition and Wellness, Lisle, IL 60532-0900. Offers MS. *Students:* 29 full-time (28 women), 44 part-time (42 women); includes 13 minority (4 Black or African American, non-Hispanic/Latino; 6 Asian, non-Hispanic/Latino; 3 Hispanic/Latino). 49 applicants, 67% accepted, 25 enrolled. In 2013, 22 master's awarded. *Entrance requirements:* Additional exam requirements/recommendations for international students: Required—TOEFL (minimum score 550 paper-based). *Application deadline:* For fall admission, 9/1 for domestic students; for winter admission, 12/1 for domestic students; for spring admission, 2/15 for domestic students. Applications are processed on a rolling basis. Application fee: $40. Electronic applications accepted. *Expenses: Tuition:* Part-time $590 per credit hour. *Financial support:* Career-related internships or fieldwork and health care benefits available. Support available to part-time students. *Faculty research:* Community and corporate wellness risk assessment, health behavior change, self-efficacy, evaluation of health program impact and effectiveness. *Total annual research expenditures:* $8,335. *Unit head:* Catherine Arnold, Director, 630-829-6534, E-mail: carnold@ben.edu. *Application contact:* Kari Gibbons, Associate Vice President, Enrollment Center, 630-829-6200, Fax: 630-829-6584, E-mail: kgibbons@ben.edu.

Boise State University, College of Health Sciences, Department of Community and Environmental Health, Boise, ID 83725-0399. Offers environmental health (MHS); evaluation and research (MHS); health policy (MHS); health promotion (MHS); health services leadership (MHS).

Boston University, School of Public Health, Social and Behavioral Sciences Department, Boston, MA 02215. Offers Dr PH. *Accreditation:* CEPH. Part-time and evening/weekend programs available. *Students:* 82 full-time (69 women), 50 part-time (44 women); includes 32 minority (9 Black or African American, non-Hispanic/Latino; 9 Asian, non-Hispanic/Latino; 10 Hispanic/Latino; 4 Two or more races, non-Hispanic/Latino), 10 international. Average age 26. 361 applicants, 59% accepted, 55 enrolled. *Degree requirements:* For doctorate, thesis/dissertation. *Entrance requirements:* For doctorate, GRE, GMAT. Additional exam requirements/recommendations for international students: Required—TOEFL (minimum score 600 paper-based; 100 iBT) or IELTS (minimum score 6). *Application deadline:* For fall admission, 2/1 priority date for domestic and international students; for spring admission, 10/15 priority date for domestic and international students. Applications are processed on a rolling basis. Application fee: $115. Electronic applications accepted. *Expenses: Tuition:* Full-time $43,970; part-time $1374 per credit hour. *Required fees:* $60 per semester. Tuition and fees vary according to class time, course level and program. *Financial support:* Career-related internships or fieldwork, Federal Work-Study, institutionally sponsored loans, scholarships/grants, and tuition waivers (partial) available. Support available to part-time students. Financial award application deadline: 3/1; financial award applicants required to submit FAFSA. *Unit head:* Dr. Mary Jane England, Interim Chair, Community Health Sciences, 617-638-5160, E-mail: asksb@bu.edu. *Application contact:* LePhan Quan, Associate Director of Admissions, 617-638-4640, Fax: 617-638-5299, E-mail: asksph@bu.edu.
Website: http://sph.bu.edu/sb

Bridgewater State University, School of Graduate Studies, School of Education and Allied Studies, Department of Movement Arts, Health Promotion, and Leisure Studies,

Health Promotion

Program in Health Promotion, Bridgewater, MA 02325-0001. Offers M Ed. Part-time and evening/weekend programs available. *Entrance requirements:* For master's, GRE General Test.

Brigham Young University, Graduate Studies, College of Life Sciences, Department of Exercise Sciences, Provo, UT 84602. Offers athletic training (MS); exercise physiology (MS, PhD); exercise science (MS); health promotion (MS, PhD); physical medicine and rehabilitation (PhD). *Faculty:* 20 full-time (3 women), 1 part-time/adjunct (0 women). *Students:* 45 full-time (20 women), 2 part-time (1 woman); includes 4 minority (2 Asian, non-Hispanic/Latino; 2 Two or more races, non-Hispanic/Latino). Average age 28. 23 applicants, 48% accepted, 8 enrolled. In 2013, 13 master's, 1 doctorate awarded. *Degree requirements:* For master's, thesis, oral defense; for doctorate, comprehensive exam, thesis/dissertation, oral defense, oral and written exams. *Entrance requirements:* For master's, GRE General Test, minimum GPA of 3.2 in last 60 hours of course work; for doctorate, GRE General Test, minimum GPA of 3.5 in last 60 hours of course work. Additional exam requirements/recommendations for international students: Required—TOEFL (minimum score 580 paper-based; 85 iBT), IELTS (minimum score 7). *Application deadline:* For fall admission, 2/1 for domestic and international students. Application fee: $50. Electronic applications accepted. *Expenses: Tuition:* Full-time $6130; part-time $340 per credit hour. Tuition and fees vary according to program and student's religious affiliation. *Financial support:* In 2013–14, 36 students received support, including 24 research assistantships with partial tuition reimbursements available (averaging $2,600 per year), 19 teaching assistantships with partial tuition reimbursements available (averaging $3,350 per year); fellowships, career-related internships or fieldwork, institutionally sponsored loans, scholarships/grants, tuition waivers (partial), unspecified assistantships, and 10 PhD full tuition scholarships also available. Financial award application deadline: 3/1. *Faculty research:* Injury prevention and rehabilitation, human skeletal muscle adaptation, cardiovascular health and fitness, lifestyle modification and health promotion. *Total annual research expenditures:* $22,117. *Unit head:* Dr. Gary Mack, Chair, 801-422-2466, Fax: 801-422-0555, E-mail: gary_mack@byu.edu. *Application contact:* Dr. William J. Myrer, Graduate Coordinator, 801-422-2690, Fax: 801-422-0555, E-mail: bill_myrer@byu.edu.
Website: http://exsc.byu.edu/

California Baptist University, Program in Public Health, Riverside, CA 92504-3206. Offers food, nutrition and health (MPH); health policy and administration (MPH); physical activity (MPH). Part-time and evening/weekend programs available. *Degree requirements:* For master's, capstone project; practicum. *Entrance requirements:* For master's, minimum undergraduate GPA of 2.75, bachelor's degree transcripts, three recommendations, 500-word essay, resume, interview. Additional exam requirements/recommendations for international students: Required—TOEFL (minimum score 80 iBT). *Application deadline:* For fall admission, 8/1 priority date for domestic students, 7/1 for international students; for spring admission, 12/1 priority date for domestic students, 11/1 for international students. Applications are processed on a rolling basis. Application fee: $45. Electronic applications accepted. *Expenses:* Contact institution. *Financial support:* Applicants required to submit CSS PROFILE or FAFSA. *Unit head:* Dr. Chuck Sands, Dean, College of Allied Health, 951-343-4619, E-mail: csands@calbaptist.edu. *Application contact:* Dr. Wayne Fletcher, Chair, Department of Health Sciences, 951-552-8724, E-mail: wfletcher@calbaptist.edu.
Website: http://www.calbaptist.edu/explore-cbu/schools-colleges/college-allied-health/health-sciences/master-public-health/

California State University, Fresno, Division of Graduate Studies, College of Health and Human Services, Department of Public Health, Fresno, CA 93740-8027. Offers health policy and management (MPH); health promotion (MPH). *Accreditation:* CEPH. Part-time and evening/weekend programs available. *Degree requirements:* For master's, thesis or alternative. *Entrance requirements:* For master's, GRE General Test, minimum GPA of 2.5. Additional exam requirements/recommendations for international students: Required—TOEFL. Electronic applications accepted. *Faculty research:* Foster parent training, geriatrics, tobacco control.

Claremont Graduate University, Graduate Programs, School of Community and Global Health, Claremont, CA 91773. Offers health promotion science (PhD); public health (MPH). *Accreditation:* CEPH. *Faculty:* 12 full-time (5 women). *Students:* 36 full-time (23 women), 29 part-time (23 women); includes 42 minority (5 Black or African American, non-Hispanic/Latino; 17 Asian, non-Hispanic/Latino; 16 Hispanic/Latino; 4 Two or more races, non-Hispanic/Latino), 4 international. Average age 30. In 2013, 21 master's awarded. *Entrance requirements:* For master's and doctorate, GRE. Additional exam requirements/recommendations for international students: Required—TOEFL (minimum score 550 paper-based; 80 iBT). *Application deadline:* For fall admission, 2/1 priority date for domestic and international students; for spring admission, 11/1 priority date for domestic students. Applications are processed on a rolling basis. Application fee: $80. Electronic applications accepted. *Expenses: Tuition:* Full-time $40,560; part-time $1690 per credit. *Required fees:* $275 per semester. Tuition and fees vary according to program. *Financial support:* Fellowships, research assistantships, teaching assistantships, Federal Work-Study, institutionally sponsored loans, and scholarships/grants available. Support available to part-time students. Financial award application deadline: 2/15; financial award applicants required to submit FAFSA. *Unit head:* Stewart Donaldson, Dean, 909-607-8235, E-mail: stewart.donaldson@cgu.edu. *Application contact:* Admissions Office, 909-607-7811, E-mail: information@cgu.edu.
Website: http://www.cgu.edu/pages/5644.asp

Cleveland University–Kansas City, Program in Health Promotion, Overland Park, KS 66210. Offers MSHP. Part-time programs available. *Entrance requirements:* Additional exam requirements/recommendations for international students: Required—TOEFL (minimum score 550 paper-based; 79 iBT). Electronic applications accepted. *Expenses:* Contact institution.

Concord University, Graduate Studies, Athens, WV 24712-1000. Offers educational leadership and supervision (M Ed); geography (M Ed); health promotion (MA); reading specialist (M Ed); special education (M Ed); teaching (MAT). Part-time and evening/weekend programs available. Postbaccalaureate distance learning degree programs offered (no on-campus study). *Degree requirements:* For master's, thesis (for some programs). *Entrance requirements:* For master's, GRE or MAT, baccalaureate degree with minimum GPA of 2.5 from regionally-accredited institution; teaching license; 2 letters of recommendation; completed disposition assessment form. Electronic applications accepted.

East Carolina University, Graduate School, College of Health and Human Performance, Department of Health Education and Promotion, Greenville, NC 27858-4353. Offers environmental health (MS); health education (MA Ed); health education and promotion (MA). *Accreditation:* NCATE. *Degree requirements:* For master's, comprehensive exam, thesis optional. *Entrance requirements:* For master's, GRE General Test or MAT. Additional exam requirements/recommendations for international students: Required—TOEFL. *Application deadline:* For fall admission, 6/1 priority date for domestic students. Applications are processed on a rolling basis. Application fee: $50. *Expenses:* Tuition, state resident: full-time $4223. Tuition, nonresident: full-time $16,540. *Required fees:* $2184. *Financial support:* Fellowships, research assistantships, teaching assistantships, and career-related internships or fieldwork available. Support available to part-time students. Financial award application deadline: 6/1. *Faculty research:* Community health education, worksite health promotion, school health education, environmental health. *Unit head:* Dr. J. Don Chaney, Chair, 252-737-4942, E-mail: chaneyj@ecu.edu. *Application contact:* Dr. J. Don Chaney, Chair, 252-737-4942, E-mail: chaneyj@ecu.edu.
Website: http://www.ecu.edu/hlth/

Eastern Kentucky University, The Graduate School, College of Health Sciences, Department of Exercise and Sport Science, Richmond, KY 40475-3102. Offers exercise and sport science (MS); exercise and wellness (MS); sports administration (MS). Part-time programs available. *Entrance requirements:* For master's, GRE General Test (minimum score 700 verbal and quantitative), minimum GPA of 2.5 (for most), minimum GPA of 3.0 (analytical writing). *Faculty research:* Nutrition and exercise.

Eastern Michigan University, Graduate School, College of Health and Human Services, School of Health Promotion and Human Performance, Ypsilanti, MI 48197. Offers MS, Graduate Certificate. Part-time and evening/weekend programs available. Postbaccalaureate distance learning degree programs offered (minimal on-campus study). *Faculty:* 29 full-time (13 women). *Students:* 66 full-time (39 women), 107 part-time (48 women); includes 52 minority (23 Black or African American, non-Hispanic/Latino; 2 American Indian or Alaska Native, non-Hispanic/Latino; 14 Asian, non-Hispanic/Latino; 8 Hispanic/Latino; 1 Native Hawaiian or other Pacific Islander, non-Hispanic/Latino; 4 Two or more races, non-Hispanic/Latino), 26 international. Average age 28. 146 applicants, 72% accepted, 68 enrolled. In 2013, 75 master's, 1 other advanced degree awarded. *Entrance requirements:* For master's, MAT (orthotics and prosthetics). Additional exam requirements/recommendations for international students: Required—TOEFL. *Application deadline:* For fall admission, 8/1 for domestic students, 5/1 for international students; for winter admission, 12/1 for domestic students, 10/1 for international students; for spring admission, 4/15 for domestic students, 3/1 for international students. Applications are processed on a rolling basis. Application fee: $35. *Expenses:* Tuition, state resident: full-time $12,300; part-time $466 per credit hour. Tuition, nonresident: full-time $23,159; part-time $918 per credit hour. *Required fees:* $71 per credit hour. $46 per semester. One-time fee: $100. Tuition and fees vary according to course level and degree level. *Financial support:* Fellowships, research assistantships with full tuition reimbursements, teaching assistantships with full tuition reimbursements, career-related internships or fieldwork, Federal Work-Study, institutionally sponsored loans, scholarships/grants, tuition waivers (partial), and unspecified assistantships available. Support available to part-time students. Financial award applicants required to submit FAFSA. *Unit head:* Dr. Christopher Herman, Director, 734-487-2185, Fax: 734-487-2024, E-mail: cherman2@emich.edu. *Application contact:* Dr. Brenda Riemer, Chair, Graduate Programs, 734-487-7120 Ext. 2745, Fax: 734-487-2024, E-mail: briemer@emich.edu.

Emory University, Rollins School of Public Health, Online Program in Public Health, Atlanta, GA 30322-1100. Offers applied epidemiology (MPH); applied public health informatics (MPH); prevention science (MPH). Part-time and evening/weekend programs available. Postbaccalaureate distance learning degree programs offered (minimal on-campus study). *Degree requirements:* For master's, thesis, practicum. *Entrance requirements:* For master's, GRE. Additional exam requirements/recommendations for international students: Required—TOEFL (minimum score 550 paper-based; 80 iBT). Electronic applications accepted.

Fairmont State University, Programs in Education, Fairmont, WV 26554. Offers digital media, new literacies and learning (M Ed); education (MAT); exercise science, fitness and wellness (M Ed); online learning (M Ed); professional studies (M Ed); reading (M Ed); special education (M Ed). *Accreditation:* NCATE. Part-time and evening/weekend programs available. Postbaccalaureate distance learning degree programs offered. *Faculty:* 18 part-time/adjunct (11 women). *Students:* 75 full-time (55 women), 120 part-time (96 women); includes 11 minority (5 Black or African American, non-Hispanic/Latino; 2 American Indian or Alaska Native, non-Hispanic/Latino; 1 Asian, non-Hispanic/Latino; 1 Hispanic/Latino; 2 Two or more races, non-Hispanic/Latino), 1 international. Average age 32. 69 applicants, 86% accepted, 45 enrolled. In 2013, 82 master's awarded. *Entrance requirements:* For master's, GRE. Additional exam requirements/recommendations for international students: Required—TOEFL. *Application deadline:* For fall admission, 5/1 for domestic and international students. Applications are processed on a rolling basis. Application fee: $40. *Expenses:* Tuition, state resident: full-time $6404; part-time $349 per credit hour. Tuition, nonresident: full-time $13,694; part-time $754 per credit hour. Part-time tuition and fees vary according to course load. *Financial support:* In 2013–14, 30 students received support. *Unit head:* Dr. Carolyn Crislip-Tacy, Interim Dean, School of Education, 304-367-4143, Fax: 304-367-4599, E-mail: carolyn.crislip-tacy@fairmontstate.edu. *Application contact:* Jack Kirby, Director of Graduate Studies, 304-367-4101, E-mail: jack.kirby@fairmontstate.edu.
Website: http://www.fairmontstate.edu/graduatestudies/default.asp

Florida Atlantic University, College of Education, Department of Exercise Science and Health Promotion, Boca Raton, FL 33431-0991. Offers MS. Part-time and evening/weekend programs available. *Faculty:* 5 full-time (1 woman), 1 (woman) part-time/adjunct. *Students:* 46 full-time (20 women), 17 part-time (9 women); includes 22 minority (6 Black or African American, non-Hispanic/Latino; 1 Asian, non-Hispanic/Latino; 14 Hispanic/Latino; 1 Two or more races, non-Hispanic/Latino), 4 international. Average age 28. 76 applicants, 43% accepted, 22 enrolled. In 2013, 20 master's awarded. *Degree requirements:* For master's, comprehensive exam, thesis optional. *Entrance requirements:* For master's, GRE General Test, minimum GPA of 3.0 during last 60 hours of course work. Additional exam requirements/recommendations for international students: Required—TOEFL (minimum score 500 paper-based; 61 iBT), IELTS (minimum score 6). *Application deadline:* For fall admission, 7/1 priority date for domestic students, 2/15 for international students; for spring admission, 11/1 priority date for domestic students, 7/15 for international students. Applications are processed on a rolling basis. Application fee: $30. *Expenses:* Tuition, state resident: full-time $6660; part-time $370 per credit hour. Tuition, nonresident: full-time $18,450; part-time $1025 per credit hour. Tuition and fees vary according to course load. *Financial support:* Research assistantships with partial tuition reimbursements, teaching assistantships with partial tuition reimbursements, and career-related internships or fieldwork available. *Faculty research:* Pulmonary limitations during exercise, metabolism regulation, determinants of performance, age-related change in functional mobility and geriatric exercise, behavioral change aimed at promoting active lifestyles. *Unit head:* Dr. Sue Graves, Chair, 954-236-1261, Fax: 954-236-1259. *Application contact:* Dr. Joseph A. O'Kroy, Graduate Coordinator, 954-236-1266, Fax: 954-236-1259, E-mail: okroy@fau.edu.
Website: http://www.coe.fau.edu/academicdepartments/eshp/

Florida International University, Robert Stempel College of Public Health and Social Work, Programs in Public Health, Miami, FL 33199. Offers biostatistics (MPH); environmental and occupational health (MPH, PhD); epidemiology (MPH, PhD); health policy and management (MPH); health promotion and disease prevention (PhD); health promotion and diseases prevention (MPH). Ph D program has fall admissions only; MPH offered jointly with University of Miami. *Accreditation:* CEPH. Part-time and evening/weekend programs available. Postbaccalaureate distance learning degree programs offered (no on-campus study). *Degree requirements:* For master's, thesis optional; for doctorate, comprehensive exam, thesis/dissertation. *Entrance requirements:* For master's, minimum GPA of 3.0, letters of recommendation; for doctorate, GRE, resume, minimum GPA of 3.0, letters of recommendation, letter of intent. Additional exam requirements/recommendations for international students: Required—TOEFL (minimum score 550 paper-based; 80 iBT). Electronic applications accepted. *Expenses:* Contact institution. *Faculty research:* Drugs/AIDS intervention among migrant workers, provision of services for active/recovering drug users with HIV.

George Mason University, College of Education and Human Development, School of Recreation, Health and Tourism, Manassas, VA 20110. Offers exercise, fitness, and health promotion (MS); sport and recreation studies (MS). *Faculty:* 31 full-time (12 women), 67 part-time/adjunct (37 women). *Students:* 24 full-time (16 women), 25 part-time (10 women); includes 13 minority (7 Black or African American, non-Hispanic/Latino; 5 Hispanic/Latino; 1 Two or more races, non-Hispanic/Latino), 1 international. Average age 27. 60 applicants, 77% accepted, 24 enrolled. In 2013, 19 master's awarded. *Degree requirements:* For master's, thesis (for some programs). *Entrance requirements:* For master's, GRE General Test or MAT, 3 letters of recommendation; official transcripts; expanded goals statement; undergraduate course in statistics and minimum GPA of 3.0 in last 60 credit hours and overall (for MS in sport and recreation studies); baccalaureate degree related to kinesiology, exercise science or athletic training (for MS in exercise, fitness and health promotion). Additional exam requirements/recommendations for international students: Required—TOEFL (minimum score 575 paper-based; 88 iBT), IELTS (minimum score 6.5), PTE. *Application deadline:* For fall admission, 4/1 priority date for domestic students; for spring admission, 11/1 priority date for domestic students. Application fee: $65 ($80 for international students). Electronic applications accepted. *Expenses:* Tuition, state resident: full-time $9350; part-time $390 per credit. Tuition, nonresident: full-time $25,754; part-time $1073 per credit. *Required fees:* $2688; $112 per credit. *Financial support:* In 2013–14, 10 students received support, including 10 research assistantships with full and partial tuition reimbursements available (averaging $10,484 per year); career-related internships or fieldwork, Federal Work-Study, scholarships/grants, unspecified assistantships, and health care benefits (for full-time research or teaching assistantship recipients) also available. Support available to part-time students. Financial award application deadline: 3/1; financial award applicants required to submit FAFSA. *Faculty research:* Informing policy; promoting economic development; advocating stewardship of natural resources; improving the quality of life of individuals, families, and communities at the local, national and international levels. *Total annual research expenditures:* $1.5 million. *Unit head:* David Wiggins, Director, 703-993-2057, Fax: 703-993-2025, E-mail: dwiggin1@gmu.edu. *Application contact:* Lindsey Olson, Office Assistant, 703-993-2098, Fax: 703-993-2025, E-mail: lolson7@gmu.edu.
Website: http://rht.gmu.edu/

Georgetown University, Graduate School of Arts and Sciences, Programs in Biomedical Sciences, Department of Microbiology and Immunology, Washington, DC 20057. Offers biohazardous threat agents and emerging infectious diseases (MS); biomedical science policy and advocacy (MS); general microbiology and immunology (MS); global infectious diseases (PhD); microbiology and immunology (PhD). Part-time programs available. *Degree requirements:* For master's, 30 credit hours of coursework; for doctorate, comprehensive exam, thesis/dissertation. *Entrance requirements:* For master's, GRE General Test, 3 letters of reference, bachelor's degree in related field; for doctorate, GRE General Test, 3 letters of reference, MS/BS in related field. Additional exam requirements/recommendations for international students: Required—TOEFL (minimum score 505 paper-based). *Application deadline:* For fall admission, 7/1 for domestic students, 6/1 priority date for international students; for winter admission, 2/2 priority date for domestic students, 1/2 priority date for international students; for spring admission, 11/1 for domestic students, 10/1 priority date for international students. Applications are processed on a rolling basis. Application fee: $75. Electronic applications accepted. *Financial support:* Fellowships with full tuition reimbursements available. *Faculty research:* Pathogenesis and basic biology of the fungus Candida albicans, molecular biology of viral immunopathological mechanisms in Multiple Sclerosis. *Unit head:* Dr. Richard A. Calderone, Chair, 202-687-1513, E-mail: calderor@georgetown.edu. *Application contact:* Kimberly Bassalian, Graduate Program Coordinator, 202-687-3422, Fax: 202-687-1800, E-mail: kdb70@georgetown.edu.
Website: http://microbiology.georgetown.edu/

Georgia College & State University, Graduate School, College of Health Sciences, Department of Kinesiology, Milledgeville, GA 31061. Offers health promotion (M Ed); human performance (M Ed); outdoor education (M Ed); physical education (MAT). *Accreditation:* NCATE (one or more programs are accredited). Part-time and evening/weekend programs available. *Students:* 31 full-time (14 women), 13 part-time (12 women); includes 11 minority (all Black or African American, non-Hispanic/Latino), 1 international. Average age 26. In 2013, 25 master's awarded. *Degree requirements:* For master's, comprehensive exam, thesis optional. *Entrance requirements:* For master's, GRE General Test or MAT, minimum GPA of 2.75 in upper-level undergraduate courses, 2 letters of reference. Additional exam requirements/recommendations for international students: Recommended—TOEFL (minimum score 550 paper-based; 79 iBT). *Application deadline:* For fall admission, 7/1 priority date for domestic students, 4/1 priority date for international students; for spring admission, 11/15 priority date for domestic students, 9/1 priority date for international students. Applications are processed on a rolling basis. Application fee: $40. Electronic applications accepted. *Financial support:* In 2013–14, 26 research assistantships with full tuition reimbursements were awarded; career-related internships or fieldwork and unspecified assistantships also available. Support available to part-time students. Financial award applicants required to submit FAFSA. *Unit head:* Dr. Lisa Griffin, Chair, 478-445-4072, Fax: 478-445-4074, E-mail: lisa.griffin@gcsu.edu. *Application contact:* 800-342-0471, E-mail: grad-admit@gcsu.edu.

Goddard College, Graduate Division, Master of Arts in Health Arts and Sciences Program, Plainfield, VT 05667-9432. Offers MA. *Degree requirements:* For master's, thesis. *Entrance requirements:* For master's, 3 letters of recommendation, study plan and resource list, interview. Electronic applications accepted.

Harvard University, Harvard School of Public Health, Department of Social and Behavioral Sciences, Boston, MA 02115-6096. Offers SM, SD. Part-time programs available. *Faculty:* 20 full-time (8 women), 28 part-time/adjunct (17 women). *Students:* 92 full-time, 10 part-time; includes 32 minority (9 Black or African American, non-Hispanic/Latino; 1 American Indian or Alaska Native, non-Hispanic/Latino; 11 Asian, non-Hispanic/Latino; 7 Hispanic/Latino; 1 Native Hawaiian or other Pacific Islander, non-Hispanic/Latino; 3 Two or more races, non-Hispanic/Latino), 14 international. Average age 27. 288 applicants, 19% accepted, 36 enrolled. In 2013, 20 master's, 17 doctorates awarded. *Degree requirements:* For doctorate, thesis/dissertation, qualifying exam. *Entrance requirements:* For master's, GRE, MCAT; for doctorate, GRE. Additional exam requirements/recommendations for international students: Required—TOEFL (minimum score 600 paper-based; 100 iBT); Recommended—IELTS (minimum score 7). *Application deadline:* For fall admission, 12/15 for domestic and international students. Application fee: $120. Electronic applications accepted. *Expenses:* *Tuition:* Full-time $38,888. *Required fees:* $958. Tuition and fees vary according to campus/location, program and student level. *Financial support:* Fellowships, research assistantships, teaching assistantships, Federal Work-Study, scholarships/grants, traineeships, and unspecified assistantships available. Support available to part-time students. Financial award application deadline: 2/15; financial award applicants required to submit FAFSA. *Faculty research:* Social determinants of health, program design and planned social change, health and social policy, heath care and community-based interventions, health effects and prevention of gender-based violence. *Unit head:* Dr. Ichiro Kawachi, Chair, 617-432-1135, Fax: 617-432-3123, E-mail: ikawachi@hsph.harvard.edu. *Application contact:* Vincent W. James, Director of Admissions, 617-432-1031, Fax: 617-432-7080, E-mail: admissions@hsph.harvard.edu.
Website: http://www.hsph.harvard.edu/social-and-behavioral-sciences/

Immaculata University, College of Graduate Studies, Program in Nutrition Education, Immaculata, PA 19345. Offers nutrition education for the registered dietitian (MA); nutrition education with dietetic internship (MA); nutrition education with wellness promotion (MA). Part-time and evening/weekend programs available. *Degree requirements:* For master's, comprehensive exam, thesis optional. *Entrance requirements:* For master's, GRE or MAT, minimum GPA of 3.0. Additional exam requirements/recommendations for international students: Required—TOEFL. *Application deadline:* Applications are processed on a rolling basis. Application fee: $50. Electronic applications accepted. *Expenses:* *Tuition:* Part-time $660 per credit. Part-time tuition and fees vary according to degree level and program. *Financial support:* Application deadline: 5/1; applicants required to submit FAFSA. *Faculty research:* Sports nutrition, pediatric nutrition, changes in food consumption patterns in weight loss, nutritional counseling. *Unit head:* Dr. Laura Frank, Chair, 610-647-4400 Ext. 3482, E-mail: lfrank@immaculata.edu.

Independence University, Program in Health Services, Salt Lake City, UT 84107. Offers community health (MSHS); wellness promotion (MSHS). Part-time and evening/weekend programs available. Postbaccalaureate distance learning degree programs offered (no on-campus study). *Degree requirements:* For master's, fieldwork, internship, final project (wellness promotion). *Entrance requirements:* For master's, previous course work in psychology.

Independence University, Program in Nursing, Salt Lake City, UT 84107. Offers community health (MSN); gerontology (MSN); nursing administration (MSN); wellness promotion (MSN).

Indiana State University, College of Graduate and Professional Studies, College of Nursing, Health and Human Services, Department of Health, Safety, and Environmental Health Sciences, Terre Haute, IN 47809. Offers community health promotion (MA, MS); health and safety education (MA, MS); occupational safety management (MA, MS). *Accreditation:* NCATE (one or more programs are accredited). *Degree requirements:* For master's, thesis or alternative. *Entrance requirements:* For master's, GRE General Test. Electronic applications accepted.

Indiana University Bloomington, School of Public Health, Department of Kinesiology, Bloomington, IN 47405. Offers applied sport science (MS); athletic administration/sport management (MS); athletic training (MS); biomechanics (MS); ergonomics (MS); exercise physiology (MS); human performance (PhD), including biomechanics, exercise physiology, motor learning/control, sport management; motor learning/control (MS); physical activity (MPH); physical activity, fitness and wellness (MS). Part-time programs available. *Faculty:* 26 full-time (9 women). *Students:* 128 full-time (45 women), 16 part-time (6 women); includes 20 minority (11 Black or African American, non-Hispanic/Latino; 2 American Indian or Alaska Native, non-Hispanic/Latino; 3 Asian, non-Hispanic/Latino; 3 Hispanic/Latino; 1 Two or more races, non-Hispanic/Latino), 28 international. Average age 28. 174 applicants, 57% accepted, 48 enrolled. In 2013, 56 master's, 8 doctorates awarded. Terminal master's awarded for partial completion of doctoral program. *Degree requirements:* For master's, thesis optional; for doctorate, variable foreign language requirement, comprehensive exam, thesis/dissertation. *Entrance requirements:* For master's, GRE General Test, minimum GPA of 2.8; for doctorate, GRE General Test, minimum graduate GPA of 3.5, undergraduate 3.0. Additional exam requirements/recommendations for international students: Required—TOEFL (minimum score 80 iBT). *Application deadline:* For fall admission, 1/1 priority date for international students; for spring admission, 9/1 priority date for international students. Applications are processed on a rolling basis. Application fee: $55 ($65 for international students). *Financial support:* Fellowships, research assistantships with full tuition reimbursements, teaching assistantships with full tuition reimbursements, career-related internships or fieldwork, Federal Work-Study, institutionally sponsored loans, scholarships/grants, health care benefits, tuition waivers (partial), unspecified assistantships, and fee remissions available. Support available to part-time students. Financial award application deadline: 3/1; financial award applicants required to submit FAFSA. *Faculty research:* Exercise physiology and biochemistry, sports biomechanics, human motor control, adaptation of fitness and exercise to special populations. *Unit head:* Dr. David M. Koceja, Chairperson, 812-855-5523, Fax: 812-855-3193, E-mail: koceja@indiana.edu. *Application contact:* Kristine M. Wasson, Administrative Assistant for Graduate Studies, 812-855-5523, Fax: 812-855-3193, E-mail: ktanksle@indiana.edu.
Website: http://www.publichealth.indiana.edu/departments/kinesiology/index.shtml

Instituto Tecnologico de Santo Domingo, Graduate School, Area of Health Sciences, Santo Domingo, Dominican Republic. Offers bioethics (M Bioethics); clinical bioethics (Certificate); clinical nutrition (Certificate); comprehensive health and the adolescent (Certificate); comrehensive adloescent health (MS); health and social security (M Mgmt).

Kent State University, Graduate School of Education, Health, and Human Services, School of Health Sciences, Program in Health Education and Promotion, Kent, OH 44242-0001. Offers M Ed, PhD. *Accreditation:* NCATE. *Faculty:* 7 full-time (6 women), 1 (woman) part-time/adjunct. *Students:* 17 full-time (14 women), 12 part-time (9 women); includes 7 minority (6 Black or African American, non-Hispanic/Latino; 1 Hispanic/Latino), 1 international. 34 applicants, 38% accepted. In 2013, 13 master's, 1 doctorate awarded. *Degree requirements:* For doctorate, comprehensive exam, thesis/dissertation. *Entrance requirements:* For master's, 2 letters of reference, goals statement; for doctorate, GRE General Test, goals statement, resume, interview. Additional exam requirements/recommendations for international students: Required—TOEFL (minimum score 550 paper-based; 80 iBT). *Application deadline:* Applications are processed on a rolling basis. Application fee: $30 ($60 for international students). Electronic applications accepted. *Financial support:* In 2013–14, 1 research assistantship with full tuition reimbursement (averaging $8,500 per year), 5 teaching assistantships with full tuition reimbursements (averaging $12,000 per year) were awarded; Federal Work-Study, scholarships/grants, and unspecified assistantships also available. Financial award application deadline: 4/1; financial award applicants required to submit FAFSA. *Faculty research:* Substance use/abuse, sexuality, community health assessment, epidemiology, HIV/AIDS. *Unit head:* Dr. Kele Ding, Coordinator, 330-672-0688, E-mail: kding@kent.edu. *Application contact:* Nancy Miller, Academic Program Director, Office of Graduate Student Services, 330-672-2586, Fax: 330-672-9162, E-mail: ogs@kent.edu.
Website: http://www.kent.edu/ehhs/Schools/hs/programs/hedp/

Lehman College of the City University of New York, School of Natural and Social Sciences, Department of Health Sciences, Program in Health Education and Promotion,

Health Promotion

Bronx, NY 10468-1589. Offers MA. *Accreditation:* CEPH; NCATE. Part-time and evening/weekend programs available. *Degree requirements:* For master's, thesis or alternative. *Entrance requirements:* For master's, minimum GPA of 2.7.

Liberty University, School of Health Sciences, Lynchburg, VA 24515. Offers biomedical sciences (MS); clinical mental health counseling (MA); global health (MPH); health promotion (MPH); human services (MA), including addictions and recovery, business, Christian ministry, criminal justice, crisis response and trauma, executive leadership, health and wellness, life coaching, marriage and family, military resilience; marriage and family therapy (MA); nurse educator (MS); nursing (MSN); nursing administration (MSN); nutrition (MPH); pastoral care and counseling (PhD); professional counseling (MA, PhD). *Students:* 2,830 full-time (2,293 women), 6,275 part-time (5,051 women); includes 1,677 minority (1,178 Black or African American, non-Hispanic/Latino; 19 American Indian or Alaska Native, non-Hispanic/Latino; 36 Asian, non-Hispanic/Latino; 278 Hispanic/Latino; 7 Native Hawaiian or other Pacific Islander, non-Hispanic/Latino; 159 Two or more races, non-Hispanic/Latino), 177 international. Average age 37. 9,147 applicants, 50% accepted, 2939 enrolled. In 2013, 2,618 master's, 11 doctorates awarded. *Degree requirements:* For master's, thesis (for some programs); for doctorate, thesis/dissertation. *Entrance requirements:* For doctorate, MAT or GRE, minimum GPA of 3.25 in master's program, 2-3 recommendations, writing samples (for some programs), letter of intent, professional vitae. Additional exam requirements/recommendations for international students: Required—TOEFL (minimum score 600 paper-based; 100 iBT). Application fee: $50. *Expenses: Tuition:* Full-time $9630; part-time $535 per credit hour. *Required fees:* $175 per term. One-time fee: $50. Tuition and fees vary according to course load, degree level, campus/location and program. *Application contact:* Jay Bridge, Director of Admissions, 800-424-9595, Fax: 800-628-7977, E-mail: gradadmissions@liberty.edu.

Loma Linda University, School of Public Health, Programs in Health Promotion and Education, Loma Linda, CA 92350. Offers MPH, Dr PH. *Accreditation:* CEPH (one or more programs are accredited). *Degree requirements:* For doctorate, thesis/dissertation. *Entrance requirements:* For doctorate, GRE General Test. Additional exam requirements/recommendations for international students: Required—Michigan English Language Assessment Battery or TOEFL.

Marymount University, School of Health Professions, Program in Health Education Management, Arlington, VA 22207-4299. Offers MS. Part-time and evening/weekend programs available. *Faculty:* 3 full-time (2 women). *Students:* 6 full-time (5 women), 13 part-time (11 women); includes 7 minority (5 Black or African American, non-Hispanic/Latino; 2 Asian, non-Hispanic/Latino), 2 international. Average age 32. 16 applicants, 100% accepted, 11 enrolled. In 2013, 22 master's awarded. *Entrance requirements:* For master's, GRE or MAT, 2 letters of recommendation, interview, resume. Additional exam requirements/recommendations for international students: Required—TOEFL (minimum score 600 paper-based; 96 iBT), IELTS (minimum score 6.5). *Application deadline:* For fall admission, 7/1 for international students. Applications are processed on a rolling basis. Application fee: $40. Electronic applications accepted. *Expenses: Tuition:* Part-time $850 per credit. *Required fees:* $10 per credit. One-time fee: $200 part-time. Tuition and fees vary according to program. *Financial support:* In 2013–14, 2 students received support, including 1 research assistantship with full and partial tuition reimbursement available; career-related internships or fieldwork, Federal Work-Study, scholarships/grants, and unspecified assistantships also available. Support available to part-time students. Financial award applicants required to submit FAFSA. *Unit head:* Dr. Michelle Walters-Edwards, Chair, 703-526-1597, Fax: 703-284-3819, E-mail: michelle.walters-edwards@marymount.edu. *Application contact:* Francesca Reed, Director, Graduate Admissions, 703-284-5901, Fax: 703-527-3815, E-mail: grad.admissions@marymount.edu.
Website: http://www.marymount.edu/academics/programs/healthPromo

Marywood University, Academic Affairs, College of Health and Human Services, Department of Nutrition and Dietetics, Scranton, PA 18509-1598. Offers dietetic internship (Certificate); human development (PhD), including health promotion; nutrition (MS); sports nutrition and exercise science (MS). *Entrance requirements:* Additional exam requirements/recommendations for international students: Required—TOEFL (minimum score 550 paper-based; 79 iBT). Application fee: $35. Electronic applications accepted. *Expenses: Tuition:* Part-time $775 per credit. Tuition and fees vary according to degree level. *Financial support:* Career-related internships or fieldwork, scholarships/grants, and unspecified assistantships available. Support available to part-time students. Financial award application deadline: 6/30; financial award applicants required to submit FAFSA. *Faculty research:* Community nutrition and the environment, wellness, human performance and sports nutrition, dietary regimens, food systems management. *Unit head:* Dr. Lee Harrison, Chairperson, 570-348-6211 Ext. 2303, E-mail: harrisonl@marywood.edu. *Application contact:* Tammy Manka, Assistant Director of Graduate Admissions, 866-279-9663, E-mail: tmanka@marywood.edu.
Website: http://www.marywood.edu/nutrition/

McNeese State University, Doré School of Graduate Studies, Burton College of Education, Department of Health and Human Performance, Lake Charles, LA 70609. Offers exercise physiology (MS); health promotion (MS); nutrition and wellness (MS). *Accreditation:* NCATE. Evening/weekend programs available. *Entrance requirements:* For master's, GRE, undergraduate major or minor in health and human performance or related field of study.

Mississippi State University, College of Agriculture and Life Sciences, Department of Food Science, Nutrition and Health Promotion, Mississippi State, MS 39762. Offers food science and technology (MS, PhD); health promotion (MS); nutrition (MS, PhD). Postbaccalaureate distance learning degree programs offered (no on-campus study). *Faculty:* 7 full-time (1 woman). *Students:* 61 full-time (43 women), 40 part-time (32 women); includes 16 minority (10 Black or African American, non-Hispanic/Latino; 2 American Indian or Alaska Native, non-Hispanic/Latino; 1 Asian, non-Hispanic/Latino; 3 Hispanic/Latino), 20 international. Average age 29. 174 applicants, 30% accepted, 38 enrolled. In 2013, 30 master's, 2 doctorates awarded. *Degree requirements:* For master's, comprehensive exam, thesis; for doctorate, comprehensive exam, thesis/dissertation. *Entrance requirements:* For master's, GRE General Test, minimum GPA of 2.75; for doctorate, GRE General Test, minimum GPA of 2.75 undergraduate, 3.0 graduate. Additional exam requirements/recommendations for international students: Required—TOEFL (minimum score 550 paper-based; 79 iBT); Recommended—IELTS (minimum score 6.5). *Application deadline:* For fall admission, 7/1 for domestic students, 5/1 for international students; for spring admission, 11/1 for domestic students, 9/1 for international students. Applications are processed on a rolling basis. Application fee: $60. Electronic applications accepted. *Financial support:* In 2013–14, 12 research assistantships with full tuition reimbursements (averaging $15,205 per year), 5 teaching assistantships with full tuition reimbursements (averaging $11,591 per year) were awarded; Federal Work-Study, institutionally sponsored loans, scholarships/grants, and unspecified assistantships also available. Financial award application deadline: 4/1; financial award applicants required to submit FAFSA. *Faculty research:* Food preservation, food chemistry, food safety, food processing, product development. *Unit head:* Dr. Sam Chang, Professor and Head, 662-325-3200, Fax: 662-325-8728, E-mail: sc1690@msstate.edu. *Application contact:* Dr. Zee Haque, Graduate Coordinator, 662-325-3200, Fax: 662-325-8728, E-mail: haque@ra.msstate.edu.
Website: http://www.fsnhp.msstate.edu

Morehouse School of Medicine, Master of Public Health Program, Atlanta, GA 30310-1495. Offers epidemiology (MPH); health administration, management and policy (MPH); health education/health promotion (MPH); international health (MPH). *Accreditation:* CEPH. Part-time programs available. *Students:* 37 full-time (27 women), 5 part-time (3 women); includes 33 minority (32 Black or African American, non-Hispanic/Latino; 1 American Indian or Alaska Native, non-Hispanic/Latino). Average age 28. In 2013, 13 master's awarded. *Degree requirements:* For master's, thesis, practicum, public health leadership seminar. *Entrance requirements:* For master's, GRE General Test, writing test, public health or human service experience. Additional exam requirements/recommendations for international students: Required—TOEFL (minimum score 550 paper-based). *Application deadline:* For fall admission, 3/1 for domestic and international students. Application fee: $50. Electronic applications accepted. *Expenses:* Contact institution. *Financial support:* Fellowships, research assistantships with partial tuition reimbursements, teaching assistantships, career-related internships or fieldwork, Federal Work-Study, institutionally sponsored loans, scholarships/grants, and unspecified assistantships available. Support available to part-time students. Financial award application deadline: 5/1; financial award applicants required to submit FAFSA. *Faculty research:* Women's and adolescent health, violence prevention, cancer epidemiology/disparities, substance abuse prevention. *Unit head:* Dr. Stephanie Miles-Richardson, Interim Director, 404-752-1944, Fax: 404-752-1051, E-mail: smiles-richardson@msm.edu. *Application contact:* Brandon Hunter, Director of Admissions, 404-752-1650, Fax: 404-752-1512, E-mail: mphadmissions@msm.edu.
Website: http://www.msm.edu/educationTraining/degreePrograms/mph.aspx

Mount St. Joseph University, Graduate Program in Religious Studies, Cincinnati, OH 45233-1670. Offers pastoral administration (Certificate); religious studies (MA); spirituality and wellness (Certificate). Part-time and evening/weekend programs available. *Faculty:* 1 (woman) full-time. *Students:* 13 part-time (10 women); includes 1 minority (Black or African American, non-Hispanic/Latino). Average age 44. 6 applicants, 83% accepted, 4 enrolled. In 2013, 6 master's awarded. *Degree requirements:* For master's, integrating project, field experience. *Entrance requirements:* For master's, 3 letters of recommendation, interview, minimum GPA of 3.0, academic transcripts, essay. Additional exam requirements/recommendations for international students: Required—TOEFL (minimum score 560 paper-based; 83 iBT). *Application deadline:* Applications are processed on a rolling basis. Application fee: $50. Electronic applications accepted. *Expenses: Tuition:* Full-time $18,400; part-time $575 per credit hour. *Required fees:* $450; $450 per year. Part-time tuition and fees vary according to course load, degree level and program. *Financial support:* In 2013–14, 10 students received support. Scholarships/grants available. Financial award application deadline: 3/1; financial award applicants required to submit FAFSA. *Faculty research:* Contextual/cultural/systematic theology, historical/spiritual theology, business/economics ethics, social justice, Biblical/cultural/pastoral theology. *Unit head:* Dr. John Trokan, Chair of Religious/Pastoral Studies, 513-244-4272, Fax: 513-244-4222, E-mail: john_trokan@mail.msj.edu. *Application contact:* Mary Brigham, Assistant Director of Graduate Recruitment, 513-244-4233, Fax: 513-244-4629, E-mail: mary_brigham@mail.msj.edu.
Website: http://www.msj.edu/academics/graduate-programs/religious-studies-programs/

National University, Academic Affairs, School of Health and Human Services, La Jolla, CA 92037-1011. Offers clinical affairs (MS); clinical informatics (Certificate); clinical regulatory affairs (MS); health and life science analytics (MS); health coaching (Certificate); health informatics (MS); healthcare administration (MHA); nurse anesthesia (MS); nursing (MS), including forensic nursing, nursing administration, nursing informatics; nursing administration (Certificate); nursing informatics (Certificate); nursing practice (DNP); public health (MPH), including health promotion, healthcare administration, mental health. Part-time and evening/weekend programs available. Postbaccalaureate distance learning degree programs offered (no on-campus study). *Faculty:* 20 full-time (12 women), 27 part-time/adjunct (16 women). *Students:* 229 full-time (176 women), 89 part-time (52 women); includes 215 minority (58 Black or African American, non-Hispanic/Latino; 1 American Indian or Alaska Native, non-Hispanic/Latino; 68 Asian, non-Hispanic/Latino; 63 Hispanic/Latino; 8 Native Hawaiian or other Pacific Islander, non-Hispanic/Latino; 17 Two or more races, non-Hispanic/Latino), 18 international. Average age 33. 118 applicants, 100% accepted, 92 enrolled. In 2013, 29 master's awarded. *Degree requirements:* For master's, thesis (for some programs). *Entrance requirements:* For master's, interview, minimum GPA of 2.5. Additional exam requirements/recommendations for international students: Required—TOEFL (minimum score 550 paper-based; 79 iBT), IELTS (minimum score 6). *Application deadline:* Applications are processed on a rolling basis. Application fee: $60 ($65 for international students). Electronic applications accepted. *Expenses: Tuition:* Full-time $13,824; part-time $1728 per course. One-time fee: $160. *Financial support:* Career-related internships or fieldwork, institutionally sponsored loans, scholarships/grants, and tuition waivers (partial) available. Support available to part-time students. Financial award application deadline: 6/30; financial award applicants required to submit FAFSA. *Faculty research:* Nursing education, obesity prevention, workforce diversity. *Unit head:* School of Health and Human Services, 800-628-8648, E-mail: shhs@nu.edu. *Application contact:* Louis Cruz, Interim Vice President for Enrollment Services, 800-628-8648, E-mail: advisor@nu.edu.
Website: http://www.nu.edu/OurPrograms/SchoolOfHealthAndHumanServices.html

Nebraska Methodist College, Program in Health Promotion Management, Omaha, NE 68114. Offers MS. Part-time and evening/weekend programs available. Postbaccalaureate distance learning degree programs offered (no on-campus study). *Faculty:* 9 part-time/adjunct (7 women). *Students:* 28 full-time (22 women), 11 part-time (9 women); includes 1 minority (Asian, non-Hispanic/Latino). Average age 35. 63 applicants, 27% accepted, 13 enrolled. In 2013, 37 master's awarded. *Degree requirements:* For master's, thesis or alternative, capstone project. *Entrance requirements:* For master's, interview. Additional exam requirements/recommendations for international students: Required—TOEFL (minimum score 550 paper-based; 80 iBT). *Application deadline:* Applications are processed on a rolling basis. Application fee: $25. *Expenses: Tuition:* Full-time $12,258; part-time $681 per credit hour. *Required fees:* $450; $450 per year. *Financial support:* Scholarships/grants available. Financial award applicants required to submit FAFSA. *Faculty research:* Congregational health promotion, fitness testing with elderly, educational assessment, statistics instruction, resilience. *Unit head:* Kara Meisinger, Academic Program Director, 402-354-7237, E-mail: kara.meisinger@methodistcollege.edu. *Application contact:* Laurel Zentner, Recruitment and Admissions Coordinator, 402-354-7170, Fax: 402-354-7020, E-mail: admissions@methodistcollege.edu.
Website: http://www.methodistcollege.edu/health-promotion-management

New York Medical College, School of Health Sciences and Practice, Department of Epidemiology and Community Health, Program in Behavioral Sciences and Health Promotion, Valhalla, NY 10595-1691. Offers advanced public health (Graduate Certificate); behavioral sciences and health promotion (MPH). Part-time and evening/weekend programs available. *Faculty:* 5 full-time, 16 part-time/adjunct. *Students:* 40 full-time, 53 part-time. Average age 32. 40 applicants, 78% accepted, 30 enrolled. In 2013,

25 master's awarded. *Degree requirements:* For master's, thesis. *Entrance requirements:* For master's, minimum undergraduate GPA of 3.0. Additional exam requirements/recommendations for international students: Required—TOEFL (minimum score 637 paper-based; 110 iBT), IELTS (minimum score 7). *Application deadline:* For fall admission, 8/1 priority date for domestic students, 5/15 for international students; for spring admission, 12/1 priority date for domestic students, 10/15 for international students. Applications are processed on a rolling basis. Application fee: $50 ($100 for international students). Electronic applications accepted. *Expenses: Tuition:* Full-time $49,170; part-time $910 per credit. Tuition and fees vary according to program. *Financial support:* Career-related internships or fieldwork, Federal Work-Study, institutionally sponsored loans, health care benefits, and tuition reimbursements available. Support available to part-time students. Financial award applicants required to submit FAFSA. *Unit head:* Dr. Penny Liberatos, Assistant Professor, 914-594-4804, Fax: 914-594-3481, E-mail: penny_liberatos@nymc.edu. *Application contact:* Pamela Suett, Director of Recruitment, 914-594-4510, Fax: 914-594-4292, E-mail: shsp_admissions@nymc.edu.
Website: http://www.nymc.edu/shsp

New York University, Steinhardt School of Culture, Education, and Human Development, Department of Applied Psychology, Program in Counseling, New York, NY 10003. Offers counseling and guidance (MA), including bilingual school counseling K-12, counseling and guidance; counseling and guidance: K-12 (Advanced Certificate); counseling for mental health and wellness (MA); counseling psychology (PhD); LGBT health, education, and social services (Advanced Certificate). *Accreditation:* APA (one or more programs are accredited). Part-time programs available. *Faculty:* 12 full-time (9 women). *Students:* 140 full-time (118 women), 48 part-time (39 women); includes 75 minority (22 Black or African American, non-Hispanic/Latino; 19 Asian, non-Hispanic/Latino; 30 Hispanic/Latino; 1 Native Hawaiian or other Pacific Islander, non-Hispanic/Latino; 3 Two or more races, non-Hispanic/Latino), 18 international. Average age 29. 715 applicants, 32% accepted, 64 enrolled. In 2013, 80 master's, 1 doctorate awarded. *Degree requirements:* For master's, thesis (for some programs); for doctorate, thesis/dissertation. *Entrance requirements:* For doctorate, GRE General Test, interview. Additional exam requirements/recommendations for international students: Required—TOEFL (minimum score 100 iBT). *Application deadline:* For fall admission, 12/1 priority date for domestic and international students. Applications are processed on a rolling basis. Application fee: $75. Electronic applications accepted. *Expenses: Tuition:* Full-time $35,856; part-time $1494 per unit. *Required fees:* $1408; $64 per unit. $473 per term. Tuition and fees vary according to course load and program. *Financial support:* Fellowships with full and partial tuition reimbursements, research assistantships, teaching assistantships with partial tuition reimbursements, career-related internships or fieldwork, Federal Work-Study, institutionally sponsored loans, scholarships/grants, tuition waivers (partial), and unspecified assistantships available. Support available to part-time students. Financial award application deadline: 2/1; financial award applicants required to submit FAFSA. *Faculty research:* Sexual and gender identities, group dynamics, psychopathy and personality, multicultural assessment, working people's lives. *Unit head:* 212-998-5555, Fax: 212-995-4358. *Application contact:* 212-998-5030, Fax: 212-995-4328, E-mail: steinhardt.gradadmissions@nyu.edu.
Website: http://steinhardt.nyu.edu/appsych/counseling

Oakland University, Graduate Study and Lifelong Learning, School of Health Sciences, Program in Complimentary Medicine and Wellness, Rochester, MI 48309-4401. Offers Certificate. *Students:* 1 (woman) part-time; minority (Hispanic/Latino). Average age 37. 2 applicants. In 2013, 6 Certificates awarded. Application fee: $35. *Unit head:* Dr. Robert Janski, Director, 248-370-4191. *Application contact:* Christina J. Grabowski, Associate Director of Graduate Study and Lifelong Learning, 248-370-3167, Fax: 248-370-4114, E-mail: grabowsk@oakland.edu.

Old Dominion University, Darden College of Education, Program in Physical Education, Exercise and Wellness Emphasis, Norfolk, VA 23529. Offers MS Ed. Part-time and evening/weekend programs available. *Faculty:* 7 full-time (2 women). *Students:* 18 full-time (8 women), 5 part-time (4 women); includes 4 minority (2 Black or African American, non-Hispanic/Latino; 1 Asian, non-Hispanic/Latino; 1 Hispanic/Latino), 1 international. Average age 27. 27 applicants, 48% accepted, 11 enrolled. In 2013, 16 master's awarded. *Degree requirements:* For master's, comprehensive exam, thesis or alternative, internship, research project. *Entrance requirements:* For master's, GRE, minimum GPA of 2.8 overall, 3.0 in major. Additional exam requirements/recommendations for international students: Required—TOEFL (minimum score 550 paper-based; 79 iBT). *Application deadline:* For fall admission, 3/1 for domestic students; for spring admission, 11/1 for domestic students. Application fee: $50. *Expenses:* Tuition, state resident: full-time $9888; part-time $412 per credit. Tuition, nonresident: full-time $25,152; part-time $1048 per credit. *Required fees:* $59 per semester. One-time fee: $50. *Financial support:* In 2013–14, 1 research assistantship (averaging $9,000 per year), 2 teaching assistantships (averaging $9,000 per year) were awarded; unspecified assistantships also available. Financial award application deadline: 4/15. *Faculty research:* Diabetes, exercise prescription, gait and balance, lower extremity biomechanics, vascular function. *Total annual research expenditures:* $581,000. *Unit head:* Dr. Lynn Ridinger, Graduate Program Director, 757-683-4353, E-mail: lridinge@odu.edu. *Application contact:* William Heffelfinger, Director of Graduate Admissions, 757-683-5554, Fax: 757-683-3255, E-mail: gradadmit@odu.edu.
Website: http://education.odu.edu/esper/academics/exsci/graduate.shtml

Oregon State University, College of Public Health and Human Sciences, Program in Public Health, Corvallis, OR 97331. Offers biostatistics (MPH); environmental and occupational health and safety (MPH, PhD); epidemiology (MPH); health management and policy (MPH); health policy (PhD); health promotion and health behavior (MPH, PhD); international health (MPH). *Accreditation:* CEPH. Part-time programs available. *Faculty:* 29 full-time (16 women), 4 part-time/adjunct (3 women). *Students:* 137 full-time (102 women), 29 part-time (18 women); includes 37 minority (4 Black or African American, non-Hispanic/Latino; 7 Asian, non-Hispanic/Latino; 17 Hispanic/Latino; 9 Two or more races, non-Hispanic/Latino), 15 international. Average age 32. 163 applicants, 58% accepted, 48 enrolled. In 2013, 39 master's, 3 doctorates awarded. Terminal master's awarded for partial completion of doctoral program. *Degree requirements:* For doctorate, one foreign language, thesis/dissertation. *Entrance requirements:* For master's and doctorate, GRE, minimum GPA of 3.0 in last 90 hours. Additional exam requirements/recommendations for international students: Required—TOEFL (minimum score 80 iBT), IELTS (minimum score 6.5). *Application deadline:* For fall admission, 12/1 for domestic students. Applications are processed on a rolling basis. Application fee: $60. *Expenses:* Contact institution. *Financial support:* Fellowships, research assistantships, teaching assistantships, career-related internships or fieldwork, Federal Work-Study, and institutionally sponsored loans available. Support available to part-time students. Financial award application deadline: 2/1. *Faculty research:* Traffic safety, health safety, injury control, health promotion. *Unit head:* Dr. Sheryl Thorburn, Professor/Co-Director, 541-737-9493. *Application contact:* Eileen Kaspar, Public Health Graduate Programs Manager, 541-737-3825, E-mail: eileen.kaspar@oregonstate.edu.

Plymouth State University, Program in Personal and Organizational Wellness, Plymouth, NH 03264-1595. Offers MA.

Portland State University, Graduate Studies, College of Urban and Public Affairs, School of Community Health, Portland, OR 97207-0751. Offers aging (Certificate); health education (MA, MS); health education and health promotion (MPH); health studies (MPA, MPH), including health administration. MPH offered jointly with Oregon Health & Science University. *Accreditation:* CEPH. Part-time programs available. *Faculty:* 21 full-time (16 women), 28 part-time/adjunct (13 women). *Students:* 39 full-time (33 women), 28 part-time (27 women); includes 13 minority (2 Black or African American, non-Hispanic/Latino; 1 American Indian or Alaska Native, non-Hispanic/Latino; 2 Asian, non-Hispanic/Latino; 4 Hispanic/Latino; 4 Two or more races, non-Hispanic/Latino), 3 international. Average age 30. 127 applicants, 40% accepted, 45 enrolled. In 2013, 45 master's awarded. *Degree requirements:* For master's, oral and written exams. *Entrance requirements:* For master's, GRE General Test, 3 letters of recommendation, minimum GPA of 3.0. Additional exam requirements/recommendations for international students: Required—TOEFL (minimum score 550 paper-based). *Application deadline:* For fall admission, 2/1 for domestic and international students. Application fee: $50. *Expenses:* Tuition, state resident: full-time $9207; part-time $341 per credit. Tuition, nonresident: full-time $14,391; part-time $533 per credit. *Required fees:* $1263; $22 per credit. $98 per quarter. One-time fee: $150. Tuition and fees vary according to program. *Financial support:* In 2013–14, 7 research assistantships with full and partial tuition reimbursements (averaging $5,695 per year), 1 teaching assistantship with full tuition reimbursement (averaging $3,186 per year) were awarded; career-related internships or fieldwork, Federal Work-Study, scholarships/grants, and unspecified assistantships also available. Support available to part-time students. Financial award application deadline: 3/1; financial award applicants required to submit FAFSA. *Total annual research expenditures:* $1.2 million. *Unit head:* Dr. Carlos J. Crespo, Director, 503-725-5120, Fax: 503-725-5100. *Application contact:* Elizabeth Bull, Assistant to the Director, 503-725-4592, Fax: 503-725-5100, E-mail: bulle@pdx.edu.
Website: http://www.healthed.pdx.edu/

Rowan University, Graduate School, College of Education, Department of Health and Exercise Science, Glassboro, NJ 08028-1701. Offers MA. *Faculty:* 2 full-time (both women), 2 part-time/adjunct (both women). *Students:* 66 part-time (55 women); includes 8 minority (4 Black or African American, non-Hispanic/Latino; 1 American Indian or Alaska Native, non-Hispanic/Latino; 1 Asian, non-Hispanic/Latino; 2 Hispanic/Latino). Average age 35. 32 applicants, 100% accepted, 21 enrolled. In 2013, 5 master's awarded. *Degree requirements:* For master's, comprehensive exam, thesis. *Entrance requirements:* For master's, GRE General Test, GRE Subject Test, interview, minimum GPA of 2.8. Additional exam requirements/recommendations for international students: Required—TOEFL. *Application deadline:* For fall admission, 9/15 for domestic and international students; for spring admission, 2/15 for domestic and international students. Applications are processed on a rolling basis. Application fee: $65. Electronic applications accepted. *Expenses: Tuition, area resident:* Part-time $638 per credit. Tuition, state resident: full-time $5742. *Required fees:* $142 per credit. Tuition and fees vary according to course level and program. *Financial support:* Career-related internships or fieldwork, Federal Work-Study, and unspecified assistantships available. Support available to part-time students. *Unit head:* Richard Fopeano, Chair, 856-256-4500 Ext. 3740, E-mail: fopeano@rowan.edu. *Application contact:* Admissions and Enrollment Services, 856-256-5435, Fax: 856-256-5637, E-mail: cgceadmissions@rowan.edu.

St. Catharine College, School of Graduate Studies, St. Catharine, KY 40061-9499. Offers leadership (MA), including community and regional studies, health promotion. *Degree requirements:* For master's, thesis or alternative. *Entrance requirements:* For master's, GRE, official transcripts. Additional exam requirements/recommendations for international students: Required—TOEFL, IELTS, or Michigan English Language Assessment Battery. Electronic applications accepted.

San Diego State University, Graduate and Research Affairs, College of Health and Human Services, Graduate School of Public Health, San Diego, CA 92182. Offers environmental health (MPH); epidemiology (MPH, PhD), including biostatistics (MPH); global emergency preparedness and response (MS); global health (PhD); health behavior (PhD); health promotion (MPH); health services administration (MPH); toxicology (MS); MPH/MA; MSW/MPH. *Accreditation:* CAHME (one or more programs are accredited); CEPH (one or more programs are accredited). Part-time programs available. *Degree requirements:* For master's, comprehensive exam (for some programs), thesis (for some programs); for doctorate, thesis/dissertation. *Entrance requirements:* For master's, GMAT (MPH in health services administration), GRE General Test; for doctorate, GRE General Test. Additional exam requirements/recommendations for international students: Required—TOEFL. *Faculty research:* Evaluation of tobacco, AIDS prevalence and prevention, mammography, infant death project, Alzheimer's in elderly Chinese.

Simmons College, School of Nursing and Health Sciences, Boston, MA 02115. Offers didactic dietetics (Certificate); dietetic internship (Certificate); health professions education (CAGS); nursing (MS); nursing practice (DNP); nutrition and health promotion (MS); physical therapy (DPT); sports nutrition (Certificate). Part-time programs available. Postbaccalaureate distance learning degree programs offered (minimal on-campus study). *Students:* 143 full-time (129 women), 347 part-time (329 women); includes 72 minority (31 Black or African American, non-Hispanic/Latino; 17 Asian, non-Hispanic/Latino; 15 Hispanic/Latino; 9 Two or more races, non-Hispanic/Latino), 4 international. 196 applicants, 56% accepted, 88 enrolled. In 2013, 70 master's, 45 doctorates awarded. *Entrance requirements:* For doctorate, GRE. Additional exam requirements/recommendations for international students: Required—TOEFL (minimum score 570 paper-based; 88 iBT). *Application deadline:* For fall admission, 6/1 for international students. Application fee: $50. Electronic applications accepted. *Financial support:* In 2013–14, 33 students received support, including 24 teaching assistantships (averaging $6,000 per year); scholarships/grants and unspecified assistantships also available. *Unit head:* Dr. Judy Beal, Dean, 617-521-2139. *Application contact:* Carmen Fortin, Assistant Dean/Director of Admission, 617-521-2651, Fax: 617-521-3137, E-mail: gshsadm@simmons.edu.
Website: http://www.simmons.edu/snhs/

Sonoma State University, School of Science and Technology, Department of Kinesiology, Rohnert Park, CA 94928. Offers adapted physical education (MA); interdisciplinary (MA); interdisciplinary pre-occupational therapy (MA); lifetime physical activity (MA), including coach education, fitness and wellness; physical education (MA); pre-physical therapy (MA). Part-time programs available. *Faculty:* 5 full-time (3 women). *Students:* 1 full-time (0 women), 11 part-time (3 women); includes 2 minority (1 Hispanic/Latino; 1 Two or more races, non-Hispanic/Latino). Average age 29. *Degree requirements:* For master's, thesis, oral exam. *Entrance requirements:* For master's, minimum GPA of 2.8. Additional exam requirements/recommendations for international students: Required—TOEFL (minimum score 500 paper-based). *Application deadline:* For fall admission, 11/30 for domestic students; for spring admission, 9/1 for domestic students. Applications are processed on a rolling basis. Application fee: $55. *Expenses:* Tuition, state resident: full-time $8500. Tuition, nonresident: full-time $12,964. *Required fees:* $1762. *Financial support:* Career-related internships or fieldwork available. Financial award application deadline: 3/2; financial award applicants required to submit

FAFSA. *Unit head:* Dr. Elaine McHugh, Chair, 707-664-2660, E-mail: elaine.mchugh@sonoma.edu. *Application contact:* Dr. Lauren Morimoto, Graduate Coordinator, 707-664-2479, E-mail: morimoto@sonoma.edu.
Website: http://www.sonoma.edu/kinesiology/

Springfield College, Graduate Programs, Programs in Exercise Science and Sport Studies, Springfield, MA 01109-3797. Offers athletic training (MS); exercise physiology (MS), including clinical exercise physiology, science and research; exercise science and sport studies (PhD); health promotion and disease prevention (MS); sport psychology (MS). Part-time programs available. *Faculty:* 17 full-time, 2 part-time/adjunct. *Students:* 85 full-time. Average age 30. 138 applicants, 59% accepted, 48 enrolled. In 2013, 27 master's awarded. Terminal master's awarded for partial completion of doctoral program. *Degree requirements:* For master's, comprehensive exam, research project or thesis; for doctorate, comprehensive exam, thesis/dissertation. *Entrance requirements:* For master's and doctorate, GRE General Test. Additional exam requirements/recommendations for international students: Required—TOEFL (minimum score 550 paper-based); Recommended—IELTS (minimum score 6). *Application deadline:* For fall admission, 1/15 for domestic and international students; for winter admission, 11/1 for domestic and international students; for spring admission, 11/1 for domestic and international students. Application fee: $50. Electronic applications accepted. *Expenses: Tuition:* Full-time $13,620; part-time $908 per credit. *Financial support:* Fellowships with partial tuition reimbursements, teaching assistantships with partial tuition reimbursements, career-related internships or fieldwork, Federal Work-Study, institutionally sponsored loans, and unspecified assistantships available. Financial award application deadline: 3/1; financial award applicants required to submit FAFSA. *Unit head:* Dr. Tracey Matthews, Director, 413-748-3397, E-mail: tmatthews@springfieldcollege.edu. *Application contact:* Evelyn Cohen, Associate Director of Graduate Admissions, 413-748-3479, Fax: 413-748-3694, E-mail: ecohen@springfieldcollege.edu.

Tennessee Technological University, College of Graduate Studies, College of Education, Department of Exercise Science, Physical Education and Wellness, Cookeville, TN 38505. Offers adapted physical education (MA); elementary/middle school physical education (MA); lifetime wellness (MA); sport management (MA). *Accreditation:* NCATE. Part-time programs available. Postbaccalaureate distance learning degree programs offered (no on-campus study). *Faculty:* 7 full-time (0 women). *Students:* 10 full-time (0 women), 38 part-time (11 women); includes 5 minority (all Black or African American, non-Hispanic/Latino). Average age 27. 38 applicants, 58% accepted, 20 enrolled. In 2013, 23 master's awarded. *Degree requirements:* For master's, comprehensive exam, thesis or alternative. *Entrance requirements:* For master's, MAT or GRE. Additional exam requirements/recommendations for international students: Required—TOEFL (minimum score 527 paper-based; 71 iBT), IELTS (minimum score 5.5), PTE (minimum score 48), or TOEIC (Test of English as an International Communication). *Application deadline:* For fall admission, 8/1 for domestic students, 5/1 for international students; for spring admission, 12/1 for domestic students, 10/1 for international students. Applications are processed on a rolling basis. Application fee: $35 ($40 for international students). Electronic applications accepted. *Expenses:* Tuition, state resident: full-time $9347; part-time $465 per credit hour. Tuition, nonresident: full-time $23,635; part-time $1152 per credit hour. *Financial support:* In 2013–14, fellowships (averaging $8,000 per year), 3 research assistantships (averaging $4,000 per year), 4 teaching assistantships (averaging $4,000 per year) were awarded; career-related internships or fieldwork also available. Financial award application deadline: 4/1. *Unit head:* Dr. John Steven Smith, Interim Chairperson, 931-372-3467, Fax: 931-372-6319, E-mail: jssmith@tntech.edu. *Application contact:* Shelia K. Kendrick, Coordinator of Graduate Studies, 931-372-3808, Fax: 931-372-3497, E-mail: skendrick@tntech.edu.

Texas A&M University–Commerce, Graduate School, College of Education and Human Services, Department of Health and Human Performance, Commerce, TX 75429-3011. Offers exercise physiology (MS); health and human performance (M Ed); health promotion (MS); health, kinesiology and sports studies (Ed D); motor performance (MS); sport studies (MS). Part-time programs available. *Degree requirements:* For master's, comprehensive exam, thesis (for some programs). *Entrance requirements:* For master's, GRE General Test. Electronic applications accepted. *Expenses:* Tuition, state resident: full-time $3630; part-time $2420 per year. Tuition, nonresident: full-time $9948; part-time $6632.16 per year. *Required fees:* $1006 per year. Tuition and fees vary according to course load. *Faculty research:* Teaching, physical fitness.

Union Institute & University, Individualized Master of Arts Program, Cincinnati, OH 45206-1925. Offers creativity studies (MA); health and wellness (MA); history and culture (MA); leadership, public policy, and social issues (MA); literature and writing (MA). Part-time programs available. *Degree requirements:* For master's, thesis. *Entrance requirements:* For master's, transcript, essay, 3 letters of recommendation. Electronic applications accepted.

Universidad del Turabo, Graduate Programs, Programs in Education, Program in Wellness, Gurabo, PR 00778-3030. Offers MPHE.

The University of Alabama, Graduate School, College of Human Environmental Sciences, Department of Health Science, Tuscaloosa, AL 35487-0311. Offers health education and promotion (PhD); health studies (MA). Part-time programs available. Postbaccalaureate distance learning degree programs offered (no on-campus study). *Faculty:* 10 full-time (6 women). *Students:* 58 full-time (47 women), 156 part-time (129 women); includes 53 minority (43 Black or African American, non-Hispanic/Latino; 2 American Indian or Alaska Native, non-Hispanic/Latino; 1 Asian, non-Hispanic/Latino; 3 Hispanic/Latino; 4 Two or more races, non-Hispanic/Latino), 1 international. Average age 33. 113 applicants, 66% accepted, 54 enrolled. In 2013, 83 master's, 3 doctorates awarded. *Degree requirements:* For master's, comprehensive exam, thesis optional; for doctorate, one foreign language, comprehensive exam, thesis/dissertation. *Entrance requirements:* For master's, minimum GPA of 3.0; for doctorate, GRE General Test, minimum GPA of 3.0, prerequisites in health education. Additional exam requirements/recommendations for international students: Required—TOEFL. *Application deadline:* For fall admission, 3/15 priority date for domestic students, 3/15 for international students. Applications are processed on a rolling basis. Application fee: $50 ($60 for international students). Electronic applications accepted. *Expenses:* Tuition, state resident: full-time $9450. Tuition, nonresident: full-time $23,950. *Financial support:* In 2013–14, 2 research assistantships with full tuition reimbursements (averaging $10,500 per year), 6 teaching assistantships with full tuition reimbursements (averaging $10,500 per year) were awarded; career-related internships or fieldwork, Federal Work-Study, institutionally sponsored loans, health care benefits, and unspecified assistantships also available. Financial award application deadline: 4/14. *Faculty research:* Program planning, substance abuse prevention, obesity prevention, nutrition, physical activity, athletic training, osteoporosis, health behavior. *Total annual research expenditures:* $49,063. *Unit head:* Dr. Lori W. Turner, Department Head and Professor, 205-348-2956, Fax: 205-348-7568, E-mail: lwturner@ches.ua.edu. *Application contact:* Dr. Stuart Usdan, Associate Professor and Doctoral Program Coordinator, 205-348-8373, Fax: 205-348-7568, E-mail: susdan@ches.ua.edu.
Website: http://ches.ua.edu/

The University of Alabama at Birmingham, School of Education, Program in Health Education and Promotion, Birmingham, AL 35294. Offers PhD. Program offered jointly with School of Public Health, School of Health Professions, and The University of Alabama (Tuscaloosa). *Accreditation:* NCATE. *Degree requirements:* For doctorate, thesis/dissertation. *Entrance requirements:* For doctorate, GRE General Test (preferred minimum scores of 156 or greater for each section), minimum GPA of 3.0, letters of recommendation. Electronic applications accepted.

The University of Alabama at Birmingham, School of Public Health, Program in Health Education and Promotion, Birmingham, AL 35294. Offers PhD. Program offered jointly with The University of Alabama (Tuscaloosa). *Entrance requirements:* For doctorate, GRE, letters of recommendation. Additional exam requirements/recommendations for international students: Recommended—TOEFL, IELTS.

University of Alberta, School of Public Health, Centre for Health Promotion Studies, Edmonton, AB T6G 2E1, Canada. Offers health promotion (M Sc, Postgraduate Diploma). Part-time programs available. Postbaccalaureate distance learning degree programs offered.

University of Arkansas, Graduate School, College of Education and Health Professions, Department of Health, Human Performance and Recreation, Program in Community Health Promotion, Fayetteville, AR 72701-1201. Offers MS, PhD.

University of Arkansas for Medical Sciences, College of Public Health, Little Rock, AR 72205-7199. Offers biostatistics (MPH); environmental and occupational health (MPH, Certificate); epidemiology (MPH, PhD); health behavior and health education (MPH); health policy and management (MPH); health promotion and prevention research (PhD); health services administration (MHSA); health systems research (PhD); public health (Certificate); public health leadership (Dr PH). Part-time programs available. *Faculty:* 37 full-time (19 women), 9 part-time/adjunct (5 women). *Students:* 56 full-time (35 women), 85 part-time (58 women); includes 54 minority (38 Black or African American, non-Hispanic/Latino; 1 American Indian or Alaska Native, non-Hispanic/Latino; 8 Asian, non-Hispanic/Latino; 3 Hispanic/Latino; 1 Native Hawaiian or other Pacific Islander, non-Hispanic/Latino; 3 Two or more races, non-Hispanic/Latino), 5 international. Average age 30. 70 applicants, 91% accepted, 33 enrolled. In 2013, 2 master's, 1 doctorate, 2 other advanced degrees awarded. *Degree requirements:* For master's, preceptorship, culminating experience, internship; for doctorate, comprehensive exam, capstone. *Entrance requirements:* For master's, GRE, GMAT, LSAT, PCAT, MCAT, DAT; for doctorate, GRE. Additional exam requirements/recommendations for international students: Required—TOEFL (minimum score 80 iBT), IELTS. *Application deadline:* For fall admission, 3/1 for domestic students, 2/1 for international students; for spring admission, 8/1 for domestic and international students; for summer admission, 2/1 for domestic and international students. Application fee: $25 ($50 for international students). Electronic applications accepted. *Expenses:* Contact institution. *Financial support:* In 2013–14, 8 research assistantships with full tuition reimbursements (averaging $13,000 per year) were awarded; scholarships/grants and tuition waivers (full and partial) also available. *Faculty research:* Health systems, tobacco prevention control, obesity prevention, environmental and occupational exposure, cancer prevention. *Unit head:* Dr. James M. Raczynski, Dean, 501-526-6600, E-mail: raczynskijameson@uams.edu. *Application contact:* Angie Choi, Director of Admission, 501-526-4620, Fax: 501-526-6750, E-mail: anchoi@uams.edu.
Website: http://publichealth.uams.edu/

University of Central Oklahoma, The Jackson College of Graduate Studies, College of Education and Professional Studies, Department of Kinesiology and Health Studies, Edmond, OK 73034-5209. Offers athletic training (MS); wellness management (MS), including exercise science, health studies. *Faculty:* 5 full-time (4 women), 8 part-time/adjunct (3 women). *Students:* 31 full-time (20 women), 43 part-time (23 women); includes 26 minority (10 Black or African American, non-Hispanic/Latino; 3 American Indian or Alaska Native, non-Hispanic/Latino; 1 Asian, non-Hispanic/Latino; 6 Hispanic/Latino; 6 Two or more races, non-Hispanic/Latino), 10 international. Average age 27. 41 applicants, 95% accepted, 22 enrolled. In 2013, 18 master's awarded. *Degree requirements:* For master's, comprehensive exam (for some programs), thesis (for some programs). *Entrance requirements:* For master's, GRE. Additional exam requirements/recommendations for international students: Required—TOEFL (minimum score 550 paper-based; 79 iBT), IELTS (minimum score 6.5). *Application deadline:* For fall admission, 12/15 priority date for domestic students, 7/1 for international students; for spring admission, 11/1 for international students. Application fee: $50. Electronic applications accepted. *Expenses:* Tuition, state resident: full-time $4137; part-time $206.85 per credit hour. Tuition, nonresident: full-time $10,359; part-time $517.95 per credit hour. *Required fees:* $481. Tuition and fees vary according to course load and program. *Financial support:* In 2013–14, 23 students received support, including 8 research assistantships with partial tuition reimbursements available (averaging $3,189 per year), 1 teaching assistantship with partial tuition reimbursement available (averaging $2,958 per year); career-related internships or fieldwork, scholarships/grants, tuition waivers (partial), and unspecified assistantships also available. Financial award application deadline: 3/31. *Unit head:* Dr. Debra T. Traywick, Chair, 405-974-5363, Fax: 405-974-3805, E-mail: dtraywick@uco.edu. *Application contact:* Dr. Richard Bernard, Dean, Graduate College, 405-974-3493, Fax: 405-974-3852, E-mail: gradcoll@uco.edu.
Website: http://www.ucogradat.net

University of Chicago, Division of Biological Sciences, Program in Health Studies, Chicago, IL 60637-1513. Offers MS, PhD. Part-time programs available. *Degree requirements:* For master's, thesis; for doctorate, comprehensive exam, thesis/dissertation, ethics class, 2 teaching assistantships. *Entrance requirements:* For doctorate, GRE General Test. Additional exam requirements/recommendations for international students: Required—TOEFL (minimum score 600 paper-based; 104 iBT), IELTS (minimum score 7). Electronic applications accepted.

University of Colorado Colorado Springs, College of Letters, Arts and Sciences, Master of Sciences Program, Colorado Springs, CO 80933-7150. Offers biology (M Sc); chemistry (M Sc); health promotion (M Sc); mathematics (M Sc); physics (M Sc); sports medicine (M Sc), including strength and conditioning; sports nutrition (M Sc). Part-time programs available. *Students:* 50 full-time (36 women), 35 part-time (23 women); includes 12 minority (1 Black or African American, non-Hispanic/Latino; 1 American Indian or Alaska Native, non-Hispanic/Latino; 3 Asian, non-Hispanic/Latino; 5 Hispanic/Latino; 2 Two or more races, non-Hispanic/Latino), 11 international. Average age 29. 122 applicants, 47% accepted, 36 enrolled. In 2013, 37 master's awarded. *Degree requirements:* For master's, thesis or alternative. *Entrance requirements:* For master's, minimum GPA of 2.75. Additional exam requirements/recommendations for international students: Required—TOEFL (minimum score 525 paper-based). *Application deadline:* For fall admission, 3/1 priority date for domestic students; for spring admission, 12/1 for domestic students. Applications are processed on a rolling basis. Application fee: $60 ($75 for international students). Electronic applications accepted. *Expenses:* Contact institution. *Financial support:* In 2013–14, 21 students received support, including 21 fellowships (averaging $2,600 per year); research assistantships, teaching assistantships, career-related internships or fieldwork, Federal Work-Study, and scholarships/grants also available. Support available to part-time students. Financial award application deadline: 3/1; financial award applicants required to submit FAFSA.

Faculty research: Biomechanics and physiology of elite athletic training, genetic engineering in yeast and bacteria including phage display and DNA repair, immunology and cell biology, synthetic organic chemistry. *Total annual research expenditures:* $38,075. *Unit head:* Dr. Peter A. Braza, Dean, 719-255-4550, Fax: 719-255-4200, E-mail: pbraza@uccs.edu. *Application contact:* Taryn Bailey, Graduate Recruitment Specialist, 719-255-3702, Fax: 719-255-3037, E-mail: gradinfo@uccs.edu.

University of Delaware, College of Health Sciences, Department of Behavioral Health and Nutrition, Newark, DE 19716. Offers health promotion (MS); human nutrition (MS). Part-time programs available. *Degree requirements:* For master's, thesis. *Entrance requirements:* For master's, GRE General Test, interview, minimum GPA of 3.0. Additional exam requirements/recommendations for international students: Required—TOEFL (minimum score 550 paper-based). Electronic applications accepted. *Faculty research:* Sport biomechanics, rehabilitation biomechanics, vascular dynamics.

University of Georgia, College of Public Health, Department of Health Promotion and Behavior, Athens, GA 30602. Offers MPH, PhD. *Accreditation:* CEPH; NCATE (one or more programs are accredited). *Degree requirements:* For master's, thesis (MA); for doctorate, thesis/dissertation. *Entrance requirements:* For master's, GRE General Test or MAT; for doctorate, GRE General Test. Electronic applications accepted.

University of Kentucky, Graduate School, College of Education, Department of Kinesiology and Health Promotion, Lexington, KY 40506-0032. Offers exercise science (PhD); health promotion (MS, Ed D); kinesiology (MS); physical education training (Ed D). Terminal master's awarded for partial completion of doctoral program. *Degree requirements:* For master's, comprehensive exam, thesis optional; for doctorate, comprehensive exam, thesis/dissertation. *Entrance requirements:* For master's, GRE General Test, minimum undergraduate GPA of 2.75; for doctorate, GRE General Test, minimum graduate GPA of 3.0. Additional exam requirements/recommendations for international students: Required—TOEFL (minimum score 550 paper-based). Electronic applications accepted.

University of Louisville, Graduate School, School of Public Health and Information Sciences, Department of Health Promotion and Behavioral Sciences, Louisville, KY 40202. Offers health promotion (PhD). *Accreditation:* CEPH. Part-time programs available. *Degree requirements:* For doctorate, comprehensive exam, thesis/dissertation. *Entrance requirements:* For doctorate, GRE or equivalent, official transcripts, statement of purpose, resume/curriculum vitae, letters of recommendation. Additional exam requirements/recommendations for international students: Required—TOEFL (minimum score 600 paper-based; 100 iBT). *Application deadline:* For fall admission, 2/1 for domestic and international students. Application fee: $60. Electronic applications accepted. *Expenses:* Tuition, state resident: full-time $10,788; part-time $599 per credit hour. Tuition, nonresident: full-time $22,446; part-time $1247 per credit hour. *Required fees:* $196. Tuition and fees vary according to program and reciprocity agreements. *Financial support:* Research assistantships with full tuition reimbursements, scholarships/grants, health care benefits, and unspecified assistantships available. Financial award applicants required to submit FAFSA. *Faculty research:* Infectious disease control, emergency preparedness, health equity, evaluation methods, tobacco prevention policy. *Total annual research expenditures:* $24,922. *Unit head:* Dr. Richard Wilson, Department Chair, 502-852-3443, Fax: 502-852-3291, E-mail: richard.wilson@louisville.edu. *Application contact:* Kathie Sacksteder, Administrative Assistant, 502-852-8040, Fax: 502-852-3291, E-mail: kathie.sacksteder@louisville.edu.
Website: http://louisville.edu/sphis/departments/health-promotion-behavioral-sciences

University of Massachusetts Lowell, College of Health Sciences, School of Nursing, PhD Program in Nursing, Lowell, MA 01854-2881. Offers PhD. *Accreditation:* AACN. *Degree requirements:* For doctorate, thesis/dissertation, qualifying examination. *Entrance requirements:* For doctorate, GRE General Test, master's degree in nursing with minimum GPA of 3.3, current MA RN license, 2 years of professional nursing experience, 3 letters of recommendation.

University of Memphis, Graduate School, College of Education, Department of Health and Sport Sciences, Memphis, TN 38152. Offers clinical nutrition (MS); exercise and sport science (MS); health promotion (MS); physical education teacher education (MS), including teacher education; sport and leisure commerce (MS). Part-time and evening/weekend programs available. *Faculty:* 22 full-time (8 women), 3 part-time/adjunct (2 women). *Students:* 83 full-time (51 women), 28 part-time (23 women); includes 37 minority (29 Black or African American, non-Hispanic/Latino; 6 Asian, non-Hispanic/Latino; 2 Two or more races, non-Hispanic/Latino), 7 international. Average age 27. 86 applicants, 67% accepted, 29 enrolled. In 2013, 35 master's awarded. *Degree requirements:* For master's, comprehensive exam, thesis. *Entrance requirements:* For master's, GRE General Test or GMAT (for sport and leisure commerce). *Application deadline:* For fall admission, 5/1 priority date for domestic students; for spring admission, 11/1 for domestic students. Applications are processed on a rolling basis. Application fee: $35 ($60 for international students). *Financial support:* In 2013–14, 59 students received support. Research assistantships with full tuition reimbursements available, teaching assistantships with full tuition reimbursements available, career-related internships or fieldwork, Federal Work-Study, scholarships/grants, tuition waivers (partial), and unspecified assistantships available. Financial award application deadline: 2/15; financial award applicants required to submit FAFSA. *Faculty research:* Sport marketing and consumer analysis, health psychology, smoking cessation, psychosocial aspects of cardiovascular disease, global health promotion. *Unit head:* Linda H. Clemens, Interim Chair, 901-678-2324, Fax: 901-678-3591, E-mail: lhclemns@memphis.edu. *Application contact:* Dr. Kenneth Ward, Graduate Studies Coordinator, 901-678-1714, E-mail: kdward@memphis.edu.
Website: http://coe.memphis.edu/hss/

University of Michigan, School of Public Health, Department of Health Behavior and Health Education, Ann Arbor, MI 48109. Offers MPH, PhD, MPH/MSW. PhD offered through the Horace H. Rackham School of Graduate Studies. *Accreditation:* CEPH (one or more programs are accredited). Terminal master's awarded for partial completion of doctoral program. *Degree requirements:* For doctorate, oral defense of dissertation, preliminary exam. *Entrance requirements:* For master's, GRE General Test (preferred); MCAT; for doctorate, GRE General Test. Additional exam requirements/recommendations for international students: Required—TOEFL (minimum score 560 paper-based; 100 iBT). Electronic applications accepted. Tuition and fees vary according to course level, course load, degree level, program and student level. *Faculty research:* Empowerment theory; structure, culture, and health; health disparities; community-based participatory research; health and medical decision-making.

University of Mississippi, Graduate School, School of Applied Sciences, Department of Health, Exercise Science, and Recreation Management, University, MS 38677. Offers exercise science (MS); health and kinesiology (PhD); health promotion (MS); park and recreation management (MA). *Faculty:* 9 full-time (3 women), 3 part-time/adjunct (1 woman). *Students:* 45 full-time (23 women), 14 part-time (9 women); includes 11 minority (8 Black or African American, non-Hispanic/Latino; 1 Asian, non-Hispanic/Latino; 2 Hispanic/Latino), 5 international. In 2013, 19 master's, 1 doctorate awarded. *Degree requirements:* For master's, thesis (for some programs); for doctorate, thesis/dissertation. *Entrance requirements:* For master's, GRE General Test, minimum GPA of 3.0; for doctorate, GRE General Test. Additional exam requirements/recommendations for international students: Required—TOEFL. *Application deadline:* For fall admission, 4/1 for domestic students; for spring admission, 10/1 for domestic students. Applications are processed on a rolling basis. *Financial support:* Scholarships/grants available. Financial award application deadline: 3/1; financial award applicants required to submit FAFSA. *Unit head:* Dr. Scott G. Owens, Chair, 662-915-5844, Fax: 662-915-5525, E-mail: dbramlett@olemiss.edu. *Application contact:* Dr. Christy M. Wyandt, Associate Dean, 662-915-7474, Fax: 662-915-7577, E-mail: cwyandt@olemiss.edu.

University of Missouri, Graduate School, Master of Public Health Program, Columbia, MO 65211. Offers global public health (Graduate Certificate); health promotion and policy (MPH); public health (Graduate Certificate); veterinary public health (MPH); DVM/MPH; MPH/MA; MPH/MPA. *Accreditation:* CEPH. *Students:* 88 full-time (67 women), 104 part-time (83 women); includes 43 minority (19 Black or African American, non-Hispanic/Latino; 9 Asian, non-Hispanic/Latino; 10 Hispanic/Latino; 5 Two or more races, non-Hispanic/Latino), 16 international. Average age 30. 133 applicants, 84% accepted, 79 enrolled. In 2013, 40 master's, 49 other advanced degrees awarded. *Entrance requirements:* Additional exam requirements/recommendations for international students: Required—TOEFL (minimum score 550 paper-based; 80 iBT). *Application deadline:* For fall admission, 6/30 priority date for domestic and international students. Applications are processed on a rolling basis. Application fee: $55 ($75 for international students). Electronic applications accepted. *Financial support:* Fellowships with tuition reimbursements, research assistantships with tuition reimbursements, teaching assistantships with tuition reimbursements, scholarships/grants, traineeships, health care benefits, and unspecified assistantships available. Support available to part-time students. *Faculty research:* Health professions, health care equality, global health, communicable diseases, public health; zoonosis and infectious diseases, medical education, inquiry-based learning, social determinants of health, violence against women, health disparities, breast cancer screening, epigenetic, nursing, environmental health, cancer and chronic diseases, environmental exposures with metals, geographical information systems, substance use disorders/addictions, mental health. *Unit head:* Lise Saffran, Interim Director, 573-884-6835, E-mail: saffranl@health.missouri.edu. *Application contact:* Sandra Gummersheimer, Academic Advisor, 573-884-6836, E-mail: gummersheimers@health.missouri.edu.
Website: http://publichealth.missouri.edu/

University of Nebraska–Lincoln, Graduate College, College of Education and Human Sciences, Department of Nutrition and Health Sciences, Lincoln, NE 68588. Offers community nutrition and health promotion (MS); nutrition (MS, PhD); nutrition and exercise (MS); nutrition and health sciences (MS, PhD). *Degree requirements:* For master's, thesis optional. *Entrance requirements:* For master's, GRE General Test. Additional exam requirements/recommendations for international students: Required—TOEFL (minimum score 550 paper-based). Electronic applications accepted. *Faculty research:* Foods/food service administration, community nutrition science, diet-health relationships.

University of North Alabama, College of Education, Department of Health, Physical Education, and Recreation, Florence, AL 35632-0001. Offers health and human performance (MS), including exercise science, kinesiology, wellness and health promotion; secondary education (MA Ed), including physical education (P-12). Part-time and evening/weekend programs available. *Faculty:* 5 full-time (2 women). *Students:* 21 full-time (11 women), 7 part-time (2 women); includes 3 minority (2 Black or African American, non-Hispanic/Latino; 1 Two or more races, non-Hispanic/Latino), 3 international. Average age 27. 30 applicants, 90% accepted, 22 enrolled. In 2013, 3 master's awarded. *Degree requirements:* For master's, comprehensive exam (for some programs), thesis optional. *Entrance requirements:* For master's, MAT or GRE, 3 letters of recommendation, essay. Additional exam requirements/recommendations for international students: Required—TOEFL (minimum score 550 paper-based; 79 iBT), IELTS (minimum score 6). *Application deadline:* For fall admission, 7/1 for domestic and international students; for spring admission, 12/1 for domestic and international students. Applications are processed on a rolling basis. Application fee: $25 ($50 for international students). Electronic applications accepted. *Expenses:* Tuition, state resident: full-time $4968; part-time $3312 per year. Tuition, nonresident: full-time $9936; part-time $6624 per year. *Required fees:* $970; $60.33 per credit. $362 per semester. *Financial support:* Application deadline: 4/1; applicants required to submit FAFSA. *Unit head:* Dr. Thomas E. Coates, Chair, 256-765-4377. *Application contact:* Russ Darracott, Graduate Admissions Counselor, 256-765-4447, E-mail: erdarracott@una.edu.
Website: http://www.una.edu/hper/docs/HPERThesisGuideliens.pdf

The University of North Carolina at Chapel Hill, Graduate School, Gillings School of Global Public Health, Public Health Leadership Program, Chapel Hill, NC 27599. Offers health care and prevention (MPH); leadership (MPH); occupational health nursing (MPH). Part-time programs available. Postbaccalaureate distance learning degree programs offered (minimal on-campus study). *Degree requirements:* For master's, comprehensive exam, thesis (MS), paper (MPH). *Entrance requirements:* For master's, GRE General Test, minimum GPA of 3.0 (recommended), public health experience. Additional exam requirements/recommendations for international students: Required—TOEFL. Electronic applications accepted. *Faculty research:* Occupational health issues, clinical outcomes, prenatal and early childcare, adolescent health, effectiveness of home visiting, issues in occupational health nursing, community-based interventions.

University of Northern Iowa, Graduate College, College of Education, School of Health, Physical Education, and Leisure Services, MA Program in Health Promotion and Education, Cedar Falls, IA 50614. Offers health education (MA); health promotion/fitness (MA); school health education (MA). Part-time and evening/weekend programs available. *Students:* 10 full-time (6 women), 6 part-time (all women); includes 1 minority (Black or African American, non-Hispanic/Latino), 2 international. 14 applicants, 79% accepted, 5 enrolled. In 2013, 9 master's awarded. *Degree requirements:* For master's, comprehensive exam, thesis or alternative. *Entrance requirements:* For master's, minimum GPA of 3.0. Additional exam requirements/recommendations for international students: Required—TOEFL (minimum score 500 paper-based; 61 iBT). *Application deadline:* For fall admission, 8/1 priority date for domestic students. Applications are processed on a rolling basis. Application fee: $50 ($70 for international students). Electronic applications accepted. *Financial support:* Career-related internships or fieldwork, Federal Work-Study, and tuition waivers (full and partial) available. Support available to part-time students. Financial award application deadline: 2/1. *Unit head:* Dr. Susan Roberts-Dobie, Coordinator, 319-273-5930, Fax: 319-273-5958, E-mail: susan.dobie@uni.edu. *Application contact:* Laurie S. Russell, Record Analyst, 319-273-2623, Fax: 319-273-2885, E-mail: laurie.russell@uni.edu.
Website: http://www.uni.edu/coe/departments/school-health-physical-education-leisure-services/health-promotion-and-education

University of Oklahoma, College of Arts and Sciences, Department of Health and Exercise Science, Norman, OK 73019. Offers exercise physiology (PhD); health promotion (MS). *Faculty:* 10 full-time (4 women). *Students:* 43 full-time (21 women), 9 part-time (6 women); includes 9 minority (2 Black or African American, non-Hispanic/Latino; 1 American Indian or Alaska Native, non-Hispanic/Latino; 1 Hispanic/Latino; 5 Two or more races, non-Hispanic/Latino), 9 international. Average age 27. 49 applicants, 57% accepted, 27 enrolled. In 2013, 9 master's, 5 doctorates awarded.

Health Promotion

Degree requirements: For master's, comprehensive exam (for some programs), thesis, minimum GPA of 3.0; for doctorate, comprehensive exam, thesis/dissertation, minimum GPA of 3.0. *Entrance requirements:* For master's and doctorate, GRE, letters of recommendation, interview. Additional exam requirements/recommendations for international students: Required—TOEFL (minimum score 79 iBT). *Application deadline:* For fall and spring admission, 2/1 for domestic and international students. Application fee: $50 ($100 for international students). Electronic applications accepted. *Expenses:* Tuition, state resident: full-time $4205; part-time $175.20 per credit hour. Tuition, nonresident: full-time $16,205; part-time $675.20 per credit hour. *Required fees:* $2745; $103.85 per credit hour. $126.50 per semester. *Financial support:* In 2013–14, 49 students received support, including 46 teaching assistantships with partial tuition reimbursements available (averaging $12,543 per year); health care benefits, tuition waivers (full), and unspecified assistantships also available. Financial award application deadline: 6/1; financial award applicants required to submit FAFSA. *Faculty research:* Aging and muscle wasting; osteoporosis and bone loss; multiple sclerosis; tobacco use prevention; diet, obesity, and nutrition; behavioral change and lifestyle intervention; cardiovascular adjustment to exercise and aging; neural aspects of muscle function; pain; functional physical performance. *Total annual research expenditures:* $90,383. *Unit head:* Dr. Michael G. Bemben, Professor/Chair, 405-325-2717, Fax: 405-325-0594, E-mail: mgbemben@ou.edu. *Application contact:* Dr. Travis Beck, Graduate Liaison, 405-325-1378, Fax: 405-325-0594, E-mail: tbeck@ou.edu.
Website: http://cas.ou.edu/hes

University of Oklahoma Health Sciences Center, Graduate College, College of Public Health, Department of Health Promotion Sciences, Oklahoma City, OK 73190. Offers MPH, MS, Dr PH, PhD. *Accreditation:* CEPH (one or more programs are accredited). Part-time programs available. *Faculty:* 7 full-time (3 women), 1 (woman) part-time/adjunct. *Students:* 8 full-time (all women), 8 part-time (all women); includes 5 minority (3 Black or African American, non-Hispanic/Latino; 1 American Indian or Alaska Native, non-Hispanic/Latino; 1 Asian, non-Hispanic/Latino), 2 international. Average age 34. 8 applicants, 13% accepted. In 2013, 4 master's, 1 doctorate awarded. *Degree requirements:* For master's, comprehensive exam, thesis (for some programs); for doctorate, 2 foreign languages, comprehensive exam, thesis/dissertation. *Entrance requirements:* For master's, letters of recommendation, resume; for doctorate, GRE, letters of recommendation. Additional exam requirements/recommendations for international students: Required—TOEFL (minimum score 570 paper-based). *Application deadline:* For fall admission, 7/1 for domestic students; for winter admission, 4/1 for domestic students; for spring admission, 12/1 for domestic students. Applications are processed on a rolling basis. Application fee: $50. *Expenses:* Tuition, state resident: full-time $3504; part-time $175.20 per credit hour. Tuition, nonresident: full-time $13,504; part-time $675.20 per credit hour. *Required fees:* $1545; $52.70 per credit hour. $245.25 per semester. Tuition and fees vary according to course load. *Financial support:* In 2013–14, 10 research assistantships (averaging $10,000 per year) were awarded; career-related internships or fieldwork, institutionally sponsored loans, traineeships, and tuition waivers (partial) also available. Support available to part-time students. Financial award application deadline: 5/1. *Faculty research:* Health education, school health, health behavior, American Indian health. *Unit head:* Dr. Gary Raskob, Chair, 405-271-2017, E-mail: gary-raskob@ouhsc.edu. *Application contact:* Robin Howell, Information Contact, 405-271-2308, E-mail: robin-howell@ouhsc.edu.

University of Pittsburgh, School of Health and Rehabilitation Sciences, Master's Programs in Health and Rehabilitation Sciences, Pittsburgh, PA 15260. Offers health and rehabilitation sciences (MS), including health care supervision and management, health information systems, occupational therapy, physical therapy, rehabilitation counseling, rehabilitation science and technology, sports medicine, wellness and human performance. *Accreditation:* APTA. Part-time and evening/weekend programs available. *Faculty:* 63 full-time (37 women), 4 part-time/adjunct (2 women). *Students:* 117 full-time (70 women), 44 part-time (27 women); includes 18 minority (8 Black or African American, non-Hispanic/Latino; 1 American Indian or Alaska Native, non-Hispanic/Latino; 6 Asian, non-Hispanic/Latino; 3 Hispanic/Latino), 52 international. Average age 30. 368 applicants, 57% accepted, 96 enrolled. In 2013, 90 master's awarded. *Degree requirements:* For master's, comprehensive exam (for some programs), thesis optional. *Entrance requirements:* For master's, minimum GPA of 3.0. Additional exam requirements/recommendations for international students: Required—TOEFL (minimum score 550 paper-based; 80 iBT), IELTS (minimum score 6.5). *Application deadline:* For fall admission, 3/1 for international students; for spring admission, 9/1 for international students. Applications are processed on a rolling basis. Application fee: $50. Electronic applications accepted. *Expenses:* Contact institution. *Financial support:* In 2013–14, 3 fellowships (averaging $20,460 per year) were awarded; Federal Work-Study, institutionally sponsored loans, scholarships/grants, traineeships, and unspecified assistantships also available. Financial award applicants required to submit FAFSA. *Faculty research:* Assistive technology, seating and wheeled mobility, cellular neurophysiology, low back syndrome, augmentative communication. *Total annual research expenditures:* $8.1 million. *Unit head:* Dr. Clifford E. Brubaker, Dean, 412-383-6560, Fax: 412-383-6535, E-mail: cliffb@pitt.edu. *Application contact:* Jessica Maguire, Director of Admissions, 412-383-6557, Fax: 412-383-6535, E-mail: maguire@pitt.edu.
Website: http://www.shrs.pitt.edu/

University of Puerto Rico, Medical Sciences Campus, Graduate School of Public Health, Department of Human Development, Program in School Health Promotion, San Juan, PR 00936-5067. Offers Certificate.

University of South Carolina, The Graduate School, Arnold School of Public Health, Department of Health Promotion, Education, and Behavior, Columbia, SC 29208. Offers health education (MAT); health promotion, education, and behavior (MPH, MS, MSPH, Dr PH, PhD); school health education (Certificate); MSW/MPH. MAT offered in cooperation with the College of Education. *Accreditation:* CEPH (one or more programs are accredited); NCATE (one or more programs are accredited). Part-time programs available. *Degree requirements:* For master's, comprehensive exam, thesis or alternative, practicum (MPH), project (MS); for doctorate, comprehensive exam, thesis/dissertation. *Entrance requirements:* For master's and doctorate, GRE General Test. Additional exam requirements/recommendations for international students: Required—TOEFL (minimum score 570 paper-based; 75 iBT). Electronic applications accepted. *Faculty research:* Health disparities and inequalities in communities, global health and nutrition, cancer and HIV/AIDS prevention, health communication, policy and program design.

University of South Carolina, The Graduate School, Arnold School of Public Health, Program in Physical Activity and Public Health, Columbia, SC 29208. Offers MPH. *Accreditation:* CEPH. Part-time programs available. *Degree requirements:* For master's, comprehensive exam, practicum. *Entrance requirements:* For master's, GRE. Additional exam requirements/recommendations for international students: Required—TOEFL (minimum score 570 paper-based). Electronic applications accepted.

University of Southern California, Keck School of Medicine and Graduate School, Graduate Programs in Medicine, Department of Preventive Medicine, Master of Public Health Program, Los Angeles, CA 90032. Offers biostatistics-epidemiology (MPH); child and family health (MPH); environmental health (MPH); global health leadership (MPH); health communication (MPH); health education and promotion (MPH); public health policy (MPH). *Accreditation:* CEPH. Part-time and evening/weekend programs available. *Faculty:* 22 full-time (12 women), 3 part-time/adjunct (0 women). *Students:* 179 full-time (136 women), 31 part-time (24 women); includes 120 minority (19 Black or African American, non-Hispanic/Latino; 64 Asian, non-Hispanic/Latino; 37 Hispanic/Latino), 36 international. Average age 24. 205 applicants, 70% accepted, 73 enrolled. In 2013, 90 master's awarded. *Degree requirements:* For master's, practicum, final report, oral presentation. *Entrance requirements:* For master's, GRE General Test, MCAT, GMAT, minimum GPA of 3.0. Additional exam requirements/recommendations for international students: Required—TOEFL (minimum score 600 paper-based; 90 iBT). *Application deadline:* For fall admission, 6/1 priority date for domestic and international students; for spring admission, 10/1 priority date for domestic and international students; for summer admission, 3/1 for domestic and international students. Applications are processed on a rolling basis. Application fee: $85. Electronic applications accepted. *Financial support:* Career-related internships or fieldwork, Federal Work-Study, institutionally sponsored loans, and scholarships/grants available. Support available to part-time students. Financial award application deadline: 5/4; financial award applicants required to submit CSS PROFILE or FAFSA. *Faculty research:* Substance abuse prevention, cancer and heart disease prevention, mass media and health communication research, health promotion, treatment compliance. *Unit head:* Dr. Louise A. Rohrbach, Director, 323-442-8237, Fax: 323-442-8297, E-mail: rohrbac@usc.edu. *Application contact:* Valerie Burris, Admissions Counselor, 323-442-7257, Fax: 323-442-8297, E-mail: valeriem@usc.edu.
Website: http://mph.usc.edu/

The University of Tennessee, Graduate School, College of Education, Health and Human Sciences, Program in Health Promotion and Health Education, Knoxville, TN 37996. Offers MS. *Accreditation:* CEPH. Part-time programs available. *Degree requirements:* For master's, thesis optional. *Entrance requirements:* For master's, minimum GPA of 2.7. Additional exam requirements/recommendations for international students: Required—TOEFL. Electronic applications accepted. *Expenses:* Tuition, state resident: full-time $9540; part-time $531 per credit hour. Tuition, nonresident: full-time $27,728; part-time $1542 per credit hour. *Required fees:* $1404; $67 per credit hour.

University of the Incarnate Word, School of Graduate Studies and Research, School of Mathematics, Science, and Engineering, Program in Nutrition, San Antonio, TX 78209-6397. Offers administration (MS); nutrition education and health promotion (MS). Part-time and evening/weekend programs available. *Faculty:* 3 full-time (2 women), 2 part-time/adjunct (both women). *Students:* 10 full-time (8 women), 19 part-time (16 women); includes 16 minority (1 Black or African American, non-Hispanic/Latino; 1 Asian, non-Hispanic/Latino; 14 Hispanic/Latino), 1 international. Average age 26. 59 applicants, 63% accepted, 17 enrolled. In 2013, 5 master's awarded. *Degree requirements:* For master's, comprehensive exam, thesis or alternative. *Entrance requirements:* For master's, two letters of recommendation. Additional exam requirements/recommendations for international students: Required—TOEFL (minimum score 560 paper-based; 83 iBT). *Application deadline:* Applications are processed on a rolling basis. Application fee: $20. Electronic applications accepted. *Expenses: Tuition:* Part-time $815 per credit hour. *Required fees:* $86 per credit hour. One-time fee: $40 part-time. Tuition and fees vary according to degree level and program. *Financial support:* In 2013–14, research assistantships (averaging $5,000 per year) were awarded; Federal Work-Study and scholarships/grants also available. Financial award applicants required to submit FAFSA. *Faculty research:* Nutrition. *Total annual research expenditures:* $109,000. *Unit head:* Dr. Beth Senne-Duff, Associate Professor, 210-829-3165, Fax: 210-829-3153, E-mail: beths@uiwtx.edu. *Application contact:* Andrea Cyterski-Acosta, Dean of Enrollment, 210-829-6005, Fax: 210-829-3921, E-mail: admis@uiwtx.edu.
Website: http://www.uiw.edu/nutrition/nutrition3.htm

The University of Toledo, College of Graduate Studies, College of Medicine and Life Sciences, Department of Public Health and Preventative Medicine, Toledo, OH 43606-3390. Offers biostatistics and epidemiology (Certificate); contemporary gerontological practice (Certificate); environmental and occupational health and safety (MPH); epidemiology (Certificate); global public health (Certificate); health promotion and education (MPH); industrial hygiene (MSOH); medical and health science teaching and learning (Certificate); occupational health (Certificate); public health administration (MPH); public health and emergency response (Certificate); public health epidemiology (MPH); public health nutrition (MPH); MD/MPH. Part-time and evening/weekend programs available. *Faculty:* 9. *Students:* 69 full-time (50 women), 88 part-time (66 women); includes 50 minority (35 Black or African American, non-Hispanic/Latino; 10 Asian, non-Hispanic/Latino; 4 Hispanic/Latino; 1 Two or more races, non-Hispanic/Latino), 6 international. Average age 30. 92 applicants, 80% accepted, 52 enrolled. In 2013, 59 master's, 15 other advanced degrees awarded. *Degree requirements:* For master's, thesis or alternative. *Entrance requirements:* For master's, GRE, minimum undergraduate GPA of 3.0, three letters of recommendation, statement of purpose, transcripts from all prior institutions attended, resume; for Certificate, minimum undergraduate GPA of 3.0, three letters of recommendation, statement of purpose, transcripts from all prior institutions attended, resume. Additional exam requirements/recommendations for international students: Required—TOEFL (minimum score 550 paper-based; 80 iBT), IELTS (minimum score 6.5). *Application deadline:* For fall admission, 6/15 for domestic students, 3/15 priority date for international students; for spring admission, 10/15 for domestic students, 6/15 for international students; for summer admission, 3/15 for domestic students, 10/15 for international students. Applications are processed on a rolling basis. Application fee: $45 ($75 for international students). Electronic applications accepted. *Financial support:* In 2013–14, 4 research assistantships with full tuition reimbursements (averaging $10,000 per year) were awarded; Federal Work-Study, institutionally sponsored loans, scholarships/grants, tuition waivers (full and partial), and unspecified assistantships also available. *Unit head:* Dr. Sheryl A. Milz, Chair, 419-383-3976, Fax: 419-383-6140, E-mail: sheryl.milz@utoledo.edu. *Application contact:* Admissions Analyst, 419-383-4112, Fax: 419-383-6140.
Website: http://nocphmph.org/

The University of Toledo, College of Graduate Studies, College of Nursing, Department of Health Promotions, Outcomes, Systems, and Policy, Toledo, OH 43606-3390. Offers MSN, DNP. *Accreditation:* CEPH. Postbaccalaureate distance learning degree programs offered (no on-campus study). *Students:* 11 full-time (9 women), 17 part-time (16 women); includes 1 minority (Hispanic/Latino), 1 international. Average age 39. 27 applicants, 70% accepted, 15 enrolled. In 2013, 1 doctorate awarded. *Degree requirements:* For doctorate, thesis/dissertation or alternative, evidence-based project. *Entrance requirements:* For doctorate, GRE (taken within the past 5 years), personal statement, resume/curriculum vitae, letters of recommendation, documented supervised clinical hours in master's program, Nursing CAS application, UT supplemental application. Additional exam requirements/recommendations for international students: Required—TOEFL (minimum score 550 paper-based; 80 iBT). Application fee: $45 ($75 for international students). Electronic applications accepted. *Financial support:* Research assistantships with full and partial tuition reimbursements and tuition waivers (full and partial) available. *Unit head:* Dr. Huey-Shys Chen, Chair, 419-383-5893, Fax: 419-383-5894, E-mail: hueyshys.chen@utoledo.edu. *Application*

contact: David Lymanstall, Nursing Advisor, 419-383-5841, E-mail: david.lymanstall@utoledo.edu.
Website: http://www.utoledo.edu/nursing/

University of Toronto, School of Graduate Studies, Dalla Lana School of Public Health, Toronto, ON M5S 1A1, Canada. Offers biostatistics (M Sc, PhD); community health (M Sc); epidemiology (MPH, PhD); health and behavioral science (PhD); health promotion (MPH); social science and health (PhD). *Accreditation:* CAHME (one or more programs are accredited); CEPH (one or more programs are accredited). Part-time programs available. *Degree requirements:* For master's, thesis (for some programs), practicum; for doctorate, comprehensive exam, thesis/dissertation, oral thesis defense. *Entrance requirements:* For master's, 2 letters of reference, relevant professional/research experience, minimum B average in final year; for doctorate, 2 letters of reference, relevant professional/research experience, minimum B+ average. Additional exam requirements/recommendations for international students: Required—TOEFL (minimum score 580 paper-based; 93 iBT), TWE (minimum score 5). Electronic applications accepted. *Expenses:* Contact institution.

University of Utah, Graduate School, College of Health, Department of Health Promotion and Education, Salt Lake City, UT 84112. Offers M Phil, MS, Ed D, PhD. Part-time and evening/weekend programs available. *Faculty:* 5 full-time (3 women), 9 part-time/adjunct (4 women). *Students:* 28 full-time (20 women), 29 part-time (21 women); includes 11 minority (2 Black or African American, non-Hispanic/Latino; 3 Asian, non-Hispanic/Latino; 3 Hispanic/Latino; 1 Native Hawaiian or other Pacific Islander, non-Hispanic/Latino; 2 Two or more races, non-Hispanic/Latino), 6 international. Average age 32. 36 applicants, 58% accepted, 18 enrolled. In 2013, 8 master's, 3 doctorates awarded. Terminal master's awarded for partial completion of doctoral program. *Degree requirements:* For master's, comprehensive exam, thesis or alternative, field experience; for doctorate, comprehensive exam, thesis/dissertation, field experience. *Entrance requirements:* For master's, GRE (for thesis option), minimum GPA of 3.0; for doctorate, GRE General Test, minimum GPA of 3.2. Additional exam requirements/recommendations for international students: Required—TOEFL (minimum score 500 paper-based). *Application deadline:* For fall admission, 2/1 for domestic and international students; for spring admission, 2/15 for domestic and international students; for summer admission, 2/1 for domestic and international students. Applications are processed on a rolling basis. Application fee: $55 ($65 for international students). Electronic applications accepted. *Expenses:* Tuition, state resident: full-time $5259. Tuition, nonresident: full-time $18,569. *Required fees:* $841. Tuition and fees vary according to course load. *Financial support:* In 2013–14, 14 students received support, including 2 research assistantships with full and partial tuition reimbursements available (averaging $12,000 per year), 4 teaching assistantships with full tuition reimbursements available (averaging $12,000 per year); career-related internships or fieldwork, Federal Work-Study, institutionally sponsored loans, and scholarships/grants also available. Financial award application deadline: 2/15; financial award applicants required to submit FAFSA. *Faculty research:* Health behavior and counseling, health service administration, evaluation of health programs. *Unit head:* Leslie K. Chatelain, Department Chair, 801-581-4512, Fax: 801-585-3646, E-mail: les.chatelain@utah.edu. *Application contact:* Dr. Justine J. Reel, Director of Graduate Studies, 801-581-3481, Fax: 801-585-3646, E-mail: justine.reel@hsc.utah.edu.
Website: http://www.health.utah.edu/healthed/index.htm

University of Wisconsin–Milwaukee, Graduate School, Zilber School of Public Health, Department of Public Health, Milwaukee, WI 53201-0413. Offers community and behavioral health promotion (PhD); public health (MPH, Graduate Certificate). *Students:* 31 full-time (23 women), 14 part-time (13 women); includes 12 minority (4 Black or African American, non-Hispanic/Latino; 6 Asian, non-Hispanic/Latino; 2 Two or more races, non-Hispanic/Latino), 4 international. Average age 31. 74 applicants, 46% accepted, 16 enrolled. *Unit head:* Amy Harley, Assistant Professor, 414-229-4342, E-mail: harley@uwm.edu. *Application contact:* Darcie K. G. Warren, Graduate Program Manager, 414-229-5633, E-mail: darcie@uwm.edu.

University of Wisconsin–Stevens Point, College of Professional Studies, School of Health Promotion and Human Development, Stevens Point, WI 54481-3897. Offers human and community resources (MS); nutritional sciences (MS). Part-time programs available. *Degree requirements:* For master's, thesis or alternative. *Entrance requirements:* For master's, minimum GPA of 2.75.

University of Wyoming, College of Health Sciences, Division of Kinesiology and Health, Laramie, WY 82071. Offers MS. *Accreditation:* NCATE. Part-time programs available. Postbaccalaureate distance learning degree programs offered (no on-campus study). *Degree requirements:* For master's, comprehensive exam (for some programs), thesis (for some programs). *Entrance requirements:* For master's, GRE General Test, minimum GPA of 3.0. Additional exam requirements/recommendations for international students: Required—TOEFL. Electronic applications accepted. *Faculty research:* Teacher effectiveness, effects of exercising on heart function, physiological responses of overtraining, psychological benefits of physical activity, health behavior.

Walden University, Graduate Programs, School of Health Sciences, Minneapolis, MN 55401. Offers clinical research administration (MS, Graduate Certificate); health education and promotion (MS); health informatics (MS); health services (PhD), including community health, healthcare administration, leadership, public health policy, self-designed; healthcare administration (MHA); public health (MPH, Dr PH, PhD), including community health and education (PhD), epidemiology (PhD). Part-time and evening/weekend programs available. Postbaccalaureate distance learning degree programs offered (minimal on-campus study). *Faculty:* 18 full-time (12 women), 236 part-time/adjunct (120 women). *Students:* 2,563 full-time (1,867 women), 1,775 part-time (1,233 women); includes 2,532 minority (1,963 Black or African American, non-Hispanic/Latino; 29 American Indian or Alaska Native, non-Hispanic/Latino; 212 Asian, non-Hispanic/Latino; 238 Hispanic/Latino; 15 Native Hawaiian or other Pacific Islander, non-Hispanic/Latino; 75 Two or more races, non-Hispanic/Latino), 97 international. Average age 39. 1,191 applicants, 94% accepted, 861 enrolled. In 2013, 723 master's, 121 doctorates, 17 other advanced degrees awarded. *Degree requirements:* For doctorate, thesis/dissertation, residency. *Entrance requirements:* For master's, bachelor's degree or higher; minimum GPA of 2.5; official transcripts; goal statement (for some programs); access to computer and Internet; for doctorate, master's degree or higher; three years of related professional or academic experience (preferred); minimum GPA of 3.0; goal statement and current resume (select programs); official transcripts; access to computer and Internet; for Graduate Certificate, relevant work experience; access to computer and Internet. Additional exam requirements/recommendations for international students: Required—TOEFL (minimum score 550 paper-based; 79 iBT), IELTS (minimum score 6.5), Michigan English Language Assessment Battery (minimum score 82), or PTE. *Application deadline:* Applications are processed on a rolling basis. Application fee: $0. Electronic applications accepted. *Expenses: Tuition:* Full-time $11,813.55; part-time $500 per credit. *Required fees:* $618.76. *Financial support:* Fellowships, Federal Work-Study, scholarships/grants, unspecified assistantships, and family tuition reduction, active duty/veteran tuition reduction, group tuition reduction, interest-free payment plans, employee tuition reduction available. Support available to part-time students. Financial award applicants required to submit FAFSA. *Unit head:* Dr. Jorg Westermann, Associate Dean, 800-925-3368. *Application contact:* Jennifer Hall, Vice President of Enrollment Management, 866-4-WALDEN, E-mail: info@waldenu.edu.
Website: http://www.waldenu.edu/colleges-schools/school-of-health-sciences

Washington State University, Graduate School, The Edward R. Murrow College of Communication, Pullman, WA 99164-2520. Offers communication and technology (MA, PhD); health communication and promotion (MA, PhD); intercultural communication (PhD); media processes and effects (PhD); political communication (MA, PhD); science communication (MA, PhD); strategic communication (MA). *Degree requirements:* For master's, comprehensive exam (for some programs), thesis optional, oral exam; for doctorate, comprehensive exam, thesis/dissertation. *Entrance requirements:* For master's, GRE General Test, minimum GPA of 3.25, 3 letters of recommendation; for doctorate, GRE General Test, minimum undergraduate GPA of 3.25, graduate 3.5; MA in communication; 3 letters of recommendation. Additional exam requirements/recommendations for international students: Required—TOEFL (minimum score 580 paper-based). Electronic applications accepted. *Faculty research:* Communication technology, health communication, science communication, political communication, intercultural communication.

West Virginia University, School of Medicine, Department of Community Medicine, Morgantown, WV 26506. Offers public health (MPH), including community health/preventative medicine; public health sciences (PhD). *Accreditation:* CEPH. Part-time and evening/weekend programs available. Postbaccalaureate distance learning degree programs offered (minimal on-campus study). *Degree requirements:* For master's, thesis (for some programs). *Entrance requirements:* For master's, minimum GPA of 3.0. Additional exam requirements/recommendations for international students: Required—TOEFL. *Faculty research:* Adolescent smoking cessation, cardiovascular disease, women's health, worker's health.

Wilfrid Laurier University, Faculty of Graduate and Postdoctoral Studies, Faculty of Science, Department of Kinesiology and Physical Education, Waterloo, ON N2L 3C5, Canada. Offers physical activity and health (M Sc). *Degree requirements:* For master's, thesis. *Entrance requirements:* For master's, honours degree in kinesiology, health, physical education with a minimum B+ in kinesiology and health-related courses. Additional exam requirements/recommendations for international students: Required—TOEFL (minimum score 89 iBT). Electronic applications accepted. *Faculty research:* Biomechanics, health, exercise physiology, motor control, sport psychology.

Wright State University, School of Medicine, Program in Public Health, Dayton, OH 45435. Offers health promotion and education (MPH); public health management (MPH); public health nursing (MPH). *Accreditation:* CEPH.

Industrial Hygiene

California State University, Northridge, Graduate Studies, College of Health and Human Development, Department of Environmental and Occupational Health, Northridge, CA 91330. Offers environmental and occupational health (MS); industrial hygiene (MS). *Degree requirements:* For master's, seminar, field experience, comprehensive exam or thesis. *Entrance requirements:* For master's, GRE General Test or minimum GPA of 3.0. Additional exam requirements/recommendations for international students: Required—TOEFL.

Montana Tech of The University of Montana, Graduate School, Department of Industrial Hygiene, Butte, MT 59701-8997. Offers MS. *Accreditation:* ABET. Part-time programs available. Postbaccalaureate distance learning degree programs offered (no on-campus study). *Faculty:* 7 full-time (2 women). *Students:* 6 full-time (1 woman), 64 part-time (30 women); includes 15 minority (3 Black or African American, non-Hispanic/Latino; 3 American Indian or Alaska Native, non-Hispanic/Latino; 1 Asian, non-Hispanic/Latino; 8 Hispanic/Latino). 31 applicants, 32% accepted, 10 enrolled. In 2013, 23 master's awarded. *Degree requirements:* For master's, comprehensive exam (for some programs), thesis. *Entrance requirements:* For master's, GRE (or 5 years' work experience for online program), minimum GPA of 3.0. Additional exam requirements/recommendations for international students: Required—TOEFL (minimum score 525 paper-based; 71 iBT). *Application deadline:* For fall admission, 4/1 priority date for domestic students; for spring admission, 10/1 priority date for domestic students. Applications are processed on a rolling basis. Application fee: $30. Electronic applications accepted. *Expenses:* Tuition, state resident: full-time $2901; part-time $242 per credit hour. Tuition, nonresident: full-time $21,066; part-time $878 per credit hour. *Required fees:* $75 per credit hour. $30 per semester. Full-time tuition and fees vary according to course load, degree level and reciprocity agreements. *Financial support:* In 2013–14, 15 students received support, including 9 teaching assistantships with partial tuition reimbursements available (averaging $2,400 per year); research assistantships with partial tuition reimbursements available, career-related internships or fieldwork, institutionally sponsored loans, and tuition waivers (full and partial) also available. Financial award application deadline: 4/1; financial award applicants required to submit FAFSA. *Faculty research:* Ergonomics, metal bioavailability, aerosols, particulate sizing, respiration protection. *Unit head:* Dr. Terry Spear, Head, 406-496-4445, Fax: 406-496-4650, E-mail: tspear@mtech.edu. *Application contact:* Fred Sullivan, Administrator, Graduate School, 406-496-4304, Fax: 406-496-4710, E-mail: fsullivan@mtech.edu.
Website: http://www.mtech.edu/academics/gradschool/degreeprograms/degrees-industrial-hygiene.htm

Murray State University, College of Health Sciences and Human Services, Program in Occupational Safety and Health, Murray, KY 42071. Offers environmental science (MS); industrial hygiene (MS); safety management (MS). *Accreditation:* ABET. Part-time programs available. *Degree requirements:* For master's, comprehensive exam, thesis optional, professional internship. Electronic applications accepted. *Faculty research:* Light effects on plant growth, ergonomics, toxic effects of pets' pesticides, traffic safety.

New York Medical College, School of Health Sciences and Practice, Department of Environmental Health Science, Graduate Certificate Program in Industrial Hygiene, Valhalla, NY 10595-1691. Offers Graduate Certificate. *Faculty:* 5 full-time, 16 part-time/

adjunct. *Students:* 15 full-time, 25 part-time. Average age 32. 20 applicants, 75% accepted, 14 enrolled. *Entrance requirements:* Additional exam requirements/ recommendations for international students: Required—TOEFL (minimum score 637 paper-based; 110 iBT), IELTS (minimum score 7). *Application deadline:* For fall admission, 8/1 for domestic students, 5/15 for international students; for spring admission, 12/1 for domestic students, 10/1 for international students. Applications are processed on a rolling basis. Application fee: $50. Electronic applications accepted. *Expenses: Tuition:* Full-time $49,170; part-time $910 per credit. Tuition and fees vary according to program. *Unit head:* Dr. Diane E. Heck, Chair, 914-594-3383, Fax: 914-594-4292, E-mail: diane_heck@nymc.edu. *Application contact:* Pamela Suett, Director of Recruitment, 914-594-4510, Fax: 914-594-4292, E-mail: shsp_admissions@ nymc.edu.
Website: http://www.nymc.edu/shsp

The University of Alabama at Birmingham, School of Public Health, Program in Environmental Health Sciences, Birmingham, AL 35294. Offers environmental health sciences research (PhD); industrial hygiene (PhD). *Degree requirements:* For doctorate, comprehensive exam, thesis/dissertation. *Entrance requirements:* For doctorate, GRE General Test, evaluation forms. Additional exam requirements/recommendations for international students: Recommended—TOEFL, IELTS. Electronic applications accepted. *Faculty research:* Aquatic toxicology, virology.

The University of Alabama at Birmingham, School of Public Health, Program in Public Health, Birmingham, AL 35294. Offers accelerated industrial hygiene (MPH); applied epidemiology (MSPH); biostatistics (MPH); clinical and translational science (MSPH); environmental health (MPH); environmental health and toxicology (MSPH); epidemiology (MPH); general theory and practice (MPH); health behavior (MPH); health care organization (MPH); health policy quantitative policy analysis (MPH); industrial hygiene (MPH, MSPH); maternal and child health policy (Dr PH); maternal and child health policy and leadership (MPH); occupational health and safety (MPH); outcomes research (MSPH, Dr PH); pharmacoepidemiology and comparative effectiveness research (MSPH); public health (PhD); public health management (Dr PH); public health preparedness management (MPH). *Accreditation:* CEPH. *Entrance requirements:* For master's and doctorate, GRE, evaluations. Additional exam requirements/ recommendations for international students: Recommended—TOEFL (minimum score 550 paper-based; 79 iBT), IELTS (minimum score 6.5).

University of Central Missouri, The Graduate School, Warrensburg, MO 6409. Offers accountancy (MA); accounting (MBA); applied mathematics (MS); aviation safety (MA); biology (MS); business administration (MBA); career and technical education leadership (MS); college student personnel administration (MS); communication (MA); computer science (MS); counseling (MS); criminal justice (MS); educational leadership (Ed D); educational technology (MS); elementary and early childhood education (MSE); English (MA); environmental studies (MA); finance (MBA); history (MA); human services/ educational technology (Ed S); human services/learning resources (Ed S); human services/professional counseling (Ed S); industrial hygiene (MS); industrial management (MS); information systems (MBA); information technology (MS); kinesiology (MS); library science and information services (MS); literacy education (MSE); marketing (MBA); mathematics (MS); music (MA); occupational safety management (MS); psychology (MS); rural family nursing (MS); school administration (MSE); social gerontology (MS); sociology (MA); special education (MSE); speech language pathology (MS); superintendency (Ed S); teaching (MAT); teaching English as a second language (MA); technology (MS); technology management (PhD); theatre (MA). Part-time programs available. *Faculty:* 233. *Students:* 890 full-time (396 women), 1,486 part-time (1,001 women); includes 192 minority (97 Black or African American, non-Hispanic/Latino; 9 American Indian or Alaska Native, non-Hispanic/Latino; 32 Asian, non-Hispanic/Latino; 40 Hispanic/Latino; 3 Native Hawaiian or other Pacific Islander, non-Hispanic/Latino; 11 Two or more races, non-Hispanic/Latino), 539 international. Average age 31. 1,953 applicants, 75% accepted. In 2013, 719 master's, 58 other advanced degrees awarded. *Degree requirements:* For master's and Ed S, comprehensive exam (for some programs), thesis (for some programs). *Entrance requirements:* Additional exam requirements/recommendations for international students: Required—TOEFL (minimum score 550 paper-based; 79 iBT). *Application deadline:* For fall admission, 6/1 for domestic students; for spring admission, 10/1 for domestic and international students. Applications are processed on a rolling basis. Application fee: $30 ($75 for international students). Electronic applications accepted. *Expenses:* Tuition, state resident: full-time $7326; part-time $276.25 per credit hour. Tuition, nonresident: full-time $13,956; part-time $552.50 per credit hour. *Required fees:* $29 per credit hour. *Financial support:* In 2013–14, 118 students received support, including 271 research assistantships with full and partial tuition reimbursements available (averaging $7,500 per year), 109 teaching assistantships with full and partial tuition reimbursements available (averaging $7,500 per year); career-related internships or fieldwork, Federal Work-Study, scholarships/ grants, and administrative and laboratory assistantships also available. Support available to part-time students. Financial award application deadline: 3/1; financial award applicants required to submit FAFSA. *Unit head:* Dr. Joseph Vaughn, Assistant Provost for Research/Dean, 660-543-4092, Fax: 660-543-4778, E-mail: vaughn@ ucmo.edu. *Application contact:* Brittany Lawrence, Graduate Student Services Coordinator, 660-543-4621, Fax: 660-543-4778, E-mail: gradinfo@ucmo.edu.
Website: http://www.ucmo.edu/graduate/

University of Cincinnati, Graduate School, College of Medicine, Graduate Programs in Biomedical Sciences, Department of Environmental Health, Cincinnati, OH 45221. Offers environmental and industrial hygiene (MS, PhD); environmental and occupational medicine (MS); environmental genetics and molecular toxicology (MS, PhD); epidemiology and biostatistics (MS, PhD); occupational safety and ergonomics (MS, PhD). *Accreditation:* ABET (one or more programs are accredited). Terminal master's awarded for partial completion of doctoral program. *Degree requirements:* For master's, thesis; for doctorate, thesis/dissertation, qualifying exam. *Entrance requirements:* For master's, GRE General Test, bachelor's degree in science; for doctorate, GRE General Test. Additional exam requirements/recommendations for international students: Required—TOEFL (minimum score 600 paper-based; 100 iBT). Electronic applications accepted. *Faculty research:* Carcinogens and mutagenesis, pulmonary studies, reproduction and development.

The University of Iowa, Graduate College, College of Public Health, Department of Occupational and Environmental Health, Iowa City, IA 52242-1316. Offers agricultural safety and health (MS, PhD); ergonomics (MPH); industrial hygiene (MS, PhD); occupational and environmental health (MPH, MS, PhD, Certificate); MS/MA; MS/MS. *Accreditation:* ABET (one or more programs are accredited); CEPH. *Degree requirements:* For master's, thesis optional, exam; for doctorate, comprehensive exam, thesis/dissertation. *Entrance requirements:* For master's and doctorate, GRE General Test, minimum GPA of 3.0. Additional exam requirements/recommendations for international students: Required—TOEFL (minimum score 600 paper-based; 100 iBT). Electronic applications accepted.

University of Massachusetts Lowell, College of Health Sciences, Department of Work Environment, Lowell, MA 01854-2881. Offers cleaner production and pollution prevention (MS, Sc D); environmental risk assessment (Certificate); epidemiology (MS, Sc D); ergonomics and safety (MS, Sc D); identification and control of ergonomic hazards (Certificate); job stress and healthy job redesign (Certificate); occupational and environmental hygiene (MS, Sc D); radiological health physics and general work environment protection (Certificate); work environment policy (MS, Sc D). *Accreditation:* ABET (one or more programs are accredited). Part-time programs available. Terminal master's awarded for partial completion of doctoral program. *Degree requirements:* For master's, thesis optional; for doctorate, thesis/dissertation. *Entrance requirements:* For master's and doctorate, GRE General Test. Additional exam requirements/ recommendations for international students: Required—TOEFL.

University of Michigan, School of Public Health, Department of Environmental Health Sciences, Ann Arbor, MI 48109. Offers environmental health sciences (MS, PhD); environmental quality and health (MPH); human nutrition (MPH); industrial hygiene (MPH, MS); nutritional sciences (MS); occupational and environmental epidemiology (MPH); toxicology (MPH, MS, PhD). *Accreditation:* CEPH (one or more programs are accredited). Part-time programs available. Terminal master's awarded for partial completion of doctoral program. *Degree requirements:* For master's, thesis (for some programs); for doctorate, thesis/dissertation, preliminary exam, oral defense of dissertation. *Entrance requirements:* For master's and doctorate, GRE General Test and/or MCAT. Additional exam requirements/recommendations for international students: Required—TOEFL (minimum score 560 paper-based; 100 iBT). Electronic applications accepted. Tuition and fees vary according to course level, course load, degree level, program and student level. *Faculty research:* Toxicology, occupational hygiene, nutrition, environmental exposure sciences, environmental epidemiology.

University of Minnesota, Twin Cities Campus, School of Public Health, Division of Environmental Health Sciences, Area in Industrial Hygiene, Minneapolis, MN 55455-0213. Offers MPH, MS, PhD. *Accreditation:* ABET (one or more programs are accredited); CEPH (one or more programs are accredited). *Degree requirements:* For doctorate, thesis/dissertation. *Entrance requirements:* For master's and doctorate, GRE General Test. Electronic applications accepted.

The University of North Carolina at Chapel Hill, Graduate School, Gillings School of Global Public Health, Department of Environmental Sciences and Engineering, Chapel Hill, NC 27599. Offers air, radiation and industrial hygiene (MPH, MS, MSEE, MSPH, PhD); aquatic and atmospheric sciences (MPH, MS, MSPH, PhD); environmental engineering (MPH, MS, MSEE, MSPH, PhD); environmental health sciences (MPH, MS, MSPH, PhD); environmental management and policy (MPH, MS, MSPH, PhD). Terminal master's awarded for partial completion of doctoral program. *Degree requirements:* For master's, comprehensive exam, thesis (for some programs), research paper; for doctorate, comprehensive exam, thesis/dissertation. *Entrance requirements:* For master's and doctorate, GRE General Test, minimum GPA of 3.0 (recommended). Additional exam requirements/recommendations for international students: Required—TOEFL. Electronic applications accepted. *Faculty research:* Air, radiation and industrial hygiene, aquatic and atmospheric sciences, environmental health sciences, environmental management and policy, water resources engineering.

University of Puerto Rico, Medical Sciences Campus, Graduate School of Public Health, Department of Environmental Health, Program in Industrial Hygiene, San Juan, PR 00936-5067. Offers MS. Part-time programs available. *Degree requirements:* For master's, thesis. *Entrance requirements:* For master's, GRE, previous course work in biology, chemistry, mathematics, and physics. *Expenses:* Contact institution.

University of South Carolina, The Graduate School, Arnold School of Public Health, Department of Environmental Health Sciences, Program in Industrial Hygiene, Columbia, SC 29208. Offers MPH, MSPH, PhD. *Accreditation:* CEPH (one or more programs are accredited). *Degree requirements:* For master's, comprehensive exam, thesis (for some programs), practicum (MPH); for doctorate, one foreign language, comprehensive exam, thesis/dissertation. *Entrance requirements:* Additional exam requirements/recommendations for international students: Required—TOEFL (minimum score 570 paper-based). Electronic applications accepted. *Faculty research:* Sampling and calibration method development, exposure and risk assessment, respirator and dermal protective equipment, ergonomics, air cleaning methods and devices.

The University of Toledo, College of Graduate Studies, College of Medicine and Life Sciences, Department of Public Health and Preventative Medicine, Toledo, OH 43606-3390. Offers biostatistics and epidemiology (Certificate); contemporary gerontological practice (Certificate); environmental and occupational health and safety (MPH); epidemiology (Certificate); global public health (Certificate); health promotion and education (MPH); industrial hygiene (MSOH); medical and health science teaching and learning (Certificate); occupational health (Certificate); public health administration (MPH); public health and emergency response (Certificate); public health epidemiology (MPH); public health nutrition (MPH); MD/MPH. Part-time and evening/weekend programs available. *Faculty:* 9. *Students:* 69 full-time (50 women), 88 part-time (66 women); includes 50 minority (35 Black or African American, non-Hispanic/Latino; 10 Asian, non-Hispanic/Latino; 4 Hispanic/Latino; 1 Two or more races, non-Hispanic/ Latino), 6 international. Average age 30. 92 applicants, 80% accepted, 52 enrolled. In 2013, 59 master's, 15 other advanced degrees awarded. *Degree requirements:* For master's, thesis or alternative. *Entrance requirements:* For master's, GRE, minimum undergraduate GPA of 3.0, three letters of recommendation, statement of purpose, transcripts from all prior institutions attended, resume; for Certificate, minimum undergraduate GPA of 3.0, three letters of recommendation, statement of purpose, transcripts from all prior institutions attended, resume. Additional exam requirements/ recommendations for international students: Required—TOEFL (minimum score 550 paper-based; 80 iBT), IELTS (minimum score 6.5). *Application deadline:* For fall admission, 6/15 for domestic students, 3/15 priority date for international students; for spring admission, 10/15 for domestic students, 6/15 for international students; for summer admission, 3/15 for domestic students, 10/15 for international students. Applications are processed on a rolling basis. Application fee: $45 ($75 for international students). Electronic applications accepted. *Financial support:* In 2013–14, 4 research assistantships with full tuition reimbursements (averaging $10,000 per year) were awarded; Federal Work-Study, institutionally sponsored loans, scholarships/grants, tuition waivers (full and partial), and unspecified assistantships also available. *Unit head:* Dr. Sheryl A. Milz, Chair, 419-383-3976, Fax: 419-383-6140, E-mail: sheryl.milz@ utoledo.edu. *Application contact:* Admissions Analyst, 419-383-4112, Fax: 419-383-6140.
Website: http://nocphmph.org/

University of Wisconsin–Stout, Graduate School, College of Technology, Engineering, and Management, MS Program in Risk Control, Menomonie, WI 54751. Offers MS. Part-time programs available. *Degree requirements:* For master's, thesis. *Entrance requirements:* For master's, minimum GPA of 3.0. Additional exam requirements/recommendations for international students: Required—TOEFL (minimum score 500 paper-based; 61 iBT). Electronic applications accepted. *Faculty research:* Environmental microbiology, water supply safety, facilities planning, industrial ventilation, bioterrorist.

West Virginia University, College of Engineering and Mineral Resources, Department of Industrial and Management Systems Engineering, Program in Industrial Hygiene, Morgantown, WV 26506. Offers MS. *Accreditation:* ABET. Part-time programs available. *Degree requirements:* For master's, thesis or alternative. *Entrance requirements:* For master's, GRE General Test, minimum GPA of 3.0. Additional exam requirements/recommendations for international students: Required—TOEFL. *Faculty research:* Safety management, ergonomics and workplace design, safety and health training, construction safety.

International Health

Arizona State University at the Tempe campus, College of Liberal Arts and Sciences, School of Human Evolution and Social Change, Tempe, AZ 85287-2402. Offers anthropology (PhD); anthropology (archaeology) (PhD); anthropology (bioarchaeology) (PhD); anthropology (museum studies) (MA); anthropology (physical) (PhD); applied mathematics for the life and social sciences (PhD); environmental social science (PhD); environmental social science (urbanism) (PhD); global health (MA); global health (health and culture) (PhD); global health (urbanism) (PhD); immigration studies (Graduate Certificate). Terminal master's awarded for partial completion of doctoral program. *Degree requirements:* For master's, thesis or alternative, interactive Program of Study (iPOS) submitted before completing 50 percent of required credit hours; for doctorate, comprehensive exam, thesis/dissertation, interactive Program of Study (iPOS) submitted before completing 50 percent of required credit hours. *Entrance requirements:* For master's and doctorate, GRE, minimum GPA of 3.0 or equivalent in last 2 years of work leading to bachelor's degree. Additional exam requirements/recommendations for international students: Required—TOEFL (minimum score 80 iBT), TOEFL, IELTS, or PTE. Electronic applications accepted.

Arizona State University at the Tempe campus, College of Nursing and Health Innovation, Phoenix, AZ 85004. Offers advanced nursing practice (DNP); child/family mental health nurse practitioner (Graduate Certificate); clinical research management (MS); community and public health practice (Graduate Certificate); community health (MS); exercise and wellness (MS), including exercise and wellness; family nurse practitioner (Graduate Certificate); healthcare innovation (MHI); international health for healthcare (Graduate Certificate); kinesiology (MS, PhD); nursing (MS, Graduate Certificate); nursing and healthcare innovation (PhD); nutrition (MS); physical activity nutrition and wellness (PhD), including physical activity, nutrition and wellness; public health (MPH); regulatory science and health safety (MS). *Accreditation:* AACN. Postbaccalaureate distance learning degree programs offered (minimal on-campus study). *Degree requirements:* For master's, comprehensive exam (for some programs), thesis (for some programs), interactive Program of Study (iPOS) submitted before completing 50 percent of required credit hours; for doctorate, comprehensive exam, thesis/dissertation, interactive Program of Study (iPOS) submitted before completing 50 percent of required credit hours. *Entrance requirements:* For master's and doctorate, GRE, minimum GPA of 3.0 or equivalent in last 2 years of work leading to bachelor's degree. Additional exam requirements/recommendations for international students: Required—TOEFL (minimum score 80 iBT), TOEFL, IELTS, or PTE. Electronic applications accepted. *Expenses:* Contact institution.

Boston University, School of Public Health, International Health Department, Boston, MA 02215. Offers MPH, Dr PH. *Accreditation:* CEPH (one or more programs are accredited). Part-time and evening/weekend programs available. *Faculty:* 29 full-time, 37 part-time/adjunct. *Students:* 180 full-time (155 women), 63 part-time (58 women); includes 54 minority (12 Black or African American, non-Hispanic/Latino; 1 American Indian or Alaska Native, non-Hispanic/Latino; 22 Asian, non-Hispanic/Latino; 11 Hispanic/Latino; 8 Two or more races, non-Hispanic/Latino), 28 international. Average age 26. 656 applicants, 54% accepted, 108 enrolled. *Degree requirements:* For doctorate, thesis/dissertation. *Entrance requirements:* For master's, GRE, DAT, MCAT, GMAT, LSAT; for doctorate, GRE, GMAT. Additional exam requirements/recommendations for international students: Required—TOEFL (minimum score 600 paper-based; 100 iBT) or IELTS (minimum score 6). *Application deadline:* For fall admission, 2/1 priority date for domestic and international students; for spring admission, 10/15 priority date for domestic and international students. Applications are processed on a rolling basis. Application fee: $115. Electronic applications accepted. *Expenses: Tuition:* Full-time $43,970; part-time $1374 per credit hour. *Required fees:* $60 per semester. Tuition and fees vary according to class time, course level and program. *Financial support:* Research assistantships with full tuition reimbursements, career-related internships or fieldwork, Federal Work-Study, institutionally sponsored loans, and scholarships/grants available. Financial award application deadline: 3/1; financial award applicants required to submit FAFSA. *Unit head:* Dr. Jonathon Simon, Chair, 617-638-5234, E-mail: ih@bu.edu. *Application contact:* LePhan Quan, Associate Director of Admissions, 617-638-4640, Fax: 617-638-5299, E-mail: asksph@bu.edu.
Website: http://sph.bu.edu/ih

Brandeis University, The Heller School for Social Policy and Management, Program in International Health Policy and Management, Waltham, MA 02454-9110. Offers MS. *Entrance requirements:* For master's, 3 letters of recommendation, curriculum vitae or resume, 5 years of international health experience. Additional exam requirements/recommendations for international students: Required—TOEFL (minimum score 600 paper-based; 100 iBT). Electronic applications accepted. *Faculty research:* International development, health financing, and health systems.

Brandeis University, The Heller School for Social Policy and Management, Program in Social Policy, Waltham, MA 02454-9110. Offers assets and inequalities (PhD); children, youth and families (PhD); global health and development (PhD); health and behavioral health (PhD). *Degree requirements:* For doctorate, comprehensive exam, thesis/dissertation, qualifying paper, 2-year residency. *Entrance requirements:* For doctorate, GRE General Test, 3 letters of recommendation, statement of purpose, writing sample, at least 3-5 years of professional experience. Additional exam requirements/recommendations for international students: Required—TOEFL (minimum score 600 paper-based; 100 iBT). Electronic applications accepted. *Faculty research:* Health; mental health; substance abuse; children, youth, and families; aging; international and community development; disabilities; work and inequality; hunger and poverty.

Cedarville University, Graduate Programs, Cedarville, OH 45314-0601. Offers business administration (MBA); curriculum (M Ed); educational administration (M Ed); family nurse practitioner (MSN); global health ministries (MSN); instruction (M Ed); pharmacy (Pharm D). Part-time programs available. Postbaccalaureate distance learning degree programs offered (no on-campus study). *Faculty:* 23 full-time (12 women), 12 part-time/adjunct (5 women). *Students:* 119 full-time (74 women), 103 part-time (73 women); includes 16 minority (11 Black or African American, non-Hispanic/Latino; 4 Asian, non-Hispanic/Latino; 1 Native Hawaiian or other Pacific Islander, non-Hispanic/Latino), 4 international. Average age 31. In 2013, 26 master's awarded. *Degree requirements:* For master's, thesis. *Entrance requirements:* For master's, GRE, 2 professional recommendations; for doctorate, PCAT, professional recommendation from a practicing pharmacist or current employer/supervisor, resume, essay, interview. Additional exam requirements/recommendations for international students: Required—TOEFL (minimum score 550 paper-based; 80 iBT). *Application deadline:* For fall admission, 5/1 priority date for domestic and international students; for spring admission, 11/1 priority date for domestic and international students. Applications are processed on a rolling basis. Application fee: $30. Electronic applications accepted. *Financial support:* Scholarships/grants and unspecified assistantships available. Support available to part-time students. Financial award applicants required to submit FAFSA. *Unit head:* Dr. Mark McClain, Dean of Graduate Studies, 937-766-7700, E-mail: mcclain@cedarville.edu. *Application contact:* Roscoe F. Smith, Associate Vice-President of Enrollment, 937-766-7700, Fax: 937-766-7575, E-mail: smithr@cedarville.edu.
Website: http://www.cedarville.edu/academics/graduate/

Central Michigan University, Central Michigan University Global Campus, Program in Health Administration, Mount Pleasant, MI 48859. Offers health administration (DHA); international health (Certificate); nutrition and dietetics (MS). Part-time and evening/weekend programs available. Postbaccalaureate distance learning degree programs offered (minimal on-campus study). Electronic applications accepted. *Financial support:* Scholarships/grants available. Support available to part-time students. Financial award applicants required to submit FAFSA. *Unit head:* Dr. Steven D. Berkshire, Director, 989-774-1640, E-mail: berks1sd@cmich.edu. *Application contact:* Off-Campus Programs Call Center, 877-268-4636, E-mail: cmuoffcampus@cmich.edu.

Duke University, Graduate School, Duke Global Health Institute, Durham, NC 27708. Offers MS. *Faculty:* 50. *Students:* 64 full-time (46 women); includes 15 minority (3 Black or African American, non-Hispanic/Latino; 11 Asian, non-Hispanic/Latino; 1 Hispanic/Latino), 19 international. 136 applicants, 53% accepted, 34 enrolled. In 2013, 27 master's awarded. *Degree requirements:* For master's, thesis. *Entrance requirements:* For master's, GRE General Test or MCAT. Additional exam requirements/recommendations for international students: Required—TOEFL (minimum score 577 paper-based; 90 iBT) or IELTS (minimum score 7). *Application deadline:* For fall admission, 1/31 priority date for domestic and international students. Application fee: $80. *Unit head:* Dr. Christopher Woods, Director of Graduate Studies, 919-613-5077, Fax: 919-681-7748, E-mail: s.martin@duke.edu. *Application contact:* Elizabeth Hutton, Director of Admissions, 919-684-3913, Fax: 919-684-2277, E-mail: grad-admissions@duke.edu.
Website: https://globalhealth.duke.edu/

Emory University, Rollins School of Public Health, Hubert Department of Global Health, Atlanta, GA 30322-1100. Offers global health (MPH); public nutrition (MSPH). *Accreditation:* CEPH. *Degree requirements:* For master's, thesis, practicum. *Entrance requirements:* For master's, GRE General Test. Additional exam requirements/recommendations for international students: Required—TOEFL (minimum score 550 paper-based; 80 iBT). Electronic applications accepted.

George Mason University, College of Health and Human Services, Department of Global and Community Health, Fairfax, VA 22030. Offers global health (MS); public health (MPH, Certificate). *Accreditation:* CEPH. *Faculty:* 12 full-time (8 women), 16 part-time/adjunct (13 women). *Students:* 70 full-time (58 women), 62 part-time (55 women); includes 58 minority (21 Black or African American, non-Hispanic/Latino; 22 Asian, non-Hispanic/Latino; 11 Hispanic/Latino; 1 Native Hawaiian or other Pacific Islander, non-Hispanic/Latino; 3 Two or more races, non-Hispanic/Latino), 9 international. Average age 29. 144 applicants, 69% accepted, 51 enrolled. In 2013, 54 master's, 1 other advanced degree awarded. *Degree requirements:* For master's, comprehensive exam (for some programs), thesis or practicum. *Entrance requirements:* For master's, GRE, 2 official transcripts; expanded goals statement; 3 letters of recommendation; resume; 1 completed course in health science, statistics, natural sciences and social science (for MPH); 6 credits of foreign language if not fluent (for MS in global health); for Certificate, 2 official transcripts; expanded goals statement; 3 letters of recommendation; resume; bachelor's degree from regionally-accredited institution with minimum GPA of 3.0; statistics and college-level algebra with minimum B grade (for Certificate in biostatistics). Additional exam requirements/recommendations for international students: Required—TOEFL (minimum score 570 paper-based; 88 iBT), IELTS (minimum score 6.5), PTE. *Application deadline:* For fall admission, 4/1 priority date for domestic students; for spring admission, 11/1 priority date for domestic students. Applications are processed on a rolling basis. Application fee: $65 ($80 for international students). Electronic applications accepted. *Expenses:* Contact institution. *Financial support:* In 2013–14, 4 students received support, including 4 research assistantships with full and partial tuition reimbursements available (averaging $14,250 per year); career-related internships or fieldwork, Federal Work-Study, scholarships/grants, unspecified assistantships, and health care benefits (for full-time research or teaching assistantship recipients) also available. Financial award application deadline: 3/1; financial award applicants required to submit FAFSA. *Faculty research:* Health issues and the needs of affected populations at the regional and global level. *Total annual research expenditures:* $21,323. *Unit head:* Keith Howell, Interim Chair, 703-993-9633, Fax: 703-993-1943, E-mail: khowell@gmu.edu. *Application contact:* Ali Weinstein, Graduate Coordinator, 703-993-9632, Fax: 703-993-1908, E-mail: aweinst2@gmu.edu.
Website: http://chhs.gmu.edu/gch/index

George Mason University, College of Humanities and Social Sciences, Program in Global Affairs, Fairfax, VA 22030. Offers MA. *Faculty:* 16 full-time (6 women), 1 part-time/adjunct (0 women). *Students:* 22 full-time (18 women), 35 part-time (25 women); includes 12 minority (3 Black or African American, non-Hispanic/Latino; 2 Asian, non-Hispanic/Latino; 6 Hispanic/Latino; 1 Two or more races, non-Hispanic/Latino), 2 international. Average age 27. 86 applicants, 55% accepted, 16 enrolled. In 2013, 19 master's awarded. *Degree requirements:* For master's, capstone seminar. *Entrance requirements:* For master's, GRE, expanded goals statement, 2 letters of recommendation, evidence of professional competency in a second language tested through Language Testing International or other means approved by the department. Additional exam requirements/recommendations for international students: Required—TOEFL (minimum score 575 paper-based; 88 iBT), IELTS (minimum score 6.5), PTE. *Application deadline:* For fall admission, 3/15 for domestic students, 2/15 for international students; for spring admission, 10/15 for domestic students, 9/15 for international students. Application fee: $65 ($80 for international students). *Expenses:* Tuition, state resident: full-time $9350; part-time $390 per credit. Tuition, nonresident: full-time $25,754; part-time $1073 per credit. *Required fees:* $2688; $112 per credit. *Financial support:* Career-related internships or fieldwork, Federal Work-Study, and health care benefits (for full-time research or teaching assistantship recipients) available. Financial award application deadline: 3/1; financial award applicants required to submit FAFSA. *Unit head:* Lisa C. Breglia, Director, 703-993-9184, Fax: 703-993-1244, E-mail: lbreglia@gmu.edu. *Application contact:* Erin McSherry, Graduate Coordinator/Academic Advisor/Program Assistant, 703-993-5056, Fax: 703-993-1244, E-mail: emcsherr@gmu.edu.

Georgetown University, Law Center, Washington, DC 20001. Offers environmental law (LL M); global health law (LL M); global health law and international institutions (LL M); individualized study (LL M); international business and economic law (LL M); law (JD, SJD); national security law (LL M); securities and financial regulation (LL M); taxation (LL M); JD/LL M; JD/MA; JD/MBA; JD/MPH; JD/PhD. *Accreditation:* ABA. Part-time and evening/weekend programs available. *Degree requirements:* For master's, thesis; for doctorate, thesis/dissertation (for some programs). *Entrance requirements:* For master's, JD, LL B, or first law degree earned in country of origin; for doctorate, LSAT (for JD). Additional exam requirements/recommendations for international students: Required—TOEFL. *Application deadline:* Applications are processed on a rolling basis. Application fee: $60. *Expenses:* Contact institution. *Financial support:* Fellowships, Federal Work-Study, and institutionally sponsored loans available. Support available to part-time students. Financial award application deadline: 3/1; financial award applicants required to submit FAFSA. *Faculty research:* Constitutional law, legal history, jurisprudence. *Unit head:* William M. Treanor, Dean, 202-662-9030. *Application contact:* William M. Treanor, Dean, 202-662-9030.
Website: http://www.law.georgetown.edu/

The George Washington University, School of Public Health and Health Services, Department of Global Health, Washington, DC 20052. Offers MPH, JD/MPH, LL M/MPH, MD/MPH. *Accreditation:* CEPH. *Faculty:* 14 full-time (8 women). *Students:* 60 full-time (53 women), 90 part-time (79 women); includes 47 minority (22 Black or African American, non-Hispanic/Latino; 2 American Indian or Alaska Native, non-Hispanic/Latino; 11 Asian, non-Hispanic/Latino; 11 Hispanic/Latino; 1 Two or more races, non-Hispanic/Latino), 7 international. Average age 29. 260 applicants, 82% accepted. In 2013, 61 master's awarded. *Degree requirements:* For master's, case study or special project. *Entrance requirements:* For master's, GMAT, GRE General Test, or MCAT. Additional exam requirements/recommendations for international students: Required—TOEFL. *Application deadline:* For fall admission, 4/15 priority date for domestic students, 4/15 for international students; for spring admission, 11/1 for domestic and international students. Applications are processed on a rolling basis. Application fee: $75. *Financial support:* In 2013–14, 24 students received support. Tuition waivers available. Financial award application deadline: 2/15. *Unit head:* Dr. James Tielsch, Chair, 202-994-0270, Fax: 202-994-1955, E-mail: jtielsch@gwu.edu. *Application contact:* Jane Smith, Director of Admissions, 202-994-0248, Fax: 202-994-1860, E-mail: sphhsinfo@gwumc.edu.

Harvard University, Harvard School of Public Health, Department of Global Health and Population, Boston, MA 02115-6096. Offers SM, SD. Part-time programs available. *Faculty:* 53 full-time (22 women), 30 part-time/adjunct (8 women). *Students:* 80 full-time (54 women), 1 (woman) part-time; includes 12 minority (4 Black or African American, non-Hispanic/Latino; 4 Asian, non-Hispanic/Latino; 3 Hispanic/Latino; 1 Two or more races, non-Hispanic/Latino), 29 international. Average age 27. 285 applicants, 19% accepted, 27 enrolled. In 2013, 26 master's, 12 doctorates awarded. *Degree requirements:* For master's, thesis; for doctorate, thesis/dissertation, qualifying exam. *Entrance requirements:* For master's, GRE, MCAT; for doctorate, GRE. Additional exam requirements/recommendations for international students: Required—TOEFL (minimum score 600 paper-based; 100 iBT); Recommended—IELTS (minimum score 7). *Application deadline:* For fall admission, 12/15 for domestic and international students. Application fee: $120. Electronic applications accepted. *Expenses: Tuition:* Full-time $38,888. *Required fees:* $958. Tuition and fees vary according to campus/location, program and student level. *Financial support:* Fellowships, research assistantships, teaching assistantships, Federal Work-Study, scholarships/grants, traineeships, and unspecified assistantships available. Support available to part-time students. Financial award application deadline: 2/15; financial award applicants required to submit FAFSA. *Faculty research:* Health systems, international health policy, economics, population and reproductive health, ecology. *Unit head:* Dr. Wafaie W. Fawzi, Chair, 617-432-2086, Fax: 617-432-2435, E-mail: mina@hsph.harvard.edu. *Application contact:* Vincent W. James, Director of Admissions, 617-432-1031, Fax: 617-432-7080, E-mail: admissions@hsph.harvard.edu.
Website: http://www.hsph.harvard.edu/global-health-and-population/

Johns Hopkins University, Bloomberg School of Public Health, Department of International Health, Baltimore, MD 21205. Offers global disease epidemiology and control (MHS, PhD); health systems (MHS, PhD); human nutrition (MHS, PhD); international health (MSPH, Dr PH); registered dietician (MSPH); social and behavioral interventions (MHS, PhD). *Faculty:* 137 full-time (82 women), 185 part-time/adjunct (63 women). *Students:* 284 full-time (212 women), 4 part-time (3 women); includes 70 minority (11 Black or African American, non-Hispanic/Latino; 1 American Indian or Alaska Native, non-Hispanic/Latino; 41 Asian, non-Hispanic/Latino; 6 Hispanic/Latino; 11 Two or more races, non-Hispanic/Latino), 73 international. Average age 28. 515 applicants, 44% accepted, 104 enrolled. In 2013, 78 master's, 24 doctorates awarded. *Degree requirements:* For master's, comprehensive exam, thesis (for some programs), 1-year full-time residency, 4-9 month internship; for doctorate, comprehensive exam, thesis/dissertation or alternative, 1.5 years' full-time residency, oral and written exams. *Entrance requirements:* For master's, GRE General Test or MCAT, 3 letters of recommendation, resume; for doctorate, GRE General Test or MCAT, 3 letters of recommendation, resume, transcripts. Additional exam requirements/recommendations for international students: Required—TOEFL (minimum score 600 paper-based; 100 iBT); Recommended—IELTS (minimum score 7). *Application deadline:* For fall admission, 1/2 priority date for domestic and international students. Applications are processed on a rolling basis. Application fee: $45. Electronic applications accepted. *Financial support:* Fellowships, Federal Work-Study, institutionally sponsored loans, scholarships/grants, traineeships, and stipends available. Financial award application deadline: 1/2. *Faculty research:* Nutrition, infectious diseases, health systems, health economics, humanitarian emergencies. *Total annual research expenditures:* $72 million. *Unit head:* Dr. David Peters, Chair, 410-955-3928, Fax: 410-955-7159, E-mail: dpeters@jhsph.edu. *Application contact:* Cristina G. Salazar, Academic Program Manager, 410-955-3734, Fax: 410-955-7159, E-mail: csalazar@jhsph.edu.
Website: http://www.jhsph.edu/dept/IH/

Liberty University, School of Health Sciences, Lynchburg, VA 24515. Offers biomedical sciences (MS); clinical mental health counseling (MA); global health (MPH); health promotion (MPH); human services (MA), including addictions and recovery, business, Christian ministry, criminal justice, crisis response and trauma, executive leadership, health and wellness, life coaching, marriage and family, military resilience; marriage and family therapy (MA); nurse educator (MS); nursing (MSN); nursing administration (MSN); nutrition (MPH); pastoral care and counseling (PhD); professional counseling (MA, PhD). *Students:* 2,830 full-time (2,293 women), 6,275 part-time (5,051 women); includes 1,677 minority (1,178 Black or African American, non-Hispanic/Latino; 19 American Indian or Alaska Native, non-Hispanic/Latino; 36 Asian, non-Hispanic/Latino; 278 Hispanic/Latino; 7 Native Hawaiian or other Pacific Islander, non-Hispanic/Latino; 159 Two or more races, non-Hispanic/Latino), 177 international. Average age 37. 9,147 applicants, 50% accepted, 2939 enrolled. In 2013, 2,618 master's, 11 doctorates awarded. *Degree requirements:* For master's, thesis (for some programs); for doctorate, thesis/dissertation. *Entrance requirements:* For doctorate, MAT or GRE, minimum GPA of 3.25 in master's program, 2-3 recommendations, writing samples (for some programs), letter of intent, professional vitae. Additional exam requirements/recommendations for international students: Required—TOEFL (minimum score 600 paper-based; 100 iBT). Application fee: $50. *Expenses: Tuition:* Full-time $9630; part-time $535 per credit hour. *Required fees:* $175 per term. One-time fee: $50. Tuition and fees vary according to course load, degree level, campus/location and program. *Application contact:* Jay Bridge, Director of Admissions, 800-424-9595, Fax: 800-628-7977, E-mail: gradadmissions@liberty.edu.

Loma Linda University, School of Public Health, Programs in Global Health, Loma Linda, CA 92350. Offers MPH. *Accreditation:* CEPH. *Entrance requirements:* Additional exam requirements/recommendations for international students: Required—Michigan English Language Assessment Battery or TOEFL.

Massachusetts School of Professional Psychology, Graduate Programs, Boston, MA 02132. Offers applied psychology in higher education student personnel administration (MA); clinical psychology (Psy D); counseling psychology (MA); counseling psychology and community mental health (MA); counseling psychology and global mental health (MA); executive coaching (Graduate Certificate); forensic and counseling psychology (MA); leadership psychology (Psy D); organizational psychology (MA); primary care psychology (MA); respecialization in clinical psychology (Certificate); school psychology (Psy D); MA/CAGS. *Accreditation:* APA. *Degree requirements:* For master's, comprehensive exam (for some programs); for doctorate, thesis/dissertation (for some programs). Electronic applications accepted.

Medical University of South Carolina, College of Health Professions, Program in Health Administration-Global, Charleston, SC 29425. Offers MHA. *Entrance requirements:* Additional exam requirements/recommendations for international students: Required—TOEFL.

Morehouse School of Medicine, Master of Public Health Program, Atlanta, GA 30310-1495. Offers epidemiology (MPH); health administration, management and policy (MPH); health education/health promotion (MPH); international health (MPH). *Accreditation:* CEPH. Part-time programs available. *Students:* 37 full-time (27 women), 5 part-time (3 women); includes 33 minority (32 Black or African American, non-Hispanic/Latino; 1 American Indian or Alaska Native, non-Hispanic/Latino). Average age 28. In 2013, 13 master's awarded. *Degree requirements:* For master's, thesis, practicum, public health leadership seminar. *Entrance requirements:* For master's, GRE General Test, writing test, public health or human service experience. Additional exam requirements/recommendations for international students: Required—TOEFL (minimum score 550 paper-based). *Application deadline:* For fall admission, 3/1 for domestic and international students. Application fee: $50. Electronic applications accepted. *Expenses:* Contact institution. *Financial support:* Fellowships, research assistantships with partial tuition reimbursements, teaching assistantships, career-related internships or fieldwork, Federal Work-Study, institutionally sponsored loans, scholarships/grants, and unspecified assistantships available. Support available to part-time students. Financial award application deadline: 5/1; financial award applicants required to submit FAFSA. *Faculty research:* Women's and adolescent health, violence prevention, cancer epidemiology/disparities, substance abuse prevention. *Unit head:* Dr. Stephanie Miles-Richardson, Interim Director, 404-752-1944, Fax: 404-752-1051, E-mail: smiles-richardson@msm.edu. *Application contact:* Brandon Hunter, Director of Admissions, 404-752-1650, Fax: 404-752-1512, E-mail: mphadmissions@msm.edu.
Website: http://www.msm.edu/educationTraining/degreePrograms/mph.aspx

New York Medical College, School of Health Sciences and Practice, Department of Health Policy and Management, Graduate Certificate Program in Global Health, Valhalla, NY 10595-1691. Offers Graduate Certificate. *Accreditation:* CEPH. Part-time and evening/weekend programs available. *Faculty:* 2 full-time, 3 part-time/adjunct. *Students:* 15 full-time, 30 part-time. 40 applicants, 75% accepted, 25 enrolled. *Entrance requirements:* Additional exam requirements/recommendations for international students: Required—TOEFL (minimum score 637 paper-based; 96 iBT), IELTS (minimum score 7). *Application deadline:* For fall admission, 8/1 priority date for domestic students, 5/15 for international students; for spring admission, 12/1 priority date for domestic students, 10/15 for international students; for summer admission, 5/1 for domestic students, 4/1 for international students. Applications are processed on a rolling basis. Application fee: $50 ($100 for international students). Electronic applications accepted. *Expenses: Tuition:* Full-time $49,170; part-time $910 per credit. Tuition and fees vary according to program. *Financial support:* Research assistantships, teaching assistantships, career-related internships or fieldwork, Federal Work-Study, institutionally sponsored loans, health care benefits, and tuition waivers (partial) available. Support available to part-time students. Financial award applicants required to submit FAFSA. *Unit head:* Dr. Padmini Murthy, Director, 914-594-3480, Fax: 914-594-3481, E-mail: mini_murthy@nymc.edu. *Application contact:* Pamela Suett, Director of Recruitment, 914-594-4510, Fax: 914-594-4292, E-mail: shsp_admissions@nymc.edu.
Website: http://www.nymc.edu/sph/

New York University, Steinhardt School of Culture, Education, and Human Development, Department of Nutrition, Food Studies, and Public Health, Program in Public Health, New York, NY 10003. Offers community and international health (MPH); global health leadership (MPH); public health nutrition (MPH). *Accreditation:* CEPH. Part-time programs available. *Faculty:* 7 full-time (5 women). *Students:* 6 full-time (all women), 2 part-time (both women); includes 3 minority (2 Asian, non-Hispanic/Latino; 1 Hispanic/Latino). Average age 32. 44 applicants, 7% accepted, 2 enrolled. In 2013, 1 degree awarded. *Degree requirements:* For master's, thesis (for some programs). *Entrance requirements:* For master's, GRE General Test. Additional exam requirements/recommendations for international students: Required—TOEFL. *Application deadline:* For fall admission, 12/1 priority date for domestic and international students; for spring admission, 11/1 for domestic and international students. Applications are processed on a rolling basis. Application fee: $75. Electronic applications accepted. *Expenses: Tuition:* Full-time $35,856; part-time $1494 per unit. *Required fees:* $1408; $64 per unit. $473 per term. Tuition and fees vary according to course load and program. *Financial support:* Fellowships with full and partial tuition reimbursements, career-related internships or fieldwork, Federal Work-Study, institutionally sponsored loans, scholarships/grants, and tuition waivers (partial) available. Support available to part-time students. Financial award application deadline: 2/1; financial award applicants required to submit FAFSA. *Faculty research:* Social epidemiology, primary health care, global health, immigrants and health, infectious disease prevention, HIV/AIDS. *Unit head:* Prof. James Macinko, Director, 212-998-5592, Fax: 212-995-4192, E-mail: james.macinko@nyu.edu.

Application contact: 212-998-5030, Fax: 212-995-4328, E-mail: steinhardt.gradadmissions@nyu.edu.
Website: http://steinhardt.nyu.edu/nutrition/public_health

North Dakota State University, College of Graduate and Interdisciplinary Studies, College of Agriculture, Food Systems, and Natural Resources, Department of Veterinary and Microbiological Sciences, Fargo, ND 58108. Offers international infectious disease (MS); microbiology (MS); molecular pathogenesis (PhD). Part-time programs available. *Faculty:* 15 full-time (8 women). *Students:* 11 full-time (6 women), 6 part-time (4 women), 5 international. Average age 30. 2 applicants, 50% accepted, 1 enrolled. In 2013, 8 master's, 1 doctorate awarded. *Degree requirements:* For master's, thesis; for doctorate, thesis/dissertation, oral and written preliminary exams. *Entrance requirements:* For master's and doctorate, GRE. Additional exam requirements/recommendations for international students: Required—TOEFL (minimum score 525 paper-based; 71 iBT). *Application deadline:* For fall admission, 2/15 priority date for domestic students. Applications are processed on a rolling basis. Application fee: $35. *Financial support:* Fellowships with full tuition reimbursements, research assistantships with full tuition reimbursements, teaching assistantships with full tuition reimbursements, Federal Work-Study, and institutionally sponsored loans available. Financial award application deadline: 4/15. *Faculty research:* Bacterial gene regulation, antibiotic resistance, molecular virology, mechanisms of bacterial pathogenesis, immunology of animals. *Unit head:* Dr. Charlene Wolf-Hall, Head, 701-231-7667, E-mail: charlene.hall@ndsu.edu. *Application contact:* Dr. John McEvoy, Associate Professor, 701-231-8530, Fax: 701-231-7514, E-mail: eugene.berry@ndsu.edu.
Website: http://vetmicro.ndsu.nodak.edu/

Northwestern University, School of Professional Studies, Program in Global Health, Evanston, IL 60208. Offers MS. Program offered in partnership with Northwestern University Feinberg School of Medicine?s Center for Global Health. Postbaccalaureate distance learning degree programs offered (no on-campus study). *Degree requirements:* For master's, practicum.

Oregon State University, College of Public Health and Human Sciences, Program in Public Health, Corvallis, OR 97331. Offers biostatistics (MPH); environmental and occupational health and safety (MPH, PhD); epidemiology (MPH); health management and policy (MPH); health policy (PhD); health promotion and health behavior (MPH, PhD); international health (MPH). *Accreditation:* CEPH. Part-time programs available. *Faculty:* 29 full-time (16 women), 4 part-time/adjunct (3 women). *Students:* 137 full-time (102 women), 29 part-time (18 women); includes 37 minority (4 Black or African American, non-Hispanic/Latino; 7 Asian, non-Hispanic/Latino; 17 Hispanic/Latino; 9 Two or more races, non-Hispanic/Latino), 15 international. Average age 32. 163 applicants, 58% accepted, 48 enrolled. In 2013, 39 master's, 3 doctorates awarded. Terminal master's awarded for partial completion of doctoral program. *Degree requirements:* For doctorate, one foreign language, thesis/dissertation. *Entrance requirements:* For master's and doctorate, GRE, minimum GPA of 3.0 in last 90 hours. Additional exam requirements/recommendations for international students: Required—TOEFL (minimum score 80 iBT), IELTS (minimum score 6.5). *Application deadline:* For fall admission, 12/1 for domestic students. Applications are processed on a rolling basis. Application fee: $60. *Expenses:* Contact institution. *Financial support:* Fellowships, research assistantships, teaching assistantships, career-related internships or fieldwork, Federal Work-Study, and institutionally sponsored loans available. Support available to part-time students. Financial award application deadline: 2/1. *Faculty research:* Traffic safety, health safety, injury control, health promotion. *Unit head:* Dr. Sheryl Thorburn, Professor/Co-Director, 541-737-9493. *Application contact:* Eileen Kaspar, Public Health Graduate Programs Manager, 541-737-3825, E-mail: eileen.kaspar@oregonstate.edu.

Park University, School of Graduate and Professional Studies, Kansas City, MO 54105. Offers adult education (M Ed); business and government leadership (Graduate Certificate); business, government, and global society (MPA); communication and leadership (MA); creative and life writing (Graduate Certificate); disaster and emergency management (MPA, Graduate Certificate); educational leadership (M Ed); finance (MBA, Graduate Certificate); general business (MBA); global business (Graduate Certificate); healthcare administration (MHA); healthcare services management and leadership (Graduate Certificate); international business (MBA); language and literacy (M Ed), including English for speakers of other languages, special reading teacher/literacy coach; leadership of international healthcare organizations (Graduate Certificate); management information systems (MBA, Graduate Certificate); music performance (ADP, Graduate Certificate), including cello (MM, ADP), piano (MM, ADP), viola (MM, ADP), violin (MM, ADP); nonprofit and community services management (MPA); nonprofit leadership (Graduate Certificate); performance (MM), including cello (MM, ADP), piano (MM, ADP), viola (MM, ADP), violin (MM, ADP); public management (MPA); social work (MSW); teacher leadership (M Ed), including curriculum and assessment, instructional leader. Part-time and evening/weekend programs available. Postbaccalaureate distance learning degree programs offered (no on-campus study). *Students:* 862 full-time (482 women); includes 55 minority (30 Black or African American, non-Hispanic/Latino; 2 American Indian or Alaska Native, non-Hispanic/Latino; 4 Asian, non-Hispanic/Latino; 14 Hispanic/Latino; 5 Two or more races, non-Hispanic/Latino), 141 international. Average age 34. 497 applicants, 62% accepted, 119 enrolled. In 2013, 281 master's, 14 other advanced degrees awarded. *Degree requirements:* For master's, comprehensive exam (for some programs), thesis (for some programs), internship (for some programs); exam (for some programs). *Entrance requirements:* For master's, GRE or GMAT (for some programs), teacher certification (for some M Ed programs), letters of recommendation, essay, resume (for some programs). Additional exam requirements/recommendations for international students: Required—TOEFL (minimum score 550 paper-based; 79 iBT), IELTS (minimum score 6). *Application deadline:* For fall admission, 8/1 priority date for domestic students, 7/15 priority date for international students; for spring admission, 1/1 priority date for domestic students, 11/1 priority date for international students. Applications are processed on a rolling basis. Application fee: $50 ($100 for international students). Electronic applications accepted. *Financial support:* In 2013–14, 2 research assistantships with full tuition reimbursements (averaging $15,760 per year) were awarded. Financial award applicants required to submit FAFSA. *Unit head:* Dr. Laurie Dipadova-Stocks, Dean of Graduate and Professional Studies, 816-559-5624, Fax: 816-472-1173, E-mail: ldipadovastocks@park.edu. *Application contact:* Judith Appollis, Director of Graduate Admissions and Internationalization, School of Graduate and Professional Studies, 816-559-5627, Fax: 816-472-1173, E-mail: gradschool@park.edu.
Website: http://www.park.edu/grad

San Diego State University, Graduate and Research Affairs, College of Health and Human Services, Graduate School of Public Health, San Diego, CA 92182. Offers environmental health (MPH); epidemiology (MPH, PhD), including biostatistics (MPH); global emergency preparedness and response (MS); global health (PhD); health behavior (PhD); health promotion (MPH); health services administration (MPH); toxicology (MS); MPH/MA; MSW/MPH. *Accreditation:* CAHME (one or more programs are accredited); CEPH (one or more programs are accredited). Part-time programs available. *Degree requirements:* For master's, comprehensive exam (for some programs), thesis (for some programs); for doctorate, thesis/dissertation. *Entrance requirements:* For master's, GMAT (MPH in health services administration), GRE General Test; for doctorate, GRE General Test. Additional exam requirements/recommendations for international students: Required—TOEFL. *Faculty research:* Evaluation of tobacco, AIDS prevalence and prevention, mammography, infant death project, Alzheimer's in elderly Chinese.

Simon Fraser University, Office of Graduate Studies, Faculty of Health Sciences, Burnaby, BC V5A 1S6, Canada. Offers global health (Graduate Diploma); health sciences (M Sc, PhD); public health (MPH). *Students:* 177 full-time (138 women), 4 part-time (2 women). 373 applicants, 39% accepted, 53 enrolled. In 2013, 66 master's, 1 other advanced degree awarded. *Degree requirements:* For master's, thesis (for some programs); for doctorate, comprehensive exam, thesis/dissertation. *Entrance requirements:* For master's, minimum GPA of 3.0 (on scale of 4.33), or 3.33 based on last 60 credits of undergraduate courses; for doctorate, minimum GPA of 3.5 (on scale of 4.33); for Graduate Diploma, minimum GPA of 2.5 (on scale of 4.33), or 2.67 based on the last 60 credits of undergraduate courses. Additional exam requirements/recommendations for international students: Recommended—TOEFL (minimum score 580 paper-based; 93 iBT), IELTS (minimum score 7), TWE (minimum score 5). Application fee: $90 ($125 for international students). Electronic applications accepted. *Expenses: Tuition, area resident:* Full-time $5084 Canadian dollars. *Required fees:* $840 Canadian dollars. *Financial support:* In 2013–14, 42 students received support, including 39 fellowships (averaging $6,250 per year), teaching assistantships (averaging $5,608 per year); research assistantships, career-related internships or fieldwork, and scholarships/grants also available. *Unit head:* Dr. Jamie Scott, Graduate Chair, 778-782-7189, Fax: 778-782-5927, E-mail: msc-phd-grad-chair@sfu.ca. *Application contact:* Jennifer Van Rassel, Graduate Secretary, 778-782-7036, Fax: 778-782-5927, E-mail: fhsgrads@sfu.ca.
Website: http://www.fhs.sfu.ca/

Stanford University, School of Humanities and Sciences, Program in International Policy Studies, Stanford, CA 94305-9991. Offers democracy, development, and rule of law (MA); energy, environment, and natural resources (MA); global health (MA); international political economy (MA); international security and cooperation (MA). *Degree requirements:* For master's, thesis optional. *Entrance requirements:* For master's, GRE General Test. Additional exam requirements/recommendations for international students: Required—TOEFL. Electronic applications accepted. *Expenses: Tuition:* Full-time $42,690; part-time $949 per credit. *Required fees:* $185.

Syracuse University, Falk College of Sport and Human Dynamics, Program in Global Health, Syracuse, NY 13244. Offers CAS. Part-time programs available. *Students:* 1 (woman) full-time; minority (Black or African American, non-Hispanic/Latino). Average age 23. 2 applicants, 100% accepted. *Entrance requirements:* For degree, bachelor's degree from accredited institution with minimum cumulative GPA of 3.0 in undergraduate coursework. Additional exam requirements/recommendations for international students: Required—TOEFL (minimum score 100 iBT). *Application deadline:* For fall admission, 3/15 priority date for domestic and international students; for spring admission, 11/15 priority date for domestic and international students. *Financial support:* Application deadline: 1/1. *Unit head:* Dr. Brooks Gump, Graduate Program Director, 315-443-2208, Fax: 315-443-2562, E-mail: bbgump@syr.edu. *Application contact:* Felicia Otero, Director of College Admissions, 315-443-5555, Fax: 315-443-2562, E-mail: falk@syr.edu.
Website: http://falk.syr.edu/HealthWellness/GlobalHealth_CAS.aspx

Trident University International, College of Health Sciences, Program in Health Sciences, Cypress, CA 90630. Offers clinical research administration (MS, Certificate); emergency and disaster management (MS, Certificate); environmental health science (Certificate); health care administration (PhD); health care management (MS), including health informatics; health education (MS, Certificate); health informatics (Certificate); health sciences (PhD); international health (MS); international health: educator or researcher option (PhD); international health: practitioner option (PhD); law and expert witness studies (MS, Certificate); public health (MS); quality assurance (Certificate). Part-time and evening/weekend programs available. Postbaccalaureate distance learning degree programs offered (no on-campus study). *Degree requirements:* For doctorate, comprehensive exam, thesis/dissertation, defense of dissertation. *Entrance requirements:* For master's, minimum GPA of 2.5 (students with GPA 3.0 or greater may transfer up to 30% of graduate level credits); for doctorate, minimum GPA of 3.4, curriculum vitae, course work in research methods or statistics. Additional exam requirements/recommendations for international students: Required—TOEFL. Electronic applications accepted.

Tufts University, The Fletcher School of Law and Diplomacy, Medford, MA 02155. Offers LL M, MA, MALD, MIB, PhD, DVM/MA, JD/MALD, MALD/MA, MALD/MBA, MALD/MS, MD/MA. Postbaccalaureate distance learning degree programs offered (minimal on-campus study). *Faculty:* 43 full-time, 42 part-time/adjunct. *Students:* 615 full-time (310 women), 12 part-time (5 women); includes 116 minority (17 Black or African American, non-Hispanic/Latino; 50 Asian, non-Hispanic/Latino; 27 Hispanic/Latino; 22 Two or more races, non-Hispanic/Latino), 211 international. Average age 31. In 2013, 313 master's, 12 doctorates awarded. *Degree requirements:* For master's, one foreign language, thesis; for doctorate, one foreign language, comprehensive exam, thesis/dissertation, dissertation defense. *Entrance requirements:* For master's and doctorate, GMAT or GRE General Test. Additional exam requirements/recommendations for international students: Required—TOEFL (minimum score 600 paper-based; 100 iBT), IELTS (minimum score 7). *Application deadline:* For fall admission, 1/10 for domestic and international students; for spring admission, 10/15 for domestic and international students. Application fee: $80. Electronic applications accepted. *Expenses:* Contact institution. *Financial support:* Career-related internships or fieldwork, Federal Work-Study, institutionally sponsored loans, scholarships/grants, and tuition waivers (partial) available. Financial award application deadline: 1/10; financial award applicants required to submit FAFSA. *Faculty research:* Negotiation and conflict resolution, international organizations, international business and economic law, security studies, development economics. *Unit head:* Dr. James Stavridis, Dean, 617-627-3050, Fax: 617-627-3712. *Application contact:* Laurie A. Hurley, Director of Admissions and Financial Aid, 617-627-3040, E-mail: fletcheradmissions@tufts.edu.
Website: http://www.fletcher.tufts.edu

Tulane University, School of Public Health and Tropical Medicine, Department of International Health and Development, New Orleans, LA 70118-5669. Offers MPH, Dr PH, PhD, MSW/MPH. *Accreditation:* CEPH (one or more programs are accredited). Part-time programs available. Terminal master's awarded for partial completion of doctoral program. *Degree requirements:* For master's, one foreign language; for doctorate, one foreign language, comprehensive exam, thesis/dissertation. *Entrance requirements:* For master's and doctorate, GRE General Test. Additional exam requirements/recommendations for international students: Required—TOEFL. Electronic applications accepted. *Faculty research:* Reproductive health, HIV/AIDS, nutrition and food security, health financing, program evaluation.

Uniformed Services University of the Health Sciences, School of Medicine, Graduate Programs in the Biomedical Sciences and Public Health, Bethesda, MD 20814. Offers emerging infectious diseases (PhD); medical and clinical psychology (PhD), including clinical psychology, medical psychology; molecular and cell biology (MS, PhD); neuroscience (PhD); preventive medicine and biometrics (MPH, MS, MSPH,

MTMH, Dr PH, PhD), including environmental health sciences (PhD), healthcare administration and policy (MS), medical zoology (PhD), public health (MPH, MSPH, Dr PH), tropical medicine and hygiene (MTMH). *Faculty:* 372 full-time (119 women), 4,044 part-time/adjunct (908 women). *Students:* 240 full-time (133 women); includes 40 minority (15 Black or African American, non-Hispanic/Latino; 13 Asian, non-Hispanic/Latino; 12 Hispanic/Latino), 30 international. Average age 25. 598 applicants, 17% accepted, 77 enrolled. In 2013, 19 master's, 50 doctorates awarded. Terminal master's awarded for partial completion of doctoral program. *Degree requirements:* For master's, comprehensive exam, thesis or alternative; for doctorate, comprehensive exam, thesis/dissertation, qualifying exam. *Entrance requirements:* For master's, GRE General Test; for doctorate, GRE General Test, minimum GPA of 3.0. Additional exam requirements/recommendations for international students: Required—TOEFL. *Application deadline:* For fall admission, 1/1 priority date for domestic and international students. Applications are processed on a rolling basis. Application fee: $0. Electronic applications accepted. *Financial support:* In 2013–14, fellowships with full tuition reimbursements (averaging $27,000 per year), research assistantships with full tuition reimbursements (averaging $27,000 per year) were awarded; career-related internships or fieldwork, scholarships/grants, health care benefits, and tuition waivers (full) also available. *Unit head:* Dr. Eleanor S. Metcalf, Associate Dean, 301-295-1104, E-mail: emetcalf@usuhs.edu. *Application contact:* Tina Finley, Administrative Officer, 301-295-3642, Fax: 301-295-6772, E-mail: netina.finley@usuhs.edu.
Website: http://www.usuhs.mil/graded

Uniformed Services University of the Health Sciences, School of Medicine, Graduate Programs in the Biomedical Sciences and Public Health, Department of Preventive Medicine and Biometrics, Program in Tropical Medicine and Hygiene, Bethesda, MD 20814-4799. Offers MTMH. *Accreditation:* CEPH. *Degree requirements:* For master's, comprehensive exam. *Entrance requirements:* For master's, GRE General Test, MD, U.S. citizenship. *Application deadline:* For fall admission, 1/1 priority date for domestic students. Applications are processed on a rolling basis. Application fee: $0. *Financial support:* Health care benefits available. *Faculty research:* Epidemiology, biostatistics, tropical public health. *Unit head:* Dr. David Cruess, Director, 301-295-3465, Fax: 301-295-1933, E-mail: dcruess@usuhs.edu. *Application contact:* Elena Marina Sherman, Program Administrative Specialist, 301-295-3913, Fax: 301-295-6772, E-mail: elena.sherman@usuhs.edu.
Website: http://www.usuhs.mil/pmb

University of Alberta, School of Public Health, Department of Public Health Sciences, Edmonton, AB T6G 2E1, Canada. Offers clinical epidemiology (M Sc, MPH); environmental and occupational health (MPH); environmental health sciences (M Sc); epidemiology (M Sc); global health (M Sc, MPH); health policy and management (MPH); health policy research (M Sc); health technology assessment (MPH); occupational health (M Sc); population health (M Sc); public health leadership (MPH); public health sciences (PhD); quantitative methods (MPH). *Accreditation:* CEPH (one or more programs are accredited). Terminal master's awarded for partial completion of doctoral program. *Degree requirements:* For master's, thesis (for some programs); for doctorate, thesis/dissertation. *Entrance requirements:* For master's, GMAT or GRE General Test. Additional exam requirements/recommendations for international students: Required—TOEFL (minimum score 550 paper-based) or IELTS (minimum score 6). Electronic applications accepted. *Faculty research:* Biostatistics, health promotion and socio-behavioral health science.

University of California, San Diego, Office of Graduate Studies, Program in Public Health, La Jolla, CA 92093-0901. Offers public health and epidemiology (PhD); public health and global health (PhD); public health and health behavior (PhD). Program offered jointly with San Diego State University. *Students:* 35 (25 women); includes 11 minority (3 Black or African American, non-Hispanic/Latino; 4 Asian, non-Hispanic/Latino; 4 Hispanic/Latino), 4 international. In 2013, 11 doctorates awarded. *Degree requirements:* For doctorate, thesis/dissertation, 2 semesters/quarters of teaching assistantship. *Entrance requirements:* For doctorate, GRE General Test, minimum GPA of 3.0. Additional exam requirements/recommendations for international students: Required—TOEFL, IELTS. *Application deadline:* For fall admission, 12/14 for domestic students. Application fee: $55. Electronic applications accepted. *Expenses:* Tuition, state resident: full-time $11,220; part-time $1870 per quarter. Tuition, nonresident: full-time $26,322; part-time $4387 per quarter. *Required fees:* $519.50 per quarter. Part-time tuition and fees vary according to course load and program. *Faculty research:* Maternal and pediatric HIV/AIDS; healthy aging and gender differences; non-parametric and semi-parametric regression, resampling, and the analysis of high-dimensional data; neighborhood correlates of physical activity in children, teens, adults and older adults; medication safety and medication therapy management through practice-based research networks. *Unit head:* John Pierce, Program Director, 858-822-2380, E-mail: jppierce@ucsd.edu. *Application contact:* Hollie Ward, Graduate Coordinator, 858-822-2382, E-mail: hward@ucsd.edu.
Website: http://publichealth.ucsd.edu/jdp/

University of Colorado Denver, Business School, Master of Business Administration Program, Denver, CO 80217. Offers bioinnovation and entrepreneurship (MBA); business intelligence (MBA); business strategy (MBA); business to business marketing (MBA); business to consumer marketing (MBA); change management (MBA); corporate financial management (MBA); enterprise technology management (MBA); entrepreneurship (MBA); health administration (MBA), including financial management, health administration, health information technologies, international health management and policy; human resources management (MBA); international business (MBA); investment management (MBA); managing for sustainability (MBA); sports and entertainment management (MBA). *Accreditation:* AACSB. Part-time and evening/weekend programs available. Postbaccalaureate distance learning degree programs offered (no on-campus study). *Students:* 611 full-time (246 women), 144 part-time (58 women); includes 102 minority (14 Black or African American, non-Hispanic/Latino; 2 American Indian or Alaska Native, non-Hispanic/Latino; 38 Asian, non-Hispanic/Latino; 42 Hispanic/Latino; 6 Two or more races, non-Hispanic/Latino), 26 international. Average age 32. 330 applicants, 64% accepted, 125 enrolled. In 2013, 398 master's awarded. *Degree requirements:* For master's, 48 semester hours, including 30 of core courses, 3 in international business, and 15 in electives from over 50 other graduate business courses. *Entrance requirements:* For master's, GMAT, resume, official transcripts, essay, two letters of recommendation, financial statements (for international applicants). Additional exam requirements/recommendations for international students: Required—TOEFL (minimum score 560 paper-based; 83 iBT); Recommended—IELTS (minimum score 6.5). *Application deadline:* For fall admission, 4/15 priority date for domestic students, 3/15 priority date for international students; for spring admission, 10/15 priority date for domestic students, 9/15 priority date for international students. Applications are processed on a rolling basis. Application fee: $50 ($75 for international students). Electronic applications accepted. *Expenses:* Contact institution. *Financial support:* In 2013–14, 62 students received support. Fellowships, research assistantships, teaching assistantships, Federal Work-Study, institutionally sponsored loans, scholarships/grants, traineeships, and unspecified assistantships available. Financial award application deadline: 4/1; financial award applicants required to submit FAFSA. *Faculty research:* Marketing, management, entrepreneurship, finance, health administration. *Unit head:* Elizabeth Cooperman, Professor of Finance and Managing for Sustainability/MBA Program Director, 303-315-8422, E-mail: elizabeth.cooperman@ucdenver.edu. *Application contact:* Shelly Townley, Admissions Director, Graduate Programs, 303-315-8202, E-mail: shelly.townley@ucdenver.edu.
Website: http://www.ucdenver.edu/academics/colleges/business/degrees/mba/Pages/MBA.aspx

University of Colorado Denver, School of Medicine, Physician Assistant Program, Aurora, CO 80045. Offers child health associate (MPAS), including global health, leadership, education, advocacy, development, and scholarship, rural health, urban/underserved populations. *Accreditation:* ARC-PA. *Students:* 132 full-time (107 women); includes 15 minority (1 American Indian or Alaska Native, non-Hispanic/Latino; 6 Asian, non-Hispanic/Latino; 8 Hispanic/Latino). Average age 27. 1,313 applicants, 3% accepted, 44 enrolled. In 2013, 43 master's awarded. *Degree requirements:* For master's, comprehensive exam, successful completion of all coursework and rotations. *Entrance requirements:* For master's, GRE General Test, minimum GPA of 2.8, 3 letters of recommendation, prerequisite courses in chemistry, biology, general genetics, psychology and statistics, interviews. Additional exam requirements/recommendations for international students: Required—TOEFL (minimum score 550 paper-based; 80 iBT). *Application deadline:* For fall admission, 9/1 for domestic students, 8/15 for international students. Application fee: $170. Electronic applications accepted. *Expenses:* Contact institution. *Financial support:* In 2013–14, 85 students received support. Fellowships, research assistantships, teaching assistantships, career-related internships or fieldwork, Federal Work-Study, institutionally sponsored loans, scholarships/grants, traineeships, and unspecified assistantships available. Financial award application deadline: 3/15; financial award applicants required to submit FAFSA. *Faculty research:* Clinical genetics and genetic counseling, evidence-based medicine, pediatric allergy and asthma, childhood diabetes, standardized patient assessment. *Unit head:* Jonathan Bowser, Program Director, 303-724-1349, E-mail: jonathan.bowser@ucdenver.edu. *Application contact:* Kay Denler, Director of Admissions, 303-724-7963, E-mail: kay.denler@ucdenver.edu.
Website: http://www.ucdenver.edu/academics/colleges/medicalschool/education/degree_programs/PAProgram/Pages/Home.aspx

University of Denver, Josef Korbel School of International Studies, Denver, CO 80210. Offers conflict resolution (MA); global finance, trade and economic integration (MA); global health affairs (Certificate); homeland security (Certificate); humanitarian assistance (Certificate); international administration (MA); international development (MA); international human rights (MA); international law and human rights (Certificate); international security (MA); international studies (MA, PhD). Part-time programs available. *Faculty:* 37 full-time (12 women), 18 part-time/adjunct (9 women). *Students:* 430 full-time (258 women), 23 part-time (11 women); includes 78 minority (14 Black or African American, non-Hispanic/Latino; 11 Asian, non-Hispanic/Latino; 43 Hispanic/Latino; 1 Native Hawaiian or other Pacific Islander, non-Hispanic/Latino; 9 Two or more races, non-Hispanic/Latino), 48 international. Average age 27. 841 applicants, 90% accepted, 227 enrolled. In 2013, 204 master's, 6 doctorates, 32 other advanced degrees awarded. *Degree requirements:* For master's, one foreign language, thesis (for some programs); for doctorate, one foreign language, comprehensive exam, thesis/dissertation, two extended research papers. *Entrance requirements:* For master's, GRE General Test, bachelor's degree, transcripts, two letters of recommendation, statement of purpose, resume or curriculum vitae; for doctorate, GRE General Test, master's degree, transcripts, three letters of recommendation, statement of purpose, resume or curriculum vitae, writing sample; for Certificate, bachelor's degree, transcripts, two letters of recommendation, statement of purpose, resume or curriculum vitae. Additional exam requirements/recommendations for international students: Required—TOEFL (minimum score 587 paper-based; 95 iBT). *Application deadline:* For fall admission, 1/15 priority date for domestic students, 12/15 priority date for international students; for winter admission, 11/1 priority date for domestic and international students. Application fee: $65. Electronic applications accepted. *Financial support:* In 2013–14, 216 students received support, including 1 research assistantship, 2 teaching assistantships with full and partial tuition reimbursements available (averaging $8,280 per year); career-related internships or fieldwork, Federal Work-Study, institutionally sponsored loans, scholarships/grants, and unspecified assistantships also available. Support available to part-time students. Financial award application deadline: 2/15; financial award applicants required to submit FAFSA. *Faculty research:* Human rights and international security, international politics and economics, economic-social and political development, international technology analysis and management. *Unit head:* Christopher R. Hill, Dean, 303-871-2359, Fax: 303-871-2456, E-mail: christopher.r.hill@du.edu. *Application contact:* Brad Miller, Director of Graduate Admissions, 303-871-2989, Fax: 303-871-2124, E-mail: brad.miller@du.edu.
Website: http://www.du.edu/korbel/

University of Florida, Graduate School, College of Public Health and Health Professions, Department of Environmental and Global Health, Gainesville, FL 32610. Offers one health (MHS). *Faculty:* 13 full-time (5 women), 5 part-time/adjunct (1 woman). *Students:* 5 full-time (4 women), 2 part-time (1 woman); includes 2 minority (both Black or African American, non-Hispanic/Latino), 1 international. Average age 32. 10 applicants, 40% accepted, 1 enrolled. *Entrance requirements:* For master's, GRE, minimum GPA of 3.0. Additional exam requirements/recommendations for international students: Required—TOEFL (minimum score 550 paper-based; 80 iBT), IELTS (minimum score 6). *Application deadline:* For fall admission, 1/1 for domestic students. Application fee: $30. *Expenses:* Tuition, state resident: full-time $12,640. Tuition, nonresident: full-time $30,000. *Financial support:* Applicants required to submit FAFSA. *Unit head:* Dr. Gregory C. Gray, MD, Chair, 352-273-9449, E-mail: gcgray@phhp.ufl.edu. *Application contact:* Office of Admissions, 352-392-1365, E-mail: webrequests@admissions.ufl.edu.
Website: http://egh.phhp.ufl.edu/

University of Michigan, School of Public Health, Department of Epidemiology, Ann Arbor, MI 48109-2029. Offers dental public health (MPH); epidemiological science (PhD); epidemiology (MS); general epidemiology (MPH); hospital and molecular epidemiology (MPH); international health (MPH). PhD and MS offered through the Horace H. Rackham School of Graduate Studies. *Accreditation:* CEPH (one or more programs are accredited). Part-time programs available. Terminal master's awarded for partial completion of doctoral program. *Degree requirements:* For master's, thesis (for some programs); for doctorate, comprehensive exam, thesis/dissertation, oral defense of dissertation, preliminary exam. *Entrance requirements:* For master's and doctorate, GRE General Test, MCAT. Additional exam requirements/recommendations for international students: Required—TOEFL (minimum score 560 paper-based; 100 iBT). Electronic applications accepted. Tuition and fees vary according to course level, course load, degree level, program and student level. *Faculty research:* Molecular virology, infectious diseases, women's health, genetics, social epidemiology.

University of Minnesota, Twin Cities Campus, School of Public Health, Division of Environmental Health Sciences, Minneapolis, MN 55455-0213. Offers environmental and occupational epidemiology (MPH, MS, PhD); environmental chemistry (MS, PhD); environmental health policy (MPH, MS, PhD); environmental infectious diseases (MPH, MS, PhD); environmental toxicology (MPH, MS, PhD); exposure sciences (MS); general environmental health (MPH, MS); global environmental health (MPH, MS, PhD);

industrial hygiene (MPH, MS, PhD); occupational health nursing (MPH, MS, PhD); occupational medicine (MPH); MPH/MS. *Accreditation:* CEPH (one or more programs are accredited). Part-time programs available. *Degree requirements:* For master's, thesis optional; for doctorate, thesis/dissertation. *Entrance requirements:* For master's and doctorate, GRE General Test. Additional exam requirements/recommendations for international students: Required—TOEFL (minimum score 600 paper-based; 100 iBT). Electronic applications accepted. *Faculty research:* Behavior/measurement of airborne particles, toxicity mechanisms of environmental contaminants, health and safety interventions, foodborne disease surveillance, measuring pesticide exposures in children.

University of Missouri, Graduate School, Master of Public Health Program, Columbia, MO 65211. Offers global public health (Graduate Certificate); health promotion and policy (MPH); public health (Graduate Certificate); veterinary public health (MPH); DVM/MPH; MPH/MA; MPH/MPA. *Accreditation:* CEPH. *Students:* 88 full-time (67 women), 104 part-time (83 women); includes 43 minority (19 Black or African American, non-Hispanic/Latino; 9 Asian, non-Hispanic/Latino; 10 Hispanic/Latino; 5 Two or more races, non-Hispanic/Latino), 16 international. Average age 30. 133 applicants, 84% accepted, 79 enrolled. In 2013, 40 master's, 49 other advanced degrees awarded. *Entrance requirements:* Additional exam requirements/recommendations for international students: Required—TOEFL (minimum score 550 paper-based; 80 iBT). *Application deadline:* For fall admission, 6/30 priority date for domestic and international students. Applications are processed on a rolling basis. Application fee: $55 ($75 for international students). Electronic applications accepted. *Financial support:* Fellowships with tuition reimbursements, research assistantships with tuition reimbursements, teaching assistantships with tuition reimbursements, scholarships/grants, traineeships, health care benefits, and unspecified assistantships available. Support available to part-time students. *Faculty research:* Health professions, health care equality, global health, communicable diseases, public health; zoonosis and infectious diseases, medical education, inquiry-based learning, social determinants of health, violence against women, health disparities, breast cancer screening, epigenetic, nursing, environmental health, cancer and chronic diseases, environmental exposures with metals, geographical information systems, substance use disorders/addictions, mental health. *Unit head:* Lise Saffran, Interim Director, 573-884-6835, E-mail: saffranl@health.missouri.edu. *Application contact:* Sandra Gummersheimer, Academic Advisor, 573-884-6836, E-mail: gummersheimers@health.missouri.edu.
Website: http://publichealth.missouri.edu/

University of Pennsylvania, Perelman School of Medicine, Master of Public Health Program, Philadelphia, PA 19129. Offers generalist (MPH); global health (MPH); DMD/MPH; JD/MPH; MD/MPH; MPH/MBE; MSCE/MPH; MSN/MPH; MSSP/MPH; MSW/MPH; PhD/MPH. Part-time and evening/weekend programs available. *Faculty:* 33 full-time (19 women), 35 part-time/adjunct (19 women). *Students:* 44 full-time (33 women), 51 part-time (43 women); includes 30 minority (12 Black or African American, non-Hispanic/Latino; 14 Asian, non-Hispanic/Latino; 2 Hispanic/Latino; 2 Two or more races, non-Hispanic/Latino). 117 applicants, 62% accepted, 41 enrolled. In 2013, 24 master's awarded. *Entrance requirements:* For master's, GRE. Additional exam requirements/recommendations for international students: Recommended—TOEFL. *Application deadline:* For fall and spring admission, 4/30 for domestic and international students. Applications are processed on a rolling basis. Application fee: $70. *Financial support:* In 2013–14, 14 students received support, including 2 fellowships with partial tuition reimbursements available (averaging $1,000 per year), 14 teaching assistantships with partial tuition reimbursements available; scholarships/grants and tuition waivers (partial) also available. Financial award application deadline: 5/15. *Faculty research:* Health disparities, health behaviors, obesity, global health, epidemiology and prevention research. *Unit head:* Dr. Jennifer A. Pinto-Martin, Director, 215-898-4726, E-mail: pinto@nursing.upenn.edu. *Application contact:* Moriah Hall, MPH Program Coordinator, 215-573-8841, E-mail: moriahh@mail.med.upenn.edu.
Website: http://www.publichealth.med.upenn.edu/

University of Southern California, Keck School of Medicine and Graduate School, Graduate Programs in Medicine, Department of Preventive Medicine, Master of Public Health Program, Los Angeles, CA 90032. Offers biostatistics-epidemiology (MPH); child and family health (MPH); environmental health (MPH); global health leadership (MPH); health communication (MPH); health education and promotion (MPH); public health policy (MPH). *Accreditation:* CEPH. Part-time and evening/weekend programs available. *Faculty:* 22 full-time (12 women), 3 part-time/adjunct (0 women). *Students:* 179 full-time (136 women), 31 part-time (24 women); includes 120 minority (19 Black or African American, non-Hispanic/Latino; 64 Asian, non-Hispanic/Latino; 37 Hispanic/Latino), 36 international. Average age 24. 205 applicants, 70% accepted, 73 enrolled. In 2013, 90 master's awarded. *Degree requirements:* For master's, practicum, final report, oral presentation. *Entrance requirements:* For master's, GRE General Test, MCAT, GMAT, minimum GPA of 3.0. Additional exam requirements/recommendations for international students: Required—TOEFL (minimum score 600 paper-based; 90 iBT). *Application deadline:* For fall admission, 6/1 priority date for domestic and international students; for spring admission, 10/1 priority date for domestic and international students; for summer admission, 3/1 for domestic and international students. Applications are processed on a rolling basis. Application fee: $85. Electronic applications accepted. *Financial support:* Career-related internships or fieldwork, Federal Work-Study, institutionally sponsored loans, and scholarships/grants available. Support available to part-time students. Financial award application deadline: 5/4; financial award applicants required to submit CSS PROFILE or FAFSA. *Faculty research:* Substance abuse prevention, cancer and heart disease prevention, mass media and health communication research, health promotion, treatment compliance. *Unit head:* Dr. Louise A. Rohrbach, Director, 323-442-8237, Fax: 323-442-8297, E-mail: rohrbac@usc.edu. *Application contact:* Valerie Burris, Admissions Counselor, 323-442-7257, Fax: 323-442-8297, E-mail: valeriem@usc.edu.
Website: http://mph.usc.edu/

University of South Florida, College of Public Health, Department of Global Health, Tampa, FL 33620-9951. Offers MPH, MSPH, Dr PH, PhD. Part-time and evening/weekend programs available. *Degree requirements:* For master's, comprehensive exam, thesis (for some programs), minimum GPA of 3.0; for doctorate, comprehensive exam, thesis/dissertation. *Entrance requirements:* For master's, GRE General Test, minimum GPA of 3.0 in upper-level course work, goal statement letter, two professional letters of recommendation, resume/curriculum vitae; for doctorate, GRE General Test, minimum GPA of 3.0 in upper-level course work, goal statement letter, three professional letters of recommendation, resume/curriculum vitae, writing sample. Additional exam requirements/recommendations for international students: Required—TOEFL (minimum score 550 paper-based; 79 iBT). Electronic applications accepted.

University of South Florida, Innovative Education Graduate Certificate Programs, Tampa, FL 33620-9951. *Unit head:* Kathy Barnes, Interdisciplinary Programs Coordinator, 813-974-8031, Fax: 813-974-7061, E-mail: barnesk@usf.edu. *Application contact:* Karen Tylinski, Metro Initiatives, 813-974-9943, Fax: 813-974-7061, E-mail: ktylinsk@usf.edu.
Website: http://www.usf.edu/innovative-education/

The University of Toledo, College of Graduate Studies, College of Medicine and Life Sciences, Department of Public Health and Preventative Medicine, Toledo, OH 43606-3390. Offers biostatistics and epidemiology (Certificate); contemporary gerontological practice (Certificate); environmental and occupational health and safety (MPH); epidemiology (Certificate); global public health (Certificate); health promotion and education (MPH); industrial hygiene (MSOH); medical and health science teaching and learning (Certificate); occupational health (Certificate); public health administration (MPH); public health and emergency response (Certificate); public health epidemiology (MPH); public health nutrition (MPH); MD/MPH. Part-time and evening/weekend programs available. *Faculty:* 9. *Students:* 69 full-time (50 women), 88 part-time (66 women); includes 50 minority (35 Black or African American, non-Hispanic/Latino; 10 Asian, non-Hispanic/Latino; 4 Hispanic/Latino; 1 Two or more races, non-Hispanic/Latino), 6 international. Average age 30. 92 applicants, 80% accepted, 52 enrolled. In 2013, 59 master's, 15 other advanced degrees awarded. *Degree requirements:* For master's, thesis or alternative. *Entrance requirements:* For master's, GRE, minimum undergraduate GPA of 3.0, three letters of recommendation, statement of purpose, transcripts from all prior institutions attended, resume; for Certificate, minimum undergraduate GPA of 3.0, three letters of recommendation, statement of purpose, transcripts from all prior institutions attended, resume. Additional exam requirements/recommendations for international students: Required—TOEFL (minimum score 550 paper-based; 80 iBT), IELTS (minimum score 6.5). *Application deadline:* For fall admission, 6/15 for domestic students, 3/15 priority date for international students; for spring admission, 10/15 for domestic students, 6/15 for international students; for summer admission, 3/15 for domestic students, 10/15 for international students. Applications are processed on a rolling basis. Application fee: $45 ($75 for international students). Electronic applications accepted. *Financial support:* In 2013–14, 4 research assistantships with full tuition reimbursements (averaging $10,000 per year) were awarded; Federal Work-Study, institutionally sponsored loans, scholarships/grants, tuition waivers (full and partial), and unspecified assistantships also available. *Unit head:* Dr. Sheryl A. Milz, Chair, 419-383-3976, Fax: 419-383-6140, E-mail: sheryl.milz@utoledo.edu. *Application contact:* Admissions Analyst, 419-383-4112, Fax: 419-383-6140.
Website: http://nocphmph.org/

University of Washington, Graduate School, School of Public Health, Department of Epidemiology, Seattle, WA 98195. Offers clinical research (MS); epidemiology (MPH, MS, PhD); global health (MPH); maternal/child health (MPH); MPH/MPA. *Accreditation:* CEPH (one or more programs are accredited). *Faculty:* 65 full-time (38 women), 39 part-time/adjunct (17 women). *Students:* 120 full-time (84 women), 30 part-time (20 women); includes 19 minority (3 Black or African American, non-Hispanic/Latino; 2 American Indian or Alaska Native, non-Hispanic/Latino; 14 Asian, non-Hispanic/Latino), 12 international. Average age 32. 234 applicants, 37% accepted, 40 enrolled. In 2013, 41 master's, 18 doctorates awarded. *Degree requirements:* For master's, comprehensive exam (for some programs), thesis; for doctorate, comprehensive exam, thesis/dissertation, general exam, dissertation proposal, final exam (dissertation defense). *Entrance requirements:* For master's, GRE (except for those holding PhD, MD, DDS, DVM, DO or equivalent from U.S. institutions); for doctorate, GRE. Additional exam requirements/recommendations for international students: Required—TOEFL (minimum score 580 paper-based, 92 iBT), IELTS (minimum score 7), or PTE (minimum score of 65). *Application deadline:* For fall admission, 12/1 for domestic students, 11/1 for international students. Application fee: $85. Electronic applications accepted. *Expenses:* Contact institution. *Financial support:* In 2013–14, 138 students received support, including 70 fellowships with partial tuition reimbursements available, 40 research assistantships with partial tuition reimbursements available, 12 teaching assistantships with partial tuition reimbursements available; career-related internships or fieldwork, Federal Work-Study, traineeships, health care benefits, tuition waivers, and unspecified assistantships also available. Support available to part-time students. Financial award application deadline: 12/1; financial award applicants required to submit FAFSA. *Faculty research:* Chronic disease, health disparities and social determinants of health, aging and neuroepidemiology, maternal and child health, molecular and genetic epidemiology. *Unit head:* Dr. Scott Davis, Chair, 206-543-1065, E-mail: epiapply@uw.edu. *Application contact:* Kate O'Brien, Student Services Manager, 206-543-1065, E-mail: epiapply@uw.edu.
Website: http://depts.washington.edu/epidem/

University of Washington, Graduate School, School of Public Health, Department of Global Health, Seattle, WA 98195. Offers global health (MPH); global health metrics and implementation science (PhD); health metrics and evaluation (MPH); leadership, policy and management (MPH); pathobiology (PhD); MPH/MAIS; MPH/MD; MPH/MN; MPH/MPA; MPH/MSW; MPH/PhD. *Faculty:* 59 full-time (25 women), 58 part-time/adjunct (27 women). *Students:* 55 full-time (29 women), 20 part-time (6 women); includes 11 minority (4 Black or African American, non-Hispanic/Latino; 7 Asian, non-Hispanic/Latino), 23 international. Average age 30. 308 applicants, 28% accepted, 40 enrolled. In 2013, 30 master's awarded. *Degree requirements:* For master's, thesis, practicum; for doctorate, comprehensive exam, thesis/dissertation. *Entrance requirements:* For master's, GRE. Additional exam requirements/recommendations for international students: Required—TOEFL (minimum score 500 paper-based; 61 iBT), IELTS (minimum score 6). *Application deadline:* For fall admission, 12/1 for domestic students, 11/1 for international students. Application fee: $85. Electronic applications accepted. *Financial support:* In 2013–14, 1 student received support, including 7 fellowships with full tuition reimbursements available, 3 research assistantships with full tuition reimbursements available, 11 teaching assistantships with full tuition reimbursements available; tuition waivers (full) also available. Financial award application deadline: 6/30; financial award applicants required to submit FAFSA. *Faculty research:* AIDS and sexually-transmitted diseases, international health, reproductive health, tuberculosis, infectious disease. *Unit head:* Dr. King K. Holmes, Chair, 206-744-8493, Fax: 206-744-3694. *Application contact:* Program Contact, 206-685-7362, Fax: 206-685-1292, E-mail: ghrc@uw.edu.
Website: http://globalhealth.washington.edu/

Washington University in St. Louis, George Warren Brown School of Social Work, St. Louis, MO 63130. Offers Alaska native/American Indian studies (MSW); children, youth and families (MSW); gerontology (MSW); mental health (MSW); public health (MPA, MPH), including epidemiology/biostatistics (MPH), global health (MPA); social and economic development (MSW); social work (MSW, PhD), including health (MSW); JD/MSW; M Arch/MSW; MBA/MSW; MPH/MBA; MSW/M Div; MSW/MAPS; MSW/MJCS; MSW/MPH. MSW/M Div and MSW/MAPS offered jointly with Eden Theological Seminary. *Accreditation:* CSWE (one or more programs are accredited). *Faculty:* 42 full-time (24 women), 81 part-time/adjunct (49 women). *Students:* 298 full-time (263 women), 5 part-time (all women); includes 78 minority (32 Black or African American, non-Hispanic/Latino; 4 American Indian or Alaska Native, non-Hispanic/Latino; 18 Asian, non-Hispanic/Latino; 9 Hispanic/Latino; 2 Native Hawaiian or other Pacific Islander, non-Hispanic/Latino; 13 Two or more races, non-Hispanic/Latino), 47 international. Average age 26. 817 applicants, 62% accepted, 303 enrolled. In 2013, 239 master's, 5 doctorates awarded. *Degree requirements:* For master's, 60 credit hours (MSW), 52 credit hours (MPH); practicum; for doctorate, comprehensive exam, thesis/dissertation. *Entrance requirements:* For master's, GRE, GMAT, LSAT, or MCAT (public health), minimum GPA of 3.0; for doctorate, GRE, MA or MSW. Additional exam requirements/recommendations for international students: Required—TOEFL (minimum

score 100 iBT). *Application deadline:* For fall admission, 3/1 priority date for domestic and international students. Applications are processed on a rolling basis. Application fee: $40. Electronic applications accepted. *Expenses:* Contact institution. *Financial support:* In 2013–14, 301 students received support. Fellowships, research assistantships, Federal Work-Study, institutionally sponsored loans, scholarships/grants, health care benefits, tuition waivers (partial), and unspecified assistantships available. Support available to part-time students. Financial award application deadline: 3/1; financial award applicants required to submit FAFSA. *Faculty research:* Mental health services, social development, child welfare, at-risk teens, autism, environmental health, health policy, health communications, obesity, violence and injury prevention, chronic disease prevention, poverty, public health, productive aging/gerontology, social work, civic engagement, school social work, program evaluation, health disparities. *Unit head:* Dr. Edward F. Lawlor, Dean/Professor, 314-935-6693, Fax: 314-935-8511, E-mail: elawlor@wustl.edu. *Application contact:* Leslie D. Duling, Admissions Counselor, 314-935-6694, Fax: 314-935-4859, E-mail: lduling@brownschool.wustl.edu.
Website: http://gwbweb.wustl.edu/

Wayne State University, School of Medicine, Graduate Programs in Medicine, Program in Global and Pediatric Health, Detroit, MI 48202. Offers Graduate Certificate. *Degree requirements:* For Graduate Certificate, international field placement in a clinical and research experience. *Entrance requirements:* For degree, MD, DO, DDS, Pharm D or equivalent degree in human health care. Additional exam requirements/recommendations for international students: Required—TOEFL (minimum score 600 paper-based; 100 iBT). Electronic applications accepted. *Expenses:* Contact institution. *Unit head:* Dr. Deepak Kamat, Director, 313-745-5870, E-mail: kamat@wayne.edu. *Application contact:* Dr. Norman Silas, Jr., Associate Dean for Admissions, Diversity and Inclusion, 313-577-1466, E-mail: admissions@med.wayne.edu.
Website: http://gradprograms.med.wayne.edu/program-spotlight.php?id-36

Yale University, School of Medicine, Yale School of Public Health, New Haven, CT 06520. Offers applied biostatistics and epidemiology (APMPH); biostatistics (MPH, MS, PhD), including global health (MPH); chronic disease epidemiology (MPH, PhD), including global health (MPH); environmental health sciences (MPH, PhD), including global health (MPH); epidemiology of microbial diseases (MPH, PhD), including global health (MPH); global health (APMPH); health management (MPH), including global health; health policy (MPH), including global health; health policy and administration (APMPH, PhD); occupational and environmental medicine (APMPH); preventive medicine (APMPH); social and behavioral sciences (APMPH, MPH), including global health (MPH); JD/MPH; M Div/MPH; MBA/MPH; MD/MPH; MEM/MPH; MFS/MPH; MM Sc/MPH; MPH/MA; MSN/MPH. MS and PhD offered through the Graduate School. *Accreditation:* CEPH. Part-time programs available. Terminal master's awarded for partial completion of doctoral program. *Degree requirements:* For master's, thesis, summer internship; for doctorate, comprehensive exam, thesis/dissertation, residency. *Entrance requirements:* For master's, GMAT, GRE, or MCAT, two years of undergraduate coursework in math and science; for doctorate, GRE General Test. Additional exam requirements/recommendations for international students: Required—TOEFL (minimum score 100 iBT). Electronic applications accepted. *Expenses:* Contact institution. *Faculty research:* Genetic and emerging infections epidemiology, virology, cost/quality, vector biology, quantitative methods, aging, asthma, cancer.

Maternal and Child Health

Bank Street College of Education, Graduate School, Program in Child Life, New York, NY 10025. Offers MS. *Degree requirements:* For master's, thesis. *Entrance requirements:* For master's, interview, essays, 100 hours of volunteer experience in a child life setting. Additional exam requirements/recommendations for international students: Required—TOEFL (minimum score 600 paper-based; 100 iBT), IELTS (minimum score 7). *Faculty research:* Therapeutic play in child life setting, child advocacy, psychosocial and educational intervention with care of sick children.

Bank Street College of Education, Graduate School, Program in Infant and Family Development and Early Intervention, New York, NY 10025. Offers infant and family development (MS Ed); infant and family early childhood special and general education (MS Ed); infant and family/early childhood special education (Ed M). *Degree requirements:* For master's, thesis. *Entrance requirements:* For master's, interview, essays. Additional exam requirements/recommendations for international students: Required—TOEFL (minimum score 600 paper-based; 100 iBT), IELTS (minimum score 7). Electronic applications accepted. *Faculty research:* Early intervention, early attachment practice in infant and toddler childcare, parenting skills in adolescents.

Boston University, School of Public Health, Maternal and Child Health Department, Boston, MA 02215. Offers maternal and child health (MPH, Dr PH). Part-time and evening/weekend programs available. *Students:* 77 full-time (74 women), 41 part-time (40 women); includes 27 minority (10 Black or African American, non-Hispanic/Latino; 7 Asian, non-Hispanic/Latino; 6 Hispanic/Latino; 4 Two or more races, non-Hispanic/Latino), 6 international. Average age 27. 215 applicants, 52% accepted, 37 enrolled. In 2013, 24 master's, 1 doctorate awarded. *Degree requirements:* For doctorate, thesis/dissertation. *Entrance requirements:* For master's, GRE, DAT, MCAT, LSAT, or GMAT; for doctorate, GRE, GMAT. Additional exam requirements/recommendations for international students: Required—TOEFL (minimum score 600 paper-based; 100 iBT) or IELTS (minimum score 6). *Application deadline:* For fall admission, 2/1 priority date for domestic and international students; for spring admission, 10/15 priority date for domestic and international students. Applications are processed on a rolling basis. Application fee: $115. Electronic applications accepted. *Expenses: Tuition:* Full-time $43,970; part-time $1374 per credit hour. *Required fees:* $60 per semester. Tuition and fees vary according to class time, course level and program. *Financial support:* In 2013–14, 10 fellowships were awarded; career-related internships or fieldwork, Federal Work-Study, institutionally sponsored loans, scholarships/grants, traineeships, and tuition waivers (partial) also available. Financial award application deadline: 3/1; financial award applicants required to submit FAFSA. *Unit head:* Dr. Deborah Bowen, Chair, Community Health Sciences, 617-638-5205, E-mail: askmch@bu.edu. *Application contact:* LePhan Quan, Associate Director of Admissions, 617-638-4640, Fax: 617-638-5299, E-mail: asksph@bu.edu.
Website: http://sph.bu.edu/mch

Columbia University, Columbia University Mailman School of Public Health, Department of Population and Family Health, New York, NY 10032. Offers MPH. *Accreditation:* CEPH. Part-time programs available. *Students:* 124 full-time (102 women), 6 part-time (all women); includes 44 minority (6 Black or African American, non-Hispanic/Latino; 17 Asian, non-Hispanic/Latino; 17 Hispanic/Latino; 4 Two or more races, non-Hispanic/Latino), 7 international. Average age 28. 303 applicants, 51% accepted, 59 enrolled. In 2013, 75 master's awarded. *Entrance requirements:* For master's, GRE General Test. Additional exam requirements/recommendations for international students: Required—TOEFL (minimum score 600 paper-based; 100 iBT). *Application deadline:* For fall admission, 12/1 priority date for domestic and international students. Application fee: $120. *Financial support:* Research assistantships, career-related internships or fieldwork, and Federal Work-Study available. Financial award application deadline: 2/1; financial award applicants required to submit FAFSA. *Faculty research:* Child and adolescent health, global health systems, health and human rights, humanitarian disasters, sexual and reproductive health. *Unit head:* Dr. John Santelli, Chairperson, 212-304-5200. *Application contact:* Dr. Joseph Korevec, Director of Admissions and Financial Aid, 212-305-8698, Fax: 212-342-1861, E-mail: ph-admit@columbia.edu.
Website: http://www.mailman.hs.columbia.edu/popfam/index.html

East Carolina University, Graduate School, Thomas Harriot College of Arts and Sciences, Department of Psychology, Program in Health Psychology, Greenville, NC 27858-4353. Offers clinical health psychology (PhD); occupational health psychology (PhD); pediatric school psychology (PhD). *Entrance requirements:* For doctorate, GRE. *Expenses:* Tuition, state resident: full-time $4223. Tuition, nonresident: full-time $16,540. *Required fees:* $2184. *Financial support:* Fellowships, research assistantships, and teaching assistantships available. *Unit head:* Dr. Samuel F. Sears, Jr., Chair, 252-328-6118, Fax: 252-328-6283, E-mail: searss@ecu.edu. *Application contact:* Dean of Graduate School, 252-328-6012, Fax: 252-328-6071, E-mail: gradschool@ecu.edu.
Website: http://www.ecu.edu/psyc/Health-Psychology-Doctoral-Program.cfm

Future Generations Graduate School, Program in Applied Community Change, Conservation, and Peacebuilding, Franklin, WV 26807. Offers conservation (MA); peacebuilding (MA). *Faculty:* 40 full-time (18 women). *Students:* 40 full-time (18 women); includes 33 minority (15 Black or African American, non-Hispanic/Latino; 1 American Indian or Alaska Native, non-Hispanic/Latino; 10 Asian, non-Hispanic/Latino; 7 Hispanic/Latino). Average age 29. 60 applicants, 50% accepted, 25 enrolled. In 2013, 18 master's awarded. *Degree requirements:* For master's, one foreign language, applied practicum research. *Entrance requirements:* For master's, bachelor's degree, community involvement. Additional exam requirements/recommendations for international students: Required—TOEFL. *Application deadline:* For winter admission, 10/11 for domestic and international students. Application fee: $0. Electronic applications accepted. *Expenses: Tuition:* Full-time $17,500. *Financial support:* In 2013–14, 40 students received support. Scholarships/grants and tuition waivers (partial) available. Financial award application deadline: 10/1; financial award applicants required to submit FAFSA. *Faculty research:* Sustainable communities, community engagement, peacebuilding, seed-scale community development. *Unit head:* Dr. Michael Rechlin, Dean, 304-358-2000, E-mail: mike@future,edu. *Application contact:* Dr. Karen Jean Edwards, Director of Admissions, 518-483-7432, E-mail: karen@future.edu.
Website: http://www.future.edu

Instituto Tecnologico de Santo Domingo, Graduate School, Area of Health Sciences, Santo Domingo, Dominican Republic. Offers bioethics (M Bioethics); clinical bioethics (Certificate); clinical nutrition (Certificate); comprehensive health and the adolescent (Certificate); comrehensive adloescent health (MS); health and social security (M Mgmt).

Oakland University, Graduate Study and Lifelong Learning, School of Health Sciences, Program in Physical Therapy, Rochester, MI 48309-4401. Offers neurological rehabilitation (Certificate); orthopedic manual physical therapy (Certificate); orthopedic physical therapy (Certificate); pediatric rehabilitation (Certificate); physical therapy (MSPT, DPT, Dr Sc PT); teaching and learning for rehabilitation professionals (Certificate). *Accreditation:* APTA. *Faculty:* 11 full-time (9 women), 1 part-time/adjunct (0 women). *Students:* 134 full-time (92 women), 36 part-time (22 women); includes 6 minority (1 Black or African American, non-Hispanic/Latino; 3 Asian, non-Hispanic/Latino; 2 Hispanic/Latino), 3 international. Average age 26. 448 applicants, 12% accepted, 47 enrolled. In 2013, 7 master's, 38 doctorates, 22 other advanced degrees awarded. *Degree requirements:* For master's, thesis (for some programs). *Entrance requirements:* For master's, minimum GPA of 3.0; for doctorate, GRE General Test. Additional exam requirements/recommendations for international students: Required—TOEFL (minimum score 550 paper-based). *Application deadline:* For fall admission, 10/15 for domestic and international students. Application fee: $0. *Expenses:* Contact institution. *Financial support:* Federal Work-Study, institutionally sponsored loans, and tuition waivers (full) available. Financial award application deadline: 3/1; financial award applicants required to submit FAFSA. *Unit head:* Dr. Kristine A. Thompson, Program Director, 248-370-4041, E-mail: marcoux@oakland.edu. *Application contact:* Christina J. Grabowski, Associate Director of Graduate Study and Lifelong Learning, 248-370-3167, Fax: 248-370-4114, E-mail: grabowsk@oakland.edu.

Syracuse University, Falk College of Sport and Human Dynamics, Program in Child and Family Health in the Global Community, Syracuse, NY 13244. Offers MS. Part-time programs available. *Students:* 7 full-time (6 women), 1 (woman) part-time. Average age 28. 11 applicants, 64% accepted, 3 enrolled. In 2013, 2 master's awarded. *Entrance requirements:* For master's, GRE. Additional exam requirements/recommendations for international students: Required—TOEFL (minimum score 100 iBT). *Application deadline:* For fall admission, 3/15 priority date for domestic students, 3/15 for international students; for spring admission, 11/15 priority date for domestic and international students. Application fee: $75. Electronic applications accepted. *Financial support:* Fellowships with full tuition reimbursements, research assistantships with partial tuition reimbursements, and teaching assistantships with partial tuition reimbursements available. Financial award application deadline: 1/15. *Unit head:* Dr. Brooks Gump, Graduate Program Director, 315-443-2206, Fax: 315-443-2562, E-mail: bbgump@syr.edu. *Application contact:* Felicia Otero, Director, College Relations, 315-443-5555, Fax: 315-443-2562, E-mail: falk@syr.edu.
Website: http://falk.syr.edu/

Troy University, Graduate School, College of Health and Human Services, Program in Nursing, Troy, AL 36082. Offers adult health (MSN); clinical nurse specialist adult health (DNP); clinical nurse specialist maternal infant (DNP); family nurse practitioner (MSN, DNP, PMC); informatics specialist (MSN); maternal infant (MSN). Part-time and evening/weekend programs available. *Faculty:* 15 full-time (8 women), 3 part-time/

adjunct (1 woman). *Students:* 61 full-time (56 women), 228 part-time (193 women); includes 97 minority (77 Black or African American, non-Hispanic/Latino; 4 American Indian or Alaska Native, non-Hispanic/Latino; 2 Asian, non-Hispanic/Latino; 5 Hispanic/Latino; 9 Two or more races, non-Hispanic/Latino). Average age 34. 138 applicants, 80% accepted, 39 enrolled. In 2013, 81 master's, 9 doctorates awarded. *Degree requirements:* For master's, comprehensive exam, minimum GPA of 3.0, candidacy; for doctorate, minimum GPA of 3.0, submission of approved comprehensive e-portfolio, completion of residency synthesis project, minimum of 1000 hours of clinical practice, score of 80% or better on qualifying exam. *Entrance requirements:* For master's, GRE (minimum score of 850 on old exam or 294 on new exam) or GMAT (minimum score of 500), minimum GPA of 3.0, BSN, current RN licensure; 2 letters of reference, undergraduate health assessment course; for doctorate, GRE (minimum score of 850 on old exam or 294 on new exam) or GMAT (minimum score of 500), BSN or MSN, minimum GPA of 3.0, 2 letters of reference, current RN licensure, essay. Additional exam requirements/recommendations for international students: Required—TOEFL (minimum score 523 paper-based; 70 iBT), IELTS (minimum score 6). *Application deadline:* Applications are processed on a rolling basis. Application fee: $50. Electronic applications accepted. *Expenses:* Tuition, state resident: full-time $6084; part-time $338 per credit hour. Tuition, nonresident: full-time $12,168; part-time $676 per credit hour. *Required fees:* $630; $35 per credit hour. $50 per semester. *Financial support:* Available to part-time students. Applicants required to submit FAFSA. *Unit head:* Dr. Diane Weed, Director, School of Nursing, 334-670-5864, Fax: 334-670-3745, E-mail: lweed@troy.edu. *Application contact:* Brenda K. Campbell, Director of Graduate Admissions, 334-670-3178, Fax: 334-670-3733, E-mail: bcamp@troy.edu.

Tulane University, School of Public Health and Tropical Medicine, Department of Community Health Sciences, Program in Maternal and Child Health, New Orleans, LA 70118-5669. Offers MPH, Dr PH, MSW/MPH. *Accreditation:* CEPH (one or more programs are accredited). *Degree requirements:* For doctorate, comprehensive exam, thesis/dissertation. *Entrance requirements:* For master's and doctorate, GRE General Test. Additional exam requirements/recommendations for international students: Required—TOEFL.

The University of Alabama at Birmingham, School of Public Health, Program in Public Health, Birmingham, AL 35294. Offers accelerated industrial hygiene (MPH); applied epidemiology (MSPH); biostatistics (MPH); clinical and translational science (MSPH); environmental health (MPH); environmental health and toxicology (MSPH); epidemiology (MPH); general theory and practice (MPH); health behavior (MPH); health care organization (MPH); health policy quantitative policy analysis (MPH); industrial hygiene (MPH, MSPH); maternal and child health policy (Dr PH); maternal and child health policy and leadership (MPH); occupational health and safety (MPH); outcomes research (MSPH, Dr PH); pharmacoepidemiology and comparative effectiveness research (MSPH); public health (PhD); public health management (Dr PH); public health preparedness management (MPH). *Accreditation:* CEPH. *Entrance requirements:* For master's and doctorate, GRE, evaluations. Additional exam requirements/recommendations for international students: Recommended—TOEFL (minimum score 550 paper-based; 79 iBT), IELTS (minimum score 6.5).

University of California, Davis, Graduate Studies, Program in Maternal and Child Nutrition, Davis, CA 95616. Offers MAS. *Degree requirements:* For master's, comprehensive exam. *Entrance requirements:* Additional exam requirements/recommendations for international students: Required—TOEFL (minimum score 550 paper-based).

University of Maryland, College Park, Academic Affairs, School of Public Health, Department of Family Science, College Park, MD 20742. Offers family studies (PhD); marriage and family therapy (MS); maternal and child health (PhD). *Accreditation:* AAMFT/COAMFTE. Part-time and evening/weekend programs available. *Faculty:* 17 full-time (13 women), 15 part-time/adjunct (14 women). *Students:* 46 full-time (39 women), 2 part-time (both women); includes 13 minority (10 Black or African American, non-Hispanic/Latino; 2 Hispanic/Latino; 1 Two or more races, non-Hispanic/Latino), 7 international. 142 applicants, 12% accepted, 14 enrolled. In 2013, 8 master's, 3 doctorates awarded. *Degree requirements:* For master's, thesis or alternative; for doctorate, comprehensive exam, thesis/dissertation, oral defense. *Entrance requirements:* For master's, GRE General Test, minimum GPA of 3.0, 3 letters of recommendation; for doctorate, GRE General Test, minimum GPA of 3.0, 3 letters of recommendation, research sample. *Application deadline:* For fall admission, 12/15 for domestic and international students. Applications are processed on a rolling basis. Application fee: $75. Electronic applications accepted. *Expenses:* Tuition, state resident: full-time $10,314; part-time $573 per credit hour. Tuition, nonresident: full-time $22,248; part-time $1236 per credit. *Required fees:* $1446; $403.15 per semester. Tuition and fees vary according to program. *Financial support:* In 2013–14, 2 fellowships with partial tuition reimbursements (averaging $11,250 per year), 1 research assistantship (averaging $17,125 per year), 29 teaching assistantships (averaging $15,907 per year) were awarded; career-related internships or fieldwork, Federal Work-Study, and scholarships/grants also available. Support available to part-time students. Financial award applicants required to submit FAFSA. *Faculty research:* Family life quality, interracial couples, child support, homeless families, family and child well-being. *Total annual research expenditures:* $983,140. *Unit head:* Elaine Anderson, Chair, 301-405-4009, Fax: 301-314-9161, E-mail: eanders@umd.edu. *Application contact:* Dr. Charles A. Caramello, Dean of Graduate School, 301-405-0358, Fax: 301-314-9305, E-mail: ccaramel@umd.edu.
Website: http://www.sph.umd.edu/fmsc/

University of Minnesota, Twin Cities Campus, School of Public Health, Major in Maternal and Child Health, Minneapolis, MN 55455-0213. Offers MPH. *Accreditation:* CEPH. Part-time programs available. *Degree requirements:* For master's, fieldwork, project. *Entrance requirements:* For master's, GRE General Test, 1 year of relevant experience. Additional exam requirements/recommendations for international students: Required—TOEFL. Electronic applications accepted. *Expenses:* Contact institution. *Faculty research:* Reproductive and perinatal health, family planning, child adolescent and family health, risk reduction and resiliency, child and family adaptation to chronic health conditions.

The University of North Carolina at Chapel Hill, Graduate School, Gillings School of Global Public Health, Department of Maternal and Child Health, Chapel Hill, NC 27599. Offers MPH, MSPH, Dr PH, PhD, MD/MSPH, MPH/MSW, MSPH/M Ed, MSPH/MSW. *Accreditation:* CEPH (one or more programs are accredited). *Degree requirements:* For master's, comprehensive exam, major paper; for doctorate, comprehensive exam, thesis/dissertation. *Entrance requirements:* For master's, GRE General Test or MCAT, minimum GPA of 3.0 (recommended), at least one year of post-BA MHCH-related work experience; for doctorate, GRE General Test, minimum GPA of 3.0, at least one year of post-BA MHCH-related work experience. Additional exam requirements/recommendations for international students: Required—TOEFL. Electronic applications accepted. *Faculty research:* Women's health, prenatal health, family planning, program evaluation, child health policy and priorities.

University of Puerto Rico, Medical Sciences Campus, Graduate School of Public Health, Department of Human Development, Program in Maternal and Child Health, San Juan, PR 00936-5067. Offers MPH. Part-time and evening/weekend programs available. *Entrance requirements:* For master's, GRE, previous course work in algebra.

University of South Florida, Innovative Education Graduate Certificate Programs, Tampa, FL 33620-9951. *Unit head:* Kathy Barnes, Interdisciplinary Programs Coordinator, 813-974-8031, Fax: 813-974-7061, E-mail: barnesk@usf.edu. *Application contact:* Karen Tylinski, Metro Initiatives, 813-974-9943, Fax: 813-974-7061, E-mail: ktylinsk@usf.edu.
Website: http://www.usf.edu/innovative-education/

University of Washington, Graduate School, School of Public Health, Department of Epidemiology, Seattle, WA 98195. Offers clinical research (MS); epidemiology (MPH, MS, PhD); global health (MPH); maternal/child health (MPH); MPH/MPA. *Accreditation:* CEPH (one or more programs are accredited). *Faculty:* 65 full-time (38 women), 39 part-time/adjunct (17 women). *Students:* 120 full-time (84 women), 30 part-time (20 women); includes 19 minority (3 Black or African American, non-Hispanic/Latino; 2 American Indian or Alaska Native, non-Hispanic/Latino; 14 Asian, non-Hispanic/Latino), 12 international. Average age 32. 234 applicants, 37% accepted, 40 enrolled. In 2013, 41 master's, 18 doctorates awarded. *Degree requirements:* For master's, comprehensive exam (for some programs), thesis; for doctorate, comprehensive exam, thesis/dissertation, general exam, dissertation proposal, final exam (dissertation defense). *Entrance requirements:* For master's, GRE (except for those holding PhD, MD, DDS, DVM, DO or equivalent from U.S. institutions); for doctorate, GRE. Additional exam requirements/recommendations for international students: Required—TOEFL (minimum score 580 paper-based, 92 iBT), IELTS (minimum score 7), or PTE (minimum score of 65). *Application deadline:* For fall admission, 12/1 for domestic students, 11/1 for international students. Application fee: $85. Electronic applications accepted. *Expenses:* Contact institution. *Financial support:* In 2013–14, 138 students received support, including 70 fellowships with partial tuition reimbursements available, 40 research assistantships with partial tuition reimbursements available, 12 teaching assistantships with partial tuition reimbursements available; career-related internships or fieldwork, Federal Work-Study, traineeships, health care benefits, tuition waivers, and unspecified assistantships also available. Support available to part-time students. Financial award application deadline: 12/1; financial award applicants required to submit FAFSA. *Faculty research:* Chronic disease, health disparities and social determinants of health, aging and neuroepidemiology, maternal and child health, molecular and genetic epidemiology. *Unit head:* Dr. Scott Davis, Chair, 206-543-1065, E-mail: epiapply@uw.edu. *Application contact:* Kate O'Brien, Student Services Manager, 206-543-1065, E-mail: epiapply@uw.edu.
Website: http://depts.washington.edu/epidem/

University of Washington, Graduate School, School of Public Health, Department of Health Services, Seattle, WA 98195. Offers clinical research (MS); community-oriented public health practice (MPH); evaluative sciences and statistics (PhD); health behavior and social determinants of health (PhD); health economics (PhD); health informatics and health information management (MHIHIM); health services (MS, PhD); health services administration (EMHA, MHA); health systems and policy (MPH); health systems research (PhD); maternal and child health (MPH); social and behavioral sciences (MPH); JD/MHA; MHA/MBA; MHA/MD; MHA/MPA; MPH/JD; MPH/MD; MPH/MN; MPH/MPA; MPH/MS; MPH/MSD; MPH/MSW; MPH/PhD. *Faculty:* 63 full-time (30 women), 56 part-time/adjunct (25 women). *Students:* 121 full-time (101 women), 19 part-time (11 women); includes 28 minority (3 Black or African American, non-Hispanic/Latino; 2 American Indian or Alaska Native, non-Hispanic/Latino; 23 Asian, non-Hispanic/Latino), 5 international. Average age 30. 242 applicants, 48% accepted, 36 enrolled. In 2013, 43 master's, 9 doctorates awarded. Terminal master's awarded for partial completion of doctoral program. *Degree requirements:* For master's, thesis (for some programs), practicum (MPH); for doctorate, comprehensive exam, thesis/dissertation. *Entrance requirements:* For master's and doctorate, GRE General Test, minimum GPA of 3.0. Additional exam requirements/recommendations for international students: Required—TOEFL (minimum score 580 paper-based; 92 iBT), IELTS (minimum score 7). *Application deadline:* For fall admission, 1/1 for domestic students, 11/1 for international students. Application fee: 85 Albanian leks. Electronic applications accepted. *Financial support:* In 2013–14, 45 students received support, including 12 fellowships with full and partial tuition reimbursements available (averaging $22,000 per year), 9 research assistantships with full and partial tuition reimbursements available (averaging $18,700 per year), 9 teaching assistantships with full and partial tuition reimbursements available (averaging $4,575 per year); institutionally sponsored loans, traineeships, and health care benefits also available. Financial award application deadline: 2/28; financial award applicants required to submit FAFSA. *Faculty research:* Public health practice, health promotion and disease prevention, maternal and child health, organizational behavior and culture, health policy. *Unit head:* Dr. Larry Kessler, Chair, 206-543-2930. *Application contact:* Kitty A. Andert, MPH/MS/PhD Programs Manager, 206-616-2926, Fax: 206-543-3964, E-mail: hservmph@u.washington.edu.
Website: http://depts.washington.edu/hserv/

Wayne State University, School of Medicine, Graduate Programs in Medicine, Program in Global and Pediatric Health, Detroit, MI 48202. Offers Graduate Certificate. *Degree requirements:* For Graduate Certificate, international field placement in a clinical and research experience. *Entrance requirements:* For degree, MD, DO, DDS, Pharm D or equivalent degree in human health care. Additional exam requirements/recommendations for international students: Required—TOEFL (minimum score 600 paper-based; 100 iBT). Electronic applications accepted. *Expenses:* Contact institution. *Unit head:* Dr. Deepak Kamat, Director, 313-745-5870, E-mail: kamat@wayne.edu. *Application contact:* Dr. Norman Silas, Jr., Associate Dean for Admissions, Diversity and Inclusion, 313-577-1466, E-mail: admissions@med.wayne.edu.
Website: http://gradprograms.med.wayne.edu/program-spotlight.php?id-36

HARVARD UNIVERSITY

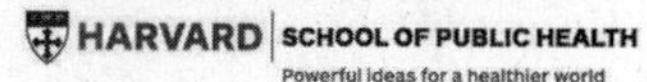

School of Public Health

Programs of Study

The Harvard School of Public Health (HSPH) offers programs leading to the graduate degrees of Master of Public Health (M.P.H.), Doctor of Public Health (Dr.P.H.), Master of Science in a specified field (S.M. in that field), and Doctor of Science in a specified field (S.D. in that field). Doctor of Philosophy (Ph.D.) degrees are offered in specific fields of study through the Graduate School of Arts and Sciences. Programs are offered in biostatistics; computational biology and quantitative genetics; environmental health; epidemiology; genetics and complex diseases; global health and population; health policy and management; immunology and infectious diseases; nutrition; and social and behavioral sciences. Some programs are designed for physicians, lawyers, managers, and other health-care professionals; some for college graduates who wish to train for health careers; and others for individuals who hold graduate degrees in medicine, law, business, government, education, and other fields who wish to apply their special skills to public health problems. Special programs include the Master of Science in maternal and child health nursing, administered jointly by HSPH and Simmons College; the combined M.D./M.P.H. program, offered in conjunction with accredited U.S. medical schools; and the J.D./M.P.H. joint-degree program offered by HSPH and Harvard Law School. The School offers residency training leading to certification by the American Board of Preventive Medicine in occupational medicine.

Research Facilities

The main buildings of the School are the Sebastian S. Kresge Educational Facilities Building at 677 Huntington Avenue, the François-Xavier Bagnoud Building at 651 Huntington Avenue, and the Health Sciences Laboratories at 665 Huntington Avenue. The School maintains well-equipped research laboratories containing sophisticated instrumentation and supporting animal facilities. Computing and data processing resources are also available to students through the Instructional Computing Facility. The Francis A. Countway Library serves the library needs of the School. It holds more than 630,000 volumes, subscribes to 3,500 current journal titles, and houses over 10,000 noncurrent biomedical journal titles in addition to its extensive collection of historical materials, making it the largest library in the country serving a medical and health-related school.

Financial Aid

Financial aid at the School of Public Health can come from a variety of sources. Some departments have training grants that offer students full tuition plus a stipend. Through need-based and merit-based programs at the School and University levels, other students are offered grants that range from half to full tuition. To supplement other aid, many students borrow through one or more of the federal educational loan programs and work at part-time jobs at Harvard and in the community.

Cost of Study

Master's program students are assessed tuition at $1,005–$1,184 per credit. Students in a one-year master's program are required to take a minimum of 42.5 credits at $50,320, while students in multiple-year master's programs typically take 40 credits their first year at $40,200. Doctoral students are assessed a flat tuition rate. The full-time rate for 2014–15 for students in their first or second year is $40,200. Health insurance and health services fee are required, which total $3,358. Books and supplies cost approximately $1,384 in 2014–15.

Living and Housing Costs

For the academic year 2014–15, it is estimated that a single student needs a minimum of $19,034 for housing and living costs: $11,475 for rent and utilities and $7,560 for other expenses. Limited housing is available in the Shattuck International House, with preference given to international students. Most students arrange for housing in the adjacent communities.

Student Group

There are 1,003 graduate students (610 women and 393 men) enrolled in 2014–15. Seventy-two nations are represented.

Student Outcomes

Graduates of the Harvard School of Public Health find employment in a variety of settings. It depends in part upon their previous experience and in part upon department and degree programs from which they graduate. Recent graduates have found positions in research institutes, with pharmaceutical companies and governmental and nongovernmental agencies, within the health-care industry, and as faculty members of universities.

Location

Boston is a heterogeneous metropolis rich in history and charm. Athletic, cultural, and recreational activities are abundant. The School is within walking distance of museums, colleges and universities, waterways, and parks.

The University and The School

Harvard College was founded in 1636; until the establishment of professorships in medicine in 1782, it composed the whole of the institution now called Harvard University. In addition to the college, ten graduate schools are now part of the University.

HSPH has just celebrated its centennial. In September 1913, the new Harvard-MIT School for Health Officers welcomed its class of 8 students. From those modest beginnings emerged HSPH and its long record of accomplishments. More information can be found at http://www.hsph.harvard.edu/centennial. The primary mission of the School is to carry out teaching and research aimed at improving the health of population groups throughout the world. The School emphasizes not only the development and implementation of disease prevention and treatment programs but also the planning and management of systems involved in the delivery of health services in this country and abroad. The School cooperates with the Medical School in teaching and research and has close ties with other Harvard faculties. The School has more than 431 full-time and part-time faculty members and nine academic departments representing major biomedical and social disciplines.

Applying

HSPH participates in the Schools of Public Health Application Service (SOPHAS), which is an online, common application service designed to provide a more efficient application process. Students should visit the SOPHAS website at http://www.sophas.org for more specific information and for access to the application for admission. All applicants to the School are required to submit scores from the GRE (ETS school code: 3456); applicants are urged to take the test no later than November, since applications are not considered without the scores. Applicants may submit the DAT, GMAT, or MCAT, as appropriate to the applicant's background, in lieu of the GRE. In addition, applicants must persuade the Committee on Admissions and Degrees of their ability to meet academic standards and of their overall qualifications to undertake advanced study at a graduate level. Students should visit the School's website (http://www.hsph.harvard.edu/) for information concerning the deadline to apply for admission and to apply online.

As a matter of policy, law, and commitment, the Harvard School of Public Health does not discriminate against any person on the basis of race, color, sexual orientation, gender identity, religion, age, national or ethnic origin, political beliefs, veteran status, or disability in admission to, access to, treatment in, or employment in its programs and activities. Members of minority groups are strongly encouraged to apply.

Correspondence and Information

Harvard School of Public Health Admissions Office
158 Longwood Avenue
Boston, Massachusetts 02115-5810
United States
Phone: 617-432-1031
Fax: 617-432-7080
E-mail: admissions@hsph.harvard.edu
Website: http://www.hsph.harvard.edu/

Counseling and program information:
Vincent W. James, Director
Kerri Noonan, Associate Director
Isabelle Bourdonné
Kelly Latendresse
Maria Maxell
Ruth Thompson
Cathy Tso

FACULTY CHAIRS AND DEPARTMENTAL ACTIVITIES

Biostatistics (617-432-1056, biostat_admissions@hsph.harvard.edu)
Chair: Victor De Gruttola, S.D. The program combines both theory and application of statistical science to analyze public health problems and further biomedical research. Students are prepared for academic and private-sector research careers. Faculty research spans both methodological developments on new statistical techniques and important subject-matter applications that lead to significant advances in the health sciences. Current departmental research on statistical and computing methods for observational studies and clinical trials includes survival analysis, missing-data problems, and causal inference. Other areas of investigation include environmental research; statistical aspects of the study of AIDS and cancer; quantitative problems in health-risk analysis, technology assessment, and clinical decision making; statistical methodology in psychiatric research and in genetic studies; and statistical genetics and computational biology.

Environmental Health (617-432-1270, envhlth@hsph.harvard.edu)
Chair: Douglas Dockery, S.D. The mission of the Department of Environmental Health is to advance the health of all people around the world through research and training in environmental health. The department emphasizes the role of air, water, the built environment, and the workplace as critical determinants of health. Faculty members in the department study the pathogenesis and prevention of environmentally produced illnesses and act as catalysts for scientifically based public health advances. Research approaches range from the molecular studies to policy evaluation. Teaching and research activities of the department are carried out through three concentrations: exposure, epidemiology, and risk; occupational health; and molecular and integrative physiological sciences.

Epidemiology (617-432-1055, jpaulson@hsph.harvard.edu)
Chair: Michelle Williams, Sc.D. Epidemiology, the study of the frequency, distribution, and determinants of disease in humans, is a fundamental science of public health. Epidemiologists use many approaches, but the ultimate aim of epidemiologic research is the prevention or effective control of human disease. Current research involves the role of viruses in the etiology of cancer; the connection between diet and risk of cancer, cardiovascular disease, and other major chronic diseases; the relationship between exposure to chemicals in the workplace and the development of cancer; the epidemiology of infectious disease; factors in early life predisposing individuals to chronic diseases; and the health effects of drugs and medical devices.

Genetics and Complex Diseases
(617-432-0054, dhasting@hsph.harvard.edu)
Chair: Gökhan Hotamisligil, M.D., Ph.D. The complex interplay of biological processes with environmental factors as they apply to chronic, multigenic, and multifactorial diseases is the emphasis of the Department of Genetics and Complex Diseases. Research programs in the department focus on molecular mechanisms of adaptive responses to environmental signals to elucidate the mechanisms underlying the intricate interaction between genetic determinants and their divergent responses to stress signals. Alterations in these integrated adaptive mechanisms have a major impact on the health of human populations. The diseases under study include nutritional and metabolic diseases (obesity, diabetes, and cardiovascular diseases), inflammatory bowel disease, cancer, and aging.

Global Health and Population
(617-432-2253, bheil@hsph.harvard.edu)
Chair: Wafaie Fawzi, M.B.B.S., D.P.H. The department seeks to improve global health through education, research, and service from a population-based perspective. Research interests span a wide spectrum of topics, including social and economic development, health policy, and demography; design and financing of health-care systems; women's health and children's health; and prevention and control of infectious and chronic diseases. The department has a special concern with questions of health equity and human rights, particularly in relation to health and population issues in developing countries.

Health Policy and Management
(617-432-4511, aocchipi@hsph.harvard.edu)
Chair: Kate Baicker, Ph.D. The department is mission oriented in its concern with improving the health-care delivery system and mitigating public health risks in the United States and abroad. It is dedicated to resolving major management and health policy problems through original research, advanced training, and dispute resolution. Research priorities are organized into seven broad areas: decision science, health care management, health economics, law and public health, quality and access, political policy, and public health policy.

Immunology and Infectious Diseases
(617-432-1023, asabarof@hsph.harvard.edu)
Chair: Dyann Wirth, Ph.D. The department focuses on the biological, immunological, epidemiological, and ecological aspects of viral, bacterial, protozoan, and helminthic diseases of animals and humans and the vectors that transmit some of these infectious agents. Emphasis is on research identifying basic pathogenic mechanisms that may lead to better diagnostic tools and the development of vaccines as well as the identification of new targets for antiviral and antiparasitic drugs.

Nutrition (617-432-1333, pbrown@hsph.harvard.edu)
Chair: Walter C. Willett, M.D., M.P.H., D.P.H. The department's mission is to improve human health through research aimed at understanding how diet influences health, the dissemination of new knowledge about nutrition to health professionals and the public, the development of nutritional strategies, and the education of researchers and practitioners. Department research ranges from molecular biology to human studies of cancer and heart disease, including the conduct of population-based intervention trials. Current research covers a wide range of topics, including large prospective studies of dietary factors in relation to heart disease, cancer, diabetes, and ophthalmologic disease; development of methods to assess nutritional status by analysis of body tissue; the interaction of nutritional factors with genetic determinants of disease; and the interaction of nutritional factors and infectious agents.

Social and Behavioral Sciences
(617-432-3761, esolomon@hsph.harvard.edu)
Chair: Ichiro Kawachi, M.D., Ph.D. The mission of the Department of Social and Behavioral Sciences is to improve health throughout the lifespan, including a special emphasis on children and adolescents. This mission is achieved through research to identify the social and behavioral determinants of health, development and evaluation of interventions and policies leading to the improvement of population health, and the preparation of professionals and researchers who fill leadership positions in advocacy and public service. The department's educational mission is to train both scholars and practitioners: scholars whose research illuminates basic social determinants of health and who identify and test innovative social policy and service interventions and practitioners who are skilled in designing, implementing, and evaluating health-enhancing interventions in action settings.

Master of Public Health Program
(617-432-0090, roberta@hsph.harvard.edu)
Director: Murray Mittleman, M.D.C.M., M.P.H., D.P.H. The program is designed to provide both a general background and flexibility of specialization in public health. The seven areas of concentration are clinical effectiveness, global health, health and social behavior, health management, health policy, occupational and environmental health, and quantitative methods.

Doctor of Public Health Program (drph@hsph.harvard.edu)
Director: Peter Berman, M.Sc., Ph.D. The Doctor of Public Health degree is for exceptional individuals with proven potential who want to accelerate their careers, lead organizations, and have an important impact on people's health and lives. The inaugural class for this new degree will enjoy unique opportunities to engage with Harvard's world-renowned faculty through rigorous teaching, interactive learning, case discussions, simulations, and field experiences in a variety of major public health organizations. This innovative, transformative educational experience has been designed so that no prior public health degree is required.

Division of Biological Sciences
(617-432-4470, bph@hsph.harvard.edu)
Director: Brendan Manning, Ph.D. The Division of Biological Sciences is an umbrella organization encompassing the HSPH Departments of Environmental Health, Genetics and Complex Diseases, Immunology and Infectious Diseases, and Nutrition. In most of these departments, two doctoral degrees are offered: the Doctor of Philosophy (Ph.D.) and the Doctor of Science (S.D.). The Ph.D. programs generally center on laboratory-based investigation in the biological sciences, whereas the S.D. programs emphasize epidemiological analysis. The Ph.D. programs are offered under the aegis of the Harvard Graduate School of Arts and Sciences and administered by the Harvard School of Public Health Division of Biological Sciences.

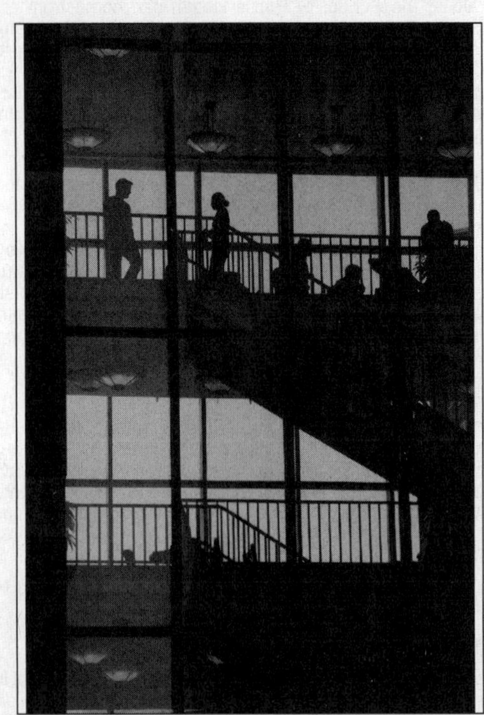

ACADEMIC AND PROFESSIONAL PROGRAMS IN THE MEDICAL PROFESSIONS AND SCIENCES

Section 25
Acupuncture and Oriental Medicine

This section contains a directory of institutions offering graduate work in acupuncture and oriental medicine. Additional information about programs listed in the directory but not augmented by an in-depth entry may be obtained by writing directly to the dean of a graduate school or chair of a department at the address given in the directory.

CONTENTS

Program Directory

Acupuncture and Oriental Medicine

Academy for Five Element Acupuncture, Graduate Program, Hallandale, FL 33009. Offers M Ac. *Accreditation:* ACAOM.

Academy of Chinese Culture and Health Sciences, Program in Traditional Chinese Medicine, Oakland, CA 94612. Offers MS. *Accreditation:* ACAOM. Part-time and evening/weekend programs available. *Degree requirements:* For master's, comprehensive exam, thesis. *Entrance requirements:* Additional exam requirements/recommendations for international students: Required—TOEFL (minimum score 500 paper-based). *Faculty research:* Herbs, acupuncture.

Acupuncture & Integrative Medicine College, Berkeley, Program in Oriental Medicine, Berkeley, CA 94704. Offers MS. *Accreditation:* ACAOM. Part-time and evening/weekend programs available. *Degree requirements:* For master's, comprehensive exam. *Entrance requirements:* For master's, interview, minimum GPA of 2.5, 60 semester units of course work at the baccalaureate level. Additional exam requirements/recommendations for international students: Required—TOEFL (minimum score 500 paper-based). *Faculty research:* Stimulus therapy, oxygen hemoglobin, acupuncture needling, classical Chinese medicine.

Acupuncture and Massage College, Program in Oriental Medicine, Miami, FL 33176. Offers MOM. *Accreditation:* ACAOM.

American College of Acupuncture and Oriental Medicine, Graduate Studies, Houston, TX 77063. Offers MAOM. *Accreditation:* ACAOM. Part-time programs available. *Entrance requirements:* For master's, 60 undergraduate credit hours. Additional exam requirements/recommendations for international students: Required—TOEFL.

American College of Traditional Chinese Medicine, Graduate Programs, San Francisco, CA 94107. Offers acupuncture and Oriental medicine (DAOM); dermatology (Certificate); shiatsu massage (Certificate); traditional Chinese medicine (MSTCM); tui na massage (Certificate). *Accreditation:* ACAOM. Part-time programs available. *Degree requirements:* For master's, one foreign language, comprehensive exam, internship; for doctorate, thesis/dissertation, clinical experience. *Entrance requirements:* For master's, minimum of 90 semester or 135 quarter units from an accredited institution, minimum GPA of 3.0, interview; for doctorate, MSTCM or equivalent, interview, state or national license. Additional exam requirements/recommendations for international students: Required—TOEFL (minimum score 550 paper-based; 79 iBT); Recommended—IELTS (minimum score 6.5).

AOMA Graduate School of Integrative Medicine, Doctor of Acupuncture and Oriental Medicine Program, Austin, TX 78757. Offers DAOM. *Faculty:* 10 full-time (4 women), 13 part-time/adjunct (7 women). *Students:* 15 full-time (9 women); includes 4 minority (3 Asian, non-Hispanic/Latino; 1 Hispanic/Latino). Average age 46. 20 applicants, 95% accepted, 17 enrolled. *Degree requirements:* For doctorate, comprehensive exam, clinical internship, clinical externship, capstone research project, portfolio. *Entrance requirements:* For doctorate, master's degree from ACAOM-accredited program in acupuncture and Oriental medicine; minimum GPA of 3.0 in master's studies; current license or eligibility to obtain a license to practice acupuncture in the state of Texas. Additional exam requirements/recommendations for international students: Required—TOEFL (minimum score 508 paper-based; 85 iBT). *Application deadline:* For fall admission, 5/20 priority date for domestic students, 5/20 for international students. Applications are processed on a rolling basis. Application fee: $75. Electronic applications accepted. Full-time tuition and fees vary according to degree level and program. *Financial support:* In 2013–14, 1 student received support. Federal Work-Study available. Financial award application deadline: 6/30; financial award applicants required to submit FAFSA. *Faculty research:* Allergy, cancer, women's health. *Unit head:* Dr. John S. Finnell, President, 512-492-3057, Fax: 512-454-7001, E-mail: jfinnell@aoma.edu. *Application contact:* Justine Meccio, Director of Admissions, 512-492-3017, Fax: 512-454-7001, E-mail: admissions@aoma.edu.
Website: https://aoma.edu/doctoral-program/

AOMA Graduate School of Integrative Medicine, Master of Acupuncture and Oriental Medicine Program, Austin, TX 78757. Offers MAcOM. *Accreditation:* ACAOM. *Faculty:* 8 full-time (3 women), 23 part-time/adjunct (14 women). *Students:* 144 full-time (110 women), 57 part-time (42 women); includes 42 minority (7 Black or African American, non-Hispanic/Latino; 17 Asian, non-Hispanic/Latino; 18 Hispanic/Latino). Average age 35. 35 applicants, 89% accepted, 20 enrolled. In 2013, 37 master's awarded. *Degree requirements:* For master's, comprehensive exam, clinical rotations (40.5 credits), portfolio. *Entrance requirements:* For master's, BA or higher or minimum of 90 credits at baccalaureate level from regionally-accredited institution with 30 credits of general education coursework; minimum GPA of 2.5. Additional exam requirements/recommendations for international students: Required—TOEFL (minimum score 508 paper-based; 85 iBT). *Application deadline:* For fall admission, 7/26 priority date for domestic students, 7/26 for international students; for winter admission, 11/4 priority date for domestic students, 11/4 for international students; for spring admission, 2/20 priority date for domestic students, 2/20 for international students. Applications are processed on a rolling basis. Application fee: $75. Electronic applications accepted. Full-time tuition and fees vary according to degree level and program. *Financial support:* Federal Work-Study and scholarships/grants available. Financial award applicants required to submit FAFSA. *Faculty research:* Acupuncture, Chinese herbal medicine, integrative medicine, pulse diagnosis. *Unit head:* Lesley Hamilton, Program Director, 512-454-3040, Fax: 512-454-7001, E-mail: info@aoma.edu. *Application contact:* Justine Meccio, Director of Admissions, 512-492-3017, Fax: 512-454-7001, E-mail: admissions@aoma.edu.
Website: https://aoma.edu/prospective-students/

Arizona School of Acupuncture and Oriental Medicine, Graduate Programs, Tucson, AZ 85712. Offers M Ac, M Ac OM. *Accreditation:* ACAOM.

Atlantic Institute of Oriental Medicine, Graduate Program, Fort Lauderdale, FL 33301. Offers MS. *Accreditation:* ACAOM. Evening/weekend programs available. *Faculty:* 8 full-time (1 woman), 18 part-time/adjunct (7 women). *Students:* 161 full-time (115 women); includes 23 minority (3 Black or African American, non-Hispanic/Latino; 7 Asian, non-Hispanic/Latino; 13 Hispanic/Latino), 7 international. *Entrance requirements:* For master's, official transcripts, professional resume, essay, two letters of reference. Additional exam requirements/recommendations for international students: Required—TOEFL (minimum score 500 paper-based). *Application deadline:* For fall admission, 7/1 for domestic students, 5/1 for international students; for spring admission, 11/30 for domestic students, 2/28 for international students. Applications are processed on a rolling basis. Application fee: $20 ($100 for international students). *Unit head:* Dr. Johanna C. Yen, President, 954-763-9840 Ext. 202, Fax: 954-763-9844, E-mail: president@atom.edu. *Application contact:* Milagros Ferreira, Registrar, 954-763-9840 Ext. 207, Fax: 954-763-9844, E-mail: registrar@atom.edu.
Website: http://www.atom.edu/graduate-programs.aspx

Bastyr University, School of Acupuncture and Oriental Medicine, Kenmore, WA 98028-4966. Offers acupuncture (MS); acupuncture and Oriental medicine (MS, DAOM); Chinese herbal medicine (Certificate). *Accreditation:* ACAOM. Evening/weekend programs available. *Students:* 116 full-time (86 women), 21 part-time (20 women); includes 45 minority (3 Black or African American, non-Hispanic/Latino; 30 Asian, non-Hispanic/Latino; 4 Hispanic/Latino; 8 Two or more races, non-Hispanic/Latino), 16 international. Average age 32. *Entrance requirements:* For master's, course work in biology, chemistry, intermediate algebra and psychology; for doctorate, MS in acupuncture or certificate and 10 years of clinical experience. Additional exam requirements/recommendations for international students: Required—TOEFL (minimum score 550 paper-based; 79 iBT). *Application deadline:* For fall admission, 3/15 priority date for domestic and international students. Applications are processed on a rolling basis. Application fee: $75. Electronic applications accepted. *Financial support:* Career-related internships or fieldwork, Federal Work-Study, and scholarships/grants available. Support available to part-time students. Financial award application deadline: 4/15; financial award applicants required to submit FAFSA. *Faculty research:* Integrative oncology, acupuncture and chemotherapy-induced peripheral neuropathy (CIPN), traditional Chinese medicine and stroke rehabilitation, acupuncture and prevention and wellness, electroacupuncture. *Unit head:* Dr. Kyo Mitchell, Interim Associate Dean and Assistant Professor, 425-602-3151, Fax: 425-823-6222, E-mail: kmitchell@bastyr.edu. *Application contact:* Admissions Office, 425-602-3330, Fax: 425-602-3090, E-mail: admissions@bastyr.edu.
Website: http://www.bastyr.edu/academics/areas-study/acupuncture-oriental-medicine

Canadian Memorial Chiropractic College, Certificate Programs, Toronto, ON M2H 3J1, Canada. Offers chiropractic clinical sciences (Certificate); chiropractic radiology (Certificate); chiropractic sports sciences (Certificate); clinical acupuncture (Certificate). *Degree requirements:* For Certificate, thesis. *Entrance requirements:* For degree, DC, board certification. *Faculty research:* Theories and concepts of chiropractic, sciences related to chiropractic, assessments of the efficacy and efficiency of chiropractic.

Colorado School of Traditional Chinese Medicine, Graduate Program, Denver, CO 80206-2127. Offers acupuncture (MS); traditional Chinese medicine (MS). *Accreditation:* ACAOM. Part-time programs available. *Faculty:* 52 part-time/adjunct (20 women). *Students:* 128 full-time (100 women), 8 part-time (7 women). 62 applicants, 100% accepted, 62 enrolled. *Entrance requirements:* For master's, 60 semester credits or 90 quarter credits from an accredited college. Additional exam requirements/recommendations for international students: Required—TOEFL (minimum score 500 paper-based; 61 iBT). *Application deadline:* For fall admission, 8/23 for domestic and international students; for winter admission, 12/24 for domestic and international students; for spring admission, 4/26 for domestic and international students. Applications are processed on a rolling basis. Application fee: $50. *Financial support:* Scholarships/grants available. Financial award applicants required to submit FAFSA. *Unit head:* Vladimir Dibrigida, Administrative Director, 303-329-6355 Ext. 11, Fax: 303-388-8165, E-mail: director@cstcm.edu. *Application contact:* Chris Duxbury-Edwards, Recruiting Director, 303-329-6355 Ext. 21, Fax: 303-388-8165, E-mail: recruiting@cstcm.edu.
Website: http://www.cstcm.edu

Dongguk University Los Angeles, Program in Oriental Medicine, Los Angeles, CA 90020. Offers MS. *Accreditation:* ACAOM. Part-time and evening/weekend programs available.

East West College of Natural Medicine, Graduate Programs, Sarasota, FL 34234. Offers MSOM. *Accreditation:* ACAOM.

Emperor's College of Traditional Oriental Medicine, Graduate Programs, Santa Monica, CA 90403. Offers MTOM, DAOM. *Accreditation:* ACAOM. Part-time and evening/weekend programs available. *Entrance requirements:* For master's, minimum 2 years of undergraduate course work, interview; for doctorate, CA acupuncture licensure. *Faculty research:* Menopause, dysmenorrhea.

Five Branches University: Graduate School of Traditional Chinese Medicine, Program in Traditional Chinese Medicine, Santa Cruz, CA 95062. Offers MTCM. *Accreditation:* ACAOM. *Degree requirements:* For master's, comprehensive exam. *Entrance requirements:* For master's, 6 units in anatomy and physiology, 9 units in basic sciences, minimum GPA of 2.5. Electronic applications accepted.

Florida College of Integrative Medicine, Graduate Program, Orlando, FL 32809. Offers MSOM. *Accreditation:* ACAOM. Evening/weekend programs available. *Entrance requirements:* For master's, minimum 60 semester hours of undergraduate coursework. Electronic applications accepted.

Hawaii College of Oriental Medicine, Graduate Programs, Kamuela, HI 96743-2288. Offers MSOM. *Accreditation:* ACAOM.

Institute of Clinical Acupuncture and Oriental Medicine, Program in Oriental Medicine, Honolulu, HI 96817. Offers MSOM. *Accreditation:* ACAOM.

Maryland University of Integrative Health, Chinese Herb Certificate Program, Laurel, MD 20723. Offers Certificate. Part-time and evening/weekend programs available. *Entrance requirements:* Additional exam requirements/recommendations for international students: Required—TOEFL.

Maryland University of Integrative Health, Program in Acupuncture, Laurel, MD 20723. Offers M Ac. *Accreditation:* ACAOM. *Degree requirements:* For master's, comprehensive exam, 500 clinical hours, oral exams. *Entrance requirements:* Additional exam requirements/recommendations for international students: Required—TOEFL. *Faculty research:* Philosophical roots of oriental medicine, meridian pathways, points, pulses.

Maryland University of Integrative Health, Program in Applied Healing Arts, Laurel, MD 20723. Offers MA. *Entrance requirements:* Additional exam requirements/recommendations for international students: Required—TOEFL. *Faculty research:* Healing habits of mind and heart, an expanded vision, bringing of one's vision and practices to a special arena.

Maryland University of Integrative Health, Program in Herbal Medicine, Laurel, MD 20723. Offers MS. *Entrance requirements:* Additional exam requirements/recommendations for international students: Required—TOEFL. *Faculty research:* Philosophical roots of holistic healing, botany, herbal pharmacology; materia medica, holistic healing.

Midwest College of Oriental Medicine, Graduate Programs, Racine, WI 53403-9747. Offers acupuncture (Certificate); oriental medicine (MSOM). *Accreditation:* ACAOM.

Part-time and evening/weekend programs available. *Degree requirements:* For master's and Certificate, comprehensive exam, thesis. *Entrance requirements:* For master's and Certificate, 60 semester credit hours from accredited school, 2 letters of recommendation, interview. Additional exam requirements/recommendations for international students: Required—TOEFL. *Faculty research:* Pharmacology.

Midwest College of Oriental Medicine, Graduate Programs-Chicago, Chicago, IL 60613. Offers acupuncture (Certificate); oriental medicine (MSOM). *Accreditation:* ACAOM. Part-time and evening/weekend programs available. *Degree requirements:* For master's and Certificate, comprehensive exam, thesis. *Entrance requirements:* For master's and Certificate, 60 semester credit hours from accredited school, 2 letters of recommendation, interview. Additional exam requirements/recommendations for international students: Required—TOEFL.

National College of Natural Medicine, School of Classical Chinese Medicine, Portland, OR 97201. Offers M Ac, MSOM. *Accreditation:* ACAOM. Evening/weekend programs available. *Degree requirements:* For master's, thesis. *Entrance requirements:* Additional exam requirements/recommendations for international students: Recommended—TOEFL. *Expenses:* Contact institution. *Faculty research:* Cases on herbs and acupuncture for asthma, diabetes, depression associated with menopause; Qi Gong to maintain weight loss.

National University of Health Sciences, College of Professional Studies, Lombard, IL 60148-4583. Offers acupuncture (MSAC); chiropractic medicine (DC); naturopathic medicine (ND); Oriental medicine (MSOM). *Accreditation:* CCE. *Degree requirements:* For master's and doctorate, comprehensive exam, internship, community service. *Entrance requirements:* For master's, bachelor's degree, character references, undergraduate transcripts; for doctorate, bachelor's degree, character references, undergraduate transcripts, written essay. Additional exam requirements/recommendations for international students: Required—TOEFL (minimum score 550 paper-based; 79 iBT). Electronic applications accepted. *Faculty research:* Discipline/whole practice research (including practice-based research networks), mechanisms of action, clinical trials, and evidence-based practice of CAM therapies; educational research in CAM teaching institutions.

New England School of Acupuncture, Program in Acupuncture and Oriental Medicine, Newton, MA 02458. Offers acupuncture (M Ac); acupuncture and Oriental medicine (MAOM). *Accreditation:* ACAOM (one or more programs are accredited). Part-time programs available. *Degree requirements:* For master's, comprehensive exam. *Entrance requirements:* For master's, previous course work in anatomy, biology, physiology, and psychology. Additional exam requirements/recommendations for international students: Required—TOEFL (minimum score 550 paper-based). *Faculty research:* Acupuncture and women's health, acupuncture and stroke rehabilitation, tai chi and cardiovascular health, tai chi and balance, cancer.

New York Chiropractic College, Finger Lakes School of Acupuncture and Oriental Medicine, Seneca Falls, NY 13148-0800. Offers acupuncture (MS); acupuncture and Oriental medicine (MS). *Accreditation:* ACAOM. *Degree requirements:* For master's, clinical internship. *Entrance requirements:* For master's, interview, three written references. Additional exam requirements/recommendations for international students: Recommended—TOEFL (minimum score 550 paper-based). *Application deadline:* Applications are processed on a rolling basis. Application fee: $60. Electronic applications accepted. *Financial support:* Fellowships with tuition reimbursements, Federal Work-Study, and scholarships/grants available. Financial award applicants required to submit FAFSA. *Faculty research:* Chinese herbal medicine, traditional Chinese medicine, cancer, gait and posture, obesity. *Unit head:* Dr. Frank J. Nicchi, President, 315-568-3268. *Application contact:* Dr. Frank J. Nicchi, President, 315-568-3268.
Website: http://aom.nycc.edu/

New York College of Health Professions, Graduate School of Oriental Medicine, Syosset, NY 11791-4413. Offers acupuncture (MS); Oriental medicine (MS). *Accreditation:* ACAOM. Part-time programs available. *Degree requirements:* For master's, thesis. *Entrance requirements:* For master's, minimum GPA of 2.5, 60 semester credits in undergraduate course work. Additional exam requirements/recommendations for international students: Required—TOEFL. *Faculty research:* Breast cancer, diabetic neuropathy hemolysis.

New York College of Traditional Chinese Medicine, Graduate Programs, Mineola, NY 11501. Offers oriental medicine (MAOM). *Accreditation:* ACAOM.

Northwestern Health Sciences University, College of Acupuncture and Oriental Medicine, Bloomington, MN 55431-1599. Offers acupuncture (M Ac); Oriental medicine (MOM). *Accreditation:* ACAOM. *Students:* 113 full-time (96 women), 22 part-time (17 women); includes 19 minority (3 Black or African American, non-Hispanic/Latino; 12 Asian, non-Hispanic/Latino; 2 Hispanic/Latino; 2 Two or more races, non-Hispanic/Latino), 1 international. Average age 33. In 2013, 42 master's awarded. *Entrance requirements:* For master's, 60 semester credits of course work with minimum GPA of 2.5. Additional exam requirements/recommendations for international students: Required—TOEFL (minimum score 540 paper-based; 76 iBT). *Application deadline:* For fall admission, 5/1 priority date for domestic and international students; for winter admission, 9/1 priority date for domestic and international students. Applications are processed on a rolling basis. Application fee: $50. Electronic applications accepted. *Expenses: Tuition:* Full-time $11,207; part-time $379 per credit. *Required fees:* $804; $402 per trimester. Tuition and fees vary according to course load, degree level and program. *Financial support:* In 2013–14, 58 students received support. Career-related internships or fieldwork, Federal Work-Study, and scholarships/grants available. Support available to part-time students. Financial award applicants required to submit FAFSA. *Unit head:* Dr. Teri Powers, Dean, 952-888-4777 Ext. 274, Fax: 952-889-1398, E-mail: tpowers@nwhealth.edu. *Application contact:* Kate DiAna, Director of Admissions, 952-888-4777 Ext. 273, Fax: 952-888-6713, E-mail: admit@nwhealth.edu.
Website: http://www.nwhealth.edu/acupuncture-oriental-medicine/

Oregon College of Oriental Medicine, Graduate Program in Acupuncture and Oriental Medicine, Portland, OR 97216. Offers M Ac OM, MAcOM, DAOM. *Accreditation:* ACAOM. Part-time programs available. *Entrance requirements:* For master's, minimum 3 years of college; course work in chemistry, biology, and psychology; for doctorate, documentation of clinical practice, 3 years of clinical experience. Additional exam requirements/recommendations for international students: Required—TOEFL (minimum score 550 paper-based).

Pacific College of Oriental Medicine, Graduate Program, San Diego, CA 92108. Offers MSTOM, DAOM. *Accreditation:* ACAOM. Part-time and evening/weekend programs available. *Entrance requirements:* For master's, 2 letters of reference, interviews, minimum GPA of 3.0. *Faculty research:* PMS, acupuncture, herbs, Tai Ji Quan, sports medicine.

Pacific College of Oriental Medicine–Chicago, Graduate Program, Chicago, IL 60601. Offers MTOM. *Accreditation:* ACAOM. Part-time and evening/weekend programs available. *Entrance requirements:* For master's, 2 letters of reference, interview, minimum GPA of 3.0. *Faculty research:* AIDS, cancer, mental health, clinical counseling.

Pacific College of Oriental Medicine-New York, Graduate Program, New York, NY 10010. Offers MSTOM. *Accreditation:* ACAOM. Part-time and evening/weekend programs available. *Entrance requirements:* For master's, 2 letters of reference, interview, minimum GPA of 3.0. *Faculty research:* Energy medicine, acupuncture in the treatment of neurological disorders.

Samra University of Oriental Medicine, Program in Oriental Medicine, Los Angeles, CA 90015. Offers MS, DAOM. Part-time and evening/weekend programs available. *Degree requirements:* For master's, comprehensive exam. *Entrance requirements:* For master's, 60 semester (90 quarter) units with a "C" average in general education from an accredited college. *Faculty research:* Herbal therapy; alleviation of AIDS symptoms, cancer, colds, flu.

Seattle Institute of Oriental Medicine, Graduate Program, Seattle, WA 98115. Offers M Ac OM. *Accreditation:* ACAOM. *Degree requirements:* For master's, one foreign language, comprehensive exam. *Entrance requirements:* For master's, course work in biology, psychology, chemistry, anatomy, physiology; CPR/first aid certification; 3 years (90 semester credits) post secondary coursework. Additional exam requirements/recommendations for international students: Recommended—TOEFL (minimum score 500 paper-based).

South Baylo University, Program in Oriental Medicine and Acupuncture, Anaheim, CA 92801-1701. Offers MS. *Accreditation:* ACAOM. Evening/weekend programs available. *Degree requirements:* For master's, 3 foreign languages, comprehensive exam. *Entrance requirements:* Additional exam requirements/recommendations for international students: Required—TOEFL (minimum score 500 paper-based). Electronic applications accepted. *Faculty research:* Effectiveness of acupuncture therapy.

Southern California University of Health Sciences, College of Acupuncture and Oriental Medicine, Whittier, CA 90609-1166. Offers MAOM. *Accreditation:* ACAOM. Part-time and evening/weekend programs available. *Entrance requirements:* For master's, 60 semester hours or 90 quarter credits of undergraduate course work, interview. Additional exam requirements/recommendations for international students: Required—TOEFL (minimum score 500 paper-based). Electronic applications accepted. *Faculty research:* Hypertension, low back pain, smoking cessation, sports medicine.

Southwest Acupuncture College, Program in Oriental Medicine, Albuquerque Campus, Albuquerque, NM 87109. Offers MS. *Accreditation:* ACAOM. Part-time programs available. *Entrance requirements:* For master's, minimum 2 years of college general education. Additional exam requirements/recommendations for international students: Required—TOEFL (minimum score 500 paper-based). Electronic applications accepted.

Southwest Acupuncture College, Program in Oriental Medicine, Boulder Campus, Boulder, CO 80301. Offers MS. *Accreditation:* ACAOM. Part-time programs available. *Entrance requirements:* For master's, minimum 2 years of college general education.

Southwest Acupuncture College, Program in Oriental Medicine, Santa Fe Campus, Santa Fe, NM 87505. Offers MS. *Accreditation:* ACAOM. Part-time programs available. *Entrance requirements:* For master's, minimum 2 years of college general education. Additional exam requirements/recommendations for international students: Required—TOEFL (minimum score 500 paper-based). Electronic applications accepted.

Swedish Institute, College of Health Sciences, Graduate Program, New York, NY 10001-6700. Offers acupuncture (MS). *Accreditation:* ACAOM. Part-time and evening/weekend programs available. *Entrance requirements:* Additional exam requirements/recommendations for international students: Required—TOEFL (minimum score 72 iBT).

Texas Health and Science University, Program in Acupuncture and Oriental Medicine, Austin, TX 78704. Offers MAOM. *Accreditation:* ACAOM. *Entrance requirements:* For master's, 60 hours applicable to bachelor's degree. Additional exam requirements/recommendations for international students: Required—TOEFL (minimum score 500 paper-based), TWE. Electronic applications accepted.

Tri-State College of Acupuncture, Program in Acupuncture, New York, NY 10011. Offers acupuncture (MS); oriental medicine (MS); traditional Chinese herbology (Certificate). *Accreditation:* ACAOM. Evening/weekend programs available. *Entrance requirements:* Additional exam requirements/recommendations for international students: Recommended—TOEFL.

University of Bridgeport, Acupuncture Institute, Bridgeport, CT 06604. Offers MS. *Accreditation:* ACAOM. Part-time programs available. *Faculty:* 2 full-time (1 woman), 8 part-time/adjunct (2 women). *Students:* 29 full-time (23 women), 11 part-time (7 women); includes 15 minority (5 Black or African American, non-Hispanic/Latino; 1 American Indian or Alaska Native, non-Hispanic/Latino; 6 Asian, non-Hispanic/Latino; 2 Hispanic/Latino; 1 Two or more races, non-Hispanic/Latino), 7 international. Average age 38. 39 applicants, 74% accepted, 13 enrolled. In 2013, 7 master's awarded. *Entrance requirements:* Additional exam requirements/recommendations for international students: Recommended—TOEFL (minimum score 550 paper-based; 80 iBT), IELTS (minimum score 6.5). *Application deadline:* For fall admission, 8/1 priority date for domestic students, 8/1 for international students; for spring admission, 12/1 priority date for domestic students, 12/1 for international students. Applications are processed on a rolling basis. Application fee: $50. Electronic applications accepted. *Expenses:* Contact institution. *Unit head:* Dr. Jennifer Brett, Director, 203-576-4122, Fax: 203-576-4107, E-mail: acup@bridgeport.edu. *Application contact:* Leanne Proctor, Director of Health Sciences Admission, 203-576-4352, Fax: 203-576-4941, E-mail: acup@bridgeport.edu.

WON Institute of Graduate Studies, Acupuncture Studies Program, Glenside, PA 19038. Offers M Ac. *Accreditation:* ACAOM. *Faculty:* 4 full-time (2 women), 17 part-time/adjunct (11 women). *Students:* 36 full-time (29 women); includes 6 minority (2 Black or African American, non-Hispanic/Latino; 3 Asian, non-Hispanic/Latino; 1 Hispanic/Latino). 24 applicants, 83% accepted, 18 enrolled. In 2013, 12 master's awarded. *Entrance requirements:* For master's, 6 prerequisite credits in anatomy and physiology, 2 letters of recommendation, essay, bachelor's degree, 3 credits of basic science (chemistry, biology, physics or botany). Additional exam requirements/recommendations for international students: Required—TOEFL (minimum score 550 paper-based; 79 iBT). *Application deadline:* For fall admission, 7/15 for domestic students. Application fee: $75. Electronic applications accepted. *Expenses: Tuition:* Full-time $16,900; part-time $400 per credit hour. *Required fees:* $400 per credit. $100 per semester. Tuition and fees vary according to program. *Faculty research:* Meditation and pulse taking, acupuncture and apprehension. *Unit head:* Dr. Janet Leidy, Chair, 215-884-8942, Fax: 215-884-8942, E-mail: janet.leidy@woninstitute.edu. *Application contact:* Zach Bremmer, Director of Enrollment Management, 215-884-8942, E-mail: zach.bremmer@woninstitute.edu.
Website: http://woninstitute.edu/index.php?page=acupuncture-studies-program

Acupuncture and Oriental Medicine

World Medicine Institute, Program in Acupuncture and Oriental Medicine, Honolulu, HI 96821. Offers M Ac OM. *Accreditation:* ACAOM. Part-time and evening/weekend programs available. *Entrance requirements:* For master's, minimum 60 college credits.

Yo San University of Traditional Chinese Medicine, Program in Acupuncture and Traditional Chinese Medicine, Los Angeles, CA 90066. Offers MATCM. *Accreditation:* ACAOM. Part-time programs available. Postbaccalaureate distance learning degree programs offered (no on-campus study). *Degree requirements:* For master's, observation and practice internships, exam. *Entrance requirements:* For master's, minimum 2 years of college, interview, minimum GPA of 2.5.

Section 26
Chiropractic

This section contains a directory of institutions offering graduate work in chiropractic. Additional information about programs listed in the directory but not augmented by an in-depth entry may be obtained by writing directly to the dean of a graduate school or chair of a department at the address given in the directory.

CONTENTS

Chiropractic

Canadian Memorial Chiropractic College, Certificate Programs, Toronto, ON M2H 3J1, Canada. Offers chiropractic clinical sciences (Certificate); chiropractic radiology (Certificate); chiropractic sports sciences (Certificate); clinical acupuncture (Certificate). *Degree requirements:* For Certificate, thesis. *Entrance requirements:* For degree, DC, board certification. *Faculty research:* Theories and concepts of chiropractic, sciences related to chiropractic, assessments of the efficacy and efficiency of chiropractic.

Canadian Memorial Chiropractic College, Professional Program, Toronto, ON M2H 3J1, Canada. Offers DC. *Entrance requirements:* For doctorate, 3 full years of university (15 full courses or 90 hours). *Faculty research:* Theories and concepts of chiropractic, sciences related to chiropractic, assessment of the efficacy and efficiency of chiropractic.

Cleveland University–Kansas City, Professional Program, Overland Park, KS 66210. Offers DC. *Accreditation:* CCE. Part-time programs available. *Degree requirements:* For doctorate, comprehensive exam. *Entrance requirements:* For doctorate, 90 semester hours of pre-professional study. Additional exam requirements/recommendations for international students: Required—TOEFL (minimum score 550 paper-based; 79 iBT). Electronic applications accepted. *Faculty research:* Effectiveness and efficacy of chiropractic care.

D'Youville College, Department of Chiropractic, Buffalo, NY 14201-1084. Offers DC. *Accreditation:* CCE. *Students:* 75 full-time (24 women), 8 part-time (2 women); includes 10 minority (1 Black or African American, non-Hispanic/Latino; 1 American Indian or Alaska Native, non-Hispanic/Latino; 3 Asian, non-Hispanic/Latino; 5 Hispanic/Latino), 26 international. Average age 27. 108 applicants, 43% accepted, 26 enrolled. In 2013, 14 doctorates awarded. *Entrance requirements:* For doctorate, minimum GPA of 2.5, 90 undergraduate credits. *Application deadline:* Applications are processed on a rolling basis. Application fee: $25. Electronic applications accepted. *Expenses:* Contact institution. *Faculty research:* Radiology diagnosis, chiropractic treatment and diagnosis. *Unit head:* Dr. Kathleen Linaker, Executive Director, Chiropractic Department, 716-829-7725 Ext. 7793, Fax: 716-829-7893. *Application contact:* Mark Pavone, Graduate Admissions Director, 716-829-8400, Fax: 716-829-7900, E-mail: graduateadmissions@dyc.edu.

Institut Franco-Européen de Chiropratique, Professional Program, 94200 Ivry-sur-Seine, France. Offers DC.

Life Chiropractic College West, Professional Program, Hayward, CA 94545. Offers DC. *Accreditation:* CCE. *Faculty:* 22 full-time (7 women), 38 part-time/adjunct (12 women). *Students:* 456 (198 women); includes 117 minority (9 Black or African American, non-Hispanic/Latino; 4 American Indian or Alaska Native, non-Hispanic/Latino; 38 Hispanic/Latino; 66 Native Hawaiian or other Pacific Islander, non-Hispanic/Latino). *Entrance requirements:* For doctorate, minimum GPA of 3.0. Additional exam requirements/recommendations for international students: Required—TOEFL (minimum score 550 paper-based). *Application deadline:* For fall admission, 8/1 priority date for domestic students, 7/1 priority date for international students; for winter admission, 10/1 priority date for domestic and international students; for spring admission, 2/1 priority date for domestic students, 1/1 priority date for international students. Applications are processed on a rolling basis. Application fee: $45. *Expenses: Tuition:* Full-time $25,140. One-time fee: $100 full-time. *Financial support:* Research assistantships, teaching assistantships, career-related internships or fieldwork, Federal Work-Study, and scholarships/grants available. Financial award application deadline: 4/1; financial award applicants required to submit FAFSA. *Faculty research:* Imaging, ergonomics, upper cervical adjusting, academics. *Unit head:* Dr. Brian Kelly, President, 800-788-4476 Ext. 2350, E-mail: bkelly@lifewest.edu. *Application contact:* Mary Flannery, Director of Enrollment, 510-780-4500 Ext. 2065, E-mail: admissions@lifewest.edu.
Website: http://www.lifewest.edu/

Life University, College of Chiropractic, Marietta, GA 30060-2903. Offers DC. *Accreditation:* CCE. Part-time programs available. *Degree requirements:* For doctorate, comprehensive exam, thesis/dissertation or alternative. *Entrance requirements:* For doctorate, minimum of 3 years of college; course work in biology, chemistry, physics, humanities, psychology, and English; minimum GPA of 2.5. Additional exam requirements/recommendations for international students: Required—TOEFL (minimum score 500 paper-based). Electronic applications accepted. *Faculty research:* Chiropractic clinical trial, spinal modeling, biomechanics, clinical evaluation studies, chiropractic technique development, sports performance.

Logan University, College of Chiropractic, Chesterfield, MO 63017. Offers DC. *Accreditation:* CCE. *Faculty:* 53 full-time (21 women), 26 part-time/adjunct (11 women). *Students:* 781 full-time (295 women), 53 part-time (18 women); includes 60 minority (26 Black or African American, non-Hispanic/Latino; 1 American Indian or Alaska Native, non-Hispanic/Latino; 11 Asian, non-Hispanic/Latino; 11 Hispanic/Latino; 11 Two or more races, non-Hispanic/Latino), 12 international. Average age 26. In 2013, 219 doctorates awarded. *Degree requirements:* For doctorate, comprehensive exam. *Entrance requirements:* For doctorate, 90 hours of pre-chiropractic including biology, chemistry, physics, and social sciences; minimum GPA of 3.0. Additional exam requirements/recommendations for international students: Required—TOEFL (minimum score 79 iBT). *Application deadline:* For fall admission, 7/15 priority date for domestic and international students; for winter admission, 11/15 priority date for domestic and international students; for spring admission, 3/15 priority date for domestic students, 3/15 for international students. Applications are processed on a rolling basis. Application fee: $50. Electronic applications accepted. *Expenses: Tuition:* Full-time $18,320. *Financial support:* In 2013–14, 61 students received support. Federal Work-Study and scholarships/grants available. Support available to part-time students. Financial award applicants required to submit FAFSA. *Faculty research:* Effects of injury on proprioception as measured by joint position sense, interventions for older adults with low back pain, interventions affecting heart rate variability, finite element computer modeling of spinal biomechanics, electrophysiological diagnosis of common neuromusculoskeletal conditions, the effects of spinal manipulation on posture and postural control. *Unit head:* Dr. Vincent DeBono, Dean of the College of Chiropractic, 636-227-2100 Ext. 2701, Fax: 636-207-2431, E-mail: vincent.debono@logan.edu. *Application contact:* Stacey Till, Director of Admissions, 636-227-2100 Ext. 1749, Fax: 636-207-2425, E-mail: admissions@logan.edu.

Logan University, College of Health Sciences, Chesterfield, MO 63017. Offers nutrition and human performance (MS); sports science and rehabilitation (MS). Part-time programs available. Postbaccalaureate distance learning degree programs offered (no on-campus study). *Faculty:* 10 full-time (3 women), 15 part-time/adjunct (8 women). *Students:* 19 full-time (9 women), 63 part-time (31 women); includes 12 minority (2 Black or African American, non-Hispanic/Latino; 5 Asian, non-Hispanic/Latino; 3 Hispanic/Latino; 2 Two or more races, non-Hispanic/Latino), 1 international. Average age 32. In 2013, 82 master's awarded. *Degree requirements:* For master's, comprehensive exam. *Entrance requirements:* For master's, GRE or National Board of Chiropractic Examiners test, minimum GPA of 2.5; specific undergraduate coursework based on program of interest. Additional exam requirements/recommendations for international students: Required—TOEFL (minimum score 79 iBT). *Application deadline:* For fall admission, 7/15 priority date for domestic and international students; for winter admission, 11/15 priority date for domestic and international students; for spring admission, 3/15 priority date for domestic students, 3/15 for international students. Applications are processed on a rolling basis. Application fee: $50. Electronic applications accepted. *Expenses:* Contact institution. *Financial support:* Federal Work-Study and scholarships/grants available. Support available to part-time students. Financial award applicants required to submit FAFSA. *Faculty research:* Ankle injury prevention in high school athletes, low back pain in college football players, short arc banding and low back pain, the effects of enzymes on inflammatory blood markers, gait analysis in high school and college athletes. *Unit head:* Dr. Sherri Cole, Vice President, Academic Affairs, 636-227-2100 Ext. 2702, Fax: 636-207-2431, E-mail: sherri.cole@logan.edu. *Application contact:* Stacey Till, Director of Admissions, 636-227-2100 Ext. 1749, Fax: 636-207-2425, E-mail: admissions@logan.edu.
Website: http://www.logan.edu

National University of Health Sciences, Chiropractic Program in Florida, Seminole, FL 33772. Offers DC. *Degree requirements:* For doctorate, comprehensive exam, internship, community service. *Entrance requirements:* For doctorate, bachelor's degree, character references, undergraduate transcripts, written essay. Additional exam requirements/recommendations for international students: Required—TOEFL (minimum score 550 paper-based; 79 iBT). Electronic applications accepted.

National University of Health Sciences, College of Professional Studies, Lombard, IL 60148-4583. Offers acupuncture (MSAC); chiropractic medicine (DC); naturopathic medicine (ND); Oriental medicine (MSOM). *Accreditation:* CCE. *Degree requirements:* For master's and doctorate, comprehensive exam, internship, community service. *Entrance requirements:* For master's, bachelor's degree, character references, undergraduate transcripts; for doctorate, bachelor's degree, character references, undergraduate transcripts, written essay. Additional exam requirements/recommendations for international students: Required—TOEFL (minimum score 550 paper-based; 79 iBT). Electronic applications accepted. *Faculty research:* Discipline/whole practice research (including practice-based research networks), mechanisms of action, clinical trials, and evidence-based practice of CAM therapies; educational research in CAM teaching institutions.

New York Chiropractic College, Doctor of Chiropractic Program, Seneca Falls, NY 13148-0800. Offers DC. *Accreditation:* CCE. *Degree requirements:* For doctorate, internship in health center. *Entrance requirements:* For doctorate, 24 credit hours of course work in science; 90 credit hours with minimum GPA of 2.5; references; interview. Additional exam requirements/recommendations for international students: Recommended—TOEFL (minimum score 550 paper-based). *Application deadline:* Applications are processed on a rolling basis. Application fee: $60. Electronic applications accepted. *Financial support:* Fellowships with full tuition reimbursements, research assistantships, Federal Work-Study, and scholarships/grants available. Financial award applicants required to submit FAFSA. *Faculty research:* Anatomy, pathophysiology, neurophysiology biomechanics, musculoskeletal pain syndrome, nutrition. *Unit head:* Dr. Karen A. Bobak, Dean, 315-568-3864, Fax: 315-568-3087. *Application contact:* Dr. Karen A. Bobak, Dean, 315-568-3864, Fax: 315-568-3087.
Website: http://www.nycc.edu/AcademicPrograms_DCprogram.htm

Northwestern Health Sciences University, College of Chiropractic, Bloomington, MN 55431-1599. Offers DC. *Accreditation:* CCE. *Students:* 620 full-time (280 women), 36 part-time (15 women); includes 47 minority (4 Black or African American, non-Hispanic/Latino; 1 American Indian or Alaska Native, non-Hispanic/Latino; 24 Asian, non-Hispanic/Latino; 11 Hispanic/Latino; 7 Two or more races, non-Hispanic/Latino), 20 international. Average age 26. In 2013, 152 doctorates awarded. *Entrance requirements:* For doctorate, 90 semester hours of course work in health or science, minimum GPA of 2.75. Additional exam requirements/recommendations for international students: Required—TOEFL (minimum score 540 paper-based; 76 iBT). *Application deadline:* For fall admission, 5/1 priority date for domestic and international students; for winter admission, 9/1 priority date for domestic and international students. Applications are processed on a rolling basis. Application fee: $50. Electronic applications accepted. *Expenses: Tuition:* Full-time $11,207; part-time $379 per credit. *Required fees:* $804; $402 per trimester. Tuition and fees vary according to course load, degree level and program. *Financial support:* In 2013–14, 245 students received support. Career-related internships or fieldwork, Federal Work-Study, and scholarships/grants available. Support available to part-time students. Financial award applicants required to submit FAFSA. *Faculty research:* Headache, low back pain, neck pain, sciatica, rehabilitative exercise. *Unit head:* Dr. Timothy Stark, Dean, 952-888-4777 Ext. 471, Fax: 952-888-6713, E-mail: tstark@nwhealth.edu. *Application contact:* Kate DiAna, Director of Admissions, 952-888-4777 Ext. 273, Fax: 952-888-6713, E-mail: admit@nwhealth.edu.
Website: http://www.nwhealth.edu/college-of-chiropractic/

Palmer College of Chiropractic, Professional Program, Davenport, IA 52803-5287. Offers DC. *Accreditation:* CCE. Part-time programs available. *Entrance requirements:* For doctorate, minimum GPA of 2.5, 90 hours of prerequisite coursework. Additional exam requirements/recommendations for international students: Required—TOEFL (minimum score 500 paper-based; 61 iBT). Electronic applications accepted. *Faculty research:* Studies to advance the understanding of chiropractic.

Palmer College of Chiropractic, Professional Program–Florida Campus, Davenport, IA 52803-5287. Offers DC. *Accreditation:* CCE. Part-time programs available. *Degree requirements:* For doctorate, clinical internship. *Entrance requirements:* For doctorate, minimum GPA of 2.5, 90 hours of prerequisite coursework. Additional exam requirements/recommendations for international students: Recommended—TOEFL (minimum score 500 paper-based; 61 iBT).

Palmer College of Chiropractic, Professional Program–West Campus, San Jose, CA 95134-1617. Offers DC. *Accreditation:* CCE. Part-time programs available. *Degree requirements:* For doctorate, clinical internship. *Entrance requirements:* For doctorate, minimum GPA of 2.5. Additional exam requirements/recommendations for international students: Required—TOEFL. Electronic applications accepted. *Faculty research:* Low back pain complaints, spinal manipulation therapy, cervical biomechanics, clinical trials, practice guidelines.

Parker University, Doctor of Chiropractic Program, Dallas, TX 75229-5668. Offers DC. *Accreditation:* CCE. Part-time programs available. *Entrance requirements:* For doctorate, minimum GPA of 2.65. Additional exam requirements/recommendations for international students: Required—TOEFL (minimum score 550 paper-based). Electronic applications accepted. *Faculty research:* Arterial tonometry, bioenergetics, outcome assessment for clinical care.

Sherman College of Chiropractic, Professional Program, Spartanburg, SC 29304-1452. Offers DC. *Accreditation:* CCE. *Faculty:* 25 full-time (14 women), 11 part-time/adjunct (5 women). *Students:* 249 full-time (112 women), 44 part-time (16 women). *Application deadline:* For fall admission, 8/18 for domestic students; for winter admission, 11/24 for domestic students, 8/28 for international students. Applications are processed on a rolling basis. Application fee: $35. Electronic applications accepted. *Expenses: Tuition:* Full-time $21,543; part-time $23.94 per hour. Part-time tuition and fees vary according to course load. *Financial support:* Career-related internships or fieldwork, Federal Work-Study, institutionally sponsored loans, and scholarships/grants available. Support available to part-time students. Financial award applicants required to submit FAFSA. *Faculty research:* Chiropractic effect of immune response, biomechanics, videofluoroscopy, dynamic motion. *Application contact:* Dr. Robert Irwin, Vice President for Academic Affairs, 864-578-8770 Ext. 223, Fax: 864-599-4860, E-mail: admissions@sherman.edu.
Website: http://www.sherman.edu

Southern California University of Health Sciences, Los Angeles College of Chiropractic, Whittier, CA 90609-1166. Offers DC. *Accreditation:* CCE. *Degree requirements:* For doctorate, clinical internship. *Entrance requirements:* For doctorate, minimum GPA of 2.5, 90 incoming units in prerequisite coursework. Additional exam requirements/recommendations for international students: Required—TOEFL (minimum score 500 paper-based). Electronic applications accepted. *Faculty research:* Low back pain, smoking cessation, sports medicine.

Texas Chiropractic College, Professional Program, Pasadena, TX 77505-1699. Offers DC. *Accreditation:* CCE. *Faculty:* 35 full-time, 4 part-time/adjunct. *Students:* 245 full-time (104 women); includes 100 minority (26 Black or African American, non-Hispanic/Latino; 4 American Indian or Alaska Native, non-Hispanic/Latino; 26 Asian, non-Hispanic/Latino; 32 Hispanic/Latino; 2 Native Hawaiian or other Pacific Islander, non-Hispanic/Latino; 10 Two or more races, non-Hispanic/Latino), 8 international. *Entrance requirements:* For doctorate, 90 semester hours at regionally-accredited college or university, minimum GPA of 3.0 (24 hours of life and physical sciences, half of which have a lab component). Additional exam requirements/recommendations for international students: Required—TOEFL. *Application deadline:* For fall admission, 9/1 priority date for domestic students; for spring admission, 12/1 priority date for domestic students; for summer admission, 5/1 priority date for domestic students. Applications are processed on a rolling basis. Application fee: $50. *Expenses: Tuition:* Full-time $32,445; part-time $902 per credit hour. *Required fees:* $1192.50. *Financial support:* Career-related internships or fieldwork, Federal Work-Study, institutionally sponsored loans, and scholarships/grants available. Financial award application deadline: 4/15; financial award applicants required to submit FAFSA. *Faculty research:* Range of motion comparison male vs. female student stress levels. *Unit head:* Lee A. Canales, Director of Admission, 281-998-6065, Fax: 281-991-5237, E-mail: lcanales@txchiro.edu.
Website: http://www.txchiro.edu/academics/dc-program

Université du Québec à Trois-Rivières, Graduate Programs, Program in Chiropractic, Trois-Rivières, QC G9A 5H7, Canada. Offers DC.

University of Bridgeport, College of Chiropractic, Bridgeport, CT 06604. Offers DC. *Accreditation:* CCE. *Faculty:* 20 full-time (4 women), 16 part-time/adjunct (5 women). *Students:* 163 full-time (60 women), 1 part-time (0 women); includes 54 minority (17 Black or African American, non-Hispanic/Latino; 18 Asian, non-Hispanic/Latino; 12 Hispanic/Latino; 7 Two or more races, non-Hispanic/Latino), 4 international. Average age 28. 80 applicants, 56% accepted, 29 enrolled. In 2013, 31 doctorates awarded. *Degree requirements:* For doctorate, thesis/dissertation, National Board of Chiropractic Exam Parts I and II. *Entrance requirements:* Additional exam requirements/recommendations for international students: Recommended—TOEFL (minimum score 550 paper-based; 80 iBT), IELTS (minimum score 6.5). *Application deadline:* For fall admission, 4/1 priority date for domestic and international students; for spring admission, 11/1 priority date for domestic and international students. Applications are processed on a rolling basis. Application fee: $75. Electronic applications accepted. *Expenses:* Contact institution. *Financial support:* In 2013–14, 50 students received support. Federal Work-Study and institutionally sponsored loans available. Support available to part-time students. Financial award application deadline: 6/1; financial award applicants required to submit FAFSA. *Unit head:* Dr. David J. Wickes, Dean, 203-576-4279, E-mail: dwickes@bridgeport.edu. *Application contact:* Leanne Proctor, Director of Health Science Admissions, 203-576-4352, Fax: 203-576-4941, E-mail: chiro@bridgeport.edu.

University of Western States, Professional Program, Portland, OR 97230-3099. Offers DC. *Accreditation:* CCE. *Degree requirements:* For doctorate, comprehensive exam, internship. *Entrance requirements:* For doctorate, 3 years of pre-chiropractic study in biological sciences, minimum GPA of 2.5. *Faculty research:* Low back pain.

Section 27
Dentistry and Dental Sciences

This section contains a directory of institutions offering graduate work in dentistry and dental sciences, followed by an in-depth entry submitted by an institution that chose to prepare a detailed program description. Additional information about programs listed in the directory but not augmented by an in-depth entry may be obtained by writing directly to the dean of a graduate school or chair of a department at the address given in the directory.

For programs offering related work, see also in this book *Allied Health.*

CONTENTS

Program Directories

Display and Close-Up

Dentistry

A.T. Still University, Missouri School of Dentistry and Oral Health, Kirksville, MO 63501. Offers dental medicine (DMD). *Faculty:* 2 full-time (1 woman), 3 part-time/adjunct (0 women). *Students:* 42 full-time (22 women); includes 13 minority (1 Black or African American, non-Hispanic/Latino; 7 Asian, non-Hispanic/Latino; 2 Hispanic/Latino; 3 Two or more races, non-Hispanic/Latino). Average age 25. 954 applicants, 5% accepted, 42 enrolled. *Degree requirements:* For doctorate, National Board exams 1 and 2. *Entrance requirements:* For doctorate, DAT, minimum GPA of 2.5 overall and science. *Application deadline:* For summer admission, 12/1 for domestic students. Applications are processed on a rolling basis. Application fee: $70. Electronic applications accepted. *Financial support:* In 2013–14, 1 student received support. Federal Work-Study and scholarships/grants available. Financial award application deadline: 5/1; financial award applicants required to submit FAFSA. *Faculty research:* Oral perception, dental education assessments, dental ethics, adverse events of dentistry, maxillary arterial variation in the dental anesthesia. *Unit head:* Dr. Christopher G. Halliday, Dean, 660-626-2800. *Application contact:* Donna Sparks, Associate Director for Admissions, 660-626-2237, Fax: 660-626-2969, E-mail: admissions@atsu.edu.
Website: http://www.atsu.edu/mosdoh/

Boston University, Henry M. Goldman School of Dental Medicine, Boston, MA 02118. Offers advanced general dentistry (CAGS); dental public health (MS, MSD, D Sc D, CAGS); dentistry (DMD); endodontics (MSD, D Sc D, CAGS); operative dentistry (MSD, D Sc D, CAGS); oral and maxillofacial surgery (MSD, D Sc D, CAGS); oral biology (MSD, D Sc, D Sc D, PhD); orthodontics (MSD, D Sc D, CAGS); pediatric dentistry (MSD, D Sc D, CAGS); periodontology (MSD, D Sc D, CAGS); prosthodontics (MSD, D Sc D, CAGS). *Accreditation:* ADA (one or more programs are accredited). *Faculty:* 119 full-time (53 women), 83 part-time/adjunct (24 women). *Students:* 818 full-time (423 women); includes 158 minority (8 Black or African American, non-Hispanic/Latino; 1 American Indian or Alaska Native, non-Hispanic/Latino; 102 Asian, non-Hispanic/Latino; 40 Hispanic/Latino; 7 Two or more races, non-Hispanic/Latino), 359 international. Average age 28. 6,681 applicants, 8% accepted, 263 enrolled. In 2013, 14 master's, 199 doctorates, 55 other advanced degrees awarded. *Degree requirements:* For master's and CAGS, thesis; for doctorate, thesis/dissertation (for some programs). *Entrance requirements:* For doctorate, DAT (for DMD), minimum recommended GPA of 3.0 (for DMD); for CAGS, National Board Dental Exam Part 1, dental degree. Additional exam requirements/recommendations for international students: Required—TOEFL. *Application deadline:* For fall admission, 12/1 for domestic and international students. Applications are processed on a rolling basis. Application fee: $75 ($105 for international students). Electronic applications accepted. *Expenses:* Contact institution. *Financial support:* In 2013–14, 480 students received support. Career-related internships or fieldwork, institutionally sponsored loans, and stipends and scholarships (for Advanced Education in General Dentistry and Oral and Maxillofacial Surgery residents) available. Financial award application deadline: 4/15; financial award applicants required to submit FAFSA. *Faculty research:* Defense mechanisms, bone-cell regulation, protein biochemistry, molecular biology, biomaterials. *Unit head:* Dr. Jeffrey W. Hutter, Dean, 617-638-4780. *Application contact:* Admissions Representative, 617-638-4787, Fax: 617-638-4798, E-mail: sdmadmis@bu.edu.
Website: http://www.bu.edu/dental

Case Western Reserve University, School of Dental Medicine, Professional Program in Dentistry, Cleveland, OH 44106. Offers DMD. *Accreditation:* ADA. *Degree requirements:* For doctorate, thesis/dissertation. *Entrance requirements:* For doctorate, DAT. Additional exam requirements/recommendations for international students: Required—TOEFL (minimum score 550 paper-based). *Expenses:* Contact institution. *Faculty research:* Periodontal disease; overall health; natural antibodies; obesity and periodontal disease; 3D cone beam computerized tomography.

Columbia University, College of Dental Medicine, Professional Program in Dental and Oral Surgery, New York, NY 10032. Offers DDS, DDS/MBA, DDS/MPH. *Accreditation:* ADA. *Entrance requirements:* For doctorate, DAT, previous course work in biology, organic chemistry, inorganic chemistry, physics, and English.

Creighton University, School of Dentistry, Omaha, NE 68178-0001. Offers DDS. *Accreditation:* ADA. *Entrance requirements:* For doctorate, DAT. *Expenses:* Contact institution. *Faculty research:* Dental implants, bone calcification, dental materials, laser usage in dentistry.

Georgia Regents University, College of Dental Medicine, Augusta, GA 30912. Offers DMD, DMD/MS, DMD/PhD. *Accreditation:* ADA. *Faculty:* 53 full-time (10 women), 14 part-time/adjunct (4 women). *Students:* 308 full-time (135 women), 3 part-time (0 women); includes 94 minority (40 Black or African American, non-Hispanic/Latino; 30 Asian, non-Hispanic/Latino; 15 Hispanic/Latino; 9 Two or more races, non-Hispanic/Latino). Average age 27. 309 applicants, 26% accepted, 70 enrolled. In 2013, 61 doctorates awarded. *Degree requirements:* For doctorate, comprehensive exam. *Entrance requirements:* For doctorate, DAT, previous course work in biology, English, organic chemistry, and general chemistry; 1 semester of course work in physics. Additional exam requirements/recommendations for international students: Required—TOEFL (minimum score 100 iBT). *Application deadline:* For fall admission, 10/15 for domestic students. Application fee: $30. Electronic applications accepted. *Expenses:* Contact institution. *Financial support:* Federal Work-Study and scholarships/grants available. Financial award application deadline: 5/1; financial award applicants required to submit FAFSA. *Faculty research:* Biocompatibility, dentin bonding, oral cancer, ceramic strengthening, resin polymerization. *Total annual research expenditures:* $1.2 million. *Unit head:* Dr. Connie Drisko, Dean, 706-721-2117, Fax: 706-721-6276, E-mail: cdrisko@georgiahealth.edu. *Application contact:* Dr. Carole M. Hanes, Associate Dean for Student and Alumni Affairs, 706-721-3587, Fax: 706-721-6276, E-mail: chanes@georgiahealth.edu.
Website: http://www.gru.edu/dentalmedicine/

Harvard University, School of Dental Medicine, Advanced Graduate Programs in Dentistry, Cambridge, MA 02138. Offers advanced general dentistry (Certificate); dental public health (Certificate); endodontics (Certificate); general practice residency (Certificate); oral biology (M Med Sc, D Med Sc); oral implantology (Certificate); oral medicine (Certificate); oral pathology (Certificate); oral surgery (Certificate); orthodontics (Certificate); pediatric dentistry (Certificate); periodontics (Certificate); prosthodontics (Certificate). *Expenses: Tuition:* Full-time $38,888. *Required fees:* $958. Tuition and fees vary according to campus/location, program and student level.

Harvard University, School of Dental Medicine, Professional Program in Dental Medicine, Cambridge, MA 02138. Offers DMD. *Accreditation:* ADA. *Entrance requirements:* For doctorate, DAT, 1 year each: biology, general chemistry, organic chemistry, physics, calculus, English. *Expenses: Tuition:* Full-time $38,888. *Required fees:* $958. Tuition and fees vary according to campus/location, program and student level.

Howard University, College of Dentistry, Washington, DC 20059-0002. Offers advanced education program general dentistry (Certificate); dentistry (DDS); general dentistry (Certificate); oral and maxillofacial surgery (Certificate); orthodontics (Certificate); pediatric dentistry (Certificate). *Accreditation:* ADA (one or more programs are accredited). *Degree requirements:* For doctorate, comprehensive exam, didactic and clinical exams. *Entrance requirements:* For doctorate, DAT, 8 semester hours of course work in each biology, inorganic chemistry, organic chemistry. *Expenses:* Contact institution. *Faculty research:* Epidemiological, biomaterial, molecular genetic, behavioral modification, and clinical trial studies.

Idaho State University, Office of Graduate Studies, Kasiska College of Health Professions, Department of Dental Sciences, Pocatello, ID 83209-8088. Offers advanced general dentistry (Post-Doctoral Certificate). First year of Idaho Dental Education Program available in conjunction with Creighton University's School of Dentistry. *Degree requirements:* For Post-Doctoral Certificate, comprehensive exam, thesis optional, 1-year residency. *Entrance requirements:* For degree, DAT, 3 dental application forms. Additional exam requirements/recommendations for international students: Required—TOEFL (minimum score 600 paper-based). Electronic applications accepted. *Expenses:* Contact institution.

Indiana University–Purdue University Indianapolis, School of Dentistry, Indianapolis, IN 46202-2896. Offers MS, MSD, DDS, PhD, Certificate. *Accreditation:* ADA (one or more programs are accredited). *Faculty:* 96 full-time (28 women). *Students:* 250,506 full-time (261 women), 51 part-time (22 women); includes 105 minority (21 Black or African American, non-Hispanic/Latino; 1 American Indian or Alaska Native, non-Hispanic/Latino; 59 Asian, non-Hispanic/Latino; 19 Hispanic/Latino; 5 Two or more races, non-Hispanic/Latino), 71 international. Average age 28. In 2013, 19 master's, 108 doctorates, 3 other advanced degrees awarded. *Degree requirements:* For master's, thesis or manuscript, qualifying exam; for doctorate, thesis/dissertation, completion of all coursework with a passing grade; minimum GPA of 3.0 and qualifying examination (for PhD); minimum GPA of 2.0 and passing scores for Part I and II of National Board of Dental Examinations (for DDS); for Certificate, thesis, completion of all coursework with passing grades, minimum GPA of 3.0. *Entrance requirements:* For master's, GRE (orthodontics); National Board Dental Exam Part I (periodontics), Parts I and II (endodontics); for doctorate, GRE (for PhD); DAT (for DDS). Additional exam requirements/recommendations for international students: Required—TOEFL (minimum score 550 paper-based; 79 iBT). *Application deadline:* For winter admission, 11/1 for domestic and international students. Applications are processed on a rolling basis. Electronic applications accepted. *Expenses:* Contact institution. *Financial support:* In 2013–14, 43 students received support. Fellowships, research assistantships, teaching assistantships, Federal Work-Study, institutionally sponsored loans, and scholarships/grants available. Financial award application deadline: 3/1; financial award applicants required to submit FAFSA. *Faculty research:* Caries research: early caries detection and management, secondary caries, remineralization, oral biofilms, fluoride, dental erosion; oral biology: molecular biology and immunobiology of streptococcus mutans, oral biofilms, infection control, actinobaccillus actinomycetemcomitans; orthodontics and oral facial genetics: orthodontics biomechanics; oral pathology and immunology: chronic inflammation and autoimmunity, innate immunity in oral pathology; periodontal disease and implants. *Total annual research expenditures:* $7.8 million. *Unit head:* John N. Williams, Dean, 317-274-7461. *Application contact:* Student Records and Admissions Office, 317-274-8173, E-mail: dsoaa@iupui.edu.
Website: http://www.iusd.iupui.edu/

Loma Linda University, School of Dentistry, Loma Linda, CA 92350. Offers MS, DDS, Certificate, DDS/MS, DDS/PhD, MS/Certificate. *Accreditation:* ADA. *Entrance requirements:* For master's, GRE, minimum GPA of 3.0; for doctorate, DAT. Additional exam requirements/recommendations for international students: Required—TOEFL (minimum score 550 paper-based). *Expenses:* Contact institution.

Louisiana State University Health Sciences Center, School of Dentistry, New Orleans, LA 70112-2223. Offers DDS. *Accreditation:* ADA. *Entrance requirements:* For doctorate, DAT, interview. *Expenses:* Contact institution. *Faculty research:* HIV/AIDS, implants, metallurgy, lipids, DNA.

Marquette University, School of Dentistry, Professional Program in Dentistry, Milwaukee, WI 53201-1881. Offers DDS. *Accreditation:* ADA. *Faculty:* 37 full-time (9 women), 131 part-time/adjunct (36 women). *Students:* 343 full-time (147 women); includes 78 minority (13 Black or African American, non-Hispanic/Latino; 4 American Indian or Alaska Native, non-Hispanic/Latino; 28 Asian, non-Hispanic/Latino; 29 Hispanic/Latino; 4 Two or more races, non-Hispanic/Latino), 2 international. Average age 25. 2,522 applicants, 6% accepted, 81 enrolled. In 2013, 82 doctorates awarded. *Degree requirements:* For doctorate, National Board Dental Exam Part 1 and 2, regional licensure exam. *Entrance requirements:* For doctorate, DAT, 1 year of course work each in biology, inorganic chemistry, organic chemistry, physics, and English. Additional exam requirements/recommendations for international students: Required—TOEFL. *Application deadline:* For fall admission, 1/1 for domestic and international students. Applications are processed on a rolling basis. Application fee: $50. *Expenses:* Contact institution. *Financial support:* In 2013–14, 292 students received support. Institutionally sponsored loans and scholarships/grants available. Financial award applicants required to submit FAFSA. *Faculty research:* Biomaterials, wound healing, diabetes, biocompatibility, cancer, aging, lasers. *Unit head:* Dr. William K. Lobb, Dean and Professor, 414-288-7485. *Application contact:* Dr. William K. Lobb, Dean and Professor, 414-288-7485.
Website: http://www.marquette.edu/dentistry

McGill University, Faculty of Graduate and Postdoctoral Studies, Faculty of Dentistry, Montréal, QC H3A 2T5, Canada. Offers forensic dentistry (Certificate); oral and maxillofacial surgery (M Sc, PhD).

McGill University, Professional Program in Dentistry, Montréal, QC H3A 2T5, Canada. Offers DMD. *Accreditation:* ADA. Electronic applications accepted.

Medical University of South Carolina, College of Dental Medicine, Charleston, SC 29425. Offers DMD, DMD/PhD. *Accreditation:* ADA. *Degree requirements:* For doctorate, National Board of Dental Examinations Part I and II. *Entrance requirements:* For doctorate, DAT, interview, 52 hours of specific pre-dental course work. Additional exam requirements/recommendations for international students: Required—TOEFL (minimum score 600 paper-based). Electronic applications accepted. *Expenses:* Contact institution. *Faculty research:* South Carolina oral health, genetics, health disparities, chlamydia, oral cancer.

Meharry Medical College, School of Dentistry, Nashville, TN 37208-9989. Offers DDS. *Accreditation:* ADA. *Entrance requirements:* For doctorate, DAT.

Midwestern University, Downers Grove Campus, College of Dental Medicine-Illinois, Downers Grove, IL 60515-1235. Offers DMD. *Accreditation:* ADA. *Entrance requirements:* For doctorate, DAT, bachelor's degree, minimum overall GPA of 2.75, three letters of recommendation.

Midwestern University, Glendale Campus, College of Dental Medicine, Glendale, AZ 85308. Offers DMD. *Accreditation:* ADA.

New York University, College of Dentistry, Advanced Placement DDS Program, New York, NY 10010. Offers DDS. *Accreditation:* ADA. *Faculty:* 242 full-time (85 women), 689 part-time/adjunct (186 women). *Students:* 741 applicants, 24% accepted, 126 enrolled. *Entrance requirements:* For doctorate, National Dental Board Exam. Additional exam requirements/recommendations for international students: Required—TOEFL (minimum score 90 iBT). *Application deadline:* For fall admission, 12/1 for domestic and international students. Applications are processed on a rolling basis. Application fee: $100. Electronic applications accepted. *Expenses: Tuition:* Full-time $35,856; part-time $1494 per unit. *Required fees:* $1408; $64 per unit. $473 per term. Tuition and fees vary according to course load and program. *Unit head:* Dr. Charles Bertolami, Dean, 212-998-9898, Fax: 212-995-4240, E-mail: charles.bertolami@nyu.edu. *Application contact:* Dr. Anthony M. Palatta, Assistant Dean for Student Affairs and Admissions, 212-998-9918, Fax: 212-995-4240, E-mail: ap16@nyu.edu.

New York University, College of Dentistry, Professional Program in Dentistry, New York, NY 10010. Offers DDS. *Accreditation:* ADA. *Faculty:* 242 full-time (85 women), 689 part-time/adjunct (186 women). *Students:* 1,442 full-time (770 women); includes 589 minority (43 Black or African American, non-Hispanic/Latino; 2 American Indian or Alaska Native, non-Hispanic/Latino; 465 Asian, non-Hispanic/Latino; 73 Hispanic/Latino; 6 Two or more races, non-Hispanic/Latino), 363 international. Average age 25. 4,585 applicants, 19% accepted, 360 enrolled. In 2013, 340 doctorates awarded. *Entrance requirements:* For doctorate, DAT, BA or 90-credit equivalent. Additional exam requirements/recommendations for international students: Required—TOEFL (minimum score 100 iBT). *Application deadline:* For fall admission, 2/2 for domestic and international students. Applications are processed on a rolling basis. Application fee: $80. Electronic applications accepted. *Expenses: Tuition:* Full-time $35,856; part-time $1494 per unit. *Required fees:* $1408; $64 per unit. $473 per term. Tuition and fees vary according to course load and program. *Financial support:* In 2013–14, 106 students received support. Application deadline: 3/1; applicants required to submit FAFSA. *Unit head:* Dr. Eugenia E. Mejia, Senior Director of Admissions, 212-998-9918, Fax: 212-995-4240, E-mail: eem1@nyu.edu. *Application contact:* Dr. Eugenia E. Mejia, Senior Director of Admissions, 212-998-9818, Fax: 212-995-4240, E-mail: dental.admissions@nyu.edu.
Website: http://www.nyu.edu/dental/

Nova Southeastern University, College of Dental Medicine, Fort Lauderdale, FL 33314-7796. Offers dental medicine (DMD); dentistry (MS, Graduate Certificate). *Accreditation:* ADA. *Faculty:* 108 full-time (37 women), 178 part-time/adjunct (42 women). *Students:* 591 full-time (311 women), 6 part-time (1 woman); includes 255 minority (10 Black or African American, non-Hispanic/Latino; 109 Asian, non-Hispanic/Latino; 120 Hispanic/Latino; 1 Native Hawaiian or other Pacific Islander, non-Hispanic/Latino; 15 Two or more races, non-Hispanic/Latino), 73 international. Average age 28. 2,328 applicants, 10% accepted, 124 enrolled. In 2013, 7 master's, 126 doctorates, 42 other advanced degrees awarded. *Degree requirements:* For master's, thesis. *Entrance requirements:* For doctorate, DAT, minimum GPA of 3.0. Additional exam requirements/recommendations for international students: Required—TOEFL (minimum score 550 paper-based). *Application deadline:* For fall admission, 12/31 for domestic students, 1/1 for international students. Applications are processed on a rolling basis. Application fee: $50. *Expenses:* Contact institution. *Financial support:* Application deadline: 4/15. *Faculty research:* Tissue engineering, dental materials. *Unit head:* Dr. Linda Niessen, Dean, 954-262-7334, Fax: 954-262-1782, E-mail: lniessen@nova.edu. *Application contact:* Su-Ann Zarrett, Associate Director of HPD Admissions, 954-262-1108, Fax: 954-262-2282, E-mail: zarrett@nsu.nova.edu.

The Ohio State University, College of Dentistry, Columbus, OH 43210. Offers dental anesthesiology (MS); dental hygiene (MDH); dentistry (DDS); endodontics (MS); oral and maxillofacial pathology (MS); oral and maxillofacial surgery (MS); oral biology (PhD); orthodontics (MS); pediatric dentistry (MS); periodontology (MS); prosthodontics (MS); DDS/PhD. *Accreditation:* ADA (one or more programs are accredited). *Faculty:* 75. *Students:* 510 full-time (220 women), 7 part-time (4 women); includes 89 minority (12 Black or African American, non-Hispanic/Latino; 51 Asian, non-Hispanic/Latino; 16 Hispanic/Latino; 10 Two or more races, non-Hispanic/Latino), 26 international. Average age 26. In 2013, 17 master's, 105 doctorates awarded. Terminal master's awarded for partial completion of doctoral program. *Degree requirements:* For master's, thesis; for doctorate, thesis/dissertation (for some programs). *Entrance requirements:* For master's, GRE General Test (for all applicants with cumulative GPA below 3.0); for doctorate, DAT (for DDS); GRE General Test, GRE Subject Test in biology recommended (for PhD). Additional exam requirements/recommendations for international students: Required—TOEFL (minimum score 550 paper-based; 79 iBT), Michigan English Language Assessment Battery (minimum score 82), IELTS (minimum score 7) for MS and PhD; TOEFL (minimum score 577 paper-based; 90 iBT), Michigan English Language Assessment Battery (minimum score 84), IELTS (minimum score 7.5) for DDS. *Application deadline:* Applications are processed on a rolling basis. Electronic applications accepted. *Expenses:* Contact institution. *Financial support:* Fellowships with tuition reimbursements, research assistantships with tuition reimbursements, teaching assistantships with tuition reimbursements, Federal Work-Study, and institutionally sponsored loans available. Financial award application deadline: 2/15. *Faculty research:* Neurobiology, inflammation and immunity, materials science, bone biology. *Total annual research expenditures:* $3.4 million. *Unit head:* Dr. Patrick M. Lloyd, Dean, 614-292-9755, E-mail: lloyd.256@osu.edu. *Application contact:* Graduate and Professional Admissions, 614-292-9444, Fax: 614-292-3656.
Website: http://www.dent.osu.edu/

Oregon Health & Science University, School of Dentistry, Professional Program in Dentistry, Portland, OR 97239-3098. Offers dentistry (DMD); oral and maxillofacial surgery (Certificate); MD/DMD. *Accreditation:* ADA. *Entrance requirements:* For doctorate, DAT. Electronic applications accepted. *Faculty research:* Dentin permeability, tooth sensations, fluoride metabolism, immunology of periodontal disease, craniofacial growth.

Roseman University of Health Sciences, College of Dental Medicine - Henderson Campus, Henderson, NV 89014. Offers business administration (MBA); dental medicine (Post-Doctoral Certificate). *Faculty:* 3 full-time (1 woman), 11 part-time/adjunct (2 women). *Students:* 29 full-time (12 women); includes 13 minority (1 Black or African American, non-Hispanic/Latino; 11 Asian, non-Hispanic/Latino; 1 Two or more races, non-Hispanic/Latino). Average age 30. 110 applicants, 9% accepted, 10 enrolled. In 2013, 10 other advanced degrees awarded. *Degree requirements:* For master's, comprehensive exam, thesis or alternative. *Entrance requirements:* For master's, National Board Dental Examination 1 and 2, graduation from U.S. or Canadian dental school, Nevada dental license. *Application deadline:* For fall admission, 9/15 for domestic students. Applications are processed on a rolling basis. Application fee: $50. *Expenses:* Contact institution. *Financial support:* In 2013–14, 1 student received support. Scholarships/grants, health care benefits, and stipends available. Financial award application deadline: 3/2; financial award applicants required to submit FAFSA. *Unit head:* Dr. Jaleh Pourhamidi, Dean, 702-968-1652, Fax: 702-968-5277, E-mail: jpourhamidi@roseman.edu. *Application contact:* Maria Doleshal, Administrative Assistant to the Dean, 702-968-1682, E-mail: mdoleshal@roseman.edu.
Website: http://www.roseman.edu

Roseman University of Health Sciences, College of Dental Medicine - South Jordan, Utah Campus, South Jordan, UT 84020. Offers DMD. *Faculty:* 31 full-time (2 women), 26 part-time/adjunct (3 women). *Students:* 223 full-time (51 women); includes 66 minority (1 Black or African American, non-Hispanic/Latino; 59 Asian, non-Hispanic/Latino; 2 Hispanic/Latino; 4 Two or more races, non-Hispanic/Latino). Average age 28. 1,835 applicants, 10% accepted, 80 enrolled. *Degree requirements:* For doctorate, comprehensive exam, thesis/dissertation or alternative, National Board Dental Examinations (NBDE). *Entrance requirements:* For doctorate, DAT. *Application deadline:* For fall admission, 12/1 for domestic and international students. Applications are processed on a rolling basis. Application fee: $75. Electronic applications accepted. *Expenses: Tuition:* Full-time $45,240. *Required fees:* $425. *Financial support:* In 2013–14, 10 students received support. Federal Work-Study available. Financial award application deadline: 3/2; financial award applicants required to submit FAFSA. *Unit head:* Dr. Frank W. Licari, Dean, College of Dental Medicine, 801-878-1400, E-mail: flicari@roseman.edu. *Application contact:* Amanda Hinton, Admissions Coordinator, 801-878-1405, E-mail: ahinton@roseman.edu.
Website: http://www.roseman.edu/dental

Rutgers, The State University of New Jersey, Newark, Rutgers School of Dental Medicine, Newark, NJ 07101-1709. Offers dental science (MS); dentistry (DMD); endodontics (Certificate); oral medicine (Certificate); orthodontics (Certificate); pediatric dentistry (Certificate); periodontics (Certificate); prosthodontics (Certificate); DMD/MPH; DMD/PhD; MD/Certificate; MS/Certificate. DMD/MPH offered jointly with New Jersey Institute of Technology, Rutgers, The State University of New Jersey, Camden. *Accreditation:* ADA (one or more programs are accredited). *Entrance requirements:* For doctorate, DAT. Electronic applications accepted. *Expenses:* Contact institution.

Saint Louis University, Graduate Education, Center for Advanced Dental Education, St. Louis, MO 63103-2097. Offers endodontics (MSD); orthodontics (MSD); periodontics (MSD). *Degree requirements:* For master's, comprehensive exam, thesis, teaching practicum. *Entrance requirements:* For master's, GRE General Test, NBDE (National Board Dental Exam), DDS or DMD, interview, letters of recommendation. Additional exam requirements/recommendations for international students: Required—TOEFL (minimum score 525 paper-based). Electronic applications accepted. *Faculty research:* Craniofacial growth.

Southern Illinois University Edwardsville, School of Dental Medicine, Alton, IL 62026. Offers DMD. *Accreditation:* ADA. *Faculty:* 15 full-time (5 women). *Students:* 205 full-time (82 women); includes 27 minority (5 Black or African American, non-Hispanic/Latino; 9 Asian, non-Hispanic/Latino; 8 Hispanic/Latino; 1 Native Hawaiian or other Pacific Islander, non-Hispanic/Latino; 4 Two or more races, non-Hispanic/Latino). 585 applicants, 12% accepted. In 2013, 40 doctorates awarded. *Entrance requirements:* For doctorate, DAT. *Application deadline:* For fall admission, 6/1 priority date for domestic and international students. Electronic applications accepted. *Expenses:* Contact institution. *Financial support:* Application deadline: 3/1; applicants required to submit FAFSA. *Unit head:* Dr. Bruce Rotter, Dean, 618-474-7000, Fax: 618-474-7249, E-mail: sdmapps@siue.edu.
Website: http://www.siue.edu/dentalmedicine

Stony Brook University, State University of New York, Stony Brook University Medical Center, Health Sciences Center, School of Dental Medicine, Professional Program in Dental Medicine, Stony Brook, NY 11794. Offers dental medicine (DDS); endodontics (Certificate); orthodontics (Certificate); periodontics (Certificate). *Accreditation:* ADA (one or more programs are accredited). *Faculty:* 29 full-time (12 women), 69 part-time/adjunct (18 women). *Students:* 184 full-time (94 women); includes 47 minority (3 Black or African American, non-Hispanic/Latino; 35 Asian, non-Hispanic/Latino; 7 Hispanic/Latino; 2 Two or more races, non-Hispanic/Latino), 2 international. Average age 25. 1,113 applicants, 7% accepted, 42 enrolled. In 2013, 36 doctorates awarded. *Entrance requirements:* For doctorate, DAT. *Application deadline:* For fall admission, 1/15 for domestic students. Application fee: $100. *Expenses:* Tuition, state resident: full-time $9870; part-time $411 per credit. Tuition, nonresident: full-time $18,350; part-time $765 per credit. *Financial support:* Research assistantships, teaching assistantships, and Federal Work-Study available. Support available to part-time students. *Total annual research expenditures:* $2.8 million. *Unit head:* Dr. Mary R. Truhlar, Interim Dean, 631-632-8950, Fax: 631-632-9105. *Application contact:* Patricia Berry, Acting Director of Admissions, 631-632-8871, Fax: 631-632-7130, E-mail: patricia.berry@stonybrook.edu.
Website: http://dentistry.stonybrookmedicine.edu/

Temple University, Kornberg School of Dentistry, Professiona[illegible]gram in Dentistry, Philadelphia, PA 19122-6096. Offers DMD, DMD/MBA. *Accreditation:* ADA. *Entrance requirements:* For doctorate, DAT, 6 credits of course work in each biology, chemistry, organic chemistry, physics, and English. *Expenses:* Contact institution.

Texas A&M Health Science Center, Baylor College of Dentistry, Professional Program in Dentistry, College Station, TX 77840. Offers DDS. *Entrance requirements:* For doctorate, DAT. *Expenses:* Contact institution. *Faculty research:* Bleaching, implants, craniofacial growth, oral oncology, pulp biology.

Tufts University, School of Dental Medicine, International Student Program in Dental Medicine, Medford, MA 02155. Offers DMD. *Accreditation:* ADA. *Entrance requirements:* For doctorate, National Dental Hygiene Board Exam Part I, BDS, DDS, or equivalent. Additional exam requirements/recommendations for international students: Required—TOEFL.

Tufts University, School of Dental Medicine, Professional Program in Dental Medicine, Medford, MA 02155. Offers DMD, DMD/PhD. *Accreditation:* ADA. *Entrance requirements:* For doctorate, DAT.

Universidad Central del Este, School of Dentistry, San Pedro de Macoris, Dominican Republic. Offers DMD.

Universidad Iberoamericana, Graduate School, Santo Domingo D.N., Dominican Republic. Offers business administration (MBA, PMBA); constitutional law (LL M); dentistry (DMD); educational management (MA); integrated marketing communication (MA); psychopedagogical intervention (M Ed); real estate law (LL M); strategic management of human talent (MM).

Universidad Nacional Pedro Henriquez Urena, School of Dentistry, Santo Domingo, Dominican Republic. Offers DDS.

Université Laval, Faculty of Dentistry, Professional Programs in Dentistry, Québec, QC G1K 7P4, Canada. Offers DMD. *Accreditation:* ADA. *Entrance requirements:* For doctorate, visual perception exam, manual dexterity exam, interview, knowledge of French. Electronic applications accepted.

Dentistry

University at Buffalo, the State University of New York, Graduate School, School of Dental Medicine, Graduate Programs in Dental Medicine, Buffalo, NY 14260. Offers advanced education in general dentistry (Certificate); biomaterials (MS); endodontics (Certificate); general practice residency (Certificate); oral and maxillofacial pathology (Certificate); oral and maxillofacial surgery (Certificate); oral biology (PhD); oral sciences (MS); orthodontics (MS, Certificate); pediatric dentistry (Certificate); periodontics (Certificate); prosthodontics (Certificate); temporomandibular disorders and oralfacial pain (Certificate). *Faculty:* 68 full-time (25 women), 124 part-time/adjunct (38 women). *Students:* 126 full-time (46 women), 24 part-time (9 women); includes 12 minority (2 Black or African American, non-Hispanic/Latino; 8 Asian, non-Hispanic/Latino; 1 Hispanic/Latino; 1 Two or more races, non-Hispanic/Latino), 84 international. Average age 30. 496 applicants, 8% accepted, 39 enrolled. In 2013, 17 master's, 4 doctorates awarded. *Degree requirements:* For master's, thesis; for doctorate, thesis/dissertation; for Certificate, comprehensive exam (for some programs). *Entrance requirements:* For master's and doctorate, GRE General Test; for Certificate, National Board Dental Exam, DDS, DMD or equivalent. Additional exam requirements/recommendations for international students: Required—TOEFL (minimum score 550 paper-based; 79 iBT). *Application deadline:* For fall admission, 10/1 for domestic and international students. Application fee: $50. Electronic applications accepted. *Expenses:* Contact institution. *Financial support:* Fellowships with full and partial tuition reimbursements, research assistantships with full and partial tuition reimbursements, Federal Work-Study, institutionally sponsored loans, scholarships/grants, traineeships, and unspecified assistantships available. Financial award applicants required to submit FAFSA. *Faculty research:* Immunology and microbiology of dental disease, surface science, saliva chemistry, bone biology. *Total annual research expenditures:* $5.8 million. *Unit head:* Dr. Heidi C. Crow, Associate Dean for Advanced Education, 716-829-2241, Fax: 716-829-3554, E-mail: hccrow@buffalo.edu. *Application contact:* Kristin Yager, Admissions Secretary, 716-829-2839, Fax: 716-829-2731, E-mail: kmyager2@buffalo.edu.

University at Buffalo, the State University of New York, Graduate School, School of Dental Medicine, Professional Program in Dental Medicine, Buffalo, NY 14260. Offers DDS. *Accreditation:* ADA. *Faculty:* 68 full-time (25 women), 124 part-time/adjunct (38 women). *Students:* 401 full-time (205 women); includes 101 minority (8 Black or African American, non-Hispanic/Latino; 3 American Indian or Alaska Native, non-Hispanic/Latino; 79 Asian, non-Hispanic/Latino; 9 Hispanic/Latino; 2 Two or more races, non-Hispanic/Latino), 33 international. Average age 26. 1,905 applicants, 10% accepted. In 2013, 108 doctorates awarded. *Degree requirements:* For doctorate, National Dental Board Exams. *Entrance requirements:* For doctorate, DAT, GRE. Additional exam requirements/recommendations for international students: Required—TOEFL (minimum score 550 paper-based; 79 iBT). *Application deadline:* For fall admission, 12/1 for domestic and international students. Applications are processed on a rolling basis. Application fee: $50. *Financial support:* Federal Work-Study, institutionally sponsored loans, and scholarships/grants available. Financial award application deadline: 3/1; financial award applicants required to submit FAFSA. *Unit head:* Dr. Michael Glick, Dean, 716-829-2836, Fax: 716-833-3517, E-mail: sdm-dean@buffalo.edu. *Application contact:* Dr. David H. Brown, Director of Admissions, 716-829-2839, Fax: 716-829-2731, E-mail: dhbrown@buffalo.edu.

The University of Alabama at Birmingham, School of Dentistry, Professional Program in Dentistry, Birmingham, AL 35294. Offers DMD. *Accreditation:* ADA. *Entrance requirements:* For doctorate, DAT, interview. Electronic applications accepted. *Faculty research:* Etiology and pathogenesis of dental diseases, dental biomaterials, therapy of dental diseases.

University of Alberta, Faculty of Medicine and Dentistry, Department of Dentistry, Professional Program in Dentistry, Edmonton, AB T6G 2E1, Canada. Offers DDS. *Accreditation:* ADA. *Entrance requirements:* For doctorate, DAT (Canadian version), interview. Additional exam requirements/recommendations for international students: Required—TOEFL. Electronic applications accepted. *Faculty research:* Oral biology, biochemistry of connective tissues, preventive dentistry, applied clinical orthodontics, biomaterials.

The University of British Columbia, Faculty of Dentistry, Professional Program in Dentistry, Vancouver, BC V6T 1Z1, Canada. Offers DMD. *Accreditation:* ADA. *Entrance requirements:* For doctorate, DAT, ACFD Eligibility Exam, interview, psychomotor assessment. Additional exam requirements/recommendations for international students: Required—IELTS. Electronic applications accepted. *Expenses:* Contact institution.

University of California, Los Angeles, School of Dentistry, Professional Program in Dentistry, Los Angeles, CA 90095. Offers DDS, Certificate, DDS/MS, DDS/PhD, MS/Certificate, PhD/Certificate. *Accreditation:* ADA (one or more programs are accredited). *Entrance requirements:* For doctorate, DAT, interview. Additional exam requirements/recommendations for international students: Required—TOEFL. Electronic applications accepted. *Expenses:* Contact institution.

University of California, San Francisco, School of Dentistry, San Francisco, CA 94143-0150. Offers DDS. *Accreditation:* ADA. *Entrance requirements:* For doctorate, DAT. *Application deadline:* For fall admission, 10/15 for domestic students. Applications are processed on a rolling basis. Application fee: $80 ($100 for international students). *Expenses:* Contact institution. *Financial support:* Fellowships, research assistantships, career-related internships or fieldwork, Federal Work-Study, and institutionally sponsored loans available. Financial award application deadline: 5/1. *Unit head:* John Featherstone, Dean, 415-476-1323, Fax: 415-476-4226. *Application contact:* John Featherstone, Dean, 415-476-1323, Fax: 415-476-4226.
Website: http://dentistry.ucsf.edu/

University of Colorado Denver, School of Dental Medicine, Aurora, CO 80045. Offers dental surgery (DDS); orthodontics (MS); periodontics (MS). *Accreditation:* ADA. *Faculty:* 86 full-time (31 women), 47 part-time/adjunct (17 women). *Students:* 422 full-time (198 women), 5 part-time (2 women); includes 108 minority (7 Black or African American, non-Hispanic/Latino; 3 American Indian or Alaska Native, non-Hispanic/Latino; 60 Asian, non-Hispanic/Latino; 33 Hispanic/Latino; 1 Native Hawaiian or other Pacific Islander, non-Hispanic/Latino; 4 Two or more races, non-Hispanic/Latino), 29 international. Average age 29. In 2013, 18 master's, 88 doctorates awarded. *Entrance requirements:* For master's, GRE, National Board Dental Exam Part I and II, three letters of recommendation, personal essay; for doctorate, DAT, prerequisite courses in microbiology, general biochemistry and English composition (1 semester each); general chemistry/lab, organic chemistry/lab, general biology/lab and general physics/lab (2 semesters each), interview, letters of recommendation, essay. Additional exam requirements/recommendations for international students: Required—TOEFL (minimum score 580 paper-based; 80 iBT); Recommended—IELTS (minimum score 6.8). *Application deadline:* For fall admission, 12/31 for domestic students, 12/15 for international students. Application fee: $50 ($75 for international students). Electronic applications accepted. *Expenses:* Contact institution. *Financial support:* In 2013–14, 83 students received support. Fellowships, research assistantships, teaching assistantships, Federal Work-Study, institutionally sponsored loans, scholarships/grants, and traineeships available. Financial award application deadline: 4/1; financial award applicants required to submit FAFSA. *Faculty research:* Pain control, materials research, geriatric dentistry, restorative dentistry, periodontics. *Total annual research expenditures:* $5 million. *Unit head:* Dr. Denise K. Kassebaum, Dean, 303-724-7100, Fax: 303-724-7109, E-mail: denise.kassebaum@ucdenver.edu. *Application contact:* Graduate Student Admissions, 303-724-7122, Fax: 303-724-7109.
Website: http://www.ucdenver.edu/academics/colleges/dentalmedicine/Pages/DentalMedicine.aspx

University of Connecticut Health Center, School of Dental Medicine, Professional Program in Dental Medicine, Farmington, CT 06030. Offers DMD, Certificate. *Accreditation:* ADA. *Entrance requirements:* For doctorate, National Board Dental Examination. Additional exam requirements/recommendations for international students: Required—TOEFL (minimum score 550 paper-based).

University of Detroit Mercy, School of Dentistry, Professional Program in Dentistry, Detroit, MI 48221. Offers DDS. *Accreditation:* ADA. *Entrance requirements:* For doctorate, DAT. *Faculty research:* Peer evaluation in teaching, evaluation of restorative materials, HIV and periodontal disease.

University of Florida, College of Dentistry, Professional Programs in Dentistry, Gainesville, FL 32611. Offers dentistry (DMD); foreign trained dentistry (Certificate). *Degree requirements:* For Certificate, National Dental Boards Parts I and II. *Entrance requirements:* For doctorate, DAT, interview; for Certificate, interview. Additional exam requirements/recommendations for international students: Required—TOEFL (minimum score 550 paper-based). *Expenses:* Tuition, state resident: full-time $12,640. Tuition, nonresident: full-time $30,000. *Faculty research:* Actinobacillus, critical thinking, DNA adenine, methylase, LJP.

University of Illinois at Chicago, College of Dentistry, Professional Program in Dentistry, Chicago, IL 60607-7128. Offers DDS, DDS/MPH, DDS/PhD. *Accreditation:* ADA. *Faculty:* 90 full-time (31 women). *Students:* 107 full-time (60 women); includes 57 minority (5 Black or African American, non-Hispanic/Latino; 36 Asian, non-Hispanic/Latino; 14 Hispanic/Latino; 2 Two or more races, non-Hispanic/Latino). Average age 27. 1,666 applicants, 5% accepted, 52 enrolled. In 2013, 110 doctorates awarded. *Entrance requirements:* For doctorate, DAT. Additional exam requirements/recommendations for international students: Required—TOEFL. *Application deadline:* For fall admission, 12/1 for domestic and international students. Applications are processed on a rolling basis. Application fee: $40 ($50 for international students). Electronic applications accepted. *Expenses:* Tuition, state resident: full-time $11,066; part-time $3689 per term. Tuition, nonresident: full-time $23,064; part-time $7688 per term. *Required fees:* $3004; $1190 per term. Tuition and fees vary according to course level and program. *Financial support:* Fellowships, research assistantships, and teaching assistantships available. *Unit head:* Dr. Bruce S. Graham, Dean, 312-996-1040, Fax: 312-996-1022. *Application contact:* Jackie Perry, Graduate College Receptionist, 312-413-2550, Fax: 312-413-0185, E-mail: gradcoll@uic.edu.
Website: http://dentistry.uic.edu/

The University of Iowa, College of Dentistry and Graduate College, Graduate Programs in Dentistry, Iowa City, IA 52242-1316. Offers endodontics (MS, Certificate); operative dentistry (MS, Certificate); oral and maxillofacial surgery (MS, PhD, Certificate); oral pathology, radiology and medicine (MS, PhD, Certificate); oral science (MS, PhD); orthodontics (MS, Certificate); pediatric dentistry (Certificate); periodontics (MS, Certificate); preventive and community dentistry (MS), including dental public health; prosthodontics (MS, Certificate). *Accreditation:* ADA. *Degree requirements:* For master's, thesis; for doctorate, thesis/dissertation. *Entrance requirements:* For master's, GRE, DDS; for Certificate, DDS. Additional exam requirements/recommendations for international students: Required—TOEFL. *Expenses:* Contact institution.

The University of Iowa, College of Dentistry, Professional Program in Dentistry, Iowa City, IA 52242-1316. Offers DDS. *Accreditation:* ADA. *Entrance requirements:* For doctorate, DAT, minimum 90 semester hours with minimum GPA of 2.5.

University of Kentucky, College of Dentistry, Lexington, KY 40506-0032. Offers DMD. *Accreditation:* ADA. *Faculty:* 63 full-time (20 women), 38 part-time/adjunct (8 women). *Students:* 233 full-time (110 women); includes 48 minority (13 Black or African American, non-Hispanic/Latino; 17 Asian, non-Hispanic/Latino; 6 Hispanic/Latino; 12 Two or more races, non-Hispanic/Latino), 3 international. Average age 28. 1,706 applicants, 7% accepted, 66 enrolled. In 2013, 56 doctorates awarded. *Entrance requirements:* For doctorate, DAT. *Application deadline:* For fall admission, 12/1 priority date for domestic students. Applications are processed on a rolling basis. Application fee: $75. Electronic applications accepted. *Financial support:* In 2013–14, 162 students received support. Fellowships, research assistantships, teaching assistantships, career-related internships or fieldwork, Federal Work-Study, institutionally sponsored loans, and scholarships/grants available. Support available to part-time students. Financial award application deadline: 4/15; financial award applicants required to submit FAFSA. *Faculty research:* Herpes virus reactivation, chronic oral infection and inflammation of periodontal disease, prevention and control programs, orofacial pain, craniofacial bone biology. *Total annual research expenditures:* $4.1 million. *Unit head:* Dr. Sharon P. Turner, Dean, 859-323-1884, Fax: 859-323-1042. *Application contact:* Melissa D. Lockard, Admissions Coordinator, 859-323-6071, Fax: 859-257-5550, E-mail: mlock2@email.uky.edu.
Website: http://www.mc.uky.edu/Dentistry/

University of Louisville, School of Dentistry, Louisville, KY 40202. Offers dentistry (DMD); oral biology (MS). *Accreditation:* ADA (one or more programs are accredited). Part-time programs available. *Students:* 514 full-time (208 women), 15 part-time (9 women); includes 109 minority (28 Black or African American, non-Hispanic/Latino; 1 American Indian or Alaska Native, non-Hispanic/Latino; 49 Asian, non-Hispanic/Latino; 13 Hispanic/Latino; 1 Native Hawaiian or other Pacific Islander, non-Hispanic/Latino; 17 Two or more races, non-Hispanic/Latino), 25 international. Average age 27. 184 applicants, 88% accepted, 142 enrolled. In 2013, 4 master's, 80 doctorates awarded. *Degree requirements:* For master's, thesis; for doctorate, National Board exams. *Entrance requirements:* For master's, DAT, GRE General Test, or National Board Dental Exam, minimum GPA of 2.75; for doctorate, DAT, 32 hours of course work in science. Additional exam requirements/recommendations for international students: Required—TOEFL (minimum score 100 iBT). *Application deadline:* For fall admission, 1/1 for domestic and international students. Applications are processed on a rolling basis. Application fee: $60. Electronic applications accepted. *Expenses:* Contact institution. *Financial support:* In 2013–14, 1 research assistantship with full tuition reimbursement (averaging $20,000 per year) was awarded. Financial award application deadline: 3/15; financial award applicants required to submit FAFSA. *Faculty research:* Inflammation and periodontitis, birth defects and developmental biology, biomaterials, oral infections, digital imaging. *Total annual research expenditures:* $7.4 million. *Unit head:* Dr. John J. Sauk, Dean, 502-852-1304, Fax: 502-852-3364, E-mail: jjsauk01@louisville.edu. *Application contact:* Robin Benningfield, Admissions Counselor, 502-852-5081, Fax: 502-852-1210, E-mail: dmdadms@louisville.edu.
Website: http://louisville.edu/dental/

The University of Manchester, School of Dentistry, Manchester, United Kingdom. Offers basic dental sciences (cancer studies) (M Phil, PhD); basic dental sciences (molecular genetics) (M Phil, PhD); basic dental sciences (stem cell biology) (M Phil, PhD); biomaterials sciences and dental technology (M Phil, PhD); dental public health/community dentistry (M Phil, PhD); dental science (clinical) (PhD); endodontology (M Phil, PhD); fixed and removable prosthodontics (M Phil, PhD); operative dentistry

(M Phil, PhD); oral and maxillofacial surgery (M Phil, PhD); oral radiology (M Phil, PhD); orthodontics (M Phil, PhD); restorative dentistry (M Phil, PhD).

University of Manitoba, Faculty of Dentistry, Professional Program in Dentistry, Winnipeg, MB R3T 2N2, Canada. Offers DMD. *Accreditation:* ADA. *Entrance requirements:* For doctorate, DAT, interview. *Faculty research:* Oral physiology, microbiology, and biochemistry of the oral cavity in health and disease; application of clinical research.

University of Maryland, Baltimore, Professional and Advanced Education Programs in Dentistry, Baltimore, MD 21201-1627. Offers advanced general dentistry (Certificate); dentistry (DDS); endodontics (Certificate); oral-maxillofacial surgery (Certificate); orthodontics (Certificate); pediatric dentistry (Certificate); periodontics (Certificate); prosthodontics (Certificate); DDS/MBA; DDS/PhD. *Accreditation:* ADA. *Students:* 587 full-time (304 women), 5 part-time (3 women); includes 223 minority (38 Black or African American, non-Hispanic/Latino; 1 American Indian or Alaska Native, non-Hispanic/Latino; 120 Asian, non-Hispanic/Latino; 43 Hispanic/Latino; 21 Two or more races, non-Hispanic/Latino), 28 international. Average age 26. In 2013, 127 doctorates, 29 Certificates awarded. *Entrance requirements:* For doctorate, DAT, coursework in science; for Certificate, National Dental Board Exams, DDS. Additional exam requirements/recommendations for international students: Required—TOEFL (minimum score 550 paper-based; 80 iBT). *Application deadline:* Applications are processed on a rolling basis. Application fee: $85. Electronic applications accepted. *Expenses:* Contact institution. *Financial support:* Career-related internships or fieldwork, Federal Work-Study, scholarships/grants, and traineeships available. Financial award application deadline: 3/1; financial award applicants required to submit FAFSA. *Faculty research:* Pain/neuroscience, oncology/molecular and cell biology, infectious disease/ microbiology, bio-material studies, health promotion and disparities. *Unit head:* Dr. Christian S. Stohler, Dean, 410-706-7461. *Application contact:* Dr. Patricia Meehan, Assistant Dean for Admissions, 410-706-7472, Fax: 410-706-0945, E-mail: ddsadmissions@umaryland.edu.
Website: http://www.dental.umaryland.edu/

University of Michigan, School of Dentistry, Professional Program in Dentistry, Ann Arbor, MI 48109. Offers DDS. *Accreditation:* ADA. *Students:* 439 full-time (195 women); includes 127 minority (13 Black or African American, non-Hispanic/Latino; 94 Asian, non-Hispanic/Latino; 12 Hispanic/Latino; 8 Two or more races, non-Hispanic/Latino). 1,963 applicants, 10% accepted, 108 enrolled. In 2013, 107 doctorates awarded. *Entrance requirements:* For doctorate, DAT, 6 credits of course work in English; 8 credits of course work each in chemistry, organic chemistry, biology, and physics; 3 credits each of biochemistry, microbiology, psychology, and sociology. *Application deadline:* For fall admission, 10/15 for domestic students. Applications are processed on a rolling basis. Application fee: $75. Electronic applications accepted. *Expenses:* Contact institution. *Financial support:* In 2013–14, 364 students received support. Fellowships, research assistantships, teaching assistantships, and scholarships/grants available. Financial award applicants required to submit FAFSA. *Unit head:* Dr. Renee Duff, Assistant Dean for Student Services, 734-763-3313, Fax: 734-764-1922, E-mail: ddsadmissions@umich.edu. *Application contact:* Patricia Katcher, Associate Director of Admissions, 734-763-3316, Fax: 734-764-1922, E-mail: ddsadmissions@umich.edu.
Website: http://www.dent.umich.edu

University of Minnesota, Twin Cities Campus, School of Dentistry, Professional Program in Dentistry, Minneapolis, MN 55455-0213. Offers DDS. *Accreditation:* ADA. *Entrance requirements:* For doctorate, DAT. Additional exam requirements/ recommendations for international students: Required—TOEFL.

University of Mississippi Medical Center, School of Dentistry, Jackson, MS 39216-4505. Offers MS, DMD, PhD. *Accreditation:* ADA. *Entrance requirements:* For doctorate, DAT (for DMD). *Expenses:* Contact institution. *Faculty research:* Bone growth factors, salivary markers of disease, biomaterial synthesis and evaluation, metabolic bone disease, periodontal disease.

University of Missouri–Kansas City, School of Dentistry, Kansas City, MO 64110-2499. Offers advanced education in dentistry (Graduate Dental Certificate); dental hygiene education (MS); dentistry (DDS); endodontics (Graduate Dental Certificate); oral and maxillofacial surgery (Graduate Dental Certificate); oral biology (MS, PhD); orthodontics and dentofacial orthopedics (Graduate Dental Certificate); periodontics (Graduate Dental Certificate). PhD (interdisciplinary) offered through the School of Graduate Studies. *Accreditation:* ADA (one or more programs are accredited). *Faculty:* 97 full-time (45 women), 61 part-time/adjunct (18 women). *Students:* 425 full-time (178 women), 50 part-time (26 women); includes 87 minority (12 Black or African American, non-Hispanic/Latino; 3 American Indian or Alaska Native, non-Hispanic/Latino; 51 Asian, non-Hispanic/Latino; 15 Hispanic/Latino; 6 Two or more races, non-Hispanic/ Latino), 3 international. Average age 27. 807 applicants, 17% accepted, 131 enrolled. In 2013, 10 master's, 106 doctorates, 17 other advanced degrees awarded. *Degree requirements:* For master's, thesis; for doctorate, thesis/dissertation (for some programs). *Entrance requirements:* For master's, DAT, letters of evaluation, personal interview; for doctorate, DAT (for DDS); for Graduate Dental Certificate, DDS. Additional exam requirements/recommendations for international students: Required—TOEFL (minimum score 550 paper-based; 80 iBT). *Application deadline:* For fall admission, 2/1 for domestic and international students. Application fee: $45 ($50 for international students). *Expenses:* Contact institution. *Financial support:* In 2013–14, 2 research assistantships (averaging $23,800 per year) were awarded; career-related internships or fieldwork, Federal Work-Study, institutionally sponsored loans, and tuition waivers (full and partial) also available. Support available to part-time students. Financial award application deadline: 3/1; financial award applicants required to submit FAFSA. *Faculty research:* Biomaterials, dental use of lasers, effectiveness of periodontal treatments, temporomandibular joint dysfunction. *Unit head:* Dr. Marsha Pyle, Dean, 816-235-2010, E-mail: pylem@umkc.edu. *Application contact:* Richard Bigham, Assistant Dean for Student Programs, 816-235-2082, E-mail: bighamr@umkc.edu.
Website: http://dentistry.umkc.edu/

University of Nebraska Medical Center, College of Dentistry, Graduate Programs in Dentistry, Omaha, NE 68198. Offers MS, PhD, Certificate. *Accreditation:* ADA. *Degree requirements:* For Certificate, thesis or alternative. *Entrance requirements:* For degree, GRE or National Board Dental Exam, DDS or DMD. *Expenses: Required fees:* $300 per semester. Tuition and fees vary according to program.

University of Nebraska Medical Center, College of Dentistry, Professional Program in Dentistry, Lincoln, NE 68583-0740. Offers DDS. *Accreditation:* ADA. *Entrance requirements:* For doctorate, DAT. *Expenses:* Contact institution.

University of New England, College of Dental Medicine, Biddeford, ME 04005-9526. Offers DMD. *Faculty:* 5 full-time (1 woman), 6 part-time/adjunct (1 woman). *Students:* 64 full-time (33 women); includes 9 minority (8 Asian, non-Hispanic/Latino; 1 Two or more races, non-Hispanic/Latino), 1 international. Average age 26. 1,135 applicants, 11% accepted, 64 enrolled. *Entrance requirements:* For doctorate, DAT, minimum 30 hours of clinical experience in dental setting. *Application deadline:* For fall admission, 11/1 for domestic and international students. Electronic applications accepted. *Financial support:* Application deadline: 5/1; applicants required to submit FAFSA. *Unit head:* Dr. James Koelbl, Provost/Senior Vice President/Founding Dean, 207-221-4700, Fax: 207-523-1915, E-mail: jkoelbl@une.edu. *Application contact:* Dr. Cynthia Forrest, Vice President for Student Affairs, 207-221-4225, Fax: 207-523-1925, E-mail: gradadmissions@ une.edu.
Website: http://www.une.edu/dentalmedicine/

The University of North Carolina at Chapel Hill, School of Dentistry, Professional Program in Dentistry, Chapel Hill, NC 27599-7450. Offers DDS, DDS/PhD. *Accreditation:* ADA. *Entrance requirements:* For doctorate, DAT, interview. Additional exam requirements/recommendations for international students: Required—TOEFL (minimum score 550 paper-based). Electronic applications accepted. *Expenses:* Contact institution.

University of Oklahoma Health Sciences Center, College of Dentistry, Advanced Education in General Dentistry Program, Oklahoma City, OK 73190. Offers Certificate. *Accreditation:* ADA. Electronic applications accepted. *Expenses:* Tuition, state resident: full-time $3504; part-time $175.20 per credit hour. Tuition, nonresident: full-time $13,504; part-time $675.20 per credit hour. *Required fees:* $1545; $52.70 per credit hour. $245.25 per semester. Tuition and fees vary according to course load.

University of Oklahoma Health Sciences Center, College of Dentistry, Professional Program in Dentistry, Oklahoma City, OK 73190. Offers DDS. *Accreditation:* ADA. *Degree requirements:* For doctorate, National Board Dental Exam Part I and Part II. *Entrance requirements:* For doctorate, DAT, minimum GPA of 2.5; course work in English, general psychology, biology, general chemistry, organic chemistry, physics, and biochemistry. Additional exam requirements/recommendations for international students: Required—TOEFL (minimum score 570 paper-based). Electronic applications accepted. *Expenses:* Tuition, state resident: full-time $3504; part-time $175.20 per credit hour. Tuition, nonresident: full-time $13,504; part-time $675.20 per credit hour. *Required fees:* $1545; $52.70 per credit hour. $245.25 per semester. Tuition and fees vary according to course load. *Faculty research:* Dental caries, microwave sterilization, dental care delivery systems, dental materials, oral health of Native Americans.

University of Pennsylvania, School of Dental Medicine, Philadelphia, PA 19104. Offers DMD, DMD/MS Ed. *Accreditation:* ADA. *Entrance requirements:* For doctorate, DAT. *Expenses:* Contact institution. *Faculty research:* Bone, teeth and extracellular matrix; craniofacial genetic anomalies; infection and host response; periodonatal diseases; stem cells; improvement of tempormandibular function.

University of Pittsburgh, School of Dental Medicine, First Professional Program In Dental Medicine, Pittsburgh, PA 15260. Offers DMD. *Accreditation:* ADA. *Faculty:* 91 full-time (38 women), 194 part-time/adjunct (52 women). *Students:* 317 full-time (137 women); includes 97 minority (12 Black or African American, non-Hispanic/Latino; 1 American Indian or Alaska Native, non-Hispanic/Latino; 71 Asian, non-Hispanic/Latino; 11 Hispanic/Latino; 2 Native Hawaiian or other Pacific Islander, non-Hispanic/Latino), 31 international. Average age 26. 2,024 applicants, 11% accepted, 80 enrolled. In 2013, 75 doctorates awarded. *Entrance requirements:* For doctorate, DAT, minimum GPA of 3.2 (science and non-science). Additional exam requirements/recommendations for international students: Recommended—TOEFL (minimum score 100 iBT). *Application deadline:* For fall admission, 11/1 for domestic and international students. Applications are processed on a rolling basis. Application fee: $50 ($75 for international students). Electronic applications accepted. *Expenses:* Contact institution. *Financial support:* In 2013–14, 93 students received support. Fellowships, teaching assistantships with full tuition reimbursements available, and scholarships/grants available. Financial award application deadline: 4/30; financial award applicants required to submit FAFSA. *Faculty research:* Human genetics, tissue engineering, public health, periodontal disease, cariology. *Total annual research expenditures:* $5.8 million. *Unit head:* Dr. Kenneth Etzel, Associate Dean for Student Services and Admissions, 412-648-8422, Fax: 412-648-9571, E-mail: kre@pitt.edu. *Application contact:* Katherine Adomitis, Student Services and Admissions Assistant, 412-648-8422, Fax: 412-648-9571, E-mail: kaa77@ pitt.edu.
Website: http://www.dental.pitt.edu

University of Pittsburgh, School of Dental Medicine, Residency Programs in Dental Medicine, Advanced Education Program in General Practice Residency, Pittsburgh, PA 15260. Offers Certificate. *Accreditation:* ADA. *Faculty:* 3 full-time (1 woman), 5 part-time/ adjunct (2 women). *Students:* 3 full-time (2 women); includes 2 minority (1 Black or African American, non-Hispanic/Latino; 1 Asian, non-Hispanic/Latino). Average age 28. 33 applicants, 9% accepted, 3 enrolled. In 2013, 3 Certificates awarded. *Application deadline:* For fall admission, 10/15 for domestic students. Application fee: $0. Electronic applications accepted. *Expenses:* Tuition, state resident: full-time $19,964; part-time $807 per credit. Tuition, nonresident: full-time $32,686; part-time $1337 per credit. *Required fees:* $740; $200. Tuition and fees vary according to program. *Unit head:* Dr. Mary Ellen Cuccaro, Program Director, 412-648-6730, Fax: 412-648-6798, E-mail: mec11@pitt.edu. *Application contact:* Andrea M. Ford, Residency Coordinator, 412-648-6801, Fax: 412-648-6835, E-mail: fordam@upmc.edu.

University of Pittsburgh, School of Dental Medicine, Residency Programs in Dental Medicine, Department of Pediatric Dentistry, Pittsburgh, PA 15260. Offers MDS, Certificate. *Accreditation:* ADA. *Faculty:* 3 full-time (all women), 4 part-time/adjunct (2 women). *Students:* 4 full-time (3 women); includes 1 minority (Hispanic/Latino). Average age 28. 46 applicants, 4% accepted, 2 enrolled. *Degree requirements:* For Certificate, clinical research project. *Entrance requirements:* For degree, National Dental Board Exam Parts I and II, U.S. or Canadian dental degree. *Application deadline:* For fall admission, 10/1 for domestic students. Application fee: $35. Electronic applications accepted. *Expenses:* Tuition, state resident: full-time $19,964; part-time $807 per credit. Tuition, nonresident: full-time $32,686; part-time $1337 per credit. *Required fees:* $740; $200. Tuition and fees vary according to program. *Financial support:* In 2013–14, 4 students received support. Stipends available. Financial award application deadline: 7/ 30; financial award applicants required to submit FAFSA. *Faculty research:* Sports dentistry, behavior management, special needs populations, adolescent oral health, infant oral health, genetics, and cariology. *Unit head:* Dr. Deborah A. Studen-Pavlovich, Chair and Professor, 412-648-8183, Fax: 412-648-8435, E-mail: das12@pitt.edu. *Application contact:* Sharon A. Hohman, Departmental Secretary, 412-648-8416, Fax: 412-648-8435, E-mail: sah10@pitt.edu.
Website: http://www.dental.pitt.edu

University of Pittsburgh, School of Dental Medicine, Residency Programs in Dental Medicine, Program in Advanced Education in General Dentistry, Pittsburgh, PA 15260. Offers Certificate. *Accreditation:* ADA. *Faculty:* 4 part-time/adjunct (1 woman). *Students:* 3 full-time (1 woman), 1 international. Average age 27. 35 applicants, 9% accepted, 3 enrolled. In 2013, 3 Certificates awarded. *Entrance requirements:* For degree, National Dental Board Parts I and II, American or Canadian DDS or DMD. *Application deadline:* For fall admission, 12/15 priority date for domestic students. Applications are processed on a rolling basis. Application fee: $50. Electronic applications accepted. *Expenses:* Tuition, state resident: full-time $19,964; part-time $807 per credit. Tuition, nonresident: full-time $32,686; part-time $1337 per credit. *Required fees:* $740; $200. Tuition and fees vary according to program. *Financial support:* In 2013–14, 3 fellowships (averaging $23,000 per year) were awarded. *Unit head:* Dr. Maribeth Krzesinski, Director, 412-648-8093, Fax: 412-383-7796, E-mail: mbk3@pitt.edu. *Application contact:* Aileen

Brasacchio, Administrator, Office of Resident Education, 412-648-8422, Fax: 412-648-8219, E-mail: amb001@pitt.edu.
Website: http://www.dental.pitt.edu/students/residency_program.php

University of Puerto Rico, Medical Sciences Campus, School of Dental Medicine, Professional Program in Dentistry, San Juan, PR 00936-5067. Offers DMD. *Accreditation:* ADA. *Entrance requirements:* For doctorate, DAT, interview. *Expenses:* Contact institution. *Faculty research:* Analgesic drugs, anti-inflammatory drugs, saliva cytoanalysis, dental material and cariology, oral health condition of school-age population.

University of Saskatchewan, College of Dentistry, Saskatoon, SK S7N 5A2, Canada. Offers DMD. *Accreditation:* ADA. *Entrance requirements:* For doctorate, DAT. Additional exam requirements/recommendations for international students: Required—TOEFL (minimum score 550 paper-based; 80 iBT), IELTS (minimum score 6.5), Michigan English Language Assessment Battery (85); CanTEST (4.0); CAEL (60); CPE (C). Electronic applications accepted. *Expenses:* Contact institution. *Faculty research:* Protein structure, oral cavity, immunology, bone densitometry, biological sciences.

University of Southern California, Graduate School, Herman Ostrow School of Dentistry, Professional Program in Dentistry, Los Angeles, CA 90089. Offers DDS, DDS/MBA, DDS/MS. *Accreditation:* ADA (one or more programs are accredited).

The University of Tennessee Health Science Center, College of Dentistry, Memphis, TN 38163-0002. Offers DDS. *Accreditation:* ADA. *Entrance requirements:* For doctorate, DAT, interview, pre-professional evaluation. Additional exam requirements/recommendations for international students: Required—TOEFL. *Application deadline:* For fall admission, 12/31 for domestic and international students. Applications are processed on a rolling basis. Application fee: $50. Electronic applications accepted. *Expenses:* Contact institution. *Financial support:* Federal Work-Study and minority scholarships available. Support available to part-time students. Financial award application deadline: 2/15; financial award applicants required to submit FAFSA. *Faculty research:* Oral cancer, proteomics, inflammation mechanisms, defensins, periopathogens, dental material. *Unit head:* Dr. Timothy L. Hottel, Dean, 901-448-6200, Fax: 901-448-1625, E-mail: thottel@uthsc.edu. *Application contact:* Dr. J. Stansill Covington, III, Associate Dean for Admissions and Student Affairs, 901-448-5560, Fax: 901-448-7772.
Website: http://www.uthsc.edu/dentistry/

The University of Texas Health Science Center at Houston, The University of Texas School of Dentistry at Houston, Houston, TX 77225-0036. Offers MS, DDS. *Accreditation:* ADA. *Faculty:* 86 full-time (38 women), 99 part-time/adjunct (41 women). *Students:* 371 full-time (203 women); includes 177 minority (17 Black or African American, non-Hispanic/Latino; 2 American Indian or Alaska Native, non-Hispanic/Latino; 85 Asian, non-Hispanic/Latino; 73 Hispanic/Latino). Average age 25. 1,454 applicants, 11% accepted, 100 enrolled. In 2013, 86 doctorates awarded. *Entrance requirements:* For doctorate, DAT, 90 semester hours of prerequisite courses. *Application deadline:* For fall admission, 10/1 for domestic students. Applications are processed on a rolling basis. Application fee: $140. Electronic applications accepted. *Expenses:* Tuition, state resident: full-time $3474; part-time $193 per credit hour. Tuition, nonresident: full-time $13,644; part-time $758 per credit hour. *Required fees:* $226.30; $87 per credit hour. *Financial support:* In 2013–14, 288 students received support. Institutionally sponsored loans and scholarships/grants available. Financial award application deadline: 3/1; financial award applicants required to submit FAFSA. *Faculty research:* Salivary diagnostics, autoimmune disease, mucosal immunity, craniofacial anomalies, molecular imaging, bioengineering. *Unit head:* Dr. John A. Valenza, Dean, 713-486-4021, Fax: 713-486-4089. *Application contact:* Dr. H. Philip Pierpont, Associate Dean for Student and Alumni Affairs, 713-486-4151, Fax: 713-486-4425.
Website: http://www.db.uth.tmc.edu

The University of Texas Health Science Center at San Antonio, Dental School, San Antonio, TX 78229-3900. Offers MS, DDS, Certificate, DDS/PhD. *Accreditation:* ADA (one or more programs are accredited). *Faculty:* 117 full-time (34 women), 76 part-time/adjunct (18 women). *Students:* 500 full-time (241 women), 41 part-time (20 women); includes 230 minority (9 Black or African American, non-Hispanic/Latino; 1 American Indian or Alaska Native, non-Hispanic/Latino; 126 Asian, non-Hispanic/Latino; 79 Hispanic/Latino; 15 Two or more races, non-Hispanic/Latino), 38 international. Average age 28. 1,874 applicants, 13% accepted, 124 enrolled. In 2013, 23 master's, 97 doctorates awarded. *Degree requirements:* For master's, thesis; for doctorate, comprehensive exam. *Entrance requirements:* For master's, GRE General Test, DDS; for doctorate, DAT; for Certificate, National Board Part 1 and Part 2, DDS. Additional exam requirements/recommendations for international students: Required—TOEFL (minimum score 92 iBT). *Application deadline:* For fall admission, 10/1 for domestic and international students. Application fee: $140. *Financial support:* In 2013–14, 265 students received support. Institutionally sponsored loans and scholarships/grants available. Financial award application deadline: 3/1; financial award applicants required to submit FAFSA. *Faculty research:* Neuropharmacology, periodontal disease, biomaterials, bone mineralization, caries prevention. *Total annual research expenditures:* $6.3 million. *Unit head:* Dr. Adriana Segura, Associate Dean for Student Affairs, 210-567-3180, Fax: 210-567-4776, E-mail: seguraa@uthscsa.edu. *Application contact:* E-mail: dsadmissions@uthscsa.edu.
Website: http://dental.uthscsa.edu/

University of the Pacific, Arthur A. Dugoni School of Dentistry, Stockton, CA 95211-0197. Offers MSD, DDS, Certificate. *Accreditation:* ADA (one or more programs are accredited). *Faculty:* 73 full-time (19 women), 197 part-time/adjunct (78 women). *Students:* 513 full-time (246 women); includes 279 minority (1 Black or African American, non-Hispanic/Latino; 1 American Indian or Alaska Native, non-Hispanic/Latino; 224 Asian, non-Hispanic/Latino; 35 Hispanic/Latino; 1 Native Hawaiian or other Pacific Islander, non-Hispanic/Latino; 17 Two or more races, non-Hispanic/Latino), 32 international. Average age 26. 3,016 applicants, 8% accepted, 141 enrolled. In 2013, 4 master's, 166 doctorates awarded. *Degree requirements:* For master's, comprehensive exam, thesis. *Entrance requirements:* For master's, GRE General Test; for doctorate, National Board Dental Exam Part I, DAT, foreign dental degree (for international students); for Certificate, DDS/DMD. Additional exam requirements/recommendations for international students: Required—TOEFL. *Application deadline:* For fall admission, 9/15 priority date for international students. Applications are processed on a rolling basis. Electronic applications accepted. *Expenses:* Contact institution. *Financial support:* Institutionally sponsored loans, scholarships/grants, and stipends available. Support available to part-time students. Financial award application deadline: 3/2; financial award applicants required to submit FAFSA. *Faculty research:* Cell kinetics, cell membrane transport, orthodontics, virus cell membrane fusion, bioenergy transduction. *Unit head:* Patrick J. Ferrillo, Jr., Dean, 415-929-6425. *Application contact:* Dr. Craig S. Yarborough, Associate Dean for Institutional Advancement and Student Services, 415-929-6431.
Website: http://dental.pacific.edu/

University of Toronto, School of Graduate Studies, Faculty of Dentistry, Professional Program in Dentistry, Toronto, ON M5S 1A1, Canada. Offers DDS. *Accreditation:* ADA. *Entrance requirements:* For doctorate, Canadian DAT or equivalent, minimum GPA of 3.0; completion of at least 2 courses in life sciences and 1 course in humanities or social sciences. Additional exam requirements/recommendations for international students: Required—TOEFL (minimum score 600 paper-based; 100 iBT), TWE (minimum score 5). Electronic applications accepted. *Expenses:* Contact institution.

University of Utah, School of Dentistry, Salt Lake City, UT 84112. Offers DDS. *Accreditation:* ADA. *Faculty:* 1 (woman) full-time, 6 part-time/adjunct (0 women). *Students:* 20 full-time (4 women); includes 2 minority (1 Hispanic/Latino; 1 Two or more races, non-Hispanic/Latino). Average age 25. 775 applicants, 3% accepted, 20 enrolled. *Entrance requirements:* For doctorate, DAT, minimum overall and science GPA of 3.3. *Application deadline:* For fall admission, 12/31 priority date for domestic students, 12/31 for international students. Application fee: $75. Electronic applications accepted. *Expenses:* Contact institution. *Financial support:* Application deadline: 4/1; applicants required to submit FAFSA. *Unit head:* Rena N. D'Souza, PhD, Dean, 801-587-1199, Fax: 801-585-6485, E-mail: rena.dsouza@hsc.utah.edu. *Application contact:* Gary W. Lowder, DDS, Office of Admissions, 801-581-8951, Fax: 801-585-6485, E-mail: dental.admissions@hsc.utah.edu.
Website: http://dentistry.utah.edu/

University of Washington, Graduate School, School of Dentistry, Program in Dental Surgery, Seattle, WA 98195. Offers DDS. *Accreditation:* ADA. *Entrance requirements:* For doctorate, DAT.

The University of Western Ontario, Schulich School of Medicine and Dentistry, School of Dentistry, Professional Program in Dentistry, London, ON N6A 5B8, Canada. Offers DDS. *Accreditation:* ADA. *Entrance requirements:* For doctorate, DAT (Canadian version), minimum B average.

Virginia Commonwealth University, Medical College of Virginia-Professional Programs, School of Dentistry, Richmond, VA 23284-9005. Offers MS, DDS, DDS/MS, DDS/PhD. *Accreditation:* ADA. *Entrance requirements:* For master's, National Board Dental Exam; for doctorate, DAT. Electronic applications accepted. *Expenses:* Contact institution.

Western University of Health Sciences, College of Dental Medicine, Pomona, CA 91766-1854. Offers DMD. *Accreditation:* ADA. *Faculty:* 34 full-time (14 women), 23 part-time/adjunct (7 women). *Students:* 283 full-time (125 women); includes 162 minority (4 Black or African American, non-Hispanic/Latino; 1 American Indian or Alaska Native, non-Hispanic/Latino; 118 Asian, non-Hispanic/Latino; 19 Hispanic/Latino; 1 Native Hawaiian or other Pacific Islander, non-Hispanic/Latino; 19 Two or more races, non-Hispanic/Latino), 8 international. Average age 28. 2,339 applicants, 9% accepted, 66 enrolled. In 2013, 64 doctorates awarded. *Entrance requirements:* For doctorate, DAT, minimum 30 hours of dental-related work experience; minimum 90 semester or 135 quarter units of undergraduate/graduate coursework; letters of recommendation. Additional exam requirements/recommendations for international students: Required—TOEFL (minimum score 550 paper-based; 79 iBT). *Application deadline:* For fall admission, 12/1 for domestic students. Applications are processed on a rolling basis. Application fee: $60. Electronic applications accepted. *Unit head:* Dr. Steven Friedrichsen, Dean, 909-706-3911, E-mail: sfriedrichsen@westernu.edu. *Application contact:* Marie Anderson, Director of Admissions, 909-469-5335, Fax: 909-469-5570, E-mail: admissions@westernu.edu.
Website: http://www.westernu.edu/dentistry/

West Virginia University, School of Dentistry, Professional Program in Dentistry, Morgantown, WV 26506. Offers DDS. *Accreditation:* ADA. *Degree requirements:* For doctorate, comprehensive exam. *Entrance requirements:* For doctorate, DAT, letters of recommendation, interview. Additional exam requirements/recommendations for international students: Required—TOEFL (minimum score 500 paper-based).

Oral and Dental Sciences

A.T. Still University, Arizona School of Dentistry and Oral Health, Mesa, AZ 85206. Offers dental medicine (DMD); orthodontics (Certificate). *Faculty:* 40 full-time (18 women), 127 part-time/adjunct (42 women). *Students:* 310 full-time (142 women), 3 part-time (2 women); includes 122 minority (13 Black or African American, non-Hispanic/Latino; 4 American Indian or Alaska Native, non-Hispanic/Latino; 71 Asian, non-Hispanic/Latino; 19 Hispanic/Latino; 2 Native Hawaiian or other Pacific Islander, non-Hispanic/Latino; 13 Two or more races, non-Hispanic/Latino). Average age 27. 3,543 applicants, 4% accepted, 76 enrolled. In 2013, 65 doctorates, 3 Certificates awarded. *Degree requirements:* For doctorate, National Board Exams I and II. *Entrance requirements:* For doctorate, DAT, minimum GPA of 2.5 overall and in science. Additional exam requirements/recommendations for international students: Recommended—TOEFL. *Application deadline:* For fall admission, 12/1 for domestic and international students; for summer admission, 11/15 for domestic students. Applications are processed on a rolling basis. Application fee: $70. Electronic applications accepted. *Expenses:* Contact institution. *Financial support:* In 2013–14, 31 students received support. Federal Work-Study and scholarships/grants available. Financial award application deadline: 5/1; financial award applicants required to submit FAFSA. *Faculty research:* Evidence-based dentistry in clinical practice, xerostomia and malnutrition in assisted living settings, medical screening in the dental office: patient attitudes, rapid oral HIV screening in the dental setting, dental public health: early childhood caries, self-efficacy and oral health. *Unit head:* Dr. Jack Dillenberg, Dean, 480-219-6000, Fax: 480-219-6110, E-mail: jdillenberg@atsu.edu. *Application contact:* Donna Sparks, Associate Director, Admissions Processing, 660-626-2117, Fax: 660-626-2969, E-mail: admissions@atsu.edu.
Website: http://www.atsu.edu/asdoh

A.T. Still University, School of Health Management, Kirksville, MO 63501. Offers dental public health (MPH); health administration (MHA, DHA); health education (DH Ed); public health (MPH). Part-time and evening/weekend programs available.

Postbaccalaureate distance learning degree programs offered (no on-campus study). *Faculty:* 20 full-time (10 women), 49 part-time/adjunct (27 women). *Students:* 164 full-time (123 women), 256 part-time (144 women); includes 143 minority (61 Black or African American, non-Hispanic/Latino; 4 American Indian or Alaska Native, non-Hispanic/Latino; 46 Asian, non-Hispanic/Latino; 25 Hispanic/Latino; 3 Native Hawaiian or other Pacific Islander, non-Hispanic/Latino; 4 Two or more races, non-Hispanic/Latino), 12 international. Average age 34. 154 applicants, 93% accepted, 114 enrolled. In 2013, 132 master's, 13 doctorates awarded. *Degree requirements:* For master's, thesis, integrated terminal project, practicum; for doctorate, thesis/dissertation. *Entrance requirements:* For master's, minimum GPA of 3.0, bachelor's degree or equivalent, background check, essay, three references; for doctorate, minimum GPA of 3.0, master's or terminal degree, background check, essay, three references. Additional exam requirements/recommendations for international students: Required—TOEFL (minimum score 550 paper-based; 80 iBT). *Application deadline:* For fall admission, 5/31 for domestic and international students; for winter admission, 8/2 for domestic and international students; for spring admission, 11/8 for domestic and international students; for summer admission, 1/24 for domestic and international students. Application fee: $70. Electronic applications accepted. *Expenses:* Contact institution. *Financial support:* Scholarships/grants available. Financial award application deadline: 5/1; financial award applicants required to submit FAFSA. *Faculty research:* Public health: influence of availability of comprehensive wellness resources online, student wellness, oral health care needs assessment of community, oral health knowledge and behaviors of Medicaid-eligible pregnant women and mothers of young children in relations to early childhood caries and tooth decay, alcohol use and alcohol related problems among college students. *Unit head:* Dr. Donald Altman, Interim Dean, 660-626-2820, Fax: 660-626-2826, E-mail: daltman@atsu.edu. *Application contact:* Sarah Spencer, Associate Director, Admissions, 660-626-2820 Ext. 2669, Fax: 660-626-2826, E-mail: sspencer@atsu.edu.
Website: http://www.atsu.edu/shm

Boston University, Henry M. Goldman School of Dental Medicine, Boston, MA 02118. Offers advanced general dentistry (CAGS); dental public health (MS, MSD, D Sc D, CAGS); dentistry (DMD); endodontics (MSD, D Sc D, CAGS); operative dentistry (MSD, D Sc D, CAGS); oral and maxillofacial surgery (MSD, D Sc D, CAGS); oral biology (MSD, D Sc, D Sc D, PhD); orthodontics (MSD, D Sc D, CAGS); pediatric dentistry (MSD, D Sc D, CAGS); periodontology (MSD, D Sc D, CAGS); prosthodontics (MSD, D Sc D, CAGS). *Accreditation:* ADA (one or more programs are accredited). *Faculty:* 119 full-time (53 women), 83 part-time/adjunct (24 women). *Students:* 818 full-time (423 women); includes 158 minority (8 Black or African American, non-Hispanic/Latino; 1 American Indian or Alaska Native, non-Hispanic/Latino; 102 Asian, non-Hispanic/Latino; 40 Hispanic/Latino; 7 Two or more races, non-Hispanic/Latino), 359 international. Average age 28. 6,681 applicants, 8% accepted, 263 enrolled. In 2013, 14 master's, 199 doctorates, 55 other advanced degrees awarded. *Degree requirements:* For master's and CAGS, thesis; for doctorate, thesis/dissertation (for some programs). *Entrance requirements:* For doctorate, DAT (for DMD), minimum recommended GPA of 3.0 (for DMD); for CAGS, National Board Dental Exam Part 1, dental degree. Additional exam requirements/recommendations for international students: Required—TOEFL. *Application deadline:* For fall admission, 12/1 for domestic and international students. Applications are processed on a rolling basis. Application fee: $75 ($105 for international students). Electronic applications accepted. *Expenses:* Contact institution. *Financial support:* In 2013–14, 480 students received support. Career-related internships or fieldwork, institutionally sponsored loans, and stipends and scholarships (for Advanced Education in General Dentistry and Oral and Maxillofacial Surgery residents) available. Financial award application deadline: 4/15; financial award applicants required to submit FAFSA. *Faculty research:* Defense mechanisms, bone-cell regulation, protein biochemistry, molecular biology, biomaterials. *Unit head:* Dr. Jeffrey W. Hutter, Dean, 617-638-4780. *Application contact:* Admissions Representative, 617-638-4787, Fax: 617-638-4798, E-mail: sdmadmis@bu.edu.
Website: http://www.bu.edu/dental

Boston University, School of Medicine, Division of Graduate Medical Sciences, Program in Oral Biology, Boston, MA 02215. Offers PhD. *Degree requirements:* For doctorate, thesis/dissertation. *Application deadline:* For fall admission, 1/15 priority date for domestic students; for spring admission, 10/15 for domestic students. *Expenses: Tuition:* Full-time $43,970; part-time $1374 per credit hour. *Required fees:* $60 per semester. Tuition and fees vary according to class time, course level and program. *Unit head:* Dr. Phillip Trackman, Director, 617-638-4942, E-mail: trackman@bu.edu. *Application contact:* GMS Admissions Office, 617-638-5255, Fax: 617-638-5740, E-mail: natashah@bu.edu.
Website: http://www.bu.edu/dental-research/student-research/phd-in-oral-biology/

Boston University, School of Medicine, Division of Graduate Medical Sciences, Program in Oral Health Sciences, Boston, MA 02118. Offers MS. *Degree requirements:* For master's, capstone project or thesis. *Entrance requirements:* For master's, DAT. Electronic applications accepted. *Expenses: Tuition:* Full-time $43,970; part-time $1374 per credit hour. *Required fees:* $60 per semester. Tuition and fees vary according to class time, course level and program. *Unit head:* Dr. Theresa A. Davies, Director, 618-638-5242, E-mail: tdavies@bu.edu. *Application contact:* GMS Office of Admissions, 617-638-5255, Fax: 617-638-5740.
Website: http://www.bumc.bu.edu/gms/oral-health-masters/

Case Western Reserve University, School of Dental Medicine and School of Graduate Studies, Advanced Specialty Education Programs in Dentistry, Cleveland, OH 44106. Offers advanced general dentistry (Certificate); endodontics (MSD, Certificate); oral surgery (Certificate); orthodontics (MSD, Certificate); pedodontics (MSD, Certificate); periodontics (MSD, Certificate). *Degree requirements:* For master's, thesis. *Entrance requirements:* For master's, National Dental Board Exam, DDS, minimum GPA of 3.0; for Certificate, DDS. Additional exam requirements/recommendations for international students: Required—TOEFL (minimum score 550 paper-based; 79 iBT). *Expenses:* Contact institution. *Faculty research:* Natural antibiotics, obesity and periodontal disease, perioninfection and CV disease, periodontal disease and overall health, 3D cone beam computerized tomography.

Columbia University, College of Dental Medicine and Graduate School of Arts and Sciences, Programs in Dental Specialties, New York, NY 10027. Offers advanced education in general dentistry (Certificate); biomedical informatics (MA, PhD); endodontics (Certificate); orthodontics (MS, Certificate); periodontics (MS, Certificate); prosthodontics (MS, Certificate); science education (MA). *Degree requirements:* For master's, thesis, presentation of seminar. *Entrance requirements:* For master's, GRE General Test, DDS or equivalent. *Expenses:* Contact institution. *Faculty research:* Analysis of growth/form, pulpal microcirculation, implants, microbiology of oral environment, calcified tissues.

Dalhousie University, Faculty of Dentistry, Department of Oral and Maxillofacial Surgery, Halifax, NS B3H 3J5, Canada. Offers MD/M Sc. Electronic applications accepted. *Expenses:* Contact institution. *Faculty research:* Cleft lip/palate, jaw biomechanics.

Georgia Regents University, The Graduate School, Program in Oral Biology and Maxillofacial Pathology, Augusta, GA 30912. Offers MS, PhD. Part-time programs available. *Degree requirements:* For master's, thesis; for doctorate, thesis/dissertation. *Entrance requirements:* For master's and doctorate, GRE General Test or DAT, DDS, DMD, or equivalent degree. Additional exam requirements/recommendations for international students: Required—TOEFL (minimum score 550 paper-based; 79 iBT). Electronic applications accepted. *Faculty research:* Oral cancer and chemoprevention, properties of biomaterials including oxidative stress, mechanical stress and shear stress responses, taurine and blood pressure in diabetes, bone and dentin biology, induction of periodontal regeneration.

Harvard University, Graduate School of Arts and Sciences, Program in Biological Sciences in Dental Medicine, Cambridge, MA 02138. Offers PhD. *Expenses: Tuition:* Full-time $38,888. *Required fees:* $958. Tuition and fees vary according to campus/location, program and student level.

Harvard University, School of Dental Medicine, Advanced Graduate Programs in Dentistry, Cambridge, MA 02138. Offers advanced general dentistry (Certificate); dental public health (Certificate); endodontics (Certificate); general practice residency (Certificate); oral biology (M Med Sc, D Med Sc); oral implantology (Certificate); oral medicine (Certificate); oral pathology (Certificate); oral surgery (Certificate); orthodontics (Certificate); pediatric dentistry (Certificate); periodontics (Certificate); prosthodontics (Certificate). *Expenses: Tuition:* Full-time $38,888. *Required fees:* $958. Tuition and fees vary according to campus/location, program and student level.

Howard University, College of Dentistry, Washington, DC 20059-0002. Offers advanced education program general dentistry (Certificate); dentistry (DDS); general dentistry (Certificate); oral and maxillofacial surgery (Certificate); orthodontics (Certificate); pediatric dentistry (Certificate). *Accreditation:* ADA (one or more programs are accredited). *Degree requirements:* For doctorate, comprehensive exam, didactic and clinical exams. *Entrance requirements:* For doctorate, DAT, 8 semester hours of course work in each biology, inorganic chemistry, organic chemistry. *Expenses:* Contact institution. *Faculty research:* Epidemiological, biomaterial, molecular genetic, behavioral modification, and clinical trial studies.

Idaho State University, Office of Graduate Studies, Kasiska College of Health Professions, Department of Dental Sciences, Pocatello, ID 83209-8088. Offers advanced general dentistry (Post-Doctoral Certificate). First year of Idaho Dental Education Program available in conjunction with Creighton University's School of Dentistry. *Degree requirements:* For Post-Doctoral Certificate, comprehensive exam, thesis optional, 1-year residency. *Entrance requirements:* For degree, DAT, 3 dental application forms. Additional exam requirements/recommendations for international students: Required—TOEFL (minimum score 600 paper-based). Electronic applications accepted. *Expenses:* Contact institution.

Jacksonville University, School of Orthodontics, Jacksonville, FL 32211. Offers Certificate. *Entrance requirements:* Additional exam requirements/recommendations for international students: Required—TOEFL. *Expenses:* Contact institution.

Loma Linda University, School of Dentistry, Program in Endodontics, Loma Linda, CA 92350. Offers MS, Certificate, MS/Certificate. *Degree requirements:* For master's, thesis. *Entrance requirements:* For master's, GRE General Test, DDS or DMD, minimum GPA of 3.0, National Boards. Additional exam requirements/recommendations for international students: Required—TOEFL (minimum score 550 paper-based).

Loma Linda University, School of Dentistry, Program in Implant Dentistry, Loma Linda, CA 92350. Offers MS, Certificate, MS/Certificate. *Degree requirements:* For master's, thesis. *Entrance requirements:* For master's, GRE General Test, DDS or DMD, minimum GPA of 3.0.

Loma Linda University, School of Dentistry, Program in Oral and Maxillofacial Surgery, Loma Linda, CA 92350. Offers MS, Certificate, MS/Certificate. *Degree requirements:* For master's, thesis. *Entrance requirements:* For master's, GRE General Test, DDS or DMD, minimum GPA of 3.0.

Loma Linda University, School of Dentistry, Program in Orthodontics, Loma Linda, CA 92350. Offers MS, Certificate, MS/Certificate. *Degree requirements:* For master's, thesis. *Entrance requirements:* For master's, GRE General Test, DDS or DMD, minimum GPA of 3.0. Additional exam requirements/recommendations for international students: Required—TOEFL (minimum score 550 paper-based).

Loma Linda University, School of Dentistry, Program in Periodontics, Loma Linda, CA 92350. Offers MS. *Degree requirements:* For master's, thesis. *Entrance requirements:* For master's, GRE General Test, DDS or DMD, minimum GPA of 3.0. Additional exam requirements/recommendations for international students: Required—TOEFL (minimum score 550 paper-based).

Marquette University, School of Dentistry and Graduate School, Graduate Programs in Dentistry, Program in Advanced Training in General Dentistry, Milwaukee, WI 53201-1881. Offers MS, Certificate. *Faculty:* 2 full-time (1 woman), 2 part-time/adjunct (0 women). *Students:* 4 full-time (2 women), 2 international. Average age 31. 27 applicants, 15% accepted, 4 enrolled. In 2013, 4 other advanced degrees awarded. *Entrance requirements:* For master's, National Board Dental Exams I and II, DDS or equivalent. Additional exam requirements/recommendations for international students: Required—TOEFL. *Application deadline:* For fall admission, 10/1 for domestic students, 9/1 for international students. Application fee: $50. *Financial support:* In 2013–14, fellowships with partial tuition reimbursements (averaging $35,000 per year) were awarded; institutionally sponsored loans also available. Financial award application deadline: 9/1; financial award applicants required to submit FAFSA. *Unit head:* Dr. T. Gerry Bradley, Professor and Chair, 414-288-5480. *Application contact:* Dr. Joseph Vitolo, Clinical Associate Professor/Director, 414-288-3640.
Website: http://www.marquette.edu/dentistry/admissions/AEGD.shtml

Marquette University, School of Dentistry and Graduate School, Graduate Programs in Dentistry, Program in Dental Biomaterials, Milwaukee, WI 53201-1881. Offers MS. Part-time programs available. *Faculty:* 1 full-time (0 women). *Students:* 1 (woman) full-time, 3 part-time (all women); all minorities (1 American Indian or Alaska Native, non-Hispanic/Latino; 3 Hispanic/Latino), 3 international. Average age 31. 15 applicants, 47% accepted, 2 enrolled. In 2013, 1 master's awarded. *Degree requirements:* For master's, thesis. *Entrance requirements:* For master's, GRE General Test. Additional exam requirements/recommendations for international students: Required—TOEFL. *Application deadline:* For spring admission, 3/1 priority date for domestic and international students. Applications are processed on a rolling basis. Application fee: $50. *Financial support:* Fellowships, career-related internships or fieldwork, institutionally sponsored loans, and tuition waivers (partial) available. Financial award application deadline: 9/1. *Faculty research:* Metallurgy, ceramics, polymers, mechanical behavior, cements. *Unit head:* Dr. T. Gerry Bradley, Professor and Chair, 414-288-5480. *Application contact:* Dr. David Berzins, Associate Professor and Director, 414-288-5690.
Website: http://www.marquette.edu/dentistry/admissions/DentalBiomaterials.shtml

Marquette University, School of Dentistry and Graduate School, Graduate Programs in Dentistry, Program in Endodontics, Milwaukee, WI 53201-1881. Offers MS, Certificate. *Faculty:* 1 full-time (0 women), 4 part-time/adjunct (0 women). *Students:* 6 full-time (3 women), 3 international. Average age 32. 46 applicants, 7% accepted, 3 enrolled. In 2013, 3 master's awarded. *Degree requirements:* For master's, research thesis or acceptance of a paper in a peer-reviewed journal. *Entrance requirements:* For master's,

National Board Dental Exams I and II, DDS or equivalent. Additional exam requirements/recommendations for international students: Required—TOEFL. *Application deadline:* For fall admission, 9/1 priority date for domestic and international students. Application fee: $50. *Expenses:* Contact institution. *Financial support:* Fellowships, institutionally sponsored loans, and tuition waivers (partial) available. Financial award application deadline: 9/1; financial award applicants required to submit FAFSA. *Faculty research:* Properties of NiTi files, prevention of post-endodontic pain. *Unit head:* Dr. T. Gerry Bradley, Professor and Chair, 414-288-5480. *Application contact:* Dr. Sheila Stover, Clinical Associate Professor, 414-288-8393.
Website: http://www.marquette.edu/dentistry/admissions/Endodontics.shtml

Marquette University, School of Dentistry and Graduate School, Graduate Programs in Dentistry, Program in Orthodontics, Milwaukee, WI 53201-1881. Offers MS, Certificate. *Faculty:* 3 full-time (0 women), 11 part-time/adjunct (0 women). *Students:* 10 full-time (7 women); includes 3 minority (1 Black or African American, non-Hispanic/Latino; 1 Asian, non-Hispanic/Latino; 1 Two or more races, non-Hispanic/Latino), 1 international. Average age 27. 145 applicants, 3% accepted, 5 enrolled. In 2013, 5 master's awarded. *Degree requirements:* For master's, thesis. *Entrance requirements:* For master's, National Board Dental Exams I and II, DDS or equivalent. Additional exam requirements/recommendations for international students: Required—TOEFL. *Application deadline:* For fall admission, 9/1 priority date for domestic and international students. Application fee: $50. *Expenses:* Contact institution. *Financial support:* Fellowships, institutionally sponsored loans, and tuition waivers (partial) available. Financial award application deadline: 9/1; financial award applicants required to submit FAFSA. *Faculty research:* In vitro and in vivo behavior of orthodontic wires, effect of orthodontic treatment on facial esthetics. *Unit head:* Dr. T. Gerry Bradley, Professor and Chair, 414-288-5480, Fax: 414-288-3586, E-mail: thomas.bradley@marquette.edu. *Application contact:* Dr. T. Gerry Bradley, Professor and Chair, 414-288-5480, Fax: 414-288-3586, E-mail: thomas.bradley@marquette.edu.
Website: http://www.marquette.edu/dentistry/admissions/Mission_000.shtml

Marquette University, School of Dentistry and Graduate School, Graduate Programs in Dentistry, Program in Prosthodontics, Milwaukee, WI 53201-1881. Offers MS, Certificate. *Faculty:* 2 full-time (1 woman), 2 part-time/adjunct (0 women). *Students:* 7 full-time (4 women); includes 1 minority (Asian, non-Hispanic/Latino), 4 international. Average age 28. 15 applicants. In 2013, 3 master's awarded. *Degree requirements:* For master's, thesis or alternative. *Entrance requirements:* For master's, National Board Dental Exams I and II, DDS or equivalent. Additional exam requirements/recommendations for international students: Required—TOEFL. *Application deadline:* For fall admission, 9/1 priority date for domestic and international students. Application fee: $50. *Financial support:* Fellowships, institutionally sponsored loans, and tuition waivers (partial) available. Financial award application deadline: 9/1; financial award applicants required to submit FAFSA. *Faculty research:* Properties of ceramic materials. *Unit head:* Dr. T. Gerry Bradley, Professor and Chair, 414-288-5480. *Application contact:* Dr. Geoffrey Thompson, Assistant Professor and Director, 414-288-8415, E-mail: arthur.hefti@marquette.edu.
Website: http://www.marquette.edu/dentistry/admissions/Prosthodontics.shtml

McGill University, Faculty of Graduate and Postdoctoral Studies, Faculty of Dentistry, Montréal, QC H3A 2T5, Canada. Offers forensic dentistry (Certificate); oral and maxillofacial surgery (M Sc, PhD).

Metropolitan State University, College of Health, Community and Professional Studies, St. Paul, MN 55106-5000. Offers advanced dental therapy (MS); leadership and management (MSN); nurse educator (MSN); nursing (DNP); psychology (MA). *Accreditation:* AACN. Part-time programs available. *Degree requirements:* For master's, thesis or alternative; for doctorate, thesis/dissertation or alternative. *Entrance requirements:* For master's, GRE General Test, minimum GPA of 3.0, RN license, BS/BA; for doctorate, minimum GPA of 3.0; RN license, MSN. Additional exam requirements/recommendations for international students: Required—TOEFL (minimum score 550 paper-based). *Expenses:* Tuition, state resident: full-time $5548. Tuition, nonresident: full-time $10,929. *Faculty research:* Women's health, gerontology.

New York University, College of Dentistry and College of Dentistry, Department of Biomaterials and Biomimetics, New York, NY 10012-1019. Offers biomaterials science (MS). *Faculty:* 5 full-time (2 women). *Students:* 229 full-time (137 women), 45 part-time (23 women); includes 47 minority (11 Black or African American, non-Hispanic/Latino; 1 American Indian or Alaska Native, non-Hispanic/Latino; 24 Asian, non-Hispanic/Latino; 10 Hispanic/Latino; 1 Two or more races, non-Hispanic/Latino), 79 international. Average age 30. 32 applicants, 100% accepted, 32 enrolled. In 2013, 28 master's awarded. *Degree requirements:* For master's, thesis. *Entrance requirements:* For master's, GRE. Additional exam requirements/recommendations for international students: Required—TOEFL. *Application deadline:* For fall admission, 5/1 for domestic and international students; for spring admission, 10/1 for domestic and international students. Application fee: $95. *Expenses: Tuition:* Full-time $35,856; part-time $1494 per unit. *Required fees:* $1408; $64 per unit. $473 per term. Tuition and fees vary according to course load and program. *Financial support:* Application deadline: 5/1; applicants required to submit FAFSA. *Faculty research:* Calcium phosphate, composite restoratives, surfactants, dental metallurgy, impression materials. *Unit head:* Dr. John L. Ricci, Director of Graduate Studies, 212-998-9703, Fax: 212-995-4244, E-mail: gsas.graduate.biomaterials@nyu.edu. *Application contact:* Carmen Chilsom, Department Administrator, 212-998-9703, Fax: 212-995-4244, E-mail: graduate.biomaterials@nyu.edu.
Website: http://www.nyu.edu/gsas/program/biomaterials/

New York University, College of Dentistry, Postgraduate Programs in Dentistry, New York, NY 10010. Offers endodontics (Advanced Certificate); oral and maxillofacial surgery (Advanced Certificate); orthodontics (Advanced Certificate); pediatric dentistry (Advanced Certificate); periodontics (Advanced Certificate); prosthodontics (Advanced Certificate). *Faculty:* 242 full-time (85 women), 689 part-time/adjunct (186 women). *Students:* 110 full-time (51 women); includes 35 minority (2 Black or African American, non-Hispanic/Latino; 22 Asian, non-Hispanic/Latino; 11 Hispanic/Latino), 30 international. Average age 31. 567 applicants, 8% accepted, 38 enrolled. In 2013, 35 Advanced Certificates awarded. *Entrance requirements:* For degree, National Dental Boards Exam Part I, DDS. Additional exam requirements/recommendations for international students: Required—TOEFL (minimum score 587 paper-based; 95 iBT). *Application deadline:* For fall admission, 12/1 for domestic students. Application fee: $100. Electronic applications accepted. *Expenses: Tuition:* Full-time $35,856; part-time $1494 per unit. *Required fees:* $1408; $64 per unit. $473 per term. Tuition and fees vary according to course load and program. *Financial support:* Scholarships/grants and unspecified assistantships available. Financial award application deadline: 3/1; financial award applicants required to submit FAFSA. *Unit head:* Dr. Andrea Schreiber, Dean, College of Dentistry, 212-998-9624, Fax: 212-995-4240, E-mail: andrea.schreiber@nyu.edu. *Application contact:* Dr. Eugenia E. Mejia, Senior Director of Admissions, 212-998-9818, Fax: 212-995-4240, E-mail: dental.admissions@nyu.edu.
Website: http://www.nyu.edu/dental/

New York University, Graduate School of Arts and Science, Department of Biology, New York, NY 10012-1019. Offers biology (PhD); biomedical journalism (MS); cancer and molecular biology (PhD); computational biology (PhD); computers in biological research (MS); developmental genetics (PhD); general biology (MS); immunology and microbiology (PhD); molecular genetics (PhD); neurobiology (PhD); oral biology (MS); plant biology (PhD); recombinant DNA technology (MS); MS/MBA. Part-time programs available. *Faculty:* 24 full-time (5 women). *Students:* 161 full-time (88 women), 28 part-time (15 women); includes 41 minority (5 Black or African American, non-Hispanic/Latino; 23 Asian, non-Hispanic/Latino; 9 Hispanic/Latino; 4 Two or more races, non-Hispanic/Latino), 80 international. Average age 27. 412 applicants, 54% accepted, 65 enrolled. In 2013, 77 master's, 9 doctorates awarded. Terminal master's awarded for partial completion of doctoral program. *Degree requirements:* For master's, thesis or alternative, qualifying paper; for doctorate, comprehensive exam, thesis/dissertation. *Entrance requirements:* For master's and doctorate, GRE General Test. Additional exam requirements/recommendations for international students: Required—TOEFL. *Application deadline:* For fall admission, 12/1 priority date for domestic students, 12/1 for international students. Application fee: $95. *Expenses: Tuition:* Full-time $35,856; part-time $1494 per unit. *Required fees:* $1408; $64 per unit. $473 per term. Tuition and fees vary according to course load and program. *Financial support:* Fellowships with tuition reimbursements, research assistantships with tuition reimbursements, teaching assistantships with tuition reimbursements, career-related internships or fieldwork, Federal Work-Study, institutionally sponsored loans, scholarships/grants, health care benefits, and unspecified assistantships available. Financial award application deadline: 12/1; financial award applicants required to submit FAFSA. *Faculty research:* Genomics, molecular and cell biology, development and molecular genetics, molecular evolution of plants and animals. *Unit head:* Stephen Small, Chair, 212-998-8200, Fax: 212-995-4015, E-mail: biology.admissions@nyu.edu. *Application contact:* Justin Blau, Director of Graduate Studies, PhD Programs, 212-998-8200, Fax: 212-995-4015, E-mail: biology.admissions@nyu.edu.
Website: http://biology.as.nyu.edu/

The Ohio State University, College of Dentistry, Columbus, OH 43210. Offers dental anesthesiology (MS); dental hygiene (MDH); dentistry (DDS); endodontics (MS); oral and maxillofacial pathology (MS); oral and maxillofacial surgery (MS); oral biology (PhD); orthodontics (MS); pediatric dentistry (MS); periodontology (MS); prosthodontics (MS); DDS/PhD. *Accreditation:* ADA (one or more programs are accredited). *Faculty:* 75. *Students:* 510 full-time (220 women), 7 part-time (4 women); includes 89 minority (12 Black or African American, non-Hispanic/Latino; 51 Asian, non-Hispanic/Latino; 16 Hispanic/Latino; 10 Two or more races, non-Hispanic/Latino), 26 international. Average age 26. In 2013, 17 master's, 105 doctorates awarded. Terminal master's awarded for partial completion of doctoral program. *Degree requirements:* For master's, thesis; for doctorate, thesis/dissertation (for some programs). *Entrance requirements:* For master's, GRE General Test (for all applicants with cumulative GPA below 3.0); for doctorate, DAT (for DDS); GRE General Test, GRE Subject Test in biology recommended (for PhD). Additional exam requirements/recommendations for international students: Required—TOEFL (minimum score 550 paper-based; 79 iBT), Michigan English Language Assessment Battery (minimum score 82), IELTS (minimum score 7) for MS and PhD; TOEFL (minimum score 577 paper-based; 90 iBT), Michigan English Language Assessment Battery (minimum score 84), IELTS (minimum score 7.5) for DDS. *Application deadline:* Applications are processed on a rolling basis. Electronic applications accepted. *Expenses:* Contact institution. *Financial support:* Fellowships with tuition reimbursements, research assistantships with tuition reimbursements, teaching assistantships with tuition reimbursements, Federal Work-Study, and institutionally sponsored loans available. Financial award application deadline: 2/15. *Faculty research:* Neurobiology, inflammation and immunity, materials science, bone biology. *Total annual research expenditures:* $3.4 million. *Unit head:* Dr. Patrick M. Lloyd, Dean, 614-292-9755, E-mail: lloyd.256@osu.edu. *Application contact:* Graduate and Professional Admissions, 614-292-9444, Fax: 614-292-3656.
Website: http://www.dent.osu.edu/

Oregon Health & Science University, School of Dentistry, Graduate Programs in Dentistry, Department of Endodontics, Portland, OR 97239-3098. Offers Certificate. *Entrance requirements:* For degree, GRE General Test. Additional exam requirements/recommendations for international students: Required—TOEFL.

Oregon Health & Science University, School of Dentistry, Graduate Programs in Dentistry, Department of Orthodontics, Portland, OR 97239-3098. Offers MS, Certificate. *Degree requirements:* For master's, thesis. *Entrance requirements:* For master's and Certificate, GRE General Test, DMD/DDS. Additional exam requirements/recommendations for international students: Required—TOEFL.

Oregon Health & Science University, School of Dentistry, Graduate Programs in Dentistry, Department of Pediatric Dentistry, Portland, OR 97239-3098. Offers Certificate.

Oregon Health & Science University, School of Dentistry, Graduate Programs in Dentistry, Department of Periodontology, Portland, OR 97239-3098. Offers MS, Certificate. *Degree requirements:* For master's, thesis. *Entrance requirements:* For master's and Certificate, GRE General Test, DMD/DDS. Additional exam requirements/recommendations for international students: Required—TOEFL.

Oregon Health & Science University, School of Dentistry, Graduate Programs in Dentistry, Department of Restorative Dentistry, Division of Biomaterials and Biomechanics, Portland, OR 97239-3098. Offers MS.

Oregon Health & Science University, School of Dentistry, Graduate Programs in Dentistry, Program in Oral Molecular Biology, Portland, OR 97239-3098. Offers MS.

Oregon Health & Science University, School of Dentistry, Professional Program in Dentistry, Portland, OR 97239-3098. Offers dentistry (DMD); oral and maxillofacial surgery (Certificate); MD/DMD. *Accreditation:* ADA. *Entrance requirements:* For doctorate, DAT. Electronic applications accepted. *Faculty research:* Dentin permeability, tooth sensations, fluoride metabolism, immunology of periodontal disease, craniofacial growth.

Rutgers, The State University of New Jersey, Newark, Rutgers School of Dental Medicine, Newark, NJ 07101-1709. Offers dental science (MS); dentistry (DMD); endodontics (Certificate); oral medicine (Certificate); orthodontics (Certificate); pediatric dentistry (Certificate); periodontics (Certificate); prosthodontics (Certificate); DMD/MPH; DMD/PhD; MD/Certificate; MS/Certificate. DMD/MPH offered jointly with New Jersey Institute of Technology, Rutgers, The State University of New Jersey, Camden. *Accreditation:* ADA (one or more programs are accredited). *Entrance requirements:* For doctorate, DAT. Electronic applications accepted. *Expenses:* Contact institution.

Saint Louis University, Graduate Education, Center for Advanced Dental Education, St. Louis, MO 63103-2097. Offers endodontics (MSD); orthodontics (MSD); periodontics (MSD). *Degree requirements:* For master's, comprehensive exam, thesis, teaching practicum. *Entrance requirements:* For master's, GRE General Test, NBDE (National Board Dental Exam), DDS or DMD, interview, letters of recommendation. Additional exam requirements/recommendations for international students: Required—TOEFL (minimum score 525 paper-based). Electronic applications accepted. *Faculty research:* Craniofacial growth.

Seton Hill University, Program in Orthodontics, Greensburg, PA 15601. Offers MS. *Faculty:* 3 full-time (0 women), 9 part-time/adjunct (1 woman). *Students:* 22 full-time (8

women); includes 3 minority (1 Black or African American, non-Hispanic/Latino; 2 Asian, non-Hispanic/Latino). Average age 31. 129 applicants, 8% accepted, 10 enrolled. *Entrance requirements:* Additional exam requirements/recommendations for international students: Required—TOEFL (minimum score 650 paper-based; 114 iBT), IELTS (minimum score 7). *Application deadline:* For fall admission, 9/15 priority date for domestic students, 9/15 for international students. *Expenses: Tuition:* Full-time $14,220; part-time $790 per credit. *Required fees:* $700; $34 per credit. $50 per semester. *Faculty research:* Biomechanics and orthodontic tooth movement, self-ligating brackets, occlusion and TMD (Temporomandibular Disorder), clear aligners used in orthodontics, perceptions of discomfort during orthodontic treatment, patient perceptions of orthodontic treatment outcomes, oral hygiene protocols in orthodontics. *Unit head:* Dr. Donald Rinchuse, Director, 724-652-2950, E-mail: rinchuse@setonhill.edu. *Application contact:* Meghan Kennedy, Orthodontic Center Business Manager, 724-652-2997, E-mail: mkennedy@setonhill.edu.
Website: http://www.setonhill.edu/academics/graduate_programs/orthodontics

Stony Brook University, State University of New York, Stony Brook University Medical Center, Health Sciences Center, School of Dental Medicine and Graduate School, Department of Oral Biology and Pathology, Stony Brook, NY 11794. Offers MS, PhD. *Faculty:* 10 full-time (5 women), 1 (woman) part-time/adjunct. *Students:* 4 full-time (3 women), 1 (woman) part-time; includes 1 minority (Asian, non-Hispanic/Latino), 3 international. Average age 34. 5 applicants, 20% accepted. *Degree requirements:* For doctorate, thesis/dissertation. *Entrance requirements:* For doctorate, GRE General Test. Additional exam requirements/recommendations for international students: Required—TOEFL. *Application deadline:* For fall admission, 1/15 for domestic students; for spring admission, 10/1 for domestic students. Application fee: $100. *Expenses:* Contact institution. *Financial support:* In 2013–14, 2 fellowships, 1 research assistantship were awarded; teaching assistantships and Federal Work-Study also available. Financial award application deadline: 3/15. *Faculty research:* Oral biology, oral diseases, pathology, dentistry, dental health and hygiene, periodontal diseases, stem cells, therapeutics, oral tissues and organs. *Total annual research expenditures:* $1.3 million. *Unit head:* Dr. Maria E. Ryan, Chair, 631-632-9529, E-mail: maria.ryan@stonybrook.edu. *Application contact:* Marguerite Baldwin, Coordinator, 631-632-9189, Fax: 631-632-9707, E-mail: marguerite.baldwin@stonybrook.edu.
Website: http://www.stonybrookmedicalcenter.org/dental/oralbiology

Stony Brook University, State University of New York, Stony Brook University Medical Center, Health Sciences Center, School of Dental Medicine, Professional Program in Dental Medicine, Stony Brook, NY 11794. Offers dental medicine (DDS); endodontics (Certificate); orthodontics (Certificate); periodontics (Certificate). *Accreditation:* ADA (one or more programs are accredited). *Faculty:* 29 full-time (12 women), 69 part-time/adjunct (18 women). *Students:* 184 full-time (94 women); includes 47 minority (3 Black or African American, non-Hispanic/Latino; 35 Asian, non-Hispanic/Latino; 7 Hispanic/Latino; 2 Two or more races, non-Hispanic/Latino), 2 international. Average age 25. 1,113 applicants, 7% accepted, 42 enrolled. In 2013, 36 doctorates awarded. *Entrance requirements:* For doctorate, DAT. *Application deadline:* For fall admission, 1/15 for domestic students. Application fee: $100. *Expenses:* Tuition, state resident: full-time $9870; part-time $411 per credit. Tuition, nonresident: full-time $18,350; part-time $765 per credit. *Financial support:* Research assistantships, teaching assistantships, and Federal Work-Study available. Support available to part-time students. *Total annual research expenditures:* $2.8 million. *Unit head:* Dr. Mary R. Truhlar, Interim Dean, 631-632-8950, Fax: 631-632-9105. *Application contact:* Patricia Berry, Acting Director of Admissions, 631-632-8871, Fax: 631-632-7130, E-mail: patricia.berry@stonybrook.edu.
Website: http://dentistry.stonybrookmedicine.edu/

Temple University, Kornberg School of Dentistry and Graduate School, Graduate Programs in Dentistry, Philadelphia, PA 19122-6096. Offers advanced education in general dentistry (Certificate); endodontology (Certificate); oral biology (MS); orthodontics (Certificate); periodontology (Certificate). *Degree requirements:* For master's, thesis; for Certificate, comprehensive exam. *Entrance requirements:* For master's, GRE; for Certificate, National Boards Parts I and II, DMD or DDS, 3 letters of recommendation. Additional exam requirements/recommendations for international students: Required—TOEFL (minimum score 650 paper-based). *Expenses:* Contact institution. *Faculty research:* Saliva and salivary glands, implantology, material science, periodontal disease, geriatric dentistry.

Texas A&M Health Science Center, Baylor College of Dentistry, Department of Diagnostic Sciences, College Station, TX 77840. Offers oral and maxillofacial pathology (MS, PhD, Certificate). Part-time programs available. Terminal master's awarded for partial completion of doctoral program. *Degree requirements:* For master's, thesis; for doctorate, thesis/dissertation. *Entrance requirements:* For master's and doctorate, GRE General Test, DDS or DMD; for Certificate, GRE General Test, National Board Dental Examination, DDS or DMD. Additional exam requirements/recommendations for international students: Required—TOEFL. *Faculty research:* Oral cancer and precancer, odontogenic tumors, stomatology.

Texas A&M Health Science Center, Baylor College of Dentistry, Department of Endodontics, College Station, TX 77840. Offers endodontics (PhD, Certificate); health professions education (MS); oral biology (MS). *Degree requirements:* For master's, thesis; for doctorate, thesis/dissertation. *Entrance requirements:* For master's and Certificate, GRE General Test, National Board Dental Examination, DDS or DMD; for doctorate, GRE General Test, DDS or DMD. Additional exam requirements/recommendations for international students: Required—TOEFL. *Faculty research:* Periradicular healing in response to a biologically inductive root-end filling material.

Texas A&M Health Science Center, Baylor College of Dentistry, Department of Oral and Maxillofacial Surgery, College Station, TX 77840. Offers MD, Certificate. MD offered jointly with Texas Tech University. *Degree requirements:* For Certificate, thesis. *Entrance requirements:* For doctorate, DAT, MCAT; for Certificate, GRE General Test, National Board Dental Examination, DDS or DMD. Additional exam requirements/recommendations for international students: Required—TOEFL. *Faculty research:* Dental implants, temporomandibular joint, recombinant BMP-2.

Texas A&M Health Science Center, Baylor College of Dentistry, Department of Orthodontics, College Station, TX 77840. Offers MS, Certificate. *Degree requirements:* For master's and Certificate, thesis. *Entrance requirements:* For master's and Certificate, GRE General Test, National Board Dental Examination, DDS or DMD. Additional exam requirements/recommendations for international students: Required—TOEFL. *Faculty research:* Craniofacial biology, distraction osteogenesis, clinical orthodontics, function and shape memory alloys.

Texas A&M Health Science Center, Baylor College of Dentistry, Department of Pediatric Dentistry, College Station, TX 77840. Offers MS, Certificate. Part-time programs available. *Degree requirements:* For master's and Certificate, thesis. *Entrance requirements:* For master's and Certificate, GRE General Test, National Board Dental Examination, DDS or DMD. Additional exam requirements/recommendations for international students: Required—TOEFL. *Faculty research:* Pulp biology, pharmacological methods of behavior management.

Texas A&M Health Science Center, Baylor College of Dentistry, Department of Periodontics, College Station, TX 77840. Offers MS, Certificate. Part-time programs available. *Degree requirements:* For master's and Certificate, thesis. *Entrance requirements:* For master's and Certificate, GRE General Test, National Board Dental Examination, DDS or DMD. Additional exam requirements/recommendations for international students: Required—TOEFL. *Faculty research:* Dental implants, quantification of &ITcandida albicans&RO in adult periodontitis: a survey, smoking, wound healing, stomatology, gingival overgrowth, diabetes mellitus.

Texas A&M Health Science Center, Baylor College of Dentistry, Department of Restorative Sciences, Field of Prosthodontics, College Station, TX 77840. Offers MS, Certificate. Part-time programs available. *Degree requirements:* For master's, thesis. *Entrance requirements:* For master's and Certificate, GRE General Test, National Board Dental Examination, DDS or DMD. Additional exam requirements/recommendations for international students: Required—TOEFL. *Faculty research:* Biomaterials, implants.

Tufts University, School of Dental Medicine, Advanced Education Programs in Dental Medicine, Medford, MA 02155. Offers dentistry (Certificate), including endodontics, oral and maxillofacial surgery, orthodontics, pediatric dentistry, periodontology, prosthodontics. *Entrance requirements:* Additional exam requirements/recommendations for international students: Required—TOEFL. *Expenses:* Contact institution.

Tufts University, School of Dental Medicine, Graduate Programs in Dental Medicine, Medford, MA 02155. Offers MS. *Degree requirements:* For master's, thesis. *Entrance requirements:* For master's, DDS, DMD, or equivalent; minimum B average. Additional exam requirements/recommendations for international students: Required—TOEFL. *Expenses:* Contact institution. *Faculty research:* Periodontal research, dental materials, salivary research, epidemiology, bone biology.

Université de Montréal, Faculty of Dental Medicine, Program in Multidisciplinary Residency, Montréal, QC H3C 3J7, Canada. Offers Certificate. Electronic applications accepted.

Université de Montréal, Faculty of Dental Medicine, Program in Oral and Dental Sciences, Montréal, QC H3C 3J7, Canada. Offers M Sc. Electronic applications accepted.

Université de Montréal, Faculty of Dental Medicine, Program in Orthodontics, Montréal, QC H3C 3J7, Canada. Offers M Sc. Electronic applications accepted.

Université de Montréal, Faculty of Dental Medicine, Program in Pediatric Dentistry, Montréal, QC H3C 3J7, Canada. Offers M Sc. Electronic applications accepted.

Université de Montréal, Faculty of Dental Medicine, Program in Prosthodontics Rehabilitation, Montréal, QC H3C 3J7, Canada. Offers M Sc. Electronic applications accepted.

Université Laval, Faculty of Dentistry, Diploma Program in Buccal and Maxillofacial Surgery, Québec, QC G1K 7P4, Canada. Offers DESS. *Degree requirements:* For DESS, comprehensive exam. *Entrance requirements:* For degree, interview, knowledge of French. Electronic applications accepted.

Université Laval, Faculty of Dentistry, Diploma Program in Gerodontology, Québec, QC G1K 7P4, Canada. Offers DESS. Part-time programs available. *Entrance requirements:* For degree, interview, good knowledge of French. Electronic applications accepted.

Université Laval, Faculty of Dentistry, Diploma Program in Multidisciplinary Dentistry, Québec, QC G1K 7P4, Canada. Offers DESS. *Entrance requirements:* For degree, interview, knowledge of French. Electronic applications accepted.

Université Laval, Faculty of Dentistry, Diploma Program in Periodontics, Québec, QC G1K 7P4, Canada. Offers DESS. *Entrance requirements:* For degree, interview, knowledge of French. Electronic applications accepted.

Université Laval, Faculty of Dentistry, Graduate Program in Dentistry, Québec, QC G1K 7P4, Canada. Offers M Sc. *Degree requirements:* For master's, thesis (for some programs). Electronic applications accepted.

University at Buffalo, the State University of New York, Graduate School, School of Dental Medicine, Graduate Programs in Dental Medicine, Department of Oral Biology, Buffalo, NY 14260. Offers PhD. *Students:* 5 full-time (4 women), 4 international. Average age 28. 19 applicants, 11% accepted, 2 enrolled. In 2013, 4 doctorates awarded. *Degree requirements:* For doctorate, thesis/dissertation. *Entrance requirements:* For doctorate, GRE General Test. Additional exam requirements/recommendations for international students: Required—TOEFL (minimum score 550 paper-based; 79 iBT). *Application deadline:* For fall admission, 2/1 priority date for domestic and international students. Application fee: $50. Electronic applications accepted. *Financial support:* Fellowships with full tuition reimbursements, research assistantships with full and partial tuition reimbursements, Federal Work-Study, institutionally sponsored loans, scholarships/grants, and traineeships available. Financial award applicants required to submit FAFSA. *Faculty research:* Oral immunology and microbiology, bone physiology, biochemistry, molecular genetics, neutrophil biology. *Unit head:* Dr. Mira Edgerton, Program Director, 716-829-2854, Fax: 716-829-3942, E-mail: edgerto@buffalo.edu. *Application contact:* Kristin Yager, Admissions Secretary, 716-829-2839, Fax: 716-829-2731, E-mail: kmyager2@buffalo.edu.

University at Buffalo, the State University of New York, Graduate School, School of Dental Medicine, Graduate Programs in Dental Medicine, Department of Orthodontics, Buffalo, NY 14260. Offers MS, Certificate. *Faculty:* 3 full-time (1 woman), 3 part-time/adjunct (1 woman). *Students:* 20 full-time (6 women); includes 2 minority (both Asian, non-Hispanic/Latino), 7 international. Average age 25. 130 applicants, 5% accepted, 6 enrolled. In 2013, 4 master's awarded. *Degree requirements:* For master's, thesis. *Entrance requirements:* For master's, GRE General Test, National Board Dental Exam, DDS or equivalent. Additional exam requirements/recommendations for international students: Required—TOEFL (minimum score 550 paper-based; 79 iBT). *Application deadline:* For fall admission, 9/1 for domestic and international students. Application fee: $50. Electronic applications accepted. *Faculty research:* Stem cell, clinical respiration, growth and development. *Unit head:* Dr. C. Brian Preston, Program Director/Chair, 716-829-2845, Fax: 716-829-2572, E-mail: cbp@buffalo.edu. *Application contact:* Kristin Yager, Admissions Secretary, 716-829-2839, Fax: 716-829-2731, E-mail: kmyager2@buffalo.edu.

University at Buffalo, the State University of New York, Graduate School, School of Dental Medicine, Graduate Programs in Dental Medicine, Program in Biomaterials, Buffalo, NY 14260. Offers MS. Part-time programs available. *Faculty:* 11 full-time (4 women), 15 part-time/adjunct (4 women). *Students:* 13 full-time (5 women); includes 1 minority (Black or African American, non-Hispanic/Latino), 8 international. Average age 28. 23 applicants, 17% accepted, 3 enrolled. In 2013, 3 master's awarded. *Degree requirements:* For master's, thesis. *Entrance requirements:* For master's, GRE General Test. Additional exam requirements/recommendations for international students: Required—TOEFL (minimum score 550 paper-based; 79 iBT). *Application deadline:* For fall admission, 4/1 priority date for domestic students, 2/1 for international students; for spring admission, 9/1 priority date for domestic students, 8/1 for international students. Applications are processed on a rolling basis. Application fee: $50. Electronic applications accepted. *Financial support:* Research assistantships with full and partial tuition reimbursements, Federal Work-Study, institutionally sponsored loans, scholarships/grants, and unspecified assistantships available. Financial award applicants required to submit FAFSA. *Faculty research:* Orofacial pain, surface science, bioadhesion, ontology, oral medicine. *Unit head:* Dr. Robert E. Baier, Program Director, 716-645-3560, Fax: 716-829-3554, E-mail: baier@buffalo.edu. *Application contact:* Dr. Anne E. Meyer, Associate Dean for Research, 716-829-3560, Fax: 716-829-3554, E-mail: aemeyer@buffalo.edu.

University at Buffalo, the State University of New York, Graduate School, School of Dental Medicine, Graduate Programs in Dental Medicine, Program in Oral Sciences, Buffalo, NY 14260. Offers MS. *Faculty:* 28 full-time (12 women), 2 part-time/adjunct (both women). *Students:* 11 full-time (5 women), 24 part-time (9 women); includes 2 minority (1 Asian, non-Hispanic/Latino; 1 Hispanic/Latino), 30 international. Average age 31. 81 applicants, 20% accepted, 14 enrolled. In 2013, 11 master's awarded. *Degree requirements:* For master's, thesis. *Entrance requirements:* For master's, DDS, DMD or equivalent foreign degree. Additional exam requirements/recommendations for international students: Required—TOEFL (minimum score 550 paper-based; 79 iBT). *Application deadline:* For fall admission, 2/1 priority date for domestic and international students. Applications are processed on a rolling basis. Application fee: $50. Electronic applications accepted. *Financial support:* Research assistantships with full and partial tuition reimbursements, scholarships/grants, and traineeships available. Financial award applicants required to submit FAFSA. *Faculty research:* Oral biology and pathology, behavioral sciences, neuromuscular physiology, facial pain, oral microbiology. *Unit head:* Dr. Ernesto DeNardin, Director, 716-829-3998, Fax: 716-829-2387, E-mail: denardin@buffalo.edu. *Application contact:* Kristin Yager, Admissions Secretary, 716-829-2839, Fax: 716-829-2731, E-mail: kmyager2@buffalo.edu.

The University of Alabama at Birmingham, School of Dentistry, Graduate Programs in Dentistry, Birmingham, AL 35294. Offers MS. *Degree requirements:* For master's, thesis.

University of Alberta, Faculty of Medicine and Dentistry, Department of Dentistry, Program in Orthodontics, Edmonton, AB T6G 2E1, Canada. Offers M Sc, PhD. *Degree requirements:* For master's, thesis; for doctorate, thesis/dissertation. *Entrance requirements:* Additional exam requirements/recommendations for international students: Required—TOEFL (minimum score 580 paper-based). Electronic applications accepted.

The University of British Columbia, Faculty of Dentistry and Faculty of Graduate Studies, Graduate/Postgraduate and Professional Specialty Programs in Dentistry, Vancouver, BC V6T 1Z1, Canada. Offers dental science (M Sc, PhD); periodontics (Diploma). *Degree requirements:* For master's, thesis; for doctorate, comprehensive exam, thesis/dissertation. *Entrance requirements:* For degree, dental license, interview. Additional exam requirements/recommendations for international students: Required—TOEFL (minimum score 580 paper-based). Electronic applications accepted. *Expenses:* Contact institution. *Faculty research:* Cell biology, oral physiology, microbiology, immunology, biomaterials.

University of California, Los Angeles, Graduate Division, College of Letters and Science and David Geffen School of Medicine, UCLA ACCESS to Programs in the Molecular, Cellular and Integrative Life Sciences, Los Angeles, CA 90095. Offers biochemistry and molecular biology (PhD); biological chemistry (PhD); cellular and molecular pathology (PhD); human genetics (PhD); microbiology, immunology, and molecular genetics (PhD); molecular biology (PhD); molecular toxicology (PhD); molecular, cellular and integrative physiology (PhD); neurobiology (PhD); oral biology (PhD); physiology (PhD). *Degree requirements:* For doctorate, thesis/dissertation, oral and written qualifying exams. *Entrance requirements:* For doctorate, GRE General Test, bachelor's degree; minimum undergraduate GPA of 3.0 (or its equivalent if letter grade system not used). Additional exam requirements/recommendations for international students: Required—TOEFL. Electronic applications accepted.

University of California, Los Angeles, School of Dentistry and Graduate Division, Graduate Programs in Dentistry, Program in Oral Biology, Los Angeles, CA 90095. Offers MS, PhD, DDS/MS, DDS/PhD, MD/PhD, MS/Certificate, PhD/Certificate. *Degree requirements:* For master's, thesis; for doctorate, thesis/dissertation, oral and written qualifying exams; 1 quarter of teaching experience. *Entrance requirements:* For master's and doctorate, GRE General Test, bachelor's degree; minimum undergraduate GPA of 3.0 (or its equivalent if letter grade system not used). Additional exam requirements/recommendations for international students: Required—TOEFL. Electronic applications accepted.

University of California, San Francisco, Graduate Division, Program in Oral and Craniofacial Sciences, San Francisco, CA 94143. Offers MS, PhD. Terminal master's awarded for partial completion of doctoral program. *Degree requirements:* For master's, thesis; for doctorate, thesis/dissertation. *Entrance requirements:* For master's and doctorate, GRE General Test. Application fee: $40. *Expenses:* Tuition, state resident: full-time $11,220. Tuition, nonresident: full-time $26,322. *Required fees:* $5204. Full-time tuition and fees vary according to degree level and program. *Financial support:* Application deadline: 1/10. *Unit head:* Peter Sargent, Associate Dean for Academic Affairs, 415-476-8922, E-mail: peter.sargent@ucst.edu. *Application contact:* Daliah Williams, Admissions Coordinator, 415-476-1749, Fax: 415-476-4226, E-mail: daliah.williams@ucst.edu.
Website: http://dentistry.ucsf.edu/science-research/ogra/oral-craniofacial-sciences-graduate-program

University of Colorado Denver, School of Dental Medicine, Aurora, CO 80045. Offers dental surgery (DDS); orthodontics (MS); periodontics (MS). *Accreditation:* ADA. *Faculty:* 86 full-time (31 women), 47 part-time/adjunct (17 women). *Students:* 422 full-time (198 women), 5 part-time (2 women); includes 108 minority (7 Black or African American, non-Hispanic/Latino; 3 American Indian or Alaska Native, non-Hispanic/Latino; 60 Asian, non-Hispanic/Latino; 33 Hispanic/Latino; 1 Native Hawaiian or other Pacific Islander, non-Hispanic/Latino; 4 Two or more races, non-Hispanic/Latino), 29 international. Average age 29. In 2013, 18 master's, 88 doctorates awarded. *Entrance requirements:* For master's, GRE, National Board Dental Exam Part I and II, three letters of recommendation, personal essay; for doctorate, DAT, prerequisite courses in microbiology, general biochemistry and English composition (1 semester each); general chemistry/lab, organic chemistry/lab, general biology/lab and general physics/lab (2 semesters each), interview, letters of recommendation, essay. Additional exam requirements/recommendations for international students: Required—TOEFL (minimum score 580 paper-based; 80 iBT); Recommended—IELTS (minimum score 6.8). *Application deadline:* For fall admission, 12/31 for domestic students, 12/15 for international students. Application fee: $50 ($75 for international students). Electronic applications accepted. *Expenses:* Contact institution. *Financial support:* In 2013–14, 83 students received support. Fellowships, research assistantships, teaching assistantships, Federal Work-Study, institutionally sponsored loans, scholarships/grants, and traineeships available. Financial award application deadline: 4/1; financial award applicants required to submit FAFSA. *Faculty research:* Pain control, materials research, geriatric dentistry, restorative dentistry, periodontics. *Total annual research expenditures:* $5 million. *Unit head:* Dr. Denise K. Kassebaum, Dean, 303-724-7100, Fax: 303-724-7109, E-mail: denise.kassebaum@ucdenver.edu. *Application contact:* Graduate Student Admissions, 303-724-7122, Fax: 303-724-7109.
Website: http://www.ucdenver.edu/academics/colleges/dentalmedicine/Pages/DentalMedicine.aspx

University of Connecticut, Graduate School, University of Connecticut Health Center, Field of Dental Science, Storrs, CT 06269. Offers M Dent Sc. *Degree requirements:* For master's, comprehensive exam. *Entrance requirements:* For master's, GRE General Test. Additional exam requirements/recommendations for international students: Required—TOEFL (minimum score 550 paper-based). Electronic applications accepted.

University of Connecticut Health Center, Graduate School, Programs in Biomedical Sciences, Combined Degree Programs in Oral Biology, Farmington, CT 06030. Offers DMD/PhD. *Entrance requirements:* Additional exam requirements/recommendations for international students: Required—TOEFL (minimum score 600 paper-based).

University of Connecticut Health Center, Graduate School, Programs in Biomedical Sciences, Program in Skeletal, Craniofacial and Oral Biology, Farmington, CT 06030. Offers PhD, DMD/PhD, MD/PhD. *Degree requirements:* For doctorate, comprehensive exam, thesis/dissertation. *Entrance requirements:* For doctorate, GRE General Test. Additional exam requirements/recommendations for international students: Required—TOEFL (minimum score 600 paper-based). Electronic applications accepted. *Faculty research:* Skeletal development and patterning, bone biology, connective tissue biology, neurophysiology of taste and smell, microbiological aspects of caries.

See Display on next page and Close-Up on page 913.

University of Connecticut Health Center, School of Dental Medicine, Program in Dental Science, Farmington, CT 06030. Offers MDS. Part-time programs available. *Degree requirements:* For master's, comprehensive exam, thesis. *Entrance requirements:* For master's, National Board Dental Examination Parts I and II. *Expenses:* Contact institution.

University of Detroit Mercy, School of Dentistry, Department of Endodontics, Detroit, MI 48221. Offers MS, Certificate. *Degree requirements:* For master's, thesis. *Entrance requirements:* For master's, DDS or DMD; for Certificate, DAT, DDS or DMD. *Faculty research:* Roof and filling materials, cavity preparations, pulp biology.

University of Detroit Mercy, School of Dentistry, Department of Orthodontics, Detroit, MI 48221. Offers MS, Certificate. *Degree requirements:* For master's, thesis. *Entrance requirements:* For master's, DDS or DMD; for Certificate, DAT, DDS or DMD. *Faculty research:* Changes in oral flora due to fixed orthodontic appliances, cranioskeletal osteogenesis.

University of Detroit Mercy, School of Dentistry, Department of Periodontology and Dental Hygiene, Detroit, MI 48221. Offers periodontics (MS, Certificate).

University of Florida, College of Dentistry and Graduate School, Graduate Programs in Dentistry, Department of Endodontics, Gainesville, FL 32611. Offers MS, Certificate. *Entrance requirements:* For master's, DAT, GRE General Test, National Board Dental Examination Parts I and II, minimum GPA of 3.0, interview; for Certificate, DAT. Additional exam requirements/recommendations for international students: Required—TOEFL (minimum score 550 paper-based). *Expenses:* Tuition, state resident: full-time $12,640. Tuition, nonresident: full-time $30,000. *Faculty research:* Canal cleanliness, antibiotics, resilon, lasers, microbes.

University of Florida, College of Dentistry and Graduate School, Graduate Programs in Dentistry, Department of Oral Biology, Gainesville, FL 32611. Offers PhD. *Degree requirements:* For doctorate, thesis/dissertation. *Entrance requirements:* For doctorate, GRE General Test, minimum GPA of 3.0. Additional exam requirements/recommendations for international students: Required—TOEFL. Electronic applications accepted. *Expenses:* Tuition, state resident: full-time $12,640. Tuition, nonresident: full-time $30,000. *Faculty research:* Bacterial genetics, cell adhesion, salivary glands, cell proliferation.

University of Florida, College of Dentistry and Graduate School, Graduate Programs in Dentistry, Department of Orthodontics, Gainesville, FL 32611. Offers MS, Certificate. *Degree requirements:* For master's, thesis. *Entrance requirements:* For master's, DAT, GRE General Test, National Board Dental Examination Parts I and II, minimum GPA of 3.0, interview. Additional exam requirements/recommendations for international students: Required—TOEFL (minimum score 550 paper-based). *Expenses:* Tuition, state resident: full-time $12,640. Tuition, nonresident: full-time $30,000. *Faculty research:* Bone biology, osteoclasts, clinical research, root resorption, pain control.

University of Florida, College of Dentistry and Graduate School, Graduate Programs in Dentistry, Department of Periodontology, Gainesville, FL 32611. Offers MS, Certificate. *Degree requirements:* For master's, thesis. *Entrance requirements:* For master's, DAT, GRE General Test, National Board Dental Examination Parts I and II, minimum GPA of 3.0, interview. Additional exam requirements/recommendations for international students: Required—TOEFL (minimum score 550 paper-based). *Expenses:* Tuition, state resident: full-time $12,640. Tuition, nonresident: full-time $30,000. *Faculty research:* Gingival grafting, periodontal plastic surgery, regenerative periodontal surgery, dental implant complications, osteogenic fibroma.

University of Florida, College of Dentistry and Graduate School, Graduate Programs in Dentistry, Department of Prosthodontics, Gainesville, FL 32611. Offers MS, Certificate. *Degree requirements:* For master's, thesis. *Entrance requirements:* For master's, DAT, GRE General Test, National Board Dental Examination Parts I and II, minimum GPA of 3.0, interview. Additional exam requirements/recommendations for international students: Required—TOEFL (minimum score 550 paper-based). *Expenses:* Tuition, state resident: full-time $12,640. Tuition, nonresident: full-time $30,000. *Faculty research:* Computer panograph, dental implants, resin provisional materials wear rate, implant surface variation, Sjorgen's Syndrome.

University of Illinois at Chicago, College of Dentistry and Graduate College, Graduate Programs in Oral Sciences, Chicago, IL 60607-7128. Offers MS, PhD. *Students:* 13 full-time (9 women), 7 part-time (3 women); includes 7 minority (1 Black or African American, non-Hispanic/Latino; 4 Asian, non-Hispanic/Latino; 2 Hispanic/Latino), 1 international. Average age 27. 34 applicants, 53% accepted, 6 enrolled. In 2013, 17 master's, 2 doctorates awarded. *Degree requirements:* For master's, thesis. *Entrance requirements:* For master's, GRE General Test, DDS, DVM, or MD. Additional exam requirements/recommendations for international students: Required—TOEFL. *Application deadline:* For fall admission, 5/15 for domestic students, 2/15 for international students; for spring admission, 11/15 for domestic students, 7/15 for international students. Application fee: $40 ($50 for international students). Electronic applications accepted. *Expenses:* Contact institution. *Financial support:* In 2013–14, 5 students received support. Fellowships, research assistantships with full tuition reimbursements available, teaching assistantships with full tuition reimbursements available, Federal Work-Study, scholarships/grants, traineeships, health care benefits, tuition waivers (full), and unspecified assistantships available. Financial award application deadline: 3/1. *Unit head:* Katherine A. Long, Assistant Director of Graduate and Research Education, 312-996-2465. *Application contact:* Jackie Perry, Graduate College Receptionist, 312-413-2550, Fax: 312-413-0185, E-mail: gradcoll@uic.edu.

The University of Iowa, College of Dentistry and Graduate College, Graduate Programs in Dentistry, Department of Endodontics, Iowa City, IA 52242-1316. Offers MS, Certificate. *Degree requirements:* For master's, thesis. *Entrance requirements:* For master's, GRE, DDS; for Certificate, DDS. Additional exam requirements/recommendations for international students: Required—TOEFL.

The University of Iowa, College of Dentistry and Graduate College, Graduate Programs in Dentistry, Department of Operative Dentistry, Iowa City, IA 52242-1316. Offers MS, Certificate. *Degree requirements:* For master's, thesis. *Entrance requirements:* For master's, GRE, DDS; for Certificate, DDS. Additional exam requirements/recommendations for international students: Required—TOEFL.

The University of Iowa, College of Dentistry and Graduate College, Graduate Programs in Dentistry, Department of Oral and Maxillofacial Surgery, Iowa City, IA 52242-1316. Offers MS, PhD, Certificate. *Degree requirements:* For master's, thesis. *Entrance requirements:* For master's, GRE, DDS; for Certificate, DDS.

The University of Iowa, College of Dentistry and Graduate College, Graduate Programs in Dentistry, Department of Oral Pathology, Radiology and Medicine, Iowa City, IA 52242-1316. Offers MS, PhD, Certificate. *Degree requirements:* For master's, thesis. *Entrance requirements:* For master's, GRE, DDS, minimum GPA of 2.7. Additional exam requirements/recommendations for international students: Required—TOEFL.

The University of Iowa, College of Dentistry and Graduate College, Graduate Programs in Dentistry, Department of Orthodontics, Iowa City, IA 52242-1316. Offers MS, Certificate. *Degree requirements:* For master's, thesis. *Entrance requirements:* For master's, GRE, DDS; for Certificate, DDS. Additional exam requirements/recommendations for international students: Required—TOEFL.

The University of Iowa, College of Dentistry and Graduate College, Graduate Programs in Dentistry, Department of Pediatric Dentistry, Iowa City, IA 52242-1316. Offers Certificate. *Entrance requirements:* For degree, DDS. Additional exam requirements/recommendations for international students: Required—TOEFL.

The University of Iowa, College of Dentistry and Graduate College, Graduate Programs in Dentistry, Department of Periodontics, Iowa City, IA 52242-1316. Offers MS, Certificate. *Degree requirements:* For master's, thesis. *Entrance requirements:* For master's, GRE, DDS; for Certificate, DDS. Additional exam requirements/recommendations for international students: Required—TOEFL.

The University of Iowa, College of Dentistry and Graduate College, Graduate Programs in Dentistry, Department of Preventive and Community Dentistry, Iowa City, IA 52242-1316. Offers dental public health (MS). *Degree requirements:* For master's, thesis. *Entrance requirements:* For master's, GRE, DDS. Additional exam requirements/recommendations for international students: Required—TOEFL.

The University of Iowa, College of Dentistry and Graduate College, Graduate Programs in Dentistry, Department of Prosthodontics, Iowa City, IA 52242-1316. Offers MS, Certificate. *Degree requirements:* For master's, thesis. *Entrance requirements:* For master's, GRE, DDS; for Certificate, DDS. Additional exam requirements/recommendations for international students: Required—TOEFL.

The University of Iowa, College of Dentistry and Graduate College, Graduate Programs in Dentistry, Oral Science Graduate Program, Iowa City, IA 52242-1316. Offers MS, PhD. *Degree requirements:* For master's, thesis; for doctorate, thesis/dissertation. *Entrance requirements:* For master's, GRE, DDS. Additional exam requirements/recommendations for international students: Required—TOEFL.

University of Kentucky, Graduate School, Graduate Program in Dentistry, Lexington, KY 40506-0032. Offers MS. *Degree requirements:* For master's, comprehensive exam, thesis. *Entrance requirements:* For master's, GRE General Test, minimum undergraduate GPA of 2.5. Additional exam requirements/recommendations for international students: Required—TOEFL (minimum score 550 paper-based). Electronic applications accepted.

University of Louisville, School of Dentistry, Louisville, KY 40202. Offers dentistry (DMD); oral biology (MS). *Accreditation:* ADA (one or more programs are accredited). Part-time programs available. *Students:* 514 full-time (208 women), 15 part-time (9 women); includes 109 minority (28 Black or African American, non-Hispanic/Latino; 1 American Indian or Alaska Native, non-Hispanic/Latino; 49 Asian, non-Hispanic/Latino; 13 Hispanic/Latino; 1 Native Hawaiian or other Pacific Islander, non-Hispanic/Latino; 17 Two or more races, non-Hispanic/Latino), 25 international. Average age 27. 184 applicants, 88% accepted, 142 enrolled. In 2013, 4 master's, 80 doctorates awarded. *Degree requirements:* For master's, thesis; for doctorate, National Board exams. *Entrance requirements:* For master's, DAT, GRE General Test, or National Board Dental Exam, minimum GPA of 2.75; for doctorate, DAT, 32 hours of course work in science. Additional exam requirements/recommendations for international students: Required—TOEFL (minimum score 100 iBT). *Application deadline:* For fall admission, 1/1 for domestic and international students. Applications are processed on a rolling basis. Application fee: $60. Electronic applications accepted. *Expenses:* Contact institution. *Financial support:* In 2013–14, 1 research assistantship with full tuition reimbursement (averaging $20,000 per year) was awarded. Financial award application deadline: 3/15; financial award applicants required to submit FAFSA. *Faculty research:* Inflammation and periodontitis, birth defects and developmental biology, biomaterials, oral infections, digital imaging. *Total annual research expenditures:* $7.4 million. *Unit head:* Dr. John J. Sauk, Dean, 502-852-1304, Fax: 502-852-3364, E-mail: jjsauk01@louisville.edu. *Application contact:* Robin Benningfield, Admissions Counselor, 502-852-5081, Fax: 502-852-1210, E-mail: dmdadms@louisville.edu.
Website: http://louisville.edu/dental/

The University of Manchester, School of Dentistry, Manchester, United Kingdom. Offers basic dental sciences (cancer studies) (M Phil, PhD); basic dental sciences (molecular genetics) (M Phil, PhD); basic dental sciences (stem cell biology) (M Phil, PhD); biomaterials sciences and dental technology (M Phil, PhD); dental public health/community dentistry (M Phil, PhD); dental science (clinical) (PhD); endodontology (M Phil, PhD); fixed and removable prosthodontics (M Phil, PhD); operative dentistry (M Phil, PhD); oral and maxillofacial surgery (M Phil, PhD); oral radiology (M Phil, PhD); orthodontics (M Phil, PhD); restorative dentistry (M Phil, PhD).

University of Manitoba, Faculty of Dentistry and Faculty of Graduate Studies, Graduate Programs in Dentistry, Department of Dental Diagnostic and Surgical Sciences, Winnipeg, MB R3T 2N2, Canada. Offers oral and maxillofacial surgery (M Dent); periodontology (M Dent). *Entrance requirements:* For master's, dental degree. *Faculty research:* Implantology, clinical trials, tobacco use, periodontal disease.

University of Manitoba, Faculty of Dentistry and Faculty of Graduate Studies, Graduate Programs in Dentistry, Department of Oral Biology, Winnipeg, MB R3T 2N2, Canada. Offers M Sc, PhD. *Degree requirements:* For master's, thesis; for doctorate, comprehensive exam, thesis/dissertation. *Entrance requirements:* For master's, B Sc or pre-M Sc. Additional exam requirements/recommendations for international students: Required—TOEFL. *Faculty research:* Oral bacterial ecology and metabolism, biofilms, saliva and oral health, secretory mechanisms.

University of Manitoba, Faculty of Dentistry and Faculty of Graduate Studies, Graduate Programs in Dentistry, Department of Preventive Dental Science, Winnipeg, MB R3T 2N2, Canada. Offers orthodontics (M Sc). *Degree requirements:* For master's, thesis. *Entrance requirements:* For master's, dental degree. Electronic applications accepted.

Oral and Dental Sciences

University of Maryland, Baltimore, Graduate School, Graduate Programs in Dentistry, Department of Oral Pathology, Baltimore, MD 21201. Offers MS, PhD. *Students:* 3 full-time (0 women), 1 part-time (0 women); includes 1 minority (Asian, non-Hispanic/Latino), 2 international. Average age 30. 11 applicants, 18% accepted. In 2013, 1 doctorate awarded. *Degree requirements:* For master's, thesis or alternative; for doctorate, comprehensive exam, thesis/dissertation. *Entrance requirements:* For master's and doctorate, GRE General Test, DDS, DMD. Additional exam requirements/recommendations for international students: Required—TOEFL (minimum score 550 paper-based; 80 iBT) or IELTS (minimum score 7). *Application deadline:* For fall admission, 5/1 for domestic students, 1/15 for international students. Application fee: $75. Electronic applications accepted. *Financial support:* Fellowships, research assistantships, and teaching assistantships available. Support available to part-time students. Financial award application deadline: 2/15; financial award applicants required to submit FAFSA. *Faculty research:* Histopathology, epidemiology of oral lesions, embryology. *Unit head:* Dr. Mark A. Reynolds, Dean and Professor, 410-706-7461, Fax: 410-706-0406, E-mail: mreynolds@umaryland.edu. *Application contact:* Dr. Bernard Levy, Director, 410-706-7342, E-mail: blevy@umaryland.edu.

University of Maryland, Baltimore, Graduate School, Graduate Programs in Dentistry, Graduate Program in Biomedical Sciences, Baltimore, MD 21201. Offers MS, PhD, DDS/PhD. *Students:* 1 full-time (0 women), all international. Average age 29. In 2013, 14 master's awarded. *Degree requirements:* For master's, thesis optional; for doctorate, comprehensive exam, thesis/dissertation. *Entrance requirements:* For master's and doctorate, GRE General Test. Additional exam requirements/recommendations for international students: Required—TOEFL (minimum score 550 paper-based; 80 iBT) or IELTS (minimum score 7). *Application deadline:* For fall admission, 5/1 for domestic students, 1/15 for international students. Application fee: $75. Electronic applications accepted. *Financial support:* In 2013–14, research assistantships with full tuition reimbursements (averaging $23,000 per year) were awarded. Financial award applicants required to submit FAFSA. *Faculty research:* Neuroscience, molecular and cell biology, infectious diseases. *Unit head:* Dr. Ronald Dubner, Professor and Chair, 410-706-0860, Fax: 410-706-0865, E-mail: rdubner@dental.umaryland.edu. *Application contact:* Dr. Pei Feng, Graduate Program Director, 410-706-7340, Fax: 410-706-0865, E-mail: pfeng@umaryland.edu.

University of Maryland, Baltimore, Professional and Advanced Education Programs in Dentistry, Baltimore, MD 21201-1627. Offers advanced general dentistry (Certificate); dentistry (DDS); endodontics (Certificate); oral-maxillofacial surgery (Certificate); orthodontics (Certificate); pediatric dentistry (Certificate); periodontics (Certificate); prosthodontics (Certificate); DDS/MBA; DDS/PhD. *Accreditation:* ADA. *Students:* 587 full-time (304 women), 5 part-time (3 women); includes 223 minority (38 Black or African American, non-Hispanic/Latino; 1 American Indian or Alaska Native, non-Hispanic/Latino; 120 Asian, non-Hispanic/Latino; 43 Hispanic/Latino; 21 Two or more races, non-Hispanic/Latino), 28 international. Average age 26. In 2013, 127 doctorates, 29 Certificates awarded. *Entrance requirements:* For doctorate, DAT, coursework in science; for Certificate, National Dental Board Exams, DDS. Additional exam requirements/recommendations for international students: Required—TOEFL (minimum score 550 paper-based; 80 iBT). *Application deadline:* Applications are processed on a rolling basis. Application fee: $85. Electronic applications accepted. *Expenses:* Contact institution. *Financial support:* Career-related internships or fieldwork, Federal Work-Study, scholarships/grants, and traineeships available. Financial award application deadline: 3/1; financial award applicants required to submit FAFSA. *Faculty research:* Pain/neuroscience, oncology/molecular and cell biology, infectious disease/microbiology, bio-material studies, health promotion and disparities. *Unit head:* Dr. Christian S. Stohler, Dean, 410-706-7461. *Application contact:* Dr. Patricia Meehan, Assistant Dean for Admissions, 410-706-7472, Fax: 410-706-0945, E-mail: ddsadmissions@umaryland.edu.
Website: http://www.dental.umaryland.edu/

University of Michigan, School of Dentistry and Rackham Graduate School, Graduate Programs in Dentistry, Endodontics Program, Ann Arbor, MI 48109-1078. Offers MS. *Students:* 12 full-time (3 women); includes 2 minority (1 Asian, non-Hispanic/Latino; 1 Hispanic/Latino), 3 international. 48 applicants, 8% accepted, 4 enrolled. In 2013, 7 master's awarded. *Degree requirements:* For master's, thesis. *Entrance requirements:* For master's, DDS. Additional exam requirements/recommendations for international students: Required—TOEFL (minimum score 84 iBT). *Application deadline:* For fall admission, 7/15 for domestic and international students. Applications are processed on a rolling basis. Application fee: $75 ($90 for international students). Electronic applications accepted. Tuition and fees vary according to course level, course load, degree level, program and student level. *Unit head:* Dr. Neville McDonald, Program Director, 734-647-3722, E-mail: somerled@umich.edu. *Application contact:* Patricia Katcher, Associate Admissions Director, 734-763-3316, Fax: 734-764-1922, E-mail: graddentinquiry@umich.edu.
Website: http://www.dent.umich.edu/crse/graduateprogram/endodontics

University of Michigan, School of Dentistry and Rackham Graduate School, Graduate Programs in Dentistry, Orthodontics Program, Ann Arbor, MI 48109-1078. Offers MS. *Students:* 21 full-time (11 women); includes 4 minority (2 Asian, non-Hispanic/Latino; 1 Hispanic/Latino; 1 Two or more races, non-Hispanic/Latino), 1 international. 185 applicants, 4% accepted, 7 enrolled. In 2013, 8 master's awarded. *Degree requirements:* For master's, thesis. *Entrance requirements:* For master's, GRE, National Dental Board Exam, DDS. Additional exam requirements/recommendations for international students: Required—TOEFL (minimum score 84 iBT). *Application deadline:* For fall admission, 8/15 for domestic and international students. Application fee: $75 ($90 for international students). Electronic applications accepted. Tuition and fees vary according to course level, course load, degree level, program and student level. *Unit head:* Dr. Sunil Kapila, Program Director, 734-764-1080, E-mail: skapila@umich.edu. *Application contact:* Patricia Katcher, Associate Admissions Director, 734-763-3316, Fax: 734-764-1922, E-mail: graddentinquiry@umich.edu.
Website: http://www.dent.umich.edu/opd/graduateprograms/ortho/about

University of Michigan, School of Dentistry and Rackham Graduate School, Graduate Programs in Dentistry, Pediatric Dentistry Program, Ann Arbor, MI 48109-1078. Offers MS. *Students:* 19 full-time (18 women); includes 6 minority (1 Black or African American, non-Hispanic/Latino; 3 Asian, non-Hispanic/Latino; 2 Two or more races, non-Hispanic/Latino), 5 international. 150 applicants, 4% accepted, 6 enrolled. In 2013, 6 master's awarded. *Degree requirements:* For master's, thesis. *Entrance requirements:* For master's, DDS. Additional exam requirements/recommendations for international students: Required—TOEFL (minimum score 84 iBT). *Application deadline:* For fall admission, 9/1 for domestic students, 10/1 for international students. Application fee: $75 ($90 for international students). Electronic applications accepted. Tuition and fees vary according to course level, course load, degree level, program and student level. *Unit head:* Dr. James Boynton, Program Director, 734-764-1522, E-mail: jboynton@umich.edu. *Application contact:* Patricia Katcher, Associate Admissions Director, 734-763-3316, Fax: 734-764-1922, E-mail: graddentinquiry@umich.edu.
Website: http://www.dent.umich.edu/opd/graduateprograms/ped/aboutus

University of Michigan, School of Dentistry and Rackham Graduate School, Graduate Programs in Dentistry, Periodontics Program, Ann Arbor, MI 48109-1078. Offers MS. *Students:* 15 full-time (5 women); includes 2 minority (1 Black or African American, non-Hispanic/Latino; 1 Two or more races, non-Hispanic/Latino), 10 international. 54 applicants, 7% accepted, 4 enrolled. In 2013, 2 master's awarded. *Degree requirements:* For master's, thesis. *Entrance requirements:* For master's, DDS. Additional exam requirements/recommendations for international students: Required—TOEFL (minimum score 84 iBT). *Application deadline:* For fall admission, 8/1 for domestic and international students. Applications are processed on a rolling basis. Application fee: $75 ($90 for international students). Electronic applications accepted. Tuition and fees vary according to course level, course load, degree level, program and student level. *Unit head:* Dr. Hom-Lay Wang, Program Director, 734-764-1948, E-mail: homlay@umich.edu. *Application contact:* Patricia Katcher, Associate Admissions Director, 734-763-3316, Fax: 734-764-1922, E-mail: graddentinquiry@umich.edu.
Website: http://www.dent.umich.edu/pom/academics/gradprograms#perio

University of Michigan, School of Dentistry and Rackham Graduate School, Graduate Programs in Dentistry, Prosthodontics Program, Ann Arbor, MI 48109-1078. Offers MS. *Students:* 14 full-time (8 women); includes 2 minority (1 Asian, non-Hispanic/Latino; 1 Hispanic/Latino), 7 international. 66 applicants, 6% accepted, 4 enrolled. In 2013, 2 master's awarded. *Degree requirements:* For master's, thesis. *Entrance requirements:* For master's, DDS. Additional exam requirements/recommendations for international students: Required—TOEFL (minimum score 84 iBT). *Application deadline:* For fall admission, 9/1 for domestic and international students. Applications are processed on a rolling basis. Application fee: $75 ($90 for international students). Electronic applications accepted. Tuition and fees vary according to course level, course load, degree level, program and student level. *Unit head:* Dr. Michael Razzoog, Program Director, 734-647-1369, E-mail: merim@umich.edu. *Application contact:* Patricia Katcher, Associate Admissions Director, 734-763-3316, Fax: 734-764-1922, E-mail: graddentinquiry@umich.edu.
Website: http://www.dent.umich.edu/bms/gradstudentsprosgradprog

University of Michigan, School of Dentistry and Rackham Graduate School, Graduate Programs in Dentistry, Restorative Dentistry Program, Ann Arbor, MI 48109-1078. Offers MS. *Students:* 18 full-time (8 women); includes 3 minority (1 Black or African American, non-Hispanic/Latino; 1 Hispanic/Latino; 1 Two or more races, non-Hispanic/Latino), 15 international. 50 applicants, 10% accepted, 5 enrolled. In 2013, 3 master's awarded. *Degree requirements:* For master's, thesis. *Entrance requirements:* Additional exam requirements/recommendations for international students: Required—TOEFL (minimum score 84 iBT). *Application deadline:* For fall admission, 9/1 for domestic and international students. Applications are processed on a rolling basis. Application fee: $75 ($90 for international students). Electronic applications accepted. Tuition and fees vary according to course level, course load, degree level, program and student level. *Unit head:* Dr. Peter Yaman, Program Director, 734-647-3722, E-mail: pyam@umich.edu. *Application contact:* Patricia Katcher, Associate Admissions Director, 734-763-3316, Fax: 734-764-1922, E-mail: graddentinquiry@umich.edu.
Website: http://www.dent.umich.edu/crse/graduateprograms/restorativedentistry

University of Michigan, School of Dentistry, Oral Health Sciences PhD Program, Ann Arbor, MI 48109-1078. Offers PhD. *Faculty:* 30 full-time (7 women). *Students:* 15 full-time (8 women); includes 6 minority (5 Asian, non-Hispanic/Latino; 1 Hispanic/Latino), 4 international. Average age 29. 21 applicants, 14% accepted, 3 enrolled. In 2013, 2 doctorates awarded. *Degree requirements:* For doctorate, thesis/dissertation, preliminary exam, oral defense of dissertation. *Entrance requirements:* For doctorate, GRE. Additional exam requirements/recommendations for international students: Required—TOEFL. *Application deadline:* For fall admission, 12/5 for domestic and international students. Applications are processed on a rolling basis. Application fee: $75 ($90 for international students). Electronic applications accepted. Tuition and fees vary according to course level, course load, degree level, program and student level. *Financial support:* In 2013–14, fellowships with full tuition reimbursements (averaging $26,000 per year), research assistantships with full tuition reimbursements (averaging $28,000 per year) were awarded; teaching assistantships, scholarships/grants, and traineeships also available. Financial award application deadline: 1/5. *Faculty research:* Craniofacial development, oral and pharyngeal cancer, mineralized tissue biology and musculoskeletal disorders, tissue engineering and regeneration, oral infectious and immunologic diseases, oral sensory systems and central circuits. *Total annual research expenditures:* $15.4 million. *Unit head:* Dr. Jan Hu, Director, 734-615-1970, E-mail: ohsphd@umich.edu. *Application contact:* Patricia E. Schultz, Manager, 734-615-1970, E-mail: ohsphd@umich.edu.

University of Minnesota, Twin Cities Campus, School of Dentistry and Graduate School, Graduate Programs in Dentistry, Advanced Education Program in Periodontology, Minneapolis, MN 55455-0213. Offers MS. *Degree requirements:* For master's, comprehensive exam, thesis. *Entrance requirements:* For master's, DDS/DMD, letter from Dental Dean, specific GGP/class rank, two letters of recommendation. Additional exam requirements/recommendations for international students: Required—TOEFL (minimum score 590 paper-based). *Faculty research:* Periodontitis, risk factors, regenerating, diabetes immunology.

University of Minnesota, Twin Cities Campus, School of Dentistry and Graduate School, Graduate Programs in Dentistry, Division of Endodontics, Minneapolis, MN 55455-0213. Offers MS, Certificate. *Degree requirements:* For master's, thesis. *Entrance requirements:* Additional exam requirements/recommendations for international students: Required—TOEFL. *Faculty research:* Pain, inflammation, neuropharmacology, neuropeptides, cytokines.

University of Minnesota, Twin Cities Campus, School of Dentistry and Graduate School, Graduate Programs in Dentistry, Division of Orthodontics, Minneapolis, MN 55455-0213. Offers MS. *Degree requirements:* For master's, thesis. *Entrance requirements:* Additional exam requirements/recommendations for international students: Required—TOEFL (minimum score 587 paper-based). *Faculty research:* Bone biology, 3-D imaging.

University of Minnesota, Twin Cities Campus, School of Dentistry and Graduate School, Graduate Programs in Dentistry, Division of Pediatric Dentistry, Minneapolis, MN 55455-0213. Offers MS. *Degree requirements:* For master's, thesis. *Entrance requirements:* Additional exam requirements/recommendations for international students: Required—TOEFL. *Faculty research:* Molecular genetics of facial growth, dental material/adhesion, expanded functions dental auxiliary utilization.

University of Minnesota, Twin Cities Campus, School of Dentistry and Graduate School, Graduate Programs in Dentistry, Division of Prosthodontics, Minneapolis, MN 55455-0213. Offers MS. *Degree requirements:* For master's, thesis, clinical. *Entrance requirements:* Additional exam requirements/recommendations for international students: Required—TOEFL.

University of Minnesota, Twin Cities Campus, School of Dentistry and Graduate School, Graduate Programs in Dentistry, Program in Oral Biology, Minneapolis, MN 55455-0213. Offers MS, PhD. *Degree requirements:* For master's, thesis. *Faculty research:* Microbiology, neuroscience, biomaterials, biochemistry, cancer biology.

University of Minnesota, Twin Cities Campus, School of Dentistry and Graduate School, Graduate Programs in Dentistry, Program in Oral Health Services for Older Adults (Geriatrics), Minneapolis, MN 55455-0213. Offers MS, Certificate. *Degree* *requirements:* For master's, thesis (for some programs). *Entrance requirements:* For master's, DDS degree or equivalent. Additional exam requirements/recommendations for international students: Required—TOEFL (minimum score 560 paper-based). Electronic applications accepted. *Faculty research:* Geriatrics dental care, long-term care dental services, oral-systemic health relationships, utilization of care by older adults.

University of Minnesota, Twin Cities Campus, School of Dentistry and Graduate School, Graduate Programs in Dentistry, Program in Temporomandibular Joint Disorders, Minneapolis, MN 55455-0213. Offers MS. *Degree requirements:* For master's, comprehensive exam, thesis. *Entrance requirements:* Additional exam requirements/recommendations for international students: Required—TOEFL. Electronic applications accepted. *Faculty research:* Clinical trials, TMJ mechanicals, diagnostic criteria, biomarkers, genetics.

University of Mississippi Medical Center, School of Dentistry, Department of Craniofacial and Dental Research, Jackson, MS 39216-4505. Offers MS, PhD.

University of Missouri–Kansas City, School of Dentistry, Kansas City, MO 64110-2499. Offers advanced education in dentistry (Graduate Dental Certificate); dental hygiene education (MS); dentistry (DDS); endodontics (Graduate Dental Certificate); oral and maxillofacial surgery (Graduate Dental Certificate); oral biology (MS, PhD); orthodontics and dentofacial orthopedics (Graduate Dental Certificate); periodontics (Graduate Dental Certificate). PhD (interdisciplinary) offered through the School of Graduate Studies. *Accreditation:* ADA (one or more programs are accredited). *Faculty:* 97 full-time (45 women), 61 part-time/adjunct (18 women). *Students:* 425 full-time (178 women), 50 part-time (26 women); includes 87 minority (12 Black or African American, non-Hispanic/Latino; 3 American Indian or Alaska Native, non-Hispanic/Latino; 51 Asian, non-Hispanic/Latino; 15 Hispanic/Latino; 6 Two or more races, non-Hispanic/Latino), 3 international. Average age 27. 807 applicants, 17% accepted, 131 enrolled. In 2013, 10 master's, 106 doctorates, 17 other advanced degrees awarded. *Degree requirements:* For master's, thesis; for doctorate, thesis/dissertation (for some programs). *Entrance requirements:* For master's, DAT, letters of evaluation, personal interview; for doctorate, DAT (for DDS); for Graduate Dental Certificate, DDS. Additional exam requirements/recommendations for international students: Required—TOEFL (minimum score 550 paper-based; 80 iBT). *Application deadline:* For fall admission, 2/1 for domestic and international students. Application fee: $45 ($50 for international students). *Expenses:* Contact institution. *Financial support:* In 2013–14, 2 research assistantships (averaging $23,800 per year) were awarded; career-related internships or fieldwork, Federal Work-Study, institutionally sponsored loans, and tuition waivers (full and partial) also available. Support available to part-time students. Financial award application deadline: 3/1; financial award applicants required to submit FAFSA. *Faculty research:* Biomaterials, dental use of lasers, effectiveness of periodontal treatments, temporomandibular joint dysfunction. *Unit head:* Dr. Marsha Pyle, Dean, 816-235-2010, E-mail: pylem@umkc.edu. *Application contact:* Richard Bigham, Assistant Dean for Student Programs, 816-235-2082, E-mail: bighamr@umkc.edu.
Website: http://dentistry.umkc.edu/

University of Missouri–Kansas City, School of Graduate Studies, Kansas City, MO 64110-2499. Offers interdisciplinary studies (PhD), including art history, cell biology and biophysics, chemistry, computer and electrical engineering, computer science and informatics, economics, education, engineering, English, entrepreneurship and innovation, geosciences, history, mathematics and statistics, molecular biology and biochemistry, music education, oral and craniofacial sciences, pharmaceutical sciences, pharmacology, physics, political science, public affairs and administration, religious studies, social science, telecommunications and computer networking; PMBA/MHA. *Students:* 80 full-time (29 women), 270 part-time (107 women); includes 29 minority (16 Black or African American, non-Hispanic/Latino; 4 Asian, non-Hispanic/Latino; 7 Hispanic/Latino; 1 Native Hawaiian or other Pacific Islander, non-Hispanic/Latino; 1 Two or more races, non-Hispanic/Latino), 155 international. Average age 35. 288 applicants, 25% accepted, 56 enrolled. In 2013, 45 doctorates awarded. *Degree requirements:* For doctorate, comprehensive exam, thesis/dissertation, residency. *Entrance requirements:* For doctorate, GRE General Test, minimum GPA of 2.75 (undergraduate), 3.0 (graduate). Additional exam requirements/recommendations for international students: Required—TOEFL (minimum score 550 paper-based; 80 iBT), TWE (minimum score 4). *Application deadline:* For fall admission, 1/15 priority date for domestic and international students. Applications are processed on a rolling basis. Application fee: $45 ($50 for international students). Electronic applications accepted. *Expenses:* Tuition, state resident: full-time $6073; part-time $337.40 per credit hour. Tuition, nonresident: full-time $15,680; part-time $871.10 per credit hour. *Required fees:* $97.59 per credit hour. Full-time tuition and fees vary according to program. *Financial support:* Career-related internships or fieldwork, Federal Work-Study, tuition waivers (partial), and unspecified assistantships available. Support available to part-time students. Financial award application deadline: 3/1; financial award applicants required to submit FAFSA. *Unit head:* Dr. Denis M. Medeiros, Dean, 816-235-1301, Fax: 816-235-1310, E-mail: medeirosd@umkc.edu. *Application contact:* Quincy Bennett Johnson, Coordinator of Admissions and Recruitment, Interdisciplinary PhD Program, 816-235-1559, Fax: 816-235-1310, E-mail: bennettq@umkc.edu.
Website: http://sgs.umkc.edu/

The University of North Carolina at Chapel Hill, School of Dentistry and Graduate School, Graduate Programs in Dentistry, Chapel Hill, NC 27599. Offers dental hygiene (MS); endodontics (MS); epidemiology (PhD); operative dentistry (MS); oral and maxillofacial pathology (MS); oral and maxillofacial radiology (MS); oral biology (PhD); orthodontics (MS); pediatric dentistry (MS); periodontology (MS); prosthodontics (MS). *Degree requirements:* For master's, thesis; for doctorate, thesis/dissertation. *Entrance requirements:* For master's, GRE General Test (for orthodontics and oral biology only); National Dental Board Part I (Part II if available), dental degree (for all except dental hygiene); for doctorate, GRE General Test. Additional exam requirements/recommendations for international students: Required—TOEFL (minimum score 550 paper-based; 79 iBT). Electronic applications accepted. *Expenses:* Contact institution. *Faculty research:* Clinical research, inflammation, immunology, neuroscience, molecular biology.

University of Oklahoma Health Sciences Center, College of Dentistry and Graduate College, Graduate Programs in Dentistry, Department of Orthodontics, Oklahoma City, OK 73190. Offers MS. *Degree requirements:* For master's, thesis. *Entrance requirements:* For master's, minimum GPA of 3.0, DDS/DMD. Additional exam requirements/recommendations for international students: Required—TOEFL. Electronic applications accepted. *Expenses:* Tuition, state resident: full-time $3504; part-time $175.20 per credit hour. Tuition, nonresident: full-time $13,504; part-time $675.20 per credit hour. *Required fees:* $1545; $52.70 per credit hour. $245.25 per semester. Tuition and fees vary according to course load. *Faculty research:* Craniofacial growth and development, biomechanical principles in orthodontics.

University of Oklahoma Health Sciences Center, College of Dentistry and Graduate College, Graduate Programs in Dentistry, Department of Periodontics, Oklahoma City, OK 73190. Offers MS. *Degree requirements:* For master's, thesis. *Entrance requirements:* For master's, DDS/DMD, minimum GPA of 3.0. Additional exam requirements/recommendations for international students: Required—TOEFL (minimum score 550 paper-based). Electronic applications accepted. *Expenses:* Tuition, state resident: full-time $3504; part-time $175.20 per credit hour. Tuition, nonresident: full-time $13,504; part-time $675.20 per credit hour. *Required fees:* $1545; $52.70 per credit hour. $245.25 per semester. Tuition and fees vary according to course load.

University of Pittsburgh, School of Dental Medicine, Residency Programs in Dental Medicine, Advanced Education Program in Prosthodontics, Pittsburgh, PA 15261. Offers MDS, Certificate. *Faculty:* 3 full-time (0 women), 4 part-time/adjunct (0 women). *Students:* 9 full-time (5 women); includes 1 minority (Asian, non-Hispanic/Latino), 2 international. Average age 28. 59 applicants, 5% accepted, 3 enrolled. In 2013, 1 master's awarded. *Degree requirements:* For master's, comprehensive exam, thesis. *Entrance requirements:* Additional exam requirements/recommendations for international students: Required—TOEFL. *Application deadline:* For fall admission, 11/1 for domestic and international students. Applications are processed on a rolling basis. Application fee: $50. Electronic applications accepted. *Expenses:* Tuition, state resident: full-time $19,964; part-time $807 per credit. Tuition, nonresident: full-time $32,686; part-time $1337 per credit. *Required fees:* $740; $200. Tuition and fees vary according to program. *Financial support:* In 2013–14, 9 students received support. Stipends available. *Faculty research:* Implant dentistry, occlusion, biomechanics, genetics, biomaterials. *Unit head:* Dr. Mohsen Azarbal, Associate Professor/Program Director, 412-648-8453, Fax: 412-648-8850, E-mail: moa5@pitt.edu. *Application contact:* Aileen Brasacchio, Administrator, Office of Resident Education, 412-648-8422, Fax: 412-648-9571, E-mail: amb001@pitt.edu.

University of Pittsburgh, School of Dental Medicine, Residency Programs in Dental Medicine, Department of Dental Anesthesia, Pittsburgh, PA 15260. Offers Certificate. *Faculty:* 3 full-time (0 women), 6 part-time/adjunct (0 women). *Students:* 10 full-time (0 women). Average age 35. 32 applicants, 13% accepted, 4 enrolled. In 2013, 2 Certificates awarded. *Entrance requirements:* For degree, National Board Dental Exam Parts I and II, DMD or DDS. *Application deadline:* For fall admission, 9/16 for domestic students. Application fee: $50. Electronic applications accepted. *Expenses:* Tuition, state resident: full-time $19,964; part-time $807 per credit. Tuition, nonresident: full-time $32,686; part-time $1337 per credit. *Required fees:* $740; $200. Tuition and fees vary according to program. *Financial support:* In 2013–14, 10 fellowships (averaging $36,000 per year) were awarded; health care benefits also available. *Faculty research:* Clinical pharmacology and random controlled trials. *Unit head:* Dr. Michael A. Cuddy, Program Director, 412-648-8609, Fax: 412-648-2591, E-mail: mc2@pitt.edu. *Application contact:* Lisa R. Lehman, Department Administrator, 412-648-8609, Fax: 412-648-2591, E-mail: lrl12@pitt.edu.
Website: http://www.dental.pitt.edu/

University of Pittsburgh, School of Dental Medicine, Residency Programs in Dental Medicine, Department of Endodontics, Pittsburgh, PA 15260. Offers MDS, Certificate. *Faculty:* 2 full-time (1 woman), 6 part-time/adjunct (1 woman). *Students:* 7 full-time (2 women); includes 2 minority (1 Asian, non-Hispanic/Latino; 1 Native Hawaiian or other Pacific Islander, non-Hispanic/Latino). Average age 29. 59 applicants, 7% accepted, 4 enrolled. In 2013, 3 Certificates awarded. *Degree requirements:* For master's, comprehensive exam, thesis. *Entrance requirements:* For master's and Certificate, National Dental Board Exams Part 1 and 2. *Application deadline:* For fall admission, 9/1 for domestic students. Application fee: $50. *Expenses:* Tuition, state resident: full-time $19,964; part-time $807 per credit. Tuition, nonresident: full-time $32,686; part-time $1337 per credit. *Required fees:* $740; $200. Tuition and fees vary according to program. *Financial support:* Application deadline: 4/15. *Faculty research:* Pulpal neurobiology, root canal therapy, root fracture/resorption repair, osseous grafts related to endodontics, endodontic surge. *Total annual research expenditures:* $10,000. *Unit head:* Dr. Herbert L. Ray, Jr., Director, 412-648-8647, Fax: 412-383-7796, E-mail: skipp@pitt.edu. *Application contact:* Aileen Brasacchio, Administrator, Office of Resident Education, 412-648-8422, Fax: 412-648-9571, E-mail: amb0001@pitt.edu.
Website: http://www.dental.pitt.edu/

University of Pittsburgh, School of Dental Medicine, Residency Programs in Dental Medicine, Department of Oral and Maxillofacial Surgery, Pittsburgh, PA 15260. Offers Certificate. *Faculty:* 10 full-time (0 women). *Students:* 15 full-time (1 woman); includes 1 minority (Asian, non-Hispanic/Latino). Average age 25. 111 applicants. In 2013, 4 Certificates awarded. *Degree requirements:* For Certificate, comprehensive exam. *Entrance requirements:* For degree, National Boards Part I, U.S. or Canadian dental degree (DDS or DMD). *Application deadline:* For fall admission, 10/15 for domestic students. Applications are processed on a rolling basis. Application fee: $0. Electronic applications accepted. *Expenses:* Contact institution. *Financial support:* In 2013–14, 8 students received support, including 4 fellowships with partial tuition reimbursements available (averaging $36,000 per year); scholarships/grants, health care benefits, and tuition waivers also available. *Faculty research:* Clefts, craniofacial anomalies, facial trauma, head and neck cancer, pain management. *Total annual research expenditures:* $2 million. *Unit head:* Dr. Bernard J. Costello, Program Director, 412-648-6801, Fax: 412-648-6835. *Application contact:* Andrea M. Ford, Residency and Fellowship Coordinator, 412-648-6801, Fax: 412-648-6835, E-mail: fordam@upmc.edu.
Website: http://www.dental.pitt.edu/

University of Pittsburgh, School of Dental Medicine, Residency Programs in Dental Medicine, Department of Orthodontics and Dentofacial Orthopedics, Pittsburgh, PA 15261. Offers orthodontics (MDS, Certificate). *Faculty:* 2 full-time (0 women), 12 part-time/adjunct (2 women). *Students:* 12 full-time (5 women); includes 5 minority (4 Asian, non-Hispanic/Latino; 1 Hispanic/Latino). Average age 27. 171 applicants, 2% accepted. In 2013, 1 master's awarded. *Degree requirements:* For master's, comprehensive exam, thesis; for Certificate, comprehensive exam. *Entrance requirements:* For master's and Certificate, National Boards Parts I and II. *Application deadline:* For fall admission, 10/1 for domestic students. *Expenses:* Tuition, state resident: full-time $19,964; part-time $807 per credit. Tuition, nonresident: full-time $32,686; part-time $1337 per credit. *Required fees:* $740; $200. Tuition and fees vary according to program. *Faculty research:* Facial form, orthodontic outcomes. *Unit head:* Dr. Joseph F. A. Petrone, Chair, Department of Orthodontics and Dentofacial Orthopedics, 412-648-8638, Fax: 412-648-8817, E-mail: jfap@pitt.edu. *Application contact:* Lauren B. Lagana, Department Administrator, 412-648-8419, Fax: 412-648-8817, E-mail: lmb111@pitt.edu.
Website: http://www.dental.pitt.edu/orthodontics/index.php

University of Pittsburgh, School of Dental Medicine, Residency Programs in Dental Medicine, Department of Periodontics, Pittsburgh, PA 15261. Offers MDS, MPH, Certificate. *Faculty:* 4 full-time (3 women), 9 part-time/adjunct (1 woman). *Students:* 9 full-time (3 women); includes 3 minority (1 Black or African American, non-Hispanic/Latino; 2 Asian, non-Hispanic/Latino). Average age 28. 36 applicants, 8% accepted, 3 enrolled. In 2013, 2 master's, 3 other advanced degrees awarded. *Degree requirements:* For master's, comprehensive exam, thesis. *Entrance requirements:* For degree, DMD, DDS. *Application deadline:* For fall admission, 8/1 priority date for domestic and international students. Applications are processed on a rolling basis. Application fee: $50. *Expenses:* Tuition, state resident: full-time $19,964; part-time $807 per credit. Tuition, nonresident: full-time $32,686; part-time $1337 per credit. *Required fees:* $740; $200. Tuition and fees vary according to program. *Financial support:* Stipends available. *Faculty research:* Periodontics, implantology, osteoporosis, perio systemic disease, diabetes. *Total annual research expenditures:* $50,000. *Unit head:* Dr. Pouran

Famili, Director/Chair, 412-648-8598, Fax: 412-648-8594, E-mail: pof@pitt.edu. *Application contact:* Aileen Brasacchio, Residency Education Administrator, 412-648-8406, Fax: 412-648-8219, E-mail: amb001@pitt.edu.

University of Puerto Rico, Medical Sciences Campus, School of Dental Medicine, Graduate Programs in Dentistry, San Juan, PR 00936-5067. Offers general dentistry (Certificate); oral and maxillofacial surgery (Certificate); orthodontics (Certificate); pediatric dentistry (Certificate); prosthodontics (Certificate). *Degree requirements:* For Certificate, comprehensive exam (for some programs). *Entrance requirements:* For degree, National Board Dental Exam I, National Board Dental Exam II, DDS or DMD, interview. Electronic applications accepted. *Expenses:* Contact institution. *Faculty research:* Analgesic drugs, anti-inflammatory drugs, saliva cytoanalysis, dental materials, oral epidemiology and dental caries.

University of Rochester, School of Medicine and Dentistry, Graduate Programs in Medicine and Dentistry, Center for Oral Biology, Rochester, NY 14627. Offers dental science (MS). *Degree requirements:* For master's, thesis. *Entrance requirements:* For master's, GRE General Test, DDS or equivalent. *Expenses: Tuition:* Full-time $44,580; part-time $1394 per credit hour. *Required fees:* $492.

University of Southern California, Graduate School, Herman Ostrow School of Dentistry and Graduate School, Department of Craniofacial Biology, Los Angeles, CA 90089. Offers MS, PhD, Graduate Certificate. Terminal master's awarded for partial completion of doctoral program. *Degree requirements:* For master's, comprehensive exam, thesis; for doctorate, comprehensive exam, thesis/dissertation. *Entrance requirements:* For master's and doctorate, GRE, undergraduate degree. Additional exam requirements/recommendations for international students: Required—TOEFL. Electronic applications accepted. *Faculty research:* Orthodontics, periodontics, tooth development, oral biology, stem cell biology.

The University of Tennessee Health Science Center, College of Graduate Health Sciences, Memphis, TN 38163-0002. Offers biomedical engineering (MS, PhD); biomedical sciences (PhD); dental sciences (MDS); epidemiology (MS); health outcomes and policy research (PhD); laboratory research and management (MS); nursing science (PhD); pharmaceutical sciences (PhD); pharmacology (MS); speech and hearing science (PhD); DDS/PhD; DNP/PhD; MD/PhD; Pharm D/PhD. *Faculty:* 318 full-time (92 women), 59 part-time/adjunct (16 women). *Students:* 220 full-time (102 women), 22 part-time (13 women); includes 194 minority (22 Black or African American, non-Hispanic/Latino; 161 Asian, non-Hispanic/Latino; 7 Hispanic/Latino; 3 Native Hawaiian or other Pacific Islander, non-Hispanic/Latino; 1 Two or more races, non-Hispanic/Latino), 106 international. Average age 25. 404 applicants, 17% accepted, 64 enrolled. In 2013, 13 master's, 25 doctorates awarded. Terminal master's awarded for partial completion of doctoral program. *Degree requirements:* For master's, comprehensive exam, thesis; for doctorate, comprehensive exam, thesis/dissertation, oral and written preliminary and comprehensive exams. *Entrance requirements:* For master's and doctorate, GRE General Test, minimum GPA of 3.0. Additional exam requirements/recommendations for international students: Required—TOEFL (minimum score 79 iBT); Recommended—IELTS (minimum score 6.5). *Application deadline:* For fall admission, 5/15 priority date for domestic students. Applications are processed on a rolling basis. Application fee: $0. Electronic applications accepted. *Financial support:* In 2013–14, 125 students received support, including 125 research assistantships (averaging $23,000 per year); career-related internships or fieldwork, Federal Work-Study, institutionally sponsored loans, and tuition waivers (full and partial) also available. Support available to part-time students. Financial award application deadline: 2/25; financial award applicants required to submit FAFSA. *Unit head:* Dr. Donald B. Thomason, Dean, 901-448-5538, E-mail: dthomaso@uthsc.edu. *Application contact:* William Carter, Director for Admissions, 901-448-1687, E-mail: wcarte17@uthsc.edu. Website: http://www.uthsc.edu/grad/

The University of Toledo, College of Graduate Studies, College of Medicine and Life Sciences, Department of Surgery, Toledo, OH 43606-3390. Offers oral biology (MSBS). *Faculty:* 12. *Students:* 6 full-time (3 women); includes 2 minority (1 Asian, non-Hispanic/Latino; 1 Hispanic/Latino). Average age 31. In 2013, 3 master's awarded. *Degree requirements:* For master's, thesis or alternative. *Entrance requirements:* For master's, DAT, minimum undergraduate GPA of 3.0, three letters of recommendation, statement of purpose, transcripts from all prior institutions attended, acceptance into Pediatric Dental Residency Program at UT. Additional exam requirements/recommendations for international students: Required—TOEFL (minimum score 550 paper-based; 80 iBT). *Application deadline:* Applications are processed on a rolling basis. Application fee: $45 ($75 for international students). Electronic applications accepted. *Financial support:* In 2013–14, 3 fellowships with full tuition reimbursements were awarded; Federal Work-Study, institutionally sponsored loans, and tuition waivers also available. *Faculty research:* Oral biology-tissue cultures. *Unit head:* Dr. Michael Nedley, Chair, 419-383-3504, E-mail: michael.nedley@utoledo.edu. *Application contact:* Brandi Hendrickson, Program Coordinator, 419-383-3504, E-mail: brandi.hendrickson@utoledo.edu. Website: http://www.utoledo.edu/med/grad/

University of Toronto, School of Graduate Studies, Faculty of Dentistry, Graduate Programs in Dentistry, Toronto, ON M5S 1A1, Canada. Offers M Sc, PhD. Part-time programs available. Terminal master's awarded for partial completion of doctoral program. *Degree requirements:* For master's, thesis; for doctorate, thesis/dissertation. *Entrance requirements:* For master's, honors B Sc, minimum B average, 2 letters of reference; for doctorate, M Sc, minimum B+ average. Additional exam requirements/recommendations for international students: Required—Michigan English Language Assessment Battery, IELTS, TOEFL or COPE. Electronic applications accepted. *Expenses:* Contact institution. *Faculty research:* Plaque, periodontal biology, biomaterials/dental implants, community dentistry, growth and development.

University of Toronto, School of Graduate Studies, Faculty of Dentistry, Specialty Master's Programs, Toronto, ON M5S 1A1, Canada. Offers dental anesthesia (M Sc); dental public health (M Sc); endodontics (M Sc); oral and maxillofacial surgery and anesthesia (M Sc); oral pathology (M Sc); oral radiology (M Sc); orthodontics (M Sc); pediatric dentistry (M Sc); periodontology (M Sc); prosthodontics (M Sc). *Degree requirements:* For master's, thesis. *Entrance requirements:* For master's, completion of professional degree of DDS/BDS, DMD, minimum B average, 2 letters of reference. Additional exam requirements/recommendations for international students: Required—TOEFL (minimum score 600 paper-based; 100 iBT), TWE (minimum score 5). *Expenses:* Contact institution. *Faculty research:* Plaque and periodontal biology, biomaterials/dental implants, community dentistry, growth development, neurophysiology.

University of Washington, Graduate School, School of Dentistry and Graduate School, Graduate Programs in Dentistry, Department of Endodontics, Seattle, WA 98195. Offers MSD, Certificate.

University of Washington, Graduate School, School of Dentistry and Graduate School, Graduate Programs in Dentistry, Department of Orthodontics, Seattle, WA 98195. Offers MSD, Certificate.

University of Washington, Graduate School, School of Dentistry, Program in Dental Surgery, Seattle, WA 98195. Offers DDS. *Accreditation:* ADA. *Entrance requirements:* For doctorate, DAT.

The University of Western Ontario, Schulich School of Medicine and Dentistry, School of Dentistry, Program in Graduate Orthodontics, London, ON N6A 5B8, Canada. Offers M Cl D. *Degree requirements:* For master's, thesis. *Entrance requirements:* For master's, GRE General Test, minimum B average, 1 year of general practice preferred. Additional exam requirements/recommendations for international students: Required—TOEFL (minimum score 600 paper-based).

West Virginia University, School of Dentistry, Division of Dental Hygiene, Morgantown, WV 26506. Offers MS. Part-time programs available. *Degree requirements:* For master's, thesis. *Entrance requirements:* For master's, GRE, MAT, BS in dental hygiene or equivalent, minimum GPA of 2.75. Additional exam requirements/recommendations for international students: Required—TOEFL. *Faculty research:* Curriculum and instruction, infection control, special patient care, diversity and cultural sensitivity, oral health disparities.

West Virginia University, School of Dentistry, Graduate Programs in Dentistry, Morgantown, WV 26506. Offers endodontics (MS); orthodontics (MS); prosthodontics (MS). *Degree requirements:* For master's, thesis. *Entrance requirements:* For master's, National Dental Board Exam Parts I and II, DDS/DMD from accredited U.S. or Canadian Dental School, minimum GPA of 3.0. Additional exam requirements/recommendations for international students: Required—TOEFL. *Expenses:* Contact institution. *Faculty research:* Growth and development, cephalographics, endodontic interpretation and therapy.

UCONN HEALTH

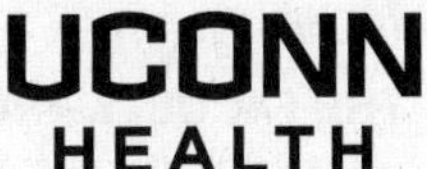

Graduate Program in Skeletal, Craniofacial, and Oral Biology

Programs of Study

The Graduate Program in Skeletal, Craniofacial, and Oral Biology provides students with interdisciplinary research training in the areas of skeletal, craniofacial, and oral biology, emphasizing contemporary research technologies in cell, molecular, and developmental biology; genetics; and biochemistry. Trainees may enter a Ph.D. program or a combined D.M.D./Ph.D., M.D./Ph.D., or dental residency/Ph.D. program. The program prepares trainees for academic or industrial careers in the basic biomedical sciences or for academic careers in medicine or dental medicine.

Areas of research include regulation of the formation, outgrowth, and patterning of the developing limb; control of cartilage differentiation, endochondral ossification, osteogenesis, and joint formation; molecular regulation of gene expression in bone; homeobox gene regulation of osteoblast differentiation; gene therapy of bone diseases; hormonal and cytokine regulation of bone growth, formation, and remodeling; control of craniofacial skeletogenesis and tooth development; signal transduction and intracellular signaling pathways; cellular and molecular aspects of the pathogenesis of inflammatory disease; microbiology, pathogenesis, and immunology of caries and periodontal disease; neural structure and function in the gustatory system; biomaterial development for tissue engineering; bone cell–implant interactions; differentiation of human embryonic stem cells into skeletal tissues; and analysis of oral and mucosal function and disease.

Research Facilities

The University complex provides excellent physical facilities for research in both basic and clinical sciences. The Lyman Maynard Stowe Library is well equipped with extensive journal and book holdings and rapid electronic access to database searching, Internet, and library holdings. The library also contains the Computer Education Center and the End User Support Center. The Center for Laboratory Animal Care contains a transgenic mouse production facility fully equipped for gene targeting studies and with special facilities for housing immunodeficient animals. Facilities include the Center for Biomaterials, the General Clinical Research Center, the Center for Cell Analysis and Modeling (confocal microscopy, low light level microscopy, two photon microscopy), the Center for Bone Histology and Histomorphometry; the Molecular Imaging Laboratory, the Fluorescence Flow Cytometry Facility, the Electron Microscopy Facility, Gene Targeting and Transgenic Facility, the Microarray Core Facility, the Molecular Core Facility, NMR Structural Biology Facility, National Resource for Cell Analysis and Modeling, and the Center for Molecular Medicine (laser capture microdissection).

Financial Aid

Support for doctoral students engaged in full-time degree programs at UConn Health is provided on a competitive basis. Graduate research assistantships for 2014–15 provide a stipend of $29,000 per year, which includes a waiver of tuition/most University fees for the fall and spring semesters and the option of participating in a student health-insurance plan. While financial aid is offered competitively, the UConn Health makes every possible effort to address the financial needs of all students during their period of training.

Cost of Study

For 2014–15, tuition is $12,202 per year for full-time students who are Connecticut residents and $32,258 per year for full-time students who are out-of-state residents. General University fees are added to the cost of tuition for students who do not receive a tuition waiver. These costs are usually met by traineeships or research assistantships for doctoral students.

Living and Housing Costs

There is a wide range of affordable housing options in the Greater Hartford area within easy commuting distance of the campus, including an extensive complex that is adjacent to UConn Health. Costs range from $700 to $1,000 per month for a one-bedroom unit; two or more students sharing an apartment usually pay less. University housing is not available on the campus.

Student Group

The Program in Skeletal, Craniofacial, and Oral Biology has approximately 20 trainees. At UConn Health there are about 500 students in the Schools of Medicine and Dental Medicine, 150 Ph.D. students, and about 50 postdoctoral fellows. Graduate students are represented on various administrative committees concerned with curricular affairs. A graduate student organization fosters social contact among graduate students at UConn Health and represents graduate students' needs and concerns to the faculty and administration.

Location

UConn Health is located in the historic town of Farmington, Connecticut. Set in the beautiful New England countryside, on a hill overlooking the Farmington Valley, it is close to ski areas, hiking trails, and facilities for boating, fishing, and swimming. Connecticut's capital city of Hartford, 7 miles east of Farmington, is the center of an urban region of approximately 800,000 people. The beaches of the Long Island Sound are about 50 minutes away to the south, and the beautiful Berkshires are a short drive to the northwest. New York City and Boston can be reached within 2½ hours by car.

Hartford is the home of the acclaimed Hartford Stage Company, TheatreWorks, the Hartford Symphony and Chamber orchestras, two ballet companies, an opera company, the Wadsworth Atheneum (the oldest public art museum in the nation), the Mark Twain house, the Hartford Civic Center, and many other interesting cultural and recreational facilities. The area is also home to several branches of the University of Connecticut, Trinity College, and the University of Hartford, which includes the Hartt School of Music. Bradley International Airport (about 30 minutes from campus) serves the Hartford/Springfield area with frequent airline connections to major cities in this country and abroad. Frequent bus and rail service is also available from Hartford.

The Health Center

The 200-acre UConn Health campus at Farmington houses a division of the University of Connecticut Graduate School, as well as the Schools of Medicine and Dental Medicine. The campus also includes the John Dempsey Hospital, associated clinics, and extensive medical research facilities, all in a centralized facility with more than 1 million square feet of floor space. The Academic Research Building, built in 1999, is an impressive eleven-story structure providing 170,000 square feet of laboratory space. In addition, renovations are underway in the main Laboratory building, converting existing lab space to state-of-the-art open lab areas. The faculty includes more than 260 full-time members. The institution has a strong commitment to graduate study within an environment that promotes social and intellectual interaction among the various educational programs. Graduate students are represented on various administrative committees concerned with curricular affairs, and the Graduate Student Organization (GSO) represents graduate students' needs and concerns to the faculty and administration, in addition to fostering social contact among graduate students at UConn Health.

Applying

Applications for admission should be submitted via the online application system and should be filed together with transcripts, three letters of recommendation, a personal statement, and recent results from the General Test of the Graduate Record Examinations. International students must take the Test of English as a Foreign Language (TOEFL) to satisfy Graduate School requirements.

The deadline for completed applications and receipt of all supplemental materials is **December 1**. Please note that GRE and TOEFL exams taken after the due date will not be accepted for consideration for admission.

Deadlines and application procedures for combined programs vary depending on the program. For further information on combined programs, prospective students should contact Dr. Mina Mina in the Department of Reconstructive Sciences.

In accordance with the laws of the state of Connecticut and of the United States, UConn Health does not discriminate against any person in its educational and employment activities on the grounds of race, color, creed, national origin, sex, age, or physical disability.

Correspondence and Information

Graduate Admissions Office
Ph.D. in Biomedical Science Program
UConn Health
263 Farmington Ave., MC 3906
Farmington, Connecticut 06030-3906
United States
Phone: 860-679-4509
E-mail: BiomedSciAdmissions@uchc.edu
Website: http://grad.uchc.edu/prospective/programs/phd_biosci/index.html

THE FACULTY AND THEIR RESEARCH

Andrew Arnold, Professor of Medicine and Murray-Heilig Chair in Molecular Medicine; M.D., Harvard. The molecular genetic underpinnings of tumors of the endocrine glands, role of the cyclin D1 oncogene, animal modeling of hyperparathyroidism.

Dashzeveg Bayarsaihan, Associate Professor; Ph.D. TFII-I family proteins.

I-Ping Chen, Assistant Professor, Oral Health and Diagnostic Sciences, D.D.S., Ph.D. Connecticut Health Center. Generation of induced pluripotent stem (iPS) cells from craniometaphyseal dysplasia (CMD) patients; investigation of osteoclast biology in the human stem cell system as well as in CMD mouse models.

Caroline N. Dealy, Associate Professor of Reconstructive Sciences, Center for Regenerative Medicine and Skeletal Development; Ph.D., Connecticut. Roles of various growth factors and signaling molecules, particularly IGF-I and insulin, in the regulation of chick limb development.

Anne Delany, Associate Professor of Medicine; Ph.D., Dartmouth. Study of noncollagenous matrix proteins and metalloproteinases important in bone remodeling, including investigation of function and posttranscriptional regulation of osteonectin or SPARC in bone and function and regulation of the metastasis-associated metalloproteinase, stromelysyin-3, in bone.

Patricia I. Diaz, Assistant Professor; Ph.D., Adelaide (Australia); D.D.S., Universidad CES (Colombia). Interspecies interactions in oral microbial communities that determine oral biofilm formation; shifts in the oral microbiome composition associated with oral diseases such as mucositis during cancer chemotherapy and periodontal diseases; interaction of oral microbial communities with the host.

Anna Dongari-Bagtzoglou, Professor, Department of Oral Health and Diagnostic Sciences, Division of Periodontology; D.D.S., Ph.D., Texas Health Science Center at San Antonio. Host-pathogen interactions, with emphasis on the pathogenesis of inflammation and the innate immune functions of oral mucosal cells.

Hicham Drissi, Associate Professor of Orthopaedic Surgery; Ph.D., University of Paris V. Molecular pathways of bone and cartilage repair.

Paul M. Epstein, Associate Professor of Cell Biology; Ph.D., Yeshiva (Einstein). Second messengers and signal transduction, with particular focus on cyclic nucleotide metabolism and protein phosphorylation, with emphasis on analysis of cyclic nucleotide phosphodiesterase (PDE).

Marion Frank, Professor of Oral Health and Diagnostic Sciences and Director, Center for Neurosciences; Ph.D., Brown. Study of the sense of taste, using basic and clinical research; development of a fundamental understanding of gustatory systems in mammals at all levels from receptors to cerebral cortex; application of basic knowledge of gustatory systems to the diagnosis and treatment of taste disorders in humans.

A. Jon Goldberg, Professor of Reconstructive Sciences, Center for Regenerative Medicine and Skeletal Development; Ph.D., Michigan. Biomaterials, with studies involving structure-property relationships, development of novel systems, clinical evaluations, and surface analysis.

Gloria Gronowicz, Professor of Surgery; Ph.D., Columbia. Effects of hormones and growth factors on the production of extracellular matrix (ECM) proteins, on the regulation of integrins (receptors for ECM proteins), and on apoptosis in bone; response of bone cells to implant biomaterials.

Arthur R. Hand, Professor of Craniofacial Sciences, Division of Pediatric Dentistry; D.D.S., UCLA. Study of gene expression in rodent salivary glands during normal growth and development and in various experimental conditions employing morphological, immunological, and biochemical methodology.

Marc Hansen, Professor of Medicine, Center for Molecular Medicine; Ph.D., Cincinnati. Molecular genetics of osteosarcoma and related bone diseases.

Marja M. Hurley, Professor of Medicine; M.D., Connecticut. Molecular mechanisms regulating the expression of fibroblast growth factors in bone, mechanisms of signal transduction by growth factors in bone cells, and role of fibroblast growth factors in bone remodeling.

Ivo Kalajzic, Assistant Professor, Department of Reconstructive Sciences and Department of Genetics and Developmental Biology; M.D., Zagreb (Croatia); Ph.D., Split (Croatia). Bone biology, differentiation of the osteoblast lineage cells.

Yusuf Khan, Assistant Professor of Orthopaedic Surgery and Chemical, Materials, and Biomolecular Engineering; Ph.D. Drexel. Strategies to synthesize scaffolds that are also capable of delivering proteins and growth factors essential for complete and adequate healing of bone defects through the use of biodegradable polymers alone and in combination with ceramic materials.

Barbara E. Kream, Professor of Medicine; Ph.D., Yale. Hormonal regulation of bone remodeling.

Liisa T. Kuhn, Associate Professor of Reconstructive Sciences, Center for Regenerative Medicine and Skeletal Development; Ph.D., California, Santa Barbara. Biomaterials for drug delivery and bone regeneration and repair.

Sangamesh Kumbar, Assistant Professor of Orthopedic Surgery; Ph.D., Karnatak (India). Synthesis and characterization of novel biomaterials/polymers for tissue engineering and drug delivery applications.

Marc Lalande, Professor and Head, Department of Genetics and Developmental Biology; Ph.D., Toronto. Genomic imprinting of human chromosome 15q.

Sun-Kyeong Lee, Assistant Professor of Medicine; Ph.D., Connecticut. Osteoclast biology and molecular and cellular regulation by cytokines in osteoclastogenesis.

Alexander Lichtler, Associate Professor of Reconstructive Sciences, Center for Regenerative Medicine and Skeletal Development; Ph.D., Florida. Hormone regulation of bone collagen synthesis.

Alan G. Lurie, Professor of Oral Health and Diagnostic Sciences and Chairperson, Division of Oral and Maxillofacial Radiology; D.D.S., UCLA; Ph.D., Rochester. Actions and interactions of radiation and chemical carcinogens during epithelial carcinogenesis, DNA mutagenesis and repair by gamma radiation in lymphoblasts from both normal and ataxia telangiectatic humans, clinical research digital imaging.

Peter Maye, Assistant Professor of Reconstructive Sciences, Ph.D., Wesleyan. Isolation, characterization, and differentiation of embryonic and adult skeletal stem cells down the osteogenic lineage.

Mina Mina, Professor of Craniofacial Sciences; Chairperson, Division of Pediatric Dentistry; and Director, Skeletal, Craniofacial, and Oral Biology Graduate Program; D.M.D., National University of Iran; Ph.D., Connecticut Health Center. Development of the mandibular arch, including the elongation and polarized outgrowth of the mandibular primordia and subsequent differentiation of the skeletal tissues in spatially defined patterns; characterization of genetic and epigenetic influences involved in the pattern formation and skeletogenesis of the chick mandible and mouse tooth germ; regulation of patterning in the developing mandible and developing teeth by mandibular epithelium, extracellular matrix molecules, growth factors, and transcription factors.

Lakshmi Nair, Assistant Professor of Orthopedic Surgery and Chemical, Materials, and Biomolecular Engineering; Ph.D., SCTIMST (India). Design and development of regenerative biomaterials to favorably modulate the responses of a variety of cell types involved in tissue regeneration and repair.

Syam P. Nukavarapu, Assistant Professor of Orthopaedic Surgery and Chemical, Materials, and Biomolecular Engineering. Ph.D, Indian Institute of Science. Scaffold-based bone-tissue engineering.

Carol C. Pilbeam, Professor of Medicine; Ph.D., Yale. Mechanisms of regulation of bone formation and resorption.

Justin D. Radolf, Professor of Medicine and Center for Microbial Pathogenesis; M.D., California, San Francisco. Molecular pathogenesis and immunobiology of spirochetal infections.

Ernst Reichenberger, Associate Professor of Reconstructive Sciences, Center for Regenerative Medicine and Skeletal Development; Ph.D., Erlangen (Germany). Study of complex processes required for generating and maintaining the skin and bones through characterization of human genetic disorders in which they are disrupted, including aplasia cutis congenita (ACC), cherubism, and craniometaphyseal dysplasia (CMD).

Blanka Rogina, Associate Professor of Genetics and Developmental Biology; Ph.D., Zagreb (Croatia). Molecular and genetic mechanisms underlying aging and cost of reproduction.

Edward F. Rossomando, Professor of Craniofacial Sciences; D.D.S., Pennsylvania; Ph.D., Rockefeller; M.S. (management), Rensselaer. Translational research, strategic management, entrepreneurship, management of innovation and technology, strategic management in the health-care industry.

David W. Rowe, Professor of Reconstructive Sciences and Director, Center for Regenerative Medicine and Skeletal Development; M.D., Vermont. Genetic and hormonal control of type I collagen production, development of strategies for somatic gene therapy for heritable diseases of bone built upon the structural and regulatory principles of collagen production.

Archana Sanjay, Assistant Professor of Orthopaedic Surgery, School of Medicine; Ph.D. Regulation of bone remodeling; examining signaling pathways that regulate osteoblast and osteoclast differentiation and function.

Section 28
Medicine

This section contains a directory of institutions offering graduate work in medicine, followed by an in-depth entry submitted by an institution that chose to prepare a detailed program description. Additional information about programs listed in the directory but not augmented by an in-depth entry may be obtained by writing directly to the dean of a graduate school or chair of a department at the address given in the directory.

CONTENTS

Program Directories

Display and Close-Up

Allopathic Medicine

Albany Medical College, Professional Program, Albany, NY 12208-3479. Offers MD. *Accreditation:* LCME/AMA. *Degree requirements:* For doctorate, United States Medical Licensing Exam Steps 1 and 2, clinical skills. *Entrance requirements:* For doctorate, MCAT, letters of recommendation, interview. Electronic applications accepted. *Expenses:* Contact institution.

Albert Einstein College of Medicine, Professional Program in Medicine, Bronx, NY 10461. Offers MD, MD/PhD. *Accreditation:* LCME/AMA. *Degree requirements:* For doctorate, independent scholars project. *Entrance requirements:* For doctorate, MCAT, interview. *Faculty research:* Cancer, diabetes mellitus, liver disease, infectious disease, neuroscience.

American University of Beirut, Graduate Programs, Faculty of Medicine, Beirut, Lebanon. Offers anatomy, cell biology and human morphology (MS); biochemistry and medical genetics (MS); biomedical sciences (PhD); experimental pathology, immunology and microbiology (MS); medicine (MD); neuroscience (MS); pharmacology and toxicology (MS). Part-time programs available. *Faculty:* 259 full-time (78 women), 93 part-time/adjunct (16 women). *Students:* 364 full-time (165 women), 62 part-time (54 women). Average age 23. In 2013, 18 master's awarded. *Degree requirements:* For master's, one foreign language, comprehensive exam, thesis (for some programs); for doctorate, one foreign language, comprehensive exam, thesis/dissertation. *Entrance requirements:* For master's, letter of recommendation; for doctorate, MCAT, bachelor's degree. Additional exam requirements/recommendations for international students: Required—TOEFL (minimum score 600 paper-based; 100 iBT), IELTS (minimum score 7.5). *Application deadline:* For fall admission, 4/30 for domestic and international students; for spring admission, 11/1 for domestic and international students. Application fee: $50. *Expenses: Tuition:* Full-time $14,724; part-time $818 per credit. *Required fees:* $692. Tuition and fees vary according to course load and program. *Financial support:* In 2013–14, 242 students received support, including 60 teaching assistantships (averaging $4,000 per year); career-related internships or fieldwork, institutionally sponsored loans, scholarships/grants, health care benefits, and unspecified assistantships also available. Financial award application deadline: 2/2. *Faculty research:* Cancer research (targeted therapy, mechanisms of leukemogenesis, tumor cell extravasation and metastasis, cancer stem cells), stem cell research (regenerative medicine, drug discovery), genetic research (neurogenetics, hereditary cardiomyopathy, hemoglobinopathies, pharmacogenomics, proteomics), neuroscience research (pain, neurodegenerative disorder), metabolism (inflammation and metabolism, metabolic disorder, diabetes mellitus), vascular and renal biology, signal transduction. *Total annual research expenditures:* $2.6 million. *Unit head:* Dr. Mohamed Sayegh, Dean, 961-1350000 Ext. 4700, Fax: 961-1744464, E-mail: msayegh@aub.edu.lb. *Application contact:* Dr. Salim Kanaan, Director, Admissions Office, 961-1-350000 Ext. 2594, Fax: 96-1-1750775, E-mail: sk00@aub.edu.lb.
Website: http://www.aub.edu.lb/fm/fm_home/Pages/index.aspx

Baylor College of Medicine, Medical School, Professional Program in Medicine, Houston, TX 77030-3498. Offers MD. *Accreditation:* LCME/AMA. *Entrance requirements:* For doctorate, MCAT, 90 hours of pre-med course work. Electronic applications accepted. *Expenses:* Contact institution.

Boston University, School of Medicine, Professional Program in Medicine, Boston, MA 02215. Offers MD, MD/JD, MD/MA, MD/MACI, MD/MBA, MD/MPH, MD/PhD. *Accreditation:* LCME/AMA. *Students:* 687 full-time (343 women), 26 part-time (14 women); includes 349 minority (40 Black or African American, non-Hispanic/Latino; 210 Asian, non-Hispanic/Latino; 75 Hispanic/Latino; 3 Native Hawaiian or other Pacific Islander, non-Hispanic/Latino; 21 Two or more races, non-Hispanic/Latino), 30 international. Average age 26. In 2013, 177 doctorates awarded. *Application deadline:* For fall admission, 11/1 for domestic students. Application fee: $95. *Expenses: Tuition:* Full-time $43,970; part-time $1374 per credit hour. *Required fees:* $60 per semester. Tuition and fees vary according to class time, course level and program. *Financial support:* Federal Work-Study available. Support available to part-time students. *Unit head:* Dr. Karen H. Antman, Dean, 617-638-5300. *Application contact:* Dr. Robert Witzburg, Associate Dean for Admissions, 617-638-4630.

Brown University, Graduate School, Division of Biology and Medicine, Program in Medicine, Providence, RI 02912. Offers MD, MD/PhD. *Accreditation:* LCME/AMA. *Expenses:* Contact institution.

Case Western Reserve University, School of Medicine, Professional Program in Medicine, Cleveland, OH 44106. Offers MD, MD/JD, MD/MA, MD/MBA, MD/MPH, MD/MS, MD/PhD. *Accreditation:* LCME/AMA. *Entrance requirements:* For doctorate, MCAT, interview. Electronic applications accepted.

Charles Drew University of Medicine and Science, Professional Program in Medicine, Los Angeles, CA 90059. Offers MD. *Entrance requirements:* For doctorate, MCAT.

Columbia University, College of Physicians and Surgeons, Professional Program in Medicine, New York, NY 10032. Offers MD, MD/DDS, MD/MPH, MD/MS, MD/PhD. *Accreditation:* LCME/AMA. Part-time programs available. *Entrance requirements:* For doctorate, MCAT.

Columbia University, School of Continuing Education, Program in Narrative Medicine, New York, NY 10027. Offers MS. Electronic applications accepted.

Creighton University, School of Medicine, Professional Program in Medicine, Omaha, NE 68178-0001. Offers MD, MD/PhD. *Accreditation:* LCME/AMA. *Faculty:* 263 full-time (76 women), 13 part-time/adjunct (3 women). *Students:* 604 full-time (302 women). Average age 25. 6,956 applicants, 5% accepted, 152 enrolled. In 2013, 123 doctorates awarded. *Entrance requirements:* For doctorate, MCAT. *Application deadline:* For fall admission, 11/1 for domestic and international students. Applications are processed on a rolling basis. Application fee: $95. Electronic applications accepted. *Expenses: Tuition:* Full-time $13,608; part-time $756 per credit hour. *Required fees:* $149 per semester. Tuition and fees vary according to course load, campus/location, program, reciprocity agreements and student's religious affiliation. *Financial support:* In 2013–14, 395 students received support. Institutionally sponsored loans and scholarships/grants available. Support available to part-time students. Financial award application deadline: 4/1; financial award applicants required to submit FAFSA. *Faculty research:* Hereditary cancer, osteoporosis, diabetes, immunology, microbiology. *Total annual research expenditures:* $21.2 million. *Unit head:* Dr. Robert W. Dunlay, Dean, 402-280-2600, Fax: 402-280-1410, E-mail: robertdunlay@creighton.edu. *Application contact:* Dr. Thomas Quinn, Assistant Dean for Admissions, 402-280-2799, Fax: 402-280-1241, E-mail: medschadm@creighton.edu.
Website: http://medicine.creighton.edu/

Dalhousie University, Faculty of Medicine, Halifax, NS B3H 4H7, Canada. Offers M Sc, MD, PhD, M Sc/PhD, MD/M Sc, MD/PhD. *Accreditation:* LCME/AMA. *Entrance requirements:* For master's, MCAT; for doctorate, MCAT (for MD). Electronic applications accepted.

Dartmouth College, Dartmouth Medical School, Hanover, NH 03755. Offers MD, MD/MBA, MD/PhD. *Accreditation:* LCME/AMA.

Drexel University, College of Medicine, Professional Program in Medicine, Philadelphia, PA 19104-2875. Offers MD, MD/PhD. *Accreditation:* LCME/AMA. *Degree requirements:* For doctorate, National Board Exam Parts I and II. *Entrance requirements:* For doctorate, MCAT. Electronic applications accepted.

Duke University, School of Medicine, Professional Program in Medicine, Durham, NC 27708-0586. Offers MD, MD/JD, MD/MALS, MD/MBA, MD/MHS, MD/MLS, MD/MMCi, MD/MPH, MD/MPP, MD/MSIS, MD/PhD. *Accreditation:* LCME/AMA. *Faculty:* 1,464 full-time (469 women). *Students:* 430 full-time (221 women); includes 218 minority (60 Black or African American, non-Hispanic/Latino; 7 American Indian or Alaska Native, non-Hispanic/Latino; 129 Asian, non-Hispanic/Latino; 22 Hispanic/Latino), 14 international. Average age 25. 4,962 applicants, 4% accepted, 113 enrolled. In 2013, 106 doctorates awarded. *Entrance requirements:* For doctorate, MCAT. *Application deadline:* For fall admission, 10/1 for domestic students. Application fee: $85. Electronic applications accepted. *Expenses:* Contact institution. *Financial support:* In 2013–14, 284 students received support. Institutionally sponsored loans and scholarships/grants available. Financial award application deadline: 5/1; financial award applicants required to submit FAFSA. *Unit head:* Dr. Edward G. Buckley, Vice Dean of Medical Education, 919-668-3381, Fax: 919-660-7040, E-mail: buckl002@mc.duke.edu. *Application contact:* Dr. Brenda Armstrong, Director of Admissions, 919-684-2985, Fax: 919-684-8893, E-mail: medadm@mc.duke.edu.
Website: http://www.dukemed.duke.edu/

East Carolina University, Brody School of Medicine, Professional Program in Medicine, Greenville, NC 27858-4353. Offers MD. *Accreditation:* LCME/AMA. *Entrance requirements:* For doctorate, MCAT, pre-med courses, interviews, faculty evaluations. *Application deadline:* For fall admission, 11/15 for domestic students. Applications are processed on a rolling basis. Application fee: $60. Electronic applications accepted. *Expenses:* Tuition, state resident: full-time $4223. Tuition, nonresident: full-time $16,540. *Required fees:* $2184. *Financial support:* Institutionally sponsored loans and scholarships/grants available. *Faculty research:* Diabetes, cardiovascular disease, cancer, neurological disorders. *Unit head:* Dr. Paul Cunningham, Dean, 252-744-2201, E-mail: cunninghamp@ecu.edu. *Application contact:* Contact Center, 252-744-1020, E-mail: somadmissions@ecu.edu.

Eastern Virginia Medical School, Professional Program in Medicine, Norfolk, VA 23501-1980. Offers MD, MD/MPH. *Accreditation:* LCME/AMA. *Students:* 556 full-time (245 women); includes 210 minority (48 Black or African American, non-Hispanic/Latino; 1 American Indian or Alaska Native, non-Hispanic/Latino; 129 Asian, non-Hispanic/Latino; 9 Hispanic/Latino; 2 Native Hawaiian or other Pacific Islander, non-Hispanic/Latino; 21 Two or more races, non-Hispanic/Latino). 5,803 applicants, 6% accepted, 146 enrolled. In 2013, 118 doctorates awarded. *Entrance requirements:* For doctorate, MCAT, bachelor's degree or equivalent, course work in sciences. *Application deadline:* For fall admission, 11/15 priority date for domestic students. Applications are processed on a rolling basis. Application fee: $95. Electronic applications accepted. *Financial support:* Applicants required to submit FAFSA. *Unit head:* Dr. Ronald W. Flenner, Associate Dean for Medicine, 757-446-5829, Fax: 757-446-5896, E-mail: flennerw@evms.edu. *Application contact:* Susan Castora, Director of Admissions, 757-446-5812, Fax: 757-446-5896, E-mail: castorsl@evms.edu.
Website: http://www.evms.edu/education/doctoral_programs/doctor_of_medicine/

East Tennessee State University, James H. Quillen College of Medicine, Professional Programs in Medicine, Johnson City, TN 37614. Offers MD. *Accreditation:* LCME/AMA. *Faculty:* 115 full-time (36 women), 35 part-time/adjunct (8 women). *Students:* 281 full-time (124 women), 1 part-time (0 women); includes 44 minority (6 Black or African American, non-Hispanic/Latino; 3 American Indian or Alaska Native, non-Hispanic/Latino; 24 Asian, non-Hispanic/Latino; 7 Hispanic/Latino; 4 Two or more races, non-Hispanic/Latino). Average age 26. 1,144 applicants, 9% accepted, 60 enrolled. In 2013, 60 doctorates awarded. *Entrance requirements:* For doctorate, MCAT. Additional exam requirements/recommendations for international students: Required—TOEFL (minimum score 550 paper-based). *Application deadline:* For fall admission, 12/1 for domestic students. Applications are processed on a rolling basis. Application fee: $25. *Expenses:* Tuition, state resident: full-time $7900; part-time $395 per credit hour. Tuition, nonresident: full-time $21,960; part-time $1098 per credit hour. *Required fees:* $1345; $84 per credit hour. *Financial support:* Career-related internships or fieldwork, Federal Work-Study, institutionally sponsored loans, and scholarships/grants available. Financial award application deadline: 5/10; financial award applicants required to submit FAFSA. *Total annual research expenditures:* $2 million. *Unit head:* Dr. Philip Bagnell, Dean, 423-439-6316, Fax: 423-439-8090, E-mail: bagnell@etsu.edu. *Application contact:* E. Doug Taylor, Assistant Dean for Admissions and Records, 423-439-2033, Fax: 423-439-2110, E-mail: dougt@etsu.edu.

Emory University, School of Medicine, Professional Program in Medicine, Atlanta, GA 30322-4510. Offers MD, MD/MA, MD/MPH, MD/MSCR, MD/PhD. *Accreditation:* LCME/AMA. *Faculty:* 2,195 full-time (802 women), 1,084 part-time/adjunct (464 women). *Students:* 550 full-time (280 women); includes 185 minority (41 Black or African American, non-Hispanic/Latino; 96 Asian, non-Hispanic/Latino; 38 Hispanic/Latino; 10 Two or more races, non-Hispanic/Latino), 17 international. Average age 25. 5,096 applicants, 7% accepted, 136 enrolled. In 2013, 139 doctorates awarded. *Degree requirements:* For doctorate, United States Medical Licensing Exam Step 1 and 2. *Entrance requirements:* For doctorate, MCAT, AMCAS application, supplemental application, interview (by invitation only). *Application deadline:* For fall admission, 10/15 for domestic and international students. Applications are processed on a rolling basis. Application fee: $120. Electronic applications accepted. *Expenses:* Contact institution. *Financial support:* In 2013–14, 311 students received support. Institutionally sponsored loans and scholarships/grants available. Financial award application deadline: 3/1; financial award applicants required to submit CSS PROFILE or FAFSA. *Faculty research:* Immunology and pathogenesis of chronic viral infections, immunological memory and vaccine development, development of antiviral agents to treat infections caused by human immunodeficiency and hepatitis viruses, development of therapeutic and diagnostic approaches to improve outcomes after transplantation genetic mechanisms of neuropsychiatric disease, Fragile X Syndrome, immune system ontogeny and phylogeny. *Total annual research expenditures:* $316.3 million. *Unit head:* Dr. John William Eley, Executive Associate Dean, Medical Education and Student Affairs, 404-727-5655, Fax: 404-727-0045, E-mail: jeley@emory.edu. *Application contact:* Dr. Ira K. Schwartz, Associate Dean of Medical Education and Student Affairs/

Director of Admissions, 404-727-5660, Fax: 404-727-5456, E-mail: medadmiss@emory.edu.
Website: http://www.med.emory.edu

Florida Atlantic University, Charles E. Schmidt College of Medicine, Boca Raton, FL 33431-0991. Offers biomedical science (MS); medicine (MD). Part-time programs available. *Faculty:* 13 full-time (5 women), 4 part-time/adjunct (0 women). *Students:* 220 full-time (120 women), 16 part-time (10 women); includes 79 minority (16 Black or African American, non-Hispanic/Latino; 26 Asian, non-Hispanic/Latino; 33 Hispanic/Latino; 4 Two or more races, non-Hispanic/Latino), 1 international. Average age 25. 3,109 applicants, 3% accepted, 78 enrolled. In 2013, 24 master's awarded. *Degree requirements:* For master's, thesis (for some programs); for doctorate, comprehensive exam. *Entrance requirements:* For master's, GRE, minimum GPA of 3.0; for doctorate, MCAT, AMCAS application, letters of recommendation, interview. *Application deadline:* For fall admission, 5/1 for domestic students, 3/15 for international students; for spring admission, 10/1 for domestic and international students. Application fee: $30. Electronic applications accepted. *Expenses:* Tuition, state resident: full-time $6660; part-time $370 per credit hour. Tuition, nonresident: full-time $18,450; part-time $1025 per credit hour. Tuition and fees vary according to course load. *Financial support:* In 2013–14, 1 student received support. Fellowships and research assistantships available. Financial award applicants required to submit FAFSA. *Faculty research:* Osteoarthritis, aging, breast cancer, HIV/AIDS, cardiometabolic risk in psychiatry. *Unit head:* Dr. David J. Bjorkman, Dean, 561-297-4341. *Application contact:* Julie Sivigny, Academic Program Specialist for Graduate Studies, 561-297-2216, E-mail: jsivigny@fau.edu.
Website: http://med.fau.edu/

Florida International University, Herbert Wertheim College of Medicine, Miami, FL 33199. Offers MPA, MD, PhD. *Entrance requirements:* For doctorate, MCAT (minimum score of 25), minimum overall GPA of 3.0; 3 letters of recommendation, 2 from basic science faculty (biology, chemistry, physics, math) and 1 from any other faculty member. Electronic applications accepted. *Expenses:* Contact institution.

Georgetown University, School of Medicine, Washington, DC 20057. Offers MD, MD/MBA, MD/PhD. *Accreditation:* LCME/AMA. *Entrance requirements:* For doctorate, MCAT, minimum 90 credit hours with 1 year of course work in biology, organic chemistry, inorganic chemistry, physics, mathematics, and English. *Application deadline:* For fall admission, 11/1 for domestic students. Applications are processed on a rolling basis. Application fee: $55. *Expenses:* Contact institution. *Unit head:* Dr. Stephen Ray Mitchell, Dean, 202-687-3922. *Application contact:* Dr. Stephen Ray Mitchell, Dean, 202-687-3922.

The George Washington University, School of Medicine and Health Sciences, Professional Program in Medicine, Washington, DC 20052. Offers MD, MD/MPH, MD/PhD. *Accreditation:* LCME/AMA. *Faculty:* 139 full-time (68 women). *Students:* 714 full-time (384 women), 2 part-time (0 women); includes 300 minority (61 Black or African American, non-Hispanic/Latino; 1 American Indian or Alaska Native, non-Hispanic/Latino; 205 Asian, non-Hispanic/Latino; 25 Hispanic/Latino; 3 Native Hawaiian or other Pacific Islander, non-Hispanic/Latino; 5 Two or more races, non-Hispanic/Latino), 23 international. Average age 26. In 2013, 158 doctorates awarded. *Entrance requirements:* For doctorate, MCAT, minimum 90 undergraduate semester hours, specific pre-med courses equal to 38 semester hours. *Application deadline:* For fall admission, 12/1 for domestic students. Applications are processed on a rolling basis. Application fee: $80. *Financial support:* Career-related internships or fieldwork, Federal Work-Study, and institutionally sponsored loans available. *Unit head:* Dr. Alan Wasserman, Chair, 202-741-2302. *Application contact:* Diane P. McQuail, Director of Admissions, 202-994-3507, E-mail: maeve@gwu.edu.

Georgia Regents University, Medical College of Georgia, Augusta, GA 30912. Offers MD, MD/PhD. *Accreditation:* LCME/AMA. *Faculty:* 438 full-time (133 women), 80 part-time/adjunct (37 women). *Students:* 908 full-time (393 women); includes 339 minority (70 Black or African American, non-Hispanic/Latino; 1 American Indian or Alaska Native, non-Hispanic/Latino; 214 Asian, non-Hispanic/Latino; 37 Hispanic/Latino; 17 Two or more races, non-Hispanic/Latino). Average age 25. 2,055 applicants, 15% accepted, 190 enrolled. In 2013, 178 doctorates awarded. *Degree requirements:* For doctorate, comprehensive exam. *Entrance requirements:* For doctorate, MCAT, minimum GPA of 3.6 in sciences, 3.64 overall. *Application deadline:* For fall admission, 11/1 for domestic students. Applications are processed on a rolling basis. Application fee: $0. *Expenses:* Contact institution. *Financial support:* Fellowships with tuition reimbursements, career-related internships or fieldwork, Federal Work-Study, institutionally sponsored loans, and scholarships/grants available. Support available to part-time students. Financial award application deadline: 5/1; financial award applicants required to submit FAFSA. *Faculty research:* Cancer, cardiovascular diseases, diabetes, neurological diseases, infection and inflammation. *Total annual research expenditures:* $59.1 million. *Unit head:* Dr. Peter Buckley, Dean, 706-721-2231, Fax: 706-721-7035, E-mail: pbuckley@georgiahealth.edu. *Application contact:* Dr. Geoffrey H. Young, Associate Dean for Admissions, 706-721-3186, Fax: 706-721-0959, E-mail: geyoung@georgiahealth.edu.
Website: http://www.gru.edu/mcg/

Harvard University, Harvard Medical School, Professional Program in Medicine, Cambridge, MA 02138. Offers MD, PhD, MD/MBA, MD/MM Sc, MD/MPH, MD/MPP, MD/PhD. *Accreditation:* LCME/AMA. Electronic applications accepted. *Expenses: Tuition:* Full-time $38,888. *Required fees:* $958. Tuition and fees vary according to campus/location, program and student level.

Hofstra University, School of Medicine, Hempstead, NY 11549. Offers medicine (MD); molecular basis of medicine (PhD); MD/PhD. *Accreditation:* LCME/AMA.

Howard University, College of Medicine, Professional Program in Medicine, Washington, DC 20059-0002. Offers MD, PhD, MD/PhD. *Accreditation:* LCME/AMA. *Faculty research:* Infectious diseases, protein modeling, neuropsychopharmacology.

Icahn School of Medicine at Mount Sinai, Department of Medical Education, New York, NY 10029-6504. Offers MD, MD/PhD. *Accreditation:* LCME/AMA. *Degree requirements:* For doctorate, comprehensive exam, United States Medical Licensing Examination Steps 1 and 2. *Entrance requirements:* For doctorate, MCAT. Additional exam requirements/recommendations for international students: Required—TOEFL. Electronic applications accepted. *Expenses:* Contact institution. *Faculty research:* Academic medicine, translational research.

Indiana University–Purdue University Indianapolis, Indiana University School of Medicine, Indianapolis, IN 46202-5114. Offers MS, MD, PhD, MD/MA, MD/MBA, MD/MS, MD/PhD. *Accreditation:* LCME/AMA. *Faculty:* 270 full-time (56 women). *Students:* 1,574 full-time (761 women), 20 part-time (13 women); includes 403 minority (108 Black or African American, non-Hispanic/Latino; 1 American Indian or Alaska Native, non-Hispanic/Latino; 183 Asian, non-Hispanic/Latino; 70 Hispanic/Latino; 1 Native Hawaiian or other Pacific Islander, non-Hispanic/Latino; 40 Two or more races, non-Hispanic/Latino), 95 international. Average age 26. 1,496 applicants, 40% accepted, 390 enrolled. In 2013, 87 master's, 334 doctorates awarded. *Degree requirements:* For doctorate, thesis/dissertation (for some programs). *Entrance requirements:* For master's, GRE General Test; for doctorate, GRE General Test (for PhD); MCAT (for MD). Additional exam requirements/recommendations for international students: Required—TOEFL. *Application deadline:* For fall admission, 8/1 priority date for domestic students. Applications are processed on a rolling basis. Application fee: $55 ($65 for international students). *Expenses:* Contact institution. *Financial support:* Fellowships with full and partial tuition reimbursements, research assistantships with full and partial tuition reimbursements, teaching assistantships with full tuition reimbursements, Federal Work-Study, institutionally sponsored loans, scholarships/grants, tuition waivers (full and partial), and stipends available. Support available to part-time students. *Total annual research expenditures:* $94.3 million. *Unit head:* Dr. Randy R. Brutkiewicz, Associate Dean for Graduate Studies, 317-274-3441. *Application contact:* Valerie Winbush, Graduate Program Assistant, 317-274-3441, E-mail: vwinbush@iupui.edu.
Website: http://www.medicine.iu.edu/

Instituto Tecnologico de Santo Domingo, School of Medicine, Santo Domingo, Dominican Republic. Offers M Bioethics, MD.

Johns Hopkins University, School of Medicine, Professional Program in Medicine, Baltimore, MD 21218-2699. Offers MD, MD/PhD. *Accreditation:* LCME/AMA. *Faculty:* 2,463 full-time (956 women), 1,267 part-time/adjunct (432 women). *Students:* 484 full-time (235 women); includes 248 minority (48 Black or African American, non-Hispanic/Latino; 3 American Indian or Alaska Native, non-Hispanic/Latino; 153 Asian, non-Hispanic/Latino; 30 Hispanic/Latino; 14 Two or more races, non-Hispanic/Latino), 20 international. Average age 25. 4,004 applicants, 7% accepted, 115 enrolled. In 2013, 115 doctorates awarded. *Entrance requirements:* For doctorate, MCAT. *Application deadline:* For fall admission, 10/15 for domestic and international students. Applications are processed on a rolling basis. Application fee: $80. Electronic applications accepted. *Financial support:* Career-related internships or fieldwork, Federal Work-Study, institutionally sponsored loans, scholarships/grants, and health care benefits available. Financial award application deadline: 3/15; financial award applicants required to submit FAFSA. *Unit head:* Dr. Paul B. Rothman, Dean of Medical Faculty and Chief Executive Officer, 410-955-3180. *Application contact:* 410-955-3182, Fax: 410-516-5188, E-mail: somadmiss@jhmi.edu.
Website: http://hopkinsmedicine.org/

Loma Linda University, School of Medicine, Loma Linda, CA 92350. Offers MS, MD, PhD. *Accreditation:* LCME/AMA. *Degree requirements:* For master's, thesis optional; for doctorate, thesis/dissertation (for some programs). *Entrance requirements:* For doctorate, MCAT (for MD). Additional exam requirements/recommendations for international students: Required—TOEFL (minimum score 550 paper-based). *Expenses:* Contact institution.

Louisiana State University Health Sciences Center, School of Medicine in New Orleans, New Orleans, LA 70112-2223. Offers MPH, MD, MD/PhD. Open only to Louisiana residents. *Accreditation:* LCME/AMA. *Entrance requirements:* For doctorate, MCAT. Electronic applications accepted. *Expenses:* Contact institution. *Faculty research:* Medical and basic sciences.

Louisiana State University Health Sciences Center at Shreveport, School of Medicine, Shreveport, LA 71130-3932. Offers MD, MD/PhD. *Accreditation:* LCME/AMA. *Entrance requirements:* For doctorate, MCAT. *Expenses:* Contact institution. *Faculty research:* Biomedical science, molecular biology, cardiovascular science.

Loyola University Chicago, Stritch School of Medicine, Maywood, IL 60153. Offers MD. *Accreditation:* LCME/AMA. *Degree requirements:* For doctorate, passing scores on U. S. Medical Licensing Exam Step 1, Step 2CS, and Step 2CK. *Entrance requirements:* For doctorate, MCAT, 1 full academic year of general biology or zoology, organic chemistry, physics and inorganic chemistry all with labs. *Expenses:* Contact institution. *Faculty research:* Cardiovascular pathophysiology, cancer biology, neuroscience, burn injury, infectious disease.

Marshall University, Joan C. Edwards School of Medicine, Professional Program in Medicine, Huntington, WV 25755. Offers MD. *Accreditation:* LCME/AMA. *Degree requirements:* For doctorate, U.S. Medical Licensing Exam, Steps 1 and 2. *Entrance requirements:* For doctorate, MCAT, 1 year of course work in biology, physics, chemistry, organic chemistry, English, and social or behavioral sciences. *Expenses:* Contact institution.

Mayo Medical School, Professional Program, Rochester, MN 55905. Offers MD, MD/Certificate, MD/PhD. MD offered through the Mayo Foundation's Division of Education; MD/PhD, MD/Certificate with Mayo Graduate School. *Accreditation:* LCME/AMA. *Entrance requirements:* For doctorate, MCAT, previous undergraduate course work in biology, chemistry, physics, and biochemistry. Electronic applications accepted.

McGill University, Faculty of Graduate and Postdoctoral Studies, Faculty of Medicine, Department of Surgery, Montréal, QC H3A 2T5, Canada. Offers M Sc, PhD.

McGill University, Professional Program in Medicine, Montréal, QC H3A 2T5, Canada. Offers MD/CM, MD/MBA, MD/PhD. *Accreditation:* LCME/AMA.

Medical College of Wisconsin, Medical School, Professional Program in Medicine, Milwaukee, WI 53226-0509. Offers MD, MD/MA, MD/MS, MD/PhD. *Accreditation:* LCME/AMA. *Entrance requirements:* For doctorate, GRE, official transcripts, three letters of recommendation. Additional exam requirements/recommendations for international students: Required—TOEFL.

Medical University of South Carolina, College of Medicine, Charleston, SC 29425. Offers MD, MD/MBA, MD/MHA, MD/MPH, MD/MSCR, MD/PhD. *Accreditation:* LCME/AMA. *Degree requirements:* For doctorate, Steps 1 and 2 of Clinical Performance Exam and U.S. Medical Licensing Examination. *Entrance requirements:* For doctorate, MCAT, interview. Electronic applications accepted. *Expenses:* Contact institution. *Faculty research:* Cardiovascular proteomics, translational cancer research, diabetes mellitus, neurodegenerative diseases, addiction.

Meharry Medical College, School of Medicine, Nashville, TN 37208-9989. Offers MD. *Accreditation:* LCME/AMA. *Entrance requirements:* For doctorate, MCAT. Electronic applications accepted. *Faculty research:* Signal transduction, membrane biology, neurophysiology, tropical medicine.

Mercer University, School of Medicine, Macon, GA 31207. Offers MFT, MPH, MSA, MD. *Accreditation:* AAMFT/COAMFTE; LCME/AMA (one or more programs are accredited). *Entrance requirements:* Additional exam requirements/recommendations for international students: Required—TOEFL. *Faculty research:* Anatomy, biochemistry/nutrition, genetics, microbiology/immunology, neuroscience.

Michigan State University, College of Human Medicine, Professional Program in Human Medicine, East Lansing, MI 48824. Offers human medicine (MD); human medicine/medical scientist training program (MD). *Accreditation:* LCME/AMA. *Entrance requirements:* Additional exam requirements/recommendations for international students: Required—TOEFL, Michigan State University ELT (minimum score 85), Michigan Michigan English Language Assessment Battery (minimum score 83). Electronic applications accepted.

Morehouse School of Medicine, Professional Program, Atlanta, GA 30310-1495. Offers MD, MD/MPH. *Accreditation:* LCME/AMA. *Students:* 287 full-time (182 women), 2 part-time (0 women). *Degree requirements:* For doctorate, U.S. Medical Licensing Exam Steps 1 and 2. *Entrance requirements:* For doctorate, MCAT. *Application deadline:* For fall admission, 12/1 for domestic students. Applications are processed on a rolling basis. Application fee: $50. Electronic applications accepted. *Expenses:* Contact institution.

Financial support: Career-related internships or fieldwork, Federal Work-Study, institutionally sponsored loans, and scholarships/grants available. Financial award application deadline: 5/1; financial award applicants required to submit FAFSA. *Faculty research:* Cardiovascular disease and related sequela, infectious diseases/HIV-AIDS, neurological diseases, cancer. *Unit head:* Dr. Ngozi Anachebe, Associate Dean for Admissions and Student Affairs, 404-752-1881, Fax: 404-752-1594. *Application contact:* Brandon Hunter, Director of Admissions, 404-752-1650, Fax: 404-752-1512, E-mail: mdadmission@msm.edu.
Website: http://www.msm.edu/EducationTraining/degreePrograms/mdProgram/MDProgram.php

New York Medical College, School of Medicine, Vahalla, NY 10595-1691. Offers MD, MD/DPT, MD/MPH, MD/PhD. *Accreditation:* LCME/AMA. *Faculty:* 1,286 full-time (498 women), 1,506 part-time/adjunct (480 women). *Students:* 809 full-time (403 women); includes 340 minority (62 Black or African American, non-Hispanic/Latino; 1 American Indian or Alaska Native, non-Hispanic/Latino; 206 Asian, non-Hispanic/Latino; 71 Hispanic/Latino), 6 international. Average age 25. 12,077 applicants, 5% accepted, 200 enrolled. In 2013, 210 doctorates awarded. *Entrance requirements:* For doctorate, MCAT, 2 semesters of course work in general biology, general chemistry, organic chemistry, physics, and English. *Application deadline:* For fall admission, 1/31 for domestic and international students. Applications are processed on a rolling basis. Application fee: $110. Electronic applications accepted. *Expenses:* Contact institution. *Financial support:* Research assistantships, Federal Work-Study, institutionally sponsored loans, and scholarships/grants available. Financial award application deadline: 4/30; financial award applicants required to submit FAFSA. *Faculty research:* Cardiovascular diseases, cancer, infectious diseases, neurosciences, renal diseases, pulmonary diseases. *Total annual research expenditures:* $20.2 million. *Unit head:* Jennifer Koestler, MD, Senior Associate Dean for Medical Education, 914-594-4500, E-mail: jennifer_koestler@nymc.edu. *Application contact:* Fern Juster, MD, Associate Dean of Admissions, 914-594-4507, Fax: 914-594-4613, E-mail: mdadmit@nymc.edu.
Website: http://www.nymc.edu/

New York University, School of Medicine, New York, NY 10016. Offers MS, MD, PhD, MD/MA, MD/MBA, MD/MPA, MD/MPH, MD/MS, MD/PhD. *Accreditation:* LCME/AMA (one or more programs are accredited). *Faculty:* 1,361 full-time (511 women), 1,162 part-time/adjunct (542 women). *Students:* 660 full-time (318 women); includes 175 minority (13 Black or African American, non-Hispanic/Latino; 13 Asian, non-Hispanic/Latino; 67 Hispanic/Latino; 71 Native Hawaiian or other Pacific Islander, non-Hispanic/Latino; 11 Two or more races, non-Hispanic/Latino), 9 international. Average age 24. 8,835 applicants, 6% accepted, 159 enrolled. In 2013, 6 master's awarded. *Degree requirements:* For master's, comprehensive exam, thesis; for doctorate, comprehensive exam (for some programs), thesis/dissertation (for some programs). *Entrance requirements:* For doctorate, MCAT (for MD). *Application deadline:* For fall admission, 10/15 for domestic students; for winter admission, 12/18 for domestic students, 12/15 for international students. Applications are processed on a rolling basis. Application fee: $100. *Expenses:* Contact institution. *Financial support:* In 2013–14, 267 students received support, including 29 fellowships with full tuition reimbursements available (averaging $31,000 per year), 47 research assistantships with full tuition reimbursements available (averaging $31,000 per year); teaching assistantships, Federal Work-Study, institutionally sponsored loans, scholarships/grants, and health care benefits also available. Financial award application deadline: 3/1; financial award applicants required to submit FAFSA. *Faculty research:* AIDS, cancer, neuroscience, molecular biology, neuroscience, cell biology and molecular genetics, structural biology, microbial pathogenesis and host defense, pharmacology, molecular oncology and immunology. *Total annual research expenditures:* $201.1 million. *Unit head:* Dr. Robert Grossman, Dean, 212-263-3269, Fax: 212-263-1828, E-mail: robert.grossman@nyumc.org. *Application contact:* Dr. Rafael Rivera, Associate Dean, Admissions and Financial Aid, 212-263-5290, Fax: 212-263-0720, E-mail: rafael.rivera@nyumc.org.
Website: http://school.med.nyu.edu/

Northeast Ohio Medical University, College of Medicine, Rootstown, OH 44272-0095. Offers MD. *Accreditation:* LCME/AMA. *Faculty:* 408 full-time (133 women), 1,778 part-time/adjunct (452 women). *Students:* 538 full-time (235 women); includes 200 minority (9 Black or African American, non-Hispanic/Latino; 2 American Indian or Alaska Native, non-Hispanic/Latino; 176 Asian, non-Hispanic/Latino; 7 Hispanic/Latino; 1 Native Hawaiian or other Pacific Islander, non-Hispanic/Latino; 5 Two or more races, non-Hispanic/Latino). Average age 24. 3,198 applicants, 15% accepted, 161 enrolled. In 2013, 107 doctorates awarded. *Degree requirements:* For doctorate, U.S. Medical Licensing Exam Step 1. *Entrance requirements:* For doctorate, MCAT, 2 semesters of course work in organic chemistry and physics. *Application deadline:* For fall admission, 8/1 priority date for domestic students; for winter admission, 10/1 for domestic students. Applications are processed on a rolling basis. Application fee: $40. Electronic applications accepted. *Expenses:* Contact institution. *Financial support:* In 2013–14, 264 students received support. Institutionally sponsored loans and scholarships/grants available. Financial award application deadline: 4/15; financial award applicants required to submit FAFSA. *Faculty research:* Lipid metabolism/cardiovascular disease, bone diseases/skeletal biology, virology/infectious diseases, clinical outcomes, sensory neurobiology. *Total annual research expenditures:* $9.1 million. *Unit head:* Dr. Jeffrey L. Susman, Dean, 330-325-6254. *Application contact:* Luke Gloeckner, Enrollment Services Specialist, 330-325-6274, E-mail: lgloeckner@neoucom.edu.
Website: http://www.neomed.edu/academics/medicine

Northwestern University, Fienberg School of Medicine, Combined MD/PhD Medical Scientist Training Program, Evanston, IL 60208. Offers MD/PhD. Application must be made to both The Graduate School and the Medical School. *Accreditation:* LCME/AMA. Electronic applications accepted. *Faculty research:* Cardiovascular epidemiology, cancer epidemiology, nutritional interventions for the prevention of cardiovascular disease and cancer, women's health, outcomes research.

The Ohio State University, College of Medicine, Professional Program in Medicine, Columbus, OH 43210. Offers MD, MD/PhD. *Accreditation:* LCME/AMA. *Faculty:* 1,487. *Students:* 843 full-time (378 women), 4 part-time (2 women); includes 346 minority (57 Black or African American, non-Hispanic/Latino; 1 American Indian or Alaska Native, non-Hispanic/Latino; 198 Asian, non-Hispanic/Latino; 69 Hispanic/Latino; 1 Native Hawaiian or other Pacific Islander, non-Hispanic/Latino; 20 Two or more races, non-Hispanic/Latino). Average age 25. In 2013, 209 doctorates awarded. *Entrance requirements:* For doctorate, MCAT. *Application deadline:* For fall admission, 11/1 for domestic and international students. Applications are processed on a rolling basis. Application fee: $80. Electronic applications accepted. *Financial support:* Fellowships, research assistantships, teaching assistantships, Federal Work-Study, institutionally sponsored loans, and scholarships/grants available. Support available to part-time students. Financial award application deadline: 2/15; financial award applicants required to submit FAFSA. *Faculty research:* Molecular genetics, stress and the immune system, molecular cardiology, transplantation biology. *Total annual research expenditures:* $39.2 million. *Unit head:* Edmund F. Funai, MD, Interim Dean, 614-292-2600, Fax: 614-292-1301. *Application contact:* Professional Admissions, 614-292-9444, Fax: 614-292-3895, E-mail: professional@osu.edu.
Website: http://medicine.osu.edu/

Oregon Health & Science University, School of Medicine, Professional Program in Medicine, Portland, OR 97239-3098. Offers MD, MD/DMD, MD/MPH, MD/PhD. *Accreditation:* LCME/AMA. *Faculty:* 1,737. *Students:* 528 full-time (271 women); includes 103 minority (6 Black or African American, non-Hispanic/Latino; 2 American Indian or Alaska Native, non-Hispanic/Latino; 65 Asian, non-Hispanic/Latino; 13 Hispanic/Latino; 1 Native Hawaiian or other Pacific Islander, non-Hispanic/Latino; 16 Two or more races, non-Hispanic/Latino). Average age 28. 5,225 applicants, 4% accepted, 132 enrolled. In 2013, 118 doctorates awarded. *Degree requirements:* For doctorate, National Board Exam Parts I and II. *Entrance requirements:* For doctorate, MCAT, 1 year of course work in biology, English, social science and physics; 2 years of course work in chemistry and genetics. *Application deadline:* For fall admission, 10/15 for domestic students. Applications are processed on a rolling basis. Application fee: $100. *Financial support:* Fellowships, research assistantships, Federal Work-Study, institutionally sponsored loans, scholarships/grants, and health care benefits available. Financial award application deadline: 3/1; financial award applicants required to submit FAFSA. *Unit head:* Dr. Molly Osborne, Associate Dean for Student Affairs, 503-494-8220, Fax: 503-494-3400. *Application contact:* Debbie Melton, Director, Admissions, 503-494-8220, Fax: 503-494-3400.
Website: http://www.ohsu.edu/som/

Penn State Hershey Medical Center, College of Medicine, Hershey, PA 17033. Offers MPH, MS, MD, PhD, MD/PhD, PhD/MBA. *Accreditation:* LCME/AMA. Terminal master's awarded for partial completion of doctoral program. *Degree requirements:* For master's, thesis optional; for doctorate, comprehensive exam (for some programs), thesis/dissertation (for some programs), minimum GPA of 3.0 (for PhD). *Entrance requirements:* For master's, GRE; for doctorate, GRE (for PhD); MCAT (for MD). Additional exam requirements/recommendations for international students: Required—TOEFL (minimum score 560 paper-based). *Application deadline:* Applications are processed on a rolling basis. Application fee: $65. Electronic applications accepted. *Expenses:* Contact institution. *Financial support:* In 2013–14, 99 students received support, including research assistantships with full tuition reimbursements available (averaging $22,260 per year); fellowships with full tuition reimbursements available, career-related internships or fieldwork, scholarships/grants, health care benefits, and unspecified assistantships also available. *Unit head:* Dr. Michael Verderame, Assistant Dean for Graduate Studies, 717-531-8892, Fax: 717-531-0786, E-mail: grad-hmc@psu.edu. *Application contact:* Dr. Michael F. Verderame, Associate Dean of Graduate Studies, 717-531-8892, Fax: 717-531-0786, E-mail: grad-hmc@psu.edu.
Website: http://www.pennstatehershey.org/web/gsa/home

Ponce School of Medicine & Health Sciences, Professional Program, Ponce, PR 00732-7004. Offers MD. *Accreditation:* LCME/AMA. *Faculty:* 102 full-time (37 women), 87 part-time/adjunct (31 women). *Students:* 268 full-time (143 women); includes 258 minority (257 Hispanic/Latino; 1 Native Hawaiian or other Pacific Islander, non-Hispanic/Latino), 1 international. Average age 25. 1,314 applicants, 10% accepted, 69 enrolled. In 2013, 72 doctorates awarded. *Degree requirements:* For doctorate, one foreign language, comprehensive exam, United States Medical Licensing Exam. *Entrance requirements:* For doctorate, MCAT, coursework in Spanish language, proficiency in Spanish/English. *Application deadline:* For fall admission, 12/15 for domestic and international students. Applications are processed on a rolling basis. Application fee: $150. *Financial support:* In 2013–14, 105 students received support. Fellowships and scholarships/grants available. Financial award application deadline: 4/30; financial award applicants required to submit FAFSA. *Unit head:* Dr. Olga Rodriguez, Interim President and Dean, 787-844-3710, Fax: 787-840-9756, E-mail: orodriguez@psm.edu. *Application contact:* Maria Colon, Admissions Officer, 787-840-2575 Ext. 2143, E-mail: mcolon@psm.edu.

Pontificia Universidad Catolica Madre y Maestra, Department of Medicine, Santiago, Dominican Republic. Offers MD.

Queen's University at Kingston, School of Medicine, Professional Program in Medicine, Kingston, ON K7L 3N6, Canada. Offers MD. *Accreditation:* LCME/AMA. *Entrance requirements:* For doctorate, MCAT.

Rosalind Franklin University of Medicine and Science, The Chicago Medical School, North Chicago, IL 60064-3095. Offers MD, MD/MS, MD/PhD. *Accreditation:* LCME/AMA. *Degree requirements:* For doctorate, clerkship, step 1 and step 2 exams. *Entrance requirements:* For doctorate, MCAT, 3 years of course work with lab in biology, physics, inorganic chemistry, and organic chemistry. *Expenses:* Contact institution. *Faculty research:* Neurosciences, structural biology, cancer biology, cell biology, developmental biology.

Rush University, Rush Medical College, Chicago, IL 60612. Offers MD. *Accreditation:* LCME/AMA. *Entrance requirements:* For doctorate, MCAT, in-person interview. Electronic applications accepted. *Expenses:* Contact institution.

Rutgers, The State University of New Jersey, Newark, New Jersey Medical School, Newark, NJ 07101-1709. Offers MD, MD/Certificate, MD/JD, MD/MBA, MD/MPH, MD/PhD. *Accreditation:* LCME/AMA. *Entrance requirements:* For doctorate, MCAT. Additional exam requirements/recommendations for international students: Required—TOEFL. Electronic applications accepted. *Expenses:* Contact institution.

Rutgers, The State University of New Jersey, New Brunswick, Robert Wood Johnson Medical School, Piscataway, NJ 08822. Offers MD, MD/JD, MD/MBA, MD/MPH, MD/MS, MD/MSJ, MD/PhD. *Accreditation:* LCME/AMA (one or more programs are accredited). *Entrance requirements:* For doctorate, MCAT. Additional exam requirements/recommendations for international students: Required—TOEFL. Electronic applications accepted. *Expenses:* Contact institution.

Saint Louis University, Graduate Education, School of Medicine, Program in Medicine, St. Louis, MO 63103-2097. Offers MD. *Accreditation:* LCME/AMA. *Degree requirements:* For doctorate, U.S. Medical Licensing Exam Steps 1 and 2. *Entrance requirements:* For doctorate, MCAT, photograph, letters of recommendation, interview. Additional exam requirements/recommendations for international students: Required—TOEFL (minimum score 525 paper-based). Electronic applications accepted. *Expenses:* Contact institution. *Faculty research:* Geriatric medicine, organ transplantation, chronic disease prevention, vaccine research.

San Juan Bautista School of Medicine, Professional Program, Caguas, PR 00726-4968. Offers MPH, MD. *Accreditation:* LCME/AMA. *Faculty:* 35 full-time (19 women), 20 part-time/adjunct (4 women). *Students:* 268 full-time (139 women); includes 253 minority (8 Black or African American, non-Hispanic/Latino; 3 Asian, non-Hispanic/Latino; 242 Hispanic/Latino). Average age 25. 1,002 applicants, 12% accepted, 63 enrolled. In 2013, 22 master's, 39 doctorates awarded. *Degree requirements:* For doctorate, comprehensive exam, United States Medical Licensing Exam Steps I and II. *Entrance requirements:* For master's, bachelor's degree from university or college accredited by the Council of Higher Education of Puerto Rico or by a renowned accrediting agency that is registered at the Federal Education Department; minimum GPA of 2.5; for doctorate, MCAT, interview. *Application deadline:* For fall admission, 12/15 priority date for domestic students. Applications are processed on a rolling basis. Application fee: $100. Full-time tuition and fees vary according to degree level. *Financial support:* Applicants required to submit FAFSA. *Faculty research:* Protein structure, CI tissue inflammations, bacterial metabolism, human hormone. *Unit head:* Dr. Yocasta Brugal,

President/Dean, 787-743-3038, Fax: 787-746-3093, E-mail: xbrugal@sanjuanbautista.edu. *Application contact:* Jaymi Sanchez, Admissions Officer, 787-743-3038 Ext. 236, Fax: 787-746-3093, E-mail: jsanchez@sanjuanbautista.edu.
Website: http://www.sanjuanbautista.edu

Stanford University, School of Medicine, Professional Program in Medicine, Stanford, CA 94305-9991. Offers MD, MD/PhD. *Accreditation:* LCME/AMA. *Entrance requirements:* For doctorate, MCAT. Electronic applications accepted. *Expenses:* Contact institution.

State University of New York Downstate Medical Center, College of Medicine, Brooklyn, NY 11203-2098. Offers MPH, MD, MD/MPH, MD/PhD. *Accreditation:* LCME/AMA. *Entrance requirements:* For doctorate, MCAT. *Expenses:* Contact institution. *Faculty research:* AIDS epidemiology, virus/host interaction, molecular genetics, developmental neurobiology, prostate cancer.

State University of New York Downstate Medical Center, School of Graduate Studies, MD/PhD Program, Brooklyn, NY 11203-2098. Offers MD/PhD. *Entrance requirements:* Additional exam requirements/recommendations for international students: Recommended—TOEFL.

State University of New York Upstate Medical University, College of Medicine, Syracuse, NY 13210-2334. Offers MD, MD/PhD. *Accreditation:* LCME/AMA. *Degree requirements:* For doctorate, comprehensive exam. *Entrance requirements:* For doctorate, MCAT. Additional exam requirements/recommendations for international students: Required—TOEFL. Electronic applications accepted. *Expenses:* Contact institution.

Stony Brook University, State University of New York, Stony Brook University Medical Center, Health Sciences Center, School of Medicine, Medical Scientist Training Program, Stony Brook, NY 11794. Offers MD/PhD. *Application deadline:* For fall admission, 1/15 for domestic students. *Expenses:* Tuition, state resident: full-time $9870; part-time $411 per credit. Tuition, nonresident: full-time $18,350; part-time $765 per credit. *Financial support:* Tuition waivers (full) available. *Unit head:* Dr. Michael A. Frohman, Director, Medical Scientist Training Program, 631-444-3219, Fax: 631-444-6229, E-mail: michael.frohman@stonybrook.edu. *Application contact:* Carron Allen, Program Administrator, 631-444-3219, Fax: 631-444-3492, E-mail: carron.kaufman@stonybrook.edu.
Website: http://www.pharm.stonybrook.edu/mstp/

Stony Brook University, State University of New York, Stony Brook University Medical Center, Health Sciences Center, School of Medicine, Professional Program in Medicine, Stony Brook, NY 11794. Offers MD, MD/PhD. *Accreditation:* LCME/AMA. *Faculty:* 715 full-time (278 women), 101 part-time/adjunct (62 women). *Students:* 506 full-time (228 women); includes 201 minority (29 Black or African American, non-Hispanic/Latino; 143 Asian, non-Hispanic/Latino; 24 Hispanic/Latino; 5 Two or more races, non-Hispanic/Latino). Average age 26. 5,196 applicants, 7% accepted, 124 enrolled. In 2013, 130 doctorates awarded. *Entrance requirements:* For doctorate, MCAT, interview. Application fee: $100. *Expenses:* Tuition, state resident: full-time $9870; part-time $411 per credit. Tuition, nonresident: full-time $18,350; part-time $765 per credit. *Financial support:* Fellowships and teaching assistantships available. *Total annual research expenditures:* $39.7 million. *Unit head:* Dr. Kenneth Kaushansky, Dean and Senior Vice President of Health Sciences, 631-444-2113, Fax: 631-444-6032, E-mail: somadmissions@stonybrook.edu. *Application contact:* Committee on Admissions, 631-444-2113, Fax: 631-444-6032, E-mail: somadmissions@stonybrookmedicine.edu.
Website: http://www.stonybrookmedicalcenter.org/som/

Temple University, School of Medicine, Doctor of Medicine Program, Philadelphia, PA 19140. Offers MD, MD/MA, MD/MPH, MD/PhD. *Accreditation:* LCME/AMA. *Faculty:* 550 full-time (184 women), 51 part-time/adjunct (19 women). *Students:* 834 full-time (384 women); includes 318 minority (55 Black or African American, non-Hispanic/Latino; 1 American Indian or Alaska Native, non-Hispanic/Latino; 164 Asian, non-Hispanic/Latino; 78 Hispanic/Latino; 1 Native Hawaiian or other Pacific Islander, non-Hispanic/Latino; 19 Two or more races, non-Hispanic/Latino). Average age 24. 10,980 applicants, 5% accepted, 215 enrolled. In 2013, 188 doctorates awarded. *Degree requirements:* For doctorate, United States Medical Licensing Exam Step 1, Step 2CK, Step 2CS. *Entrance requirements:* For doctorate, MCAT. *Application deadline:* For fall admission, 12/15 for domestic students. Applications are processed on a rolling basis. Application fee: $75. Electronic applications accepted. *Expenses:* Contact institution. *Financial support:* In 2013–14, 313 students received support, including 13 fellowships with full and partial tuition reimbursements available (averaging $15,865 per year), 9 research assistantships with full tuition reimbursements available (averaging $26,500 per year); Federal Work-Study, institutionally sponsored loans, and scholarships/grants also available. Financial award application deadline: 3/1; financial award applicants required to submit FAFSA. *Faculty research:* Translational medicine, molecular biology and immunology of autoimmune diseases and cancer, cardiovascular and pulmonary disease pathophysiology, biology of substance abuse, causes and consequences of obesity, molecular mechanisms of neurological dysfunction. *Total annual research expenditures:* $66.1 million. *Unit head:* Dr. Larry R. Kaiser, Dean, 215-707-8773, E-mail: larry.kaiser@temple.edu. *Application contact:* Information Contact, 215-707-3656, Fax: 215-707-6932, E-mail: medadmissions@temple.edu.
Website: http://www.temple.edu/medicine/

Texas Tech University Health Sciences Center, School of Medicine, Lubbock, TX 79430-0002. Offers MD, JD/MD, MD/MBA, MD/PhD. Open only to residents of Texas, eastern New Mexico, and southwestern Oklahoma; MD/PhD offered jointly with Texas Tech University; JD/MD with School of Law. *Accreditation:* LCME/AMA. *Entrance requirements:* For doctorate, MCAT. Additional exam requirements/recommendations for international students: Required—TOEFL. Electronic applications accepted. *Expenses:* Contact institution.

Thomas Jefferson University, Jefferson Graduate School of Biomedical Sciences, MD/PhD Program, Philadelphia, PA 19107. Offers MD/PhD. *Students:* 16 full-time (6 women); includes 3 minority (2 Asian, non-Hispanic/Latino; 1 Native Hawaiian or other Pacific Islander, non-Hispanic/Latino), 1 international. 170 applicants, 5% accepted, 5 enrolled. *Entrance requirements:* Additional exam requirements/recommendations for international students: Required—TOEFL (minimum score 100 iBT) or IELTS. *Application deadline:* For fall admission, 11/1 for domestic and international students. Applications are processed on a rolling basis. Application fee: $0. Electronic applications accepted. *Financial support:* In 2013–14, 16 fellowships with full tuition reimbursements were awarded; Federal Work-Study and institutionally sponsored loans also available. Financial award application deadline: 5/1; financial award applicants required to submit FAFSA. *Faculty research:* Signal transduction, tumorigenesis, apoptosis, molecular immunology, structural biology. *Unit head:* Dr. Scott A. Waldman, Academic Director, 215-955-6086, Fax: 215-955-5681, E-mail: scott.waldman@jefferson.edu. *Application contact:* Marc E. Stearns, Director of Admissions, 215-503-0155, Fax: 215-503-3433, E-mail: jgsbs-info@jefferson.edu.
Website: http://www.jefferson.edu/university/jmc_jgsbs/md_phd.html.html

Thomas Jefferson University, Sidney Kimmel Medical College, Philadelphia, PA 19107. Offers MD, MD/PhD. *Accreditation:* LCME/AMA. *Faculty:* 1,100 full-time (366 women), 59 part-time/adjunct (29 women). *Students:* 1,061 full-time (529 women); includes 329 minority (14 Black or African American, non-Hispanic/Latino; 4 American Indian or Alaska Native, non-Hispanic/Latino; 245 Asian, non-Hispanic/Latino; 66 Hispanic/Latino), 50 international. Average age 23. 10,118 applicants, 4% accepted, 260 enrolled. In 2013, 252 doctorates awarded. *Entrance requirements:* For doctorate, MCAT. *Application deadline:* For fall admission, 11/15 for domestic and international students. Applications are processed on a rolling basis. Application fee: $80. Electronic applications accepted. *Expenses:* Contact institution. *Financial support:* In 2013–14, 753 students received support. Federal Work-Study, institutionally sponsored loans, and scholarships/grants available. Financial award application deadline: 3/1; financial award applicants required to submit FAFSA. *Faculty research:* Translational medicine, Alzheimer's research, pancreatic cancer, oncology and endocrinology. *Total annual research expenditures:* $47.1 million. *Unit head:* Dr. Mark Tykowcinski, Interim Dean, 215-955-6980, Fax: 215-923-6939. *Application contact:* Dr. Clara Callahan, Dean for Admissions, 215-955-6983, Fax: 215-955-5151, E-mail: clara.callahan@jefferson.edu.
Website: http://www.jefferson.edu/university/jmc.html

Tufts University, School of Medicine, Professional Program in Medicine, Medford, MA 02155. Offers MD, MD/MA, MD/MBA, MD/MPH, MD/PhD. MD/PhD offered jointly with Sackler School of Graduate Biomedical Sciences; MD/MBA with Brandeis University. *Accreditation:* LCME/AMA. *Students:* 805 full-time (400 women), 3 part-time (all women); includes 254 minority (29 Black or African American, non-Hispanic/Latino; 2 American Indian or Alaska Native, non-Hispanic/Latino; 155 Asian, non-Hispanic/Latino; 35 Hispanic/Latino; 2 Native Hawaiian or other Pacific Islander, non-Hispanic/Latino; 31 Two or more races, non-Hispanic/Latino), 6 international. Average age 27. 8,647 applicants, 6% accepted, 204 enrolled. In 2013, 200 doctorates awarded. *Entrance requirements:* For doctorate, MCAT. *Application deadline:* For fall admission, 1/15 for domestic students. Applications are processed on a rolling basis. Application fee: $105. Electronic applications accepted. *Expenses:* Contact institution. *Financial support:* Federal Work-Study, institutionally sponsored loans, and scholarships/grants available. Financial award application deadline: 3/28; financial award applicants required to submit FAFSA. *Unit head:* Dr. Harris Berman, Dean, 617-636-6565. *Application contact:* Thomas Slavin, Director of Admissions, 617-636-6571, E-mail: med-admissions@tufts.edu.
Website: http://medicine.tufts.edu/

Tulane University, School of Medicine, Professional Programs in Medicine, New Orleans, LA 70118-5669. Offers MD, MD/MBA, MD/MPH, MD/MPHTM, MD/MSPH, MD/PhD. *Accreditation:* LCME/AMA. *Entrance requirements:* For doctorate, MCAT.

Universidad Autonoma de Guadalajara, School of Medicine, Guadalajara, Mexico. Offers MD.

Universidad Central del Caribe, School of Medicine, Bayamón, PR 00960-6032. Offers MA, MS, MD, PhD. *Accreditation:* LCME/AMA. *Degree requirements:* For doctorate, variable foreign language requirement. *Entrance requirements:* For doctorate, MCAT (for MD). *Faculty research:* Membrane neurotransmitter receptors, brain neurotransmission, cocaine toxicology, membrane transport, antimetabolite pharmacology.

Universidad Central del Este, Medical School, San Pedro de Macoris, Dominican Republic. Offers MD.

Universidad de Ciencias Medicas, Graduate Programs, San Jose, Costa Rica. Offers dermatology (SP); family health (MS); health service center administration (MHA); human anatomy (MS); medical and surgery (MD); occupational medicine (MS); pharmacy (Pharm D). Part-time programs available. *Degree requirements:* For master's, thesis; for doctorate and SP, comprehensive exam. *Entrance requirements:* For master's, MD or bachelor's degree; for doctorate, admissions test; for SP, admissions test, MD.

Universidad de Iberoamerica, Graduate School, San Jose, Costa Rica. Offers clinical neuropsychology (PhD); clinical psychology (M Psych); educational psychology (M Psych); forensic psychology (M Psych); hospital management (MHA); intensive care nursing (MN); medicine (MD).

Universidad Iberoamericana, School of Medicine, Santo Domingo D.N., Dominican Republic. Offers MD.

Universidad Nacional Pedro Henriquez Urena, School of Medicine, Santo Domingo, Dominican Republic. Offers MD.

Université de Montréal, Faculty of Medicine, Professional Program in Medicine, Montréal, QC H3C 3J7, Canada. Offers MD. Open only to Canadian residents. *Accreditation:* LCME/AMA. *Entrance requirements:* For doctorate, proficiency in French. Electronic applications accepted.

Université de Sherbrooke, Faculty of Medicine and Health Sciences, Professional Program in Medicine, Sherbrooke, QC J1K 2R1, Canada. Offers MD. *Accreditation:* LCME/AMA. Electronic applications accepted.

Université Laval, Faculty of Medicine, Post-Professional Programs in Medical Studies, Québec, QC G1K 7P4, Canada. Offers anatomy–pathology (DESS); anesthesiology (DESS); cardiology (DESS); care of older people (Diploma); clinical research (DESS); community health (DESS); dermatology (DESS); diagnostic radiology (DESS); emergency medicine (Diploma); family medicine (DESS); general surgery (DESS); geriatrics (DESS); hematology (DESS); internal medicine (DESS); maternal and fetal medicine (Diploma); medical biochemistry (DESS); medical microbiology and infectious diseases (DESS); medical oncology (DESS); nephrology (DESS); neurology (DESS); neurosurgery (DESS); obstetrics and gynecology (DESS); ophthalmology (DESS); orthopedic surgery (DESS); oto-rhino-laryngology (DESS); palliative medicine (Diploma); pediatrics (DESS); plastic surgery (DESS); psychiatry (DESS); pulmonary medicine (DESS); radiology–oncology (DESS); thoracic surgery (DESS); urology (DESS). *Degree requirements:* For other advanced degree, comprehensive exam. *Entrance requirements:* For degree, knowledge of French. Electronic applications accepted.

Université Laval, Faculty of Medicine, Professional Program in Medicine, Québec, QC G1K 7P4, Canada. Offers MD. *Accreditation:* LCME/AMA. *Entrance requirements:* For doctorate, interview, proficiency in French. Electronic applications accepted.

University at Buffalo, the State University of New York, Graduate School, School of Medicine and Biomedical Sciences, Professional Program in Medicine, Buffalo, NY 14260. Offers MD, MD/MBA, MD/MPH, MD/PhD. *Accreditation:* LCME/AMA. *Students:* 576 full-time (251 women); includes 197 minority (20 Black or African American, non-Hispanic/Latino; 5 American Indian or Alaska Native, non-Hispanic/Latino; 142 Asian, non-Hispanic/Latino; 30 Hispanic/Latino). Average age 24. 4,090 applicants, 10% accepted, 140 enrolled. In 2013, 141 doctorates awarded. *Entrance requirements:* For doctorate, MCAT, interview. *Application deadline:* For fall admission, 11/15 for domestic students. Applications are processed on a rolling basis. Application fee: $65. Electronic applications accepted. *Financial support:* In 2013–14, 101 students received support. Career-related internships or fieldwork, Federal Work-Study, institutionally sponsored loans, and scholarships/grants available. Financial award application deadline: 3/1; financial award applicants required to submit FAFSA. *Faculty research:* Microbial

pathogenesis, neuronal plasticity, structural biology of ion channels, structural development, cell biology of development. *Unit head:* Dr. Charles Severin, Dean for Admissions, 716-829-2803, Fax: 716-829-2798, E-mail: severin@buffalo.edu. *Application contact:* James J. Rosso, Admissions Advisor, 716-829-3466, Fax: 716-829-3849, E-mail: jjrosso@buffalo.edu.
Website: http://medicine.buffalo.edu/education/md.html

The University of Alabama at Birmingham, School of Medicine, Birmingham, AL 35294-3412. Offers MD. *Accreditation:* LCME/AMA. *Entrance requirements:* For doctorate, MCAT (minimum score of 24), AMCAS application, letters of recommendation, interview. *Expenses:* Contact institution.

The University of Arizona, College of Medicine, Professional Programs in Medicine, Tucson, AZ 85721. Offers MD, MD/PhD. MD program open only to state residents. *Accreditation:* LCME/AMA. *Faculty:* 1,600. *Students:* 724 full-time (356 women); includes 171 minority (10 Black or African American, non-Hispanic/Latino; 1 American Indian or Alaska Native, non-Hispanic/Latino; 48 Asian, non-Hispanic/Latino; 41 Hispanic/Latino; 71 Two or more races, non-Hispanic/Latino). Average age 30. 280 applicants, 71% accepted, 191 enrolled. In 2013, 162 doctorates awarded. *Entrance requirements:* For doctorate, MCAT, previous course work in general chemistry, organic chemistry, biology/zoology, physics, and English. Application fee: $0. *Expenses:* Tuition, state resident: full-time $11,526. Tuition, nonresident: full-time $27,398. *Financial support:* Fellowships, research assistantships, teaching assistantships, career-related internships or fieldwork, Federal Work-Study, institutionally sponsored loans, and tuition waivers (full and partial) available. *Faculty research:* Developmental biology, cellular structure and function, immunology, clinical cancer research, heart and respiratory disease. *Total annual research expenditures:* $160.2 million. *Unit head:* Dr. Steven Goldschmid, Dean, 520-626-4555, E-mail: lupeo@email.arizona.edu. *Application contact:* Dr. Shirley Nickols Fahey, Associate Dean for Admissions, 520-621-2211.
Website: http://medicine.arizona.edu/

The University of Arizona, College of Medicine, Program in Medical Sciences, Tucson, AZ 85721. Offers MS, PhD. *Students:* 5 full-time (1 woman), 6 part-time (4 women); includes 5 minority (2 Black or African American, non-Hispanic/Latino; 2 Hispanic/Latino; 1 Two or more races, non-Hispanic/Latino), 1 international. Average age 29. 13 applicants, 69% accepted, 3 enrolled. In 2013, 1 master's, 1 doctorate awarded. *Degree requirements:* For doctorate, comprehensive exam, thesis/dissertation. *Application deadline:* For fall admission, 5/5 for domestic students. Application fee: $75. *Expenses:* Tuition, state resident: full-time $11,526. Tuition, nonresident: full-time $27,398. *Financial support:* Traineeships, health care benefits, and unspecified assistantships available. *Unit head:* Diane Poskus, Coordinator, 520-626-3972, E-mail: dposkus@surgery.arizona.edu. *Application contact:* Kathy Detloff, Associate Dean for Admissions, 520-626-3972, E-mail: kdetloff@surgery.arizona.edu.
Website: http://surgery.arizona.edu/education/medical-sciences-graduate-program

University of Arkansas for Medical Sciences, College of Medicine, Little Rock, AR 72205-7199. Offers MD, MD/PhD. *Accreditation:* LCME/AMA. *Faculty:* 832 full-time (327 women), 191 part-time/adjunct (86 women). *Students:* 677 full-time (236 women); includes 137 minority (29 Black or African American, non-Hispanic/Latino; 2 American Indian or Alaska Native, non-Hispanic/Latino; 70 Asian, non-Hispanic/Latino; 25 Hispanic/Latino; 11 Two or more races, non-Hispanic/Latino). Average age 29. 1,149 applicants, 18% accepted, 173 enrolled. In 2013, 159 doctorates awarded. *Entrance requirements:* For doctorate, MCAT. *Application deadline:* For fall admission, 11/1 for domestic students. Application fee: $100. Electronic applications accepted. *Expenses:* Contact institution. *Financial support:* Federal Work-Study available. *Unit head:* Dr. G. Richard Smith, Dean, 501-686-5350, E-mail: smithgrichard@uams.edu. *Application contact:* Linda Dupuy, Director of Medical Student Recruitment and Admissions, 501-686-5355, E-mail: dupuylinda@uams.edu.
Website: http://www.uams.edu/com/

The University of British Columbia, Faculty of Medicine, Department of Surgery, Vancouver, BC V6T 1Z1, Canada. Offers M Sc. Part-time programs available. *Degree requirements:* For master's, thesis. *Entrance requirements:* Additional exam requirements/recommendations for international students: Required—TOEFL. Electronic applications accepted. *Expenses: Tuition, area resident:* Full-time $8000 Canadian dollars. *Faculty research:* Photodynamic therapy, transplantation immunobiology, isolated cell culture, neurophysiology.

The University of British Columbia, Faculty of Medicine, Professional Program in Medicine, Vancouver, BC V6T 1Z1, Canada. Offers MD, MD/PhD. *Accreditation:* LCME/AMA. *Entrance requirements:* For doctorate, MCAT. *Expenses: Tuition, area resident:* Full-time $8000 Canadian dollars.

University of Calgary, Cumming School of Medicine, MD Program, Calgary, AB T2N 1N4, Canada. Offers MD. *Accreditation:* LCME/AMA. *Students:* 497 full-time (288 women). Average age 25. 1,642 applicants, 17% accepted, 155 enrolled. In 2013, 172 doctorates awarded. *Entrance requirements:* For doctorate, MCAT. *Application deadline:* For fall admission, 10/1 for domestic students. Application fee: $150. Electronic applications accepted. *Financial support:* Career-related internships or fieldwork available. *Unit head:* Dr. Bruce Wright, Associate Dean, Medical Education, 403-220-3843, Fax: 403-270-2681, E-mail: umeadm4@ucalgary.ca. *Application contact:* Adele Meyers, Coordinator, Admissions and Student Affairs, 403-220-4357, Fax: 403-210-8148, E-mail: meyers@ucalgary.ca.
Website: http://medicine.ucalgary.ca

University of California, Berkeley, Graduate Division, School of Public Health, Group in Health and Medical Sciences, Berkeley, CA 94720-1500. Offers MD/MS. Program offered jointly with University of California, San Francisco.

University of California, Davis, School of Medicine, Sacramento, CA 95817. Offers MD, MD/MBA, MD/MPH, MD/MS, MD/PhD. *Accreditation:* LCME/AMA. *Faculty:* 740 full-time (248 women), 133 part-time/adjunct (58 women). *Students:* 415 full-time (221 women); includes 242 minority (26 Black or African American, non-Hispanic/Latino; 3 American Indian or Alaska Native, non-Hispanic/Latino; 152 Asian, non-Hispanic/Latino; 60 Hispanic/Latino; 1 Native Hawaiian or other Pacific Islander, non-Hispanic/Latino), 1 international. Average age 27. 5,863 applicants, 4% accepted, 104 enrolled. In 2013, 106 doctorates awarded. *Degree requirements:* For doctorate, comprehensive exam. *Entrance requirements:* For doctorate, MCAT, 1 year each of English, biological science (lower-division with lab), general chemistry (with lab), organic chemistry (with lab), physics, and college-level math, plus 1/2 year upper-division biology. *Application deadline:* For fall admission, 10/1 for domestic and international students. Applications are processed on a rolling basis. Application fee: $80. Electronic applications accepted. *Expenses:* Contact institution. *Financial support:* In 2013–14, 405 students received support, including 12 fellowships with full tuition reimbursements available (averaging $22,833 per year), 6 research assistantships with full tuition reimbursements available (averaging $38,988 per year), 3 teaching assistantships with partial tuition reimbursements available (averaging $2,828 per year); institutionally sponsored loans and scholarships/grants also available. Support available to part-time students. Financial award application deadline: 3/2; financial award applicants required to submit FAFSA. *Faculty research:* Cancer biology, cardiovascular disease, clinical and translational research, neuroscience, regenerative medicine. *Total annual research expenditures:* $168.3 million. *Unit head:* Dr. Julie Ann Freischlag, Dean/Vice Chancellor, Human Health Sciences, 916-734-7131, Fax: 916-734-7055, E-mail: julie.freischlag@ucdmc.ucdavis.edu. *Application contact:* Joanna Garcia, Director of Admissions, 916-734-4663, Fax: 916-734-4050, E-mail: joanna.garcia@ucdmc.ucdavis.edu.
Website: http://www.ucdmc.ucdavis.edu/medschool/

University of California, Irvine, School of Medicine, Professional Program in Medicine, Irvine, CA 92697. Offers MD, MD/MBA, MD/MPH, MD/PhD. *Accreditation:* LCME/AMA. *Students:* 419 full-time (221 women), 25 part-time (9 women); includes 65 minority (2 Black or African American, non-Hispanic/Latino; 1 American Indian or Alaska Native, non-Hispanic/Latino; 45 Asian, non-Hispanic/Latino; 16 Hispanic/Latino; 1 Native Hawaiian or other Pacific Islander, non-Hispanic/Latino). Average age 26. *Entrance requirements:* For doctorate, MCAT. Additional exam requirements/recommendations for international students: Required—TOEFL (minimum score 550 paper-based). *Application deadline:* For fall admission, 11/1 for domestic students. Application fee: $80 ($100 for international students). Electronic applications accepted. *Financial support:* Fellowships, institutionally sponsored loans, traineeships, health care benefits, and unspecified assistantships available. Financial award application deadline: 3/1; financial award applicants required to submit FAFSA. *Unit head:* Prof. Ralph Victor Clayman, Dean and Professor, 949-824-5926, Fax: 949-824-2676, E-mail: rclayman@uci.edu. *Application contact:* Prof. Alan L. Goldin, Senior Associate Dean and Professor, 949-824-5334, Fax: 949-824-8504, E-mail: agoldin@uci.edu.

University of California, Los Angeles, David Geffen School of Medicine, Professional Program in Medicine, Los Angeles, CA 90095. Offers MD, MD/MBA, MD/PhD. *Accreditation:* LCME/AMA. *Entrance requirements:* For doctorate, MCAT, interview. *Expenses:* Contact institution.

University of California, San Diego, School of Medicine, Professional Program in Medicine, La Jolla, CA 92093. Offers MD, MD/PhD. *Accreditation:* LCME/AMA. *Entrance requirements:* For doctorate, MCAT. *Expenses:* Tuition, state resident: full-time $11,220; part-time $1870 per quarter. Tuition, nonresident: full-time $26,322; part-time $4387 per quarter. *Required fees:* $519.50 per quarter. Part-time tuition and fees vary according to course load and program.

University of California, San Francisco, School of Medicine, San Francisco, CA 94143-0410. Offers MD, PhD, MD/MPH, MD/MS, MD/PhD. *Accreditation:* LCME/AMA (one or more programs are accredited). *Faculty:* 2,031 full-time (678 women), 128 part-time/adjunct (41 women). *Students:* 632 full-time (341 women); includes 331 minority (44 Black or African American, non-Hispanic/Latino; 124 Asian, non-Hispanic/Latino; 100 Hispanic/Latino; 24 Native Hawaiian or other Pacific Islander, non-Hispanic/Latino; 39 Two or more races, non-Hispanic/Latino). Average age 24. 6,926 applicants, 4% accepted, 149 enrolled. In 2013, 163 doctorates awarded. *Entrance requirements:* For doctorate, MCAT (for MD), interview (for MD). *Application deadline:* For fall admission, 10/15 for domestic students. Applications are processed on a rolling basis. Application fee: $60 ($80 for international students). Electronic applications accepted. *Expenses:* Contact institution. *Financial support:* In 2013–14, 543 students received support. Federal Work-Study, institutionally sponsored loans, scholarships/grants, and tuition waivers (partial) available. Financial award application deadline: 2/1; financial award applicants required to submit FAFSA. *Faculty research:* Neurosciences, human genetics, developmental biology, social/behavioral/policy sciences, immunology. *Total annual research expenditures:* $414.4 million. *Unit head:* Dr. Sam Hawgood, Dean, 415-476-2342, Fax: 415-476-0689, E-mail: sam.hawgood@ucsf.edu. *Application contact:* Hallen Chung, Director of Admissions, 415-476-8090, Fax: 415-476-5490, E-mail: chungh@medsch.ucsf.edu.
Website: http://www.medschool.ucsf.edu/

University of Central Florida, College of Medicine, Orlando, FL 32816. Offers MS, MD, PhD. *Accreditation:* LCME/AMA. *Financial support:* Fellowships, research assistantships, and teaching assistantships available. *Unit head:* Dr. Deborah C. German, Vice President for Medical Affairs/Dean, 407-266-1000, E-mail: deborah.german@ucf.edu. *Application contact:* Barbara Rodriguez, Director, Admissions and Registration, 407-823-2766, Fax: 407-823-6442, E-mail: gradadmissions@ucf.edu.
Website: http://www.med.ucf.edu

University of Chicago, Pritzker School of Medicine, Chicago, IL 60637-1513. Offers MD, MD/PhD. *Accreditation:* LCME/AMA. *Faculty:* 1,075 full-time (410 women), 239 part-time/adjunct (99 women). *Students:* 397 full-time (187 women); includes 157 minority (32 Black or African American, non-Hispanic/Latino; 1 American Indian or Alaska Native, non-Hispanic/Latino; 84 Asian, non-Hispanic/Latino; 28 Hispanic/Latino; 2 Native Hawaiian or other Pacific Islander, non-Hispanic/Latino; 10 Two or more races, non-Hispanic/Latino), 2 international. 5,713 applicants, 4% accepted, 87 enrolled. In 2013, 82 doctorates awarded. *Entrance requirements:* For doctorate, MCAT, one year of each with lab: chemistry, physics, biology and organic chemistry. *Application deadline:* For fall admission, 10/15 for domestic and international students. Applications are processed on a rolling basis. Application fee: $85. Electronic applications accepted. *Financial support:* In 2013–14, 354 students received support. Career-related internships or fieldwork, Federal Work-Study, institutionally sponsored loans, and scholarships/grants available. Financial award application deadline: 4/1; financial award applicants required to submit FAFSA. *Faculty research:* Human genetics, diabetes, developmental biology, structural biology, neurobiology. *Total annual research expenditures:* $262.6 million. *Application contact:* Sylvia Robertson, Assistant Dean for Admissions and Financial Aid, 773-702-1937, Fax: 773-834-5412, E-mail: pritzkeradmissions@bsd.uchicago.edu.
Website: http://pritzker.bsd.uchicago.edu/

University of Cincinnati, Graduate School, College of Allied Health Sciences, Program in Transfusion and Transplantation Sciences, Cincinnati, OH 45221. Offers blood transfusion medicine (MS); cellular therapies (MS). *Degree requirements:* For master's, comprehensive exam, thesis. *Entrance requirements:* For master's, GRE General Test. Additional exam requirements/recommendations for international students: Required—TOEFL (minimum score 570 paper-based). Electronic applications accepted. *Faculty research:* Preservation of red cells, red cell oxidation and delivery to tissues, cellular therapies, coagulopathies.

University of Cincinnati, Graduate School, College of Medicine, Physician Scientist Training Program, Cincinnati, OH 45221. Offers MD/PhD. *Entrance requirements:* Additional exam requirements/recommendations for international students: Required—TOEFL. Electronic applications accepted.

University of Cincinnati, Graduate School, College of Medicine, Professional Program in Medicine, Cincinnati, OH 45221. Offers MD. *Accreditation:* LCME/AMA. *Entrance requirements:* For doctorate, MCAT. Electronic applications accepted. *Faculty research:* Molecular genetics, environmental health, neuroscience and cell biology, cardiovascular science, developmental biology.

University of Colorado Denver, School of Medicine, Professional Program in Medicine, Aurora, CO 80045. Offers MD, MD/MBA, MD/PhD. *Students:* 631 full-time (305 women); includes 126 minority (17 Black or African American, non-Hispanic/Latino; 3 American Indian or Alaska Native, non-Hispanic/Latino; 61 Asian, non-Hispanic/

Latino; 42 Hispanic/Latino; 3 Two or more races, non-Hispanic/Latino), 6 international. Average age 27. 647 applicants, 26% accepted, 160 enrolled. In 2013, 164 doctorates awarded. *Entrance requirements:* For doctorate, MCAT, application completed through both AMCAS and the Colorado Med school program, essay, interviews, prerequisite coursework in biology (with lab), general chemistry (with lab), organic chemistry (with lab), general physics (with lab), English literature/composition, college-level mathematics (algebra and above). Additional exam requirements/recommendations for international students: Required—TOEFL (minimum score 550 paper-based; 80 iBT). *Application deadline:* For fall admission, 11/1 for domestic students, 10/1 for international students. Application fee: $100 ($125 for international students). Electronic applications accepted. *Expenses:* Contact institution. *Financial support:* In 2013–14, 321 students received support. Fellowships, research assistantships, teaching assistantships, Federal Work-Study, institutionally sponsored loans, scholarships/grants, traineeships, health care benefits, and unspecified assistantships available. Financial award application deadline: 4/1; financial award applicants required to submit FAFSA. *Unit head:* Dr. Ozzie Grenardo, Interim Associate Dean for Admissions, 303-724-0882, E-mail: ozzie.a.grenardo@ucdenver.edu. *Application contact:* Ashley Ehlers, Office of Admissions Medical Program Assistant, 303-724-8025, E-mail: somadmin@ucdenver.edu.
Website: http://www.ucdenver.edu/academics/colleges/medicalschool/Pages/somWelcome.aspx

University of Connecticut Health Center, School of Medicine, Farmington, CT 06030. Offers MD, MD/MBA, MD/MPH, MD/PhD. *Accreditation:* LCME/AMA. *Entrance requirements:* For doctorate, MCAT. Electronic applications accepted. *Expenses:* Contact institution.

University of Florida, College of Medicine, Professional Program in Medicine, Gainesville, FL 32611. Offers MD, MD/PhD. *Accreditation:* LCME/AMA. *Entrance requirements:* For doctorate, MCAT, 8 semester hours of course work in biology, general chemistry, and general physics; 4 semester hours of course work in geochemistry and organic chemistry. Electronic applications accepted. *Expenses:* Tuition, state resident: full-time $12,640. Tuition, nonresident: full-time $30,000. *Faculty research:* Neurobiology, gene therapy and genetic imaging technologies, diabetes and autoimmune diseases, transplantation.

University of Hawaii at Manoa, John A. Burns School of Medicine, Professional Program in Medicine, Honolulu, HI 96822. Offers MD. *Accreditation:* LCME/AMA. *Entrance requirements:* For doctorate, MCAT. Electronic applications accepted. *Expenses:* Contact institution.

University of Illinois at Chicago, College of Medicine, Professional Program in Medicine, Chicago, IL 60607-7128. Offers MD, MD/MS, MD/PhD. Part-time programs available. *Faculty:* 357 full-time (148 women), 145 part-time/adjunct (43 women). *Students:* 1,385 full-time (645 women); includes 738 minority (122 Black or African American, non-Hispanic/Latino; 4 American Indian or Alaska Native, non-Hispanic/Latino; 347 Asian, non-Hispanic/Latino; 231 Hispanic/Latino; 3 Native Hawaiian or other Pacific Islander, non-Hispanic/Latino; 31 Two or more races, non-Hispanic/Latino). Average age 26. 5,837 applicants, 11% accepted, 396 enrolled. In 2013, 299 doctorates awarded. *Entrance requirements:* For doctorate, MCAT. *Application deadline:* For fall admission, 12/15 for domestic students. Applications are processed on a rolling basis. Application fee: $40 ($50 for international students). Electronic applications accepted. *Expenses:* Tuition, state resident: full-time $11,066; part-time $3689 per term. Tuition, nonresident: full-time $23,064; part-time $7688 per term. *Required fees:* $3004; $1190 per term. Tuition and fees vary according to course level and program. *Financial support:* Fellowships, research assistantships, and teaching assistantships available. *Faculty research:* Biomedical and clinical sciences. *Total annual research expenditures:* $24.8 million. *Unit head:* Dr. Dimitri T. Azar, Dean, 312-996-3500, Fax: 312-996-9006, E-mail: dazar@uic.edu. *Application contact:* Jackie Perry, Graduate College Receptionist, 312-413-2550, Fax: 312-413-0185, E-mail: gradcoll@uic.edu.

University of Illinois at Urbana–Champaign, Graduate College, Medical Scholars Program, Urbana, IL 61801. Offers MD/MBA, MD/PhD. *Students:* 122 full-time (59 women); includes 41 minority (2 Black or African American, non-Hispanic/Latino; 30 Asian, non-Hispanic/Latino; 9 Hispanic/Latino). Average age 23. 108 applicants, 14% accepted, 10 enrolled. *Application deadline:* For fall admission, 12/31 for domestic students. Application fee: $0. Electronic applications accepted. *Expenses:* Contact institution. *Financial support:* In 2013–14, 28 fellowships with full tuition reimbursements (averaging $10,000 per year), 25 research assistantships with full tuition reimbursements (averaging $15,000 per year), 23 teaching assistantships with full tuition reimbursements (averaging $15,000 per year) were awarded; traineeships, health care benefits, and unspecified assistantships also available. Financial award applicants required to submit FAFSA. *Unit head:* James W. Hall, EdD, Associate Dean, 217-333-8146, Fax: 217-333-2640. *Application contact:* Jennifer L. Crum, Coordinator, 217-333-8146, Fax: 217-333-2640, E-mail: jlcrum@illinois.edu.
Website: https://www.med.illinois.edu/mdphd/

The University of Iowa, Roy J. and Lucille A. Carver College of Medicine and Graduate College, Medical Scientist Training Program, Iowa City, IA 52242-1316. Offers MD/PhD. *Faculty:* 155 full-time (36 women), 2 part-time/adjunct (0 women). *Students:* 72 full-time (26 women); includes 25 minority (1 Black or African American, non-Hispanic/Latino; 2 American Indian or Alaska Native, non-Hispanic/Latino; 15 Asian, non-Hispanic/Latino; 6 Hispanic/Latino; 1 Native Hawaiian or other Pacific Islander, non-Hispanic/Latino). Average age 24. 200 applicants, 16% accepted, 13 enrolled. *Application deadline:* For fall admission, 12/15 priority date for domestic students. Applications are processed on a rolling basis. Electronic applications accepted. Application fee is waived when completed online. *Financial support:* In 2013–14, 43 students received support, including 12 fellowships with full tuition reimbursements available (averaging $22,032 per year), 43 research assistantships with full tuition reimbursements available (averaging $3,468 per year); scholarships/grants, traineeships, health care benefits, unspecified assistantships, and travel awards also available. *Faculty research:* Structure and function of ion channels, molecular genetics of human disease, neurobiology of pain, viral immunology and immunopathology, epidemiology of aging and cancer, human learning and memory, structural enzymology. *Total annual research expenditures:* $2 million. *Unit head:* Dr. Steven R. Lentz, Director, 319-356-4048, Fax: 319-335-6634, E-mail: steven-lentz@uiowa.edu. *Application contact:* Leslie Harrington, Administrative Director, 319-335-8304, Fax: 319-335-6634, E-mail: mstp@uiowa.edu.
Website: http://www.medicine.uiowa.edu/mstp

The University of Iowa, Roy J. and Lucille A. Carver College of Medicine, Professional Program in Medicine, Iowa City, IA 52242-1316. Offers MD, MD/JD, MD/MBA, MD/MPH, MD/PhD. *Accreditation:* LCME/AMA. *Faculty:* 891 full-time (254 women). *Students:* 588 full-time (255 women); includes 136 minority (20 Black or African American, non-Hispanic/Latino; 2 American Indian or Alaska Native, non-Hispanic/Latino; 62 Asian, non-Hispanic/Latino; 34 Hispanic/Latino; 18 Two or more races, non-Hispanic/Latino). Average age 26. 3,489 applicants, 8% accepted, 152 enrolled. In 2013, 137 doctorates awarded. *Degree requirements:* For doctorate, U.S. Medical Licensing Examination Steps 1 and 2. *Entrance requirements:* For doctorate, MCAT, course work in biology, chemistry, organic chemistry, biochemistry, physics, mathematics, English, and social sciences; bachelor's degree. *Application deadline:* For fall admission, 11/1 for domestic students. Applications are processed on a rolling basis. Application fee: $60. Electronic applications accepted. *Expenses:* Contact institution. *Financial support:* In 2013–14, 350 students received support. Institutionally sponsored loans, scholarships/grants, and unspecified assistantships available. Support available to part-time students. Financial award applicants required to submit FAFSA. *Unit head:* Dr. Christopher Cooper, Associate Dean, 319-335-8435, Fax: 319-335-8643. *Application contact:* Kathi J. Huebner, Director of Admissions, 319-335-6703, Fax: 319-335-8049, E-mail: medical-admissions@uiowa.edu.
Website: http://www.medicine.uiowa.edu/md/

The University of Kansas, University of Kansas Medical Center, School of Medicine, MD/PhD Program, Kansas City, KS 66160. Offers MD/PhD. *Students:* 32 full-time (13 women); includes 6 minority (2 Black or African American, non-Hispanic/Latino; 3 Asian, non-Hispanic/Latino; 1 Two or more races, non-Hispanic/Latino). Average age 28. 79 applicants, 6% accepted, 3 enrolled. *Application deadline:* For fall admission, 11/15 priority date for domestic students. Applications are processed on a rolling basis. Application fee: $50. Electronic applications accepted. *Financial support:* Fellowships with full tuition reimbursements, research assistantships with full tuition reimbursements, and teaching assistantships with full tuition reimbursements available. Financial award application deadline: 3/1; financial award applicants required to submit FAFSA. *Faculty research:* Neuroscience, cancer biology, stem cell biology, reproductive biology. *Unit head:* Dr. Timothy A. Fields, Director, 913-588-7169, E-mail: tfields@kumc.edu. *Application contact:* Janice Fletcher, Administrative Manager, 913-588-5241, Fax: 913-945-6848, E-mail: jfletcher@kumc.edu.
Website: http://www.kumc.edu/md-phd-program.html

The University of Kansas, University of Kansas Medical Center, School of Medicine, MD Program, Kansas City, KS 66160. Offers MD. *Students:* 800 full-time (344 women); includes 173 minority (30 Black or African American, non-Hispanic/Latino; 3 American Indian or Alaska Native, non-Hispanic/Latino; 67 Asian, non-Hispanic/Latino; 45 Hispanic/Latino; 28 Two or more races, non-Hispanic/Latino). Average age 26. 2,899 applicants, 9% accepted, 208 enrolled. In 2013, 160 doctorates awarded. *Degree requirements:* For doctorate, comprehensive exam. *Entrance requirements:* For doctorate, MCAT, bachelor's degree. *Application deadline:* For fall admission, 10/15 for domestic students. Applications are processed on a rolling basis. Application fee: $50. Electronic applications accepted. *Faculty research:* Reproductive biology (fertility, ovulation, embryo implantation, pregnancy maintenance), multidisciplinary research on the basic mechanisms of cancer, renal research, neurological research, liver research. *Unit head:* Dr. Robert Simari, Executive Dean, 913-588-5200, E-mail: rsimari@kumc.edu. *Application contact:* Amy Meara, Director, Premed Programs, 913-588-5280, Fax: 913-588-5259, E-mail: premedinfo@kumc.edu.
Website: http://www.kumc.edu/school-of-medicine/office-of-medical-education.html

University of Kentucky, College of Medicine, Lexington, KY 40506-9983. Offers MD, MD/MBA, MD/MPH, MD/PhD. *Degree requirements:* For doctorate, comprehensive exam (for some programs), thesis/dissertation (for some programs). *Entrance requirements:* For doctorate, MCAT (for MD). Electronic applications accepted. *Expenses:* Contact institution. *Faculty research:* Aging, cancer, cardiovascular disease, infectious disease, women's maternal and child health.

University of Louisville, School of Medicine, Professional Programs in Medicine, Louisville, KY 40292-0001. Offers MD, MD/MBA, MD/MS, MD/PhD. *Accreditation:* LCME/AMA. *Students:* 645 full-time (281 women), 3 part-time (2 women); includes 127 minority (38 Black or African American, non-Hispanic/Latino; 1 American Indian or Alaska Native, non-Hispanic/Latino; 66 Asian, non-Hispanic/Latino; 14 Hispanic/Latino; 2 Native Hawaiian or other Pacific Islander, non-Hispanic/Latino; 6 Two or more races, non-Hispanic/Latino). Average age 26. 3,206 applicants, 9% accepted, 162 enrolled. In 2013, 162 doctorates awarded. *Entrance requirements:* For doctorate, MCAT. Additional exam requirements/recommendations for international students: Required—TOEFL (minimum score 550 paper-based; 79 iBT). *Application deadline:* For fall admission, 1/28 for domestic students. Applications are processed on a rolling basis. Application fee: $60. Electronic applications accepted. *Expenses:* Tuition, state resident: full-time $10,788; part-time $599 per credit hour. Tuition, nonresident: full-time $22,446; part-time $1247 per credit hour. *Required fees:* $196. Tuition and fees vary according to program and reciprocity agreements. *Faculty research:* Environmental effects on the cardiovascular system, diabetes, obesity and metabolics, molecular targets for cancer chemotherapy, plasticity of neural tissue, stem cells in repair of damaged cardiovascular tissue. *Total annual research expenditures:* $49 million. *Unit head:* Dr. Toni Michelle Ganzel, Dean, 502-852-1499, Fax: 502-852-1484, E-mail: meddean@louisville.edu. *Application contact:* Director of Admissions, 502-852-5793, Fax: 502-852-6849.

University of Maryland, Baltimore, School of Medicine, Professional Program in Medicine, Baltimore, MD 21201. Offers MD, MD/PhD. *Accreditation:* LCME/AMA. *Students:* 651 full-time (383 women), 12 part-time (7 women); includes 242 minority (43 Black or African American, non-Hispanic/Latino; 1 American Indian or Alaska Native, non-Hispanic/Latino; 158 Asian, non-Hispanic/Latino; 24 Hispanic/Latino; 16 Two or more races, non-Hispanic/Latino), 2 international. Average age 25. 4,941 applicants, 7% accepted, 172 enrolled. In 2013, 158 doctorates awarded. *Entrance requirements:* For doctorate, MCAT, AMCAS application, science coursework. *Application deadline:* For fall admission, 11/1 for domestic students. Applications are processed on a rolling basis. Application fee: $70. Electronic applications accepted. *Expenses:* Contact institution. *Financial support:* Federal Work-Study and scholarships/grants available. Financial award application deadline: 3/15; financial award applicants required to submit FAFSA. *Unit head:* Dr. E. Albert Reece, Dean and Vice President for Medical Affairs, 410-706-7410, Fax: 410-706-0235, E-mail: deanmed@som.umaryland.edu. *Application contact:* Dr. Milford M. Foxwell, Jr., Associate Dean for Admissions, 410-706-7478, Fax: 410-706-0467, E-mail: admissions@som.umaryland.edu.

University of Massachusetts Worcester, School of Medicine, Worcester, MA 01655-0115. Offers MD, MD/PhD. *Accreditation:* LCME/AMA. *Faculty:* 1,388 full-time (521 women), 309 part-time/adjunct (198 women). *Students:* 518 full-time (282 women); includes 145 minority (23 Black or African American, non-Hispanic/Latino; 1 American Indian or Alaska Native, non-Hispanic/Latino; 101 Asian, non-Hispanic/Latino; 19 Hispanic/Latino; 1 Native Hawaiian or other Pacific Islander, non-Hispanic/Latino). Average age 26. 1,172 applicants, 16% accepted, 125 enrolled. In 2013, 122 degrees awarded. *Median time to degree:* Of those who began their doctoral program in fall 2005, 98% received their degree in 8 years or less. *Degree requirements:* For doctorate, U.S. Medical Licensing Examination Step 1 and Step 2 (CS and CK). *Entrance requirements:* For doctorate, MCAT, state residency; bachelor's degree. *Application deadline:* For fall admission, 12/15 for domestic students. Applications are processed on a rolling basis. Application fee: $100. Electronic applications accepted. *Expenses:* Contact institution. *Financial support:* In 2013–14, 436 students received support. Institutionally sponsored loans, scholarships/grants, health care benefits, tuition waivers (partial), and unspecified assistantships available. Financial award application deadline: 4/16; financial award applicants required to submit FAFSA. *Faculty research:* RNA interference, cell dynamics, immunology and virology, chemical biology, stem cell research. *Total annual research expenditures:* $245.9 million. *Unit head:* Dr. Terence R. Flotte, Dean/Provost/Executive Deputy Chancellor, 508-856-8000, E-mail: terry.flotte@

umassmed.edu. *Application contact:* Karen Lawton, Director of Admissions, 508-856-2323, Fax: 508-856-3629, E-mail: admissions@umassmed.edu.
Website: http://www.umassmed.edu/som

University of Miami, Graduate School, Miller School of Medicine, Professional Program in Medicine, Coral Gables, FL 33124. Offers MD. *Accreditation:* LCME/AMA. *Entrance requirements:* For doctorate, MCAT, 90 pre-med semester hours. Electronic applications accepted. *Faculty research:* AIDS, cancer, diabetes, neuroscience, wound healing.

University of Michigan, Medical School and Rackham Graduate School, Medical Scientist Training Program, Ann Arbor, MI 48109. Offers MD/PhD. *Accreditation:* LCME/AMA. *Students:* 91 full-time (30 women); includes 39 minority (4 Black or African American, non-Hispanic/Latino; 35 Asian, non-Hispanic/Latino). 360 applicants, 11% accepted, 15 enrolled. *Application deadline:* For fall admission, 10/15 for domestic students. Applications are processed on a rolling basis. Application fee: $160. Electronic applications accepted. Tuition and fees vary according to course level, course load, degree level, program and student level. *Financial support:* In 2013–14, 91 students received support, including 72 fellowships with full tuition reimbursements available (averaging $28,500 per year), 16 research assistantships with full tuition reimbursements available (averaging $28,500 per year), 3 teaching assistantships with full tuition reimbursements available (averaging $28,500 per year); scholarships/grants, traineeships, and health care benefits also available. *Unit head:* Dr. Ronald J. Koenig, Director, 734-764-6176, Fax: 734-764-8180, E-mail: rkoenig@umich.edu. *Application contact:* Laurie Koivupalo, Administrative Associate, 734-764-6176, Fax: 734-764-8180, E-mail: lkoivupl@umich.edu.
Website: http://www.med.umich.edu/medschool/mstp/

University of Michigan, Medical School, Professional Program in Medicine, Ann Arbor, MI 48109. Offers MD, MD/MA Edu, MD/MBA, MD/MPH, MD/MPP, MD/MS, MD/MSI, MD/PhD. *Accreditation:* LCME/AMA. *Entrance requirements:* For doctorate, MCAT. Electronic applications accepted. Tuition and fees vary according to course level, course load, degree level, program and student level.

University of Minnesota, Duluth, Medical School, Professional Program in Medicine, Duluth, MN 55812-2496. Offers MD. Program offered jointly with University of Minnesota, Twin Cities Campus. *Entrance requirements:* For doctorate, MCAT. Electronic applications accepted.

University of Minnesota, Twin Cities Campus, Medical School, Minneapolis, MN 55455-0213. Offers MA, MS, DPT, MD, PhD, JD/MD, MD/MBA, MD/MHI, MD/MPH, MD/MS, MD/PhD. Part-time and evening/weekend programs available. *Expenses:* Contact institution.

University of Mississippi Medical Center, School of Medicine, Jackson, MS 39216-4505. Offers MD, MD/PhD. *Accreditation:* LCME/AMA. *Entrance requirements:* For doctorate, MCAT. *Faculty research:* Cardiovascular physiology (computer simulation), transplant immunology, reproductive endocrinology, protein structure, neurotransmitter vesicle structure.

University of Missouri, School of Medicine, Professional Program in Medicine, Columbia, MO 65211. Offers MD, MD/PhD. *Accreditation:* LCME/AMA. *Faculty:* 330 full-time (88 women), 78 part-time/adjunct (15 women). *Entrance requirements:* For doctorate, MCAT, minimum GPA of 3.49. *Application deadline:* For fall admission, 11/1 for domestic students. Applications are processed on a rolling basis. *Financial support:* Career-related internships or fieldwork, institutionally sponsored loans, and scholarships/grants available. Financial award application deadline: 8/15; financial award applicants required to submit FAFSA. *Faculty research:* Basic and clinical biomedical sciences. *Unit head:* Leslie W. Hall, Interim Dean, 573-884-9080, E-mail: halllw@missouri.edu. *Application contact:* Alison Martin, Student Support Services Manager II, 573-882-8047, E-mail: martinat@missouri.edu.
Website: http://som.missouri.edu/

University of Missouri–Kansas City, School of Medicine, Kansas City, MO 64110-2499. Offers anesthesia (MS); bioinformatics (MS); health professions education (MS); medicine (MD); physician assistant (MMS); MD/PhD. *Accreditation:* LCME/AMA. *Faculty:* 49 full-time (20 women), 13 part-time/adjunct (6 women). *Students:* 462 full-time (241 women), 16 part-time (8 women); includes 253 minority (33 Black or African American, non-Hispanic/Latino; 2 American Indian or Alaska Native, non-Hispanic/Latino; 196 Asian, non-Hispanic/Latino; 14 Hispanic/Latino; 1 Native Hawaiian or other Pacific Islander, non-Hispanic/Latino; 7 Two or more races, non-Hispanic/Latino), 3 international. Average age 24. 1,070 applicants, 11% accepted, 94 enrolled. In 2013, 12 master's, 88 doctorates awarded. *Degree requirements:* For doctorate, one foreign language, United States Medical Licensing Exam Step 1 and 2. *Entrance requirements:* For doctorate, interview. *Application deadline:* For fall admission, 11/15 for domestic and international students. Application fee: $50. *Expenses:* Contact institution. *Financial support:* In 2013–14, 4 fellowships (averaging $38,964 per year), 4 research assistantships (averaging $17,373 per year) were awarded; career-related internships or fieldwork, Federal Work-Study, institutionally sponsored loans, scholarships/grants, and tuition waivers (partial) also available. Financial award application deadline: 3/1; financial award applicants required to submit FAFSA. *Faculty research:* Cardiovascular disease, women's and children's health, trauma and infectious diseases, neurological, metabolic disease. *Unit head:* Dr. Betty Drees, Dean, 816-235-1808, E-mail: dreesb@umkc.edu. *Application contact:* Janine Kluckhohn, Admissions Coordinator, 816-235-1870, Fax: 816-235-6579, E-mail: kluckhohnj@umkc.edu.
Website: http://www.med.umkc.edu/

University of Nebraska Medical Center, College of Medicine, Omaha, NE 68198-5527. Offers MD, Certificate, MD/MPH, MD/PhD. *Accreditation:* LCME/AMA. *Faculty:* 653 full-time, 107 part-time/adjunct. *Students:* 510 full-time (206 women); includes 56 minority (11 Black or African American, non-Hispanic/Latino; 22 Asian, non-Hispanic/Latino; 6 Hispanic/Latino; 17 Two or more races, non-Hispanic/Latino), 3 international. Average age 22. 1,568 applicants, 11% accepted, 124 enrolled. In 2013, 123 doctorates awarded. *Entrance requirements:* For doctorate, MCAT. *Application deadline:* For fall admission, 11/1 for domestic students. Applications are processed on a rolling basis. Application fee: $70. Electronic applications accepted. *Expenses:* Contact institution. *Financial support:* Career-related internships or fieldwork, Federal Work-Study, institutionally sponsored loans, and tuition waivers (full) available. Support available to part-time students. Financial award application deadline: 2/1; financial award applicants required to submit FAFSA. *Unit head:* Dr. Bradley E. Britigan, Dean, 402-559-4283, Fax: 402-559-4148, E-mail: bradley.britigan@unmc.edu. *Application contact:* Gigi R. Rogers, Program Coordinator, 402-559-2259, Fax: 402-559-6840, E-mail: comadmissions@unmc.edu.
Website: http://www.unmc.edu/COM/admissions.htm

University of New Mexico, School of Medicine, Professional Program in Medicine, Albuquerque, NM 87131-2039. Offers MD. *Degree requirements:* For doctorate, comprehensive exam, research. *Entrance requirements:* For doctorate, MCAT, general biology, general chemistry, organic chemistry, biochemistry and physics; minimum GPA of 3.0. *Application deadline:* For fall admission, 11/1 for domestic students. Applications are processed on a rolling basis. Electronic applications accepted. *Expenses:* Contact institution. *Financial support:* Institutionally sponsored loans and scholarships/grants available. Financial award application deadline: 3/1; financial award applicants required to submit FAFSA. *Faculty research:* Cancer, infectious disease, brain and behavioral illness, children's health, cardiovascular and metabolic disease.
Website: http://hsc.unm.edu/som/admissions

The University of North Carolina at Chapel Hill, School of Medicine, Professional Program in Medicine, Chapel Hill, NC 27599. Offers MD, MD/MPH, MD/PhD. *Accreditation:* LCME/AMA. *Entrance requirements:* For doctorate, MCAT.

University of North Dakota, School of Medicine and Health Sciences, Professional Program in Medicine, Grand Forks, ND 58202. Offers MD, MD/PhD. *Accreditation:* LCME/AMA. *Entrance requirements:* For doctorate, MCAT, minimum GPA of 3.0. Additional exam requirements/recommendations for international students: Required—TOEFL (minimum score 550 paper-based; 79 iBT), IELTS (minimum score 6.5). Electronic applications accepted.

University of Oklahoma Health Sciences Center, College of Medicine, Professional Program in Medicine, Oklahoma City, OK 73190. Offers MD, MD/PhD. *Accreditation:* LCME/AMA. *Faculty:* 92 full-time (26 women), 13 part-time/adjunct (4 women). *Students:* 658 full-time (268 women), 2 part-time (1 woman); includes 174 minority (3 Black or African American, non-Hispanic/Latino; 15 American Indian or Alaska Native, non-Hispanic/Latino; 98 Asian, non-Hispanic/Latino; 12 Hispanic/Latino; 46 Two or more races, non-Hispanic/Latino). Average age 25. 1,143 applicants, 17% accepted, 164 enrolled. In 2013, 156 doctorates awarded. *Entrance requirements:* For doctorate, MCAT. *Application deadline:* For fall admission, 10/31 for domestic students. Application fee: $25 ($50 for international students). *Expenses:* Tuition, state resident: full-time $3504; part-time $175.20 per credit hour. Tuition, nonresident: full-time $13,504; part-time $675.20 per credit hour. *Required fees:* $1545; $52.70 per credit hour. $245.25 per semester. Tuition and fees vary according to course load. *Financial support:* Fellowships available. *Faculty research:* Behavior and drugs, structure and function of endothelium, genetics and behavior, gene structure and function, action of antibiotics. *Unit head:* Dr. Dewayne Andrews, Executive Dean, 405-271-2265. *Application contact:* Dr. Herman Jones, Associate Dean, 405-271-2316, E-mail: herman-jones@ouhsc.edu.

University of Ottawa, Faculty of Graduate and Postdoctoral Studies, Faculty of Medicine, Ottawa, ON K1N 6N5, Canada. Offers M Sc, MD, PhD. *Accreditation:* LCME/AMA. *Degree requirements:* For master's, thesis; for doctorate, thesis/dissertation (for some programs). *Entrance requirements:* For master's, honors degree or equivalent, minimum B average. Electronic applications accepted.

University of Pennsylvania, Perelman School of Medicine, Professional Program in Medicine, Philadelphia, PA 19104. Offers MD, MD/JD, MD/MBA, MD/MBE, MD/MS, MD/MSCE, MD/PhD. *Accreditation:* LCME/AMA. *Faculty:* 2,719 full-time (1,028 women), 1,257 part-time/adjunct (577 women). *Students:* 806 full-time (365 women); includes 346 minority (69 Black or African American, non-Hispanic/Latino; 161 Asian, non-Hispanic/Latino; 88 Hispanic/Latino; 28 Two or more races, non-Hispanic/Latino), 18 international. Average age 25. 5,740 applicants, 5% accepted, 168 enrolled. *Entrance requirements:* For doctorate, MCAT. *Application deadline:* For fall admission, 10/15 for domestic and international students. Application fee: $80. Electronic applications accepted. *Financial support:* In 2013–14, 650 students received support. Fellowships, research assistantships, teaching assistantships, career-related internships or fieldwork, Federal Work-Study, institutionally sponsored loans, and scholarships/grants available. Financial award application deadline: 5/1; financial award applicants required to submit FAFSA. *Unit head:* Dr. Gail Morrison, MD, Senior Vice Dean, 215-898-8034, E-mail: morrisog@mail.med.upenn.edu. *Application contact:* Gaye Sheffler, Director, Admissions, 215-898-8001, Fax: 215-898-0833, E-mail: sheffler@mail.med.upenn.edu.

University of Pittsburgh, School of Medicine, Professional Program in Medicine, Pittsburgh, PA 15261. Offers MD. *Accreditation:* LCME/AMA. *Faculty:* 2,262 full-time (785 women), 59 part-time/adjunct (39 women). *Students:* 602 full-time (274 women); includes 291 minority (47 Black or African American, non-Hispanic/Latino; 1 American Indian or Alaska Native, non-Hispanic/Latino; 184 Asian, non-Hispanic/Latino; 41 Hispanic/Latino; 18 Two or more races, non-Hispanic/Latino). Average age 25. 4,982 applicants, 7% accepted, 162 enrolled. In 2013, 144 doctorates awarded. *Degree requirements:* For doctorate, comprehensive exam, U.S. Medical Licensing Examination Steps 1 and 2, scholarly project. *Entrance requirements:* For doctorate, MCAT, at least one full-year of undergraduate education in the United States or Canada. Additional exam requirements/recommendations for international students: Required—TOEFL (minimum score 600 paper-based; 100 iBT), IELTS. *Application deadline:* For fall admission, 10/15 for domestic and international students. Applications are processed on a rolling basis. Application fee: $85. Electronic applications accepted. *Expenses:* Contact institution. *Financial support:* In 2013–14, 362 students received support. Institutionally sponsored loans and scholarships/grants available. Financial award application deadline: 4/16; financial award applicants required to submit FAFSA. *Faculty research:* Drug discovery and design; vaccine development; comparative effectiveness research; organ transplantation/immunology; stem cell biology and tissue engineering; medical device development; vascular biology; cancer research and therapy; cardiology and cardiovascular biology; bioinformatics and computational biology; psychiatry, neurobiology, systems neuroscience, and neurological surgery; structural biology; developmental biology; precision medicine; clinical research/clinical trials. *Total annual research expenditures:* $497.1 million. *Unit head:* Dr. Beth Piraino, Associate Dean, 412-648-9891, Fax: 412-648-8768, E-mail: admissions@medschool.pitt.edu. *Application contact:* Cynthia May Bonetti, Executive Director for Admissions and Financial Aid, 412-648-9891, Fax: 412-648-8768, E-mail: admissions@medschool.pitt.edu.
Website: http://www.medschool.pitt.edu/

University of Puerto Rico, Medical Sciences Campus, School of Medicine, Professional Program in Medicine, San Juan, PR 00936-5067. Offers MD. *Accreditation:* LCME/AMA. *Degree requirements:* For doctorate, one foreign language. *Entrance requirements:* For doctorate, MCAT, minimum GPA of 2.5, computer literacy.

University of Rochester, School of Medicine and Dentistry, Professional Program in Medicine, Rochester, NY 14627. Offers MD, MD/MPH, MD/MS, MD/PhD. *Accreditation:* LCME/AMA. *Entrance requirements:* For doctorate, MCAT. *Expenses: Tuition:* Full-time $44,580; part-time $1394 per credit hour. *Required fees:* $492.

University of Saskatchewan, College of Medicine, Professional Program in Medicine, Saskatoon, SK S7N 5A2, Canada. Offers MD. *Accreditation:* LCME/AMA. *Expenses: Tuition, area resident:* Full-time $3585 Canadian dollars; part-time $585 Canadian dollars per course. Tuition, nonresident: part-time $877 Canadian dollars per course. *International tuition:* $5377 Canadian dollars full-time. *Required fees:* $889.51 Canadian dollars.

University of South Alabama, College of Medicine, Professional Program in Medicine, Mobile, AL 36688. Offers MD, MD/PhD. *Accreditation:* LCME/AMA. *Faculty:* 33 full-time (7 women). *Students:* 292 full-time (119 women); includes 53 minority (19 Black or African American, non-Hispanic/Latino; 26 Asian, non-Hispanic/Latino; 5 Native Hawaiian or other Pacific Islander, non-Hispanic/Latino; 3 Two or more races, non-Hispanic/Latino). In 2013, 73 doctorates awarded. *Entrance requirements:* For doctorate, MCAT. Additional exam requirements/recommendations for international students: Required—TOEFL. *Application deadline:* For fall admission, 11/15 for domestic and international students. Application fee: $75. Electronic applications accepted. *Expenses:* Tuition, state resident: full-time $8976; part-time $374 per credit hour. Tuition, nonresident: full-time $17,952; part-time $748 per credit hour. *Financial support:* Scholarships/grants available. Financial award applicants required to submit FAFSA. *Unit head:* Mark Scott, Dean, USA College of Medicine, 251-460-7176, E-mail: mscott@usouthal.edu. *Application contact:* Peggy Terrell, Academic Advisor/Director of Admissions, 251-460-7176, Fax: 251-461-1513, E-mail: mscott@usouthal.edu.

University of South Carolina, School of Medicine, Professional Program in Medicine, Columbia, SC 29208. Offers MD, MD/MPH, MD/PhD. *Accreditation:* LCME/AMA. *Entrance requirements:* For doctorate, MCAT. Electronic applications accepted. *Faculty research:* Cardiovascular diseases, oncology, reproductive biology, vision, neuroscience.

The University of South Dakota, Graduate School, School of Medicine, Professional Program in Medicine, Vermillion, SD 57069-2390. Offers MD. *Accreditation:* LCME/AMA. *Degree requirements:* For doctorate, U.S. Medical Licensing Exam-Step 1 & 2, CK OSCE. *Entrance requirements:* For doctorate, MCAT, previous course work in biology, chemistry, organic chemistry, mathematics and physics. Electronic applications accepted.

University of Southern California, Keck School of Medicine, Professional Program in Medicine, Los Angeles, CA 90089. Offers MD, MD/MBA, MD/MPH, MD/PhD. *Accreditation:* LCME/AMA. *Students:* 716 full-time (339 women); includes 363 minority (33 Black or African American, non-Hispanic/Latino; 1 American Indian or Alaska Native, non-Hispanic/Latino; 239 Asian, non-Hispanic/Latino; 88 Hispanic/Latino; 2 Native Hawaiian or other Pacific Islander, non-Hispanic/Latino), 5 international. Average age 24. 7,859 applicants, 6% accepted, 186 enrolled. In 2013, 157 doctorates awarded. *Entrance requirements:* For doctorate, MCAT, 2 semesters or 3 quarters of course work in biology, chemistry, organic chemistry, physics (all with lab); 1 course in molecular biology; 30 units of course work in social sciences. *Application deadline:* For fall admission, 11/1 for domestic and international students. Applications are processed on a rolling basis. Application fee: $90. Electronic applications accepted. *Expenses:* Contact institution. *Financial support:* In 2013–14, 134 students received support, including 12 research assistantships (averaging $25,000 per year); institutionally sponsored loans and scholarships/grants also available. Financial award application deadline: 4/15; financial award applicants required to submit FAFSA. *Unit head:* Dr. Raquel Arias, Associate Dean for Admissions, 323-442-2552, Fax: 323-442-2433, E-mail: medadmit@usc.edu. *Application contact:* Susan Wong, Admissions Coordinator, 323-442-2552, Fax: 323-442-2433, E-mail: medadmit@usc.edu.
Website: http://keck.usc.edu/

University of South Florida, Morsani College of Medicine, Tampa, FL 33620-9951. Offers MSB, MSBCB, MSHI, MSMS, DPT, MD, PhD, DPT/MPH, MS/MA, PhD/MD. *Accreditation:* LCME/AMA. Part-time programs available. *Faculty:* 108 full-time (29 women), 31 part-time/adjunct (11 women). *Students:* 591 full-time (357 women), 1,033 part-time (543 women); includes 652 minority (143 Black or African American, non-Hispanic/Latino; 8 American Indian or Alaska Native, non-Hispanic/Latino; 275 Asian, non-Hispanic/Latino; 201 Hispanic/Latino; 3 Native Hawaiian or other Pacific Islander, non-Hispanic/Latino; 22 Two or more races, non-Hispanic/Latino), 32 international. Average age 25. 3,799 applicants, 9% accepted, 178 enrolled. In 2013, 191 master's, 152 doctorates awarded. Terminal master's awarded for partial completion of doctoral program. *Degree requirements:* For master's, comprehensive exam, thesis; for doctorate, comprehensive exam (for some programs), thesis/dissertation (for some programs). *Entrance requirements:* For master's, GRE General Test (minimum preferred scores of 500 Verbal and 500 Quantitative) or GMAT (minimum score of 500), BA or equivalent degree from regionally-accredited university with minimum GPA of 3.0 in upper-division coursework; for doctorate, GRE General Test (minimum score of 600 quantitative on old scoring), BA or equivalent degree from regionally-accredited university with minimum GPA of 3.0 in upper-division sciences coursework; three letters of recommendation; personal interview; one- to two-page personal statement. Additional exam requirements/recommendations for international students: Required—TOEFL (minimum score 550 paper-based; 79 iBT). *Application deadline:* For fall admission, 2/15 for domestic students, 1/2 for international students. Application fee: $30. Electronic applications accepted. *Faculty research:* Allergy, immunology, and infectious diseases; cancer biology; cardiovascular research; neuroscience research; biomedical engineering; nanomedicine; neuromusculoskeletal disorders; pharmacogenomics; regenerative medicine; sport's medicine; women's health. *Total annual research expenditures:* $4.1 million. *Unit head:* Dr. Charles J. Lockwood, Dean, 813-974-0533, Fax: 813-974-4990, E-mail: cjlockwood@health.usf.edu. *Application contact:* Dr. Michael Barber, Associate Dean/Professor, 813-974-9702, Fax: 813-974-4990, E-mail: mbarber@health.usf.edu.
Website: http://health.usf.edu/medicine/index.htm

The University of Tennessee Health Science Center, College of Medicine, Memphis, TN 38163-0002. Offers MD, MD/PhD. *Accreditation:* LCME/AMA. *Entrance requirements:* For doctorate, MCAT. *Application deadline:* For fall admission, 11/15 for domestic students. Applications are processed on a rolling basis. Application fee: $50. Electronic applications accepted. *Expenses:* Contact institution. *Financial support:* Career-related internships or fieldwork, Federal Work-Study, and institutionally sponsored loans available. Support available to part-time students. Financial award application deadline: 2/28. *Unit head:* Dr. David M. Stern, Executive Dean, 901-448-5529, Fax: 901-448-7683, E-mail: dstern@uthsc.edu. *Application contact:* E. Nelson Strother, Assistant Dean for Admissions, 901-448-2747, Fax: 901-448-7772, E-mail: nstrother@uthsc.edu.
Website: http://uthsc.edu/Medicine/

The University of Texas Health Science Center at Houston, University of Texas Medical School at Houston, Houston, TX 77225-0036. Offers MD, MD/MPH, MD/PhD. *Accreditation:* LCME/AMA. *Entrance requirements:* For doctorate, MCAT. Electronic applications accepted. *Expenses:* Contact institution. *Faculty research:* Stroke, infectious diseases, cardiovascular disease, neoplastic disease (cancer), molecular medicine for the prevention of diseases.

The University of Texas Health Science Center at San Antonio, School of Medicine, San Antonio, TX 78229-3900. Offers deaf education and hearing (MS); medicine (MD); MPH/MD. *Accreditation:* LCME/AMA. *Faculty:* 838 full-time (348 women), 394 part-time/adjunct (142 women). *Students:* 876 full-time (420 women), 20 part-time (all women); includes 392 minority (41 Black or African American, non-Hispanic/Latino; 152 Asian, non-Hispanic/Latino; 179 Hispanic/Latino; 20 Two or more races, non-Hispanic/Latino), 1 international. Average age 26. 4,100 applicants, 17% accepted, 220 enrolled. In 2013, 12 master's, 228 doctorates awarded. *Degree requirements:* For master's, comprehensive exam, practicum assignments. *Entrance requirements:* For master's, minimum GPA of 3.0, interview, 3 professional letters of recommendation; for doctorate, MCAT. *Application deadline:* For fall admission, 10/1 for domestic and international students. Applications are processed on a rolling basis. Application fee: $140. Electronic applications accepted. *Expenses:* Contact institution. *Financial support:* In 2013–14, 599 students received support. Federal Work-Study, institutionally sponsored loans, tuition waivers (full and partial), and stipends, department payments available. Financial award application deadline: 6/1; financial award applicants required to submit FAFSA. *Faculty research:* Geriatrics, diabetes, cancer, AIDS, obesity. *Total annual research expenditures:* $117.4 million. *Unit head:* Dr. Francisco Gonzalez-Scarano, Dean, 210-567-4432, Fax: 210-567-3435, E-mail: scarano@uthscsa.edu. *Application contact:* Dr. David J. Jones, Senior Associate Dean for Admissions, 210-567-6080, Fax: 210-567-6962, E-mail: jonesd@uthscsa.edu.
Website: som.uthscsa.edu

The University of Texas Medical Branch, School of Medicine, Galveston, TX 77555. Offers MD. *Accreditation:* LCME/AMA. *Entrance requirements:* For doctorate, MCAT. *Expenses:* Contact institution.

The University of Texas Southwestern Medical Center, Southwestern Medical School, Dallas, TX 75390. Offers MD, MD/PhD. *Accreditation:* LCME/AMA. *Faculty:* 2,076 full-time, 647 part-time/adjunct. *Students:* 940 full-time (430 women); includes 475 minority (37 Black or African American, non-Hispanic/Latino; 1 American Indian or Alaska Native, non-Hispanic/Latino; 314 Asian, non-Hispanic/Latino; 101 Hispanic/Latino; 22 Two or more races, non-Hispanic/Latino), 33 international. Average age 26. 3,483 applicants, 12% accepted, 228 enrolled. In 2013, 227 doctorates awarded. *Entrance requirements:* For doctorate, MCAT. *Application deadline:* For fall admission, 10/15 for domestic students. Applications are processed on a rolling basis. Application fee: $65. Electronic applications accepted. *Expenses:* Contact institution. *Financial support:* In 2013–14, 700 students received support. Federal Work-Study and institutionally sponsored loans available. Financial award application deadline: 3/15; financial award applicants required to submit FAFSA. *Faculty research:* Endocrinology, molecular biology, immunology, cancer biology, neuroscience. *Total annual research expenditures:* $206,000. *Unit head:* Dr. Greg Fitz, Dean, 214-648-2509. *Application contact:* Anne Mclane, Associate Director of Admissions, 214-648-5617, Fax: 214-648-3289, E-mail: admissions@utsouthwestern.edu.
Website: http://www.utsouthwestern.edu/

University of Toronto, Faculty of Medicine, Toronto, ON M5S 1A1, Canada. Offers M Sc, M Sc BMC, M Sc OT, M Sc PT, MH Sc, MD, PhD, MD/PhD. *Accreditation:* LCME/AMA. *Entrance requirements:* For doctorate, MCAT (for MD). Electronic applications accepted. *Expenses:* Contact institution.

University of Utah, School of Medicine, MD/PhD Program in Medicine, Salt Lake City, UT 84112-1107. Offers MD/PhD. Part-time programs available. Electronic applications accepted. *Expenses:* Tuition, state resident: full-time $5259. Tuition, nonresident: full-time $18,569. *Required fees:* $841. Tuition and fees vary according to course load. *Faculty research:* Molecular biology, biochemistry, cell biology, immunology, bioengineering.

University of Utah, School of Medicine, Professional Program in Medicine, Salt Lake City, UT 84112-1107. Offers MD. *Accreditation:* LCME/AMA. *Entrance requirements:* For doctorate, MCAT, 2 years chemistry with lab, 1 year physics with lab, writing/speech, 2 courses biology, 1 course cell biology or biochemistry, 1 course humanities, 1 course diversity, 1 course social science. Electronic applications accepted. *Expenses:* Contact institution. *Faculty research:* Molecular biology, genetics, immunology, cardiology, endocrinology.

University of Vermont, College of Medicine, Professional Program in Medicine, Burlington, VT 05405. Offers MD, MD/MS, MD/PhD. *Accreditation:* LCME/AMA. *Students:* 458 (224 women); includes 138 minority (7 Black or African American, non-Hispanic/Latino; 83 Asian, non-Hispanic/Latino; 36 Hispanic/Latino; 12 Two or more races, non-Hispanic/Latino), 1 international. 5,346 applicants, 5% accepted, 114 enrolled. In 2013, 106 doctorates awarded. *Entrance requirements:* For doctorate, MCAT. Additional exam requirements/recommendations for international students: Required—TOEFL (minimum score 550 paper-based; 80 iBT). *Application deadline:* For fall admission, 11/1 for domestic and international students. Applications are processed on a rolling basis. Application fee: $95. Electronic applications accepted. *Expenses:* Contact institution. *Financial support:* In 2013–14, 340 students received support. Institutionally sponsored loans and scholarships/grants available. Support available to part-time students. Financial award application deadline: 2/28; financial award applicants required to submit FAFSA. *Unit head:* Dr. Christa H. Zehle, Associate Dean for Student Affairs, 802-656-2150, Fax: 802-656-9377. *Application contact:* Janice M. Gallant, Associate Dean for Admissions, 802-656-2150.

University of Virginia, School of Medicine, Charlottesville, VA 22903. Offers MPH, MS, MD, PhD, JD/MD, JD/MPH, MD/MBA, MD/PhD, MPP/MPH. *Accreditation:* LCME/AMA. *Faculty:* 944 full-time (310 women), 89 part-time/adjunct (64 women). *Students:* 918 full-time (437 women), 10 part-time (7 women); includes 307 minority (46 Black or African American, non-Hispanic/Latino; 4 American Indian or Alaska Native, non-Hispanic/Latino; 145 Asian, non-Hispanic/Latino; 76 Hispanic/Latino; 1 Native Hawaiian or other Pacific Islander, non-Hispanic/Latino; 35 Two or more races, non-Hispanic/Latino), 53 international. Average age 25. 5,326 applicants, 11% accepted, 223 enrolled. In 2013, 61 master's, 188 doctorates awarded. *Entrance requirements:* For doctorate, MCAT (for MD). Additional exam requirements/recommendations for international students: Required—TOEFL. *Application deadline:* Applications are processed on a rolling basis. Application fee: $80. Electronic applications accepted. *Expenses:* Tuition, state resident: part-time $334 per credit hour. Tuition, nonresident: part-time $1224 per credit hour. *Financial support:* Institutionally sponsored loans and scholarships/grants available. Financial award applicants required to submit FAFSA. *Unit head:* Nancy E. Dunlap, Vice President and Dean, 434-924-5118. *Application contact:* John J. Densmore, Associate Dean for Admissions and Student Affairs, 434-924-5571, Fax: 434-982-2586, E-mail: jjd2q@virginia.edu.
Website: http://www.medicine.virginia.edu/

University of Washington, Graduate School, School of Medicine, Professional Program in Medicine, Seattle, WA 98195. Offers MD, MD/MPH, MD/PhD. *Accreditation:* LCME/AMA. *Entrance requirements:* For doctorate, MCAT or GRE, minimum 3 years of college. Electronic applications accepted.

The University of Western Ontario, Faculty of Graduate Studies, Biosciences Division, Department of Family Medicine, London, ON N6A 5B8, Canada. Offers M Cl Sc. *Accreditation:* LCME/AMA. Part-time programs available. Postbaccalaureate distance learning degree programs offered (minimal on-campus study). *Degree requirements:* For master's, thesis. *Entrance requirements:* For master's, medical degree, minimum B average. Additional exam requirements/recommendations for international students: Required—TOEFL. *Faculty research:* Family medicine education, dietary counseling, alcohol problems, palliative care support, multicultural health care.

The University of Western Ontario, Schulich School of Medicine and Dentistry, Professional Program in Medicine, London, ON N6A 5B8, Canada. Offers MD. *Accreditation:* LCME/AMA.

University of Wisconsin–Madison, School of Medicine and Public Health, Professional Program in Medicine, Madison, WI 53705. Offers MD. *Accreditation:* LCME/AMA. *Students:* 699 full-time (330 women); includes 144 minority (27 Black or African American, non-Hispanic/Latino; 4 American Indian or Alaska Native, non-Hispanic/Latino; 77 Asian, non-Hispanic/Latino; 21 Hispanic/Latino; 15 Two or more races, non-Hispanic/Latino). Average age 25. 5,045 applicants, 6% accepted, 175 enrolled. *Entrance requirements:* For doctorate, MCAT. *Application deadline:* For fall admission, 11/1 for domestic students. Applications are processed on a rolling basis.

Application fee: $56. Electronic applications accepted. *Expenses:* Tuition, state resident: full-time $10,728; part-time $790 per credit. Tuition, nonresident: full-time $24,054; part-time $1623 per credit. *Required fees:* $1130; $119 per credit. *Financial support:* In 2013–14, 244 students received support. Scholarships/grants available. Financial award applicants required to submit FAFSA. *Faculty research:* Biomedical research: population health, medical ethics, cancer research, neurosciences. *Unit head:* Dr. Robert N. Golden, Dean, 608-263-4910, Fax: 608-265-3286, E-mail: rngolden@wisc.edu. *Application contact:* Becky Duffy, MD Admissions Advisor, 608-263-8228, Fax: 608-262-4226, E-mail: rlduffy@wisc.edu.
Website: http://www.med.wisc.edu/education/main/100

Vanderbilt University, School of Medicine, Nashville, TN 37240-1001. Offers MDE, MMP, MPH, MS, MSCI, Au D, DMP, MD, PhD, MD/PhD. *Accreditation:* LCME/AMA (one or more programs are accredited). *Entrance requirements:* For doctorate, MCAT (for MD). Electronic applications accepted. *Expenses:* Contact institution.

Virginia Commonwealth University, Medical College of Virginia-Professional Programs, School of Medicine, Professional Program in Medicine, Richmond, VA 23284-9005. Offers MD, MD/MHA, MD/MPH, MD/PhD. *Accreditation:* LCME/AMA. *Entrance requirements:* For doctorate, MCAT. Electronic applications accepted. *Expenses:* Contact institution.

Wake Forest University, School of Medicine, Professional Program in Medicine, Winston-Salem, NC 27109. Offers MD, MD/MA, MD/MBA, MD/MS, MD/PhD. *Accreditation:* LCME/AMA. *Entrance requirements:* For doctorate, MCAT, 32 hours of course work in science. Electronic applications accepted. *Faculty research:* Cancer, stroke, infectious diseases, membrane biology, nutrition.

Washington University in St. Louis, School of Medicine, Professional Program in Medicine, St. Louis, MO 63130-4899. Offers MD, MD/MA, MD/MS, MD/PhD. *Accreditation:* LCME/AMA. *Faculty:* 1,862 full-time (624 women), 145 part-time/adjunct (86 women). *Students:* 602 full-time (293 women); includes 261 minority (42 Black or African American, non-Hispanic/Latino; 3 American Indian or Alaska Native, non-Hispanic/Latino; 198 Asian, non-Hispanic/Latino; 18 Hispanic/Latino), 6 international. Average age 24. 4,445 applicants, 8% accepted, 122 enrolled. In 2013, 119 doctorates awarded. *Degree requirements:* For doctorate, thesis/dissertation (for some programs). *Entrance requirements:* For doctorate, MCAT (for MD). *Application deadline:* For fall admission, 12/31 for domestic and international students. Applications are processed on a rolling basis. Application fee: $80. Electronic applications accepted. *Expenses:* Contact institution. *Financial support:* Career-related internships or fieldwork and institutionally sponsored loans available. *Unit head:* Dr. Larry Shapiro, Dean, 314-362-6827. *Application contact:* Dr. Valerie Ratts, Associate Dean, 314-362-6848, Fax: 314-362-4658, E-mail: wumscoa@msnotes.wustl.edu.

Wayne State University, School of Medicine, Professional Program in Medicine, Detroit, MI 48202. Offers MD, MD/PhD. *Accreditation:* LCME/AMA. *Students:* 1,172 full-time (544 women), 47 part-time (24 women); includes 348 minority (61 Black or African American, non-Hispanic/Latino; 4 American Indian or Alaska Native, non-Hispanic/Latino; 242 Asian, non-Hispanic/Latino; 18 Hispanic/Latino; 5 Native Hawaiian or other Pacific Islander, non-Hispanic/Latino; 18 Two or more races, non-Hispanic/Latino), 62 international. Average age 25. 4,952 applicants, 11% accepted, 290 enrolled. In 2013, 251 doctorates awarded. *Degree requirements:* For doctorate, Steps 1 and 3 of National Board examinations and sit for the Step 2 examination. *Entrance requirements:* For doctorate, MCAT, bachelor's degree or equivalent, strong background in basic sciences, 2 semesters each of inorganic chemistry with labs, biology/zoology with labs, college English, organic chemistry with labs, physics with labs, at least 21 years old and exhibit good moral character, be suitable for the practice of medicine. Additional exam requirements/recommendations for international students: Required—TOEFL (minimum score 600 paper-based; 100 iBT), TWE (minimum score 6). *Application deadline:* For fall admission, 6/1 for domestic and international students. Application fee: $100. Electronic applications accepted. *Expenses:* Contact institution. *Financial support:* In 2013–14, 487 students received support. Scholarships/grants available. Financial award application deadline: 3/1; financial award applicants required to submit FAFSA. *Unit head:* Dr. Valerie M. Parisi, Dean, 313-577-1335, E-mail: valerie.parisi@wayne.edu. *Application contact:* Dr. Silas Norman, Associate Dean for Admissions, 313-577-1466, Fax: 313-577-9420, E-mail: admissions@med.wayne.edu.
Website: http://home.med.wayne.edu/

West Virginia University, School of Medicine, Professional Program in Medicine, Morgantown, WV 26506. Offers MD, MD/PhD. *Accreditation:* LCME/AMA. *Entrance requirements:* For doctorate, MCAT.

Wright State University, School of Medicine, Professional Program in Medicine, Dayton, OH 45435. Offers MD. *Accreditation:* LCME/AMA. *Entrance requirements:* For doctorate, MCAT.

Yale University, School of Medicine, Professional Program in Medicine, New Haven, CT 06510. Offers MD. *Accreditation:* LCME/AMA. *Degree requirements:* For doctorate, thesis/dissertation. *Entrance requirements:* For doctorate, MCAT. Electronic applications accepted.

Bioethics

Albany Medical College, Alden March Bioethics Institute, Albany, NY 12208. Offers bioethics (MS, DPS); clinical ethics (Certificate); clinical ethics consultation (Certificate). Part-time and evening/weekend programs available. Postbaccalaureate distance learning degree programs offered (no on-campus study). *Degree requirements:* For master's, thesis. *Entrance requirements:* For master's and Certificate, GRE, GMAT, LSAT, or MCAT (if no graduate degree), essay, official transcripts, 2 letters of reference. Additional exam requirements/recommendations for international students: Recommended—TOEFL. Electronic applications accepted. *Expenses:* Contact institution. *Faculty research:* Ethics in nanotechnology, ethics in genetics, ethics in transplants, philosophy and bioethics, the states and bioethics.

Boston University, School of Public Health, Health Law, Bioethics and Human Rights Department, Boston, MA 02215. Offers MPH. Part-time and evening/weekend programs available. *Faculty:* 5 full-time, 16 part-time/adjunct. *Students:* 10 full-time (all women), 7 part-time (6 women); includes 1 minority (Asian, non-Hispanic/Latino). Average age 26. 86 applicants, 56% accepted, 9 enrolled. *Entrance requirements:* For master's, GRE, MCAT, LSAT, GMAT, DAT. Additional exam requirements/recommendations for international students: Required—TOEFL (minimum score 600 paper-based; 100 iBT) or IELTS (minimum score 6). *Application deadline:* For fall admission, 2/1 priority date for domestic and international students; for spring admission, 10/15 priority date for domestic and international students. Applications are processed on a rolling basis. Application fee: $115. Electronic applications accepted. *Expenses: Tuition:* Full-time $43,970; part-time $1374 per credit hour. *Required fees:* $60 per semester. Tuition and fees vary according to class time, course level and program. *Financial support:* In 2013–14, 1 fellowship was awarded; career-related internships or fieldwork, Federal Work-Study, institutionally sponsored loans, scholarships/grants, and tuition waivers (partial) also available. Support available to part-time students. Financial award application deadline: 3/1; financial award applicants required to submit FAFSA. *Unit head:* Prof. George Annas, Chair, 617-638-4626, E-mail: hld@bu.edu. *Application contact:* LePhan Quan, Associate Director of Admissions, 617-638-4640, Fax: 617-638-5299, E-mail: asksph@bu.edu.
Website: http://sph.bu.edu

Case Western Reserve University, Frances Payne Bolton School of Nursing, Nursing/Bioethics Program, Cleveland, OH 44106. Offers MSN/MA. *Students:* 1 full-time (0 women). *Application deadline:* For fall admission, 6/1 for domestic and international students; for spring admission, 10/1 for domestic and international students. Applications are processed on a rolling basis. Application fee: $75. *Financial support:* Fellowships, research assistantships, and teaching assistantships available. Financial award application deadline: 6/30; financial award applicants required to submit FAFSA. *Unit head:* Dr. Barbara Daly, Head, 216-368-5994, E-mail: barbara.daly@case.edu. *Application contact:* Donna Hassik, Admissions Coordinator, 216-368-5253, Fax: 216-368-0124, E-mail: dmh7@case.edu.
Website: http://fpb.case.edu/MSN/

Case Western Reserve University, School of Medicine and School of Graduate Studies, Graduate Programs in Medicine, Department of Bioethics, Cleveland, OH 44106. Offers MA, JD/MA, MA/MD, MA/MPH, MA/PhD, MSN/MA, MSSA/MA. *Entrance requirements:* For master's, GRE General Test or MCAT or MAT or LSAT or GMAT. Additional exam requirements/recommendations for international students: Required—TOEFL (minimum score 550 paper-based). Electronic applications accepted. *Faculty research:* Ethical issues in genetics, conflicts of interest, organ donation, end-of-life decision making, clinical ethics consultation.

Cleveland State University, College of Graduate Studies, College of Liberal Arts and Social Sciences, Department of Philosophy and Comparative Religion, Cleveland, OH 44115. Offers bioethics (MA, Certificate), including bioethics (MA); philosophy (MA), including philosophy. Part-time and evening/weekend programs available. *Faculty:* 4 full-time (all women), 2 part-time/adjunct (1 woman). *Students:* 1 full-time (0 women), 13 part-time (4 women). Average age 33. 13 applicants, 92% accepted, 3 enrolled. In 2013, 9 master's, 1 other advanced degree awarded. *Degree requirements:* For master's, comprehensive exam, thesis optional, 32 credit hours of coursework; for Certificate, 12 credit hours of coursework. *Entrance requirements:* For master's, BA or BS or equivalent degree with minimum GPA of 2.75; for Certificate, BA, BS, or equivalent degree with minimum GPA of 2.75. Additional exam requirements/recommendations for international students: Required—TOEFL (minimum score 525 paper-based). *Application deadline:* For fall admission, 5/1 priority date for domestic and international students. Applications are processed on a rolling basis. Application fee: $30. *Expenses:* Tuition, state resident: full-time $8335; part-time $521 per credit hour. Tuition, nonresident: full-time $15,670; part-time $979 per credit hour. *Required fees:* $50; $25 per semester. *Financial support:* In 2013–14, 5 students received support, including 5 teaching assistantships with full tuition reimbursements available (averaging $4,000 per year); health care benefits, tuition waivers (full), and unspecified assistantships also available. Support available to part-time students. *Faculty research:* Ethics, early modern philosophy, bioethics, social and political philosophy, history of women philosophers. *Unit head:* Dr. Mary Ellen Waithe, Chairperson, 216-687-3900, Fax: 216-523-7482, E-mail: m.waithe@csuohio.edu. *Application contact:* Deborah L. Brown, Interim Assistant Director, Graduate Admissions, 216-523-7572, Fax: 216-687-5400, E-mail: d.l.brown@csuohio.edu.
Website: http://www.csuohio.edu/class/philosophy-religion/philosophy-religion

Columbia University, School of Continuing Education, Program in Bioethics, New York, NY 10027. Offers MS. Part-time programs available. *Degree requirements:* For master's, thesis. Electronic applications accepted.

Drew University, Caspersen School of Graduate Studies, Program in Medical Humanities, Madison, NJ 07940-1493. Offers MMH, DMH, CMH. Programs conducted jointly with Saint Barnabas Medical Center. Part-time and evening/weekend programs available. *Degree requirements:* For master's, thesis; for doctorate, thesis/dissertation. *Entrance requirements:* For master's and doctorate, transcripts, writing sample, personal statement, recommendations. Additional exam requirements/recommendations for international students: Required—TOEFL (minimum score 585 paper-based; 95 iBT), TWE (minimum score 4). *Expenses:* Contact institution. *Faculty research:* Biomedical ethics, medical narrative, history of medicine, medicine and the arts.

Duke University, Graduate School, Program in Bioethics and Science Policy, Durham, NC 27708-0141. Offers MA. *Faculty:* 15. *Entrance requirements:* For master's, GRE General Test. Additional exam requirements/recommendations for international students: Required—TOEFL (minimum score 577 paper-based; 90 iBT) or IELTS (minimum score 7). *Application deadline:* For fall admission, 1/31 priority date for domestic and international students. Application fee: $80. *Unit head:* Nita Farahany, Chair, 919-613-8514, E-mail: farahany@duke.edu. *Application contact:* Elizabeth Hutton, Director of Admissions, 919-684-3913, Fax: 919-684-2277, E-mail: grad-admissions@duke.edu.
Website: http://scienceandsociety.duke.edu/learn/ma/

Duquesne University, Graduate School of Liberal Arts, Program in Health Care Ethics, Pittsburgh, PA 15282-0001. Offers MA, DHCE, PhD, Certificate. Part-time programs available. Postbaccalaureate distance learning degree programs offered (no on-campus study). *Faculty:* 3 full-time (0 women), 2 part-time/adjunct (both women). *Students:* 52 full-time (31 women), 1 (woman) part-time; includes 9 minority (7 Black or African American, non-Hispanic/Latino; 2 Asian, non-Hispanic/Latino), 15 international. Average age 38. 25 applicants, 56% accepted, 10 enrolled. In 2013, 1 master's, 6 doctorates awarded. Terminal master's awarded for partial completion of doctoral program. *Degree requirements:* For doctorate, 2 foreign languages, comprehensive exam, thesis/dissertation. *Entrance requirements:* For master's, GRE General Test; for doctorate, GRE General Test, master's degree in health care ethics. Additional exam requirements/recommendations for international students: Required—TOEFL. *Application deadline:* For fall admission, 8/1 for domestic students, 5/1 for international

students. Applications are processed on a rolling basis. Electronic applications accepted. *Expenses: Tuition:* Full-time $18,162; part-time $1009 per credit. *Required fees:* $1728; $96 per credit. Tuition and fees vary according to program. *Financial support:* In 2013–14, 6 teaching assistantships (averaging $18,000 per year) were awarded; Federal Work-Study and tuition waivers (full and partial) also available. Support available to part-time students. Financial award application deadline: 5/1. *Unit head:* Dr. Henk ten Have, Director, 412-396-1585. *Application contact:* Linda Rendulic, Assistant to the Dean, 412-396-6400, Fax: 412-396-5265, E-mail: rendulic@duq.edu.
Website: http://www.duq.edu/academics/schools/liberal-arts/graduate-school/programs/healthcare-ethics

Emory University, Laney Graduate School, Emory Center for Ethics, Atlanta, GA 30322-1100. Offers bioethics (MA). Terminal master's awarded for partial completion of doctoral program. *Degree requirements:* For master's, practicum experience, capstone project. *Entrance requirements:* Additional exam requirements/recommendations for international students: Recommended—TOEFL. Electronic applications accepted.

Icahn School of Medicine at Mount Sinai, The Bioethics Program, New York, NY 10029-6504. Offers MS. Program offered jointly with Union Graduate College.

Indiana University–Purdue University Indianapolis, School of Liberal Arts, Department of Philosophy, Indianapolis, IN 46202-2896. Offers American philosophy (Certificate); bioethics (Certificate); philosophy (MA); JD/MA; MD/MA. Part-time programs available. *Faculty:* 13 full-time (2 women), 1 part-time/adjunct (0 women). *Students:* 11 full-time (4 women), 9 part-time (5 women); includes 2 minority (1 Black or African American, non-Hispanic/Latino; 1 Asian, non-Hispanic/Latino), 2 international. Average age 32. 15 applicants, 87% accepted, 10 enrolled. In 2013, 8 master's, 1 other advanced degree awarded. *Degree requirements:* For master's, thesis optional. *Entrance requirements:* For master's, GRE. Additional exam requirements/recommendations for international students: Required—TOEFL. *Application deadline:* For fall admission, 3/1 priority date for domestic and international students; for spring admission, 11/15 for domestic and international students. Applications are processed on a rolling basis. Application fee: $55 ($65 for international students). Electronic applications accepted. *Financial support:* Fellowships, research assistantships with full tuition reimbursements, and teaching assistantships available. Financial award application deadline: 1/15; financial award applicants required to submit FAFSA. *Faculty research:* American philosophy, Peirce bioethics, metaphysics, ethical theory. *Unit head:* Dr. Timothy Lyons, 317-278-7768, E-mail: tdlyons@iupui.edu. *Application contact:* Dr. Chad Carmichael, 317-278-5825, E-mail: crcarmic@iupui.edu.
Website: http://liberalarts.iupui.edu/philosophy/index.php/programs/

Instituto Tecnologico de Santo Domingo, Graduate School, Area of Health Sciences, Santo Domingo, Dominican Republic. Offers bioethics (M Bioethics); clinical bioethics (Certificate); clinical nutrition (Certificate); comprehensive health and the adolescent (Certificate); comrehensive adloescent health (MS); health and social security (M Mgmt).

Johns Hopkins University, Bloomberg School of Public Health, Department of Health Policy and Management, Baltimore, MD 21205-1996. Offers bioethics and policy (PhD); health and public policy (PhD); health care management and leadership (Dr PH); health economics (MHS); health economics and policy (PhD); health finance and management (MHA); health policy (MSPH); health services research and policy (PhD); public policy (MPP). *Accreditation:* CAHME (one or more programs are accredited). Part-time programs available. *Faculty:* 60 full-time (32 women), 178 part-time/adjunct (66 women). *Students:* 204 full-time (152 women), 107 part-time (56 women); includes 81 minority (12 Black or African American, non-Hispanic/Latino; 1 American Indian or Alaska Native, non-Hispanic/Latino; 45 Asian, non-Hispanic/Latino; 14 Hispanic/Latino; 1 Native Hawaiian or other Pacific Islander, non-Hispanic/Latino; 8 Two or more races, non-Hispanic/Latino), 92 international. Average age 31. 550 applicants, 42% accepted, 113 enrolled. In 2013, 55 master's, 34 doctorates awarded. *Degree requirements:* For master's, thesis (for some programs), internship (for some programs); for doctorate, comprehensive exam, thesis/dissertation, 1-year full-time residency (for some programs), oral and written exams. *Entrance requirements:* For master's, GRE General Test or GMAT, 3 letters of recommendation, curriculum vitae/resume; for doctorate, GRE General Test or GMAT, 3 letters of recommendation, curriculum vitae, transcripts. Additional exam requirements/recommendations for international students: Recommended—TOEFL (minimum score 600 paper-based; 100 iBT), IELTS. *Application deadline:* For fall admission, 12/1 for domestic and international students. Applications are processed on a rolling basis. Application fee: $45. Electronic applications accepted. *Financial support:* Fellowships, research assistantships, teaching assistantships, career-related internships or fieldwork, Federal Work-Study, institutionally sponsored loans, scholarships/grants, traineeships, and stipends available. Support available to part-time students. Financial award application deadline: 3/15; financial award applicants required to submit FAFSA. *Faculty research:* Quality of care and health outcomes, health care finance and technology, health disparities and vulnerable populations, injury prevention, health policy and health care policy. *Total annual research expenditures:* $14.2 million. *Unit head:* Dr. Ellen J. MacKenzie, Chairman, 410-955-3625, E-mail: emackenz@jhsph.edu. *Application contact:* Mary Sewell, Coordinator, 410-955-2489, Fax: 410-614-9152, E-mail: msewell@jhsph.edu.
Website: http://www.jhsph.edu/hpm/

Kansas City University of Medicine and Biosciences, College of Biosciences, Kansas City, MO 64106-1453. Offers bioethics (MA); biomedical sciences (MS). Part-time programs available. *Degree requirements:* For master's, comprehensive exam, thesis (for some programs). *Entrance requirements:* For master's, MCAT, GRE.

Loma Linda University, Faculty of Religion, Program in Biomedical and Clinical Ethics, Loma Linda, CA 92350. Offers MA, Certificate. *Degree requirements:* For master's, comprehensive exam, thesis optional. *Entrance requirements:* For master's, GRE General Test, baccalaureate degree. Additional exam requirements/recommendations for international students: Required—TOEFL. Electronic applications accepted.

Loyola Marymount University, College of Liberal Arts, The Bioethics Institute, Program in Bioethics, Los Angeles, CA 90045. Offers MA. Part-time programs available. In 2013, 6 master's awarded. *Entrance requirements:* For master's, GRE or MAT, personal statement, interview, letters of recommendation. Additional exam requirements/recommendations for international students: Required—TOEFL (minimum score 600 paper-based; 100 iBT). *Application deadline:* For fall admission, 3/1 for domestic students; for spring admission, 10/1 for domestic students. Applications are processed on a rolling basis. Application fee: $50. Electronic applications accepted. *Financial support:* In 2013–14, 2 students received support. Scholarships/grants and unspecified assistantships available. Support available to part-time students. Financial award application deadline: 6/1; financial award applicants required to submit FAFSA. *Unit head:* Robert V. Doyle, Program Director, 310-258-2621, E-mail: robert.doyle@lmu.edu. *Application contact:* Chake H. Kouyoumjian, Associate Dean of the Graduate Division, 310-338-2721, E-mail: ckouyoum@lmu.edu.
Website: http://bellarmine.lmu.edu/bioethics

Loyola University Chicago, Graduate School, Program in Bioethics, Chicago, IL 60660. Offers D Be. Postbaccalaureate distance learning degree programs offered (minimal on-campus study). *Entrance requirements:* For doctorate, master's degree in bioethics or health care ethics. *Expenses: Tuition:* Full-time $16,740; part-time $930 per credit. *Required fees:* $135 per semester. *Unit head:* Dr. Samuel Attoh, Dean, 773-508-8948, Fax: 773-508-2460, E-mail: sattoh@luc.edu. *Application contact:* Ron Martin, Assistant Director of Enrollment Management, 312-915-8950, Fax: 312-915-8905, E-mail: gradapp@luc.edu.

Loyola University Chicago, Graduate School, Program in Bioethics and Health Policy, Chicago, IL 60660. Offers D Be, Certificate, MD/MA. Postbaccalaureate distance learning degree programs offered (no on-campus study). *Students:* 13 full-time (9 women), 94 part-time (56 women); includes 13 minority (7 Black or African American, non-Hispanic/Latino; 4 Asian, non-Hispanic/Latino; 2 Hispanic/Latino), 1 international. Average age 47. 55 applicants, 67% accepted, 31 enrolled. In 2013, 8 doctorates, 4 Certificates awarded. *Expenses: Tuition:* Full-time $16,740; part-time $930 per credit. *Required fees:* $135 per semester. *Financial support:* Scholarships/grants available. *Unit head:* Dr. Samuel Attoh, Dean, 773-508-8948, Fax: 773-508-2460, E-mail: sattoh@luc.edu. *Application contact:* Ron Martin, Assistant Director of Enrollment Management, 312-915-8950, Fax: 312-915-8905, E-mail: gradapp@luc.edu.

McGill University, Faculty of Graduate and Postdoctoral Studies, Faculty of Arts, Department of Philosophy, Montréal, QC H3A 2T5, Canada. Offers bioethics (MA); philosophy (PhD).

McGill University, Faculty of Graduate and Postdoctoral Studies, Faculty of Law, Montréal, QC H3A 2T5, Canada. Offers air and space law (LL M, DCL, Graduate Certificate); bioethics (LL M); comparative law (LL M, DCL, Graduate Certificate); law (LL M, DCL). Applications for LL M with specialization in bioethics are made initially through the Biomedical Ethics Unit in the Faculty of Medicine.

McGill University, Faculty of Graduate and Postdoctoral Studies, Faculty of Medicine, Department of Medicine, Montréal, QC H3A 2T5, Canada. Offers experimental medicine (M Sc, PhD), including bioethics (M Sc), experimental medicine.

Medical College of Wisconsin, Graduate School of Biomedical Sciences, Center for Bioethics and Medical Humanities, Milwaukee, WI 53226-0509. Offers bioethics (MA); clinical bioethics (Graduate Certificate); research ethics (Graduate Certificate). Part-time programs available. *Degree requirements:* For master's, thesis. *Entrance requirements:* For master's and Graduate Certificate, GRE, official transcripts, three letters of recommendation. Additional exam requirements/recommendations for international students: Required—TOEFL. *Faculty research:* Ethics committees and consultation, ethics of managed care, discussion of code status by physicians.

New York University, Graduate School of Arts and Science, Program in Bioethics, New York, NY 10012-1019. Offers MA. Part-time programs available. *Students:* 15 full-time (8 women), 15 part-time (7 women); includes 10 minority (2 Black or African American, non-Hispanic/Latino; 7 Asian, non-Hispanic/Latino; 1 Hispanic/Latino), 2 international. Average age 26. 22 applicants, 82% accepted, 14 enrolled. In 2013, 17 master's awarded. *Degree requirements:* For master's, one foreign language. *Entrance requirements:* For master's, GRE General Test. Additional exam requirements/recommendations for international students: Required—TOEFL. *Application deadline:* For fall admission, 5/1 for domestic and international students; for spring admission, 11/1 for domestic and international students. Application fee: $95. *Expenses: Tuition:* Full-time $35,856; part-time $1494 per unit. *Required fees:* $1408; $64 per unit. $473 per term. Tuition and fees vary according to course load and program. *Financial support:* Application deadline: 5/1. *Unit head:* S. Matthew Liao, Director of Graduate Studies, 212-992-7999, Fax: 212-995-4157, E-mail: bioethics@nyu.edu. *Application contact:* Amanda Anjum, Graduate Program Administrator, 212-992-7999, Fax: 212-995-4157, E-mail: bioethics@nyu.edu.

Northeast Ohio Medical University, College of Graduate Studies, Rootstown, OH 44272-0095. Offers bioethics (Certificate); health-system pharmacy administration (MS); integrated pharmaceutical medicine (MS, PhD); public health (MS). *Faculty:* 80 part-time/adjunct (26 women). *Students:* 38 full-time (21 women); includes 4 minority (3 Asian, non-Hispanic/Latino; 1 Hispanic/Latino). Average age 28. 45 applicants, 84% accepted, 38 enrolled. In 2013, 9 master's, 1 doctorate awarded. *Application deadline:* For fall admission, 9/1 priority date for domestic students; for winter admission, 1/5 priority date for domestic students. Applications are processed on a rolling basis. Application fee: $45. Electronic applications accepted. Full-time tuition and fees vary according to program. Part-time tuition and fees vary according to degree level. *Unit head:* Dr. Walter E. Horton, Jr., Dean of the College of Graduate Studies. *Application contact:* Luke Gloeckner, Associate Director for Enrollment Services and Registration, 330-325-6274, E-mail: lgloeckner@gmail.com.
Website: http://www.neomed.edu/academics/graduatestudies

Rush University, College of Health Sciences, Program in Healthcare Ethics, Chicago, IL 60612-3832. Offers MA, Graduate Certificate. Part-time programs available. *Degree requirements:* For master's, oral presentation of thesis. *Entrance requirements:* For master's, GRE General Test, minimum GPA of 3.0. Electronic applications accepted. *Faculty research:* Daily spirituality in the disease process, training psychiatry residents in spirituality, defining and screening for spiritual struggle.

Saint Louis University, Graduate Education, Center for Health Care Ethics, St. Louis, MO 63103-2097. Offers clinical health care ethics (Certificate); health care ethics (PhD). *Degree requirements:* For doctorate, comprehensive exam, thesis/dissertation. *Entrance requirements:* For doctorate, GRE General Test, master's degree in ethics or a field related to health care, basic competencies in philosophical and applied ethics, transcripts. Additional exam requirements/recommendations for international students: Required—TOEFL (minimum score 525 paper-based). Electronic applications accepted. *Faculty research:* Health policy, clinical ethics, research ethics, empirical bioethics, ethics education and assessment.

Stony Brook University, State University of New York, Stony Brook University Medical Center, Health Sciences Center, School of Medicine, Center for Medical Humanities, Compassionate Care, and Bioethics, Stony Brook, NY 11794. Offers MD/MA. *Students:* 5 full-time (2 women), 5 part-time (1 woman); includes 2 minority (1 Black or African American, non-Hispanic/Latino; 1 Asian, non-Hispanic/Latino), 1 international. *Entrance requirements:* Additional exam requirements/recommendations for international students: Required—TOEFL. *Application deadline:* For fall admission, 7/1 for domestic students, 5/15 for international students; for spring admission, 11/1 for domestic students, 10/1 for international students. *Expenses:* Tuition, state resident: full-time $9870; part-time $411 per credit. Tuition, nonresident: full-time $18,350; part-time $765 per credit. *Unit head:* Dr. Stephen G. Post, Director, 631-444-9797, E-mail: michael.ortega@stonybrookmedicine.edu. *Application contact:* Michael Ortega, 631-444-8029, E-mail: michael.ortega@stonybrookmedicine.edu.
Website: http://www.stonybrook.edu/bioethics/index.shtml

Trinity International University, Trinity Graduate School, Deerfield, IL 60015-1284. Offers bioethics (MA); communication and culture (MA); counseling psychology (MA); instructional leadership (M Ed); teaching (MA). Part-time and evening/weekend programs available. Postbaccalaureate distance learning degree programs offered (minimal on-campus study). *Degree requirements:* For master's, comprehensive exam. *Entrance requirements:* For master's, GRE General Test or MAT, minimum undergraduate GPA of 3.0. Additional exam requirements/recommendations for international students: Required—TOEFL (minimum score 580 paper-based), TWE (minimum score 4). Electronic applications accepted.

Union Graduate College, Center for Bioethics and Clinical Leadership, Schenectady, NY 12308-3107. Offers bioethics (MS); clinical ethics (AC); clinical leadership in health management (MS); health, policy and law (AC); research ethics (AC). Part-time and evening/weekend programs available. Postbaccalaureate distance learning degree programs offered (minimal on-campus study). *Faculty:* 2 full-time (0 women), 9 part-time/adjunct (7 women). *Students:* 2 full-time (both women), 59 part-time (39 women); includes 17 minority (3 Black or African American, non-Hispanic/Latino; 8 Asian, non-Hispanic/Latino; 2 Hispanic/Latino; 4 Two or more races, non-Hispanic/Latino), 4 international. Average age 36. In 2013, 19 master's, 3 other advanced degrees awarded. *Entrance requirements:* For master's, letters of recommendation. Additional exam requirements/recommendations for international students: Required—TOEFL (minimum score 550 paper-based). *Application deadline:* Applications are processed on a rolling basis. Electronic applications accepted. *Expenses:* Contact institution. *Financial support:* Federal Work-Study, scholarships/grants, health care benefits, and tuition waivers (partial) available. Support available to part-time students. Financial award applicants required to submit FAFSA. *Faculty research:* Bioethics education, clinical ethics consultation, research ethics, history of biomedical ethics, international bioethics/research ethics. *Unit head:* Dr. Sean Philpott, Director, 518-631-9860, Fax: 518-631-9903, E-mail: philpotts@uniongraduatecollege.edu. *Application contact:* Ann Nolte, Assistant Director, 518-631-9860, Fax: 518-631-9903, E-mail: noltea@uniongraduatecollege.edu.

Université de Montréal, Faculty of Medicine, Programs in Bioethics, Montréal, QC H3C 3J7, Canada. Offers MA, DESS. Electronic applications accepted.

Université de Montréal, Faculty of Theology and Sciences of Religions, Montréal, QC H3C 3J7, Canada. Offers health, spirituality and bioethics (DESS); practical theology (MA, PhD); religious sciences (MA, PhD); theology (MA, D Th, PhD, L Th); theology-Biblical studies (PhD). *Degree requirements:* For master's, one foreign language; for doctorate, 2 foreign languages, thesis/dissertation, general exam. Electronic applications accepted.

University of Pennsylvania, Perelman School of Medicine, Department of Medical Ethics and Health Policy, Philadelphia, PA 19104. Offers MBE, DMD/MBE, JD/MBE, LL M/MBE, MD/MBE, MS Ed/MBE, MSN/MBE, MSW/MBE, PhD/MBE. Part-time and evening/weekend programs available. *Faculty:* 12 full-time (4 women), 10 part-time/adjunct (4 women). *Students:* 46 full-time (24 women), 35 part-time (20 women); includes 18 minority (5 Black or African American, non-Hispanic/Latino; 10 Asian, non-Hispanic/Latino; 3 Hispanic/Latino). Average age 31. 46 applicants, 96% accepted, 40 enrolled. In 2013, 60 master's awarded. *Degree requirements:* For master's, thesis. *Application deadline:* Applications are processed on a rolling basis. Application fee: $70. *Unit head:* Dr. Autumn Fiester, Director, 215-573-2602, Fax: 215-573-3036.
Website: http://medicalethics.med.upenn.edu/

University of Pittsburgh, Dietrich School of Arts and Sciences, Center for Bioethics and Health Law, Pittsburgh, PA 15260. Offers bioethics (MA). Part-time programs available. *Faculty:* 4 full-time (1 woman), 3 part-time/adjunct (1 woman). *Students:* 13 part-time (10 women), 1 international. Average age 28. 11 applicants, 27% accepted, 3 enrolled. In 2013, 1 master's awarded. *Degree requirements:* For master's, thesis. *Entrance requirements:* For master's, GRE General Test, letters of recommendation, writing sample. Additional exam requirements/recommendations for international students: Required—TOEFL. *Application deadline:* For fall admission, 3/31 for domestic students, 6/30 for international students. Applications are processed on a rolling basis. Application fee: $50. Electronic applications accepted. *Expenses:* Tuition, state resident: full-time $19,964; part-time $807 per credit. Tuition, nonresident: full-time $32,686; part-time $1337 per credit. *Required fees:* $740; $200. Tuition and fees vary according to program. *Financial support:* Tuition waivers (partial) available. *Faculty research:* End of life care, ethics and genetics, health law and policy, organ donation and transplantation, research ethics. *Unit head:* Dr. Lisa S. Parker, Director of Graduate Education, 412-648-7007, Fax: 412-648-2649, E-mail: lisap@pitt.edu. *Application contact:* Janet E. Malis, Administrative Assistant, 412-648-7007, Fax: 412-648-2649, E-mail: bioethic@pitt.edu.
Website: http://www.bioethics.pitt.edu

University of South Florida, Innovative Education Graduate Certificate Programs, Tampa, FL 33620-9951. *Unit head:* Kathy Barnes, Interdisciplinary Programs Coordinator, 813-974-8031, Fax: 813-974-7061, E-mail: barnesk@usf.edu. *Application contact:* Karen Tylinski, Metro Initiatives, 813-974-9943, Fax: 813-974-7061, E-mail: ktylinsk@usf.edu.
Website: http://www.usf.edu/innovative-education/

The University of Tennessee, Graduate School, College of Arts and Sciences, Department of Philosophy, Knoxville, TN 37996. Offers medical ethics (MA, PhD); philosophy (MA, PhD); religious studies (MA). Part-time programs available. *Degree requirements:* For master's, thesis or alternative; for doctorate, one foreign language, thesis/dissertation. *Entrance requirements:* For master's and doctorate, GRE General Test, minimum GPA of 2.7. Additional exam requirements/recommendations for international students: Required—TOEFL. Electronic applications accepted. *Expenses:* Tuition, state resident: full-time $9540; part-time $531 per credit hour. Tuition, nonresident: full-time $27,728; part-time $1542 per credit hour. *Required fees:* $1404; $67 per credit hour.

University of Toronto, Faculty of Medicine, Institute of Medical Science, Toronto, ON M5S 1A1, Canada. Offers bioethics (MH Sc); biomedical communications (M Sc BMC); medical radiation science (MH Sc); medical science (M Sc, PhD). *Degree requirements:* For master's, thesis; for doctorate, thesis/dissertation, thesis defense. *Entrance requirements:* For master's, minimum GPA of 3.7 in 3 of 4 years (M Sc), interview; for doctorate, M Sc or equivalent, defended thesis, minimum A- average, interview. Additional exam requirements/recommendations for international students: Required—TOEFL (minimum score 600 paper-based; 93 iBT), TWE (minimum score 5). Electronic applications accepted.

University of Washington, Graduate School, School of Medicine, Graduate Programs in Medicine, Department of Medical History and Ethics, Seattle, WA 98195. Offers bioethics (MA).

Naturopathic Medicine

Bastyr University, School of Naturopathic Medicine, Kenmore, WA 98028-4966. Offers ND. *Accreditation:* CNME; MEAC. Part-time programs available. *Students:* 564 full-time (117 women), 27 part-time (7 women); includes 136 minority (18 Black or African American, non-Hispanic/Latino; 3 American Indian or Alaska Native, non-Hispanic/Latino; 63 Asian, non-Hispanic/Latino; 17 Hispanic/Latino; 35 Two or more races, non-Hispanic/Latino), 47 international. Average age 30. *Degree requirements:* For doctorate, comprehensive exam. *Entrance requirements:* For doctorate, 1 year of course work in biology, chemistry, organic chemistry and physics. Additional exam requirements/recommendations for international students: Required—TOEFL (minimum score 550 paper-based; 79 iBT). *Application deadline:* For fall admission, 2/1 priority date for domestic and international students. Applications are processed on a rolling basis. Application fee: $75. Electronic applications accepted. *Financial support:* Career-related internships or fieldwork, Federal Work-Study, and scholarships/grants available. Support available to part-time students. Financial award application deadline: 4/15; financial award applicants required to submit FAFSA. *Faculty research:* Integrative oncology, integrative care for neurodegenerative diseases, vitamin D supplementation, sauna (hyperthermia-based) detoxification, intranasal glutathione (nasal spray) for Parkinson's disease. *Unit head:* Dr. Jane Guiltinan, Dean, 425-823-1300, Fax: 425-823-6222. *Application contact:* Alexis Rush, Associate Director of Admissions, 425-602-3330, Fax: 425-602-3090, E-mail: ndadvise@bastyr.edu.
Website: http://www.bastyr.edu/academics/areas-study/study-naturopathic-medicine/

Canadian College of Naturopathic Medicine, Bachelor of Naturopathy Program, Toronto, ON M2K 1E2, Canada. Offers BN. *Accreditation:* CNME. *Faculty:* 16 full-time, 105 part-time/adjunct. *Students:* 383 full-time (287 women), 216 part-time (162 women). Average age 26. 196 applicants, 73% accepted, 103 enrolled. In 2013, 127 degrees awarded. *Degree requirements:* For BN, 12-month internship. *Entrance requirements:* For degree, 1 year of course work in general biology, humanities and physiology; 1 semester of course work in organic chemistry and psychology. Additional exam requirements/recommendations for international students: Recommended—TOEFL (minimum score 580 paper-based; 86 iBT), IELTS (minimum score 6.5). *Application deadline:* For fall admission, 12/31 priority date for domestic and international students; for winter admission, 5/1 priority date for domestic and international students. Applications are processed on a rolling basis. Application fee: $115. Electronic applications accepted. *Expenses: Tuition:* Full-time $21,010 Canadian dollars. *Required fees:* $635 Canadian dollars. Tuition and fees vary according to student level. *Financial support:* In 2013–14, 85 students received support. Institutionally sponsored loans, scholarships/grants, and health care benefits available. Support available to part-time students. Financial award application deadline: 10/31; financial award applicants required to submit FAFSA. *Faculty research:* Natural health products for lung cancer; the use of habanero chili pepper for cancer; melatonin as an anticancer agent with and without chemotherapy; interactions between natural health products and pharmaceuticals; the use of selenium for patients with HIV/AIDS. *Unit head:* Bob Bernhardt, President/CEO, 416-498-1255, Fax: 416-498-3197, E-mail: bbernhardt@ccnm.edu. *Application contact:* Student Services and Admissions Department, 416-498-1225 Ext. 245, Fax: 416-498-3197, E-mail: info@ccnm.edu.
Website: http://www.ccnm.edu/

See Display on next page and Close-Up on page 931.

National College of Natural Medicine, School of Naturopathic Medicine, Portland, OR 97201. Offers integrative medicine research (MS); naturopathic medicine (ND). *Accreditation:* CNME. *Entrance requirements:* For master's, GRE. Additional exam requirements/recommendations for international students: Recommended—TOEFL. *Faculty research:* Diet and diabetes, whole practice research, cruciferous vegetables and cancer, natural medicine and immune function, taraxacum and diuretics.

National University of Health Sciences, College of Professional Studies, Lombard, IL 60148-4583. Offers acupuncture (MSAC); chiropractic medicine (DC); naturopathic medicine (ND); Oriental medicine (MSOM). *Accreditation:* CCE. *Degree requirements:* For master's and doctorate, comprehensive exam, internship, community service. *Entrance requirements:* For master's, bachelor's degree, character references, undergraduate transcripts; for doctorate, bachelor's degree, character references, undergraduate transcripts, written essay. Additional exam requirements/recommendations for international students: Required—TOEFL (minimum score 550 paper-based; 79 iBT). Electronic applications accepted. *Faculty research:* Discipline/whole practice research (including practice-based research networks), mechanisms of action, clinical trials, and evidence-based practice of CAM therapies; educational research in CAM teaching institutions.

Southwest College of Naturopathic Medicine and Health Sciences, Program in Naturopathic Medicine, Tempe, AZ 85282. Offers ND. *Accreditation:* CNME. *Faculty:* 17 full-time (9 women), 55 part-time/adjunct (37 women). *Students:* 405 full-time (297 women), 7 part-time (5 women); includes 37 minority (11 Black or African American, non-Hispanic/Latino; 9 Asian, non-Hispanic/Latino; 12 Hispanic/Latino; 5 Two or more races, non-Hispanic/Latino), 7 international. Average age 31. 182 applicants, 74% accepted, 76 enrolled. In 2013, 71 doctorates awarded. *Entrance requirements:* For doctorate, minimum GPA of 3.0, letters of recommendation, in-person interview. Additional exam requirements/recommendations for international students: Required—TOEFL (minimum score 637 paper-based; 110 iBT). *Application deadline:* For fall admission, 3/1 priority date for domestic and international students; for winter admission, 7/1 priority date for domestic students, 7/1 for international students; for spring admission, 11/1 for domestic students. Applications are processed on a rolling basis. Application fee: $115. Electronic applications accepted. *Expenses: Tuition:* Full-time $28,128; part-time $293 per credit. *Financial support:* Federal Work-Study and scholarships/grants available. Support available to part-time students. Financial award application deadline: 5/1; financial award applicants required to submit FAFSA. *Faculty research:* Anti-microbial botanicals, immune-modulatory botanicals, characterization of colloidal silver, ozone therapy, threat of bioterrorism. *Unit head:* Dr. Christine Girard, Executive Vice President, 480-858-9100 Ext. 241, E-mail: c.girard@scnm.edu. *Application contact:* Eve Bilotas, Director of Admissions, 480-858-9100 Ext. 213, Fax: 480-222-9413, E-mail: e.bilotas@scnm.edu.
Website: http://www.scnm.edu

Universidad del Turabo, Graduate Programs, School of Health Sciences, Program in Naturopathy, Gurabo, PR 00778-3030. Offers ND.

University of Bridgeport, College of Naturopathic Medicine, Bridgeport, CT 06604. Offers ND. *Accreditation:* CNME. *Faculty:* 6 full-time (3 women), 19 part-time/adjunct (7 women). *Students:* 104 full-time (82 women), 4 part-time (all women); includes 39 minority (16 Black or African American, non-Hispanic/Latino; 1 American Indian or

Alaska Native, non-Hispanic/Latino; 8 Asian, non-Hispanic/Latino; 8 Hispanic/Latino; 6 Two or more races, non-Hispanic/Latino), 1 international. Average age 32. 144 applicants, 42% accepted, 27 enrolled. In 2013, 34 doctorates awarded. *Degree requirements:* For doctorate, NPLEX Part I. *Entrance requirements:* For doctorate, minimum GPA of 2.5. Additional exam requirements/recommendations for international students: Recommended—TOEFL (minimum score 550 paper-based; 80 iBT), IELTS. *Application deadline:* For fall admission, 8/1 priority date for domestic and international students; for spring admission, 12/1 for domestic students, 2/1 priority date for international students. Applications are processed on a rolling basis. Application fee: $75. Electronic applications accepted. *Expenses: Tuition:* Part-time $755 per credit. *Required fees:* $200 per semester. Tuition and fees vary according to program. *Financial support:* In 2013–14, 40 students received support. Federal Work-Study, institutionally sponsored loans, and scholarships/grants available. Financial award application deadline: 4/1; financial award applicants required to submit FAFSA. *Unit head:* Dr. Marcia Prenguber, Dean, 203-576-4110, Fax: 203-574-4107, E-mail: mprengub@bridgeport.edu. *Application contact:* Leanne Proctor, Director of Health Science Admissions, 203-576-4352, Fax: 203-576-4941, E-mail: natmed@bridgeport.edu.

Osteopathic Medicine

A.T. Still University, Kirksville College of Osteopathic Medicine, Kirksville, MO 63501. Offers biomedical sciences (MS); osteopathic medicine (DO). *Accreditation:* AOsA. *Faculty:* 37 full-time (5 women), 36 part-time/adjunct (6 women). *Students:* 702 full-time (282 women), 10 part-time (3 women); includes 132 minority (13 Black or African American, non-Hispanic/Latino; 1 American Indian or Alaska Native, non-Hispanic/Latino; 69 Asian, non-Hispanic/Latino; 18 Hispanic/Latino; 31 Two or more races, non-Hispanic/Latino), 6 international. Average age 26. 4,110 applicants, 10% accepted, 172 enrolled. In 2013, 13 master's, 177 doctorates awarded. *Degree requirements:* For master's, thesis; for doctorate, Level 1 and 2 COMLEX-PE and CE exams. *Entrance requirements:* For master's, GRE, MCAT, or DAT, minimum undergraduate GPA of 2.65 (cumulative and science); for doctorate, MCAT, bachelor's degree with minimum GPA of 2.8 (cumulative and science) or 90 semester hours with minimum GPA of 3.5 (cumulative and science). Additional exam requirements/recommendations for international students: Recommended—TOEFL. *Application deadline:* For fall admission, 2/1 for domestic and international students; for summer admission, 2/1 for domestic students. Applications are processed on a rolling basis. Application fee: $70. Electronic applications accepted. *Expenses:* Contact institution. *Financial support:* In 2013–14, 230 students received support, including 23 fellowships with full tuition reimbursements available (averaging $49,817 per year); Federal Work-Study and scholarships/grants also available. Financial award application deadline: 5/1; financial award applicants required to submit FAFSA. *Faculty research:* Practice-based research network, antibiotic resistance, staphylococcus aureus, bacterial virulence and environmental survival, excitability of the exercise pressor reflex, clinical trials. *Total annual research expenditures:* $243,048. *Unit head:* Dr. Margaret WIlson, Dean, 660-626-2354, Fax: 660-626-2080, E-mail: mwilson@atsu.edu. *Application contact:* Donna Sparks, Associate Director, Admissions Processing, 660-626-2117, Fax: 660-626-2969, E-mail: admissions@atsu.edu.
Website: http://www.atsu.edu/kcom/

A.T. Still University, School of Osteopathic Medicine in Arizona, Mesa, AZ 85206. Offers DO. *Accreditation:* AOsA. *Faculty:* 33 full-time (12 women), 33 part-time/adjunct (11 women). *Students:* 429 full-time (206 women), 2 part-time (1 woman); includes 178 minority (2 Black or African American, non-Hispanic/Latino; 1 American Indian or Alaska Native, non-Hispanic/Latino; 122 Asian, non-Hispanic/Latino; 27 Hispanic/Latino; 26 Two or more races, non-Hispanic/Latino). Average age 28. 4,569 applicants, 5% accepted, 108 enrolled. In 2013, 104 doctorates awarded. *Degree requirements:* For doctorate, Level 1 and 2 COMLEX-PE and CE exams. *Entrance requirements:* For doctorate, MCAT, minimum undergraduate GPA of 2.8 (cumulative and science) with bachelor's degree. *Application deadline:* For fall admission, 3/1 for domestic students; for summer admission, 3/1 for domestic students. Applications are processed on a rolling basis. Application fee: $70. Electronic applications accepted. *Financial support:* In 2013–14, 29 students received support, including 2 fellowships (averaging $47,567 per year); Federal Work-Study and scholarships/grants also available. Financial award application deadline: 5/1; financial award applicants required to submit FAFSA. *Faculty research:* Medical education research, osteopathic medicine research, practice-based research network. *Total annual research expenditures:* $52,443. *Unit head:* Dr. Kay Kalousek, Dean, 480-219-6000, Fax: 480-219-6110, E-mail: kkalousek@atsu.edu. *Application contact:* Donna Sparks, Associate Director for Admissions, 660-626-2117, Fax: 660-626-2969, E-mail: admissions@atsu.edu.
Website: http://www.atsu.edu/soma

Des Moines University, College of Osteopathic Medicine, Des Moines, IA 50312-4104. Offers DO. *Accreditation:* AOsA. *Degree requirements:* For doctorate, National Board of Osteopathic Medical Examiners Exam Level 1 and 2. *Entrance requirements:* For doctorate, MCAT, minimum GPA of 3.0; 8 hours of course work in biology, chemistry, organic chemistry, and physics; 3 hours of biochemistry; 6 hours of course work in English; interview. Electronic applications accepted. *Expenses:* Contact institution. *Faculty research:* Cardiovascular, infectious disease, cancer immunology, cell signaling nociception.

Edward Via College of Osteopahtic Medicine–Virginia Campus, Graduate Program, Blacksburg, VA 24060. Offers DO. *Accreditation:* AOsA. *Degree requirements:* For doctorate, thesis/dissertation. *Entrance requirements:* For doctorate, MCAT, 8 hours of biology, general chemistry, and organic chemistry; 6 hours each of additional science and English; minimum overall science GPA of 2.75. *Faculty research:* Nanobiology of aging, calcium transport regulation, prescription drug abuse, oxidative stress and inflammation, immune protection.

Edward Via College of Osteopathic Medicine–Carolinas Campus, Graduate Program, Spartanburg, SC 29303. Offers DO.

Georgia Campus–Philadelphia College of Osteopathic Medicine, Doctor of Osteopathic Medicine Program, Suwanee, GA 30024. Offers DO. *Accreditation:* AOsA. *Students:* 473 full-time (264 women); includes 196 minority (45 Black or African

American, non-Hispanic/Latino; 69 Asian, non-Hispanic/Latino; 7 Hispanic/Latino; 1 Native Hawaiian or other Pacific Islander, non-Hispanic/Latino; 74 Two or more races, non-Hispanic/Latino), 4 international. 3,533 applicants, 6% accepted, 135 enrolled. In 2013, 79 doctorates awarded. *Degree requirements:* For doctorate, comprehensive exam. *Entrance requirements:* For doctorate, MCAT. Additional exam requirements/recommendations for international students: Required—TOEFL (minimum score 79 iBT). *Application deadline:* For fall admission, 3/1 for domestic and international students. Applications are processed on a rolling basis. Application fee: $50. Electronic applications accepted. *Financial support:* Application deadline: 3/15; applicants required to submit FAFSA. *Unit head:* Deborah Benvenger, Chief Admissions Officer, 215-871-6700, Fax: 215-871-6719. *Application contact:* Deborah Benvenger, Chief Admissions Officer.
Website: http://web.pcom.edu/Academic_Programs/aca_do/aca_do.html

Kansas City University of Medicine and Biosciences, College of Osteopathic Medicine, Kansas City, MO 64106-1453. Offers DO, DO/MA, DO/MBA. *Accreditation:* AOsA. *Degree requirements:* For doctorate, comprehensive exam, National Board Exam - COMLEX. *Entrance requirements:* For doctorate, MCAT, on-campus interview. *Faculty research:* 2-Chloroadenine in DNA use in controlling leukemia, dietary isoprenoids role in tumor cell control, preventive medicine and public health research of maternal and child health, nonenzymatic glycosylation in cardiac tissue.

Lake Erie College of Osteopathic Medicine, Professional Programs, Erie, PA 16509-1025. Offers biomedical sciences (Postbaccalaureate Certificate); medical education (MS); osteopathic medicine (DO); pharmacy (Pharm D). *Accreditation:* ACPE; AOsA. *Degree requirements:* For doctorate, comprehensive exam, National Osteopathic Medical Licensing Exam, Levels 1 and 2; for Postbaccalaureate Certificate, comprehensive exam, North American Pharmacist Licensure Examination (NAPLEX). *Entrance requirements:* For doctorate, MCAT, minimum GPA of 3.2, letters of recommendation; for Postbaccalaureate Certificate, PCAT, letters of recommendation, minimum GPA of 3.5. Electronic applications accepted. *Faculty research:* Cardiac smooth and skeletal muscle mechanics, chemotherapeutics and vitamins, osteopathic manipulation.

Lincoln Memorial University, DeBusk College of Osteopathic Medicine, Harrogate, TN 37752-1901. Offers DO. *Accreditation:* AOsA. *Entrance requirements:* For doctorate, MCAT. Additional exam requirements/recommendations for international students: Required—TOEFL (minimum score 600 paper-based; 100 iBT).

Marian University, College of Osteopathic Medicine, Indianapolis, IN 46222-1997. Offers DO. *Faculty:* 23 full-time (7 women). *Students:* 162 full-time (79 women); includes 27 minority (2 Black or African American, non-Hispanic/Latino; 18 Asian, non-Hispanic/Latino; 7 Hispanic/Latino). Average age 25. 3,352 applicants, 8% accepted, 162 enrolled. *Degree requirements:* For doctorate, comprehensive exam, cognitive and performance evaluations. *Entrance requirements:* For doctorate, MCAT. Additional exam requirements/recommendations for international students: Required—TOEFL. *Application deadline:* For fall admission, 3/1 for domestic and international students. Applications are processed on a rolling basis. Application fee: $100. Electronic applications accepted. *Expenses: Tuition:* Part-time $400 per credit hour. Full-time tuition and fees vary according to degree level and program. *Faculty research:* Biochemical mechanisms of immunology, antibiotic resistance, comparative anatomy, development of population genetic models, evaluation of human and non-human primates, infection pathology signaling networks in human physiology. *Unit head:* Dr. Paul Evans, Vice President/Founding Dean, 317-955-6700, E-mail: pevans@marian.edu. *Application contact:* Bryan Moody, Director of Enrollment Management, 317-955-6284, Fax: -, E-mail: bmoody@marian.edu.
Website: http://www.marian.edu/osteopathic-medical-school

Michigan State University, College of Osteopathic Medicine, Professional Program in Osteopathic Medicine, East Lansing, MI 48824. Offers DO. *Accreditation:* AOsA. Electronic applications accepted.

Midwestern University, Downers Grove Campus, Chicago College of Osteopathic Medicine, Downers Grove, IL 60515-1235. Offers DO. *Accreditation:* AOsA. *Entrance requirements:* For doctorate, MCAT, 1 year course work each in organic chemistry, general chemistry, biology, physics, and English. *Expenses:* Contact institution. *Faculty research:* Cadmium toxicity, amino acid transport, metabolic actions of vanadium, diabetes and obesity.

Midwestern University, Glendale Campus, Arizona College of Osteopathic Medicine, Glendale, AZ 85308. Offers DO. *Accreditation:* AOsA. *Entrance requirements:* For doctorate, MCAT. Electronic applications accepted. *Expenses:* Contact institution.

New York Institute of Technology, College of Osteopathic Medicine, Old Westbury, NY 11568-8000. Offers medical/healthcare simulation (MS); osteopathic medicine (DO); DO/MBA; DO/MS. *Accreditation:* AOsA. *Faculty:* 58 full-time (19 women), 26 part-time/adjunct (7 women). *Students:* 1,199 full-time (592 women), 18 part-time (11 women); includes 568 minority (59 Black or African American, non-Hispanic/Latino; 1 American Indian or Alaska Native, non-Hispanic/Latino; 447 Asian, non-Hispanic/Latino; 57 Hispanic/Latino; 3 Native Hawaiian or other Pacific Islander, non-Hispanic/Latino; 1 Two or more races, non-Hispanic/Latino), 2 international. Average age 27. 6,200 applicants, 7% accepted, 315 enrolled. In 2013, 13 master's, 287 doctorates awarded. *Degree requirements:* For doctorate, comprehensive exam. *Entrance requirements:* For doctorate, MCAT, 6 semester hours of English; 8 semester hours each of biology, general chemistry, organic chemistry, and physics; minimum GPA of 2.75. *Application deadline:* For fall admission, 2/1 for domestic students. Applications are processed on a rolling basis. Application fee: $80. Electronic applications accepted. *Expenses:* Contact institution. *Financial support:* Fellowships with partial tuition reimbursements and tuition waivers (full and partial) available. Financial award application deadline: 4/1; financial award applicants required to submit FAFSA. *Faculty research:* Osteopathic manipulation therapy, paleodiet of fossil horses, osteopathic treatment of muscle with compromised innervation, biomedical science. *Unit head:* Dr. Wolfgang Gilliar, Dean, 516-686-3722, Fax: 516-686-3830, E-mail: wgilliar@nyit.edu. *Application contact:* Rodika Zaika, Director of Admissions, 516-686-3792, Fax: 516-686-3831, E-mail: rzaika@nyit.edu.
Website: http://www.nyit.edu/medicine

Nova Southeastern University, College of Osteopathic Medicine, Fort Lauderdale, FL 33328. Offers biomedical informatics (MS, Graduate Certificate), including biomedical informatics (MS), clinical informatics (Graduate Certificate), public health informatics (Graduate Certificate); disaster and emergency preparedness (MS); osteopathic medicine (DO); public health (MPH). *Accreditation:* AOsA. *Faculty:* 107 full-time (55 women), 1,235 part-time/adjunct (297 women). *Students:* 1,036 full-time (439 women), 171 part-time (101 women); includes 537 minority (81 Black or African American, non-Hispanic/Latino; 247 Asian, non-Hispanic/Latino; 168 Hispanic/Latino; 41 Two or more races, non-Hispanic/Latino), 31 international. Average age 28. 4,012 applicants, 12% accepted, 246 enrolled. In 2013, 70 master's, 215 doctorates, 1 other advanced degree awarded. *Entrance requirements:* For master's, GRE, licensed healthcare professional or GRE; for doctorate, MCAT, biology, chemistry, organic chemistry, physics (all with labs), and English. *Application deadline:* For fall admission, 1/15 for domestic students. Applications are processed on a rolling basis. Application fee: $50. Electronic applications accepted. *Expenses:* Contact institution. *Financial support:* In 2013–14, 39 students received support, including 24 fellowships (averaging $45,593 per year); research assistantships, teaching assistantships, Federal Work-Study, and scholarships/grants also available. Financial award application deadline: 6/1; financial award applicants required to submit FAFSA. *Faculty research:* Teaching strategies, simulated patient use, HIV/AIDS education, minority health issues, managed care education. *Unit head:* Anthony J. Silavgni, DO, Dean, 954-262-1407, E-mail: silvagni@hpd.nova.edu. *Application contact:* Monica Sanchez, Admissions Counselor, College of Osteopathic Medicine, 954-262-1110, Fax: 954-262-2282, E-mail: mh1156@nova.edu.
Website: http://www.medicine.nova.edu/

Ohio University, Heritage College of Osteopathic Medicine, Athens, OH 45701-2979. Offers DO, DO/MA, DO/MBA, DO/MHA, DO/MPH, DO/MS, DO/PhD. *Accreditation:* AOsA. *Faculty:* 93 full-time (37 women), 24 part-time/adjunct (8 women). *Students:* 536 full-time (268 women); includes 113 minority (46 Black or African American, non-Hispanic/Latino; 6 American Indian or Alaska Native, non-Hispanic/Latino; 40 Asian, non-Hispanic/Latino; 20 Hispanic/Latino; 1 Two or more races, non-Hispanic/Latino). Average age 26. 4,129 applicants, 4% accepted, 141 enrolled. In 2013, 111 doctorates awarded. *Degree requirements:* For doctorate, comprehensive exam, National Board Exam Parts I and II, COMLEX-PE. *Entrance requirements:* For doctorate, MCAT, interview; course work in English, physics, biology, general chemistry, organic chemistry, and behavioral sciences. *Application deadline:* For fall admission, 2/1 for domestic students. Applications are processed on a rolling basis. Application fee: $60. Electronic applications accepted. *Expenses:* Contact institution. *Financial support:* In 2013–14, 155 students received support, including 12 fellowships with full tuition reimbursements available (averaging $10,233 per year); Federal Work-Study, institutionally sponsored loans, scholarships/grants, and tuition waivers (partial) also available. Financial award applicants required to submit FAFSA. *Faculty research:* Diabetes, healthy aging, pain management, neuroscience, global health. *Total annual research expenditures:* $2.5 million. *Unit head:* Dr. Kenneth Johnson, Executive Dean, 740-593-9350, Fax: 740-593-0761, E-mail: wilcox@ohio.edu. *Application contact:* Jill Harman, Director of Admissions, 740-593-2147, Fax: 740-593-2256, E-mail: harmanj@ohio.edu.
Website: http://www.oucom.ohiou.edu/

Oklahoma State University Center for Health Sciences, College of Osteopathic Medicine, Tulsa, OK 74107. Offers DO, DO/MS, DO/PhD. *Accreditation:* AOsA. *Faculty:* 100 full-time (38 women), 659 part-time/adjunct (140 women). *Students:* 67 full-time (39 women), 627 part-time (134 women); includes 117 minority (20 Black or African American, non-Hispanic/Latino; 42 American Indian or Alaska Native, non-Hispanic/Latino; 37 Asian, non-Hispanic/Latino; 16 Hispanic/Latino; 2 Two or more races, non-Hispanic/Latino). Average age 27. 2,189 applicants, 6% accepted, 112 enrolled. In 2013, 87 doctorates awarded. *Entrance requirements:* For doctorate, MCAT (minimum score 21), interview, minimum 90 hours of college course work, minimum GPA of 3.0. *Application deadline:* For fall admission, 2/1 for domestic students. Applications are processed on a rolling basis. Application fee: $40. Electronic applications accepted. *Expenses:* Tuition, state resident: full-time $22,127; part-time $178 per credit hour. Tuition, nonresident: full-time $43,572; part-time $728 per credit hour. *Required fees:* $910.79; $200 per semester. *Financial support:* In 2013–14, 139 students received support. Federal Work-Study, institutionally sponsored loans, scholarships/grants, and tuition waivers available. Financial award application deadline: 4/1; financial award applicants required to submit FAFSA. *Faculty research:* Neuroscience, artificial vision, mechanisms of hormone action, vaccines and immunotherapy, pathogenic free-living amoebae. *Total annual research expenditures:* $1.7 million. *Unit head:* Dr. Kayse M. Shrum, Provost and Dean, Center for Health Sciences, 918-561-8201, Fax: 918-561-8413, E-mail: lana.rusch@okstate.edu. *Application contact:* Lindsey Kirkpatrick, Assistant Director of Admissions and Recruitment, 800-677-1972, Fax: 918-561-8243, E-mail: lindsey.kirkpatrick@okstate.edu.

Philadelphia College of Osteopathic Medicine, Graduate and Professional Programs, Doctor of Osteopathic Medicine Program (Philadelphia Campus), Philadelphia, PA 19131. Offers DO, DO/MA, DO/MBA, DO/MPH, DO/MS, DO/PhD. *Accreditation:* AOsA. *Faculty:* 77 full-time (38 women), 1,293 part-time/adjunct (257 women). *Students:* 1,086 full-time (542 women); includes 278 minority (67 Black or African American, non-Hispanic/Latino; 69 Asian, non-Hispanic/Latino; 18 Hispanic/Latino; 1 Native Hawaiian or other Pacific Islander, non-Hispanic/Latino; 123 Two or more races, non-Hispanic/Latino), 11 international. Average age 28. 7,700 applicants, 5% accepted, 270 enrolled. In 2013, 263 doctorates awarded. *Entrance requirements:* For doctorate, MCAT, minimum GPA of 3.2; premedical prerequisite coursework; biochemistry (recommended). Additional exam requirements/recommendations for international students: Required—TOEFL (minimum score 79 iBT). *Application deadline:* For fall admission, 2/1 for domestic students. Applications are processed on a rolling basis. Application fee: $50. Electronic applications accepted. *Financial support:* In 2013–14, 870 students received support, including 14 fellowships with partial tuition reimbursements available; Federal Work-Study, institutionally sponsored loans, and scholarships/grants also available. Financial award application deadline: 3/15; financial award applicants required to submit FAFSA. *Faculty research:* Neuroscience and neurodegenerative disorders, inflammation and allergic response to food allergens, cardiovascular function and disease, bone and joint disorders, cancer biology. *Total annual research expenditures:* $533,489. *Unit head:* Dr. Kenneth J. Veit, Dean, 215-871-6770, Fax: 215-871-6781, E-mail: kenv@pcom.edu. *Application contact:* Kari A. Shotwell, Director of Admissions, 215-871-6700, Fax: 215-871-6719, E-mail: karis@pcom.edu.
Website: http://www.pcom.edu

Rowan University, School of Osteopathic Medicine, Stratford, NJ 08084-1501. Offers DO, DO/MA, DO/MBA, DO/MPH, DO/MS, DO/PhD, JD/DO. *Accreditation:* AOsA. *Faculty:* 181 full-time (87 women), 44 part-time/adjunct (25 women). *Students:* 632 full-time (309 women), 2 part-time (0 women); includes 323 minority (50 Black or African American, non-Hispanic/Latino; 2 American Indian or Alaska Native, non-Hispanic/Latino; 229 Asian, non-Hispanic/Latino; 42 Hispanic/Latino). Average age 26. 4,714 applicants, 6% accepted, 162 enrolled. In 2013, 124 degrees awarded. *Median time to degree:* Of those who began their doctoral program in fall 2005, 97% received their degree in 8 years or less. *Degree requirements:* For doctorate, comprehensive exam. *Entrance requirements:* For doctorate, MCAT. *Application deadline:* For fall admission, 2/1 for domestic and international students. Applications are processed on a rolling basis. Application fee: $90. Electronic applications accepted. *Expenses:* Contact institution. *Financial support:* Federal Work-Study and scholarships/grants available. Financial award applicants required to submit FAFSA. *Unit head:* Dr. Thomas A. Cavalieri, Dean, 856-566-6996, Fax: 856-566-6865, E-mail: cavalita@umdnj.edu. *Application contact:* Paula Watkins, Director of Enrollment Management, 856-566-7050, Fax: 856-566-6895, E-mail: fennerpa@rowan.edu.
Website: http://www.rowan.edu/som/

Touro University, Graduate Programs, Vallejo, CA 94592. Offers education (MA); medical health sciences (MS); osteopathic medicine (DO); pharmacy (Pharm D); public health (MPH). *Accreditation:* AOsA; ARC-PA. Part-time and evening/weekend programs available. *Faculty:* 103 full-time (54 women), 57 part-time/adjunct (33 women). *Students:* 1,390 full-time (841 women), 27 part-time (20 women). *Degree requirements:* For master's, comprehensive exam, thesis; for doctorate, comprehensive exam. *Entrance requirements:* For doctorate, BS/BA. *Application deadline:* For fall admission, 3/15 for domestic students; for winter admission, 12/1 for domestic students. Applications are processed on a rolling basis. Application fee: $100. Electronic applications accepted. *Financial support:* Fellowships, research assistantships, teaching assistantships, Federal Work-Study, and scholarships/grants available. Support available to part-time students. Financial award applicants required to submit FAFSA. *Faculty research:* Cancer, heart disease. *Application contact:* Steve Davis, Director of Admissions, 707-638-5270, Fax: 707-638-5250, E-mail: steven.davis@tu.edu.

University of New England, College of Osteopathic Medicine, Program in Osteopathic Medicine, Biddeford, ME 04005-9526. Offers DO. *Faculty:* 38 full-time (18 women), 32 part-time/adjunct (14 women). *Students:* 523 full-time (298 women); includes 73 minority (4 Black or African American, non-Hispanic/Latino; 51 Asian, non-Hispanic/Latino; 3 Hispanic/Latino; 15 Two or more races, non-Hispanic/Latino), 16 international. Average age 27. 4,234 applicants, 8% accepted, 175 enrolled. In 2013, 118 doctorates awarded. *Degree requirements:* For doctorate, clinical clerkships. *Entrance requirements:* For doctorate, MCAT. *Application deadline:* For fall admission, 2/1 for domestic students. Applications are processed on a rolling basis. Electronic applications accepted. *Financial support:* Institutionally sponsored loans available. Financial award application deadline: 5/1; financial award applicants required to submit FAFSA. *Unit head:* Dr. Douglas L. Wood, Dean, College of Osteopathic Medicine, 207-602-2807, E-mail: deanunecom@une.edu. *Application contact:* Dr. Cynthia Forrest, Vice President for Student Affairs, 207-221-4225, Fax: 207-523-1925, E-mail: gradadmissions@une.edu. Website: http://www.une.edu/com

University of North Texas Health Science Center at Fort Worth, Texas College of Osteopathic Medicine, Fort Worth, TX 76107-2699. Offers osteopathic medicine (DO); physician assistant studies (MPAS); DO/MPH; DO/MS; DO/PhD; MPAS/MPH. DO/MPH offered jointly with University of North Texas. *Accreditation:* AOsA. *Entrance requirements:* For doctorate, MCAT, 1 year course work in each biology, physics and English; 2 years course work in chemistry. Electronic applications accepted. *Faculty research:* Tuberculosis, aging, cardiovascular disease, cancer.

University of Pikeville, Kentucky College of Osteopathic Medicine, Pikeville, KY 41501. Offers DO. *Accreditation:* AOsA. *Faculty:* 19 full-time (6 women), 45 part-time/adjunct (25 women). *Students:* 430 full-time (205 women); includes 39 minority (7 Black or African American, non-Hispanic/Latino; 5 American Indian or Alaska Native, non-Hispanic/Latino; 14 Asian, non-Hispanic/Latino; 7 Hispanic/Latino; 6 Native Hawaiian or other Pacific Islander, non-Hispanic/Latino). Average age 26. 3,121 applicants, 9% accepted, 134 enrolled. In 2013, 78 doctorates awarded. *Degree requirements:* For doctorate, COMLEX Level 1 and COMLEX Level 2CE and 2PE. *Entrance requirements:* For doctorate, MCAT. *Application deadline:* For fall admission, 5/1 for domestic students. Applications are processed on a rolling basis. Application fee: $75. *Expenses: Tuition:* Full-time $4740; part-time $395 per credit hour. *Financial support:* In 2013–14, 3 students received support, including 3 fellowships with full tuition reimbursements available (averaging $38,950 per year); scholarships/grants also available. Financial award application deadline: 8/1; financial award applicants required to submit FAFSA. *Faculty research:* Primary care in medically underserved areas. *Unit head:* Dr. Boyd Buser, Dean, 606-218-5410, Fax: 606-218-8442, E-mail: boydbuser@upike.edu. *Application contact:* Dr. Linda Dunatov, Associate Dean for Student Affairs, 606-218-5408, Fax: 606-218-5442, E-mail: lindadunatov@upike.edu.
Website: http://www.upike.edu/College-of-Osteopathic-Medicine

Western University of Health Sciences, College of Osteopathic Medicine of the Pacific, Pomona, CA 91766-1854. Offers DO. *Accreditation:* AOsA. *Faculty:* 65 full-time (23 women), 25 part-time/adjunct (10 women). *Students:* 1,215 full-time (563 women); includes 524 minority (12 Black or African American, non-Hispanic/Latino; 2 American Indian or Alaska Native, non-Hispanic/Latino; 390 Asian, non-Hispanic/Latino; 52 Hispanic/Latino; 2 Native Hawaiian or other Pacific Islander, non-Hispanic/Latino; 66 Two or more races, non-Hispanic/Latino), 19 international. Average age 27. 3,521 applicants, 18% accepted, 332 enrolled. In 2013, 215 doctorates awarded. *Entrance requirements:* For doctorate, MCAT, minimum GPA of 3.3, interview, letters of recommendation. *Application deadline:* For fall admission, 3/1 for domestic students. Application fee: $65. Electronic applications accepted. *Financial support:* Fellowships, research assistantships, teaching assistantships, institutionally sponsored loans, scholarships/grants, tuition waivers (full), unspecified assistantships, and veterans educational benefits available. Financial award application deadline: 3/2; financial award applicants required to submit FAFSA. *Unit head:* Dr. Paula Crone, Dean, 541-259-0206, Fax: 541-259-0201, E-mail: pcrone@westernu.edu. *Application contact:* Susan Hanson, Director of Admissions, 909-469-5335, Fax: 909-469-5570, E-mail: admissions@westernu.edu.
Website: http://www.westernu.edu/osteopathy/

West Virginia School of Osteopathic Medicine, Professional Program, Lewisburg, WV 24901-1196. Offers DO. *Accreditation:* AOsA. *Degree requirements:* For doctorate, comprehensive exam, Comlex Level 1 and 2 (PE and CE). *Entrance requirements:* For doctorate, MCAT, 3 hours of English; 8 hours each of biology, physics, inorganic chemistry, and organic chemistry. Electronic applications accepted. *Faculty research:* OMT response bio-markers, linking muscle energy use to power production in primates.

Podiatric Medicine

Barry University, School of Podiatric Medicine, Podiatric Medicine and Surgery Program, Miami Shores, FL 33161-6695. Offers DPM, DPM/MBA, DPM/MPH. *Accreditation:* APMA. *Entrance requirements:* For doctorate, MCAT, GRE General Test, previous course work in science and English. Additional exam requirements/recommendations for international students: Required—TOEFL. Electronic applications accepted. *Expenses:* Contact institution.

California School of Podiatric Medicine at Samuel Merritt University, Professional Program, Oakland, CA 94609. Offers DPM. *Accreditation:* APMA. *Entrance requirements:* For doctorate, MCAT (less than 3 years old), at least 90 semester hours of undergraduate course work; 1 year of course work in organic chemistry or biochemistry, inorganic chemistry, physics, biological sciences (all courses must come with a lab), and English/communications. *Expenses:* Contact institution. *Faculty research:* Glycation in diabetes and protein dysfunction, lower extremity biomechanics, diabetic wound care, plantar warts among HIV-infected patients, interdisciplinary equity and inclusion issues.

Des Moines University, College of Podiatric Medicine and Surgery, Des Moines, IA 50312-4104. Offers DPM. *Accreditation:* APMA. *Entrance requirements:* For doctorate, MCAT, interview; minimum GPA of 2.5; 1 year of organic chemistry, inorganic chemistry, physics, biology, and English. Electronic applications accepted. *Expenses:* Contact institution. *Faculty research:* Physics of equines, gait analysis.

Kent State University, College of Podiatric Medicine, Kent, OH 44242-0001. Offers DPM. *Accreditation:* APMA. *Degree requirements:* For doctorate, comprehensive exam, clinical competencies; NBPME Boards 1 & 2. *Entrance requirements:* For doctorate, MCAT, satisfactory course work in biology, chemistry, English and physics; background check, drug test. Additional exam requirements/recommendations for international students: Recommended—TOEFL (minimum score 81 iBT). Electronic applications accepted. *Faculty research:* Diabetic foot ulcers, plantar shear stresses, nonvisual foot examinations, treatment modalities for onychomycosis.

Midwestern University, Glendale Campus, College of Health Sciences, Arizona Campus, Program in Podiatric Medicine, Glendale, AZ 85308. Offers DPM. *Accreditation:* APMA. *Entrance requirements:* For doctorate, MCAT or PCAT, 90 semester hours at an accredited college or university, minimum GPA of 2.75. *Expenses:* Contact institution.

New York College of Podiatric Medicine, Professional Program, New York, NY 10035. Offers DPM, DPM/MPH. *Accreditation:* APMA. *Degree requirements:* For doctorate, comprehensive exam. *Entrance requirements:* For doctorate, MCAT or DAT, 1 year course work in biology, physics, English, and general and organic chemistry. Additional exam requirements/recommendations for international students: Required—TOEFL.

Rosalind Franklin University of Medicine and Science, The Dr. William M. Scholl College of Podiatric Medicine, North Chicago, IL 60064-3095. Offers DPM. *Accreditation:* APMA. *Entrance requirements:* For doctorate, MCAT (or GRE on approval), 12 semester hours of biology; 8 semester hours of inorganic chemistry, organic chemistry and physics; 6 semester hours of English. Additional exam requirements/recommendations for international students: Required—TOEFL.

Temple University, School of Podiatric Medicine, Philadelphia, PA 19107-2496. Offers DPM, DPM/MBA, DPM/PhD. DPM/PhD offered jointly with Drexel University, University of Pennsylvania. *Accreditation:* APMA. *Degree requirements:* For doctorate, National Board Exam. *Entrance requirements:* For doctorate, MCAT, GRE, or DAT, interview, 8 hours of organic chemistry, inorganic chemistry, physics, biology. *Faculty research:* Gait analysis, infectious diseases, diabetic neuropathy, peripheral vascular disease.

THE CANADIAN COLLEGE OF NATUROPATHIC MEDICINE

Bachelor of Naturopathy Program

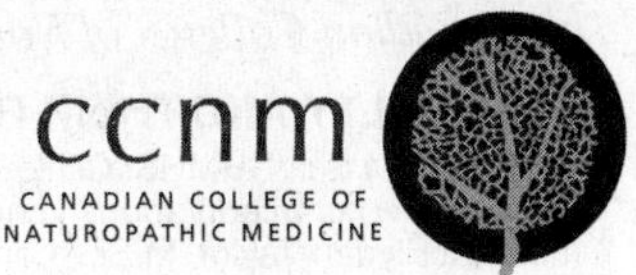

Programs of Study

The Canadian College of Naturopathic Medicine (CCNM) is Canada's premier institute for education and research in naturopathic medicine. CCNM offers a rigorous four-year, full-time bachelor of naturopathy program. The program involves more than 4,200 hours of classroom and clinical instruction, including a twelve-month supervised internship.

As of May 2014, the CCNM naturopathic program became the first such program in Canada to be able to award degrees to graduates. The consent provided by the Ontario Minister of Training, Colleges, and Universities is the result of an extensive process involving three reviews of CCNM's program and its operations. Ontario's Post-Secondary Quality Assessment Board (PEQAB) recommended approval to the Minister based upon its assessment of the level of the program and the quality and security of the operations of the College.

In addition, the naturopathic medicine program at CCNM is accredited by the Council on Naturopathic Medical Education (CNME). CNME accreditation enables CCNM students to write the Naturopathic Physicians Licensing Examinations (NPLEX), offered by the North American Board of Naturopathic Examiners (NABNE). Passage of the NPLEX is required for licensure in most regulated jurisdictions in North America.

The curriculum involves three major areas of study: basic sciences, clinical sciences, and naturopathic disciplines. Students take courses in the basic sciences of anatomy, histopathology, physiology, biochemistry, microbiology, and immunology. Development of problem-solving skills in applied basic life sciences is achieved through lectures, case discussion, tutorial groups, and clinical simulations. Laboratory resources include diagnostic test kits and access to human cadavers for gross anatomy study. Clinical science disciplines include physical and clinical diagnosis, differential and laboratory diagnosis, advanced imaging, physical assessment, health psychology, primary care, and pathology. The principles and philosophy of naturopathic medicine form the bridgework between the academic and clinical parts of the curriculum. Six major disciplines define the areas of naturopathic practice: acupuncture/traditional Chinese medicine (TCM), botanical medicine, physical medicine (massage, hydrotherapy, etc.), clinical nutrition, homeopathic medicine, and lifestyle counseling.

Research Facilities

CCNM has collaborated with many major medical research institutions, including McMaster University, University of Oxford, the Hospital for Sick Children, the University of Toronto, the Ottawa Regional Cancer Centre, the Ottawa General Hospital, the Centre for Addiction and Mental Health, the Mayo Clinic, and the Johns Hopkins University, to advance the state of knowledge in naturopathic medicine. Researchers from CCNM have published numerous systematic reviews and research articles on naturopathic therapies in a wide variety of peer-reviewed journals, including *BMJ, JAMA, Lancet Oncology, the Archives of Internal Medicine,* and *PloS One.*

CCNM's Ottawa Integrative Cancer Centre (OICC), which opened in 2011, is a model multidisciplinary flagship centre providing whole-person integrative care to people with cancer, cancer survivors, and those seeking both primary and secondary cancer prevention. The OICC is the first integrative oncology and research centre in Eastern Canada to provide care, advocacy, and education for the use of whole-person care to the cancer community and health-care practitioners, regionally and nationally.

Research department faculty members educate students in their first years in epidemiology, encouraging them to investigate evidence-based medicine throughout their years at the college and to consider a research project of their own. This commitment to evidence-based medicine cultivates research initiatives within the CCNM community, including student and faculty initiatives, through teaching, experiential learning, and mentorship. By fostering this culture of research, CCNM has become a leader in naturopathic and complementary medicine worldwide, investigating topics that not only improve naturopathic treatment practices but also have widespread relevance and international impact.

Financial Aid

Canadian students enrolled in the bachelor of naturopathy program may be eligible for federal and provincial financial assistance. For more information, students can contact their provincial loan office or Student Services.

American students attending CCNM may be eligible for U.S.-based financial assistance such as unsubsidized Direct Loans.

Students may also be eligible for scholarships and bursaries and should contact Student Services for more information.

Bank loans through major Canadian Banks are another possibility. As policies at financial institutions are subject to change, students should contact their institution of choice to confirm details).

Cost of Study

In-state and out-of-state tuition for the 2014–15 academic year is Can$21,010; international tuition is Can$21,990. Books, materials, and miscellaneous expenses cost approximately Can$1,500–$3,000.

Living and Housing Costs

On-campus residence is $495 per month.

Student Group

Currently, nearly 600 students are enrolled at CCNM. Students come from every province in Canada; with significant numbers from the United States and abroad. The ratio of women to men at CCNM is approximately 4:1. Student ages range from 20 to 50 years and older.

Student Outcomes

Naturopathic Doctors (N.D.'s) are trained as primary-care providers. They learn to treat all aspects of family health and wellness, from pediatrics to geriatrics. Their scope of practice may include everything from nutrition and botanical medicine to clinical diagnosis and pharmacology. Other possible career options include education; public health; research; and serving as consultants to insurance companies, public service, political, and other organizations.

Location

CCNM's 4.43-acre, 176,000-square-foot campus is conveniently located in Toronto's North York region at the Leslie subway station. It is also close to major highways. Toronto is Canada's largest city, with a population of 4.4 million. Toronto is well maintained, with excellent public transportation and comparatively low living costs. Rated the safest large North American city, Toronto is a welcoming multicultural mosaic. Toronto offers students a wealth of entertainment, leisure, and cultural activities. Whether tastes lead to exotic cuisines, multicultural festivals, sports events, or the theatre district, there is always something to capture interest in Toronto.

The College

The Canadian College of Naturopathic Medicine (CCNM) is Canada's premier institute for education and research in naturopathic medicine. CCNM offers a rigorous four-year, full-time naturopathic medicine program.

CCNM is also home to the Robert Schad Naturopathic Clinic, a dynamic naturopathic teaching clinic where senior clinicians and N.D. supervisors conduct more than 26,000 patient visits per year.

Applying

CCNM is committed to excellence in naturopathic education and to the success of its graduates. All candidates for admission are evaluated based on their academic history and personal interview, as well as their motivation for becoming a naturopathic doctor, leadership skills, problem-solving and critical-thinking skills, and specific personal qualities and characteristics. The admission decision is based primarily on the applicant's undergraduate grade point average, but additional criteria may include the applicant's academic history, essay, references, autobiographical sketch, and interview. Historically, the average cumulative GPA of accepted students has been 3.3 on a 4.0 scale, encompassing a range of 2.7 to 4.0.

Applicants must have completed a baccalaureate degree. Prerequisite courses include biology, organic chemistry, psychology, physiology, and humanities, as well as recommended courses in anatomy, environmental science, microbiology, physics, sociology, and statistics.

Correspondence and Information

Student Services
The Canadian College of Naturopathic Medicine
1255 Sheppard Avenue East
Toronto, Ontario M2K 1E2
Canada
Phone: 416-498-1255 Ext. 245
866-241-2266 Ext. 245 (toll-free)
E-mail: info@ccnm.edu.
Website: http://www.ccnm.edu

THE FACULTY AND THEIR RESEARCH

Nadia Bakir, M.Sc., DHMHS; Clinic supervisor, Associate Professor. http://www.ccnm.edu/about_ccnm/faculty_profiles/nadia_bakir

Kimberlee Blyden-Taylor, M.Sc.; Clinic supervisor, Associate Professor. http://www.ccnm.edu/about_ccnm/faculty_profiles/kimberlee_blyden_taylor

Kieran Cooley, M.Sc.; Associate Director, Research, Assistant Professor. http://www.ccnm.edu/about_ccnm/faculty_profiles/kieran_cooley

Ian Fraser, Ph.D.; Instructor. http://www.ccnm.edu/about_ccnm/faculty_profiles/ian_fraser

Neemez Kassam, M.Sc.; Instructor. http://www.ccnm.edu/about_ccnm/faculty_profiles/neemez_kassam_0

Daniel Lander, N.D., FABNO; Clinic supervisor, Assistant Professor. http://www.ccnm.edu/about_ccnm/faculty_profiles/daniel_lander

Jonathan E. Prousky, M.Sc.; Chief Naturopathic Medical Officer, Professor. http://www.ccnm.edu/about_ccnm/faculty_profiles/jonathan_e_prousky

Paul Saunders, Ph.D.; Instructor. http://www.ccnm.edu/about_ccnm/faculty_profiles/paul_saunders

Ljubisa Terzic, M.D.; Associate Professor. http://www.ccnm.edu/about_ccnm/faculty_profiles/ljubisa_terzic

Jonathan Wilde, M.B.A.; Director, Institutional Advancement, Assistant Professor. http://www.ccnm.edu/about_ccnm/faculty_profiles/jonathan_wilde

PRIMARY RESEARCH PROJECTS

Primary Research—Clinical Trials:

Randomized clinical trial to assess the effect of melatonin on lung cancer recurrence and mortality (AMPLCaRe). A large five-year multicentred trial that is being conducted in partnership with the Canadian Association of Thoracic Surgeons.

Pragmatic randomized clinical trial of naturopathic medicine's ability to treat and prevent cardiovascular disease. A multicentre study supported by a joint project from the Canada Post Corporation and the Canadian Union of Postal Workers.

Pilot study to assess the safety and effectiveness of a compound natural health product in children with attention deficit hyperactivity disorder. A randomized trial to explore nutritional deficiencies associated with ADHD. This trial will also test a compound NHP for treatment in this population.

Randomized clinical trial to test the efficacy of cinnamon as an aid in diabetes to reduce blood sugar levels.

Pilot study to explore the effect of three common homeopathic remedies on chronic whiplash. A small-scale pilot study supported by the Homeonet Research Network of Canada, slated to be completed in 2014.

Pilot study to test the effect of using classical homeopathy on insufficient lactation. A small-scale pilot study supported by the Homeonet Research Network of Canada.

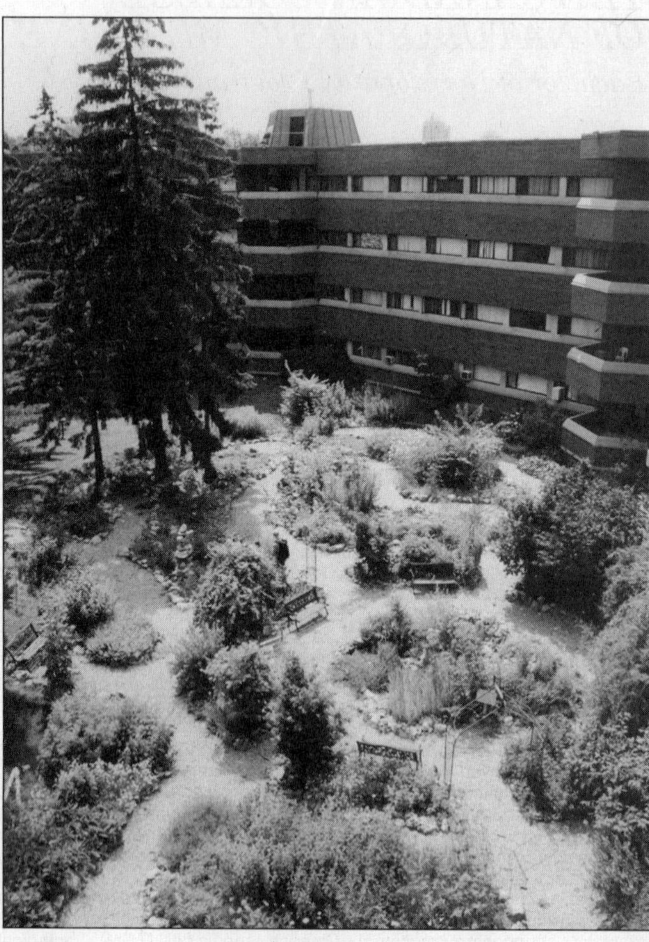

Section 29
Optometry and Vision Sciences

This section contains a directory of institutions offering graduate work in optometry and vision sciences. Additional information about programs listed in the directory may be obtained by writing directly to the dean of a graduate school or chair of a department at the address given in the directory.

In the other guides in this series:

Graduate Programs in the Humanities, Arts & Social Sciences
See *Psychology and Counseling*

Graduate Programs in the Physical Sciences, Mathematics, Agricultural Sciences, the Environment & Natural Resources
See *Physics*

Graduate Programs in Engineering & Applied Sciences
See *Biomedical Engineering* and *Biotechnology*

CONTENTS

Program Directories

Optometry

Ferris State University, Michigan College of Optometry, Big Rapids, MI 49307. Offers OD. *Accreditation:* AOA. *Faculty:* 18 full-time (5 women), 98 part-time/adjunct (34 women). *Students:* 150 full-time (89 women); includes 18 minority (1 Black or African American, non-Hispanic/Latino; 3 Asian, non-Hispanic/Latino; 9 Hispanic/Latino; 5 Two or more races, non-Hispanic/Latino), 5 international. Average age 24. 319 applicants, 17% accepted, 34 enrolled. In 2013, 33 doctorates awarded. *Degree requirements:* For doctorate, comprehensive exam, research project. *Entrance requirements:* For doctorate, OAT. Additional exam requirements/recommendations for international students: Required—TOEFL (minimum score 500 paper-based; 61 iBT). *Application deadline:* For fall admission, 2/15 for domestic and international students. Applications are processed on a rolling basis. Application fee: $150. Electronic applications accepted. *Expenses:* Contact institution. *Financial support:* In 2013–14, 77 students received support. Career-related internships or fieldwork, Federal Work-Study, and scholarships/grants available. Financial award application deadline: 3/15; financial award applicants required to submit FAFSA. *Faculty research:* Corneal reshaping, spatial vision and vision science, reading disabilities, vision development, vision care access. *Unit head:* Dr. David Damari, Dean, 231-591-3706, Fax: 231-591-2394, E-mail: damarid@ferris.edu. *Application contact:* Colleen Olson, Assistant to the Associate Dean, 231-591-3703, Fax: 231-591-2394, E-mail: olsonc@ferris.edu.
Website: http://www.ferris.edu/mco/

Illinois College of Optometry, Professional Program, Chicago, IL 60616-3878. Offers OD. *Accreditation:* AOA. *Entrance requirements:* For doctorate, OAT. Electronic applications accepted. *Faculty research:* Eye disease treatment, binocular vision, cataract development, pediatric vision, genetic eye disease.

Indiana University Bloomington, School of Optometry, Bloomington, IN 47405-3680. Offers MS, OD, PhD. *Accreditation:* AOA (one or more programs are accredited). *Faculty:* 36 full-time (11 women), 7 part-time/adjunct (5 women). *Students:* 327 full-time (189 women), 5 part-time (1 woman); includes 36 minority (7 Black or African American, non-Hispanic/Latino; 1 American Indian or Alaska Native, non-Hispanic/Latino; 16 Asian, non-Hispanic/Latino; 6 Hispanic/Latino; 6 Two or more races, non-Hispanic/Latino), 32 international. Average age 25. 348 applicants, 44% accepted, 92 enrolled. In 2013, 10 master's, 73 doctorates awarded. Terminal master's awarded for partial completion of doctoral program. *Degree requirements:* For master's, thesis; for doctorate, comprehensive exam, thesis/dissertation. *Entrance requirements:* For master's, GRE, BA in science; for doctorate, GRE; OAT (for OD), BA in science (master's degree preferred). Additional exam requirements/recommendations for international students: Required—TOEFL (minimum score 550 paper-based; 80 iBT). *Application deadline:* For fall admission, 1/15 for domestic students; for winter admission, 2/1 for domestic and international students; for spring admission, 9/1 for domestic students. Applications are processed on a rolling basis. Application fee: $55 ($65 for international students). Electronic applications accepted. *Expenses:* Contact institution. *Financial support:* Fellowships with full tuition reimbursements, research assistantships with full tuition reimbursements, Federal Work-Study, institutionally sponsored loans, scholarships/grants, and health care benefits available. Support available to part-time students. Financial award application deadline: 12/1; financial award applicants required to submit FAFSA. *Faculty research:* Corneal physiology, contact lenses, adaptive optics, dry eye, low vision, refractive anomalies, ophthalmic imaging, glaucoma, ocular physiology, infant vision, retinal disease. *Total annual research expenditures:* $5.6 million. *Unit head:* Dr. Joseph Bonanno, Dean, E-mail: jbonanno@indiana.edu. *Application contact:* Josie Gingrich, Associate Director of Financial Aids and Records, 812-856-4247, Fax: 812-855-4389, E-mail: jmgingri@indiana.edu.
Website: http://www.opt.indiana.edu/

Inter American University of Puerto Rico School of Optometry, Professional Program, Bayamn, PR 00957. Offers OD. *Accreditation:* AOA. *Degree requirements:* For doctorate, thesis/dissertation, research project. *Entrance requirements:* For doctorate, OAT, interview, minimum GPA of 2.5, 2 letters of recommendation. Electronic applications accepted. *Expenses:* Contact institution. *Faculty research:* Visual characteristics of special populations, contact lenses, refraction and diabetes.

Marshall B. Ketchum University, Graduate and Professional Programs, Fullerton, CA 92831-1615. Offers optometry (OD); vision science (MS). *Accreditation:* AOA. *Degree requirements:* For doctorate, thesis/dissertation. *Entrance requirements:* For doctorate, OAT. Electronic applications accepted. *Faculty research:* Structure and function of the human visual system.

Midwestern University, Glendale Campus, Arizona College of Optometry, Glendale, AZ 85308. Offers OD. *Accreditation:* AOA. *Entrance requirements:* For doctorate, OAT, bachelor's degree, minimum overall cumulative and science GPA of 2.75, 2 letters of recommendation.

The New England College of Optometry, Graduate and Professional Programs, Boston, MA 02115-1100. Offers optometry (OD); vision science (MS). *Accreditation:* AOA. *Entrance requirements:* For doctorate, OAT. Electronic applications accepted.

Northeastern State University, College of Optometry, Tahlequah, OK 74464. Offers OD. Applicants must be a resident of Oklahoma, Arkansas, Kansas, Colorado, New Mexico, Missouri, Texas, or Nebraska. *Accreditation:* AOA. *Faculty:* 16 full-time (6 women), 1 part-time/adjunct (0 women). *Students:* 111 full-time (62 women); includes 33 minority (1 Black or African American, non-Hispanic/Latino; 11 American Indian or Alaska Native, non-Hispanic/Latino; 8 Asian, non-Hispanic/Latino; 6 Hispanic/Latino; 7 Two or more races, non-Hispanic/Latino). Average age 26. In 2013, 28 doctorates awarded. *Degree requirements:* For doctorate, research project. *Entrance requirements:* For doctorate, OAT. *Application deadline:* For fall admission, 2/1 for domestic students. Applications are processed on a rolling basis. Application fee: $45. Electronic applications accepted. *Expenses:* Contact institution. *Financial support:* Federal Work-Study, institutionally sponsored loans, scholarships/grants, tuition waivers (partial), and residencies available. Financial award application deadline: 5/1; financial award applicants required to submit FAFSA. *Unit head:* Dr. Douglas Penisten, Dean of Oklahoma College of Optometry, 918-444-4025, E-mail: penisten@nsuok.edu. *Application contact:* Natalie Batt, Student and Alumni Affairs, 918-456-5511 Ext. 4036, Fax: 918-458-2104, E-mail: batt@nsuok.edu.
Website: http://optometry.nsuok.edu

Nova Southeastern University, College of Optometry, Fort Lauderdale, FL 33328. Offers clinical vision research (MS); optometry (OD). *Accreditation:* AOA. Postbaccalaureate distance learning degree programs offered (no on-campus study). *Students:* 425 full-time (280 women), 5 part-time (4 women); includes 190 minority (29 Black or African American, non-Hispanic/Latino; 1 American Indian or Alaska Native, non-Hispanic/Latino; 92 Asian, non-Hispanic/Latino; 56 Hispanic/Latino; 12 Two or more races, non-Hispanic/Latino), 41 international. Average age 26. In 2013, 1 master's, 97 doctorates awarded. *Degree requirements:* For master's, comprehensive exam (for some programs), thesis; for doctorate, comprehensive exam. *Entrance requirements:* For master's, OAT or GRE, BA; for doctorate, OAT, minimum GPA of 3.0. Additional exam requirements/recommendations for international students: Required—TOEFL (minimum score 79 iBT). *Application deadline:* For fall admission, 4/1 for domestic and international students. Applications are processed on a rolling basis. Application fee: $50. Electronic applications accepted. *Expenses:* Contact institution. *Financial support:* Federal Work-Study, institutionally sponsored loans, and scholarships/grants available. Support available to part-time students. Financial award applicants required to submit FAFSA. *Faculty research:* Retinal disease, low vision, binocular vision, contact lenses, accommodation. *Unit head:* Dr. David Loshin, Dean, 954-262-1404, Fax: 954-262-1818. *Application contact:* Juan Saavedra, Admissions Counselor, 954-262-1132, Fax: 954-262-2282, E-mail: jsaavedra@nova.edu.
Website: http://optometry.nova.edu/

The Ohio State University, College of Optometry, Columbus, OH 43210. Offers optometry (OD); vision science (MS, PhD); OD/MS. *Accreditation:* AOA (one or more programs are accredited). *Faculty:* 32. *Students:* 257 full-time (161 women), 4 part-time (2 women); includes 38 minority (3 Black or African American, non-Hispanic/Latino; 24 Asian, non-Hispanic/Latino; 9 Hispanic/Latino; 2 Two or more races, non-Hispanic/Latino), 2 international. Average age 25. In 2013, 5 master's, 59 doctorates awarded. *Degree requirements:* For master's, thesis; for doctorate, thesis/dissertation. *Entrance requirements:* For master's, GRE; for doctorate, GRE (for PhD); OAT (for OD). Additional exam requirements/recommendations for international students: Required—TOEFL (minimum score 550 paper-based, 79 iBT), Michigan English Language Assessment Battery (minimum score 82), IELTS (minimum score 7) for MS and PhD; TOEFL (minimum score 577 paper-based; 90 iBT), Michigan English Language Assessment Battery (minimum score 84), IELTS (minimum score 7.5) for OD. *Application deadline:* For fall admission, 3/31 for domestic and international students; for spring admission, 12/1 for domestic students, 11/1 for international students. Applications are processed on a rolling basis. Application fee: $60 ($70 for international students). Electronic applications accepted. *Expenses:* Contact institution. *Financial support:* Research assistantships with full tuition reimbursements, teaching assistantships with full tuition reimbursements, Federal Work-Study, institutionally sponsored loans, and scholarships/grants available. Financial award application deadline: 2/1; financial award applicants required to submit FAFSA. *Unit head:* Dr. Karla Zadnik, Dean, 614-292-6603, E-mail: zadnik.4@osu.edu. *Application contact:* Graduate Admissions, 614-292-9444, Fax: 614-292-3895, E-mail: gradadmissions@osu.edu.
Website: http://www.optometry.osu.edu/

Salus University, College of Optometry, Elkins Park, PA 19027-1598. Offers OD, OD/MS. *Accreditation:* AOA. *Degree requirements:* For doctorate, comprehensive exam (for some programs). *Entrance requirements:* For doctorate, OAT, interview. Additional exam requirements/recommendations for international students: Required—TOEFL. Electronic applications accepted. *Faculty research:* Vision research, visual perception, ocular motility, electrodiagnosis, photobiology glaucoma, myopia, keratoconus.

Southern College of Optometry, Professional Program, Memphis, TN 38104-2222. Offers OD. *Accreditation:* AOA. *Degree requirements:* For doctorate, clinical experience. *Entrance requirements:* For doctorate, OAT, 3 years of undergraduate pre-optometry course work.

State University of New York College of Optometry, Professional Program, New York, NY 10036. Offers OD, OD/MS, OD/PhD. *Accreditation:* AOA. *Entrance requirements:* For doctorate, OAT. Additional exam requirements/recommendations for international students: Required—TOEFL (minimum score 550 paper-based; 80 iBT). Electronic applications accepted. *Faculty research:* Optometry, vision research.

Université de Montréal, School of Optometry, Professional Program in Optometry, Montréal, QC H3C 3J7, Canada. Offers OD. Open only to Canadian residents. *Accreditation:* AOA. *Degree requirements:* For doctorate, thesis/dissertation. Electronic applications accepted.

The University of Alabama at Birmingham, School of Optometry, Professional Program in Optometry, Birmingham, AL 35294. Offers OD. *Entrance requirements:* For doctorate, OAT, composite evaluation or letters or recommendation, interview. Additional exam requirements/recommendations for international students: Required—TOEFL.

University of California, Berkeley, School of Optometry, Berkeley, CA 94720-1500. Offers OD, Certificate. *Accreditation:* AOA. *Entrance requirements:* For doctorate, OAT. Additional exam requirements/recommendations for international students: Required—TOEFL (minimum score 570 paper-based). Electronic applications accepted. *Faculty research:* Low vision, spatial vision, psychophysics of vision, clinical optics, patient care.

University of Houston, College of Optometry, Professional Program in Optometry, Houston, TX 77204. Offers OD. *Accreditation:* AOA. *Faculty research:* Refractive error development, corneal physiology, low vision, binocular vision.

The University of Manchester, Faculty of Life Sciences, Manchester, United Kingdom. Offers adaptive organismal biology (M Phil, PhD); animal biology (M Phil, PhD); biochemistry (M Phil, PhD); bioinformatics (M Phil, PhD); biomolecular sciences (M Phil, PhD); biotechnology (M Phil, PhD); cell biology (M Phil, PhD); cell matrix research (M Phil, PhD); channels and transporters (M Phil, PhD); developmental biology (M Phil, PhD); Egyptology (M Phil, PhD); environmental biology (M Phil, PhD); evolutionary biology (M Phil, PhD); gene expression (M Phil, PhD); genetics (M Phil, PhD); history of science, technology and medicine (M Phil, PhD); immunology (M Phil, PhD); integrative neurobiology and behavior (M Phil, PhD); membrane trafficking (M Phil, PhD); microbiology (M Phil, PhD); molecular and cellular neuroscience (M Phil, PhD); molecular biology (M Phil, PhD); molecular cancer studies (M Phil, PhD); neuroscience (M Phil, PhD); ophthalmology (M Phil, PhD); optometry (M Phil, PhD); organelle function (M Phil, PhD); pharmacology (M Phil, PhD); physiology (M Phil, PhD); plant sciences (M Phil, PhD); stem cell research (M Phil, PhD); structural biology (M Phil, PhD); systems neuroscience (M Phil, PhD); toxicology (M Phil, PhD).

University of Missouri–St. Louis, College of Optometry, Professional Program in Optometry, St. Louis, MO 63121. Offers OD. *Accreditation:* AOA. *Faculty:* 23 full-time (6 women), 14 part-time/adjunct (4 women). *Students:* 172 full-time (113 women); includes 20 minority (3 Black or African American, non-Hispanic/Latino; 1 American Indian or Alaska Native, non-Hispanic/Latino; 12 Asian, non-Hispanic/Latino; 4 Hispanic/Latino). Average age 23. 402 applicants, 32% accepted, 46 enrolled. In 2013, 38 doctorates awarded. *Entrance requirements:* For doctorate, OAT, 90 hours of undergraduate course work. *Application deadline:* For fall admission, 2/15 for domestic and international students. Applications are processed on a rolling basis. Application fee: $50. Electronic applications accepted. *Expenses:* Tuition, state resident: full-time

$7364; part-time $409.10 per credit hour. Tuition, nonresident: full-time $19,162; part-time $1008.50 per credit hour. *Financial support:* In 2013–14, 140 students received support, including 3 research assistantships (averaging $500 per year), 3 teaching assistantships (averaging $500 per year); Federal Work-Study, institutionally sponsored loans, and scholarships/grants also available. Financial award application deadline: 2/15; financial award applicants required to submit FAFSA. *Faculty research:* Visual psychophysics and perception, noninvasive assessment of visual processing, aging and Alzheimer's disease, orthokeratology. *Unit head:* Dr. Edward S. Bennett, Director, Student Services, 314-516-6263, Fax: 314-516-6708, E-mail: optstuaff@umsl.edu. *Application contact:* Linda Stein, Administrative Assistant, 314-516-5905, Fax: 314-516-6708, E-mail: steinli@umsl.edu.
Website: http://www.umsl.edu/divisions/optometry/Academic%20Programs/opt_curric.html

University of the Incarnate Word, School of Optometry, San Antonio, TX 78209-6397. Offers OD. *Accreditation:* AOA. *Faculty:* 20 full-time (8 women), 7 part-time/adjunct (2 women). *Students:* 254 full-time (150 women); includes 128 minority (7 Black or African American, non-Hispanic/Latino; 1 American Indian or Alaska Native, non-Hispanic/Latino; 97 Asian, non-Hispanic/Latino; 21 Hispanic/Latino; 1 Native Hawaiian or other Pacific Islander, non-Hispanic/Latino; 1 Two or more races, non-Hispanic/Latino), 15 international. Average age 26. 108 applicants, 97% accepted, 105 enrolled. *Degree requirements:* For doctorate, clinical contact hours. *Entrance requirements:* For doctorate, OAT, 90 credit hours of prerequisite course work; letters of recommendation; interview. Additional exam requirements/recommendations for international students: Required—TOEFL (minimum score 560 paper-based; 83 iBT). *Application deadline:* For fall admission, 5/15 for domestic students. Application fee: $50. Electronic applications accepted. *Expenses:* Contact institution. *Financial support:* In 2013–14, 5 fellowships (averaging $4,000 per year) were awarded; Federal Work-Study and scholarships/grants also available. Financial award applicants required to submit FAFSA. *Faculty research:* Computer-based color vision, contrast sensitivity, and Amsler grid testing; response time in color deficiency; binocular enhancement of color vision; interactive instructional tools for teaching gross anatomy. *Total annual research expenditures:* $130,000. *Unit head:* Dr. Andrew Buzzelli, Founding Dean, 210-883-1195, Fax: 210-283-6890, E-mail: buzzelli@uiwtx.edu. *Application contact:* Kristine Benne, Director of Admissions and Student Services, School of Optometry, 210-883-1190, Fax: 210-883-1191, E-mail: optometry@uiwtx.edu.
Website: http://optometry.uiw.edu/

University of Waterloo, Graduate Studies, Faculty of Science, School of Optometry, Waterloo, ON N2L 3G1, Canada. Offers optometry (OD); vision science (M Sc, PhD). *Accreditation:* AOA. Part-time programs available. *Degree requirements:* For master's, thesis; for doctorate, thesis/dissertation. *Entrance requirements:* For master's, honors degree, minimum B average; for doctorate, master's degree, minimum B average. Additional exam requirements/recommendations for international students: Required—TOEFL (minimum score 580 paper-based), TWE (minimum score 4). Electronic applications accepted. *Faculty research:* Vision science, fundamental and clinical vision, physiological optics, psycho-physics, perception.

Western University of Health Sciences, College of Optometry, Pomona, CA 91766-1854. Offers OD. *Accreditation:* AOA. *Faculty:* 27 full-time (12 women), 4 part-time/adjunct (2 women). *Students:* 346 full-time (237 women); includes 236 minority (12 Black or African American, non-Hispanic/Latino; 1 American Indian or Alaska Native, non-Hispanic/Latino; 162 Asian, non-Hispanic/Latino; 32 Hispanic/Latino; 29 Two or more races, non-Hispanic/Latino), 21 international. Average age 27. 542 applicants, 37% accepted, 91 enrolled. In 2013, 73 doctorates awarded. *Degree requirements:* For doctorate, comprehensive exam (for some programs). *Entrance requirements:* For doctorate, OAT, letters of recommendation; BS or BA (recommended). Additional exam requirements/recommendations for international students: Required—TOEFL (minimum score 550 paper-based; 79 iBT). *Application deadline:* For fall admission, 6/1 for domestic and international students. Application fee: $65. Electronic applications accepted. *Unit head:* Dr. Elizabeth Hoppe, Dean, 909-706-3497, E-mail: ehoppe@westernu.edu. *Application contact:* Marie Anderson, Director of Admissions, 909-469-5335, Fax: 909-469-5570, E-mail: admissions@westernu.edu.
Website: http://www.westernu.edu/optometry/

Vision Sciences

Eastern Virginia Medical School, Ophthalmic Technology Program, Norfolk, VA 23501-1980. Offers Certificate. *Faculty:* 2 full-time (both women). *Students:* 34 full-time (26 women); includes 12 minority (5 Black or African American, non-Hispanic/Latino; 6 Asian, non-Hispanic/Latino; 1 Two or more races, non-Hispanic/Latino). 11 applicants, 64% accepted, 7 enrolled. *Application deadline:* For fall admission, 4/1 for domestic students. Applications are processed on a rolling basis. Application fee: $60. Electronic applications accepted. *Expenses:* Contact institution. *Unit head:* Lori J. Wood, Director, 757-446-5104, Fax: 757-446-6179, E-mail: optech@evms.edu. *Application contact:* Rose Mwayungu, Admissions and Enrollment Manager, 757-446-7153, Fax: 757-446-6179, E-mail: mwayunra@evms.edu.

Marshall B. Ketchum University, Graduate and Professional Programs, Fullerton, CA 92831-1615. Offers optometry (OD); vision science (MS). *Accreditation:* AOA. *Degree requirements:* For doctorate, thesis/dissertation. *Entrance requirements:* For doctorate, OAT. Electronic applications accepted. *Faculty research:* Structure and function of the human visual system.

The New England College of Optometry, Graduate and Professional Programs, Boston, MA 02115-1100. Offers optometry (OD); vision science (MS). *Accreditation:* AOA. *Entrance requirements:* For doctorate, OAT. Electronic applications accepted.

Nova Southeastern University, College of Optometry, Fort Lauderdale, FL 33328. Offers clinical vision research (MS); optometry (OD). *Accreditation:* AOA. Postbaccalaureate distance learning degree programs offered (no on-campus study). *Students:* 425 full-time (280 women), 5 part-time (4 women); includes 190 minority (29 Black or African American, non-Hispanic/Latino; 1 American Indian or Alaska Native, non-Hispanic/Latino; 92 Asian, non-Hispanic/Latino; 56 Hispanic/Latino; 12 Two or more races, non-Hispanic/Latino), 41 international. Average age 26. In 2013, 1 master's, 97 doctorates awarded. *Degree requirements:* For master's, comprehensive exam (for some programs), thesis; for doctorate, comprehensive exam. *Entrance requirements:* For master's, OAT or GRE, BA; for doctorate, OAT, minimum GPA of 3.0. Additional exam requirements/recommendations for international students: Required—TOEFL (minimum score 79 iBT). *Application deadline:* For fall admission, 4/1 for domestic and international students. Applications are processed on a rolling basis. Application fee: $50. Electronic applications accepted. *Expenses:* Contact institution. *Financial support:* Federal Work-Study, institutionally sponsored loans, and scholarships/grants available. Support available to part-time students. Financial award applicants required to submit FAFSA. *Faculty research:* Retinal disease, low vision, binocular vision, contact lenses, accommodation. *Unit head:* Dr. David Loshin, Dean, 954-262-1404, Fax: 954-262-1818. *Application contact:* Juan Saavedra, Admissions Counselor, 954-262-1132, Fax: 954-262-2282, E-mail: jsaavedra@nova.edu.
Website: http://optometry.nova.edu/

Salus University, College of Education and Rehabilitation, Elkins Park, PA 19027-1598. Offers education of children and youth with visual and multiple impairments (M Ed, Certificate); low vision rehabilitation (MS, Certificate); orientation and mobility therapy (MS, Certificate); vision rehabilitation therapy (MS, Certificate); OD/MS. Part-time programs available. Postbaccalaureate distance learning degree programs offered. *Entrance requirements:* For master's, GRE or MAT, letters of reference (3), interviews (2). Additional exam requirements/recommendations for international students: Required—TOEFL, TWE. *Expenses:* Contact institution. *Faculty research:* Knowledge utilization, technology transfer.

State University of New York College of Optometry, Graduate Programs, New York, NY 10036. Offers PhD, OD/MS, OD/PhD. Part-time programs available. Terminal master's awarded for partial completion of doctoral program. *Degree requirements:* For doctorate, comprehensive exam, thesis/dissertation, specialty exam. *Entrance requirements:* For doctorate, GRE General Test. Additional exam requirements/recommendations for international students: Required—TOEFL (minimum score 550 paper-based; 80 iBT). *Expenses:* Contact institution. *Faculty research:* Oculomotor systems, perception, physiological optics, ocular biochemistry, accommodation, color and motion.

Université de Montréal, School of Optometry, Graduate Programs in Optometry, Montréal, QC H3C 3J7, Canada. Offers vision sciences (M Sc); visual impairment intervention-orientation and mobility (DESS); visual impairment intervention-readaptation (DESS). Part-time programs available. *Degree requirements:* For master's, thesis. *Entrance requirements:* For master's, OD or appropriate bachelor's degree, minimum GPA of 2.7. Electronic applications accepted. *Faculty research:* Binocular vision, visual electrophysiology, eye movements, corneal metabolism, glare sensitivity.

The University of Alabama at Birmingham, School of Optometry, Graduate Program in Vision Science, Birmingham, AL 35294. Offers sensory impairment (PhD); vision science (MS, PhD). Terminal master's awarded for partial completion of doctoral program. *Degree requirements:* For master's, thesis; for doctorate, thesis/dissertation. *Entrance requirements:* For master's and doctorate, GRE General Test, interview.

University of Alberta, Faculty of Medicine and Dentistry and Faculty of Graduate Studies and Research, Graduate Programs in Medicine, Department of Ophthalmology, Edmonton, AB T6G 2E1, Canada. Offers M Sc, PhD. Part-time programs available. Terminal master's awarded for partial completion of doctoral program. *Degree requirements:* For master's, thesis; for doctorate, comprehensive exam, thesis/dissertation. *Faculty research:* Ocular genetics.

University of California, Berkeley, Graduate Division, Group in Vision Science, Berkeley, CA 94720-1500. Offers MS, PhD. *Degree requirements:* For master's, thesis; for doctorate, thesis/dissertation. *Entrance requirements:* For master's and doctorate, GRE General Test, GRE Subject Test, minimum GPA of 3.0, 3 letters of recommendation. *Faculty research:* Visual neuroscience, bioengineering, computational vision, molecular cell biology, basic and clinical psychophysics.

University of Chicago, Division of Biological Sciences, Department of Ophthalmology and Visual Science, Chicago, IL 60637-1513. Offers PhD. *Degree requirements:* For doctorate, thesis/dissertation, ethics class, 2 teaching assistantships. *Entrance requirements:* For doctorate, GRE General Test. Additional exam requirements/recommendations for international students: Required—TOEFL (minimum score 600 paper-based; 104 iBT), IELTS (minimum score 7). *Faculty research:* Visual psychophysics, visual molecular biology, immunology, transplantation, infections.

University of Guelph, Ontario Veterinary College and Graduate Studies, Graduate Programs in Veterinary Sciences, Department of Clinical Studies, Guelph, ON N1G 2W1, Canada. Offers anesthesiology (M Sc, DV Sc); cardiology (DV Sc, Diploma); clinical studies (Diploma); dermatology (M Sc); diagnostic imaging (M Sc, DV Sc); emergency/critical care (M Sc, DV Sc, Diploma); medicine (M Sc, DV Sc); neurology (M Sc, DV Sc); ophthalmology (M Sc, DV Sc); surgery (M Sc, DV Sc). *Degree requirements:* For master's, thesis; for doctorate, comprehensive exam, thesis/dissertation. *Entrance requirements:* Additional exam requirements/recommendations for international students: Required—TOEFL (minimum score 550 paper-based), IELTS (minimum score 6.5). Electronic applications accepted. *Faculty research:* Orthopedics, respirology, oncology, exercise physiology, cardiology.

University of Houston, College of Optometry, Program in Physiological Optics/Vision Science, Houston, TX 77204. Offers physiological optics (MS, PhD). *Faculty research:* Space perception, amblyopia, binocular vision, development of visual skills, strabismus, visual cell biology, refractive error.

The University of Manchester, Faculty of Life Sciences, Manchester, United Kingdom. Offers adaptive organismal biology (M Phil, PhD); animal biology (M Phil, PhD); biochemistry (M Phil, PhD); bioinformatics (M Phil, PhD); biomolecular sciences (M Phil, PhD); biotechnology (M Phil, PhD); cell biology (M Phil, PhD); cell matrix research (M Phil, PhD); channels and transporters (M Phil, PhD); developmental biology (M Phil, PhD); Egyptology (M Phil, PhD); environmental biology (M Phil, PhD); evolutionary biology (M Phil, PhD); gene expression (M Phil, PhD); genetics (M Phil, PhD); history of science, technology and medicine (M Phil, PhD); immunology (M Phil, PhD); integrative neurobiology and behavior (M Phil, PhD); membrane trafficking (M Phil, PhD); microbiology (M Phil, PhD); molecular and cellular neuroscience (M Phil, PhD); molecular biology (M Phil, PhD); molecular cancer studies (M Phil, PhD); neuroscience (M Phil, PhD); ophthalmology (M Phil, PhD); optometry (M Phil, PhD); organelle function (M Phil, PhD); pharmacology (M Phil, PhD); physiology (M Phil, PhD); plant sciences (M Phil, PhD); stem cell research (M Phil, PhD); structural biology (M Phil, PhD); systems neuroscience (M Phil, PhD); toxicology (M Phil, PhD).

University of Waterloo, Graduate Studies, Faculty of Science, School of Optometry, Waterloo, ON N2L 3G1, Canada. Offers optometry (OD); vision science (M Sc, PhD). *Accreditation:* AOA. Part-time programs available. *Degree requirements:* For master's, thesis; for doctorate, thesis/dissertation. *Entrance requirements:* For master's, honors degree, minimum B average; for doctorate, master's degree, minimum B average. Additional exam requirements/recommendations for international students: Required—TOEFL (minimum score 580 paper-based), TWE (minimum score 4). Electronic applications accepted. *Faculty research:* Vision science, fundamental and clinical vision, physiological optics, psycho-physics, perception.

Section 30
Pharmacy and Pharmaceutical Sciences

This section contains a directory of institutions offering graduate work in pharmacy and pharmaceutical sciences, followed by in-depth entries submitted by institutions that chose to prepare detailed program descriptions. Additional information about programs listed in the directory but not augmented by an in-depth entry may be obtained by writing directly to the dean of a graduate school or chair of a department at the address given in the directory.

For programs offering related work, see also in this book *Allied Health, Biochemistry, Biological and Biomedical Sciences, Nutrition, Pharmacology and Toxicology,* and *Physiology.* In the other guides in this series:

Graduate Programs in the Physical Sciences, Mathematics, Agricultural Sciences, the Environment & Natural Resources

See *Chemistry*

Graduate Programs in Engineering & Applied Sciences

See *Biomedical Engineering and Biotechnology,* and *Chemical Engineering*

CONTENTS

Program Directories

Displays and Close-Ups

Medicinal and Pharmaceutical Chemistry

Cleveland State University, College of Graduate Studies, College of Sciences and Health Professions, Department of Chemistry, Cleveland, OH 44115. Offers analytical chemistry (MS); clinical chemistry (MS); clinical/bioanalytical chemistry (PhD), including cellular and molecular medicine, clinical chemistry, clinical/bioanalytical chemistry; environmental chemistry (MS); inorganic chemistry (MS); pharmaceutical/organic chemistry (MS); physical chemistry (MS). Part-time and evening/weekend programs available. *Faculty:* 12 full-time (0 women). *Students:* 17 full-time (10 women), 95 part-time (43 women); includes 6 minority (5 Black or African American, non-Hispanic/Latino; 1 Asian, non-Hispanic/Latino), 73 international. Average age 27. 121 applicants, 55% accepted. In 2013, 19 master's, 9 doctorates awarded. *Degree requirements:* For master's, thesis optional; for doctorate, comprehensive exam, thesis/dissertation. *Entrance requirements:* For master's and doctorate, GRE General Test. Additional exam requirements/recommendations for international students: Required—TOEFL (minimum score 525 paper-based; 65 iBT). *Application deadline:* For fall admission, 1/15 priority date for domestic and international students. Applications are processed on a rolling basis. Application fee: $30. Electronic applications accepted. *Expenses:* Tuition, state resident: full-time $8335; part-time $521 per credit hour. Tuition, nonresident: full-time $15,670; part-time $979 per credit hour. *Required fees:* $50; $25 per semester. *Financial support:* In 2013–14, 44 students received support, including 5 fellowships with full tuition reimbursements available (averaging $22,500 per year), 13 research assistantships with full tuition reimbursements available (averaging $22,500 per year), 24 teaching assistantships with full tuition reimbursements available (averaging $21,000 per year); scholarships/grants and unspecified assistantships also available. Financial award application deadline: 1/15. *Faculty research:* Bioanalytical techniques and molecular diagnostics, glycoproteomics and antithrombotic agents, drug discovery and innovation, analytical pharmacology, inflammatory disease research. *Total annual research expenditures:* $3 million. *Unit head:* Dr. David W. Ball, Chair, 216-687-2467, Fax: 216-687-9298, E-mail: d.ball@csuohio.edu. *Application contact:* Richelle P. Emery, Administrative Coordinator, 216-687-2457, Fax: 216-687-9298, E-mail: r.emery@csuohio.edu.
Website: http://www.csuohio.edu/sciences/dept/chemistry/index.html

Duquesne University, Mylan School of Pharmacy, Graduate School of Pharmaceutical Sciences, Program in Medicinal Chemistry, Pittsburgh, PA 15282-0001. Offers MS, PhD. *Faculty:* 5 full-time (0 women). *Students:* 25 full-time (10 women), all international. Average age 27. 34 applicants, 24% accepted, 5 enrolled. In 2013, 1 master's, 2 doctorates awarded. *Degree requirements:* For master's, thesis; for doctorate, comprehensive exam, thesis/dissertation. *Entrance requirements:* For master's and doctorate, GRE General Test. Additional exam requirements/recommendations for international students: Required—TOEFL or IELTS (minimum score 7). *Application deadline:* For fall admission, 2/1 priority date for domestic and international students; for spring admission, 10/1 priority date for domestic and international students. Applications are processed on a rolling basis. Application fee: $50. Electronic applications accepted. *Expenses: Tuition:* Full-time $18,162; part-time $1009 per credit. *Required fees:* $1728; $96 per credit. Tuition and fees vary according to program. *Financial support:* In 2013–14, 21 students received support, including 9 research assistantships with full tuition reimbursements available, 12 teaching assistantships with full tuition reimbursements available. *Unit head:* Dr. Aleem Gangjee, Head, 412-396-6070. *Application contact:* Information Contact, 412-396-1172, E-mail: gsps-adm@duq.edu.
Website: http://www.duq.edu/academics/schools/pharmacy/graduate-school-of-pharmaceutical-sciences

Florida Agricultural and Mechanical University, Division of Graduate Studies, Research, and Continuing Education, College of Pharmacy and Pharmaceutical Sciences, Graduate Programs in Pharmaceutical Sciences, Tallahassee, FL 32307-3200. Offers environmental toxicology (PhD); medicinal chemistry (MS, PhD); pharmaceutics (MS, PhD); pharmacology/toxicology (MS, PhD); pharmacy administration (MS). *Accreditation:* CEPH. *Degree requirements:* For master's, comprehensive exam, thesis, publishable paper; for doctorate, comprehensive exam, thesis/dissertation, publishable paper. *Entrance requirements:* For master's and doctorate, GRE General Test, minimum GPA of 3.0 in last 60 hours. Additional exam requirements/recommendations for international students: Required—TOEFL. *Faculty research:* Anticancer agents, anti-inflammatory drugs, chronopharmacology, neuroendocrinology, microbiology.

Idaho State University, Office of Graduate Studies, College of Pharmacy, Department of Biomedical and Pharmaceutical Sciences, Pocatello, ID 83209-8334. Offers biopharmaceutical analysis (PhD); drug delivery (PhD); medicinal chemistry (PhD); pharmaceutical sciences (MS); pharmacology (PhD). Part-time programs available. *Degree requirements:* For master's, one foreign language, comprehensive exam, thesis, thesis research, classes in speech and technical writing; for doctorate, comprehensive exam, thesis/dissertation, written and oral exams, classes in speech and technical writing. *Entrance requirements:* For master's, GRE General Test, minimum GPA of 3.0, 3 letters of recommendation; for doctorate, GRE General Test, BS in pharmacy or related field, minimum GPA of 3.0, 3 letters of recommendation. Additional exam requirements/recommendations for international students: Required—TOEFL (minimum score 550 paper-based; 80 iBT). Electronic applications accepted. *Expenses:* Contact institution. *Faculty research:* Metabolic toxicity of heavy metals, neuroendocrine pharmacology, cardiovascular pharmacology, cancer biology, immunopharmacology.

Long Island University–LIU Post, School of Health Professions and Nursing, Department of Biomedical Sciences, Brookville, NY 11548-1300. Offers cardiovascular perfusion (MS); clinical laboratory management (MS); medical biology (MS), including hematology, immunology, medical biology, medical chemistry, medical microbiology. Part-time and evening/weekend programs available. Postbaccalaureate distance learning degree programs offered. *Degree requirements:* For master's, thesis. *Entrance requirements:* For master's, minimum GPA of 2.75 in major. Electronic applications accepted.

Medical University of South Carolina, College of Graduate Studies, Department of Pharmaceutical and Biomedical Sciences, Charleston, SC 29425. Offers cell injury and repair (PhD); drug discovery (PhD); medicinal chemistry (PhD); toxicology (PhD); DMD/PhD; MD/PhD; Pharm D/PhD. *Degree requirements:* For doctorate, thesis/dissertation, oral and written exams, teaching and research seminar. *Entrance requirements:* For doctorate, GRE General Test, interview, minimum GPA of 3.0. Additional exam requirements/recommendations for international students: Required—TOEFL (minimum score 600 paper-based; 100 iBT). Electronic applications accepted. *Faculty research:* Drug discovery, toxicology, metabolomics, cell stress and injury.

New Jersey Institute of Technology, College of Science and Liberal Arts, Newark, NJ 07102. Offers applied mathematics (MS); applied physics (M Sc, PhD); applied statistics (MS); biology (MS, PhD); biostatistics (MS); chemistry (MS, PhD); computational biology (MS); environmental science (MS, PhD); history (MA, MAT); materials science and engineering (MS, PhD); mathematical and computational finance (MS); mathematics science (PhD); pharmaceutical chemistry (MS); professional and technical communications (MS). Part-time and evening/weekend programs available. *Faculty:* 150 full-time (33 women), 76 part-time/adjunct (27 women). *Students:* 245 full-time (97 women), 115 part-time (49 women); includes 75 minority (26 Black or African American, non-Hispanic/Latino; 1 American Indian or Alaska Native, non-Hispanic/Latino; 35 Asian, non-Hispanic/Latino; 12 Hispanic/Latino; 1 Native Hawaiian or other Pacific Islander, non-Hispanic/Latino), 189 international. Average age 30. 754 applicants, 59% accepted, 109 enrolled. In 2013, 104 master's, 29 doctorates awarded. Terminal master's awarded for partial completion of doctoral program. *Degree requirements:* For master's, thesis optional; for doctorate, thesis/dissertation. *Entrance requirements:* For master's, GRE General Test; for doctorate, GRE General Test, minimum graduate GPA of 3.5. Additional exam requirements/recommendations for international students: Required—TOEFL (minimum score 550 paper-based; 79 iBT). *Application deadline:* For fall admission, 6/1 priority date for domestic students, 5/1 priority date for international students; for spring admission, 11/15 priority date for domestic and international students. Applications are processed on a rolling basis. Application fee: $65. Electronic applications accepted. *Expenses:* Tuition, state resident: full-time $17,384; part-time $945 per credit. Tuition, nonresident: full-time $25,404; part-time $1341 per credit. *Required fees:* $2396; $118 per credit. *Financial support:* Fellowships with full tuition reimbursements, research assistantships with full tuition reimbursements, and teaching assistantships with full tuition reimbursements available. Financial award application deadline: 1/15. *Total annual research expenditures:* $6.9 million. *Unit head:* Dr. Fadi P. Deek, Dean, 973-596-3676, Fax: 973-565-0586, E-mail: fadi.deek@njit.edu. *Application contact:* Kathryn Kelly, Director of Admissions, 973-596-3300, Fax: 973-596-3461, E-mail: admissions@njit.edu.
Website: http://csla.njit.edu/

Purdue University, College of Pharmacy and Pharmacal Sciences and Graduate School, Graduate Programs in Pharmacy and Pharmacal Sciences, Department of Medicinal Chemistry and Molecular Pharmacology, West Lafayette, IN 47907. Offers biophysical and computational chemistry (PhD); cancer research (PhD); immunology and infectious disease (PhD); medicinal biochemistry and molecular biology (PhD); medicinal chemistry and chemical biology (PhD); molecular pharmacology (PhD); neuropharmacology, neurodegeneration, and neurotoxicity (PhD); systems biology and functional genomics (PhD). *Faculty:* 23 full-time (3 women), 6 part-time/adjunct (1 woman). *Students:* 50 full-time (21 women), 3 part-time (2 women); includes 1 minority (Asian, non-Hispanic/Latino), 30 international. Average age 26. 147 applicants, 20% accepted, 13 enrolled. In 2013, 12 doctorates awarded. *Degree requirements:* For doctorate, thesis/dissertation. *Entrance requirements:* For doctorate, GRE General Test; GRE Subject Test in biology, biochemistry, and chemistry (recommended), minimum undergraduate GPA of 3.0. Additional exam requirements/recommendations for international students: Required—TOEFL (minimum score 550 paper-based; 77 iBT); Recommended—TWE. *Application deadline:* For fall admission, 2/1 for domestic and international students. Applications are processed on a rolling basis. Application fee: $60 ($75 for international students). Electronic applications accepted. *Financial support:* Fellowships, research assistantships, teaching assistantships, and traineeships available. Support available to part-time students. Financial award applicants required to submit FAFSA. *Faculty research:* Drug design and development, cancer research, drug synthesis and analysis, chemical pharmacology, environmental toxicology. *Unit head:* Dr. Richard F. Borch, Head, 765-494-1403, E-mail: borch@purdue.edu. *Application contact:* Dr. Janine C. Mott, Graduate Contact, 765-494-1269, E-mail: jmott@purdue.edu.

Rutgers, The State University of New Jersey, New Brunswick, Ernest Mario School of Pharmacy, Program in Medicinal Chemistry, Piscataway, NJ 08854-8097. Offers MS, PhD. Part-time programs available. *Degree requirements:* For master's, comprehensive exam, thesis; for doctorate, comprehensive exam, thesis/dissertation. *Entrance requirements:* For master's and doctorate, GRE General Test. Additional exam requirements/recommendations for international students: Required—TOEFL (minimum score 600 paper-based; 90 iBT). Electronic applications accepted. *Faculty research:* Synthesis and design of anticancer drugs, synthesis of pro-drugs for prostate cancer, natural product synthesis, natural product isolation and structure elucidation, computational chemistry.

Temple University, School of Pharmacy, Department of Pharmaceutical Sciences, Philadelphia, PA 19140. Offers medicinal chemistry (MS, PhD); pharmaceutics (MS, PhD); pharmacodynamics (MS, PhD); quality assurance/regulatory affairs (MS). Part-time programs available. Postbaccalaureate distance learning degree programs offered. *Faculty:* 18 full-time (4 women). *Students:* 33 full-time (15 women), 205 part-time (137 women); includes 35 minority (8 Black or African American, non-Hispanic/Latino; 2 American Indian or Alaska Native, non-Hispanic/Latino; 20 Asian, non-Hispanic/Latino; 4 Hispanic/Latino; 1 Two or more races, non-Hispanic/Latino), 35 international. 121 applicants, 50% accepted, 43 enrolled. In 2013, 59 master's, 7 doctorates awarded. *Degree requirements:* For master's, comprehensive exam (for some programs), thesis (for some programs); for doctorate, 2 foreign languages, comprehensive exam, thesis/dissertation. *Entrance requirements:* For master's, GRE General Test, minimum undergraduate GPA of 3.0; for doctorate, GRE General Test, minimum GPA of 3.0. Additional exam requirements/recommendations for international students: Required—TOEFL (minimum score 550 paper-based; 82 iBT). *Application deadline:* For fall admission, 1/15 for domestic students, 12/15 for international students. Application fee: $60. Electronic applications accepted. *Expenses:* Contact institution. *Financial support:* In 2013–14, 2 fellowships with full tuition reimbursements (averaging $23,000 per year), 6 research assistantships with full tuition reimbursements (averaging $22,000 per year), 11 teaching assistantships with full tuition reimbursements (averaging $22,000 per year) were awarded. Financial award application deadline: 1/15; financial award applicants required to submit FAFSA. *Faculty research:* Pharmacokinetics, synthesis of medicinals, protein research, biopharm-formulation. *Unit head:* Dr. Daniel Canney, Director of Graduate Studies, 215-707-4948, E-mail: phscgrad@temple.edu. *Application contact:* Sophon Din, Administrative Assistant, 215-204-4948, E-mail: tuspgrad@temple.edu.

University at Buffalo, the State University of New York, Graduate School, College of Arts and Sciences, Department of Chemistry, Buffalo, NY 14260. Offers chemistry (MA, PhD); medicinal chemistry (MS, PhD). Part-time programs available. *Faculty:* 28 full-time (4 women), 1 (woman) part-time/adjunct. *Students:* 159 full-time (58 women), 1 part-time (0 women); includes 20 minority (11 Black or African American, non-Hispanic/Latino; 9 Hispanic/Latino), 31 international. Average age 26. 187 applicants, 37% accepted, 37 enrolled. In 2013, 9 master's, 21 doctorates awarded. Terminal master's awarded for partial completion of doctoral program. *Degree requirements:* For master's, thesis or alternative, project; for doctorate, thesis/dissertation, synopsis proposal.

Entrance requirements: For master's and doctorate, GRE General Test. Additional exam requirements/recommendations for international students: Required—TOEFL (minimum score 550 paper-based; 79 iBT). *Application deadline:* For fall admission, 3/1 priority date for domestic students, 3/1 for international students; for spring admission, 11/1 priority date for domestic students. Applications are processed on a rolling basis. Application fee: $75. Electronic applications accepted. *Financial support:* In 2013–14, 7 students received support, including 7 fellowships with full tuition reimbursements available (averaging $22,080 per year), 33 research assistantships with full tuition reimbursements available (averaging $22,080 per year), 95 teaching assistantships with full tuition reimbursements available (averaging $22,080 per year); Federal Work-Study, institutionally sponsored loans, and unspecified assistantships also available. Financial award application deadline: 6/15; financial award applicants required to submit FAFSA. *Faculty research:* Synthesis, measurements, structure theory, translation. *Total annual research expenditures:* $8 million. *Unit head:* Dr. Michael R. Detty, Chairman, 716-645-6824, Fax: 716-645-6963, E-mail: chechair@buffalo.edu. *Application contact:* Dr. Diana S. Aga, Director of Graduate Studies, 716-645-4220, Fax: 716-645-6963, E-mail: dianaaga@buffalo.edu.
Website: http://www.chemistry.buffalo.edu/

University of California, Irvine, College of Health Sciences, Program in Medicinal Chemistry and Pharmacology, Irvine, CA 92697. Offers PhD. *Students:* 8 full-time (5 women); includes 3 minority (2 Asian, non-Hispanic/Latino; 1 Hispanic/Latino), 2 international. Average age 26. 95 applicants, 22% accepted, 8 enrolled. Application fee: $80 ($100 for international students). *Unit head:* Richard Chamberlin, Chair, 949-824-7089, Fax: 949-824-9920, E-mail: richard.chamberlin@uci.edu. *Application contact:* Geneva Lopez-Sandoval, Student Affairs Office, 949-824-0878, E-mail: lopezg@uci.edu.
Website: http://www.pharmsci.uci.edu/graduate/index.php

University of California, San Francisco, School of Pharmacy and Graduate Division, Chemistry and Chemical Biology Graduate Program, San Francisco, CA 94143. Offers PhD. *Degree requirements:* For doctorate, thesis/dissertation. *Entrance requirements:* For doctorate, GRE General Test, minimum GPA of 3.0, bachelor's degree. Additional exam requirements/recommendations for international students: Required—TOEFL (minimum score 550 paper-based; 80 iBT). *Application deadline:* For fall admission, 12/1 for domestic and international students. Applications are processed on a rolling basis. Application fee: $80 ($100 for international students). Electronic applications accepted. *Expenses:* Tuition, state resident: full-time $11,220. Tuition, nonresident: full-time $26,322. *Required fees:* $5204. Full-time tuition and fees vary according to degree level and program. *Financial support:* In 2013–14, fellowships with full tuition reimbursements (averaging $32,500 per year), research assistantships with full tuition reimbursements (averaging $32,500 per year) were awarded; teaching assistantships with partial tuition reimbursements, institutionally sponsored loans, scholarships/grants, traineeships, and tuition waivers (full) also available. Financial award application deadline: 5/15. *Faculty research:* Macromolecular structure function and dynamics, computational chemistry and biology, biological chemistry and synthetic biology, chemical biology and molecular design, nanomolecular design. *Unit head:* Dr. Charles S. Craik, Director, 415-476-8146, E-mail: craik@cgl.ucsf.edu. *Application contact:* Julia Molla, Administrator, 415-476-1914, Fax: 415-514-1546, E-mail: julia.molla@ucsf.edu.
Website: http://ccb.ucsf.edu/

University of Connecticut, Graduate School, School of Pharmacy, Department of Pharmaceutical Sciences, Program in Medicinal Chemistry, Storrs, CT 06269. Offers MS, PhD. Terminal master's awarded for partial completion of doctoral program. *Degree requirements:* For master's, comprehensive exam, thesis; for doctorate, thesis/dissertation. *Entrance requirements:* Additional exam requirements/recommendations for international students: Required—TOEFL (minimum score 550 paper-based). Electronic applications accepted.

University of Florida, Graduate School, College of Pharmacy and Graduate School, Graduate Programs in Pharmacy, Department of Medicinal Chemistry, Gainesville, FL 32610. Offers medicinal chemistry (MSP, PhD); pharmaceutical chemistry (MSP). Part-time and evening/weekend programs available. Postbaccalaureate distance learning degree programs offered (minimal on-campus study). *Faculty:* 9 full-time (3 women), 2 part-time/adjunct (0 women). *Students:* 49 full-time (33 women), 281 part-time (193 women); includes 65 minority (32 Black or African American, non-Hispanic/Latino; 3 American Indian or Alaska Native, non-Hispanic/Latino; 11 Asian, non-Hispanic/Latino; 19 Hispanic/Latino), 26 international. Average age 32. 68 applicants, 12% accepted, 7 enrolled. In 2013, 129 master's, 5 doctorates awarded. Terminal master's awarded for partial completion of doctoral program. *Degree requirements:* For master's, thesis optional; for doctorate, comprehensive exam, thesis/dissertation. *Entrance requirements:* For master's and doctorate, GRE General Test, minimum GPA of 3.0. Additional exam requirements/recommendations for international students: Required—TOEFL (minimum score 550 paper-based; 80 iBT), IELTS (minimum score 6). *Application deadline:* For fall admission, 5/1 priority date for domestic students, 5/1 for international students; for winter admission, 10/1 for domestic and international students. Applications are processed on a rolling basis. Application fee: $30. Electronic applications accepted. *Expenses:* Tuition, state resident: full-time $12,640. Tuition, nonresident: full-time $30,000. *Financial support:* In 2013–14, 14 students received support, including 3 research assistantships (averaging $20,010 per year), 11 teaching assistantships (averaging $19,200 per year). Financial award application deadline: 4/15; financial award applicants required to submit CSS PROFILE or FAFSA. *Faculty research:* Drug metabolism and toxicology, discovery of biologically active natural products, chelator chemistry and biochemistry, anti-cancer drug and pro-drug discovery, discovery of neuroactive drugs. *Unit head:* Dr. Margaret O. James, Professor and Chair, 352-273-7707, Fax: 352-392-9455, E-mail: mojames@ufl.edu. *Application contact:* Hendrik Luesch, PhD, Graduate Coordinator, 352-273-7738, Fax: 352-392-9455, E-mail: luesch@cop.ufl.edu.
Website: http://pharmacy.ufl.edu/mc/

The University of Iowa, College of Pharmacy, Iowa City, IA 52242-1316. Offers clinical pharmaceutical sciences (PhD); medicinal and natural products chemistry (PhD); pharamaceutics (PhD); pharmaceutical socioeconomics (PhD); pharmaceutics (MS); pharmacy (Pharm D); Pharm D/MPH. *Accreditation:* ACPE (one or more programs are accredited). *Degree requirements:* For master's, thesis optional, exam; for doctorate, comprehensive exam, thesis/dissertation. *Entrance requirements:* For master's and doctorate, GRE General Test, minimum GPA of 3.0. Additional exam requirements/recommendations for international students: Required—TOEFL (minimum score 550 paper-based; 81 iBT). Electronic applications accepted.

The University of Kansas, Graduate Studies, School of Pharmacy, Department of Medicinal Chemistry, Lawrence, KS 66045. Offers MS, PhD. *Faculty:* 14. *Students:* 34 full-time (13 women); includes 1 minority (Asian, non-Hispanic/Latino), 16 international. Average age 26. 75 applicants, 11% accepted, 6 enrolled. In 2013, 4 master's, 3 doctorates awarded. Terminal master's awarded for partial completion of doctoral program. *Degree requirements:* For master's, comprehensive exam, thesis (for some programs); for doctorate, comprehensive exam, thesis/dissertation, cumulative exams. *Entrance requirements:* For master's and doctorate, GRE General Test. Additional exam requirements/recommendations for international students: Required—TOEFL. *Application deadline:* For fall admission, 2/1 for domestic and international students. Application fee: $55 ($65 for international students). Electronic applications accepted. *Financial support:* Fellowships with full tuition reimbursements, research assistantships with full tuition reimbursements, teaching assistantships with full tuition reimbursements, health care benefits, and unspecified assistantships available. Financial award application deadline: 3/1. *Faculty research:* Cancer, neuroscience, synthetic methods, natural products, biochemistry. *Unit head:* Dr. Thomas Prisinzano, Professor/Chair, 785-864-4495, Fax: 785-864-5326, E-mail: prisinza@ku.edu. *Application contact:* Norma Henley, Administrative Associate, 785-864-4495, Fax: 785-864-5326, E-mail: nah@ku.edu.
Website: http://www.medchem.ku.edu/

The University of Kansas, Graduate Studies, School of Pharmacy, Department of Pharmaceutical Chemistry, Lawrence, KS 66047. Offers MS, PhD. Part-time and evening/weekend programs available. Postbaccalaureate distance learning degree programs offered (no on-campus study). *Faculty:* 14. *Students:* 36 full-time (12 women), 19 part-time (11 women); includes 10 minority (7 Asian, non-Hispanic/Latino; 1 Hispanic/Latino; 2 Two or more races, non-Hispanic/Latino), 20 international. Average age 29. 74 applicants, 19% accepted, 10 enrolled. In 2013, 12 master's, 5 doctorates awarded. Terminal master's awarded for partial completion of doctoral program. *Degree requirements:* For master's, thesis, qualifying exam; for doctorate, comprehensive exam, thesis/dissertation, qualifying exam. *Entrance requirements:* For master's, GRE General Test, bachelor's degree in biological sciences, chemical engineering, chemistry, or pharmacy; official transcripts from all universities/institutions in which the applicant has studied; personal statement; resume; for doctorate, GRE General Test, official transcripts from all universities/institutions in which the applicant has studied, personal statement, resume. Additional exam requirements/recommendations for international students: Required—TOEFL. *Application deadline:* For fall admission, 1/15 for domestic and international students. Applications are processed on a rolling basis. Application fee: $55 ($65 for international students). Electronic applications accepted. *Financial support:* Fellowships with full tuition reimbursements, research assistantships with full and partial tuition reimbursements, career-related internships or fieldwork, scholarships/grants, traineeships, and unspecified assistantships available. Financial award application deadline: 1/15. *Faculty research:* Physical pharmacy, biotechnology, bioanalytical chemistry, biopharmaceutics and pharmacokinetics, nanotechnology. *Unit head:* Dr. Christian Schoneich, Chair, 785-864-4880, Fax: 785-864-5736, E-mail: schoneic@ku.edu. *Application contact:* Nancy Helm, Administrative Associate, 785-864-4822, Fax: 785-864-5736, E-mail: nhelm@ku.edu.
Website: http://www.pharmchem.ku.edu/

University of Michigan, College of Pharmacy and University of Michigan, Department of Medicinal Chemistry, Ann Arbor, MI 48109. Offers PhD. *Students:* 47 full-time (19 women); includes 6 minority (2 Black or African American, non-Hispanic/Latino; 2 Asian, non-Hispanic/Latino; 2 Hispanic/Latino), 6 international. Average age 27. 90 applicants, 24% accepted, 9 enrolled. In 2013, 5 doctorates awarded. *Degree requirements:* For doctorate, thesis/dissertation, oral defense of dissertation, preliminary exam. *Entrance requirements:* For doctorate, GRE. Additional exam requirements/recommendations for international students: Required—TOEFL (minimum score 560 paper-based; 84 iBT) or IELTS (minimum score 6.5). *Application deadline:* For fall admission, 12/31 for domestic and international students. Application fee: $60 ($75 for international students). Electronic applications accepted. *Expenses:* Contact institution. *Financial support:* In 2013–14, 47 students received support, including 21 fellowships (averaging $46,107 per year), 15 research assistantships (averaging $46,107 per year), 11 teaching assistantships (averaging $46,107 per year); career-related internships or fieldwork, institutionally sponsored loans, scholarships/grants, traineeships, health care benefits, and unspecified assistantships also available. *Unit head:* Dr. George A. Garcia, Chair, 734-764-2202, Fax: 734-647-8430, E-mail: gagarcia@med.umich.edu. *Application contact:* Sarah Lloyd, Executive Secretary, 734-647-8429, Fax: 734-647-8430, E-mail: sarlloyd@med.umich.edu.
Website: https://pharmacy.umich.edu/medchem

University of Minnesota, Twin Cities Campus, College of Pharmacy and Graduate School, Graduate Programs in Pharmacy, Graduate Program in Medicinal Chemistry, Minneapolis, MN 55455. Offers MS, PhD. *Faculty:* 27 full-time (4 women), 6 part-time/adjunct (2 women). *Students:* 40 full-time (12 women); includes 5 minority (1 Black or African American, non-Hispanic/Latino; 3 Asian, non-Hispanic/Latino; 1 Two or more races, non-Hispanic/Latino), 15 international. Average age 26. 65 applicants, 17% accepted, 4 enrolled. In 2013, 3 master's, 6 doctorates awarded. Terminal master's awarded for partial completion of doctoral program. *Degree requirements:* For master's, comprehensive exam, thesis; for doctorate, comprehensive exam, thesis/dissertation. *Entrance requirements:* For doctorate, GRE General Test, BS in biology, chemistry, or pharmacy. Additional exam requirements/recommendations for international students: Required—TOEFL (minimum score 550 paper-based). *Application deadline:* For fall admission, 1/5 priority date for domestic and international students. Application fee: $75 ($95 for international students). Electronic applications accepted. *Financial support:* In 2013–14, 30 students received support, including 28 fellowships with full and partial tuition reimbursements available (averaging $8,000 per year), 24 research assistantships with full tuition reimbursements available (averaging $26,000 per year), 7 teaching assistantships with full tuition reimbursements available (averaging $15,171 per year); health care benefits and unspecified assistantships also available. Financial award application deadline: 1/5. *Faculty research:* Drug design and synthesis, molecular modeling, chemical aspects of drug metabolism and toxicity. *Total annual research expenditures:* $5.1 million. *Unit head:* Dr. Gunda I. Georg, Department Head of Medicinal Chemistry, 612-626-6320, Fax: 612-626-3114, E-mail: georg@umn.edu. *Application contact:* Information Contact, 612-625-3014, Fax: 612-625-6002, E-mail: gsquest@umn.edu.
Website: http://www.pharmacy.umn.edu/medchem/graduate/

University of Mississippi, Graduate School, School of Pharmacy, Graduate Programs in Pharmacy, University, MS 38677. Offers medicinal chemistry (PhD); pharmaceutical sciences (MS); pharmaceutics (PhD); pharmacognosy (PhD); pharmacology (PhD); pharmacy administration (PhD). *Faculty:* 41 full-time (17 women), 14 part-time/adjunct (7 women). *Students:* 81 full-time (27 women), 8 part-time (5 women); includes 4 minority (2 Black or African American, non-Hispanic/Latino; 2 Asian, non-Hispanic/Latino), 61 international. In 2013, 5 master's, 16 doctorates awarded. Application fee: $40. *Unit head:* Dr. David Allen, Dean, 662-915-7267, Fax: 662-915-5118, E-mail: sop@olemiss.edu. *Application contact:* Dr. Christy M. Wyandt, Associate Dean, 662-915-7474, Fax: 662-915-7577, E-mail: cwyandt@olemiss.edu.

The University of Montana, Graduate School, College of Health Professions and Biomedical Sciences, Skaggs School of Pharmacy, Department of Biomedical and Pharmaceutical Sciences, Missoula, MT 59812-0002. Offers biomedical sciences (PhD); medicinal chemistry (MS, PhD); molecular and cellular toxicology (MS, PhD); neuroscience (PhD); pharmaceutical sciences (MS). *Accreditation:* ACPE. *Degree requirements:* For master's, oral defense of thesis; for doctorate, research dissertation defense. *Entrance requirements:* For master's and doctorate, GRE General Test. Additional exam requirements/recommendations for international students: Required—TOEFL (minimum score 540 paper-based). *Application deadline:* For fall admission, 3/1

priority date for domestic and international students. Applications are processed on a rolling basis. Application fee: $45. Electronic applications accepted. *Financial support:* Teaching assistantships with full and partial tuition reimbursements, Federal Work-Study, scholarships/grants, and tuition waivers (full and partial) available. Financial award application deadline: 3/1. *Faculty research:* Cardiovascular pharmacology, medicinal chemistry, neurosciences, environmental toxicology, pharmacogenetics, cancer. *Unit head:* Dr. Richard Bridges, Chair, 406-243-4972, E-mail: richard.bridges@umontana.edu. *Application contact:* Information Contact, E-mail: gradschl@mso.umt.edu.
Website: http://www.umt.edu/pharmsci/

University of Rhode Island, Graduate School, College of Pharmacy, Department of Biomedical and Pharmaceutical Sciences, Kingston, RI 02881. Offers medicinal chemistry and pharmacognosy (MS, PhD); pharmaceutics and pharmacokinetics (MS, PhD); pharmacology and toxicology (MS, PhD). Part-time programs available. *Faculty:* 21 full-time (7 women). *Students:* 37 full-time (14 women), 15 part-time (7 women); includes 3 minority (1 Black or African American, non-Hispanic/Latino; 1 Asian, non-Hispanic/Latino; 1 Two or more races, non-Hispanic/Latino), 29 international. In 2013, 3 master's, 18 doctorates awarded. *Entrance requirements:* For master's and doctorate, GRE (minimum new/old format scores: Verbal 350/143; Quantitative 550/146; Analytical, 3.0), 2 letters of recommendation. Additional exam requirements/recommendations for international students: Required—TOEFL (minimum score 550 paper-based). *Application deadline:* For fall admission, 7/15 for domestic students, 2/1 for international students. Application fee: $65. Electronic applications accepted. *Expenses:* Tuition, state resident: full-time $11,532; part-time $641 per credit. Tuition, nonresident: full-time $23,606; part-time $1311 per credit. *Required fees:* $1388; $36 per credit. $35 per semester. One-time fee: $130. *Financial support:* In 2013–14, 8 research assistantships with full and partial tuition reimbursements (averaging $12,147 per year), 13 teaching assistantships with full and partial tuition reimbursements (averaging $13,579 per year) were awarded. Financial award application deadline: 2/1; financial award applicants required to submit FAFSA. *Faculty research:* Chemical carcinogenesis with a major emphasis on the structural and synthetic aspects of DNA-adduct formation, drug-drug/herb interaction, drug-genetic interaction, signaling of nuclear receptors, transcriptional regulation, oncogenesis. *Total annual research expenditures:* $5.8 million. *Unit head:* Dr. Bingfang Yan, Chair, 401-874-5032, Fax: 401-874-2181, E-mail: byan@uri.edu. *Application contact:* Graduate Admissions, 401-874-2872, E-mail: gradadm@etal.uri.edu.
Website: http://www.uri.edu/pharmacy/departments/bps/index.shtml

The University of Texas at Austin, Graduate School, College of Pharmacy, Graduate Programs in Pharmacy, Austin, TX 78712-1111. Offers health outcomes and pharmacy practice (PhD); health outcomes and pharmacy practice (MS); medicinal chemistry (PhD); pharmaceutics (PhD); pharmacology and toxicology (PhD); pharmacotherapy (MS, PhD); translational science (PhD). PhD in translational science offered jointly with The University of Texas Health Science Center at San Antonio and The University of Texas at San Antonio. *Degree requirements:* For master's, thesis; for doctorate, thesis/dissertation. *Entrance requirements:* For master's and doctorate, GRE General Test. Electronic applications accepted. *Faculty research:* Synthetic medical chemistry, synthetic molecular biology, bio-organic chemistry, pharmacoeconomics, pharmacy practice.

University of the Sciences, College of Graduate Studies, Program in Chemistry, Biochemistry and Pharmacognosy, Philadelphia, PA 19104-4495. Offers biochemistry (MS, PhD); chemistry (MS, PhD); pharmacognosy (MS, PhD). Part-time programs available. *Faculty:* 10 full-time (1 woman), 1 part-time/adjunct (0 women). *Students:* 30 full-time (15 women), 15 part-time (10 women); includes 7 minority (4 Black or African American, non-Hispanic/Latino; 3 Asian, non-Hispanic/Latino), 6 international. Average age 28. 52 applicants, 83% accepted, 9 enrolled. In 2013, 4 master's, 2 doctorates awarded. *Degree requirements:* For master's, thesis, qualifying exams; for doctorate, comprehensive exam, thesis/dissertation, qualifying exams. *Entrance requirements:* For master's and doctorate, GRE General Test, GRE Subject Test. Additional exam requirements/recommendations for international students: Required—TOEFL, TWE. *Application deadline:* For fall admission, 5/1 for international students; for winter admission, 10/1 for international students; for spring admission, 3/1 for international students. Applications are processed on a rolling basis. Application fee: $50. *Expenses:* Contact institution. *Financial support:* In 2013–14, 17 students received support, including 1 fellowship with full tuition reimbursement available, 2 research assistantships with full tuition reimbursements available (averaging $13,884 per year), 11 teaching assistantships with full tuition reimbursements available (averaging $18,836 per year); institutionally sponsored loans, scholarships/grants, and tuition waivers (full) also available. Financial award application deadline: 5/1. *Faculty research:* Organic and medicinal synthesis, mass spectroscopy use in protein analysis, study of analogues of taxol, cholesteryl esters. *Unit head:* Dr. Shenaz Tejani-Butt, Associate Dean, Graduate Studies, E-mail: graduate@usciences.edu. *Application contact:* Christopher Miciek, Associate Director, Graduate Admissions, 215-596-8597, E-mail: c.miciek@usciences.edu.

The University of Toledo, College of Graduate Studies, College of Pharmacy and Pharmaceutical Sciences, Program in Medicinal and Biological Chemistry, Toledo, OH 43606-3390. Offers MS, PhD. Terminal master's awarded for partial completion of doctoral program. *Degree requirements:* For master's, thesis; for doctorate, thesis/dissertation. *Entrance requirements:* For master's and doctorate, GRE General Test. Additional exam requirements/recommendations for international students: Required—TOEFL (minimum score 550 paper-based; 80 iBT). Electronic applications accepted. *Faculty research:* Neuroscience, molecular modeling, immunotoxicology, organic synthesis, peptide biochemistry.

University of Utah, Graduate School, College of Pharmacy, Department of Medicinal Chemistry, Salt Lake City, UT 84112-5820. Offers MS, PhD. *Faculty:* 7 full-time (0 women), 4 part-time/adjunct (2 women). *Students:* 11 full-time (4 women); includes 2 minority (1 Asian, non-Hispanic/Latino; 1 Hispanic/Latino), 4 international. Average age 29. 9 applicants, 11% accepted, 1 enrolled. In 2013, 1 doctorate awarded. *Degree requirements:* For doctorate, thesis/dissertation. *Entrance requirements:* For doctorate, GRE, minimum GPA of 3.0. Additional exam requirements/recommendations for international students: Required—TOEFL (minimum score 550 paper-based; 80 iBT), IELTS (minimum score 6.5). *Application deadline:* For fall admission, 12/15 for domestic and international students. Application fee: $55 ($65 for international students). Electronic applications accepted. *Expenses:* Tuition, state resident: full-time $5259. Tuition, nonresident: full-time $18,569. *Required fees:* $841. Tuition and fees vary according to course load. *Financial support:* In 2013–14, 11 students received support, including fellowships with full tuition reimbursements available (averaging $25,000 per year), research assistantships with full tuition reimbursements available (averaging $25,000 per year); health care benefits, tuition waivers (full), and unspecified assistantships also available. *Faculty research:* Anticancer and anti-infective drug discovery, assays for high-throughput screening, neuroactive peptides, bioinorganic chemistry, structure-based drug design and modeling. *Total annual research expenditures:* $3.4 million. *Unit head:* Dr. Darrell R. Davis, Chair, 801-581-7063, Fax: 801-581-7087, E-mail: darrell.davis@utah.edu. *Application contact:* Dr. Thomas E. Cheatham, Director of Graduate Studies, 801-587-9652, Fax: 801-581-7087, E-mail: tom.cheatham@pharm.utah.edu.
Website: http://www.pharmacy.utah.edu/medchem/

University of Utah, Graduate School, College of Pharmacy, Department of Pharmaceutics and Pharmaceutical Chemistry, Salt Lake City, UT 84112. Offers MS, PhD. *Faculty:* 5 full-time (1 woman), 8 part-time/adjunct (2 women). *Students:* 20 full-time (9 women), 6 part-time (5 women); includes 2 minority (both Asian, non-Hispanic/Latino), 17 international. Average age 28. 68 applicants, 4% accepted, 2 enrolled. In 2013, 5 doctorates awarded. Terminal master's awarded for partial completion of doctoral program. *Degree requirements:* For master's, thesis; for doctorate, comprehensive exam, thesis/dissertation, peer-reviewed scientific publications and oral presentations. *Entrance requirements:* For master's and doctorate, GRE. Additional exam requirements/recommendations for international students: Required—TOEFL (minimum score 550 paper-based). *Application deadline:* For fall admission, 12/1 priority date for domestic and international students. Applications are processed on a rolling basis. Application fee: $55 ($65 for international students). Electronic applications accepted. *Expenses:* Tuition, state resident: full-time $5259. Tuition, nonresident: full-time $18,569. *Required fees:* $841. Tuition and fees vary according to course load. *Financial support:* In 2013–14, 26 students received support, including 26 research assistantships (averaging $25,000 per year); scholarships/grants, health care benefits, tuition waivers (full), and unspecified assistantships also available. *Faculty research:* Delivery of therapeutic genes, trafficking mechanisms for drugs within cells, combination devices and local drug release from implants, anti-cancer polymer-based therapeutics and vaccines, nanotechnology for drug carriers. *Total annual research expenditures:* $1.8 million. *Unit head:* Dr. David W. Grainger, Chairperson, 801-581-7831, Fax: 801-581-3674, E-mail: david.grainger@utah.edu. *Application contact:* Office of Admissions, 801-581-7281, Fax: 801-585-3034, E-mail: admissionweb_grad@saff.utah.edu.
Website: http://www.pharmacy.utah.edu/pharmaceutics/

University of Washington, School of Pharmacy, Department of Medicinal Chemistry, Seattle, WA 98195. Offers PhD. *Faculty:* 8 full-time (1 woman). *Students:* 22 full-time (9 women); includes 8 minority (1 Black or African American, non-Hispanic/Latino; 1 American Indian or Alaska Native, non-Hispanic/Latino; 4 Asian, non-Hispanic/Latino; 2 Hispanic/Latino), 3 international. 46 applicants, 15% accepted, 4 enrolled. In 2013, 6 doctorates awarded. *Degree requirements:* For doctorate, thesis/dissertation. *Entrance requirements:* For doctorate, GRE General Test, minimum GPA of 3.0, 3 letters of recommendation, statement of purpose, transcripts, resume. Additional exam requirements/recommendations for international students: Required—TOEFL. *Application deadline:* For fall admission, 12/15 for domestic and international students. Application fee: $85. Electronic applications accepted. *Financial support:* Fellowships, research assistantships, Federal Work-Study, and institutionally sponsored loans available. *Faculty research:* Chemical and molecular aspects of drug action, metabolism and drug toxicity, theoretical studies on protein folding, nuclear magnetic resonance (NMR) of macromolecules and biomedical mass spectrometry. *Unit head:* Dr. Allan E. Rettie, Chairman, 206-685-0615, E-mail: rettie@uw.edu. *Application contact:* Meg Running, Graduate Program Assistant, 206-543-2224, E-mail: medchem@uw.edu.
Website: http://sop.washington.edu/medchem

Virginia Commonwealth University, Medical College of Virginia-Professional Programs, School of Pharmacy, Department of Pharmaceutics, Richmond, VA 23284-9005. Offers medicinal chemistry (MS); pharmaceutical sciences (PhD); pharmaceutics (MS); pharmacotherapy and pharmacy administration (MS). Terminal master's awarded for partial completion of doctoral program. *Degree requirements:* For master's, thesis; for doctorate, thesis/dissertation. *Entrance requirements:* For master's and doctorate, GRE General Test. Additional exam requirements/recommendations for international students: Required—TOEFL. Electronic applications accepted. *Faculty research:* Drug delivery systems, drug development.

Wayne State University, Eugene Applebaum College of Pharmacy and Health Sciences, Department of Pharmaceutical Sciences, Detroit, MI 48202. Offers medicinal chemistry (MS, PhD); pharmaceutics (MS, PhD); pharmacology/toxicology (MS, PhD). *Accreditation:* ACPE (one or more programs are accredited). Part-time programs available. *Faculty:* 17 full-time (3 women). *Students:* 33 full-time (15 women), 2 part-time (1 woman); includes 3 minority (1 American Indian or Alaska Native, non-Hispanic/Latino; 2 Asian, non-Hispanic/Latino), 29 international. Average age 25. 205 applicants, 8% accepted, 9 enrolled. In 2013, 1 master's, 3 doctorates awarded. *Degree requirements:* For master's, thesis; for doctorate, thesis/dissertation. *Entrance requirements:* For master's, GRE General Test, admission to the Graduate School, bachelor's degree, three letters of recommendation, personal statement; for doctorate, GRE General Test, admission to the Graduate School; bachelor's or master's degree in one of the behavioral, biological, pharmaceutical or physical sciences; minimum undergraduate GPA of 3.0; three letters of recommendation. Additional exam requirements/recommendations for international students: Required—TOEFL (minimum score 550 paper-based; 79 iBT), Michigan English Language Assessment Battery (minimum score 85); Recommended—IELTS (minimum score 6.5), TWE (minimum score 5.5). *Application deadline:* For fall admission, 3/1 for domestic and international students. Application fee: $0. Electronic applications accepted. *Expenses:* Contact institution. *Financial support:* In 2013–14, 13 students received support, including 2 fellowships with tuition reimbursements available (averaging $24,272 per year), 11 research assistantships with full tuition reimbursements available (averaging $24,565 per year); scholarships/grants, health care benefits, and unspecified assistantships also available. Financial award application deadline: 3/31; financial award applicants required to submit FAFSA. *Faculty research:* Mechanisms of resistance of bacteria to anti-microbial agents, drug metabolism and disposition in children, treatment strategies for stroke/neurovascular disease, prevalence and treatment of diabetes in Arab-Americans, ethnic variability in development of osteoporosis. *Unit head:* Dr. George Corcoran, Chair and Professor, 313-577-1737, E-mail: corcoran@wayne.edu. *Application contact:* 313-577-1047, E-mail: pscgrad@wayne.edu.
Website: http://www.cphs.wayne.edu/psc/index.php

West Virginia University, School of Pharmacy, Program in Pharmaceutical and Pharmacological Sciences, Morgantown, WV 26506. Offers administrative pharmacy (PhD); behavioral pharmacy (MS, PhD); biopharmaceutics/pharmacokinetics (MS, PhD); industrial pharmacy (MS); medicinal chemistry (MS, PhD); pharmaceutical chemistry (MS, PhD); pharmaceutics (MS, PhD); pharmacology and toxicology (MS); pharmacy (MS); pharmacy administration (MS). Part-time programs available. Terminal master's awarded for partial completion of doctoral program. *Degree requirements:* For master's, thesis; for doctorate, one foreign language, comprehensive exam, thesis/dissertation. *Entrance requirements:* For master's and doctorate, GRE General Test, minimum GPA of 2.75. Additional exam requirements/recommendations for international students: Required—TOEFL; Recommended—TWE. Electronic applications accepted. *Expenses:* Contact institution. *Faculty research:* Pharmaceutics, medicinal chemistry, biopharmaceutics/pharmacokinetics, health outcomes research.

Pharmaceutical Administration

Columbia University, Graduate School of Business, MBA Program, New York, NY 10027. Offers accounting (MBA); decision, risk, and operations (MBA); entrepreneurship (MBA); finance and economics (MBA); healthcare and pharmaceutical management (MBA); human resource management (MBA); international business (MBA); leadership and ethics (MBA); management (MBA); marketing (MBA); media (MBA); private equity (MBA); real estate (MBA); social enterprise (MBA); value investing (MBA); DDS/MBA; JD/MBA; MBA/MIA; MBA/MPH; MBA/MS; MD/MBA. *Entrance requirements:* For master's, GMAT, 2 letters of recommendation. Additional exam requirements/ recommendations for international students: Required—TOEFL. Electronic applications accepted. *Expenses:* Contact institution. *Faculty research:* Human decision making and behavioral research; real estate market and mortgage defaults; financial crisis and corporate governance; international business; security analysis and accounting.

Duquesne University, Mylan School of Pharmacy, Graduate School of Pharmaceutical Sciences, Program in Pharmaceutical Administration, Pittsburgh, PA 15282-0001. Offers pharmacy administration (MS). *Faculty:* 4 full-time (1 woman). *Students:* 6 full-time (3 women), 4 international. Average age 27. 27 applicants, 7% accepted, 2 enrolled. In 2013, 2 master's awarded. *Degree requirements:* For master's, thesis. *Entrance requirements:* For master's, GRE General Test. Additional exam requirements/ recommendations for international students: Required—TOEFL or IELTS (minimum score 7). *Application deadline:* For fall admission, 2/1 priority date for domestic and international students. Applications are processed on a rolling basis. Application fee: $50. Electronic applications accepted. *Expenses: Tuition:* Full-time $18,162; part-time $1009 per credit. *Required fees:* $1728; $96 per credit. Tuition and fees vary according to program. *Financial support:* In 2013–14, 5 students received support, including 5 teaching assistantships with full tuition reimbursements available. *Unit head:* Dr. Khalid Kamal, Head, 412-396-1926. *Application contact:* Information Contact, 412-396-1172, E-mail: gsps-adm@duq.edu.
Website: http://www.duq.edu/academics/schools/pharmacy/graduate-school-of-pharmaceutical-sciences

Emmanuel College, Graduate Studies, Graduate Programs in Management, Boston, MA 02115. Offers biopharmaceutical leadership (MSM, Graduate Certificate); human resource management (MSM, Graduate Certificate); management (MSM); management and leadership (Graduate Certificate); research administration (MSM, Graduate Certificate). Part-time and evening/weekend programs available. Postbaccalaureate distance learning degree programs offered (no on-campus study). *Faculty:* 1 (woman) full-time, 41 part-time/adjunct (15 women). *Students:* 5 full-time (4 women), 152 part-time (123 women); includes 49 minority (31 Black or African American, non-Hispanic/ Latino; 1 American Indian or Alaska Native, non-Hispanic/Latino; 4 Asian, non-Hispanic/ Latino; 13 Hispanic/Latino). Average age 36. In 2013, 82 master's, 4 other advanced degrees awarded. *Degree requirements:* For master's, thesis or alternative, 36 credits, including 6-credit capstone project. *Entrance requirements:* For master's and Graduate Certificate, transcripts from all regionally-accredited institutions attended (showing proof of bachelor's degree completion), 2 letters of recommendation, essay, resume, interview. Additional exam requirements/recommendations for international students: Required—TOEFL (minimum score 600 paper-based; 106 iBT) or IELTS (minimum score 6.5). *Application deadline:* For fall admission, 7/31 priority date for domestic students; for spring admission, 11/30 priority date for domestic students. Applications are processed on a rolling basis. Application fee: $0. Electronic applications accepted. *Financial support:* Applicants required to submit FAFSA. *Unit head:* Sandy Robbins, Dean of Enrollment, 617-735-9700, Fax: 617-507-0434, E-mail: graduatestudies@ emmanuel.edu. *Application contact:* Enrollment Counselor, 617-735-9700, Fax: 617-507-0434, E-mail: graduatestudies@emmanuel.edu.
Website: http://www.emmanuel.edu/graduate-studies-nursing/academics/ management.html

Fairleigh Dickinson University, Metropolitan Campus, Silberman College of Business, Program in Pharmaceutical Studies, Teaneck, NJ 07666-1914. Offers chemical studies (Certificate); pharmaceutical studies (MBA, Certificate).

Florida Agricultural and Mechanical University, Division of Graduate Studies, Research, and Continuing Education, College of Pharmacy and Pharmaceutical Sciences, Graduate Programs in Pharmaceutical Sciences, Tallahassee, FL 32307-3200. Offers environmental toxicology (PhD); medicinal chemistry (MS, PhD); pharmaceutics (MS, PhD); pharmacology/toxicology (MS, PhD); pharmacy administration (MS). *Accreditation:* CEPH. *Degree requirements:* For master's, comprehensive exam, thesis, publishable paper; for doctorate, comprehensive exam, thesis/dissertation, publishable paper. *Entrance requirements:* For master's and doctorate, GRE General Test, minimum GPA of 3.0 in last 60 hours. Additional exam requirements/recommendations for international students: Required—TOEFL. *Faculty research:* Anticancer agents, anti-inflammatory drugs, chronopharmacology, neuroendocrinology, microbiology.

Idaho State University, Office of Graduate Studies, College of Pharmacy, Department of Pharmacy Practice and Administrative Sciences, Pocatello, ID 83209-8333. Offers pharmacy (Pharm D); pharmacy administration (MS, PhD). *Accreditation:* ACPE (one or more programs are accredited). Part-time programs available. *Degree requirements:* For master's, one foreign language, comprehensive exam, thesis, thesis research, speech and technical writing classes; for doctorate, comprehensive exam, thesis/dissertation, oral and written exams, speech and technical writing classes. *Entrance requirements:* For master's, GRE General Test, minimum GPA of 3.0, 3 letters of recommendation; for doctorate, GRE General Test, BS in pharmacy or related field, minimum GPA of 3.0, 3 letters of recommendation. Additional exam requirements/recommendations for international students: Required—TOEFL (minimum score 550 paper-based; 80 iBT). Electronic applications accepted. *Expenses:* Contact institution. *Faculty research:* Pharmaceutical care outcomes, drug use review, pharmacoeconomics.

Long Island University–LIU Brooklyn, Arnold and Marie Schwartz College of Pharmacy and Health Sciences, Graduate Programs in Pharmacy, Division of Social and Administrative Sciences, Brooklyn, NY 11201-8423. Offers drug regulatory affairs (MS); pharmacy administration (MS). Part-time and evening/weekend programs available. *Degree requirements:* For master's, thesis optional. *Entrance requirements:* For master's, minimum GPA of 3.0.

New Jersey Institute of Technology, Newark College of Engineering, Newark, NJ 07102. Offers biomedical engineering (MS, PhD); chemical engineering (MS, PhD); computer engineering (MS, PhD); electrical engineering (MS, PhD); engineering management (MS); healthcare systems management (MS); industrial engineering (MS, PhD); Internet engineering (MS); manufacturing engineering (MS); mechanical engineering (MS, PhD); occupational safety and health engineering (MS); pharmaceutical bioprocessing (MS); pharmaceutical engineering (MS); pharmaceutical systems management (MS); power and energy systems (MS); telecommunications (MS); transportation (MS, PhD). Part-time and evening/weekend programs available. *Faculty:* 133 full-time (18 women), 101 part-time/adjunct (14 women). *Students:* 823 full-time (222 women), 535 part-time (130 women); includes 361 minority (92 Black or African American, non-Hispanic/Latino; 4 American Indian or Alaska Native, non-Hispanic/Latino; 142 Asian, non-Hispanic/Latino; 123 Hispanic/Latino), 605 international. Average age 29. 2,800 applicants, 68% accepted, 523 enrolled. In 2013, 471 master's, 32 doctorates awarded. Terminal master's awarded for partial completion of doctoral program. *Degree requirements:* For master's, thesis optional; for doctorate, thesis/dissertation. *Entrance requirements:* For master's, GRE General Test; for doctorate, GRE General Test, minimum graduate GPA of 3.5. Additional exam requirements/recommendations for international students: Required—TOEFL (minimum score 550 paper-based; 79 iBT). *Application deadline:* For fall admission, 6/1 priority date for domestic students, 5/1 priority date for international students; for spring admission, 11/15 priority date for domestic and international students. Applications are processed on a rolling basis. Application fee: $65. Electronic applications accepted. *Expenses:* Tuition, state resident: full-time $17,384; part-time $945 per credit. Tuition, nonresident: full-time $25,404; part-time $1341 per credit. *Required fees:* $2396; $118 per credit. *Financial support:* Fellowships with full and partial tuition reimbursements, research assistantships with full and partial tuition reimbursements, and teaching assistantships with full and partial tuition reimbursements available. Financial award application deadline: 1/15. *Total annual research expenditures:* $16 million. *Unit head:* Dr. Basil Baltzis, Dean, 973-596-3000, E-mail: sunil.saigal@njit.edu. *Application contact:* Stephen Eck, Director of Admissions, 973-596-3300, Fax: 973-596-3461, E-mail: admissions@njit.edu.
Website: http://engineering.njit.edu/

Northeast Ohio Medical University, College of Graduate Studies, Rootstown, OH 44272-0095. Offers bioethics (Certificate); health-system pharmacy administration (MS); integrated pharmaceutical medicine (MS, PhD); public health (MS). *Faculty:* 80 part-time/adjunct (26 women). *Students:* 38 full-time (21 women); includes 4 minority (3 Asian, non-Hispanic/Latino; 1 Hispanic/Latino). Average age 28. 45 applicants, 84% accepted, 38 enrolled. In 2013, 9 master's, 1 doctorate awarded. *Application deadline:* For fall admission, 9/1 priority date for domestic students; for winter admission, 1/5 priority date for domestic students. Applications are processed on a rolling basis. Application fee: $45. Electronic applications accepted. Full-time tuition and fees vary according to program. Part-time tuition and fees vary according to degree level. *Unit head:* Dr. Walter E. Horton, Jr., Dean of the College of Graduate Studies. *Application contact:* Luke Gloeckner, Associate Director for Enrollment Services and Registration, 330-325-6274, E-mail: lgloeckner@gmail.com.
Website: http://www.neomed.edu/academics/graduatestudies

The Ohio State University, College of Pharmacy, Columbus, OH 43210. Offers MS, PhD, Pharm D, Pharm D/MBA, Pharm D/MPH. *Accreditation:* ACPE (one or more programs are accredited). Part-time programs available. *Faculty:* 44. *Students:* 561 full-time (336 women), 3 part-time (1 woman); includes 136 minority (20 Black or African American, non-Hispanic/Latino; 1 American Indian or Alaska Native, non-Hispanic/ Latino; 97 Asian, non-Hispanic/Latino; 14 Hispanic/Latino; 4 Two or more races, non-Hispanic/Latino), 56 international. Average age 25. In 2013, 12 master's, 133 doctorates awarded. *Degree requirements:* For doctorate, thesis/dissertation (for some programs). *Entrance requirements:* For master's, GRE General Test, minimum GPA of 3.0; for doctorate, GRE General Test; PCAT (for Pharm D), minimum GPA of 3.0. Additional exam requirements/recommendations for international students: Required—TOEFL (minimum score 600 paper-based; 100 iBT), Michigan English Language Assessment Battery (minimum score 84). *Application deadline:* For fall admission, 12/15 priority date for domestic students, 12/15 for international students. Application fee: $60 ($70 for international students). Electronic applications accepted. *Expenses:* Contact institution. *Financial support:* Fellowships with full tuition reimbursements, research assistantships with full tuition reimbursements, teaching assistantships with full tuition reimbursements, career-related internships or fieldwork, Federal Work-Study, institutionally sponsored loans, scholarships/grants, and traineeships available. *Unit head:* Dr. Henry J. Mann, Dean, 614-292-5711, Fax: 614-292-2588, E-mail: odmail@pharmacy.ohio-state.edu. *Application contact:* Mary Kivel, Graduate Program Coordinator, 614-292-6822, Fax: 614-292-2588, E-mail: gradprogram@pharmacy.ohio-state.edu.
Website: http://www.pharmacy.osu.edu

Purdue University, College of Pharmacy and Pharmacal Sciences and Graduate School, Graduate Programs in Pharmacy and Pharmacal Sciences, Department of Industrial and Physical Pharmacy, West Lafayette, IN 47907. Offers pharmaceutics (PhD); regulatory quality compliance (MS, Certificate). *Faculty:* 8 full-time (3 women), 35 part-time/adjunct (8 women). *Students:* 29 full-time (13 women), 27 part-time (21 women); includes 11 minority (2 Black or African American, non-Hispanic/Latino; 8 Asian, non-Hispanic/Latino; 1 Hispanic/Latino), 23 international. Average age 31. 86 applicants, 27% accepted, 13 enrolled. In 2013, 6 master's, 6 doctorates, 13 other advanced degrees awarded. *Degree requirements:* For doctorate, thesis/dissertation. *Entrance requirements:* For master's, minimum GPA of 3.0; for doctorate, GRE General Test, minimum GPA of 3.0. Additional exam requirements/recommendations for international students: Required—TOEFL (minimum score 580 paper-based; 77 iBT). *Application deadline:* For fall admission, 1/1 for domestic and international students. Applications are processed on a rolling basis. Application fee: $60 ($75 for international students). Electronic applications accepted. *Financial support:* Fellowships, research assistantships, teaching assistantships, and traineeships available. Support available to part-time students. Financial award applicants required to submit FAFSA. *Faculty research:* Controlled drug delivery systems, liposomes, antacids, coating technology. *Unit head:* Dr. Elizabeth Topp, Graduate Head, 765-496-7760, E-mail: topp@ purdue.edu. *Application contact:* Dr. Kenneth R. Morris, Graduate Committee Chair, 765-496-3387, E-mail: morris@pharmacy.purdue.edu.

St. John's University, College of Pharmacy and Health Sciences, Graduate Programs in Pharmaceutical Sciences, Program in Pharmacy Administration, Queens, NY 11439. Offers MS. Part-time and evening/weekend programs available. Postbaccalaureate distance learning degree programs offered (no on-campus study). *Students:* 21 full-time (8 women), 5 part-time (4 women); includes 4 minority (1 Black or African American, non-Hispanic/Latino; 3 Asian, non-Hispanic/Latino), 20 international. Average age 26. 51 applicants, 41% accepted, 2 enrolled. In 2013, 7 master's awarded. *Degree requirements:* For master's, comprehensive exam, thesis optional, one-year residency. *Entrance requirements:* For master's, GRE General Test, bachelor's degree in pharmacy, minimum GPA of 3.0, 2 letters of recommendation. Additional exam requirements/recommendations for international students: Required—TOEFL (minimum score 600 paper-based; 100 iBT), IELTS (minimum score 5.5). *Application deadline:* For fall admission, 3/1 priority date for domestic students, 5/1 priority date for international students; for spring admission, 11/1 priority date for domestic and international students.

Pharmaceutical Administration

Applications are processed on a rolling basis. Application fee: $70. Electronic applications accepted. *Expenses:* Contact institution. *Financial support:* Fellowships, research assistantships, and career-related internships or fieldwork available. Support available to part-time students. Financial award application deadline: 3/1; financial award applicants required to submit FAFSA. *Unit head:* Dr. Wenchen Wu, Chair, 718-990-6640, E-mail: wuw@stjohns.edu. *Application contact:* Robert Medrano, Director of Graduate Admissions, 718-990-1601, Fax: 718-990-5686, E-mail: gradhelp@stjohns.edu.
Website: http://www.stjohns.edu//academics/schools-and-colleges/college-pharmacy-and-health-sciences/programs-and-majors/pharmacy-administration-master-science

San Diego State University, Graduate and Research Affairs, College of Sciences, Program in Regulatory Affairs, San Diego, CA 92182. Offers MS. *Degree requirements:* For master's, thesis. *Entrance requirements:* For master's, GRE General Test, 3 letters of recommendation, employment/volunteer experience list. Additional exam requirements/recommendations for international students: Required—TOEFL. Electronic applications accepted.

Temple University, Fox School of Business, MBA Programs, Philadelphia, PA 19122-6096. Offers accounting (MBA); business management (MBA); financial management (MBA); healthcare and life sciences innovation (MBA); human resource management (MBA); international business (IMBA); IT management (MBA); marketing management (MBA); pharmaceutical management (MBA); strategic management (EMBA, MBA). EMBA offered in Philadelphia, PA and Tokyo, Japan. *Accreditation:* AACSB. Part-time and evening/weekend programs available. Postbaccalaureate distance learning degree programs offered (minimal on-campus study). *Entrance requirements:* For master's, GMAT, minimum undergraduate GPA of 3.0. Additional exam requirements/recommendations for international students: Required—TOEFL (minimum score 600 paper-based; 100 iBT), IELTS (minimum score 7.5).

University of Florida, Graduate School, College of Pharmacy and Graduate School, Graduate Programs in Pharmacy, Department of Pharmaceutical Outcomes and Policy, Gainesville, FL 32610. Offers medication therapy management (MSP); pharmaceutical outcomes and policy (MSP, PhD). Part-time programs available. Postbaccalaureate distance learning degree programs offered (minimal on-campus study). *Faculty:* 9 full-time (4 women), 5 part-time/adjunct (3 women). *Students:* 33 full-time (20 women), 142 part-time (88 women); includes 54 minority (26 Black or African American, non-Hispanic/Latino; 1 American Indian or Alaska Native, non-Hispanic/Latino; 19 Asian, non-Hispanic/Latino; 8 Hispanic/Latino), 20 international. Average age 39. 112 applicants, 53% accepted, 51 enrolled. In 2013, 78 master's, 4 doctorates awarded. *Degree requirements:* For doctorate, thesis/dissertation. *Entrance requirements:* For master's, GRE General Test, minimum GPA of 3.0; for doctorate, GRE General Test, minimum GPA of 3.0. Additional exam requirements/recommendations for international students: Required—TOEFL (minimum score 550 paper-based; 80 iBT), IELTS (minimum score 6). *Application deadline:* For fall admission, 1/15 priority date for domestic students. Applications are processed on a rolling basis. Application fee: $30. Electronic applications accepted. *Expenses:* Tuition, state resident: full-time $12,640. Tuition, nonresident: full-time $30,000. *Financial support:* In 2013–14, 18 students received support, including 2 fellowships (averaging $32,625 per year), 1 research assistantship (averaging $16,122 per year), 17 teaching assistantships (averaging $21,910 per year); tuition waivers (full) also available. Financial award applicants required to submit FAFSA. *Faculty research:* Pharmaceutical care, drug use systems, drug-related morbidity. *Unit head:* Richard Segal, PhD, Chair, 352-273-6265, Fax: 352-273-6270, E-mail: segal@cop.health.ufl.edu. *Application contact:* Almut Winterstein, PhD, Professor and Graduate Program Director, 352-273-6258, Fax: 352-273-6270, E-mail: almut@cop.ufl.edu.
Website: http://www.cop.ufl.edu/education/graduate-programs/pharmaceutical-outcomes-and-policy/

University of Georgia, College of Pharmacy, Department of Clinical and Administrative Pharmacy, Athens, GA 30602. Offers clinical and experimental therapeutics (PhD); pharmacy care administration (PhD).

University of Houston, College of Pharmacy, Houston, TX 77204. Offers pharmaceutics (MSPHR, PhD); pharmacology (MSPHR, PhD); pharmacy (Pharm D); pharmacy administration (MSPHR, PhD). *Accreditation:* ACPE. Part-time programs available. Terminal master's awarded for partial completion of doctoral program. *Entrance requirements:* For doctorate, PCAT (for Pharm D). Additional exam requirements/recommendations for international students: Required—TOEFL. Electronic applications accepted. *Faculty research:* Drug screening and design, cardiovascular pharmacology, infectious disease, asthma research, herbal medicine.

University of Illinois at Chicago, College of Pharmacy and Graduate College, Graduate Programs in Pharmacy, Chicago, IL 60607-7128. Offers biopharmaceutical sciences (PhD); forensic science (MS), including forensic toxicology; medicinal chemistry (MS, PhD); pharmacognosy (MS, PhD); pharmacy administration (MS, PhD). *Faculty:* 81 full-time (31 women), 16 part-time/adjunct (3 women). *Students:* 122 full-time (62 women), 12 part-time (9 women); includes 23 minority (6 Black or African American, non-Hispanic/Latino; 15 Asian, non-Hispanic/Latino; 2 Hispanic/Latino), 68 international. Average age 27. 331 applicants, 18% accepted, 29 enrolled. In 2013, 12 master's, 22 doctorates awarded. Terminal master's awarded for partial completion of doctoral program. *Degree requirements:* For master's, variable foreign language requirement, thesis; for doctorate, variable foreign language requirement, thesis/dissertation. *Entrance requirements:* For master's and doctorate, GRE General Test. Additional exam requirements/recommendations for international students: Required—TOEFL. *Application deadline:* For fall admission, 2/1 for domestic students. Applications are processed on a rolling basis. Application fee: $40 ($50 for international students). Electronic applications accepted. *Expenses:* Contact institution. *Financial support:* In 2013–14, 122 students received support, including 2 fellowships with full tuition reimbursements available; research assistantships with full tuition reimbursements available, teaching assistantships with full tuition reimbursements available, career-related internships or fieldwork, Federal Work-Study, institutionally sponsored loans, traineeships, tuition waivers (full), and unspecified assistantships also available. Financial award application deadline: 3/1; financial award applicants required to submit FAFSA. *Unit head:* Janet P. Engle, Executive Associate Dean for Academic Affairs, 312-996-6212. *Application contact:* Jackie Perry, Graduate College Receptionist, 312-413-2550, Fax: 312-413-0185, E-mail: gradcoll@uic.edu.

University of Maryland, Baltimore, Graduate School, Graduate Programs in Pharmacy, Department of Pharmaceutical Health Service Research, Baltimore, MD 21201. Offers epidemiology (MS); pharmacy administration (PhD); Pharm D/PhD. *Degree requirements:* For doctorate, comprehensive exam, thesis/dissertation. *Entrance requirements:* For doctorate, GRE General Test. Additional exam requirements/recommendations for international students: Required—TOEFL, IELTS. Electronic applications accepted. *Faculty research:* Pharmacoeconomics, outcomes research, public health policy, drug therapy and aging.

University of Maryland, Baltimore, Graduate School, Graduate Programs in Pharmacy, Program in Regulatory Science, Baltimore, MD 21201. Offers MS.

University of Michigan, College of Pharmacy and Rackham Graduate School, Department of Social and Administrative Sciences, Ann Arbor, MI 48109. Offers PhD. *Students:* 9 full-time (6 women); includes 1 minority (Asian, non-Hispanic/Latino), 5 international. Average age 28. Terminal master's awarded for partial completion of doctoral program. *Degree requirements:* For doctorate, thesis/dissertation, oral defense of dissertation, preliminary exam. *Entrance requirements:* For doctorate, GRE. Additional exam requirements/recommendations for international students: Required—TOEFL (minimum score 560 paper-based; 84 iBT) or IELTS (minimum score 6.5). *Application deadline:* For fall admission, 2/1 priority date for domestic and international students. Applications are processed on a rolling basis. Application fee: $60 ($75 for international students). Electronic applications accepted. *Expenses:* Contact institution. *Financial support:* In 2013–14, 9 students received support, including 6 fellowships (averaging $46,107 per year), 2 research assistantships (averaging $46,107 per year), 1 teaching assistantship (averaging $46,107 per year); career-related internships or fieldwork, institutionally sponsored loans, scholarships/grants, traineeships, health care benefits, and unspecified assistantships also available. *Unit head:* Dr. James G. Stevenson, Chair, 734-763-6629, Fax: 734-763-4480, E-mail: jimsteve@med.umich.edu. *Application contact:* Antoinette Hopper, Student Services Program Coordinator, 734-615-6326, Fax: 734-763-4480, E-mail: acast@med.umich.edu.
Website: https://pharmacy.umich.edu/csas

University of Minnesota, Twin Cities Campus, College of Pharmacy and Graduate School, Graduate Programs in Pharmacy, Graduate Program in Social and Administrative Pharmacy, Minneapolis, MN 55455-0213. Offers MS, PhD. Part-time programs available. Terminal master's awarded for partial completion of doctoral program. *Degree requirements:* For master's, thesis (for some programs); for doctorate, thesis/dissertation. *Entrance requirements:* For master's, GRE General Test, BS in science; for doctorate, GRE General Test or Pharm D. Additional exam requirements/recommendations for international students: Required—TOEFL (minimum score 100 iBT). Electronic applications accepted. *Faculty research:* Pharmaceutical economics, pharmaceutical policy, pharmaceutical social/behavioral sciences.

University of Mississippi, Graduate School, School of Pharmacy, Graduate Programs in Pharmacy, University, MS 38677. Offers medicinal chemistry (PhD); pharmaceutical sciences (MS); pharmaceutics (PhD); pharmacognosy (PhD); pharmacology (PhD); pharmacy administration (PhD). *Faculty:* 41 full-time (17 women), 14 part-time/adjunct (7 women). *Students:* 81 full-time (27 women), 8 part-time (5 women); includes 4 minority (2 Black or African American, non-Hispanic/Latino; 2 Asian, non-Hispanic/Latino), 61 international. In 2013, 5 master's, 16 doctorates awarded. Application fee: $40. *Unit head:* Dr. David Allen, Dean, 662-915-7267, Fax: 662-915-5118, E-mail: sop@olemiss.edu. *Application contact:* Dr. Christy M. Wyandt, Associate Dean, 662-915-7474, Fax: 662-915-7577, E-mail: cwyandt@olemiss.edu.

University of Southern California, Graduate School, School of Pharmacy, Program in Healthcare Decision Analysis, Los Angeles, CA 90089. Offers MS. Part-time programs available. Postbaccalaureate distance learning degree programs offered (no on-campus study).

University of the Sciences, College of Graduate Studies, Program in Pharmaceutical Business, Philadelphia, PA 19104-4495. Offers MBA. Part-time and evening/weekend programs available. Postbaccalaureate distance learning degree programs offered (minimal on-campus study). *Faculty:* 4 full-time (1 woman), 15 part-time/adjunct (2 women). *Students:* 17 full-time (11 women), 33 part-time (14 women); includes 15 minority (5 Black or African American, non-Hispanic/Latino; 10 Asian, non-Hispanic/Latino), 1 international. Average age 31. In 2013, 11 master's awarded. *Entrance requirements:* Additional exam requirements/recommendations for international students: Required—TOEFL, TWE. *Application deadline:* For fall admission, 5/1 for international students; for winter admission, 10/1 for international students; for spring admission, 3/1 for international students. Applications are processed on a rolling basis. Application fee: $50. *Expenses:* Contact institution. *Financial support:* In 2013–14, 8 students received support. Tuition waivers (partial) available. *Unit head:* Dr. Shenaz Tejani-Butt, Associate Dean, Graduate Studies, 215-596-8597, E-mail: graduate@usciences.edu. *Application contact:* Christopher Miciek, Associate Director, Graduate Admissions, 215-596-8597, E-mail: c.miciek@usciences.edu.
Website: http://www.usip.edu/graduate/

University of the Sciences, College of Graduate Studies, Program in Pharmacy Administration, Philadelphia, PA 19104-4495. Offers MS. Part-time programs available. *Faculty:* 1 full-time (0 women). *Students:* 11 full-time (7 women), 9 part-time (7 women); includes 1 minority (Asian, non-Hispanic/Latino), 4 international. Average age 25. 117 applicants, 13% accepted, 5 enrolled. In 2013, 7 master's awarded. *Entrance requirements:* Additional exam requirements/recommendations for international students: Required—TOEFL, TWE. *Application deadline:* For fall admission, 5/1 for international students; for winter admission, 10/1 for international students; for spring admission, 3/1 for international students. Applications are processed on a rolling basis. Application fee: $50. *Expenses:* Contact institution. *Financial support:* In 2013–14, 8 students received support, including 1 research assistantship with full tuition reimbursement available; teaching assistantships, institutionally sponsored loans, traineeships, tuition waivers (partial), and unspecified assistantships also available. Financial award application deadline: 5/1. *Faculty research:* Cost-effect analysis, pharmaceutical economics, pharmaceutical care, marketing research, health communications. *Unit head:* Dr. Shenaz Tejani-Butt, Associate Dean, Graduate Studies, 215-596-8597, E-mail: graduate@usciences.edu. *Application contact:* Christopher Miciek, Associate Director, Graduate Studies, 215-596-8597, E-mail: c.miciek@usciences.edu.

The University of Toledo, College of Graduate Studies, College of Pharmacy and Pharmaceutical Sciences, Program in Pharmaceutical Sciences, Toledo, OH 43606-3390. Offers administrative pharmacy (MSPS); industrial pharmacy (MSPS); pharmacology toxicology (MSPS). *Degree requirements:* For master's, thesis. *Entrance requirements:* For master's, GRE General Test. Additional exam requirements/recommendations for international students: Required—TOEFL (minimum score 550 paper-based; 80 iBT). Electronic applications accepted.

University of Utah, Graduate School, College of Pharmacy, Department of Pharmacotherapy, Salt Lake City, UT 84112. Offers health system pharmacy administration (MS); outcomes research and health policy (PhD). *Faculty:* 5 full-time (3 women), 28 part-time/adjunct (17 women). *Students:* 7 full-time (4 women), 5 international. Average age 27. 26 applicants, 19% accepted, 2 enrolled. In 2013, 4 master's awarded. Terminal master's awarded for partial completion of doctoral program. *Degree requirements:* For master's, comprehensive exam, thesis or alternative, project; for doctorate, comprehensive exam, thesis/dissertation. *Entrance requirements:* For doctorate, GRE. Additional exam requirements/recommendations for international students: Required—TOEFL (minimum score 550 paper-based; 80 iBT). *Application deadline:* For fall admission, 1/10 for domestic students, 12/15 for international students. Application fee: $55 ($65 for international students). *Expenses:* Tuition, state resident: full-time $5259. Tuition, nonresident: full-time $18,569. *Required fees:* $841. Tuition and fees vary according to course load. *Financial support:* In 2013–14, 7 students received support, including 5 research assistantships with full tuition reimbursements available (averaging $21,400 per year); health care benefits and

unspecified assistantships also available. Financial award application deadline: 12/15. *Faculty research:* Outcomes in pharmacy, pharmacotherapy. *Total annual research expenditures:* $131,217. *Unit head:* Dr. Diana I. Brixner, Department Chair and Professor, 801-581-6731. *Application contact:* Sara Ray, Academic Program Manager, 801-581-5984, Fax: 801-585-6160, E-mail: sara.ray@pharm.utah.edu.
Website: http://www.pharmacy.utah.edu/pharmacotherapy/

University of West Florida, College of Professional Studies, Department of Research and Advanced Studies, Pensacola, FL 32514-5750. Offers administration (MSA), including acquisition and contract administration, biomedical/pharmaceutical, criminal justice administration, database administration, education leadership, healthcare administration, human performance technology, leadership, nursing administration, public administration, software engineering and administration; college student personnel administration (M Ed), including college personnel administration, guidance and counseling; curriculum and instruction (M Ed, Ed S); educational leadership (M Ed); middle and secondary level education and ESOL (M Ed). Part-time and evening/weekend programs available. *Entrance requirements:* For master's, GRE or MAT, official transcripts; minimum undergraduate GPA of 3.0; letter of intent; three letters of recommendation; resume. Additional exam requirements/recommendations for international students: Required—TOEFL (minimum score 550 paper-based).

University of Wisconsin–Madison, School of Pharmacy and Graduate School, Graduate Programs in Pharmacy, Madison, WI 53706-1380. Offers pharmaceutical sciences (PhD); social and administrative sciences in pharmacy (MS, PhD). Terminal master's awarded for partial completion of doctoral program. *Degree requirements:* For master's, thesis (for some programs); for doctorate, comprehensive exam (for some programs), thesis/dissertation. *Entrance requirements:* For master's and doctorate, GRE. Additional exam requirements/recommendations for international students: Required—TOEFL. Electronic applications accepted. *Expenses:* Contact institution.

Virginia Commonwealth University, Medical College of Virginia-Professional Programs, School of Pharmacy, Department of Pharmaceutics, Richmond, VA 23284-9005. Offers medicinal chemistry (MS); pharmaceutical sciences (PhD); pharmaceutics (MS); pharmacotherapy and pharmacy administration (MS). Terminal master's awarded for partial completion of doctoral program. *Degree requirements:* For master's, thesis; for doctorate, thesis/dissertation. *Entrance requirements:* For master's and doctorate, GRE General Test. Additional exam requirements/recommendations for international students: Required—TOEFL. Electronic applications accepted. *Faculty research:* Drug delivery systems, drug development.

West Virginia University, School of Pharmacy, Program in Pharmaceutical and Pharmacological Sciences, Morgantown, WV 26506. Offers administrative pharmacy (PhD); behavioral pharmacy (MS, PhD); biopharmaceutics/pharmacokinetics (MS, PhD); industrial pharmacy (MS); medicinal chemistry (MS, PhD); pharmaceutical chemistry (MS, PhD); pharmaceutics (MS, PhD); pharmacology and toxicology (MS); pharmacy (MS); pharmacy administration (MS). Part-time programs available. Terminal master's awarded for partial completion of doctoral program. *Degree requirements:* For master's, thesis; for doctorate, one foreign language, comprehensive exam, thesis/dissertation. *Entrance requirements:* For master's and doctorate, GRE General Test, minimum GPA of 2.75. Additional exam requirements/recommendations for international students: Required—TOEFL; Recommended—TWE. Electronic applications accepted. *Expenses:* Contact institution. *Faculty research:* Pharmaceutics, medicinal chemistry, biopharmaceutics/pharmacokinetics, health outcomes research.

Pharmaceutical Sciences

Albany College of Pharmacy and Health Sciences, School of Pharmacy and Pharmaceutical Sciences, Albany, NY 12208. Offers health outcomes research (MS); pharmaceutical sciences (MS), including pharmaceutics, pharmacology; pharmacy (Pharm D). *Accreditation:* ACPE. *Students:* 527 full-time (308 women), 15 part-time (10 women); includes 138 minority (19 Black or African American, non-Hispanic/Latino; 95 Asian, non-Hispanic/Latino; 13 Hispanic/Latino; 1 Native Hawaiian or other Pacific Islander, non-Hispanic/Latino; 10 Two or more races, non-Hispanic/Latino), 64 international. Average age 24. 1,209 applicants, 15% accepted, 78 enrolled. In 2013, 6 master's, 283 doctorates awarded. *Degree requirements:* For master's, thesis; for doctorate, practice experience. *Entrance requirements:* For master's, GRE, minimum GPA of 3.0; for doctorate, PCAT, minimum GPA of 2.5. Additional exam requirements/recommendations for international students: Required—TOEFL (minimum score 84 iBT). *Application deadline:* For fall admission, 3/1 for domestic and international students. Applications are processed on a rolling basis. Application fee: $75. Electronic applications accepted. *Financial support:* In 2013–14, 20 students received support. Federal Work-Study and scholarships/grants available. Support available to part-time students. Financial award application deadline: 3/1; financial award applicants required to submit FAFSA. *Faculty research:* Therapeutic use of drugs, pharmacokinetics, drug delivery and design. *Unit head:* Dr. Angela Dominelli, Dean, School of Pharmacy and Pharmaceutical Sciences, 518-694-7333. *Application contact:* Ann Bruno, Coordinator, Graduate Programs, 518-694-7130, E-mail: graduate@acphs.edu.
Website: http://www.acphs.edu/academics/schools-departments/school-pharmacy-pharmaceutical-sciences

Auburn University, Harrison School of Pharmacy and Graduate School, Graduate Program in Pharmacy, Auburn University, AL 36849. Offers pharmacal sciences (MS, PhD); pharmaceutical sciences (PhD); pharmacy care systems (MS, PhD). Part-time programs available. *Faculty:* 50 full-time (28 women), 1 (woman) part-time/adjunct. *Students:* 30 full-time (13 women), 5 part-time (2 women); includes 2 minority (both Asian, non-Hispanic/Latino), 24 international. Average age 28. 109 applicants, 11% accepted, 10 enrolled. In 2013, 5 master's, 2 doctorates awarded. *Degree requirements:* For master's, thesis; for doctorate, thesis/dissertation. *Entrance requirements:* For master's and doctorate, GRE General Test. *Application deadline:* For fall admission, 7/7 for domestic students; for spring admission, 11/24 for domestic students. Applications are processed on a rolling basis. Application fee: $50 ($60 for international students). Electronic applications accepted. *Expenses:* Tuition, state resident: full-time $8262; part-time $459 per credit hour. Tuition, nonresident: full-time $24,786; part-time $1377 per credit hour. Tuition and fees vary according to degree level and program. *Financial support:* Fellowships, research assistantships, and teaching assistantships available. *Faculty research:* Communications, facilities design, substance abuse. *Total annual research expenditures:* $600,000. *Unit head:* Dr. R. Lee Evans, Dean and Professor, Harrison School of Pharmacy, 334-844-8348, Fax: 334-844-8353. *Application contact:* Dr. George Flowers, Dean of the Graduate School, 334-844-2125.

Boston University, School of Medicine, Division of Graduate Medical Sciences, Department of Pharmacology and Experimental Therapeutics, Boston, MA 02118. Offers MA, PhD, MD/PhD. Terminal master's awarded for partial completion of doctoral program. *Degree requirements:* For master's, thesis; for doctorate, thesis/dissertation. *Application deadline:* For fall admission, 1/15 for domestic students; for spring admission, 10/15 for domestic students. *Expenses: Tuition:* Full-time $43,970; part-time $1374 per credit hour. *Required fees:* $60 per semester. Tuition and fees vary according to class time, course level and program. *Unit head:* Dr. David H. Farb, Chairman, 617-638-4300, Fax: 617-638-4329, E-mail: dfarb@bu.edu. *Application contact:* Dr. Carol T. Walsh, Graduate Director, 617-638-4326, Fax: 617-638-4329, E-mail: ctwalsh@bu.edu.
Website: http://www.bumc.bu.edu/busm-pm/

Butler University, College of Pharmacy and Health Sciences, Indianapolis, IN 46208-3485. Offers pharmaceutical science (MS, Pharm D); physician assistance studies (MS). *Accreditation:* ACPE (one or more programs are accredited). Part-time and evening/weekend programs available. *Faculty:* 6 full-time (2 women). *Students:* 296 full-time (196 women), 12 part-time (7 women); includes 24 minority (7 Black or African American, non-Hispanic/Latino; 1 American Indian or Alaska Native, non-Hispanic/Latino; 10 Asian, non-Hispanic/Latino; 4 Hispanic/Latino; 2 Two or more races, non-Hispanic/Latino), 11 international. Average age 24. 52 applicants, 6% accepted, 2 enrolled. In 2013, 50 master's awarded. *Degree requirements:* For master's, research paper or thesis. *Application deadline:* For fall admission, 8/1 priority date for domestic students; for spring admission, 12/15 for domestic students. Applications are processed on a rolling basis. Application fee: $35. Electronic applications accepted. *Expenses:* Contact institution. *Financial support:* Applicants required to submit FAFSA. *Unit head:* Dr. Mary Andritz, Dean, 317-940-8056, E-mail: mandritz@butler.edu. *Application contact:* Diane Dubord, Graduate Student Services Specialist, 317-940-8107, E-mail: ddubord@butler.edu.
Website: http://www.butler.edu/academics/graduate-cophs/

Campbell University, Graduate and Professional Programs, School of Pharmacy, Buies Creek, NC 27506. Offers clinical research (MS); pharmaceutical science (MS); pharmacy (Pharm D). *Accreditation:* ACPE. Part-time and evening/weekend programs available. *Entrance requirements:* For master's, MCAT, PCAT, GRE, bachelor's degree in health sciences or related field; for doctorate, PCAT. Additional exam requirements/recommendations for international students: Required—TOEFL (minimum score 550 paper-based; 79 iBT). Electronic applications accepted. *Expenses:* Contact institution. *Faculty research:* Immunology, medicinal chemistry, pharmaceutics, applied pharmacology.

Creighton University, School of Medicine and Graduate School, Graduate Programs in Medicine, Department of Pharmacology, Omaha, NE 68178-0001. Offers pharmaceutical sciences (MS); pharmacology (MS, PhD); Pharm D/MS. *Faculty:* 10 full-time (3 women). *Students:* 7 full-time (4 women); includes 1 minority (Asian, non-Hispanic/Latino), 2 international. Average age 25. 20 applicants, 10% accepted, 2 enrolled. In 2013, 1 doctorate awarded. Terminal master's awarded for partial completion of doctoral program. *Degree requirements:* For master's, comprehensive exam, thesis; for doctorate, comprehensive exam, thesis/dissertation, oral and written preliminary exams. *Entrance requirements:* For master's and doctorate, GRE General Test, minimum GPA of 3.0, undergraduate degree in sciences. Additional exam requirements/recommendations for international students: Required—TOEFL. *Application deadline:* For spring admission, 4/1 priority date for domestic and international students. Applications are processed on a rolling basis. Application fee: $35. Electronic applications accepted. *Expenses: Tuition:* Full-time $13,608; part-time $756 per credit hour. *Required fees:* $149 per semester. Tuition and fees vary according to course load, campus/location, program, reciprocity agreements and student's religious affiliation. *Financial support:* In 2013–14, 6 fellowships with full tuition reimbursements (averaging $23,868 per year) were awarded; institutionally sponsored loans and tuition waivers (full and partial) also available. Financial award application deadline: 4/1. *Faculty research:* Pharmacology secretion, cardiovascular-renal pharmacology, adrenergic receptors, signal transduction, genetic regulation of receptors. *Total annual research expenditures:* $2.3 million. *Unit head:* Dr. Thomas F. Murray, Chair, 402-280-2983, Fax: 402-280-2142, E-mail: tfmurray@creighton.edu. *Application contact:* Dr. Margaret A. Scofield, Associate Professor, 402-280-2245, Fax: 402-280-2142, E-mail: mscof@creighton.edu.
Website: http://medschool.creighton.edu/medicine/departments/pharmacology/

Creighton University, School of Pharmacy and Health Professions and Department of Pharmacology, Program in Pharmaceutical Sciences, Omaha, NE 68178-0001. Offers MS, Pharm D/MS. *Degree requirements:* For master's, thesis. *Entrance requirements:* For master's, GRE, three recommendations. Additional exam requirements/recommendations for international students: Required—TOEFL (minimum score 550 paper-based; 80 iBT). Electronic applications accepted. *Expenses: Tuition:* Full-time $13,608; part-time $756 per credit hour. *Required fees:* $149 per semester. Tuition and fees vary according to course load, campus/location, program, reciprocity agreements and student's religious affiliation.

Dartmouth College, Program in Experimental and Molecular Medicine, Molecular Pharmacology, Toxicology and Experimental Therapeutics Track, Hanover, NH 03755. Offers PhD.

Drexel University, College of Medicine, Biomedical Graduate Programs, Program in Drug Discovery and Development, Philadelphia, PA 19104-2875. Offers MS. *Degree requirements:* For master's, thesis.

Duquesne University, Mylan School of Pharmacy, Graduate School of Pharmaceutical Sciences, Program in Pharmaceutics, Pittsburgh, PA 15282-0001. Offers MS, PhD, MBA/MS. *Faculty:* 6 full-time (1 woman), 1 part-time/adjunct (0 women). *Students:* 21 full-time (7 women), 1 part-time (0 women); includes 1 minority (Asian, non-Hispanic/Latino), 15 international. Average age 27. 71 applicants, 6% accepted, 3 enrolled. In 2013, 1 master's, 1 doctorate awarded. *Degree requirements:* For master's, thesis; for doctorate, comprehensive exam, thesis/dissertation. *Entrance requirements:* For master's and doctorate, GRE General Test. Additional exam requirements/recommendations for international students: Required—TOEFL or IELTS (minimum score 7). *Application deadline:* For fall admission, 2/1 priority date for domestic and international students; for spring admission, 10/1 priority date for domestic and international students. Applications are processed on a rolling basis. Application fee: $50. Electronic applications accepted. *Expenses: Tuition:* Full-time $18,162; part-time $1009 per credit. *Required fees:* $1728; $96 per credit. Tuition and fees vary according

to program. *Financial support:* In 2013–14, 20 students received support, including 1 research assistantship with full tuition reimbursement available, 19 teaching assistantships with full tuition reimbursements available; unspecified assistantships also available. *Unit head:* Dr. Wilson S. Meng, Head, 412-396-6366. *Application contact:* Information Contact, 412-396-1172, E-mail: gsps-adm@duq.edu.
Website: http://www.duq.edu/academics/schools/pharmacy/graduate-school-of-pharmaceutical-sciences

East Tennessee State University, James H. Quillen College of Medicine, Department of Biomedical Sciences, Johnson City, TN 37614. Offers anatomy (PhD); biochemistry (PhD); microbiology (PhD); pharmaceutical sciences (PhD); pharmacology (PhD); physiology (PhD); quantitative biosciences (PhD). *Faculty:* 43 full-time (11 women), 1 (woman) part-time/adjunct. *Students:* 31 full-time (17 women), 4 part-time (1 woman); includes 6 minority (2 Black or African American, non-Hispanic/Latino; 3 Asian, non-Hispanic/Latino; 1 Hispanic/Latino), 9 international. Average age 29. 53 applicants, 17% accepted, 8 enrolled. In 2013, 6 doctorates awarded. *Degree requirements:* For doctorate, thesis/dissertation, comprehensive qualifying exam. *Entrance requirements:* For doctorate, GRE General Test, GRE Subject Test. Additional exam requirements/recommendations for international students: Required—TOEFL (minimum score 550 paper-based; 79 iBT). *Application deadline:* For fall admission, 3/15 priority date for domestic students, 3/1 priority date for international students. Application fee: $35 ($45 for international students). Electronic applications accepted. *Expenses:* Contact institution. *Financial support:* In 2013–14, 30 students received support, including 30 research assistantships with full tuition reimbursements available (averaging $19,000 per year); career-related internships or fieldwork, institutionally sponsored loans, scholarships/grants, and unspecified assistantships also available. Financial award application deadline: 7/1; financial award applicants required to submit FAFSA. *Faculty research:* Cardiovascular, infectious disease, neurosciences, cancer, immunology. *Unit head:* Dr. Mitchell E. Robinson, Associate Dean/Program Director, 423-439-2031, Fax: 423-439-2140, E-mail: robinson@etsu.edu. *Application contact:* Shella Bennett, Graduate Specialist, 423-439-4708, Fax: 423-439-5624, E-mail: bennetsg@etsu.edu.
Website: http://www.etsu.edu/com/dbms/

Florida Agricultural and Mechanical University, Division of Graduate Studies, Research, and Continuing Education, College of Pharmacy and Pharmaceutical Sciences, Graduate Programs in Pharmaceutical Sciences, Tallahassee, FL 32307-3200. Offers environmental toxicology (PhD); medicinal chemistry (MS, PhD); pharmaceutics (MS, PhD); pharmacology/toxicology (MS, PhD); pharmacy administration (MS). *Accreditation:* CEPH. *Degree requirements:* For master's, comprehensive exam, thesis, publishable paper; for doctorate, comprehensive exam, thesis/dissertation, publishable paper. *Entrance requirements:* For master's and doctorate, GRE General Test, minimum GPA of 3.0 in last 60 hours. Additional exam requirements/recommendations for international students: Required—TOEFL. *Faculty research:* Anticancer agents, anti-inflammatory drugs, chronopharmacology, neuroendocrinology, microbiology.

Idaho State University, Office of Graduate Studies, College of Pharmacy, Department of Biomedical and Pharmaceutical Sciences, Pocatello, ID 83209-8334. Offers biopharmaceutical analysis (PhD); drug delivery (PhD); medicinal chemistry (PhD); pharmaceutical sciences (MS); pharmacology (PhD). Part-time programs available. *Degree requirements:* For master's, one foreign language, comprehensive exam, thesis, thesis research, classes in speech and technical writing; for doctorate, comprehensive exam, thesis/dissertation, written and oral exams, classes in speech and technical writing. *Entrance requirements:* For master's, GRE General Test, minimum GPA of 3.0, 3 letters of recommendation; for doctorate, GRE General Test, BS in pharmacy or related field, minimum GPA of 3.0, 3 letters of recommendation. Additional exam requirements/recommendations for international students: Required—TOEFL (minimum score 550 paper-based; 80 iBT). Electronic applications accepted. *Expenses:* Contact institution. *Faculty research:* Metabolic toxicity of heavy metals, neuroendocrine pharmacology, cardiovascular pharmacology, cancer biology, immunopharmacology.

Johns Hopkins University, Zanvyl Krieger School of Arts and Sciences, Advanced Academic Programs, Program in Regulatory Science, Washington, DC 20036. Offers MS. Part-time and evening/weekend programs available. Postbaccalaureate distance learning degree programs offered (no on-campus study). *Faculty:* 8 full-time (4 women), 99 part-time/adjunct (21 women). *Students:* 15 full-time (0 women), 59 part-time (44 women); includes 26 minority (10 Black or African American, non-Hispanic/Latino; 14 Asian, non-Hispanic/Latino; 1 Hispanic/Latino; 1 Two or more races, non-Hispanic/Latino), 5 international. Average age 37. 25 applicants, 96% accepted, 30 enrolled. In 2013, 59 master's awarded. *Degree requirements:* For master's, practicum. *Entrance requirements:* For master's, undergraduate degree in the life sciences or engineering with minimum GPA of 3.0 from a four-year college. Additional exam requirements/recommendations for international students: Required—TOEFL (minimum score 100 iBT). Application fee: $75. *Financial support:* Scholarships/grants available. Financial award applicants required to submit FAFSA. *Unit head:* Kirsty Gharavi, Director, 301-294-7162, E-mail: kgharavi@jhu.edu. *Application contact:* Melissa Edwards, Admissions Manager, 202-452-1941, Fax: 202-452-1970, E-mail: aapadmissions@jhu.edu.
Website: http://advanced.jhu.edu/academics/graduate-degree-programs/regulatory-science/

Long Island University–Hudson at Rockland, Graduate School, Program in Pharmaceutics, Orangeburg, NY 10962. Offers cosmetic science (MS); industrial pharmacy (MS). Part-time programs available. *Entrance requirements:* For master's, college transcripts, 2 letters of recommendation. Additional exam requirements/recommendations for international students: Required—TOEFL.

Long Island University–LIU Brooklyn, Arnold and Marie Schwartz College of Pharmacy and Health Sciences, Graduate Programs in Pharmacy, Division of Pharmaceutical Sciences, Brooklyn, NY 11201-8423. Offers cosmetic science (MS); industrial pharmacy (MS); pharmaceutics (PhD); pharmacology/toxicology (MS). Part-time and evening/weekend programs available. Terminal master's awarded for partial completion of doctoral program. *Degree requirements:* For master's, thesis optional; for doctorate, thesis/dissertation, candidacy exam. *Entrance requirements:* For master's and doctorate, minimum GPA of 3.0.

MCPHS University, Graduate Studies, Program in Pharmaceutics/Industrial Pharmacy, Boston, MA 02115-5896. Offers MS, PhD. Terminal master's awarded for partial completion of doctoral program. *Degree requirements:* For master's, thesis, oral defense of thesis; for doctorate, one foreign language, comprehensive exam, thesis/dissertation, oral defense of dissertation, qualifying exam. *Entrance requirements:* For master's and doctorate, GRE General Test, minimum QPA of 3.0. Additional exam requirements/recommendations for international students: Required—TOEFL (minimum score 550 paper-based; 79 iBT). *Faculty research:* Pharmacokinetics and drug metabolism, pharmaceutics and physical pharmacy, dosage forms.

Memorial University of Newfoundland, School of Graduate Studies, School of Pharmacy, St. John's, NL A1C 5S7, Canada. Offers MSCPharm, PhD. Part-time programs available. *Degree requirements:* For master's, thesis, seminar; for doctorate, comprehensive exam, thesis/dissertation, oral defense of thesis. *Entrance requirements:* For master's, B Sc in pharmacy or related area. Electronic applications accepted. *Faculty research:* Pharmaceutics, medicinal chemistry, physical pharmacy, pharmacology, toxicology.

Mercer University, Graduate Studies, Cecil B. Day Campus, College of Pharmacy, Macon, GA 31207-0003. Offers pharmaceutical sciences (PhD); pharmacology (PhD); pharmacy (Pharm D); Pharm D/MBA; Pharm D/PhD. *Accreditation:* ACPE (one or more programs are accredited). *Faculty:* 24 full-time (15 women). *Students:* 653 full-time (421 women), 7 part-time (4 women); includes 291 minority (110 Black or African American, non-Hispanic/Latino; 1 American Indian or Alaska Native, non-Hispanic/Latino; 137 Asian, non-Hispanic/Latino; 15 Hispanic/Latino; 28 Two or more races, non-Hispanic/Latino), 47 international. Average age 26. 1,895 applicants, 18% accepted, 176 enrolled. In 2013, 137 doctorates awarded. *Degree requirements:* For doctorate, comprehensive exam (for some programs), thesis/dissertation (for some programs). *Entrance requirements:* For doctorate, GRE; PCAT (for Pharm D), Pharm D or BS in pharmacy or science, minimum GPA of 3.0. Additional exam requirements/recommendations for international students: Required—TOEFL. *Application deadline:* Applications are processed on a rolling basis. Electronic applications accepted. *Expenses:* Contact institution. *Financial support:* In 2013–14, 350 students received support. Teaching assistantships with tuition reimbursements available, career-related internships or fieldwork, Federal Work-Study, institutionally sponsored loans, scholarships/grants, tuition waivers, and unspecified assistantships available. Support available to part-time students. Financial award application deadline: 5/1; financial award applicants required to submit FAFSA. *Faculty research:* Stability and compatibility of steroids, synthesis of antihypertensives, disposition of cyclosporine, synthesis of enzyme inhibitors. *Unit head:* Dr. Hewitt W. Matthews, Dean, 678-547-6306, Fax: 678-547-6315, E-mail: matthews_h@mercer.edu. *Application contact:* Dr. James W. Bartling, Associate Dean for Student Affairs and Admissions, 678-547-6181, Fax: 678-547-6518, E-mail: bartling_jw@mercer.edu.
Website: http://pharmacy.mercer.edu/

North Dakota State University, College of Graduate and Interdisciplinary Studies, College of Pharmacy, Nursing and Allied Sciences, Department of Pharmaceutical Sciences, Fargo, ND 58108. Offers MS, PhD. *Accreditation:* ACPE. Part-time programs available. *Faculty:* 11 full-time (2 women). *Students:* 16 full-time (8 women), 6 part-time (3 women), 18 international. Average age 29. 47 applicants, 9% accepted, 4 enrolled. In 2013, 9 doctorates awarded. Terminal master's awarded for partial completion of doctoral program. *Degree requirements:* For master's, thesis; for doctorate, thesis/dissertation. *Entrance requirements:* For master's and doctorate, GRE General Test. Additional exam requirements/recommendations for international students: Required—TOEFL. *Application deadline:* For fall admission, 3/15 priority date for domestic students; for spring admission, 11/15 priority date for domestic students. Applications are processed on a rolling basis. Application fee: $35. Electronic applications accepted. *Financial support:* In 2013–14, 19 research assistantships with full tuition reimbursements (averaging $14,000 per year) were awarded; institutionally sponsored loans also available. Financial award application deadline: 4/15. *Faculty research:* Subcellular pharmacokinetics, cancer, cardiovascular drug design, iontophonesis, neuropharmacology. *Unit head:* Dr. Jagdish Singh, Chair, 701-231-7943, E-mail: jagdishsingh@ndsu.edu. *Application contact:* Assistant Professor.
Website: http://www.ndsu.edu/pharmsci/

Northeastern University, Bouvé College of Health Sciences, Boston, MA 02115-5096. Offers audiology (Au D); biotechnology (MS); counseling psychology (MS, PhD, CAGS); counseling/school psychology (PhD); exercise physiology (MS), including exercise physiology, public health; health informatics (MS); nursing (MS, PhD, CAGS), including acute care (MS), administration (MS), anesthesia (MS), primary care (MS), psychiatric mental health (MS); pharmaceutical sciences (PhD); pharmaceutics and drug delivery systems (MS); pharmacology (MS); physical therapy (DPT); physician assistant (MS); school psychology (PhD, CAGS); school/counseling psychology (PhD); speech language pathology (MS); urban public health (MPH); MS/MBA. *Accreditation:* ACPE (one or more programs are accredited). Part-time and evening/weekend programs available. *Degree requirements:* For doctorate, thesis/dissertation (for some programs); for CAGS, comprehensive exam.

Northeast Ohio Medical University, College of Graduate Studies, Rootstown, OH 44272-0095. Offers bioethics (Certificate); health-system pharmacy administration (MS); integrated pharmaceutical medicine (MS, PhD); public health (MS). *Faculty:* 80 part-time/adjunct (26 women). *Students:* 38 full-time (21 women); includes 4 minority (3 Asian, non-Hispanic/Latino; 1 Hispanic/Latino). Average age 28. 45 applicants, 84% accepted, 38 enrolled. In 2013, 9 master's, 1 doctorate awarded. *Application deadline:* For fall admission, 9/1 priority date for domestic students; for winter admission, 1/5 priority date for domestic students. Applications are processed on a rolling basis. Application fee: $45. Electronic applications accepted. Full-time tuition and fees vary according to program. Part-time tuition and fees vary according to degree level. *Unit head:* Dr. Walter E. Horton, Jr., Dean of the College of Graduate Studies. *Application contact:* Luke Gloeckner, Associate Director for Enrollment Services and Registration, 330-325-6274, E-mail: lgloeckner@gmail.com.
Website: http://www.neomed.edu/academics/graduatestudies

Oregon State University, College of Pharmacy, Program in Pharmaceutical Research, Corvallis, OR 97331. Offers MS, PhD. Part-time programs available. *Faculty:* 29 full-time (14 women), 4 part-time/adjunct (1 woman). *Students:* 25 full-time (10 women), 3 part-time (0 women); includes 1 minority (Hispanic/Latino), 19 international. Average age 29. 73 applicants, 15% accepted, 7 enrolled. In 2013, 3 master's, 7 doctorates awarded. *Median time to degree:* Of those who began their doctoral program in fall 2005, 95% received their degree in 8 years or less. *Entrance requirements:* For master's and doctorate, GRE. Additional exam requirements/recommendations for international students: Required—TOEFL (minimum score 80 iBT), IELTS (minimum score 6.5). *Application deadline:* For fall admission, 1/1 for domestic students. *Expenses:* Tuition, state resident: full-time $11,664; part-time $432 per credit hour. Tuition, nonresident: full-time $19,197; part-time $711 per credit hour. *Required fees:* $1446; $443 per quarter. One-time fee: $300. Tuition and fees vary according to course load and program. *Unit head:* Dr. Mark Zabriskie, Dean and Professor, 541-737-5781, E-mail: mark.zabriskie@oregonstate.edu. *Application contact:* Debra Peters, Pharmacy Advisor, 541-737-8743, E-mail: debra.peters@oregonstate.edu.
Website: http://pharmacy.oregonstate.edu/

Purdue University, College of Pharmacy and Pharmacal Sciences and Graduate School, Graduate Programs in Pharmacy and Pharmacal Sciences, Department of Pharmacy Practice, West Lafayette, IN 47907. Offers clinical pharmacy (MS, PhD); pharmacy administration (MS, PhD). *Faculty:* 16 full-time (5 women), 13 part-time/adjunct (4 women). *Students:* 11 full-time (9 women), 3 part-time (0 women); includes 2 minority (1 Black or African American, non-Hispanic/Latino; 1 Hispanic/Latino), 8 international. Average age 29. 39 applicants, 13% accepted, 2 enrolled. In 2013, 1 master's, 3 doctorates awarded. Terminal master's awarded for partial completion of doctoral program. *Degree requirements:* For master's, thesis optional; for doctorate, thesis/dissertation. *Entrance requirements:* For master's, GRE General Test, minimum undergraduate GPA of 3.0 or equivalent; for doctorate, GRE General Test, minimum undergraduate GPA of 3.0 or equivalent; master's degree with minimum GPA of 3.0 or equivalent. Additional exam requirements/recommendations for international students:

Required—TOEFL (minimum score 550 paper-based; 77 iBT), TWE (recommended for MS, required for PhD). *Application deadline:* Applications are processed on a rolling basis. Application fee: $60 ($75 for international students). Electronic applications accepted. *Financial support:* In 2013–14, teaching assistantships with tuition reimbursements (averaging $20,000 per year) were awarded; fellowships, research assistantships, career-related internships or fieldwork, and traineeships also available. Support available to part-time students. Financial award applicants required to submit FAFSA. *Faculty research:* Clinical drug studies, pharmacy education advancement, administrative studies. *Unit head:* Dr. James E. Tisdale, Interim Head, 317-613-2315 Ext. 306, E-mail: jtisdale@purdue.edu. *Application contact:* Dr. Janine C. Mott, Graduate Contact, 765-494-1362, E-mail: jmott@purdue.edu.

Queen's University at Kingston, School of Graduate Studies, Faculty of Health Sciences, Department of Anatomy and Cell Biology, Kingston, ON K7L 3N6, Canada. Offers biology of reproduction (M Sc, PhD); cancer (M Sc, PhD); cardiovascular pathophysiology (M Sc, PhD); cell and molecular biology (M Sc, PhD); drug metabolism (M Sc, PhD); endocrinology (M Sc, PhD); motor control (M Sc, PhD); neural regeneration (M Sc, PhD); neurophysiology (M Sc, PhD). Part-time programs available. *Degree requirements:* For master's, thesis; for doctorate, one foreign language, comprehensive exam, thesis/dissertation. *Entrance requirements:* Additional exam requirements/recommendations for international students: Required—TOEFL. Electronic applications accepted. *Faculty research:* Human kinetics, neuroscience, reproductive biology, cardiovascular.

Rush University, Graduate College, Division of Pharmacology, Chicago, IL 60612-3832. Offers clinical research (MS); pharmacology (MS, PhD); MD/PhD. Terminal master's awarded for partial completion of doctoral program. *Degree requirements:* For master's, thesis; for doctorate, thesis/dissertation. *Entrance requirements:* For master's and doctorate, GRE General Test, interview. Additional exam requirements/recommendations for international students: Required—TOEFL (minimum score 550 paper-based). *Faculty research:* Dopamine neurobiology and Parkinson's disease; cardiac electrophysiology and clinical pharmacology; neutrophil motility, apoptosis, and adhesion; angiogenesis; pulmonary vascular physiology.

Rutgers, The State University of New Jersey, New Brunswick, Ernest Mario School of Pharmacy, Program in Pharmaceutical Science, Piscataway, NJ 08854-8097. Offers MS, PhD. Part-time programs available. Terminal master's awarded for partial completion of doctoral program. *Degree requirements:* For master's, thesis; for doctorate, thesis/dissertation. *Entrance requirements:* For master's and doctorate, GRE General Test, 3 letters of recommendation. Additional exam requirements/recommendations for international students: Required—TOEFL (minimum score 550 paper-based; 83 iBT). Electronic applications accepted. *Faculty research:* Drug delivery, drug transport and drug metabolism; pharmacokinetics and pharmacodynamics; cancer chemoprevention and dietary phytochemicals; pharmacogenomics and personalized medicine; bioinformatics and computational pharmaceutical sciences.

St. John's University, College of Pharmacy and Health Sciences, Graduate Programs in Pharmaceutical Sciences, Program in Pharmaceutical Sciences, Queens, NY 11439. Offers MS, PhD. Part-time and evening/weekend programs available. *Students:* 105 full-time (39 women), 39 part-time (26 women); includes 19 minority (4 Black or African American, non-Hispanic/Latino; 13 Asian, non-Hispanic/Latino; 1 Hispanic/Latino; 1 Two or more races, non-Hispanic/Latino), 107 international. Average age 28. 250 applicants, 31% accepted, 17 enrolled. In 2013, 22 master's, 3 doctorates awarded. Terminal master's awarded for partial completion of doctoral program. *Degree requirements:* For master's, comprehensive exam, thesis optional, one-year residency; for doctorate, comprehensive exam, thesis/dissertation, qualifying exams, residency. *Entrance requirements:* For master's, GRE General Test, minimum GPA of 3.0, 2 letters of recommendation, statement of goals; for doctorate, GRE General Test, minimum GPA of 3.5 (undergraduate), 3.0 (graduate); 2 letters of recommendation. Additional exam requirements/recommendations for international students: Required—TOEFL (minimum score 600 paper-based; 100 iBT), IELTS (minimum score 5.5). *Application deadline:* For fall admission, 3/1 priority date for domestic students, 5/1 priority date for international students; for spring admission, 11/1 priority date for domestic and international students. Applications are processed on a rolling basis. Application fee: $70. Electronic applications accepted. *Expenses:* Contact institution. *Financial support:* Fellowships, research assistantships, career-related internships or fieldwork, and scholarships/grants available. Support available to part-time students. Financial award application deadline: 3/1; financial award applicants required to submit FAFSA. *Faculty research:* Neurotoxicology, biochemical toxicology, molecular pharmacology, neuropharmacology, intermediary metabolism. *Unit head:* Dr. Louis Trombetta, Chair, 718-990-6025, E-mail: trombetl@stjohns.edu. *Application contact:* Robert Medrano, Director of Graduate Admission, 718-990-1601, Fax: 718-990-5686, E-mail: gradhelp@stjohns.edu.
Website: http://www.stjohns.edu/academics/schools-and-colleges/college-pharmacy-and-health-sciences/programs-and-majors

South Dakota State University, Graduate School, College of Pharmacy, Department of Pharmaceutical Sciences, Brookings, SD 57007. Offers biological science (MS); pharmaceutical sciences (PhD). *Degree requirements:* For master's, thesis, oral exam; for doctorate, comprehensive exam, thesis/dissertation, oral exam. *Entrance requirements:* For master's and doctorate, GRE General Test. Additional exam requirements/recommendations for international students: Required—TOEFL (minimum score 550 paper-based). *Faculty research:* Drugs of abuse, anti-cancer drugs, sustained drug delivery, drug metabolism.

Stevens Institute of Technology, Graduate School, Charles V. Schaefer Jr. School of Engineering, Department of Mechanical Engineering, Program in Pharmaceutical Manufacturing, Hoboken, NJ 07030. Offers M Eng, MS, Certificate.

Stevens Institute of Technology, Graduate School, Wesley J. Howe School of Technology Management, Program in Business Administration, Hoboken, NJ 07030. Offers engineering management (MBA); financial engineering (MBA); information management (MBA); information technology in financial services (MBA); information technology in the pharmaceutical industry (MBA); information technology outsourcing (MBA); pharmaceutical management (MBA); project management (MBA); technology management (MBA); telecommunications management (MBA).

Temple University, School of Pharmacy, Department of Pharmaceutical Sciences, Program in Quality Assurance/Regulatory Affairs, Fort Washington, PA 19054. Offers MS. Part-time and evening/weekend programs available. Postbaccalaureate distance learning degree programs offered (minimal on-campus study). *Students:* 5 full-time (3 women), 188 part-time (127 women); includes 31 minority (8 Black or African American, non-Hispanic/Latino; 2 American Indian or Alaska Native, non-Hispanic/Latino; 16 Asian, non-Hispanic/Latino; 4 Hispanic/Latino; 1 Two or more races, non-Hispanic/Latino), 8 international. 68 applicants, 68% accepted, 34 enrolled. In 2013, 58 master's awarded. *Degree requirements:* For master's, thesis optional. *Entrance requirements:* For master's, minimum undergraduate GPA of 3.0. Additional exam requirements/recommendations for international students: Required—TOEFL (minimum score 550 paper-based; 82 iBT). *Application deadline:* For fall admission, 8/1 for domestic students, 12/15 for international students; for spring admission, 12/15 for domestic students, 8/1 for international students. Applications are processed on a rolling basis. Application fee: $60. Electronic applications accepted. *Financial support:* Application deadline: 1/15; applicants required to submit FAFSA. *Unit head:* Dr. Daniel Canney, Director of Graduate Studies, 215-707-4948, E-mail: canney@temple.edu. *Application contact:* Sophon Din, Administrative Assistant, 215-707-4922, E-mail: tuspgrad@temple.edu.
Website: http://www.temple.edu/pharmacy_QARA

Texas Southern University, College of Pharmacy and Health Sciences, Department of Pharmaceutical Sciences, Houston, TX 77004-4584. Offers MS, PhD. Postbaccalaureate distance learning degree programs offered. *Faculty:* 10 full-time (5 women), 4 part-time/adjunct (1 woman). *Students:* 16 full-time (12 women), 4 part-time (1 woman); includes 18 minority (12 Black or African American, non-Hispanic/Latino; 6 Asian, non-Hispanic/Latino), 2 international. Average age 31. 13 applicants, 15% accepted, 2 enrolled. In 2013, 2 doctorates awarded. *Entrance requirements:* For master's, PCAT; for doctorate, GRE General Test. *Application deadline:* For fall admission, 2/15 for domestic and international students. Applications are processed on a rolling basis. Application fee: $50 ($75 for international students). Electronic applications accepted. *Financial support:* In 2013–14, 2 research assistantships (averaging $28,000 per year) were awarded; fellowships, teaching assistantships, career-related internships or fieldwork, scholarships/grants, and tuition waivers (partial) also available. Financial award application deadline: 5/1; financial award applicants required to submit FAFSA. *Unit head:* Dr. Dong Liang, Chair, 713-313-1885, E-mail: liang_dx@tsu.edu. *Application contact:* Dr. Gregory Maddox, Dean of the Graduate School, 713-313-7011, E-mail: maddox_gh@tsu.edu.
Website: http://www.tsu.edu/academics/colleges__schools/College_of_Pharmacy_and_Health_Sciences/Departments_Programs/default.php

Texas Tech University Health Sciences Center, Graduate School of Biomedical Sciences, Program in Pharmaceutical Sciences, Lubbock, TX 79430. Offers MS, PhD. *Accreditation:* ACPE. Terminal master's awarded for partial completion of doctoral program. *Degree requirements:* For master's, thesis; for doctorate, thesis/dissertation. *Entrance requirements:* For master's and doctorate, GRE General Test, minimum GPA of 3.0. Additional exam requirements/recommendations for international students: Required—TOEFL (minimum score 550 paper-based; 79 iBT). Electronic applications accepted. *Faculty research:* Drug design and delivery, pharmacology, pharmacokinetics, drug receptor modeling, molecular and reproductive biology.

Université de Montréal, Faculty of Pharmacy, Montréal, QC H3C 3J7, Canada. Offers drugs development (DESS); pharmaceutical care (DESS); pharmaceutical practice (M Sc); pharmaceutical sciences (M Sc, PhD); pharmacist-supervisor teacher (DESS). Part-time programs available. Terminal master's awarded for partial completion of doctoral program. *Degree requirements:* For master's, thesis; for doctorate, thesis/dissertation. *Entrance requirements:* For master's and doctorate, proficiency in French. Electronic applications accepted. *Faculty research:* Novel drug delivery systems, immunoassay development, medicinal chemistry of CNS compounds, pharmacokinetics and biopharmaceutical compounds.

Université Laval, Faculty of Pharmacy, Program in Hospital Pharmacy, Québec, QC G1K 7P4, Canada. Offers M Sc. *Entrance requirements:* For master's, knowledge of French, interview. Electronic applications accepted.

Université Laval, Faculty of Pharmacy, Programs in Community Pharmacy, Québec, QC G1K 7P4, Canada. Offers DESS. Part-time programs available. *Entrance requirements:* For degree, knowledge of French. Electronic applications accepted.

Université Laval, Faculty of Pharmacy, Programs in Pharmacy, Québec, QC G1K 7P4, Canada. Offers M Sc, PhD. Part-time programs available. Terminal master's awarded for partial completion of doctoral program. *Degree requirements:* For master's, thesis; for doctorate, comprehensive exam, thesis/dissertation. *Entrance requirements:* For master's and doctorate, knowledge of French. Electronic applications accepted.

University at Buffalo, the State University of New York, Graduate School, School of Pharmacy and Pharmaceutical Sciences, Department of Pharmaceutical Sciences, Buffalo, NY 14260. Offers MS, PhD, Pharm D/MS, Pharm D/PhD. *Faculty:* 17 full-time (5 women), 4 part-time/adjunct (0 women). *Students:* 60 full-time (34 women), 6 part-time (5 women); includes 12 minority (1 Black or African American, non-Hispanic/Latino; 11 Asian, non-Hispanic/Latino), 26 international. Average age 28. 304 applicants, 8% accepted, 19 enrolled. In 2013, 8 master's, 8 doctorates awarded. Terminal master's awarded for partial completion of doctoral program. *Degree requirements:* For master's, comprehensive exam (for some programs), thesis optional, project; for doctorate, comprehensive exam, thesis/dissertation. *Entrance requirements:* For master's, GRE, BS, B Eng, or Pharm D; for doctorate, GRE, BS, MS, B Eng, M Eng, or Pharm D. Additional exam requirements/recommendations for international students: Required—TOEFL (minimum score 550 paper-based; 79 iBT); Recommended—IELTS, TSE. *Application deadline:* For fall admission, 2/15 for domestic and international students. Applications are processed on a rolling basis. Application fee: $50. Electronic applications accepted. *Financial support:* In 2013–14, 39 students received support, including 39 research assistantships with full tuition reimbursements available (averaging $23,500 per year); health care benefits and unspecified assistantships also available. Financial award application deadline: 3/1; financial award applicants required to submit FAFSA. *Faculty research:* Pharmacokinetics, biopharmaceutics, drug delivery systems, pharmacodynamics, drug metabolism and analysis. *Total annual research expenditures:* $4.3 million. *Unit head:* Dr. William J. Jusko, Chair, 716-645-2855 Ext. 225, Fax: 716-645-3693, E-mail: wjjusko@acsu.buffalo.edu. *Application contact:* Dr. Murali Ramanathan, Director of Graduate Studies, 716-645-4846, Fax: 716-645-3690, E-mail: murali@buffalo.edu.
Website: http://pharmacy.buffalo.edu/departments-offices/pharmaceutical-sciences.html

University of Alberta, Faculty of Graduate Studies and Research, Department of Pharmacy and Pharmaceutical Sciences, Edmonton, AB T6G 2E1, Canada. Offers M Sc, PhD. Terminal master's awarded for partial completion of doctoral program. *Degree requirements:* For master's, thesis; for doctorate, thesis/dissertation. *Entrance requirements:* Additional exam requirements/recommendations for international students: Required—Michigan English Language Assessment Battery or IELTS. Electronic applications accepted. *Faculty research:* Radiopharmacy, pharmacokinetics, bionucleonics, medicinal chemistry, microbiology.

The University of Arizona, College of Pharmacy, Program in Pharmaceutical Sciences, Tucson, AZ 85721. Offers medicinal and natural products chemistry (MS, PhD); pharmaceutical economics (MS, PhD); pharmaceutics and pharmacokinetics (MS, PhD). *Faculty:* 9 full-time (3 women), 2 part-time/adjunct (0 women). *Students:* 36 full-time (18 women), 4 part-time (1 woman); includes 9 minority (5 Asian, non-Hispanic/Latino; 3 Hispanic/Latino; 1 Two or more races, non-Hispanic/Latino), 11 international. Average age 30. 65 applicants, 9% accepted, 6 enrolled. In 2013, 2 master's, 10 doctorates awarded. *Degree requirements:* For master's, thesis; for doctorate, one foreign language, thesis/dissertation. *Entrance requirements:* For master's, GRE General Test, 3 letters of recommendation, bachelor's degree in related field; for doctorate, GRE General Test, 3 letters of recommendation, statement of purpose, bachelor's degree in related field. Additional exam requirements/recommendations for international students: Required—TOEFL (minimum score 550 paper-based; 79 iBT). *Application deadline:* For fall admission, 1/1 for domestic students, 12/1 for international

students. Applications are processed on a rolling basis. Application fee: $75. Electronic applications accepted. *Expenses:* Tuition, state resident: full-time $11,526. Tuition, nonresident: full-time $27,398. *Financial support:* In 2013–14, 40 research assistantships with full tuition reimbursements (averaging $24,000 per year) were awarded; scholarships/grants, health care benefits, tuition waivers (full), and unspecified assistantships also available. Financial award application deadline: 3/1. *Faculty research:* Drug design, natural products isolation, biological applications of NMR and mass spectrometry, drug formulation and delivery, pharmacokinetics. *Total annual research expenditures:* $3.6 million. *Unit head:* Dr. Terrence Monks, Department Head, 520-626-9906, Fax: 520-626-4063, E-mail: monks@pharmacy.arizona.edu. *Application contact:* Sonya Basurto, Information Contact, 520-626-7265, Fax: 520-626-2466, E-mail: basurto@pharmacy.arizona.edu.
Website: http://grad.arizona.edu/live/programs/description/129

The University of British Columbia, Faculty of Pharmaceutical Sciences, Vancouver, BC V6T 1Z3, Canada. Offers M Sc, PhD, Pharm D. *Students:* 59 full-time (28 women), 1 part-time (0 women). Average age 26. 99 applicants, 14% accepted, 12 enrolled. In 2013, 3 master's, 5 doctorates awarded. *Degree requirements:* For master's, thesis, seminar; for doctorate, comprehensive exam, thesis/dissertation, seminar. *Entrance requirements:* Additional exam requirements/recommendations for international students: Required—TOEFL (minimum score 600 paper-based; 100 iBT), IELTS (minimum score 6.5). *Application deadline:* For fall admission, 3/15 for domestic students, 2/15 for international students. Application fee: $95 Canadian dollars ($153 Canadian dollars for international students). Electronic applications accepted. *Expenses: Tuition, area resident:* Full-time $8000 Canadian dollars. *Financial support:* In 2013–14, 60 students received support, including 10 fellowships (averaging $19,000 per year), 45 research assistantships (averaging $8,000 per year), 28 teaching assistantships (averaging $12,000 per year); career-related internships or fieldwork, institutionally sponsored loans, scholarships/grants, traineeships, and unspecified assistantships also available. *Faculty research:* Pharmacology and cellular pharmacology, neuropharmacology, toxicology, nanomedicines and drug delivery, pharmacogenomics and personalized medicine, health outcomes research and evaluation, pharmacoepidemiology, and medicinal chemistry. *Unit head:* Dr. Michael Coughtrie, Dean, 604-822-2343, Fax: 604-822-3035, E-mail: michael.coughtrie@ubc.ca. *Application contact:* Rachel Wu, Graduate Programs Manager, 604-827-0188, Fax: 604-822-3035, E-mail: rachel.wu@ubc.ca.
Website: http://www.pharmacy.ubc.ca

University of California, San Francisco, School of Pharmacy and Graduate Division, Pharmaceutical Sciences and Pharmacogenomics Program, San Francisco, CA 94158-0775. Offers PhD. *Degree requirements:* For doctorate, comprehensive exam, thesis/dissertation. *Entrance requirements:* For doctorate, GRE General Test, bachelor's degree, 3 letters of recommendation, personal statement. Additional exam requirements/recommendations for international students: Required—TOEFL. *Application deadline:* For fall admission, 12/1 for domestic and international students. Application fee: $80 ($100 for international students). Electronic applications accepted. *Expenses:* Tuition, state resident: full-time $11,220. Tuition, nonresident: full-time $26,322. *Required fees:* $5204. Full-time tuition and fees vary according to degree level and program. *Financial support:* In 2013–14, fellowships with full tuition reimbursements (averaging $32,500 per year), research assistantships with full tuition reimbursements (averaging $32,500 per year), teaching assistantships with full tuition reimbursements (averaging $32,500 per year) were awarded; career-related internships or fieldwork, institutionally sponsored loans, scholarships/grants, traineeships, tuition waivers (full), and unspecified assistantships also available. Financial award application deadline: 4/6. *Faculty research:* Drug development sciences, molecular pharmacology, therapeutic bioengineering, pharmacogenomics and functional genomics, quantitative and systems pharmacology, computational genomics. *Unit head:* Dr. Deanna L. Kroetz, Director, 415-476-1159, Fax: 415-476-6022, E-mail: deanna.kroetz@ucsf.edu. *Application contact:* Debbie Acoba-Idlebi, Administrator, 415-476-1947, Fax: 415-476-6022, E-mail: debbie.acoba@ucsf.edu.
Website: http://pspg.ucsf.edu/

University of Cincinnati, College of Pharmacy, Division of Pharmaceutical Sciences, Cincinnati, OH 45221. Offers MS, PhD. *Degree requirements:* For master's, thesis; for doctorate, thesis/dissertation. *Entrance requirements:* For master's and doctorate, GRE General Test, minimum GPA of 3.0. Additional exam requirements/recommendations for international students: Required—TOEFL.

University of Colorado Denver, School of Pharmacy, Doctor of Pharmacy Program, Aurora, CO 80045. Offers Pharm D. Postbaccalaureate distance learning degree programs offered (no on-campus study). *Students:* 644 full-time (369 women), 195 part-time (129 women); includes 308 minority (49 Black or African American, non-Hispanic/Latino; 9 American Indian or Alaska Native, non-Hispanic/Latino; 197 Asian, non-Hispanic/Latino; 48 Hispanic/Latino; 5 Two or more races, non-Hispanic/Latino), 34 international. Average age 30. 235 applicants, 89% accepted, 189 enrolled. In 2013, 198 doctorates awarded. *Degree requirements:* For doctorate, final-year experience in pharmacy setting. *Entrance requirements:* For doctorate, PCAT, minimum GPA of 2.5, 2.75 in the sciences; prerequisite coursework in general chemistry with lab, organic chemistry with lab, general biology with lab, microbiology with lab, biochemistry, human anatomy and physiology with lab, general physics, calculus, English composition, public speaking, and microeconomics. Additional exam requirements/recommendations for international students: Required—TOEFL (minimum score 550 paper-based; 80 iBT). *Application deadline:* For fall admission, 12/1 for domestic students, 11/1 for international students. Application fee: $150. Electronic applications accepted. *Expenses:* Contact institution. *Financial support:* In 2013–14, 278 students received support. Fellowships, research assistantships, teaching assistantships, career-related internships or fieldwork, Federal Work-Study, institutionally sponsored loans, scholarships/grants, traineeships, and unspecified assistantships available. Financial award application deadline: 3/15; financial award applicants required to submit FAFSA. *Faculty research:* Mechanistic studies of viral assembly, synthetic gene delivery systems for use in gene therapy, mechanisms of toxicity, pulmonary drug delivery. *Unit head:* Douglas Fish, Chair of PharmD Program, 303-724-2615, E-mail: doug.fish@ucdenver.edu. *Application contact:* Admissions, 303-724-2882, E-mail: pharmd.info@ucdenver.edu.
Website: http://www.ucdenver.edu/academics/colleges/pharmacy/AcademicPrograms/PharmDProgram/Pages/PharmDProgram.aspx

University of Colorado Denver, School of Pharmacy, Program in Pharmaceutical Sciences, Aurora, CO 80045. Offers clinical pharmaceutical sciences (PhD); pharmaceutical biotechnology (PhD); pharmaceutical outcomes research (PhD). *Students:* 27 full-time (12 women), 1 part-time (0 women); includes 6 minority (1 Black or African American, non-Hispanic/Latino; 5 Asian, non-Hispanic/Latino), 13 international. Average age 30. 50 applicants, 12% accepted, 6 enrolled. In 2013, 5 doctorates awarded. *Degree requirements:* For doctorate, comprehensive exam, thesis/dissertation, minimum 60 credit hours of upper-level courses, 30 of which are thesis research, research rotations and thesis defense. *Entrance requirements:* For doctorate, GRE, minimum undergraduate GPA of 3.0; prior coursework in general chemistry, organic chemistry, calculus, biology, and physics. Additional exam requirements/recommendations for international students: Required—TOEFL (minimum score 550 paper-based; 80 iBT). *Application deadline:* For fall admission, 1/15 for domestic students, 12/15 for international students. Application fee: $50 ($75 for international students). Electronic applications accepted. *Expenses:* Contact institution. *Financial support:* In 2013–14, 24 students received support. Fellowships, research assistantships, teaching assistantships, Federal Work-Study, institutionally sponsored loans, scholarships/grants, traineeships, health care benefits, tuition waivers (full), and unspecified assistantships available. Financial award application deadline: 3/15; financial award applicants required to submit FAFSA. *Faculty research:* Pharmaceutical biotechnology, molecular toxicology, cancer pharmacology, drug discovery, clinical and translational sciences. *Unit head:* Dr. David Ross, Chair/Professor of Toxicology, 303-724-7265, E-mail: david.ross@ucdenver.edu. *Application contact:* Jackie Milowski, Graduate Admissions, 303-724-7263, E-mail: jackie.milowski@ucdenver.edu.
Website: http://www.ucdenver.edu/academics/colleges/pharmacy/AcademicPrograms/PhDPrograms/PhDPharmaceuticalSciences/Pages/PhDPharmaceuticalSciences.aspx

University of Connecticut, Graduate School, School of Pharmacy, Department of Pharmaceutical Sciences, Program in Pharmaceutics, Storrs, CT 06269. Offers MS, PhD. Terminal master's awarded for partial completion of doctoral program. *Degree requirements:* For master's, comprehensive exam, thesis; for doctorate, thesis/dissertation. *Entrance requirements:* For master's and doctorate, GRE General Test. Additional exam requirements/recommendations for international students: Required—TOEFL (minimum score 550 paper-based). Electronic applications accepted.

University of Florida, Graduate School, College of Pharmacy and Graduate School, Graduate Programs in Pharmacy, Department of Pharmaceutics, Gainesville, FL 32610. Offers clinical and translational sciences (PhD); pharmaceutical sciences (MSP, PhD); pharmacy (MSP, PhD). *Faculty:* 11 full-time (2 women), 10 part-time/adjunct (1 woman). *Students:* 18 full-time (9 women), 2 part-time (1 woman); includes 1 minority (Asian, non-Hispanic/Latino), 17 international. Average age 30. 234 applicants, 48% accepted, 86 enrolled. In 2013, 1 master's, 9 doctorates awarded. *Degree requirements:* For doctorate, comprehensive exam, thesis/dissertation. *Entrance requirements:* For master's and doctorate, GRE General Test, minimum GPA of 3.0. Additional exam requirements/recommendations for international students: Required—TOEFL (minimum score 550 paper-based; 80 iBT), IELTS (minimum score 6). *Application deadline:* For fall admission, 2/1 priority date for domestic students, 2/1 for international students; for spring admission, 9/1 for domestic students, 10/1 for international students. Applications are processed on a rolling basis. Application fee: $30. Electronic applications accepted. *Expenses:* Tuition, state resident: full-time $12,640. Tuition, nonresident: full-time $30,000. *Financial support:* In 2013–14, 18 students received support, including 4 research assistantships (averaging $13,785 per year), 16 teaching assistantships (averaging $15,745 per year); tuition waivers (full) and unspecified assistantships also available. Financial award applicants required to submit FAFSA. *Faculty research:* Basic, applied, and clinical investigations in pharmacokinetics/biopharmaceutics; pharmaceutical analysis, pharmaceutical biotechnology and drug delivery; herbal medicine. *Unit head:* Hartmut Derendorf, PhD, Professor and Chair, 352-273-7856, Fax: 352-392-4447, E-mail: hartmut@ufl.edu. *Application contact:* Dr. Anthony Palmieri, III, Graduate Coordinator, 352-273-7868, E-mail: palmieri@cop.ufl.edu.
Website: http://www.cop.ufl.edu/pc/

University of Florida, Graduate School, College of Pharmacy and Graduate School, Graduate Programs in Pharmacy, Department of Pharmacotherapy and Translational Research, Gainesville, FL 32610. Offers clinical pharmaceutical sciences (PhD); clinical pharmacy (MSP). *Faculty:* 8 full-time (3 women), 4 part-time/adjunct (2 women). *Students:* 7 full-time (3 women), 5 international. Average age 31. *Entrance requirements:* For master's and doctorate, GRE General Test, minimum GPA of 3.0. Additional exam requirements/recommendations for international students: Required—TOEFL (minimum score 550 paper-based; 80 iBT), IELTS (minimum score 6). *Application deadline:* For fall admission, 1/15 for domestic and international students. Application fee: $30. Electronic applications accepted. *Expenses:* Tuition, state resident: full-time $12,640. Tuition, nonresident: full-time $30,000. *Financial support:* In 2013–14, 5 students received support, including 5 teaching assistantships (averaging $22,185 per year). Financial award application deadline: 1/15; financial award applicants required to submit FAFSA. *Faculty research:* Understanding genetic and non-genetic factors that contribute to variability in drug response, cardiology, transplant/immunology, asthma/pulmonary, psychiatry, clinical pharmacology/drug metabolism. *Unit head:* Dr. Reginald F. Frye, Professor and Chair, 352-273-5453, Fax: 352-273-6242, E-mail: frye@cop.ufl.edu. *Application contact:* Dr. Taimour Langaee, Associate Research Professor/Graduate Coordinator, 352-273-6357, Fax: 352-273-6242, E-mail: langaee@cop.ufl.edu.
Website: http://www.cop.ufl.edu/research/pharmacotherapy-and-translational-research/

University of Georgia, College of Pharmacy, Department of Pharmaceutical and Biomedical Sciences, Athens, GA 30602. Offers PhD. *Degree requirements:* For doctorate, one foreign language, thesis/dissertation. *Entrance requirements:* For doctorate, GRE General Test, minimum GPA of 3.0. Additional exam requirements/recommendations for international students: Required—TOEFL. Electronic applications accepted. *Faculty research:* Cancer and infectious diseases, drug delivery, neuropharmacology, cardiovascular pharmacology, bioanalytical chemistry, structural biology.

University of Hawaii at Hilo, Program in Pharmaceutical Sciences, Hilo, HI 96720-4091. Offers PhD. *Students:* 9 full-time (6 women), 1 part-time (0 women); includes 9 minority (4 Asian, non-Hispanic/Latino; 2 Hispanic/Latino; 3 Two or more races, non-Hispanic/Latino), 2 international. Average age 28. *Entrance requirements:* Additional exam requirements/recommendations for international students: Required—TOEFL. *Application deadline:* For fall admission, 5/1 for domestic students. Application fee: $50. Electronic applications accepted. *Expenses:* Tuition, state resident: full-time $4668. Tuition, nonresident: full-time $10,704. Tuition and fees vary according to course load and program. *Financial support:* Application deadline: 3/1; applicants required to submit FAFSA. *Application contact:* PhD Program Admissions, 808-932-7700, Fax: 808-933-3889, E-mail: pharmacy@hawaii.edu.
Website: http://pharmacy.uhh.hawaii.edu/academics/graduate/

University of Houston, College of Pharmacy, Houston, TX 77204. Offers pharmaceutics (MSPHR, PhD); pharmacology (MSPHR, PhD); pharmacy (Pharm D); pharmacy administration (MSPHR, PhD). *Accreditation:* ACPE. Part-time programs available. Terminal master's awarded for partial completion of doctoral program. *Entrance requirements:* For doctorate, PCAT (for Pharm D). Additional exam requirements/recommendations for international students: Required—TOEFL. Electronic applications accepted. *Faculty research:* Drug screening and design, cardiovascular pharmacology, infectious disease, asthma research, herbal medicine.

University of Illinois at Chicago, College of Pharmacy and Graduate College, Graduate Programs in Pharmacy, Chicago, IL 60607-7128. Offers biopharmaceutical sciences (PhD); forensic science (MS), including forensic toxicology; medicinal chemistry (MS, PhD); pharmacognosy (MS, PhD); pharmacy administration (MS, PhD). *Faculty:* 81 full-time (31 women), 16 part-time/adjunct (3 women). *Students:* 122 full-time (62 women), 12 part-time (9 women); includes 23 minority (6 Black or African American, non-Hispanic/Latino; 15 Asian, non-Hispanic/Latino; 2 Hispanic/Latino), 68 international.

Average age 27. 331 applicants, 18% accepted, 29 enrolled. In 2013, 12 master's, 22 doctorates awarded. Terminal master's awarded for partial completion of doctoral program. *Degree requirements:* For master's, variable foreign language requirement, thesis; for doctorate, variable foreign language requirement, thesis/dissertation. *Entrance requirements:* For master's and doctorate, GRE General Test. Additional exam requirements/recommendations for international students: Required—TOEFL. *Application deadline:* For fall admission, 2/1 for domestic students. Applications are processed on a rolling basis. Application fee: $40 ($50 for international students). Electronic applications accepted. *Expenses:* Contact institution. *Financial support:* In 2013–14, 122 students received support, including 2 fellowships with full tuition reimbursements available; research assistantships with full tuition reimbursements available, teaching assistantships with full tuition reimbursements available, career-related internships or fieldwork, Federal Work-Study, institutionally sponsored loans, traineeships, tuition waivers (full), and unspecified assistantships also available. Financial award application deadline: 3/1; financial award applicants required to submit FAFSA. *Unit head:* Janet P. Engle, Executive Associate Dean for Academic Affairs, 312-996-6212. *Application contact:* Jackie Perry, Graduate College Receptionist, 312-413-2550, Fax: 312-413-0185, E-mail: gradcoll@uic.edu.

The University of Iowa, College of Pharmacy, Iowa City, IA 52242-1316. Offers clinical pharmaceutical sciences (PhD); medicinal and natural products chemistry (PhD); pharamaceutics (PhD); pharmaceutical socioeconomics (PhD); pharmaceutics (MS); pharmacy (Pharm D); Pharm D/MPH. *Accreditation:* ACPE (one or more programs are accredited). *Degree requirements:* For master's, thesis optional, exam; for doctorate, comprehensive exam, thesis/dissertation. *Entrance requirements:* For master's and doctorate, GRE General Test, minimum GPA of 3.0. Additional exam requirements/recommendations for international students: Required—TOEFL (minimum score 550 paper-based; 81 iBT). Electronic applications accepted.

The University of Kansas, Graduate Studies, School of Pharmacy, Department of Pharmacy Practice, Lawrence, KS 66047. Offers MS. *Faculty:* 7. *Students:* 3 full-time (1 woman), 4 part-time (3 women); includes 3 minority (all Asian, non-Hispanic/Latino). Average age 26. 3 applicants, 100% accepted, 3 enrolled. In 2013, 3 master's awarded. *Degree requirements:* For master's, thesis. *Entrance requirements:* For master's, GRE General Test, Pharm D, Kansas pharmacy license. Additional exam requirements/recommendations for international students: Recommended—TOEFL. *Application deadline:* For fall admission, 2/1 priority date for domestic students. Application fee: $55 ($65 for international students). Electronic applications accepted. *Financial support:* Fellowships with partial tuition reimbursements, health care benefits, and residencies available. Financial award application deadline: 2/15. *Faculty research:* Drug trials, drug stability, pharmacoeconomics, education, outcomes. *Total annual research expenditures:* $42,000. *Unit head:* David Henry, Chair, 785-864-6066, Fax: 785-864-2399, E-mail: dhenry@kumc.edu. *Application contact:* Dr. Dennis Grauer, Graduate Director, 785-864-3262, Fax: 785-864-2399, E-mail: dgrauer@kumc.edu.
Website: http://pharmpractice.ku.edu/

University of Kentucky, Graduate School, Graduate Programs in Pharmaceutical Sciences, Lexington, KY 40506-0032. Offers MS, PhD. Terminal master's awarded for partial completion of doctoral program. *Degree requirements:* For master's, thesis optional; for doctorate, comprehensive exam, thesis/dissertation. *Entrance requirements:* For master's, GRE General Test, minimum undergraduate GPA of 3.2; for doctorate, GRE General Test, minimum graduate GPA of 3.2. Additional exam requirements/recommendations for international students: Required—TOEFL (minimum score 550 paper-based; 79 iBT). Electronic applications accepted. *Faculty research:* Drug development, biotechnology, medicinal chemistry, cardiology, pharmacokinetics, CNS pharmacology, clinical pharmacology, pharmacotherapy and health outcomes, pharmaceutical policy.

The University of Manchester, School of Pharmacy and Pharmaceutical Sciences, Manchester, United Kingdom. Offers M Phil, PhD.

University of Manitoba, Faculty of Graduate Studies, Faculty of Pharmacy, Winnipeg, MB R3T 2N2, Canada. Offers M Sc, PhD. *Degree requirements:* For master's, one foreign language, thesis.

University of Maryland, Baltimore, Graduate School, Graduate Programs in Pharmacy, Department of Pharmaceutical Sciences, Baltimore, MD 21201. Offers PhD. *Degree requirements:* For doctorate, comprehensive exam, thesis/dissertation. *Entrance requirements:* For doctorate, GRE General Test. Additional exam requirements/recommendations for international students: Required—TOEFL (minimum score 600 paper-based), IELTS. Electronic applications accepted. *Faculty research:* Drug delivery, cellular and biological chemistry, clinical pharmaceutical sciences, biopharmaceutics, neuroscience.

University of Michigan, College of Pharmacy and Rackham Graduate School, Department of Pharmaceutical Sciences, Ann Arbor, MI 48109. Offers PhD. *Students:* 47 full-time (25 women); includes 13 minority (3 Black or African American, non-Hispanic/Latino; 7 Asian, non-Hispanic/Latino; 2 Hispanic/Latino; 1 Two or more races, non-Hispanic/Latino), 12 international. Average age 25. 111 applicants, 16% accepted, 13 enrolled. In 2013, 9 doctorates awarded. Terminal master's awarded for partial completion of doctoral program. *Degree requirements:* For doctorate, thesis/dissertation, oral defense of dissertation, preliminary exam. *Entrance requirements:* For doctorate, GRE. Additional exam requirements/recommendations for international students: Required—TOEFL (minimum score 560 paper-based; 84 iBT) or IELTS (minimum score 6.5). *Application deadline:* For fall admission, 1/6 for domestic and international students. Applications are processed on a rolling basis. Application fee: $60 ($75 for international students). Electronic applications accepted. *Expenses:* Contact institution. *Financial support:* In 2013–14, 47 students received support, including 27 fellowships (averaging $46,107 per year), 10 research assistantships (averaging $46,107 per year), 10 teaching assistantships (averaging $46,107 per year); career-related internships or fieldwork, institutionally sponsored loans, scholarships/grants, traineeships, tuition waivers, health care benefits, and unspecified assistantships also available. *Faculty research:* New drug design, new drug delivery systems, new biotechnology, pharmacy and the public sector. *Unit head:* Dr. Steven P. Schwedeman, Chair, 734-647-8339, Fax: 734-615-6162, E-mail: schwende@med.umich.edu. *Application contact:* Patrina Hardy, Executive Secretary, 734-615-3749, Fax: 734-615-6162, E-mail: thardy@med.umich.edu.
Website: https://pharmacy.umich.edu/pharmsci

University of Minnesota, Twin Cities Campus, College of Pharmacy and Graduate School, Graduate Programs in Pharmacy, Graduate Program in Experimental and Clinical Pharmacology, Minneapolis, MN 55455-0213. Offers MS, PhD. *Degree requirements:* For doctorate, thesis/dissertation.

University of Minnesota, Twin Cities Campus, College of Pharmacy and Graduate School, Graduate Programs in Pharmacy, Graduate Program in Pharmaceutics, Minneapolis, MN 55455. Offers PhD. *Faculty:* 10 full-time (3 women), 11 part-time/adjunct (2 women). *Students:* 19 full-time (11 women); includes 2 minority (both Asian, non-Hispanic/Latino), 15 international. Average age 26. 61 applicants, 13% accepted, 3 enrolled. In 2013, 4 doctorates awarded. Terminal master's awarded for partial completion of doctoral program. *Degree requirements:* For doctorate, comprehensive exam, thesis/dissertation. *Entrance requirements:* For doctorate, GRE General Test (preferred minimum score: Analytical Writing 3.5), bachelor's degree. Additional exam requirements/recommendations for international students: Required—TOEFL (minimum score 600 paper-based; 100 iBT), IELTS (minimum score 6.5). *Application deadline:* For fall admission, 12/31 for domestic and international students. Application fee: $75 ($95 for international students). Electronic applications accepted. *Expenses:* Contact institution. *Financial support:* In 2013–14, 19 students received support, including 5 fellowships with full tuition reimbursements available (averaging $22,500 per year), 10 research assistantships with full tuition reimbursements available (averaging $22,500 per year), 4 teaching assistantships with full tuition reimbursements available (averaging $22,500 per year); career-related internships or fieldwork, health care benefits, unspecified assistantships, and summer internships with pharmaceutical companies also available. Financial award application deadline: 12/31. *Faculty research:* Drug delivery, drug metabolism, molecular biopharmaceutics, pharmacokinetics and pharmacodynamics, crystal engineering, biophysical chemistry. *Total annual research expenditures:* $2.8 million. *Unit head:* Prof. William F. Elmquist, PhD, Professor and Head of the Department, 612-625-0097, Fax: 612-626-2125, E-mail: elmqu011@umn.edu. *Application contact:* Candice McDermott, Assistant to the Director of Graduate Studies, 612-624-5153, Fax: 612-626-2125, E-mail: mcder002@umn.edu.
Website: http://www.pharmacy.umn.edu/pharmaceutics/

University of Mississippi, Graduate School, School of Pharmacy, Graduate Programs in Pharmacy, University, MS 38677. Offers medicinal chemistry (PhD); pharmaceutical sciences (MS); pharmaceutics (PhD); pharmacognosy (PhD); pharmacology (PhD); pharmacy administration (PhD). *Faculty:* 41 full-time (17 women), 14 part-time/adjunct (7 women). *Students:* 81 full-time (27 women), 8 part-time (5 women); includes 4 minority (2 Black or African American, non-Hispanic/Latino; 2 Asian, non-Hispanic/Latino), 61 international. In 2013, 5 master's, 16 doctorates awarded. Application fee: $40. *Unit head:* Dr. David Allen, Dean, 662-915-7267, Fax: 662-915-5118, E-mail: sop@olemiss.edu. *Application contact:* Dr. Christy M. Wyandt, Associate Dean, 662-915-7474, Fax: 662-915-7577, E-mail: cwyandt@olemiss.edu.

University of Missouri–Kansas City, School of Pharmacy, Kansas City, MO 64110-2499. Offers pharmaceutical sciences (PhD); pharmacology and toxicology (PhD); pharmacy (Pharm D). PhD offered through School of Graduate Studies. *Accreditation:* ACPE (one or more programs are accredited). Postbaccalaureate distance learning degree programs offered (minimal on-campus study). *Faculty:* 54 full-time (26 women), 6 part-time/adjunct (3 women). *Students:* 424 full-time (252 women); includes 77 minority (14 Black or African American, non-Hispanic/Latino; 2 American Indian or Alaska Native, non-Hispanic/Latino; 43 Asian, non-Hispanic/Latino; 10 Hispanic/Latino; 1 Native Hawaiian or other Pacific Islander, non-Hispanic/Latino; 7 Two or more races, non-Hispanic/Latino), 1 international. Average age 26. 365 applicants, 37% accepted, 136 enrolled. In 2013, 122 doctorates awarded. *Degree requirements:* For doctorate, comprehensive exam (for some programs), thesis/dissertation (for some programs). *Entrance requirements:* For doctorate, PCAT (for Pharm D). Additional exam requirements/recommendations for international students: Required—TOEFL (minimum score 550 paper-based; 80 iBT). *Application deadline:* For fall admission, 3/1 for domestic and international students. Applications are processed on a rolling basis. Application fee: $45 ($50 for international students). Electronic applications accepted. *Expenses:* Contact institution. *Financial support:* In 2013–14, 26 research assistantships with full and partial tuition reimbursements (averaging $11,585 per year), 26 teaching assistantships with full tuition reimbursements (averaging $14,213 per year) were awarded; career-related internships or fieldwork, Federal Work-Study, institutionally sponsored loans, tuition waivers (full and partial), and unspecified assistantships also available. Financial award application deadline: 3/1; financial award applicants required to submit FAFSA. *Faculty research:* Bio-organic and medicinal chemistry, drug delivery, pharmaceutics, molecular neurobiology, neurology. *Unit head:* Dr. Russell B. Melchert, Dean, 816-235-1609, Fax: 816-235-5190, E-mail: melchertr@umkc.edu. *Application contact:* Shelly M. Janasz, Director, Student Services, 816-235-2400, Fax: 816-235-5190, E-mail: janaszs@umkc.edu.
Website: http://pharmacy.umkc.edu/

The University of Montana, Graduate School, College of Health Professions and Biomedical Sciences, Skaggs School of Pharmacy, Department of Biomedical and Pharmaceutical Sciences, Missoula, MT 59812-0002. Offers biomedical sciences (PhD); medicinal chemistry (MS, PhD); molecular and cellular toxicology (MS, PhD); neuroscience (PhD); pharmaceutical sciences (MS). *Accreditation:* ACPE. *Degree requirements:* For master's, oral defense of thesis; for doctorate, research dissertation defense. *Entrance requirements:* For master's and doctorate, GRE General Test. Additional exam requirements/recommendations for international students: Required—TOEFL (minimum score 540 paper-based). *Application deadline:* For fall admission, 3/1 priority date for domestic and international students. Applications are processed on a rolling basis. Application fee: $45. Electronic applications accepted. *Financial support:* Teaching assistantships with full and partial tuition reimbursements, Federal Work-Study, scholarships/grants, and tuition waivers (full and partial) available. Financial award application deadline: 3/1. *Faculty research:* Cardiovascular pharmacology, medicinal chemistry, neurosciences, environmental toxicology, pharmacogenetics, cancer. *Unit head:* Dr. Richard Bridges, Chair, 406-243-4972, E-mail: richard.bridges@umontana.edu. *Application contact:* Information Contact, E-mail: gradschl@mso.umt.edu.
Website: http://www.umt.edu/pharmsci/

University of Nebraska Medical Center, Department of Pharmaceutical Sciences, Omaha, NE 68198-6000. Offers MS, PhD. Terminal master's awarded for partial completion of doctoral program. *Degree requirements:* For master's, thesis; for doctorate, comprehensive exam, thesis/dissertation. *Entrance requirements:* For master's, GRE General Test; for doctorate, GRE. Additional exam requirements/recommendations for international students: Required—TOEFL (minimum score 550 paper-based). Electronic applications accepted. *Expenses: Required fees:* $300 per semester. Tuition and fees vary according to program. *Faculty research:* Pharmaceutics, medicinal chemistry, toxicology, chemical carcinogenesis, pharmacokinetics.

University of New Mexico, Graduate School, College of Pharmacy, Graduate Programs in Pharmaceutical Sciences, Albuquerque, NM 87131-2039. Offers MS, PhD. Part-time programs available. *Degree requirements:* For master's, comprehensive exam, thesis; for doctorate, comprehensive exam, thesis/dissertation. *Entrance requirements:* For master's and doctorate, GRE General Test (for some concentrations), 3 letters of recommendation, letter of intent, resume. Additional exam requirements/recommendations for international students: Required—TOEFL (minimum score 580 paper-based; 93 iBT). Electronic applications accepted. *Faculty research:* Pharmaceutical research, cancer research, pharmacy administration, radiopharmacy, toxicology.

The University of North Carolina at Chapel Hill, Eshelman School of Pharmacy, Chapel Hill, NC 27599. Offers MS, PhD. *Accreditation:* ACPE (one or more programs are accredited). *Faculty:* 101 full-time (43 women), 345 part-time/adjunct (184 women). *Students:* 93 full-time (45 women), 1 part-time (0 women); includes 16 minority (3 Black or African American, non-Hispanic/Latino; 1 American Indian or Alaska Native, non-Hispanic/Latino; 9 Asian, non-Hispanic/Latino; 1 Hispanic/Latino; 2 Two or more races,

non-Hispanic/Latino), 22 international. Average age 26. 221 applicants, 12% accepted, 26 enrolled. In 2013, 8 master's, 24 doctorates awarded. Terminal master's awarded for partial completion of doctoral program. *Degree requirements:* For master's, comprehensive exam, thesis; for doctorate, comprehensive exam, thesis/dissertation. *Entrance requirements:* For master's and doctorate, GRE General Test, minimum GPA of 3.0. Additional exam requirements/recommendations for international students: Required—TOEFL (minimum score 550 paper-based). *Application deadline:* For fall admission, 12/17 priority date for domestic and international students. Applications are processed on a rolling basis. Application fee: $85. Electronic applications accepted. *Financial support:* In 2013–14, 13 students received support, including 32 fellowships with full tuition reimbursements available (averaging $27,500 per year), 32 research assistantships with full tuition reimbursements available (averaging $27,500 per year), 13 teaching assistantships with full tuition reimbursements available (averaging $27,500 per year); career-related internships or fieldwork, Federal Work-Study, institutionally sponsored loans, scholarships/grants, traineeships, health care benefits, and unspecified assistantships also available. Financial award application deadline: 4/1. *Faculty research:* Health services research, pharmacokinetics, molecular modeling, infectious disease, genomics and proteomics, translational research. *Total annual research expenditures:* $27.7 million. *Unit head:* Dr. Robert A. Blouin, Dean, 919-966-1122, Fax: 919-966-6919, E-mail: bob_blouin@unc.edu. *Application contact:* Mimi Lewis, Assistant Director of Admissions, 919-962-0097, Fax: 919-966-9428, E-mail: mimi_lewis@unc.edu.
Website: http://pharmacy.unc.edu/

University of Oklahoma Health Sciences Center, College of Pharmacy and Graduate College, Graduate Programs in Pharmacy, Oklahoma City, OK 73190. Offers MS, PhD, MS/MBA. MS/MBA offered jointly with Oklahoma State University and University of Oklahoma. *Faculty:* 11 full-time (5 women), 1 part-time/adjunct (0 women). *Students:* 7 full-time (4 women), 12 part-time (2 women); includes 4 minority (2 Asian, non-Hispanic/Latino; 1 Hispanic/Latino; 1 Two or more races, non-Hispanic/Latino), 8 international. Average age 33. 43 applicants, 9% accepted, 3 enrolled. In 2013, 1 master's, 4 doctorates awarded. Terminal master's awarded for partial completion of doctoral program. *Degree requirements:* For master's, comprehensive exam, thesis; for doctorate, comprehensive exam, thesis/dissertation. *Entrance requirements:* For master's and doctorate, GRE General Test. Additional exam requirements/recommendations for international students: Required—TOEFL. *Application deadline:* For fall admission, 4/1 priority date for domestic students. Application fee: $50. *Expenses:* Tuition, state resident: full-time $3504; part-time $175.20 per credit hour. Tuition, nonresident: full-time $13,504; part-time $675.20 per credit hour. *Required fees:* $1545; $52.70 per credit hour. $245.25 per semester. Tuition and fees vary according to course load. *Financial support:* In 2013–14, 9 research assistantships (averaging $17,000 per year) were awarded; fellowships, teaching assistantships, career-related internships or fieldwork, and institutionally sponsored loans also available. *Faculty research:* Medicinal chemistry, pharmacokinetics/biopharmaceutics, nuclear pharmacy, pharmacy administration, pharmacodynamics and toxicology. *Unit head:* Dr. Nathan Shankar, Graduate Liaison, 405-271-6598. *Application contact:* Director of Student Services.

University of Pittsburgh, School of Pharmacy, Graduate Program in Pharmaceutical Sciences, Pittsburgh, PA 15260. Offers MS, PhD. Part-time programs available. *Faculty:* 39 full-time (11 women). *Students:* 86 full-time (42 women), 3 part-time (2 women); includes 5 minority (2 Black or African American, non-Hispanic/Latino; 3 Asian, non-Hispanic/Latino), 68 international. Average age 30. 95 applicants, 39% accepted, 24 enrolled. In 2013, 9 master's, 4 doctorates awarded. Terminal master's awarded for partial completion of doctoral program. *Degree requirements:* For master's, comprehensive exam (for some programs), thesis (for some programs); for doctorate, comprehensive exam, thesis/dissertation, 72 credits. *Entrance requirements:* For master's and doctorate, GRE General Test. Additional exam requirements/recommendations for international students: Required—TOEFL (minimum score 590 paper-based; 96 iBT). *Application deadline:* For fall admission, 12/15 priority date for domestic and international students. Applications are processed on a rolling basis. Application fee: $50. Electronic applications accepted. *Expenses:* Contact institution. *Financial support:* In 2013–14, 43 students received support, including 5 fellowships with full tuition reimbursements available (averaging $24,000 per year), 22 research assistantships with full tuition reimbursements available (averaging $28,665 per year), 16 teaching assistantships with full tuition reimbursements available (averaging $23,763 per year); career-related internships or fieldwork, scholarships/grants, health care benefits, and unspecified assistantships also available. Financial award application deadline: 12/15. *Faculty research:* Drug delivery and targeting; neuroendocrine pharmacology; genomics, proteomics, and drug discovery; clinical pharmaceutical sciences. *Unit head:* Dr. M. Maggie Folan, Chair, Graduate Program Council, 412-648-8555, Fax: 412-383-9996, E-mail: folanm@pitt.edu. *Application contact:* Lori M. Schmotzer, Graduate Program Coordinator, 412-648-1014, Fax: 412-383-9996, E-mail: schmotze@pitt.edu.
Website: http://www.pharmacy.pitt.edu

University of Puerto Rico, Medical Sciences Campus, School of Pharmacy, San Juan, PR 00936-5067. Offers industrial pharmacy (MS); pharmaceutical sciences (MS); pharmacy (Pharm D). The MS in Pharmacy program is not admitting students in the academic year 2010-2011. *Accreditation:* ACPE. Part-time and evening/weekend programs available. *Degree requirements:* For master's, thesis; for doctorate, portfolio, research project. *Entrance requirements:* For master's, GRE, interview; for doctorate, PCAT, interview. Electronic applications accepted. *Expenses:* Contact institution. *Faculty research:* Controlled release, solid dosage form, screening of anti-HIV drugs, pharmacokinetic/pharmacodynamic of drugs.

University of Rhode Island, Graduate School, College of Pharmacy, Department of Biomedical and Pharmaceutical Sciences, Kingston, RI 02881. Offers medicinal chemistry and pharmacognosy (MS, PhD); pharmaceutics and pharmacokinetics (MS, PhD); pharmacology and toxicology (MS, PhD). Part-time programs available. *Faculty:* 21 full-time (7 women). *Students:* 37 full-time (14 women), 15 part-time (7 women); includes 3 minority (1 Black or African American, non-Hispanic/Latino; 1 Asian, non-Hispanic/Latino; 1 Two or more races, non-Hispanic/Latino), 29 international. In 2013, 3 master's, 18 doctorates awarded. *Entrance requirements:* For master's and doctorate, GRE (minimum new/old format scores: Verbal 350/143; Quantitative 550/146; Analytical, 3.0), 2 letters of recommendation. Additional exam requirements/recommendations for international students: Required—TOEFL (minimum score 550 paper-based). *Application deadline:* For fall admission, 7/15 for domestic students, 2/1 for international students. Application fee: $65. Electronic applications accepted. *Expenses:* Tuition, state resident: full-time $11,532; part-time $641 per credit. Tuition, nonresident: full-time $23,606; part-time $1311 per credit. *Required fees:* $1388; $36 per credit. $35 per semester. One-time fee: $130. *Financial support:* In 2013–14, 8 research assistantships with full and partial tuition reimbursements (averaging $12,147 per year), 13 teaching assistantships with full and partial tuition reimbursements (averaging $13,579 per year) were awarded. Financial award application deadline: 2/1; financial award applicants required to submit FAFSA. *Faculty research:* Chemical carcinogenesis with a major emphasis on the structural and synthetic aspects of DNA-adduct formation, drug-drug/herb interaction, drug-genetic interaction, signaling of nuclear receptors, transcriptional regulation, oncogenesis. *Total annual research expenditures:* $5.8 million. *Unit head:* Dr. Bingfang Yan, Chair, 401-874-5032, Fax: 401-874-2181, E-mail: byan@uri.edu. *Application contact:* Graduate Admissions, 401-874-2872, E-mail: gradadm@etal.uri.edu.
Website: http://www.uri.edu/pharmacy/departments/bps/index.shtml

University of Rhode Island, Graduate School, College of Pharmacy, Department of Pharmacy Practice, Kingston, RI 02881. Offers pharmaceutical sciences (MS, PhD), including pharmacoepidemiology and pharmacoeconomics; pharmacy practice (Pharm D); MS/PhD; PhD/MBA. *Accreditation:* ACPE. *Faculty:* 29 full-time (24 women). *Students:* 727 full-time (452 women), 1 (woman) part-time; includes 123 minority (22 Black or African American, non-Hispanic/Latino; 58 Asian, non-Hispanic/Latino; 31 Hispanic/Latino; 12 Two or more races, non-Hispanic/Latino), 36 international. In 2013, 97 doctorates awarded. *Entrance requirements:* For master's and doctorate, 2 letters of recommendation. Additional exam requirements/recommendations for international students: Required—TOEFL (minimum score 550 paper-based). *Application deadline:* For fall admission, 2/1 for domestic and international students. Application fee: $65. Electronic applications accepted. *Expenses:* Tuition, state resident: full-time $11,532; part-time $641 per credit. Tuition, nonresident: full-time $23,606; part-time $1311 per credit. *Required fees:* $1388; $36 per credit. $35 per semester. One-time fee: $130. *Financial support:* Application deadline: 2/1; applicants required to submit FAFSA. *Faculty research:* Treatment, virulence inhibition (toxin and biofilm), colonization and control of Methicillin-resistant Staphylococcus aureus (MRSA); investigating activity of catheter lock solutions against biofilm producing bacteria. *Total annual research expenditures:* $464,501. *Unit head:* Dr. Marilyn Barbour, Chair, 401-874-5842, Fax: 401-874-2181, E-mail: mbarbourri@aol.com.
Website: http://www.uri.edu/pharmacy/departments/php/index.shtml

University of Saskatchewan, College of Graduate Studies and Research, College of Pharmacy and Nutrition, Saskatoon, SK S7N 5A2, Canada. Offers M Sc, PhD. *Degree requirements:* For master's, thesis; for doctorate, thesis/dissertation. *Entrance requirements:* Additional exam requirements/recommendations for international students: Required—TOEFL. *Expenses: Tuition, area resident:* Full-time $3585 Canadian dollars; part-time $585 Canadian dollars per course. Tuition, nonresident: part-time $877 Canadian dollars per course. *International tuition:* $5377 Canadian dollars full-time. *Required fees:* $889.51 Canadian dollars.

University of South Carolina, South Carolina College of Pharmacy and The Graduate School, Department of Basic Pharmaceutical Sciences, Columbia, SC 29208. Offers MS, PhD. PhD offered jointly with Medical University of South Carolina. Part-time programs available. Terminal master's awarded for partial completion of doctoral program. *Degree requirements:* For master's, one foreign language, comprehensive exam, thesis; for doctorate, one foreign language, comprehensive exam, thesis/dissertation. *Entrance requirements:* For master's, GRE General Test, BS in biology, chemistry, pharmacy, or related field; for doctorate, GRE General Test, BS in biology, chemistry, or related field. Additional exam requirements/recommendations for international students: Required—TOEFL. Electronic applications accepted. *Faculty research:* Cancer treatment and prevention, Ion channels, DNA damage repair, inflammation.

University of Southern California, Graduate School, School of Pharmacy, Department of Pharmacology and Pharmaceutical Sciences, Los Angeles, CA 90089. Offers MS, PhD. Terminal master's awarded for partial completion of doctoral program. *Degree requirements:* For master's, comprehensive exam, thesis, 24 units of formal course work, excluding research and seminar courses; for doctorate, comprehensive exam, thesis/dissertation, 24 units of formal course work, excluding research and seminar courses. *Entrance requirements:* For master's and doctorate, GRE. Additional exam requirements/recommendations for international students: Required—TOEFL (minimum score 603 paper-based; 100 iBT). Electronic applications accepted. *Faculty research:* Drug design, drug delivery, pharmaceutical sciences.

University of Southern California, Graduate School, School of Pharmacy, Graduate Programs in Pharmaceutical Economics and Policy, Los Angeles, CA 90033. Offers MS, PhD. Terminal master's awarded for partial completion of doctoral program. *Degree requirements:* For master's, comprehensive exam, thesis, 24 units of formal course work, excluding research and seminar courses; for doctorate, comprehensive exam, thesis/dissertation, 24 units of formal course work, excluding research and seminar courses. *Entrance requirements:* For master's and doctorate, GRE. Additional exam requirements/recommendations for international students: Required—TOEFL (minimum score 603 paper-based; 100 iBT). Electronic applications accepted. *Faculty research:* Cost-effective analyses/modeling, retrospective data analysis of comparative effectiveness, quality of life measurement, competitive pricing systems in health care.

University of Southern California, Graduate School, School of Pharmacy, Program in Clinical and Experimental Therapeutics, Los Angeles, CA 90089. Offers PhD. Terminal master's awarded for partial completion of doctoral program. *Degree requirements:* For doctorate, comprehensive exam, thesis/dissertation, 24 units of course work, excluding research and dissertation courses. *Entrance requirements:* For doctorate, GRE, minimum overall GPA of 3.0, three letters of recommendation. Additional exam requirements/recommendations for international students: Required—TOEFL (minimum score 625 paper-based; 100 iBT). Electronic applications accepted. *Faculty research:* Pharmacology and therapeutics: inflammation, tissue regeneration, myelosuppression, bacterial resistance and virulence, alcoholism, CNS disorders, metabolomics and lipidomics.

University of Southern California, Graduate School, School of Pharmacy, Regulatory Science Programs, Los Angeles, CA 90089. Offers clinical research design and management (Graduate Certificate); food safety (Graduate Certificate); patient and product safety (Graduate Certificate); preclinical drug development (Graduate Certificate); regulatory and clinical affairs (Graduate Certificate); regulatory science (MS, DRSc). Part-time and evening/weekend programs available. Postbaccalaureate distance learning degree programs offered (minimal on-campus study). Terminal master's awarded for partial completion of doctoral program. *Degree requirements:* For master's, thesis optional; for doctorate, comprehensive exam, thesis/dissertation. *Entrance requirements:* For master's, GRE. Additional exam requirements/recommendations for international students: Required—TOEFL (minimum score 603 paper-based; 100 iBT). Electronic applications accepted.

The University of Tennessee Health Science Center, College of Graduate Health Sciences, Memphis, TN 38163-0002. Offers biomedical engineering (MS, PhD); biomedical sciences (PhD); dental sciences (MDS); epidemiology (MS); health outcomes and policy research (PhD); laboratory research and management (MS); nursing science (PhD); pharmaceutical sciences (PhD); pharmacology (MS); speech and hearing science (PhD); DDS/PhD; DNP/PhD; MD/PhD; Pharm D/PhD. *Faculty:* 318 full-time (92 women), 59 part-time/adjunct (16 women). *Students:* 220 full-time (102 women), 22 part-time (13 women); includes 194 minority (22 Black or African American, non-Hispanic/Latino; 161 Asian, non-Hispanic/Latino; 7 Hispanic/Latino; 3 Native Hawaiian or other Pacific Islander, non-Hispanic/Latino; 1 Two or more races, non-Hispanic/Latino), 106 international. Average age 25. 404 applicants, 17% accepted, 64 enrolled. In 2013, 13 master's, 25 doctorates awarded. Terminal master's awarded for partial completion of doctoral program. *Degree requirements:* For master's, comprehensive exam, thesis; for doctorate, comprehensive exam, thesis/dissertation, oral and written preliminary and comprehensive exams. *Entrance requirements:* For master's and doctorate, GRE General Test, minimum GPA of 3.0. Additional exam requirements/recommendations for international students: Required—TOEFL (minimum score 79 iBT); Recommended—IELTS (minimum score 6.5). *Application deadline:* For fall admission, 5/15 priority date for domestic students. Applications are processed on a rolling basis. Application fee: $0. Electronic applications accepted. *Financial support:* In 2013–14, 125 students received support, including 125 research assistantships (averaging $23,000 per year); career-related internships or fieldwork, Federal Work-Study, institutionally sponsored loans, and tuition waivers (full and partial) also available. Support available to part-time students. Financial award application deadline: 2/25; financial award applicants required to submit FAFSA. *Unit head:* Dr. Donald B. Thomason, Dean, 901-448-5538, E-mail: dthomaso@uthsc.edu. *Application contact:* William Carter, Director for Admissions, 901-448-1687, E-mail: wcarte17@uthsc.edu. Website: http://www.uthsc.edu/grad/

The University of Texas at Austin, Graduate School, College of Pharmacy, Graduate Programs in Pharmacy, Austin, TX 78712-1111. Offers health outcomes and pharmacy practice (PhD); health outcomes and pharmacy practice (MS); medicinal chemistry (PhD); pharmaceutics (PhD); pharmacology and toxicology (PhD); pharmacotherapy (MS, PhD); translational science (PhD). PhD in translational science offered jointly with The University of Texas Health Science Center at San Antonio and The University of Texas at San Antonio. *Degree requirements:* For master's, thesis; for doctorate, thesis/dissertation. *Entrance requirements:* For master's and doctorate, GRE General Test. Electronic applications accepted. *Faculty research:* Synthetic medical chemistry, synthetic molecular biology, bio-organic chemistry, pharmacoeconomics, pharmacy practice.

University of the Pacific, Thomas J. Long School of Pharmacy and Health Sciences, Pharmaceutical and Chemical Sciences Graduate Program, Stockton, CA 95211-0197. Offers MS, PhD. *Faculty:* 7 full-time (1 woman). *Students:* 5 full-time (3 women), 53 part-time (28 women); includes 12 minority (1 Black or African American, non-Hispanic/Latino; 9 Asian, non-Hispanic/Latino; 2 Hispanic/Latino), 39 international. Average age 27. 89 applicants, 21% accepted, 19 enrolled. In 2013, 2 master's, 2 doctorates awarded. *Entrance requirements:* Additional exam requirements/recommendations for international students: Required—TOEFL (minimum score 475 paper-based). Application fee: $75. *Financial support:* In 2013–14, 18 teaching assistantships were awarded. Financial award application deadline: 3/1; financial award applicants required to submit FAFSA. *Unit head:* Dr. Xiaolin Li, Head, 209-946-3163, E-mail: xli@pacific.edu. *Application contact:* Ron Espejo, Recruitment Specialist, 209-946-3957, Fax: 209-946-3147, E-mail: respejo@pacific.edu.

University of the Sciences, College of Graduate Studies, Program in Pharmaceutics, Philadelphia, PA 19104-4495. Offers MS, PhD. Part-time programs available. *Faculty:* 3 full-time (0 women). *Students:* 10 full-time (7 women), 27 part-time (15 women); includes 4 minority (all Asian, non-Hispanic/Latino), 7 international. Average age 33. In 2013, 3 doctorates awarded. Terminal master's awarded for partial completion of doctoral program. *Degree requirements:* For master's, thesis (for some programs); for doctorate, comprehensive exam, thesis/dissertation, oral defense. *Entrance requirements:* For master's and doctorate, GRE General Test. Additional exam requirements/recommendations for international students: Required—TOEFL, TWE. *Application deadline:* For fall admission, 5/1 for international students; for winter admission, 10/1 for international students; for spring admission, 3/1 for international students. Applications are processed on a rolling basis. Application fee: $50. *Expenses: Tuition:* Part-time $1447 per credit. Tuition and fees vary according to campus/location and program. *Financial support:* In 2013–14, 13 students received support, including 1 fellowship with full tuition reimbursement available, 1 research assistantship with full tuition reimbursement available, 9 teaching assistantships with full tuition reimbursements available (averaging $18,996 per year); institutionally sponsored loans and tuition waivers (full and partial) also available. Financial award application deadline: 3/1. *Faculty research:* Pharmacodynamics, disperse systems, peptide-biomembranes interactions, in vitro/in vivo correlations, cellular drug delivery. *Unit head:* Dr. Shenaz Tejani-Butt, Associate Dean, Graduate Studies, 215-596-8591, E-mail: graduate@usciences.edu. *Application contact:* Christopher Miciek, Associate Director, Graduate Admissions, 215-596-8597, E-mail: c.miciek@usciences.edu.

The University of Toledo, College of Graduate Studies, College of Pharmacy and Pharmaceutical Sciences, Program in Pharmaceutical Sciences, Toledo, OH 43606-3390. Offers administrative pharmacy (MSPS); industrial pharmacy (MSPS); pharmacology toxicology (MSPS). *Degree requirements:* For master's, thesis. *Entrance requirements:* For master's, GRE General Test. Additional exam requirements/recommendations for international students: Required—TOEFL (minimum score 550 paper-based; 80 iBT). Electronic applications accepted.

University of Toronto, School of Graduate Studies, Leslie Dan Faculty of Pharmacy, Toronto, ON M5S 1A1, Canada. Offers M Sc, PhD, Pharm D. Part-time programs available. *Degree requirements:* For master's, thesis, poster presentation, oral thesis defense; for doctorate, thesis/dissertation (for some programs). *Entrance requirements:* For master's, minimum B average in last 2 years of full-time study, 3 letters of reference, resume. Additional exam requirements/recommendations for international students: Required—TOEFL (600 paper-based), Michigan English Language Assessment Battery (88) or IELTS (7); GRE General Test. Electronic applications accepted.

University of Utah, Graduate School, College of Pharmacy, Department of Pharmacotherapy, Salt Lake City, UT 84112. Offers health system pharmacy administration (MS); outcomes research and health policy (PhD). *Faculty:* 5 full-time (3 women), 28 part-time/adjunct (17 women). *Students:* 7 full-time (4 women), 5 international. Average age 27. 26 applicants, 19% accepted, 2 enrolled. In 2013, 4 master's awarded. Terminal master's awarded for partial completion of doctoral program. *Degree requirements:* For master's, comprehensive exam, thesis or alternative, project; for doctorate, comprehensive exam, thesis/dissertation. *Entrance requirements:* For doctorate, GRE. Additional exam requirements/recommendations for international students: Required—TOEFL (minimum score 550 paper-based; 80 iBT). *Application deadline:* For fall admission, 1/10 for domestic students, 12/15 for international students. Application fee: $55 ($65 for international students). *Expenses:* Tuition, state resident: full-time $5259. Tuition, nonresident: full-time $18,569. *Required fees:* $841. Tuition and fees vary according to course load. *Financial support:* In 2013–14, 7 students received support, including 5 research assistantships with full tuition reimbursements available (averaging $21,400 per year); health care benefits and unspecified assistantships also available. Financial award application deadline: 12/15. *Faculty research:* Outcomes in pharmacy, pharmacotherapy. *Total annual research expenditures:* $131,217. *Unit head:* Dr. Diana I. Brixner, Department Chair and Professor, 801-581-6731. *Application contact:* Sara Ray, Academic Program Manager, 801-581-5984, Fax: 801-585-6160, E-mail: sara.ray@pharm.utah.edu. Website: http://www.pharmacy.utah.edu/pharmacotherapy/

University of Washington, School of Pharmacy, Department of Pharmaceutics, Seattle, WA 98195. Offers MS, PhD, Pharm D/PhD. *Faculty:* 15 full-time (7 women). *Students:* 23 full-time (12 women); includes 6 minority (3 Asian, non-Hispanic/Latino; 3 Hispanic/Latino), 5 international. Average age 30. 69 applicants, 10% accepted, 5 enrolled. In 2013, 1 master's, 4 doctorates awarded. Terminal master's awarded for partial completion of doctoral program. *Degree requirements:* For master's, thesis; for doctorate, thesis/dissertation. *Entrance requirements:* For master's and doctorate, GRE General Test. Additional exam requirements/recommendations for international students: Required—TOEFL. *Application deadline:* For fall admission, 1/15 for domestic and international students. Application fee: $75. Electronic applications accepted. *Financial support:* In 2013–14, 22 students received support, including 6 fellowships with full tuition reimbursements available (averaging $27,900 per year), 16 research assistantships with full tuition reimbursements available (averaging $27,900 per year); career-related internships or fieldwork, institutionally sponsored loans, scholarships/grants, traineeships, health care benefits, tuition waivers, and unspecified assistantships also available. *Faculty research:* Pharmacokinetics, drug delivery, drug metabolism, pharmacogenetics, transporters. *Unit head:* Dr. Kenneth E. Thummel, Chair, 206-543-9434, Fax: 206-543-3204, E-mail: thummel@u.washington.edu. *Application contact:* Dr. Yvonne Lin, Graduate Program Director, 206-616-2797, Fax: 206-543-3204, E-mail: pceut@u.washington.edu. Website: http://sop.washington.edu/pharmaceutics

University of Wisconsin–Madison, School of Pharmacy and Graduate School, Graduate Programs in Pharmacy, Pharmaceutical Sciences Division, Madison, WI 53706-1380. Offers PhD. Terminal master's awarded for partial completion of doctoral program. *Degree requirements:* For doctorate, comprehensive exam, thesis/dissertation. *Entrance requirements:* For doctorate, GRE. Additional exam requirements/recommendations for international students: Required—TOEFL. Electronic applications accepted. *Expenses:* Tuition, state resident: full-time $10,728; part-time $790 per credit. Tuition, nonresident: full-time $24,054; part-time $1623 per credit. *Required fees:* $1130; $119 per credit. *Faculty research:* Drug action, drug delivery, drug discovery.

University of Wisconsin–Madison, School of Pharmacy and Graduate School, Graduate Programs in Pharmacy, Social and Administrative Sciences in Pharmacy Division, Madison, WI 53706-1380. Offers MS, PhD. Terminal master's awarded for partial completion of doctoral program. *Degree requirements:* For master's, comprehensive exam (for some programs), thesis optional; for doctorate, comprehensive exam, thesis/dissertation. *Entrance requirements:* For master's and doctorate, GRE. Additional exam requirements/recommendations for international students: Required—TOEFL. Electronic applications accepted. *Expenses:* Tuition, state resident: full-time $10,728; part-time $790 per credit. Tuition, nonresident: full-time $24,054; part-time $1623 per credit. *Required fees:* $1130; $119 per credit. *Faculty research:* Patient-provider communication, economics, patient care systems.

Virginia Commonwealth University, Medical College of Virginia-Professional Programs, School of Pharmacy, Department of Pharmaceutics, Richmond, VA 23284-9005. Offers medicinal chemistry (MS); pharmaceutical sciences (PhD); pharmaceutics (MS); pharmacotherapy and pharmacy administration (MS). Terminal master's awarded for partial completion of doctoral program. *Degree requirements:* For master's, thesis; for doctorate, thesis/dissertation. *Entrance requirements:* For master's and doctorate, GRE General Test. Additional exam requirements/recommendations for international students: Required—TOEFL. Electronic applications accepted. *Faculty research:* Drug delivery systems, drug development.

Washington State University Spokane, Graduate Program in Pharmaceutical Sciences, Spokane, WA 99210-1495. Offers PhD. Terminal master's awarded for partial completion of doctoral program. *Degree requirements:* For doctorate, comprehensive exam, thesis/dissertation. *Entrance requirements:* For doctorate, GRE, BS, minimum GPA of 3.0. Additional exam requirements/recommendations for international students: Required—TOEFL. Electronic applications accepted. *Faculty research:* Cancer biology and therapy, gene therapy and delivery, diabetes and novel approaches to its clinical management, pharmacokinetics, proteomics, reproductive biology and neuropharmacology.

Wayne State University, Eugene Applebaum College of Pharmacy and Health Sciences, Department of Pharmaceutical Sciences, Detroit, MI 48202. Offers medicinal chemistry (MS, PhD); pharmaceutics (MS, PhD); pharmacology/toxicology (MS, PhD). *Accreditation:* ACPE (one or more programs are accredited). Part-time programs available. *Faculty:* 17 full-time (3 women). *Students:* 33 full-time (15 women), 2 part-time (1 woman); includes 3 minority (1 American Indian or Alaska Native, non-Hispanic/Latino; 2 Asian, non-Hispanic/Latino), 29 international. Average age 25. 205 applicants, 8% accepted, 9 enrolled. In 2013, 1 master's, 3 doctorates awarded. *Degree requirements:* For master's, thesis; for doctorate, thesis/dissertation. *Entrance requirements:* For master's, GRE General Test, admission to the Graduate School, bachelor's degree, three letters of recommendation, personal statement; for doctorate, GRE General Test, admission to the Graduate School; bachelor's or master's degree in one of the behavioral, biological, pharmaceutical or physical sciences; minimum undergraduate GPA of 3.0; three letters of recommendation. Additional exam requirements/recommendations for international students: Required—TOEFL (minimum score 550 paper-based; 79 iBT), Michigan English Language Assessment Battery (minimum score 85); Recommended—IELTS (minimum score 6.5), TWE (minimum score 5.5). *Application deadline:* For fall admission, 3/1 for domestic and international students. Application fee: $0. Electronic applications accepted. *Expenses:* Contact institution. *Financial support:* In 2013–14, 13 students received support, including 2 fellowships with tuition reimbursements available (averaging $24,272 per year), 11 research assistantships with full tuition reimbursements available (averaging $24,565 per year); scholarships/grants, health care benefits, and unspecified assistantships also available. Financial award application deadline: 3/31; financial award applicants required to submit FAFSA. *Faculty research:* Mechanisms of resistance of bacteria to anti-microbial agents, drug metabolism and disposition in children, treatment strategies for stroke/neurovascular disease, prevalence and treatment of diabetes in Arab-Americans, ethnic variability in development of osteoporosis. *Unit head:* Dr. George Corcoran, Chair and Professor, 313-577-1737, E-mail: corcoran@wayne.edu. *Application contact:* 313-577-1047, E-mail: pscgrad@wayne.edu. Website: http://www.cphs.wayne.edu/psc/index.php

Western University of Health Sciences, College of Pharmacy, Program in Pharmaceutical Sciences, Pomona, CA 91766-1854. Offers MS. *Faculty:* 12 full-time (4 women), 1 part-time/adjunct (0 women). *Students:* 9 full-time (5 women), 3 part-time (2 women); includes 6 minority (all Asian, non-Hispanic/Latino), 3 international. Average age 25. 36 applicants, 11% accepted, 4 enrolled. In 2013, 9 master's awarded. *Entrance requirements:* For master's, GRE, minimum overall GPA of 2.5; BS in pharmacy, chemistry, biology or related scientific area, letters of recommendation, curriculum vitae. Additional exam requirements/recommendations for international students: Required—TOEFL (minimum score 550 paper-based; 79 iBT). *Application deadline:* For fall admission, 3/1 for domestic and international students; for spring admission, 1/1 for domestic and international students. Application fee: $40. Electronic applications accepted. *Expenses:* Contact institution. *Financial support:* Institutionally sponsored loans and scholarships/grants available. Financial award application deadline: 3/2; financial award applicants required to submit FAFSA. *Unit head:* Jeffrey Wang, Chair, 909-469-5413, Fax: 909-469-5539, E-mail: jwang@westernu.edu. *Application contact:*

Kathryn Ford, Director of Admissions, 909-469-5335, Fax: 909-469-5570, E-mail: admissions@westernu.edu.
Website: http://www.westernu.edu/pharmacy-dpp_message

West Virginia University, School of Medicine, Graduate Programs at the Health Sciences Center, Interdisciplinary Graduate Programs in Biomedical Sciences, Program in Pharmaceutical and Pharmacological Sciences, Morgantown, WV 26506. Offers MS, PhD, MD/PhD. *Degree requirements:* For doctorate, comprehensive exam, thesis/dissertation. *Entrance requirements:* For doctorate, GRE General Test, minimum GPA of 3.0. Additional exam requirements/recommendations for international students: Required—TOEFL. Electronic applications accepted. *Faculty research:* Medicinal chemistry, pharmacokinetics, nano-pharmaceutics, polymer-based drug delivery, molecular therapeutics.

West Virginia University, School of Pharmacy, Program in Pharmaceutical and Pharmacological Sciences, Morgantown, WV 26506. Offers administrative pharmacy (PhD); behavioral pharmacy (MS, PhD); biopharmaceutics/pharmacokinetics (MS, PhD); industrial pharmacy (MS); medicinal chemistry (MS, PhD); pharmaceutical chemistry (MS, PhD); pharmaceutics (MS, PhD); pharmacology and toxicology (MS); pharmacy (MS); pharmacy administration (MS). Part-time programs available. Terminal master's awarded for partial completion of doctoral program. *Degree requirements:* For master's, thesis; for doctorate, one foreign language, comprehensive exam, thesis/dissertation. *Entrance requirements:* For master's and doctorate, GRE General Test, minimum GPA of 2.75. Additional exam requirements/recommendations for international students: Required—TOEFL; Recommended—TWE. Electronic applications accepted. *Expenses:* Contact institution. *Faculty research:* Pharmaceutics, medicinal chemistry, biopharmaceutics/pharmacokinetics, health outcomes research.

Pharmacy

Albany College of Pharmacy and Health Sciences, School of Pharmacy and Pharmaceutical Sciences, Albany, NY 12208. Offers health outcomes research (MS); pharmaceutical sciences (MS), including pharmaceutics, pharmacology; pharmacy (Pharm D). *Accreditation:* ACPE. *Students:* 527 full-time (308 women), 15 part-time (10 women); includes 138 minority (19 Black or African American, non-Hispanic/Latino; 95 Asian, non-Hispanic/Latino; 13 Hispanic/Latino; 1 Native Hawaiian or other Pacific Islander, non-Hispanic/Latino; 10 Two or more races, non-Hispanic/Latino), 64 international. Average age 24. 1,209 applicants, 15% accepted, 78 enrolled. In 2013, 6 master's, 283 doctorates awarded. *Degree requirements:* For master's, thesis; for doctorate, practice experience. *Entrance requirements:* For master's, GRE, minimum GPA of 3.0; for doctorate, PCAT, minimum GPA of 2.5. Additional exam requirements/recommendations for international students: Required—TOEFL (minimum score 84 iBT). *Application deadline:* For fall admission, 3/1 for domestic and international students. Applications are processed on a rolling basis. Application fee: $75. Electronic applications accepted. *Financial support:* In 2013–14, 20 students received support. Federal Work-Study and scholarships/grants available. Support available to part-time students. Financial award application deadline: 3/1; financial award applicants required to submit FAFSA. *Faculty research:* Therapeutic use of drugs, pharmacokinetics, drug delivery and design. *Unit head:* Dr. Angela Dominelli, Dean, School of Pharmacy and Pharmaceutical Sciences, 518-694-7333. *Application contact:* Ann Bruno, Coordinator, Graduate Programs, 518-694-7130, E-mail: graduate@acphs.edu.
Website: http://www.acphs.edu/academics/schools-departments/school-pharmacy-pharmaceutical-sciences

Appalachian College of Pharmacy, Doctor of Pharmacy Program, Oakwood, VA 24631. Offers Pharm D.

Auburn University, Harrison School of Pharmacy, Professional Program in Pharmacy, Auburn University, AL 36849. Offers Pharm D. *Accreditation:* ACPE. Part-time programs available. *Faculty:* 50 full-time (28 women), 1 (woman) part-time/adjunct. *Students:* 584 full-time (393 women), 6 part-time (5 women); includes 103 minority (47 Black or African American, non-Hispanic/Latino; 7 American Indian or Alaska Native, non-Hispanic/Latino; 45 Asian, non-Hispanic/Latino; 4 Hispanic/Latino), 3 international. Average age 24. 539 applicants, 44% accepted, 150 enrolled. In 2013, 147 doctorates awarded. Application fee: $0. *Expenses:* Contact institution. *Financial support:* Federal Work-Study available. Support available to part-time students. Financial award applicants required to submit FAFSA. *Unit head:* Dr. R. Lee Evans, Dean and Professor, Harrison School of Pharmacy, 334-844-8348, Fax: 334-844-8353. *Application contact:* Dr. George Flowers, Dean of the Graduate School, 334-844-2125.

Belmont University, College of Pharmacy, Nashville, TN 37212-3757. Offers Pharm D. *Accreditation:* ACPE. *Faculty:* 29 full-time, 6 part-time/adjunct. *Students:* 290 full-time (172 women), 1 part-time (0 women); includes 43 minority (12 Black or African American, non-Hispanic/Latino; 22 Asian, non-Hispanic/Latino; 8 Hispanic/Latino; 1 Two or more races, non-Hispanic/Latino), 3 international. Average age 25. 806 applicants, 20% accepted, 78 enrolled. *Degree requirements:* For doctorate, comprehensive exam. *Entrance requirements:* For doctorate, PCAT. Additional exam requirements/recommendations for international students: Required—TOEFL. *Application deadline:* For fall admission, 8/31 priority date for domestic students; for spring admission, 3/1 for domestic students. Applications are processed on a rolling basis. Application fee: $50. Electronic applications accepted. *Financial support:* Applicants required to submit FAFSA. *Faculty research:* Academic innovation, cultural competency, medication errors, patient safety. *Unit head:* Dr. Phil Johnston, Dean, 615-460-6746, Fax: 615-460-6741, E-mail: phil.johnston@belmont.edu. *Application contact:* Dr. Elinor Gray, Dean of Enrollment Services, 615-460-6747, Fax: 615-460-6741, E-mail: elinor.gray@belmont.edu.
Website: http://www.belmont.edu/pharmacy

Butler University, College of Pharmacy and Health Sciences, Indianapolis, IN 46208-3485. Offers pharmaceutical science (MS, Pharm D); physician assistance studies (MS). *Accreditation:* ACPE (one or more programs are accredited). Part-time and evening/weekend programs available. *Faculty:* 6 full-time (2 women). *Students:* 296 full-time (196 women), 12 part-time (7 women); includes 24 minority (7 Black or African American, non-Hispanic/Latino; 1 American Indian or Alaska Native, non-Hispanic/Latino; 10 Asian, non-Hispanic/Latino; 4 Hispanic/Latino; 2 Two or more races, non-Hispanic/Latino), 11 international. Average age 24. 52 applicants, 6% accepted, 2 enrolled. In 2013, 50 master's awarded. *Degree requirements:* For master's, research paper or thesis. *Application deadline:* For fall admission, 8/1 priority date for domestic students; for spring admission, 12/15 for domestic students. Applications are processed on a rolling basis. Application fee: $35. Electronic applications accepted. *Expenses:* Contact institution. *Financial support:* Applicants required to submit FAFSA. *Unit head:* Dr. Mary Andritz, Dean, 317-940-8056, E-mail: mandritz@butler.edu. *Application contact:* Diane Dubord, Graduate Student Services Specialist, 317-940-8107, E-mail: ddubord@butler.edu.
Website: http://www.butler.edu/academics/graduate-cophs/

Campbell University, Graduate and Professional Programs, School of Pharmacy, Buies Creek, NC 27506. Offers clinical research (MS); pharmaceutical science (MS); pharmacy (Pharm D). *Accreditation:* ACPE. Part-time and evening/weekend programs available. *Entrance requirements:* For master's, MCAT, PCAT, GRE, bachelor's degree in health sciences or related field; for doctorate, PCAT. Additional exam requirements/recommendations for international students: Required—TOEFL (minimum score 550 paper-based; 79 iBT). Electronic applications accepted. *Expenses:* Contact institution. *Faculty research:* Immunology, medicinal chemistry, pharmaceutics, applied pharmacology.

Cedarville University, Graduate Programs, Cedarville, OH 45314-0601. Offers business administration (MBA); curriculum (M Ed); educational administration (M Ed); family nurse practitioner (MSN); global health ministries (MSN); instruction (M Ed); pharmacy (Pharm D). Part-time programs available. Postbaccalaureate distance learning degree programs offered (no on-campus study). *Faculty:* 23 full-time (12 women), 12 part-time/adjunct (5 women). *Students:* 119 full-time (74 women), 103 part-time (73 women); includes 16 minority (11 Black or African American, non-Hispanic/Latino; 4 Asian, non-Hispanic/Latino; 1 Native Hawaiian or other Pacific Islander, non-Hispanic/Latino), 4 international. Average age 31. In 2013, 26 master's awarded. *Degree requirements:* For master's, thesis. *Entrance requirements:* For master's, GRE, 2 professional recommendations; for doctorate, PCAT, professional recommendation from a practicing pharmacist or current employer/supervisor, resume, essay, interview. Additional exam requirements/recommendations for international students: Required—TOEFL (minimum score 550 paper-based; 80 iBT). *Application deadline:* For fall admission, 5/1 priority date for domestic and international students; for spring admission, 11/1 priority date for domestic and international students. Applications are processed on a rolling basis. Application fee: $30. Electronic applications accepted. *Financial support:* Scholarships/grants and unspecified assistantships available. Support available to part-time students. Financial award applicants required to submit FAFSA. *Unit head:* Dr. Mark McClain, Dean of Graduate Studies, 937-766-7700, E-mail: mcclain@cedarville.edu. *Application contact:* Roscoe F. Smith, Associate Vice-President of Enrollment, 937-766-7700, Fax: 937-766-7575, E-mail: smithr@cedarville.edu.
Website: http://www.cedarville.edu/academics/graduate/

Chicago State University, College of Pharmacy, Chicago, IL 60628. Offers Pharm D. *Accreditation:* ACPE. *Entrance requirements:* For doctorate, PCAT, minimum cumulative GPA of 2.5.

Creighton University, School of Pharmacy and Health Professions, Professional Program in Pharmacy, Omaha, NE 68178-0001. Offers Pharm D. *Accreditation:* ACPE. Postbaccalaureate distance learning degree programs offered (no on-campus study). *Entrance requirements:* For doctorate, PCAT. Additional exam requirements/recommendations for international students: Required—TOEFL. Electronic applications accepted. *Expenses: Tuition:* Full-time $13,608; part-time $756 per credit hour. *Required fees:* $149 per semester. Tuition and fees vary according to course load, campus/location, program, reciprocity agreements and student's religious affiliation. *Faculty research:* Patient safety in health services research, health information technology and health services research, nanotechnology and drug development, pharmacy practice outcomes research, cross-cultural care of patients in pharmacy practice.

Drake University, College of Pharmacy and Health Sciences, Des Moines, IA 50311-4516. Offers pharmacy (Pharm D); Pharm D/JD; Pharm D/MBA; Pharm D/MPA. *Accreditation:* ACPE. *Faculty:* 37 full-time (16 women), 1 part-time/adjunct (0 women). *Students:* 446 full-time (302 women), 3 part-time (1 woman); includes 67 minority (3 Black or African American, non-Hispanic/Latino; 1 American Indian or Alaska Native, non-Hispanic/Latino; 50 Asian, non-Hispanic/Latino; 5 Hispanic/Latino; 8 Two or more races, non-Hispanic/Latino), 2 international. Average age 22. In 2013, 122 doctorates awarded. *Degree requirements:* For doctorate, rotations. *Entrance requirements:* For doctorate, PCAT, interview. Additional exam requirements/recommendations for international students: Required—TOEFL. *Application deadline:* For fall admission, 2/1 priority date for domestic students. Application fee: $135. Electronic applications accepted. *Expenses:* Contact institution. *Financial support:* In 2013–14, 10 teaching assistantships (averaging $3,200 per year) were awarded; career-related internships or fieldwork, Federal Work-Study, institutionally sponsored loans, and scholarships/grants also available. Support available to part-time students. Financial award application deadline: 3/1; financial award applicants required to submit FAFSA. *Faculty research:* Cost-benefit and cost-analysis of pharmaceutical products and services, patient satisfaction, community health planning and development, nutrition, ambulatory care. *Total annual research expenditures:* $163,164. *Unit head:* Dr. Wendy Duncan, Dean, 515-271-1814, Fax: 515-271-4171, E-mail: wendy.duncan@drake.edu. *Application contact:* Dr. Renae J. Chesnut, Associate Dean for Student Affairs, 515-271-3018, Fax: 515-271-4171, E-mail: renae.chesnut@drake.edu.
Website: http://pharmacy.drake.edu/

Duquesne University, Mylan School of Pharmacy, Professional Program in Pharmacy, Pittsburgh, PA 15282. Offers Pharm D. Students enter program as first-year undergraduates. *Accreditation:* ACPE. Evening/weekend programs available. *Faculty:* 45 full-time (19 women), 4 part-time/adjunct (0 women). *Students:* 721 full-time (445 women), 63 part-time (39 women); includes 69 minority (20 Black or African American, non-Hispanic/Latino; 1 American Indian or Alaska Native, non-Hispanic/Latino; 34 Asian, non-Hispanic/Latino; 9 Hispanic/Latino; 5 Two or more races, non-Hispanic/Latino), 11 international. Average age 23. 355 applicants, 69% accepted, 226 enrolled. In 2013, 205 doctorates awarded. *Entrance requirements:* For doctorate, PCAT (for professional phase). Additional exam requirements/recommendations for international students: Required—TOEFL. *Application deadline:* For fall admission, 12/1 priority date for domestic and international students. Applications are processed on a rolling basis. Application fee: $100. Electronic applications accepted. *Expenses: Tuition:* Full-time $18,162; part-time $1009 per credit. *Required fees:* $1728; $96 per credit. Tuition and fees vary according to program. *Financial support:* In 2013–14, 800 students received support. Federal Work-Study and scholarships/grants available. Financial award application deadline: 5/1; financial award applicants required to submit FAFSA. *Unit head:* Dr. Thomas J. Mattei, Associate Dean for Professional Programs, 412-396-6393.

Application contact: Scott Copley, Director of Admission and Data Management, 412-396-6393, Fax: 412-396-4375, E-mail: pharmadmission@duq.edu.
Website: http://www.duq.edu/academics/schools/pharmacy/become-a-student/doctor-of-pharmacy

D'Youville College, School of Pharmacy, Buffalo, NY 14201-1084. Offers Pharm D. *Accreditation:* ACPE. *Students:* 259 full-time (121 women), 7 part-time (3 women); includes 38 minority (8 Black or African American, non-Hispanic/Latino; 21 Asian, non-Hispanic/Latino; 4 Hispanic/Latino; 5 Two or more races, non-Hispanic/Latino), 18 international. Average age 24. *Unit head:* Dr. Canio Marasco, Assistant Dean of Faculty and Student Affairs, 716-829-7846, Fax: 716-829-7760, E-mail: pharmacyadmissions@dyc.edu. *Application contact:* Mark Pavone, Graduate Admissions Director, 716-829-8400, Fax: 716-829-7900, E-mail: graduateadmissions@dyc.edu.
Website: http://www.dyc.edu/academics/pharmacy/

East Tennessee State University, Bill Gatton College of Pharmacy, Johnson City, TN 37614. Offers Pharm D. *Accreditation:* ACPE. Part-time programs available. *Students:* 326 full-time (181 women), 3 part-time (0 women); includes 37 minority (10 Black or African American, non-Hispanic/Latino; 16 Asian, non-Hispanic/Latino; 6 Hispanic/Latino; 5 Two or more races, non-Hispanic/Latino). Average age 25. In 2013, 74 doctorates awarded. *Expenses:* Tuition, state resident: full-time $7900; part-time $395 per credit hour. Tuition, nonresident: full-time $21,960; part-time $1098 per credit hour. *Required fees:* $1345; $84 per credit hour. *Unit head:* Dr. Larry D. Calhoun, Dean, 423-439-2068, Fax: 423-439-6310, E-mail: calhoun@etsu.edu. *Application contact:* Admissions and Records Office, 423-439-6300, Fax: 423-439-6320, E-mail: pharmacy@etsu.edu.
Website: http://www.etsu.edu/pharmacy/

Ferris State University, College of Pharmacy, Big Rapids, MI 49307. Offers Pharm D. *Accreditation:* ACPE. *Faculty:* 36 full-time (20 women), 4 part-time/adjunct (3 women). *Students:* 552 full-time (297 women), 36 part-time (14 women); includes 48 minority (8 Black or African American, non-Hispanic/Latino; 1 American Indian or Alaska Native, non-Hispanic/Latino; 20 Asian, non-Hispanic/Latino; 13 Hispanic/Latino; 6 Two or more races, non-Hispanic/Latino), 18 international. Average age 24. 663 applicants, 28% accepted, 141 enrolled. In 2013, 116 doctorates awarded. *Degree requirements:* For doctorate, 6 clerkships during 4th professional year which equals 1,740 hours of clerkship. *Entrance requirements:* For doctorate, PCAT, 3 years or more of pre-pharmacy course work. *Application deadline:* For fall admission, 12/1 for domestic and international students. Application fee: $150. *Expenses:* Contact institution. *Financial support:* Career-related internships or fieldwork, Federal Work-Study, institutionally sponsored loans, and scholarships/grants available. Financial award applicants required to submit FAFSA. *Faculty research:* Diabetes, rural health education, managed care practice, antimicrobial pharmacotherapy, medicinal flora. *Unit head:* Dr. Stephen Durst, Dean, 231-591-2254, Fax: 231-591-3829, E-mail: dursts@ferris.edu. *Application contact:* Tara M. Lee, Administrative Specialist, Admissions, 231-591-3780, Fax: 231-591-3829, E-mail: leet@ferris.edu.
Website: http://www.ferris.edu/colleges/pharmacy/

Florida Agricultural and Mechanical University, Division of Graduate Studies, Research, and Continuing Education, College of Pharmacy and Pharmaceutical Sciences, Professional Program in Pharmacy and Pharmaceutical Sciences, Tallahassee, FL 32307-3200. Offers Ex Doc, Pharm D. *Accreditation:* ACPE. *Entrance requirements:* Additional exam requirements/recommendations for international students: Required—TOEFL.

Georgia Campus–Philadelphia College of Osteopathic Medicine, School of Pharmacy, Suwanee, GA 30024. Offers Pharm D. *Faculty:* 29 full-time (12 women), 174 part-time/adjunct (99 women). *Students:* 365 full-time (192 women); includes 174 minority (57 Black or African American, non-Hispanic/Latino; 1 American Indian or Alaska Native, non-Hispanic/Latino; 37 Asian, non-Hispanic/Latino; 1 Native Hawaiian or other Pacific Islander, non-Hispanic/Latino; 78 Two or more races, non-Hispanic/Latino), 15 international. Average age 27. 1,047 applicants, 18% accepted, 102 enrolled. *Degree requirements:* For doctorate, capstone. *Entrance requirements:* For doctorate, PCAT. Additional exam requirements/recommendations for international students: Required—TOEFL (minimum score 79 iBT). *Application deadline:* For fall admission, 3/1 for domestic students. Applications are processed on a rolling basis. Application fee: $50. Electronic applications accepted. *Financial support:* In 2013–14, 129 students received support. Federal Work-Study, institutionally sponsored loans, and scholarships/grants available. Financial award application deadline: 3/15; financial award applicants required to submit FAFSA. *Total annual research expenditures:* $533,489. *Unit head:* Dr. Mark Okamoto, Dean, 678-407-7330, Fax: 678-407-7339. *Application contact:* Marsha Williams, Associate Director of Admissions, 215-871-6700, E-mail: marshawi@pcom.edu.
Website: http://www.pcom.edu/Academic_Programs/aca_pharmd/pharmd_curriculum.html

See Display on this page and Close-Up on page 963.

Hampton University, School of Pharmacy, Hampton, VA 23668. Offers Pharm D. *Accreditation:* ACPE.

Harding University, College of Pharmacy, Searcy, AR 72147-2230. Offers Pharm D. *Accreditation:* ACPE. *Faculty:* 34 full-time (18 women), 1 part-time/adjunct (0 women). *Students:* 231 full-time (134 women), 4 part-time (2 women); includes 69 minority (23 Black or African American, non-Hispanic/Latino; 2 American Indian or Alaska Native, non-Hispanic/Latino; 42 Asian, non-Hispanic/Latino; 1 Hispanic/Latino; 1 Two or more races, non-Hispanic/Latino), 10 international. Average age 27. 294 applicants, 35% accepted, 62 enrolled. In 2013, 54 doctorates awarded. *Degree requirements:* For doctorate, licensure as a pharmacy intern in AR, completion of 300 hours of introductory pharmacy practice experience and 1,440 hours of advanced pharmacy practice experience. *Entrance requirements:* For doctorate, PCAT, 90 semester hours of undergraduate work. Additional exam requirements/recommendations for international students: Required—TOEFL (minimum score 550 paper-based). *Application deadline:* For fall admission, 3/1 priority date for domestic and international students. Applications are processed on a rolling basis. Application fee: $50. Electronic applications accepted. *Expenses:* Contact institution. *Financial support:* In 2013–14, 35 students received support. Scholarships/grants available. Financial award applicants required to submit FAFSA. *Faculty research:* Field stable molecular diagnostics reagent development; the impact of UGT2B17 genetic polymorphisms on the disposition and action exemestane in healthy volunteers; optimization of 5-FU cancer chemotherapy, evaluation of issues associated with pediatric eosing; exploration of the physiologic impact of salmonella toxins; clinical study evaluating a novel point of care device as compared to the current industry standard for measurement of prothrombin time. *Total annual research expenditures:* $49,750. *Unit head:* Dr. Julie Ann Hixson-Wallace, Dean, 501-279-5205, Fax: 501-279-5525, E-mail: jahixson@harding.edu. *Application contact:* Carol Jones, Director of Admissions, 501-279-5523, Fax: 501-279-5525, E-mail: ccjones@harding.edu.
Website: http://www.harding.edu/pharmacy/

Howard University, College of Pharmacy, Washington, DC 20059-0002. Offers Pharm D, Pharm D/MBA. *Accreditation:* ACPE. Postbaccalaureate distance learning degree programs offered (minimal on-campus study). *Degree requirements:* For doctorate, comprehensive exam. *Entrance requirements:* For doctorate, PCAT, minimum GPA of 2.5. Electronic applications accepted. *Expenses:* Contact institution. *Faculty research:* Kinetics of drug absorption, stealth liposomes, synthesis, opiate analgesics.

Husson University, School of Pharmacy, Bangor, ME 04401-2999. Offers Pharm D. *Expenses: Tuition:* Full-time $5556; part-time $463 per credit. One-time fee: $100. Tuition and fees vary according to course load, degree level and program.

Idaho State University, Office of Graduate Studies, College of Pharmacy, Department of Pharmacy Practice and Administrative Sciences, Pocatello, ID 83209-8333. Offers pharmacy (Pharm D); pharmacy administration (MS, PhD). *Accreditation:* ACPE (one or more programs are accredited). Part-time programs available. *Degree requirements:* For master's, one foreign language, comprehensive exam, thesis, thesis research, speech and technical writing classes; for doctorate, comprehensive exam, thesis/dissertation, oral and written exams, speech and technical writing classes. *Entrance requirements:* For master's, GRE General Test, minimum GPA of 3.0, 3 letters of recommendation; for doctorate, GRE General Test, BS in pharmacy or related field, minimum GPA of 3.0, 3 letters of recommendation. Additional exam requirements/recommendations for international students: Required—TOEFL (minimum score 550 paper-based; 80 iBT). Electronic applications accepted. *Expenses:* Contact institution. *Faculty research:* Pharmaceutical care outcomes, drug use review, pharmacoeconomics.

Lake Erie College of Osteopathic Medicine, Professional Programs, Erie, PA 16509-1025. Offers biomedical sciences (Postbaccalaureate Certificate); medical education (MS); osteopathic medicine (DO); pharmacy (Pharm D). *Accreditation:* ACPE; AOsA. *Degree requirements:* For doctorate, comprehensive exam, National Osteopathic Medical Licensing Exam, Levels 1 and 2; for Postbaccalaureate Certificate, comprehensive exam, North American Pharmacist Licensure Examination (NAPLEX). *Entrance requirements:* For doctorate, MCAT, minimum GPA of 3.2, letters of recommendation; for Postbaccalaureate Certificate, PCAT, letters of recommendation, minimum GPA of 3.5. Electronic applications accepted. *Faculty research:* Cardiac smooth and skeletal muscle mechanics, chemotherapeutics and vitamins, osteopathic manipulation.

Lebanese American University, School of Pharmacy, Beirut, Lebanon. Offers Pharm D. *Accreditation:* ACPE.

Lipscomb University, College of Pharmacy, Nashville, TN 37204-3951. Offers Pharm D. *Accreditation:* ACPE. *Faculty:* 34 full-time (15 women), 3 part-time/adjunct (2 women). *Students:* 302 full-time (167 women), 2 part-time (1 woman); includes 49 minority (14 Black or African American, non-Hispanic/Latino; 23 Asian, non-Hispanic/Latino; 5 Hispanic/Latino; 2 Native Hawaiian or other Pacific Islander, non-Hispanic/Latino; 5 Two or more races, non-Hispanic/Latino). Average age 26. 703 applicants, 19% accepted, 74 enrolled. In 2013, 70 doctorates awarded. *Entrance requirements:* For doctorate, PCAT (minimum 45th percentile), 66 pre-professional semester hours, minimum GPA of 2.5, interview, PharmCAS application (for international students). Additional exam requirements/recommendations for international students: Required—TOEFL (minimum score 550 paper-based; 80 iBT). *Application deadline:* For fall admission, 2/7 for domestic students. Applications are processed on a rolling basis. Application fee: $50 ($75 for international students). Electronic applications accepted. *Expenses: Tuition:* Full-time $15,570; part-time $865 per credit hour. Tuition and fees vary according to degree level and program. *Financial support:* Application deadline: 2/15; applicants required to submit FAFSA. *Unit head:* Dr. Roger Davis, Dean/Professor of Pharmacy Practice, 615-966-7161. *Application contact:* Laura Ward, Director of Admissions and Student Affairs, 615-966-7173, E-mail: laura.ward@lipscomb.edu.
Website: http://lipscomb.edu/pharmacy

Loma Linda University, School of Pharmacy, Loma Linda, CA 92350. Offers Pharm D. *Accreditation:* ACPE. *Degree requirements:* For doctorate, intern pharmacist license.

Manchester University, Graduate Programs, Doctor of Pharmacy Program, Fort Wayne, IN 46845. Offers Pharm D. *Faculty:* 28 full-time (15 women). *Students:* 135 full-time (80 women); includes 61 minority (20 Black or African American, non-Hispanic/Latino; 35 Asian, non-Hispanic/Latino; 4 Hispanic/Latino; 2 Native Hawaiian or other Pacific Islander, non-Hispanic/Latino). 760 applicants, 14% accepted, 73 enrolled. *Degree requirements:* For doctorate, service learning, portfolio, competency assessments. *Entrance requirements:* For doctorate, minimum GPA of 2.5 (cumulative and prerequisites), minimum C grade on all prerequisite courses, U.S. citizenship or permanent residency, PharmCAS and supplemental application, 3 letters of recommendation. *Application deadline:* For fall admission, 3/1 for domestic students. Application fee: $230. *Unit head:* Dr. Joseph K. Bonnarens, Associate Dean for Student Affairs, 260-470-2655, E-mail: jkbonnarens@manchester.edu. *Application contact:* Dr. Mark Huntington, Associate Dean for Academic Affairs, 260-982-5033, E-mail: mwhuntington@manchester.edu.
Website: http://pharmacy.manchester.edu/

Marshall University, Academic Affairs Division, School of Pharmacy, Huntington, WV 25755. Offers Pharm D. *Faculty:* 10 full-time (5 women). *Students:* 145 part-time (84 women); includes 34 minority (12 Black or African American, non-Hispanic/Latino; 16 Asian, non-Hispanic/Latino; 3 Hispanic/Latino; 3 Two or more races, non-Hispanic/Latino). Average age 26. *Unit head:* Dr. Kevin W. Yingling, Founding Dean, 304-696-7302, E-mail: pharmacy@marshall.edu. *Application contact:* Dr. Tammy Johnson, Graduate Admissions, 304-746-1900, Fax: 304-746-1902, E-mail: services@marshall.edu.
Website: http://www.marshall.edu/wpmu/pharmacy/

MCPHS University, Graduate Studies, Doctoral Programs in Pharmacy–Boston, Doctor of Pharmacy Program - Boston, Boston, MA 02115-5896. Offers Pharm D. Students enter program as undergraduates. Postbaccalaureate distance learning degree programs offered. *Entrance requirements:* For doctorate, SAT (if fewer than 30 semester hours completed), minimum GPA of 2.5, interview. Additional exam requirements/recommendations for international students: Required—TOEFL (minimum score 550 paper-based; 79 iBT). Electronic applications accepted.

MCPHS University, Graduate Studies, Doctoral Programs in Pharmacy–Boston, Postbaccalaureate Doctor of Pharmacy Pathway Program, Boston, MA 02115-5896. Offers Pharm D. Part-time programs available. Postbaccalaureate distance learning degree programs offered (minimal on-campus study). *Entrance requirements:* For doctorate, registered pharmacist status in the U.S.; working at or have access to a site that provides opportunities to practice pharmaceutical care; curriculum vitae; letter of recommendation. Additional exam requirements/recommendations for international students: Required—TOEFL (minimum score 550 paper-based; 79 iBT). Electronic applications accepted.

MCPHS University, School of Pharmacy–Worcester/Manchester, Boston, MA 02115-5896. Offers Pharm D. *Entrance requirements:* Additional exam requirements/recommendations for international students: Required—TOEFL (minimum score 550 paper-based; 79 iBT).

Medical University of South Carolina, South Carolina College of Pharmacy, Charleston, SC 29425. Offers Pharm D. *Accreditation:* ACPE. *Entrance requirements:* For doctorate, PCAT, 2 years of pre-professional course work, interview, minimum GPA of 2.5. Additional exam requirements/recommendations for international students: Required—TOEFL (minimum score 550 paper-based). Electronic applications accepted. *Expenses:* Contact institution. *Faculty research:* Rational and computer aided drug design; drug metabolism and transport; molecular immunology and cellular toxicology; cell injury, death and regeneration; outcome sciences.

Mercer University, Graduate Studies, Cecil B. Day Campus, College of Pharmacy, Macon, GA 31207-0003. Offers pharmaceutical sciences (PhD); pharmacology (PhD); pharmacy (Pharm D); Pharm D/MBA; Pharm D/PhD. *Accreditation:* ACPE (one or more programs are accredited). *Faculty:* 24 full-time (15 women). *Students:* 653 full-time (421 women), 7 part-time (4 women); includes 291 minority (110 Black or African American, non-Hispanic/Latino; 1 American Indian or Alaska Native, non-Hispanic/Latino; 137 Asian, non-Hispanic/Latino; 15 Hispanic/Latino; 28 Two or more races, non-Hispanic/Latino), 47 international. Average age 26. 1,895 applicants, 18% accepted, 176 enrolled. In 2013, 137 doctorates awarded. *Degree requirements:* For doctorate, comprehensive exam (for some programs), thesis/dissertation (for some programs). *Entrance requirements:* For doctorate, GRE; PCAT (for Pharm D), Pharm D or BS in pharmacy or science, minimum GPA of 3.0. Additional exam requirements/recommendations for international students: Required—TOEFL. *Application deadline:* Applications are processed on a rolling basis. Electronic applications accepted. *Expenses:* Contact institution. *Financial support:* In 2013–14, 350 students received support. Teaching assistantships with tuition reimbursements available, career-related internships or fieldwork, Federal Work-Study, institutionally sponsored loans, scholarships/grants, tuition waivers, and unspecified assistantships available. Support available to part-time students. Financial award application deadline: 5/1; financial award applicants required to submit FAFSA. *Faculty research:* Stability and compatibility of steroids, synthesis of antihypertensives, disposition of cyclosporine, synthesis of enzyme inhibitors. *Unit head:* Dr. Hewitt W. Matthews, Dean, 678-547-6306, Fax: 678-547-6315, E-mail: matthews_h@mercer.edu. *Application contact:* Dr. James W. Bartling, Associate Dean for Student Affairs and Admissions, 678-547-6181, Fax: 678-547-6518, E-mail: bartling_jw@mercer.edu.
Website: http://pharmacy.mercer.edu/

Midwestern University, Downers Grove Campus, Chicago College of Pharmacy, Downers Grove, IL 60515-1235. Offers Pharm D. *Accreditation:* ACPE. Part-time programs available. Postbaccalaureate distance learning degree programs offered (minimal on-campus study). *Entrance requirements:* For doctorate, PCAT. *Expenses:* Contact institution.

Midwestern University, Glendale Campus, College of Pharmacy-Glendale, Glendale, AZ 85308. Offers Pharm D. *Accreditation:* ACPE. *Entrance requirements:* For doctorate, PCAT. *Expenses:* Contact institution.

Northeast Ohio Medical University, College of Pharmacy, Rootstown, OH 44272-0095. Offers Pharm D. *Accreditation:* ACPE. *Faculty:* 53 full-time (21 women), 444 part-time/adjunct (230 women). *Students:* 268 full-time (156 women); includes 48 minority (7 Black or African American, non-Hispanic/Latino; 1 American Indian or Alaska Native, non-Hispanic/Latino; 33 Asian, non-Hispanic/Latino; 4 Hispanic/Latino; 3 Two or more races, non-Hispanic/Latino). Average age 26. 422 applicants, 36% accepted, 76 enrolled. In 2013, 71 doctorates awarded. *Entrance requirements:* For doctorate, PCAT. *Application deadline:* For fall admission, 9/1 priority date for domestic students; for winter admission, 1/5 for domestic students. Applications are processed on a rolling basis. Application fee: $50. Electronic applications accepted. *Expenses:* Contact institution. *Financial support:* In 2013–14, 112 students received support. Scholarships/grants available. Financial award application deadline: 4/15; financial award applicants required to submit FAFSA. *Total annual research expenditures:* $415,414. *Unit head:* Dr. Charles Taylor, Dean, 330-325-6461, Fax: 330-325-5930. *Application contact:* Luke Gloeckner, Enrollment Services Specialist, 330-325-6274, E-mail: lgloeckner@neoucom.edu.
Website: http://www.neomed.edu/academics/pharmacy

Nova Southeastern University, College of Pharmacy, Fort Lauderdale, FL 33314-7796. Offers PhD, Pharm D. *Accreditation:* ACPE. *Faculty:* 57 full-time (26 women), 3 part-time/adjunct (2 women). *Students:* 930 full-time (600 women), 27 part-time (9 women); includes 644 minority (64 Black or African American, non-Hispanic/Latino; 164 Asian, non-Hispanic/Latino; 401 Hispanic/Latino; 1 Native Hawaiian or other Pacific Islander, non-Hispanic/Latino; 14 Two or more races, non-Hispanic/Latino), 88 international. Average age 27. 1,237 applicants, 33% accepted, 255 enrolled. In 2013, 237 doctorates awarded. *Degree requirements:* For doctorate, comprehensive exam (for some programs), thesis/dissertation (for some programs). *Entrance requirements:* For doctorate, PCAT (for Pharm D); GRE (for PhD). Additional exam requirements/recommendations for international students: Required—TOEFL (minimum score 550 paper-based) or IELTS. *Application deadline:* For fall admission, 3/1 for domestic students, 2/1 for international students. Applications are processed on a rolling basis. Application fee: $50. Electronic applications accepted. *Expenses:* Contact institution. *Financial support:* In 2013–14, 47 students received support, including 10 teaching assistantships with full tuition reimbursements available; career-related internships or fieldwork, Federal Work-Study, institutionally sponsored loans, and scholarships/grants also available. Financial award application deadline: 4/15; financial award applicants required to submit FAFSA. *Faculty research:* Neovascularization, health care delivery, pharmacoeconomics, cardiovascular/metabolic metastasis. *Total annual research expenditures:* $711,286. *Unit head:* Dr. Lisa Deziel, Dean, 954-262-1304, Fax: 954-262-2278, E-mail: copdean@nova.edu. *Application contact:* Kori Desiderio, Pharmacy Admissions Counselor, 954-262-1112, Fax: 954-262-2282, E-mail: desideri@nova.edu.
Website: http://pharmacy.nova.edu/

See Display on next page and Close-Up on page 961.

Ohio Northern University, Raabe College of Pharmacy, Ada, OH 45810-1599. Offers Pharm D. Students enter the program as undergraduates. *Accreditation:* ACPE. *Faculty:* 26 full-time (12 women), 3 part-time/adjunct (2 women). *Students:* 646 full-time (409 women), 8 part-time (5 women); includes 44 minority (10 Black or African American, non-Hispanic/Latino; 22 Asian, non-Hispanic/Latino; 2 Hispanic/Latino; 10 Two or more races, non-Hispanic/Latino), 16 international. Average age 22. 719 applicants, 37% accepted, 160 enrolled. In 2013, 164 doctorates awarded. *Degree requirements:* For doctorate, 9 clinical rotations, capstone course. *Entrance requirements:* For doctorate, ACT or SAT. Additional exam requirements/recommendations for international students: Required—TOEFL (minimum score 550 paper-based; 80 iBT). *Expenses:* Contact institution. *Financial support:* Federal Work-Study, institutionally sponsored loans, and scholarships/grants available. Financial award applicants required to submit FAFSA. *Faculty research:* Alcohol and substance abuse, women in pharmacy, non-traditional educations, continuing pharmaceutical education, medicinal chemistry. *Unit head:* Dr. Tom Kier, Interim Dean, 419-772-2282, Fax: 419-772-2282, E-mail: t-kier@onu.edu. *Application contact:* Dr. Kelly Shields, Assistant Dean of Student Services, 419-772-2752, Fax: 419-772-2752, E-mail: k-shields@onu.edu.
Website: http://www.onu.edu/pharmacy/

The Ohio State University, College of Pharmacy, Columbus, OH 43210. Offers MS, PhD, Pharm D, Pharm D/MBA, Pharm D/MPH. *Accreditation:* ACPE (one or more

programs are accredited). Part-time programs available. *Faculty:* 44. *Students:* 561 full-time (336 women), 3 part-time (1 woman); includes 136 minority (20 Black or African American, non-Hispanic/Latino; 1 American Indian or Alaska Native, non-Hispanic/Latino; 97 Asian, non-Hispanic/Latino; 14 Hispanic/Latino; 4 Two or more races, non-Hispanic/Latino), 56 international. Average age 25. In 2013, 12 master's, 133 doctorates awarded. *Degree requirements:* For doctorate, thesis/dissertation (for some programs). *Entrance requirements:* For master's, GRE General Test, minimum GPA of 3.0; for doctorate, GRE General Test; PCAT (for Pharm D), minimum GPA of 3.0. Additional exam requirements/recommendations for international students: Required—TOEFL (minimum score 600 paper-based; 100 iBT), Michigan English Language Assessment Battery (minimum score 84). *Application deadline:* For fall admission, 12/15 priority date for domestic students, 12/15 for international students. Application fee: $60 ($70 for international students). Electronic applications accepted. *Expenses:* Contact institution. *Financial support:* Fellowships with full tuition reimbursements, research assistantships with full tuition reimbursements, teaching assistantships with full tuition reimbursements, career-related internships or fieldwork, Federal Work-Study, institutionally sponsored loans, scholarships/grants, and traineeships available. *Unit head:* Dr. Henry J. Mann, Dean, 614-292-5711, Fax: 614-292-2588, E-mail: odmail@pharmacy.ohio-state.edu. *Application contact:* Mary Kivel, Graduate Program Coordinator, 614-292-6822, Fax: 614-292-2588, E-mail: gradprogram@pharmacy.ohio-state.edu.
Website: http://www.pharmacy.osu.edu

Oregon State University, College of Pharmacy, Pharmacy Doctoral Program, Corvallis, OR 97331. Offers Pharm D. *Faculty:* 29 full-time (14 women), 4 part-time/adjunct (1 woman). *Students:* 344 full-time (205 women), 18 part-time (10 women); includes 173 minority (3 Black or African American, non-Hispanic/Latino; 1 American Indian or Alaska Native, non-Hispanic/Latino; 128 Asian, non-Hispanic/Latino; 14 Hispanic/Latino; 2 Native Hawaiian or other Pacific Islander, non-Hispanic/Latino; 25 Two or more races, non-Hispanic/Latino), 10 international. Average age 26. 95 applicants, 100% accepted, 83 enrolled. In 2013, 85 doctorates awarded. *Application deadline:* For fall admission, 11/1 for domestic students. Application fee: $60. *Expenses:* Contact institution. *Unit head:* Dr. Mark Zabriskie, Dean and Professor, 541-737-5781, E-mail: mark.zabriskie@oregonstate.edu. *Application contact:* Angela Austin Haney, Director of Student Services/Head Advisor, 541-737-5784, E-mail: angela.austinhaney@oregonstate.edu.
Website: http://pharmacy.oregonstate.edu/

Pacific University, School of Pharmacy, Forest Grove, OR 97116-1797. Offers Pharm D. *Accreditation:* ACPE. *Entrance requirements:* Additional exam requirements/recommendations for international students: Required—TOEFL (minimum score 600 paper-based). Electronic applications accepted. *Expenses:* Contact institution. *Faculty research:* Informatics, enzyme metabolism, apostosis/cell cycle, neurophysiology of chronic pain, neurophysiology of Alzheimer's.

Palm Beach Atlantic University, Gregory School of Pharmacy, West Palm Beach, FL 33416-4708. Offers Pharm D. *Accreditation:* ACPE. *Faculty:* 24 full-time (17 women), 11 part-time/adjunct (5 women). *Students:* 303 full-time (180 women), 12 part-time (7 women); includes 152 minority (31 Black or African American, non-Hispanic/Latino; 1 American Indian or Alaska Native, non-Hispanic/Latino; 50 Asian, non-Hispanic/Latino; 59 Hispanic/Latino; 2 Native Hawaiian or other Pacific Islander, non-Hispanic/Latino; 9 Two or more races, non-Hispanic/Latino), 9 international. Average age 26. 665 applicants, 26% accepted, 79 enrolled. In 2013, 69 doctorates awarded. *Entrance requirements:* For doctorate, PCAT, minimum GPA of 2.75. Additional exam requirements/recommendations for international students: Required—TOEFL (minimum score 550 paper-based; 79 iBT). *Application deadline:* For fall admission, 2/3 priority date for domestic and international students. Applications are processed on a rolling basis. Application fee: $150. Electronic applications accepted. *Expenses:* Contact institution. *Financial support:* In 2013–14, 31 students received support. Application deadline: 5/1; applicants required to submit FAFSA. *Unit head:* Dr. Mary Ferrill, Dean, 561-803-2700, E-mail: mary_ferrill@pba.edu. *Application contact:* Lucas Whittaker, Director of Pharmacy Admissions, 561-803-2751, E-mail: lucas_whittaker@pba.edu.
Website: http://www.pba.edu/school-of-pharmacy

Philadelphia College of Osteopathic Medicine, Graduate and Professional Programs, Program in Pharmacy, Philadelphia, PA 19131-1694. Offers Pharm D. *Unit head:* Kari A. Shotwel, Director of Admissions, 215-871-6700, Fax: 215-871-6719, E-mail: karis@pcom.edu. *Application contact:* Kari A. Shotwell, Director of Admissions, 215-871-6700, Fax: 215-871-6719, E-mail: karis@pcom.edu.

Purdue University, College of Pharmacy and Pharmacal Sciences, Professional Program in Pharmacy and Pharmacal Sciences, West Lafayette, IN 47907. Offers Pharm D. *Accreditation:* ACPE. *Students:* 625 full-time (220 women), 2 part-time (1 woman); includes 144 minority (28 Black or African American, non-Hispanic/Latino; 2 American Indian or Alaska Native, non-Hispanic/Latino; 89 Asian, non-Hispanic/Latino; 13 Hispanic/Latino; 12 Two or more races, non-Hispanic/Latino), 23 international. Average age 23. 697 applicants, 24% accepted, 155 enrolled. In 2013, 169 doctorates awarded. *Entrance requirements:* For doctorate, minimum 2 years of pre-pharmacy course work, interview. *Application deadline:* For fall admission, 12/2 for domestic and international students. Application fee: $60 ($75 for international students). *Expenses:* Contact institution. *Financial support:* Career-related internships or fieldwork, Federal Work-Study, and scholarships/grants available. Financial award application deadline: 3/15; financial award applicants required to submit FAFSA. *Faculty research:* Medicinal chemistry, pharmacology, pharmaceutics, clinical pharmacy, pharmacy administration. *Unit head:* Dr. C. L. Svensson, Dean, 765-494-1368, Fax: 765-494-7880, E-mail: svensson@purdue.edu. *Application contact:* G. Marc Loudon, Associate Dean for Research and Graduate Programs, 765-494-1362.

Regis University, Rueckert-Hartman College for Health Professions, School of Pharmacy, Denver, CO 80221-1099. Offers Pharm D. *Faculty:* 29 full-time (18 women), 4 part-time/adjunct (2 women). *Students:* 226 full-time (127 women); includes 104 minority (8 Black or African American, non-Hispanic/Latino; 1 American Indian or Alaska Native, non-Hispanic/Latino; 69 Asian, non-Hispanic/Latino; 14 Hispanic/Latino; 12 Two or more races, non-Hispanic/Latino), 2 international. Average age 34. 786 applicants, 24% accepted, 56 enrolled. In 2013, 48 doctorates awarded. *Entrance requirements:* For doctorate, PharmCAS application. Additional exam requirements/recommendations for international students: Required—TOEFL (minimum score 550 paper-based; 82 iBT). *Application deadline:* For fall admission, 3/1 for domestic students, 2/1 for international students. Application fee: $0. Electronic applications accepted. *Expenses:* Contact institution. *Financial support:* In 2013–14, 22 students received support. Federal Work-Study and scholarships/grants available. Financial award application deadline: 4/15; financial award applicants required to submit FAFSA. *Unit head:* Dr. Rodney Carter, Dean, 303-625-1301, Fax: 303-625-1305. *Application contact:* Sarah Engel, Director of Admissions, 303-458-4900, Fax: 303-964-5534, E-mail: regisadm@regis.edu.
Website: http://www.regis.edu/RHCHP/Schools/School-of-Pharmacy.aspx

Roosevelt University, Graduate Division, College of Pharmacy, Chicago, IL 60605. Offers Pharm D. *Accreditation:* ACPE.

Roseman University of Health Sciences, College of Pharmacy, Henderson, NV 89014. Offers Pharm D. *Accreditation:* ACPE. *Faculty:* 59 full-time (28 women), 11 part-time/adjunct (2 women). *Students:* 775 full-time (403 women); includes 389 minority (27 Black or African American, non-Hispanic/Latino; 2 American Indian or Alaska Native, non-Hispanic/Latino; 283 Asian, non-Hispanic/Latino; 34 Hispanic/Latino; 7 Native Hawaiian or other Pacific Islander, non-Hispanic/Latino; 36 Two or more races, non-Hispanic/Latino), 2 international. Average age 28. 826 applicants, 44% accepted, 260 enrolled. In 2013, 220 doctorates awarded. *Degree requirements:* For doctorate,

comprehensive exam. *Entrance requirements:* For doctorate, PCAT. *Application deadline:* For fall admission, 12/1 for domestic and international students. Applications are processed on a rolling basis. Application fee: $60. *Expenses: Tuition:* Full-time $45,240. *Required fees:* $425. *Financial support:* In 2013–14, 82 students received support. Federal Work-Study and scholarships/grants available. Financial award application deadline: 3/1; financial award applicants required to submit FAFSA. *Unit head:* Dr. Scott Stolte, Dean, 702-968-5944, Fax: 702-990-4435, E-mail: sstolte@roseman.edu. *Application contact:* Dr. Helen Park, Director of Admissions and Student Affairs, 702-968-5248, Fax: 702-968-1644, E-mail: hpark@roseman.edu.
Website: http://www.roseman.edu

Rutgers, The State University of New Jersey, New Brunswick, Ernest Mario School of Pharmacy, Piscataway, NJ 08854-8097. Offers medicinal chemistry (MS, PhD); pharmaceutical science (MS, PhD); pharmacy (Pharm D). *Accreditation:* ACPE. *Degree requirements:* For doctorate, variable foreign language requirement. *Entrance requirements:* For doctorate, SAT or PCAT (for Pharm D), interview, criminal background check (for Pharm D). Additional exam requirements/recommendations for international students: Recommended—TOEFL (minimum score 550 paper-based). Electronic applications accepted. *Expenses:* Contact institution. *Faculty research:* Pharmacokinetics, cancer prevention, cardiology, neurology, pharmacodynamics.

St. John Fisher College, Wegmans School of Pharmacy, Doctor of Pharmacy Program, Rochester, NY 14618-3597. Offers Pharm D. *Accreditation:* ACPE. *Faculty:* 31 full-time (21 women), 2 part-time/adjunct (1 woman). *Students:* 318 full-time (174 women), 2 part-time (1 woman); includes 65 minority (14 Black or African American, non-Hispanic/Latino; 2 American Indian or Alaska Native, non-Hispanic/Latino; 38 Asian, non-Hispanic/Latino; 5 Hispanic/Latino; 6 Two or more races, non-Hispanic/Latino), 8 international. Average age 25. 792 applicants, 23% accepted, 84 enrolled. In 2013, 73 doctorates awarded. *Degree requirements:* For doctorate, advanced pharmacy practice experience. *Entrance requirements:* For doctorate, PCAT, 2 letters of recommendation, interview, minimum of 62 credit hours of specific undergraduate courses. Additional exam requirements/recommendations for international students: Required—TOEFL (minimum score 575 paper-based; 80 iBT). *Application deadline:* For fall admission, 3/1 for domestic students. Applications are processed on a rolling basis. Application fee: $50. Electronic applications accepted. *Expenses:* Contact institution. *Financial support:* In 2013–14, 55 students received support. Scholarships/grants available. Financial award applicants required to submit FAFSA. *Faculty research:* Opioid pharmacology, heavy metal toxicology. *Unit head:* Dr. Scott A. Swigart, Dean of the School of Pharmacy, 585-385-8201, Fax: 585-385-8453, E-mail: sswigart@sjfc.edu. *Application contact:* Jose Perales, Director of Graduate Admissions, 585-385-8067, E-mail: jperales@sjfc.edu.
Website: http://www.sjfc.edu/pharmacy/

St. Louis College of Pharmacy, Professional Program, St. Louis, MO 63110-1088. Offers Pharm D. *Accreditation:* ACPE. *Faculty:* 55 full-time (34 women), 25 part-time/adjunct (18 women). *Students:* 620 full-time (367 women), 7 part-time (3 women); includes 72 minority (8 Black or African American, non-Hispanic/Latino; 1 American Indian or Alaska Native, non-Hispanic/Latino; 58 Asian, non-Hispanic/Latino; 5 Hispanic/Latino), 2 international. Average age 22. *Entrance requirements:* For doctorate, PCAT, 2 letters of recommendation. Additional exam requirements/recommendations for international students: Required—TOEFL (minimum score 550 paper-based). Application fee: $55. Electronic applications accepted. *Expenses: Tuition:* Full-time $27,619; part-time $885 per credit hour. *Required fees:* $373. Full-time tuition and fees vary according to student level. *Financial support:* Federal Work-Study and scholarships/grants available. Financial award application deadline: 12/15; financial award applicants required to submit FAFSA. *Faculty research:* Geriatrics, cardiology, psychobiology, infectious diseases. *Application contact:* Penny Bryant, Director of Admissions/Registrar, 314-446-8313, Fax: 314-446-8310, E-mail: pbryant@stlcop.edu.

Samford University, McWhorter School of Pharmacy, Birmingham, AL 35229. Offers Pharm D. *Accreditation:* ACPE. *Faculty:* 25 full-time (16 women), 1 part-time/adjunct (0 women). *Students:* 484 full-time (326 women), 15 part-time (10 women); includes 61 minority (31 Black or African American, non-Hispanic/Latino; 2 American Indian or Alaska Native, non-Hispanic/Latino; 20 Asian, non-Hispanic/Latino; 6 Hispanic/Latino; 2 Two or more races, non-Hispanic/Latino), 9 international. Average age 24. 511 applicants, 25% accepted, 126 enrolled. In 2013, 125 doctorates awarded. *Degree requirements:* For doctorate, comprehensive exam, thesis/dissertation. *Entrance requirements:* For doctorate, PCAT, minimum GPA of 2.75. Additional exam requirements/recommendations for international students: Required—TOEFL (minimum score 550 paper-based; 80 iBT). *Application deadline:* For fall admission, 2/1 for domestic students. Applications are processed on a rolling basis. Application fee: $50. Electronic applications accepted. *Expenses:* Contact institution. *Financial support:* In 2013–14, 194 students received support. Career-related internships or fieldwork, Federal Work-Study, and institutionally sponsored loans available. Financial award application deadline: 5/2; financial award applicants required to submit FAFSA. *Faculty research:* Biotechnology, transdermal drug delivery, vaccines, human skin models, genetic mapping of disease, determination of pharmacokinetics of new drug candidates, impact of herbal supplements on administered chemotherapeutic drugs, stability of compounded drug formulations, novel ophthalmic drug delivery systems, icon channel, cystic fibrosis novel drug discovery (protein misfolding). *Total annual research expenditures:* $45,000. *Unit head:* Dr. Michael D. Hogue, Interim Dean, 205-726-2820, Fax: 205-726-2759, E-mail: mdhogue@samford.edu. *Application contact:* C. Bruce Foster, Director of Pharmacy Admissions, 205-726-2982, Fax: 205-726-4141, E-mail: cbfoster@samford.edu.
Website: http://pharmacy.samford.edu

Shenandoah University, Bernard J. Dunn School of Pharmacy, Winchester, VA 22601-5195. Offers Pharm D. *Accreditation:* ACPE. Part-time programs available. Postbaccalaureate distance learning degree programs offered (minimal on-campus study). *Faculty:* 39 full-time (24 women), 10 part-time/adjunct (7 women). *Students:* 409 full-time (261 women), 123 part-time (79 women); includes 212 minority (54 Black or African American, non-Hispanic/Latino; 1 American Indian or Alaska Native, non-Hispanic/Latino; 140 Asian, non-Hispanic/Latino; 17 Hispanic/Latino), 20 international. Average age 30. 1,074 applicants, 24% accepted, 144 enrolled. In 2013, 111 doctorates awarded. *Degree requirements:* For doctorate, scholarly project, minimum GPA of 2.0, 142 credit hours in didactic and experiential curriculum (not including prerequisite courses), clerkship. *Entrance requirements:* For doctorate, PCAT, BS in pharmacy (or foreign equivalent), essay, interview, minimum GPA of 2.5, 3 letters of recommendation. Additional exam requirements/recommendations for international students: Required—TOEFL (minimum score 550 paper-based; 79 iBT), IELTS (minimum score 6.5), Sakae Institute of Study Abroad (SISA) test (minimum score 15). *Application deadline:* For fall admission, 3/1 for domestic and international students; for spring admission, 10/15 for domestic and international students. Application fee: $30. Electronic applications accepted. *Expenses:* Contact institution. *Financial support:* In 2013–14, 10 students received support. Career-related internships or fieldwork and scholarships/grants available. Support available to part-time students. Financial award application deadline: 3/15; financial award applicants required to submit FAFSA. *Faculty research:* Drug metabolism, pharmacogenomics, pharmacokinetics, natural products, gene expression. *Total annual research expenditures:* $6,065. *Unit head:* Dr. Alan McKay, Dean, 540-665-1282, Fax: 540-665-1283, E-mail: amckay@su.edu. *Application contact:* Andrew Woodall, Executive Director of Recruitment and Admissions, 540-665-4581, Fax: 540-665-4627, E-mail: admit@su.edu.
Website: http://www.pharmacy.su.edu

South Dakota State University, Graduate School, College of Pharmacy, Professional Program in Pharmacy, Brookings, SD 57007. Offers Pharm D. *Accreditation:* ACPE. *Entrance requirements:* For doctorate, ACT or PCAT, bachelor's degree in pharmacy. Additional exam requirements/recommendations for international students: Required—TOEFL (minimum score 550 paper-based). *Faculty research:* Geriatric medicine, drugs of abuse, anti-cancer drugs, drug metabolism, sustained drug delivery.

Southern Illinois University Edwardsville, School of Pharmacy, Edwardsville, IL 62026. Offers Pharm D. *Accreditation:* ACPE. *Faculty:* 18 full-time (6 women). *Students:* 325 full-time (201 women); includes 38 minority (11 Black or African American, non-Hispanic/Latino; 15 Asian, non-Hispanic/Latino; 8 Hispanic/Latino; 4 Two or more races, non-Hispanic/Latino). 310 applicants, 43% accepted. In 2013, 79 doctorates awarded. *Entrance requirements:* For doctorate, PCAT. *Application deadline:* For fall admission, 11/1 for domestic and international students. Application fee: $40. Electronic applications accepted. *Expenses:* Tuition, state resident: full-time $3551. Tuition, nonresident: full-time $8378. *Financial support:* Career-related internships or fieldwork, Federal Work-Study, institutionally sponsored loans, scholarships/grants, and traineeships available. Support available to part-time students. Financial award application deadline: 3/1; financial award applicants required to submit FAFSA. *Unit head:* Dr. Gireesh V. Gupchup, Dean, 618-650-5150, Fax: 618-650-5152, E-mail: pharmacy@siue.edu. *Application contact:* Melissa K. Mace, Assistant Director of Graduate and International Admissions, 618-650-2756, Fax: 618-650-3618, E-mail: mmace@siue.edu.
Website: http://www.siue.edu/pharmacy

South University, Graduate Programs, School of Pharmacy, Savannah, GA 31406. Offers Pharm D/MBA. *Accreditation:* ACPE.

South University, Program in Pharmacy, Columbia, SC 29203. Offers Pharm D.

Southwestern Oklahoma State University, College of Pharmacy, Weatherford, OK 73096-3098. Offers Pharm D. *Accreditation:* ACPE. *Entrance requirements:* For doctorate, PCAT.

Temple University, School of Pharmacy, Professional Program in Pharmacy, Philadelphia, PA 19140. Offers Pharm D. *Accreditation:* ACPE. *Faculty:* 40 full-time (20 women), 2 part-time/adjunct (0 women). *Students:* 591 full-time (328 women); includes 203 minority (34 Black or African American, non-Hispanic/Latino; 1 American Indian or Alaska Native, non-Hispanic/Latino; 151 Asian, non-Hispanic/Latino; 13 Hispanic/Latino; 4 Two or more races, non-Hispanic/Latino), 37 international. 791 applicants, 32% accepted, 158 enrolled. In 2013, 145 doctorates awarded. *Entrance requirements:* For doctorate, PCAT. *Application deadline:* For winter admission, 2/1 for domestic and international students. Application fee: $60. *Expenses:* Contact institution. *Financial support:* Scholarships/grants available. *Unit head:* Dr. Ina Calligaro, Associate Dean for Education, Faculty Development, and Experiential Education, 215-707-4967, Fax: 215-707-3678, E-mail: ina.calligaro@temple.edu. *Application contact:* Dr. Marquette Cannon-Babb, PharmD, Assistant Dean, 215-707-4900, Fax: 215-707-3678.
Website: http://www.temple.edu/pharmacy/programs/PharmD.html

Texas A&M Health Science Center, Irma Lerma Rangel College of Pharmacy, College Station, TX 77840. Offers Pharm D. *Accreditation:* ACPE. *Entrance requirements:* For doctorate, PCAT, minimum GPA of 2.75, transcripts from each college/university attended.

Texas Southern University, College of Pharmacy and Health Sciences, Department of Pharmacy Practice, Houston, TX 77004-4584. Offers Pharm D. Postbaccalaureate distance learning degree programs offered. *Faculty:* 13 full-time (7 women), 6 part-time/adjunct (3 women). *Students:* 359 full-time (214 women), 86 part-time (49 women); includes 385 minority (207 Black or African American, non-Hispanic/Latino; 158 Asian, non-Hispanic/Latino; 20 Hispanic/Latino), 30 international. Average age 29. 117 applicants, 100% accepted, 116 enrolled. In 2013, 139 doctorates awarded. *Entrance requirements:* For doctorate, GRE General Test, PCAT. *Application deadline:* For fall admission, 2/15 for domestic and international students. Applications are processed on a rolling basis. Application fee: $50 ($75 for international students). Electronic applications accepted. *Financial support:* Fellowships, research assistantships, teaching assistantships, career-related internships or fieldwork, scholarships/grants, and tuition waivers (partial) available. Financial award application deadline: 5/1; financial award applicants required to submit FAFSA. *Unit head:* Dr. Inyang Osemene, Chair, 713-313-1887, E-mail: osemene_in@tsu.edu. *Application contact:* Dr. Gregory Maddox, Dean of the Graduate School, 713-313-7011, E-mail: maddox_gh@tsu.edu.
Website: http://www.tsu.edu/academics/colleges__schools/College_of_Pharmacy_and_Health_Sciences/Departments_Programs/default.php

Thomas Jefferson University, Jefferson School of Pharmacy, Philadelphia, PA 19107. Offers Pharm D. *Accreditation:* ACPE. *Students:* 290 full-time (165 women), 2 part-time (1 woman); includes 126 minority (12 Black or African American, non-Hispanic/Latino; 1 American Indian or Alaska Native, non-Hispanic/Latino; 106 Asian, non-Hispanic/Latino; 7 Hispanic/Latino), 10 international. Average age 27. 834 applicants, 18% accepted, 55 enrolled. In 2013, 56 doctorates awarded. *Entrance requirements:* For doctorate, PCAT. Additional exam requirements/recommendations for international students: Required—TOEFL. *Application deadline:* For fall admission, 3/1 for domestic and international students. Applications are processed on a rolling basis. Application fee: $25. Electronic applications accepted. *Expenses:* Contact institution. *Financial support:* In 2013–14, 144 students received support. Federal Work-Study, institutionally sponsored loans, and scholarships/grants available. Financial award application deadline: 4/1; financial award applicants required to submit FAFSA. *Unit head:* Dr. Rebecca S. Finley, Dean, 215-955-6300. *Application contact:* Niki M. Kelley, Associate Director of Admissions, 215-503-1041, E-mail: niki.kelley@jefferson.edu.
Website: http://www.jefferson.edu/pharmacy

Touro University, Graduate Programs, Vallejo, CA 94592. Offers education (MA); medical health sciences (MS); osteopathic medicine (DO); pharmacy (Pharm D); public health (MPH). *Accreditation:* AOsA; ARC-PA. Part-time and evening/weekend programs available. *Faculty:* 103 full-time (54 women), 57 part-time/adjunct (33 women). *Students:* 1,390 full-time (841 women), 27 part-time (20 women). *Degree requirements:* For master's, comprehensive exam, thesis; for doctorate, comprehensive exam. *Entrance requirements:* For doctorate, BS/BA. *Application deadline:* For fall admission, 3/15 for domestic students; for winter admission, 12/1 for domestic students. Applications are processed on a rolling basis. Application fee: $100. Electronic applications accepted. *Financial support:* Fellowships, research assistantships, teaching assistantships, Federal Work-Study, and scholarships/grants available. Support available to part-time students. Financial award applicants required to submit FAFSA. *Faculty research:* Cancer, heart disease. *Application contact:* Steve Davis, Director of Admissions, 707-638-5270, Fax: 707-638-5250, E-mail: steven.davis@tu.edu.

Universidad de Ciencias Medicas, Graduate Programs, San Jose, Costa Rica. Offers dermatology (SP); family health (MS); health service center administration (MHA); human anatomy (MS); medical and surgery (MD); occupational medicine (MS); pharmacy (Pharm D). Part-time programs available. *Degree requirements:* For master's, thesis; for doctorate and SP, comprehensive exam. *Entrance requirements:* For master's, MD or bachelor's degree; for doctorate, admissions test; for SP, admissions test, MD.

University at Buffalo, the State University of New York, Graduate School, School of Pharmacy and Pharmaceutical Sciences, Professional Program in Pharmacy, Buffalo, NY 14260. Offers Pharm D, Pharm D/JD, Pharm D/MBA, Pharm D/MPH, Pharm D/MS, Pharm D/PhD. *Accreditation:* ACPE. *Faculty:* 27 full-time (12 women), 9 part-time/adjunct (3 women). *Students:* 497 full-time (290 women); includes 190 minority (21 Black or African American, non-Hispanic/Latino; 1 American Indian or Alaska Native, non-Hispanic/Latino; 160 Asian, non-Hispanic/Latino; 8 Hispanic/Latino), 16 international. Average age 24. 766 applicants, 22% accepted, 131 enrolled. In 2013, 111 doctorates awarded. *Degree requirements:* For doctorate, project. *Entrance requirements:* For doctorate, PCAT. Additional exam requirements/recommendations for international students: Required—TOEFL (minimum score 550 paper-based; 79 iBT); Recommended—IELTS, TSE. *Application deadline:* For fall admission, 2/1 priority date for domestic and international students. Applications are processed on a rolling basis. Application fee: $50. Electronic applications accepted. *Financial support:* In 2013–14, 292 students received support, including 5 fellowships (averaging $43,000 per year); scholarships/grants and health care benefits also available. Financial award application deadline: 3/1; financial award applicants required to submit FAFSA. *Faculty research:* Pharmacokinetics, pharmacoepidemiology, Attention Deficit Hyperactivity Disorder (ADHD), HIV/AIDS, oncology, critical care, renal transplantation, pharmacometrics. *Total annual research expenditures:* $4.5 million. *Unit head:* Dr. Edward M. Bednarczyk, Chairman, 716-645-2828 Ext. 357, Fax: 716-829-6568, E-mail: eb@buffalo.edu. *Application contact:* Dr. Jennifer M. Hess, Assistant Dean, 716-645-2825 Ext. 1, Fax: 716-829-6568, E-mail: prepharm@buffalo.edu.
Website: http://pharmacy.buffalo.edu/academic-programs/pharmd.html

University of Alberta, Faculty of Graduate Studies and Research, Department of Pharmacy and Pharmaceutical Sciences, Edmonton, AB T6G 2E1, Canada. Offers M Sc, PhD. Terminal master's awarded for partial completion of doctoral program. *Degree requirements:* For master's, thesis; for doctorate, thesis/dissertation. *Entrance requirements:* Additional exam requirements/recommendations for international students: Required—Michigan English Language Assessment Battery or IELTS. Electronic applications accepted. *Faculty research:* Radiopharmacy, pharmacokinetics, bionucleonics, medicinal chemistry, microbiology.

The University of Arizona, College of Pharmacy, Pharmacy Professional Program, Tucson, AZ 85721. Offers Pharm D. *Accreditation:* ACPE. Part-time programs available. *Faculty:* 38 full-time (7 women). *Students:* 392 full-time (243 women), 3 part-time (0 women); includes 197 minority (4 Black or African American, non-Hispanic/Latino; 2 American Indian or Alaska Native, non-Hispanic/Latino; 75 Asian, non-Hispanic/Latino; 35 Hispanic/Latino; 81 Two or more races, non-Hispanic/Latino), 4 international. Average age 30. In 2013, 95 doctorates awarded. *Entrance requirements:* For doctorate, PCAT, 4-6 months of pharmacy experience. Additional exam requirements/recommendations for international students: Required—TOEFL (minimum score 550 paper-based; 79 iBT). Application fee: $75. Electronic applications accepted. *Expenses:* Tuition, state resident: full-time $11,526. Tuition, nonresident: full-time $27,398. *Financial support:* In 2013–14, 11 research assistantships (averaging $20,700 per year) were awarded; career-related internships or fieldwork, scholarships/grants, health care benefits, and unspecified assistantships also available. *Faculty research:* Health/service administrative pharmacy education, geriatric pharmacy, social and behavioral pharmacy management and economics. *Total annual research expenditures:* $11.8 million. *Unit head:* Dr. Marie A. Chisholm-Burns, Head, 520-626-2298, E-mail: chilholm@pharmacy.arizona.edu. *Application contact:* General Information Contact, 520-626-4311, E-mail: admissionsinfo@pharmacy.arizona.edu.
Website: http://www.pharmacy.arizona.edu/programs/pharmd-program

University of Arkansas for Medical Sciences, College of Pharmacy, Little Rock, AR 72205-7199. Offers MS, Pharm D. *Accreditation:* ACPE (one or more programs are accredited). *Faculty:* 56 full-time (27 women), 6 part-time/adjunct (0 women). *Students:* 477 full-time (303 women), 2 part-time (1 woman); includes 74 minority (24 Black or African American, non-Hispanic/Latino; 2 American Indian or Alaska Native, non-Hispanic/Latino; 18 Asian, non-Hispanic/Latino; 12 Hispanic/Latino; 18 Two or more races, non-Hispanic/Latino). Average age 23. 536 applicants, 27% accepted, 121 enrolled. In 2013, 125 doctorates awarded. *Degree requirements:* For master's, thesis. *Entrance requirements:* For master's, GRE; for doctorate, PCAT. Additional exam requirements/recommendations for international students: Recommended—TOEFL. *Application deadline:* For fall admission, 2/3 for domestic students. Applications are processed on a rolling basis. Application fee: $100. Electronic applications accepted. *Expenses:* Contact institution. *Financial support:* Research assistantships available. Support available to part-time students. *Unit head:* Dr. Stephanie Gardner, Dean, 501-686-5558. *Application contact:* Dr. Kim Light, Graduate Program Director, 501-686-6496, E-mail: kelight@uams.edu.
Website: http://pharmcollege.uams.edu/

The University of British Columbia, Faculty of Pharmaceutical Sciences, Vancouver, BC V6T 1Z3, Canada. Offers M Sc, PhD, Pharm D. *Students:* 59 full-time (28 women), 1 part-time (0 women). Average age 26. 99 applicants, 14% accepted, 12 enrolled. In 2013, 3 master's, 5 doctorates awarded. *Degree requirements:* For master's, thesis, seminar; for doctorate, comprehensive exam, thesis/dissertation, seminar. *Entrance requirements:* Additional exam requirements/recommendations for international students: Required—TOEFL (minimum score 600 paper-based; 100 iBT), IELTS (minimum score 6.5). *Application deadline:* For fall admission, 3/15 for domestic students, 2/15 for international students. Application fee: $95 Canadian dollars ($153 Canadian dollars for international students). Electronic applications accepted. *Expenses: Tuition, area resident:* Full-time $8000 Canadian dollars. *Financial support:* In 2013–14, 60 students received support, including 10 fellowships (averaging $19,000 per year), 45 research assistantships (averaging $8,000 per year), 28 teaching assistantships (averaging $12,000 per year); career-related internships or fieldwork, institutionally sponsored loans, scholarships/grants, traineeships, and unspecified assistantships also available. *Faculty research:* Pharmacology and cellular pharmacology, neuropharmacology, toxicology, nanomedicines and drug delivery, pharmacogenomics and personalized medicine, health outcomes research and evaluation, pharmacoepidemiology, and medicinal chemistry. *Unit head:* Dr. Michael Coughtrie, Dean, 604-822-2343, Fax: 604-822-3035, E-mail: michael.coughtrie@ubc.ca. *Application contact:* Rachel Wu, Graduate Programs Manager, 604-827-0188, Fax: 604-822-3035, E-mail: rachel.wu@ubc.ca.
Website: http://www.pharmacy.ubc.ca

University of California, San Diego, School of Pharmacy and Pharmaceutical Sciences, La Jolla, CA 92093. Offers Pharm D. *Accreditation:* ACPE. *Expenses:* Tuition, state resident: full-time $11,220; part-time $1870 per quarter. Tuition, nonresident: full-time $26,322; part-time $4387 per quarter. *Required fees:* $519.50 per quarter. Part-time tuition and fees vary according to course load and program.

University of California, San Francisco, School of Pharmacy, Program in Pharmacy, San Francisco, CA 94143. Offers Pharm D. *Accreditation:* ACPE. *Degree requirements:* For doctorate, comprehensive exam, supervised practice experience. *Entrance requirements:* For doctorate, 2 years of preparatory course work in basic sciences. *Application deadline:* For fall admission, 11/3 for domestic and international students. Application fee: $80 ($100 for international students). Electronic applications accepted. *Expenses:* Tuition, state resident: full-time $11,220. Tuition, nonresident: full-time $26,322. *Required fees:* $5204. Full-time tuition and fees vary according to degree level and program. *Financial support:* Teaching assistantships, career-related internships or fieldwork, Federal Work-Study, institutionally sponsored loans, and scholarships/grants available. Financial award application deadline: 2/1; financial award applicants required to submit FAFSA. *Faculty research:* Drug delivery, drug metabolism and chemical toxicology, macromolecular structure, molecular parasitology, pharmacokinetics. *Unit head:* Cynthia B. Watchmaker, Associate Dean of Student Affairs and Education Services, 415-476-8025, Fax: 415-476-6805, E-mail: watchmakerc@pharmacy.ucsf.edu. *Application contact:* Joel Gonzales, Admissions Director, 415-502-5368, Fax: 415-476-6805, E-mail: osaca@pharmacy.ucsf.edu.
Website: http://pharmacy.ucsf.edu/pharmd

University of Charleston, School of Pharmacy, Charleston, WV 25304-1099. Offers Pharm D. *Accreditation:* ACPE. *Faculty:* 25 full-time (16 women), 1 (woman) part-time/adjunct. *Students:* 314 full-time (166 women); includes 72 minority (24 Black or African American, non-Hispanic/Latino; 2 American Indian or Alaska Native, non-Hispanic/Latino; 32 Asian, non-Hispanic/Latino; 6 Hispanic/Latino; 2 Native Hawaiian or other Pacific Islander, non-Hispanic/Latino; 6 Two or more races, non-Hispanic/Latino), 7 international. Average age 25. In 2013, 75 doctorates awarded. *Degree requirements:* For doctorate, passing grade in all coursework, minimum cumulative GPA of 2.3 for all courses. *Entrance requirements:* For doctorate, PCAT (taken within 3 years of the date of application), criminal background check, proof of health insurance, immunizations and health clearance, minimum undergraduate GPA of 2.75, two letters of recommendation, interview. Additional exam requirements/recommendations for international students: Required—TOEFL. *Application deadline:* For fall admission, 2/1 for domestic and international students. Applications are processed on a rolling basis. Electronic applications accepted. *Financial support:* Career-related internships or fieldwork and scholarships/grants available. Financial award application deadline: 3/1; financial award applicants required to submit FAFSA. *Unit head:* Dr. Michelle Easton, Dean, 304-357-4889, Fax: 304-357-4868, E-mail: michelleeaston@ucwv.edu. *Application contact:* Jamie Bero, Director of Student Affairs, School of Pharmacy, 304-357-4889, Fax: 304-357-4868, E-mail: pharmacy@ucwv.edu.
Website: http://www.ucwv.edu/Pharmacy/

University of Cincinnati, College of Pharmacy, Division of Pharmacy Practice, Cincinnati, OH 45221. Offers Pharm D. *Accreditation:* ACPE. *Entrance requirements:* For doctorate, GRE General Test, BS in pharmacy or equivalent, minimum GPA of 3.0. Additional exam requirements/recommendations for international students: Required—TOEFL.

University of Connecticut, Graduate School, School of Pharmacy, Professional Program in Pharmacy, Storrs, CT 06269. Offers Pharm D.

The University of Findlay, Office of Graduate Admissions, Findlay, OH 45840-3653. Offers athletic training (MAT); business (MBA), including health care management, hospitality management, organizational leadership, public management; education (MA Ed), including administration, children's literature, early childhood, human resource development, reading, science, special education, technology; environmental, safety and health management (MSEM); health informatics (MS); occupational therapy (MOT); pharmacy (Pharm D); physical therapy (DPT); physician assistant (MPA); rhetoric and writing (MA); teaching English to speakers of other languages (TESOL) and bilingual education (MA). Part-time and evening/weekend programs available. Postbaccalaureate distance learning degree programs offered (no on-campus study). *Faculty:* 209 full-time (98 women), 69 part-time/adjunct (38 women). *Students:* 551 full-time (332 women), 457 part-time (276 women); includes 77 minority (37 Black or African American, non-Hispanic/Latino; 1 American Indian or Alaska Native, non-Hispanic/Latino; 15 Asian, non-Hispanic/Latino; 23 Hispanic/Latino; 1 Native Hawaiian or other Pacific Islander, non-Hispanic/Latino), 135 international. Average age 28. 637 applicants, 66% accepted, 241 enrolled. In 2013, 267 master's, 91 doctorates awarded. *Degree requirements:* For master's, thesis, cumulative project, capstone project. *Entrance requirements:* For master's, GRE/GMAT, bachelor's degree from accredited institution, minimum undergraduate GPA of 2.5 in last 64 hours of course work; for doctorate, GRE, minimum cumulative GPA of 3.0. Additional exam requirements/recommendations for international students: Required—TOEFL (minimum score 80 iBT). *Application deadline:* Applications are processed on a rolling basis. Application fee: $25. Electronic applications accepted. *Expenses: Required fees:* $146 per semester. Tuition and fees vary according to degree level and program. *Financial support:* In 2013–14, 11 research assistantships with full and partial tuition reimbursements (averaging $4,000 per year), 10 teaching assistantships with full and partial tuition reimbursements (averaging $3,600 per year) were awarded; career-related internships or fieldwork, Federal Work-Study, health care benefits, and unspecified assistantships also available. Financial award application deadline: 4/1; financial award applicants required to submit FAFSA. *Unit head:* Christopher M. Harris, Director of Admissions, 419-434-4347, E-mail: harrisc1@findlay.edu. *Application contact:* Emily Ickes, Graduate Admissions Counselor, 419-434-6933, Fax: 419-434-4898, E-mail: ickese@findlay.edu.
Website: http://www.findlay.edu/admissions/graduate/Pages/default.aspx

University of Florida, Graduate School, College of Pharmacy and Graduate School, Graduate Programs in Pharmacy, Department of Pharmaceutics, Gainesville, FL 32610. Offers clinical and translational sciences (PhD); pharmaceutical sciences (MSP, PhD); pharmacy (MSP, PhD). *Faculty:* 11 full-time (2 women), 10 part-time/adjunct (1 woman). *Students:* 18 full-time (9 women), 2 part-time (1 woman); includes 1 minority (Asian, non-Hispanic/Latino), 17 international. Average age 30. 234 applicants, 48% accepted, 86 enrolled. In 2013, 1 master's, 9 doctorates awarded. *Degree requirements:* For doctorate, comprehensive exam, thesis/dissertation. *Entrance requirements:* For master's and doctorate, GRE General Test, minimum GPA of 3.0. Additional exam requirements/recommendations for international students: Required—TOEFL (minimum score 550 paper-based; 80 iBT), IELTS (minimum score 6). *Application deadline:* For fall admission, 2/1 priority date for domestic students, 2/1 for international students; for spring admission, 9/1 for domestic students, 10/1 for international students. Applications are processed on a rolling basis. Application fee: $30. Electronic applications accepted. *Expenses:* Tuition, state resident: full-time $12,640. Tuition, nonresident: full-time $30,000. *Financial support:* In 2013–14, 18 students received support, including 4 research assistantships (averaging $13,785 per year), 16 teaching assistantships (averaging $15,745 per year); tuition waivers (full) and unspecified assistantships also available. Financial award applicants required to submit FAFSA. *Faculty research:* Basic, applied, and clinical investigations in pharmacokinetics/biopharmaceutics; pharmaceutical analysis, pharmaceutical biotechnology and drug delivery; herbal medicine. *Unit head:* Hartmut Derendorf, PhD, Professor and Chair, 352-273-7856, Fax:

352-392-4447, E-mail: hartmut@ufl.edu. *Application contact:* Dr. Anthony Palmieri, III, Graduate Coordinator, 352-273-7868, E-mail: palmieri@cop.ufl.edu.
Website: http://www.cop.ufl.edu/pc/

University of Florida, Graduate School, College of Pharmacy, Professional Program in Pharmacy, Gainesville, FL 32610. Offers Pharm D, MBA/Pharm D, Pharm D/MPH, Pharm D/PhD. *Accreditation:* ACPE. Part-time programs available. Postbaccalaureate distance learning degree programs offered (no on-campus study). *Entrance requirements:* For doctorate, PCAT, minimum GPA of 2.5. Additional exam requirements/recommendations for international students: Required—TOEFL. *Application deadline:* For fall admission, 3/1 for domestic and international students. Applications are processed on a rolling basis. Application fee: $30. Electronic applications accepted. *Expenses:* Tuition, state resident: full-time $12,640. Tuition, nonresident: full-time $30,000. *Financial support:* Federal Work-Study and institutionally sponsored loans available. Support available to part-time students. Financial award applicants required to submit FAFSA. *Faculty research:* Drug discovery, drug delivery, pharmacodynamics, socioeconomics of pharmacy, neurobiology of aging. *Unit head:* Michael W. McKenzie, PhD, Associate Dean for Professional Affairs, 352-273-6217, Fax: 352-273-6219, E-mail: mckenzie@cop.ufl.edu. *Application contact:* Mary Beth Yokomi, Admissions Coordinator, 352-273-6216, E-mail: yokomi@cop.ufl.edu.
Website: http://pharmacy.ufl.edu/education/doctor-of-pharmacy-degree-pharmd/

University of Georgia, College of Pharmacy, Athens, GA 30602. Offers MS, PhD, Pharm D, Certificate. *Accreditation:* ACPE (one or more programs are accredited). *Degree requirements:* For doctorate, variable foreign language requirement, thesis/dissertation (for some programs). *Entrance requirements:* For master's, GRE General Test, minimum GPA of 3.0; for doctorate, GRE General Test (for PhD), minimum GPA of 3.0 (for PhD). Additional exam requirements/recommendations for international students: Required—TOEFL (minimum score 80 iBT). Electronic applications accepted. *Expenses:* Contact institution.

University of Hawaii at Hilo, Program in Pharmacy, Hilo, HI 96720-4091. Offers Pharm D. *Students:* 343 full-time (180 women), 1 part-time (0 women); includes 279 minority (12 Black or African American, non-Hispanic/Latino; 199 Asian, non-Hispanic/Latino; 13 Hispanic/Latino; 6 Native Hawaiian or other Pacific Islander, non-Hispanic/Latino; 49 Two or more races, non-Hispanic/Latino), 3 international. Average age 27. In 2013, 84 degrees awarded. *Application deadline:* For fall admission, 2/1 priority date for domestic students. Applications are processed on a rolling basis. Application fee: $50. Electronic applications accepted. *Expenses:* Tuition, state resident: full-time $4668. Tuition, nonresident: full-time $10,704. Tuition and fees vary according to course load and program. *Financial support:* Application deadline: 3/1; applicants required to submit FAFSA. *Unit head:* John Pezzuto, Dean, 808-933-2909, Fax: 808-933-2974, E-mail: pezzuto@hawaii.edu. *Application contact:* Pharm D Program Admissions, 808-932-7700, Fax: 808-933-3889, E-mail: pharmacy@hawaii.edu.
Website: http://pharmacy.uhh.hawaii.edu/academics/pharmd/

University of Houston, College of Pharmacy, Houston, TX 77204. Offers pharmaceutics (MSPHR, PhD); pharmacology (MSPHR, PhD); pharmacy (Pharm D); pharmacy administration (MSPHR, PhD). *Accreditation:* ACPE. Part-time programs available. Terminal master's awarded for partial completion of doctoral program. *Entrance requirements:* For doctorate, PCAT (for Pharm D). Additional exam requirements/recommendations for international students: Required—TOEFL. Electronic applications accepted. *Faculty research:* Drug screening and design, cardiovascular pharmacology, infectious disease, asthma research, herbal medicine.

University of Illinois at Chicago, College of Pharmacy, Department of Biopharmaceutical Sciences, Chicago, IL 60607-7173. Offers PhD. *Faculty:* 15 full-time (4 women), 8 part-time/adjunct (0 women). *Students:* 28 full-time (20 women), 4 part-time (3 women); includes 4 minority (1 Black or African American, non-Hispanic/Latino; 3 Asian, non-Hispanic/Latino), 21 international. Average age 28. 73 applicants, 16% accepted, 6 enrolled. In 2013, 5 doctorates awarded. *Expenses:* Tuition, state resident: full-time $11,066; part-time $3689 per term. Tuition, nonresident: full-time $23,064; part-time $7688 per term. *Required fees:* $3004; $1190 per term. Tuition and fees vary according to course level and program. *Total annual research expenditures:* $2 million. *Unit head:* Prof. William T. Beck, Head, 312-996-0888, Fax: 312-996-0098, E-mail: wtbeck@uic.edu.
Website: http://www.uic.edu/pharmacy/depts/Biopharmaceutical_Sciences/index.php

University of Illinois at Chicago, College of Pharmacy, Professional Program in Pharmacy, Chicago, IL 60607-7128. Offers Pharm D. *Accreditation:* ACPE. *Faculty:* 81 full-time (31 women), 16 part-time/adjunct (3 women). *Students:* 806 full-time (497 women); includes 406 minority (53 Black or African American, non-Hispanic/Latino; 292 Asian, non-Hispanic/Latino; 36 Hispanic/Latino; 2 Native Hawaiian or other Pacific Islander, non-Hispanic/Latino; 23 Two or more races, non-Hispanic/Latino), 25 international. Average age 26. 718 applicants, 34% accepted, 204 enrolled. In 2013, 167 doctorates awarded. *Entrance requirements:* For doctorate, PCAT. Application fee: $40 ($50 for international students). *Expenses:* Tuition, state resident: full-time $11,066; part-time $3689 per term. Tuition, nonresident: full-time $23,064; part-time $7688 per term. *Required fees:* $3004; $1190 per term. Tuition and fees vary according to course level and program. *Financial support:* Fellowships available. *Unit head:* Jerry Bauman, Dean, 312-996-7240, E-mail: jbauman@uic.edu. *Application contact:* Jackie Perry, Graduate College Receptionist, 312-413-2550, Fax: 312-413-0185, E-mail: gradcoll@uic.edu.
Website: http://www.uic.edu/pharmacy/education/professional_degree_prog.php

The University of Iowa, College of Pharmacy, Iowa City, IA 52242-1316. Offers clinical pharmaceutical sciences (PhD); medicinal and natural products chemistry (PhD); pharamaceutics (PhD); pharmaceutical socioeconomics (PhD); pharmaceutics (MS); pharmacy (Pharm D); Pharm D/MPH. *Accreditation:* ACPE (one or more programs are accredited). *Degree requirements:* For master's, thesis optional, exam; for doctorate, comprehensive exam, thesis/dissertation. *Entrance requirements:* For master's and doctorate, GRE General Test, minimum GPA of 3.0. Additional exam requirements/recommendations for international students: Required—TOEFL (minimum score 550 paper-based; 81 iBT). Electronic applications accepted.

University of Kentucky, Professional Program in Pharmacy, Lexington, KY 40506-0032. Offers Pharm D. *Accreditation:* ACPE. *Entrance requirements:* For doctorate, PCAT, interview, minimum GPA of 2.5. Additional exam requirements/recommendations for international students: Required—TOEFL (minimum score 527 paper-based). Electronic applications accepted. *Expenses:* Contact institution. *Faculty research:* Innovations in pharmacy practice and education; policy and outcomes research; drug discovery and development; drug delivery and nanotechnology; natural products and computational chemistry.

University of Louisiana at Monroe, Graduate School, College of Health and Pharmaceutical Sciences, School of Pharmacy, Monroe, LA 71209-0001. Offers pharmacy (PhD); toxicology (PhD). *Accreditation:* ACPE. *Degree requirements:* For doctorate, comprehensive exam, thesis/dissertation. *Entrance requirements:* For doctorate, GRE General Test, minimum undergraduate GPA of 2.5. Additional exam requirements/recommendations for international students: Required—TOEFL (minimum score 500 paper-based; 61 iBT). *Application deadline:* For fall admission, 3/1 for domestic and international students; for winter admission, 12/14 for domestic students; for spring admission, 9/1 for domestic and international students. Applications are processed on a rolling basis. Application fee: $20 ($30 for international students). Electronic applications accepted. *Expenses:* Tuition, state resident: full-time $6607. Tuition, nonresident: full-time $17,179. Full-time tuition and fees vary according to program. *Financial support:* Research assistantships, Federal Work-Study, and unspecified assistantships available. Financial award application deadline: 4/1; financial award applicants required to submit FAFSA. *Unit head:* Dr. Benny L. Blaylock, Dean, 318-342-1603, E-mail: blaylock@ulm.edu. *Application contact:* Dr. Paul W. Sylvester, Director, Research and Graduate Studies, 318-342-1958, Fax: 318-342-1606, E-mail: sylvester@ulm.edu.
Website: http://www.ulm.edu/pharmacy/

The University of Manchester, School of Pharmacy and Pharmaceutical Sciences, Manchester, United Kingdom. Offers M Phil, PhD.

University of Maryland, Baltimore, Graduate School, Graduate Programs in Pharmacy, Baltimore, MD 21201. Offers pharmaceutical health service research (MS, PhD), including epidemiology (MS), pharmacy administration (PhD); pharmaceutical sciences (PhD); Pharm D/PhD. *Accreditation:* ACPE (one or more programs are accredited). *Degree requirements:* For doctorate, comprehensive exam, thesis/dissertation. *Entrance requirements:* For doctorate, GRE General Test. Additional exam requirements/recommendations for international students: Required—TOEFL (minimum score 550 paper-based), IELTS. Electronic applications accepted. *Faculty research:* Drug discovery, pharmacokinetics, drug delivery, pharmaceutical outcomes and policy, pharmaceutical sciences.

University of Maryland, Baltimore, Professional Program in Pharmacy, Baltimore, MD 21201. Offers Pharm D, JD/Pharm D, Pharm D/MBA, Pharm D/MPH, Pharm D/PhD. *Accreditation:* ACPE. *Faculty:* 77 full-time (41 women), 8 part-time/adjunct (3 women). *Students:* 67 full-time (44 women), 79 part-time (54 women); includes 313 minority (74 Black or African American, non-Hispanic/Latino; 233 Asian, non-Hispanic/Latino; 6 Hispanic/Latino). Average age 25. 1,007 applicants, 26% accepted, 162 enrolled. In 2013, 77 doctorates awarded. *Entrance requirements:* For doctorate, PCAT, 65 hours in pre-pharmacy course work, on-site interview. Additional exam requirements/recommendations for international students: Required—TOEFL (minimum score 550 paper-based; 80 iBT). *Application deadline:* For fall admission, 1/6 for domestic and international students. Application fee: $45. Electronic applications accepted. *Financial support:* In 2013–14, 308 students received support. Career-related internships or fieldwork, Federal Work-Study, institutionally sponsored loans, and scholarships/grants available. Support available to part-time students. Financial award application deadline: 3/1; financial award applicants required to submit FAFSA. *Faculty research:* Pharmaceutics, molecular biology, pharmacology, pharmacoepidemiology, pharmacoeconomics. *Total annual research expenditures:* $18.1 million. *Unit head:* Dr. Cherokee Layson-Wolf, Associate Dean for Student Affairs, 410-706-1067, Fax: 410-706-2158, E-mail: cwolf@rx.umaryland.edu. *Application contact:* Patrice Sharp, Admissions Officer, 410-706-0732, Fax: 410-706-2158, E-mail: pharmdhelp@umaryland.edu.
Website: http://www.pharmacy.umaryland.edu

University of Michigan, College of Pharmacy, Professional Program in Pharmacy, Ann Arbor, MI 48109. Offers Pharm D, Pharm D/PhD. *Accreditation:* ACPE. *Entrance requirements:* For doctorate, PCAT. *Application deadline:* For fall admission, 2/1 for domestic students. Tuition and fees vary according to course level, course load, degree level, program and student level. *Financial support:* Applicants required to submit FAFSA. *Unit head:* Frank J. Ascione, Dean, 734-764-7144, Fax: 734-763-2022, E-mail: fascione@umich.edu. *Application contact:* Mark S. Nelson, Director, Admissions and Student Counseling Services, 734-764-7312, E-mail: mnelson@med.umich.edu.
Website: https://pharmacy.umich.edu/prospective-students/programs/doctor-pharmacy-pharmd-degree

University of Minnesota, Duluth, Medical School, Department of Biochemistry, Molecular Biology and Biophysics, Duluth, MN 55812-2496. Offers biochemistry, molecular biology and biophysics (MS); biology and biophysics (PhD); social, administrative, and clinical pharmacy (MS, PhD); toxicology (MS, PhD). Terminal master's awarded for partial completion of doctoral program. *Degree requirements:* For master's, comprehensive exam, thesis; for doctorate, comprehensive exam, thesis/dissertation. *Entrance requirements:* For master's and doctorate, GRE General Test. Additional exam requirements/recommendations for international students: Required—TOEFL. Electronic applications accepted. *Faculty research:* Intestinal cancer biology; hepatotoxins and mitochondriopathies; toxicology; cell cycle regulation in stem cells; neurobiology of brain development, trace metal function and blood-brain barrier; hibernation biology.

University of Minnesota, Twin Cities Campus, College of Pharmacy, Professional Program in Pharmacy, Minneapolis, MN 55455-0213. Offers Pharm D. *Accreditation:* ACPE. *Degree requirements:* For doctorate, paper and seminar presentation. *Entrance requirements:* For doctorate, 2 years of pharmacy-related course work.

University of Mississippi, Graduate School, School of Pharmacy, Professional Program in Pharmacy, University, MS 38677. Offers Pharm D. *Accreditation:* ACPE. *Faculty:* 13 full-time (5 women). *Students:* 231 full-time (145 women), 1 part-time (0 women); includes 48 minority (16 Black or African American, non-Hispanic/Latino; 1 American Indian or Alaska Native, non-Hispanic/Latino; 22 Asian, non-Hispanic/Latino; 6 Hispanic/Latino; 3 Two or more races, non-Hispanic/Latino), 2 international. In 2013, 94 doctorates awarded. *Application deadline:* For fall admission, 4/1 for domestic students. Applications are processed on a rolling basis. Application fee: $40. *Expenses:* Contact institution. *Financial support:* Scholarships/grants available. Financial award application deadline: 3/1; financial award applicants required to submit FAFSA. *Unit head:* Dr. David Allen, Dean, 662-915-7265, Fax: 662-915-5704, E-mail: pharmacy@olemiss.edu. *Application contact:* Dr. Marvin Wilson, Associate Dean, 662-915-7265, Fax: 662-915-5704.

University of Missouri–Kansas City, School of Pharmacy, Kansas City, MO 64110-2499. Offers pharmaceutical sciences (PhD); pharmacology and toxicology (PhD); pharmacy (Pharm D). PhD offered through School of Graduate Studies. *Accreditation:* ACPE (one or more programs are accredited). Postbaccalaureate distance learning degree programs offered (minimal on-campus study). *Faculty:* 54 full-time (26 women), 6 part-time/adjunct (3 women). *Students:* 424 full-time (252 women); includes 77 minority (14 Black or African American, non-Hispanic/Latino; 2 American Indian or Alaska Native, non-Hispanic/Latino; 43 Asian, non-Hispanic/Latino; 10 Hispanic/Latino; 1 Native Hawaiian or other Pacific Islander, non-Hispanic/Latino; 7 Two or more races, non-Hispanic/Latino), 1 international. Average age 26. 365 applicants, 37% accepted, 136 enrolled. In 2013, 122 doctorates awarded. *Degree requirements:* For doctorate, comprehensive exam (for some programs), thesis/dissertation (for some programs). *Entrance requirements:* For doctorate, PCAT (for Pharm D). Additional exam requirements/recommendations for international students: Required—TOEFL (minimum score 550 paper-based; 80 iBT). *Application deadline:* For fall admission, 3/1 for domestic and international students. Applications are processed on a rolling basis. Application fee: $45 ($50 for international students). Electronic applications accepted.

Expenses: Contact institution. *Financial support:* In 2013–14, 26 research assistantships with full and partial tuition reimbursements (averaging $11,585 per year), 26 teaching assistantships with full tuition reimbursements (averaging $14,213 per year) were awarded; career-related internships or fieldwork, Federal Work-Study, institutionally sponsored loans, tuition waivers (full and partial), and unspecified assistantships also available. Financial award application deadline: 3/1; financial award applicants required to submit FAFSA. *Faculty research:* Bio-organic and medicinal chemistry, drug delivery, pharmaceutics, molecular neurobiology, neurology. *Unit head:* Dr. Russell B. Melchert, Dean, 816-235-1609, Fax: 816-235-5190, E-mail: melchertr@umkc.edu. *Application contact:* Shelly M. Janasz, Director, Student Services, 816-235-2400, Fax: 816-235-5190, E-mail: janaszs@umkc.edu.
Website: http://pharmacy.umkc.edu/

The University of Montana, Graduate School, College of Health Professions and Biomedical Sciences, Skaggs School of Pharmacy, Missoula, MT 59812-0002. Offers biomedical and pharmaceutical sciences (MS, PhD), including biomedical sciences (PhD), medicinal chemistry, molecular and cellular toxicology, neuroscience (PhD), pharmaceutical sciences (MS); pharmacy (Pharm D). *Application deadline:* Applications are processed on a rolling basis. Electronic applications accepted. *Financial support:* Teaching assistantships with full and partial tuition reimbursements, career-related internships or fieldwork, Federal Work-Study, institutionally sponsored loans, scholarships/grants, and tuition waivers (full and partial) available. Financial award applicants required to submit FAFSA. *Faculty research:* Neuroendocrinology, neuropharmacology, molecular biochemistry, cardiovascular pharmacology, pharmacognosy. *Unit head:* Reed Humphrey, Dean, 406-243-4341, E-mail: reed.humphrey@umontana.edu. *Application contact:* Information Contact, E-mail: gradschl@mso.umt.edu.
Website: http://www.umt.edu/pharmacy/

University of Nebraska Medical Center, College of Pharmacy, Omaha, NE 68198-6000. Offers Pharm D. *Accreditation:* ACPE. *Entrance requirements:* For doctorate, PCAT, 90 semester hours of pre-pharmacy work. Electronic applications accepted. *Expenses:* Contact institution. *Faculty research:* Biopharmaceutics, nanomedicine, drug design, pharmaceutics, pharmacokinetics.

University of New England, College of Pharmacy, Biddeford, ME 04005-9526. Offers Pharm D. *Accreditation:* ACPE. *Faculty:* 26 full-time (10 women), 3 part-time/adjunct (0 women). *Students:* 390 full-time (245 women); includes 127 minority (21 Black or African American, non-Hispanic/Latino; 3 American Indian or Alaska Native, non-Hispanic/Latino; 85 Asian, non-Hispanic/Latino; 10 Hispanic/Latino; 4 Native Hawaiian or other Pacific Islander, non-Hispanic/Latino; 4 Two or more races, non-Hispanic/Latino), 6 international. Average age 26. 670 applicants, 28% accepted, 102 enrolled. In 2013, 86 doctorates awarded. *Entrance requirements:* For doctorate, PCAT. *Application deadline:* For fall admission, 2/1 for domestic students. Applications are processed on a rolling basis. Electronic applications accepted. *Financial support:* Application deadline: 5/1; applicants required to submit FAFSA. *Unit head:* Dr. Gayle A. Brazeau, Dean, College of Pharmacy, 207-221-4500, Fax: 207-523-1927, E-mail: gbrazeau@une.edu. *Application contact:* Dr. Cynthia Forrest, Vice President for Student Affairs, 207-221-4225, Fax: 207-523-1925, E-mail: gradadmissions@une.edu.
Website: http://www.une.edu/pharmacy/

University of New Mexico, Graduate School, College of Pharmacy, Professional Program in Pharmacy, Albuquerque, NM 87131-2039. Offers Pharm D. *Accreditation:* ACPE. *Entrance requirements:* For doctorate, PCAT, 3 letters of recommendation, interview, 91 credit hours of prerequisites, letter of intent, Pharmcas application. Electronic applications accepted. *Expenses:* Contact institution.

University of Oklahoma Health Sciences Center, College of Pharmacy, Professional Program in Pharmacy, Oklahoma City, OK 73190. Offers Pharm D. *Accreditation:* ACPE. *Faculty:* 42 full-time (27 women), 2 part-time/adjunct (1 woman). *Students:* 423 full-time (242 women), 5 part-time (4 women); includes 167 minority (19 Black or African American, non-Hispanic/Latino; 16 American Indian or Alaska Native, non-Hispanic/Latino; 85 Asian, non-Hispanic/Latino; 13 Hispanic/Latino; 34 Two or more races, non-Hispanic/Latino), 8 international. Average age 26. 452 applicants, 37% accepted, 95 enrolled. In 2013, 107 doctorates awarded. Application fee: $25 ($50 for international students). *Expenses:* Tuition, state resident: full-time $3504; part-time $175.20 per credit hour. Tuition, nonresident: full-time $13,504; part-time $675.20 per credit hour. *Required fees:* $1545; $52.70 per credit hour. $245.25 per semester. Tuition and fees vary according to course load. *Unit head:* Dr. JoLaine Drauglais, Dean, 405-271-6484, E-mail: jolaine-draugalis@ouhsc.edu. *Application contact:* Jennifer Richardson, Director of Student Services, 405-271-6598, E-mail: jennifer-richardson@ouhsc.edu.

University of Pittsburgh, School of Pharmacy, Professional Program in Pharmacy, Pittsburgh, PA 15260. Offers Pharm D. *Accreditation:* ACPE. *Faculty:* 75 full-time (35 women), 6 part-time/adjunct (3 women). *Students:* 435 full-time (261 women); includes 65 minority (19 Black or African American, non-Hispanic/Latino; 42 Asian, non-Hispanic/Latino; 3 Hispanic/Latino; 1 Two or more races, non-Hispanic/Latino), 4 international. Average age 23. 598 applicants, 26% accepted, 113 enrolled. In 2013, 106 doctorates awarded. *Entrance requirements:* For doctorate, PCAT. *Application deadline:* For fall admission, 12/1 for domestic students. Application fee: $215. Electronic applications accepted. *Expenses:* Tuition, state resident: full-time $19,964; part-time $807 per credit. Tuition, nonresident: full-time $32,686; part-time $1337 per credit. *Required fees:* $740; $200. Tuition and fees vary according to program. *Financial support:* In 2013–14, 181 students received support. Career-related internships or fieldwork, Federal Work-Study, and scholarships/grants available. Financial award application deadline: 10/1. *Faculty research:* Drug delivery and targeting; neuroendocrine pharmacology; genomics, proteomics, and drug discovery; clinical pharmaceutical sciences. *Unit head:* Dr. Sharon Corey, Assistant Dean of Students, 412-648-9157, Fax: 412-383-9996, E-mail: coreys@pitt.edu. *Application contact:* Marcia L. Borrelli, Director of Student Services, 412-383-9000, Fax: 412-383-9996, E-mail: borrelli@pitt.edu.
Website: http://www.pharmacy.pitt.edu

University of Puerto Rico, Medical Sciences Campus, School of Pharmacy, San Juan, PR 00936-5067. Offers industrial pharmacy (MS); pharmaceutical sciences (MS); pharmacy (Pharm D). The MS in Pharmacy program is not admitting students in the academic year 2010-2011. *Accreditation:* ACPE. Part-time and evening/weekend programs available. *Degree requirements:* For master's, thesis; for doctorate, portfolio, research project. *Entrance requirements:* For master's, GRE, interview; for doctorate, PCAT, interview. Electronic applications accepted. *Expenses:* Contact institution. *Faculty research:* Controlled release, solid dosage form, screening of anti-HIV drugs, pharmacokinetic/pharmacodynamic of drugs.

University of Rhode Island, Graduate School, College of Pharmacy, Department of Pharmacy Practice, Kingston, RI 02881. Offers pharmaceutical sciences (MS, PhD), including pharmacoepidemiology and pharmacoeconomics; pharmacy practice (Pharm D); MS/PhD; PhD/MBA. *Accreditation:* ACPE. *Faculty:* 29 full-time (24 women). *Students:* 727 full-time (452 women), 1 (woman) part-time; includes 123 minority (22 Black or African American, non-Hispanic/Latino; 58 Asian, non-Hispanic/Latino; 31 Hispanic/Latino; 12 Two or more races, non-Hispanic/Latino), 36 international. In 2013, 97 doctorates awarded. *Entrance requirements:* For master's and doctorate, 2 letters of recommendation. Additional exam requirements/recommendations for international students: Required—TOEFL (minimum score 550 paper-based). *Application deadline:* For fall admission, 2/1 for domestic and international students. Application fee: $65. Electronic applications accepted. *Expenses:* Tuition, state resident: full-time $11,532; part-time $641 per credit. Tuition, nonresident: full-time $23,606; part-time $1311 per credit. *Required fees:* $1388; $36 per credit. $35 per semester. One-time fee: $130. *Financial support:* Application deadline: 2/1; applicants required to submit FAFSA. *Faculty research:* Treatment, virulence inhibition (toxin and biofilm), colonization and control of Methicillin-resistant Staphylococcus aureus (MRSA); investigating activity of catheter lock solutions against biofilm producing bacteria. *Total annual research expenditures:* $464,501. *Unit head:* Dr. Marilyn Barbour, Chair, 401-874-5842, Fax: 401-874-2181, E-mail: mbarbourri@aol.com.
Website: http://www.uri.edu/pharmacy/departments/php/index.shtml

University of Saint Joseph, School of Pharmacy, West Hartford, CT 06117-2700. Offers Pharm D. *Application deadline:* Applications are processed on a rolling basis. Electronic applications accepted. *Financial support:* Career-related internships or fieldwork available. *Unit head:* Dr. Joseph R. Ofosu, Dean, 860-231-5858. *Application contact:* Graduate Admissions Office, 860-231-5261, E-mail: graduate@usj.edu.
Website: http://www.usj.edu/academics/schools/school-of-pharmacy/

University of South Carolina, South Carolina College of Pharmacy, Professional Program in Pharmacy, Columbia, SC 29208. Offers Pharm D. *Degree requirements:* For doctorate, one foreign language. *Entrance requirements:* For doctorate, PCAT, 2 years of preprofessional study, interview. Electronic applications accepted. *Faculty research:* Cancer treatment and prevention, Ion channels, DNA damage repair, inflammation.

University of Southern California, Graduate School, School of Pharmacy, Professional Program in Pharmacy, Los Angeles, CA 90089. Offers Pharm D, Pharm D/MBA, Pharm D/MS, Pharm D/PhD. *Accreditation:* ACPE. Electronic applications accepted. *Faculty research:* Infectious diseases, health services research, geriatric pharmacology, clinical psychopharmacology.

University of South Florida, College of Pharmacy, Tampa, FL 33620-9951. Offers Pharm D. *Faculty:* 6 full-time (1 woman). *Students:* 225 part-time (126 women); includes 91 minority (24 Black or African American, non-Hispanic/Latino; 36 Asian, non-Hispanic/Latino; 28 Hispanic/Latino; 3 Two or more races, non-Hispanic/Latino). Average age 26. 598 applicants, 34% accepted, 109 enrolled. *Total annual research expenditures:* $236,853. *Unit head:* Dr. Karen D. Liller, Dean, 813-974-7359, Fax: 813-974-5762, E-mail: kliller@usf.edu. *Application contact:* Francisco Vera, Assistant Director for Admissions, 813-974-8800, E-mail: fvera@usf.edu.

University of South Florida, Innovative Education Graduate Certificate Programs, Tampa, FL 33620-9951. *Unit head:* Kathy Barnes, Interdisciplinary Programs Coordinator, 813-974-8031, Fax: 813-974-7061, E-mail: barnesk@usf.edu. *Application contact:* Karen Tylinski, Metro Initiatives, 813-974-9943, Fax: 813-974-7061, E-mail: ktylinsk@usf.edu.
Website: http://www.usf.edu/innovative-education/

The University of Tennessee Health Science Center, College of Pharmacy, Memphis, TN 38163-0002. Offers MS, PhD, Pharm D, Pharm D/PhD. *Accreditation:* ACPE (one or more programs are accredited). Terminal master's awarded for partial completion of doctoral program. *Degree requirements:* For master's, thesis; for doctorate, thesis/dissertation (for some programs). *Entrance requirements:* For doctorate, PCAT, minimum GPA of 3.0. Additional exam requirements/recommendations for international students: Required—TOEFL. *Application deadline:* For fall admission, 2/1 for domestic students. Applications are processed on a rolling basis. Application fee: $50. Electronic applications accepted. *Expenses:* Contact institution. *Financial support:* Fellowships, research assistantships, teaching assistantships, career-related internships or fieldwork, Federal Work-Study, institutionally sponsored loans, and tuition waivers (full) available. Support available to part-time students. Financial award application deadline: 2/15. *Unit head:* Marie A. Chisholm-Burns, Dean, 901-448-6036, Fax: 901-528-7053, E-mail: mchisho3@uthsc.edu. *Application contact:* Angela S. Finerson, Director of Admissions, 901-448-7172, Fax: 901-448-7772, E-mail: afinerso@uthsc.edu.
Website: http://www.uthsc.edu/pharmacy/

The University of Texas at Austin, Graduate School, College of Pharmacy, Professional Program in Pharmacy, Austin, TX 78712-1111. Offers Pharm D, Pharm D/PhD. Program offered jointly with The University of Texas Health Science Center at San Antonio. *Accreditation:* ACPE. *Entrance requirements:* For doctorate, GRE General Test.

University of the Incarnate Word, Feik School of Pharmacy, San Antonio, TX 78209-6397. Offers Pharm D. *Accreditation:* ACPE. *Faculty:* 17 full-time (11 women), 1 (woman) part-time/adjunct. *Students:* 399 full-time (255 women), 10 part-time (7 women); includes 265 minority (28 Black or African American, non-Hispanic/Latino; 102 Asian, non-Hispanic/Latino; 125 Hispanic/Latino; 1 Native Hawaiian or other Pacific Islander, non-Hispanic/Latino; 9 Two or more races, non-Hispanic/Latino), 21 international. Average age 27. 146 applicants, 100% accepted, 97 enrolled. In 2013, 94 doctorates awarded. *Entrance requirements:* For doctorate, PCAT, 80 hours of documented pharmacy observational experience; on-site interview (if selected); critical thinking assessment and writing sample during interview process; minimum GPA of 2.5 and 64 hours (71 hours for financial aid) in accredited pre-pharmacy course. Additional exam requirements/recommendations for international students: Required—TOEFL (minimum score 560 paper-based; 83 iBT). *Application deadline:* For fall admission, 12/1 for domestic and international students. Application fee: $100. Electronic applications accepted. *Expenses:* Contact institution. *Financial support:* Federal Work-Study and scholarships/grants available. Financial award applicants required to submit FAFSA. *Unit head:* Dr. Arcelia Johnson-Fannin, Founding Dean, 210-883-1015, Fax: 210-822-1516, E-mail: johnsonf@uiwtx.edu. *Application contact:* Dr. Kevin Lord, Assistant Dean, Student Affairs/Assistant Professor, Pharmaceutical Sciences, 210-883-1060, Fax: 210-822-1521, E-mail: lord@uiwtx.edu.
Website: http://www.uiw.edu/pharmacy

University of the Pacific, Thomas J. Long School of Pharmacy and Health Sciences, Professional Program in Pharmacy, Stockton, CA 95211-0197. Offers Pharm D. *Accreditation:* ACPE. *Faculty:* 38 full-time (19 women), 4 part-time/adjunct (1 woman). *Students:* 621 full-time (399 women), 10 part-time (8 women); includes 500 minority (7 Black or African American, non-Hispanic/Latino; 3 American Indian or Alaska Native, non-Hispanic/Latino; 425 Asian, non-Hispanic/Latino; 47 Hispanic/Latino; 18 Two or more races, non-Hispanic/Latino), 5 international. Average age 24. 1,598 applicants, 19% accepted, 208 enrolled. In 2013, 197 doctorates awarded. *Entrance requirements:* Additional exam requirements/recommendations for international students: Required—TOEFL. *Application deadline:* For fall admission, 2/1 for domestic students. Application fee: $75. *Financial support:* In 2013–14, 27 teaching assistantships were awarded; career-related internships or fieldwork, Federal Work-Study, institutionally sponsored loans, and tuition waivers (partial) also available. Support available to part-time students. Financial award application deadline: 3/1; financial award applicants required to submit FAFSA. *Unit head:* Dr. Philip Oppenheimer, Dean, 209-946-2561, Fax: 209-

946-2410. *Application contact:* Ron Espejo, Recruitment Specialist, 209-946-3957, Fax: 209-946-3147, E-mail: respejo@pacific.edu.
Website: http://www.pacific.edu/pharmacy/

University of the Sciences, Philadelphia College of Pharmacy, Philadelphia, PA 19104-4495. Offers MS, PhD, Pharm D. *Accreditation:* ACPE. *Faculty:* 9 full-time (0 women). *Students:* 37 full-time (24 women), 41 part-time (28 women); includes 7 minority (all Asian, non-Hispanic/Latino), 16 international. Average age 31. 556 applicants, 6% accepted, 16 enrolled. In 2013, 8 master's, 5 doctorates awarded. *Entrance requirements:* Additional exam requirements/recommendations for international students: Required—TOEFL, TWE. *Application deadline:* For fall admission, 4/15 for domestic students; for spring admission, 10/24 for domestic students. Application fee: $50. *Expenses: Tuition:* Part-time $1447 per credit. Tuition and fees vary according to campus/location and program. *Financial support:* In 2013–14, 3 students received support, including 1 fellowship (averaging $22,000 per year), 2 research assistantships (averaging $17,550 per year), 17 teaching assistantships (averaging $20,265 per year); career-related internships or fieldwork also available. Support available to part-time students. Financial award application deadline: 4/15; financial award applicants required to submit FAFSA. *Faculty research:* Pharmacokinetics, oncology, critical care, pediatrics, cardiology. *Unit head:* Dr. Lisa Lawson, Dean, 215-596-8939, Fax: 215-596-8977, E-mail: l.lawson@usciences.edu. *Application contact:* Christopher Miciek, Associate Director, Graduate Admissions, 215-596-8597, Fax: 215-895-1185, E-mail: graduate@usciences.edu.
Website: http://www.usciences.edu/academics/collegesDepts/pcp

University of Utah, Graduate School, College of Pharmacy, Professional Program in Pharmacy, Salt Lake City, UT 84112-5820. Offers Pharm D. *Accreditation:* ACPE. *Faculty:* 10 full-time (4 women), 36 part-time/adjunct (19 women). *Students:* 235 full-time (109 women), 5 part-time (3 women); includes 54 minority (2 Black or African American, non-Hispanic/Latino; 37 Asian, non-Hispanic/Latino; 9 Hispanic/Latino; 6 Two or more races, non-Hispanic/Latino), 2 international. Average age 28. 299 applicants, 20% accepted, 60 enrolled. In 2013, 57 doctorates awarded. *Entrance requirements:* For doctorate, PCAT. Additional exam requirements/recommendations for international students: Required—TOEFL (minimum score 80 iBT). *Application deadline:* For fall admission, 12/1 for domestic and international students. Application fee: $55 ($65 for international students). Electronic applications accepted. *Expenses:* Contact institution. *Financial support:* In 2013–14, 96 students received support, including 31 teaching assistantships (averaging $1,500 per year). Financial award application deadline: 2/4. *Faculty research:* Anti-convulsing drug development, natural drug development, pharmacogenomics, pharmacogenetics, tissue engineering. *Total annual research expenditures:* $15.8 million. *Unit head:* Dr. Chris M. Ireland, Dean, 801-581-6731. *Application contact:* Heidi Bates, Academic Advising Coordinator, 801-581-7046, E-mail: pharmd.admissions@pharm.utah.edu.
Website: http://www.pharmacy.utah.edu/

University of Washington, School of Pharmacy and Graduate School, Department of Pharmacy, Seattle, WA 98195-7630. Offers MS, PhD. *Faculty:* 15 full-time (5 women), 3 part-time/adjunct (1 woman). *Students:* 19 full-time (11 women); includes 5 minority (4 Asian, non-Hispanic/Latino; 1 Hispanic/Latino), 4 international. 63 applicants, 6% accepted, 4 enrolled. In 2013, 4 master's, 3 doctorates awarded. *Degree requirements:* For master's, thesis; for doctorate, thesis/dissertation. *Entrance requirements:* For master's and doctorate, GRE General Test. Additional exam requirements/recommendations for international students: Required—TOEFL. *Application deadline:* For fall admission, 12/31 priority date for domestic and international students; for winter admission, 1/1 for domestic and international students. Application fee: $75 ($100 for international students). Electronic applications accepted. *Financial support:* In 2013–14, 8 students received support, including 3 fellowships with full tuition reimbursements available (averaging $14,751 per year), 5 research assistantships with full tuition reimbursements available (averaging $14,751 per year), 3 teaching assistantships with full tuition reimbursements available (averaging $14,751 per year); institutionally sponsored loans, scholarships/grants, and tuition waivers (full) also available. *Faculty research:* Pharmacoeconomics, pharmacoepidemiology, drug policy, outcomes research. *Total annual research expenditures:* $1.2 million. *Unit head:* Dr. Peggy Odegard, Chair, 206-543-6788, Fax: 206-543-3835, E-mail: podegard@uw.edu. *Application contact:* Dr. David Veenstra, Director, 206-543-6788, Fax: 206-543-3835, E-mail: veenstra@uw.edu.
Website: http://sop.washington.edu/porpp

University of Washington, School of Pharmacy, Professional Program in Pharmacy, Seattle, WA 98195-7631. Offers Pharm D, Pharm D/Certificate. *Accreditation:* ACPE. *Students:* 372 full-time (237 women); includes 218 minority (4 Black or African American, non-Hispanic/Latino; 4 American Indian or Alaska Native, non-Hispanic/Latino; 178 Asian, non-Hispanic/Latino; 10 Hispanic/Latino; 2 Native Hawaiian or other Pacific Islander, non-Hispanic/Latino; 20 Two or more races, non-Hispanic/Latino). Average age 26. 413 applicants, 32% accepted, 96 enrolled. In 2013, 81 doctorates awarded. *Entrance requirements:* For doctorate, PCAT. Additional exam requirements/recommendations for international students: Required—TOEFL (minimum score 100 iBT). *Application deadline:* For fall admission, 1/6 for domestic and international students. Application fee: $45. Electronic applications accepted. *Financial support:* In 2013–14, 185 students received support. Career-related internships or fieldwork and scholarships/grants available. Financial award application deadline: 7/12; financial award applicants required to submit FAFSA. *Unit head:* Dr. Nanci Murphy, Associate Dean, Academic and Student Programs, 206-685-2715, Fax: 206-616-2740. *Application contact:* Cher Espina, Advisor, 206-543-6100, Fax: 206-616-2740, E-mail: pharminf@u.washington.edu.
Website: http://sop.washington.edu/students

University of Wisconsin–Madison, School of Pharmacy, Professional Program in Pharmacy, Madison, WI 53706-1380. Offers Pharm D. *Accreditation:* ACPE. *Expenses:* Tuition, state resident: full-time $10,728; part-time $790 per credit. Tuition, nonresident: full-time $24,054; part-time $1623 per credit. *Required fees:* $1130; $119 per credit.

University of Wyoming, College of Health Sciences, School of Pharmacy, Laramie, WY 82071. Offers Pharm D. *Accreditation:* ACPE. *Entrance requirements:* For doctorate, PCAT. Additional exam requirements/recommendations for international students: Required—TOEFL.

Virginia Commonwealth University, Medical College of Virginia-Professional Programs, School of Pharmacy, Professional Program in Pharmacy, Richmond, VA 23284-9005. Offers Pharm D, Pharm D/MBA, Pharm D/MPH, Pharm D/PhD. *Accreditation:* ACPE. Part-time programs available. *Degree requirements:* For doctorate, research project. *Entrance requirements:* For doctorate, PCAT. Electronic applications accepted. *Faculty research:* Oncology, cardiology, infectious diseases, epilepsy, connective tissue.

Washington State University, Graduate School, College of Pharmacy, Pullman, WA 99164. Offers dietetics, nutrition, and exercise physiology (MS); pharmacy (PhD, Pharm D). *Accreditation:* ACPE (one or more programs are accredited). *Degree requirements:* For master's, comprehensive exam, thesis, oral exam; for doctorate, comprehensive exam, thesis/dissertation, oral exam (for PhD). *Entrance requirements:* For master's, GRE General Test, minimum GPA of 3.0, interview; for doctorate, GRE General Test, minimum GPA of 3.0, interview, minimum 60 hours of documented pharmacy experience. *Faculty research:* Hormonal carcinogenesis, drug metabolism/transport, toxicology of chlorinated compounds, alcohol effects on immune system, effects of cocaine on neuronal function.

Washington State University Spokane, Program in Pharmacy, Spokane, WA 99210. Offers Pharm D. *Degree requirements:* For doctorate, comprehensive exam, thesis/dissertation. *Entrance requirements:* For doctorate, PCAT, 2 letters of recommendation, pharmacy CAS form, interview. Electronic applications accepted. *Expenses:* Contact institution. *Faculty research:* Infectious disease, neuropsychopharmacology, biotechnology/gene therapy.

Wayne State University, Eugene Applebaum College of Pharmacy and Health Sciences, Department of Pharmaceutical Sciences, Detroit, MI 48202. Offers medicinal chemistry (MS, PhD); pharmaceutics (MS, PhD); pharmacology/toxicology (MS, PhD). *Accreditation:* ACPE (one or more programs are accredited). Part-time programs available. *Faculty:* 17 full-time (3 women). *Students:* 33 full-time (15 women), 2 part-time (1 woman); includes 3 minority (1 American Indian or Alaska Native, non-Hispanic/Latino; 2 Asian, non-Hispanic/Latino), 29 international. Average age 25. 205 applicants, 8% accepted, 9 enrolled. In 2013, 1 master's, 3 doctorates awarded. *Degree requirements:* For master's, thesis; for doctorate, thesis/dissertation. *Entrance requirements:* For master's, GRE General Test, admission to the Graduate School, bachelor's degree, three letters of recommendation, personal statement; for doctorate, GRE General Test, admission to the Graduate School; bachelor's or master's degree in one of the behavioral, biological, pharmaceutical or physical sciences; minimum undergraduate GPA of 3.0; three letters of recommendation. Additional exam requirements/recommendations for international students: Required—TOEFL (minimum score 550 paper-based; 79 iBT), Michigan English Language Assessment Battery (minimum score 85); Recommended—IELTS (minimum score 6.5), TWE (minimum score 5.5). *Application deadline:* For fall admission, 3/1 for domestic and international students. Application fee: $0. Electronic applications accepted. *Expenses:* Contact institution. *Financial support:* In 2013–14, 13 students received support, including 2 fellowships with tuition reimbursements available (averaging $24,272 per year), 11 research assistantships with full tuition reimbursements available (averaging $24,565 per year); scholarships/grants, health care benefits, and unspecified assistantships also available. Financial award application deadline: 3/31; financial award applicants required to submit FAFSA. *Faculty research:* Mechanisms of resistance of bacteria to anti-microbial agents, drug metabolism and disposition in children, treatment strategies for stroke/neurovascular disease, prevalence and treatment of diabetes in Arab-Americans, ethnic variability in development of osteoporosis. *Unit head:* Dr. George Corcoran, Chair and Professor, 313-577-1737, E-mail: corcoran@wayne.edu. *Application contact:* 313-577-1047, E-mail: pscgrad@wayne.edu.
Website: http://www.cphs.wayne.edu/psc/index.php

Wayne State University, Eugene Applebaum College of Pharmacy and Health Sciences, Department of Pharmacy Practice, Detroit, MI 48202. Offers pharmacy (Pharm D); Pharm D/PhD. *Faculty:* 26 full-time (16 women), 1 part-time/adjunct (0 women). *Students:* 344 full-time (207 women), 27 part-time (18 women); includes 57 minority (3 Black or African American, non-Hispanic/Latino; 52 Asian, non-Hispanic/Latino; 2 Two or more races, non-Hispanic/Latino), 33 international. Average age 25. 375 applicants, 41% accepted, 97 enrolled. In 2013, 79 doctorates awarded. *Entrance requirements:* For doctorate, PharmCAS application (submit by 11/1), interview, criminal background check, minimum GPA of 3.0 in required preprofessional courses and overall. Additional exam requirements/recommendations for international students: Required—TOEFL (minimum score 550 paper-based; 79 iBT), Michigan English Language Assessment Battery (minimum score 85); Recommended—IELTS (minimum score 6.5), TWE (minimum score 5.5). *Application deadline:* For fall admission, 11/1 for domestic and international students. Electronic applications accepted. *Expenses:* Contact institution. *Financial support:* In 2013–14, 98 students received support. Scholarships/grants available. Financial award application deadline: 3/31; financial award applicants required to submit FAFSA. *Faculty research:* Pharmacodynamics and pharmacokinetics of anti-infective agents, efficacy of drug treatments for traumatic head injury and stroke, cultural difference in Arab-Americans related to diabetes treatment and prevention, drug disposition and effect in pediatrics, evaluation of anticoagulation regimens. *Total annual research expenditures:* $3.7 million. *Unit head:* Dr. Brian L. Crabtree, Chair and Professor, 313-577-0827, E-mail: brian.crabtree@wayne.edu. *Application contact:* 313-577-1716, E-mail: cphsinfo@wayne.edu.
Website: http://www.cphs.wayne.edu/practice/index.php

Western New England University, College of Pharmacy, Springfield, MA 01119. Offers Pharm D, Pharm D/MBA. *Faculty:* 28 full-time (14 women). *Students:* 223 full-time (128 women); includes 51 minority (13 Black or African American, non-Hispanic/Latino; 35 Asian, non-Hispanic/Latino; 3 Hispanic/Latino). Average age 24. 447 applicants, 30% accepted, 76 enrolled. *Entrance requirements:* For doctorate, PCAT, PharmCAS application, two letters of recommendation. Additional exam requirements/recommendations for international students: Required—TOEFL (minimum score 80 iBT). *Application deadline:* For fall admission, 2/1 for domestic students. Applications are processed on a rolling basis. Electronic applications accepted. Tuition and fees vary according to program. *Financial support:* Scholarships/grants available. Financial award application deadline: 4/15; financial award applicants required to submit FAFSA. *Unit head:* Dr. Evan T. Robinson, Dean, 413-796-2323, E-mail: evan.robinson@wne.edu. *Application contact:* Bonnie Mannix, Assistant Director of Pharmacy Admissions, 413-796-2073, E-mail: rxadmissions@wne.edu.
Website: http://www1.wne.edu/pharmacy/index.cfm?selection-doc.8399

Western University of Health Sciences, College of Pharmacy, Program in Pharmacy, Pomona, CA 91766-1854. Offers Pharm D. *Accreditation:* ACPE. *Faculty:* 26 full-time (11 women), 1 part-time/adjunct (0 women). *Students:* 535 full-time (393 women); includes 384 minority (13 Black or African American, non-Hispanic/Latino; 1 American Indian or Alaska Native, non-Hispanic/Latino; 295 Asian, non-Hispanic/Latino; 49 Hispanic/Latino; 26 Two or more races, non-Hispanic/Latino), 12 international. Average age 28. 1,193 applicants, 19% accepted, 132 enrolled. In 2013, 141 doctorates awarded. *Degree requirements:* For doctorate, comprehensive exam (for some programs). *Entrance requirements:* For doctorate, minimum GPA of 2.75, interview, letters of recommendation; BS in pharmacy or equivalent (recommended). Additional exam requirements/recommendations for international students: Required—TOEFL (minimum score 550 paper-based; 79 iBT). *Application deadline:* For fall admission, 10/1 for domestic and international students. Application fee: $65. Electronic applications accepted. *Expenses:* Contact institution. *Financial support:* Institutionally sponsored loans and scholarships/grants available. Financial award application deadline: 3/2; financial award applicants required to submit FAFSA. *Unit head:* Dr. Daniel Robinson, Dean, 909-469-5533, Fax: 909-469-5539, E-mail: drobinson@westernu.edu. *Application contact:* Kathryn Ford, Admission Director, 909-469-5335, Fax: 909-469-5570, E-mail: admissions@westernu.edu.
Website: http://www.westernu.edu/pharmacy-dpp_message

West Virginia University, School of Pharmacy, Professional Program in Pharmacy, Morgantown, WV 26506. Offers clinical pharmacy (Pharm D). Students enter program as undergraduates. *Accreditation:* ACPE. *Degree requirements:* For doctorate, 100 hours of community service. *Entrance requirements:* For doctorate, PCAT, minimum GPA of 3.1. Electronic applications accepted.

West Virginia University, School of Pharmacy, Program in Pharmaceutical and Pharmacological Sciences, Morgantown, WV 26506. Offers administrative pharmacy (PhD); behavioral pharmacy (MS, PhD); biopharmaceutics/pharmacokinetics (MS, PhD); industrial pharmacy (MS); medicinal chemistry (MS, PhD); pharmaceutical chemistry (MS, PhD); pharmaceutics (MS, PhD); pharmacology and toxicology (MS); pharmacy (MS); pharmacy administration (MS). Part-time programs available. Terminal master's awarded for partial completion of doctoral program. *Degree requirements:* For master's, thesis; for doctorate, one foreign language, comprehensive exam, thesis/dissertation. *Entrance requirements:* For master's and doctorate, GRE General Test, minimum GPA of 2.75. Additional exam requirements/recommendations for international students: Required—TOEFL; Recommended—TWE. Electronic applications accepted. *Expenses:* Contact institution. *Faculty research:* Pharmaceutics, medicinal chemistry, biopharmaceutics/pharmacokinetics, health outcomes research.

Wilkes University, College of Graduate and Professional Studies, Nesbitt College of Pharmacy and Nursing, School of Pharmacy, Wilkes-Barre, PA 18766-0002. Offers Pharm D. *Students:* 288 full-time (177 women); includes 24 minority (2 Black or African American, non-Hispanic/Latino; 9 Asian, non-Hispanic/Latino; 3 Hispanic/Latino; 10 Two or more races, non-Hispanic/Latino), 1 international. Average age 23. In 2013, 69 doctorates awarded. *Entrance requirements:* For doctorate, PCAT. Additional exam requirements/recommendations for international students: Required—TOEFL (minimum score 550 paper-based; 79 iBT). *Financial support:* Application deadline: 3/1; applicants required to submit FAFSA. *Unit head:* Dr. Bernard Graham, Dean, 570-408-4280, Fax: 570-408-7729, E-mail: bernard.graham@wilkes.edu. *Application contact:* Joanne Thomas, Interim Director of Graduate Education, 570-408-4234, Fax: 570-408-7846, E-mail: joanne.thomas1@wilkes.edu.
Website: http://www.wilkes.edu/pages/390.asp

Wingate University, School of Pharmacy, Wingate, NC 28174-0159. Offers Pharm D. *Accreditation:* ACPE. *Degree requirements:* For doctorate, comprehensive exam. *Entrance requirements:* For doctorate, PCAT. Electronic applications accepted. *Expenses:* Contact institution. *Faculty research:* Stress response in aging, arthritis therapy educational processes, professional development, sarcopenia in aging, geriatric-psych drug therapy.

Xavier University of Louisiana, College of Pharmacy, New Orleans, LA 70125-1098. Offers Pharm D. *Accreditation:* ACPE. *Entrance requirements:* Additional exam requirements/recommendations for international students: Required—TOEFL. Electronic applications accepted. *Expenses:* Contact institution.

NOVA SOUTHEASTERN UNIVERSITY

College of Pharmacy

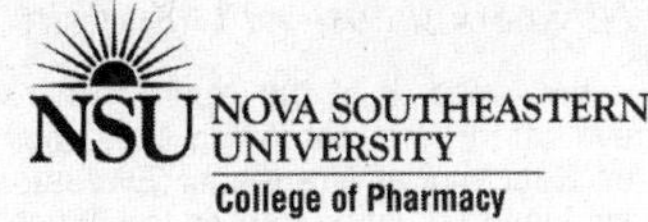

Programs of Study

Nova Southeastern University (NSU) offers an innovative program of graduate study and research leading to the Doctor of Philosophy degree (Ph.D.). Students can choose to pursue the Ph.D. degree in one of three distinct sequences: Molecular Medicine and Pharmacogenomics (Drug Discovery), Drug Development (Pharmaceutics), or Social and Administrative Pharmacy (Determinants of Drug Use). Also available is the dual degree, Doctor of Pharmacy/Master of Business Administration (Pharm.D./M.B.A.).

At the completion of the Ph.D. sequences, students are able to demonstrate the knowledge base expected at the Ph.D. level in a pharmacy specialty; design and conduct independent research that adds to the understanding of their pharmacy specialty; prepare and defend rational and structured proposals seeking support for research efforts; and prepare and present lucid reports on their own research, as well as the research of others.

Programs in the College of Pharmacy (COP) are taught primarily by multilingual, multicultural, full-time faculty members. Clinical and applied research is delivered at sites in Fort Lauderdale and Palm Beach, Florida, and San Juan, Puerto Rico. Both live and online lectures are used.

Research Facilities

NSU is one of the few colleges of pharmacy in the United States with a full-service community pharmacy (on the main campus) and a full-service hospital pharmacy.

The research laboratories in the COP occupy approximately 3,000 square feet of the Library/Research Building in the Health Professions Division (HPD). Each individual laboratory space ranges from 300 to 750 square feet and is equipped with general biochemistry and/or tissue culture equipment. Some laboratories include specialized equipment for pharmaceutical preparations, radioligand binding assays, molecular biological applications, and proteomics applications. There are also common laboratory facilities for shared equipment. Two FluorChem E digital darkroom systems are available for use, along with a fully equipped darkroom and a fully equipped laboratory designed for studies using radioactive chemicals. All common use laboratories are located in close proximity to the College of Pharmacy laboratories and are fully accessible to all HPD researchers.

The animal facility is also located within the research area of the Library/Laboratory Building, and it complies with the minimum standards for use of rats and mice. The College of Pharmacy also has access to an OLAW approved animal facility at the Rumbaugh-Goodwin Institute for Cancer Research (RGICR), located near the main campus. This facility has two holding rooms to house rodents and separate cage wash and storage areas. The RGICR animal facility is maintained by a full-time caretaker who also oversees the animal rooms in the HPD Library and Research Building. Both facilities are governed by an Institutional Animal Care and Use Committee (IACUC). The RGICR facility is fully compliant with OLAW standards and is available for use by all NSU researchers. A consulting veterinarian is responsible for oversight of the health of animals in both facilities.

NSU maintains an extensive information technology network for teaching, learning, research, and administrative computing. Comprehensive fiber-optic and wireless networks provide connectivity for user access. A dedicated wide area network (WAN) supports high-speed connections from all campuses. The research facility has computers for data collection, data processing, and analysis. The COP researchers all have access to modern computers in their offices as well as in their laboratories, equipped with the necessary software for word processing, routine data analysis, and photo processing. Researchers also have easy access to NSU's four computer labs that house more than 200 Pentium 200 MHz PCs with ready access to the Internet and Ovid online database.

Financial Aid

Top candidates are eligible for scholarships, which consist of a tuition waiver and teaching assistantships. Non-scholarship students can apply for a variety of loans.

Cost of Study

Tuition for 2014–15 is $26,265 (subject to change by the board of trustees without notice). An HPD general access fee of $145 is required each year. An NSU student services fee of $1,050 is also required annually.

Living and Housing Costs

The Rolling Hills Graduate Apartments, which opened in 2008, are approximately 1 mile west of the NSU main campus and offer housing for approximately 373 students. Each single and quad room is fully furnished and features a kitchen, bathroom, and living room. Married housing is also available. Costs range between $2,641 and $6,513 per semester or between $1,165 and $15,691 for a twelve-month contract. All rates include unlimited laundry, NSU-secured wireless Internet, furnishings, utilities, air conditioning, cable TV, and local telephone service. More information about student housing is available at http://www.nova.edu/housing/.

Student Group

NSU's College of Pharmacy has consistently led the nation in the level of enrollment of Hispanic doctoral pharmacy students. Students are actively involved in local, national, and international community-based health clinics; the legislative processes; and humanitarian missions in countries abroad.

Student Outcomes

Graduate passing rates for NSU students on pharmacy licensing exams are at rates near or above 93 percent, consistent with national pass rates.

Location

Davie, a city of more than 80,000, maintains a sense of small-town intimacy while its location between major highways is near both an international airport and a seaport, which offers access to the state's metropolitan centers. The area is famous for its wide expanses of sandy beaches and its tropical climate. Nearby Fort Lauderdale is home to numerous museums, art galleries, and a performing arts center.

NSU's main campus consists of 300 acres with general-purpose athletic fields and NCAA-qualifying soccer and baseball fields. The residence halls on the main campus serve undergraduate, graduate, health professions, and law students. The College of Pharmacy also has branch campuses in Palm Beach, Florida and San Juan, Puerto Rico.

The University and The College

Founded in 1964 as Nova University, the institution merged with Southeastern University of the Health Sciences in 1994, creating Nova Southeastern University. NSU offers a wide range of undergraduate, graduate, and professional degree programs to more than 29,000 students every year. It is the seventh-largest independent institution in the nation and the largest independent not-for-profit university in the Southeast. NSU is experiencing a sustained period of academic growth, fiscal strength, and commitment to the challenges of the twenty-first century.

The NSU College of Pharmacy has experienced the fastest growth among colleges of pharmacy. Since 1986, it has graduated more than 2,900 pharmacists.

Applying

Students are recruited for the Ph.D. program from the NSU College of Pharmacy; other U.S. schools/colleges of pharmacy; and graduates with degrees in fields related to social, economic, behavioral, and administrative pharmacy, as well as chemistry, biology, and other related scientific fields. Students are also recruited from international institutions, especially pharmacy graduates from India, Saudi Arabia, China, Europe, Canada, Latin America and the Caribbean. Successful applicants, whether foreign or domestic, are required to comply with the following guidelines. All applicants must have an earned baccalaureate degree, with a GPA equivalent to a B or better, from an accredited institution of higher education in pharmacy or a related scientific area or in a discipline related to social, economic, behavioral, or administrative pharmacy. Application materials must include GRE results, proof of proficiency in English, a formal application form, three letters of reference, transcripts received directly from the degree granting institution, and a brief written essay on the goals of the applicant.

Applicants may apply for matriculation into the fall semester. The Office of Admissions processes applications on a rolling admissions basis; therefore, it is in the best interest of the applicant to apply as early as possible. To be considered for admission, students must complete the application form and submit supporting documents and a nonrefundable fee of $50 by March 1. Official transcripts of all work attempted at all colleges and universities must be forwarded by the institutions attended to Enrollment Processing Services (EPS), College of Pharmacy, Office of Admissions, 3301 College Ave, P.O. Box 299000, Ft. Lauderdale, FL 33329-9905. It is the responsibility of the applicant to ensure that arrangements are made for these transcripts to be sent. A final transcript covering all of the applicant's work must be forwarded to EPS prior to matriculation. Three individual letters of evaluation from professors or supervisors in the applicant's major field of study are required. All applicants are required to submit official Graduate Record Examination (GRE) scores. The NSU code is 5522. GRE scores must be less than five years old prior to the candidate's matriculation. Undergraduate course work taken at an international institution must be evaluated for U.S. institution equivalence. It is the applicant's responsibility to have the course work evaluated by either World Education Services, Josef Silney & Associates, or Educational Credential Evaluators, Inc. A complete course-by-course evaluation must be sent to the Office of Admissions.

Upon receipt of the completed application and required credentials, the Ph.D. Committee on Admissions selects those applicants to receive personal interviews on the NSU Fort Lauderdale campus or via telephone. The Office of Admissions notifies those who are selected of the interview date and time. Being granted an interview does not guarantee admission.

Applications forms are available and can be submitted online at http://www.nova.edu/apply/index.html. Applicants may also have an application mailed to them by request.

Correspondence and Information

Dr. Michelle A. Clark
Interim Associate Dean, Research and Graduate Education
Health Professions Division
College of Pharmacy
Nova Southeastern University
Fort Lauderdale, Florida 78249
United States
E-mail: copphd@nova.edu

Health Professions Admissions Office
Attention: Kori Desiderio
Nova Southeastern University
Phone: 954-262-1112
877-640-0218 (toll-free)
Website: http://www.nova.edu

THE FACULTY AND THEIR RESEARCH

Drug Development and Molecular Medicine and Pharmacogenomics (Drug Discovery) Sequences

Michelle A. Clark, Interim Associate Dean, Research and Graduate Education; Associate Professor and Chairperson, Department of Pharmaceutical Sciences; Ph.D., South Florida, 1996. Central signaling pathways for blood pressure regulation and control, role of the central renin angiotensin system in the regulation of cardiovascular and other diseases.

Rais A. Ansari, Assistant Professor, Pharmaceutical Sciences; Ph.D., Kanpur (India), 1985. Mechanism of alcohol-mediated hypertension, transcriptional regulation of human angiotensinogen gene after ethanol and environmental toxicants exposure.

Ana Maria Castejon, Associate Professor, Pharmaceutical Sciences; Ph.D., Central University (Venezuela), 1997. Oxidative stress and autism, diabetes mellitus, effects of statins in vascular smooth muscle cells, genetics of salt sensitivity in human subjects.

Luigi Cubeddu, Professor, Pharmaceutical Sciences; M.D., Central University (Venezuela); Ph.D., Colorado. Mechanisms and treatment of hypertension associated with obesity, salt-sensitive hypertension, early detection of insulin resistance and abnormalities in glucose metabolism, statin withdrawal syndrome.

Young M. Kwon, Assistant Professor, Pharmaceutical Sciences, Ph.D., Utah, 2003. Targeted delivery and triggered release system for therapeutic macromolecules; bioconjugate chemistry and PEGylation; nonviral gene carriers and intracellular drug delivery; protein stability and release from biodegradable polymer.

Jean J. Latimer, Associate Professor, Pharmaceutical Sciences; Ph.D., Buffalo, SUNY, 1989. Loss of DNA repair as causative factor in cancer formation; breast tissue engineering; ancestral disparity in breast cancer development and pharmacogenomics; drug resistance (via cancer stem cells) in childhood leukemia.

Anastasios Lymperopoulos, Assistant Professor, Pharmaceutical Sciences; Ph.D., Patras (Greece), 2004. Cardiovascular biology/pharmacology and gene therapy, with a focus on adrenergic system regulation in heart failure; novel roles of G-protein coupled receptor kinases and their cofactors, beta-arrestins, in regulation of various important cardiovascular G-protein coupled receptors; roles of G-protein coupled receptor kinases and their cofactors, beta-arrestins, in adrenal gland physiology and biology.

Enrique A. Nieves, Assistant Professor, Pharmaceutical Sciences; Ph.D., Florida, 1982. Applications of nanotechnology in drug product development and pharmaceutical process designs, development of co-excipients for improved drug formulations, nanotechnology applications in the extraction and isolation of new drugs from natural sources.

Hamid Omidian, Associate Professor, Pharmaceutical Sciences; Ph.D., Brunel (London), 1997. Hydrogels for pharmaceutical and biomedical applications, hydrogel-based controlled delivery systems and technologies, hydrogel-based gastroretentive drug delivery platforms, hydrogel-based platforms for cell culture and proliferation.

Mutasem Rawas-Qalaji, Associate Professor, Pharmaceutical Sciences; Ph.D., Manitoba (Canada), 2006. Enhancing the permeability and the relative bioavailability of poorly absorbed drugs by nanotechnology, formulation and delivery of drug-loaded nanoparticles through noninvasive and user-friendly routes of administration, formulation and evaluation of sublingual ODT tablets as an alternative noninvasive dosage form.

Syed A. A. Rizvi, Assistant Professor, Pharmaceutical Sciences; Ph.D., Mercer, 2010. Cocrystallization and formulation strategies for low bioavailability drugs; micellar electrokinetic chromatography.

Robert C. Speth, Professor, Pharmaceutical Sciences; Ph.D., Vanderbilt, 1976. Brain renin-angiotensin system pharmacology and functionality.

Richard C. Deth, Professor, Pharmaceutical Sciences, Ph.D., Miami (Florida), 1975. Role of redox and methylation status in neurodevelopmental disorders.

Social and Administrative Pharmacy (Determinants of Drug Use) Sequence

Barry A. Bleidt, Professor, Sociobehavioral and Administrative Pharmacy; Pharm.D., Xavier of Louisiana, 1994; Ph.D., Florida, 1982. Cultural competency/diversity/health disparities; assessment of student achievement; faculty workload and performance measures; peer teaching evaluation strategies; Internet, technology and medical information; and pharmacoeconomics.

Manuel J. Carvajal, Professor and Chairperson, Department of Sociobehavioral and Administrative Pharmacy; Ph.D., Florida, 1974. Applied econometrics geared to problem solving; various areas of human capital including fertility, migration, poverty, and discrimination; gender and ethnic differences in labor market outcomes and job satisfaction.

Catherine A. Harrington, Associate Professor, Sociobehavioral and Administrative Pharmacy; Ph.D., Michigan, 1993; Pharm.D., Michigan, 1987. Developing databases and information systems that assist in evaluation of drug therapy, use of meta-analysis techniques to obtain evidence from literature.

Nile M. Khanfar, Assistant Professor, Sociobehavioral and Administrative Pharmacy; Ph.D., Louisiana at Monroe, 2005; M.B.A., Louisiana at Monroe, 2001. Management leadership, strategic management/marketing business cases, direct-to-consumer advertising of prescription medication and its influence on consumer behavior.

L. Leanne Lai, Professor, Sociobehavioral and Administrative Pharmacy; Ph.D., Maryland, Baltimore, 1996. Pharmacoeconomics and outcomes research, pharmacoepidemiology and secondary data analysis, international education.

Ioana Popovici, Assistant Professor, Sociobehavioral and Administrative Pharmacy; Ph.D., Florida International, 2007. Economic evaluation of substance abuse treatment interventions, relationship between addictive substance use or abuse and its economic consequences.

Sylvia E. Rabionet, Associate Professor, Sociobehavioral and Administrative Pharmacy; Ed.D., Harvard, 2002. Health disparities, public health issues.

Jesus Sanchez, Assistant Professor, Sociobehavioral and Administrative Pharmacy; Ph.D., Miami (Florida), 2001. HIV reduction among high-risk migrant workers; building capacity and infrastructure in the migrant farm worker communities in South Florida; prevalence of HIV, hepatitis B and C, and associated risk factors among Hispanic injection drug users.

PHILADELPHIA COLLEGE OF OSTEOPATHIC MEDICINE

School of Pharmacy–Georgia Campus

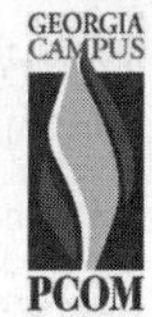

Program of Study

The Philadelphia College of Osteopathic Medicine (PCOM) School of Pharmacy–Georgia Campus (GA–PCOM) offers a four-year Doctor of Pharmacy (Pharm.D.) program, tailored to the needs of students seeking the comprehensive education necessary to develop a generalist pharmacist capable of practicing in many different health-care environments. Faculty members conduct research in basic, clinical, and administrative sciences, sharing their expertise and scholarly work with students. Each student in the program is assigned to a group of their peers for team- and case-based learning to foster team-building skills in clinical case discussions. Each student is also assigned a faculty adviser to assist with their academic needs and guide them as they progress through the curriculum and prepare for a career in pharmacy.

The PCOM School of Pharmacy–Georgia Campus's curriculum is consistent with the applied emphasis of PCOM's graduate and medical programs. The mission of the program is to educate caring, proactive pharmacists according to a model of patient-centered care, a practice of pharmacy in which the practitioner assumes responsibility for a patient's medication-related needs and is held accountable for this commitment.

While preparing pharmacy practitioners is the primary mission of the Pharm.D. program, it also provides an avenue by which students may explore a broad range of career opportunities. The program is designed to prepare a well-rounded student capable of practicing in many areas of pharmacy. The program also aspires to develop analytical and life-long learning skills to help students excel after graduation in the rapidly changing and evolving field of health care.

Research Facilities

PCOM's campus features large lecture halls, small classrooms, labs for teaching and research, a state-of-the-art library, and scenic landscaping, in a suburban environment. An Information Commons integrates library and student computer lab functions. The facility houses sufficient computers to support extensive use of electronic resources available through the PCOM Digital Library.

The PCOM Digital Library provides access to a wealth of licensed Internet resources, including over 10,000 full-text e-journals, electronic textbooks, bibliographic databases, streaming videos, clinical simulations, diagnostic decision support programs, and evidence-based clinical information systems, as well as subject access to selected Internet resources. Print subscriptions to a number of core journal titles constitute a reading room collection for the Information Commons. The PCOM library electronically provides articles from any print-only titles in its collection to GA–PCOM users. GA–PCOM and the School of Pharmacy are committed to the advancement of knowledge and intellectual growth through teaching and research, and to the well-being of the community through leadership and service.

Financial Aid

PCOM's Office of Financial Aid provides comprehensive assistance to all admitted students. Financial assistance can be provided through the Federal Direct Loan program, institutional grants, and various alternative private loan programs.

Cost of Study

Tuition and fees for the Pharm.D. program for the 2014–15 academic year are $34,985.

Living and Housing Costs

Suwanee and the neighboring communities of Lawrenceville and Duluth offer a less hurried lifestyle with all the necessary amenities, yet with easy access to all Atlanta has to offer: shopping, professional sports, the arts, and more. Picturesque mountains and spring-fed rivers are only a short drive away and the Georgia seashore is easily accessible for a weekend getaway. There is no on-campus housing so students live off-campus. Room and board costs vary based each student's arrangements.

Student Group

PCOM enrolled 79 students in its inaugural class in August, 2010. For the 2013–14 academic year, PCOM School of Pharmacy enrolled 100 new students with a diverse cultural makeup. Current enrollment projections call for approximately 100 new students to be admitted to the Pharm.D. program each year.

Location

The GA–PCOM campus is located in a suburban setting in Suwanee, Georgia, approximately 30 minutes from the city of Atlanta. The campus is also close to a myriad of outdoor recreational opportunities, including Stone Mountain Park, the North Georgia mountains, and scenic Lake Lanier, which offers boating, fishing, water parks, canoeing, and horseback riding.

The College

PCOM is one of the largest of thirty osteopathic colleges in the United States, with campuses in Philadelphia and suburban Atlanta. Georgia Campus–Philadelphia College of Osteopathic Medicine was chartered in 2005, and is committed to educating responsive medical professionals prepared to practice in the twenty-first century. Supported by the latest in medical and educational technology, the Georgia Campus shares the PCOM mission and also articulates a focus of improving the quality of life for residents of Georgia and the southeast by preparing healthcare practitioners and professionals to address the social, economic, and health-care needs of the region. Since joining the established community of students, faculty, and staff in Georgia in 2010, the School of Pharmacy's focus has been to train students for entry-level careers with the right combination of skills, knowledge, and attitudes to develop and grow in the ever-changing field.

Applying

Admission to the Pharm.D. program is competitive and selective. Students are evaluated on a variety of criteria. Academic performance in science courses, as well as overall academic performance, as determined by grade point average (GPA) are the major criteria used by the Admissions Committee. Competitive scores on the Pharmacy College Admissions Test (PCAT) are also considered. Professional preparedness, motivation, decision-making skills, and written and verbal communication skills are also evaluated. Prior degrees earned and previous pharmacy-related work experiences are additional considerations. Qualified applicants who have satisfactorily completed all prerequisite coursework but have not earned a bachelor's degree can apply and enroll at PCOM. Qualified applicants may also apply and be offered admission without having completed all prerequisite course work. However, all applicants must successfully complete prerequisite coursework before matriculating to the School of Pharmacy. Note also, that while a bachelor's degree is not required, the Admissions Committee gives preference to those students who have earned a bachelor's degree.

PCOM School of Pharmacy participates in the PharmCAS application service (http://www.pharmcas.org). The School participates in the Early Decision program, with a primary application deadline of September 2nd. The application deadline for regular decision candidates is March 2nd. Supplemental applications are due no later than April 1st.

Prospective students can find additional information about the application process, including prerequisite coursework requirements, at http://admissions.pcom.edu/app-process/pharmacy-pharmd/.

Correspondence and Information

Office of Admissions
Georgia Campus–Philadelphia College of Osteopathic Medicine
625 Old Peachtree Road NW
Suwanee, Georgia 30024
Phone: 678-225-7500
866-282-4544 (toll-free)
Fax: 678-225-7509
E-mail: pharmdadmissions@pcom.edu
Website: http://www.pcom.edu

THE FACULTY

Shari Allen, Pharm.D., Assistant Professor of Pharmacy Practice.
Yun Bai, Ph.D., Assistant Professor of Pharmaceutical Sciences.
Vishakha Bhave, Ph.D., Assistant Professor of Pharmaceutical Sciences.
Bonnie Chan, Pharm.D., Assistant Professor of Pharmacy Practice.
Carmen Echols, Pharm.D., Assistant Professor of Pharmacy Practice.
Jennifer Elliot, Pharm.D., Assistant Professor of Pharmacy Practice.
Dee Fanning, Pharm.D., Assistant Professor of Pharmacy Practice.
Naushad Khan Ghilzai, Ph.D., Associate Dean for Academics and Assessment, Professor of Pharmaceutical Sciences.
Jennifer Gooch, Ph.D., Associate Professor of Pharmaceutical Sciences.
Adina Hirsch, Pharm.D., Assistant Professor of Pharmacy Practice.
Christopher (Shawn) Holaway, Pharm.D., Assistant Professor of Pharmacy Practice.
Yue-Qiao (George) Huang, Ph.D., Assistant Professor of Pharmaceutical Sciences.
Samuel M. John, Pharm.D., Assistant Professor of Pharmacy Practice.
Michael Lee, Ph.D., Assistant Dean of Professional and Student Affairs, Assistant Professor of Pharmaceutical Sciences.
Dusty Lisi, Pharm.D., Assistant Professor of Pharmacy Practice.
Mark Okamoto, Pharm.D., Dean & Chief Academic Officer, Professor of Pharmacy.
Harish S. Parihar, R.Ph., Ph.D., Assistant Professor of Pharmaceutical Science.
Sonia Patel, Pharm.D., Assistant Professor of Pharmacy Practice.
Srujana Rayalam, Ph.D., Assistant Professor in Pharmaceutical Sciences.
Mandy Reece, Pharm.D., BC-ADM, CDE, Assistant Professor of Pharmacy Practice.
Brent Rollins, R.Ph., Ph.D., Assistant Professor of Pharmacy Administration.
Rangaiah Shashidharamurthy, Ph.D., Assistant Professor of Pharmaceutical Sciences.
Avadhesh C. Sharma, Pharm.D., Ph.D., Chair and Professor, Department of Pharmaceutical Science.
Kinjal Sidhpura, Pharm.D., Assistant Professor of Pharmacy Practice.
Gregory Smallwood, Pharm.D., Chair and Associate Professor, Department of Pharmacy Practice.
Desuo Wang, Ph.D., Associate Professor of Pharmaceutical Science.
Julie Wickman, Pharm.D., Director of Experiential Education, Assistant Professor of Pharmacy Practice.
Xinyu (Eric) Wang, Ph.D., Assistant Professor of Pharmaceutical Science.
Zhiqian (James) Wu, Ph.D., Assistant Professor of Pharmaceutical Sciences.
Hongjun Yin, Ph.D., Assistant Professor of Pharmacy Practice.

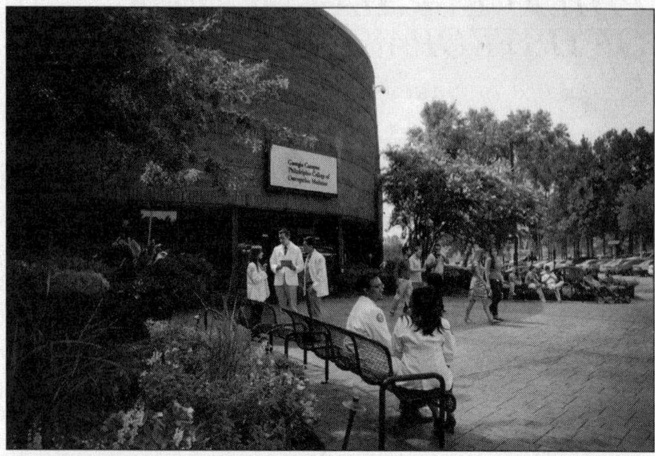

The PCOM School of Pharmacy–Georgia Campus provides students a collaborative learning environment.

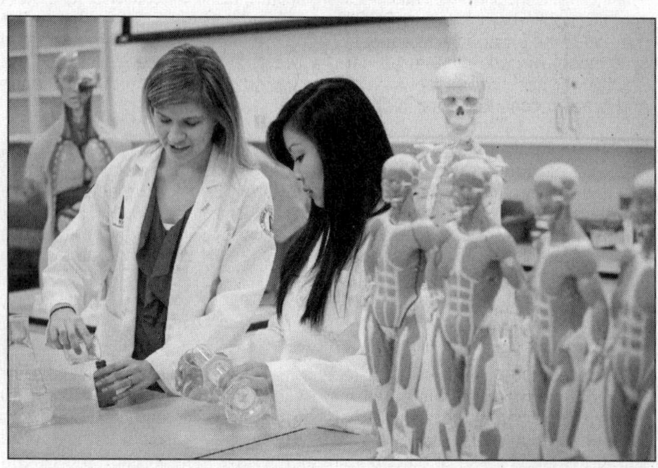

Pharmacy students learn in state-of-the-art high-tech labs.

Section 31
Veterinary Medicine and Sciences

This section contains a directory of institutions offering graduate work in veterinary medicine and sciences. Additional information about programs listed in the directory may be obtained by writing directly to the dean of a graduate school or chair of a department at the address given in the directory.

For programs offering related work, see also in this book *Biological and Biomedical Sciences* and *Zoology*. In the other guides in this series:

Graduate Programs in the Humanities, Arts & Social Sciences
See *Economics (Agricultural Economics and Agribusiness)*

Graduate Programs in the Physical Sciences, Mathematics, Agricultural Sciences, the Environment & Natural Resources
See *Agricultural and Food Sciences, Marine Sciences and Oceanography,* and *Natural Resources*

Graduate Programs in Engineering & Applied Sciences
See *Agricultural Engineering and Bioengineering* and *Biomedical Engineering and Biotechnology*

CONTENTS

Program Directories

Veterinary Medicine

Auburn University, College of Veterinary Medicine, Professional Program in Veterinary Medicine, Auburn University, AL 36849. Offers DVM, DVM/MS. *Accreditation:* AVMA. *Faculty:* 100 full-time (41 women), 4 part-time/adjunct (1 woman). *Students:* 445 full-time (351 women), 37 part-time (27 women); includes 23 minority (6 Black or African American, non-Hispanic/Latino; 2 American Indian or Alaska Native, non-Hispanic/Latino; 6 Asian, non-Hispanic/Latino; 9 Hispanic/Latino). Average age 25. 1,132 applicants, 11% accepted, 120 enrolled. In 2013, 91 doctorates awarded. *Degree requirements:* For doctorate, preceptorship. *Application deadline:* For fall admission, 7/7 for domestic students; for spring admission, 11/24 for domestic students. Applications are processed on a rolling basis. Application fee: $50 ($60 for international students). *Expenses:* Contact institution. *Financial support:* Fellowships available. Financial award application deadline: 3/15; financial award applicants required to submit FAFSA. *Unit head:* Dr. Calvin Johnson, Dean, 334-844-4546. *Application contact:* Dr. George Flowers, Interim Dean of the Graduate School, 334-844-2125.

Colorado State University, College of Veterinary Medicine and Biomedical Sciences, Professional Program in Veterinary Medicine, Fort Collins, CO 80523-1601. Offers DVM, DVM/PhD, MBA/DVM. *Accreditation:* AVMA. *Students:* 547 full-time (438 women); includes 94 minority (3 American Indian or Alaska Native, non-Hispanic/Latino; 28 Asian, non-Hispanic/Latino; 42 Hispanic/Latino; 1 Native Hawaiian or other Pacific Islander, non-Hispanic/Latino; 20 Two or more races, non-Hispanic/Latino), 3 international. Average age 27. 1,540 applicants, 9% accepted, 141 enrolled. In 2013, 140 doctorates awarded. *Entrance requirements:* For doctorate, GRE General Test, transcripts, VMCAS (Veterinary Medical College Application Service), letters of recommendation. Additional exam requirements/recommendations for international students: Required—TOEFL. *Application deadline:* For fall admission, 10/3 for domestic and international students. Application fee: $60. Electronic applications accepted. *Expenses:* Tuition, state resident: full-time $9075.40; part-time $504 per credit. Tuition, nonresident: full-time $22,248; part-time $1236 per credit. *Required fees:* $1819; $60 per credit. *Financial support:* In 2013–14, 3 students received support, including 3 fellowships (averaging $57,908 per year); research assistantships and teaching assistantships also available. Financial award application deadline: 3/1; financial award applicants required to submit FAFSA. *Faculty research:* Animal reproduction, infectious diseases, cancer biology, musculoskeletal research, neurobiology. *Total annual research expenditures:* $1.1 million. *Unit head:* Dr. Dean Hendrickson, Associate Dean, 970-491-2009, E-mail: dean.hendrickson@colostate.edu. *Application contact:* Dr. Sherry Stewart, Assistant Dean of Admissions and Student Affairs, 970-297-4246, Fax: 970-491-2250, E-mail: sherry.stewart@colostate.edu.
Website: http://csu-cvmbs.colostate.edu/dvm-program/Pages/default.aspx

Cornell University, College of Veterinary Medicine, Ithaca, NY 14853-0001. Offers DVM. *Accreditation:* AVMA. *Faculty:* 179 full-time (71 women). *Students:* 384 full-time (310 women); includes 72 minority (10 Black or African American, non-Hispanic/Latino; 3 American Indian or Alaska Native, non-Hispanic/Latino; 24 Asian, non-Hispanic/Latino; 27 Hispanic/Latino; 8 Two or more races, non-Hispanic/Latino), 3 international. Average age 26. 958 applicants. In 2013, 89 doctorates awarded. *Entrance requirements:* For doctorate, GRE General Test or MCAT, animal or veterinary experience, letters of recommendation. Additional exam requirements/recommendations for international students: Required—TOEFL. *Application deadline:* For fall admission, 10/2 for domestic and international students. Application fee: $65. Electronic applications accepted. *Expenses:* Contact institution. *Financial support:* In 2013–14, 318 students received support. Federal Work-Study, institutionally sponsored loans, and scholarships/grants available. Financial award application deadline: 2/1; financial award applicants required to submit CSS PROFILE or FAFSA. *Faculty research:* Biomedical research, comparative cancer, infectious diseases/host response, reproductive biology, genetics/epigenetics. *Total annual research expenditures:* $46.5 million. *Unit head:* Dr. Michael Kotlikoff, Dean, 607-253-3771, Fax: 607-253-3701. *Application contact:* Jennifer A. Mailey, Director of Admissions, 607-253-3700, Fax: 607-253-3709, E-mail: jam333@cornell.edu.
Website: http://www.vet.cornell.edu/

Iowa State University of Science and Technology, Department of Veterinary Diagnostic and Production Animal Medicine, Ames, IA 50011. Offers veterinary preventative medicine (MS). *Accreditation:* AVMA. *Degree requirements:* For master's, thesis or alternative. *Entrance requirements:* For master's, GRE General Test. Additional exam requirements/recommendations for international students: Required—TOEFL (minimum score 550 paper-based; 79 iBT), IELTS (minimum score 6.5). Electronic applications accepted.

Kansas State University, College of Veterinary Medicine, Professional Program in Veterinary Medicine, Manhattan, KS 66506. Offers DVM. *Accreditation:* AVMA. *Faculty:* 8 full-time (6 women), 4 part-time/adjunct (3 women). *Students:* 462 full-time (348 women); includes 50 minority (5 Black or African American, non-Hispanic/Latino; 4 American Indian or Alaska Native, non-Hispanic/Latino; 17 Asian, non-Hispanic/Latino; 18 Hispanic/Latino; 1 Native Hawaiian or other Pacific Islander, non-Hispanic/Latino; 5 Two or more races, non-Hispanic/Latino). Average age 25. 1,225 applicants, 9% accepted, 112 enrolled. In 2013, 108 doctorates awarded. *Entrance requirements:* Additional exam requirements/recommendations for international students: Required—TOEFL. *Application deadline:* For fall admission, 10/1 for domestic students. Application fee: $50 ($80 for international students). *Expenses:* Contact institution. *Financial support:* Research assistantships, teaching assistantships, Federal Work-Study, institutionally sponsored loans, and scholarships/grants available. Financial award application deadline: 3/15; financial award applicants required to submit FAFSA. *Faculty research:* Surgery and medicine, epithelial function, infectious disease of animals, neuroscience, analytical pharmacology. *Total annual research expenditures:* $301,950. *Unit head:* Dr. Ronnie G. Elmore, DVM, Associate Dean for Academic Programs, Admissions and Diversity, 785-532-5660, E-mail: elmore@vet.k-state.edu. *Application contact:* Janel Koonz, Administrative Assistant, 785-532-5660, Fax: 785-532-5884, E-mail: jksu@ksu.edu.
Website: http://www.vet.k-state.edu/admit/dvm.htm

Louisiana State University and Agricultural & Mechanical College, School of Veterinary Medicine, Professional Program in Veterinary Medicine, Baton Rouge, LA 70803. Offers DVM. Program is limited to state and contract students and a limited number of highly qualified out-of-state applicants. *Students:* 341 full-time (262 women), 1 (woman) part-time; includes 33 minority (5 Black or African American, non-Hispanic/Latino; 2 Asian, non-Hispanic/Latino; 22 Hispanic/Latino; 4 Two or more races, non-Hispanic/Latino), 3 international. Average age 25. 98 applicants, 100% accepted, 95 enrolled. In 2013, 81 doctorates awarded. *Entrance requirements:* For doctorate, GRE General Test or MCAT. Additional exam requirements/recommendations for international students: Required—TOEFL. *Application deadline:* For fall admission, 3/1 priority date for domestic students. Applications are processed on a rolling basis. *Expenses:* Contact institution. *Financial support:* In 2013–14, 287 students received support. Fellowships with full and partial tuition reimbursements available, research assistantships with full and partial tuition reimbursements available, teaching assistantships with full and partial tuition reimbursements available, Federal Work-Study, institutionally sponsored loans, health care benefits, tuition waivers (full and partial), and unspecified assistantships available. Financial award applicants required to submit FAFSA. *Faculty research:* Veterinary microbiology, pathology, immunology, anatomy, epidemiology. *Unit head:* Dr. Peter Haynes, Dean, 225-578-9903, E-mail: pfhaynes@vetmed.lsu.edu. *Application contact:* Dr. James E. Miller, Associate Dean, 225-578-9652, E-mail: jmille1@lsu.edu.
Website: http://www.vetmed.lsu.edu/

Michigan State University, College of Veterinary Medicine, Professional Program in Veterinary Medicine, East Lansing, MI 48824. Offers veterinary medicine (DVM); veterinary medicine/medical scientist training program (DVM). *Accreditation:* AVMA. *Entrance requirements:* Additional exam requirements/recommendations for international students: Required—TOEFL. Electronic applications accepted. *Expenses:* Contact institution.

Mississippi State University, College of Veterinary Medicine, Professional Program in Veterinary Medicine, Mississippi State, MS 39762. Offers DVM. *Accreditation:* AVMA. *Faculty:* 48 full-time (18 women), 3 part-time/adjunct (0 women). *Students:* 330 full-time (251 women); includes 27 minority (7 Black or African American, non-Hispanic/Latino; 4 Asian, non-Hispanic/Latino; 13 Hispanic/Latino; 3 Two or more races, non-Hispanic/Latino), 1 international. Average age 25. 92 applicants, 100% accepted, 88 enrolled. *Entrance requirements:* For doctorate, VCAT, GRE, minimum GPA of 3.5 in math and science coursework and overall; letter of recommendation. Additional exam requirements/recommendations for international students: Required—TOEFL. *Application deadline:* For fall admission, 10/1 for domestic students. Application fee: $60. Electronic applications accepted. *Expenses:* Contact institution. *Faculty research:* Veterinary education, advancing research in veterinary medicine and biomedical fields. *Unit head:* Dr. Margaret Kern, Associate Dean for Academic Affairs, 662-325-1326, Fax: 662-325-8714, E-mail: kern@cvm.msstate.edu. *Application contact:* Missy Hadaway, Admissions Coordinator, 662-325-9065, Fax: 662-325-8714, E-mail: hadaway@cvm.msstate.edu.
Website: http://www.cvm.msstate.edu/

North Carolina State University, College of Veterinary Medicine, Professional Program, Raleigh, NC 27695. Offers DVM. *Entrance requirements:* For doctorate, GRE. Additional exam requirements/recommendations for international students: Required—TOEFL.

North Carolina State University, College of Veterinary Medicine, Program in Specialized Veterinary Medicine, Raleigh, NC 27695. Offers MSpVM. *Accreditation:* AVMA. *Degree requirements:* For master's, thesis optional. *Entrance requirements:* For master's, GRE General Test. Additional exam requirements/recommendations for international students: Required—TOEFL (minimum score 550 paper-based). Electronic applications accepted. *Faculty research:* Cell biology, infectious diseases, pharmacology and toxicology, genomics, pathology and population medicine.

North Carolina State University, College of Veterinary Medicine, Program in Veterinary Public Health, Raleigh, NC 27695. Offers MVPH. *Degree requirements:* For master's, thesis optional. Electronic applications accepted.

Oklahoma State University, Center for Veterinary Health Sciences, Professional Program in Veterinary Medicine, Stillwater, OK 74078. Offers DVM. *Accreditation:* AVMA. *Entrance requirements:* For doctorate, GRE General Test, GRE Subject Test (biology). Electronic applications accepted. *Expenses:* Tuition, state resident: full-time $4272; part-time $178 per credit hour. Tuition, nonresident: full-time $17,472; part-time $709 per credit hour. *Required fees:* $2413.20; $100.55 per credit hour. One-time fee: $50 full-time. Part-time tuition and fees vary according to course load and campus/location. *Faculty research:* Infectious diseases, physiology, toxicology, biomedical lasers, clinical studies.

Oregon State University, College of Veterinary Medicine, Veterinary Medicine Professional Program, Corvallis, OR 97331. Offers DVM. Program admissions open only to residents of Oregon and other states participating in the Western Interstate Commission for Higher Education. *Accreditation:* AVMA. *Faculty:* 40 full-time (19 women), 3 part-time/adjunct (all women). *Students:* 222 full-time (195 women), 1 (woman) part-time; includes 27 minority (4 American Indian or Alaska Native, non-Hispanic/Latino; 9 Asian, non-Hispanic/Latino; 8 Hispanic/Latino; 1 Native Hawaiian or other Pacific Islander, non-Hispanic/Latino; 5 Two or more races, non-Hispanic/Latino), 2 international. Average age 27. 61 applicants, 100% accepted, 57 enrolled. In 2013, 55 doctorates awarded. *Entrance requirements:* For doctorate, GRE. *Application deadline:* For fall admission, 10/2 for domestic students. Application fee: $60. *Expenses:* Contact institution. *Financial support:* Federal Work-Study, institutionally sponsored loans, and scholarships/grants available. Support available to part-time students. Financial award application deadline: 2/1. *Unit head:* Dr. Susan J. Tornquist, Interim Dean, 541-737-2098, Fax: 541-737-4245, E-mail: susan.tornquist@oregonstate.edu. *Application contact:* Admissions, 541-737-2098, E-mail: cvmproginfo@oregonstate.edu.
Website: http://oregonstate.edu/vetmed/students/future/dvm

Purdue University, School of Veterinary Medicine, Professional Program in Veterinary Medicine, West Lafayette, IN 47907. Offers DVM, DVM/MS, DVM/PhD. *Accreditation:* AVMA. *Entrance requirements:* For doctorate, GRE General Test. Additional exam requirements/recommendations for international students: Required—TOEFL. Electronic applications accepted.

Texas A&M University, College of Veterinary Medicine and Biomedical Sciences, Professional Program in Veterinary Medicine, College Station, TX 77843. Offers DVM. *Accreditation:* AVMA. *Students:* 584 full-time (440 women), 4 part-time (3 women); includes 87 minority (4 Black or African American, non-Hispanic/Latino; 3 American Indian or Alaska Native, non-Hispanic/Latino; 25 Asian, non-Hispanic/Latino; 49 Hispanic/Latino; 6 Two or more races, non-Hispanic/Latino), 3 international. Average age 26. 185 applicants, 98% accepted, 178 enrolled. *Entrance requirements:* For doctorate, GRE. *Application deadline:* For fall admission, 9/1 for domestic students. Application fee: $100. *Expenses:* Contact institution. *Financial support:* Application deadline: 4/1; applicants required to submit FAFSA. *Faculty research:* Reproductive biology, theriogenology, genetics, endocrinology, animal behavior. *Unit head:* Dr. Eleanor M. Green, Dean, 979-845-5053, E-mail: emgreen@tamu.edu. *Application contact:* Yolanda Brinkman, Academic Coordinator, 979-458-0379, Fax: 979-845-5088, E-mail: ymbrinkman@cvm.tamu.edu.
Website: http://vetmed.tamu.edu/dvm

Texas A&M University, College of Veterinary Medicine and Biomedical Sciences, Program in Laboratory Animal Medicine, College Station, TX 77843. Offers MS. *Faculty:* 5. *Students:* 13 full-time (10 women), 4 part-time (all women); includes 1 minority (Hispanic/Latino), 2 international. Average age 30. 2 applicants, 100% accepted, 2 enrolled. In 2013, 4 master's awarded. *Degree requirements:* For master's, thesis (for some programs). *Entrance requirements:* For master's, GRE General Test. Additional exam requirements/recommendations for international students: Required—TOEFL. Application fee: $50 ($75 for international students). *Expenses:* Tuition, state resident: full-time $4078; part-time $226.55 per credit hour. Tuition, nonresident: full-time $10,450; part-time $580.55 per credit hour. *Required fees:* $2328; $278.50 per credit hour. $642.45 per semester. *Financial support:* In 2013–14, fellowships with tuition reimbursements (averaging $37,500 per year), research assistantships (averaging $30,700 per year), teaching assistantships (averaging $37,500 per year) were awarded. Financial award application deadline: 4/1; financial award applicants required to submit FAFSA. *Faculty research:* Epidemiology, including environmental and food safety; veterinary clinical studies. *Unit head:* Dr. Allen Roussel, Head, 979-845-9127, Fax: 979-847-8863, E-mail: aroussel@tamu.edu. *Application contact:* Dr. James A. Thompson, Graduate Advisor, 979-845-3541, Fax: 979-847-8863, E-mail: jthompson@cvm.tamu.edu.
Website: http://vetmed.tamu.edu/vlcs

Tufts University, Cummings School of Veterinary Medicine, North Grafton, MA 01536. Offers animals and public policy (MS); biomedical sciences (PhD), including digestive diseases, infectious diseases, neuroscience and reproductive biology, pathology; conservation medicine (MS); veterinary medicine (DVM); DVM/MPH; DVM/MS. *Accreditation:* AVMA (one or more programs are accredited). *Faculty:* 98 full-time (45 women), 13 part-time/adjunct (7 women). *Students:* 426 full-time (364 women); includes 60 minority (5 Black or African American, non-Hispanic/Latino; 1 American Indian or Alaska Native, non-Hispanic/Latino; 32 Asian, non-Hispanic/Latino; 20 Hispanic/Latino; 2 Two or more races, non-Hispanic/Latino), 4 international. Average age 25. 899 applicants, 29% accepted, 119 enrolled. In 2013, 85 master's, 2 doctorates awarded. *Degree requirements:* For master's, thesis (for some programs); for doctorate, comprehensive exam, thesis/dissertation (for some programs). *Entrance requirements:* For master's and doctorate, GRE General Test. Additional exam requirements/recommendations for international students: Required—TOEFL or IELTS. *Application deadline:* For fall admission, 11/1 for domestic and international students. Application fee: $70. Electronic applications accepted. *Expenses:* Contact institution. *Financial support:* In 2013–14, 230 students received support, including 7 research assistantships with full tuition reimbursements available (averaging $25,000 per year), 6 teaching assistantships (averaging $5,000 per year); career-related internships or fieldwork, Federal Work-Study, institutionally sponsored loans, scholarships/grants, and institutional aid awards, health care benefits for PhD students also available. Financial award application deadline: 4/15; financial award applicants required to submit FAFSA. *Faculty research:* Oncology, veterinary ethics, international veterinary medicine, veterinary genomics, pathogenesis of Clostridium difficile, wildlife fertility control. *Unit head:* Dr. Deborah T. Kochevar, Dean, 508-839-5302, Fax: 508-839-2953, E-mail: deborah.kochevar@tufts.edu. *Application contact:* Rebecca Russo, Director of Admissions, 508-839-7920, Fax: 508-887-4820, E-mail: vetadmissions@tufts.edu.
Website: http://www.tufts.edu/

Tuskegee University, Graduate Programs, College of Veterinary Medicine, Nursing and Allied Health, School of Veterinary Medicine, Tuskegee, AL 36088. Offers MS, DVM. *Degree requirements:* For master's, thesis. *Entrance requirements:* For master's, GRE General Test; for doctorate, VCAT. Additional exam requirements/recommendations for international students: Required—TOEFL (minimum score 500 paper-based). *Application deadline:* For fall admission, 7/15 for domestic students. Applications are processed on a rolling basis. Application fee: $25 ($35 for international students). *Financial support:* Application deadline: 4/15. *Unit head:* Dr. Tsegaye Habtemariam, Dean, 334-727-8174, Fax: 334-727-8177. *Application contact:* Dr. Cynthia Sellers-Simon, Vice President for Student Affairs and Enrollment Management, 334-724-4746, Fax: 334-727-5750, E-mail: sellersc@mytu.tuskegee.edu.

Université de Montréal, Faculty of Veterinary Medicine, Professional Program in Veterinary Medicine, Montréal, QC H3C 3J7, Canada. Offers DES. Open only to Canadian residents. *Accreditation:* AVMA. Part-time programs available. Electronic applications accepted. *Faculty research:* Animal reproduction, infectious diseases of swine, physiology of exercise in horses, viral diseases of cattle, health management and epidemiology.

University of California, Davis, School of Veterinary Medicine, Program in Veterinary Medicine, Davis, CA 95616. Offers DVM, DVM/MPVM. *Accreditation:* AVMA. *Entrance requirements:* For doctorate, GRE General Test. Additional exam requirements/recommendations for international students: Required—TOEFL. Electronic applications accepted.

University of Florida, College of Veterinary Medicine, Professional Program in Veterinary Medicine, Gainesville, FL 32611. Offers DVM. *Accreditation:* AVMA. *Entrance requirements:* For doctorate, GRE General Test. *Expenses:* Tuition, state resident: full-time $12,640. Tuition, nonresident: full-time $30,000.

University of Georgia, College of Veterinary Medicine, Athens, GA 30602. Offers MAM, MFAM, MS, DVM, PhD. *Accreditation:* AVMA (one or more programs are accredited). *Degree requirements:* For doctorate, variable foreign language requirement, thesis/dissertation (for some programs). *Entrance requirements:* For master's, GRE General Test; for doctorate, GRE General Test; GRE Subject Test in biology (for DVM). Electronic applications accepted. *Expenses:* Contact institution.

University of Guelph, Ontario Veterinary College and Graduate Studies, Graduate Programs in Veterinary Sciences, Department of Clinical Studies, Guelph, ON N1G 2W1, Canada. Offers anesthesiology (M Sc, DV Sc); cardiology (DV Sc, Diploma); clinical studies (Diploma); dermatology (M Sc); diagnostic imaging (M Sc, DV Sc); emergency/critical care (M Sc, DV Sc, Diploma); medicine (M Sc, DV Sc); neurology (M Sc, DV Sc); ophthalmology (M Sc, DV Sc); surgery (M Sc, DV Sc). *Degree requirements:* For master's, thesis; for doctorate, comprehensive exam, thesis/dissertation. *Entrance requirements:* Additional exam requirements/recommendations for international students: Required—TOEFL (minimum score 550 paper-based), IELTS (minimum score 6.5). Electronic applications accepted. *Faculty research:* Orthopedics, respirology, oncology, exercise physiology, cardiology.

University of Illinois at Urbana–Champaign, College of Veterinary Medicine, Professional Program in Veterinary Medicine, Champaign, IL 61820. Offers veterinary medical science (DVM). *Accreditation:* AVMA. *Students:* 486. *Expenses:* Contact institution. *Unit head:* Peter Constable, Dean, 217-333-2760, Fax: 217-333-4628, E-mail: constabl@illinois.edu. *Application contact:* Nikki Hausmann, Office Administrator, 217-333-4291, Fax: 217-333-4628, E-mail: nhausman@illinois.edu.
Website: http://vetmed.illinois.edu/

University of Maryland, College Park, Academic Affairs, College of Agriculture and Natural Resources, Maryland Campus of VA/MD Regional College of Veterinary Medicine, Professional Program in Veterinary Medicine, College Park, MD 20742. Offers DVM. *Students:* 122 full-time (102 women); includes 17 minority (1 Black or African American, non-Hispanic/Latino; 9 Asian, non-Hispanic/Latino; 6 Hispanic/Latino; 1 Native Hawaiian or other Pacific Islander, non-Hispanic/Latino). 30 applicants, 100% accepted, 30 enrolled. In 2013, 25 doctorates awarded. *Degree requirements:* For doctorate, thesis/dissertation, oral exam, public seminar. Application fee: $75. *Expenses:* Tuition, state resident: full-time $10,314; part-time $573 per credit hour. Tuition, nonresident: full-time $22,248; part-time $1236 per credit. *Required fees:* $1446; $403.15 per semester. Tuition and fees vary according to program. *Unit head:* Dr. Siba K. Samal, Chair, 301-314-6830, Fax: 301-314-6855, E-mail: ssamal@umd.edu. *Application contact:* Dr. Charles A. Caramello, Dean of Graduate School, 301-405-0358, Fax: 301-314-9305.

University of Minnesota, Twin Cities Campus, College of Veterinary Medicine, Professional Program in Veterinary Medicine, Minneapolis, MN 55455-0213. Offers DVM, DVM/PhD. *Accreditation:* AVMA. *Entrance requirements:* For doctorate, GRE General Test. Electronic applications accepted. *Expenses:* Contact institution. *Faculty research:* Infectious toxic diseases of animals, zoonotic animal models of human disease, epidemiologic and preventive medicine.

University of Missouri, College of Veterinary Medicine, Professional Program in Veterinary Medicine, Columbia, MO 65211. Offers DVM. *Accreditation:* AVMA. *Entrance requirements:* For doctorate, VCAT, minimum GPA of 2.5 (for state residents), 3.0 (for nonresidents). *Application deadline:* For fall admission, 11/1 for domestic students. Electronic applications accepted. *Financial support:* Fellowships, research assistantships, career-related internships or fieldwork, institutionally sponsored loans, tuition waivers (full), and research associateships available. *Faculty research:* Cardiovascular physiology, food safety, infectious diseases, laboratory animal medicine, ophthalmology. *Unit head:* Dr. Neil C. Olson, Dean, 573-882-3768, E-mail: olsonne@missouri.edu. *Application contact:* Dr. Claud B. Chastain, Associate Dean of Academic Affairs, 573-882-9594, E-mail: chastainc@missouri.edu.
Website: http://vetmed.missouri.edu/

University of Pennsylvania, School of Veterinary Medicine, Philadelphia, PA 19104. Offers VMD, VMD/MBA, VMD/PhD. *Accreditation:* AVMA. *Faculty:* 114 full-time (57 women), 31 part-time/adjunct (11 women). *Students:* 468 full-time (378 women), 7 part-time (6 women); includes 58 minority (6 Black or African American, non-Hispanic/Latino; 1 American Indian or Alaska Native, non-Hispanic/Latino; 32 Asian, non-Hispanic/Latino; 12 Hispanic/Latino; 7 Two or more races, non-Hispanic/Latino). Average age 24. 1,533 applicants, 11% accepted, 118 enrolled. In 2013, 115 doctorates awarded. *Entrance requirements:* For doctorate, GRE. Additional exam requirements/recommendations for international students: Required—TOEFL. *Application deadline:* For fall admission, 10/1 for domestic students. Application fee: $0. *Expenses:* Contact institution. *Financial support:* Career-related internships or fieldwork, Federal Work-Study, and institutionally sponsored loans available. *Total annual research expenditures:* $25 million. *Unit head:* Dr. Joan C. Hendricks, Dean, 215-898-8841, Fax: 215-573-8837, E-mail: vetdean@vet.upenn.edu. *Application contact:* School of Veterinary Medicine Office of Admissions, 215-898-5434, E-mail: admissions@vet.upenn.edu.
Website: http://www.vet.upenn.edu

University of Prince Edward Island, Atlantic Veterinary College, Professional Program in Veterinary Medicine, Charlottetown, PE C1A 4P3, Canada. Offers DVM. *Accreditation:* AVMA. *Entrance requirements:* For doctorate, GRE. Additional exam requirements/recommendations for international students: Required—TOEFL (minimum score 550 paper-based; 80 iBT), Canadian Academic English Language Assessment, Michigan English Language Assessment Battery, Canadian Test of English for Scholars and Trainees. *Faculty research:* Shellfish toxicology, animal nutrition, fish health, toxicology, animal health management.

University of Saskatchewan, Western College of Veterinary Medicine and College of Graduate Studies and Research, Graduate Programs in Veterinary Medicine, Department of Large Animal Clinical Sciences, Saskatoon, SK S7N 5A2, Canada. Offers M Sc, M Vet Sc, PhD. *Degree requirements:* For master's, thesis (for some programs); for doctorate, comprehensive exam (for some programs), thesis/dissertation. *Entrance requirements:* Additional exam requirements/recommendations for international students: Required—TOEFL (minimum score 80 iBT); Recommended—IELTS (minimum score 6.5). Electronic applications accepted. *Expenses: Tuition, area resident:* Full-time $3585 Canadian dollars; part-time $585 Canadian dollars per course. Tuition, nonresident: part-time $877 Canadian dollars per course. *International tuition:* $5377 Canadian dollars full-time. *Required fees:* $889.51 Canadian dollars. *Faculty research:* Reproduction, infectious diseases, epidemiology, food safety.

University of Saskatchewan, Western College of Veterinary Medicine and College of Graduate Studies and Research, Graduate Programs in Veterinary Medicine, Department of Small Animal Clinical Sciences, Saskatoon, SK S7N 5A2, Canada. Offers small animal clinical sciences (M Sc, PhD); veterinary anesthesiology, radiology and surgery (M Vet Sc); veterinary internal medicine (M Vet Sc). *Degree requirements:* For master's, thesis (for some programs); for doctorate, comprehensive exam (for some programs), thesis/dissertation. *Entrance requirements:* Additional exam requirements/recommendations for international students: Required—TOEFL (minimum score 80 iBT); Recommended—IELTS (minimum score 6.5). Electronic applications accepted. *Expenses: Tuition, area resident:* Full-time $3585 Canadian dollars; part-time $585 Canadian dollars per course. Tuition, nonresident: part-time $877 Canadian dollars per course. *International tuition:* $5377 Canadian dollars full-time. *Required fees:* $889.51 Canadian dollars. *Faculty research:* Orthopedics, wildlife, cardiovascular exercise/myelopathy, ophthalmology.

University of Saskatchewan, Western College of Veterinary Medicine, Professional Program in Veterinary Medicine, Saskatoon, SK S7N 5A2, Canada. Offers DVM. *Accreditation:* AVMA. *Degree requirements:* For doctorate, thesis/dissertation. *Expenses: Tuition, area resident:* Full-time $3585 Canadian dollars; part-time $585 Canadian dollars per course. Tuition, nonresident: part-time $877 Canadian dollars per course. *International tuition:* $5377 Canadian dollars full-time. *Required fees:* $889.51 Canadian dollars.

The University of Tennessee, Graduate School, College of Veterinary Medicine, Knoxville, TN 37996. Offers DVM. *Accreditation:* AVMA. *Entrance requirements:* For doctorate, VCAT, interview, minimum GPA of 2.7. Additional exam requirements/recommendations for international students: Required—TOEFL. *Expenses:* Contact institution.

University of Wisconsin–Madison, School of Veterinary Medicine, Madison, WI 53706-1380. Offers MS, DVM, PhD. *Accreditation:* AVMA (one or more programs are accredited). Terminal master's awarded for partial completion of doctoral program. *Degree requirements:* For master's, thesis; for doctorate, thesis/dissertation (for some programs). *Entrance requirements:* For doctorate, GRE General Test (for DVM). *Expenses:* Contact institution. *Faculty research:* Infectious disease, ophthalmology, orthopedics, food animal production, oncology, cardio-respiratory.

Virginia Polytechnic Institute and State University, Virginia-Maryland Regional College of Veterinary Medicine, Blacksburg, VA 24061. Offers biomedical and veterinary sciences (MS, PhD); public health (MPH); research in translational medicine (Certificate); veterinary medicine (DVM). *Accreditation:* AVMA (one or more programs

are accredited). *Faculty:* 105 full-time (45 women), 1 (woman) part-time/adjunct. *Students:* 573 full-time (428 women), 44 part-time (35 women); includes 67 minority (17 Black or African American, non-Hispanic/Latino; 13 Asian, non-Hispanic/Latino; 13 Hispanic/Latino; 1 Native Hawaiian or other Pacific Islander, non-Hispanic/Latino; 23 Two or more races, non-Hispanic/Latino), 32 international. Average age 26. 102 applicants, 69% accepted, 47 enrolled. In 2013, 14 master's, 104 doctorates awarded. *Degree requirements:* For master's, comprehensive exam (for some programs), thesis (for some programs); for doctorate, comprehensive exam (for some programs), thesis/dissertation (for some programs). *Entrance requirements:* For master's and doctorate, GRE/GMAT (may vary by department). Additional exam requirements/recommendations for international students: Required—TOEFL (minimum score 550 paper-based). *Application deadline:* For fall admission, 8/1 for domestic students, 4/1 for international students; for spring admission, 1/1 for domestic students, 9/1 for international students. Applications are processed on a rolling basis. Application fee: $75. Electronic applications accepted. *Expenses:* Contact institution. *Financial support:* In 2013–14, 1 fellowship (averaging $39,777 per year), 14 research assistantships with full tuition reimbursements (averaging $23,189 per year), 44 teaching assistantships with full tuition reimbursements (averaging $21,977 per year) were awarded. Financial award application deadline: 3/1; financial award applicants required to submit FAFSA. *Total annual research expenditures:* $6.6 million. *Unit head:* Dr. Cyril R. Clark, Dean, 540-231-7666, Fax: 540-231-7367, E-mail: cvmdean@vt.edu. *Application contact:* Shelia Steele, Executive Assistant, 540-231-7910, Fax: 540-231-7367, E-mail: ssteele@vt.edu.
Website: http://www.vetmed.vt.edu

Washington State University, College of Veterinary Medicine, Professional Program in Veterinary Medicine, Pullman, WA 99164-7010. Offers DVM, DVM/MS, DVM/PhD. *Accreditation:* AVMA. *Faculty:* 43 full-time (8 women), 27 part-time/adjunct (7 women). *Students:* 447 full-time (344 women); includes 53 minority (4 American Indian or Alaska Native, non-Hispanic/Latino; 13 Asian, non-Hispanic/Latino; 21 Hispanic/Latino; 1 Native Hawaiian or other Pacific Islander, non-Hispanic/Latino; 14 Two or more races, non-Hispanic/Latino), 2 international. Average age 25. 1,169 applicants, 16% accepted, 133 enrolled. In 2013, 98 doctorates awarded. *Entrance requirements:* For doctorate, GRE General Test. Additional exam requirements/recommendations for international students: Required—TOEFL. *Application deadline:* For fall admission, 10/2 for domestic and international students. Application fee: $60. Electronic applications accepted. *Financial support:* In 2013–14, 326 students received support. Research assistantships, teaching assistantships, career-related internships or fieldwork, Federal Work-Study, institutionally sponsored loans, scholarships/grants, traineeships, and tuition waivers (partial) available. Support available to part-time students. Financial award application deadline: 2/15; financial award applicants required to submit FAFSA. *Faculty research:* Biotechnology, immunology, pathology, neurosciences, clinical sciences. *Unit head:* Dr. Patricia Talcott, Director of Admissions, 509-355-1532. *Application contact:* Barbara Hodson, Program Coordinator, 509-335-1532, Fax: 509-335-6133, E-mail: bhodson@vetmed.wsu.edu.
Website: http://www.vetmed.wsu.edu/

Washington State University, College of Veterinary Medicine, Program in Immunology and Infectious Diseases, Pullman, WA 99164. Offers veterinary science (MS, PhD). *Faculty:* 26 full-time (10 women), 22 part-time/adjunct (5 women). *Students:* 41 full-time (27 women); includes 2 minority (both Hispanic/Latino), 18 international. Average age 31. 52 applicants, 10% accepted, 5 enrolled. In 2013, 4 master's, 6 doctorates awarded. Terminal master's awarded for partial completion of doctoral program. *Degree requirements:* For master's, thesis, oral exam; for doctorate, thesis/dissertation, oral exam. *Entrance requirements:* For master's and doctorate, minimum GPA of 3.0. Additional exam requirements/recommendations for international students: Required—TOEFL (minimum score 550 paper-based; 80 iBT). *Application deadline:* Applications are processed on a rolling basis. Application fee: $75. Electronic applications accepted. *Financial support:* In 2013–14, 15 fellowships, 26 research assistantships were awarded; institutionally sponsored loans, scholarships/grants, traineeships, health care benefits, and unspecified assistantships also available. Financial award application deadline: 3/1. *Faculty research:* Microbial pathogenesis, veterinary and wildlife parasitology, laboratory animal pathology, immune responses to infectious diseases. *Unit head:* Dr. Michele E. Hardy, Chair, 509-335-6030, Fax: 509-335-8529, E-mail: mhardy@vetmed.wsu.edu. *Application contact:* Sue Zumwalt, Graduate Coordinator, 509-335-6027, Fax: 509-335-8529, E-mail: szumwalt@vetmed.wsu.edu.
Website: http://www.vetmed.wsu.edu/depts-vmp/graduate/MSPhD.aspx

Western University of Health Sciences, College of Veterinary Medicine, Pomona, CA 91766-1854. Offers DVM. *Accreditation:* AVMA. *Faculty:* 54 full-time (28 women), 5 part-time/adjunct (1 woman). *Students:* 416 full-time (335 women); includes 147 minority (7 Black or African American, non-Hispanic/Latino; 1 American Indian or Alaska Native, non-Hispanic/Latino; 59 Asian, non-Hispanic/Latino; 62 Hispanic/Latino; 4 Native Hawaiian or other Pacific Islander, non-Hispanic/Latino; 14 Two or more races, non-Hispanic/Latino), 5 international. Average age 27. 794 applicants, 22% accepted, 103 enrolled. In 2013, 97 doctorates awarded. *Degree requirements:* For doctorate, comprehensive exam (for some programs). *Entrance requirements:* For doctorate, MCAT or GRE General Test, minimum GPA of 2.75, letters of recommendation, BA or BS (recommended), 500 hours of hands-on animal-related experience. Additional exam requirements/recommendations for international students: Required—TOEFL (minimum score 550 paper-based). *Application deadline:* For fall admission, 10/15 for domestic students. Application fee: $50. Electronic applications accepted. *Expenses:* Contact institution. *Financial support:* Institutionally sponsored loans, scholarships/grants, and veterans educational benefits available. Financial award application deadline: 3/2; financial award applicants required to submit FAFSA. *Unit head:* Dr. Phil Nelson, Dean, 909-469-5661, Fax: 909-469-5635, E-mail: pnelson@westernu.edu. *Application contact:* Karen Hutton-Lopez, Director of Admissions, 909-469-5335, Fax: 909-469-5570, E-mail: admissions@westernu.edu.
Website: http://www.westernu.edu/veterinary

Veterinary Sciences

Auburn University, College of Veterinary Medicine and Graduate School, Graduate Programs in Veterinary Medicine, Auburn University, AL 36849. Offers biomedical sciences (MS, PhD), including anatomy, physiology and pharmacology (MS), biomedical sciences (PhD), clinical sciences (MS), large animal surgery and medicine (MS), pathobiology (MS), radiology (MS), small animal surgery and medicine (MS); DVM/MS. Part-time programs available. *Faculty:* 100 full-time (41 women), 4 part-time/adjunct (1 woman). *Students:* 24 full-time (16 women), 38 part-time (25 women); includes 5 minority (1 Black or African American, non-Hispanic/Latino; 1 American Indian or Alaska Native, non-Hispanic/Latino; 2 Asian, non-Hispanic/Latino; 1 Hispanic/Latino), 22 international. Average age 30. 36 applicants, 44% accepted, 13 enrolled. In 2013, 12 master's, 8 doctorates awarded. *Degree requirements:* For doctorate, thesis/dissertation. *Entrance requirements:* For master's, GRE General Test; for doctorate, GRE General Test, GRE Subject Test. *Application deadline:* For fall admission, 7/7 for domestic students; for spring admission, 11/24 for domestic students. Applications are processed on a rolling basis. Application fee: $50 ($60 for international students). Electronic applications accepted. *Expenses:* Tuition, state resident: full-time $8262; part-time $459 per credit hour. Tuition, nonresident: full-time $24,786; part-time $1377 per credit hour. Tuition and fees vary according to degree level and program. *Financial support:* Research assistantships, teaching assistantships, and Federal Work-Study available. Support available to part-time students. Financial award application deadline: 3/15; financial award applicants required to submit FAFSA. *Unit head:* Dr. Calvin Johnson, Acting Dean, 334-844-2650. *Application contact:* Dr. George Flowers, Dean of the Graduate School, 334-844-2125.

Clemson University, Graduate School, College of Agriculture, Forestry and Life Sciences, Department of Animal and Veterinary Sciences, Clemson, SC 29634. Offers animal and veterinary sciences (MS, PhD). Part-time programs available. *Faculty:* 9 full-time (5 women), 2 part-time/adjunct (0 women). *Students:* 12 full-time (10 women), 2 part-time (0 women), 2 international. Average age 25. 8 applicants, 63% accepted, 5 enrolled. In 2013, 4 master's, 1 doctorate awarded. *Degree requirements:* For master's, comprehensive exam, thesis (for some programs); for doctorate, comprehensive exam, thesis/dissertation. *Entrance requirements:* For master's and doctorate, GRE General Test. Additional exam requirements/recommendations for international students: Required—TOEFL. *Application deadline:* For fall admission, 4/15 for international students; for spring admission, 9/15 for international students. Applications are processed on a rolling basis. Application fee: $70 ($80 for international students). Electronic applications accepted. *Expenses:* Contact institution. *Financial support:* In 2013–14, 9 students received support, including 2 fellowships with full and partial tuition reimbursements available (averaging $10,000 per year), 6 research assistantships with partial tuition reimbursements available (averaging $14,571 per year), 5 teaching assistantships with partial tuition reimbursements available (averaging $13,328 per year); career-related internships or fieldwork, Federal Work-Study, institutionally sponsored loans, scholarships/grants, and unspecified assistantships also available. Financial award applicants required to submit FAFSA. *Total annual research expenditures:* $684,353. *Unit head:* Dr. James R. Strickland, Chair, 864-656-3138, Fax: 864-656-3131, E-mail: jrstric@clemson.edu. *Application contact:* Dr. Peter A. Skewes, Associate Dean for Research and Graduate Studies, 864-656-4026, E-mail: pskewes@clemson.edu.
Website: http://www.clemson.edu/avs

Colorado State University, College of Veterinary Medicine and Biomedical Sciences, Department of Clinical Sciences, Fort Collins, CO 80523-1678. Offers MS, PhD. Part-time programs available. *Faculty:* 63 full-time (27 women), 1 part-time/adjunct (0 women). *Students:* 23 full-time (17 women), 47 part-time (32 women); includes 1 minority (Asian, non-Hispanic/Latino), 17 international. Average age 34. 23 applicants, 78% accepted, 17 enrolled. In 2013, 11 master's, 5 doctorates awarded. *Degree requirements:* For master's, comprehensive exam (for some programs), thesis (for some programs), exam; for doctorate, comprehensive exam, thesis/dissertation, exam. *Entrance requirements:* For master's, minimum GPA of 3.0, DVM or other equivalent medical degree, 3 letters of recommendation; for doctorate, DVM or other equivalent medical degree, 3 letters of recommendation, biographical statement. Additional exam requirements/recommendations for international students: Recommended—TOEFL (minimum score 550 paper-based; 80 iBT). *Application deadline:* For fall admission, 6/1 priority date for domestic students, 4/1 for international students; for spring admission, 11/1 for domestic students, 9/1 for international students. Applications are processed on a rolling basis. Application fee: $50. Electronic applications accepted. *Expenses:* Tuition, state resident: full-time $9075.40; part-time $504 per credit. Tuition, nonresident: full-time $22,248; part-time $1236 per credit. *Required fees:* $1819; $60 per credit. *Financial support:* In 2013–14, 54 students received support, including 42 fellowships (averaging $32,842 per year), 12 research assistantships with full and partial tuition reimbursements available (averaging $23,471 per year); Federal Work-Study, institutionally sponsored loans, and unspecified assistantships also available. Financial award application deadline: 2/15; financial award applicants required to submit FAFSA. *Faculty research:* Orthopedics, oncology, epidemiology, critical care/emergency medicine, equine medicine. *Total annual research expenditures:* $5.4 million. *Unit head:* Dr. Christopher Orton, Interim Department Head, 970-297-1250, Fax: 970-297-1275, E-mail: chris.orton@colostate.edu. *Application contact:* Morna J. Mynard, Information Contact, 970-297-4030, Fax: 970-297-1275, E-mail: morna.mynard@colostate.edu.
Website: http://csu-cvmbs.colostate.edu/academics/clinsci/graduate-programs/Pages/default.aspx

Drexel University, College of Medicine, Biomedical Graduate Programs, Program in Laboratory Animal Science, Philadelphia, PA 19104-2875. Offers MLAS. Part-time programs available. *Degree requirements:* For master's, comprehensive exam. *Entrance requirements:* For master's, GRE General Test, minimum GPA of 3.0. Additional exam requirements/recommendations for international students: Required—TOEFL. Electronic applications accepted. *Faculty research:* Laboratory animal medicine, experimental surgery, development of animal models for human diseases.

Iowa State University of Science and Technology, Department of Veterinary Clinical Sciences, Ames, IA 50011. Offers MS. *Degree requirements:* For master's, thesis or alternative. *Entrance requirements:* For master's, GRE. Additional exam requirements/recommendations for international students: Required—TOEFL (minimum score 550 paper-based; 79 iBT), IELTS (minimum score 6.5). Electronic applications accepted. *Faculty research:* Theriogenology, veterinary medicine, veterinary surgery, extracorporeal shock waves, therapy, orthopedic research in animals.

Iowa State University of Science and Technology, Department of Veterinary Microbiology and Preventive Medicine, Ames, IA 50011. Offers veterinary microbiology (MS, PhD). *Entrance requirements:* For master's and doctorate, GRE General Test. Additional exam requirements/recommendations for international students: Required—TOEFL (minimum score 550 paper-based; 79 iBT), IELTS (minimum score 6.5). Electronic applications accepted. *Faculty research:* Bacteriology, immunology, virology, public health and food safety.

Kansas State University, College of Veterinary Medicine, Department of Clinical Sciences, Manhattan, KS 66506. Offers MPH. *Faculty:* 58 full-time (21 women), 16 part-time/adjunct (10 women). *Students:* 47 full-time (34 women), 27 part-time (18 women); includes 5 minority (2 Black or African American, non-Hispanic/Latino; 2 Asian, non-Hispanic/Latino; 1 Hispanic/Latino), 5 international. Average age 32. 42 applicants, 50% accepted, 16 enrolled. In 2013, 26 master's awarded. *Degree requirements:* For master's, thesis. *Entrance requirements:* For master's, GRE, DVM. Additional exam requirements/recommendations for international students: Required—TOEFL (minimum score 550 paper-based). *Application deadline:* For fall admission, 2/1 priority date for domestic and international students; for spring admission, 8/1 priority date for domestic and international students. Applications are processed on a rolling basis. Application fee: $50 ($75 for international students). Electronic applications accepted. *Financial support:* In 2013–14, 11 research assistantships (averaging $30,118 per year) were awarded; institutionally sponsored loans and scholarships/grants also available. Financial award application deadline: 3/1; financial award applicants required to submit FAFSA. *Faculty research:* Clinical trials, equine gastrointestinal ulceration, leptospirosis, food animal pharmacology, equine immunology, diabetes. *Total annual research expenditures:* $1.2 million. *Unit head:* Dr. Michael Cates, Director and Professor, 785-532-2042, E-mail: cates@ksu.edu. *Application contact:* Barta Stevenson, Program Assistant, 785-532-2042, E-mail: bstevens@vet.k-state.edu.
Website: http://www.vet.k-state.edu/depts/ClinicalSciences/

Louisiana State University and Agricultural & Mechanical College, School of Veterinary Medicine and Graduate School, Department of Comparative Biomedical Sciences, Baton Rouge, LA 70803. Offers MS, PhD. *Faculty:* 13 full-time (1 woman). *Students:* 12 full-time (3 women), 2 part-time (1 woman); includes 1 minority (Asian, non-Hispanic/Latino), 9 international. Average age 30. 3 applicants, 33% accepted. In 2013, 2 doctorates awarded. *Degree requirements:* For master's, thesis; for doctorate, thesis/dissertation, final exam. *Entrance requirements:* For master's and doctorate, GRE, minimum GPA of 3.0. Additional exam requirements/recommendations for international students: Required—TOEFL (minimum score 550 paper-based; 79 IBT), IELTS (minimum score 6.5), or PTE (minimum score 59). *Application deadline:* For fall admission, 5/15 for international students; for spring admission, 10/15 for international students. Electronic applications accepted. *Financial support:* In 2013–14, 13 students received support, including 1 fellowship with full and partial tuition reimbursement available (averaging $41,274 per year), 10 research assistantships with full and partial tuition reimbursements available (averaging $21,600 per year); teaching assistantships, Federal Work-Study, institutionally sponsored loans, scholarships/grants, health care benefits, and unspecified assistantships also available. Support available to part-time students. Financial award applicants required to submit FAFSA. *Faculty research:* Gene therapy, metastasis, DNA repair, cytokines in cardiovascular function, aquatic toxicology. *Total annual research expenditures:* $1.3 million. *Unit head:* Dr. James Mathis, Chair, 225-578-9759, Fax: 225-578-9895, E-mail: jmathis@lsu.edu. *Application contact:* Dr. Masami Yoshimura, Graduate Coordinator, 225-578-9759, Fax: 225-578-9895, E-mail: myoshimura@vetmed.lsu.edu.
Website: http://www.vetmed.lsu.edu/van/

Louisiana State University and Agricultural & Mechanical College, School of Veterinary Medicine and Graduate School, Department of Pathobiological Sciences, Baton Rouge, LA 70803. Offers MS, PhD. *Faculty:* 29 full-time (8 women). *Students:* 25 full-time (14 women), 9 part-time (3 women); includes 5 minority (3 Asian, non-Hispanic/Latino; 1 Hispanic/Latino; 1 Two or more races, non-Hispanic/Latino), 9 international. Average age 29. 10 applicants, 60% accepted, 5 enrolled. In 2013, 1 master's, 4 doctorates awarded. *Degree requirements:* For doctorate, thesis/dissertation. *Entrance requirements:* Additional exam requirements/recommendations for international students: Required—TOEFL (minimum score 550 paper-based; 79 IBT), IELTS (minimum score 6.5), or PTE (minimum score 59). *Application deadline:* For fall admission, 5/15 for international students; for spring admission, 10/15 for international students. Application fee: $50 ($70 for international students). Electronic applications accepted. *Financial support:* In 2013–14, 34 students received support, including 5 fellowships with full tuition reimbursements available (averaging $37,533 per year), 25 research assistantships with full and partial tuition reimbursements available (averaging $23,613 per year); teaching assistantships with full and partial tuition reimbursements available, Federal Work-Study, scholarships/grants, health care benefits, and unspecified assistantships also available. Support available to part-time students. Financial award applicants required to submit FAFSA. *Faculty research:* Infectious disease, host-pathogen interaction, vaccinology. *Total annual research expenditures:* $5.9 million. *Unit head:* Dr. Ronald Thune, Chair, 225-578-9684, Fax: 225-578-9701, E-mail: rthune@lsu.edu. *Application contact:* Dr. Kevin Macaluso, Graduate Adviser, 225-578-9677, Fax: 225-578-9701, E-mail: kmacaluso@vetmed.lsu.edu.
Website: http://www1.vetmed.lsu.edu//PBS/index.html

Louisiana State University and Agricultural & Mechanical College, School of Veterinary Medicine and Graduate School, Department of Veterinary Clinical Sciences, Baton Rouge, LA 70803. Offers MS, PhD. *Faculty:* 32 full-time (15 women). *Students:* 4 full-time (2 women), 6 part-time (2 women); includes 1 minority (Hispanic/Latino), 6 international. Average age 31. 9 applicants, 33% accepted, 1 enrolled. In 2013, 1 master's, 2 doctorates awarded. *Entrance requirements:* For master's and doctorate, GRE, DVM or equivalent degree. Additional exam requirements/recommendations for international students: Required—TOEFL (minimum score 550 paper-based; 79 IBT), IELTS (minimum score 6.5), or PTE (minimum score 59). *Application deadline:* For fall admission, 5/15 for domestic and international students; for spring admission, 10/15 for international students. Application fee: $50 ($70 for international students). Electronic applications accepted. *Financial support:* In 2013–14, 8 students received support, including 3 research assistantships with full and partial tuition reimbursements available (averaging $19,667 per year); fellowships, teaching assistantships, Federal Work-Study, institutionally sponsored loans, scholarships/grants, health care benefits, and unspecified assistantships also available. Support available to part-time students. Financial award applicants required to submit FAFSA. *Faculty research:* Urology/nephrology, equine arthroscopy orthopedics and laser surgery, physical rehabilitation on companion animals, cardiology, gastroenterology, infectious diseases, medical oncology, mare infertility. *Total annual research expenditures:* $385,117. *Unit head:* Dr. Dale Paccamonti, Head, 225-578-9551, Fax: 225-578-9559, E-mail: pacc@lsu.edu. *Application contact:* Dr. Susan Eades, Graduate Adviser, 225-578-9512, Fax: 225-578-9559, E-mail: sceades@vetmed.lsu.edu.
Website: http://www.vetmed.lsu.edu/vcs/

Michigan State University, College of Veterinary Medicine and The Graduate School, Graduate Programs in Veterinary Medicine, East Lansing, MI 48824. Offers comparative medicine and integrative biology (MS, PhD), including comparative medicine and integrative biology, comparative medicine and integrative biology–environmental toxicology (PhD); food safety and toxicology (MS), including food safety; integrative toxicology (PhD), including animal science–environmental toxicology, biochemistry and molecular biology–environmental toxicology, chemistry–environmental toxicology, crop and soil sciences–environmental toxicology, environmental engineering–environmental toxicology, environmental geosciences–environmental toxicology, fisheries and wildlife–environmental toxicology, food science–environmental toxicology, forestry–environmental toxicology, genetics–environmental toxicology, human nutrition–environmental toxicology, microbiology–environmental toxicology, pharmacology and toxicology–environmental toxicology, zoology–environmental toxicology; large animal clinical sciences (MS, PhD); microbiology and molecular genetics (MS, PhD), including industrial microbiology, microbiology, microbiology and molecular genetics, microbiology–environmental toxicology (PhD); pathobiology and diagnostic investigation (MS, PhD), including pathology, pathology–environmental toxicology (PhD); pharmacology and toxicology (MS, PhD); pharmacology and toxicology–environmental toxicology (PhD); physiology (MS, PhD); small animal clinical sciences (MS). Electronic applications accepted. *Faculty research:* Molecular genetics, food safety/toxicology, comparative orthopedics, airway disease, population medicine.

Mississippi State University, College of Veterinary Medicine, Office of Research and Graduate Studies, Mississippi State, MS 39762. Offers environmental toxicology (PhD); veterinary medical sciences (MS, PhD). Part-time programs available. *Faculty:* 85 full-time (30 women), 46 part-time/adjunct (16 women). *Students:* 45 full-time (22 women), 32 part-time (19 women); includes 9 minority (5 Black or African American, non-Hispanic/Latino; 2 Asian, non-Hispanic/Latino; 1 Hispanic/Latino; 1 Two or more races, non-Hispanic/Latino), 24 international. Average age 31. 27 applicants, 48% accepted, 13 enrolled. In 2013, 9 master's, 11 doctorates awarded. Terminal master's awarded for partial completion of doctoral program. *Degree requirements:* For master's, thesis (for some programs); for doctorate, thesis/dissertation. *Entrance requirements:* For master's, minimum undergraduate GPA of 3.0, bachelor's degree; for doctorate, minimum undergraduate GPA of 3.0. Additional exam requirements/recommendations for international students: Required—TOEFL (minimum score 550 paper-based; 79 iBT); Recommended—IELTS (minimum score 6.5). *Application deadline:* For fall admission, 7/1 priority date for domestic students, 5/1 priority date for international students; for spring admission, 11/1 priority date for domestic students, 9/1 priority date for international students; for summer admission, 4/1 priority date for domestic and international students. Applications are processed on a rolling basis. Application fee: $60. Electronic applications accepted. *Expenses:* Contact institution. *Financial support:* In 2013–14, 24 students received support, including 27 research assistantships with partial tuition reimbursements available (averaging $19,593 per year); career-related internships or fieldwork, institutionally sponsored loans, scholarships/grants, and unspecified assistantships also available. Financial award application deadline: 4/1; financial award applicants required to submit FAFSA. *Faculty research:* Food animal health (poultry and warm-water aquaculture) using immunology, microbiology, molecular biology, parasitology, pathology, pharmacology, and environmental toxicology. *Total annual research expenditures:* $4.2 million. *Unit head:* Dr. Mark L. Lawrence, Associate Dean of Research and Graduate Studies, 662-325-1205, Fax: 662-325-1193, E-mail: lawrence@cvm.msstate.edu. *Application contact:* Barbara E. Perrigin, Coordinator, Graduate Studies, 662-325-1417, Fax: 662-325-1193, E-mail: bperrigin@cvm.msstate.edu.
Website: http://www.cvm.msstate.edu/index.php/academics/degree-programs-research/office-of-research-graduate-studies-orgs

North Carolina State University, College of Veterinary Medicine, Program in Comparative Biomedical Sciences, Raleigh, NC 27695. Offers cell biology (MS, PhD); infectious disease (MS, PhD); pathology (MS, PhD); pharmacology (MS, PhD); population medicine (MS, PhD). Part-time programs available. *Degree requirements:* For master's, thesis; for doctorate, thesis/dissertation. *Entrance requirements:* For master's and doctorate, GRE General Test. Additional exam requirements/recommendations for international students: Required—TOEFL (minimum score 550 paper-based). Electronic applications accepted. *Expenses:* Contact institution. *Faculty research:* Infectious diseases, cell biology, pharmacology and toxicology, genomics, pathology and population medicine.

North Dakota State University, College of Graduate and Interdisciplinary Studies, College of Agriculture, Food Systems, and Natural Resources, Department of Veterinary and Microbiological Sciences, Fargo, ND 58108. Offers international infectious disease (MS); microbiology (MS); molecular pathogenesis (PhD). Part-time programs available. *Faculty:* 15 full-time (8 women). *Students:* 11 full-time (6 women), 6 part-time (4 women), 5 international. Average age 30. 2 applicants, 50% accepted, 1 enrolled. In 2013, 8 master's, 1 doctorate awarded. *Degree requirements:* For master's, thesis; for doctorate, thesis/dissertation, oral and written preliminary exams. *Entrance requirements:* For master's and doctorate, GRE. Additional exam requirements/recommendations for international students: Required—TOEFL (minimum score 525 paper-based; 71 iBT). *Application deadline:* For fall admission, 2/15 priority date for domestic students. Applications are processed on a rolling basis. Application fee: $35. *Financial support:* Fellowships with full tuition reimbursements, research assistantships with full tuition reimbursements, teaching assistantships with full tuition reimbursements, Federal Work-Study, and institutionally sponsored loans available. Financial award application deadline: 4/15. *Faculty research:* Bacterial gene regulation, antibiotic resistance, molecular virology, mechanisms of bacterial pathogenesis, immunology of animals. *Unit head:* Dr. Charlene Wolf-Hall, Head, 701-231-7667, E-mail: charlene.hall@ndsu.edu. *Application contact:* Dr. John McEvoy, Associate Professor, 701-231-8530, Fax: 701-231-7514, E-mail: eugene.berry@ndsu.edu.
Website: http://vetmicro.ndsu.nodak.edu/

The Ohio State University, College of Veterinary Medicine, Program in Comparative and Veterinary Medicine, Columbus, OH 43210. Offers MS, PhD. *Faculty:* 116. *Students:* 102 full-time (71 women), 4 part-time (all women); includes 5 minority (1 Black or African American, non-Hispanic/Latino; 1 Asian, non-Hispanic/Latino; 3 Hispanic/Latino), 37 international. Average age 30. In 2013, 17 master's, 13 doctorates awarded. *Entrance requirements:* For master's and doctorate, GRE (for graduates of institutions not accredited by the AVMA). Additional exam requirements/recommendations for international students: Required—TOEFL (minimum score 550 paper-based; 79 iBT), Michigan English Language Assessment Battery (minimum score 82). *Application deadline:* Applications are processed on a rolling basis. Application fee: $60 ($70 for international students). Electronic applications accepted. *Unit head:* Lonnie King, Dean, 614-688-8749, Fax: 614-292-3544, E-mail: king.1518@osu.edu. *Application contact:* Graduate Admissions, 614-292-6031, Fax: 614-292-3656, E-mail: gradadmissions@osu.edu.
Website: http://vet.osu.edu/education/graduate-programs

Oklahoma State University, Center for Veterinary Health Sciences and Graduate College, Graduate Program in Veterinary Biomedical Sciences, Stillwater, OK 74078. Offers MS, PhD. Postbaccalaureate distance learning degree programs offered (no on-campus study). Terminal master's awarded for partial completion of doctoral program. *Degree requirements:* For master's, thesis; for doctorate, comprehensive exam, thesis/dissertation. *Entrance requirements:* For master's and doctorate, GRE General Test. Additional exam requirements/recommendations for international students: Required—TOEFL (minimum score 80 iBT). Electronic applications accepted. *Expenses:* Contact institution. *Faculty research:* Infectious and parasitic diseases, physiology, toxicology, biomedical lasers, clinical studies.

Oregon State University, College of Veterinary Medicine, Program in Veterinary Science, Corvallis, OR 97331. Offers MS, PhD. *Faculty:* 18 full-time (9 women), 6 part-time/adjunct (4 women). *Students:* 15 full-time (10 women); includes 3 minority (2 Black or African American, non-Hispanic/Latino; 1 Hispanic/Latino), 3 international. Average

age 31. 2 applicants, 100% accepted, 2 enrolled. In 2013, 1 master's awarded. *Degree requirements:* For master's, one foreign language, thesis. *Entrance requirements:* For master's, minimum GPA of 3.0 in last 90 hours of course work. Additional exam requirements/recommendations for international students: Required—TOEFL. *Application deadline:* For fall admission, 11/1 for domestic students. Application fee: $50. *Expenses:* Tuition, state resident: full-time $11,664; part-time $432 per credit hour. Tuition, nonresident: full-time $19,197; part-time $711 per credit hour. *Required fees:* $1446; $443 per quarter. One-time fee: $300. Tuition and fees vary according to course load and program. *Financial support:* Fellowships, research assistantships, Federal Work-Study, and institutionally sponsored loans available. Support available to part-time students. Financial award application deadline: 2/1. *Faculty research:* Microbiology, virology, toxicology. *Unit head:* Dr. Luiz E. Bermudez, Department Head, 541-737-6532, Fax: 541-737-8035, E-mail: cvm.biomed@oregonstate.edu. *Application contact:* Dr. Susan J. Tornquist, Associate Dean, 541-737-2098, Fax: 541-737-4245, E-mail: susan.tornquist@oregonstate.edu.

Penn State Hershey Medical Center, College of Medicine, Graduate School Programs in the Biomedical Sciences, Graduate Program in Laboratory Animal Medicine, Hershey, PA 17033. Offers MS. *Students:* 4 full-time (3 women); includes 1 minority (Black or African American, non-Hispanic/Latino). 2 applicants, 100% accepted, 2 enrolled. In 2013, 1 master's awarded. *Degree requirements:* For master's, thesis or alternative. *Entrance requirements:* For master's, GRE, DVM. Additional exam requirements/recommendations for international students: Required—TOEFL (minimum score 550 paper-based). *Application deadline:* For fall admission, 1/31 priority date for domestic students, 2/1 priority date for international students. Applications are processed on a rolling basis. Application fee: $65. Electronic applications accepted. *Financial support:* In 2013–14, 2 students received support. Fellowships with full tuition reimbursements available, research assistantships with full tuition reimbursements available, scholarships/grants, traineeships, health care benefits, and unspecified assistantships available. Financial award applicants required to submit FAFSA. *Faculty research:* Veterinary pathology; pain, analgesia and anesthesia of lab animals; genetically modified animal models of cancer; transgenic animals. *Unit head:* Dr. Ronald P. Wilson, Chair, 717-531-8460, Fax: 717-531-5001, E-mail: grad-hmc@psu.edu. *Application contact:* Nannette Kirst, Program Aide, 717-531-8460, Fax: 717-531-5001, E-mail: nkirst@psu.edu.
Website: http://www.pennstatehershey.org/web/comparativemedicine/programs

Penn State University Park, Graduate School, College of Agricultural Sciences, Department of Veterinary and Biomedical Sciences, University Park, PA 16802. Offers pathobiology (MS, PhD). *Unit head:* Dr. Barbara J. Christ, Interim Dean, 814-865-2541, Fax: 814-865-3103, E-mail: ebf@psu.edu. *Application contact:* Cynthia E. Nicosia, Director of Graduate Enrollment Services, 814-865-1834, Fax: 814-863-4627, E-mail: cey1@psu.edu.
Website: http://vbs.psu.edu/

Purdue University, School of Veterinary Medicine and Graduate School, Graduate Programs in Veterinary Medicine, Department of Basic Medical Sciences, West Lafayette, IN 47907. Offers anatomy (MS, PhD); pharmacology (MS, PhD); physiology (MS, PhD). Part-time programs available. Terminal master's awarded for partial completion of doctoral program. *Degree requirements:* For master's, thesis; for doctorate, thesis/dissertation. *Entrance requirements:* For master's and doctorate, GRE General Test. Additional exam requirements/recommendations for international students: Required—TOEFL. Electronic applications accepted. *Faculty research:* Development and regeneration, tissue injury and shock, biomedical engineering, ovarian function, bone and cartilage biology, cell and molecular biology.

Purdue University, School of Veterinary Medicine and Graduate School, Graduate Programs in Veterinary Medicine, Department of Comparative Pathobiology, West Lafayette, IN 47907-2027. Offers comparative epidemiology and public health (MS); comparative epidemiology and public heath (PhD); comparative microbiology and immunology (MS, PhD); comparative pathobiology (MS, PhD); interdisciplinary studies (PhD), including microbial pathogenesis, molecular signaling and cancer biology, molecular virology; lab animal medicine (MS); veterinary anatomic pathology (MS); veterinary clinical pathology (MS). Terminal master's awarded for partial completion of doctoral program. *Degree requirements:* For master's, thesis (for some programs); for doctorate, thesis/dissertation. *Entrance requirements:* For master's and doctorate, GRE General Test. Additional exam requirements/recommendations for international students: Required—TOEFL (minimum score 575 paper-based), IELTS (minimum score 6.5), TWE (minimum score 4). Electronic applications accepted.

Purdue University, School of Veterinary Medicine and Graduate School, Graduate Programs in Veterinary Medicine, Department of Veterinary Clinical Sciences, West Lafayette, IN 47907. Offers MS, PhD. Degrees offered are post-DVM. Terminal master's awarded for partial completion of doctoral program. *Degree requirements:* For master's, thesis (for some programs); for doctorate, thesis/dissertation. *Entrance requirements:* For master's and doctorate, DVM. *Faculty research:* Flow cytometry, chemotherapy, biologic response modifiers, broncho-alveolar lavage, lithotripsy.

South Dakota State University, Graduate School, College of Agriculture and Biological Sciences, Department of Veterinary and Biomedical Sciences, Brookings, SD 57007. Offers biological sciences (MS, PhD). Part-time and evening/weekend programs available. *Degree requirements:* For master's, thesis (for some programs), oral exam; for doctorate, comprehensive exam, thesis/dissertation, preliminary oral and written exams. *Entrance requirements:* Additional exam requirements/recommendations for international students: Required—TOEFL (minimum score 525 paper-based; 71 iBT). *Faculty research:* Infectious disease, food animal, virology, immunology.

Texas A&M University, College of Veterinary Medicine and Biomedical Sciences, Program in Science and Technology Journalism, College Station, TX 77843. Offers MS. *Faculty:* 4. *Students:* 13 full-time (4 women), 3 part-time (2 women); includes 2 minority (both Hispanic/Latino), 7 international. Average age 32. 3 applicants, 100% accepted, 3 enrolled. *Degree requirements:* For master's, thesis. *Entrance requirements:* For master's, GRE General Test. Additional exam requirements/recommendations for international students: Required—TOEFL. Application fee: $50 ($75 for international students). *Expenses:* Tuition, state resident: full-time $4078; part-time $226.55 per credit hour. Tuition, nonresident: full-time $10,450; part-time $580.55 per credit hour. *Required fees:* $2328; $278.50 per credit hour. $642.45 per semester. *Financial support:* In 2013–14, research assistantships with full tuition reimbursements (averaging $13,800 per year) were awarded; fellowships and teaching assistantships also available. Financial award application deadline: 3/1; financial award applicants required to submit FAFSA. *Faculty research:* Gastroenterology, anesthesiology, nephrology and urology, cardiology, nutrition. *Unit head:* Dr. Sandee Hartsfield, Head, 979-845-9051, Fax: 979-845-6978, E-mail: shartsfield@tamu.edu. *Application contact:* Graduate Admissions, 979-845-1044, E-mail: admissions@tamu.edu.
Website: http://vetmed.tamu.edu/vscs/

Tuskegee University, Graduate Programs, College of Veterinary Medicine, Nursing and Allied Health, School of Veterinary Medicine, Tuskegee, AL 36088. Offers MS, DVM. *Degree requirements:* For master's, thesis. *Entrance requirements:* For master's, GRE General Test; for doctorate, VCAT. Additional exam requirements/recommendations for international students: Required—TOEFL (minimum score 500 paper-based). *Application deadline:* For fall admission, 7/15 for domestic students. Applications are processed on a rolling basis. Application fee: $25 ($35 for international students). *Financial support:* Application deadline: 4/15. *Unit head:* Dr. Tsegaye Habtemariam, Dean, 334-727-8174, Fax: 334-727-8177. *Application contact:* Dr. Cynthia Sellers-Simon, Vice President for Student Affairs and Enrollment Management, 334-724-4746, Fax: 334-727-5750, E-mail: sellersc@mytu.tuskegee.edu.

Université de Montréal, Faculty of Veterinary Medicine and Faculty of Graduate Studies, Graduate Programs in Veterinary Sciences, Montréal, QC H3C 3J7, Canada. Offers M Sc, PhD. *Degree requirements:* For master's, one foreign language, thesis optional. Electronic applications accepted. *Faculty research:* Animal reproduction, infectious diseases of swine, physiology of exercise in horses, viral diseases of cattle, health management and epidemiology.

University of California, Davis, School of Veterinary Medicine and Graduate Studies, Program in Preventive Veterinary Medicine, Davis, CA 95616. Offers MPVM, DVM/MPVM. Part-time programs available. *Degree requirements:* For master's, thesis. *Entrance requirements:* For master's, DVM or equivalent. Additional exam requirements/recommendations for international students: Required—TOEFL (minimum score 550 paper-based). *Faculty research:* Epidemiology, zoonoses, veterinary public health, wildlife and ecosystem health.

University of California, Davis, School of Veterinary Medicine, Residency Training Program, Davis, CA 95616. Offers Certificate. *Entrance requirements:* For degree, DVM or equivalent, 1 year of related experience. *Faculty research:* Small animal and large animal medicine, surgery, infectious diseases, pathology.

University of Florida, College of Veterinary Medicine, Graduate Program in Veterinary Medical Sciences, Gainesville, FL 32611. Offers forensic toxicology (Certificate); veterinary medical sciences (MS, PhD), including forensic toxicology (MS). Postbaccalaureate distance learning degree programs offered (no on-campus study). Terminal master's awarded for partial completion of doctoral program. *Degree requirements:* For master's, thesis; for doctorate, thesis/dissertation. *Entrance requirements:* For master's and doctorate, GRE General Test, minimum GPA of 3.0. Additional exam requirements/recommendations for international students: Required—TOEFL (minimum score 550 paper-based). Electronic applications accepted. *Expenses:* Contact institution.

University of Georgia, College of Veterinary Medicine, Department of Large Animal Medicine, Athens, GA 30602. Offers MS. Application fee is waived when completed online.

University of Georgia, College of Veterinary Medicine, Department of Population Health, Athens, GA 30602. Offers food animal medicine (MFAM); population health (MAM). *Entrance requirements:* For master's, GRE General Test. Electronic applications accepted.

University of Georgia, College of Veterinary Medicine, Department of Small Animal Medicine and Surgery, Athens, GA 30602. Offers MS.

University of Guelph, Ontario Veterinary College and Graduate Studies, Graduate Programs in Veterinary Sciences, Guelph, ON N1G 2W1, Canada. Offers M Sc, DV Sc, PhD, Diploma. *Accreditation:* AVMA (one or more programs are accredited). *Degree requirements:* For master's, thesis; for doctorate, comprehensive exam, thesis/dissertation. *Entrance requirements:* Additional exam requirements/recommendations for international students: Required—TOEFL. *Faculty research:* Veterinary and comparative medicine, biomedical sciences, population medicine, pathology, microbiology.

University of Idaho, College of Graduate Studies, College of Agricultural and Life Sciences, Department of Animal and Veterinary Science, Moscow, ID 83844-2330. Offers animal physiology (PhD); animal science (MS), including production. *Faculty:* 6 full-time. *Students:* 15 full-time, 12 part-time. Average age 30. In 2013, 3 master's, 2 doctorates awarded. *Degree requirements:* For doctorate, thesis/dissertation. *Entrance requirements:* For master's, GRE General Test, minimum GPA of 2.8; for doctorate, minimum undergraduate GPA of 2.8, graduate 3.0. *Application deadline:* For fall admission, 8/1 for domestic students; for spring admission, 12/15 for domestic students. Applications are processed on a rolling basis. Application fee: $60. Electronic applications accepted. *Expenses:* Tuition, state resident: full-time $5596; part-time $363 per credit hour. Tuition, nonresident: full-time $18,672; part-time $1089 per credit hour. *Financial support:* Research assistantships and teaching assistantships available. Financial award applicants required to submit FAFSA. *Faculty research:* Reproductive biology, muscle and growth physiology, meat science, aquaculture, ruminant nutrition. *Unit head:* Dr. Mark A. McGuire, Interim Department Head, 208-885-6345, E-mail: avs-students@uidaho.edu. *Application contact:* Stephanie Thomas, Graduate Recruitment Coordinator, 208-885-4001, Fax: 208-885-4406, E-mail: gadms@uidaho.edu.
Website: http://www.uidaho.edu/cals/avs

University of Illinois at Urbana–Champaign, College of Veterinary Medicine, Department of Comparative Biosciences, Urbana, IL 61802. Offers comparative biosciences (MS, PhD); DVM/PhD. *Students:* 12 (8 women). *Degree requirements:* For doctorate, thesis/dissertation. Application fee: $75 ($90 for international students). *Unit head:* Dr. Duncan Ferguson, Head, 217-333-2506, Fax: 217-244-1652, E-mail: dcf@illinois.edu. *Application contact:* Alice Finnigan-Bunick, Research Specialist, 217-244-5967, Fax: 217-244-1652, E-mail: abunick@illinois.edu.
Website: http://vetmed.illinois.edu/cb/

University of Illinois at Urbana–Champaign, College of Veterinary Medicine, Department of Pathobiology, Urbana, IL 61802. Offers MS, PhD, DVM/PhD. *Students:* 21 (8 women). Terminal master's awarded for partial completion of doctoral program. *Degree requirements:* For doctorate, thesis/dissertation. Application fee: $75 ($90 for international students). *Unit head:* Mark S. Kuhlenschmidt, Head, 217-333-9039, Fax: 217-244-7421, E-mail: kuhlensc@illinois.edu. *Application contact:* Paula Moxley, Administrative Aide, 217-244-8924, Fax: 217-244-7421, E-mail: pkm@illinois.edu.
Website: http://vetmed.illinois.edu/path/

University of Illinois at Urbana–Champaign, College of Veterinary Medicine, Department of Veterinary Clinical Medicine, Urbana, IL 61801. Offers MS, PhD, DVM/PhD. *Students:* 30 (22 women). *Degree requirements:* For doctorate, thesis/dissertation. Application fee: $75 ($90 for international students). *Unit head:* Karen L. Campbell, Head, 217-333-5310, Fax: 217-244-1475, E-mail: klcampbe@illinois.edu. *Application contact:* Theresa Schafroth, Office Manager, 217-244-7434, Fax: 217-244-1475, E-mail: schafrot@illinois.edu.
Website: http://vetmed.illinois.edu/vcm/

University of Kentucky, Graduate School, College of Agriculture, Food and Environment, Program in Veterinary Science, Lexington, KY 40506-0032. Offers MS, PhD. *Degree requirements:* For master's, comprehensive exam, thesis; for doctorate, comprehensive exam, thesis/dissertation. *Entrance requirements:* For master's, GRE General Test, minimum undergraduate GPA of 2.75; for doctorate, GRE General Test, minimum graduate GPA of 3.0. Additional exam requirements/recommendations for international students: Required—TOEFL (minimum score 550 paper-based). Electronic applications accepted. *Faculty research:* Microbiology, reproductive physiology, genetics, pharmacology/toxicology, parasitology.

University of Louisville, Graduate School, College of Business, Program in Equine Business, Louisville, KY 40292-0001. Offers Graduate Certificate. *Students:* 2 full-time (both women), 1 part-time (0 women). Average age 32. *Expenses:* Tuition, state resident: full-time $10,788; part-time $599 per credit hour. Tuition, nonresident: full-time $22,446; part-time $1247 per credit hour. *Required fees:* $196. Tuition and fees vary according to program and reciprocity agreements. *Unit head:* Timothy T. Capps, Director, 502-852-4846, E-mail: ttcapp01@louisville.edu. *Application contact:* Susan E. Hildebrand, Program Director, 502-852-7257, Fax: 502-852-4901, E-mail: s.hildebrand@louisville.edu.
Website: http://business.louisville.edu/equine/

University of Maryland, College Park, Academic Affairs, College of Agriculture and Natural Resources, Maryland Campus of VA/MD Regional College of Veterinary Medicine, Veterinary Medical Sciences Program, College Park, MD 20742. Offers MS, PhD. *Students:* 22 full-time (9 women); includes 1 minority (Hispanic/Latino), 15 international. 19 applicants, 32% accepted, 6 enrolled. In 2013, 4 master's, 3 doctorates awarded. *Degree requirements:* For master's, thesis, oral exam; for doctorate, thesis/dissertation, oral exam, public seminar. *Entrance requirements:* For doctorate, GRE General Test. *Application deadline:* For fall admission, 5/1 for domestic students, 2/1 for international students; for spring admission, 9/1 for domestic students, 6/1 for international students. Applications are processed on a rolling basis. Application fee: $75. Electronic applications accepted. *Expenses:* Tuition, state resident: full-time $10,314; part-time $573 per credit hour. Tuition, nonresident: full-time $22,248; part-time $1236 per credit. *Required fees:* $1446; $403.15 per semester. Tuition and fees vary according to program. *Financial support:* In 2013–14, 2 fellowships with partial tuition reimbursements (averaging $25,000 per year), 7 research assistantships (averaging $17,908 per year), 9 teaching assistantships (averaging $17,627 per year) were awarded. *Unit head:* Dr. Xiaoping Zhu, Director, 301-314-6814, Fax: 301-314-6855, E-mail: xzhu1@umd.edu. *Application contact:* Dr. Charles A. Caramello, Dean of Graduate School, 301-405-0358, Fax: 301-314-9305, E-mail: ccaramel@umd.edu.

University of Minnesota, Twin Cities Campus, College of Veterinary Medicine and Graduate School, Graduate Programs in Veterinary Medicine, Program in Comparative and Molecular Bioscience, Minneapolis, MN 55455-0213. Offers MS, PhD, DVM/PhD. Terminal master's awarded for partial completion of doctoral program. *Degree requirements:* For master's, comprehensive exam, thesis; for doctorate, comprehensive exam, thesis/dissertation. *Entrance requirements:* For master's and doctorate, GRE. Additional exam requirements/recommendations for international students: Required—TOEFL (minimum score 550 paper-based; 79 iBT). Electronic applications accepted. *Faculty research:* Molecular regulation of immunity; mechanisms of bacterial, viral, and parasite pathogenesis; structural and functional comparative physiology and pathology.

University of Minnesota, Twin Cities Campus, College of Veterinary Medicine and Graduate School, Graduate Programs in Veterinary Medicine, Program in Veterinary Medicine, Minneapolis, MN 55455-0213. Offers MS, PhD, DVM/PhD. Terminal master's awarded for partial completion of doctoral program. *Degree requirements:* For master's, comprehensive exam, thesis; for doctorate, comprehensive exam, thesis/dissertation. *Entrance requirements:* Additional exam requirements/recommendations for international students: Required—TOEFL (minimum score 550 paper-based; 79 iBT). Electronic applications accepted. *Faculty research:* Infectious diseases, internal medicine, population medicine, surgery/radiology/anesthesiology, theriogenology.

University of Missouri, College of Veterinary Medicine and Graduate School, Graduate Programs in Veterinary Medicine, Columbia, MO 65211. Offers biomedical sciences (MS, PhD), including biomedical sciences, comparative medicine (MS); veterinary medicine and surgery (MS); veterinary pathobiology (MS, PhD), including comparative medicine (MS), pathobiology; DVM/MS; DVM/PhD. *Faculty:* 112 full-time (41 women), 12 part-time/adjunct (4 women). *Students:* 43 full-time (25 women), 37 part-time (24 women); includes 9 minority (1 Black or African American, non-Hispanic/Latino; 3 Asian, non-Hispanic/Latino; 4 Hispanic/Latino; 1 Two or more races, non-Hispanic/Latino), 7 international. Average age 31. 70 applicants, 39% accepted, 23 enrolled. In 2013, 5 master's, 7 doctorates awarded. *Degree requirements:* For master's, thesis; for doctorate, 2 foreign languages, comprehensive exam, thesis/dissertation. *Entrance requirements:* For master's and doctorate, GRE General Test, minimum GPA of 3.0. Additional exam requirements/recommendations for international students: Required—TOEFL (minimum score 600 paper-based; 100 iBT). Application fee: $55 ($75 for international students). Electronic applications accepted. *Expenses:* Contact institution. *Financial support:* Fellowships with full tuition reimbursements, research assistantships with full tuition reimbursements, teaching assistantships with full tuition reimbursements, institutionally sponsored loans, scholarships/grants, traineeships, health care benefits, and unspecified assistantships available. Support available to part-time students. *Faculty research:* Exercise physiology, cardiovascular science, comparative medicine, biodefense-related organisms, vector borne infectious diseases. *Unit head:* Dr. Ronald Terjung, Associate Dean for Research and Postdoctoral Studies, 573-882-2635, E-mail: terjungr@missouri.edu. *Application contact:* Brenda Klemme, Office Support Staff III, 573-882-7305, E-mail: klemmeb@missouri.edu.
Website: http://vetmed.missouri.edu/departments.htm

University of Nebraska–Lincoln, Graduate College, College of Agricultural Sciences and Natural Resources, School of Veterinary Medicine and Biomedical Sciences, Lincoln, NE 68588. Offers veterinary science (MS). MS, PhD offered jointly with University of Nebraska Medical Center. Postbaccalaureate distance learning degree programs offered (minimal on-campus study). *Degree requirements:* For master's, thesis optional; for doctorate, comprehensive exam, thesis/dissertation. *Entrance requirements:* For master's, GRE General Test; for doctorate, GRE General Test, MCAT, or VCAT. Additional exam requirements/recommendations for international students: Required—TOEFL (minimum score 550 paper-based). Electronic applications accepted. *Faculty research:* Virology, immunobiology, molecular biology, mycotoxins, ocular degeneration.

University of Prince Edward Island, Atlantic Veterinary College, Graduate Program in Veterinary Medicine, Charlottetown, PE C1A 4P3, Canada. Offers anatomy (M Sc, PhD); bacteriology (M Sc, PhD); clinical pharmacology (M Sc, PhD); clinical sciences (M Sc, PhD); epidemiology (M Sc, PhD), including reproduction; fish health (M Sc, PhD); food animal nutrition (M Sc, PhD); immunology (M Sc, PhD); microanatomy (M Sc, PhD); parasitology (M Sc, PhD); pathology (M Sc, PhD); pharmacology (M Sc, PhD); physiology (M Sc, PhD); toxicology (M Sc, PhD); veterinary science (M Vet Sc); virology (M Sc, PhD). Part-time programs available. *Degree requirements:* For master's, thesis; for doctorate, thesis/dissertation. *Entrance requirements:* For master's, DVM, B Sc honors degree, or equivalent; for doctorate, M Sc. Additional exam requirements/recommendations for international students: Required—TOEFL (minimum score 550 paper-based; 80 iBT). *Expenses:* Contact institution. *Faculty research:* Animal health management, infectious diseases, fin fish and shellfish health, basic biomedical sciences, ecosystem health.

University of Saskatchewan, Western College of Veterinary Medicine and College of Graduate Studies and Research, Graduate Programs in Veterinary Medicine, Saskatoon, SK S7N 5A2, Canada. Offers large animal clinical sciences (M Sc, M Vet Sc, PhD); small animal clinical sciences (M Sc, M Vet Sc, PhD), including small animal clinical sciences (M Sc, PhD), veterinary anesthesiology, radiology and surgery (M Vet Sc), veterinary internal medicine (M Vet Sc); veterinary biomedical sciences (M Sc, M Vet Sc, PhD), including veterinary anatomy (M Sc), veterinary biomedical sciences (M Vet Sc), veterinary physiological sciences (M Sc, PhD); veterinary medicine (M Sc, PhD); veterinary microbiology (M Sc, M Vet Sc, PhD); veterinary pathology (M Sc, M Vet Sc, PhD). *Degree requirements:* For master's, comprehensive exam, thesis (for some programs); for doctorate, comprehensive exam, thesis/dissertation. *Entrance requirements:* Additional exam requirements/recommendations for international students: Required—TOEFL (minimum score 80 iBT) or IELTS (minimum score 6.5). Electronic applications accepted. *Expenses:* Contact institution. *Faculty research:* Reproduction, toxicology, wildlife diseases, food animal medicine, equine health.

University of Washington, Graduate School, School of Medicine, Graduate Programs in Medicine, Department of Comparative Medicine, Seattle, WA 98195. Offers MS.

University of Wisconsin–Madison, School of Veterinary Medicine, Madison, WI 53706-1380. Offers MS, DVM, PhD. *Accreditation:* AVMA (one or more programs are accredited). Terminal master's awarded for partial completion of doctoral program. *Degree requirements:* For master's, thesis; for doctorate, thesis/dissertation (for some programs). *Entrance requirements:* For doctorate, GRE General Test (for DVM). *Expenses:* Contact institution. *Faculty research:* Infectious disease, ophthalmology, orthopedics, food animal production, oncology, cardio-respiratory.

Utah State University, School of Graduate Studies, College of Agriculture, Department of Animal, Dairy and Veterinary Sciences, Logan, UT 84322. Offers animal science (MS, PhD); bioveterinary science (MS, PhD); dairy science (MS). Part-time programs available. *Degree requirements:* For master's, thesis (for some programs); for doctorate, comprehensive exam, thesis/dissertation. *Entrance requirements:* For master's and doctorate, GRE General Test, minimum GPA of 3.0. Additional exam requirements/recommendations for international students: Required—TOEFL. Electronic applications accepted. *Faculty research:* Monoclonal antibodies, antiviral chemotherapy, management systems, biotechnology, rumen fermentation manipulation.

Virginia Polytechnic Institute and State University, Virginia-Maryland Regional College of Veterinary Medicine, Blacksburg, VA 24061. Offers biomedical and veterinary sciences (MS, PhD); public health (MPH); research in translational medicine (Certificate); veterinary medicine (DVM). *Accreditation:* AVMA (one or more programs are accredited). *Faculty:* 105 full-time (45 women), 1 (woman) part-time/adjunct. *Students:* 573 full-time (428 women), 44 part-time (35 women); includes 67 minority (17 Black or African American, non-Hispanic/Latino; 13 Asian, non-Hispanic/Latino; 13 Hispanic/Latino; 1 Native Hawaiian or other Pacific Islander, non-Hispanic/Latino; 23 Two or more races, non-Hispanic/Latino), 32 international. Average age 26. 102 applicants, 69% accepted, 47 enrolled. In 2013, 14 master's, 104 doctorates awarded. *Degree requirements:* For master's, comprehensive exam (for some programs), thesis (for some programs); for doctorate, comprehensive exam (for some programs), thesis/dissertation (for some programs). *Entrance requirements:* For master's and doctorate, GRE/GMAT (may vary by department). Additional exam requirements/recommendations for international students: Required—TOEFL (minimum score 550 paper-based). *Application deadline:* For fall admission, 8/1 for domestic students, 4/1 for international students; for spring admission, 1/1 for domestic students, 9/1 for international students. Applications are processed on a rolling basis. Application fee: $75. Electronic applications accepted. *Expenses:* Contact institution. *Financial support:* In 2013–14, 1 fellowship (averaging $39,777 per year), 14 research assistantships with full tuition reimbursements (averaging $23,189 per year), 44 teaching assistantships with full tuition reimbursements (averaging $21,977 per year) were awarded. Financial award application deadline: 3/1; financial award applicants required to submit FAFSA. *Total annual research expenditures:* $6.6 million. *Unit head:* Dr. Cyril R. Clark, Dean, 540-231-7666, Fax: 540-231-7367, E-mail: cvmdean@vt.edu. *Application contact:* Shelia Steele, Executive Assistant, 540-231-7910, Fax: 540-231-7367, E-mail: ssteele@vt.edu.
Website: http://www.vetmed.vt.edu

Washington State University, College of Veterinary Medicine, Program in Veterinary Clinical Sciences, Pullman, WA 99164-7010. Offers MS. Part-time programs available. *Faculty:* 37 full-time (15 women). *Students:* 27 full-time (20 women), 7 international. Average age 30. 5 applicants, 100% accepted, 5 enrolled. In 2013, 6 master's awarded. *Degree requirements:* For master's, thesis, oral exam. *Entrance requirements:* For master's, GRE General Test, minimum GPA of 3.0, DVM or equivalent. *Application deadline:* For fall admission, 12/31 priority date for domestic students. Application fee: $75. Electronic applications accepted. *Financial support:* In 2013–14, research assistantships with full tuition reimbursements (averaging $27,816 per year) were awarded. Financial award application deadline: 3/1. *Faculty research:* Oncology, mastitis, nuclear medicine, neuroanesthesia, exercise physiology. *Total annual research expenditures:* $500,000. *Unit head:* Dr. William Dernell, Chair, 509-335-0738, Fax: 509-335-0880. *Application contact:* Kathy L. Dahmen, Administrative Manager, 509-335-4156, Fax: 509-335-0880, E-mail: dahmen@vetmed.wsu.edu.
Website: http://www.vetmed.wsu.edu/graduate/VCS/

APPENDIXES

Institutional Changes Since the 2014 Edition

Following is an alphabetical listing of institutions that have recently closed, merged with other institutions, or changed their names or status. In the case of a name change, the former name appears first, followed by the new name.

Alderson-Broaddus College (Philippi, WV): *name changed to Alderson Broaddus University*

American InterContinental University London (London, United Kingdom): *merged into Regent's University London (London, United Kingdom)*

The American University of Athens (Athens, Greece): *no longer accredited by agency recognized by USDE or CHEA*

Arizona State University (Tempe, AZ): *name changed to Arizona State University at the Tempe campus*

Armstrong Atlantic State University (Savannah, GA): *name changed to Armstrong State University*

The Art Institute of Dallas (Dallas, TX): *name changed to The Art Institute of Dallas, a campus of South University*

A.T. Still University of Health Sciences (Kirksville, MO): *name changed to A.T. Still University*

Bangor Theological Seminary (Bangor, ME): *closed*

BryanLGH College of Health Sciences (Lincoln, NE): *name changed to Bryan College of Health Sciences*

Caldwell College (Caldwell, NJ): *name changed to Caldwell University*

Calvary Baptist Theological Seminary (Landsdale, PA): *closed*

Catholic Theological Union at Chicago (Chicago, IL): *name changed to Catholic Theological Union*

Central Baptist Theological Seminary of Virginia Beach (Virginia Beach, VA): *name changed to Virginia Beach Theological Seminary*

Central State University (Wilberforce, OH): *no longer offers graduate degrees*

Chancellor University (Cleveland, OH): *closed*

Cleveland Chiropractic College–Kansas City Campus (Overland Park, KS): *name changed to Cleveland University–Kansas City*

Coe College (Cedar Rapids, IA): *no longer offers graduate degrees*

College of Mount St. Joseph (Cincinnati, OH): *name changed to Mount St. Joseph University*

Collège universitaire de Saint-Boniface (Saint-Boniface, MB, Canada): *name changed to Université de Saint-Boniface*

Colorado Technical University Sioux Falls (Sioux Falls, SD): *closed*

Conservatorio de Musica (San Juan, PR): *name changed to Conservatorio de Musica de Puerto Rico*

Conway School of Landscape Design (Conway, MA): *name changed to The Conway School*

Corcoran College of Art and Design (Washington, DC): *merged into a single entry for The George Washington University (Washington, DC)*

Davenport University (Warren, MI): *merged into a single entry for Davenport University (Grand Rapids, MI)*

DeVry University (Lincolnshire, IL): *closed*

Franklin College Switzerland (Sorengo, Switzerland): *name changed to Franklin University Switzerland*

Graduate School and University Center of the City University of New York (New York, NY): *name changed to The Graduate Center, City University of New York*

Gwynedd-Mercy College (Gwynedd Valley, PA): *name changed to Gwynedd Mercy University*

ICR Graduate School (Santee, CA): *name changed to Institute for Creation Research*

Instituto Tecnológico y de Estudios Superiores de Monterrey, Campus Mazatlán (Mazatlán, Mexico): *closed*

Jamestown College (Jamestown, ND): *name changed to University of Jamestown*

Jewish University of America (Skokie, IL): *closed*

The Johns Hopkins University (Baltimore, MD): *name changed to Johns Hopkins University*

King College (Bristol, TN): *name changed to King University*

Kona University (Kailúa-Kona, HI): *no longer accredited by agency recognized by USDE or CHEA*

Laurel University, Spanish Academic Division (Miami, FL): *closed*

Logan University–College of Chiropractic (Chesterfield, MO): *name changed to Logan University*

Long Island University–Brooklyn Campus (Brooklyn, NY): *name changed to Long Island University–LIU Brooklyn*

Long Island University–C. W. Post Campus (Brookville, NY): *name changed to Long Island University–LIU Post*

Louisiana State University and Agricultural and Mechanical College (Baton Rouge, LA): *name changed to Louisiana State University and Agricultural & Mechanical College*

Maranatha Baptist Bible College (Watertown, WI): *name changed to Maranatha Baptist University*

Mars Hill College (Mars Hill, NC): *name changed to Mars Hill University*

Massachusetts College of Pharmacy and Health Sciences (Boston, MA): *name changed to MCPHS University*

Mount Mary College (Milwaukee, WI): *name changed to Mount Mary University*

Mount Sinai School of Medicine (New York, NY): *name changed to Icahn School of Medicine at Mount Sinai*

Newschool of Architecture & Design (San Diego, CA): *name changed to NewSchool of Architecture and Design*

North Shore–LIJ Graduate School of Molecular Medicine (Manhasset, NY): *name changed to Elmezzi Graduate School of Molecular Medicine*

Northwestern College (St. Paul, MN): *name changed to University of Northwestern–St. Paul*

Oglethorpe University (Atlanta, GA): *no longer offers graduate degrees*

Perelandra College (La Mesa, CA): *no longer accredited by agency recognized by USDE or CHEA*

Polytechnic Institute of New York University (Brooklyn, NY): *Polytechnic School of Engineering now profiled as a unit of New York University (New York, NY)*

Polytechnic Institute of NYU, Long Island Graduate Center (Melville, NY): *Polytechnic School of Engineering now profiled as a unit of New York University (New York, NY)*

Polytechnic Institute of NYU, Westchester Graduate Center (Hawthorne, NY): *Polytechnic School of Engineering now profiled as a unit of New York University (New York, NY)*

Regent's American College London (London, United Kingdom): *name changed to Regent's University London*

Rockford College (Rockford, IL): *name changed to Rockford University*

Schiller International University (Strasbourg, France): *closed*

Southern California College of Optometry (Fullerton, CA): *name changed to Marshall B. Ketchum University*

Spertus Institute of Jewish Studies (Chicago, IL): *name changed to Spertus Institute for Jewish Learning and Leadership*

Tai Sophia Institute (Laurel, MD): *name changed to Maryland University of Integrative Health*

Teacher Education University (Winter Park, FL): *no longer accredited by agency recognized by USDE or CHEA*

University of Atlanta (Atlanta, GA): *no longer accredited by agency recognized by USDE or CHEA*

University of Medicine and Dentistry of New Jersey (Newark, NJ): *merged into Rutgers School of Health Related Professions with programs at Rutgers, The State University of New Jersey, Camden (Camden, NJ); Rutgers, The State University of New Jersey, Newark (Newark, NJ); Rutgers, The State University of New Jersey, New Brunswick (Piscataway, NJ); and Rowan University (Glassboro, NJ)*

University of Phoenix–Central Florida Campus (Maitland, FL): *closed*

University of Phoenix–Fairfield County Campus (Norwalk, CT): *closed*

University of Phoenix–Harrisburg Campus (Harrisburg, PA): *closed*

University of Phoenix–Metro Detroit Campus (Troy, MI): *closed*

University of Phoenix–Northern Nevada Campus (Reno, NV): *closed*

University of Phoenix–Northern Virginia Campus (Reston, VA): *closed*

University of Phoenix–Phoenix Main Campus (Tempe, AZ): *name changed to University of Phoenix–Phoenix Campus*
University of Phoenix–Raleigh Campus (Raleigh, NC): *closed*
University of Phoenix–Richmond Campus (Richmond, VA): *name changed to University of Phoenix–Richmond-Virginia Beach Campus*
University of Phoenix–Washington Campus (Tukwila, WA): *name changed to University of Phoenix–Western Washington Campus*
University of Phoenix–West Michigan Campus (Walker, MI): *closed*
University of Puerto Rico, Río Piedras (San Juan, PR): *name changed to University of Puerto Rico, Río Piedras Campus*
The University of Tennessee Space Institute (Tullahoma, TN): *merged into a single entry for The University of Tennessee (Knoxville, TN)*
University of Tulsa (Tulsa, OK): *name changed to The University of Tulsa*
Victory University (Memphis, TN): *closed*
Western State University College of Law at Argosy University (Fullerton, CA): *name changed to Western State College of Law at Argosy University*
World Medicine Institute of Acupuncture and Herbal Medicine (Honolulu, HI): *name changed to World Medicine Institute*

Abbreviations Used in the Guides

The following list includes abbreviations of degree names used in the profiles in the 2015 edition of the guides. Because some degrees (e.g., Doctor of Education) can be abbreviated in more than one way (e.g., D.Ed. or Ed.D.), and because the abbreviations used in the guides reflect the preferences of the individual colleges and universities, the list may include two or more abbreviations for a single degree.

DEGREES

A Mus D	Doctor of Musical Arts
AC	Advanced Certificate
AD	Artist's Diploma
	Doctor of Arts
ADP	Artist's Diploma
Adv C	Advanced Certificate
Adv M	Advanced Master
AGC	Advanced Graduate Certificate
AGSC	Advanced Graduate Specialist Certificate
ALM	Master of Liberal Arts
AM	Master of Arts
AMBA	Accelerated Master of Business Administration
	Aviation Master of Business Administration
AMRS	Master of Arts in Religious Studies
APC	Advanced Professional Certificate
APMPH	Advanced Professional Master of Public Health
App Sc	Applied Scientist
App Sc D	Doctor of Applied Science
AstE	Astronautical Engineer
Au D	Doctor of Audiology
B Th	Bachelor of Theology
CAES	Certificate of Advanced Educational Specialization
CAGS	Certificate of Advanced Graduate Studies
CAL	Certificate in Applied Linguistics
CALS	Certificate of Advanced Liberal Studies
CAMS	Certificate of Advanced Management Studies
CAPS	Certificate of Advanced Professional Studies
CAS	Certificate of Advanced Studies
CASPA	Certificate of Advanced Study in Public Administration
CASR	Certificate in Advanced Social Research
CATS	Certificate of Achievement in Theological Studies
CBHS	Certificate in Basic Health Sciences
CBS	Graduate Certificate in Biblical Studies
CCJA	Certificate in Criminal Justice Administration
CCSA	Certificate in Catholic School Administration
CCTS	Certificate in Clinical and Translational Science
CE	Civil Engineer
CEM	Certificate of Environmental Management
CET	Certificate in Educational Technologies
CGS	Certificate of Graduate Studies
Ch E	Chemical Engineer
CM	Certificate in Management
CMH	Certificate in Medical Humanities
CMM	Master of Church Ministries
CMS	Certificate in Ministerial Studies
CNM	Certificate in Nonprofit Management
CPASF	Certificate Program for Advanced Study in Finance
CPC	Certificate in Professional Counseling
	Certificate in Publication and Communication
CPH	Certificate in Public Health
CPM	Certificate in Public Management
CPS	Certificate of Professional Studies
CScD	Doctor of Clinical Science
CSD	Certificate in Spiritual Direction
CSS	Certificate of Special Studies
CTS	Certificate of Theological Studies
CURP	Certificate in Urban and Regional Planning
D Admin	Doctor of Administration
D Arch	Doctor of Architecture
D Be	Doctor in Bioethics
D Com	Doctor of Commerce
D Couns	Doctor of Counseling
D Div	Doctor of Divinity
D Ed	Doctor of Education
D Ed Min	Doctor of Educational Ministry
D Eng	Doctor of Engineering
D Engr	Doctor of Engineering
D Ent	Doctor of Enterprise
D Env	Doctor of Environment
D Law	Doctor of Law
D Litt	Doctor of Letters
D Med Sc	Doctor of Medical Science
D Min	Doctor of Ministry
D Miss	Doctor of Missiology
D Mus	Doctor of Music
D Mus A	Doctor of Musical Arts
D Phil	Doctor of Philosophy
D Prof	Doctor of Professional Studies
D Ps	Doctor of Psychology
D Sc	Doctor of Science
D Sc D	Doctor of Science in Dentistry
D Sc IS	Doctor of Science in Information Systems
D Sc PA	Doctor of Science in Physician Assistant Studies
D Th	Doctor of Theology
D Th P	Doctor of Practical Theology
DA	Doctor of Accounting
	Doctor of Arts
DA Ed	Doctor of Arts in Education
DAH	Doctor of Arts in Humanities
DAOM	Doctorate in Acupuncture and Oriental Medicine
DAT	Doctorate of Athletic Training
DATH	Doctorate of Art Therapy
DBA	Doctor of Business Administration
DBH	Doctor of Behavioral Health
DBL	Doctor of Business Leadership
DBS	Doctor of Buddhist Studies
DC	Doctor of Chiropractic
DCC	Doctor of Computer Science
DCD	Doctor of Communications Design

DCL	Doctor of Civil Law
	Doctor of Comparative Law
DCM	Doctor of Church Music
DCN	Doctor of Clinical Nutrition
DCS	Doctor of Computer Science
DDN	Diplôme du Droit Notarial
DDS	Doctor of Dental Surgery
DE	Doctor of Education
	Doctor of Engineering
DED	Doctor of Economic Development
DEIT	Doctor of Educational Innovation and Technology
DEL	Doctor of Executive Leadership
DEM	Doctor of Educational Ministry
DEPD	Diplôme Études Spécialisées
DES	Doctor of Engineering Science
DESS	Diplôme Études Supérieures Spécialisées
DFA	Doctor of Fine Arts
DGP	Diploma in Graduate and Professional Studies
DH Ed	Doctor of Health Education
DH Sc	Doctor of Health Sciences
DHA	Doctor of Health Administration
DHCE	Doctor of Health Care Ethics
DHL	Doctor of Hebrew Letters
	Doctor of Hebrew Literature
DHS	Doctor of Health Science
DHSc	Doctor of Health Science
Dip CS	Diploma in Christian Studies
DIT	Doctor of Industrial Technology
DJ Ed	Doctor of Jewish Education
DJS	Doctor of Jewish Studies
DLS	Doctor of Liberal Studies
DM	Doctor of Management
	Doctor of Music
DMA	Doctor of Musical Arts
DMD	Doctor of Dental Medicine
DME	Doctor of Music Education
DMEd	Doctor of Music Education
DMFT	Doctor of Marital and Family Therapy
DMH	Doctor of Medical Humanities
DML	Doctor of Modern Languages
DMP	Doctorate in Medical Physics
DMPNA	Doctor of Management Practice in Nurse Anesthesia
DN Sc	Doctor of Nursing Science
DNAP	Doctor of Nurse Anesthesia Practice
DNP	Doctor of Nursing Practice
DNP-A	Doctor of Nursing PracticeAnesthesia
DNS	Doctor of Nursing Science
DO	Doctor of Osteopathy
DOT	Doctor of Occupational Therapy
DPA	Doctor of Public Administration
DPC	Doctor of Pastoral Counseling
DPDS	Doctor of Planning and Development Studies
DPH	Doctor of Public Health
DPM	Doctor of Plant Medicine
	Doctor of Podiatric Medicine
DPPD	Doctor of Policy, Planning, and Development
DPS	Doctor of Professional Studies
DPT	Doctor of Physical Therapy
DPTSc	Doctor of Physical Therapy Science
Dr DES	Doctor of Design
Dr NP	Doctor of Nursing Practice
Dr PH	Doctor of Public Health
Dr Sc PT	Doctor of Science in Physical Therapy
DRSc	Doctor of Regulatory Science
DS	Doctor of Science
DS Sc	Doctor of Social Science
DSJS	Doctor of Science in Jewish Studies
DSL	Doctor of Strategic Leadership
DSW	Doctor of Social Work
DTL	Doctor of Talmudic Law
DV Sc	Doctor of Veterinary Science
DVM	Doctor of Veterinary Medicine
DWS	Doctor of Worship Studies
EAA	Engineer in Aeronautics and Astronautics
EASPh D	Engineering and Applied Science Doctor of Philosophy
ECS	Engineer in Computer Science
Ed D	Doctor of Education
Ed DCT	Doctor of Education in College Teaching
Ed L D	Doctor of Education Leadership
Ed M	Master of Education
Ed S	Specialist in Education
Ed Sp	Specialist in Education
EDB	Executive Doctorate in Business
EDM	Executive Doctorate in Management
EE	Electrical Engineer
EJD	Executive Juris Doctor
EMBA	Executive Master of Business Administration
EMFA	Executive Master of Forensic Accounting
EMHA	Executive Master of Health Administration
EMIB	Executive Master of International Business
EML	Executive Master of Leadership
EMPA	Executive Master of Public Administration
EMS	Executive Master of Science
EMTM	Executive Master of Technology Management
Eng	Engineer
Eng Sc D	Doctor of Engineering Science
Engr	Engineer
Ex Doc	Executive Doctor of Pharmacy
Exec Ed D	Executive Doctor of Education
Exec MBA	Executive Master of Business Administration
Exec MPA	Executive Master of Public Administration
Exec MPH	Executive Master of Public Health
Exec MS	Executive Master of Science
G Dip	Graduate Diploma
GBC	Graduate Business Certificate
GCE	Graduate Certificate in Education
GDM	Graduate Diploma in Management
GDPA	Graduate Diploma in Public Administration
GDRE	Graduate Diploma in Religious Education
GEMBA	Global Executive Master of Business Administration
GEMPA	Gulf Executive Master of Public Administration
GM Acc	Graduate Master of Accountancy
GMBA	Global Master of Business Administration
GP LL M	Global Professional Master of Laws
GPD	Graduate Performance Diploma
GSS	Graduate Special Certificate for Students in Special Situations

IEMBA	International Executive Master of Business Administration
IM Acc	Integrated Master of Accountancy
IMA	Interdisciplinary Master of Arts
IMBA	International Master of Business Administration
IMES	International Master's in Environmental Studies
Ingeniero	Engineer
JCD	Doctor of Canon Law
JCL	Licentiate in Canon Law
JD	Juris Doctor
JSD	Doctor of Juridical Science
	Doctor of Jurisprudence
	Doctor of the Science of Law
JSM	Master of Science of Law
L Th	Licenciate in Theology
LL B	Bachelor of Laws
LL CM	Master of Laws in Comparative Law
LL D	Doctor of Laws
LL M	Master of Laws
LL M in Tax	Master of Laws in Taxation
LL M CL	Master of Laws (Common Law)
M Ac	Master of Accountancy
	Master of Accounting
	Master of Acupuncture
M Ac OM	Master of Acupuncture and Oriental Medicine
M Acc	Master of Accountancy
	Master of Accounting
M Acct	Master of Accountancy
	Master of Accounting
M Accy	Master of Accountancy
M Actg	Master of Accounting
M Acy	Master of Accountancy
M Ad	Master of Administration
M Ad Ed	Master of Adult Education
M Adm	Master of Administration
M Adm Mgt	Master of Administrative Management
M Admin	Master of Administration
M ADU	Master of Architectural Design and Urbanism
M Adv	Master of Advertising
M Aero E	Master of Aerospace Engineering
M AEST	Master of Applied Environmental Science and Technology
M Ag	Master of Agriculture
M Ag Ed	Master of Agricultural Education
M Agr	Master of Agriculture
M Anesth Ed	Master of Anesthesiology Education
M App Comp Sc	Master of Applied Computer Science
M App St	Master of Applied Statistics
M Appl Stat	Master of Applied Statistics
M Aq	Master of Aquaculture
M Arc	Master of Architecture
M Arch	Master of Architecture
M Arch I	Master of Architecture I
M Arch II	Master of Architecture II
M Arch E	Master of Architectural Engineering
M Arch H	Master of Architectural History
M Bioethics	Master in Bioethics
M Biomath	Master of Biomathematics
M Ch	Master of Chemistry
M Ch E	Master of Chemical Engineering
M Chem	Master of Chemistry
M Cl D	Master of Clinical Dentistry
M Cl Sc	Master of Clinical Science
M Comp	Master of Computing
M Comp Sc	Master of Computer Science
M Coun	Master of Counseling
M Dent	Master of Dentistry
M Dent Sc	Master of Dental Sciences
M Des	Master of Design
M Des S	Master of Design Studies
M Div	Master of Divinity
M Ec	Master of Economics
M Econ	Master of Economics
M Ed	Master of Education
M Ed T	Master of Education in Teaching
M En	Master of Engineering
	Master of Environmental Science
M En S	Master of Environmental Sciences
M Eng	Master of Engineering
M Eng Mgt	Master of Engineering Management
M Engr	Master of Engineering
M Ent	Master of Enterprise
M Env	Master of Environment
M Env Des	Master of Environmental Design
M Env E	Master of Environmental Engineering
M Env Sc	Master of Environmental Science
M Fin	Master of Finance
M Geo E	Master of Geological Engineering
M Geoenv E	Master of Geoenvironmental Engineering
M Geog	Master of Geography
M Hum	Master of Humanities
M Hum Svcs	Master of Human Services
M IBD	Master of Integrated Building Delivery
M IDST	Master's in Interdisciplinary Studies
M Kin	Master of Kinesiology
M Land Arch	Master of Landscape Architecture
M Litt	Master of Letters
M Mat SE	Master of Material Science and Engineering
M Math	Master of Mathematics
M Mech E	Master of Mechanical Engineering
M Med Sc	Master of Medical Science
M Mgmt	Master of Management
M Mgt	Master of Management
M Min	Master of Ministries
M Mtl E	Master of Materials Engineering
M Mu	Master of Music
M Mus	Master of Music
M Mus Ed	Master of Music Education
M Music	Master of Music
M Nat Sci	Master of Natural Science
M Oc E	Master of Oceanographic Engineering
M Pet E	Master of Petroleum Engineering
M Pharm	Master of Pharmacy
M Phil	Master of Philosophy
M Phil F	Master of Philosophical Foundations
M Pl	Master of Planning
M Plan	Master of Planning
M Pol	Master of Political Science
M Pr Met	Master of Professional Meteorology
M Prob S	Master of Probability and Statistics
M Psych	Master of Psychology

M Pub	Master of Publishing
M Rel	Master of Religion
M Sc	Master of Science
M Sc A	Master of Science (Applied)
M Sc AC	Master of Science in Applied Computing
M Sc AHN	Master of Science in Applied Human Nutrition
M Sc BMC	Master of Science in Biomedical Communications
M Sc CS	Master of Science in Computer Science
M Sc E	Master of Science in Engineering
M Sc Eng	Master of Science in Engineering
M Sc Engr	Master of Science in Engineering
M Sc F	Master of Science in Forestry
M Sc FE	Master of Science in Forest Engineering
M Sc Geogr	Master of Science in Geography
M Sc N	Master of Science in Nursing
M Sc OT	Master of Science in Occupational Therapy
M Sc P	Master of Science in Planning
M Sc Pl	Master of Science in Planning
M Sc PT	Master of Science in Physical Therapy
M Sc T	Master of Science in Teaching
M SEM	Master of Sustainable Environmental Management
M Serv Soc	Master of Social Service
M Soc	Master of Sociology
M Sp Ed	Master of Special Education
M Stat	Master of Statistics
M Sys E	Master of Systems Engineering
M Sys Sc	Master of Systems Science
M Tax	Master of Taxation
M Tech	Master of Technology
M Th	Master of Theology
M Tox	Master of Toxicology
M Trans E	Master of Transportation Engineering
M Urb	Master of Urban Planning
M Vet Sc	Master of Veterinary Science
MA	Master of Accounting
	Master of Administration
	Master of Arts
MA Comm	Master of Arts in Communication
MA Ed	Master of Arts in Education
MA Ed Ad	Master of Arts in Educational Administration
MA Ext	Master of Agricultural Extension
MA Islamic	Master of Arts in Islamic Studies
MA Min	Master of Arts in Ministry
MA Miss	Master of Arts in Missiology
MA Past St	Master of Arts in Pastoral Studies
MA Ph	Master of Arts in Philosophy
MA Psych	Master of Arts in Psychology
MA Sc	Master of Applied Science
MA Sp	Master of Arts (Spirituality)
MA Th	Master of Arts in Theology
MA-R	Master of Arts (Research)
MAA	Master of Administrative Arts
	Master of Applied Anthropology
	Master of Applied Arts
	Master of Arts in Administration
MAAA	Master of Arts in Arts Administration
MAAAP	Master of Arts Administration and Policy
MAAE	Master of Arts in Art Education
MAAT	Master of Arts in Applied Theology
	Master of Arts in Art Therapy
MAB	Master of Agribusiness
MABC	Master of Arts in Biblical Counseling
	Master of Arts in Business Communication
MABE	Master of Arts in Bible Exposition
MABL	Master of Arts in Biblical Languages
MABM	Master of Agribusiness Management
MABMH	bioethics and medical humanities
MABS	Master of Arts in Biblical Studies
MABT	Master of Arts in Bible Teaching
MAC	Master of Accountancy
	Master of Accounting
	Master of Arts in Communication
	Master of Arts in Counseling
MACC	Master of Arts in Christian Counseling
	Master of Arts in Clinical Counseling
MACCM	Master of Arts in Church and Community Ministry
MACCT	Master of Accounting
MACD	Master of Arts in Christian Doctrine
MACE	Master of Arts in Christian Education
MACFM	Master of Arts in Children's and Family Ministry
MACH	Master of Arts in Church History
MACI	Master of Arts in Curriculum and Instruction
MACIS	Master of Accounting and Information Systems
MACJ	Master of Arts in Criminal Justice
MACL	Master of Arts in Christian Leadership
MACM	Master of Arts in Christian Ministries
	Master of Arts in Christian Ministry
	Master of Arts in Church Music
	Master of Arts in Counseling Ministries
MACN	Master of Arts in Counseling
MACO	Master of Arts in Counseling
MAcOM	Master of Acupuncture and Oriental Medicine
MACP	Master of Arts in Christian Practice
	Master of Arts in Counseling Psychology
MACS	Master of Applied Computer Science
	Master of Arts in Catholic Studies
	Master of Arts in Christian Studies
MACSE	Master of Arts in Christian School Education
MACT	Master of Arts in Christian Thought
	Master of Arts in Communications and Technology
MAD	Master of Art and Design
MAD-Crit	Master of Arts in Design Criticism
MADR	Master of Arts in Dispute Resolution
MADS	Master of Animal and Dairy Science
	Master of Applied Disability Studies
MAE	Master of Aerospace Engineering
	Master of Agricultural Economics
	Master of Agricultural Education
	Master of Architectural Engineering
	Master of Art Education
	Master of Arts in Education
	Master of Arts in English
MAEd	Master of Arts Education
MAEL	Master of Arts in Educational Leadership
MAEM	Master of Arts in Educational Ministries
MAEN	Master of Arts in English
MAEP	Master of Arts in Economic Policy

MAES	Master of Arts in Environmental Sciences
MAET	Master of Arts in English Teaching
MAF	Master of Arts in Finance
MAFE	Master of Arts in Financial Economics
MAFLL	Master of Arts in Foreign Language and Literature
MAFM	Master of Accounting and Financial Management
MAFS	Master of Arts in Family Studies
MAG	Master of Applied Geography
MAGU	Master of Urban Analysis and Management
MAH	Master of Arts in Humanities
MAHA	Master of Arts in Humanitarian Assistance
	Master of Arts in Humanitarian Studies
MAHCM	Master of Arts in Health Care Mission
MAHG	Master of American History and Government
MAHL	Master of Arts in Hebrew Letters
MAHN	Master of Applied Human Nutrition
MAHSR	Master of Applied Health Services Research
MAIA	Master of Arts in International Administration
	Master of Arts in International Affairs
MAIB	Master of Arts in International Business
MAIDM	Master of Arts in Interior Design and Merchandising
MAIH	Master of Arts in Interdisciplinary Humanities
MAIOP	Master of Arts in Industrial/Organizational Psychology
MAIPCR	Master of Arts in International Peace and Conflict Management
MAIS	Master of Arts in Intercultural Studies
	Master of Arts in Interdisciplinary Studies
	Master of Arts in International Studies
MAIT	Master of Administration in Information Technology
	Master of Applied Information Technology
MAJ	Master of Arts in Journalism
MAJ Ed	Master of Arts in Jewish Education
MAJCS	Master of Arts in Jewish Communal Service
MAJE	Master of Arts in Jewish Education
MAJPS	Master of Arts in Jewish Professional Studies
MAJS	Master of Arts in Jewish Studies
MAL	Master in Agricultural Leadership
MALA	Master of Arts in Liberal Arts
MALD	Master of Arts in Law and Diplomacy
MALER	Master of Arts in Labor and Employment Relations
MALM	Master of Arts in Leadership Evangelical Mobilization
MALP	Master of Arts in Language Pedagogy
MALPS	Master of Arts in Liberal and Professional Studies
MALS	Master of Arts in Liberal Studies
MAM	Master of Acquisition Management
	Master of Agriculture and Management
	Master of Applied Mathematics
	Master of Arts in Ministry
	Master of Arts Management
	Master of Avian Medicine
MAMB	Master of Applied Molecular Biology
MAMC	Master of Arts in Mass Communication
	Master of Arts in Ministry and Culture
	Master of Arts in Ministry for a Multicultural Church
	Master of Arts in Missional Christianity
MAME	Master of Arts in Missions/Evangelism
MAMFC	Master of Arts in Marriage and Family Counseling
MAMFCC	Master of Arts in Marriage, Family, and Child Counseling
MAMFT	Master of Arts in Marriage and Family Therapy
MAMHC	Master of Arts in Mental Health Counseling
MAMI	Master of Arts in Missions
MAMS	Master of Applied Mathematical Sciences
	Master of Arts in Ministerial Studies
	Master of Arts in Ministry and Spirituality
MAMT	Master of Arts in Mathematics Teaching
MAN	Master of Applied Nutrition
MANT	Master of Arts in New Testament
MAOL	Master of Arts in Organizational Leadership
MAOM	Master of Acupuncture and Oriental Medicine
	Master of Arts in Organizational Management
MAOT	Master of Arts in Old Testament
MAP	Master of Applied Psychology
	Master of Arts in Planning
	Master of Psychology
	Master of Public Administration
MAP Min	Master of Arts in Pastoral Ministry
MAPA	Master of Arts in Public Administration
MAPC	Master of Arts in Pastoral Counseling
	Master of Arts in Professional Counseling
MAPE	Master of Arts in Political Economy
MAPM	Master of Arts in Pastoral Ministry
	Master of Arts in Pastoral Music
	Master of Arts in Practical Ministry
MAPP	Master of Arts in Public Policy
MAPPS	Master of Arts in Asia Pacific Policy Studies
MAPS	Master of Arts in Pastoral Counseling/Spiritual Formation
	Master of Arts in Pastoral Studies
	Master of Arts in Public Service
MAPT	Master of Practical Theology
MAPW	Master of Arts in Professional Writing
MAR	Master of Arts in Reading
	Master of Arts in Religion
Mar Eng	Marine Engineer
MARC	Master of Arts in Rehabilitation Counseling
MARE	Master of Arts in Religious Education
MARL	Master of Arts in Religious Leadership
MARS	Master of Arts in Religious Studies
MAS	Master of Accounting Science
	Master of Actuarial Science
	Master of Administrative Science
	Master of Advanced Study
	Master of Aeronautical Science
	Master of American Studies
	Master of Applied Science
	Master of Applied Statistics
	Master of Archival Studies
MASA	Master of Advanced Studies in Architecture
MASD	Master of Arts in Spiritual Direction
MASE	Master of Arts in Special Education

MASF	Master of Arts in Spiritual Formation
MASJ	Master of Arts in Systems of Justice
MASLA	Master of Advanced Studies in Landscape Architecture
MASM	Master of Aging Services Management
	Master of Arts in Specialized Ministries
MASP	Master of Applied Social Psychology
	Master of Arts in School Psychology
MASPAA	Master of Arts in Sports and Athletic Administration
MASS	Master of Applied Social Science
	Master of Arts in Social Science
MAST	Master of Arts in Science Teaching
MASW	Master of Aboriginal Social Work
MAT	Master of Arts in Teaching
	Master of Arts in Theology
	Master of Athletic Training
	Master's in Administration of Telecommunications
Mat E	Materials Engineer
MATCM	Master of Acupuncture and Traditional Chinese Medicine
MATDE	Master of Arts in Theology, Development, and Evangelism
MATDR	Master of Territorial Management and Regional Development
MATE	Master of Arts for the Teaching of English
MATESL	Master of Arts in Teaching English as a Second Language
MATESOL	Master of Arts in Teaching English to Speakers of Other Languages
MATF	Master of Arts in Teaching English as a Foreign Language/Intercultural Studies
MATFL	Master of Arts in Teaching Foreign Language
MATH	Master of Arts in Therapy
MATI	Master of Administration of Information Technology
MATL	Master of Arts in Teacher Leadership
	Master of Arts in Teaching of Languages
	Master of Arts in Transformational Leadership
MATM	Master of Arts in Teaching of Mathematics
MATS	Master of Arts in Theological Studies
	Master of Arts in Transforming Spirituality
MATSL	Master of Arts in Teaching a Second Language
MAUA	Master of Arts in Urban Affairs
MAUD	Master of Arts in Urban Design
MAURP	Master of Arts in Urban and Regional Planning
MAWSHP	Master of Arts in Worship
MAYM	Master of Arts in Youth Ministry
MB	Master of Bioinformatics
	Master of Biology
MBA	Master of Business Administration
MBA-AM	Master of Business Administration in Aviation Management
MBA-EP	Master of Business Administration–Experienced Professionals
MBA/MGPS	Master of Business Administration/Master of Global Policy Studies
MBAA	Master of Business Administration in Aviation
MBAE	Master of Biological and Agricultural Engineering
	Master of Biosystems and Agricultural Engineering
MBAH	Master of Business Administration in Health
MBAi	Master of Business Administration–International
MBAICT	Master of Business Administration in Information and Communication Technology
MBATM	Master of Business Administration in Technology Management
MBC	Master of Building Construction
MBE	Master of Bilingual Education
	Master of Bioengineering
	Master of Bioethics
	Master of Biological Engineering
	Master of Biomedical Engineering
	Master of Business and Engineering
	Master of Business Economics
	Master of Business Education
MBEE	Master in Biotechnology Enterprise and Entrepreneurship
MBET	Master of Business, Entrepreneurship and Technology
MBIOT	Master of Biotechnology
MBiotech	Master of Biotechnology
MBL	Master of Business Law
	Master of Business Leadership
MBLE	Master in Business Logistics Engineering
MBMI	Master of Biomedical Imaging and Signals
MBMSE	Master of Business Management and Software Engineering
MBOE	Master of Business Operational Excellence
MBS	Master of Biblical Studies
	Master of Biological Science
	Master of Biomedical Sciences
	Master of Bioscience
	Master of Building Science
	Master of Business and Science
MBST	Master of Biostatistics
MBT	Master of Biblical and Theological Studies
	Master of Biomedical Technology
	Master of Biotechnology
	Master of Business Taxation
MC	Master of Communication
	Master of Counseling
	Master of Cybersecurity
MC Ed	Master of Continuing Education
MC Sc	Master of Computer Science
MCA	Master of Arts in Applied Criminology
	Master of Commercial Aviation
MCAM	Master of Computational and Applied Mathematics
MCC	Master of Computer Science
MCCS	Master of Crop and Soil Sciences
MCD	Master of Communications Disorders
	Master of Community Development
MCE	Master in Electronic Commerce
	Master of Christian Education
	Master of Civil Engineering
	Master of Control Engineering
MCEM	Master of Construction Engineering Management

MCH	Master of Chemical Engineering
MCHE	Master of Chemical Engineering
MCIS	Master of Communication and Information Studies
	Master of Computer and Information Science
	Master of Computer Information Systems
MCIT	Master of Computer and Information Technology
MCJ	Master of Criminal Justice
MCJA	Master of Criminal Justice Administration
MCL	Master in Communication Leadership
	Master of Canon Law
	Master of Comparative Law
MCM	Master of Christian Ministry
	Master of Church Music
	Master of City Management
	Master of Communication Management
	Master of Community Medicine
	Master of Construction Management
	Master of Contract Management
	Master of Corporate Media
MCMP	Master of City and Metropolitan Planning
MCMS	Master of Clinical Medical Science
MCN	Master of Clinical Nutrition
MCOL	Master of Arts in Community and Organizational Leadership
MCP	Master of City Planning
	Master of Community Planning
	Master of Counseling Psychology
	Master of Cytopathology Practice
	Master of Science in Quality Systems and Productivity
MCPC	Master of Arts in Chaplaincy and Pastoral Care
MCPD	Master of Community Planning and Development
MCR	Master in Clinical Research
MCRP	Master of City and Regional Planning
MCRS	Master of City and Regional Studies
MCS	Master of Christian Studies
	Master of Clinical Science
	Master of Combined Sciences
	Master of Communication Studies
	Master of Computer Science
	Master of Consumer Science
MCSE	Master of Computer Science and Engineering
MCSL	Master of Catholic School Leadership
MCSM	Master of Construction Science/ Management
MCST	Master of Science in Computer Science and Information Technology
MCTP	Master of Communication Technology and Policy
MCTS	Master of Clinical and Translational Science
MCVS	Master of Cardiovascular Science
MD	Doctor of Medicine
MDA	Master of Development Administration
	Master of Dietetic Administration
MDB	Master of Design-Build
MDE	Master of Developmental Economics
	Master of Distance Education
	Master of the Education of the Deaf
MDH	Master of Dental Hygiene
MDM	Master of Design Methods
	Master of Digital Media
MDP	Master in Sustainable Development Practice
	Master of Development Practice
MDR	Master of Dispute Resolution
MDS	Master of Dental Surgery
	Master of Design Studies
ME	Master of Education
	Master of Engineering
	Master of Entrepreneurship
	Master of Evangelism
ME Sc	Master of Engineering Science
MEA	Master of Educational Administration
	Master of Engineering Administration
MEAP	Master of Environmental Administration and Planning
MEBT	Master in Electronic Business Technologies
MEC	Master of Electronic Commerce
MECE	Master of Electrical and Computer Engineering
Mech E	Mechanical Engineer
MED	Master of Education of the Deaf
MEDS	Master of Environmental Design Studies
MEE	Master in Education
	Master of Electrical Engineering
	Master of Energy Engineering
	Master of Environmental Engineering
MEEM	Master of Environmental Engineering and Management
MEENE	Master of Engineering in Environmental Engineering
MEEP	Master of Environmental and Energy Policy
MEERM	Master of Earth and Environmental Resource Management
MEH	Master in Humanistic Studies
	Master of Environmental Horticulture
MEHP	Master of Education in the Health Professions
MEHS	Master of Environmental Health and Safety
MEIM	Master of Entertainment Industry Management
MEL	Master of Educational Leadership
	Master of English Literature
MELP	Master of Environmental Law and Policy
MEM	Master of Ecosystem Management
	Master of Electricity Markets
	Master of Engineering Management
	Master of Environmental Management
	Master of Marketing
MEME	Master of Engineering in Manufacturing Engineering
	Master of Engineering in Mechanical Engineering
MENG	Master of Arts in English
MENVEGR	Master of Environmental Engineering
MEP	Master of Engineering Physics
MEPC	Master of Environmental Pollution Control
MEPD	Master of EducationNProfessional Development
	Master of Environmental Planning and Design
MER	Master of Employment Relations
MERE	Master of Entrepreneurial Real Estate

MES	Master of Education and Science
	Master of Engineering Science
	Master of Environment and Sustainability
	Master of Environmental Science
	Master of Environmental Studies
	Master of Environmental Systems
	Master of Special Education
MESM	Master of Environmental Science and Management
MET	Master of Educational Technology
	Master of Engineering Technology
	Master of Entertainment Technology
	Master of Environmental Toxicology
METM	Master of Engineering and Technology Management
MEVE	Master of Environmental Engineering
MF	Master of Finance
	Master of Forestry
MFA	Master of Fine Arts
MFAM	Master in Food Animal Medicine
MFAS	Master of Fisheries and Aquatic Science
MFAW	Master of Fine Arts in Writing
MFC	Master of Forest Conservation
MFCS	Master of Family and Consumer Sciences
MFE	Master of Financial Economics
	Master of Financial Engineering
	Master of Forest Engineering
MFG	Master of Functional Genomics
MFHD	Master of Family and Human Development
MFM	Master of Financial Management
	Master of Financial Mathematics
MFMS	Master's in Food Microbiology and Safety
MFPE	Master of Food Process Engineering
MFR	Master of Forest Resources
MFRC	Master of Forest Resources and Conservation
MFS	Master of Food Science
	Master of Forensic Sciences
	Master of Forest Science
	Master of Forest Studies
	Master of French Studies
MFST	Master of Food Safety and Technology
MFT	Master of Family Therapy
	Master of Food Technology
MFWB	Master of Fishery and Wildlife Biology
MFWCB	Master of Fish, Wildlife and Conservation Biology
MFWS	Master of Fisheries and Wildlife Sciences
MFYCS	Master of Family, Youth and Community Sciences
MG	Master of Genetics
MGA	Master of Global Affairs
	Master of Governmental Administration
MGC	Master of Genetic Counseling
MGD	Master of Graphic Design
MGE	Master of Geotechnical Engineering
MGEM	Master of Global Entrepreneurship and Management
MGIS	Master of Geographic Information Science
	Master of Geographic Information Systems
MGM	Master of Global Management
MGP	Master of Gestion de Projet
MGPS	Master of Global Policy Studies
MGPS/MA	Master of Global Policy Studies/Master of Arts
MGPS/MPH	Master of Global Policy Studies/Master of Public Health
MGREM	Master of Global Real Estate Management
MGS	Master of Gerontological Studies
	Master of Global Studies
MH	Master of Humanities
MH Ed	Master of Health Education
MH Sc	Master of Health Sciences
MHA	Master of Health Administration
	Master of Healthcare Administration
	Master of Hospital Administration
	Master of Hospitality Administration
MHAD	Master of Health Administration
MHB	Master of Human Behavior
MHCA	Master of Health Care Administration
MHCI	Master of Health Care Informatics
	Master of Human-Computer Interaction
MHCL	Master of Health Care Leadership
MHE	Master of Health Education
	Master of Human Ecology
MHE Ed	Master of Home Economics Education
MHEA	Master of Higher Education Administration
MHHS	Master of Health and Human Services
MHI	Master of Health Informatics
	Master of Healthcare Innovation
MHIIM	Master of Health Informatics and Information Management
MHIS	Master of Health Information Systems
MHK	Master of Human Kinetics
MHL	Master of Hebrew Literature
MHM	Master of Healthcare Management
MHMS	Master of Health Management Systems
MHP	Master of Health Physics
	Master of Heritage Preservation
	Master of Historic Preservation
MHPA	Master of Heath Policy and Administration
MHPE	Master of Health Professions Education
MHR	Master of Human Resources
MHRD	Master in Human Resource Development
MHRIR	Master of Human Resources and Industrial Relations
MHRLR	Master of Human Resources and Labor Relations
MHRM	Master of Human Resources Management
MHS	Master of Health Science
	Master of Health Sciences
	Master of Health Studies
	Master of Hispanic Studies
	Master of Human Services
	Master of Humanistic Studies
MHSA	Master of Health Services Administration
MHSM	Master of Health Systems Management
MI	Master of Information
	Master of Instruction
MI Arch	Master of Interior Architecture
MIA	Master of Interior Architecture
	Master of International Affairs
MIAA	Master of International Affairs and Administration
MIAM	Master of International Agribusiness Management

MIAPD	Master of Interior Architecture and Product Design
MIB	Master of International Business
MIBA	Master of International Business Administration
MICM	Master of International Construction Management
MID	Master of Industrial Design
	Master of Industrial Distribution
	Master of Interior Design
	Master of International Development
MIDC	Master of Integrated Design and Construction
MIE	Master of Industrial Engineering
MIH	Master of Integrative Health
MIHTM	Master of International Hospitality and Tourism Management
MIJ	Master of International Journalism
MILR	Master of Industrial and Labor Relations
MiM	Master in Management
MIM	Master of Industrial Management
	Master of Information Management
	Master of International Management
MIMLAE	Master of International Management for Latin American Executives
MIMS	Master of Information Management and Systems
	Master of Integrated Manufacturing Systems
MIP	Master of Infrastructure Planning
	Master of Intellectual Property
	Master of International Policy
MIPA	Master of International Public Affairs
MIPER	Master of International Political Economy of Resources
MIPP	Master of International Policy and Practice
	Master of International Public Policy
MIPS	Master of International Planning Studies
MIR	Master of Industrial Relations
	Master of International Relations
MIRHR	Master of Industrial Relations and Human Resources
MIS	Master of Industrial Statistics
	Master of Information Science
	Master of Information Systems
	Master of Integrated Science
	Master of Interdisciplinary Studies
	Master of International Service
	Master of International Studies
MISE	Master of Industrial and Systems Engineering
MISKM	Master of Information Sciences and Knowledge Management
MISM	Master of Information Systems Management
MIT	Master in Teaching
	Master of Industrial Technology
	Master of Information Technology
	Master of Initial Teaching
	Master of International Trade
	Master of Internet Technology
MITA	Master of Information Technology Administration
MITM	Master of Information Technology and Management
MITO	Master of Industrial Technology and Operations
MJ	Master of Journalism
	Master of Jurisprudence
MJ Ed	Master of Jewish Education
MJA	Master of Justice Administration
MJM	Master of Justice Management
MJS	Master of Judicial Studies
	Master of Juridical Science
MKM	Master of Knowledge Management
ML	Master of Latin
ML Arch	Master of Landscape Architecture
MLA	Master of Landscape Architecture
	Master of Liberal Arts
MLAS	Master of Laboratory Animal Science
	Master of Liberal Arts and Sciences
MLAUD	Master of Landscape Architecture in Urban Development
MLD	Master of Leadership Development
MLE	Master of Applied Linguistics and Exegesis
MLER	Master of Labor and Employment Relations
MLHR	Master of Labor and Human Resources
MLI Sc	Master of Library and Information Science
MLIS	Master of Library and Information Science
	Master of Library and Information Studies
MLM	Master of Library Media
MLRHR	Master of Labor Relations and Human Resources
MLS	Master of Leadership Studies
	Master of Legal Studies
	Master of Liberal Studies
	Master of Library Science
	Master of Life Sciences
MLSP	Master of Law and Social Policy
MLT	Master of Language Technologies
MLTCA	Master of Long Term Care Administration
MM	Master of Management
	Master of Ministry
	Master of Missiology
	Master of Music
MM Ed	Master of Music Education
MM Sc	Master of Medical Science
MM St	Master of Museum Studies
MMA	Master of Marine Affairs
	Master of Media Arts
	Master of Musical Arts
MMAE	Master of Mechanical and Aerospace Engineering
MMAL	Master of Maritime Administration and Logistics
MMAS	Master of Military Art and Science
MMB	Master of Microbial Biotechnology
MMBA	Managerial Master of Business Administration
MMC	Master of Manufacturing Competitiveness
	Master of Mass Communications
	Master of Music Conducting
MMCM	Master of Music in Church Music
MMCSS	Master of Mathematical Computational and Statistical Sciences
MME	Master of Manufacturing Engineering
	Master of Mathematics Education
	Master of Mathematics for Educators
	Master of Mechanical Engineering
	Master of Medical Engineering

	Master of Mining Engineering
	Master of Music Education
MMF	Master of Mathematical Finance
MMFT	Master of Marriage and Family Therapy
MMG	Master of Management
MMH	Master of Management in Hospitality
	Master of Medical Humanities
MMI	Master of Management of Innovation
MMIS	Master of Management Information Systems
MMM	Master of Manufacturing Management
	Master of Marine Management
	Master of Medical Management
MMME	Master of Metallurgical and Materials Engineering
MMP	Master of Management Practice
	Master of Marine Policy
	Master of Medical Physics
	Master of Music Performance
MMPA	Master of Management and Professional Accounting
MMQM	Master of Manufacturing Quality Management
MMR	Master of Marketing Research
MMRM	Master of Marine Resources Management
MMS	Master of Management Science
	Master of Management Studies
	Master of Manufacturing Systems
	Master of Marine Studies
	Master of Materials Science
	Master of Medical Science
	Master of Medieval Studies
MMSE	Master of Manufacturing Systems Engineering
	Multidisciplinary Master of Science in Engineering
MMSM	Master of Music in Sacred Music
MMT	Master in Marketing
	Master of Music Teaching
	Master of Music Therapy
	Master's in Marketing Technology
MMus	Master of Music
MN	Master of Nursing
	Master of Nutrition
MN NP	Master of Nursing in Nurse Practitioner
MNA	Master of Nonprofit Administration
	Master of Nurse Anesthesia
MNAL	Master of Nonprofit Administration and Leadership
MNAS	Master of Natural and Applied Science
MNCM	Master of Network and Communications Management
MNE	Master of Network Engineering
	Master of Nuclear Engineering
MNL	Master in International Business for Latin America
MNM	Master of Nonprofit Management
MNO	Master of Nonprofit Organization
MNPL	Master of Not-for-Profit Leadership
MNpS	Master of Nonprofit Studies
MNR	Master of Natural Resources
MNRES	Master of Natural Resources and Environmental Studies
MNRM	Master of Natural Resource Management
MNRS	Master of Natural Resource Stewardship
MNS	Master of Natural Science
MO	Master of Oceanography
MOD	Master of Organizational Development
MOGS	Master of Oil and Gas Studies
MOH	Master of Occupational Health
MOL	Master of Organizational Leadership
MOM	Master of Oriental Medicine
MOR	Master of Operations Research
MOT	Master of Occupational Therapy
MP	Master of Physiology
	Master of Planning
MP Ac	Master of Professional Accountancy
MP Acc	Master of Professional Accountancy
	Master of Professional Accounting
	Master of Public Accounting
MP Aff	Master of Public Affairs
MP Aff/MPH	Master of Public Affairs/Master of Public Health
MP Th	Master of Pastoral Theology
MPA	Master of Physician Assistant
	Master of Professional Accountancy
	Master of Professional Accounting
	Master of Public Administration
	Master of Public Affairs
MPAC	Master of Professional Accounting
MPAID	Master of Public Administration and International Development
MPAP	Master of Physician Assistant Practice
	Master of Public Affairs and Politics
MPAS	Master of Physician Assistant Science
	Master of Physician Assistant Studies
MPC	Master of Pastoral Counseling
	Master of Professional Communication
	Master of Professional Counseling
MPCU	Master of Planning in Civic Urbanism
MPD	Master of Product Development
	Master of Public Diplomacy
MPDS	Master of Planning and Development Studies
MPE	Master of Physical Education
	Master of Power Engineering
MPEM	Master of Project Engineering and Management
MPH	Master of Public Health
MPHE	Master of Public Health Education
MPHTM	Master of Public Health and Tropical Medicine
MPI	Master of Product Innovation
MPIA	Master in International Affairs
	Master of Public and International Affairs
MPM	Master of Pastoral Ministry
	Master of Pest Management
	Master of Policy Management
	Master of Practical Ministries
	Master of Project Management
	Master of Public Management
MPNA	Master of Public and Nonprofit Administration
MPO	Master of Prosthetics and Orthotics
MPOD	Master of Positive Organizational Development
MPP	Master of Public Policy
MPPA	Master of Public Policy Administration

	Master of Public Policy and Administration
MPPAL	Master of Public Policy, Administration and Law
MPPM	Master of Public and Private Management
	Master of Public Policy and Management
MPPPM	Master of Plant Protection and Pest Management
MPRTM	Master of Parks, Recreation, and Tourism Management
MPS	Master of Pastoral Studies
	Master of Perfusion Science
	Master of Planning Studies
	Master of Political Science
	Master of Preservation Studies
	Master of Professional Studies
	Master of Public Service
MPSA	Master of Public Service Administration
MPSRE	Master of Professional Studies in Real Estate
MPT	Master of Pastoral Theology
	Master of Physical Therapy
	Master of Practical Theology
MPVM	Master of Preventive Veterinary Medicine
MPW	Master of Professional Writing
	Master of Public Works
MQM	Master of Quality Management
MQS	Master of Quality Systems
MR	Master of Recreation
	Master of Retailing
MRA	Master in Research Administration
MRC	Master of Rehabilitation Counseling
MRCP	Master of Regional and City Planning
	Master of Regional and Community Planning
MRD	Master of Rural Development
MRE	Master of Real Estate
	Master of Religious Education
MRED	Master of Real Estate Development
MREM	Master of Resource and Environmental Management
MRLS	Master of Resources Law Studies
MRM	Master of Resources Management
MRP	Master of Regional Planning
MRS	Master of Religious Studies
MRSc	Master of Rehabilitation Science
MS	Master of Science
MS Cmp E	Master of Science in Computer Engineering
MS Kin	Master of Science in Kinesiology
MS Acct	Master of Science in Accounting
MS Accy	Master of Science in Accountancy
MS Aero E	Master of Science in Aerospace Engineering
MS Ag	Master of Science in Agriculture
MS Arch	Master of Science in Architecture
MS Arch St	Master of Science in Architectural Studies
MS Bio E	Master of Science in Bioengineering
	Master of Science in Biomedical Engineering
MS Bm E	Master of Science in Biomedical Engineering
MS Ch E	Master of Science in Chemical Engineering
MS Chem	Master of Science in Chemistry
MS Cp E	Master of Science in Computer Engineering
MS Eco	Master of Science in Economics
MS Econ	Master of Science in Economics
MS Ed	Master of Science in Education
MS El	Master of Science in Educational Leadership and Administration
MS En E	Master of Science in Environmental Engineering
MS Eng	Master of Science in Engineering
MS Engr	Master of Science in Engineering
MS Env E	Master of Science in Environmental Engineering
MS Exp Surg	Master of Science in Experimental Surgery
MS Int A	Master of Science in International Affairs
MS Mat E	Master of Science in Materials Engineering
MS Mat SE	Master of Science in Material Science and Engineering
MS Met E	Master of Science in Metallurgical Engineering
MS Mgt	Master of Science in Management
MS Min	Master of Science in Mining
MS Min E	Master of Science in Mining Engineering
MS Mt E	Master of Science in Materials Engineering
MS Otal	Master of Science in Otalrynology
MS Pet E	Master of Science in Petroleum Engineering
MS Phys	Master of Science in Physics
MS Poly	Master of Science in Polymers
MS Psy	Master of Science in Psychology
MS Pub P	Master of Science in Public Policy
MS Sc	Master of Science in Social Science
MS Sp Ed	Master of Science in Special Education
MS Stat	Master of Science in Statistics
MS Surg	Master of Science in Surgery
MS Tax	Master of Science in Taxation
MS Tc E	Master of Science in Telecommunications Engineering
MS-R	Master of Science (Research)
MS/CAGS	Master of Science/Certificate of Advanced Graduate Studies
MSA	Master of School Administration
	Master of Science Administration
	Master of Science in Accountancy
	Master of Science in Accounting
	Master of Science in Administration
	Master of Science in Aeronautics
	Master of Science in Agriculture
	Master of Science in Anesthesia
	Master of Science in Architecture
	Master of Science in Aviation
	Master of Sports Administration
MSA Phy	Master of Science in Applied Physics
MSAA	Master of Science in Astronautics and Aeronautics
MSAAE	Master of Science in Aeronautical and Astronautical Engineering
MSABE	Master of Science in Agricultural and Biological Engineering
MSAC	Master of Science in Acupuncture
MSACC	Master of Science in Accounting
MSAE	Master of Science in Aeronautical Engineering
	Master of Science in Aerospace Engineering
	Master of Science in Applied Economics
	Master of Science in Applied Engineering
	Master of Science in Architectural Engineering
MSAH	Master of Science in Allied Health

MSAL	Master of Sport Administration and Leadership
MSAM	Master of Science in Applied Mathematics
MSANR	Master of Science in Agriculture and Natural Resources Systems Management
MSAPM	Master of Security Analysis and Portfolio Management
MSAS	Master of Science in Applied Statistics
	Master of Science in Architectural Studies
MSAT	Master of Science in Accounting and Taxation
	Master of Science in Advanced Technology
	Master of Science in Athletic Training
MSB	Master of Science in Bible
	Master of Science in Biotechnology
	Master of Science in Business
	Master of Sustainable Business
MSBA	Master of Science in Business Administration
	Master of Science in Business Analysis
MSBAE	Master of Science in Biological and Agricultural Engineering
	Master of Science in Biosystems and Agricultural Engineering
MSBC	Master of Science in Building Construction
MSBCB	bioinformatics and computational biology
MSBE	Master of Science in Biological Engineering
	Master of Science in Biomedical Engineering
MSBENG	Master of Science in Bioengineering
MSBIT	Master of Science in Business Information Technology
MSBM	Master of Sport Business Management
MSBME	Master of Science in Biomedical Engineering
MSBMS	Master of Science in Basic Medical Science
MSBS	Master of Science in Biomedical Sciences
MSC	Master of Science in Commerce
	Master of Science in Communication
	Master of Science in Computers
	Master of Science in Counseling
	Master of Science in Criminology
MSCC	Master of Science in Christian Counseling
	Master of Science in Community Counseling
MSCD	Master of Science in Communication Disorders
	Master of Science in Community Development
MSCE	Master of Science in Civil Engineering
	Master of Science in Clinical Epidemiology
	Master of Science in Computer Engineering
	Master of Science in Continuing Education
MSCEE	Master of Science in Civil and Environmental Engineering
MSCF	Master of Science in Computational Finance
MSCH	Master of Science in Chemical Engineering
MSChE	Master of Science in Chemical Engineering
MSCI	Master of Science in Clinical Investigation
	Master of Science in Curriculum and Instruction
MSCIS	Master of Science in Computer and Information Systems
	Master of Science in Computer Information Science
	Master of Science in Computer Information Systems
MSCIT	Master of Science in Computer Information Technology
MSCJ	Master of Science in Criminal Justice
MSCJA	Master of Science in Criminal Justice Administration
MSCJS	Master of Science in Crime and Justice Studies
MSCLS	Master of Science in Clinical Laboratory Studies
MSCM	Master of Science in Church Management
	Master of Science in Conflict Management
	Master of Science in Construction Management
MScM	Master of Science in Management
MSCM	Master of Supply Chain Management
MSCNU	Master of Science in Clinical Nutrition
MSCP	Master of Science in Clinical Psychology
	Master of Science in Community Psychology
	Master of Science in Computer Engineering
	Master of Science in Counseling Psychology
MSCPE	Master of Science in Computer Engineering
MSCPharm	Master of Science in Pharmacy
MSCPI	Master in Strategic Planning for Critical Infrastructures
MSCR	Master of Science in Clinical Research
MSCRP	Master of Science in City and Regional Planning
	Master of Science in Community and Regional Planning
MSCRP/MP Aff	Master of Science in Community and Regional Planning/Master of Public Affairs
MSCRP/MSSD	Master of Science in Community and Regional Planning/Master of Science in Sustainable Design
MSCRP/MSUD	Master of Science in Community and Regional Planning/Masters of Science in Urban Design
MSCS	Master of Science in Clinical Science
	Master of Science in Computer Science
MSCSD	Master of Science in Communication Sciences and Disorders
MSCSE	Master of Science in Computer Science and Engineering
MSCTE	Master of Science in Career and Technical Education
MSD	Master of Science in Dentistry
	Master of Science in Design
	Master of Science in Dietetics
MSE	Master of Science Education
	Master of Science in Economics
	Master of Science in Education
	Master of Science in Engineering
	Master of Science in Engineering Management
	Master of Software Engineering
	Master of Special Education
	Master of Structural Engineering
MSECE	Master of Science in Electrical and Computer Engineering
MSED	Master of Sustainable Economic Development
MSEE	Master of Science in Electrical Engineering
	Master of Science in Environmental Engineering
MSEH	Master of Science in Environmental Health
MSEL	Master of Science in Educational Leadership

MSEM	Master of Science in Engineering Management
	Master of Science in Engineering Mechanics
	Master of Science in Environmental Management
MSENE	Master of Science in Environmental Engineering
MSEO	Master of Science in Electro-Optics
MSEP	Master of Science in Economic Policy
MSEPA	Master of Science in Economics and Policy Analysis
MSES	Master of Science in Embedded Software Engineering
	Master of Science in Engineering Science
	Master of Science in Environmental Science
	Master of Science in Environmental Studies
MSESM	Master of Science in Engineering Science and Mechanics
MSET	Master of Science in Educational Technology
	Master of Science in Engineering Technology
MSEV	Master of Science in Environmental Engineering
MSEVH	Master of Science in Environmental Health and Safety
MSF	Master of Science in Finance
	Master of Science in Forestry
	Master of Spiritual Formation
MSFA	Master of Science in Financial Analysis
MSFAM	Master of Science in Family Studies
MSFCS	Master of Science in Family and Consumer Science
MSFE	Master of Science in Financial Engineering
MSFOR	Master of Science in Forestry
MSFP	Master of Science in Financial Planning
MSFS	Master of Science in Financial Sciences
	Master of Science in Forensic Science
MSFSB	Master of Science in Financial Services and Banking
MSFT	Master of Science in Family Therapy
MSGC	Master of Science in Genetic Counseling
MSH	Master of Science in Health
	Master of Science in Hospice
MSHA	Master of Science in Health Administration
MSHCA	Master of Science in Health Care Administration
MSHCI	Master of Science in Human Computer Interaction
MSHCPM	Master of Science in Health Care Policy and Management
MSHE	Master of Science in Health Education
MSHES	Master of Science in Human Environmental Sciences
MSHFID	Master of Science in Human Factors in Information Design
MSHFS	Master of Science in Human Factors and Systems
MSHI	Master of Science in Health Informatics
MSHP	Master of Science in Health Professions
	Master of Science in Health Promotion
MSHR	Master of Science in Human Resources
MSHRL	Master of Science in Human Resource Leadership
MSHRM	Master of Science in Human Resource Management
MSHROD	Master of Science in Human Resources and Organizational Development
MSHS	Master of Science in Health Science
	Master of Science in Health Services
	Master of Science in Health Systems
	Master of Science in Homeland Security
MSHT	Master of Science in History of Technology
MSI	Master of Science in Information
	Master of Science in Instruction
	Master of System Integration
MSIA	Master of Science in Industrial Administration
	Master of Science in Information Assurance and Computer Security
MSIB	Master of Science in International Business
MSIDM	Master of Science in Interior Design and Merchandising
MSIDT	Master of Science in Information Design and Technology
MSIE	Master of Science in Industrial Engineering
	Master of Science in International Economics
MSIEM	Master of Science in Information Engineering and Management
MSIID	Master of Science in Information and Instructional Design
MSIM	Master of Science in Information Management
	Master of Science in International Management
MSIMC	Master of Science in Integrated Marketing Communications
MSIR	Master of Science in Industrial Relations
MSIS	Master of Science in Information Science
	Master of Science in Information Studies
	Master of Science in Information Systems
	Master of Science in Interdisciplinary Studies
MSIS/MA	Master of Science in Information Studies/ Master of Arts
MSISE	Master of Science in Infrastructure Systems Engineering
MSISM	Master of Science in Information Systems Management
MSISPM	Master of Science in Information Security Policy and Management
MSIST	Master of Science in Information Systems Technology
MSIT	Master of Science in Industrial Technology
	Master of Science in Information Technology
	Master of Science in Instructional Technology
MSITM	Master of Science in Information Technology Management
MSJ	Master of Science in Journalism
	Master of Science in Jurisprudence
MSJC	Master of Social Justice and Criminology
MSJE	Master of Science in Jewish Education
MSJFP	Master of Science in Juvenile Forensic Psychology
MSJJ	Master of Science in Juvenile Justice
MSJPS	Master of Science in Justice and Public Safety
MSJS	Master of Science in Jewish Studies
MSK	Master of Science in Kinesiology
MSL	Master of School Leadership

	Master of Science in Leadership
	Master of Science in Limnology
	Master of Strategic Leadership
	Master of Studies in Law
MSLA	Master of Science in Landscape Architecture
	Master of Science in Legal Administration
MSLD	Master of Science in Land Development
MSLFS	Master of Science in Life Sciences
MSLP	Master of Speech-Language Pathology
MSLS	Master of Science in Library Science
MSLSCM	Master of Science in Logistics and Supply Chain Management
MSLT	Master of Second Language Teaching
MSM	Master of Sacred Ministry
	Master of Sacred Music
	Master of School Mathematics
	Master of Science in Management
	Master of Science in Organization Management
	Master of Security Management
MSMA	Master of Science in Marketing Analysis
MSMAE	Master of Science in Materials Engineering
MSMC	Master of Science in Mass Communications
MSME	Master of Science in Mathematics Education
	Master of Science in Mechanical Engineering
MSMFE	Master of Science in Manufacturing Engineering
MSMFT	Master of Science in Marriage and Family Therapy
MSMIS	Master of Science in Management Information Systems
MSMIT	Master of Science in Management and Information Technology
MSMLS	Master of Science in Medical Laboratory Science
MSMOT	Master of Science in Management of Technology
MSMS	Master of Science in Management Science
	Master of Science in Medical Sciences
MSMSE	Master of Science in Manufacturing Systems Engineering
	Master of Science in Material Science and Engineering
	Master of Science in Mathematics and Science Education
MSMT	Master of Science in Management and Technology
MSMus	Master of Sacred Music
MSN	Master of Science in Nursing
MSN-R	Master of Science in Nursing (Research)
MSNA	Master of Science in Nurse Anesthesia
MSNE	Master of Science in Nuclear Engineering
MSNED	Master of Science in Nurse Education
MSNM	Master of Science in Nonprofit Management
MSNS	Master of Science in Natural Science
	Master of Science in Nutritional Science
MSOD	Master of Science in Organizational Development
MSOEE	Master of Science in Outdoor and Environmental Education
MSOES	Master of Science in Occupational Ergonomics and Safety
MSOH	Master of Science in Occupational Health
MSOL	Master of Science in Organizational Leadership
MSOM	Master of Science in Operations Management
	Master of Science in Oriental Medicine
MSOR	Master of Science in Operations Research
MSOT	Master of Science in Occupational Technology
	Master of Science in Occupational Therapy
MSP	Master of Science in Pharmacy
	Master of Science in Planning
	Master of Science in Psychology
	Master of Speech Pathology
MSPA	Master of Science in Physician Assistant
	Master of Science in Professional Accountancy
MSPAS	Master of Science in Physician Assistant Studies
MSPC	Master of Science in Professional Communications
	Master of Science in Professional Counseling
MSPE	Master of Science in Petroleum Engineering
MSPG	Master of Science in Psychology
MSPH	Master of Science in Public Health
MSPHR	Master of Science in Pharmacy
MSPM	Master of Science in Professional Management
	Master of Science in Project Management
MSPNGE	Master of Science in Petroleum and Natural Gas Engineering
MSPS	Master of Science in Pharmaceutical Science
	Master of Science in Political Science
	Master of Science in Psychological Services
MSPT	Master of Science in Physical Therapy
MSpVM	Master of Specialized Veterinary Medicine
MSR	Master of Science in Radiology
	Master of Science in Reading
MSRA	Master of Science in Recreation Administration
MSRC	Master of Science in Resource Conservation
MSRE	Master of Science in Real Estate
	Master of Science in Religious Education
MSRED	Master of Science in Real Estate Development
MSRLS	Master of Science in Recreation and Leisure Studies
MSRMP	Master of Science in Radiological Medical Physics
MSRS	Master of Science in Rehabilitation Science
MSS	Master of Science in Software
	Master of Security Studies
	Master of Social Science
	Master of Social Services
	Master of Software Systems
	Master of Sports Science
	Master of Strategic Studies
MSSA	Master of Science in Social Administration
MSSCP	Master of Science in Science Content and Process
MSSD	Master of Science in Sustainable Design
MSSE	Master of Science in Software Engineering
	Master of Science in Space Education
	Master of Science in Special Education
MSSEM	Master of Science in Systems and Engineering Management

MSSI	Master of Science in Security Informatics
	Master of Science in Strategic Intelligence
MSSL	Master of Science in School Leadership
	Master of Science in Strategic Leadership
MSSLP	Master of Science in Speech-Language Pathology
MSSM	Master of Science in Sports Medicine
MSSP	Master of Science in Social Policy
MSSPA	Master of Science in Student Personnel Administration
MSSS	Master of Science in Safety Science
	Master of Science in Systems Science
MSST	Master of Science in Security Technologies
MSSW	Master of Science in Social Work
MSSWE	Master of Science in Software Engineering
MST	Master of Science and Technology
	Master of Science in Taxation
	Master of Science in Teaching
	Master of Science in Technology
	Master of Science in Telecommunications
	Master of Science Teaching
MSTC	Master of Science in Technical Communication
	Master of Science in Telecommunications
MSTCM	Master of Science in Traditional Chinese Medicine
MSTE	Master of Science in Telecommunications Engineering
	Master of Science in Transportation Engineering
MSTM	Master of Science in Technical Management
	Master of Science in Technology Management
	Master of Science in Transfusion Medicine
MSTOM	Master of Science in Traditional Oriental Medicine
MSUD	Master of Science in Urban Design
MSW	Master of Social Work
MSWE	Master of Software Engineering
MSWREE	Master of Science in Water Resources and Environmental Engineering
MSX	Master of Science in Exercise Science
MT	Master of Taxation
	Master of Teaching
	Master of Technology
	Master of Textiles
MTA	Master of Tax Accounting
	Master of Teaching Arts
	Master of Tourism Administration
MTCM	Master of Traditional Chinese Medicine
MTD	Master of Training and Development
MTE	Master in Educational Technology
MTESOL	Master in Teaching English to Speakers of Other Languages
MTHM	Master of Tourism and Hospitality Management
MTI	Master of Information Technology
MTIM	Master of Trust and Investment Management
MTL	Master of Talmudic Law
MTM	Master of Technology Management
	Master of Telecommunications Management
	Master of the Teaching of Mathematics
MTMH	Master of Tropical Medicine and Hygiene
MTOM	Master of Traditional Oriental Medicine
MTP	Master of Transpersonal Psychology
MTPC	Master of Technical and Professional Communication
MTR	Master of Translational Research
MTS	Master of Theatre Studies
	Master of Theological Studies
MTSC	Master of Technical and Scientific Communication
MTSE	Master of Telecommunications and Software Engineering
MTT	Master in Technology Management
MTX	Master of Taxation
MUA	Master of Urban Affairs
MUCD	Master of Urban and Community Design
MUD	Master of Urban Design
MUDS	Master of Urban Design Studies
MUEP	Master of Urban and Environmental Planning
MUP	Master of Urban Planning
MUPDD	Master of Urban Planning, Design, and Development
MUPP	Master of Urban Planning and Policy
MUPRED	Master of Urban Planning and Real Estate Development
MURP	Master of Urban and Regional Planning
	Master of Urban and Rural Planning
MURPL	Master of Urban and Regional Planning
MUS	Master of Urban Studies
MUSA	Master of Urban Spatial Analytics
MVM	Master of VLSI and Microelectronics
MVP	Master of Voice Pedagogy
MVPH	Master of Veterinary Public Health
MVS	Master of Visual Studies
MWC	Master of Wildlife Conservation
MWE	Master in Welding Engineering
MWPS	Master of Wood and Paper Science
MWR	Master of Water Resources
MWS	Master of Women's Studies
	Master of Worship Studies
MZS	Master of Zoological Science
Nav Arch	Naval Architecture
Naval E	Naval Engineer
ND	Doctor of Naturopathic Medicine
NE	Nuclear Engineer
Nuc E	Nuclear Engineer
OD	Doctor of Optometry
OTD	Doctor of Occupational Therapy
PBME	Professional Master of Biomedical Engineering
PC	Performer's Certificate
PD	Professional Diploma
PGC	Post-Graduate Certificate
PGD	Postgraduate Diploma
Ph L	Licentiate of Philosophy
Pharm D	Doctor of Pharmacy
PhD	Doctor of Philosophy
PhD Otal	Doctor of Philosophy in Otalrynology
PhD Surg	Doctor of Philosophy in Surgery
PhDEE	Doctor of Philosophy in Electrical Engineering
PMBA	Professional Master of Business Administration
PMC	Post Master Certificate

PMD	Post-Master's Diploma
PMS	Professional Master of Science
	Professional Master's
Post-Doctoral MS	Post-Doctoral Master of Science
Post-MSN Certificate	Post-Master of Science in Nursing Certificate
PPDPT	Postprofessional Doctor of Physical Therapy
Pro-MS	Professional Science Master's
PSM	Professional Master of Science
	Professional Science Master's
Psy D	Doctor of Psychology
Psy M	Master of Psychology
Psy S	Specialist in Psychology
Psya D	Doctor of Psychoanalysis
Rh D	Doctor of Rehabilitation
S Psy S	Specialist in Psychological Services
Sc D	Doctor of Science
Sc M	Master of Science
SCCT	Specialist in Community College Teaching
ScDPT	Doctor of Physical Therapy Science
SD	Doctor of Science
	Specialist Degree
SJD	Doctor of Juridical Science
SLPD	Doctor of Speech-Language Pathology
SM	Master of Science
SM Arch S	Master of Science in Architectural Studies
SMACT	Master of Science in Art, Culture and Technology
SMBT	Master of Science in Building Technology
SP	Specialist Degree
Sp C	Specialist in Counseling
Sp Ed	Specialist in Education
Sp LIS	Specialist in Library and Information Science
SPA	Specialist in Arts
SPCM	Specialist in Church Music
Spec	Specialist's Certificate
Spec M	Specialist in Music
SPEM	Specialist in Educational Ministries
Spt	Specialist Degree
SPTH	Specialist in Theology
SSP	Specialist in School Psychology
STB	Bachelor of Sacred Theology
STD	Doctor of Sacred Theology
STL	Licentiate of Sacred Theology
STM	Master of Sacred Theology
TDPT	Transitional Doctor of Physical Therapy
Th D	Doctor of Theology
Th M	Master of Theology
VMD	Doctor of Veterinary Medicine
WEMBA	Weekend Executive Master of Business Administration
XMA	Executive Master of Arts

INDEXES

Displays and Close-Ups

Directories and Subject Areas

Following is an alphabetical listing of directories and subject areas. Also listed are cross-references for subject area names not used in the directory structure of the guides, for example, "City and Regional Planning (*see* Urban and Regional Planning)."

Graduate Programs in the Humanities, Arts & Social Sciences

Transpersonal and Humanistic Psychology
Urban and Regional Planning
Urban Design
Urban Planning (*see* Architecture; Urban and Regional Planning; Urban Design; Urban Studies)
Urban Studies
Video (*see* Film, Television, and Video Production)
Visual Arts (*see* Applied Arts and Design; Art/Fine Arts; Film, Television, and Video Production; Graphic Design; Illustration; Photography)
Western European Studies
Women's Studies
World Wide Web (*see* Internet and Interactive Multimedia)
Writing

Graduate Programs in the Biological/Biomedical Sciences & Health-Related Medical Professions

Acupuncture and Oriental Medicine
Acute Care/Critical Care Nursing Administration (*see* Health Services Management and Hospital Administration; Nursing and Healthcare Administration; Pharmaceutical Administration)
Adult Nursing
Advanced Practice Nursing (*see* Family Nurse Practitioner Studies)
Allied Health—General
Allied Health Professions (*see* Clinical Laboratory Sciences/Medical Technology; Clinical Research; Communication Disorders; Dental Hygiene; Emergency Medical Services; Occupational Therapy; Physical Therapy; Physician Assistant Studies; Rehabilitation Sciences)
Allopathic Medicine
Anatomy
Anesthesiologist Assistant Studies
Animal Behavior
Bacteriology
Behavioral Sciences (*see* Biopsychology; Neuroscience; Zoology)
Biochemistry
Bioethics
Biological and Biomedical Sciences—General Biological Chemistry (*see* Biochemistry)
Biological Oceanography (*see* Marine Biology)
Biophysics
Biopsychology
Botany
Breeding (*see* Botany; Plant Biology; Genetics)
Cancer Biology/Oncology
Cardiovascular Sciences
Cell Biology
Cellular Physiology (*see* Cell Biology; Physiology)
Child-Care Nursing (*see* Maternal and Child/Neonatal Nursing)
Chiropractic
Clinical Laboratory Sciences/Medical Technology
Clinical Research
Community Health
Community Health Nursing
Computational Biology
Conservation (*see* Conservation Biology; Environmental Biology)
Conservation Biology
Crop Sciences (*see* Botany; Plant Biology)
Cytology (*see* Cell Biology)
Dental and Oral Surgery (*see* Oral and Dental Sciences)
Dental Assistant Studies (*see* Dental Hygiene)
Dental Hygiene
Dental Services (*see* Dental Hygiene)
Dentistry
Developmental Biology Dietetics (*see* Nutrition)
Ecology
Embryology (*see* Developmental Biology)
Emergency Medical Services
Endocrinology (*see* Physiology)
Entomology
Environmental Biology
Environmental and Occupational Health
Epidemiology
Evolutionary Biology
Family Nurse Practitioner Studies
Foods (*see* Nutrition)
Forensic Nursing
Genetics
Genomic Sciences
Gerontological Nursing
Health Physics/Radiological Health
Health Promotion
Health-Related Professions (*see* individual allied health professions)
Health Services Management and Hospital Administration
Health Services Research
Histology (*see* Anatomy; Cell Biology)
HIV/AIDS Nursing
Hospice Nursing
Hospital Administration (*see* Health Services Management and Hospital Administration)
Human Genetics
Immunology
Industrial Hygiene
Infectious Diseases
International Health
Laboratory Medicine (*see* Clinical Laboratory Sciences/Medical Technology; Immunology; Microbiology; Pathology)
Life Sciences (*see* Biological and Biomedical Sciences)
Marine Biology
Maternal and Child Health
Maternal and Child/Neonatal Nursing
Medical Imaging
Medical Microbiology
Medical Nursing (*see* Medical/Surgical Nursing)
Medical Physics
Medical/Surgical Nursing
Medical Technology (*see* Clinical Laboratory Sciences/Medical Technology)
Medical Sciences (*see* Biological and Biomedical Sciences)
Medical Science Training Programs (*see* Biological and Biomedical Sciences)
Medicinal and Pharmaceutical Chemistry
Medicinal Chemistry (*see* Medicinal and Pharmaceutical Chemistry)
Medicine (*see* Allopathic Medicine; Naturopathic Medicine; Osteopathic Medicine; Podiatric Medicine)
Microbiology
Midwifery (*see* Nurse Midwifery)
Molecular Biology
Molecular Biophysics
Molecular Genetics
Molecular Medicine
Molecular Pathogenesis
Molecular Pathology
Molecular Pharmacology
Molecular Physiology
Molecular Toxicology
Naturopathic Medicine
Neural Sciences (*see* Biopsychology; Neurobiology; Neuroscience)
Neurobiology
Neuroendocrinology (*see* Biopsychology; Neurobiology; Neuroscience; Physiology)
Neuropharmacology (*see* Biopsychology; Neurobiology; Neuroscience; Pharmacology)
Neurophysiology (*see* Biopsychology; Neurobiology; Neuroscience; Physiology)
Neuroscience
Nuclear Medical Technology (*see* Clinical Laboratory Sciences/Medical Technology)
Nurse Anesthesia
Nurse Midwifery
Nurse Practitioner Studies (*see* Family Nurse Practitioner Studies)
Nursing Administration (*see* Nursing and Healthcare Administration)
Nursing and Healthcare Administration
Nursing Education
Nursing—General
Nursing Informatics

Graduate Programs in the Physical Sciences, Mathematics, Agricultural Sciences, the Environment & Natural Resources

Graduate Programs in Engineering & Applied Sciences

Graduate Programs in Business, Education, Information Studies, Law & Social Work

Directories and Subject Areas in This Book

NOTES

NOTES

NOTES

NOTES

NOTES

NOTES

NOTES

NOTES